W9-APT-444

Third Edition

PHARMACOTHERAPY

A Pathophysiologic Approach

Editors

Joseph T. DiPiro, PharmD, FCCP
Professor, College of Pharmacy, Head, Department of Pharmacy Practice, University of Georgia;
Clinical Professor of Surgery, Medical College of Georgia, Augusta, Georgia

Robert L. Talbert, PharmD, FCCP, BCPS
Professor and Division Head, College of Pharmacy, University of Texas at Austin, Austin;
Professor, Departments of Medicine and Pharmacology, University of Texas
Health Science Center at San Antonio, San Antonio, Texas

Gary C. Yee, PharmD, FCCP
Associate Professor, Department of Pharmacy Practice, College of Pharmacy,
University of Florida Health Science Center, Gainesville, Florida

Gary R. Matzke, PharmD, FCP, FCCP
Professor, Department of Pharmacy and Therapeutics, Center for Clinical Pharmacology,
Schools of Pharmacy and Medicine, University of Pittsburgh; Clinical Pharmacy Specialist–Nephrology,
Department of Pharmacy, University of Pittsburgh Medical Center, Pittsburgh, Pennsylvania

Barbara G. Wells, PharmD, FASHP, FCCP
Professor and Dean, Idaho State University College of Pharmacy, Pocatello, Idaho

L. Michael Posey, RPh
President, Pharmacy/Association Services, Athens, Georgia

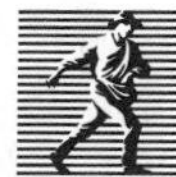

APPLETON & LANGE
Stamford, Connecticut

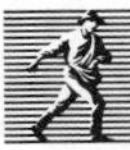

97 98 99 00 01 / 10 9 8 7 6 5 4

Prentice Hall International (UK) Limited, *London*
Prentice Hall of Australia Pty. Limited, *Sydney*
Prentice Hall Canada, Inc., *Toronto*
Prentice Hall Hispanoamericana, S.A., *Mexico*
Prentice Hall of India Private Limited, *New Delhi*
Prentice Hall of Japan, Inc., *Tokyo*
Simon & Schuster Asia Pte. Ltd., *Singapore*
Editora Prentice Hall do Brasil Ltda., *Rio de Janeiro*
Prentice Hall, *Upper Saddle River, New Jersey*

Library of Congress Cataloging-in-Publication Data

Pharmacotherapy : a pathophysiologic approach / editors, Joseph Dipiro
. . . [et al.]. — 3rd ed.
p. cm.
Includes bibliographical references and index.
ISBN 0-8385-7892-6 (case : alk. paper)
1. Chemotherapy. 2. Physiology, Pathological. I. DiPiro, Joseph
T.
[DNLM: 1. Drug Therapy. WB 330 P5357 1996]
RM263.P56 1996
615.5'8—dc20
DNLM/DLC 95-25685
for Library of Congress CIP

Executive Editor: Cheryl L. Mehalik
Editorial Assistant: Virginia Allen
Production: Spectrum Publisher Services
Designer: Mary Skudlarek

ISBN 0-8385-7892-6
90000
9 780838 578926

PRINTED IN THE UNITED STATES OF AMERICA

To those pharmacists who had the courage and perseverance to take the early steps that were needed to develop personally and professionally in the clinical practice of pharmacy

To our mentors, whose vision provided educational and training programs that encouraged the professional growth of their students

And to our families and faculty colleagues for their efforts and support for our endeavors

Contents

Foreword to the Third Edition

In 1988, introducing the first edition of this successful textbook, Professor Charles Walton celebrated the profound maturation of the profession of pharmacy since the mid-1970s. He applauded pharmacy's dramatic change of focus from trade protection issues to an organization of interests that included scientific and technological questions and ethical issues promoting the best interests of its patients. Professor Walton believed firmly that the profession of pharmacy was ready for schools and colleges to train students with special knowledge and skills so as to function as competent specialists in drug therapy. He also held that within *Pharmacotherapy: A Pathophysiologic Approach* the reader will find the scientific foundation for the knowledge needed by pharmacists who aspire to practice as pharmacotherapists.

Publication of the second edition of *Pharmacotherapy: A Pathophysiologic Approach* again found a broad audience receptive to the efforts of the editors. The Board of Pharmaceutical Specialties had recently recognized pharmacotherapy as a pharmacy practice specialty, and 139 pharmacists were board certified. Hundreds of others would seek to secure that distinction.

The buzz word, *pharmaceutical care,* had captured the imagination of the profession and remarkably facilitated the development of a vision for the future mission of pharmacy practice. The goal was to change the focus of practice from an emphasis on drug distribution to the provision of integrated drug information to enhance the sensible use of drugs in patients. For the first time in history, the profession ringingly declared that the pharmacist, like the doctor and nurse, was also responsible for the patient's care.

Introducing the second edition of *Pharmacotherapy: A Pathophysiologic Approach,* Dr. William A. Miller observed that the American Association of Colleges of Pharmacy had urged schools and colleges to emphasize problem-solving, communications, and practice skills and to make curricular changes that assure the preparation of graduates who can render pharmaceutical care. The need for *Pharmacotherapy: A Pathophysiologic Approach* to provide an underpinning to this rigorous course of study was considerable.

Today, times have changed but our goals have not, and the third edition of *Pharmacotherapy: A Pathophysiologic Approach* is again most welcome. The idea of pharmaceutical care continues to enjoy near universal support in the profession, yet we have had critical lapses in organizational and academic leadership. Those who feared and prophesied that the path to fulfillment of pharmacy's future mission might be strewn with obstacles calling for careful strategy were ridiculed and ignored. Now, we inherit the wind.

Milo Gibaldi
University of Washington
Seattle, Washington
June 1996

Preface

The publication of the third edition of *Pharmacotherapy: A Pathophysiologic Approach* continues the standards and philosophies set forth by the previous editions. More than any other book in its field, *Pharmacotherapy* seeks to advance the level of pharmaceutical care. We believe that this textbook will stimulate the pharmacy student to achieve a higher level of learning; motivate the young practitioner to perform more advanced patient care; challenge established pharmacists to learn concepts missed during years of practice; and inform the profession at large about the standards of pharmaceutical care toward which all should strive.

The authors and editors have attempted to impart a process of thinking about pharmacotherapy for the student and developing practitioner. The key to this process is the pathophysiology sections, which identify mechanisms of disease as a foundation for applying pharmacotherapeutic principles and strategies. By understanding pathophysiology and principles of therapy, the student and practitioner can assess more rigorously the place of new drugs or new therapeutic approaches.

As with the previous two editions, this third edition demonstrates the geographic diversity of expertise in pharmaceutical care. More than 200 individuals, representing numerous institutions, served as contributors. We have welcomed the addition of a new editor, Barbara G. Wells, Dean of the College of Pharmacy at Idaho State University. Dr. Wells continues the superb contributions of Peggy E. Hayes in Neurologic Disorders and Psychiatric Disorders.

The editors have revised the current edition to meet the continually expanding needs of students and practitioners. The third edition includes 136 chapters, a net increase of 7 chapters. The following chapters have been added:

Chapter 1: Pharmacoeconomics: Principles, Methods, and Application to Pharmacotherapy
Chapter 30: Evaluation of the Gastrointestinal Tract
Chapter 45: Renal Transplantation
Chapter 46: Principles and Practice of Chronic Renal Replacement Therapy
Chapter 61: Assessment of Psychiatric Illness
Chapter 92: Hematopoiesis
Chapter 128: Melanoma
Chapter 130: Assessment of Nutrition Status and Nutrition Requirements

The contributors have added a section entitled "Evaluation of Therapeutic Outcomes" to some of their chapters to stress the increasing recognition of measures, such as quality of life and pharmacoeconomic assessments, which are of ultimate importance to determining success or failure of pharmacotherapy. Other new features of this edition include the use of color to provide clarity and focus for many tables and figures, and the inclusion of tables of drug pharmacokinetic and pharmacodynamic data.

To many readers, the most exciting development is the availability of a companion book, *Pharmacotherapy: A Patient-Focused Approach,* which presents more than 100 extensive patient cases to develop the clinical problem-solving skills of students. This book was developed by Terry L. Schwinghammer in collaboration with the editors of *Pharmacotherapy: A Pathophysiologic Approach* and numerous pharmacy professionals throughout the United States.

The overall organization of the book is retained from previous editions. The first nine chapters in the book again provide primers on important fundamental topics, such as pharmacoeconomics, health outcomes, pharmacokinetics, drug interactions, and molecular biology. Most of the remaining chapters in this textbook specifically focus on disease states and maintain a standard format including epidemiology, pathophysiology, clinical presentation, therapeutic management, and evaluation of therapeutic outcomes. Whenever possible, tables or flow diagrams have been added to the chapters to provide thorough recommendations for pharmacotherapy.

The editors recognize that many areas of this text will rapidly become outdated as our understanding of disease processes increases or as new therapies are adopted. The challenge for the student and the practitioner is to integrate information from a variety of sources, form a basis for application in pharmacotherapy, and be receptive to new information as it appears in the literature or as it is gained by personal experience. We are hopeful that new publishing technologies, such as CD-ROM versions of the text or distribution of updated material through the Internet, will allow more timely dissemination of new information in the future.

The editors are deeply indebted to the contributors for the hours spent preparing accurate, thorough, and relevant discussions of each topic. A heartfelt thank you is well earned by the personnel at Appleton & Lange, especially Cheryl Mehalik, who shepherded the third edition from first outline to the final editing and printing.

The Editors
June 1996

Contributors

Paul A. Abraham, MD
Associate Professor, School of Medicine, University of Minnesota; Chief of Nephrology, St. Paul–Ramsey Medical Center, St. Paul, Minnesota

Colin G. Adair, PhD
Assistant Director of Post Graduate Pharmaceutical Education, Pharmaceutical Branch, Department of Health, Belfast, United Kingdom

Val Adams, PharmD
Post Doctoral Fellow, Department of Pharmacy Practice, College of Pharmacy, University of Florida Health Science Center, Gainesville, Florida

J. V. Anandan, PharmD
Assistant Director, Department of Pharmacy, Henry Ford Hospital; Adjunct Associate Professor, College of Pharmacy and Allied Health Professions, Wayne State University, Detroit, Michigan

Jan Dalke Anderson, PharmD, BCNSP
Assistant Professor of Pharmacy Practice, University of Colorado Health Sciences Center, Denver, Colorado

Edward P. Armstrong, PharmD, BCPS
Associate Professor, Pharmacy Practice, College of Pharmacy, The University of Arizona, Tucson, Arizona

George R. Bailie, MSc, PharmD, PhD, FCCP
Professor of Pharmacy, Albany College of Pharmacy, Union University, Albany, New York

Carol Balmer, PharmD
Associate Professor and Oncology Clinical Pharmacist, Department of Pharmacy Practice, University of Colorado School of Pharmacy, Denver, Colorado

Steven L. Barriere, PharmD, FCCP
Associate Director, Anti-Infectives, Rhône-Poulenc Rorer, Collegeville, Pennsylvania

Larry A. Bauer, PharmD, FCP, FCCP
Associate Professor, Department of Pharmacy, School of Pharmacy, and Department of Laboratory Medicine, School of Medicine, University of Washington, Seattle, Washington

Jerry L. Bauman, PharmD, FCCP, FACC
Professor, Departments of Pharmacy Practice and Medicine, University of Illinois at Chicago, Chicago, Illinois

Terry J. Baumann, PharmD
Clinical Manager, Department of Pharmacy, Munson Medical Center, Traverse City, Michigan

Steven F. Bauwens, PharmD, FASCP
Director, Professional Services, The Center for Long Term Care Research and Education, Chesapeake, Virginia

Eula D. Beasley, PharmD
Clinical Manager, Department of Pharmacy Services, The Washington Hospital Center, Washington, DC

Brian E. Beckett, PharmD
Associate Professor of Pharmacy Practice, Department of Pharmacy Practice, Samford University, Birmingham, Alabama; Assistant Director for Clinical Pharmacy Services, Lloyd Noland Hospital, Fairfield, Alabama

William H. Benefield, Jr., PharmD, FASCP
Clinical Assistant Professor of Pharmacy, College of Pharmacy, The University of Texas at Austin, Austin, Texas; Clinical Assistant Professor of Pharmacology, Department of Pharmacology, Clinical Pharmacy Programs, The University of Texas Health Science Center at San Antonio, San Antonio, Texas; Clinical Pharmacologist, San Antonio State School, San Antonio, Texas

Rosemary R. Berardi, PharmD, FASHP
Professor of Pharmacy, College of Pharmacy and Clinical Pharmacist in Gastroenterology, Department of Pharmacy Services, University of Michigan Medical Center, The University of Michigan, Ann Arbor, Michigan

Richard C. Berchou, PharmD
Clinical Neuroscience Program, Sinai Hospital, Detroit, Michigan

Joseph S. Bertino, Jr., PharmD, FCCP
Co-Director, Clinical Pharmacology Research Center, Assistant Director, Clinical Pharmacy Service, Bassett Healthcare, Cooperstown, New York; Associate Professor of Clinical Pharmacology, College of Physicians and Surgeons, Columbia University, New York, New York

Larry E. Boh, MS, RPh
Professor and Chair, Pharmacy Practice Division, School of Pharmacy, University of Wisconsin, Madison, Wisconsin

John A. Bosso, PharmD, FCCP
Professor, Department of Pharmaceutical Sciences, Medical University of South Carolina, Charleston, South Carolina

Bradley A. Boucher, PharmD
Associate Professor and Director of Research, Department of Clinical Pharmacy, University of Tennessee, Memphis, Tennessee

Talmadge A. Bowden, Jr., MD
Professor of Surgery, Medical College of Georgia, Augusta, Georgia

J. Chris Bradberry, PharmD
Professor and Chair, Department of Pharmacy Practice, College of Pharmacy, University of Oklahoma Health Sciences Center, Oklahoma City, Oklahoma

Rex O. Brown, PharmD
Professor, Clinical Pharmacy, College of Pharmacy, University of Tennessee, Memphis, Tennessee

Kathryn K. Bucci, PharmD, BCPS
Associate Professor of Family Medicine, Clinical Associate Professor of Pharmacy Practice, Medical University of South Carolina, Charleston, South Carolina; Self Memorial Hospital, Family Practice Residency Program, Greenwood, South Carolina

Gilbert J. Burckart, PharmD, FCCP
Professor, Pharmacy and Therapeutics, School of Pharmacy, University of Pittsburgh, Pittsburgh, Pennsylvania

Mark B. Burlingame, PharmD
Clinical Coordinator, Pharmacy Services, Department of Veterans Affairs Medical Center; Clinical Assistant Professor, Department of Pharmacy Practice, College of Pharmacy, University of Florida Health Science Center, Gainesville, Florida

Henry I. Bussey, PharmD
Associate Professor of Pharmacy, University of Texas at Austin, Austin, Texas; Associate Professor of Pharmacology, University of Texas Health Science Center, San Antonio, Texas

Deborah Stier Carson, PharmD, BCPS
Associate Professor of Pharmacy Practice, Assistant Professor of Family Medicine, Medical University of South Carolina, Charleston, South Carolina

Peggy L. Carver, PharmD
Clinical Pharmacist, Infectious Diseases, University of Michigan, Ann Arbor, Michigan

Daniel T. Casto, PharmD, FCCP
Associate Professor, College of Pharmacy, University of Texas at Austin, Austin, Texas; Associate Professor of Pediatrics, University of Texas Health Science Center, San Antonio, Texas

Katherine Hammond Chessman, PharmD, BCNSP, BCPS
Assistant Professor of Hospital Pharmacy Practice and Administration, College of Pharmacy, Medical University of South Carolina, Charleston, South Carolina

Marie A. Chisholm, PharmD
Clinical Assistant Professor, Pharmacy Practice, The University of Georgia College of Pharmacy; Assistant Adjunct Professor, Internal Medicine, Medical College of Georgia, Augusta, Georgia

Kerri K. Chitwood-Dagner, PharmD, BCPS
Manager, Pharmacoeconomic and Outcomes Research, Diversified Pharmaceutical Services, Inc.; Clinical Assistant Professor, College of Pharmacy, University of Minnesota, Minneapolis, Minnesota

Ann C. Collier, MD
Associate Professor, Department of Medicine, University of Washington, Seattle, Washington

Thomas J. Comstock, PharmD
Associate Professor, Department of Pharmacy and Pharmaceutics, School of Pharmacy, Medical College of Virginia/Virginia Commonwealth University, Richmond, Virginia

Stephen Joel Coons, PhD
Director, Center for Pharmaceutical Economics; Associate Professor, Department of Pharmacy Practice, College of Pharmacy, University of Arizona, Tucson, Arizona

Brian L. Crabtree, PharmD
Associate Professor of Clinical Pharmacy Practice, Clinical Pharmacy Practice, University of Mississippi School of Pharmacy, Jackson, Mississippi

M. Lynn Crismon, PharmD, FCCP
Professor and Head, Clinical Division at Austin, College of Pharmacy, The University of Texas at Austin; Director of Neuropsychiatric Research, Center for Clinical Research of the Austin Diagnostic Clinic, Austin, Texas

Clarence E. Curry, Jr., PharmD
Associate Professor, Clinical and Administrative Pharmacy Sciences, College of Pharmacy and Pharmaceutical Sciences, Howard University, Washington, DC

Christina Dalmady-Israel, PharmD, BCPS
Clinical Associate, MedOutcomes, Inc., Richmond, Virginia

Larry H. Danziger, PharmD
Professor of Pharmacy Practice, College of Pharmacy, University of Illinois, Chicago, Illinois

Lisa E. Davis, PharmD
Associate Professor of Clinical Pharmacy, Department of Pharmacy Practice and Pharmacy Administration, Philadelphia College of Pharmacy and Science, Philadelphia, Pennsylvania

Jeffrey C. Delafuente, MS
Professor and Associate Chairman, Department of Pharmacy Practice, College of Pharmacy, University of Florida Health Science Center, Gainesville, Florida

Mariela Diaz-Linares, PharmD
Clinical Assistant Professor, Department of Pharmacy Practice, College of Pharmacy, University of Illinois, Chicago, Illinois

Joseph T. DiPiro, PharmD, FCCP
Professor, College of Pharmacy, Head, Department of Pharmacy Practice, University of Georgia; Clinical Professor of Surgery, Medical College of Georgia, Augusta, Georgia

Julie A. Dopheide, PharmD
Assistant Professor of Clinical Pharmacy, Department of Pharmacy Practice, University of Southern California, Los Angeles, California

Peter G. Dorson, PharmD
Clinical Assistant Professor, College of Pharmacy, University of Texas at Austin; Director of Clinical Pharmacology Service, Austin State Hospital, Austin, Texas

Michael Doukas, MD
Associate Professor, Department of Internal Medicine, College of Medicine, University of Kentucky, Lexington, Kentucky

Michael N. Dudley, PharmD, FCCP
Professor and Director, Antiinfective Pharmacology Research Unit; Chairman, Department of Pharmacy Practice, University of Rhode Island College of Pharmacy and Roger Williams Medical Center, Providence, Rhode Island

Steven C. Ebert, PharmD
Clinical Specialist, Infectious Diseases, Department of Pharmacy, Meriter Hospital; Clinical Associate Professor, School of Pharmacy, University of Wisconsin, Madison, Wisconsin

Andrea Eggert, PharmD
Clinical Assistant Professor of Pharmacy, University of Texas at Austin, Austin, Texas; Clinical Assistant Professor of Pharmacology and Psychiatry, University of Texas Health Science Center at San Antonio, San Antonio, Texas

Maha A. Elkordy, MD
Associate in Medicine, Bone Marrow Transplant Program, Department of Medicine, Duke University Medical Center, Durham, North Carolina

Victor A. Elsberry, PharmD, BCNSP
Assistant Professor, Pharmacy Practice, College of Pharmacy, The University of Arizona, Tucson, Arizona

Sharon M. Erdman, PharmD
Loyola Medical Center, Department of Pharmacy, Chicago, Illinois

Larry Ereshefsky, PharmD, FCCP
Romeo Barchand Professor of Pharmacy, Pharmacology, and Psychiatry, University of Texas Health Science Center at San Antonio, and College of Pharmacy, The University of Texas at Austin; Assistant Director of Research, Clinical Research Unit, San Antonio State Hospital, San Antonio, Texas

W. Gary Erwin, PharmD
Professor and Associate Vice President, Office of Professional Programs, Philadelphia College of Pharmacy and Science, Philadelphia, Pennsylvania

Martha P. Fankhauser, MS
Clinical Associate Professor, Department of Pharmacy Practice, College of Pharmacy, University of Arizona, Tucson, Arizona

Timothy A. Feger, MD
Section of Allergy and Immunology, Department of Pediatrics, Medical College of Georgia, Augusta, Georgia

Rebecca S. Finley, PharmD, MS
Head, Section of Pharmacy Services, University of Maryland Cancer Center; Pharmacy School Associate Professor, Department of Pharmacy Practice and Science, University of Maryland School of Pharmacy, Baltimore, Maryland

Richard Fiscella, RPh, MPH
Assistant Professor of Pharmacy Practice, Pharmacy Practice, University of Illinois at Chicago, Chicago, Illinois

Douglas N. Fish, PharmD
Assistant Professor, Department of Pharmacy Practice, University of Colorado School of Pharmacy, Denver, Colorado

Courtney V. Fletcher, PharmD
Associate Professor, Department of Pharmacy Practice, University of Minnesota, Minneapolis, Minnesota

William R. Friedenberg, MD
Department of Hematology and Oncology, Marshfield Clinic, Marshfield, Wisconsin

Reginald F. Frye, PharmD, PhD
Research Assistant Professor, Department of Pharmacy and Therapeutics, School of Pharmacy; Member, Center for Clinical Pharmacology, School of Medicine, University of Pittsburgh, Pittsburgh, Pennsylvania

Peter Gal, PharmD, FCCP, BCPS
Director, Pharmacy Education and Research, Greensboro AHEC, Moses Cone Health System, Greensboro, North Carolina; Clinical Professor, School of Pharmacy, University of North Carolina, Chapel Hill, North Carolina

William R. Garnett, PharmD
Professor of Pharmacy and Pharmaceutics, Professor of Neurology, Virginia Commonwealth University/Medical College of Virginia, Richmond, Virginia

Carlos A. Garza, MA, CRRT, CPFT
Director, Respiratory Care Unit, Audie L. Murphy Veterans Memorial Hospital, San Antonio, Texas

Mark A. Gill, PharmD
Professor of Clinical Pharmacy, School of Pharmacy, University of Southern California, Los Angeles, California

Barry R. Goldspiel, PharmD
Oncology Clinical Pharmacy Specialist, Department of Pharmacy, National Institutes of Health Clinical Center, Bethesda, Maryland

S. Diane Goodwin, PharmD
Manager, HIV/Herpes Program Development, Case Management Division, Glaxo Wellcome, Inc., Research Triangle Park, North Carolina

Sean P. Gorman, PhD
Reader in Pharmaceutical Microbiology, School of Pharmacy, The Queen's University of Belfast, United Kingdom

David R. P. Guay, PharmD, FCP
Associate Professor of Pharmacy, College of Pharmacy, University of Minnesota, Minneapolis; Clinical Specialist in Geriatrics Pharmacy Program, St. Paul–Ramsey Medical Center, St. Paul, Minnesota

Margaret L. Guill, MD
Associate Professor of Pulmonology, Depart-

ment of Pediatrics, Medical College of Georgia, Augusta, Georgia

John G. Gums, PharmD
Associate Professor of Pharmacy and Medicine, Departments of Pharmacy Practice and Family Medicine, University of Florida, Gainesville, Florida

Philip D. Hall, PharmD
Assistant Professor, Department of Pharmaceutical Sciences, College of Pharmacy, Medical University of South Carolina, Charleston, South Carolina

Erkan Hassan, PharmD
Associate Professor, Department of Clinical Pharmacy, University of Maryland, Baltimore, Maryland

David W. Hawkins, PharmD
Professor and Assistant Dean of Pharmacy, University of Georgia, Athens, Georgia; Clinical Professor of Medicine and Assistant Dean for Clinical Pharmacy, Medical College of Georgia, Augusta, Georgia

Peggy E. Hayes, PharmD
Senior Associate Director–CNS, Sandoz Research Institute, East Hanover, New Jersey

Karen Heim-Duthoy, PharmD, FCCP
Clinical Scientist, Drug Evaluation Unit, Division of Nephrology, Hennepin County Medical Center; Associate Professor, College of Pharmacy, University of Minnesota, Minneapolis, Minnesota

Lisa M. Henderson, PharmD
Glaxo Pharmacy Fellow in Gastroenterology and Clinical Assistant Professor of Pharmacy, College of Pharmacy, The University of Michigan, Ann Arbor, Michigan

Eileen G. Holland, PharmD
Assistant Professor, Clinical Pharmacy Practice, Auburn University School of Pharmacy; Adjunct Assistant Professor, Department of Family Practice and Community Medicine, University of South Alabama College of Medicine; Adjunct Assistant Professor, Department of Pharmacology, University of South Alabama College of Medicine, Mobile, Alabama

Mark W. Jackson, MD
Assistant Professor of Medicine, Section of Gastroenterology, Medical College of Georgia, Augusta, Georgia

Stephen W. Janning, PharmD
Clinical Coordinator, Department of Pharmacy, Duke University Medical Center, Durham, North Carolina

Douglas D. Janson, PharmD
Nutrition Support Specialist, Department of Pharmacy, University of Pittsburgh Medical Center; Assistant Professor, Department of Pharmacy and Therapeutics, School of Pharmacy, University of Pittsburgh, Pittsburgh, Pennsylvania

Stephen G. Jenkinson, MD
Chief, Division of Pulmonary Diseases and Critical Care Medicine, Audie L. Murphy Veterans Memorial Hospital; Professor of Medicine, The University of Texas Health Science Center at San Antonio, San Antonio, Texas

Julie A. Johnson, PharmD
Associate Professor, Department of Clinical Pharmacy, University of Tennessee, Memphis, Tennessee

Steven B. Johnson, MD
Associate Professor of Surgery, Section of General Surgery and Trauma; Chief, Surgical Critical Care, University of Arizona, Tucson, Arizona

Lori A. Jones, PharmD
Clinical Assistant Professor, College of Pharmacy, University of Texas at Austin, Austin, Texas; Clinical Pharmacy Program, University of Texas Health Science Center, San Antonio, Texas

Alan K. Kamada, PharmD
Assistant Professor, Clinical Pharmacology Division, Department of Pediatrics, National Jewish Center for Immunology and Respiratory Medicine, Denver, Colorado

Peter W. Kazakoff, PharmD
Assistant Professor, Department of Pharmacy Practice, School of Pharmacy, University of Colorado Health Sciences Center, Denver, Colorado

H. William Kelly, PharmD
Professor, Pharmacy and Pediatrics, College of Pharmacy and Department of Pediatrics, S.O.M., University of New Mexico Health Sciences Center, Albuquerque, New Mexico

Robert A. Kilroy, PharmD, BCPS
Clinical Associate Professor, Department of Pharmacy Services, Shands Hospital at the University of Florida; Supervisor, Clinical Pharmacy Services, Shands Hospital, Gainesville, Florida

William R. Kirchain, PharmD
Associate Professor of Clinical Pharmacy, Pharmacy Practice and Administration, Philadelphia College of Pharmacy and Science, Philadelphia, Pennsylvania

Cynthia K. Kirkwood, PharmD
Assistant Professor, School of Pharmacy, Virginia Commonwealth University, Richmond, Virginia

Leroy C. Knodel, PharmD
Associate Professor, Pharmacology Department, University of Texas Health Science Center at San Antonio, San Antonio, Texas; Clinical Associate Professor, College of Pharmacy, University of Texas at Austin, Austin, Texas

Jim Koeller, MS
Professor, College of Pharmacy, University of Texas at Austin, Austin, Texas, and University of Texas Health Science Center, San Antonio, Texas

Jill M. Kolesar, PharmD
Clinical Science Fellow, University of Texas Health Science Center at San Antonio, San Antonio, Texas; Clinical Instructor, College of Pharmacy, University of Texas, Austin, Texas

Motria M. Krawczeniuk, PharmD
Assistant Professor of Clinical Pharmacy, Department of Pharmacy Practice and Pharmacy Administration, Philadelphia College of Pharmacy and Science, Philadelphia, Pennsylvania

Maura A. Kraynak, PharmD
Director, Investigational Drug Section, Cancer Therapy and Research Center, San Antonio, Texas

John G. Kuhn, PharmD, FCCP
Professor, College of Pharmacy, University of Texas at Austin, Austin, Texas, and University of Texas Health Science Center, San Antonio, Texas

Kathleen D. Lake, PharmD, BCPS
Clinical Associate Professor, College of Pharmacy, University of Minnesota; Program Director, Division of Cardiothoracic Transplantation, Abbott Northwestern Hospital/Minneapolis Heart Institute Foundation, Minneapolis, Minnesota

Richard L. Lalonde, PharmD
Senior Director, Scientific Affairs and Clinical Pharmacology, Phoenix International Life Sciences, Inc., Montreal, Quebec, Canada

Lawrence J. Lambrecht, PharmD, BCPS
Research Fellow, The Drug Evaluation Unit, Division of Nephrology, Hennepin County Medical Center, Minneapolis, Minnesota

Tom A. Larson, PharmD
Associate Professor, Pharmacy Rural Education Program, Pharmacy Practice, College of Pharmacy, University of Minnesota, Minneapolis, Minnesota

Alan H. Lau, PharmD, FCCP
Associate Professor of Pharmacy Practice, College of Pharmacy, University of Illinois at Chicago, Chicago, Illinois

Marc LeBel, PharmD, FCCP, FCSHP
Professor, Ecole de Pharmacie, Universite Laval; President, Anapharm, Inc., Québec, Canada

Timothy S. Lesar, PharmD
Director of Pharmacy, Department of Pharmaceutical Services, Albany Medical Center, Albany, New York

Peter A. LeWitt, MD
Associate Professor of Neurology, Clinical Neuroscience Program, Sinai Hospital; Wayne State University, Detroit, Michigan

Celeste Lindley, PharmD, MS, FCCP, FASHP
Associate Professor, Department of Pharmacy Practice, School of Pharmacy, University of North Carolina, Chapel Hill, North Carolina

R. Leon Longe, PharmD
Professor, Department of Pharmacy Practice, University of Georgia, Athens, Georgia

Larry M. Lopez, PharmD, FCCP
Professor of Pharmacy, Department of Pharmacy Practice, College of Pharmacy, University of Florida, Gainesville, Florida

William L. Macias, MD, PhD
Clinical Pharmacologist, Eli Lilly and Company; Clinical Associate Professor of Medicine, Nephrology Division, Department of Medicine, Indiana University School of Medicine, Indianapolis, Indiana

Karl J. Madaras-Kelly, PharmD
Assistant Professor, Department of Pharmacy Practice and Administrative Sciences, Idaho State University, Pocatello, Idaho

Laura A. Mandos, PharmD
Associate Professor, Department of Pharmacy Practice, Philadelphia College of Pharmacy and Science; Clinical Assistant Professor, Department of Psychiatry, University of Pennsylvania School of Medicine, Philadelphia, Pennsylvania

Patricia A. Marken, BSPharm, PharmD
Associate Professor of Pharmacy Practice and Psychiatry, Schools of Pharmacy and Medicine, Division of Pharmacy Practice, University of Missouri at Kansas City, Kansas City, Missouri

Todd W. Mattox, PharmD, BCNSP
Nutrition Support Pharmacist, Department of Pharmacy, H. Lee Moffitt Cancer Center and Research Institute, Tampa, Florida

Gary R. Matzke, PharmD, FCP, FCCP
Professor, Department of Pharmacy and Therapeutics, Center for Clinical Pharmacology, Schools of Pharmacy and Medicine, University of Pittsburgh; Clinical Pharmacy Specialist–Nephrology, Department of Pharmacy, University of Pittsburgh Medical Center, Pittsburgh, Pennsylvania

J. Russell May, PharmD
Associate Director of Pharmacy, Department of Pharmacy, Medical College of Georgia Hospital and Clinics, Augusta, Georgia; Adjunct Associate Professor, Department of Pharmacy Practice, College of Pharmacy, University of Georgia, Athens, Georgia

Janet McCombs, PharmD
Clinical Assistant Professor, Department of Pharmacy Practice, College of Pharmacy, University of Georgia, Athens, Georgia

Margaret E. McGuinness, PharmD
Assistant Professor, College of Pharmacy, Oregon State University, Portland, Oregon

Timothy R. McGuire, PharmD
Associate Professor, Department of Pharmacy Practice, University of Nebraska College of Pharmacy, Omaha, Nebraska

Scott W. Mihalovic, PharmD, BCPS
Staff Pharmacist, Unity Pharmacy, St. Francis Medical Center, La Crosse, Wisconsin

Jay M. Mirtallo, MS, RPh, FASHP, BCNSP
Specialty Practice Pharmacist, Nutrition Support, Department of Pharmacy, The Ohio State University Medical Center; Clinical Associate Professor, Pharmacy Practice, College of Pharmacy, The Ohio State University, Columbus, Ohio

Andrea O. Moore, PharmD
Vice President of Clinical Operations, Advance Paradigm, Inc., Dallas, Texas

Robert M. Mowers, PharmD, BCPS
Coordinator, Drug Information Service, Department of Pharmaceutical Services, University of California at Davis Medical Center, Sacramento, California; Associate Clinical Professor, School of Pharmacy, Division of Clinical Pharmacy, University of California at San Francisco, San Francisco, California; Assistant Clinical Professor, School of Medicine, Division of Pulmonary and Critical Care Medicine, University of California at Davis, Davis, California

Patricia Moynahan Mullins, PharmD
National DUR Director, First Health Services Corporation, Richmond, Virginia

Bruce A. Mueller, PharmD, BCPS
Associate Professor of Clinical Pharmacy, Department of Pharmacy Practice, Purdue University School of Pharmacy and Pharmacal Sciences, West Lafayette, Indiana

Timothy A. Mullenix, PharmD, MS
Associate Professor, Pharmacy Practice, University of South Carolina College of Pharmacy, Columbia, South Carolina

Becky A. Nagle, PharmD, BCPS
Assistant Professor, Pharmacy Practice and Science, University of Maryland, Baltimore, Maryland

Milap C. Nahata, PharmD, FCCP
Professor of Pharmacy and Pediatrics, Colleges of Pharmacy and Medicine, Ohio State University; Director, Infectious Disease Research Laboratory, Wexner Institute for Pediatric Research, Children's Hospital, Columbus, Ohio

Jean Nappi, PharmD, FCCP, BCPS
Professor, College of Pharmacy, Medical University of South Carolina, Charleston, South Carolina

Warren A. Narducci, PharmD
Associate Professor of Pharmacy Practice and Department Chairman, College of Pharmacy, University of Nebraska Medical Center, Omaha, Nebraska

Merlin V. Nelson, PharmD, MD
Resident in Neurology, Department of Neurology, Henry Ford Hospital, Detroit, Michigan

Phillip A. Nowakowski, PharmD
Clinical Assistant Professor, Pharmacy Practice, College of Pharmacy, University of Illinois, Chicago, Illinois

Margaret A. Noyes, PharmD, BCPS
Assistant Professor, Department of Clinical Sciences and Administration, College of Pharmacy, University of Houston, Houston, Texas

Mary Beth O'Connell, PharmD, BCPS, FASHP, FCCP
Associate Professor, Pharmacy Practice, College of Pharmacy, University of Minnesota, Minneapolis, Minnesota

Beth E. Ostergaard, PharmD
Research Fellow, Infectious Diseases, Clinical Pharmacy, University of Minnesota/St. Paul–Ramsey Medical Center, St. Paul, Minnesota

Michael D. Parr, PharmD
Assistant Director, Department of Pharmacy, The University Hospital of Arkansas, Little Rock, Arkansas

William P. Petros, PharmD
Clinical Associate, Bone Marrow Transplant Program, Department of Medicine, Duke University Medical Center, Durham, North Carolina

Stephanie J. Phelps, PharmD, FCCP
Professor, Department of Clinical Pharmacy, University of Tennessee, Memphis, Tennessee

Denise Walbrandt Pigarelli, PharmD
Clinical Pharmacist, Department of Pharmacy, Carl T. Hayden Veterans Affairs Medical Center, Phoenix, Arizona

Ron E. Polk, PharmD
Professor of Pharmacy and Medicine, School of Pharmacy, Medical College of Virginia/Virginia Commonwealth University, Richmond, Virginia

Alexis Polles, MD
Research Fellow, National Institute on Aging, National Institutes of Health, U.S. Public Health Service, Bethesda, Maryland

L. Michael Posey, RPh
President, Pharmacy/Association Services, Athens, Georgia

Randall A. Prince, PharmD
Professor, Clinical Sciences and Administration, University of Houston College of Pharmacy, Texas Medical Center, Houston, Texas

L. Michael Prisant, MD
Professor of Medicine, Medical College of Georgia, Augusta, Georgia

Marc R. Pritzker, MD
Medical Director, Division of Cardiothoracic Transplantation, Abbott Northwestern Hospital/Minneapolis Heart Institute, Minneapolis, Minnesota

Richard J. Ptachcinski, PharmD, FCCP, BCPS
Director of Pharmacy, Ambulatory Care, Department of Pharmacy, University of Pittsburgh Medical Center; Associate Professor, Department of Pharmacy and Therapeutics, School of Pharmacy, University of Pittsburgh, Pittsburgh, Pennsylvania

Mark C. Pugh, PharmD
Pharmacist Manager, First Health Services Corporation, Richmond, Virginia

Marsha A. Raebel, PharmD, FCCP, BCPS
Clinical Pharmacy Services Manager, Department of Pharmacy Services, Kaiser Permanente of Colorado, Aurora, Colorado

Daniel W. Rahn, MD
Professor of Medicine; Vice Dean for Clinical Affairs, Medical College of Georgia, Augusta, Georgia

Robert P. Rapp, PharmD
Professor and Director, Division of Pharmacy Practice and Science, College of Pharmacy, University of Kentucky, Lexington, Kentucky

Charles A. Reasner, MD, FACE
Associate Professor, Department of Medicine, Division of Clinical Endocrinology, University of Texas Health Science Center, San Antonio, Texas

Kenneth E. Record, PharmD
Associate Professor of Pharmacy, Division of Pharmacy Practice and Science, College of Pharmacy, University of Kentucky, Chandler Medical Center, Lexington, Kentucky

Michael D. Reed, PharmD
Professor of Pediatrics, Department of Pediatrics, School of Medicine, Case Western Reserve University; Pediatric Pharmacology and Critical Care, Rainbow Babies and Childrens Hospital, Cleveland, Ohio

Monique Richer, PharmD, BCPS
Assistant Professor, Ecole de Pharmacie, Université Laval, Québec, Canada

Dennis H. Robinson, PhD
Associate Professor of Pharmaceutical Sciences, University of Nebraska College of Pharmacy, Omaha, Nebraska

Keith A. Rodvold, PharmD, FCCP, BCPS
Professor, Department of Pharmacy Practice, College of Pharmacy; Associate Professor, Section of Infectious Diseases, College of Medicine, University of Illinois, Chicago, Illinois

David A. Rogers, MD
Assistant Professor of Surgery, Department of Surgery, Medical College of Georgia, Augusta, Georgia

John C. Rotschafer, PharmD, FCCP
Professor, University of Minnesota/St. Paul–Ramsey Medical Center, Section of Clinical Pharmacy, St. Paul, Minnesota

Jean A. Rumsfield, PharmD
Clinical Assistant Professor, Department of Dermatology, College of Medicine, University of Illinois, Chicago, Illinois

Michael J. Rybak, PharmD, FCCP, BCPS
Professor of Pharmacy Practice, College of Pharmacy, Wayne State University; Director, The Anti-Infective Research Laboratory, Department of Pharmacy Services, Detroit Receiving Hospital and University Health Center, Detroit, Michigan

Gordon S. Sacks, PharmD
Nutrition Support Specialist, Clinical Pharmacy, Huntsville Hospital, Huntsville, Alabama

Lisa A. Sanchez, PharmD
Vice President, Department of Health Economics, Emron, Inc., Boston, Massachusetts

Michael J. Schmidt, PharmD
Clinical Pharmacist, Pharmacy Department, Clement Zablocki Veterans Affairs Medical Center, Milwaukee, Wisconsin

Mark E. Schneiderhan, BSPharm, PharmD
Pharmacotherapist, Department of Pharmacy, Michael Reese Hospital, Chicago, Illinois

Marieke Dekker Schoen, PharmD
Clinical Assistant Professor, Departments of Pharmacy Practice and Medicine, University of Illinois at Chicago, Chicago, Illinois

Nathan J. Schultz, PharmD, BCPS
Vice President, Pharmaceutical Industry Operations and Formulary Strategies, Diversified Pharmaceutical Services, Inc.; Clinical Assistant Professor, College of Pharmacy, University of Minnesota, Minneapolis, Minnesota

Arthur A. Schuna, MS, FASHP
Clinical Professor, School of Pharmacy, University of Wisconsin, Madison, Wisconsin

Rowena N. Schwartz, PharmD
Associate Professor, Department of Pharmacy and Therapeutics, School of Pharmacy, University of Pittsburgh, Pittsburgh, Pennsylvania

Russell E. Seay, PharmD
Clinical Assistant Professor, College of Pharmacy, University of Minnesota; Clinical Pharmacy Specialist, Pediatric Intensive Care Unit, Children's Health Care–Minneapolis, Minneapolis, Minnesota

John K. Siepler, PharmD, BCNSD
Nutrition Support Pharmacist, Department of Pharmaceutical Services, University of California at Davis Medical Center, Sacramento, California; Associate Clinical Professor, School of Pharmacy, Division of Clinical Pharmacy, University of California at San Francisco, San Francisco, California

Charles L. Smith, MD
Assistant Professor, School of Medicine, University of Minnesota; Department of Medicine, Hennepin County Medical Center, Minneapolis, Minnesota

Steven P. Smith, PharmD, BCPS
Clinical Assistant Professor, Department of Pharmacy Practice, University of Florida College of Pharmacy; Adult Oncology Clinical Specialist, Department of Pharmacy Services, Shands Hospital, Gainesville, Florida

Roger W. Sommi, PharmD
Associate Professor of Pharmacy Practice and Psychiatry, Schools of Pharmacy and Medicine, Division of Pharmacy Practice, University of Missouri at Kansas City, Kansas City, Missouri

Rakesh K. Sood, MD
Associate Professor, Department of Psychiatry, Virginia Commonwealth University, Richmond, Virginia

William J. Spruill, PharmD
Associate Professor, Department of Pharmacy Practice, College of Pharmacy, University of Georgia, Athens, Georgia

Wendy L. St. Peter, PharmD, BCPS
Assistant Professor, College of Pharmacy, University of Minnesota; Clinical Scientist, The Drug Evaluation Unit, Division of Nephrology, Hennepin County Medical Center, Minneapolis, Minnesota

Chester T. Stafford, MD
Professor of Medicine and Pediatrics, Allergy/Immunology Section, Medical College of Georgia, Augusta, Georgia

Condit F. Steil, PharmD, CDE
Associate Professor of Pharmacy Practice, Department of Pharmacy Practice, School of Pharmacy, Samford University, Birmingham, Alabama

Mark A. Stratton, PharmD, BCPS, FASHP
Professor and Chair, Department of Clinical Sciences and Administration, College of Pharmacy, University of Houston, Houston, Texas

Kathleen A. Stringer, PharmD, FCCP
Assistant Professor of Pharmacy, Department of Pharmacy Practice, College of Pharmacy, University of Colorado, Health Science Center, Denver, Colorado

Edward Sypniewski, Jr., PharmD
School of Pharmacy, Virginia Commonwealth University, Richmond, Virginia

Robert L. Talbert, PharmD, FCCP, BCPS
Professor and Division Head, College of Pharmacy, University of Texas at Austin; Professor, Departments of Medicine and Pharmacology, University of Texas Health Science Center at San Antonio, San Antonio, Texas

Joseph A. Tami, PharmD
Operations Manager, ISIS Pharmaceuticals, San Diego, California

Ignatius Y. S. Tang, PharmD, BCPS
Clinical Assistant Professor of Pharmacy Practice, College of Pharmacy, University of Illinois; Pharmacotherapist–Nephrology, University of Illinois at Chicago, Chicago, Illinois

A. Thomas Taylor, PharmD
Associate Professor, Department of Pharmacy Practice, University of Georgia College of Pharmacy; Associate Clinical Professor, Department of Family Medicine, Medical College of Georgia School of Medicine, Augusta, Georgia

Kathleen M. Teasley-Strausburg, MS, RPh, BCNSP
Nutrition Support Pharmacist, Lakewood, Colorado

Mary E. Teresi, PharmD
Assistant Professor, Division of Clinical and Administrative Pharmacy, The University of Iowa College of Pharmacy, Iowa City, Iowa

Karen A. Theesen, PharmD
Associate Professor of Pharmacy Practice and Psychiatry, Department of Pharmacy Practice, Creighton University, Omaha, Nebraska

Philip Toltzis, MD
Assistant Professor of Pediatrics, Department of Pediatrics, School of Medicine, Case Western Reserve University, Cleveland, Ohio

Clarence T. Ueda, PharmD, PhD
Professor and Dean, Department of Pharmaceutical Sciences, College of Pharmacy, University of Nebraska College of Pharmacy, Omaha, Nebraska

Amy Wells Valley, PharmD
Oncology Pharmacy Specialist, Audie L. Murphy Memorial Veterans' Hospital; Clinical Assistant Professor, Clinical Pharmacy Programs, University of Texas Health Science Center at San Antonio, San Antonio, Texas

Marigel Vargas-Ruiz, RPh, MS
Clinical Manager, Internal Medicine/Nephrology, University of Texas Medical Branch at Galveston; Assistant Professor, University of Texas, Galveston, Texas

Raman Venkataramanan, PhD, FCP
Professor, Pharmaceutical Sciences, School of Pharmacy, University of Pittsburgh, Pittsburgh, Pennsylvania

William E. Wade, PharmD
Associate Professor, Department of Pharmacy Practice, College of Pharmacy, University of Georgia, Athens, Georgia

Sharon M. Watling, PharmD, BCPS
Clinical Specialist, Critical Care; Assistant Professor of Medicine, Department of Pharmacy and Medicine, University of Missouri, Columbia, Missouri

Lynda S. Welage, PharmD
Associate Professor of Pharmacy, College of Pharmacy, University of Michigan; Clinical Pharmacist, Surgery–Trauma, University of Michigan Medical Center, Ann Arbor, Michigan

Barbara G. Wells, PharmD, FASHP, FCCP
Professor and Dean, Idaho State University College of Pharmacy, Pocatello, Idaho

Dennis P. West, PhD, FCCP
Professor, Department of Dermatology, Northwestern University Medical School, Chicago, Illinois

Dianne B. Williams, PharmD
Drug Information Specialist, Medical College of Georgia Hospital and Clinics; Adjunct Assistant Professor, College of Pharmacy, University of Georgia, Augusta, Georgia

Vickie M. Wilt, PharmD
Clinical Assistant Professor of Pharmacy, Department of Pharmacy Practice, University of Florida, Gainesville, Florida

Madolin K. Witte, MD
Assistant Professor of Pediatrics, Department of Pediatrics, School of Medicine, University of Utah, Salt Lake City, Utah

Shawn E. Wright, MD
American Lung Association Fellow in Pulmonary Diseases, The University of Texas Health Science Center, San Antonio, Texas

Gary C. Yee, PharmD, FCCP
Associate Professor, Department of Pharmacy Practice, College of Pharmacy, University of Florida Health Science Center, Gainesville, Florida

William C. Zamboni, PharmD
Research Fellow, Department of Pharmaceutical Sciences, St. Jude Children's Research Hospital, Memphis, Tennessee

Mario Zarama, MD
Nephrology Fellow, School of Medicine, University of Minnesota, Minneapolis, Minnesota

Illustrations

PART ONE

Basic Concepts of Pathophysiology and Pharmacotherapy

Chapter 1

Pharmacoeconomics: Principles, Methods, and Application to Pharmacotherapy

Lisa A. Sanchez, PharmD

Today's cost-sensitive health care environment has created a competitive and challenging workplace for clinicians of the 1990s. Competition for diminishing resources has necessitated that the appraisal of health care goods and services extend beyond evaluations of safety and efficacy and consider the economic impact of these goods and services on the cost of health care. A challenge for health care professionals of the 1990s is to provide quality patient care with minimal resources.

An interest in defining the "value" of medicine is a common thread joining today's health care professionals, especially pharmacists. With serious concerns about rising medication costs and consistent pressure to decrease pharmacy expenditures and budgets, pharmacists must answer the question, "What is the value of the pharmaceutical goods and services I provide?" *Pharmacoeconomics,* or the discipline of placing a value on drug therapy,[1] has evolved to provide an answer to this question.

Challenged to provide high-quality patient care in the least expensive way, pharmacists have developed strategies aimed at containing costs. However, most of these strategies focus solely on determining the least expensive alternative rather than the alternative that possesses the best value for the money. The "cheapest" alternative—with respect to drug acquisition cost—is not always the best value for patients, departments, institutions, and health care systems.

Quality patient care must not be compromised while attempting to contain costs. The products and services delivered by today's pharmacists should demonstrate "pharmacoeconomic value," that is, a balance of both economic *and* clinical outcomes. Pharmacoeconomics can provide the systematic means for this quantification. This chapter discusses the principles and methods of pharmacoeconomics and how they can be applied to clinical pharmacy practice, and thereby how they can assist in evaluating the value of pharmacotherapy and other modalities of treatment in clinical practice.

Principles of Pharmacoeconomics

Pharmacoeconomics has been defined as the description and the analysis of the cost of drug therapy to health care systems and society.[2] More specifically, pharmacoeconomic research is the process of identifying, measuring, and comparing the costs, risks, and benefits of programs, services, or therapies and determining which alternative produces the best health outcome for the resource invested.[3] For most pharmacists this translates into weighing the cost of providing a pharmacy product or service against the consequences (outcomes) realized by using the product or service, to determine which alternative yields the optimal outcome per dollar spent. This information can assist clinical decision makers in choosing the most cost-effective treatment options.[4]

Pharmacoeconomics is not synonymous with outcomes research. Although pharmacoeconomics is a division of outcomes research, not all outcomes research is pharmacoeconomic research. Outcomes research is defined more broadly as studies that attempt to identify, measure, and evaluate the results of health care services in general.[5] Outcomes research is discusssed further in Chapter 2.

Cost is defined as the value of the resources consumed by a program or drug therapy of interest. *Consequence* is defined as the effects, outputs, or outcomes of the program of drug therapy of interest. Consideration of both costs and consequences differentiates most pharmacoeconomic evaluation methods from traditional cost-containment strategies and drug-use evaluations.

Assessing costs and consequences—the value of a pharmaceutical product or service—depends heavily on the perspective of the evaluation. Perspectives include the following:

- Patient
- Provider
- Hospital or health system

- Third-party payer or managed-care organization
- Government
- Society

A pharmacoeconomic evaluation can assess the value of a product or service from single or multiple perspectives. However, clarification of the perspective is critical since the results of a pharmacoeconomic evaluation depend heavily on the perspective taken. For example, if comparing the value of alteplase (tPA) to streptokinase, from a patient or societal perspective tPA may be the best value alternative because a 1% reduction in mortality rates is observed in this large population. Yet, from a small community hospital's perspective, streptokinase may represent a better value because it provides similar outcomes for less money.

Once the perspective is clear, a full evaluation of the relevant costs and consequences can begin. Health care costs or economic outcomes can be grouped into several categories[6]:

- Direct medical
- Direct nonmedical
- Indirect nonmedical
- Intangible costs

Direct medical costs are those incurred for medical products and services used to prevent, detect, and/or treat a disease (e.g., drugs, labs, hospitalizations).[6] *Direct nonmedical* costs are any costs for nonmedical services that are results of illness but do not involve purchasing medical services (e.g., costs of transportation and hotel rooms near a treatment center).[5] *Indirect nonmedical* costs are the costs of reduced productivity (e.g., morbidity and mortality costs).[6–8] *Intangible* costs are those costs incurred that represent other nonfinancial outcomes of disease and medical care, which are not appropriately expressed in a dollar value (e.g., pain, suffering, grief).[5] Costs can also be measured as "opportunity costs." Opportunity costs represent the economic benefit forgone when using one therapy instead of the next best alternative therapy,[8] that is, the greatest possible benefit that might have been obtained by using the resources elsewhere.[8] Table 1.1 contains examples of these costs.

Consequences (or outcomes) can also be categorized. Types of outcomes include economic (discussed previously), clinical, and humanistic outcomes. Clinical outcomes are the medical events that occur as a result of disease or treatment.[9] Humanistic outcomes are the consequences of disease or treatment on patient functional status or quality of life along several dimensions (e.g., physical function, social function, general health and well-being, life satisfaction).[9] These consequences (outcomes) can also be categorized as positive or negative. An example of a positive outcome is a desired effect of a drug, possibly manifested as an efficacy or effectiveness measure of a drug. A negative outcome is an undesired or adverse effect of a drug, possibly manifested as a treatment failure or an adverse drug reaction (ADR). Pharmacoeconomic evaluations should include assessments of both positive and negative outcomes. Evaluating only positive outcomes may be misleading because of the detriment and expense associated with negative outcomes.

TABLE 1.1. EXAMPLE OF HEALTH CARE COST CATEGORIES

Cost Category	Costs
Direct medical costs	Drugs Supplies Laboratory tests Health care professionals' time Hospitalization
Direct nonmedical costs	Transportation Food Family care Home aides
Indirect nonmedical costs	Patient lost wages (morbidity) Spouse, family, or friend lost wages Income forgone due to premature death (mortality)
Intangible costs	Pain Suffering Grief
Opportunity costs	Lost opportunity Revenue forgone

(From Ref. 15.)

Methods of Pharmacoeconomics

The pharmacoeconomic methods of evaluation are listed in Fig. 1.1. These methods or tools can be separated into two distinct categories, economic and humanistic evaluation techniques. These methods have been used in a variety of fields and are being applied increasingly to health care.[10] Those most commonly used by pharmacists are discussed in the following sections and briefly summarized in Table 1.2.

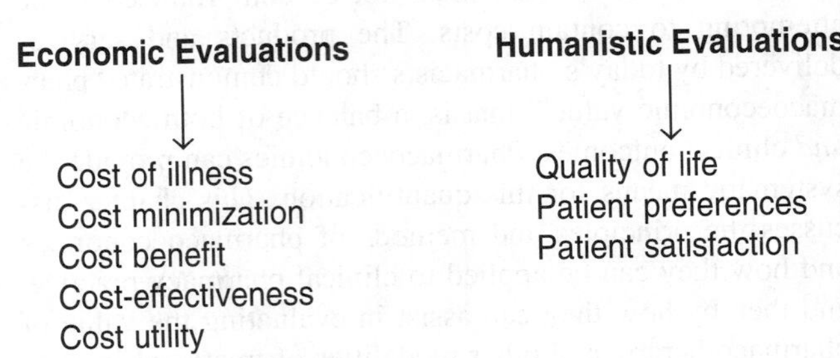

Figure 1.1. Components of pharmacoeconomics. *(From Ref. 45.)*

TABLE 1.2. SUMMARY OF PHARMACOECONOMIC METHODOLOGIES

Method	Description	Application	Cost Unit	Outcome Unit
COI	Estimates the cost of a disease on a defined population	Use to provide baseline to compare prevention/treatment options against	$$$	NA
CMA	Finds the least expensive cost alternative	Use when benefits are the same	$$$	Assume to be equivalent in comparative groups
CBA	Measures benefit in monetary units and computes a net gain	Can compare programs with different objectives	$$$	$$$
CEA	Compares alternatives with therapeutic effects measured in physical units and computes a C/E ratio	Can compare drugs/programs that differ in clinical outcomes and use same units of benefit	$$$	Natural units (mm Hg blood pressure, mg/dL blood sugar)
CUA	Measures therapeutic consequences in utility units rather than physical units; computes a C/U ratio	Use to compare drugs/programs that are life extending with serious side effects or those producing reductions in morbidity	$$$	Quality adjusted life years (QALYs) or other utilities
QOL	Physical, social, and emotional aspects of patient's well being that are relevant and important to the patient	Examines drug effects in areas not covered by laboratory or physiologic measurements	NA	QOL score

Key: CBA = cost-benefit analysis; CEA = cost-effectiveness analysis; CMA = cost-minimization analysis; COI = cost-of-illness evaluation; CUA = cost-utility analysis; QOL = quality-of-life assessment. (Compiled from Refs. 7, 20, and 45.)

ECONOMIC EVALUATION METHODS

The basic task of economic evaluations is to identify, measure, value, and compare the costs and consequences of the alternatives being considered. The two distinguishing characteristics of economic evaluations are as follows: (1) Is there a comparison of two or more alternatives? and (2) Are both costs and consequences of the alternatives examined?[12] A full economic evaluation encompasses both characteristics, while a partial economic evaluation addresses only one of these characteristics.

Application of economic evaluation methods to health care products and services, especially pharmaceuticals, may increase their acceptance by health care professionals and society.[13] Popular economic evaluation methods include cost-of-illness evaluation, and cost-minimization, cost-benefit, cost-effectiveness, and cost-utility analyses. Each method, except cost-of-illness evaluation, is used to compare competing programs or treatment alternatives. The methods are all similar in the way they measure cost (dollars) and different in their measurement of outcomes. A brief discussion of each method is provided.

Cost-of-Illness Evaluation

A cost-of-illness (COI) evaluation identifies and estimates the overall cost of a particular disease on a defined population.[7] This evaluation method is often referred to as "burden-of-illness" and involves measuring the direct and indirect costs attributable to a specific disease. The cost of various diseases, including peptic ulcer disease, mental disorders, and cancer, in the United States have been estimated.

By successfully identifying direct and indirect costs of an illness, one can determine the relative value of a treatment or prevention strategy. For example, by determining the cost of a particular disease to society, the cost of a prevention strategy could be subtracted from this to yield the benefit of implementing this strategy nationwide. COI is not used to compare competing treatment alternatives, but to provide an estimation of the financial burden of a disease. Thus, the value of prevention and treatment strategies can be measured against this illness cost.

Cost-Minimization Analysis

Cost-minimization analysis (CMA) involves the determination of the least costly alternative when comparing two or more treatment alternatives. With CMA, the alternatives must have an assumed or demonstrated equivalency in safety and efficacy (i.e., the two alternatives must be therapeutically equivalent). Once this equivalency in outcome is confirmed, the costs can be identified, measured, and compared in monetary units (dollars).

CMA is a relatively straightforward and simple method for comparing competing programs or treatment alternatives, as long as the therapeutic equivalence of the alternatives being compared has been established. If no evidence exists to support this, then a more comprehensive method such as cost-effectiveness analysis should be employed. Remember, CMA shows only a “cost savings” of one program or treatment over another.[14]

Employing CMA is appropriate when comparing two or more therapeutically equivalent agents or alternate dosing regimens of the same agent.[14] For example, if drugs A and B are antiulcer agents, documented to be equal in efficacy and incidence of ADRs, then the costs of using these drugs could be compared using CMA. These costs should extend beyond a comparison of drug acquisition costs and include costs of preparation, administration, and storage. The least expensive agent, considering all of these costs, should be preferred.

Cost-Benefit Analysis

Cost-benefit analysis (CBA) is a method that allows for the identification, measurement, and comparison of the benefits and costs of a program or treatment alternative. The benefits realized from a program or treatment alternative are compared with the costs of providing the program or treatment alternative. Both the costs and the benefits are measured and converted into equivalent dollars in the year in which they will occur.[6,10] Future cost and benefits are discounted or reduced to their current value.

These costs and benefits are expressed as a ratio (a benefit-to-cost ratio [B/C]), a net benefit, or a net cost. A clinical decision maker would choose the program or treatment alternative with the highest net benefit or the greatest B/C ratio.[8] Guidelines for the interpretation of this ratio are indicated.[11,14,15]

If $B/C > 1$, the program or treatment is of value (i.e., benefits realized by the program/treatment alternative outweigh the cost of providing the program/treatment alternative).

If $B/C = 1$, the benefits equal the cost (i.e., the benefits realized by the program/treatment alternative are equivalent to the cost of providing the program/treatment alternative).

If $B/C < 1$, the program or treatment is not economically beneficial (i.e., cost of providing the program/treatment alternative outweighs the benefits realized by the program/treatment alternative).

CBA should be employed when comparing treatment alternatives in which the costs and benefits do not occur simultaneously. CBA may also be used when comparing programs with different objectives, because all benefits are converted into dollars. CBA can also be used to evaluate a single program or compare multiple programs. However, valuing health benefits in monetary terms can be difficult and controversial. The expression of some health benefits as monetary units is neither appropriate nor widely accepted. Therefore, unless the benefits of a program or treatment alternative are appropriately expressed in dollars, CBA should not be employed.[14]

CBA may be an appropriate method to use in justifying and documenting the value of an existing pharmacy service or the potential worth of a new one. For example, when competing for institutional resources, CBA can provide data to document that a clinical pharmacy service yields a high return on investment compared with other institutional services competing for the same resources. However, the relative magnitude of the costs and benefits for the service must be considered when making this resource allocation decision. If a service costs $100 to implement and results in a benefit to the hospital of $1000, and a service that costs $100,000 to implement results in a benefit of $1,000,000, both have a B/C ratio of 10.[14] Thus, caution should be exercised when using B/C ratios and CBA as a comparison tool.

Cost-Effectiveness Analysis

Cost-effectiveness analysis (CEA) is a way of summarizing the health benefits and resources used by competing health care programs so that policymakers can choose among them.[12] CEA involves comparing programs or treatment alternatives with different safety and efficacy profiles. Cost is measured in dollars, and outcomes in terms of obtaining a specific therapeutic outcome. These outcomes are often expressed in physical units, natural units, or nondollar units (i.e., lives saved, cases cured, life expectancy, or mm Hg drop in blood pressure).[7,16,17]

The results of CEA are also expressed as a ratio—either as an average cost-effectiveness ratio (ACER) or as an incremental cost-effectiveness (C/E) ratio. An ACER represents the total cost of a program or treatment alternative divided by the clinical outcome of the program or treatment alternative to yield a ratio representing the dollar cost per specific clinical outcome gained, independent of comparators. The AC/E ratio can be summarized as follows.[6,14,17]

$$AC/E = \frac{\text{Health care costs (\$)}}{\text{Clinical outcome (not in \$)}}$$

This allows the costs and outcomes to be reduced to a single value to allow for comparison. Using this ratio, the clinician would choose the alternative with the least cost per outcome gained.[8]

The most cost-effective alternative is not always the least costly alternative for obtaining a specific therapeutic objective. In this regard, cost effectiveness need not be cost reduction, but rather cost optimization.[18]

Often clinical effectiveness is gained at an increased cost. Is the increased benefit worth the increased cost? Incremental cost-effectiveness analysis may be used to determine the additional cost and effectiveness gained when one treatment alternative is compared with the next best treatment alternative.[6] Thus, instead of comparing the average C/E ratios of each treatment alternative, the additional cost that a treatment alternative imposes over another treatment is compared with the additional effect, benefit, or outcome it provides. The incremental C/E ratio (ICER) can be summarized as follows:

$$\text{ICER} = \frac{\text{Cost (\$)}_a - \text{Cost (\$)}_b}{\text{Effect (\%)}_a - \text{Effect (\%)}_b}$$

This formula yields the additional cost required to obtain the additional effect gained by switching from drug A to drug B.

CEA is particularly useful in balancing cost with patient outcome, determining which treatment alternatives represent the best health outcome per dollar spent, and when it is appropriate to measure outcome in terms of obtaining a specific therapeutic objective. In addition, CEA may provide data to support drug policy, formulary management, and individual patient treatment decisions. Globally, CEA is being used to set public policies regarding the use of pharmaceutical products (national formularies) in countries such as Australia,[19] New Zealand, and Canada.[20]

When comparing antiemetic agents for development of a policy for the prevention of chemotherapy-induced emesis (CIE), CEA can be employed. Many of these agents differ with respect to effectiveness, safety, and cost. By performing a thorough CEA, these variables can be reduced into a single number (C/E ratio), which will allow for a meaningful comparison. The treatment alternative with a better C/E ratio than the others (i.e., lower cost per unit of outcome) would be selected and promoted for use.

Cost-Utility Analysis

Cost-utility analysis (CUA) is another method for comparing treatment alternatives. CUA integrates patient preferences and health-related quality of life (QOL). Cost is measured in dollars and therapeutic outcome in patient-weighted utilities, rather than in physical units. Often the utility measure used is a "quality-adjusted-life-year" (QALY) gained. QALY is a common measure of health status used in CUA, combining morbidity and mortality data.

Results of CUA are also expressed in a ratio, a cost-utility (C/U) ratio. Most often, this ratio is translated as the "cost per quality-adjusted-life-year (QALY) gained."[7,11] The preferred treatment alternative is that with the lowest cost per QALY (or other health status utility).

CUA is the most appropriate method to use when comparing programs and treatment alternatives that are life extending with serious side effects (e.g., cancer chemotherapy), those that produce reductions in morbidity rather than mortality (e.g., medical treatment of arthritis),[18] and when QOL is the most important health outcome being examined. CUA is employed less frequently than other economic evaluation methods because of lack of agreement in measuring utilities, difficulty comparing QALYs across patients and populations, and difficulty quantifying patient preferences. Thus, CUA should be reserved for comparing treatment alternatives whose primary goal is improving QOL, and caution should be exercised when using this method.

HUMANISTIC EVALUATION METHODS

Pharmacoeconomic evaluations may also focus on humanistic concerns. Methods for evaluating the impact of disease and treatment of disease on patient's health-related QOL, patient preferences, and patient satisfaction are all growing in popularity and application to pharmacotherapy decisions. These methods can also assist clinicians in quantifying the value of pharmaceuticals.

QOL has been defined as the assessment of the functional effects of illness and its consequent therapy as perceived by the patient.[21] These effects are often displayed as physical, emotional, and social effects on the patient.[13] Measurement of health-related QOL is usually achieved through the use of patient-completed questionnaires. Many questionnaires are available, and most are either disease-specific or generic measures of health status.[22,23] Various overviews on QOL and its application to pharmacy have been published.[24–26] For further discussion, refer to Chapter 2.

APPLICATION OF PHARMACOECONOMICS TO PHARMACOTHERAPY

BENEFITS OF PHARMACOECONOMICS

Pharmacists, regardless of practice setting, can benefit from using pharmacoeconomics. Various benefits of pharmacoeconomics are listed in Table 1.3. Many pharmacists have been called on to quantify the value of the products and services they provide. The appropriate application of the principles and methods of pharmacoeconomics provides the means for this valuation.

One of the primary uses of pharmacoeconomics in clinical practice is to aid clinical and policy decision making. Complete pharmacotherapy decisions should contain three basic evaluation components: clinical, economic, and

TABLE 1.3. BENEFITS OF PHARMACOECONOMICS FOR CLINICIANS

- Pharmacoeconomics can assess the value of the products and services that pharmacists provide.
- Pharmacoeconomics can assist in choosing between competing treatment alternatives.
- Pharmacoeconomics can provide data necessary to make better medication use decisions.
- Pharmacoeconomics can assist pharmacists in balancing cost with quality and patient outcome.

(Compiled from Refs. 14 and 15.)

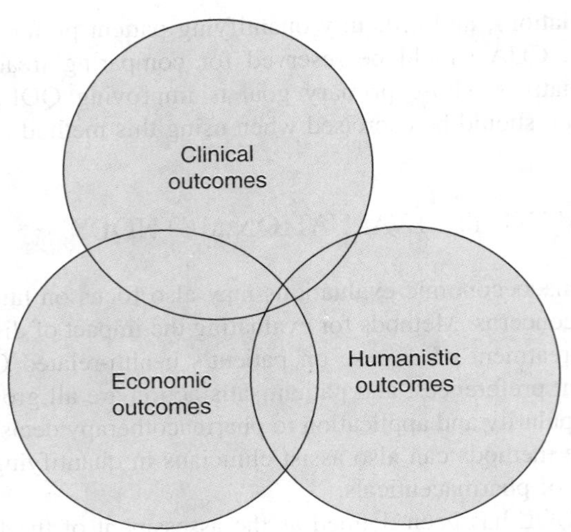

Figure 1.2. Components of contemporary clinical decision making. *(From Kozma CM, Reeder CE, Shulz RM. Economic, clinical, and humanistic outcomes: A planning model for pharmacoeconomic research. Clin Ther, 1993;15(6):112–1132.)*

humanistic outcomes; that is, pharmacoeconomic value of a drug or service,[1,10,14] as illustrated in Fig. 1.2. No longer can drug selection decisions be based solely on acquisition costs. This strategy is misleading because of the inability to capture potential costs associated with diminished safety and efficacy profiles. Through the appropriate application of pharmacoeconomic principles and methods, incorporating these three critical components into clinical decisions can be accomplished.

Pharmacoeconomic data can be a poweful tool to support various clinical decisions, including effective formulary management, individual patient treatment, medication policy, and resource allocation.[14,17] For example, pharmacoeconomics can provide critical cost-effectiveness data to support formulary addition or removal. In fact, the pharmacoeconomic assessment of formulary actions is becoming a standardized part of many pharmacy and therapeutic (P&T) committees. A drug-use policy decision may have a greater impact on prescribing behavior, if based on sound pharmacoeconomic data. When competing for hospital resources, pharmacoeconomics can provide the data necessary to justify that a pharmacy service maximizes the resources allocated to it by hospital administration. Evaluating the impact a drug has on a patient's health-related quality of life can be useful when deciding between two agents for an individual patient treatment decision.

In the past, inclusion of economic outcomes (costs) in clinical decisions seemed to necessitate a compromise in the quality of care delivered. However, when used appropriately, pharmacoeconomics can assist in balancing cost with patient outcome (quality of care), often resulting in maintaining or improving quality of care, at potential cost-savings (see Fig. 1.3). Best-valued drugs will be those with optimal patient outcome per dollar spent compared to competitors.

STRATEGIES TO INCORPORATE PHARMACOECONOMICS INTO PHARMACOTHERAPY

Various strategies are available to incorporate pharmacoeconomics into pharmacotherapy decisions. Popular strategies for using pharmacoeconomics to assess the value of pharmaceuticals include using the results of published pharmacoeconomic evaluations, using economic modeling, or conducting pharmacoeconomic research.[27] Some advan-

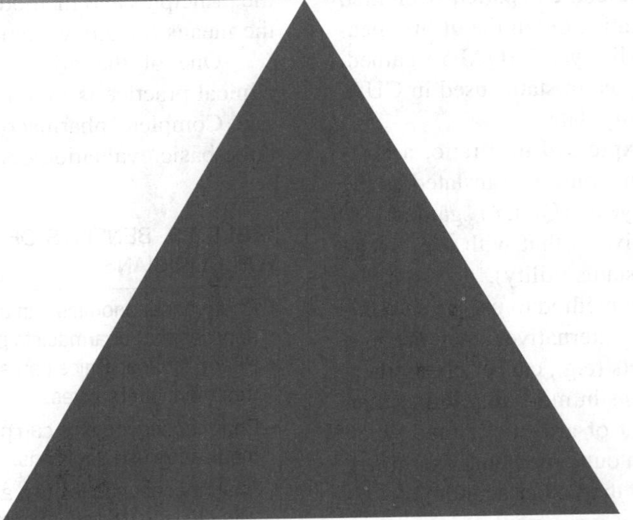

Figure 1.3. Cost and consequence balance.

TABLE 1.4. ADVANTAGES AND DISADVANTAGES OF STRATEGIES TO PUT PHARMACOECONOMICS INTO PRACTICE

Strategy	Advantage	Disadvantage
Use published literature	Inexpensive Readily available Provides data quickly Subject to peer review Results may be from a large population randomized, controlled trial	Data may be from a randomized, controlled trial (protocol-driven) Difficult to generalize results May not be comparative Variations in quality of analyses published
Build an economic model	Relatively inexpensive Provides data quickly Can bridge efficacy and effectiveness Can be plan or institution specific	Results are dependent on assumptions Researcher bias may be introduced Controversial
Conduct an institution or plan-specific study	Usually comparative Data will be plan or institution specific Designed to reflect "usual care" Can be prospective or retrospective	Expensive Time consuming Can be difficult to randomize and highly control Patient selection bias may be introduced Potential for small sample size

Adapted from Sanchez LA. In Principles of Pharmacoeconomics. 2nd ed. Cincinnati OH, Harvey Whitney Books, 1991.

tages and disadvantages of these strategies are summarized in Table 1.4.

Use of Pharmacoeconomic Literature

Quantifying the value of pharmaceuticals through pharmacoeconomics has increased in popularity. Many pharmacoeconomic analyses have been published in primary medical and pharmacy literature sources. However, the eagerness to conduct pharmacoeconomic evaluations of drugs has often exceeded the quality of these evaluations. Variations in quality and indiscriminate use of pharmacoeconomic terminology have been documented in medical and pharmacy literature sources.[4,28–30] To use this literature to aid in clinical decision making, it must be (1) critically evaluated for quality and (2) interpreted correctly.

It can be difficult to generalize the results of a published pharmacoeconomic study to other sites. This primarily is due to differences in patient populations, practice techniques, and acquistion costs between hospitals and organizations. Therefore, prior to using pharmacoeconomic data to make the decisions about whether to use the data to support clinical or policy decisions, those who make the decisions should recognize its limitations.

Various guidelines or criteria for evaluating, conducting, and reporting pharmacoeconomic literature have been published.[6,12,20,31–36] These guidelines and criteria have been combined and summarized into 11 categories most pertinent to pharmacotherapy.[34] A summary of these 11 criteria and pertinent questions for each category are contained in Table 1.5. Each evaluation criterion is briefly discussed next.

Study Objective

A clear statement of the purpose of the study should be given. This objective should be clear, concise, well defined, and measurable.

Study Perspective

The researcher must select one or more perspectives (e.g., patient, provider, payer, or society) from which the analysis will be conducted.[8] This perspective should be appropriate given the scope of the pharmacoeconomic problem identified. An evaluation may be conducted from single or multiple perspectives, as long as the costs and consequences identified are relevant to the perspective(s) chosen.

Study Method

It should be clear which pharmacoeconomic method was employed (CEA, CMA, CBA, or CUA), and this method should be appropriate given the problem (e.g., CMA is appropriate if comparing two alternatives equivalent in therapeutic outcome, but not if the alternatives differ in therapeutic outcome). Also, a researcher may claim a specific method was employed (e.g., CEA) but actually employ another method (e.g., CMA).

Study Design

Pharmacoeconomic evaluations can be prospective or retrospective. Although prospective designs are usually preferred, retrospective evaluations can be rich with information and reflective of usual care. Many pharmacoeconomic evaluations today are conducted as a part of randomized, controlled, clinical trials. Two cautions for interpreting pharmacoeconomic data collected in this manner include (1) costs can be protocol driven, not necessarily reflective of using a drug in common practice,[39] and (2) control of subjects and decreased complications may yield greater costs and benefits than those observed in common practice.[31]

Choice of Interventions

All relevant and available treatment options should be completely described or mentioned. The treatment alternatives

TABLE 1.5. CRITERIA FOR THE EVALUATION OF PHARMACOECONOMIC LITERATURE

Objective
What is the question(s) being considered?
Is the question clear, defined, and measurable?
Perspective
What is the perspective(s) of the analysis?
Is it appropriate given the scope of the problem?
Type of Analysis
What pharmacoeconomic tool was used?
Is it appropriate given the problem?
Is it actually what was conducted?
Study Design
What was the study design?
What were the data sources?
Is the evaluation suitable if carried out in a clinical trial?
Choice of Interventions
Were all appropriate alternatives considered and described?
Were any appropriate alternatives omitted?
Are the alternatives relevant to the perspective and clinical nature of the study?
Is there evidence that the alternatives' effectiveness has been established?
Costs and Consequences
What are the costs and consequences (outcomes) included?
Are the costs and outcomes relevant to the perspective chosen?
Do they include negative outcomes (failures, ADRs)?
How were they valued?
Were cost and consequences measured in the appropriate physical units?
Discounting
Was the study performed over time?
Were costs and consequences which occur in the future discounted to their present value?
Was any justification given for discount rate used?
Results
Are the results accurate and practical for medical decision makers?
Were the appropriate statistical analyses performed?
Was an incremental analysis performed?
Are all the assumptions and limitations of study discussed?
Sensitivity Analysis
Are cost ranges for significant variables tested for sensitivity?
Are the appropriate and relevant variables varied?
Do the findings follow the anticipated trend?
Conclusions
Are the conclusions of the study justified?
Is it possible to extrapolate the conclusions to daily clinical practice?
Sponsorship
Was there any bias due to sponsorship of the study?

(Compiled from Refs. 3, 4, 7, 12, 28, 30–34, 37, and 38.)

and dosages being compared should be those used in common practice, and evidence of their effectiveness should be established. Since pharmacoeconomic methods are tools to aid in choosing between treatment alternatives, assessing the cost of a single alternative is considered a partial economic evaluation.

Costs and Consequences

All the important and relevant costs and consequences for each program or treatment alternative should be identified. The cost and consequences identified must be relevant to the study perspective(s), and measured in suitable terms, using the appropriate physical units. Costs should include direct, indirect, and intangible costs and consequences should include the positive and negative clinical and humanistic outcomes associated with the program or treatment alternative. All of these costs and consequences must be valued credibly, with the data sources clearly identified.

Discounting

The comparison of programs or treatment alternatives should be made at one point in time, thus any costs and consequences not occurring in the present must be addressed. "Discounting," or adjusting for differential timing, is the process of reducing any costs and consequences that may occur in the future back to their present value. If a study is performed over time (more than one year), or if future cost savings are projected, discounting should be done using an appropriate discount rate. The rate typically used is 4–8%, representing annual inflation or bank interest rates. However, many researchers use a discount rate of 5%.

Study Results

A full discussion of the study assumptions, limitations, and how to interpret the results in the context of different practice settings[12] should be provided. This discussion should include all relevant issues of concern to potential users of the study. The results should reflect that the appropriate statistical analyses were performed. Also, it may be appropriate to express the study results in terms of increases, that is, to use incremental cost analysis (additional cost of gaining an additional benefit by using one drug over another).

Sensitivity Analysis

It is imperative that researchers test the sensitivity of study results using sensitivity analysis. Sensitivity analysis (SA) is the process of testing the robustness of an economic evaluation by examining changes in results. Specific variables such as percent effectiveness, incidence of ADRs, and dominant resources can be varied over a range of plausible values and the results recalculated. SA is of paramount importance because of the very common need for investigators to use assumptions and estimates for unknown variables.[30]

Study Conclusions

Researchers should assist the reader in extrapolating study conclusions to clinical practice. The conclusions drawn from the study results should be justified (internal validity) and able to be generalized (external validity).[31] Also, conclusions drawn from results that were "statistically" significant may or may not be "clinically" significant, and vice versa.

Sponsorship

Similar to evaluating the quality of a clinical trial, sponsorship of a study should be considered when evaluating the quality and usefulness of a pharmacoeconomic study.[32] Quality of studies conducted or sponsored by pharmaceutical companies will vary by company, product, or evaluation and the potential for bias should be neither ignored nor assumed. Many of the studies sponsored or conducted by the pharmaceutical industry to date have been academically rigorous as well as informative. A clear understanding of how to evaluate, critique, and use the pharmacoeconomic literature appropriately will minimize any potential effects of this criteria on clinical decision making.

Build an Economic Model

Modeling studies use existing clinical and/or epidemiological data to project future cost savings.[38] Use of economic models can provide support for various clinical decisions, especially those that are time contingent.[27] Identifying assumptions regarding the treatment alternatives being compared, the patient outcomes under study, and the probability of those outcomes occurring can provide the basis for an economic simulation to assist in the medication decision-making process.

Economic modeling often employs decision analysis, which has been defined as an explicit, quantitative, and prescriptive approach to choosing among alternative outcomes.[41,42] The tool used in decision analysis is a decision tree. A decision tree provides a framework to display graphically primary variables including treatment options, outcomes associated with those treatment options, and probabilities of the outcomes. The researcher can then algebraically reduce all of these factors into a single value, allowing for comparison.

Building an economic model can help the clinician to forecast the impact of medication-use decisions on a patient, institution, or health care system. Also, as new drugs are marketed that can displace older agents, an economic model can expedite the reappraisal process for formulary management and drug-use policy decisions.[41] For building an economic model to assist in clinical decision making, various published examples can be considered.[42,43]

Conduct a Pharmacoeconomic Evaluation

Clinicians may need to conduct a pharmacoeconomic evaluation if there is insufficient literature, if published results cannot be extrapolated to clinical practice, or if building a model is not appropriate. Before conducting a pharmacoeconomic evaluation, clinicians should be familiar with the similarities, differences, and appropriate application of pharmacoeconomic methods, discussed earlier in this chapter.

The decision to conduct a local pharmacoeconomic study is not without its own costs. Because both time and monetary resources are consumed by these evaluations, specific pharmacy products and services for pharmacoeconomic evaluation should be targeted. Thus this strategy should be reserved for pharmacy decisions that may have a significant impact on cost or quality of care.

Conducting pharmacoeconomic research in a hospital or managed care environment can be challenging. Lack of institutional resources, small sample sizes, difficulty randomizing, inability to compare with placebo, and difficulty generalizing results may all be limitations. For example, when asked to determine and recommend the most cost-effective antihypertensive agent for a formulary management decision, clinicians may lack monetary and time resources to conduct a scientifically rigorous study.

Conducting a pharmacoeconomic evaluation should be guided by the criteria for quality economic evaluations,[7,12,20,31–34] a 10-step process identified by Jolicoeur et al.,[43] and four additional steps identified by the author can provide readers with guidance for conducting a local pharmacoeconomic study.[27] Table 1.6 contains 14 steps to guide a pharmacoeconomic evaluation. Many of these steps are

TABLE 1.6. GUIDELINES FOR PERFORMING PHARMACOECONOMIC RESEARCH IN MANAGED CARE/HOSPITAL SETTINGS

1. Define the pharmacoeconomic problem.
2. Create a cross-functional project team.
3. Determine the study's perspective.
4. Determine the treatment alternatives and outcomes.
5. Select the appropriate pharmacoeconomic method.
6. Place monetary values on the outcomes.
7. Identify resources.
8. Establish the probabilities of the outcome events.
9. Use decision analysis.
10. Discount costs or perform a sensitivity or incremental cost analysis.
11. Present the results.
12. Develop an intervention or policy.
13. Implement intervention or policy and educate key professionals.
14. Document quality of care and potential cost savings through follow-up.

(Compiled from Refs. 34 and 44.)

similar to the evaluation criterion discussed earlier in this chapter but they are discussed briefly in the following paragraphs.

Step 1: Define the Pharmacoeconomic Problem

A broad problem might be "Which antiemetic regimen represents the best value for the prevention of chemotherapy-induced emesis (CIE)?" However, a more succinct and measurable problem would be "Which regimen is the best value for preventing acute CIE in patients receiving highly emetogenic chemotherapy?"

Step 2: Assemble a Cross-Functional Study Team

This team can provide early "buy-in" and additional resources for a pharmacoeconomic evaluation. Team members vary depending on the analysis, but may include representatives from medicine, nursing, pharmacy, hospital administration, and information systems.

Step 3: Define the Appropriate Study Perspective

Choose a study perspective(s) most relevant to the problem. For example, if the problem is as listed in step 1, then the perspective of the institution may be most appropriate.

Step 4: Identify Treatment Alternatives and Outcomes Associated with Alternatives

Treatment alternatives can include pharmacologic and nonpharmacologic options, but should include all clinically relevant alternatives. The outcomes identified should include both positive and negative clinical outcomes.

Step 5: Identify the Appropriate Pharmacoeconomic Method to Employ

Methods to choose from include cost-minimization, cost-benefit, cost-effectiveness, and cost-utility analyses. Employing the incorrect method can adversely affect medication decisions influencing both cost and quality of care.

Step 6: Place a Monetary Value on Treatment Alternatives and Outcomes

This includes not only drug administration and acquisition costs but also the cost of positive and negative clinical outcomes, for example, determining the cost of ADRs and treatment failures. This can be measured prospectively or retrospectively or estimated using comprehensive databases or expert panels.

Step 7: Identify Resources to Conduct Study in an Efficient Manner

Resources necessary will vary by study but may include access to medical or computerized records, average medical personnel wages, and specialty medical staff.

Step 8: Identify Probabilities That Outcomes May Occur in Study Population

What are the probabilities of the outcomes identified in step 4 actually occurring in clinical practice? Using primary literature and expert opinion, these probabilities can be obtained and may be manifested as efficacy rates and incidence of ADRs.

Step 9: Employ Decision Analysis

The use of decision analysis can assist in conducting various economic evaluations, including CEA. Through a decision tree, treatment alternatives, outcomes, and probabilities may be graphically presented and algebraically reduced to a single value for comparison (i.e., C/E ratio).

Step 10: Discount Costs or Perform a Sensitivity or Incremental Cost Analysis

Costs and consequences that occur in the future must be discounted back to their present value. Sensitive variables must be tested over a clinically relevant range and results recalculated. If appropriate, an incremental analysis of the costs and consequences should be performed.

Step 11: Present Study Results

Results should be presented to the cross-functional team and the appropriate committees.

Step 12: Develop a Policy or an Intervention

Take the study results and develop a policy or an intervention that can improve or maintain quality of care, possibly at a cost savings.

Step 13: Implement Policy and Educate Professionals

Spend adequate time and resources strategically implementing the policy or intervention. Educate those health care professionals most likely to be affected by this policy, using various strategies including verbal, written, and online communication.

Step 14: Follow-Up Documentation

Once the intervention or policy has been implemented for a reasonable period of time, collect follow-up data. These data will provide feedback on the success and quality of the policy or intervention.

CONCLUSION

The principles and methods of pharmacoeconomics provide the means to quantify the value of pharmacotherapy through balancing costs and outcomes. Providing quality care with minimal resources is the future and the future is here. By understanding the principles, methods, and application of pharmacoeconomics, pharmacists will be prepared to determine and quantify the value of pharmacotherapy to the health care system and society.

REFERENCES

1. Sanchez LA. Expanding the pharmacists role in pharmacoeconomics: How and why? PharmacoEconomics 1994;5(5):367–375.
2. Townsend RJ. Post-marketing drug research and development. DICP 1987;21:134–136.
3. Drummond M, Smith GT, Wells N. Economic Evaluation in the Development of Medicines. London, England, Office of Health Economics, 1988, p 33.
4. Lee JT, Sanchez LA. Interpretation of cost-effective and soundness of economic evaluations in the pharmacy literature. Am J Hosp Pharm 1991;48:2622–2627.
5. Bootman JL. Pharmacoeconomics and outcomes research. Am J Health-System Pharm 1995;52(suppl 3):S16–S19.
6. Eisenberg JM. Clinical economics. A guide to economic analysis of clinical practices. JAMA 1989;262:2879–2886.
7. Bootman JL, Townsend RJ, McGhan WF. Principles of Pharmacoeconomics. Cincinnati OH, Harvey Whitney Books, 1991.
8. Freund DA, Dittus RS. Principles of pharmacoeconomic analysis of drug therapy. PharmacoEconomics 1992;1(1): 20–32.
9. Glossary of terms used in pharmacoeconomic and quality of life analysis. PharmacoEconomics 1992;1(2):151.
10. Kozma CM, Reeder CE, Schulz RM. Economic, clinical, and humanistic outcomes: A planning model for pharmacoeconomic research. Clin Ther 1993;15(6):1121–1132.
11. Draugalis JR, Bootman LJ, Larson LN, McGhan WF. Current Concepts: Pharmacoeconomics. Kalamazoo, MI, The Upjohn Co., 1989.
12. Drummond MF, Stoddart GL, Torrance GW. Methods for the Economic Evaluation of Health Care Programmes. Oxford, Oxford University Press, 1986, pp 5–38,74–111.
13. McGhan WF. Pharmacoeconomics and the evaluation of drugs and services. Hosp Formul 1993;28(4):365–378.
14. Sanchez LA, Lee JT. Use and misuse of pharmacoeconomic terms. Top Hosp Pharm Manage 1994;13(4):11–22.
15. Sanchez LA. Pharmacoeconomic principles and methods: An introduction for hospital pharmacists. Hosp Pharm 1994;29(11):1035–1040.
16. Bootman JL, Larson LN, McGhan WF, Townsend RJ. Pharmacoeconomic research and clinical trials: Concepts and issues. DICP Ann Pharmacother 1989;23:693–697.
17. Detsky AS, Nagiie IG. A clinician's guide to cost-effectiveness analysis. Ann Intern Med 1990;113:147–154.
18. Bootman JL. The basics of pharmacoeconomic analysis. Pharm Rep 1993;23(5):14–15.
19. Langley PC. The role of pharmacoeconomic guidelines for formulary approval: The Australian experience. Clin Ther 1993;15(6):1154–1176.
20. Detsky AS. Guidelines for economic analysis of pharmaceutical products: A draft document for Ontario and Canada. PharmacoEconomics 1993;3:354–361.
21. Schipper H, Clinch J, Powell V. Definitions and conceptual issues, in Spilker B (ed): Quality of Life Assessments in Clinical Trials. New York, Raven Press, 1990.
22. Spilker B. Quality of Life Assessments in Clinical Trials. New York, Raven Press, 1990.
23. Spilker B, et al. Quality of Life Bibliography and Indexes–1990 update. Clin Pharmacoepidemiology 1992;6(2):57–158.
24. Coons SJ. Quality of life assessment: Understanding its use as an outcome measure. Hosp Formul 1993;28(5): 486–498.
25. Jaeschke R, Guyatt GH, Cook D. Quality of life instruments in the evaluation of new drugs. PharmacoEconomics 1992;1(2):84–94.
26. Mackeigan LD, Pathak DS. Overview of health-related quality-of-life measures. Am J Hosp Pharm 1992;49:2236–2245.
27. Sanchez LA. Pharmacoeconomic principles and methods: Including pharmacoeconomics into hospital pharmacy practice. Hosp Pharm 1994;29(11):1035–1040.
28. Doubilet P, et al. The use and misuse of the term "cost effective" in medicine. N Engl J Med 1986;314(4): 253–256.
29. Bradley CA, Iskedjian M, Lanctot KL, et al. Quality assessment of economic evaluation in selected pharmacy, medical, and health economic journals. Ann Pharmacother 1995;29: 681–689.
30. Udvarhelyi S, Colditz GA, Rai A, et al. Cost effectiveness and cost benefit analyses in the medical literature. Ann Intern Med 1992;116:238–244.
31. Sacristan JA, Soto J, Galende I. Evaluation of pharmacoeconomic studies: Utilization of a checklist. Ann Pharmacother 1993;27:1126–1133.
32. Hillman AL, Eisenberg JM, Pauly MV, et al. Avoiding bias in the conduct and reporting of cost-effectiveness research sponsored by pharmaceutical companies. N Engl J Med 1991;324:1362–1365.
33. McGhan WF, Lewis JV. Guidelines for pharmacoeconomic studies. Clin Ther 1992;14:486–494.
34. Sanchez LA. Pharmacoeconomic principles and methods: Evaluating the quality of published pharmacoeconomic evaluations. Hosp Pharm 1995;30(2): (in press).
35. Clemans K, Townsend R, Luscombe F, et al. Methodological and conduct principles for pharmacoeconomic research. Pharmacoeconomics 1995;8(2):169–174.
36. Task Force on Principles for Economic Analysis of Health Care Technology. Economic analysis of health care technology: A report on principles. Ann Intern Med 1995;122:61–70
37. Eisenberg JM, Glick H, Koffer H. Pharmacoeconomics: Economic evaluation of pharmaceuticals, in Strom BL (ed): Pharmacoepidemiology. New York, Churchill Livingstone, 1989, pp 325–350.
38. Milne RJ. Evaluation of the pharmacoeconomic literature. PharmacoEconomics 1994;6(4):337–345.
39. Sackett DL, Haynes RB, Tugwell P. Clinical Epidemiology: A Basic Science for Clinical Medicine. Boston, Little Brown and Company, 1985, p 126.
40. Barr JT, Schumacher GE. Applying decision analysis to pharmacy management and practice decisions. Top Hosp Pharm Manage 1994;13:60–71.

41. Schecter CB. Decision analysis in formulary decision making. PharmacoEconomics 1993;3(6): 454–461.
42. Crane VS. Economic aspects of clinical decision making: Applications of clinical decision analysis. Am J Hosp Pharm 1988;45:548–553.
43. Mutnick AH, Szymusiak-Mutnick B, Schumacher GE, Barr JT. Using decision analysis in the evaluation of drug therapy. Pharm Times 1990;59–66.
44. Jolicoeur LM, Jones-Grizzle AJ, Boyer JG. Guidelines for performing a pharmacoeconomic analysis. Am J Hosp Pharm 1992;49:1741–1747.
45. Sanchez LA. Pharmacoeconomics in pharmacy practice. Pharm Manage Adv 1994;1(5):3–11.

Chapter 2

Health Outcomes and Quality of Life

Stephen Joel Coons, PhD

The United States has entered the third era of modern medical care: the *Era of Assessment and Accountability.*[1] This era follows the *Era of Expansion* (i.e., the late 1940s through the 1960s) and the *Era of Cost Containment* (i.e., the 1970s and 1980s). During the *Era of Expansion,* in an effort to improve access to medical care, a great number of hospitals and health care facilities were built and/or better equipped. In addition, financial access was increased by the rapid growth of private health insurance and through the enactment of Medicare and Medicaid legislation in 1965.

During the *Era of Cost Containment,* containing costs was an explicit goal of most stakeholders in health care. Nevertheless, no substantial cost containment occurred. Primarily, costs were shifted from one payer to another or from one component of health care delivery to another. The excesses or failures of these earlier eras led to the *Era of Assessment and Accountability.* An essential element of this third era is the effort to maximize the net health benefit derived from the utilization of finite health care resources. However, there is a serious lack of critical information as to what value is received for the tremendous amount of resources expended on medical care. This lack of critical information as to the outcomes produced is an obstacle to optimal health care decision making at all levels.

Health Outcomes

Although the implicit objective of medical care is to improve health outcomes, there is minimal evidence of the true effectiveness of many current health care practices.[2] In addition, measures of the overall quality of the U.S. health care system, such as access to primary health care, health indicators (e.g., infant mortality and life expectancy), and public satisfaction in relation to costs, provide evidence that we trail other countries that spend significantly less than the United States does on medical care.[3]

Outcome is one of the three components of the conceptual framework articulated by Donabedian for assessing and assuring the quality of health care: *structure, process,* and *outcome.*[4] Traditionally, the approach to evaluating health care has emphasized the *structure* and *processes* involved in medical care delivery rather than the *outcomes.* However, health care regulators, payers, providers, manufacturers, and patients are placing increasing emphasis on the *outcomes* that medical care products and services produce.[5] As stated by Ellwood, outcomes research is "designed to help patients, payers, and providers make rational medical care-related choices based on better insight into the effect of these choices on the patient's life."[6]

TYPES OF OUTCOMES

The types of outcomes that result from medical care interventions can be described in a number of ways. One classic list of health outcomes, called "the five D's," appears in Table 2.1. The five D's, although quite negatively worded, capture a wide range of outcomes that have been used in assessing the quality of medical care.[7]

A more comprehensive conceptual framework, the ECHO model, places outcomes into the three categories shown in Table 2.2.[8] The model covers the five D's within the clinical and humanistic outcomes domains, and provides an added economic outcomes dimension. As described by Kozma and associates, *clinical outcomes* are the medical events that occur as a result of the condition or its treatment. *Economic outcomes* are the direct, indirect, and intangible costs compared with the consequences of a medical intervention. Along with patient satisfaction, an essential *humanistic outcome* is patient function and well-

TABLE 2.1. OUTCOMES: THE FIVE D'S

- Death
- Disease
- Disability
- Discomfort
- Dissatisfaction

TABLE 2.2. OUTCOMES IN THE ECHO MODEL

- Economic outcomes
- Clinical outcomes
- Humanistic outcomes

(From Ref. 8.)

being, or health-related quality of life. This chapter focuses on health-related quality of life as an outcome of pharmacotherapeutic interventions.

QUALITY OF LIFE

DEFINITION

As discussed earlier, one of the essential elements of outcomes research is the assessment of patient *health-related quality of life*. However, there is no consensus on the definition of quality of life or its overall conceptual framework.[9] In the literature, the term *quality of life* has been used in a variety of ways. It has been proposed that studies of health outcomes use the term *health-related quality of life* to distinguish health effects from the effects of job satisfaction, environment, and other factors on overall quality of life.[10] Only health outcomes are discussed in this chapter, so the terms *quality of life* and *health-related quality of life* are used interchangeably. In addition, another term that will be used interchangeably with *health-related quality of life* is *health status*.

Quality of life, like other aspects of the human experience, is hard to define. In much of the empiric literature, explicit definitions of *quality of life* are rare; readers must deduce the implicit definition of *quality of life* from the manner in which it is measured. However, some authors have provided definitions. For example, Schron and Shumaker define quality of life as "a multidimensional concept referring to a person's total well-being including his or her psychological, social, and physical health status."[11] Patrick and Erickson propose that quality of life is "the value assigned to duration of life as modified by the impairments, functional states, perceptions, and social opportunities that are influenced by disease, injury, treatment, or policy."[12] Although the two definitions differ in certain respects, a conceptual characteristic they share is the multidimensionality of quality of life. Although the terminology may vary with the author, commonly measured dimensions of health-related quality of life include:

- Physical health
- Emotional health
- Social and role functioning
- Perceptions of general well-being
- Disease- and/or treatment-related symptomatology

RELEVANCE OF QUALITY OF LIFE AS AN OUTCOME

For medical care providers, quality of life is increasingly viewed as a therapeutic endpoint. An overriding factor leading to this has been the gradual shift in the focus of primary medical care from limiting mortality to limiting morbidity and the patient-reported impact of that morbidity. The pattern of illness in U.S. society has shifted from mostly acute disease to one in which chronic conditions predominate. In the early part of this century, many individuals died from infectious diseases for which cures (e.g., antibiotics) and/or effective preventive measures (e.g., increased sanitation, vaccines) were unavailable or underused. Although many diseases currently remain that may shorten life expectancy, it is more likely that a disease will have adverse health consequences leading to dysfunction and decreased well-being. For those conditions that shorten life expectancy and for which there are no cures, managing symptoms and maintaining function and well-being should be the primary objectives of medical care.

Since therapeutic interventions such as medications can enhance as well as decrease quality of life, medical care providers must strive to achieve enhanced quality of life as an outcome of therapy. Although it must be assumed that quality of life has always played an implicit role in the provision of health care, it has not always been viewed as equal in importance to the more clinical or biological outcome parameters (e.g., blood pressure). The subjective nature of quality of life assessment has made many people uneasy with it as a measure of the patient outcomes produced by medical treatment.[13] However, there is growing awareness that in certain diseases, quality of life may be the most important health outcome to consider in assessing treatment.[14] Physiologic measures may change without improving functioning and well-being. Likewise, patients may feel better without measurable change in physiologic values.

QUALITY OF LIFE AND PHARMACOTHERAPY

Four possible quality of life outcomes are associated with pharmacotherapeutic interventions:[15]

1. Quality of life is improved.
2. Quality of life is actively maintained.
3. Quality of life decreases.
4. Quality of life remains unaffected.

Nevertheless, the quality of life impact of pharmaceutical products and services has not been routinely measured and has only recently become recognized as a therapeutic outcome.[16,17] A study by Croog and colleagues[18] was one of the first in a growing body of literature reporting the quality of life impact of pharmacotherapy, specifically the use of antihypertensive agents. Hypertension is one condition that is receiving much attention about quality of life implications of the disease and its treatment.[19–21] Other therapeutic areas that are receiving increasing attention are cancer, asthma, HIV infection, and arthritis.[22–26]

Information about the impact of pharmacotherapy on quality of life can provide additional data for making medication-use policy decisions. Pharmacy and therapeutics committees should incorporate quality of life data into the formulary and practice guideline decision-making process. Quality of life as an input to clinical decision making at the patient level is also very important. For example, alternative treatments may have equal efficacy based on traditional clinical parameters (e.g., blood pressure reduction) but produce very different effects on the patient's quality of life. Thus, a provider's selection among competing alternatives may hinge on documented differential impact on quality of life. A perceived decrease in quality of life attributed by the patient to an adverse effect of the drug may lead to a decrease in adherence to the medication regimen.[15]

MEASURING QUALITY OF LIFE

TYPES OF INSTRUMENTS

Hundreds of health-related quality of life instruments are available.[27–31] Table 2.3 provides a taxonomy of the different types of instruments.[32] A primary distinction among quality of life instruments is whether they are generic or specific.

Generic Instruments

Generic quality of life instruments are designed to be applicable across all diseases or conditions, across different medical interventions, and across a wide variety of populations.[33] Table 2.4 lists the dimensions or domains that comprise four generic instruments. In choosing or evaluating the use of an instrument, the dimensions of functioning and well-being must be considered. The instruments in Table 2.4 share common dimensions but they also reflect the diversity and range of dimensions covered.

TABLE 2.3. TAXONOMY OF QUALITY OF LIFE INSTRUMENTS

Generic Instruments
Health profiles
Utility-based measures
Specific Instruments
Disease specific (e.g., diabetes)
Population specific (e.g., frail elderly)
Function specific (e.g., sexual functioning)
Condition or problem specific (e.g., pain)

(From Ref. 32.)

TABLE 2.4. DOMAINS AND DIMENSIONS OF SELECTED GENERIC INSTRUMENTS

NHP—Nottingham Health Profile[34]	
Part I: Distress within the following domains:	
Emotions	Energy
Sleep	Pain
Social isolation	Mobility
Part II: Health-related problems within the following domains:	
Occupation	Sex life
Housework	Hobbies
Social life	Holidays
Home life	
QWB—Quality of Well-Being Scale[35]	
Symptoms/problems	Physical activity
Mobility	Social activity
SIP—Sickness Impact Profile[36]	
Sleep and rest	Home management
Eating	Recreation and pastimes
Work	Body care and movement
Ambulation	Alertness behavior
Mobility	Emotional behavior
Communication	Social interaction
HUI—Health Utilities Index (Mark III)[37]	
Vision	Dexterity
Hearing	Cognition
Speech	Pain and discomfort
Ambulation	Emotion

The two main types of generic instruments are health profiles and utility-based measures.

Health Profiles

Health profiles provide an array of scores representing individual dimensions or domains of quality of life or health status. An advantage of a health profile is that it provides multiple outcome scores that may be useful to clinicians and/or researchers who are attempting to measure differential effects of a condition or its treatment on various quality of life domains. A commonly used profile instrument is the Medical Outcomes Study Short Form-36 (SF-36). The SF-36 is also known and distributed as the RAND 36-Item Health Survey 1.0. The SF-36/RAND 36-Item Health Survey 1.0 grew out of the Medical Outcomes Study (MOS) conducted by researchers from the RAND Corporation.[38,39] The instrument includes nine health concepts or dimensions as shown in Table 2.5. The SF-36/RAND 36-Item Health Survey 1.0 can be self-administered or administered by a trained interviewer (face to face or via telephone). This instrument has several advantages. For example, it is brief (i.e., takes about 5 to 10 minutes to complete) and its reliability and validity have been demonstrated in many clinical situations and disease states.[39–41]

TABLE 2.5. DIMENSIONS OF RAND 36-ITEM HEALTH SURVEY 1.0/SF-36 SCALES

- General health perceptions
- Physical functioning
- Social functioning
- Role limitations attributed to physical problems
- Role limitations attributed to emotional problems
- Bodily pain
- General mental health
- Energy/fatigue (vitality)
- Health transition

(Compiled from Refs. 38 and 39.)

A copy of the RAND 36-Item Health Survey 1.0 is provided in the appendix to this chapter.

Utility-Based Measures

Quality of life as measured by utility-based instruments is on a continuum from death (0.0) to perfect health (1.0). This approach incorporates the measurement of an individual's health status with an adjustment for the value (e.g., utility) of that health state. The values or utilities are empirically measured or assigned through a variety of procedures.

Utility-based measures are useful in pharmacoeconomic research, specifically cost-utility analysis (CUA).[42] (CUA is an economic technique discussed in Chapter 1.) CUA involves comparing the costs of an intervention (e.g., a medication) with its outcomes expressed in units such as quality-adjusted life years (QALYs) gained.[43] *QALYs gained* is an outcome measure that incorporates both quantity and quality of life. This can be a key outcome measure, especially in diseases where the treatment itself can have a major impact on patient functioning and well-being (e.g., cancer).

QALYs can be produced by increases in quality of life and/or length of life. Figure 2.1 represents a case in which QALYs were gained through an increase in quality of life alone. The top curve represents the hypothetical life course of a cohort of individuals receiving a specific health care intervention compared with the life course of a cohort (i.e., lower curve) that did not receive the intervention. Average age at death did not differ between the two cohorts, but the intervention led to improvements in quality of life in the treatment cohort. The area between the curves represents the QALYs gained through the intervention. This hypothetical case reflects a chronic disease, such as arthritis, in which functioning and well-being are increased but survival remains unchanged. Other hypothetical combinations of quality and quantity of life can be graphed in this manner. For example, an alternative scenario could reflect a

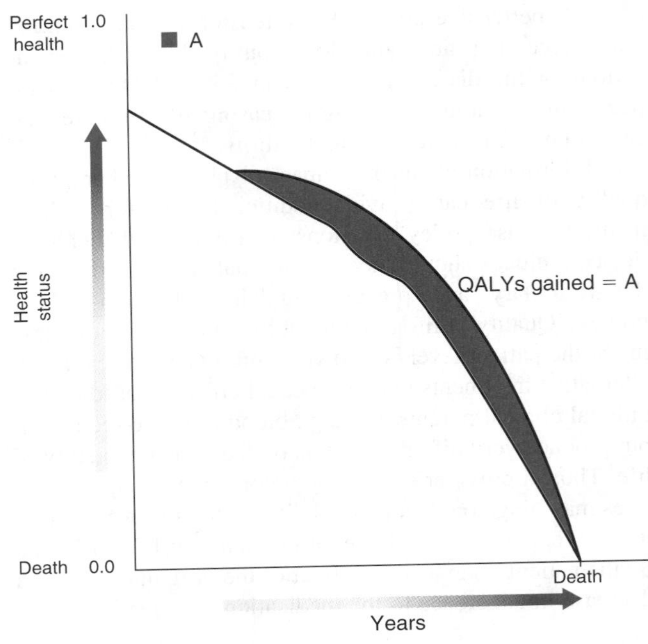

Figure 2.1. QALYs gained secondary to a hypothetical health care intervention, such as a drug.

decrease in quality of life but an increase in survival that may result from a chemotherapeutic regimen for cancer.

Direct Measures of Health State Values/Utilities. The most commonly used direct measurement techniques include visual analog scales, standard gamble, and time trade-off.[44]

Visual analog scales. The visual analog scale is a line, typically 100 centimeters in length, with the endpoints well defined (e.g., 0 = "worst imaginable health state" and 100 = "best imaginable health state"). The respondent is asked to mark the line where they would place one or more health states in relation to the two endpoints. If the subject were to rate their health state, or a health state described to them in a scenario, at the midpoint between 0 and 100 on the scale, the value for that health state would be 0.5.

Standard gamble. The standard gamble offers a choice between two alternatives: choice A—living in health state *i* with certainty, or choice B—taking a gamble on a new treatment for which the outcome is uncertain. Figure 2.2 shows this gamble.[45] The subject is told that a hypothetical treatment will lead to perfect health with a probability of *p* or immediate death with a probability of $1-p$. They can choose between remaining in state *i*, which is intermediate between healthy and dead, or taking the gamble and trying the new treatment. The probability *p* is varied until the subject is indifferent between choices A and B. For example, if a subject is indifferent between

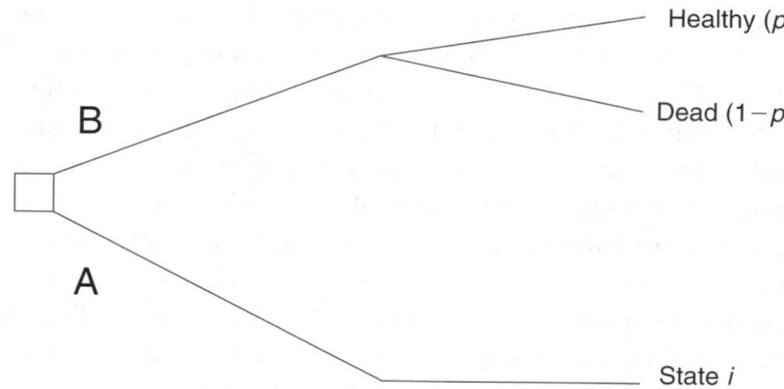

Figure 2.2. Standard gamble for a chronic health state *i*. Patients respond to various probabilities *p* of living after intervention A, which would cure them of condition *i*. The probability *p* at which the patient is indifferent between living with condition *i* and dying from treatment B represents the utility of state *i*.

the choices A and B when $p = 0.75$, the utility of state *i* is 0.75.

Time trade-off. Figure 2.3 represents the time trade-off technique for a chronic disease state.[46] Here, the subject is offered a choice of living for a defined amount of time *(x)* in perfect health or a variable amount of time *(t)* in an alternative state *(i)* that is less desirable. By reducing the time *x* of being healthy (i.e., at 1.0) and leaving the time *t* in the suboptimal health state fixed, an indifference point can be determined ($h_i = x/t$). For example, a subject may indicate that undergoing chronic hemodialysis for 2 years is equivalent to perfect health for 1 year. Therefore, the value of that health state would be 0.5 (i.e., $h_i = 1/2$).

Multiattribute Utility Systems. In addition to direct measures, instruments are available for which the utilities and values have been empirically derived through population studies. The instruments are administered to measure respondents' health status, which is then mapped onto a multiattribute health status system. Examples of such instruments include the Quality of Well-being Scale (QWB)[35] and the Health Utilities Index (HUI).[36]

The QWB is a generic quality of life instrument that includes symptoms or problems plus three dimensions of functional health status (Table 2.4). Standardized preference values for the QWB have been measured (via the category rating scale method, a technique related to visual analog scales) and validated on a general population in San Diego, California.[47] Other investigators have reweighted the symptoms or problems and function levels of the QWB in specific populations such as arthritis patients[48] and HIV-infected subjects[49] and have found the generalizability of the original values to be very high.

The HUI is another generic instrument that describes the health status of a person at a point in time in terms of his or her ability to function on a set of attributes or dimensions of health status. The measurements of the preferences or utilities for the health status classification system were made with visual analog scales and the standard gamble technique. The dimensions covered in the most recent version of the HUI (Mark III) are listed in Table 2.4.[37]

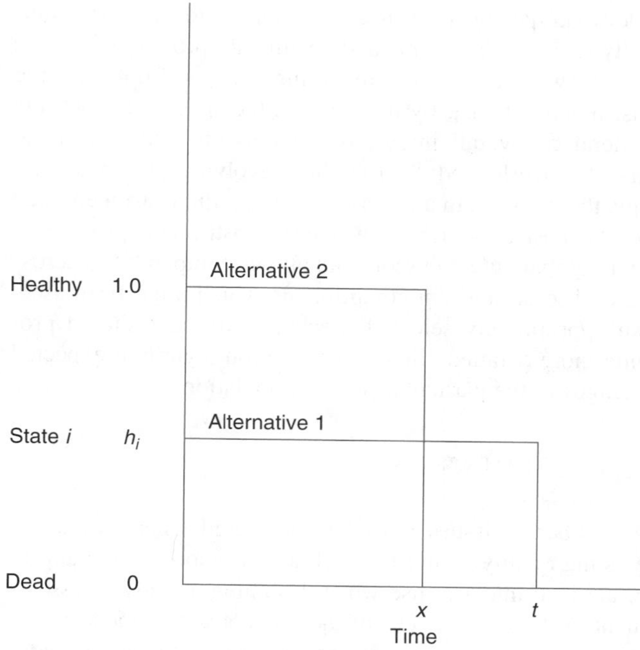

Figure 2.3. Time trade-off for a chronic health state. The subject chooses between living for a shorter amount of time in perfect health *(x)* or a longer amount of time *(t)* with state *i*. The length of time in perfect health is shortened until the subject is indifferent between the two choices. The value of health state *i* (h_i) is then calculated by dividing x/t.

Specific Instruments

Specific instruments are intended to provide greater detail concerning particular outcomes, in terms of functioning and well-being, uniquely associated with a condition or its treatment. Several selected examples of disease-specific instruments are shown in Table 2.6.

Disease or condition-specific instruments may be more sensitive than a generic measure to particular changes in quality of life secondary to the disease or its treatment. In

TABLE 2.6. SELECTED DISEASE-SPECIFIC QUALITY OF LIFE INSTRUMENTS

- Arthritis Impact Measurement Scale (AIMS)[50]
- Asthma Quality of Life Questionnaire (AQLQ)[51]
- Diabetes Quality of Life (DQOL)[52]
- Kidney Disease Quality of Life (KDQOL)[53]
- Quality of Life in Epilepsy (QOLIE)[54]
- HIV Overview of Problems—Evaluation System (HOPES)[55]

addition, specific measures may appear to be more clinically relevant to patients and health care providers.[32]

However, a concern regarding the use of only specific instruments is that, by focusing on the specific impact, the general or overall impact on functioning and well-being may be overlooked.[56] In studies involving pharmacotherapy, the use of both a generic and a specific instrument may be the best approach. The generic instrument provides a more global outcome score and allows comparability across other disease states or conditions in which it has been used. An appropriately selected specific instrument should provide more detailed clinical information regarding expected changes in the particular patient population.

MEASUREMENT ISSUES

A number of issues must be considered when evaluating existing quality of life research and/or choosing the appropriate instrument to use when designing a study or assessment. A thorough review of these is not within the scope of this chapter. More in-depth reviews of methodologic considerations are available in the literature.[32,57–59] The two issues discussed in this section are measurement or psychometric properties of instruments and respondent or investigator burden. Successful assessment of quality of life will depend on appropriate consideration of these two issues.

Psychometric Properties

Of particular concern are the psychometric properties of a chosen instrument. Psychometrics refers to the measurement of psychologic constructs, such as quality of life. Instruments are developed and tested such that one can place confidence in the measurement made. Psychometric properties include the reliability and validity of measurements.

Reliability: Consistent Results Among Items and Over Time

Reliability refers to the extent to which measures give consistent or accurate results.[60] The purpose of evaluating the reliability of a quality of life instrument is to estimate how much of the variation in a score is real as opposed to random. The two reliability assessment methods most often discussed in the quality of life literature are internal consistency and test–retest reliability. *Internal consistency* is an assessment of the performance of items within a scale. It is a function of the number of items and their covariation.[61] Internal consistency is commonly measured using Cronbach's alpha coefficient. Alpha coefficients above 0.90 are needed for making comparisons between individuals and above 0.70 for comparisons between groups.[62]

Test–retest reliability refers to the relationship between scores obtained from the same instrument on two or more separate occasions when all pertinent conditions remain relatively unchanged.[61] It is usually evaluated using a Pearson product–moment correlation coefficient. However, quality of life is not assumed to be constant over the course of time. In fact, most clinical studies attempt to assess how quality of life changes. Test–retest reliability estimates may have limited value in evaluating measures that are designed to assess a dynamic process. Table 2.7 shows the internal consistency and test–retest reliability estimates for the multi-item scales of the U.K. developmental version of the SF-36 in a sample of general practice patients.[63] The reliability estimates for the SF-36 scales in this sample were quite acceptable, with scores for only two domains falling below 0.90 for internal consistency and test–retest values all at 0.60 or above.

Inter-rater reliability and *equivalent-forms reliability* are two other approaches to reliability assessment that are not as commonly used in quality of life research. More in-depth discussions of these and the other reliability assessment methods are found elsewhere.[61,64]

Validity: True Reflection of Reality

Reliability is necessary, but not sufficient for valid measurement.[61] Validity is an estimation of the extent to which the instrument is measuring what it is supposed to be measuring. It defines the range of inferences that is justifiable on the basis of a score or measure. Validity is not absolute

TABLE 2.7. RELIABILITY ESTIMATES FOR SF-36 SCALES (U.K. DEVELOPMENTAL VERSION)

	Internal Consistency	Test–Retest
General health perceptions	0.95	0.80
Physical functioning	0.93	0.81
Social functioning	0.73	0.60
Role limitations—physical problems	0.96	0.69
Role limitations—emotional problems	0.96	0.63
Bodily pain	0.85	0.78
General mental health	0.95	0.75
Energy/fatigue (vitality)	0.96	0.80

(From Ref. 63.)

but is relative to the domain under study. Three types of validity commonly considered are criterion, content, and construct.

Criterion validity is achieved when a new measure corresponds to an established measure or observation that accurately reflects the phenomenon of interest. By definition, the criterion must be a superior measure of the phenomenon if it is to serve as a comparative norm.[47] However, in quality of life assessment, gold standards or criterion measures rarely exist against which a new measure can be compared.

Content validity, which is infrequently tested statistically, refers to how adequately the sampling of questions reflects the aims of the measure.

Construct validity refers to the relationship between measures purporting to measure the same underlying theoretical construct (i.e., convergent evidence) or purporting to measure a different construct (i.e., discriminant evidence). For example, convergent evidence for the validity of role performance items is established by showing associations between the responses to the items and observed verifiable functioning. Evidence for the construct validity of other aspects of the measure might be established through comparisons with physiologic measures, organ pathology, or clinical signs. Construct validity is not absolute. A measure is not "valid," but rather data support its validity through research findings. Ware and colleagues[60] have provided a substantial amount of data supporting the validity of the SF-36.

Another aspect of a measure that supports its validity is responsiveness or sensitivity to change. Responsiveness is the ability or power of the measure to detect clinically important change when it occurs.[65] Although some authors have suggested that responsiveness is a psychometric property of a measure distinct from validity,[66] others argue that responsiveness is an aspect of validity rather than a separate property.[61,67]

Respondent Burden: Taking as Little Time as Possible

A practical aspect of the measurement of quality of life is length of the instrument or the administration time involved. Instruments should be as brief as possible without severely compromising the validity and reliability of the measurement. The longer an instrument, the greater the respondent burden that can lead to unwillingness or refusal to complete the instrument or incomplete responses.

Another practical consideration is the means of administration.[68] Many quality of life measures can be administered in different ways. The primary modes of administration are (1) interviewer administered, either in person or over the telephone, or (2) self-administered.[32] Also used, but not recommended, are surrogate responders (i.e., using a health care provider, family member, or friend to respond for the subject when the subject is unable to complete the instrument). Because quality of life is such a subjective concept, patients must have the opportunity to provide their perspective on the impact of medical care on their functioning and well-being. The patient's perspective has been shown to be quite different from that of outside observers, including physicians and other health professionals providing direct care to the patient.[69]

Conclusion

The concept of quality of life has gained increasing attention in the evaluation of the outcomes associated with medical care, including pharmacotherapy. In fact, in certain diseases, quality of life may be the most important outcome to consider in assessing the effectiveness of health care interventions. Health care practitioners and policymakers must remember that efforts to increase quantity of life must not outstrip the ability to maintain or improve quality of life.

As might be expected in a relatively new field of endeavor, a number of theoretical and methodologic issues remain unresolved. However, some general concepts in the measurement of quality of life outcomes should be carefully considered when designing a study, evaluating existing research, or evaluating new programs or services. This chapter has provided only a brief overview of the concepts in an effort to sensitize students and current health care practitioners to the complexity of the area as well as to provide insight as to how these concepts can and should be incorporated into their practices.

References

1. Relman AS. Assessment and accountability: The third revolution in medical care. N Engl J Med 1988;319:1220–1221.
2. Roper WL, Winkenwerder W, Hackbarth GM, Krakauer H. Effectiveness in health care: An initiative to evaluate and improve medical practice. N Engl J Med 1988;319:1197–1202.
3. Starfield B. Primary care and health: A cross-national comparison. JAMA 1991;266:2268–2271.
4. Donabedian A. Explorations in Quality Assessment and Monitoring, Vol I: The Definition of Quality and Approaches to Its Assessment. Ann Arbor, MI, Health Administration Press, 1980.
5. Zitter M. Outcomes assessment: True customer focus comes to health care. Med Interface 1992(May);5(5):32–37.
6. Ellwood PM. Outcomes management: A technology of patient experience. N Engl J Med 1988;318:1551.
7. Lohr KN. Outcome measurement: Concepts and questions. Inquiry 1988;25:37–50.
8. Kozma CM, Reeder CE, Schulz RM. Economic, clinical, and humanistic outcomes: A planning model for pharmacoeconomic research. Clin Ther 1993;15:1121–1132.

9. Stewart AL. Conceptual and methodologic issues in defining quality of life: State of the art. Prog Cardiovasc Nurs 1992;7(1):3–11.
10. Kaplan RM, Bush JW. Health-related quality of life measurement for evaluation research and policy analysis. Health Psychol 1982;1:61–80.
11. Schron EB, Shumaker SA. The integration of health quality of life in clinical research: Experience from cardiovascular clinical trials. Prog Cardiovasc Nurs 1992;7(2):21.
12. Patrick DL, Erickson P. Health Status and Health Policy: Allocating Resources to Health Care. New York, Oxford University Press, 1993, p 22.
13. Schipper H, Clinch J, Powell V. Definitions and conceptual issues, in Spilker B (ed.): Quality of Life Assessments in Clinical Trials. New York, Raven Press, 1990, pp 11–24.
14. Staquet M, Aaronson NK, Ahmedzai S, et al. Health-related quality of life research [editorial]. Qual Life Res 1992;1:3.
15. Smith M. Medication, quality of life and compliance: The role of the pharmacist. PharmacoEconomics 1992;1:225–230.
16. Patrick DL. Health-related quality of life in pharmaceutical evaluation: Forging progress and avoiding pitfalls. PharmacoEconomics 1992;1:76–78.
17. Revicki DA, Rothman M, Luce B. Health-related quality of life assessment and the pharmaceutical industry. PharmacoEconomics 1992;1:394–408.
18. Croog SH, Levine S, Testa MA, et al. The effects of antihypertensive therapy on quality of life. N Engl J Med 1988;319:1220–1221.
19. Hollenberg NK, Testa M, Williams GH. Quality-of-life as a therapeutic end-point: An analysis of therapeutic trials in hypertension. PharmacoEconomics 1991;6:83–93.
20. Beto JA, Bansal VK. Quality of life in the treatment of hypertension: A meta-analysis of clinical trials. Am J Hypertens 1992;5:125–133.
21. Bulpitt CJ, Fletcher AE. Quality-of-life instruments in hypertension. PharmacoEconomics 1994;6:523–535.
22. Osoba D. Measuring the effect of cancer on health-related quality of life. PharmacoEconomics 1995;7:308–319.
23. Cassileth BR. Principles of quality-of-life assessment in cancer chemotherapy. PharmacoEconomics 1992;2:279–284.
24. Lenderking WR, Gelber RD, Cotton DJ. Evaluation of the quality of life associated with zidovudine treatment in asymptomatic human immunodeficiency infection. N Engl J Med 1994;330:738–743.
25. Kaplan RM, Anderson JP, Wu AW, Mathews WC, Kozin F, Orenstein D. The Quality of Well-being Scale: Applications in AIDS, cystic fibrosis, and arthritis. Med Care 1989;27: S27–S43.
26. Testa MA, Lenderking WR. Interpreting pharmacoeconomic and quality-of-life clinical trial data for use in therapeutics. PharmacoEconomics 1992;2:107–117.
27. Spilker B, Molinek FR, Johnston KA, Simpson RL, Tilson HH. Quality of life bibliography and indexes. Med Care 1990;28(suppl 12):DS1–DS77.
28. Spilker B, White WSA, Simpson RL, Tilson HH. Quality of life bibliography and indexes: 1990 update. J Clin Res Pharmacoepidemiol 1992;6:87–156.
29. Spilker B, Simpson RL, Tilson HH. Quality of life bibliography and indexes: 1991 update. J Clin Res Pharmacoepidemiol 1992;6:205–266.
30. Berzon RA, Simeon GP, Simpson RL, Tilson HH. Quality of life bibliography and indexes: 1992 update. J Clin Res Drug Dev 1993;7:203–242.
31. Berzon RA, Simeon GP, Simpson RL, Donnelly MA, Tilson HH. Quality of life bibliography and indexes: 1993 update. Qual Life Res 1995;4:53–74.
32. Guyatt GH, Feeny DH, Patrick DL. Measuring health-related quality of life. Ann Intern Med 1993;118:622–629.
33. Patrick DL, Deyo RA. Generic and disease-specific measures in assessing health status and quality of life. Med Care 1989;27:S217–S232.
34. Hunt SM, McKewan J, McKenna SP. Measuring health status: A new tool for clinicians and epidemiologists. J R Coll Gen Prac 1985;35:185–188.
35. Kaplan RM, Anderson JP. The general health policy model: An integrated approach, in Spilker B (ed.): Quality of Life Assessments in Clinical Trials. New York, Raven Press, 1990, pp 131–149.
36. Bergner M, Bobbitt RA, Carter WB, Gilson BS. The Sickness Impact Profile: Development and final revisions of a health status measure. Med Care 1976;14:57–67.
37. Feeny D, Torrance GW, Goldsmith CH, Furlong W, Boyle M. A multi-attribute approach to health status. McMaster University Centre for Health Economics and Policy Analysis Working Paper Series (Paper 94–5). Toronto, Ontario, McMaster University, 1994 (Feb).
38. Hays RD, Sherbourne CD, Mazel RM. The RAND 36-Item Health Survey 1.0. Health Econ 1993;2:217–227.
39. Ware JE Jr, Sherbourne CD. The MOS 36-Item Short-Form Health Survey (SF-36): I. Conceptual framework and item selection. Med Care 1992;30:473–483.
40. McHorney CA, Ware JE Jr, Raczek AE. The MOS 36-Item Short-Form Health Survey (SF-36): II. Psychometric and clinical tests of validity in measuring physical and mental health constructs. Med Care 1993;31:247–263.
41. McHorney CA, Ware JE Jr, Raczek AE. The MOS 36-Item Short-Form Health Survey (SF-36): III. Tests of data quality, scaling assumptions, and reliability across diverse patient groups. Med Care 1994;32:40–66.
42. Kongpatanakul S, Strom BL. Quality of life, health status and clinical drug research. PharmacoEconomics 1992;2:8–14.
43. Coons SJ, Kaplan RM. Cost-utility analysis, in Bootman JL, Townsend RJ, McGhan WF, (eds.): Principles of Pharmacoeconomics, 2nd ed. Cincinnati, OH, Harvey Whitney Books Company (in press).
44. Revicki DA. Relationships between health utility and psychometric health status measures. Med Care 1992;30:MS274–MS282.
45. Drummond MF, Stoddart GL, Torrance GW. Methods for the Economic Evaluation of Health Care Programmes. Oxford, Oxford University Press, 1987.
46. Torrance GW, Thomas WH, Sackett DL. Utility maximization model for evaluation of health care programmes. Health Serv Res 1972;7:118–133.
47. Kaplan RM, Bush JW, Berry CC. Health status: Types of validity and the Index of Well-being. Health Serv Res 1976;11:478–507.
48. Balaban DJ, Fagi PC, Goldfarb NI, Nettler S. Weights for scoring the quality of well-being instrument among rheumatoid arthritics. Med Care 1986;24:973–980.

49. Hughes TE, Coons SJ, Kaplan RM, Draugalis JR. Reweighting the Quality of Well-being Scale in HIV-infected subjects. Presented at the Inaugural Meeting of the International Society for Health-Related Quality of Life, Brussels, Belgium, 1994 (Feb 3).
50. Meenan RF, Gertman PM, Mason JH. Measuring health status in arthritis: The Arthritis Impact Measurement Scales. Arthr Rheum 1980;23:146–152.
51. Juniper EF, Guyatt GH, Epstein RS, Ferrie PJ, Jaeschke R, Hiller TK. Evaluation of impairment of health-related quality of life in asthma: Development of a questionnaire for use in clinical trials. Thorax 1992;47:76–83.
52. Parkerson GR, Connis RT, Broadhead WE, Patrick DL, Taylor TR, Tse C-KJ. Disease-specific versus generic measurement of health-related quality of life in insulin-dependent diabetic patients. Med Care 1993;7:629–639.
53. Hays RD, Kallich JD, Mapes DL, Coons SJ, Carter WB. Development of the Kidney Disease Quality of Life (KDQOL^{TM}) instrument. Qual Life Res 1994;3:329–338.
54. Perrine KR. A new quality of life inventory for epilepsy patients: Interim results. Epilepsia 1993;34(suppl 4):S28–S33.
55. Ganz PA, Schag CAC, Kahn B, Petersen L, Hirji K. Describing the health-related quality of life impact of HIV infection: Findings from a study using the HIV Overview of Problems—Evaluation System (HOPES). Qual Life Res 1993;2:109–119.
56. Coons SJ, Kaplan RM. Assessing health-related quality of life: Application to drug therapy. Clin Ther 1992;14:850–858.
57. Ware JE Jr. Standards for validating health measures: Definition and content. J Chron Dis 1987;40:473–480.
58. Pathak DS, MacKeigan LD. Assessment of quality of life and health status: Selected observations. J Res Pharm Econ 1992;4(4):31–52.
59. Smith ND. Quality of life studies from the perspective of an FDA reviewing statistician. Drug Info J 1993;27:617–623.
60. Ware JE Jr, Snow KK, Kosinski M, Gandek B. SF-36 Health Survey: Manual and Interpretation Guide. Boston, The Health Institute, 1993.
61. Hays RD, Anderson R, Revicki D. Psychometric considerations in evaluating health-related quality of life measures. Qual Life Res 1993;2:441–449.
62. Nunnally J. Psychometric Theory, 2nd ed. New York, McGraw-Hill, 1978.
63. Brazier JE, Harper R, Jones NM, et al. Validating the SF-36 health survey questionnaire: New outcome measure for primary care. Br Med J 1992;305:160–164.
64. Kaplan RM, Saccuzzo DP. Psychological Testing: Principles, Applications, and Issues, 3rd ed. Pacific Grove, CA, Brooks/Cole, 1993.
65. Jaeschke R, Guyatt GH. How to develop and evaluate a new quality of life instrument, in Spilker B (ed.): Quality of Life Assessments in Clinical Trials. New York, Raven Press, 1990, pp 47–57.
66. Guyatt G, Walter S, Norman G. Measuring change over time: Assessing the usefulness of evaluative instruments. J Chron Dis 1987;40:171–178.
67. Hays RD, Hadorn D. Responsiveness to change: An aspect of validity, not a separate dimension. Qual Life Res 1992;1: 73–75.
68. Cook DJ, Guyatt GH, Juniper E, et al. Interviewer versus self-administered questionnaires in developing a disease-specific, health-related quality of life instrument for asthma. J Clin Epidemiol 1993;46:529–534.
69. Jachuck SJ, Brierly H, Jachuck S, Wilcox PM. The effect of hypotensive drugs on the quality of life. J R Coll Gen Prac 1982;32:103–105.

RAND 36-Item Health Survey 1.0

1. In general, would you say your health is:

(Circle One Number)

Excellent	1
Very Good	2
Good	3
Fair	4
Poor	5

2. **Compared to one year ago,** how would you rate your health in general **now**?

(Circle One Number)

Much better now than one year ago	1
Somewhat better now than one year ago	2
About the same	3
Somewhat worse now than one year ago	4
Much worse now than one year ago	5

The following items are about activities you might do during a typical day. Does **your health now limit you** in these activiites? If so, how much?

(Circle One Number on Each Line)

	Yes, Limited a Lot	Yes, Limited a Little	No, Not Limited at All
3. **Vigorous activities,** such as running, lifting heavy objects, participating in strenuous sports	1	2	3
4. **Moderate activities,** such as moving a table, pushing a vacuum cleaner, bowling, or playing golf	1	2	3
5. Lifting or carrying groceries	1	2	3
6. Climbing **several** flights of stairs	1	2	3
7. Climbing **one** flight of stairs	1	2	3
8. Bending, kneeling, or stooping	1	2	3
9. Walking **more than a mile**	1	2	3
10. Walking **several blocks**	1	2	3
11. Walking **one block**	1	2	3

For additional information on the *RAND 36-Item Health Survey 1.0* contact: RAND, 1700 Main Street, PO Box 2138, Santa Monica, CA 90407-2138, TEL: 310/451-7002, FAX: 310/451-6915.

12. Bathing or dressing yourself	1	2	3

During the **past 4 weeks,** have you had any of the following problems with your work or other regular daily activities **as a result of your physical health?**

(Circle One Number on Each Line)

	Yes	No
13. Cut down the **amount of time** you spent on work or other activities	1	2
14. **Accomplished less** than you would like	1	2
15. Were limited in the **kind** of work or other activities	1	2
16. Had **difficulty** performing the work or other activities (for example, it took extra effort)	1	2

During the **past 4 weeks,** have you had any of the following problems with your work or other regular daily activities **as a result of any emotional problems** (such as feeling depressed or anxious)?

(Circle One Number on Each Line)

	Yes	No
17. Cut down the **amount of time** you spent on work or other activities	1	2
18. **Accomplished less** than you would like	1	2
19. Didn't do work or other activities as **carefully** as usual	1	2

20. During the **past 4 weeks,** to what extent has your physical health or emotional problems interfered with your normal social activities with family, friends, neighbors, or groups?

(Circle One Number)

Not at all	1
Slightly	2
Moderately	3
Quite a bit	4
Extremely	5

21. How much **bodily** pain have you had during the **past 4 weeks?**

(Circle One Number)

None	1
Very mild	2
Mild	3
Moderate	4
Severe	5
Very severe	6

22. During the **past 4 weeks,** how much did **pain** interfere with your normal work (including both work outside the home and housework)?

(Circle One Number)

Not at all 1
A little bit 2
Moderately 3
Quite a bit 4
Extremely 5

These questions are about how you feel and how things have been with you **during the past 4 weeks.** For each question, please give the one answer that comes closest to the way you have been feeling.

How much of the time during the **past 4 weeks. . .**

(Circle One Number on Each Line)

	All of the Time	Most of the Time	A Good Bit of the Time	Some of the Time	A Little of the Time	None of the Time
23. Did you feel full of pep?	1	2	3	4	5	6
24. Have you been a very nervous person?	1	2	3	4	5	6
25. Have you felt so down in the dumps that nothing could cheer you up?	1	2	3	4	5	6
26. Have you felt calm and peaceful?	1	2	3	4	5	6
27. Did you have a lot of energy?	1	2	3	4	5	6
28. Have you felt downhearted and blue?	1	2	3	4	5	6
29. Did you feel worn out?	1	2	3	4	5	6
30. Have you been a happy person?	1	2	3	4	5	6
31. Did you feel tired?	1	2	3	4	5	6

32. During the **past 4 weeks,** how much of the time has your **physical health or emotional problems** interfered with your social activities (like visiting with friends, relatives, etc.)?

(Circle One Number)

All of the time 1
Most of the time 2
Some of the time 3
A little of the time 4
None of the time 5

How TRUE or FALSE is each of the following statements for you?

(Circle One Number on Each Line)

	Definitely True	Mostly True	Don't Know	Mostly False	Definitely False
33. I seem to get sick a little easier than other people	1	2	3	4	5
34. I am as healthy as anybody I know	1	2	3	4	5
35. I expect my health to get worse	1	2	3	4	5
36. My health is excellent	1	2	3	4	5

Chapter 3

Individualization of Drug Therapy: Clinical Pharmacokinetics and Pharmacodynamics

Larry A. Bauer, PharmD, FCP, FCCP

Pharmacokinetic concepts have been used successfully to individualize patient drug therapy. Laboratories routinely measure patient serum or plasma samples for many drugs including antibiotics (aminoglycosides, vancomycin), theophylline, antiepileptics (phenytoin, phenobarbital, ethosuximide, carbamazepine), methotrexate, lithium, and antiarrhythmics (lidocaine, procainamide, quinidine, digoxin). Combined with a knowledge of the disease states and conditions that influence the disposition of a particular drug, kinetic concepts can be used to modify doses to produce serum drug concentrations that produce desirable pharmacologic effects without unwanted side effects. This narrow range of concentrations within which the pharmacologic response is produced and the adverse effects prevented in most patients is defined as the *therapeutic range* of the drug. Table 3.1 lists the therapeutic ranges for commonly used medications.

Although most individuals experience favorable effects with serum drug concentrations in the therapeutic range, the effects of a given serum concentration can vary widely among individuals. Clinicians should never assume that a serum concentration within the therapeutic range will be safe and effective for every patient. The response to the drug, such as number of seizures a patient experiences while taking an antiepileptic agent, should always be assessed when serum concentrations are measured.

Throughout this chapter, abbreviations for various pharmacokinetic parameters are used frequently. Pharmacists should be able to recognize these abbreviations as easily as they do the full terms. Commonly used abbreviations—ones that pharmacists should recognize—are listed in Table 3.2.

TABLE 3.1. SELECTED THERAPEUTIC RANGES

Drug	Therapeutic Range
Digoxin	0.9–2 ng/mL
Lidocaine	1.5–5 μg/mL
Procainamide/*N*-acetylprocainamide	10–30 μg/mL
Quinidine	2–5 μg/mL
Amikacin[a]	20–30 μg/mL (peak) <5 μg/mL (trough)
Gentamicin, tobramycin, netilmicin[a]	5–10 μg/mL (peak) <2 μg/mL (trough)
Chloramphenicol	10–20 μg/mL
Lithium	0.6–1.4 mEq/L
Carbamazepine	4–12 μg/mL
Ethosuximide	40–100 μg/mL
Phenobarbital	15–40 μg/mL
Phenytoin	10–20 μg/mL
Primidone	5–12 μg/mL
Valproic acid	50–100 μg/mL
Theophylline	10–20 μg/mL

[a]Using a multiple dose per day dosage schedule, single daily dose therapeutic concentrations not yet established.

Clinical Pharmacokinetics

Clinical pharmacokinetics is the discipline that describes the absorption, distribution, metabolism, and elimination of drugs in patients requiring drug therapy. When a drug is administered extravascularly to patients, it must be absorbed across biologic membranes to reach the systemic circulation. If the drug is given orally, the drug molecules must pass through the gastrointestinal tract wall into capillaries. For transdermal patches, the drug must penetrate the skin to enter the vascular system. In general, the pharmacologic effect of the drug is delayed when it is given extravascularly because time is required for the drug absorption into the vascular system.

The vascular system generally provides the "transportation" for the drug molecule to its site of activity. After

TABLE 3.2. PHARMACOKINETIC ABBREVIATIONS

Abbreviation	Definition
CL	Clearance
k_0	Intravenous infusion rate
C_{ss}	Steady-state concentration
D	Dose
τ	Dosage interval
F	Fraction of drug absorbed into the systemic circulation
Q	Blood flow
E	Extraction ratio
C_{out}	Concentration of drug in blood coming out of an organ
C_{in}	Concentration of drug in blood going into an organ
f_b	Fraction of drug in the blood that is unbound
f_t	Fraction of drug in the tissues that is unbound
CL_{int}	Intrinsic clearance
$C_{ss,u}$	Steady-state concentration of unbound drug
V_D	Volume of distribution
LD	Loading dose
MD	Maintenance dose
V_b	Volume of blood
V_t	Volume of tissue
$t_{1/2}$	Half-life
A_i	y intercept of ith line
k_i	Rate constant for ith line
k	Elimination rate constant
k_a	Absorption rate constant
α	Distribution rate constant
β	Terminal rate constant
$V_{D,\beta}$	V_D during phase of curve
$V_{D,ss}$	V_D at steady state
k_{12}, k_{21}, k_{10}	Microconstants
t'	Postinfusion time
T	Duration of infusion
AUC	Area under serum or blood concentration-versus-time curve
AUMC	Area under the first moment curve
C_{last}	Last serum or blood concentration
t_{last}	Time at which C_{last} was obtained
V_{max}	Maximum rate of drug metabolism
K_m	Serum concentration at which the rate of metabolism equals $V_{max}/2$
C_{max}	Maximum serum or blood concentration
C_{min}	Minimum serum or blood concentration
DR	Dosage rate
C_{est}	Estimated serum or blood concentration
C_{act}	Actual serum or blood concentration
Cr CL_{est}	Estimated creatinine clearance
S_{cr}	Serum creatinine

the drug reaches the systemic circulation, it can leave the vasculature and penetrate the various tissues or remain in the blood. If the drug remains in the blood it may bind to endogenous proteins such as albumin or α_1-acid glycoprotein. This binding is usually reversible, and an equilibrium is created between protein-bound drug and unbound drug. Unbound drug in the blood provides the driving force for distribution of the agent to body tissues. If unbound drug leaves the bloodstream and distributes to tissue it may become tissue-bound, it may remain unbound in the tissue, or, if the tissue can metabolize or eliminate the drug, it may be rendered inactive and/or eliminated from the body. If the drug becomes tissue bound, it may bind to the receptor that causes its pharmacologic or toxic effect or to a nonspecific binding site that causes no effect. Again, tissue binding is usually reversible so that the tissue-bound drug is in equilibrium with unbound drug in the tissue.

Certain organs—such as the liver and lung—possess enzymes that metabolize drugs. The resulting metabolite may be inactive or have a pharmacologic effect of its own. The blood also contains esterases, which cleave ester bonds in drug molecules and generally render them inactive.

Drug metabolism usually occurs in the liver through one or both of two types of reactions. Phase I reactions generally make the drug molecule more polar and water soluble so that it is prone to elimination by the kidney. Phase I modifications include oxidation, hydrolysis, and reduction. Phase II reactions involve conjugation to form glucuronides, acetates, or sulfates. These reactions generally inactivate the pharmacologic activity of the drug and may make it more prone to elimination by the kidney.

Other organs have the ability to eliminate drugs or metabolites from the body. The kidney can excrete drugs by glomerular filtration or by such active processes as proximal tubular secretion. Drugs can also be eliminated via bile produced by the liver or air expired by the lungs.

CONCEPTS

Most drugs follow linear pharmacokinetics: Serum drug concentrations change proportionally with long-term daily dosing. As an example, if the drug dose were doubled from 300 to 600 mg/d, the patient's serum drug concentration would double.

When a drug is given by continuous intravenous infusion, the clinical goal is to increase the serum concentrations until an equilibrium is established between the drug dosage rate and the rate of drug elimination. At that point, a maintenance dose is given such that the rate of drug administration equals the rate of drug elimination and the serum concentrations therefore remain constant (Fig. 3.1). For example, if a patient were receiving a continuous intravenous infusion at 40 mg/h, the serum drug concentration would increase until the patient's body was eliminating the

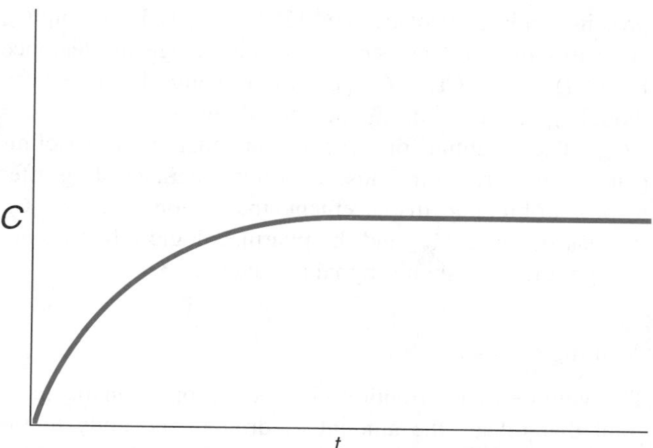

Figure 3.1. Normal serum concentration–time curve following a continuous intravenous infusion.

drug at 40 mg/h. When serum drug concentrations reach a constant value, steady state is achieved.

If the drug is given at intermittent dosage intervals, such as 250 mg every 6 hours, steady state is achieved when the serum concentration-versus-time curves for each dosage interval are superimposable. The amount of drug eliminated during the dosage interval equals the dose.

Clearance

Clearance (CL) is the most important pharmacokinetic parameter because it determines the steady-state concentration for a given dosage rate. When a drug is given at a continuous intravenous infusion rate equal to k_0 the steady-state concentration (C_{ss}) is determined by the quotient of k_0 and CL ($C_{ss} = k_0/\text{CL}$). If the drug is administered as individual doses *(D)* at a given dosage interval (τ), the average steady-state concentration (C_{ss}) over the dosage interval is given by the equation[1]:

$$C_{ss} = [F(D/\tau)]/\text{CL}$$

where F is the fraction of dose absorbed into the systemic vascular system. The average steady-state concentration over the dosage interval is the steady-state concentration that would have occurred had the same dose been given as a continuous intravenous infusion (e.g., 300 mg every 6 hours at an infusion rate of 50 mg/h).

Physiologically, clearance is determined by (1) blood flow *(Q)* to the organ that metabolizes or eliminates the drug and (2) the efficiency of the organ in extracting the drug from the bloodstream.[2] Efficiency is measured using an extraction ratio *(E),* calculated by subtracting the concentration in the blood leaving the extracting organ (C_{out}) from the concentration in the blood entering the organ (C_{in}) and then dividing the result by C_{in}:

$$E = (C_{in} - C_{out})/(C_{in})$$

Clearance for that organ is calculated by taking the product of Q and E: ($\text{CL} = QE$). For example, if liver blood flow equals 1.5 L/min and the drug's extraction ratio is 0.33, hepatic clearance equals 0.5 L/min. Total clearance is computed by summing all of the individual organ clearance values. Clearance changes occur in patients when the blood flow to extracting organs changes or when the extraction ratio changes. Vasodilators like hydralazine or nifedipine increase liver blood flow, whereas congestive heart failure and hypotension can decrease hepatic blood flow. Extraction ratios can increase when enzyme inducers increase the amount of drug-metabolizing enzyme. Extraction ratios may decrease if enzyme inhibitors inhibit drug metabolizing enzymes or necrosis causes loss of parenchyma.

Intrinsic Clearance

The extraction ratio can also be thought of in terms of the unbound fraction of drug in the blood (f_b), the intrinsic ability of the extracting organ to clear unbound drug from the blood (CL_{int}), and blood flow to the organ (Q)[3,4]:

$$E = [f_b(\text{CL}_{int})]/\{Q + [f_b(\text{CL}_{int})]\}$$

By substituting this equation for E, the clearance equation becomes:

$$\text{CL} = Q[f_b(\text{CL}_{int})]/\{Q + [f_b(\text{CL}_{int})]\}$$

Clearance changes will occur when blood flow to the clearing organ changes (e.g., in conditions where blood flow is reduced [shock, congestive heart failure] or when medications such as vasodilators increase blood flow), binding in the blood changes (e.g., if highly protein-bound drugs are displaced), or intrinsic clearance of unbound drug changes (e.g., when metabolizing enzymes are induced or inhibited).

If CL_{int} is large (i.e., enzymes have a high capacity to metabolize the drug), the product of f_b and CL_{int} is much larger than Q. When $f_b(\text{CL}_{int})$ is much greater than Q, the sum of Q and $f_b(\text{CL}_{int})$ in the denominator of the clearance equation almost equals $f_b(\text{CL}_{int})$:

$$f_b(\text{CL}_{int}) \approx Q + f_b(\text{CL}_{int})$$

Substituting this expression in the denominator of the clearance equation and canceling common terms leads to the following expression for drugs with a large CL_{int}: $\text{CL} \approx Q$. In this case the clearance of the drug is equal to blood flow to the organ; such drugs are called *high-clearance drugs* and have large extraction ratios. Propranolol, verapamil, morphine, and lidocaine are examples of high-clearance drugs.

If CL_{int} is small (i.e., enzymes have a limited capacity to metabolize the drug), Q is much larger than the product of f_b and CL_{int}. When Q is much greater than $f_b(\text{CL}_{int})$, the sum of Q and $f_b(\text{CL}_{int})$ in the denominator of the clearance equation becomes almost equal to Q: $Q \approx Q + f_b(\text{CL}_{int})$. Substituting this expression in the denominator of the clearance equation and canceling common terms leads to the following expression for drugs with a small CL_{int}: $CL \approx f_b(CL_{int})$. In this case, clearance of the drug is equal to the product of the fraction unbound in the blood and the intrinsic ability of the organ to clear unbound drug from the blood; such drugs are known as *low-clearance drugs* and have small extraction ratios. Warfarin, theophylline, diazepam, and phenobarbital are examples of low-clearance drugs.

As previously mentioned, the concentration of unbound drug in the blood is probably more important pharmacologically than the total (bound plus unbound) concentration. The unbound drug in the blood is in equilibrium with the unbound drug in the tissues and reflects the concentration of drug at its site of action. Therefore, the pharmacologic effect of a drug is thought to be a function of the concentration of unbound drug in the blood. The unbound steady-state concentration ($C_{ss,u}$) can be calculated by multiplying C_{ss} and f_b: $C_{ss,u} = C_{ss}f_b$. The effect that changes in Q, f_b, and CL_{int} have on $C_{ss,u}$ and therefore on the pharmacologic response of a drug depends on whether a high- or low-clearance drug is involved. Because $CL = Q$ for high-clearance drugs, a change in f_b or CL_{int} does not change CL or C_{ss} ($C_{ss} = k_0/CL$). However, a change in unbound drug fraction does alter $C_{ss,u}$ ($C_{ss,u} = f_bC_{ss}$), thereby affecting the pharmacologic response. Plasma protein binding displacement drug interactions are thus very important clinically, but they are also dangerous because the changes in $C_{ss,u}$ are not reflected in changes in C_{ss}. Since laboratories usually measure only total concentrations (concentrations of unbound drug are difficult to determine), the interaction is hard to detect. If CL_{int} changes for high-clearance drugs, CL, C_{ss}, $C_{ss,u}$, and pharmacologic response do not change. Changes in Q cause a change in CL; changes in C_{ss}, $C_{ss,u}$, and drug response are indirectly proportional to changes in CL.

For low-clearance drugs, total clearance is determined by unbound drug fraction and intrinsic clearance: $CL = f_b(CL_{int})$. A change in Q does not change CL, C_{ss}, $C_{ss,u}$, or pharmacologic response. However, a change in f_b or CL_{int} does alter CL and C_{ss} ($C_{ss} = k_0/CL$). Changes in CL_{int} will cause a proportional change in CL. Changes in C_{ss}, $C_{ss,u}$, and drug response are indirectly proportional to changes in CL. Altering f_b for low-clearance drugs produces interesting results. A change in f_b alters CL and C_{ss} ($C_{ss} = k_0/CL$). As CL and C_{ss} change in opposite directions with changes in f_b, $C_{ss,u}$ ($C_{ss,u} = f_bC_{ss}$), and pharmacologic responses do not change with alterations in the fraction of unbound drug in the blood. For example, a low-clearance drug is administered to a patient until steady-state is achieved:

$$CL = f_b(CL_{int})$$

$$C_{ss} = k_0/CL$$

Suppose another drug is administered to the patient that displaces the first drug from plasma protein binding sites and doubles f_b (f_b now equals $2f_b$). CL doubles because of the protein binding displacement [$2CL = 2f_b(CL_{int})$], and C_{ss} decreases by one-half because of the change in clearance [$1/2(C_{ss}) = k_0/(2CL)$]. $C_{ss,u}$ does not change because even though f_b is doubled, C_{ss} decreased by one-half ($C_{ss,u} = f_bC_{ss}$). The potential for error in this situation is that clinicians may increase the dose of a low-clearance drug after a protein-binding displacement interaction because C_{ss} decreased. Since $C_{ss,u}$ and the pharmacologic effect do not change, the dose should remain unaltered.

Volume of Distribution

The volume of distribution (V_D) is a proportionality constant that relates the amount of drug in the body to the serum concentration (amount in body = CV_D). V_D is used to calculate the loading dose (LD) of a drug that will immediately achieve a desired C_{ss} ($LD = C_{ss}V_D$). However, in practice the patient's own V_D is not known at the time the loading dose is administered. In this case an average V_D is assumed and used to calculate a loading dose. Because the patient's V_D is almost always different from the average V_D for the drug, a loading dose does not attain the calculated C_{ss}, but it hopefully achieves a therapeutic concentration.

The numeric value for the volume of distribution is determined by the physiologic volume of blood and tissues and how the drug binds in blood and tissues[5]:

$$V_D = V_b + (f_b/f_t)V_t$$

where V_b and V_t are the volumes of blood and tissues, respectively, and f_b and f_t are the fractions of unbound drug in blood and tissues, respectively.

Half-Life

Half-life ($t_{1/2}$) is the time required for serum concentrations to decrease by one-half after absorption and distribution are complete. It takes the same amount of time for serum concentrations to drop from 200 to 100 mg/L as it does for concentrations to decline from 2 to 1 mg/L.

Half-life is important because it determines the time required to reach steady state and the dosage interval. It takes approximately three to five $t_{1/2}$ to reach steady-state concentrations during continuous dosing. In three $t_{1/2}$, serum concentrations are at about 90% of their ultimate steady-state values. Because most serum drug assays have about a 10% error, it is difficult to differentiate concentrations that are within 10% of each other. For this reason, many clinicians consider concentrations obtained after three $t_{1/2}$ to be C_{ss}.

Half-life is also used to determine the dosage interval for a drug. For instance, it may be desirable to maintain maximum steady-state concentrations at 20 mg/L and minimum steady-state concentrations at 10 mg/L. In this case it would be necessary to administer the drug every $t_{1/2}$

because the minimum desirable concentration is one-half the maximum desirable concentration.

Half-life is a *dependent* kinetic variable because its value depends on the values of CL and V_D.[5] The equation that describes the relationship among the three variables is $t_{1/2} = 0.693V_D/\text{CL}$. Changes in $t_{1/2}$ can result from a change in either V_D or CL; a change in $t_{1/2}$ does not necessarily indicate that CL has changed. Half-life can change solely because of changes in V_D.

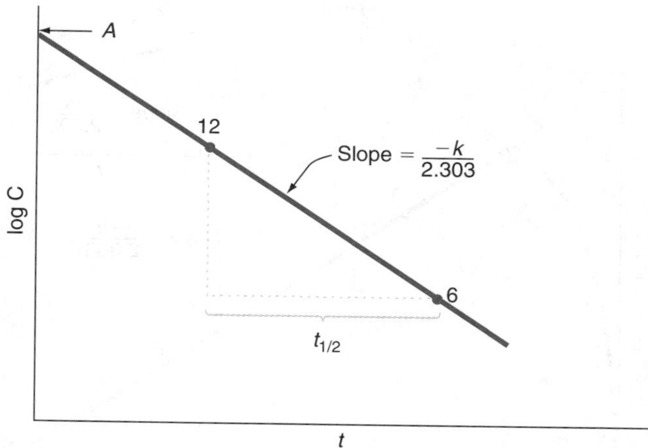

Figure 3.2. Calculation of the half-life of a drug following intravenous bolus dosing.

DETERMINISTIC MODELS

Pharmacokinetic models are useful to describe data sets, predict serum concentrations after several doses or different routes of administration, and calculate pharmacokinetic constants such as CL, V_D, and $t_{1/2}$.[6] Two methods have been devised to accomplish these goals. In the first, multiexponential equations are used to describe the data. The other method uses compartmental models that depict the body as one or more discrete compartments to which drug is distributed and/or from which drug is eliminated. In both cases the shape of the serum concentration-versus-time curve determines the number of exponents in the equation or the number of compartments, leading to the term *deterministic model.*

Exponential Equations

In serum concentration-versus-time graphs, concentrations often appear to change according to an exponential equation of the form $C = \Sigma(A_i e^{-k_i t})$ where C is the serum concentration at any time t and A_i is the y intercept of the ith line with a slope equal to $-k_i/2.303$. CL, V_D, and $t_{1/2}$ can easily be calculated using the A_i and k_i values of the individual lines.[7,8]

Monoexponential Equations

The simplest situation occurs when the logarithm of the serum concentrations after a single intravenous bolus declines in a straight line with time (Fig. 3.2). In this case the equation that describes the data is $C = Ae^{-kt}$. A is obtained from the graph by extrapolating the line back to the y intercept. The terminal elimination rate constant (k) can be computed using the slope of the line: slope = $-k/2.303$. Alternatively, $t_{1/2}$ can be obtained from the graph by determining the time it takes for serum concentrations to decrease by one-half, and the following formula can be used to compute k: $k = 0.693/t_{1/2}$. CL and V_D are calculated using the equations $\text{CL} = D/(A/k)$ and $V_D = \text{CL}/k$.[9–11]

More complex situations occur when drugs are given by different routes of administration. When a dose is given extravascularly, serum concentrations usually increase while the drug is being absorbed, reaching a maximum concentration (C_{max}), and then declining in a straight line when plotted on semilogarithmic coordinates (Fig. 3.3). The multiexponential equation that describes this data set is $C = Ae^{-kt} - Ae^{-k_a t}$, where k is the terminal rate constant (slope = $-k/2.303$), A is the y intercept of the terminal slope, k_a is the absorption rate constant, and t is time. This equation represents the difference between two lines. When plotted on semilogarithmic paper, the first line has a y intercept of A and a slope equal to $-k/2.303$. The other line has the same y intercept (A) but a slope equal to $-k_a/2.303$.

The method of residuals is used to obtain the slopes and intercepts of the two lines (Fig. 3.2). A is determined by extrapolating the terminal slope to the y axis; k can be obtained by calculating the slope or $t_{1/2}$ and using the formulas given for the intravenous bolus case. At each time point in the absorption portion of the curve, the concentration value from the extrapolated line is noted and called the extrapolated concentration. For each point the actual concentration is subtracted from the extrapolated concentration to compute the residual concentration. When the residual concentrations are plotted on semilogarithmic coordinates, a line with y intercept equal to A and slope equal to $-k_a/2.303$ is obtained. When these values are calculated, they can be placed into the equation ($C = Ae^{-kt} - Ae^{-k_a t}$) and used to compute the serum concentration at any time after the extravascular dose. The slopes and rate constants can also be used to compute CL and V_D: $\text{CL} = FD/(A/k - A/k_a)$ and $V_D = \text{CL}/k$, where F is the fraction of the dose absorbed into the systemic circulation.

Continuous Intravenous Infusion

During a continuous intravenous infusion, C_{ss} is achieved after three to five half-lives (Fig. 3.4). C_{ss} is used to calculate CL ($\text{CL} = k_0/C_{ss}$). If the infusion is discontinued, k and $t_{1/2}$ can be calculated from the terminal slope. The volume of distribution is computed once CL and k are known ($V_D = \text{CL}/k$).

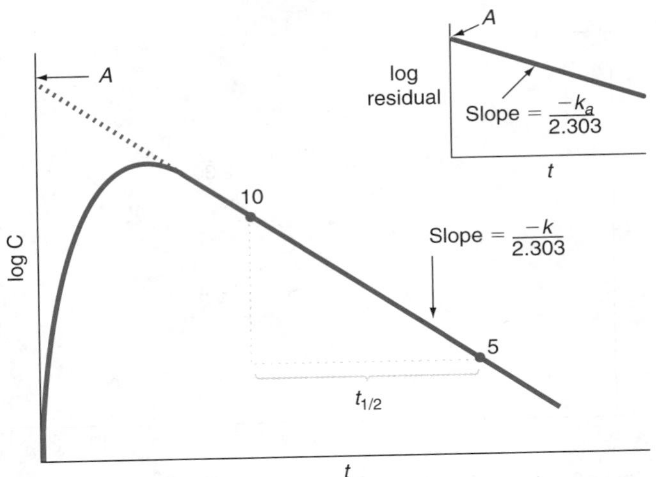

Figure 3.3. Calculation of the half-life of a drug following oral, intramuscular, or other extravascular dosing route.

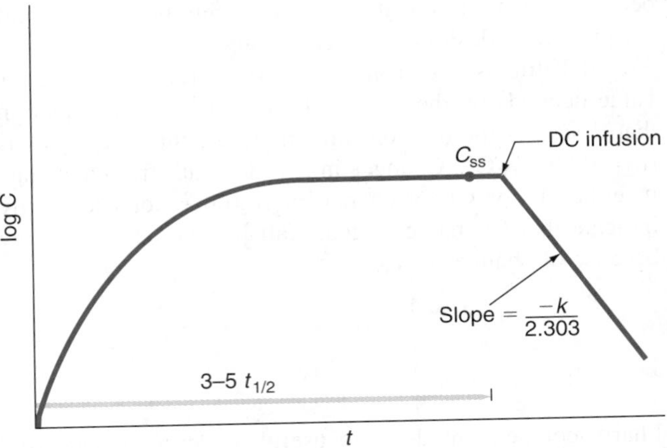

Figure 3.4. Achievement of steady-state serum concentrations after three to five half-lives of a drug. Note the elimination phase after discontinuance of the infusion.

Multiexponential Equations

After an intravenous bolus dose, serum concentrations often decline in two or more phases. During the early phases, drug leaves the bloodstream by two mechanisms: distribution into tissues and metabolism and/or elimination. Because the drug is leaving the bloodstream through these two mechanisms, serum concentrations decline rapidly. After tissues and blood are in equilibrium, only metabolism and/or elimination remove drug from the blood. During this terminal phase serum concentrations decline more slowly. The half-life is measured during the terminal phase by determining the time required for concentrations to decline by one half.

Biexponential Equations

For the simplest case the serum concentration-versus-time curve decreases in two phases and is described by the equation $C = Ae^{-\alpha t} + Be^{-\beta t}$, where β is computed from the terminal slope (slope $= -\beta/2.303$ or $\beta = 0.693/t_{1/2}$) and is called the terminal rate constant, B is the y intercept of the terminal extrapolated line, α is computed from the slope of the residual line, and A is the y intercept of the residual line (Fig. 3.5).

The residual line is calculated as before using the method of residuals. The terminal line is extrapolated to the y axis, and extrapolated concentrations are determined for each time point. Because actual concentrations are greater in this case, residual concentrations are calculated by subtracting the extrapolated concentrations from the actual concentrations. When plotted on semilogarithmic paper the residual line has a y intercept equal to A.The slope of the residual line is used to compute α (slope $= -\alpha/2.303$). With the rate constants (α and β) and the intercepts (A and B), concentrations can be calculated for any time after the intravenous bolus dose ($C = Ae^{-\alpha t} + Be^{-\beta t}$) or pharmacokinetic constants can be computed: $CL = D/[(A/\alpha) + (B/\beta)]$, $V_{D,\beta} = CL/\beta$, $V_{D,ss} = D[(A/\alpha^2) + (B/\beta^2)]/[(A/\alpha) + (B/\beta)]^2$.

Volumes of Distribution in Multiexponential Equations

Two different V_D values are needed as proportionality constants for drugs that require multiexponential equations to describe the serum concentration-time curve. The V_D that is used to compute the amount of drug in the body during the terminal (β) portion of the curve is called $V_{D,\beta}$ (amount of drug in body $= V_{D,\beta}C$). During a continuous intravenous infusion at steady state, $V_{D,ss}$ is used to compute the amount of drug in the body (amount of drug in body $= V_{D,ss}C$). $V_{D,ss}$ is also the V_D that can be computed using the physiologic volumes of blood and tissues and the ratio of unbound drug in blood to that in tissues [$V_{D,ss} = V_b + (f_b/f_t)V_t$]. Because the

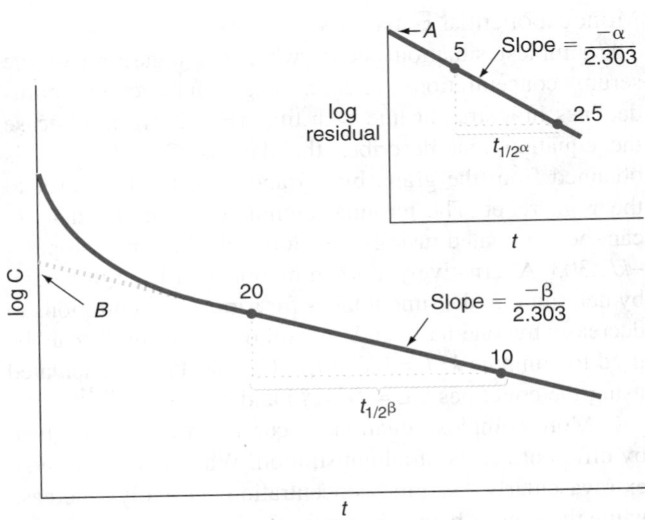

Figure 3.5. Calculation of α and β half-lives following intravenous dosing.

value of $V_{D,\beta}$ changes when CL changes, $V_{D,ss}$ should be used to indicate if drug distribution changes during pharmacokinetic or drug interaction experiments.

Compartmental Models

Compartmental models can also be used to describe pharmacokinetic data sets.[12,13] As mentioned previously, these models depict the body as one or more compartments from which drug is eliminated and/or to which drug is distributed (Fig. 3.6). First-order rate constants, known as microconstants, describe the rate of transfer from one compartment to another. Each compartment also has its own V_D. In all situations, the equations derived from compartmental models are very similar to those derived using intercepts and rate constants.

One-Compartment Model

The simplest case uses a single compartment to represent the entire body (Fig. 3.6). Drug enters the compartment by continuous intravenous infusion (k_0), absorption from an extravascular site with an absorption rate constant of k_a, or intravenous bolus *(D)*. After an intravenous bolus, serum concentrations decline in a straight line when plotted on semilogarithmic coordinates. As before, the slope of the line is $-k/2.303$; $t_{1/2}$ can be computed by determining the time required for concentrations to decrease by one-half ($t_{1/2} = 0.693/k$). The equation that describes the data is $C = (D/V_D)\, e^{-kt}$. V_D is calculated by dividing the intravenous dose by the *y* intercept (the concentration at time zero, C_0) of the graph. CL is computed by taking the product of *k* and V_D. Once V_D and *k* are known, concentrations at any time after the dose can be computed [$C = (D/V_D)\, e^{-kt}$].

When an extravascular dose is given, one-compartment model serum concentrations rise during absorption, reach C_{max}, and then decrease in a straight line with a slope equal to $-k/2.303$. The equation that describes the data is $C = [(FDk_a)/V_D(k_a-k)](e^{-kt} - e^{-k_a t})$, where *F* is the fraction of the dose absorbed into the systemic circulation. The absorption rate constant (k_a) is obtained using the method of residuals. The *y* intercept (*A*) of the terminal phase and the residual line is $A = FDk_a/[V_D(k_a - k)]$. If *F* is known, V_D can be calculated using *A*, k_a, and *k*. CL is computed by taking the product of *k* and V_D.

During a continuous intravenous infusion, the serum concentrations in a one-compartment model change according to the following function: $C = (k_0/\text{CL})(1 - e^{-kt})$. If the infusion has been running for more than three to five half-lives, the patient will be at steady state and CL can be calculated ($\text{CL} = k_0/C_{ss}$). When the infusion is discontinued, serum concentrations appear to decline in a straight line when plotted on semilogarithmic paper with a slope of $-k/2.303$. V_D is computed by dividing CL by *k*.

Multicompartment Model

After an intravenous bolus dose, serum concentrations decrease as if the drug were being injected into a central compartment that not only metabolizes and eliminates drug, but also distributes drug to one or more other compartments. Of these multicompartment models, the two-compartment model is most commonly encountered (Fig. 3.6). After an intravenous bolus injection, serum concentrations decrease in two distinct phases described by the equation:

$$C = D(\alpha - k_{21})/[V_{D1}(\alpha - \beta)]e^{-\alpha t} + D(k_{21} - \beta)/[V_{D1}(\alpha - \beta)]e^{-\beta t}$$

where k_{21} is the first-order rate constant that reflects the transfer of drug from compartment 2 to compartment 1 and V_{D1} is the V_D of compartment 1. As previously explained, *A*, *B*, α, and β are obtained using the method of residuals. Once these have been computed the following equations are used to calculate kinetic constants:

$$k_{21} = (A\beta + B\alpha)/(A + B)$$

$$k_{10} = \alpha\beta/k_{21}$$

$$k_{12} = \alpha + \beta - k_{21} - k_{10}$$

$$V_{D1} = D/(A + B)$$

$$V_{D,\beta} = D/\{\beta[(A/\alpha) + (B/\beta)]\}$$

$$V_{D,ss} = V_{D1}[(k_{21} + k_{12})/k_{21}]$$

$$\text{CL} = V_{D1}k_{10}$$

$$t_{1/2} = 0.693/\beta$$

If serum concentrations of a drug given as a continuous intravenous infusion decline in a biphasic manner after the infusion is discontinued, a two-compartment model describes the data set[14,15] (Fig. 3.7). In this instance the postinfusion concentrations decrease according to the equation: $C = Re^{-t'} + Se^{-t'}$, where t' is the postinfusion time ($t' = 0$ when infusion is discontinued) and *R*, *S*, α, and β are determined from the postinfusion concentrations using the method of residuals with the *y* axis set at $t' = 0$. *R* and *S* are

1 compartment

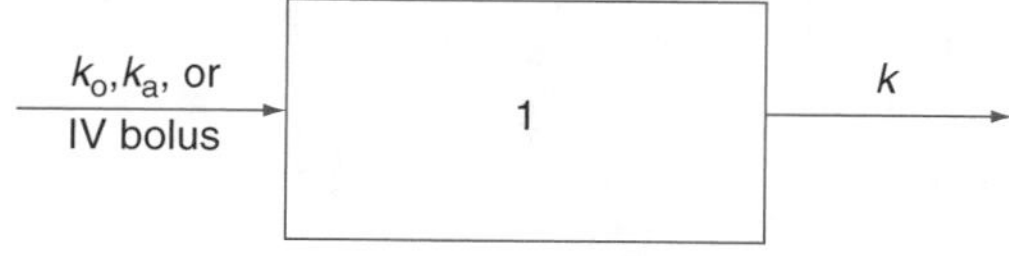

2 compartments

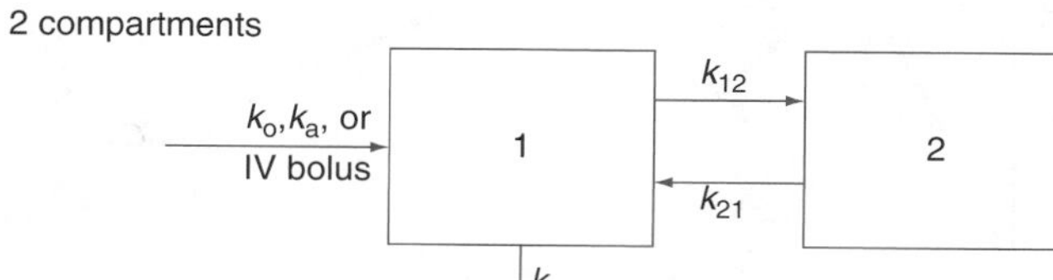

Figure 3.6. Visual representations of one- and two-compartment drug-distribution models.

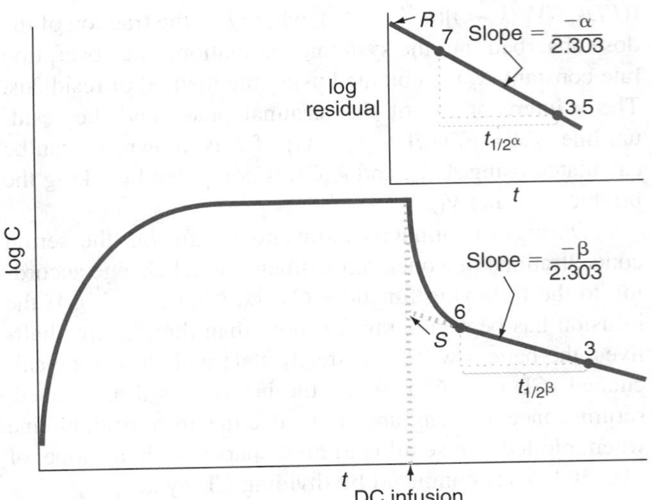

Figure 3.7. Calculation of α and β half-lives following a steady-state infusion.

used to compute A and B. A and B are the y intercepts that would have occurred had the total dose given during the infusion ($D = k_0T$) been administered as an intravenous bolus dose:

$$A = RD\alpha/[k_0(1 - e^{-\alpha T})]$$

$$B = SD\beta/[k_0(1 - e^{-\beta T})]$$

where T is the duration of infusion. Once A, B, α, and β are known, the equations for an intravenous bolus are used to compute the pharmacokinetic constants. Often, when a drug is given as an intravenous bolus or continuous intravenous infusion, a two-compartment model is used to describe the data, but when the same agent is given extravascularly, a one-compartment model applies.[7] In this case, distribution occurs during the absorption phase so a distribution phase is not observed.

Multiple Dosing

Any of these equations can be used to determine serum concentrations after multiple doses. The multiple dosing factor, $(1 - e^{-nK})/(1 - e^{-K})$, where n is the number of doses, K is the appropriate rate constant, and is the dosage interval, is simply multiplied by each exponential term in the equation, substituting the rate constant of each exponent for K. Time (t) is set at 0 at the beginning of each dosage interval. For example, a single-dose biexponential intravenous bolus is calculated as follows: $C = Ae^{-\alpha t} + Be^{-\beta t}$. The equation for a multiple dose biexponential intravenous bolus is therefore

$$C = Ae^{-\alpha t}[(1 - e^{-n\alpha\tau})/(1 - e^{-\alpha\tau})] + Be^{-\beta t}[(1 - e^{-n\beta\tau})/(1 - e^{-\beta\tau})]$$

A single-dose one-compartment intravenous bolus is calculated as $C = (D/V_D)e^{-kt}$. For a multiple-dose one-compartment intravenous bolus the concentration is $C = (D/V_D)e^{-kt}[(1 - e^{-nk\tau})/(1 - e^{-k\tau})]$.

Noncompartmental Analysis

Pharmacokinetic constants and serum concentrations after several doses can be calculated without deterministic models.[16–18] This approach requires the measurement of areas under curves. The area under the serum concentration-versus-time curve (AUC) and the area under the first moment curve (serum concentration × time-versus-time curve, AUMC) are determined and used in computations. The trapezoidal rule is among the easiest methods used to calculate areas under curves (area of trapezoid = $[(C_1 + C_2)/2](t_2 - t_1)$, Fig. 3.8). First, the times and serum concentrations are written down in tabular form and the first moments (time multiplied by respective concentration) are calculated as shown here:

Time (h)	Concentration (mg/L)	Time × Concentration (mg × h/L)
0	100	0
0.5	80	40
1.0	60	60
3.0	30	60
.	.	.
.	.	.
.	.	.
7.0	7.5	52.5
9.0	3.7	32.6

Individual trapezoids are made for each consecutive time-concentration pair to compute AUC {first trapezoid =

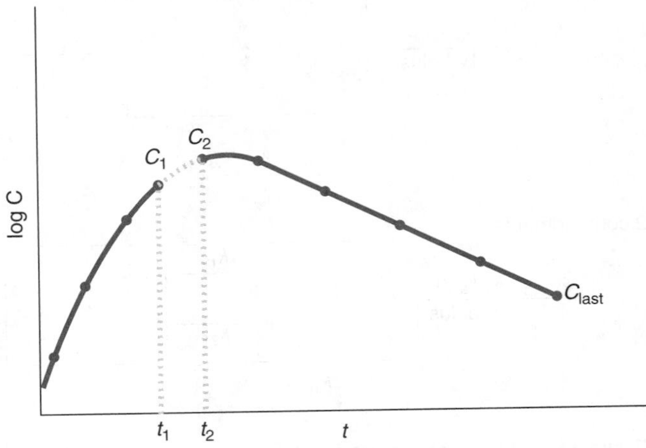

Figure 3.8. Representation of sampling intervals and the trapezoidal rule.

[(100 mg/L + 80 mg/L)/2](0.5 h – 0 h), second trapezoid = [(80 mg/L + 60 mg/L)/2](1 h – 0.5 h), etc.} and for each consecutive time-time × concentration pair to compute AUMC (first trapezoid = [(0 mg × h/L + 40 mg × h/L)/2](0.5 h – 0 h), second trapezoid = [(40 mg × h/L + 60 mg × h/L)/2](1 h – 0.5 h), etc). Individual trapezoids for AUC and AUMC, respectively, are added together to compute the AUC and AUMC from $t = 0$ to the time (t_{last}) the last serum concentration (C_{last}) is obtained ($AUC_{0-t_{last}}$ and $AUMC_{0-t_{last}}$). The following equations calculate the AUC and AUMC from t_{last} to infinity:

$$AUC_{t_{last}-\infty} = C_{last}/k$$

$$AUMC_{t_{last}-\infty} = (t_{last}\, C_{last}/k) + (C_{last}/k^2)$$

where k is the terminal rate constant calculated from the slope of the postdistribution serum concentration line or calculated using $t_{1/2}$ (slope = $-k/2.303$ or $k = 0.693/t_{1/2}$). The equations used to compute the total AUC and AUMC from zero to infinity are:

$$AUC_{0-\infty} = AUC_{0-t_{last}} + AUC_{t_{last}-\infty}$$

$$AUMC_{0-\infty} = AUMC_{0-t_{last}} + AUMC_{t_{last}-\infty}$$

Intravenous Bolus

After an intravenous bolus dose pharmacokinetic constants are calculated as follows[16,18]:

$$V_{D,\beta} = D/[k(AUC_{0-\infty})]$$

$$V_{D,ss} = [D(AUMC_{0-\infty})]/(AUC_{0-\infty})^2$$

$$CL = D/(AUC_{0-\infty})$$

$$t_{1/2} = 0.693/k$$

$$MRT = AUMC_{0-\infty}/AUC_{0-\infty}$$

MRT (mean residence time) is the time the average drug molecule stays in the body. Sixty-three percent of an intravenous dose is eliminated during the MRT.

Continuous Intravenous Infusion

After a continuous intravenous infusion pharmacokinetic constants are computed using the following equations[17,18]:

$$V_{D,\beta} = D/[k(AUC_{0-\infty})]$$

$$V_{D,ss} = \{[D(AUMC_{0-\infty})]/(AUC_{0-\infty})^2\} - \{(DT)/[2(AUC_{0-\infty})]\}$$

$$CL = D/AUC_{0-\infty}$$

$$t_{1/2} = 0.693/k$$

where T is the duration of infusion and D is the total dose infused ($D = k_0T$). k is calculated from the terminal slope after the infusion has been discontinued.

Extravascular Dosing

After an extravascular dose, kinetic constants are computed using similar equations[18]:

$$V_{D,\beta} = FD/[k(AUC_{0-\infty})]$$

$$V_{D,ss} = [FD(AUMC_{0-\infty})/(AUC_{0-\infty})^2] - [FD/k_a(AUC_{0-\infty})]$$

$$CL = FD/AUC_{0-\infty}$$

$$t_{1/2} = 0.693/k$$

where k_a is the absorption rate constant calculated using the method of residuals and F is the fraction of the dose absorbed systemically.

Clearances for Different Routes of Elimination and Metabolic Pathways

Clearances for individual organs can be computed if the excretion the organ produces can be obtained. For example, renal clearance can be calculated if urine is collected during a pharmacokinetic experiment. The patient empties his or her bladder immediately before the dose is given. Subsequent urine production is collected until the last serum concentration (C_{last}) is obtained. Renal clearance (CL_R) is computed by dividing the amount of drug excreted in the urine by $AUC_{0-t_{last}}$. Biliary and other clearance values are computed in a similar fashion.

Clearances can also be calculated for each metabolite that is formed from the parent drug. This computation is particularly useful in drug interaction studies to determine which metabolic pathway is stimulated or inhibited. In the following metabolic scheme, the parent drug (D) is metabolized into two different metabolites (M_1, M_2), which are subsequently eliminated by the kidney (M_{1R}, M_{2R}):

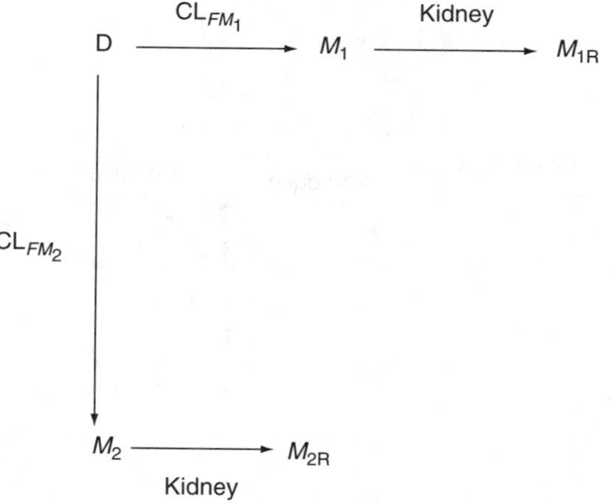

To compute the formation clearance of M_1 and M_2 (CL_{FM_1}, CL_{FM_2}), urine would be collected for five or more half-lives after a single dose or during a dosage interval at steady state. The amount of metabolite eliminated in the urine is then determined. The fraction of the dose (in moles, since the molecular weight of the parent drug and metabolites are not equal) eliminated by each metabolic pathway ($f_{M_1} = M_{1R}/D$ and $f_{M_2} = M_{2R}/D$) can then be computed. Formation clearance for each pathway can be calculated using the following equations: $CL_{FM_1} = f_{M_1}CL_M$ and $CL_{FM_2} = f_{M_2}CL_M$, where CL_M is the metabolic clearance for the parent drug.

Multiple Dosing

Serum concentrations after multiple doses can be computed from single-dose data using the principle of superposition.[6] According to the definition of linear pharmacokinetics, C_{ss} and $AUC_{0-\infty}$ change proportionally with dose. Therefore, serum concentration-versus-time curves can be added to or subtracted from each other. For example, if an intravenous bolus dose of 250 mg is administered to a patient and serum concentrations are obtained, the concentration that would occur 6 hours after the third dose (250 mg intravenous bolus every 8 hours) can be calculated using the data from the single-dose experiment. First, the single-dose curve would be replicated every 8 hours as if no other doses were given (Fig. 3.9). The concentration contributed from each individual dose would be obtained from the graph at 22 hours (6 hours after the third dose given on an 8-hour schedule) and added together to derive the concentration from all three doses. Using this technique serum concentrations after very complex dosage regimens can be calculated.

Because addition of several concentration curves using superposition can become quite tedious, a mathematical solution has been derived. It assumes that all doses are given after absorption and distribution are complete. The single-dose curve is drawn, the slope of the terminal postabsorption, postdistribution phase is determined (slope = $-k/2.303$), and the terminal phase is extrapolated to determine the y intercept (B). The following equation is used to calculate the serum concentration t hours after the nth dose (C_n) once the serum concentration t hours after the first dose (C_1) is known:

$$C_n = C_1 + Be^{-k\tau}\{[1 - e^{-k\tau(n-1)}]/(1 - e^{-kt}\,e^{-k\tau}\}$$

where τ is the dosage interval.

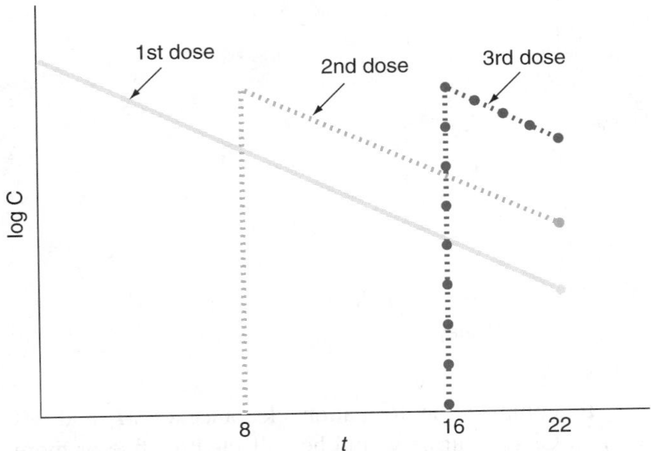

Figure 3.9. Superposition can be used to compute serum concentrations after multiple doses. Serum concentrations from each dose are added to determine the actual concentration at 22 hours.

BIOAVAILABILITY AND BIOEQUIVALENCE

The fraction of drug absorbed into the systemic circulation (F) after extravascular administration can be calculated after single intravenous and extravascular doses as[19]

$$F = D_{iv}(AUC_{0-\infty})/D(AUC_{iv_{0-\infty}})$$

where D and D_{iv} are the extravascular and intravenous doses, respectively, and $AUC_{iv_{0-\infty}}$ and $AUC_{0-\infty}$ are the intravenous and extravascular AUC, respectively, from time zero to infinity.

When the extravascular dose is administered orally, part of the dose may be metabolized by the liver before it reaches the systemic circulation.[20] This commonly occurs when drugs have a high liver extraction ratio because, after oral administration, almost all of the drug must pass through the portal circulation into the liver. For example, if an orally administered drug is 100% absorbed from the gastrointestinal tract but has a hepatic extraction ratio of 0.75, only 25% of the original dose enters the systemic circulation. This "first-pass" effect through the liver is avoided when the drug is given by other routes of administration. The computation of F does not separate loss of oral drug metabolized by the first-pass effect and drug not absorbed by the gastrointestinal tract. Special techniques are needed to determine the fraction of drug absorbed orally for drugs with high liver extraction ratios.

Two different dosage forms of the same drug are considered to be bioequivalent when they produce $AUC_{0-\infty}$, C_{max}, and t_{max} values that are neither clinically nor statistically different. When this occurs, the serum concentration-versus-time curves for the two dosage forms should be superimposable. Bioequivalence studies have become very important as many expensive drugs have recently become available in generic form. Most bioequivalence studies involve 18 to 25 healthy adults who are given the brand-name product and the generic product in a randomized, crossover study design.

STEADY-STATE PHARMACOKINETICS

Up to this point in this discussion, pharmacokinetic experiments have involved single-dose trials. It is possible and sometimes desirable to conduct kinetic experiments while the patient is at steady state. Fortunately, if the same dose is administered, the area under the serum concentration-versus-time curve over a dosage interval at steady state (AUC_{ss}) is equal to the $AUC_{0-\infty}$ after a single dose. This means that either AUC can be used in any of the noncompartmental model kinetic equations. However, the $AUMC_{0-\infty}$ after a single dose is not equivalent to the AUMC over a dosage interval at steady state.[21] Superposition can be used to construct a single-dose curve from steady-state serum concentrations (Fig. 3.9). The single-dose curve can then be used to compute $AUMC_{0-\infty}$. AUC_{ss} and $AUMC_{0-\infty}$ can be substituted in noncompartmental model equations to compute kinetic constants.

NONLINEAR PHARMACOKINETICS

Michaelis–Menten Kinetics

Some drugs do not follow the rules of linear pharmacokinetics. Instead of C_{ss} and AUC increasing proportionally with dose, serum concentrations change more or less than expected (Fig. 3.10). One explanation for the greater-than-expected increase in C_{ss} and AUC after an increase in dose is that the enzymes responsible for the metabolism or elimination of the drug may start to become saturated. When this occurs the maximum rate of metabolism (V_{max}) for the drug is approached. This is called Michaelis–Menten kinetics. The serum concentration at which the rate of metabolism equals $V_{max}/2$ is K_m. Practically speaking, K_m is the serum concentration at which nonproportional changes in C_{ss} and AUC start to occur when dose is increased. The Michaelis–Menten constants (V_{max} and K_m) determine the dosage rate (DR) needed to maintain a given C_{ss}: $DR = V_{max}C_{ss}/(K_m + C_{ss})$. Most drugs eliminated by the liver are metabolized by enzymes but still appear to follow linear kinetics. The reason for this disparity is that the therapeutic range for most drugs is well below the K_m of the enzyme system that metabolizes the agent. The therapeutic range is higher than K_m for some commonly used drugs. The average K_m for phenytoin is about 4 mg/L. The therapeutic range for phenytoin is usually 10–20 mg/L. Most patients experience Michaelis–Menten kinetics while taking phenytoin.

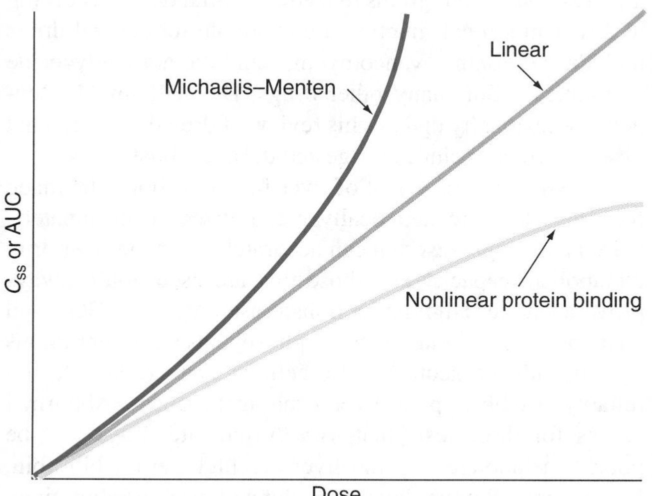

Figure 3.10. Relationship of dose and C_{ss} or AUC under linear and nonlinear conditions.

Nonlinear Protein Binding

Another type of nonlinear kinetics can occur if C_{ss} and AUC increase less than expected after an increase in dose of a low-clearance drug. This usually indicates that plasma protein binding sites are starting to become saturated so that f_b increases with increases in dose (Fig. 3.10). For a low-clearance drug, CL is dependent on the values of f_b and CL_{int}($CL = f_bCL_{int}$). When a dosage increase takes place, f_b increases because nearly all plasma protein binding sites are occupied and no binding sites are available. If f_b increases, CL increases and C_{ss} increases less than expected with the dosage change ($C_{ss} = k_0/CL$). However, $C_{ss,u}$ increases proportionally with dose since $C_{ss,u}$ depends on CL_{int} for low-clearance drugs ($C_{ss,u} = k_0/CL_{int}$). Valproic acid[22] and disopyramide[23] both follow saturable protein binding pharmacokinetics.

USE OF PHARMACOKINETIC CONCEPTS FOR INDIVIDUALIZATION OF DRUG THERAPY

Many factors must be taken into consideration when deciding on the best drug dose for a patient. For example, the age of the patient is important because the dose (in mg per kg) for pediatric patients may be higher, and for geriatric patients may be lower, than the typically prescribed dose for young adults. Gender can also be a factor because males and females metabolize and eliminate some drugs differently. Patients who are significantly obese or cachectic may also require different drug doses because of clearance and volume of distribution changes. Other drug therapy that could cause drug interactions needs to be considered. Disease states and conditions may alter the drug-dosage regimen for a patient. Three disease states that deserve special mention are congestive heart failure, renal disease, and hepatic disease. Renal and hepatic disease cause loss of organ function and decreased drug elimination and metabolism. Congestive heart failure causes decreased blood flow to organs that clear the drug from the body.

Many drug compounds are racemic mixtures of stereoisomers. In most cases, one of the isomers is more pharmacologically active than the other isomer, and each isomer may exhibit different pharmacokinetic properties. Propranolol, verapamil, and ibuprofen are all racemic mixtures of stereoisomers. Some drug interactions inhibit or increase the elimination of only one stereoisomer. The importance of the drug interaction depends on which isomer is affected. Other drugs, such as dextromethorphan and diltiazem, are composed of just one stereoisomer.

Genetics also plays a role in drug metabolism. Cytochrome P-450 is a generic term for the group of enzymes that are responsible for most drug metabolism oxidation reactions. Several P-450 isozymes have been identified that are responsible for the metabolism of many important drugs. P450IIC18 (CYP2C18, P-450_{mp}; formerly included in P450IIC9) is responsible for aromatic hydroxylation of mephenytoin and P450IID6 (CYP2D6, P-450_{db}) oxidizes debrisoquine.[24] These subsets of the P-450 enzyme family are also responsible for the metabolism of several other drugs (e.g., P450IID6: most tricyclic antidepressants, encainide, metoprolol). Both of these isozymes appear to be under genetic control. As a consequence, there are "poor metabolizers" who lack the gene for the isozyme, cannot manufacture the isozyme and, therefore, cannot metabolize the drug substrate very well. "Extensive metabolizers" have the gene for the isozyme and metabolize the drugs normally. Poor metabolizers usually are a minority of the general population. They may achieve toxic concentrations of drug when usual doses are prescribed for them, or if the active drug moiety is a metabolite, may fail to have any pharmacologic effect from the drug. Different ethnic backgrounds can have a different incidence of poor metabolizers.[24] For example, the incidence of poor metabolizers for P450IID6 is about 5–10% for Caucasians and about 0–1% for Asians, while for P450IIC18 poor metabolizers make up about 3–6% of the Caucasian population and about 20% of the Asian population.

Other P-450 isozymes have been isolated.[24] P450IA2 (CYP1A2) is the enzyme that is responsible for the demethylation of caffeine and theophylline, P450IIC9 (CYP2C9) metabolizes phenytoin and tolbutamide, cyclosporine and nifedipine are metabolized by P450IIIA4 (CYP3A4), and ethanol is a substrate for P450IIE1 (CYP2E1). It is important to recognize that a drug may be metabolized by more than one P-450 isozyme. While most tricyclic antidepressants are hydroxylated by P450IID6, *N*-demethylation is probably mediated by P450IIC18. Acetaminophen appears to be metabolized by both P450IA2 and P4502E1. The 4-hydroxy metabolite of propranolol is produced by P450IID6, but side chain oxidation of propranolol is probably a product of P450IIC18.

Understanding which P-450 isozyme is responsible for the metabolism of a drug is extraordinarily useful when predicting and understanding drug interactions. Some drug metabolism inhibitors and inducers are highly selective for certain P-450 isozymes.[24] Quinidine is an extremely potent inhibitor of the P450IID6 enzyme system[24]; a single 50-mg dose of quinidine can change a rapid metabolizer of debrisoquine into a poor metabolizer. Verapamil and diltiazem inhibit, while tobacco or marijuana smoke induce P450IA2. Some drugs that are enzyme inhibitors are also substrates for that same enzyme system and appear to cause drug interactions by being a competitive inhibitor. For example, erythromycin is both a substrate for, and inhibitor of, P450IIIA4. Obviously, if one knows that a new drug is metabolized by a given P-450 enzyme system, it is logical to assume that the new drug will exhibit drug interactions with the known inducers and inhibitors of that P-450 isozyme.

SELECTION OF INITIAL DRUG DOSES

When deciding on initial doses for drugs that are renally eliminated, the patient's renal function should be assessed. A common, useful way to do this is to measure the patient's serum creatinine concentration and convert this value into an estimated creatinine clearance (Cr CL_{est}). Serum creatinine values alone should not be used to assess renal function because they do not include the effects of age, body weight, or gender. The Cockcroft–Gault equation[25] is probably the most widely used method to estimate creatinine clearance in adults (18 years or older) who are within about 30% of their ideal body weight:

$$\text{Male, Cr } CL_{est} \text{ (in mL/min)} = \frac{(140 - \text{age})BW}{72 \cdot S_{cr}}$$

$$\text{Female, Cr } CL_{est} \text{ (in mL/min)} = \frac{0.85(140 - \text{age})BW}{72 \cdot S_{cr}}$$

where BW is body weight (in kg), age is the patient's age (in yr), 0.85 is a correction factor to account for lower muscle mass in females, and S_{cr} is serum creatinine (in mg/dL). Other methods to determine Cr CL_{est} for children,[26] obese adults,[27] and patients with rapidly changing renal function[28] are available. Nomograms that adjust initial doses according to a patient's renal function are available for several drugs including digoxin,[29] vancomycin,[30] and the aminoglycoside antibiotics.[31] For many other drugs, Dr. William M. Bennett[32] occasionally updates his review of drug dosing in renal disease, which includes suggested dosage adjustments.

A similar assessment of liver function should be made for drugs that are hepatically metabolized. Unfortunately, there is no single test that can accurately estimate liver drug metabolism capacity and those that are used don't always prove accurate. High aminotransferase (AST or SGOT and ALT or SGPT) and alkaline phosphatase concentrations usually indicate acute hepatic cellular damage and do not reliably establish poor liver drug metabolism. Abnormal values for three tests that *usually* indicate drugs will be poorly metabolized by the liver are high serum bilirubin, low serum albumin, and a prolonged prothrombin time. Bilirubin is metabolized by the liver, and albumin and clotting factors are manufactured by the liver, so aberrant values for all three of these tests are a more reliable indicator of abnormal liver drug metabolism. The Child–Pugh score,[33] a widely used clinical classification for liver disease which incorporates clinical signs and symptoms (ascites and hepatic encephalopathy) in addition to these three laboratory tests, can be used as an indicator of a patient's ability to metabolize drugs that are eliminated by the liver. A score in excess of 10 suggests very poor liver function. As a general rule, patients with cirrhosis have the most severe decreases in liver drug metabolism. Patients with acute or chronic hepatitis often retain relatively normal or slightly decreased hepatic drug metabolism capacity.

Heart failure is often overlooked as a disease state that can alter drug disposition. Severe heart failure decreases cardiac output and, therefore, reduces liver blood flow. Theophylline,[34] lidocaine,[35] and drugs with high extraction ratios are compounds whose clearance declines with decreased liver blood flow. Initial dosages of these drugs should be reduced in patients with moderate to severe heart failure by 25–50% until steady-state concentrations and response can be determined.

USE OF STEADY-STATE DRUG CONCENTRATIONS

Serum drug concentrations are readily available to clinicians to use as guides for the individualization of drug therapy. The therapeutic ranges for several drugs have been identified, and it is likely that new drugs will also be monitored using serum concentrations. Although several individualization methods have been advocated for specific drugs, one simple, reliable method is commonly used. For drugs that exhibit linear pharmacokinetics, C_{ss} changes proportionally with dose. To adjust a patient's drug therapy, a reasonable starting dose is administered for an estimated three to five half-lives. A serum concentration is obtained assuming that it will reflect C_{ss}. Independent of the route of administration, the new dose (D_{new}) needed to attain the desired $C_{ss}(C_{ss,new})$ is calculated: $D_{new} = C_{ss,new}(D_{old}/C_{ss,old})$, where D_{old} and $C_{ss,old}$ are the old dose and old C_{ss}, respectively. To use this method $C_{ss,old}$ must reflect steady-state conditions. Often, patients are noncompliant with regard to their drug dosage and, therefore, are not at steady state. This occurs not only in outpatients, but in hospital inpatients as well. Inpatients can spit out oral doses or alter the infusion rates on intravenous pumps after the nurse leaves the hospital room. If $C_{ss,old}$ is much larger or smaller than expected for the D_{old} the patient is taking, one should suspect noncompliance and repeat the serum concentration after another three to five $t_{1/2}$ or change the patient's dose cautiously and monitor for signs of toxicity or lack of effect.

If it is necessary to determine the kinetic constants for a patient, a small kinetic experiment could be conducted in the individual. With the methods outlined under Noncompartmental Analysis and Steady-State Pharmacokinetics, CL, V_D, and $t_{1/2}$ can be calculated and used to individualize dose for any drug. Alternately, several methods for specific drugs have been derived that assume specific kinetic models and clinical situations.

AMINOGLYCOSIDES

Although aminoglycoside pharmacokinetics follow multicompartment models,[36] a one-compartment model appears sufficient to individualize doses in patients.[37] Aminoglycosides are usually given as short-term intermittent intravenous infusions and administered as a single daily dose or multiple doses per day. When this is the case, kinetic parameters can be calculated at any point in therapy. Serum aminoglycoside concentrations are obtained before a dose (C_{min}), after a dose administered as an intravenous infusion of about 1 hour (C_{max}), and at two or more times before the next dose (C_3, C_4, etc.). C_{max}, C_3, and C_4 are plotted on semilogarithmic paper; $t_{1/2}$ and k are obtained from the graph. Assuming a one-compartment model, the following equation is used to compute V_D[37]:

$$V_D = [(D/T)(1 - e^{-kT})]/\{k[C_{max} - (C_{min}e^{-kT})]\}$$

where D is dose and T is duration of infusion. Once these are known, the dose and dosage interval (t) can be calculated for any desired maximum $C_{ss}(C_{ss,\,max})$ and minimum $C_{ss}(C_{ss,\,min})$:

$$\tau = -\{[\ln(C_{ss,\,min}/C_{ss,\,max})]/k\} + T$$

$$D = \tau k V_D C_{ss,\,max}[1 - e^{-k\tau})/(1 - e^{-kT})]$$

The dose and dosage interval should be rounded to provide clinically accepted values (e.g., every 8, 12, 24, 48 hours for dosage interval, nearest 5–10 mg for dose). This method has also been used to individualize intravenous theophylline dosage regimens.[38]

THEOPHYLLINE

Theophylline disposition is most accurately described by nonlinear kinetics.[39,40] However, at the usual doses, theophylline acts as if it obeys linear kinetics in most patients. Continuous intravenous infusions of theophylline (or its salt, aminophylline) can be rapidly individualized by determining the patient's CL.[41] Assuming the patient receives theophylline only by continuous intravenous infusion (previous doses of sustained-release oral theophylline are completely absorbed), two serum theophylline concentrations are obtained 4 or more hours apart. The infusion rate (k_0) cannot be changed between the times the concentrations are drawn. With one-compartment model equations, the first

(C_1) and second (C_2) theophylline concentrations are used to calculate theophylline CL:

$$CL = 2k_0/(C_1 + C_2) + [2V_D(C_1 - C_2)/(C_1 + C_2)(t_2 - t_1)]$$

V_D is assumed to be 0.5 L/kg and t_1 and t_2 are the times at which C_1 and C_2, respectively, are obtained. Once CL is known, k_0 can be easily computed for any desired C_{ss}($C_{ss} = k_0$/CL).

This method can probably be applied to other drugs that are administered as continuous intravenous infusions, such as intravenous antiarrhythmics, when rapid individualization of drug dosage is desirable.

PHENYTOIN

Phenytoin doses are very difficult to individualize because the drug follows Michaelis–Menten kinetics, and there is a large amount of interpatient variability in V_{max} and K_m. The methods used to individualize phenytoin doses involve rearrangements of the Michaelis–Menten equation [DR = $V_{max}C_{ss}/(K_m + C_{ss})$, in which DR is the dosage rate at steady state] so that two or more doses and C_{ss} values can be used to obtain graphic solutions for V_{max} and K_m. One rearrangement[42] is DR = $-K_m$(DR/C_{ss}) + V_{max}. When DR is plotted on the *y* axis and DR/C_{ss} is plotted on the *x* axis of Cartesian graph paper, a straight line with a *y* intercept of V_{max} and slope equal to $-K_m$ is found (Fig. 3.11). To use this method, patients are prescribed an initial phenytoin dose and C_{ss} is obtained. The phenytoin dose is then changed and a second C_{ss} from the new dose is obtained. Each dose is divided by its respective C_{ss} to derive DR/C_{ss} values. The DR/C_{ss} and C_{ss} values are plotted on the graph to calculate V_{max} (*y* intercept) and K_m (-slope). The steady-state Michaelis–Menten equation can be used to compute C_{ss} for a given DR or a DR for any C_{ss}.

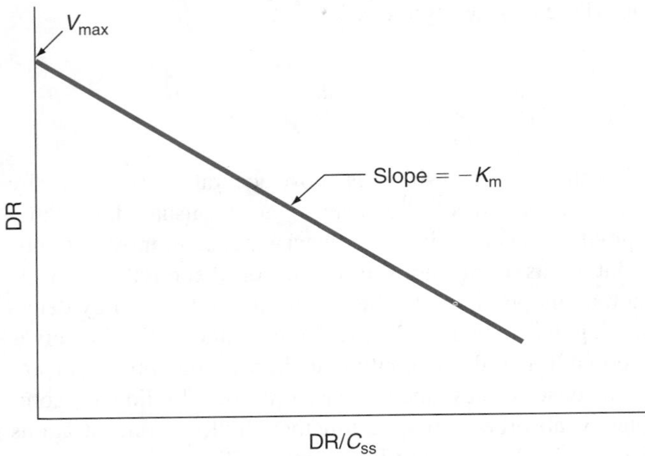

Figure 3.11. Relationship between dosage rate (DR) and steady-state serum concentrations (C_{ss}).

COMPUTER PROGRAMS

Computer programs that aid in the individualization of therapy are available for many different drugs. The most sophisticated programs use nonlinear regression to fit CL and V_D to actual serum concentrations obtained in a patient.[43] After drug doses and serum concentrations are entered into the computer, nonlinear regression programs adjust CL and V_D until the sum of the squared error between actual (C_{act}) and computer-estimated concentrations (C_{est}) is at a minimum [$\Sigma(C_{est} - C_{act})^2$]. Once estimates of CL and V_D are available, doses are easily calculated.

Many programs also take into account what the CL and V_D should be on the basis of disease states and conditions present in the patient.[44] Incorporation of expected population-based parameters allows the computer to use a limited number of serum concentrations (one or two) to provide estimates of CL and V_D. This type of computer program is called "Bayesian" because it incorporates portions of Bayes' theorem during the fitting routine.[45]

PHARMACODYNAMICS

Pharmacodynamics is the study of the relationship between the concentration of a drug and the response obtained in a patient. Originally, investigators examined the dose–response relationship of drugs in humans, but found that the same dose of a drug usually resulted in different concentrations in individuals because of pharmacokinetic differences in clearance and volume of distribution. Examples of quantifiable pharmacodynamic measurements include changes in blood pressure during antihypertensive drug therapy and decreases in heart rate during β-blocker treatment.

For drugs that exhibit a direct and reversible effect, the following diagram describes what occurs at the level of the drug receptor:

Drug + Receptor ⟷ Drug-receptor complex ⟷ Response

According to this scheme, there is a drug receptor located within the target organ or tissue. When a drug molecule "finds" the receptor, it forms a complex that causes the pharmacologic response to occur. The drug and receptor are in dynamic equilibrium with the drug-receptor complex.

THE E_{max} AND SIGMOID E_{max} MODELS

The mathematical model that comes from the classic drug receptor theory shown previously is known as the E_{max} model:

$$E = \frac{E_{max} \times C}{EC_{50} + C}$$

where E is the pharmacologic effect elicited by the drug, E_{max} is the maximum effect the drug can cause, EC_{50} is the concentration causing one-half of the maximum drug effect ($E_{max}/2$), and C is the concentration of drug at the receptor site. EC_{50} can be used as a measure of drug potency (a lower EC_{50} indicating a more potent drug), whereas E_{max} reflects the intrinsic efficacy of the drug (a higher E_{max} indicating greater efficacy). If pharmacologic effect is plotted versus concentration in the E_{max} equation, a hyperbola results with an asymptote equal to E_{max} (Fig. 3.12). At a concentration of zero, no measurable effect is present.

When dealing with human studies where a drug is administered to a patient and pharmacologic effect is measured, it is very difficult to determine the concentration of drug at the receptor site. Because of this, serum concentrations (total or unbound) are usually used as the concentration parameter in the E_{max} equation. Therefore, the values of E_{max} and EC_{50} are much different than if the drug were added to an isolated tissue contained in a laboratory beaker.

The result is that a much more empiric approach is used to describe the relationship between concentration and effect in clinical pharmacology studies. After a pharmacodynamic experiment has been conducted, concentration–effect plots are generated. The shape of the concentration–effect curve is used to determine which pharmacodynamic model will be used to describe the data. Because of this, the pharmacodynamic models used in a clinical pharmacology study are *deterministic* in the same way that the shape of the serum concentration-versus-time curve determines which pharmacokinetic model is used in clinical pharmacokinetic studies.

Sometimes a hyperbolic function does not adequately describe the concentration–effect relationship at lower concentrations. When this is the case, the sigmoid E_{max} equation may be superior to the E_{max} model:

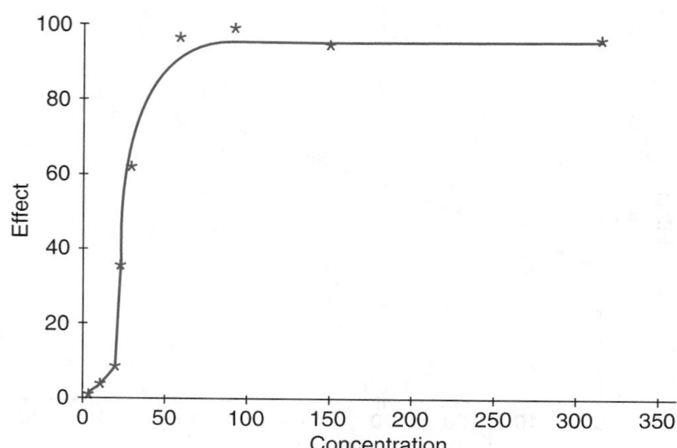

Figure 3.13. The sigmoid E_{max} model $[E = (E_{max} \times C^n)/(EC_{50}{}^n + C^n)]$ has an S-shaped curve at lower concentrations. In this example, E_{max} and EC_{50} have the same values as in Fig. 3.2.

$$E = \frac{E_{max} \times C^n}{EC_{50}^n + C^n}$$

where n is an exponent that changes the shape of the concentration–effect curve. When $n > 1$, the concentration–effect curve is S or sigmoid shaped at lower serum concentrations. When $n < 1$, the concentration–effect curve has a steeper slope at lower concentrations (Fig. 3.13).

With both the E_{max} and sigmoid E_{max} models, the largest changes in drug effect occur at the lower end of the concentration scale. Small changes in low serum concentrations cause large changes in effect. As serum concentrations become larger, further increases in serum concentration result in smaller changes in effect. Using the E_{max} model as an example and setting E_{max} = 100 units and EC_{50} = 20 mg/L, doubling the serum concentration from 5 to 10 mg/L increases the effect from 20 to 33 units (a 67% increase), whereas doubling the serum concentration from 40 to 80 mg/L only increases the effect from 67 to 80 units (a 19% increase). This is an important concept for clinicians to remember when doses are being titrated in patients.

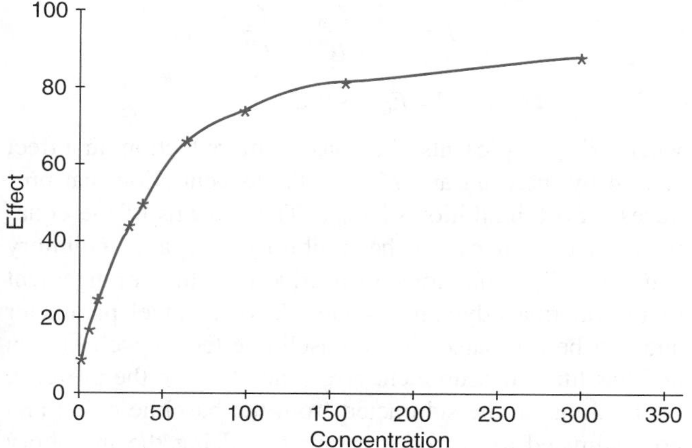

Figure 3.12. The E_{max} model $[E = (E_{max} \times C)/(EC_{50} + C)]$ has the shape of a hyperbola with an asymptote equal to $E_{max} \times EC_{50}$ is the concentration where effect = $E_{max}/2$.

LINEAR MODELS

When serum concentrations obtained during a pharmacodynamic experiment are between 20–80% E_{max}, the concentration–effect curve may appear to be linear (Fig. 3.14). This occurs often because lower drug concentrations may not be detectable with the analytic technique used to assay serum samples and higher drug concentrations may be avoided to prevent toxic side effects. The equation used is

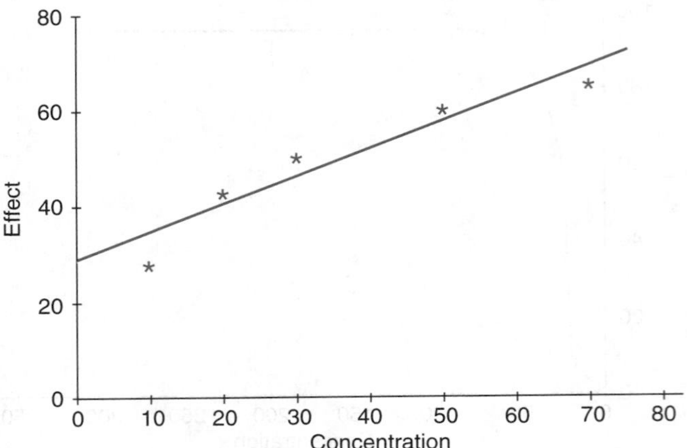

Figure 3.14. The linear model ($E = S \times C + I$) is often used as a pharmacodynamic model when the measured pharmacologic effect is 20–80% of E_{max}. In this situation, the determination of E_{max} and EC_{50} is not possible. To illustrate this, effect measurements from Fig. 3.2 between 20–80% of E_{max} are graphed using the linear pharmacodynamic model.

that of a simple line: $E = S \times C + I$, where E is the drug effect, C is the drug concentration, S is the slope of the line, and I is the y intercept. In this situation, the value of S can be used as a measure of drug potency (the larger the value of S, the more potent the drug). The linear model can be derived from the E_{max} model. When EC_{50} is much greater than C, $E = (E_{max}/EC_{50})C = S \times C$, where $S = E_{max}/EC_{50}$.

The linear model allows a nonzero value for effect when the concentration equals zero. This may be a baseline value for the effect that is present without the drug, the result of measurement error when determining effect, or model misspecification. Also, this model does not allow the prediction of a maximum response.

Some investigators have used a log–linear model in pharmacodynamic experiments: $E = S \times (\log C) + I$, where the symbols have the same meaning as the linear model. The advantages of this model are that the concentration scale is compressed on concentration-effect plots for experiments where wide concentration ranges were used, and the concentration values are transformed so that linear regression can be used to compute model parameters. The disadvantages are that the model cannot predict a maximum effect or an effect when the concentration equals zero. With the increased availability of nonlinear regression programs that can easily compute the parameters of nonlinear functions such as the E_{max} model, the use of the log–linear model has been discouraged.[46]

BASELINE EFFECTS

At times, the effect measured during a pharmacodynamic study has a value before the drug is administered to the patient. In these cases, the drug changes the patient's baseline value. Examples of these types of measurements are heart rate or blood pressure. In addition, a given drug may increase or decrease the baseline value. Two basic techniques are used to incorporate baseline values into pharmacodynamic data. One way incorporates the baseline value into the pharmacodynamic model; the other way transforms the effect data to take baseline values into account.

Incorporation of the baseline value into the pharmacodynamic model involves the addition of a new term to the previous equations. E_0 is the symbol used to denote the baseline value of the effect that will be measured. The form that these equations takes depends on whether the drug increases or decreases the pharmacodynamic effect. When the drug increases the baseline value, E_0 is added to the equations:

$$E = E_0 + \frac{E_{max} \times C}{EC_{50} + C}$$

$$E = E_0 + \frac{E_{max} \times C^n}{EC_{50}^n + C^n}$$

$$E = S \times C + E_0$$

When E_0 is not known with any better certainty than any other effect measurement, it should be estimated as a model parameter similar to the way that one would estimate the values of E_{max}, EC_{50}, S, or n.[46,47] If the baseline effect is well known and has only a small amount of measurement error, it can be subtracted from the effect determined in the patient during the experiment and not estimated as a model parameter. This approach can lead to better estimates of the remaining model parameters.[47] Using the linear model as an example, the equation used would be $E - E_0 = S \times C$.

If the drug decreases the baseline value, the drug effect is subtracted from E_0 in the pharmacodynamic models:

$$E = E_0 - \frac{E_{max} \times C}{IC_{50} + C}$$

$$E = E_0 - \frac{E_{max} \times C^n}{IC_{50}^n + C^n}$$

$$E = E_0 - S \times C$$

where E_{max} represents the maximum reduction in effect caused by the drug and IC_{50} is the concentration that produces a 50% inhibition of E_{max}. These forms of the equations have been called the inhibitory E_{max} and inhibitory sigmoidal E_{max} equations, respectively. In this arrangement of the pharmacodynamic model, E_0 is a model parameter and can be estimated. If the baseline effect is well known and has little measurement error, the effect in the presence of the drug can be subtracted from the baseline effect and not estimated as a model parameter. Using the inhibitory E_{max} model as an example, the formula would be $E_0 - E = (E_{max} \times C)/(IC_{50} + C)$.

When using the inhibitory E_{max} model, a special situation occurs if the baseline effect can be completely obliterated by the drug (e.g., decreased premature ventricular contractions during antiarrhythmic therapy). In this situation, $E_{max} = E_0$ and the equation simplifies to a rearrangement known as the fractional E_{max} equation:

$$E = E_0\left(1 - \frac{C}{IC_{50} + C}\right)$$

This form of the model relates drug concentration to the fraction of the maximum effect.

An alternative approach to the pharmacodynamic modeling of drugs that alter baseline effects is to transform the effect data so that it represents a percent increase or decrease from the baseline value.[47] For drugs that increase the effect, the following transformation equation would be used: percent effect$_t$ = [(treatment$_t$ − baseline)/baseline] × 100. For drugs that decrease the effect, the following formula would be applied to the data: percent inhibition$_t$ = [(baseline − treatment$_t$)/baseline] × 100. The subscript indicates the treatment, effect, or inhibition that occurred at time t during the experiment. If the study included a placebo control phase, baseline measurements made at the same time as treatment measurements (i.e., heart rate determined 2 hours after placebo and 2 hours after drug treatment) could be used in the appropriate transformation equation.[47] The appropriate model (excluding E_0) would then be used.

HYSTERESIS

Concentration–effect curves do not always follow the same pattern when serum concentrations increase as they do when serum concentrations decrease. In this situation the concentration–effect curves form a loop that is known as *hysteresis*. With some drugs, the effect is greater when serum concentrations are increasing, while with other drugs the effect is greater while serum concentrations are decreasing (Fig. 3.15). When individual concentration–effect pairs are joined in time sequence, this results in clockwise and counterclockwise hysteresis loops.

Clockwise hysteresis loops are usually caused by the development of tolerance to the drug. In this situation, the longer the patient is exposed to the drug, the smaller the pharmacologic effect for a given concentration. Therefore, after an extravascular or short-term infusion dose of the drug, the effect is smaller when serum concentrations are decreasing compared with the time when serum concentrations are increasing during the infusion or absorption phase. Accumulation of a drug metabolite that acts as an antagonist can also cause clockwise hysteresis.

Counterclockwise hysteresis loops can be caused by the accumulation of an active metabolite, sensitization to the drug, or delay in time in equilibration between serum concentration and concentration of drug at the site of action. Combined pharmacokinetic–pharmacodynamic models have been devised that allow equilibration lag times to be taken into account.

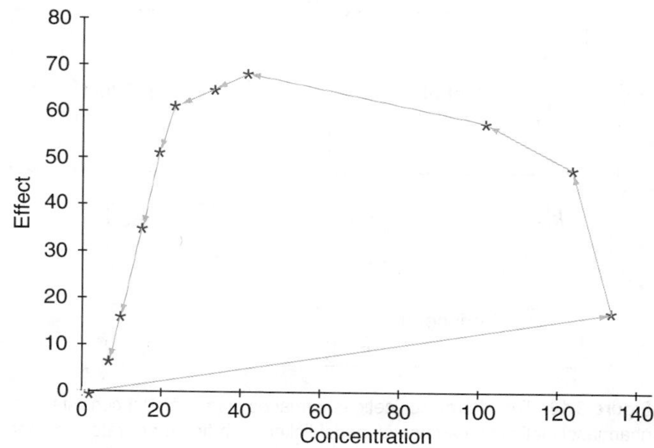

Figure 3.15. Hysteresis occurs when effect measurements are different at the same concentration. This is commonly seen after short-term intravenous infusions or extravascular doses where concentrations increase and subsequently decrease. Counterclockwise hysteresis loops are found when concentration–effect points are joined as time increases (shown by arrows) and effect is larger at the same concentration but at a later time. Clockwise hysteresis loops are similar, but the concentration–effect points are joined in clockwise order and the effect is smaller at a later time.

PHARMACOKINETIC–PHARMACODYNAMIC MODELS

When counterclockwise hysteresis occurs, a possible explanation for the lag between serum concentration and effect is a time delay in equilibration between serum concentration and concentration at the site of action. Using a linked pharmacokinetic–pharmacodynamic model, it is possible to use the time course of effect to define the rate of drug movement to the site of action. The linked pharmacokinetic–pharmacodynamic model is shown in general terms in Fig. 3.16.

The principle behind this model is to treat the effect site as a discreet pharmacokinetic compartment that communicates directly with the central compartment. The rate of drug movement from central compartment to the effect compartment is controlled by a first-order rate constant, k_{e1}. Drug is irreversibly removed from the effect compartment via the first-order rate constant k_{e0}. To justify this, it is assumed that the amount of drug that enters the effect compartment is negligible and k_{e1} is very small compared with the other rate constants in the pharmacokinetic model.[48]

Just as with pharmacokinetic models, the rate constant that controls the accumulation of drug in the effect compartment and the onset of effect is the removal rate constant

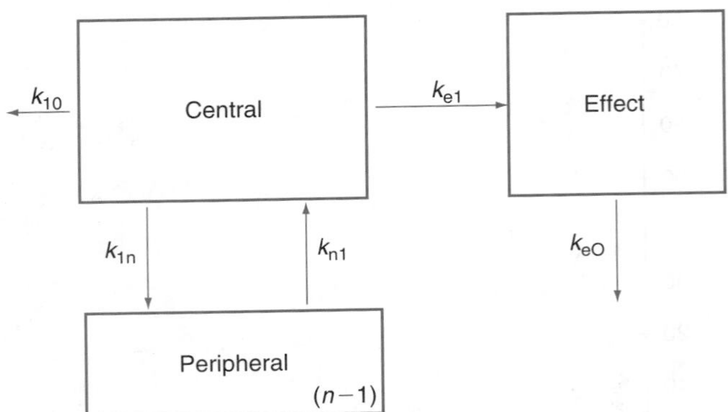

Figure 3.16. The pharmacokinetic–pharmacodynamic model consists of a pharmacokinetic compartmental model linked by a first-order rate constant (k_{e1}) to a pharmacodynamic model. The pharmacokinetic model has a sufficient number of compartments to describe the concentration–time data. The effect compartment concentration–response data is used to select the best pharmacodynamic model.

from the effect compartment (k_{e0}). The concentration of drug in the effect compartment is used as the concentration on the concentration–effect curve. This process allows the hysteresis loop to be collapsed so that the concentration–effect relationship can be modeled.

Two steps are involved in the analysis of linked pharmacokinetic–pharmacodynamic models. First, the appropriate pharmacokinetic compartmental model is used in a nonlinear regression computer program to fit the observed serum concentration-versus-time data. Once this has been done, the equation for the concentration in the effect compartment can be easily derived.[46] Pharmacokinetic parameters derived from the serum concentration–time curve are then used to generate effect site concentrations. The second step involves determination of the appropriate pharmacodynamic model (e.g., E_{max}, sigmoid E_{max}, linear) and computation of pharmacodynamic constants using the effect compartment concentration and effect data in a nonlinear regression computer program. Usually, small data sets prohibit simultaneous fitting of pharmacokinetic–pharmacodynamic models.[48]

NONPARAMETRIC PHARMACOKINETIC–PHARMACODYNAMIC MODELS

Nonparametric pharmacodynamic models[49] and nonparametric pharmacokinetic-pharmacodynamic models[50] that retain the first-order link between serum concentration and effect-site concentration have been recently proposed. The nonparametric approach involves a minimum of assumptions and does not require the selection of specific pharmacokinetic compartmental model and/or pharmacodynamic model. The nonparametric pharmacodynamic model approach involves the iterative solution of a value for k_{e0} that collapses the effect-site concentration/effect curve.[49] The effect-site concentration is determined using a pharmacokinetic compartmental model as described earlier. The combined nonparametric pharmacokinetic–pharmacodynamic model approach combines an iterative solution for k_{e0} and linear interpolation of serum concentration-time data.[50]

FIXED-EFFECT MODELS

Fixed-effect pharmacodynamic models use a predefined fixed response to examine the concentration–response relationship. Examples of fixed effects would be a 70% reduction in premature ventricular contractions during antiarrhythmic therapy or living versus dead after the administration of an anticancer agent. In these cases, a patient is classified as a responder or nonresponder to drug treatment. The cumulative percent of the total population that responded to drug therapy as stated by the predefined fixed effect is plotted versus concentration (Fig. 3.17). Although a sigmoid curve is often the result of this plot, the basis for this type of curve is the cumulative distribution function of statistical theory and not the sigmoid E_{max} model.[46]

COMPUTER METHODS

Pharmacodynamic models are deterministic because the shape of the concentration–response curve determines the model that is used. The first step in the analysis of pharmacodynamic data is plotting the concentration–response

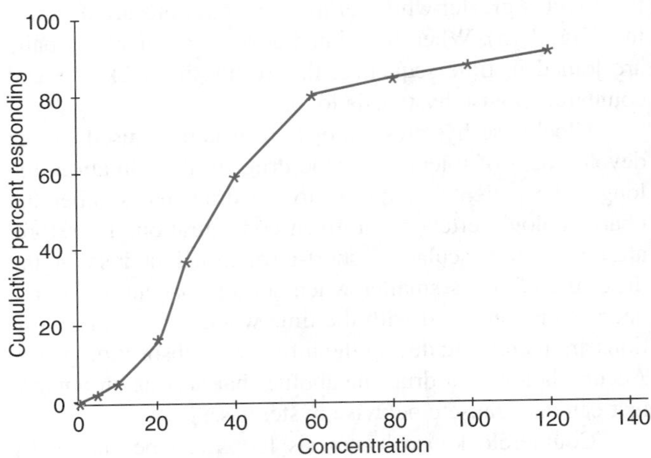

Figure 3.17. The fixed-effect pharmacodynamic model plots the cumulative percent response versus concentration. The shape of the plot is usually a sigmoid curve. Although it resembles the sigmoid E_{max} model, the basis for this curve is statistical theory.

points on graph paper. After the appropriate model is chosen by visual inspection, initial parameter estimates are made from the graph. A nonlinear regression computer program is then used to calculate the final parameter estimates.

If a combined pharmacokinetic–pharmacodynamic model is used, the pharmacokinetic data need to be analyzed first using the methods in the Clinical Pharmacokinetics section. Effect site concentrations are generated using the appropriate equation.[46] Effect site concentration–effect data are then fitted to the appropriate pharmacodynamic model using a nonlinear regression program. Simultaneous fitting of the pharmacokinetic–pharmacodynamic model can also be attempted, but enough data may not be available for the program to converge on final parameter estimates.[46]

CONCLUSION

The availability of inexpensive, rapidly available serum drug concentrations has changed the way clinicians monitor drug therapy in patients. The therapeutic range for many drugs is known, and it is likely that more drugs will be monitored using serum concentrations in the future. Clinicians need to remember that the therapeutic range is merely an average guideline and to take into account interindividual pharmacodynamic variability when treating patients. Individual patients may respond to smaller concentrations or require concentrations that are much greater to obtain a therapeutic effect. Conversely, patients may show toxic effects at concentrations within or below the therapeutic range. Serum concentrations should never replace clinical judgment.

Three kinetic constants determine the dosage requirements of patients. Clearance determines the maintenance dose ($MD = CLC_{ss}$), volume of distribution determines the loading dose ($LD = V_DC_{ss}$) and half-life determines the time to steady state and the dosage interval. Several methods are available to compute these parameters.

Methods available to individualize drug therapy range from clinical pharmacokinetic techniques using simple mathematical relationships that hold for all drugs that obey linear pharmacokinetics and very complex computer programs that are specific to one drug to pharmacodynamic techniques that monitor patient response to treatment. New techniques for monitoring serum drug concentrations are available on an experimental basis and may revolutionize clinical pharmacokinetics in the future.

REFERENCES

1. Wagner JG, Northam JI, Alway CD, et al. Blood levels of drug at the equilibrium state after multiple dosing. Nature 1965;207:1301–1302.
2. Rowland M, Benet LZ, Graham GG. Clearance concepts in pharmacokinetics. J Pharmacokinet Biopharm 1973;1 :123–136.
3. Wilkinson GR, Shand DG. A physiological approach to hepatic drug clearance. Clin Pharmacol Ther 1975;18:377–390.
4. Nies AS, Shand DG, Wilkinson GR. Altered hepatic blood flow and drug disposition. Clin Pharmacokinet 1976;1: 135–155.
5. Gibaldi M, Koup JR. Pharmacokinetic concepts—drug binding, apparent volume of distribution and clearance. Eur J Clin Pharmacol 1981;20:299–305.
6. Gibaldi M, Perrier D. Pharmacokinetics, 2nd ed. New York, Marcel Dekker, 1980.
7. Wagner JG. Model-independent linear pharmacokinetics. Drug Intell Clin Pharm 1976;10:179–180.
8. Wagner JG. Linear pharmacokinetic equations allowing direct calculation of many needed pharmacokinetic parameters from the coefficients and exponents of polyexponential equations which have been fitted to the data. J Pharmacokinet Biopharm 1976;4:443–467.
9. Riegelman S, Loo J, Rowland M. Concept of a volume of distribution and possible errors in evaluation of this parameter. J Pharm Sci 1968;57:128–133.
10. Gibaldi M, Nagashima R, Levy G. Relationship between drug concentration in plasma or serum and amount of drug in the body. J Pharm Sci 1969;58:193–197.
11. Gibaldi M, Perrier D. Drug elimination and apparent volume of distribution in multicompartment systems. J Pharm Sci 1972;61: 952–954.
12. Riegelman S, Loo JCK, Rowland M. Shortcomings in pharmacokinetic analysis by conceiving the body to exhibit properties of a single compartment. J Pharm Sci 1968;57: 117–123.
13. Benet LZ. General treatment of linear mamillary models with elimination from any compartment as used in pharmacokinetics. J Pharm Sci 1972;61:536–541.
14. Gibaldi M. Estimation of the pharmacokinetic parameters of the two-compartment open model from post-infusion plasma concentration data. J Pharm Sci 1969;58: 1133–1135.
15. Loo JCK, Riegelman S. Assessment of pharmacokinetic constants from postinfusion blood curves obtained after IV infusion. J Pharm Sci 1970;59:53–55.
16. Benet LZ, Galeazzi RL. Noncompartmental determination of the steady state volume of distribution. J Pharm Sci 1979;68:1071–1074.
17. Lee CS, Brater DC, Gambertoglio JG, et al. Disposition kinetics of ethambutol in man. J Pharmacokinet Biopharm 1980;8:335–346.
18. Perrier D, Mayersohn M. Noncompartmental determination of the steady state volume of distribution for any mode of administration. J Pharm Sci 1982;71:372–373.
19. Koup JR, Gibaldi M. Some comments on the evaluation of bioavailability data. Drug Intell Clin Pharm 1980;14: 327–330.
20. Gibaldi M, Boyes RN, Feldman S. Influence of first pass effect on availability of drugs on oral administration. J Pharm Sci 1971;60:1338–1340.
21. Bauer LA, Gibaldi M. Computation of model independent pharmacokinetic parameters during multiple dosing. J Pharm Sci 1983;72:978–979.

22. Bowdle TA, Patel IH, Levy RH, et al. Valproic acid dosage and plasma protein binding and clearance. Clin Pharmacol Ther 1980;28:486–492.
23. Lima JJ, Boudonlas H, Blanford M. Concentration-dependence of disopyramide binding to plasma protein and its influence on kinetics and dynamics. J Pharmacol Exp Ther 1981;219:741–747.
24. Brosen K. Recent developments in hepatic drug oxidation—implications for clinical pharmacokinetics. Clin Pharmacokin 1990;18:220–239.
25. Cockcroft DW, Gault MH. Prediction of creatinine clearance from serum creatinine. Nephron 1976;16:31–41.
26. Traub SL, Johnson CE. Comparison of methods of estimating creatinine clearance in children. Am J Hosp Pharm 1980;37:195–201.
27. Salazar DE, Corcoran GB. Predicting creatinine clearance and renal drug clearance in obese patients from estimated fat-free body mass. Am J Med 1988;84:1053–1060.
28. Jelliffe RW, Jelliffe SM. A computer program for estimation of creatinine clearance from unstable serum creatinine levels, age, sex, and weight. Math Biosci 1972;14:17–24.
29. Koup JR, Jusko WJ, Elwood CM, Kohli RK. Digoxin pharmacokinetics—role of renal failure in dosage regimen design. Clin Pharmacol Ther 1975;18:9–21.
30. Matzke GR, McGory RW, Halstenson CE, Keane WF. Pharmacokinetics of vancomycin in patients with various degrees of renal function. Antimicrob Agents Chemother 1984;25:433–437.
31. Sarubbi FA, Hull JH. Amikacin serum concentrations—predictions of levels and dosage guidelines. Ann Intern Med 1978;89:612–618.
32. Sivan SK, Bennett WM. Drug dosing guidelines in patients with renal failure. West J Med 1992;156:633–638.
33. Pugh RNH, Murray-Lyon IM, Dawson JL, Pietroni MC, Williams R. Transection of the oesophagus for bleeding oesophageal varices. Br J Surg 1973;60:646–649.
34. Jusko WJ, Gardner MJ, Mangione A, et al. Factors affecting theophylline clearances—age, tobacco, marijuana, cirrhosis, congestive heart failure, obesity, oral contraceptives, benzodiazepines, barbiturates, and ethanol. J Pharm Sci 1979;68:1358–1366.
35. Thomson PD, Melmon KL, Richardson JA, et al. Lidocaine pharmacokinetics in advanced heart failure, liver disease, and renal failure in humans. Ann Intern Med 1973;78:499–508.
36. Schentag JJ, Jusko WJ. Renal clearance and tissue accumulation of gentamicin. Clin Pharmacol Ther 1977;22:364–370.
37. Sawchuk RJ, Zaske DE, Cipolle RJ, et al. Kinetic model for gentamicin dosing with the use of individual patient parameters. Clin Pharmacol Ther 1977;21:362–369.
38. Pancorbo S, Sawchuk RJ, Dashe C, et al. Use of a pharmacokinetic model for individual intravenous doses of aminophylline. Eur J Clin Pharmacol 1979;16:251–254.
39. Sarrazin E, Hendeles L, Weinberger M, et al. Dose-dependent kinetics for theophylline—observations among ambulatory asthmatic children. J Pediatr 1980;97:825–828.
40. Tang-Liu DDS, Williams RL, Riegelman S. Nonlinear theophylline elimination. Clin Pharmacol Ther 1982;31:358–369.
41. Vozeh S, Kewitz G, Wenk M, et al. Rapid prediction of steady-state serum theophylline concentrations in patients treated with intravenous aminophylline. Eur J Clin Pharmacol 1980;18:473–477.
42. Ludden TM, Allen JP, Valutsky WA, et al. Individualization of phenytoin dosage regimens. Clin Pharmacol Ther 1977;21:287–293.
43. Koup JR, Killen T, Bauer LA. Multiple-dose nonlinear regression analysis program—aminoglycoside dose prediction. Clin Pharmacokinet 1983;8:456–462.
44. Sheiner LB, Beal S, Rosenberg B, et al. Forecasting individual pharmacokinetics. Clin Pharmacol Ther 1979;26:294–305.
45. Sheiner LB, Beal SL: Bayesian individualization of pharmacokinetics—simple implementation and comparison with non-Bayesian methods. J Pharm Sci 1982;71:1344–1348.
46. Holford NHG, Sheiner LB. Understanding the dose–effect relationship—clinical application of pharmacokinetic–pharmacodynamic models. Clin Pharmacokinet 1981;6:429–453.
47. Schwinghammer TL, Kroboth PD. Basic concepts in pharmacodynamic modeling. J Clin Pharmacol 1988;28:388–394.
48. Sheiner LB, Stanski DR, Vozeh S, et al. Simultaneous modeling of pharmacokinetics and pharmacodynamics—application to *d*-tubocurarine. Clin Pharmacol Ther 1979;25:358–371.
49. Fuseau E, Sheiner LB. Simultaneous modeling of pharmacokinetics and pharmacodynamics with a nonparametric pharmacodynamic model. Clin Pharmacol Ther 1984;35:733–741.
50. Unadkat J, Bartha F, Sheiner LB. Simultaneous modeling of pharmacokinetics and pharmacodynamics with nonparametric kinetic and dynamic models. Clin Pharmacol Ther 1986;40:86–93.

Chapter 4

Drug Delivery and Administration

Dennis H. Robinson, PhD, Warren A. Narducci, PharmD, and Clarence T. Ueda, PharmD, PhD

Drugs are administered in delivery systems designed to (1) provide accurate and convenient drug administration, (2) obtain the desired therapeutic response with minimum side effects, and (3) maximize patient compliance. In determining the most clinically effective and safe method of drug delivery, three major factors should be considered. First, the most appropriate route of administration will depend on whether a local or systemic drug effect is desired. Localized drug administration has the advantage of concentrating drug at the desired site of action and minimizing systemic side effects. The systemic approach is used when the target tissue is inaccessible by direct administration or application. Second, the properties of the delivery system will frequently dictate the route by which the dosage form can be given or a device used. Finally, while the desired pharmacologic effect will govern the choice of drug used, the physicochemical and pharmacokinetic properties of the drug may restrict its use to certain dosage forms or routes of administration. Other factors that affect the method and route of drug administration include the age and status of the patient, convenience, desired onset time, and duration of drug treatment.

Tables 4.1 and 4.2 summarize the principal factors known to influence the bioavailability characteristics of a drug and the approach that should be used in the design of a dosage form, respectively. A list of the most common routes of administration is given in Table 4.3.

An important factor to consider when assessing the therapeutic performance of a drug is patient adherence to the medication regimen. All attempts made to obtain an optimal therapeutic response through the selection of the most desirable drug delivery system and route of administration may be negated if the patient is noncompliant. Further, patient education is important to ensure that the

TABLE 4.1. FACTORS THAT INFLUENCE DRUG BIOAVAILABILITY

Physicochemical Properties of the Drug
Solubility in aqueous and organic solvents
pH–solubility profile
Lipid–water partition coefficient
pK_a
Particle size and size distribution
Crystalline and polymorphic forms
Solvation and hydration
Salt form
Stability in solid state and solution
Molecular weight
Physiologic Factors
pH
Temperature
Surface area
Surface tension
Volume and composition of biological fluid
Disease state
Sex
Age
Manufacturing Variables
Added diluents
Manufacturing factors (e.g., force of compression)
Manufacturing method
Packaging
Environmental Factors
Humidity
Temperature

TABLE 4.2. STEPWISE APPROACH TO DOSAGE FORM DESIGN

1. Select route of administration including systemic or local therapy, chronic or acute treatment, convenience, and patient factors.
2. Select dosage form design including drug content, desired release rate, duration of release, and site of release.
3. Select method of manufacture.
4. Formulate with compatible additives.
5. Preliminary *in vitro* and *in vivo* evaluations to optimize release.
6. *In vitro* testing.
7. *In vivo* testing.
8. Establish quality assurance criteria and validate bioavailability and other clinical testing.

TABLE 4.3. ROUTES OF DRUG ADMINISTRATION AND COMMON DOSAGE FORMS

Route	Site	Common Dosage Form
Oral	Mouth, gastrointestinal tract	Solution, suspension, powder, capsule, tablet, troche, lozenge
Sublingual	Under the tongue	Tablet, aerosol
Buccal	Oral mucosa	Tablet, lozenge
Parenteral	Other than gastrointestinal tract	Solution, suspension, implant, device
Intravenous	Vein	
Intra-arterial	Artery	
Intra-articular	Joints	
Intracisternal	Cerebrospinal column	
Intracardiac	Heart	
Intradermal	Dermal layer of the skin	
Intraspinal	Spinal column	
Intraosseous	Bone	
Intrasynovial	Joint fluid	
Intrathecal	Spinal fluid	
Intramuscular	Muscle	
Subcutaneous	Beneath the skin	
Topical/transdermal	Skin surface	Ointment, cream, paste, gel, powder, solution, suspension, aerosol, device, transdermal patch
Intraocular	Eye	Solution, suspension, ointment, aerosol
Intrarespiratory	Lung	Solution, suspension, aerosol, inhaler, nebulizer
Rectal	Rectum	Solution, ointment, suppository
Intravaginal	Vagina	Solution, ointment, foam, tablet, suppository, insert
Intrauterine	Uterus	Insert
Urethral	Urethra	Suppository

TABLE 4.4. FACTORS CONTRIBUTING TO PATIENT NONCOMPLIANCE AND COMPLIANCE

Factors Contributing to Noncompliance
- Failure to comprehend the importance of therapy
- Poor understanding of the instructions
- Multiple drug therapy
- Frequency of administration
- Duration of therapy
- Adverse effects
- Fear of becoming drug dependent
- Patients may be asymptomatic or the symptoms may subside
- Unpleasant taste of medication
- Waiting to see the physician or pharmacist
- Illness
- Cost of the medication
- Measurement of medication

Steps to Improve Patient Compliance
- Identification of risk factors that may contribute to noncompliance
- Development of treatment plan with recognition of patient's normal pattern of activities
- Designation of specific times of day at which medication is to be taken
- Educating the patient—recognition of the need for effective verbal and written communication with the patient
- Monitoring therapy

(From Gourley DR, Ueda CT. Patient factors that influence dosage form selection, in Banker GS, Chalmers RK (eds), Pharmaceutics and Pharmacy Practice. Philadelphia, JB Lippincott, 1982, p 144, with permission.)

medications are correctly administered or applied.[1] Factors contributing to patient noncompliance and steps to improve compliance are listed in Table 4.4.

Drug-delivery systems for systemic and localized drug administration are discussed in the following sections. The major factors to consider for each delivery system and associated routes of administration are discussed with respect to the effects on the therapeutic performance of drugs.

Parenteral Administration

While parenteral drug administration can be interpreted literally to mean giving a drug by any nonoral route, the term is used most commonly to refer to an injection directly into an internal body compartment or cavity to bypass the protective effects of the skin and mucous membranes. The most common parenteral routes of drug administration are intravenous, intramuscular, and subcutaneous. Other more specialized parenteral routes of administration are listed in Table 4.3. The principal advantages and disadvantages of parenteral drug administration are summarized in Table 4.5.

When a drug is administered parenterally, proper injection techniques must be used. An improper injection can cause injuries to nerves, muscle, bone and/or blood vessels. Thus, when an injection is to be self-administered, the

TABLE 4.5. ADVANTAGES AND DISADVANTAGES OF PARENTERAL DRUG ADMINISTRATION

Advantages

Drugs can be administered to uncooperative, unconscious, or nauseous patients.
Drugs that are normally ineffective, poorly absorbed, or inactive orally can be effectively administered.
Intravenous route provides immediate onset of drug action when needed during emergency situations.
Other parenteral routes can be used to slow onset and/or prolong duration of drug action.
Localized and systemic drug effects can be produced depending on the route of administration and product formulation.
Patient compliance problems are largely avoided.
Aside from drug administration the parenteral route can be used to correct patient fluid and electrolyte imbalance, and provide nutrient and calorific requirements.

Disadvantages

Parenteral preparations are usually administered by trained personnel.
Strict adherence to aseptic procedures is required.
Some degree of pain is inevitable.
Drug effects are difficult to reverse.
Parenteral administration may be inconvenient when frequent dosing is required.

patient must be properly instructed on the use of the parenteral dosage form and injection procedure.

PREPARATIONS

Parenteral drug delivery systems include drug formulations in solutions, suspensions, emulsions, or as drug powders for reconstitution immediately before use. Although all products for parenteral drug administration must be sterile, pyrogen-free, and, in the case of solutions, meet United States Pharmacopeia standards for particulate matter, the properties of some preparations are influenced by the route of administration. For example, intraocular, intraspinal, intracisternal, and intrathecal drug administration require formulations of the highest purity because of the sensitivity of nerve tissue to irritant and toxic substances. Suspensions cannot be administered intravenously because of the possibility of insoluble particles blocking the capillaries. Subcutaneous injections should be isotonic to prevent unnecessary irritation and pain.

Solutions are the most common form of injectable products. Most are aqueous, but nonaqueous solvents such as polyethylene glycol, vegetable oils, or surfactant–castor oil–alcohol vehicles (e.g., tacrolimus and cyclosporine solutions) may be used. Further, some aqueous solutions may contain varying proportions of water-miscible liquids such as propylene glycol or glycerol to increase drug solubility and/or stability. Water-immiscible oils such as sesame, corn, or peanut oil are used as an alternate method to enhance drug solubility or stability or to prolong the rate of drug release to obtain a sustained effect. The ideal parenteral vehicle should be nonirritating, nontoxic, nonsensitizing, and physiologically inert. In addition, it should be easy to purify and sterilize (i.e., be heat-stable).

Parenteral suspensions are prepared with drugs that possess low water solubility. For this type of parenteral preparation, the particle size and size distribution must be carefully controlled to ensure that they can be accurately drawn into syringes. They should also have reliable and reproducible drug bioavailability. Further, surfactants and suspending agents are usually added to aid wetting and dispersion of the solid drug.

Parenteral emulsions are usually of the oil-in-water type and are used as vehicles for parenteral drug administration for the following principal reasons[2]:

- To solubilize water-insoluble drugs
- To stabilize hydrolytically susceptible compounds
- To prevent drug uptake by infusion sets
- To reduce irritation or toxicity
- To provide sustained-release or site-specific drug delivery

The particle size range of oil-in-water emulsions is generally 0.025 to 1 μm. An example of this type of preparation is the intravenous lipid emulsion that is used as a source of calories and essential fatty acids for parenteral nutrition. Emulsions are not used more widely because of the inherent difficulties associated with producing stable emulsion drops of the desired size of less than 5 μm.

Unstable drugs are prepared in dry powder form to be reconstituted as a solution or suspension immediately before use by the addition of an appropriate diluent such as water for injection, 0.9% sodium chloride injection (normal saline), or 5% dextrose injection. More detailed information about these and other more specialized parenteral formulations such as total parenteral nutrition, radiopharmaceuticals, and biologicals can be found in the literature.[3]

BIOPHARMACEUTICAL CONSIDERATIONS

Drugs administered intravenously are often injected into a large proximal forearm vein and provide rapid action. The intensity and duration of drug activity depends on several factors:

- Dose administered
- Degree of binding to plasma proteins
- Extent of distribution throughout the body
- Rate of elimination by metabolism and/or excretion

Intravenous infusion is commonly used to give drugs with short elimination half-lives.

Intramuscular injections are administered deep into skeletal muscles away from major nerves and blood vessels. The principal sites of injection are the gluteal (buttocks), deltoid (upper arm), and vastus lateralis (lateral thigh) muscles. Essentially all injectable products can be given intramuscularly including aqueous or oleaginous solutions and suspensions, emulsions, and reconstituted powders. Intramuscular injections form a "depot" in the muscle, and therefore generally produce a slower onset of action and longer duration of effect relative to an intravenous injection. Although the extent of drug absorption after intramuscular administration is usually complete, the rate of absorption may vary widely because of factors such as the physicochemical properties of the drug, formulation variables, and various physiologic factors such as blood perfusion rate.

Long-acting preparations have been designed for intramuscular administration to provide slow, sustained drug release over an extended period. Most of these preparations act by retarding the rate of drug release and/or dissolution from the finished product via a physical or chemical mechanism.[4]

Subcutaneous administration most frequently involves the injection of a small volume (<2 mL) of aqueous solution or suspension into the loose interstitial tissue beneath the skin of the arm, forearm, thigh, abdomen, or buttocks. However, implants, which are solid-drug-delivery systems, may be inserted subcutaneously for long-term drug effect (e.g., Norplant for contraception). Subcutaneous implants should be inserted (and removed) by a trained physician. When drugs are given by subcutaneous injection, the injection site should be varied when repeated daily dosing is required. Subcutaneous administration should not be confused with the intradermal mode of administration, which involves the injection of a small volume (<0.1 mL) of diagnostic, desensitizing, or immunizing products into the vascular dermis layer of the skin.

Some current drug-delivery systems are being investigated as prolonged-release parenterals for site-specific delivery; these include magnetic and nonmagnetic microspheres, microcapsules, liposomes, multiple infusions, magnetic emulsions, biocompatible carriers, and prodrugs.[5]

THERAPEUTIC CONSIDERATIONS

The most important factors to consider when administering a parenteral medication are the route and injection site, injection volume, needle gauge and length, intended therapeutic effect, and special administration/injection techniques to be used.[6] A summary of these factors is provided in Table 4.6.

The most frequent local adverse effects of parenteral administration are pain at the injection site, infiltration, extravasation and phlebitis after intravenous injection, infection, formation of sterile abscesses from irritating drugs following subcutaneous administration, and the possibility of bleeding and peripheral nerve damage from inappropriately placed intramuscular injections. Each of these undesirable effects can be avoided or minimized by using proper injection technique and the utmost caution in the selection and care of the injection site.

The onset and intensity of a drug's pharmacologic effect(s) can be predetermined by selecting the route and method of administration best suited for the condition and therapeutic requirements of the patient. An intravenous bolus provides rapid onset of action but may be undesirable because of the toxicity of the drug or the vehicle (e.g., phenytoin and diazepam injections). The subcutaneous route provides a more sustained effect for water-soluble drugs, and intramuscular injections are most appropriate for irritating drugs, aqueous suspensions, and for injection volumes of 1.5–5.0 mL. Intramuscular injections usually produce a more rapid onset of effect than do subcutaneous injections.

The patient's age and physical condition are major considerations when selecting intravenous and intramuscular injection sites. In elderly, nonambulatory or emaciated patients, muscle mass is likely to be diminished in the gluteus medius and vastus lateralis. Large intramuscular injections should be administered in the gluteus maximus muscle in these patients. Infants and small children should receive intramuscular injections in their thigh muscles, which are developed better than the gluteal muscles.

With the increasing trend toward provision of care in patients' homes, self-administration of parenteral medications has become routine, and patient education by a health care professional is essential. Specifically, instruction for site preparation, aseptic technique, injection technique, and self-monitoring of drug therapy is required.

PARENTERAL INFUSION

A variety of external and implantable infusion devices are available for long-term controlled drug delivery via subcutaneous, intramuscular, intravenous, and intraperitoneal routes of administration.[7] These devices include gravity flow controllers, rotary or linear peristaltic pumps, motorized syringe pumps, cassette systems, and elastomeric reservoirs.[8] Infusion pumps should normally be used when conventional treatment methods have failed to control the disease satisfactorily or to allow patients greater mobility and freedom. Most of the experience with the use of these devices has been in the treatment of ambulatory patients with insulin-dependent diabetes.

Other therapeutic applications of infusion devices include patient-controlled analgesia, and continuous or intermittent administration of analgesics, anticoagulants, antineoplastics, antimicrobial agents, and nutritional fluids.[9] The use of implantable pumps has become more prevalent in the administration of subcutaneous and intra-arterial infusions. Implantable pumps decrease risks of infection,

TABLE 4.6. CHARACTERISTICS OF ROUTES OF INJECTION

Injection Sites	Usual Needles	Range (mL)	Common Medications
Epidural (use: systemic analgesia, regional anesthesia)			
L3–L4 vertebrae into space above dura mater	16–17 G Tuohy needle, catheters	1–25	Anesthetics, narcotics
Intra-arterial (use: regional therapy of organ, tissue, tumor)			
Patent artery perfusing target area	Catheters	10–50	Antineoplastics
Intra-articular (use: treat afflicted joint or synovium)			
Ankle, elbow, knee, shoulder, wrist	21–23 G × 1–1.5 in.	0.1–2	Anesthetics, antimicrobials, corticosteroids
Finger, toe	25 G × 1 in.	0.1–0.5	Same
Hip	20–22 G × 3 in.	1–3	Same
Intracardiac (use: rare as emergency cardiac stimulation)			
Through left chest into right ventricle	18–20 G × 3–6 in.	1–10	Epinephrine
Intradermal (use: diagnose allergy, give vaccine)			
In skin of ventral forearm and midscapular area	25–28 G × 3/8–1/2 in.	0.01–0.1	Antibiotics and other allergens, smallpox vaccine, tuberculin
Intralesional (use: local therapy)			
Acne cysts, psoriatic and lichenous plaques, tumors, recluse spider bites	25–26 G × 1/2–5/8 in.	0.1–1	Antineoplastics, corticosteroids
Intramuscular (use: rapid, multiple daily, and depot systemic therapy)			
Deltoid	22–25 G × 1–1.5 in.	0.1–2	Epinephrine, haloperidol, lidocaine, sedatives, vaccines, vitamin B_{12}
Gluteus maximus (dorsogluteal)	20–23 G × 1.5–3 in.	0.1–5	Antibiotics, antiemetics, hormones, iron dextran, narcotics, sedatives
Gluteus minimus and medius (ventrogluteal)	Same	Same	Same
Vastus lateralis (outer midthigh)	Pediatric, infant: 23–26 G × 1/2–1 in.	0.1–1	Same, vitamin K
	Adult: 20–23 G × 1.5–2 in.	0.1–5	Same
Intrathecal (use: treat CNS infections, pain, and tumors)			
L3–L4 vertebrae through dura mater into spinal canal, into a lateral ventricle	Pediatric: 25–27 G × 0.5–1.5 in. Adult: 20–22 G × 3.5 in.	1–10	Antimicrobials, antineoplastics, narcotics
Intravenous (use: chronic, emergency, or high-volume systemic therapy)			
Adults and children: basilic and cephalic veins in forearm	Needles: 18–23 G × 1–1.5 in. Catheters: 16–22 G × 2–12 in.	0.1–1000 hourly	Analgesics, antimicrobials, antineoplastics, bronchodilators, corticosteroids, electrolytes, hormones, immune modulators
Infants: basilic, cephalic, marginal, and small saphenous veins	22–26 G × 5/8–1 in.	0.1–10	Nutrients, thrombolytics, vasopressors
Subcutaneous (use: chronic systemic therapy, epinephrine in emergencies)			
Lateral abdomen, upper back, hips below beltline, lateral proximal arms	25–27 G × 0.5–1 in.	0.1–1.5	Analgesics, aqueous epinephrine solution and suspension, heparin sodium, hormones, immune modulators, insulin, tetanus toxoid, vaccines

(Adapted from Newton DW, Newton M. Route, site, and technique: three key decisions in giving parenteral medication. Nursing 1979;9:18–25, with permission.)

restrict fewer patient activities, and enable more targeted drug delivery. Some examples of these types of pumps include the Infusaid, Medtronic SynchroMed, and Alzet systems.[8]

Some issues related to administration of medications via an infusion device include physical and/or chemical stability of the drug, drug solubility and potency in relatively small infusion volumes, ease of use by the patient, and patient education to ensure safe and effective operation. Pharmacists who provide infusion devices to patients and other health care personnel must establish comprehensive evaluation, maintenance, education, and quality control programs that address these issues.

DEVICES

The successful treatment of wide individual variation in pain medication requirements using patient-controlled analgesia (PCA) has resulted in a proliferation of marketed infusion devices. Future developments in this area will include the following[8–10]:

1. Programmed or biofeedback controlled systems with implantable sensors to meet complicated drug demands
2. Miniaturization of the infusion devices to allow for easier implantation
3. Administration of a wider range of drugs via alternative routes of administration
4. Sophisticated microprocessor-controlled devices able to generate hardcopy for permanent records of drug administration
5. Controllers with multiple rate or multiple solution programming

Many available devices have no demonstrated evidence of safety in long-term patient care, and pharmacists must monitor for possible hazards during prolonged use.[11]

BIOPHARMACEUTICAL CONSIDERATIONS

Ideally, the flow rate of an infusion device should be adjustable and capable of delivering both a priming dose and a constant zero-order maintenance dose. The subcutaneous route of administration is usually preferred because of the large surface area available for injection sites, ease of access, and low potential for complications. As with PCA, the onset and duration of drug effect can be controlled. Although intravenous infusion produces a rapid onset of action, there are serious disadvantages that preclude widespread use (e.g., septicemia and thromboembolism). The intraperitoneal route may be used more extensively in the future because drug absorption from the peritoneal cavity has been shown to be complete and predictable.[12]

THERAPEUTIC CONSIDERATIONS

Use of portable intravenous and subcutaneous infusion devices will increase as a result of new technologies, improvements in design, and the trend toward ambulatory health care. However, this route of drug administration is not appropriate for all patients. In general, pediatric and geriatric patients are less suited for this form of drug administration than are adolescent or adult patients.

Infusion therapy is ideal for the highly motivated patient with the capability to care for the injection site, administer the infusion, and maintain and program the pump. Patient acceptance of an infusion device will depend largely on its perceived benefits, such as freedom of movement and fewer hospitalizations, compared with the risks and inconveniences of carrying a device that requires care and attention to maintain its effectiveness.

An important factor in the selection of an infusion device as an alternative method of drug delivery is drug stability. Very little is known about the stability of drugs in these devices. Consequently, drugs should be assumed to be unstable in an infusion device unless stability tests have proven otherwise.

The most common and serious undesirable effects from infusion therapy occur at the site of injection. These effects include pain, inflammation, and, to a lesser extent, infection. Inflammation, particularly with subcutaneous infusion pumps, may affect patient compliance and necessitate removal of the infusion catheter.

ORAL ADMINISTRATION

Oral administration is the most convenient and economical method for systemic drug delivery. Some drugs administered orally exert a local effect on the gastrointestinal system, but most are absorbed through the mucosa into the blood and lymphatic circulatory systems and exert a systemic effect. Absorption can occur in the mouth (buccal and sublingual), small intestine, and to a lesser extent, the stomach and large intestine.

LIQUID ORAL PREPARATIONS

When solid dosage forms are unavailable or inappropriate for oral administration, liquids are the preferred dosage form. The most common liquid oral preparations include aqueous solutions and suspensions. Oil-in-water emulsions and oral aerosols are less commonly used.

Syrups and elixirs, both aqueous solutions, are particularly useful for the administration of drugs to pediatric patients. These sweetened vehicles effectively mask drug taste. However, the concentration of sucrose in syrups is high (85% wt/vol), which can compromise drug dissolution. Drugs are usually more soluble in elixirs than in syrups; however, the alcohol content of elixirs may preclude the use of this vehicle in some patients.

Oral suspensions are frequently prepared with drugs that are insoluble, unstable, or unpleasant tasting in solution. Many oral suspensions are formulated as powders or granules that are reconstituted with purified water before dispensing. Oral extemporaneously prepared suspensions can be manufactured from bulk drug products, tablets, or the contents of a capsule incorporated in a sweetened, flavored vehicle such as simple or cherry syrup, or commercial products such as Ora Sweet and Ora Plus.

The administration of liquid preparations through a nasogastric (NG) tube may be necessary for some institutionalized patients. The most common method of drug delivery through an NG tube is the preparation of a suspension or slurry of the drug using a commercial tablet or capsule. Appropriate vehicles for this form of drug administration include diluted syrups (which provide greater viscosity) and water.

A number of drug products and dosage forms should not be crushed and administered as a liquid suspension because of local drug toxicity or the characteristics of the dosage form. These products include controlled-release and enteric-coated tablets, drugs with extremely unpleasant tastes or odors, and drugs that are irritating to mucosal membranes.[13] Alternatives to crushing tablets include emptying the contents of a capsule into soft food, using an injectable solution of the drug in juice or other suitable liquid, or substituting a similar therapeutic agent.

Poor patient acceptance and inaccurate drug delivery have limited the use of oil-in-water emulsions to laxatives and vitamin supplements. Oral aerosol devices can be used for drugs such as nitroglycerin that have limited stability in solution.

SOLID ORAL PREPARATIONS

Solid oral dosage forms, primarily tablets and capsules, confer greater drug stability and provide a more accurate drug dosage. Nevertheless, they may be less preferable than liquids for patients such as those in the pediatric or geriatric age ranges. Tablets are the most preferred dosage form because they are generally the least expensive delivery system to manufacture and they possess the greatest flexibility in formulation and design.

Buccal and sublingual tablets may be used for local or systemic drug administration. Saliva is usually available to dissolve the drug, and the vascular lining of the buccal cavity and tongue provide sites for drug absorption. Buccal tablets are either designed to dissolve slowly in the buccal cavity or directly on the affected area (e.g., mouth ulcer); or they employ a mucoadhesive to prolong drug release. They are not to be dissolved under the tongue, chewed, or swallowed. Hot liquids will accelerate the dissolution of a buccal tablet. Sublingual tablets are placed under the tongue for rapid drug absorption and onset of action and usually contain drugs that have poor oral bioavailability characteristics or high first-pass (hepatic) metabolism. Troches and lozenges are usually sucrose-based solid dosage forms that slowly dissolve in saliva, releasing drug into the mouth for an immediate, local effect, such as nystatin lozenges for oral thrush.

Chewable tablets are available for patients who have difficulty swallowing. Frequently, mannitol is used as the tablet base to provide a sweet, pleasant taste, and a cooling sensation within the mouth. Most chewable tablets do not contain disintegrants; therefore, chewing before swallowing is essential to optimize drug bioavailability. Effervescent tablets rely on the reaction between alkaline (e.g., sodium bicarbonate) and acidic (e.g., tartaric acid) substances to provide rapid disintegration and dissolution of a drug or to improve palatability. Effervescent tablets must be protected against moisture during storage.

Hard gelatin capsules usually contain 65–1000 mg of drug and appropriate excipients contained within a hard-gelatin capsule shell. This dosage form is suitable for drugs that are unstable in solution, that cannot readily be compressed, or that have an unpleasant taste or odor. However, they should not be used for extremely water-soluble drugs or highly efflorescent or deliquescent compounds. Although the vulnerability of hard-gelatin capsules to tampering has resulted in new standards for tamper-resistant packaging, the use of these capsules has increased significantly in the last decade largely because of their relatively good bioavailability characteristics. Gelcaps, which are seamless, one-piece, hard gelatin shells, have reduced the likelihood of tampering. The release, dissolution, and absorption of a drug from a capsule is generally more rapid than from a tablet.

Soft gelatin capsules contain a liquid solution or suspension in a water-immiscible or water-miscible vehicle such as mineral oil and glycols surrounded by a soft, plasticized, gelatin shell. This one-piece sealed capsule is usually intended for oral use but may also be used for rectal, vaginal, topical, ophthalmic, or otic drug delivery.[14] Soft gelatin capsules are ideal for accurate delivery of drugs in oils and other liquids, but cannot be used for low molecular weight compounds or for liquids that dissolve or migrate freely through the capsule.

BIOPHARMACEUTICAL CONSIDERATIONS

Despite limitations in the design and performance of oral drug delivery systems because of intrasubject and intersubject variation as well as the physiologic constraints and variations within the gastrointestinal tract, the oral route remains the most popular route of drug administration.

Drug bioavailability from oral dosage forms in decreasing order is generally as follows: solutions, suspensions, oil-in-water emulsions, capsules, tablets, and modified-release capsules and tablets.

Aqueous solutions rapidly reach the duodenum and absorption commences almost immediately. Suspension particles must first dissolve in the gastrointestinal secretions before absorption can occur. Absorption from oral emulsions occurs by pinocytosis and may be relatively rapid, especially if digestible oils are used.

Conventional tablets and capsules must disintegrate in the stomach or small intestine before drug dissolution and absorption can occur. Disintegration, dissolution, and bioavailability are greatly influenced by formulation variables, method of manufacture, and the physicochemical properties of the drug. Many examples of the influence of these factors causing variable drug release, absorption, and bioavailability may be found in the literature as it relates to the subject of bioequivalence.[15,16]

THERAPEUTIC CONSIDERATIONS

Key factors in selecting the optimal oral dosage form include drug availability, patient age and disease state, environmental conditions, and biopharmaceutic considerations. After the appropriate dosage form has been selected, other factors such as whether the drug should be administered in the presence or absence of food should also be considered.

Pediatric and geriatric patients generally prefer oral liquid dosage forms. Patient-specific doses are more easily administered. Moreover, solid dosage forms are not swallowed very easily by patients in these age groups, which may result in erratic drug absorption, patient noncompliance, and esophageal trauma or irritation.[17] Chewable tablets are an alternative dosage form in these patients, but these are not widely available for many drugs and do not mask drug taste as well as flavored liquids. Some components of a liquid vehicle (e.g., ethanol) may limit its usefulness in certain patients, including children and those with diabetes or peptic ulcer disease.

An alternative route of administration may be required for patients who are unwilling or unable to swallow oral dosage forms. These patients include the blind, comatose, mentally or physically impaired, and those with local gastrointestinal diseases such as peptic ulcer or ulcerative colitis.

The presence of food in the gastrointestinal tract may alter pH, motility, gastric-emptying time, and the rate and extent of drug absorption. In general, drugs that cause gastrointestinal irritation should be taken with food. Drugs that should be taken on an empty stomach include those that are acid labile or known to exhibit decreases in their rates and/or extent of absorption when taken with food. Anticholinergic drugs should be taken 15–30 minutes before meals so they can exert their antispasmodic effect before food ingestion.[18]

General patient instructions related to oral drug administration include the following:

1. Most tablets and capsules should be swallowed whole with plenty of water.
2. Liquids are preferred for children and elderly patients but may require special storage precautions to maximize drug stability and prevent accidental poisonings.
3. Specialty oral dosage forms such as sublingual, buccal, and chewable tablets, as well as capsules used as "carriers" (i.e., those intended to be emptied into food or beverages), require specific and complete patient instructions to ensure optimal drug delivery.
4. Patients should always be given a schedule for taking their medications, with particular reference to meals and nighttime administration.

ORAL MODIFIED-RELEASE DOSAGE FORMS

Depending on the desired effect, the rate of drug release from a dosage form may be enhanced or retarded by modifying its design and composition. A modified-release formulation can delay, prolong, sustain, or target drug delivery.[19] The aim of a modified-release, drug-delivery preparation is to maintain plasma drug concentrations for prolonged periods above the minimum effective concentration and below the minimum toxic concentration.

To produce and maintain a constant plasma drug concentration, the rate-limiting step for drug bioavailability must be controlled by the drug-delivery system. Further, drug delivery into the body should ideally be at a constant rate and equal to the rate of drug elimination. Few drug-delivery systems, however, are able to achieve this ideal situation. Most modified-delivery systems release the drug at a constantly declining (first-order) rate. Some potential advantages of modified-release pharmaceuticals when compared to conventional dosage forms include a reduction in dosing frequency, a decrease in the incidence and/or intensity of undesirable effects, greater selectivity of pharmacological activity, more constant therapeutic effect, and improved patient compliance.[20]

Although various chemical and biological methods have been employed, physical methods are most commonly used in the design of modified-release drug-delivery systems. To achieve constant plasma concentrations, modified-release preparations are usually formulated to provide a rapidly available dose to establish an initial therapeutic plasma level, and a controlled-release component that maintains the desired concentration.

PREPARATIONS

Dissolution-controlled systems are usually encapsulated or matrix formulations. Encapsulation methods involve coating drug particles or granules (microencapsulation) with a slowly dissolving wall material. These coated particles can subsequently be formulated into tablets or capsules. Repeat-action capsules can be obtained by coating granules with multiple coats of the same or different wall materials. Alternatively, the rate of dissolution can be modified by compressing the drug into a slowly dissolving matrix. In these types of modified-release preparations, drug-release rate is influenced by such factors as tablet porosity, surface area, compressional force, soluble additives and wettability of the delivery system.

Diffusion-controlled systems are either reservoir or matrix devices. Reservoir devices consist of a water-insoluble, semipermeable, polymeric coating surrounding a drug core reservoir. Drug release is governed by Fick's law of diffusion. Matrix systems contain the drug homogeneously dispersed in an inert, insoluble, nondisintegrating matrix consisting of polymeric or fatty materials. In practice, drug release from many oral modified-release systems is both dissolution- and diffusion-controlled.

Ion-exchange resins have long been used in attempts to control drug delivery. However, the success rate of these preparations has been limited because of variations in the ionic content of the gastrointestinal tract secondary to diet, pH, water intake, and composition of the gastrointestinal contents. An improved form of the delivery system is the Pennkinetic system, in which the drug is bound to a nonabsorbable, ion-exchange polymer, a portion of which is coated within a semipermeable membrane to provide 12 hours of sustained delivery.[21] Drug molecules are released when displaced by ions from the gastrointestinal fluid. The release of drug from both liquid and solid oral formulations that have been prepared using this approach is reportedly independent of gastrointestinal pH, temperature, and content.

Osmotically actuated dosage forms have been used to deliver drugs via a variety of routes.[22] The oral osmotic system Oros consists of an osmotically active drug in a tablet core coated with a semipermeable membrane in which a small delivery orifice has been drilled (Fig. 4.1A). When in contact with body fluid, water enters the core secondary to an osmotic pressure difference across the membrane and dissolves the drug. The increase in hydrostatic pressure inside the tablet core forces the drug in solution out through the orifice. The rate of drug release depends on the rate at which water enters the core and is essentially independent of the nature of the gastrointestinal environment. Osmotic control

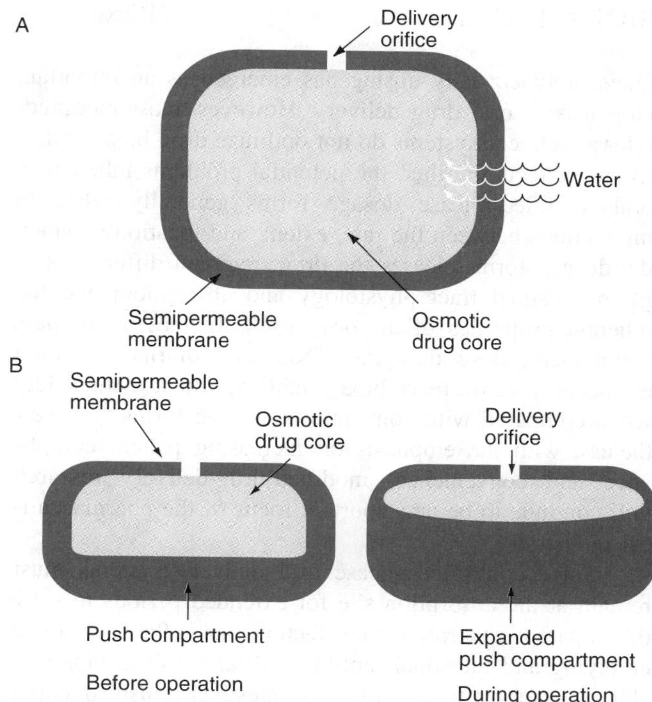

Figure 4.1. (A) Simple osmotic delivery system. (B) Push–pull osmotic delivery system. *(Modified from Theeuwes F. Oral dosage form design: Status and goals of oral osmotic systems technology. Pharm Int 1984;5(12):293–296, with permission.)*

provides constant zero-order drug release for approximately 70% of the drug contained in the formulation.

The nifedipine gastrointestinal therapeutic system, GITS, operates on a push–pull osmotic principle (Fig. 4.1B) and extends the simple oral osmotic pump principle.[23,24] For effective delivery rates using the simple osmotic pump principle, drugs should have an intrinsic water solubility of 50–300 mg/mL; otherwise, release will be too slow or too fast. However, effective release may be obtained with drugs that are otherwise poor candidates by modulating the solubility of these drugs within the core.[25]

The duration of drug release from oral modified-release systems is usually restricted by the limited residence time in the vicinity of the absorption site. Hence, attempts have recently been made to prolong the residence time of the drug-delivery systems in the gastrointestinal tract through the use of floating and inflatable tablets and capsules, and unfolding multilaminated, hydrodynamic-pressure-controlled and bioadhesive devices. Perhaps the most important developments in oral controlled delivery in recent years have occurred with the application of bioadhesives for both buccal and gastrointestinal delivery as well as the continued advances in osmotically driven delivery systems. Since bioadhesives have been shown to be useful for drug delivery via numerous routes, their use is described in the following section.

BIOPHARMACEUTICAL CONSIDERATIONS

Once or twice daily dosing has emerged as an important emphasis in oral drug delivery. However, most modified-release delivery systems do not optimize drug bioavailability and effects. Further, the potential problems inherent in oral modified-release dosage forms generally relate to interactions between the rate, extent, and location at which the dosage form releases the drug; regional differences in gastrointestinal tract physiology and absorption; and the inherent properties of the drug itself. Increased first-pass metabolism, dose dumping, food, and diurnal variation effects may all decrease bioavailability, efficacy, and safety when compared with conventional dosage forms.[26] Nevertheless, with the emphasis on increasing patient compliance and convenience, modified-drug-delivery research will continue to be an important focus of the pharmaceutical industry.

Since controlled-release oral delivery systems must remain at the absorption site for extended periods to slow the apparent absorption rate, factors that influence gastric emptying and intestinal motility will affect drug bioavailability. Attempts to control gastrointestinal transit time and attain site-specific release of a drug at its "absorption window" are alternative approaches that are currently being investigated in the design of modified-release oral drug-delivery systems.

Drugs that possess low aqueous solubility or an elimination half-life of greater than 10 hours should not be delivered in a modified-release system since the duration of their pharmacologic effects is inherently long. Other drug properties such as dose size, stability, pH-dependent absorption, first-pass metabolism, or excessive protein binding usually restrict rather than prohibit the formulation of a drug in a modified-release delivery system.[27]

THERAPEUTIC CONSIDERATIONS

All solid modified-release preparations must be swallowed whole, preferably with a glass of water. Damage to the tablet matrix or other release-controlling mechanism, for example by chewing, can result in potentially serious dose dumping. Some oral modified-release formulations may be unsuitable for the young or elderly patient because of the dose size necessary to sustain therapeutic drug levels. At present, there is controversy over whether solid oral or multiparticulate modified-release dosage forms provide a more predictable clinical effect. Another potential problem is that coated and matrix tablets may adhere to or become trapped in the folds of the gastrointestinal tract, causing localized irritation, obstruction, and/or ulceration.

RECTAL ADMINISTRATION

The rectal route is used for both local and systemic drug administration. It is an alternative to oral administration in children, psychiatric patients who will not take oral medications, bedridden patients, or patients with nausea and vomiting. Drugs that cause excessive gastrointestinal irritation or that have a high hepatic first-pass metabolism may be effectively administered rectally. In Anglo-Saxon countries, rectal suppository administration accounts for only 1–2% of all drugs that are given for their systemic effects. However, suppositories account for approximately 15–20% of all products used in many European and Latin American countries.[28] When used for their systemic effects, rectally administered drugs are generally given in doses of one half to twice the oral dose.

PREPARATIONS

Drugs intended for rectal administration are most commonly formulated in solid suppository dosage forms. After insertion, the suppositories dissolve or melt in the rectal secretions, releasing the drug to produce a local effect or to be absorbed through the rectal mucosa to produce a systemic effect. Enemas are solutions or suspensions that can be used for the delivery of drugs locally or systemically, but they are most commonly given to stimulate the evacuation of the bowel or to instill radiologic contrast media.

For rapid and complete drug release from a suppository, lipophilic drugs should be formulated in hydrophilic bases and water-soluble compounds in lipophilic bases. A variety of natural and synthetic substances of widely differing physical and chemical properties are available for use as suppository bases.[29] The ideal suppository base should melt or dissolve at 37°C, be nonirritating, nontoxic, nonsensitizing, and compatible with a wide range of drugs.

BIOPHARMACEUTICAL CONSIDERATIONS

The human rectum consists of the terminal 15- to 20-cm segment of the large intestine. It contains approximately 2–3 mL of mucous fluid secretions of pH of 7–8 and no buffering capacity or enzymatic activity. Because of the absence of villi and microvilli such as those in the small intestine, the available surface area for absorption in the rectum is very limited (200–400 cm^2). The luminal pressure, degree of rectal motility, and presence of fecal material affect the extent of dispersion of the dosage form after it has dissolved or melted. These factors are altered with age, trauma, hemorrhoids, or concomitant diseases.[28]

The availability of drug following rectal administration may be limited by the rate at which the drug is released from the suppository or the absorption rate of the drug across the rectal mucosa. In general, the absorption of drugs from the rectal area is slower, less complete, and more erratic in comparison to drugs given orally. The major source of blood to the rectum is provided by the superior rectal artery. Venous return is via the superior, middle, and inferior hemorrhoidal veins. Since the superior hemorrhoid vein drains directly into the portal vein, the extent of hepatic drug metabolism from a first-pass effect increases with the depth of rectal insertion. The middle and inferior veins drain directly into the general circulation via the iliac vein and vena cava.

THERAPEUTIC CONSIDERATIONS

Cocoa butter and synthetic oil base suppositories should be stored under refrigeration and warmed in the patient's hand to increase comfort during insertion. For similar reasons, polyethylene glycol base suppositories should be moistened with warm tap water before insertion. All suppositories should be retained in the rectum for at least 20–30 minutes to ensure melting or dissolution of the base, as well as release of the drug from the liquefied base. A slight laxative effect may be observed after the use of cocoa butter or synthetic oil base suppositories.

With an enema, the tip of the applicator and the contents should be warmed in the patient's hands before inserting. Low-volume enemas should be used for children to avoid stimulation of defecation when a systemic effect is desired.

TOPICAL AND TRANSDERMAL ADMINISTRATION

Although the multilayered structure and heterogeneous composition of the skin provide an effective barrier to the passage of substances into and out of the body, drugs are applied to the skin in various dosage forms for their local and systemic effects. With the exception of drugs used for their superficial topical effects (e.g., zinc oxide and sulfur), drugs applied to the skin must penetrate to the appropriate skin layer to produce their desired therapeutic effects, as summarized in Table 4.7. Of the three main skin layers—stratum corneum, epidermis, and dermis—the rate-limiting barrier for drug absorption through intact skin is the dense, keratinized stratum corneum outer layer. Variations in skin drug permeability at various places on the body result primarily from differences in the structure and thickness of this layer. The target areas for drugs applied topically for their "local" effects are the skin surface, stratum corneum, viable epidermis and dermis, and the appendages (e.g., nails, sebaceous and sweat glands, and hair follicles). The presence of an efficient vascular network in the dermis (or corium) enables drugs that penetrate the stratum corneum and viable epidermis to be readily absorbed systemically. Detailed descriptions of the structure, composition, and function of the skin are available in the literature.[30,31]

Improved understanding of the physiology of the skin and the process of percutaneous drug absorption has enabled topically applied drugs to be administered for their systemic effects. Initially, when ointments were applied topically, based on the observations with nitroglycerin,[32] systemic drug absorption was unpredictable because of the variability in skin permeation, imprecise dosage, and unreliable drug delivery.[33] Modern transdermal delivery systems appear to have overcome these problems by controlling the rate of drug release onto the skin surface. With these systems, drug availability is independent of the rate at which it permeates the skin into the general circulation.

Assuming that the drug is absorbed in sufficient quantities, transdermal systemic drug delivery offers several advantages. The risks and inconveniences of intravenous therapy are avoided, the variable drug bioavailability seen after oral therapy is eliminated, and drugs with narrow therapeutic indices or short biologic half-lives may be administered safely and for prolonged periods. As side effects and the frequency of dosing are reduced, patient compliance improves. Rapid termination of drug effect also is possible simply by removing the delivery device from the skin.

PREPARATIONS

Topical preparations, as opposed to transdermal drug-delivery systems, are used primarily for their local effects and usually contain the following constituents in addition to active drug: buffer, preservative, one or more cosolvents, emulsifying agent, viscosity-enhancing agent, antioxidant, permeation enhancer, and/or propellants. Transdermal drug-delivery systems are used exclusively for the production of a systemic effect. Usually adhesive patches, these products are multiphasic.

Liquid dosage forms include low viscosity solutions, suspensions, and dilute emulsions designed to cover a large area of the body uniformly with the medicament. Generally, aqueous vehicles are used for this purpose. However, other solvents such as glycerol may be included in the formulation to promote adhesion of powders to the skin and skin hydration. Ethanol may be added as a cosolvent or to promote a cooling effect.

Semisolids include ointments, creams, gels, and pastes. Ointments, usually anhydrous, are greasy and contain the drug dissolved or suspended in one of four types of bases. Paraffin is the main component of hydrocarbon bases that possess occlusive properties. The water-repellant char-

TABLE 4.7. COMMON DRUG TREATMENTS AND ASSOCIATED SKIN LAYERS

Skin Layer	Principal Structural Characteristic	Common Drugs and Conditions
Skin surface	Acid mantle, pH 4.2–5.6	Antiseptic Antiperspirant Acne Sunburn
Stratum corneum (<10 μm)	Densely packed, dead keratinized cells	Emollient Keratolytic Psoriasis Dandruff
Viable epidermis (<200 μm)	Four cell layers	Antiinflammatory Antihistamine Anesthetic Antipuritic
Dermis (2000–5000 μm) Capillaries	Fibrous collagen Reach to within 200 μm of the skin surface	Systemic drug therapy (angina, kinetosis, osteoporosis, menopause, hypertension)

(From Barry BW. Structure, function, diseases and topical treatment of human skin, in Swarbrick J (ed): Dermatological Formulations: Percutaneous Absorption. New York, Marcel Dekker, 1983, p 32, with permission.)

acteristics of a base are enhanced by the inclusion of silicone polymers such as dimethicone. Absorption bases such as anhydrous lanolin, Polysorb, and Aquaphor are able to absorb water to form water-in-oil (w/o) emulsions. The two remaining types of bases are the water-miscible emulsifying bases and water-soluble bases. The latter is especially useful for incorporating aqueous drug solutions into topical preparations.

Creams are most often emollient water-in-oil emulsions or oil-in-water (o/w) emulsions used as water-washable bases or vanishing creams. Newer formulations of steroids in fatty alcohol–propylene glycol cream bases have demonstrated superior bioavailability and efficacy.[34] Gels are used for application of benzoyl peroxide and tretinoin to the face. Pastes are not commonly used for topical drug delivery. Drugs can also be administered as solutions, suspensions, foams, or semisolids directly onto the damaged area as an aerosol. Topical powders are especially useful in drying wound exudates.

All topical preparations should maximize drug availability from the finished dosage form, facilitate easy and uniform application, and adhere to the skin while not being too greasy or difficult to remove. The most important factor that influences the rate and extent of percutaneous drug absorption is the occlusive effect of oily vehicles that softens and swells the skin, thereby altering skin permeability dramatically. The general relationship between the type of vehicle and skin hydration and skin permeability is oily base > w/o emulsion > o/w emulsion.

Although numerous designs have been investigated, transdermal drug-delivery systems can be classified into four general categories.[35] All are multilayered films with a common backing of drug-impermeable metallic plastic film. To ensure that transdermal systemic drug bioavailability is independent of variations in skin permeability, the rate of drug delivery from the device to the skin surface must be the rate-limiting step in transdermal absorption.

Membrane-moderated systems consist of four layers with the drug dispersed or suspended in a solid or liquid reservoir compartment. A rate-controlling polymeric membrane of defined drug permeability is covered with a drug-compatible, hypoallergenic adhesive polymer to maintain skin contact. As seen with the scopolamine therapeutic system, ideally the delivery systems should contain a primary dose to achieve therapeutic plasma concentrations rapidly while the membrane controls the availability of the maintenance dose from the reservoir.[19]

Adhesive-diffusion-controlled systems are a simplified three-layered device in which the drug is adsorbed and dissolved in a water-insoluble, polymeric adhesive base that functions as both the drug reservoir and release-control element. The constant thickness of these systems provides diffusion-controlled drug delivery.

Matrix-diffusion systems contain the drug homogeneously dispersed in a disk-shaped, cross-linked, hydrophilic polymer matrix of controlled surface area and thickness.[35] Skin contact is maintained by an adhesive rim around the perimeter of the drug matrix; hence, drug does not pass through an adhesive layer.

Microreservoir systems use a combination of the reservoir and matrix dispersion approaches. The drug is dispersed within microscopic aqueous, polymer solution droplets (5–50 μm) entrapped in a cross-linked silicone elastomer matrix of controlled thickness and surface area. The rim of adhesive foam pad ensures skin contact.[33] No universal transdermal system design for systemic drug delivery exists. Each system is uniquely formulated to meet specific biopharmaceutical and functional criteria, which in turn dictate the materials of construction, configuration, and combination of drug with the proper solvents, excipients, and penetration enhancers to optimize adhesive properties and drug-delivery requirements. Topical application of drugs has recently focused attention on (1) skin permeability and the use of chemical enhancers to decrease the barrier function of the stratum corneum, (2) iontophoresis (i.e., the migration of charged drug molecules through the skin by the use of an electric field), and (3) phonophoresis or sonophoresis (i.e., the migration of drug molecules through the skin by the use of ultrasound).

BIOPHARMACEUTICAL CONSIDERATIONS

The principal transport mechanism across mammalian skin is passive diffusion. Percutaneous drug absorption is much slower and more selective than gastrointestinal absorption since the stratum corneum is relatively impermeable to drug molecules. The heterogeneous multilayered structure of the skin provides a complex diffusional barrier to drug transport either through the skin or via hair follicles and sweat glands that act as diffusional shunts. Thus, drug absorption through intact skin can occur via a transepidermal route that allows drugs to penetrate by intercellular and/or intracellular diffusion through cells of the stratum corneum and the transappendageal (transfollicular) route where drugs penetrate by diffusion down hair follicles, in the secretions of the sebaceous and/or eccrine glands.[30,31]

In general, because of ability to partition into the dead stratum corneum, the transdermal route is favored by nonelectrolytes that possess both hydrophilic and hydrophobic properties. The transappendageal route is said to be favored by electrolytes, polar molecules, and large molecules such as steroids and antibiotics.[30] Nevertheless, a particular drug will penetrate the skin by the route that offers the least resistance to passive diffusion. Therefore, there are many physicochemical properties of the drug, dosage form, and skin condition that not only determine which absorption pathway predominates, but also the rate and extent of percutaneous absorption. Absorption may continually change as the vehicle, skin secretions, and disease state modify the skin barrier.

With the exception of the extremities below the knee or elbow, transdermal systems for the delivery of drug to the systemic circulation may be generally applied to any clean, dry, hairless skin area on the body. The site used should be varied between applications, avoiding areas where cuts and abrasions are present. Hair interfering with application of the system should be removed by clipping but not shaving.

One specifically designed preparation for application behind the ear is the scopolamine therapeutic system.

The rate of drug release from transdermal delivery systems remains constant as long as the diffusion gradient between the system and the skin is maintained. Drug diffusion begins as soon as the system is applied to the skin. After saturation of the binding sites in the skin, constant drug release establishes therapeutically active plasma concentrations. After removal of the transdermal patch, plasma concentrations decrease at a rate determined by the half-life of the drug.[35] Since the size of the therapeutic system determines the amount of drug absorbed per unit time, plasma drug concentrations are linearly proportional to the drug-releasing surface of the transdermal system in contact with the skin. The quantity of drug in the reservoir determines the duration of action.

For transdermally administered drugs to be clinically effective, they must be therapeutically potent in daily doses of less than about 10 mg, able to permeate the skin in sufficient quantities to exert systemic effects, nonirritating and nonsensitizing to the skin, and unaffected by enzymes in the epidermis. Drugs successfully marketed or being developed for transdermal delivery include nitroglycerin, scopolamine, clonidine, estradiol, isosorbide dinitrate, fentanyl, testosterone, nicotine, and papaverine. Evidence of interest in this area is demonstrated by the increasing number of devices and therapeutic agents being investigated for transdermal delivery. These developments have focused on penetration-enhancing agents, iontophoresis, and phonophoresis.

Because of the low skin permeability of most drugs, further research is required before transdermal delivery is a realistic alternative for a wide range of drugs. Chemical penetration enhancers can be classified into a wide variety of chemical classes including surfactants, lipophilic and hydrophilic solvents, and macrocyclic compounds such as macrocyclic ketones/lactones.[36] Penetration enhancers also have application in nasal and rectal delivery.[37]

In the presence of an increasing electric field, iontophoresis has been shown to deliver systemically small and large drug molecules such as thyrotropin-releasing hormone, vasopressin, insulin, and leuprolide, through the skin of various animal models and human volunteers.[38,39] The efficacy of iontophoresis is affected by current density, ionic strength, buffer type, duration of application of current, and whether a constant or pulsed current is used.

Phonophoretic delivery systems are still in the developmental stage and many questions remain regarding how ultrasonic energy improves drug penetration through the skin. Phonophoresis is thought to enhance skin penetration by inducing thermal, mechanical, and chemical alterations of biological tissues. Iontophoresis and phonophoresis are similar in that, with both systems, periosteal burns can result if either technique is incorrectly applied and drugs must be ionized to be electrically transported. The two systems differ in that ultrasonic waves can penetrate up to 5 cm below the skin, whereas iontophoresis penetrates to only approximately 1 cm; in addition, the usual treatment time for phonophoresis is 10 minutes, compared with 20–30 minutes for iontophoresis.[40]

THERAPEUTIC CONSIDERATIONS

The affected area of the skin should be cleansed thoroughly before applying a topical preparation. This will also hydrate the skin and thus enhance drug penetration. Preparations intended for a local effect, such as steroids and benzoyl peroxide, should be applied as a thin film and covered with a nonocclusive dressing to ensure that the area remains clean and to prevent staining of the clothing.

However, preparations intended for a superficial protective or irritant effect, such as calamine lotion or zinc oxide ointment for diaper rash, should be applied liberally, and also covered with a nonocclusive dressing. Occlusion also enhances percutaneous drug absorption. Although drugs are usually distributed rapidly by the capillary network, certain drugs such as corticosteroids remain in the subcutaneous tissues for extended periods.[35]

Skin penetration is greatly enhanced when the stratum corneum is damaged. Dangers of systemic toxicity can arise when a medication is applied liberally to broken skin or over a large surface area.

Effective adhesion of the transdermal delivery system to the skin surface is critical to maintaining the diffusion gradient needed for drug delivery. Adhesive cover patches may be used over the delivery system to maintain effective contact for prolonged periods and during day-to-day activity. Since transdermal systems deliver the drug at a controlled rate per unit area, most systems are available in more than one size so the dosage of the drug can be varied. Cutting transdermal devices in an attempt to manipulate the dosage should be avoided since this may damage the drug reservoir or rate-controlling element—or destroy the ability of the device to make effective adhesive contact with the skin surface. Further, since the aluminum-containing backing of transdermal patches may cause arcing when defibrillation is attempted during cardiopulmonary resuscitation, these types of patches should be removed before defibrillating.[41] With nitroglycerin patches, it may also be reasonable to consider removing the transdermal delivery system before an ECG examination since small explosions have been reported.

Although the *in vitro* release characteristics of nitroglycerin from the four types of transdermal system designs are different,[35] bioavailability studies in humans indicate that, when the daily nitroglycerin dose correlates with the amount released per unit area for each device, the systems are clinically interchangeable.[42,43] Because nitrate tolerance develops, intermittent use of these systems is recommended to maintain effective long-term angina prophylaxis.[44–46]

OPHTHALMIC ADMINISTRATION

The eye, with its unique structure and function, is an extremely sensitive organ that often requires prompt medical treatment upon injury or in the presence of a disease. Drugs are most commonly applied directly to the eye in the form of eyedrops or an ointment. The treatment of diseases of the eye via topical application or systemic administration may be ineffective and/or inefficient because of various factors known to affect the distribution of drug into the eye (Fig. 4.2).[47]

Ocular injections are used when a drug is unable to penetrate to the desired intraocular site after topical administration, or when it is not possible to obtain therapeutic concentration of drug in the posterior portion of the eye following direct application. Subconjunctival injections are used in the emergency management of acute infections of the anterior eye. A retrobulbar injection may be used for the treatment of optic nerve damage or for anesthesia prior to surgery.[48] In general, intraocular injections should be avoided because of the dangers and high risks for complications.

PREPARATIONS

Ophthalmic drops are usually aqueous, sterile, buffered solutions that frequently contain a preservative and viscosity-enhancing agent. Although the pH of an ophthalmic solution should be in the range of 5–9 to avoid corneal damage and pain, they need not be isotonic since the solutions undergo rapid dilution following instillation. The eye is able to tolerate an osmotic pressure equivalent to 0.6–1.8% wt/vol sodium chloride.

Ophthalmic suspensions may be employed when a drug is insoluble, unstable, or when a prolonged action is desired. With suspension formulations, drug particle size is critical since it will influence the rate and extent of drug absorption as well as patient comfort. All suspensions must be shaken before instillation.

Ophthalmic ointments contain drug dissolved or suspended in a petroleum-based vehicle that melts near body temperature. Lanolin may be added to facilitate the inclusion of water-soluble drugs. Although ophthalmic ointments may prolong drug release and contact time, they often blur the vision and therefore should be limited for use just before bedtime.

Ophthalmic preparations for injection must meet all of the requirements for a parenteral solution, such as being sterile and particle-free.

The relatively frequent dosing required with the present ophthalmic preparations is a major shortcoming of the currently available ophthalmic drug-delivery systems. To overcome this deficiency and optimize ophthalmic drug

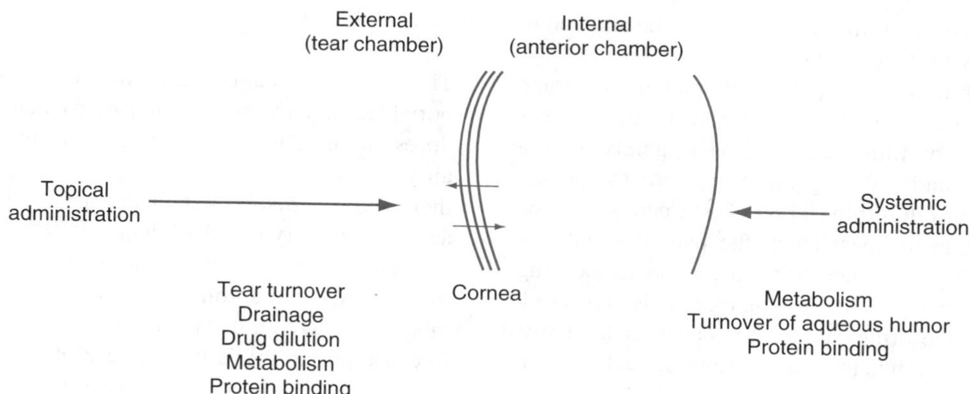

Figure 4.2. Schematic representation of the sites and factors that influence the effectiveness of a drug in the eye. *(From Robinson JR, Gosham LM. Topical drug-delivery systems (eye, ears, nose), in Banker GS, Chalmers RK (eds): Pharmaceutics and Pharmacy Practice, Philadelphia, JB Lippincott, 1982, pp 312–352, with permission.)*

delivery, efforts are being made to reduce ocular drainage using viscosity-enhancing agents, suspensions, emulsions, ointments, biodegradable and nonbiodegradable inserts and to improve corneal drug penetration using ionophores, ion-pairs, liposomes, and prodrugs.[48] For example, to reduce drug loss secondary to drainage in the nasal lacrimal ducts, the use of soft lenses and soluble and nonbiodegradable ophthalmic inserts have produced an improvement in ocular drug penetration. However, patient acceptance of these drug-delivery systems has been poor because they can be uncomfortable and may be dislodged or dispelled.

Drug-soaked collagen shields that resemble soft contact lenses have been tested to treat corneal ulcers and iridocyclitis.[49] By varying the extent of collagen cross-linking, different drug release rates can be produced. In addition, collagen shields are more comfortable, less traumatic, and less costly than subconjunctival injections.

Attempts to improve ocular absorption have proven to be more successful. For example, dipivalylepinephrine, a lipophilic prodrug of epinephrine, has been shown to penetrate the cornea approximately 17 times more readily than epinephrine; it thereby produces a more sustained drug effect with fewer systemic side effects.[50]

BIOPHARMACEUTICAL CONSIDERATIONS

The human eye is protected by the sclera and cornea, and drug penetration to intraocular target sites is hindered by the presence of various blood–eye "barriers" (Fig. 4.2). When drops are instilled into the eye, usually 90–99% of the drug is lost because of the limited capacity of the precorneal area (10–20 μL) in comparison with an average drop size of 50 μL.[47,51] This loss is accentuated by blinking and when patients rub their eyes. Thus, the instillation of multiple drops is wasteful.

Human tears are continuously replaced at a rate of approximately 15% per minute, resulting in limited contact time for drug absorption and rapid dilution of drug concentration. Because of the small volume of medication used, protein binding may significantly decrease absorption, and enzymes located in the tears, cornea, and aqueous humor may extensively metabolize drugs before absorption takes place.

The cornea is a unique biological barrier consisting of a thick aqueous stroma sandwiched between the lipid epithelium and endothelium layers. Therefore, only drugs that are both hydrophilic and lipophilic can pass across the cornea from the external tear chamber into the anterior chamber of the eye by passive diffusion. Further, corneal penetration is greatly affected by the lipid solubility characteristics and molecular weight of the drug. Properties of the delivery system also influence corneal penetration, especially when a surfactant is added to decrease surface tension and promote wetting, and when a viscosity-enhancing agent is used to prolong the contact time of the drug. A series of articles examined the kinetics, pathways, and molecular transport mechanisms of corneal drug penetration.[52–54]

THERAPEUTIC CONSIDERATIONS

Preserving the sterility of the ophthalmic preparation and integrity of all its components are of utmost importance. Patients should be instructed to inspect their ophthalmic solutions for cloudiness or discoloration and to discard the preparation if either exists.

Ideally, someone other than the patient should instill an ophthalmic preparation into the patient's eye to avoid product contamination, ensure accurate drug delivery, and promote compliance. The tip of the drug applicator (i.e., dropper, squeeze bottle, or tube) should never be allowed to come in contact with the eyelid or lashes.

The administration technique for all ophthalmic dosage forms is similar. The solution, suspension, or ointment is instilled in the eye by tilting the head back, gently pulling out the lower lid, and instilling the drops into the pocket formed in the lower lid. A thin ribbon of ointment should be applied in the same manner. Then, the patient should be instructed to blink gently once or twice to spread the drug product across the eye. If multiple drug therapy is to be used, the instillation of the drugs should be spaced at least five minutes apart to maximize the contact time of each drug in the eye.

Patients receiving ophthalmic drug therapy may experience blurring of their vision as a result of either a drug effect (e.g., adrenergics) or the dosage form itself (e.g., ointments). Systemic drug absorption of ophthalmic beta blockers may be a potential problem for patients with heart failure, bradyarrhythmias, and asthma. Patients with eye trauma should be immediately referred to a physician for emergency medical treatment.

RESPIRATORY INHALATION ADMINISTRATION

Drug administration by inhalation provides a rapid and convenient means of introducing drugs directly into the respiratory tract for the treatment of bronchopulmonary diseases.[55,56] The main advantages offered by this route and method of administration include the localized delivery of small doses of drug for rapid onset of action and the minimization of systemic side effects. However, patient education about the disease, drug therapy, inhalation devices, and inhalation techniques is essential for optimal therapeutic effect.

Respiratory delivery may be intended for local and/or systemic activity, including the administration of peptides and proteins.[57] The effectiveness of an inhaled therapeutic aerosol depends on the distribution of the deposited particles within the respiratory tract, lung pathology, mucociliary and alveolar clearance rate of the particle after deposition, and the extent of drug metabolism by the lungs.[58,59] While peptide delivery via the respiratory tract offers a potential alternative to parenteral administration, high metabolic instability and low bioavailability of these drugs remain major obstacles. Examples of medications administered by inhalation for obstructive or bronchospastic pulmonary disease include beta agonists (e.g., albuterol), corticosteroids (e.g., beclomethasone), anticholinergics (e.g., ipratropium bromide), and mast cell inhibitors (e.g., cromolyn sodium).[60] Additional drugs administered by inhalation for treatment of infectious diseases include amphotericin B and pentamidine isethionate for fungal[61] and *Pneumocystis carini*[62,63] infections, respectively.

PREPARATIONS

The ideal inhalation drug-delivery device should be portable, easy to operate, and reproducibly deliver precise doses of drug into the central and peripheral respiratory airways. Three types of delivery devices are used for therapeutic aerosols: nebulizers, pressurized metered-dose aerosols, and dry powder inhalers.[55,64,65]

Nebulizers convert a drug solution into a fine aerosol mist usually using compressed air or oxygen. The patient inhales the aerosol from a mouthpiece or preferably a mask. Because portability is limited, use of a nebulizer is primarily restricted to the treatment of severe bronchopulmonary diseases in the home or hospital.

Pressurized metered-dose aerosols consist of the drug either dissolved or suspended in a mixture of liquefied chlorofluorocarbon propellants hermetically sealed within a metal container at high pressures. The mixture may also contain cosolvents, an antioxidant, dispersant, and surfactant. Mixtures of propellants are used to produce the desired pressures to aerosolize the drug, solution, or suspension (approximately 400 kPa at 20°C). Although large doses or repeated inhalations of chlorofluorocarbons may be cardiotoxic, the dose from therapeutic aerosols is generally considered too small to produce adverse effects.[55] The metering chamber, usually 25–50 μL in capacity, is contained in the valve assembly and when actuated, delivers up to 400 individual metered doses. Patients should be advised that metered-dose aerosols are designed to operate at normal room temperature, and when not in regular use, the devices should be actuated once or twice before use to ensure that the metering chamber is full.

A comparison of compressor nebulization and metered-dose inhaler administration of terbutaline suggests that equivalent bronchodilation is achieved and that the cost of metered-dose inhaler therapy is less.[66] Therefore, it may be preferable to use the more convenient and widely available metered-dose inhalers in ambulatory patients.

An important adjunct to inhalation therapy in recent years has been the use of spacer attachments designed to decrease drug deposition in the oropharyngeal mucosa by allowing more time for the propellant to evaporate and the particle velocity to decrease.[67–70] These auxiliary delivery devices include portable telescopic extension tubes or larger pear- or cone-shaped reservoirs. Further, because as many as 50% of patients experience difficulty in coordinating actuation of the metered-dose aerosol with inspiration,[68] the reservoir attachments reduce the need for this requirement by the patient. Ideal spacer/extension devices have the following characteristics: compact size, portability, minimal coordination needed to attach to the inhaler, system for monitoring the rate of inhalation, and the presence of a one-way valve to prevent exhalation of inhaled particles into the spacer. The one-way valve also enables the patient to actuate the inhaler, and then place the mouthpiece in the mouth for inhalation.

Dry powder delivery systems are breath-activated inhalation devices such as the Spinhaler or Rotohaler.[71] Micronized solid drug particles are mixed with a more coarse lactose or glucose carrier contained in a hard gelatin capsule. After the capsule is pierced or broken in the delivery device, the powder is then withdrawn from the capsule in a turbulent airstream when the patient inhales. Because dry powder devices are activated when the patient inhales, operation is relatively simple. The main advantage of dry powder inhalers is that they can be used by patients who lack the coordination necessary to use metered-dose aerosols correctly. The primary disadvantage is local irritation from deposition of the filler on the oropharyngeal mucosa.

BIOPHARMACEUTICAL CONSIDERATIONS

The lungs provide a multibranching tortuous route for the passage of inhaled drug particles. Further, the distribution, deposition, and retention of particles in the lung cannot be predicted because the inhaled particle size and velocity change with the distance traveled, the dimensions of the respiratory airways change, and the airway characteristics and patterns of breathing vary between patients and with the disease state. Controversy also still exists as to whether the open- or closed-mouth technique is more effective. The following are important considerations for this route of administration[55,64,67]:

1. Assuming that the correct inhalation technique is used, aerosol droplet size is probably the most important factor in determining the site of deposition. For optimum deposition in the respiratory airways, the mass median diameter of inhaled particles or droplets should be between 1 and 8 μm.
2. Even with particles of optimum size distribution and using the ideal inhalation technique, only about 10% of the total dose reaches the respiratory airways after oral inspiration. The majority of drug is lost by inertial impaction in the inhalation device, or the mouth and/or oropharyngeal region and is then swallowed.
3. Deposition of particles 1–8 μm occurs by a combination of inertial impaction in the large central airways and gravitational sedimentation in the smaller airways and alveoli. Particles less than 1 μm are either exhaled or deposited by Brownian diffusion in the alveoli; however, this mechanism of deposition is generally insignificant for therapeutic aerosols. Particles greater than 8 μm in diameter are deposited by impaction almost exclusively in the oropharynx and therefore do not reach the lungs.
4. Greater deposition after inhalation occurs with slower inspiration rates (25–30 L/min) and longer breath holding (10 seconds). Directions for the proper use of metered-dose aerosols are given in Table 4.8.

TABLE 4.8. PROPER USE OF METERED-DOSE INHALERS

Steps for Determining How Much Medication Is in the Canister

1. If the canister is new, it is full.
2. If the canister has been used repeatedly, it might be empty. Check product label to see how many inhalations should be in each canister. To check how much medication is left, put the canister (not the mouth piece) in a cup of water. If the canister sinks to the bottom, it is full. If the canister floats sideways on the surface, it is empty.

Steps for Using the Inhaler

1. Remove the cap and hold inhaler upright.
2. Shake the inhaler.
3. Tilt your head back slightly and breath out.
4. Position the inhaler in one of the following ways:
   Open mouth with inhaler 1 to 2 inches away.
   Use spacer (recommended especially for young children).
   Place in mouth.
5. Press down on inhaler to release medication as you start to breathe in slowly.
6. Breathe in slowly (3 to 5 seconds).
7. Hold breath for 10 seconds to allow medication to reach deeply into lungs.
8. Repeat puffs as directed. Waiting 1 minute between puffs may permit the second puff to penetrate the lungs better.

Note: Inhaled dry powder capsules require a different inhalation technique. To use a dry powder inhaler, it is important to close the mouth tightly around the mouthpiece of the inhaler and to inhale rapidly. (Reprinted from the National Asthma Education Program's *Expert Panel Report: Guidelines for the Diagnosis and Management of Asthma*. Bethesda, MD, National Heart, Lung, and Blood Institute, 1991, with permission.)

THERAPEUTIC CONSIDERATIONS

Dry powder inhalers or metered-dose aerosols fitted with spacers or reservoirs, with or without meters, are recommended for the elderly, physically and mentally disabled, those patients with poor coordination, and for children 3 to 7 years of age. The nebulizer is recommended in patients with severe bronchopulmonary diseases and for young children less than 3 years of age. Metered-dose aerosols can be managed by most adults and children older than 7 years of age.

A problem associated with the use of ambulatory inhalation equipment is the potential contamination of the solutions and/or devices with pathogenic microorganisms.[72] An example is the potential for *Pseudomonas aeruginosa* contamination of nebulizers used by cystic fibrosis patients.

Other cases of fungal and bacterial growth as a result of poorly cleaned metered-dose inhalers and aerosol products have occurred. Scrupulous cleaning of the equipment as directed by the manufacturer is absolutely essential to prevent these problems from occurring.

Patients using multiple inhalers (bronchodilators, corticosteroids, anticholinergics, and/or mast cell inhibitors) should be instructed to use the bronchodilator first, and then the other inhaler(s) 5–10 minutes later. This regimen will enhance the effectiveness of the therapy by increasing the availability of the drugs administered following the bronchodilation at the target site of action (i.e., bronchioles and alveoli).

The specific type of bronchopulmonary disease will have an impact on the effectiveness of the drug regimen. For example, emphysema patients are able to inhale, but have difficulty exhaling. It is imperative that these patients are instructed to take small, shallow breaths, followed by complete exhalations, before drug administration. This technique will maximize air exchange and allow more inhaled particles to reach the small airways.

Provided that the patient's condition is stable and the correct inhalation technique is used, similar clinical effects are obtained with the various types of inhalation devices. However, a significant limitation of inhalation therapy is that inhaled particles are frequently poorly delivered to diseased, badly ventilated areas. Regardless of the particular device used, maximum therapeutic benefit is possible only when the patient is educated about the disease, the drug therapy program, and is instructed in the correct use of the particular inhalation device.

Intranasal Administration

Most drugs administered into the nasal cavity are used for their local effects. Research is now focusing on intranasal administration of systemically acting drugs that are unstable in the gastrointestinal tract or possess high presystemic hepatic clearances.

The nasal cavity is highly vascularized and consists, in part, of the following anatomical regions: (1) central septum, (2) turbinates—projections that extend into the nasal cavity and increase nasal surface area, (3) mucus—a continuously produced, thin liquid layer that traps foreign bodies, and (4) epithelial cilia, which remove these foreign bodies by moving the mucus into the nasopharynx. In general, drug absorption following topical nasal administration occurs from the mucosal surfaces in the posterior region of the cavity. A wide range of drugs—including beta blockers (e.g., propranolol), steroids (e.g., progesterone, estradiol), and peptides and proteins (e.g., insulin, interferon, vasopressin, oxytocin, leutinizing hormone release factor analogues, nafarelin acetate)—are known to be absorbed from the nasal mucosa.

PREPARATIONS

The majority of the currently available nasal preparations are isotonic, buffered (pH 5.5–6.5), aqueous solutions containing a preservative and/or stabilizing agent. These preparations are administered as drops or fine sprays from a plastic dropper bottle, mechanical pump, or aerosol spray container. Suspensions are not normally used owing to the limited amount of water available in the nasal passages to dissolve the drug. In addition, insoluble drugs are treated as foreign bodies and are therefore propelled to the back of the throat and swallowed.

Nasal sprays are the preferred form for the delivery of drugs intranasally because of their ability to cover a large surface area with a fine mist. Nasal drops are preferentially used in infants and small children. Mechanical metered-dose spray devices work better than previously available devices. With the increased interest in the intranasal route for systemic drug administration,[73] metered-dose mechanical pump nebulizers and metered-dose aerosols are used increasingly to facilitate deeper nasal penetration of the drug solution.

Nasal ointments and gels can only be used for the application of drugs in the anterior regions of the nose.

BIOPHARMACEUTICAL CONSIDERATIONS

Nasal airflow and nasal valve constriction cause the deposition of most aerosols and fine powders in the anterior area of the nose. For drugs with a high first-pass effect, intranasal drug administration offers an alternative to parenteral drug administration. For example, plasma propranolol concentrations obtained following intranasal drug administration were comparable with the concentration–time profile obtained following intravenous administration.[74]

Several factors known to affect plasma drug concentrations following intranasal administration are summarized in Table 4.9. For some drugs—such as insulin—absorption promoters increase plasma concentrations to levels obtained with intravenous and subcutaneous administration.[75,76] Physicochemical, biopharmaceutical, pharmacokinetic, and toxicologic considerations in nasal systemic absorption as well as the intranasal delivery of peptides, proteins, nonpeptide molecules, and diagnostic agents have been reviewed.[77]

THERAPEUTIC CONSIDERATIONS

Contamination of nasal preparations occurs routinely as a result of contact of the applicator or dropper with the nasal mucosal surface. Patients should be instructed to wash the tip of the dropper in hot water before replacing it in the bottle. This procedure should also be used with squeeze bottles

TABLE 4.9. FACTORS THAT MAY INFLUENCE DRUG BIOAVAILABILITY FOLLOWING INTRANASAL ADMINISTRATION

Physiologic Conditions of the Nasal Passages
Rate of mucus flow
Infection
Atmospheric conditions
Formulation Factors
Drug concentration
Volume administered
Viscosity
pH and tonicity
Excipients
Administration Technique
Device used
Position of head
Droplet size and volume
Site of deposition
Drug loss (e.g., into the esophagus)

(Adapted from Colaizzi JL. Pharmacokinetics of intranasal drug administration, in Chien YW (ed): Transnasal Systemic Medications. New York, Elsevier, 1985, pp 115–116, with permission.)

containing nasal sprays. Before instilling the preparation, the patient should inspect the solution for cloudiness or discoloration and dispose of the preparation if either exists.

Nasal drops are the preferred dosage form for infants with congestion. Before applying, parents should clear excessive mucus from the nasal passages of infants using a specially designed nasal bulb syringe.

Rebound congestion (i.e., chronic edema of the nasal mucosa) may occur in some patients who use nasal decongestants above the recommended doses for more than 3 to 4 days. Proper use of all nasal preparations is essential to ensure optimal therapeutic effect and to minimize adverse effects.

OTIC ADMINISTRATION

The human ear consists of three distinct anatomic regions: the external, middle, and inner ear. Drugs instilled in the external ear canal by direct local application are used almost exclusively for their local effects. Agents that are commonly used as otics include antibiotics, anti-inflammatory agents, and anesthetics. Systemic drug administration is necessary for conditions affecting the middle and inner ear.

PREPARATIONS

Otic preparations should be manufactured in a nonaqueous, water-miscible vehicle such as glycerol or propylene glycol that will not support bacterial growth and will mix with the cerumen in the ear. The addition of a surfactant is desirable to promote mixing of the solution with the oily secretions of the sebaceous and cerumen glands. Warming of otic solutions, suspensions, and ointments will also promote mixing with these secretions, and increase patient comfort. The use of an otic suspension is less desirable than a solution since the particles of the suspension may compact with the ear cerumen.

BIOPHARMACEUTICAL CONSIDERATIONS

The ideal method of drug administration into the ear canal is direct local application. Because the surfaces of the canal are lined with a thin layer of cerumen, this region is able to tolerate most drugs and chemical substances that may be placed in the ear, provided the tympanic membrane is intact. The surfaces of the external ear are essentially extensions of the skin. Therefore, the factors affecting drug absorption in the ear are identical to those governing percutaneous drug absorption. If the tympanic membrane is perforated, drug absorption would be similar to that seen across mucous membranes.

THERAPEUTIC CONSIDERATIONS

Before an otic preparation is used, the ear should be thoroughly cleansed, using an ear syringe if necessary. Sharp objects should never be used to remove cerumen. In most cases, 1–4 drops of the otic preparation is instilled in the ear canal. The preparation should remain in contact with the ear canal for a minimum of 15–20 minutes. This can be facilitated by gently occluding the ear canal with a cotton plug.

The use of eardrops at extreme temperatures should be avoided. Patients should be instructed to warm the preparation by holding the bottle tightly in their hands prior to instillation. Under no circumstances should an otic preparation be warmed in boiling or very hot water. Patients with fever, severe ear pain, or drainage from the ear should be referred to a physician.

VAGINAL ADMINISTRATION

The vaginal epithelium is permeable to a wide variety of both organic and inorganic compounds. With the exception of extemporaneous formulations of progesterone used for infertility and to maintain pregnancy, drugs administered vaginally are used primarily for their local effects. The vaginal route is generally considered inappropriate for the delivery of drugs for their systemic effects due to the influences of the menstrual cycle on the characteristics of the vaginal tissue as well as the composition and volume of the vaginal secretions.

PREPARATIONS

Vaginal products include semisolid vaginal suppositories, vaginal tablets, creams, ointments, gels, liquids, and aerosol foams. Vaginal sponges, rings, foaming tablets, and water-soluble films have been used or are currently being investigated as delivery systems for contraceptive agents.[78] Vaginal applicators are usually needed to insert the dosage forms into the vagina.

Vaginal suppositories are usually oval or oblong in shape, weighing approximately 5 grams. They are prepared by fusion using a mold or by cold compression. Solid wedge-shaped vaginal tablets are prepared in the same manner as conventional compressed tablets. After insertion, the vaginal preparations soften, melt, or dissolve, and spread over the vaginal surfaces to produce a localized effect. As previously mentioned, systemic drug absorption may also occur following vaginal administration. In theory, intravaginal controlled-released drug delivery would be an effective means to achieve continuous long-term delivery of therapeutic agents—such as progesterone and estradiol—that are poorly absorbed after oral administration because of extensive first-past hepatic metabolism. Two intravaginal delivery systems for controlled-drug release are vaginal rings and biodegradable microcapsules. Extemporaneously compounded progesterone vaginal suppositories have become popular in the treatment of luteal phase defect and infertility.

BIOPHARMACEUTICAL CONSIDERATIONS

The human vagina is a thin-walled, fibromuscular cavity 6–8.5 cm in length with a rich blood supply. Numerous microridges on the vaginal epithelium provide a surface well suited for drug absorption. The vaginal surface is usually covered with a film of moisture.

Drugs are absorbed from the vagina by both active and passive mechanisms. Further, drug absorption depends on the physicochemical and pharmacokinetic properties of the drug. For example, most steroids are readily absorbed from the vagina, and the extent of absorption is usually greater than that seen after oral administration because of a reduced first-pass effect. Absorption of high molecular weight substances such as proteins and nonoxynol-9 has been observed. In addition, therapeutic blood levels of progesterone have been achieved in patients with luteal phase defect following administration of vaginal progesterone suppositories.

Environmental factors within the vagina known to affect the rate and/or extent of drug absorption include the rate of blood perfusion, vaginal pH (3.5–4.2 in women of child-bearing age), volume and composition of the vaginal secretions, and the physiologic status of the vaginal mucosal layer.[79,80]

THERAPEUTIC CONSIDERATIONS

The primary vaginal dosage forms prescribed are creams, tablets, and suppositories. Foams and jellies are the dosage forms used most often as nonprescription contraceptives. Effective vaginal drug administration usually requires appropriate use of an applicator, especially with anti-infectives and contraceptives.

Tablets and suppositories should be moistened before insertion to hasten their mixing with the vaginal mucosal fluid. Local irritation is the most common undesirable effect seen with vaginal products; it is usually temporary and tolerable. However, severe cases of vaginal inflammation may necessitate medical intervention. Pregnant patients have aborted spontaneously while receiving vaginal drug therapy.

Because current knowledge of the effects of drugs administered by this route is limited, complete instructions must be given to patients, including administration techniques, possible adverse effects, and the importance of total compliance with the prescribed dosage regimen.

INTRAUTERINE ADMINISTRATION

As a result of the extensive use of intrauterine devices (IUDs) in China, this form of contraception is now the world's most commonly used.[81] Medicated IUDs are inserted and retained in the uterus, where they deliver directly to the endometrium low controlled-rate contraceptive doses. Therefore, not only can systemic side effects of synthetic steroids be avoided, but also the method is simple, readily reversible, it uses drugs with a short biological half-life, and can be used to deliver the drug at a constant rate.

PREPARATIONS

Two examples of extensively studied medicated IUDs are Progestasert and Cu-7. The T-shaped Progestasert is a membrane rate-controlled delivery system that delivers 65 μg of progesterone per day for one year. Cu-7 is a polypropylene 7-shaped device that releases 9.87 μg of copper per day for up to 40 months.

Although serious complications are preventable, the main disadvantage of this form of drug delivery is numerous side effects with both medicated and nonmedicated IUDs.[82] However, because of the simplicity of the method and the potential for long-term contraception, research continues in an attempt to develop the ideal intrauterine device. Approaches include encapsulated drug-delivery devices and biodegradable and nonbiodegradable matrix technologies.[83]

BIOPHARMACEUTICAL CONSIDERATIONS

The principal reason for using a medicated IUD is to deliver a low dose of drug directly to the target organ. Thus, IUDs are formulated to minimize systemic drug absorption. For example, progesterone is absorbed rapidly by the endometrium to achieve localized effects with minimal systemic side effects.[84] Although the uterus undergoes dynamic changes in size and shape during different phases of the menstrual cycle, this appears to have little effect on clinical efficacy. However, the lack of structural adaptability may lead to expulsion and uterine bleeding, infection, perforation, and pain.

THERAPEUTIC CONSIDERATIONS

Intrauterine devices are inserted by physicians to ensure proper placement. However, medical/ethical problems associated with IUD use such as septic abortion and congenital anomalies require a strong emphasis on patient education in the areas of risk–benefit analysis, self-monitoring of therapy, and precautions to ensure safe use of these devices. This method of drug delivery is contraindicated in patients with a history of pelvic inflammatory disease, spontaneous abortions, genital bleeding of unknown etiology, venereal disease, previous ectopic pregnancy, or other uterine abnormalities. Patient package inserts and complete patient instructions are available with these products.

INNOVATIVE DRUG-DELIVERY SYSTEMS

New drug-delivery systems have become much more available during the last 20 years, largely as a result of the high cost of developing new drug entities and the advances that have been made in polymer science and engineering technology. Many of these delivery systems attempt to achieve some level of drug targeting. The following is a brief description of recent innovations. In-depth reviews of these delivery systems can be found in the literature.[5,85–88]

BIOADHESIVES

Mucus, which represents a potential site of attachment of a bioadhesive delivery system, is normally found in the gastrointestinal tract, urogenital tract, lungs, nose, ears, and eyes. In addition to acting as platforms for controlled drug-delivery systems, bioadhesive polymers can exert some control over the rate and extent of drug release and improve therapeutic efficacy. Examples of the use of bioadhesives in the design and performance of drug delivery systems for various routes of administration have been summarized.[89,90] The potential advantages of bioadhesive drug delivery include prolonged delivery of drug via all noninjectable routes of administration, localized delivery for regional therapy, permeability modification, protease and other enzyme inhibition and modulation of immunologic response, and improved viability of noninjectable, nonoral routes of drug administration.[91]

PRODRUGS

The term *prodrug* is used to describe an agent that must undergo chemical or enzymatic transformation to the active or parent drug after administration, so that the metabolic product or parent drug can subsequently exhibit the desired pharmacologic response.[92] Prodrugs, delivered via all routes of administration, have been widely exploited for many years to modify a physical property of a drug, such as solubility, stability, taste, or smell; modify a biological property such as metabolism, distribution, toxicity, or bacterial resistance; reduce pain or irritation at an injection site; protect a reactive functional group such as alkylating agents, carcinogens, and toxins; and achieve prolonged or site-specific delivery. Conversion of a prodrug to an active agent usually occurs either enzymatically (esterases, amidases, phosphatases, peptidases, or reductases) or nonenzymatically via ester hydrolysis (Fig. 4.3). Numerous examples of the design and performance of prodrugs are available.[93,94]

A recent development is the retrometabolic drug-design approach.[95] An example is the novel chemical redox prodrug that uses the hydrophobic, reduced drug form, which is converted to the free oxidized, active form of the

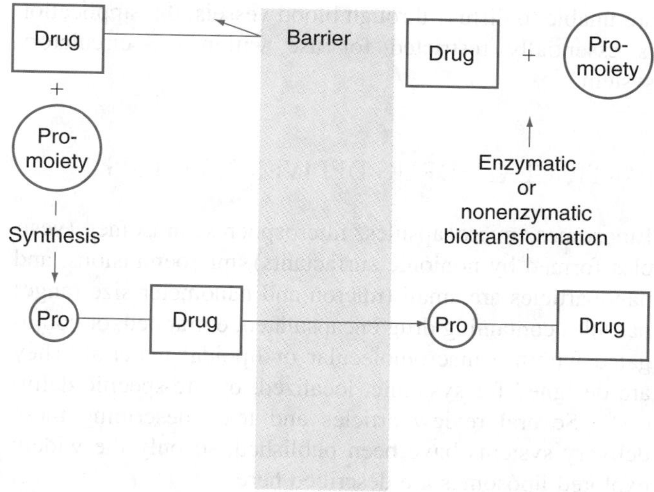

Figure 4.3. Schematic illustration of a prodrug. *(From Stella VJ, Himmelstein KJ. Prodrugs and site-specific drug delivery. J Med Chem 1980;23:1275–1282, with permission.)*

drug once the physiologic barrier is overcome.[95] Examples of this type of prodrug are the hydrophobic dihydronicotinic acid derivatives that have been used to target the central nervous system. After penetrating the blood–brain barrier, the prodrug is enzymatically oxidized to the hydrophilic species, and is thus "locked-in" the brain.

MACROMOLECULAR DRUG CARRIERS

Macromolecular drug complexes can be prepared with a wide range of steric and physicochemical properties to bypass or penetrate various barriers, and thereby improve drug delivery to receptor sites. Future understanding of transport mechanisms will help make these systems more practical. A variety of carriers have been used including proteins and protein conjugates (albumin, glycoproteins, antibodies, lipoproteins), lectins, hormones, dextran, and other polysaccharides, DNA, and water-soluble or water-insoluble biodegradable and nonbiodegradable synthetic polymers.[96,97] The design of polymeric prodrugs using natural and synthetic macromolecules and their effect on pharmaceutical, pharmacokinetic, and pharmacodynamic phases of drug action, including drug targeting, have been described in the literature.[98]

CELLULAR DRUG CARRIERS

Cellular elements such as erythrocytes, leukocytes, and fibroblasts can be "loaded" with drug or enzymes for controlled release or enzyme replacement therapy. Since a patient's own cells can be used in this approach, it has the advantage that the delivery system (i.e., cells) is biocompatible, is nonantigenic, and may be targeted by labeling with immunoglobulins. Because the cellular carriers are unable to diffuse through blood vessels, this application is essentially restricted for use within the circulatory system.

PARTICULATE DRUG DELIVERY SYSTEMS

Liposomes, microcapsules, microspheres, niosomes (vesicles formed by nonionic surfactants), microemulsions, and nanoparticles are small (micron and nanometer size range) particles containing drug encapsulated, entrapped, or conjugated within a macromolecular or lipoidal material. They are designed for systemic, localized, or site-specific delivery.[99] Several review articles and texts describing these delivery systems have been published, so only the widely explored liposomes are described here.

Liposomes have received more attention as drug carriers than any other particulate carrier system. They are discrete, artificial vesicles that form one or more concentric lipid bilayers enclosing an equal number of aqueous spaces (Fig. 4.4). Drug may be encapsulated within the aqueous or the lipid layer, with selective absorption and distribution theoretically possible by modifying both the size and surface characteristics, particularly surface charge, of the liposomes. Despite problems of instability, liposomes continue to be used as a mechanism to deal with or optimize many drug-delivery problems. Liposomes have also been widely researched for targeted drug delivery. However, with the exception of cells of the liver, the targeting ability of liposomes is limited by their inability to cross capillary endothelial cells.

Although the clearance of liposomes depends on their size, nature of the lipid, surface charge, type and amount of drug, and stability, they are usually removed by the reticuloendothelial system, especially macrophages in the liver and spleen.[99] When liposomes reach cells intact, drugs can reach intracellular sites by adsorption, endocytosis, lipid exchange, or fusion mechanisms.[100] The lipophilic nature of liposomes has been exploited to enhance membrane penetration of drugs, and they have demonstrated promise in the treatment of *Candida* infections of the eye,[101] delivery of pulmonary drugs,[102] and monoclonal antibody therapy of tumors.[103] Many texts have been written on the preparation, application, and biological interactions of liposomes.[104] In addition, the preparation and application of immunoliposomes—liposomes with an antibody covalently bound to their surface—for targeted drug delivery as well as immunodiagnostic assays have also been reviewed.[105] Cationic liposomes have been shown to deliver genes in cell tissue cultures.[106]

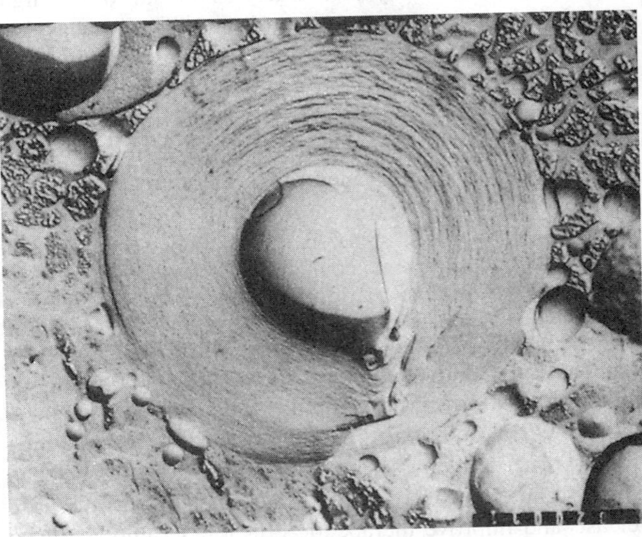

Figure 4.4. Photomicrograph of a liposome. *(Kindly supplied by the Liposome Company, Inc., Princeton, NJ.)*

PROTEINS AND PEPTIDES

The advent of hybridoma technology and genetic engineering has led to the development of various novel therapeutic peptides, polypeptides, and protein drugs, including monoclonal antibodies, toxins, cytokines, enzymes, growth factors, biologic-response modifiers, immunotoxins, and tumor-infiltrating lymphocytes that may be useful in treating a wide variety of diseases including cancer. Numerous biotechnologically derived products are already in the marketplace, including the following:

- Human insulin
- Human growth hormone
- Human alpha interferon
- Human tissue plasminogen activator
- Colony stimulating factors
- OKT-3 monoclonal antibody
- Erythropoietin

Many others are in different phases of experimental and clinical trials.

Because peptides and proteins are (1) prone to proteolytic degradation, (2) large (molecular weight typically 600 to >100,000 daltons in the nonaggregated state), and (3) possess complex secondary, tertiary, and sometimes quaternary structures, they pose major packaging, shipping, storage, and administration problems. Allied with chemical instability problems, their plasma half-lives are sometimes expressed in seconds. Because of their hydrophilic nature and high molecular weight, proteins and peptides exhibit low permeabilities across biological membranes.[107] To improve their transport properties, and thereby their systemic bioavailability, several strategies have been applied, such as the synthesis of stabilized lipophilic analogues, the concomitant use of absorption enhancers and protease inhibitors, and the design of alternative dosage forms. Several authors have reviewed the developments directed toward the effective delivery of proteins and peptides, which remains a major foreseeable challenge to drug-delivery research.[108,109]

MOLECULAR CARRIERS IN GENE THERAPY

Various molecular and particulate carriers have been proposed for site-specific delivery.[5,97,110] Cell surface receptors offer a natural mechanism by which drugs, including genes, may be selectively delivered and internalized within cells. A large number of mammalian cells express cell surface sugar-binding proteins called *membrane lectins.* Numerous membrane lectins with different sugar specifications have been characterized.[111] For example, asialoglycoprotein receptors on normal hepatocytes have been used to target DNA specifically to these cells. More recently, normal genes in the form of targetable protein–DNA complexes have been introduced by intravenous injection into animals possessing inherited metabolic disorders.[112] The choice of a particular carrier in drug targeting is based on several factors[111]: cell selectivity, immunogenicity, feasibility of scale-up production, and ability to target genes, antisense DNA, and RNA *in vivo.*

VIRAL VECTORS IN GENE DELIVERY

Viral vectors have been effective for gene delivery because they are extremely stable, which facilitates scale-up and commercialization. A wide range of virus vectors have been developed for research purposes based on murine retroviruses, adenoviruses, herpes viruses, and pox viruses. To date, viral vectors used for clinical studies have been limited to those derived from murine retroviruses and adenoviruses.

RECOMBINANT RETROVIRUSES AND RETROVIRAL-MEDIATED GENE TRANSFER

Most retroviral-mediated gene transfer systems are based on modification of the Moloney murine leukemia virus (Mo-MLV). Retroviral-mediated gene transfer provides a mechanism for the efficient and safe introduction and expression of stable gene copies into the chromosomal DNA contained in large numbers of cells.[113] Potential limitations of retroviral delivery systems are their inability to introduce genes only into nondividing cells and the physical size limitation of the gene that can be packaged.

Examples of clinical trials where gene therapy has been used include the following: adenosine deaminase (ADA) deficiency, hypercholesterolemia, and cancers, specifically melanoma, ovarian cancer, and glioblastoma.

ADENOVIRAL VECTORS

Adenovirus-associated vectors (AAVs) have emerged in gene therapy because they are nonpathogenic, stable, and readily purified.[114,115] AAVs offer potential as delivery vehicles for immunization strategies and gene therapy for the correction of inherited and acquired diseases. In contrast to retroviruses, adenoviruses rarely integrate into the host cell's genetic material. Cellular uptake and release of the virus occurs by endosmolysis.[114] The adenoviral genome is transported into the cell nucleus where the adenoviral genetic program unfolds.

Natural AAVs have been tested in humans, but recent interest has focused on their use as gene transfer vehicles because of the wide range of recombinant adenoviral vectors available.[114] These vectors have successfully been used to transfer genes into multiple organs in preclinical animal studies. Because recombinant adenoviral vectors are able to transduce dividing and nondividing cells, they will likely find multiple applications in gene therapy.

POLYCATIONIC LIPOSOMES

The delivery of gene sequences to tissue culture cells, without the use of retroviruses, has been accomplished using polycationic liposomes consisting of a liposome/polynucleotide complex.[106,116] Virtually all biological surfaces possess a net negative charge. Therefore, positively charged vesicles such as polycationic liposomes spontaneously react with the negative surfaces of cells.

BIORESPONSIVE AND SELF-REGULATING DELIVERY SYSTEMS

Delivery systems can be optimized by pulsed or self-regulated delivery of drug in direct response to physiologic need. Examples of clinical conditions for which this would be desirable include diabetes mellitus, arrhythmias, angina pectoris, hormone replacement, and immunization.

Bioresponsive polymeric delivery systems are externally regulated by magnetic fields, ultrasound, heat, electricity, microwaves, or photochemical control.[117]

Self-regulating systems have been developed that use pH-sensitive polymers, enzyme-substrate reaction, pH-sensitive drug solubility, competitive binding, and metal concentration-dependent hydrolysis. An example of feedback control of drug delivery is the glucose oxidase-controlled-release system of insulin from ethylene vinyl acetate copolymer. The enzymatic conversion of glucose to gluconic acid results in a decrease in pH within the polymer microenvironment, which greatly enhances the solubility of insulin. In turn, this causes an increase in the release rate of insulin from the polymer in response to elevated glucose concentrations.[118]

TARGETED OR SITE-SPECIFIC DELIVERY

The concept of targeted or site-directed prodrug delivery can be separated into two processes: (1) site-directed, in which the prodrug is transported and distributed preferentially to tissues or cells according to the physicochemical properties of the prodrug and the nature of the barriers encountered in the transport process within the organism, and (2) site activation, in which the prodrug or drug-carrier conjugate is taken up by the cell and transformed into active drug species. However, to achieve true site-specific delivery, the time profile of drug at the target organ must be optimized, and the burden of drug delivered to other tissues must be minimized.

MONOCLONAL ANTIBODIES

Since they were first used experimentally in humans in the early 1980s, monoclonal antibodies have been regarded as the prototypical magic bullet for either drug therapy or diagnosis because of their inherent specificity. Monoclonal antibodies that bind to specific antigens could be used alone or as conjugates with drugs (immunoconjugates) to reach target cells selectively. However, despite some promising results, many obstacles to the use of immunoconjugates in treating diseases still remain, including undesirable side effects, generation of antigen–antibody complexes, interference by the drug on cell specificity, and limitation in the number of drug molecules that can be conjugated to each antibody (i.e., amount that can be delivered).[119,120] Current interest continues to focus on the development of new chemical linkages and spacer molecules in an attempt to improve the efficacy of antibody–drug conjugates.

CONTROLLED DRUG DELIVERY INSERTS, IMPLANTS, AND DEVICES

The literature contains a diverse array of delivery systems designed to be inserted into a variety of cavities (ophthalmic, rectal, vaginal, uterus), for localized application to body membranes and tissues (nasal, buccal, skin), or for implantation into subcutaneous and other tissue cavities. Controlled-delivery implants and inserts may be formulated to maintain localized or systemic therapeutic drug concentrations for days to years, diminishing the extent of patient noncompliance and decreasing drug side effects. Potential disadvantages of these preparations include their cost relative to conventional delivery systems, need for surgical implantation, pain or irritation after insertion, bioincompatibility, and burst effects secondary to the breakdown of the rate-controlling mechanism.

Many of the developments in modern drug delivery have resulted from applied polymer science and technology. For example, polymers can be synthesized to be biodegradable or nonbiodegradable with well-defined aqueous solubility, swelling, adhesive, permeability, and biological stability characteristics. Typical nonbiode-gradable polymers include silicone polymers, poly-methyl-methacrylates, ethylene-vinyl acetate copolymers, polyamides, and polyurethane. More recently, emphasis has been directed toward the use of biodegradable polymers in drug delivery, including aliphatic polyesters (polylactic and polyglycolic acid copolymers, polyhydroxybutyrates, polyhydroxyvalerates), polycaprolactones, polyamino acids, polyorthoesters, polyanhydrides, and polyphosphazenes. The various types of polymers used in drug-delivery systems and their use have been described in the literature.[121] Norplant is an example of a nonbiodegradable subdermal, silicone-based implant designed to deliver the contraceptive levonorgestrel for up to 5 years.

A more recent developmental implant is the biodegradable, polyanhydride wafer used to deliver the carmustine derivative, BCNU, for the treatment of a universally fatal form of brain cancer, glioblastoma multiform.[122] Other implant therapeutic opportunities exist for the delivery of proteins, peptides, cancer therapy, immunizations, ophthalmic agents, and dental therapy.

FUTURE CONSIDERATIONS

Advances in polymer science and technology have accelerated the interest in controlled-release dosage forms. Alternative routes of administration are being researched. Delivery systems using biofeedback, computer-controlled, complex rate programs will be able to adapt blood levels to circadian or other variations. However, just as there is no ideal drug, there is no ideal drug-delivery system or route of administration. Emphasis on drug-delivery system design and pharmacodynamics will continue in an attempt to optimize drug therapy. Because of their selective application or prohibitive cost, many innovative drug-delivery systems will never be widely used or marketed. Many of the issues associated with testing and regulatory approval are just beginning to be addressed. Existing technologies need to be intelligently applied to meet specific clinical needs with products that are cost effective and well received by patients.

REFERENCES

1. Gourley DR, Ueda CT. Patient factors that influence dosage from selection, in Banker GS, Chalmers RK (eds): Pharmaceutics and Pharmacy Practice. Philadelphia, JB Lippincott, 1982, pp 131–154.
2. Prankerd RJ, Stella VA. The use of oil-in-water emulsions as a vehicle for parenteral drug administration. J Parent Sci Technol 1990;44:139–149.
3. Turco S, King RE. Sterile Dosage Forms: Their preparation and Clinical Application, 4th ed. Philadelphia, Lea & Febiger, 1994.
4. Avis KE. Sterile products, in Lachman L, Lieberman HA, Kanig JL (eds): The Theory and Practice of Industrial Pharmacy, 3rd ed. Philadelphia, Lea & Febiger, 1986, pp 639–677.
5. Kreuter J (ed). Colloidal Drug Delivery Systems. Drugs and the Pharmaceutical Sciences. New York, Marcel Dekker, 1994.
6. Newton DW, Newton M. Route, site, and technique: Three key decisions in giving parenteral medication. Nursing 1979;9:18–25.
7. Leung SHS, Robinson JR, Lee VHL. Parenteral products, in Robinson JR, Lee VHL (eds): Controlled Drug Delivery: Fundamentals and Application, 2nd ed. New York, Marcel Dekker, 1987, pp 433–480.
8. Kwan JW. High-technology i.v. infusion devices. Am J Hosp Pharm 1989;49:320–325.
9. Tyle, P. (ed): Drug Delivery Devices: Fundamentals and Applications. New York, Marcel Dekker. 1994; Chaps 5–8.
10. Bulhwald H, Rohde TD. Implantable drug-delivery systems for chronic drug administration: current status. Intern Med 1989;10:182–210.
11. Rapp RP, Bivins BA, Littrell RA, Foster TS. A review of the effectiveness of therapy and evaluation of currently available devices. DICP 1989;23:899–904.
12. Franetzki F. Drug delivery by program or sensor controlled infusion devices. Pharm Res 1984;1:237–244.
13. Mitchell JF, Pawlicki KS. Oral dosage forms that should not be crushed. Hosp Pharm 1994;29:666–675.
14. Ebert WR. Soft elastic gelatin capsules: a unique dosage form. Pharm Technol 1987;11:44–56.
15. Strom BL. Generic drug substitution revisited. N Engl J Med 1987;316:1456–1462.
16. Riley TN, Ravis WR. Key concepts in drug bioequivalence. US Pharm 1987;12:40–56.
17. Kikendall JW, Friedman AC, Oyewole MA, et al. Pill-induced esophageal injury: Case reports and review of the medical literature. Digest Dis Sci 1983;28:174–182.
18. Bates E, Menkis H, Tiefenbach S, Jones J. Medication administration and its relationship to meals. Fla J Hosp Pharm 1987;7:51–57.
19. Heilmann K. Therapeutic Systems: Rate-Controlled Drug Concept and Development, 2nd ed. Stuttgard, Thieme-Stratton, 1984.
20. Robinson JR, Lee VH (eds). Controlled Drug Delivery: Fundamentals and Applications, 2nd ed. New York, Marcel Dekker, 1987.
21. Amsel L. Pennkinetic: A flexible delivery system, in Controlled-Release Drug Delivery and Pennkinetic. Symposium Proceedings. Springfield, Omega Communications, 1983, pp 32–37.
22. Eckenhoff B, Theeuwes F, Urquhart J. Osmotically actuated dosage forms for rate-controlled drug delivery. Pharm Technol 1987;11:96–105.
23. Swanson DR, Barclay BL, Wong PSL, Theeuwes F. Nifedipine gastrointestinal therapeutic system. Am J Med 1987;83(suppl 6B):3–9.
24. Chung M, Reitberg DP, Gaffney M, Singleton W. Clinical pharmacokinetics of nifedipine gastrointestinal therapeutic system. Am J Med 1987;83(suppl 6B):10–14.
25. McClelland GA, Sutton SC, Engle K, Zentner GM. The solubility-modulated osmotic pump: In vitro/in vivo release of dithiazem hydrochloride. Pharm Res 1991;8:88–92.
26. Bogentoft C. Oral controlled-release dosage forms in perspective. Pharm Int 1982;3:366–369.
27. Li VHK, Robinson JR, Lee VH. Influence of drug properties and routes of drug administration on the design of sustained and oral controlled release systems, in Robinson JR, Lee

WHL (eds): Controlled Drug Delivery: Fundamentals and Applications, 2nd ed. New York, Marcel Dekker, 1987, pp 3–94.

28. Roller L. Rectal and vaginal routes of administration. Aust J Hosp Pharm 1980;10:36–40.
29. Coben LJ, Leiberman HA. Suppositories, in The Theory and Practice of Industrial Pharmacy, 3rd ed. Philadelphia, Lea & Febiger, 1986, pp 564–588.
30. Barry BW. Dermatological formulations: percutaneous absorption, in Swarbrick J (ed): Structure, Function, Diseases and Topical Treatment of Human Skin. New York, Marcel Dekker, 1983, pp 1–48.
31. Flynn GL. Cutaneous and transdermal delivery: Processes and systems of delivery, in Banker GS, Rhodes CT (eds): Modern Pharmaceutics, 3rd ed. New York, Marcel Dekker, Inc., 1996, pp 239–298.
32. Elkayam H, Aronow WS. Glyceryl trinitrate ointment and isosorbide dinitrate: A review of their pharmacological properties and therapeutic uses. Drugs 1982;23:165–194.
33. Karim A. Transdermal absorption: Unique opportunity for constant delivery of nitroglycerin. Drug Dev Indust Pharm 1983;9:671–689.
34. Ostrenga J, Halebian J, Poulsen B, et al. Vehicle design for a new topical steroid, fluocinonide. J Invest Derm 1971;56:392–399.
35. Chien YW. Transdermal therapeutic systems, in Robinson JR, Lee VHL (eds): Controlled Drug Delivery: Fundamentals and Applications, 2nd ed. New York, Marcel Dekker, 1987, pp 523–552.
36. Pfister WR, Hsieh DST. Permeation enhancers compatible with transdermal drug delivery systems. Part I: Selection and formulation considerations. Pharm Technol 1990;14(9):132–140.
37. de Boer AG, VanHoogalem EJ, Breimer DD. Improvement of drug absorption through enhancers. Eur J Drug Metab Pharmacokin 1990;15:155–157.
38. Chein YW, Siddiqui O, Sun Y, et al. Transdermal iontophoretic delivery of peptides/proteins I: Insulin. Ann NY Acad Sci 1987;507:32–51.
39. Lee VHL. Trends in peptide and protein delivery. Biopharm 1991;4(3):22–25.
40. Tyle P, Agrawala P. Drug delivery by phonophoresis. Pharm Res 1989;6:355–361.
41. Black CD. Update: Programmed drug delivery system. US Pharm 1983;146:533–540.
42. Chien YW. Pharmaceutical considerations of transdermal nitroglycerin delivery: The various approaches. Am Heart J 1984;1:207–216.
43. Wolff M, Cordes G, Luckow V. In vitro and in vivo release of nitroglycerin from a new transdermal therapeutic system. Pharm Res 1985;2:23–29.
44. Abrams J. The brief saga of transdermal nitroglycerin discs: Paradise lost? Am J Cardiol 1984;54:220–224.
45. Reichek N, Priest C, Zimrin D, et al. Antianginal effects of nitroglycerin patches. Am J Cardiol 1984;54:1–7.
46. Parker JO, Fung HL. Transdermal nitroglycerin in angina pectoris. Am J Cardiol 1984;54:471–476.
47. Robinson JR, Goshman LM. Topical drug-delivery systems (eye, ears, nose), in Banker GS, Chalmers RK (eds): Pharmaceutics and Pharmacy Practice. Philadelphia, JB Lippincott, 1982, pp 312–352.
48. Chiou GCY, Watanabe K. Drug delivery to the eye, in Ihler EM (ed): Methods of Drug Delivery. International Encyclopedia of Pharmacology and Therapeutics. New York, Pergamon Press, 1986, pp 203–212.
49. Polard PE, Kaufman HE. Clinical use of collagen shields. J Cataract Refract Surg 1988;14:489–491.
50. Kohn AN, Moss AP, Hargett NA, et al. Clinical comparison of dipivalyl epinephrine and epinephrine in the treatment of glaucoma. Am J Ophthalmol 1979;87:196–201.
51. Akers MJ. Ocular bioavailability of topically applied ophthalmic drugs. Am Pharm 1983;NS23:33–37.
52. Grass GM, Robinson JR. Mechanism of corneal drug penetration I: In vivo and in vitro kinetics. J Pharm Sci 1988;77:3–14.
53. Grass GM, Robinson JR. Mechanism of corneal drug penetration II: Ultrastructural analysis of potential pathways for drug movement. J Pharm Sci 1988;77:15–23.
54. Grass GM, Robinson JR. Mechanism of corneal drug penetration III: Modeling of molecular transport. J Pharm Sci 1986;77:24–26.
55. Lourenco RV, Cotromanes E. Clinical aerosols I. Characterization of aerosols and their diagnostic uses. Arch Intern Med 1982;142:2163–2172.
56. Lourenco RV, Cotromanes E. Clinical aerosols II. Therapeutic aerosols. Arch Inter Med 1982;142:2299–2308.
57. Byron PR. Respiratory drug delivery. Boca Raton, FL, CRC Press, 1990.
58. Gerrity TR. Pathophysiological and disease constraints on aerosol delivery, in Byron PR (ed): Respiratory Drug Delivery. Boca Raton, FL, CRC Press, 1990, pp 1–38.
59. Crooks PA, Damani LA. Drug application to the respiratory tract: Metabolic and pharmacokinetic considerations, in Byron PR (ed): Respiratory Drug Delivery. Boca Raton, FL, CRC Press, 1990, pp 61–91.
60. Johnson CE. Principles of nebulizer-delivered drug therapy for asthma. Am J Hosp Pharm 1989;1845–1855.
61. Conneally E, Cafferkey MT, Daly PA, et al. Nebulized amphotericin B as prophylaxis against invasive aspergillosis in granulocytopenic patients. Bone Marrow Transpl 1990;5:403–406.
62. Montgomery AB, Debs RJ, Luce JM, et al. Aerosolized pentamidine as sole therapy for *Pneumocystis carinii* pneumonia in patients with the acquired immunodeficiency syndrome. Lancet 1978;2:480–483.
63. Conte JE, Hollander H, Golden JA. Inhaled or reduced-dose intravenous pentamidine for *Pneumocystis carinii* pneumonia. Ann Intern Med 1987;107:495–498.
64. Newman SP. Production of radioaerosols, in Clarke SW, Pavia D (eds): Aerosols and the lung: Clinical and experimental aspects. London, Butterworth, 1984, pp 71–91.
65. Medication Teaching Manual, 5th ed. Bethesda, MD, American Society of Hospital Pharmacists, 1991, p 528.
66. Summer W, Elston R, Tharpe L, et al. Aerosol bronchodilator delivery methods: relative impact on pulmonary function and cost of respiratory care. Arch Intern Med 1989;149:618–623.

67. Newman SP. Deposition and Effects of Inhalation Aerosols. Lund, Sweden, Rahm Si Lund Tryckeri, 1983.
68. McFadden Jr ER. Inhaled Aerosol Bronchodilators. Baltimore, Williams & Wilkins, 1986, p 29.
69. Newman SP. Therapeutic aerosols, in Clarke SW, Pavia D (eds): Aerosols and the Lung: Clinical and Experimental Aspects. London, Butterworth, 1984, 197–224.
70. Byron PR. Aerosol formulation, generation and delivery using metered systems, in Byron, PR (ed): Respiratory Drug Delivery. Boca Raton, FL, CRC Press, 1990, pp 167–205.
71. Ganderton D, Kassem NM. Drug powder inhalers. Adv Pharm Sci 1992;16:165–191.
72. Pritchard KC, Corey M, Highsmith AK, et al. *Pseudomonas* species contamination of cystic fibrosis patients' home inhalation equipment. J Pediatr 1987;111:212–216.
73. Chien YW (ed). Transnasal Systemic Medications: Fundamental, Developmental Concepts and Biomedical Assessments. New York, Elsevier, 1985.
74. Hussain AA, Harai S, Bawarshi R. Nasal absorption of propranolol in rats. J Pharm Sci 1979;68:1196.
75. Colaizzi JL. Pharmacokinetics of intranasal drug administration, in Chien YW (ed): Transnasal Systemic Medications: Fundamental, Developmental Concepts and Biomedical Assessments. New York, Elsevier, 1985, pp 107–119.
76. Yokosuka T, Omori Y, Hirata Y, Hirai S. Nasal and sublinqual administration of insulin in man. J Japn Diab Soc 1977;20:146–152.
77. Chien YW, Su KSE, Chang SF. Nasal systemic drug delivery. New York, Marcel Dekker, 1989.
78. Chien YW. Intravaginal controlled-release drug administration, in Chien YW (ed): Novel Drug Delivery Systems. New York, Marcel Dekker, 1982.
79. Ansel HC, Popovich NG, Allen Jr LV. Pharmaceutical Dosage Forms and Drug Delivery Systems, 6th ed. Philadelphia, Lea & Febiger, 1995, pp 437–442.
80. Benziger DP, Edelson J. Absorption from the vagina. Drug Metab Rev 1983;14:137–168.
81. Hatcher RA, Guest F, Stewart F, et al. Intrauterine devices, in Contraception Technology, 12th ed. New York, Irvington Publishers, 1984, pp 78–105.
82. Edelman DA, Berger GS, Keith LG. Intrauterine Devices and Their Complications. Boston, G.K. Hall & Co, 1979.
83. Chien YW, Intrauterine controlled-release drug administration, in Chien YW (ed): Novel Drug Delivery Systems. New York, Marcel Dekker, 1982, 97–147.
84. Chien YW. Implantable therapeutic systems, in Robinson JR, Lee VHL (eds): Controlled Drug Delivery: Fundamentals and Application, 2nd ed. New York, Marcel Dekker, 1987, pp 481–522.
85. Chien YW. Novel Drug Delivery Systems, 2nd ed. New York, Marcel Dekker, 1992.
86. Tyle P. Specialized Drug Delivery Systems: Manufacturing and Production Technology. New York, Marcel Dekker, 1994.
87. Rolland A. Pharmaceutical Particulate Carriers: Therapeutic Applications. New York, Marcel Dekker, 1993.
88. Ihler GM. Methods of Drug Delivery. International Encyclopedia of Pharmacology and Therapeutics. New York, Pergamon Press, 1986.
89. Gurny R, Junginger HE (eds): Bioadhesion—Possibilities and Future Trends. Stuttgart, Wissenschaftiche Vertagsges schaft, 1990.
90. Lenaerts V, Gurny R (eds): Bioadhesive Drug Delivery Systems. Boca Raton, FL, CRC Press, 1990.
91. Robinson JR. Rationale of bioadhesion/mucoadhesion, in Gurny R, Junginger HE (eds): Bioadhesion—Possibilities and Future Trends. Stuttgart, Wissenschaftiche Vertagsges schaft, 1990, pp 13–15.
92. Stella VJ, Himmelstein KJ. Prodrugs and site-specific drug delivery. J Med Chem 1980;23:1275–1282.
93. Stella VJ, Charman WNA, Naringrekar VH. Prodrugs: do they have the advantage in clinical practice. Drugs 1985;29:255–273.
94. Sloan KB. Prodrugs: Topical and Ocular Drug Delivery. New York, Marcel Dekker, 1992.
95. Bodor, N. Redox drug delivery systems for targeting drugs to the brain. Ann NY Acad Sci 1988;507:289–306.
96. Tirrell DA, Donaruma LG, Turek AB (eds): Macromolecules as drugs and as carriers for biologically active materials. Ann NY Acad Sci 1985;446:1–458.
97. Juliano RL. Targeted Drug Delivery. Handbook of Experimental Pharmacology. Berlin, Springer-Verlag, 1991.
98. Joshi HE. Recent advances in drug delivery systems: polymeric prodrugs. Pharm Technol 1988;12:118–129.
99. O'Mullane JE, Artursson P, Thomlinson E. Biopharmaceutics of microparticulate drug carriers. Ann NY Acad Sci 1987;507:120–140.
100. Ostro MJ. Liposomes. Sci Am 1987;256:102–111.
101. Ostro MJ, Cullis PR. Use of liposomes as injectable-drug delivery systems. Am J Hosp Pharm 1989;46:1576–1587.
102. Taylor KMG, Taylor G, Kellaway IW, Stevens J. The influence of liposomal encapsulation on sodium chromoglygate pharmacokinetics in man. Pharm Res 1989;6:633–636.
103. Paphadjopoulos D, Gabizon A. Targeting of liposomes to tumor cells in vivo. Ann NY Acad Sci 1987;507:64–74.
104. Gregoriadis G. Liposome Technology, 2nd ed. Boca Raton, FL, CRC Press, 1993. Vol. I: Liposomal Preparation and Related Techniques. Boca Raton, FL, CRC Press, 1988. Vol. II: Entrapment of Drugs and Other Materials, 2nd ed. Boca Raton, FL, CRC Press, 1993. Vol. III: Interactions of Liposomes with the Biological Millieu. Boca Raton, FL, CRC Press, 1993.
105. Sullivan SM, Connor J, Huang L. Immunoliposomes: preparation, properties and applications. Med Res Rev 1986;6:171–195.
106. Felgner PL. Particulate systems and polymers for in vitro and in vivo delivery of polynucleotides. Adv Drug Del Rev 1990;5:163–187.
107. Audus KL, Raub TL. Biological Barriers to Protein Delivery. Pharmaceutical Biotechnology. New York, Plenum Press, 1993.
108. Davis SS, Illim L, Tomlinson E (eds): Delivery Systems for Peptide Drugs. New York, Plenum Press, 1986.
109. Sanders LM. Drug delivery systems and routes or administration for peptide and protein drugs. Eur J Drug Metab Pharmacokinet 1990;15:95–102.
110. Guyer RL, Koshland DE. Molecule of the year. Sci 1990;250:1640–1643.

111. Monsigny M, Roche AC, Midoux P, Mayer R. Glycoconjugates as carriers for specific delivery of therapeutic drugs and genes. Adv Drug Del Rev 1994;14:1–24.
112. Wu GY, Wu CH. Liver directed gene delivery. Adv Drug Del Rev 1993;12:159–167.
113. Morgan JR, Tompkins RG, Yarmush ML. Advances in recombinant retroviruses for gene delivery. Adv Drug Del Rev 1993;12:143–158.
114. Trapnell BC. Adenoviral vectors for gene transfer. Adv Drug Del Rev 1993;12:185–199.
115. Xiao X, deVlaminck W, Monahan J. Adeno-associated virus mediated gene transfer. Adv Drug Del Rev 1993;12:201–215.
116. Crommelin DJA, Schrier H. Liposomes, in Kruter J (ed): Colloidal Drug Delivery Systems. New York, Marcel Dekker, 1994, pp 73–190.
117. Kost J, Langer R. Responsive polymeric delivery systems. Adv Drug Del Rev 1990;6:19–50.
118. Fischel-Ghodsian F, Brown L, Mathiowitz E, et al. Enzymatically controlled drug delivery. Proc Natl Acad Sci 1988;85:2403–2406.
119. Brodsky FM. Monoclonal antibodies as magic bullets. Pharm Res 1988;5:1–9.
120. Ram BP, Tyle P. Immunoconjugates: application in targeted drug delivery for cancer therapy. Pharm Res 1987;4:181–188.
121. Chasin M, Langer R. Biodegradable Polymers as Drug Delivery Systems. New York, Marcel Dekker, 1990.
122. Chasin M, Hollenbeck G, Brem H, et al. Interstitial drug therapy for brain tumors: a case study. Drug Dev Ind Pharm 1990;16:2579–2594.

Chapter 5

Pediatrics

Milap C. Nahata, PharmD, FCCP

Remarkable progress has been made in the management of pediatric patients. This chapter highlights important principles of pediatric drug therapy that must be considered when the diseases discussed in other chapters of this textbook occur in pediatric patients, defined as those less than 18 years of age. Covered are notable examples of problems in pediatrics, pharmacokinetic differences in pediatric patients, drug efficacy and toxicity in this patient group, and various factors affecting pediatric pharmacotherapy. Specific examples of problems and special considerations in pediatric patients are cited to enhance understanding.

Special Problems in Pediatric Pharmacotherapy

Infant mortality has declined from 200 per 1000 births in the nineteenth century to 75 per 1000 births in 1925 to 8.9 per 1000 births in 1991.[1] This success has resulted largely from improvements in identification, prevention, and treatment of diseases once common during delivery and the neonatal period (the first month of life). Although most marketed drugs are used in pediatric patients, only one-fourth of the drugs approved by the Food and Drug Administration have indications specific for use in the pediatric population. Data on the pharmacokinetics, pharmacodynamics, efficacy, and safety of drugs in infants and children are scarce. Lack of this type of information led to such disasters as gray baby syndrome from chloramphenicol, phocomelia from thalidomide, and kernicterus from sulfonamide therapy.

Gray syndrome was first reported in two neonates who died after excessive chloramphenicol doses (100–300 mg/kg/d); the serum concentrations of chloramphenicol immediately before death were 75 and 100 µg/mL. Patients with gray syndrome usually have abdominal distension, vomiting, diarrhea, a characteristic gray color, respiratory distress, hypotension, and progressive shock.

Thalidomide is well known for its teratogenic effects. Clearly implicated as the cause of multiple congenital fetal abnormalities (particularly limb deformities), it can also cause polyneuritis, nerve damage, and mental retardation. Isotretinoin (Accutane) is another teratogen. Since it is used to treat acne vulgaris, common in teenage patients who may be sexually active but unmarried, isotretinoin has presented a difficult problem in patient education during the 1980s and 1990s.

Kernicterus was reported in infants receiving sulfonamides, which displaced bilirubin from protein-binding sites in the blood to cause a hyperbilirubinemia. This results in deposition of bilirubin in the brain and induces encephalopathy in infants. Another area of concern in pediatrics is identifying an optimal dosage. Dosage regimens cannot be based simply on body weight or surface area of a pediatric patient extrapolated from adult data. Bioavailability, pharmacokinetics, pharmacodynamics, efficacy, and adverse effects information can markedly differ between pediatric and adult patients as well as among pediatric patients because of differences in age, organ function, and disease state. Significant progress has been made in the area of pediatric pharmacokinetics during the last two decades, but few such studies have correlated pharmacokinetics with pharmacodynamics.

Several additional factors should be considered in optimizing pediatric drug therapy. Many drugs widely prescribed for infants and children are not available in suitable dosage forms. For example, extemporaneous liquid dosage forms of acetazolamide, captopril, rifampin, and spironolactone are prepared for infants and children who cannot swallow tablets or capsules; and parenteral dosage forms of aminophylline, methylprednisolone, morphine, and phenobarbital are diluted to measure accurately small doses for infants. Alteration (dilution or reformulation) of dosage forms intended for adult patients raises questions about the stability and compatibility of these drugs. Because of low fluid volume requirements and limited access to intravenous sites, special methods must be used for the delivery of intravenous drugs to infants and children. As simple as it may seem, administration of oral drugs to young patients continues to be a difficult task for nurses and parents. Similarly, assuring compliance with drug therapy in pediatric patients poses a special challenge.

Finally, the need for additional pharmacologic or therapeutic research brings up the issue of ethical justification for conducting research. The investigators proposing studies and institutional review committees approving human studies must assess the risk–benefit ratio of each study to be fair to children who are not in a position to accept or reject the opportunity to participate in the research project.

Pharmacokinetic Principles

Enormous progress has been made in characterization of drug pharmacokinetics in pediatric patients. Two factors have contributed to this progress: (1) the availability of sensitive and specific analytic methods to measure drugs and their metabolites in small volumes of biologic fluids and (2) awareness of the importance of clinical pharmacokinetics in optimization of drug therapy. Absorption, distribution, metabolism, and elimination of many drugs are different in premature infants, full-term infants, and older children.

ABSORPTION

Gastrointestinal Tract

Two factors affecting the absorption of drugs from the gastrointestinal tract are pH-dependent passive diffusion and gastric-emptying time. Both processes are strikingly different in premature infants compared with older children and adults. In a full-term infant, gastric pH ranges from 6 to 8 at birth, but declines to 1 to 3 within 24 hours.[2] In contrast, the gastric pH is elevated in premature infants because of immature acid secretion.[3]

Higher serum concentrations of acid-labile drugs such as penicillin,[4] ampicillin,[5] and nafcillin[6] and lower serum concentrations of a weak acid such as phenobarbital[7] in premature infants can be explained by the higher gastric pH. Because of a lack of extensive data comparing serum concentration–time profiles after oral versus intravenous drug administration, differences in the bioavailability of drugs in premature infants are poorly understood. Studies have also shown that gastric emptying is slow in a premature infant.[8] Thus, drugs with limited absorption in adults may be efficiently absorbed in a premature infant because of prolonged contact time with gastrointestinal mucosa.

Erratic gastrointestinal absorption of chloramphenicol occurs from use of the oral prodrug chloramphenicol palmitate in premature infants, an interesting phenomenon given the previously discussed gray baby syndrome. Because premature infants cannot metabolize the inactive chloramphenicol palmitate to active chloramphenicol in the gastrointestinal tract, the absorption of chloramphenicol is erratic and incomplete.[9]

Intramuscular Sites

Drug absorption from an intramuscular site may also be altered in premature infants. Differences in relative muscle mass, blood flow to various muscles, peripheral vasomotor instability, and insufficient muscular contractions in premature infants compared with older children and adults can influence drug absorption from the intramuscular site. The net effect of these factors on drug absorption is impossible to predict thus, specific studies are needed. Phenobarbital has been reported to be rapidly absorbed,[10] whereas diazepam absorption may be delayed.[11]

Skin

Percutaneous absorption may be substantially increased in newborn infants because of an underdeveloped epidermal barrier (i.e., stratum corneum) and increased skin hydration. The increased permeability can produce toxic effects after the topical use of hexachlorophene soaps and powders,[12] salicylic acid ointment, and rubbing alcohol.[13] Interestingly, a recent study has shown that a therapeutic serum concentration of theophylline can be achieved to control apnea in premature infants of less than 30 weeks' gestation after a topical application of gel containing a standard dose of theophylline.[14] The use of this route of administration may minimize the unpredictability of oral and intramuscular absorption and complications of intravenous drug administration for certain drugs.

DISTRIBUTION

Drug distribution is determined by the physicochemical properties of the drug itself (e.g., pK_a, molecular weight, partition coefficient), and the physiologic factors specific for the patient. Although the physicochemical properties of the drug are constant, the physiologic functions often vary in different patient populations. Some important patient-specific factors include extracellular and total body water, protein binding by the drug in plasma, and presence of pathologic conditions modifying physiologic function. Total body water, as a percentage of total body weight, has been estimated to be 94% in the fetus, 85% in premature infants, 78% in full-term infants, and 60% in adults.[15] Extracellular fluid volume is also markedly different in premature infants compared with older children and adults; the extracellular fluid volume may account for 50% of body weight in premature infants, 35% in 4- to 6-month-old infants, 25% in children 1 year of age, and 19% in adults.[15] This conforms to the observed gentamicin distribution volumes of 0.48 L/kg in neonates and 0.20 L/kg in adults.[16] Recent studies have shown that the distribution volume of tobramycin is largest in the most premature infants and decreases with increases in the gestational age and birth weight of the infant.[17]

Binding of drugs to plasma proteins is also decreased in newborn infants, because of the decreased plasma protein concentration, lower binding capacity of protein, decreased affinity of proteins for drug binding, and competition for certain binding sites by endogenous compounds such as bilirubin. The plasma protein binding of many drugs—including phenobarbital, salicylates, phenytoin, theophylline, propranolol, lidocaine, penicillin, nafcillin, and chloramphenicol—is significantly less in the neonate than in the adult.[18] The decrease in plasma protein binding of drugs can increase their apparent volumes of distribution. Therefore, premature infants require a larger loading dose than older children and adults to achieve a therapeutic serum concentration of such drugs as aminoglycosides,[16,17] phenobarbital,[19] phenytoin,[20] and theophylline.[21]

The consequences of increased concentrations of free or unbound drug in the serum and tissues must be considered. Pharmacologic and toxic effects are directly related to the concentration of free drug in the body. Increases in free drug concentrations may result directly from decreases in plasma protein binding or indirectly from, for example, drug displacement from binding sites. The increased mortality from the development of kernicterus secondary to displacement of bilirubin by sulfisoxazole in neonates has been well documented.[22] However, because drug bound to plasma proteins cannot be eliminated by the kidney, an increase in free drug concentration may also increase its clearance.[23]

The amount of body fat is substantially lower in neonates compared with adults, which may affect drug therapy. Certain highly lipid-soluble drugs are distributed less widely in infants than in adults. The apparent volume of distribution of diazepam has ranged from 1.4–1.8 L/kg in neonates and from 2.2–2.6 L/kg in adults.[24] In recent years, the numbers of mothers breast-feeding their infants has climbed. Thus, certain drugs distributed in breast milk may pose problems for the infants. The American Academy of Pediatrics recommends that amethopterin, bromocriptine, cimetidine, clemastine, cyclophosphamide, ergotamine, gold salts, methimazole, phenindione, and thiouracil be contraindicated during breast-feeding. Further, metronidazole and radiopharmaceuticals should be temporarily stopped during breast-feeding.[25] Note that these recommendations are based on limited data; other drugs taken over a prolonged period by the mother may also be toxic to the infant. Ideally, the use of any drug should be avoided by the mother during pregnancy and while breast-feeding.

METABOLISM

Drug metabolism is substantially slower in infants compared with older children and adults. There are important differences in the maturation of various pathways of metabolism within a premature infant. For example, the sulfation pathway is well developed, but the glucuronidation pathway has not developed in infants.[26] Although acetaminophen metabolism by glucuronidation is impaired in an infant compared with adults, it is partly compensated for by the sulfation pathway. The tragedy of the chloramphenicol-induced gray baby syndrome in newborn infants is directly related to a decreased metabolism of chloramphenicol by glucuronyl transferases to the inactive glucuronide metabolite.[27] This metabolic pathway appears to be age-related[28] and may take several months to a year to develop fully. Evidence for this is the increase in clearance with age up to 1 year.[29]

Interestingly, higher serum concentrations of morphine are required to achieve efficacy in a premature infant than in an adult, because the infant is not able to metabolize morphine adequately to its 6-glucuronide (20 times more active than morphine).[30]

Metabolism of drugs such as theophylline, phenobarbital, and phenytoin by oxidation is also impaired in newborn infants. The rate of metabolism, however, is more rapid with phenobarbital and phenytoin than with theophylline. Total clearance of phenytoin surpasses adult values by 2 weeks of age, whereas theophylline clearance is not fully developed for several months.[18] Two additional observations should be noted about theophylline metabolism in pediatric patients. First, in premature infants receiving theophylline for the treatment of apnea, a significant amount of its active metabolite caffeine may be present, unlike in older children and adults.[18] Second, theophylline clearance in children 1 to 9 years of age exceeds the values in young infants as well as adults. Thus, a child with asthma often requires markedly higher doses on a weight basis of theophylline compared with an adult.[31] Because of decreased metabolism, doses of such drugs as theophylline, phenobarbital, phenytoin, and diazepam should be decreased in premature infants.

ELIMINATION

Drugs and their metabolites are often eliminated by the kidney. The processes of glomerular filtration, tubular secretion, and tubular reabsorption determine the efficiency of renal excretion. These processes may take several weeks to 1 year after birth to develop fully.

Recent studies in infants have shown that tobramycin clearance during the first postnatal week may increase with an increase in gestational age.[17] Netilmicin studies in infants up to 1 month after birth have suggested that postnatal age is also directly correlated with netilmicin clearance.[29] Thus, premature infants require a lower daily dose of drugs eliminated by the kidney during the first week of life; the dosage requirement then increases with age.

Because of immature renal elimination, chloramphenicol succinate can accumulate in premature infants. Although chloramphenicol succinate is inactive, this accumulation may be the reason for an increased bioavailability of chloramphenicol in premature infants compared with older children.[28] These data indicate that dose-related toxicity may result from an underdeveloped glucuronidation pathway as well as increased bioavailability of chloramphenicol in premature infants.

Drug Efficacy and Toxicity

In addition to pharmacokinetic differences previously identified between pediatric and older patients, factors related to drug efficacy and toxicity should also be considered in planning pediatric pharmacotherapy. Unique pathophysiologic changes occur in pediatric patients with some disease states.

Examples of these pathophysiologic and pharmacodynamic differences are numerous. Clinical presentation of chronic asthma differs in children and adults.[32] Children present almost exclusively with a reversible extrinsic type of asthma, whereas adults have nonspecific, nonatopic bronchial irritability.[32] This explains the value of adjunctive-hyposensitization therapy in the management of pediatric patients with extrinsic asthma.[33,34]

The maintenance dose of digoxin is substantially higher in an infant than in an adult. This is explained by a lower binding affinity of receptors in the myocardium for digoxin and increased digoxin-binding sites on neonatal erythrocytes, compared with adult erythrocytes.[35] Insulin requirement is highest during adolescence because of the individual's rapid growth.

Certain adverse effects of drugs are most common in the newborn period, whereas other toxic effects may continue to be important for many years of childhood. Chloramphenicol toxicity is increased in a newborn infant because of immature metabolism and enhanced bioavailability. Similarly, propylene glycol—added to many injectable drugs, including phenytoin, phenobarbital, digoxin, diazepam, vitamin D, and hydralazine, to increase their stability—can cause hyperosmolality in infants.[36] Benzyl alcohol was a popular preservative in intravascular flush solutions until a syndrome of metabolic acidosis, seizures, neurologic deterioration, gasping respirations, hepatic and renal abnormalities, cardiovascular collapse, and death was described in premature infants. A 1986 study showed a decline in both mortality and the incidence of major intraventricular hemorrhage after the use of solutions containing benzyl alcohol was stopped in low-birth-weight infants.[37]

Tetracyclines are also contraindicated in pregnant women, nursing mothers, and children less than 8 years of age because they can cause dental staining and defects in enamelization of deciduous and permanent teeth as well as a decrease in bone growth.[38]

The antibiotics of the fluoroquinolone class (e.g., ciprofloxacin) are not recommended for children or pregnant women, because of an association between these drugs and development of permanent lesions of the cartilage of weight-bearing joints and other signs of arthropathy in immature animals of various species.[39]

Certain drugs may be less toxic in pediatric patients than in adults. Aminoglycosides appear to be less toxic in infants than in adults. In adults, aminoglycoside toxicity is related to both peripheral compartment accumulation and the individual patient's inherent sensitivity to these tissue concentrations.[40] Although neonatal peripheral tissue compartments for gentamicin have been reported to resemble closely those of adults with similar renal function,[16] gentamicin is rarely nephrotoxic in infants. This dissimilarity in the incidence of nephrotoxicity implies that newborn infants may have less inherent tissue sensitivity for toxicity than adults.

The differences in efficacy, toxicity, and protein binding of drugs in pediatric versus adult patients raise an important question about the acceptable therapeutic range in children. Therapeutic ranges for drugs are first established in adults and are often directly applied to pediatric patients, but specific studies should be conducted in pediatric patients to define optimal therapeutic ranges of drugs. As an example, a therapeutic range of chloramphenicol peak serum concentration of 10–20 µg/mL was established in adults and is widely used in all patients. Experience at my institution as well as a recent study suggests that some children with peak serum chloramphenicol concentrations exceeding 50 µg/mL may exhibit no apparent toxicity.[41]

Factors Affecting Pediatric Therapy

DISEASE STATES

Because most drugs are either metabolized by the liver or eliminated by the kidney, hepatic and renal disease are expected to decrease the dosage requirements in patients. Nevertheless, not all diseases require lower doses of drugs; for instance, patients with cystic fibrosis require larger doses of certain drugs to achieve therapeutic concentrations.[42]

Liver Disease

Because the liver is the main organ for drug metabolism, drug clearance is usually decreased in patients with hepatic disease; however, most studies on the influence of liver disease on dosage requirements have been carried out in adults, and these data may not be extrapolated uniformly to pediatric patients.

Drug metabolism by the liver depends on complex interactions among hepatic blood flow, ability of the liver to extract the drug from the blood, drug binding in the blood, and both type and severity of liver disease. Routine liver function tests—such as determination of serum aspartate transaminase, serum alanine transaminase, alkaline phosphatase, and bilirubin levels—have not consistently correlated with drug pharmacokinetics. Further, because of different pathologic changes in various types of liver diseases, patients with acute viral hepatitis may have different abilities to metabolize drugs compared with patients with alcoholic cirrhosis.[43]

On the basis of hepatic extraction characteristics, drugs can be divided into two categories. The first category consists of drugs with a high hepatic extraction ratio (>0.7; e.g., morphine, meperidine, lidocaine, and propranolol). Clearance of these drugs is affected by hepatic blood flow. A decreased hepatic blood flow in the presence of such disease states as cirrhosis and congestive heart failure is expected to decrease the clearance of drugs with high extraction ratios. The second category comprises drugs with a low extraction ratio (<0.2), and a low affinity for plasma proteins. Metabolism of these drugs (e.g., theophylline, chloramphenicol, and acetaminophen) is influenced mainly by hepatocellular function and not as much by changes in hepatic blood flow or plasma protein binding. One report suggested that theophylline clearance may decrease by 45% in a child with acute viral hepatitis.[44] Because of a lack of specific data on dosage adjustment in liver disease, drug therapy should be closely monitored in pediatric patients to avoid potential toxicity from excessive doses, particularly for drugs with narrow therapeutic indices.

Renal Disease

Renal failure decreases the dosage requirement of drugs eliminated by the kidney. Once again, because of limited studies, dosage adjustments in pediatric patients are based largely on data obtained in adults. For many important drugs—such as aminoglycoside antibiotics—renal clearance or rate of elimination is directly proportional to the glomerular filtration rate as measured by endogenous renal creatinine clearance. Serum drug concentrations should be monitored for drugs with narrow therapeutic indices and eliminated largely by the kidney (e.g., aminoglycosides and vancomycin) to optimize therapy in pediatric patients with renal dysfunction. For drugs with wide therapeutic ranges (e.g., penicillins and cephalosporins), dosage adjustment may be necessary only in moderate to severe renal failure.

Cystic Fibrosis

Drug therapy in pediatric patients with cystic fibrosis has been reviewed.[45] For unknown reasons, these patients require increased doses of certain drugs. Studies have reported higher clearance of drugs including gentamicin, tobramycin, netilmicin, amikacin, dicloxacillin, cloxacillin, azlocillin, piperacillin, and theophylline in patients with cystic fibrosis compared with those without this disease; the apparent distribution volume of certain drugs may also be altered in cystic fibrosis.[45] Severity of the illness may influence the change in dosage requirements, but this is not certain. Chapter 29 reviews these changes in detail.

Other Diseases

Although specific dosage guidelines are not available, pediatric patients with gastrointestinal disease (e.g., celiac disease, gastroenteritis, and severe malabsorption) may require dosage adjustments.[42] Hypoxemia has also been shown to decrease the elimination of amikacin in low-birth-weight infants.[46] Critically ill adult and pediatric patients with severe head trauma require higher than normal doses of phenytoin, but specific pharmacokinetics data in infants and children are not available.

DRUG ADMINISTRATION

Drugs are often given by the intravenous route to seriously ill patients. Flow rates and injection sites vary widely with pediatric intravenous drug-delivery sets. Effective serum concentrations are expected to be achieved rapidly after drug infusion. In 1979, a therapeutic drug monitoring service was made available at my institution. Soon thereafter, lower-than-predicted peak and higher-than-predicted trough serum concentrations of aminoglycosides and chloramphenicol were noted. In fact, in some patients, trough exceeded peak serum concentration. Subsequently, several studies demonstrated that the method of drug infusion has a profound influence on peak serum concentration and time to attain peak concentrations of chloramphenicol and tobramycin.[47,48] This has practical implications for routine therapeutic drug monitoring in that anticipated serum concentrations may be inaccurate, leading to unjustified, costly, and potentially harmful alterations in doses. Proper recommendations for obtaining patient specimens can be made only with the knowledge of drug characteristics and infusion method.

Intravenous drugs can be infused either by an antegrade or a retrograde technique. Drugs are commonly infused in an antegrade fashion. By this method, the doses injected at various sites of the intravenous set (e.g., flashball, Y-site, and a volumetric chamber such as Metriset or Buretrol) are expected to move directly toward the patient (Fig. 5.1).

In vitro studies with gentamicin and aminophylline have shown that the delivery of these drugs may be delayed substantially depending on the flow rate and injection site.[49]

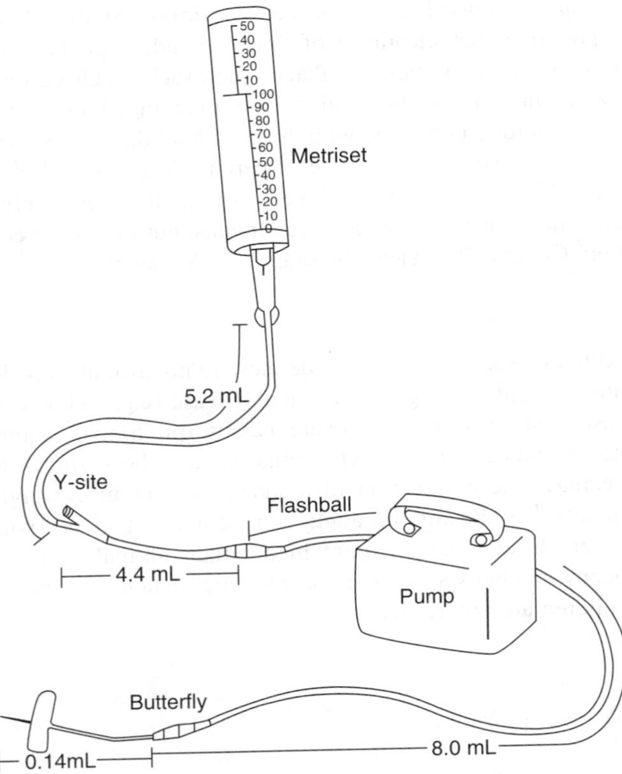

Figure 5.1. Schematic diagram of an intravenous set with a volumetric chamber (Metriset or Buretrol), Y-site, flashball, and butterfly. Values shown for the various components of the system are volume capacities. *(From Gould T, Roberts RJ. Therapeutic problems arising from the use of intravenous route for drug administration. J Pediatr 1979;95:465–471, with permission.)*

These observations were confirmed with infusion of chloramphenicol succinate[47] and tobramycin.[48] These studies have clearly demonstrated that the variables of intravenous drug infusion systems (e.g., flow rate, injection site, volume of drug, and fluid volume of the tubing) can markedly affect the serum concentrations of drugs after antegrade infusions into pediatric patients. For example, mean peak serum concentrations of chloramphenicol can be 5 μg/mL higher and occur 1 hour earlier after flashball injection compared with Buretrol injection in infants and children.[47] Similarly, the mean serum concentrations of tobramycin can be 2.3–2.5 μg/mL higher and occur 1–1.5 hours earlier after an infusion from a syringe pump compared with infusions from the Y-site of a system similar to that of Fig. 5.1.[48] These differences can be very important because of the narrow therapeutic indices of chloramphenicol and tobramycin. Furthermore, a lack of knowledge of these variables may result in inappropriate timing and interpretation of blood level data, leading to unnecessary dosage adjustments.

The retrograde infusion method was first described in 1973. This infusion system consists of extension tubing inserted between two four-way stopcocks. When a drug is administered, the stopcock closest to the patient is turned off to the patient end of the system. Diluted drug is then introduced through the stopcock and forced to move in the direction opposite the usual direction of fluid flow (i.e., retrograde, away from the patient). Simultaneously, the distal stopcock is turned off to the pump end of the system, and a syringe is attached to accept displaced maintenance fluid from the extension tubing. This fluid is then discarded. After the drug is introduced into the line, the stopcocks are repositioned to allow normal fluid flow, and the dose infuses at the rate set for the maintenance fluid.

In vitro studies have found this infusion system predictable for delivery of drugs.[50–52] Some practical limitations of the retrograde infusion system exist: (1) Drug delivery may be delayed with this system and (2) the drug volume should not exceed 50% of the volume of the extension tubing to ensure that only displaced maintenance fluid is discarded.[53] Retrograde drug infusion systems have not been adequately evaluated in patients.

Specific gravity can also influence drug delivery at slow infusion rates.[54] For example, *in vitro* studies have indicated that drugs with a specific gravity lower than that of the maintenance fluid may layer at the top of the tubing where delivery would be prolonged by laminar-flow characteristics.[54] Similarly, injections into a filter chamber, Y-site, or T-site with dead space can also prolong drug delivery.

No infusion system is ideal for drug delivery in all institutions. Each facility must be cognizant of problems of drug delivery and develop specific guidelines for intravenous infusions. At my institution, specific guidelines are provided for administration of each drug. These guidelines take into account various infusion rates and provide consistency of delivery with each dose. As long as the time for actual delivery can be anticipated, times to obtain blood samples can be adjusted accordingly to generate meaningful data.

ALTERATION OF DOSAGE FORMS

Many drugs used in pediatric patients are not available in suitable dosage forms. This necessitates dilution of high concentrations of drugs intended for adult patients. Examples of these drugs include atropine, carbamazepine, diazepam, digoxin, epinephrine, hydralazine, insulin, morphine, phenobarbital, and phenytoin. Volumes ranging from 0.001 to 0.1 mL must be measured to dispense these drugs for use in infants. This can obviously be associated with large errors in measurements, and such errors have caused intoxication with digoxin[55] and morphine[56] in infants. One solution to this problem is to dilute these concentrated products, but such alterations can influence the stability or compatibility of these drugs. Because of limited data, pharmacists may justifiably be reluctant to alter dosage forms of certain drugs.

Selection of the appropriate vehicle to dilute the adult dosage forms for use in pediatric patients can also be difficult. Phenobarbital sodium contains propylene glycol in the original product to improve drug stability. Because propylene glycol can cause hyperosmolality in infants,[36] further addition of this vehicle may not be wise. Because of limited access to intravenous sites in pediatric patients, drugs must be administered through the same site; however, data on their compatibility are often missing. Newborn infants often require aminoglycosides for presumed or proven sepsis and calcium gluconate to correct hypocalcemia. Tobramycin and calcium gluconate have been found to be compatible at least during a 1-hour period of administration at the same site.[57]

Administration of oral drugs continues to challenge parents and nurses. Alteration of these drugs by crushing or mixing, refusal of patients to accept the medication, and loss of drug during administration are some factors that can affect pediatric therapy. A common practice is to mix medications in applesauce, syrup, ice cream, or other vehicles to make the drugs palatable.

A variety of extemporaneous formulations for oral, intravenous, and rectal administration are included in a recent publication for use in pediatric patients.[58] A specific reference on the stability of many drugs in these formulations, however, is still lacking. This emphasizes the need for continued research in this area. Drug administration into the middle ear, nose, and eye of a child requires special attention. Certain drugs (e.g., sodium valproate and morphine) can be administered rectally to infants who have limited access for intravenous drug administration or if oral drug administration cannot be accomplished.

Transdermal drug delivery can be used in pediatric patients (1) to avoid problems of drug absorption from the oral route and complications from the intravenous route and (2) to maximize duration of effect and minimize adverse effects of drugs. Unfortunately, the commercially available transdermal dosage forms (e.g., clonidine, scopolamine) are not intended for pediatric patients; these would deliver doses much higher than those needed for infants and children. Favorable results with percutaneous theophylline in infants with apnea[14] and with subcutaneous morphine in pediatric patients with cancer[59] form the basis for studies with additional drugs.

MEDICATION COMPLIANCE

The issue of medication compliance is more complex in pediatric patients than in adults. The parents must appreciate the importance of following the prescribing information. Among the factors that can negatively affect compliance are poor communication between the physician and patient or parent, insufficient prescribing information, lack of understanding about the severity of illness by the patient or parent, fear of side effects, failure of the patient or parent to remember to administer the drugs, inconvenient dosage forms or dosing schedules, and unpalatability of drug products.[60] Studies in adults have reported significant differences in palatability of antibiotics and antacids.[61,62] These data may have important implications for compliance in children.

Future Developments

Although tremendous progress has been made in the area of pediatric pharmacotherapy, many questions remain unanswered. The pharmacokinetics of many important drugs have been elucidated, but correlation between pharmacokinetics and pharmacodynamics has not been explored fully. Similarly, effect of disease states, patient characteristics such as genetic status, and protein-binding alterations have not been studied for most drugs. Although pharmacokinetics studies are generally conducted once during therapy, data for certain drugs suggest that serum concentrations may change during a typical course of therapy in a patient receiving the same dose. Implications of such changes on patient outcome are unknown.

There will be a continued need to develop new methods and refine present techniques for measuring drug concentrations in small volumes of various body fluids of pediatric patients. These analytic methods should be easy to use, accurate, precise, sensitive, and specific for measuring drugs in biologic specimens.

The development of new drugs has contributed to improved patient care. However, greater emphasis should be placed on disease prevention. Millions of children die because of preventable diseases, particularly in developing countries of the world. Administration of vaccines and control of diarrhea alone could save millions of these lives annually. However, the developed countries face different problems. The infant mortality rate in the United States is nearly twice as high among blacks as with whites. In some cities, more than 30% of the infants admitted to neonatal intensive care units were born to cocaine-abusing mothers.[63] Improved prenatal care and educational programs, and avoidance of alcohol, smoking, and drugs of abuse during pregnancy may decrease mortality as well as morbidity from illnesses, including acquired immunodeficiency syndrome.

Another exciting development is an identification of the genetic cause of common serious diseases such as cystic fibrosis. Nearly 70% of the gene mutations in cystic fibrosis are caused by the loss of a single trinucleotide codon, and the protein therefore lacks only one amino acid, phenylalanine. One day soon it may be possible to offer gene therapy to correct the gene defects that cause a multitude of diseases.[64] Finally, new procedures (e.g., extracorporeal membrane oxygenation and organ transplantation) and new drugs (e.g., colony stimulating factors, dornase alfa, epoetin alfa, immunoglobulins, surfactants, and growth hormones) may improve quality of life or survival in patients in certain situations.

Although much needs to be learned about the optimization of pediatric therapy, it is encouraging to witness the continued growth in knowledge of this area.

References

1. CDC. Infant mortality—United States, 1991. MMWR 1993;42:926–930.
2. Avery GB, Randolph JG, Weaver T. Gastric acidity in the first day of life. Pediatrics 1966;37:1005–1007.
3. Agunod M, Yamaguchi N, Lopex R, et al. Correlative study of hydrochloric acid, pepsin, and intrinsic factor secretion in newborns and infants. Am J Dig Dis 1969;14:400–414.
4. Huang NN, High RN. Comparison of serum levels following the administration of oral and parenteral preparations of penicillin to infants and children of various age groups. J Pediatr 1953;42:657–668.
5. Silverio J, Poole JW. Serum concentrations of ampicillin in newborn infants after oral administration. Pediatrics 1973;51:578–580.
6. O'Connor WJ, Warren GH, Edrada LS, et al. Serum concentrations of sodium nafcillin in infants during the perinatal period. Antimicrob Agents Chemother 1965:220–222.
7. Jalling B. Plasma concentrations of phenobarbital in the treatment of seizures in newborns. Acta Paediatr Scand 1975;64:514–524.
8. Signer E, Fridrich R. Gastric emptying in newborns and young infants. Acta Paediatr Scand 1975;64:525–530.
9. Shankaran S, Kauffman RE. Use of chloramphenicol palmitate in neonates. J Pediatr 1984;105:113–116.
10. Boreus IO. Plasma concentrations of phenobarbital in mother and child after combined prenatal and postnatal administration for prophylaxis of hyperbilirubinemia. J Pediatr 1978;93:695.
11. Morselli PL. Serum levels and pharmacokinetics of anticonvulsants in the management of seizure disorders, in Merkin B (ed): Clinical Pharmacology. Chicago, Year Book Medical Publishers, 1978, p 89.
12. Tyrala FF, Hillman LS, Hillman RE, et al. Clinical pharmacology of hexachlorophene in newborn infants. J Pediatr 1977;91:481–486.
13. McFadden S, Haddow JE. Coma produced by topical application of isopropanol. Pediatrics 1969;43:622–623.
14. Evans NJ, Rutter N, Hadgraft J, et al. Percutaneous administration of theophylline in preterm infant. J Pediatr 1985;107:307–311.
15. Friis-Hansen B. Body water compartments in children: Changes during growth and related changes in body composition. Pediatrics 1961;28:169–181.
16. Haughey DB, Hilligoss DM, Grassi A, et al. Two-compartment gentamicin pharmacokinetics in premature neonates: A comparison to adults with decreased glomerular filtration rates. J Pediatr 1980;96:325–330.
17. Nahata MC, Powell DA, Durrell DE, et al. Effect of gestational age and birth weight on tobramycin kinetics in newborn infants. J Antimicrob Chemother 1984;14:59–65.
18. Roberts RJ. Pharmacologic principles in therapeutics in infants, in Drug Therapy in Infants. Philadelphia, WB Saunders, 1984, pp 3–12.
19. Pitlick W, Painter M, Pippenger C. Phenobarbital pharmacokinetics in neonates. Clin Pharmacol Ther 1978;23:346–350.
20. Painter MJ, Pippenger C, MacDonald H, et al. Phenobarbital and diphenylhydantoin levels in neonates with seizures. J Pediatr 1978;92:315–319.
21. Giacoia G, Jusko WJ, Menke J, et al. Theophylline pharmacokinetics in premature infants with apnea. J Pediatr 1976;89:829–832.
22. Silverman WA, Anderson DH, Blanc WA, et al. A difference in mortality rate and incidence of kernicterus among premature infants allotted to two prophylactic antibacterial regimens. Pediatrics 1956;18:614–624.
23. Odell GB. The dissociation of bilirubin from albumin and its clinical implications. J Pediatr 1959;55:268–279.
24. Morselli PL. Clinical pharmacokinetics in neonates. Clin Pharmacokinet 1976;1:81–98.
25. Committee on Drugs, American Academy of Pediatrics. The transfer of drugs and other chemicals into human breast milk. Pediatrics 1983;72:375–383.
26. Rane A. Basic principles of drug disposition and action in infants and children, in Yaffe JF (ed): Pediatric Pharmacology: Therapeutic Principles in Practice. New York, Grune and Stratton, 1980, pp 7–28.
27. Weiss CF, Glazko AJ, Weston JK. Chloramphenicol in the newborn infant. A physiologic explanation of its toxicity when given in excessive doses. N Engl J Med 1960; 262:787–794.
28. Nahata MC, Powell DA. Comparative bioavailability and pharmacokinetics of chloramphenicol after intravenous chloramphenicol succinate in premature infants and older patients. Dev Pharmacol Ther 1983;6:23–32.
29. Kuhn R, Nahata MC, Powell DA, et al. Netilmicin pharmacokinetics in newborn infants. Eur J Clin Pharmacol 1986;29:635–637.
30. Chay PCW, Duffy BJ, Walker JS. Pharmacokinetic–pharmacodynamic relationships of morphine in neonates. Clin Pharmacol Ther 1992;51:334–342.
31. Edwards DJ, Zarowitz BJ, Slaughter RL. Theophylline, in Evans WE, Schentag JJ, Jusko WJ (eds): Applied Pharmacokinetics, 3rd ed. Vancouver, WA, Applied Therapeutics, 1992, pp 1–47.
32. Leffert FL. The management of chronic asthma. J Pediatr 1980;97:875–885.
33. Johnston DE. Immunotherapy in children: Past, present, and future. Part I. Ann Allergy 1981;46:1–7.
34. Johnston DE. Immunotherapy in children: Past, present, and future. Part II. Ann Allergy 1981;46:59–66.
35. Kearin M, Kelly JG, O'Malley K. Digoxin "receptors" in neonates: An explanation of less sensitivity to digoxin than in adults. Clin Pharmacol Ther 1980;28:346–349.

36. Glasgow AM, Boeckx RL, Miller MK, et al. Hyperosmolality in small infants due to propylene glycol. Pediatrics 1983; 72:353–355.
37. Hiller JL, Benda GI, Rahatzad M, et al. Benzyl alcohol toxicity: Impact of mortality and intraventricular hemorrhage among very low birth weight infants. Pediatrics 1986;77: 500–506.
38. Grossman ER, Walchek A, Freedman H. Tetracyclines and permanent teeth: The relation between dose and tooth color. Pediatrics 1971;47:567–570.
39. Walker RC, Wright AJ. The quinolones. Mayo Clin Proc 1987;62:1007–1012.
40. Schentag JJ, Plaut ME, Cerra FB, et al. Aminoglycoside nephrotoxicity in critically ill surgical patients. J Surg Res 1979;26:270–279.
41. Shann F, Linnemann V, MacKenzie A, et al. Absorption of chloramphenicol sodium succinate after intramuscular administration in children. N Engl J Med 1985;313:410–414.
42. Kauffman RE, Habersange R. Modification of dosage regimens in disease states of childhood, in Mirkin BL (ed): Clinical Pharmacology and Therapeutics: A Pediatric Perspective. Chicago, Year Book Medical Publishers, 1978, pp 73–88.
43. Roberts RJ. Special considerations in drug therapy in infants, in Drug Therapy in Infants. Philadelphia, WB Saunders, 1984, pp 25–35.
44. Feinstein RA, Miles MV. The effect of acute viral hepatitis on theophylline clearance. Clin Pediatr 1985;24:357–358.
45. Wallace CS, Hall M, Kuhn RJ. Pharmacologic management of cystic fibrosis. Clin Pharm 1993;12:657–674.
46. Myers MG, Roberts JF, Mirhig NJ. Effect of gestational age, birth weight, and hypoxemia on the pharmacokinetics of amikacin in serum of infants. Antimicrob Agents Chemother 1977;11:1027.
47. Nahata MC, Powell DA, Glazer JP, et al. Effect of intravenous flow rate and infection site on in vitro delivery of chloramphenicol succinate and in vivo kinetics. J Pediatr 1981;99:463–466.
48. Nahata MC, Powell DA, Durrell DE, et al. Effect of infusion methods on tobramycin serum concentrations in newborn infants. J Pediatr 1984;104:136–138.
49. Gould T, Roberts RJ. Therapeutic problems arising from the use of intravenous route for drug administration. J Pediatr 1979;95:465–471.
50. Leff R, Roberts RJ. Methods for intravenous drug administration in the pediatric patient. J Pediatr 1981;98:631–635.
51. Benzing G, Loggie J. A new retrograde method for administering drugs intravenously. Pediatrics 1973;52:420–425.
52. Eling RF, Brissie EO. Intravenous infusion of drugs by a retrograde technique. Am J Hosp Pharm 1974;31:740–742.
53. Roberts RJ. Intravenous administration of medication in pediatric patients: Problems and solutions. Pediatr Clin North Am 1981;28:23–34.
54. Rajchgot P, Radde IC, MacLeod SM. Influence of specific gravity on intravenous drug delivery. J Pediatr 1981; 99:658–661.
55. Berman W, Whitman V, Marks KH, et al. Inadvertent overadministration of digoxin to low birthweight infants. J Pediatr 1978;92:1024.
56. Zenk KE, Anderson S. Improving the accuracy of mini-volume injections. Infusion 1982;(Jan/Feb):7–11.
57. Nahata MC, Durrell DE. Stability of tobramycin sulfate in admixtures containing calcium gluconate. Am J Hosp Pharm 1985;42:1987–1988.
58. Nahata MC, Hipple TF. Pediatric Drug Formulations, 2nd ed. Cincinnati, OH, Harvey Whitney Books, 1992, 1–79.
59. Nahata MC, Miser A, Miser J, et al. Analgesic plasma concentrations of morphine in children with terminal malignancy receiving a continuous subcutaneous infusion of morphine sulfate to control severe pain. Pain 1984;18: 109–114.
60. Boreus LO. Drug compliance, in Yaffe SJ (ed): Principles of Pediatric Pharmacology. New York, Churchill Livingstone, 1982, pp 176–192.
61. Demers DM, Chan DS, Bass JW. Antimicrobial drug suspensions: a blinded comparison of taste of twelve common pediatric drugs including cefixime, cefpodoxime, cefprozil and loracarbef. Pediatr Infect Dis J 1994;13:87–89.
62. Bahal O'Mara N, Force RW, Nahata MC. Comparative palatability of antacids in healthy adults. Am Pharm 1994;NS34:31–35.
63. Cherukuri R, Minkoff H, Feldman J, et al. A cohort study of alkaloidal cocaine (crack) in pregnancy. Obstet Gynecol 1988;72:147–151.
64. Nahata MC. Discovery of the gene defect in cystic fibrosis: Implications for diagnosis and treatment. Clin Pharm 1990;9:716–717.

Chapter 6

Geriatrics

Becky A. Nagle, PharmD, BCPS, and W. Gary Erwin, PharmD

The population of the elderly increased in the United States significantly in the last half of the twentieth century. Recognition of problems that complicate the health of older individuals has grown. The elderly experience a higher incidence of disease, hospitalization, physical impairment, medication use, and adverse drug effects than younger adults. The interrelated disciplines of *gerontology,* defined as the study of aging, and *geriatrics,* defined as the health and social care of the elderly, have expanded our knowledge of the older adult. Interdisciplinary health care teams emerged during this period to better serve the complex needs of the elderly.

Aging or senescence in the human organism begins in the mid-20s and proceeds at varying rates. Aging processes contribute to disease processes that change healthy individuals into frail individuals—those elderly individuals with complex medical and psychosocial impairment and functional disability.

Chronologic age and physiologic age may differ. Not all individuals older than 65 are frail. Many elderly have single organ disease or no disease at all. Historically, demographers, insurers, and employers have described the elderly as those persons older than age 65, but today we recognize that this heterogeneous population of individuals older than 65 is not so easily defined.

Coexistence of multiple medical and psychosocial problems plagues many geriatric patients. These problems in the geriatric patient result in blurring of diagnostic categories. In addition, nonspecific or atypical presentation and clinical course of disease occur frequently. Geriatrics is often described as management of special problem complexes called the five I's:

- Iatrogenic disease
- Incompetence (mental)
- Incontinence
- Immobility
- Impaired homeostasis

Management of these medical problems frequently involves medication use. Consequently, the elderly consume multiple medications. Use of multiple medications frequently increases the development of adverse events. Age-related changes in organ system functioning or diseases that affect compliance, pharmacokinetics, and pharmacodynamics can cause adverse events. To maximize drug appropriateness, effectiveness, and safety while providing pharmaceutical care for the elderly, the pharmacist must be aware of the previously mentioned changes to employ strategies to avoid adverse outcomes that could result from these changes. This chapter focuses primarily on effects of aging organ systems and how they relate to medication use.

Demographics and Epidemiology

The number of individuals older than 65 is the most rapidly increasing segment of the U.S. population. The life expectancy of the entire U.S. population at birth has risen from 62.9 years in 1940 to 75.8 years in 1992.[1] In 1900, 1 in 25 Americans was 65 or older. In 1984, the proportion had increased to 1 in 8. Currently, those people 65 and older constitute 12.4% of the population. The projection for the year 2050 is 21.8%.[2]

Mortality

Historically, race and gender influence life expectancy; white women have the longest projected life span and black men the shortest. In 1992, life expectancy for white women was 5.9 years higher than that of black women and 8.2 years higher for white men than for black men. In addition, the life expectancy at birth reached 79.8 for white women, 73.9 for black women, 73.2 for white men, and 65.0 for black men.

The most common cause of death in elderly individuals 65 and older is heart disease. In the subset of elderly persons 65–74 years of age, malignant neoplasms cause death more frequently than heart disease. The most common causes of death and age-specific death rates in the total U.S. population in 1992 are depicted in Table 6.1.[3]

TABLE 6.1. DEATH RATES FOR THE 15 LEADING CAUSES OF DEATH IN THE TOTAL POPULATION AND INCIDENCE RATES IN THE ELDERLY IN 1992

	Deaths/100,000 People (Order of Incidence)			
	All Ages[a]	**65–74 Years**[b]	**75–84 Years**[b]	**85+ Years**[b]
All causes	853	2589	5775	14,973
Heart disease	281 (1)	848 (2)	2147 (1)	6513 (1)
Malignant neoplasm	204 (2)	873 (1)	1351 (2)	1787 (2)
Cerebrovascular disease	56 (3)	135 (4)	468 (3)	1566 (3)
Pulmonary disease	36 (4)	155 (3)	326 (4)	461 (5)
Accidental death	34 (5)	44 (7)	96 (7)	255 (7)
Pneumonia/influenza	30 (6)	55 (6)	227 (5)	1023 (4)
Diabetes mellitus	20 (7)	76 (5)	143 (6)	254 (8)
HIV infection	13 (8)	5	2	<1
Suicide	12 (9)	16	23	22
Homicide	10 (10)	4	4	4
Liver disease	10 (11)	34 (8)	32	24
Renal disease	9 (12)	25 (9)	70 (8)	207 (9)
Septicemia	8 (13)	21 (10)	58 (9)	178 (10)
Atherosclerosis	7 (14)	11	46 (10)	278 (6)
Perinatal causes	6 (15)	0	0	0
All other causes	117			

[a]Deaths per 100,000 in all ages and order of incidence ( ) for the most common causes of mortality.
[b]Deaths per 100,000 in specified age group and order of incidence ( ) of the most common causes of mortality. (From National Center for Health Statistics. Monthly Vital Statistics Report, 1994;43(6).)

MORBIDITY

The presence of multiple chronic conditions increases with advancing age. In 1984, 35% of men and 45% of women 60–69 years of age reported two or more chronic conditions. In the older than 80 population, 53% of men and 70% of women reported two or more chronic conditions. These figures are reported from noninstitutionalized elderly.[4] The most common chronic conditions afflicting the elderly include arthritis, hypertension, hearing difficulties, and heart disease.[3] See Table 6.2 for rates and other causes of disease in the elderly. Heart disease is also responsible for more physician office visits, hospital days, and deaths than any other problem experienced by the elderly.[5]

Elderly persons have fewer psychiatric problems in terms of incidence, with the exception of the dementias, than other age groups. Alzheimer's disease (AD) is the leading cause and the primary mental health problem of the elderly. Advancing age correlates clearly with development of AD. Prevalence figures for AD are 3.0% for those 65–74, 18.7% for those 75–84, and 47.2% for persons 85 and older.[6]

Delirium, defined as an acute confusional state, often plagues the elderly. Delirium was present on hospital admission in approximately 15% of patients admitted to a general medical service.[7] Delirium subsequently develops in approximately 5–10% of patients who are not delirious on admission.

Depression is the other major mental health problem of the elderly. Approximately 20% of the healthy elderly report at least one depressive episode after age 65.[8] Individuals older than 65 years comprise only 12.4% of the total U.S. population, yet they are responsible for 25% of completed suicides.[9]

FUNCTIONAL STATUS

Most elderly people view their own health as good; 69% of the elderly persons living in the community considered their own health as good to excellent compared with others their own age. Only 31% reported their health as being fair or poor.[10] A full 60% had no limitation in activity. Only 25% had some mild degree of functional disability. As age increases, so do disabilities, such that by age 85, limitations in activity occur more commonly. Still, only 50% of those older than 85 report some mild degree of functional disability. The relatively good health of most elders living within the community differs dramatically from the small minority residing in nursing homes. Approximately 5% of individuals older than 65 are in nursing homes. About 40% of all elderly experience some difficulty with at least one *activity of daily living* (ADL) (Table 6.3). Nearly 75% of elderly with impairment in four or more ADLs resided in nursing homes in 1987.[11]

TABLE 6.2. INCIDENCE OF COMMON CHRONIC CONDITIONS REPORTED BY GENDER AND AGE IN THE NONINSTITUTIONALIZED POPULATION PER 100,000 PERSONS IN 1991

	Number of People with Condition/100,000 Population					
	Men			Women		
Condition	45–64	65–74	≥75	45–64	65–74	≥75
Arthritis	193.2	335.5	481.3	284.7	498.4	630.9
Chronic bronchitis	41.6	56.2	40.3	65.2	56.2	50.5
Asthma	33.7	34.1	30.2	47.2	41.2	39.4
Emphysema	17.2	52.8	50.3	8.6	16.5	20.9
Hearing loss	178.5	330.6	436.6	107.0	214.1	383.9
Vision loss	63.5	72.6	133.8	32.7	44.0	101.2
Speech impairment	9.6	8.6	19.9	10.5	4.2	14.6
Paralysis of extremities (complete or partial)	9.5	8.8	23.3	4.8	7.8	22.6
Hypertension	242.4	319.4	281.0	254.4	422.8	415.6
Heart disease	152.7	290.4	324.2	116.9	229.1	372.2
Cerebrovascular disease	12.9	63.4	77.0	19.0	54.1	66.3
Ulcer 25.2	26.0	43.0	27.1	23.1	23.8	
Frequent constipation	8.1	29.6	71.4	29.3	50.9	97.4
Thyroid disease	4.4	13.1	14.8	50.4	71.8	47.9
Diabetes	57.9	97.3	95.1	57.0	109.0	91.1
Kidney disease	16.7	18.0	23.7	17.9	27.9	29.9

(From National Center for Health Statistics. Vital and Health Statistics, 1992:10(184)84).

Thus, the majority of elderly in the United States are functioning without assistance. In 1985, 80% of adults reported no impairment in ADLs. This is expected to decrease to 70% as the population ages.[12] The most affected ADL is continence of urine. Incontinence is reported in approximately 9% of individuals 65–74 and in 17% of individuals older than 75.[13] Impairment of the remaining ADLs occurs less frequently, in this order: bathing, dressing, transferring, using the toilet, and eating. (See Table 6.3 for rates of impairment for these ADLs.)

PHYSIOLOGIC AGING VERSUS PATHOLOGIC AGING

Normal aging in the absence of disease is a remarkably benign process. The process occurs as a continuum with marked individual variability. Whether a particular manifestation in an elderly individual represents physiologic aging or a pathologic consequence is often impossible to determine. For instance, senescence reflects the expression of a variety of interacting influences including genetic pre-

TABLE 6.3. SELF-REPORTED DEFICITS IN PERSONS 65 YEARS AND OLDER IN THE UNITED STATES

	Number of People/1000 Population	
Activities of Daily Living	Age 65–74 Years	Age 75 Years or More
Bathing	35.2	106.5
Dressing	29.3	66.0
Using the toilet	12.4	39.3
Continence of urine	92.2	172.9
Getting in and out of bed or chair	17.7	46.6
Eating	6.3	17.5

(From National Center for Health Statistics, Vital and Health Statistics, 1989:10(167)7.)

implicated in drug-induced ulcerations.[28] An age-related component to the chronic constipation that afflicts so many elderly is unclear. Last, the incidence of diverticulum formation in the colon increases with age.

GENITOURINARY SYSTEMS

The genitourinary tract atrophies during aging. In women, decreased estrogen causes atrophy of the vagina. Symptoms of atrophic vaginitis such as itching, discomfort, burning, dyspareunia, and even vaginal bleeding as the epithelium thins may develop. Loss of uterine support with subsequent uterine descensus may also occur. Estrogen-replacement therapy effectively treats most of these symptoms. In men, prostate hypertrophy is a common consequence of aging that parallels age-associated alterations in androgens and dihydrotestosterone concentrations. By the eighth decade, 90% experience hypertrophy, and about 25% of these men will require treatment.[29]

Age-related changes in the genitourinary tract may predispose older individuals to incontinence. Inability to control voiding is pathologic and warrants medical attention. Incontinence afflicts 15–30% of community-dwelling elderly and approximately 50% of nursing home residents.[30]

HEPATIC SYSTEM

Liver size, weight, and blood flow decline with age. Older subjects experience a 41% decrease in liver volume per kilogram of total body weight and a 47% reduction in weight-adjusted hepatic blood flow.[31] Age-related decreases in albumin concentrations have been reported. Controversy exists over whether activity of the metabolic enzyme systems of the liver decreases with age. Antipyrine, a drug with low hepatic extraction metabolized exclusively by oxidative pathways, is frequently used to quantify hepatic enzyme function. Studies of drug metabolism have documented decreased antipyrine clearance with aging, suggesting a decrease in phase I reactions (oxidation–reduction reactions) in the elderly.[33] Little or no change occurs during phase II reactions (conjugation reactions) as a result of normal aging.[34]

IMMUNE SYSTEM AND INFECTIONS

Infections are a major cause of morbidity and mortality in the elderly. A variety of changes occur in the aging immune system. In addition, changes may vary with the health status of the individual. Cell-mediated immunity declines with aging. Alterations in cell-mediated immunity may result in negative antigen skin tests, reduced contact sensitivity, and increased tumor incidence. Zoster (shingles—an eruption of herpes zoster) is a common problem in the elderly, and diminished cellular immunity is believed contributory. Changes in humoral immunity occur but do not appear to be clinically important. Response to vaccines does not decline in healthy elderly. However, elderly with some diseases experience altered antibody responses to vaccines. They exhibit a delay in rise in titers, lower maximum responses, an earlier decline in titers, and decreases in seroconversion.[35]

Aging of the immune system may contribute to the increased susceptibility of the elderly to infectious diseases and cancer. Impaired immunity in itself cannot explain the increased incidence of infections in the elderly. Other factors contributing to the increased susceptibility of infections include decreased pulmonary function and cough reflex, decreased gastric activity and gastrointestinal motility, atherosclerosis and decreased capillary blood flow, thin skin, decreased mobility, inadequate nutrition and hydration, lack of recent immunizations, cognitive impairment, chronic disease, institutionalization, and placement of invasive devices (i.e., urinary catheters, nasogastric tubes).[36]

RENAL SYSTEM

The total number of glomeruli decreases by 30–40% by the eighth decade.[37] There is a continuous loss of glomeruli with aging, which has substantial impact on renal function. A cross-sectional study demonstrated a 46% decline in insulin clearance from ages 20 to 90.[38] Similarly, a longitudinal study demonstrated a decline in creatinine clearance but without an increase in serum creatinine.[39] No alteration in serum creatinine suggests that decreasing muscle mass with aging parallels decreasing creatinine clearance. This finding emphasizes the necessity of estimating creatinine clearance as opposed to simply following serum creatinine measurements in the elderly. A decline in creatinine clearance of 0.75 mL/min/yr was observed in men with no underlying renal disease.[40] Of particular interest was identification of three distinct groups:

- Those with significantly decreased creatinine clearance
- Those with small but significantly decreased creatinine clearance
- Those with no decrease in creatinine clearance

Other important physiologic changes in the kidney include decreased renal blood flow, decreased tubular function, and decreased ability to concentrate. Basal renin is diminished by 30–50% in older individuals. Renin alterations and other renal changes diminish the capability of the older adult to maintain sodium and water balance especially in the presence of stresses.[41]

RESPIRATORY SYSTEM

Normal aging of the lungs includes decreased total alveolar surface, loss of elastic recoil, decline in chest wall compliance, and decreased respiratory muscle strength. Forced vital capacity (FVC) decreases by 14–30 mL/yr, and forced expiratory volume at 1 second (FEV_1) decreases by 23–32 mL/yr in men who have never smoked. The decline in women is slightly less.[42] These alterations produce generally insignificant abnormalities in pulmonary function under normal conditions. However, these changes increase the risk of pulmonary disease and compromise pulmonary function when the lungs are stressed. In addition, loss of an effective cough reflex may occur with aging.

SENSES

A variety of visual changes occur as a person ages. A diminution of accommodation of the lens of the eye (presbyopia) occurs normally during aging, producing farsightedness, which can be improved with corrective lenses. Night vision is diminished in part because of the failure of pupils to dilate, crystalline lens discoloration and opacification, increased light scatter, slower dark adaptation, increased reaction time, and perceptual delays. Although many changes occur in the aging eye in the absence of disease, visual acuity declines very little, visual fields remain full, and night vision declines only slightly. Serious visual impairment is usually a function of disease as opposed to normal aging. Most commonly, cataracts, glaucoma, and diabetes mellitus are contributory in the elderly with major visual deficits.[43]

Loss of auditory acuity (presbycusis) also plagues many elderly individuals. Men suffer more frequently than women.[44] The elderly more often complain of difficulty understanding speech in contrast to difficulty hearing sounds. Speech understanding diminishes as well as pure tone sensitivity.[45]

Alterations in taste include a diminished ability to taste sweetness, sourness, and bitterness, but not saltiness. Touch sensitivity decreases with age. The elderly often experience a decreased thirst response, which may contribute to an increase in dehydration in aging.

SKELETAL SYSTEM

A progressive, linear loss of average skeletal bone mass (osteopenia) accompanies aging. Osteoporosis, a loss of trabecular mass primarily of the axial skeleton, occurs frequently in aging. The vertebral bodies and the bones of the wrist and hip are most affected. The loss of bone mass accelerated in postmenopausal women occurs at a rate of 1–2% per year. Approximately 50% of bone mass is lost by the eighth decade.[46] Osteoporosis predisposes the older patients to fractures from falls.

SKIN AND SOFT TISSUES

The major gross morphologic changes in the aging skin are dryness, wrinkling, and uneven pigmentation. The epithelial layer of the skin becomes thin and the support tissues lose their elasticity. There is a 20% loss in dermal thickness. The remaining skin is relatively avascular and acellular. The turnover of epidermal cells is reduced by 50% between the third and eighth decade.[47]

Vitamin D synthesis in the skin is markedly reduced. Vitamin D deficiencies in the elderly are often exacerbated by decreased time spent in sunlight and decreased dairy product intake.

The number of hair follicles decrease with aging, as do the number of melanocytes with each hair bulb, the result being thinner, gray or white hair. Long-term sun exposure can accelerate these age-related changes and is also responsible for 90% of skin cancers. Minor trauma is more likely to break the integrity of the skin in the older individual. Scratching to ameliorate itching secondary to senile pruritus may further diminish the integrity of the skin. Immobility produces stress on the skin surfaces and frequently results in pressure ulcers. Decreased dermal thickness also contributes to the elderly patient's diminished thermoregulatory capacity.

EFFECTS OF AGING ON PHARMACOTHERAPY

The elderly are particularly vulnerable to the effects of drugs because of the changes that accompany aging and are more likely to experience adverse effects[48,49] that can lead to worsening health and decreased quality of life. Adverse drug reactions may result in hospitalization[50,51] or death.[52] Drug therapy should be appropriate, effective, and safe to avoid adverse outcomes. Physiologic changes in aging make these goals more difficult to attain. Knowledge of the impact of physiologic changes that occur with aging is necessary to prevent adverse outcomes in the elderly. The elderly are susceptible to problems associated with drug-taking behavior (compliance), pharmacokinetics, and pharmacodynamics. An understanding of the interrelationships between these influences is essential to the development of rational drug therapy. Table 6.4 summarizes selected age-related changes in functioning organ systems and their impact on compliance, pharmacokinetics, and pharmacodynamics that are described in the following sections.

COMPLIANCE

The most appropriate and effective therapy has little utility if medication is not taken as prescribed. Thus, careful monitoring must focus on compliance issues. Compliance rates in the elderly vary from 26–59%.[53] The elderly are at great risk for noncompliance. Although age alone is a poor predictor of

TABLE 6.4. SELECTED AGE-RELATED CHANGES THAT AFFECT PHARMACOTHERAPY

Factor	Potential Age-Related Influences
Compliance	Cognitive impairment
	Decreased vision
	Decreased hearing
	Diminished strength
Pharmacokinetics	
Absorption	Increased GI pH
	Decreased gastric blood flow
	Decreased active transport mechanisms
	Decreased GI motility
	Decreased first-pass metabolism
Distribution	Decreased total body water
	Increased adipose tissue
	Decreased lean muscle mass
	Decreased albumin
	Increased α-1-acid glycoprotein
Metabolism	Decreased liver blood flow
	Decreased liver size
	Decreased phase I metabolism
Excretion	Decreased glomerular filtration rate
	Decreased renal blood flow
	Decreased tubular function
Pharmacodynamics	Decreased sensitivity of beta receptors
	Decreased sensitivity of baroreceptors
	Increased warfarin response
	Increased benzodiazepine response

such behavior, other characteristics common to this population are good predictors. Factors associated with noncompliance include female sex, lower socioeconomic status, living alone, lack of a support system, multiple drug use, complicated drug regimens, and multiple diseases.[54] Factors associated with noncompliance-related hospitalization in the elderly included poor recall of drug regimens, seeing numerous physicians, using numerous drugs, and believing that drugs are expensive.[51] Strategies to simplify the regimen and improve communication are of paramount importance in improving compliance. The fewest number of drugs and fewest number of doses per day should be used whenever possible. Drugs no longer needed should be discontinued.

In addition, physical impairments can complicate compliance with medications. Cognitive, hearing, and visual impairment can limit many patients' abilities to comply. Providing written materials can emphasize and clarify oral directives. Grip strength in the elderly can be diminished from stroke, arthritis, or generalized frailty, creating problems with opening medication containers. Disorders that cause tremors can also interfere with successful medication administration. Inability to open containers can lead to inappropriate storage, keeping multiple drugs in one container, and mislabeling from storage of drugs in old containers, all of which can produce adverse outcomes through subsequent noncompliance.

Further, older patients may experience difficulty breaking tablets, measuring liquids, shaking liquids, administering eyedrops, using metered-dose inhalers, measuring and injecting insulin, and using home-monitoring equipment because of a variety of physical and cognitive deficits secondary to aging or comorbid conditions. Patient demonstration of bottle opening and label reading should be used to assess patient capabilities.[55] Ability to use difficult dosage forms such as metered-dose inhalers should also be demonstrated and evaluated.

PHARMACOKINETICS

Once compliance is optimized, success is not guaranteed. Physiologic changes of aging can affect drug absorption, distribution, metabolism, and elimination, resulting in adverse events. An in-depth review is beyond the scope of the chapter, and the reader is encouraged to seek previously published information.[28] A major goal of drug therapy in the elderly is the attainment of a desired steady-state drug concentration within a proven therapeutic range established specifically for the elderly population, as follows:

$$C_{ss} = \frac{\text{Dose} \times F}{\text{CL} \times \tau} \quad (1)$$

where C_{ss} = steady-state drug concentration, F = fraction of drug, CL = clearance, and τ = dosing interval. If this goal is accomplished, there is a greater potential for beneficial effects than adverse effects. The clinician seeks a dose that adjusts for age-related changes and produces the desired steady-state concentration. Aging can affect this equation in several ways.

The bioavailability (F) of a drug can be altered by decreasing or increasing the absorption. Bioavailability alterations will produce parallel changes in steady-state concentrations if other parameters remain constant. Little information exists regarding age and absorption from routes of administration other than oral drug administration. Consequently, this discussion refers only to drugs administered orally. As mentioned previously, several aging changes occur within the GI tract that could affect the extent (peak concentration) and rate (time to peak concentration) of absorption of drugs. Although a delay in gastric emptying time would be expected to produce a decreased rate in absorption, the extent of absorption would not likely be decreased. Generally, the age-related GI changes in absorption are not clinically important other than for some drug product formulation and chemical characteristics. For example, decreased acidity associated with aging would probably have an adverse effect on the dissolution rates of acidic drugs (e.g., ketoconazole). Drugs less stable in an acidic environment may experience less degradation (e.g., penicillin, erythromycin).

Splanchnic blood flow—including portal and hepatic arterial flow—is decreased in aging.[56] Diminished blood flow may affect absorption of drugs that undergo extensive first-pass hepatic metabolism. For example, the systemic bioavailability of levodopa,[57] propranolol,[58] and lidocaine[59] is greater in the elderly because of decreased first-pass hepatic metabolism. In conclusion, with the exception of drugs with extensive first-pass metabolism, alterations in absorption are usually not clinically important. To avoid adverse outcomes that may not be anticipated practitioners should start with low doses and titrate doses slowly in the elderly.

Volume of distribution (V_D) can be substantially affected by age. V_D may be affected by plasma protein binding, lipid–water solubility, and drug binding in the tissues. Changes in body composition with aging result in decreased V_D for water-soluble drugs and increased V_D for lipid-soluble drugs. Changes in V_D can influence concentration, and elimination half-life ($t_{1/2}$) as follows:

$$V_D = \frac{\text{Dose}}{C_{ss}} \tag{2}$$

$$t_{1/2} = \frac{0.693\ (V_D)}{\text{CL}} \tag{3}$$

Lipophilic drugs such as diazepam have a significantly increased V_D because of the increase in adipose tissue that occurs with normal aging. Hydrophilic drugs such as acetaminophen have a reduced V_D secondary to the age-related decrease in total body water.[60]

The decrease in albumin with aging is important because albumin is a major site of drug binding. This decrease is even more pronounced in frail elderly. With aging, serum albumin is diminished and thus the potential is increased for decreased binding of certain drugs and resultant increased plasma free (unbound) fraction. The importance of this increased free fraction is questionable because, while more free drug is available for receptor binding, more free drug is also available for metabolism and elimination. As a result, a new equilibrium in drug disposition is quickly reached. Important to note is that exceptions may occur. Certain drugs (e.g., naproxen) may exhibit an increased plasma free fraction and decreased total clearance.[61]

Alpha-1-acid glycoprotein (AAG) also binds to some drugs. An acute-phase reactant, AAG can be increased with age, but especially so in persons who are acutely ill. Clinically important alterations have been reported in lidocaine[62] and propranolol.[63,64] In these circumstances, decreased protein binding can potentially influence pharmacologic activity. Other protein-binding factors—such as displacement by other drugs or displacement by drug metabolites—may also contribute to changes in binding that occur with aging. Half-life ($t_{1/2}$) may change if altered protein-binding effects are not compensated for by clearance and V_D. Dosage adjustments may be necessary when drugs have a narrow therapeutic index.

Total clearance, a biologically independent variable, characterizes the ability of body organs to remove a drug from the blood. It is expressed as the amount of blood from which a drug is completely removed per unit of time. The rate of clearance is determined from the amount of blood that can be delivered to a clearing organ, as well as the intrinsic ability of the organ to remove the drug from the blood. Physiologic changes that decrease delivery of blood to an organ—such as a decrease in cardiac output—can decrease the amount of drug cleared. Clearance can be calculated from V_D and $t_{1/2}$ by rearranging equation 3. The pharmokinetic variable $t_{1/2}$ depends on both CL and V_D. Aging affects this variable mainly through changes in the intrinsic function of the major drug-clearing organs, the liver and the kidney. As stated previously, phase I enzymatic reactions are subject to greater age-related changes than phase II enzymatic reactions. Drugs with increased V_D and decreased hepatic CL secondary to oxidative biotransformation (e.g., diazepam) may significantly prolong $t_{1/2}$ in the elderly.[65] Consequently, diazepam, chlordiazepoxide, and flurazepam should be avoided. If a benzodiazepine is required, lorazepam, oxazepam, or temazepam is generally preferred in the elderly. Gender and environmental influences such as smoking also contribute to age-related changes in $t_{1/2}$.

Aging can affect renal clearance and subsequently $t_{1/2}$ when drugs are eliminated via the kidneys. Prediction of the effect of age-related changes in renal function upon drug clearance is difficult because of the great degree of individuality in changes in renal function. As a result, no prediction of renal function can be made on the basis of age alone. The renal function of each elderly individual must be measured or appropriately estimated using nomograms or equations that take into account the patient's age. The generally accepted method for estimating creatinine clearance (CL_{cr}) is the Cockcroft–Gault equation as follows[66]:

$$\text{CL}_{cr} = \frac{(140 - \text{Age}) \times \text{WT}}{72 \times S_{cr}} \tag{4}$$

where S_{cr} = serum creatinine concentration (in mg/mL) and WT = weight in kilograms. The CL_{cr} for women is obtained by multiplying the results of this calculation by 0.85.

In general, the otherwise healthy aging kidney is capable of maintaining normal acid–base status, electrolyte balance, and drug clearance. For example, no significant differences in V_D, CL, or $t_{1/2}$ were determined in bacteremia of otherwise healthy young patients versus old patients receiving gentamicin.[67] Despite these findings, the aging kidney is at greater risk for nephrotoxicity because it has fewer functioning nephrons; it has lost a portion of its reserve capacity.

To avoid adverse outcomes from drugs that are renally eliminated, clinicians are referred to the product labeling or drug information texts that contain specific dosage recommendations for different levels of renal impairment. For example, if a patient is to receive ranitidine, the creatinine clearance should be calculated using the Cockcroft–Gault equation to estimate renal function because ranitidine is significantly eliminated via the kidneys. The product labeling suggests decreasing the dose of ranitidine from 150 mg twice daily to 150 mg once daily when the creatinine clearance is less than 50 mL/min.[68] Adjusting the dose will prevent accumulation and potential adverse events from decreased clearance (drug in is reduced to equal drug out). In dosage adjustments for renal impairment the dosage interval is usually increased, as opposed to decreasing the dose and keeping the interval constant.

For some drugs, this interval can become prolonged and calculated dosage intervals may become impractical, such as every 18 to 36 hours. Generally compliance is best when dosage regimens conform to once daily, once every 2 or 3 days, or once on certain days of the week.

PHARMACODYNAMICS

Despite dosage adjustments for age-related pharmacokinetic changes and attainment of desired therapeutic drug concentrations, alterations in drug effects can occur secondary to altered pharmacodynamics in aging. Simply stated, equal concentrations of drug at receptor sites in young and old individuals produce differing effects. With aging, changes can occur because of increased or decreased receptor sensitivity, decreased cellular viability, or decreased homeostatic mechanisms.[69]

The etiology of such pharmacodynamic changes is unclear but probably relates to altered receptor function or decreased numbers of receptors. Examples of pharmacodynamic changes in the elderly include an increased depression of the central nervous system with diazepam,[70] increased warfarin effects from a decreased production of vitamin K-dependent clotting factors,[71] decreased sensitivity to the short-term effects of verapamil on cardiac conduction,[72] and decreased sensitivity to β-adrenergic stimulation and blockade.[73] Age-related alterations in pharmacodynamics have not been well-studied. As with age-related pharmacokinetics the effects of age appear to vary. To avoid adverse outcomes from unknown effects, the rule of starting with low doses and titrating slowly upward until the desired effect is achieved applies once again.

Greater knowledge of the compliance, pharmacokinetic, and pharmacodynamic effects of age-related changes should lower the incidence of adverse events. Some resulting general rules for geriatric pharmacotherapy can be developed:

1. Start low and increase slowly.
2. Remember that $t_{1/2}$ of many drugs is often prolonged in the elderly.
3. Rapid dose escalations do not allow for evaluation of the maximal response because the patient has not reached steady state.
4. Use the fewest number of drugs possible.
5. Look for toxicity.
6. As with atypical presentation of the disease, adverse drug events may be atypical in the elderly.
7. Pay particular attention to CNS changes because they may be a marker for toxicity.

GERIATRIC PATIENT CARE ISSUES

GERIATRIC ASSESSMENT

Despite effective treatment, the frail elderly often experience a cascade of events during acute care hospitalization. These individuals often develop physical and cognitive impairment associated with confusion, immobility, incontinence, and malnutrition. In attempting to interrupt the downward spiral of impairment in these patients, geriatric assessment teams have been developed. Comprehensive geriatric assessment is defined as a multidisciplinary evaluation in which the multiple problems of an older person are uncovered, described, and explained if possible, and in which the resources and strengths of the person are catalogued, the need for services assessed, and a coordinated care plan developed to focus interventions on each person's problems.

The goals of geriatric assessment are

1. To improve in diagnostic accuracy
2. To guide the selection of interventions to restore or preserve health
3. To recommend an optimal environment for care
4. To predict outcomes
5. To monitor clinical change over time

The core of the geriatric assessment team consists, at a minimum, of a physician, nurse, and social worker. Other participating professions often include dentistry, occupational therapy, pharmacy, physical therapy, podiatry, psychiatry/psychology, and speech therapy.[74] Roles for the pharmacist to fulfill in the geriatric assessment team include drug-regimen review, which is required under federal law for all nursing home patients on a monthly basis. Pharmacists screen patients for potential age-related changes that affect compliance, pharmacokinetics, and pharmacodynamics of drugs and make recommendations to avoid or minimize adverse outcomes related to pharmacotherapy. In addition, patient and/or caregiver assessment and counseling are paramount to ensuring compliance with medication regimens.

In the hospitalized elderly, the movement away from the traditional medical model of curing disease to an interdisciplinary evaluative model of managing disease has been demonstrated to improve function, decrease the risk of nursing home placement, and improve survival.[75,76] Assessment should include evaluation of the several domains, most commonly physical, cognitive, psychosocial, environmental, and economic.[77] Multiple tests are available to quantify these domains. A few of the commonly encountered tools are listed as follows.

Physical functioning is commonly measured by the Katz ADLs,[78] Instrumental ADLs,[79] and the Timed "Up and Go" Test.[80] Brief mental status assessments include the Folstein's Mini-Mental State Exam (MMSE)[81] and the Pfeiffer Short-Portable Mental Status Questionnaire (SP-MSQ).[82] Examples of quality of life assessment tools include the Medical Outcomes Study Short Form-36 (MOS-36)[83] and the Geriatric Depression Scale (GDS).[84] In the nursing home patient, regulations mandate that a minimum data set (MDS) be maintained on each resident. The purpose of the MDS is to screen and document the patient assessment information from various disciplines regarding cognitive functioning, ADLs, skin condition, drug use, and so on.[85]

The impact of medications on an elderly individual's domains is important. When a medication is used to treat chronic disease, not only must it produce the desired therapeutic effect, but it should also enhance or maintain the patient's quality of life and functional status. The results of these monitoring and screening tools can provide invaluable information about the patient's functional ability. For example, if a patient has a MMSE of 20 (scores less than 24 usually represent significant cognitive impairment), alternative arrangements for medication self-administration will be needed. In addition, results of tests may assist with monitoring the safety and efficacy of drug therapy. Adverse effects such as incontinence can be detected with routine monitoring of ADLs. Finally, effectiveness of antidepressants can be measured by improvements in quality of life scales.

LONG-TERM CARE

Although only 5% of the elderly population resides in a long-term care facility (LTCF), most in nursing homes, this number is expected to increase substantially as the population ages and becomes more disabled. The impact of geographically dispersed families and working women will also contribute to the need for more LTCF beds.

Historically, the care of LTCF patients has been substandard. Fewer than 10% of all physicians see patients in nursing homes. The physician visits are infrequent and often brief. Medical records are scanty. Many medical problems are often underdiagnosed and misdiagnosed. In addition, the care provided to LTCF residents is often provided by unlicensed nursing personnel with limited education.[86]

LTCF residents are older (median age 83), women, and white. In 1985, 22% of all individuals 85 years and older were residing in LTCFs.[87] Nearly 75% of the elderly LTCF residents receive three or more drugs, and 45% receive five or more drugs.[88] Psychotropic overuse and misuse occur frequently.[89] Regulations and legislation have been enacted to resolve some of these problems. The role of the pharmacist was increased in 1987 to require monthly drug-regimen review in all nursing home residents. Multiple studies of pharmacist-conducted drug-regimen review have demonstrated benefits. Findings have included a decrease in number of medications per patient, nursing time spent on drug administration, hospitalizations, cost of medications, and antipsychotic drug use.[90] The reader interested in consultant pharmacy practice is referred elsewhere for guidelines for drug-regimen review, indicators for drug-regimen review, survey methodology for detecting medication errors, and regulations from the Omnibus Budget Reconciliation Act (OBRA) of 1987.[91]

HOSPITALIZATION OF THE ELDERLY PATIENT

Although it is generally assumed hospitals help sick people to recover, in the case of the elderly patient, hospitalization may be hazardous to the patient's health. For many persons, hospitalization can lead to an often irreversible decline in functional status and quality of life. Iatrogenic illness is common among hospitalized elderly. Bedrest may be contributory. Bedrest can lead to orthostatic intolerance, decreased exercise capacity, atelectasis, pneumonia, decreased muscle strength and contractures, osteoporosis, pressure ulcers, compression neuropathy, constipation, hypercalcemia, functional urinary incontinence, depression, and anxiety.[92] The risk of nosocomial infections is increased in this population and may be partially explained by increased length of hospitalization.

Multiple medication use is common in this setting as well. Medication has been implicated in the development of iatrogenic illnesses in 18% of hospitalized elderly.[93] This finding is not surprising since elderly hospitalized patients receive an average of eight medications.[94] Adverse effects from drug use during hospitalization occur, in part from inaccurate or incomplete drug histories, addition of problematic "routine" medications, and altered physiologic changes in pharmacokinetics and pharmacodynamics.[92]

CONCLUSION

The contribution of aging toward health status is an issue that all health care practitioners now face. Important to understand are physiologic age-related changes and common diseases that affect compliance, pharmacokinetics, and pharmacodynamics of drug therapy in the elderly to ensure that drug therapy is appropriate, safe, and effective in this population. In addition, the clinician must remember that this population is heterogeneous and therapy must be individualized in the elderly. Aging is but another increasingly common, confounding variable in our efforts to meet this responsibility.

References

1. Monthly Vital Statistics Report. Hyattsville, MD, National Center for Health Statistics, 1994;43(6).
2. U.S. Senate Special Committee on Aging. Aging America. Trends and projections. Washington, DC, U.S. Department of Health and Human Services, 1985–86.
3. Monthly Vital Statistics Report. Hyattsville, MD, National Center for Health Statistics, 1994;43(6).
4. Vital and Health Statistics. Hyattsville, MD, National Center for Health Statistics Advanced Data, 1989(May);17.
5. Public Health Service. Hyattsville, MD, U.S. Department of Health and Human Services, 1990. DHHS Pub. No. (PHS) 91-1232.
6. Evans DA, Funkenstein HH, Albert MS, et al. Prevalence of Alzheimer's disease in a community of older persons: Higher than previously reported. JAMA 1989;262:2551–2556.
7. Francis J, Kapoor WN. Delirium in hospitalized elderly. J Gen Intern Med 1990;5:65–79.
8. The Families USA Foundation. Three Year Report, 1986–1987–1988. Washington, DC.
9. Sendbuehler J, Goldstein S. Attempted suicides among the aged. J Am Geriatr Soc 1977;25:245–248.
10. Aging America. Trends and Projections. Washington, DC, U.S. Department of Health and Human Services, 1987–88.
11. Feinleib S, Cunningham P, Short P. Use of nursing and personal care homes by the civilian population, 1987. National Medical Expenditure Survey Findings 23, Agency for Health Care Policy and Research. Rockville, MD, Public Health Service. AHCPR Pub. No. 94-0096.
12. Manton KG. Epidemiological, demographic, and social correlates of disability among the elderly. Milbank Q 1989;67:13–58.
13. Vital and Health Statistics. Hyattsville, MD, National Center for Health Statistics, 1989(Mar);10(107).
14. Evans JG, Williams TG (eds): Oxford Textbook of Geriatric Medicine. New York, Oxford University Press, 1992.
15. Hazzard WR, Bierman EL, Blass FP, et al. (eds): Principles of Geriatric Medicine and Gerontology, 3rd ed. New York, McGraw-Hill, 1994.
16. Fulop T, Worum I, Csongor J, Foris G, Leovey A. Body composition in elderly people. Gerontology 1985;31:6–14.
17. Rodeheffer RJ, Gerstenblith G, Becker LC, et al. Exercise cardiac output is maintained with advance age in healthy subjects. Cardiac dilation and increased stroke volume compensate for a diminished heart rate. Circulation 1984;69:202–213.
18. Lakatta EG. Alterations in circulatory function, in Hazzard WR, Bierman EL, Blass FP, et al. (eds): Principles of Geriatric Medicine and Gerontology, 3rd ed. New York, McGraw-Hill, 1994, pp 493–508.
19. Lipsitz LA. Orthostatic hypotension in the elderly. N Engl J Med 1989;321:952–957.
20. Albert MS. Cognition and aging, in Hazzard WR, Bierman EL, Blass FP, et al. (eds): Principles of Geriatric Medicine and Gerontology, 3rd ed. New York, McGraw-Hill, 1994, pp 1013–1019.
21. Davis PJ, Katz PR. Disorders of the thyroid gland, in Evans JG, Williams TG (eds): Oxford Textbook of Geriatric Medicine. New York, Oxford University Press, 1992, pp 140–148.
22. Marshburn PB, Carr BR. The menopause and hormone replacement therapy, in Hazzard WR, Bierman EL, Blass FP, et al. (eds): Principles of Geriatric Medicine and Gerontology, 3rd ed. New York, McGraw-Hill, 1994, 867–878.
23. Morrow LA, Herman WH, Halter JB. Diabetes mellitus, in Evans JG, Williams TG, (eds): Oxford Textbook of Geriatric Medicine. New York, Oxford University Press, 1992, pp 131–140.
24. Wolfson LI. Gait and mobility, in Evans JG, Williams TG (eds.): Oxford Textbook of Geriatric Medicine. New York, Oxford University Press, 1992, p 585.
25. Overstall PW, Exton-Smith AN, Imms FJ, Johnson AL. Falls in the elderly related to postural imbalance. Br Med J 1977;1:261–264.
26. Miller AJ, Brunelle JA, Carlos JP, et al. The National Survey of Oral Health in US Adults: 1985–1986. US Department of Health and Human Services, Public Health Service, National Institutes of Health. NIH Pub. No. 87-2868. Washington, DC, US Government Printing Office, 1987.
27. Baum BJ. Saliva secretion and composition, In Fergoson DB (ed): The Aging Mouth. Basel, Switzerland, Karger, 1987, p 126.
28. Mayersohn MB. Special pharmacokinetic considerations for the elderly, in Evans WE, Schentag JJ, Jusko WJ (eds): Applied Pharmacokinetics, 3rd ed. Vancouver WA, Applied Therapeutics, 1992, p 9-1–9-44.
29. Brendler CB. Disorders of the prostate, in Hazzard WR, Bierman EL, Blass FP, et al. (eds): Principles of Geriatric Medicine and Gerontology, 3rd ed. New York, McGraw-Hill, 1994, 657–664.
30. Diokno AD, Brock BM, Brown MB, Herzog AR. Prevalence of urinary incontinence and other urologic symptoms in the noninstitutionalized elderly. J Urol 1986;136:1022–1025.
31. Wynne HA, Cope LH, Mutch E, et al. The effect of age upon liver volume and apparent liver blood flow in healthy men. Hepatology 1989;9:297–301.
32. Greenblatt DJ. Reduced serum albumin concentration in the elderly: A report from the Boston Collaborative Drug Surveillance Program. J Am Geriatr Soc 1979;27:20–22.
33. Vestal RE, Norris AH, Tobin JD, et al. Antipyrine metabolism in man: influence of age, alcohol, caffeine, and smoking. Clin Pharmacol Ther 1975;18:425–432.
34. Greenblatt DJ, Divoll M, Harmatz JS, et al. Oxazepam kinetics: Influence and effects of age and sex. J Pharmacol Exp Ther 1980;215:86–91.
35. Fox RA. Immunology and ageing, in Evans JG, Williams TG (eds): Oxford Textbook of Geriatric Medicine. New York, Oxford University Press, 1992, pp 51–56.

36. Adler WH, Nagel JE. Clinical immunology and aging, in Hazzard WR, Bierman EL, Blass FP, et al. (eds): Principles of Geriatric Medicine and Gerontology, 3rd ed. New York: McGraw-Hill, 1994, pp 61–76.
37. Darmady EM, Offer J, Woodhouse MA. The parameters of the aging kidney. J Pathol 1973;109:195–207.
38. Davies DF, Shock NW. Age changes in glomerular filtration rate, effective renal plasma flow and tubular excretory capacity in adult males. J Clin Invest 1950;29:496–507.
39. Rowe JW, Andres R, Tobin JD, et al. The effects of age on creatinine clearance in man: A cross-sectional and longitudinal study. J Gerontol 1976;31:155–163.
40. Lindeman RD, Tobin J, Shock NW. Longitudinal studies on the rate of decline in renal function with age. J Am Geriatr Soc 1985;33:278–285.
41. Rowe JW. Nephrology and the genitourinary system, in Hazzard WR, Bierman EL, Blass FP, et al. (eds): Principles of Geriatric Medicine and Gerontology, 3rd ed. New York, McGraw-Hill, 1994, pp 425–431.
42. Ware JH, Dockery DW, Louis TA, et al. Longitudinal and cross-sectional estimates of pulmonary function decline in never-smoking adults. Am J Epidemiol 1992;132:685–700.
43. Michaels DD. The eye, in Hazzard WR, Bierman EL, Blass FP, et al (eds): Principles of Geriatric Medicine and Gerontology, 3rd ed. New York, McGraw-Hill, 1994, pp 441–456.
44. Gates GA. Hearing in the elderly: The Framingham cohort, 1983–1985. Ear Hear 1990;11:247.
45. Jerger J. Speech understanding in the elderly. Adv Otorhinolaryngol 1973;20:115–124.
46. Marshburn PB, Carr BR. The menopause and hormone replacement therapy, in Hazzard WR, Bierman EL, Blass FP, et al. (eds): Principles of Geriatric Medicine and Gerontology, 3rd ed. New York, McGraw-Hill, 1994, pp 867–878.
47. Lavker RM, Zheng P, Dong G. Morphology of aged skin. Clin Geriatr Med 1989;5:53–67.
48. Lindley CM, Tully MP, Paramsothy V, Tallis RC. Inappropriate medication is a major cause of adverse drug reactions in elderly patients. Age Ageing 1992;21:294–300.
49. Francis J, Martin D, Kapoor WN. A prospective study of delirium hospitalized elderly. JAMA 1990;263:1097–1101.
50. Gosney M, Tallis R. Prescriptions of contraindicated and interacting drugs in elderly patients admitted to hospital. Lancet 1984;2:564–567.
51. Col N, Fanale JE, Kronholm P. The role of medication noncompliance and adverse drug reactions in hospitalization of the elderly. Arch Intern Med 1990;150:841–845.
52. Williamson J, Chopin JM. Adverse reactions to prescribed drugs in the elderly: A multicenter investigation. Age Ageing 1980;9(2):73–80.
53. Coons SJ, Sheahan SL, Martin SS, et al. Predictors of medication noncompliance in a sample of older adults. Clin Ther 1994;16:110–118.
54. Fedder DO. Drug use in the elderly: Issues of noncompliance. Drug Intell Clin Pharm 1984;18:158–162.
55. Kazis LE, Friedman RH. Improving medication compliance in the elderly. Strategies for the health care provider. J Am Geriatr Soc 1988;36:1161–1162.
56. Sherlock S, Bearn AG, Billing GH, Paterson JCS. Splanchnic blood flow in man by bromsulfalein method: The relation of peripheral plasma by bromsulfalein level to the calculated flow. J Lab Clin Med 1950;35:923–932.
57. Robertson DRC, Wood ND, Everest H, et al. The effects of age on the pharmacokinetics of levodopa administration administered alone and in the presence of carbidopa. Br J Clin Pharmacol 1989;28:61–69.
58. Castledon CM, George CF. The effect of aging on the hepatic clearance of propranolol. Br J Clin Pharmacol 1979;7:49–54.
59. Cusack B, O'Malley K, Lavan J, Noel J, Kelly JG. Protein binding and disposition lignocaine in the elderly. Eur J Clin Pharmacol 1985;29:323–329.
60. Divoll M, Abernethy DR, Ameer B, Greenblatt DJ. Acetaminophen kinetics in the elderly. Clin Pharmacol Ther 1982;31:151–156.
61. Upton RA, Williams RL, Kelly J, Jones RM. Naproxen pharmacokinetics in the elderly. Br J Clin Pharmacol 1984;18:207–214.
62. Davis D, Grossman SH, Kitchell BB, Shand DC, Rutledge PA. Age related changes in the plasma protein binding of lidocaine and diazepam. Clin Res 1980;28:234A.
63. Lalonde RL, Tenero DM, Burlew BS, et al. Effects of age on protein binding and disposition of propranolol stereoisomer. Clin Pharmacol Ther 1990;47:447–455.
64. Paxton JW, Briant RH. Alpha-1-acid glycoprotein concentrations and propranolol binding in elderly patients with acute illness. Br J Clin Pharmacol 1984;18:806–810.
65. Klotz U, Avant GR, Hoyumpa A, et al. The effects of age and liver disease on the disposition and elimination of diazepam in adult man. J Clin Invest 1975;55:347–359.
66. Crockcroft DW, Gault MH. Prediction of creatinine clearance from serum creatinine. Nephron 1976;16:31–41.
67. Bauer LA, Blouin RA. Gentamicin pharmacokinetics: Effect of aging in patients with normal renal function. J Am Geriatr Soc 1982;30:309–311.
68. Semla TP, Beizer JL, Higbee MD (eds): Geriatric Dosing Handbook 1993–1994. Hudson, OH, Lexi-comp, 1993, p 624.
69. Feely J, Coakley D. Altered pharmacodynamics in the elderly. Clin Geriatr Med 1990;6:269–283.
70. Clinical depression of the central nervous system due to diazepam and chlordiazepoxide in relation to cigarette smoking and age: A report from the Boston Collaborative Drug Surveillance Program. N Engl J Med 1973;288:277–280.
71. Sheperd AMM, Hewick DS, Moreland TZ, Stevenson IH. Age as a determinant of sensitivity to warfarin. Br J Clin Pharmacol 1977;4:315–320.
72. Abernethy DR, Schwartz JB, Todd EL, et al. Verapamil pharmacodynamics and disposition in young and elderly hypertensive patients. Ann Intern Med 1986;105:329–336.
73. Vestal RE, Wood AJJ, Shand DG. Reduced β-adrenoreceptor sensitivity in the elderly. Clin Pharmacol Ther 1979;26:181–186.
74. National Institutes of Health Consensus Development Conference Panel. Geriatric assessment methods for clinical decision-making. J Am Geriatr Soc 1988;36:342–347.
75. Applegate WB, Miller ST, Graney MJ, et al. A randomized controlled trial of a geriatric assessment unit in a community rehabilitation hospital. N Engl J Med 1990;322:1572–1578.

76. Hogan DB, Fox RA. A prospective controlled trial of a geriatric consultation team. Age Ageing 1990;19:107–113.
77. Rubenstein LV, Calkins DR, Grainfield S, et al. Health status assessment for elderly patients. Report of the Society of General Internal Medicine task force on health assessment. J Am Geriatr Soc 1988;37:562–569.
78. Katz S, Ford AB, Moskowitz RW, et al. Studies of illness in the aged. The index of ADL: A standardized measure of biological and psychosocial function. JAMA 1963;185:914–919.
79. Lawton MP, Brody EM. Assessment of older people: Self-monitoring and instrumental activities of daily living. Gerontologist 1969;9:179–186.
80. Podsiadlo D, Richardson S. The timed "up and go": A test of basic functional mobility for frail elderly persons. J Am Geriatr Soc 1991;39:142–146.
81. Folstein MF, Folstein S, McHugh PR. Mini-mental state: A practical method for grading cognitive state of patients for the clinician. J Psychol Res 1975;12:189–198.
82. Pfeiffer E. A short portable mental status questionnaire for the assessment of organic brain deficit in elderly patients. J Am Geriatr Soc 1975;23:433–441.
83. Ware JE, Sherbourne CD. The MOS 36-item short-form health survey. I. Conceptual framework and item selection. Med Care 1992;30:473–483.
84. Shiekh JL. Yesavage JA. Geriatric depression scale (GDS): Recent evidence and development of a shorter version. Clin Gerontol 1986;5:165.
85. Gore MJ. Resident assessment and minimum data sets: What have they wrought? Consult Pharm 1992;7:1159–1164.
86. Ouslander JG. Nursing home care, in Hazzard WR, Bierman EL, Blass FP, et al. (eds): Principles of Geriatric Medicine and Gerontology, 3rd ed. New York, McGraw-Hill, 1994, pp 357–374.
87. Hing E, Sekscenski E, Strahan G. The national nursing home survey: 1985 summary for the United States. Vital & Health Statistics, Hyattsville, MD, National Center for Health Statistics, 1990, 13(97).
88. National Disease and Therapeutic Index. A medical profile of the over-65 population. Philadelphia, IMS America, 1991.
89. Beers M, Avorn J, Soumerai SH, et al. Psychoactive medication use in intermediate care facility residents. JAMA 1988;260:3016–3020.
90. Kidder SW. Cost-benefit of pharmacist-conducted drug-regimen reviews. Consult Pharm 1987;2:394–398.
91. Erwin WG (ed). Drug regimen review: A process guide for pharmacists. Alexandria, VA, American Society of Consultant Pharmacists, 1996.
92. Gorbien MJ, Bishop J, Beers MH, et al. Iatrogenic illness in hospitalized elderly people. J Am Geriatr Soc 1992;40:1021–1042.
93. Steel K, Gertman PM, Crescenzi C, Anderson J. Iatrogenic illness on a general medical service at a university hospital. N Engl J Med 1981;304:639–642.
94. May FE, Stewart RB, Cluff LE. Drug interactions and multiple drug administration. Clin Pharmacol Ther 1977;22:322–328.

Chapter 7

Adverse Drug Reactions and Interactions

J. Russell May, PharmD, FASHP

Adverse drug reactions and drug interactions represent the negative consequences of pharmacotherapy. A thorough knowledge of how the adverse reactions and drug interactions occur will aid in our ability to provide the best patient care possible. This chapter reviews the magnitude of this problem and provides some historical perspective. Adverse drug reactions and drug interactions are defined and mechanisms of how they occur are discussed; ways to identify, assess, manage, and report these reactions are presented. The importance of postmarketing surveillance is highlighted.

Magnitude of the Problem

Drug-related adverse events represent an alarming problem that must be addressed by health care practitioners. Adverse drug reactions are responsible for a significant number of hospital admissions, with reported ranges from 0.3% to as high as 7%.[1,2] In a large study of more than 10,000 emergency room patients, 293 (2.9%) had drug-related illness, with 71 (24%) requiring hospitalization.[3] Some have estimated that up to 15% of hospitalized patients suffer at least one adverse drug reaction during their hospital stays.[4] In a study of more than 30,000 hospital records, nearly 4% of patients received disabling injuries caused by medical treatment.[5] Drug complications were the most common cause for injuries, accounting for 19% of the total.

Table 7.1 lists the drug classes responsible for adverse events in order of frequency. The most troublesome classes were antibiotics and antitumor agents, responsible for the recorded adverse effects in approximately 16% and 15% of cases, respectively. Table 7.2 lists the types of drug-related adverse events in order of frequency. The most common complications were bone-marrow suppression (16%), bleeding (15%), central nervous system effects (15%), and allergic/cutaneous reactions (14%).

TABLE 7.1. DRUG CLASSES RESPONSIBLE FOR ADVERSE EFFECTS

Drug Class	Frequency
Antibiotics	Most frequent
Antitumor agents	↓
Anticoagulants	
Cardiovascular agents	
Anticonvulsant agents	
Diabetes therapy	
Antihypertensives	
Analgesics	
Antiasthmatics	
Sedative–hypnotics	
Antidepressants	
Antipsychotics	
Peptic ulcer therapy	Least frequent

(Adapted from Ref. 5.)

Trying to determine the prevalence of adverse drug reactions in the outpatient setting is difficult due to the different methods used to collect data. Reported rates range from 2.6–50.6%, with the lower rates coming from physician data collection and the higher rates coming from patient surveys.[6] The elderly are at special risk because of number of medications they consume and the complicated clinical states they often present. An estimated 75% of elderly patients are receiving prescription drugs, while 82% use nonprescription drugs regularly; polypharmacy is a particular problem in this age group.[7]

Most definitions for adverse drug reactions are broad enough to encompass drug interactions. In 1972, the Boston Collaborative Drug Surveillance Program reported a study of 9900 patients with 83,200 drug exposures and found 3600 adverse drug reactions, 234 (6.5%) of which were attributable to drug interactions.[8] Durrence and associates[9] reviewed drug profiles of 1825 surgical patients and found at least one potential drug interaction in 17% of the patients. A study of nursing home patients revealed that

TABLE 7.2. TYPES OF DRUG-RELATED ADVERSE EFFECTS BY FREQUENCY

Type of Adverse Event	Frequency
Marrow suppression	Most frequent
Bleeding	↓
Central nervous system	
Allergic/cutaneous	
Metabolic	
Cardiac	
Gastrointestinal	
Renal	
Respiratory	Least frequent

(Adapted from Ref. 5.)

19% of patients were receiving combinations of drugs with known interactions.[10] A slightly higher percentage, 23%, was found in a similar study of an outpatient clinic population.[11] Borda et al.[12] reported that 22% of the adverse reactions on medical wards resulted from drug interactions. Certainly, drug interactions represent an important challenge for pharmacists.

The magnitude of this problem increases significantly in certain patient populations. One study documented an exponential increase in the incidence of adverse drug reactions in relationship to the number of drugs given.[13] Average hospital stay and mortality rates were also higher in relation to the number of drugs administered. Several population groups have been singled out as having a high potential for adverse drug reactions because of the large number of drugs used. These include the elderly,[14] critical care patients,[15] and patients undergoing complicated surgical procedures.[16]

Not only do drug interactions represent a danger to the patient, but they also can greatly increase health care costs. A study of drug interactions' impact on costs and other outcomes for hospitalized patients revealed an increased length of stay of 3.14 days for patients receiving warfarin with a potentially interacting drug compared with a control group.[17] Patients on the combination also required more laboratory tests. Certainly, an important goal in health care should be to maximize therapeutic outcomes using the fewest number of drugs possible.

Historical Perspective

Early recognition of a drug's potential adverse reaction profile is critical. During safety and efficacy studies (before a drug is introduced to the market), an attempt is made to identify any adverse reactions. Unfortunately, only a relatively small number of patients are evaluated. Exclusion criteria for many of these studies eliminate patients with multiple disease states or other complicating factors. Also, the very young and the very old are often not well studied. To complicate matters further, most of the studies are short term, thus eliminating the ability to recognize any adverse reactions associated with long-term use. This process sets up the potential for long lag times between the commercial release of a drug and the emergence of a true picture of its adverse reaction profile.

Table 7.3 lists some classic adverse drug reactions and the lag time, in years, until the adverse reaction was first reported.[18] This table illustrates how long it can take until the medical community is alerted to an adverse reaction via the medical literature. Recognition at this point depends on the information reaching the medical community. Further delays are encountered as the reaction is verified and some regulatory action is taken, such as adding the adverse drug reaction warning to the product label. In the case of lactic acidosis with phenformin, the first case report appeared in the late 1950s, with numerous reports during the 1960s and early 1970s, followed by the drug's withdrawal from the market in the late 1970s.[18] Many people were exposed to the risk of this adverse reaction because of the lag time.

To illustrate this process, Figs. 7.1 and 7.2 show the cumulative number of case reports over time for two classic adverse drug reactions, pseudomembranous colitis with clindamycin and coagulation defects associated with moxalactam. In Fig. 7.1, the 3-year delay from the time clindamycin was released in the United States to the first case report of pseudomembranous colitis is shown. During the next 4 years, the cumulative number of case reports rose rapidly. At this point, the number leveled, indicating that the reaction was well recognized and no longer "reportable." The time between clindamycin's release and the wide recognition of the adverse drug reaction could be considered 7 years. Figure 7.2 shows the more recent example of moxalactam and its association with coagulation defects.

TABLE 7.3. SUMMARY OF TIME LAGS AFTER U.S. MARKETING BEFORE ADVERSE DRUG REACTIONS WERE WIDELY RECOGNIZED

Adverse Reaction	Drug	Time Lag (yr)
Pulmonary embolism	Oral contraceptives	3
Myocardial infarction	Oral contraceptives	5
Deaths from asthma	Sympathomimetic aerosols	4
Jaundice	Halothane	7
Colitis	Lincomycin	6
Colitis	Clindamycin	5
Aplastic anemia	Phenylbutazone	6

(Adapted from Ref. 18.)

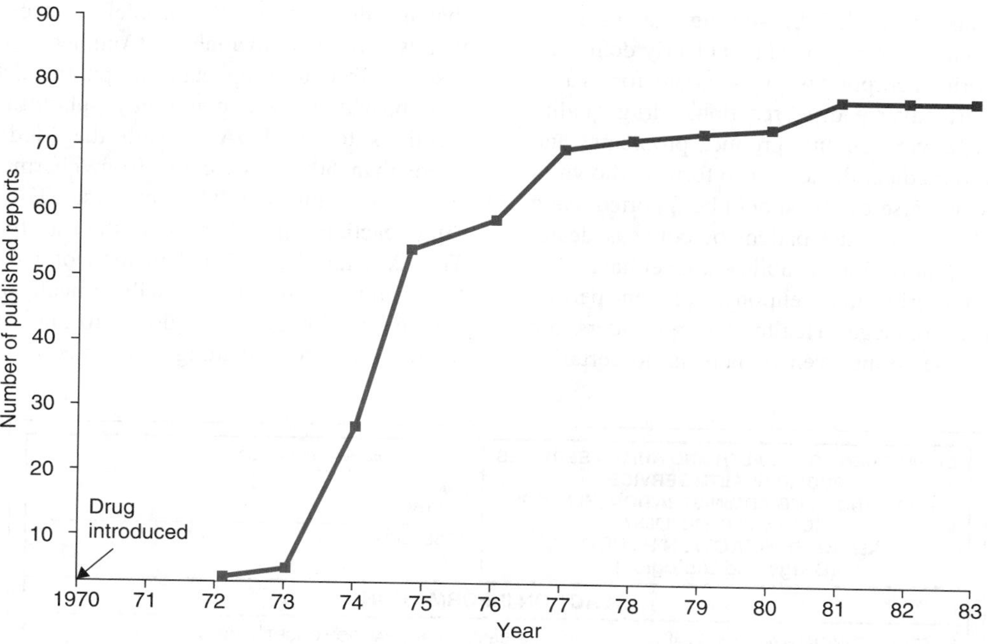

Figure 7.1. Cumulative number of published reports of pseudomembranous colitis with clindamycin.

These examples should point out the importance of reporting adverse drug reactions. Upon a drug's commercial release, postmarketing surveillance—whether formally organized or through spontaneous individual practitioner reports—is critical to gaining a rapid picture of a drug's true adverse reaction profile. Clinical trials can detect adverse events with a frequency of 1 per 1000 patients or higher[19]; less common effects will not likely be identifiable until after marketing. Once the drug reaches the market, patients may be taking other drugs in combination with the new drug, resulting in interactions not detected in premarketing studies.[20] Understanding methods for monitoring adverse drug reactions and drug interactions is important and is discussed later in this chapter.

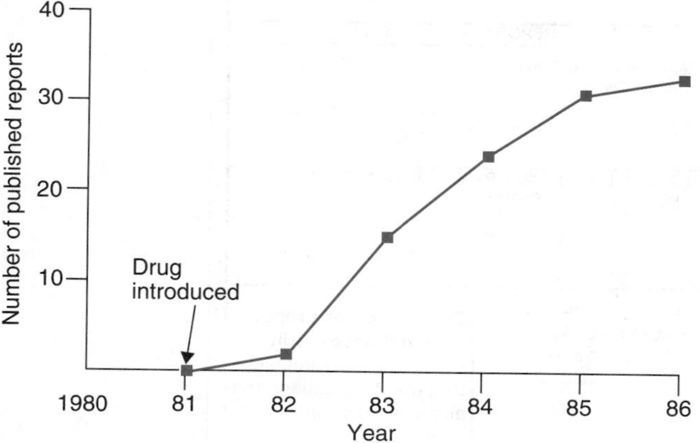

Figure 7.2. Cumulative number of published reports of hypoprothrombinemia with moxalactam.

Definitions

The first step in setting up a system to monitor adverse drug reactions is to establish a working definition to determine what parameters will be recorded and reported. The two most commonly cited definitions, from the World Health Organization[21] and Karch and Lasagna,[22] are as follows:

> *WHO:* Any response to a drug which is noxious and unintended, and which occurs at doses normally used in man for prophylaxis, diagnosis, or therapy of disease, or for the modification of physiological function.
>
> *Karch & Lasagna:* Any response to a drug which is noxious and unintended, and that occurs at doses used in humans for prophylaxis, diagnosis, or therapy, excluding failure to accomplish the intended purpose.

To aid in the development of a working definition, the American Society of Health-System Pharmacists recommends including any undesirable or unexpected event that requires discontinuing a drug, modifying a dose, prolonging hospitalization, or administering supportive treatment.[2] This modification expands the above definitions to include drug overdoses and drug interactions.

Some guidance should be given to those health care providers monitoring patients' drug therapies as to what adverse drug reactions should be reported. All reactions that fit the clinician's working definition should be reported within the institution's adverse drug reaction monitoring system (see further discussion later in this chapter). In 1993, the approach to reporting adverse effects to the Food and Drug Administration (FDA)—through a program known as MedWatch—was improved and clearly defined.[23] The MedWatch form incorporates the separate forms that were used to report adverse drug reactions, drug quality product problems, device quality product problems, and adverse reactions to medical devices. The form is shown in Fig. 7.3. "Serious" adverse events should be reported using the form and include when the patient outcome is death, life-threatening, hospitalization, disability, congenital anomaly, or a reaction requiring intervention to prevent permanent impairment or damage. Health care providers are encouraged to use the forms even if there is no certainty that the drug caused the problem and even when all the details are not available. Complete confidentiality is assured. To date, it appears that pharmacists are the health care providers most commonly submitting adverse drug reactions to the FDA through the MedWatch system.[24] More than 50% have come from pharmacists, with 20% from physicians, and 7% from nurses. Historically, adverse drug reactions have been classified as type A or type B. This is a fairly simplified method of viewing these reactions, and not all reactions will fit neatly into one of these categories. However, it is useful to know these definitions to aid in the understanding this subject.

DEPARTMENT OF HEALTH AND HUMAN SERVICES
PUBLIC HEALTH SERVICE
FOOD AND DRUG ADMINISTRATION (HFN-730)
ROCKVILLE, MD 20857
ADVERSE REACTION REPORT
(Drugs and Biologics)

Form Approved: 0910-0230.

FDA CONTROL NO.

ACCESSION NO.

I. REACTION INFORMATION

1. PATIENT ID/INITIALS *(In Confidence)*
2. AGE YRS.
3. SEX
4.-6. REACTION ONSET — MO. DA. YR.
8.-12. CHECK ALL APPROPRIATE:
☐ PATIENT DIED
☐ REACTION TREATED WITH Rx DRUG
☐ RESULTED IN, OR PROLONGED, INPATIENT HOSPITALIZATION
☐ RESULTED IN PERMANENT DISABILITY
☐ NONE OF THE ABOVE

7. DESCRIBE REACTION(S)

13. RELEVANT TESTS/LABORATORY DATA

II. SUSPECT DRUG(S) INFORMATION

14. SUSPECT DRUG(S) *(Give manufacturer and lot no. for vaccines/biologics)*
20. DID REACTION ABATE AFTER STOPPING DRUG? ☐ YES ☐ NO ☐ NA
15. DAILY DOSE
16. ROUTE OF ADMINISTRATION
21. DID REACTION REAPPEAR AFTER REINTRODUCTION? ☐ YES ☐ NO ☐ NA
17. INDICATION(S) FOR USE
18. DATES OF ADMINISTRATION *(From/To)*
19. DURATION OF ADMINISTRATION

III. CONCOMITANT DRUGS AND HISTORY

22. CONCOMITANT DRUGS AND DATES OF ADMINISTRATION *(Exclude those used to treat reaction)*

23. OTHER REVELANT HISTORY *(e.g. diagnoses, allergies, pregnancy with LMP, etc.)*

IV. ONLY FOR REPORTS SUBMITTED BY MANUFACTURER

24. NAME AND ADDRESS OF MANUFACTURER *(Include Zip Code)*
24a. IND/NDA. NO. FOR SUSPECT DRUG
24b. MFR CONTROL NO.
24c. DATE RECEIVED BY MANUFACTURER
24d. REPORT SOURCE *(Check all that apply)* ☐ FOREIGN ☐ STUDY ☐ HEALTH PROFESSIONAL ☐ LITERATURE ☐ CONSUMER
25. 15 DAY REPORT? ☐ YES ☐ NO
25a. REPORT TYPE ☐ INITIAL ☐ FOLLOWUP
NOTE: Required of manufacturers by 21 CFR 314.80

V. INITIAL REPORTER *(in confidence)*

26.-26a. NAME AND ADDRESS OF REPORTER *(Include Zip Code)*
26b. TELEPHONE NO. *(include area code)*
26c. HAVE YOU ALSO REPORTED THIS REACTION TO THE MANUFACTURER? ☐ YES ☐ NO
26d. ARE YOU A HEALTH PROFESSIONAL? ☐ YES ☐ NO

Submission of a report does not necessarily constitute an admission that the drug caused the adverse reaction.

FORM FDA 1639 (7 86) PREVIOUS EDITIONS MAY BE USED

Figure 7.3. FDA MedWatch adverse drug reaction report form.

Type A (augmented) reactions are normal pharmacologic effects of the drug exaggerated to the point of being undesirable. Therefore, they are usually dose dependent and fairly predictable. Examples include warfarin causing bruising, diazepam-induced drowsiness, and orthostatic hypotension from an antihypertensive medication. These represent adverse reactions secondary to the drug's desired pharmacologic effect at its desired site of action. Type A reactions also include reactions from a drug's desired pharmacologic effect occurring at an undesired location. A good example are effects from antineoplastic drugs. Although their desired effect is to destroy rapidly proliferating tumor cells, other fast-growing cells are killed as well: hair (alopecia), bone marrow (myelosuppression), and oral mucosa (mucositis).

Another form of type A reaction involves a drug's recognized pharmacologic property other than the primary desired one. β-adrenergic blocking agents elicit their effect on β receptors other than those in the heart and vasculature leading to the potential of bronchospasm due to β-blockade in the pulmonary tree. Many other common adverse drug effects fall into this category. Dry mouth, urinary retention, and other anticholinergic effects can be seen secondary to antihistamines and tricyclic antidepressants because of their anticholinergic properties. Antibiotics altering normal bowel flora can result in moderate to severe diarrhea. By reviewing a drug's pharmacologic properties, one can often predict likely type A reactions, allowing the health care practitioner to prevent or minimize the reaction. This principle is important when establishing prospective adverse drug reaction monitoring programs.

Type B (bizarre) adverse drug reactions are effects unrelated to the known pharmacologic action of the drug. These reactions are unpredictable and may or may not be dose dependent. Type B reactions are particularly dangerous. Their incidence is low, but mortality may be high. An anaphylactic reaction to penicillin and most other immunologic reactions fall in the type B category. Other examples include agranulocytosis secondary to chloramphenicol and malignant hyperthermia from anesthetic agents. The term "idiosyncratic" has been used in many texts as a label for type B reactions. Because these are less predictable, type B reactions are even more important to report so that widespread knowledge of them will be available as quickly as possible.

Drug interactions may be included in an institution's adverse drug reaction definition. The term *drug interaction* is used when administration of, or exposure to, a substance modifies a patient's response to a drug. The substance may be another drug (drug–drug interaction), a food (drug–food interaction), or other substances such as alcohol or tobacco. Although drug interactions are usually thought of as detrimental, some may actually be beneficial. Drug interactions are discussed in depth later in this chapter.

Problems That Can Occur When Drugs Are Administered

Although the purpose of administering a medication to a patient is to relieve symptoms, speed recovery from illness, or cure or prevent diseases, many things can go wrong and result in an adverse event. Some causes are drug-related factors, such as the wrong dose prescribed, while others are patient related, such as hemolytic anemia after sulfonamide administration in a patient with glucose-6-phosphate dehydrogenase deficiency. Some adverse drug reactions occur because of a combination of the two (i.e., dose of a renally eliminated drug too high in a patient with renal disease). Understanding the general principles of things that can go wrong, both drug related and patient related, will aid in the provision of good pharmaceutical care.

DRUG-RELATED PROBLEMS

Dose

Determining the proper dose for any particular patient is crucial in preventing type A reactions. The drug must be dosed in such a way that an adequate concentration is reached to elicit the desired therapeutic response. Dosing the drug too low results in therapeutic failures and dosing too high results in adverse reactions and other toxic effects. For some drugs the range in which the drug is effective without evidence of toxicity is wide. Drugs with this wide therapeutic window are generally considered safer and easier to dose than drugs with a narrow therapeutic window. This principle is shown in Fig. 7.4. Careful attention must be paid to how the drug is dosed. Agents with narrow therapeutic windows are usually good selections for therapeutic drug monitoring programs. Examples include the aminoglycosides, phenytoin, theophylline, and digoxin.

Route

Adverse drug reactions may be closely associated with the route of administration. Undesired effects result from administering a drug via an unintended route, such as accidental intra-arterial injection of an intravenous drug preparation. Local extravasation during intravenous infusion of highly irritating agents, such as with cytotoxic drugs, may result in extensive tissue necrosis.

Confusion over the proper dose for a given route of administration may result in undesired effects. An oral dose of a drug may be quite different from the intravenous dose due to several reasons. Doses of oral morphine need to be six times higher than the dose given parenterally because of absorption problems. Propranolol undergoes substantial first-pass metabolism when taken orally, resulting in required doses 10–40 times higher than the intravenous dose. The intravenous route of drug administration is often

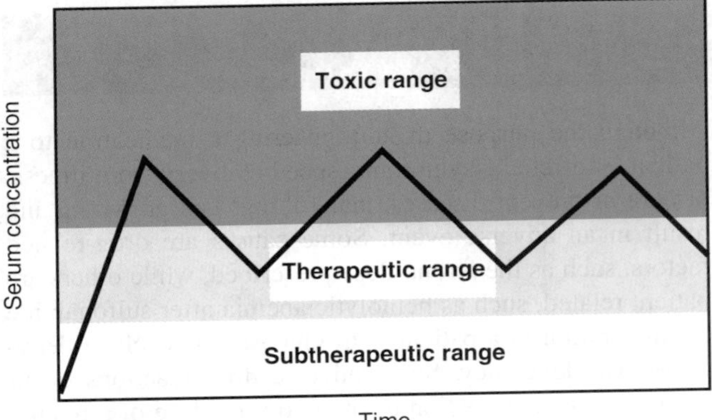

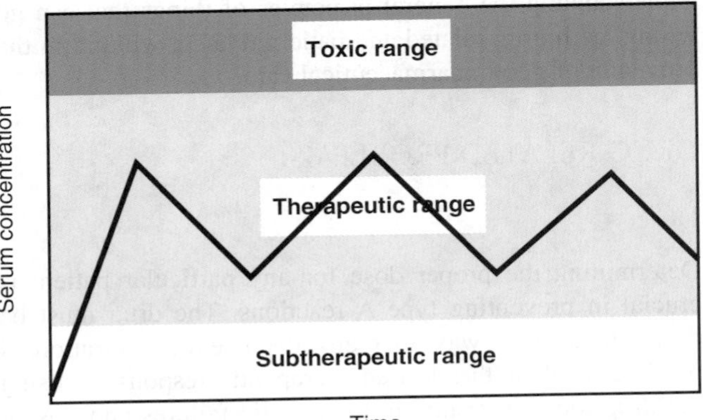

Figure 7.4. Comparison of wide (bottom) versus narrow (top) therapeutic window.

associated with adverse events, many of which are preventable. A common problem is infusing the drug too fast, resulting in a serum concentration that is too high. Local irritation and erythema may result from infusing antibiotics too fast or not sufficiently diluted, a problem associated with several β-lactam antibiotics. For example, nafcillin 1 g in less than 50 mL of solution administered in less than 10 minutes is much more likely to result in local irritation than the same dose in 50 mL of solution given over 30 minutes. "Red man" or "red neck" syndrome is a well-known adverse effect from administering vancomycin too fast. This syndrome is characterized by a sudden and possibly profound drop in blood pressure, usually accompanied by a maculopapular rash over the face, neck, upper chest, and extremities.

Duration

Examples of things that can go wrong must include this obvious one—duration of therapy. When drug therapy continues longer than needed, the patient is exposed to unnecessary risks. Many examples exist. Extending antibiotic therapy may lead to overgrowth of resistant organisms or fungal superinfections. Prolonged administration of benzodiazepine hypnotics is not recommended because of the potential for addiction and because insomnia may be a symptom of other disorders. This would lead to a delay in treatment of the underlying disease. This logic holds true for many other drugs used to treat symptoms. Extended use of corticosteroids exposes the patient to a long list of potential adverse drug reactions including adrenal suppression, increased susceptibility to infection, and fluid and electrolyte imbalance. Other chapters cover specific drug-induced diseases.

Preparation-Related Problems

Adverse reactions specifically related to the product being administered are often overlooked, but in many cases can be preventable. Preparations intended for use in the eye must be properly buffered, isotonic, and sterile to prevent potential adverse events. The nasal mucosa is highly sensitive to some vehicles such as alcohol and glycerin. Nasal vehicles should also be buffered and isotonic. Intravenous preparations that are hypo-osmotic can result in hemolysis, while hyperosmotic solutions can cause local irritation. The pH of these solutions may also contribute to local adverse reactions if it is too high or too low.

Excipients in some pharmaceutical preparations are known to cause problems in sensitive individuals. Serious adverse reactions, primarily allergic in nature, have occurred in sensitive individuals receiving products containing dyes (tartrazine or FD&C yellow no. 5), preservatives (sodium metabisulfite), or antiseptics (thimerosal). Reactions to other excipients can occur. A thorough patient history and knowledge of the excipients contained in various preparations are necessary for identifying this problem as the source of an adverse reaction.

Problems associated with a drug's release from its dosage form would fall into this category. A wide range of examples exists. A prescription for a sustained-release theophylline written with instructions for a nonsustained release product (e.g., theophylline sustained release 300 mg every 6 hours) would result in the drug being administered too frequently, with expected toxicities. If the opposite occurred (i.e., the nonsustained product ordered twice daily), subtherapeutic concentrations would result and the patient would not receive the desired benefit from the drug. Variations in drug release between brand name and generic products have caused problems with a number of drugs such as digoxin, theophylline, and phenytoin. The sustained-release dosage form has been useful in decreasing adverse reactions in some cases. Potassium chloride tablets are associated with a high incidence of gastrointestinal irritation; however, sustained-release products have helped avoid high local concentrations of potassium in the gastrointestinal tract.

Size of a tablet has been a source of problems. Following seven reports of patients having difficulty swallowing cholestyramine tablets, including two choking episodes, the manufacturer withdrew the tablets from the market.[25]

The action was taken only a few months after the product's approval and release.

Extension of Therapeutic Effect

This example of things that can go wrong was previously described under the definition for a type A adverse drug reaction. These reactions can be predicted, minimized, and, in many cases, avoided if there is a thorough knowledge of the drug being prescribed and of the patient receiving the drug.

PATIENT-RELATED PROBLEMS

Pharmacokinetic Variables

Patient variability in drug absorption, distribution, metabolism, and elimination can lead to adverse drug reactions, particularly type A reactions. Each pharmacokinetic parameter plays a role in how the patient handles the medication. Variations may lead to subtherapeutic responses or higher than desired drug concentrations and the associated adverse reactions. Again, knowledge of a given drug's pharmacokinetic characteristics and the patient's potential variation from normal may help prevent these adverse reactions. Another potential factor leading to pharmacokinetic variations is drug interactions. These are addressed later in this chapter. Differences in the rate and extent of absorption may have serious therapeutic consequences. Several factors may vary among patients including gastrointestinal motility, the absorptive capacity of the gastric mucosa, mucosal blood flow, and the ability of the gastrointestinal wall and liver to destroy drugs before they reach the systemic circulation.

How and where drugs are distributed in the body can be influenced by individual patient factors. Many drugs are highly bound to plasma proteins. Since only the drug's unbound portion contributes to its pharmacologic action, variation in the degree of plasma protein binding can greatly influence a drug's actions. An inverse relationship between the concentration of albumin in serum and adverse reactions to a highly protein-bound drug has been described.[26] Although this association seems logical, the relationship between protein binding and drug activity is much more complex (see Chapter 3 for a complete discussion). Increased free drug is also available for metabolism and elimination. Disease states such as uremia may decrease a drug's protein binding. This can be clinically relevant with drugs having a small volume of distribution, such as phenytoin, salicylates, sulfonamides, and others.

A drug's metabolism and elimination from the body depend on patient-specific variables. Patients with decreased hepatic or renal function may have drastic changes in drug disposition, leading to adverse drug reactions unless proper dosage adjustments are made. Numerous dosing guides are available to aid in adjusting doses in these patients. Unfortunately, these recommended adjustments are not always made by prescribers, probably because of a lack of knowledge of the need to adjust the doses.[27]

Age

Closely related to the pharmacokinetic principles is the patient-related factor of age. How a patient handles drugs varies greatly from birth to old age. Hydrophilic and lipophilic drugs may be affected by the patient's lean body mass or the amount of adipose tissue. The ability of the liver to metabolize certain drugs may be reduced in the very young and the very old. Renal function tends to decrease with increasing age. A drug's volume of distribution varies greatly between infant, child, adult, and elderly patients. These differences are detailed in Chapters 5 and 6. Dosage guidelines based on age must be closely adhered to so as to prevent adverse reactions. Psychotropics and diuretics have been implicated as risk factors for falls that result in hip fractures in the elderly.[28] Another important point related to age is that the elderly are more likely to be taking multiple drugs, therefore increasing the possibility of drug interactions.

Genetics

Idiosyncratic reactions to drugs result from an abnormal susceptibility to the drug by a patient. These reactions occur in genetically abnormal subjects and are dose related. One of the best known examples is a drug-induced hemolytic anemia in patients with glucose-6-phosphate dehydrogenase deficiency. This genetic enzyme deficiency in erythrocytes causes weaknesses in the cell membrane. Certain drugs are capable of affecting the integrity of the cell membrane and causing it to hemolyze. These drugs include doxorubicin, furazolidone, methylene blue, nalidixic acid, nitrofurantoin, phenazopyridine, primaquine, and sulfamethoxazole. Blacks, persons of Jewish descent, and other dark-hued Caucasian groups (such as persons of Greek or Iranian descent) tend to have a greater incidence of this deficiency.[29]

Another well-recognized example is the recessive autosomal trait affecting an individual's ability to acetylate isoniazid. Slow acetylators develop high serum concentration of isoniazid when given normal doses and show a much higher incidence of dose-related adverse effects such as peripheral neuropathy. Interestingly, the incidence of isoniazid-induced hepatitis is higher in fast acetylators, probably secondary to a faster rate of formation of toxic metabolites.[30] Other adverse drug reactions may be idiosyncratic in nature; however, these need to be investigated for their genetic links. Some of the reactions that appear to be idiosyncratic are nausea and vomiting, renal and hepatic reactions, gastrointestinal reactions, and fever.

Allergy

True allergic reactions are immunologically mediated, nonpharmacologic effects. These types of reactions may vary from mild, such as a nonserious rash, to life-threatening bronchospasm and hypotension associated with anaphylaxis.

Many factors influence the development of allergic reactions. A patient's predisposition toward the development of hypersensitivity reactions to common allergens (e.g., those with allergic rhinitis) may be at much greater risk for drug allergies.[4] Older patients, who may be sensitized by more frequent exposure to drugs, are more likely to develop allergic reactions.[31] Route of administration is also important, with the topical route being the most sensitizing, the parenteral route being the most hazardous, and the oral route being the safest.[4]

Anticipating the possibility of allergic reactions offers the best opportunity for prevention or early treatment to minimize effects. A thorough drug allergy history is essential. Patients should be observed for 20–30 minutes after receiving potentially antigenic drugs. Patients predisposed to anaphylaxis should carry warning identification and should be taught to self-administer epinephrine.

The Uninformed Patient

An uninformed patient is a serious—but preventable—patient-related risk factor for the development of adverse drug reactions. The patient must be carefully instructed on the proper use of his or her medications.

Potential adverse drug reactions should be discussed with the patient. They must be put in the proper perspective to prevent making patients reluctant to take their medications for fear of adverse effects. Adverse reactions transient in nature should be identified for the patient as well as reactions about which the patient should notify his or her physician or pharmacist immediately.

Educating patients about their drug therapy can aid in preventing or minimizing drug interactions. If patients are more attentive to the development of excessive or unexpected responses to their drug therapy, problems may be identified earlier. The use of nonprescription medications should be discussed with the patient. Interactions with these agents are often overlooked.

Finally, patients should be encouraged to ask questions about their drug therapy. Potential drug–drug and drug–food interactions should be discussed with the patient. All instructions for appropriate administration must be fully understood by the patient.

Drug–Drug Interactions

An important type of adverse drug reaction is drug interaction. Thousands of drug–drug interactions have been described in the literature, but only a relatively small number are clinically important. In this section, the three categories of drug–drug interactions—pharmacokinetic, pharmacodynamic, and pharmaceutic—are described and clinically relevant examples are given.

PHARMACOKINETIC INTERACTIONS

A pharmacokinetic interaction may occur by several mechanisms. Generally, one drug alters the absorption, distribution, metabolism, or elimination of another drug, resulting in a change in drug concentration in the body and an altered response. Numerous controlled studies have described various types of pharmacokinetic interactions; however, such controlled trials are typically performed in healthy volunteers and do not always give a true perspective of the potential for an interaction. Data from pharmacokinetic or epidemiologic studies of actual patients are generally more helpful in determining the clinical importance of a pharmacokinetic interaction.

Absorption

Absorption interactions result in an increase or decrease in the relative rate of absorption or in the amount of the drug absorbed. A decrease in the rate of absorption may result in failure of a drug to reach a therapeutic concentration even if the total amount of drug absorbed is unchanged. Absorption rate can be slowed by any drug that slows gastric motility, such as anticholinergic drugs (e.g., propantheline) and opiates (e.g., codeine). Because the small intestine provides the largest surface area for absorption, it is the major site of absorption for most orally administered drugs. Any drug that decreases the speed at which another drug passes from the stomach to the small intestine will induce a decrease in absorption rate. However, drugs that increase gastric motility, such as metoclopramide, can increase the absorption rate. Although these agents can produce marked effects on absorption rate, few clinically important drug–drug interactions have been reported. Interactions resulting in a decrease in the total amount of one drug's absorption are usually more important clinically.

Decreases in the amount of drug absorbed may be caused by the formation of insoluble complexes or by changes in gastrointestinal pH. The quantity of drug absorbed may also be affected by agents that decrease gastric motility as previously described. Tetracycline's interactions with antacids and dairy products are well known. Divalent or trivalent cations (aluminum, calcium, iron, and magnesium) combine with tetracycline to form a nonabsorbable complex, greatly reducing serum tetracycline concentrations. These interactions can be prevented by separating administration time of the interacting agents by 2 hours. The absorption of ketoconazole appears to be reduced when the gastrointestinal pH is increased.[32] A significant reduction in plasma ketoconazole concentrations occurred when it was given concurrently with antacids or cimetidine.[32,33] Many other absorption interactions have been reported. The clinical importance of most of these is not well documented.

Drug–food interactions that affect absorption may be important and are discussed later in this chapter.

Distribution

Two types of distribution interactions are most common: protein-binding/displacement interactions and cellular distribution interactions. Once absorbed, drugs are distributed via the blood as both free drug and plasma protein-bound drug. Because only the free or unbound fraction of the drug is active, any change in the percentage bound can lead to a change in a drug's availability to receptor sites and its metabolism and excretion. When two or more highly protein-bound drugs are administered concurrently, competitive binding by one may increase the free fraction of the other.

Drug–drug interactions in this class are complex and probably in some cases overstated. For example, much has been published about the use of nonsteroidal anti-inflammatory agents (NSAIDs) in combination with warfarin. Many NSAIDs may decrease warfarin's protein binding. The traditional view is that because NSAIDs are highly protein bound, they displace warfarin, thereby increasing its anticoagulant effect; however, a review of the literature reveals that much of the evidence is based on *in vitro* data, and *in vivo* studies have downplayed this effect.[34] Other reasons exist for the occasionally observed increase in anticoagulation such as the effect of NSAIDs on warfarin metabolism and their independent effect on hemostasis.[35] Whatever the cause, the interaction between warfarin and NSAIDs is clinically relevant and should be monitored. The risk of developing hemorrhagic peptic ulcer disease in patients receiving concomitant warfarin and NSAIDs is increased 13-fold.[36]

Rolan[37] challenged the clinical importance of most protein-binding/displacement interactions. Displacement produces a minor transient increase in free drug, and the mean steady-state concentration remains unchanged. Drugs most likely to result in clinically important interactions were greater than 90% protein bound, have a narrow therapeutic index, have a high hepatic extraction ratio, and are given intravenously. Still, caution should be exercised in the administration of any two highly protein bound drugs when one or both have a narrow therapeutic index. Interactions involving cellular distribution are unusual but can be clinically relevant. Tricyclic antidepressants displace guanethidine from its intracellular site of action, resulting in a markedly reduced antihypertensive effect.[38] This combination should probably be avoided.

Metabolism

Many interactions involve the effect of one drug on the metabolism of another drug, and these can be clinically important. The metabolic rate may be increased or decreased. Certain drugs, such as barbiturates, are known to induce hepatic enzymes, resulting in shortened plasma half-lives for some drugs. A well-documented and clinically important example is seen with administration of barbiturates and warfarin[39]; higher than usual dosages of warfarin are needed to produce suitable anticoagulation. When a patient stabilized on warfarin discontinues barbiturate therapy, hemorrhage often results. Other drugs that may act as enzyme inducers include carbamazepine, phenytoin, rifampin, and phenylbutazone.

Many drugs are metabolized in hepatic microsomes by an enzyme system called the mixed-function oxidase system (cytochrome P-450 system). Drugs that inhibit the cytochrome P-450 system (e.g., cimetidine, influenza vaccine, allopurinol, disulfiram) may affect the metabolic rate of many drugs (e.g., warfarin, theophylline, some benzodiazepines, phenytoin). Drug metabolism rate is affected by genetic background, age, nutritional state, diseases, hormonal state, and endogenous chemicals. Considerable interpatient and intrapatient variation occurs with this type of interaction, making prediction of the extent of the interaction difficult. Cimetidine, a histamine H_2-receptor antagonist widely prescribed for the treatment and prevention of gastrointestinal ulcers, has been shown to have inhibitory effects on the cytochrome P-450 enzyme system. This has resulted in several well-documented drug interactions (e.g., cimetidine's effect on the metabolism of theophylline). One study described a 39% mean decrease in theophylline clearance in young healthy volunteers after 2 days of cimetidine therapy.[40] This interaction was later confirmed in case reports.[41–43]

This type of interaction has also been reported with terfenadine.[44] A specific P-450 enzyme converts terfenadine to an active metabolite. Increased concentrations of the parent drug may exert a quinidine-like action, leading to torsades de pointes.[45] Erythromycin and ketoconazole interfere with this enzyme and lead to increased terfenadine plasma levels.[46] Other risk factors for this cardiotoxicity include overdose and serious hepatic dysfunction. Because torsades de pointes has been reported following overdoses of another antihistamine (astemizole), similar concerns apply.[46] More work is needed to document the potential interaction between erythromycin or ketoconazole and astemizole. Coadministration of loratadine with erythromycin resulted in increased serum concentrations of loratadine and its metabolite, but no clinically relevant changes in electrocardiographic parameters were noted.[47]

Given the unpredictability of these reactions, caution is advised in prescribing two drugs metabolized by the P-450 enzyme system.

Elimination

Most interactions involving elimination or excretion occur in the kidneys. A change in glomerular filtration rate, tubular secretion, or urine pH can alter the excretion of some drugs. Fortunately, only a handful of these interactions results in clinically relevant changes and some of these are beneficial.

A potentially dangerous interaction in this category is that between diuretics and lithium. Prolonged thiazide therapy has been shown to cause a compensatory increase in proximal tubule reabsorption of sodium, resulting in increased lithium reabsorption as well.[48] This interaction has resulted in serious lithium toxicity.[49]

PHARMACODYNAMIC INTERACTIONS

Pharmacodynamic interactions generally fall into four categories on the basis of the effects produced: antagonistic, synergistic therapeutic, synergistic adverse, and indirect effect.

Antagonistic Effects

Antagonistic interactions occur when two drugs with opposing pharmacologic effects are given together. For example, a nonspecific β-adrenergic blocking agent such as propranolol may induce bronchoconstriction because of its effect on the β receptors in the bronchi of a patient taking theophylline for bronchodilation. This interaction may also be beneficial, for instance, when the opiate antagonist naloxone is given to reverse the effects of opiate analgesics.

Synergistic or Additive Therapeutic Effects

Two drugs with similar therapeutic effects may interact. For example, coadministration of two central nervous system depressants, such as diazepam for anxiety and chloral hydrate for insomnia, may result in oversedation.

Administration of a drug that inhibits platelet aggregation (such as aspirin) together with warfarin increases the anticoagulant effects, possibly to the point of bleeding.

Synergistic or Additive Side Effects

This interaction is similar to the preceding one, except it involves the side effects rather than the therapeutic effects of the drugs. For example, administration of an antihistamine with a skeletal muscle relaxant such as cyclobenzaprine, both of which cause drowsiness, may result in additive sedation. Administering two drugs with anticholinergic side effects, such as disopyramide and a tricyclic antidepressant, may produce intolerable effects. Drug interactions involving antiviral agents primarily involve shared toxicities (e.g., neutropenia with ganciclovir and zidovudine).[50] Designing antiviral drugs that selectively inhibit viruses without damaging the cells they infect is difficult. The result is drugs that may be teratogenic, mutagenic, and carcinogenic.

Indirect Pharmacodynamic Effects

In this type of interaction, the pharmacologic effect of one drug indirectly affects another drug's action. Diuretics that decrease body potassium concentrations may alter the therapeutic effects of digoxin and some other antiarrhythmics. The effect of digoxin is enhanced by potassium depletion, whereas the effects of some antiarrhythmics, such as lidocaine and quinidine, are decreased.

PHARMACEUTIC INTERACTIONS

Pharmaceutic interactions occur when two drugs are mixed in the same intravenous fluid, resulting in physical or chemical incompatibility (chemical inactivation or precipitation). Incompatibility can occur for a variety of reasons. For example, drugs known to be alkali labile should not be mixed in intravenous solutions containing aminophylline, which has an alkaline pH. Such drugs include epinephrine, erythromycin gluceptate, and cephalothin sodium.[51] Incompatibility is common with the use of intravenous phenytoin, because crystallization or precipitation may result if the drug's vehicle is altered or the pH lowered.[52,53] Therefore, phenytoin sodium injection should not be mixed in the same intravenous fluid with other drugs.

BENEFICIAL INTERACTIONS

Drug–drug interactions are generally thought of as detrimental, but many are actually clinically desirable. Epinephrine is added to some common local anesthetics, such as lidocaine, to produce local vasoconstriction and slow anesthetic absorption; this reduces the risk of lidocaine toxicity and prolongs the localized action of the anesthetic. Carbidopa prevents the metabolism of levodopa by inhibiting dopa decarboxylase, thereby allowing levodopa to cross the blood–brain barrier before it is converted to dopamine. Probenecid inhibits secretion of penicillins into the proximal tubule, thus reducing the rate of penicillin excretion; this combination results in a twofold higher and more prolonged blood penicillin concentration.[54] Trimethoprim and sulfamethoxazole sequentially inhibit two steps in an essential bacterial biosynthetic pathway, resulting in synergistic antibacterial activity.

DRUG–FOOD INTERACTIONS

Administration of drugs with food may result in an interaction that modifies the activity of the drug or the nutritional effect of the food (decreased drug response, increased drug response, or impairment of nutritional status).

EFFECT OF FOOD ON DRUG ABSORPTION

The most frequently observed type of drug–food interaction affects drug absorption. The primary reason for decreased drug response with drug–food interactions is the effect food has on the absorption of some orally administered drugs. As with drug–drug absorption interactions, the result may be a decreased drug absorption rate or a decreased amount of drug absorbed. Drugs whose absorption may be delayed or reduced by food include most penicillins, tetracycline, digoxin, acetaminophen, levodopa, and aspirin. It may be best for patients to take these medications 1 hour before or 2 hours after meals. Absorption of some drugs—for example, spironolactone[55] and griseofulvin[56]—is increased when the drugs are taken with certain foods.

PHARMACOLOGIC INTERACTIONS

Food can interact with drugs in a variety of ways other than that affecting absorption. The most clinically important of these occurs with monoamine oxidase inhibitors (MAOIs). Monoamine oxidase normally metabolizes tyramine in food before it reaches the systemic circulation. If a person is taking an MAOI, large amounts of tyramine may reach the systemic circulation, resulting in an excessive pressor effect that may lead to seriously acute hypertension. Table 7.4 lists foods to be avoided by patients taking MAOIs.

Other examples involve vitamin K and pyridoxine (vitamin B_6). Foods rich in vitamin K may antagonize the effect of warfarin. This rarely results in problems if patients avoid the extreme types of food. Examples of vitamin K–rich foods are leafy green vegetables, liver, green tea, tomatoes, and coffee. Pyridoxine can enhance the metabolism of levodopa, decreasing the amount of levodopa available to cross the blood–brain barrier and reach its site of action. Patients taking levodopa should be warned not to eat excessive amounts of pyridoxine-rich foods such as avocados, beans, bacon, beef liver, peas, pork, sweet potatoes, and tuna. Also, many nonprescription vitamin preparations contain pyridoxine.

TABLE 7.4. FOODS HIGH IN TYRAMINE

Avocados (especially if overripe)
Bananas
Bean pods
Canned figs
Cheese (especially aged)
Chicken livers
Chocolate
Coffee
Cola beverages
Fermented meats (salami, pepperoni, summer sausage)
Herring (pickled or dry)
Raspberries
Soy sauce
Wines (especially red)
Yeast preparations
Yogurt

EFFECT OF DRUGS ON NUTRITION

The most common form of drug-induced nutritional deficiency is mineral depletion in the elderly.[57] Diuretics frequently cause potassium deficiency. This problem can be compounded in patients who also use laxatives frequently. Elderly patients may have an inadequate dietary intake of calcium, magnesium, and zinc, and depletion may be accentuated by some drugs.

Many drugs affect a patient's nutritional status indirectly. Drugs that cause nausea, vomiting, gastrointestinal upset, constipation, or diarrhea have an impact on a patient's food intake. As one might guess, this list of drugs is quite long. Oral decongestants, such as phenylpropanolamine and pseudoephedrine, may also result in decreased food intake because they can suppress appetite. Many other drug–food interactions have been reported.

ETHANOL/TOBACCO–DRUG INTERACTIONS

Technically, interactions of drugs with alcohol or tobacco should be considered drug–drug interactions but, in the medical literature, they are addressed separately.

TOBACCO–DRUG INTERACTIONS

The effect of smoking on drug metabolism is well established in the medical literature.[58,59] The primary mechanism for this interaction appears to be enhanced drug metabolism resulting from induction of hepatic microsomal enzymes by the constituents of tobacco smoke; however, in many cases, the exact mechanism has not been established. The interaction results in lowered plasma drug concentrations for some drugs (Table 7.5). Of the drugs listed in Table 7.5, the most clinically important interactions appear to be with the oral contraceptives, other estrogen compounds, and theophylline.

TABLE 7.5. DRUGS AFFECTED BY EXPOSURE TO TOBACCO SMOKE

Antidiabetics, oral	Pentazocine
Benzodiazepines	Propoxyphene
Chlordiazepoxide	Propranolol
Diazepam	Theophylline
Chlorpromazine	Tricyclic antidepressants
Contraceptives, oral	Amitriptyline
Estrogens	Desipramine
Heparin	Imipramine
Lidocaine	Nortriptyline

Tobacco–Estrogen Adverse Effects

Epidemiologic studies indicate that the risk of cardiovascular adverse effects such as stroke, myocardial infarction, and thromboembolism, which are associated with oral contraceptive use, are increased in smokers.[60] The risk increases with age and the number of cigarettes smoked per day. The exact mechanism for this interaction is unclear. Women taking oral contraceptives should not smoke. If they will not stop smoking, they should be encouraged to use alternative birth control methods, such as condoms and contraceptive foam.

Tobacco–Theophylline Effects

Smoking significantly affects theophylline pharmacokinetics.[61,62] Smoking stimulates the hepatic metabolism of theophylline, resulting in increased theophylline clearance, a shorter serum half-life, and lower serum concentrations. Some heavy smokers may require as much as two times the usual maintenance dose of theophylline.

ETHANOL–DRUG INTERACTIONS

Several drug interactions involving ethanol are clinically important. Often overlooked and not viewed as the potent drug it actually is, ethanol is involved in both straightforward and complex interactions. The effects of short- and long-term ethanol consumption on drug metabolism have been studied.[63] Long-term ethanol consumption may increase the clearance of a drug by induction of oxidative metabolism, whereas short-term consumption may decrease clearance. Clearance by hepatic *N*-acetylation appears to increase after just a single drink. Conjugation with glucuronide is inhibited for some drugs in the presence of ethanol. For drugs cleared by multiple pathways, the change in total clearance caused by alcohol is unknown. The importance of the H_2-receptor antagonists' effect on blood alcohol concentrations is unsettled. In a review of the controversy, Gugler[64] described studies showing an effect and studies with no effect. He concluded that the interaction is probably minor and limited to young, nonalcoholic, non-Asian men when the alcohol is given in small, concentrated doses after meals.

Additive Central Nervous System Effects

A dangerous drug interaction may occur when ethanol is combined with other central nervous system (CNS) depressants such as antihistamines, barbiturates, tranquilizers, or other psychotropic drugs. The CNS depressant effect may be additive or synergistic. With some agents (e.g., benzodiazepines), the interaction involves more than just an additive side effect. Ethanol may increase the absorption[65] and decrease the metabolism[66] of diazepam. Also, patients with alcoholic liver disease may eliminate benzodiazepines more slowly than those with normal liver function.[67]

Other Effects

Ethanol interacts with a variety of other drugs. One clinically relevant example is the antagonism by ethanol of the oral antidiabetic agents (e.g., chlorpropamide and tolbutamide), for which several mechanisms are possible. Ethanol itself may produce hypoglycemia.[68] To confuse matters, ethanol may also increase the metabolism of some oral antidiabetics.[69] This action may counteract ethanol's hypoglycemic effect, but it is unpredictable.

Chlorpropamide and possibly other sulfonylureas may also interact with ethanol by producing the "disulfiram reaction" (flushing, hypotension, nausea, tachycardia, vertigo, dyspnea, and blurred vision).[70] Disulfiram, which produces hypersensitivity to alcohol, is used as an alcohol deterrent to help maintain alcohol abstinence. Most researchers believe this reaction occurs because of disulfiram's effect on ethanol metabolism, which results in increased production of acetaldehyde; however, other theories exist. Unfortunately, as previously mentioned, other drugs can produce this reaction.

ADVERSE DRUG REACTION MONITORING AND REPORTING PROGRAMS

The clinician must have a thorough understanding of the pharmacology of the drugs he or she administers to patients in the practice setting. This knowledge aids in identifying adverse reactions and interactions when they occur and is also helpful in detecting a previously unreported adverse drug reaction.

A comprehensive adverse drug reaction monitoring and reporting program includes multiple systems for identifying reactions. Once the potential reaction is identified, it must be assessed and appropriately managed. The reactions should be reported in an organized and predefined fashion. Methods to prevent future adverse reactions should be established and educational feedback given to prescribers.

This entire process constitutes a good adverse drug reaction monitoring and reporting program.

IDENTIFICATION, ASSESSMENT, AND MANAGEMENT

Several mechanisms are used to detect a potential adverse drug reaction. Steps taken from this point are illustrated in Fig. 7.5. The first step taken is to determine if the effect seen is drug related. Published literature on the drug is reviewed to determine if such an effect has been previously described. This includes reviewing known reactions to the drug, drug–drug interactions, and drug–disease interactions that might be responsible, and the characteristics of these published effects. It may also be helpful to contact the manufacturer of the suspected drug for any unpublished data. At the same time, information about the patient is gathered on the details of the reaction. A complete review of the patient's medical history is done to determine other drugs or disease states that could be responsible. A chronological sequence of events is established to see if there is a temporal relationship between drug administration and the reaction, as previously described for drug interaction detection. If a reaction is related to a changing laboratory parameter, drug–laboratory test interactions should be ruled out. The patient-specific information is compared with the medical literature to determine the likelihood of a drug cause. If the reaction is severe enough and there is enough evidence pointing to the drug, the medication is discontinued or changed to an alternate therapy. This is called *dechallenge.* The patient can then be observed to determine if the adverse effect improves or goes away. If the consequences of readministering are not serious or if the suspected agent is still indicated and the reaction is thought to be dose related, the patient may be rechallenged with a smaller dose while being carefully observed.

Management of drug interactions usually consists of monitoring specific parameters and then taking the appropriate action. For example, a serum drug assay may be needed, or a particular laboratory value may need to be monitored closely. In many cases, potentially interacting

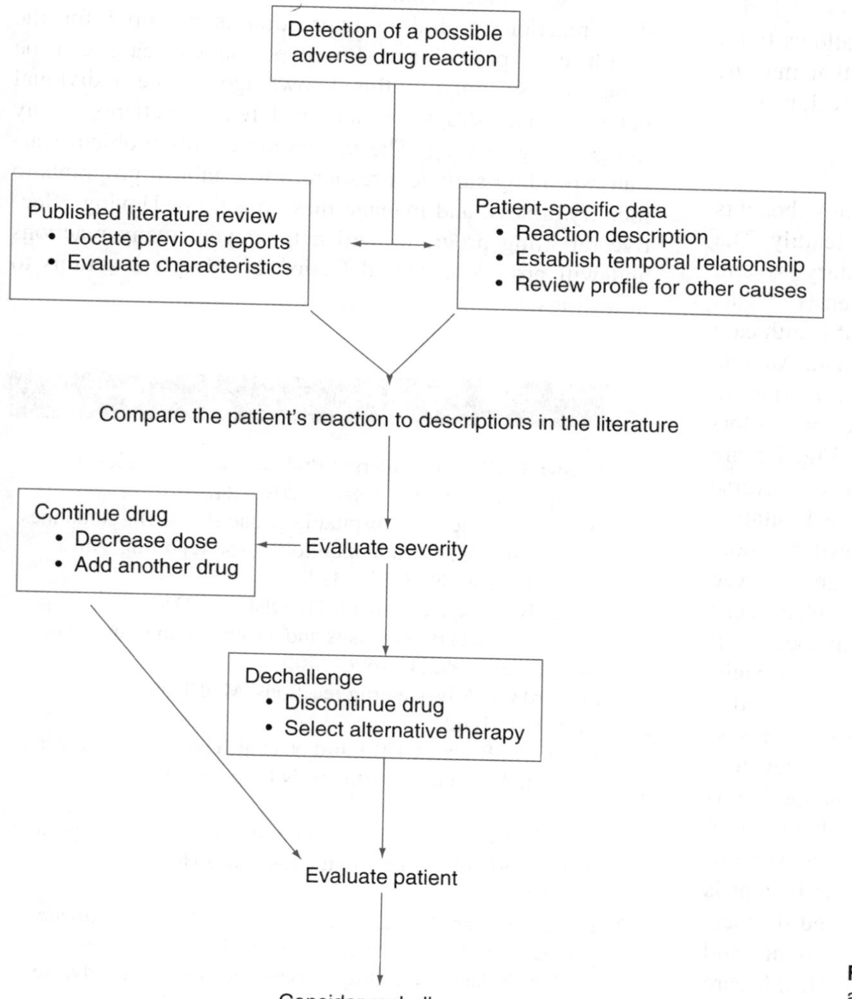

Figure 7.5. Flowchart of assessment and management of an adverse drug reaction. *(Adapted from Ref. 71.)*

drugs can be administered concurrently as long as appropriate patient or laboratory assessments are performed.

METHODS FOR MONITORING AND DETECTING

Several methods are available for monitoring and detecting adverse drug reactions. Each of the methods has strengths and weaknesses. The best system should incorporate multiple methods based on the resources available.

Retrospective Systems

Patient charts can be reviewed retrospectively by a random or selective process. Chart screening can be performed by supportive personnel and may generate more reports than voluntary methods. However, retrospective reviews rely solely on the written record, and all the surrounding circumstances because the patient has already been discharged. Also, this method provides no benefit to the patient who experienced the reaction. An alternative to random screening is to preselect high-risk drugs or high-risk patients to be monitored retrospectively. This allows fairly rapid identification of the types of problems that may be encountered so prospective programs can be developed.

Prospective or Concurrent Monitoring Systems

Formalized prospective monitoring offers many benefits because patients can be identified and treated readily. The most commonly used method is the voluntary system because it is easy to implement and inexpensive. This method is based on the voluntary cooperation of health care providers who come into contact with the patient. Anyone suspecting an adverse reaction voluntarily fills out an adverse drug reaction report form. Typically the form is forwarded to a pharmacy and the steps given in Fig. 7.5 are initiated. Although widely used, the number of adverse reactions reported voluntarily may be small. This limitation can be overcome by the pharmacist. When questions about a potential adverse drug reaction or interaction are received in the pharmacy or drug information center, the pharmacist should determine whether the question is patient specific. If so, the management steps are initiated and the pharmacist follows up by ensuring that the report form is completed.

Setting up prospective or concurrent surveillance system for drugs and patients with a high risk for the development of an adverse drug reaction or drug interaction is highly desirable. Drugs with known serious adverse drug reaction profiles should be targeted for ongoing surveillance. Profiles need to be reviewed to see if the patient is currently receiving any drugs commonly involved in interactions. Other risk factors—such as tobacco smoking and alcohol consumption—should be documented. Health care personnel should be educated on the potential problems with these drugs. As new drugs are marketed, their use should be closely watched until their adverse reaction profile is well defined. Patients at high risk for adverse effects should also be the focus of ongoing surveillance.

A formalized drug interaction screening program should be used in all pharmacies. This can be a simple manual system using patient drug profiles and a drug interaction reference book or a computerized system. Because of their growing use in pharmacy, computers can be expected to play a greater role in the screening and analysis of individual drug regimens.

These prospective systems benefit the patients who experience a reaction because they are recognized earlier and future patients benefit from information learned from past patients. Other benefits could include the economic impact of reduced hospitalization, efficient and economical drug use, and minimized organizational liability.[2]

CONCLUSION

A thorough understanding of the mechanisms of adverse drug reactions and drug interaction is essential for the health care practitioner. Improved patient care can be achieved by applying this knowledge to the individual patient. When drugs are administered to patients, many things can go wrong. The magnitude of this problem warrants spending sufficient resources to establish programs to identify, assess, and manage these reactions. Having effective reporting programs will help prevent many reactions and will provide earlier detection of adverse reactions to new drugs.

REFERENCES

1. DeSwarte RD. Drug allergy: Problems and strategies. J Allergy Clin Immunol 1984;74:209–224.
2. American Society of Hospital Pharmacists. ASHP guidelines on adverse drug reaction monitoring and reporting. Am J Hosp Pharm 1989;46:336–337.
3. Prince BS, Goetz CM, Rihn TL, Olsky M. Drug-related emergency department visits and hospital admissions. Am J Hosp Pharm 1992;49:1696–1700.
4. Stafford CT. Adverse drug reactions. Med Times 1988;116:31–42.
5. Leape LL, Brennan TA, Laird N, et al. The nature of adverse events in hospitalized patients. N Engl J Med 1991;324:337–384.
6. Schneider JK, Mion LC, Frengley JD. Adverse drug reactions in an elderly outpatient population. Am J Hosp Pharm 1992;49:90–96.
7. Honig PK, Cantilena LR. Polypharmacy: Pharmacokinetic perspectives. Clin Pharmacokinet 1994;26:85–90.
8. Boston Collaborative Drug Surveillance Program. Adverse drug interactions. JAMA 1972;220:1238–1239.

9. Durrence CW, DiPiro JT, May JR, et al. Potential drug interactions in surgical patients. Am J Hosp Pharm 1985;42:1553–1555.
10. Blaschke TF, Cohen SN, Tatro DS. Drug–drug interactions and aging, in Jarvik LF, Greenblatt DJ, Harman D (eds): Clinical Pharmacology in the Aged Patient. New York, Raven, 1981.
11. Stanaszek WF, Franklin CE. Survey of potential drug interaction incidence in an outpatient clinic population. Hosp Pharm 1978;13:255–263.
12. Borda IT, Slone D, Hick H. Assessment of adverse reactions within a drug surveillance program. JAMA 1968;205:645–647.
13. Smith JW, Seidl LG, Cluff LE. Studies on the epidemiology of adverse drug reactions. V. Clinical factors influencing susceptibility. Ann Intern Med 1966;65:629–640.
14. D'Arcy PF. Drug reactions and interactions in the elderly patient. Drug Intell Clin Pharm 1982;16:925–929.
15. Zarowitz B, Conway W, Popvich J. Adverse interactions of drugs in critical care patients. Henry Ford Hosp Med J 1985;33:48–55.
16. Nagashima H. Drug interactions in the recovery room. Int Anesthesiol Clin 1983;21:93–105.
17. Jankel CA, McMillan JA, Martin BC. Effects of drug interactions on outcomes of patients receiving warfarin or theophylline. Am J Hosp Pharm 1994;51:661–666.
18. Venning GR. Identification of adverse reactions to new drugs II. (continued): How were 18 important adverse reactions discovered and with what delays. Br Med J 1983;286:365–368.
19. Norrby Sr, Lietman PS. Safety and tolerability of fluoroquinolones. Drugs 1993;45(suppl 3):59–64.
20. Peck CC, Temple CR, Collins JM. Understanding consequences of concurrent therapy. JAMA 1993;269:1550–1552.
21. Requirements for adverse drug reaction reporting. Geneva, Switzerland, World Health Organization, 1975.
22. Karch FE, Lasagna L. Adverse drug reactions—a critical review. JAMA 1975;234:1236–1241.
23. Kessler DA. Introducing MedWatch: A new approach to reporting medication and device adverse effects and product problems. JAMA 1993;269:2765–2768.
24. Anonymous. MedWatch update: Pharmacists submit over half of product problem reports. Am J Hosp Pharm 1993;50:2478.
25. Anonymous. Bristol-Myers-Squibb withdrawing Questran tablets. F-D-C Reports—The Pink Sheet 1994;56:T&G-3.
26. Greenblatt DJ, Koch-Weser J. Clinical toxicology of chlordiazepoxide and diazepam in relation to serum albumin concentration: A report from the Boston Collaborative Drug Surveillance Program. Eur J Clin Pharmacol 1974;7:259–262.
27. May JR, Barbree CD. Communicating DUE results via a service specific newsletter. P&T 1991;16(10):803–819.
28. Cumming RG, Kineberg RJ. Psychotropics, thiazide diuretics and hip fractures. Med J Aust 1993;158:414–417.
29. Kirkman HN. Glucose-6-phosphate dehydrogenase variants and drug-induced hemolysis. Ann NY Acad Sci 1968;151:753.
30. Lunde PKM, Frislid K, Hansteen V. Disease and acetylation polymorphism. Clin Pharmacokinet 1977;2:182–187.
31. DeSwarte RD. Drug allergy, in Patterson R (ed): Allergic Diseases, Diagnosis and Management. Philadelphia, JB Lippincott, 1985.
32. Van der Meer JWM, Scheijgrond HW, Heykants J, et al. The influence of gastric acidity on the bioavailability of ketoconazole. J Antimicrob Chemother 1980;6:552–554.
33. Blum RA, D'Andrea DT, Florentino BM, et al. Increased gastric pH and the bioavailability of fluconazole and ketoconazole. Ann Intern Med 1991;114:755–757.
34. O'Callaghan JW, Thompson RN, Russell AS. Combining NSAIDs with anticoagulants: yes and no. Can Med Assoc J 1984;131:857–858.
35. O'Reilly RA, Trager WF, Motley CH, et al. Stereoselective interaction of phenylbutazone with (12c-13c) warfarin pseudoracemates in man. J Clin Invest 1980;65:746–753.
36. Shorr RI, Ray WA, Daughery JR, Griffin MR. Concurrent use of nonsteroidal anti-inflammatory drugs and oral anticoagulants places elderly persons at high risk for hemorrhagic peptic ulcer disease. Arch Intern Med 1993;153:1665–1670.
37. Rolan PE. Plasma protein binding displacement interactions—why are they still regarded as clinically important? Br J Clin Pharmacol 1994;37:125–128.
38. Mitchell JR, Arias L, Oates JA. Antagonism of the antihypertensive action of guanethidine sulfate by desipramine hydrochloride. JAMA 1967;202:973–976.
39. O'Reilly RA. Interaction of secorbarbital with warfarin pseudoracemates. Clin Pharmacol Ther 1980;28:187.
40. Jackson JE, Powell JR, Wandell M, et al. Cimetidine decreases theophylline clearance. Am Rev Resp Dis 1981;123:615–617.
41. Weinberger MM, Smith G, Milavetz G, et al. Decreased theophylline clearance due to cimetidine [letter]. N Engl J Med 1981;304:672.
42. Campbell MA, Plachetka JR, Jackson JE, et al. Cimetidine decreases theophylline clearance: A case report. Ann Intern Med 1981;95:68–69.
43. Fenje PC, Isles AF, Baltodano A, et al. Interaction of cimetidine and theophylline in two infants [letter]. Can Med Assoc J 1982;126:1178.
44. Honig PK, Wortham DC, Zamani K, Conner DP, Mullin JC, Cantilena LR. Terfenadine–ketoconazole interaction: Pharmacokinetic and electrocardiographic consequences. JAMA 1993;269:1513–1518.
45. Woolsey RL, Chen Y, Freiman JP, Gillis RA. Mechanism of the cardiotoxic actions of terfenadine. JAMA 1993;269:1532–1536.
46. Nightingale SL. Warnings issued on nonsedating antihistamines terfenadine and astemizole. JAMA 1992;268:705.
47. Data on File. Schering-Plough Research Institute. 1994.
48. Peterson V, Hvidts S, Thomsen K, et al. Effect of prolonged thiazide treatment on renal lithium clearance. Br Med J 1974;2:143–145.
49. Mehta BR, Robinson BHB. Lithium toxicity induced by triamterene–hydrochlorothiazide. Postgrad Med J 1980;56:783–784.
50. Morris DJ. Adverse effects and drug interactions of clinical importance with antiviral drugs. Drug Safety 1994;10:281–291.
51. Trissel LA. Handbook of Injectable Drugs, 4th ed. Bethesda, MD, American Society of Hospital Pharmacists, 1986.
52. Sachtles G. Dilantin for I.V. use [letter]. Drug Intell Clin Pharm 1973;7:418.

53. Burke WA. I.V. drug incompatibilities—Dilantin. Am J IV Ther 1975;2:16.
54. Weiner IM, Mudge GH. Inhibitors of tubular transport of organic compounds, in Gilman AG, Goodman LS, Rall TW, et al. (eds): The Pharmacological Basis of Therapeutics, 7th ed. New York, Macmillan, 1985, p 923.
55. Melander A, Danielson K, Schersten B, et al. Enhancement by food of canrenone bioavailability from spironolactone. Clin Pharmacol Ther 1977;22:100–103.
56. Crounse RG. Human pharmacology of griseofulvin: The effect of fat intake on gastrointestinal absorption. J Invest Dermatol 1961;37:529–533.
57. Roe DA. Therapeutic significance of drug–nutrient interactions in the elderly. Pharmacol Rev 1984;36:S109–S122.
58. Jusko WJ. Role of tobacco smoking in pharmacokinetics. J Pharmacokinet Biopharm 1978;6:7–39.
59. Vestal RE, Wood AJJ. Influence of age and smoking on drug pharmacokinetics in man—studies using model compounds. Clin Pharmacokinet 1980;5:309–319.
60. Collaborative Group for the Study of Stroke in Young Women. Oral contraceptives and stroke in young women. JAMA 1978;231:718–722.
61. Jusko WJ, Schentag JJ, Clark JH, et al. Enhanced biotransformation of theophylline in marijuana and tobacco smokers. Clin Pharmacol Ther 1978;24:406–410.
62. Hunt SN, Jusko JW, Yurchak AM. Effect of smoking on theophylline disposition. Clin Pharmacol Ther 1976;19:546–551.
63. Lane EA, Guthrie S, Linnoila M. Effects of ethanol on drug and metabolite pharmacokinetics. Clin Pharmacokinet 1985;10:228–247.
64. Gugler R. H_2-antagonists and alcohol: Do they interact? Drug Safety 1994;10:271–280.
65. Hayes SL, Pablo G, Radomski T, et al. Ethanol and oral diazepam absorption. N Engl J Med 1977;296:186–189.
66. Sellers EM, Naranjo CA, Giles HG, et al. Intravenous diazepam and oral ethanol interaction. Clin Pharmacol Ther 1980;28:638–645.
67. Juhl RP, Van Thiel DH, Dittert LW, et al. Alprazolam pharmacokinetics in alcoholic liver disease. J Clin Pharmacol 1984;24:113–119.
68. Baruh S, Sherman L, Kolodny HD, et al. Fasting hypoglycemia. Med Clin North Am 1973;57:1441–1462.
69. Kater RMH, Tobon F, Iber FL. Increased rate of metabolism in alcoholic patients. JAMA 1969;207:363–365.
70. Fitzgerald MG, Gaddie R, Malins JM, et al. Alcohol sensitivity in diabetics receiving chlorpropamide. Diabetes 1962;2:40–43.
71. Garnett WR. Adverse drug reactions: Detection, assessment, reporting, and prevention, in Ray MD (ed): Basic Skills in Clinical Pharmacy Practice. Bethesda, MD, American Society of Hospital Pharmacists, 1983, pp 209–245.

Chapter 8

Molecular Biology and Biotechnology Drugs

Jim Koeller, MS, and Gary C. Yee, PharmD, FCCP

The structure of DNA was elucidated in 1953 by Drs. James D. Watson and Francis Crick.[1] During the decades following this scientific accomplishment, molecular biologists have learned how to manipulate DNA and other genetic machinery in order to accomplish many practical achievements and to continue expansion of this body of knowledge. Numerous scientific disciplines, including the medical sciences, have benefited from the information and techniques supplied by molecular biologists and geneticists. The development of molecular biologic techniques that facilitate the evaluation of genetic material and expression allows medical science to attain a much greater knowledge of the pathogenesis of disease and its treatment. Techniques provided by the molecular biologist also provide powerful tools for the diagnosis of disease that has a genetic origin or entails a genetic realignment. In addition, this expansion of biotechnology enables the production of new therapeutic agents in a sufficient quantity for clinical use. As the number of such diagnostic tools and therapeutic interventions increases, so will the responsibility of the clinician expand to competently handle these new technologies as they apply to patient care.

This chapter acquaints the reader with the salient aspects of the basic sciences upon which molecular biologic methods are based, to provide an introduction to some of the commonly used techniques and terminologies, and to briefly discuss biotechnology drugs.

Basic Principles: DNA, RNA, and Protein Synthesis

Cellular DNA contains the blueprint that provides the information necessary for daily function and viability of cells. Normally, genetic information is faithfully conserved during replication of the DNA molecule and during cellular division.[2] Expression of genetic information provides the endocrine proteins, structural proteins, and enzymes necessary for cellular growth, reproduction, differentiation, and daily function. To accomplish this, genes made of deoxynucleic acid (DNA) determine the nucleotide sequences of ribonucleic acids (RNA) made by the cell. The RNA then delivers the code to the ribosome which dictates the specific type of polypeptide to be synthesized by the cell (Fig. 8.1). Every unique polypeptide is formed from the genetic information contained on a single gene. There are two major classifications of organisms that carry out DNA, RNA, and protein synthesis; they are prokaryotes and eukaryotes (Table 8.1). Prokaryotes are simple, generally single-celled organisms. Bacteria would fit into this category. Eukaryotes, on the other hand, are more complexed-celled organisms and are generally multicellular. Plants, fungus, and animals fit into this category.

Cellular genes are aligned on double-stranded, helical molecules of DNA. The basic building blocks of DNA are (1) phosphoric acid; (2) a sugar; and (3) four nitrogen-containing bases, which include two purines, adenine (A) and guanine (G), and two pyrimidines, thymine (T) and cytosine (C) (Fig. 8.2). The four nucleotides (base pairs) bind to each other in a very specific manner. Chargaff's rule states that adenine will always form a double hydrogen bond with thymine, whereas cytosine will always form a triple hydrogen bond with guanine. It is the covalent bonding of one molecule of phosphoric acid, one molecule of deoxyribose, and one of the four base pairs that comprises a nucleotide.

The orientation of nucleotides within the RNA strand is illustrated in Fig. 8.3. The structure of RNA is very similar to DNA except that (1) ribonucleic acid is the sugar component and (2) uracil replaces thymine as the complementary base for adenine. Triphosphorylated RNA nucleotides are considered activated and, therefore, ready to be transcribed into a RNA molecule.[2]

Each group of three successive nucleotide bases provides the code for a particular amino acid to be utilized for the translation of a specific protein (polypeptide). Therefore, the organization of nucleotide base triplets, known as codons, determines the character and function of the pro-

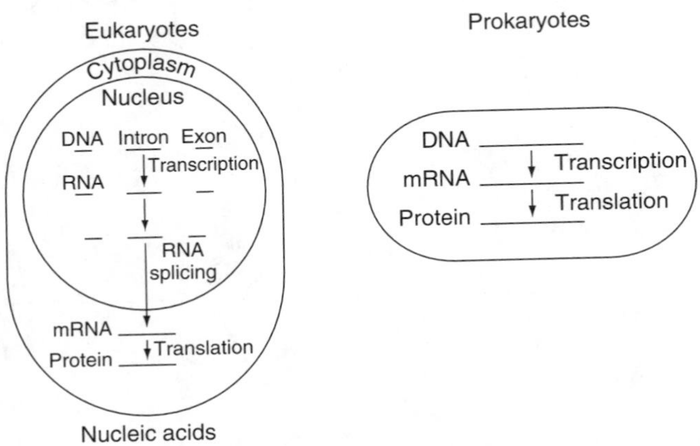

Figure 8.1. Protein synthesis in eukaryotic and prokaryotic organisms. *(From Alberts B, Bray D, Lewis J, et al [eds]. Molecular Biology of the Cell, 2nd ed. New York, Garland Publishing, 1989, p 101, with permission.)*

teins which evolve from expression of DNA (Fig. 8.4). This is known as the genetic code. The genetic code has remained highly conserved during evolution, and with a few minor exceptions it is the same for diverse species of both the animal and plant world.[2]

DNA FUNCTION

The complete set of instructions for making an organism is called its genome. A genome includes tightly coiled threads of DNA and associated protein molecules. Chromosomes are made up of DNA and histones (basic, positively charged proteins that neutralize the DNA acidity). Therefore, each chromosome has DNA; the difference is in the sequence of nucleotides. The human genome is approximately 3 billion base pairs long. The nucleus of most human cells contains two sets of chromosomes (one set from each parent). Each set would thus have 23 single chromosomes (22 autosomes and 1 sex chromosome, e.g., X or Y). An autosome is simply a chromosome not involved in sex determination. Thus the human genome consists of 46 chromosomes (22 pairs of autosomes and 1 pair of sex chromosomes. Females would have a pair X chromosomes and males would have one X and one Y. All genes are arranged linearly along the chromosomes. A gene is a specific sequence of nucleotide bases, whose sequences carry the information required for manufacturing proteins. The human genome is estimated to have approximately 100,000 genes.

DNA carries out two critical functions (Fig. 8.2). First, it must be able to duplicate itself in order to pass along its genetic information from generation to generation. Second, it must translate its genetic code in such a way that all functional components of life's processes are created.

MOLECULAR BIOLOGY TECHNIQUES

Before a human protein can be recombinantly produced, it must first be isolated and its amino acid sequence deciphered. Up until the 1970s there was no precise way to cut up DNA fragments in an ordered fashion such that individual gene identification was possible. Instead, medicinal chemists had to laboriously manufacture a protein. Amino acid sequencing by this method was most difficult and explained why there were no human-manufactured proteins available for commercial use. In the coming section, we explain in general terms the process of protein identification.

RESTRICTION ENDONUCLEASES

The ability to characterize DNA and isolate specific amino acid sequences has been greatly enhanced by the use of

TABLE 8.1. COMPARISON OF PROKARYOTIC AND EUKARYOTIC ORGANISMS

	Prokaryotes	Eukaryotes
Organisms	Bacteria and cyanobacteria	Protists, fungi, plants, animals
Cell size	Generally 1 to 10 μm in linear dimension	Generally 10 to 100 μm in linear dimension
Metabolism	Anaerobic or aerobic	Aerobic
Organelles	Few or none	Nucleus, mitochondria, chloroplasts, endoplasmic reticulum, etc.
DNA	Circular DNA in cytoplasm	Very long linear DNA molecules containing many noncoding regions; bounded by nuclear envelope
RNA and protein	RNA and protein synthesized in same compartment	RNA synthesized and processed in nuclease; proteins synthesized in cytoplasm
Cytoplasm	No cytoskeleton; cytoplasmic streaming, endocytosis, and exocytosis all absent	Cytoskeleton composed of protein filaments; cytoplasmic streaming; endocytosis and exocytosis
Cell division	Chromosomes pulled apart by attachments to plasma membrane	Chromosomes pulled apart by cytoskeletal spindle apparatus
Cellular organization	Mainly unicellular	Mainly multicellular, with differentiation of many cell types

(From Watson JD, Hopkins NH, Roberts JW, et al (eds). Molecular Biology of the Gene, 4th ed. Menlo Park, CA, Benjamin/Cummings, 1987, p 97, with permission.)

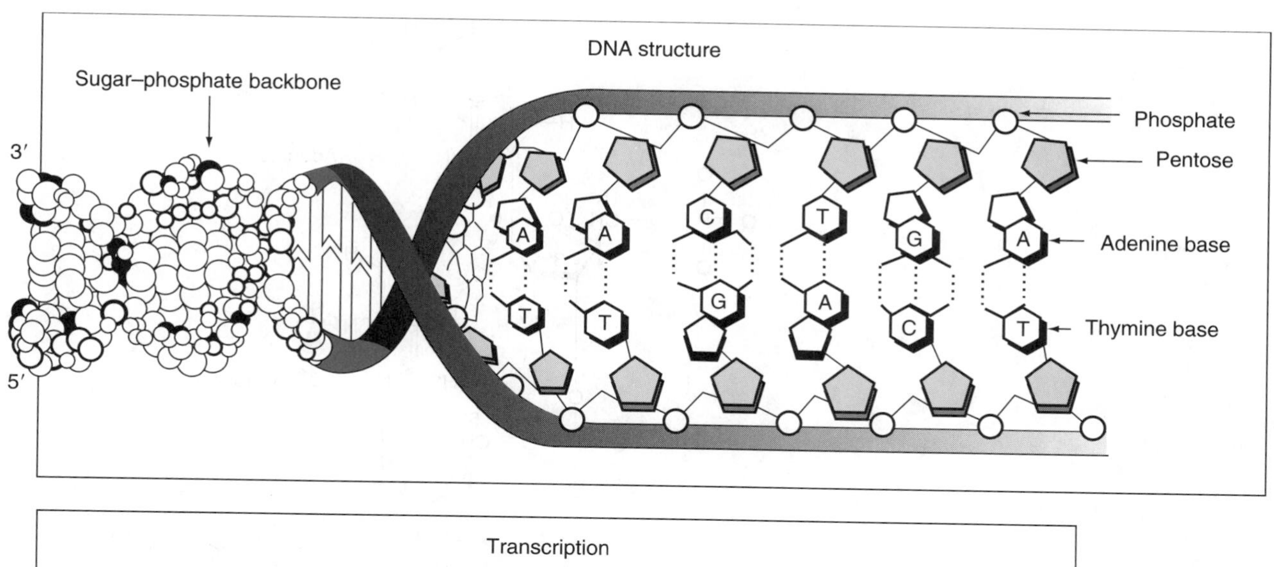

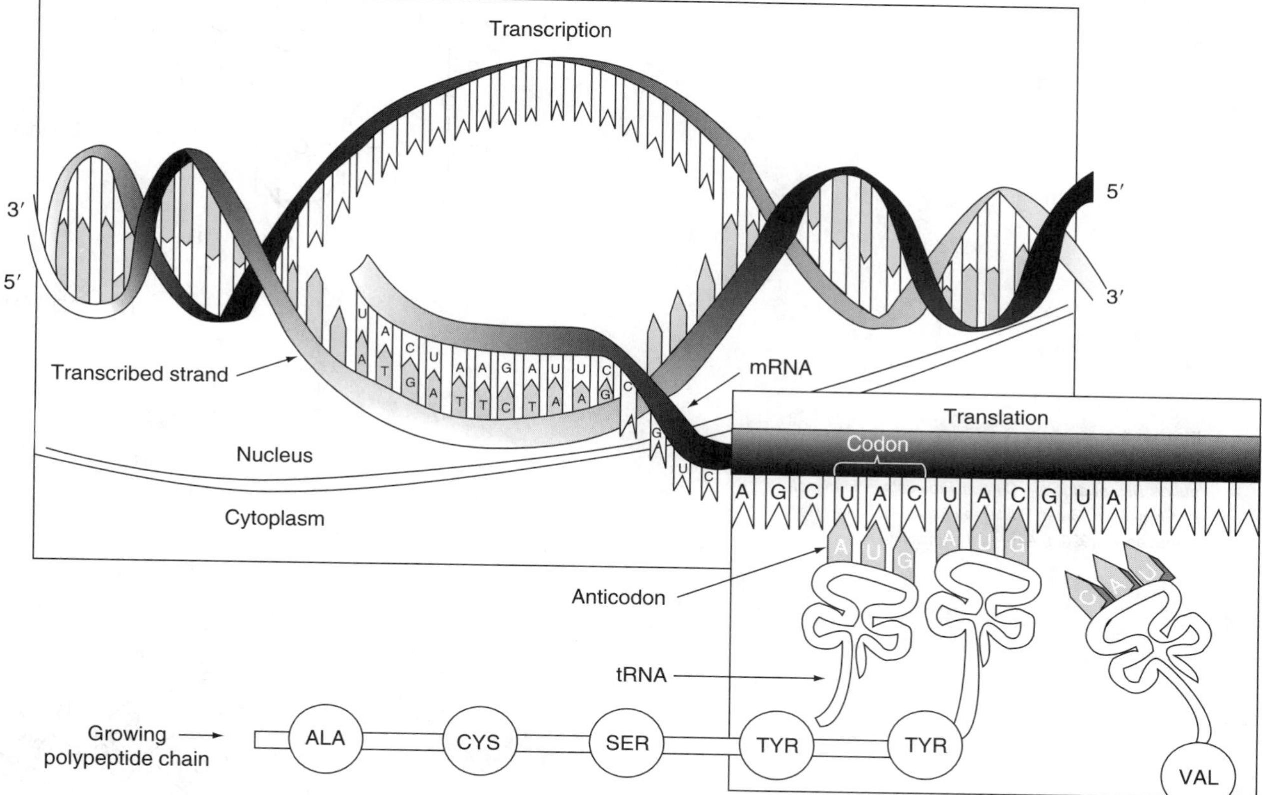

Figure 8.2. The DNA double helix and the flow of genetic information. The top panel shows the sequence of four bases (guanine, adenine, thymine, and cytosine), which determines the specificity of genetic information. The bases face inward from the sugar–phosphate backbone and form pairs (dashed lines) with complementary bases on the opposing strand. In the larger bottom panel, transcription in the nucleus creates a complementary nucleic acid copy (mRNA) from one of the DNA strands in the double helix. The mRNA leaves the nucleus and associates with ribosomes in the cytoplasm, where it is translated into protein (smaller bottom panel). Special transfer RNAs (tRNA) align the corresponding amino acids along the mRNA, using the three-base genetic code to transform the nucleic acid sequence into a protein sequence. *(From Rosenthal, N. DNA and the genetic code. N Engl J Med 1994;331:39–41, Massachusetts Medical Society, with permission.)*

restriction endonucleases called "cutters." These enzymes, which are isolated from bacteria, will cleave double-stranded DNA into well-defined fragments known as restriction fragments. Bacteria produce these enzymes as a self-defense mechanism to protect themselves from invaders such as viruses. Sequences in the bacterias' DNA, which may be cut by these same endonucleases, are protected by methyl groups such that hydrolysis cannot take place. Many restriction endonuclease enzymes are available commercially; a few of these are listed in Table 8.2.[3] The

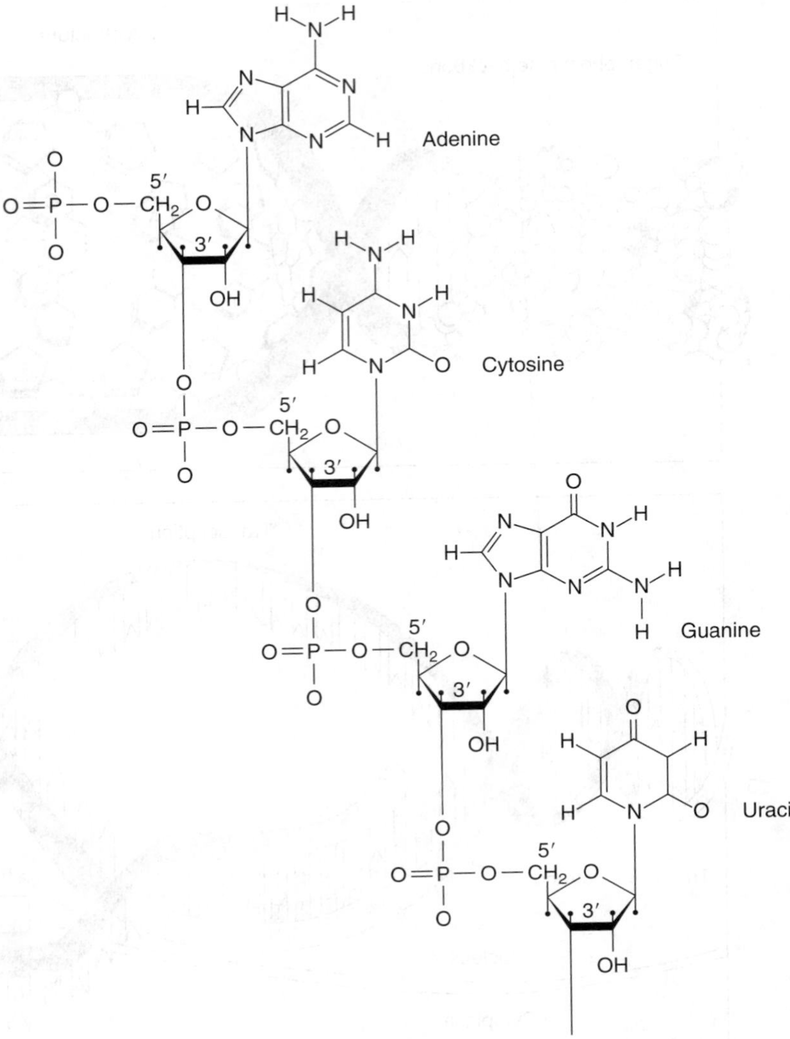

Figure 8.3. A portion of a polyribonucleotide (RNA) chain. *(From Coligan JE, Kruisbeek AM, Margulies DH, et al [eds]. Current Protocols in Immunology. New York, Green Publishing Associates and Wiley-Interscience, 1990, p A15, with permission.)*

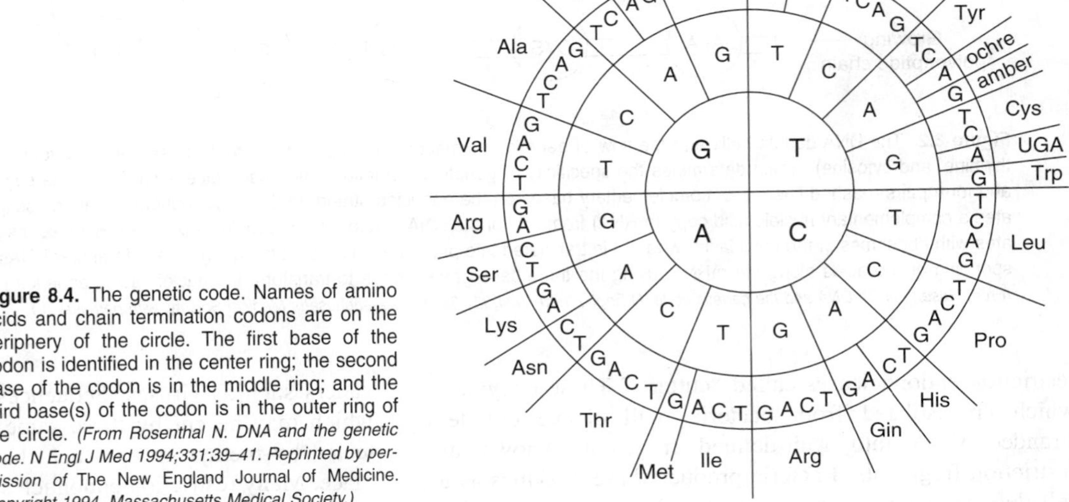

Figure 8.4. The genetic code. Names of amino acids and chain termination codons are on the periphery of the circle. The first base of the codon is identified in the center ring; the second base of the codon is in the middle ring; and the third base(s) of the codon is in the outer ring of the circle. *(From Rosenthal N. DNA and the genetic code. N Engl J Med 1994;331:39–41. Reprinted by permission of* The New England Journal of Medicine. *Copyright 1994, Massachusetts Medical Society.)*

TABLE 8.2. RECOGNITION SEQUENCES OF VARIOUS RESTRICTION ENZYMES

Enzyme	Recognition Site (Axis; Cut bond)	Enzyme	Recognition Site (Axis of symmetry; Cut bond)
Eco RI	↓ 5′-GAA | TTC CTT | AAG ↑	*Hin* dII	↓ 5′-CTPy | PuAC CAPu | PytG ↑
Hin dIII	↓ AAG | CTT TTC | GAA ↑	*Hpa* I	↓ GTT | AAC CAA | TTG ↑
Hpa II	↓ CC | GG GG | CC ↑	*Hae* III	↓ GG | CC CC | GG ↑
Acy I	↓ GPuC | GPyC CPyG | CPuG ↑	*Afl* III	↓ ACPu | PyGT TGPy | PuCA ↑
Aha II	↓ GPuC | GPyC CPyG | CPuG ↑	*Ava* I	↓ CPyC | GPuG CPuG | CPyC ↑
Cfr I	↓ PyGG | CCPu PuCC | GGPy ↑	*Gdi* II	↓ PyGG | CCG PuCC | GGC ↑
Hae II	↓ PuGG | GCPy PyCG | CGPu ↑	*Hgi* CI	↓ GGPy | PuCC CCPu | PyGG ↑
Hgi III	↓ GPuG | CPyC CPyC | GPuG ↑	*Nsp* CI	↓ PuCA | TGPy PyGT | ACPu ↑
Alu I	↓ AG | CT TC | GA ↑	*Asu* II	↓ TTC | GAA AAG | CTT ↑
Cla I	↓ ATC | GAT TAG | CTA ↑	*Bse* PI	↓ GCG | CGC CGC | GCG ↑

Arrows denote the site of cleavage. All base sequences are known with the 5′ end of the upper strand at the left. Pu, purine; Py, pyrimidine. *(From Watson JD, Hopkins NH, Roberts JW, et al (eds). Molecular Biology of the Gene, 4th ed. Menlo Park, CA, Benjamin/Cummings, 1987, p 289, with permission.)*

signal for a particular restriction endonuclease to cut DNA is provided by a specific 4- or 6-base pair sequence that acts as a recognition site for the enzyme. These 4- and 6-base pair recognition sites occur every several hundred to every several thousand base pairs, respectively. Cleavage that occurs from restriction endonucleases will yield either two blunt-end DNA fragments or two short uneven ends (Fig. 8.5). The uneven ends are called "sticky" or cohesive ends because they are capable of forming complementary base pairs with the uneven ends of another fragment produced by the same enzyme. Different endonucleases known as isoschizomers may recognize the same nucleotide sequences. Isoschizomers do not always cleave DNA identically and therefore may produce different types of ends. However, isoschizomers or restriction endonucleases that recognize different nucleotide sequences can produce identical DNA fragment termini, which are termed compatible ends.[4,5]

To get DNA coupled from different sources (recombinant DNA or rDNA) restriction endonucleases can be used to cut DNA in a way that would allow other pieces of DNA to be inserted.

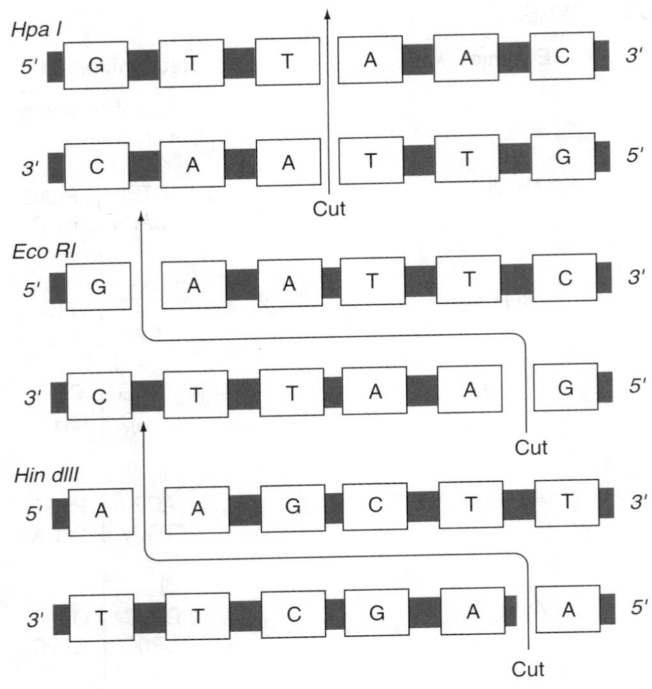

Figure 8.5. Types of cleavage produced by restriction endonucleases: (top figure) blunt cut and (bottom two figures) sticky cut. *(From Alberts B, Bray D, Lewis J, et al [eds]. Molecular Biology of the Cell, 2nd ed. New York, Garland Publishing, 1989, p 182, with permission.)*

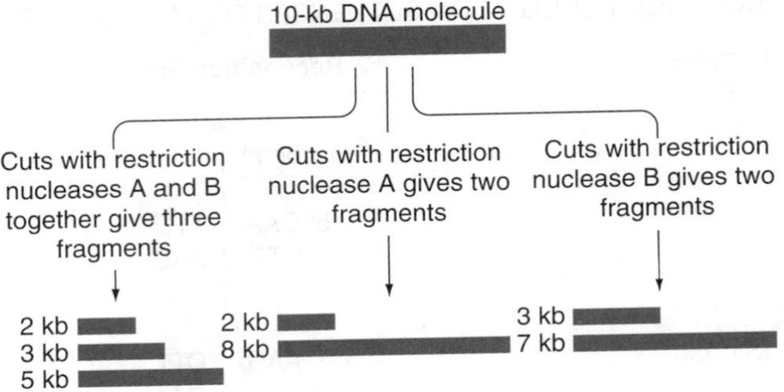

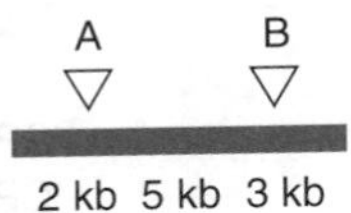

Figure 8.6. Restriction mapping of DNA. *(From Alberts B, Bray D, Lewis J, et al [eds]. Molecular Biology of the Cell, 2nd ed. New York, Garland Publishing, 1989, p 182, with permission.)*

RESTRICTION MAPPING

The cleavage of a DNA segment by a restriction endonuclease will yield several DNA fragments which can be used to construct a map to identify the sizes of the various fragments (Fig. 8.6). To accomplish this, the individual fragments produced by the use of a cutter are placed in an agarose (polysaccharide) gel, and then a current is run across the gel. The DNA fragments will move toward the positive pole, with small fragments able to move faster than larger fragments. Ethidium bromide present in the gel mixture will stain the migrating fragments and allow visualization with ultraviolet light. This process is called gel electrophoresis and allows the fragment sizes in the gel to be compared with known DNA fragment sizes. This process is called restriction mapping. Restriction mapping provides important information for sequence analysis of DNA and certain DNA cloning procedures.[6] A mutation in the DNA could affect the results of a restriction map. Differences in DNA among individuals would be referred to as a polymorphism. Common polymorphisms would be a point mutation (e.g., a "G" replacing an "A" in the DNA strand), DNA repeats (e.g., "ATATAT"), or an insertion or deletion of a segment of DNA. Most polymorphisms occur outside of the coding region of DNA.

Each human has a distinct pattern of nucleotide sequencing. Comparison of restriction fragments from two different individuals is a technique used to detect the presence of genetic differences or aberrations. This is possible because DNA variations would have different nucleotide sequences and the number and size of restriction fragments produced by endonucleases would be different. The presence of such aberrations is known as restriction fragment length polymorphisms (RFLP). This process is used in genetic linkage studies to evaluate the genetic makeup of individuals (forensic applications), families with inherited traits, or other genetic diseases. Once a specific RFLP has been identified, it can be used to identify an individual or screen family members and establish inheritance patterns.[7]

SOUTHERN BLOTTING AND HYBRIDIZATION

Southern blotting and hybridization is a method that can detect the presence of specific nucleotide sequences from fragments of DNA.[8] Once DNA fragments have been separated by size using agarose gel electrophoresis, they must be transferred to a solid media support so that further evaluation can be performed. The process of transferring the DNA fragments from the gel to a solid nitrocellulose filter that immobilizes the fragments is called Southern blotting (Fig. 8.7).

Once the fragments have been transferred to a solid base, they are treated with sodium hydroxide to denature (separate) the DNA strands. The single DNA strand can then be exposed to a radiolabeled DNA probe. Sections of the fragment with sequences complementary to the sequence of interest are targeted with the radioactive isotope which will hybridize (join together). Hybridization reactions using DNA probes are sensitive and selective and can detect one fragment of complementary DNA per cell. The most commonly used isotope for labeling nucleotide is ^{32}P. Its short half-life (14 days) and inability to alter enzymatic activity make it quite popular. The radiolabeled nitrocellulose filter paper is exposed to x-ray film (called autoradiography) which shows off dark bands where the probe attached (Fig. 8.7).[9] Southern blotting can be used for the detection and diagnosis of single-gene diseases such as cystic fibrosis, Huntington's disease, and Duchenne's muscular dystrophy.

Where Southern blotting can be used to analyze DNA, RNA can be analyzed using an analogous technique called Northern blotting. With this technique, cellular RNA or mRNA is separated by size using agarose gel electrophoresis. Enzymatic digestion of RNA is not necessary prior to electrophoresis because most RNA is already small enough to migrate through agarose gel. A denaturing agent such as formaldehyde or methyl mercury is added to the gel to prevent the formation of secondary structures. The fragments are then transferred to a solid matrix and fixed. Hybridization with an appropriately labeled probe is performed after which autoradiography will produce dark bands, once again corresponding to the probes located on the RNA strands. Northern blotting is used to confirm the accuracy of cloned cDNA. It also is used to measure the level of gene expression in specific tissues.

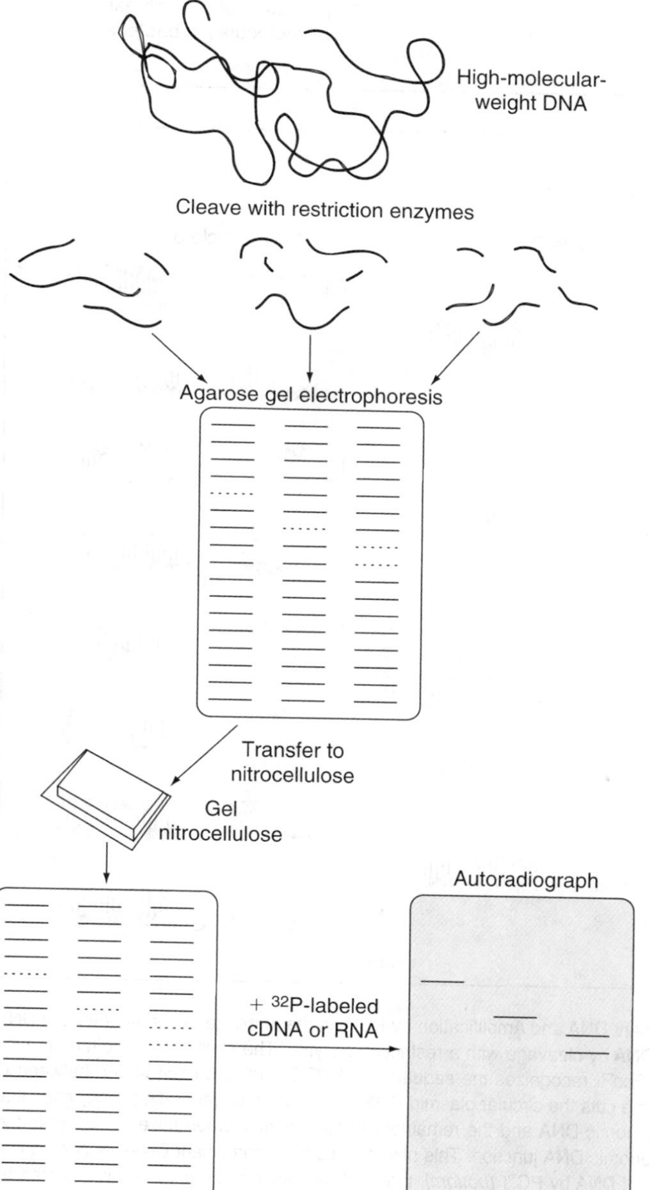

Figure 8.7. Southern blotting. *(From Watson JD, Tooze J, Kurtz DT [eds]. Recombinant DNA: A Short Course. New York, WH Freeman, 1983, p 83, with permission.)*

Western blotting is a technique used to analyze proteins and other polypeptides. It is also called sodium dodecyl sulfate polyacrylamide-gel electrophoresis (SDS–PAGE). When polyacrylamide is polymerized, it provides an inert matrix through which proteins will migrate. To facilitate the separation of proteins based on molecular weight, samples are first solubilized in a solution of sodium dodecyl sulfate (SDS), which is a strong negatively charged detergent. This causes protein–protein and protein–lipid binding to be disrupted. Thus, the proteins migrate unfolded through the polyacrylamide gel. Due to the negative charge inferred by the SDS–protein complex, the proteins will migrate toward the positive charge of a gel when current is applied. As with DNA fragments, smaller proteins will move faster than the larger ones. A single protein band may represent more than one type of protein as all proteins of a given molecular weight will move to a single band. Overlapping of bands can also occur.[10,11] The bands are stained for detection purposes. Generally, SDS–PAGE is capable of separating samples containing fewer than 50 proteins. As with the other techniques, the proteins are transferred to a solid matrix and probed using either a radioisotope, antibody-directed enzyme, or fluorescent-labeled dye.

When a two-dimensional gel electrophoresis (separation by weight and electrical charge) is used, it is possible to separate more than 1000 proteins.[12]

POLYMERASE CHAIN REACTION

One of the more recent applications of new molecular biology techniques includes polymerase chain reaction (PCR). This is a process that efficiently amplifies specific DNA sequences *in vitro* for characterization and analysis. This method makes it possible to increase a targeted DNA sequence geometrically even when the starting amount is extremely small.

The reaction is performed by heating and cooling the DNA in the presence of a mixture containing the four DNA bases, two DNA primers, and a buffer solution. The DNA primers are pieces of DNA that are synthesized, under precise conditions, to match up exactly with and attach to a stretch of DNA before and after the DNA sequence being

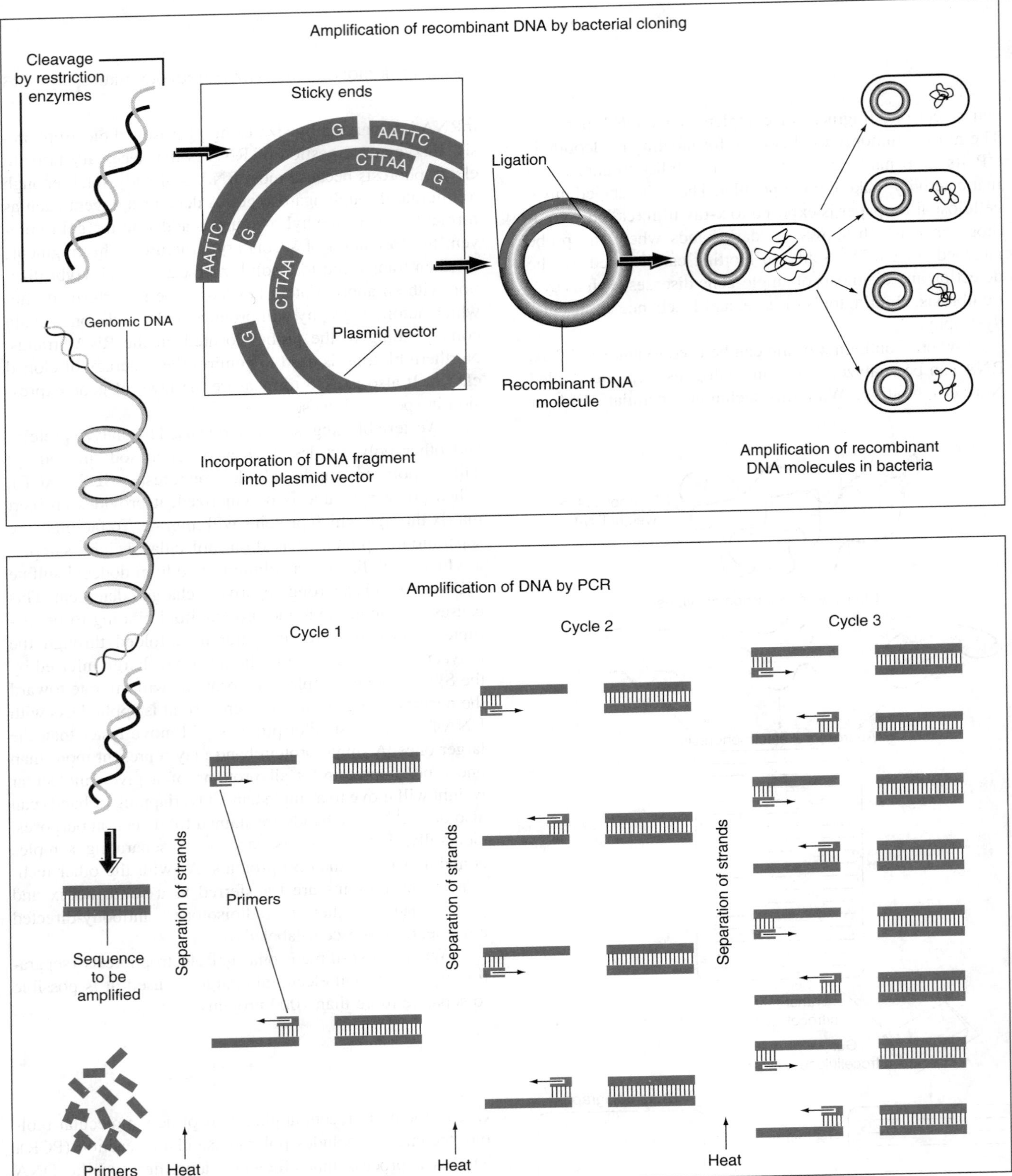

Figure 8.8. Polymerase chain reaction (PCR) process. Amplification of Recombinant DNA and Amplification by PCR. In the amplification of recombinant DNA (top), the DNA segment to be amplified is separated from surrounding genomic DNA by cleavage with a restriction enzyme. The enymatic cuts often produce staggered or "sticky" ends. In the example shown here, the restriction enzyme *Eco*RI recognizes the sequence GAATTC and cuts each strand between G (guanine) and A (adenine) (C = cytosine, T = thymine). The same restriction enzyme cuts the circular plasmid DNA at a single site, generating sticky ends that are complementary to the sticky ends of the genomic DNA fragment. The cut genomic DNA and the remainder of the plasmid, when mixed together in the presence of a ligase enzyme, form smooth joints on each side of the plasmid–genomic DNA junction. This new molecule—recombinant DNA—is carried into bacteria, which replicate the plasmid as they grow in culture. In the amplification of DNA by PCR *(bottom),* the DNA sequence to be amplified is selected by primers, which are short, synthetic oligonucleotides that correspond to sequences flanking the DNA to be amplified. After an excess of primers is added to the DNA, together with a heat-stable DNA polymerase, the strands of both the genomic DNA and the primers are separated by heating and then allowed to cool. A heat-stable polymerase elongates the primers on either strand, thus generating two new identical double-stranded DNA molecules and doubling the number of DNA fragments. Each cycle takes only a few minutes and doubles the number of copies of the original DNA fragment. *(From Rosenthal, N. Molecular medicine tools of the trade recombinant DNA. N Engl J Med 1994;331:316, Massachusetts Medical Society, with permission.)*

TABLE 8.3. SINGLE-GENE DISEASES DETECTABLE BY USING POLYMERASE CHAIN REACTION

Sickle cell disease
β-Thalassemia
Duchenne's muscular dystrophy
Cystic fibrosis
Tay–Sachs disease
Huntington's disease

(From Watson JD, Hopkins NH, Roberts JW, et al. (eds). Molecular Biology of the Gene, 4th ed. Menlo Park, CA, Benjamin/Cummings, 1987, p 268, with permission.)

amplified. The mixture is heated to separate the strands of double-stranded DNA and then slightly cooled to allow the primers to align and attach to their complementary sequences on the separated strands. Once this happens the reaction temperature is changed to allow the *Taq polymerase* to begin its work of adding the appropriate DNA bases in order to synthesize a new strand of DNA.

PCR is utilized in several clinical and research applications (Fig. 8.8). Diagnosis of many single-gene disorders is possible using PCR (Table 8.3). Samples of prenatal chorion obtained during the first trimester have been used to diagnosis certain genetic disorders such as sickle cell anemia and β-thalassemia. Retroviruses, including human immunodeficiency virus, are detectable using PCR. PCR analysis of major histocompatability (MHC) class II protein can provide a marker for such diseases as insulin-dependent diabetes, rheumatoid arthritis, Reiter's disease, and ankylosing spondolytis.

Recombinant DNA Technology

Recombinant DNA (rDNA) technology utilizes several molecular biologic techniques for the isolation and cloning of a gene to produce large amounts of protein. To achieve this, rDNA is constructed from the gene of interest and inserted into an appropriate vector or carrier (Fig. 8.8). The most common vectors used are plasmids (bacterial) and bacteriophage (viral). Plasmid vectors are capable of transporting rDNA into a host cell by a process known as transfection. Following the transfection of rDNA, the host cells are grown in a favorable culture medium and subsequently produce millions of copies of the recombinant gene for translation into large amounts of protein.[13]

RECOMBINANT DNA SOURCES

Screening the entire human genome for a single gene is not practical. Instead, one can isolate the cells that make a specific protein, knowing that in nature cells express only a limited number of their genes. For example, if one wishes to isolate the protein interleukin-2 (IL-2), activated T cells (which produce IL-2) would be isolated. If IL-2 is being produced by a cell, the gene for IL-2 of that cell would have to be transcribed into mRNA. Copies of the mRNA for IL-2 should then be able to be isolated from the cytoplasm of the activated T cells. In the presence of a reverse transcriptase enzyme, mRNA can be used to produce a complementary copy of DNA, called cDNA. This cDNA can then be used for cloning. This process is initiated by the addition of an oligodeoxythymidine molecule to the complementary tail of DNA synthesis. DNA polymerase will synthesize cDNA until it reaches the 3′ end of the mRNA template. At this point, most DNA polymerase enzymes will make a hairpin turn and continue cDNA synthesis using the DNA strand as a template. Following completion of DNA synthesis, the single-stranded DNA loop resultant from the turning of DNA polymerase may be cleaved by nuclease enzymes specific for single-stranded DNA.[14] Further enzymatic modification by transferase or ligase activity will facilitate the insertion of this newly synthesized cDNA into a host cell for cloning and amplification.[14,15] The cloning (producing exact copies) of cDNA will produce a cDNA library. The cDNA library contains only copies of actively expressed genes. This allows for the indefinite storage of the DNA that will express a specific gene.[16]

VECTORS

Vectors are small circular pieces of extrachromosomal DNA which are used as carriers of the human gene fragment for placement into the host cell for growth. The bacterial plasmid, the virus bacteriophage λ, and a hybrid of bacteriophage λ (called a cosmid) are the most common vectors used.

Plasmid vectors must be quite small to ensure that they are taken up by the host bacteria (a process called transformation). Due to their size, the plasmid can only carry DNA fragments of up to 10 kilobase (kb) pairs. For this reason, the plasmid is most often used to create gene libraries of smaller DNA fragments.[17] The most common plasmid vector used is the artificially constructed pBR322. Even at their greatest efficiency, plasmids will be transformed (taken up) by a host such as *E. coli* at a rate of only 0.01%.

For DNA fragments larger than 10 kb, the viral vector bacteriophage λ or its hybrid, the cosmid, must be used.[18] The bacteriophage λ can transport DNA fragments up to 21 kb. The bacteriophage λ has a "head" and "tail" and will in fact attach to the outer membrane of the host cell; the linear DNA is then injected into the cell. Once inside, the DNA circularizes. By injecting its DNA into the host, the bacteriophage λ bypasses the transformation step required with plasmids and thus allows the uptake of larger DNA fragments. The cosmid vector is a bacteriophage λ hybrid which is used to carry DNA fragments between 32 and 47 kb in length.

The circular DNA vectors are opened using restriction enzymes, so that the human DNA fragments can be added. The vector is then closed with the enzyme DNA ligase. The end product of combining the genetic material from two different species is called recombinant DNA.

HOST CELLS

Several different host cells are used as cloning factories for the various vectors described previously. The prokaryote *E. coli* is commonly used. *Escherichia coli* have a well-characterized genome, are generally easy to maintain, grow rapidly (genetic material reproduced every 20 minutes), and are also relatively inexpensive. However, there are certain limitations with the use of prokaryotes such as *E. coli.* Prokaryotes are unable to process pre-mRNA by extracting the introns (noncoding nucleotides) from the RNA. Consequently, it is necessary to use cDNA in the prokaryote host for the synthesis of a functional protein.[13] Prokaryotes also lack the ability to carry out several post-translational processes such as glycosylation and proteolysis. Most human proteins are glycosylated, that is, they contain sugars. If the sugars are necessary for biologic function (e.g., erythropoietin), then a prokaryote could not be used for production. The human protein insulin is converted from proinsulin to insulin through proteolysis carried out post-translationally. In addition, prokaryotes cannot excrete their proteins. For example, *E. coli* would have to be lysed to remove the protein cloned during the recombinant process. This could allow contaminants (e.g., endotoxin) to become part of the final product.

When a more complex-celled organism is needed as a host, a eukaryote is generally used.[19] The yeast *Saccharomyces cerevisiae* is commonly used.[20] They are well characterized, grow faster than both plant and animal cells, and are generally nonpathogenic. Yeast are also able to partially glycosylate the proteins they produce. In addition, yeast excrete the proteins they produce, eliminating the need for cell lysis. As with prokaryotes, yeast cannot remove introns from pre-mRNA; thus cDNA must also be used as the genetic material. Yeast are, however, harder to grow and more expensive to work with than *E. coli.* Higher eukaryotic organisms that have been used include the African green monkey kidney cell (COS), mouse 3T3 fibroblast cell (WOP), and the Chinese hamster ovary (CHO) cell. These are the most difficult of the eukaryotic cells to grow, requiring elaborate culture systems which are time consuming and expensive.

Recombinant DNA technology has contributed extensively to the ability of scientists to characterize genes and gene products. Furthermore, many therapeutic agents are available in sufficient quantities for clinical use due to recombinant DNA technology (Table 8.4).

TABLE 8.4. APPROVED BIOTECHNOLOGY DRUGS

Drug	Trade Name (Company)	Year Approved
Insulin	Humulin (Eli Lilly)	1982
Somatrem (growth hormone)	Protropin (Genentech)	1985
Interferon alfa-2b	Intron A (Schering-Plough)	1986
Interferon alfa-2a	Roferon (Hoffmann-La Roche)	
Muromonab-CD3	Orthoclone OKT3 (Ortho)	1986
Hepatitis B vaccine	Recombivax HB (Merck)	1986
Somatropin (growth hormone)	Humatrope (Eli Lilly)	1987
Alteplase (tPA)	Activase (Genentech)	1987
Epoetin alfa	Epogen (Amgen)	1989
Hepatitis B vaccine	Engerix B (SmithKline Beecham)	1989
Interferon alfa-n3	Alferon (Interferon Sciences)	1989
Epoetin alfa	Procrit (Ortho)	1990
Interferon gamma-1b	Actimmune (Genentech)	1990
Filgrastim (G-CSF)	Neupogen (Amgen)	1991
Sargramostim (GM-CSF)	Leukine (Immunex)	1991
Insulin	Novolin (Novo Nordisk)	1991
Aglucerase	Ceredase (Genzyme)	1991
Aldesleukin (interleukin-2)	Proleukin (Chiron)	1992
Factor VIII	RECOMBINATE (Genetics Institute/Baxter)	1992
Staumonab pendetide	OncoScint CR/OV (Cytogen)	1992
Factor VIII	KoGENate (Miles)	1993
Interferon beta-1b	Betaseron (Chiron/Berlex)	1993
Dornase alfa (DNase)	Pulmozyme (Genentech)	1993
Somatropin (growth hormone)	Nutropin (Genentech)	1994
Imiglucerase	Cerezyme (Genzyme)	1994
Abciximab (7E3 Fab)	ReoPro (Centocor/Eli Lilly)	1994
Somatropin (growth hormone)	Norditropin (Novo Nordisk)	1995
Somatropin (growth hormone)	Bio-Tropin (Bio-Technology General)	1995

Biotechnology Drugs

One of the most important applications of molecular biology is the use of recombinant DNA techniques to make biotechnology drugs. Although experts define a biotechnology drug differently, most agree that a biotechnology drug is made with living cells. The Food and Drug Administration defines biotechnology as a "technique that uses living organisms or a part of a living organism to produce or modify a product, to improve a plant or animal, or to develop a microorganism to be used for a specific purpose." But if we use that definition, then biotechnology drugs are not new because antibiotics have been made with microorganisms for many years. Most biotechnology drugs are protein drugs made in living cells by either monoclonal antibody or rDNA technology. However, some experts will also include drugs such as liposomal drugs that are not made in living cells. In addition to different manufacturing processes, biotechnology drugs differ from nonbiotechnology drugs in other ways. Biotechnology drugs are of great concern to pharmacy because of their high acquisition costs and questionable reimbursement. In many hospitals, biotechnology drugs comprise about 15–20% of the total drug budget. Another difference is that most biotechnology drugs are manufactured by small biotechnology companies, although they are often marketed by a large pharmaceutical company. Most have narrow FDA-approved indications but a wide range of potential indications. Biotechnology companies pursue this strategy because many have limited resources and because of pressure by investors to bring a drug to market quickly. After the drug becomes commercially available, the company tries to increase sales by promoting clinical use of the drug in non-FDA-approved indications. Finally, biotechnology drugs raise many complex patent issues. For example, two biotechnology drugs may have the same biological activity but differ in their amino acid structure.

Biotechnology drugs have had a major impact on the treatment of many diseases. Prior to the availability of rDNA technology, it was difficult to obtain protein drugs in sufficient quantities for clinical use. Sources of human proteins were limited; protein drugs could only be obtained from plasma or other biological fluids (e.g., urine) or cadavers. Animals represent another possible source but were less desirable because of the problems associated with administration of an animal protein. Even when protein drugs could be obtained from these sources, quantities were limited and purity was often a concern. It should be noted that many biotechnology drugs could not be made by any method other than by rDNA technology.

Table 8.4 lists the currently available biotechnology drugs. The first biotechnology drug, recombinant human insulin, was introduced in 1982. That number grew to 11 by the end of 1989 and to nearly 30 by mid-1995. All but five of the drugs are made by recombinant DNA technology; three of these five are made with monoclonal antibody technology (muromonab-CD3, staumonab pendetide, abciximab) and the remaining two are made in living cells but not with monoclonal antibody or rDNA technology (interferon alfa [Alferon] and aglucerase). Recombinant proteins can be categorized into several major categories. The first category is *hormones* such as insulin or growth hormone; epoetin alfa is also sometimes categorized as a hormone. Another category of recombinant proteins is *cytokines,* which are soluble mediators produced by mononuclear cells (i.e., lymphocytes or monocytes/macrophages) that regulate the immune response (discussed in Chapter 80). Examples of cytokines include the interferons (alfa, gamma, and beta), filgrastim, sargramostim, and interleukin-2. Filgrastim, sargramostim, and epoetin alfa are also referred to as colony-stimulating factors or hematopoietic growth factors (discussed in Chapter 119). *Enzymes* such as alteplase, imiglucerase, and dornase alfa are another major category of proteins. Finally, recombinant factor VIII is an example of a *clotting factor* and the recombinant hepatitis B vaccine is an example of a *subunit vaccine.*

It is also useful to categorize biotechnology drugs as either endogenous proteins or "designer" proteins. Endogenous proteins are usually given for one of several clinical indications: as replacement therapy in a deficiency state, to augment a normal physiologic response, or to suppress a normal physiologic response. "Designer" proteins are not endogenous proteins but are often based on the known structure of a protein. Monoclonal antibodies, for example, are used to inhibit the activity of a specific protein, cell, or microorganism. Another example of a "designer" protein is a subunit vaccine, which is given to elicit an immune response against a specific antigen made with rDNA technology.

Many other biotechnology drugs are currently in clinical trials. According to the 1995 Pharmaceutical Research and Manufacturers of America (PhRMA) report entitled "Biotechnology Medicines in Development," 234 biotechnology drugs are in clinical trials. Fourteen of these products are awaiting approval at the FDA and 49 are in phase III clinical trials. Monoclonal antibodies represent the largest category of biotechnology drugs, accounting for about 30% of the drugs in clinical trials. Other major categories include vaccines (43), gene therapy (17), interleukins (13), growth factors (11), and interferons (10). It is interesting to note that gene therapy is included in this list. In gene therapy, the "drug" may be genetically altered cells or DNA itself, encapsulated in a fatty envelope and injected directly into the patient. Although cancer is the disease most often targeted by these biotechnology drugs, products are also being tested to treat AIDS, amyotrophic lateral sclerosis (Lou Gehrig's disease), asthma, diabetes, heart disease, Lyme disease, multiple sclerosis, rheumatoid arthritis, stroke, and viral infections. Other products are being tested to reduce bleeding from surgical procedures, aid wound healing, and prevent or treat graft rejection following solid organ transplantation.

FUTURE APPLICATIONS

The highly conserved organization of cellular genetic information combined with the high degree of transcriptional specificity provides a valuable tool for the development of diagnostic and therapeutic techniques. In addition to the detection of inherited disease, genetic technology holds the promise for cure of hereditary disease through the development of sophisticated gene therapy. It is currently possible to identify and characterize the genetic qualities of diseases that often do not have a formal distribution. This is evident by the expanding information describing characteristics of oncogenes of cells. Advances in genetic technology will also provide significant breakthroughs in the treatment of pathogenic microorganisms which are not sensitive to current antiinfective therapy. The optimum treatment of disease caused by viruses, fungi, and mycobacteria may be genetically engineered and/or genetically targeted.

The number of biotechnology drugs will continue to increase, and sales of biotechnology drugs are expected to grow at a rate higher than that of nonbiotechnology drugs. Biotechnology drugs have had a major impact on pharmacy practice. Because many biotechnology drugs are expensive, pharmacists at many institutions are being asked to serve as gatekeepers to ensure that these drugs are used appropriately. Many institutions have developed clinical use guidelines for their use and monitor their use with utilization review. Moreover, many payers want to see the results of effectiveness and pharmacoeconomic studies before they approve widespread use of these expensive drugs.

REFERENCES

1. Watson JD, Hopkins NH, Roberts JW, et al (eds). Molecular Biology of the Gene, 4th ed. Menlo Park, CA, Benjamin/Cummings, 1987, p 74.
2. Alberts B, Bray D, Lewis J, et al (eds). Molecular Biology of the Cell, 2nd ed. New York, Garland Publishing, 1989, pp 96–115.
3. Roberts RJ. Restriction enzymes and their isoschizomers. Nucleic Acids Res 1983;(suppl)16r:271–313.
4. Bloch KD, Bartos B. Digestion of DNA with restriction endonucleases, in Current Protocols Molecular Biology. New York, Green Publishing Associates and Wiley Interscience, 1990, pp 3.03–3.1.17.
5. Fuchs R, Blakesley R. Guide to use of type II restriction endonuclease. Methods Enzymol 1983;100:3–38.
6. Alberts B, Bray D, Lewis J, et al (eds). Molecular Biology of the Cell, 2nd ed. New York, Garland Publishing, 1989, p 182.
7. Watkins PC. Restriction fragment length polymorphism (RFLP): Application in human chromosome mapping and genetic disease research. Biotechnology 1988;6:310–320.
8. Southern EM. Detection of specific sequences among DNA fragments separated by gel electrophoresis. J Mol Biol 1975;98:503–517.
9. Meinkoth J, Wahl G. Hybridization of nucleic acids immobilized on solid supports. Anal Biochem 1984;138:267–284.
10. Hunkapillar MW, Lujan E, Ostrander F, et al. Isolation of microgram quantities of proteins from polyacrylamide gels for amino acids sequences analysis. Methods Enzymol 1983;91:227–236.
11. Alberts B, Bray D, Lewis J, et al (eds). Molecular Biology of the Cell, 2nd ed. New York, Garland Publishing, 1989, pp 170–172.
12. O'Farrell PH. High-resolution two-dimensional electrophoresis of proteins. J Biol Chem 1975;250:4007–4021.
13. Watson JD, Hopkins NH, Roberts JW, et al (eds). Molecular Biology of the Gene, 4th ed. Menlo Park, CA, Benjamin/Cummings, 1987, pp 609–615.
14. Okayama H, Berg P. High-efficiency cloning of full-length cDNA. Mol Cell Biol 1982;2:161–170.
15. Hedrick SM, Cohen DI, Nielsen EA, et al. Isolation of cDNA clones encoding T cell-specific membrane associated proteins. Nature 1984;308:149–153.
16. Klickstein LB. Amplification of a bacteriophage library, in Ausubel FM, Brent R, Kingston RE, et al (eds): Current Protocols in Molecular Biology. New York, Greene Publishing Associates and Wiley Interscience, 1990, pp 5.9–2.3.
17. Seed B, Parker RC, Davidson N. Representation of DNA sequences in recombinant DNA libraries prepared by restriction enzyme partial digestion. Gene 1982;9:201–209.
18. Moore DD. Construction of recombinant DNA libraries, in Ausubel FM, Brent R, Kingston RE, et al (eds): Current Protocol in Molecular Biology. New York, Green Publishing Associates and Wiley Interscience, 1990, pp 5.1–1.3.
19. Kaufmann RJ. Overview of protein expression in mammalian cells, in Ausubel FM, Brent R, Kingston RE, et al (eds): Current Protocol in Molecular Biology. New York, Green Publishing Associates and Wiley Interscience, 1990, p 16.12.1–6.
20. Lundland V. *Saccharomyces cerevisiae,* in Ausubel FM, Brent R, Kingston RE, et al (eds): Current Protocol in Molecular Biology. New York, Green Publishing Associates and Wiley Interscience, 1990, p 13.0.3–5.

Chapter 9

Overview of Transplantation

Gilbert J. Burckart, PharmD, FCCP, Raman Venkataramanan, PhD, FCP, and Richard J. Ptachcinski, PharmD, FCCP, BCPS

Organ transplantation is currently an accepted mode of therapy for diseases that lead to irreversible failure of the kidney, heart, lung, and liver. As the surgical techniques, organ preservation, and immunosuppressive regimens have improved over the years, an expanding number of patients are being treated by transplantation of the pancreas, small bowel, or multiple organs. The objective of the following discussion is to provide a general background for the understanding of transplantation immunology, the rejection process, pharmacologic and nonpharmacologic methods of transplant immunosuppression, and continuing problems with long-term graft survival in transplantation.

History and Current Status of Transplantation in The United States

An increased number of transplantation procedures in the United States has been documented by the United Network for Organ Sharing (UNOS), established in 1987 under a contract with the U.S. Department of Health and Human Services. The UNOS Scientific Registry provides comprehensive information on all liver, heart, heart–lung, lung, pancreas, kidney–pancreas, and kidney donors and recipients in the United States, and recently documented 16,509 solid organ transplants for the period of January through November 1994. Although this figure represents greater than a 15% increase in the number of kidney transplants above the 1988 figures, the number of kidney transplants in the United States appears to have plateaued (10,361 in 1993, 10,363 in 1994). With more than 28,000 people registered with UNOS waiting for a kidney transplant and approximately 15,000 new registrants per year, the plateau in the number of kidney transplant operations represents a shortage of organs donated for transplantation rather than meeting the needs of the potential recipients. In 1988, the U.S. Congress passed legislation compelling hospitals to promptly ask next of kin about the donation of the cadaver's organs, but compliance still depends on the cooperation of the health professionals involved with the family.

Liver transplantation is the second most common solid organ transplant procedure, with 3643 operations being performed in 1994, followed by heart transplantation with 2340 operations in 1994. The 3-year graft survival rates for liver and heart transplants are 61 and 75%, respectively (UNOS 1994 figures). Some transplant operations, such as intestinal transplantation, are still classified as experimental procedures but may be more widely accepted as improvements in drug therapy and in our understanding of transplantation immunology increase patient survival rates. While the less common transplant procedures are still increasing in numbers, the only change in the more common procedures is that the distribution of the donated organs among transplant centers has changed due to the current system for allocation.

Most transplant recipients receive organs from a cadaveric donor. Living-related donors contributed 26% of kidney transplants performed in 1994, and are a special facet of kidney transplantation that is rarely observed in other types of solid organ transplants. While the 3-year graft survival rate for cadaveric kidneys is 69%, the 3-year graft survival for living-related kidneys is 84%. Living-related donor operations are now occurring infrequently for segmental liver and lung transplant operations. While transplantation is becoming more accessible worldwide, inhibiting factors include the lack of advanced supportive technology, lack of knowledge concerning organ transplantation, and religious beliefs that prevent cadaveric organ donation. The cost of these procedures and the therapeutic interventions necessary to improve their success is considerable and continues to rise as biotechnologic advances produce new agents for use in transplantation.

The organ shortage has continued to promote research in cellular transplantation, segmental organ transplantation, artificial organs, and xenogeneic (originating from another species) transplantation. While organ transplantation has traditionally been considered within the realm of the practice of medicine, which the Food and Drug Administration (FDA) does not regulate, some of these new practices have attracted the attention of the FDA and will most likely be regulated by the federal government.

Table 9.1 lists several experimental approaches to cellular transplantation for end-stage organ failure. Xenotransplantation has been attempted unsuccessfully with kidney, liver, and heart grafts, but the possibility for success has improved as newer methods to control the complement activation system have been devised. The temporary use of an animal organ as a "bridge" while the critically ill patient awaits a human cadaveric donor has also been reported.

The origin of solid organ transplantation is multifaceted, and a complete historical time line is available.[1] The present success of organ transplant procedures would not have been possible if the techniques of vascular anastomosis had not been studied and refined to allow experimental and clinical work. In 1902, Alex Carrel published a paper that is the basis for modern techniques of suturing. Mathieu Jaboulay, Carrel's teacher, attempted the first human kidney transplant in 1906 using a pig as a donor. Although this initial trial of transplantation was unsuccessful, Carrel continued his work in the United States and was awarded the Nobel prize in 1912 for his work with vascular anastomosis.

Interest in kidney transplantation was revived in the early 1950s when several human kidneys were transplanted without immunosuppression and without long-term success. The understanding of the immune mechanisms of organ rejection improved rapidly, and the first successful kidney transplant with prolonged survival was performed between identical twins in Boston in 1954.

The need for immunosuppression soon became clear, but the means were crude and difficult to control. Table 9.2 provides a historical time line for the development of immunosuppressive therapy in organ transplantation. Total body irradiation was used on 12 kidney graft recipients in Boston between 1958 and 1962 with only one survivor. The development of 6-mercaptopurine and derivatives for testing by Hitchings and Elion of Burroughs Wellcome offered drug therapy as an alternative to total body irradiation. Stimulated by animal studies performed by Schwartz and Dameshek, British investigator Roy Calne first used 6-mercaptopurine and later its derivative, azathioprine, in humans and demonstrated that pharmacologic immunosuppression was possible in renal transplantation. Thomas Starzl further refined these immunosuppressive regimens to routinely include corticosteroids, which significantly improved kidney graft survival and encouraged the practice of organ transplantation in the 1960s.

TABLE 9.1. EXPERIMENTAL APPROACHES TO CELLULAR TRANSPLANTATION

- Injection of cells (e.g., pancreatic islets) into the thymus to promote immune tolerance to the cells
- Injection of cells from pigs' brains into the brain of a Parkinson's disease patient
- Injection of pancreatic islet T cells from pigs for glucose control
- Injection of human cadaveric hepatocytes to reconstitute hepatic function
- Injection of pancreatic islets that have been transfected with a gene for producing an endogenous immunomodulator (IL-10)

TABLE 9.2. HISTORICAL TIME LINE FOR THE DEVELOPMENT OF TRANSPLANT IMMUNOSUPPRESSION

Year	Event
1908	Total body irradiation
1958	Total body irradiation used
1959	6-Mercaptopurine used
1961	Azathioprine used
1965	Corticosteroids used, multidrug regimens initiated
1967	Antilymphocyte sera used
1969	Mycophenolic acid developed
1976	Cyclosporine developed
1980	OKT3 clinical trials
1983	Cyclosporine approved in the United States
1987	Tacrolimus and deoxyspergualin developed
1989	Rapamycin developed for transplantation
1994	Tacrolimus approved in the United States
1995	Mycophenolate mofetil approved in the United States

The 1970s was a quiescent period during which several important accomplishments in the area of organ transplantation occurred. Methods of tissue typing and organ sharing schemes were developed and improved. The concept of "brain death" was established and would be critical for organ procurement. Most important, cyclosporine was developed by Jean Borel at Sandoz, Inc., in Switzerland and would dramatically change the approach to immunosuppression in the 1980s. Cyclosporine (CyA), then called cyclosporin A, had a totally different mechanism of action on the immune system when compared with other agents available at that time, and encouraged the expansion of human organ transplantation to heart, liver, pancreas, and heart–lung.

Immunosuppressive therapy in solid organ transplantation has undergone rapid changes from 1980 to the present time. Our understanding of new agents and their mechanisms has advanced rapidly during the 1990s, but the place of these new agents in clinical practice remains unclear. To appreciate the role of these newer drugs in immunosuppressive therapy, let's look at the underlying principles of transplantation immunology.

TRANSPLANTATION IMMUNOLOGY

The normal immune response to foreign material is incompletely understood. Much of the progress made in our understanding of the immune system in the past 30 years has been based on the study of transplantation and tissue rejection. As we have learned more about the immune system, the method by which engrafted tissues are rejected has become increasingly difficult to comprehend. A basic background in the current concepts in immunology is essential for understanding transplantation immunology and drug therapy.

HISTOCOMPATIBILITY

Much of the study of transplantation immunology has been directed toward the examination of histocompatibility antigens. The transplantation antigens are produced under the direction of the major histocompatibility complex (MHC), called human leukocyte antigens (HLA), which is a cluster of closely related genes responsible for the production of these antigenic proteins. The human genes coding for the MHC is located on the short arm of chromosome 6 and encodes for two major classes of transplantation antigens. Class I antigens are encoded by HLA-A, HLA-B, and HLA-C loci and occur virtually on all cell surfaces except red blood cells. Registries of these class I antigens are being continually updated as considerable variation in their antigenic structure is recognized. Although the simpler serologic typing system was still in use as of 1995, the system of nomenclature for the HLA system has become complex with the application of molecular biologic tools for identifying HLA alleles. In March 1994, the WHO Nomenclature Committee on HLA accepted two new HLA genes, HLA-K and HLA-L, which are novel class I pseudogenes located near HLA-A. Hundreds of HLA alleles are now recognized.[2] The HLA class I antigens share distinct antigenic determinants called public epitopes, regions with structural similarity to other class I molecules. Transplant patients who are said to be highly sensitized often have antibodies against these public class I antigens, and will therefore have more difficulty in obtaining a nonreactive cross-match.

Class II HLA antigens are the second group of molecules encoded by the HLA-D region of the human MHC. The HLA-D region has been further subdivided into three primary subregions called HLA-DP, HLA-DQ, and HLA-DR. Class II antigens are present on a restricted cell repertoire that includes B lymphocytes, monocytes, macrophages, and activated T lymphocytes. Certain lymphokines (subcellular messengers secreted by lymphocytes) such as γ-interferon (IFNγ) can induce class II antigens on certain endothelial, epithelial, and other types of cells.[3] The class II antigens are polymorphic in nature, and more than 100 alleles of HLA-DR, more than 40 alleles of HLA-DQ, and more than 50 alleles of HLA-DP have been identified.

Both class I and class II antigens play an important role in transplantation immunology and cell–cell interactions with T lymphocytes. Helper T cells recognize class II molecules, whereas cytotoxic T cells recognize class I antigens. The importance of either determinant is best demonstrated by the significant improvement in the survival of renal grafts with HLA antigen matching. In the studies to date that have not considered all of the specificities of the HLA determinants, the strongest positive effect for survival of a renal graft is compatibility of the HLA-DR component, followed by HLA-B and HLA-A. Tissue matching should not be considered uniformly beneficial for all patients. For example, in liver transplant patients matching may make the patient more susceptible to attack on the graft by recipient T cells previously sensitized to cytomegalovirus (CMV), an event less likely to occur with unmatched donor antigen-presenting cells (APCs) in the graft.

A number of questions about the importance of the MHC antigens in transplant survival still exist.[4] For example, the recipient of a kidney transplant from an HLA-identical sibling will still require immunosuppressive therapy, and complete graft survival is not assured. Genes outside the MHC can clearly act as transplantation antigens, and include ABO and Lewis blood groups, vascular endothelial cell antigens, or tissue-specific antigens. The importance of these so-called "minor" antigens has been clearly demonstrated in the production of graft-versus-host disease in identical siblings, in which transplanted immunocompetent T cells attack an immunologically incompetent host, and in the rejection of solid organs transplanted in animal models. The precise factors that cause one antigen or one MHC determinant to be more immunogenic than another are as yet unknown.

ABO blood group compatibility is considered an essential criterion for matching donor and recipient. The risk of hyperacute rejection after an incompatible ABO transplant was recognized in the early studies of kidney transplantation (see section on Hyperacute Rejection). Even in liver transplantation, which appears to be relatively resistant to hyperacute rejection, the successful engraftment rate of ABO-incompatible transplants is very low. Compatible but nonidentical kidney and liver grafts (O to any non-O; A or B to AB) have about a 10% lower long-term graft survival rate when compared with identical ABO matching.[5] The only solid organ transplant in which ABO matching has not been essential is in corneal grafting.

IMMUNE SENSITIZATION

The precise point of stimulation of the recipient's immune response to donor tissue is uncertain. An increased expression of MHC class I antigens within engrafted tissue is observed shortly after transplantation as is the induction of expression of MHC class II antigens on special cells such as the endothelium. An important factor in sensitization of the recipient may be the exposure to donor leukocytes, which are either monocytes or tissue macrophages such as dendritic cells within the transplanted tissue. The dendritic cell is a very potent stimulator of the immune response, and increasing evidence points to the importance of these "passenger" leukocytes. Depletion of dendritic cells from the donor graft using monoclonal antibodies has been reported to improve transplant survival, and graft survival has been correlated with the number of passenger dendritic cells in some animal models. Dendritic cells from the graft have been shown to migrate to the recipient spleen, which provides some evidence that a central sensitization process, rather than a peripheral process within the graft, is active in the immune response to the donor graft. A third possibility for sensitization involves the release of soluble MHC donor antigens from the graft, but these molecules are weakly antigenic by themselves.

A recent concept related to recipient sensitization to donor cells is the direct and indirect presentation of donor MHC peptides to recipient T lymphocytes. The direct presentation of foreign MHC molecules to recipient T lymphocytes evokes a stronger response than against other foreign antigens, and may elicit an early and rapid rejection of transplanted donor tissue. The indirect presentation of donor MHC material would involve processing of the material by the recipient's APCs with the subsequent presentation to recipient T lymphocytes. The T cell's helper function for driving a B-cell response and antibody formation secondary to the indirect presentation pathway is very poorly inhibited by drugs such as cyclosporine.[6] Therefore while the drugs typically used in transplant immunosuppression protocols may be targeted at the T-lymphocyte response to direct antigen presentation, the indirect response may result in a chronic rejection process, a major clinical problem. New drug therapy strategies directed against the indirect antigen presentation response must be developed to facilitate long-term graft survival.

THE IMMUNE RESPONSE

While T lymphocytes are clearly recognized as the mediators of the rejection process, the importance of each of the T-lymphocyte subsets involved in the rejection process cannot be precisely defined. Specific depletion of CD4+ T helper cells or CD8+ cytotoxic T cells is possible in animal models; this suggests that the suppression or deletion of CD4+ cells plays a predominant role in maintaining organ engraftment (CD stands for clusters of differentiation, or groups of cells with the same surface markers). Some role for CD8+ lymphocytes is inevitable, however, particularly in the highly sensitized host. While natural killer (NK) cells are important in tumor surveillance, their role in organ transplant rejection remains uncertain. The influence of each of the lymphocyte subsets is unclear in part because these cells have overlapping roles (e.g., CD4+ cells can be cytotoxic). Suppressor cells may carry either the CD4+ or the CD8+ marker. Suppressor cells demonstrated soon after transplantation are frequently CD4+ and after long-term maintenance of a graft are CD8+. The suppressor T lymphocytes are not considered to be a separate population of cells, and the factors that encourage their emergence are not currently understood. The usefulness of inducing T suppressor cells as a strategy to clinically promote long-term graft survival is being actively explored through the use of an investigational agent called SK&F 105685, which induces suppressor cells in animal models.

The complex interactions of cells that define the immune response to transplanted tissue may eventually become clear when the activities of the subcellular messengers of cell action are completely understood. These messengers are soluble products elaborated by cells to communicate with other cells. Approximately 20 of these subcellular messengers have been identified, including the interleukins (IL) and cytokines that play a critical role in cell growth and differentiation. The number of interleukins identified is rapidly expanding, and IL-1 through IL-15 have been recognized. Each interleukin interacts with a specific receptor expressed at the cell surface, and monoclonal antibodies can be specifically directed at some component of each IL receptor. Some components of IL receptors are shared by multiple cytokines; for example, the chain of the IL-2 receptor (IL-2R) also binds IL-4, IL-7, IL-9, IL-13, and IL-15.

Of the identified cytokines, IL-1 and IL-2 have been most frequently studied in transplantation immunology. IL-1 is produced by macrophages in response to a T-cell interaction or an immune complex and is also known as endogenous pyrogen. IL-1 produces a number of inflammatory actions such as the initiation of fever and chemotaxis, but its ability to induce the IL-2R and IL-2 production is particularly important in transplantation. Two types of IL-1 receptors have now been identified separately on T and B cells and have provided the opportunity to produce IL-1 receptor antagonists. These antagonists have been shown to be effective in animal models of systemic inflammation and transplantation.

The secretion of IL-2 is a critical step in the process of continuing the immune response leading to the rejection of a transplanted organ. IL-2 is synthesized by CD4+ cells and to a lesser extent by CD8+ cells, but IL-1 is necessary for maximal IL-2 secretion. IL-2 acts on activated T cells causing those cells to proliferate and demonstrate their differentiated function such as cytotoxicity. Activated T lymphocytes express both a high-affinity and a low-affinity IL-2R, and IL-2R blockade can antagonize the proliferative actions of IL-2. While the therapeutic use of IL-2 as an immunostimulatory compound is finding its way in cancer therapy, IL-2R is the focus of direct investigation in the development of immunosuppressive monoclonal antibodies. Clinical trials with a murine anti-IL-2R monoclonal antibody have been successful in delaying the onset of acute rejection episodes and in suppressing the presence of soluble IL-2R in serum, but have not been demonstrated to have any effect on kidney graft survival. A humanized antibody against the IL-2R is in clinical trials (see section on Investigational Agents). Receptor blockade should not be considered a simple process, since multiple cytokine interactions take place. For example, IL-4, a T-cell-derived B-cell growth factor, inhibits monocyte production of IL-1, tumor necrosis factor (TNF), and IL-6 (a B-cell differentiation factor) *in vitro*. Another problem in predicting the activity of a cytokine analogue or its receptor antagonist is the possibility of natural structural variation. For example, 21 known subtypes of α-interferon have been identified in humans. Therefore, the clinical application of our knowledge about cytokines in transplantation is expected to be very slow.

The interest in the interactions of cytokines involved in allograft rejection has been heightened by the recognition that subsets of T helper cells produce different cytokines, may be antagonistic to one another, and drive different responses within the immune system. T helper cells have now been classified on the basis of their general phenotypic pattern of cytokine production: Th0 cells produce IL-2, IL-4, and IFNγ, Th1 cells produce IL-2, tumor necrosis factor (TNFβ) and IFNγ, and Th2 cells produce IL-4, IL-5, IL-6, and IL-10 (Fig. 9.1).[7] A primary response to an antigen results in an IL-2 response, whereas a secondary response is associated with an IL-2, IL-4, and IFNγ response. The groups of cytokines from Th1 and Th2 cells are generally antagonistic to one another, and the predominance of one type of response versus the other may have important implications for graft rejection and tolerance of the graft.

An additional concept related to cell proliferation and tolerance is costimulation, or the necessity to have more than just T-cell receptor (TCR) binding to the APC to initiate cell proliferation. Figure 9.2 presents several of the costimulatory molecules found on the T cell and the APC. One of the most important sets of costimulatory molecules is the B7/CD28 combination. If the TCR is stimulated and B7/CD28 costimulation is blocked, immune tolerance rather than a proliferative response develops.[8] Blocking costimulation of the T cell could become a major therapeutic strategy (see section on Investigational Agents).

MECHANISMS OF GRAFT REJECTION

The general sequence of events that underlies graft rejection is (1) recognition of the donor's histocompatibility differences by the recipient's immune system, (2) recruitment of activated lymphocytes, (3) initiation of immune effector mechanisms, and (4) destruction of the graft. These processes can take place at varying rates and may involve differing effector mechanisms. Rejection of the transplanted tissue can therefore take place at any time following surgery and is clinically classified as hyperacute rejec-

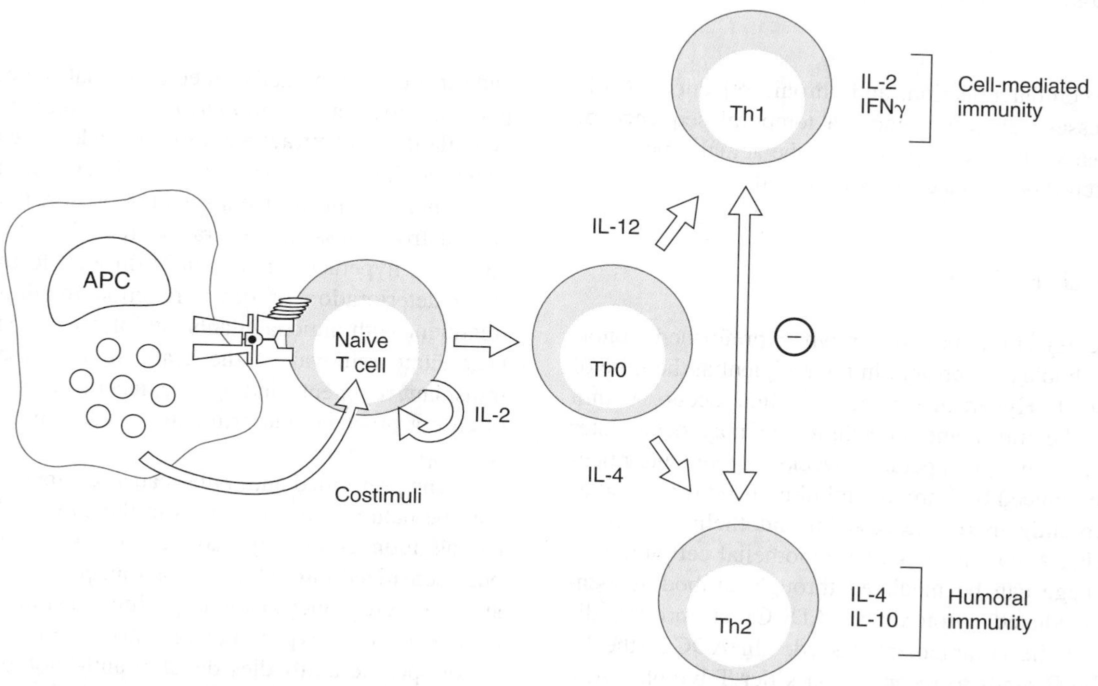

Figure 9.1. The production of T helper subsets, their differential cytokines, and the resulting immune response. APC, antigen presenting cell. *(From Steele AW, Strom TB. Cytokines and the Th1/Th2 paradigm in transplantation. Curr Opin Immunol 1994;6:757–764, with permission.)*

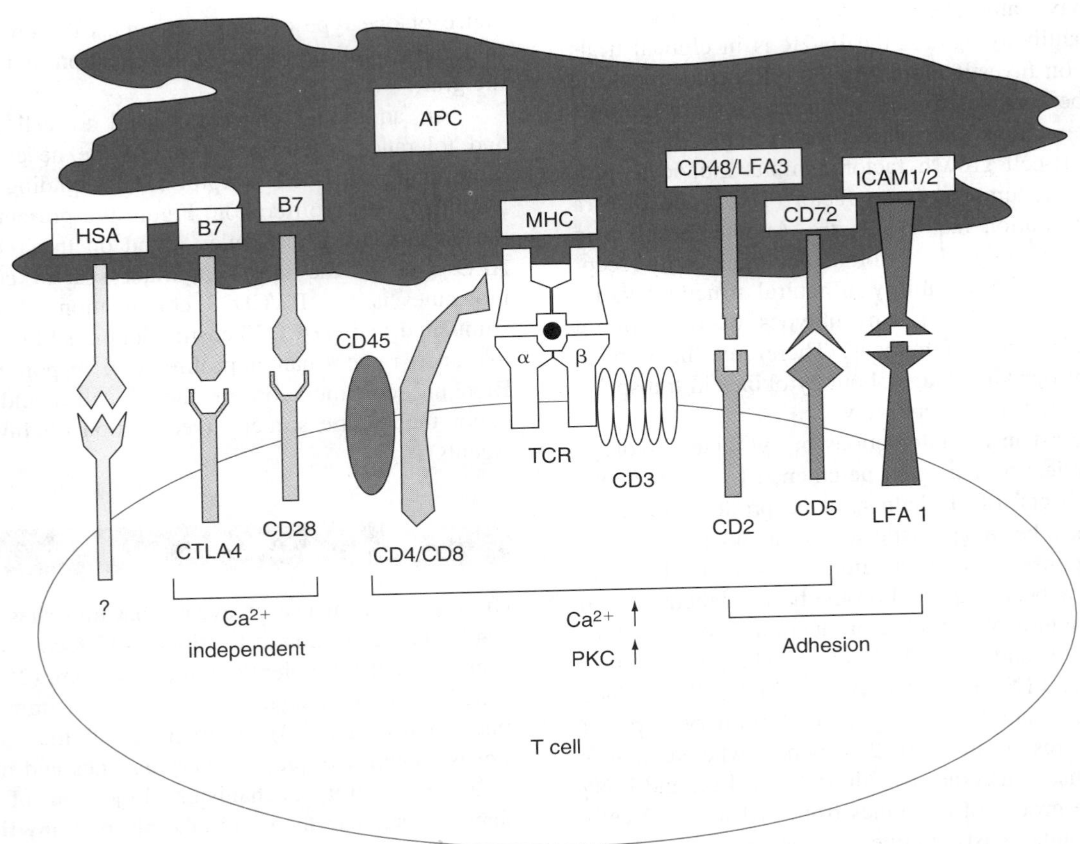

Figure 9.2. The cell surface interactions that take place between the T cell and the antigen presenting cell (APC). PKC, protein kinase C; HSA, heat stable antigen. *(From Nickerson PW, Steurer W, Steiger J, Strom TB. In pursuit of the "Holy Grail": Allograft tolerance. Kidney Int 1994;45(suppl 44):S40–S49, with permission.)*

tion, acute cellular rejection, and chronic rejection. While these processes generally denote a temporal sequence of events, considerable overlap exists in the actual time frame of when each type of rejection is observed.

HYPERACUTE REJECTION

Hyperacute rejection may occur when preformed donor-specific antibodies are present in the recipient at the time of the transplant. Hyperacute rejection often occurs within minutes of the transplant procedure, but may occur later within the first two postoperative weeks. Hyperacute rejection can be induced by immunoglobulin G (IgG) antibodies that bind to antigens on the vascular endothelium, such as class I MHC, ABO, and vascular endothelial cell antigens. Tissue damage can be mediated through antibody-dependent, cell-mediated cytotoxicity (ADCC) or through the activation of the complement cascade. In ADCC, the Fc portion of IgG binds to receptors on killer T lymphocytes, which directly damage the transplanted tissue. When the antigen–antibody complex activates the complement cascade it produces bioactive mediators that increase vascular permeability, cause smooth muscle contraction, trigger coagulation, and attract polymorphonuclear leukocytes. The ischemic damage to the microvasculature rapidly produces tissue necrosis in most transplanted organs, but the liver is spared from classical hyperacute rejection. In the clinical situation, hyperacute rejection is difficult to manage since rapid deterioration of organ function requires immediate treatment with anticoagulants, antiplatelet agents, and may necessitate removal of the graft. In the case of a heart transplant recipient, finding a replacement organ quickly is often not practical and artificial organs provide a bridge to retransplantation.

The preformed antibodies causing hyperacute rejection may be naturally occurring, as in the case of the ABO isohemagglutinins, or they may develop in a patient who has been sensitized through previous transplants, blood transfusions, or pregnancy. Donor-specific sensitization may not always lead to hyperacute rejection. Some patients with donor-specific antibodies develop anti-idiotypic antibodies that can neutralize donor-specific cytotoxic antibodies. This concept has been proposed to explain the beneficial effect of donor-specific blood transfusions to improve graft survival (see Nonpharmacologic Immunosuppression). Hyperacute rejection has become uncommon because transplant donors are matched for ABO blood groups, and cross-match testing is done to determine the presence of donor-specific lymphocytotoxic antibodies. A positive cross-match presents a serious risk factor for graft failure even if hyperacute rejection does not occur. A negative lymphocytotoxicity cross-match does not entirely rule out the possibility of hyperacute rejection because non-MHC antigens on the vascular endothelium can serve as targets of donor-specific antibodies.

ACUTE CELLULAR REJECTION

The cellular rejection process is referred to as acute rejection. Although the earliest episodes have been observed within days postoperatively, acute rejection may occur at any time after transplantation. Cellular rejection is mediated by alloreactive T lymphocytes that appear in circulation and infiltrate the allograft through the vascular endothelium. Because only class I HLA antigens are expressed on the vascular endothelium, class I-specific T cells, presumably CD8+ cytotoxic cells, should initially be involved in cellular rejection. Lymphokines such as IFNγ released by these lymphocytes induce the expression of class II MHC antigens on the vascular endothelium, which are subsequently recognized by class II-specific lymphocytes of the CD4+ phenotype. The upregulation of class II MHC antigens on vascular endothelium may occur in other situations. Local processes such as inflammation and infection in the graft may produce class II MHC antigen expression without the prior infiltration of class I-sensitive lymphocytes. Once the graft is infiltrated by lymphocytes, the cytotoxic cells can specifically kill allograft targets, whereas the local release of lymphokines will attract and stimulate macrophages to produce tissue damage through a delayed hypersensitivity-like mechanism.

The diagnosis of graft rejection is frequently difficult in patients following transplantation. This is particularly true when attempting to differentiate renal graft rejection from drug-induced nephrotoxicity or hepatic graft rejection from drug-induced hepatotoxicity. Rejection of a transplanted organ is frequently associated with fever, malaise, and graft enlargement. The biochemical changes that occur during graft rejection are those associated with abnormal function of the transplanted organ. Patients with renal allograft rejection have a decreased urine output, accompanied by a rapidly rising serum creatinine, blood urea nitrogen, and decreased blood flow on renal scan. Liver graft rejection is suspected in patients with a rise in their serum bilirubin, alkaline phosphatase, and serum transaminase concentrations. Rejection in patients following cardiac transplantation may present in a very subtle manner, and only in the later stages is manifest by changes on electrocardiogram or signs of congestive heart failure.

Graft rejection is frequently confirmed by examining a graft biopsy. A biopsy specimen with a diffuse infiltrate of lymphocytes is consistent with acute cellular rejection. The absolute usefulness of histologically grading the extent of cellular infiltration is as yet unclear. For example, lymphocytes activated against donor tissue can be grown from biopsy specimens that have no apparent cellular infiltrate. After the diagnosis of rejection has been confirmed, the potential risks and benefits of antirejection therapy must be evaluated.

CHRONIC REJECTION

Chronic rejection is perhaps the most important problem to be addressed in transplantation over the next decade. While major strides have been made in the management of acute rejection, the half-life of organ survival after transplantation remains unchanged over the past 15 years. The process of chronic rejection is poorly understood. While chronic rejection may simply be a slow and indolent form of cellular rejection, the involvement of the humoral immune system and antibodies against the vascular endothelium may play a role. The pathogenesis of chronic rejection is difficult to dissect because of prolonged exposure to multiple drugs, and because of the presence of other abnormalities such as hyperlipidemia that may predispose the patient to similar pathologic changes in organ function.

The clinical presentation of chronic rejection depends on which organ was grafted and is more completely discussed in the individual transplant chapters (see Chapters 18, 41, 45, and 129). In liver transplant patients, chronic rejection may be manifested by the disappearance of bile ducts due to their necrosis and replacement with fibrous tissue. In lung transplant patients, bronchiolitis obliterans presents a major problem with graft function and is now felt to be due primarily to a chronic rejection process. In heart transplant patients, accelerated arteriosclerotic coronary artery disease is considered to be one manifestation of chronic rejection. These processes are very difficult to treat because their presentation is slow and indolent, and the changes in organ function are usually not reversible.

An improved understanding of cell activation/reactivation may change the therapeutic approach to chronic rejection. Since T cells directed against the graft can be reactivated by cytokines produced locally in response to a viral infection such as CMV or in response to other activated T cells, aggressive regimens to prevent viral infections or acute rejection may result in less chronic rejection and graft and patient loss.

PREVENTING OR REDUCING REJECTION

Rejection of the transplanted donor graft by a recipient should not be viewed as an inevitable process. The goal of immunomodulatory therapy in transplantation should be to promote the acceptance of the donor tissue, while maintaining the functional status of the immune system with respect to all other foreign material. The goal of true tolerance (nonreactivity only to the donor tissue) will be difficult to achieve for all but fetal transplantation, but considerable progress has been made through better preservation of the donor tissue and through both nonpharmacologic and pharmacologic means of immunosuppression.

ORGAN PRESERVATION

Cadaveric donors constitute the major source of organs for transplantation. Organs harvested from donors undergo a period of warm ischemia during organ removal and cold ischemia during organ storage before being transplanted into a patient. Individual organs differ in their susceptibility to warm ischemic damage at 37°C, and irreversible damage will occur in 3–5 minutes for brain, 15–20 minutes for liver, 30–40 minutes for heart and lungs, 50–100 minutes for kidney, and about 6 hours for skin. The ultimate objective of organ preservation is immediate graft function after transplantation. Development of an ideal organ preservation solution will achieve those benefits outlined in Table 9.3. In preservation of an organ for transplantation, the preservation process must avoid hypoxic damage to the cells, excessive hydrogen ion accumulation in the cell, osmotic shock, and the accumulation of metabolic waste while meeting the nutritional requirements of the organ. Hypothermia is the single most important method of organ preservation. Although not uniformly successful, hyperbaric oxygen has been used in combination with hypothermia to preserve organ function. Continuous perfusion of an organ maintained under hypothermic conditions provides oxygen to the organ and minimizes ischemia, but this method is expensive and technically complex. Techniques that involve freezing have been successful for isolated cells but are not practical for whole organs at the present time.

TABLE 9.3. CLINICAL GOALS FOR IDEAL ORGAN PRESERVATION

1. Increase the number of organs available for transplantation.
2. Increase the efficiency of organ utilization by organ sharing between centers.
3. Make organ transplantation a semielective procedure.
4. Decrease the number of individuals necessary to carry out transplant surgery.
5. Provide sufficient time for cross-matching and use of organs in the most suitable donor.
6. Reduce delayed graft function or primary nonfunction of the transplanted organs.
7. Provide an opportunity to alter the immunologic status of the organ.
8. Reduce the cost of organ procurement.

Until recently, Euro–Collin's solution (Table 9.4) was most commonly used for cold storage of the kidney, liver, and pancreas. Use of this solution typically resulted in a storage time of 24 hours for kidneys and 6 hours for livers and pancreases. The development of UW solution (Table 9.4) at the University of Wisconsin has significantly increased the cold preservation time to up to 3 days for kidney, 12 hours for liver, and 11 hours for pancreas. The components of the preservation solution generally accomplish one of seven functions: (1) minimize any cellular swelling, which necessitates the use of certain impermeant ions; (2) prevent intracellular acidosis due to the accumulation of lactic acid and hydrogen ions by the use of buffers; (3) prevent expansion of the interstitial space during flush out by using colloids to provide osmotic pressure; (4) prevent injury from oxygen free radicals by the use of free radical scavengers or by directly preventing formation of oxygen free radicals; (5) minimize cell damage secondary to calcium accumulation; (6) suppress the activity of phospholipases and stabilize lysosomes by the use of cytoprotective agents; and (7) provide substrates for regenerating high-energy phosphates during reperfusion since ATP degrades during hypothermic storage. Further increases in preservation time are possible with a combination of initial cold storage followed by hypothermic perfusion of the kidney. Hearts and lungs are typically stored in cardioplegic solu-

TABLE 9.4. ORGAN PRESERVATION SOLUTIONS

Constituent	Collins'	UW Solution	Use[a]
Sodium (mM)	10	30	
Potassium (mM)	105	120	
as lactobionate		(100)	1
Magnesium (mM)	30	5	
Bicarbonate (mM)	10		2
Hydroxyethyl starch (g/dL)		5	1,3
Adenosine (mM)		5	7
Raffinose (mM)		30	
Dexamethasone (mg/dL)		0.86	
Allopurinol (mM)		1	4
Glutathione (mM)		3	4
Insulin (U/mL)		0.1	7
pH at 25°C	7.2	7.4	
Osmolality (mOsm/L)	304	320	

[a]1 = minimize cellular swelling; 2 = prevent acidosis; 3 = prevent edematous changes; 4 = prevent free radical injury; 7 = provide energy substrates.

tion for a maximum period of 6 hours. The use of cryopreservation for long-term storage (1 to 2 weeks) requires additional studies on safety, methods of addition and removal of various cryoprotectants, and a thorough understanding of the freezing characteristics of vascularized organs.

NONPHARMACOLOGIC IMMUNOSUPPRESSION

Early methods of transplant immunosuppression included total body irradiation and lymphocyte depletion through thoracic duct drainage of lymph. These methods often yielded unreliable results, but led to continued research in radiotherapy and lymphocyte depletion as immunosuppressive strategies.

A recent concept that may influence drug therapy is that of a stable microchimerism, or a state in which the donor cells are tolerated by the host.[9] This concept emerged after it became possible to identify small numbers of donor cells in the skin biopsies of long-term survivors of renal or liver allografts. The development of microchimerism requires that a certain number of donor cells migrate out of the graft to establish a mutual natural immunosuppression with recipient T cells. Having too few donor migratory cells from an organ with little lymphatic tissue (e.g., kidney or heart) might lead to classic host-versus-graft rejection, while having too much lymphatic tissue (e.g., lung or intestine) might lead to graft-versus-host disease. Therefore, a stable balance of donor cell and recipient cell interaction might be necessary for long-term graft survival. If microchimerism is important to long-term graft survival in an organ transplant patient, this state may be facilitated by (1) supplementing some solid organ transplants with bone marrow from the donor, and (2) an adjustment in drug therapy so that the donor–recipient interaction in the immediate post-transplant period is not totally suppressed.

Total lymphoid irradiation (TLI) is considered an alternative immunosuppressive therapy for highly sensitized patients who have received prior organ transplantation. By targeting x-rays to lymphoid tissues, using small fractionated doses to minimize side effects, and discontinuing therapy with the appearance of adverse effects, TLI has been used successfully in renal transplant patients in combination with low doses of immunosuppressive drugs. Leukopenia and thrombocytopenia occur in the majority of patients who receive TLI, and localized herpes zoster infections are also common. Therapy with TLI has induced donor-specific tolerance in animals and humans, and may do so through inducing suppressor T-cell activity. With the rapid development of other forms of immunosuppressive therapy, the place of TLI in immunosuppressive regimens in transplantation is unclear, but its long-term safety in Hodgkin's disease suggests that TLI might have a place in the therapy of sensitized patients or in the induction of tolerance.

Donor-specific blood transfusions have also served as a means of mild immunosuppressive therapy. This treatment arose from observations during the 1940s that erythrocyte infusions did not promote rejection of skin grafts but rather enhanced their survival. The controversy of the effectiveness of therapy with either donor-specific or third-party blood transfusions was most vocal before the widespread availability of newer T-cell-specific immunosuppressive drugs such as CyA. With the clinical use of these newer agents in the 1980s, the risk of blood transfusion outweighed the minimal potential benefits conferred by this therapy. The development of the concept of chimerism has renewed interest in similar approaches, and newer strategies have used donor bone marrow infusions with or without antilymphocytic globulin for solid organ recipients. Some success at improving renal and liver allograft survival has been claimed with the attendant risk of graft-versus-host disease. Continued attempts at nonpharmacologic manipulation of the immune system are warranted in transplantation, but these must be administered in combination with pharmacologic therapy that has proven to be successful.

PHARMACOLOGIC IMMUNOSUPPRESSION

Immunosuppression with drugs or biologic agents following organ transplantation appears complex because of the large number of varying protocols used by transplant centers throughout the world. The most commonly used agents in those protocols came into use in transplantation in the 1960s (corticosteroids, azathioprine, and the antilymphocytic globulins). The more T-cell-specific agents of the 1980s (CyA and OKT3 monoclonal antibodies) complete the set of the five agents used extensively in transplant patients. Two new agents have recently been approved for use by the FDA (tacrolimus and mycophenolate), which will further complicate the regimens used within specific transplant centers. Newer agents in clinical trials or under investigation could produce dramatic changes in immunosuppressive protocols in the next decade.

The mechanisms of action of the immunosuppressive compounds, increasingly understood, are complex and highly interactive with other immunomodulatory compounds. While surface receptors on cells have been available for study, the transcription of receptor binding to drug action through cytoplasmic and nuclear events within the lymphocyte is poorly understood. New information about glucocorticoid-receptor complexes in the nucleus or CyA binding to enzymes in the cytoplasm does not have direct clinical application, but it does explain the diverse effects of steroids on multiple cytokines and CyA interactions with the newer macrocyclic immunosuppressants. Understanding these interactions should allow the pharmacotherapist to combine agents in such a manner as to produce selective immunosuppression with minimal adverse drug effects. Figure 9.3 presents the general scheme of drug action on the immune system.

Drug combinations hold the greatest promise for managing transplant-related immunosuppression. While protocols using some of the newer agents alone (CyA, tacrolimus) have been as effective as older drug combinations, multiple drug therapy represents the most logical approach to transplant immunosuppression. As discussed previously, the transplant rejection process involves both T and B cells, multiple cytokines, and inflammatory mediators. Selective drug combinations that prevent compensatory immune mechanisms from avoiding suppression and that take advantage of proven synergism between agents should provide the most effective therapy. Drug combinations also allow the use of minimal effective doses of immunosuppressive agents so that drug toxicity is diminished.

The development of immunosuppressive regimens since the mid-1960s has resulted in the current use of "triple therapy" or "quadruple therapy" as the standard regimen in most transplant centers. Triple therapy—low-dose CyA or tacrolimus, azathioprine, and steroids—takes advantage of the immunosuppressive effects of CyA or tacrolimus while minimizing their adverse effects. Quadruple therapy adds antilymphocyte globulin (ALG) or muromonab-CD3 (OKT3) to triple therapy with a delay in the start of CyA until adequate renal function is established.[10] To achieve initial immunosuppression, patients receive loading regimens of methylprednisolone (250–1000 mg), azathioprine (3–5 mg/kg), and CyA (8–17 mg/kg) or tacrolimus (0.1–0.3 mg/kg). To avoid the nephrotoxic effects of CyA, initial therapy may include corticosteroids, azathioprine, and either ALG or OKT3. Cyclosporine therapy is then started 1–2 weeks after transplantation.[11] The advantage of new potent agents such as tacrolimus (FK-506) is that the corticosteroid therapy can generally be eliminated in the long-term regimen, reducing hypertension and many of the adverse effects of prolonged corticosteroid therapy.

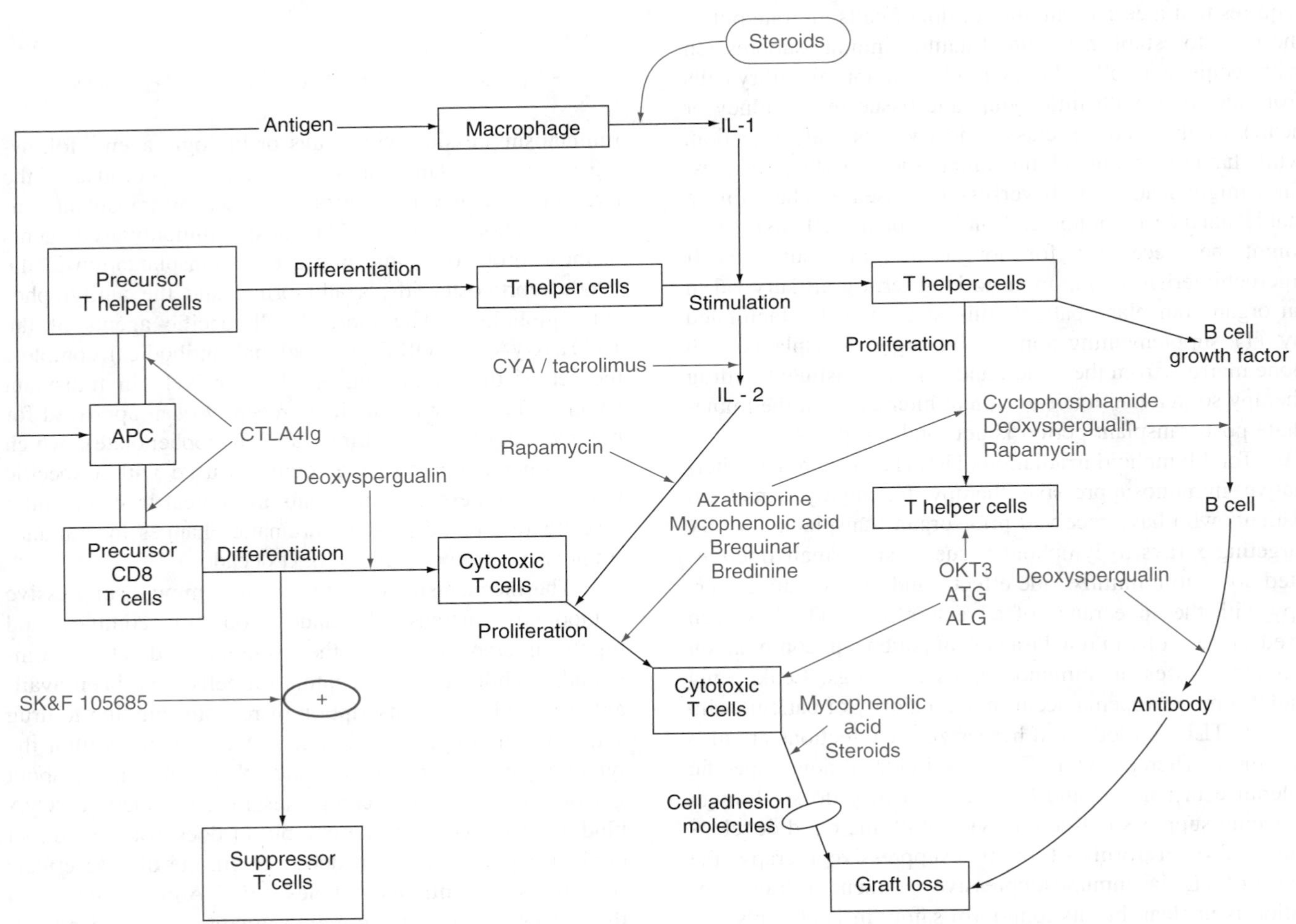

Figure 9.3. Stimulation of the T-cell system by an antigen-presenting cell with subsequent attack on the graft by the immune system. Points of blockade by pharmacologic agents are noted. Agents have a negative effect on the process indicated with the exception of SK&F 105685.

CURRENTLY USED IMMUNOSUPPRESSIVE AGENTS IN TRANSPLANTATION

Steroid Therapy

The corticosteroids used in transplantation most frequently include methylprednisolone and prednisone, which is converted to active prednisolone in the body. Corticosteroids have multiple effects on the immune system, including blocking lymphocyte proliferation through inhibition of production of IL-1 and IL-6 in macrophages. Other actions of corticosteroids include reduction in the formation of other cytokines such as IL-2, IL-4 and IFNγ, of the inflammatory eicosanoids, and of adhesion molecules on endothelial cells necessary for leukocytes to migrate out of the blood stream. The anti-inflammatory activity of steroids may contribute to the beneficial effects of these agents when administered in high doses for the treatment of acute rejection.

Corticosteroid doses vary according to protocols established at each transplant center. The doses of steroids are highest immediately following the transplant procedure and during treatment of acute rejection. After a preoperative dose of methylprednisolone (250–1000 mg), oral prednisone doses of 20–200 mg are used during the first postoperative week. The doses of steroids are tapered according to individual treatment protocols at each transplant center, and the goal is to decrease steroid doses in adults to less than 15 mg of prednisone per day by 6 months after transplantation. Long-term maintenance doses of prednisone are less than 10 mg/d in most patients. The use of alternate-day steroid therapy has been successful in some transplant centers. Most patients are maintained on a small dose of corticosteroids long term to prevent graft rejection, but complete discontinuation of steroids has become a more frequent practice in many transplant centers. Recent evidence suggests that the quality of life for transplant patients may be improved by the discontinuation of corticosteroid therapy.

The first-line therapy for the treatment of acute graft rejection is high-dose (250–1000 mg/d) intravenous methylprednisolone for 3 days. Some transplant centers treat rejection with a cycle of oral prednisone starting at a dose of 200 mg/d orally, which is tapered over the 5-day treatment course to 20 mg/d. Oral steroid regimens are less costly and easier to administer than intravenous therapy, and are considered equally efficacious. The half-life of prednisolone in transplant patients is 2.9–4.3 hours, but the coadministration of rifampin, phenobarbital, or phenytoin will increase prednisolone clearance and could precipitate a rejection episode.

Corticosteroid doses are a special concern in children, and growth rates in children requiring steroid therapy are slowed in a manner similar to that in children with chronic renal, hepatic, or cardiac disease. Some transplant centers withhold prednisone therapy in children until their first rejection episode. Alternate-day steroids improve growth rates in patients who require corticosteroids to maintain allograft function.[12]

In addition to the usual concerns of suppression of the hypothalamic–pituitary–adrenal axis, slow discontinuation of steroid therapy is advisable in transplant patients because of a potential rebound in the cytokine effect. Corticosteroid therapy may suppress cytokine production, but receptors for cytokines are up-regulated in the presence of glucocorticosteroids. Therefore a rebound in the cell proliferative response driven by cytokines may follow the discontinuation of corticosteroids with a resultant episode of acute rejection.

ANTIPROLIFERATIVE AGENTS

Azathioprine Therapy

Azathioprine is a thiopurine analogue structurally related to 6-mercaptopurine. Azathioprine must be metabolized in erythrocytes and in the liver to the pharmacologically active agents 6-mercaptopurine, 6-thioinosinic acid, and 6-thioguanine. Azathioprine inhibits DNA and RNA synthesis by preventing the formation of adenylic and guanylic acids from inosinic acid, and functions as an effective antiproliferative agent against both B and T lymphocytes. The immunosuppressive effect of azathioprine lasts for 12–24 hours following a dose, making once-daily dosing possible.

Azathioprine is used for the prevention of rejection following transplantation so that lifelong therapy is indicated. Azathioprine is not used as a treatment for acute graft rejection. The dosing of azathioprine following transplantation is empiric and varies substantially among transplant centers. A "loading dose" of oral or intravenous azathioprine (3–5 mg/kg) is often administered perioperatively, and the daily dose is tapered to a maintenance dose of 2–3 mg/kg/d for combination therapy with prednisone. When azathioprine is included as part of "triple therapy" the maintenance dose may be as low as 0.25–0.5 mg/kg/d.

The dose of azathioprine is adjusted in response to changes in white blood count (WBC) and platelet count. In the early postoperative period, daily WBC and platelet monitoring is essential for adequate dosage adjustments. If the WBC decreases to 4000/mm^3 or less, careful consideration must be given to making a dosage reduction. A WBC higher than 3000/mm^3 should be maintained during azathioprine therapy, but other factors may decrease the WBC in transplant patients such as CMV infection. Following a dosage reduction of azathioprine, the WBC should stabilize for several days before any additional adjustments are made.

Impaired renal function does not affect the response to azathioprine or 6-mercaptopurine. In patients with hepatic dysfunction, decreased hepatic conversion of azathioprine to its active metabolites will decrease the pharmacologic response to the drug. Azathioprine is also metabolized by xanthine oxidase, so concurrent therapy with azathioprine and allopurinol results in a significant increase in the immunosuppressive and toxic effects of the drug. If combination therapy with azathioprine and allopurinol is required, a decrease in the azathioprine dose by 50–75% is necessary to avoid toxicity.

Mycophenolate Mofetil

Mycophenolate mofetil is a pro-drug of mycophenolic acid recently approved for the prevention and treatment of allograft rejection following renal transplantation. *In vitro* and *in vivo,* mycophenolic acid blocks the proliferative responses to T and B lymphocytes and inhibits antibody formation and the generation of cytotoxic T cells. While the drug has many similarities to azathioprine as an antiproliferative agent, its mechanism of action is more specific for the pathway of purine metabolism involved in lymphocyte proliferation. Mycophenolate blocks the *de novo* synthesis of purines by inhibiting the enzyme inosine monophosphate dehydrogenase, which in turn inhibits lymphocyte proliferation. Mycophenolate may also act by inhibiting the glycosylation of adhesion molecules on endothelial cells, which is necessary for the leukocytes to migrate out of the bloodstream. This agent has been shown to have synergistic immunosuppressive activity when combined with CyA and prednisone.

Clinical studies with mycophenolate mofetil are limited. Mycophenolate has demonstrated potential for primary maintenance immunosuppression and as a rescue therapy for patients undergoing renal, liver, or heart transplantation. The dose of mycophenolate mofetil required for optimal immunosuppression appears to be 2 g/d, administered in two divided doses every 12 hours. After oral administration, mycophenolate mofetil is rapidly hydrolyzed to mycophenolic acid. Mycophenolic acid is excreted unchanged and as a glucuronide conjugate that is eliminated in bile and urine. Dosage adjustments of the drug do not appear to be necessary in patients with liver or renal dysfunction. Therapeutic monitoring of this drug is not routinely used in clinical practice.

Adverse effects associated with mycophenolate mofetil include neutropenia and thrombocytopenia. However, these effects appear to be less common and severe compared with azathioprine. Infectious complications, including candid CMV, herpes, and bacterial pneumonia, occur at a similar rate in patients receiving mycophenolate mofetil and other immunosuppressive regimens. Central nervous system effects such as headache, weakness, dizziness, and insomnia have also been reported. Gastrointestinal effects including nausea and diarrhea may occur early in therapy and respond to dosage reductions of the drug. Other rare adverse effects include pancreatitis, burning on urination and urinary frequency, hepatotoxicity, ocular effects, rash, and myalgias.

The exact role of this drug in clinical transplantation is yet to be defined. The usefulness of mycophenolate in patients unable to tolerate maximum doses of azathioprine appears to be established. Whether mycophenolate will replace azathioprine in "triple" immunosuppressive regimens will depend on long-term experience with the drug and on cost considerations.

ANTI-T-CELL BIOLOGICAL PRODUCTS

Muromonab-CD3 (OKT3)

OKT3 is a monoclonal antibody preparation that reacts with the CD3 receptor on lymphocytes. While a number of monoclonal antibodies have been manufactured for clinical and diagnostic purposes, only OKT3 is commercially available for use as an immunosuppressant in transplant patients. The other monoclonal antibodies against other T cell or cytokine receptors are discussed under Investigational Agents.

Within minutes of an infusion of OKT3, circulating T cells become virtually undetectable and this depletion of T cells appears to be essential for effective immunosuppression. OKT3 therapy is used as induction therapy following transplantation, as a first-line treatment of acute cellular rejection, and as a second-line therapy for the treatment of acute rejection unresponsive to high-dose corticosteroids. The dose of OKT3 used for induction therapy or to treat acute rejection is 5 mg/d in adults and 2.5 mg/d in children. Occasionally, doses of OKT3 as high as 10–25 mg have been used to treat rejection. These large doses would be required by patients who have been previously treated with OKT3 and who have developed antimurine antibodies. The duration of OKT3 therapy ranges from 5–14 days, and its rapid intravenous administration is an advantage in comparison with ALG/ATG.

Some controversy exists regarding dose adjustments of other immunosuppressants during OKT3 therapy. Many clinicians prefer to decrease the doses of other immunosuppressants to minimize the potential infectious complications of overimmunosuppression. If the doses of other agents are lowered, an increase in the other immunosuppressants should be made several days before completion of OKT3 therapy with an overlap of 2 full days of therapeutic CyA concentrations. Other investigators have suggested that maintaining full doses of azathioprine and prednisone during OKT3 therapy will decrease the formation of human antimurine antibodies.

The initial administration of OKT3 is associated with the risk of a first-dose reaction. This reaction to OKT3 may occur within an hour of the first injection and may include chills, fever, chest tightness, and wheezing. First-dose reactions can be minimized by premedication with antipyretics, antihistamines, and corticosteroids. Pulmonary edema and cardiac arrest have been reported in patients clinically fluid overloaded before receiving the drug. A chest x-ray and an accurate assessment of weight and volume status should be made before initiating OKT3 therapy.

A syndrome of aseptic meningitis presenting as fever, headache, and neck stiffness has been reported during OKT3 therapy.[13] In addition, patients may experience visual hallucinations, acute psychosis, and severe depression with the drug. While the central nervous system toxicity of OKT3 is self-limited, some patients may require discontinuation of the drug. The most severe complications of OKT3 therapy are those associated with overimmunosuppression. Viral infections with CMV and lymphoproliferative disorders have been attributed to OKT3, but the incidence of these disorders is unlikely to be different than in patients overimmunosuppressed with other agents.

The effects of OKT3 are monitored through clinical signs of allograft function, infection, and drug toxicity. Immunologic monitoring including a sequential analysis of T-cell subsets, identification of peripheral lymphocytes coated with antibody, and serum concentrations of the monoclonal and antimurine antibodies may allow a better assessment of efficacy of OKT3, but an improvement in patient outcome through the use of these techniques has not yet been clearly demonstrated. Current recommendations suggest that monitoring based on these methods should be individualized to the transplant center because of considerations of concurrent immunosuppressive protocol, analytic methods available, and cost.[14]

Antilymphocyte/Antithymocyte Globulin (ALG/ATG) Therapy

ALG/ATG is a sterile, nonpyrogenic solution of immunoglobulins (IgG). ALG or ATG is obtained from horses, rabbits, or goats immunized with human lymphoid cells. Product availability is frequently the primary factor in product selection, and no specific product has been proven to be the most efficacious. Currently the only commercial product in the United States is an equine product, but a rabbit-derived thymoglobulin is in clinical trials. Substantial batch-to-batch variability in ALG/ATG preparations occurs and is a problem associated with the clinical use of these products.

The primary effect of ALG or ATG is the elimination of T cells and a decrease in the proliferation of newly formed lymphocytes. Upon cessation of therapy, the number of circulating T cells gradually returns to normal while the proliferative response of lymphocytes remains impaired. This antiproliferative action is responsible for the long-lasting immunosuppressive effects of ALG/ATG.[15]

ALG/ATG is used for induction therapy immediately following transplantation and for the treatment of an acute cellular rejection. The dose and duration of ALG/ATG therapy varies among transplant centers. Doses range from 10–30 mg/kg/d for 5–14 days in adults, whereas doses in children range from 5–25 mg/kg/d. ALG/ATG dosage and duration is typically adjusted according to the clinical status of the patient with consideration for other immunosuppressive therapy, infection, or toxicity.

Chills and febrile reactions are frequently reported during and following an infusion of ALG/ATG. First-dose reactions can be minimized by premedication with antipyretics, antihistamines, and/or a single dose of corticosteroids. Chemical phlebitis and hypotension associated with ALG/ATG administration can usually be avoided by administering the product intravenously via a central line over 4–6 hours. Serum sickness with arthralgia, fever, and general malaise can occur at any time during the first few weeks after administration of ALG/ATG. Thrombocytopenia is a dose-related complication of ALG/ATG therapy. Patients treated with ALG/ATG are also at high risk for developing bacterial, fungal, and viral infections.

IMMUNOPHILIN-BINDING AGENTS

Cyclosporine

Cyclosporine is a cyclic polypeptide that inhibits T-lymphocyte proliferation by inhibiting the production of IL-2 and other cytokines by T cells. Cyclosporine produces this effect by binding to a cytoplasmic immunophilin called cyclophyllin.[16] This drug-immunophilin complex can then block the action of a cytoplasmic phosphatase enzyme called calcineurin (Fig. 9.4). *In vitro* studies with cell lines deficient in immunophilin suggest that CyA is inactive in the absence of this intracytoplasmic protein.

Cyclosporine may be administered orally or as an intravenous infusion. A wide range of doses are used for CyA depending on the clinical status of the patient (early versus late postoperative period, open versus closed T tube in bile duct) and the use of other drugs (alone versus triple or quadruple therapy, coadministration of drugs that affect CyA metabolism). The normal dose range for intravenous CyA is 2–5 mg/kg/d as a continuous infusion since rapid intravenous administration of CyA has been associated with hypotension, tachycardia, severe headache, bronchospasm, flushing, and nausea. The oral bioavailability of CyA is about 30% and the initial oral doses are 8–17 mg/kg/d. Lower initial oral CyA doses and dosage reduction long term to less than 5 mg/kg/d are strategies used to minimize nephrotoxicity, but dosage reductions below 4 mg/kg/d have been associated with chronic rejection.

The nephrotoxicity of CyA is the major factor limiting the usefulness of CyA following transplantation. Following renal transplantation, nephrotoxicity must be distinguished from allograft rejection. Rejection and nephrotoxicity from

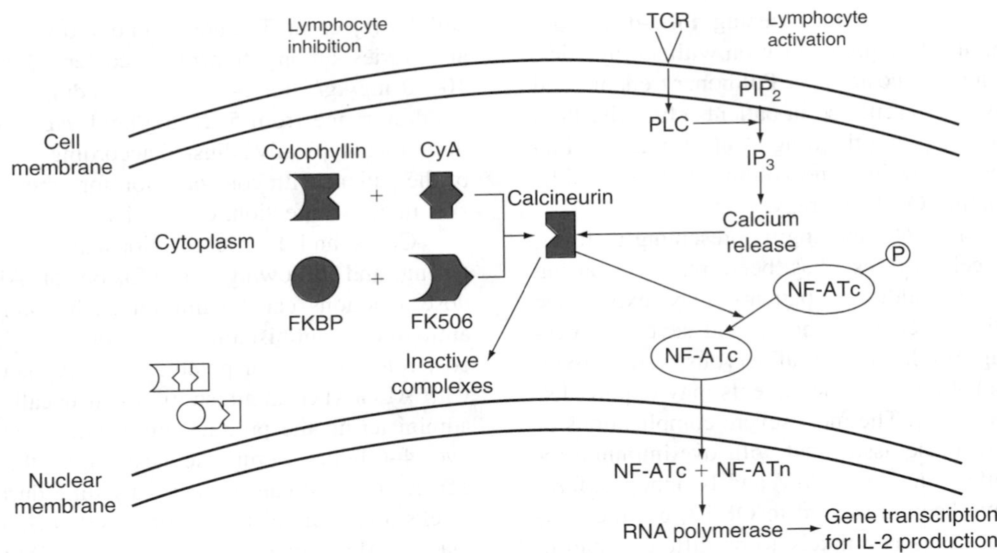

Figure 9.4. Model of the proposed actions of CyA and FK-506 on lymphocyte proliferation. Stimulation of the T-cell receptor (TCR) phosphorylates phospholipase C (PLC) causes formation of inositol triphosphate (IP_3) through phosphatyl inositol diphosphate (PIP_2), which produces the intracellular release of calcium ions. Calcium activates the phosphatase calcineurin, which dephosphorylates cytoplasmic nuclear factor of activated T cells (NF-ATc). NF-ATc translocates into the nucleus of the cell where it combines with its intranuclear cofactor (NF-ATn) to activate RNA polymerase, which regulates the transcription of genes that control production of IL-2 and other cytokines.

CyA may occur simultaneously in the patient, making differentiation of the processes difficult. Clinical signs of graft rejection, radiologic studies, and CyA blood or plasma concentrations are all used to distinguish between nephrotoxicity and rejection in renal transplant patients. While the exact cause of CyA nephrotoxicity is not known, several forms of renal toxicity have been described, and ischemia associated with a deterioration in renal blood flow may be a major contributor. Clinical syndromes of CyA nephrotoxicity include prolongation of acute tubular necrosis following renal transplantation, the chronic deterioration of renal function, and a rare form of hemolytic–uremic syndrome within the first week following transplantation. Renal function is adversely affected by the administration of cyclooxygenase inhibitors in patients on CyA, and the administration of misoprostil has been suggested as having a beneficial effect on renal function in CyA-treated patients. Management of CyA-induced nephrotoxicity primarily involves reducing or discontinuing the drug, but renal transplantation has been necessary in some patients who could not be exposed to the greater risk of rejection of the transplanted organ (liver, heart) posed by a reduction in CyA dosage.

Cyclosporine blood or plasma concentration monitoring is useful in making dosage adjustments for the drug.[17] While only a weak correlation exists between high CyA concentrations and drug toxicity or between low concentrations and allograft rejection, monitoring is a useful guide to dosing in patients with poor absorption, hepatic dysfunction, and drug interactions. Significantly higher incidences of graft rejection have been reported in patients who have poor absorption of CyA. Chromatographic assays and immunoassays for CyA are both useful for clinical monitoring, but therapeutic ranges depend on assay method and whether the biologic specimen is blood or plasma. Newer immunoassay techniques using monoclonal antibodies yield results closer to those of high-performance liquid chromatographic assays. Methodologic problems will be encountered with assays for new immunosuppressants that have immunoreactive metabolites.

A new product formulation of CyA called Neoral was approved in 1995. Neoral is a microemulsion of cyclosporine and has improved and more reliable absorption of the drug. The need for intravenous CyA immediately following liver transplantation or during periods of T-tube drainage may be decreased or eliminated by this product. The choice of oral CyA formulations may however depend on cost considerations since CyA will be available as a much less expensive generic product.

Tacrolimus (FK-506)

Tacrolimus is indicated for the prevention and treatment of allograft rejection in patients undergoing liver transplantation. The usefulness of tacrolimus as an immunosuppressant following kidney, heart, heart–lung, lung, pancreas, and intestinal transplantation has also been demonstrated. Tacrolimus prevents rejection of the transplanted organ by inhibiting the production of IL-2 in T cells, thereby inhibiting growth and proliferation of those cells. This activity occurs as a result of tacrolimus binding to the cytoplasmic immunophilin, FK-binding protein (FKBP), with subsequent inhibition of the activity of calcineurin.

Tacrolimus has been evaluated in clinical trials at major transplantation centers in the United States, Japan, and Europe. Patient and graft survival rates for various transplant procedures under tacrolimus are not significantly different than those achieved under "conventional" immunosuppression with CyA, prednisone, and azathioprine (Table 9.5).[18] However, many factors, including surgical advances, better postoperative care for the transplant patient, new agents such as ganciclovir for CMV infection, and improvements in organ preservation during organ transportation, have all had a positive influence on graft and patient survival. A major benefit of tacrolimus as compared with CyA relates to an enhanced ability in patients to discontinue corticosteroids. Shorter hospitalizations and reduced hospital costs have been reported for patients receiving tacrolimus.[19]

The pharmacokinetics of tacrolimus is influenced by a number of factors. Following oral administration, the bioavailability of tacrolimus ranges from 5–67% with a mean of 29% in liver, kidney, and small bowel transplant patients. The poor oral bioavailability of tacrolimus necessitates the use of three to four times higher oral doses than intravenous doses to obtain similar blood concentrations. Meals with moderate fat content appear to reduce the extent and rate of absorption of orally administered tacrolimus. Unlike CyA, the oral absorption of tacrolimus does not appear to be decreased in patients with liver dysfunction or in patients with a T tube.

Tacrolimus is extensively distributed throughout the body with a steady-state volume of distribution of 5–65 L/kg. The drug is highly distributed into erythrocytes. The partitioning of tacrolimus between erythrocytes and plasma depends on the tacrolimus concentration, the hematocrit, the temperature of separation of plasma, and the plasma protein concentration. The whole blood concentration of tacrolimus in transplant patients is 10 to 30 times higher than the corresponding plasma concentration. In plasma, tacrolimus is associated with 1-acid glycoprotein, an acute-phase protein.

TABLE 9.5. COMPARISON OF CYCLOSPORINE AND TACROLIMUS PATIENT- AND GRAFT-SURVIVAL RATES

	1-Year Survival Rates (%)			
	Tacrolimus		Cyclosporine	
Transplant	Patient	Graft	Patient	Graft
Liver	88	82	68	79
Renal				
Living related	90	100	97	91
Cadaver	90	74	93	80
Heart	92	92	82	82
Lung	80	80	69	69

(From Ref. 18.)

Tacrolimus is primarily eliminated from the body by hepatic and intestinal metabolism resulting in its conversion to at least nine metabolites. Strong evidence suggests that cytochrome P450-3A is primarily involved in the metabolism of tacrolimus, but information that additional subsets of cytochrome P450 enzymes are involved has also been reported. Since tacrolimus is primarily eliminated by metabolism, alterations in hepatic function are expected to influence its elimination. Higher trough tacrolimus concentrations, decreased clearance, and longer half-lives of tacrolimus have been reported in transplant patients with impaired liver function. Liver transplant recipients with significant perioperative graft dysfunction have higher tacrolimus plasma concentrations in spite of dose reductions in comparison to liver transplant recipients with normal or improving graft function.

Pediatric transplant patients clear the drug more rapidly than do adult transplant patients on a body weight basis. Therefore, pediatric patients require as much as two to four times higher doses of tacrolimus based on mg/kg body weight than do adults to maintain similar plasma tacrolimus concentrations.

The renal clearance of tacrolimus is less than 1% of the total body clearance. Therefore, dosage adjustments of the drug are not required in patients with renal dysfunction or in patients receiving dialysis treatments.

The management of patients receiving tacrolimus may be complicated by a number of potential drug interactions. *In vitro* studies indicate that the tacrolimus concentration in a solution is significantly decreased in the presence of magnesium oxide and sodium bicarbonate secondary to pH-mediated drug degradation. These pH-altering compounds should, therefore, be administered at least 2 hours apart from tacrolimus oral administration. Aluminum hydroxide gel physically adsorbs tacrolimus. Magnesium chloride, aluminum hydroxide powder, aluminum hydroxide dried gel, and calcium carbonate do not alter tacrolimus concentrations in simulated gastric fluid.

Since tacrolimus appears to be metabolized primarily by cytochrome P450-3A, an enzyme known to metabolize CyA, drugs known to alter CyA concentrations are likely to alter tacrolimus concentrations in patients. Administration of erythromycin, clotrimazole, fluconazole, methylprednisolone, and danazole can increase tacrolimus concentrations in transplant patients. While other drug interactions are not well documented in humans, ketoconazole, itraconazole, diltiazem, verapamil, cimetidine, and other macrolide antibiotics should be used cautiously with tacrolimus.

Phenobarbital, phenytoin, rifampin, and dexamethasone may lower tacrolimus concentrations in patients. The addition of nephrotoxic drugs such as NSAIDs, aminoglycosides, or amphotericin B to tacrolimus therapy may result in an increased risk of nephrotoxicity in transplant patients and should warrant more intensive monitoring. The combined use of CyA and tacrolimus results in synergistic immunosuppression, but also increased nephrotoxicity. Synergistic hyperkalemia may be observed in patients receiving tacrolimus in combination with potassium supplements or angiotensin-converting enzyme inhibitors. Therefore potassium concentrations should be closely monitored in individuals receiving these combinations.

Dosing of tacrolimus is highly variable. Initial intravenous doses range from 0.05–0.1 mg/kg/d, administered as a continuous infusion. Oral doses range from 0.1–0.3 mg/kg/d, administered in two divided doses every 12 hours. Tacrolimus doses are adjusted based on a patient's clinical response, adverse effects, and tacrolimus blood concentration.

Therapeutic monitoring of tacrolimus concentrations is routinely employed for patients receiving the drug. The currently available method for tacrolimus quantification uses a microparticulate enzyme immunoassay (MEIA) assay. Unchanged tacrolimus and its metabolites cross-react with the antibody used in the ELISA assay. Whole blood concentration monitoring avoids the variability in plasma concentrations associated with concentration-dependent changes in erythrocyte binding, temperature-dependent alterations in the distribution of the drug, and changes in hematocrit frequently observed following transplantation. The therapeutic range for tacrolimus is not well established. As a general rule, target whole blood tacrolimus concentrations in the first 6 months following transplantation are 10–20 ng/mL. Several months later patients may be maintained at concentrations of 5–15 ng/mL.

Adverse effects experienced by patients receiving tacrolimus as their primary immunosuppression are similar to those experienced in patients receiving CyA. The most common side effects observed with tacrolimus are neurologic in nature. Minor neurologic side effects have included insomnia, mild tremors, headaches, photophobia, nightmares, and hyperesthesias, and major neurologic side effects have included confusion, seizures, coma, dysarthrias (expressive aphasia), psychosis, and encephalopathy. The incidence of neurologic side effects has been reported as 10–20% for minor side effects and 8–21% for major side effects. The incidence and severity of these neurologic effects may be dose and dosing route related.

Tacrolimus has been shown to adversely affect glomerular filtration rate, renal blood flow, and renal vascular resistance. Direct comparisons of the nephrotoxicity of tacrolimus and CyA have not been performed. Dialysis treatment has been required in patients with severe renal toxicity resulting from the use of tacrolimus. Tacrolimus produces significantly smaller increases in systolic blood pressure, diastolic blood pressure, and systemic vascular resistance in liver transplant recipients when compared with CyA. Serum potassium, serum magnesium, and serum bicarbonate levels are affected similarly in tacrolimus- and CyA-treated patients, with mean serum potassium levels being reported in the high normal range and mean serum magnesium levels being reported in the low normal range. Abnormally high serum potassium levels can be treated with diet changes, potassium-binding resins, or fludrocortisone therapy. Low serum magnesium levels can be corrected with magnesium supplements.

CMV infection is the primary infectious complication in patients receiving tacrolimus. The incidence of CMV infections in patients receiving tacrolimus and CyA appear to be similar (28 vs. 20%, respectively). Lymphoproliferative disorders are strongly associated with Epstein–Barr virus infection and occur in less than 2% of transplant patients receiving tacrolimus. Other adverse effects—including glucose intolerance sometimes requiring insulin therapy, nausea, rash, itching, and anemia—have been observed in patients receiving tacrolimus.

The role of tacrolimus in clinical transplantation is yet to be defined. The success of liver and intestinal transplants suggests that tacrolimus may become the immunosuppressive agent of choice for new patients undergoing these procedures or for patients failing therapy with CyA. The role of tacrolimus in primary renal transplantation is less well defined considering the high success rates routinely achieved under CyA immunosuppression. If the steroid-sparing potential of tacrolimus is established in long-term clinical trials, tacrolimus could be considered a major advance in the long-term treatment of organ transplant patients.

INVESTIGATIONAL IMMUNOSUPPRESSIVE AGENTS IN TRANSPLANTATION

As new immunologic pathways are discovered, their true role in the complex functioning of the immune system is often revealed in animal models in which that component of the immune system can be deleted or blocked. New immunosuppressive agents that are developed should improve our understanding of the immune system and may improve patient care. Several investigational methods of pharmacologically inhibiting the rejection response are detailed in this section.

Rapamycin

Rapamycin is an investigational macrolide immunosuppressant structurally related to tacrolimus. Rapamycin binds to FKBP in the cytoplasm with a higher affinity than does tacrolimus, but appears to have a different pharmacologic action. Unlike tacrolimus and CyA, rapamycin blocks lymphocyte proliferation induced by IL-2, and affects lymphocyte proliferation at a later step (after promotion of IL-2 formation) than CyA or tacrolimus. Rapamycin appears to directly affect B-cell function in a manner that is not seen for CyA or tacrolimus, so that therapy with this new agent may provide information about the clinical importance of B-cell suppression concurrent with T-cell suppression in preventing chronic rejection in transplant patients. Some investigators feel that the ability of rapamycin to prevent chronic rejection and to halt the progression of preexisting vascular graft disease could be the most important contribution of rapamycin to transplantation pharmacotherapy. Clinical trials with rapamycin in transplant patients are currently being conducted.

Fusion Proteins

Fusion proteins are the products of connecting two separate entities. These include the chimeric and humanized monoclonal antibodies discussed earlier, the immunoligands, and bispecific antibodies. The most developed of the immunoligands is CTLA4Ig, which takes advantage of CTLA4's 20-fold higher affinity for binding B7 than that of CD28 (Fig. 9.2). By blocking the costimulation of the TCR, CTLA4Ig could theoretically induce tolerance to donor tissue, and trials of preventing graft-versus-host disease in animal models of bone marrow transplantation have been attempted. CTLA4Ig actually holds more promise presently for solid organ transplantation, and multicenter trials of CTLA4Ig are being initiated.

HLA Peptide Fragments

Peptides derived from the α-helix of Class I HLA molecules, called Allotrap peptides, appear to have immunosuppressive activity. While this activity was initially thought to result from interference with antigen presentation to the TCR, more recent studies have shown that this function may be caused by binding to heat shock proteins intracellularly. The D-isomers of some of the Allotrap peptides are as effective in animal transplant models as the L-isomers, but are not susceptible to degradation by serum proteases. The Allotrap peptide investigation may reveal new knowledge about transplantation immunology and may find a place in clinical use since so many amino acid combinations are possible in the formulation of these peptide fragments.

New Antiproliferative Agents

Bredinine, also called misoribine, is a nucleoside antibiotic shown to prolong kidney graft survival in dogs and humans. Its mechanism of action appears to be similar to that of azathioprine, but bredinine does not possess any hepatotoxicity or myelotoxicity. The lymphocytotoxic effect of the drug is conferred by its ability to interfere with purine synthesis, but bredinine does not inhibit the production of IL-2. Most human studies with this drug have been conducted in Japan, and the drug is not currently being pursued for marketing in the United States.

Leflunomide is an isoxazole derivative with demonstrated immunosuppressive activity in animal models of transplantation and in clinical trials in rheumatoid arthritis. Leflunomide was originally thought to be the first immunosuppressive agent used clinically that demonstrated activity against the tyrosine kinases, which are an important early event in the signal transduction cascade. More recent work has suggested that leflunomide acts as a pyrimidine antagonist, and its development as an agent for transplantation patients is now in question.

The only other pyrimidine antagonist to be studied in transplantation, brequinar sodium, is not currently being pursued for clinical trials in transplantation. While cyclophosphamide is used primarily in oncology, renewed interest in the drug for transplantation has come about in the area of xenotransplantation because of cyclophosphamide's potent anti-B-cell effect.

Cyclosporine Derivatives

Early enthusiasm for derivatives of CyA centered on cyclosporin G (CyG), also called Nva2-cyclosporine and OG 37-325, which was considered to have less nephrotoxic potential. Early trials demonstrated that CyG was equally effective in renal transplantation to CyA, but adverse effects related to increased liver enzymes and nephrotoxicity were observed. While enthusiasm for this agent has waned, the recognition of the significant immunosuppressive activity of CyG and of some of the metabolites of CyA demonstrates that new products of this nature are possible. Another CyA derivative in clinical trials is SDZ IMM 125.

Deoxyspergualin

Deoxyspergualin is a guanidine-like compound used as an anticancer agent. Its mechanism of action appears to be very different from that of CyA, tacrolimus, or mycophenolate, and may involve binding to heat shock proteins within the cell important for antigen processing and other cell functions. Deoxyspergualin affects the activity of APCs, T cells, and B cells. Initial trials in renal transplant patients have found the drug to be effective in early episodes of rejection and in steroid-resistent rejection. Deoxyspergualin may find a place in transplant protocols as adjunctive therapy for the treatment of refractory rejection or for induction therapy.

SK&F 105685

This azaspirane derivative is unique in that it enhances suppressor cell activity in animal models of autoimmune disease and transplantation. This activity has been compared with benefit derived from lymphoid irradiation while maintaining an excellent safety profile of the drug in animals. The clinical usefulness of this approach in organ transplantation is unknown at present.

Monoclonal Antibodies

An extensive list of murine monoclonal antibodies that can block T cell or adhesion molecule function has been studied in animals, but the slow progress of these products to clinical application dampens any encouragement for this class of drugs. One change that revived clinical interest in the monoclonal antibodies is the availability of the technology to make chimeric or human monoclonal antibodies. For example, earlier clinical investigation of a murine monoclonal antibody that blocks IL-2R showed the biologic effectiveness of this approach, but the overall clinical outcome in transplant patients treated with the mouse-derived product did not change. A newer agent against the same portion of the IL-2R, also called Tac, is a humanized anti-Tac or HAT antibody. This product has a long half-life in humans and is now in clinical trials in transplant patients.

Numerous other monoclonal antibodies are now under study. Anti-CD4 monoclonal antibodies have been used in animal models with particular success at inducing tolerance to skin, islet, and cardiac allografts, and clinical trials are now being conducted with a humanized product. A human/mouse chimeric antibody (antibody with fragments from different species) with anti-CD7 specificity is undergoing clinical testing and will provide information on patient antibody production to the chimeric product. Attacking the CD7 antigen is of interest since it is a cell-activation antigen whose exact function remains unknown. Campath-1 is another monoclonal antibody that binds to an antigen found on all mature T cells and on some B cells, and has been studied in patients receiving kidney–pancreas and liver allografts. Adhesion molecules are blocked by either an anti-ICAM-1 monoclonal antibody or by an anti-LFA-1 antibody, and they appear to confer some protection against delayed graft function of kidneys.

Anti-Inflammatory Agents

Inflammatory mediators have effects on T-cell function clearly identified in *in vitro* studies, but these have been difficult to document in clinical trials. Prostaglandin analogues have been reported to improve graft function and diminish CyA toxicity in animal studies, and preliminary information with the use of misoprostil in renal transplant patients appears to be encouraging. Thromboxane receptor antagonists hold similar promise, as do platelet-activating factor antagonists. Free oxygen radical scavengers such as superoxide dismutase have a theoretical place in preventing reperfusion injury of transplanted organs, but limited clinical trials have not yet been successful.

Local Immunosuppression

Providing intense immunosuppressive therapy locally has proven effective in animal studies and more recently in human transplantation. This procedure may be accomplished by either directed local administration of a drug or by using gene therapy to get T cells to produce their own immunosuppressive substances. Cyclosporine is currently being aerosolized and inhaled by lung transplant patients as one method of delivering the drug in high concentrations to the graft and avoiding some of the risk of systemic drug toxicity. An example of gene therapy-induced immunosuppression would be getting pancreatic islet T cells to produce TGF-β or IL-10, which are immunosuppressive in nature. As technologic devices improve that can provide long-term local drug infusions, or as organs with direct access (lungs, small bowel) become transplanted more frequently, local immunosuppression may give rise to the need for agents with different biopharmaceutical properties than those agents used systemically at present.

DRUG THERAPY CONSIDERATIONS IN TRANSPLANT PATIENTS

Improved immune monitoring is essential for successful immunosuppressive therapy. Unless donor-specific tolerance becomes a reality, the pharmacotherapist will always be balancing adequate immunosuppression to prevent rejection against overimmunosuppression and its attendant risks. Markers of organ function are important monitoring tools, but reflect an immunologic process that has already occurred. Histopathologic studies of organ biopsies provide the accepted standard in transplantation today, but findings that immune-competent T lymphocytes can be cultured from biopsies demonstrating no rejection cast doubt on their value as a prospective monitoring tool of subtle rejection. Markers of immune cell activation such as serum IL-2R and IL-6 concentrations can be misleading because of their nonspecific elevation during infection. A panel of plasma cytokines and soluble adhesion molecules may eventually assist in the assessment of the transplant patient. Drug concentrations are important as general guides to drug dosing in the organ transplant patient, but their relationship to immunosuppression has not been clearly established. Flow cytometric studies of T-cell subsets have been of primary value when conducted on tissue from the graft itself. Because no direct measure of the recipient's immune reactivity to donor tissue is available, the pharmacotherapists must take into account all of the above measures of organ function, immune function, and biopharmaceutical considerations to optimize therapy for each individual transplant patient.

The preceding discussion concentrated on immunosuppressive therapy, but many other pharmacologic agents are often required for the adequate management of a transplant patient. In some instances, such as in the use of diuretics and anti-infectives, the use of these agents parallels the use in other patient populations. Even then, special considerations must be given to the biopharmaceutical properties of drugs in kidney, liver, and heart transplant patients with recovering organ function.

Hypertension continues to be a serious problem in transplant patients. Until the exact mechanism of hypertension is determined in transplant patients, its treatment remains empiric and highly individualized from one transplant center to another. The use of newer protocols with tacrolimus and low or no dose corticosteroids should significantly diminish the problem of hypertension in liver transplant patients.

Anti-infective prophylaxis (antibiotic, antifungal, antiviral) and therapy are carried out in transplant patients in the same manner as other immunocompromised hosts. There are patient populations within transplantation that appear to be much more susceptible to infectious disease, such as the recipient who lacks antibodies to CMV but receives an organ from a CMV-positive donor. The antibiotics chosen for surgical prophylaxis and for the preoperative cleansing of the gastrointestinal tract remain empiric choices.

Another drug-related problem in transplant patients is the development of post-transplant lymphomas. Lymphomas develop in 1–5% of transplant patients, with the greatest frequency being in nonrenal transplant patients. This difference is most likely the result of the intensity of the immunosuppressive therapy in organ transplant patients who do not have an alternative to graft survival, as do the renal patients with dialysis. Individual agents such as OKT3 have been implicated in the production of lymphomas, but these agents are almost always used in combination with other immunosuppressive drugs. Additional evidence that immunosuppression alone is associated with the production of lymphomas comes from patients with primary immunodeficiency and acquired immunodeficiency syndrome, both of which are associated with lymphomas that share the characteristics of those in transplant patients. Transplant patients do have the alternative of decreasing or stopping immunosuppressive therapy, which can produce complete regression of lymphomatous changes in some patients. Additional discussion of this problem is found in Chapter 18, Cardiac Transplantation.

Conclusion

The pharmacotherapist can make significant contributions to the care of organ transplant patients. These contributions can be made through the management of complex drug regimens by managing drug dosing, toxicity, and drug interactions; by managing special dosing considerations in patients with rapidly changing renal, hepatic, and cardiac disease; by assessing the pharmacoeconomic impact of new biotechnology-derived agents; and by the investigation of new immunosuppressive agents and new pharmacodynamic monitoring techniques for transplant patients.

References

1. Kahan BD. Transplantation time-line. Transplantation 1991;51:1–21.
2. Bodmer JG, Marsh SGE, Albert ED, et al. Nomenclature for factors of the HLA system, 1994. Hum Immunol 1994;41:1–20.
3. Duquesnoy RJ, Cramer DV. Immunologic mechanisms of cardiac transplant rejection. Cardiovasc Clin 1990;20:87–103.
4. Morris PJ. Rejection—unanswered questions. Hum Immunol 1990;28:104–111.
5. Port FK, Held PJ, Wolfe RA, et al. The impact of nonidentical ABO cadaveric renal transplantation on waiting times and graft survival. Am J Kidney Dis 1991;17:519–523.
6. Shoskes DA, Wood KJ. Indirect presentation of MHC antigens in transplantation. Immunol Today 1994;15:32–38.
7. Steele AW, Strom TB. Cytokines and the Th1/Th2 paradigm in transplantation. Curr Opin Immunol 1994;6:757–764.
8. Nickerson PW, Steurer W, Steiger J, Strom TB. In pursuit of the "Holy Grail": Allograft tolerance. Kidney Int 1994;45(suppl 44):S40–S49.
9. Starzl TE, Demetris AJ, Murase N, et al. Donor cell chimerism permitted by immunosuppressive drugs: A new view of organ transplantation. Immunol Today 1993;14:326–332.
10. Deierhoi MH, Sollinger HW, Kalayogly M, et al. Quadruple immunosuppression in 305 consecutive cadaver renal allografts. Clin Transpl 1987;1:71–74.
11. Walker AM (ed). Transplant Protocols. Chestnut Hill, MA, Epidemiology Resources, 1990.
12. Tejani A, Butt KMH, Rajpoot D, et al. Strategies for optimizing growth in children with kidney transplantation. Transplantation 1989;47:229–233.
13. Thisethwaite JR, Stuart JK, Mayes JT, et al. Complications and monitoring of OKT3 therapy. Am J Kidney Dis 1988;11:112–119.
14. Rossi SJ. Immunologic monitoring of OKT3 therapy, in Transplant Pharmacy Newsletter, American College of Clinical Pharmacy, Winter 1995, pp 2–5.
15. Thomas JM, Carver FM, Haisch CE, et al. Suppressor cells in rhesus monkey treated with antilymphocyte globulin. Transplantation 1982;34:83–89.
16. Touchette N. Immune suppressants signal surprises in T cell activation. J NIH Res 1991;3:70–74.
17. Critical issues in cyclosporine monitoring: Report of the Task Force on Cyclosporine Monitoring. Clin Chem 1987;33:1269–1288.
18. Kelly PA, Burckart GJ, Venkataramanan R. Review of the new immunosuppressant tacrolimus (FK506). Am J Health-Syst Pharmacy 1995:52;1521–1535.
19. Staschak S, Wagner S, Block G, et al. A cost comparison of liver transplantation with FK-506 or CyA as the primary immunosuppressive agent. Transplant Proc 1990;22:47–49.

PART TWO

Disorders of Organ Systems

Section 1
Cardiovascular Disorders

Chapter 10
Cardiovascular Testing

Margaret E. McGuinness, PharmD,
and Robert L. Talbert, PharmD, FCCP

The physical examination and history taking remain the most important elements of patient assessment.[1–6] The advent of sophisticated diagnostic tests for any disease state does not obviate the need to complete a thorough physical examination and obtain a patient history.[1,2] (Tables 10.1 and 10.2). Technologically advanced tests (e.g., echocardiography, cardiac catheterization) are additive and supplementary to the physical examination and do not replace it.

The physical examination and history provide valuable insight into the patient's condition and help in the planning and interpretation of tests performed at a later date. The physical examination and history are cost effective, because they are obtained directly with no lag time for results and evaluation.[1–3] History taking enables the examiner to establish a relationship with the patient and develop an awareness of the patient's perception of problems. It also allows assessment of the acuteness or chronicity and severity of a problem, identification of the current versus past level of activity, and determination of whether or not quality of life is impaired by the problem. History taking covers elements such as chief complaint, present problems, past medical history, review of systems, and social and family history. Physical examination of the cardiovascular system includes observation, palpation, percussion, and auscultation of the heart and related structures.

Signs and Symptoms[1,2]

The primary signs and symptoms of cardiovascular disease include chest pain, dyspnea with or without orthopnea, paroxysmal nocturnal dyspnea, cyanosis, fatigue, palpitations, cough, edema, and syncope. The physical exam and history allow identification of these signs and symptoms and provide information on their severity.

Physical Examination[1,3–5]

The physical examination may be divided into four categories: (1) measurement of parameters of cardiovascular function (pulse, blood pressure), (2) observation and assessment of physical findings (e.g., jugular venous pressure), (3) auscultation and palpation of the chest and review of all body systems, and (4) examination of the entire patient for signs of cardiovascular disease.[1] Factors such as skin color, condition, and temperature are just as important as the finding of an elevated blood pressure. Each physical finding allows the clinician to direct more specific questioning in order to define the differential diagnosis more clearly (e.g., dyspnea may be a symptom of either pulmonary or cardiovascular disease). Accompanying symptoms and relief measures can help elucidate its etiology and relevance to cardiovascular disease. Chest pain, for example, may be a nonspecific indicator of cardiovascular disease and requires careful localization plus other factors, as outlined in Table 14.4 in Chapter 14, Ischemic Heart Disease.

Prior to auscultation of the heart, the precordium should be inspected (observed) and palpated for normal impulses, thrills (humming vibrations like the throat of a purring cat), and heaves (lifting of the chest wall). The apical pulse (also known as the point of maximum impulse or

TABLE 10.1. TYPES OF TESTS USED TO EVALUATE THE CARDIOVASCULAR SYSTEM

	Cardiac Function			
	Myocardial Perfusion	**Pump**	**Electrical Rhythm**	**Anatomy**
Type of Test	Stress tests Nuclear imaging Angiography Echocardiography	Angiography MUGA Echocardiography	ECG Electrophysiologic studies (EPS) Holter monitoring	Echocardiography Angiography
Parameters Evaluated	Coronary anatomy and blood flow Myocardial perfusion	Cardiac output Ejection fraction Valvular function Shunts	Rhythm Rate Conduction pathways	Chamber size Wall motion Valve function Valve structure Pericardium Coronary anatomy

Key: MUGA, multigated acquisition; ECG, electrocardiogram.
Note: Not all tests under any one cardiac function are used to evaluate all parameters listed.

PMI) is helpful to estimate heart size and rotation. This is usually located in the fifth intercostal space, 7–9 centimeters from the midsternal line, and radiates in an arc of 1–2 centimeters. Heightened intensity is suggestive of left or right ventricle enlargement while reduced intensity may be a sign of fluid overload or pericardial effusion. Factors such as obesity, large breasts, muscularity, and pulmonary disease can interfere with determination of the apical pulse. Other characteristics which are examined by inspection and palpation include thrills, which may accompany murmurs (e.g., aortic stenosis), and heaves, which may indicate enlargement of one of the heart chambers or an abnormal vessel such as an aneurysm. The carotid pulse, located just below the angle of the jaw, can be examined for its intensity and timing concurrently with the apical pulse to identify its concordance within the cardiac cycle. Decreased carotid pulsations may be due to reduced stroke volume or atherosclerotic narrowing of the carotid artery.

HEART SOUNDS[1–5]

Auscultation is listening to the heart throughout the cardiac cycle with a stethoscope to characterize the location, timing, duration, pitch, and intensity of the normal heart sounds, S_1 (first heart sound) and S_2 (second heart sound), and to determine the presence or absence of other sounds, such as S_3 (third heart sound) and S_4 (fourth heart sound) and murmurs. The diaphragm is better at picking up high-pitched sounds such as S_1 and S_2, the murmurs of aortic and mitral regurgitation, and pericardial friction rubs. The bell is preferred for low-pitched sounds such as S_3 and S_4. When the bell is pressed firmly against the skin, it becomes more like the diaphragm and low-pitched sounds may disappear as it is pressed more firmly. Auscultation proceeds in a systematic manner to ensure that all sites where normal and abnormal sounds are typically heard are reviewed (Table 10.3). Initially the patient is asked to roll partly onto the left side and the bell is placed on the apical impulse. This is done to accentuate left-sided S_3 and S_4 and mitral murmurs. Next the patient sits up, leans forward, exhales completely, and is asked to stop breathing for a few seconds. This helps to bring out aortictic murmurs. The other areas which are auscultated are the apex or base of the heart (mitral sounds), lower left sternal border (tricuspid sounds), second left interspace (pulmonic sounds), and second right interspace (aortic sounds). At each of these locations, S_1 and S_2 should be heard. Heart sounds are characterized by pitch, intensity, duration and timing within the cardiac cycle.

S_1 is the click heard as the mitral and tricuspid valves close at the end of diastole and is usually synchronous with

TABLE 10.2. TYPES OF TESTS FOR DIFFERENT DISORDERS

Disorder	CXR	Echocardiography	Angiography	Nuclear Scans	CT	MRI
Ischemic	+	++	++++	+++	++	++
Valvular	++	++++	++++	++	+++	+++
Congenital	++	++++	++++	++	+++	+++
Cardiomyopathy	+	++++	+++	++	+++	+++
Pericardial	+	+++	++	—	++++	++++
Endocarditis	+	++++	++	—	++	+++
Masses	—	++++	+++	—	++++	+++

TABLE 10.3. CHARACTERISTICS OF HEART SOUNDS

Heart Sound	Cardiac Event	Location for Auscultation	Pitch	Patient Position	Stethoscope End Piece
S_1	Closure of tricuspid and mitral valves	Apex Tricuspid—split S_1	High	Any position	Diaphragm
S_2	Closure of pulmonic and aortic valves	2nd RICS (A) 2nd LICS (P) Base Pulmonic—split S_2	High	Sitting or supine	Diaphragm
S_3	Rapid ventricular filling	Apex	Low	Supine or left lateral	Bell
S_4	Atrial ejection into distended ventricle	Apex	Low	Supine	Bell

Key: A, aortic valve; P, pulmonic valve; RICS, right intercostal space; LICS, left intercostal space.

the apical pulse. The sound may be split, should the valves not close in a synchronous manner. The intensity of S_1 can be increased if systole begins prior to the mitral valve closing, which may occur in high output states (exercise, tachycardia, anemia, or hyperthyroidism) and mitral valve stenosis. S_1 intensity is decreased in first-degree heart block, mitral regurgitation, states of reduced myocardial contractility such as congestive heart failure or coronary artery disease, in obesity (difficult to hear), and in systemic or pulmonary hypertension. S_2 is heard as the aortic and pulmonary valves close (as a snap) at the end of systole and is best heard at the tricuspid and mitral areas. Most of the sound arises from aortic valve closure. Conditions that alter either pulmonic or aortic valve closure will alter the intensity of S_2. Increased intensity of P_2 is seen in pulmonary hypertension, dilated pulmonary arteries, and atrial septal defect. Decreased or absent P_2 may be seen in aging and pulmonic stenosis. S_2 is frequently heard as a split sound because the aortic valve (A_2 component) closes before the pulmonic valve (P_2 component) and is most predominant at the height of inspiration.

Physiologic splitting of S_1 or S_2 is accentuated by inspiration and may disappear with expiration. Although S_1 may also be split, this is often difficult to hear. Pathological splitting of S_2 during expiration is described as wide splitting, fixed splitting, and paradoxical or fixed splitting and may be indicative of both stenosis and regurgitation, indicating that the valves did not close completely or synchronously with each cardiac cycle. The timing and characteristics of the heart sounds are important because they have diagnostic implications; for example, an S_1 heard as a opening snap is characteristic of mitral stenosis. Because the S_1 sound is thought to be generated by the close of the valvular leaflet, the loud snap heard in mitral stenosis indicates the valve is pliable but does not close as rapidly as a normal valve. A soft or absent S_1 may also be heard in mitral valve stenosis if the valve is so calcified that it is unable to snap shut, or in mitral regurgitation due to the backflow of blood through the valve. S_1 and S_2 intensity also varies inversely to the PR interval length due to atrial and ventricle dyschronous contraction. The shorter the PR, the louder S_1 becomes. In the presence of right heart overload (pulmonary edema), right bundle branch block, pulmonic stenosis, and atrial septal defects, the S_2 sound may be split as closure of the pulmonic valve is delayed. In the presence of right heart overload (pulmonary edema), right bundle branch block, pulmonic stenosis, and atrial septal defects, the S_2 sound may be split as closure of the pulmonic valve is delayed. Fixed splitting of S_2 may not be affected by respiration, and this is associated with large atrial-septal defects and right ventricular failure.

Extra heart sounds in systole include early systolic ejection sounds and clicks. Early ejection sounds such as aortic or pulmonic ejection sounds are often associated with valvular disease. Midsystolic to late systolic clicks are usually due to mitral valve prolapse. Mitral valve prolapse (MVP) affects about 5% of young adults and is more common in women. MVP is best heard at or medial to the apex but may also be heard at the left lower sternal border.

The S_3 heart sound, or ventricular gallop, is an abnormal, low-pitched sound, usually heard at the apex of the heart. It is thought to be due to rapid filling and stretching of the left ventricle where the left ventricle is somewhat noncompliant, or when there is extremely rapid filling of the left ventricle. This heart sound is characteristic of congestive heart failure (especially left-sided heart failure), or in the presence of volume overloading associated with tricuspid or mitral valve insufficiency and in atrial and/or ventricular septal defects. A physiologic S_3 is commonly heard in children and may persist into young adulthood. Localization of the S_3 is helpful for determining heart rotation within the chest cavity.

The S_4 diastolic sound is a dull, low-pitched postsystolic atrial gallop (rapid blood flow), usually due to reduced ventricular compliance. It is best heard at the apex in the left lateral position. Like the S_3, it occurs with reduced ventricular compliance, and so is present in conditions such as aortic stenosis, hypertension, hypertrophic cardiomyopathies, and coronary artery disease. It is not as specific for congestive heart failure as is the S_3.

Respiratory pattern, various maneuvers such as handgrip or the valsalva maneuver, sitting versus standing, and pharmacologic agents (e.g., amyl nitrate) may also be used in the evaluation of heart sounds to accentuate or diminish the intensity of these sounds. Auscultation is an acquired art and requires considerable practice to become competent.

Various other heart sounds may also be heard, such as ejection clicks (early systole) and midsystolic clicks. These are suggestive of valvular abnormalities and their timing (systolic versus midsystolic) indicates the valve involved.

HEART MURMURS[1,3]

Murmurs are auditory vibrations heard on auscultation and they are divided into systolic, diastolic, and continuous. Most murmurs occur because of turbulent blood flow within the heart chambers or through the valves. Some murmurs are considered innocent or physiologic and result from rapid, turbulent flow of blood into the left ventricle during atrial systole and through the aorta during ventricular systole. These murmurs have a gap between the murmur and S_2 that is useful in differentiating midsystolic from pansystolic murmurs. Fever, anxiety, anemia, hyperthyroidism, and pregnancy exacerbate physiologic murmurs, and these murmurs need to be distinguished from those suggestive of valvular abnormalities. As with heart sounds, accurate determination of murmurs requires practice. Murmurs are classified by their location, timing and duration in the cardiac cycle, intensity, shape (configuration or pattern), pitch (frequency), quality, and radiation (Table 10.4). The intensity or loudness or a murmur is graded using a scale of grade I to VI. Grade I is so faint that it is heard only with special effort. Grade VI may be heard with the stethoscope just off the chest wall. Determinants of the grade include the amount of blood ejected across a valve, severity of the lesion, and chest anatomy.

Systolic murmurs begin with or after S_1 and end at or before S_2 on its side of origin. Systolic murmurs are classified based on time of onset and termination as midsystolic, holosystolic, early systolic, or late systolic. Pathologic midsystolic murmurs are associated with pulmonic stenosis, aortic stenosis, and hypertrophic cardiomyopathy. Holosystolic (pansystolic) murmurs occur when blood flows from a chamber of higher pressure to one of lower pressure, such as mitral or tricuspid regurgitation, ventricular septal defects, and, at times, aortopulmonary connections. Early systolic murmurs are decrescendo and may be associated with ventricular septal defects, mitral regurgitation, or tricuspid regurgitation. A late systolic murmur preceded by one or more midsystolic to late systolic clicks is the hallmark of mitral valve prolapse. Atherosclerotic obstruction of the carotid, subclavicular, or iliofemoral arteries can give rise to a crescendo–decrescendo extracardiac systolic arterial murmur. Midsystolic murmurs include obstruction to ventricular outflow, dilatation of the aortic root or pulmonary trunk, an increased flow in the great arteries, anatomic changes in the semilunar valves, and some forms of regurgitation.

Early diastolic murmurs are commonly heard with aortic regurgitation. This murmur begins with A_2, and is generally decrescendo, reflecting the progressive decline in volume and rate of regurgitant flow during diastole. Aortic regurgitation is best heard by having the patient lean forward while holding his breath and listening with the diaphragm at the midleft sternal border. Handgrip intensifies the murmur. Pulmonary hypertension (Graham Steell's murmur) may also cause an early diastolic murmur. Middiastolic murmurs occur across the atrioventricular valves during rapid filling and are consistent with pure mitral stenosis or mitral stenosis along with a ventricular septal defect or tricuspid regurgitation with an atrial septal defect. The Austin Flint murmur may be middiastolic or presystolic and results from antegrade flow across the mitral valve that is closing rapidly because of simultaneous left ventricular filling from aortic regurgitation.

Continuous murmurs begin in systole and continue without interruption through S_2 into all or part of diastole. Such murmurs are mainly due to aortopulmonary connections (e.g., patent ductus arteriosus), arteriovenous connections (e.g., arteriovenous fistula, coronary artery fistula), and disturbances of flow patterns in arteries or veins.

TABLE 10.4. CHARACTERIZATION OF MURMURS

Type of Murmur	Example Conditions	Location	Pitch	Radiation	Quality
Midsystolic	Aortic stenosis	2nd RICS	Medium	Neck, left sternal border	Harsh
	Pulmonic stenosis	2nd and 3rd LICS	Medium	Left shoulder and neck	Harsh
	Hypertrophic cardiomyopathy	3rd and 4th LICS	Medium	Left sternal border to apex	Harsh
Pansystolic	Mitral regurgitation	Apex	Medium to high	Left axilla	Blowing
	Tricuspid regurgitation	Lower left sternal border	Medium	Right sternum, xiphoid	Blowing
	Ventricular septal defect	3rd, 4th, and 5th LICS	High	Often wide	Often harsh
Diastolic	Aortic regurgitation	2nd to 4th LICS	High	Apex	Blowing
	Mitral stenosis	Apex	Low	Little or none	

Key: RICS, right intercostal space; LICS, left intercostal space.

Anatomic correlation of murmurs may require cardiac catheterization or echocardiography where direct visualization of the blood flow abnormality and calculation of flow and chamber pressures can be obtained.

JUGULAR VENOUS PRESSURE[1–5]

The jugular venous pressure (JVP) reflects right atrial pressure. The JVP is observed in a normal patient in the right internal jugular vein with the patient supine at 30° or less. In the presence of an elevated central venous pressure (CVP), the JVP is measured at 60–90°.[3] In patients with poor myocardial function, the accuracy of the JVP as a measure of CVP is reduced, and is best measured directly by means of a Swan–Ganz catheter.

The JVP is described for its quality and character, effects of respiration, and patient position-induced changes. Both the degree of elevation of the JVP and its wave flow in conjunction with the heart beat are noted. The first wave, or *A wave,* represents atrial contraction and occurs just prior to S_1, giving rise to an increased pressure. It is seen as an undulating pulsation in the internal jugular vein. The second and much larger wave, *V wave,* represents the increased venous pressure that occurs during venous filling. To interpret the JVP accurately, the carotid pulse is concurrently palpated. The A wave occurs just before the pulse and the V wave just after. The JVP is measured in centimeters from the sternal angle and is best visualized with the patient's head rotated to the left. The normal JVP is a V wave 1–2 cm above the sternal ridge. If it is greater than halfway to the jaw angle, there is elevated CVP. When reporting a JVP, both the measure and the patient position must be reported. The JVP can be reported as actual centimeters above the manubrium or this value plus 5–7 cm to indicate the rise of the JVP above the right ventricle.

PERIPHERAL CIRCULATION[1–5]

Besides characterization of the peripheral pulses, the patient's overall peripheral circulation should be noted. Presence and degree of edema and signs of venous or arterial insufficiency are noted. Color, condition, and integrity of the skin are also recorded including signs of thrombophlebitis, tenderness, or swelling. Capillary refill may be delayed (>2 seconds) if intravascular volume is reduced. This is assessed by depressing the nail bed until it blanches, then releasing pressure and watching for the return of color indicating blood flow.

HEART RATE[1–5]

During routine physical examination the pulse is taken as an arterial pulse at an extremity, most commonly the radial pulse. This is an accurate measure of the ventricular rate in the healthy person with good ventricular function.

In patients with a rapid ventricular rate, either because of supraventricular tachyarrhythmias such as atrial flutter or fibrillation or rapid ventricular rates (e.g., ventricular tachycardia or premature ventricular beats [PVCs]), the radial pulse may be considerably slower than the true ventricular rate. The pulse deficit is a measure of the difference in true ventricular rate and peripheral pulse rate. A more accurate ventricular rate is determined by listening to the ventricles with the stethoscope (usually at the apex) or counted from an electrocardiogram. In patients with atrial fibrillation and a fast ventricular rate the pulse deficit may be significant, 10–20 beats/min, and in these patients one must be careful to record whether a pulse is a radial or apical pulse. This is important because the ventricular rate is a measure of success of drug therapy and its control is essential for adequate cardiac output and tissue and organ perfusion. Obviously, as the ventricular rate decreases the pulse deficit will be reduced.

In recording a heart rate, both the rate and rhythm should be reported. In healthy individuals, the heart rate is usually assessed by counting the radial pulse for 15 seconds and multiplying by four. In patients with irregular rhythms, the pulse should be taken over an extended period, approximately 1–2 minutes, to try to determine the patient's average pulse and rhythm, because a 10- to 15-second measure may result in inaccurate estimates of the pulse rate.

Although the radial pulse is most frequently used to determine heart rate, all arterial pulses should be evaluated bilaterally by observation, palpation, and auscultation for presence, character, pattern, and rhythm. Auscultation allows characterization of blood flow through the artery, and bruits and thrills are detected using the heel of the hand to sense the vibrations. Various arterial pulse patterns are described such as pulsus alterans (variation in amplitude beat to beat), bisferans pulse (increased arterial pulse with a double systolic peak), bigeminal pulse (reduced amplitude associated with premature ventricular beats), and paradoxical pulse (decrease in amplitude with inspiration). Although each may be associated with certain disorders (e.g., bigeminal pulse in premature ventricular contractions), none is sensitive or specific enough to be diagnostic.

CHEST X-RAY[1,5–9]

The chest x-ray (CXR) is useful in detecting cardiac and noncardiac abnormalities. Standing posterior–anterior (PA) and lateral views are taken at maximal inspiration to provide the best resolution. Portable CXRs are often less than satisfactory due to penetration difficulties and patient rotation. Initial assessment of the CXR evaluates the quality of film for patient rotation, inspiratory effort, and penetration. Rotation is assessed by evaluating symmetry of the clavicles and central placement of the carina. Inspiratory effect is considered adequate if the diaphragm is pulled below the ninth rib. Lack of inspiratory effort and obesity lead to poor quality CXR and make it difficult to assess for pleural effusions and fluid in the costophrenic angles. If possible, comparison with previous or baseline films should be made to determine both quality of film and comparison of structures.

The CXR provides supplemental information to the physical examination and is usually the first diagnostic test in a cardiac workup. It does not provide details of internal cardiac structures but gives global information about position and size of the heart and chambers, and surrounding anatomy. The PA CXR outlines the superior vena cava, right atrium on the right side and on the left, the aortic knob, main pulmonary artery, left atrial appendage (especially if enlarged), and the left ventricle. In the lateral view, the CXR visualizes the right ventricle, inferior vena cava, and left ventricle. These structures are visualized as shadows of differing density rather than discrete structures.

The CXR examination can be approached from two perspectives: objective observation and clinical correlation. Objective observation notes gross anatomic features such as size and placement of the cardiac silhouette, chamber enlargement, pulmonary vasculature, air fluid levels, and definition of cardiac border and diaphragm. Cardiac enlargement is determined by the cardiothoracic (CT) ratio, which is the maximal transverse diameter of the heart divided by the maximal transverse diameter of the thorax of a PA view. Normal averages 0.45 but may be up to 0.55 in some normal patients with large stroke volumes (e.g., highly trained athletes). A normal cardiac silhouette size is not always commensurate with normal cardiac function. Heart conditions such as ischemic heart disease do not alter cardiac size unless accompanied by other disorders such as congestive heart failure or hypertension. Individual chamber enlargement can be evaluated from the CXR. Right ventricle enlargement is best seen on the lateral film where if the right ventricle is enlarged, the heart appears to occupy the retrosternal space. Left atrial enlargement is suspected if there is elevation of the left bronchus, or there is an increase in the atrial appendage bulge. Left ventricular enlargement is the most common feature identified on CXR and is seen as an elongation and downward displacement of the apex of the heart. Sometimes a characteristic boot outline is seen.

The pulmonary vessels are examined for plumpness and definition of vessel walls. Decreased pulmonary flow (e.g., tetralogy of Fallot) causes central and peripheral vessels to be decreased in size. Increased pulmonary flow is associated with high output states such as hyperthyroidism and atrial septal defects. This may lead to enlargement and tortuosity of the central and peripheral vessels. Pulmonary arterial hypertension (increased pulmonary resistance) is identified by enlargement of the central vessels and diminished peripheral vessels. Pulmonary venous hypertension is usually due to mitral stenosis or left ventricular failure. This is characterized by larger than normal vessels in the upper lung zones due to recruitment of upper vessels from blood diverted from the lower constricted vessels (cephalization of flow).

Heart failure causes Kerley B lines (edema of interlobular septa), which appear as thin horizontal reticular lines in the costophrenic angles. At higher pressures, alveolar edema and pleural effusions appear. Pericardial effusions may also appear as a large heart but because it usually occurs rapidly there is no evidence of pulmonary venous congestion. Fluoroscopy may be useful to detect pulsation and calcification of either the cardiac shadow or valves.

ELECTROCARDIOGRAM[10–13]

Measurement of electrical activity in the heart was introduced about 75 years ago by Willem Einthoven. The electrocardiogram (ECG, EKG) is the most frequently used cardiovascular test and is the only practical and noninvasive method to the record electrical activity of the heart.[12] The ECG also provides information about the anatomy, blood flow, and hemodynamics of the cardiovascular system.

Few ECG recordings are highly specific or sensitive to a disease state. Sensitivity and specificity of ECG changes primarily depend on the clinical setting, recording technique, and the skill of interpreters. ECG reading requires considerable skill and practice. Computer interpretation of the ECG provides a standardized reading of the normal ECG and identifies waveform abnormalities but does not identify arrhythmias well. Physicians are advised to read the ECG independently prior to acknowledging the computerized ECG diagnosis. Serial ECGs obtained from a patient during an acute event significantly increase the sensitivity and specificity of the diagnostic accuracy of ECG findings. As an example, initial ECGs in patients with myocardial infarction are normal in about 10% of patients, and abnormal but not diagnostic in 40%, but over time more than 80% of patients will develop changes highly suggestive or diagnostic of myocardial ischemia.[12] If at all possible, one should obtain and compare prior ECGs before calling new diagnostic findings on a current ECG. This is particularly important in patients with significant cardiac disease, and for medications that can alter the ECG. The ECG is not only used as a stand-alone diagnostic test but is combined with almost all other cardiovascular tests to monitor the patient and identify if abnormalities detected during the test relate to ECG changes. Many tests are "gated" to the ECG to allow correlation of cardiac cycle events with the ECG. Multiple cardiac cycles are overlayed, thus increasing the sensitivity to detect abnormalities of wall motion, valvular activity, etc.

The normal ECG reflects the electrical activity of the heart, whereas arrhythmias frequently arise from abnormal impulse generation and conduction through the heart and create abnormal waveforms or patterns on the ECG. Arrhythmias are described in terms of their automaticity and conduction pathways. While the ECG is sensitive enough to detect rhythm abnormalities, it does not record the actual activity of the conduction tissue, nor does it identify if multiple abnormalities give rise to the findings.

The ECG is used as both a diagnostic and prognostic tool. In epidemiologic studies, the ECG is used to assess physical fitness, document the prevalence of ischemic heart disease, and identify subclinical heart disease. Because the sensitivity and specificity of ECG changes are highly dependent on the pretest probability for heart disease, rarely are ECG findings from epidemiologic studies prognostic for a population. Considerable debate has been given to the use and value of the ECG as a screening tool; it is rarely used as such, except in certain professions, where the diagnosis of heart disease would preclude active employment. ECG findings obtained during a clinical workup are much more likely to have prognostic significance than those found on a routine screening examination. In the elderly there is a greater correlation of ECG abnormalities and the presence of heart disease, because there is a much higher incidence of heart disease in this population.

Electrocardiography is based on the measurement of change in summated, three-dimensional electrical vectors or forces, which result from depolarization and repolarization of cells in the conduction system and heart muscle. The standard external 12-lead ECG uses two sets of leads: limb and chest. The six limb leads look at the heart in a single frontal plane. Limb lead nomenclature is as follows: lead I, right arm/left arm; lead II, right arm/left leg; lead III, left arm/left leg. Altering resistances create the augmented limb leads, which are called aVR, aVL, and aVF. Unipolar chest leads are positioned across the chest, and labeled V_1 to V_6. V_1 is positioned slightly to the right of the midline and V_6 is positioned in the left midaxillary line. Leads aVR and V_1 are considered right-sided leads and appear as inverted leads on the ECG. Leads aVL, I, II, and $V_{5,6}$ are left-sided leads. Leads II, III, and aVF are inferior leads and leads V_1 to V_4 are anterior wall leads. ECG patterns found on consecutive leads can help identify where a particular conduction defect or impulse generation is occurring or anatomic problem is located; e.g., ST elevation in V_2 to V_6 is indicative of anterior wall myocardial infarction from occlusion of the left anterior descending coronary artery. Abnormalities in one lead may have no clinical significance and could occur with poor lead placement or the position of the patient, or they could be recording artifacts.

Recording of the ECG has several standard features. The paper is divided into squares of 1 mm, each 10 mm (10 small boxes) is equivalent to 1 mV. Paper speed is 25 mm/s, each small box on the tracing paper equals 0.04 seconds, and each big box is 0.2 seconds.

The ECG pattern is as follows: Electrical activation of the right and then left atria due to discharge from the sinoatrial (SA) nodes causes an upward or positive deflection in lead II called the P wave. The normal duration of the P wave is ≤0.12 seconds and has an amplitude of ≤0.25 mV (i.e., 2.5 small boxes). The PR segment, created by passage of the impulse through the atrioventricular (AV) node and the bundle of His and its branches, has a duration of 0.12–0.21 seconds. The QRS complex primarily traces the electrical depolarization and repolarization of the ventricles. Initially there is a negative deflection, the Q wave, followed by a positive deflection, the R wave, and finally a negative deflection, the S wave. Q-wave duration is normally 0.4 seconds or less and the amplitude is 25% or less of the overall height of the QRS complex. Normal duration of the QRS complex is ≤0.12 seconds and the normal axis is −30° (above the horizontal) to +110° (away from the horizontal). The QRS complex is positive in left-sided leads and negative in right-sided leads, because the left ventricle is much thicker than the right, and the forces going left during depolarization dominate. The QT interval is measured from the start of the QRS complex to the end of the T wave. This varies with heart rate and is therefore corrected (QTc) for heart rates greater than 60 beats/min, to allow for comparisons between ECGs. The corrected QT is less than 0.42 seconds in men and 0.43 seconds in women.

Following the QRS is a plateau phase called the ST segment, which extends from the end of the QRS complex (called the J-point) to the beginning of the T wave. The ST segment is evaluated for its position relevant to the baseline, configuration, and lead location of any changes. The ST segment is normally on the baseline or slightly above it. Configuration changes, convexity upward or downward, in the ST segment are common and identify the presence of myocardial ischemia. ST elevation may be seen in persons with no known coronary disease but is usually indicative of hyperacute ischemia. ST depression is never considered a normal finding. Lead localization of ST changes indicates the area of ischemic myocardium. Repolarization of the ventricle leads to the T wave. The T wave usually goes in the same direction as the QRS complex. T wave changes are the most frequent and most sensitive abnormality on the ECG but are also the least specific. They are frequently found in persons with no heart disease. Peaked T waves are characteristic of hyperkalemia and warrant immediate attention. Comparing ST segments between ECGs is very important, because many persons may have what appear on a single record to be abnormal ST segments. ST segments should not be evaluated from a rhythm strip or a monitor.

The ECG is evaluated in a systematic manner, the first items noted being the rate and rhythm. The P-wave rate and regularity are used to classify the regularity of the rhythm, and can be used to calculate the rate. Usually the QRS is used to determine rate, because the ventricular rate is most important, and helps identify any degree of heart block. Because the paper is moving at a set speed, the QRS relationship to rate is as follows: one QRS per 6 big boxes (6 × 0.20 seconds) gives a heart rate of 50 beats/min, while one QRS per big box is a heart rate of 300 beats/min.

When reading the ECG for rhythm, the following items are identified: (1) the rate of the QRS, with >100 per minute being tachycardia, and <60 being bradycardia. (2) The regularity of the QRS; the presence or absence of the QRS complex with each P wave helps identify if the rhythm is atrial or ventricular in origin, and if each atrial beat (P wave) is being conducted to the ventricles. The regularity of the QRS identifies conditions such as atrial fibrillation and extra beats. (3) Configuration of the QRS; wide or narrow, indicating if it is generated from electrical activity that arose in the atria or ventricles.

Other items consistently identified are the measurement of the PR, QRS, and QT intervals; and duration, magnitude, and configuration of the P waves, QRS complexes, ST segments, T waves, and U waves help to identify specific abnormalities. Short PR intervals are associated with the Wolff–Parkinson–White, and the Lown–Ganong–Levine syndromes, and reflect the presence of accessory pathways. Long PR intervals are measures of heart block. The presence of a Q wave is a marker of loss of electrically functioning myocardium, and suggests a prior myocardial infarction. It may also be present in congenital heart disorders, hypertrophic cardiomyopathy, left ventricular hypertrophy, conduction defects such as Wolff–Parkinson–White syndrome and intraventricular conduction defects and nonischemic myocardial disease. U waves are relatively nonspecific, the most common cause being hypertension.

Abnormalities of ECG include various forms of heart block, changes due to ischemia and infarction, atrial and ventricular enlargement and hypertrophy, atrial and ventricular rhythm disorders, pericarditis, metabolic abnormalities, drug-induced changes, and pacemaker-related changes.

Bundle branch blocks are very common findings, and indicate there is a conduction defect in one of the bundles of His. These give rise to characteristic changes on the ECG. Their presence makes it difficult to identify some of the more common and important ECG findings such as ischemia. Right bundle branch block is associated with an R′ wave and the following abnormalities: QRS complex greater than or equal to 12 milliseconds; delayed right ventricular forces resulting in terminal R waves in the right-sided leads and S wave in the left-sided lead; and right-sided ST segment depression and T-wave inversion. Left bundle branch block is characterized by the following: QRS complex greater than or equal to 12 milliseconds; delayed left ventricular activation; loss of the normal "septal Q wave" in the left-sided leads; and left-sided ST depression and T-wave inversion. Intraventricular conduction delay usually causes a wide QRS complex and generally there are ST-T wave abnormalities.

Myocardial ischemia results in T-wave changes, injury causes ST abnormalities, and damage or necrosis and scarring result in changes in the QRS complex. Myocardial infarction results in a typical pattern of ECG changes, which begins with tall peaked T waves persisting up to several hours, followed by ST segment elevation with a coved (convexity upward) configuration, and inverted T waves. Development of a new Q wave has a high specificity but low sensitivity for acute myocardial ischemia. Q waves, which are 4 milliseconds or longer in duration and 25% or greater of the overall QRS height, are considered diagnostic, and occur within minutes to hours of occlusion. ST segment elevation frequently returns to baseline in about 1 week but Q waves persist indefinitely in 80–90% of myocardial infarctions. The location of Q waves identifies the region of myocardium affected and the coronary artery blocked (e.g., inferior infarction will result in Q waves in II, III, and aVF, associated with blockage in the right coronary artery). Non-Q-wave (subendocardial) myocardial infarction is detected by enzyme elevation and history rather than the ECG, because the ECG changes usually do not meet the diagnostic criteria for Q-wave infarction, although ST segment depression may be present. Poor R-wave progression (increases in size of the R wave moving from V_1 to V_6) can lead to an inappropriate diagnosis of anterior myocardial infarction, because smaller R waves can be due to other causes (e.g., chronic obstructive pulmonary disease).

Left atrial enlargement is indicated by a P wave that is ≥12 mV in lead II or, in lead V_1 the negative component of the biphasic P is ≥4 mV in duration and 0.1 mV in depth. In right atrial enlargement, the P wave in lead II can exceed 0.25 mV and usually has a vertical axis. Ventricular hypertrophy results in increased deflection of the QRS because of the increased muscle mass. Left ventricular hypertrophy (LVH) is diagnosed from the ECG using several different sets of criteria; none is considered highly sensitive or specific. Voltage criteria indicating LVH commonly used are summation of the S wave in V_1 and the R wave in V_5 or the S wave in V_2 and the R wave in V_6 ≥3.5 mV (35 small boxes); or the R wave in lead aVL exceeds 1.1 mV (11 small boxes). Associated ST-T-wave abnormalities are required to make the diagnosis more specific. LVH significantly increases cardiovascular risk and its presence should be considered in the treatment of hypertension (see Chapter 12). Right ventricular hypertrophy is characterized by an R wave in V_1 that is equal to or greater than the S wave in that lead. In persons who are obese, increased voltage may not be apparent, making voltage criteria a less useful tool to identify hypertrophy.

ST segment changes are very common, and should always be compared to a previous ECG. As noted previously, ST depression is never normal, but ST elevation may not be abnormal. ST segment scooping (convexity downward) may be normal but coving (convexity upward) is abnormal. Exertion in normal individuals may cause J-point depression with rapid rise of the ST segment and this may be confused with ST depression due to the configuration. Depression of the ST segment that does not quickly return to normal and changes in multiple leads suggest clinically significant heart disease. Diffuse ST segment elevation in all leads except V_1 and aVR suggests the diagnosis of pericarditis. Pericardial effusion limits the amount of voltage, which is measured on the skin surface, and QRS voltage is reduced. Large effusions may allow the heart to swing on a beat-to-beat basis, causing rapid changes in the positive to negative deflection of the QRS or electrical alternans.

Electrolyte abnormalities have characteristic signs on the ECG and can be used as monitoring parameters in the critically ill to reduce the number of blood draws. Hypokalemia increases ventricular ectopy and is seen as ST segment depression, T-wave flattening, and appearance of a U wave (usually when serum potassium is ≤3.0 mEq/L). Hyperkalemia results in very characteristic changes in the ECG. Potassium concentrations ≥6.0 mEq/L produce tall peaked T waves. As the concentration rises further, intraventricular conduction blocks, widening of the QRS complex, and, ultimately, a sine wave appearance develop. Calcium or bicarbonate administration rapidly provides a temporary reversal of these effects. Hypercalcemia causes a short QT interval and, occasionally, ST segment depression, sinus arrest, and AV conduction blocks. Hypocalcemia causes a long QT interval and some broadening of the T wave.

Ambulatory Electrocardiographic (Holter) Monitoring[14–16]

Ambulatory electrocardiographic monitoring (AEM), commonly referred to as Holter monitoring after its inventor, is an aid to the detection, documentation, characterization and evaluation of arrhythmias and other abnormalities such as ischemia.[14] In any 24-hour period, even in a healthy individual, there will be a number of ECG changes that could be interpreted as abnormal. As a diagnostic or screening tool there is considerable controversy as to AEM's value because of low sensitivity and specificity. As a prognostic tool it is primarily used to evaluate patients with known cardiovascular disease (higher prior probability for disease) who have symptoms which may be associated with an arrhythmia or in whom cardiovascular disease needs to be ruled out as the etiology for symptoms (e.g., syncope due to neurologic disease). Few ECG abnormalities are pathognomic of a specific cardiovascular disorder; thus the chance finding of an abnormal ECG at some point during the recording period is fairly frequent and difficult to interpret. A patient's history and the results of other diagnostic tests increase the probability that observed ECG changes are correlated with disease.[5,14,16]

The American Heart Association (AHA) and American College of Cardiology (ACC) in 1993 published guidelines as to the recommended uses of Holter monitoring. Justification for use of AEM is based on available evidence[14] (Table 10.5). Class I indications are defined as general agreement that ambulatory ECG monitoring is useful and reliable. Class II is defined as divergence of opinion as to the usefulness of AEM. Conditions suitable for evaluation with AEM include detection of myocardial ischemia in patients with chest pain, assessment of symptoms possibly related to arrhythmias, evaluation of antiarrhythmic devices or drugs, and assessing risk of future cardiac events in patients with certain cardiovascular conditions known to be associated with sudden cardiac death. The main goals of AEM are to document and characterize occurrences of random and spontaneous arrhythmias and to define a temporal relationship to symptoms and activities. AEM is used to evaluate patients who present with symptoms that could be related to arrhythmias, such as syncope or dizziness, with no other cause. Long-term AEM can detect potentially serious arrhythmias, which occur with no symptoms, although as a

TABLE 10.5. INDICATIONS FOR AMBULATORY ECG MONITORING

Class I Indications	Class II Indications
Evaluation of palpitations, syncope, dizziness	Shortness of breath, chest pain or fatigue not explained by other causes
Sleep apnea (evaluate for R-R interval)	Patients with Wolff–Parkinson–White syndrome
Idiopathic hypertrophic cardiomyopathy	Patients with long QT intervals
Postmyocardial infarction with LV dysfunction	Assessment of proarrhythmias
Patients with baseline arrhythmias suggestive of risk for sudden death (e.g., sustained PVCs, VT)	Assessment of drug-induced arrhythmias
Evaluation of paroxysmal symptoms in patients with pacemakers	Evaluation of pacemaker activity
Detection of pacemaker-mediated tachycardia	Evaluation of SVTs in patients with implantable defibrillators
Evaluation of antitachycardia pacing devices	Documentation of ST changes in patients unable to be tested with stress testing
Evaluation of Patients with Prinztmetal's angina	Evaluation of efficacy of anti-ischemic therapy to suppress asymptomatic ischemia

(Adapted from Refs. 14 and 15.)

screening test for potentially lethal arrhythmias it is not a very sensitive test without a suggestive history. It may also be used to evaluate the success of antiarrhythmic therapy if a specific arrhythmia can be identified. It has been shown that with repeated AEM in a patient on two occasions with no intervention, there may be as much as a 90% difference in the number of PVCs recorded.[16] Follow-up monitoring should demonstrate a 75–85% reduction in PVCs, and a 70% reduction in the frequency of complex ventricular before the intervention can be said to be successful.

AEM is also used in patients with ischemic heart disease to identify the frequency and pattern of ischemic changes and the response to therapy. This application of AEM is very controversial. Although abnormalities can be detected with Holter monitoring during ischemic events, such as down-sloping or up-sloping of the ST segment, these findings may not be diagnostic for ischemia. Correlation with the patient's clinical history and other test results is necessary for proper interpretation of this diagnostic study.

AEM requires the patient to wear a portable electrocardiographic recorder with two to four thoracic leads for up to 24 hours. It is recommended that at least two leads are used to reduce aberrant and artifact recordings being interpreted as ECG abnormalities and increase the sensitivity to identify ST abnormalities. Three types of monitors are available. Continuous monitors record an ECG strip over the duration of the test. Event or intermittent recorders are preprogrammed to record abnormal ECG events or the patient activates the recorder based on occurrence of symptoms. Real-time analytical recorders record throughout the monitoring period and analyze each beat as it occurs. They digitize, encode, and store the information in a solid-state memory. These types of recorders allow for on-line analysis. Parameters such as the number of PVCs and heart rate are some of the frequently used predetermined parameters for event recorders. During monitoring the patient maintains a diary in which the occurrence, duration, and severity of symptoms (e.g., lightheadedness, chest pain) are recorded, plus any specific activities undertaken, development of symptoms with the activity, and any interventions such as taking of medication. A clocking device in the recorder allows later correlation of the patient's diary and the recorded ECG.

Computer-assisted interpretation is used to scan the ECG and identify irregular rhythms, rates, and ST-T-wave changes. Sections identified by the computer as abnormal or those correlating with patient symptoms are then evaluated by technical personnel and physicians. The main advantages of computer analysis are to reduce interpretation of artifact recordings and to identify those areas of the ECG warranting closer inspection. Confounding factors when utilizing AEM can arise from the patient and the device (Table 10.6). The success of AEM depends on whether or not arrhythmias occur during the recording time interval. Patients who are symptomatic are more likely to demonstrate ECG changes than those who are asymptomatic or have only transient symptoms. The most important features of the rhythm strip are the pattern of the rhythm, its duration, and identification of potentially pathologic patterns.

TABLE 10.6. CONFOUNDING FACTORS IN AMBULATORY ECG MONITORING

Patient Factors	Equipment Factors
Electrolyte abnormalities	Battery failure
Hyperventilation	Loose lead
Medications	Mechanical failure of recorder
Patient activities, e.g., sudden exercise	Motor failure
Lead interference by patient	Overrecording
Physiologic variations in ECG waveforms	Computer inability to detect arrhythmias
Presence of atrial fibrillation	

(Adapted from Ref. 14.)

Improved understanding of arrhythmias and their lethality and advancing technology for recording, and interpreting the ECGs from AEM will increase its utility and contribution to management of cardiac disorders.

Exercise Stress Testing (Tolerance) Testing[17–20]

Exercise stress testing is a noninvasive test used to evaluate clinical and cardiovascular responses to exercise. Many patients with ischemic heart disease (IHD) are asymptomatic and/or have no ECG changes suggestive of ischemia at rest. Provocation which increases myocardial oxygen demand or decreases myocardial oxygen supply may produce symptoms or undesirable hemodynamic changes suggestive of heart disease. It is assumed that in the presence of IHD, affected arteries and arterioles are drawing on coronary reserve to maintain an adequate nutrient and oxygen flow to distal tissues under resting conditions. When stress (exercise) is applied there is a demand for increased myocardial blood flow, ventricular wall tension increases, there is insufficient coronary reserve to maintain adequate coronary blood flow, and the patient develops symptoms.

Exercise tolerance testing (ETT) can be used to determine adequacy of cardiovascular function, assess an individual patient's functional capacity, and provide prognostic and diagnostic information. ETT is a controlled method to assess the balance between myocardial oxygen demand and coronary blood flow. The principle behind ETT is to increase myocardial oxygen demand above myocardial oxygen supply and coronary reserve, thereby provoking ischemia. Patient symptoms, changes in blood pressure, heart rate, and the ECG (rhythm, configuration, and rate) are used as endpoints for the test.[5] In addition, exercise tolerance provides an index of the degree of coronary artery disease. The type of ECG changes and leads affected can be used as an index of severity and location of disease. Final interpretation of the test requires correlation with the patient's history (e.g., age, gender, concurrent risk factors, diseases), motivation, ability to exercise, and concomitant therapy. Results of exercise stress testing can be used as a guide to future patient management, including suitability for interventional cardiology and selection of pharmacotherapy.[18,20,21]

Essentially the exercise stress test aims to quantitate the maximum oxygen uptake (Vo_{2max}) or amount of oxygen used in metabolism before symptoms suggestive of ischemia. From a practical viewpoint, metabolic equivalents (METs) are used as a measure of Vo_{2max}. A MET is a measure of resting oxygen uptake. Activity energy demands can then be calculated in terms of METS; e.g., 4 METS is equivalent to walking at 4 mph. The number of METS a patient can undertake without symptoms of ischemia correlates with prognosis and helps guide appropriate management strategies.[20] Refer to Table 10.7 for examples of METS and activity correlations.

ETT is relatively simple to perform and not demanding of personnel time. Specialized and calibrated equipment is necessary for the test result to be meaningful, and reproducible.[18–20] For tests to be useful, there should be a clear indication for the test, and patients should be carefully selected and prescreened for risk factors for cardiovascular disease. The specificity of ETT to detect the presence of IHD, compared to angiography, is 84% for an ETT test, which demonstrates 0.1-mV horizontal or down-sloping ST segment depression. Sensitivity ranges from 40–90% depending on the number of vessels affected, with a mean of 66%.[20] There are no data to substantiate the ETT as a screening tool for IHD or its effectiveness in detecting early coronary artery disease in asymptomatic subjects.[21] The objective parameters used in ETT have relatively low specificity and sensitivity, and poor predictive value of 1-mm ST segment depressions in subjects with no cardiovascular disease. For such subjects, combinations of abnormal responses, e.g., 2-mm ST depression with abnormal hemodynamic abnormalities, would be necessary to call a test positive.

TABLE 10.7. MET RELATIONSHIP TO ACTIVITY AND PROGNOSIS

METs	Level of Activity	ETT Result
1	Resting	**<6 METS**
2	Level walking at 2 mph	Symptom limited lifestyle
4	Level walking at 4 mph	Poor prognosis
10	Climbing stairs (slowly)	**10 METS** Good prognosis
13	Cycling 9–10 mph	**>13 METS** Little or no activity limited lifestyle Excellent prognosis, even if IHD
20	Shoveling heavy snow	

TABLE 10.8. FORMS OF STRESS TESTING

Physical Stresses	Pharmacologic Stresses
Bicycle ergometer	Dipyridamole
Treadmill	Adenosine
Atrial pacing[a]	Dobutamine
Cold water[a]	Isoproterenol[b]
	Papaverine[c]

[a]Not used in stress testing.
[b]Investigational.
[c]Used for evaluation of coronary flow reserve in studies.

Exercise stress testing is conducted on a treadmill or bicycle ergometer or by means of a handgrip. Dynamic forms of exercise, such as the treadmill are preferred to assess exercise tolerance, because they induce a volume pressure on the heart and can be delivered in a graded and calibrated manner. Treadmill walking is also preferred over the other two modalities because it involves more muscle mass. However, it may not be employed in patients with disabilities. In this instance, pharmacologic stress testing with dipyridamole or other agents may be useful. The Vo_{2max} achieved with cycle ergometer is 10–15% lower than with the treadmill.[20] Many patients cannot exercise to full capacity on the cycle ergometer because of leg fatigue. Other forms of stress testing are listed in Table 10.8.

The AHA and the ACC guidelines and indications for exercise testing are listed in Table 10.9.[18–20] Additional indications for stress testing include assessment of patients' functional capacity, and assessment of symptoms such as chest pain or breathlessness. Indications for ETT can be classified into three groups according to the relative usefulness of the test based on clinical experience. Class I indications are those for which an ETT has unequivocally been shown to provide useful information about the patient's condition. Examples of such subjects are males older than the age of 40 who have atypical symptoms suggestive of IHD, or where functional capacity needs to be assessed to determine prognosis in a patient with confirmed IHD. Class II indications are those where there is some disagreement as to the usefulness of ETT, and includes patients with variant angina, or women with a history of typical or atypical chest pain. Class III conditions are those where ETT has not been shown to be of any value or the patient's condition precludes successful or safe testing. Examples of Class III indications are patients with simple PVCs on a resting ECG, with no other signs or symptoms of IHD.[18,20]

Five specific clinical groups have been identified as appropriate to be evaluated using ETT:

1. For patients with diagnosed IHD or with symptoms or signs suggestive of IHD,[18] the ETT is used to confirm the diagnosis, assess the patient's functional capacity, and provide prognostic information.
2. In patients considered to be at risk for IHD, an ETT can be used as a screening tool in certain situations. Males older than the age of 40 with symptoms suggestive of IHD and risk factors for coronary artery disease are the most suitable patients. Screening ETTs may also be used in sedentary males older than 40 who are considering embarking on a vigorous exercise or activity program, or those who have high-risk occupations, such as pilots and firemen. False-positive tests are common in most other subjects and especially in women. The reason for the high rate of false-positives in woman is unclear but may relate to a "digoxin"-like effect on the ECG from estrogen.[20]
3. In postmyocardial infarction, the ETT is of benefit to evaluate ventricular function, assess cardiovascular functional status, and determine the degree of rehabilitation the patient has achieved. This provides guidance for reentry into the workforce and resumption of normal activities. The ETT is also of value in these patients prognostically as an indicator for future cardiac events.[22]
4. The ETT is essentially a functional assessment of cardiovascular performance, and can be employed before and after cardiac interventions to assess patient status.
5. The ETT is also used to assess exercise capability in patients with mitral or aortic valvular disease.[18]

The ETT is conducted according to an established protocol to decrease inter- and intrapatient variability and allow for standardization in the interpretation of the tests. Numerous protocols have been developed, but the two most common are the Bruce and Naughton. An example of a protocol is given in Table 10.10. Protocols indicate when and what degree of gradient and speed changes will be made during the test. Patients are fasted for a minimum of 3 hours prior to the test, may not exercise 12 hours prior to the test, and must be dressed appropriately for exercise. A history and physical and baseline parameters (blood pressure, heart rate, and ECG) are measured prior to testing. The test begins with a 1-minute warm-up period to orient the patient to the equipment. Each stage of the test is maintained for at least 3 minutes. Blood pressure, heart rate, and ECG are recorded at 2 minutes into each stage. Patients are also questioned 2–3 minutes into each stage of the test about symptoms such as headache, dizziness, and specifically about chest pain, and are observed for signs and symptoms of ischemia. During the test, patients are encouraged to exercise as vigorously as they can to ensure an adequate test to assess the ECG and symptom responses. Patient comments regarding the level of fatigue they experience have been shown to be reliable between tests to assess the level of fatigue the patient is experiencing. Onset, nature, and duration of all changes are noted. Following the test there is a cool-down period during which the patient is seated or lying and is observed for changes as described above.[17–20]

Interpretation of the ETT requires correlation of clinical, ECG, and other parameters measured during the test with the patient's history and physical and risk factors for IHD. Clinical symptoms assessed include color of skin, level of perspiration, and evidence of peripheral cyanosis and lightheadedness. A patient's exercise capacity provides prognostic and therapy information. An optimal test lasts 6–10 minutes, with a heart rate response to 85–90% of maximum predicted, and a maximal effort by the patient.[18–20] Exercise capacities of less than 5 METS are associated with poor prognosis; those greater than 13 METS have a good prognosis, despite presence of disease.[23]

Endpoints for ETT are either open or close ended; the latter are more commonly used. Tests are continued to the predetermined endpoint(s) unless the patient tires or certain characteristics are noted (Table 10.11). Open-ended tests are terminated by the patient for increasing symptoms, exhaustion, or chest pain. The investigator may also termi-

TABLE 10.9. AMERICAN COLLEGE OF CARDIOLOGY AND AMERICAN HEART ASSOCIATION GUIDELINES FOR EXERCISE STRESS TESTING

Indications for Exercise Testing	Guidelines for Exercise Testing
1. To aid in the diagnosis of ischemic heart disease.	Class I: Conditions for which there is general agreement that exercise testing is justified.
2. To evaluate prognostic implications of ischemic heart disease.	Class II: Conditions for which there is divergence of opinion about the value of exercise testing.
3. To determine a patient's functional capacity.	Class III: Conditions for which there is general agreement that exercise testing is of little value.
4. To evaluate efficacy of medical and surgical therapy.	
5. To plan additional medical or surgical interventions.	

(Adapted from Ref. 18.)

TABLE 10.10. EXAMPLE OF EXERCISE STRESS TEST PROTOCOL: NAUGHTON PROTOCOL

Stage	Speed (mph)	Elevation (% grade)	Duration (min)	Approximate Vo_2/kg/min O_2 (mL)
1	3.0	0.0	2.0	10
2	3.0	2.5	2.0	14
3	3.0	5.0	2.0	18
4	3.0	7.5	2.0	21
5	3.0	10.0	2.0	24
6	3.0	12.5	2.0	28
7	3.0	15.0	2.0	32
8	3.0	17.5	2.0	35
9	3.0	20.0	2.0	38
10	3.0	22.5	2.0	42

(From Seceri S, Michelassi C. Prognostic impact of stress testing in coronary artery disease. Circulation 1991;83(5 suppl III):III82–89, with permission.)

nate them because of excessive blood pressure changes, significant ST segment changes indicative of ischemia or development of ventricular arrhythmias, or because a predetermined endpoint has been achieved without symptomatology. Close-ended testing is the use of fixed endpoints such as time on the treadmill.[17–20] The most common predetermined endpoint is a maximal heart rate—usually 85–90% of the maximally predicted heart rate for a given age, sex, and physical training.[17] This is the most objective endpoint, and is usually the goal of the test—if the patient can tolerate the level of exercise. Usually these tests are of a lower intensity than open-ended tests, and results must be interpreted with caution, to avoid false-negatives, because conditions optimal to produce an ischemic response may not be present.[17]

During exercise the body responds with an increase in heart rate, cardiac output, and systolic blood pressure. Inappropriate or inadequate responses in blood pressure and/or heart rate to exercise suggest heart disease.[23] The product of blood pressure and heart rate (double product) is a measure of myocardial oxygen demand (see Chapter 14, Ischemic Heart Disease).[17,23] In patients with stable angina, the double product is reproducible on repeat ETTs, thus it is used as an objective parameter to follow a patient's disease.

TABLE 10.11. COMMON ENDPOINTS USED IN EXERCISE STRESS TESTING

Clinical	Hemodynamic Changes	ECG Changes	Physical Examination
Pain	Blood pressure	ST changes	Gallops
Fatigue	Heart rate	Ectopic beats	Murmurs
Cool		U waves	Light headedness
Perspiring			Vertigo
Ashen/cyanosis			

A reduction in heart rate or a flat response (failure to increase heart rate above 120) with increasing levels of stress has a poor prognosis.[17,22] Likewise, failure to increase the systolic blood pressure or the finding of a sustained decrease of more than 10 mm Hg are also associated with a worse prognosis. Such responses indicate the heart has an inadequate reserve to respond to stress. The duration of symptom-free exercise time, the level of stress (of the ETT) at which symptoms occur, and the heart rate and blood pressure responses relate to the positivity or negativity of the test. Patients who are unable to progress beyond stage II of the Bruce protocol have a poor prognosis and more severe IHD.

A number of specific ECG changes (e.g., ST depression) evident only on the exercise ECG are also noted to be associated with IHD. Electrocardiographic changes are primarily ST segment changes. Ischemia produces ST segment depression. Depression of 1 mm or greater is considered a significant change. Numerous factors can produce such ST segment changes so these findings are not specific to diagnose IHD. ST segment depression of 2 mm or more, especially in conjunction with heart rates of less than 120 beats/min, low levels of stress, or depression persisting for up to 6 minutes after the cessation of the ETT, is associated with a poor prognosis.[22] Depression of the ST segment in multiple leads is also significant. Other electrocardiographic changes include development of U waves and increased complexity and/or frequency of PVCs or beats, especially if associated with bigeminy or periods of ventricular tachycardia. Finding simple PVCs on an exercise ECG is not diagnostic of IHD and does not relate to prognosis. Suppression of PVCs on subsequent tests also is not useful to judge efficacy of therapy, because the occurrence of such rhythms is highly variable and can occur in healthy people without IHD. During an ETT, the patient may not reach a heart rate that is correlated with a maximal hyperemic response; however, ischemia may still result. It is recommended that patients attempt to reach the predetermined heart rate to minimize interpretation of the test as negative; this occurs only because the stress applied was insufficient to exceed coronary reserve.[17,24]

Although it is hoped a patient will complete the ETT, there are certain absolute and relative indicators which necessitate terminating the ETT early. These are listed in Table 10.12. Patients in whom the ETT is contraindicated are those who are unable or who should not exercise because of physiologic or psychologic limitations. Patients with comorbid diseases such as chronic obstructive pulmonary disease (COPD) or peripheral vascular disease (PVD) may be limited in their exercise capacity, while lower limb amputees are unable to perform the standard treadmill test. Unstable angina is usually a contraindication to ETT, because of the instability of the patient's disease state and patients cannot exercise to a satisfactory level for the test to be considered adequate. The test does not pro-

TABLE 10.12. CONTRAINDICATIONS FOR EXERCISE STRESS TESTING

Absolute	Relative
Unstable angina	Left main coronary artery disease
Syncope	Tachy or brady arrhythmias
<72 hours post AMI	Electrolyte abnormalities
Uncontrolled CHF	Hypertension (SBP > 220 mm Hg)
Uncontrolled arrhythmias	High degree AV block
Acute systemic illness	
Acute pulmonary embolism	
Acute myocarditis	
Thrombosis of lower extremity	

vide any useful data; the patient was already known to have functionally limiting disease. In patients with untreated life-threatening arrhythmias or congestive heart failure, the ETT is also contraindicated. ETT is relatively safe with an estimated risk of myocardial infarction (MI) or death of 10 per 10,000 tests overall.[20] Patients post-MI and those with ventricular arrhythmias have a higher rate of complications. Most adverse effects are cardiac in nature including arrhythmias, primarily bradyarrhythmias, sudden death, hypotension, and myocardial infarction.

There are a number of limitations to the use of ETT as indicated above; lack of fitness is also a limiting factor. The ETT requires considerable effort, with many patients requiring encouragement to perform to the best of their ability, although some patients use the test as a personal challenge, so they perform better on repeated attempts and as they learn how to use the equipment in an optimal manner. This is referred to as a training effect and may be a confounding factor in using ETT to assess the effect of drug therapy or after interventions for IHD in clinical trials, if ETT is performed frequently over a relatively short period of time. Silent ischemia may also confound the interpretation of ETT because blood pressure and ECG changes may occur in the absence of symptoms. In post-MI patients, the ETT is often used to expedite hospital discharge. It can be used as a screening test to determine functional capacity, assess the degree of rehabilitation, and identify those patients at risk of further cardiovascular events. A modified protocol is used; termination of the test occurs when a heart rate of 70–75% of age and gender predicted maximum is reached (e.g., 140 beats/min for those <40, and 130 for those >40 years), or a MET level of 5 for patients >40 and a MET level of 7 for those <40 years of age.[20] There is considerable controversy as to the best time to perform the test but most tests are done prior to discharge or at least within the first 6 weeks postinfarction. Risks associated with post-MI ETT do not differ greatly from the non-MI patient populations. Mortality and morbidity are 0.02 and 0.05%, respectively. Patients may be stratified into low-, intermediate-, and high-risk categories, dependent on evidence of ischemia and the level of exercise tolerance.

Drug therapy is rarely discontinued for the test primarily because little data exist to support better test results off drug therapy. Some interferences are known to occur, the most common being a decreased maximum heart rate and systolic blood pressure product for patients on β blockers or calcium channel blockers. While these patients may not achieve the maximal heart rates, the ETT may demonstrate that patients have adequate exercise capacity on drug therapy. While it might seem prudent to discontinue these medications, this is rarely done with β blockers because of risks of rebound angina. Calcium antagonists may be stopped 24 hours prior to the procedure to allow a more accurate interpretation of the test. Nitrates do not alter exercise capacity directly so need not be discontinued. Digoxin interferes with interpretation of ST segment changes, and patients rarely achieve ST segment changes greater than 1 mm even in the face of significant ischemia. Exercise-induced ST segment depression persists for prolonged periods following digoxin discontinuation, so it is usually impractical to stop the drug unless a trial without digoxin is warranted.[20]

ECHOCARDIOGRAPHY[25–29]

Echocardiography is the use of ultrasound to examine and visualize structures within the heart, including valves, and to estimate wall thickness and ejection fraction, assess ventricular function, detect pericardial effusions, and observe wall motion.[25–29] When used in cardiovascular medicine, the transducer is both the transmitter and receiver of the sound waves. It is a simple noninvasive test and is the procedure of choice in the diagnosis and evaluation of a number of conditions such as valvular dysfunction (aortic and mitral stenosis and regurgitation, endocarditis), wall motion abnormalities associated with ischemia, and congenital abnormalities, such as ventricular or atrial septal defects (Table 10.13). Echocardiography is also used to assess the presence and regression of vegetations in endocarditis.

Echocardiography is based on the principle of differential acoustic impedance (or tissue density) and the laws of reflection and refraction. Sound waves directed across tissues from a transducer will reflect back sound waves of

TABLE 10.13. ADVANTAGES AND DISADVANTAGES OF ECHOCARDIOGRAPHY

Advantages	Disadvantages
Noninvasive	Difficult to use in obesity
Image generated as test performed	Lung disease
Safe	Requires skilled personnel to interpret test

different frequencies. The ability of the ultrasonic beam to penetrate chest wall structures is inversely proportional to the frequency of the signal. In adults, frequencies of 2.0–5.0 MHz are commonly used while in children frequencies of 3.5–10.0 Mhz are used. Corrections for impedance of the ultrasound wave through structures which are not part of the test, and for depth of structures which are part of the test, improve the image viewed on the oscilloscope. This allows for better visualization of anatomic structures. The theory of echocardiography is simple, but performance and interpretation of results require considerable skill.

Various types of echocardiography are used. They include M-mode (motion) echocardiography, two-dimensional (2-D), Doppler and color flow Doppler, and transesophageal echocardiography (TEE). Newer but less commonly used forms are contract and epicardial echocardiography. Most echocardiography is done with the patient at rest to allow for best visualization of heart structures. Echocardiography can be linked with the various stress tests (ETT, dipyridamole, etc.) to assess stress-induced structural or functional abnormalities (e.g., changes in wall motion). Both M-mode and 2-D echocardiography provide visualization of heart structures and can indicate numerous structural abnormalities such as aneurysms, wall thickness abnormalities, chamber collapse (e.g., tamponade), and valvular stenosis. Echocardiography can thus be used as a tool in evaluating coronary artery disease in the face of stress. Echocardiography is also of great value in diagnosing pericardial effusions and cardiac tumors, although it does not differentiate between tumors and other solid lesions (e.g., thrombus).

In M-mode, the transducer is placed at a single site on the chest (usually along the sternal border) with the ultrasound being directed posteriorly. M-mode echocardiography provides a single picture of a small region of the heart or an "ice-pick" view. The results depend on the exact placement of the transducer with respect to the underlying structures. M-mode echocardiography records only static objects in one plane, which limits its usefulness. An improved method for M-mode echocardiography is to sweep the transducer in an arc from the apex to the base of the heart. In this way, virtually the whole heart can be visualized, although essentially it is still a one-dimensional image. Conventional M-mode echo provides visualization of the right ventricle, left ventricle, and posterior left ventricular wall and pericardium; the use of an arc allows inclusion of the valves and left atrium. It was the first diagnostic procedure available for mitral stenosis and still is the primary evaluation method for this condition. It is possible to compute the degree of mitral stenosis and chamber volumes with M-mode echocardiography but improved accuracy is achieved using other modalities of echocardiography.

2-D echocardiography uses the same principles as M-mode but multiple views (windows) of the heart are recorded, each view providing a wedge-shaped view. Windows most commonly used include parasternal long and short axis, and apical two- and four-chamber views. These views can be collected on videotape to produce a motion picture of the heart. Apart from improved visualization of structures with 2-D echocardiography, there is increased accuracy in calculating ventricular volumes, wall thickness, and degree of valvular stenosis. Doppler echocardiography is more accurate in estimating valvular stenosis than 2-D echocardiography and Doppler is very useful in assessing hemodynamic information such as pressure gradients across a stenotic valve. Color Doppler is used to assess valvular regurgitation or insufficiency because it provides different colors for antegrade and retrograde flow.

Calculated parameters such as ejection fraction and wall thickness are compared to standardized values. These are of limited use, because standard values are population based and so encompass either a wide range of persons or a very select group, and are not adjusted for disease or age. Serial determinations may provide more information than single evaluations, and thus be of greater use in following the course of disease.

TEE is becoming extremely popular because of higher resolution and improved visualization of structures within the heart.[30,31] TEE visualizes the heart posteriorly and at closer range than conventional transthoracic echocardiography. Interference of ribs, lungs, and subcutaneous tissues is minimized, enabling TEE to be more useful in patients where the conventional transthoracic approach has been limited because of pulmonary disease, mechanical ventilation, or obesity. Better resolution is also obtained by using a higher frequency transducer (5 MHz for adults). The closer proximity of the transducer to the heart allows visualization of structures not readily seen on transthoracic echocardiography. These structures include the pulmonary veins, thoracic aorta heart chambers, and valves. TEE essentially has the same indications as transthoracic echocardiography but improved image resolution gives it wider clinical application. Visualization of the heart valves, in particular, the mitral valve, is superior, allowing more accurate evaluation of both native and prosthetic valves.[25,27] Visualization of vegetations is significantly improved with TEE, with a sensitivity of 100% versus 63% with transthoracic echocardiography in one study.[30] In a study of 80 patients with infective endocarditis, TEE detected vegetations in 90% of patients compared to 58% with transthoracic echocardiography. Visualization of small vegetations (less than 5 mm) on both native and prosthetic valves can be readily seen on TEE.[32] TEE can detect vegetations of less than 5 mm on both native and prosthetic valves.[33] It can also help define complications of endocarditis such as thrombosis or valve leakages.[33,34] In aortic dissection, TEE is able to identify the initial flap and origin of dissection. The overall sensitivity and specificity for this method are 97% and 100%, respectively.[30,31] While computerized tomography remains the diagnostic method of choice for aortic dissection, TEE is a popular, sensitive, and fast test which can be conducted in the emergency room.

Other uses of TEE include identification of cardiac thrombus, especially those in the left atrium and assessment of atrial dilation. After transient ischemic attacks or cerebrovascular accident, TEE may enable identification of the site of cardiac emboli by providing excellent images of likely sources of such, namely, cardiac tumors, valvular vegetation, ventricular or atrial thrombus, cardiac shunts, or atrial and ventricular septal defects. In particular, TEE provides good visualization of the left atrial appendage. In a study of almost 1500 patients with cerebral ischemia or nonvalvular atrial fibrillation, atrial thrombi were seen in 183 patients when evaluated by TEE versus only 2 patients using transthoracic echocardiography.[30] Recent observations of dense spontaneous echo contrast which are thought to be due to platelet or red blood cell aggregation, may provide prognostic indicators for patients at higher risk of thromboembolism than patients with less dense or no spontaneous contrast.[31] With TEE, it is possible to visualize proximal coronary artery anatomy to aid in the diagnosis of coronary artery disease. Intraoperative TEE with Doppler flow during valvular surgery is useful in planning and monitoring surgical corrections. TEE is the most sensitive technique currently available for detecting air embolism.

In TEE the transducer is advanced into the esophagus and allowed to rest just behind the heart. Images are obtained in either horizontal or vertical planes. There is also some experience with passing the transducer into the fundus of the stomach to obtain better images of the ventricles. The procedure is considered to be a low-risk, invasive procedure by the AHA, and does not require routine antibiotic prophylaxis for patients at risk of developing endocarditis. Some physicians still choose to use prophylaxis, with amoxicillin being the drug of choice. Premedication of the patient requires sedation with a short-acting benzodiazepine and pharyngeal anaesthesia.

TEE rarely causes complications. Esophageal tears or perforation might occur, but in one series of 10,218 studies only one death (0.0098%) was reported, comparable to that with esophageal gastroduodenoscopy (0.004%).[30] Esophageal burns, transient ventricular tachycardia, minor throat irritations, and transient vocal cord paralysis have rarely been reported. The only contraindications are in those patients with esophageal abnormalities such as strictures or varices which would limit passage of the transducer.

The Doppler principle involves reflecting sound off a moving object, in the case of echocardiography, the red blood cell.[26–28] As the red cell moves in relation to the transducer, a frequency shift occurs in the reflected wave and the velocity of intracardiac blood flow can be used to determine blood flow and intracardiac pressures. Turbulence associated with valvular abnormalities and wall motion abnormalities can be clearly visualized and quantified. Conventional echocardiography provides structural and anatomic information, but it does not indicate how blood flow is altered by structural abnormalities. Assessment with Doppler echocardiography combines both structural image and hemodynamic monitoring. Thus, it is possible to evaluate the impact of structural disease on cardiac function and quantify the associated hemodynamics. This is particularly important in valvular disease such as aortic stenosis and regurgitation. Doppler echocardiography allows measurement of transvalvular pressure gradients, valve area, and pressure changes on either side of the valve.

Doppler echocardiography is either continuous or pulsed; the former is used to assess pressure changes, while pulsed is used to localize points of origin and creation of turbulent and high blood flow. In aortic regurgitation, Doppler echocardiography is the best noninvasive technique to assess the pressure and severity of regurgitation. Color flow mapping allows tracing of the jet direction and an indication of its volume, point of wall contact, and width. Because Doppler echocardiography distinguishes different types of turbulence, it can simultaneously identify more than one type of valvular abnormality (e.g., aortic regurgitation and mitral stenosis) and the source of concomitant heart murmur. Diastolic performance can be visualized with Doppler echocardiography, with the peak early and late diastolic flow velocities being the main indicators of performance, but these methods have yet to be standardized.

In coronary artery disease it is possible to visualize areas affected by ischemia as wall motion abnormalities, seen as altered thickness of various segments of the heart and decreased anterior and septal wall movement between diastolic and systolic contraction. Wall motion abnormalities may be graded with increasing severity going from hypokinetic to akinetic to dyskinetic movement. Loss of myocardial thickness is also indirect evidence of scar formation. Linkage of echocardiography with dipyridamole infusion or other stress tests allows comparison of the resting and stressed states. Post-MI echocardiography is a useful noninvasive diagnostic tool for detection of ventricular aneurysms and can be used serially for diagnostic and prognostic information. Because it is possible to visualize the complete ventricle with echocardiography (in segments), both global left ventricular function and regional function can be assessed with calculation of ejection fractions. The valve of epicardial echocardiography in evaluating atherosclerotic lesions in the coronary arteries is yet to be determined.

COMPUTED AXIAL TOMOGRAPHY[35–37]

Tomographic imaging techniques (Table 10.14) have overcome constraints of earlier techniques by providing

TABLE 10.14. PARAMETERS OF CARDIAC FUNCTION AND USES FOR NEWER DIAGNOSTIC METHODS

	Magnetic Resonance Imaging (MRI)	Computerized Axial Tomography[a] (CT)	Positron Emission Tomography (PET)
Cardiac anatomy	++++	++++	++
Cardiac and paracardiac masses	++++	++++	++
Pericardial disease	++++	++++	—
Coronary artery anatomy	++	++	—
Graft patency	++	+++	++
Ventricular function	+++	++++	++
Tissue characterization	++	+	+++
Myocardial metabolism	—	—	++++
Myocardial blood flow	+	++	++++

Scale: ++++, highly effective method; +++, useful method; ++, some usefulness; —, no usefulness.
[a]Includes both ultrafast (cine) CT and regular CT scanning. (Adapted from Grover-McKay M, Skorton DJ. Comparative aspects of modern imaging techniques, in Zipes DP, Rowland DJ (eds): Progress in Cardiology. Philadelphia, Lea & Febiger; 1990, p 3.)

enhanced resolution of structures and three-dimensional images. Tomographic images provide excellent contrast and spatial resolution of tissues and structures. This overcomes the constraints of planar imaging techniques such as scintigraphy (e.g., thallium-201), overlapping of structures, and lack of sharp definition of individual tissues and organs. More accurate determination of chamber volume and size, and mass calculations of myocardial wall thickness, can be obtained from tomographic imaging than with other methods such as echocardiography or angiography because of better edge definition of structures and reduced background interference.

The success of tomographic methods depends on the position of the camera with respect to the organ of primary interest, and the accuracy of the computerized collimator which assesses the incoming images and computes the final three-dimensional image. Accurate axes must be calculated to ensure appropriate orientation of final images. Despite the high resolution of images produced by tomography, the advanced technology requires considerable skill and attention to detail.

Computerized axial tomography (CT) is not a primary diagnostic procedure in the evaluation of cardiovascular disease and function, because it primarily identifies structural abnormalities which are well defined and visualized by other diagnostic procedures. However, there are now several areas in which CT imaging is clearly more definitive and accurate than echocardiography such as diagnosis of aortic dissection and accurate determination of heart chamber volumes.

Until recently, CT scanning of the heart was also limited by cardiac motion and the need to, in some way, correlate the CT scan slices with the cardiac cycle. "Gating," or the linkage of and simultaneous recording of an ECG and the CT scan, has largely overcome the above problem. Gating is either prospective where a certain portion of the cardiac cycle is predetermined as the time during which the CT scan is obtained, or retrospective, where the ECG and CT are recorded simultaneously but independently and later matched for concurrent events. Ultrafast (cine) scanners are now available, which can obtain images with millisecond exposure times, so scans are obtained as real time images.[35,36] Gating is not required for ultrafast CT scanners, but a set event within the cardiac cycle (determined by ECG) is usually used as initiator for imaging to ensure standardization. Ultrafast CT obtains scans with an exposure time of 50 milliseconds and 10-mm slices at 10 to 14 tomographic levels will completely scan the heart. Cine scanners can be operated in three different modes: cine, triggered, and volume; the choice is dependent on the information to be obtained.

The most popular uses of CT scanning in cardiovascular disease are in the diagnosis of pericardial disease and assessment of presence of paracardiac or cardiac masses. The pericardium is visualized as a distinct entity allowing both the presence and type of pericardial disease to be defined. It is currently the most sensitive technique for identifying cardiac and pericardial calcification and to differentiate and document constrictive and effusive constrictive pericarditis and pericardial fluid volume. CT scanning compares well with echocardiographic imaging for pericardial abnormalities and may be better for defining loculated and hemorrhagic effusions. Because the pericardium is specifically visualized, it is possible to visualize and measure pericardial thickening (defined as thickness greater than 4 mm). Other features suggestive of pericardial disease such as dilated atria and inferior vena cava and small ventricular chambers are also readily seen on CT. CT is also useful in identifying congenital abnormalities and cysts of the pericardium.

In the evaluation of cardiac masses, the main advantage that CT provides is that the mass is visualized as a distinct space-occupying entity. The shape, density, and tissue type may also be delineated, aiding in the determination of the nature of masses. This degree of detail is not available using echocardiography.

CT scanning is also used in the diagnosis and as follow-up evaluation of thoracic and abdominal aortic aneurysms. Diagnostic accuracy of aortic dissections with CT scanning is at least 90%. Clear definition of the edges of the intimal flap of the dissection and true and false channels can be seen.

CT scanning provides clear definition of the components of the myocardial wall; from the inner endocardial wall through to the epicardial surface and pericardium. This allows precise visualization of abnormalities within and on either side of the wall; such as aneurysms, thrombi, and observation of areas which are thickened or thinned or have abnormal motion. Detection of the presence of a thrombus on CT is comparable in accuracy to 2-D echocardiography.

Although not yet in common practice, CT scans have been used as a diagnostic tool in ischemic heart disease, to localize areas of infarction and abnormal perfusion, to identify wall-motion abnormalities, and to quantify the extent and density of coronary artery calcification. One of the advantages of CT scanning in this situation is its unequivocal spatial separation of cardiac anatomic regions, which allows more precise delineation and distribution of areas of wall thinning/thickening and/or the dynamics of wall-motion abnormalities. When images are linked to the cardiac cycle, it is possible to observe and contrast differences in the extent of wall thickening in both diastole and systole. It has been shown that both gated and cine CT scanning have a 94% sensitivity and 87% specificity when compared to left ventricular cineangiography from catheterization to detect regional wall abnormalities.[35] The three-dimensional image of CT also allows determination of the extent and distribution of left ventricular hypertrophy in patients with hypertrophic or congestive cardiomyopathy.

Although still in its infancy, cine-CT has been proposed as a screening tool for evaluating the risk of developing obstructive coronary artery disease. Cine-CT is more sensitive and specific than fluoroscopy to identify the extent and density of coronary artery calcification. The calcium score (calcium density and volume of calcium) in patients older than 30–70 years of age with known coronary artery disease is significantly higher than subjects with no coronary artery disease, and appears to correlate well with the degree of coronary artery occlusion.[35]

CT perfusion scanning for assessment of coronary and myocardial perfusion or assessment of patency of coronary bypass grafting is not as popular as nuclear imaging or coronary angiography primarily because of lack of data and availability of equipment. Although accuracy to detect patency of grafts has been shown to be 90%, CT scans do not provide information regarding degree of stenosis or adequacy of blood flow. The sensitivity of CT scanning postcoronary artery bypass graft appears good but is highly variable. Factors affecting sensitivity include the criteria used to judge graft patency and the contrast-enhancement technique. Like radionuclide assessment (MUGA), contrast angiography and echocardiography, CT scanning can be used to calculate ejection fraction, left ventricular volume, and stroke volume. The blood pool is identified using IV iodinated contrast material, which provides a good contrast with anatomic structures. Ventricular volumes, ejection fraction, and stroke volume are determined directly from the blood pool on each image and not from a geometric model as in the other methods, providing a more accurate value than those obtained on angiography and echocardiography. A high degree of reproducibility between observers and studies has been shown for these volume determinations with CT scanning.

CT scanning has proven to be an effective noninvasive method to visualize congenital heart disease. However, its role is challenged by the high-resolution capacity of magnetic resonance imaging. For measuring parameters in some congenital disorders, such as evaluation of ventricular function and estimation of the volume of cardiac shunts, CT scanning still remains the evaluation method of choice.

In summary, CT scanning has been shown to be equal to echocardiography in identification of wall-motion abnormalities, and superior in cardiac mass imaging, pericardial disease, and aortic dissections and, perhaps, congenital heart disease.

NUCLEAR MAGNETIC RESONANCE[38–40]

Magnetic resonance imaging (MRI) is a relatively new diagnostic testing method that produces three-dimensional images with excellent anatomic resolution, and differentiation between tissues, including different soft tissues (refer to Table 10.13). It readily differentiates blood from tissues and structures, so no radionuclide or contrast media is required; thus it is a noninvasive technique. Although a number of radioactive elements could theoretically be used, only proton imaging has been used clinically.

The principle of MRI is to use an external magnetic field to pick up the magnetic properties of nuclei or protons. The nuclei of atoms with unpaired protons have a magnetic resonance when placed in a magnetic field and exposed to electromagnetic radiation of an appropriate frequency. They are elevated to a higher energy state and will emit energy, causing magnetic resonance. The frequency of the electromagnetic radiation used must be proportional to the local magnetic field and specific nucleus being imaged. The magnetic field used in MRI is very strong, being on the order of 0.15 to 2 T, as compared to the earth's magnetic field of 0.0003 to 0.0007 T. To obtain these strengths, a very small internal diameter (as little as 60 cm) is used in the machine. Lack of motion is essential to the success of an MRI image; in cardiovascular evaluation, gating to the ECG is essential. The patient must be able to cooperate by being completely motionless throughout the scanning procedure; many patients require sedation. Magnetic field imaging is contraindicated in patients with pacemakers, ferromagnetic intracerebral clips, and for patients with unstable conditions, who cannot remain motionless, or who suffer from claustrophobia. At present, the main factors limiting the use of MRI are cost, time, the requirement for specialized equipment and environment, and the lack of comparative data with other techniques.

In cardiovascular disease, MRI is primarily used to assess anatomic and contractile function. Its primary advantages are that it is a noninvasive technique and the resultant images provide excellent contrast between a wide variety of soft tissues and blood. Although excellent images are produced, there are few specific indications for MRI. Echocardiography, especially computer-assisted echocardiography and other less expensive techniques provide comparable information to MRI.

In thoracic aortic aneurysms and aortic dissection, MRI has been shown to be at least comparable to CT scanning, echocardiography, and angiography (aortic aneurysm).[39] Advantages for MRI in these acute situations are the lack of contrast dye needed and the high resolution of images. In abdominal aortic aneurysms, MRI has been shown to be superior to ultrasound, but because ultrasound is portable it remains the preferred screening technology because it too is able to clearly depict aneurysm and branch involvement.

In ischemic heart disease, MRI is easily able to differentiate between viable and nonviable myocardium and clearly show where myocardium has been replaced by fibrous tissue. It cannot distinguish between ischemic and normal myocardium. It also provides excellent resolution between the endocardial and epicardial interfaces so can readily identify areas of wall thickening or thinning. At present it remains a research tool in IHD, because there are few studies providing comparative data to other diagnostic methods.

MRI has been used in cardiomyopathy to detect the presence and distribution of ventricular hypertrophy, and to assess myocardial mass and wall thickness. MRI is not superior to echocardiography or CT scanning in identifying pericardial disease, but because of soft tissue resolution, it may be able to characterize the type of fluid in a pericardial effusion. In the evaluation of cardiac and paracardiac masses, MRI is able to identify mediastinal or pulmonary mass invasion into the heart because of soft tissue delineation.

An investigational use of MRI has been to indirectly assess the presence and extent of rejection of cardiac transplantation by detecting abnormal relaxation properties and evidence of reduced high-energy phosphate levels. The obvious advantage of this technique is to avoid the invasive nature of transvenous endomyocardial biopsy, which is the current state-of-the-art method. MRI remains an investigational and research tool in this area; only two studies in humans thus far have been published.[39]

POSITRON EMISSION TOMOGRAPHY[41,42]

Positron emission tomography (PET) is an advanced technology which developed from simple nuclear imaging. In the latter, radioactively labeled compounds emitting α, γ, or β rays are used to evaluate perfusion and/or uptake of the radiopharmaceuticals in various tissues. The assumption is that the uptake of radiopharmaceuticals is primarily dependent on blood flow to the organ in question, or that some specific property of the compound produces the ideal conditions for a high extraction ratio into the organ system. The radiopharmaceutical's radioactivity (concentration) is detected by a specific camera and, with the aid of a computer, a planar image is produced.

In the case of PET, radioactivity is generated from positron-emitting substances and multiple simultaneous images are taken by a rotating camera. The final PET image is produced with the aid of CT. Significant advances in computer technology and instrumentation have enabled PET to become a reality, and despite the newness of this technique, there is considerable interest in using it as an imaging technique in clinical cardiology. At present, PET remains experimental, because validation and comparison with other established imaging techniques are not yet complete. The primary advantages of PET are its noninvasive nature, the ability to do repeat scans within a short period of time, such as pre- and postpercutaneous transluminal coronary angioplasty, and the reproducibility of images over time.

PET is a physiologic imaging technique and is currently primarily used to assess myocardial tissue perfusion and to characterize physiologic and metabolic activity within the myocardium. Positron-emitting elements are linked with a substance which is to be used as the marker of perfusion or metabolic activity. A number of positron-emitting tracers are used, the choice being dependent on the type of evaluation to be undertaken. For myocardial perfusion studies, ^{82}rubidium, ^{13}N ammonia, and ^{15}O-labeled water have been used. In myocardial substrate metabolism studies, ^{11}C palmitate, ^{11}C acetate, and ^{18}F 2-deoxyglucose (FDG) are used. Tracers must remain in the tissue long enough for appropriate images to be taken and the kinetics of the traces should be known so kinetic modeling can be used to compute perfusion and substrate metabolism. PET scanning has been used to measure regional myocardial uptake of exogeneous glucose and fatty acids, quantitate free fatty acid metabolism, and define perfused myocardium energy source(s), and evaluate myocardial chemoreceptor sites.

PET scanning can be used clinically to detect coronary artery disease and assess and follow the physiologic significance of stenotic lesions. Postinfarction, myocardial substrate metabolism studies with PET are used to evaluate the amount and activity of viable tissue around the infarcted area. PET scanning has also been linked with physiologic (exercise) or pharmacologic (dipyridamole) stress. Such studies allow assessment of the myocardium under various conditions and so better plan interventional and therapeutic strategies to protect and salvage at risk of ischemia. The ideal agent to assess blood flow in the heart will accurately mimic perfusion, have minimal noncardiac tissue uptake, and not have altered extraction ratios in adverse clinical conditions (e.g., acidosis). Rubidium-82 uptake occurs preferentially in viable tissue, although uptake tends to decrease at high myocardial blood flows. Tissue resolving from an ischemic insult has reduced net uptake, with irreversibly injured tissue demonstrating a net loss of the agent after its first pass uptake. Hence, viable tissue demonstrates an overall accumulation of ^{82}Rb shown as increased density on the tomograph. Although ^{82}Rb is primarily used to evaluate myocardial blood flow, it is also a marker of tissue viability, with viable tissue continuing to accumulate the compound.

Nitrogen-13 ammonia is extracted into myocardium by glutamine synthetase. Although its uptake is metabolically dependent, animal studies have not demonstrated that different metabolic conditions alter the uptake. The overall uptake is still dependent on blood flow and, like rubidium, uptake decreases at high flow rates. Oxygen-15-labeled water has a high extraction ratio into myocardial tissue, which appears to be independent of blood flow or the metabolic state of the myocardium. Correction is required for this background activity and is achieved by repeat studies using ^{15}O carbon monoxide, which labels red blood cells in the vascular space. The activity from this study is subtracted from the ^{15}O study.[41]

Tracers used for assessment of myocardial metabolism are selected based on the type of metabolism of interest; FDG traces glucose metabolism; ^{11}C palmitate, mitochondrial fatty acid metabolism; and ^{11}C acetate is an indirect marker for myocardial oxygen consumption. Carbon-11 palmitate is a useful marker for normal myocardial oxygen consumption, because baseline energy needs of the myocardium are met through fatty acid oxidation. Clearance of ^{11}C palmitate follows a biexponential pattern, the initial fast clearance reflective of the rate of free fatty acid oxidation. Studies in animals and in healthy men have shown clearance to be proportional to cardiac workload and myocardial oxygen consumption. Increased cardiac workload increases the first phase of clearance, reflecting an increased rate of fatty acid oxidation and decreases in the endogenous lipid pool. The second clearance phase is unrelated to cardiac workload, and is believed to merely represent uptake of ^{11}C palmitate into the endogenous lipid pool. In the postprandial state, the increase in fatty acid oxidation is less marked, as glucose is used as a fuel of choice. The use of ^{11}C palmitate to assess myocardial metabolism in ischemic tissue is limited because there is altered transport and storage of the compound, and significant back diffusion of the agent into the vascular space, and it needs to be given by intracoronary injection. FDG is taken up more avidly into ischemic tissue and its uptake is dependent on the metabolic state of the myocardium.[42]

Clinically, PET has been used to detect coronary artery disease, ischemic versus nonischemic cardiomyopathy, and site and extent of myocardial infarction, and to assess the myocardium for signs of acute and chronic ischemia. Limited studies in patients with more than 50% stenosis on angiography suggest that dipyridamole-stress single photon emission computerized tomography (SPECT) and ^{13}N ammonia PET are comparable tests to assess coronary artery perfusion, with respective sensitivities of 98% and 96% and specificity of 88% and 81%. Rubidium-82, with its short half-life, is likely to prove a useful test to assess efficacy of thrombolytic therapy in terms of tissue salvage. FDG studies will help identify the affected vascular bed and allow evaluation as to whether angioplasty or surgery might be used. Because PET scanning is able to assess perfusion and/or metabolic states of tissue, it provides a useful noninvasive technique to assess cardiomyopathy pathophysiology. In ischemic cardiomyopathy, PET imaging reveals discrete regional ischemia as a patchy nonhomogeneous uptake of the tracers. Assessment of metabolic activity is a useful marker especially for hypoperfused but still viable tissue. Studies with FDG have shown it to be accurate in distinguishing hypoperfused yet viable tissue (active glucose metabolism) from hypoperfused scarred tissue. This gives a more definitive evaluation of overall myocardial function, especially in patients postinfarction, where revascularization is being considered, as it identifies the degree of hibernating myocardium which on perfusion studies may show up as poorly perfused tissue. Patients with a significant degree of jeopardized or hibernating myocardium identified on PET scanning could then undergo vascularization procedures with restoration to functional myocardium. Based on perfusion scans this option would not have been considered.

The future of PET appears promising. Improved tomographic scanners, development of new radiopharmaceuticals, and improved understanding of substrate metabolism and its relationship to myocardial tissue viability will provide new dimensions to assess and evaluate myocardial function. It is even possible that receptors may be labeled to improve insight into cardiovascular physiology and how altered receptor function, biochemical abnormalities, substrate metabolism, or other as-yet unrecognized abnormalities impair cardiac function.

Cardiac Catheterization and Angiography[43–53]

The development of the cardiac catheterization technique was a major milestone in the diagnosis and management of cardiovascular disease, because it provided a physiologic and anatomic approach to assess patency of coronary vessels and hemodynamic parameters of cardiac function. Although cardiac catheterization is commonly referred to as the test a patient is to undergo, this is only a description of the method of approach; i.e., catheterization of the coronary arteries or heart chambers. Once the catheters are placed, other procedures are undertaken, be it angiography (ventriculography or arteriography) or determination of cardiac performance parameters.[43–46]

There are many applications for cardiac catheterization, but this procedure is primarily undertaken as an aid to diagnosis or to confirm the presence of coronary artery disease, define the anatomy of the coronary arteries, evaluate cardiac performance using angiographic evidence by measuring cardiac chamber pressures, blood flow, and to visualize valvular abnormalities. Cardiac catheterization with arteriography is now the "gold standard" in the diagnosis and assessment of coronary artery disease against which all new noninvasive methods, such as dipyridamole-thallium scintigraphy, are measured.[47] Unlike most other procedures, catheterization determines the morphology of a stenotic lesion.

Cardiac catheterization is also used for therapeutic maneuvers such as balloon angioplasty and for evaluation of success of thrombolytic therapy in MI.[43,48–49] Other therapeutic uses include nonsurgical closure of patent ductus arteriosus and transverse pulmonary embolectomy. Catheterization can be utilized for intracoronary administration of pharmacologic agents, but at the present time intracoronary administration is only used in clinical trials to document artery patency of thrombolysis, in the treatment of intercurrent events during catheterization (e.g., nitroglycerin for chest pain or spasm), or for diagnostic purposes (e.g., ergonovine).[43,46,47] Patients who present with chest pain of less than 6 hours duration may be sent to the catheterization laboratory for angioplasty and intracoronary thrombolytics but this is not routine practice and requires a 24-hour aid in the prognostic evaluations of patients with IHD. Placement of cardiac pacemarkers, selective internal mammary artery angiography, and aortic root angiography may also be completed during angiography.[47,48,50]

Catheterization allows determination of chamber pressures during both diastole and systole, determination of flow rates across the heart valves, and direct measurement or calculation of cardiac performance parameters, such as cardiac output, stroke volume, and systemic vascular resistance. Measured and observed parameters obtained during catheterization are used to determine cardiac performance. Contractility, as judged by wall motion and ejection fraction, can be used to assess global cardiac performance and to plan and evaluate or assess therapy. Further applications of cardiac catheterization are listed in Table 10.15.[47]

The ACC and AHA have developed guidelines for the appropriate use of and criteria for cardiac catheterization, coronary angiography and percutaneous transluminal coronary angioplasty (PTCA).[47–49] They classify patients into three groups: Class I includes patients in whom the procedure is justified based on findings from previous tests, risk factors, and the clinical presentation. Class II includes patients for whom the test may be justified but where there is divergence of opinion among physicians concerning the need for the procedure (e.g., post-MI patient with normal LV function, evidence of ischemia and a positive ETT but no history of heart disease). Class III is made up of patients in whom the test would not be considered justified but in certain circumstances may become the procedure of choice. Patients in this category would include those who have had a coronary bypass graft and currently have no evidence of ischemia. If these patients were to develop new or worsening symptoms, angiography would be an appropriate test, but it is not used as a screening test for coronary artery patency in the face of no symptoms.[47–49] Prevention of infection is essential, with monitoring for febrile reactions during and postprocedure being routine.

TABLE 10.15. INDICATIONS FOR CARDIAC CATHETERIZATION

Angiography	Catheterization
Arteriography	Left and right heart catheterization
Selective internal mammary angiography	Hemodynamic assessments
Pharmacologic studies	Atrial septostomy
Digital subtraction angiography	Electrophysiologic studies
Intracoronary drug administration	Endomyocardial biopsy
Pulmonary angiography	Left ventricular puncture
Retrieval of intravascular foreign bodies	Cardiac pacing
Percutaneous transluminal angioplasty	Arrhythmia ablation
Atherectomy	Transseptal catheterization
Aortic root angiography	Valvuloplasty

(Adapted from Refs. 47–49.)

Venous catheterization enables the right heart, coronary sinus pulmonary arteries, and pulmonary wedge position to be reached. Left-sided heart catheterization is usually achieved by crossing through the atrial or ventricular septum. High pressures in the left heart and the necessity of a retrograde catheter approach may make left-sided heart catheterization difficult from an arterial approach. This is especially so in patients with aortic stenosis or prosthetic aortic valves. Left-sided catheterization is necessary if left ventriculography or arteriography is to be performed. Right-sided catheterization is primarily used for determination of cardiac performance parameters. Hemodynamic measurements are useful in patients with congestive heart failure, and in this setting they may be obtained with a Swan–Ganz flow-directed catheter.[43–46]

The technique of catheterization varies, depending on the center, type of catheter used, and the reason for catheterization. Brachial and femoral vascular access are the most commonly used. Venous access is obtained first, and the guidewire and venous catheter advanced prior to arterial catheterization, should this be required for ateriography. Catheter advancement is achieved either fluoroscopically or by pressure monitoring. Visualization of catheter placement is essential to safe and effective catheterization.[43,47–50]

Prior to the procedure the patient is given nothing by mouth (after midnight) except for oral medications. It is not necessary to stop any medications except warfarin prior to catheterization. Patients requiring warfarin prior to the procedure should be switched to heparin about 1–2 days prior to the procedure. Heparin is used during the procedure to prevent thrombosis and, if given prior to the procedure (e.g., unstable angina, warfarin patients), is stopped about 6 hours before the procedure to allow normalization of coagulation. Depending on the procedure undertaken, heparin is either discontinued almost immediately following the procedure, or continued for 12–24 hours. Patients frequently develop chest pain and/or vasospasm during introduction and manipulation of catheters and injection of angiography dyes. Nitroglycerin and/or morphine may be given for chest pain. Nitroglycerin (NTG) can be used sublingually or by intravenous infusion. Most units routinely give this prior to the procedure to prevent vasospasm as the catheter is introduced. For patients undergoing PTCA, aspirin and calcium channel blockers are also used. Sedatives, such as midazolam or other short-acting benzodiazepines, are frequently given to ensure patient comfort and safety, but the patient is awake and aware of the procedure because patient cooperation is necessary to obtain the angiographic views and assess symptoms. The patient may even be able to view the procedure on a television screen. To reduce bleeding complications, the sheath is removed several hours after the procedure; and the patient remains still in bed for about 8 hours.[47–49] Despite the invasive nature of the procedure, there is some controversy as to the need for prophylactic antibiotics in patients at risk for bacterial endocarditis because of valvular protheses or postrheumatic fever.[47] Current recommendations include ampicillin and gentamicin (see Chapter 104, Infective Endocarditis).

Measurements taken during catheterization are done after hemodynamic stabilization whether at baseline, after movement of the catheter, or during pharmacologic intervention.[47,50] In this way accurate parameters can be obtained and early attention to acute changes in the patient's status, such as electrical instability, hypotension, and severe vagal reactions, can be attended to. During the procedure, hemodynamic parameters are continuously monitored, as well as blood pressure and heart rate. The patient is also on continuous electrocardiographic monitoring, with 12-lead ECG repeated at intervals throughout the procedure. Observations noted during angiography are those present at the time of the procedure only. It is assumed that these reflect the ongoing status of the coronary circulation; however, the presence of vasospasm may be misleading as the catheter itself is a powerful stimulus for spasm. In patients with a history suggestive of vasospasm, the likelihood of finding vasospasm at angiography is increased.[43,47,50]

The ACC and the AHA guidelines for catheterization, angiography, and PTCA also include such items as technique, procedures, facilities, personnel, and training.[47–49] They recommend that patients who undergo any type of interventional procedure during catheterization should be treated as outpatients. Uncomplicated cases (e.g., arteriography) can be managed on an outpatient basis. There is concern that outpatient treatments may preclude close liaison with a cardiothoracic surgery unit, an essential component of any successful and safe cardiac catheterization unit.[47–49]

The incidence of complications is related to the expertise and experience of the operator, with case load being a good indicator of the latter. The AHA/ACC guidelines on catheterization and angioplasty include a description of the number of procedures necessary to maintain a minimum competence. The incidence of significant complications is reported to be 1.8%, with mortality ranging from 0.05–2.37%, based on the experience among operators. The AHA guidelines state that the risk to life should be less than 0.2% and the risk of adverse effects less than 0.5%. Various risk factors have been identified as being associated with an increased incidence of complications, some of which are considered direct contraindications to the procedure.[19,20] A list of contraindications is given in Table 10.16.[47–49]

Complication rates increase with the duration of catheterization, in particular, thrombotic complications. The major complication during and after cardiac catheterization is the development of an arterial thrombosis, although bleeding complications postprocedure are also of concern. The use of heparin during the procedure and immediately after has not been shown to definitively reduce thrombotic complications, but it is commonly given, especially in the

TABLE 10.16. CONTRAINDICATIONS OF CARDIAC CATHETERIZATION AND OTHER PROCEDURES[a]

Contraindications	
Recent stroke	Patient noncompliance[b]
Advanced physiologic age	Digoxin intoxication
Severe anemia	Anaphylaxis to radiographic dyes
Severe hypertension	Active infection
Active gastrointestinal bleed	Severe electrolyte imbalances
Fever	Unstable condition[e]
Other comorbid illnesses, e.g., COPD[c,d]	

[a]Primarily contraindications to procedures such as arteriography and PTCA.
[b]Patient not willing to undergo further treatment, e.g., surgery based on results of catheterization.
[c]COPD, chronic obstructive pulmonary disease.
[d]Disease states that may prohibit or increase risk of other interventions, e.g., surgery.
[e]Patients in whom emergency cardiac surgery would pose a high risk, e.g., during acute asthma or acute exacerbation of COPD.

face of arteriography, left-sided heart catheterization, and angioplasty. To reduce bleeding complications, patients should have a normal prothrombin time or international normalized ratio. Bleeding postprocedure is prevented by maintaining the patient at bedrest for several hours, and by frequent and careful observation of the entry site. In the event of a bleeding complication, direct pressure is required with sandbags, and should there be no resolution, emergency surgery may be necessary to prevent further complications. Heart perforation is an uncommon but potentially lethal complication. Emergency surgical intervention would be necessary. Dwell time of catheters is the major feature in thrombotic complications. The thrombogenicity of a catheter is determined primarily by the material, with factors such as hardness, friction coefficient, and moisture retention being important. During the procedure patients may experience a vagal reflex with development of hypotension, bradycardia, and nausea. This most frequently occurs in conjunction with patient anxiety and can be prevented or treated with atropine. An increased predisposition to MI during and after the procedure is seen in patients with unstable angina, recent subendocardial infarction, and in patients with insulin-dependent diabetes mellitus. Postcatheterization, patients may have elevated creatine phosphokinase due to tissue damage during the procedure, but usually this does not interfere with serial enzymes for detection of a myocardial infarction.[48,49,51]

Coronary angiography is still the most common indication for cardiac catheterization. Arteriography (injection of radiopaque dye into an artery) assesses the size of the artery, presence of collateral circulation, and the presence of dynamic abnormalities such as vasospasm. This does allow visualization of the coronary artery and accurate localization of lesions and their severity, but the physiologic significance, functional impact, and complex geometry may be underestimated. This is well demonstrated in diabetic patients, who may have significant microvascular coronary artery disease with apparently clean arteries at arteriography.[44,48]

During angiography, there is an attempt to assess the severity of the lesion by visual comparison with surrounding vessels. There are inherent difficulties with such a method, because it assumes that surrounding vessels are in fact normal, which may not be so, especially if the patient has diffuse disease. Calipers can be used to actually document physical size, but generally the degree of stenosis is reported as a percent narrowing. Various grading scales are used to record the percent narrowing (25–100%) and a severity score assigned from 1 to 32 (see Chapter 14, Ischemic Heart Disease).[43,47,48] Another method for determining the size of the lesion and its impact on blood flow is to use videodensitometry of the radiopaque dye, this being reduced over the site of the lesion. Anatomic problems compound these methods as vessels may travel down into the myocardium for a time, leaving the epicardial surface appearing as narrowed; or two vessels may overlie one another, distorting the image obtained. Multiple views are required to obtain a good image of the vessel, the right anterior oblique planes most commonly used (two views at 90° to each other). Lesions may be described as concentric and smooth (simple lesions) or eccentric and broad with a rough surface (complicated lesions).[44]

Angiography is able to detect lesions that occlude the vessel by as little as 20%. Occlusions of 75% or more are almost always seen on angiography. Significant narrowing is usually assumed to be 50% or more, although some studies use 75% narrowing as the cutoff point. The number of lesions is also considered of importance to the severity and prognosis of IHD, although there is considerable variation in the accuracy of such predictions, because angiographic and pathologic correlation of lesions is imperfect. The occurrence of spasm, variants in anatomy, and collateral filling also complicate interpretation of the angiogram. The angiographic films are used to plan interventions. Arteriography is considered standard care prior to interventional cardiography to ensure the best procedure is undertaken with a good outcome. The angiographic films may be used during both surgery and PTCA to guide the procedure. The operating room is not the place to discover difficult anatomy or that there is indeed no place for a bypass graft.[44,46,48]

Ventriculography studies may be performed during cardiac catheterization to obtain information about the contours of the heart and to assess the global and segmental function. Regional wall motion, filling defects, and presence of mural thrombi may also be visualized. During this procedure, contrast dye is injected into the heart chambers and serial films are taken following the dye's passage.[43,46,50] Left ventricular angiography is a routine part of left-sided catheterization unless ventricular function information is already available from other noninvasive studies or there are specific contraindications to the procedure. Prevention of infection is essential, with monitoring for febrile reactions during the postprocedure being routine.

Invasive cardiology is growing rapidly not only in terms of the numbers of patients undergoing such procedures, but the diversity of procedures. The development of electrophysiologic studies for the assessment and treatment of arrhythmias was made possible because of catheterization. The diversity of techniques is "limited only by the imagination of the physician and inventiveness of the microtechnologist."[53]

NUCLEAR CARDIOLOGY[54–58]

Nuclear cardiology has been a major breakthrough in terms of noninvasive testing methods. Development of new radionuclides with short half-lives which can be either used alone, such as ^{99m}Tc, or combined with other substances to form agents with particular properties, such as ^{99m}Tc-pyrophosphate, has expanded the role for nuclear imaging in cardiology. Factors important in extending the utility of nuclear medicine in cardiovascular medicine include cost and availability of equipment, personnel, and the sensitivity and specificity of such tests in comparison to the current gold standard testing methods.

Potentially, radionuclides may be linked with pharmaceutical agents; such a concept would allow assessment of any parameter of cardiovascular function which can be manipulated pharmacologically. The main limitation of nuclear cardiology is the availability of suitable radionuclides and correlation of nuclear images with cardiovascular function.

Despite the availability of many new radionuclides, ^{99m}Tc is the most commonly used radionuclide. It is widely used because its characteristics are ideal for clinical imaging. It has a short half-life of about 6 hours, has a single 140-keV photon peak which is suitable for available imaging systems, emits primarily γ rays, and is able to be combined with multiple pharmaceuticals. It is generated "inhouse" by a bench-top generator which helps to reduce transportation costs and provides immediate availability.

Other radionuclides used in nuclear cardiology include thallium-201, which is primarily used to assess coronary and myocardial perfusion. It has a relatively long half-life of 73 hours, which prevents the use of multiple doses close together, but this property allows for delayed imaging. The energy from thallium-201 is x-ray, with an energy level of 69–83 keV. Production of thallium requires a cyclotron production. Images are obtained with a conventional gamma camera. Thallium scanning may also be done using alternate scanning techniques, such as SPECT, which yield better images in terms of spatial orientation (Table 10.17).

The gamma camera is still the most widely used in nuclear imaging techniques and provides good images for most studies.

TABLE 10.17. RADIOPHARMACEUTICALS USED IN PERFUSION IMAGING

Property	Thallium (Tl^{201})	Technetium (Tm^{99m})
$T_{1/2}$ (hours)	73.1	6
Emission type	X ray and γ-ray	γ-ray
Emission energy	69–83 keV	140 keV
Comments	Behaves like K+ Significant redistribution over 4 hours Significant uptake by other tissues (e.g., lungs)	Used as pertechnetate Little redistribution over time

THALLIUM SCANNING[55,57–59]

Thallium is a potassium analogue which is taken up into normal myocardium by passive diffusion and possibly by active transport via the Na^+/K^+-ATPase pump. Update is dependent on regional blood flow and occurs in a linear fashion up to very high blood flow rates. Thallium uptake primarily occurs in perfused myocardium. Thallium uptake into ischemic myocardium occurs at a reduced rate. This gives disparity of radionuclide distribution on scans of the heart between normally perfused and infarcted or ischemic areas. Scans taken during ischemia (e.g., stress testing with thallium) or infarction will show areas of poor or nil distribution of thallium. Areas of nil distribution are called "cold spots," and reflect infarcted myocardium. Scans taken 4–6 hours after the initial scan may show a redistribution of the thallium into areas which previously appeared as cold spots. These defects are then referred to as partial defects and demonstrate areas of hypoperfused but viable myocardium. Cold spots that do not "refill" on repeated scanning are fixed defects and reflect infarcted areas. Redistribution occurs because there is delayed (compared to normal tissue) washout of thallium from poorly perfused myocardium, resulting in less contrast between the density of thallium in different areas of the heart. This gives the appearance of "redistribution" of the radionuclide into the previously ischemic area when viewed on the scan. Repeat scans are usually done about 4 hours after the initial scan. However, the delayed images can be obtained at 24 hours, especially if a second injection of thallium is used to heighten the redistribution defects from fixed defects and highlight areas of hypoperfused myocardium in contrast to normally perfused or infarcted areas as in thallium scanning.[56,57]

Thallium scanning with the aid of computer analysis segregates the images into anatomic regions and specifically localizes areas of dead/necrotic myocardial tissue. In conjunction with echocardiography, thallium scans can correlate areas of abnormal wall motion with areas of poor perfusion. The sensitivity of thallium scanning to detect IHD disease is about 75%.[56,59] Sensitivity to detect IHD can be increased by combining thallium scans with ECG or ETT results.

Thallium scanning is most frequently used in conjunction with exercise stress testing. Thallium is injected at the peak of the exercise test. Images are taken after another 30–60 seconds of exercise and then at 3–4 hours. Such testing allows detection of lower levels of ischemia than may be determined from ECG abnormalities or patient symptoms.[56,57,59]

Thallium scanning is useful in patients with atypical chest pain and ambiguous or false-positive ETT to determine if IHD is the cause of symptoms and the ETT abnormalities. Thallium scanning is also used for postoperative evaluation revascularization or angioplasty procedures, and for preoperative evaluation for prognostic stratification for persons with IHD. A normal thallium scan heralds a benign outcome, even in patients who have angiographically evident coronary disease. The finding of redistribution is a marker of jeopardized but viable myocardium and has been shown to have important prognostic value. Major cardiac events such as myocardial infarction in patients with normal thallium-201 studies average less than 1% per year. The best predictor of coronary events, which correlate thallium scans with clinical significance, are the number of myocardial segments with transient (redistribution) defects. Transient defects increase 6 to 12 times the risk of cardiac death or myocardial infarction compared to normal studies.

PHARMACOLOGIC STRESS TESTING[56,57,60–64]

Pharmacologic stress testing is an alternative to exercise stress testing in patients who are unable or unwilling to undergo ETT. A pharmacologic agent produces the stress by a hyperemic (vasodilator) response. Dipyridamole thallium scanning was approved by the Food and Drug Administration (FDA) in 1990 to be used in the diagnosis of coronary artery disease. The principle of dipyridamole thallium imaging is related to the coronary arteriolar vasodilator properties of dipyridamole. Dipyridamole is an indirect agonist and inhibits the intracellular uptake of adenosine, resulting in an increase in interstitial levels of this potent coronary vasodilator. The hyperemic response to dipyridamole occurs primarily in the coronary arterial system. Areas distal to a coronary artery obstruction show hypoperfusion relative to more normal coronary arteries and this is manifested by lack of perfusion followed by redistribution on repeat thallium scanning if the area is viable but jeopardized myocardium.

Like exercise thallium scanning, dipyridamole scanning is used to detect IHD, evaluate prognosis of patients with known disease, assess patients post-MI, and as a risk stratification method prior to vascular, cardiac, and noncardiac surgery.[60] Using planar scanning and dipyridamole, sensitivity to detect IHD is 90% with a 70% specificity, which is comparable to exercise thallium scanning.[56] It may be used in conjunction with exercise testing, echocardiography, or the newer tomographic imaging techniques like SPECT.[61,62] Dipyridamole testing has been shown to be safe and effective in the elderly and in those with unstable angina immediately post-MI (within days). It may also be used to assess the status of revascularization procedures.[62]

Thallium is given during the last minute or at the end of dipyridamole infusion or in the last minute in a dose of 2.5–3 Ci.[56] The maximum effect of dipyridamole occurs about 5 minutes after postintravenous infusion. The heart is scanned about 5 minutes after thallium administration with repeat scans done 4 hours later. Some centers perform the delayed images after 24 hours as in thallium scanning to heighten the redistribution defects from fixed or partial defects.[56,62]

Adverse effects with dipyridamole thallium testing are minimal, the main adverse effects being chest pain (with or without ischemic changes on the ECG), headache, dizziness, and nausea. Chest pain may not only be due to ischemia; not all patients demonstrate ECG changes.[62] Although systolic blood pressure decreases and heart rate increases during the test, these hemodynamic changes are not felt to interfere significantly with interpretation of the test to assess coronary blood flow. Adverse effects are related to the increased adenosine activity and can be ameliorated by xanthine compounds such as theophylline and caffeine. Xanthines are direct competitive antagonists of adenosine at the receptor level. Their use in dipyridamole testing to offset adverse effects is of questionable value, because adverse effects are rapidly ameliorated on completion of dipyridamole infusion. Pentoxifylline, also a methylxanthine, has been shown not to interfere with the test.

The current dosage recommendations for dipyridamole stem from investigational work in dogs, which demonstrated the maximum hyperemic response occurred with doses of 0.56 mg/kg given as a 4-minute intravenous infusion.[56,60,62] This dose has been shown to increase baseline coronary blood flow in the normal tissues up to four to five times over control. Some studies have used doses up to 0.84 mg/kg, because it is unclear if the standard dose does indeed achieve a maximal vasodilation.[56,63] At the higher dose, adverse effects such as chest pain are more common, but are also related to drug administration, and cease within a few minutes of the end of the infusion.[56,61,62]

Other agents such as papveratum, dobutamine, and norepinephrine have also been used as pharmacologic stimuli.[56] The ability of the agent to elicit a maximal coronary vasodilatory response is the major factor influencing choice of agent. Exogenous adenosine is currently under investigation and the subject of many studies. Studies are promising and correlate well with the experience of dipyridamole and coronary angiography.[61,64] The main advantage of adenosine is its short duration of action (approximately 10 seconds); however, the incidence of adverse effects is considerably higher, especially chest pain, but like its pharmacologic action these too are transient. The sensitivity and specificity of adenosine to detect IHD are greater than dipyridamole (85% and 90% respectively), but no head-to-head trials comparing the two have been completed.[56] Dobutamine, in doses of 20–40 μg/kg/min can also be used. It is an investigational agent and is felt to reflect the effects of exercise-induced stress better than dipyridamole or adenosine as it increases heart rate, blood pressure, and myocardial contracility. However, the increase in coronary blood flow is less than with dipyridamole or adenosine.[56] It has been compared with the other agents in small studies and results are comparable.[56,63] Neither adenosine or dobutamine is licensed for pharmacologic stress testing. In a recent study, exercise dobutamine and dipyridamole testing were compared with coronary angiography for diagnostic accuracy in patients with IHD. Overall accuracy was 87% for exercise, 82% for dobutamine, and 77% for dipyridamole. Only exercise versus dipyridamole were statistically significantly different.[63]

TECHNETIUM SCANNING[65,66] (Table 10.18)

Technetium scanning is used in specific situations as an infarct-avid agent to identify damaged myocardium in post-MI, suspected myocardial contusion, and for evaluation of right (versus left) heart infarction and following chest wall injuries. Technetium (^{99m}Tc) may also be used to assess the blood pool to give estimates of right and left ventricle ejection fractions, ventricular volumes, and pulmonary blood volumes in the face of stress, and to assess wall motion.[56] Technetium-pyrophosphate (^{99m}Tc-PYP) attaches to calcium deposited in the infarcted area, thus, ^{99m}Tc-PYP scanning is known as “hot spot” scanning.[54,55,58] Its uptake into infarcted tissue depends on regional blood flow, myocardial calcium concentration, the degree of irreversible myocardial injury, and time after infarction. Because these factors are not specific to an acute MI due to thrombosis, false “hot spots” may occur where there is necrotic myocardial tissue due to etiologies such as myocarditis, myocardial abscesses, and old myocardial infarctions. Trauma to the myocardium will also be seen as a “hot spot” with ^{99m}Tc-PYP imaging. It has a high-dose extraction (approximately 50%) and is rapidly cleared by the kidneys; only about 5% of the dose remains at 90 minutes.[10,30]

Calcium concentration appears to play the major role in the localizing of ^{99m}Tc-PYP in infarcted tissue (and bone).[58,65,66] There is a direct relationship between the moles of calcium and radiopharmaceutical uptake. In infarcted tissue, ^{99m}Tc-PYP levels can be as high as 18 to 20 times that of normal myocardium.[58] The central core of infarcted myocardium may have a lower density of radiopharmaceutical due to absence of blood flow, but locational of ^{99m}Tc-PYP requires only minimal blood flow.[65,66] This factor gives rise to very distinct borders between the infarcted and normal myocardium, where the ratio of ^{99m}Tc-PYP may be as high as 50 times the normal myocardium. Although sensitivity and specificity of ^{99m}Tc-PYP for necrotic tissue is high, there are reports of myocardial uptake in unstable angina at sites of ventricular aneurysms and during ventricular dyskinesia, presumably because there may be marked ischemia occurring in such conditions.[66] An important practical point with ^{99m}Tc-PYP imaging is that uptake into necrotic myocardium is somewhat delayed, increasing after about 4 hours of coronary occlusion. Scans during the first hours postinfarction are usually negative, becoming positive after 12 hours or more. Peak intensity is reached at 48 hours, with washout occurring over 5–7 days. Like lactate dehydrogenase levels, ^{99m}Tc-PYP is a useful late marker of infarction, especially in patients who present late or with a silent infarction.[58,65] With a 95% sensitivity, ^{99m}Tc-PYP is a sensitive indicator of transmural infarction.[66] Unfortunately, in nontransmural infarction (non-Q-wave, subendocardial), specificity is not high and it is in these infarctions that ^{99m}Tc-PYP would be of most value, because they are more difficult to diagnose based on ECG changes. Most commonly, planar imaging is undertaken, with qualitative assessment and the grading system to determine quantitative interpretation being institution and operator dependent. Essentially, the images are viewed by comparing sternum and rib uptake to that seen in the myocardium. SPECT imaging with ^{99m}Tc-PYP should markedly improve the sensitivity and accuracy of the test, and may aid greatly in quantification of the infarcted area.

After coronary artery bypass surgery, ^{99m}Tc-PYP imaging could be used to assess graft patency. Such a test could add considerably to the current standard of assessment of clinical and ECG variables. Certain characteristics of the images obtained have been linked with various prognostic values, but as yet these remain observations and have not stood the test of comparative and long-term prognostic trials.

Other agents using technetium include labeled red blood cells for detection of regional wall-motion abnormalities or intravascular shunts, technetium *t*-butyl isonitrile (^{99m}Tc-TIBI), technetium carboxy isopropyl isonitrile (^{99m}Tc-CPI), technetium sestabmibi, also known as methoxy-isobutyl isonitrile (^{99m}Tc-MIBI), and technetium-teboroxime. The ^{99m}Tc-TIBI and ^{99m}Tc-CPI agents are predecessor agents to ^{99m}Tc-MIBI.[58,65,66] Like ^{99m}Tc-MIBI their myocardial uptake patterns are similar to thallium but they generate much higher photon yields, which improves image quality. The ^{99m}Tc-CPI has reduced and delayed lung and liver activity compared to ^{99m}Tc-TIBI, and ^{99m}Tc-CPI does not redistribute into regions of transient ischemia so imaging does not need to be undertaken immediately postinfusion as with thallim. There is also considerable interest in using ^{99m}Tc-MIBI to assess left ventricular function, with phase III trials now under way. Unlike previous

TABLE 10.18. USE OF NUCLEAR IMAGING IN CARDIOLOGY

Diagnosis	Prognosis and Assessment
AMI	Pharmacotherapy response
Unstable angina	Post-CABG
Ischemic heart disease	Post-PTCA
Myocarditis	Perfusion defects in LBBB
Cardiomyopathy	Cardiac status before surgery
Valve dysfunction	Localization of infarction
	Size of infarction

Key: AMI, acute myocardial infarction; CABG, coronary artery bypass graft; PTCA, percutaneous transluminal coronary angioplasty; LBBB, Left bundle branch block.

uses of ^{99m}Tc-MIBI, this assessment uses the principle of first-pass determination and requires that imaging be undertaken almost immediately after infarction. The ^{99m}Tc-MIBI scanning shows good correlation with thallium scanning. The ^{99m}Tc-teboroxime agent is in phase I, II, and III trials to assess its safety and efficacy and to compare it to thallium-201. Its primary advantage appears to be the ability to complete imaging within a very short time period.

The main advantages of the newer technetium compounds are their lack of redistribution perfusion and they allow for delayed imaging.[66] This is particularly useful in an acute setting, where the radiopharmaceutical can be injected in the acute event, and imaging can take place when the patient is more stable. Thus the image obtained still reflects the perfusion defect at time of injection. The short half-life and favorable pharmacokinetic profile allow for individual high doses with repeat injections to evaluate efficacy of interventional therapy.[58,66]

A number of other radiopharmaceuticals have found some use in cardiovascular testing, such as labeled animyosin antibodies.[66] Theoretically, these antibodies should be more specific markers of myocyte necrosis. The currently used antibodies are a murine Fab fragment. While phase I, II, and III trials suggest these are highly specific for irreversibly injured myocytes, they have their limitations. The uptake into myocardial tissues is very slow, with a prolonged blood pool activity seen for at least 24 hours. In clinical use, the antibody is given within 24 hours of the infarction, and planar or SPECT imaging undertaken 24–48 hours later. Despite the supposed specificity of the antibody to myosin, localization is more dependent on blood flow than myosin concentration, which limits the uptake, so accurate measurement of infarction size appears not to be feasible at this time. An investigational agent, ^{123}-I-phenylpentadecanoic acid, is able to assess both myocardial perfusion and metabolism by virtue of its affinity for fatty acid metabolism.[66]

References

1. Braunwald E. Physical examination, in Braunwald E (ed): Heart Disease: A Textbook of Cardiovascular Medicine, 4th ed. Philadelphia, WB Saunders, 1992, pp 13–42.
2. Peeples D, Fowkes VK, Andreoli KG. Patient assessment: History and physical, in Anreoli KG, Zipes DP, Wallace AG, et al (eds): Comprehensive Cardiac Care, 6th ed. St Louis, CV Mosby, 1987, pp 27–57.
3. Alert JS, Rippie JM. Physical examination of the heart, in Manual of Cardiovascular Diagnosis and Therapy, Vol 1. Introduction to the Cardiovascular System, 3rd ed. Toronto/Boston, Little, Brown, 1988, pp 3–13.
4. O'Rourke RA, Braunwald E. Physical examination of the cardiovascular system, in Isselbacher KJ, Braunwald E, Wilson JD, et al (eds): Harrison's Principles of Internal Medicine, 13th ed. New York, McGraw-Hill, 1994, pp 947–954.
5. Come PC, Lee RT, Braunwald E. Noninvasive methods of cardiac examination, in Isselbacher KJ, Braunwald E, Wilson JD, et al (eds): Harrison's Principles of Internal Medicine, 13th ed. New York, McGraw-Hill, 1994, pp 966–972.
6. Naccarelli GV, Nishikawa A, Giebel RA. Patient assessment: Laboratory studies, in Anreoli KG, Zipes DP, Wallace AG, et al. (eds): Comprehensive Cardiac Care, 6th ed. St Louis, CV Mosby, 1987, pp 58–81.
7. AHA medical/scientific statement. Classification of functional capacity and objective assessment of patients with diseases of the heart. Circulation 1994;90:644–645.
8. Bernstein SJ, Hilborne LH, Leape LL, et al. The appropriateness of use of cardiovascular procedures in women and men. Arch Intern Med 1994;1554:2759–2765.
9. Walton S, Underwood SR, Hunter GJ. The chest x-ray, in Color Atlas of Diagnostic Investigation in Cardiology. Dobbs Ferry, NY, Sheridan Medical Books, 1989, pp 37–48.
10. Goldberger AL. 189. Electrocardiography, in Isselbacher KJ, Braunwald E, Wilson JD, et al (eds): Harrison's Principles of Internal Medicine, 13th ed. New York, McGraw-Hill, 1994, pp 954–966.
11. Zipes DP, Andreoli KG. Introduction to electrocardiography, in Comprehensive Cardiac Care, 6th ed. St Louis, CV Mosby, 1987, pp 82–113.
12. Fisch C. Evolution of the clinical electrocardiogram. J Am Coll Cardiol 1989;14:1127–1138.
13. Garland JL, Wolfson AB. Routine admission electrocardiography in emergency department patients. Ann Emerg Med 1994;23:275–280.
14. Clinical competance in ambulatory electrocardiography. A statement for physicians from the ACP/ACC/AHA task force on clinical privileges in cardiology. J Am Coll Cardiol 1993;22:331–335.
15. DiMarco JP, Philbrick JT. Ambulatory electrocardiographic (Holter) monitoring. Ann Intern Med 1990;113:77–79.
16. Fisch C, DeSanctis RW, Dodge HT, et al. Guidelines for ambulatory electrocardiography. J Am Coll Cardiol 1989;13:249–258.
17. Chaitman B. Exercise stress testing, in Braunwald (ed): Heart Disease: A Textbook of Cardiovascular Medicine, 4th ed. Philadelphia, WB Saunders, 1992, pp 161–179.
18. Report of the American College of Cardiology/American Heart Association Task Force on assessment of diagnostic and therapeutic cardiovascular procedures (Subcommittee on Exercise Stress Testing). Guidelines for exercise testing. J Am Coll Cardiol 1986;8:725–738.
19. Pina IL, Balady GJ, Hanson P, et al. Guidelines for clinical exercise testing laboratories: A statement for healthcare professionals from the Committee on Exercise and Cardiac Rehabilitation, American Heart Association. Circulation 1995;91:912–921.
20. Fletcher GF, Balady G, Froelicher VF, et al. Exercise standards: A statement for healthcare professionals from the American Heart Association. Circulation 1995;91:580–615.
21. Mark D, Prognostic value of a treadmill exercise score in outpatients with suspected coronary artery disease. New Engl J Med 1991;325:849–853.
22. Seceri S, Michelassi C. Prognostic impact of stress testing in coronary artery disease. Circulation 1991;83(5 suppl III):III82–89.

23. Gobel FL, Nordstrom LA, Nelson RR, et al. The rate pressure product as an index of myocardial oxygen consumption during exercise in patients with angina pectoris. Circulation 1978;57:549–556.
24. Singh BN, Nademanee K, Figueras J, et al. Hemodynamic and electrocardiographic correlates of symptomatic and silent myocardial ischemia: Pathophysiologic and therapeutic implications. Am J Cardiol 1986;56:3B–10B.
25. Crawford MH. Noninvasive techniques, in Stein JH (ed): Internal Medicine, Vol 2. Diseases of the Heart and Blood Vessels. II Laboratory Tests and Diagnosis, 2nd ed. Toronto/Boston, Little, Brown, 1987, pp 356–369.
26. Albert JS, Rippie JM. Noninvasive examination of the heart, in Manual of Cardiovascular Diagnosis and Therapy, Vol 1. Introduction to the Cardiovascular System, 3rd ed. Toronto/Boston, Little, Brown, 1988, pp 14–21.
27. Feigenbaum H. Echocardiography, in Braunwald (ed): Heart Disease: A Textbook of Cardiovascular Medicine, 4th ed. Philadelphia, WB Saunders, 1992, pp 64–115.
28. Come PC, Lee RT, Braunwald E. Noninvasive methods of cardiac examination, in Isselbacher KJ, Braunwald E, Wilson JD, et al (eds): Harrison's Principles of Internal Medicine, 13th ed. New York, McGraw-Hill, 1994, pp 966–972.
29. Ewy GA, Appleton CP, DeMaria AN, et al. ACC/AHA guidelines for the clinical application of echocardiography. A report of the American College of Cardiology/American Heart Association Task Force on assessment of diagnostic and therapeutic cardiovascular procedures. J Am Coll Cardiol 1990;16:1505–1528.
30. Fisher EA, Stahl JA, Budd JH, et al. Transesophageal echocardiography: Procedures and clinical application. J Am Coll Cardiol 1991;18:1333–1348.
31. Seward JB, Khandheria BK, Oh JK, et al. Critical appraisal of transesophageal echocardiography: Limitations, pitfalls, and complications. J Am Soc Echocardiogr 1992;5:288–305.
32. Shively BK, Gurule FT, Roldan CA, et al. Diagnostic value of transesophageal compared with transthoracic echocardiography in infective endocarditis. J Am Coll Cardiol 1991;18:391–397.
33. Birmingham GD, Rahko PS, Ballantyne F III. Improved detection of infective endocarditits with transesophageal echocardiography. Am Heart J 1992;123:774–781.
34. Mugge A, Daniel WG, Frank G, et al. Echocardiography in infective endocarditis: Reassessment of the prognostic implications of vegetation size determined by the transthoracic and transesophageal approach. J Am Coll Cardiol 1989;14:631–638.
35. Higgins CB. Newer cardiac imaging techniques: CT, MRI, in Braunwald (ed): Heart Disease: A Textbook of Cardiovascular Medicine, 4th ed. Philadelphia, WB Saunders, 1992, pp 312–341.
36. Higgins CB. New cardiac imaging techniques, in Isselbacher KJ, Braunwald E, Wilson JD, et al (eds): Harrison's Principles of Internal Medicine, 13th ed. New York, McGraw-Hill, 1994, pp 972–979.
37. Walton S, Underwood SR, Hunter GJ. Computerised x-ray tomography, in Color Atlas of Diagnostic Investigation in Cardiology. Dobbs Ferry, NY, Sheridan Medical Books, 1989, pp 125–129.
38. Bittner VV, Cranney GB, Lotan CS, et al. Overview of cardiovascular nuclear magnetic resonance imaging. Cardiol Clin 1989;7:631–649.
39. Report of the magnetic resonance imaging panel, Jacobson HG (sect. ed). Magnetic resonance imaging of the cardiovascular system: Present state of the art and future potential. JAMA 1988;259:253–259.
40. Walton S, Underwood SR, Hunter GJ. Magnetic resonance imaging, in Color Atlas of Diagnostic Investigation in Cardiology. Dobbs Ferry, NY, Sheridan Medical Books, 1989, pp 137–148.
41. Schwaiger M, Muzik O. Assessment of myocardial perfusion by perfusion emission tomography. Am J Cardiol 1991;67:35D–43D.
42. Brunken RC, Schelbert HR. Positron emission tomography in clinical cardiology. Cardiol Clin 1989;7:607–629.
43. Grossman W, Barry WH. Cardiac catheterization, in Braunwald (ed): Heart Disease: A Textbook of Cardiovascular Medicine, 4th ed. Philadelphia, WB Saunders, 1992, pp 180–205.
44. Levin DC, Gardiner GA. Cardiac arteriography, in Braunwald (ed): Heart Disease: A Textbook of Cardiovascular Medicine, 4th ed. Philadelphia, WB Saunders, 1992, pp 235–275.
45. Walton S, Underwood SR, Hunter GJ. Cardiac catheterization, in Color Atlas of Diagnostic Investigation in Cardiology. Dobbs Ferry, NY, Sheridan Medical Books, 1989, pp 49–68.
46. Mungo JP, Humphrey SH, Craig WH. Cardiac catheterization and angiography, in Stein JH (ed): Internal Medicine, Vol. 2. Diseases of the Heart and Blood Vessels. II Laboratory Tests and Diagnosis, 2nd ed. Toronto/Boston, Little, Brown, 1987, pp 356–359.
47. Report of the American College of Cardiology/American Heart Association Task Force on assessment of diagnostic and therapeutic cardiovascular procedures (Subcommittee on Cardiac Catheterization). Guidelines for cardiac catheterization and cardiac catheterization laboratories. J Am Coll Cardiol 1991;18:1149–1182.
48. Report of the American College of Cardiology/American Heart Association Task Force on assessment of diagnostic and therapeutic cardiovascular procedures (Subcommittee on Coronary Angiography). Guidelines for coronary angiography. J Am Coll Cardiol 1987;10:935–950.
49. Ryan TJ, Bauman WB, Kennedy JW, et al. Guidelines for percutaneous transluminal coronary angioplasty: A report of the ACC/AHA Task Force on assessment of diagnostic and therapeutic cardiovascular procedures (Committee on Percutaneous Transluminal Coronary Angioplasty). J Am Coll Cardiol 1993;22:2033–2054.
50. Grossman W, Baim DS. Diagnostic cardiac catheterization and angiography, in Isselbacher KJ, Braunwald E, Wilson JD, et al (eds): Harrison's Principles of Internal Medicine, 13th ed. New York, McGraw-Hill, 1994, pp 979–985.
51. Landau C, Lange RA, Hillis LD. Percutaneous transluminal coronary angioplasty. New Engl J Med 1994;330:981–993.
52. Walder LA, Schaller FA. Diagnostic cardiac catheterization. When is it appropriate? Postgrad Med 1995;97:37–42.
53. Gorlin R. Perspectives on invasive cardiology: The 24th Louis F Bishop Lecture. J Am Coll Cardiol 1994;23:525–532.

54. Zaret BL, Wachers FJ, Soufer R. Nuclear cardiology, in Braunwald (ed): Heart Disease: A Textbook of Cardiovascular Medicine, 4th ed. Philadelphia, WB Saunders, 1992, pp 276–311.
55. Come PC, Lee RT, Braunwald E. Noninvasive methods of cardiac examination, in Isselbacher KJ, Braunwald E, Wilson JD, et al (eds): Harrison's Principles of Internal Medicine, 13th ed. New York, McGraw-Hill, 1994, pp 966–972.
56. Report of the American College of Cardiology/American Heart Association Task Force on assessment of diagnostic and therapeutic cardiovascular procedures (Committee on Radionuclide Imaging, developed in collaboration with the American Society of Nuclear Cardiology). Guidelines for clinical use of cardiac radionuclide imaging. Circulation 1995;91:1278–1303.
57. Zaret BL, Wackers FJ. Nuclear imaging in cardiology. New Engl J Med 1993;329:775–783.
58. Zaret BL, Wackers FJ. Nuclear imaging in cardiology. New Engl J Med 1993;329:855–863.
59. Mahmarian JJ, Verani MS. Exercise thallium-201 perfusion scintigraphy in the assessment of coronary artery disease. Am J Cardiol 1991;67:2D–11D.
60. Stratmann HG, Kennedy HL. Evaluation of coronary artery disease in the patient unable to exercise: Alternatives to exercise stress testing. Am Heart J 1989;117(6)1344–1365.
61. Beller GA. Pharmacological stress testing. JAMA 1991;265(5):633–638.
62. Iskandrian AS, Heo J, Askenase A, et al. Dipyridamole cardiac imaging. Am Heart J 1988;115(2):432–443.
63. Beleslin BD, Ostojic M, Stepanovic J, et al. Stress echocardiography in the detection of myocardial ischemia. Head to toe comparison of exercise, dobutamine, and dipyridamole test. Circulation 1994;90:1168–1176.
64. Verani MS. Adenosine thallium-201 myocardial perfusion scintigraphy. Am Heart J 1991;122(1, part I):269–277.
65. Kahn JK, Pippin JJ, Corbett JR. New radionuclide agents for cardiac imaging: Descriptive application. Cardio Clin 1989;7(3):589–531.
66. Khan BA, Heber E. Imaging necrotic myocardium with ^{99m}technetium-pyrophosphate and radiolabeled antimyosin. Cardiol Clin 1989;7(3):577–588.

Chapter 11

Pharmacotherapy of Cardiopulmonary Resuscitation

Lori A. Jones, PharmD

Sudden death has been described as the leading medical emergency in the United States.[1] Of the 300,000 to 750,000 individuals in the United States who experience a cardiac arrest each year, approximately 200,000 receive artificial resuscitation.[2,3] By definition, cardiopulmonary arrest occurs when spontaneous and effective ventilation and circulation abruptly terminate following a cardiac or respiratory event.[4] Cardiac dysrhythmias, such as ventricular tachycardia and ventricular fibrillation, are the usual cause of sudden cardiac death. For individuals possessing underlying coronary artery disease, sudden death most often happens outside the hospital and within hours of developing related symptoms.[1] Other presenting dysrhythmias include bradyarrhythmias, asystole, and pulseless electrical activity (PEA). Primary respiratory arrests, however, occur most commonly in children. Respiratory arrests can occur subsequent to any of the following: sudden infant death syndrome, drowning, drug overdose, stroke, chronic obstructive pulmonary disease, infection, foreign-body aspiration, and electrocution.

Resuscitation attempts are thought to date back to Egyptian mythology and the biblical era.[5] These early efforts at restoring life centered around the sole provision of artificial resuscitation. The modern era of CPR began in the late 1950s and early 1960s.[1,4] In 1958, Safar and colleagues[6] demonstrated that adequate artificial ventilation could be provided using a mouth-to-mouth resuscitation technique. Later in 1960, Kouwenhoven and colleagues proved in animal models that administering closed-chest compressions enabled successful defibrillation following prolonged ventricular fibrillation.[7] Subsequently, resuscitation methods combining variations of mouth-to-mouth ventilation and closed-chest compressions led to the development of modern CPR techniques.

Since the mid-1960s, organized committees have convened periodically to encourage widespread competency in CPR techniques. In 1966, the National Academy of Sciences—National Research Council (NAS–NRC) recommended that all health care professionals be proficient in current CPR procedures. Since that time, four additional conferences have been organized by the American Heart Association (AHA) to update philosophies for providing CPR and emergency cardiac care (ECC) to the general population. The most recent guidelines are the result of the 1992 National Conference on CPR and ECC.[1] In addition to developing guidelines for providing basic life support (BLS) and advanced cardiac life support (ACLS), the committee recognized the importance of increasing public education on the prevention of cardiovascular and cerebrovascular disease. Likewise, emphasis has been placed on educating patients to identify early warning signs and symptoms so that medical care could be accessed earlier. Committee recommendations for all therapeutic interventions are classified into three categories according to the significance of available scientific literature.[1] Class I recommendations are considered to be appropriate and efficacious. Class II recommendations are subdivided into the following: IIa, probably beneficial and efficacious; and IIb, possibly beneficial without causing harm. Recommendations in Class III are considered to be inappropriate and potentially harmful. These recommendations have additionally been organized into treatment algorithms based on the underlying arrhythmia.

As discussed above, the guidelines supplied by the National Conference on CPR and ECC primarily address the provision of BLS and ACLS for adults, children, and neonates. BLS is based on the assessment and application of the ABCs: airway, breathing, and circulation. Initially, an unconscious victim should be assessed for the presence of spontaneous breathing. If absent, the airway should be opened and rescue breathing attempted. After successfully securing the airway, the individual should be examined for the presence of a palpable carotid or femoral pulse. A series of closed-chest compressions combined with rescue breathing should be performed only if the victim is deemed pulseless. Once begun, BLS should be continued until return of spontaneous circulation (ROSC) is achieved, ACLS is obtained, or exhaustion prohibits continued efforts. Contrary to BLS, ACLS incorporates all of the following: CPR, electrical defibrillation, airway management, electrocardiograph (ECG) monitoring, and drug administration.

How successful are resuscitation efforts for cardiopulmonary arrest? This question has been extensively researched, unfortunately with varying results. Hospital discharge rates for patients experiencing out-of-hospital cardiac arrest have been reported between 2 and 33%.[8,9] In comparison, an average of 15% of patients resuscitated in-hospital survive to discharge.[10] To reduce morbidity and costs associated with futile resuscitation attempts, a growing interest has developed in identifying factors predictive for successful resuscitation. Factors proven to enhance prehospital survival include the following: occurrence of a witnessed arrest, presence of ventricular tachycardia or ventricular fibrillation, rapid implementation of bystander CPR, early administration of defibrillation therapy for ventricular fibrillation, and early application of prehospital ACLS.[11,12] Considerable controversy, however, surrounds the identification of patient-specific factors affecting resuscitation survival. Much of the disagreement is probably related to the relatively small populations examined, many of which are not generalizable due to specific inclusion and exclusion criteria applied. In an effort to highlight crucial components for successful resuscitation, the National Council on CPR and ECC has orchestrated the "chain of survival."[13] Based on the concept of "a chain is only as strong as its weakest link," each element incorporated into the chain is essential for improving resuscitation outcomes. The four components in the "chain of survival" are swift emergency system entry (e.g., enhanced 911), prompt bystander CPR, early defibrillation, and rapid ACLS.[13]

One avenue for implementing the "chain of survival" concept is through the development of in-hospital cardiac resuscitation teams. The idea of a team approach toward cardiac resuscitation has existed since the early 1960s.[14] It was not until the late 1960s, however, that pharmacists began participating as cardiac resuscitation team members.[15] By defining roles for specific health care professionals, it is hoped that resuscitation attempts become more efficient and subsequently more effective. A representative code team may consist of the following persons: a physician-in-charge, surgeon, anesthesiologist, respiratory therapist, nurse, and pharmacist.[16] Team composition varies though among institutions. Typical roles for each team member are listed in Table 11.1.[16] Overall, the physician-in-charge coordinates the cardiac resuscitation effort and decides which therapeutic interventions are appropriate for the given situation. In addition, the physician-in-charge directs and oversees the actions of all other team members. With regard to pharmacist participation, their roles have greatly expanded from the primary drug preparation focus prevalent in the late 1960s.[15] Unfortunately, in a recent survey conducted in 1597 United States hospital-based pharmacies, only 30% of all hospitals possessing cardiac resuscitation teams included pharmacists.[17]

TABLE 11.1. RESPONSIBILITIES FOR CARDIAC RESUSCITATION TEAM MEMBERS

Team Member	Responsibilities
Physician-in-charge	Team leader; determines appropriate therapy; directs and oversees order implementation including provision of CPR, electrical therapy, endotracheal intubation, intravenous access, ECG monitoring, and drug administration; arranges postresuscitation care
Surgeon	Identifies surgically correctable causes for arrest
Anesthesiologist	Performs endotracheal intubation; provides adequate oxygenation; may assist with obtaining vascular access
Respiratory therapist	Maintains adequate oxygenation and ventilation
Nurse	Records timing and outcome of therapeutic interventions; may assist with chest compressions, obtaining peripheral venous access, administering fluids and medications, and acquiring blood samples for laboratory determination
Pharmacist	Prepares medications for administration; provides drug information; documents medication administration including name, dose, route, and time; may assist with chest compressions

(Adapted from Ref. 16.)

Pathophysiology and Outcome Measures of CPR

Two theories exist regarding the mechanism of blood flow in CPR.[4,18] The initial theory, known as the *cardiac pump theory,* explains forward blood flow based on active compression of the heart between the sternum and vertebrae. During compression, an "artificial systole" is produced in which intraventricular pressure increases, the atrioventricular valves close, the aortic valve opens, and blood is forced from the right and left ventricles. When ventricular compression ends, the atrioventricular valves reopen to allow blood to fill the ventricles passively during an analogous diastole. Alternatively, the *thoracic pump theory* gained prominence in the late 1970s after the discovery of cough CPR.[18] The thoracic pump theory is founded on the belief that blood flow during CPR results from intrathoracic pressure alterations induced by chest compressions. During compression, or systole, a pressure gradient develops between the intrathoracic arteries and extrathoracic veins, causing forward blood flow from the lungs into the systemic circulation. Retrograde blood flow is inhibited by the operation of venous valves. After compression ends, or diastole, intrathoracic pressure declines. This, subsequently, reverses the pressure gradient and results in blood return to the lungs. Therefore, in the thoracic pump theory, the heart acts merely as a passive organ through which blood flows.

Both the cardiac pump and the thoracic pump theories have been challenged since their inception. In reality, components of both theories may operate during CPR.[4,18] Despite the controversy, experimental methods of performing CPR have been developed based on the assertions of these divergent theories. As discussed previously, cough CPR follows the thoracic pump theory.[19] This technique is primarily used within closely monitored situations, such as the cardiac catheterization laboratory, in which ventricular fibrillation occurs. During vigorous coughing, intrathoracic pressures increase secondary to contraction of the diaphragm, abdominal, and intracostal muscles while the glottis remains closed. During this "cough systole," forward blood flow is achieved, which maintains cerebral perfusion. "Cough diastole" is initiated upon inhalation. At this time, declining intrathoracic and intra-abdominal pressures promote ventricular filling, coronary perfusion, and venous return. By increasing cerebral blood flow, consciousness can be maintained until definitive therapy can be given.[19] Three additional investigational methods for providing CPR utilize either a pneumatic vest, interposed abdominal compression, or active compression–decompression.[20] Preliminary studies suggest that each of these three techniques achieves significantly higher initial resuscitation rates than standard CPR techniques.[21–23] Adequately performed standard CPR techniques provide cerebral and myocardial blood flow rates comparable to 30% and 10% of their prearrest values, respectively.[2] Further research, however, is necessary to document the relative advantages and disadvantages of each investigational technique before their use can be endorsed on a widespread basis.

This brings us to the issue of outcome measures. Up to now, a myriad of outcome measures have been selected as endpoints for published CPR research. Due to the variability in definitions assigned to these endpoints, great difficulty exists in comparing results obtained by different investigators.[24] The most obvious endpoint of CPR is survival. Although seemingly unambiguous, survival has been defined in terms of initial resuscitation, 24-hour survival, hospital discharge, and 1-year survival. Neurologic outcome is similarly determined at varying timepoints and by nonstandard methods. Two hemodynamic parameters often studied are coronary and cerebral perfusion pressure. Coronary perfusion pressure is defined as aortic diastolic pressure minus right atrial diastolic pressure. Physiologically, raising aortic diastolic pressure shunts blood toward the heart and brain. Paradis and colleagues demonstrated that obtaining coronary perfusion pressures above 15 mm Hg is a positive predictor of ROSC in humans.[25] The final parameter, ROSC, is currently one of the most frequently employed outcome measures, but is unfortunately the most obscure. Arbitrary definitions for ROSC have included the attainment of either a predetermined heart rate and/or blood pressure measurement for varying lengths of time (e.g., 1–5 minutes).[26] Recently, increasing pressure has been placed on investigators to standardize research practices so that data obtained from multiple institutions will be comparable.[24,26] One method suggested to achieve more continuity is through developing standardized resuscitation definitions and data collection forms.[24,26]

Pharmacotherapy for Ventricular Fibrillation and Pulseless Ventricular Tachycardia

Approximately 80–90% of all nontraumatic cardiac arrests are initiated by either ventricular tachycardia (VT) or ventricular fibrillation (VF).[27] In contrast, only 35–55% of all patients suffering out-of-hospital cardiac arrests are actually found to be in VF or VT.[28] In addition, the percentage of patients with VT or VF as their presenting rhythm significantly declines as patient age increases.[29] The importance of this issue is based on improved survival rates for VT and/or VF compared to other presenting dysrhythmias. Approximately 20% of patients found initially in VF or VT survive to hospital discharge versus 1–7% of those in asystole or PEA.[11] Therefore, it is imperative that patients receive early BLS and ACLS to potentially reduce the number of cardiac rhythms from degenerating into less treatable dysrhythmias.

Cardiac arrest victims found in either pulseless ventricular tachycardia (PVT) or VF should receive immediate electrical defibrillation using up to three countershocks. The initial defibrillation attempt should begin with 200 J. If PVT or VF persists, a second and third attempt is recommended using 200–300 J and 360 J, respectively. If unsuccessful, a setting of 360 J should be used for all subsequent defibrillation attempts. Following unsuccessful defibrillation, the patient should receive CPR, endotracheal intubation, and intravenous (IV) access. Once an airway is achieved, patients should be ventilated with 100% oxygen. Pharmacologic agents, such as sympathomimetics and antiarrhythmics, are not recommended until an airway is obtained and IV access is attempted.

SYMPATHOMIMETICS

The goal of using adrenergic agonist agents is to augment both coronary and cerebral blood flow present during the low flow state associated with CPR.[2] Animal studies have demonstrated that coronary perfusion pressure averages between 10 and 15 mm Hg with CPR alone following 10 minutes of ventricular fibrillation.[30] This inability to raise coronary perfusion pressure results from the fact that standard CPR is unable to increase aortic diastolic pressure significantly. Following administration of epinephrine or norepinephrine, aortic diastolic pressure significantly increases without altering right atrial diastolic pressure.[30] Therefore, by definition, these agents successfully raise coronary perfusion pressure. In addition, agents possessing α-adrenergic activity prevent carotid artery collapse, thereby, increasing cerebral blood flow.[18]

Although cardiac arrest is associated with high concentrations of endogenous catecholamines, aortic diastolic pressure, myocardial blood flow, and cerebral blood flow remain low.[31] Several theories addressing the need for exogenous catecholamine administration during CPR include reduced myocardial sensitivity with acidosis or hypoxemia, decreased number of available receptors, and reduced receptor affinity.[32–38] As of yet, the optimal adrenergic agent has not been identified. Currently, epinephrine (an α_1, α_2, β_1, and β_2 agonist) is recommended as first-line pharmacologic therapy in the treatment of VF, PVT, asystole, and PEA. A multitude of studies, however, have compared sympathomimetic agents during CPR in order to distinguish desirable properties.[31] Pure α_1-agonist agents, such as phenylephrine and methoxamine, have been compared with epinephrine in order to determine whether β-agonist-related increases in myocardial oxygen demand impact negatively on cardiac arrest outcome. To date, superiority of these agents over epinephrine has not been demonstrated in human studies.[39] One reason for this finding may be related to the postsynaptic α_2 activity of epinephrine. Postsynaptic α_1 receptors, which reside in the adventitia-medial border of vascular smooth muscle, respond primarily to neuronally released norepinephrine.[40] Conversely, postsynaptic α_2 receptors are located extrajunctionally on the intimal region of the vessel lumen.[40] Since IV medications are in contact with the intimal blood vessel layer, it is thought that postsynaptic α_2 receptors may be responsible for mediating much of the vasopressor response from exogenous catecholamine administration.[40] Furthermore, during ischemia, the number of postsynaptic α_1 receptors decreases, which suggests a greater role for postsynaptic α_2-agonist activity during CPR.[31]

Another agent possessing postsynaptic α_2-agonist activity is norepinephrine (an α_1, α_2, β_1 agonist). Since it has been hypothesized that β_2-agonist-induced vasodilation might counteract the efficacy of α-agonist-induced vasoconstriction, investigators have compared exogenous administration of epinephrine and norepinephrine to determine the impact of β_2-agonist activity during CPR.[30,41–44] In 1989, Robinson and colleagues[30] conducted a study comparing the effects of epinephrine (200 mcg/kg) and norepinephrine (80 mcg/kg, 120 mcg/kg, and 160 mcg/kg) in a swine model of ventricular fibrillation. These investigators found trends in improved myocardial blood flow and successful defibrillation with the two highest norepinephrine doses as compared with epinephrine. Following these conclusions, Lindner and colleagues[41] examined the effects of epinephrine (45 mcg/kg) and norepinephrine (45 mcg/kg) on myocardial oxygen delivery and consumption in a swine model. These investigators discovered that norepinephrine reduced myocardial oxygen consumption, thereby creating a more favorable profile between myocardial oxygen supply and demand versus epinephrine. Similarly, Brown and colleagues[42] compared the effect of epinephrine (200 mcg/kg) and three doses of norepinephrine (80, 120, and 160 mcg/kg) on cerebral blood flow in a swine model. Statistically significant increases in aortic diastolic pressure and coronary perfusion pressure were achieved with epinephrine and the two highest doses of norepinephrine.

With regard to cerebral blood flow, norepinephrine doses of 120 and 160 mcg/kg significantly increased blood flow to the left cortex, pons, and medulla regions in comparison to 80 mcg/kg of norepinephrine. These authors concluded that agents, such as norepinephrine, may be preferred during CPR to improve regional cerebral blood flow and potentially increase neuronal viability.[42] Callaham and colleagues[44] performed the only large-scale randomized, double-blind, prospective trial comparing the efficacy of norepinephrine and epinephrine in the prehospital cardiac arrest setting. In this study, 816 adults were randomized to receive either standard-dose epinephrine (1 mg), high-dose epinephrine (15 mg), or high-dose norepinephrine (11 mg) after failing initial defibrillation attempts. Study endpoints were ROSC (measurable blood pressure or pulse for at least 5 minutes), hospital discharge, and neurologic status (cerebral performance criteria). Thirty-seven of 286 patients (12.9%) receiving 15 mg of epinephrine achieved ROSC prior to reaching the hospital versus 21 of 260 patients (8.1%) randomized to 1 mg of epinephrine ($p < 0.01$). ROSC was not statistically different for either high-dose epinephrine or norepinephrine. Overall, only 1.8% of all patients enrolled survived to hospital discharge. Due to the small numbers involved, statistical analysis was not performed on hospital discharge or neurologic status on discharge. The percentage of patients discharged for the standard-dose epinephrine, high-dose epinephrine, and high-dose norepinephrine groups were 1.2, 1.7, and 2.6%, respectively. Neurologic survival was most favorable in the standard-dose epinephrine group.[44] Therefore, it appears that although norepinephrine demonstrates preferred effects over epinephrine on myocardial oxygen balance and regional cerebral blood flow in animals, human studies have not confirmed this beneficial effect. Consequently, epinephrine remains the first-line adrenergic agent for CPR until more definitive information becomes available.

Considerable controversy surrounds the idea of the optimal epinephrine dose in CPR. Currently, the standard epinephrine dose recommended is 1 mg (10 mL of 1:10,000 solution) administered by IVP every 3–5 minutes.[27] This epinephrine dose, derived from animal studies, equates to approximately 0.015 mg/kg for a 70-kg human. Gonzalez and coworkers[45] demonstrated a dose-dependent vasopressor effect for epinephrine (1 mg–3 mg–5 mg) administered late in adult prehospital cardiac arrest victims. Along with published case reports suggesting increased efficacy resulting from higher epinephrine doses, the current ACLS guidelines offer suggestions for alternative dosing if the initial 1-mg dose is unsuccessful.[27] These recommendations, classified as IIb, are as follows: 2–5 mg IVP every 3–5 minutes, 1 mg–3 mg–5 mg IVP given 3 minutes apart, or 0.1 mg/kg IVP every 3–5 minutes. Table 11.2 contains the results from published studies comparing standard-dose epinephrine (SDE) and high-dose epinephrine (HDE) in adult cardiac arrest victims.[44,46–50] In these studies, SDE represents either 1 mg or 0.02 mg/kg epinephrine administered every 5 minutes. HDE implies administration of epinephrine doses greater than 1 mg or 0.02 mg/kg. Collectively, these studies[44,46–50] demonstrate that although higher doses of epinephrine may increase the initial resuscitation success rate, the percentage of patients surviving to hospital discharge is not significantly different. Furthermore, a trend for improved neurologic outcome is present for the SDE group.[44] Investigators have explained this phenomena by inferring that HDE promotes ROSC in patients who otherwise would not be resuscitated using SDE.[44] These individuals, often with prolonged resuscitation times, subsequently have worsened neurologic outcome.[44,49] The reason HDE does not appear more beneficial for adult cardiac arrest victims might be related to the increased presence of coronary artery disease in this population.[49] Consequently, the beneficial effects derived from raising aortic diastolic pressure and cerebral blood flow may be outweighed by increasing myocardial oxygen demand with higher epinephrine doses.[49]

ANTIARRHYTHMICS

Antiarrhythmic agents are administered in the treatment of persistent PVT or VF following unsuccessful defibrillation with initial epinephrine administration. Due to the scarcity of randomized, placebo controlled trials examining the efficacy of antiarrhythmic agents during CPR, these agents received a IIa classification in the 1992 ACLS guidelines.[27] The first-line antiarrhythmic agent in the treatment of PVT or VF is lidocaine, followed by bretylium. Procainamide remains a third-line agent due to the length of time necessary for drug administration. Current recommendations suggest administering successive doses of antiarrhythmic agents at a more frequent interval during cardiac arrest in an effort to increase the circulating blood concentrations and subsequently improve their efficacy.[27]

Lidocaine

Currently, AHA guidelines suggest that lidocaine therapy be initiated with a 1.5 mg/kg IVP bolus.[27] If defibrillation is unsuccessful, an additional 1.5 mg/kg bolus can be administered in 3–5 minutes (total dose of 3 mg/kg). A continuous

TABLE 11.2. SUMMARY OF ADULT HIGH-DOSE EPINEPHRINE STUDIES

Author	Design[a]	Epinephrine Dosing[b] SDE vs HDE	N	Initial Resuscitation[c] SDE vs HDE (*p* value)	Hospital Discharge SDE vs HDE (*p* value)	Discharge Neurologic Status SDE vs HDE
Lindner et al.[46]	P, R, DB	1 mg vs 5 mg, then 1-mg doses	68	6/40 vs 16/28 ($p < 0.001$)	2/40 vs 4/28	Not addressed
Callaham et al.[47]	Ret (Survived 6 h)	HDE: ≥50 µg/kg bolus or total dose >2.8 µg/kg/min	68	N/A	11/35 vs 6/33 ($p = 0.32$)	#Intact 8/11 vs 4/6[d] Impaired 2/11 vs 2/6 Vegetative 1/11 vs 0/6
Stiell et al.[48]	P, R, DB	1 mg vs 7 mg up to 5 doses	650	76/333 vs 56/317 ($p = 0.12$)	16/333 vs 10/317 ($p = 0.38$)	Best CPC[e] 94% vs 90%
Brown et al.[49]	P, R, DB, MC	0.02 mg/kg vs 0.2 mg/kg	128	217/648 vs 190/632	31/648 vs 26/632	CPC[e] 1–3: 29/31 vs 24/26 4–5: 2/31 vs 2/26
Callaham et al.[44]	P, R, DB	1 mg vs 15 mg	546	22/270 vs 37/286 ($p < 0.01$)	3/270 vs 5/286	Mean CPC[e] 2.3 vs 3.2
Lipman et al.[50]	P, R, DB	1 mg vs 10 mg up to 3 doses	35	11/16 vs 15/19	1/16 vs 0/19	Not addressed

[a]P, prospective; R, randomized; DB, double-blind; MC, multicenter; Ret, retrospective.
[b]SDE, standard dose epinephrine; HDE, high-dose epinephrine.
[c]Defined by investigators: Lindner et al.: systolic blood pressure ≥80 mm Hg for 12 hours with or without dopamine; Stiell et al.: regain pulse and blood pressure for ≥1 hour; Brown et al.: palpable pulse and blood pressure for ≥1 minute after first epinephrine dose; Callaham et al.: palpable pulse or blood pressure for ≥5 minutes; Lipman et al.: regain spontaneous rhythm.
[d]Unknown criteria.
[e]Cerebral performance category: 1 = normal; 2 = moderate disability; 3 = severe disability, dependent; 4 = coma; 5 = brain death.

lidocaine infusion of 2–4 mg/min should be started once the arrhythmia is suppressed. Although lidocaine is considered to be the first-line antiarrhythmic agent in the treatment of PVT or VF, superiority over bretylium has not been demonstrated in human clinical trials.[51,52] The selection of lidocaine over bretylium is based on the increased familiarity and preferred adverse effect profile of lidocaine.[27]

Evidence suggests that lidocaine may reduce arrhythmia recurrence following successful defibrillation.[27] Chow and colleagues found that plasma lidocaine concentrations >6 μg/mL may be necessary for antifibrillatory effects in an animal model.[53] In this study, they demonstrated that lidocaine (2 mg/kg) raised the ventricular fibrillation threshold (VFT) within 5 minutes of drug administration compared to the 10 minutes required for bretylium (5 mg/kg). The duration of effect, however, was greater for bretylium. In a similar animal model, Hanyok and colleagues demonstrated that a combination of bretylium (5 mg/kg) and lidocaine (2 mg/kg) possessed both a rapid onset of action and prolonged duration of VFT elevation.[54] Therefore, combination therapy may be rational for persistent or recurrent VF. Controversy continues to exist, however, regarding the effect of lidocaine on defibrillation energy requirements for VF.[55]

The pharmacokinetic characteristics of lidocaine, a type Ib antiarrhythmic agent, have not been extensively studied during cardiac arrest.[56] It is known, however, that hepatic blood flow is the primary determinant for the rate of hepatic lidocaine metabolism. Therefore, as cardiac output and hepatic blood flow decline during cardiac arrest, lidocaine clearance is reduced.[56] Additionally, during myocardial ischemia, lidocaine protein binding increases as α_1-acid glycoprotein is released. Consequently, while total plasma lidocaine concentrations are elevated, the percentage of unbound lidocaine (free fraction) may be reduced.[56] With more aggressive lidocaine loading as recommended by the AHA guidelines, increased toxicity may be encountered.[27] Dosage reductions are suggested for lidocaine maintenance infusions in patients with reduced cardiac output (e.g., myocardial infarction, congestive heart failure, cardiogenic shock), hepatic dysfunction, or age greater than 70 years.[27] With prolonged maintenance infusions, plasma concentrations should be monitored and patients should be assessed for adverse effects such as slurred speech, altered consciousness, muscle twitching, and seizures.[27]

Bretylium Tosylate

Bretylium is classified as a type III antiarrhythmic agent. As discussed previously, two randomized controlled trials comparing the efficacy of lidocaine and bretylium in prehospital cardiac arrests found no statistical difference.[51,52] In one study, composed of 146 cardiac arrests, 60% of patients treated with lidocaine were successfully resuscitated compared with 58% in the bretylium-treated group.[51] Hospital discharge rates were 26 and 34% for the lidocaine and bretylium groups, respectively. In a study of 91 prehospital cardiac arrest victims, Olson and colleagues[52] found that 56% of lidocaine-treated patients achieved ROSC in contrast to 35% in the bretylium group. In this study, 10% of patients receiving lidocaine survived to hospital discharge compared with 5% receiving bretylium. Therefore, in the absence of efficacy differences, the choice of bretylium as a second-line antiarrhythmic agent is based largely on the preferred adverse effect profile of lidocaine. For those patients nonresponsive to lidocaine, early administration of bretylium is desirable in order to increase the chance of successful defibrillation given the time required to raise VFT.[53–55]

In the 1950s, bretylium was used as an antihypertensive agent due to its adrenergic blocking properties. With the discovery of its antifibrillatory properties in the 1960s, there was a renewed interest in bretylium.[57] The antiarrhythmic actions of bretylium result from a complex combination of direct myocardial and indirect adrenergic effects. Apart from its ability to raise the ventricular fibrillation threshold, bretylium reduces differences in action potential duration and refractory periods between infarcted and noninfarcted myocardium.[57] In addition, bretylium improves the conduction velocity within infarcted areas, which may reduce the development of VF.[57] As for effects on adrenergic nerve terminals, these vary with the time course following drug administration. Initially, bretylium administration potentiates norepinephrine release, which can be manifested clinically by increases in blood pressure, heart rate, and cardiac output. It is hypothesized that this sympathomimetic response may be important in achieving ROSC with bretylium since coronary blood flow may be augmented.[55] Approximately 15–20 minutes following administration, bretylium blocks further release of norepinephrine. Clinically, hypotension may occur, which requires the administration of fluids and vasopressors.[57] This profound hypotensive effect, however, may have a detrimental effect on coronary perfusion pressure.[55] In addition, bretylium blocks norepinephrine reuptake into adrenergic nerve endings, which may intensify effects obtained from exogenous catecholamine administration.[57]

In the treatment of PVT or VF, the AHA guidelines recommend initiating bretylium with a 5 mg/kg IVP bolus.[27] The drug should then be allowed to circulate 1 or 2 minutes prior to defibrillation. If the defibrillation attempt is unsuccessful, subsequent bolus doses of 10 mg/kg may be administered at 5-minute intervals up to a total dose of 30–35 mg/kg. A continuous infusion may be initiated at 1–2 mg/min once arrhythmia suppression is achieved.[27] For the treatment of persistent VT, 5–10 mg/kg of bretylium should be diluted in 50 mL of fluid and infused over 8–10 minutes. Since the occurrence of nausea and vomiting are related to peak serum concentrations, intravenous infusions should be used in conscious patients.[56] Serum concentration monitoring is not useful with bretylium therapy because antifibrillatory activity correlates better with myocardial concentrations.[56]

Procainamide

Procainamide is a third-line agent in the treatment of VF or PVT after failure of lidocaine and bretylium. In the cardiac arrest setting, rapid achievement of therapeutic serum concentrations is limited by the development of hypotension. This hypotensive effect results from both the ganglionic blocking activity and direct negative inotropic effects of procainamide.[57] Consequently, when infusing procainamide, special attention should be given to patients with known or suspected left ventricular dysfunction. The degree of hypotension is related to both the procainamide infusion rate and serum concentration.[56] Therefore, in nonemergent situations, procainamide infusions should not exceed 20 mg/min in order to decrease the risk of hypotension.[56] However, current ACLS guidelines suggest that procainamide infusion rates up to 30 mg/min may be used in the treatment of VF or PVT.[27] To assess patients for procainamide toxicity, blood pressure and ECG changes should be monitored throughout the infusion. Procainamide administration should continue until one of the following four events occurs: (1) the arrhythmia is suppressed, (2) the patient becomes hypotensive, (3) the QRS widens 50% above baseline ECG measurements, or (4) a dose of 17 mg/kg is infused.[27] If hypotension or QRS widening occurs during procainamide administration, the infusion should be decreased or discontinued. Procainamide is contraindicated in patients with either preexisting prolongation of the QT interval or torsades de pointes since its use may lengthen the QT interval.[27] Once arrhythmia suppression is achieved, a continuous procainamide infusion may be started at a rate of 1–4 mg/min.[27]

Procainamide is metabolized equally by hepatic and renal routes. The active metabolite, *N*-acetylprocainamide (NAPA), is primarily renally eliminated. Subsequently, dosage reductions have been suggested for patients with renal or cardiac impairment.[58] In patients with severe renal or cardiac dysfunction, it has been recommended to decrease the initial procainamide loading dose to 12 mg/kg. The normal maintenance infusion (2.8 mg/kg/h) should also be reduced by one-third with moderate or two-thirds with severe organ impairment.[58] If infusions are continued for greater than 24 hours, plasma procainamide and NAPA concentrations should be monitored.

Therapeutic Alternatives for Refractory VF or VT

Patients with persistent or recurrent VT or VF following antiarrhythmic administration should be assessed for underlying electrolyte abnormalities as a cause for their refractory dysrhythmia. Ideally, therapeutic decisions should be based on the patient's measured electrolyte concentrations. The primary electrolyte abnormalities associated with refractory ventricular arrhythmias include hyperkalemia, hypokalemia, and hypomagnesemia.[27] Patients with known or suspected hyperkalemia ([K+] >6.0 mEq/L) should receive 4 mg/kg IV of a 10% calcium chloride solution.[27] Sodium bicarbonate (1 mEq/kg) may also be given to drive potassium intracellularly until more definitive therapy is available.[27]

In one study of prehospital cardiac arrests, 49% of resuscitated patients were found to be hypokalemic ([K+] <3.6 mEq/L) on hospital admission.[59] Although frequently debated, it is unknown whether the hypokalemia most often precedes cardiac arrest or is a consequence of cardiac resuscitation.[59–63] Preexisting hypokalemia is primarily associated with diuretic usage.[60,62,63] Hypokalemia identified during cardiac arrest may also result from conditions present during resuscitation. For example, intracellular potassium shifts may occur secondarily to metabolic derangements or elevated circulating catecholamine concentrations.[59–61] With the association of hypokalemia and sudden death, it has been recommended to administer potassium (10 mEq IV over 30 minutes) to patients with refractory VF in whom hypokalemia is known or suspected.[27] Similarly, hypomagnesemia has been associated with ventricular arrhythmias.[64] Investigators have found that in hospitalized patients, approximately 40% of hypokalemic patients have coexisting hypomagnesemia.[65,66] This is important since uncorrected hypomagnesemia may prevent successful potassium repletion.[65] It is recommended that patients in refractory VF with either known ($[Mg^{+2}]$ < 1.4 mEq/L) or suspected hypomagnesemia receive 1–2 g of magnesium sulfate diluted in 10 mL of fluid over 1–2 minutes.[27] Caution should be used since rapid magnesium supplementation may produce significant hypotension or asystole.[55]

PHARMACOTHERAPY FOR ASYSTOLE AND PEA

As discussed previously, hospital discharge rates are usually <5% for patients presenting with either asystole or PEA.[2,4] Asystole is defined by the presence of "flat line" on the ECG monitor. Although it usually signals degeneration of a ventricular arrhythmia, asystole may occur from increased parasympathetic tone. Rarely, fine VF can resemble asystole if the patient is monitored with a single ECG lead. If this occurs, a second lead should be selected to confirm the cardiac rhythm.[27] It is important to rule out fine VF because it is a much more treatable rhythm. Asystolic patients should receive the following: CPR, intubation, and IV access. If available, attempts should be made to pace the heart using transcutaneous pacing.[27] Isoproterenol (a β_1, β_2 agonist) is contraindicated as a means of pharmacologic pacing in the cardiac arrest setting since it greatly increases myocardial oxygen demand.[27] Furthermore, coronary perfusion pressure is significantly reduced by β_2-induced vasodilation.[27] The primary pharmacologic agents used in the treatment of asystole are epinephrine and atropine. Recommended epinephrine dosing is identical to that used with VF/PVT.[27] Similarly, higher doses of epinephrine may be used if the initial 1-mg dose fails. The use of atropine in asystole will be discussed below. Defibrillation should be avoided because it may increase parasympathetic tone, which, in turn, might worsen survival from asystole.[27]

PEA encompasses all pulseless rhythms associated with electrical activity other than VT or VF.[27] Since these rhythms may result from underlying treatable conditions, it is first necessary to exclude all possible causes. Specifically, these include hypoxia, hypovolemia, cardiac tamponade, tension pneumothorax, hypothermia, pulmonary embolism, drug overdose, hyperkalemia, acidosis, and acute myocardial infarction.[27] If correction of potential underlying disorders is unsuccessful, epinephrine administration should be initiated.[27] Atropine may be used in PEA in the presence of absolute bradycardia (i.e., heart rate <60 beats/min).[27]

ATROPINE

Atropine, an antimuscarinic agent, improves sinus node and atrioventricular node conduction by inhibiting vagal activity. Possible reasons for high vagal tone during cardiac arrest include (1) oropharyngeal stimulation with endotracheal intubation, (2) the presence of hypoxia and acidosis, and (3) alterations in the contribution of parasympathetic and sympathetic control.[67] To date, there have not been any large randomized trials demonstrating benefit from atropine in the treatment of asystole. The majority of human data was compiled from either small cases series or retrospective studies.[67–73]

Gupta and colleagues[68] published four case reports in which atropine was used for "cardiac standstill." The response time for treating asystole in these patients was ≤22.5 seconds. Although all patients survived, only one patient was in asystole at the time of atropine administration.[68] In 1978, Iseri and colleagues[69] published a retrospective case series of 33 patients with prehospital bradyasystole. Of the 15 asystolic patients, only two received atropine (0.5-mg dose). None of the patients with asystole survived.[69] Brown and colleagues[67] reported results from 8 asystolic cases receiving atropine. The initial atropine dose ranged from 0.5–1 mg, with a maximum dose limit of 2 mg. In this case series, 3 of 8 (37.5%) survived to hospital discharge. It should be noted, however, that asystole was related to cardiac catheterization in two of these surviving patients.[67] In 1981, Coon and associates[70] published a prospective study of 21 prehospital patients with either asystole or pulseless idioventricular rhythm. Of the 10 patients who received atropine, none survived to hospital discharge. In comparison, 1 of 11 patients in the control group was discharged.[70] Stueven and colleagues[71] compared the results of patients receiving atropine (n = 43) with control (n = 41) patients in the treatment of prehospital refractory asystole. The atropine dose used was not specified by the investigators. Although 6 of 43 (14%) of atropine-treated patients achieved ROSC, none survived to hospital discharge. In contrast, ROSC was not obtained for any patients in the control group.[71] In 1985, Ornato and associates[72] published a retrospective study containing 24 prehospital patients with asystole as the presenting rhythm. The purpose of this study was to identify the ability of defibrillation and medications to transform the cardiac rhythm. Of the 22 patients receiving atropine, asystole was abolished in 4. Unfortunately, none of these patients was discharged from the hospital.[72] Lastly, Tortolani and colleagues[73] conducted a retrospective study of 123 in-hospital cardiac arrest patients with asystole as their initial cardiac rhythm. Atropine was administered in 101 of these patients. For those receiving atropine, 24 were alive 24 hours postresuscitation. It is unclear how many of these patients were eventually discharged.[74] Therefore, with little documentation of efficacy, atropine remains to be recommended for the treatment of asystole.[27,74]

Until recently, it was recommended that atropine be initiated with a 1-mg IV bolus in the treatment of asystole. If unsuccessful, a second 1-mg bolus could be administered.[57] Although not well substantiated in the medical literature, 2 mg of atropine has been touted to be a maximally vagolytic dose for the majority of adults.[74] With the most recent revision of the ACLS guidelines, the dosing of atropine was changed based on previous scientific evidence.[27] In 1967, Chamberlain and colleagues[74] published a prospective study of 10 healthy volunteers that examined the effects of heart rate and blood pressure to incremental dosage increases of atropine. Prior to receiving atropine, these individuals were given propranolol as a means to achieve chemical sympathetic denervation. For these 10 subjects, maximal heart rate increases were obtained with the following total atropine doses: 1.8 mg (3 patients), 2.4 mg (4 patients), and 3.0 mg (3 patients). On a weight basis, the maximum vagolytic dose for atropine in these healthy individuals ranged from 0.025–0.04 mg/kg. The authors did note, however, that the maximum vagolytic dose was higher for those subjects with lower baseline heart rates.[74] Subsequently, the 1992 ACLS guidelines, reflect the information identified by the above clinical studies and recommended that atropine be initiated at a dose of 1 mg. This dose should be repeated, if necessary, at 3- to 5-minute intervals up to a total dose of 0.04 mg/kg (approximately 3 mg in a 70-kg adult).[27] In comparison, for the treatment of bradycardia, atropine dosing should begin with 0.5–1 mg although the total dose remains 0.04 mg/kg.[27] It is important, however, to avoid administering atropine in doses <0.5 mg, because a paradoxical vagotonic effect may result.[57]

CALCIUM CHLORIDE

Although once encouraged, calcium administration during cardiac resuscitation has declined during the past decade. Calcium is a positive inotropic agent. Released in response to electrical stimulation of the muscle, calcium interacts with actin and myosin filaments to augment myocardial contractility.[57] Although initially advocated for the treatment of asystole and electromechanical dissociation, investigators have demonstrated no beneficial effects from using calcium in these disorders.[75,76] Furthermore, calcium administration has been associated with causing reperfusion injury and postischemic cerebral hypoperfusion.[77–80] As a result, the indications for calcium administration during cardiac arrest are limited. Calcium is only recommended (Class IIa) for the following: hyperkalemia, hypocalcemia, and calcium antagonist toxicity.[27]

ACID–BASE MANAGEMENT DURING CARDIOPULMONARY RESUSCITATION

During cardiac arrest, acid–base imbalances result from decreased perfusion and ineffective ventilation. As established previously, approximately 30% of the baseline cardiac output is achieved during standard CPR.[2] In the presence of reduced tissue perfusion and oxygen delivery, anaerobic metabolism predominates, thereby, raising P_{CO_2} concentrations. Elimination of P_{CO_2} is hampered by this state of diminished blood flow. Subsequently, attempts to correct the acidosis should be directed at improving blood flow (i.e., optimizing cardiac compressions) and ventilation.

SODIUM BICARBONATE

Sodium bicarbonate ($NaHCO_3$) administration was recommended during cardiac resuscitation in order to correct systemic acidosis. It was believed that alkali administration would improve detrimental effects associated with acidosis such as reduced myocardial contractility and VF threshold.[81] The majority of available data, however, do not support sodium bicarbonate use in CPR.[27,81,82] Aside from the inability to improve survival,[27,82] administration of sodium bicarbonate can have detrimental results.[58,82] For example, sodium bicarbonate can generate CO_2 production by the following equation:

$$[H^+] + [HCO_3^-] \longleftrightarrow H_2CO_3 \longleftrightarrow CO_2 + H_2O$$

thereby worsening acidosis. In the absence of effective CO_2 elimination, rapid intracellular diffusion of CO_2 can result in the development of intracellular acidosis. Likewise, cerebrospinal and central venous acidosis can occur with sodium bicarbonate administration. Other possible adverse effects include decreased oxygen release secondary to alterations in the oxyhemoglobin dissociation curve, and production of hyperosmolality and hypernatremia.[57]

Currently, sodium bicarbonate has a limited role during cardiac resuscitation attempts.[27] A proportion of patients, however, may benefit from bicarbonate therapy (class IIa).[27] These individuals include those with (1) known bicarbonate-responsive acidosis, (2) hyperkalemia, or (3) tricyclic antidepressant or phenobarbital overdose. The remaining indication (class IIb) for sodium bicarbonate administration involves cases with prolonged arrest times (i.e., >10 minutes).[27] In this situation, patients should first receive adequate CPR, intubation, ventilation, and multiple epinephrine doses prior to considering sodium bicarbonate administration. If the decision is made to institute bicarbonate therapy, the initial recommended dose is 1 mEq/kg.[27] If necessary, subsequent doses of 0.5 mEq/kg can be administered at 10-minute intervals. To reduce the adverse effects associated with alkalosis, it is recommended that results from blood gas analysis guide bicarbonate administration.[27]

GUIDELINES FOR DRUG ADMINISTRATION DURING EMERGENCY SITUATIONS

During cardiac resuscitation, several routes for drug administration are available. Each route, however, is associated with various advantages and disadvantages. Ideally, the drug administration route should be easily accessible during CPR and provide rapid entry into the central circulation. Although central venous administration results in both earlier and higher peak drug concentrations compared with peripheral venous administration,[83,84] it may be unavailable early in the cardiac arrest event. Additionally, attempts to obtain central access may necessitate unwanted interruptions in performing CPR. Peripheral venous access, using the antecubital vein, is acceptable if central access is unavailable. It is recommended that all peripheral IV injections be followed immediately with a 20-mL fluid bolus and elevation of the extremity in an effort to speed drug entry into the central circulation.[27,85] If ROSC is not achieved following the first peripherally administered dose, central access should be attempted.[27]

In the event that neither central nor peripheral access is available, endotracheal administration of epinephrine, lidocaine, and atropine may be utilized. It is not recommended to administer either sodium bicarbonate or bretylium endotracheally.[86] Within the medical literature, great debate surrounds the optimal dose conversion from IV to endotracheal administration. Recommendations for the endotracheal dose have varied from equivalent doses to as much as 10 times the intravenous dose.[86] The 1992 ACLS guidelines suggest that endotracheal doses of 2–2.5 times the recommended IV dose be used.[27] Since endotracheal administration is associated with delayed onset and prolonged duration of action, rescuers should be aware that increased drug effects may be seen if spontaneous circulation is achieved.[86] The recommended method for endotracheal administration is as follows: (1) dilution of the dose in 10 mL of distilled water or normal saline, (2) interruption of CPR, (3) rapid drug administration beyond the tip of the endotracheal tube, (4) three to five quick insufflations using a bag-valve device to aerosolize the drug, and (5) resumption of CPR.[27] In pediatric patients, the intraosseous route may be used temporarily if no other routes of drug administration are available. Lastly, intracardiac drug administration is not recommended during closed-chest CPR.

Related to the issue of drug administration, the current 1992 AHA guidelines address the appropriateness of administering various IV fluids.[27] For years, dextrose-containing solutions have been used during cardiac resuscitation to keep IV lines patent as well as provide a drug delivery vehicle. Concern over the use of dextrose-containing fluids during ischemic events stems from information linking hyperglycemia with worsened neurologic survival.[87] Controversy exists, however, regarding whether hyperglycemia produces neurologic deficits or whether it is merely a marker of prolonged resuscitative efforts.[87–89] Until further clarification is available, dextrose solutions should be reserved for patients with documented or suspected hypoglycemia.[27] Use of normal saline or lactated Ringer's is suggested for all other intravenous infusions.[27,87]

Ethics in CPR

Should CPR be instituted on demand? Are physicians required to initiate CPR in terminally ill patients? Can resuscitation efforts be terminated prior to reaching the hospital? These are among the many questions currently facing emergency care providers. Most agree that attaining "neurologic survival" is the primary objective of cardiac resuscitation. Since this often is not attainable, many health care professionals are attempting to identify patients unlikely to benefit from cardiac resuscitation. The initial obstacle to accomplishing this task is defining the term "medical futility." The current AHA guidelines suggest that futility occurs only when there are no reported survivors for a population subgroup.[90] Others object to the stringent nature of this definition, recommending instead that medical futility be defined by an acceptable threshold value (e.g., <0.1, 1, 2% survivors) determined from outcome data in the medical literature.[91,92] By withholding CPR in futile cases, the following benefits may be achieved: (1) reduced number of suboptimal outcomes, (2) decreased injuries incurred while delivering rapid emergency care, and (3) provision of more cost-effective health care.[93] For example, investigators have shown that victims not regaining a pulse with ACLS prior to hospital arrival rarely survive, with the exception of those patients with refractory VT or VF.[93] Furthermore, it has been estimated that in the United States, yearly costs incurred for continued ER resuscitation efforts in these individuals approaches half a billion dollars.[93]

To decrease the number of futile resuscitation attempts, information must be gathered that documents the probabilities of successful resuscitation in given population subsets. As discussed previously, current attempts to accomplish this objective include standardizing resuscitation definitions[24,26] and developing prearrest morbidity indices.[94] Once survival probabilities are known, patients should be presented with information specific to their situation. In the meantime, efforts to establish resuscitation status prior to hospitalization should be continued, especially in the elderly and terminally ill.

Evaluation of Therapeutic Outcomes

In the most basic sense, successful CPR is often described as the restoration of a stable heart rate, cardiac rhythm, and blood pressure (SBP >70 mm Hg). However, to truly be successful, patients should remain neurologically intact with minimal morbidity following resuscitation. To gauge the success of resuscitation outcomes, therapeutic outcome monitoring should occur during the resuscitation attempt and in the postresuscitation phase. For all patient's undergoing CPR, the following parameters should be assessed and documented throughout the resuscitation attempt and subsequent to each intervention: respiratory rate, heart rate, cardiac rhythm, and blood pressure. Determination of the presence or absence of respirations, heart rate, and the associated cardiac rhythm is paramount to deciding which interventions may be appropriate. In addition, nonresponse to an array of suitable interventions may signal a patient incapable of being resuscitated. Determination of coronary and cerebral perfusion pressure during the resuscitation attempt is desirable although not realistic in most institutions. Since there are not as yet standardized resuscitation definitions for various CPR outcomes, documentation of resuscitation events and corresponding patient parameters is essential. Once developed, these definitions could be applied retrospectively in order to make assumptions regarding overall response to interventions in specific patient categories.

Following successful resuscitation, the primary goals include optimizing tissue oxygenation, identifying the precipitating cause(s) of the arrest, and preventing subsequent episodes of cardiopulmonary arrest. In an effort to determine causation, a prearrest history should be obtained, which includes documentation of any prescribed medications. During the postresuscitation period, patients should receive the following: a 12-lead ECG, CXR, ABG, blood chemistry determinations, frequent vital signs, continuous ECG monitoring, and ventilatory support if necessary. Special attention should be given to altered liver and renal function resulting from ischemic damage during the cardiopulmonary arrest. Assessment of neurologic function should be completed prior to discharge. Currently, there are no guidelines on when this assessment should occur and how it should be performed. In an attempt to document neurologic function, investigators have used the cerebral performance category, modified Mini-mental status exam, and Glasgow scale.[44,48,49] We hope that in the future we will have more definitive information regarding appropriate neurologic testing procedures in the postresuscitated patient.

References

1. Emergency Cardiac Care Committee and Subcommittees, American Heart Association. Guidelines for cardiopulmonary resuscitation and emergency cardiac care, I: Introduction. JAMA 1992;269:2172–2183.
2. O'Nunain S, Ruskin J. Cardiac arrest. Lancet 1993;341:1641–1647.
3. Madl C, Grimm G, Kramer L, et al. Early prediction of individual outcome after cardiopulmonary resuscitation. Lancet 1993;341:855–858.
4. Niemann JT. Cardiopulmonary resuscitation. N Engl J Med 1992;327(15):1075–1080.
5. Varon J, Sternbach GL. Cardiopulmonary resuscitation: Lessons from the past. J Emerg Med 1991;9:503–507.
6. Safar P, Escarraga L, Elam JO. A comparison of the mouth-to-mouth and mouth-to-airway methods of artificial respiration with the chest-pressure arm-lift method. N Engl J Med 1958;258:671–677.
7. Kouwenhoven WB, Jude JR, Knickerbocker GG. Closed-chest cardiac massage. JAMA 1960;173:1064–1067.
8. Weaver WD. Resuscitation outside the hospital—what's lacking? N Engl J Med 1991;325(20):1437–1439.
9. Eisenberg MS, Horwood BT, Cummins RO, et al. Cardiac arrest and resuscitation: A tale of 29 cities. Ann Emerg Med 1990;19:179–186.
10. Schneider AP, Nelson DJ, Brown DD. In-hospital cardiopulmonary resuscitation: A 30-year review. J Am Board Fam Pract 1993;6:91–101.
11. Joslyn SA, Pomrehn PR, Brown DD. Survival from out-of-hospital cardiac arrest: Effects of patient age and presence of 911 emergency medical services phone access. Am J Emerg Med 1993;11:200–206.
12. Kellermann AL, Hackman BB, Somes G. Predicting the outcome of unsuccessful prehospital advanced cardiac life support. JAMA 1993;270:1433–1436.
13. Emergency Cardiac Care Committee and Subcommittees, American Heart Association. Guidelines for cardiopulmonary resuscitation and emergency cardiac care, IX: Ensuring effectiveness of communitywide emergency cardiac care. JAMA 1992;269:2289–2295.
14. Ayers SM. Preventing cardiac arrest. Crit Care Med 1994;22(2):189–191.
15. Edwards GA, Samuels TM. The role of the hospital pharmacist in emergency situations. Am J Hosp Pharm 1968;25:128–133.
16. Bardas SL. Demystifying the cardiopulmonary code team response. J Pharm Technol 1992;8:151–154.
17. Bond CA, Raehl CL, Pitterle ME. 1992 national clinical pharmacy services study. Pharmacotherapy 1994;14(3):282–304.
18. Berkowitz ID, Rogers MC. The physiology of cerebral blood flow during cardiopulmonary resuscitation. Can J Anaesth 1988;35(3):S23–S29.
19. Eorgan PA, Greer JL. Cough CPR: A consideration for high-risk cardiac patient discharge teaching. Crit Care Nurse 1992;12(6):21–27.
20. Halperin HR, Weisfeldt ML. New approaches to CPR: Four hands, a plunger, or a vest. JAMA 1992;267(21):2940–2941.
21. Sack JB, Kesselbrenner MB, Anwar J. Interposed abdominal compression-cardiopulmonary resuscitation and outcome during asystole and electromechanical dissociation. Circulation 1992;86:1692–1700.
22. Cohen TJ, Goldner BG, Maccaro PC, et al. A comparison of active compression-decompression cardiopulmonary resuscitation with standard cardiopulmonary resuscitation for cardiac arrests occurring in the hospital. N Engl J Med 1993;329:1918–1921.
23. Halperin HR, Tsitlik JE, Gelfand M, et al. A preliminary study of cardiopulmonary resuscitation by circumferential compression of the chest with use of a pneumatic vest. N Engl J Med 1993;329:762–768.
24. Task Force of the American Heart Association, the European Resuscitation Council, the Heart and Stroke Foundation of Canada, and the Australian Resuscitation Council. Recommended guidelines for uniform reporting of data from out-of-hospital cardiac arrest: The Utstein style. Ann Emerg Med 1991;20(8):861–874.
25. Paradis NA, Martin GB, Rivers EP, et al. Coronary perfusion pressure and the return of spontaneous circulation in human cardiopulmonary resuscitation. JAMA 1990;263:1106–1113.
26. Becker LB, Pepe PE. Ensuring the effectiveness of community-wide emergency cardiac care. Ann Emerg Med 1993;22(2, part 2):354–365.
27. Emergency Cardiac Care Committee and Subcommittees, American Heart Association. Guidelines for cardiopulmonary resuscitation and emergency cardiac care, III: Adult advanced cardiac life support. JAMA 1992;269:2199–2241.
28. Pepe PE, Levine RL, Fromm R. Cardiac arrest presenting with rhythms other than ventricular fibrillation: Contribution of resuscitative efforts toward total survivorship. Crit Care Med 1993;21(12):1838–1843.
29. Bonnin MJ, Pepe PE, Clark PS. Survival in the elderly after out-of-hospital cardiac arrest. Crit Care Med 1993;21:1645–1651.
30. Robinson LA, Brown CG, Jeckins J, et al. The effect of norepinephrine versus epinephrine on myocardial hemodynamic during CPR. Ann Emerg Med 1989;18:336–340.
31. Brown CG, Weman HA. Collective review. Adrenergic agonists during cardiopulmonary resuscitation. Resuscitation 1990;1:1–16.
32. Darby TD, Aldinger EE, Gadsen RH, et al. Effects of metabolic acidosis on ventricular isometric systolic tension and the response to epinephrine and levarterenol. Circ Res 1980;8:1242–1253.
33. Houle OB, Weil MH, Brown EB, et al. Influence of respiratory acidosis on ECG and pressor response to epinephrine,

norepinephrine, and metaraminol. Proc Soc Exp Biol Med 1957;94:561–564.

34. Camilton de Hurtado MC, Argel MI, Cingolani HE. Influence of acid–base alterations on myocardial sensitivity to catecholamines. Arch Pharmacol 1981;317:219–224.
35. Burget DE, Visscher MB. Variations of the pH of the blood and the response of the vascular system to adrenalin. Am J Physiol 1927;81:113–123.
36. Motulsky HJ, Insel PA. Adrenergic receptors in man. Direct identification, physiologic regulation, and clinical alterations. N Engl J Med 1982;307:18–29.
37. Lefkowitz RJ, Caron MG, Stiles GI. Mechanisms of membrane-receptor regulation. Biochemical, physiological, and clinical insights derived from studies of the adrenergic receptor. N Eng J Med 1984;310;1570–1579.
38. Leftowitz RJ. Beta-adrenergic receptors: Recognition and regulation. N Engl J Med 1976;295:323–328.
39. Ornato JP. Use of adrenergic agonists during CPR in adults. Ann Emerg Med 1993;22(part 2):411–416.
40. Langer SZ, Shepperson NB. Postjunctional α_1- and α_2-adrenoceptors: Preferential innervation of α_1-adrenoceptors and the role of neuronal uptake. J Cardiovasc Pharmacol 1982;4:S8–S13.
41. Lindner KH, Ahnefeld FW, Schuermann W, et al. Epinephrine and norepinephrine in cardiopulmonary resuscitation. Chest 1990;97:1458–1462.
42. Brown CG, Robinson LA, Jenkins J, et al. The effect of norepinephrine on regional cerebral blood flow during cardiopulmonary resuscitation. Am J Emerg Med 1989;7:278–282.
43. Lindner KH, Ahnefeld FW, Grünert A. Epinephrine versus norepinephrine in prehospital ventricular fibrillation. Amer J Cardiol 1991;678:427–428.
44. Callaham M, Barton CW, Saunders, et al. A randomized clinical trial of high-dose epinephrine and norepinephrine versus standard-dose epinephrine in prehospital cardiac arrest. JAMA 1992;268:2667–2672.
45. Gonzalez ER, Ornato JP, Garnett AR, et al. Dose-dependent vasopressor response to epinephrine during CPR in human beings. Ann Emerg Med 1989;18(9):920–925.
46. Lindner KH, Ahnefeld FW, Prengel AW. Comparison of standard and high-dose adrenaline in the resuscitation of asystole and electromechanical dissociation. Acta Anaesthes Scand 1991;35:253–256.
47. Callaham M, Barton CW, Kayser S. Potential complications of high-dose epinephrine therapy in patients resuscitated from cardiac arrest. JAMA 1991;265:1117–1122.
48. Stiell IG, Hebert PC, Weitzman BN, et al. High-dose epinephrine in adult cardiac arrest. N Engl J Med 1992;327:1045–1050.
49. Brown CG, Martin DR, Pepe PE, et al. A comparison of standard-dose and high-dose epinephrine in cardiac arrest outside the hospital. N Engl J Med 1992;327:1051–1055.
50. Lipman J, Wilson W, Kobilski S, et al. High-dose adrenaline in adult in-hospital asystolic cardiopulmonary resuscitation: A double-blind randomised trial. Anaesth Intens Care 1993;21:192–196.
51. Haynes RE, Chinn TI, Copass MK, et al. Comparison of bretylium tosylate and lidocaine in the management of out-of-hospital ventricular fibrillation: A randomized clinical trial. Am J Cardiol 1981;48:353–356.
52. Olson DW, Thompson BM, Daqrin JC, et al. A randomized comparison study of bretylium tosylate and lidocaine in the resuscitation of patients with out-of-hospital ventricular fibrillation in a paramedic system. Ann Emerg Med 1984;13:807–810.
53. Chow MSS, Kluger J, DiPersio DM, et al. Antifibrillatory effects of lidocaine and bretylium immediately post cardiopulmonary resuscitation. Am Hear J 1985;110:938–943.
54. Hanyok JJ, Chow MSS, Kluger J, et al. Antifibrillatory effects of high dose bretylium and a lidocaine–bretylium combination during cardiopulmonary resuscitation. Crit Care Med 1988;16:691–694.
55. Jaffe AS. The use of antiarrhythmics in advanced cardiac life support. Ann Emerg Med 1993;22(2, part 2):307–316.
56. Pentel P, Benowitz N. Pharmacokinetic and pharmacodynamic considerations in drug therapy of cardiac emergencies. Clin Pharmacokin 1984;9:273–308.
57. Advanced Cardiac Life Support Working Group. Cardiovascular pharmacology I, in Jaffe AS (ed): Textbook of Advanced Cardiac Life Support. Dallas, American Heart Association, 1987, pp 97–113.
58. Coyle JD, Lima JJ. Procainamide, in Evans WE, Schentag JJ, Jusko WJ (eds): Applied Pharmacokinetics: Principles of Therapeutic Drug Monitoring. Spokane, WA, Applied Therapeutics, 1992.
59. Thompson RG, Cobb LA. Hypokalemia after resuscitation from out-of-hospital ventricular fibrillation. JAMA 1982;248(21):2860–2863.
60. Ornato JP, Gonzalez ER, Starke H, et al. Incidence and causes of hypokalemia associated with cardiac resuscitation. Am J Emerg Med 1985;3:503–506.
61. Higham PD, Adams PC, Murray, et al. Plasma potassium, serum magnesium and ventricular fibrillation: A prospective study. Q J Med 1993;86:609–617.
62. Singh BN, Hollenberg NK, Poole-Wilson PA, et al. Diuretic-induced potassium and magnesium deficiency: Relation to drug-induced QT prolongation, cardiac arrhythmias and sudden death. J Hyperten 1992;10:301–316.
63. McInnes, GT, Yeo WW, Ramsay LE, et al. Cardiotoxicity and diuretics: Much speculation—little substance. J Hyperten 1992;10:317–335.
64. Eisenberg MJ. Magnesium deficiency and sudden death. Amer Heart J 1992;124(2):544–549.
65. Whang R, Flink EB, Dyckner T, et al. Magnesium depletion as a cause of refractory potassium repletion. Arch Intern Med 1985;145:1686–1689.
66. Boyd JC, Bruns DE, Wills MR. Occurrence of hypomagnesemia in hypokalemic states. Clin Chem 1983;29:178–179.
67. Brown DC, Lewis AJ, Criley JM. Asystole and its treatment: The possible role of the parasympathetic nervous system in cardiac arrest. JACEP 1979;8(11):448–452.
68. Gupta PK, Lichstein E, Chadda KD. Transient atrioventricular standstill: Etiology and management. JAMA 1975;234:1038–1042.
69. Iseri LT, Humphrey SB, Siner EJ. Prehospital brady-asystolic cardiac arrest. Ann Intern Med 1978;88(6):741–745.
70. Coon GA, Clinton JE, Ruiz E. Use of atropine for brady-asystolic prehospital cardiac arrest. Ann Emerg Med 1981;10(9):462–467.

71. Stueven HA, Tonsfeldt DJ, Thompson BM, et al. Atropine in asystole: Human studies. Ann Emerg Med 1984(Part2):13(9):815–817.
72. Ornato JP, Gonzalez ER, Morkunas AR, et al. Treatment of presumed asystole during prehospital cardiac arrest: Superiority of electrical countershock. Am J Emerg Med 1985;3:395–399.
73. Tortolani AJ, Risucci DA, Powell SR, et al. In-hospital cardiopulmonary resuscitation during asystole: Therapeutic factors associated with 24-hours survival. Chest 1989;96:622–626.
74. Chamberlain DA, Turner P, Sneddon JM. Effects of atropine on heart-rate in healthy man. Lancet 1967;2(1):12–15.
75. Stueven HA, Thompson B, Aprahamian C, et al. Lack of effectiveness of calcium chloride in refractory asystole. Ann Emerg Med 1985;14:630–632.
76. Harrison EE, Arney BD. Use of calcium in electromechanical dissociation. Ann Emerg Med 1984;13(part 2):844–845.
77. Dembo DH. Calcium in advanced life support. Crit Care Med 1981;9(5):358–359.
78. Schanne FAX, Kane AB, Young EE, et al. Calcium dependence of toxic cell death: A final common pathway. Science 1979;206:700–702.
79. Kirsch JR, Dean JM, Rogers MC. Current concepts in brain resuscitation. Arch Intern Med 1986;146:1413–1419.
80. Follette DM, Key K, Buckberg GD, et al. Reducing postischemic damage by temporary modification of reperfusate calcium, potassium, pH, and osmolarity. J Thorac Cardiovasc Surg 1981;82:221–238.
81. Bleske BE, Chow MSS, Zhao H, et al. Effects of different dosages and modes of sodium bicarbonate administration during cardiopulmonary resuscitation. Am J Emerg Med 1992;10:525–532.
82. von Planta M, Bar-Joseph G, Wiklund L, et al. Pathophysiologic and therapeutic implications of acid–base changes during CPR. Ann Emerg Med 1993;22(part 2):404–410.
83. Kuhn GJ, White BC, Swetnam RE, et al. Peripheral vs central circulation time during CPR: A pilot study. Ann Emerg Med 1981;10:417–419.
84. Barsan WG, Levy RC, Weir H. Lidocaine levels during CPR: Differences after peripheral venous, ventral venous, and intracardiac injection. Ann Emerg Med 1981;10:73–78.
85. Emerman CL, Pinchak AC, Hancock D, et al. The effect of bolus injection on circulation times during cardiac arrest. Am J Emerg Med 1990;8:190–193.
86. Raehl CL. Endotracheal drug therapy in cardiopulmonary resuscitation. Clin Pharm 1986;5:572–579.
87. Grillo JA, Gonzalez ER. Changes in the pharmacotherapy of CPR. Heart Lung 1993;22:548–553.
88. Longstreth WT, Diehr P, Cobb LA, et al. Neurologic outcome and blood glucose levels during out-of-hospital cardiopulmonary resuscitation. Neurology 1986;36:1186–1191.
89. Martin GB, O'Brien JF, Best R, et al. Insulin and glucose levels during CPR in the canine model. Ann Emerg Med 1985;14:293–297.
90. Emergency Cardiac Care Committee and Subcommittees, American Heart Association. Guidelines for cardiopulmonary resuscitation and emergency cardiac care, VIII: Ethical considerations in resuscitation. JAMA 1992;269:2282–2288.
91. Murphy DF, Finucan TE. New do-not-resuscitate policies: A first step in cost control. Arch Intern Med 1993;153:1641–1648.
92. Jecker NS, Schneiderman LJ. Ceasing futile resuscitation in the field: Ethical considerations. Arch Intern Med 1992;152:2392–2397.
93. Bonnin MJ, Pepe PE, Kimball KT, et al. Distinct criteria for termination of resuscitation in the out-of-hospital setting. JAMA 1993;270:1457–1462.
94. George AL, Folk BP, Crecelius PK, et al. Pre-arrest morbidity and other correlates of survival after in-hospital cardiopulmonary arrest. Am J Med 1989;87:28–34.

Chapter 12

Hypertension

David W. Hawkins, PharmD, Henry I. Bussey, PharmD, and L. Michael Prisant, MD

Arterial blood pressure is generated by the interplay between blood flow and the resistance to blood flow. It reaches a peak during cardiac systole (systolic pressure) and a nadir at the end of diastole (diastolic pressure).[1,2] Arterial blood pressure is conventionally measured in millimeters of mercury and recorded as systolic pressure over diastolic pressure (e.g., 120/80 mm Hg). The difference between systolic and diastolic pressure, pulse pressure, is an indicator of the tone of arterial walls. The mean arterial pressure is the average pressure throughout the cardiac cycle. Mean arterial pressure (MAP) can be estimated by adding one-third of the pulse pressure (PP) to the diastolic blood pressure (DBP): $MAP = 1/3PP + DBP$.

Under normal physiologic conditions, the arterial blood pressure stays within narrow limits. It may reach its height during physical or emotional stress and it usually falls to its lowest level during sleep. Blood pressure tends to be lower in women than men, it tends to be higher in blacks than whites, and it rises with age.

Arterial blood pressure (BP) can be defined hemodynamically as the product of cardiac output (CO) and total peripheral resistance (TPR): $BP = CO \times TPR$. Cardiac output is the major determinant of systolic pressure while total peripheral resistance largely determines the level of diastolic pressure. In turn, cardiac output is a function of stroke volume, heart rate, and venous capacitance. Factors that increase stroke volume or heart rate may increase cardiac output and, consequently, systolic blood pressure. Venous capacitance affects the volume of blood (or preload) that is returned to the heart through the central venous circulation. Venous dilatation increases venous capacitance and decreases preload and systolic pressure. Contraction of the peripheral veins, of course, would cause the opposite effect.

Total peripheral resistance is regulated chiefly by contraction and dilation of the arterioles. Arteriolar constriction increases peripheral resistance and thus diastolic blood pressure. Other factors that affect intravascular resistance include the elasticity of aortic and arterial walls and blood viscosity.

Definition

Because arterial blood pressure is a continuous variable, it is impossible to define a cutoff point below which the blood pressure is normal and above which the pressure is abnormally high. Nevertheless, evidence from epidemiologic studies clearly indicates a strong correlation between blood pressure and cardiovascular morbidity and mortality.[3,4] The higher the pressure, the more likely it is that an individual will experience stroke, myocardial infarction, angina, heart failure, renal failure, or early death from a cardiovascular cause. In addition, large-scale clinical studies have shown that the increased risk of stroke and heart failure and death associated with elevated blood pressure is substantially reduced by interventions that lower blood pressure.[5–10]

It is therefore reasonable to classify hypertension based on the impact on risk, as was done by the Fifth Joint National Committee on the Detection, Evaluation, and Treatment of High Blood Pressure (JNC-V).[11] According to JNC-V, adult blood pressure is classified as follows:

Category	Systolic (mm Hg)	Diastolic (mm Hg)
Normal	<130	<85
High normal	130–139	85–89
Hypertension		
Stage 1 (mild)	140–159	90–99
Stage 2 (moderate)	160–179	100–109
Stage 3 (severe)	180–209	110–119
Stage 4 (very severe)	>209	>119

If the diastolic blood pressure is less than 90 mm Hg and the systolic blood pressure is 140 mm Hg or higher, then the term *isolated systolic hypertension* is applicable. Isolated systolic hypertension is believed to result from the pathophysiology of aging and portends an increased risk of cardiovascular morbidity and mortality.

A marked or sharp increase in diastolic blood pressure is considered a hypertensive crisis. Hypertensive crises represent either a hypertensive emergency or a hypertensive urgency. If the elevation of diastolic blood pressure is accompanied by acute target organ injury, then a hypertensive emergency exists. Examples of acute target organ injury include encephalopathy, intracranial hemorrhage, acute left ventricular failure with pulmonary edema, dissecting aortic aneurysm, unstable angina, and eclampsia or severe hypertension associated with pregnancy. Such hypertensive situations require an immediate but gradual reduction in blood pressure over a period of several minutes to several hours. A reasonable goal is to lower the diastolic blood pressure gradually down to 100–110 mm Hg. Hypertensive urgencies, on the other hand, usually signify severe hypertension without signs or symptoms of acute target organ complications. In these situations, reduction in blood pressure may proceed safely over several hours to several days.

PREVALENCE

Based on data provided by the Centers for Disease Control and Prevention, National Center for Health Statistics, as many as 50 million Americans have high blood pressure (≥140/90 mm Hg.)[11] Blood pressure increases with age, but the onset of hypertension most often occurs during the third, fourth, and fifth decades of life. The prevalence of hypertension is 17% among white women, 26% among white men, 37% among black women, and 44% among black men 35–45 years of age.[12] In the elderly population (age >65 years), sexual differences in blood pressure are less marked, and the prevalence of hypertension is approximately 63% in whites and 76% in blacks.

ETIOLOGY[3,4,13–17]

Hypertension is a heterogenous disorder that may result from either a specific cause (secondary hypertension) or some underlying pathophysiologic mechanism stemming from an unknown etiology (primary or essential hypertension). Fewer than 5% of people who suffer from high blood pressure have secondary hypertension. In most of these, chronic renal disease or renovascular disease is the cause of hypertension. Other conditions that are known to cause secondary hypertension include pheochromocytoma, Cushing's syndrome, primary aldosteronism, and coarctation of the aorta. In some instances, exposure to various exogenous substances may produce hypertension. The most notable of these are estrogens, glucocorticoids, licorice, sympathomimetic amines, nonsteroidal anti-inflammatory agents, chronic alcohol use, and tyramine-containing foods in combination with monoamine oxidase (MAO) inhibitors.

In the vast majority of individuals with high blood pressure, a specific cause of sustained hypertension cannot be found. A vigorous search for a single underlying abnormality that eventuates into high blood pressure has led to the discovery of numerous mechanisms that may contribute to the pathogenesis of hypertension.

The fact that hypertension often runs in families suggests that genetic factors may play an important pathogenic role in the development of essential hypertension. There is even some evidence that single genes might be responsible for specific subtypes of hypertension. These include genetic traits for high sodium–lithium countertransport, a low urinary kallikrein excretion, increased aldosterone and other adrenal steroids, and high angiotensinogen levels (16–17). Identifying individuals with these traits could lead to more direct approaches for preventing or treating hypertension.

PATHOPHYSIOLOGY[3,4,13–15,18–25]

Multiple factors may contribute to the development of primary hypertension including abnormal neural mechanisms; defects in peripheral autoregulation; disturbances in sodium, calcium, and natriuretic hormone; and malfunctions in either humoral or vasodepressor mechanisms.

NEURAL COMPONENTS

Both the central (CNS) and the autonomic nervous systems are intricately involved in the maintenance of arterial blood pressure.

Stimulation of certain areas within the CNS (nucleus tractus solitarius, vagal nuclei, vasomotor center, and the area postrema) can result in either an increase or a decrease in blood pressure. For example, α-adrenergic stimulation within the CNS decreases blood pressure through an inhibitory effect on the vasomotor center. Increased angiotensin II, however, increases sympathetic outflow from the vasomotor center, which eventuates in an increase in blood pressure.

Located on the presynaptic surface of sympathetic terminals are a variety of receptors that either enhance or inhibit norepinephrine release. The α and β presynaptic receptors play a role in negative and positive feedback to the norepinephrine-containing vesicles located near the neuronal ending. Stimulation of presynaptic α (α_2) receptors exerts a negative inhibition on norepinephrine release. Stimulation of presynaptic β receptors facilitates further release of norepinephrine.

The α and β receptors are also located on the surface of effector cells innervated by sympathetic neuronal fibers. Stimulation of postsynaptic α (α_1) receptors on arterioles and venules results in vasoconstriction. There are two types of postsynaptic β receptors, β_1 and β_2. Both types of β-adrenergic receptors are present in all tissue innervated by the sympathetic nervous system; however, the distribution of β_1 and β_2 receptors is such that in some tissue β_1 receptors predominate and in other tissue β_2 receptors predominate. Stimulation of β_1 receptors in the heart results in an increase in heart rate and contractility. When β_2 receptors in the arterioles and venules are stimulated, vasodilation occurs.

The major negative-feedback mechanism controlling sympathetic activity is the system of baroreceptor reflexes. Baroreceptors are nerve endings lying in the walls of large arteries, especially in the carotid arteries and aortic arch. The baroreceptors respond extremely rapidly to changes in arterial pressure. Baroreceptor impulses are transmitted to the brainstem primarily through the ninth cranial nerve and vagus nerves. In this reflex system, an acute elevation in arterial pressure increases the rate of baroreceptor discharge, which results in vasodilation throughout the peripheral circulatory system and a decrease in heart rate and myocardial contractility. Conversely, low pressure has the opposite effect, causing reflex vasoconstriction and increase in heart rate and force of contraction. These baroreceptor reflex mechanisms may be blunted in elderly individuals.

A pathologic disturbance in any of these neural components that modulate arterial blood pressure could conceivably lead to a sustained elevation in blood pressure. It is reasonable to postulate that the primary defect can occur in any of the four major components: CNS, autonomic nerve fibers, adrenergic receptors, or baroreceptors. Also, because they are so physiologically interrelated, a defect in one component may disturb the normal function in another, and the combined abnormalities may then cause hypertension.

PERIPHERAL AUTOREGULATORY COMPONENTS

Abnormalities in either the renal or tissue autoregulatory processes could cause hypertension. In fact, it seems reasonable to postulate that individuals may first develop a renal defect for sodium excretion and then reset their tissue autoregulatory processes to a higher arterial blood pressure.

Normally, the volume–pressure adaptive mechanism of the kidney works well to maintain a normal blood pressure. When the blood pressure drops, the kidneys adapt by retaining more sodium and water. This leads to plasma volume expansion, which increases blood pressure. Conversely, when blood pressure rises above normal, sodium and water excretion are increased, plasma volume and cardiac output are reduced, and the blood pressure returns to normal.

Local autoregulatory processes operate to maintain adequate tissue oxygenation. When oxygen demand is low, the arteriolar bed is in a relatively constricted state. Peripheral vascular resistance is maintained at a sufficient level to regulate adequate blood flow (flow = pressure/resistance). An increase in metabolic demand triggers arteriolar vasodilation through autoregulation. This then lowers peripheral vascular resistance to increase blood flow and oxygen delivery.

An initial defect in the renal adaptive mechanism could lead to plasma volume expansion and increase blood flow to peripheral tissues even when blood pressure is normal. To offset the increase in blood flow, local tissue autoregulatory processes would induce arteriolar constriction to raise the peripheral vascular resistance. In time, a thickening of the arteriolar walls may occur, resulting in a sustained elevation in peripheral vascular resistance. An increase in total peripheral vascular resistance is a common underlying problem in patients with primary hypertension.

HUMORAL MECHANISMS

At least three possible humoral abnormalities may be responsible for causing primary hypertension in some individuals. One involves the renin–angiotensin–aldosterone system (RAS), which has been well described. Another entails the presence of a natriuretic hormone that modulates sodium transport. A third is associated with the possible link between hyperinsulinemia and hypertension.

The RAS is important to the regulation of sodium, potassium, and fluid balance, and it significantly influences vascular tone and sympathetic nervous system activity. Of course, all of these factors contribute to blood pressure homeostasis.

In the kidney, renin is synthesized and stored in the juxtaglomerular cells, which are located primarily in the media of the renal afferent arterioles. Several factors are known to control renin release. These can be grouped into intrarenal factors (such as perfusion pressure, catecholamines, angiotensin II) and extrarenal factors (such as sodium, chloride, and potassium).

The juxtaglomerular cell functions as a baroreceptor sensing device in the afferent arteriole. Decreased perfusion pressure leads to an increase in renin secretion. The juxtaglomerular apparatus also contains a group of specialized distal tubule cells referred to collectively as the macula densa. The flux of sodium and chloride across the cells influences renin release. A decrease in the amount of sodium and chloride delivered in the distal tubule stimulates renin release.

Angiotensin II has been shown to directly inhibit the release of renin through negative feedback. Catecholamines increase renin release probably by directly stimulating the juxtaglomerular cells through an action involving the formation of cyclic AMP. Both potassium and calcium may also play a direct role in renin release. Decreased serum potassium or intracellular calcium stimulates renin release by the juxtaglomerular cells.

In blood, renin catalyzes the conversion of angiotensinogen to angiotensin I, which is then converted to angiotensin II by angiotensin-converting enzyme (ACE). Angiotensin II exerts its biological effects in various tissues following binding to specific receptors classified as AT1 or

AT2 subtypes. The AT1 receptor is located in brain, renal, myocardial, vascular, and adrenal tissue. The AT2 receptor is located in adrenal medullary tissue, uterus, and brain. AT1 receptors mediate the majority of responses critical to cardiovascular and renal function. An increase in circulating angiotensin II can cause an elevation in blood pressure through both pressor and volume effects. The pressor effects of angiotensin II include direct vasoconstriction, stimulation of catecholamine release from the adrenal medulla, and a centrally mediated increase in sympathetic nervous system activity. Angiotensin II also stimulates the release of aldosterone from the adrenal gland, which leads to retention of both sodium and fluid, with a resultant increase in plasma volume and blood pressure. Clearly, any disturbance in the RAS that leads to an increase in any or all three components could produce hypertension.

The kidney is not the only organ involved in the activation of the RAS. Recent studies have shown that other organs and tissues have the capacity to produce and secrete biologically active forms of angiotensin peptides.

Both the heart and brain contain a local RAS. In the heart, angiotensin II is also generated by a second enzyme, angiotensin I convertase (human chymase), which is not blocked by ACE inhibition. Activation of the myocardial RAS leads to increased cardiac contractility and stimulation of cardiac hypertrophy. The brain RAS has at least two functions. Angiotensin II modulates the production and release of hypothalamic and pituitary hormones. Angiotensin II also enhances sympathetic outflow from the medulla oblongata.

Local generation of biologically active angiotensin peptides in peripheral tissues may play an important role in the increased vascular resistance often observed in hypertensive individuals. There is also some evidence that angiotensin produced by local tissue may interact with other humoral regulators and endothelium-derived growth factors to stimulate vascular smooth muscle growth and metabolism. This *in situ* generation of angiotensin peptides may, in fact, underlie the development of increased vascular resistance in forms of hypertension that are associated with low plasma renin activity. Components of tissue RAS may be responsible for long-term adaptation to hypertension (i.e., left ventricular hypertrophy, smooth muscle hypertrophy of blood vessels, and glomerular hypertrophy).

Another humoral factor that may be involved in the development of primary hypertension is the increased concentration of natriuretic hormone. The proposed role of natriuretic hormone is to inhibit Na^+/K^+-ATPase and, thus, to interfere with sodium transport across cell membranes. It has been suggested that an inherited defect in the kidney's ability to eliminate sodium would cause an increase in extracellular fluid and plasma volume as discussed earlier. This may cause a compensatory increase in the concentration of circulating natriuretic hormone, which would increase urinary excretion of sodium and water. This same hormone, however, is also thought to block the active transport of sodium out of arteriolar smooth muscle cells. The increased intracellular concentration of sodium would ultimately lead to increased vascular tone and hypertension.

Evidence linking insulin resistance and hyperinsulinemia to the development of hypertension is mounting. Several possibilities by which hyperinsulinemia may lead to hypertension include renal sodium retention, enhanced sympathetic nervous system activity, and induction of vascular smooth muscle hypertrophy. Another possible way by which insulin could raise blood pressure is by increasing intracellular calcium concentration, which leads to increased vascular resistance. Hyperinsulinemia often accompanies upper body obesity, but even nonobese hypertensive individuals have been shown to be insulin resistant, glucose intolerant, and hyperinsulinemic. The mechanism by which insulin resistance and hyperinsulinemia occur in hypertension is unknown. Hyperinsulinemia is also associated with hypertriglyceridemia, which results in a decreased concentration of HDL cholesterol.

VASCULAR ENDOTHELIAL MECHANISMS

The vascular endothelium plays an important role in regulating blood vessel tone. These regulating functions are mediated through a variety of vasoactive substances synthesized by the endothelial cells including prostacyclin, bradykinin, endothelium-derived relaxing factor (nitric oxide), angiotensin II, and endothelin I.

It has been postulated that a deficiency in the local synthesis of vasodilating substances such as prostacyclin, bradykinin, and nitric oxide, or an increase in the production of vasoconstricting substances such as angiotensin II and endothelin I contribute to the pathogenesis of hypertension, atherosclerosis, and other diseases.

INFLUENCE OF DIETARY SODIUM, CALCIUM, AND POTASSIUM ON BLOOD PRESSURE

The evidence linking excess sodium to the development of hypertension is based on both epidemiologic studies and clinical experiments. In general, population studies indicate that high salt intake is associated with a high prevalence of stroke and hypertension and low salt intake is associated with a low prevalence of hypertension. Clinical studies have consistently shown that restriction of salt intake in the diet lowers blood pressure in many (but not all) subjects with hypertension. The exact mechanism by which excess sodium leads to hypertension is not known, but it is thought to be linked to the natriuretic hormone hypothesis discussed before. It has been proposed that an increased sodium intake together with an inherited defect in the kidney's ability to excrete sodium leads to a substantial increase in circulating natriuretic hormone. As previously mentioned, natriuretic hormone inhibits intracellular sodium transport, which causes increased vascular reactivity and, consequently, a rise in blood pressure.

Altered calcium homeostasis may also play an important role in the pathogenesis of hypertension. The calcium hypothesis states that a lack of calcium in the diet leads to a disturbance in the balance between intracellular and extracellular calcium. This imbalance is characterized by an increased intracellular concentration of calcium, which leads to altered vascular smooth muscle function and increased peripheral vascular resistance. Some studies have shown that supplementing the diet with calcium results in a modest decrease in the blood pressure of hypertensive subjects. More research is needed to clarify the role of altered calcium homeostasis in causing hypertension in humans.

The role of potassium fluctuations is also inadequately understood. Potassium depletion may cause an increase in peripheral vascular resistance, but the clinical impact of small changes in the serum potassium concentration is not clearly defined. Furthermore, very limited data have suggested that potassium supplementation is associated with a reduced incidence of stroke, but this issue needs further study before supplementation can be endorsed.

Clinical Presentation[3,4,11,15,26]

Patients with uncomplicated, primary hypertension are usually asymptomatic initially. While a complete history and physical examination may help identify concerns that warrant further evaluation, a few basic tests should be performed in all hypertensive patients prior to initiating drug therapy. These include hemoglobin and hematocrit, urinalysis, serum potassium and creatinine, liver function tests, and electrocardiogram. Total and high-density-lipoprotein cholesterol, plasma glucose, and serum uric acid are indicated to assess other risk factors and to develop baseline data for monitoring drug-induced metabolic changes. As the hypertension progresses, however, symptoms characteristic of cardiovascular, cerebrovascular, or renal disease may occur as the patient develops target organ damage. Patients with secondary hypertension usually complain of symptoms suggestive of the underlying disorder. For example, many patients with pheochromocytoma have a history of paroxysmal headaches, sweating, tachycardia, and palpitations occurring singly or in combinations. More than half of the patients with this form of secondary hypertension suffer episodes of orthostatic dizziness or syncope. In primary aldosteronism, hypokalemic symptoms usually manifest including muscle cramps and muscle weakness. Patients who present with hypertension secondary to Cushing's syndrome may complain of weight gain, polyuria, edema, menstrual irregularities, recurrent acne, or muscular weakness.

Frequently, the only sign of primary hypertension is an elevated blood pressure. The rest of the physical examination may be completely normal. Again, as the hypertension progresses, signs of end-organ damage begin to appear. These are chiefly related to pathologic changes in the eye, brain, heart, kidneys, and peripheral blood vessels.

The funduscopic exam may reveal arteriolar narrowing reflective of increased peripheral vascular resistance and/or arteriovenous nicking, which is a consequence of long-standing arteriosclerosis. Retinal hemorrhages and infarcts reflect serious vasculitis secondary to high arterial blood pressure indicative of accelerated hypertension. Papilledema in hypertensive patients suggests a malignant stage of high blood pressure requiring rapid treatment.

The neurologic examination will reveal gross neurologic deficits in patients with previous cerebral infarcts or occasional encephalopathy. A slight hemiparesis with some incoordination and hyperreflexia may also be found upon careful neurologic examination.

Auscultation of the heart may identify an accentuated second heart sound (S_2) created by a high intra-aortic diastolic pressure, a systolic ejection murmur caused by a hyperdynamic state, an S_4 gallop rhythm indicative of decreased ventricular compliance, or an S_3 gallop sound associated with congestive heart failure.

The physical examination may provide clues for diagnosing secondary hypertension. For example, patients with coarctation of the aorta may have diminished or even absent femoral pulses and patients with renal artery stenosis may have an abdominal systolic–diastolic bruit. Of course, patients with Cushing's syndrome may have the classic physical features (i.e., moon face, buffalo hump, hirsutism, abdominal striae, etc.) that characterize individuals with this endocrine disorder.

Certain routine laboratory tests may help identify patients with secondary hypertension. A low serum potassium before antihypertensive therapy is begun may suggest mineralocorticoid-induced hypertension. The presence of protein, blood cells, and casts in the urine may indicate an underlying parenchymal kidney disease as the cause of hypertension.

More specific laboratory tests are used to diagnose secondary hypertension. These include plasma norepinephrine and urinary metanephrine for pheochromocytoma, plasma and urinary aldosterone levels for primary aldosteronism, and plasma renin activity, captopril stimulation test, renal vein renins, and renal artery angiography for renovascular disease.

BLOOD PRESSURE MEASUREMENT

The usual, indirect method of measuring blood pressure is with the sphygmomanometer cuff on the patient's arm at the level of the heart. It is important to use a proper size cuff to avoid overestimating the actual pressure when the cuff is too small. The inflatable rubber bag should encircle at least 80% of the arm and the width of the cuff should be at least two-thirds the length of the upper arm.

Proper technique requires rapid inflation of the cuff to about 30 mm Hg above the point at which the radial pulse disappears, and then released at a rate of 2 to 3 mm Hg per second. As the pressure falls, the Korotkoff sounds become audible through the bell of the stethoscope applied over the brachial artery in the antecubital fossa. The first sounds consist of clear tapping sounds. Systolic blood pressure should be recorded at the level the first tapping sound is heard. Diastolic blood pressure should be read at the moment all sounds disappear (i.e., at the fifth Korotkoff phase).

It should be emphasized that a single reading of blood pressure elevation does not constitute a diagnosis of hypertension. If the blood pressure taken on two or more subsequent days is 140/90 mm Hg or higher, then a diagnosis of hypertension is confirmed.

Several factors, in addition to those mentioned previously, may give misleading blood pressure measurements. A falsely high blood pressure may be recorded in elderly patients with a rigid, calcified brachial artery. This is one cause of pseudohypertension, because the actual pressure as determined by direct intra-arterial measurement is much lower than that obtained by the indirect cuff method. To test for this cause of pseudohypertension, the blood pressure cuff should be inflated above peak systolic blood pressure. If the radial artery remains palpable, the patient has rigid arteries. This is known as a positive Osler's maneuver.

The occurrence of an "auscultatory gap" in some patients may result in an erroneous underestimation of systolic or overestimation of diastolic measurement. As the cuff pressure falls from the true systolic value, the Korotkoff sound may sequentially disappear (a false diastolic measurement), "reappear" (a false systolic measurement), and then disappear again at the true diastolic value. A third factor that may produce misleading values is an irregular ventricular rate. Because systolic and diastolic pressures may vary from one heartbeat to the next, the correct recording of the patient's blood pressure requires that the highest and lowest systolic and diastolic values be carefully identified and then averaged to yield a "mean" systolic and a "mean" diastolic value. In all instances, it is recommended that the stethoscope bell, rather than the diaphragm, be used. Otherwise, the low-frequency Korotkoff sounds may not be heard clearly and accurately, especially if the patient has faint or "distant" sounds.

Blood pressure varies with environmental temperature, the time of day, the timing of meals, physical activity, posture, and emotions. An individual who exhibits a defense reflex in a medical setting may experience a rise in blood pressure that returns to normal outside the medical setting. This is known as "white coat" or "office" hypertension. White coat hypertension appears to occur in approximately 20% of newly diagnosed hypertensive patients. Interestingly, such a rise in blood pressure gradually dissipates over several hours after leaving the office and usually is not precipitated by other stresses in the patient's daily life. "Office" hypertension is more likely to occur in young, female patients who do not have a long history of hypertension. Suspected "office" hypertension is one of a limited number of indications for which ambulatory blood pressure monitoring may be warranted. Recently the National High Blood Pressure Education Program Coordinating Committee published a report from their working group on ambulatory blood pressure monitoring. This report reviewed the technical, logistic, and financial constraints of utilizing currently available 24-hour blood pressure monitoring systems. Although it appears that a patient's 24-hour blood pressure profile correlates better with end-organ damage than do casual office measurements, current limitations prohibit routine use of such technology. For a more thorough discussion of this area, the reader is referred to the committee's report.[27]

NATURAL COURSE

Early in the course of primary hypertension, the blood pressure may fluctuate between abnormal and normal levels. This stage of the disease is usually referred to as labile hypertension. It may begin as early as the second decade of life. During this stage, many patients have a hyperdynamic circulation with increased cardiac output and normal or even low peripheral vascular resistance.

As the disease progresses, peripheral vascular resistance increases and patients develop a sustained increase in blood pressure. In most cases the diastolic blood pressure does not exceed 115 mm Hg. Individuals with secondary hypertension are more likely to experience severe elevations in blood pressure. Only a small proportion of patients suffering from primary hypertension develop accelerated or severe hypertension.

The main causes of death in hypertensive subjects are cerebrovascular accidents, cardiovascular events, and renal failure. The probability of premature death from any of these causes increases with increasing systolic or diastolic blood pressure.

Hypertension accelerates atherosclerosis and stimulates left ventricular and vascular hypertrophy. These pathologic changes are thought to be secondary to both a chronic pressure overload and a variety of nonhemodynamic stimuli. Some of the nonhemodynamic disturbances that have been implicated in the pathogenesis of cardiac and vascular hypertrophy include the adrenergic and renin–angiotensin systems, increased synthesis and secretion of endothelin I, and a decreased production of prostacyclin and endothelial-derived relaxing factor. The mechanisms of accelerated atherogenesis in hypertension include proliferation of smooth muscle cells, lipid infiltration into the vascular endothelium, and an enhancement of vascular calcium accumulation.

The target organ damage secondary to chronic hypertension principally involves the brain, the eye, the heart, and the kidney.

Hypertension is the major cause of stroke. The types of cerebrovascular lesions most commonly seen in hypertensive individuals include lacunar infarcts caused by thrombotic occlusion of small vessels, intracerebral hemorrhage resulting from ruptured microaneurysms, and transient ischemic attacks secondary to atherosclerotic diseases in the carotid arteries.

The damage hypertension does to the eye is characterized by a variety of retinopathies. Nonspecific changes include an increased light reflex, increased tortuosity of vessels, and arteriovenous nicking. These are all associated with the accelerated arteriosclerosis that accompanies hypertension. Focal arteriolar narrowing, retinal infarcts, and flame-shaped hemorrhages are usually pathognomonic of an accelerated or malignant phase of hypertension and are associated with increased arteriolar resistance and fibrinoid necrosis. Papilledema is a swelling of the optic disc and is caused by a breakdown in autoregulation of capillary blood flow in the presence of high pressure.

The principal cardiac complications of hypertension are left ventricular hypertrophy, coronary heart disease, and congestive heart failure. These complications may lead to cardiac arrhythmias, angina, myocardial infarction, and sudden death. Coronary heart disease is the most common cause of death in hypertensive patients.

The renal damage caused by hypertension is pathologically characterized by hyaline arteriosclerosis, hyperplastic arteriosclerosis, arteriolar hypertrophy, fibrinoid necrosis, and atheroma of the major renal arteries. Glomerular hyperfiltration and intraglomerular hypertension may be the earliest stage of hypertensive nephropathy followed by microalbuminuria and a gradual decline in renal function. It is also associated with a greater likelihood of left ventricular hypertrophy and may, therefore, be an indication for echocardiographic evaluation. Frank renal failure is rare unless accelerated hypertension occurs in which fibrinoid necrosis of renal arterioles is the pathologic hallmark. The primary renal complication in hypertension is nephrosclerosis, which is secondary to accelerated arteriosclerosis. Atheromatous disease of a major renal artery may give rise to renal artery stenosis. Although renal failure is an uncommon complication of essential hypertension, it remains an important cause of end-stage renal disease, especially in blacks.

TREATMENT

The treatment plan for hypertension should include measures to minimize contributing factors and to reduce or prevent other known risk factors. Obesity, hyperlipidemia, glucose intolerance, excessive salt intake, cigarette smoking, and alcohol consumption are important risk factors that should be addressed in formulating a rational antihypertensive treatment program.

It seems reasonable that the first step in the treatment of hypertension would consist of a carefully constructed, aggressively promoted modification in lifestyle. A sensible dietary program should be designed for gradual weight reduction, if appropriate, and for reducing the saturated fat and salt content of the diet. The rationale for dietary treatment of hypertension is based on the following observations and facts:

1. Hypertension is two to three times more prevalent in overweight as compared to lean persons.
2. Sixty percent of hypertensive persons are overweight.
3. Weight loss, even as little as 10 pounds, decreases blood pressure in 60–80% of hypertensive, overweight individuals.
4. Upper body obesity is associated with insulin resistance and hyperinsulinemia. Hyperinsulinemia may be involved in the pathogenesis of hypertension as well as hyperlipidemia.
5. Diets low in total fat intake and a high polyunsaturated/saturated ratio have been shown to lower blood pressure in hypertensive individuals. Moreover, reducing the saturated fat and cholesterol content of the diet is indicated as the initial step in the management of hyperlipidemia. Hyperlipidemia is a major independent risk factor in coronary heart disease. This risk is compounded in hypertensive people.
6. Thirty to 60% of hypertensive patients are salt sensitive. In this group, blood pressure will fall by an average of 10 mm Hg if salt intake is reduced from 12 g daily to 6 g daily.

In addition to these dietary measures, it is also important to reduce the intake of alcohol, because excessive alcohol intake may either cause or worsen hypertension. Hypertensive patients who drink alcoholic beverages should restrict their intake to one ounce or less per day. One ounce of alcohol is contained in 2 ounces of 100 proof whiskey, 8 ounces of wine, or 24 ounces of beer. Since cigarette smoking is another major independent risk factor of coronary heart disease, patients who smoke should undergo counseling and take advantage of any available smoking cessation programs.

Another useful lifestyle modification for hypertensive patients is a carefully designed program of regular physical exercise. Studies have shown that aerobic exercise, such as jogging, swimming, walking, and bicycling, can reduce blood pressure even in the absence of weight loss. Patients should consult their physicians before starting an exercise program.

The coexistence of hypertension and diabetes mellitus occurs more than chance alone would predict. This fact has led some to propose that these two chronic conditions may share a common etiologic factor. As stated earlier, insulin resistance may play a role in the pathogenesis of hypertension. Insulin resistance is, of course, an important pathogenic lesion in non-insulin-dependent diabetes mellitus. Just what causes insulin resistance to occur in the first place in either diabetes or hypertension is not known. Any intervention that increases insulin resistance or glucose intolerance may adversely affect control of blood pressure. Conversely, measures that ameliorate insulin resistance or reduce glucose intolerance should help in the overall management of hypertension.[28]

One of the major independent risk factors associated with the development of coronary heart disease, congestive heart failure, and sudden death in hypertensive patients is left ventricular hypertrophy (LVH). In past years, the prevalence of LVH was considerably underestimated because its detection depended on electrocardiographic interpretation. The electrocardiogram is a very insensitive method for detecting LVH. The echocardiogram, however, is a much more sensitive way to identify LVH, and estimates in untreated mildly to moderately hypertensive patients exceed 50%. The presence of LVH in hypertensive patients is associated with a fourfold or greater risk of cardiovascular events and death. No study has shown that regression of LVH is associated with decreased mortality.[29,30]

The results of prospective, randomized trials have shown conclusively that control of blood pressure reduces the incidence of stroke and congestive heart failure, but failed to confirm a reduction in coronary heart disease morbidity and mortality. Since hypertension is a major independent risk factor for coronary heart disease, there must be some explanation as to why controlling blood pressure has not reduced the incidence of cardiac disease and death. It is tempting to speculate that either adverse drug effects or inadequate attention to controlling other risk factors, or both, are responsible for this unexpected pharmacologic failure. With regard to adverse drug effects, the negative impact that diuretics and β blockers have on serum lipids and glucose tolerance may be sufficient to offset their beneficial effects on blood pressure. It is interesting to note that to date all major clinical trials have employed either a diuretic or β blocker as the initial antihypertensive pharmacologic treatment. It is not known whether or not other antihypertensive agents will confer either a reduction in coronary heart disease mortality or the incidence of stroke and CHF. Proper controlled trials are needed to address this important question. ACE inhibitors have been shown to decrease mortality in post-MI patients.[31]

In summary, the treatment of hypertension should be designed to reduce the blood pressure and other risk factors of coronary heart disease. A rational therapeutic regimen begins with effective lifestyle modifications including a sensible diet, smoking cessation, and abstinence from or restriction of alcoholic beverages. Pharmacologic therapy should be individualized based on a patient's age, race, known pathophysiologic variables, and concurrent conditions. Treatment should be designed not only to lower blood pressure safely and effectively, but also to avoid or reverse hyperlipidemia, glucose intolerance, and left ventricular hypertrophy.

Antihypertensive drugs may be divided into eight classes: diuretics, central α_2 agonists, adrenergic inhibitors, β blockers, ACE inhibitors, calcium channel blockers, vasodilators, and postganglionic sympathetic inhibitors. Drug selection should be based on safety, efficacy, cost, and the presence of concomitant diseases and other risk factors.

DIURETICS[3,4,19–21,32–34]

There are four classes of diuretics: carbonic anhydrase inhibitors, thiazide and thiazide-like agents, loop diuretics, and potassium-sparing diuretics. In general, carbonic anhydrase inhibitors are weak antihypertensive agents and therefore are not used in the treatment of hypertension. The potassium-sparing diuretics are also weak antihypertensive agents when used alone, but provide an additive hypotensive effect when used in combination with thiazide or loop diuretics. Moreover, they counteract the potassium- and magnesium-losing properties of other diuretic agents.

In patients with adequate renal function (i.e., a glomerular filtration rate greater than 30 mL/min), thiazide diuretics appear to be more effective hypotensive agents than loop diuretics such as furosemide. As renal function declines, however, sodium and fluid accumulate and the use of a more potent diuretic is necessary to counter the effects that volume and sodium expansion have on arterial blood pressure.

All thiazide diuretics are equally effective in lowering blood pressure. The major differences between the various thiazides are the serum half-life and the duration of diuretic effect. These differences may not be clinically relevant, however, because the serum half-life of most antihypertensive agents does not correlate with the hypotensive duration of action. Moreover, diuretics may lower blood pressure primarily through extrarenal mechanisms.

Mechanism of Action

The exact hypotensive mode of action of diuretics is not known. Of course, acutely, diuretics lower blood pressure by causing a diuresis. The reduction in plasma volume and stroke volume associated with a diuresis decreases cardiac output and, consequently, blood pressure. The initial drop in cardiac output produced by the diuresis causes a compensatory increase in peripheral vascular resistance. With continuing diuretic therapy, the extracellular fluid volume and plasma volume return almost to pretreatment levels, and peripheral vascular resistance falls below its pretreatment baseline. It is the reduction in peripheral vascular resistance that accompanies chronic use of diuretics that is responsible for their long-term hypotensive effectiveness.

Evidently, diuretic-induced total body sodium depletion is necessary for blood pressure reduction, because a high dietary sodium intake can reverse the antihypertensive effect and a low salt intake will potentiate the effect of diuretics on blood pressure.

It has been postulated that thiazide diuretics lower blood pressure by mobilizing sodium and water from arteriolar walls. This action would lessen the amount of physical encroachment on the lumen of the vessel created by excessive accumulation of intracellular fluid. Of course, as the diameter of the lumen increases (opens up), there is less resistance to the flow of blood through the vessel (i.e., peripheral vascular resistance drops).

Another postulated hypotensive mechanism of action stems from the possible association between changes in the electrolyte composition of intra-arteriolar walls and vascular responsiveness. The alterations in sodium, potassium, calcium, and magnesium intracellular concentrations may decrease vascular response to pressor substances and increase vascular response to depressor substances.

Still another possible antihypertensive mode of action of the thiazide diuretics is direct relaxation of vascular smooth muscle. This theory is based on the known mechanism of action of diazoxide, a chemical closely related to the thiazide diuretics. Diazoxide is a direct vasodilator, and it is possible that the thiazide diuretics exert a similar action.

When diuretics are used in combination with other antihypertensive agents, an additive hypotensive effect is usually observed. This occurs as a result of two independent pharmacodynamic properties. First, it is a well-known pharmacologic principle that when two drugs cause the same effect through different mechanisms of action, their combined use results in an additive or synergistic response. Second, many nondiuretic antihypertensive agents induce salt and water retention, which, of course, is counteracted by the concurrent use of a diuretic.

Side Effects

The side effects of thiazide diuretics include hypokalemia, hypomagnesemia, hypercalcemia, hyperuricemia, hyperglycemia, hyperlipidemia, and sexual dysfunction. Loop diuretics may cause the same side effects, although the effect on serum lipids and glucose is not as significant and hypocalcemia may occur. Short-term studies indicate that indapamide does not adversely effect lipids or glucose tolerance, or cause sexual dysfunction.

The hypokalemia and hypomagnesemia caused by diuretics may lead to cardiac arrhythmias in susceptible patients. Patients at greatest risk are those receiving digitalis therapy, those with left ventricular hypertrophy, and those with ischemic heart disease. There is considerable controversy as to whether or not diuretic-induced electrolyte disturbances in patients with uncomplicated hypertension are clinically significant.

A couple of measures can be taken to help prevent the development of hypokalemia in patients on diuretic therapy. The first measure is the use of low doses of diuretic, such as 12.5–25 mg of hydrochlorothiazide daily or 25 mg of chlorthalidone daily. The propensity for diuretics to cause hypokalemia is dose dependent. A second measure is reduction of the amount of sodium and augmentation of the amount of potassium in the diet. Low-sodium diets alone result in a marked increase in renal conservation of potassium. A number of foods and beverages rich in potassium (e.g., spinach, banana, dried apricots, and orange juice) can be generously incorporated into the diet as a further measure to prevent diuretic-induced hypokalemia. Another source of increased potassium and decreased sodium derives from the use of salt substitutes. Salt substitutes should be used with caution in patients who are on potassium-sparing diuretics, ACE inhibitors, or nonsteroidal anti-inflammatory drugs (NSAIDs).

If hypokalemia occurs despite these preventive measures, the use of a potassium chloride supplement or a potassium-sparing diuretic is indicated. Most clinicians prefer potassium chloride when aggressive repletion is indicated. For chronic management of milder degrees of hypokalemia, however, either approach may be employed. Whether a given patient will respond better to potassium chloride or a potassium-sparing diuretic is not predictable; but individual responses may be partially influenced by the ability of potassium-sparing diuretics to conserve magnesium as well.

A variety of potassium supplements are available; some are better tolerated than others. The appropriate use of potassium supplements to correct diuretic-induced hypokalemia calls for the chloride salt, 40–60 mEq of potassium per day, and, of course, the patient's compliance with the regimen. One of the sustained-release potassium chloride preparations is generally better tolerated than the liquid preparations.

It may take several months to correct completely a diuretic-induced total body potassium deficit, despite the fact that the serum potassium rapidly returns to normal. It seems prudent to continue the daily supplement of 40–60 mEq for 2 to 3 months while monitoring the serum potassium concentration. In some cases, the same daily dose of potassium chloride can be continued as long as the patient is on diuretics. In other cases, it may be possible to reduce the dosage.

Diuretic-induced hyperuricemia may produce gouty arthritis or uric acid stones, especially in individuals who are predisposed to gout. In patients with no previous history of gout, acute gouty arthritis and nephrolithiasis are extremely unlikely consequences of diuretic-induced hyperuricemia. If some manifestation of gout does occur in a patient who requires diuretic therapy for effective treatment of hypertension, allopurinol or a uricosuric agent can be given to prevent recurrent gouty attacks without compromising the antihypertensive effects of the diuretic.

Chronic use of thiazide diuretic therapy may alter glucose metabolism in at least two ways. First, a diuretic-induced deficiency of potassium and magnesium may lead to a reduction in postprandial insulin secretion. Second, long-term diuretic therapy may result in the development of insulin resistance. Either of these mechanisms may contribute to the production of diabetes in prediabetic individuals and worsening of metabolic control in diabetic patients. Since glucose intolerance is an additional risk factor in coronary heart disease, diuretic therapy in prediabetic or diabetic hypertensives must be used with caution.

The effect thiazide diuretics have on serum lipid concentrations is debatable. Some studies show only a transient increase in total cholesterol and triglycerides. Others show a persistent adverse effect. There are two proposed mechanisms by which diuretics may increase serum lipids. One involves the production of insulin resistance. Insulin resistance leads to basal hyperinsulinemia, which, in turn, leads to an increased synthesis and release of triglycerides. The other mechanism is related to the fact that diuretics may increase serum catecholamine concentrations. Catecholamines enhance the hepatic synthesis of cholesterol. If further research indicates that these adverse lipid effects of thiazide diuretics are persistent, then their routine use in the treatment of hypertension will have to be seriously questioned.

Potassium-sparing diuretics have the potential for causing hyperkalemia, especially in patients with renal insufficiency or diabetes, and in patients receiving concurrent treatment with an ACE inhibitor, NSAIDs, or potassium supplements. The potassium-sparing drug spironolactone may cause gynecomastia.

CENTRAL α_2-RECEPTOR AGONISTS[13–15,19,20,32]

Clonidine, guanabenz, guanfacine, and methyldopa all lower blood pressure primarily by stimulating α_2-adrenergic receptors in the brain. Such action leads to a reduction in sympathetic outflow from the vasomotor center in the brain and an associated increase in vagal tone. It is also possible that stimulation of presynaptic α_2 receptors peripherally may contribute to the reduction in sympathetic tone. As a consequence of reduced sympathetic activity together with some enhancement of parasympathetic activity, heart rate is decreased, cardiac output decreases slightly, total peripheral resistance is lowered, plasma renin activity is reduced, and baroreceptor reflexes are blunted.

Chronic use of the centrally acting α agonists results in sodium and fluid retention, which appears to be most prominent with methyldopa. Low doses of either clonidine, guanfacine, or guanabenz can be used to treat mild hypertension without the addition of a diuretic; however, methyldopa, even at low doses, usually leads to enough sodium and fluid accumulation that tolerance to its hypotensive effect soon develops in the absence of concurrent diuretic therapy.

Sedation and dry mouth are common side effects of these antihypertensive agents. These symptoms may diminish or completely abate with chronic use of low doses. As with other centrally acting antihypertensive drugs, these agents may cause depression.

Abrupt cessation of any antihypertensive agent may lead to rebound hypertension or overshoot hypertension. Rebound hypertension is characterized by a sudden increase in blood pressure to the pretreatment level, whereas overshoot implies an increase in excess of the pretreatment level. In most cases, abrupt withdrawal of antihypertensive therapy leads to a gradual increase in blood pressure. Rebound hypertension may rarely occur when a central α-receptor agonist is stopped. This is thought to occur secondary to a compensatory increase in norepinephrine release that follows a discontinuation of presynaptic α-receptor stimulation. The propensity for this is increased in patients receiving concurrent β-blocker therapy due to unopposed α-receptor stimulation.

In addition to the side effects already mentioned, methyldopa rarely may cause hepatitis or hemolytic anemia. A transient elevation in liver function tests is occasionally associated with methyldopa therapy and is clinically unimportant. But a persistent increase in serum transaminases or alkaline phosphatase may herald the onset of a fulminant hepatitis, which can be fatal. A Coombs'-positive hemolytic anemia occurs in less than 1% of patients receiving methyldopa, although 20% exhibit a positive direct Coombs' test without anemia.

One recent pharmaceutical advance that may be associated with fewer side effects and increased compliance is the transdermal delivery system for clonidine. This device, which is applied to the skin and left in place 1 week before being replaced, appears to reduce blood pressure while avoiding the high peak serum drug concentrations that are seen with oral dosing and are thought to contribute to the adverse effects. The delivery system is ideal for patients who cannot take medication by mouth, such as the perioperative patient. The disadvantages of this system are cost, a 20% incidence of local skin rash or irritation, and a 2- or 3-day delay of onset of effect so that oral medications should be overlapped for this period of time when patch therapy is first started. A similar delay in "offset" of action also may be seen when the patch is removed and the blood pressure returns to pretreatment values over a 2- or 3-day period.

PERIPHERAL α_1-RECEPTOR BLOCKERS[3,4,13–15,19,20,32]

Prazosin, terazosin, and doxazosin are selective α_1-receptor blockers. These selective α_1 blockers differ from phentolamine and phenoxybenzamine in that the latter block both α_1 and α_2 receptors. The severe reflex tachycardia associated with the use of nonselective α blockers renders them of no value in the treatment of essential hypertension. They are, however, useful for the initial management of pheochromocytoma. Since the selective α blockers do not alter α_2-receptor activity, they do not usually cause reflex tachycardia.

At low doses, selective α blockers may be used as monotherapy in the treatment of mild hypertension. At higher doses, and sometimes with chronic administration of even low doses, fluid and sodium accumulate and concurrent diuretic therapy is then required to maintain the hypotensive efficacy of the α-receptor blocker.

Even though the antihypertensive effect of these drugs is achieved through a peripheral mechanism of action, they do cross the blood–brain barrier and may cause CNS side effects such as lassitude, vivid dreams, and depression. The most interesting side effect of selective α_1 blockers is the so-called "first-dose phenomenon." This is characterized by transient dizziness or faintness, palpitations, and even syncope occurring within 1–3 hours of the first dose, or subsequently after the first increased dose. These episodes are accompanied by orthostatic hypotension and can be obviated by having the patient take the first dose, and first increased dose, at bedtime. Occasionally, orthostatic dizziness persists with chronic administration. α_1 Blockers are rarely associated with urinary incontinence and may be of value in patients with prostatic hypertrophy.

β-ADRENOCEPTOR BLOCKERS[3,4,13–15,19,20,32–36]

The hypotensive mechanism of β-adrenoceptor blockers (β blockers) is not exactly known. Several mechanisms of action have been proposed, but none of them has been shown to be consistently associated with a reduction in arterial blood pressure.

Beta blockers reduce cardiac output through their negative chronotropic and inotropic effects on the heart. It is reasonable to postulate that drugs that lower cardiac output lower blood pressure, because blood pressure is the product of cardiac output and peripheral vascular resistance; however, even though cardiac output is reduced after both intravenous and oral administration of propranolol therapy, blood pressure falls only when propranolol is given orally. Furthermore, cardiac output falls to the same degree in patients whose blood pressure is not lowered by these drugs as in patients who respond with a fall in blood pressure. Finally, β blockers with intrinsic sympathomimetic activity do not reduce cardiac output in the resting state and yet they lower blood pressure and decrease peripheral resistance.

Another possible explanation of the hypotensive action of β blockers is related to a central action. Within the brain there are both α and β receptors. Stimulation of α_2-adrenergic receptors causes a reduction in sympathetic outflow from the vasomotor center. It seems plausible that blocking β-adrenergic receptors in the brain might produce the same effect. All β blockers traverse the blood–brain barrier, but the extent to which they enter the brain depends on their degree of lipophilicity. At one end of the spectrum is propranolol, a highly lipophilic drug; at the other end is atenolol, which is weakly lipophilic. One would therefore expect a much higher concentration of propranolol in the brain than atenolol after equivalent doses of the two drugs are given, and this indeed is the case. Despite this difference in CNS concentration, there is no difference in their hypotensive effectiveness. Of course, one cannot rule out the possibility that CNS β blockade is optimally achieved with atenolol even though it penetrates the blood–brain barrier much more poorly than propranolol.

Blockade of β adrenoceptors located on the surface membranes of juxtaglomerular cells leads to a reduction in the release of renin. This, in turn, may result in the attenuation of the RAS, which should reduce blood pressure. Some studies, in fact, have shown a correlation between pretreatment plasma renin activity and reduction in blood pressure by β-blocker therapy. The higher the plasma renin activity, the greater the reduction in blood pressure. Other studies, however, have not shown an association between pretreatment plasma renin activity and degree of blood pressure reduction achieved by β blockers. Furthermore, some β blockers (e.g., pindolol, acebutolol) lower blood pressure without reducing plasma renin levels. Therefore, alternative or additional mechanisms need to be invoked to account for the antihypertensive effect of β-adrenoceptor blocking agents.

It has been suggested that a peripheral mechanism common to all β blockers may be responsible for the long-term reduction in blood pressure. The proposed peripheral mechanism involves the possible presence of β adrenoceptors on the surface of sympathetic neuronal endings. Blocking these presynaptic β receptors could lead to a reduction in the release of norepinephrine into the synaptic cleft. This intriguing hypothesis is based on the theory that norepinephrine release from neuronal endings is regulated to some extent by presynaptic adrenergic feedback loops. Stimulation of presynaptic α_2 receptors would provoke a negative inhibition on the release of norepinephrine, whereas stimulation of presynaptic β receptors would engender a positive-feedback increase in norepinephrine release. If presynaptic β receptors do indeed exist, blocking them would interrupt the positive-feedback loop and thus reduce the release of norepinephrine from the neuronal ending. A diminution in the release of norepinephrine from peripheral sympathetic nerve endings should lower blood pressure.

Pharmacodynamics/Pharmacokinetics

Even though there are important pharmacodynamic and pharmacokinetic differences among the various β blockers (Table 12.1), there is no difference in their clinical antihypertensive efficacy. Three pharmacodynamic properties of the β blockers differentiate them to some extent. The first of these is cardioselectivity. Beta blockers that possess a much greater affinity for β_1 receptors than β_2 receptors are said to be *cardioselective*. The β_1 and β_2 adrenoceptors are distributed throughout the body, but in certain organs and tissues β_1 receptors predominate and in other organs and tissues β_2 receptors predominate. There is a preponderance of β_1 receptors in the heart and kidney and a preponderance of β_2 receptors in the lungs, liver, pancreas, and arteriolar smooth muscle. Stimulation of β_1 receptors produces an increase in heart rate, contractility, and renin release. β_2-Receptor stimulation results in bronchodilation and vasodilation. Beta-adrenergic blockers that bind more avidly to β_1 receptors than to β_2 receptors are therefore less likely to provoke bronchospasm and vasoconstriction. Also, because both insulin secretion and glycogenolysis are adrenergically mediated, blockade of β_2 receptors may reduce either process and cause hyperglycemia or blunt recovery from hypoglycemia, respectively.

At low doses, bisoprolol, metoprolol, atenolol, and acebutolol are cardioselective β blockers. For this reason they may be safer than nonselective β blockers to use in patients with asthma, chronic obstructive pulmonary disease (COPD), peripheral vascular disease, and diabetes; however, it should be pointed out that cardioselectivity is a dose-dependent phenomenon. At higher doses, metoprolol, bisoprolol, atenolol, and acebutolol lose their relative selectivity for β_1 receptors and block β_2 receptors as effectively as they block β_1 receptors. The dose at which cardioselectivity is lost varies from patient to patient.

Another pharmacodynamic difference among the β blockers is the intrinsic sympathomimetic activity (ISA) that pindolol, penbutolol, carteolol, and acebutolol possess. These four β blockers are partial β-receptor agonists and are capable therefore of maintaining normal basal sympathetic tone while blocking the effects of excessive adrenergic stimulation. Unlike cardioselectivity, this property is manifested at all dosage levels and varies in significance only with the intrinsic sympathetic tone. When sympathetic tone is low, as it is during resting states, β receptors are partially stimulated. Therefore, resting heart rate, cardiac output, and peripheral blood flow are not reduced when receptors are blocked. Theoretically, pindolol, penbutolol, carteolol, and acebutolol would be less hazardous β blockers to use in patients with borderline congestive heart failure, sinus bradycardia, or perhaps even peripheral vascular disease; however, clinical studies have not confirmed a clear-cut advantage in patients with the aforementioned disorders.

All β blockers are capable of exerting a membrane-stabilizing action on cardiac cells if large enough doses are given. It was once thought that this membrane-stabilizing or quinidine-like effect was responsible for the antidysrhythmic effect of β blockers (see Chapter 16). It is now known that the effectiveness of β blockers in treating or preventing cardiac dysrhythmias is due primarily to their β-blockade property. Only propranolol, sotolol, and acebutolol are indicated for arrhythmias. The dose of β blockers

TABLE 12.1. PHARMACODYNAMIC AND PHARMACOKINETIC PROPERTIES OF THE β-ADRENOCEPTOR BLOCKING AGENTS

	α_1 Blockade	β_1 Selectivity	MSA[a]	ISA[a]	Lipid Solubility	% Bioavailability	Half-Life (hours)
Acebutolol	0	+	+	+	Low	20–60	3–4
Atenolol	0	+	0	0	Low	50	6–9
Betaxolol	0	+	±	0	Low	100	14–24
Bisoprololol	0	+++	0	0	Low	85	10–12
Carteolol	0	0	0	+	Low	50	6
Labetalol	+	0	+	0	Moderate	40	3–5
Metoprolol	0	+	0	0	Moderate	50	3–4
Nadolol	0	0	0	0	Low	30	14–24
Penbutolol	0	0	0	+	High	100	5
Pindolol	0	0	+	+++	Moderate	100	3–4
Propranolol	0	0	+	0	High	35	4–6
Timolol	0	0	0	0	Low	75	3–4

[a]MSA, membrane stabilizing activity; ISA, intrinsic sympathomimetic activity.

required to achieve membrane-stabilizing activity usually greatly exceeds that used in treating hypertension or cardiac arrhythmias.

Pharmacokinetic differences among β blockers can be found in first-pass metabolism, serum half-lives, degree of lipophilicity, and route of elimination. Propranolol and metoprolol undergo extensive first-pass metabolism. Therefore, the dose required to achieve β blockade with either drug is quite variable from patient to patient. Atenolol and nadolol, which have relatively long half-lives, are renally excreted and the dosage of each may need to be adjusted in patients with renal insufficiency. Even though the half-lives of the other β blockers are much shorter, once-daily administration may still be effective. As is the case with most other antihypertensive agents, the serum half-life does not correlate with the drug's hypotensive duration of action. Beta blockers also vary in terms of their lipophilic properties and thus CNS penetration. One might expect that the more water-soluble β blockers would be less likely to cause CNS side effects. But studies have shown that relative lipid solubility does not reliably predict the neurologic effects of β blockers.[36]

Numerous trials have shown a reduction in mortality and nonfatal reinfarction using β blockers following an acute myocardial infarction. Beta blockers with ISA (with the exception of acebutolol) do not afford this protection and, in fact, may lead to an increased risk of mortality. Thus, in hypertensive patients surviving an acute myocardial infarction, the use of β blockers without ISA may be beneficial not only in reducing blood pressure but also in reducing the risk of myocardial reinfarction and mortality.

Studies in hypertensive patients with LVH show that β blockers reduce blood pressure and produce LVH regression. All β blockers, with the possible exception of pindolol, appear to reduce left ventricular mass, irrespective of their different pharmacodynamic properties. Recent evidence also indicates that β blockers may exhibit antiatherosclerotic effects. Whether such effects are due to a reduction in stress forces at artery bifurcations, alteration in cholesterol binding in the arterial wall, an antiplatelet effect, or other mechanisms is not known at this time.

Side Effects

Most of the side effects of β blockers represent physiologic consequences of antagonizing β adrenoceptors in various organs and tissues. For example, β blockade in the myocardium can be associated with bradycardia, atrioventricular conduction abnormalities, and the development of congestive heart failure. Antagonism of β_2 receptors in the lung may lead to acute exacerbations of bronchospasm in patients with asthma or COPD. Blocking β_2 receptors in arteriolar smooth muscle may aggravate intermittent claudication or Raynaud's phenomenon and may cause cold extremities as a result of decreased peripheral blood flow. In addition, an increase of sympathetic tone during periods of acute stress (or hypoglycemia) may result in a significant increase in blood pressure because of unopposed α-receptor-mediated vasoconstriction.

Abrupt cessation of β-blocker therapy may produce unstable angina, myocardial infarction, or even death in patients predisposed to ischemic myocardial events. For this reason, it is always prudent to gradually taper the dose of β blocker over 14 days before eventually discontinuing the drug. The acute withdrawal syndrome is believed to be secondary to a combination of factors, including progression of underlying coronary artery disease, hypersensitivity of β-adrenergic receptors, and failure to recognize the need to restrict physical activity upon withdrawal of a drug that decreases myocardial oxygen requirements. The hypersensitivity of β receptors results partly from an increased synthesis of β receptors that occurs in the presence of long-term β-receptor antagonism. In patients without coronary artery disease, abrupt discontinuation of β-blocker therapy may be associated with sinus tachycardia, increased sweating, and generalized malaise.

The adverse effects β blockers have on serum lipids and glucose tolerance may unfortunately offset some of their beneficial effects on cardiovascular morbidity and mortality. Beta blockers increase serum triglyceride levels and decrease HDL cholesterol levels. These adverse lipid effects are brought on by the inhibitory effect that unopposed alpha stimulation has on the activity of lipoprotein lipase and lecithin cholesterol acyltransferase. Lipoprotein lipase enhances VLDL and triglyceride catabolism. HDL cholesterol is one of the by-products of VLDL catabolism. Lecithin cholesterol acyltransferase is also involved in the production of HDL cholesterol. Beta blockers with α-blocking properties produce no appreciable change in serum lipid concentration. Also, β blockers with ISA do not adversely affect serum lipids and may even increase HDL cholesterol.

Beta blockers may induce glucose intolerance by inhibiting insulin secretion and by generating insulin resistance. As in the case with lipids, these adverse effects on glucose tolerance usually are not associated with the use of β blockers that possess ISA or α-receptor blocking properties.

ANGIOTENSIN-CONVERTING ENZYME INHIBITORS[3,4,13–15,19,20,32,37]

Currently, there are seven ACE inhibitors on the U.S. market. Several other ACE inhibitors are in development. Enalapril is metabolized to enalaprilat, which has a long half-life and duration of hypotensive action, and is therefore given once daily in the treatment of hypertension. Lisinopril has an even longer duration of action but does not require metabolic conversion to exert its effect. Captopril, which has a much shorter half-life than enalapril, is usually administered two to three times daily. Recent studies, however, indicate that once-daily administration of captopril may be adequate for the treatment of hypertension in salt-restricted patients. All three of these drugs are excreted in the urine and therefore an adjustment in dosage may be necessary in patients with renal dysfunction. The absorption of captopril, but not enalapril or lisinopril, is reduced 30–40% by the presence of food in the stomach.

The four newest ACE inhibitors, benazepril, fosinopril, quinapril, and ramipril all have relatively long half-lives and can provide 24-hour blood pressure reduction with once-daily dosing. It is not known whether any of the three offers a particular advantage over enalapril or lisinopril. Quinapril is the most lipophilic. Benazepril, quinapril, and ramipril have the greatest effect on tissue ACE.

ACE is widely distributed in many tissues. It is present in several different cell types, but its principal location is in endothelial cells. Since the vascular endothelium covers a large surface area, the major site for angiotensin II production in the body is the blood vessels, not the kidney. ACE inhibitors block the conversion of angiotensin I to angiotensin II. This latter substance is a potent vasoconstrictor and stimulator of aldosterone secretion. ACE inhibitors also block the degradation of bradykinin and stimulate the synthesis of other vasodilating substances including prostaglandin E_2 and prostacyclin. It is conceivable that different ACE inhibitors exert different effects on these various local vasoactive substances, but that remains to be proven. The observation that ACE inhibitors lower blood pressure in patients with normal plasma renin and ACE activity clearly indicates the importance of tissue production of ACE as a cause of increased vascular resistance.

Recent experiments and clinical studies have demonstrated that the blockade of angiotensin II production by ACE inhibitors increased the compliance of large arteries. The distensibility of these vessels determines the impedance of ventricular ejection, which is important in determining end-systolic ventricular wall stress. Increased wall stress gives rise to left ventricular hypertrophy and failure. Therefore, by increasing compliance of large arteries ACE inhibitors may effectively prevent or reverse left ventricular hypertrophy. They may also help prevent or slow down the rate of arteriosclerosis in these large vessels, which is the major cause of cardiovascular complications.

The most worrisome adverse effects of the ACE inhibitors are neutropenia and agranulocytosis, proteinuria, glomerulonephritis, and angioedema. Fortunately, these serious adverse effects are rare, occurring in less than 1% of patients exposed. Patients with preexisting renal or connective tissue diseases appear to be most vulnerable to the renal and hematologic side effects. Patients with bilateral renal artery stenosis or unilateral stenosis of a solitary functioning kidney and patients dependent on the vasoconstrictive effect of angiotensin II on the efferent arteriole are particularly susceptible to developing acute renal failure on ACE inhibitors.

Approximately 10% of patients who receive captopril develop a skin rash. In most cases the rash is transient and disappears despite continued treatment with the drug. Another fairly common side effect of captopril is a reversible loss of taste or taste disturbance (dysgeusia), which has been reported in about 6% of patients who receive the drug. The higher incidence of skin rash, dysgeusia, and proteinuria with captopril has been attributed to its sulfhydryl group, which is not present on enalapril or lisinopril. Approximately 10–20% of patients will develop a persistent cough while on ACE inhibitors. Some may even develop acute bronchospasm.

Acute hypotension may occur at the onset on ACE inhibitor therapy, especially in patients who are severely sodium or volume depleted. It may be necessary to discontinue diuretics and reduce the dosage of other antihypertensive agents before initiating therapy with either captopril, enalapril, or lisinopril. One may also choose to begin ACE inhibitors at the lowest dose possible and administer the first dose at bedtime.

ACE inhibitors are absolutely contraindicated in pregnancy because serious neonatal problems, including renal failure and death, have been reported when mothers took these agents during the second and third trimesters of pregnancy.[38]

Finally, hyperkalemia has been observed in patients treated with ACE inhibitors. This propensity for hyperkalemia is seen primarily in patients with renal disease or diabetes mellitus (especially with type IV renal tubular acidosis), or patients on concomitant NSAIDs, potassium supplements, or potassium-sparing diuretics. A uricosuric effect may warrant measures to decrease the risk of uric acid precipitation in patients with hyperuricemia or gout.

Another type of renin inhibitor, angiotensin receptor antagonists, will soon be available for clinical use. These compounds are angiotensin analogues that inhibit the renin system by directly competing with angiotensin II for tissue binding sites. Therefore, they block the effects of angiotensin II generated by either ACE or the enzyme chymase. One such compound, losartan, has already received FDA approval. Losartan appears to have effects on blood pressure and systemic and renal hemodynamics that are comparable to the ACE inhibitors. However, unlike ACE inhibitors, losartan does not cause a nonproductive cough and is less likely to cause hyperkalemia.

Vasodilators[3,4,13–15,19,20,32]

Hydralazine and minoxidil cause direct arteriolar smooth muscle relaxation through mechanisms that increase the intracellular concentration of cyclic GMP. They exert little effect, if any, on the venous side of the circulation. By decreasing the amount of systemic pressure in the arterial system, they reduce impedance to myocardial contractility. Hence, hydralazine and minoxidil are also known as afterload-reducing agents and may be used in the management of congestive heart failure.

The reduction in perfusion pressure brought on by direct arteriolar vasodilation activates the baroreceptor reflexes, which results in an increase in sympathetic outflow from the vasomotor center. This leads to an increase in heart rate, cardiac output, and renin release. Consequently, the hypotensive effectiveness of direct vasodilators diminishes in time unless the patient is also taking a sympathetic inhibitor and a diuretic to counteract the compensatory changes created by the baroreceptor reflexes. In older patients, however, baroreceptor mechanisms may be blunted enough that blood pressure may be lowered with vasodilatory therapy without causing sympathetic overactivity.

Direct vasodilator use can precipitate angina in patients with underlying coronary artery disease unless the baroreceptor reflex mechanism is completely blocked. To accomplish this, any sympathetic inhibitor may work, but the β-adrenergic blocking agents are most effective.

One side effect that is unique to hydralazine is a lupus-like syndrome. This adverse effect is associated with a chronic accumulation of hydralazine and is therefore dose related. The elimination of hydralazine involves hepatic *N*-acetyltransferase activity. As the activity of this enzyme system is predetermined genetically, the rate of acetylation may vary considerably. "Slow" acetylators are especially prone to develop a lupus-like reaction to hydralazine. The syndrome, which is more common in women, seldom progresses to the extent that systemic lupus erythematosus does, and it is reversible upon discontinuation of the drug. By keeping the total daily dose below 200 mg, lupus-like reactions can usually be avoided. Other side effects associated with hydralazine include dermatitis, drug fever, peripheral neuropathy, hepatitis, and vascular headaches.

Because minoxidil is a more potent vasodilator, the compensatory increases in heart rate, cardiac output, renin release, and sodium retention are even more dramatic than those observed with hydralazine. It therefore may be necessary to coadminister a β-adrenergic blocker and a loop diuretic with minoxidil. Other sympathetic inhibitors and thiazide diuretics may prove inadequate in counteracting the minoxidil-induced baroreceptor reflex and intrarenal compensatory mechanisms.

A very troublesome side effect of minoxidil is hypertrichosis. Increased hair growth occurs on the face, arms, back, and chest. This drug-induced hirsutism ceases with discontinuation of the drug. Other minoxidil side effects include pericardial effusion and a nonspecific T-wave change on the electrocardiogram.

CALCIUM CHANNEL ANTAGONISTS[3,4,13–15,19,20,32,39,40]

An increase in the level of free intracellular calcium from the extracellular fluid is required for the contraction of cardiac and smooth muscle cells, but not skeletal muscle cells. When cardiac or vascular smooth muscle is stimulated, voltage-sensitive channels in the cell membrane are opened, allowing calcium to enter the cells. The influx of extracellular calcium into the cell initiates a release of stored calcium from the sarcoplasmic reticulum. As the intracellular concentration of free calcium increases, it binds to a protein, calmodulin, which then activates myosin kinase. Activation of myosin kinase enables myosin to interact with actin to induce contraction. Calcium channel antagonists cause relaxation of cardiac and smooth muscle by blocking voltage-sensitive calcium channels thereby reducing the entry of extracellular calcium into the cells. Vascular smooth muscle relaxation leads to vasodilation and a corresponding reduction in blood pressure.

Currently there are seven calcium channel antagonists in use for the treatment of hypertension: verapamil, diltiazem, and five dihydropyridines—amlodipine, felodipine, nifedipine, nicardipine, and isradipine. They are all similar in their antihypertensive effectiveness, but they differ somewhat in other pharmacologic effects. For example, verapamil decreases heart rate and slows atrioventricular nodal conduction. These unique properties make it an excellent drug for the treatment of supraventricular tachyarrhythmias. Verapamil also produces a negative inotropic effect that is responsible for its propensity to cause heart failure in subjects with borderline cardiac reserve. Diltiazem also decreases atrioventricular conduction and heart rate, but to a lesser extent than verapamil. Nifedipine, because of its potent peripheral vasodilating effects, causes a baroreceptor-mediated reflex increase in heart rate. It does not usually alter conduction through the atrioventricular node. The reason that pharmacologic differences exist among the three major classes of calcium channel antagonists—verapamil, diltiazem, and the dihydropyridines—is that they all act at specific receptors. The density and distribution of these receptors varies from tissue to tissue.

Nifedipine rarely may cause an increase in the frequency, intensity, and duration of angina in association with acute hypotension. This effect may be obviated by the administration of nifedipine with meals or by using sustained-released formulations of nifedipine. Other side effects of nifedipine include dizziness, flushing, headache, peripheral edema, mood changes, and various gastrointestinal complaints.

Diltiazem and verapamil rarely cause cardiac conduction abnormalities such as bradycardia, atrioventricular block, and congestive heart failure. Both can cause anorexia, nausea, peripheral edema, and hypotension. Verapamil causes constipation in about 7% of patients.

Verapamil, diltiazem, felodipine, nicardipine, and nifedipine are now marketed in sustained-release formulations. These new formulations allow for less frequent daily dosing and may result in fewer adverse drug reactions. Amlodipine is given once daily due to its long half-life.

POSTGANGLIONIC SYMPATHETIC INHIBITORS[3,4,13–15,19,20,32]

Guanethidine and guanadrel deplete norepinephrine from postganglionic sympathetic nerve terminals and they inhibit the release of norepinephrine in response to sympathetic nerve stimulation.

Hemodynamic studies indicate that the fall in blood pressure produced by postganglionic inhibitors is associated with a reduction in cardiac output and peripheral vascular resistance. Because reflex-mediated vasoconstriction is blocked by these drugs, a much greater hypotensive effect occurs in the upright posture, and postural hypotension is common. The use of postganglionic sympathetic inhibitors is associated with many other unwarranted side effects including impotence, diarrhea, and weight gain. The gastrointestinal side effects occur as a result of unopposed parasympathetic activity.

Long-term norepinephrine depletion leads to postsynaptic receptor supersensitivity. Therefore, the administration of drugs that compete with postganglionic inhibitors for uptake into the nerve terminals (such as tricyclic antidepressants and sympathomimetics) may occasionally provoke acute severe hypertensive episodes.

Because of their potential to cause explosive diarrhea, impotence, and orthostatic hypotension and syncope, the postganglionic sympathetic inhibitors are usually restricted to use in patients with refractory hypertension.

RESERPINE[3,4,32]

Reserpine lowers blood pressure through several different mechanisms. It depletes norepinephrine from sympathetic nerve endings and it blocks the transport of norepinephrine into its storage granules. When the nerve is stimulated, less than the usual amount of norepinephrine is released into the synapse. This causes diminution in sympathetic tone with a resulting decrease in peripheral vascular resistance and blood pressure.

Reserpine also depletes catecholamines from the brain and the myocardium. Consequently, the use of reserpine may lead to sedation and depression and decreased cardiac output.

Reserpine is a very long-acting drug and it may take 2–6 weeks before the maximal effect of the drug is realized. Its use is associated with significant sodium and fluid retention and therefore it should be administered in combination with a diuretic.

Reserpine's strong inhibition of sympathetic activity allows increased parasympathetic activity to occur, which is responsible for some of its side effects including nasal stuffiness, increased gastric acid secretion, diarrhea, and bradycardia.

The most important side effect of reserpine, however, is mental depression, which is a consequence of CNS depletion of catecholamines and serotonin. Patients may complain of sadness, loss of appetite, loss of self-confidence, gradual loss of energy, impotence, and early morning awakening. The incidence of reserpine-induced depression is dose related. The problem can be minimized by not exceeding a dose of 0.25 mg daily. At low doses the rate of depression with reserpine is equivalent to that of β blockers, diuretics, or placebo.[41]

Reserpine is an inexpensive antihypertensive agent and has enjoyed the distinction of being chosen as the sympathetic inhibitor in many of the major clinical trials that have documented the benefit in treating hypertension.

DIFFERENTIAL APPROACH TO THE MANAGEMENT OF HYPERTENSION

Hypertension is a heterogeneous disorder that poses special therapeutic problems in several specific clinical situations. These situations are discussed briefly in this section, which attempts to integrate the pathophysiology of hypertension in certain subgroups of patients with the pharmacology of the various antihypertensive agents. Table 12.2 summarizes some of the key points.

HYPERTENSION IN CHILDHOOD[4,41–43]

The Report of the National Heart, Lung, and Blood Institute Second Task Force on Blood Pressure Control in Children is recommended for those seeking a more detailed discussion of this topic.[43]

In most cases, the factors associated with hypertension in children are identical to those in adults. Hypertensive children often have a family history of high blood pressure. There is, however, one important distinction between hypertension in children and in adults: Secondary hypertension is much more common in children than in adults.

Renal disease is the most common cause of secondary hypertension in children. Pyelonephritis, glomerulonephritis, renal artery stenosis, and renal cysts may all produce hypertension in children. Medical or surgical management of the underlying renal disorder usually restores normal blood pressure. Pheochromocytoma and coarctation of the aorta are more often discovered during childhood and are fortunately amenable to corrective surgery. Less common

TABLE 12.2. DIFFERENTIAL ANTIHYPERTENSIVE THERAPY IN SPECIFIC CLINICAL SITUATIONS

	Advantageous	Disadvantageous
CHF[a]	ACE inhibitor, diuretic, hydralazine	β Blocker, reserpine, Ca channel antagonist
Angina	β Blocker, Ca channel antagonist	Hydralazine, minoxidil
Elderly	Diuretic, α agonist, Ca channel antagonist	
Black	Diuretic, Ca channel antagonist	β blocker as initial therapy
Young	β Blocker, α agonist, ACE inhibitor	Diuretic
Diabetes	α Agonist, ACE inhibitor, Ca channel antagonist	β Blocker, diuretic
Asthma, COPD	Ca channel antagonist	β Blocker, ACE inhibitor
Pregnancy	Methyldopa, hydralazine, labetolol	Diuretic, β blocker
Renal insufficiency	α Agonist, Ca channel antagonist, minoxidil, hydralazine, loop diuretic	Thiazide diuretic
Tachycardia	β Blocker, α agonist, reserpine, verapamil, diltiazem	Nifedipine, hydralazine, minoxidil
Hyperlipidemia	α Blocker, ACE inhibitor, Ca channel antagonist	Diuretic, β blocker
Gout/hyperuricemia	α Agonist, α blocker, Ca channel antagonist, ACE inhibitor[b]	Diuretic, β blocker, ACE inhibitor[b]

[a]CHF, congestive heart failure; ACE, angiotensin-converting enzyme; COPD, chronic obstructive pulmonary disease.
[b]ACE inhibitors may increase urinary clearance of uric acid thereby reducing hyperuricemia but increasing the risk of uric acid deposition in the urine or kidneys.

causes of secondary hypertension in children include congenital defects of adrenal steroid synthesis, Wilms' tumor, and neuroblastoma.

Primary hypertension is much more common in children than was once thought. In many young people, primary hypertension is associated with an increased cardiac output and a normal plasma volume and total peripheral vascular resistance. This is often referred to as a hyperdynamic or a hyperkinetic circulatory state. It would seem that this form of hypertension would best be treated with a β-adrenergic blocking agent. An alternative treatment might be clonidine, guanfacine, or guanabenz, which are known to lower serum norepinephrine levels and thus reduce hyperadrenergic activity.

HYPERTENSION IN PREGNANCY[13,14,44–48]

In 1990, the National High Blood Pressure Education Program Working Group Report on High Blood Pressure in Pregnancy was published. This report clearly emphasizes the importance of separating preeclampsia from chronic or transient hypertension of pregnancy since preeclampsia can lead rapidly to life-threatening complications for both the mother and fetus. Preeclampsia usually presents after 20 weeks' gestation in primigravid women. The diagnosis of preeclampsia is based on the appearance of hypertension, or a significant increase in blood pressure, with proteinuria, edema, or both. An increase of 30 mm Hg systolic or 15 mm Hg diastolic is also considered diagnostic even if the measured values do not exceed 140/90 mm Hg. Since the diastolic blood pressure usually decreases by 7–10 mm Hg during the early weeks of pregnancy, preeclampsia patients may demonstrate the required increase in blood pressure without achieving hypertensive readings. The hypertension and other signs of preeclampsia are thought to reflect pathophysiologic changes that induce vasospasm and may cause hematologic, renal, hepatic, brain, and uteroplacental damage. It is important to realize that it is the underlying pathology, not simply the blood pressure elevation, that is responsible for the terrible complications of this condition. It is uncertain whether blood pressure reduction is of any benefit in reducing the complications of preeclampsia.

Definitive treatment of preeclampsia is delivery or abortion, and this is clearly indicated if pending or frank eclampsia (preeclampsia plus convulsions) is present. Otherwise, such measures as restriction of activity, bed rest, and close monitoring are in order. Salt restriction, or any other measures that may contract blood volume, should not be employed. If drug treatment of hypertension is indicated (DBP >100 mm Hg), methyldopa (or perhaps another α-agonist) is still the recommended drug of choice; and ACE inhibitors are specifically contraindicated because of reports of animal teratogenicity and acute renal failure in neonates. Beta blockers appear safe and effective in simple hypertension of pregnancy even though there is some concern about effects on fetal heart rate, glucose intolerance, and growth retardation. Since preeclampsia is thought to involve vasospasm, it would seem logical to avoid blockade of β receptors in the vascular system since this could potentiate such vasospasm. Calcium channel blockers have been used extensively in Europe and would seem to be a good choice except, perhaps, for nifedipine. Nifedipine may induce proteinuria and has been shown to be teratogenic in rats. These agents also have been used successfully to treat preterm labor.

In 1989, two placebo-controlled studies reported beneficial results with either 60 or 100 mg of aspirin per day in pregnant women at risk of preeclampsia. The study using the lower dose started therapy at week 12 of gestation and continued until delivery. In the other study, therapy was started around week 30 of gestation and continued until 10 days before anticipated delivery. Pregnancy-induced hypertension, proteinuria, length of pregnancy, and fetal outcome were improved with aspirin therapy.[47] In a more recent study, low-dose aspirin was shown to decrease the incidence of preeclampsia among nulliparous women, primarily through its effect in those who have elevated systolic blood pressure initially.[48] However, in a multicenter study involving 9364 women, the use of aspirin was associated with a reduction of only 12% in the incidence of preeclampsia, which was not significant.[49] Until more data confirm the efficacy of low-dose aspirin in the general pregnant population, it should be reserved for high-risk patients.

HYPERTENSION IN THE ELDERLY[8–10,50–56]

The elderly may present with either isolated systolic hypertension or an elevation in both systolic and diastolic blood pressure. Epidemiologic data indicate that cardiovascular morbidity and mortality are more closely related to systolic blood pressure than to diastolic blood pressure. In a double-blind placebo-controlled trial, the Systolic Hypertension in the Elderly Program (SHEP), active treatment of isolated systolic hypertension resulted in a 36% reduction in the incidence of total stroke and a 27% reduction in the total number of cardiovascular events.

In another placebo-controlled trial, the European Working Party Hypertension in the Elderly (EWPHE) study, a subgroup analysis of patients with isolated systolic hypertension revealed that treatment reduced overall mortality by 25% and cardiovascular mortality by 27%. However, these results were obtained from a small number of subjects in that trial and statistical analysis of the result was not reported.

The Joint National Committee on Detection, Evaluation, and Treatment of High Blood Pressure recommends a reduction in the systolic blood pressure (SBP) to less than 160 mm Hg for those with a SBP greater than 180 mm Hg and a reduction in blood pressure by 20 mm Hg for those with SBP between 160 and 179 mm Hg.

Elderly patients are usually more sensitive to volume depletion and sympathetic inhibition than their younger counterparts. Therefore, antihypertensive treatment should be initiated with smaller-than-usual dosages. Most authorities agree that the initial drug should be a diuretic. The starting dose should be low (e.g., 12.5 mg of hydrochlorothiazide) and gradually increased, but probably not to the maximum dosage. If diuretic therapy alone does not achieve the desired reduction in systolic blood pressure, a sympathetic inhibitor can be added. Again, it is best to start off with a low dose and slowly increase the dose, if necessary, but avoid excessive doses. Calcium channel blockers or beta blockers should be considered in elderly patients with hypertension and angina, and ACE inhibitors might be preferred for hypertensive patients with congestive heart failure. The pharmacologic management of diastolic hypertension in the elderly should be similar to that outlined for isolated systolic hypertension.

HYPERTENSION IN BLACKS[3,11,32,57]

Hypertension is common in all races, but it affects blacks at a disproportionately higher rate. It is also more severe in blacks than nonblacks. The reasons for the increased prevalence and severity of hypertension in blacks are not fully understood. Differences in electrolyte homeostasis, glomerular filtration rate, sodium excretion and transport mechanisms, plasma renin activity, and blood pressure response to plasma volume expansion have been noted. These differences may help explain the propensity for blacks to develop hypertension, but they do not account for the increased severity of hypertension in blacks as compared with whites. Further investigations in this area are needed.

Although dietary sodium intake is similar in blacks and whites, blacks ingest less potassium and calcium than whites. Supplemental potassium and calcium have both been shown to cause a modest reduction in blood pressure in some studies. It would therefore seem reasonable to assess the effect of increasing the amount of potassium and calcium in the diet as part of the nonpharmacologic management of hypertension in blacks.

The lower plasma renin activity and increased blood pressure response to sodium and fluid loading observed in blacks suggest a more sodium- and volume-dependent hypertension than exists in nonblacks. Several clinical studies have shown that blacks are hyperresponsive to diuretic therapy, a finding that is entirely consistent with the previously mentioned physiologic observations. These findings also point out the rationale of using diuretic therapy or calcium antagonist as the initial treatment of hypertension in blacks.

If diuretic therapy alone does not adequately control blood pressure in black hypertensives, then the addition of a sympathetic inhibitor is appropriate. Some clinicians have the misconception that β blockers and ACE inhibitors are not effective in blacks. Although diuretics may be more effective as the initial treatment, diuretic therapy combined with β blockers or ACE inhibitors is equally efficacious in hypertensive blacks and whites.

Controlled clinical trials have shown that calcium channel antagonists are as effective as diuretics in the initial pharmacologic treatment of hypertension in blacks. Thus, an alternative to diuretic therapy for this group is available and might, under certain conditions, be preferable.

HYPERTENSION AND CONCOMITANT DISORDERS[11,18,19,58–62]

When hypertension is associated with other medical problems, the approach to its treatment should reflect proper consideration for the interactions that may occur between the antihypertensive drug regimen and the other disease states. These interactions consist of both positive and negative effects.

Asthma, COPD

Beta blockers, even those with β_1 selectivity, should be avoided in hypertensive patients with asthma, COPD, and peripheral vascular disease.

Glucose Intolerance

If at all possible, diuretics and β blockers should not be used to treat the diabetic hypertensive patient. Both classes of drugs cause insulin resistance and glucose intolerance. Also, as pointed out earlier, insulin resistance leads to hyperinsulinemia, which, in turn, contributes to the development of both hypertension and hyperlipidemia. There is some controversy as to the clinical importance of the metabolic consequences of diuretics and β blockers. Some argue that effects on lipids are transient and return to baseline with continuous therapy. But there is also evidence that the effects may persist. Clearly, more research is needed to resolve this controversy. If glucose intolerance or an elevation in lipids occurs in a patient already receiving either a diuretic or β blocker, it would seem prudent to switch treatment to an alternative antihypertensive therapy.

Other problems posed by β-blocker therapy in the diabetic hypertensive stem from the effects β-adrenergic blockade produces during hypoglycemic episodes. Since most of the symptoms of hypoglycemia (tremor, tachycardia, palpitations) are mediated through the sympathetic nervous system, these signs and symptoms are masked in the presence of β-adrenergic blockade. Sweating, another symptom of hypoglycemia, is cholinergically mediated, and therefore increases during a hypoglycemic episode. Since recovery of hypoglycemia depends on various compensatory mechanisms, including those produced by catecholamine input, then another consequence of β-adrenergic blockade is a delay in recovery time. Finally, hypertensive patients may experience marked elevations in blood pressure due to vasoconstrictor caused by unopposed α-receptor stimulation during the hypoglycemic recovery phase.

Other antihypertensive agents that may pose a problem in the diabetic hypertensive patient are the α-adrenergic antagonists and the centrally acting α agonists. The α_1 antagonists may increase the risk of orthostatic hypotension and the α_2 agonists may cause a paradoxical increase in blood pressure. Both of these effects appear to be secondary to a more sensitive autonomic nervous system in patients with diabetic neuropathy.

Some evidence indicates that ACE inhibitors may increase insulin sensitivity, and there are a few case reports of hypoglycemia resulting from the combination of an ACE inhibitor and an oral hypoglycemic agent. While such interactions may occur and could be detrimental in some patients, the fact that ACE inhibitors improve insulin sensitivity could be taken advantage of in the diabetic patient inadequately controlled. Another potential benefit of ACE inhibitors in diabetic patients may be their purported renal protective effects. In animal studies, ACE inhibitors and nondihydropyridine calcium channel antagonists have been shown to reduce intraglomerular hypertension. An increased glomerular pressure, hyperfiltration, and the accompanying microalbuminuria appear to be the earliest signs of diabetic nephropathy. Recent clinical studies support the renal protective effect of ACE inhibitors.[63] Thus these agents may be considered the preferred pharmacologic treatment of hypertension in the diabetic subject. One possible adverse side effect that may attend the use of ACE inhibitors in diabetics is hyperkalemia. This is particularly likely to occur in diabetic patients with type 4 renal tubular acidosis, or in any diabetic on potassium supplements or potassium-sparing diuretics.

Hyperlipidemia

As with glucose intolerance, hyperlipidemia compounds the risk of coronary artery disease attributed to hypertension. Therefore, every effort should be made to not only control high blood pressure but also to effectively manage or prevent hyperlipidemia. As discussed earlier, some antihypertensive agents may adversely affect serum lipids, namely, thiazide diuretics and β blockers without ISA or α-blocking properties. It would therefore seem prudent to avoid diuretics and β blockers at least in hypertensive patients with hyperlipidemia, and to consider alternative agents in patients who develop lipid abnormalities while on diuretic or β-blocker therapy.

Left Ventricular Hypertrophy

LVH is another independent risk factor for coronary artery disease. LVH is present in about 50% of hypertensive patients. With the exception of vasodilators, most classes of antihypertensive agents have been shown to prevent or regress LVH. Prevention or regression of LVH should be considered an important objective in the overall management of hypertension. One study showed that diuretics caused the most regression.[64]

Smoking

Smoking essentially doubles the cardiovascular risks associated with hypertension. Data from the MRC trial demonstrated that smoking eliminated any beneficial effect of propranolol in reducing cardiac events. Smoking induces catecholamine release, which, in the presence of β_2-receptor blockade, may lead to an increase in vascular resistance and therefore blood pressure and cardiac workload. The α-agonist clonidine has been shown to be useful in smoking cessation (particularly in women) and this may provide cause to consider this antihypertensive agent in smokers who are trying to kick the habit. Otherwise, there is little guidance in the literature as to how best to treat hypertension in patients who smoke.

Coronary Artery Disease

For hypertensive patients with ischemic heart disease, β blockers and calcium channel antagonists offer the advantage of lowering blood pressure and reducing myocardial oxygen demand. The cardiac stimulation that may occur with nifedipine or β blockers with ISA, however, may make these agents less desirable in this clinical setting.

In patients with coronary artery disease, overtreating high blood pressure may bring about more harm than good. Since coronary blood flow occurs during diastole, the rate of flow is directly influenced by the diastolic blood pressure. Reducing the diastolic blood pressure excessively may therefore compromise coronary perfusion, especially in patients with fixed coronary artery stenosis, and lead to myocardial infarction. Thus in hypertensive patients with preexisting coronary artery disease, the risk of infarction increases at high diastolic blood pressures, decreases as diastolic blood pressure is lowered, then increases again at less than optimal diastolic blood pressures. This phenomenon is referred to as the "J curve." A recent meta-analysis of several published studies showed that the break point in this J-curve relationship between diastolic blood pressure and cardiac events occurs at a pressure of 85 mm Hg.[65]

For secondary prevention of infarction in hypertensive patients, calcium channel blockers do not afford the same degree of benefit as β blockers. Diltiazem has been shown to reduce reinfarction in patients with non-Q-wave infarcts and may reduce cardiac events in post-MI patients who do not have CHF. However, diltiazem was shown to be harmful if pulmonary congestion was present. Similarly, verapamil offers some protection to post-MI patients with normal left ventricular ejection fractions. Studies evaluating the use of calcium channel antagonists post-MI were not carried out in hypertensive patients per se, although one would expect the same degree of protection for such patients.

Congestive Heart Failure

In patients with congestive heart failure (CHF), captopril, enalapril, and ramipril have been shown to improve symptomatology and reduce mortality. Although CHF, not hypertension, was the focus of these studies, it seems logical to use ACE inhibitors to treat hypertension in the setting of concomitant CHF. Because of the high renin and angiotensin II status of patients with CHF, therapy with an ACE inhibitor should be initiated at low doses to avoid a profound drop in blood pressure.

A β-blocker or nondihydropyridine calcium channel antagonist may improve left ventricular filling and cardiac output in patients with reduced cardiac output due to diastolic dysfunction. On the other hand, these agents may worsen CHF in patients with systolic decompensation (see Chapter 13).

Renovascular Disease

In managing patients with hypertension due to renal artery stenosis or renal artery hyperplasia, ACE inhibitors may be particularly advantageous. This is due to the fact that these conditions are associated with an increase in plasma renin and angiotensin activity. Two important cautions, however, are that patients may experience a rapid and profound drop in blood pressure or acute renal failure. The potential for ACE inhibitors to produce acute renal failure is particularly noted in patients with bilateral renal artery stenosis or a solitary functioning kidney with stenosis. Functional renal failure may occur in patients whose kidneys are dependent on angiotensin II for perfusion.

ACE inhibitors have also been shown to be effective for controlling the accelerated hypertension of sclerodermal renal crisis. If treatment is begun early, progressive deterioration in renal function can be prevented and occasional improvement in renal function results.

HYPERTENSIVE URGENCIES AND EMERGENCIES[3,4,11,20,66–69]

Oral antihypertensive loading with clonidine, nifedipine, or captopril has been found to be effective in treating hypertensive urgencies. With oral clonidine loading, 0.2 mg of clonidine is given initially followed by 0.1 mg hourly until the diastolic pressure falls below 110 mm Hg or a total of 0.7 mg of clonidine has been administered. A single dose may be all that is necessary. Rapid nifedipine effect is accomplished by having the patient swallow a perforated capsule. Since nifedipine is not absorbed well across the buccal mucosa, there is no need to administer nifedipine sublingually. Captopril is usually administered in doses of 25–50 mg orally at 1- to 2-hour intervals. The onset of action of oral captopril is 15–30 minutes, and a marked fall in blood pressure is unlikely to occur if no hypotensive response is observed within 30–60 minutes.

There are no data confirming that the rapid reduction of blood pressure in patients with severe asymptomatic hypertension is more beneficial than the gradual reduction of blood pressure in these patients. Since autoregulation of blood flow in chronically hypertensive patients occurs at a much higher range of pressure than in normotensive persons, there are some inherent risks in reducing blood pressure too precipitously, resulting in cerebrovascular accidents, myocardial infarction, and acute renal failure.

A hypertensive emergency is defined as a severe elevation in diastolic blood pressure, usually higher than 120 mm Hg, in the presence of target organ damage. Immediate treatment with an intravenous antihypertensive agent is needed to salvage viable tissue. These events are thought to be precipitated by an abrupt increase in vascular resistance as a result of an acute rise in circulating or local tissue levels of vasoconstricting substances. The marked elevation in blood pressure leads to arteriolar fibrinoid necrosis, endothelial damage, platelet and fibrin deposition in the media of smooth muscle, and loss of autoregulatory function. The end result is end-organ ischemia, which triggers a vicious cycle of further release of vasoactive substances, vasoconstriction, and endothelial proliferation. The goal in treatment is to interrupt this vicious cycle by lowering the diastolic blood pressure.

Just how rapidly to lower the pressure and to what level is somewhat controversial. Most authorities agree that the diastolic blood pressure should not be lowered below 100–110 mm Hg over several minutes to several hours depending on the clinical situation. Precipitous drops in blood pressure to the normotensive range or lower may lead to end-organ ischemia or infarction. After the goal diastolic blood pressure is reached, treatment should be designed to hold that level of pressure for several days to allow physiologic adjustments in autoregulatory function. Then, the blood pressure can be further reduced to normotensive levels.

The treatment of hypertensive emergencies can be accomplished with any one of several antihypertensive agents. The clinical situation may dictate which agent is preferred and which is contraindicated.

Nitroprusside is widely considered the agent of choice for the minute-to-minute control in most cases of severe hypertension. It is a direct-acting vasodilator that decreases peripheral vascular resistance, but does not increase cardiac output unless left ventricular failure is present. It is usually given as a continuous intravenous infusion at a rate of 0.5–8.0 μg/kg/min. Its onset of hypotensive action is immediate and its effect disappears within 2–5 minutes of discontinuation of the infusion. Nitroprusside can be given to treat any hypertensive emergency, but in aortic dissection propranolol should be given first to prevent reflex sympathetic activation. Nitroprusside is metabolized to cyanide and then to thiocyanate and eliminated by the kidneys. When the infusion must be continued longer than 72 hours, serum thiocyanate levels should be measured, and the infusion should be discontinued if the level exceeds 12 mg/dL. The risk of thiocyanate toxicity is increased in patients with impaired renal function. Other side effects of nitroprusside include fatigue, nausea, anorexia, disorientation, psychotic behavior, muscle spasms, and, rarely, hypothyroidism. Nitroprusside administration requires constant intra-arterial pressure monitoring.

Intravenous nitroglycerin shares many of the advantages of sodium nitroprusside. In large doses, nitroglycerin dilates both arterioles and venous capacitance vessels, thereby producing both afterload and preload reducing effects. By reducing end-diastolic volume and pressure, the drug decreases myocardial oxygen demand. It also dilates collateral coronary blood vessels and improves perfusion to ischemic myocardium. These properties make intravenous nitroglycerin particularly beneficial in the management of severe hypertension in the presence of myocardial ischemia. The dose of intravenous nitroglycerin is 5–100 μg/min. As in the case with oral nitrates, intravenous nitroglycerin is associated with tolerance over 24–48 hours.

Diazoxide is also a direct-acting arteriolar vasodilator that decreases peripheral resistance, increases cardiac output, and maintains or increases renal plasma flow. Because diazoxide increases plasma volume, it is common practice to give a diuretic concurrently unless the patient is volume depleted. It has quick onset and a duration of action ranging from 4–12 hours. Diazoxide occasionally causes overshoot hypotension, which can be reversed by pressor agents. To avoid the precipitous fall in pressure that occurs when diazoxide is given as a 300-mg rapid bolus, smaller bolus doses (50–100 mg every 5–10 minutes) or slow infusion over 15–30 minutes should be used. Other side effects of diazoxide include nausea, vomiting, tachycardia, hyperglycemia, and hyperuricemia.

Trimethaphan camsylate is a ganglionic blocking agent. It dilates both arterioles and veins, with hypotension potential in the upright position. It reduces cardiac output and renal plasma flow and increases plasma volume. Trimethaphan is particularly useful for treating hypertension in patients with acute aortic dissection. Like nitroprusside, trimethaphan is administered by continuous intravenous infusion, which requires constant or frequent intra-arterial pressure monitoring. The initial infusion rate is 1 mg/min and the dose can be adjusted up to 10 mg/min. Its onset of action is immediate and its effects disappear within 10 minutes of discontinuation of the infusion. Besides profound orthostatic hypotension, trimethaphan may cause ileus, urinary retention, dry mouth, and visual impairment. Respiratory arrest has been reported at infusion rates greater than 5 mg/min.

Labetolol is a combination nonselective β-adrenergic and α-adrenergic blocker. It reduces blood pressure by decreasing peripheral vascular resistance. It does not significantly affect heart rate or cardiac output. The initial dose is 20 mg by slow intravenous injection over a 2-minute period, followed by repeated injections of 40–80 mg at 10-minute intervals, up to a total dose of 300 mg. Alternatively, the drug can be administered by continuous infusion at an initial rate of 2 mg/min and adjusted according to blood pressure response. Because of its α-blocking effects, labetolol can cause orthostatic hypotension. Other side effects include nausea, vomiting, paresthesias, sweating, dizziness, flushing, and headaches.

Hydralazine is an arteriolar vasodilator. It causes a marked reflex tachycardia and an increase in myocardial oxygen demand, which can cause ischemic chest pain in patients with coronary artery disease. Its onset of action ranges from 10–30 minutes and its effects last 2–4 hours. When given intravenously, 10–20 mg is diluted in 20 mL of 5% dextrose in water (D_5W) and administered at a rate of 0.5–1.0 mL/min. Because the hypotensive response is less predictable than with other parenteral agents, its major role is in the treatment of eclampsia or hypertensive encephalopathy associated with renal insufficiency. It has a good track record in the treatment of these two types of hypertensive emergencies.

An intravenous form of nicardipine has recently been approved for short-term treatment of hypertension. It is administered at 5 to 15 mg/h, which is adjusted by 1 to 2.5 mg/h after 15 minutes. Headaches, nausea, and vomiting are common side effects, and the use of the agent increases heart rate by 8 to 18 beats per minute.

CONCLUSION

Hypertension is a very common chronic medical disorder. It affects more than 50 million Americans. In more than 90% of cases the etiology of hypertension is unknown. Several pathophysiologic mechanisms have been proposed in the causation of hypertension. These include central and peripheral nervous system abnormalities, autoregulatory dysfunction, renal defects, humoral aberrancies, and deficiencies in various endogenous vasodepressor substances.

Untreated or inadequately controlled hypertension is a major risk factor in the morbidity and mortality of cardiovascular, cerebrovascular, and renovascular diseases.

TABLE 12.3. THE ANTIHYPERTENSIVE AGENTS

Drug	Dose Range (mg/d)	
	Initial	**Maximum**
Diuretics		
Thiazides and related sulfonamide diuretics		
Bendroflumethiazide	2.5	5
Benzthiazide	25	50
Chlorothiazide sodium	250	500
Chlorthalidone	25	50
Cyclothiazide	1	2
Hydrochlorothiazide	25	50
Hydroflumethiazide	25	50
Indapamide	2.5	5
Methyclothiazide	2.5	5
Metolazone	2.5	5
Polythiazide	2	4
Quinethazone	50	100
Trichlormethiazide	2	4
Loop diuretics		
Bumetanide	0.5	10
Ethacrynic acid	50	200
Furosemide	80	480
Potassium-sparing agents		
Amiloride hydrochloride	5	10
Spironolactone	50	100
Triamterene	50	100
Adrenergic Inhibitors		
β-Adrenergic blockers		
Acebutolol	400	1200
Atenolol	25	100
Betaxolol	10	40
Bisoprolol	5	20
Carteolol	2.5	10
Metoprolol tartrate	50	300
Nadolol	20	120
Oxprenolol hydrochloride	160	480
Penbutolol	20	80
Pindolol	20	60
Propranolol hydrochloride	40	480
Propranolol, long-acting (LA)	80	480
Timolol maleate	20	60
Adrenergic Inhibitors (cont.)		
Central-acting adrenergic inhibitors		
Clonidine hydrochloride	0.2	1.2
Guanabenz acetate	8	32
Guanfacine	1	3.0
Methyldopa	500	2000
Peripheral-acting adrenergic antagonists		
Guanadrel sulfate	10	150
Guanethidine monosulfate	10	300
Rauwolfia alkaloids		
Rauwolfia (whole root)	50	100
Reserpine	0.05	0.25
α_1-Adrenergic blocker		
Doxazosin	1	16
Prazosin hydrochloride	2	20
Terazosin	1	5.0
Combined α- and β-adrenergic blockers		
Labetolol	200	1200
Vasodilators		
Hydralazine hydrochloride	50	300
Minoxidil	5	100
Angiotensin-converting enzyme inhibitors		
Benazepril	10	20
Captopril	25	150
Enalapril maleate	10	40
Fosinopril	10	80
Lisinopril	10	80
Quinapril	10	80
Ramipril	1.25	20
Calcium channel antagonists		
Amlodipine	5	10
Diltiazem hydrochloride	120	240
Isradipine	5	20
Nicardipine	60	120
Nifedipine	30	180
Nitrendipine	10	40
Verapamil hydrochloride	240	480

Antihypertensive drug therapy should be individualized according to various patient characteristics and underlying pathophysiologic circumstances. Table 12.3 provides a list of agents currently available for the treatment of hypertension in the United States.

REFERENCES

1. Guyton AC. The relationship of cardiac output and arterial pressure control. Circulation 1981;64:1079–1088.
2. Dustan HP. Physiologic regulation of arterial pressure: An overview. Hypertension 1982;4(suppl 3):62–67.
3. Caris TN. A Clinical Guide to Hypertension. Littleton, MA, PSG Publishing, 1985.
4. Kaplan MN. Clinical Hypertension, 4th ed. Baltimore, Williams & Wilkins, 1986.
5. Hypertension Detection and Follow-up Program Cooperative Group. Five year findings of the Hypertension Detection and Follow-up Program. 1: Reduction in mortality of persons with high blood pressure, including mild hypertension. JAMA 1979;242:2567–2571.
6. Veterans Administration Cooperative Study Group on Antihypertensive Agents. Effects of treatment on morbidity in hypertension. JAMA 1967;202:1028–1034.
7. Management Committee. The Australian therapeutic trial in mild hypertension. Lancet 1980;1:1261–1269.
8. SHEP Cooperative Research Group. Prevention of stroke by antihypertensive drug treatment in older persons with isolated systolic hypertension. JAMA 1991;265:3255–3264.
9. Dahöf B, Lindholm FH, Hansson L, et al. Morbidity and mortality in the Swedish trial in old patients with hypertension (STOP–Hypertension). Lancet 1991;338:1281–1285.
10. MRC Working Party. Medical Research Council trial of treatment of hypertension in older adults: Principal results. Br Med J 1992;304:405–412.
11. The Fifth Report of the National Committee on detection, evaluation, and treatment of high blood pressure (JNC-V). Arch Intern Med 1993;153:154–183.
12. Final Report of the Subcommittee on Definition and Prevalence of the Joint National Committee on Detection, Evaluation, and Treatment of High Blood Pressure, 1984.
13. Genest J, Kuchel O, Hamet P, et al. Hypertension, Physiopathology and Treatment, 2nd ed. New York, McGraw-Hill, 1983.
14. Kincaid-Smith PS, Whitworth JA. Hypertension: Mechanisms and Management. New York, ADIS Health Science Press, 1980.
15. Meyer P. Hypertension Mechanisms and Clinical and Therapeutic Aspects. Oxford, Oxford University Press, 1980.
16. Williams RR, Hunt SC, Hopkins PN, et al. Evidence for single gene contributions to hypertension and lipid disturbances: Definition, genetics, and clinical significance. Clin Genet 1994;46:80–87.
17. Caulfield M, Lavender P, Farrall M, et al. Linkage of the angiotensinogen gene to essential hypertension. N Engl J Med 1994;330:1629–1633.
18. Messerli FH, Ventura HO. Cardiovascular pathophysiology of essential hypertension: A clue to therapy. Drugs 1985;30(suppl 1):25–34.
19. McCarron DA. Management of hypertension: Pathophysiologic and therapeutic perspectives. J Cardiovasc Pharmacol 1984;6(suppl 6);5:465–545.
20. Chobanian AV. Hypertension. Clin Symposia 1982;34(5):3–32.
21. Sonnenblick EH. Hypertension and hemodynamics: Therapeutic implications. Am J Med 1983;75(4A):1–114.
22. Ferrario CM: Importance of the renin–angiotensin–aldosterone system (RAS) in the physiology and pathology of hypertension. Drugs 1990;39(suppl 2):1–8.
23. Reaven GM. Role of insulin resistance in human disease. Diabetes 1988;37:1595–1607.
24. Marigliano A, Tedde R, Sechi LA, et al. Insulinemia and blood pressure. Am J Hypertens 1990;3:521–526.
25. Vane JR, Änggard EE, Botting RM. Regulatory functions of the vascular endothelium. N Engl J Med 1990;323:27–36.
26. Prisant LM, Carr AA. Initial evaluation of the hypertensive patient. Postgrad Med 1988;84(8):197–217.
27. The National High Blood Pressure Education Program Coordinating Committee. National High Blood Pressure Education Program Working Group report on ambulatory blood pressure monitoring. Arch Intern Med 1990;150:2270–2280.
28. Epstein M, Sowers JR. Diabetes mellitus and hypertension. Hypertension 1992;19:403–418.
29. Eselin JA, Carter BC. Hypertension and left ventricular hypertrophy: Is drug therapy beneficial? Pharmacotherapy 1994;14:60–88.
30. Masserli FH, Aristizabal D, Soria F. Reduction of left ventricular hypertrophy: How beneficial? Am Heart J 1993;125:1520–1524.
31. The Acute Infarction Ramipril Efficacy (AIRE) Study Investigators. Effect of ramipril on mortality and morbidity of survivors of acute myocardial infarction with clinical evidence of heart failure. Lancet 1993;342:821–828.
32. McMahon FG. Management of Essential Hypertension: The New Low-Dose Era, 2nd ed. Mount Kisco, NY, Futura Publishing, 1984.
33. Lardinois CK, Neuman. The effects of antihypertensive agents on serum lipids and lipoproteins. Arch Intern Med 1988;148:1280–1288.
34. Houston MC. The effects of antihypertensive drugs on glucose intolerance in hypertensive nondiabetics and diabetics. Am Heart J 1988;115(3):640–656.
35. Nadelmann J, Frishman WH. Clinical use of β-adrenoceptor blockade in systemic hypertension. Drugs 1990;39(6):862–876.
36. Gengo FM, Fagan SC, de Padova A, et al. The effect of β-blockers on mental performance on older hypertensive patients. Arch Intern Med 1988;148:779–784.
37. Dzau VJ. Mechanism of action of angiotensin-converting enzyme (ACE) inhibitors in hypertension and heart failure: Role of plasma versus tissue ACE. Drugs 1990;39(suppl 2):11–16.
38. Hanssens M, Keirse MJNC, Vankelecom F, et al. Fetal and neonatal effects of treatment with angiotensin-converting-enzyme inhibitors in pregnancy. Obstet Gynecol 1991;78:128–135.
39. Kaplan NM. Calcium entry blockers in the treatment of hypertension. JAMA 1989;262:817–823.
40. Robinson BF. Calcium-entry blocking agents in the treatment of systemic hypertension. Am J Cardiol 1985;55(3):102B–106B.

41. Prisant LM, Spruill WJ, Fincham J, et al. Depression associated with antihypertensive drugs. J Fam Pract 1991;33:481–485.
42. Ingelfinger J. Pediatric Hypertension. Philadelphia, WB Saunders, 1982.
43. Report of the Second Task Force on Blood Pressure Control in Children—1987. Pediatrics 1987;79:1–25.
44. Naden RP, Redman CWG. Antihypertensive drugs in pregnancy. Clin Perinatol 1985;12:521–538.
45. Lindheimer MD, Katz AL. Hypertension in pregnancy. N Engl J Med 1985;313:675–680.
46. Cunningham FG, Lindheimer MD. Hypertension in pregnancy. N Engl J Med 1992;326:927–932.
47. National High Blood Pressure Education Program Working Group report on high blood pressure in pregnancy. Am J Obstet Gynecol 1990;163:1689–1712.
48. Sibai BM, Caritis SN, Thom E, et al. Prevention of preeclampsia with low-dose aspirin in healthy, nulliparous pregnant women. N Engl J Med 1993;329:1213–1218.
49. CLASP: A randomized trial of low-dose aspirin for the prevention and treatment of preeclampsia among 9364 pregnant women. Lancet 1994;343:619–629.
50. Gavras H, Gavras I. Hypertension in the Elderly. Boston, John Wright–PSG, 1983.
51. Franklin SS. Geriatric hypertension. Med Clin North Am 1983;67:395–416.
52. O'Malley K, O'Brien E. Management of hypertension in the elderly. N Engl J Med 1980;302:1397–1401.
53. Chobanian AV. Pathophysiologic considerations in the treatment of the elderly hypertensive patient. Am J Cardiol 1983;52:39D–53D.
54. Weber MA, Neutel JM, Cheung DG. Hypertension in the aged: A pathophysiologic basis for treatment. Am J Cardiol 1989;63:25H–32H.
55. Amery A, Birkenhager W. Brixko P, et al. Mortality and morbidity results from the European Working Party on High Blood Pressure in the Elderly trial. Lancet 1985;1:1349–1354.
56. Insug JT, Sacks HS, Lau Tai-Shing, et al. Drug treatment of hypertension in the elderly: A meta-analysis. Ann Intern Med 1994;121:355–362.
57. Hall WD, Saunders E, Shulman NB. Hypertension in Blacks: Epidemiology, Pathophysiology, and Treatment. Chicago, Year Book Medical Publishers, 1985.
58. Kaplan NM. Initial therapy in hypertension. Am J Cardiol 1983:51:619–660.
59. Frohlich ED. Role of calcium entry-blocking drugs in hypertension. Am J Cardiol 1985;56(16):1H–111H.
60. Christlieb AR. Treatment section considerations for the hypertensive diabetic patient. Arch Intern Med 1990;150:1167–1174.
61. National High Blood Pressure Education Program Working Group report on hypertension in diabetes. Hypertension 1994;23:145–158.
62. Houston MC. New insights and approaches to reduce end-organ damage in the treatment of hypertension: Subsets of hypertension approach. Am Heart J 1992;123:1337–1367.
63. Lebovitz H, Wiegmann T, Canan A, et al. Renal protective effects of enalapril in hypertensive NIDDM: Role of baseline albuminuria. Kidney Int 1994;45:S150–S155.
64. Neaton JD, Grimm RH, Prineas RJ, et al. Treatment of mild hypertension study (TOHMS). Final results. JAMA 1993;270:713–721.
65. Farnett L, Mulrow CD, Linn WD, et al. The J-curve phenomenon and the treatment of hypertension. JAMA 1991;265:489–495.
66. Zeller KR, Kuhnert LLV, Matthews C. Rapid reduction of severe asymptomatic hypertension. Arch Intern Med 1989;149:2186–2189.
67. Garcia JY, Vidt DG. Current management of hypertensive emergencies. Drugs 1987;34:263–278.
68. Calhoun DA, Oparil S. Treatment of hypertensive crisis. N Engl J Med 1990;323:1177–1183.
69. Prisant LM, Car AA, Hawkins DW. Treating hypertensive emergencies. Postgrad Med 1993;93:92–110.

Chapter 13

Congestive Heart Failure

Julie A. Johnson, PharmD, and Richard L. Lalonde, PharmD

Congestive heart failure (CHF) is a pathophysiologic state in which the heart is unable to pump blood at a rate sufficient to meet the metabolic needs of the body.[1] It is not a specific disease entity, but rather a clinical syndrome that may be caused by numerous different cardiac disorders. The normal cardiac cycle is comprised of two main components, ventricular diastole and ventricular systole, and diseases that adversely affect either component may lead to CHF. Filling of the ventricle occurs during ventricular diastole while ventricular contraction and ejection of blood occur during ventricular systole. For many years it was believed that reduced myocardial contractility, or systolic dysfunction, was the sole disturbance in cardiac function responsible for heart failure.[2] Although reduced myocardial contractility is the cause of CHF in many patients, the importance of disturbances in relaxation (lusitropic) properties of the heart has recently been recognized, because several studies have shown that 30–40% of patients with CHF symptoms have normal systolic function.[3] It is now clear that CHF may be the result of systolic dysfunction, diastolic dysfunction, or both.

It is estimated that approximately 4 million Americans have been diagnosed with CHF, and approximately 400,000 new cases are diagnosed each year.[4] The incidence of CHF increases with age, and CHF is the most common hospital discharge diagnosis in individuals older than age 65. CHF is more common in men than in women, which is thought to be due to the greater incidence of ischemic heart disease in men. Median survival from the time of diagnosis is 1.7 years in men and 3.2 years in women. When those who survive less than 90 days from the time of diagnosis are excluded, 1-year survival rates are 79% and 88% in men and women, respectively, and 5-year survival rates are 35% and 53%, respectively.[4] Death is classified as sudden in 20–50% of patients,[5–7] implicating serious ventricular arrhythmias as the underlying cause of death in many patients with CHF.

PATHOPHYSIOLOGY/ETIOLOGY

CHF is a pathophysiologic state that can result from many cardiac diseases or disorders; common causes of heart failure are shown in Table 13.1.[1,8] Many of the common cardiovascular diseases cause both systolic and diastolic dysfunction, thus many patients have CHF as a result of reduced ventricular filling and reduced myocardial contractility.

Systolic contractile dysfunction is a cardinal feature of dilated cardiomyopathies. Although the cause of reduced contractility is frequently unknown, abnormalities such as interstitial fibrosis, cellular infiltrates, cellular hypertrophy, and myocardial cell degeneration are commonly seen on histologic examination.[8] Dilated cardiomyopathies are discussed in detail in Chapter 17.

Pressure or volume overload causes ventricular hypertrophy, which helps return contractility to a near normal state. However, if the pressure or volume overload persists, the hypertrophied myocardial cells eventually become fibrotic, and contractility decreases. Ventricular hypertrophy also increases the stiffness of the ventricle and slows ventricular relaxation, therefore impairing diastolic function as well.[1] Examples of pressure overload include systemic or pulmonary hypertension and aortic or pulmonic valve stenosis. Volume overload may occur in the presence of valvular regurgitation, shunts, or high-output states such as anemia or pregnancy.

TABLE 13.1. CAUSES OF HEART FAILURE

Systolic Dysfunction (Decreased Contractility)
1. Dilated cardiomyopathies
2. Ventricular hypertrophy
   a. Pressure overload (e.g., systemic or pulmonary hypertension, aortic or pulmonic valve)
   b. Volume overload (e.g., valvular regurgitation, shunts, high-output states)
3. Reduction in muscle mass (e.g., myocardial infarction)

Diastolic Dysfunction (Restriction in Ventricular Filling)
1. Increased ventricular stiffness
   a. Ventricular hypertrophy (e.g., hypertrophic cardiomyopathy, other examples above)
   b. Infiltrative myocardial diseases (e.g., amyloidosis, sarcoidosis, endomyocardial fibrosis)
   c. Myocardial ischemia and infarction
2. Mitral or tricuspid valve stenosis
3. Pericardial disease (e.g., pericarditis, pericardial tamponade)

(Compiled from References 1 and 8.)

Another cause of systolic dysfunction is reduction in muscle mass due to acute myocardial infarction. Myocardial infarction leads to death of affected myocardial cells, and the degree to which contractility is decreased will depend on the size of the infarction. Myocardial ischemia and infarction also affect the diastolic properties of the heart by slowing ventricular relaxation and increasing ventricular stiffness. Thus, myocardial infarction frequently results in systolic and diastolic dysfunction. Less common causes of diastolic dysfunction are listed in Table 13.1 and include infiltrative myocardial diseases, mitral or tricuspid valve stenosis, and pericardial disease.

The most recently published Framingham study suggests that ischemic heart disease is the underlying etiology in 47% of females and 59% of males with CHF. Hypertension is the suspected etiology in 37% of females and 30% of males.[4] Other less common etiologies of CHF include cardiomyopathies (e.g., idiopathic dilated, viral, alcoholic, hypertrophic) and valvular heart disease.[4,8]

COMPENSATORY MECHANISMS

To understand the pathophysiologic processes in CHF, a basic understanding of normal cardiac function is necessary. Cardiac output (CO) is defined as the volume of blood ejected per unit time (L/min) and is described mathematically as the product of heart rate (HR) and stroke volume (SV).

$$CO = HR \times SV \qquad (1)$$

Heart rate is controlled by the autonomic nervous system. Stroke volume, or the volume of blood ejected during systole, is dependent on preload, afterload, and contractility.[1,9] Preload is commonly defined as ventricular filling pressure, although it is more accurately described as left ventricular end diastolic volume (LVEDV). As defined by the Frank–Starling mechanism, the ability of the heart to alter the force of contraction is dependent on changes in preload. As myocardial sarcomere length is stretched, the number of cross bridges between thick and thin myofilaments increases, resulting in an increase in the force of contraction. The length of the sarcomere is determined primarily by the volume of blood in the ventricle, therefore LVEDV is the primary determinant of preload. Because of the relationship between pressure and volume in the heart, left ventricular end diastolic pressure (LVEDP) is often used in the clinical setting to estimate preload. The hemodynamic measurement used to estimate LVEDP is the pulmonary capillary wedge pressure (PCWP) (see Chapter 10). Afterload is defined as the forces that resist shortening of the myocardial fibers and thus the forces against which the left ventricle must work to eject blood into the systemic circulation. In patients with left ventricular systolic dysfunction, an inverse relationship exists between afterload and stroke volume such that increasing afterload causes a decrease in stroke volume (Fig. 13.1). Systemic vascular resistance (SVR) is commonly used clinically to approximate left ventricular afterload. Contractility is the intrinsic property of cardiac muscle describing fiber shortening and tension development; it is difficult to measure accurately in the clinical setting. Finally, the determinants of mean arterial pressure (MAP) are:

$$MAP = CO \times SVR \qquad (2)$$

As cardiac function decreases secondary to one or more of the disorders previously described, the heart relies on three major compensatory mechanisms to maintain an adequate cardiac output: (1) increased sympathetic nervous system activity; (2) the Frank–Starling mechanism, whereby an increase in preload results in an increase in stroke volume; and (3) ventricular hypertrophy. These compensatory responses are highlighted in Fig. 13.2. Although these compensatory responses maintain cardiac function at normal levels for a period of time, they all have limited capacity. If the burden (e.g., reduced contractility or diastolic dysfunction) that initiated these compensatory responses persists, the heart will eventually fail.

The sympathetic nervous system is activated within seconds of a change in cardiac output and serves as an immediate support mechanism in patients with heart failure. Norepinephrine released from myocardial adrenergic nerve terminals serves an important compensatory role in maintaining cardiac output by increasing both contractility and heart rate. Norepinephrine release in vascular beds rich with α_1-adrenergic receptors causes vasoconstriction and

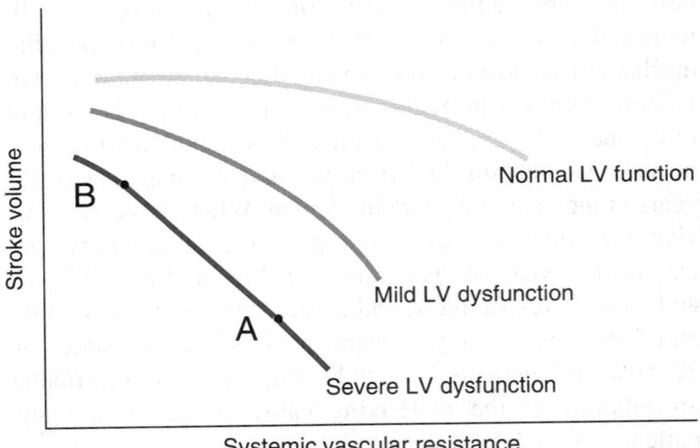

Figure 13.1. Relationship between stroke volume and systemic vascular resistance. In an individual with normal left ventricular (LV) function, increasing systemic vascular resistance has little effect on stroke volume. As the extent of LV dysfunction increases, the negative, inverse relationship between stroke volume and systemic vascular resistance becomes more important (B to A).

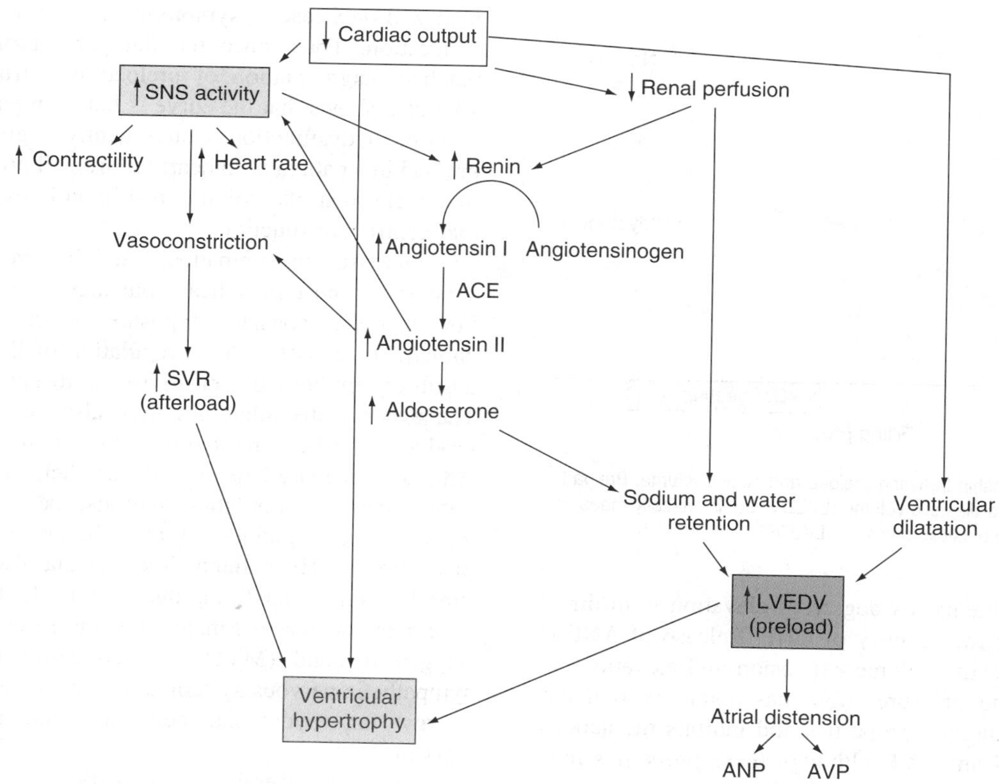

Figure 13.2. Compensatory responses to decreased cardiac output. The three major mechanisms by which the body can enhance cardiac output are (1) increased sympathetic nervous system (SNS) activity, (2) increased preload, and (3) ventricular hypertrophy. *Key:* SVR, systemic vascular resistance, ACE, angiotensin-converting enzyme; LVEDV, left ventricular end diastolic volume; ANP, atrial natriuretic peptide; AVP, arginine vasopressin.

helps to redistribute blood flow away from nonessential organs to coronary and cerebral circulations. In addition, increased sympathetic tone causes peripheral vasoconstriction and helps to support blood pressure, which may be reduced secondary to a decrease in cardiac output (Equation 2).[1] Plasma norepinephrine concentrations are elevated in correlation with the degree of heart failure and patients with the highest plasma norepinephrine concentrations have the poorest prognosis.[1]

Augmentation of preload is another important compensatory response that is rapidly activated in patients with heart failure. Renal perfusion in heart failure is reduced due to both a reduction in cardiac output and redistribution of blood away from nonvital organs. The kidney detects the reduced perfusion as an ineffective blood volume, thus stimulating sodium and water retention. Reduced renal perfusion and increased sympathetic tone also stimulate renin release from juxtaglomerular cells in the kidney. Renin is responsible for conversion of angiotensinogen to angiotensin I. Angiotensin I is converted to angiotensin II by angiotensin-converting enzyme (ACE). Angiotensin II feeds back on the adrenal gland to stimulate aldosterone release, thereby providing an additional mechanism for sodium and water retention in the kidney. As intravascular volume increases secondary to sodium and water retention, left ventricular volume and pressure (preload) increase, sarcomeres are stretched, and the force of contraction is enhanced, according to the Frank–Starling mechanism.[1,10] The relationship between filling pressure (preload) and stroke volume is shown in Fig. 13.3.

Angiotensin II also plays a direct compensatory role in CHF as a potent vasoconstrictor that increases systemic vascular resistance. As described previously, systemic vasoconstriction may help support blood pressure in CHF patients. Angiotensin II also facilitates release of norepinephrine from adrenergic nerve terminals, adding to the level of sympathetic activation. Finally, angiotensin II in cardiac tissue appears to be a proto-oncogene, which plays an important role in left ventricular hypertrophy and dilatation, which leads to progressively worsening heart failure.

Arginine vasopressin (AVP) is an antidiuretic hormone that is frequently elevated in patients with CHF.[1] It has potent vasoconstrictor properties, although the clinical importance of this hormone in CHF is unclear. Atrial natriuretic factor (ANF) is another hormone that is ele-

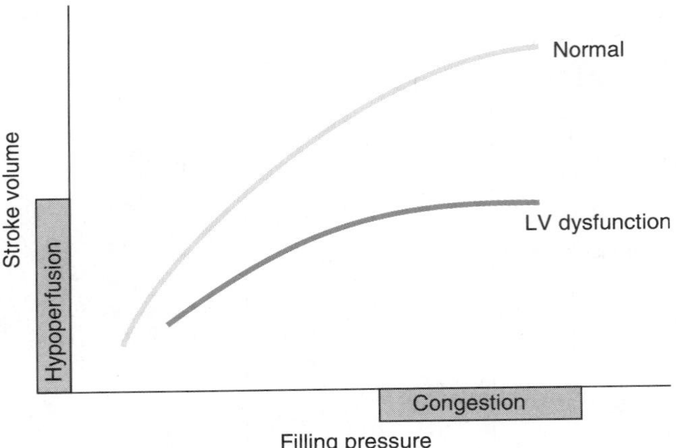

Figure 13.3. Relationship between preload and stroke volume. Preload is the left ventricular end diastolic volume (LVEDV) but is typically measured as left ventricular end diastolic pressure (LVEDP).

vated in CHF patients; its degree of elevation is in direct relationship with the severity of CHF. Release of ANF is stimulated by plasma volume expansion and elevations in atrial volume and pressure. ANF has potent vasodilator, natriuretic, and diuretic properties and inhibits the actions of angiotensin II and AVP, although these properties may be attenuated in CHF patients. Its role as a counter-regulatory hormone in CHF is unclear at this time.[1,10] There is also interest in harnessing ANF as a therapeutic agent, and a recent, small study with an inhibitor of the enzyme responsible for ANF's breakdown showed promising results.[11] The release and feedback inhibition of ANF and AVP, respectively, are controlled in part by atrial stretch receptors.

Whereas sympathetic activation and increased preload are compensatory responses with rapid onset, ventricular hypertrophy occurs more slowly. An increase in ventricular muscle mass (ventricular hypertrophy) may be stimulated by increases in preload or afterload or by decreases in contractility or myocardial muscle mass. Ventricular hypertrophy provides an important mechanism for improving contractile function but, as described previously, hypertrophied cells that are exposed to continued stress eventually become fibrotic. Thus, ventricular hypertrophy is an important compensatory response in CHF, but is eventually inadequate in maintaining cardiac function.[1]

The compensatory mechanisms previously described all play important roles in maintaining cardiac function, but detrimental overshoot of these mechanisms usually occurs. A summary of the beneficial and detrimental effects of the compensatory mechanisms of CHF are shown in Table 13.2. For example, sodium and water retention leads to an increase in preload with a consequential increase in stroke volume by the Frank–Starling mechanism. However, as can be seen in Fig. 13.3, increases in preload will increase stroke volume only to a certain point, after which the flat portion of the curve is reached and further increases in preload will only lead to symptoms of pulmonary or systemic congestion. Thus, once the flat portion of the curve is reached, augmentation of preload is detrimental. Figure 13.3 also shows that the curve is flatter in patients with left ventricular dysfunction. Consequently, a given increase in preload in a patient with heart failure will produce a smaller increment in stroke volume than in an individual with normal ventricular function.

Increases in sympathetic activity provide important support for the failing heart, but may also be detrimental. For example, constant exposure of the heart to catecholamines causes a down-regulation of β receptors, with a subsequent loss of sensitivity to receptor stimulation.[1] The excess catecholamines may also be cardiotoxic and produce further reductions in contractile function. Although increased heart rate may help maintain cardiac output, cardiac stimulation may also be an important factor in the precipitation of arrhythmias, which are often observed in CHF patients. Tachycardia also decreases the time for ventricular filling during diastole, thus stroke volume may decrease. Finally, the increases in myocardial oxygen demand (MVO_2), which result from increased sympathetic nervous system activation, consume additional energy for myocardial cells that are already energy starved.[12]

The peripheral vasoconstriction, mediated by increased sympathetic activity, angiotensin II, and other possible mechanisms such as AVP, causes an increase in systemic vascular resistance or afterload. Increased afterload resists myocardial fiber shortening and causes a further decrease in cardiac output, which leads to further increases in sodium and water retention and sympathetic nervous system activity. Thus, the compensatory mechanisms in CHF eventually initiate vicious cycles, which lead to continued worsening and downward spiraling of the CHF state.

PRECIPITATING FACTORS

Patients may have a diagnosis of CHF, yet appropriate therapy can maintain them in a state of "compensated" heart failure, indicating they are relatively symptom free. However, there are many aggravating or precipitating factors that may cause a previously compensated patient to decompensate. The relative frequency of precipitating factors in compensated chronic heart failure was evaluated prospectively in 101 consecutive patients admitted with CHF to the study hospital.[13] The results from the study are shown in Table 13.3. Note that more than one factor could be identified in a given patient. These investigators found that noncompliance with diet, drug therapy, or both was the most common precipitating factor, identified in 64% of patients. Uncontrolled hypertension despite antihypertensive therapy was also identified as a precipitating factor in 44% of patients. Arrhythmias,

TABLE 13.2. BENEFICIAL AND DETRIMENTAL EFFECTS OF THE COMPENSATORY MECHANISMS IN CHF

Compensatory Response	Mechanism(s) of Compensation	Beneficial Effects of Compensation	Detrimental Effects of Compensation
Na^+ and water retention	Decreased renal perfusion Aldosterone release	Optimize stroke volume through Frank–Starling mechanism	Pulmonary and systemic congestion and edema
Vasoconstriction	Increased SNS activity Angiotensin II Arginine vasopressin (?)	Maintain BP in face of reduced CO	Increased MVO_2 Increased afterload, which decreases stroke volume and further activates the compensatory mechanisms
Tachycardia	Increased SNS activity Baroreceptor-mediated response to decreased BP	Help maintain CO	Increased MVO_2 Precipitation of ventricular arrhythmias (?) Shortened diastolic filling time β_1-receptor down-regulation, decreased receptor sensitivity
Ventricular hypertrophy	Increased afterload Decreased cardiac output Increased preload	Help maintain CO Reduced myocardial wall stress Decreased MVO_2	Diastolic dysfunction Hypertrophied ventricle does not have normal function Risk of myocardial cell death

Key: SNS, sympathetic nervous system; BP, blood pressure; MVO_2, myocardial oxygen demand; CO, cardiac output.

especially atrial fibrillation and flutter, were also common findings. Other less common factors include pulmonary or systemic infection, myocardial infarction, chordae tendineae rupture, pulmonary embolism, emotional or environmental stress, high-output states (e.g., thyrotoxicosis, anemia, pregnancy), and development of unrelated illnesses.[13,14] Iatrogenic causes for decompensation are also important and preventable precipitants of CHF. Administration of drugs with negative inotropic, cardiotoxic, or sodium-retaining properties may exacerbate or precipitate CHF. Examples are given in Table 13.4. Similarly, blood transfusion or excess administration of sodium-containing intravenous fluids can also precipitate CHF.

Inspection of the various factors that may aggravate or precipitate CHF reveals that many are preventable. Thus, the value of careful and repeated education of patients about the importance of dietary and drug therapy compliance should not be underestimated.

TABLE 13.3. PRECIPITATING FACTORS IN CHRONIC HEART FAILURE

Factor	% of Patients
Lack of compliance	64.3
With diet	21.8
With drugs	5.9
With both diet and drugs	36.6
Uncontrolled hypertension	43.6
Cardiac arrhythmias	28.7
Atrial fibrillation	19.8
Atrial flutter	6.9
Multifocal atrial tachycardia	1.0
Ventricular tachycardia	1.0
Environmental factors	18.8
Inadequate therapy	16.8
Pulmonary infection	11.9
Emotional stress	6.9
Administration of inappropriate medications or fluid overload	4.0
Myocardial infarction/ruptured chordae tendinae	5.9
Endocrine disorders (thyrotoxicosis)	1.0

(Adapted from Reference 13.)

CLINICAL PRESENTATION[14]

An understanding of the pathophysiologic processes and compensatory mechanisms in CHF makes it relatively easy to understand the clinical signs and symptoms. The underlying pathophysiology in CHF typically causes a reduction in cardiac output. In an attempt to compensate for reduced cardiac output, stimulation of the sympathetic nervous system occurs along with activation of mechanisms that cause an increase in preload (Fig. 13.2). However, an overshoot of the mechanisms that increase preload and an inability of the heart to accept or eject the increased blood volume efficiently results in systemic and/or pulmonary congestion, the most common causes of CHF signs and symptoms. Peripheral hypoperfusion and increases in sympathetic ner-

TABLE 13.4. DRUGS THAT MAY PRECIPITATE OR EXACERBATE CONGESTIVE HEART FAILURE

Negative Inotropic Effect
- Antiarrhythmics (e.g., disopyramide, flecainide, and others)
- β Blockers (e.g., propranolol, metoprolol, atenolol, and others)
- Calcium channel blockers (e.g., verapamil and others)

Cardiotoxic
- Doxorubicin
- Daunomycin
- Cyclophosphamide

Sodium and Water Retention
- Glucocorticoids
- Androgens
- Estrogens
- Nonsteroidal anti-inflammatory agents
- Salicylates (high dose)
- Sodium-containing drugs (e.g., carbenicillin disodium, ticarcillin disodium)

TABLE 13.5. SIGNS AND SYMPTOMS OF CONGESTIVE HEART FAILURE

Symptoms	Signs
Right Ventricular Dysfunction	
Abdominal pain	Peripheral edema
Anorexia	Jugular venous distension
Nausea	Hepatojugular reflux
Bloating	Hepatomegaly
Constipation	
Ascites	
Left Ventricular Dysfunction	
Dyspnea on exertion	Bibasilar rales
Paroxysmal nocturnal dyspnea	Pulmonary edema
Orthopnea	S3 gallop
Tachypnea	Pleural effusion
Cough	Cheyne–Stokes respiration
Hemoptysis	
Nonspecific Findings	
Exercise intolerance	Tachycardia
Fatigue	Pallor
Weakness	Cyanosis of digits
Nocturia	Cardiomegaly
CNS symptoms	

(Adapted from Covinsky JO, Willett MS. Congestive heart failure, in DiPiro JT, Talbert RL, Hayes PE, et al (eds): Pharmacotherapy: A Pathophysiologic Approach. New York, Elsevier, 1989, pp 115–149.)

vous system activity are responsible for the remaining clinical findings in CHF patients. Table 13.5 contains a summary of the signs and symptoms of CHF.

Symptoms of congestion develop behind the failing ventricle such that left ventricular failure causes signs and symptoms of pulmonary congestion whereas right ventricular failure causes signs and symptoms consistent with systemic congestion. Most patients initially have left ventricular failure. However, because the ventricles share a septal wall and failure of the left ventricle will increase the workload of the right ventricle, both ventricles eventually fail. Many CHF patients will therefore present with symptoms of both systemic and pulmonary congestion.

Signs and Symptoms of Left Ventricular Failure

When the left ventricle fails, it is unable to accept and eject the increased blood volume that is delivered to it. Consequently, pulmonary venous and capillary pressures rise, leading to interstitial edema, increased airway resistance, and dyspnea. The associated signs and symptoms may include (1) dyspnea on exertion (DOE), (2) orthopnea, (3) paroxysmal nocturnal dyspnea (PND), (4) dyspnea at rest, or (5) pulmonary edema. Dyspnea with exertion occurs in normal individuals, but exertional dyspnea is a symptom of CHF when there is a reduction in the level of exertion that causes breathlessness. This is typically described by patients as more breathlessness than was previously associated with a specific activity (e.g., vacuuming, stair climbing). As CHF progresses, the degree of exertion that produces breathlessness declines until the patient eventually has dyspnea at rest.

Orthopnea is dyspnea that occurs with assumption of the supine position. It occurs within minutes of recumbency and is due to reduced pooling of blood in the lower extremities and abdomen. Orthopnea is relieved almost immediately by sitting upright on the edge of the bed and is typically prevented by elevating the head with pillows. A change in the number of pillows required to prevent orthopnea (e.g., a change from "two-pillow" to "three-pillow" orthopnea) suggests worsening heart failure. Pulmonary congestion may also cause a nonproductive cough, either with exertion or at night. Attacks of paroxysmal nocturnal dyspnea typically occur 2 to 4 hours after being asleep; they awaken the patient from sleep with the feeling of suffocation. The attacks are due to severe pulmonary and bronchial congestion, leading to shortness of breath and wheezing (thus the alternate name "cardiac asthma"). Unlike orthopnea, the patient may have to sit upright for 30 minutes or more to obtain relief from an attack of paroxysmal nocturnal dyspnea. The reasons these attacks occur at night are unclear but may include (1) reduced pooling of blood in the lower extremities and abdomen (as in orthopnea), (2) slow resorption of interstitial fluid from sites of dependent edema, (3) normal reduction in sympathetic activity that occurs with sleep (e.g., less support for the failing ventricle), and (4) normal depression in respiratory drive that occurs with sleep.

Pulmonary edema is the most severe form of pulmonary congestion, and is caused by accumulation of fluid in the interstitial space and alveoli. In CHF patients, it is the result of increased pulmonary venous pressure. The patient experiences extreme breathlessness, anxiety, and may expectorate a pink, frothy liquid. Pulmonary edema can be terrifying for the patient, causing a feeling of suffocation or drowning.

Rales (clicking or crackling sounds heard on auscultation) are heard in the lung bases in patients with left-sided CHF due to transudation of fluid into alveoli. The rales are typically bibasilar, but if heard unilaterally, are usually heard on the right side. Pulmonary edema and pleural effusion are also signs of left-sided heart failure. A third heart sound, or S3 gallop, is frequently heard in patients with left ventricular failure and may be due to elevated atrial pressure and altered distensibility of the ventricle. Patients with severe CHF occasionally have Cheyne–Stokes respiration, which alternates between hyperventilation and apnea.

The chest roentgenogram (CXR) provides a relatively specific but insensitive measure of the degree of pulmonary congestion. When pulmonary capillary pressures are in the range of 18 to 23 mm Hg, upper lobe vessels become prominent due to redistribution of blood from the congested lower lobes. Interstitial edema develops when pulmonary capillary pressures are between 20 to 25 mm Hg and may be seen on CXR as "Kerley" lines (sharp, linear densities of interlobular interstitial edema). Pulmonary capillary pressures in excess of 25 mm Hg result in a "butterfly pattern" of bilateral perihilar infiltrates on CXR.

Signs and Symptoms of Right Ventricular Failure

Signs and symptoms of right ventricular failure are the result of systemic venous congestion. Examination of the right jugular vein with the patient at a 45° angle is a simple method for assessing jugular venous pressure. Elevation of jugular venous pressure more than 4 cm above the sternal angle suggests systemic venous congestion. In patients with mild heart failure, jugular venous distension may be normal at rest but application of pressure to the abdomen will cause an elevation of jugular venous pressure. This is known as the hepatojugular reflux. An elevation in jugular venous pressure in this setting is due to abdominal (especially hepatic) congestion and an inability of the right ventricle to accept or eject the increased blood volume returning to it. Development of ascites uncommonly occurs in patients with long-standing systemic venous congestion.

Peripheral edema is a cardinal finding in right-sided heart failure. Edema usually occurs in dependent parts of the body, thus is seen as ankle or pedal edema in ambulatory patients but may be manifested as sacral edema in bedridden patients. Adults typically have a 10-lb fluid weight gain before trace peripheral edema is evident, therefore patients with acute heart failure may have no clinical evidence of peripheral edema except weight gain.

Symptoms that are associated with right-sided heart failure are less common than those of left-sided heart failure. These symptoms are related to hepatic and intestinal congestion and may include abdominal pain, anorexia, nausea, bloating, and constipation.

Nonspecific Findings in CHF

Physical examination and CXR findings that suggest cardiomegaly are found in most patients with CHF but are considered nonspecific findings. There are no specific electrocardiographic (ECG) findings that are associated with CHF. Many patients will, however, have left ventricular hypertrophy, which will be evident on ECG. The remaining nonspecific signs and symptoms of CHF are due primarily to reduced cardiac output or elevated sympathetic nervous system activity. Weakness, fatigue, and exercise intolerance are found in most patients with CHF and are related in part to inadequate oxygen delivery to skeletal muscles in patients with reduced cardiac output. It must be kept in mind, however, that these symptoms may also be seen in many noncardiac disorders. Symptoms of central nervous system (CNS) hypoperfusion such as confusion, hallucinations, nightmares, insomnia, and headache may occur in patients with severe CHF, especially if they have underlying cerebral arteriosclerosis.

Increased sympathetic nervous system activity is responsible for the tachycardia often observed in CHF. As previously described, sympathetic activation produces peripheral vasoconstriction, which may be manifested as pallor, cool extremities, or cyanosis of the digits. Sympathetically mediated vasoconstriction also serves to shunt blood away from nonvital organs such as the kidney. Nocturia is frequently noted in CHF patients because with rest there are reductions in sympathetic activation and cardiac output demands. Consequently, renal vasoconstriction diminishes, resulting in increased renal blood flow and urine formation.

CLASSIFICATION OF CONGESTIVE HEART FAILURE PATIENTS

Systems that classify patients according to their level of disability are useful from several perspectives. They can be used to follow the progress of the patient longitudinally, to assess the impact of therapeutic maneuvers, or to provide a reference point with which they can be compared with other patients. The most widely used classification system is the New York Heart Association (NYHA) Functional Classification System.[15] This classification system divides patients into four categories (see Table 13.6). Functional class (FC)-I patients have no limitation of physical activity, FC-II patients have slight limitation of physical activity, FC-III patients have marked limitation of physical activity, and FC-IV patients are unable to carry on physical activity without discomfort. There are obvious limitations to assigning a numerical score to subjective findings; however, this system is fairly useful for monitoring patients and is widely utilized in CHF studies. A system that allows assignment of scores for specific activities (shown in Chapter 14) has been developed but this system has not gained widespread popularity.

TABLE 13.6. NEW YORK HEART ASSOCIATION FUNCTIONAL CLASSIFICATION

Functional class	
I	Patients with cardiac disease but without limitations of physical activity. Ordinary physical activity does not cause undue fatigue, dyspnea, or palpitation.
II	Patients with cardiac disease that results in slight limitations of physical activity. Ordinary physical activity results in fatigue, palpitation, dyspnea, or angina.
III	Patients with cardiac disease that results in marked limitation of physical activity. Although patients are comfortable at rest, less than ordinary activity will lead to symptoms.
IV	Patients with cardiac disease that results in an inability to carry on physical activity without discomfort. Symptoms of congestive heart failure are present even at rest. With any physical activity, increased discomfort is experienced.

Compiled from Reference 15.

TREATMENT OF ACUTE/SEVERE HEART FAILURE

Certain causes of heart failure lead to a slow progressive decrease in cardiac function over many months or years. Such patients will usually present initially with mild symptoms of heart failure and can be treated on an outpatient basis. However, other individuals will present with more severe and/or sudden cardiac dysfunction and will require hospitalization and aggressive therapy with intensive monitoring. Severe heart failure may progress to cardiogenic shock, a clinical syndrome that results when cardiac dysfunction leads to circulatory collapse and inadequate blood flow to vital organ systems. This may be a manifestation of end-stage chronic heart failure, cardiac arrhythmias, valvular dysfunction, and/or acute myocardial infarction. A low cardiac output syndrome is also a common postoperative complication of cardiopulmonary bypass surgery. The most common cause of acute heart failure and cardiogenic shock is a single massive myocardial infarction or the cumulative damage from several smaller infarcts (see Chapter 15). Despite advances in pharmacologic and nonpharmacologic therapies, patients with cardiogenic shock have a dismal prognosis (mortality of 70–95%).[16]

PRINCIPLES OF THERAPY BASED ON HEMODYNAMIC SUBSETS

During the past 25 years, invasive hemodynamic monitoring using a balloon-tipped, flow-directed pulmonary artery catheter has become a critically important tool in the management of patients with severe heart failure (see Chapter 10). Invasive hemodynamic monitoring helps in the selection of appropriate medical therapy and also in the classification of patients into specific subsets. These *hemodynamic subsets* were first proposed for patients with left ventricular dysfunction following an acute myocardial infarction but are also applicable to patients with acute or severe heart failure from other causes (Fig. 13.4).[17] The hemodynamic classification has four subsets and is based on whether a patient has a cardiac index above or below 2.2 L/min/m^2 and a PCWP above or below 18 mm Hg. Similarly, a *clinical* classification can be used based on signs and symptoms of hypoperfusion (associated with a low cardiac index) and pulmonary congestion (associated with a high PCWP). A general treatment algorithm for the four hemodynamic subsets is shown in Fig. 13.5 and discussed as follows.

Subset I

Patients in hemodynamic subset I have a cardiac index and PCWP within generally acceptable ranges and have the lowest mortality of any subset. These patients do not need immediate specific interventions other than standard treatment and monitoring. It should be emphasized that patients with significant left ventricular dysfunction may still present in subset I because normal compensatory mechanisms and/or appropriate drug therapy may at least partially correct an otherwise abnormal hemodynamic profile.

Subset II

As shown in Fig. 13.4, patients in subset II have an adequate cardiac index but a PCWP higher than 18 mm Hg. These patients are likely to have pulmonary congestion secondary to increased hydrostatic pressure in the pulmonary capillaries but no evidence of peripheral hypoperfusion. The elevated PCWP may be the result of normal

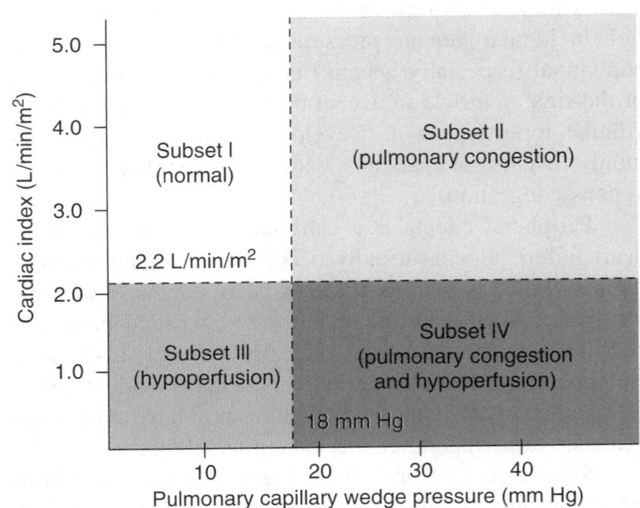

Figure 13.4. Hemodynamic subsets of heart failure patients based on cardiac index and pulmonary capillary wedge pressure. *(Adapted from Reference 17 with permission from N Engl J Med 1976;295:1356–1362).*

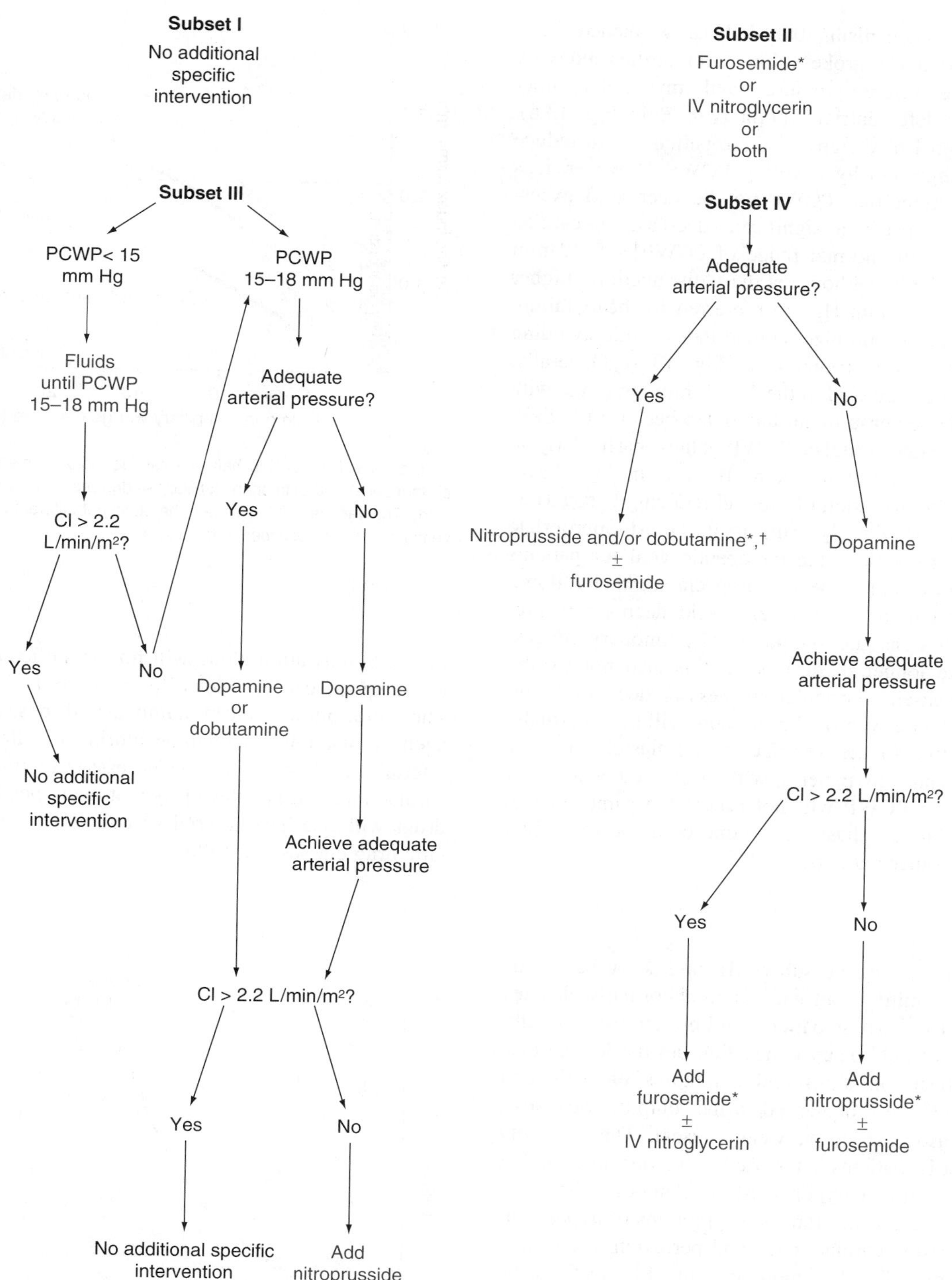

Figure 13.5. General treatment algorithm for acute/severe heart failure based on hemodynamic subsets. This is a suggested approach which may need to be modified for certain patients (see text). *Usual goals for hemodynamic parameters: cardiac index (CI) > 2.2 L/min/m^2, PCWP 15–18 mm Hg while maintaining adequate blood pressure and perfusion to essential organs. †Amrinone or milrinone are alternative agents.

compensatory mechanisms that help a weakened heart maintain an adequate stroke volume and cardiac index by increasing the filling pressure (and myocardial fiber stretch) of the left ventricle (point A to B in Fig. 13.6). The primary goal of therapy in these patients is to reduce pulmonary congestion by lowering PCWP. However, it is critically important that PCWP not be decreased excessively so as to cause a significant decrease in cardiac index. Although the normal range of PCWP is 5–12 mm Hg for individuals without cardiac dysfunction, higher pressures of 15–18 mm Hg are preferred for heart failure patients in order to optimize cardiac index while avoiding pulmonary congestion (point C in Fig. 13.6). Generally, the PCWP can be lowered to the 15–18 mm Hg range with relatively little decrease in cardiac index because the Starling curve is flatter at higher PCWP values, particularly in patients with heart failure (point B to C in Fig. 13.6). Intravenous administration of preload reducing agents (i.e., loop diuretics or nitroglycerin) is the most appropriate acute therapy to achieve the therapeutic goal for patients in subset II (see under specific drug classes that follow). These agents will produce a very rapid decrease in preload, although signs and symptoms of pulmonary congestion may take longer to disappear. It is also noteworthy that with increased ventricular stiffness or decreased ventricular compliance, ventricular pressure will be abnormally elevated relative to the ventricular end-diastolic volume (Fig. 13.7). Thus, in patients with decreased ventricular compliance, the PCWP will not reflect the same preload (i.e., ventricular end diastolic volume or myocardial fiber stretch) as in other patients.

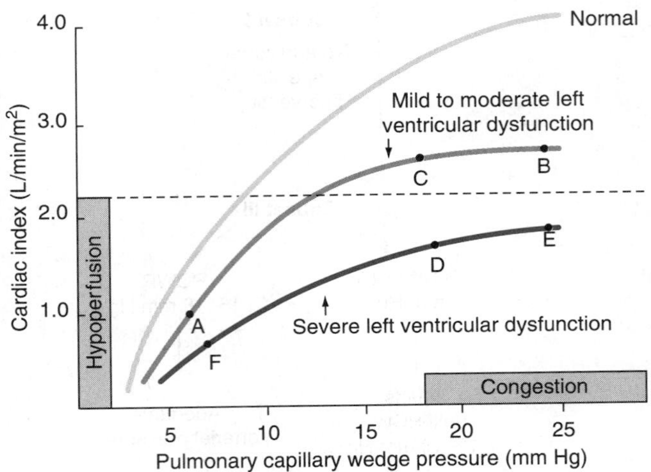

Figure 13.6. Relationship between cardiac index (a measure of cardiac performance) and pulmonary capillary wedge pressure (a measure of preload). The various points illustrate the effects of different therapeutic interventions and are described in the text.

Subset III

Patients in hemodynamic subset III have a cardiac index less than 2.2 L/min/m^2 but without an abnormally elevated PCWP (Fig. 13.4). These patients will present usually without evidence of pulmonary congestion but the low cardiac index will result in signs and symptoms of peripheral hypoperfusion (i.e., decreased urine output, weakness, peripheral vasoconstriction, weak pulses). The mortality rate of subset III patients is reported to be four times higher than patients without hypoperfusion.[17] Although the treatment goal is to alleviate signs and symptoms of hypoperfusion by increasing cardiac index and perfusion to essential organs, therapy will differ among patients (Fig. 13.5). If the PCWP is significantly below 15 mm Hg, initial therapy will be to administer intravenous fluids in order to provide a more optimal ventricular filling pressure of 15–18 mm Hg and consequently improve cardiac index. When there is only mild left ventricular dysfunction, intravenous fluid administration may be all that is necessary to achieve a cardiac index above 2.2 L/min/m^2 (point A to C in Fig. 13.6). However, many patients will have significant left ventricular dysfunction and a depressed Starling relationship so that fluid administration alone will not be sufficient to achieve an adequate cardiac index (point F to D in Fig. 13.6). Therefore, intravenously administered positive inotropic agents (dopamine, dobutamine, amrinone, milrinone) and/or arterial vasodilators may be necessary to further increase cardiac index. It is noteworthy that many positive inotropic drugs will also have arterial vasodilating activity (see specific drug classes that follow).

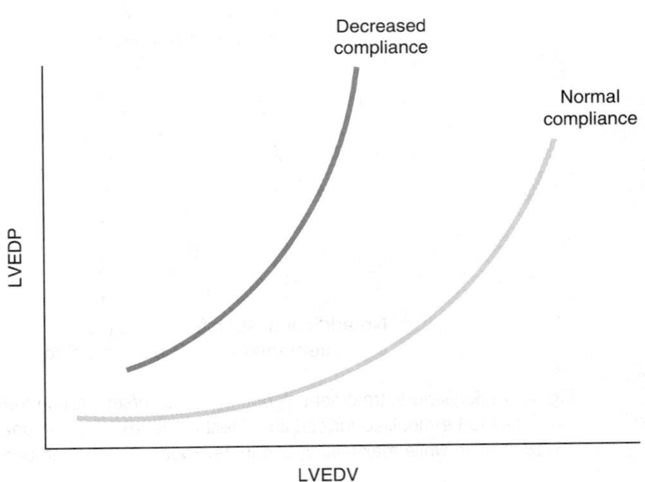

Figure 13.7. Relationship between left ventricular end diastolic volume (LVEDV) and pressure (LVEDP). A fixed increase in volume produces a larger increase in pressure when the LVEDV is elevated. Various disease states will decrease ventricular compliance and cause a shift in the curve and yield higher LVEDP for any given LVEDV.

Positive inotropic agents and arterial vasodilators will cause an upward shift in the Starling curve and produce higher cardiac indices for every level of filling pressure (point D to C in Fig. 13.6). The positive inotropic agents produce this shift through their direct effect on myocardial contractility, whereas the effect of arterial vasodilators is indirect. Figure 13.1 illustrates the inverse relationship between stroke volume and systemic vascular resistance in patients with left ventricular dysfunction. Arterial vasodilators will directly decrease systemic vascular resistance, which will lead to an increase in stroke volume and cardiac index (point A to B in Fig. 13.1). Because mean arterial pressure equals the product of cardiac output and systemic vascular resistance (Equation 2), the compensatory increase in cardiac output will tend to minimize any decrease in blood pressure that would otherwise be produced by the decrease in systemic vascular resistance. Nevertheless, a variable decrease in blood pressure will often be associated with the use of arterial vasodilators and will be an important dose-limiting adverse effect (see section on Positive Inotropic Agents Versus Arterial Vasodilators). Many clinicians would elect to use nitroprusside, a mixed arterial-venous vasodilator, because its hemodynamic effects can be titrated more easily than the longer acting hydralazine. However, special caution must be used to adjust the rate of intravenous fluid administration and prevent an excessive drop in PCWP because of the preload reducing effect of nitroprusside (see as follows).

Subset IV

Patients with a cardiac index less than 2.2 L/min/m^2 and a PCWP higher than 18 mm Hg are in hemodynamic subset IV and have the worst prognosis of any subset. Severe pump failure is evidenced by the fact that these patients cannot maintain an adequate cardiac index despite the elevated left ventricular filling pressure and increased myocardial fiber stretch. These patients will present with signs and symptoms of pulmonary congestion (subset II) and peripheral hypoperfusion (subset III). The treatment goals are to alleviate these signs and symptoms by increasing cardiac index higher than 2.2 L/min/m^2 and reducing PCWP to 15–18 mm Hg, while maintaining an adequate mean arterial pressure. Thus therapy will involve a combination of agents used for subset II and subset III patients in order to achieve these goals (point E to C in Fig. 13.6). These targets may be difficult to achieve and will necessitate careful monitoring and individualization of drug therapy. Nitroprusside is a particularly useful agent in this setting because of its mixed arterial-venous vasodilating effects. In the presence of significant hypotension, inotropic agents with vasopressor activity will need to be used initially in order to achieve an adequate perfusion pressure to essential organs, and can then be combined, if necessary, with diuretics and/or vasodilators to obtain the desired hemodynamic effects and clinical response (Fig. 13.6).

POSITIVE INOTROPIC AGENTS VERSUS ARTERIAL VASODILATORS

Both positive inotropes and arterial vasodilators will usually increase cardiac index in patients with heart failure. The choice between these two drug classes will depend on several factors. Arterial vasodilators may be particularly useful in patients with a significant elevation in systemic vascular resistance. The presence of cardiac arrhythmias and/or myocardial ischemia makes the use of inotropic agents more hazardous whereas significant hypotension precludes the use of vasodilators (Fig. 13.5). Significant hypotension must be avoided because the resulting decrease in coronary perfusion pressure could lead to ischemia and a further decrease in myocardial contractility. In patients with coronary artery disease, coronary perfusion pressure decreases across each stenotic lesion, making it impossible to predict the relationship between aortic pressure and perfusion to ischemic myocardium. Nonetheless, an inotropic agent with pressor activity (i.e., dopamine) is usually recommended when the systolic arterial pressure falls below 90–100 mm Hg or the mean arterial pressure falls below 70–75 mm Hg. In some patients with severe ventricular dysfunction, combination therapy with an arterial vasodilator and an inotropic agent may be necessary to achieve a cardiac index above 2.2 L/min/m^2 (see as follows and Fig. 13.6).

POSITIVE INOTROPIC AGENTS

Positive inotropic agents can be divided into four different classes[18]: (1) agents that increase intracellular cyclic adenosine monophosphate (e.g., adrenergic agents, phosphodiesterase inhibitors); (2) agents that affect sarcolemmal ion pumps and channels (e.g., digitalis glycosides); (3) agents that increase intracellular calcium release or sensitize contractile proteins to calcium (currently there are no marketed agents from this class); and (4) agents with multiple mechanisms of action (e.g., the investigational agents pimobendan and vesnarinone). Positive inotropic drugs may also vary in some of their ancillary properties (e.g., vasodilation, chronotropic, antiarrhythmic, etc.). Despite its limitations, this classification system helps in the understanding of the potential benefits and adverse effects of the different positive inotropic agents during both short-term and long-term therapy (see the section on Drugs Proven to Increase Mortality in Heart Failure Patients).

This discussion focuses on drugs that increase intracellular cyclic adenosine monophosphate (cAMP) since only positive inotropic agents from this class are generally used for the treatment of acute/severe heart failure. Although digoxin is used for the treatment of chronic heart failure, it has little if any place in the treatment of patients with acute heart failure who are hemodynamically unstable.

The delay in peak inotropic effect of digoxin (up to a few hours) even after an appropriate intravenous loading dose and its long duration of action are major disadvantages for the treatment of patients who require frequent dose adjustments in response to rapidly changing clinical conditions. Furthermore, other positive inotropic agents such as dobutamine produce much larger increases in cardiac index than digoxin in patients with acute heart failure and myocardial infarction. Therapeutic use of digoxin is discussed under Treatment of Chronic Heart Failure.

Adrenergic Agents

Several different adrenergic agents have been used for the treatment of patients with severe heart failure. These compounds vary in their affinities for adrenergic receptors in the heart and peripheral tissues and consequently lead to different pharmacologic effects (Table 13.7). It should be emphasized that hemodynamic effects in patients will be the result of both direct effects on adrenergic receptors and reflex-mediated actions. These compounds have half-lives of only a few minutes, a quick onset of action, a short duration of action, and consequently must be administered by continuous intravenous infusion. Although potentially useful in special circumstances, isoproterenol, epinephrine, and norepinephrine are less commonly used in the treatment of severe heart failure and have largely been replaced by dopamine and dobutamine.

Dopamine

Dopamine is the endogenous precursor of norepinephrine and exerts its effects by directly stimulating adrenergic receptors as well as causing release of norepinephrine from adrenergic nerve terminals.[19] The major advantages of dopamine, as compared to isoproterenol, are less tachycardia, fewer arrhythmias, less decrease in diastolic blood pressure, and consequently more beneficial effects on the balance between myocardial oxygen demand and supply. Nevertheless, dopamine and other positive inotropic agents can, under certain circumstances, adversely affect the critical balance between myocardial oxygen supply and demand in patients with coronary artery disease and lead to myocardial ischemia.[20,21]

TABLE 13.7. RELATIVE EFFECTS OF ADRENERGIC DRUGS ON RECEPTORS

Drug	α_1	β_1	β_2	Dopamine$_1$
Norepinephrine	++++	++++	0	0
Epinephrine	++++	++++	++	0
Dopamine[a]	++++	++++	++	++
Isoproterenol	0	++++	++++	0
Dobutamine[b]	+	++++	++	0

[a]See text for a more detailed description of the dose-dependent hemodynamic effects.
[b]Combined effects of the commercially available recemic mixture (see text).

Dopamine produces dose-dependent hemodynamic effects because of its relative affinity for α_1, β_1, and β_2 receptors as well as D_1 (dopaminergic) receptors (Table 13.7).[20,22] At low doses (0.5–3 mcg/kg/min), stimulation of D_1 receptors tends to predominate and leads to selective dilatation of renal, mesenteric, cerebral, and coronary vascular beds. The result is an increase in renal blood flow, glomerular filtration, urine output, natriuresis, and kaliuresis. These effects may be particularly beneficial because oliguria is a relatively common consequence of severe heart failure. Dopamine's beneficial renal effects are also due in part to an increase in cardiac index, which may be evident even with low doses of dopamine (Table 13.8).[22]

Positive inotropic effects mediated primarily by β_1 receptors become more prominent with dopamine doses of 3–10 mcg/kg/min. Cardiac index is increased because of an increase in stroke volume (due to the positive inotropic effect) and a variable increase in heart rate, which is more significant at higher doses (Table 13.8).[22] There is relatively little change in systemic vascular resistance, presumably because neither vasodilation (D_1 and β_2 mediated) nor vasoconstriction (α_1 mediated) predominates. Beneficial renal effects of dopamine may still be evident at these higher doses and are probably caused by a combination of D_1-mediated renovascular effects, increased cardiac index, and altered sodium tubular reabsorption.[22] As the dose of dopamine is increased to more than 10 mcg/kg/min, chronotropic and α_1-mediated vasoconstricting effects become more prominent. Mean arterial pressure is usually increased because of an increase in both cardiac index and systemic vascular resistance (Table 13.8). These doses of dopamine are particularly indicated in patients with severe heart failure and hypotension. However, the vasoconstricting effects of higher doses could indirectly limit the increase in cardiac index (see the inverse relation between stroke volume and systemic vascular resistance in Fig. 13.1) and cause an increase in PCWP, thus complicating the management of patients with an already elevated preload. In such patients, alternative agents (dobutamine, amrinone, milrinone) or addition of diuretics and/or vasodilators may be necessary. We also emphasize that dopamine, particularly at higher doses, will alter several parameters that increase myocardial oxygen demand (increased heart rate, contractility, and systolic pressure) and potentially decrease myocardial blood flow (coronary vasoconstriction and increased PCWP). Increased myocardial anaerobic metabolism, as evidenced by increased lactate production, and worsening angina have been documented in some patients with coronary artery disease receiving dopamine.[21] Increased arrhythmogenesis is also more common at higher doses of dopamine.

Dobutamine

Dobutamine is a synthetic catecholamine that has a chiral center in its structure and is commercially available as a

TABLE 13.8. USUAL HEMODYNAMIC EFFECTS OF INTRAVENOUS AGENTS COMMONLY USED FOR THE TREATMENT OF ACUTE/SEVERE HEART FAILURE[a]

Drug	Dose	HR	MAP	PCWP	CO	SVR
Dopamine	1–3 μg/kg/min	0	0	0	0/+	–
Dopamine	3–10 μg/kg/min	+	+	0	+	0
Dopamine	>10 μg/kg/min	+	+	+	+	+
Dobutamine	2.5–15 μg/kg/min	0/+	0	–	+	–
Amrinone	5–10 μg/kg/min	0/+	0/–	–	+	–
Milrinone	0.375–0.75 μg/kg/min	0/+	0/–	–	+	–
Nitroprusside	0.25–3 μg/kg/min	0/+	0/–	–	+	–
Nitroglycerin	5–200 μg/min	0/+	0/–	–	0/+	0/–
Furosemide	20–80 mg, repeated as needed up to 4–6 times/d	0	0	–	0	0

[a]See text for a more detailed description of the interpatient variability in response. *Key:* +, increase; –, decrease; 0, no change; HR, heart rate; MAP, mean arterial pressure; PCWP, pulmonary capillary wedge pressure; CO, cardiac output; SVR, systemic vascular resistance.

racemic mixture of its two enantiomers. Unlike dopamine, dobutamine does not act indirectly by releasing norepinephrine from nerve terminals.[19] However, there are important differences in the direct effects of each dobutamine enantiomer on adrenergic receptors.[19] (+)-dobutamine is a potent β_1- and β_2-receptor agonist but only a partial agonist at α_1 receptors (i.e., it binds to the receptor but has weak activity). Conversely, (–)-dobutamine is a more potent α_1-receptor agonist with weaker effects on β receptors. The overall hemodynamic effects of the racemic compound in patients are the result of a complex interaction of the two enantiomers with adrenergic receptors and reflex-mediated actions. Because the two enantiomers have similar affinities for α_1 receptors, the partial agonist activity of (+)-dobutamine tends to block or at least decrease the vasoconstricting effects of the more potent α_1-receptor agonist, (–)-dobutamine. In addition, β_2-receptor-mediated vasodilation will tend to offset any residual α_1-receptor-mediated vasoconstriction. Thus, the net vascular effect is usually vasodilation.[23] The positive inotropic effects are due to the β_1-receptor agonist effects of (+)-dobutamine and to a lesser extent (–)-dobutamine. Additional positive inotropic effects may also be mediated through stimulation of cardiac α_1 receptors by (–)-dobutamine.[23] Cardiac α_1-receptor stimulation by (–)-dobutamine causes an increase in contractility but no significant change in heart rate and may provide an explanation for the apparently more modest chronotropic effects of dobutamine compared to dopamine.[24]

The overall hemodynamic effects of racemic dobutamine are those of a potent inotropic agent with vasodilating action (Table 13.8).[25] Initial doses are usually 2.5–5 mcg/kg/min and can be progressively increased to 15 mcg/kg/min or higher based on clinical and hemodynamic responses. Cardiac index is increased because of an increase in stroke volume and a variable increase in heart rate.[24] Controlled studies that have compared dobutamine and dopamine indicate that both agents can cause an increase in heart rate, particularly at higher infusion rates.[26] These studies reveal that dobutamine tends to cause a smaller increment in heart rate but the difference between the two agents is variable and may often be clinically insignificant. In patients with heart failure, the decrease in systemic vascular resistance caused by dobutamine can be advantageous because it provides another mechanism to increase cardiac index. Because of the offsetting changes in systemic vascular resistance and cardiac index, dobutamine will usually cause relatively little change in mean arterial pressure (Equation 2) compared to the more consistent increase observed with dopamine.[26] This smaller effect on blood pressure will be beneficial in patients with heart failure and ischemic heart disease because it will minimize the increase in myocardial oxygen demand. However, the absence of a consistent hypertensive effect with dobutamine will be a disadvantage in patients with heart failure and hypotension for whom restoration of blood pressure will be a primary goal (Fig. 13.5).[24] Because of its vasodilating effects, dobutamine will usually decrease PCWP, as opposed to the increase observed with dopamine, and will be particularly useful for patients with a low cardiac index and an elevated PCWP (subset IV). Dobutamine does not bind to D_1 receptors and does not cause selective renal vasodilation. Nonetheless, the increase in cardiac index can lead to an increase in renal blood flow, urine output, and natriuresis in some patients. In view of the selective effects of dopamine on the renal circulation, some clinicians have advocated the combination of low-dose dopamine for its renovascular effects and dobutamine for its inotropic and systemic effects.[21]

The combined effects of dobutamine on myocardial contractility, heart rate, blood pressure, PCWP, and coronary blood flow suggest that it produces its desired hemodynamic effects while not adversely affecting the balance between myocardial oxygen demand and supply.[24] Thus, dobutamine can usually be used safely in patients with chronic ischemic heart disease or during the acute phase of a myocardial infarction.[21] Nevertheless, worsening angina and evidence of ischemia (i.e., increased myocardial lactate production) have been reported during dobutamine therapy.[21] These adverse effects are more likely when there is an excessive increase in heart rate or blood pressure. Although one study indicated that dobutamine was less arrhythmogenic than dopamine, it is noteworthy that both agents can produce cardiac arrhythmias, presumably through β-receptor-mediated effects on conduction/refractoriness in various cardiac tissues and a decrease in plasma potassium concentrations.[21]

Attenuation of dobutamine's hemodynamic effects has been reported after 72 hours of continuous infusion and may be a consequence of down-regulation of β-adrenergic receptors or uncoupling of the receptors from adenylate cyclase.[27] Although it is unclear if there is also attenuation of dopamine's hemodynamic effects with continuous infusions of similar duration, receptor down-regulation should occur during long-term therapy with any β-agonist. Based on the usual time course of β-receptor down-regulation, full sensitivity to β-agonists should be restored 7–10 days after drug withdrawal.[27] Furthermore, one would predict that there should be cross-tolerance with all agents that work through the same receptors. It is also noteworthy that the maximum inotropic effects of dobutamine are diminished in patients with severe heart failure compared to those without heart failure.[28] This decreased responsiveness to dobutamine in patients with heart failure is apparently the result of decreased myocardial β-receptor density caused by elevated circulating catecholamine concentrations.

Despite the fact that dobutamine has a half-life of approximately 2.5 minutes, some patients may have sustained hemodynamic and clinical benefits for several days and up to several months after a short-term infusion.[25] Three small placebo-controlled studies have reported that short-term infusions of dobutamine produced long-term improvements in functional class, exercise capacity, and left ventricular ejection fraction.[29–31] These beneficial effects have been associated with widely different dobutamine dosage regimens (i.e., a single 72-hour infusion at a mean rate of 25.3 mcg/kg/min[30] versus 7.4–8.7 mcg/kg/min for 4 h/wk for 24 weeks[29] versus 9.25 mcg/kg/min for 24 h, every 3 days for 4 weeks[31]). The mechanism of this prolonged effect is unclear but it has been proposed that dobutamine may promote cardiovascular conditioning analogous to exercise training.[29] These data led to the more widespread use of intermittent dobutamine infusions for the treatment of patients with severe refractory heart failure. However, a randomized placebo-controlled multicenter trial in outpatients with chronic heart failure was stopped prematurely because there was a trend toward increased mortality in patients who received dobutamine infusions (mean dose of 8.1 mcg/kg/min for 48 h/wk) compared to those receiving placebo (15/38 on dobutamine versus 5/30 on placebo; $p = 0.08$).[32] Thus despite apparent clinical and hemodynamic benefits, the potential for increased mortality raises serious concerns about the chronic use of intermittent dobutamine infusions. It is noteworthy that long-term therapy with oral β-agonists has also been associated with increased mortality (see Drugs Proven to Increase Mortality in Heart Failure Patients).

Phosphodiesterase Inhibitors

Drugs from this class produce their hemodynamic effects by inhibiting phosphodiesterase fraction III, an intracellular enzyme that causes the breakdown of cAMP. In myocardial cells, inhibition of phosphodiesterase III increases cAMP concentration, which leads to increased calcium entry and subsequent storage in the sarcoplasmic reticulum. During systole, more calcium is released from intracellular storage sites and available to contractile proteins to increase the force of contraction. The higher concentration of cAMP also increases reuptake of calcium during diastole to improve myocardial cell relaxation and diastolic function.[33] Conversely, in vascular smooth muscle cells, the increase in cAMP produces muscle relaxation probably by stimulating calcium extrusion and decreasing intracellular calcium concentrations.[33] Drugs from this class will therefore have positive inotropic and vasodilating effects and are sometimes called inodilators. We emphasize that β-adrenergic agonists ultimately produce a similar response but their effect is due to β-receptor-mediated activation of adenylate cyclase and increased production of cAMP. Although several phosphodiesterase inhibitors have undergone clinical investigation, the intravenous formulations of amrinone and milrinone are the only agents from this class currently approved in the United States.

Amrinone and Milrinone

The bipyridine derivatives, amrinone and milrinone, have very similar pharmacological and hemodynamic effects after intravenous administration.[21,33–35] Although there has been some debate concerning the relative importance of the positive inotropic and vasodilating effects of these drugs, it has now been clearly established that both effects contribute to the observed therapeutic response in heart failure patients.[33,35–38] By comparing the hemodynamic effects after intracoronary and intravenous administration of milrinone, Ludmer et al.[36] demonstrated that vasodilation was mainly due to a direct effect of the drug, as opposed to reflex withdrawal of sympathetic tone secondary to its positive inotropic effect. Similarly, two studies have shown that, as compared to nitroprusside, amrinone and milrinone produced a greater increase in cardiac index than predicted from their vasodilating effects alone.[37,38] The relative importance of arterial/venous vasodilation versus positive inotropic effects in a particular patient may vary depending on the dose as well as the type and extent of the underlying cardiac dysfunction.

The hemodynamic effects of amrinone and milrinone in patients with heart failure are generally similar to those produced by dobutamine or nitroprusside.[21,33,34,39–41] After intravenous administration of amrinone or milrinone to patients with severe heart failure, there is an increase in cardiac index, which is caused primarily by an increase in stroke volume because there is generally little change in heart rate (Table 13.8). Despite the increase in cardiac index, mean arterial pressure generally remains fairly constant because of the concomitant decrease in systemic vascular resistance. However, the vasodilating effects may predominate in certain patients and lead to a decrease in blood pressure and an increase in heart rate, particularly at higher doses.[38,39] Amrinone and milrinone cause a decrease in PCWP and thus are particularly useful in patients with a low cardiac index and an elevated PCWP (subset IV). Such a decrease in preload, however, can be hazardous for patients without an elevated PCWP (subset III) because it could lead to a decrease in cardiac index or at least blunt the increase that would otherwise be produced by the positive inotropic and arterial vasodilating actions. Amrinone and milrinone should not be used as single agents in heart failure patients with moderate or severe hypotension because they will not increase, and may even decrease, arterial blood pressure.

The results of controlled studies that have compared dobutamine to amrinone or milrinone indicate that these agents produce generally similar hemodynamic effects.[40,41] A greater increase in heart rate with dobutamine is the most consistent difference in these studies, although the difference may not be clinically significant in many patients. The combination of dobutamine and amrinone or milrinone produces additive effects on cardiac index and PCWP.[40,41] Intracoronary administration of milrinone has also been used to demonstrate that phosphodiesterase inhibition potentiates the positive inotropic actions of dobutamine.[28] Thus, combination of a β-receptor agonist (dobutamine, dopamine) and a phosphodiesterase inhibitor (amrinone, milrinone) may offer advantages in selected patients who have dose-limiting adverse effects with either class of drugs. It is unclear, however, if this drug combination represents a therapeutic advantage over the combination of a positive inotropic agent and a vasodilator (nitroprusside, ACE inhibitor).

Amrinone and milrinone produce relatively little change in myocardial oxygen demand. Although myocardial contractility is increased, there is a decrease in wall tension and little change in heart rate.[42] Generally, these drugs do not adversely affect the balance between myocardial oxygen demand and supply in patients with heart failure and ischemic heart disease. Amrinone and milrinone have been used in patients with ischemic heart disease without causing myocardial ischemia.[33,34] Nevertheless, caution should be used to avoid any unusual hemodynamic responses such as hypotension and tachycardia, which could be particularly hazardous in such patients.

Although it is often assumed that phosphodiesterase inhibitors will avoid the pharmacodynamic tolerance associated with dobutamine (and other β agonists) infusions of >72 hours, there is relatively little published data on the effects of such prolonged infusions with this class of drugs. Most of the hemodynamic effects of enoximone, another phosphodiesterase inhibitor, were maintained after 7 days of continuous infusion.[43] However, tolerance to the hemodynamic effects of amrinone have been reported after 72 hours of continuous infusion.[44] It is interesting to note that tolerance to amrinone was associated with a down-regulation of β-receptors and sequestration or uncoupling of β-receptors from adenylate cyclase, similar to the effects of β-agonists. This effect of amrinone was apparently mediated by an increase in circulating catecholamines (probably in response to vasodilation), which led to the alterations in β-receptor responses in cardiac and other tissues.[44] Tolerance to oral amrinone has also been reported after 2 weeks of therapy. Until more data become available, the issue of tolerance during prolonged continuous infusions of phosphodiesterase inhibitors must be considered an unresolved issue.

Compared to the intravenously administered β-agonists discussed previously, amrinone and milrinone have a much longer terminal half-life. The mean terminal half-life of milrinone in patients with heart failure is 2.3 hours while that of amrinone ranges from 2–4 hours in healthy subjects and up to 12 hours in patients with severe heart failure.[45] A long half-life is a major disadvantage because a loading dose is necessary to obtain a faster onset of action and the duration of action is in the order of hours compared to a few minutes for dopamine, dobutamine, and nitroprusside. Therefore, if adverse effects such as arrhythmias or hypotension develop, they will persist much longer after discontinuation of amrinone or milrinone, compared to the shorter acting agents. Peak hemodynamic effects are generally obtained within 5–15 minutes after the loading dose. The usual loading dose of amrinone is 0.75 mg/kg administered over 2–3 minutes, followed by a continuous infusion of 5–10 mcg/kg/min. If the therapeutic response is inadequate, an additional loading dose of 0.75 mg/kg may be repeated after 30 minutes. Other loading dose regimens and higher continuous infusion rates have been used, but maintenance doses higher than 20 mcg/kg/min may not produce additional hemodynamic benefits.[34] The recommended loading dose of milrinone is 50 mcg/kg administered over 10 minutes, followed by a continuous infusion of 0.5 mcg/kg/min (range: 0.375–0.75 mcg/kg/min). Dose/concentration-related increases in hemodynamic effects have been reported with milrinone; however, this relationship may be relatively flat at the usual doses.[38,39] More than 80% of a dose of milrinone is excreted unchanged in urine and, unlike amrinone, its infusion rate should be decreased in patients with renal impairment.

The intravenous formulations of milrinone and amrinone are usually well tolerated, unlike the relatively high incidence of adverse effects associated with chronic use of oral amrinone. In addition to undesirable hemodynamic effects, the most notable adverse effects are cardiac arrhythmias and thrombocytopenia. For example, ventricular arrhythmias including ventricular tachycardia were associated with milrinone therapy during controlled clinical trials.[46] However, it should be emphasized that these patients often had important risk factors (severe heart failure, ischemic heart disease, diuretics, digoxin) for the development of cardiac arrhythmias. Furthermore, there is little if any information on the relative risk of proarrhythmia between milrinone, amrinone, and β agonists. Thrombocytopenia is reported to occur in 2.4% of patients who have received intravenous amrinone (compared to about 20% for oral amrinone).[34] Decreased platelet survival due to nonimmunologic platelet damage is the postulated mechanism. This adverse effect is dose dependent and generally completely reversible within 5–7 days after discontinuation of amrinone. The incidence of thrombocytopenia associated with milrinone therapy is very low (< 0.5%) presumably because it is used at a dose that is much lower than that of amrinone.[46] In this respect, milrinone is preferable to amrinone. Patients who received amrinone should be monitored for signs of bleeding and have platelet counts determined before and during therapy.

Generally, milrinone or amrinone should be considered only in patients who have not responded adequately to dobutamine, dopamine, intravenous vasodilators, or a combination of these agents. Their hemodynamic effects are similar to those of dobutamine or nitroprusside. A combination of amrinone or milrinone with dopamine or dobutamine may be helpful in patients with dose-limiting adverse effects. The longer duration of action of amrinone and milrinone, compared to other agents, is a disadvantage for the treatment of unstable patients who require rapid adjustment of inotropic/vasodilator therapy.

Vasodilators

Activation of the sympathetic nervous system, the renin angiotensin aldosterone system, and arginine vasopressin all cause vasoconstriction and an increase in systemic vascular resistance (Fig. 13.2). In patients with heart failure, stroke volume varies inversely with systemic vascular resistance (Fig. 13.1), such that increases in systemic vascular resistance (a measure of afterload) will lead to a decline in stroke volume and cardiac output. Thus it was proposed that vasodilators might interrupt this cycle. Since the first report of the use of trimethaphan in 1956 and phentolamine in 1971, vasodilators have become an integral part of the drug therapy of heart failure.[21]

Vasodilators are typically described by their prominent site of action (arterial or venous). Arterial vasodilators (e.g., hydralazine) act as afterload-reducing agents and typically cause an increase in cardiac output. Venous vasodilators (e.g., nitroglycerin, isosorbide dinitrate) act as preload reducers by affecting venous capacitance. They reduce symptoms of pulmonary congestion in patients with high cardiac filling pressures. Mixed vasodilators (e.g., nitroprusside, angiotensin-converting enzyme inhibitors) act on both arterial resistance and venous capacitance vessels, and can therefore reduce congestive symptoms and increase cardiac output. Nitroprusside and nitroglycerin are the most widely studied and commonly used intravenous vasodilating agents in acute/severe heart failure. Use of oral vasodilators is discussed under Treatment of Chronic Heart Failure.

Nitroprusside

Sodium nitroprusside is a mixed arterial-venous vasodilator and was among the first vasodilators used in the treatment of acute heart failure. It acts directly on vascular smooth muscle to produce its balanced vasodilating action. Because of its mixed effects, it causes both an increase in cardiac index and a decrease in PCWP (point E to C in Fig. 13.6). Nitroprusside's effects on these parameters are qualitatively similar to those produced by dobutamine and amrinone/milrinone, despite the fact that it has no direct inotropic activity (Table 13.8). However, it generally causes a greater decrease in PCWP and systemic vascular resistance than dobutamine. Mean arterial pressure may remain fairly constant but often decreases depending on the relative increase in cardiac output and decrease in systemic vascular resistance (Equation 2). As discussed previously (Positive Inotropic Agents Versus Arterial Vasodilators), the decrease in blood pressure is an important dose-limiting adverse effect of nitroprusside and other vasodilators. Therefore, nitroprusside is particularly useful for the treatment of patients who are in subset IV and have a significantly elevated systemic vascular resistance but who are not hypotensive (Fig. 13.5).

Patients with normal left ventricular function will not have a compensatory increase in stroke volume and cardiac index when systemic vascular resistance is decreased (Fig. 13.1). Consequently, these patients experience a significant decrease in blood pressure after administration of arterial vasodilators (Equation 2). This important distinction explains why nitroprusside is a potent antihypertensive agent in patients without heart failure and yet leads to a much smaller decrease in blood pressure in patients with heart failure. Because of this difference, use of nitroprusside in heart failure causes less reflex tachycardia. Nonetheless, even a modest increase in heart rate could have adverse consequences in patients with ischemic heart disease and close monitoring is necessary.

Nitroprusside has been extensively studied and was demonstrated to be effective in the short-term management of patients with severe heart failure in a variety of settings (i.e., acute myocardial infarction, mitral and/or aortic valvular regurgitation, postcoronary bypass surgery, acute exacerbation of chronic heart failure).[21] It is often considered the prototype vasodilator to which other oral or intravenous agents are compared. There is also extensive experience with the combination of nitroprusside and dopamine or dobutamine.[21] Such combinations are particularly useful for patients in hemodynamic subset IV who fail to respond to nitroprusside or positive inotropic agents alone (Fig. 13.5). Furthermore, if the initial blood pressure is relatively low (a contraindication to nitroprusside and other vasodilators) or if significant hypotension develops during nitroprusside therapy, an infusion of dopamine to raise mean arterial pressure will allow optimal use of both inotropic and vasodilator drugs. Generally, nitroprusside will not adversely affect and may improve the balance between myocardial oxygen demand and supply. This effect is mainly due to a decrease in oxygen demand caused by the lowering of left ventricular wall tension and a possible increase in subendocardial blood flow secondary to the decrease in left ventricular filling pressure. However, an excessive decrease in systemic arterial pressure can decrease coronary perfusion and worsen ischemia. Despite the proven hemodynamic benefits of nitroprusside, a multicenter trial failed to demonstrate a decrease in short-term mortality when it was administered for 48 hours to patients with acute myocardial infarction and left ventricular failure.[47]

Nitroprusside has a rapid onset of action and a duration of action of less than 10 minutes; consequently, it must be administered by continuous intravenous infusion. This is advantageous because it allows for precise dose titration based on measured clinical and hemodynamic parameters. Nitroprusside, like other vasodilators used in heart failure, should be initiated at a low dose (i.e., 0.1–0.25 mcg/kg/min) to avoid an excessive drop in arterial pressure, and then increased by small increments (i.e., 0.1–0.2 mcg/kg/min) every 5–10 minutes as needed and tolerated. The endpoints of therapy vary between patients, but usually effective doses range from 0.5–3.0 mcg/kg/min. A rebound phenomenon has been reported after abrupt withdrawal of nitroprusside in patients with heart failure and is apparently due to reflex neurohumoral activation during therapy.[48] Although the cause and extent of any rebound effect is somewhat controversial, it is nevertheless prudent to taper doses slowly when stopping nitroprusside therapy and switching to oral drugs.[21] Nitroprusside can cause cyanide and thiocyanate toxicity but these are very unlikely when doses less than 3 mcg/kg/min are administered for less than 3 days.[49] Thiocyanate is excreted by the kidneys and its toxicity is more likely in patients with renal impairment or when plasma concentrations exceed 10 mg/dL.[49]

Nitroglycerin

The intravenous formulation of nitroglycerin is used in patients with severe heart failure to allow for precise dosage titration based on hemodynamic and clinical response. Other nitrate preparations used in the management of chronic heart failure are discussed in a separate section. Because of its short half-life and duration of action, intravenous nitroglycerin is administered by continuous infusion. The major hemodynamic effect of nitroglycerin is a decrease in preload and PCWP caused by its venous vasodilating action. However, it is now recognized that nitroglycerin also has mild arterial vasodilating effects, which may be particularly evident in patients with heart failure and an elevated systemic vascular resistance (Table 13.8).[50] This small decrease in systemic vascular resistance generally leads to a relatively small increase in cardiac index compared to that produced by inotropic agents.[51] Thus intravenous nitroglycerin is used primarily as a preload reducer for patients in hemodynamic subset II or in combination with inotropic agents for patients in subset IV (Fig. 13.5). Combination therapy with nitroglycerin and dobutamine or dopamine is appealing because of complementary effects to increase cardiac index and decrease PCWP.[51] As indicated previously, PCWP should not be reduced excessively but should be kept in the 15–18 mm Hg range in order to provide an optimal ventricular filling pressure and maintain cardiac index while relieving symptoms of pulmonary congestion (point B to C or E to D in Fig. 13.6). Because of its coronary vasodilating properties and overall beneficial effects on myocardial oxygen demand and supply, nitroglycerin is especially useful for vasodilator therapy of patients with severe heart failure and ischemic heart disease.

Nitroglycerin should be initiated at a dose of 5–10 mcg/min (0.1 mcg/kg/min) and increased progressively every 5–10 minutes as necessary and tolerated. Hypotension and an excessive decrease in PCWP are important dose-limiting side effects. Maintenance doses usually vary from 35–200 mcg/min (0.5–3.0 mcg/kg/min), although doses of more than 1000 mcg/min (15 mcg/kg/min) have been used in rare cases.[50] Tolerance to some of the hemodynamic effects of intravenous nitroglycerin develops in most patients over 12–72 hours.[52,53] However, there are subgroups of patients who seem to have a sustained response.[53] It should be noted that nitroglycerin may inhibit the anticoagulant effects of heparin. Therefore, activated partial thromboplastin times (aPTT) should be monitored more closely when nitroglycerin is added or discontinued in patients receiving heparin.

Hydralazine and Enalaprilat

Although intravenous formulations of hydralazine and enalaprilat are available, these drugs have a relatively long duration of action. This is an important disadvantage for the treatment of unstable patients for whom rapid dosage adjustments are often required. Thus, nitroprusside or nitroglycerin will generally be preferred in unstable patients. Hydralazine is an arterial vasodilator widely used as maintenance therapy for chronic heart failure (see Treatment of Chronic Heart Failure). Compared to the oral dosage form, intravenous hydralazine has not been extensively studied in patients with heart failure. The results of a short-term study in patients with acute heart failure indicate that intravenous hydralazine plus isosorbide dinitrate produce a similar decrease in preload and afterload, but a larger increase in heart rate, compared to enalaprilat.[54]

Enalaprilat is the active diacid metabolite of enalapril. Similar to other angiotensin-converting enzyme inhibitors, enalaprilat is a mixed arterial-venous vasodilator but generally has a shorter onset of action than oral drugs from the same class. The hemodynamic response to bolus and continuous infusions of enalaprilat has been documented in several studies.[54,55] Intravenous hydralazine or enalaprilat should be used mainly for the short-term management of relatively stable patients who cannot take oral medications.

DIURETICS

The use of diuretics is discussed extensively under Treatment of Chronic Heart Failure. This section focuses specifically on the use of intravenous loop diuretics in the management of acute/severe heart failure. These drugs include furosemide, ethacrynic acid, bumetanide, and torsemide; however, furosemide is by far the most widely used and studied loop diuretic in patients with severe heart failure. Diuretics decrease intravascular volume and preload, thereby improving pulmonary congestion. They are particularly useful for patients in subset II and in combination with vasodilators/inotropes for patients in subset IV (Fig. 13.5). It is important to note that unlike afterload reducers and inotropic agents, diuretics do not cause an upward shift in the Starling curve or increase cardiac index (Table 13.8). Because the curve is rather flat in patients with severe heart failure, lowering of PCWP to the optimal range of 15–18 mm Hg produces very little if any decrease in cardiac index (point B to C in Fig. 13.6). As noted previously, however, an excessive decrease in preload will lower cardiac index (point C to A in Fig. 13.6).

Intravenous bolus administration of loop diuretics also produces short-term hemodynamic effects independent of natriuresis. One widely quoted study in patients with heart failure demonstrated that furosemide caused a decrease in PCWP within 5–15 minutes, prior to any significant increase in urine output.[56] The effect was attributed to an increase in venous capacitance. More recently, however, other investigators have reported that furosemide causes an initial elevation in PCWP and systemic vascular resistance, which is associated with an acute increase in plasma renin activity, as well as norepinephrine and arginine vasopressin plasma concentrations.[57] Vasodilators and neurohumoral antagonists may prevent this initial vasoconstriction.[58] Despite the controversy over these short-term (i.e., 5–20 minutes) effects of intravenous furosemide, the diuretic effects predominate after 20 minutes and lead to a consistent decrease in PCWP and an improvement in pulmonary congestion.[57,58] While intravenous bolus administration is most commonly used and is the optimal method to produce a fast therapeutic response, there is some evidence that continuous infusion of furosemide may be more effective at maintaining the desired therapeutic response than intermittent bolus administration.[59] Regardless of the method of administration, intravenous loop diuretics continue to be extremely valuable agents in the therapy of acute/severe heart failure.

MECHANICAL CIRCULATORY SUPPORT

The intra-aortic balloon pump (IABP) is the most widely used form of mechanical circulatory assistance and is typically used in patients with acute/severe heart failure who do not respond adequately to positive inotropic agents and vasodilators. The IABP can be introduced percutaneously into the femoral artery and advanced into the descending thoracic aorta. "Counterpulsation" with the IABP refers to inflation of the balloon during diastole, which results in the displacement of blood and thereby increases aortic diastolic pressure and coronary perfusion. In systole, the balloon is deflated just prior to opening of the aortic valve and causes a sudden decrease in aortic pressure, thus allowing the left ventricle to pump against a reduced arterial impedance. Use of the IABP usually results in an increase in cardiac index and coronary perfusion while decreasing myocardial oxygen demand. Consequently, the IABP is particularly useful for patients with acute/severe heart failure in the setting of myocardial ischemia (evolving infarction, patients awaiting emergency coronary bypass surgery) but it is also used for patients with end-stage chronic heart failure who are awaiting cardiac transplantation.[60] Intravenously administered vasodilators and inotropic agents are generally used in conjunction with the IABP in an effort to maximize hemodynamic and clinical benefits.

Several different ventricular assist devices and "total artificial hearts" (or ventricles) are currently under investigation for the circulatory support of patients who cannot be sustained with pharmacologic therapy and an IABP. The devices are often used as a temporary bridge to transplantation because of the usual delay of several weeks in finding a suitable donor heart (see Chapter 18). Investigations also continue in the permanent use of artificial hearts for the long-term management of selected patients (see Reference 60 for a more complete discussion of this topic).

TREATMENT OF CHRONIC HEART FAILURE

The goals of therapy in management of chronic heart failure are to improve the patient's quality of life by reducing symptoms, reduce hospitalizations, slow progression of the disease process, and prolong survival. Drug therapies aimed at all of these goals are discussed in this section. We also discuss investigational therapies that may be useful in management of heart failure, therapies that are clearly detrimental in heart failure, and therapies aimed at preventing the development of symptomatic heart failure. Clinical practice guidelines for the management of patients with left ventricular dysfunction were published by the U.S. Public Health Service in 1994 and can be obtained by contacting the USPHS and requesting AHCPR Publication No. 94-0612.

The first step in management of chronic heart failure is to determine the etiology (Table 13.1) and/or precipitating factors (Table 13.3) of the syndrome. Treatment of underlying disorders such as anemia or hyperthyroidism may obviate the need for treatment of heart failure. Patients with valvular diseases may derive significant benefit from surgical replacement or repair of the valve. Revascularization or anti-ischemic therapy in patients with ischemia may reduce many of the signs and symptoms of CHF. Drugs that aggravate or precipitate heart failure (Table 13.4) should be discontinued if possible.

Restriction of physical activity helps to reduce the work load of the heart and is recommended for virtually all patients with symptoms of congestion. However, once the patient's heart failure symptoms have been stabilized and excess fluid removed, it is recommended that the patient be mobilized. Recent data suggest that cardiac rehabilitation programs for patients with stable heart failure will improve conditioning and increase exercise tolerance.[61]

One of the major compensatory responses to heart failure is sodium and water retention, therefore restriction of dietary sodium is an important nonpharmacologic approach to the management of CHF. The typical American diet contains 3 to 6 g of sodium per day, and it is recommended that CHF patients reduce their daily sodium intake by about half (e.g., 1.5 to 3 g of sodium per day). This can be accomplished by not adding salt to prepared foods and eliminating foods high in sodium (e.g., salt-cured meats, potato chips, pretzels, salted nuts, pickles, delicatessen meats). Further reductions in dietary sodium can be achieved by eliminating salt from cooking. However, this is not recommended for most CHF patients because excessive sodium restriction produces an unpalatable diet, which frequently results in poor dietary compliance and may compromise the patient's nutritional status. In addition, the availability of potent diuretics makes excessive sodium restriction unnecessary in most cases. Although dietary sodium restriction should be instituted in all CHF patients, pharmacologic management of their condition is usually necessary. A summary of the drugs commonly used in the management of chronic heart failure is shown in Table 13.9.

DIURETICS

The compensatory mechanisms in CHF stimulate excessive sodium and water retention, leading to signs and symptoms of systemic and pulmonary congestion. Diuretic therapy thus forms a cornerstone in the management of CHF. The primary goal of diuretic therapy is to decrease edema and pulmonary congestion by reduction of preload. Although preload is a determinant of cardiac output, the left ventricular function curve in Fig. 13.6 shows that a patient with symptoms of congestion has reached the flat portion of the curve. A reduction in filling pressure reduces symptoms but has relatively little effect on the patient's stroke volume or cardiac output (point B to C in Fig. 13.6) until it again reaches the steep portion of the curve (point C to A in Fig.

TABLE 13.9. COMPARATIVE HEMODYNAMIC EFFECTS OF DRUGS ROUTINELY USED IN THE MANAGEMENT OF CHRONIC HEART FAILURE

Drug	Daily Dose (mg)[a]	Usual Frequency	HR	MBP	PCWP	CO	SVR
Diuretics							
Furosemide	20–120	qd or bid	0	0	↓	0	0
Bumetanide	0.5–10	qd or bid	0	0	↓	0	0
ACE Inhibitors							
Captopril	37.5–300	tid	↓	↓	↓	↑	↓
Enalapril	5–40	bid	↓	↓	↓	↑	↓
Lisinopril	5–40	qd	↓	↓	↓	↑	↓
Hydralazine	100–400	qid	0/↑	0/↓	0	↑	↓
Isosorbide dinitrate	80–240	qid	0/↑	0/↓	↓	0/↑	0/↓
Digoxin	0.125–0.5	qd	↓	0	0/↓	↑	0/↓

[a]For many of the drugs, the low end of the dosage range represents appropriate starting doses with upward titration to the target dose. *Key:* HR, heart rate; MBP, mean blood pressure; PCWP, pulmonary capillary wedge pressure; CO, cardiac output; SVR, systemic vascular resistance; 0, no change; ↑, increase; ↓, decrease.

13.6). Once diuretic therapy is initiated, dosage adjustments are based on symptomatic improvement and daily body weight. Change in body weight is a sensitive marker of fluid status, which can reflect excess fluid retention or fluid loss.

Thiazide Diuretics

Thiazide diuretics such as hydrochlorothiazide act by blocking sodium and chloride reabsorption in the distal convoluted tubule. Sodium is avidly reabsorbed prior to reaching the distal convoluted tubule, with only 5–8% of the filtered sodium load being reabsorbed at this site.[62] The thiazides are therefore relatively weak diuretics and may be effective in the early stages of CHF; more potent diuretics are commonly needed in the management of CHF patients.

Loop Diuretics

Loop diuretics are the most widely utilized diuretics in the CHF population. Loop diuretics such as furosemide and bumetanide act in the thick ascending limb of the loop of Henle where they increase fractional excretion of sodium by 20–25%.[62] Because loop diuretics are highly bound to plasma proteins, they are not highly filtered at the glomerulus. They reach the tubular lumen by active transport via the organic acid transport pathway. Competitors for the organic acid pathway (such as probenecid or organic products of uremia) can inhibit delivery of loop diuretics to their site of action and therefore decrease effectiveness. The loop diuretics also induce a prostaglandin-mediated increase in renal blood flow, which contributes to their natriuretic effect. Coadministration of nonsteroidal anti-inflammatory drugs (e.g., indomethacin, ibuprofen) blocks this prostaglandin-mediated effect and can diminish response to loop diuretics.[62,63] Unlike thiazide diuretics, loop diuretics maintain their effectiveness in the presence of impaired renal function although higher doses will often be necessary. The diuretic dosage used in a CHF patient is typically that which maintains the patient at a stable weight. For furosemide this will typically range from 40 to 240 mg/day given on a once or twice daily basis.

Diuretic-Induced Hypokalemia in CHF

Diuretics are responsible for causing a variety of metabolic abnormalities and, in general, the severity of the metabolic disturbance can be related to the potency of the diuretic. The reader is referred to Chapter 12 for a detailed discussion on the adverse effects associated with diuretic therapy.

The most common metabolic disturbance associated with both thiazide and loop diuretics is hypokalemia. In patients with CHF, hypokalemia may be exacerbated by hyperaldosteronism. Hypokalemia is especially worrisome in CHF patients because it can precipitate ventricular arrhythmias, a common mode of death for these patients. Many CHF patients are also taking digoxin, which is associated with an increased incidence of ventricular arrhythmias in the presence of hypokalemia. Hypomagnesemia is also common with diuretic therapy and it also increases the risk of arrhythmias. Concomitant ACE inhibitor therapy may help minimize the incidence of diuretic-induced hypokalemia because these drugs tend to increase serum potassium through their effects on aldosterone. Nonetheless, potassium supplementation or administration of a potassium-sparing diuretic (e.g., triamterene, amiloride, spironolactone) may still be necessary. Clinicians should closely monitor potassium in CHF patients, caution patients about the use of salt substitutes, which are commonly potassium chloride, and add potassium supplementation only when necessary.

Diuretic Resistance

Occasionally, patients respond poorly to large doses of loop diuretics, and CHF is the most common clinical setting in which diuretic resistance is observed.[63] The mechanisms responsible for diuretic resistance in CHF patients appear to be both pharmacokinetic and pharmacodynamic in nature. Furosemide, the most widely used diuretic, has widely variable bioavailability which ranges from 10–80%. It has been suggested that CHF patients have reduced oral bioavailability of loop diuretics due to gut edema, Brater and colleagues[63] have shown that the problem is not with the extent of drug absorption but rather with the rate of absorption. They showed that bioavailability is normal but the rate of absorption is prolonged approximately twofold and peak concentrations are about one-half normal. Because loop diuretics have a sigmoid-shaped urine concentration-response curve, CHF patients with prolonged absorption may not attain concentrations that reach the steep portion of this curve. This may explain the diminished response observed in heart failure patients. Diuretic resistance with oral therapy can be overcome by administering the diuretic intravenously or by giving larger oral doses.

In spite of normal pharmacokinetics following intravenous administration, diuretic resistance is also observed with intravenous administration. This suggests that there is also an important pharmacodynamic component to diuretic resistance in CHF patients. The mechanism for suppressed responses in CHF patients is unclear, but may be related to increased proximal and distal tubular sodium reabsorption. Several maneuvers can be attempted to overcome the abnormal response. Treatment of the primary disease by other maneuvers (i.e., afterload reduction) may improve diuresis. Administration of low doses of dopamine may enhance diuresis by improving renal blood flow. Larger IV bolus doses may be given to achieve concentrations closer to the top of the concentration-response curve, or a continuous IV infusion may be administered to maintain more constant concentrations in the steep portion of the concentration-response curve. Recent studies of continuous infusion furosemide suggest greater natriuretic effect and no difference in metabolic adverse effects when compared to the same total daily dose given by IV bolus.[59,64]

Another commonly employed mechanism for overcoming diuretic resistance is to add a second diuretic with a different mechanism of action. The combination of a loop diuretic with an agent which acts on the distal convoluted tubule (most commonly metolazone, a thiazide-type diuretic, or hydrochlorothiazide) produces a synergistic diuretic effect, thus such a combination is commonly employed in this setting.[62,63] The distal tubule blockers have no effect on the pharmacokinetics of loop diuretics, therefore the synergistic effect is due to a pharmacodynamic interaction.[62,63] Most current literature suggests that the mechanism of the synergistic effect is related to the increased delivery of sodium to the distal convoluted tubule. As sodium reabsorption is blocked by loop diuretics in the ascending limb of the loop of Henle, the delivery of sodium to the distal tubule is markedly increased. Because mechanisms for sodium transport in the distal tubule are not normally saturated, sodium reabsorption is greater than normal in the distal tubule in a patient receiving a loop diuretic. This is especially true in disease states such as CHF in which sodium reabsorption is avid. When thiazide-type diuretics are added to the loop diuretic, they block more than their normal 5–8% of filtered sodium and the loop diuretic–thiazide combination results in a synergistic effect.[62,63]

Use of the loop diuretic–thiazide combination should generally be reserved for the inpatient setting where the patient can be closely monitored. This is because the combination can induce a profound diuresis, resulting in severe sodium, potassium, and volume depletion. When used in the outpatient setting, very low doses or only occasional doses of the thiazide-type diuretic should be utilized to avoid serious adverse events.

VASODILATORS

Use of vasodilator therapy in years past was reserved for patients with severe heart failure. However, in the past decade, several studies have documented that, in addition to producing sustained symptomatic improvement, ACE inhibitors or the combination of hydralazine/isosorbide dinitrate are also effective in decreasing mortality.[6,7,65,66] This section focuses on use of these vasodilators for the management of chronic CHF and also briefly describes vasodilators, which are not recommended for CHF management.

Nitrates and Hydralazine

The nitrates all activate guanylate cyclase to increase cyclic guanosine monophosphate (cyclic GMP) in vascular smooth muscle, with preferential effects in the venous bed. The predominant hemodynamic effect of nitrates is to reduce preload (Table 13.9), although a slight reduction in systemic vascular resistance may be seen.[67]

The nitrate product most extensively studied in the treatment of chronic congestive heart failure is isosorbide dinitrate (ISDN).[65–67] Oral nitroglycerin products are probably equally effective, however transdermal nitroglycerin products (patch or paste) are not recommended in CHF because of the tolerance associated with their use.[68] Effective doses of ISDN range from 20–80 mg every 6 hours and most studies have utilized a dose of 40 mg every 6 hours.[65–67] The controlled studies in CHF[67] show that in spite of favorable hemodynamic effects, ISDN has no effect on exercise tolerance following a single dose. However, 2–3 months of therapy result in significant improvements in resting and exercise hemodynamics, exercise tolerance, and clinical status.

Tolerance to the effects of nitrates is seen during both CHF and antianginal therapy. Intravenous and transdermal nitroglycerin administration result in relatively constant plasma concentrations and tolerance appears to be a particular problem with these routes of administration.[52,68] However, the literature is equivocal with regards to development of tolerance to oral ISDN in CHF therapy.[67,69] Most of the clinical trials with ISDN have utilized every-6-hours administration and have continued to show symptomatic improvements after months to years of therapy.[65–67] In general, nitrate tolerance does not appear to be as problematic in the management of CHF as when nitrates are used for antianginal effects. The mechanism of nitrate tolerance is still poorly understood. When it develops in a heart failure patient the best alternative, at present, for minimizing nitrate tolerance appears to be 8- to 12-hour nitrate-free intervals. A more complete discussion of nitrate tolerance can be found in Chapter 14.

Hydralazine is a direct-acting vasodilator that acts predominantly on arterial smooth muscle. It causes a significant reduction in systemic vascular resistance with resultant increases in stroke volume index and cardiac index (Fig. 13.1 and Table 13.9); effects on preload are minimal.[70,71] By reducing afterload, hydralazine theoretically interrupts the vicious cycle of worsening cardiac function. The doses of hydralazine required in CHF are often much higher than those for treatment of hypertension. Average doses range from 200 to 300 mg/d but doses as high as 3000 mg have been utilized.[70] Results from studies evaluating the role of hydralazine without a venous vasodilator in CHF are conflicting. Some studies have shown that hydralazine is associated with long-term improvements in hemodynamic parameters, symptoms, and exercise tolerance.[71,72] Other studies have shown an attenuation of the hemodynamic effects with time[73] and a lack of symptomatic or exercise tolerance improvement.[74]

To achieve both preload and afterload reduction, hydralazine is frequently given in combination with ISDN;

a combination that has been shown to reduce mortality significantly in CHF patients.[65,66] The Veterans Administration Cooperative Study (Vasodilators in Heart Failure Trial, VHeFT-I) was a placebo-controlled trial that compared the effects of hydralazine 300 mg/d plus ISDN 160 mg/d, prazosin 20 mg/d, and placebo on mortality in NYHA FC-II and FC-III patients. Compared to placebo, mortality in the hydralazine/nitrate treated patients was reduced by 38% after 1 year, 25% at 2 years, and 23% at 3 years. Similar mortality figures with hydralazine–isosorbide dinitrate were obtained in a follow-up study (VHeFT-II).[66]

Adverse effects to both nitrates and hydralazine are common, which limits use of this combination in many patients. In VHeFT-I, one or both drugs were discontinued in 19% of patients due to side effects, and only 55% of the patients could tolerate full doses of both drugs.[65]

Angiotensin-Converting Enzyme Inhibitors

A number of angiotensin-converting enzyme (ACE) inhibitors are currently available in the United States with many, but not all of them, having Food and Drug Administration approval for use in CHF. A table summarizing the available ACE inhibitors can be found in Chapter 12. The major differences in the ACE inhibitors are not in their pharmacologic properties but with their pharmacokinetic properties. While not all of the ACE inhibitors are currently approved for use in CHF, the beneficial effects of these agents in heart failure probably represent a drug class effect.

ACE inhibitors cause arterial and venous dilatation, thus reducing both preload and afterload (Table 13.9). The vasodilation produced by ACE inhibitors appears to be due to both reduced activation of angiotensin II, a potent vasoconstrictor, and reduced breakdown of bradykinin, a vasodilator (see Fig. 13.8). Bradykinin, which is inactivated by ACE (identical to kininase II), also enhances release of vasodilatory prostaglandins and histamine.

Numerous placebo-controlled trials have documented the favorable effects of ACE inhibitor therapy on hemodynamic variables, clinical status, and symptoms in heart failure.[75,76] Hemodynamic effects observed with long-term therapy include significant increases in cardiac index, stroke work index, and stroke volume index as well as significant reductions in left ventricular filling pressure, systemic vascular resistance, mean arterial pressure, and heart rate. Significant improvements in clinical status, functional class, exercise tolerance, and left ventricular size with ACE inhibition are also well documented. When compared with placebo, patients treated with ACE inhibitors have fewer treatment failures, fewer hospitalizations, fewer increases in diuretic dosages, and fewer ventricular premature beats on ambulatory electrocardiographic monitoring.[6,7,75,76] The acute response to ACE inhibitor therapy is greater in patients with high levels of plasma renin activity. However, long-term hemodynamic and clinical response to ACE inhibition cannot be predicted from the plasma renin activity or from response to the initial dose of ACE inhibitor.[77]

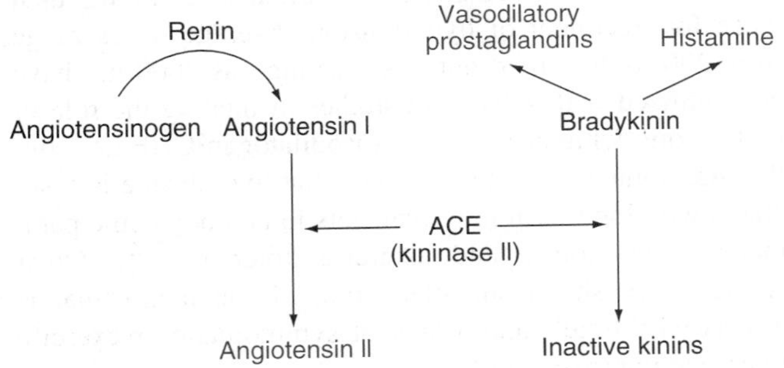

Figure 13.8. Activity of ACE, which is identical to kininase II, on angiotensin and bradykinin.

The beneficial effect of ACE inhibitor therapy on mortality has also been documented. The Cooperative North Scandinavian Enalapril Survival Study (CONSENSUS) was a study of patients with NYHA FC-IV heart failure randomized to enalapril or placebo.[6] It was stopped prematurely because of the clear beneficial effect of enalapril therapy on survival. There were 40% and 25% reductions in mortality in the enalapril-treated patients at 6 months and 1 year, respectively. A placebo-controlled study of enalapril (Studies of Left Ventricular Dysfunction, SOLVD), in which most patients were in NYHA FC-II or FC-III heart failure, also revealed significant reductions in mortality in enalapril-treated patients.[7] Differences in mortality were noted over a 48-month period, although these differences were most marked in the first 24 months of therapy. Although not documented in a large-scale study, a favorable effect on survival in patients with symptomatic CHF has also been suggested with captopril.[75] Finally, a comparative trial (VHeFT-II) of enalapril versus hydralazine–isosorbide dinitrate showed that enalapril therapy resulted in significantly lower mortality than the hydralazine–nitrate combination.[66] Mortality in enalapril-treated patients was 33.6% lower at 1 year and 28.2% lower after 2 years as compared to the hydralazine–nitrate group. Trends toward lower mortality with enalapril were also observed at 3 and 4 years but were not statistically significant. Secondary endpoints in this study, left ventricular ejection fraction and exercise tolerance, favored the hydralazine–nitrate combination over enalapril. However, these data are difficult to interpret because of the different mortality rates in the two groups.

The mechanism by which ACE inhibitors reduce mortality is not entirely clear. Increasing basic and clinical literature support the role of cardiac tissue angiotensin II as a proto-oncogene, which plays an important role in the hypertrophy and ventricular dilatation associated with progressive heart failure.[78–81] The ACE inhibitor treatment trials (CONSENSUS[6] and SOLVD[7]) and the prevention trials (SAVE,[79] AIRE,[80] and SOLVD Prevention[81]) all suggest that ACE inhibitors reduce mortality by preventing the progression of CHF. Thus, ACE inhibitor therapy appears to play an important role in preventing progressive worsening of myocardial function for which angiotensin II appears to play a critical role. However, lower mortality with enalapril compared to hydralazine–isosorbide dinitrate in VHeFT-II was due to a reduction in the incidence of sudden death; death due to progression of CHF was similar in the two groups.[66] The VHeFT-II data suggest that vasodilation (with a hydralazine-nitrate combination or with an ACE inhibitor) improves CHF survival by slowing progression of the syndrome, and the added benefit of enalapril on survival may be an indirect antiarrhythmic effect due to reduction in circulating catecholamines and elevation of serum potassium concentrations. However, no effect on sudden death has been documented in the enalapril placebo-controlled trials (CONSENSUS and SOLVD). Thus, the precise mechanism(s) by which ACE inhibitors reduce mortality remains controversial.

Adverse Effects of ACE Inhibitors in CHF

The primary adverse effects of ACE inhibitor therapy in CHF are hypotension and functional renal insufficiency. Hypotension may be manifested as dizziness, lightheadedness, presyncope, or syncope. It occurs most commonly with the first dose, although it may occur at any time during therapy.[6,76] Patients at increased risk of developing hypotension are those with hyponatremia (serum sodium <130 mmol/L) and recent increases in diuretic dose. The occurrence of hypotension may be minimized by initiating therapy with lower doses.

Functional renal insufficiency is manifested as increases in serum creatinine and blood urea nitrogen. As cardiac output and renal blood flow decline, renal perfusion is maintained by angiotensin II's vasoconstrictor effect on the efferent arteriole. Patients most dependent on this system for maintenance of renal perfusion (and therefore most likely to develop functional renal insufficiency with ACE inhibitors) are those with severe heart failure, hyponatremia, and dehydration.[6] Sodium depletion (usually secondary to diuretic therapy) is the most important factor in development of functional renal insufficiency with ACE inhibitor therapy. Renal insufficiency can therefore be minimized in many cases by reduction in diuretic dosage or liberalization of sodium intake.[82] Retention of potassium with ACE inhibitor therapy is common and is due to the reduced feedback of angiotensin II to stimulate aldosterone release. Hyperkalemia rarely develops, although caution is necessary in patients with renal insufficiency, concomitant potassium supplementation, patients using potassium containing salt substitutes, or potassium-sparing diuretic therapy.[6,76]

Rash and dysgeusia are troublesome side effects of ACE inhibitor therapy, which appear to be more common with high doses; the rash may resolve with continued therapy. A dry, hacking cough occurs with a similar frequency with all the agents and may be related to accumulation of tissues kinins. Cough occurs in up to 40% of patients with heart failure, independent of ACE inhibitor use, although ACE inhibitors significantly increase its incidence. However, in large clinical trial, only about 1% of participants discontinue ACE inhibitor therapy because of cough.

Vasodilators That Are Not Recommended for CHF Management

Prazosin is an α_1-adrenergic receptor antagonist that causes both arterial and venous dilation. It is not used in the management of CHF because long-term prazosin therapy in VHeFT-I failed to produce any long-term beneficial hemodynamic effects or have any impact on mortality.[65]

Minoxidil is an arterial vasodilator that produces hemodynamic effects similar to hydralazine. However, in spite of hemodynamic and left ventricular function improvement, studies revealed no improvement in exercise tolerance and worsening of pulmonary artery pressures and clinical status of patients.[83] Because minoxidil may have detrimental effects on the clinical course of CHF patients, its use in this setting is generally not recommended.

Calcium channel blockers cause direct vasodilation in arterial resistance vessels, but are also associated with varying degrees of direct negative inotropic activity. Similar to many other vasodilators, their short-term hemodynamic effects have not been translated into symptomatic benefits with long-term therapy. In fact, some trials suggest that long-term calcium channel blocker therapy may cause deleterious effects in CHF patients.[84–86] The Multicenter Diltiazem Postinfarction Trial randomized patients to diltiazem or placebo, with a mean follow-up of 25 months.[84] In patients with evidence of left ventricular dysfunction upon entry into the study (e.g., presence of pulmonary congestion, ejection fraction <0.40), diltiazem therapy was associated with a significantly higher cardiac event rate (cardiac death, nonfatal reinfarction) as compared to placebo. Diltiazem-treated patients with underlying left ventricular dysfunction were also significantly more likely than placebo-treated patients to develop CHF during follow-up.[85] Another study compared ISDN, nifedipine, or the combination using a crossover design in patients with FC-II or FC-III heart failure. The three regimens were associated with similar improvements in exercise performance. However, treatment with nifedipine alone and nifedipine plus ISDN resulted in a significantly higher incidence of worsening CHF than in ISDN-treated patients.[86] Worsening heart failure in these studies may be related to the negative inotropic effects of calcium channel blockers, activation of the sympathetic nervous system and renin-angiotensin-aldosterone system as well as other unidentified mechanisms.[85,86] Based on the results of these studies, it has been suggested that the use of calcium channel blockers in patients with left ventricular dysfunction may be inappropriate. However, several trials of second-generation calcium channel blockers in CHF are currently under way.[87] Calcium channel blockers may be of greater value in patients with pure diastolic dysfunction; this is discussed in greater detail in Chapter 17.

Place of Vasodilators in the Therapy of Patients with Symptomatic Heart Failure

Vasodilator therapy with an ACE inhibitor or hydralazine–nitrate combination is now clearly considered to be a cornerstone of therapy for the management of congestive heart failure.[88] Four well-conducted mortality studies[6,7,65,66] have documented that treatment with either of these regimens improves survival in patients with symptomatic heart failure. The superiority in mortality reduction with enalapril over hydralazine–isosorbide dinitrate in VHeFT-II suggests that ACE inhibitors represent the vasodilator of first choice for the treatment of congestive heart failure. Thus, all patients with symptomatic heart failure should be taking chronic ACE inhibitor therapy. Patients unable to tolerate or with a contraindication to an ACE inhibitor should be treated with a hydralazine–nitrate combination.

DIGITALIS GLYCOSIDES

In 1785, William Withering was the first to report extensively on the use of foxglove or *Digitalis purpurea* for the treatment of dropsy (i.e., edema). Although digitalis glycosides have been in clinical use for more than 200 years, not until the 1920s was it clearly demonstrated that these compounds have a positive inotropic effect on the heart.[89] Furthermore, it was not until the 1980s that most of the controlled trials were conducted to evaluate critically the place of digoxin in the therapy of chronic heart failure. The flaws and inconsistent results of these controlled trials, the controversy over the long-term use of positive inotropes, and the documented benefits of vasodilators, have raised important questions about the role of digoxin in heart failure.[89–91] Some of these questions should be answered when the results of the large Digitalis Investigators Group trial become available in the mid-1990s.[91] The following discussion focuses on digoxin because it is by far the most widely studied and frequently prescribed digitalis glycoside in the United States.

Digitalis glycosides exert their positive inotropic effects by binding to sodium-and-potassium-activated adenosine triphosphatase (NaK-ATPase or sodium pump).[89] Inhibition of NaK-ATPase decreases outward transport of sodium and leads to increased intracellular sodium concentrations. Higher intracellular sodium concentrations favor calcium entry and reduce calcium extrusion from the cell through effects on the sodium-calcium exchanger.[89] The result is increased storage of intracellular calcium in the sarcoplasmic reticulum and, with each action potential, a greater release of calcium to activate contractile elements.

Digitalis glycosides have several other notable direct and indirect pharmacologic effects, which are potentially beneficial in patients with heart failure. They increase vagal tone and lead to a variable decrease in heart rate, which may increase diastolic filling. These vagal effects are also largely responsible for the decrease in conduction and prolongation of refractoriness in the atrioventricular node, which in turn causes a slowing of the ventricular response in atrial fibrillation. Since atrial fibrillation is a common complication of heart failure, the combined positive inotropic and negative dromotropic effects of digitalis glycosides can be particularly important for such patients. There is also evidence that digitalis glycosides, unlike positive inotropes that increase intracellular cAMP, blunt the excessive neurohumoral activation that is characteristic of heart failure patients.[92] These desirable neurohumoral effects may result from direct actions and/or reflex withdrawal caused by increased cardiac performance.[21,92] Modulations of the sympathetic nervous system and the renin-angiotensin system are thus potentially important mechanisms by which digitalis glycosides could have positive long-term effects in patients with left ventricular dysfunction.[92,93] The overall response to digoxin is usually an increase in cardiac index, a decrease in systemic vascular resistance and PCWP, but relatively little change in arterial blood pressure.[89,94] The diuretic effect is presumably mediated by both an increase in cardiac index and a decrease in renin-angiotensin-aldosterone activity.[89]

PHARMACOKINETICS

Numerous studies of digoxin pharmacokinetics have been published during the past 25 years and their results are extensively reviewed elsewhere (Table 13.10).[21,95–97] Estimates of the absolute bioavailability of conventional digoxin tablets range from 50–90%. There is significant intersubject variability in the bioavailability of digoxin oral dosage forms and this contributes (along with the variability in clearance) to the observed variability in steady-state serum digoxin concentrations (SDCs) among patients receiving the same dose. Encapsulated gel preparations of digoxin (Lanoxicaps) have a bioavailability of 90–100% but the available doses are approximately equivalent to the tablets after accounting for the difference in bioavailability. Digoxin has a large volume of distribution and is extensively bound to various tissues, most notably to NaK-ATPase in skeletal and cardiac muscles. Because it does not distribute appreciably to body fat, loading doses of digoxin should be calculated based on estimates of lean body weight. There is a significant "distribution phase" after administration of oral or intravenous digoxin. Delayed distribution to the site of action explains the lag time before maximum pharmacologic response even after intravenous administration (Table 13.10). After a pseudoequilibrium is reached with the site of action (3–12 hours after the dose), the time course of cardiac effects becomes consistent with SDCs. Transiently elevated SDCs during the distribution phase are not associated with increased desired or adverse effects, although they can mislead the clinician who is unaware of when the blood sample was collected relative to the previous digoxin dose. Consequently, blood samples for measurement of SDCs should be collected at least 6 hours and preferably 12 hours or more after the last dose.

In patients with normal renal function, 60–80% of a dose of digoxin is eliminated unchanged in urine via glomerular filtration and tubular secretion. The latter is an active process, which can be affected by several different drugs (Table 13.11). Because total clearance is equal to the sum of renal and nonrenal clearances, patients with renal impairment will be relatively more dependent on nonrenal elimination of digoxin (i.e., metabolism, biliary secretion, etc.). It is important to emphasize that most studies of digoxin pharmacokinetics have used immunoassays to measure digoxin concentrations in serum and urine. Lack of specificity with the immunoassays leads to variable cross-reactivity with certain metabolites as well as endogenous digoxin-like immunoreactive substance(s) and probably affected the estimates of certain pharmacokinetic parameters.[96] The terminal half-life of digoxin is approximately 1.5 days in subjects with normal renal function and approximately 5 days in anuric patients (Table 13.10). Digitoxin pharmacokinetic parameters are compared with those of digoxin in Table 13.10. Numerous pharmacokinetic/pharmacodynamic drug interactions have been reported with digoxin and Table 13.11 summarizes those considered to be most clinically important.

Optimal Range of Serum Digoxin Concentrations

The optimal range of SDCs for heart failure patients in normal sinus rhythm has been the subject of a long controversy. A review of approximately 40 different studies demonstrated that patients without evidence of digoxin toxicity had mean SDCs of about 1.4 ng/mL compared to values two to three times higher for patients with toxicity.[97,98] However, there is very significant overlap between observed SDCs in patients with and without toxicity, so that SDCs should only be used in conjunction with thorough clinical evaluation of each patient before determining that certain signs/symptoms are due to digoxin toxicity.

The relationship between SDCs and efficacy in heart failure is no less tenuous because of the difficulty in precisely quantitating clinical response. The fact that some patients with heart failure have little or no clinical improvement even with desired SDCs makes the determination of an "optimal" range even more difficult (see section on Clinical Efficacy and Place in Therapy). With these limitations in mind, the desired range of SDCs is generally quoted as 0.8–2.0 ng/mL. Controlled studies that have demonstrated some benefits of digoxin in patients with chronic heart failure have used a similar range of SDCs, thus lending at least some general support for its use.[76,94,99–102] However, a more conservative target of 1.0–1.5 ng/mL has been advocated[97] and can be supported

TABLE 13.10. CLINICAL PHARMACOKINETICS OF DIGOXIN AND DIGITOXIN

	Digoxin	Digitoxin
Oral bioavailability		
Tablets	0.5–0.9 (0.65)[a]	0.9–1.0
Elixir	0.75–0.85 (0.80)	
Capsules	0.9–1.0 (0.95)	
Onset of action		
Oral	1.5–6 h	3–6 h
Intravenous	15–30 min	30–120 min
Peak effect		
Oral	4–6 h	6–12 h
Intravenous	1.5–4 h	4–6 h
Terminal half-life		
Normal renal function	36 h	7 d
Anuric patients	5 d	7 d
Volume of distribution at steady state	7.3 L/kg	0.6 L/kg
Fraction unbound in plasma	0.75–0.80	0.05–0.10
Principal route of elimination	Renal	Hepatic

[a]Range and mean value in parentheses. (Compiled from References 21 and 95 through 97.)

TABLE 13.11. POTENTIALLY SIGNIFICANT PHARMACOKINETIC/PHARMACODYNAMIC DRUG INTERACTIONS WITH DIGOXIN

Drug	Mechanism/Effect	Suggested Clinical Management
Amiodarone	Decrease in renal and nonrenal clearance; can increase SDC by 70–100%.	Monitor SDC and anticipate the need to reduce the dose by 50%.
Antacids	Concurrent administration may decrease digoxin bioavailability by 20–35%.	Space doses at least 2 h apart to avoid concurrent use if possible.
Neomycin, Sulfasalazine	Decrease in bioavailability by 20–25%.	Space doses at least 2 h apart to avoid concurrent use if possible.
Erythromycin, tetracycline	Alter gut bacterial flora; bioavailability and SDC increase 40–100% in about 10% of patients who extensively metabolize digoxin in the gut.	Monitor SDC and anticipate the need to reduce the dose; avoid concurrent use if possible.
Cholestrayramine, Colestipol	Bind digoxin in gut and decrease bioavailability 20–35%; may also decrease enterohepatic recycling.	Space doses at least 2 h apart to avoid concurrent use if possible.
Diuretics	Thiazides or loop diuretics may cause hypokalemia and hypomagnesemia thereby increasing the risk of digitalis toxicity.	Monitor and replace electrolytes if necessary.
Kaolin-pectin	Large dose (30–60 mL) may decrease digoxin bioavailability by about 60%.	Space drugs at least 2 h apart or avoid concurrent use if possible.
Metoclopramide	Increase in gut mobility may decrease bioavailability of slow-dissolving tablets; unknown significance.	Effect is minimized by administration of digoxin capsules.
Propantheline	Decrease in gut mobility may increase bioavailability of slow-dissolving tablets; unknown significance.	Effect is minimized by administration of digoxin capsules.
Quinidine	Decrease in renal and nonrenal clearance; also displacement of digoxin from tissue binding and decrease in the volume of distribution; SDC generally increase about twofold.	Monitor SDC and adverse effects; anticipate the need to reduce the dose by 50%.
Spironolactone	Decrease in renal and nonrenal clearance; also interference with some digoxin assays thus increasing apparent SDC.	Monitor SDC and anticipate the need to reduce dose; check assay for interference.
Verapamil	Decrease in renal and nonrenal clearance; SDC may increase 70–100%.	Monitor SDC and anticipate the need to reduce the dose by 50%; consider using another calcium channel blocker.
Propafenone	Decrease in renal clearance; SDC may increase 30–40%.	Monitor SDC and anticipate the need to reduce the dose.

with the following arguments: (1) The mean or target SDCs in the previously mentioned controlled studies with positive benefits were usually in this lower range. (2) There may be smaller increments in myocardial contractility at higher SDCs. (3) There is no clear evidence that SDCs >1.5 ng/mL provide additional benefits for patients with heart failure and normal sinus rhythm.[94] (4) SDCs above 1.5 ng/mL expose the patient to an increased risk of toxicity. (5) Other agents at least as effective if not more effective than digoxin are available. Thus a more conservative optimal range of SDCs could be used until there is more information on the risk-to-benefit ratio of higher concentrations. Finally, we must emphasize that the above data on the optimal range of SDCs are based on clinical efficacy measures (e.g., exercise capacity) but with unknown effects on mortality.[91]

Dosage

Usual maintenance doses with digoxin tablets range from 0.125–0.5 mg/day. Lower doses are usually necessary in patients with significant renal impairment. Several different equations and nomograms have been proposed to estimate digoxin maintenance doses, based on an estimate of renal function for a particular patient and population pharmacokinetic parameters. These methods are extensively reviewed elsewhere.[96,103] Heart failure patients in normal sinus rhythm do not generally need a loading dose. The necessity of a loading dose should be based on the clinical status of the patient, with the understanding that digoxin is a mild inotropic agent that will produce gradual effects over several hours, even after a loading dose. In some circumstances it may be necessary to achieve desired SDCs (and clinical benefits) before the 6 to 10 days that are normally required to approach steady state with maintenance doses. Recommended loading doses with oral digoxin tablets range from 10 to 20 mcg/kg of lean body weight, and a midrange dose of 15 mcg/kg is appropriate for most patients. Lower intravenous loading doses should be used (e.g., 10 mcg/kg of lean body weight) to compensate for the difference in bioavailability.

ADVERSE EFFECTS

Digoxin and other digitalis glycosides may produce a variety of cardiac and noncardiac adverse effects (Table 13.12).[21,98] Noncardiac adverse effects include nonspecific symptoms such as anorexia, nausea, and occasionally vomiting. Although usually described as gastrointestinal adverse effects, nausea and vomiting are primarily due to a central effect of digoxin on the chemoreceptor trigger zone in the medulla. Cardiac manifestations include numerous different arrhythmias caused by enhanced automaticity, slowed conduction, or delayed afterdepolarizations (Table 13.12). It is noteworthy that cardiac arrhythmias may be the first evidence of toxicity in a patient (before any noncardiac symptoms occur). Rhythm disturbances are of particular concern because patients with chronic heart failure are already at increased risk for sudden cardiac death presumably due to ventricular arrhythmias. Hypokalemia, hypercalcemia, and hypomagnesemia will predispose patients to cardiac manifestations of digoxin toxicity. Concomitant therapy with diuretics may lead to electrolyte abnormalities and increase the likelihood of cardiac arrhythmias. Similarly, hypothyroidism, myocardial ischemia, and acidosis will increase the risk of cardiac adverse effects. Usual treatment of digoxin toxicity includes drug withdrawal or lowering of the dose, and treatment of cardiac arrhythmias or electrolyte abnormalities. In patients with life-threatening digoxin toxicity, purified digoxin-specific Fab antibody fragments provide reversal of adverse effects within 1 hour in more than 90% of cases.[104]

TABLE 13.12. SIGNS AND SYMPTOMS OF DIGITALIS TOXICITY

Noncardiac (Mostly CNS) Adverse Effects[a]
Anorexia, nausea, vomiting, abdominal pain
Visual disturbances: halos, photophobia, problems with color perception (i.e., red-green or yellow-green vision), scotomata
Fatigue, weakness, dizziness, headache, neuralgia, confusion, delirium, psychosis
Cardiac Adverse Effects[a,b]
Ventricular arrhythmias
Premature ventricular depolarizations, bigeminy, trigeminy, ventricular tachycardia, ventricular fibrillation
Atrioventricular (AV) block
First degree, second degree (Mobitz type I), third degree
AV junctional escape rhythms, junctional tachycardia
Atrial arrhythmias with slowed AV conduction or AV block
Particularly paroxysmal atrial tachycardia with AV block
Sinus bradycardia

[a]Some adverse effects may be difficult to distinguish from the signs/symptoms of heart failure.

[b]Digitalis toxicity has been associated with almost every known rhythm abnormality (only the more common manifestations are listed). (Compiled from References 21 and 98.)

Despite the general perception that digoxin is often poorly tolerated, recent multicenter randomized double-blind trials indicate that digoxin is relatively well tolerated compared to milrinone, captopril, and even placebo.[76,100,101,105] It should be emphasized that some bias in favor of digoxin may have occurred in the previous studies because patients already receiving (and tolerating) digoxin were often selected for inclusion.

Retrospective analyses have suggested that digoxin therapy may increase mortality in patients with ischemic heart disease, particularly within a few months after a myocardial infarction. However, these conclusions have been challenged on statistical grounds and other retrospective studies have indicated that the difference in mortality may be caused by other prognostic factors associated with the use of digoxin but not with the drug itself (e.g., degree of left ventricular dysfunction).[91] There is clear evidence that drugs that exert a positive inotropic effect by increasing intracellular cAMP also increase mortality in patients with heart failure (see section on Drugs Proven to Increase Mortality in Heart Failure Patients).[93] However, it is currently unknown if this adverse effect will be shared by other positive inotropic agents with a different mechanism of action, such as digitalis glycosides.[93] This question is currently being investigated in a large multicenter trial.[91]

Clinical Efficacy and Place in Therapy

The efficacy of digoxin in patients with heart failure and supraventricular tachyarrhythmias such as atrial fibrillation is relatively well established and widely accepted.[89] However, until the 1980s, most data supporting efficacy of digitalis glycosides in heart failure patients with normal sinus rhythm came from anecdotal evidence and seriously flawed or uncontrolled studies. Since 1980, larger more rigorous clinical studies have provided some important information on the efficacy of digoxin. It has now been established that digoxin exerts a positive inotropic effect, which is sustained after chronic administration in patients with heart failure.[94] These effects correspond to an upward shift in the Starling curve (point E to C in Fig. 13.6).

A more important issue, however, is whether digoxin's hemodynamic effects lead to benefits in terms of decreased symptoms, increased exercise capacity, improved quality of life, and decreased mortality in patients with chronic heart failure. The Milrinone Multicenter Trial[100] was a randomized double-blind study that compared the efficacy of digoxin, milrinone, digoxin plus milrinone, and placebo in 230 patients who continued to receive stable doses of diuretics (see following discussion of milrinone's efficacy). Most patients were in NYHA FC-II and FC-III. Digoxin therapy (mean SDC of 1.1 ng/mL) was associated with an increase in treadmill exercise time, a reduced frequency of worsening heart failure, and a small but statistically significant increase in left ventricular ejection fraction compared to placebo. The German and Austrian Xamoterol Study Group[105] compared the effects of digoxin, xamoterol, and placebo in 433 patients with chronic heart failure, most of whom were in NYHA FC-II and approximately 20% of whom were treated with diuretics (see below for discussion of xamoterol's efficacy). In this 3-month randomized double-blind study, digoxin (mean SDC of 0.9 ng/mL) produced a small increase in exercise capacity which was not statistically different from placebo. There was also a trend for improvement in certain signs or symptoms of heart failure and some of these changes (i.e., breathlessness, tiredness, peripheral edema, rales, and body weight) were statistically different between digoxin and placebo. The Captopril-Digoxin Multicenter Research Group performed a double-blind study to compare the efficacy of digoxin, captopril, and placebo in 300 (almost all NYHA FC-II) patients receiving diuretic therapy.[76] Mean SDC in the digoxin group was not reported but doses were adjusted to achieve trough SDC greater than 0.7 ng/mL and less than 2.5 ng/mL. Digoxin therapy was associated with small improvements in exercise tolerance and functional class but neither effect was statistically different from placebo. However, there was a significant increase in left ventricular ejection fraction with digoxin. Conversely, captopril therapy produced significant increases in exercise tolerance and functional class but no change in ejection fraction, compared to placebo. The results emphasize that changes in ejection fraction do not necessarily lead to changes in functional class or exercise capacity. Both the digoxin and captopril groups had fewer treatment failures, hospitalizations, and increases in diuretic dosages than the placebo group.

The results of the three large multicenter studies and four other smaller controlled studies (all published before 1990) were evaluated by meta-analysis.[106] Overall results indicated there was a statistically significant decrease in the risk of heart failure deterioration during digoxin therapy, compared to placebo. Since that time, the Prospective Randomized Study of Ventricular Failure and Efficacy of Digoxin (PROVED)[102] and the Randomized Assessment of Digoxin on Inhibitors of Angiotensin Converting Enzyme (RADIANCE)[101] have also reported positive benefits of digoxin in patients with NYHA FC-II and FC-III heart failure and systolic dysfunction (ejection fraction <0.35). The latter study is noteworthy because it documented that digoxin decreased the risk of clinical deterioration and increased exercise capacity in patients receiving a diuretic and an ACE inhibitor. The results of these and other digoxin efficacy studies have been reviewed by Kelly and Smith[90] and Yusuf et al.[91] It must be emphasized that all studies of digoxin efficacy that have been completed were too short or too small to properly determine if mortality is increased, decreased, or unchanged by digoxin.

Almost all controlled studies of digoxin's efficacy involved withdrawal of the drug in patients who were already taking it before inclusion into the study. In addition to the potential bias of such studies, it is not possible to evaluate the impact of starting digoxin compared with placebo.[91] Unlike certain vasodilators that decrease mortality of patients with heart failure, there is no proven beneficial effect of digoxin therapy on mortality. There is actually concern that digoxin, like several other inotropic agents, could have an adverse effect on the natural progression of the disease and/or the risk of sudden death and increase mortality (see sections on Adverse Effects and Drugs Proven to Increase Mortality in Heart Failure Patients). Conversely, digoxin could have beneficial effects on mortality by, for example, altering the progression of the disease through its neurohumoral effects. The National Heart, Lung, and Blood Institute and the Veterans Administration are conducting a multicenter randomized double-blind placebo-controlled study to help answer this and other important questions (Digitalis Investigators Group trial).[91] The results of this landmark study of more than 7000 patients are expected by the mid-1990s.

Based on these studies and until the results of the Digitalis Investigators Group trial are available, the following conclusions and recommendations can be made concerning the use of digoxin. Digoxin exerts a sustained but modest positive inotropic effect, which is clinically more evident in patients with moderate-to-severe left ventricular systolic dysfunction. Patients more likely to have a beneficial response to digoxin include the following[89,107–109]: (1) patients with significant left ventricular systolic dysfunction (low ejection fraction) and supraventricular tachyarrhythmias such as atrial fibrillation with a rapid ventricular response (usually considered first-line drug); and (2) symptomatic patients with moderate-to-severe heart failure (NYHA FC-III and FC-IV) and a dilated left ventricle with systolic dysfunction (often with a third heart sound). This latter category of patients should generally be first treated with diuretics and vasodilators, then digoxin added if the clinical response is not adequate. Diuretics, with the addition of vasodilators if necessary, should be the initial drug therapy for patients with mild-to-moderate heart failure (NYHA FC-II). Digoxin can be considered an alternative to vasodilators for patients at risk of developing clinically significant hypotension or other adverse effects from vasodilators. However, digoxin is less likely to be effective and should not be used in patients whose heart failure is largely the result of diastolic dysfunction.

ANTIARRHYTHMIC THERAPY

Sudden cardiac death, presumably due to ventricular arrhythmias, is the mode of death in up to 50% of CHF patients.[5–7] The value of antiarrhythmic therapy in reducing CHF mortality is therefore an issue of interest. Unfortunately, no therapy can be recommended for reduction of sudden death in this population. Based on data from the Cardiac Arrhythmia Suppression Trials (CAST)[110,111] (see Chapter 16 for details), class I antiarrhythmics should probably be avoided in all patients with left ventricular dysfunction.[112] Most CHF patients who have experienced life-threatening arrhythmias or who have symptomatic arrhythmias are currently managed with either amiodarone therapy or implantation of an automatic implantable cardiovertor defibrillator (AICD). However, the current literature is equivocal for both of these therapeutic modalities.

Several studies with amiodarone have yielded conflicting results. A pilot study in which 100 patients with NYHA FC-III and -IV heart failure were treated with low-dose amiodarone or placebo showed that amiodarone had no effect on 1-year mortality.[113] The GESICA study randomized 516 patients with moderate to severe heart failure to amiodarone 300 mg daily or placebo.[113a] All patients were receiving standard heart failure therapies and were enrolled independent of the presence or absence of nonsustained ventricular tachycardia. The study was stopped prematurely by the steering committee because amiodarone produced a 28% risk reduction in death. Sudden death and death due to progressive heart failure were reduced by a similar magnitude in amiodarone-treated patients. Conversely, a Veterans Administration study of 674 patients with NYHA FC-III or -IV heart failure, ejection fractions of <0.40, and greater than 10 PVCs/hour derived no reduction in mortality from treatment with amiodarone.[113b] Thus, the role of amiodarone therapy for patients with CHF remains unclear.

Regarding AICDs, a case series in patients with ejection fractions of <30% who had AICD implantation showed that the incidence of sudden death was only 4, 9, and 18% at 1, 2, and 3 years, respectively. However, survival at these same time points was 82, 69, and 57%, respectively.[114] These survival statistics are essentially identical to CHF epidemiologic data,[4] suggesting that implantation of AICDs in patients with left ventricular dysfunction does not prolong survival, but merely changes the mode of death. Thus, until the results from large, ongoing clinical trials are published, no antiarrhythmic regimen can be routinely recommended for patients with CHF.

POTENTIALLY USEFUL DRUGS FOR THE MANAGEMENT OF CHF

β-Blockers

It may seem somewhat paradoxical that, within this chapter, β-blockers are listed as drugs that may exacerbate or worsen CHF (Table 13.4), and as drugs that may be useful in the management of chronic heart failure. Nonetheless, both of these are true. There is no question that administration of normal doses of β-blockers to patients with heart failure can lead to a worsening or exacerbation of their symptomatology. However, there is mounting clinical evidence that if stable patients are initiated on low doses of a β-blocker (e.g., metoprolol 6.25 mg bid) with upward dose titration over 4 to 6 weeks, they may derive significant benefits from such therapy.[115,116] There have been at least 16 randomized, controlled trials to date of β blockers in heart failure[116] and at least four other large-scale trials (>350 patients) are ongoing.[87] The largest trial published to date is the Metoprolol in Dilated Cardiomyopathy (MDC) trial, which involved 383 patients with idiopathic dilated cardiomyopathy.[115] Patients on typical CHF therapy (diuretic, ACE inhibitor, digoxin) with ejection fractions of <0.40 were randomized to metoprolol or placebo. The initial metoprolol dose of 5 mg twice daily was increased every week for 6 to 7 weeks until the patient reached the target of 100–150 mg per day. Patients were followed for a minimum of 12 months. The primary endpoint of the study was death or the need for heart transplantation. Twenty percent of placebo patients and 13% of metoprolol patients reached the primary endpoint ($p = 0.058$). Although total mortality was similar in the two groups, metoprolol caused a dramatic reduction in the number of patients needing transplantation (1% of metoprolol treated patients versus 10% of placebo-treated patients, $p < 0.0001$). Metoprolol was also associated with a number of other significant benefits compared to placebo including improved quality of life, increased exercise capacity, and improved NYHA classification. Significant hemodynamic improvements associated with metoprolol were increases in ejection fraction, cardiac index, systolic blood pressure, stroke volume, and stroke work index and decreases in heart rate and pulmonary capillary wedge pressure.[115] These findings are consistent with the smaller, controlled trials with β blockers.[116]

There is some literature to suggest that the response of heart failure patients to β-blocker therapy may depend in part on the etiology of their heart failure. Most of the clinical trials to date have involved patients with idiopathic dilated cardiomyopathies (IDCM).[116] One report suggested that patients with heart failure due to ischemic heart disease derived significantly less benefit from β blockers than patients with IDCM.[117] However, more recent reports suggest that patients with ischemic cardiomyopathies derive benefit from β blockade and that the magnitude of benefit may be similar to that observed in patients with IDCM.[118,119] Further studies will be necessary to determine if the etiology of heart failure is an important determinant of response to β-blocker therapy.

A number of potential mechanisms have been suggested to explain the beneficial effects of β blockers in heart failure patients. Potential mechanisms include blockade of the detrimental effects of sympathetic stimulation, β-receptor up-regulation, decreased sympathetic stimulation due to decreased plasma norepinephrine, and antiarrhythmic effects.[116] β blockers may also improve diastolic dysfunction by prolonging diastolic filling time. It is not clear if one or many of these mechanisms is responsible for the improvements seen in patients.

In summary, the clinical trials with β blockers in heart failure consistently report improvements in a number of hemodynamic parameters as well as symptomatic improvements. However, the effect on mortality has not been clearly documented. Until the results of the ongoing mortality trials are published, it is not possible to recommend β-blocker therapy as a routine part of the management of patients with heart failure. Nonetheless, if a patient remains symptomatic on diuretics, vasodilator therapy and digoxin, it seems reasonable to consider the addition of a β-blocker in an attempt to improve the patient's quality of life.[112]

Vesnarinone

Vesnarinone is a quinolone derivative classified as a positive inotropic agent. It possesses a number of pharmacologic properties, including mild phosphodiesterase III inhibition, increases in intracellular sodium by prolongation of opening of sodium channels, and decreases in the delayed outward and inward rectifying potassium currents.[120,121] Electrophysiologic studies suggest that it behaves like a class III antiarrhythmic (i.e., prolongs the action potential duration), which is probably attributable to its effects on potassium currents.[120] Unlike other phosphodiesterase inhibitors, vesnarinone slows, rather than increases, heart rate. It is not clear, however, if any of these pharmacologic effects are responsible for the therapeutic effects of vesnarinone.

A recent double-blind, placebo-controlled trial was conducted in which patients already treated with an ACE inhibitor, diuretic, and digoxin were given vesnarinone. Vesnarinone 120 mg per day was shown to increase mortality threefold compared to placebo, leading to early termination of the 120-mg arm of the study.[120] However, the study was continued with vesnarinone 60 mg per day versus placebo, with a total of 477 patients randomized to this portion of the trial. Opposite from the results with 120 mg per day, vesnarinone 60 mg per day produced a 62% reduction in mortality at 6 months. This degree of mortality reduction is two to three times greater than that shown in the vasodilator trials.[6,7,65,66] In spite of the reduction in mortality, vesnarinone 60 mg per day has no effect on NYHA class, or ejection fraction and marginal effects on quality of life and exercise tolerance.[120,121] It remains unclear why vesnarinone 120 mg per day increased mortality while 60 mg per day decreased mortality.

More information is needed about vesnarinone before it can be considered for widespread clinical use. First, vesnarinone's apparent narrow therapeutic-toxic range makes it essential that the pharmacokinetics of this drug, and the drugs or disease states that alter its pharmacokinetics, be well understood. Vesnarinone is also associated with a 2–4% incidence of reversible neutropenia, necessitating weekly hematologic monitoring.[120,121] Although the most recent study suggests that neutropenia is confined to the first 16 weeks of therapy[120] additional data are needed to fully characterize how long the intensive monitoring is necessary. Finally, the clinical studies to date have been short in duration (3 to 6 months), thus longer trials will be needed to fully understand vesnarinone's effects in heart failure. The FDA has requested that a larger population be studied in the mortality trial before FDA approval will be considered. The pharmaceutical company anticipates that it will resubmit to the FDA for approval in 1997.

DRUGS PROVEN TO INCREASE MORTALITY IN HEART FAILURE PATIENTS

Clinical trials of therapeutic modalities for the management of CHF have revealed drugs that improve symptoms and decrease mortality, namely, the ACE inhibitors and the combination of hydralazine–nitrate. Clinical trials have also proven a number of drugs to increase mortality in CHF. Because of the negative effects of the various compounds, most of them never received FDA approval and therefore are not available for clinical use. Nonetheless, an understanding of the types of drugs that have been shown to increase mortality provides some insight into the pathophysiologic processes in CHF.

Phosphodiesterase III Inhibitors and β-Adrenergic Agonists

Reduced contractility is the underlying pathophysiology for many patients with CHF. This fact, coupled with the dramatic hemodynamic improvements produced by β-agonists and phosphodiesterase inhibitors in acute CHF, stimulated research with these agents for management of chronic CHF. These drug classes are similar in that they act to increase intracellular levels of the second messenger cyclic adenosine monophosphate (AMP), although by different mechanisms. β-agonists increase intracellular cyclic AMP by stimulating its production while phosphodiesterase III inhibitors do so by preventing its breakdown. There was much interest, in the past, in the use of these compounds for the management of chronic heart failure. However, a lack of sustained beneficial effects and consistent data showing increased mortality have led to the virtual abandonment of research in chronic heart failure with drugs from these classes.

Oral amrinone was the first phosphodiesterase inhibitor to be tested in chronic CHF, but was withdrawn from investigation because of a lack of beneficial effects and a high rate of adverse reactions, which necessitated discontinuation of the drug.[122] Milrinone, a bipyridine derivative of amrinone, and enoximone, an imidazole derivative, were better tolerated and clinical trials with these drugs proceeded. Enoximone was compared to placebo in 102 heart failure patients. It produced no significant improvements beyond 1 month of therapy, and was associated with a significantly higher mortality rate.[123] Similarly, a comparison of milrinone and digoxin to placebo in 230 CHF patients showed that milrinone provided no advantage over digoxin, increased ventricular arrhythmias, and showed a trend toward increased mortality.[100] A subsequent study in 1088 patients with NYHA FC-III and -IV heart failure showed that milrinone was associated with a 28% increase in all-cause mortality and a 34% increase in cardiovascular mortality as compared to placebo.[124] Milrinone exerted an adverse effect on all subgroups analyzed, but patients with class IV heart failure had the greatest adverse response to milrinone, with a 53% increase in all cause mortality. Thus the clinical trials with phosphodiesterase inhibitors consistently showed that they provide marginal symptomatic benefits and increase mortality.

Studies of chronic β-agonist therapy have resulted in similarly disappointing results. In spite of favorable symptomatic and hemodynamic responses with short-term therapy, most controlled trials have shown a loss of responsiveness (tolerance) with long-term therapy. This is believed to be due in part to further down-regulation of β-receptors induced by chronic β-agonist therapy. Unlike other partial β-agonists, symptomatic and hemodynamic improvements were sustained with chronic xamoterol therapy.[105] However, enthusiasm for this agent was also dampened by a study in 516 class III and IV heart failure patients which showed a 2.54-fold increase in mortality with xamoterol compared to placebo.[125] In this study, xamoterol appeared to increase both sudden death and death due to progressive heart failure. Additional evidence that prolonged β-agonist therapy may adversely affect survival comes from the study of intermittent dobutamine therapy (see discussion on dobutamine under Pharmacotherapy of Acute/Severe Heart Failure).[32]

Finally, a meta-analysis of β agonists and phosphodiesterase III inhibitors, published prior to the large milrinone trial, supports the negative effects of these drugs on mortality.[126] The authors reviewed 21 randomized, placebo-controlled trials involving a total of 1124 patients in phosphodiesterase inhibitor studies and 1234 patients in β-agonist studies. The analysis revealed an overall 58% increase in mortality with phosphodiesterase inhibitors and a greater than twofold increase in mortality with β agonists.[126] While increasing myocardial contractility in patients with heart failure seems theoretically sound, the clinical trials suggest that doing so by increasing intracellular cyclic AMP negatively affects patient survival.

Flosequinan

Flosequinan is a direct acting arterial and venous vasodilator whose exact mechanism of action has not been elucidated, although it may involve inhibition of inositol triphosphate or protein kinase C activity. Typical hemodynamic responses to flosequinan include significant increases in cardiac index and heart rate and decreases in blood pressure, left ventricular filling pressure, and systemic vascular resistance.[127] Flosequinan was shown to produce long-term symptomatic benefits, even when added to a regimen of diuretic, ACE inhibitor and digoxin,[127,128] and the drug was approved by the FDA for use in CHF in early 1993. However, interim analysis of a mortality trial, performed shortly after the drug was marketed, did not reveal favorable results. The interim analysis showed a 39% higher mortality rate in the patients randomized to flosequinan compared to placebo.[129] Hospitalization for CHF was also higher with flosequinan than placebo. Based on the results of this trial, flosequinan was voluntarily withdrawn from the market by the manufacturer within months of its release. The increase in heart rate commonly noted with flosequinan suggests that the sympathetic nervous system may have been activated in response to the drop in blood pressure. If this is the case, sympathetic nervous system activation would provide a feasible explanation for the detrimental effects on survival.

Prostacyclin

Prostacyclin is an endogenous substance that produces both arterial and venous vasodilation, along with other potentially beneficial effects in heart failure.[130] Encouraging preliminary, short-term studies of prostacyclin in patients with heart failure led to a large-scale trial to investigate the effects on survival of prolonged prostacyclin infusion to patients with severe, refractory heart failure. This trial was stopped prematurely because of increased mortality in the prostacyclin group.[112] Again, activation of the sympathetic nervous system may have played a role in the increased mortality because early studies showed that prostacyclin increased heart rate and increased plasma concentrations of epinephrine.[130]

Prevention of Congestive Heart Failure With ACE Inhibitors

The role of ACE inhibitors in reducing morbidity and mortality associated with symptomatic CHF has been well established. However, in spite of treatment advances, CHF associated mortality remains high and recent interest has focused on therapies aimed at preventing the development of symptomatic CHF.

Four multicenter studies recently evaluated the role of ACE inhibitor therapy in preventing CHF and its associated morbidity and mortality. The Prevention Trial arm of the Studies of Left Ventricular Dysfunction[81] (SOLVD) included 4,228 patients with known heart disease and left ventricular ejection fractions of 0.35 or less, but who did not exhibit symptoms of congestive heart failure. These patients with asymptomatic left ventricular dysfunction were randomized to placebo or enalapril (target dose 10 mg bid) and were followed for an average of 37.4 months. Enalapril therapy decreased all cause mortality by 8% and cardiovascular mortality by 12%, neither of which were significantly different from placebo. Enalapril therapy did, however, produce significant reductions in morbid events associated with congestive heart failure. For example, enalapril therapy significantly prolonged the time to development of symptomatic congestive heart failure (22.3 months versus 8.3 months for placebo) and prolonged the time to first hospitalization for congestive heart failure (27.8 months versus 13.2 months for placebo). Subgroup analysis of the data revealed that the patients deriving the most benefit from enalapril therapy were those with the lowest baseline ejection fractions (<0.28).

The most common etiology of heart failure is ischemic heart disease and the left ventricular dilatation and remodeling that occur after myocardial infarction (MI) are thought to be important determinants in the development of CHF. Thus, several studies have focused on the role of ACE inhibitors in the prevention of heart failure postmyocardial infarction. In the Survival and Ventricular Enlargement (SAVE) Trial, patients were considered for study inclusion between 3 and 16 days post MI if they had a left ventricular ejection fraction ≤40%.[79] A total of 2231 patients were randomized to placebo or captopril (target dose 50 mg tid) and were followed for an average of 42 months. Captopril therapy significantly reduced all cause mortality by 19%, cardiovascular mortality by 21%, and death due to progressive heart failure by 36%. The effect of captopril on mortality became apparent after 1 year of therapy. Captopril therapy also produced significant reductions in the development of severe CHF, CHF requiring hospitalization, and recurrent MI.

The Acute Infarction Ramipril Efficacy (AIRE) study randomized post-MI patients with clinical evidence of heart failure (even if transient) to ramipril (target dose 5 mg twice daily) or placebo.[80] Enrollment occurred between days 3 and 10 after the acute MI and patients were followed for an average of 15 months. Ramipril reduced all cause mortality by 27% and reduced the development of severe/resistant heart failure by 24%. The effect of ramipril on mortality was nearly significant ($p = 0.053$) within 30 days, thus benefit in this study was apparent much earlier than in the SAVE trial.

Consistent with SAVE and AIRE, two other post-MI trials that selected patients at high risk of developing heart failure showed significant benefit from ACE inhibitor therapy. The Survival of Myocardial Infarction Long-term Evaluation (SMILE) study enrolled 1556 patients with anterior wall MI who did not receive thrombolytic therapy.[131] Patients were randomized to zofenapril or placebo, starting within 24 hours of the onset of symptoms and continuing therapy for 6 weeks. At 1 year, mortality was 29% lower in zofenapril-treated patients, in spite of therapy being continued for only 6 weeks post-MI. Preliminary results from the Trandolapril Cardiac Evaluation (TRACE) study revealed a 25% reduction in risk of cardiovascular death and a 26% reduction in risk of sudden death.[132] In this study, patients with reduced left ventricular function shortly after MI were randomized to trandolopril or placebo, starting 3 to 7 days post-MI.

All four post-MI ACE inhibitor studies described above selected patients at high risk of developing CHF post-MI. Conversely, three other studies have randomized all patients with MI to ACE inhibitor or placebo. In GISSI-2, 19,394 patients were randomized to lisinpril or placebo within 24 hours of the onset of chest pain and treated for 6 weeks, resulting in a significant, 11% decease in all cause mortality.[133] In ISIS-4, 58,050 patients with a working diagnosis of MI were randomized to captopril or placebo, with therapy continued for 28 days.[134] There was a significant, 7% decrease in mortality at 5 weeks, with mortality differences remaining different at one year. Finally, CONSENSUS-II randomized 6090 patients to enalapril or placebo within 24 hours of the onset of chest pain, with the first dose being given as intravenous enalaprilat.[135] This study was halted prematurely because of little likelihood of showing benefit, and out of concern about the possibility of adverse effects of enalapril on survival. Of particular concern was a nonsignificant trend of increased mortality in patients who experienced hypotension during the initial IV enalaprilat infusion.

In summary, the post-MI ACE inhibitor studies have clearly documented that development of CHF and mortality can be reduced by initiation of ACE inhibitor therapy in the early post-MI course. Clearly, the greatest benefit is observed in those patients who are at high risk of developing heart failure, although all patients may derive some benefit from such therapy. The variety of ACE inhibitors that have been studied clearly document that this effect is a drug class effect, although clinicians should be encouraged to use agents that have been studied because their effective dosage is documented. The mechanism of benefit in this setting probably is related largely to the ability of ACE inhibitors to prevent the growth-promoting effects of angiotensin II, rather than to the hemodynamic effects of ACE inhibitors. Specifically, ACE inhibitors prevent (or minimize) the left ventricular dilatation and hypertrophy that is crucial to the development of heart failure in the post-MI patient.

When the SOLVD Prevention Trial data are considered along with these other studies, they suggest that if patients are not treated with ACE inhibitors immediately post-MI, the mortality reducing effects may be minimal. However, such therapy may still slow the progression and onset of symptomatic CHF. Thus, although it is optimal to initiate ACE inhibitor therapy in the immediate post-MI period, significant benefit may still be derived from starting therapy in patients with asymptomatic left ventricular dysfunction at any time.

EVALUATION OF THERAPEUTIC OUTCOMES

Some of the more important therapeutic outcomes in CHF management, such as prolonged survival or prevention or slowing of the progression of heart failure, cannot be measured in an individual patient. However, symptomatic improvement is readily measurable in the heart failure patient. The cardinal signs and symptoms of heart failure are caused by excess fluid retention and symptomatic improvement can be documented by the disappearance of these signs and symptoms (see Table 13.5). Specifically, in a patient with pulmonary congestion, the patient should be monitored for the disappearance of rales and pulmonary edema, and a decrease in severity or disappearance of dyspnea on exertion, orthopnea and paroxysmal nocturnal dyspnea. For patients with systemic congestion, the patient should be monitored for a decrease or disappearance in peripheral edema, jugular venous distension, and a positive hepatojugular reflex. Other therapeutic outcomes that should be monitored include an improvement in the patient's exercise tolerance and fatigue, decreased nocturia, and a decrease in heart rate. Clinicians will also want to monitor blood pressure to ensure that the patient is not hypotensive as a result of drug therapy. Monitoring patient weight is a sensitive marker for determining fluid loss or fluid retention, and patients should be counseled to monitor their weight on a daily basis and report changes to a health care provider.

For patients with acute or severe heart failure, many of these signs and symptoms can be monitored to document therapeutic efficacy; however, there are additional parameters that will typically be assessed. In place of, or in addition to monitoring of patient weight, it is often advisable to monitor fluid intake and output by the patient. For patients with a pulmonary artery catheter in place, the clinician should also monitor cardiac index, pulmonary capillary wedge pressure, systemic vascular resistance, and blood pressure. The goals are typically to maintain cardiac index above 2.2 L/min/m^2, PCWP between 15 and 18 mm Hg, systemic vascular resistance between 800 and 1200 dyne•sec/cm^3, and systolic blood pressure > 90 mm Hg or mean arterial pressure > 70 mm Hg. Improved peripheral perfusion, as a consequence of an increase in cardiac index, can be evaluated by an increase in urine output, a decrease in peripheral vasoconstriction and stronger peripheral pulses.

CONCLUSION

Goals for the pharmacologic management of CHF now include (1) improvement of symptoms and the patient's quality of life, (2) reduced mortality, (3) alteration of the natural history of the heart failure once symptoms are present, and (4) prevention of heart failure. Studies published in the past decade have clearly revealed that it is possible to reduce mortality with either ACE inhibitors or a combination of hydralazine–nitrate in patients with symptomatic CHF.[6,7,65,66] In many cases, the reduction in morbidity and mortality is believed to be related to a slowing of the progression of left ventricular dysfunction. More recent data suggest that ACE inhibitor therapy, initiated prior to the onset of symptoms, may slow or prevent the development of symptomatic heart failure. Because heart failure typically results from another disease process, the ultimate goal is prevention of heart failure through treatment and prevention of the diseases that cause it.

The typical approach to management of a patient with symptomatic heart failure is initiation of vasodilator therapy in all patients. Because ACE inhibitors are superior to hydralazine–nitrate in mortality reduction, they represent the vasodilator of first choice. The combination of hydralazine–nitrate should be instituted in patients with contraindications to or who are unable to tolerate ACE inhibitors. Either of these therapies will reduce mortality and improve the patient's symptoms and quality of life. Diuretic therapy has not been shown to provide mortality benefits but is an important agent for controlling symptoms of heart failure and will be used in many patients in combination with a vasodilator regimen. Patients who remain symptomatic on optimal doses of vasodilator and diuretic, and who have systolic dysfunction, should be started on digoxin therapy. In patients who remain symptomatic after the addition of digoxin, clinicians may consider adding another vasodilator or a trial of low-dose β blocker.

ADDENDUM

β-BLOCKERS IN HEART FAILURE

Carvedilol, a β-blocker with alpha$_1$-receptor blocking properties and anti-oxidant effects, was recently compared to placebo in 1052 patients with FC-II to -IV heart failure who were already receiving ACE inhibitor, diuretic, amd digoxin therapy.[136] Carvedilol produced a 67% reduction in mortality. This degree of mortality reduction was noted in patients with mild (FC-II) and moderate to severe (FC-III–IV) heart failure and was irrespective of heart failure etiology (ischemic vs. nonischemic). Substudies within the mortality trial revealed that mortality reduction was dose-dependent, with the highest tested dose producing the greatest mortality reduction,[137] and carvedilol was associated with hemodynamic, symptomatic and quality of life improvements that have been documented in numerous other β-blocker trials.[138] It is unclear whether the dramatic reductions in mortality with carvedilol are related exclusively to its β-blocking properties, or whether its other pharmacologic effects contributed to its mortality-reducing effects. The results of large-scale trials with other β-blockers will help to clarify this issue.

References

1. Braunwald E. Pathophysiology of congestive heart failure, in Braunwald E (ed): Heart Disease. Philadelphia, WB Saunders, 1992, pp 393–418.
2. Litwin SE, Grossman W. Diastolic dysfunction as a cause of heart failure. J Am Coll Cardiol 1993;22(suppl A):49A–55A.
3. Johnson JA. Diastolic dysfunction in congestive heart failure. Clin Pharm 1991;10:850–861.
4. Ho KKL, Pinsky JL, Kannel WB, Levy D. The epidemiology of heart failure: The Framingham study. J Am Coll Cardiol 1993:22(suppl A):6A–13A.
5. Goldman S, Johnson G, Cohn JN, et al. for the V-HeFT VA Cooperative Studies Group. Mechanisms of death in heart failure. The Vasodilator-Heart Failure Trials. Circulation 1993;87 (suppl VI):24–31.
6. The CONSENSUS Trial Study Group. Effects of enalapril on mortality in severe congestive heart failure. Results of the Cooperative North Scandinavian Enalapril Survival Study (CONSENSUS). N Engl J Med 1987;316:1429–1435.
7. The SOLVD Investigators. Effect of enalapril on survival in patients with reduced left ventricular ejection fractions and congestive heart failure. N Engl J Med 1991;325:293–302.
8. Wynne J, Braunwald E. The cardiomyopathies and myocarditides, in Braunwald E (ed): Heart Disease. Philadelphia, WB Saunders, 1992, pp 1394–1450.
9. Braunwald E, Sonnenblick EH, Ross J. Mechanisms of cardiac contraction and relaxation, in Braunwald E (ed): Heart Disease. Philadelphia, WB Saunders, 1992, pp 351–392.
10. Pastan SO, Braunwald E. Renal disorders and heart disease, in Braunwald E, (ed): Heart Disease. Philadelphia, WB Saunders, 1992, pp 1856–1874.
11. Munzel T, Kurz S, Holtz J, et al. Neurohormonal inhibition and hemodynamic unloading during prolonged inhibition of ANF degradation in patients with severe chronic heart failure. Circulation 1992;86:1089–1098.
12. Katz AM. Cardiomyopathy of overload. A major determinant of prognosis in congestive heart failure. N Engl J Med 1990;322:100–110.
13. Ghali JK, Kadakia S, Cooper R, et al. Precipitating factors leading to decompensation of heart failure. Arch Intern Med 1988;148:2013–2016.
14. Braunwald E. Clinical aspects of heart failure, in Braunwald E (ed): Heart Disease. Philadelphia, WB Saunders, 1992, pp 444–463.
15. Criteria Committee, New York Heart Association, Inc. Diseases of the Heart and Blood Vessels. Nomenclature and Criteria for Diagnosis, 7th ed. Boston, Little, Brown, 1973.
16. Califf RM, Bengtson JR. Cardiogenic shock. N Engl J Med 1994;330:1724–1730.
17. Forrester JS, Diamond G, Chatterjee K, et al. Medical therapy of acute myocardial infarction by application of hemodynamic subsets. N Engl J Med 1976;295:1356–1362.
18. Feldman, AM. Classification of positive inotropic agents. J Am Coll Cardiol 1993;22:1223–1227.
19. Hoofman BB, Lefkowitz RJ. Catecholamines and sympathomimetic agents, in Gillman AG, Rall TW, Nies AS, Taylor P (eds): The Pharmacological Basis of Therapeutics, 8th ed. New York, Pergamon, 1990, pp 187–220.
20. Goldberg LI, Hsieh YY, Resnekov L. Newer catecholamines for treatment of heart failure and shock: An update on dopamine and a first look at dobutamine. Prog Cardiovasc Dis 1977;19:327–340.
21. Smith TW, Braunwald E, Kelly RA. The management of heart failure, in Braunwald E (ed): Heart Disease. Philadelphia, WB Saunders, 1992, pp 464–519.
22. Beregovich J, Bianchi C, Rubler S, et al. Dose-related hemodynamic and renal effects of dopamine in congestive heart failure. Am Heart J 1974;87:550–557.
23. Ruffolo RR, Yaden EL. Vascular effects of the stereoisomers of dobutamine. J Pharmacol Exp Ther 1983;224:46–50.
24. Leier CV, Unverferth DV. Dobutamine. Ann Intern Med 1983;99:490–496.
25. Majerus TC, Dasta JF, Bauman JL, et al. Dobutamine: Ten years later. Pharmacotherapy 1989;9:245–259.
26. Loeb HS, Bredakis J, Gunnar RM. Superiority of dobutamine over dopamine for augmentation of cardiac output in patients with chronic low output cardiac failure. Circulation 1977;55:375–381.
27. Unverferth DV, Blanford M, Kates RE, et al. Tolerance to dobutamine after a 72 hour continuous infusion. Am J Med 1980;69:262–266.
28. Colucci WS, Denniss AR, Leatherman GF, et al. Intracoronary infusion of dobutamine to patients with and without severe heart failure. J Clin Invest 1988;81:1103–1110.
29. Leier CV, Huss P, Lewis RP, Unverferth DV. Drug-induced conditioning in congestive heart failure. Circulation 1982;65:1382–1387.
30. Liang CS, Sherman LG, Doherty JU, et al. Sustained improvement of cardiac function in patients with congestive heart failure after short-term infusion of dobutamine. Circulation 1984;69:113–119.
31. Erlemeier HH, Kupper W, Bleifeld W. Intermittent infusion of dobutamine in the therapy of severe congestive heart failure—Long-term effects and lack of tolerance. Cardiovasc Drugs Ther 1992;6:391–398.
32. Dies F, Krell MJ, Whitlow P, et al. Intermittent dobutamine in ambulatory outpatients with chronic cardiac failure [abstract]. Circulation 1986;74(suppl II):II-38.
33. Arnold JM. The role of phosphodiesterase inhibitors in heart failure. Pharmac Ther 1993;57:161–170.

34. Bottorff MB, Rutledge DR, Pieper JA. Evaluation of intravenous amrinone: The first of a new class of positive inotropic agents with vasodilator properties. Pharmacotherapy 1985;5:227–237.
35. Colucci WS. Cardiovascular effects of milrinone. Am Heart J 1991;121:1945–1947.
36. Ludmer PL, Wright RF, Arnold JMO, et al. Separation of the direct myocardial and vasodilator actions of milrinone administered by an intracoronary infusion technique. Circulation 1986;73:130–137.
37. Konstam MA, Cohen SR, Weiland DS, et al. Relative contribution of inotropic and vasodilator effects to amrinone-induced hemodynamic improvement in congestive heart failure. Am J Cardiol 1986;57:242–248.
38. Jaski BE, Fifer MA, Wright RF, et al. Positive inotropic and vasodilator actions of milrinone in patients with severe congestive heart failure. J Clin Invest 1985;75:643–649.
39. Anderson JL and the United States Milrinone Multicenter Investigators. Hemodynamic and clinical benefits with intravenous milrinone in severe chronic heart failure: Results of a multicenter study in the United States. Am Heart J 1991;121:1956–1964.
40. Gage J, Rutman H, Lucido D, et al. Additive effects of dobutamine and amrinone on myocardial contractility and ventricular performance in patients with severe heart failure. Circulation 1986;74:367–373.
41. Meissner A, Herrmann G, Gerdesmeyer L, Simon R. Additive effects of milrinone and dobutamine in patients with congestive heart failure. Z Kardiol 1992;81:266–271.
42. Monrad ES, Baim DS, Smith HS, et al. Effects of milrinone on coronary hemodynamics and myocardial energetics in patients with congestive heart failure. Circulation 1985;71:972–979.
43. Gibelin P, Dadoun-Dybal M, Candito M, et al. Hemodynamic effects of prolonged enoximone infusion (7 days) in patients with severe heart failure. Cardiovasc Drug Ther 1993;7:333–336.
44. Amisel AS, Wright CM, Carter SM, et al. Tachyphylaxis with amrinone therapy: Association with sequestration and down-regulation of lymphocyte β-adrenergic receptors. Ann Intern Med 1989;110:195–201.
45. Park GB, Kershner RP, Angellotti J, et al. Oral bioavailability and intravenous pharmacokinetics of amrinone in humans. J Pharm Sci 1983;72:817–819.
46. Pflugfelder PW, O'Neill BJ, Ogilvie RI, et al. A Canadian multicentre study of a 48 h infusion of milrinone in patients with severe heart failure. Can J Cardiol 1991;7:5–10.
47. Cohn JN, Francioso JA, Francis GS, et al. Effect of short-term infusion of sodium nitroprusside on mortality rate in acute myocardial infarction complicated by left ventricular failure. New Engl J Med 1982;306:1129–1135.
48. Packer M, Meller J, Medina N, et al. Rebound hemodynamic events after abrupt withdrawal of nitroprusside in patients with severe heart failure. New Engl J Med 1979;301:1193–1197.
49. Cohn JN, Burke LP. Nitroprusside. Ann Intern Med 1979;91:752–757.
50. Sorkin EM, Brogden RN, Romankiewicz JA. Intravenous glyceryl trinitrate: A review of its pharmacological properties and therapeutic efficacy. Drugs 1984;27:45–80.
51. Gagnon RM, Fortin L, Boucher R, et al. Combined hemodynamic effects of dobutamine and IV nitroglycerin in congestive heart failure. Chest 1980;78:694–698.
52. Packer M, Lee WH, Kessler PD, et al. Prevention and reversal of nitrate tolerance in patients with congestive heart failure. N Engl J Med 1987;317:799–804.
53. Elkayam U, Kulick D, McIntosh N, et al. Incidence of early tolerance to hemodynamic effects of continuous infusion of nitroglycerin in patients with coronary heart disease and heart failure. Circulation 1987;76:577–588.
54. Prakash S, Silke B, Reynolds GW, et al. Vasodilator therapy of acute heart failure: Hemodynamic comparison of hydralazine-isosorbide, alpha-adrenoceptor blockade and angiotensin-converting enzyme inhibition. J Cardiovasc Pharmacol 1992;20:274–281.
55. MacFadyen RJ, Lees KR, Reid JL. Double blind controlled study of low dose intravenous perindoprilat or enalaprilat infusion in elderly patients with heart failure. Br Heart J 1993;69:293–297.
56. Dikshit K, Vyden JK, Forrester JS, et al. Renal and extrarenal hemodynamic effects of furosemide in congestive heart failure after acute myocardial infarction. New Engl J Med 1973;288:1087–1090.
57. Francis GS, Siegel RM, Goldsmith SR, et al. Acute vasoconstrictor response to intravenous furosemide in patients with chronic congestive heart failure. Ann Intern Med 1985;103:1–6.
58. Kraus PA, Lipman J, Becker PJ. Acute preload effects of furosemide. Chest 1990;98:124–128.
59. Lahav M, Regev A, Ra'anani P, et al. Intermittent administration of furosemide vs continuous infusion preceded by a loading dose for congestive heart failure. Chest 1992;102:725–731.
60. Pennington DG, Swartz M. Assisted circulation and mechanical hearts, in Braunwald E (ed): Heart Disease. Philadelphia, WB Saunders, 1992, pp 535–550.
61. Coats AJS. Exercise rehabilitation in chronic heart failure. J Am Coll Cardiol 1993;22 (suppl A):172A–177A.
62. Ellison DH. The physiologic basis of diuretic synergism: Its role in treating diuretic resistance. Ann Intern Med 1991;114–886–894.
63. Brater DC. Resistance to loop diuretics. Why it happens and what to do about it. Drugs 1985;30:427–443.
64. van Meyel JJM, Smits P, Russel FGM, et al. Diuretic efficiency of furosemide during continuous administration versus bolus injection in healthy volunteers. Clin Pharmacol Ther 1992;51:440–444.
65. Cohn JN, Archibald DG, Ziesche S, et al. Effect of vasodilator therapy on mortality in chronic congestive heart failure. N Engl J Med 1986;314:1547–1552.
66. Cohn JN, Johnson G, Ziesche S, et al. A comparison of enalapril with hydralazine–isosorbide dinitrate in the treatment of chronic congestive heart failure. N Engl J Med 1991;325:303–310.
67. Leier CV, Huss P, Magorien RD, et al. Improved exercise capacity and differing arterial and venous tolerance during chronic isosorbide dinitrate therapy for congestive heart failure. Circulation 1983;67:817–822.
68. Jordan RA, Seth L, Henry DA, et al. Dose requirements and hemodynamic effects of transdermal nitroglycerin compared

with placebo in patients with congestive heart failure. Circulation 1985;71:980–986.
69. Packer M. Are nitrates effective in the treatment of chronic heart failure? Antagonist's viewpoint. Am J Cardiol 1990;66:458–461.
70. Packer M, Meller J, Medina N, et al. Dose requirements of hydralazine in patients with severe chronic congestive heart failure. Am J Cardiol 1980;45:655–660.
71. Magorien RD, Unverferth DV, Leier CV. Hydralazine therapy in chronic congestive heart failure. Am J Med 1984;77:267–274.
72. Conradson TB, Ryden L, Ahlmark G, et al. Clinical efficacy of hydralazine in chronic heart failure. One-year double-blind placebo-controlled study. Am Heart J 1984;108:1001–1006.
73. Packer M, Meller J, Medina N, et al. Hemodynamic characterization of tolerance to long-term hydralazine therapy in severe chronic heart failure. N Engl J Med 1982;306:57–62.
74. Franciosa JA, Weber KT, Levine TB, et al. Hydralazine in the long-term treatment of chronic heart failure. Lack of difference from placebo. Am Heart J 1982;104:587–594.
75. Deedwania PC. Angiotensin-converting enzyme inhibitors in congestive heart failure. Arch Intern Med 1990;150:1798–1805.
76. The Captopril-Digoxin Multicenter Research Group. Comparative effects of therapy with captopril and digoxin in patients with mild to moderate heart failure. JAMA 1988;259:539–544.
77. Packer M, Medina N, Yushak M, et al. Usefulness of plasma renin activity in predicting haemodynamic and clinical responses and survival during long-term converting enzyme inhibition in severe chronic heart failure. Br Heart J 1985;54:298–304.
78. Katz AM. Angiotensin II: Hemodynamic regulator or growth factor? J Mol Cell Cardiol 1990;22:739–747.
79. Pfeffer MA, Braunwald E, Moye LA, et al. Effect of captopril on mortality and morbidity in patients with left ventricular dysfunction after myocardial infarction. Results of the Survival and Ventricular Enlargement Trial. N Engl J Med 1992;327:669–677.
80. The Acute Infarction Ramipril Efficacy (AIRE) Study Investigators. Effect of ramipril on mortality and morbidity of survivors of acute myocardial infarction with clinical evidence of heart failure. Lancet 1993;342:821–828.
81. The SOLVD Investigators. Effect of enalapril on mortality and the development of heart failure in asymptomatic patients with reduced left ventricular ejection fractions. N Engl J Med 1992;327:685–691.
82. Packer M, Lee WH, Medina N, et al. Functional renal insufficiency during long-term therapy with captopril and enalapril in severe chronic heart failure. Ann Intern Med 1987;106:346–354.
83. Franciosa JA, Jordan RA, Wilen MW, et al. Minoxidil in patients with chronic left heart failure contrasting hemodynamic and clinical effects in a controlled trial. Circulation 1984;70:63–68.
84. The Multicenter Diltiazem Postinfarction Trial Research Group. The effect of diltiazem on mortality and reinfarction after myocardial infarction. N Engl J Med 1988;319:385–392.
85. Goldstein RE, Boccuzzi SJ, Cruess D, et al. Diltiazem increases late-onset congestive heart failure in postinfarction patients with early reduction in ejection fraction. Circulation 1991;83:52–60.
86. Elkayam U, Amin J, Mehra A, et al. A prospective, randomized, double-blind, crossover study to compare the efficacy and safety of chronic nifedipine therapy with that of isosorbide dinitrate and their combination in the treatment of chronic congestive heart failure. Circulation 1990;82:1954–1961.
87. Garg R, Yusuf S. Current and ongoing randomized trials in heart failure and left ventricular dysfunction. J Am Coll Cardiol 1993;22 (Suppl A):194A–197A.
88. Braunwald E. ACE inhibitors. A cornerstone of the treatment of heart failure [editorial]. N Engl J Med 1991;325:351–353.
89. Smith TW. Digitalis. Mechanism of action and clinical use. New Engl J Med 1988;318:358–365.
90. Kelly RA, Smith TW. Digoxin in heart failure: Implications of recent trials. J Am Coll Cardiol 1993;22 (Suppl. A):107A–112A.
91. Yusuf S, Garg R, Held P, Gorlin R. Need for a large randomized trial to evaluate the effects of digitalis on morbidity and mortality in congestive heart failure. Am J Cardiol 1992;69:64G–70G.
92. Gheorghiade M, Ferguson D. Digoxin. A neurohormonal modulator in heart failure. Circulation 1991; 84:2181–2186.
93. Packer M. The development of positive inotropic agents for chronic heart failure: How have we gone astray? J Am Coll Cardiol 1993;22 (suppl. A):119A–126A.
94. Arnold SB, Byrd R, Meister W, et al. Long-term digitalis therapy improves ventricular function in heart failure. N Engl J Med 1980;303:1443–1448.
95. Mooraddian AD. Digitalis. An update of clinical pharmacokinetics, therapeutic monitoring techniques and treatment recommendations. Clin Pharmacokin 1988;15:165–179.
96. Reuning RH, Geraets GR, Rocci ML, Vlasses PH. Digoxin, in Evans WE, Schentag JJ, Jusko WJ (eds): Applied Pharmacokinetics: Principles of Therapeutic Drug Monitoring, 3rd ed. Spokane, WA, Applied Therapeutics, 1992, pp 20-1–20-48.
97. Smith TW. Pharmacokinetics, bioavailability and serum levels of cardiac glycosides. J Am Coll Cardiol 1985;5:43A–50A.
98. Smith TW, Antman EA, Friedman PL, et al. Digitalis glycosides: Mechanism and manifestations of toxicity. Prog Cardiovasc Dis 1984;26:413–441; 26:495–523; 27:21–56.
99. Lee DCS, Johnson RA, Bingham JB, et al. Heart failure in outpatients. A randomized trial of digoxin and placebo. N Engl J Med 1982;306:699–705.
100. DiBianco R, Shabertai R, Kostuk W, et al. A comparison of oral milrinone, digoxin, and their combination in the treatment of patients with chronic heart failure. N Engl J Med 1989;320:677–683.
101. Packer M, Gheorghiade M, Young JB, et al. Withdrawal of digoxin from patients with chronic heart failure treated with angiotensin-converting-enzyme inhibitors. N Engl J Med 1993;329:1–7.

102. Uretsky B, Young JB, Shahidi FE, et al. Randomized study assessing the effect of digoxin withdrawal in patients with mild to moderate chronic congestive heart failure: Results of the PROVED trial. J Am Coll Cardiol 1993;22:955–962.
103. Lalonde RL, Pao D. Correlation coefficient versus prediction error in assessing the accuracy of digoxin dosing methods. Clin Pharm 1984;3:178–183.
104. Antman EM, Wenger TL, Butler VP, et al. Treatment of 150 cases of life-threatening intoxication with digoxin-specific Fab antibody fragments. Final report of a multicenter trial. Circulation 1990;81:1744–1752.
105. The German and Austrian Xamoterol Study Group. Double-blind placebo-controlled comparison of digoxin and xamoterol in chronic heart failure. Lancet 1988;1:489–493.
106. Jaeschke R, Oxman A, Guyatt GH. To what extent do congestive heart failure patients in sinus rhythm benefit from digoxin therapy? A systematic overview and meta-analysis. Am J Med 1990;88:279–286.
107. Parmley WW. Should digoxin be the drug of first choice after diuretics in chronic congestive heart failure? I. Introduction. J Am Coll Cardiol 1988;12:265–267.
108. Smith TW. Should digoxin be the drug of first choice after diuretics in chronic congestive heart failure? II. Protagonist's viewpoint. J Am Coll Cardiol 1988;12:267–271.
109. Pitt B. Should digoxin be the drug of first choice after diuretics in chronic congestive heart failure? III. Antagonist's viewpoint. J Am Coll Cardiol 1988;12:271–273.
110. Echt DS, Liebson PR, Mitchell LB, et al. Mortality and morbidity in patients receiving encainide, flecainide or placebo. The Cardiac Arrhythmia Suppression Trial. N Engl J Med 1991;324:781–788.
111. The Cardiac Arrhythmia Suppression Trial II Investigators. Effect of the antiarrhythmic agent moricizine on survival after myocardial infarction. N Engl J Med 1992;327:227–233.
112. Armstrong PW, Moe GW. Medical advances in the treatment of congestive heart failure. Circulation 1994;88:2941–2952.
113. Nicklas JM, McKenna WJ, Stewart RA, et al. Prospective, double-blind, placebo-controlled trial of low-dose amiodarone in patients with severe heart failure and asymptomatic frequent ventricular ectopy. Am Heart J 1991;122:1016–1021.
113a. Doval HC, Nul DR, Grancelli HO, et al. Randomised trial of low-dose amiodarone in severe congestive heart failure. Lancet 1994;344:493–498.
113b. Singh SN, Fletcher RD, Fisher SG, et al. Results of the congestive heart failure survival trial of antiarrhythmic therapy (Veterans Affairs Cooperative Study Program #320) [abstract]. Circulation 1994;90:I–546.
114. Kim SG, Fisher JD, Choue CW, et al. Influence of left ventricular function on outcome of patients treated with implantable defibrillators. Circulation 1992;85:1304–1310.
115. Waagstein F, Bristow MR, Swedberg K, et al. Beneficial effects of metoprolol in idiopathic dilated cardiomyopathy. Lancet 1993;342:1441–1446.
116. Doughty RN, MacMahon S, Sharpe N. β-blockers in heart failure: Promising or proved? J Am Coll Cardiol 1994;23:814–821.
117. Woodley SL, Gilbert EM, Anderson JL, et al. β-blockade with bucindolol in heart failure caused by ischemic versus idiopathic dilated cardiomyopathy. Circulation 1991;84:2426–2441.
118. Fisher ML, Gottlied SS, Plotnick GD, et al. Beneficial effects of metoprolol in heart failure associated with coronary artery disease: A randomized trial. J Am Coll Cardiol 1994;23:943–950.
119. Bristow MR, O'Connell JB, Gilbert EM, et al. Dose-response of chronic β-blocker treatment in heart failure from either idiopathic dilated or ischemic cardiomyopathy. Circulation 1994;89:1632–1642.
120. Feldman AM, Bristow MR, Parmley WW, et al. Effects of vesnarinone on morbidity and mortality in patients with heart failure. N Engl J Med 1993;329:149–155.
121. Feldman AM, Baughman KL, Lee WK, et al. Usefulness of OPC-8212, a quinolone derivative, for chronic congestive heart failure in patients with ischemic heart disease or idiopathic dilated cardiomyopathy. Am J Cardiol 1991;68:1203–1210.
122. Massie B, Bourassa M, DiBianco R, et al. Long-term administration of amrinone for congestive heart failure. Lack of efficacy in a multicenter controlled trial. Circulation 1985;71:963–971.
123. Uretsky BF, Jessup M, Konstam MA, et al. Multicenter trial of oral enoximone in patients with moderate to moderately severe congestive heart failure. Lack of benefit compared with placebo. Circulation 1990;82:774–780.
124. Packer M, Carver JR, Rodeheffer RJ, et al. Effect of oral milrinone on mortality in severe chronic heart failure. N Engl J Med 1991;325:1468–1475.
125. The Xamoterol in Severe Heart Failure Study Group. Xamoterol in severe heart failure. Lancet 1990;336:1–6.
126. Yusuf S, Teo K. Inotropic agents increase mortality in patients with congestive heart failure [abstract]. Circulation 1990;82:III–673.
127. Gottlieb SS, Kukin ML, Penn J, et al. Sustained hemodynamic response to flosequinan in patients with heart failure receiving angiotensin-converting enzyme inhibitors. J Am Coll Cardiol 1993;22:963–967.
128. Massie BM, Berk MR, Brozena SC, et al. Can further benefit be achieved by adding flosequinan to patients with congestive heart failure who remain symptomatic on diuretic, digoxin and an ACE inhibitor? Circulation 1993;88:492–501.
129. Anonymous. Higher mortality risk with 100 mg dose of Manoplax®. FDA Medical Bulletin 1993; (June):3.
130. Yui Y, Nakajima H, Kawai C, Murakami T. Prostacyclin therapy in patients with congestive heart failure. Am J Cardiol 1982;50:320–324.
131. Ambrosioni E, Borghi C, Magnani B, et al. The effect of the angiotensin-converting-enzyme inhibitor zofenopril on mortality and morbidity after anterior myocardial infarction. N Engl J Med 1995;332:80–85.
132. TRACE Study Group. Reduction in sudden death by the ACE inhibitor trandolapril in the Trandolapril Cardiac Evaluation Study. (Abstract) Circulation 1995;(Suppl I):I–197.
133. Gruppo Italiano per lo Studio della Sopravvivenza nell'Infarto Miocardico. GISSI-3: effects of lisinopril and

transdermal glyceryl trinitrate singly and together on 6-week mortality and ventricular function after acute myocardial infarction. Lancet 1994;343:1115–1122.

134. ISIS-4 Collaborative Group. ISIS-4: A randomized factorial trial assessing early oral captopril, oral mononitrate, and intravenous magnesium sulphate in 58,050 patients with suspected acute myocardial infarction. Lancet 1995; 345:669–85.

135. Swedburg K, Held P, Kjekshus J, et al. Effects of the early administration of enalapril on mortality in patients with acute myocardial infarction. Results of the Cooperative New Scandinavian Enalapril Survival Study II. N Engl J Med 1992;327:678–684.

136. Packer M, Bristow MR, Cohn JN, et al. Effect of carvedilol on the survival of patients with chronic heart failure. (Abstact) Circulation 1995;(Suppl I):I–142.

137. Bristow MR, Gilbert EM, Abraham WT, et al. Multicenter oral carvedilol heart failure assessment (MOCHA): A six month dose-response evaluation in Class II–IV patients. (Abstract) Circulation 1995;(Suppl I):I–142.

138. Packer M, Colucci WS, Sackner-Bernstein J, et al. Prospective randomized evaluation of carvedilol on the symptoms and exercise tolerance in chronic heart failure: Results of the PRECISE Trial. (Abstract) Circulation 1995;(Suppl I):I–143.

Chapter 14

Ischemic Heart Disease

Robert L. Talbert, PharmD, FCCP

Historical Aspects

There is a disorder of the breast, marked with strong and peculiar symptoms, considerable for the kind of danger belonging to it, and not extremely rare, of which I do not recollect any mention among medical authors. The seat of it and sense of strangling and anxiety with which it is attended may make it not improper to be called angina pectoris.

Some Account of a Disorder of the Breast,
William Heberden, 1768

Heberden, in a lecture given in Latin before the Royal College of Physicians of London, vividly described the symptoms of ischemic heart disease, and he is credited with naming the clinical syndrome of angina pectoris.[1] Although Heberden gave an accurate and complete description of this disorder, he had no idea of the origin of the symptoms or of appropriate therapy for the disease. Symptoms similar to those described by Heberden can be found in the writings of Pliny and other authors of antiquity; however, Jenner was the first to suggest during a postmortem examination that angina was due to a morbid change in the heart structure, probably ossification, or some similar disease.[2]

In 1867, Lauder Brunton first described the use of inhaled amyl nitrite to terminate an acute anginal attack, noting an onset of action of 30 to 60 seconds and "simultaneously with the flushing of the face the pain completely disappeared, and did not return."[3] He knew from the experiments of Dr. Gamgee that amyl nitrite reduces blood pressure in animals and man and that the actions are similar to bleeding, both forms of preload reduction in contemporary terminology. Of interest, Brunton noted that repeated application of amyl nitrite causes less of an effect or that more needs to be used to obtain the same effect. In other words, nitrate tolerance was described with the first account of its therapeutic use for angina pectoris. William Murrell provided four reports detailing the use of nitroglycerin to alleviate chest pain in patients with angina in 1879.[2] Additional insight into the mechanism of nitrate action was provided by Francois-Franck when he found that these drugs were coronary vasodilating agents.[2]

Following the development of the string galvanometer by Ader and, subsequently, the electrocardiograph by Einthoven in 1900, Bousfield published the first electrocardiographic (ECG) recording obtained during an attack of angina in 1918. Although suggested in earlier literature, the diagnosis of myocardial infarction in life and its association with a clot in the coronary artery is mainly credited to Herrick.[2]

The landmark work of Ahlquist in 1948 at the University of Georgia proposed the existence of adrenotropic receptors of different types, the α and β receptors.[4] At the time, he thought of these receptors only in an abstract form to explain observed responses of tissues produced by chemicals rather than discrete protein entities that would be studied by numerous others and the subject of thousands of future publications. In fact, his observations remained unnoticed for nearly 15 years until Black and Stephenson suggested that β blockade should be useful in treating heart disease through a reduction in the work of the heart and in treating arrhythmias.[5] Later trials demonstrated that pronethalol, an early β blocker, was effective in the treatment of angina, and thus began a revolution in the management of angina that culminated in a host of drugs in this category.

In 1967, Professor Fleckenstein discovered a class of drugs that altered the transmembrane flux of calcium and interfered with energetics of the myocardium and function of vascular smooth muscle. Initially it was thought that these drugs might be β blockers, but it was soon realized that entry of calcium through channels in the cell membrane was antagonized and the class of drugs to be known as calcium channel antagonists or blockers was born. Calcium channel blockers have become valuable agents in the treatment of ischemic heart disease as well as useful tools for further understanding of cellular physiology and pathophysiology.

Epidemiology

The syndrome of angina pectoris is reported to occur with an average annual incidence rate (number of new cases per time period/total number of persons in the population for the same time period) of about 1.5% (range 0.1–5/1000) depending on the patient's age, gender, and risk factor profile[6,7] (see Figs. 14.1 and 14.2). The presenting manifestation in women is more commonly angina while men more frequently have myocardial infarction as the initial event. Estimates of the incidence and prevalence of angina are not entirely accurate due to waxing and waning of symptoms; angina may disappear in up to 30% of patients with angina that is less severe and of recent onset.[7]

Data from the Framingham study show that the prevalence was 5.9% for the 16-year period studied.[6] Others have reported a range of 0.4% in men age 40–49 years with no ECG changes to 34% in elderly men (60–64 years) with positive ECG findings. The Health Insurance Plan (HIP) of New York found prevalence rates for women and men aged 55 years to be 1.5 and 3.5%, respectively. The risk of developing ischemic heart disease (IHD) is not the same worldwide. Countries such as Japan and France are on the low end of the spectrum while Finland, Northern Ireland, Scotland, and South Africa have very high rates of IHD.

Death due to IHD continues to be a major contributing source of mortality in the United States (Table 14.1). IHD was responsible for 22.1% of total mortality while acute myocardial infarction (AMI) caused 10.5% of all deaths; other major cardiovascular disease was responsible for 42% of total mortality in 1992. Men die earlier from IHD and AMI than women, and aging of both sexes is associated with a higher incidence of these afflictions. The disparity in mortality from IHD between men and women decreases with age, going from about 4.7 times more common in men from ages of the mid-thirties to a preponderance of female deaths in the very elderly.

The average annual mortality from angina is 4%; however, the risk of death is related to coronary artery anatomy, age, gender, risk factors present and their gradation, and the functional class of angina as well as the clinical syndrome with which the patient presents.

Angina may be classified according to symptom severity, disability induced, or according to a specific activity scale (Tables 14.2 and 14.3). The specific activity scale developed by Goldman and coworkers[8] may be preferable as it has been shown to be equal to or better than the New York Heart Association or Canadian Cardiovascular Society functional classifications for reproducibility and provides better agreement with treadmill testing.

An important determinate of outcome for the angina patient is the extent of coronary artery obstruction (Fig. 14.3). As the number of coronary vessels involved and the extent of narrowing (greater than 75% for critical narrowing) in the obstructive process increases, the annual mortal-

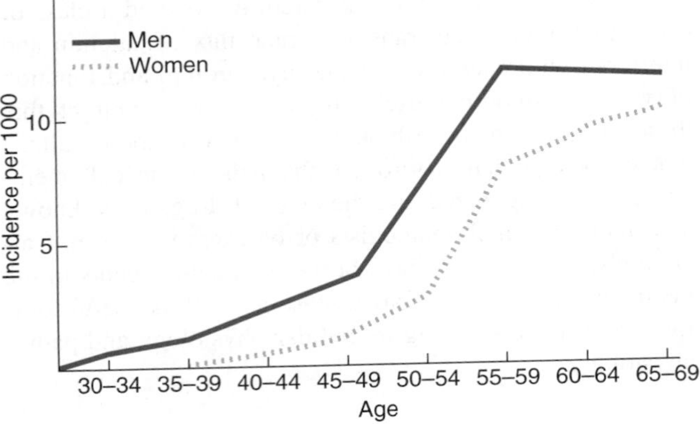

Figure 14.1. Smoothed average annual incidence of angina pectoris as a presenting complaint. Men and women aged 33 to 69 from the Framingham study. *(From Kannel WB, Feinleib M. Natural history of angina pectoris in the Framingham study. Prognosis and survival. Am J Cardiol 1972;29:157, with permission.)*

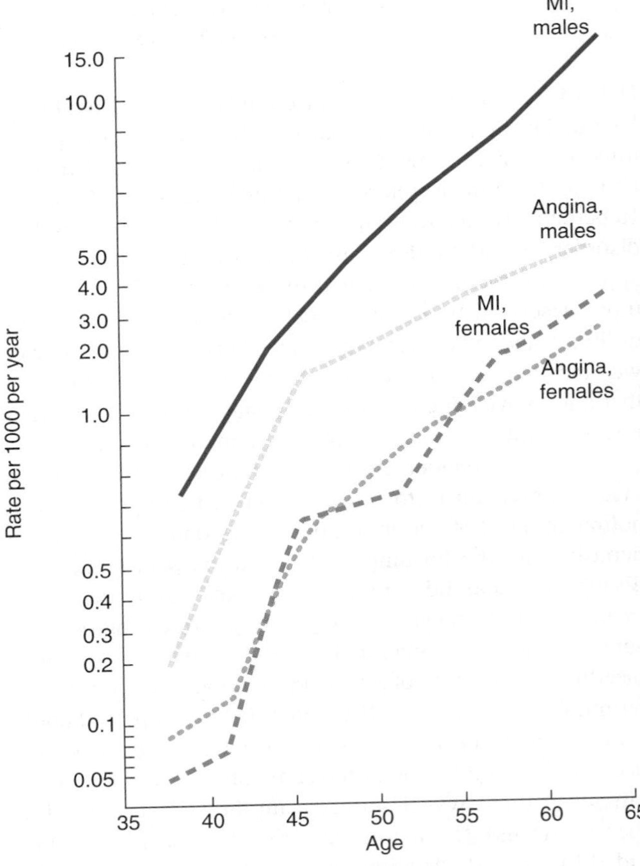

Figure 14.2. Average annual incidence of myocardial infarction (MI) and angina pectoris, by age and sex. *(From Shapiro S et al. Incidence of coronary heart disease in a population insured for medical care (HIP). Myocardial infarction, angina pectoris, and possible myocardial infarction. Am J Public Health 1969;59(6):11, with permission.)*

TABLE 14.1. CAUSES OF DEATH IN THE UNITED STATES, 1992

		All Ages	35–44 yr	45–54 yr	55–64 yr	65–74 yr	75+ yr
Death from all causes	Total	2,175,613	91,290	125,030	240,991	477,916	1,097,298
	Male	1,122,335					
	Female	1,053,277					
Major cardiovascular disease	Total	913,908	15,996	37,637	86,241	192,844	573,724
	Male	439,307					
	Female	474,601					
Ischemic heart disease	Total	480,051	6789	19,820	48,169	108,143	295,835
	Male	246,913					
	Female	233,138					
Acute myocardial infarction	Total	229,383	3868	11,703	27,435	57,323	128,323
	Male	123,121					
	Female	106,262					

(From Monthly Vital Statistics Report, Volume 43, No. 6, Supplement, Centers for Disease Control and Prevention, National Center for Health Statistics, March 22, 1995.)

ity is proportional from 1–2% for one-vessel disease, to 2–4% for two-vessel disease, to 10–12% for three-vessel involvement. Of particular note, patients with left main artery involvement are at extremely high risk (7–25% annual mortality) and constitute a unique group for therapeutic consideration.[9] The Veterans Administration Coronary Artery Bypass Surgery Cooperative Study Group (CASS) 11-year survival rates are 57% and 58% for the medical treatment and surgery groups, respectively.[9] Additional information from subgroup analyses is useful in predicting the outcome of patients managed medically or surgically. Patients at high angiographic risk (three-vessel

TABLE 14.2. CRITERIA FOR DETERMINATION OF THE SPECIFIC ACTIVITY SCALE FUNCTIONAL CLASS

	Any Yes	No
1. Can you walk down a flight of steps without stopping (4.5–5.2 mets[a])?	Go to #2	Go to #4
2. Can you carry anything up a flight of eight steps without stopping (5–5.5 mets)? Or can you: a. Have sexual intercourse without stopping (5–5.5 mets)? b. Garden, rake, weed (5.6 mets)? c. Roller skate, dance fox trot (5–6 mets)? d. Walk at a 4-mph rate on level ground (5–6 mets)?	Go to #3	Class III
3. Can you carry at least 24 pounds up eight steps (10 mets)? Or can you: a. Carry objects that weigh at least 80 pounds (18 mets)? b. Do outdoor work—shovel snow, spade soil (7 mets)? c. Engage in recreational activities such as skiing, basketball, touch football, squash, handball (7–10 mets)? d. Jog/walk 5 mph (9 mets)?	Class I	Class II
4. Can you shower without stopping (3.6–4.2 mets)? Or can you: a. Strip and make bed (3.9–5 mets)? b. Mop floors (4.2 mets)? c. Hang washed clothes (4.4 mets)? d. Clean windows (3.7 mets)? e. Walk 2.5 mph (3–3.5 mets)? f. Bowl (3–4.4 mets)? g. Play golf—walk and carry clubs (4.5 mets)? h. Push power lawn mower (4 mets)?	Class III	Go to #5
5. Can you dress without stopping because of symptoms (2–2.3 mets)?	Class III	Class IV

[a]mets, metabolic equivalents of activity. (From Goldman L, Hashimoto B, Cook F, et al. Comparative reproducibility and validity of systems for assessing cardiovascular functional class. Advantages of a new specific activity scale. Circulation 1981;64:1228.)

TABLE 14.3. CHARACTERISTICS OF ANGINA PECTORIS

Quality
- Sensation of pressure or heavy weight on the chest
- Burning sensation
- Feeling of tightness
- Shortness of breath with feeling of constriction about the larynx or upper trachea
- Visceral quality (deep, heavy, squeezing, aching)
- Gradual increase in intensity followed by gradual fading away

Location
- Over the sternum or very near to it
- Anywhere between epigastrium and pharynx
- Occasionally limited to left shoulder and left arm
- Rarely limited to right arm
- Limited to lower jaw
- Lower cervical or upper thoracic spine
- Left interscapular or suprascapular area

Duration
- 0.5–30 minutes

Precipitating Factors
- Relationship to exercise
- Effort that involves use of arms above the head
- Cold environment
- Walking against the wind
- Walking after a large meal
- Emotional factors involved with physical exercise
- Fright, anger
- Coitus

Nitroglycerin Relief
- Relief of pain occurring within 45 seconds to 5 minutes of taking nitroglycerin

Radiation
- Medical aspect of left arm
- Left shoulder
- Jaw
- Occasionally right arm

(From Helfant RH, Banka VS. A Clinical and Angiographic Approach to Coronary Heart Disease. Philadelphia, FA Davis, 1978, p 47, with permission.)

disease and impaired left ventricular function) (Fig. 14.4), high clinical risk [defined as at least two of the following: resting ST depression; history of myocardial infarction (MI); or history of hypertension] when combined with angiographic risk considerations, exercise-inducible ischemia resulting in a decline in ejection fraction, and low exercise capacity comprise a group with a high probability of death if medical management alone is instituted.[9] Patients screened but not randomized to CASS had similar survival rates suggesting that results from randomized patients may be applicable to more generalized populations as a measure of external reliability.[10]

PATHOPHYSIOLOGY[11,12]

IHD has many clinical expressions including the following syndromes: stable exertional angina; unstable (rest, preinfarction, crescendo) angina; silent myocardial ischemia; acute coronary insufficiency; coronary vasomotion or vasospasm associated with atypical, variant, or Prinzmetal's angina; and myocardial infarction. The pathophysiology that underlies this disease process is dynamic, evolutionary, and complex. To better understand the rationale for the selection and use of pharmacotherapy for IHD, one must appreciate the importance of the determinants of myocardial oxygen demand (MVO_2), regulation of coronary blood flow, the effects of ischemia on the mechanical and metabolic function of the myocardium, and how ischemia may be recognized so that treatment may be instituted.

Ischemia may be defined as lack of oxygen and decreased or no blood flow in the myocardium. In contrast, anoxia, defined as the absence of oxygen to the myocardium, results in continued perfusion with washout of acid by-products of glycolysis, thereby preserving the mechanical and metabolic status of the heart to a greater extent than ischemia for short periods of time.

DETERMINANTS OF OXYGEN DEMAND

The major determinants of MVO_2 are (1) heart rate, (2) contractility, and (3) intramyocardial wall tension. Overall, intramyocardial wall tension is thought to be the most important among these three factors. Because the consequences of IHD are due to increased demand in the face of a fixed supply of oxygen in most situations, alterations in MVO_2 are critically important in producing ischemia and for interventions intended to alleviate ischemia. MVO_2 cannot be directly measured in patients; however, an indirect assessment that correlates reasonably well with MVO_2 as determined in experimental animal models is the tension–time index (TTI). This is a measure of the area under the curve of the left ventricular (LV) pressure curve. Tension in the ventricle wall is a function of the radius of the LV and intraventricular pressure. These factors are related through Laplace's law, which states that wall stress is related directly to the product of intraventricular pressure and internal radius and inversely to wall thickness multiplied by a factor of two. Increasing systemic blood pressure or ventricular dilation would increase wall tension and oxygen demand while ventricular hypertrophy would tend to minimize increasing MVO_2. Clinical application of these principles has lead to the use of the double product (DP), which is heart rate (HR) multiplied by systolic blood pressure (SBP) ($DP = HR \times SBP$). While this is a clinically useful indirect estimate of MVO_2, it does not consider changes in contractility (an independent variable), and because only changes in pressure are considered with the double product, volume loading of the LV and increased MVO_2 related to ventricular dilation are underestimated.

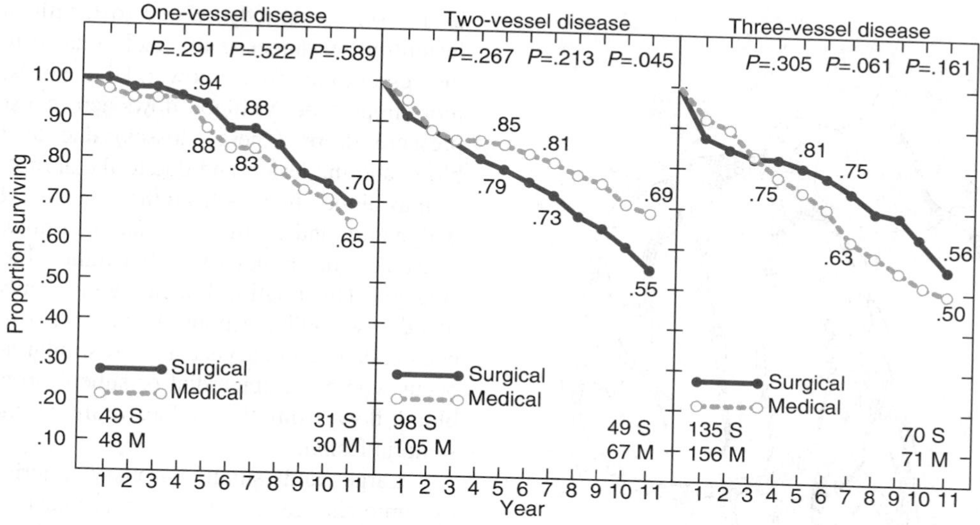

Figure 14.3. Eleven-year survival rates for patients without left main coronary artery disease who had single-, double-, or triple-vessel disease, from the VA study. M, medical; S, surgical. *(From the Veterans Administration Coronary Artery Bypass Surgery Cooperative Study Group. Eleven-year survival in the Veterans Administration randomized trial of coronary bypass surgery for stable angina. N Engl J Med 1984;311:1335, with permission.)*

REGULATION OF CORONARY BLOOD FLOW

Coronary blood flow is influenced by multiple factors; however, the caliber of the resistance vessels delivering blood to the myocardium and MV_{O_2} are the prime determinants in the occurrence of ischemia. The anatomy of the vascular bed will affect oxygen supply and, subsequently, myocardial metabolism and mechanical function.

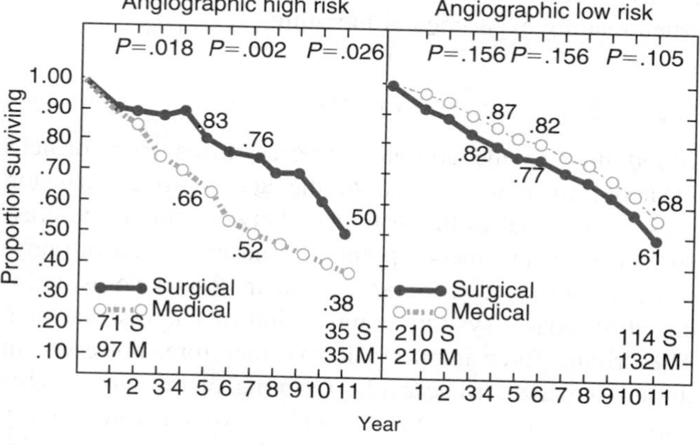

Figure 14.4. Eleven-year cumulative survival for patients without left main coronary artery disease according to angiographic risk, from the VA study. High risk was defined as three-vessel disease plus impaired left ventricular function, and low risk as one-, two-, or three-vessel disease plus normal left ventricular function or one- or two-vessel disease plus impaired left ventricular function. M, medical; S, surgical. *(From the Veterans Administration Coronary Artery Bypass Surgery Cooperative Study Group. Eleven-year survival in the Veterans Administration randomized trial of coronary bypass surgery for stable angina. N Engl J Med 1984;311:1336, with permission.)*

Anatomic Factors

The normal coronary system (Fig. 14.5) consists of large epicardial or surface vessels (R_1) that normally offer little intrinsic resistance to myocardial flow and intramyocardial arteries and arterioles (R_2), which branch into a dense capillary network (about 4000 capillaries/mm^2) to supply basal blood flow of 60–90 mL/min per 100 g of myocardium (Fig. 14.6). R_1 and R_2 are in series and total resistance is the algebraic sum; however, under normal circumstances, the resistance in R_2 is much greater. Myocardial blood flow is inversely related to arteriolar resistance and directly related to the coronary driving pressure. The arterioles dynamically alter their intrinsic tone in response to demands for oxygen and other factors and, as a result, myocardial oxygen delivery and myocardial oxygen demand are tightly coupled in a rapidly responsive system.

Atherosclerotic lesions encroaching on the luminal cross-sectional area of the larger epicardial vessels (R_1) transform the relationships among R_1, R_2, and blood flow. As resistance increases in R_1 due to occlusion, R_2 can vasodilate to maintain coronary blood flow (Fig. 14.6). This response is inadequate with greater degrees of obstruction and the coronary flow reserve afforded by R_2 vasodilation is insufficient to meet oxygen demand (also referred to as autoregulation). This scenario is depicted in Fig. 14.7, assuming a linear model for these effects. It has been determined that this simplistic approach does not account for the

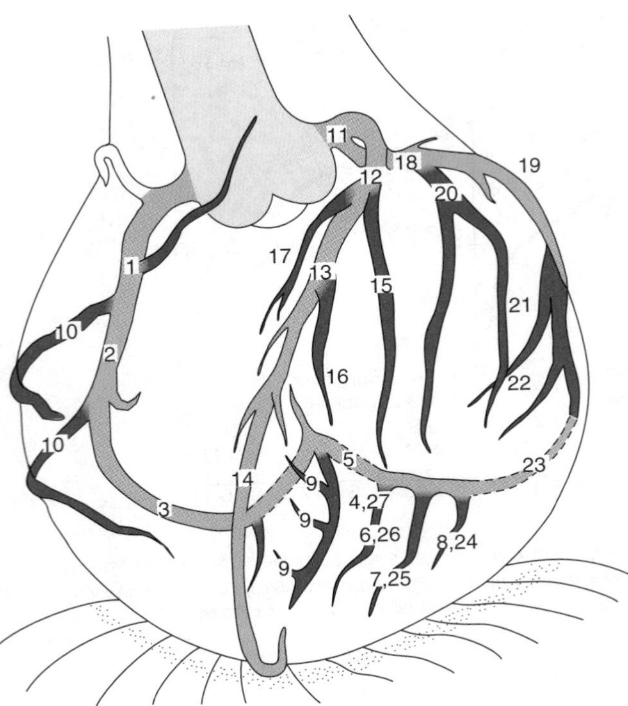

Figure 14.5. Coronary artery anatomy visualized at angiography, as defined by cooperating centers in the Coronary Artery Surgery Study. (1) Proximal right, (2) midright, (3) distal right, (4) right posterior descending, (5) right posterior lateral segment, (6) first right posterior lateral, (7) second right posterior lateral, (8) third right posterior lateral, (9) inferior septal, (10) acute marginal, (11) left main, (12) proximal left anterior descending, (13) mid left anterior descending, (14) distal left anterior descending, (15) first diagonal, (16) second diagonal, (17) first septal, (18) proximal circumflex, (19) distal circumflex, (20) first obtuse marginal, (21) second obtuse marginal, (22) third obtuse marginal, (23) left atrioventricular, (24) first left posterior lateral, (25) second left posterior lateral, (26) third left posterior lateral, (27) left posterior descending. *(From the Principal Investigators of CASS and their associates. The National Heart, Lung, and Blood Institute coronary artery surgery study (CASS). Circulation 1981;62(suppl I):I-1, with permission.)*

complex geometry of atherosclerotic lesions, collateral blood flow, and so on, but it is useful to describe the basic problem. Obviously, the extent of functional obstruction is important in the limitation of coronary blood flow, and the presence of relatively severe stenosis (80–85%) may provoke ischemia and symptoms at rest while less severe stenosis may allow a reserve of coronary blood flow for exertion.[13]

The diameter of the lesion impeding blood flow through a vessel is important but other factors such as length of the lesion and the influence of pressure drop across an area of stenosis also affect coronary blood flow and function of the collateral circulation. Resistance to flow in a vessel is directly related to length of the obstructing lesion but resistance is inversely related to the diameter of the vessel to the fourth power. Diameter is, therefore, much more important. As blood flows across a stenotic lesion the pressure drops (energy losses) due to friction between blood and the lesion and due to the abrupt turbulent expansion as blood emerges from the stenosis. This pressure drop is dynamic and is directly related to flow, giving rise to a resistance that is not fixed, but rather fluctuates as flow is changed. This relationship can dramatically affect collateral blood flow and its response to exercise resulting in what has been called "coronary steal."[13] A similar situation may also occur where the epicardial or subepicardial vessels "steal" blood flow from the endocardium in the presence of a stenotic lesion.

Large and small coronary arteries may undergo dynamic changes in coronary vascular resistance and coronary blood flow. Dynamic coronary obstruction can occur in normal vessels and vessels with stenosis in which vasomotion or spasm may be superimposed on a fixed stenosis. While it is possible that these changes may be "active" in small coronary arteries, it is also possible that the observed changes may reflect collapse due to poststenotic intraluminal pressure drop or increased intramyocardial compressive forces associated with inadequate ventricular relaxation.

Collateral blood flow exists to a certain extent from birth as native collaterals, but persisting ischemia may promote collateral growth as developed collaterals. These two types of collaterals differ in anatomy and in their ability to regulate coronary blood flow. Collateral patency is dependent upon MV_{O_2}, flow pressures, and anatomical considerations as discussed previously. Collateral development is highly species dependent and this should be considered when reading experimental literature.

Factors Extrinsic to the Vascular Bed

Blood flow to the coronary arteries arises from orifices located immediately distal to the aorta valve. Perfusion pressure is equal to the difference between the aortic pressure at an instantaneous point in time minus the intramyocardial pressure. Coronary vascular resistance is influenced by phasic systolic compression of the vascular bed. The driving force for perfusion is, therefore, not constant throughout the cardiac cycle. Opening of the aortic valve may also lead to a venturi effect, which can slightly decrease perfusion pressure. If perfusion pressure is elevated for a period of time, coronary vascular resistance declines and blood flow increases; however, continued perfusion pressure increases, within limits, lead to a return of coronary blood flow back toward baseline levels through autoregulation.

Alterations in intramyocardial wall tension throughout the cardiac cycle will also impose significant changes in

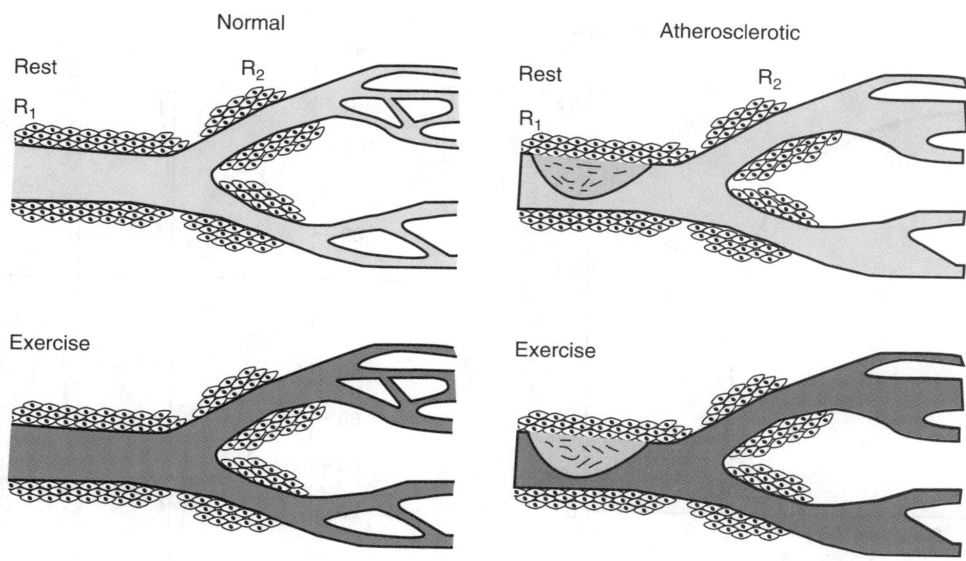

Figure 14.6. The coronary circulation with large epicardial conductance vessels (R_1) that offer little intrinsic resistance to myocardial blood flow and intramyocardial resistance arterioles (R_2). Resistance to flow equals $R_1 + R_2$ and R_2 resistance is normally much greater than R_1; hence flow is equal to the driving pressure across the coronary bed divided by the resistance in R_2. Dilatation in R_2 normally occurs in response to exercise or increased myocardial oxygen demand. When an atherosclerotic lesion narrows the conductance vessel, the arterioles dilate under resting conditions to prevent ischemia; however, with stress, the vasodilator reserve becomes limited. *(From Epstein SE, Talbot TL. Dynamic coronary tone in precipitation, exacerbation and relief of angina pectoris. Am J Cardiol 1981;48:798, with permission.)*

coronary blood flow. Diastole is the period during which coronary artery filling can occur due to these pressure differences and little or no coronary blood flow occurs to the left ventricle during systole (Fig. 14.8). The extent of pressure development in the ventricle and heart rate have a major effect on the development of wall tension, time for diastolic coronary artery filling, and myocardial oxygen demand.

Under normal conditions, the average global distribution of blood flow between the epicardial and endocardial layer is about 1 : 1 at rest and remains approximately even during exercise secondary to autoregulatory changes. Regional disparity of blood flow distribution does exist normally, and these disparities may be magnified in the presence of diseased coronary arteries and with increased cardiac work as the vasodilator reserve in the resistance vessels of the subendocardium layers is exhausted. Factors that favor a reduction in subendocardial blood flow include decreased perfusion pressure due to decreased diastolic blood pressure or coronary artery obstruction by atherosclerotic plaques with or without vasomotion, abbreviation of diastole (increased heart rate), and increased intraventricular diastolic pressure (e.g., valvular obstruction to flow).

Extravascular resistance may decrease coronary blood flow, primarily during systole. This effect is much more pronounced in the LV compared with the right ventricle (RV). When the effect of increased contractility is separated from the effect of ventricular pressure, approximately 75% of extravascular resistance is accounted for by passive stretch in equilibrium with ventricular pressure, while only 25% results from active myocardial contraction.

Factors Intrinsic to the Vascular Bed

Metabolic factors, myogenic responses, neural reflexes, and humoral substances within the vascular bed of the coronary circulation function in an orchestrated fashion to maintain relative consistency in blood flow to the myocardium in face of imposed changes in perfusion pressures. Autoregulation, mediated primarily through the effects of myogenic responses and metabolic factors, is thought to be responsible for maintaining regional blood flow in a narrow range while systemic pressure varies over a range of approximately 50–150 mm Hg.

Myogenic control (also known as the Bayliss effect) of coronary artery tone occurs when the vessel is stretched secondary to an increase in pressure and it contracts to return blood flow to normal. It is thought that the myogenic response to stretching in coronary arteries is a modest one, and that metabolic factors play a much larger role in autoregulation.

There are three well-studied metabolic factors that have the ability to modify coronary artery resistance and blood flow at the local level. Basal coronary blood flow

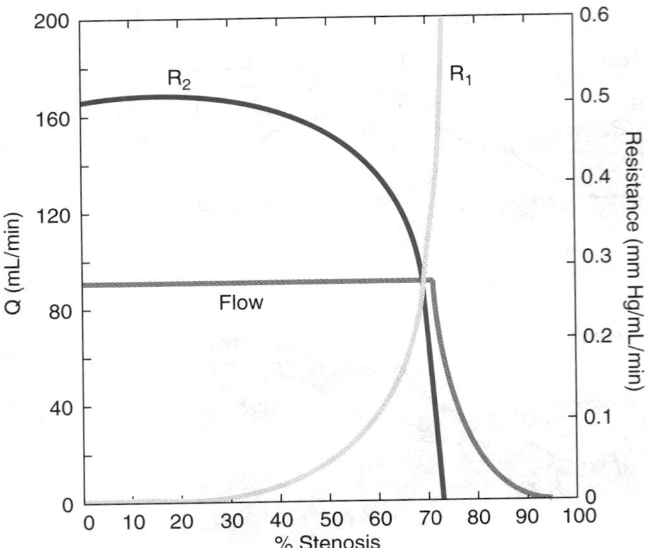

Figure 14.7. Influence of degree of stenosis on autoregulatory mechanisms that maintain appropriate levels of myocardial oxygen delivery. As epicardial coronary resistance (R_1) increases because of increased stenosis severity, arteriolar resistance (R_2) decreases, thereby maintaining total resistance (and thus flow) at normal levels. Once the vasodilator reserve of R_2 is exhausted, however, further increases in R_1 lead to decreases in flow. *(From Epstein SE et al. Hemodynamic principles in the control of coronary blood flow. Am J Cardiol 1985;56:5E, with permission.)*

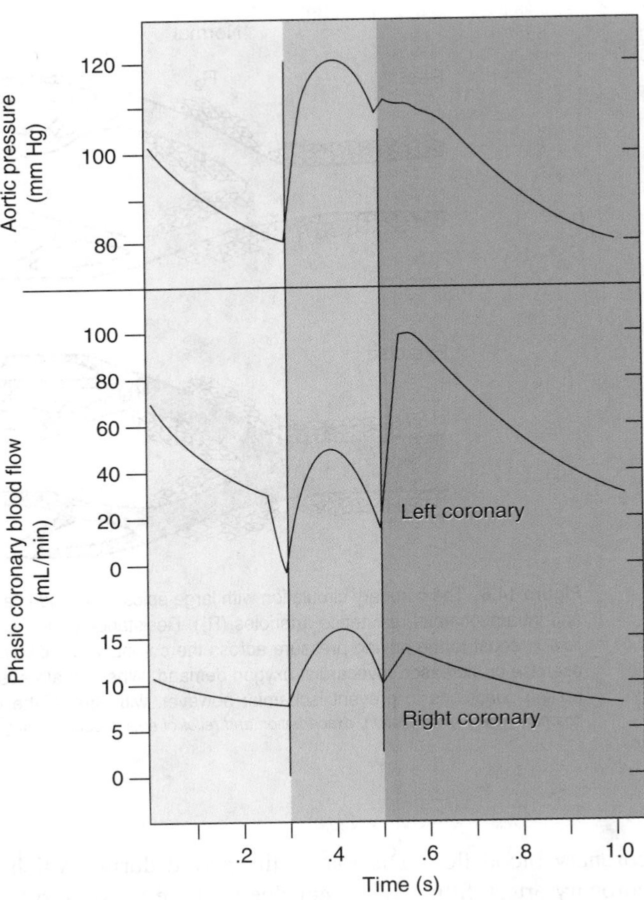

Figure 14.8. Phasic right and left coronary artery blood flow in relation to aortic blood pressure. *(From Berne RM, Levy MD. Cardiovascular Physiology, 2nd ed. St. Louis, CV Mosby, 1972, p 210, with permission.)*

meets oxygen demands of 8–10 mL/min per 100 g of myocardium with essentially complete extraction of oxygen from the blood. As cardiac output or mean arterial blood pressure increases, the increased demand for oxygen is met by increasing blood flow (Fig. 14.9) because little additional oxygen is available from hemoglobin. Decreased oxygen availability causes vasodilation of vascular smooth muscle and relaxation of precapillary sphincters, which increase tissue oxygen and help maintain blood flow on a regional basis. It is not known if these changes are due to a direct effect of hypoxia in altering the electromechanical potential of muscle cells (possibly mediated by potassium) or if vasodilating substances are produced locally in response to hypoxia.

The vascular endothelium of the coronary arteries synthesizes large molecules such as fibronectin, interleukin-1, tissue plasminogen activator, and various growth factors. Small molecules that are also produced include prostacyclin, platelet-activating factor, endothelin-1, and endothelium-derived relaxing factor (EDRF), which is now characterized as nitric oxide. EDRF is synthesized from 1-arginine and released by shear force on the endothelium as well as through interaction with many biochemical stimuli such as acetylcholine, histamine, arginine, catecholamines, arachidonic acid, ADP, serotonin, and thrombin. EDRF or nitric oxide then causes relaxation of the underlying smooth muscle and may be thought of as a paracrine homeopathic defense mechanism against noxious stimuli. Denudation or loss of the vascular endothelium results in loss of EDRF and this protective mechanism.[14] Loss of the endothelial cell layer and function may occur secondary to physical disruption (PTCA), factors impinging from the vascular side (cyanide from smoke), or disruption of the intimal-medial layers (oxidized low density lipoprotein).

At perfusion pressures less than 60 mm Hg, as the coronary arteries are maximally dilated and the buffering effect of autoregulation has reached its capacity, further reduction in coronary blood flow will decrease perfusion pressure and tissue oxygenation. It is thought that autoregulation works more efficiently in the epicardial layers than in subendocardial layers, and this may contribute to coronary steal.

Neural components that participate in the regulation of coronary blood flow include the sympathetic nervous

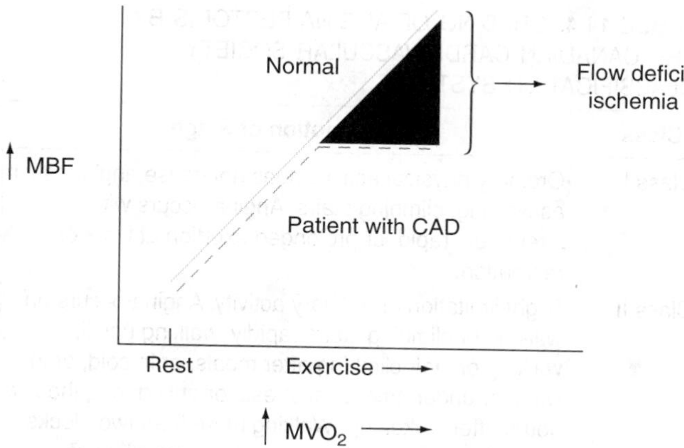

Figure 14.9. The relation between myocardial oxygen demand (MVo_2) and myocardial oxygen supply. In a normal person, myocardial blood flow (MBF) increases in proportion to the increase in MVo_2. In a patient with a fixed obstruction resulting from coronary artery disease (CAD) in R_1 as shown in Fig. 14.6, flow increases with increased oxygen demand until the ceiling for arteriolar dilatation (R_2 in Fig. 14.7) is reached. At this time, flow can no longer increase despite the continued increase in myocardial oxygen demand. A flow deficit results, leading to myocardial ischemia and angina pectoris. *(From Epstein SE, Talbot TL. Dynamic coronary tone in precipitation, exacerbation and relief of angina pectoris. Am J Cardiol 1981;48:799, with permission.)*

system, the parasympathetic nervous system, coronary reflexes, and, possibly, central control of coronary blood flow. Within the sympathetic system, stimulation of the stellate ganglion elicits coronary vasodilation, which is associated with tachycardia and enhanced contractility. This indirect coronary vasodilation is secondary to increased MVo_2 related to increased heart rate, contractility, and aortic pressure, which occurs following stellate stimulation. The direct effect of the sympathetic system is α_1-mediated vasoconstriction at rest and during exercise. Other receptor types, α_2 and β_1, have little influence on tone while β_2 stimulation produces a modest vasodilatory effect. Although coronary atherosclerosis may decrease blood flow secondary to obstruction, severe coronary atherosclerosis and obstruction may also increase the sensitivity of coronary arteries to the effects of α_1 stimulation and vasoconstriction.

Vagal stimulation within the parasympathetic system produces a small to moderate increase in coronary blood flow, which involves the coronary efferent and afferent parasympathetic components (Bezold–Jarish reflex). Indirectly, vasoconstriction may result with vagal stimulation as the result of bradycardia and decreased contractility reducing myocardial oxygen demand.

Coronary reflexes have an undetermined role in the regulation of coronary blood flow. Based on experimental data, coronary reflexes that may be important include the baroreceptor, the chemoreceptor, Bezold–Jarish reflex, and the pulmonary inhalation reflex.

Factors Limiting Coronary Perfusion

During exercise and pacing, as MVo_2 increases, coronary vascular resistance can be reduced to about 25% of basal values, which results in a fourfold to fivefold increase in coronary blood flow. The cross-sectional area can be reduced by about 80% prior to any mechanical or biochemical changes in the myocardium reflecting a margin of safety for coronary blood flow. The extent of cross-sectional obstruction, the length of the lesion, lesion composition, and the geometry of the obstructing lesion can each affect flow across coronary arteries with atherosclerosis. Bernoulli's theorem states that the pressure drop across a lesion is directly related to the length of the lesion and inversely related to the radius of the lesion to the fourth power; critical stenosis occurs when the obstructing lesion encroaches on the luminal diameter and exceeds 70–80%. Lesions creating obstruction of 50–70% may reduce blood flow; however, these obstructions are not consistent and vasospasm and thrombosis superimposed on a "noncritical" lesion may lead to clinical events such as myocardial infarction. If the lesion enlarges from 80 to 90%, resistance in that vessel is tripled. Coronary reserve is diminished at about 85% obstruction due to vasoconstriction. Exaggerated responsiveness can be seen when coronary stenosis reaches this critical level, and the role of vasoactive substances such as prostaglandins, thromboxanes, and serotonin may play more of a role in the regulation of coronary vascular tone and thrombosis.

Little reserve exists for coronary blood flow and a relatively small reduction of 10–20% results in decreased myocardial fiber shortening as the first evidence for abnormal function. The subendocardial layers are affected to a greater extent than the epicardium by ischemia considering changes in fibers shortening, arteriovenous (AV) difference in oxygen saturation, and lactate production. A reduction of 80% gives rise to akinesis, and a 95% reduction of coronary blood flow produces dyskinesis during contraction of the ventricles. Although these abnormalities of contraction are associated with transient impaired function, depletion of high-energy phosphate compounds and ultrastructural changes may last for days even after transient ischemia; this has been referred to as "stunned myocardium." Regional loss of contractility may impose a burden on the remaining myocardial tissue resulting in heart failure, increased MVo_2, and rapid depletion of oxygen stores. Consequently, zones of tissue with marginal blood flow may develop in a lateral or transmural fashion; such development puts this tissue at risk for more severe damage if the ischemic episode persists or becomes more severe. Nonischemic areas of myocardium may compensate for the severely ischemic and border zones of ischemia by developing more tension than usual in an attempt to maintain cardiac output. At the cellular level, ischemia and the attendant acidosis are thought to alter calcium release from storage sites such as the sarcolemma and the sarcoplasmic reticulum as well as inhibiting the binding of calcium to troponin, thereby impairing the association of actin and myosin. The clinical correlates of these cellular biochemical events leading to the development of LV or RV dysfunction include an S3, dyspnea, orthopnea, tachycardia, fluctuating blood pressure, transient murmurs, and mitral or tricuspid regurgitation.

Calcium accumulation and overload secondary to ischemia impairs ventricular relaxation as well as contraction. This is apparently due to impaired calcium uptake after systole from the myofilaments leading to a less negative decline of the pressure in the ventricle over time. Impaired relaxation is associated with enhanced diastolic stiffness, decreased rate of wall thinning, and slowed pressure decay producing an upward shift in the ventricular pressure–volume relationship; put more simply, MVo_2 is likely to be increased secondary to increased wall tension. Impairment of both diastolic and systolic function leads to elevation of the filling pressure of the left ventricle.

TABLE 14.4. GRADING OF ANGINA PECTORIS BY THE CANADIAN CARDIOVASCULAR SOCIETY CLASSIFICATION SYSTEM

Class	Description of Stage
Class I	Ordinary physical activity does not cause angina, such as walking, climbing stairs. Angina occurs with strenuous, rapid, or prolonged exertion at work or recreation.
Class II	Slight limitation of ordinary activity. Angina occurs on walking or climbing stairs rapidly, walking uphill, walking or stair climbing after meals, or in cold, or in wind, or under emotional stress, or only during the few hours after wakening. Walking more than two blocks on the level and climbing more than one flight of ordinary stairs at a normal pace and in normal condition.
Class III	Marked limitations of ordinary physical activity. Angina occurs on walking one to two blocks on the level and climbing one flight of stairs in normal conditions and at a normal pace.
Class IV	Inability to carry on any physical activity without discomfort—anginal symptoms may be present at rest.

(From Campeau, L. Grading of angina [letter]. *Circulation* 1976:54:522–523.)

Clinical Presentation and Diagnosis

The classic symptoms associated with typical chest pain and angina due to IHD appear in Table 14.3. Important aspects of the clinical history for chest pain in patients with angina include the nature or quality of the pain, precipitating factors, duration, pain radiation, and the response to nitroglycerin or rest. Because there can be considerable variation in the manifestations of angina, it is more accurate to refer to these symptoms as an anginal syndrome. For some patients with significant coronary disease, their presenting symptoms may differ from the classical symptoms, yet the symptoms are due to ischemic pain, and these are often referred to as anginal equivalents. Obtaining an accurate and detailed family history is useful in placing symptoms in perspective. Significant positive information would include death, especially any early one, from myocardial infarction as well as the presence of nonfatal MI or hypertension, familial lipid disorders, and diabetes mellitus. These are also obviously important in the assessment of the patient under consideration because they and smoking are major risk factors for coronary disease. Typical pain radiation patterns include anterior chest pain (96%), left upper arm pain (83.7%), left lower arm pain (29.3%), and neck pain at some time (22%). Pain from other areas is less common. Patients suffering from variant or Prinzmetal's angina secondary to coronary spasm are more likely to experience pain at rest and in the early morning hours, and the pain is not usually brought on by exertion or emotional stress nor relieved by rest; the ECG pattern is that of current of injury with ST elevation rather than depression.[15]

It is also important to differentiate the pattern of pain for stable angina from that of unstable angina. The definition of unstable angina is controversial, but includes the presence of one or more of the following: (1) new onset (<2 months) exertional angina of at least Canadian Cardiovascular Society Classification (CCSC) class III (Table 14.4) in severity; (2) recent (<2 months) acceleration of angina as reflected by an increase in severity of at least one CCSC class to at least CCSC class III; or (3) pain at rest which lasts for >20 minutes.[16] Ischemia may also be painless or "silent" in 60–100% of patients depending on the series cited and the patient population.[17] In patients with myocardial ischemia, approximately 70% of the episodes of documented ischemia are painless as determined by ambulatory ECG monitoring, and the ST-segment changes associated with these episodes can be ST elevation or depression. The mechanism of silent ischemia is unclear, but studies have shown that patients not experiencing pain have altered pain perception with the threshold and tolerance for pain being higher than patients who have pain more frequently. Silent ischemia is more common in diabetic patients, perhaps due to their neuropathy and inability to sense pain. The role of altered enkephalin or endorphin concentrations remains to be clarified.

Lastly, it should be recognized that the threshold for pain due to exertion is fixed in some patients and variable in others and that the amount of exercise or stress necessary to provoke symptoms can change over time. A fixed threshold for the induction of pain or ECG evidence of ischemia means these indicators of ischemia occur at the same, or nearly so, double rate–pressure product. This is apparently due to at least two factors. Over long periods of time atherosclerosis may progress, leading to more severe stenosis, reduced oxygen supply, and less of an increase in demand to precipitate ischemic symptoms. Once stenotic lesions reach a critical level of about 80% or greater, vasomotion, vasospasm, and thrombotic occlusion become significant factors impairing blood flow to the myocardium. Consequently, anatomic considerations and vasoactive substances may interact to provide an environment amenable to changing thresholds for the production of angina.

There appears to be little relationship between the historical features of angina and the severity or extent of coronary artery vessel involvement. Therefore, one may speculate that severe symptoms might be associated with multivessel disease, but no predictive markers exist on a routine basis.

Chest pain may resemble pain arising from a variety of noncardiac sources and the differential diagnosis of anginal pain from other etiologies may be quite difficult based on history alone. Table 14.5 outlines other common problems that may present with episodic chest pain. Although much less common, nonatherosclerotic etiologies of coronary artery disease do exist and they are outlined in Table 14.6.

There are few signs apparent on physical examination to indicate the presence of coronary artery disease and usually only the cardiovascular system reveals any useful information. Elevated heart rate or blood pressure can yield an increased double product and may be associated with angina, and it would be important to correct extreme tachycardia or hypertension if present. Other noncardiac physical findings that suggest that significant cardiovascular disease may be associated with angina include abdominal aortic aneurysms or peripheral vascular disease. A controversial finding is that of a diagonal ear lobe crease, which is said by some to be associated with significant coronary disease. Findings on the cardiac examination that may be seen in patients with coronary artery disease are noted in Table 14.7. During an angina attack these findings may appear or become more prominent, making them more valuable if present.

Other than risk-factor screening, there are no specific laboratory tests that are useful in diagnosing coronary artery disease. Lipid profiling with total cholesterol, high density cholesterol, lipoprotein (a), and triglycerides will identify individuals susceptible to atherosclerosis. Of particular importance, total cholesterol concentrations of greater than 280 mg/dL are associated with multivessel disease and should be aggressively treated with diet and possibly drug therapy (see Chapter 21, Hyperlipidemia). Knowledge of other lipoprotein fractions is useful to select appropriate therapy but they have little predictive value for IHD. Future trends may include nuclear probes

TABLE 14.5. DIFFERENTIAL DIAGNOSIS OF EPISODIC CHEST PAIN RESEMBLING ANGINA PECTORIS

	Duration	Quality	Provocation	Relief	Location	Comment
Effort angina	5–15 min	Visceral (pressure)	During effort or emotion	Rest, NTG	Substernal, radiates	First episode vivid
Rest angina	5–15 min	Visceral (pressure)	Spontaneous (? with exercise)	NTG	Substernal, radiates	Often nocturnal
Mitral prolapse	Minute–hour	Superficial (rarely visceral)	Spontaneous (no pattern)	Time	Left anterior	No pattern, variable
Esophageal reflux	10 min–1 h	Visceral	Spontaneous, cold liquids, exercise	Foods, antacids, H_2 blockers, and proton pump inhibitors	Substernal, radiates	Mimics angina
Peptic ulcer	Hour	Visceral, burning	Lack of food, “acid” foods	Foods, antacids, H_2 blockers, and proton pump inhibitors	Epigastric, substernal	
Biliary disease	Hour	Visceral (wax and wane)	Spontaneous, food	Time, analgesia	Epigastric, radiates	Colic
Cervical disc	Variable (gradually subsides)	Superficial	Head and neck, movement and palpation	Time, analgesia	Arm, neck	Not relieved by rest
Hyperventilation	2–3 min	Visceral	Emotion, tachypnea	Stimulus removed	Substernal	Facial paraesthesia
Musculoskeletal	Variable	Superficial	Movement, palpation	Time, analgesia	Multiple	Tenderness
Pulmonary	30 min	Visceral (pressure)	Often spontaneous	Rest, time bronchodilator	Substernal	Dyspneic

(From Christie LG Jr, Conti CR. Systemic approach to the evaluation of angina-like chest pain. Am Heart J 1981;102:897, with permission.)

TABLE 14.6. ETIOLOGIES OF NONATHEROSCLEROTIC ARTERY DISEASE

I. Congenital disorders of the coronary arteries
   A. Anomalous origin of a coronary artery from the pulmonary artery
   B. Anomalous origin of a coronary artery from the aorta or other coronary artery
   C. Coronary arteriovenous fistula
   D. Coronary artery aneurysm

II. Hereditary metabolic derangements with coronary artery involvement
   A. Diseases causing aortic dissection
      1. Marfan's syndrome
      2. Ehlers–Danlos syndrome
   B. Pseudoxanthoma
   C. Gargoylism (Hurler's syndrome)
   D. Homocystinuria

III. Acquired disorders of the coronary arteries
   A. Embolization
   B. Dissection
   C. Syphilitic
   D. Infiltrative
      1. Tumors
      2. Amyloidosis
   E. Connective tissue diseases
      1. Periarteritis nodosa
      2. Rheumatoid arthritis
      3. Systemic lupus erythematosus
   F. Miscellaneous
      1. Irradiation
      2. Chest trauma
      3. Nitrate withdrawal

(From Cohn PF (ed). Diagnosis and Therapy of Coronary Artery Disease, 2nd ed. Boston, Martinus Nijhoff, 1985, p 496, with permission.)

for diagnosis of apolipoprotein abnormalities, and these technologies hold great promise. Fasting glucose determinations to exclude diabetes and glucose monitoring for concurrent diabetes should be performed routinely. Cardiac enzymes, creatine phosphokinase (CPK), lactate dehydrogenase (LDH), and serum glutamic-oxaloacetic transaminase (SGOT), should all be normal in the angina patient.

Chest x-ray findings of coronary artery calcification will be associated with critical stenosis in 90% of patients, but there is little correlation to clinical manifestations. Fluoroscopy has been used to detect coronary artery calcifications and these seem to be a strong marker for stenosis if patients are less than 50 years old.

DIAGNOSTIC TESTS (SEE ALSO CHAPTER 10, CARDIOVASCULAR TESTING)

Electrocardiogram

The ECG is normal in about one-half of patients with angina who are not experiencing an acute attack. Typical ST-T-wave changes include depression, T-wave inversion, and ST-segment elevation. Forms of ischemia other than exertional angina may have ECG manifestations that are different; variant angina is associated with ST-segment elevation, whereas silent ischemia may produce elevation or depression. Significant ischemia is associated with ST-segment depression of greater than 2 mm, exertional hypotension, and reduced exercise tolerance.

Exercise Tolerance Testing

Exercise tolerance (stress) testing (ETT) is useful for a history of chest pain that is equivocal, for risk stratification, implementation of medical versus surgical therapy, and to assess the efficacy of treatment. Although the ETT is insensitive for predicting coronary artery anatomy, it does correlate well with outcome due to IHD such as the likelihood of progressing to angina, the occurrence of acute MI and cardiovascular death.[16] Ischemic ST depression that occurs during ETT is an independent risk factor for cardiac events and cardiovascular mortality. Thallium (^{201}Tl) myocardial perfusion scintigraphy may be used in conjunction with ETT to detect reversible and irreversible defects in blood flow to the myocardium.

Cardiac Imaging

Radionuclide angiocardiography (performed with technetium-99*m*, a radioisotope) is used to measure ejection fraction, regional ventricular performance, cardiac output, ventricular volumes, valvular regurgitation, asynchrony or wall motion abnormalities, and intracardiac shunts. Technectium pyrophosphate scans are used routinely for detection and quantification of acute myocardial infarction (see Chapter 15, Acute Myocardial Infarction). Positron emission tomography (PET) is useful for quantifying ischemia with metabolically important substrates such as oxygen, carbon, and nitrogen. Other metabolic probes utilize radiolabeled fatty acids and glucose to study metabolic processes that may be deranged during ischemia in animals and for investigative purposes in man.

Echocardiography

Echocardiography has been shown to be useful for direct visualization of lesions in the left main coronary artery and in providing information concerning some of the complications of IHD including the presence of ventricular aneurysms and assessing ejection fraction and detecting regional or global LV function abnormalities that occur during ischemia episodes.

Ambulatory Electrocardiographic (Holter Monitoring)

Ambulatory ECG monitoring is useful in detecting ischemia during symptomatic and asymptotic episodes and provides information for an extended period of time. This approach allows estimation of the total ischemic burden of the myocardium rather than only reported episodes of angina.

TABLE 14.7. CARDIAC FINDINGS IN PATIENTS WITH CORONARY ARTERY DISEASE

Sign	Clinical Significance	Frequency
Abnormal precordial systolic bulge	Left ventricular wall motion abnormality	Not usually present unless patient has sustained a prior MI[a] (especially anterior wall) or is experiencing angina at time of examination
Decreased intensity of S_1[a]	Decrease in left ventricular contractility	Difficult to evaluate in resting state, but can be commonly demonstrated during angina
Paradoxical splitting of S_2	Left ventricular wall motion abnormality	Very uncommon but occasionally noted during angina
S_3 (ventricular gallop)	Increased left ventricular diastolic pressure, with or without clinical CHF	Not usually present unless patient sustained extensive MI; may occasionally be present during angina
S_4 (atrial gallop)	Reduced ventricular compliance ("stiff heart")	Common; very common in patients who have sustained a prior MI as well as during angina
Apical systolic murmur (in absence of rheumatic mitral regurgitation or Barlow's syndrome)	Papillary muscle dysfunction	Not usually present unless patient has sustained prior MI
Diastolic murmur (in absence of aortic regurgitation)	Coronary artery stenosis	Rare

[a]S_1, first heart sound; S_2, second heart sound; S_3, third heart sound; S_4, fourth heart sound; MI, myocardial infarction. (From Cohn PF (ed). Diagnosis and Therapy of Coronary Artery Disease, 2nd ed. Boston, Martinus Nijhoff, 1985, p 101, with permission.)

Cardiac Catheterization and Coronary Arteriography

Cardiac catheterization and angiography in patients with suspected coronary artery disease are used diagnostically to document the presence and severity of disease as well as for prognostic purposes. Interventional catheterization is used for thrombolytic therapy in patients with acute myocardial infarction and for the management of patients with significant coronary artery disease to relieve obstruction through percutaneous transluminal coronary angioplasty (PTCA), atherectomy, or stent placement. Catheterization and arteriography may be done after coronary artery bypass grafting (CABG) to determine if the graft has closed or if coronary artery disease has progressed.

MANAGEMENT OF ISCHEMIC HEART DISEASE

MODIFICATION OF RISK FACTORS

Primary prevention of ischemic heart disease through the identification and modification of risk factors prior to the initial morbid event would be the optimal management approach and should result in a significant impact on the prevalence of IHD. However, early recognition of some risk factors may not be possible in all cases, and in others, the patient may not be willing to undertake intervention until overt evidence of coronary disease is apparent. Secondary intervention continues to be more commonly pursued by both health care professionals and patients and it is important to recognize this type of intervention as effective in reducing subsequent morbidity and mortality. The presence of risk factors in individual patients plays a major role in determining the occurrence and severity of IHD. Risk factors are additive in nature and can be classified as alterable or unalterable (Table 14.8). Unalterable risk factors include gender; age; family history or genetic composition; environmental influences such as climate, air pollution, trace metal composition of drinking water; and, to some extent, diabetes mellitus. Improved glycemic control reduces the microvascular complications of diabetes mellitus (see Chapter 72, Diabetes Mellitus) but it is not known if macrovascular complications such as IHD can be reduced with better glycemic control. Risk factors that can be altered include smoking, hypertension, hyperlipidemia, obesity, sedentary lifestyle, hyperuricemia, psychosocial factors such as stress and type A behavior patterns, and the use of certain drugs that may be detrimental including progestins, corticosteroids, cyclosporine, thiazide diuretics, and β-adrenergic blocking agents.

Cigarette smoking is common; some 50 million people are regular smokers in the United States, and the evidence for increased coronary mortality of smokers over nonsmokers of twofold to threefold is unequivocal. Of the 325,000 premature deaths each year due to smoking, one-third are due to coronary heart disease. Risk due to smoking is related to the number of cigarettes smoked per day and the duration of smoking; however, even nonsmokers may be affected because passive smoking in angina pectoris patients has been shown to decrease exercise time. Pipe and cigar smokers are at increased risk compared with nonsmokers, but their risk is somewhat less than cigarette

TABLE 14.8. BASELINE QUINTILES OF SYSTOLIC BLOOD PRESSURE, CHOLESTEROL, AND CIGARETTE SMOKING STATUS FOR THE MULTIPLE RISK FACTOR INTERVENTION TRIAL (MRFIT)

	Serum Cholesterol (mg/dL)				
SBP[a] (mm Hg)	<182	182–202	203–220	221–244	245+
Nonsmokers					
<118	31[b]	49	54	70	125
118–124	41	61	68	96	134
125–131	55	90	90	93	166
132–141	63	81	112	126	212
142+	147	176	197	245	349
Smokers					
<118	114	106	152	199	262
118–124	107	135	167	231	318
125–131	151	189	211	235	360
132–141	157	218	291	535	422
142+	304	359	443	571	642

[a]SBP, systolic blood pressure.
[b]Rate per 100,000 person-years adjusted by direct method for age; average follow-up is 11.6 years. (From Stamler J, Stamler R, Neaton JD. Blood pressure, systolic and diastolic, and cardiovascular risks. Arch Intern Med 1993;153:601.)

smokers. The direct effects of cigarette smoke that are detrimental to patients with angina include (1) elevated heart rate and blood pressure from nicotine, which increases MVO_2 and impaired myocardial oxygen delivery due to carboxyhemoglobin generation from carbon monoxide inhalation in smoke; (2) the negative inotropic effect of carboxyhemoglobin; (3) increased platelet adhesiveness and promotion of aggregation resulting in thrombotic tendencies due to nicotine and carboxyhemoglobin; and (4) lowered threshold for ventricular fibrillation during ischemia due to carboxyhemoglobin. Similar changes have been noted for marijuana smoking as well. Smoking also accelerates the risk for myocardial infarction, sudden death, cerebrovascular disease, peripheral vascular disease, and hypertension, and it reduces high-density lipoprotein concentrations. Clearly, primary prevention is needed for this risk factor and much of the education effort to discourage initiation of smoking should be targeted for teenagers. Techniques for cessation of smoking that may be useful include aversive conditioning, group programs, self-help programs, hypnosis, "cold turkey," and the use of nicotine substitutes (lobeline) or other sources of nicotine (Nicorette chewing gum and transdermal nicotine systems) for short-term substitution during withdrawal syndrome. Cessation of smoking reduces the incidence of coronary events to about one-half of that associated with continued smoking and these benefits are noted within 2 years of cessation.

Hypertension, whether labile or fixed, borderline or definite, casual or basal, systolic or diastolic, at any age regardless of gender, is the most common and a powerful contributor to atherosclerotic coronary vascular disease. Morbidity and mortality increase progressively with the degree of blood pressure elevation of either systolic or diastolic pressure and no discernible critical value exists (see Chapter 12, Hypertension). Numerous trials have documented the reduction in risk associated with blood pressure lowering; however, most of these studies show that mortality and morbidity reduction is due to fewer strokes, less renal failure and heart failure, and the reduction in coronary heart disease endpoints is not as dramatic. The reasons for this are unclear but perhaps relate to the multifactorial etiology of IHD.

Hypercholesterolemia is a significant cardiovascular risk factor and risk is directly related to the degree of cholesterol elevation. As with hypertension, there is no critical value that defines risk, but rather, risk is incrementally related to the degree of elevation and the presence of other risk factors (see Chapter 21, Hyperlipidemia). The role of triglycerides in coronary artery disease remains a controversial issue; however, most would agree that gross elevations, greater than 500 mg/dL, should be treated. In addition to total cholesterol determination, high-density lipoprotein, low-density protein, and very low-density lipoprotein concentration determinations are useful in identifying the specific lipid disorder type and for prognostic purposes. Primary intervention with diet therapy has resulted in reduced mortality in some but not all trials. Simvastatin (a HMGCo-A reductase inhibitor), cholestyramine, niacin, and gemfibrozil have been shown to reduce nonfatal myocardial infarction. Niacin and simvastatin have also been shown to reduce total and CHD mortality. Regression of atherosclerosis with diet and drug therapy has also been demonstrated in several trials as described in Chapter 21. Secondary intervention in patients with clinically apparent coronary artery disease and those with multiple risk factors should be initiated with the intent of correcting abnormal lipid levels or lowering LDL cholesterol to <100 mg/dL for secondary intervention and <130 mg/dL with ≥130 mg/dL with two or more risk factors with nutritional and pharmacologic intervention. The goals for lipid reduction in secondary intervention are described in Chapter 21.

The prevalence of obesity, defined as greater than 20% over ideal body weight, ranges from 7.4–17% in men and from 9.6–34.7% in women in the United States. Body mass index, weight (kg) divided by height (m) squared, greater than about 32 is associated with an increased mortality ratio compared with individuals of normal body weight, and the objective for patients with IHD is to maintain or reduce to a normal body weight. This may be accomplished through dietary modification, exercise, pharmacologic therapy, or surgical therapy. Frequently associated with obesity is a sedentary lifestyle, and inactivity may contribute to higher blood pressure, elevated blood lipid levels, and insulin resistance associated with glucose intolerance in diabetics (insulin resistance syndrome). Exercise to the level of about 300 kcal three times a week is useful in improving maximal oxygen uptake, improving cardiorespiratory efficiency, promoting collateral artery formation, and promoting potential alterations in the risk of ventricular fibrillation, coronary thrombosis, and improved tolerance to stress. Although a regular exercise program may not prevent the occurrence of IHD, participants feel better and their overall cardiovascular risk may be reduced.

Competitiveness, intense striving for achievement, easily provoked hostility, a sense of urgency about doing things quickly and being punctual, impatience, abrupt and rapid speech and gestures, and concentration on self-selected goals to the point of not perceiving and attending to other aspects of the environment are traits that characterize the behavioral pattern known as the type A or coronary-prone personality. Although the issue is somewhat controversial, type A individuals may have increased cardiovascular risk with risk ratios ranging from insignificant to three times that of a matched population. The mechanism by which personality affects the cardiovascular system is not understood, but may reflect the activity of the sympathetic system and enhanced responsiveness of other stress hormones when compared with non-type A personalities. Gout or hyperuricemia appears to be indirectly atherogenic, an effect most likely mediated through associated hypertension, hyperlipidemia, and obesity. Attempts at normalizing uric acid levels are rational and may alter the risk of cardiovascular disease.

Alcohol ingestion in small to moderate amounts (<40 g/d of pure ethanol) reduces the risk of coronary heart disease; however, consumption of large amounts (>50 g/d) or binge drinking of alcohol are associated with increased mortality from stroke, malignant neoplasms, and cirrhosis. The mechanisms for the presumed protective effects of alcohol are not known but the effects may be related to increased high-density lipoprotein levels, impaired platelet function, or associations between the amount of alcohol ingested and personality type. Whatever the relationship, it is well to remember that alcohol drinking is implicated in more than 40% of all fatal automobile accidents and consumption of alcohol predisposes to hepatic cirrhosis, the sixth to seventh most common cause of death in middle age in the United States. With this in mind, it seems illogical to suggest alcohol ingestion as a prophylactic measure for coronary disease but rather advise moderation of alcohol consumption, if it is the preference of the individual.

Thiazide diuretics have been shown to elevate serum cholesterol and triglyceride levels while β blockers tend to lower HDL and raise LDL slightly; however, a direct association between these drugs and cardiovascular risk is tenuous and based on aggregating results rather than randomized clinical trials. Conjugated equine strogen alone or in combination with a progestin lowers LDL and raises HDL based on the Postmenopausal Estrogen/Progestin Interventions (PEPI) study.[18] Unopposed estrogen is the optimal regimen for elevation of HDL, but the high rate of endometrial hyperplasia restricts use to women without a uterus. In women with a uterus, estrogen with cyclic medroxyprogesterone has the most favorable effect on HDL and no excess risk of endometrial hyperplasia. Oral contraceptives in smoking women over the age of 35 years increases the risk of myocardial infarction, stroke, and venous thromboembolism by threefold or higher. Alternative forms of contraception and cessation of smoking should be promoted in these patients. The risk for nonsmoking oral contraceptive users under the age of 35 is very small. Estrogens given to postmenopausal women do not appear to increase relative risk of death compared with nonusers; in particular, risk for users versus nonusers was 0.54 for gynecologically intact women, 0.34 for hysterectomized women, 0.12 for bilaterally oophorectomized women, and 0.37 overall.[19] Others, however, have shown postmenopausal use to be associated with either increased or decreased risk for death from cardiovascular events, and the use of postmenopausal estrogens remains controversial.[20,21] Recent conflicting studies have raised concern about the risk of breast cancer with estrogen use with or without progestins.[22–24] While this issue remains unresolved, the benefit of estrogen may outweigh the risk and the results of the Women's Health Initative study are needed before firm recommendations can be made.[24] Coffee consumption has also been linked to coronary heart disease and caffeine does transiently elevate blood pressure, however, the overall risk, if any, appears to be low.[25] Although thiazide diuretics and β blockers (nonselective without intrinsic sympathomimetic activity) may elevate both cholesterol and triglycerides by some 10–20%, and these effects may be detrimental, no objective evidence exists from prospective well-controlled studies to support avoiding these drugs at this time. This controversy is most pertinent in the treatment of mild hypertension and it is discussed in greater detail in Chapter 12.

PHARMACOLOGIC MANAGEMENT

Placebo Effect

Historically, about 30% of anginal syndrome symptoms have responded regardless of which therapy was instituted. Examples of these placebo responses include drug therapies such as xanthines and khellin, as well as surgical procedures such as ligation of the internal mammary artery. These observations stem from two problems inherent in clinical trials undertaken to assess the efficacy of any therapy for angina: (1) adequate trial design incorporating appropriate controls and washout periods, and (2) assessment of treatment effects utilizing objective measures of efficacy including improvement in exercise performance, resting and ambulatory ECG improvement in ischemic changes, or other objective tests to address other aspects of myocardial function or metabolism. The use of pain episode frequency and nitroglycerin consumption are subjective and their use as sole measures of efficacy should be avoided. Objective assessment using ETT has shown placebo does not provide improvement in patients with exertional angina, substantiating this as a valid means to assess efficacy.[26]

Nitrate Therapy

Nitroglycerin has a well-documented role in the alleviation of anginal attacks when used as rapidly absorbed and readily available preparations by the oral and intravenous routes. Sublingual, buccal, or spray products would be the products of choice for this indication. Prevention of symptoms may be accomplished by the prophylactic use of oral or transdermal products; however, recent concern has been expressed over the long-term efficacy of many of these preparations due to the development of tolerance.

Nitrates have multiple potential mechanisms of action and for a given patient it is not always clear which of these is most important.[27] In general, the major action appears to be indirectly mediated through a reduction of myocardial oxygen demand secondary to venodilation and arterial–arteriolar dilation, leading to a reduction in wall stress from reduced ventricular volume and pressure (Table 14.9). Systemic venodilation also promotes increased flow to deep myocardial muscle by reducing the gradient between intraventricular pressure and coronary arteriolar (R_2) pressure. Direct actions on the coronary circulation include dilation of large and small intramural coronary arteries, collateral dilation, coronary artery stenosis dilation, abolition of normal tone in narrowed vessels, and relief of spasm; these actions occur even if the endothelium is denuded or dysfunctional. It is likely that, depending on the underlying pathophysiology, different mechanisms become operative. For example, in the presence of a 60–70% stenosis, venodilation and MVO_2 reduction are most important; however, with higher grade lesions, direct

TABLE 14.9. EFFECT OF DRUG THERAPY ON MYOCARDIAL OXYGEN DEMAND[a]

			LV Wall Tension	
	Heart Rate	**Myocardial Contractility**	**Systolic Pressure**	**LV Volume**
Nitrates	↑	0	↓	↓↓
β Blockers	↓↓	↓	↓	↑
Nifedipine	↑	0 or ↓	↓↓	0 or ↓
Verapamil	↓	↓	↓	0 or ↓
Diltiazem	↓↓	0 or ↓	↓	0 or ↓

Key: LV, left ventricular.
[a]Calcium channel antagonists and nitrates may also increase myocardial oxygen supply through coronary vasodilation. Diastolic function may also be improved with verapamil, nifedipine, and, perhaps, diltiazem. These effects may vary from those indicated in the table depending on individual patient baseline hemodynamics.

effects on the coronary circulation and vessel tone are the predominant effects. Although the cellular mechanism of vasodilation by nitrates is not entirely understood, organic nitrates are converted intracellularly to nitric oxide (EDRF) and 5-nitrosothiol via interaction with sulfhydryl groups. Nitric oxide and perhaps 5-nitrosothiol activate soluble guanylate cyclase to increase intracellular concentrations of cyclic GMP. Increased cyclic GMP induces a sequence of protein phosphorylation associated with reduced intracellular calcium release from the sarcoplasmic reticulum or reduced permeability to extracellular calcium and, consequently, smooth muscle relaxation.[28]

Pharmacokinetic characteristics common to the organic nitrates used for angina include a large first-pass effect of hepatic metabolism, short to very short half-lives (except for isosorbide mononitrate), large volumes of distribution, high clearance rates, and large interindividual variations in plasma or blood concentrations.[29] Pharmacodynamic–pharmacokinetic relationships for the entire class remain poorly defined, presumably due to methodologic difficulty in characterizing the parent drug and metabolite concentrations at or within vascular smooth muscle and secondary to counterregulatory or adaptive mechanisms from the drug's effects as well as the occurrence of tolerance. Nitroglycerin is extracted by a variety of tissues and metabolized locally; differential extraction and metabolite generation occur depending on the tissue site. There are also numerous technical problems limiting the generation of reliable pharmacokinetic parameter estimates including the following: assay sensitivity; arterial–venous extraction gradients and, therefore, extrahepatic metabolism; *in vitro* degradation; drug adsorption to polyvinyl chloride tubing and syringes; potentially saturable metabolism; accumulation of metabolites (some of which are active) with multiple doses; postural and exercise-induced changes in pharmacokinetics; a variety of variables associated with transdermal delivery including the delivery system (matrix, membrane-limited, ointment), vehicle used, the surface area and thickness of application, the site application, and other skin variables (temperature, moisture content, etc.).

Nitroglycerin concentrations are affected by the route of administration. The highest concentrations are usually obtained with intravenous administration, and the lowest are seen with lower oral doses. Peak concentrations with sublingual nitroglycerin appear within 2–4 minutes with the oral route producing peaks at about 15–30 minutes and by the transdermal route at 1–2 hours. The half-life of nitroglycerin is 1–5 minutes regardless of route, hence the potential advantage of sustained-release and transdermal products. Transdermal nitroglycerin does produce sufficient concentrations for acute hemodynamic effects to occur and these concentrations are maintained for long intervals; however, the hemodynamic and antianginal effects are minimal after 1 week or less on chronic, continuous (i.e., 24 hours per day) therapy.

Isosorbide dinitrate (ISDN) is metabolized to isosorbide 2 mono- and 5-mononitrate (isosorbide mononitrate, ISMN). ISMN has a half-life of about 5 hours and may be given once or twice daily depending on the product chosen. Multiple, larger doses of ISDN lead to disproportionate increases in the area under the plasma time profile, suggesting that metabolic pathways are being saturated or that metabolite accumulation may influence the disposition of ISDN. Little pharmacokinetic information is available for other nitrate compounds.

Nitrate therapy may be used to terminate an acute anginal attack, prevent effort- or stress-induced attacks, or for long-term prophylaxis. Sublingual nitroglycerin 0.3–0.4 mg will relieve pain in about 75% of patients within 3 minutes with another 15% becoming pain free in 5–15 minutes. Pain persisting beyond about 20–30 minutes following the use of two or three nitroglycerin tablets is suggestive of evolving myocardial infarction or unstable angina and the patient should be instructed to seek emergency aid. Patients should be instructed to keep nitroglycerin in the original, tightly closed glass container and to avoid mixing with other medication, which may reduce nitroglycerin adsorption and vaporization. Additional counseling should include the facts that nitroglycerin is not an analgesic but rather it partially corrects the underlying problem and that repeated use is not harmful or addicting. Patients should also be aware that enhanced venous pooling in the sitting or standing positions may improve the effect as well as the symptoms of postural hypotension, and that inadequate saliva may slow or prevent tablet disintegration and dissolution. An acceptable albeit expensive alternative is lingual spray, which may be more convenient and has a shelf-life of 3 years compared with 6 months or so for some forms of nitroglycerin tablets.

Chewable, oral and transdermal products are acceptable for the long-term prophylaxis of angina; however, considerable controversy surrounds their use and it appears that the development of tolerance or adaptive mechanisms limits the efficacy of all chronic nitrate therapies regardless of route (Table 14.10). Dosing of the longer acting preparations should be adjusted to provide a hemodynamic response. As an example, this may require doses of oral ISDN ranging from 10–60 mg as often as every 3–4 hours due to tolerance or first-pass metabolism, and similar large doses are required for other products. Nitroglycerin ointment seems to have a duration of up to 6 hours, but it is difficult to apply in a cosmetically acceptable fashion over a consistent surface area and response varies depending on the epidermal thickness, vascularity, and the amount of hair. Percutaneous adsorption of nitroglycerin ointment may occur unintentionally if someone other than the patient applies the ointment and limiting exposure through the use of gloves or some other means is advisable. Peripheral edema may also impair the response to nitroglycerin as venodilation cannot increase capacitance to a maximum and pooling may be reduced. Transdermal patch delivery systems were approved on the basis of sustained

TABLE 14.10. NITRATE PRODUCTS

Product	Onset (min)	Duration (min/h)	Initial Dose
Nitroglycerin			
IV	1–2	3–5	5 μg/min
SL/lingual	1–3	30–60	0.3 mg
PO	40	3–6	2.5–9 mg TID
Ointment	20–60	2–8	0.5–1 inch
Patch	40–60	>8	1 patch
Erythritol tetranitrate	5–30	4–6	5–10 mg TID
Penterythritol tetranitrate	30	4–8	10–20 mg TID
Isosorbide dinitrate			
SL/chewable	2–5	1–2	2.5–5 mg TID
PO	20–40	4–6	5–20 mg TID
Isosorbide mononitrate	30–60	6–8	20 mg QD, BID[a]

[a]Product dependent.

and equivalent plasma concentrations to other forms of therapy. Trials required by the Food and Drug Administration using transdermal patches as a continuous 24-hour delivery system revealed a lack of efficacy for improved exercise tolerance. Subsequently, a large, randomized, double-blind, placebo-controlled trial of intermittent (12 hours on; 12 hours off) transdermal nitroglycerin therapy in chronic stable angina demonstrated modest but significant improvement in exercise time after 4 weeks for the highest doses at 8 hours after patch placement.[30] Subjective assessment methods for nitrate effects include reduction in the number of painful episodes and the amount of nitroglycerin consumed. Objective assessment includes the resolution of ECG changes at rest, during exercise, or with ambulatory ECG monitoring. Because nitrates work primarily through a reduction in MVO_2, the double product can be used to optimize the dose of sublingual and oral nitrate products. It is important to realize that reflex tachycardia may offset the beneficial reduction in systolic blood pressure and calculation of the observed changes is necessary. The double product is best assessed in the sitting position and at intervals of 5–10 minutes and 30–60 minutes following sublingual and oral therapy, respectively. Due to the placebo effect, the unpredictable and variable course of angina, numerous pharmacologic effects of nitroglycerin, diurnal variation in pain patterns, stringent investigative protocols, and interindividual sensitivity to nitroglycerin, assessment with transdermal and sustained-release products is difficult. ETT provides valuable information concerning efficacy and mechanism of action for nitrates but its use is usually reserved for clinical investigation rather than routine patient care. Most ETT studies have shown nitrates to delay the onset of ischemia (ST-segment changes or initial chest discomfort) at submaximal exercise but the threshold for maximal exercise is unaltered, which suggests a reduction in oxygen demand rather than an improved oxygen supply. More sophisticated studies of myocardial function such as wall motion abnormalities and myocardial metabolism could be used to document efficacy; however, these studies are generally only for investigative purposes.

Adverse effects of nitrates are related most commonly to an extension of their pharmacologic effects and include postural hypotension with associated central nervous system symptoms, headaches and flushing secondary to vasodilation, and occasional nausea from smooth muscle relaxation. If hypotension is excessive, coronary filling may be compromised and myocardial infarction can result as well as underfilling of the cerebral circulation and stroke. While reflex tachycardia is most common, bradycardia with nitroglycerin has been reported. Other noncardiovascular adverse effects include rash with all products but particularly with transdermal nitroglycerin, the production of methemoglobinemia with high doses given for extended periods, and measurable concentrations of ethanol (intoxication has been reported) and propylene glycol (found in the diluent) with intravenous nitroglycerin.

Tolerance with nitrate therapy was first described by Brunton[3] with the initial experience using amyl nitrate for angina and later widely recognized in munition workers who underwent withdrawal reactions during periods of absence from exposure. Tolerance to nitrates is associated with a reduction in tissue cyclic GMP, which results from decreased production (guanylate cyclase) and increased breakdown via cyclic GMP-phosphodiesterase.[27,28] One proposed mechanism for the lack of cyclic GMP is lack of conversion of organic nitrates to nitric oxide due to depletion of intracellular sulfhydryl cofactors (cysteine) in cells following chronic exposure to nitrates. This effect is more pronounced on the venous system than the arterial system. Activation of neurohormonal systems following vasodilation with nitrates may result in vasoconstriction and sodium retention. The major systems thought to be involved in this second mechanism are the sympathoadrenal axis and the renin–angiotensin system. Lastly, nitroglycerin administration is accompanied by a fall in hematocrit (due to hemodilution rather than renal water conservation), and intravascular volume expansion, minimizing the ability of nitrates to decrease ventricular filling pressures, may be a third mechanism of tolerance. Most of the published information from controlled trials examining nitrate tolerance have been done with either ISDN or transdermal nitroglycerin, and these studies demonstrate the development of tolerance within as little as 24 hours of therapy. While the onset of tolerance is rapid, the offset may be just as rapid, and one alternative dosing strategy to circumvent or minimize tolerance is to provide a daily nitrate-free interval of 6–8 hours. Studies with a variety of nitrate preparations and dosing schedules demonstrate that this approach is useful and the nitrate-free interval should be a minimum of 8 hours and perhaps 12 hours for even better effects. ISDN, for example, should not be used more often than three times per day if tolerance is to be avoided. Other strategies that have been used to circumvent tolerance include supplying sulfhydryl groups though the administration of acetylcysteine and methionine. This should allow nitrates to be converted to nitric oxide, and studies supporting and refuting this approach have appeared in the literature. Other approaches include interfering with the renin–angiotensin system by the use of angiotensin-converting enzyme (ACE) inhibitors that contain sulfhydryl groups and bradykinin accumulation seen with ACE inhibitors stimulates nitric oxide synthesis. Minimizing volume expansion with diuretics is another approach. ACE inhibition with both captopril and enalapril have been reported to work, but this has not been consistently reported in all studies. Diuretics do not routinely prevent the development of tolerance. Interestingly, hemodynamic tolerance does not always coincide with antianginal efficacy, but this is not well studied.

Nitrates may be combined with other drugs for anginal therapy including β-adrenergic blocking agents and calcium channel antagonists.[31] These combinations are usually instituted for chronic prophylactic therapy based on complimentary or offsetting mechanisms of action (Table 14.9). Combination therapy is generally used in patients with more severe symptoms not responding to nitrates alone (nitrates plus β blockers or calcium blockers) and in patients having an element of vasospasm leading to decreased supply (nitrates plus calcium blockers).

β-Adrenergic Blocking Agents

Decreased heart rate, decreased contractility, and a slight to moderate decrease in blood pressure with β-adrenergic receptor antagonism reduce MVO_2. The predominant receptor type in the heart is the β_1 receptor, and competitive blockade minimizes the influence of endogenous catecholamines on the chronotropic and inotropic state of the myocardium. These beneficial effects may be countered to some measure with increased ventricular volume and ejection time seen with β blockade; however, the overall effect of β blockers in patients with effort-induced angina is a reduction in oxygen demand. The β blockers do not improve oxygen supply and, in certain instances, unopposed α-adrenergic stimulation following the use of β blockers may lead to coronary vasoconstriction. For patients with chronic exertional stable angina, β blockers improve symptoms about 80% of the time and objective measures of efficacy demonstrate improved exercise duration and delay in the time at which ST-segment changes and initial or limiting symptoms occur. Beta blockers do not alter the rate pressure product (double product) for maximal exercise, therefore substantiating reduced demand rather than improved supply as the major consequence of their actions. Reflex tachycardia from nitrate therapy can be blunted with β-blocker therapy, making this a common and useful combination. Some patients with preexisting LV dysfunction who would be prone to heart failure may receive digitalis glycosides to maintain cardiac output if β blockade is necessary for IHD. Although β blockade may decrease exercise capacity in healthy individuals or in patients with hypertension, it may allow angina patients previously limited by symptoms to perform more exercise and ultimately improve overall cardiovascular performance through a training effect.[32]

Pertinent pharmacokinetics for the β blockers include half-life and route elimination, which are reviewed in Chapter 12. Drugs with longer half-lives need to be dosed less frequently than ones with shorter half-lives; however, disparity exists between half-life and duration of action for several β blockers (e.g., metoprolol) and this may reflect attenuation of the central nervous system mediated effects on the sympathetic system as well as the direct effects of this category on heart rate and contractility. Renal and hepatic dysfunction can affect the disposition of β blockers, but these agents are dosed to effect, either hemodynamic or symptomatic, and route of elimination is not a major consideration in drug selection.

Guidelines for the use of β blockers in treating angina would include the objective of lowering resting heart rate to 50 to 60 beats per minute and limiting maximal exercise heart rate to about 100 beats per minute or less. It has also been suggested that exercise heart rate should be no more than about 20 beats per minute or a 10% increment over resting heart rate with modest exercise. Because β blockade is competitive and circulating catecholamine concentrations vary depending on the intensity of exercise and other factors, and cholinergic tone may be important in controlling heart rate in some patients, these guidelines are general in nature. These effects are generally dose- and plasma concentration-related and for propranolol, plasma concentrations of 30 ng/mL are needed for a 25% reduction of anginal frequency. Initial doses of β blockers should be at the lower end of the usual dosing range and titrated to response as indicated above.

There is little evidence to suggest superiority of any β blocker; however, the duration of β blockade is dependent partially on the half-life of the agent used, and those with longer half-lives may be dosed less frequently.[33–35] Of note, propranolol may be dosed twice a day in most patients with angina and the efficacy is similar to that seen with more frequent dosing. The ancillary property of membrane stabilizing activity is irrelevant in the treatment of angina, and intrinsic sympathomimetic activity appears to be detrimental in patients with rest or severe angina because the reduction in heart rate would be minimized, therefore limiting a reduction in MVO_2.[36] Cardioselective β blockers may be used in some patients to minimize adverse effects such as bronchospasm in asthmatic or chronic obstructive pulmonary disease patients, intermittent claudication, and sexual dysfunction. It should be remembered that cardioselectivity is a relative property and the use of larger doses (e.g., metoprolol 200 mg/d) is associated with the loss of selectivity and adverse effects. Post-acute-MI patients with angina are particularly good candidates for β blockade because both anginal symptoms may be treated as well as reducing the risk of post-MI reinfarction, and mortality has been demonstrated with timolol, propranolol, and metoprolol (see Chapter 15, Acute Myocardial Infarction). Combined β (nonselective) and α blockade with labetolol may be useful in some patients with marginal LV reserve, and fewer deleterious effects are seen when compared with other β blockers on coronary blood flow.

Extension of pharmacologic effect is the underlying reason for many of the adverse effects seen with β blockade. Hypotension, heart failure, bradycardia and heart block, bronchospasm, peripheral vasoconstriction and intermittent claudication, and altered glucose metabolism are directly related to β-adrenoreceptor antagonism. Patients with preexisting LV dysfunction and the use of other negative inotropic agents are most prone to developing overt heart failure; in the absence of these, heart failure is uncommon (less than 5%). Other drugs that depress conduction are additive to β blockade, and intrinsic conduction system disease predisposes the patient to conduction abnormalities. Altered glucose metabolism is most likely to be seen in insulin-dependent diabetics and β blockade obscures the symptom of hypoglycemia except for sweating. Beta blockers may also aggravate the lipid abnormalities seen in patients with diabetes. One of the more common reasons for discontinuation of β-blocker therapy is related to central nervous system adverse effects of fatigue, malaise, and depression. Although some suggest these effects may be avoided or minimized by the use of hydrophilic rather than lipophilic β-blocking agents, recent evidence suggests differential use may not be possible.[37] In a review of prescription use, Avorn et al.[38] found antidepressants more commonly used in patients receiving β blockers with a relative risk of 1.5 to 2 regardless of the type of β blocker used. Abrupt withdrawal of β-blocker therapy in patients with angina has been associated with increased severity and number of pain episodes and myocardial infarction. The mechanism of this effect is unknown but may be related to increased receptor sensitivity or disease progression during therapy, which becomes apparent following discontinuation of β blockade. In any event, tapering of β-blocker therapy over about 2 days should minimize the risk of withdrawal reactions for those patients in whom therapy is being discontinued.

Beta-adrenoreceptor blockade is effective in chronic exertional angina as monotherapy and in combination with nitrates and/or calcium channel antagonists. Following the institution of nitrate therapy, β blockers are frequently the second line of therapy for patients with inadequate control of symptoms. This is justified based on the pharmacologic interaction between these two classes of drugs, the cost of therapy, and the tolerability of β blockers. Patients with severe angina, rest angina, or variant angina may be better treated with nitrates and, increasingly, calcium channel blockers.[39]

Calcium Channel Antagonists

Modulation of calcium entry into vascular smooth muscle and myocardium as well as a variety of other tissues is the principal action of the calcium antagonists. The cellular mechanism of these drugs is not completely understood and it differs among the available classes of the phenylalkylamines (verapamil-like), dihydropyridines (nifedipine-like), benzothiazepines (diltiazem-like), and bepridil. Receptor-operated channels stimulated by norepinephrine and other neurotransmittors, and potential-dependent channels activated by membrane depolarization control the entry of calcium, and consequently the cytosolic concentration of calcium responsible for activation of actin-myosin complex leading to contraction of vascular smooth muscle and myocardium. In the myocardium, calcium entry triggers the release of intracellular stores of calcium to increase cytosolic calcium, whereas in smooth muscle calcium derived from the extracellular fluid may do this directly. Binding proteins within the cell, calmodulin and troponin, after binding with calcium participate in phosphorylation reactions leading to contraction. Decreased calcium availability, through the actions of calcium antagonists, inhibits these reactions.

Direct actions of the calcium antagonists include vasodilation of systemic arterioles and coronary arteries leading to a reduction of arterial pressure and coronary vascular resistance as well as depression of the myocardial contractility and conduction velocity of the sinoatrial and atrioventricular nodes (see Chapter 16, Arrhythmias). Reflex β-adrenergic stimulation overcomes much of the negative inotropic effect and depression of contractility becomes clinically apparent only in the presence of LV dysfunction and when other negative inotropic drugs are used concurrently. Verapamil and diltiazem cause less peripheral vasodilation than nifedipine and, consequently, the risk of myocardial depression is greater with these two agents. Conduction through the AV node is predictably depressed with verapamil and to some extent with diltiazem, and they must be used with caution in patients with preexisting conduction abnormalities or in the presence of other drugs with negative chronotropic properties. Bepridil, in addition to having calcium channel-blocking properties, also has class I and III antiarrhythmic activity. MVO_2 is reduced with all of the calcium channel antagonists because of reduced wall tension secondary to reduced arterial pressure and, to a minor extent, depressed contractility (Table 14.9). Heart rate changes are dependent on the drug used and the state of the conduction system. Nifedipine generally increases heart rate or causes no change while either no change or decreased heart rate is seen with verapamil and diltiazem because of the interaction of these direct and indirect effects. In contrast to the β blockers, calcium channel antagonists have the potential to improve coronary blood flow through areas of fixed coronary obstruction and by inhibiting coronary artery vasomotion and vasospasm. Beneficial redistribution of blood flow from well-perfused myocardium to ischemic areas and from epicardium to endocardium may also contribute to improvement in ischemic symptoms. Overall, the benefit provided by calcium channel antagonists is related to reduced MVO_2 rather than improved oxygen supply based on lack of alteration in the rate pressure product at maximal exercise in most studies performed to date. However, as coronary artery disease progresses and vasospasm becomes superimposed on critical stenotic lesions, improved oxygen supply through coronary vasodilation may become more important.

The absorption of the three available calcium channel antagonists is characterized by excellent absorption and large, variable first-pass metabolism resulting in oral bioavailability ranging from about 20–50% or greater.[40] Saturation of this effect may occur with verapamil and diltiazem, resulting in greater amounts of drug being absorbed with chronic dosing. Nifedipine may have slow or fast absorption patterns and the ingestion of food delays and impairs its absorption as well as potential enhanced absorption in elderly patients. This variability in absorption produces fluctuation in the hemodynamic response with nifedipine. Sublingual nifedipine is frequently used to provide a more rapid response; however, the rationale for this application is suspect because little nifedipine is absorbed from the buccal mucosa and the swallowed drug is responsible for the observed plasma concentrations. Absorption of verapamil in sustained-release products may be influenced by food, and when used in the fasted state, dose dumping may occur resulting in high peak concentrations with some products. The approved sustained-release products for nifedipine, verapamil, and diltiazem are approved primarily for the treatment of hypertension (see Chapter 12). The presence of severe liver disease (e.g., alcoholic liver disease with cirrhosis) has been shown to reduce the first-pass metabolism of verapamil, and this shunting of drug around the liver gives rise to higher plasma concentrations and lower dose requirements in these patients. Interestingly, this effect appears to be stereoselective for the more active isomer of verapamil. Verapamil may also reduce liver blood flow; however, evidence for this reduction is based primarily on animal experiments. Few data are available regarding the influence of liver disease on the kinetics of nifedipine or diltiazem. These three drugs undergo extensive hepatic metabolism with little unchanged drug being renally excreted. Nifedipine has no active metabolites whereas norverapamil possesses 20% or less activity of the parent compound. Desacetyldiltiazem has not been studied in man but canine studies suggest its potency ranges from 100–40% of the parent compound for various cardiovascular effects; the clinical importance of these observations remains to be determined. With chronic dosing of verapamil and diltiazem, apparent saturation of metabolism occurs, producing higher plasma concentrations of each drug than those seen with single-dose administration. Consequently, the elimination half-life for verapamil is prolonged, and less frequent dosing intervals may be used in some patients. The elimination half-life for diltiazem is also somewhat prolonged and the half-life of desacetyldiltiazem is longer than the parent drug, but it is not clear if less frequent dosing may be used. Bepridil also undergoes hepatic elimination and an active metabolite, 4-hydroxyphenyl bepridil, is produced; the parent compound has a long half-life of 30–40 hours. Nifedipine does not accumulate with chronic dosing; however, it is eliminated via oxidative pathways that may be polymorphic, and slow and fast metabolizers have been described for nifedipine. Because oxidative pathways are important for the elimination of these drugs, inhibition or induction by drugs such as cimetidine or rifampin can alter the kinetics and pharmacodynamic response. Conversely, inhibition of hepatic microsomal drug metabolism by diltiazem and verapamil has been demonstrated and interactions with drugs (i.e., theophylline) eliminated through oxidation may be expected. Renal insufficiency has little or no effect on the pharmacokinetics of these three drugs. Although disease alterations in kinetics have been described, the most important quantitative alteration is the influence of liver disease on bioavailability and elimination. Aging has been shown to reduce the clearance of verapamil and diltiazem and dosing in this population should be done with caution. Altered protein binding due to renal disease, decreased protein concentration or increased α_1-acid glycoprotein has been noted, but the clinical import of these changes is unknown.

Management of Stable Exertional Angina Pectoris[12,16,41,43]

After assessing and manipulating the alterable risk factors as discussed previously, the next intervention that could be undertaken is the institution of a regular exercise program. Training is possible in many patients with angina and the observed benefits include decreased heart rate and systolic blood pressure as well as increased ejection fraction and duration of exercise. Although the mechanism of these effects has been debated, improved overall cardiovascular and muscular condition are probably most important. Obviously, an exercise program should be undertaken with caution and in a graded fashion with adequate supervision.

Nitrate therapy should be the first step in managing acute attacks for patients with chronic stable angina. The frequency of therapy depends on the number of episodes of chest pain reported by the patient. In general, if angina occurs no more often than once every few days, then sublingual nitroglycerin or the spray or buccal products may be sufficient to allow the patient to maintain an adequate lifestyle. For episodes of "first-effort" angina occurring in a predictable fashion, nitroglycerin may be used in a prophylactic manner with the patient taking 0.3–0.4 mg sublingually about 5 minutes prior to the anticipated time of activity. Nitroglycerin spray may be useful when inadequate saliva is produced to rapidly dissolve SL nitroglycerin or if a patient has difficulty opening the container. Most patients have a response that lasts about 30 minutes or so, but this is subject to interindividual variability. Obtaining the appropriate dose for a particular patient can be facilitated by the use of the double product to assess the hemodynamic effect of nitroglycerin. Patient-specific situations may dictate the use of other therapy that may benefit IHD, for example, a β blocker for hypertension, and angina may be improved with this intervention; however, most authorities recommend nitrates as the initial therapy of choice.

When angina occurs more frequently than once a day, a chronic prophylactic regimen using nitrates or β blockers should be considered. Chronic prophylactic therapy with long-acting forms of nitroglycerin (oral or transdermal), isosorbide dinitrate, 5-mononitrate, and pentaerythritol trinitrate may be effective; however, the development of tolerance is a major limiting step in their continued effectiveness. As described previously, providing a nitrate-free interval of 8 hours per day or longer appears to be the most promising approach to maintaining the efficacy of chronic nitrate therapy. Oral administration of nitrates is susceptible to a saturable first-pass effect; therefore, larger doses can produce a measurable hemodynamic effect and dose titration should be based on these changes in the double product. There are few well-controlled studies comparing oral or sublingual nitrate efficacy and the choice among these products should be based on familiarity with the preparation, cost, and patient acceptance.

Chronic prophylactic therapy for patients with more than one angina episode per day may also be instituted with β-adrenergic blocking agents and in many instances β blockers may be preferable because of less frequent dosing and other properties inherent in β blockade (e.g., potential cardioprotective effects, antiarrhythmic effects, lack of tolerance, and antihypertensive effects, as well as their antianginal effects). Patients who continue to smoke have reduced antianginal efficacy of β blockers and this may be due to enhanced hepatic metabolism of drugs that are eliminated through this route or related to the effects of smoking on MVo_2 and oxygenation. As discussed previously, ancillary properties such as cardioselectivity are useful in patients with concurrent problems, but these properties do not contribute to the antianginal efficacy of β blockers. The one characteristic that is relevant is the duration of effect on the double product. In normal volunteers nadolol produces a reduction in double product for a longer period compared with several other β blockers, however, the intensity of effect (maximal effect) was similar among the drugs tested and related to dose. In patients with angina, Jones and Mir[35] compared nadolol, atenolol, and propranolol (regular and sustained release) on exercise duration. Nadolol increased exercise duration to the greatest extent in the doses that were used in this study and no difference was noted between the efficacy of the two propranolol preparations. In contrast to these studies, other investigators have not detected any significant differences among β blockers for the treatment of chronic stable angina.[34] The choice of β blocker for angina rests on choosing the appropriate dose to achieve the goals outlined for heart rate and double product, and choosing an agent that is well tolerated by individual patients and cost. Selective use may incorporate ancillary properties but these are secondary considerations in overall drug product selection. Patients most likely to respond well to β blockade are those who have a high resting heart rate and those having a relatively fixed anginal threshold. In other words, their symptoms appear at the same level of exercise or workload on a consistent basis. Symptoms appearing with variable workloads suggest fluctuations in myocardial oxygen supply, perhaps due to coronary artery vasomotion, and these patients are more likely to respond to calcium channel antagonists.[41]

Calcium channel antagonists have the potential advantage of improving coronary blood flow through coronary artery vasodilation as well as decreasing MVo_2, and may be used instead of β blockers for chronic prophylactic therapy. They are as effective as β blockers and are most useful in patients who have a variable threshold for exertional angina. Calcium antagonists may provide better skeletal muscle oxygenation, resulting in decreased fatigue and better exercise tolerance. Additionally, if contraindications exist to β-blocker therapy, calcium antagonists can be safely used in many patients. Nifedipine, verapamil, and diltiazem have similar efficacy in the management of chronic stable angina. Differences in their electrophysiology, peripheral and central hemodynamic effects, and adverse effect profiles are useful in selecting the appropriate agent. Patients with conduction abnormalities and moderate to severe LV dysfunction (ejection fraction <35%) should be treated cautiously with verapamil while nifedipine may be safely used in many of these patients. Diltiazem has significant effects on the AV node and can produce heart block in patients with preexisting conduction disease or when other drugs, such as digoxin or β blockers, with effects on conduction are used concurrently. Nifedipine may cause excessive heart rate elevation, especially if the patient is not receiving a β blocker, and this may offset the beneficial effect it has on MVo_2. Gingival hyperplasia has also been reported with nifedipine and some dental authorities say this may be seen in as many as 20% of patients on nifedipine. Bepridil prolongs the QT interval in certain patients (hypokalemia, elderly, preexisting QT interval prolongation) and because of this potential proarrhythmic effect, it is indicated only in patients who have been inadequately controlled with other antianginal therapy. The hemodynamic effect of calcium antagonists is complimentary to β blockade and, consequently, combination therapy is rational.

Studies examining combination therapy have shown that calcium channel blockers when used with β blockers provide objective evidence of improvement by increasing exercise duration and decreasing ECG evidence of ischemia. The addition of a calcium antagonist to β-blocker therapy may be more useful than the addition of nitrates considering exercise duration, and changes in global and regional ejection fraction in ischemic and nonischemic myocardium. Because both β blockers and calcium antagonists have the potential for depressing contractility, this combination should be used with care in patients with poor ventricular function; however, in well-preserved ventricular function, the combination is well tolerated.

MANAGEMENT OF UNSTABLE ANGINA PECTORIS[16]

Clinical and autopsy studies indicate that most patients who present with unstable angina or acute myocardial infarction have significant underlying coronary atherosclerosis. Precipitation of these acute ischemic syndromes are thought to be due to progression of atherosclerosis, acute coronary thrombosis, coronary artery spasm, and platelet aggregation.[16] The interrelationship of these mechanisms is outlined in Fig. 14.10. Potential points of intervention in these mechanisms by naturally occurring and pharmacologic means follow the presumed pathogenesis (Fig. 14.11). Patients at high risk of death or nonfatal MI are those presenting with prolonged ongoing (>20 minutes) rest pain, pulmonary edema related to ischemia, angina at rest with dynamic ST changes of ≥1 mm, angina with new or worsening mitral regurgitation, S_3 or rales, and angina with hypotension.[16] Unstable angina differs from stable angina in that the primary event is thought to be a reduction in coronary blood flow rather than an increase in MV_{O_2} with corresponding ischemic changes in the ECG occurring prior to changes in heart rate and blood pressure.

Initial management of the patient should include history, physical examination, electrocardiogram (within 20 minutes), bed rest with continuous monitoring for ischemia and arrhythmia detection, supplemental oxygen if cyanotic or hypoxemic, and immediate consideration of the use of aspirin, heparin, β blockers, and narcotics if pain is not relieved by nitrates and β blockers.[16] Since aspirin and heparin are used in AMI, their use is not contraindicated in unstable angina. Aspirin should be dosed at 160–325 mg and heparin is given as a bolus of 80 units/kg followed by a continuous infusion of 18 units/kg/h to maintain the activated partial thromboplastin time at 1.5–2.5 times control and continued for 2–5 days or until revascularization is performed. Based on anectodal observations, this dosing regimen for heparin may overdose very obese patients and these doses should be used with caution in the very obese patient. Acutely heparin may be useful to prevent further thrombosis formation and aspirin acutely and chronically inhibits platelet aggregation. The combination of heparin and nitroglycerin has been shown in earlier studies to result in heparin resistance and more than typical heparin doses may be needed, however, more recent information suggest this interaction is not significant.[44] Low molecular weight heparin (e.g., nadroparin) may be useful along with aspirin instead of unfractionated heparin.[45] Thrombolysis is not indicated in patients who do not have evidence of acute ST-segment elevation or left bundle branch block on ECG. Long-term antiplatelet therapy with aspirin has been unequivocally shown to reduce the occurrence of mortality and nonfatal infarction in unstable angina by about 50% in doses ranging from 324–1300 mg/d in two well-controlled studies.[46,47] The Canadian multicenter study[47] also examined the effect of sulfinpyrazone alone and in combination with aspirin and found no benefit from sulfinpyrazone. Ticlopidine (250 mg two times per day) may be considered in patients with aspirin hypersensitivity or recent major gastrointestinal bleeding.

If three doses of sublingual nitroglycerin do not relieve the patient's pain, then intravenous nitroglycerin

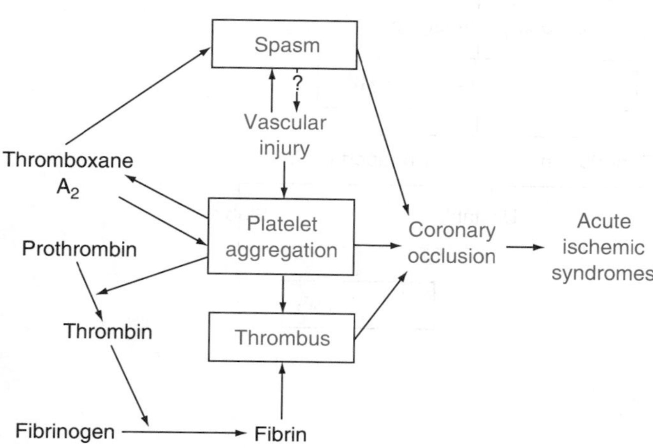

Figure 14.10. The interrelationship of dynamic mechanisms that may cause or contribute to the clinical presentation of acute ischemic syndromes. *(From Epstein SE, Palmeri ST. Mechanisms contributing to precipitation of unstable angina and acute myocardial infarction: Implications regarding therapy. Am J Cardiol 1984;54:1247, with permission.)*

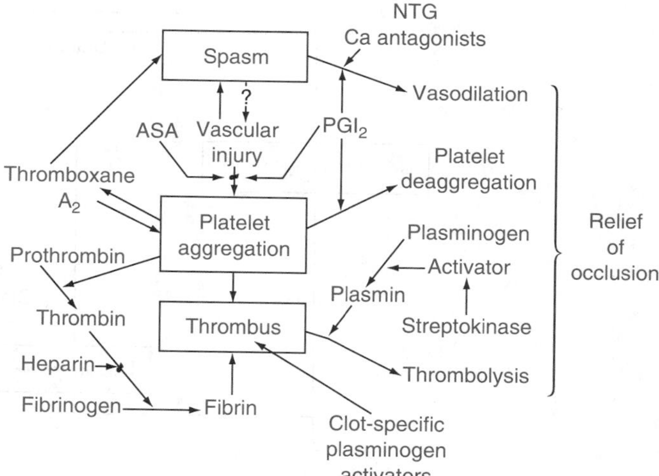

Figure 14.11. Several possible dynamic mechanisms that may cause acute ischemic syndromes, as well as naturally occurring mechanisms and pharmacologic interventions that may relieve the degree of coronary obstruction. ASA, acetylsalicylic acid; NTG, nitroglycerin. *(From Epstein SE, Palmeri ST. Mechanisms contributing to precipitation of unstable angina and acute myocardial infarction: Implications regarding therapy. Am J Cardiol 1984;54:1247, with permission.)*

provides a convenient method of titrating the dose and avoids uncertainty concerning drug delivery (Fig. 14.12). Dosing should be started low (5–10 μ/kg/min) and titrated upward by 10 μg/min every 5–10 minutes until symptoms are relieved or limiting adverse effects occur. A reduction in systolic blood pressure is expected and should be about 15 mm Hg or to a systolic pressure of 100–110 mm Hg. Caution is necessary in preload-dependent patients (right ventricular infarct, hypovolemia, pericardial constriction or effusion) to avoid hypotension and decreased coronary perfusion pressure as well as excessive heart rate elevation if the patient is not receiving β blockers. After 24 hours free of symptoms, patients may be switched over to oral or topical nitrates.

Intravenous β blockers are recommended for high-risk patients (oral for intermediate- and low-risk patients) in the absence of contraindications. Regimens are similar to those used in AMI. Unstable patients with persisting or recurring pain while on nitrates and β blockers should receive a calcium antagonist. Beta blockers in unstable angina reduce the risk of progression to MI by 13% but have not been shown to reduce mortality.[16] Beta blockers do have strong evidence supporting their use in AMI and in post-MI patients and this is sufficient evidence to recommend their routine use. Beta-blocker therapy may prevent ischemia due to tachycardia and reduce cardiac work. Patients should be screened for contraindications to therapy (see Chapter 15, Acute Myocardial Infarction).

Several studies suggest efficacy of calcium channel blockers in unstable angina and their effects are mediated via inhibition of increased coronary tone and through reduction in MVo_2. Calcium antagonists may be added to nitrates and β blockers, and some authors suggest that they are most useful in combination with pretreatment β block-

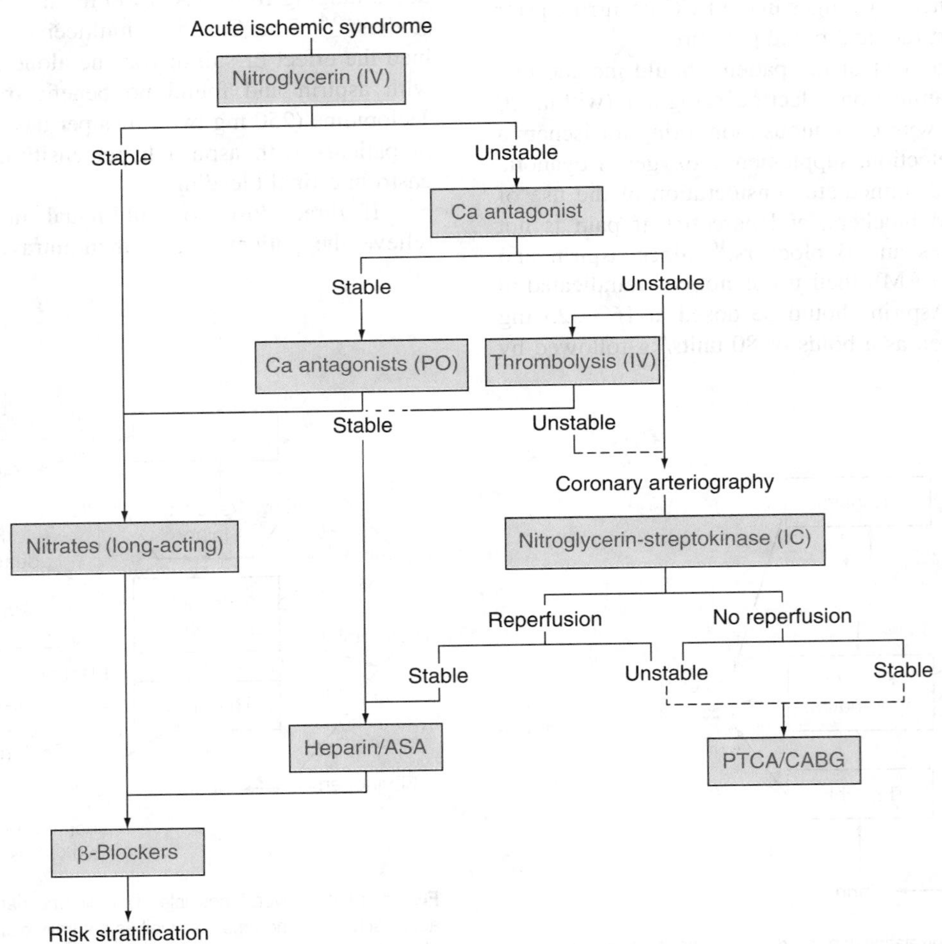

Figure 14.12. Therapeutic guidelines for managing patients who present with acute ischemic syndromes. ASA, acetylsalicylic acid; CABG, coronary artery bypass graft; IC, intracoronary; IV, intravenous; PO, orally; PTCA, percutaneous transluminal coronary angioplasty. *(From Epstein SE, Palmeri ST. Mechanisms contributing to precipitation of unstable angina and acute myocardial infarction: Implications regarding therapy. Am J Cardiol 1984;54:1250, with permission.)*

ade. ST-segment elevation appears to respond better than depression to calcium antagonism. Calcium channel blockers should be avoided in patients with pulmonary edema or evidence of left ventricular dysfunction. Nifedipine should not be used in the absence of concurrent β blockade. The largest randomized trial with nifedipine and metoprolol found metoprolol to be more effective than placebo while nifedipine increased the risk of MI and recurrent angina compared to placebo; the combination was no better than metoprolol alone.[48] Diltiazem may be more useful than other agents in the setting of unstable angina and non-Q-wave myocardial infarction because it has been shown to reduce reinfarction and refractory angina (see Chapter 15, Acute Myocardial Infarction).

Other interventions that have been shown to provide benefit in short-term studies include the prostanoids PGE_1 and prostacyclin. A search for reversible or initiating factors such as anemia, thyroid dysfunction, infection, tachyarrhythmias, or increasing heart failure should be undertaken and corrected.

Cardiac catheterization should be considered in the following groups of patients: (1) patients with prior angioplasty, bypass surgery, or MI; (2) patients who fail to stabilize on medical therapy; (3) patients opting for early invasive strategy [coronary artery bypass surgery (CABG) or percutaneous transluminal angioplasty (PTCA)]; (4) patients with high-risk clinical findings (described previously) or noninvasive test results; or (5) patients with significant congestive heart failure or left ventricular dysfunction.[16] CABG is recommended for patients found to have ≥50% occulsion of the left main artery or ≥70% three-vessel disease with depressed LV function (EF <0.50). Patients with two-vessel disease with proximal LAD stenosis ≥95% and depressed LV function should be referred promptly for CABG or PTCA. Patients with significant CAD who fail to stabilize on medical therapy or have symptoms with low levels of exertion or have ischemia accompanied by CHF should have prompt revascularization. In patients with significant CAD not falling into the categories described previously, early invasive or early conservative therapy may be chosen. Revascularization would then be performed only in medical failures in the early conservative therapy group.

If cardiac catheterization is not indicated, noninvasive exercise or pharmacologic stress testing should be performed in low- and intermediate-risk patients who have been free of angina and CHF for 48 hours. An exercise treadmill test should be used in patients with a normal ECG and not taking digoxin. Patients with significant resting ECG changes should be tested with an imaging modality. Those with physical limitations should undergo pharmacologic stress testing.

CABG can be safely performed in patients with unstable angina; however, results from the National Cooperative Unstable Angina Study Group show that early or late infarction is not significantly improved compared with medical therapy.[49] This study, which excluded patients with left main stenosis, suggests that most patients should receive intensive medical management initially; however, long term, about 36% of the medically treated patients crossed over to surgery due to inadequate symptom control. Those patients with a previous MI or hypertension, resting ST abnormalities, or greater than 3-mm ST segment depression on exercise are likely to fail maximal medical therapy (about 3%) and become candidates for surgery as well as those initially controlled with high-risk factors including left main stem stenosis, triple or proximal left anterior descending and right coronary stenoses. Additional candidates for surgery are patients with decreased left ventricular function, three vessel disease, and rest angina.

PTCA has been used successfully in the management of unstable angina.[50] This procedure involves the insertion of a guidewire and inflatable balloon into the affected coronary artery and enlarging the lumen of the artery by stretching the vessel wall. Unfortunately, this may cause atheroma plaque fracture by stretching inelastic components and denudation of the endothelium resulting in loss of EDRF.[28] Consequently, immediate vascular recoil, platelet adhesion and aggregation, mural thrombus formation, and smooth muscle proliferation and synthesis of extracellular matrix may give rise to acute occlusion and early or late restenosis.[51] The presence of coronary artery spasm and intraluminal thrombus, common occurrences in unstable angina, increases the hazard of these complications.[52] Patients best suited for PTCA are those with recent onset of worsening of angina without a long history of symptoms. Angiographic characteristics associated with these clinical findings that allow the greatest probability of success for PTCA are severe, discrete, proximal lesions found in a large epicardial vessel. Candidates for PTCA must also be suited for CABG because a small percentage of procedures results in emergency CABG. Following a period of stabilization, patients receive IV nitroglycerin with or without calcium channel blockers prior to the procedure, and follow-up treatment includes heparin acutely and warfarin chronically to prevent coronary thrombosis. Heparin has been shown to reduce the incidence of postprocedural vessel closure. Other methods have been tried recently to prevent post-PTCA late restenosis (see discussion later). Fish oil has not been as effective as anticipated in preventing reocclusion and does not seem to have a strong effect on regression of atherosclerosis.[52a,53] Initial patency rate is approximately 70% for single-vessel involvement in the hands of experienced operators; however, a restenosis rate of 15–30% or higher (e.g., variant angina) in selected patient populations remains a problem.

In the event of prolonged chest pain and ischemic ECG changes unrelieved by nitrate therapy or calcium channel antagonists, one may assume total occlusion of a coronary vessel and steps should be taken to restore blood flow. Thrombolytic therapy given by the intracoronary or intravenous route either alone or preceding PTCA has been shown in some centers to an effective management approach for unstable angina. Thrombolytic therapy for evolving myocardial infarction is further described in Chapter 15. Intra-aortic balloon counterpulsation is a mechanical assistance device introduced into the femoral artery and advanced to the thoracic aorta. The balloon is triggered by the patient's R wave to inflate in diastole and deflate at the onset of systole, which provides the hemodynamic effects of decreasing systemic vascular resistance and increasing diastolic pressure to improve coronary artery blood flow. Although the balloon pump appears to be effective in patients resistant to medical therapy, this device has a high rate of complications including thromboembolic episodes and ischemia of lower limbs, and few properly controlled trials exist to evaluate its role in therapy. One prospective randomized trial comparing intravenous nitrate therapy and counterpulsation found no difference in symptom control or mortality.[53a]

Coronary Artery Spasm and Variant Angina Pectoris[54]

Prinzmetal, in his original description of variant angina pectoris, noted the waxing and waning course of this syndrome.[15] This has been observed by others and it appears that the most severe symptoms and the greatest risk for mortality and morbidity occur within the first 6 months after the onset of symptoms. Following this initial rocky course, spontaneous remissions have been reported to occur and the cyclic nature of variant angina create difficulties in assessing the value of any therapeutic intervention.

The merit of any intervention may be assessed by several methods and a combination of these most likely will provide information for rational decisions concerning therapy. Reduction in symptoms and nitroglycerin consumption as documented by a patient diary can assist the interpretation of objective data obtained from ambulatory ECG recordings. This method may underestimate the number of ischemic episodes due to the variable nature of variant angina and serial recordings may be of great value. Evidence of efficacy includes the reduction of ischemic events, both ST-segment depression and elevation, which may be symptomatic or asymptomatic with the latter being more common overall. Additional evidence would be a reduced number of attacks of angina requiring hospitalization, absence of myocardial infarction, and sudden death. Ergonovine provocative testing has been suggested by some as a means for determining the effectiveness of therapy; however, not all investigators have found this method to be reliable because of the fluctuating course of variant angina and provocation may be associated with drug-resistant vasospasm and ventricular arrhythmias.

Optimization of therapy includes dose titration using sufficiently high doses to obtain clinical efficacy without unacceptable adverse effects in individual patients. All patients should be treated for acute attacks and maintained on prophylactic treatment for 6–12 months following the initial episode. The occurrence of serious arrhythmias during attacks is associated with a greater risk of sudden death and these patients should be treated more aggressively and for prolonged periods.[55] In patients without arrhythmias who become asymptomatic and remain so for several months after treatment has been instituted, withdrawal of therapy may be safe after first ascertaining that disease activity is quiescent. Aggravating factors such as alcohol and cigarette smoking should be eliminated when instituting treatment.

Nitrates have been the mainstay of therapy for the acute attacks of variant angina and coronary artery spasm for many years. Most patients respond rapidly to SL nitroglycerin or isosorbide dinitrate; however, intravenous and intracoronary nitroglycerin may be very useful for patients not responding to SL preparations. In particular, vasospasm provoked by ergonovine may require intracoronary nitroglycerin. Other nitrate products including intravenous isosorbide dinitrate and nitroglycerin ointment have been shown to be effective for acute attacks of variant angina. The efficacy of chronic nitrate therapy has not been extensively investigated in variant angina; however, isosorbide dinitrate in doses of 40–120 (mean 65) mg/d has been shown to decrease anginal frequency by 50% in 71% of patients treated by Hill et al.[56] They found ISDN to be similar in efficacy to nifedipine as did Ginsburg et al.,[57] but nifedipine was better tolerated in the latter study. Waters et al.[58] found nitrates to be less effective than calcium antagonists for improving survival without infarction. Because calcium antagonists may be more effective, have few serious adverse effects in effective doses, and can be given less frequently than nitrates, some consider them the agents of choice for variant angina.

Nifedipine, verapamil, and diltiazem are all equally effective as single agents for the initial management of variant angina and coronary artery spasm. Dose titration is important to maximize the response with calcium antagonists. Comparative trials, which are few in number, do not reveal significant differences among these three drugs for variant angina. In patients unresponsive to calcium antagonists alone, nitrates may be added with a good response. Combination therapy with nifedipine–diltiazem or nifedipine–verapamil has been reported useful in patients unresponsive to single-drug regimens. This is probably rational because, at the cellular level, the drugs have different receptors but the combination of verapamil–diltiazem should be used cautiously due to their potential additive effects on contractility and conduction.

Beta-adrenergic blockade has little or no role in the management of variant angina according to most authorities.[39,59] Although not all studies report increased painful episodes of variant angina with the addition of β blockers, they may induce coronary vasoconstriction and prolong ischemia as documented by continuous ECG monitoring.

Other approaches to therapy have attempted modification of α-adrenergic tone by α antagonists such as phentolamine, phenoxybenzamine, or prazosin. The overall response to α blockers is variable and long-term results are discouraging. Anticholinergic agents have also been administered to diminish enhanced parasympathetic activity leading to stimulation of sympathetic nerves and coronary vasospasm; however, only parenteral atropine has been studied and the role for chronic therapy is undetermined. Labetalol, because of its α-blocking properties, may be useful, but very little information is available. Adverse effects limit the utility of amiodarone and perhexilene, and only small numbers of patients with variant angina have been treated with these agents. Plexectomy, surgical interruption of the sympathetic innervation of the heart, with and without CABG has been reported to benefit a few patients.

Agents to modify platelet aggregation and arachidonic acid metabolism have undergone preliminary clinical trials and, as sole interventions, dramatic responses have not been seen. The effects of aspirin in variant angina have not been as successful as in unstable angina, perhaps reflecting differences in the underlying pathophysiology. The role of thromboxane synthesis inhibition, thromboxane receptor antagonism, prostacyclin, lipoxygenase inhibition, and ticlopidine are being clarified through ongoing studies, but they do not occupy a major place in therapy at the present time. Dietary supplementation with fish oil can influence lipid levels, platelet aggregation and possibly cardiovascular mortality, but because most of the available studies are either in animals or are of an epidemiologic nature, routine use cannot be recommended for the prevention or treatment of variant angina.

MANAGEMENT OF SILENT MYOCARDIAL ISCHEMIA[60-62]

The objective in the treatment of silent myocardial ischemia is to reduce the total number of ischemic episodes, both symptomatic and asymptomatic, regardless of the direction of ST-segment shift. The incidence of silent ischemia in the general, asymptomatic population is not known. Significant day-to-day variability in the number of episodes, the duration of ischemia, and the amount of ST-segment deviation complicate both the understanding of this process as well as the utility of various therapeutic interventions. Silent ischemia in patients with known CAD is common and associated with the extent of disease as well as a high risk for myocardial infarction and sudden death when compared with painful episodes of ischemia. Although the underlying mechanisms for silent ischemia are continuing to be defined, increased physical activity, activation of the sympathetic nervous system, increased cortisol secretion, increased coronary artery tone, and enhanced platelet aggregation due to the loss of EDRF leading to intermittent coronary obstruction, may be additive in lowering the threshold for ischemia. Platelet aggregability is increased in the morning hours (7 to 11 AM), corresponding to circadian rhythms noted for the peak frequency of ischemia, acute myocardial infarction, and sudden death.[63] Silent ischemia is associated with ST-segment elevation or depression and frequently occurs without antecedent changes in heart rate or blood pressure, suggesting that this form of ischemia is due to primary reduction in oxygen supply in many instances while at other times in the same patient oxygen demand is increased prior to the onset ischemia.[64] Patients with silent ischemia have a defective warning system for angina pain that may encourage excessive myocardial demand. Regardless of the exact mechanism, there is increasing concern that painless ischemia carries considerable risk for myocardial perfusion defects, detrimental hemodynamic changes, arrhythmogenesis, and sudden death. Silent ischemia is associated with reduced survival, and increased need for PTCA and CABG as well as increased risk of AMI. Because it is apparently very common in some settings, major emphasis should be placed on its management. A consensus has not been reached for the most appropriate method of detecting and quantifying the magnitude of silent ischemia; however, ambulatory ECG monitoring is felt by many to be the most useful tool at the present time.

The initial step in management is to modify the major risk factors for IHD, hypertension, hypercholesterolemia, and smoking, and data from the Multiple Risk Factor Intervention Trial (MRFIT) show these interventions to be useful in patients with silent ischemia.[65] In a subset of the study population who had abnormal baseline exercise ECG responses, the special intervention group had a 57% reduction in coronary heart disease death (22.2/1000 versus 51.8/1000) and a reduction in sudden death resulting from cessation of smoking, and lowering of blood pressure and cholesterol when compared with the usual care group.

Several studies with β blockers have shown improvement in the number of ischemic episodes, primarily ST-segment depression and those associated with effort, compared with placebo; however, this benefit is not seen with all β blockers. The largest controlled trial to date, the Atenolol Silent Ischemia Study (ASIST), has demonstrated that atenolol treatment reduced daily life ischemia and was associated with reduced risk for adverse outcome in asymptomatic and mildly symptomatic patients compared with placebo.[66] Another trial, ACIP (Asymptomatic Cardiac Ischemia Pilot), has completed the pilot phase and coronary revascularization was superior to angina- or ischemia-guided strategies at 1 year for silent ischemia.[67] This pilot study demonstrated that cardiac ischemia can be suppressed in 40–55% of patients with either low or moderate doses of medication or revascularization and that a large trial is feasible. Post-MI patients and those with a high level of sympathetic nervous system activity are perhaps the best candidates for β-blocker therapy. Reductions in the number and duration of ischemic episodes have been noted with β blockers that are nonselective and cardioselective; however, the property of intrinsic sympathomimetic activity has been found to be detrimental in patients with severe angina.[36] Perhaps because it does not alter coronary artery tone compared with other β blockers, labetalol has been shown to reduce the number of episodes of ST-segment depression (3.4 versus 1.5) and duration of ischemia (80 versus 22 minutes) when compared with placebo.[68]

Calcium channel antagonists alone and in combination have been shown to be effective in reducing symptomatic and asymptomatic ischemia; however, they do not interrupt the diurnal surge in ischemia observed on ambulatory monitoring and, in general, they are somewhat less effective than β blockers for silent ischemia. Nifedipine in particular seems to provide less protection and provides wide fluctuations in response with approximate reductions in the number of episodes ranging from 0–93% and in duration from 23–65% unless combined with β blockers. Fewer studies are available with diltiazem and verapamil, but they seem to provide slightly greater reductions in the number and duration of ischemic episodes. Subramanian et al.[69] compared verapamil (360 mg/d) and propranolol (240 mg/d) alone and in combination and found the number of ST segments with a greater than 1-mm depression to be decreased with either single agent compared with placebo; however, the combination gave a further reduction. The maximum depth of ST depression was significantly reduced with the combination but unaffected by the drugs singly. In patients with variant angina, Johnson et al.[70] found that verapamil 240–480 mg/d in a 9-month study reduced the number of ST-segment deviations per week to 7.7 from 33.1 during the placebo phases.

Nitrates, given by various routes, have demonstrated efficacy for silent ischemia and this is related to their effects on MVO_2 as well as coronary artery vasodilation and redistribution of myocardial blood flow. Average reduction in the number of episodes is about 60% with nitrates, but the overall quality of the available studies is not good. In a study by Dargie et al.[71] using nifedipine 30 or 60 mg/d or propranolol 240 or 480 mg/d or in combination demonstrated the combination to be more effective in reducing the area of ST-segment depression and the number of ST-depression episodes when compared with placebo or with either drug alone. They also noted little benefit from using the higher dose of propranolol.

Comparative studies generally show that β blockers are better than calcium channel antagonists for silent ischemia as demonstrated by a comparison of atenolol and nifedipine[72] and within the category of calcium antagonists, verapamil and diltiazem seem to be better than nifedipine. Combination therapy with calcium antagonists and β blockers or two calcium antagonists usually show the combination to be better than monotherapy[71] or that the addition of a calcium antagonist to β-blocker therapy does not add significantly to the overall effect.

Surgical intervention using CABG does not appear warranted in asymptomatic patients without significant coronary artery disease. Based on the CASS 12-year follow-up results, survival following CABG was enhanced in men with three-vessel disease compared to medical therapy (61 versus 46%) but not for women (45 versus 50%) with silent ischemia.[73] The role for PTCA is promising in silent ischemia and improvement in exercise tolerance and freedom from MI, CABG, and PTCA for new lesions or death may be seen in patients becoming aymptomatic after PTCA. However, exercise-induced silent myocardial ischemia is frequently seen early after successful PTCA and is more prevalent in patients undergoing multivessel angioplasty and incomplete revascularization. Both silent and symptomatic ischemia early after PTCA are predictors of an unfavorable prognosis.[74]

SYNDROME X

Syndrome X refers to the occurrence of effort angina and exercise-induced ECG changes with a normal coronary arteriogram with no evidence of structural (stenosis) or functional (spasm) abnormalities.[75] Although the basis for this syndrome is not yet established, it is thought that syndrome X may be due to inducible myocardial ischemia due to impaired functional coronary reserve at the microvascular level of intramural prearteriolar vessels. Maseri et al.[76] have proposed that this defect is due to defective prearteriolar regulation of blood flow into the arteriolar bed with subsequent focal, sustained, compensatory release of adenosine; excessive local concentrations of adenosine are then responsible for the pain seen in this syndrome. Prearteriolar constriction may be the result of insufficient vasodilation or inappropriate vasoconstriction, or resetting of myogenic control on a segmental or generalized distribution basis.[77] Cardiomyopathy and left bundle block may result from ischemia in some patients. Follow-up studies have shown that the occurrence of left bundle branch block in response to stress is associated with a greater likelihood of deterioration of left ventricular performance whereas stress-induced ST-segment depression does not predict a detrimental outcome in ventricular function.

Beta-adrenergic blockers are much less effective in many studies in syndrome X than in exertional angina, and one characteristic, if present, that may predict a good response to β blockers is increased sympathetic nervous system activity.[78] Calcium channel antagonists have produced inconsistent responses, suggesting that generalized vasodilation is not the optimal approach in this disorder. Alpha-adrenergic blockade with clonidine and prazosin and α-receptor challenge with phenylephrine did not produce a response or evidence that this mechanism is important in this syndrome. Evidence supporting the role of adenosine has been provided by Emdin et al.[79] by giving an aminophylline infusion (6 mg/kg) to syndrome X patients. Exercise time increased significantly (5.6–7.7 minutes) compared with placebo, and they postulated that the beneficial effects were due to theophylline-antagonizing adenosine-mediated maldistribution of myocardial blood flow at the level of small intramural coronary arteries and prevention of "transmural steal."

Coronary Artery Bypass Grafting

Following the introduction of saphenous vein graft replacement for the severely occluded coronary arteries by Favorolo and Garrett in 1967, CABG became an accepted and commonly used alternative approach for the management of IHD.[80] The objectives in performing CABG are twofold: (1) reduce the number of symptomatic anginal attacks not controlled with medical management or angioplasty and improve the lifestyle of the patient, and (2) reduce the mortality associated with coronary artery disease. Surgery is effective in providing pain relief in large numbers of patients with about 70–95% being pain free at 1 year and 46–55% being pain free at 5 years. This compares favorably with medical management with only about 30% being free of symptoms at 5 years. The second objective is met in certain patients and this has been addressed in three large, well-controlled trials of bypass surgery.[9,81–83] These three studies, the Veterans Administration (VA), European Cooperative Surgery Study (ECSS), and the Coronary Artery Surgery Study (CASS), are not directly comparable because the inclusion and exclusion criteria for entry into each study were different and patients were followed for different periods of time. They have also been criticized for not being representative of the population that may be candidates for surgery, lacking women or late-middle age or elderly patients, and for crossover of medically managed patients to the surgical group. There have also been changes in medical and surgery practice as well as new technologies that did not exist at the time these trials were initiated.[84] Consequently, the validity of generalizing the results from these studies to routine practice has been questioned, but these studies are useful for providing a basis for decisions concerning surgery. Tables 14.11 to 14.13 summarize survival at various time intervals and for several subgroups from each of these studies. In general, those patients who have left main stem stenosis of greater than 70%, proximal stenosis of the left anterior descending artery greater than 70–75%, poor left ventricular function, or severe three-vessel disease are most likely to have improved survival with surgical therapy. A notable exception to these observations is the lack of difference in any subgroup for CASS, and although trends suggesting improved survival were observed, no significant ($p < 0.05$) differences were found. This is probably related to patient selection with patients in CASS having less severe disease compared with the other studies. As these studies have been

TABLE 14.11. VETERANS ADMINISTRATION CORONARY ARTERY BYPASS SURGERY STUDY

	Survival Rates (%)					
	5 yr		7 yr		11 yr	
	M[a]	S[a]	M	S	M	S
All patients	78	83	70	77[f]	57	58
All non-LMD[b]	80	82	72	77	58	58
1 Vessel	88	94	83	88	65	70
2 Vessels	85	79	81	73	69[f]	55
3 Vessels	75	81	63	75	50	56
Impaired LVF[c]	73	80	63	74[f]	49	53
Normal LVF	90	85	84	80	71	64
Angio high risk[d]	66	83[f]	52	76[f]	38	50[f]
Angio low risk	87	82	82	77	68	61
Clinical risk—high[e]	63	86[f]	52	72	36	49[f]
Clinical risk—mid	80	82	71	79	61	62
Clinical risk—low	93[f]	82	88	81	73	63

[a]M, medically treated patients; S, surgically treated patients.
[b]All patients without left main stem coronary artery disease (LMD).
[c]Left ventricular function; impaired LVF was global ejection fraction <50% or minimal hypokinesis or akinesis of 25–75% of the heart board or greater.
[d]Angiographic high-risk patients are those with three-vessel disease and impaired LVF.
[e]Two or more of the following: resting ST-segment depression; history of MI; history of hypertension.
[f]$P < 0.05$.

TABLE 14.12. EUROPEAN CORONARY SURGERY STUDY GROUP

	Survival Rates (%)			
	5 yr		8 yr	
	M[a]	S[a]	M	S
All patients	83.6	92.4[d]	79.9	88.6[d]
LMD[b]	67.9	85.7	63.6	81.7
2 Vessels	88.2	91.2	87.4	85.0
3 Vessels	82.4	94.0[d]	76.7	91.8[d]
LAD[b] negative	92.1	93.3	88.0	62.1
LAD positive	82.0	92.7[d]	78.7	87.8[d]
ETT with ST ↓ >1.5 mm[c]	79.0	91.7[d]	76.6	89.6[d]

[a]M, medically treated patients; S, surgically treated patients.
[b]LMD, left main stem coronary artery disease; LAD, left anterior descending coronary artery disease.
[c]ST, segment depression greater than 1.5 mm on exercise tolerance testing (ETT).
[d]$P < 0.05$.

TABLE 14.13. CORONARY ARTERY SURGERY STUDY

	Survival Rates (%)[a]			
	1 yr		5 yr	
	M[b]	S[b]	M	S
All patients	98	98	90	92
1 Vessel	99	98	93	96
2 Vessels	99	98	94	95
3 Vessels	98	99	89	93
Group A[c]	99	98	95	96
Group B	98	100	85	96[d]
Group C	96	99	89	89
All EF <0.5	99	99	84	92[d]
EF <0.5 + 1 vessel	100	100	81	100
EF <0.5 + 2 vessels	100	100	88	92
EF <0.5 + 3 vessels	97	98	80	90[d]

[a]Ejection fraction (EF) >0.5 with 1, 2, 3 vessels; no significant differences noted in any group.
[b]M, medically treated patients; S, surgically treated patients.
[c]Group A, angina and ejection fraction >0.5; group B, angina and ejection fraction <0.5; group C, free of angina after MI.
[d]$P < 0.1$ trend toward significant difference. No significant differences were noted in any subgroup analysis for 1 or 5 years.

followed out to 15 years or more, the difference in survival for any subgroup including left main or left main equivalent coronary artery disease becomes insignificant. In addition to survival, other aspects evaluated include exercise capacity, evidence of ischemia, need for drugs to treat angina, and quality of life, including employment status. Exercise capacity may be improved early after CABG; however, at 5 years no significant difference was noted between the medical and surgical groups in CASS and ECSS. The need for nitrates and β blockers is clearly reduced by surgery with only 30% of CABG patients requiring chronic medication while 70% of their medical counterparts received anginal drugs. Employment status after surgery has been shown in CASS to be more dependent on the pretreatment status than an effect induced by the treatment arm, and about 70% of patients are employed before and after surgery.

Indications for bypass surgery should not be rigidly defined although general recommendations can be made based on the available data.[41] Indications may be based on symptoms, coronary anatomy, ventricular function, or evidence for myocardial ischemia with noninvasive stress testing. Based on symptoms, patients with unacceptable limitation of lifestyle because of symptoms despite optimum medical treatment or inability to tolerate drug therapy because of side effects are considered candidates.[83] Classification of the indications for CABG are shown in Tables 14.14 to 14.17. Regardless of symptoms, patients with significant stenosis (>50–70%) of left main coronary artery or triple-vessel disease when the proximal left anterior descending coronary has >70% stenosis or left ventricular function is impaired should be considered. High-risk clinical variables include early positive (>1.5-mm depression) exercise test, fall in ejection fraction >5% on exercise, large exercise-induced wall motion abnormality, or large or multiple thallium perfusion defects. In patients 65 years of age or older, surgical benefit is greatest in high-risk patients, 62% surviving compared with 33% in the medical group at 6 years' follow-up, while significant improvement was also seen overall (surgical 79% versus medical 64%). Corresponding differences were also noted in patients with chest pain.[85] Left main stem disease or left main equivalent (combined proximal left anterior descending and proximal left circumflex) coronary disease are clearly benefited by surgical intervention.[86,87] Mortality is related to the severity of stenosis in this situation and perioperative mortality is also increased. Survival at 3 years in the surgical group averages about 85–90%, while in the medical group survival is significantly lower, about 60–70%. In left main equivalent disease, survival at 5 years in CASS was reported to be 85% in the surgical group versus 55% in the medical group, and those patients with ejection fraction less than 50% were the patients with the greatest improvement in survival (69 versus 26%). Similar trends have been noted in patients with three-vessel disease and abnormal ventricular function with 4-year survival rates of 89 and 55% in the surgical and medical groups, respectively.

TABLE 14.14. CLASSIFICATION OF INDICATIONS FOR THE CORONARY BYPASS GRAFT OPERATION

Treatment Class	Description
I	Conditions for which the operation is indicated on the basis of a demonstrated advantage over medical treatment in terms of longevity or relief of symptoms or both
II	Conditions for which the operation is acceptable treatment but for which its advantages over medical treatment have not yet been fully defined
III	Condition for which the operation is not generally considered to be indicated, because of lack of demonstrated advantage over medical treatment

(From Kirklin JW, Akins CW, Blackstone EH, et al. ACC/AHA guidelines and indications for coronary artery bypass graft surgery. A report of the American College of Cardiology/American Heart Association Task Force on Assessment of Diagnostic and Therapeutic Cardiovascular Procedures (Subcommittee on Coronary Artery Bypass Graft Surgery). Circulation 1991;83:1125–1173, with permission.)

TABLE 14.15. TREATMENT CLASS OF THE CORONARY ARTERY BYPASS OPERATION IN ASYMPTOMATIC PATIENTS

	Left Ventricular Dysfunction			
CAD[a]	None	Mild	Moderate	Severe (but EF >0.20)
A. No or mild myocardial ischemia with noninvasive street testing				
Left main	I	I	I	I
3 Vessels	II[b]	II[b]	I	I
2 Vessels	III[c]	III[c]	II	II
1 Vessel	III[c]	III[c]	III[c]	III[c]
B. Moderate or severe myocardial ischemia with noninvasive stress testing				
Left main	I	I	I	I
3 Vessels	II[d]	III[d]	I	I
2 Vessels	III[d]	III[d]	III[d]	III[d]
1 Vessel	III[d]	III[d]	III[d]	III[d]

[a]CAD, coronary artery disease.
[b]Class I if there are severe proximal left anterior descending and left circumflex coronary artery stenoses.
[c]Class II if there is severe proximal stenosis in a large left anterior descending coronary artery.
[d]Class I if there is a severe proximal stenosis in a large left anterior descending coronary artery. (From Kirklin JW, Akins CW, Blackstone EH, et al. ACC/AHA guidelines and indications for coronary artery bypass graft surgery. A report of the American College of Cardiology/American Heart Association Task Force on Assessment of Diagnostic and Therapeutic Cardiovascular Procedures (Subcommittee on Coronary Artery Bypass Graft Surgery). Circulation 1991;83:1125–1173, with permission.)

Operative mortality is reported to range from 1–3% and is related to the number of vessels involved and preoperative ventricular function. Patients in CASS with one-, two-, or three-vessel disease had operative mortalities of 1.4, 2.1, and 2.8%, respectively. The relationship to left ventricular ejection fraction follows a similar trend with ejection fractions of greater than 50%, 20–40%, and less than 20% having operative mortality rates of 1.9, 4.4, and 6.7%, respectively. Perioperative infarction averages 5% depending on the sensitivity of the method for assessment, and the occurrence of an infarct reduces long-term survival. Neurologic dysfunction is relatively common postoperatively in CABG patients, but many of the deficits are clinically insignificant and resolve with time. Fatal brain damage occurs in 0.3–0.7%, stroke in about 5%, and ophthalmological defects occur in 25%, but only 3% have clinically apparent field defects. Peripheral nerve lesions (12%) and brachial plexopathy (7%) are also reported to occur. Other complications include constrictive pericarditis (0.2%), cellulitis at the site of vein graft and mediastinal infections.

Graft patency influences the success for symptom control and survival and the mechanism for graft early occlusion is probably different from that associated with late clo-

TABLE 14.16. TREATMENT CLASS OF THE CORONARY ARTERY BYPASS OPERATION IN PATIENTS WITH CHRONIC STABLE CLASS I OR II ANGINA

	Left Ventricular Dysfunction			
CAD[a]	None	Mild	Moderate	Severe (but EF >0.20)
A. No or mild myocardial ischemia with noninvasive street testing				
Left main	I	I	I	I
3 Vessels	II[b]	II[b]	I	I
2 Vessels	II[b]	II[b]	II[b]	II[b]
1 Vessel	III[c]	III[c]	II[b]	II[b]
B. Moderate or severe myocardial ischemia with noninvasive stress testing				
Left main	I	I	I	I
3 Vessels	I	I	I	I
2 Vessels	II[b]	II[b]	II[b]	II[b]
1 Vessel	III[c]	III[c]	II[b]	II[b]

[a]CAD, coronary artery disease.
[b]Class I if there are severe proximal stenoses in a large left anterior descending coronary artery.
[c]Class II if there is severe proximal stenosis in a large left anterior descending coronary artery. (From Kirklin JW, Akins CW, Blackstone EH, et al. ACC/AHA guidelines and indications for coronary artery bypass graft surgery. A report of the American College of Cardiology/American Heart Association Task Force on Assessment of Diagnostic and Therapeutic Cardiovascular Procedures (Subcommittee on Coronary Artery Bypass Graft Surgery). Circulation 1991;83:1125–1173, with permission.)

TABLE 14.17. TREATMENT CLASS OF THE CORONARY ARTERY BYPASS OPERATION IN PATIENTS WITH CHRONIC STABLE CLASS III OR IV ANGINA

	Left Ventricular Dysfunction			
CAD[a]	**None**	**Mild**	**Moderate**	**Severe (but EF >0.20)**
A. No or mild myocardial ischemia with noninvasive street testing				
Left main	I	I	I	I
3 Vessels	I	I	I	I
2 Vessels	II[b]	II[b]	II[b]	II[b]
1 Vessel	II[b]	II[b]	II[b]	II[b]
B. Moderate or severe myocardial ischemia with noninvasive stress testing				
Left main	I	I	I	I
3 Vessels	I	I	I	I
2 Vessels	II[b]	II[b]	II[b]	II[b]
1 Vessel	II[b]	II[b]	II[b]	II[b]

[a]CAD, coronary artery disease.
[b]Class I if there are severe proximal stenoses in a large left anterior descending coronary artery. (From Kirklin JW, Akins CW, Blackstone EH, et al. ACC/AHA guidelines and indications for coronary artery bypass graft surgery. A report of the American College of Cardiology/American Heart Association Task Force on Assessment of Diagnostic and Therapeutic Cardiovascular Procedures (Subcommittee on Coronary Artery Bypass Graft Surgery). Circulation 1991;83:1125–1173, with permission.)

sure. Early occlusion is related to platelet adhesion and aggregation, whereas late occlusion may be related to endothelial proliferation and progression of atherosclerosis. Patency of grafts early on after the CABG are reported to range from 88–97% in at least one graft and 58–81% in all grafts at 1 year. Long-term patency based on the CASS Montreal Heart Institute experience suggests that 60–67% of all grafts remain patent at 5–11 years. Antiplatelet therapy has been demonstrated to improve early and late patency rates and should probably be used in all patients who do not have any contraindications. Chesebro et al.[88] used aspirin (325 mg three times a day) and dipyridamole (100 mg four times a day) to reduce the late development of vein-graft occlusions from 27% in the placebo group to 16% in the treated group at 12 months. Using lower doses of aspirin others have shown similar results. Other studies have also shown that aspirin (325 mg/d) alone is effective in preventing early graft closure.[83] Late graft closure is related to elevated lipid levels and the progression of atherosclerosis in the grafted vessels as well as the native circulation. Elevation of very low-density lipoprotein (VLDL), low-density lipoprotein (LDL), and LDL apolipoprotein B is correlated to disease progression and graft closure. Recently it has been shown that this process can be delayed by instituting lipid-lowering therapy in CABG patients with colestipol and niacin, and this should be considered if excessive elevations of cholesterol occur in the bypass patient.[89] Cessation of smoking is an important preoperative and postoperative objective as well as in the management of other coronary risk factors (e.g., hypertension) and institution of a supervised, daily exercise program is recommended.

Internal mammary artery grafts should be used for revascularizing the left anterior descending artery system when possible.[83] Recent evidence demonstrates better survival rates with the internal mammary artery graft compared with saphenous vein grafts, as well as fewer postoperative infarctions and recurrent episodes of angina.

Valvular heart disease can coexist with coronary heart disease, although this is relatively uncommon with rheumatic valve disease, usually the mitral valve, and more common with aortic stenosis and regurgitation.[12] Angina may occur in 35–65% of patients with aortic stenosis or regurgitation and, if severe, may be the cause of angina in the absence of coronary artery disease. Patients being evaluated for possible CABG should also be evaluated for valvular disease to determine if valve replacement needs to be performed along with bypass grafting.

Percutaneous Transluminal Coronary Angioplasty[50]

Since the introduction into clinical cardiology of PTCA by Gruentzig in 1977, this procedure has gained rapid acceptance as a safe and effective means of managing coronary artery disease. It has been estimated that the number of procedures performed in this country during 1984 was about 63,000, nearly double that for 1983. The proposed mechanisms for reduced stenosis with PTCA include (1) compression and redistribution of the atherosclerotic plaque, (2) embolization of plaque contents, (3) aneurysm formation, and (4) disruption of the plaque and arterial wall with distortion and tearing of the intima and media, which leads to denudation of the endothelium, platelet adhesion and aggregation, thrombus formation, and smooth muscle proliferation.[50] Of these mechanisms, the last one is felt to be the most important, but the others may contribute to opening of the lesions in some situations.

The indications for PTCA are outlined in Table 14.18 and are based on the recommendations of Vlietstra and

Holmes.[50] Note that only about 10–20% of all patients with coronary artery disease are candidates for PTCA.[12] PTCA alone or when used in conjunction or sequentially with thrombolysis for acute myocardial infarction is discussed in Chapter 15.

Assessment of outcome with PTCA can be based on several clinical and functional factors. It is important to remember that the success of PTCA is dependent on the experience of the operator, complicating factors for the patient including the number of vessels to be dilated, and on technical advances in the equipment used (e.g., steerable and low profile catheters). The initial success rate for immediate opening of stenotic lesions averages 80–90% in experienced hands, and there is usually a significant reduction in the amount of stenosis. Mortality at 1 year is 1% and 3% for single-vessel disease and multiple-vessel involvement, respectively, reflecting the good prognosis associated with this degree of coronary artery disease. At 6 years, survival is 98 and 92%, respectively, for single and multiple disease.[87] Most patients remain event-free (no death, MI, or CABG) for an extended period (74 months). Symptomatic status, as measured by the New York Heart Association (NYHA) classification, is improved in many patients. Gruentzig et al.[90] found that 84 of 133 patients prior to PTCA were in NYHA class III or IV, but after PTCA only 8 of 133 remained in these classes. Pre-PTCA, 97% of the patients in this study had positive ETT, and post-PTCA 2 of 61 with single-vessel disease and 7 of 30 with multiple-vessel disease continued to have positive ETT. Exercise capacity was also improved with only 47% reaching their predicted capacity before PTCA, while 78% did so after PTCA. Restenosis is noted in about 30% of patients at 6 months, and two-thirds of these patients will have angina associated with restenosis. A few late restenotic events occur, but most restenosis occurs within the first 6 months. Factors that predict restenosis include little improvement (<5%) in ejection fraction post-PTCA, continuing wall motion abnormalities, continued smoking, high cholesterol, diabetes, and positive exercise thallium scintigraphy. Increased likelihood for failure or complications with PTCA include female gender, age over 60 years, duration of angina more than 6 months, operator experience with fewer than 50 cases, eccentric stenosis, stenosis severity greater than 90%, calcified stenosis, intraluminal thrombus, involvement of branch vessels, and stenosis located on acute bend in vessel.[50]

TABLE 14.18. CORONARY ANATOMIC INDICATIONS FOR PTCA

- Widely accepted
  - Single-vessel disease
    - Proximal subtotal stenosis
    - Recent total occlusion
  - Multivessel disease
    - Severe (70% or more)
    - Subtotal stenoses in two or three major vessels (if complete revascularization is possible)
    - Severe (70% or more) subtotal stenoses in one major vessel and moderate (50–69%) stenoses in other vessels
  - Restenosis
- Evolving
  - Occlusion during acute myocardial infarction
  - Angina after coronary artery bypass grafting
  - Operation is relatively contraindicated
  - Revascularization is likely to be incomplete

(From Vlietstra RE, Holmes DR Jr. PTCA. Philadelphia, FA Davis, 1989, p 52, with permission.)

The overall complication rate based on PTCA Registry data is 21.1%.[91] Coronary occlusion, dissection, or spasm occur in 10.4% of patients, while myocardial infarction occurs in 5.5%. Prolonged angina and ventricular tachycardia or fibrillation occurs in 6.9 and 2.3%, respectively. Mortality was reported to be 0.9% overall and high-risk events for mortality included ventricular arrhythmias and myocardial infarction. The frequency of urgent CABG because of complications should be less than 5%.

During PTCA patients are usually heparinized to prevent immediate thrombus formation during the procedure, and systemic anticoagulation is continued for up to 24 hours.[92] Some authors have advocated heparin alternatives such as hirudin or hirulog but there is no apparent long-term advantage with these agents.[93,94] In addition to anticoagulation with heparin, abciximab (RheoPro, a IIb/IIIa platelet glycoprotein inhibitor) given as a bolus and constant infusion has been shown in the EPIC trial (Evaluation of 7E3 for the Prevention of Ischemic Complications) to reduce the need for urgent repeat PTCA.[95] Abciximab works by preventing platelet binding to adhesive glycoproteins such as fibrinogen, von Willebrand factor, and others. This improvement, however, came at the cost of a twofold increase in major bleeding complications (from 7 to 14%) and this drug costs more than $1000 per treatment course. Mechanisms that result in restenosis include acute lumen loss due to "recoil," mural thrombosis formation, and smooth muscle cell proliferation with synthesis of extracellular matrix.[51] Approaches to prevent restenosis may be aimed at altering the underlying mechanisms. Recoil and loss of luminal diameter may be reduced by the use of stent placement; however, this beneficial effect is offset by an increased number of vascular complications. Cracking of the plaque leads to severe damage to the arterial wall, exposure of collagen and endothelial dysfunction. These factors promote mural thrombi and the propensity for thrombus formation is related, in part, to the compostion of the plaque as well as the depth of injury. Heparin has been the traditional antithrombotic used to prevent thrombosis in this setting and recently abciximab has been approved as well; the results of the EPIC trial are described previously. Aspirin is typically used post-PTCA to minimize the platelet contribution to thrombosis formation and the usual dose is 325 mg/d. Long-term warfarin has not been shown useful in preventing restenosis, and it is not indicated unless other indications exist.[96] An investigational drug, trapidil, has shown very promising results in trials recently completed.[97]

Smooth muscle activation leads to late restenosis (2 weeks to 3 months), which occurs in three waves. The first wave is medial smooth muscle activation, followed by medial smooth muscle cell migration secondary to the liberation of various chemoattractants and, finally, intimal proliferation and synthesis of extracellular matrix. Most of the pharmacologic interventions to prevent the third phase of restenosis have not been effective with the exception of trapidil, which is a platelet-derived growth factor antagonist as well as an inhibitor of platelet aggregation and smooth muscle cell proliferation.[97] Other approaches include local drug delivery through double balloon techniques or through barophoretic and inotophoretic methods. Future approaches may include altering gene expression with specific growth factor inhibitors, cyclin regulators or antisense nucleotides, enhancement of re-endothelialization with gene transfer or natural endothelial derived inhibitors, and photodynamic therapy to produce locally active oxygen species to alter smooth muscle cell function.

Other agents such as thromboxanes A_2 synthetase inhibitor or receptor antagonists, ticlopidine, and others might be useful. Some studies with fish oil are positive while others are negative and lovastatin does not alter restenosis. Corticosteroids and nonsteroidal agents may inhibit inflammation involved in restenosis but no large randomized trials exist supporting their use. Calcium antagonists may also be given to prevent coronary artery spasm during PTCA, and some centers also pretreat patients with antiplatelet therapy for PTCA. Following PTCA, calcium antagonists are given for 2–4 weeks to prevent coronary artery spasm and for their other anti-ischemic effects, and some believe they may also prevent restenosis; however, studies with follow-up at 10 months have shown little difference between placebo and calcium antagonists on restenosis rates. Antiplatelet therapy with aspirin or aspirin plus dipyridamole does not reduce or prevent restenosis, but the combination may reduce the incidence of acute complications during or immediately after angioplasty. Antiplatelet therapy with aspirin with or without dipyridamole is recommended by some for 1 year following PTCA to delay or prevent restenosis.[98] Trials to test the effectiveness of cilazapril in preventing intimal proliferation after angioplasty demonstrated no benefit on restenosis or clinical endpoints.[99]

Alternatives to PTCA include directional coronary atherectomy (DCA), excimer laser, rotational atherectomy (rotablator), and intracoronary stents.[84] Based on three randomized trials, DCA produces greater initial luminal diameter but results in a higher rate of postprocedural complications such as non-Q-wave MI and death and is more expensive. Consequently, PTCA is considered to be superior to DCA for most patients. The use of abciximab may improve these results. Based on the preliminary results of the Excimer Laser Rotational Atherectomy Balloon Angioplasty Complications (ERBAC) study, laser and rotablator atherectomy do not seem to have any advantages over PTCA. Intracoronary stents result in larger initial minimal lumen diameter, improved clinical outcome, and less restenosis than PTCA; however, these benefits are offset by loss of luminal diameter differences later and a two- to four-fold increase in bleeding and vascular complications due to the need for anticoagulation.[100,101]

When compared with CABG, PTCA has been shown to be better in patients with less severe disease while CABG is better for patients with more severe or multiple-vessel disease (see Fig. 14.13 and Table 14.19). Early outcome for death and MI is generally better with PTCA while

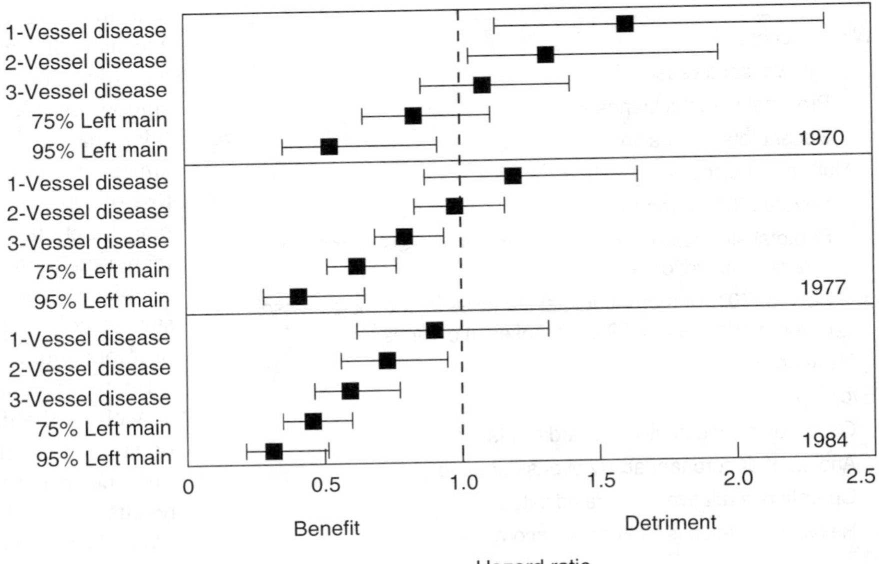

Figure 14.13. Comparison of medical and surgical average hazard ratios for patients treated in 1970, 1977, and 1984 grouped according to extent of coronary artery disease. Closed squares represent point estimates; bars represent 95% confidence intervals of average hazard ratios. *(From Califf R, Harrell FJ, Lee K et al. The evolution of medical and surgical therapy for coronary artery disease. JAMA 1989;261:2077–2086, with permission.)*

TABLE 14.19. PTCA VERSUS CABG TRIALS: CLINICAL OUTCOME (% OF PATIENTS)

	RITA[a]		GABI		CABRI		EAST	
	PTCA	CABG	PTCA	CABG	PTCA	CABG	PTCA	CABG
Randomized (*N*)	510	501	182	177	541	513	198	194
Early outcome								
Death	0.8	1.2	1.1	2.3	1.7	0.9	1.0	1.0
MI	3.5	2.4	2.3	8.1	3.1	2.9	3.0	10.3
Reintervention	6.7	NA	11.0	1.7	10.1	1.6	10.1	0
Late outcome								
Death	3.1	3.6	2.2	5.1	3.9	2.1	7.1	6.2
MI	6.7	5.3	3.8	7.3	2.9	3.3	14.6	19.6
PTCA	18.2	0.8	27.5	1.1	20.1	7.2	40	13
CABG	18.8	3.2	22.5	4.0	20.2	1.4	21.2	0.5
Angina-free	69	78	71	74	85	91	80	88
Event-free survival	62	89	56	94	60	85	46	70

[a]RITA, randomized intervention treatment of angina; GABI, German angioplasty versus bypass surgery investigation; CABRI, coronary angioplasty versus bypass revascularization investigation; EAST, Emory angioplasty surgery trial; MI, myocardial infarction; PTCA, percutaneous transluminal angioplasty; CABG, coronary artery bypass grafting.

late outcomes (>1 year) such as being angina free and survival are better with CABG. A number of other atherectomy devices and stents are being investigated and they may hold promise for improving the technology of revascularization.[102]

Evaluation of Therapeutic Outcomes

Subjective and objective measures of therapeutic outcome are routinely used to assess patients on medical therapy for ischemic heart disease and angina pectoris. The subjective measures of drug response include symptoms of chest pain, nitroglycerin and concurrent drug consumption, and patient-reported alterations in activities of daily living (e.g., time to walk two blocks, number of stairs). Patients on nitrate productions such as nitroglycerin may also report headache and mucosal burning after ingesting nitroglycerin until they develop tolerance to these effects.

Clinical measures of response that are more objective include heart rate and blood pressure and their product [double product (DP) = SBP × HR] as a measure of myocardial oxygen demand (Table 14.9). Since nitrates may increase HR but lower SBP, measuring both is useful. Calcium channel blockers and β blockers should both reduce the DP. Combination therapy may also be monitored with the DP. Monitoring for adverse effects of each drug is described in the chapter, but the major effects include headache and dizziness with nitrates, fatigue and lassititude with β blockers, and peripheral edema, constipation, and dizziness with the calcium blockers. ECG is very useful, particularly if the patient is experiencing chest pain or other symptoms thought to be potentially of ischemic origin (Tables 14.3 and 14.5). ST-segment deviations are very important and the extent of their deviation is related to the severity of ischemia. Other physical findings tend to be less reliable and less common but their appearance such as an S_3 or precordial bulge along with chest pain can be ominous findings (Table 14.7).

Exercise stress testing may also be used to evaluate the response to anti-ischemic therapy, but the expense and time needed to perform this test precludes routine use for monitoring response to therapy. Rather, ETT is more commonly used in risk stratification in strategic decisions concerning therapeutic interventions such as PTCA, CABG, or some other procedure rather than or in addition to medical management. Other types of tests such as cardiac catheterization, radionuclide scans, and echocardiography are also used primarily for risk stratification and selecting patients for more invasive procedures rather than monitoring therapy. As an example, if patients experience unstable angina, often a catheterization is done to determine anatomy, worsening stenosis, and ventricular function, however, the decision to use or not use medications such as nitroglycerin or β blockers is made on clinical grounds rather than a diagnostic test.

Ancillary monitoring to ensure that a comprehensive plan has been set into place would include lipid profiles, fasting plasma glucose, thyroid function tests, hemoglobin/hematocrit determinations, and electrolyte measurements.

References

1. Heberden W. Some account of a disorder of the breast. Med Tran R Coll Phys Lond 1772;2:59–67.
2. Matthews MB. Historical background, in Julian DG (ed): Angina Pectoris, 2nd ed. New York, Churchill Livingstone, 1985, pp 3–12.

3. Brunton TL. On the use of nitrate of amyl in angina pectoris. Lancet 1867;2:628–629.
4. Ahlquist RP. A study of the adrenotropic receptors. Am J Physiol 1948;153:583–600.
5. Black JW, Stephenson JS. Pharmacology of a new adrenergic β-receptor-blocking compound (nethalide). Lancet 1962;2:311–314.
6. Kannel WB, Feinleib M. Natural history of angina pectoris in the Framingham study: Prognosis and survival. Am J Cardiol 1972;29:154–163.
7. Greig M, Pemberton J, Hay I, et al. A prospective study of the development of coronary heart disease in a group of 1202 middle-aged men. J Epidemiol Community Health 1980;34:23–30.
8. Goldman L, Hashimoto B, Cook F, et al. Comparative reproducibility and validity of systems for assessing cardiovascular functional class: Advantages of a new specific activity scale. Circulation 1981;64:1227–1234.
9. Veterans Administration Coronary Artery Bypass Surgery Cooperative Study Group. Eleven-year survival in the Veterans Administration randomized trial of coronary bypass surgery for stable angina. N Engl J Med 1984;311:1333–1339, 1339–1345.
10. Chaitman BR, Ryan TJ, Kronmal RA, et al. Coronary Artery Surgery Study (CASS): Comparability of 10-year survival in randomized and randomizable patients. J Am Coll Cardiol 1990;16:1071–1078.
11. Braunwald E (ed). Heart Disease. A Textbook of Cardiovascular Medicine. Philadelphia, WB Saunders, 1992.
12. Cohn PF (ed). Diagnosis and Therapy of Coronary Artery Disease, 2nd ed. Boston, Martinus Nijhoff Publishing, 1985.
13. Epstein SE, Cannon RO III, Talbot TL. Hemodynamic principles in the control of coronary blood flow. Am J Cardiol 1985;56:4E–10E.
14. Vane JR, Anggard E, Botting RM. Regulatory functions of the vascular endothelium. N Engl J Med 1990;323:27–36.
15. Prinzmetal M, Kennamer R, Merliss R, et al. Angina pectoris. I. A variant form of angina pectoris. Am J Med 1959;27:375–388.
16. Braunwald E, Mark DB, Jones RH, Cheitline MD, et al. Unstable angina: Diagnosis and management, Rockville, MD, U.S. Department of Health and Human Service, Public Health Service, Agency for Health Care Policy and Research, Clinical Practice Guideline No. 10, National Heart, Lung, and Blood Institute, 1994.
17. Cohen P (ed). Silent Myocardial Ischemia. New York, Marcel Dekker, 1986.
18. Anonymous. Effects of estrogen or estrogen/progestin regimens on heart disease risk factors in postmenopausal women. The Postmenopausal Estrogen/Progestin Interventions (PEPI) trial. JAMA 1995;273:199–208
19. Bush TL, Cowan LD, Barrett-Connor E, et al. Estrogen use and all-cause mortality. Preliminary results from the Lipid Research Clinics Program follow-up study. JAMA 1983;249:903–906.
20. Stamper MJ, Willett WC, Colditz GA, et al. A prospective study of postmenopausal estrogen therapy and coronary heart disease. N Engl J Med 1985;313:1044–1049.
21. Wilson PWF, Garrison RJ, Castelli WP. Post-menopausal estrogen use, cigarette smoking, and cardiovascular morbidity in women over 50. The Framingham Study. N Engl J Med 1985;313:1038–1049.
22. Colditz GA, Hankinson SE, Hunter DJ, et al. The use of estrogens and progestins and the risk of breast cancer in postmenopausal women. N Engl J Med 1995;332:1589–1593.
23. Stanford JL, Weiss NS, Voigt LF, et al. Combined estrogen and progestin hormone replacement therapy in relation to risk of breast cancer in middle-aged women. JAMA 1995;274:137–142.
24. Knopp RH, Zhu X, Bonet B. Effects of estrogens on lipoprotein metabolism and cardiovascular disease in women. Atherosclerosis 1994;110(suppl):S83–S91.
25. Chou TM, Benowitz NL. Caffeine and coffee: Effects on health and cardiovascular disease. Comp Biochem Physiol 1994;109:173–189.
26. Khurmi NS, Bowles MJ, Kohli RS, et al. Does placebo improve indexes of effort-induced myocardial ischemia? An objective study in 150 patients with chronic stable angina pectoris. Am J Cardiol 1986;57:907–911.
27. Torfgard KE, Ahlner J. Mechanisms of action of nitrates. Cardiovasc Drug Ther 1994;8:701–717.
28. Dusting GJ. Nitric oxide in cardiovascular disorders. J Vasc Res 1995;32:143–161.
29. Bogaert MG. Clinical pharmacokinetics of nitrates. Cardiovasc Drug Ther 1994;8:693–699.
30. DeMots H, Glasser SP on behalf of the Transderm-Nitro Trial Study Group. Intermittent transdermal nitroglycerin therapy in the treatment of chronic stable angina. J Am Coll Cardiol 1989;13:786–793.
31. Thadani U, Lipicky RJ. Short and long-acting nitrates for stable angina pectoris. Cardiovasc Drug Ther 1994;8:611–624.
32. Pratt CM, Welton DE, Squires WG, Jr, et al. Demonstration of training effect during chronic β-adrenergic blockade in patients with coronary artery disease. Circulation 1981;64:1125–1129.
33. Thadani U, Davidson C, Singleton W, et al. Comparison of five β-adrenoreceptor antagonists with different ancillary properties during sustained twice daily therapy in angina pectoris. Am J Med 1980;68:243–250.
34. Miller LA, Crawford MH, O'Rourke RA. Nadolol compared to propranolol for treating chronic stable angina pectoris. Chest 1984;86:189–193.
35. Jones GR, Mir MA. Comparison of antianginal efficacy of one conventional and three long acting β-adrenoreceptor blocking agents in stable angina pectoris. Br Heart J 1981;46:503–507.
36. Quyyumi AA, Wright C, Mockus L, et al. Effect of partial agonist activity in β-blockers in severe angina pectoris: A double blind comparison of pindolol and atenolol. Br Med J 1984;289:951–953.
37. Gengo FM, Huntoon L, McHugh WB. Lipid-soluble and water-soluble β-blockers. Comparison of CNS depressant effects. Arch Intern Med 1987;147:39–43.
38. Avorn J, Everitt DE, Weiss S. Increased antidepressant use in patients prescribed β-blockers. JAMA 1986;255:357–360.
39. Parodi O, Simonetti I, L'Abbate A, et al. Verapamil versus propranolol for angina at rest. Am J Cardiol 1982;50:923–928.

40. Kelly JG, O'Malley K. Clinical pharmacokinetics of calcium antagonists. An update. Clin Pharmacokinet 1992;22:416–433.
41. Dargie HJ. Investigation and management of chronic stable angina, in Fox KM (ed): Ischaemic Heart Disease. Boston, MTP Press Limited, 1987, pp 149–217.
42. Lorimer AR. Medical management, in Julian DG (ed): Angina Pectoris, 2nd ed. New York, Churchill Livingstone, 1985, pp 164–187.
43. Kloster FE, Bristow JD. Management of stable and unstable angina, in Connor WE, Bristow JD (eds): Coronary Heart Disease. Prevention, Complications, and Treatment. Philadelphia, JB Lippincott, 1985, pp 231–250.
44. Koh KK, Park GS, Song JH, Moon TH, et al. Interaction of intravenous heparin and organic nitrates in acute ischemic syndromes. Am J Cardiol 1995;76:706–709.
45. Gurfinkel EP, Manos EJ, Majail RI, et al. Low molecular weight heparin versus regular heparin or aspirin in the treatment of unstable angina and silent ischemia. J Am Coll Cardiol 1995;26:313–318.
46. Lewis HD, Davis JW, Archibald DA, et al. Protective effect of aspirin against acute myocardial infarction and death in men with unstable angina. N Engl J Med 1983;309:396–405.
47. Cairns JA, Gent M, Singer J, et al. Aspirin, sulfinpyrazone, or both in unstable angina. Results of a Canadian multicenter trial. N Engl J Med 1985;313:1369–1375.
48. Lubsen J, Tijssen JG. Efficacy of nifedipine and metoprolol in the early treatment of unstable angina in the coronary care unit: Findings from the Holland Interuniversity Nifedipine/metoprolol Trial (HINT). Am J Cardiol 1987;60:18A–25A.
49. Unstable Angina Pectoris Study Group. Unstable Angina Pectoris National Cooperative Study Group to compare medical and surgical therapy. IV. Results in patients with left anterior descending coronary artery disease. Am J Cardiol 1981;48:517–524.
50. Vlietstra RE, Holmes DR Jr (eds). PTCA (Percutaneous Transluminal Coronary Angioplasty). Philadelphia, FA Davis, 1987.
51. Fuster V, Falk E, Fallon JT, Badimon L, et al. The three processes leading to post PTCA restenosis: Dependence on the lesion substrate. Throm Haemost 1995;74:552–559.
52. Mabin TA, Holmes DR Jr, Smith HC, et al. Intracoronary thrombus: Role in coronary occlusion complicating percutaneous transluminal coronary angioplasty. J Am Coll Cardiol 1985;5:198–202.
52a. Flaherty JT, Becker LC, Weiss JL, et al. Results of a randomized trial of intraaortic balloon counterpulsation and intravenous nitroglycerin in patients with acute myocardial infarction. J Am Coll Cardiol 1985;6:434–446.
53. Sassen LMA, Lamers JMJ, Verdouw PD. Fish oil and the prevention and regression of atherosclerosis. Cardiovasc Drugs Ther 1994;8:179–191.
53a. Sacks FM, Stone PH, Gibson M, et al. Controlled trial of fish oil for regression of human coronary atherosclerosis. J Am Coll Cardiol 1995;25:1492–1498.
54. Conti CR (ed). Coronary Artery Spasm. Pathophysiology, Diagnosis, and Treatment. New York, Marcel Dekker, 1986.
55. Weiss JN, Nademanee K, Stevenson WG, et al. Ventricular arrhythmias in ischemic heart disease. Ann Intern Med 1991;114:784–797.
56. Hill JA, Feldman RL, Pepine CJ, et al. Randomized double-blind comparison of nifedipine and isosorbide dinitrate in patients with coronary arterial spasm. Am J Cardiol 1982;49:431–438.
57. Ginsburg R, Lamb IH, Schroeder JS, et al. Randomized double-blind comparison of nifedipine and isosorbide dinitrate therapy in variant angina pectoris due to coronary artery spasm. Am Heart J 1982;103:44–48.
58. Waters DD, Miller DD, Szlachcic J, et al. Factors influencing the long-term prognosis of treated patients with variant angina. Circulation 1983;68:258–265.
59. Robertson RM, Bernard Y, Carr RK, et al. Exacerbation of vasotonic angina pectoris by propranolol. Circulation 1982;65:281–285.
60. Singh N, Langer A. Current status of silent myocardial ischemia. Can J Cardiol 1995;11:286–289.
61. Cohn PF (ed). Silent Myocardial Ischemia, 2nd ed. New York, Marcel Dekker, 1989.
62. Bertolet BD, Hill JA, Pepine CJ. Treatment strategies for daily life silent myocardial ischemia: A correlation with potential pathogenic mechanisms. Prog Cardiovasc Dis 1992;35:97–118.
63. Muller JE, Ludmer PL, Willich SN, et al. Circadian variation in the frequency of sudden cardiac death. Circulation 1987;75:131–138.
64. Pepine CJ. Circadian variations in myocardial ischemia. JAMA 1991;265:386–390.
65. Multiple Risk Factor Intervention Trial Research Group. Exercise electrocardiogram and coronary heart disease mortality in the Multiple Risk Factor Intervention Trial. Am J Cardiol 1985;55:16–24.
66. Pepine CJ, Cohn P, Deedwania PC, et al. Effects of treatment on outcome in mildly symptomatic patients with ischemia during daily life. The Atenolol Silent Ischemia Study (ASIST). Circulation 1994;90:762–768.
67. Rogers WJ, Bourassa MA, Andrews TC, et al. Asymptomatic Cardiac Ischemia Pilot (ACIP) study: Outcome at 1 year for patients with asymptomatic cardiac ischemia randomized to medical therapy or revascularization. J Am Coll Cardiol 1995;26:594–605.
68. Quyyumi AA, Wright C, Mockus L, et al. Effects of combined α- and β-adrenoceptor blockade in patients with angina pectoris. A double blind study comparing labetalol with placebo. Br Heart J 1985;53:47–52.
69. Subramanian VB, Bowles MJ, Davis AB, et al. Combined therapy with verapamil and propranolol in angina pectoris. Am J Cardiol 1982;49:125–132.
70. Johnson SM, Mauritson DR, Willerson JT, et al. A controlled trial of verapamil for Prinzmetal's variant angina. N Engl J Med 1981;304:862–866.
71. Dargie HJ, Lynch PG, Krikler D, et al. Nifedipine and propranolol: A beneficial drug interaction. Am J Med 1981;71:676–682.
72. Deedwania PC, Carbajal EV, Nelson JR, et al. Antiischemic effects of atenolol versus nifedipine in patients with coronary artery disease and ambulatory silent ischemia. J Am Coll Cardiol 1991;17:963–969.

73. Ryan TJ, Parsons L, Fisher LD, et al. Significance of silent myocardial ischemia during exercise testing in women: Report from the Coronary Artery Surgery Study. Am Heart J 1995;129:465–470.
74. Kaul U, Dev V, Manchanda SC, Wasir HS. Silent myocardial ischemia after percutaneous transluminal coronary angioplasty and its prognostic significance. Clin Cardiol 1991;14:563–566.
75. Henderson AH. Syndrome X. Cardiovasc Drugs Ther 1989;3:271.
76. Maseri A, Crea F, Kaski JC, et al. Mechanism of angina pectoris in syndrome X. J Am Coll Cardiol 1991;17:499–506.
77. Sax FL, Cannon RO, Hanson C, et al. Impaired forearm vasodilator reserve in patients with microvascular angina. N Engl J Med 1987;317:1366–1370.
78. Bugiardini R, Borghi A, Biagetti L, et al. Comparison of verapamil versus propranolol therapy in syndrome X. Am J Cardiol 1989;63:286–290.
79. Emdin M, Picano E, Lattanzi F, et al. Improved exercise capacity with acute aminophylline administration in patients with syndrome X. J Am Coll Cardiol 1989;14:1450–1453.
80. Favaloro RG. Saphenous vein autograft replacement of severe segmental coronary artery occlusion. Ann Thorac Surg 1968;5:334–339.
81. European Coronary Surgery Study Group. Long-term results of prospective randomized study of coronary artery bypass surgery in stable angina pectoris. Lancet 1982;2:1173–1180.
82. CASS Principal Investigators and their Associates. Coronary Artery Surgery Study (CASS): A randomized trial of coronary artery bypass surgery. Survival data. Circulation 1983;68:939–950.
83. Kirklin JW, Akins CW, Blackstone EH, et al. ACC/AHA guidelines and indications for coronary artery bypass graft surgery. A report of the American College of Cardiology/American Heart Association Task Force on Assessment of Diagnostic and Therapeutic Cardiovascular Procedures (Subcommittee on Coronary Artery Bypass Graft Surgery). Circulation 1991;83:1125–1173.
84. Moliterno DJ, Elliott JM, Topol EJ. Randomized trials of myocardial revascularization. Curr Prob Cardiol 1995;20:125–190.
85. Gersh BJ, Kronmal RA, Schaff HV, et al. Comparison of coronary artery bypass surgery and medical therapy in patients 65 years of age or older. N Engl J Med 1985;313:217–224.
86. Caracciolo EA, Davis KB, Sopko G, et al. Comparison of surgical and medical group survival in patients with left main coronary artery disease. Long-term CASS experience. Circulation 1995;91:2325–2334.
87. Caracciolo EA, Davis KB, Sopko G, et al. Comparison of surgical and medical group survival in patients with left main equivalent coronary artery disease. Long-term CASS experience. Circulation 1995;91:2335–2344.
88. Chesebro JH, Fuster V, Elveback LR, et al. Effect of dipyridamole and aspirin on late vein-graft patency after coronary bypass operations. N Engl J Med 1984;310:209–214.
89. Blankenhorn DH, Nessim SA, Johnson RL, et al. Beneficial effects of combined colestipol–niacin therapy on coronary atherosclerosis and coronary venous bypass grafts. JAMA 1987;257:3233–3240.
90. Gruentzig AR, King SB III, Schlumpf M, et al. Long-term follow-up after percutaneous transluminal coronary angioplasty. The early Zurich experience. N Engl J Med 1987;316:1127–1132.
91. National Heart, Lung and Blood Institute PTCA Registry. Percutaneous transluminal coronary angioplasty. University of Pittsburgh, Data Coordinating Center, November 1983.
92. Laskey MA, Deutsch E, Barnathan E, Laskey WK. Influence of heparin therapy on percutaneous transluminal coronary angioplasty outcome in unstable angina pectoris. Am J Cardiol 1990;65:1425–1429.
93. Serruys PW, Herrman JP, Simon R, et al. A comparison of hirudin with heparin in the prevention of restenosis after coronary angioplasty. N Eng J Med 1995;333:757–763.
94. Bittl JA, Strony J, Brinker JA, et al. Treatment with bivalirudin (hirulog) as compared with heparin during coronary angioplasty for unstable or postinfarction angina. N Engl J Med 1995;333:764–769.
95. EPIC investigators. Use of monoclonal antibody directed against the platelet glycoprotein IIb/IIIa receptor in high-risk coronary angioplasty. N Engl J Med 1994;330:956–961.
96. Thornton MA, Gruentzig AR, Hollman J, et al. Coumadin and aspirin in prevention of recurrence after transluminal coronary angioplasty: A randomized study. Circulation 1984;69:721–727.
97. Maresta A, Balducelli M, Cantini L, et al. Trapidil (triazolopyrimidine), a platelet-derived growth factor antagonist, reduces restenosis after percutaneous transluminal coronary angioplasty. Results of the randomized, double-blind STARC study. Studio Trapidil versus Aspirin nella Restenosi Coronarica. Circulation 1994;90:2710–2715.
98. Holmes DR Jr, Vlieststra RE, Smith HC, et al. Restenosis after percutaneous transluminal angioplasty (PTCA): A report from the PTCA registry of the National Heart, Lung and Blood Institute. Am J Cardiol 1984;53:77C–81C.
99. Faxon DP. Effect of high dose angiotensin-converting enzyme inhibition on restenosis: Final results of the MARCATOR Study, a multicenter, double-blind, placebo-controlled trial of cilazapril. The Multicenter American Research Trial with Cilazapril After Angioplasty to Prevent Transluminal Coronary Obstruction and Restenosis (MARCATOR) Study Group. J Am Coll Cardiol 1995;25:362–369.
100. Serruys PW, de Jaegere P, Kiemeneij F, et al. A comparison of balloon-expandable stent implantation with balloon angioplasty in patients with coronary artery disease. N Engl J Med 1994;331:489–495.
101. Fischman DL, Leon MB, Baim DS, et al. A randomized comparison of coronary-stent placement and balloon angioplasty in the treatment of coronary artery disease. N Engl J Med 1994;331:496–501.
102. Dean LS, Roubin GS (eds.). Preface. Contemporary interventional techniques. Cardiol Clin 1994;12:543–737.

Chapter 15

Acute Myocardial Infarction

Kathleen A. Stringer, PharmD, FCCP,
and Larry M. Lopez, PharmD, FCCP

Myocardial infarction is the number one killer of both men and women in the United States. Of the 1.5 million Americans that will have an acute myocardial infarction (MI) this year, more than 500,000 will die.[1] The majority of these patients (60%) will either die before they reach a hospital or in the emergency department.[1]

The cardiac mortality during hospitalization for first MI patients is 7–12% and approximately 6% per year thereafter.[2] Patients with larger MI such as anterior wall infarction, left ventricular dysfunction, and complex ventricular ectopy carry the highest 1-year mortality post-MI (22%).

The financial consequence of MI to the U.S. health care system is severe, approximately $50 billion annually.[3] Therefore, therapeutic interventions that reduce mortality and improve morbidity, as well as primary and secondary prevention strategies, will have a significant impact on the U.S. health care system.

Drug therapy and the approach to the management of MI patients has changed and improved dramatically since the mid-1980s. Technological and therapeutic advancements have provided the progress and development of pharmacotherapy for MI. One of the most important advancements has been the introduction of thrombolytic therapy. Though initially suggested as a potential therapeutic tool in the 1950s, thrombolytic therapy was not evaluated in clinical trials until the early 1980s. This delay was most likely due to the controversy that surrounded the etiology of MI.

Although it was suggested as early as 1912 that thrombus formation played a critical role in the pathophysiology of MI, it was not until 1980, when, using acute angiography, DeWood,[4] definitively demonstrated that thrombus formation was indeed the primary etiology of MI. Once this pathology was established, a flurry of intracoronary thrombolytic trials followed. Subsequently, the feasibility and usefulness of peripherally administered intravenous (IV) thrombolytic therapy was demonstrated and is now widely accepted. Progress continues in the development of new thrombolytic agents, anticoagulants, and antiplatelet drugs in order to enhance patient care and outcome.

This chapter provides the clinician with an in-depth overview of the pathophysiology and current pharmacotherapeutic management of patients with MI. Also included is a discussion of the principles of secondary prevention and the management of the post-MI patient.

PATHOPHYSIOLOGY

ETIOLOGY

Coronary artery disease (CAD) is the primary underlying process that, in many cases, leads to MI.[5–8] The process of CAD begins early in life, usually within the first decade. Fatty streaks deposit on coronary artery endothelium and may progress to form atherosclerotic plaques depending on the absence or presence of specific risk factors. These include hypertension, diabetes mellitus, smoking, and hyperlipidemia. If progression occurs, plaques develop, proliferate, and eventually disrupt the integrity and function of the endothelium. Subsequently, myocardial ischemia may occur due to the narrowing of one or more coronary arteries. However, coronary artery narrowing is not the etiology of MI. Thrombus formation is believed to be the cause of more than 85% of acute MIs.[5–8] The precipitating event is most often attributed to a disruption of a coronary plaque, which initiates a thrombotic process. "Lipid-rich" plaques, upon exposure of the lipid core, are particularly thrombogenic. The thrombotic process involves activation of platelets, thrombin, and fibrin and subsequently formation of a thrombus, which completely occludes the coronary vessel.

To understand completely the pathophysiology of MI, knowledge of the relationship between myocardial oxygen supply and demand is critical.[9] In addition, an understanding of the difference between myocardial ischemia and MI is important.

The primary determinant of myocardial oxygen supply is coronary blood flow. Coronary blood flow depends on coronary perfusion pressure, which, in turn, varies directly with systemic arterial pressure, left ventricular end-diastolic pressure, and diastolic filling time, which is inversely related to heart rate. Heart rate, myocardial contractility, and intraventricular wall tension are the major determinants of myocardial oxygen demand (MVo_2). Of these, intraventricular wall tension is considered to be the most important. Wall tension is directly related to intraventricular pressure and radius and indirectly influenced by ventricular wall thickness. Based on this relationship, an increase in systemic blood pressure or ventricular filling pressure (preload) results in an increase in MVo_2. However, patients with MI may have an elevated wall tension even if systemic pressure and preload are normal. As a result of myocardial injury and/or ischemia, there is a reduction in ventricular compliance (a "stiff" ventricle), which impairs both ventricular filling and emptying.

When there is an inadequate supply of oxygen to meet myocardial oxygen demand, ischemia occurs. Myocardial ischemia often occurs in patients with CAD who experience an increase in myocardial demand secondary to an increase in physical activity. In patients with CAD, blood supply is unable to meet the increase in demand. Therefore, ischemia occurs and a localized area of myocardium may become dysfunctional and/or the patient may experience chest pain or discomfort. Typically, ischemia and the associated consequences of ischemia are reversed when myocardial oxygen demand is reduced. Therefore, ischemic myocardium is considered salvageable and viable even though ventricular function may be compromised during ischemia.

Myocardial ischemia most likely precedes MI, but there are two distinct characteristics that differentiate MI from myocardial ischemia. First, MI is precipitated by a sudden interruption of blood supply to an area of myocardium due to complete, or near complete, occlusion of a coronary artery. Second, the occlusion persists long enough that myocardial function is compromised and myocardium becomes necrotic (nonviable). Infarction is characterized by a "wavefront" of ischemia that progresses from the endocardium to the epicardium (Fig. 15.1).[10] Subsequently, if coronary blood flow is not restored, myocardium dies, the time course for which is approximately 3 hours in animal models. Therefore, the primary difference between ischemia and infarction is viable myocardium. However, despite this rapid time course, it has been demonstrated that a significant percentage of myocardium "hibernates" in response to ischemia and is salvageable after as long as 12–24 hours of ischemia. This phenomenon may also be due in part to the presence of collateral blood flow within the infarcted area.[11,12] These features of MI have important implications on the therapeutic management, prognosis, and outcome of patients with MI.

Vasospasm has also been proposed as the etiology of MI in most patients. Although vasospasm is a component of and can cause MI, it is not accepted as the primary etiology. Circumstances that may contribute to coronary vasospasm include excessive physical exertion, abrupt exposure to extreme cold, and drugs, specifically catecholamines and cocaine.[13–15] Furthermore, it has been demonstrated that cocaine significantly alters both myocardial oxygen supply and demand and that this deleterious effect is exacerbated by concomitant cigarette smoking.[15]

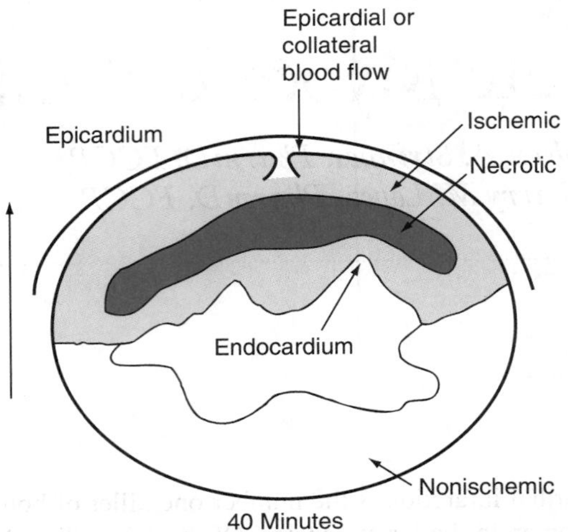

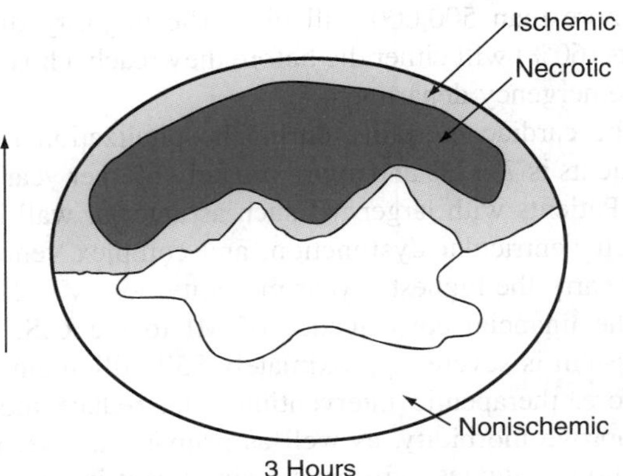

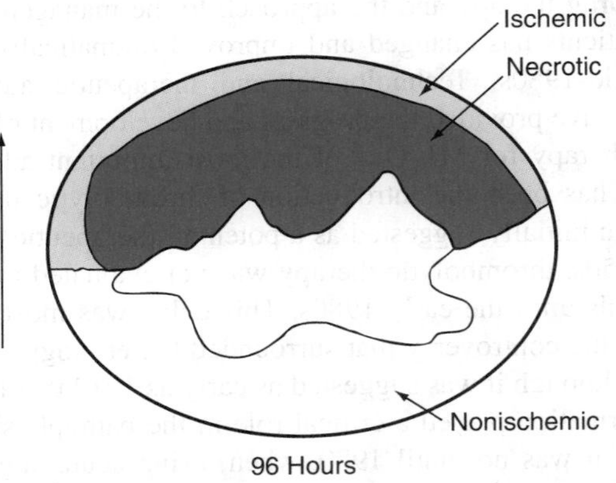

Figure 15.1. Wavefront of myocardial ischemia.

INFARCT LOCATION AND TYPE

The type and location of MI play a very important role in determining the therapeutic management and predicting the prognosis of the patient. Anterior wall MI (AWMI) involves the anterior wall of the left ventricle and most often represents occlusion of the left anterior descending artery (LAD).[16] Location of the occlusion within the LAD determines whether or not other areas of the myocardium, such as the lateral wall or septum, are involved. Typically, AWMI involves a much larger area of myocardium than inferior wall MI (IWMI) and, consequently, there is a risk of a greater loss of myocardium and myocardial function. Patients with AWMI typically have the highest mortality of MI patients.

The clinical significance of a right ventricular MI was not considered important until recently. Although isolated right ventricular infarction accounts for less than 3% of all MI, infarction of the right ventricle occurs in nearly 50% of the patients with IWMI.[17] The right ventricle is supplied by the right coronary artery (RCA). Although the oxygen demands of the right ventricle are considerably less, the incidence of atherosclerotic disease is similar to that of the left circulation. Due to the lower oxygen demand of the right ventricle there tends to be a lower incidence of right ventricular MI. However, this may not be the case in as many as 30–40% of the population in whom the RCA is a large, dominant vessel that not only supplies the right ventricle but also supplies a significant portion of inferior wall of the left ventricle. Therefore, in these individuals, occlusion of the RCA may result in an IWMI or the combination of an IWMI and right ventricular MI depending on where the occlusion in the RCA occurs. In left dominant individuals, the occlusion of the circumflex artery can result in right ventricular infarction. Because approximately 50% of IWMI patients may have right ventricular involvement, a right-sided electrocardiogram (ECG) should be obtained and assessed in all patients who present with IWMI. The presence of ST-segment elevation in V4R supports the diagnosis of right ventricular infarction as does the presence of right bundle branch block or complete heart block.[17]

Patients with right ventricular MI may be differentiated from patients with left ventricular MI by their initial presentation and clinical course.[17] Hypotension, clear lung fields, and an elevated jugular venous pressure in a patient with an IWMI is an indication of right ventricular involvement. Patients with right ventricular MI may present with or quickly develop hemodynamic compromise or cardiogenic shock. Due to right ventricular dysfunction, there is inadequate filling of the left ventricle. Therefore, patients with right ventricular MI usually require IV volume loading with normal saline to maintain right ventricular preload and cardiac output. If several liters of IV fluid are not effective in improving hypotension, patients may require inotropic support with dobutamine or dopamine. Medications such as nitroglycerin, diuretics, and other drugs that either reduce preload or blood pressure should be avoided in patients with right ventricular MI. In patients with right ventricular infarction that is accompanied by left ventricular dysfunction, IV nitroprusside may be needed to decrease the afterload of the left ventricle, and in severe cases where nitroprusside is not effective or tolerated, placement of an intra-aortic balloon pump (IABP) may be necessary.

Other than these exceptions, patients with right ventricular infarction should be managed in the same manner as patients with left ventricular infarction, particularly with regard to thrombolytic therapy, which is discussed later in this chapter. In general, the prognosis of patients with right ventricular infarction is favorable. Though patients with IWMI and right ventricular involvement may have an in-hospital mortality as high as 31%, long-term survival is usually good and, as with left ventricular infarction, depends primarily on left ventricular function.

In addition to location, the type of MI also has implications for therapeutic management. Transmural, referred to as Q-wave MI, results in injury that penetrates the entire thickness of the myocardial wall.[18] Subsequently, these patients develop significant "Q waves" on the ECG. Non-transmural, referred to as non-Q-wave MI, only involves the subendocardial myocardium. These patients present differently from patients with Q-wave MI in that their ECG may not show ST-segment elevation but may only have subtle findings such as T-wave inversion, non-specific ST-T-wave changes, or ST-segment depression. To confirm the diagnosis, cardiac enzymes are needed. More importantly, the prognosis and therapeutic management of patients with non-Q-wave MI is different from patients with Q-wave MI. This chapter focuses primarily on the pharmacotherapy of Q-wave MI and briefly discusses the management of non-Q-wave MI when applicable.

POSTINFARCTION CHANGES IN THE LEFT VENTRICLE

One of the most serious complications of MI is congestive heart failure (CHF). Enlargement of the left ventricle plays a critical role in the development of post-MI heart failure and subsequent mortality.[19–24] Heart failure following MI is directly related to the size of the MI and the amount of myocardial contractile function lost. However, the evolution of CHF appears to involve additional processes other than loss of viable tissue. Following MI, a series of events occurs that relate to the response of the left ventricle to injury. This process is called *ventricular remodeling.*[19–24] Activation of neurohumoral and renin–angiotensin systems and the release of vasopressin ensue once a decrease in cardiac output occurs. Sinus tachycardia, mediated by activation of the adrenergic system, occurs first as a response to a drop in cardiac output and, within hours of infarction, expansion of the infarcted area occurs due to thinning and stretching of the infarcted segment, which is followed by acute dilatation and hypertrophy of the noninfarcted myocardium. This initial process precipitates chronic changes in ventricular volume leading to further ventricular dilatation and hypertrophy and eventually the development of left ventricular failure and ultimately death. Scar formation and healing follow these early events with the entire process taking up to several months. Recently, clinical trials evaluating the impact of early drug therapy intervention on this remodeling process and the subsequent development of CHF have been completed.[22–24] These trials are reviewed later in this chapter.

PROGNOSIS

For patients who have experienced their first MI, the prognosis for survival is generally good.[2] However, patients with a second or third MI have approximately a twofold higher incidence of early mortality compared to patients with first MI. Furthermore, long-term survival is substantially better in first-time MI patients than in those who have had more than one MI.

Several factors have been implicated in predicting outcome of patients with MI. Baseline characteristics such as the presence of CHF and age have been shown to be predictive of outcome in MI patients.[2] However, the most predictive variables are not baseline characteristics but rather those that relate to the extent of myocardial damage after the infarction. These include heart size; peak and total cardiac enzyme release, which corresponds to infarct size; and left ventricular function.[2] In patients with first MI, age has also been shown to be the most important outcome factor followed by left ventricular function and the infarct location. Anterior wall infarction tends to be larger and therefore associated with a poorer outcome than inferior wall infarction or right ventricular infarction. Low-risk patients (a 2.5% 1-year cardiac mortality) are those patients less than 71 years of age with a left ventricular ejection fraction of at least 40%. Subsequently, patients who develop CHF post-MI have approximately a 50% 5-year mortality.

Interestingly, the overall prognosis for patients with non-Q-wave MI is not significantly different than for those with Q-wave MI; however, non-Q-wave MI is associated with a higher incidence of post-MI angina and reinfarction. Otherwise, similar outcome factors apply to non-Q-wave patients as they do to Q-wave MI.[2,18] Location of the infarct may play an important role in this circumstance. For instance, patients with inferior wall non-Q-wave MI have a significantly lower mortality rate and rate of reinfarction than do patients with anterior wall non-Q-wave MI.

Thus, careful evaluation of post-MI patients, including an assessment of left ventricular function, plays a key role in the therapeutic management and prognosis of these patients. To address these issues, aspects of secondary prevention and other post-MI management are discussed.

CLINICAL PRESENTATION

Chest pain is the predominant symptom that brings a patient with MI to the emergency department.[7,8] Patients will, however, frequently describe their symptom as chest pressure or a squeezing sensation rather than pain. Unfortunately, the presence of chest pain alone is not sufficient to make the diagnosis of MI, particularly since it may be difficult to distinguish it from a variety of other cardiac and noncardiac events such as angina, mitral valve prolapse, pericarditis, esophageal reflux or spasm, hiatal hernia, indigestion, peptic ulcer disease, costochondritis, or pleuritis. In addition, absence of pain has been reported in as many as 15–25% of patients with MI, particularly in patients with diabetes mellitus who may have autonomic dysfunction.[25] Consequently, additional criteria are necessary to confirm the diagnosis of MI.

In addition to chest pain, patients may present with physical findings such as diaphoresis, nausea and vomiting, arm tingling/numbness, and shortness of breath.[8] These symptoms too are not specific enough to confirm the diagnosis. Therefore, objective criteria must be used to confirm the diagnosis. These parameters include the 12-lead electrocardiogram (ECG), and characteristic changes in concentrations of the cardiac enzymes creatine kinase (CK), its MB isoenzyme fraction (CK-MB), and lactate dehydrogenase (LDH) and its corresponding subfractions.

The electrocardiographic diagnostic feature of MI is the Q wave associated with a pattern of ST-segment changes.[16,18] It is critical not to base the diagnosis on a single ECG but to obtain serial ECG to assess changes accurately. This strategy significantly enhances the sensitivity of the ECG in making the diagnosis. The earliest change in the ECG is associated with the T wave; it may be prolonged, peaked, or inverted. T-wave alterations are soon followed by ST-segment elevation (Fig. 15.2). A Q wave may or may not be present on the initial ECG or may appear hours or sometimes days after MI. Significant Q waves are those that are approximately one-third as deep the size of the QRS complex and are at least 1 mm (0.04 second) wide.

Serial blood samples for the determination of cardiac enzyme concentrations should be obtained from patients who present with suspected MI.[8,26] Peak concentrations of CK usually occur within 24 hours after MI followed by a decline and return to baseline by the third or fourth day. Peak LDH concentrations usually occur between 3 and 4 days after MI and return to normal by day 14. There must be an elevation of the total CK with at least a 4% CK-MB

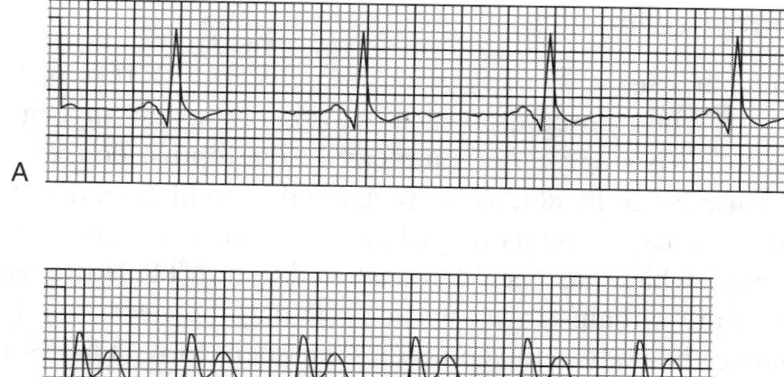

Figure 15.2. (A) Normal (isoelectric) ST segment with normal cardiac complexes and (B) ST-segment elevation with pathologic Q waves. Both rhythm strips are lead II.

fraction to confirm the diagnosis of Q-wave MI. The higher the total CK and percent MB, the larger the infarct. Patients with non-Q-wave MI do not have as high a rise in total CK and may not have much more than a 4% MB fraction. Though the utility of LDH is limited and probably unnecessary in patients who present within 24 hours of the onset of symptoms, it may be useful in patients who present late (>24 hours).[26,27] Peak concentrations should be at least two times above normal with an increase in the LDH-1 fraction that dominates in the heart. Typically, LDH-1 will peak sooner than total LDH. Ultimately, the LDH-1 concentration will exceed the concentration of the LDH-2 fraction. This change is commonly referred to as the LDH "flip." Notably, administration of a thrombolytic agent is associated with higher and earlier peaks in concentrations of cardiac enzymes, due to "washout" from ischemic and/or necrotic tissue.

Ultimately, the diagnosis of Q-wave MI is made if the following criteria are met: the presence of ischemic chest pain for at least 30 minutes, and/or ST-segment elevation on the ECG with the subsequent development of significant Q waves. The diagnosis is then confirmed by a rise in cardiac enzymes as described above.

Pharmaceutical Care of Patients with Uncomplicated Q-Wave Myocardial Infarction

GOALS OF THERAPY

The primary goals of therapy for patients with MI are to (1) minimize infarct size, (2) salvage ischemic myocardium, (3) prevent or minimize complications, and (4) improve outcome.

Admission to an intensive care or coronary care unit is mandatory for close observation and the acute care of MI patients. Close monitoring of vital signs, symptoms, and the ECG is recommended for the first 48–72 hours after MI in uncomplicated patients.[28] This includes patients who have received thrombolytic therapy or have undergone primary percutaneous transluminal coronary angioplasty (PTCA). Continued intensive monitoring is recommended beyond 72 hours if the patient is hemodynamically unstable and has persistent ischemia and/or hemodynamically significant cardiac arrhythmias. The highest incidence of MI complications and death is during the first 12–24 hours after the onset of symptoms.

In addition to intensive care, a number of other factors related to myocardial oxygen consumption should be aggressively controlled. Activity should be restricted for the first 3–4 days and gradually increased as tolerated by the patient. The hospital diet should include use of multiple small meals, sodium restriction, and reduced content of saturated fats and cholesterol. To avoid the stress associated with defecation, a stool softener, either docusate sodium 100 mg or docusate calcium 240 mg once or twice a day, is recommended.

In the following section, a treatment plan for the management of acute MI is discussed. Even though therapies are presented sequentially, most interventions for MI are "acute" in nature and frequently occur simultaneously or in close proximity to each other. Patients should be considered candidates for each therapy described based on a careful assessment of the risk and potential benefit of each intervention.

TREATMENT PLAN

Clinical Laboratories

Patients with presumed acute MI should, if possible, have three large-bore (18-gauge) peripheral intravenous (IV) lines placed upon admission to the emergency department. Early establishment of IV access ensures prompt therapy with important drugs that impact on the morbidity and mortality of the patient. In addition, IV access facilitates collection of blood for tests that are imperative to the diagnosis and assessment of a patient's suitability for thrombolytic therapy. One IV line should be reserved, if possible, for obtaining the frequent blood samples required. Pertinent laboratory tests on admission should include, but are not limited to, complete blood count (CBC) with platelet count, CK, CK-MB, activated partial thromboplastin time (aPTT), and prothrombin time (PT). Serial CK and CK-MB should be obtained every 6–8 hours for 24 hours. The utility of serial LDH determinations is limited unless that patient presents late (beyond 24 hours) from the onset of symptoms.[27] If this is the case, determination of serial LDH concentrations every 6–8 hours may be useful in confirming the diagnosis. If the patient receives thrombolytic therapy, a regular assessment of hemoglobin, hematocrit, and platelets should also be obtained. Details regarding appropriate laboratory monitoring of drug therapy are given in the following discussions of each agent when applicable.

Oxygen

Patients may be moderately hypoxic even during an uncomplicated MI. This may be due, in part, to a ventilation–perfusion mismatch.[28] Therefore, for the first few hours of MI, supplemental oxygen (2–4 L/min by nasal cannula) should be administered. Use of oxygen is even more important for patients with pulmonary edema or evidence of CHF because these patients will be more hypoxic. In severe cases of pulmonary edema or CHF, the patient may require mechanical ventilation.

Analgesia

Pain control and relief of anxiety are the most immediate objectives in the management of acute MI. Notably, recent experience with thrombolytic agents strongly suggests that pain associated with MI is due mainly to continuing ischemia of viable myocardium rather than to necrosis.[29]

IV morphine sulfate is the drug of choice for acute management of pain associated with MI.[28–30] Morphine blocks sympathetic efferent discharge from the central nervous system, resulting in peripheral arteriolar dilation, making it particularly effective in the setting of acute MI. Overall, morphine reduces myocardial oxygen demand (MVO_2) by decreasing systemic vascular resistance and afterload and decreasing circulating concentrations of catecholamines, which may, in turn, reduce the likelihood of ventricular arrhythmias.

Meperidine and hydromorphone are other analgesics that may also be useful for pain relief in MI. However, neither has been shown to be superior to morphine. Use of meperidine may be preferable in patients with IWMI because it is less vagotonic than morphine, but it has not been shown to be any more advantageous than morphine in this situation.

Dosing Guidelines

IV morphine should be administered slowly in small doses of 2–5 mg every 5–15 minutes as needed for pain. Dosage is often guided by blood pressure in that patients who are normotensive or hypertensive will tolerate higher morphine doses. A small number of patients whose pain persists may require maintenance doses of 4–8 mg every 4–6 hours.

Evaluation of Therapeutic Outcomes

Morphine therapy should be continued until pain relief is achieved or an unacceptable endpoint, such as hypotension (SBP <90 mm Hg), is reached. While receiving morphine, patients should be monitored closely for adverse effects such as hypotension, respiratory depression, and allergic reactions as well as the primary outcome, pain relief.

Nitroglycerin

The purpose of therapy with nitroglycerin (NTG) is to relieve chest discomfort and salvage ischemic myocardium.[28,31] Nitroglycerin is preferred to nitroprusside (NTP) because NTG, in addition to peripheral venodilation, dilates the coronary circulation without resulting in coronary "steal," which has been demonstrated with NTP. However, there are circumstances when NTP may be necessary to manage hemodynamic compromise associated with MI (see section on infarct location and section on complications). Pain relief by NTG is not due to analgesia but rather to an improvement in myocardial oxygen supply due to the dilation of epicardial and collateral vessels that improve blood supply to ischemic myocardium. In addition, NTG reduces MVO_2 by decreasing myocardial wall tension. Therefore, it is important that NTG not be used as a substitute for appropriate analgesic.

The benefit of NTG has been established in several clinical trials during the prethrombolytic era.[31,32] NTG reduces susceptibility to ventricular arrhythmias, specifically ventricular fibrillation; limits infarct size; and reduces mortality by 10–30%, although this effect appears to be restricted to patients with large MI. These benefits are attributed primarily to the ability of NTG to enhance collateral and epicardial blood flow, subsequently salvaging ischemic myocardium that may otherwise have infarcted. However, recent data from the Third Gruppo Italiano per lo Studio della Sopravvivenza nell'Infarto Miocardico (GISSI-3) suggest that IV NTG administered for 24 hours followed by transdermal NTG (10 mg) for 6 weeks, has no impact on mortality.[24] Therefore, though NTG appears to be useful in managing ischemic chest pain associated with MI, there is no apparent benefit to its long-term use alone (see section on angiotensin-converting enzyme inhibitors). Long-term NTG use (beyond the peri-infarction period) may only be necessary in patients with persistent angina.

Dosing Guidelines and Evaluation of Therapeutic Outcomes

Patients whose systolic blood pressure is less than 90 mm Hg should receive NTG cautiously or not at all. Tachycardiac (heart rate >100 beats/min) or bradycardic (heart rate <60 beats/min) patients, particularly if in combination with hypotension (systolic blood pressure <90 mm Hg), should not receive NTG. Furthermore, use of NTG should be avoided in patients with right ventricular MI and should be used cautiously in patients who present with bradycardia associated with IWMI.

Sublingual (SL) NTG (0.4 mg) is frequently used to determine whether chest pain is due to either MI or ischemia. Typically, 0.4 mg SL NTG is administered and chest pain intensity and the ECG are assessed. For the purpose of diagnosis, this dose of NTG may be repeated three times, once every 5 minutes, as long as heart rate and blood pressure are stable.

Following SL administration, heart rate and blood pressure should be closely monitored and the ECG should be evaluated. It is possible that SL NTG will relieve some or all of the patient's initial chest pain, but the ST segment elevation on the ECG may remain. If the ECG changes persist despite relief of chest pain, the diagnosis is MI.

IV NTG, rather than oral or transdermal, is preferred in the management of MI because it is easily titrated.[27] Therapy may be initiated with a 15-μg bolus followed by a initial infusion rate of 5–10 μg/min via an infusion pump, though a bolus dose may not be necessary due to the very brief elimination half-life of NTG. The NTG infusion may be increased every 5–10 minutes by 5–10 μg/min based on the therapeutic endpoints described below. Duration of IV NTG therapy is variable but a patient with an uncomplicated MI may only require 24–48 hours of therapy before switching to an oral or transdermal dosage form.

During IV NTG administration, it is also critical that heart rate and blood pressure be monitored. The NTG infusion may be increased every 5–10 minutes by 5–10 μg/min increments for chest pain relief, resolution of ECG abnormalities, or until the systolic blood pressure is between 90 and 100 mm Hg. One or more of these therapeutic endpoints should be expected within 30 minutes of initiating therapy.

Reduction of the systolic blood pressure to less than 90 mm Hg is not recommended since a low systolic pressure will compromise coronary perfusion pressure resulting in extension of the infarcted area. If a patient develops hypotension, the rate of the NTG infusion should be reduced or gradually discontinued. If upon discontinuation, the patient remains hypotensive, IV fluids should be administered.

NTG administration may be associated with either tachycardia or bradycardia. If the patient becomes either symptomatically tachycardiac or bradycardic, the NTG infusion rate should be decreased. The ECG should also be closely monitored for reemergence of ischemia even if the patient does not have recurrent chest pain.

Headache associated with NTG administration is common (>50%), and a small percentage of patients (<5%) may experience intolerable headache, which may require discontinuation of the drug. The willingness of the patient to accept headache as a consequence of therapy may need to be discussed as well as the potential benefits of NTG. Decreasing the infusion rate and acetaminophen may be effective in relieving NTG headache and should be given consideration prior to discontinuation of the NTG infusion.

Lidocaine

Cardiac arrhythmias, specifically, ventricular tachycardia (VT) and ventricular fibrillation (VF), are the most common consequences of MI.[8,33,34] The mechanism is believed to be extremely high levels of catecholamines secondary to the level of stress MI patients experience. However, the incidence of VT/VF declines almost linearly to zero within the first 24 hours after MI.[34] Since the incidence of VF is approximately 11% with a mortality rate of nearly 50%, it would seem reasonable to administer prophylactic antiarrhythmic therapy to these patients.

Lidocaine is the drug of choice for management of ventricular arrhythmias associated with MI. However, the use of prophylactic lidocaine is not widely accepted. The assumption made with prophylactic lidocaine is that suppression of premature ventricular contractions (PVCs) may decrease or eliminate the likelihood of VT or VF. However, despite suppression of PVCs with lidocaine, ventricular arrhythmias still may occur. A recent meta-analysis of prophylactic lidocaine studies showed that prehospital use of lidocaine did not result in a reduction in mortality and that in-hospital lidocaine actually resulted in an increase in mortality.[35] Thus, the risks of lidocaine, such as an increase in the incidence of asystole and central nervous system toxicity, appear to outweigh any benefit. Therefore, the use of prophylactic lidocaine in patients with MI is not recommended.

In patients who manifest ventricular arrhythmias, IV lidocaine is considered the drug of choice. It is now believed, however, that lidocaine should be reserved for patients who manifest either sustained or symptomatic ventricular arrhythmias or in patients who have received thrombolytic therapy and develop the following since the incidence of reperfusion arrhythmias is high[35,36]:

1. PVCs occurring >6/min
2. Closely coupled (R on T) PVCs
3. Multiform PVCs
4. Short bursts of ≥3 in succession
5. Ventricular tachycardia/fibrillation in association with CPR and electrical cardioversion if necessary.

The duration of lidocaine therapy should not exceed 48 hours since the incidence of ventricular arrhythmias associated with MI declines to nearly zero by 24–36 hours after MI. Typically, ventricular arrhythmias associated with acute MI are shortlived and responsive to drug therapy. There will be, however, a small subset of patients (approximately 10%) who will have persistent arrhythmias beyond 24 hours and who may or may not respond to lidocaine.[8,37] These patients represent a high-risk subgroup with post-MI arrhythmias that potentially have a more serious underlying cardiac problem that requires further evaluation. The management of post-MI arrhythmias is discussed in detail in the cardiac arrhythmia chapter (Chapter 16).

Dosing Guidelines

Patients who require lidocaine therapy must be dosed appropriately in order to maximize antiarrhythmic efficacy and minimize the risk of toxicity. Therapy should be initiated with an IV bolus dose of 1 mg/kg, which should not exceed 100 mg. Additional bolus doses may be given every

8–10 minutes up to a total loading dose of 4 mg/kg. Simultaneously, upon administration of the initial bolus dose, a constant infusion of 22–50 μg/kg/min should be started. Doses of lidocaine may need to be reduced in patients with CHF and/or liver disease.

Evaluation of Therapeutic Outcomes

The goal of lidocaine therapy is suppression of ventricular arrhythmias. Therefore, the ECG should be closely observed for PVCs and VT/VF. Recurrent arrhythmias may indicate the need for additional lidocaine or alternative therapy.

Patients who receive lidocaine should also be carefully monitored for adverse effects such as nausea, drowsiness, perioral numbness, dizziness, confusion, hypotension, bradycardia, asystole, and seizures. This requires regular assessment of the ECG, heart rate, blood pressure, and the mental status of the patient. Determination of serum lidocaine concentrations may not be useful in this situation because of the short duration of therapy and alteration of lidocaine pharmacokinetics in association with MI. The use of lidocaine concentrations in the setting of MI may only be appropriate if the patient is not responding to therapy or develops signs and symptoms of toxicity that may not clearly be due to lidocaine. Patients whose ventricular arrhythmias do not respond to lidocaine should be switched to IV procainamide. The reader is referred to Chapter 16 of this text for details regarding the use of other antiarrhythmic drugs in the management of VT/VF.

Early Administration of β-Adrenergic Blockers

As many as 32 clinical trials have established that early administration (within 12 hours of the onset of chest pain) of β blockers reduces the incidence of ventricular arrhythmias, recurrent ischemia, and reinfarction, and, most importantly, mortality in patients with acute MI.[38–43] It is believed that this benefit is derived from the ability of β blockers to reduce MVO_2 by slowing heart rate, lowering blood pressure, and reducing myocardial contractility.[44] The benefit of β blockers appears to be particularly significant in tachycardiac and/or hypertensive patients.[28]

Though many studies have been conducted evaluating the use of β blockers in MI, these studies were conducted prior to the thrombolytic era. Until recently, the usefulness of a β blocker in patients receiving thrombolytic therapy was not known. The Thrombolysis in Myocardial Infarction (TIMI) IIB study, however, showed that patients who receive early therapy with IV metoprolol have a lower incidence of reinfarction and/or ischemia than patients who do not.[43] Consequently, it appears that the benefits of β-blocker therapy are sustained in patients who receive thrombolytic therapy.

The choice of β blocker does not appear to be an issue when treating MI patients; the benefit of early administration has been demonstrated with several different agents. However, β blockers with intrinsic sympathomimetic activity (ISA) should be avoided in this setting; they have not been shown to be of benefit.[28,44]

Dosing Guidelines and Evaluation of Therapeutic Outcomes

Beta-blocker therapy is recommended for hemodynamically stable patients who are tachycardiac and/or hypertensive whether or not they receive thrombolytic therapy. Before β-blocker therapy is initiated, an assessment of the patient should be made to determine whether relative or absolute contraindications to β blockers exist. Patients who have one or more of the following, should not receive β blockers (absolute contraindications): a heart rate of less than 50 beats/min, systolic blood pressure of less than 100 mm Hg, moderate to severe left ventricular dysfunction, signs of peripheral hypoperfusion, a PR interval >0.26 second, or severe chronic obstructive pulmonary disease (COPD). A risk–benefit assessment should be made in patients who have *relative* contraindications to β-blocker therapy, such as a history of asthma and/or current use of either a β blocker or calcium channel blocker. Patients with signs of mild heart failure should still be considered candidates since this group of patients has been shown to benefit from β-blocker therapy.

Prior to starting a β blocker, heart rate and blood pressure should be determined. Blood pressure and heart rate should be at least 100 mm Hg and 55 beats/min, respectively. After each IV dose, heart rate and blood pressure should be carefully reassessed and the ECG reviewed for AV block. The patient should be carefully observed for signs of worsening heart failure. It may require more than 5–10 minutes between doses to assess fully the hemodynamic and electrocardiographic response of the patient. If the heart rate falls below 55 beats/min and/or blood pressure falls below 90 mm Hg, or if the PR interval prolongs beyond 0.26 second, IV administration of β blockers should be discontinued while hemodynamic and electrocardiographic assessment continues. In some cases, bradycardia, hypotension, and AV block may be transient. If this is the case, the IV regimen can be resumed, but if it persists, the IV regimen should be stopped. Approximately 10–15% of patients may not tolerate the full IV regimen.[43] This difficulty, however, does not preclude any patient from continuing with an oral regimen that can be initiated 6–12 hours after the last IV dose depending on the β blocker used. An algorithm outlining the decision-making process for acute β-blocker therapy is outlined in Fig. 15.3.

Late Administration of β-Adrenergic Blockers

The goal of late oral administration (at least 24 hours after MI) of β-blocker therapy is secondary prevention. Patients who are not eligible for early IV β-blocker therapy should still be considered candidates for late administration.

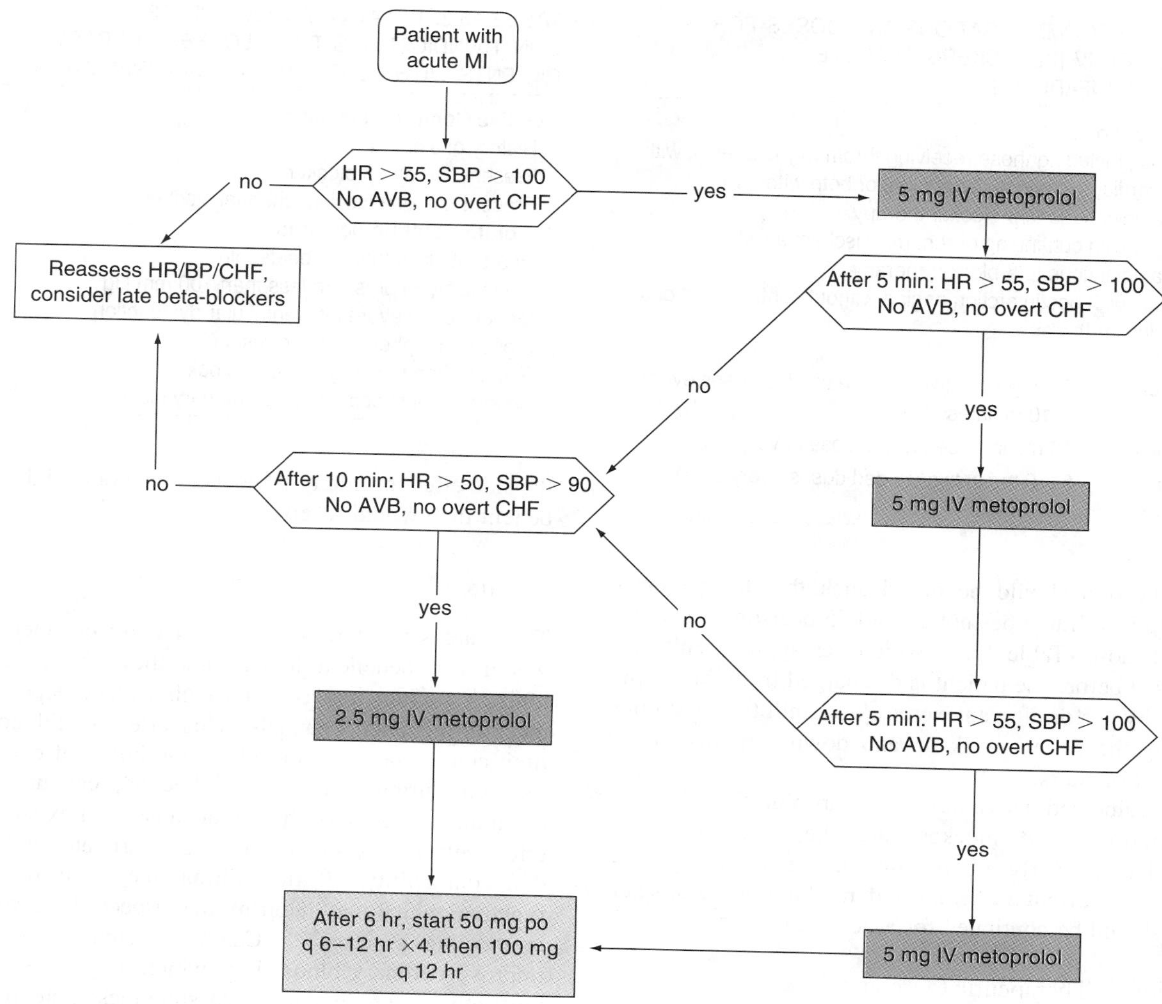

Figure 15.3. Algorithm for the administration of early IV metoprolol to patients with acute myocardial infarction. HR, heart rate; SBP, systolic blood pressure; AVB, atrioventricular block; CHF, congestive heart failure.

Approximately 16 studies of the long-term efficacy of β blockers in acute MI have been conducted, the benefit of which was first demonstrated with propranolol.[38,45] These studies demonstrated an improvement in survival and a reduction in reinfarction when β-blocker therapy is initiated between 24 and 72 hours after MI. Interestingly, patients with mild CHF appeared to benefit as much and, in some cases, to a greater extent, than patients with normal or near-normal left ventricular function.[45–47] Specifically, use of a β blocker in such patients with mild to moderate CHF was associated with a lower incidence of sudden cardiac death compared with similar patients who did not receive a β blocker. Data from two long-term studies have shown a marked (47 and 43%) reduction in sudden cardiac death in patients with left ventricular dysfunction treated with β blockers, illustrating the importance of this class of drugs in this patient population.[46,47]

In patients with uncomplicated MI, benefits of long-term β blockade are less obvious. These patients would include those with good left ventricular function (>40% ejection fraction), no postinfarction angina or arrhythmias, and those with no evidence of ischemia during exercise testing. Such patients have a very favorable prognosis for the first year after MI and adverse effects of β blockade may be bothersome enough in this group to outweigh benefit.[48]

Dosing Guidelines

As with early administration, many β-blocking agents have been evaluated and those with ISA should not be used. The FDA-approved β blockers for use in MI are propranolol, timolol, and metoprolol. Though some patients may not tolerate recommended doses (Tables 15.1 and 15.2) this should not preclude a patient from receiving a β blocker.

TABLE 15.1. RECOMMENDATIONS AND DOSES FOR EARLY USE OF IV β BLOCKERS IN ACUTE MYOCARDIAL INFARCTION

Recommendations

1. Patients, including those receiving thrombolytic agents, with tachycardia, systolic hypertension, or both without contraindications to β-blocker therapy
2. Patients with continuing or recurrent ischemia without contraindications to β-blocker therapy
3. Patients with postinfarction angina without contraindications to β-blocker therapy

IV Doses

Propranolol	0.1 mg/kg in two to three divided doses every 10 minutes
Metoprolol	15 mg in three divided doses every 5 minutes
Atenolol	5–10 mg in two divided doses every 5–10 minutes

The medication should be dosed such that the patient's exercising heart rate does not exceed 75 beats/min or to the maximum dose (Table 15.3), whichever applies. This can be assessed before the patient is discharged from the hospital either by performing an exercise treadmill test or simply by having the patient walk up and down a hallway or a short flight of stairs.

Contraindications (relative and absolute) to the late administration of β blockers are the same as those described under early administration. For secondary prevention of recurrent ischemia and reinfarction, β-blocker therapy should be continued for at least 2 years.[27]

Evaluation of Therapeutic Outcomes

As mentioned under dosing guidelines, heart rate is an important tool in assessing a patient's response to β-blocker therapy. In addition, the patient should be followed closely for the development of CHF and/or hypotension. Although patients who leave the hospital with some degree of ventricular compromise (ejection fraction <40%) derive the greatest mortality benefit from β blockers, they also may be more prone to these adverse effects. If they occur, β-blocker dosage should either be decreased or therapy should be discontinued. Patients should also be monitored for symptomatic bradycardia and for long-term adverse reactions such as impotence, hyperlipidemia, depression, and claudication. In low-risk patients, those that have had a small MI (IWMI and/or a CK enzyme peak <1000 ng/mL), the side effect profile of β blockers may outweigh the small benefit they would receive.

TABLE 15.2. BETA BLOCKERS FOR LATE ADMINISTRATION IN ACUTE MYOCARDIAL INFARCTION

Oral Doses

Propranolol	180–240 mg/d in four divided doses
Metoprolol	220 mg/d in two divided doses
Atenolol	100 mg/d as a single dose
Timolol	22 mg/d in two divided doses

TABLE 15.3. RELATIVE AND ABSOLUTE CONTRAINDICATIONS TO β-BLOCKER THERAPY IN PATIENTS WITH ACUTE MYOCARDIAL INFARCTION

Relative Contraindications

- History of asthma
- Present use of a β blocker
- Present use of a calcium channel blocker

Absolute Contraindications

- Heart rate less than 50 beats/min
- Systolic blood pressure less than 100 mm Hg
- Moderate or severe left ventricular dysfunction
- Signs of peripheral hypoperfusion
- Greater than first degree heart block
- Severe chronic obstructive pulmonary disease

Calcium Channel Antagonists

There are several reasons why calcium channel blockers would seem beneficial in MI. First, they inhibit the entry of ionized calcium into cells through voltage-dependent and receptor-mediated channels. This effect could potentially limit cell damage by controlling the influx of calcium into the cell during ischemia.[44,49] Second, calcium blockers (with the exception of those that cause a reflex tachycardia) effectively reduce blood pressure, heart rate, and myocardial contractility.[44,49] In addition, they improve diastolic function, which may interrupt that aspect of the ventricular remodeling process.[44,49] Calcium channel blockers also improve coronary blood flow, which may be beneficial in preventing infarct extension. Despite these potential advantages, several studies have shown that the benefits of calcium channel blockers are minimal at best and, specifically, nifedipine actually worsens outcome.[50–52]

To date, two studies, the Multicenter Diltiazem Postinfarction Trial (MDPIT) and the second Danish Study Group on Verapamil in Myocardial Infarction (DAVITII), have shown that when initiated within 1–2 weeks of MI, verapamil or diltiazem reduces the incidence of cardiac events and mortality.[50,51] This benefit however was only observed in patients who did not have pulmonary congestion at the time of MI or study drug initiation. The absolute reduction in cardiac events was modest, 3% in the MDPIT and 5% in the DAVITII. Furthermore, these studies were conducted prior to the era of thrombolytic therapy.

Nifedipine has also been studied in MI. Interestingly, the SPRINT (Secondary Prevention Reinfarction Israeli Nifedipine Trial) study was conducted concomitantly with streptokinase.[52] However, nifedipine did not enhance myocardial salvage, improve ventricular function, or reduce the incidence of myocardial ischemia. The lack of benefit of nifedipine is most likely due to excessive blood pressure lowering coupled with a decrease in coronary perfusion pressure and reflex tachycardia. Thus, the use of calcium channel antagonists is not routinely recommended in patients with Q-wave MI.

Calcium Channel Antagonists in the Management of Non-Q-Wave MI

An estimated 25–40% of patients admitted for presumed MI suffer a non-Q-wave MI.[8,53,54] Typically, non-Q-wave MI is associated with a lower in-hospital mortality rate than Q-wave MI. However, long-term survival is not as favorable for non-Q-wave patients as it is for Q-wave patients. This is believed to be primarily due to a higher incidence of recurrent ischemia in non-Q-wave patients. Hence, the need for aggressive preventative intervention has been established.

During the past 10 years, a number of clinical trials have been conducted evaluating the efficacy of calcium channel antagonists in MI.[44] However, only two prospective, randomized studies, have been conducted to address the use of calcium channel blockers in non-Q-wave MI.[50,53,55] In the Diltiazem Reinfarction Study, the incidence of recurrent MI was 5.2% in diltiazem-treated patients versus 9.3% in patients treated with placebo. Though from the initial analysis this translated into a 24-month reinfarction rate reduction of 51.2% ($p < 0.029$), the benefit was neither sustained in long-term follow-up nor by data generated from the Multicenter Diltiazem Postinfarction Trial. Diltiazem has also been shown to be effective in reducing post-MI refractory angina by 49.7% ($p = 0.035$) and angina associated with ECG changes by 28% ($p = 0.005$). However, no data show that diltiazem has any impact on mortality in these patients. Thus, diltiazem is recommended for patients with non-Q-wave MI for the prevention of post-MI angina and reinfarction.

Dosing Guidelines

The contraindications to calcium channel blockers are similar to those of β blockers. Patients with evidence of compromised left ventricular dysfunction should be treated cautiously if not at all with diltiazem, and diltiazem should be avoided in patients with heart block and/or hypotension. In patients with non-Q-wave MI, who do not have contraindications to a calcium antagonist, diltiazem 90 mg every 6 hours should be initiated between 24 and 72 hours after the onset of MI and continued for 2 years.

Evaluation of Therapeutic Outcomes

Heart rate and blood pressure should be monitored closely in patients receiving diltiazem. In particular, patients should be questioned about signs and symptoms of bradycardia, heart failure, and the frequency and severity of anginal episodes. The most common side effects of diltiazem include constipation, nausea, and dizziness.

Secondary Prevention with Calcium Channel Antagonists

When evaluating the role of calcium antagonists in secondary prevention of MI, one must keep in mind important intrinsic differences between the agents. With regard to mortality, the trend with nifedipine is clearly negative, while diltiazem and verapamil appear to provide some benefit. However, this effect is small and is limited to patients who have no evidence of CHF. Therefore, routine use of calcium channel blockers for secondary prevention of MI is currently not recommended.

Amiodarone

Post-MI patients who continue to manifest frequent premature ventricular contractions (PVCs) and/or ventricular arrhythmias represent a subgroup of patients at high risk for sudden cardiac death, the etiology of which is believed to be VT/VF.[56–58] Recently, the Cardiac Arrhythmia Suppression Trial (CAST) evaluated the efficacy of encainide, flecainide, and moricizine in this subgroup of post-MI patients.[59,60] This study clearly showed that antiarrhythmic therapy was associated with a significantly higher mortality than placebo. However, since CAST only evaluated the efficacy of class IC drugs, the possibility exists that other antiarrhythmic agents have different effects.

Amiodarone, a class III antiarrhythmic drug, possesses unique characteristics such as mild calcium channel and β-blocking properties that suggest that it may be useful in post-MI patients at high risk for sudden cardiac death. During the last 5 years, several studies have been conducted to determine the effect of amiodarone on mortality in these patients. One study, the Spanish Study on Sudden Death, compared low-dose amiodarone (200 mg/d) to metoprolol (100–200 mg/d) in 368 patients with asymptomatic ventricular arrhythmias with left ventricular ejection fractions of 22–45%.[61] This preliminary study suggests that in this subgroup of patients, amiodarone is effective in suppressing ventricular arrhythmias and was associated with a lower mortality rate than patients treated with metoprolol. However, this small study is only suggestive (the difference in mortality between amiodarone and metoprolol was not statistically significant) and given the established benefit of β blockers in post-MI patients, particularly those with mild-to-moderate heart failure, these data need to be interpreted cautiously. A larger study will need to be conducted to confirm these findings.

Recently, a meta-analysis of four prospective, randomized, placebo-controlled studies of amiodarone was published.[62] In the studies evaluated, low doses of amiodarone (220–400 mg/d) in a total of 1140 patients resulted in a significant reduction in sudden cardiac death (3.1%) and mortality (6.1%) when compared to placebo (6.9 and 11.2%, respectively; $p < 0.01$). Furthermore, there was no significant difference between placebo- and amiodarone-treated patients with left ventricular dysfunction (ejection fraction <45%; $p = 0.30$). Although amiodarone appears to be beneficial in post-MI patients by meta-analysis, the role of amiodarone compared to β blockers and in patients with left ventricular dysfunction will not be clarified until large, ongoing, randomized trials are completed.

Magnesium

The use of IV magnesium has been evaluated as part of the continuing search for new therapeutic modalities for the management of MI. Though magnesium was used as an antiarrhythmic in management of MI in the 1960s, only small studies were conducted. With the attention of most clinicians focused on thrombolytic and antithrombotic therapy, the potential role of magnesium was not aggressively pursued until recently. Several small studies have been conducted and a meta-analysis of them shows that when compared with placebo, IV magnesium significantly reduces the mortality associated with MI.[63] As a note of caution, however, this meta-analysis included trials that were performed prior to the routine use of thrombolytic therapy and aspirin. Regardless, this triggered a renewed interest in the potential benefit of magnesium in MI and as a result a large prospective study was conducted.

More than 4500 patients with suspected MI were randomized to either magnesium or placebo in the Second Leicester IV Magnesium Intervention Trial (LIMIT-2).[64] Magnesium-treated patients received 8 mmol of IV $MgSO_4$ over 5 minutes followed by a constant infusion of 65 mmol over 24 hours. As a result of this regimen serum magnesium concentration increased approximately twofold over the 24-hour period and returned to normal within 48 hours of randomization. In patients who received magnesium, the 28-day mortality rate was 7.8 versus 10.3% for placebo treated patients ($p = 0.04$), a relative reduction in mortality of 24%. This benefit could not be attributed to an antiarrhythmic effect of magnesium. However, it was suggested that it could be due, in part, to a reduction in peripheral and coronary vascular resistance, which resulted in an improvement in cardiac output and coronary blood flow. Side effects of magnesium were minimal and included transient flushing during the bolus injection and a slightly higher incidence of bradycardia in patients who received magnesium (10.8 versus 8%). The study concluded that magnesium is a safe, effective, and inexpensive therapeutic agent for patients with MI. However, they stopped short of recommending its routine use because the confidence intervals in the mortality analysis overlapped, suggesting that a larger sample size would be needed to determine definitively the significance of their finding.

The Fourth International Study of Infarct Survival (ISIS-4) was a much larger trial than LIMIT-2, evaluating the usefulness of magnesium in the management of MI.[65] In this study, more than 50,000 patients with suspected MI were randomized to receive either captopril, nitrates, or IV magnesium. The mortality rate of patients who received magnesium differed insignificantly from that observed in patients who did not (7.28 versus 6.92%, respectively). So, despite a large difference in mortality in early studies, the results of ISIS-4 do not support routine use of magnesium in patients with MI. Whether subgroups of patients benefit from magnesium is not known and further analysis of ISIS-4 data is expected.

Thrombolytic Therapy

Thrombolytic therapy probably represents the most important advancement in the treatment of MI in the last decade. Currently, three agents are approved for use by the FDA in patients with MI in the United States: streptokinase (SK [Streptase/Kabikinase]), recombinant tissue-type plasminogen activator (tPA, alteplase [Activase]), and anisoylated plasminogen streptokinase activator complex (APSAC, anistreplase [Eminase]). These agents do not alter myocardial oxygen demand. Instead, they improve myocardial oxygen supply by dissolving the thrombus associated with acute MI, reestablishing blood flow to ischemic myocardium. Consequently, the extent of myocardial necrosis and infarct size are limited and the likelihood of survival is significantly improved if thrombolysis is achieved in a timely fashion.

All of these agents are plasminogen activators.[66,67] They act by converting, either directly or indirectly, plasminogen to the nonspecific proteolytic enzyme, plasmin (Fig. 15.4). Plasmin is the enzyme responsible for clot lysis, which results in the liberation of fibrin(ogen) degradation products. In addition, clotting factors I, II, V, and VIII break down and fibrinogen is depleted, resulting in a "lytic" state that inhibits further clotting (Fig. 15.4). Streptokinase, a protein isolated from β-hemolytic streptococci, interacts with both circulating and fibrin bound plasminogen to form a SK–plasminogen complex. This complex subsequently acts on circulating and fibrin-bound plasminogen converting it to plasmin. Anistreplase (ASTP), a second-generation thrombolytic, is a modified inactive derivative of the SK–plasminogen complex. The catalytic site of the SK–plasminogen complex is an anisoyl group. After IV administration, activation begins immediately with the enzymatic cleavage of the anisoyl group and subsequent release of the SK–plasminogen complex into the systemic circulation.

Unlike SK and ASTP, tPA acts directly on plasminogen to form plasmin. In addition, tPA has a higher affinity for fibrin-bound plasminogen than circulating plasminogen. It was originally believed that this property of tPA would produce less of a systemic lytic state than SK, thereby reducing the risk of hemorrhagic complications. However, a modest systemic lytic state does accompany tPA and risk of hemorrhage associated with its use is indistinguishable

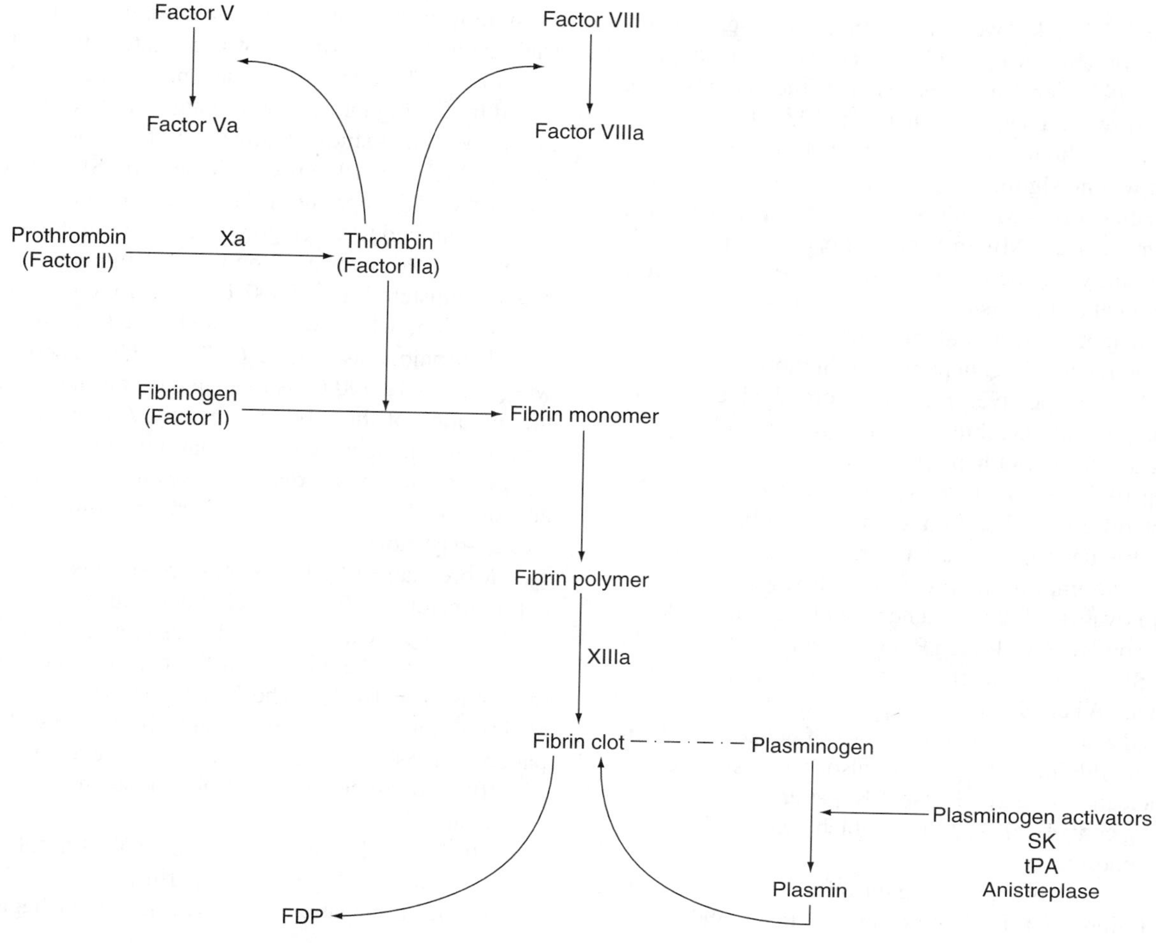

Figure 15.4. Clot formation and thrombolysis. SK, streptokinase; tPA, tissue plasminogen activator; FDP, fibrin degradation products.

from other thrombolytic agents. In fact, the incidence of cerebral bleeds is somewhat higher in tPA-treated patients than in SK-treated patients.

Many clinical trials have established the efficacy, safety, and mortality benefit of thrombolytic therapy in patients with MI.[68] However, controversy arose regarding the superiority of one agent over the others. Subsequently, the focus of most recent studies has been the direct comparison of the agents to one another. The first of these large trials, the Second Gruppo Italiano per lo Studio della Streptochinasi nell'Infarto Miocardio (GISSI-2) in combination with the International Study group (GISSI-2/Int), randomized nearly 23,000 patients presenting within 12 hours of onset of symptoms to either to SK 1.5 million units over 1 hour or tPA 100 mg over 3 hours.[69,70] Patients were also randomized to either receive 12,500 U subcutaneous (SQ) heparin every 12 hours starting 12 hours after the beginning of the thrombolytic infusion or to no heparin at all. There was no significant difference in mortality rate between patients who received SK or tPA (8.5 versus 8.9%, respectively), regardless of SQ heparin administration (8.5% heparin versus 8.9% no heparin). Furthermore, in patients who received tPA, the frequency of stroke was higher than in the SK group (1.33 versus 0.94%, respectively; p = 0.008) while major hemorrhages occurred more frequently in the SK group than in the tPA group (0.9 versus 0.6%, respectively). Notably, major hemorrhage occurred more often in patients who received SQ heparin than in those who did not (1 versus 0.5%, respectively; p = 0.0057) and SQ heparin did not alter the incidence of stroke or reinfarction. In addition to showing no significant difference between SK and tPA, the results of GISSI-2 raised important questions about the role of heparin in patients receiving thrombolytic therapy; this issue is discussed later in this chapter.

The Third International Study of Infarct Survival (ISIS-3) is another large trial that compared thrombolytic agents.[71] This trial randomized more than 41,000 patients with suspected MI within 24 hours of the onset of chest pain to receive either IV SK (1.5 MU over 1 hour), tPA

(Duteplase, 0.6 MU/kg over 4 hours [not alteplase, which is the "tPA" available in the United States]), or anistreplase (Eminase, 30 U over 3 minutes). Half of the patients were also randomized to receive SQ heparin, 12,500 U every 12 hours, starting 4 hours after the start of thrombolytic therapy. There was no significant difference in 35-day mortality between patients treated with SK or ASTP, although there were fewer recurrent MIs in patients treated with tPA. The 35-day mortality rate between the SK and tPA groups were nearly identical (10.6 versus 10.3%, respectively). The incidence of major, noncerebral hemorrhage was greater in patients who received SQ heparin than in those who did not (1 versus 0.8%, respectively). Furthermore, the incidence of definite or probable cerebral hemorrhage was also significantly higher in the SQ heparin group than in the nonheparin group (0.56 versus 0.4%, respectively; $p < 0.05$). No significant difference between groups was observed with respect to frequency of stroke. Overall, the addition of SQ heparin had no impact on 35-day mortality.

There was a slightly higher incidence of stroke in patients who received ASTP compared to those who received SK. This difference was attributed to cerebral hemorrhage. When SK was compared to tPA, tPA-treated patients had a slightly higher incidence of noncerebral hemorrhage. In addition, tPA patients also had a significantly higher incidence of stroke than SK patients (1.39 versus 1.04%, respectively; $p < 0.01$), which was attributed to cerebral hemorrhage.

Finally, a study that has again raised controversy, the GUSTO (Global Utilization of Streptokinase and Tissue Plasminogen Activator for Occluded Coronary Arteries) trial, evaluated the efficacy of accelerated tPA (bolus of 15 mg, 0.75 mg/kg over 30 minutes, not to exceed 50 mg followed by 0.5 mg/kg over 60 minutes, not to exceed 35 mg) in an open-label study, compared to three other strategies: SK, 1.5 MU over 1 hour with IV heparin; SK, 1.5 MU over 1 hour with SQ heparin; or the combination of SK, 1.5 MU over 1 hour, and tPA (1 mg/kg over 1 hour not to exceed 90 mg with 10% given as a bolus).[72,73] Intravenous heparin was administered as a 5000 U bolus followed by a 1000 U/h infusion, which was adjusted based on the activated partial thromboplastin time (aPTT). Subcutaneous heparin was given as 12,500 units twice a day starting 4 hours after the initiation of thrombolytic therapy. All patients received aspirin and patients without contraindications received 5 mg IV atenolol in two divided doses followed by oral therapy of 50–100 mg/d. The primary endpoint of the study was 30-day mortality.

More than 41,000 patients were enrolled into GUSTO, approximately 10,000 in each treatment arm. The 30-day mortality significantly favored accelerated tPA (Fig. 15.5) and there was no significant difference between the two SK regimens ($p = 0.731$). The benefit observed with accelerated tPA translates to approximately 10 lives saved per 1000 patients, a risk reduction of 14%. However, there was a slightly higher incidence of stroke in patients who received accelerated tPA.

Stroke of all types occurred in 1.6% of accelerated tPA patients and 1.4% of SK/IV heparin patients and 1.2% of SK/SQ heparin patients. However, hemorrhagic stroke

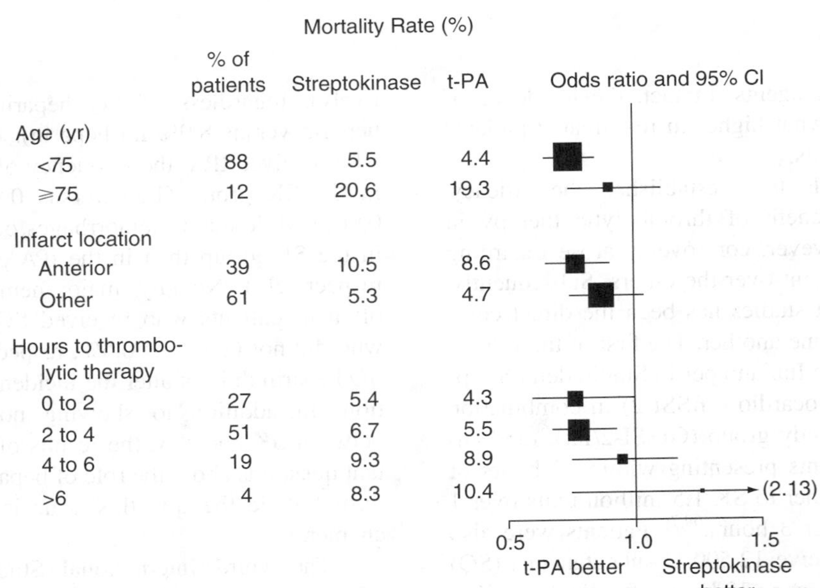

Figure 15.5. Mortality rates (%) of streptokinase- and tPA-treated patients in the GUSTO trial. Odds ratios and 95% confidence intervals (CI) for 30-day mortality in the prespecified subgroups defined by age, infarct location, and time to thrombolytic therapy. See text for revised data. *(Adapted with permission from Ref. 72.)*

occurred more often in patients who received accelerated tPA than either of the SK groups (0.72% versus 0.54% SK/IV versus 0.49% SK/SQ). Though there was no significant difference in severe or life-threatening bleeding between the treatment groups, moderate bleeding was slightly higher in the SK groups.

Additional important findings made in the GUSTO trial (Fig. 15.5) included the incidence of hemorrhagic stroke. In patients more than 75 years of age, there was a 71% higher incidence of hemorrhagic stroke in accelerated tPA-treated patients versus those treated with SK. Furthermore, the mortality rate of patients greater than age 75 was approximately fourfold higher than those age 75 or less, regardless of the thrombolytic agent they received (SK: 22.6 versus 5.5%, respectively, $p < 0.05$; tPA: 23.3 versus 4.4%, respectively, $p < 0.05$). In addition, only patients who presented within 4 hours from the onset of chest pain significantly benefited from accelerated tPA. The mortality rate of patients who presented between 4 and 6 hours from symptom onset was not different between the accelerated tPA and SK groups (9.3 versus 8.9%, respectively). However, these data were later refuted during further analysis. There is no significant difference between SK and tPA based on hours to thrombolytic therapy. Finally, only patients with AWMI experienced a benefit from accelerated tPA. These observations suggest that the choice of thrombolytic drug should be based on time of presentation, the age of the patient, and the infarct location.

Patient Eligibility

Patients who present within the first 12 hours after the onset of chest pain should be evaluated as candidates for thrombolytic therapy.[71,74] There are data, however, to support administration of thrombolytic therapy as far out as 24 hours after the onset of chest pain.[71,74] Patients who present after 24 hours should not be considered eligible for thrombolytic therapy. Patients who present between 12 and 24 hours are typically only considered for thrombolytic therapy if they have signs and symptoms of ongoing ischemia such as persistent ST-segment elevation and chest pain. Some of these patients may give a history of "stuttering" chest pain that has come and gone and come again in the last 6–12 hours. These patients represent a unique subgroup and need to be carefully evaluated. The risks and benefits of thrombolytic therapy need to be weighed before the decision to treat the patient with a lytic agent can be made.[75] Currently, the recommendation for consideration of thrombolytic therapy is 12 hours from the onset of chest pain.

Contraindications need to be carefully considered when determining whether an MI patient should receive thrombolytic therapy. So that therapy is not delayed, evaluation of potential contraindications needs to be made quickly. The sooner patients are treated with thrombolytic therapy, the better the outcome.[72,74,75] Good outcome is optimally achieved if eligible patients are treated with thrombolytic therapy within 70 minutes from the time of emergency department admission.[76] Furthermore, patients who are treated within 4 hours from the onset of their chest pain have a better outcome in regard to infarct artery patency and preservation of left ventricular function.[72,73]

Absolute and relative contraindications to thrombolytic therapy are outlined in Table 15.4. The decision to administer thrombolytic therapy should be made on a timely assessment of risks and benefits. The presence of more than one relative contraindication is considered an *absolute* contraindication to therapy. Of significant importance is the issue of the patient's age. Age is neither an absolute nor relative contraindication.[75] Certainly, older individuals, particularly those over the age of 75, have a significantly higher mortality from MI than younger individuals regardless of whether they are treated with thrombolytic therapy or not. However, older patients still gain a mortality benefit from thrombolytic therapy. Therefore, in the absence of an absolute contraindication, older patients (>65 years) should not be excluded as candidates for thrombolytic therapy.

The choice of thrombolytic agent is another consideration in the decision-making process. A 1% mortality benefit of accelerated tPA compared to SK is supported by data from the GUSTO study. However, as mentioned previously, it appears that only a subset of patients clearly benefits from

TABLE 15.4. RELATIVE AND ABSOLUTE CONTRAINDICATIONS TO THROMBOLYTIC THERAPY

Relative
- Recent trauma or surgery (i.e., <2 weeks)
- History of cerebrovascular accident
- History of GI or GU surgery or stroke within last 6 months
- Active peptic ulcer
- History of chronic severe HTN with or without drug therapy
- Significant liver dysfunction
- Prior exposure to streptokinase or anistreplase
- Known bleeding diathesis

Absolute
- Possible aortic dissection
- Acute pericarditis
- Active internal bleeding
- Severe uncontrolled hypertension (BP >220/110 mm Hg)
- Recent head trauma or known intracranial neoplasm
- History of hemorrhagic cerebrovascular accident
- Diabetic hemorrhagic retinopathy or other hemorrhagic ophthalmic condition
- Previous allergic reaction to streptokinase or anistreplase; use tPA
- Prolonged cardiopulmonary resuscitation with evidence of chest trauma
- Pregnancy

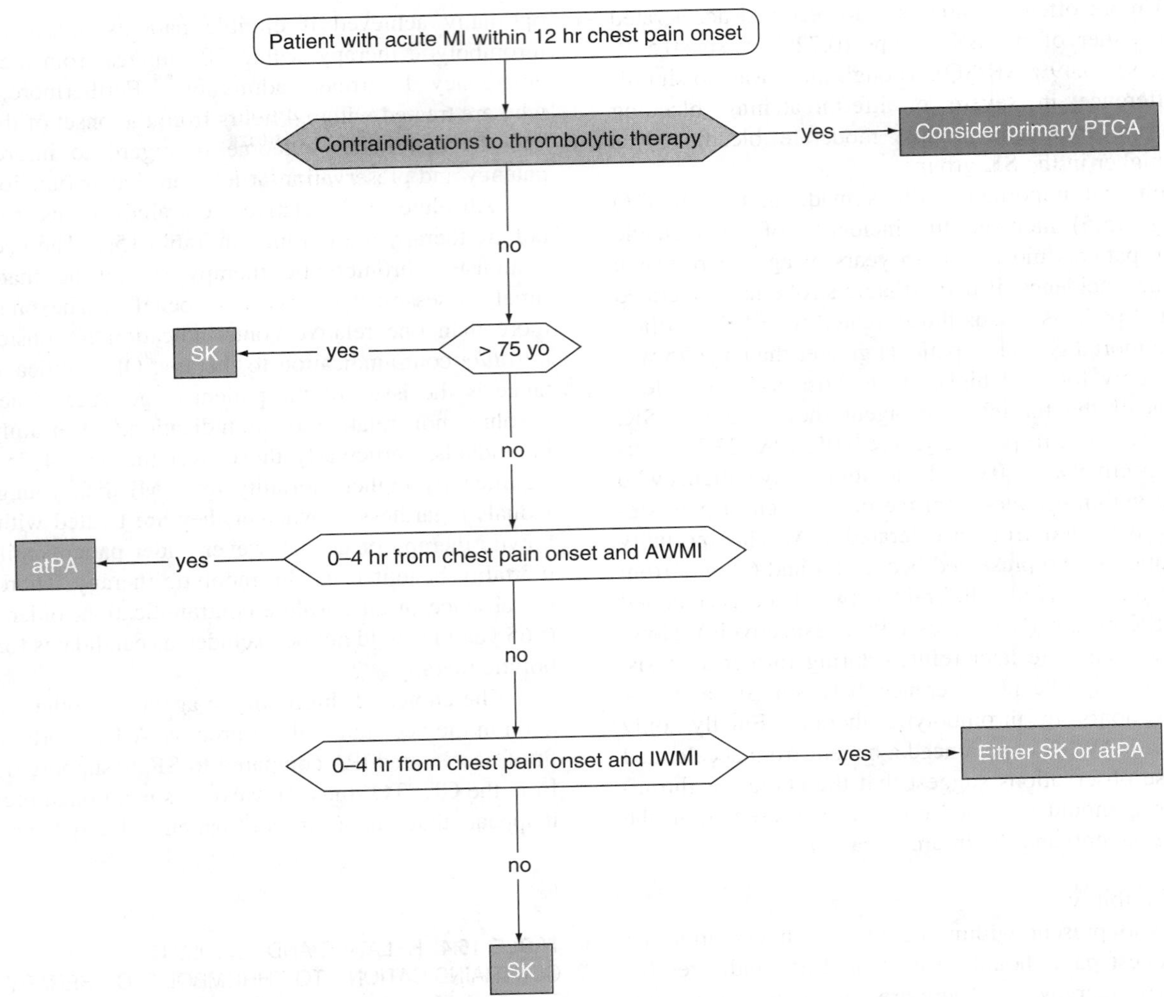

Figure 15.6. Algorithm for the administration of either streptokinase or accelerated tissue plasminogen to patients with acute myocardial infarction. AWMI, anterior wall myocardial infarction; IWMI, inferior wall myocardial infarction; SK, streptokinase, 1.5 million units over 60 minutes; atPA, accelerated tissue plasminogen activator, 100 mg over 1.5 hours.

accelerated tPA. When deciding between SK and tPA, these factors should be taken into consideration (Fig. 15.6). In addition, a component of the decision process should also include cost. On average, tPA costs approximately \$2400 for 100 mg compared to SK, which is about \$220 for 1.5 million units. Is the 1% mortality benefit observed with accelerated tPA worth the difference in cost between the two agents? Though a complete economic analysis of GUSTO has not yet been published, speculation about the cost to the U.S. health care system has been made. For example, the cost of the 1% 30-day mortality advantage of accelerated tPA projected over several years would amount to approximately \$22,000 per year of life saved.[77] Another estimate assumes that of the MIs that occur annually in the United States, 500,000 would receive thrombolytic therapy.[78] Based on this analysis, the cost of SK for 500,000 patients is 110 million dollars versus 1.1 billion dollars for tPA. The cost difference between the two is \$1,098,900,000 per year, resulting in a cost for one life saved of \$223,780 for tPA-treated patients. Though these estimates are not formal economic analyses, and do not take into account other factors besides cost, they do shed some light on the impact that the price difference between SK and tPA could have on the U.S. health care system. However, until more formal evaluations are done, it is more important that a thrombolytic drug be given in a timely manner to eligible patients. Rapid administration of thrombolytic therapy can be facilitated, in part, by the availability of pharmacy services in the emergency room. Alternatively, pharmacists can assist in the development of thrombolytic therapy "kits" that contain the agent, diluent, and instructions for preparation and administration.

Dosing Guidelines

Though controversy still surrounds which thrombolytic agent is the drug of choice, it is not as important an issue as the underutilization of these drugs. Less than 30% of patients who are eligible for thrombolytic therapy actually receive it.[79] It has been suggested that increasing this number could save an additional 5000 lives annually. Therefore, the current recommendations call for the administration of thrombolytic therapy to patients with electrocardiographic evidence of Q-wave MI who present within 12 hours of the onset of chest pain without contraindications to therapy. Patients who present beyond 12 hours still may benefit from thrombolytic therapy but this subgroup of patients still needs to be more clearly defined.

Eligible patients should be treated as soon as possible, but preferably within 70 minutes from the time they present to the emergency department, with one of the following regimens:

1. Tissue plasminogen activator (Activase, Genentech), 15 mg bolus followed by 0.75 mg/kg infusion (not to exceed 50 mg) over 30 minutes followed by 0.5 mg/kg infusion (not to exceed 35 mg)
2. Streptokinase, 1.5 million units in 50 mL of normal saline or D_5W over 60 minutes
3. Anistreplase (Eminase, SmithKline Beecham), 30 mg IVP over 2 minutes.

Evaluation of Therapeutic Outcomes

Following thrombolytic therapy administration, the patient should be carefully monitored for adverse events as well as signs and symptoms of reperfusion. A lytic state develops rapidly after administration and may persist for up to 24 hours. It may be somewhat longer in patients who receive ASTP. During this time, the risk of bleeding is the greatest. The lytic state is characterized clinically by a fall in fibrinogen concentration, an increase in fibrin degradation products and prolongation of the aPTT.[66] If the patient begins to bleed during this period, timely management is essential. Utilization of the algorithm outlined in Fig. 15.7, for the management of bleeding that is not immediately life threatening, provides guidelines for intervention and assists in the decision-making process. Hemorrhagic stroke is the most serious and concerning adverse effect associated with thrombolytic therapy.[80] However, this concern should not preclude the administration of thrombolytic therapy to an eligible candidate. The incidence of stroke due to thrombolytic therapy is approximately 1% with tPA having a small but significant excess incidence of stroke compared to SK (1.33 versus 0.94; $p < 0.05$). Other adverse effects for which patients should be monitored include hypotension and allergic reactions that occur more frequently with SK and ASTP than with tPA.

Successful reperfusion with thrombolytic therapy can be assessed by (1) evaluation of ECG; ST-segment elevation should normalize when reperfusion occurs; (2) relief of chest pain; initially chest discomfort may actually become worse at the time of reperfusion but should ultimately be relieved; and (3) abrupt onset of arrhythmias, usually ventricular in nature.[81] Management of reperfusion arrhythmias should follow the guidelines outlined in the lidocaine section of this chapter. These arrhythmias are usually self-limiting or quite responsive to drug therapy or direct current cardioversion. Normalization of the ECG, relief of chest pain, and reperfusion arrhythmias are noninvasive ways to assess whether thrombolysis has been successful. Unfortunately, presence or absence of these observations may not always be an accurate assessment of thrombolytic success or failure since thrombolytic therapy is unsuccessful in approximately 22–30% of patients.[82] In addition, approximately 5–10% of patients will spontaneously reperfuse. This explains the difference in rates between patency and reperfusion in that patency rates tend to be approximately 5–10% higher than reperfusion rates.

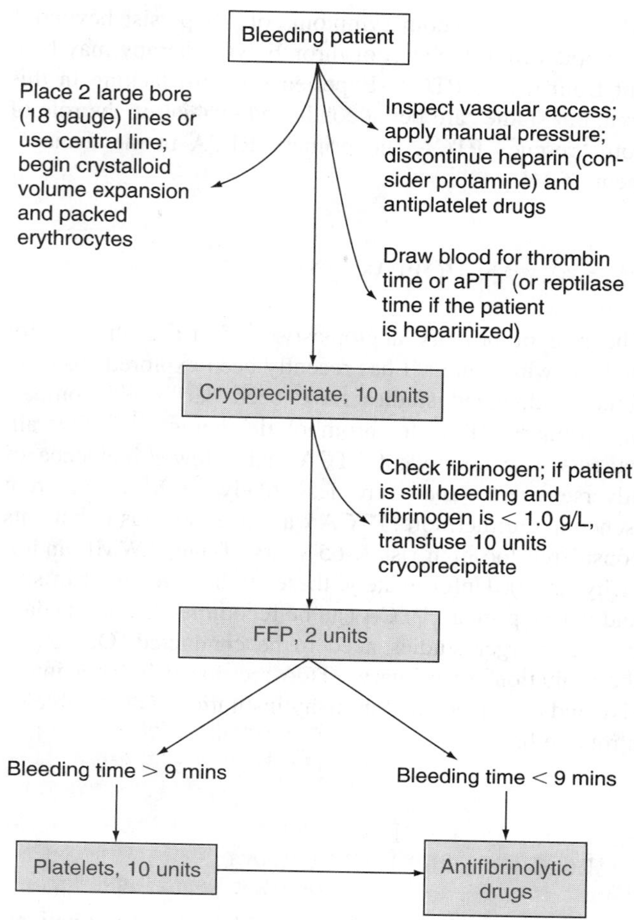

Figure 15.7. Algorithm for the management of bleeding associated with the administration of thrombolytic therapy. FFP, fresh frozen plasma. *(Adapted with permission from Ref. 80.)*

Patients in whom symptoms of MI persist beyond 1 to 2 hours from the start of thrombolytic therapy may benefit from rescue PTCA. Experience is still lacking in this area, but studies are being conducted evaluating the role of both "rescue" PTCA and primary PTCA in the management of MI.

PRIMARY ANGIOPLASTY

The role of primary angioplasty as first-line therapy for patients with acute MI has recently been explored. To date, three randomized studies have been performed comparing primary PTCA to thrombolytic therapy.[83–86] Overall, patients who underwent PTCA had a lower incidence of adverse events and were less likely to have recurrent ischemia. Furthermore, PTCA was advantageous in patients considered too high risk (>65 years of age, AWMI, and/or tachycardic). Unfortunately, these studies are small in size and before primary PTCA can be recommended as standard practice, larger studies need to be conducted. Obviously, the limitations of primary PTCA are that it is labor intensive and expensive, and in many institutions not feasible on a routine basis.[87]

ANGIOPLASTY FOLLOWING THROMBOLYTIC THERAPY

Though thrombolytic is effective in the majority of patients with acute MI, approximately 75–90% of patients will have a residual stenosis following clot lysis.[87–90] PTCA has been shown to be very effective in reducing this residual stenosis. However, several studies have shown that PTCA immediately following thrombolytic therapy is not beneficial and actually may contribute to morbidity and mortality. Subsequently, two large studies, the Should we Intervene Following Thrombolysis (SWIFT) study and the TIMI IIB, showed that patients treated conservatively rather than having angioplasty 1–2 days following thrombolytic therapy had a better outcome.[90–92] Patients randomized to the conservative treatment arm only underwent PTCA if they experienced recurrent ischemia or had provocable ischemia during exercise testing. Thus, PTCA following thrombolytic therapy should be reserved for patients who have symptomatic or objective evidence of ischemia.

ANTITHROMBOTIC THERAPY

Aspirin

Antithrombotic therapy with agents such as aspirin, heparin, and oral anticoagulants such as warfarin, have played an important role in the management of patients with acute MI. Aspirin, in particular, has become a critical component of acute MI therapy. Aspirin is a potent inhibitor of platelet cyclooxygenase, inhibiting the enzyme in a dose-dependent manner.[93] An advantageous property of aspirin is its rapid onset, usually before aspirin concentrations are detectable in the systemic circulation. Also, aspirin is an irreversible platelet inhibitor that elicits its effect for the life span of the platelet (8–10 days). Though many studies have been conducted evaluating the efficacy of aspirin in cardiovascular disease, none is probably as important as the Second International Study of Infarct Survival (ISIS-2) trial.[74] This study randomized 17,187 patients with suspected MI to receive in a double-blind fashion either IV SK (1.5 million units over 1 hour), aspirin (160 mg daily for 1 month), both aspirin and SK, or placebo. Compared with placebo, use of aspirin for 35 days in this study was associated with a highly significant ($p < 0.00001$) 23% reduction in mortality. Furthermore, in patients assigned to receive both aspirin and streptokinase, the mortality rate was 39% lower than that observed in the placebo group ($p < 0.00001$). This study clearly established the importance of early aspirin administration with concomitant thrombolytic therapy as well as the involvement of platelets in the thrombotic process.

Aspirin for Secondary Prevention

Several studies have been conducted that support the use of aspirin for secondary prevention of recurrent cardiovascular events follow acute MI.[94] Aspirin, when started within days or years of MI, significantly reduces recurrent events. More recently, the Antiplatelet Trialists' Collaboration has shown that the use of aspirin following MI reduces the risk of death from cardiovascular causes (including MI and stroke) by one-sixth, while the risk of a second nonfatal MI is reduced by one-third.[94]

Eight studies involving more than 16,000 MI patients have demonstrated that aspirin (300–1500 mg/d) alone or in combination with dipyridamole, decreases the risk of recurrent MI by 30–49%.[94] Table 15.5 shows the relative risk reduction from three different studies, all of which evaluated different daily aspirin doses. Furthermore, the benefit of aspirin is independent of age, gender, and cardiovascular risk factors. Current studies are evaluating the utility of the combination of aspirin and ticlopidine or dipyridamole or low-dose warfarin.

TABLE 15.5. RELATIVE RISK REDUCTION

ASA Dosage (mg)	At 3 Months (%)	At 1 Year (%)
1300	NA	30
324	41	NA
75	64	48

NA, not applicable.

Heparin in Combination with Thrombolytic Therapy

The goal of heparin therapy in combination with thrombolytic therapy is to prevent rethrombosis as well as possibly influence fibrinolysis.[67,95] Unfortunately, when thrombolytic trials began in the early 1980s, it was assumed that concomitant administration of heparin was necessary in order to prevent rethrombosis. Consequently, the use and role of heparin was never prospectively evaluated. Recent studies, specifically GISSI-2 and ISIS-3 as described previously, have shown that heparin (high-dose SQ) confers a small added benefit to thrombolytic therapy, however, this tends to be at the expense of an increased risk of bleeding.[69,70] The role of IV heparin is less clear. Though heparin has not been shown to influence 90-minute infarct artery patency, it appears to be important in maintaining patency in patients treated with tPA.[67] To date, however, there are no data to show that heparin has a favorable impact on mortality regardless of the thrombolytic agent used.[96]

Part of the difficulty in assessing the role of heparin has been the lack of use of weight-adjusted dosing (U/kg) and appropriate monitoring of the drug. Several studies have now been done that clearly demonstrate the importance of using weight-adjusted heparin dosing and the benefit of a standardized nomogram for consistent infusion rate adjustments.[97,98] Thus, ongoing trials and future studies are moving toward use of a weight-based dosing regimen and established guidelines for the adjustment of heparin based on the aPTT.

Interestingly, independent of the anticoagulant activity of heparin, there are data to suggest that heparin may effect fibrinolysis.[95] Specifically, heparin appears to interact with plasminogen activators. There is evidence that tPA binds to heparin, subsequently enhancing the catalytic activity of tPA. However, heparin binding to tPA actually attenuates tPA–fibrin binding resulting in diminished thrombolytic activity. This interaction has not been demonstrated with SK. In addition, the clinical significance of this finding is not yet known but ultimately could be important in clarifying the role of heparin in the management of patients treated with thrombolytic therapy.

Heparin in the Prevention of Thromboembolism

In addition to concomitant use with thrombolytic therapy, heparin is important in the prevention of left ventricular mural thrombus associated with MI. The incidence of mural thrombus in patients with AWMI may be as high as 70%.[99] Appropriate use of heparin and warfarin in these patients has been shown to reduce frequency of this complication to approximately 22%. However, recent data suggest that patients who are not treated with early IV heparin have a higher incidence of left ventricular thrombus regardless of warfarin therapy.[100] Thus, the greatest benefit is gained if IV heparin is given early to patients with AWMI since formation of left ventricular thrombus occurs within the first 10 days after MI.

When anticoagulation is continued for 1 to 3 months with oral warfarin therapy, systemic thromboembolism, such as cerebral embolism, has been shown to be reduced from 3% to 1%.[100] Most embolic complications occur within 3 days of MI. The risk of thromboembolism is enhanced in patients with heart failure or cardiogenic shock, massive or recurrent MI, patients more than 70 years of age, or those immobilized for a prolonged period of time. Therefore, early initiation (within 12–18 hours) of low-dose heparin (5000 U SQ BID), has been shown to diminish frequency of deep vein thrombosis from 23% in 145 patients assigned to a control group to 4% in 138 heparin-treated patients.[101]

Secondary Prevention with Warfarin

Whether or not anticoagulant therapy with warfarin should be continued indefinitely to prevent recurrent ischemia or reinfarction is controversial. Though many clinical trials have been conducted to resolve this controversy most have been too small or poorly designed and controlled. Recently, however, two studies, the Warfarin Re-Infarction Study (WARIS) and the Antithrombotics in the Prevention of Reocclusion in Coronary Thrombolysis (APRICOT) study, have shed some light on the role of warfarin in secondary prevention.

The WARIS evaluated whether warfarin, in a randomized, double-blind, placebo-controlled study, reduced the risk of death, reinfarction, and thromboembolic morbidity over a 3-year period.[102] More than 1200 patients were enrolled into the study all of whom were less than 75 years of age. Twenty percent of the placebo patients died compared to 15% in the warfarin group, equalling a risk reduction of 24% ($p = 0.026$). Warfarin therapy also reduced the incidence of recurrent MI by 43% while the incidence of major bleeding was 0.6% annually in warfarin-treated patients. Though this study concluded that warfarin is safe and effective in reducing post-MI thromboembolic complications, aspirin, currently the standard therapy for secondary prevention, was not included as part of the study. Therefore, it is difficult to interpret these results.

The APRICOT study was designed to compare aspirin, warfarin, and placebo in MI patients successfully treated with thrombolytic therapy in regard to recurrent ischemic events, left ventricular function, and infarct artery patency, 3 months after MI.[103] Patients were randomized to either 325 mg aspirin daily, or placebo, or warfarin dosed to achieve an INR of 2.8–4.0. After 3 months of therapy, infarct artery reocclusion rates were not significantly different between the groups (25% with aspirin, 30% with warfarin, and 32% with placebo). Reinfarction was observed in approximately 30% of the patients regardless of antithrombotic therapy. However, aspirin did significantly reduce the incidence of reinfarction when compared to placebo ($p < 0.025$). A 3-month event-free clinical course was observed in 93% of the aspirin patients, 82% of the warfarin patients, and 76% of the placebo patients (aspirin versus placebo, $p < 0.001$; aspirin versus warfarin, $p < 0.05$). The mortality rate was 2% and did not differ between groups. From these results it appears that despite antithrombotic therapy, reocclusion occurs in approximately 30% of post-MI patients. Though aspirin significantly reduced the reinfarction rate, clinical events, and mortality, warfarin is less beneficial than aspirin. These data support the need for a larger, randomized trial to delineate the role of warfarin in secondary prevention.

Though aspirin provides a benefit post-MI, there is still a high incidence of reinfarction. Thus, the search for new antithrombotic agents continues. In addition, several ongoing studies are evaluating combined therapy such as aspirin and ticlopidine, and aspirin and low-dose warfarin. To more clearly decipher the role of combined aspirin and warfarin therapy, a large multicenter trial, Coumadin-Aspirin Reinfarction Study (CARS), which will enroll 6000 post-MI patients, is ongoing. This study will evaluate and compare effects of aspirin (160 mg daily) with the combination of low-dose warfarin (1 or 3 mg daily) and aspirin (80 mg daily) in post-MI patients over a 4-year period. Preliminary data suggest that the warfarin–aspirin combination is safe. This study will provide useful information as to whether the addition of warfarin to aspirin is more beneficial than aspirin alone in the long-term management of these patients. Until more data are available, routine use of warfarin is not yet considered standard practice.

Dosing Guidelines

Aspirin as Adjunctive Therapy to Thrombolytic Therapy. Current recommendations for aspirin therapy in patients with acute MI call for immediate initiation of aspirin 160–325 mg at the time the patient presents to the emergency department whether or not the patient is considered a candidate for thrombolytic therapy. The only exceptions to this guideline are an aspirin allergy or aspirin intolerance due to gastrointestinal (GI) problems. When given, aspirin (160–325 mg) should be chewed and swallowed as soon as possible after the onset of symptoms.

Aspirin for Secondary Prevention. To achieve an immediate antiplatelet effect, aspirin should be given as a single loading dose of 300–325 mg in patients not already receiving aspirin as part of their MI care. Subsequently, long-term aspirin therapy should consist of 160–325 mg/d. This recommendation is based on the studies that have been conducted to date evaluating the role of aspirin in secondary prevention. Enteric-coated aspirin should be used because it helps reduce the incidence of GI side effects.

Concomitant Heparin and Thrombolytic Therapy. Until more information is acquired, the current recommendation for concomitant heparin administration with thrombolytic therapy is as follows[104]: Patients who receive tPA (accelerated or standard) should also receive a 75 U/kg bolus of heparin followed by a 1000 U/h infusion at the time the tPA infusion is initiated. For patients who receive SK, a heparin bolus should not be given, rather a maintenance infusion of 1000 U/h should be initiated 1–3 hours after the start of the SK infusion. Concomitant heparin administration is currently recommended for those patients who receive ASTP. Given the lack of strong evidence to support heparin use with SK, it may also be unnecessary with ASTP. To date though, this issue has not been prospectively evaluated so the current recommendation for heparin therapy with ASTP is the same as that for SK. In all cases, heparin should be titrated to maintain the aPTT at 1.5 to 2 times control and continued for approximately 48 hours. The patient can then be switched to low-dose subcutaneous heparin (5000 U BID) until ambulatory. If the patient is at high risk for systemic embolism then he/she should remain on full-dose IV heparin while oral anticoagulation with warfarin is initiated. Patients at high risk for systemic embolism are discussed later in the text.

Heparin for Anterior Wall Myocardial Infarction. Use of either full-dose IV heparin as described previously or high-dose subcutaneous heparin (12,500 units subcutaneously every 12 hours) is recommended for short-term prevention of mural thrombus in patients with AWMI. Heparin therapy should be followed by warfarin therapy. The warfarin dose should be titrated to prolong the prothrombin time (PT) to an International Normalized Ratio (INR) of 2.0 to 3.0.

Heparin for Prevention of Thromboembolism. In those patients not receiving full-dose IV or SQ heparin, low-dose heparin (5000 units subcutaneously every 8–12 hours) should be started within 12–18 hours after onset of chest pain to prevent thromboembolic complications of MI. This regimen should be continued for 24–72 hours or until the patient is ambulatory.

Evaluation of Therapeutic Outcomes

Aspirin. Following acute MI, patients should be followed on a regular basis and evaluated for signs and symptoms of recurrent ischemia. Though aspirin is very effective in preventing recurrent ischemia, as many as 30–40% of patients will experience recurrent ischemia or reinfarction despite aspirin therapy.

Bleeding and GI side effects of aspirin are the most common and concerning. However, the risk of these adverse events is dose dependent; with low doses of aspirin (≤325 mg/d) the incidence of adverse events is no different from placebo. The incidence of GI complications such as stomach pain, heartburn, and nausea is as high as 40–60% in patients receiving 900–1300 mg/d of aspirin, while the incidence of these side effects is 4–13% in patients receiving 75 mg/d. The overall incidence of hemorrhagic stroke with low-dose aspirin is 0.3%, which increases as the dose of aspirin increases.

As noted previously, the use of enteric-coated aspirin reduces the incidence of GI side effects.

Heparin. During continuous IV or high-dose SQ heparin therapy, patients should be monitored closely for signs and symptoms of bleeding and recurrent ischemia. Keep in mind that just because a patient is anticoagulated on heparin, reinfarction can still occur.

The aPTT is the coagulation test most commonly used to assess the level of heparin anticoagulation. Since therapeutic heparin concentrations correlate well to aPTT levels, the aPTT should not be measured until at least 6 hours after initiating a heparin infusion and, due to delayed distribution of SQ heparin, 12 hours after an SQ dose.[105] So-called therapeutic aPTTs vary substantially between institutions due to the number and variety of aPTT reagents and instruments available. The clinical laboratory should be contacted to determine the aPTT that corresponds to therapeutic levels of heparin (0.2–0.4 U/mL).[105] On average, this usually corresponds to an aPTT of 60–80 seconds but can range to as low as 50 seconds to as high as 110 seconds. Thus, arbitrarily assuming a therapeutic aPTT as 60–80 seconds may place patients at risk for either overcoagulation or undercoagulation.

Once an infusion rate is established, the aPTT should be checked once a day and at 6 hours following an infusion rate change.

Angiotensin-Converting Enzyme Inhibitors

The primary goal of an angiotensin-converting enzyme inhibitor (ACEI) after MI is to limit postinfarction left ventricular dilatation and hypertrophy so that pump function is preserved or improved. Substantial data show that this remodeling process initially improves hemodynamics by maintaining stroke volume and cardiac output.[19,23,24,106,107] Ultimately, however, this benefit is lost and deterioration ensues. The progression to ventricular hypertrophy leads to CHF and probably plays a role in angina and sudden cardiac death post-MI.

During the past several years, studies have shown that ACEIs are effective in reducing the likelihood of post-MI CHF.[22–24] This effect is most likely due to a reduction in myocardial demand, a reduction in angiotensin-mediated vasoconstriction, and modification of endothelial control of vascular tone, ultimately leading to an improvement in hemodynamics and, subsequently, cardiac output. Though data are still forthcoming, several studies have evaluated the use of ACEI in MI. The CONSENSUS II (Cooperative New Scandinavian Enalapril Survival Study) trial is the largest of these studies.[22] More than 6000 patients were enrolled into CONSENSUS II while the SAVE (Survival and Ventricular Enlargement) trial entered more than 2200 patients.[23] Both of these studies enrolled patients who had survived an MI and had left ventricular ejection fractions of less than 40%. The primary difference between these two studies was time to randomization. Patients in CONSENSUS II were randomized to either enalaprilat (IV enalapril) or placebo within 24 hours of MI. Patients enrolled in SAVE, however, were not eligible for randomization to either captopril or placebo until 72 hours and up to 16 days after MI. Patients in CONSENSUS II randomized to ACEI received enalaprilat 1 mg over 2 hours followed by oral enalapril 2.5 mg twice daily for 6 months with a target enalapril dose of 22 mg daily. SAVE patients randomized to captopril received a test dose of 6.25 mg followed by a starting dose of 12.5 mg, which was titrated up to 25 mg three times a day for inpatients and 50 mg three times a day for outpatients. Patients in both trials were followed for up to 36 months.

CONSENSUS II was stopped prematurely due to a higher mortality rate in the enalapril group as compared with placebo at 1 and 6 months (6.3 and 10.2% in the placebo group versus 7.2 and 11.0% in the enalapril group; $p = 0.26$). In addition, unacceptable adverse effects, primarily hypotension, occurred more frequently in the enalapril group than in the placebo group (12 versus 3%; $p < 0.001$) even though patients treated with enalapril were less likely to develop heart failure than patients in the placebo group (28 versus 25%; $p = 0.012$). The investigators hypothesized that hypotension associated with early use of enalapril may have exacerbated ischemia, which increased the likelihood of mortality.

The SAVE study revealed quite a different effect of ACEIs after MI than the CONSENSUS II trial. The reduction in risk of death from any cause or risk of cardiovascular death in captopril-treated patients was 19% ($p = 0.019$) and 21% ($p = 0.014$) lower, respectively, than placebo patients. Use of captopril in this study was associated with a reduction in likelihood of death from heart failure by 36% and from atherosclerotic disease by 23%. Furthermore, captopril-treated patients had a significantly lower frequency of hospitalization due to heart failure than the placebo patients. However, adverse effects such as dizziness, altered taste, cough, and diarrhea were more common in patients receiving captopril than in those receiving placebo.

More recently, data from the GISSI-3 study show that mortality and the combined endpoint of mortality and severe left ventricular dysfunction are significantly reduced in MI patients treated with lisinopril (5 mg initially followed by 10 mg/d) within 24 hours of the onset of symptoms (odds ratio 0.88 [95% CI 0.79–0.99] and

0.9 [0.84–0.98], respectively).[32] In addition, the combination of lisinopril and NTG also produced significant decreases in mortality and the combined endpoint (0.83 [0.70–0.94] and 0.85 [0.76–0.94], respectively).

Dosing Guidelines

The findings of the SAVE and GISSI-3 trials are striking. However, not all captopril-treated patients in the SAVE trial benefited from therapy. Specifically, younger patients (<55 years old) derived no reduction in cardiovascular morbidity or mortality or in death from all causes; neither did women nor patients who received thrombolytic therapy. Despite this subgroup analysis, the study was not designed to prospectively evaluate these groups, so these data should be interpreted cautiously. In the GISSI-3 trial, prespecified subgroups consisted of patients over the age of 70 years and women. In the elderly group, there was a significant decrease in the combined endpoint with lisinopril (12%, $2p = 0.0039$) or NTG (9%, $2p = 0.048$). A similar benefit was shown in female patients. Furthermore, there was an even more dramatic benefit with the combination of lisinopril and NTG: Both elderly patients and women experienced a 21% reduction ($2p = 0.0004$ and $2p = 0.0051$, respectively) for the combined endpoint.

Since studies have not yet been completed to address discrepancies between patient subgroups, it is difficult to make definitive recommendations about the use of ACEI in patients after MI. However, it appears that patients with a first MI who have a left ventricular ejection fraction of less than 40% and who are not hypotensive (systolic blood pressure <100 mm Hg) may derive the greatest benefit from either lisinopril or long-term oral captopril therapy. Captopril should be initiated no sooner than 72 hours after MI with a test dose of 6.25 mg followed by 12.5 mg. The dose should be titrated, if possible, up to 50 mg three times a day. Lisinopril should be initiated within 24 hours of the onset of symptoms at 5 mg/d then increased to 10 mg/d. Future studies and further subgroup analysis will help clarify specific patient populations that may or may not benefit from ACEI therapy post-MI and determine whether there are intrinsic pharmacologic differences between ACEI that may explain the discrepancy between the SAVE, GISSI-3, and CONSENSUS II study results.

Evaluation of Therapeutic Outcomes

When initiating ACEI therapy, blood pressure should be monitored closely. Usually if patients are going to have a hypotensive response to ACEI, they have it on the initial dose. Patients who are hyponatremic and/or hypertensive tend to be at greater risk for a hypotensive response to ACEI. Blood pressure should continue to be monitored regularly on an outpatient basis during therapy.

Other monitoring parameters for ACEI therapy include signs and symptoms of worsening heart failure, renal function, and serum potassium, particularly if the patient is concomitantly taking a diuretic and potassium supplementation. Common side effects of ACEI that patients should be questioned about and observed for are altered taste, dizziness, cough, and diarrhea. Captopril and lisinopril contain sulfhydryl groups and may predispose patients to allergic side effects.

Pharmacotherapeutic Management of Complications Associated with Acute Myocardial Infarction

Despite the advancements in the pharmacotherapy of acute MI, approximately 5–9% of patients treated with thrombolytic therapy die.[68–71] Interestingly, the majority of these patients die during the first 24 hours following MI, suggesting that thrombolytic therapy may not prevent early death, and other factors may contribute to the demise of these patients.[108] The most common etiology of early death in MI patients is pump failure. Another etiology, reinfarction, also contributes to morbidity and mortality. Patients who leave the hospital with an occluded infarct-related artery have a substantially higher long-term mortality rate than those whose infarct-related artery is patent. Thus, drug therapy during the early course of MI should be directed toward preventing and limiting early pump failure and maintaining infarct artery patency.

The most common complication associated with acute MI is ventricular arrhythmias, which subsequently predispose the patient to sudden cardiac death.[8,33,34,57] The therapeutic management of ventricular arrhythmias is discussed in detail in Chapter 16.

POST-MI ANGINA/REOCCLUSION

Long-term outcome is primarily determined by infarct size, which is directly related to myocardial viability and function.[2] Therefore, limitation of infarct size and patency of the infarct-related artery are of utmost importance in the management of MI. Encompassing this task is prevention of reinfarction, which can occur if the patient reoccludes the infarct-related artery during the first 24 hours after the initial event. Though β blockers and calcium antagonists may be effective in the management of postinfarction angina, if the pain is associated with ECG changes, PTCA is indicated.

For patients who have persistent pain during the peri-infarction period without ECG changes, initial therapy should consist of IV β blockade as described earlier in the chapter. This can be followed by increasing the NTG infusion rate to lower the systolic blood pressure to 90–100 mm Hg. In addition, IV morphine sulfate 2–5 mg can be given for pain relief. If angina persists, then therapy with a calcium channel blocker, either diltiazem or verapamil, is an option. However, these drugs should be used with extreme caution, if at all, in patients who have received β blockers. Though calcium channel blockers are an option for recurrent angina, patients who do not respond to β blockers, morphine, and IV NTG, are often referred for coronary angiography to assess the infarct-related artery. This is most often the case in patients who have received thrombolytic therapy who have not shown clinical signs of reperfusion.

Therapeutic management of chest pain beyond 12–24 hours of the initial MI should be managed as unstable angina (see Chapter 14). If pain is associated with ECG changes consistent with ischemia, coronary angiography is indicated. Evaluation of exercise capacity and left ventricular function as described under post-MI management will assist in guiding antianginal therapy, the need for invasive procedures such as PTCA, and will also determine the patient's prognosis.

PUMP FAILURE/CARDIOGENIC SHOCK

Acute MI patients who present with signs and symptoms of congestive heart failure have a higher mortality based on the severity of left ventricular dysfunction (Table 15.6). The mortality rate of patients who present in cardiac arrest or in cardiogenic shock (Killip class IV) may be in excess of 85%.[28,108]

Cardiogenic shock occurs in 10–15% of patients with MI and is the most frequent cause of in-hospital mortality.[28,108] In-hospital mortality rate has been reported to vary between 85 and 95% and, unfortunately, 50% of survivors die within the following 2 years. Signs and symptoms of pump failure and shock include weak pulse, poor peripheral perfusion, obtundation, and oliguria (urine output is <22 mL/h). Typically the systolic blood pressure is less than 80 mm Hg, the skin is cool and moist with evidence of cyanosis, cardiac output is depressed (<1.8 L/min/m^2), there is pulmonary congestion, and the left ventricular filling pressure is elevated (>18 mm Hg).

The management of pump failure should be based on the patient's hemodynamic status.[28] For example, if the systolic blood pressure is greater than 100 mm Hg, the left ventricular filling pressure is more than 15 mm Hg, but the cardiac index is less than 2.5 L/min/m^2, then afterload reduction should be considered as first-line therapy. However, if the patient is markedly hypotensive (arterial pressure less than 90 mm Hg), intra-aortic balloon pump insertion and mobilization to the cardiac catheterization laboratory for PTCA is indicated; these patients have the worse prognosis. If hypotension is severe (systolic pressure <70 mm Hg), IV norepinephrine, 2–4 μg/min, titrated to a systolic pressure of 80–90 mm Hg, is the agent of choice. Once this blood pressure goal is achieved, norepinephrine can be switched to IV dopamine. If systolic pressure is 70–90 mm Hg, dopamine is the preferred agent at an infusion rate of 5–15 μg/kg/min. To reduce systemic vascular resistance and improve cardiac output as well as to minimize the increase in myocardial oxygen demand due to dopamine, IV nitroprusside may be initiated at a low dose of 0.25–0.5 μg/min and increased cautiously by no more than 0.5 μg/min. Concomitant use of a venodilator such as IV NTG or IV furosemide and/or a positive inotrope like dobutamine may be especially useful in patients with pulmonary congestion associated with a marked elevation in left ventricular end-diastolic pressure. More details pertaining to hemodynamic subsets and the choice of drug therapy are given in the chapter on congestive heart failure (Chapter 13).

Patients who initially present to the emergency department in cardiogenic shock due to acute MI should also be considered for emergent PTCA.[109] When angioplasty is performed early after onset of symptoms, survival has been reported to be as high as 50%, a figure that represents a major improvement over that associated with vasopressors and vasodilators.

If primary PTCA is unavailable, or if the patient needs to be transported to another facility for the procedure, pharmacologic therapy should be used to attempt to reduce pulmonary congestion, support blood pressure, and improve cardiac output. The appropriate use of pharmacologic interventions is dependent on an accurate assessment of hemodynamic status: cardiac output/index, left ventricular filling pressure, blood pressure, systemic vascular resistance, and heart rate. This requires insertion of a Swan–Ganz catheter. Once these hemodynamic parameters are known, therapy can then be individualized.

TABLE 15.6. KILLIP CLASSIFICATION OF PATIENTS WITH ACUTE MYOCARDIAL INFARCTION

Mortality Rate (%)		Classification
0–5	I:	No signs of pulmonary or venous congestion
10–22	II:	Moderate heart failure as evidenced by pulmonary rales at lung bases, a third heart sound (S_3), tachypnea, or signs of right-sided heart failure such as venous or hepatic congestion
35–45	III:	Severe heart failure with pulmonary edema
85–100	IV:	Cardiogenic shock; systolic BP < 90 mm Hg, evidence of peripheral constriction, diaphoresis, peripheral cyanosis, mental confusion, and a decrease in urine output

Finally, if myocardial dysfunction is felt to be irreversible, a left ventricular assist device may be used only if the patient is considered a candidate for cardiac transplantation.

POST-MI MANAGEMENT

Patients with uncomplicated MI are usually discharged from the hospital within 1 week. Now in the era of cost containment, patients can be safely discharged after an uncomplicated course within 3–4 days. Although in-hospital management plays a critical role in the outcome of MI patients, what happens after hospital discharge is also important. At the time of or near the time of hospital discharge, patients should be carefully evaluated to ensure the appropriate plan for rehabilitation.[2,110] Typically, patients after their first MI have a very good prognosis. Therefore, ensuring that all aspects of their post-MI care are discussed and understood is important. Prior to discharge, a discussion between health care practitioners, the patient, and the patient's family regarding medications, particularly secondary prevention; modification of risk factors such as smoking, cholesterol, and hypertension; an exercise program; and diet should be held. Guidelines for safe resumption of customary activities, such as returning to work or recreational activities, should be discussed in detail. All questions should be answered to the patient's satisfaction.

In addition to post-MI counseling, an objective assessment of a patient's prognosis and stratification for risk of recurrent cardiovascular events should be made. This usually includes an evaluation of the patient's exercise tolerance and determination of left ventricular function. These parameters will assist in guiding further evaluation and treatment. A multitude of procedures and tests is available to assist in the stratification of post MI patients.[110] However, many have limited utility and are extremely expensive. It is important to select a procedure/test that is cost effective and will provide useful and prognostic information about the patient.

Probably the most common noninvasive test that is performed post-MI is the exercise tolerance test.[2,110] This is typically done using a treadmill or bicycle and continuous ECG and blood pressure monitoring. This procedure will determine the patient's overall exercise capacity, blood pressure response to exercise, and if angina occurs, at what point during exercise it occurs, as well as if activity precipitates arrhythmias. Submaximal exercise testing can usually be performed just prior to hospital discharge and can then be followed by a full exercise test 1 month after infarction.

High-risk patients are easily identified by their low exercise capability, failure of the systolic blood pressure to rise above the resting value during exercise (frequently referred to as an inadequate blood pressure response to exercise), and chest pain associated with ischemic changes on the ECG.[2,110] In some cases, these patients may experience ventricular ectopy during or shortly after exercise. These patients require further evaluation by invasive means (coronary angiography) to assess coronary anatomy. In patients without these findings, no further diagnostic evaluation is necessary and the risk of a subsequent cardiac event is very low. Current guidelines recommend that post-MI patients undergo exercise testing annually following acute MI.

Many procedures exist to evaluate left ventricular function. Though no one test is considered the "gold standard," the type of test used depends on the expertise that exists at the given institution. Echocardiography, coronary angiography, and radionuclear ventriculograms are a few examples of methods to assess left ventricular function.

CONCLUSION

Though many pharmacotherapeutic advances have been made that have substantially lowered the mortality associated with MI, acute MI is still a leading cause of death in the United States today. A better understanding of the pathophysiology of MI has provided the basis for the advancement in therapeutic interventions such as thrombolytic therapy. Other therapies, β blockers, aspirin, and nitroglycerin also contribute to an improved outcome.

Probably the most significant advance made in the last decade has been thrombolytic therapy. These drugs have become the cornerstone of management for patients with MI. Unfortunately, only a fraction of eligible patients is treated with thrombolytic drugs. Continuing to educate the general public as well as health care providers as to the importance of quickly recognizing and responding to MI will hopefully improve the utilization of these important drugs. Though the battle of the clot busters will most likely continue, enhanced utilization of any one of the thrombolytic drugs will save lives.

Over the next few years, large multicenter trials will be conducted to delineate the role of primary PTCA in acute MI and how it compares to thrombolytic therapy. Research will continue to evaluate a multitude of investigational agents and other modalities for the treatment of MI. Studies are ongoing to further assess the role of ACEI in postinfarction patients, the utilization of new thrombolytic agents, and antithrombotic drugs. This continuum of information will surely provide new treatments and approaches to the therapeutic management of MI patients.

Though the management of MI has changed and improved dramatically over the last decade, progress continues. In the next 10 years, more therapies and strategies will be evaluated and become available. Insight as to the most appropriate management of patients with cardiogenic shock and postinfarction heart failure will be delineated. So, just as such advances have been made during the last several years, they will continue and the management of these patients will remain a dynamic process.

REFERENCES

1. American Heart Association data, 1992.
2. Moss AJ, Benhorin J. Prognosis and management after a first myocardial infarction. N Engl J Med 1990;322:743–753.
3. Wittels EH, Hay JW, Gotto AM. Medical costs of coronary artery disease in the United States. Am J Cardiol 1990;65:432–440.
4. DeWood MA, Spores J, Notske R, et al. Prevalence of total coronary occlusion during the early hours of transmural myocardial infarction. N Engl J Med 1980;303:897–902.
5. Fuster V, Badimon L, Badimon JJ, Chesebro JH. The pathogenesis of coronary artery disease and the acute coronary syndromes (first of two parts). N Engl J Med 1992;326:242–250.
6. Fuster V, Badimon L, Badimon JJ, Chesebro JH. The pathogenesis of coronary artery disease and the acute coronary syndromes (second of two parts). N Engl J Med 1992;326:310–318.
7. Kawai C. Pathogenesis of acute myocardial infarction. Novel regulatory systems of bioactive substances in the vessel wall. Circulation 1994;90:1033–1043.
8. Lavie CJ, Gersh BJ. Acute myocardial infarction: Initial manifestations, management, and prognosis. Mayo Clin Proc 1990;65:531–538.
9. Braunwald E, Sobel BE. Coronary blood flow and myocardial ischemia, in Braunwald E (ed): Heart Disease, 4th ed. Philadelphia, PA, WB Saunders, 1992, pp 1161–1239.
10. Reimer KA, Jennings RB. The wavefront phenomenon of myocardial ischemic cell death II. Transmural progression of necrosis within the framework of ischemic bed size (myocardium at risk) and collateral flow. Lab Invest 1979;40:633–644.
11. Sabia PJ, Powers ER, Ragosta M, et al. An association between collateral blood flow and myocardial viability in patients with recent myocardial infarction. N Engl J Med 1992;327:1825–1831.
12. Charney R, Cohen M. The role of the coronary collateral circulation in limiting myocardial ischemia and infarct size. Am Heart J 1993;126:937–945.
13. Willich SN, Lewis M, Lowel H, et al. Physical exertion as a trigger of acute myocardial infarction. N Engl J Med 1993;329:1684–1690.
14. Mittleman MA, Maclure M, Tofler GH, et al. Triggering of acute myocardial infarction by heavy physical exertion. N Engl J Med 1993;329:1677–1683.
15. Moliterno DJ, Willard JE, Lange RA, et al. Coronary-artery vasoconstriction induced by cocaine, cigarette smoking, or both. N Engl J Med 1994;330:454–459.
16. Antaloczy Z, Barcsak J, Magyar E. Correlation of electrocardiographic and pathologic findings in 100 cases of Q wave and non-Q wave myocardial infarction. J Electrocardiol 1988;23:331–335.
17. Kinch JW, Ryan TJ. Right ventricular infarction. N Engl J Med 1994;330:1211–1217.
18. Klein LW, Helfant RH. The Q-wave and non Q-wave myocardial infarction: Differences and similarities. Prog Cardiovasc Dis 1986;29:205–220.
19. Pfeffer MA, Braunwald E. Ventricular remodeling after myocardial infarction. Experimental observations and clinical implications. Circulation 1990;81:1161–1172.
20. Gaudron P, Eilles C, Kugler I, Ertl G. Progressive left ventricular dysfunction and remodeling following myocardial infarction: Potential mechanism and early predictors. Circulation 1993;87:755–763.
21. Gaudron P, Eilles C, Ertl G, Kochsiek K. Compensatory and non-compensatory left ventricular dilatation after myocardial infarction: Time course and hemodynamic consequences at rest and during exercise. Am Heart J 1992;123:377–385.
22. Swedberg K, Held P, Kjekshus J, et al. Effects of the early administration of enalapril on mortality in patients with acute myocardial infarction. N Engl J Med 1992;327:678–684.
23. Pfeffer MA, Braunwald E, Moye LA, et al. Effect of captopril on mortality and morbidity in patients with left ventricular dysfunction after myocardial infarction. N Engl J Med 1992;327:669–677.
24. Gruppo Italian per lo Stuido della Sopravvievenza nel'Infarto Miocardico (GISSI-3): Effects of lisinopril and transdermal glyceryl trinitrate singly and together on 6-week mortality and ventricular function after acute myocardial infarction. Lancet 1994;343:1115–1122.
25. Niakan E, Harati Y, Rolak LA, et al. Silent myocardial infarction and diabetic cardiovascular autonomic neuropathy. Arch Intern Med 1986;146:2229–2230.
26. Fisher ML, Kelemen MH, Collins D, et al. Routine serum enzyme tests in the diagnosis of acute myocardial infarction. Cost effectiveness. Arch Intern Med 1983;143:1541–1543.
27. Reis GJ, Kaufman HW, Horowitz GL, Pasternak RC. Usefulness of lactate dehydrogenase and lactate dehydrogenase isoenzymes for diagnosis of acute myocardial infarction. Am J Cardiol 1988;61:754–758.
28. A report of the American College of Cardiology/American Heart Association Task Force on assessment of diagnostic and therapeutic cardiovascular procedures. ACC/AHA guidelines for the early management of patients with acute myocardial infarction. Circulation 1990;82:664–707.
29. Malliani A, Lombardi F. Consideration of the fundamental mechanisms eliciting cardiac pain. Am Heart J 1982;103:575–578.
30. Herlitz J, Hjalmarson A, Waagstein F. Treatment of pain in acute myocardial infarction. Br Heart J 1989;61:9–13.
31. Jugdutt BI, Warnica W. Intravenous nitroglycerin therapy to limit myocardial infarct size, expansion, and complications: Effect of timing, dosage, and infarct location. Circulation 1988;78:906–919.
32. Yusuf S, Slight P, Held P, McMahon S. Routine medical management of acute myocardial infarction. Lessons from overviews of recent randomized controlled trials. Circulation 1990;82(suppl II):117–134.
33. Weinberg B, Zipes D. Strategies to manage the post-myocardial infarction patient with ventricular arrhythmias. Clin Cardiol 1989;12(suppl III):86–90.

34. Meltzer LE, Cohen HE. The incidence of arrhythmias associated with acute myocardial infarction, in Meltzer LE, Dunning AJ (eds): Textbook of Coronary Care. Philadelphia, Charles Press, 1972.
35. Hine LK, Laird N, Hewitt P, Chalmers TC. Meta-analytic evidence against prophylactic use of lidocaine in acute myocardial infarction. Arch Intern Med 1989;149:2694–2698.
36. Wyse DG, Kellen J, Rademaker AW. Prophylactic versus selective lidocaine for early ventricular arrhythmias of myocardial infarction. J Am Coll Cardiol 1988;12:507–513.
37. Bigger JT, Fleiss JL, Rolnitzky LM. Prevalence, characteristics and significance of ventricular tachycardia detected by 24-hour continuous electrocardiographic recordings in the late hospital phase of acute myocardial infarction. Am J Cardiol 1986;58:1151–1160.
38. Yusuf S, Peto R, Lewis J, Sleight P. Beta blockade during and after myocardial infarction: An overview of the randomized trials. Prog Cardiovasc Dis 1985;17:335–371.
39. The MIAMI (Metoprolol in Acute Myocardial Infarction) Trial Research Group. A randomized placebo controlled international trial. Eur Heart J 1985;6:199–226.
40. ISIS-1 (First International Study of Infarct Survival) Collaborative Group. Randomized trial of intravenous atenolol among 16,027 cases of suspected acute myocardial infarction: ISIS-1. Lancet 1986;ii:57–66.
41. Held PH, Hjalmarson A, Ryden L, et al. Central haemodynacie effects of metoprolol early in acute myocardial infarction. A placebo controlled randomized study in patients with low heart rate. Eur Heart J 1986;7:937–944.
42. Roque R, Amuchastegue LM, Lopez Morillos MA, et al. and the TIARA Study Group. Beneficial effects of timolol on infarct size and late ventricular tachycardia in patients with acute myocardial infarction. Circulation 1987;76:610–617.
43. Roberts R, Rogers WJ, Mueller HS, et al. Immediate versus deferred beta-blockade following thrombolytic therapy patients with acute myocardial infarction. Results of the Thrombolysis in Myocardial Infarction (TIMI) II-B Study. Circulation 1991;83:422–437.
44. Held PH, Yusuf S. Effects of beta-blockers and calcium channel blockers in acute myocardial infarction. Eur Heart J 1993;14(suppl F):18–25.
45. Held P. Effects of beta blockers on ventricular dysfunction after myocardial infarction: Tolerability and survival effects. Am J Cardiol 1993;71:39C–44C.
46. Chadda K, Goldstein S, Byington R, Burb JD. Effect of propranolol after acute myocardial infarction in patients with congestive heart failure. Circulation 1986;73:503–510.
47. Gundersen T. Influence of heart size on mortality and reinfarction in patients treated with timolol after myocardial infarction. Br Heart J 1983;50:135–139.
48. Burris JR. Beta-blockers, dyslipidemia, and coronary artery disease: A reassessment. Arch Intern Med 1993;153:2085–2092.
49. Schartl M. Calcium antagonists in the treatment early after myocardial infarction. J Cardiovasc Pharmacol 1992;20(suppl 5):S79–S81.
50. The Multicenter Diltiazem Postinfarction Trial Research Group. The effect of diltiazem on mortality and reinfarction after myocardial infarction. N Engl J Med 1988;319:385–392.
51. The Danish Study Group on Verapamil in Myocardial Infarction. Effect of verapamil on mortality and major events after acute myocardial infarction. Am J Cardiol 1990;66:779–785.
52. The Israel Sprint Study Group. Secondary Prevention Reinfarction Israeli Nifedipine Trial (SPRINT). A randomized intervention trial of nifedipine in patients with acute myocardial infarction. Eur Heart J 1988;9:354–364.
53. Wong S-C, Greenberg H, Hager WD, Dwyer EM. Effects of diltiazem on recurrent myocardial infarction in patients with non-Q wave myocardial infarction. J Am Coll Cardiol 1992;19:1421–1425.
54. Gibson RS, Beller GA, Gheorghiade M, et al. The prevalence and clinical significance of residual myocardial ischemia 2 weeks after uncomplicated non-Q wave infarction: A prospective natural history study. Circulation 1986;73:1186–1198.
55. Gibson RS, Boden WE, Theroux P, et al. Diltiazem and reinfarction in patients with non-Q-wave myocardial infarction. N Engl J Med 1986;315:423–429.
56. Marcus RI, Cobb LA, Edwards JE, et al. Mechanism of death and prevalence of myocardial ischemic symptoms in the terminal event after acute myocardial infarction. Am J Cardiol 1988;61:8–15.
57. Bigger JT, Fleiss JL, Kleiger R, et al. The relationships among ventricular arrhythmias, left ventricular dysfunction, and mortality in the 2 years after myocardial infarction. Circulation 1984;69:250–258.
58. Kremers MS, Black WH, Wells PJ. Sudden cardiac death: Etiologies, pathologies, and treatment. Dis Mon 1989;35:383–385.
59. Echt DS, Liebson PR, Mitchell B, et al. Mortality and morbidity in patients receiving encainide, flecainide, or placebo. N Engl J Med 1991;324:781–788.
60. The Cardiac Arrhythmia Suppression Trial II Investigators. Effect of the antiarrhythmic agent moricizine on survival after myocardial infarction. N Engl J Med 1992;327:227–233.
61. Navarro-Lopez F, Cosin J, Marrugat J, et al. Comparison of the effects of amiodarone versus metoprolol on the frequency of ventricular arrhythmias and on mortality after myocardial infarction. SSSD Investigators. Spanish Study on Sudden Death. Am J Cardiol 1993;72:1243–1248.
62. Zarembski DG, Nolan PE, Slack MK, Caruso AC. Empiric long-term amiodarone prophylaxis following myocardial infarction. Arch Intern Med 1993;153:2661–2667.
63. Teo KK, Yusuf S, Collins R, et al. Effects of intravenous magnesium in suspected acute myocardial infarction: Overview of randomized trials. Br Med J 1991;303:1499–1503.
64. Woods KL, Fletcher S, Roffe C, Haider Y. Intravenous magnesium sulphate in suspected acute myocardial infarction: Results of the second Leicester Intravenous Magnesium Intervention Trial (LIMIT-2). Lancet 1992;339:1553–1558.
65. ISIS-4. Effects of intravenous magnesium sulfate in suspected acute myocardial infarction on acute arrhythmias and long-term outcome. Int J Cardiol 1995;49:143–151.

66. Sherry S. Thrombolytic agents for acute myocardial infarction. Cardiovasc Drug Rev 1988;6:1–19.
67. Anderson HV, Willerson JT. Thrombolysis in acute myocardial infarction. N Engl J Med 1993;329:703–709.
68. Sherry S, Marder VJ. Streptokinase and recombinant tissue plasminogen activator (rt-PA) are equally effective in treating acute myocardial infarction. Ann Intern Med 1991;114:417–423.
69. Gruppo Italiano per lo Studio Della Sopravvivenza Nell'Infarto Miocardico (GISSI-2): A factorial randomised trial of alteplase versus streptokinase and heparin versus no heparin among 12,490 patients with acute myocardial infarction. Lancet 1990;336:65–71.
70. The International Study Group. In-hospital mortality and clinical course of 20,891 patients with suspected acute myocardial infarction randomised between alteplase and streptokinase with or without heparin. Lancet 1990;336:71–75.
71. Third International Study of Infarct Survival Collaborative Group (ISIS-3): A randomised comparison of streptokinase vs tissue plasminogen activator vs anistreplase and of aspirin plus heparin vs aspirin alone among 41,299 cases of suspected acute myocardial infarction. Lancet 1992;339:753–770.
72. The GUSTO Investigators. An international randomized trial comparing four thrombolytic strategies for acute myocardial infarction. N Engl J Med 1993;329:673–682.
73. The GUSTO Angiographic Investigators. The effect of tissue plasminogen activator, streptokinase, or both on coronary-artery patency, ventricular function, and survival after acute myocardial infarction. N Engl J Med 1993;329:1615–1622.
74. Second International Study of Infarct Survival (ISIS-2): Randomised trial of intravenous streptokinase, oral aspirin, both, or neither among 17,187 cases of suspected acute myocardial infarction: ISIS-2. Lancet 1988;ii:349–360.
75. Wasserman AG, Ross AM. Patient selection for thrombolytic therapy. Am J Cardiol 1989;64:17B–21B.
76. Weaver WD, Cerqueira M, Hallstrom AP, et al. Prehospital-initiated vs hospital-initiated thrombolytic therapy: The myocardial infarction triage and intervention trial. JAMA 1993;270:1211–1216.
77. Pepine CJ. GUSTO trial results: Optimizing thrombolytic strategies. J Myocard Ischem 1993;5:10–11.
78. Conti CR. Myocardial infarction, thrombolytic therapy, and economics. Clin Cardiol 1993;16:635.
79. Pfeffer MA, Moye LA, Braunwald E, et al. Selection bias in the use of thrombolytic therapy in acute myocardial infarction. JAMA 1991;266:528–532.
80. Sane DC, Califf RM, Topol EJ, et al. Bleeding during thrombolytic therapy for acute myocardial infarction: Mechanisms and management. Ann Int Med 1989;111:1010–1022.
81. Shah PK, Cercek B, Lew AS, Ganz W. Angiographic validation of bedside markers of reperfusion. J Am Coll Cardiol 1993;21:55–61.
82. Lincoff AM, Topol EJ. Illusion of reperfusion. Does anyone achieve optimal reperfusion during acute myocardial infarction? Circulation 1993;88:1361–1374.
83. Grines CL, Browne KF, Marco J, et al. A comparison of immediate angioplasty with thrombolytic therapy for acute myocardial infarction. N Engl J Med 1993;328:673–679.
84. Zijlstra F, de Boer MJ, Hoorntje JCA, et al. A comparison of immediate coronary angioplasty with intravenous streptokinase in acute myocardial infarction. N Engl J Med 1993;328:680–684.
85. Gibbons RJ, Holmes DR, Reeder GS, et al. Immediate angioplasty compared with the administration of a thrombolytic agent followed by conservative treatment for myocardial infarction. N Engl J Med 1993;328:685–691.
86. Landau C, Glamann DB, Willard JE, et al. Coronary angioplasty in the patient with acute myocardial infarction. Am J Med 1994;96:536–543.
87. Landau C, Lange RA, Hillis LD. Percutaneous transluminal coronary angioplasty. N Engl J Med 1994;330:981–993.
88. Neuhaus KL, Von Essen R, Tebbe U, et al. Improved thrombolysis in acute myocardial infarction wavefront-loaded administration of alteplase: Results of the rt-PA-APSAC patency study (TAPS). J Am Coll Cardiol 1992;19:885–891.
89. Topol EJ, Califf RM, George BE, et al. A randomized trial of immediate versus delayed elective angioplasty after intravenous tissue plasminogen activator in acute myocardial infarction. N Engl J Med 1987;317:581–588.
90. TIMI Research Group. Immediate vs delayed catheterization and angioplasty following thrombolytic therapy for acute myocardial infarction: TIMI IIA results. JAMA 1988;260:2849–2858.
91. SWIFT (Should We Intervene Following Thrombolysis?) Trial Study Group. SWIFT trial of delayed elective intervention v conservative treatment after thrombolysis with anistreplase in acute myocardial infarction. BMJ 1991;302:555–560.
92. TIMI Study Group. Comparison of invasive and conservative strategies after treatment with intravenous tissue plasminogen activator in acute myocardial infarction: Results of the Thrombolysis in Myocardial Infarction (TIMI) phase II trial. N Engl J Med 1989;320:618–627.
93. Patrono C. Aspirin as an antiplatelet drug. N Engl J Med 1994;330:1287–1294.
94. Antiplatelet Trialists' Collaboration. Collaborative overview of randomised trials of antiplatelet therapy—I: Prevention of death, myocardial infarction, and stroke by prolonged antiplatelet therapy in various categories of patients. BMJ 1994;308:81–106.
95. Fears R, Esmail AF, Greenwood HC. Effect of heparin on the fibrinolytic response to plasminogen activators. Semin Thromb Hemost 1991;17:389–393.
96. Ridker PM, Hebert PR, Fuster V, Hennekens CH. Are both aspirin and heparin justified as adjuncts to thrombolytic therapy for acute myocardial infarction? Lancet 1993;341:1574–1577.
97. Cruickshank MK, Levine MN, Hirsh J, et al. A standard heparin nomogram for the management of heparin therapy. Arch Intern Med 1991;151:333–337.
98. Raschke RA, Reilly BM, Guidry JR, et al. The weight-based heparin dosing nomogram compared with a "standard care" nomogram: A randomized controlled trial. Ann Intern Med 1993;119:874–881.

99. Davis MJE, Ireland MA. Effect of early anticoagulation on the frequency of left ventricular thrombi after anterior wall acute myocardial infarction. Am J Cardiol 1986;57:1244–1247.
100. Kontny F, Dale J, Abildgaard U, et al. Adverse effect of warfarin in acute MI: Increased left ventricular thrombus formation in patients not treated with high dose heparin. Eur Heart J 1993;14:1040–1043.
101. Clagett GP, Salzman EW, Wheller HB, et al. Prevention of venous thromboembolism. Chest 1992;102:391S–407S.
102. Smith P, Arnesen H, Holme I. The effect of warfarin on mortality and reinfarction after myocardial infarction. N Engl J Med 1990;323:147–152.
103. Meijer A, Verheugt FWA, Werter CJPJ, et al. Aspirin versus coumadin in the prevention of reocclusion and recurrent ischemia after successful thrombolysis: A prospective placebo-controlled angiographic study. Results of the APRICOT study. Circulation 1993;87:1524–1530.
104. Cairns JA, Fuster V, Kennedy JW. Coronary thrombolysis. Chest 1992;102:482S–507S.
105. Hirsh J, Fuster V. Guide to anticoagulant therapy Part 1: Heparin. Circulation 1994;89:1449–1468.
106. Sabbah HN, Goldstein S. Ventricular remodeling: Consequences and therapy. Eur Heart J 1993;14(suppl C):24–29.
107. Ertl G. Angiotensin converting enzyme inhibitors in angina and myocardial infarction: What role will they play in the 1990s? Drugs 1993;46:209–218.
108. Kleiman NS, Terrin M, Mueller H, et al. Mechanisms of early death despite thrombolytic therapy: Experience from the thrombolysis in myocardial infarction phase II (TIMI II) study. J Am Coll Cardiol 1992;19:1129–1135.
109. Hibbard MD, Holmes DR, Bailey KR, et al. Percutaneous transluminal coronary angioplasty in patients with cardiogenic shock. J Am Coll Cardiol 1992;19:639–646.
110. DeBusk RF. Specialized testing after recent myocardial infarction. Ann Intern Med 1989;110:470–481.

Chapter 16

The Arrhythmias

Jerry L. Bauman, PharmD, FCCP, FACC, and Marieke Dekker Schoen, PharmD

The heart has two basic properties, an electrical property and a mechanical property. The synchronous interaction between these two properties is complex, precise, and relatively enduring. The study of the electrical properties of the heart has grown at a slow steady rate, interrupted by salvos of information due to paroxysmal scientific breakthroughs. Einthoven's pioneering work has allowed graphic electrical tracings of cardiac rhythm and probably represents the first of these breakthroughs. This discovery of the surface electrocardiogram (ECG) has remained the cornerstone of diagnostic tools for cardiac rhythm disturbances. However, one must be aware that, prior to the availability of the ECG, meticulous clinical observation of venous and arterial pulsations provided a relatively sophisticated classification of many cardiac arrhythmias. More recently, intracardiac recordings and programmed cardiac stimulation have led to a wealth of both basic and clinical data. Microelectrode, voltage clamp, and patch clamping techniques have allowed considerable insight into the electrophysiologic actions and mechanisms of antiarrhythmic drugs. In terms of drug therapy, the use of digitalis and later quinidine were important first steps. The 1980s led to a considerable number of new agents. The theme of drug discovery initially was to find orally absorbed lidocaine-congeners and later other drugs that had extremely potent effects on conduction (i.e., flecainide-like agents). Unfortunately, the initial promise of a "magic bullet" in terms of antiarrhythmic drug therapy has gone unfulfilled. It is noteworthy that many of the problems associated with these new agents became clear after they were approved and marketed. Indeed, the overall volume of antiarrhythmic drug usage in the United States has declined in the past 4 years. The reasons for this are severalfold. First, awareness of the significance of drug-related proarrhythmia has been heightened. As highlighted by the Cardiac Arrhythmias Suppression Trial (CAST), proarrhythmia is an important side effect and has a potential effect on patient mortality. The CAST is perhaps the most important study ever performed regarding the treatment of rhythm disorders and continues to have a far-reaching impact on the clinical use of drugs and drug discovery. Second, technical advances have been made in the development of nondrug therapies. For instance, it is quite possible that interrupting reentry circuits by radiofrequency ablation could render long-term antiarrhythmic drug use obsolete in certain arrhythmias. Further, refinement of internal cardioverter/defibrillators continues to advance at an impressive rate, and this combined with the now known hazards of drugs have led some to choose this form of therapy as the first-line treatment of serious, recurrent ventricular arrhythmias.

What does the future hold for the use of antiarrhythmic drugs? Certainly new knowledge and technological advances have forced investigators and clinicians to rethink the concept of traditional membrane-active drugs. The current focus of investigational antiarrhythmic drugs is the potassium-channel blockers with sotalol being the first approved in the United States. Although considerable enthusiasm exists currently, the overall impact of these efforts has yet to be determined.

This chapter reviews the principles involved in both normal and abnormal cardiac conduction and addresses the pathophysiology and treatment of the more commonly encountered arrhythmias. Certainly, many volumes of complete text could be (and have been) devoted to basic and clinical electrophysiology. Therefore, this chapter briefly addresses those principles necessary for clinical pharmacists.

ARRHYTHMOGENESIS

NORMAL CONDUCTION

Electrical activity is initiated by the sinoatrial (SA) node and courses through cardiac tissue by a treelike conduction network. The SA node initiates cardiac rhythm under normal circumstances because this tissue possesses the highest degree of automaticity or rate of spontaneous impulse generation. The degree of automaticity of the SA node is largely influenced by the autonomic nervous system in that both cholinergic and sympathetic innervation control sinus rate. Most tissues within the conduction system also possess varying degrees of inherent automatic properties. However, the rates of spontaneous impulse generation of these tissues are less than that of the SA node. Thus, these latent automatic pacemakers are continuously excited and overdriven by impulses arising from the SA node (primary pacemaker) and do not become clinically apparent.

From the SA node, electrical activity moves in a wavefront through an atrial specialized conducting system and eventually gains entrance to the ventricle via an atrioventricular (AV) node and a large bundle of conducting tissue referred to as the bundle of His. Aside from this AV nodal–Hisian pathway, the atria and ventricles are separated by a fibrous AV ring that will not permit electrical stimulation. The conducting tissues bridging the atria and ventricles are referred to as the junctional areas. Again, this area of tissue (junction) is largely influenced by autonomic input, and it possesses a relatively high degree of inherent automaticity (but still less than that of the SA node). From the bundle of His, the cardiac conduction system bifurcates into several (usually three) bundle branches: one right bundle and two left bundles. These bundle branches further arborize into a conduction network referred to as the Purkinje system. The conduction system as a whole innervates the mechanical myocardium and serves to initiate excitation–contraction coupling and the contractile process. When a cell or group of cells within the heart is electrically stimulated, a brief period of time follows in which those cells cannot again be excited. This time period is referred to as the refractory period. As the electrical wavefront moves down the conduction system, the impulse eventually encounters tissue refractory to stimulation (recently excited) and subsequently dies. Then the SA node recovers, fires spontaneously, and begins the process again.

Prior to cellular excitation, an electrical gradient exists between the inside and the outside of the cell membrane. At this time, the cell is said to be polarized. In atrial and ventricular conducting tissue, the intracellular space is about 80–90 mV negative with respect to the extracellular environment. The electrical gradient just prior to excitation is referred to as resting membrane potential (RMP) and is the result of differences in ion concentrations between the inside and the outside of the cell. At RMP, the cell is polarized primarily by the action of active membrane ion pumps, the most notable of these being the sodium–potassium pump. For example, this specific pump (in addition to other systems) attempts to maintain the intracellular sodium concentration at 5–15 mEq/L and the extracellular sodium at 135–142 mEq/L; the intracellular potassium concentration at 135–140 mEq/L and the extracellular potassium concentration at 3–5 mEq/L. RMP can be calculated by means of the Nernst equation:

$$\text{RMP} = -61.5 \log \frac{[\text{ion outside}]}{[\text{ion inside}]}$$

Electrical stimulation (or depolarization) of the cell will result in changes in membrane potential over time or a characteristic action potential curve (Fig. 16.1). The action

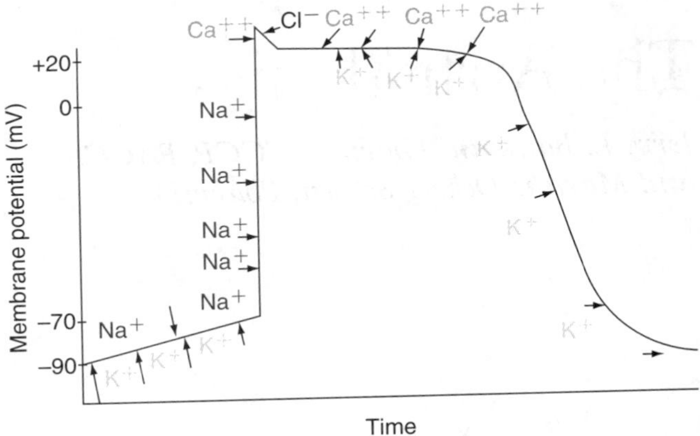

Figure 16.1. Purkinje fiber action potential showing specific ion flux responsible for the change in membrane potential.

potential curve results from the transmembrane movement of specific ions and is divided into different phases. Phase 0 (rapid depolarization) of atrial and ventricular tissues is due to an abrupt increase in the permeability of the membrane to sodium influx. This rapid depolarization more than equilibrates (overshoots) the electrical potential, resulting in passive chloride influx (initial repolarization) and phase 1. Calcium begins to move into the intracellular space at about −60 mV (during phase 0), causing a slower depolarization. Calcium influx continues throughout phase 2 of the action potential (plateau phase) and is balanced to some degree by potassium efflux. Calcium entrance distinguishes cardiac conducting cells from nerve tissue, and provides the critical ionic link to excitation–contraction coupling and the mechanical properties of the heart as a pump (see Chapter 13). The membrane remains permeable to potassium efflux during phase 3, resulting in cellular repolarization. Phase 4 of the action potential is the gradual depolarization of the cell and is related to a constant sodium leak into the intracellular space balanced by a decreasing (over time) efflux of potassium. The slope of phase 4 depolarization determines, in large part, the automatic properties of the cell. As the cell is slowly depolarized during phase 4, an abrupt increase in sodium permeability is encountered, allowing the rapid cellular depolarization of phase 0. The juncture of phase 4 and phase 0 where rapid sodium influx is initiated is referred to as the threshold potential of the cell. The level of threshold potential also regulates the degree of cellular automaticity.

Not all cells in the cardiac conduction system rely on sodium influx for initial depolarization. Some tissues depolarize in response to a slower inward ionic current caused by calcium influx. These "calcium-dependent" tissues are found primarily in the SA and AV nodes and possess distinct conduction properties in comparison to "sodium-dependent" fibers. Calcium-dependent cells generally have a less negative RMP (−40 to −60 mV) and a slower conduction velocity. Furthermore, in calcium-dependent tissues, recovery of excitability outlasts full repolarization, whereas in sodium-dependent tissue, recovery is prompt after repolarization. These two types of electrical fibers also differ dramatically in how drugs modify their conduction properties (see later in the chapter).

Ion conductance across the lipid bilayer of the cell membrane occurs via the formation of membrane pores or "channels" (Fig. 16.2). Selective ion channels probably form in response to specific electrical potential differences between the inside and the outside of the cell (voltage dependence). The membrane itself is composed of both organized and disorganized lipids and phospholipids in a dynamic sol–gel matrix. During ion flux and electrical excitation, changes in this sol–gel equilibrium occur and permit the formation of activated ion channels. Besides channel formation and membrane composition, the transmembrane movement of ions is also regulated by intrachannel proteins or phospholipids referred to as gates. These gates are believed to be positioned strategically within the channel to modulate ion flow (Fig. 16.2). Each ion channel conceptually has two types of gates: an activation gate and an inactivation gate. The activation gate opens during depolarization to allow the ion current to enter or exit from the cell and the inactivation gate closes to stop ion movement. When the cell is in a rested state, the activation gates are closed and the inactivation gates are open. The activation gates then open to allow ion movement through the channel and the inactivation gates later close to stop ion conductance. Therefore, the cell cycles between three states: resting, activation, and inactivation. Therefore, the activation of SA and AV nodal tissue depends on a slow depolarizing current through calcium channels and gates, whereas the activation of atrial and ventricular tissue depends on a rapid depolarizing current through sodium channels and gates. Sometimes these types of conduction tissues are referred to as slow and fast fibers, respectively.

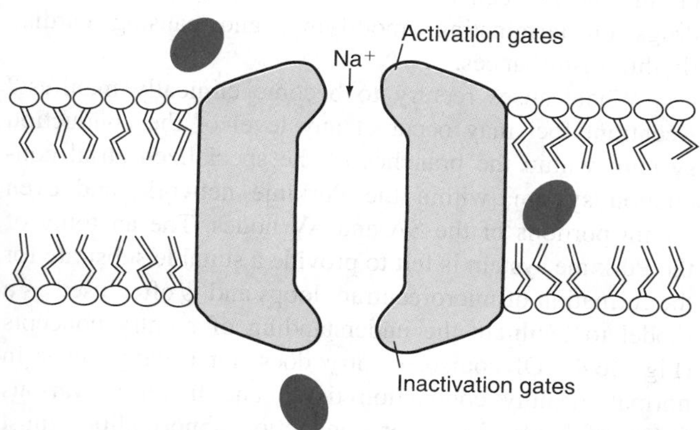

Figure 16.2. Lipid bilayer, sodium channel, and possible sites of action of the type I agents (colored circles). Type I antiarrhythmic drugs may theoretically inhibit sodium influx at an extracellular, intramembrane, or intracellular receptor site. However, all approved agents appear to block sodium conductance at a single receptor site by gaining entrance to the interior of the channel from an intracellular route. Active ionized drugs block the channel predominantly during the activated or inactivated state and bind and unbind with specific time constraints (described as fast on–off, slow on–off, and intermediate).

ABNORMAL CONDUCTION

The mechanisms of tachyarrhythmias have been classically divided into two general categories—those resulting from an abnormality in impulse generation or *automatic tachycardias* and those resulting from an abnormality in impulse conduction or *reentrant tachycardias.*

Automatic tachycardias depend on spontaneous impulse generation in latent pacemakers and may be due to several different mechanisms. Experimentally, chemicals such as digitalis glycosides or catecholamines and conditions such as hypoxemia, electrolyte abnormalities (e.g., hypokalemia), or fiber stretch (e.g., cardiac dilatation) may lead to an increased slope of phase 4 depolarization in tissues other than the SA node. These factors, which experimentally lead to abnormal automaticity, are also known to be arrhythmogenic in clinical situations. The increased slope of phase 4 causes heightened automaticity of these tissues and competition with the SA node for dominance of cardiac rhythm. If the rate of spontaneous impulse generation of the abnormally automatic tissue exceeds that of the SA node, then an automatic tachycardia may result. Automatic tachycardias have the following characteristics: (1) The onset of the tachycardia is not related to an initiating event such as a premature beat; (2) the initiating beat is usually identical to subsequent beats of the tachycardia; (3) the tachycardia cannot be initiated by programmed cardiac stimulation; (4) the tachycardia often occurs in association with digitalis toxicity, high degrees of sympathetic tone, hypokalemia, and/or severe pulmonary disease; and (5) onset of the tachycardia is usually preceded by a gradual acceleration in rate and termination by a deceleration in rate.

Triggered automaticity is also a possible mechanism for abnormal impulse generation. Briefly, triggered automaticity refers to transient membrane depolarizations that occur during repolarization (early after-depolarizations) or after repolarization (delayed after-depolarizations) but prior to phase 4 of the action potential. After-depolarizations may be related to abnormal calcium and sodium influx during or just after full cellular repolarization. Experimentally, early after-depolarizations may be precipitated by hypokalemia, type Ia antiarrhythmic drugs, or slow stimulation rates and have been implicated as a cause of torsades de pointes. Late after-depolarizations may be precipitated by digitalis or catecholamines and suppressed by calcium channel inhibitors, and have been suggested as the mechanism for multifocal atrial tachycardia and exercise-provoked ventricular tachycardia. Triggered automatic rhythms possess some of the characteristics of automatic tachycardias and some of the characteristics of reentrant tachycardias.

As previously mentioned, the impulse originating from the SA node in an individual with sinus rhythm eventually meets previously excited and thus refractory tissue. Reentry is a concept that involves indefinite propagation of the impulse and continued activation of previously refractory tissue.[1,2] Three conduction requirements must be met for the formation of a viable reentrant focus: (1) two pathways for impulse conduction, (2) an area of unidirectional block (prolonged refractoriness) in one of these pathways, and (3) slow conduction in the other pathway (Fig. 16.3). Usually a critically timed premature beat initiates reentry. This premature impulse enters both conduction pathways but encounters refractory tissue in one of the pathways at the area of unidirectional block. The impulse dies out because it is still refractory from the previous (sinus) impulse. Although it fails to propagate in one pathway, the impulse may still proceed in a forward direction (antegrade) through the other pathway because of this pathway's relatively shorter refractory period. The impulse may then proceed through a loop of tissue and "reenter" the area of unidirectional block in a backward direction (retrograde). Because the antegrade pathway has slow conduction characteristics, the area of unidirectional block has time to recover its excitability. The impulse can proceed retrogradely through this (previously refractory) tissue and continue around the loop of tissue in a circular fashion. Thus, the key to the formation of a reentrant focus is crucial conduction discrepancies in the electrophysiologic characteristics of the two pathways. The reentrant focus may excite surrounding tissue at a rate greater than that of the SA node, and a clinical tachycardia results. The previously mentioned model is anatomically determined in that there is only one pathway for impulse conduction with a fixed circuit length. Another model of reentry, referred to as a functional reentrant loop or leading circle model, may also occur (Fig. 16.4).[3] In a functional reentrant focus, the length of the circuit may vary depending on the conduction velocity and recovery characteristics of the impulse. The area in the middle of the loop is continually kept refractory by the inwardly moving impulse. The length of the circuit is not fixed, but is the smallest circle possible, such that the leading edge of the wavefront is continuously exciting tissue just as it recovers; the head of the impulse chases its tail. It differs from the anatomic model in that the leading edge of the impulse is not preceded by an excitable gap of tissue, and it does not have an obstacle in the middle or a fixed anatomic circuit. Clinically, many reentrant foci probably have both anatomic and functional characteristics. In the figure 8 model, a zone of unidirectional block is present, allowing for two impulse loops, which join and reenter the area of block in a retrograde fashion to form a pretzel-shaped reentrant circuit.[4] This model combines functional characteristics with an excitable gap. All of these theoretical models require a critical balance of refractoriness and conduction velocity within the circuit and as such have helped to explain the effects of drugs on terminating, modifying, and causing cardiac rhythm disturbances.

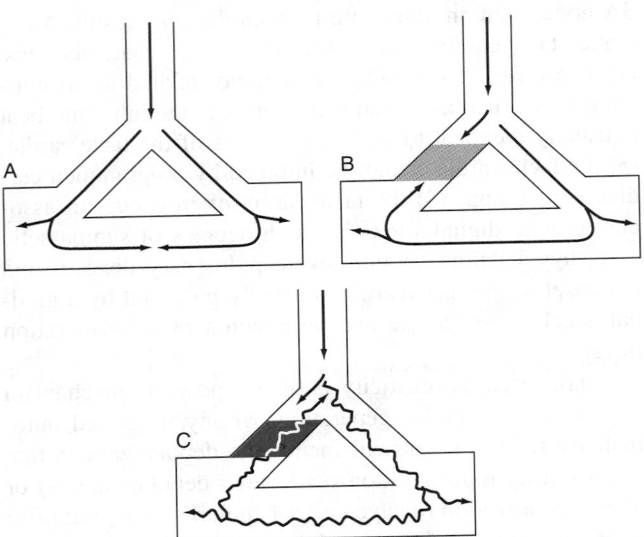

Figure 16.3. Process of reentry into a loop of tissue in an anatomically determined model of reentry. (A) Normal conduction process. (B) Area of unidirectional block caused by prolonged tissue refractoriness. (C) Reentrant loop is formed with necessary ingredients: an area of unidirectional block and a loop of tissue with slowed conduction velocity. *(From Bauman JL. Understanding and treating supraventricular arrhythmias. Clin Pharm 1983;2:313, with permission.)*

What causes reentry to become clinically manifest? Reentrant foci may occur at any level of the conduction system: within the branches of the specialized atrial conduction system, within the Purkinje network, and even within portions of the SA and AV nodes. The anatomy of the Purkinje system is felt to provide a suitable substrate for the formation of microreentrant loops and is often used as a model to facilitate the understanding of reentry concepts (Fig. 16.4). Of course, reentry does not usually occur in normal, healthy conduction tissue and therefore various forms of heart disease or conduction abnormalities must usually be present before reentry becomes manifest. In other words, the various forms of heart disease can result in changes in conduction in the pathways of a suitable reentrant substrate. An often-used example is reentry occurring as a consequence of ischemic or hypoxic damage: With inadequate cellular oxygen, cardiac tissue resorts to anaerobic glycolysis for ATP production. As the high-energy phosphate concentration diminishes, the activity of the trans-

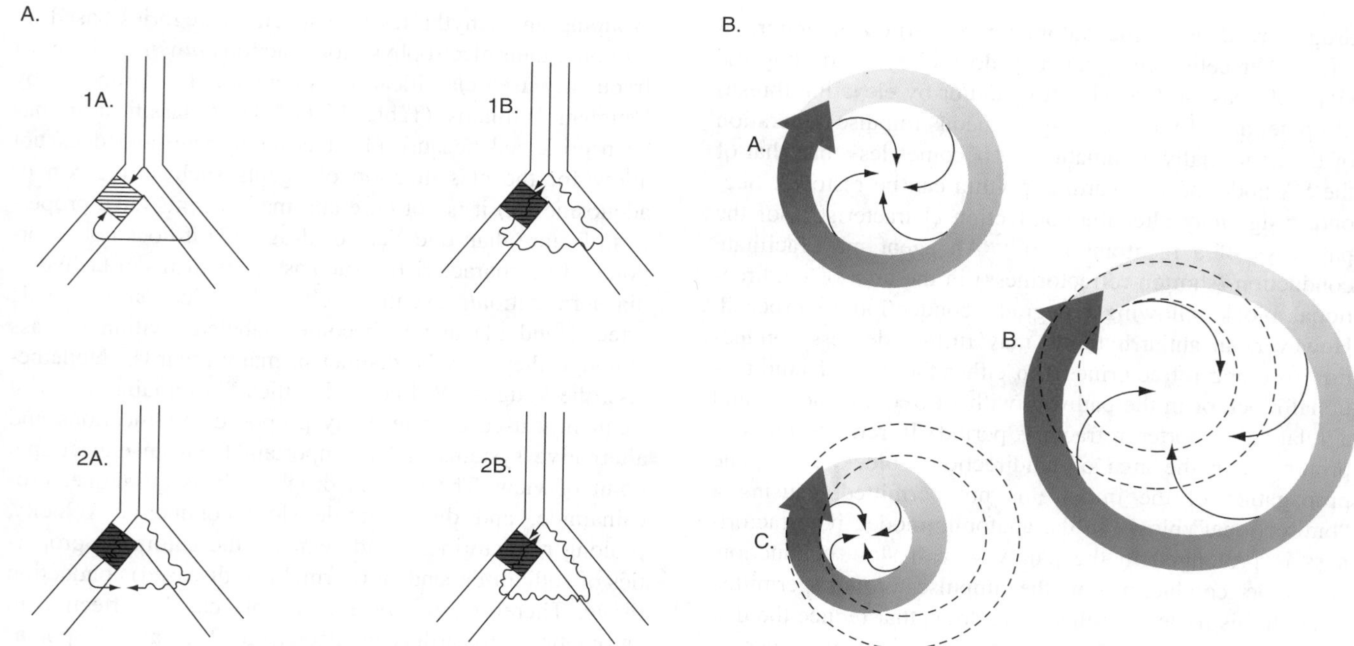

Figure 16.4. A. Possible mechanism of proarrhythmia in the anatomic model of reentry. (1A) Nonviable reentrant loop due to bidirectional block (shaded area). (1B) Instance where a drug slows conduction velocity without significantly prolonging the refractory period. The impulse is now able to reenter the area of unidirectional block (shaded area) because slowed conduction through the contralateral limb allows recovery of the block. A new reentrant tachycardia may result. (2A) Nonviable reentrant loop due to a lack of a unidirectional block. (2B) Instance where a drug prolongs the refractory period without significantly slowing conduction velocity. The impulse moving antegrade meets refractory tissue (shaded area) allowing for unidirectional block. A new reentrant tachycardia may result. **B.** Mechanism of reentry and proarrhythmia. (A) Functionally determined (leading circle) reentrant circuit. This model should be contrasted with anatomic reentry: Here the circuit is not fixed (it does not necessarily move around an anatomic obstacle) and there is no excitable gap. All tissue inside is held continuously refractory. (B) Instance where a drug prolongs the refractory period without significantly slowing conduction velocity. The tachycardia may terminate or slow in rate as shown due to a greater circuit length. The dashed lines represent the original reentrant circuit prior to drug treatment. (C) Instance where a drug slows conduction velocity without significantly prolonging the refractory period (i.e., type Ic agents) and accelerates the tachycardia. The tachycardia rate may increase (proarrhythmia) as shown due to a shorter circuit length. The dashed lines represent the original reentrant circuit prior to drug treatment. *(From McCollam PL et al. Proarrhythmia: A paradoxic response to antiarrhythmic agents. Pharmacotherapy 1989;9:146, with permission.)*

membrane ion pumps declines and RMP rises. This rise in RMP causes inactivation in the voltage-dependent sodium channel and the tissue begins to assume slow conduction characteristics. If changes in conduction parameters occur in a discordant manner due to varying degrees of ischemia or hypoxia, then a reentry circuit may become manifest. Furthermore, an ischemic, dying cell liberates intracellular potassium, which also causes a rise in RMP. In other cases, reentry may occur due to anatomic or functional variants in the normal conduction system. Patients, for example, may possess two (instead of one) conduction pathways within the AV node or have an anomalous, extranodal AV pathway that possesses different electrophysiologic characteristics from the normal AV nodal pathway. Reentry in these cases may occur within the AV node or encompass both atrial and ventricular tissue (see section entitled "Paroxysmal Superventricular Tachycardia Due to Reentry"). Reentrant tachycardias have the following characteristics: (1) the onset of the tachycardia is usually related to an initiating event (i.e., premature beat), (2) the initiating beat is usually different in morphology from subsequent beats of the tachycardia, (3) initiation of the tachycardia is usually possible with programmed cardiac stimulation, and (4) the initiation and termination of the tachycardia is usually abrupt without an acceleration or deceleration phase.

MECHANISM OF ANTIARRHYTHMIC DRUGS

In a theoretical sense, drugs may have antiarrhythmic activity by directly altering conduction in several ways. First, a drug may depress the automatic properties of abnormal pacemaker cells. An agent may do this by decreasing the slope of phase 4 depolarization and/or by elevating threshold potential. If the rate of spontaneous impulse generation of the abnormally automatic foci becomes less than that of the SA node, normal cardiac rhythm can be restored. Second, drugs may alter the conduction characteristics of the pathways of a reentrant loop.[1,2] An agent may facilitate conduction (shorten refractoriness) in the area of unidirectional block, allowing antegrade conduction to proceed. However, an antiarrhythmic may further depress conduction (prolong refractoriness) in either the area of unidirectional block or in the pathway with slowed conduction and a relatively shorter refractory period. If refractoriness is prolonged in the area of unidirectional block, retrograde propagation of the impulse is not permitted, causing a "bidirectional" block. In the anatomic model, if refractoriness is prolonged in the pathway with slow conduction, antegrade conduction of the impulse is not permitted through this route. In either case, drugs that reduce the discordance and cause a uniformity in conduction properties of the two pathways may suppress the reentrant substrate. In the functionally determined model, if refractoriness is prolonged without significantly slowing conduction velocity, the tachycardia may terminate or slow in rate due to a greater circuit length (Fig. 16.4). According to another theoretically possible mechanism, a drug may eliminate the critically timed premature impulse that triggers reentry.

Antiarrhythmic drugs have specific electrophysiologic actions that alter cardiac conduction in patients with or without heart disease. These actions form the basis of grouping antiarrhythmics into specific categories based on grouping their electrophysiologic actions *in vitro*. The most frequently used classification system was first proposed by Vaughan Williams (Table 16.1).[5] This classification has been criticized because (1) it is incomplete and does not allow for the classification of agents such as digoxin or adenosine; (2) it is not pure and many agents have properties of more than one class of drugs; (3) it does not incorporate drug characteristics such as mechanisms of tachycardia termination/prevention, clinical indications, or side effects; and (4) agents become "labeled" within a class although they may be distinct in many regards.[6] Nonetheless, the Vaughan Williams classification remains the most frequently used despite many proposed modifications and alternative systems and is important from an educational point of view. The type Ia drugs such as quinidine, procainamide, and disopyramide slow conduction velocity, prolong refractoriness, and decrease the automatic properties of sodium-dependent (normal and diseased) conduction tissue. Therefore, the type Ia agents can be effective in automatic tachycardias by decreasing the rate of spontaneous impulse generation of atrial or ventricular foci. In reentrant tachycardias, these drugs generally depress conduction and prolong refractoriness, theoretically transforming the area of unidirectional block into a bidirectional block. Clinically, type Ia drugs are broad-spectrum antiarrhythmics, being effective for both supraventricular and ventricular arrhythmias.

Historically, lidocaine and phenytoin were categorized separately from quinidine-like drugs. This was due to early work demonstrating that lidocaine had distinctly different

TABLE 16.1. CLASSIFICATION OF ANTIARRHYTHMIC DRUGS

Type	Drug	Conduction Velocity[a]	Refractory Period	Automaticity	Ion Block
Ia	Quinidine Procainamide Disopyramide	↓	↑	↓	Sodium (intermediate)
Ib	Lidocaine Mexiletine Tocainide	0/↓	↓	↓	Sodium (fast on–off)
Ic	Flecainide Propafenone[b] Moricizine[c]	↓↓	0	↓	Sodium (slow on–off)
II[d]	Beta blockers	↓	↑	↓	Calcium (indirect)
III	Amiodarone[b,e] Bretylium[b] Sotolol[b]	0	↑↑	0	Potassium
IV[d]	Verapamil Diltiazem	↓	↑	↓	Calcium

Key: ↑, increase; ↓, decrease.
[a]Variables for normal tissue models in ventricular tissue.
[b]Also has type II β-blocking actions.
[c]Classification controversial.
[d]Variables for SA and AV nodal tissue only.
[e]Amiodarone also blocks calcium and sodium channels (fast on–off).

electrophysiologic actions. In normal tissue models, lidocaine generally had facilitative actions on cardiac conduction by shortening refractoriness and having little effect on conduction velocity. Thus, it was postulated that these agents could improve antegrade conduction, eliminating the area of unidirectional block. Of course, arrhythmias do not usually arise from normal tissue, leading investigators to study the actions of lidocaine and phenytoin in ischemic and hypoxic tissue models. Interestingly, studies have shown these drugs to possess quinidine-like properties in diseased tissues.[7] Therefore, it is probable that lidocaine acts in clinical tachycardias in a fashion similar to the type Ia drugs (i.e., accentuated effects in diseased tissues leading to bidirectional block in a reentrant circuit). Lidocaine and similar agents have accentuated effects in ischemic tissue due to the local acidosis and potassium shifts that occur during cellular hypoxia. Changes in pH alter the time that local anesthetics occupy the sodium channel receptor and, therefore, affect the agent's electrophysiologic actions.[8] For phenytoin (but not lidocaine), other researchers[9] have suggested a novel mechanism of action mediated through the central nervous system. The type Ib agents such as lidocaine (and structural analogues such as tocainide or mexiletine) are considerably more effective in ventricular arrhythmias than supraventricular arrhythmias.

The third group of type I drugs, type Ic, includes propafenone, flecainide, and moricizine. These agents profoundly slow conduction velocity while leaving refractoriness relatively unaltered. Type Ic drugs theoretically eliminate reentry by slowing conduction to a point where the impulse is extinguished and cannot propagate further. Although effective for both ventricular and supraventricular arrhythmias, their use for ventricular arrhythmias has been limited by the risk of proarrhythmia (see section entitled "Proarrhythmia").

Type I drugs exert their effects on a subcellular basis by inhibiting the transmembrane influx of sodium. In essence, type I agents can be referred to as sodium channel blockers. The receptor site for the antiarrhythmics is probably inside the sodium channel so that, in effect, the drug plugs the pore. The agent may gain access to the receptor either via the intracellular space through the membrane lipid bilayer or directly through the channel.[10] Several principles are inherent in antiarrhythmic-sodium channel receptor theories[11]:

1. Type I antiarrhythmics have predominant affinity for a particular state of the channel (e.g., during activation or inactivation). For example, lidocaine and flecainide block sodium current primarily when the cell is in the inactivated state, whereas quinidine is predominantly an open (or activated) channel blocker.
2. Type I antiarrhythmics have specific binding and unbinding characteristics to the receptor. For example, lidocaine binds to and dissociates from the channel receptor quickly (termed fast on–off) but flecainide has very slow on–off properties. This explains why flecainide has such potent effects on slowing ventricular conduction but lidocaine has little effect on normal tissue. In general, the type Ic drugs are slow on–off, the type Ib drugs are fast on–off, and the type Ia drugs are intermediate in their binding kinetics.
3. Type I antiarrhythmics possess rate dependence (i.e., sodium-channel blockade and slowed conduction are greatest at fast heart rates and least during bradycardia). For slow on–off drugs, sodium channel blockade is evident at normal rates (60–100 beats/min) but for fast on–off agents, slowed conduction is only apparent at rapid rates of stimulation.
4. Type I antiarrhythmics (except phenytoin) are weak bases with a $pK_a > 7.0$, and they block the sodium channel in their ionized form. Therefore, pH will alter these actions: Acidosis will accentuate and alkalosis will diminish sodium-channel blockade.
5. Type I antiarrhythmics appear to share a single receptor site in the sodium channel.

These principles are important in understanding additive drug combinations (e.g., quinidine and mexiletine), antagonistic combinations (e.g., flecainide and lidocaine), and potential antidotes to excess sodium-channel blockade (e.g., sodium bicarbonate or propranolol).

The β-adrenergic antagonists are classified as type II antiarrhythmic drugs. For the most part, the clinically relevant antiarrhythmic mechanisms of the β blockers result from their antiadrenergic actions. Because the SA and AV nodes are heavily influenced by adrenergic innervation, β blockers would be most useful in tachycardias in which these nodal tissues are abnormally automatic or are a portion of a reentrant loop. These agents are also helpful in slowing ventricular response in atrial tachycardias (e.g., atrial fibrillation) by their effects on the AV node. Furthermore, some tachycardias are exercise related or precipitated by states of high sympathetic tone (perhaps through triggered activity), and β blockers may be useful in these instances. Beta-adrenergic stimulation results in increased conduction velocity, shortened refractoriness, and increased automaticity of the nodal tissues; β-adrenergic blockers will antagonize these effects. Propranolol is often noted to have "local anesthetic" or quinidine-like activity; however, suprapharmacologic concentrations are usually required to elicit this action. In the nodal tissues, β blockers interfere with calcium entry into the cell by altering catecholamine-dependent channel integrity and gating kinetics. In sodium-dependent atrial and ventricular tissue, β blockers shorten repolarization somewhat, but otherwise have little direct effect.

Type III antiarrhythmics include those agents that specifically prolong refractoriness in atrial and ventricular fibers. This class includes three very different drugs—bretylium, amiodarone, and sotalol. These drugs share the common effect of delaying repolarization by blocking potassium channels. The electrophysiologic actions of bretylium are related to its multifaceted pharmacology. Bretylium is structurally similar to guanethidine and can, likewise, cause an initial increase in catecholamine release from the adrenergic neuron. This action may potentially affect arrhythmogenesis by indirectly increasing coronary blood flow and myocardial perfusion, which reverses ischemia-related arrhythmias (similar to epinephrine's action in a patient with ventricular fibrillation). After causing catecholamine release, bretylium then causes an uncoupling of autonomic nerve stimulation from the release step, resulting in antiadrenergic effects. Theoretically, bretylium may also be antiarrhythmic by these sympatholytic actions. Nonetheless, bretylium prolongs repolarization due to blockade of potassium conductance, independent of the sympathetic nervous system, and many researchers believe these direct actions account for its clinical effectiveness. Importantly, bretylium increases the ventricular fibrillation threshold and seems to have selective antifibrillatory but not antitachycardic effects. In other words, bretylium can be effective in ventricular fibrillation, whereas it is rarely effective in ventricular tachycardia.

In contrast, amiodarone and sotalol are effective in a wide variety of tachycardias. Amiodarone actually displays electrophysiologic characteristics consistent with each class within the Vaughan Williams scheme; it is a sodium-channel blocker with relatively fast on–off kinetics, has β-blocking actions, blocks potassium channels, and also has a small degree of calcium antagonist activity. At normal heart rates, its predominant effect is to prolong repolarization. Theoretically, amiodarone, like type I agents, may interrupt the reentrant substrate by transforming an area of unidirectional block into one of bidirectional block. However, electrophysiologic studies utilizing programmed cardiac stimulation imply that amiodarone may leave the reentrant loop intact.[12] Rather, it is possible that amiodarone abolishes the premature impulse that usually triggers the reentry process. Although amiodarone may have the most impressive side effect profile of all of the antiarrhythmics, it also seems that it is the most highly effective agent available. Sotalol is a potent inhibitor of outward potassium movement during repolarization and also possesses β-blocking actions. Indeed, it was first synthesized as a nonselective β antagonist but now has evolved into the prototype type III agent upon which most investigational agents are based. Pure potassium current blockers display *reverse use-dependence* (i.e., their effects on repolarization are greatest at low heart rates). Sotalol and similar drugs also appear to be much more effective in preventing ventricular fibrillation (in dog models) than the traditional sodium blockers. They also decrease defibrillation threshold in contrast to type I agents, which tend to increase this parameter. This could be important in patients with automatic internal defibrillators. Although most of the excitement surrounding antiarrhythmic drug therapy currently centers around sotalol-like agents, most, if not all, of these agents may cause proarrhythmia in the form of torsades de pointes. More long-term data regarding safety and efficacy are necessary in order to ascertain their true place in therapy.

The calcium channel antagonists (verapamil and diltiazem) comprise the type IV antiarrhythmic category. Because calcium-dependent tissue and slow channels are found primarily in the SA and AV nodes, one may expect these agents to manifest their activity primarily against tachycardias at these sites. By inhibiting calcium entry into the cell, verapamil and diltiazem slow conduction, prolong refractoriness, and decrease automaticity of the SA and AV nodes. Therefore, these agents are effective in automatic or reentrant tachycardias, which arise from or utilize the SA or AV nodes. In atrial tachycardias these drugs can slow ventricular response (e.g., atrial fibrillation) by slowing AV nodal conduction. Furthermore, because calcium entry seems to be integral to exercise-related tachycardias and/or tachycardias due to some forms of triggered automaticity, preliminary evidence shows effectiveness in these types of arrhythmias. In all likelihood, verapamil and diltiazem work at different receptor sites because of their dissimilar chemical structures and pharmacologic actions. Nifedipine (or any of the dihydropyridine calcium antagonists) does not have significant antiarrhythmic activity because a reflex increase in sympathetic tone due to vasodilation counteracts this agent's direct negative dromotropic action. Calcium antagonists can slightly shorten repolarization in normal sodium-dependent tissue but otherwise have little effect. The pharmacokinetics of the antiarrhythmic agents are summarized in Table 16.2.

Supraventricular Arrhythmias

The common supraventricular tachycardias that often require drug treatment are (1) atrial fibrillation or atrial flutter, (2) paroxysmal supraventricular tachycardia, and (3) automatic atrial tachycardias. Other common supraventricular arrhythmias that usually do not require drug therapy include premature atrial complexes (PACs), wandering atrial pacemaker, sinus arrhythmia, and sinus tachycardia. As an example, PACs rarely cause symptoms, never cause hemodynamic compromise, and drug therapy, therefore, is not indicated. Similarly, sinus tachycardia is usually the result of underlying metabolic or hemodynamic disorders

TABLE 16.2. PHARMACOKINETICS OF ANTIARRHYTHMIC DRUGS

Drug	Bioavailability (%)	Primary Route of Elimination[a]	$V_{D,ss}$ (L/kg)	Protein Binding (%)	$t_{1/2}$	Therapeutic Range (mg/L)
Quinidine	70–80	H	2.0–3.5	80–90	5–9 h	2–6
Procainamide	75–95	H/R	1.5–3.0	10–20	2.5–5.0 h	4–15
Disopyramide	70–95	H/R	0.8–2.0	50–80	4–8 h	2–6
Lidocaine	20–40	H	1–2	65–75	60–180 min	1.5–5.0
Mexiletine	80–95	H	5–12	60–75	6–12 h	0.8–2.0
Tocainide	90–95	H	1.5–3.0	10–30	12–15 h	4–10
Moricizine	34–38	H	6–11	92–95	1–6 h	—
Flecainide	90–95	H/R	8–10	35–45	13–20 h	0.3–2.5
Propafenone[b]						
Poor	11–39	H	2.5–4.0	85–95	12–32 h	—
Extensive					2–10 h	
Amiodarone	22–88	H	70–150	95–99	15–100 d	1.0–2.5
Sotolol	90–95	R	1.2–2.4	30–40	12–20 h	—
Bretylium	15–20	R	4–8	Negligible	5–10 h	0.5–2.0
Verapamil	20–40	H	1.5–5.0	95–99	4–12 h	>0.05
Diltiazem	35–50	H	3–5	70–85	4–10 h	>0.05

[a]H, hepatic; R, renal.
[b]Variables for parent compound (not 5–OH, propafenone).

(e.g., infection, dehydration, hypotension, etc.), and therapy should be directed at the underlying cause not the tachycardia per se. Of course, there are exceptions to these suggestions. For example, sinus tachycardia may be deleterious in patients after cardiac surgery or myocardial infarction or in those with an unusual rhythm termed nonparoxysmal sinus tachycardia, so that antiarrhythmic drugs may be indicated. Stated in another way, although many arrhythmias generally do not require therapy, clinical judgment and patient-specific variables play an important role in this decision. Nevertheless, for the purpose of this discussion, only the tachycardias usually requiring antiarrhythmic drug therapy as listed previously are addressed.

Supraventricular tachycardias may cause a variety of symptoms. Some patients may be totally asymptomatic or only complain of minor palpitations and/or irregular pulse. In contrast, severe and even life-threatening symptoms can sometimes result. Patients may experience dizziness or acute syncopal episodes associated with the onset of their tachycardia, because of an abrupt drop in cardiac output, blood pressure, and cerebral perfusion. This drop in forward cardiac output occurs due to the rapid ventricular rate with resultant poor ventricular filling and asynchronous AV contraction. Heart failure symptoms may also occur and patients tolerate the tachycardia particularly poorly if preexisting left ventricular dysfunction is present. Furthermore, patients may experience anginal chest pain if underlying coronary obstruction is present, due to altered coronary perfusion (low cardiac output) and elevated myocardial oxygen demand (rapid heart rate). More often, patients complain of a choking or pressure sensation during the tachycardia episode, which can be confused with angina pectoris. Note also that symptoms such as palpitations and even syncope correlate rather poorly with documented recurrences of the tachycardia.

ATRIAL FIBRILLATION AND ATRIAL FLUTTER

Atrial fibrillation and atrial flutter are common supraventricular tachycardias. These tachycardias occur more often in men and elderly persons. The overall incidence of atrial fibrillation is about 2% (independent of gender and age), and this approximately doubles in elderly men.[13] These arrhythmias may present as a chronic, established tachycardia; an acute tachycardia; or a self-terminating, paroxysmal form. Atrial fibrillation is characterized as an extremely rapid (400–600 atrial beats/min) and disorganized atrial activation. With this disorganized atrial activity, there is a loss of the contribution of atrial contraction (atrial kick) to forward cardiac output. Supraventricular impulses penetrate the AV conduction system in variable degrees, resulting in an irregular activation of the ventricles and an irregularly irregular pulse. The AV junction will not conduct most of the supraventricular impulses, causing ventricular response to be considerably slower (120–180 beats/min) than the atrial rate. Atrial flutter occurs less frequently than atrial fibrillation, but is similar in its precipitating factors, consequences, and drug therapy approach. This arrhythmia is characterized by rapid (270–330 atrial beats/min) but regular atrial activation. The slower and regular electrical activity results in a regular ventricular response and pulse that is in approximate multiples of 300 beats/min (i.e., 1 : 1 AV conduction = ventricular rate 300 beats/min; 2 : 1 AV conduction = ventricular rate 150 beats/min; 3 : 1 AV conduction = ventricular rate 100 beats/min). Atrial flutter may occur in two distinct forms (type I and type II). Type I flutter is the more common classic form with atrial rates of approximately 300 beats/min and the typical "sawtooth" pattern of atrial activation as shown by the surface electrocardiogram. Type II flutter tends to be faster, being somewhat of a hybrid between classic atrial flutter and atrial fibrillation. Although the ventricular response usually has a regular pattern, atrial flutter with varying degrees of AV block or that occur with episodes of atrial fibrillation ("fib-flutter") can cause an irregular ventricular rate and pulse.

It is generally accepted that the predominant mechanism of atrial fibrillation and atrial flutter is reentry. Atrial fibrillation appears to result from multiple atrial reentrant loops (or wavelets), and atrial flutter is due to a single, dominant reentrant substrate. Atrial fibrillation or flutter usually occurs in association with forms of organic heart disease that cause atrial distention. Forms of heart disease that commonly lead to atrial stretch and precipitate atrial fibrillation or flutter include ischemia or infarction, hypertensive heart disease, valvular disorders such as mitral stenosis, mitral insufficiency, congenital abnormalities such as septal defects, and primary myocardial disease such as congestive or obstructive cardiomyopathy. Disorders that cause right atrial stretch and are associated with atrial fibrillation or flutter include acute pulmonary embolus and chronic lung disease, resulting in pulmonary hypertension and cor pulmonale. These arrhythmias may also occur in association with states of high adrenergic tone such as thyrotoxicosis, alcohol withdrawal, sepsis, or excessive physical exertion. Established or paroxysmal atrial fibrillation occurring without identifiable heart disease or known precipitating factors is termed "lone" atrial fibrillation. Other states in which patients are predisposed to episodes of atrial fibrillation are the presence of an anomalous AV pathway (i.e., Kent bundle) and sinus node dysfunction (i.e., tachy–brady or sick sinus syndrome).

Patients with atrial fibrillation or flutter may experience the entire range of symptoms associated with other supraventricular tachycardias, although syncope as a presenting symptom is uncommon. Since atrial kick is lost with the onset of atrial fibrillation, severe low output states may result in forms of heart disease that rely heavily on atrial contraction to maintain cardiac output (e.g., mitral stenosis or hypertrophic obstructive cardiomyopathy). An additional complication of atrial fibrillation is arterial embolization resulting from atrial stasis and poorly adherent mural thrombi. Of course, the most devastating complication in this regard is the occurrence of an embolic stroke.[14] The overall incidence of stroke in patients with atrial fibrillation not receiving antithrombotic therapy is about 3–6%.[15] Patients with concurrent mitral stenosis or severe systolic heart failure and atrial fibrillation are at particularly high risk for cerebral embolism. In addition, stroke can precede the onset of documented atrial fibrillation, probably due to undetected paroxysms prior to the onset of established atrial fibrillation.[14] In contrast, patients with atrial fibrillation in whom precipitating factors cannot be identified (i.e., lone atrial fibrillation) and patients with only atrial flutter have a low risk of embolic stroke.[16]

The ultimate treatment goals of atrial fibrillation or flutter are the restoration of sinus rhythm, the prevention of thromboembolic complications, and the prevention of further recurrences (Fig. 16.5). However, the methods by which to attain these goals vary and often raise ill-defined areas of controversy. First, consider the patient with new onset atrial fibrillation or flutter. If presenting symptoms are severe (as detailed previously), patients may require direct-current cardioversion (DCC) in an attempt to restore sinus rhythm immediately. Atrial flutter often requires relatively low energy levels of countershock (i.e., 25–50 W/s), whereas atrial fibrillation often requires higher energy levels (i.e., greater than 200 W/s). However, if tolerable symptoms are present, no such emergency measures are necessary. Type Ia antiarrhythmic agents may restore sinus rhythm but should not be administered initially. These agents may paradoxically increase ventricular response in the absence of drugs that slow AV nodal conduction. Traditionally, this observation has been attributed to the vagolytic action of quinidine, procainamide, or disopyramide despite the fact that only disopyramide displays major anticholinergic side effects. Therefore, a more likely alternative explanation exists: All of these agents slow atrial conduction, decreasing the number of impulses reaching the AV node and, as a result, the AV node paradoxically allows more impulses to gain entrance to the ventricular conduction system (increasing ventricular rate). Because of this phenomenon and the lack of need for immediate restoration of sinus rhythm, drugs that slow conduction and increase refractoriness in the AV node should be used as initial therapy. Traditionally, loading dosages of digoxin have been used due to time-proven effectiveness and the high incidence of concurrent heart failure. However, digoxin's place in therapy has been questioned in both the acute and chronic setting.[17] Digoxin is sometimes ineffective and often slow in onset; although an initial decrease in ventricular response can sometimes be observed within 1 hour of intravenous administration, full control (heart rate less than 100 beats/min) is usually not achieved for 24–48 hours. Digoxin will not restore sinus rhythm although spontaneous termination of atrial fibrillation may occur in some patients during the loading procedure.[18]

As mentioned previously, patients can present at two ends of the spectrum (i.e., either severely symptomatic or

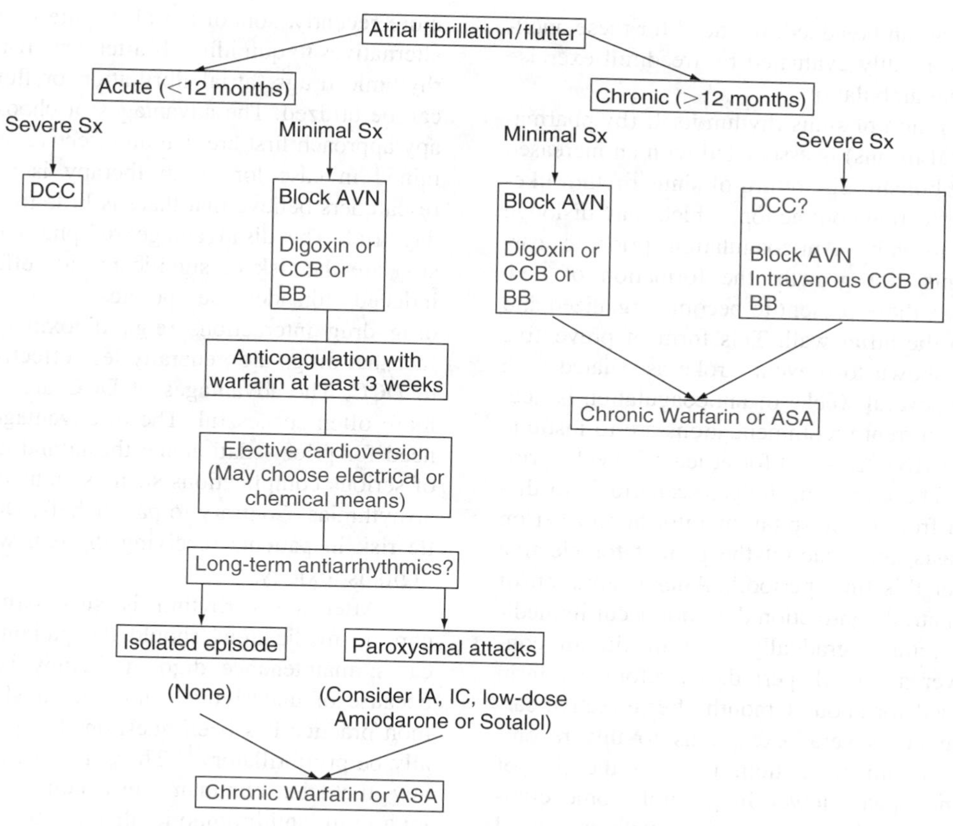

Figure 16.5. Algorithm for the treatment of atrial fibrillation and atrial flutter. Sx, symptoms; AVN, AV node; DCC, direct-current cardioversion; CCB, calcium channel antagonist (verapamil or diltiazem); BB, beta blocker; ASA, aspirin. *(From Bauman JL et al. Tachycardias, in Carter B, Angaran D, Lake K, Raebel M [eds]: Pharmacotherapy Self-Assessment Program, 2nd ed. Kansas City, MO, ACCP, 1995, with permission.)*

with no or mild symptoms) and often they present somewhere in between. Consequently, clinical judgment is necessary in choosing the proper treatment strategy. For example, intravenous calcium antagonists (diltiazem or verapamil) provide an alternative approach, allowing for a rapid decrease in ventricular rate and symptomatic relief without the need for DCC.[19,20] Because control of ventricular response can be transient, verapamil and diltiazem can be given as an initial intravenous bolus followed by a continuous infusion titrated to heart rate. Although digoxin previously has been the drug of first choice to slow ventricular rate, many clinicians now choose calcium antagonists in most patients with atrial fibrillation or flutter. Further, atrial fibrillation or flutter precipitated by states of high adrenergic tone, such as thyrotoxicosis, is often resistant to digoxin therapy (digoxin slows AV nodal conduction primarily through vagotonic mechanisms). In these cases, intravenous β blockers (propranolol, esmolol) can be highly effective. Note, however, that at this time, there are no direct comparative studies between calcium antagonists, β blockers, and/or digoxin.[18]

Patients may present with a slow ventricular response (in the absence of AV nodal-blocking drugs) and thus do not require therapy with digoxin, verapamil, or propranolol. This type of presentation should alert the clinician to the possibility of preexisting SA or AV nodal conduction disease such as sick sinus syndrome. DCC should not be attempted in these patients without a temporary pacemaker in place (see section entitled "Atrioventricular Block").

After treatment with AV nodal blocking agents and a subsequent decrease in ventricular response, the patient should be evaluated for the possibility of restoring sinus rhythm. Within the context of this evaluation, several factors should be considered. First, maintenance of sinus rhythm for a significant length of time is usually not feasible in some patients [e.g., those with a history of chronic (more than 1 year), established atrial fibrillation or those with large atrial size (greater than 45 mm determined by echocardiography)]. Therefore, cardioversion may not even be attempted and these patients can remain in atrial fibrillation, chronically treated with AV nodal-blocking agents to control ventricular response. Often, long-term therapy with digoxin alone for this purpose will not control exercise-related increases in ventricular response and tachycardia symptoms. In these patients, small doses of calcium antagonists or β blockers can be added; the need for these ancillary agents can be readily evaluated by treadmill exercise testing or by simple ambulation.

Second, restoration of sinus rhythm itself (by pharmacologic or electrical means) is associated with an increased risk of thromboembolism. The return of sinus rhythm likewise restores an effective contraction, which may dislodge poorly adherent thrombi. Anticoagulation prior to cardioversion prevents clot growth, the formation of new thrombi, and allows those present to become organized and to adhere well to the atrial wall. This form of preventive therapy has been shown to prevent stroke associated with cardioversion but several weeks of anticoagulation is necessary. Therefore, current recommendations are to institute warfarin treatment (INR 2.0–3.0) for at least 3 weeks prior to cardioversion. The common clinical scenario is to discharge the patient from the hospital, monitor him or her on an ambulatory basis, and readmit the patient for elective cardioversion after this time period.[15] After restoration of sinus rhythm, full atrial contraction does not occur immediately. Rather, it returns gradually to a maximum contractible force over a 3-week period. Therefore, warfarin should be continued for about 1 month after effective cardioversion. There are several exceptions to this recommended process of anticoagulation. Because the risk of thromboembolism appears lower in general, some clinicians do not routinely anticoagulate patients with only atrial flutter [unless concurrent risks for thrombosis are present (e.g., severe left ventricular dysfunction or mitral valve disease)] or lone atrial fibrillation. Also, in patients with atrial fibrillation of less than 48 hours' duration, anticoagulation prior to cardioversion is probably not necessary because there has not been sufficient time to form atrial thrombi. However, in most presentations of atrial fibrillation, the exact time of onset is unclear. Transesophageal echocardiography (TEE) is being investigated as a tool to stratify which patients may require anticoagulation prior to DCC from those who may not. If an atrial thrombus or severe stasis is not noted on TEE, then perhaps these patients can be cardioverted without the mandatory 3 weeks of warfarin pretreatment. However, conclusive data have not been published, and some researchers believe that DCC itself promotes thrombogenesis, necessitating anticoagulation regardless.

After prior anticoagulation, the methods available to restore sinus rhythm can be considered. There are two methods of restoring sinus rhythm in patients with atrial fibrillation or flutter—pharmacologic cardioversion and DCC. Choosing the method to use is a matter of clinical preference. With pharmacologic cardioversion, antiarrhythmic drugs such as quinidine, procainamide, flecainide, propafenone, or sotalol can be used. The time-honored method is to begin oral quinidine therapy; maintenance dosages are sufficient and oral loading schedules are unnecessary. Intravenous procainamide, oral flecainide, and, more recently, sotalol are also quite effective and suitable alternatives to quinidine. If after a short-term trial of antiarrhythmic drugs, atrial fibrillation or flutter persists, DCC can be utilized. The advantages of choosing the drug therapy approach first are that an effective agent may be determined in case long-term therapy is required and many researchers believe that there is little to lose with a 2- to 3-day trial. The disadvantages of pharmacologic cardioversion are the risk of significant side effects such as drug-induced torsades de pointes,[21] the inconvenience of drug–drug interactions (e.g., digoxin–quinidine), and the fact that drugs are generally less effective when compared to DCC. The advantages of DCC are that it is quick and more often successful. The disadvantages of DCC are the need for prior sedation/anesthesia and a risk (albeit small) of serious complications such as sinus arrest or ventricular arrhythmias. Contrary to past beliefs, DCC carries very little risk in patients receiving digoxin without evidence of digitalis toxicity.[22]

After sinus rhythm is successfully restored, what chronic medications should the patient receive? In many cases, maintenance digoxin therapy is continued simply because of underlying ventricular dysfunction. This common practice has been questioned; digoxin may occasionally be profibrillatory.[17] There are two other forms of therapy that the clinician must consider in each patient: long-term antithrombotic therapy to prevent stroke and long-term antiarrhythmic drugs to prevent recurrences of atrial fibrillation. Consider the issue of antithrombotic therapy first. In the past, patients with atrial fibrillation were not routinely anticoagulated (unless there was a history of stroke or concurrent mitral valve disease) because it was believed that the risk of warfarin exceeded its potential (although unknown) benefit. In the past several years, five major trials designed to evaluate this issue have been published. All possess very similar findings and all were terminated prematurely because of a significant effect in the treatment group (warfarin). Perhaps the best known of these trials was the Stroke Prevention in Atrial Fibrillation (SPAF) study.[23] This study, similar to the other four studies, found warfarin to reduce significantly the incidence of stroke in patients with atrial fibrillation (not associated with prior thromboembolic episodes or mitral valve disease) with an acceptable risk of bleeding complications. In all, these studies culminated in the American College of Chest Physicians Consensus Conference[15] on antithrombotic therapy to strongly recommend that all patients with atrial fibrillation receive chronic warfarin treatment (INR 2.0–3.0). Exceptions may include young (<60 years of age) patients with "lone" atrial fibrillation, those with only atrial flutter, and unreliable/poorly compliant patients. In lieu of warfarin, these patients may receive daily aspirin. Indeed, the use of aspirin (versus warfarin) is one of the remaining controversies. The original SPAF study (SPAF I) found aspirin (325 mg/d) to be effective in preventing stroke but could not directly compare it to warfarin because of sample size and study design. The debate of aspirin use for this indication was complicated by the second SPAF trial (SPAF II).[24] In this study, warfarin tended to be more effective than aspirin (although not statistically different) but it was also associated with a higher risk of intracranial hemorrhage, particularly in elderly patients. This study also identified major risk factors for stroke in atrial fibrillation—the presence of hypertension, recent heart failure, and prior thromboembolism. Young patients (<75 years) had an extremely low incidence of stroke if these risk factors were absent. Because of the findings of SPAF II, it appears that strong consideration should be given to the use of aspirin (325 mg/d) instead of warfarin in patients with atrial fibrillation not associated with the identified risk factors. Nevertheless, studies are ongoing to clarify the aspirin versus warfarin debate. In the meantime, all patients with atrial fibrillation should receive a form of antithrombotic therapy; the majority of published evidence for efficacy is in regards to warfarin.

The second form of chronic therapy to be considered is antiarrhythmic drugs to prevent recurrences of AF. With some exceptions (thyrotoxicosis, postoperative situations) atrial fibrillation usually recurs after initial cardioversion because most patients have irreversible, underlying heart disease. Historically, many clinicians would prescribe oral antiarrhythmic drugs (usually quinidine) to prevent these recurrences despite the fact that only small studies with conflicting results existed that evaluated this approach. To evaluate the efficacy of quinidine in preventing atrial fibrillation, a meta-analysis of the existing literature was completed.[25] This meta-analysis demonstrated that indeed more patients remain in sinus rhythm with quinidine therapy (compared to placebo), although approximately 50% have recurrences of atrial fibrillation within a year despite quinidine. However, this reported effectiveness was at the cost of an associated increase in mortality (presumably due, in part, to proarrhythmia) in the quinidine-treated patients. These disturbing results became widely quoted and highly visible, making clinicians question the wisdom of long-term prevention of recurrences of atrial fibrillation with antiarrhythmic drugs. Although the results were questioned because some of the reported causes of death in the treated patients could not be directly attributed to quinidine, a subanalysis of the SPAF study[26] tended to support the findings of the meta-analysis.

It is possible that the newer antiarrhythmic agents such as the type Ic and the type III agents may provide alternatives to quinidine. Flecainide and propafenone tend to be better tolerated than the type Ia agents and have been shown to be highly effective in the termination and prevention of atrial fibrillation.[27,28] However, the major fear with the type Ic agents is the risk of ventricular proarrhythmia. The CAST[29] and other studies[30] demonstrate that patients being treated for ventricular arrhythmias with coexisting ischemic heart disease and poor left ventricular function are at increased risk of proarrhythmia. Patients with atrial fibrillation often possess these risks. Also, there is evidence to indicate that other patient types (i.e., those with supraventricular arrhythmias and preserved left ventricular function) may be at risk as well.[31] Recent data regarding antiarrhythmic drug prescribing trends[32] show a large increase in the use of the type III agents (sotalol and amiodarone). Initial studies[33] indicate that low doses of amiodarone (100–200 mg/d) are highly effective in preventing the recurrence of atrial fibrillation, perhaps at a lower risk of serious toxicity than that associated with higher doses (400 mg/d). Another alternative, sotalol, has been shown to be at least as effective as quinidine in preventing recurrences of atrial fibrillation.[34] However, treatment with either quinidine or sotalol is associated with a similar incidence of torsades de pointes. Since this form of proarrhythmia primarily occurs with higher doses of sotalol (compared to the non-dose-related torsades de pointes due to quinidine), it may be more easily predicted and therefore avoided. One advantage to the use of amiodarone or sotalol as an alternative to long-term quinidine is that recurrences of atrial fibrillation during therapy will result in a relatively slow ventricular response because of the β-blocking activity of these drugs.

At this time and in view of newer studies implying increased mortality due to the time-honored approach of prescribing long-term quinidine, we suggest the following approach: Reserve chronic antiarrhythmic drugs for only those patients with documented symptomatic recurrences or symptomatic paroxysmal atrial fibrillation. Those with an isolated episode should not receive chronic preventive therapy. In terms of drug choice, most clinicians will resort more frequently and earlier to the use of low-dose amiodarone and sotalol. Whereas in the past these agents were reserved for drug-refractory patients, their use as first-line agents will be more frequent. The reader should also note that current studies are under way to compare the use of long-term antiarrhythmic drugs to prevent atrial fibrillation/flutter and the use of drugs that simply control ventricular rate (e.g., digoxin and/or calcium antagonists) with mortality as the primary endpoint. These studies should more clearly define the long-term approach to these arrhythmias. It is possible that, in the future, most patients can be managed by strategies to control rate (drugs, ablation) without chronic antiarrhythmic drug therapy.

PAROXYSMAL SUPRAVENTRICULAR TACHYCARDIA DUE TO REENTRY

Paroxysmal supraventricular tachycardia (PSVT) arising by reentrant mechanisms includes those arrhythmias caused by AV nodal reentry, AV reentry incorporating an anomalous AV pathway, SA nodal reentry, and intra-atrial reentry. AV nodal reentry and AV reentry are by far the most common of these tachycardias.

The underlying substrate of AV nodal reentry is the functional division of the AV node into two (or more) longitudinal conduction pathways or "dual" AV nodal pathways.[35] Although there is some disagreement, most electrophysiologists now believe that there are not two distinct, anatomic pathways inside the AV node itself. Rather, it is likely that a fanlike network of perinodal fibers inserts into the AV node and represents the second pathway. The two pathways possess key differences in conduction characteristics: One is a fast conducting pathway with a relatively long refractory period (β or fast pathway) and the other is a slower conducting pathway with a shorter refractory period (α or slow pathway). The presence of dual pathways does not necessarily imply that the patient will have clinical PSVT. In fact, it is estimated that between 10 and 46% of patients have discernable dual pathways but the incidence of PSVT is considerably lower.[35] Sustenance of the tachycardia depends on the critical electrophysiologic discrepancies and the ability of one pathway (usually the slow one) to allow repetitive antegrade conduction and the ability of the other pathway (usually the fast one) to allow repetitive retrograde conduction. During sinus rhythm, a patient with dual pathways conducts supraventricular impulses antegradely through both pathways. Electrical activity reaches the distal common pathway at the level of or above the bundle of His and continues to depolarize the ventricles in an antegrade direction. Conduction proceeds via the two pathways but reaches the distal common pathway first through the fast AV nodal route (Fig. 16.6). For this reason, a short PR interval is sometimes observed during sinus rhythm.

PSVT due to AV nodal reentry may occur by the following sequence of events. The occurrence of an appropriately timed premature impulse penetrates the AV node, but is blocked in the fast pathway, which is still refractory from the previous beat. However, the slow pathway, which has a shorter refractory period, permits antegrade conduction of the premature impulse. By the time the impulse has reached the distal common pathway, the fast pathway has recovered its excitability and now will permit retrograde conduction. The impulse reaches the common proximal pathway, preceded by an excitable gap of tissue, and reenters the slow pathway. A reentrant circuit that does not require atrial or ventricular tissue is completed within (or nearly so) the AV node and a tachycardia is thereby initiated (Fig. 16.6). The common form of this tachycardia uses the slow pathway for antegrade conduction and the fast pathway for retrograde conduction. Lown–Ganong–Levine syndrome (LGL) is defined by paroxysms of a narrow QRS tachycardia associated with a short PR interval on surface electrocardiograms (during sinus rhythm) and is commonly due to AV nodal reentry.[36]

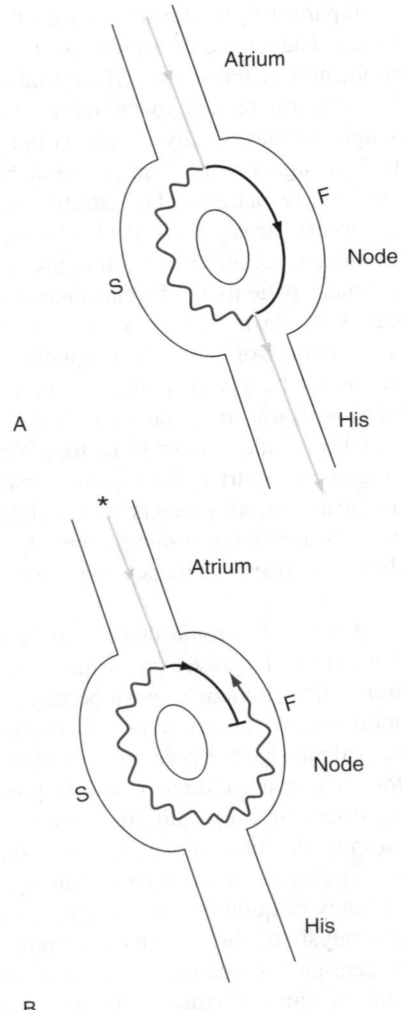

Figure 16.6. Reentry mechanism of dual-AV-nodal-pathway PSVT. (A) Sinus rhythm: The impulse travels from the atrium through the fast pathway (F) and then to the His–Purkinje system. The impulse also travels through the slow pathway (S) but is stopped when refractory tissue is encountered. (B) Dual-AV-nodal reentry: A critically timed premature impulse (*) is stopped in the fast pathway (because of prolonged refractoriness) but is able to travel antegrade down the slow pathway and retrograde through the fast pathway. *(From Bauman JL. Understanding and treating supraventricular arrhythmias. Clin Pharm 1983;2:314, with permission.)*

AV reentrant tachycardia depends on the presence of an anomalous, or accessory, extranodal pathway that bypasses the normal AV conduction pathway. Several different types of accessory pathways have been described, depending on the specific anatomic areas they connect (e.g., atrioventricular bundles or nodoventricular tracts); some are also referred to as eponyms, such as the Kent bundle. A Kent bundle is an extranodal AV connection that is associated with the Wolff–Parkinson–White syndrome (WPW).[37] During sinus rhythm (Fig. 16.7) patients with WPW depo-

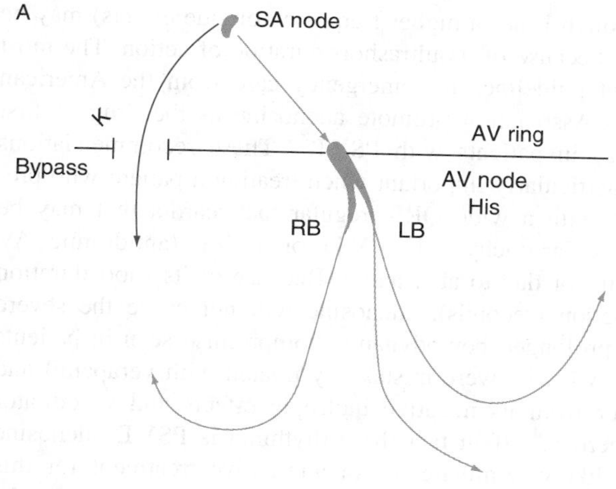

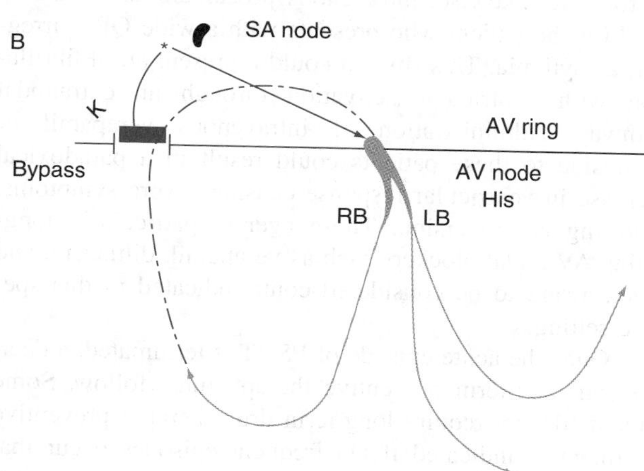

Figure 16.7. Reentry mechanism for AV-accessory-pathway PSVT in WPW syndrome. (A) Sinus rhythm: The impulse travels from the atrium to the ventricle by two pathways—the AV node and an accessory bypass tract (K, Kent bundle). (B) AV reentry: A critically timed premature impulse (*) is stopped in the Kent bundle (because of prolonged refractoriness) but travels antegrade through the AV node and retrograde through the Kent bundle. *(From Bauman JL. Understanding and treating supraventricular arrhythmias. Clin Pharm 1983;2:314, with permission.)*

larize the ventricles simultaneously through both AV pathways (AV nodal pathway and the Kent bundle), creating a fusion pattern on the early portion of the QRS complex (delta wave). The degree of ventricular "preexcitation" depends on the contribution of antegrade ventricular activation through the accessory pathway. Patients may have an accessory pathway that is not evident on surface electrocardiograms or a "concealed" Kent bundle. These concealed accessory pathways are often incapable of antegrade conduction and can only accept electrical stimulation in a retrograde fashion. The electrocardiographic expression of preexcitation (delta wave) depends on the location of the accessory pathway, the distance from the wavefront of sinus activation, and the conduction characteristics of the various structures involved. It should be noted that (similar to patients with dual AV nodal pathways) not all patients with preexcitation due to an accessory AV pathway are capable of having clinical PSVT.

Patients with an accessory AV pathway may have three forms of supraventricular tachycardia: orthodromic reentry, antidromic reentry, and/or atrial fibrillation or flutter. AV reentrant PSVT usually occurs by the following sequence of events. Analogous to AV nodal reentry, two pathways (the normal AV nodal pathway and the accessory AV pathway) exist that have different electrophysiologic characteristics. The AV nodal pathway usually has a relatively slower conduction velocity and shorter refractory period, and the accessory pathway has a faster conduction velocity and a longer refractory period. A critically timed premature impulse may block the accessory pathway because it is still refractory from the previous sinus beat. However, the AV nodal pathway with a relatively shorter refractory period may accept antegrade conduction of the premature impulse. Meanwhile, the accessory pathway may recover its excitability and now allow retrograde conduction. A macroreentrant tachycardia is thereby initiated in which the antegrade pathway is the AV nodal pathway; the distal common pathway is the ventricle; the retrograde pathway is the accessory pathway; and the proximal common pathway is the atrium (Fig. 16.7). This sequence of events (down node, up Kent), termed orthodromic PSVT, is the common variety of reentry in patients with an accessory AV pathway, resulting in a narrow QRS tachycardia. In the uncommon variety (down Kent, up node), conduction proceeds in the opposite direction, resulting in a wide QRS tachycardia, termed antidromic PSVT. Patients with WPW can have a third type of tachycardia, namely, atrial fibrillation. The mechanism for its occurrence is unknown, but the occurrence of this arrhythmia can be very serious and sudden death is well described. Because atrial fibrillation is an extremely rapid atrial tachycardia, conduction can proceed down the accessory AV pathway resulting in a very fast ventricular response or even ventricular fibrillation.[38] Unlike the AV nodal pathway, the refractory period of the accessory bundle shortens in response to rapid stimulation rates.

Sinus node reentry and intra-atrial reentry occur less commonly and are not as well described as AV nodal or AV reentry.[39] Aside from a characteristic abrupt onset and termination coupled with subtle changes in P-wave morphology, these tachycardias can be difficult to diagnose. Electrophysiologic studies may be necessary to determine the ultimate mechanism of the PSVT.

Both pharmacologic and nonpharmacologic methods have been used to treat patients with PSVT. Drugs used in the treatment of PSVT can be divided into three broad categories: (1) those that directly or indirectly increase vagal tone to the AV node such as edrophonium, vasopressors, and digoxin; (2) those that depress conduction through slow, calcium-dependent tissue such adenosine, β blockers, and calcium channel blockers; and (3) those that depress conduction through fast, sodium-dependent tissue such as quinidine, procainamide, disopyramide, and flecainide. Drugs within these categories alter the electrophysiologic characteristics of the reentrant substrate so that PSVT cannot be sustained.[40,41] In PSVT due to AV nodal reentry, type I antiarrhythmic drugs such as procainamide act primarily on the retrograde fast pathway. Digoxin and propranolol may work on either the retrograde fast or the antegrade slow limb. Verapamil, diltiazem, and adenosine prolong conduction time and increase refractoriness primarily in the slow antegrade pathway of the reentrant loop. In PSVT due to AV reentry incorporating an extranodal pathway, type I drugs increase refractoriness in the fast accessory pathway or within the His–Purkinje system. Propranolol, digoxin, adenosine, and verapamil all act by their effects on the AV nodal (antegrade, slow) portion of the reentrant circuit. Regardless of the mechanism, treatment measures are directed at first terminating an acute episode of PSVT and then (if necessary) preventing symptomatic recurrences of PSVT.

As in any rapid reentrant tachycardia resulting in severe symptoms (syncope, near syncope, anginal chest pain, severe heart failure), synchronized DCC is the treatment of choice. Even at low energy levels (such as 25 W/s), DCC for PSVT is almost always effective in quickly restoring sinus rhythm and correcting severe hemodynamic compromise. Patients with only mild to moderate symptoms usually do not require DCC and nondrug measures that increase vagal tone to the AV node can be utilized first. Carotid sinus massage, valsalva maneuver, ice-water facial immersion, induced retching, and other more elaborate vagomimetic measures are often successful in terminating PSVT, although carotid massage and valsalva maneuver are the simplest, least obtrusive, and most frequently used of these techniques.

In the event that these methods fail, drug therapy is the next option. A therapeutic approach to the acute therapy of the different forms of reentrant PSVT is presented in Fig. 16.8. This approach is based on analysis of the electrocardiographic characteristics of the rhythm because PSVT is not always discernible from other arrhythmias, and some forms of PSVT require different treatment. In patients with a narrow QRS, regular arrhythmia (AV nodal reentry or orthodromic AV reentry), intravenous verapamil (5–10 mg) or adenosine (6–12 mg) is equally efficacious; either may be chosen as agents of first choice. About 80–90% of PSVT episodes will revert to sinus rhythm within 5 minutes of intravenous verapamil or adenosine therapy.[42] Verapamil has the advantage in terms of cost, being available in generic formulations; whereas adenosine (although it has a higher frequency of side effects) may be safer because of its ultrashort duration of action. The most recent guidelines for emergency care from the American Heart Association promote adenosine as the drug of first choice in patients with PSVT.[43] These recommendations are particularly important when treating a patient who presents with a wide QRS, regular tachycardia that may be ventricular tachycardia (VT) or PSVT (antidromic AV reentry or due to aberrancy). Because of its short duration of action (seconds), adenosine will not cause the severe and prolonged hemodynamic compromise seen in patients with VT who were mistakenly treated with verapamil and suffer from its negative inotropic effects and vasodilator properties.[44] If in fact the arrhythmia is PSVT, adenosine will likely terminate it. An alternative treatment for this type of patient is intravenous procainamide, which works on the fast, sodium-dependent extranodal pathway as well as for VT. Likewise, intravenous procainamide should be used for the patient who presents with a wide QRS, irregular arrhythmia. This rhythm could represent atrial fibrillation with ventricular activation through an extranodal pathway. Administration of intravenous verapamil or adenosine to these patients could result in a paradoxical increase in ventricular response causing severe symptoms, requiring cardioversion. These agents (particularly long-acting AV nodal blockers such as verapamil, diltiazem, and digoxin) are to be considered contraindicated in this specific setting.

Once the acute episode of PSVT is terminated, a decision on long-term preventive therapy must follow. Some patients do not require long-term drug therapy; preventive treatment is indicated if (1) frequent episodes occur that necessitate therapeutic intervention (i.e., emergency room visits or interference with the patient's lifestyle), or (2) infrequent but severely symptomatic symptoms occur. Also, effective vagal maneuvers can sometimes be taught to the patient, obviating the need for chronic drug therapy. For those patients in whom a preventive drug therapy regimen is deemed necessary, three traditional treatment strategies are available. First, clinicians may use a trial and error approach on an ambulatory basis for those patients with frequently recurrent, mildly symptomatic PSVT. Ambulatory electrocardiographic recordings (Holter) or telephonic transmissions of cardiac rhythm (event monitors) can be used to document objectively the efficacy or failure of drug therapy. How should one choose empiric drug regimens? A combination of digoxin and propranolol or verapamil is often effective so that the clinician can try one of these agents first, and then add the other drug if monotherapy fails. Maintenance digoxin therapy should be used with caution in patients with manifest preexcitation (i.e., delta wave on ECG during sinus rhythm). If atrial fibrillation occurs in such a patient, one consequence is ventricular fibrillation by rapid AV conduction through the accessory bundle. Digoxin is safest in patients with concealed Kent

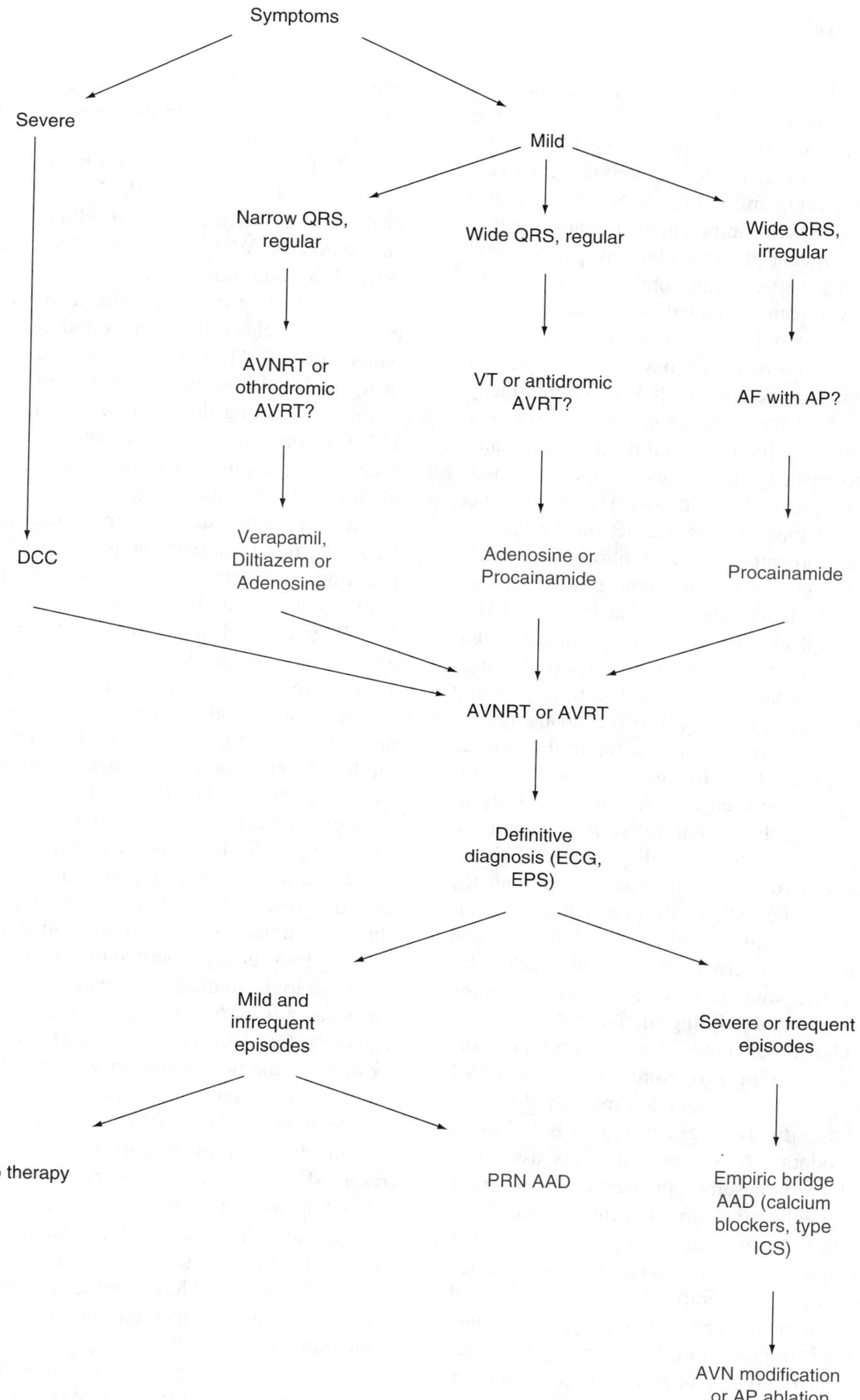

Figure 16.8. Algorithm for the treatment of acute (top portion) PSVT and chronic prevention of recurrences (bottom portion). DCC, direct current cardioversion; AVNT, AV nodal reentrant tachycardia; VT, ventricular tachycardia; AF, atrial fibrillation; AP, accessory pathway; ECG, electrocardiographic monitoring; EPS, electrophysiologic studies; PRN, as needed; AAD, antiarrhythmic drugs. Note that for empiric bridge therapy prior to radiofrequency ablation procedures, calcium antagonists (or other AV nodal blockers) should not be used if the patient has AV reentry with preexcitation. *(From Bauman JL et al. Tachycardias, in Carter B,Angaran D, Lake K, Raebel M [eds] : Pharmacotherapy Self-Assessment Program, 2nd ed. Kansas City, MO, ACCP, 1995, with permission.)*

pathways or AVN reentry. One may assume that the agent that was successful in terminating the acute episode of PSVT will also provide effective preventive therapy, but actually there is little evidence to support this approach. Indeed, chronic oral verapamil is often ineffective in those patients who responded to intravenous therapy. This is probably due to significant pharmacodynamic and pharmacokinetic differences between the oral and intravenous dosage forms of verapamil coupled with stereoselective first-pass metabolism with the oral racemate.[45]

Bauernfeind and coworkers[46] have studied the patterns of drug response in patients with AV reentrant tachycardia, which may help the clinician choose empiric therapy. These investigators found a significant concordance of responses between drugs that work on the slow antegrade limb (e.g., propranolol and digoxin), a concordance of drug responses for those agents that act on the fast retrograde limb (e.g., procainamide and quinidine), and a discordance of response between these two groups of drugs. In other words, if quinidine is effective, it is likely that procainamide will also be effective but unlikely that propranolol or digoxin will be effective. These findings imply that there is a "weak link" in the reentrant pathway that is susceptible to drug therapy. The second method to find effective long-term therapy is to use the trial-and-error method during hospitalization. In this case, Holter monitoring or telemetry can be used to assess drug efficacy or failure objectively. Initially, all antiarrhythmics should be discontinued and attacks detected and quantified. Following this drug-free control period in which the frequency and characteristics of the tachycardia are defined, antiarrhythmic agents are administered in a serial fashion and evaluated for efficacy. It is crucial to determine drug efficacy (abolition of symptomatic PSVT) with consideration to the tachycardia frequency during the control period.

The trial-and-error methods for determining drug effectiveness have inherent shortcomings. If the PSVT episodes are infrequent, a considerable time period may be consumed before an effective regimen is realized. Also, if the patient has moderate to severe symptoms associated with PSVT, several troublesome episodes may be experienced by the patient before the correct agent(s) is identified. Serial testing of antiarrhythmic agents by invasive electrophysiologic techniques can be a valuable method in determining effective long-term therapy in those patients with sporadic and/or symptomatic PSVT. Basically, the patient's clinical tachycardia is replicated in the laboratory by inserting appropriately timed, premature extra stimuli via a transvenous right heart catheter. The patient is first studied off of antiarrhythmic therapy; induction of the tachycardia by premature stimuli by programmed stimulation serves as a control study. Then, over a period of several days specific drugs are administered in a serial fashion and tested for efficacy in preventing the induction of PSVT.[40,41] Inability to induce PSVT or induction of only brief, self-terminating episodes usually predicts that drug regimen will be effective long-term therapy.

Electrophysiologic drug testing has several advantages over the trial-and-error methods. First, the actual mechanism of the tachycardia (e.g., PSVT versus ventricular tachycardia or AV reentry versus AV nodal reentry) can be defined. Second, this technique is time efficient and probably cost effective in that an efficacious agent can be determined in a relatively short period of time. Third, if the patient has PSVT associated with severe symptoms, the tachycardia will be induced in a well-equipped laboratory setting, preventing the potentially serious consequences of PSVT recurrence at home or in a car. Fourth, a patient-specific drug regimen and therapeutic concentration can be identified. Fifth, patients with drug refractory PSVT can be readily identified and appropriate measures can be taken. However, this is an invasive procedure and, although complications are uncommon, candidates for programmed stimulation must be carefully chosen.

Regardless of the method for choosing long-term therapy, chronic antiarrhythmic drug treatment in these often young, otherwise healthy patients is problematic. Besides the necessity of taking daily medication possibly for life, antiarrhythmic drugs are not well tolerated, sometimes precipitate severe side effects, and are commonly ineffective. For these reasons, nondrug therapies have been pioneered. One such procedure, namely, transcutaneous catheter ablation using radio-frequency (rf) current of the PSVT substrate, has dramatically altered traditional treatment of these patients (Fig. 16.9). Radio-frequency energy delivered through a transvenous or arterial catheter causes small, discrete lesions through thermal energy. During invasive electrophysiologic studies, portions of the reentrant circuit can be located (or "mapped") by the use of a number of catheters. Once this is completed, rf energy is applied to kill or damage the tissue necessary for reentry. In this way the substrate for reentry is destroyed, "curing" the patient of recurrent episodes of PSVT and obviating the need for chronic drug therapy. Historically, ablation procedures were reserved for drug-refractory patients because they necessitated open-heart surgery. However, breakthroughs in technology have allowed, first, transvenous catheter approaches and then later the use of rf (rather than direct current) energy. These procedures can be lengthy depending on the experience of the operator and may involve significant radiation exposure (fluoroscopy) to both the patient and the physician. Complications, although unusual, include tamponade, pericarditis, valvular insufficiency, and AV block. However, rf ablation is highly effective, preventing the recurrence of PSVT in 85–98% of patients.[47,48] The procedure was originally pioneered in patients with WPW syndrome.[47] Here, the extranodal pathway is often located at the left lateral free wall of the left ventricle

(Fig. 16.9). After the pathway is located, the catheter is put as close to the site as possible and rf current applied to make small burns in the tissue. Ablation of the extranodal connection occurs promptly and evidence of preexcitation (delta waves) disappears. Later, a similar approach was developed for patients with AV nodal reentry.[48] The preferred method in these individuals is to apply small amounts of rf current to the slow pathway of the reentrant circuit in order to modify its properties enough so that PSVT cannot recur.

Although rf catheter ablation is a relatively new technique, and long-term follow-up of potential late complications remains necessary, it has been suggested that *all* patients with symptomatic PSVT undergo the procedure.[49] This is because it is highly effective and curative, rarely results in complications, and obviates the need for chronic antiarrhythmic drug therapy. In other words, no longer should rf ablation be reserved only for drug-refractory patients; it should be considered in any patient who would previously be considered for chronic antiarrhythmic drug treatment (effective or ineffective).

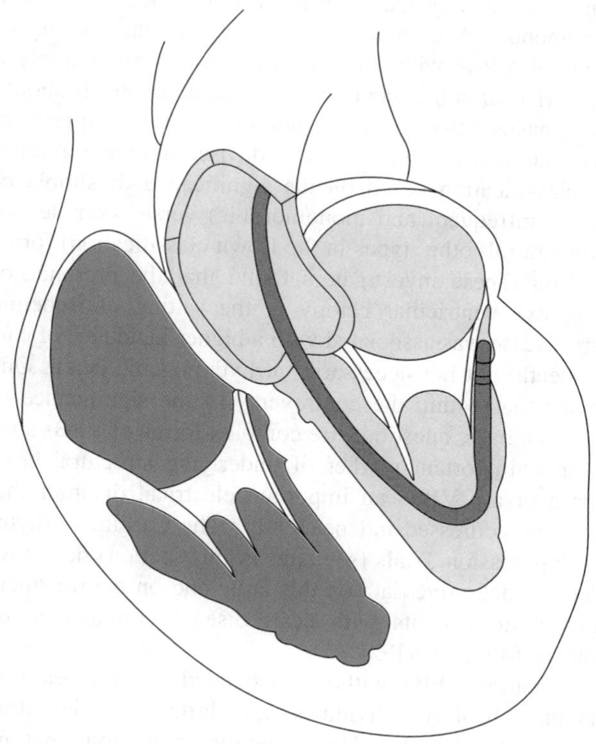

Figure 16.9. Drawing showing catheter placement for radiofrequency ablation of left free wall accessory pathway. Here, the retrograde arterial approach is taken although a venous (atrial) trans-septal puncture has also been used. *(From Scheinman MM. Catheter ablation. Present role and projected impact on health care for patients with cardiac arrhythmias. Circulation 1991;83:1489–1498, with permission.)*

AUTOMATIC ATRIAL TACHYCARDIAS

Automatic atrial tachycardias such as multifocal atrial tachycardia appear to arise from supraventricular foci, which have enhanced automatic properties.[50,51] It is presumed that multifocal atrial tachycardia (sometimes referred to as chaotic atrial tachycardia) is the result of multiple ectopic atrial pacemakers, which account for the variable and differing P-wave morphology. In unifocal atrial tachycardia (sometimes referred to as ectopic atrial tachycardia) a single P-wave morphology different from that of sinus rhythm is recorded. In either case, the underlying, precipitating disorder present in the majority (60–80%) of these patients is severe pulmonary disease. Other disease states associated with these arrhythmias include acute infection (pneumonia and sepsis) and dilated congestive cardiomyopathy. Note that young patients without associated precipitating factors may rarely present with rapid atrial tachycardias from unknown etiologies. In these cases, long-standing tachycardias *cause* a cardiomyopathic state. Effective treatment of the tachycardia may result in reversal of left ventricular dysfunction. Traditionally, many factors (i.e., electrolyte disturbances, hypoxia, catecholamines, tissue stretch) may cause an elevated slope of phase 4 depolarization and theoretically result in abnormal heightened automaticity. Many of these factors are often clinically present in patients with concurrent pulmonary disease and automatic atrial tachycardia. However, recent information implies that triggered activity is a more likely mechanism in the genesis of these tachycardias. Atrial tachycardias with AV block or a slow ventricular response should alert the clinician to the possibility of digitalis toxicity.

The first step in the treatment of automatic atrial tachycardia is to correct the underlying, precipitating factors.[51] One should ensure proper oxygenation and ventilation and correct acid–base or electrolyte disturbances. These measures alone may result in the return of sinus rhythm, but in some cases, the tachycardia will persist. Patients with an asymptomatic atrial tachycardia and a relatively slow ventricular response usually require no drug therapy. In symptomatic patients, medical therapy can be tailored to either control ventricular response or to restore sinus rhythm. Type I antiarrhythmic drugs such as procainamide or quinidine are occasionally effective in restoring sinus rhythm, presumably by their ability to decrease the automatic properties of latent pacemakers, but these agents are usually not considered first-line therapy. Direct-current cardioversion is usually ineffective in restoring sinus rhythm, and the use of programmed stimulation will not replicate the clinical tachycardia so that serial drug testing is of no value. Beta blockers, to slow ventricular response, are usually contraindicated because of the frequent coexistence of severe pulmonary disease or heart failure. Digoxin has been utilized but is controversial because of its ability to increase the automatic properties of atrial tissue, and the high sympathetic state of these patients frequently overrides the vagotonic effects of digoxin, rendering it ineffective. Calcium antagonists such as verapamil are most effective and may now be considered first-line drug therapy.[52] Surprisingly, verapamil seems to decrease ventricular response by altering atrial automaticity, not by slowing AV nodal conduction.[52] Recent information suggests that intravenous magnesium (independent of serum magnesium) can also be effective.[51] Both verapamil and parenteral magnesium probably act by suppressing calcium-mediated triggered activity.

Ventricular Arrhythmias

The common ventricular arrhythmias include (1) ventricular premature beats (VPBs), (2) ventricular tachycardia (VT), and (3) ventricular fibrillation (VF). Again, these arrhythmias may result in a wide variety of symptoms. VPBs often cause no symptoms or only mild palpitations. VT may be a life-threatening situation associated with hemodynamic collapse or be totally asymptomatic. VF, by definition, is an acute medical emergency necessitating cardiopulmonary resuscitation.

VENTRICULAR PREMATURE BEATS

VPBs are very common ventricular rhythm disturbances that occur in patients with or without heart disease. Experimental models have shown that premature ventricular depolarizations may be elicited by abnormal automaticity, triggered activity or by reentrant mechanisms. It has become well known that VPBs can be commonly observed in apparently healthy individuals. However, VPBs occurring in overtly normal subjects without discernable heart disease seem to have little if any prognostic significance. VPBs seem to occur more frequently and in more complex forms (see later in this section) in patients with detectable heart disease than in healthy individuals. The prognostic meaning of VPBs has been well studied in patients with myocardial infarction (acute or remote) with several consistent themes.[53] Less is known about the significance of VPBs occurring in association with forms of heart disease (other than ischemic heart disease) such as hypertension, mitral valve prolapse, or primary myocardial disease.

Some investigators have promoted the concept that patients in the acute phase of myocardial infarction may have types of VPBs that are predictive of VF and sudden cardiac death.[54] These types of VPBs were referred to as "warning arrhythmias" and include frequent ectopy (more than 5 per minute), multiform configuration (different morphology), couplets (two in a row), and R-on-T phenomenon (VPBs occurring during the repolarization phase of the preceding sinus beat in the vulnerable period of ventricular recovery). However, utilizing sophisticated monitoring techniques, it has become apparent that almost all patients have VPBs (often warning arrhythmias) in the acute infarct setting. Furthermore, in those patients who experience VF, warning arrhythmias are no more common than in those without VF. Therefore, warning arrhythmias observed during acute myocardial infarction are neither a sensitive nor specific predictive tool in determining which patients will have VF.

However, data strongly imply that VPBs documented in the convalescence period of myocardial infarction do carry long-term prognostic significance.[53] VPBs occurring after a myocardial infarction seem to be a risk factor for patient death that is independent of the degree of left ventricular dysfunction or the extent of coronary atherosclerosis. Lown and Wolf[55] have developed a grading scale for classifying different types of VPBs. The grading scale is as follows: grade 0, no ectopy; grade I, less than 30 VPBs/h of uniform morphology; grade II, more than 30 VPBs/h of uniform morphology; grade III, multiform VPBs; grade IVa, couplets; grade IVb, three or more consecutive VPBs (nonsustained ventricular tachycardia); grade V, R-on-T phenomenon. A common assumption is that the higher grades of VPBs within this classification system imply a higher risk of subsequent arrhythmogenic death. It should be emphasized that this assumption has never been proven. Ruberman and coworkers[53] have devised a simple alternative classification based on the significance of simple or benign (infrequent and monomorphic) versus complex or malignant (all other types in the Lown classification) forms of VPBs. These investigators found that the presence of "complex" ventricular ectopy in the setting of ischemic heart disease was associated with a higher incidence of cardiac death, but not necessarily arrhythmogenic death. One can see that within the controversy of the significance of VPBs is a basic question: Are complex forms of VPBs simply an unimportant marker of underlying structural heart disease or are VPBs an important electrical disorder that should be addressed independently? The Cardiac Arrhythmia Suppression Trials (see later in this section) have provided the definitive data on this issue and on the treatment approach to patients with heart disease complicated by complex forms of VPBs.

Because VPBs without associated heart disease in apparently healthy individuals carry little or no risk, drug therapy is unnecessary. Uncommonly, palpitations that are bothersome to the patient occur in association with the VPBs. The clinician should attempt to reassure the patient of the generally excellent prognosis and avoid antiarrhythmic drugs if possible. If drug therapy is necessary, β blockers are the drugs of choice because they are generally better tolerated than type I antiarrhythmic agents and, particularly in patients with prior myocardial infarction, beta blockers decrease mortality. The endpoint of drug therapy in this case should not necessarily be a quantitative reduction in VPB frequency but rather a symptomatic relief of bothersome palpitations. It is interesting to note that β blockers decrease the incidence of sudden death (presumable arrhythmogenic) after an infarct but do not necessarily alter VPB frequency. In patients with acute myocardial infarction, there is little need to direct drug therapy (usually lidocaine) specifically at VPB suppression. Studies have shown that effective prevention of VF in the acute infarct setting may be achieved without the abolition of VPBs. The inability of VPBs (warning arrhythmias) to predict the occurrence of VF coupled with the lack of correlation between a drug's effectiveness in preventing VF and suppressing VPBs form the basis of suggesting antiarrhythmic drug prophylaxis (e.g., lidocaine, magnesium) for all patients with an uncomplicated acute myocardial infarction.

A major area of controversy is the chronic antiarrhythmic drug treatment of VPBs in patients with associated heart disease (usually postmyocardial infarction). Traditionally, some suggested aggressive antiarrhythmic drug therapy designed to suppress a high percentage of VPBs, based on the Lown grading system. The underlying premise of this approach is to attempt to eliminate a risk factor for cardiac death in patients with coronary disease, namely, the presence of complex VPBs. However, others have favored a more conservative approach and disregarded drug therapy in the absence of significant symptoms. The release of the initial CAST results[29] clearly supports the later conservative approach but it is worthwhile to review the issues involved in this controversy.

First, the frequency of VPBs is sporadic and extremely variable, making it difficult to determine effective drug therapy. Winkle,[56] by evaluating continuous ECGs and VPB frequency, found a marked spontaneous variability that often mimicked drug efficacy or drug-induced aggravation of VPBs. Morganroth and coworkers[57] analyzed the variations in VPB frequency on 24-hour Holter recordings. These investigators estimated that in order to attribute a reduction in VPB frequency to drug effectiveness instead of spontaneous variability, a decrease in VPB frequency of greater than 83% was necessary. Despite this finding, many clinicians and published studies judged drug efficacy by a 50% reduction in VPB frequency or simply a statistically significant reduction in the number of VPBs by serial Holter monitors. These criteria obviously do not account for the spontaneous variability in VPB frequency. Other investigators[58] have noted an impressive discordance between the drug concentrations necessary for 83% reduction in VPBs frequency and those necessary to prevent VT or VF. In other words, a high degree of VPB suppression is not a necessary prerequisite for the successful prevention of VT or VF.

Second, all antiarrhythmic agents currently available have an impressive side-effect profile (Table 16.3). A considerable percentage of patients cannot tolerate long-term therapy with these drugs and chances are good that an agent will have to be discontinued because of side effects. In one trial,[59] more than 50% of patients had to discontinue long-term procainamide (mostly due to a lupuslike syndrome) after myocardial infarction. In another study,[60] disopyramide caused anticholinergic side effects in about 70% of patients. Flecainide and disopyramide may precipitate congestive heart failure in a significant number of patients with underlying left ventricular dysfunction.[61] The type Ib agents such as tocainide and mexiletine cause neurologic and/or gastrointestinal toxicity in a high percentage of patients. Tocainide, specifically, has been reported to cause both pulmonary fibrosis and leukopenia, the significance of which came to light after FDA approval. Long-term therapy with amiodarone frequently causes multisystem toxicity including occasional cases of hepatitis and pulmonary fibrosis.[12,62] Clearly the most frightening adverse effects related to antiarrhythmic drugs are the aggravation of underlying ventricular arrhythmias or the precipitation of new (and life-threatening) ventricular arrhythmias.[21,63]

Despite these issues, the prevailing assumption among many clinicians historically was to suppress asymptomatic ectopy in postinfarct patients with antiarrhythmic drug therapy in an effort to decrease the risk of sudden cardiac death. However, the results of the CAST indicate that although good intentioned, this approach is flawed: Ectopy was suppressed but the risk of death increased.

The CAST[29,64] was initiated by the National Institutes of Health (NIH) in 1987 to determine if suppression of ventricular ectopy with encainide, flecainide, or moricizine could decrease the incidence of death from arrhythmia in patients who had suffered a myocardial infarction. Entrance criteria included documented myocardial infarction between 6 days and 2 years prior to enrollment, and six or more VPBs per hour without runs of ventricular tachycardia greater than 15 beats in length. Also, patients were required to have an ejection fraction of ≤55% if recruited within 90 days of myocardial infarction or ≤40% if recruited 90 days or more after infarction. Patients with an ejection fraction <30% were randomized only to encainide or moricizine. Patients were randomized to receive drug therapy or placebo after demonstrating VPB suppression with one of the agents. The drug and dose were determined during an open-label dose titration phase that preceded randomization.

In April 1989, a routine, preliminary review of the study by the Safety and Monitoring Board revealed alarming results and the study was interrupted. The results show that compared to placebo, treatment with encainide or fle-

TABLE 16.3. SIDE EFFECTS OF ANTIARRHYTHMIC DRUGS

Quinidine	Cinchonism, diarrhea, GI,[a] hypotension, torsades de pointes, aggravation of underlying heart failure, conduction disturbances or ventricular arrhythmias, hepatitis, thrombocytopenia, hemolytic anemia
Procainamide	Systemic lupus erythematosus, GI, torsades de pointes, aggravation of underlying heart failure, conduction disturbances or ventricular arrhythmias, agranulocytosis
Disopyramide	Anticholinergic symptoms, GI, torsades de pointes, heart failure, aggravation of underlying conduction disturbances and/or ventricular arrhythmias, hypoglycemia, hepatic cholestasis
Lidocaine	CNS,[b] seizures, psychosis, sinus arrest, aggravation of underlying conduction disturbances
Mexiletine	CNS, psychosis, GI, aggravation of underlying conduction disturbances or ventricular arrhythmias
Tocainide	CNS, psychosis, GI, aggravation of underlying conduction disturbances or ventricular arrhythmias, rash/arthralgias, pulmonary infiltrates, agranulocytosis, thrombocytopenia
Moricizine	Dizziness, headache, GI, aggravation of underlying conduction disturbances or ventricular arrhythmias
Flecainide, propafenone	Blurred vision, dizziness, headache, GI, bronchospasm,[c] aggravation of underlying heart failure, conduction disturbances or ventricular arrhythmias
Amiodarone	CNS, corneal microdeposits/blurred vision, GI, aggravation of underlying ventricular arrhythmias, torsades de pointes, bradycardia or AV block, bruising without thrombocytopenia, pulmonary fibrosis, hepatitis, hypothyroidism, hyperthyroidism, photosensitivity, blue-gray skin discoloration, myopathy
Sotolol	Fatigue, GI, depression, torsades de pointes, bronchospasm, aggravation of underlying heart failure, conduction disturbances or ventricular arrhythmias
Bretylium	Hypotension, GI

[a]GI = nausea, anorexia.
[b]CNS = confusion, paresthesias, tremor, ataxia, etc.
[c]Propafenone only.

cainide was associated with a significantly higher rate of total mortality and death due to arrhythmia, presumably due to proarrhythmia (Fig. 16.10). Analysis of the moricizine arm indicated neither harm nor benefit from this therapy, therefore, only this portion of the study was allowed to continue as CAST II. However, later (July 1991), CAST II was also prematurely stopped; there was a trend toward an increase in mortality in moricizine-treated patients. This was particularly true during the initiation of moricizine therapy (dose titration phase) but was not observed during the chronic treatment phase. The overall results of the two CASTs conclusively prove that patients with VPBs post myocardial infarction do not benefit from chronic antiarrhythmic drug therapy (beyond the general use of β-blocking agents) and, in fact, this type of therapy is detrimental. The study also puts into perspective the risk associated with the use of antiarrhythmic therapy and the need to select carefully only those patients with a defined therapeutic benefit.

The CAST is already considered one of the most important trials ever undertaken by the NIH and has had a tremendous influence on the overall approach to the treatment of tachycardias in addition to a far-reaching impact on new drug development. The results have colored the long-term use of all antiarrhythmics, causing broad skepticism regarding the risk–benefit of this class of drugs. Pharmaceutical companies, as a result, have shifted their drug discovery and investigative efforts away from potent sodium channel blockers. As immediate fallout, encainide was pulled from the market by the pharmaceutical company, and another pharmaceutical manufacturer decided not to market the type Ic agent, indecainide, despite Federal Drug Administration (FDA) approval. These findings also provided additional fuel for the pursuit of nondrug therapies for tachycardias such as ablation and implantable devices.

Despite the discouraging results of the CAST, post myocardial infarction patients with complex ventricular ectopy remain at risk for death, and other forms of therapy (besides β blockers) designed to decrease this risk require investigation. Of the currently available antiarrhythmic drugs, low-dose amiodarone may hold the greatest promise. Although preliminary trials imply that amiodarone may decrease mortality in these patients,[65] this practice cannot be universally recommended until the results of larger, multicenter randomized studies are available.

VENTRICULAR TACHYCARDIA

Ventricular tachycardia (VT) is a wide QRS tachycardia that may acutely occur as a result of metabolic abnormalities, ischemia, or drug toxicity; or it may chronically recur as a paroxysmal form. On electrocardiographic inspection, VT may appear as either repetitive monomorphic or polymorphic ventricular complexes. The strict definition of VT is three or more repetitive VPBs occurring at a rate greater than 100 beats/min. An acute episode of VT may be precipitated by severe electrolyte abnormalities (hypokalemia), hypoxemia, or digitalis toxicity, or (most commonly) may

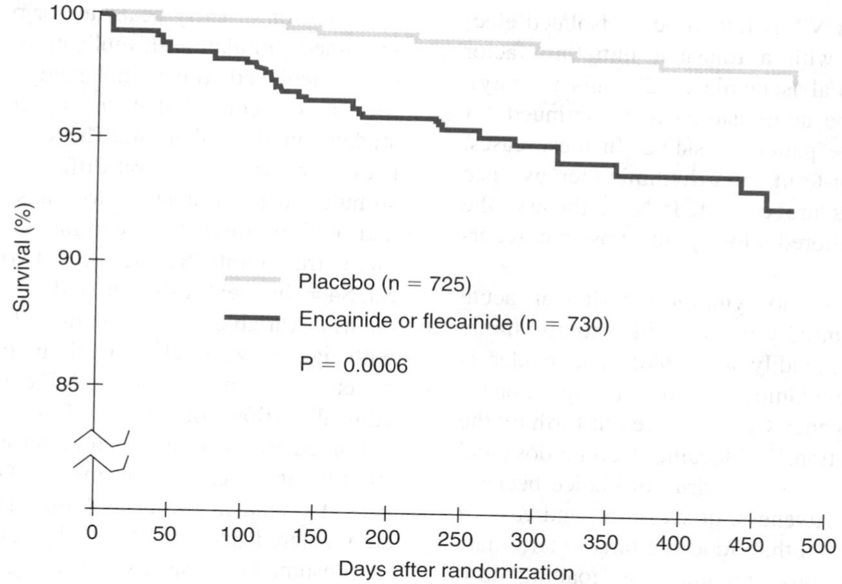

Figure 16.10. Life table curves from the CAST, specifically for patients receiving encainide or flecainide (light line) and matching placebo (heavy line). Note the divergent slopes of each line, implying sustained risk of death (presumed proarrhythmia). *(From The CAST Investigators. Preliminary report: Effect of encainide and flecainide on mortality in a randomized trial of arrhythmia suppression after myocardial infarction. N Engl J Med 1989;321:406–412, with permission.)*

occur during an acute myocardial infarction. In these cases, correction of the underlying precipitating factors will usually prevent further recurrences of VT. As an example, if VT occurs during an acute myocardial infarction and is effectively treated, it will probably not reappear on a chronic basis after the infarcted area has healed or ischemia has resolved. This form of acute VT may be due to either enhanced automatic properties of a ventricular focus or reentrant mechanisms within the ischemic ventricle. In contrast, some patients have a chronic recurrent form of VT that is almost always associated with some type of underlying organic heart disease. Common examples are paroxysmal VT associated with idiopathic dilated congestive cardiomyopathy or remote myocardial infarction with a left ventricular aneurysm. Indeed, left ventricular dysfunction and aneurysm formation are risk factors for the development of VT on a recurrent basis after myocardial infarction. In chronic, recurrent VT, microreentry within the distal Purkinje network is presumed to be responsible for the underlying substrate in a large majority of patients.[66] Theoretically, electrophysiologic discrepancies occur as a result of structural damage and heart disease within the ventricular conducting system. The reentrant circuit may possess both anatomically determined and functional properties coursing through normal, damaged (but not dead) and islands of necrosed tissue. In a minority of patients, macroreentrant circuits may be responsible for recurrent ventricular tachycardia, including reentry incorporating the bundle branches.

Patients with acute VT associated with a precipitating factor often suffer severe symptoms requiring immediate treatment measures. Chronic recurrent VT may also cause severe hemodynamic compromise, but sometimes only mild symptoms, which are generally well tolerated, result. Different varieties of VT may occur and require some definition. Sustained VT is that which requires therapeutic intervention to restore a stable rhythm or lasts a relatively long time (usually greater than 30 seconds). Nonsustained VT (NSVT) is that which self-terminates after a brief duration (usually less than 30 seconds). If the patient has VT more frequently than sinus rhythm (VT is the dominant rhythm), this is referred to as incessant VT. Exercise-induced VT is that which occurs during times of high sympathetic tone such as physical exertion. Monomorphic VT has a consistent QRS configuration, whereas polymorphic VT has varying QRS complexes. A characteristic type of polymorphic VT, in which the QRS complexes appear to undulate around a central axis and which is associated with evidence of delayed ventricular repolarization (long QT interval or prominent U waves), is referred to as torsades de pointes (see later).

Like other rapid tachycardias, the initial management of an acute episode of VT requires a quick assessment of the patient's status and symptoms. If severe symptoms are present, then DCC should be instituted to restore sinus rhythm immediately. An investigation should be made into possible precipitating factors and these should be corrected if possible. The diagnosis of acute myocardial infarction should be entertained. If VT is felt to be an isolated electrical event associated with a transient initiating factor (such as acute myocardial ischemia or digitalis toxicity), then lidocaine should be administered and continued for 24–48 hours or until the patient is stable. In these cases, there is no need for long-term antiarrhythmic therapy once the precipitating factors are corrected. Nevertheless, the patient should be monitored closely for possible recurrences of VT.

Patients with mild or no symptoms during an acute episode of VT can be initially treated with antiarrhythmic drugs (DCC should be readily available). The reader is referred to the most recent Guidelines for Cardiopulmonary Resuscitation and Emergency Cardiac Care put forth by the American Heart Association.[43] Lidocaine (loading dose and infusion) is usually considered the drug of choice because of a high degree of effectiveness, quick onset, and ease of administration. In the event that lidocaine fails to terminate the tachycardia, intravenous procainamide (loading dose and infusion) can be tried next. DCC should be instituted if the patient's status deteriorates, VT degenerates to VF, or drug therapy fails. As an alternative to DCC, a transvenous pacing wire can be inserted and VT terminated by overdrive pacing methods. There is basically no reason to allow the patient to remain in VT without intervention even if symptoms are minimal.

Once an acute episode of sustained VT has been successfully terminated by electrical or pharmacologic means and an acute myocardial infarction ruled out, the possibility of paroxysmal VT reappearing on a recurrent basis should be considered. This possibility can often be confirmed by the use of invasive electrophysiologic study using programmed ventricular stimulation. The management of the patient with chronic recurrent sustained VT deserves considerable attention. Because these patients are at extremely high risk for death, trial-and-error attempts to find effective therapy is unwarranted. Two methods using surrogate endpoints have been used: (1) suppression of ventricular ectopy by serial 24-hour continuous electrocardiographic (Holter) monitoring and (2) inability to induce sustained VT with programmed extrastimuli by invasive electrophysiologic studies.

Electrophysiologic studies utilizing programmed stimulation incorporate the concepts of reentry in order to replicate the patient's clinical tachycardia in a controlled laboratory setting.[67] The patient is admitted to the hospital (often an intensive care setting) and strips of the clinical tachycardia are carefully analyzed. All antiarrhythmic drugs are discontinued and (after the systemic elimination of these drugs) the patient is brought to the electrophysiology laboratory in the nonsedated state. Transvenous multipolar catheters, which can both pace the heart and record electrical activity, then are inserted into the right heart. Next, attempts to replicate the clinical tachycardia are made by the insertion of early beats and/or pacing methods via programmed stimulation. If replication of the clinical tachycardia is achieved, this initial study (without drug therapy) serves as a control that can be compared to subsequent studies on drug therapy. The electrophysiologist usually uses a protocol of several different grades of programmed stimulation from at least two sites (right ventricular apex and outflow tract): S1 = continuous pacing train; S1, S2 = one extra stimuli; S1, S2, S3 = two extra stimuli; S1, S2, S3, S4 = three extra stimuli; and rapid ventricular pacing (V burst) at variable rates. Induction of polymorphic VT or VF with aggressive grades of stimulation (V burst, S4) in a patient with a monomorphic VT can be viewed as a "nonclinical" artifact of the test. Once VT is induced by programmed stimulation, it can be terminated by programmed stimulation, overdrive pacing, or DCC depending on the patient's status. Antiarrhythmic drugs are then serially administered and the electrophysiologic study is repeated (at presumed drug steady state) (Fig. 16.11). If a patient has sustained VT induced during the control study, then the inability to reproduce VT or the induction of only brief, self-terminating episodes of VT (usually less than 15 beats) generally predicts that the drug will be effective in preventing recurrent episodes on a long-term basis. When VT is rendered noninducible with drug therapy, a serum drug level should be obtained immediately. This serum level then serves as the patient's target level for chronic oral therapy (Fig. 16.11). Efforts should be directed to keep the serum level at or above this target to prevent recurrence of the arrhythmia.[68]

Although this method is efficacious in determining effective antiarrhythmic drug therapy in patients with recurrent VT, it has several drawbacks besides its invasive nature. Foremost in this regard is that the yield for finding

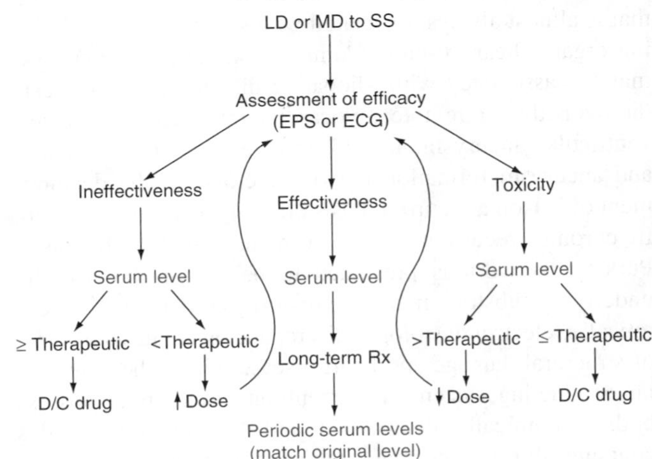

Figure 16.11. Algorithm for the clinical approach to therapeutic drug monitoring of antiarrhythmic drugs. EPS, electrophysiologic study; ECG, continuous electrocardiographic monitoring; D/C, discontinue drug.

an effective drug is low. Sustained monomorphic VT can be rendered noninducible or nonsustained in only 20–25% of patients.[69] Therefore, the clinician frequently must search for other therapeutic options or settle for less optimal treatment endpoints. Some clinicians believe that a lower grade of stimulation (e.g., S4 induction on control versus S2 induction on drug therapy) will make the clinical tachycardia less likely or that the induction of sustained VT of a considerably slower rate will make the tachycardia better tolerated. Nevertheless, these options are not well studied, and many centers will not consistently rely on these responses in the electrophysiology laboratory. Sometimes combination therapy is tried for patients refractory to single agents. The combination of a type Ia drug with a type Ib drug (i.e., quinidine and mexiletine) is effective in some patients that are resistant to either drug used alone.[70] Amiodarone is clearly the most effective (about 50%/2 years) agent in patients with recurrent VT. Although a matter of continuing controversy, many clinicians believe that electrophysiologic drug testing does not predict the clinical efficacy of amiodarone.[71] Patients may have continued inducibility of VT on amiodarone despite long-term success. For this reason, sometimes amiodarone is given empirically without repeat electrophysiologic studies.

The second method in these patients is the use of serial Holter monitors with drug testing. The surrogate endpoint in this case is the suppression of ventricular ectopy (>83%) and total abolition of NSVT compared to control (drug-free) recordings. This method was not used routinely in the United States; initial small studies[72] demonstrated a superiority of invasive electrophysiologic testing over serial Holter recordings. Nonetheless, enough controversy was generated to initiate a large study to compare the two methods of drug testing. The ESVEM (electrophysiologic study versus electrocardiographic monitoring)[73,74] trial enrolled patients with documented clinical VT/VF, inducible ventricular tachycardia and frequent ventricular ectopy. These patients were randomized to electrophysiologic studies or serial Holter recordings to test up to 7 antiarrhythmic drugs (imipramine, mexiletine, pirmenol, procainamide, quinidine, propafenone, or sotalol). Holter testing had a greater yield of identifying effective agents, and there was no statistical difference between this method and electrophysiologic testing in terms of VT recurrence or sudden death. Although patients with poor left ventricular systolic function could not receive it in ESVEM, sotalol proved to be the most effective drug in the trial. The study has been criticized to some extent because of the methods of using programmed stimulation and patient selection so that many invasive electrophysiologists remain unconvinced about the relative merits of serial Holter testing. Further, because there was no placebo group in ESVEM (for ethical reasons) one cannot be sure that either method is truly effective. Perhaps suppression of ectopy by Holter criteria or noninducibility during serial electrophysiologic studies in and of themselves portend an overall good prognosis, independent of any drug effect. This debate therefore continues and regardless of the methods of drug testing, the recurrence rate of VT in ESVEM was high (20–50% per year depending on the drug chosen). These findings and the impressive side-effect profiles of antiarrhythmic agents have led investigators to study nondrug approaches to the treatment of recurrent VT/VF.[75]

Some centers have had excellent results with the surgical excision of the VT focus in appropriate candidates for this extensive procedure. With the aid of endocardial mapping techniques, procedures such as ventricular aneurysmectomy, encircling ventriculotomy, and cryo, laser, or rf ablation can successfully abolish the arrhythmogenic substrate. However, the introduction and advances in the implantable automatic cardioverter defibrillator (ICD) have made it one of the more frequent forms of current therapy for patients with recurrent, sustained VT/VF (Fig. 16.12). Early ICDs required a thoracotomy for placement and were programmed to tachycardia rate. Once the patient's rate rose to a certain level, a series of internal defibrillations was delivered. Although effective in terminating VT/VF, inappropriate shocks were sometimes delivered for SVTs or NSVTs. Further, a pulse generator was placed in the abdomen with a relatively short battery life in these early models. ICD technology is rapidly expanding so that now the newer devices employ a "tiered therapy approach." New ICDs provide, in a sequential fashion, programmed stimulation, overdrive pacing, and low-energy cardioversion before internal defibrillation is employed as a last step. In addition, backup bradycardia pacing and extended battery lives have made these devices much more attractive. Importantly, transvenous insertion techniques not requiring a thoracotomy are now being utilized at many institutions (Fig. 16.12).

Most would agree that the ICD is highly effective in preventing sudden death due to recurrent VT or VF,[76] although several problems do remain. First, the device and implantation are expensive. The approximate cost for the ICD device alone is $18,000 to $20,000. Total cost for the device, hospitalization, and physician fees is about $40,000. Second, many patients (as high as 50%) end up receiving antiarrhythmic drugs (usually amiodarone) in addition to the ICD. Here, the endpoint of drug therapy is different than without the ICD (i.e., the drugs do not necessarily need to prevent all sustained recurrences). Antiarrhythmic drugs are prescribed in this instance to decrease the frequency of VT/VF episodes and NSVT, minimize patient discomfort, and save battery life. Some immediately couple antiarrhythmic drugs with the ICD implantation but we do not recommend this approach. Rather, each patient should be individualized and antiarrhythmic drugs administered in those with frequent VT and shocks. If antiarrhythmic drugs

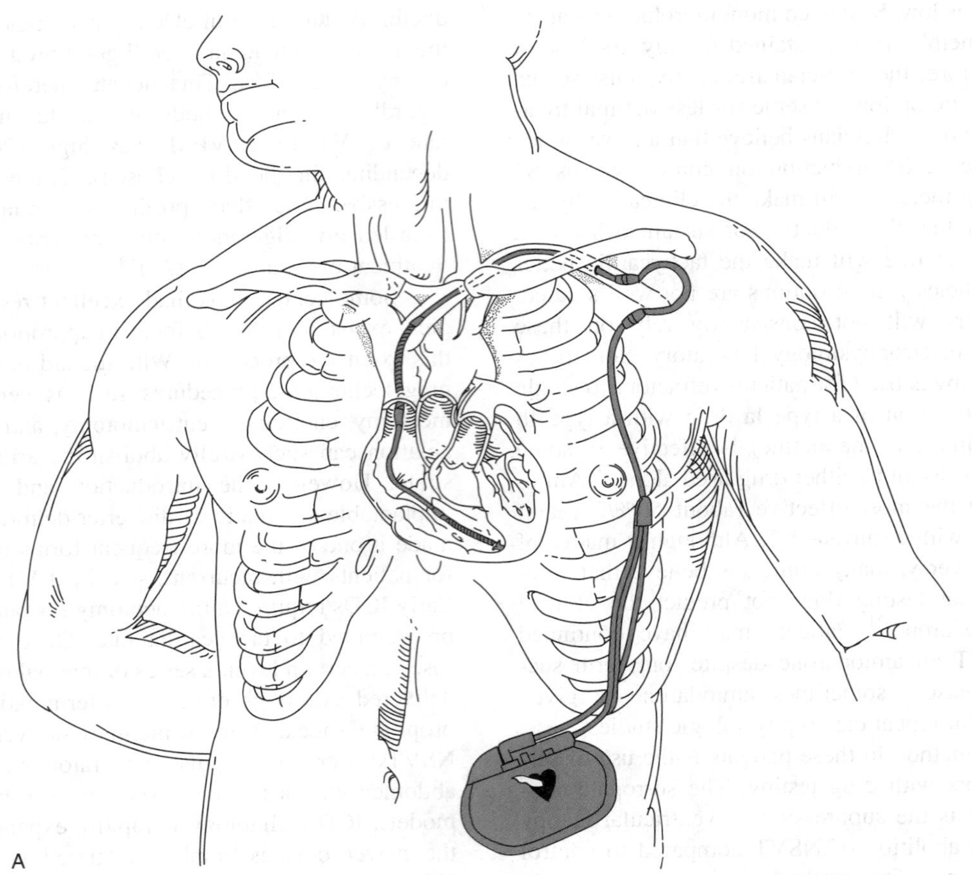

Figure 16.12. Drawings showing automatic implantable cardioverter defibrillators with two currently possible methods of device placement. (A) An endocardial lead system where the leads are placed transvenously without the need for a thoracotomy. (B) An epicardial lead system where the leads (patches) are sewn directly on the epicardial surface, necessitating surgery. In both instances, the pulse generator is placed in the anterior abdominal wall and connected to the leads by wires tunneled subcutaneously. *(Courtesy of Cardiac Pacemakers, Inc., St. Paul, MN, with permission.)*

are added to ICD therapy, one should note that many agents alter defibrillation thresholds and therefore the device should be reprogrammed.[77] Third, it remains unclear if the ICD decreases overall mortality in patients with recurrent VT/VF.[78] Perhaps the ICD alters the cause of death without decreasing all-cause mortality.

At this time it is clear that patients with complex ventricular ectopy should not be treated with traditional (type I) antiarrhythmic drugs and those with recurrent, sustained VT definitely require some form of preventative treatment (drugs and/or devices), but the approach to NSVT is a current area of considerable controversy. Obviously, those patients with long, symptomatic episodes require drug therapy but most have asymptomatic NSVT. Epidemiologic data indicate that patients with NSVT and coronary disease are at increased risk for sudden death.[79] However, due in part to the results of the CAST, clinicians have sought more clear risk stratification before initiating drug therapy. Wilber et al.[80] have suggested that electrophysiologic studies may provide a useful (but costly and invasive) tool to stratify patients at increased risk. This study found that post-MI patients with NSVT who had inducible sustained VT were at increased risk for subsequent arrhythmia or sudden death. Alternatively, those without inducible sustained tachycardias were at low risk for subsequent spontaneous sustained arrhythmias. In patients with inducible sustained VT in whom the tachycardia was rendered noninducible by drugs, the risk of death was similar to those who had no inducible arrhythmias at all. Perhaps patients with NSVT should undergo programmed stimulation and those found to have inducible sustained VT should be treated aggressively with antiarrhythmic drugs. Those with no inducible sustained tachycardia can then be followed closely without drug therapy (Fig. 16.13). However,

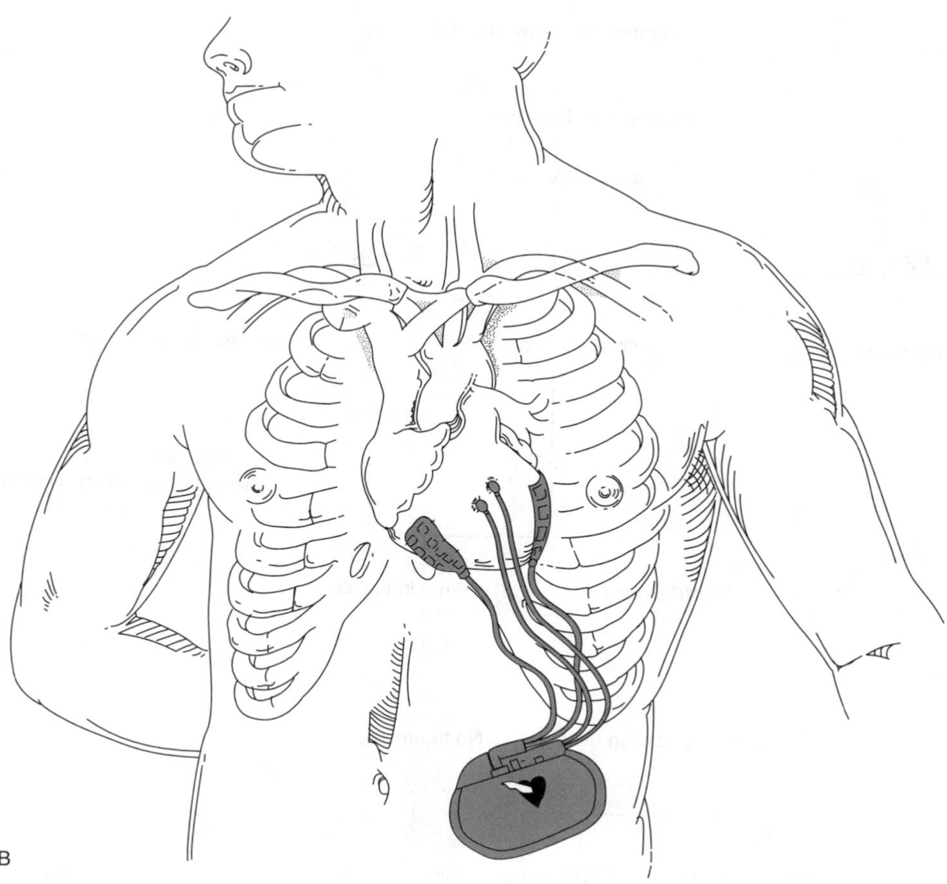

Wilber's study was unable to demonstrate that electrophysiologic-guided drug therapy decreased long-term mortality.

Another approach to risk stratification involves the use of noninvasive tools. Gomes et al.[81] evaluated the predictive utility of Holter monitoring, left ventricular ejection fraction assessment, and signal-averaged electrocardiogram (SAECG) for determining prognosis after myocardial infarction. The SAECG detects "late potentials" believed to be due to areas in the ventricle that possess slow and fragmented conduction, promoting the proper substrate for VT. The results indicate that the presence of high-grade ectopy, decreased ejection fraction (<40%), and abnormal SAECG are all significant risk factors for subsequent arrhythmia (sustained VT) or sudden death. Further, the more risk factors a patient has, the greater the risk. It has been proposed that those individuals with two or more risk factors undergo electrophysiologic studies and possible serial drug testing for further risk stratification based on the inducibility of sustained ventricular tachycardia. It should be pointed out that this approach, with the final step being invasive programmed stimulation, represents an aggressive treatment strategy. Many clinical electrophysiologists choose to ignore most cases of brief, asymptomatic episodes of NSVT. Others use empiric or Holter guided therapy, generally with amiodarone or sotalol. Again, there are no data to suggest that these approaches decrease overall mortality. Another confounding factor is the underlying form of heart disease associated with NSVT. Patients with idiopathic dilated cardiomyopathy and NSVT also appear to be a high risk for sudden death yet usually do not have inducible sustained VT with invasive studies (unlike those with coronary disease). Clearly, further large prospective trials are necessary (and currently ongoing) to discern the proper approach to NSVT. One such study referred to as the MUSTT (Multicenter UnSustained Tachycardia Trial) is in progress. This trial will evaluate the value of electrophysiologic-guided therapy (including the ICD) in patients with NSVT and coronary disease.

PROARRHYTHMIA

All antiarrhythmic agents have the potential to aggravate existing arrhythmias or to cause new arrhythmias. It is believed that antiarrhythmic drugs may cause proarrhythmia in 5–20% of patients.[63] Although drug-induced arrhythmias

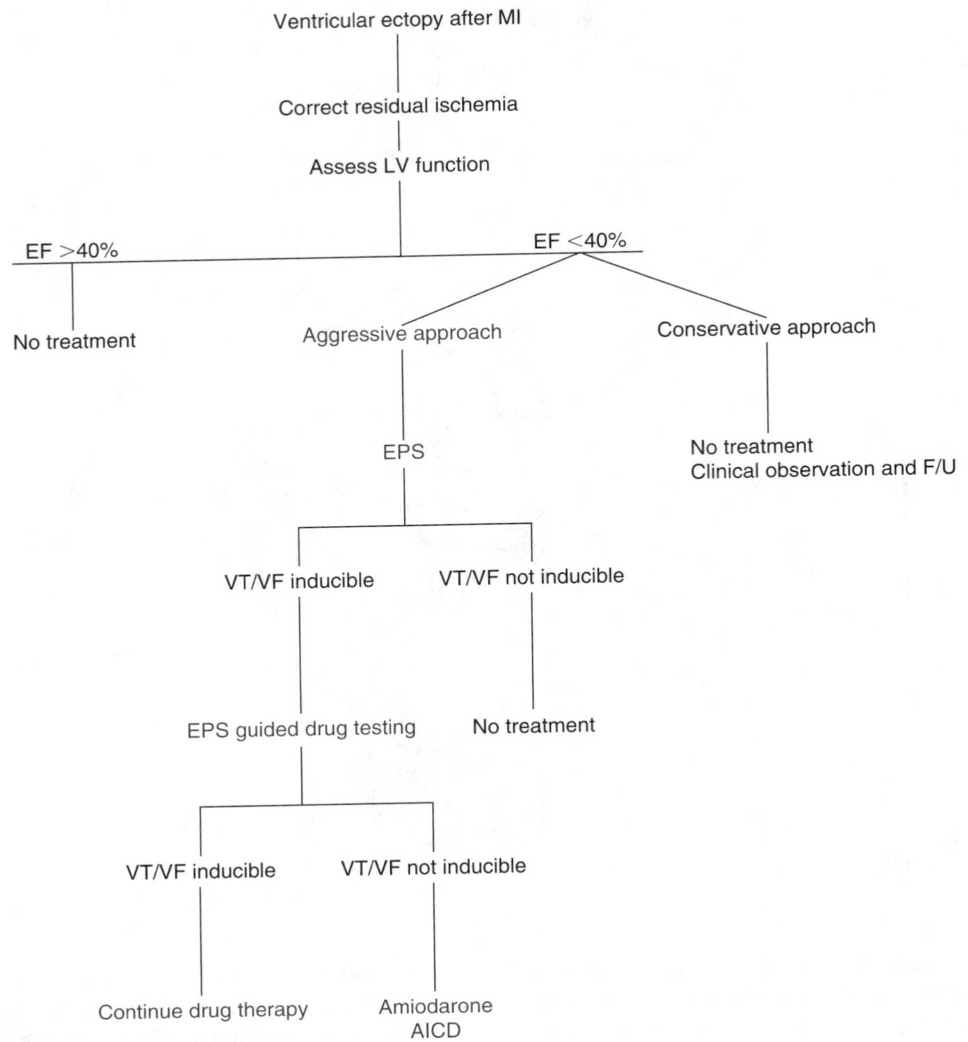

Figure 16.13. An algorithm for management of patients with ventricular ectopy after myocardial infarction. Correction of residual ischemia may include treatment with antianginal drug therapy, percutaneous transluminal coronary angioplasty, or bypass surgery. No treatment indicates that antiarrhythmic therapy (either pharmacologic or nonpharmacologic therapy) is not indicated. EF, ejection fraction; EPS, electrophysiologic studies; VT/VF, ventricular tachycardia/ventricular fibrillation; ICD, automatic implantable cardioverter–defibrillator; F/U, follow-up. *(From Bauman JL et al. Tachycardias, in Carter B, Angaran D, Lake K, Raebel M [eds]: Pharmacotherapy Self-Assessment Program, 2nd ed. Kansas City, MO, ACCP, 1995, with permission.)*

have been recognized for several years, it has only been recently that this adverse effect has gained widespread attention. Many definitions for proarrhythmia have been proposed; however, in simplest terms it indicates the development of a significant new arrhythmia (such as VT, VF, or torsades de pointes) or worsening of an existing arrhythmia (episodes are longer, faster, or more frequent). As with all arrhythmias, the consequences of proarrhythmia are varied. Some patients who develop proarrhythmia may be totally asymptomatic, others may notice a worsening of symptoms, while some may die suddenly from this side effect. The development of proarrhythmia results from the same mechanisms that cause arrhythmias in general (e.g., quinidine-induced torsades de pointes due to early after-depolarizations) or from an alteration in the underlying substrate due to the antiarrhythmic agent (e.g., development of an accelerated tachycardia due to flecainide, which decreases conduction velocity without significantly altering the refractory period).[63] The diagnosis of proarrhythmia is sometimes difficult to make due to the variable nature of the underlying arrhythmias. However, in all cases, the agent should be discontinued if proarrhythmia is detected or suspected.

The issue of proarrhythmia, particularly from type Ic agents, has gained considerable publicity due to the results of the CAST. Flecainide and encainide have been known to cause a rapid, sustained, monomorphic VT with a characteristic sinusoidal QRS pattern, which is resistant to resuscitation with cardioversion or overdrive pacing. This arrhythmia was thought to occur within the first several days of drug initiation; however, the results of the CAST indicate that the risk may exist as long as the agent is continued. Patient factors that definitely predispose to this form of proarrhythmia are the presence of underlying ventricular arrhythmias, ischemic heart disease, and poor left ventricular function. Provocation of proarrhythmia due to the type Ic drugs is frequently reported during exercise. This is more than likely due to augmented slowed conduction at rapid heart rates (i.e., rate-dependent sodium blockade). The incidence of proarrhythmia is greatest in patients with all three risk factors (approximately 10–20%) and considerably less (less than 5%) in those without risks, such as patients with good left ventricular function and supraventricular tachycardias. Other factors that have a less-defined association with proarrhythmia are elevated antiarrhythmic serum concentrations (and rapid dosage escalation) and recent therapy with a type Ia antiarrhythmic. It has been proposed that the presence of underlying ventricular conduction delays may also pose a risk.[82] Interestingly, in this study, the incidence of death due to proarrhythmia from encainide and flecainide was approximately the same as the chance of long-term effectiveness. As mentioned earlier, this arrhythmia is resistant to resuscitation; however, some clinicians have had success with intravenous lidocaine or the administration of sodium bicarbonate.

TORSADES DE POINTES

Torsades de pointes (TdP) is a rapid form of polymorphic VT (Fig. 16.14) and is associated with evidence of delayed ventricular repolarization (long QT interval or prominent U waves) on surface ECGs. It is important to note that polymorphic VT, occurring in the setting of a normal QT interval, is similar to monomorphic VT in terms of etiology and treatment strategies.[83] TdP may occur in association with hereditary syndromes or as acquired forms. The underlying etiology in both cases is delayed ventricular repolarization due to blockade or abnormal potassium conductance. Two well-described heritable forms are Romano and Ward syndrome (long QT, TdP, and high incidence of sudden death) and Jervell and Lange–Neilson syndrome (long QT, TdP, high incidence of sudden death, and congenital deaf-mutism). It is possible that many individuals have a partially expressed form of these congenital syndromes but never suffer TdP unless some other external factor (drugs, diseases) further delays ventricular repolarization. Acquired forms of TdP are associated with electrolyte disturbances (hypokalemia or hypomagnesemia), subarachnoid hemorrhage, myocarditis, liquid protein diets, arsenic poisoning, hypothyroidism, or drug therapy (notably phenothiazines, antihistamines, tricyclic or tetracyclic antidepressants, and antiarrhythmics) (Table 16.14). The type Ia drugs (especially quinidine) are most notorious for precipitating torsades de pointes but the type Ib and Ic drugs rarely ever cause it. The syndrome often referred to as "quinidine syncope" is, in most cases, due to drug-induced TdP. Quinidine syncope occurs in 4–8% of patients treated with this agent. Associated features, most of which are shared with other forms of drug-induced TdP are as follows[21]: (1) low to "therapeutic" quinidine serum concentrations without other evidence of quinidine-related toxicity such as prolonged QRS duration; (2) concurrent organic heart disease, commonly ischemic; (3) evidence of mild delayed repolarization prior to quinidine therapy; (4) documentation usually within 1 week of initiating therapy; (5) high incidence of cross-sensitivity (recurrence of TdP) with other type Ia antiarrhythmic agents but not type Ib or Ic drugs, or amiodarone; (6) frequent coexisting electrolyte disturbances such as hypo-

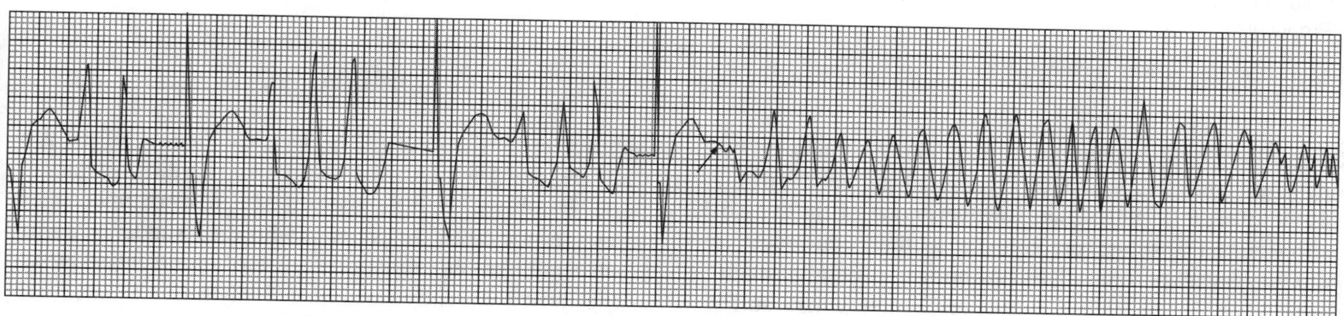

Figure 16.14. Torsades de pointes due to quinidine. Note the couplet and two triplets that follow each extra systolic pause. The pause gets progressively longer until it is long enough to result in an episode of sustained torsades de pointes (labeled ↑). Also as the pause lengthens, discernible U waves (EADs?) begin to appear. The amplitude of the U wave is somewhat greater with the longest pause. *(From Bauman JB: Drug safety: Cardiac arrhythmias. Antihistamine update symposium. Hospital Medicine 1995;31:24, with permission.)*

TABLE 16.4. REPORTED CAUSES OF QT PROLONGATION AND TORSADES DE POINTES

Conditions
Congenital long QT syndromes
Myocarditis
Myocardial ischemia/infarction
Severe bradycardia due to AV block; <50 beats/min
Hypokalemia
Severe hypothermia
Hypomagnesemia
Hypothyroidism
Cardiomyopathy
Subarachnoid hemorrhage
Drugs
Antiarrhythmic/vasodilating drugs
Quinidine
Procainamide
Disopyramide
Amiodarone
Sotalol
Bepridil
N-acetylprocainamide
Psychotropics
Phenothiazines
Tricyclic and tetracyclic antidepressants
Haloperidol
Toxins
Organophosphate insecticides
Arsenic
Antihistamines
Terfenadine
Astemizole
Antibiotics
Pentamidine
Erythromycin
Trimethoprim-sulfamethoxazole
Miscellaneous
Liquid protein diets[a]
Corticosteroids[a]
Diuretics[a]
Vasopressin
Quinine
Chloroquine
Chloral hydrate
Probucol

[a]Due, more than likely, to severe electrolyte imbalance.

kalemia or hypomagnesemia; and (7) a characteristic long–short initiating sequence ("pause" dependence) of the episode of TdP (Fig. 16.14). However, none of these associations is an absolute prerequisite to the occurrence of quinidine syncope and TdP. Although generally documented early in the course of therapy, patients may suffer TdP during chronic quinidine treatment.[84] Other drug-related causes of TdP occur more frequently with high concentrations and doses (e.g., terfenidine, sotalol, *N*-acetylprocainamide). Amiodarone is an infrequent cause of TdP.

The electrophysiologic etiology of TdP has not been fully elucidated. It has been suggested that TdP may be due to discrepancies in ventricular repolarization and inhomogeneous ventricular recovery, allowing the formation of multiple reentrant circuits. More likely, recent investigations have suggested that TdP is likely due to triggered activity (early after depolarizations) caused by a delay in ventricular repolarization. For an acute episode of TdP, most patients will require and respond to DCC. However, TdP tends to be paroxysmal in nature and often will rapidly recur after countershock. Therefore, after the initial restoration of a stable rhythm, therapy designed to prevent recurrences of TdP should be instituted. Almost all antiarrhythmics have been reported to be successful in isolated case reports, but because of the unpredictable and self-terminating nature of TdP, it is difficult to establish a cause-and-effect relationship. Drugs that further prolong repolarization such as intravenous procainamide are absolutely contraindicated. Lidocaine is usually ineffective. It is now well established that preventive therapy should increase heart rate and thereby shorten ventricular repolarization. Therefore, the initial treatments (after DCC) include either temporary transvenous pacing (105–120 beats/min) or pharmacologic pacing (isoproterenol or epinephrine infusion). Intravenous magnesium sulfate, independent of serum magnesium concentration, also provides valuable adjunctive therapy (probably by suppression of triggered activity).[85] All agents that prolong QT interval should be discontinued and exacerbating factors (such as hypokalemia) corrected.

The heritable long-QT syndromes may possibly be due to a basic derangement in centrally mediated autonomic control of cardiac rhythm. For this reason, propranolol has been shown to prevent recurrences of TdP and prevent sudden death.[86] In refractory patients, phenytoin or ICD placement have been utilized. In acquired long-QT syndromes, correction of the underlying cause is the key to long-term preventive therapy. No drug agents need be utilized on a chronic basis. In the case of quinidine syncope, type Ia agents should be avoided for the future treatment of the patient's underlying arrhythmias.

VENTRICULAR FIBRILLATION

Ventricular fibrillation (VF) is electrical anarchy of the ventricle, resulting in no cardiac output and cardiovascular collapse. Death will ensue rapidly if effective treatment measures are not taken. In patients who died suddenly during electrocardiographic monitoring, VF often preceded by VT is the most frequently documented rhythm.[87] Sudden cardiac death accounts for about 400,000 deaths per year or 1000 deaths per day in the United States. Sudden cardiac death occurs most commonly in patients with ischemic heart disease and primary myocardial disease; less commonly in WPW, mitral valve prolapse, and occasionally those without associated heart disease. Patients who have sudden cardiac death (not associated with acute myocardial infarction) but survive because of appropriate cardiopulmonary resuscitation usually have inducible sustained VT and/or VF during electrophysiologic studies.[88] These individuals are at high risk for the recurrence of VT and/or VF.

In contrast, patients who have VF associated with acute myocardial infarction usually have little risk of recurrence. Of all patients who die due to an acute MI, approximately 50% die suddenly prior to hospitalization, presumably due to VF. VF associated with acute myocardial infarction (MI) can be subdivided into two types: primary VF and complicated or secondary VF. Primary VF occurs in an uncomplicated MI not associated with heart failure; secondary VF occurs in an MI complicated by heart failure. The time course, incidence, mechanisms, treatment, and complications of these two forms of VF are different. For example, about 2–11% patients with acute MI suffer primary VF within 24 hours of chest pain but the risk of VF declines rapidly over time and is very low after the initial 24-hour period. Complicated VF does not follow such a predictable time course and may occur in the late infarction period. Moreover, the value of prophylactic therapy has been best studied in the prevention of primary VF with very little information in patients with heart failure complicating the infarction. The premise of prophylactic antiarrhythmic drugs administered to all patients with uncomplicated MI is based on the inability to predict which patients are at risk for primary VF and the predictable time course of primary VF (in contrast to complicated VF). Of the prophylactic therapies utilized, lidocaine has been the most widely debated and studied. Lie and coworkers[89] performed the classic study showing the effectiveness of lidocaine in preventing primary VF. Although lidocaine significantly reduced the incidence of VF compared to placebo, there was not a decrease in mortality due to VF between the groups. This fact and the effectiveness of rapidly instituted DCC in modern coronary care units with sophisticated monitoring techniques have caused many to reject the notion of prophylactic lidocaine administration for all patients with uncomplicated myocardial infarction. Two recent meta-analyses[90,91] also conclude against the routine use of prophylactic lidocaine due to a possible increase in mortality in lidocaine-treated patients[90] and the declining incidence of primary VF documented in recent years.[91]

More recently, the use of intravenous magnesium sulfate has been entertained for the prevention of VF during the acute infarct period. Small trials implying effectiveness were subsequently incorporated into a meta-analysis.[92] This meta-analysis found a decrease in the incidence of VT/VF and a reduction in total mortality with magnesium therapy. A subsequent large multicenter trial[93] found similar results, although most of the decrease in mortality was (surprisingly) attributed to heart failure deaths rather than deaths due to ventricular arrhythmias. These results would lead one to conclude that magnesium sulfate should be routinely administered to patients with suspected MI because of its ease of administration and safety. However, preliminary data from another large trial (ISIS-4) apparently has verified no such effectiveness of magnesium therapy in this setting. Hence, prophylactic magnesium cannot be recommended at this time; indeed, no therapies (lidocaine, magnesium, or other antiarrhythmic drugs) have shown a conclusive benefit to prevent VF in the acute infarct period (at least for now).

A patient with VF (with or without associated myocardial ischemia) should be managed according to the American Heart Association's recommendations for advanced cardiac life support.[43] Summarizing, DCC should be immediately instituted and repeated twice (if unsuccessful) prior to drug therapy. If DCC does not restore a stable rhythm, epinephrine (intravenous or intratracheal if a line is not established) should be administered prior to the next DCC. It has been debated whether the standard dose of epinephrine (1.0 mg) is sufficient. Recently, a large multicenter trial[94] found that "high-dose" epinephrine (0.2 mg/kg) did not affect success or survival (compared to 0.02 mg/kg) of patients with cardiac arrest (including VF). Nevertheless, if epinephrine (coupled with DCC) is unsuccessful, lidocaine then bretylium should be given and DCC repeated as necessary. Bear in mind that the onset of action of bretylium can be delayed (10–20 minutes), presumably due to slow distribution to the myocardium. Procainamide can be tried in the event that the first two agents fail.

Once the patient is successfully resuscitated, antiarrhythmics should be continued until the patient's rhythm and overall status is stable. If the episode of VF was associated with acute ischemia, long-term antiarrhythmic drugs are probably unnecessary but the patient should be monitored closely for recurrence of VT and/or VF. If, however, VF was not associated with acute MI (or a known precipitating factor), the patient should undergo invasive electrophysiologic studies and (depending on the results) serial drug testing by programmed stimulation for inducible VT/VF (Fig. 16.15).

BRADYARRHYTHMIAS

The previous sections reviewed the pathophysiology and treatment of tachyarrhythmias, and this section serves to consider the bradyarrhythmias briefly. For the most part, the symptoms of bradyarrhythmias result from a decline in cardiac output. Because cardiac output increases as heart rate increases (to a point), patients experience symptoms in association with hypotension such as dizziness, syncope, fatigue, and confusion. If left ventricular dysfunction exists, patients may have an exacerbation of congestive heart failure symptoms. Except in the case of recurrent syncope, these symptoms are often subtle and nonspecific.

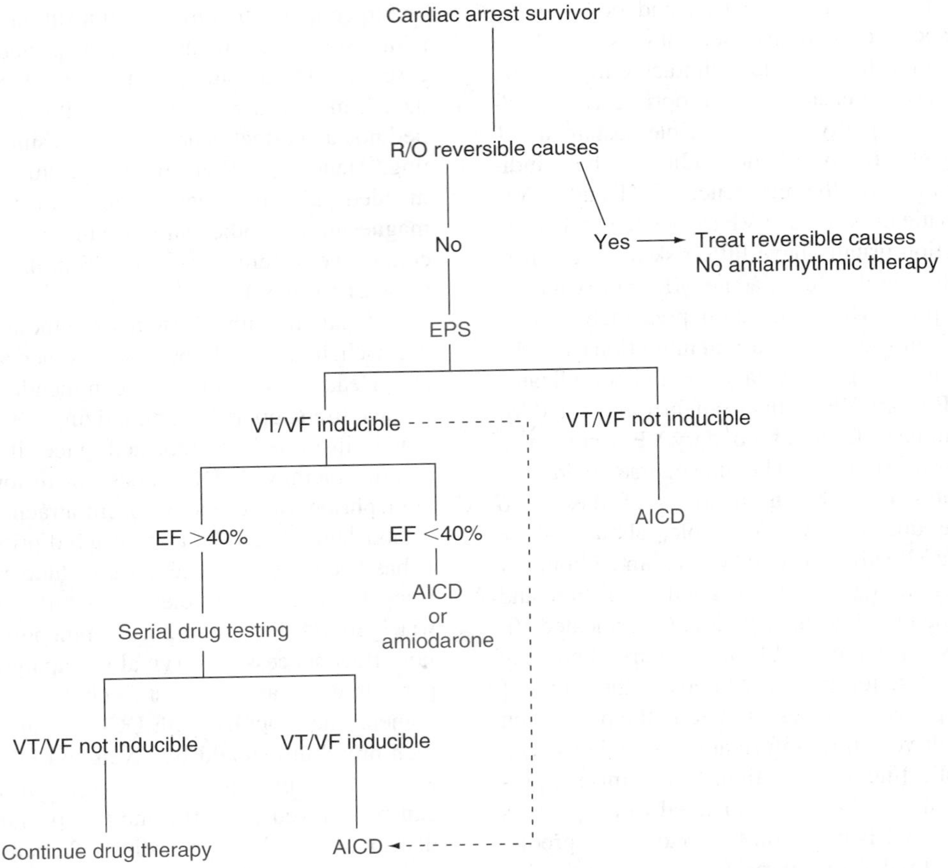

Figure 16.15. Example of an approach to the management of survivors of cardiac arrest. Reversible causes of cardiac arrest (e.g., electrolyte abnormalities, acute phase of MI) should be treated with specific therapy. The hatched line represents the approach of some clinicians who would proceed directly to ICD implantation in patients with inducible VT/VF regardless of the ejection fraction. *(From Bauman JL et al. Tachycardias, in Carter B, Angaran D, Lake K, Raebel M [eds]: Pharmacotherapy Self-Assessment Program, 2nd ed. Kansas City, MO, ACCP, 1995, with permission.)*

SINUS NODE DYSFUNCTION

Sinus bradyarrhythmias (heart rate less than 60 beats/min) is a common finding especially in young, athletically active individuals and usually is not symptomatic and does not require therapeutic intervention. However, some patients, particularly the elderly, have sinus node dysfunction. This may be the result of underlying organic heart disease and the normal aging process, which, over time, attenuates SA nodal function. Sick sinus syndrome refers to this process, resulting in symptomatic sinus bradycardia and/or periods of sinus arrest.[95] Sinus node dysfunction is usually representative of diffuse conduction disease, and accompanying AV block is not uncommon. Furthermore, symptomatic bradyarrhythmias may be accompanied by paroxysmal tachycardias such as atrial fibrillation. Because of diffuse conduction disease, atrial fibrillation sometimes presents with a rather slow ventricular response (in the absence of AV nodal blocking drugs). The occurrence of alternating bradyarrhythmias and tachyarrhythmias is referred to as the "tachy–brady syndrome."[95,96] The occurrence of paroxysmal atrial fibrillation in a patient with sinus node dysfunction may be due to underlying heart disease with atrial dysfunction or to atrial escape in response to reduced sinus node automaticity. In fact, because the rate of impulse generation by the sinus node is generally depressed or may fail altogether, other automatic pacemakers within the conduction system may "rescue" the sinus node. These rescue rhythms may present as paroxysmal atrial rhythms or as a junctional escape rhythm.

The treatment of sinus node dysfunction involves the elimination of symptomatic bradycardia and the possibility of managing alternating tachycardias such as atrial fibrillation. In general, the long-term therapy of choice is a permanent ventricular pacemaker. Pacemaker therapy, however, should be reserved for patients with significant symptoms. In other words, the aim of pacing is not to correct electrocardiographic findings but to improve the patient's symptoms and quality of life.

Drugs that are commonly employed to treat supraventricular tachycardias should be used with caution, if at all, in the absence of a functioning pacemaker.[96] Type I agents such as quinidine can suppress the escape or rescue rhythms that appear in severe sinus bradycardia or sinus arrest. In this way they may transform an asymptomatic patient with bradycardia into a symptomatic one. It is also important to remember that the addition of type I antiarrhythmic agents can affect pacemaker threshold and result in loss of capture if the pacemaker is not appropriately interrogated and adjusted.[77] Other drugs that depress SA or AV nodal function such as β blockers or calcium channel antagonists may significantly exacerbate bradycardia. Even agents with indirect sympatholytic actions such as α-methyldopa or clonidine may worsen sinus node dysfunction. Digitalis use in these patients is controversial, but in most cases, it can be used safely.

Another reason for paroxysmal bradycardia and sinus arrest that is not due directly to sinus node dysfunction is carotid-sinus hypersensitivity.[97,98] Again, this syndrome occurs commonly in the aged with underlying heart disease. Symptoms occur when the carotid sinus is stimulated, resulting in an accentuated baroreceptor reflex. Thus, the patient may experience paroxysmal episodes of dizziness or syncope because of sinus arrest due to increased vagal tone and sympathetic withdrawal (cardioinhibitory type), drop in systemic blood pressure due to sympathetic withdrawal (vasodepressor type), or both (mixed cardioinhibitory and vasodepressor types). The diagnosis can be confirmed by performing carotid sinus massage with electrocardiographic and blood pressure monitoring in controlled conditions.

Carotid-sinus hypersensitivity can also be treated with permanent pacemaker therapy.[97] However, some patients, particularly those with a significant vasodepressor component, still experience syncope or dizziness. In these cases, α-adrenergic stimulants such as ephedrine, sometimes in combination with β blockers to achieve maximal α-sympathetic stimulation, can be tried in addition to the pacemaker.[98]

Another syndrome, vasovagal syncope, is believed to be the cause of syncope in many patients who present with recurrent syncope of unknown origin.[99,100] This reaction is presumed to be a neurally mediated, paradoxical reaction involving stimulation of cardiac mechanoreceptors (i.e., Bezold–Jarisch reflex). Forceful contraction of the ventricle coupled with low ventricular volumes provides a powerful stimulus for cardiac mechanoreceptors. Syncope results from the spontaneous development of transient hypotension (sympathetic withdrawal) and bradycardia (vagotonia). Patients believed to have frequent episodes of vasovagal syncope have been evaluated and diagnosed using the upright body tilt test, a potent stimulus for the development of vasovagal symptoms. Although commonly used, the sensitivity and reproducibility of this test has been questioned.

Vasovagal syncope can usually be successfully treated with oral β blockers. Although these agents may seem inappropriate to treat a syndrome resulting from vasodilation and bradycardia, the therapeutic approach is designed to block an inappropriate vasovagal reaction. Beta blockers act by inhibiting the sympathetic surge that causes forceful ventricular contraction and precedes the onset of hypotension and bradycardia. Drug testing with IV esmolol or metoprolol during repeat head-up tilt tests has been used to predict the long-term response of oral beta blockers. Other drugs that have been used successfully (with or without β blockers) include scopolamine patches, α-adrenergic agonists, theophylline, dipyridamole, and disopyramide. More information is required, particularly comparative trials with effective agents, in order to make definitive conclusions regarding the place of these alternatives to β blockers in this disorder.

ATRIOVENTRICULAR BLOCK

Conduction delay or block may occur in any area of the AV conduction system: the AV node, the His bundle, or the bundle branches. AV block is usually categorized into three different types based on surface electrocardiographic findings (Table 16.5). First-degree AV block is 1 : 1 AV conduction with a prolonged PR interval. Second-degree AV block is divided into two forms: Mobitz I AV block (Wenkebach periodicity) is less than 1 : 1 AV conduction with progressively lengthening PR intervals until a ventricular complex is dropped; Mobitz II AV block is intermittently dropped ventricular beats in a random fashion without progressive PR lengthening. Third-degree AV block is complete heart block where AV conduction is totally absent (AV dissociation). By utilizing intracardiac His bundle electrocardiograms, the actual site of conduction delay/block can be correlated to the previous diagnosis. First-degree AV block usually represents conduction block within the AV node. Mobitz I, second-degree AV block is also usually due to prolonged conduction in the AV node. Indeed, Wenkebach periodicity is a normal AV nodal response to rapid supraventricular stimulation or high vagal tone. In contrast,

TABLE 16.5. FORMS OF ATRIOVENTRICULAR BLOCK

Type	Criteria
First-degree block	Prolonged PR interval (>0.2 s), 1 : 1 AV conduction
Second-degree block	
Mobitz I	Progressive PR prolongation until QRS is dropped, <1 : 1 AV conduction
Mobitz II	Random nonconducted beats (absence of QRS), <1 : 1 AV conduction
Third-degree block	AV dissociation, absence of AV conduction

Mobitz II AV block is usually due to conduction disease below the AV node (i.e., His bundle). Third-degree AV block may be due to disease at any level of the AV conduction system: complete AV nodal block, His bundle block, or trifascicular block. The ventricle will beat independently of the atria (AV dissociation), and the rates of ventricular activation and QRS configuration are determined by the site of AV block. The usual degree of automaticity of ventricular pacemakers progressively declines as impulses move down the conduction system. Therefore, the ventricular escape rate in cases of trifascicular block will be significantly less than complete AV nodal block.

AV block may be found in patients without underlying heart disease such as trained athletes or during sleep when vagal tone is high. Also, AV block may be transient where the underlying etiology is reversible such as in myocarditis, myocardial ischemia, after cardiovascular surgery, or during drug therapy. Beta blockers, digitalis, or calcium antagonists may cause AV block, primarily in the AV nodal area. Type I antiarrhythmic agents may exacerbate conduction delays below the level of the AV node (sodium-dependent tissue). In other cases, AV block may be irreversible such as that due to acute myocardial infarction, rare degenerative diseases, primary myocardial disease, or congenital forms.

The cornerstone to the acute treatment of symptomatic bradycardia or AV block is temporary, transvenous pacing.[43] However, since it takes time for the insertion of a right ventricular lead, bridge therapy with transcutaneous pacing devices or drugs that improve sinus and AV nodal conduction (e.g., atropine, epinephrine infusion) should be used. In the past, isoproterenol infusion was frequently chosen for this purpose but is now not recommended because of its vasodilating properties and its ability to increase myocardial oxygen consumption (particularly during acute infarction). Pharmacologic therapies such as atropine or sympathomimetics may improve symptoms and conduction in sinus bradycardia/arrest and AV nodal block. These agents will not help when the site of AV block is below the AV node (e.g., Mobitz II or trifascicular AV block).

Patients with chronic symptomatic AV block should be treated with the insertion of a permanent pacemaker. Patients without symptoms can usually be followed closely without the need for a pacemaker. Because symptoms often correlate with the ventricular rate and the ventricular rate corresponds to the site of block, pacemaker therapy is usually necessary in distal AV blocks such as that occurring in the His bundle or the bundle branches. Patients with acute myocardial infarction and evidence of new AV block or conduction disturbances will often require the insertion of a temporary transvenous pacemaker. AV block more commonly occurs as a complication of inferior wall infarcts because of high vagal innervation at this site, and the coronary blood flow to the nodal areas usually supplies the inferior wall. However, the AV block may be only transient, obviating the need for permanent pacing. In patients with chronic AV conduction disturbances, intracardiac recordings (His bundle electrocardiograms) are sometimes utilized to document the actual site of block and define the potential need for and specific type of pacemaker therapy.

EVALUATION OF THERAPEUTIC OUTCOMES

Generally, patients who suffer from tachyarrhythmias can be monitored for one or several possible therapeutic outcomes. Obviously, the presence or recurrence of any arrhythmia can be documented by electrocardiographic means (e.g., surface ECG, Holter monitor, or event monitor). Further, patients may experience a decrease in blood pressure that may result in symptoms from lightheadedness to abrupt syncope depending on the rate of the arrhythmia and the status of the underlying heart disease. For some patients, the potential alteration in hemodynamics may result in death if the arrhythmia is not detected and treated immediately. Besides these clinical outcomes, many patients with tachyarrhythmias experience alterations in quality of life due to recurrent symptoms of the arrhythmia or from side effects of therapy. Finally, there are the economic considerations of medical or surgical intervention, continued medical care, and chronic drug or nondrug treatment.

Some therapeutic outcomes are unique to certain arrhythmias. For instance, patients with atrial fibrillation or flutter need to be monitored for thromboembolism and for complications of anticoagulation therapy (bleeding, drug interactions) prescribed to prevent it. However, the most important monitoring parameters for most patients fall into the following categories: (1) mortality (total and arrhythmic), (2) arrhythmia recurrence (duration, frequency, symptoms), (3) hemodynamic consequences (rate, blood pressure, symptoms), and (4) treatment complications (need for alternative or additional drugs, devices, surgery) (Table 16.6).

TABLE 16.6. OUTCOMES—ARRHYTHMIAS

- Mortality
  - Total, all-cause
  - Arrhythmic death (i.e., sudden)
- Recurrences documented by ECG
  - Time to recurrence
  - Frequency of recurrences
- Tolerance
  - Symptoms
  - Blood pressure
  - Rate of tachycardia
- Necessity of nondrug interventions (e.g., ICD)
- Side effects of drugs/treatment complications
- Quality of life
- Economics
- Outcomes specific to tachycardia (e.g., ventricular rate, systemic embolism in atrial fibrillation)

REFERENCES

1. Wit AL, Rosen MR, Hoffman BF. Electrophysiology and pharmacology of cardiac arrhythmias. II. Relationship of normal and abnormal electrical activity of cardiac fibers to the genesis of arrhythmias. B. Reentry section I. Am Heart J 1974;88:664–670.
2. Wit AL, Rosen MR, Hoffman BF. Electrophysiology and pharmacology of cardiac arrhythmias. II. Relationship of normal and abnormal electrical activity in cardiac fibers to the genesis of arrhythmias. B. Reentry section II. Am Heart J 1974;88:798–806.
3. Allessie MA, Bonke FIM, Schopman FJG. Circus movement in rabbit atrial muscle as a mechanism of tachycardia III. The "leading circle" concept: A new model of circus movement in cardiac tissue without the involvement of an anatomic obstacle. Circ Res 1977;41:9–18.
4. El-Sherif N. The figure 8 model of reentrant excitation in the canine postinfarction heart, in Zipes DP, Jalife J (eds): Cardiac Electrophysiology and Arrhythmias. Orlando, FL, Grune and Stratton, 1985, pp 363–378.
5. Vaughn Williams EM. A classification of antiarrhythmic actions reassessed after a decade of new drugs. J Clin Pharmacol 1984;24:129–147.
6. Working Group on Arrhythmias of the European Society of Cardiology. The Sicilian Gambit. A new approach to the classification of antiarrhythmic drugs based upon their actions on arrhythmogenic mechanisms. Circulation 1991;84:1831–1851.
7. El-Sherif N, Scherlag BJ, Lazzara R, et al. Reentrant ventricular arrhythmias in the late myocardial infarction period 4. Mechanism of action of lidocaine. Circulation 1977;56:395–402.
8. Grant AO, Strauss LJ, Wallace AG, Strauss HC. The influence of pH on the electrophysiological effects of lidocaine in guinea pig ventricular myocardium. Circ Res 1980;47:542–550.
9. Evans DE, Gillis RA. Effect of diphenylhydantoin and lidocaine on cardiac arrhythmias induced by hypothalamic stimulation. J Pharmacol Exp Ther 1974;191:506–517.
10. Glicklich JI, Hoffman BF. Sites of action and active forms of lidocaine and some derivatives on cardiac Purkinje fibers. Am J Cardiol 1978;43:638–651.
11. Hondeghem LM, Katzung BG. Antiarrhythmic agents: The modulated receptor mechanism of action of sodium and calcium channel-blocking drugs. Ann Rev Pharmacol Toxicol 1984;24:387–423.
12. Heger JJ, Prystowsky EN, Jackman WM, et al. Amiodarone. Clinical efficacy and electrophysiology during long-term therapy for recurrent ventricular tachycardia or ventricular fibrillation. N Engl J Med 1981;305:539–545.
13. Kannel WB, Abbott RD, Savage DD, et al. Epidemiologic features of chronic atrial fibrillation. The Framingham study. N Engl J Med 1982;306:1018–1022.
14. Wolf PA, Dauber TA, Thomas EH, et al. Epidemiologic assessment of chronic atrial fibrillation and risk of stroke: The Framingham study. Neurology 1978;28:973–977.
15. Laupacia A, Albers G, Dunn M, Feinberg W. Antithrombotic therapy in atrial fibrillation. Chest 1992;102:426S–433S.
16. Kopecky SL, Gersh BJ, McGoon MD, et al. The natural history of lone atrial fibrillation: A population-based study over three decades. N Engl J Med 1987;317:669–674.
17. Falk RH, Leavitt JI. Digoxin for atrial fibrillation: A drug whose time has gone? Ann Intern Med 1991;114:573–575.
18. Roberts SA, Diaz C, Nolan PE, et al. Effectiveness and costs of digoxin treatment for atrial fibrillation and flutter. Am J Cardiol 1993;72:567–573.
19. Ellenbogen KA, Dias VC, Plumb VJ, et al. A placebo-controlled trial of continuous intravenous diltiazem infusion for 24-hour heart rate control during atrial fibrillation and atrial flutter. A multicenter study. J Am Coll Cardiol 1991;18:891–897.
20. Barbarash R, Bauman JL, Srebro J, et al. Verapamil infusions in the treatment of atrial tachyarrhythmias. Crit Care Med 1986;14:886–888.
21. Bauman JL, Bauernfeind RA, Hoff JV, et al. Torsades de pointes due to quinidine: Observations in 31 patients. Am Heart J 1984;107:425–430.
22. Mann DL, Maisel AS, Atwood JE, et al. Absence of cardioversion-induced ventricular arrhythmias in patients with therapeutic digoxin levels. J Am Coll Cardiol 1985;5:882–890.
23. The Stroke Prevention in Atrial Fibrillation Investigators. Stroke prevention in atrial fibrillation: Final results. Circulation 1991;84:527–539.
24. The Stroke Prevention in Atrial Fibrillation Investigators. Warfarin versus aspirin for prevention of thromboembolism in atrial fibrillation: Stroke Prevention in Atrial Fibrillation II Study. Lancet 1994;343:687–691.
25. Coplen SE, Antman EM, Berlin JA, et al. Efficacy and safety of quinidine therapy for maintenance of sinus rhythm after cardioversion: A meta-analysis of randomized control trials. Circulation 1990;82:1106–1116.
26. Flaker GC, Blackshear JL, McBride R, et al. Antiarrhythmic drug therapy and cardiac mortality in atrial fibrillation. J Am Coll Cardiol 1992;20:527–532.
27. Anderson JL, Gilbert EM, Alpert BL, et al. Prevention of symptomatic recurrences of paroxysmal atrial fibrillation in patients initially tolerating therapy. A multicenter, double-blind, crossover study of flecainide and placebo with trans-telephonic monitoring. Circulation 1989;80:1557–1570.
28. Antman EM, Beamer AD, Cantillion C, et al. Long-term oral propafenone therapy for suppression of refractory symptomatic atrial fibrillation and atrial flutter. J Am Coll Cardiol 1988;12:1005–1011.
29. Echt DS, Liebson PR, Mitchell B, et al. Mortality and morbidity in patients receiving encainide, flecainide, or placebo. The cardiac arrhythmia suppression trial. N Engl J Med 1991;324:781–788.
30. Morganroth J, Horowitz LN. Flecainide: Its proarrhythmic effect and expected changes on the surface electrocardiogram. Am J Cardiol 1984;53:89B–94B.
31. Falk RH. Flecainide-induced ventricular tachycardia and fibrillation in patients treated for atrial fibrillation. Ann Intern Med 1989;111:107–111.
32. Phillips BG, Bauman JL. Prescribing trends and pharmacoeconomic considerations of antiarrhythmic drugs: A focus on atrial fibrillation and flutter. Pharmacoecon 1995;7:521–533.

33. Gosselink ATM, Crijns HJM, VanGelder IC, et al. Low-dose amiodarone for maintenance of sinus rhythm after cardioversion of atrial fibrillation or flutter. JAMA 1992;267:3289–3292.
34. Juul-Moller S, Edvardsson N, Rehnqvist-Ahlberg N. Sotalol versus quinidine for the maintenance of sinus rhythm after direct current conversion of atrial fibrillation. Circulation 1990;82:1932–1939.
35. Sung RJ, Lauer MR, Chun H. Atrioventricular node reentry: Current concepts and new perspectives. PACE 1994;17:1413–1430.
36. Lown B, Ganong WF, Levine SA. Syndrome of short PR interval, normal QRS complex and paroxysmal rapid heart action. Circulation 1952;5:693–706.
37. Wolff L, Parkinson J, White PD. Bundle branch block with short PR interval in healthy young people prone to paroxysmal tachycardia. Am Heart J 1930;51:685–704.
38. Klein GJ, Bashore TM, Sellers TD, et al. Ventricular fibrillation in the Wolff–Parkinson–White syndrome. N Engl J Med 1979;301:1080–1085.
39. Wu D, Amat-y-Leon F, Denes P, et al. Demonstration of sustained sinus and atrial reentry as a mechanism of paroxysmal supraventricular tachycardia. Circulation 1975;51:234–243.
40. Bauernfeind RA, Wyndham CR, Dhingra RC, et al. Serial electrophysiologic testing of multiple drugs in patients with atrioventricular nodal reentrant paroxysmal tachycardia. Circulation 1980;62:1341–1349.
41. Wu D, Amat-y-Leon F, Simpson R, et al. Electrophysiological studies with multiple drugs in patients with atrioventricular reentrant tachycardias utilizing an extra nodal pathway. Circulation 1977;56:727–736.
42. DiMarco JP, Miles W, Akhtar M, et al. Adenosine for paroxysmal supraventricular tachycardia: Dose ranging and comparison with verapamil. Assessment in placebo-controlled, multicenter trials. Ann Intern Med 1990;1113:104–110.
43. Emergency Cardiac Care Committee and Subcommittee, American Heart Association. Guidelines for cardiopulmonary resuscitation and emergency care. JAMA 1992;268:2199–2241.
44. Rankin AC, McGovern BA. Adenosine or verapamil for the acute treatment of supraventricular tachycardia? Ann Intern Med 1991;114:513–515.
45. Hoon TJ, Bauman JL, Rodvold KA, et al. The pharmacodynamic and pharmacokinetic differences of the *d*- and *l*-isomers of verapamil: Implications in the treatment of PSVT. Am Heart J 1986;112:396–403.
46. Bauernfeind RA, Swiryn S, Petropolous AT, et al. Concordance and discordance of drug responses in atrioventricular reentrant tachycardia. J Am Coll Cardiol 1983;2:345–350.
47. Jackman WM, Wang Z, Friday KJ, et al. Catheter ablation of accessory atrioventricular pathways (Wolff–Parkinson–White syndrome) by radiofrequency current. N Engl J Med 1991;324:1605–1611.
48. Jackman WM, Beckman KJ, McClelland JH, et al. Treatment of supraventricular tachycardia due to atrioventricular nodal reentry by radiofrequency catheter ablation of slow pathway conduction. N Engl J Med 1992;327:313–318.
49. Scheinman MM. Radiofrequency catheter ablation for patients with supraventricular tachycardia. PACE 1993;16:671–679.
50. Scheinman MM, Basu D, Hollenburg M. Electrophysiologic studies in patients with persistent atrial tachycardia. Circulation 1974;50:266–273.
51. Kastor JA. Multifocal atrial tachycardia. N Engl J Med 1990;322:1713–1717.
52. Levine JH, Michael JR, Guarnier T. Treatment of multifocal atrial tachycardia with verapamil. N Engl J Med 1985;312:21–25.
53. Ruberman W, Weinblatt E, Goldberg JD, et al. Ventricular premature beats and mortality after myocardial infarction. N Engl J Med 1977;297:750–757.
54. Lown B, Fakhro AM, Hood WB, et al. The coronary care unit. JAMA 1967;199:156–166.
55. Lown B, Wolf M. Approaches to sudden death from coronary heart disease. Circulation 1971;44:130–142.
56. Winkle RA. Antiarrhythmic drug effect mimicked by spontaneous variability of ventricular ectopy. Circulation 1978;57:1116–1121.
57. Morganroth J, Michelson EL, Horowitz LN, et al. Limitations of routine electrocardiographic monitoring to assess ventricular ectopic frequency. Circulation 1978;58:408–414.
58. Myerburg RJ, Conde C, Sheps DS, et al. Antiarrhythmic drug therapy in survivors of hospital cardiac arrest: Comparison of effects on chronic ventricular arrhythmias and recurrent cardiac arrest. Circulation 1979;59:855–863.
59. Kosowsky BD, Taylor J, Lown B, et al. Long-term procaine amide following acute myocardial infarction. Circulation 1973;47:1204–1210.
60. Bauman JL, Gallastegui J, Strasberg B, et al. Long-term therapy with disopyramide phosphate: Side effects and effectiveness. Am Heart J 1986;111:654–660.
61. Podrid PJ, Schoeneburger A, Lown B. Congestive heart failure caused by oral disopyramide. N Engl J Med 1980;302:614–617.
62. Dusman RE, Stanton MS, Miles WM, et al. Clinical features of amiodarone-induced pulmonary toxicity. Circulation 1990;82:51–59.
63. McCollam PL, Parker RB, Beckman KJ, et al. Proarrhythmia: A paradoxic response to antiarrhythmic agents. Pharmacotherapy 1989;9:144–153.
64. The Cardiac Arrhythmia Suppression Trial II Investigators. Effect of the antiarrhythmic agent moricizine on survival after myocardial infarction. N Engl J Med 1992;327:227–233.
65. Ceremuzynski L, Kleczar E, Drzeminska-Pakula M, et al. Effect of amiodarone on mortality after myocardial infarction: A double-blind, placebo-controlled, pilot study. J Am Coll Cardiol 1992;20:1056–1062.
66. Wellens HJJ, Duren DR, Lie KI. Observations on mechanisms of ventricular tachycardia in man. Circulation 1976;54:237–244.
67. Horowitz LN, Josephson ME, Farshidi A, et al. Recurrent sustained ventricular tachycardia 3. Role of electrophysiologic study in selection of antiarrhythmic regimens. Circulation 1978;58:986–997.
68. Bauman JL, Schoen MD, Hoon TJ. Practical optimization of antiarrhythmic drug therapy using pharmacokinetic principles. Clin Pharmacokinet 1991;20:151–166.
69. Wellens HJJ, Brugada P, Stevenson LUG. Programmed electrical stimulation of the heart in patients with life-

threatening arrhythmias: What is the significance of induced arrhythmias and what is the correct stimulation protocol? Circulation 1985;72:1–7.

70. Greenspan AM, Spielman SR, Webb CR, et al. Efficacy of combination therapy with mexiletine and a type Ia agent for inducible ventricular tachyarrhythmias secondary to coronary artery disease. Am J Cardiol 1985;56:277–284.
71. Winkle RA: Amiodarone and the American way. J Am Coll Cardiol 1985;6:822–824.
72. Mitchell LB, Duff HJ, Manyari DE, et al. A randomized clinical trial of the noninvasive and invasive approaches to drug therapy of ventricular tachycardia. N Engl J Med 1987;317:1681–1687.
73. Mason JW and the Electrophysiologic Study versus Electrocardiographic Monitoring Investigators. A comparison of electrophysiologic testing with Holter monitoring to predict antiarrhythmic drug efficacy for ventricular tachyarrhythmias. N Engl J Med 1993;329:445–451.
74. Mason JW and the Electrophysiologic Study versus Electrocardiographic Monitoring Investigators. A comparison of seven antiarrhythmic drugs in patients with ventricular tachyarrhythmias. N Engl J Med 1993;329:452–458.
75. Zipes DP. Cardiac electrophysiology: Promises and contributions. J Am Coll Cardiol 1989;13:1329–1352.
76. Powell AC, Fuchs T, Finklestein DM, et al. Influence of implantable cardioverter–defibrillators on long-term prognosis of survivors of out-of-hospital cardiac arrest. Circulation 1993;88:1083–1092.
77. Tworek DA, Nazari J, Ezri M, Bauman JL. Interference by antiarrhythmic agents with the function of electrical cardiac devices. Clin Pharm 1992;11:48–56.
78. Kim SG, Fisher JD, Furman S, et al. Benefits of implantable defibrillators are overestimated by sudden death rates and better represented by the total arrhythmic death rate. J Am Coll Cardiol 1991;17:1587–1592.
79. Mitra RI, Buxton AE. The clinical significance of nonsustained ventricular tachycardia. J Cardiovasc Electrophys 1993;4:490–496.
80. Wilber DJ, Olshansky B, Moran JF, et al. Electrophysiological testing and nonsustained ventricular tachycardia. Use and limitations in patients with coronary artery disease and impaired ventricular function. Circulation 1990;82:350–358.
81. Gomes JA, Winters SL, Stewart D, et al. A new noninvasive index to predict sustained ventricular tachycardia and sudden death in the first year after myocardial infarction: Based on signal-averaged electrocardiogram, radionuclide ejection fraction and holter monitoring. J Am Coll Cardiol 1987;10:349–357.
82. Herre JM, Titus C, Oeff M, et al. Inefficacy and proarrhythmic effects of flecainide and encainide for sustained ventricular tachycardia and ventricular fibrillation. Ann Intern Med 1990;113:671–676.
83. Soffer J, Dreifus LS, Michelson EL, et al. Polymorphous ventricular tachycardia associated with normal and long QT intervals. Am J Cardiol 1982;49:2021–2029.
84. Oberg KC, O'Toole MF, Gallastegui JL, Bauman JL. "Late" proarrhythmia due to quinidine. Am J Cardiol 1994;74:192–194.
85. Tzivoni D, Banai S, Schuger C, et al. Treatment of torsades de pointes with magnesium sulfate. Circulation 1987;77:392–397.
86. Schwartz PJ. Idiopathic long QT syndrome: Progress and questions. Am Heart J 1985;109:399–415.
87. Zipes DP, Heger JJ, Prystowsky EN. Sudden cardiac death. Am J Med 1981;70:1151–1153.
88. Ruskin JN, DiMarco JP, Garan H. Out-of-hospital cardiac arrest. Electrophysiologic observation and selection of long-term antiarrhythmic therapy. N Engl J Med 1980;303:607–613.
89. Lie KI, Wellens HJJ, Van Capelle FJ. Lidocaine in the prevention of primary ventricular fibrillation. N Engl J Med 1974;291:1324–1326.
90. MacMahon S, Collin R, Peto R, et al. Effects of prophylactic lidocaine in suspected acute myocardial infarction. An overview of results from the randomized controlled trials. JAMA 1988;260:1910–1916.
91. Antman EM, Berlin JA. Declining incidence of ventricular fibrillation in myocardial infarction. Implications for the prophylactic use of lidocaine. Circulation 1992;86:764–773.
92. Horner SM. Efficacy of intravenous magnesium in acute myocardial infarction in reducing arrhythmias and mortality. Meta-analysis of magnesium in acute myocardial infarction. Circulation 1992;86:774–779.
93. Woods KL, Fletcher S, Roffe C, Haider Y. A randomized trial of intravenous magnesium sulfate in suspected acute myocardial infarction: Results of the second Leicester Intravenous Magnesium Intervention Trial (LIMIT-2). Lancet 1992;339:1553–1558.
94. Brown CG, Martin DR, Pepe PE, et al. A comparison of standard-dose and high dose epinephrine in cardiac arrest outside the hospital. N Engl J Med 1992;327:1051–1055.
95. Ferrer MI. The sick sinus syndrome. Circulation 1973;47:635–647.
96. Talano JV, Euler D, Randall WC, et al. Sinus node dysfunction. An overview with emphasis on autonomic and pharmacologic consideration. Am J Med 1978;64:773–781.
97. Sugrue DD, Gersh BJ, Holmes DR, et al. Symptomatic "isolated" carotid sinus hypersensitivity: Natural history and results of treatment with anticholinergic drugs or pacemaker. J Am Coll Cardiol 1986;7:158–162.
98. Strasberg B, Sagie A, Erdman S, et al. Carotid sinus hypersensitivity and the carotid sinus syndrome. Prog Cardiovasc Dis 1989;31:379–391.
99. Milstein S, Reyes WJ, Benditt DG. Upright body tilt for evaluation of patients with recurrent, unexplained syncope. PACE 1989;12:117–124.
100. Almquist A, Goldenberg I, Milstein S. Provocation of bradycardia and hypotension by isoproterenol and upright posture in patients with unexplained syncope. N Engl J Med 1990;320:346–351.

Chapter 17

The Cardiomyopathies

Jean Nappi, PharmD, FCCP, BCPS

The cardiomyopathies represent a variety of diseases affecting the myocardium in either a diffuse or multifocal manner that frequently results in heart failure. The terminology and classification used for the cardiomyopathies have undergone change over the years and can be confusing because there is some overlap among the diseases and/or classification schemes. In the truest sense, a patient with cardiomyopathy has a heart muscle disease of unknown cause. However, cardiomyopathies are sometimes defined according to etiology, as primary or secondary forms. Primary cardiomyopathies are those disorders where either the structure or the function of the myocardium is affected in the *absence* of other known causes of heart disease or systemic diseases known to affect the heart. Secondary forms of cardiomyopathy are conditions where the myocardial abnormality is due to a recognized factor. Infectious agents, inflammation, metabolic disorders, infiltrative diseases, and toxins are a few of the causative factors of secondary cardiomyopathy. In some cases, secondary cardiomyopathy is also referred to as "specific heart muscle disease."[1,2]

Many times a specific etiology is not evident. Therefore, another commonly used categorization of the cardiomyopathies is made on the basis of the structural and/or functional abnormalities present. The three groups of cardiomyopathies are usually described as dilated (congestive), hypertrophic, and restrictive (obliterative) (Fig. 17.1). An understanding of the pathophysiologic basis for each type of cardiomyopathy leads to a rational selection of drug therapy or other treatment modality. The characteristics for each type of cardiomyopathy are presented in Table 17.1. The distinction among the cardiomyopathies is not absolute and there is some overlap in the functional abnormalities.

In dilated cardiomyopathy (DCM) the cardinal feature is dilatation of the ventricles. Systolic function is typically abnormal, leading to a decreased cardiac output. In the past, the term congestive cardiomyopathy was frequently used. In those patients with hypertrophic cardiomyopathy (HCM), the ventricular cavity is not dilated and the ventricular muscle mass is increased. Ventricular cavity size is normal or decreased and systolic function is often preserved. Patients with HCM may have an obstructive or nonobstructive form. Patients with restrictive or obliterative cardiomyopathy have inadequate ventricular compliance causing abnormal ventricular filling or diastolic dysfunction due to endocardial and/or myocardial disease. The clinical presentation is similar to one with constrictive pericarditis.

Other terms are frequently encountered in discussions of patients with cardiomyopathy. Familial cardiomyopathy is used to denote a condition found in more than one family member. Genetic predisposition may occur in all three functional types. Ischemic cardiomyopathy is another frequently used term. Patients with occlusive atherosclerotic coronary artery disease and left ventricular dysfunction are said to have ischemic cardiomyopathy. Ischemic cardiomyopathy is not a true cardiomyopathy since there is an identifiable cause of the ventricular muscle dysfunction.

Myocardial hypertrophy is one of the most important adaptive measures that the failing heart uses to compensate for pressure and volume overload conditions. However, these hypertrophied cells are not normal and this "cardiomyopathy of overload" may eventually lead to myocardial cell deterioration and death.[3] The role of altered gene expression in the hypertrophied myocardium is an area of extensive research.

Dilated Cardiomyopathy

Dilated cardiomyopathy is the most common of the cardiomyopathies. DCM occurs in people of all ages worldwide, however it is more frequent in African Americans and men, particularly those of middle age.[4,5] In the majority of patients the cause is unknown, however there are over 75 specific diseases of the heart muscle that can lead to DCM. DCM is characterized by systolic pump failure (ejection fraction <0.4) and dilatation of the ventricles. Mural thrombi frequently occur in the left ventricle or atrial appendages. In many patients there is no known cause and in that case, the term *idiopathic dilated cardiomyopathy* is

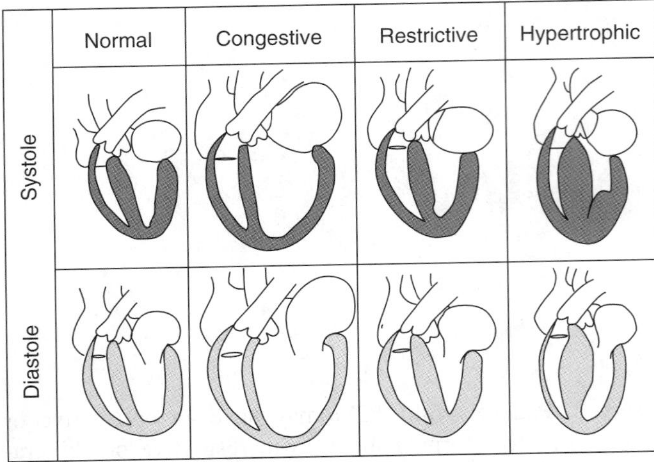

Figure 17.1. Illustration of the 50° left anterior oblique views of the heart in the different types of cardiomyopathy at end-systole and end-diastole. The radionuclide features of each type are discussed in the text. *(From Goldman MR, Boucher CA. Value of radionuclide imaging techniques in assessing cardiomyopathy. Am J Cardiol 1980;46:1232–1236, with permission.)*

used. There are, however, many known conditions that are associated with the development of DCM. Some of these conditions are chronic alcoholism (alcoholic cardiomyopathy), pregnancy or the postpartal period (peripartum or postpartum cardiomyopathy), the administration of anthracyclines (anthracycline cardiomyopathy), selenium deficiency (Keshan disease), and occlusive coronary artery disease (ischemic cardiomyopathy).[6]

PATHOPHYSIOLOGY

In addition to dilatation of the ventricles and poor ventricular contractility, patients with DCM have an increase in myocardial mass and elevated left (and sometimes right) ventricular pressures. The pathophysiologic changes seen in patients with DCM are the same as those in patients with heart failure from other known causes (see Chapter 13). There are short-term and long-term compensatory responses to the decrease in cardiac performance. What may be beneficial to sustain cardiac output for a short period of time may be detrimental if sustained over a prolonged period.

There are several proposed mechanisms whereby the compensatory responses may ultimately cause harm.[3] First, the neurohormonal stimulation that leads to an increase in cytosolic calcium concentrations may overload the systems responsible for removing calcium. Calcium is actively taken from the myofibrils and cardiac muscle sarcoplasm and pumped back into the sarcoplasmic reticulum and extracellularly during diastole. This intracellular calcium overload may impair normal relaxation of the ventricle and impair filling during diastole. In addition, the increase in intracellular calcium may play a role in the genesis of arrhythmias. The increase in calcium would also lead to an increase in energy expenditure by the heart, which is already imbalanced in the setting of heart failure.

The failing heart also loses its ability to respond to sympathetic neurotransmitters. This is partially explained by the decrease in total β-adrenergic receptor density (also known as down-regulation).[3,7] The human heart contains both β_1 and β_2 receptors in a ratio of approximately 80 : 20 ($\beta_1 : \beta_2$). The β_1-adrenergic receptor density is decreased by approximately 60–70% in the failing heart, changing the $\beta_1 : \beta_2$ ratio to 60 : 40. Although the density of the β_2 receptor is unchanged, the receptor is partially "uncoupled" from the adenylate cyclase enzyme. While desensitization of the β-adrenergic system blunts the response of the failing heart to sympathetic stimulation, other biochemical processes leading to increased inotropy are intact. It is not clear whether the desensitization of the β-adrenergic receptors is beneficial or harmful in patients with heart failure.

TABLE 17.1. CHARACTERISTICS OF THE CARDIOMYOPATHIES

	Dilated	Hypertrophic	Restrictive
Myocardial mass	↑ → ↑↑	↑↑↑	nl → ↑
Ventricular cavity size	↑↑ → ↑↑↑↑	↓↓ → nl	nl → ↓
Contractile function	↓↓↓	↑↑ → ↓	nl → ↓
LV filling pressure	↑↑	nl → ↑	↑
Chest x-ray	Moderate to marked cardiac enlargement	Mild to moderate cardiac enlargement	Mild cardiac enlargement
Electrocardiogram	ST- and T-wave abnormalities	ST- and T-wave abnormalities, left ventricular hypertrophy	Low voltage, conduction defects
Echocardiogram	LV dilatation and dysfunction	Asymmetric septal hypertrophy, systolic anterior motion of the mitral valve	Increased LV wall thickness possible
Radionuclide studies	LV dilatation and dysfunction	Vigorous systolic function	Normal systolic function

Key: ↑, increased; ↓, decreased; nl, normal; LV, left ventricular. (Modified from Refs. 1 and 4.)

Although it was thought that the adaptive mechanism of hypertrophy was intended to preserve myocardial function, it may ultimately be detrimental. The hypertrophy that occurs in response to heart failure can exacerbate the energy production and energy expenditure imbalance. The distance between the capillaries and the impaired diffusion of substrates is particularly problematic in underperfused regions such as the subendocardial portion of the left ventricle. Myofibrils, which are energy consumers, take up a larger portion of the cell relative to the energy providing mitochondria. This further leads to the chronic energy deprivation of the myocardium. Myocyte necrosis stimulates the proliferation of fibroblasts, which replace myocardial tissue with connective tissue. Patients with DCM have an increase in intramyocardial fibrillar collagen that may adversely affect ventricular compliance.[8] Measuring extracellular matrix turnover, which may be derived from fibrosis of the myocardium, may be used in the future for risk stratification and prognosis of patients with DCM.[9]

At the molecular level, there is a growing body of knowledge that suggests changes in gene expression occur by the cells of the failing myocardium. It has been suggested that up to 20% of the cases of idiopathic DCM may be familial. Autosomal dominant, autosomal recessive, and X-linked transmission have been reported.[10] An increased frequency of the angiotensin-converting enzyme (ACE) *DD* genotype has been noted in patients with IDC. DCM is also commonly seen in patients with Duchenne muscular dystrophy and may be related to specific mutations of the Xp21 locus of the dystrophin gene. In addition, in patients with chronic heart failure, the synthesis of the myosin heavy chains, which determine ATPase activity, is altered. Interestingly, the abnormal gene responsible for HCM is located on chromosome 14, where the cardiac myosin heavy chains map.[3]

It has also been noted that there is a 30–40% increase in the activity of the inhibitory guanine nucleotide-binding protein (G_i proteins) in myocardial cells in failing hearts. The change in the G_i protein blunts the response of the failing heart to sympathetic stimulation.[3,7] Furthermore, there is increasing evidence for the existence of anti-β-receptor antibodies that inhibit adenylate cylase activity in some patients with DCM.[11] The presence of these antibodies has been linked to specific human leukocyte antigen (HLA) phenotypes. Further studies are needed to clarify these findings.

Alcohol consumption causes an acute depressant effect on myocardial contractility, even in normal subjects.[12] Impaired early filling of the left ventricle due to delayed relaxation has been noted in asymptomatic alcoholics.[13] This diastolic dysfunction may be one of the earliest signs of alcoholic cardiomyopathy. Although a direct causal relation between alcohol ingestion and heart disease is well supported, the mechanism by which chronic alcohol consumption may cause progressive cardiomyopathy is not known. Alcoholic cardiomyopathy is indistinguishable from idiopathic dilated cardiomyopathy except that it may be reversible if alcohol consumption is completely stopped.[1] The amount of alcohol necessary to cause permanent damage is highly variable. Other factors, such as concomitant nutritional deficiencies, may also play a role.

Selenium deficiency has been noted to cause cardiomyopathy (Keshan disease) in China and may also be a cause of increased platelet aggregation. Selenium appears to be required for normal immune function in some species. In the United States, selenium deficiency might occur in the setting of prolonged total parenteral nutrition.[6] Hypophosphatemia, hypocalcemia, beriberi, pellagra, scurvy, and carnitine deficiency have also been identified as affecting cardiac function.[1,2]

Both myocarditis and DCM may present as new and unexplained symptoms of heart failure or ventricular arrhythmias.[14,15] Some patients who have viral myocarditis go on to develop DCM. An autoimmune response triggered by aberration in the induction of the major histocompatibility complex-antigen expression could be responsible for the acute insult as well as disease progression.[5] Serologic studies have shown that patients with myocarditis or DCM have a higher incidence of antibodies to a variety of viruses, particularly coxsackie virus B.[14] Some patients with myocarditis may also have antibodies against myosin.[16] Many viral, bacterial, protozoal and fungal organisms have been identified as potential causes of myocarditis.[17] The incidence of DCM following biopsy-proven myocarditis has been estimated to be as high as 25–50%. However, this incidence may be overestimated since many cases of myocarditis are asymptomatic and never diagnosed. The true natural history of myocarditis is poorly defined. It has been suggested that there are immunoregulatory defects (abnormalities in suppressor T-cell function and reduction in natural killer cells) in patients with DCM or myocarditis. These defects could lead to an exaggerated immune response and unchecked myocardial inflammation.

It is well known that there is a relationship between certain drugs and the development of cardiomyopathy. Doxorubicin (Adriamycin) produces a dose-related cardiomyopathy. Although it is frequently cited that the dose of doxorubicin should not exceed 550 mg/m^2, this upper limit can and should be individualized based on cardiac catheterization and endomyocardial biopsy findings. There is considerable amount of variability among patients with regard to the damage seen and the dose received. In addition to the cumulative anthracycline dose, radiation to the mediastinal area will also influence the predisposition to cardiomyopathy, such that patients receiving prior radiation will have an upper limit doxorubicin dose of approximately 250 mg/m^2.[18] The degree of myocardial cell damage found with biopsy is proportional to the dose received; however, myocardial function is preserved until a threshold dose or critical amount of damage occurs. This means that a certain amount of myocardial damage must occur before cardiac function is affected. Once this deterioration process begins, however, it will proceed quite rapidly. There have been rare reports of reversibility of the left ventricular dysfunction. The latency period from the time that the doxorubicin is given until patient presents with signs of heart failure can be quite variable. Usually the cardiomyopathy occurs 1 to 6 months following the cessation of therapy; however, it has been described as occurring as late as 7 years after treatment.[19]

It has been suggested that rest and exercise evaluations of left ventricular ejection fraction be performed in order to assess risk for anthracycline cardiomyopathy. In patients with no risk factors (i.e., no radiation, heart disease, hypertension, or advanced age), these assessments may be delayed until the patient has received a doxorubicin dose of 450 mg/m^2.[20] In patients with risk factors present, an assessment of left ventricular ejection fraction should be made at rest and during exercise at periodic intervals with the first assessment prior to the third dose.

A number of methods are available that attempt to decrease the incidence of anthracycline cardiotoxicity. Alterations in dosing schedules have increased the cumulative amount of anthracycline that patients can tolerate. It appears that the risk of cardiotoxicity of doxorubicin is related to the peak serum drug concentrations, whereas the antitumor effect is related to the area under the curve.[21] Although the optimal dosing schedule has yet to be established, there is evidence that short-term intravenous infusions given over 4–5 days have decreased toxicity and maintained or enhanced the antitumor effect of the drug.[22] Infusions given over 96 hours have allowed more patients to receive higher amounts of doxorubicin. The mechanism by which the anthracyclines cause cardiac toxicity is thought to result from drug-induced free radical formation. Doxorubicin is able to chelate iron and the resulting iron complex can bind to DNA and cell membranes and catalyze the cleavage of hydrogen peroxide to the hydroxyl radical.[21] Bispiperazinedione (ICRF-187), an iron chelator, may offer protection against the cardiotoxicity of doxorubicin.[21,23] There are many newer anthracycline analogs being investigated, some of which are reported to have less cardiotoxicity than doxorubicin.

Those patients with ischemic cardiomyopathy may have a form of DCM that is characterized by discrete but multifocal sites of myocardial damage. Coronary artery disease is usually severe and widespread. Necrosis due to infarction places a demand on the surviving tissue to sustain cardiac function. This is done through the process of hypertrophy of the myocytes and hyperplasia of the interstitial fibroblasts and endothelial cells.[24] Unfortunately, there is usually inadequate growth of the vascular beds to sustain this hypertrophied tissue, leading to continued ischemia and necrosis. Pump function is generally reduced in direct proportion to the amount of necrosed myocardium. It remains to be determined if the hypertrophy that develops is a compensatory process or just another step in the progression of cardiac failure. Additionally, data suggest that patients with ischemic cardiomyopathy have impaired responsiveness to stimulation by isoproteranol that is disproportionate to the degree of β-receptor down-regulation. This increased uncoupling of the β-adrenergic receptor pathway may be the result of an increase in the activity of inhibitory G proteins.[7] Persistent left ventricular dysfunction in the absence of tissue necrosis is referred to as "hibernating myocardium."[25] Improvement in ventricular function is possible, even after years of impairment, if revascularization is successful.

The cardiomyopathy associated with pregnancy frequently develops during the latter part of pregnancy or within the first few months after delivery. Some women will spontaneously recover whereas others will have a rapidly fatal course. In one study of 26 matched female patients, significant differences between patients with idiopathic DCM and patients with peripartum cardiomyopathy were described.[26] Both groups of women had high elevated filling pressures. Right-sided filling pressures tended to be higher in the dilated cardiomyopathy group but the difference was not statistically significant. The patients with peripartum cardiomyopathy had a higher mean cardiac index, with three patients having a cardiac index level above the upper limit of normal. The patients with peripartum cardiomyopathy had a significantly lower mean systemic vascular resistance and lower right ventricular stroke work index when compared to the women with DCM. It would appear that peripartum cardiomyopathy does not have a homogenous hemodynamic presentation. There is a subset of patients with peripartum cardiomyopathy who have high output cardiac failure. Prior myocarditis may play a role in some patients. Women who recover should be encouraged to avoid further pregnancies, especially if cardiomegaly persists.[1]

CLINICAL PRESENTATION

The signs and symptoms are similar to those seen in patients with congestive heart failure (see Chapter 13). The onset of heart failure is frequently insidious and commonly manifests initially as dyspnea. Fatigue, orthopnea, paroxysmal nocturnal dyspnea, peripheral edema, tachycardia, and palpitations gradually appear in most patients. Chest pain occurs in one-fourth to one-half of patients consistent with myocardial ischemia despite normal coronary arteries.[4] Typical auscultatory findings include systolic murmurs secondary to mitral regurgitation and a third heart sound or a summation gallop. Although the heart is increased in weight, the thickness of the left ventricular free wall is diminished due to the ventricular dilatation.

Blood gases will show a reduced oxygen saturation of the mixed venous blood sample, resulting in a high arteriovenous oxygen difference. Elevated pulmonary artery pressure may ultimately lead to right-sided heart failure. Patients may suffer from thromboembolic complications as a result of the mural thrombi that form in either the left or right side of the heart.

The chest roentgenogram demonstrates cardiac enlargement due to dilatation of both ventricles. The atria may also be enlarged. There may be pulmonary vascular redistribution changes and pleural and pericardial effusions. The electrocardiogram may have nonspecific ST-T-wave changes. Sinus tachycardia is frequently present. Atrial fibrillation is common, as is left bundle branch block. Frequent ventricular ectopy and nonsustained ventricular tachycardia have been noted.[4] Gated blood pool scans (radionuclide angiography) will show that the ventricles have a global or homogeneous reduction in wall motion. The ejection fraction may be as low as 10%. Myocardial imaging with thallium or positron emission tomography are helpful in distinguishing nonischemic dilated cardiomyopathy from congestive heart failure due to repeated myocardial infarction (ischemic cardiomyopathy).[27]

DIAGNOSIS

The diagnosis of dilated cardiomyopathy is usually one of exclusion. The differential diagnosis includes other causes of congestive heart failure, specifically atherosclerotic heart disease, hypertensive heart disease, valvular disease, and heart muscle disease secondary to other systemic disease. Ischemic cardiomyopathy is more commonly seen in the United States than idiopathic cardiomyopathy. The opposite is true in the underdeveloped nations of the world. In Central and South America, Chagas' disease, which can present as DCM, is caused by *Trypanosoma cruzi.* Other infectious agents known to cause DCM include coxsackievirus B, coxsackievirus A, echovirus, poliovirus, arboviruses, *Toxoplasma gondii, Mycoplasma pneumoniae,* varicella, influenza, rabies, cytomegalovirus, *Cryptococcus neoformans, Candida albicans, Trichinella spiralis, Schistosoma mansoni, Corynbacterium diphtheriae,* and *Neisseria meningitidis* among others.[28]

Echocardiography is the most useful initial diagnostic tool.[5] Left ventricular dilatation and global hypokinesis are common. An ejection fraction below 45% is generally required for diagnosis. Hemodynamic studies will reveal a reduced cardiac output that does not increase normally with exercise. Left ventricular end-diastolic, left atrial, and pulmonary capillary wedge pressures are usually elevated. When right-sided heart failure is present, the right ventricular end-diastolic, right atrial, and central venous pressures will be elevated. The coronary arteries are usually normal. Coronary angiography may be necessary to differentiate idiopathic DCM from ischemic cardiomyopathy.[4]

The results of an endomyocardial biopsy tend to be nonspecific in most cases of DCM. Biopsy may be helpful if there is a suspicion of active myocarditis and specific inflammatory changes are seen. Other indications for endomyocardial biopsy are for the detection of anthracycline cardiotoxicity, cardiac involvement in systemic diseases like amyloidosis and sarcoidosis, and for the diagnosis of rejection following cardiac transplantation.[15]

NATURAL HISTORY/PROGNOSIS

Approximately 20,000 new cases of DCM are diagnosed each year in the United States.[7] The natural history of DCM can be quite variable. Survival data from tertiary referral centers estimated that 25–30% of patients die within 1 year, whereas stabilization or even improvement may be seen in 20–50% of patients. More recent data suggest a 5-year mortality rate closer to 20%.[5] The usual course for DCM is steadily downhill until death from progressive pump failure. Some patients will die suddenly, presumably from ventricular tachycardia/fibrillation. The prognosis depends primarily on the severity of left ventricular dysfunction at the time of diagnosis. Left bundle branch block has been found to be an adverse prognostic indicator by some investigators. Ventricular arrhythmias are common in patients with DCM, but their significance is unclear. The severity of left ventricular dysfunction seems to be a more accurate and consistent predictor of sudden cardiac death than are studies using ambulatory electrocardiographic recordings (Holter monitoring), programmed electrical stimulation (electrophysiologic testing), or signal-averaged electrocardiograms.[7,29]

TREATMENT

When a patient first presents with the signs and symptoms of cardiomyopathy, other causes or conditions associated with cardiomyopathy should first be excluded. A systemic disorder with myocardial involvement can usually be excluded by a thorough history and physical examination with appropriate laboratory studies. Pericardial disease can be identified by echocardiography or other cardiac imaging studies. Ischemic cardiomyopathy is determined by performing a coronary angiogram. It may be more appropriate to treat the underlying cause or condition rather than the patient's symptoms.

Specific therapy for DCM is not available since the cause of the condition is usually not known. Patients with DCM are generally treated in the same manner as those with congestive heart failure (see Chapter 13). Therapy is aimed at improving the signs and symptoms of heart failure manifested by the patient. This would include sodium restriction, diuretics, vasodilators, and inotropic agents, which are not discussed in detail in this chapter. Nonpharmacologic therapy includes avoiding strenuous activity. Alcohol should be completely avoided (particularly in the case of alcoholic cardiomyopathy). Pregnancy is not advised in women with a history of peripartal cardiomyopathy.[1]

Immunosuppression

When a patient presents with the recent onset of the signs and symptoms of heart failure and no apparent cause, the differential diagnosis is frequently between myocarditis and the early phase of DCM.[15] This distinction is important if one believes that treating myocarditis with immunosuppression could be beneficial. The exact relationship between myocarditis and DCM has yet to be established. However, endomyocardial biopsy findings consistent with the diagnosis of myocarditis can be found in some patients (ranging from 0–67%) with recent onset of symptoms suggesting DCM.[17] The large range among studies may be due to a variety of factors; two important ones being different diagnostic criteria used and the length of time from the onset of symptoms to the time of biopsy. Although specific criteria for endomyocardial biopsy (Dallas Classification System) have been established for making the diagnosis of myocarditis, the true incidence of the disease is difficult to assess. There is a possibility that patchy or focal myocarditis may exist and that due to sampling error, the diagnosis is missed when performing endomyocardial biopsy. There is controversy as to whether the right or the left ventricle is the preferred sight of biopsies and how many samples are necessary to ensure adequate sampling.[15] The natural history of viral myocarditis is ill defined. Patients with active myocarditis may sometimes present with ventricular arrhythmias, electrocardiographic changes, or pericarditis instead of heart failure.[14] Persistent inflammation following myocardial infection has been thought to be a common cause of DCM for decades. Patients with myocarditis are usually younger, and the left ventricular dysfunction less severe when compared to those with DCM.[14] In the majority of cases, the clinical course is benign and complete recovery without sequelae is expected. In those with residual left ventricular dysfunction after the acute illness, 50% will show gradual improvement.[30]

Viral myocarditis has two distinct phases. The first phase is one of viral replication, which lasts 3–14 days from the day of infection.[14,31] The second phase occurs later and is characterized by an inflammatory infiltrate found in the myocardium. In one study, heart reactive-antibodies (immunoglobulin G) have been observed in 59% of myocarditis samples, 20% in cardiomyopathy samples, and in no control samples.[32] Therefore, there is evidence to suggest that the myocardial damage that occurs after viral myocarditis is due to an immune-related mechanism rather than the virus itself. The presence of enterovirus RNA and symptomatic heart failure have been shown to be independent prognostic variables for mortality in one series of 120 patients.[33] Animal studies have shown that giving immunosuppressive agents during the viral replication stage can be detrimental.[14,30]

The results of studies using immunosuppressives have been conflicting. The number of patients with biopsy-proven myocarditis showing improvement after receiving immunosuppression have varied greatly. This is not surprising given the difficulty in making the diagnosis and the variability in the clinical course of the disease. In addition, many of the studies published have not been randomized and/or controlled. The results of a randomized, multicenter study of patients with myocarditis sponsored by the National Institutes of Health (Myocarditis Treatment Trial) did not demonstrate any difference in outcome measurements between patients with biopsy-proven myocarditis who were randomized to either conventional therapy for heart failure or conventional therapy plus immunosuppression with cyclosporin and/or prednisone.[17,34,35] Although overall there was no demonstrable benefit from immunosuppression, there may be some subsets of patients who respond favorably. It is not known if antiviral therapy would be beneficial in patients with documented viral cardiomyopathy.

Beta Blockade

As described earlier, cardiac contractility is regulated by the autonomic nervous system. Sympathetic (excitatory) nerves innervate the ventricles, resulting in a potent inotropic effect. Although there are other receptors in the myocardium, the β-adrenergic pathway is the most potent in terms of stimulating cardiac contractility. Both β_1- and β_2-adrenergic receptors are coupled to adenylate cyclase stimulation and myocardial contractility. Norepinephrine, by virtue of its higher affinity for β_1 receptors, acts as a relatively selective β_1 agonist.[7,36] In the setting of heart failure, circulating levels of norepinephrine are increased and correlate with the severity of the disease. Patients with a high plasma norepinephrine level have a less favorable prognosis. Norepinephrine is a potent vasoconstrictor and increased levels lead to an increase in systemic vascular resistance. The failing heart already has an imbalance between energy expenditure versus energy production and excessive sympathetic stimulation may lead to a further imbalance. There is also the possibility that excessive sympathetic stimulation results in arrhythmogenesis and sudden cardiac death. Excessive catecholamines may also have a direct toxic effect on the myocardium, resulting in intracellular calcium overload. Clinical trials with the inotropes milrinone and intermittent dobutamine were stopped prematurely due to the higher mortality rate in treated patients.

Therefore, it has been proposed that the β_1-adrenergic receptors be "down-regulated" as a protective mechanism from overstimulation by the sympathetic nervous system in the failing heart.

Changes occur in the ratio of β_1- and β_2-adrenergic receptors in the setting of heart failure. Because the β_1 receptors are down-regulated to the point where they represent about 60% of the total β receptors, stimulation by a selective β_1 agonist will have minimal clinical effect. If maximum inotropic effect is desired, a nonselective agonist is required.[36] Table 17.2 describes how the altered adrenergic receptors may influence the pharmacotherapy of heart failure.

Beta-blocking drugs act competitively by binding to β-adrenergic receptors. Because of their high affinity, they occupy a high percentage of the receptors, making them unavailable for occupancy by agonists of lower affinity.[36] This may be one mechanism whereby β blockers are protective and potentially beneficial in patients with heart failure. For years, clinicians have been taught that β-blocking agents are contraindicated in patients with heart failure. It was believed that the heart required the increase in sympathetic activity in order to compensate for the decrease in myocardial function. This concept was first questioned in the mid- to late 1970s, when β blockers were used clinically in patients with heart failure and tachycardia and were reported to have beneficial effects.

Results from clinical trials using β blockers have been inconsistent. Most of the clinical trials have been small in number (less than 30 patients), and many were not randomized or lacked prospective controls. The studies are difficult to compare due to differences in patient populations (disease state and its severity), the drugs and dosage regimens used, length of treatment, and the endpoints considered. Some studies have demonstrated a positive or beneficial response to β blockers. Improvements in hemodynamic variables, symptoms, and functional class, as well as reports of patients deteriorating after withdrawal of β blockade, have been reported.[37]

TABLE 17.2. IMPACT OF ALTERED ADRENERGIC RECEPTOR FUNCTION ON THERAPY OF HEART FAILURE

β_1-Selective partial agonists will not be as effective as inotropic agents and will function as antagonists.

β_2-Selective partial agonists could be used as inotropic agents.

Nonselective agonists (isoproterenol, dopamine, dobutamine) will be the most effective inotropic agents.

β_1 Antagonists may have less negative inotropic effects than nonselective antagonists.

β_1 Antagonists may lead to up-regulation of β_1 receptors and "paradoxical" restoration of endogenous or exogenous β-agonist response.

(Adapted from Ref. 36.)

The largest trial to date has evaluated metoprolol in idiopathic DCM (the MDC trial).[38] This trial involved 383 patients with idiopathic DCM who were randomized to either placebo or metoprolol in addition to conventional medication for heart failure. The primary endpoints were all-cause mortality or clinical deterioration requiring heart transplantation. Secondary endpoints were cardiac function, exercise capacity, hospitalizations, and quality of life. There was a 34% risk reduction in the combined primary endpoints in the metoprolol group. There were a similar number of deaths in the two groups; however, 19 patients in the placebo group versus two patients in the metoprolol group required transplantation. There was also a statistically significant increase in ejection fraction and exercise time in the metoprolol group.

Several characteristics have been noted in those trials where patients receiving β blockade have shown improvement. The initial dose of the β blocker has been very small (i.e., 5–6.25 mg for metoprolol) and the dose has been increased in a gradual fashion over 1–2 months. In addition, the hemodynamic or functional improvement occurred over a period of months in most patients. Several of the studies showing a poor response to β blockade evaluated the patients after a short duration of treatment (i.e., 1 month) or started therapy with a "usual" maintenance dose of the drug instead of a gradual titration.

The mechanism responsible for the improvement observed in patients with cardiomyopathy receiving β blockers is not clearly defined. Studies in patients with idiopathic DCM and ischemic cardiomyopathy using β blockade have shown improvement in left ventricular ejection fraction and other hemodynamic variables as well as symptomatic improvement.[7,39–41] Beta-adrenergic receptor density may be increased following treatment with metoprolol when measured by endomyocardial biopsy[37]; however, the use of measuring lymphocyte β receptors to predict cardiac β-receptor density is quite limited.[42] The effect of β blockers on circulating catecholamines has been inconsistent.

Newer β-adrenergic blockers with different pharmacologic properties are also being investigated in patients with cardiomyopathy. Bucindolol is a nonselective β-blocking agent with vasodilating properties. In studies in patients with cardiomyopathy, bucindolol has been used in doses starting at 12.5 mg BID gradually titrated to 100 mg BID. Small placebo-controlled trials have shown improvements in the majority of bucindolol-treated patients.[43,44] The results on exercise duration were inconsistent. However, improvements in heart failure symptoms and hemodynamic measurements at rest and exercise were demonstrated in both studies in the bucindolol-treated patients. Carvedilol, a mildly selective β_1 blocker with vasodilating properties, has also been useful in patients with ischemic and idiopathic cardiomyopathy.[45,46]

Beta-blocking agents appear to hold promise for some patients with idiopathic and ischemic cardiomyopathy. It is not clear how certain pharmacologic properties may influence the effectiveness of β blockade. Are cardioselective β blockers more advantageous than nonselective β blockers or vice versa? Should β blockers with intrinsic sympathomimetic activities be avoided? Would a β blocker with the additional property of α-adrenergic blockade be advantageous? Are there different outcomes in patients with ischemic cardiomyopathy versus idiopathic dilated cardiomyopathy or other types of cardiomyopathy? Further studies are needed to define the precise mechanism of action of the β blockers and to better identify those patients who are most likely to benefit. Table 17.3 outlines some of the proposed mechanisms through which β blockers may benefit patients with DCM.

Vasodilators

The use of vasodilators, including calcium channel blockers, nitrates, angiotensin-converting enzyme (ACE) inhibitors, and others, in the treatment of heart failure is discussed in detail in Chapter 13. Patients with heart failure due to various types of cardiomyopathy are frequently included in other clinical heart failure trials using a variety of treatment modalities. The rationale for the use of calcium channel blockers in patients with heart failure includes their vasodilatory and anti-ischemic effects and their ability to reduce diastolic dysfunction.[47] By decreasing systemic vascular resistance, which results in afterload reduction, cardiac output is often enhanced. However, some calcium channel blockers also have the propensity to cause a decrease in myocardial contractility. This negative inotropic property may offset any potential benefit from the vasodilatation. More recent and ongoing trials in patients with heart failure are using the second-generation dihydropyridine calcium channel blockers (amlodipine, felodipine, and nisoldipine).[48] These newer agents have less direct effects on myocardial contractility and are sometimes referred to as being vasoselective. Combination therapy with ACE inhibitors is currently under investigation. It has also been suggested that cardiomyopathy may be the result of microvascular spasm.[49] If this is the case, a beneficial effect may occur if an antispasmotic agent is given early in the course of the disease to prevent myocardial cell loss (Fig. 17.2). Calcium channel blockers may be appropriate for those patients with ongoing ischemia. Verapamil had a modest beneficial effect in a small trial of 20 men with abnormal left ventricular diastolic filling and normal systolic function.[50]

TABLE 17.3. POTENTIAL MECHANISMS FOR BENEFIT FROM β BLOCKADE IN DCM

Up-regulation of β-adrenergic receptors
Protection from catecholamine toxicity
Reduction in heart rate
Reduction in myocardial oxygen demand
Reduction in sudden death
Improved diastolic function

Controversy exists regarding the chronic use of nitrates in the management of heart failure including those patients with cardiomyopathy.[51,52] Nitrates act by reducing systemic and coronary vascular resistance and by minimizing left ventricular dilation through their effects on the venous capacitance vessels. In addition, coronary blood flow is shifted to enhance endocardial perfusion. Nitrates are frequently used in conjunction with hydralazine or other arterial vasodilators for CHF. Large clinical trials specifically designed to evaluate the effectiveness of nitrate therapy alone do not exist. Concern has been raised regarding the tolerance known to develop to some of the hemodynamic effects of nitrates, although this can be overcome by allowing a nitrate-free interval. However, it is unlikely that

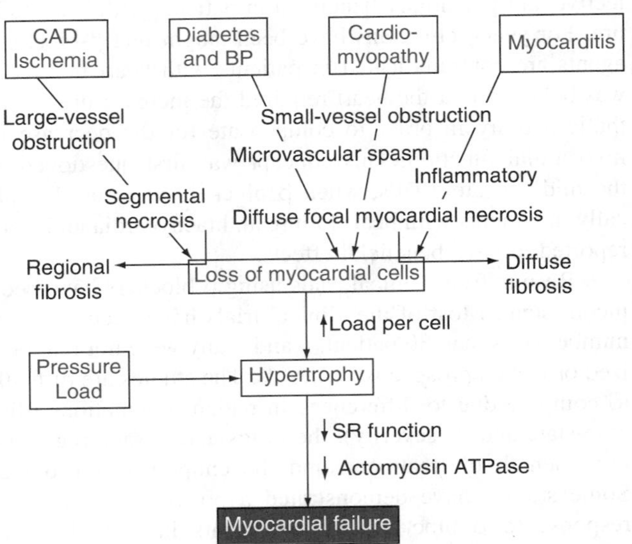

Figure 17.2. Conceptual view of myocardial failure. Many different processes, including ischemic coronary artery disease (CAD), diabetes mellitus, hypertension (BP), and some forms of cardiomyopathy, including that seen in the hamster and myocarditis, may lead to loss of myocardial cells. This cell loss can develop from large-vessel obstruction producing segmental necrosis, as in acute myocardial infarction, microvascular spasm causing focal necrosis, and inflammatory processes of unknown nature that may affect microcirculation or myocardial cells directly. Resultant loss of myocytes increases the load per cell, stimulating hypertrophy of unaffected myocardium. End-stage of myocardial failure results from inadequate numbers of cells to pump effectively, stiffening of myocardium due to connective tissue deposition, and decreased function associated with pathologic cellular hypertrophy. Although myocardial failure may occur rapidly with myocardial infarction, in cardiomyopathy these processes may take years to develop and they may not be clinically apparent until the patient presents with congestive heart failure. ATPase, adenosine triphosphatase; SR, sarcoplasmic reticulum. *(From Sonnenblick EH, Fein F, Capasso JM, et al. Microvascular spasm as a cause of cardiomyopathies and the calcium-blocking agent verapamil as potent primary therapy. Am J Cardiol 1985;55:179B–184B, with permission.)*

any patient with cardiomyopathy or heart failure from any cause will be treated with nitrates alone.

One of the most significant advances in the therapy of heart failure has been the demonstration of a decrease in mortality and morbidity secondary to the use of ACE inhibitors (refer to Chapter 13 for a detailed discussion). In most studies with symptomatic patients, an ACE inhibitor has been added to a regimen of digitalis and diuretic. As mentioned previously, combination therapy with calcium channel blockers is also under investigation. It is not known at this time whether there are significant differences among the different ACE inhibitors in terms of patient outcomes.

Inotropic Agents

In addition to digitalis compounds, which are not discussed in this chapter, investigations with β-adrenergic agonists and phosphodiesterase inhibitors have been carried out in patients with cardiomyopathy. The β-adrenergic agonists enhance contractility by stimulating either β_1 and/or β_2 receptors, which, in turn, stimulate adenylate cyclase to produce cyclic AMP. Cyclic AMP is active until it is destroyed by cytoplasmic phosphodiesterase. In general, the use of β-adrenergic agonist agents, such as pirbuterol, albuterol, and prenaterol, has been disappointing. Down-regulation of β-adrenergic receptors is exacerbated with chronic dosing of these agents. Despite initial beneficial hemodynamic effects, chronic dosing leads to tachyphylaxis and loss of effectiveness.[53]

Phosphodiesterase inhibitors such as amrinone, milrinone, and enoximone increase myocardial contractility by inhibiting the phosphodiesterase enzyme, which is responsible for the breakdown of cyclic AMP. Short-term beneficial hemodynamic effects have been observed with the phosphodiesterase inhibitors. Increases in cardiac output and ejection fraction along with decreases in systemic vascular resistance and left- and right-sided filling pressures have been noted. Unfortunately, proarrhythmia is associated with the use of these agents. Interestingly, in one study, mortality due to sudden cardiac death was higher in patients with ischemic heart disease when compared to patients with nonischemic dilated cardiomyopathy.[54] A retrospective analysis of 21 trials with either β-adrenergic agonists (9 trials) or phosphodiesterase inhibitors (12 trials) has shown an excess mortality for both types of agents when compared to controls.[55] It is not clear if the optimal doses of either of these agents were used in these studies. It is possible that excess mortality may be due to using doses that were too high.

Vesnarinone is a unique agent since it exhibits some phosphodiesterase inhibition in addition to prolonging action potential duration. In a 6-month trial, heart failure patients receiving vesnarinone 60 mg daily had lower morbidity and mortality as compared to a placebo group.[56] However, patients who received the higher dose of vesnarinone (120 mg daily) experienced a higher mortality. The mechanism through which the beneficial effect of vesnarinone was produced is unclear.

Antiarrhythmic Agents

Sudden cardiac death occurs in a significant number of patients with hypertrophic and dilated cardiomyopathy. Although the presence of complex ventricular arrhythmias in patients with DCM is a poor prognostic indicator, it has not been shown that suppression of ventricular ectopy with antiarrhythmic agents will alter mortality rates. In patients with cardiomyopathy, the exact relationship between non-sustained ventricular tachycardia and sudden cardiac death is controversial, as is the use of antiarrhythmic drugs.[57] It is also unclear as to the best way to assess drug efficacy in cardiomyopathy patients. Electrophysiologic studies have been less useful in patients with cardiomyopathy when compared to patients with arrhythmias in the presence of coronary artery disease.[58] The predictive value of ambulatory electrocardiographic monitoring and signal-averaged electrocardiography is also debated.

Many factors should be considered in evaluating a patient with cardiomyopathy and arrhythmias. Can the sympathetic stimulation known to occur in heart failure be attenuated? Is there a problem with ongoing ischemia? Is the patient receiving a drug known to have proarrhythmic effects? Is the patient receiving a drug known to adversely affect electrolyte balance? Before initiating therapy with an antiarrhythmic agent, any reversible factor known to cause an arrhythmia or heart failure should first be corrected. Treatment with an ACE inhibitor and/or a β blocker should be considered. If antiarrhythmic agents are used, those that decrease contractility should be avoided. Patients with DCM and symptomatic ventricular arrhythmias should be evaluated and treated with conventional methods. There is preliminary evidence that the use of amiodarone may prevent sudden death.[59] Early cardiac transplantation or implantation of an automatic defibrillator are other options to be considered. Patient selection criteria have not yet been well defined.

Anticoagulants

Systemic embolization is a possible complication of DCM. The presence of a left ventricular mural thrombus has been associated with a greater risk of thromboembolism and as a predictor of increased mortality.[60] There may be important differences between the mural thrombus formation found after myocardial infarction and dilated cardiomyopathy. For example, the risk of embolization is high in the early weeks after myocardial infarction and lessens after 3–6 months, whereas the risk in patients with DCM is fairly constant over time.[61] Furthermore, the thrombi found in cardiomyopathy patients may have a smaller area of attachment to the endomyocardial surface. Some clinicians use anticoagulation in patients with ejection fractions of 20% or less, unless a contraindication exists.[7] Lower than normal doses may be adequate for patients with cardiomyopathy because hepatic clearance of the drug may be compromised. A large, randomized controlled trial of anticoagulation versus placebo would be useful in determining the risk–benefit ratio of warfarin in this patient population.

Nonpharmacologic Therapy

Because short-term responses to drug therapy do not always predict long-term effects, improvements in hemodynamic measurements and exercise capacity do not always translate into improved survival. Other nonpharmacologic modes of therapy are also being investigated. Improvements in left ventricular ejection fraction, New York Heart Association class, and left atrial and right ventricular size have been reported following dual-chamber (atrioventricular-sequential) pacing.[62] The mechanism by which pacing improves cardiomyopathy is probably related to factors influencing preload or afterload rather than heart rate or myocardial contractility. Ventricular filling may be improved by a controlled atrioventricular delay leading to an improved "atrial kick." As more data become available, the role of pacemakers in the setting of dilated cardiomyopathy will be evaluated.

Surgical Therapy

For those patients with ischemic cardiomyopathy, coronary artery bypass grafts (CABGs) may offer improvement in myocardial function. However, this procedure would not be helpful in patients with ischemic cardiomyopathy whose lesions are diffuse. A new surgical procedure, dynamic cardiomyoplasty, may be helpful in some patients with dilated cardiomyopathy.[63] In this procedure, skeletal muscle (latissimus dorsi) is wrapped around the heart and then stimulated to contract in synchrony with the heart. Lastly, cardiac transplantation is an option. The survival rate following cardiac transplantation has improved dramatically with the advent of improved immunosuppression (see Chapter 18). However, due to the limited supply of donors, relatively few patients with cardiomyopathy will be able to receive a new heart.

Hypertrophic Cardiomyopathy

Hypertrophic cardiomyopathy (HCM) is a primary myocardial disorder characterized by a hypertrophied and nondilated left ventricle, existing in the absence of known causes of left ventricular hypertrophy.[64] The distribution of the hypertrophy is usually asymmetric, meaning segments of the left ventricle are thickened to varying degrees. There may also be enlargement of the atria, thickening of the mitral valve leaflets and fibrotic areas within the ventricular wall. Hypertrophic cardiomyopathy has also been termed idiopathic hypertrophic subaortic stenosis (IHSS) and hypertrophic obstructive cardiomyopathy. These latter terms are used less frequently now because it is felt they overemphasize the obstructive component of the disease, which is present in a minority of patients.[65]

PATHOPHYSIOLOGY

The genetic predisposition to HCM is thought to be an autosomal dominant trait with variable penetrance.[65,66] Due to the wide variability of presentation, not all cases in a family may be detected. One is less likely to find a detectable inheritance pattern in patients who are diagnosed later in life. Familial HCM can be caused by mutations in the genes for β cardiac myosin heavy chain, α-tropomyosin, or cardiac troponin T.[67] Hypertrophic cardiomyopathy appears to have several different pathophysiologic mechanisms leading to similar clinical manifestations, although the prognoses for the different subsets of patients will vary. Overall, it is a rare disease with an estimated prevalence in the United States of less than 0.3%.

The pathophysiology of HCM is a complex relationship among several factors including (1) asymmetric left ventricular hypertrophy, (2) diastolic dysfunction, (3) dynamic obstruction of the outflow tract, and (4) myocardial ischemia. Each of these components contributes to the overall presentation of the patient to a varying degree (Fig. 17.3).

Left Ventricular Hypertrophy

The hypertrophy seen in HCM is usually diffuse and involves the septum and left ventricular anterolateral free wall to a greater degree than the posterior segment. Asymmetric septal hypertrophy (ASH) is a sensitive marker for HCM but is not specific for this disorder. In patients with outflow obstruction, the basal septum is usually markedly thickened at the level of the mitral valve. In patients with nonobstructive HCM, the outflow tract is larger and the septal hypertrophy that occurs has a more distal or apical distribution.[64]

Cellular disorganization is a common histologic finding of HCM. Morphologic abnormalities are found at the gross, microscopic, and ultrastructural levels. It has been estimated that 90–95% of patients with HCM have focal myocardial fiber disarray in 5% or more of the myocardium. In other cardiac disorders that have associated disorganization, the abnormal cells are in small numbers. The clinical consequences of this disordered architecture are not clearly defined, but it may contribute to impaired diastolic and/or systolic function or serve as a nidus for ventricular arrhythmias.[64]

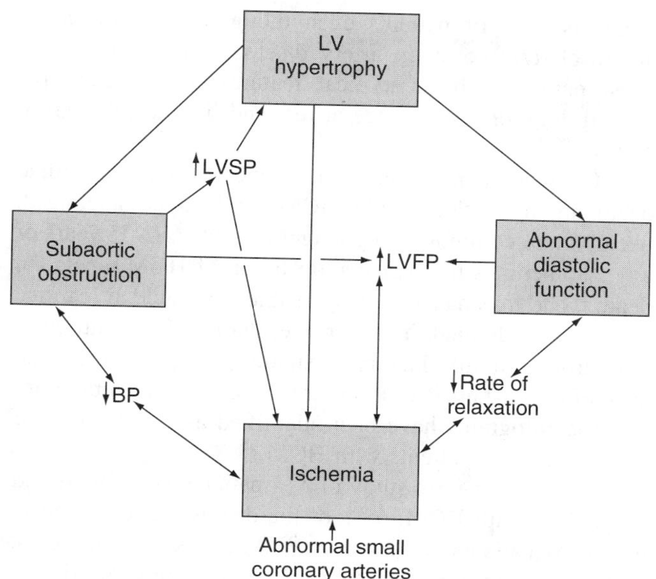

Figure 17.3. Pathophysiologic and hemodynamic interrelations between left ventricular (LV) hypertrophy, subaortic obstruction, diastolic dysfunction, and myocardial ischemia in hypertrophic cardiomyopathy. The symptoms in any given patient reflect the complex interaction among these pathophysiologic mechanisms. LVSP, left ventricular systolic pressure; LVFP, left ventricular filling pressure; BP, blood pressure. *(Reprinted with permission from* The New England Journal of Medicine, *vol. 316, page 845, 1987.)*

It appears that the degree of left ventricular hypertrophy is associated with a worse clinical course. Patients with severe and diffuse hypertrophy are predisposed to symptoms of heart failure and lethal arrhythmias and sudden death.[65]

Diastolic Dysfunction

Diastolic dysfunction is the most common abnormality found in patients with HCM. Approximately 80% of patients will exhibit symptoms associated with diastolic dysfunction. Studies of the left ventricle have led to the realization that diastolic dysfunction is the result of abnormalities in relaxation, distensibility (compliance), and filling. The abnormalities of diastolic function can be both regional and global and lead to an incoordination of contraction and relaxation. Abnormal relaxation is manifested by a prolonged isovolumic relaxation period and a reduced rate of decline in left ventricular pressure. Filling of the left ventricle is prolonged in most patients. The presence of mitral regurgitation tends to normalize these abnormalities. Beta-adrenergic stimulation can aggravate these abnormalities whereas β blockade may diminish them.[64,66]

Myocardial relaxation is an energy-dependent process that is sensitive to episodes of ischemia. Calcium ions are inactivated by being taken up by the sarcoplasmic reticulum. In the event of ischemia, the sequestration of calcium is inhibited, allowing the calcium to continue its interaction with the myofibrillar contractile proteins. Calcium channel blocking drugs have been used with some success in patients with diastolic dysfunction.[64]

Abnormalities in filling are also related to the chamber stiffness that occurs in HCM. This stiffness may be the result of myocardial fibrosis, cellular disorganization, or the increase in myocardial mass. The decreased distensibility leads to an abnormally steep slope of the diastolic pressure–volume curve, such that an increase in left ventricular volume results in a disproportionate increase in diastolic pressure.[64]

Systolic Function and Outflow Tract Obstruction

Abnormalities of systolic function also occur in patients with HCM. The hypertrophied left ventricle may cause a powerful but sometimes uncoordinated contraction presumably due to the abnormal architecture of the myocardium. The increase seen in the left ventricular wall thickness results in decreased wall stress during systole. Therefore, the left ventricle contracts against a decreased afterload, so that the left ventricle should be described as being hyperdynamic rather than hypercontractile.[64] Ejection fraction is often increased.

Considerable controversy has surrounded the issue of the importance of outflow tract obstruction in conjunction with HCM. The presence of a gradient is indicative of a dynamic obstruction of the left ventricular outflow tract. Outflow tract gradients occur in about 25% of patients with HCM.[66] The obstruction that occurs usually shows spontaneous variability, and may be reduced by interventions that decrease myocardial contractility. The gradient can be augmented by factors that increase contractility[64,65] (Table 17.4).

Enhanced contraction, apposition of the anterior mitral leaflet to the hypertrophied septum impeding aortic flow, large papillary muscles, and reduced left ventricular cavity size are factors that may contribute to the production of a systolic pressure gradient. The ventricle ejects 75% (versus 70% under normal conditions) of its stroke volume in the first third of the systolic ejection period in patients with HCM. Some argue that blood flow cannot be impeded in a ventricle where so much of the stroke volume is ejected before the gradient reaches its maximum. Others believe that portions of the mitral valve that move anteriorly across the outflow tract constitute a true mechanical obstruction to left ventricular ejection. This systolic anterior motion (SAM) of the mitral valve leads to increased intraventricular systolic pressures, which, in turn, increases myocardial oxygen demand.[64] The importance of the pressure gradient remains controversial because there is a poor correlation between the presence of a gradient and the clinical symptoms or prognosis of a patient.

TABLE 17.4. FACTORS KNOWN TO AFFECT GRADIENTS

Factors that Diminish Gradients
Decreasing myocardial contractility
β-blocking drugs
Verapamil
Increasing ventricular volume
Increasing arterial pressure
Factors that Enhance Gradients
Increasing myocardial contractility
Exercise
Inotropic agents
Decreasing ventricular volume
Decreasing arterial pressure

Myocardial Ischemia

Chest pain, in the absence of coronary artery disease, is a common symptom of patients with HCM. Several mechanisms have been proposed for the myocardial ischemia seen in this patient population. There may be inadequate capillary density in relation to the increased left ventricular muscle mass. The small intramural coronary arteries may be abnormally narrowed or excessively compressed during systole. Impaired relaxation during diastole may inhibit blood flow to the subendocardium. Once myocardial ischemia develops, further increases in left ventricular filling pressure may occur, which, in turn, leads to more ischemia.[64] Repeated episodes of ischemia may be responsible for progressive myocyte loss and fibrosis. The subendocardium is at greatest risk for ischemic damage due to the lower capillary density and higher oxygen demand secondary to wall tension.[66]

CLINICAL PRESENTATION

The clinical presentation of patients with HCM varies widely, ranging from no symptoms to severe symptoms of angina, heart failure, and/or sudden cardiac death. The most common symptoms are chest pain, dyspnea, fatigue, palpitations, presyncope, and syncope. In general, the severity of symptoms corresponds to the degree of left ventricular hypertrophy, but this relationship is not absolute. Some patients with mild or localized hypertrophy will have severe symptoms, whereas other patients with marked hypertrophy will have minimal symptoms. Furthermore, the presence or absence of a dynamic obstruction does not seem to play a role in the patient's presentation.[64]

The symptoms of fatigue, orthopnea, and dyspnea are usually due to the elevated pressures secondary to diastolic dysfunction. However, some patients may develop dyspnea due to systolic dysfunction secondary to myocardial ischemia and fibrosis. Chest pain is seen in as many as 75% of patients even though the incidence of atherosclerotic coronary artery disease is much less. The chest pain may have atypical features including a prolonged duration, occurrence at rest and limited relief from nitrates.[66]

Of major concern is the incidence of sudden cardiac death among patients with HCM. Sudden cardiac death occurs more commonly in younger patients (10–35 years of age). Sometimes the first manifestation of HCM is sudden death. The mechanisms responsible for sudden cardiac death are ill defined. Younger age, marked left ventricular hypertrophy, family history of sudden death, and the presence of nonsustained ventricular tachycardia on ambulatory electrocardiograms have been identified as risk factors for sudden death in patients with HCM.[65]

In one long-term study of 314 patients with HCM and 82 patients with DCM, 68% of the deaths that occurred in the HCM patients were sudden.[68] Age less than 30 years, fractional shortening less than 35%, and left ventricular end-diastolic pressures greater than 20 mm HG were factors associated with sudden cardiac death. Patients who were less than 30 years of age rarely (5%) had ventricular tachycardia on Holter monitoring. It was suggested that young patients with hypertrophic cardiomyopathy may die suddenly as a result of exercise-induced ischemia rather than ventricular arrhythmias.

A variety of other rhythm abnormalities may be seen including supraventricular and ventricular tachyarrhythmias, bradyarrhythmias, aberrant atrioventricular nodal pathways, and complete heart block.[64] In 25 children with HCM, 6 (24%) were found to have a prolonged QT interval.[69] Either DCM or HCM may be a cause of QT prolongation.

Less often, sudden death may be the result of hemodynamic changes. The onset of atrial fibrillation, in the face of severe left ventricular diastolic dysfunction, may result in a significant decrease in stroke volume. This decrease in cardiac output could lead to acute left ventricular failure, myocardial infarction, or sudden death.

DIAGNOSIS

The diagnosis of HCM may be a difficult one. It is often confused with coronary artery disease, mitral regurgitation, and aortic stenosis. Patients with HCM are often physically active. The physical signs of the cardiac examination depend on the presence of a systolic pressure gradient within the left ventricle. If a gradient is present, a late-onset systolic murmur is often heard. The murmur is intensified by standing and the Valsalva maneuver and lessened with squatting or handgrip. Some patients develop an end-stage left ventricular dilatation and a declining left ventricular ejection fraction, which is often confused with idiopathic DCM.[66]

A chest roentgenogram is usually not helpful, because the cardiac silhouette is often normal. Signs consistent with an increase in left atrial pressure may be present. With severe disease the cardiac silhouette may be enlarged due to hypertrophy, pericardial effusion, or dilatation of the ventricle secondary to myocardial infarction. The electrocardiogram is usually characteristic for the increase in QRS voltage and T-wave inversion seen with left ventricular hypertrophy. The ECG may have Q waves that may be either the result of septal hypertrophy or myocardial infarction.[1]

Doppler echocardiography is needed to confirm the diagnosis. Findings consistent with HCM include a low normal or decreased end-diastolic dimension, a septal wall thickness of ≥15 mm, and a septal to posterior wall thickness ratio of ≥1.3 : 1. The presence of a hyperdynamic left ventricle and systolic anterior motion of the anterior mitral leaflet (SAM) increases the likelihood of the diagnosis. The coexistence of hypertension, congenital heart disease, and hyperthyroidism complicate the diagnostic process, since some of these patients will have asymmetric hypertrophy and similar clinical findings.[66] Radionuclide imaging techniques with thallium-201 will demonstrate myocardial perfusion abnormalities. Angiography is indicated prior to surgery.[1]

NATURAL HISTORY/PROGNOSIS

The natural history of HCM is quite variable, ranging from an asymptomatic form to a severe life-threatening illness. As mentioned previously, there is no relation between the presence or absence of an outflow tract gradient and clinical presentation or prognosis. The development or increase of a murmur suggests progression of disease, but disappearance of a murmur does not suggest improvement. In fact, disappearance of a murmur may herald further impairment of systolic function. Some patients will progress to congestive heart failure due to atrial fibrillation, mitral regurgitation, or myocardial infarction. If heart failure develops, the patient has a poor prognosis.[64]

Presentation of HCM in latter decades of life is common. Patients who present with HCM at an advanced age (>65 years) in general have a prognosis no different than age- and gender-matched controls.[70] It is not clear whether this elderly patient subgroup had a better prognosis compared to patients presenting at a younger age as a result of a different pathophysiologic process. Elderly patients presenting with New York Heart Association functional class III dyspnea had a higher mortality rate when compared to a control group. Increased left atrial size was associated with reduced survival.

Sudden death is a common complication, especially in young athletes with HCM. It is recommended that young patients with HCM refrain from competitive athletics.

TREATMENT

Since there are no known means available to prevent HCM, methods to minimize the consequences of disease prevail. The treatment of HCM is designed to reduce symptoms, improve exercise tolerance, retard disease progression, and improve prognosis. Agents that decrease contractility, improve diastolic dysfunction, and suppress arrhythmias have been used with some success.

Beta-Blocking Agents

Beta-blocking agents have been used in obstructive and nonobstructive forms of HCM since the 1960s. It has been estimated that one-third to over one-half of patients with angina, dyspnea, lightheadedness, or syncope will have a favorable response to these agents.[64] Most patients require doses of 320 mg/d of propranolol or its equivalent, although it is recommended that maximally tolerated doses be used.[66] Standing heart rate should be 60 beats/min and the maximum exercise heart rate should be <130 beats/min. The mechanism by which β blockade is thought to be helpful is by inhibiting sympathetic stimulation of the heart. Myocardial oxygen demand is reduced by decreasing heart rate, left ventricular contractility, and myocardial wall stress during systole. Outflow tract obstruction may be minimized with β blockade, especially under conditions of stress or exercise, when sympathetic stimulation is high. Furthermore, consequences of a decreased resting and exercise heart rate include an increase in left ventricular diastolic filling time, reduction of the abnormally prolonged isovolumic relaxation period, and lengthening of early rapid filling. Cardioselective β-blocking drugs are thought to be less desirable since their effect on outflow tract gradient is less. It has been suggested that they should be reserved for those patients with COPD. Furthermore, β-blocking agents with intrinsic sympathomimetic activity (ISA) may not reduce resting heart rate sufficiently.[64,66]

Calcium Channel Blocking Agents

There are a number of reasons why calcium channel blocking agents may be of benefit to patients with HCM. Increased calcium concentrations have been shown to play a role in prolonging the ventricular action potential and also the duration of isometric contraction and relaxation. As described earlier, patients with HCM have a hyperdynamic ventricle in systole and delayed relaxation and decreased compliance in diastole. Preliminary work in patients with HCM has shown an increased number of calcium antagonist receptors in myocardial tissue, which likely reflects an increase in the number of voltage-dependent calcium channels.[71] It has been suggested that an increase in the number of calcium channels is a primary defect in HCM patients rather than a response to the hypertrophy. It has also been suggested that the increase in calcium channels may be part of a generalized disorder and not limited to the myocardium. Therefore, there are a number of reasons why a calcium channel blocker may be beneficial in a patient with HCM. Calcium channel blocking drugs decrease the myocardial oxygen determinants, resulting in an improved balance between oxygen supply and demand. In addition, diastolic function may also be improved.

Most patients with HCM who have been treated with a calcium channel blocker have received verapamil, although diltiazem and some of the dihydropyridines have also been used. In one study of 101 patients, 85% of previously symptomatic patients reported improvement or complete relief of symptoms when treated with a calcium channel blocker.[72] Intravenous verapamil has been noted to reduce the outflow tract gradient in those patients with obstructive HCM. The mechanism may be a decrease in systolic function as well as an increase in left ventricular volumes due to an enhanced left ventricular diastolic filling. Propranolol and verapamil increase exercise duration to a similar degree.[73]

The adverse effects associated with the use of verapamil are usually manifestations of the drug's pharmacologic action. Adverse effects include sinus node dysfunction, prolongation of the PR interval, atrioventricular dissociation, hypotension, and pulmonary congestion.[64,72] The risks may outweigh the benefits in those patients with (1) a pulmonary capillary wedge pressure of >20 mm HG, (2) a history of paroxysmal nocturnal dyspnea or orthopnea, (3) sick sinus syndrome or significant atrioventricular nodal disease in the absence of a permanent pacemaker, and (4) low systolic blood pressure.[73]

Studies using other calcium channel blockers are limited. Improvement in diastolic dysfunction may occur, however, the dihydropyridines may cause a reflex increase in heart rate, cause hypotension, or worsen the outflow tract gradient. It has been suggested that a combination of a β blocker with a calcium channel blocker may be useful. In that situation, a β blocker should be initiated prior to starting a dihydropyridine.[66] If verapamil has been used first, additional benefit has been reported with the addition of pindolol.[74] Trials using combination therapy are extremely limited.

Antiarrhythmic Agents

The incidence of sudden cardiac death in patients with HCM is a cause of great concern among clinicians. Disopyramide has been used in treating both the supraventricular and ventricular arrhythmias occurring in patients with HCM. In addition, disopyramide's negative inotropic effect and its ability to increase peripheral vascular resistance has been used to reduce outflow tract obstruction.[64,72] The number of patients receiving disopyramide is small and there are few controlled trials available. The anticholinergic side effects (blurred vision, dry mouth, and urinary retention) make disopyramide a less desirable agent for long-term therapy.

Amiodarone has also been used in the management of HCM. Amiodarone is a complex agent with α-, β-, and calcium blocking effects. As a result, it has negative chronotropic, inotropic, and coronary vasodilating properties. Amiodarone may relieve symptoms and prolong exercise duration in some patients, independent of its antiarrhythmic actions.[64,75] Unfortunately, sudden death may occur, despite the abolishment of ventricular tachycardia determined by ambulatory Holter monitoring.

In one trial where 35 patients with HCM were assessed by electrophysiologic study, amiodarone prevented or made it more difficult to induce ventricular tachycardia in 31% of patients that were inducible off drug.[76] Ventricular tachycardia was easier to induce or inducible only while the patient was taking amiodarone in 51% of patients. During a follow-up period, 4 of 18 patients in whom amiodarone facilitated ventricular tachycardia died or received appropriate electrical shocks from implantable defibrillators. None of the 17 patients taking amiodarone in whom ventricular tachycardia was rendered more difficult to induce died. Amiodarone may be proarrhythmic in some patients and electrophysiologic studies may help identify those patients who will do poorly if placed on amiodarone for long-term therapy.

Electrophysiologic guided therapy is probably warranted in those patients who are symptomatic, have documented sustained ventricular tachycardia, or who have survived a cardiac arrest. Large controlled trials are needed to assess the effectiveness of antiarrhythmic agents, β blockers, and calcium channel blockers, alone or in combination, and implantation of automatic defibrillators on the incidence of sudden cardiac death.

In those patients who present with chronic atrial fibrillation, digitalis may be useful despite the fact that it has positive inotropic properties. Anticoagulation should also be considered since these patients are at risk for systemic embolization and stroke. If amiodarone is added to a patient receiving warfarin, the prothrombin time or INR should be closely monitored.[64] There is no clear indication for anticoagulation if the patient with HCM is in normal sinus rhythm.

Surgical Therapy

Surgical treatment is generally reserved for those patients who are refractory to medical management, have an outflow gradient of 50 mm HG or more, a very thick ventricular septum, and high left ventricular pressures. Surgical intervention is designed to relieve the outflow obstruction and the elevated left ventricular pressures. This is accomplished by performing a partial septal resection and/or incision (ventricular myotomy–myectomy). Surgery does not stop the progression of disease nor has it been shown to affect long-term survival. Complications may include septal perforation and late occurrence of congestive heart failure. Mitral valve replacement has also been used to abolish the subaortic gradient that occurs due to the anterior motion of the mitral leaflets during systole. This procedure is generally reserved for patients with severe mitral regurgitation or those with mild ventricular septal hypertrophy where myotomy–myectomy may cause perforation.[64–66]

Restrictive Cardiomyopathy

Restrictive cardiomyopathy is the cardiomyopathy encountered least frequently. Restrictive cardiomyopathy is associated with normal or near-normal systolic function, but elevated filling pressures in the absence of coronary artery disease, valvular disease, and HCM. Restrictive cardiomyopathy is one type of diastolic dysfunction where there is rapid completion of ventricular filling of a poorly compliant ventricle in the early phase of diastole. The abnormality in ventricular filling rather than relaxation may be the result of morphologic changes in the endocardium and/or myocardium. Several cardiomyopathies have restrictive characteristics at some phase in their development.[77,78]

PATHOPHYSIOLOGY

The major hemodynamic abnormality in restrictive cardiomyopathy is a limitation of ventricular filling leading to increased filling pressures. Thrombi are frequently found in the cardiac chambers. Patients have signs and symptoms consistent with congestive heart failure. The abnormality is similar to what is seen in pericardial disease causing constriction or tamponade. In the early stages of the disease, systolic function is usually normal. Atrial dimensions are often increased.

Restrictive cardiomyopathies may be either idiopathic or secondary to an infiltrative disease. Amyloidosis, hemochromatosis, scleroderma, carcinoid, sarcoidosis, pseudoxanthoma elasticum, and endomyocardial fibrosis have been known to cause restrictive cardiomyopathy.[79]

CLINICAL PRESENTATION

Patients present with dyspnea, orthopnea, fatigue, edema, and at times chest pain. The heart is either normal in size or has atrial enlargement. Significant jugular venous distension is quite common. Mitral and/or tricuspid regurgitant murmurs may be heard. The electrocardiogram may show atrial arrhythmias, tachy-brady syndrome or conduction abnormalities. Recordings of ventricular pressure may show a characteristic dip and plateau (square root sign). This is a result of rapid completion of ventricular filling early in diastole. The square root sign is not always present because it can be affected by heart rate, degree of hydration, and the severity of disease.[77,79]

DIAGNOSIS

The diagnosis of restrictive cardiomyopathy should be considered in the patient who presents with signs and symptoms of congestive heart failure but has only mild cardiomegaly. Differentiation from constrictive pericarditis is important since pericardectomy is an effective form of treatment for constrictive pericarditis.

Restrictive cardiomyopathy may be due to a variety of causes. In tropical parts of the world, restrictive cardiomyopathy occurs as a result of endomyocardial fibrosis. The endocardium becomes scarred and thickened, which leads to abnormal ventricular filling and diastolic dysfunction. The subendocardium and atrioventricular valves may also become involved. A similar disease associated with eosinophilia (Loeffler's endocardial fibrosis) occurs in developed countries.[78]

In Western societies, cardiac symptoms resembling a restrictive cardiomyopathy are often seen as a result of amyloidosis, hemochromatosis, sarcoidosis, Fabry's disease, neoplasms, scleroderma, carnitine deficiency, and radiation. Endomyocardial biopsy is helpful in establishing the diagnosis and cause of restrictive cardiomyopathy and distinguishing it from constrictive pericarditis.[78,79]

NATURAL HISTORY/PROGNOSIS

Because of the rare occurrence of restrictive cardiomyopathy, the natural course of the disease is not well characterized and reports on prognosis have been highly variable. The cause of the disease, the severity of heart failure symptoms, and the presence of cardiac thrombi and arrhythmias are factors that affect long-term survival. Children diagnosed with restrictive cardiomyopathy have a worse prognosis than adults and should be considered for early cardiac transplantation.[80]

TREATMENT

The treatment of restrictive cardiomyopathy is complex because of the heterogeneity of the pathophysiologic abnormalities. Diuretics and vasodilators are used for the symptoms of congestive heart failure in the presence of restrictive cardiomyopathy but caution is advised since these patients require high filling pressures to maintain an adequate stroke volume cardiac output. Hypotension and cardiogenic shock may occur as a result of the use of these drugs. Because systolic function is often normal, digitalis may be of little or no benefit. Anticoagulation may be helpful in decreasing the risk of systemic embolization. Calcium channel blockers have not been studied in a systematic fashion, but might improve diastolic compliance. In the case of hemachromatosis, chelation therapy and/or repeated phlebotomy may be of benefit.[77–79]

Evaluation of Therapeutic Outcomes

Patients with DCM should be treated no differently than patients with known causes of congestive heart failure (see Chapter 13). Therapy should include an ACE inhibitor and a diuretic. Blood pressure should be closely monitored to ensure that the patient has adequate perfusion yet at the same time reducing systemic resistance. Some basilar rales or mild pedal edema may be tolerated in order to ensure an adequate filling pressure. Generally loop diuretics are necessary to achieve an adequate diuresis. Patients should be instructed to weigh themselves on a regular basis and to contact their health care provider if their weight increases by five or more pounds or if their symptoms worsen. Potassium and magnesium serum concentrations should be monitored and supplements administered if needed. Digoxin should be added to the regimen in order to enhance myocardial contractility. If the patient remains symptomatic, a trial of β-blocker therapy may be initiated; however, this therapy is considered to be investigational. The dose of metoprolol should be gradually titrated over a period of several weeks with the heart rate, blood pressure, and patient's symptoms carefully monitored. The usual intial dose is 6.25 mg twice daily titrated up to 50 mg twice daily if tolerated.

If the patient has an ejection fraction <20% or if a mural thrombus is suspected, a trial of anticoagulation may be warranted if the benefit is thought to outweigh the risk in the individual patient. If the patient experiences an episode of sudden death or has sustained ventricular tachycardia, an antiarrhythmic agent is usually prescribed. Selection of the agent may be based on the results of an electrophysiologic study (EPS), or amiodarone may be empirically prescribed. If the patient continues to deteriorate, cardiac transplantation may be a viable alternative.

The goal of treatment for patients with HCM is primarily to reduce their symptoms of dyspnea and exercise intolerance. Either β blockers or calcium channel blockers may be used. If a β blocker is chosen, it is best to use an agent that does not have intrinsic sympathomimetic activity. Doses of propranolol are usually 320 mg daily or more. The dose should be increased until the resting standing heart rate is 60 beats/min or less and the exercise heart rate is less than 130 beats/min. If the patient does not tolerate a β blocker or has a contraindication to the use of a β blocker, then a calcium channel blocker may be tried. The most commonly used calcium channel blocker is verapamil. Doses of 360 mg daily are frequently used. Resolution of symptoms may take months to occur. Patients should be monitored for resolution of symptoms and an increase in exercise tolerance. In addition, both β blockers and calcium channel blockers may cause hypotension and conduction abnormalities. Beta blockers may worsen pulmonary function. Combination therapy with a β blocker and calcium channel blocker may be tried if the desired therapeutic response is not achieved with either agent alone. If dyspnea continues with maximal doses of a β blocker and calcium channel blocker, a diuretic agent or a nitrate may be added.

Those patients who have demonstrated the presence of potentially lethal arrhythmias or syncope should undergo an electrophysiologic study. Selection of an antiarrhythmic should be based on the results of this study. Frequently, combination therapy with a type IA, IB, or IC agent and a β blocker is effective. Amiodarone may also be prescribed but careful monitoring is required due to the many side effects associated with its use. If patients are in atrial fibrillation, anticoagulation therapy should be considered.

For those patients with a significant obstruction to left ventricular outflow that do not respond to medical management, a surgical approach may be necessary. Septal myotomy–myectomy has been employed. Surgical therapy is generally reserved for those patients who have an outflow gradient of >50 mm Hg and/or severe symptoms and who have failed an adequate trial of medical therapy.

The first step in assessing and treating a patient with restrictive cardiomyopathy is to rule out constrictive pericarditis because the two conditions have a similar presentation. Constrictive pericarditis is easily treated with surgery, whereas patients with restrictive cardiomyopathy have a varied approach to therapy dependent on the etiology of their disorder. The treatment is aimed at relieving the symptoms associated with high filling pressures. This is generally achieved through the use of diuretics. Diuretic therapy should be initiated with low doses. Normalization of filling pressures is not possible or desirable. Patient symptoms should be monitored for improvement. Overdiuresis will result in an inadequate cardiac output. Chelation therapy has been advocated for patients with hemochromatosis. Prednisone has been suggested for patients with sarcoidosis. There is no curative treatment for restrictive cardiomyopathy.

Conclusion

The cardiomyopathies are classified into dilated, hypertrophic, and restrictive types. There may be some overlap among the types as patients progress through the different stages of their specific disorder. Treatment is varied and can be either symptomatic or aimed at altering the disease process.

The dilated cardiomyopathies are characterized by a large dilated ventricle and congestive symptoms that may respond to conventional treatment of diuretics and vasodilators. The relationship between myocarditis and dilated cardiomyopathy continues to be explored as does the use of immunosuppressive therapy. The beneficial use of β blockers in some patients has caused us to look carefully at changes that occur at the receptor level. Further study is warranted in this area. Antiarrhythmic agents and anticoagulation may also be beneficial. Cardiac transplantation may be curative but is limited by donor availability.

The patient with HCM has a variety of structural and functional abnormalities. Left ventricular and septal hypertrophy, diastolic dysfunction, and outflow tract obstruction are factors that affect patient presentation and treatment. Beta-blocking agents, calcium channel blocking agents, antiarrhythmic drugs, and surgery may be used in the management of the patient with HCM.

Restrictive cardiomyopathy is the least common form of cardiomyopathy seen in the United States. Many of the patients with restrictive cardiomyopathy may be suffering from an infiltrative disease that is difficult to treat. Therapy is often directed at symptoms and the use of diuretics and vasodilators should be judicious. Cardiac transplantation is warranted in children.

REFERENCES

1. Wynne J, Braunwald E. The cardiomyopathies and myocarditidies, in Isselbacher KJ, Braunwald E, Wilson JD, et al. (eds): Harrison's Principles of Internal Medicine, 13th ed. New York, McGraw-Hill, 1994, pp 1088–1094.
2. Mason JW. Classification of cardiomyopathy, in Schlant RC, Alexander RW (eds): Hurst's The Heart, 8th ed. New York, McGraw-Hill, 1994, pp 1585–1590.
3. Katz AM. Cardiomyopathy of overload. N Engl J Med 1990;322:100–110.
4. Wynne J, Braunwald E. The cardiomyopathies and myocarditides: Toxic, chemical and physical damage to the heart, in Braunwald E (ed): Heart Disease, 4th ed. Philadelphia, WB Saunders, 1992, pp 1394–1450.
5. Dec GW, Fuster V. Idiopathic dilated cardiomyopathy. N Engl J Med 1994;331:1564–1575.
6. Ferrans VJ. Pathologic anatomy of the dilated cardiomyopathies. Am J Cardiol 1989;64:9C–11C.
7. Gilbert EM, Bristow MR. Idiopathic dilated cardiomyopathy, in Schlant RC, Alexander RW (eds): Hurst's The Heart, 8th ed. New York, McGraw-Hill, 1994, pp 1609–1619.
8. Marijianowski MMH, Teeling P, Mann J, et al. Dilated cardiomyopathy is associated with an increase in the type I/type III collagen ratio: A quantitative assessment. J Am Coll Cardiol 1995;25:1263–1272.
9. Klappacher G, Franzen P, Haab D, et al. Measuring extracellular matrix turnover in the serum of patients with idiopathic or ischemic dilated cardiomyopathy and impact on diagnosis and prognosis. Am J Cardiol 1995;75:913–918.
10. Marian AJ, Roberts R. Molecular basis of hypertrophic and dilated cardiomyopathy. Texas Heart Institute J 1994;21:6–15.
11. Limas C, Limas CJ, Boudoulas H, et al. Anti-β-receptor antibodies in familial cardiomyopathy: Correlation with HLA-DR and HLA-DQ gene polymorphisms. Am Heart J 1994;127:382–386.
12. Lang RM, Borow KM, Neumann A, Feldman T. Adverse cardiac effects of acute alcohol ingestion in young adults. Ann Intern Med 1985;102:742–747.
13. Kupari M, Koskinen P, Suokas A, Ventila M. Left ventricular filling impairment in asymptomatic chronic alcoholics. Am J Cardiol 1990;66:1473–1477.
14. Lee HR, O'Connell JB, Mason JW. Immunosuppression and beta-blockade in heart failure. Cardiol Clin 1989;7:171–181.
15. Shabetai, R. Myocarditis and dilated cardiomyopathy: Twins or distant relatives. Cardiology 1989;76:332–337.
16. Lauer B, Padberg K, Schultheiss H, Strauer B. Autoantibodies against human ventricular myosin in sera of patients with acute and chronic myocarditis. J Am Coll Cardiol 1994;23:146–153.
17. O'Connell JB, Renlund DG. Myocarditis and specific myocardial diseases, in Schlant RC, Alexander RW (eds): Hurst's The Heart, 8th ed. New York, McGraw-Hill, 1994, pp 1591–1607.
18. Bristow MR, Mason JW, Billingham ME, Daniels JR. Dose-effect and structure-function relationships in doxorubicin cardiomyopathy. Am Heart J 1981;102:709–718.
19. Freter CE, Lee TC, Billingham ME, et al. Doxorubicin cardiac toxicity manifesting seven years after treatment. Am J Med 1986;80:483–485.
20. McKillop JH, Bristow MR, Goris ML, et al. Sensitivity and specificity of radionuclide ejection fractions in doxorubicin cardiotoxicity. Am Heart J 1983;106:1048–1056.
21. Myers CE, Chabner BA. Anthracyclines, in Chabner BA, Collins JM (eds): Cancer Chemotherapy: Principles and Practice. Philadelphia, JB Lippincott, 1990, pp 356–375.
22. Legha SS, Hortobagyi GN, Benjamin RS. Anthracyclines, in Lokich JJ (ed): Cancer Chemotherapy by Infusion. Chicago, Precept Press, 1987, pp 130–144.
23. Speyer JL, Green MD, Kramer E, et al. Protective effect of the bispiperazedione ICRF-187 against doxorubicin-induced cardiac toxicity in women with advanced breast cancer. N Engl J Med 1988;319:745–752.
24. Anversa P, Sonnenblick EH. Ischemic cardiomyopathy: Pathophysiologic mechanisms. Prog Cardiovasc Dis 1990;33:49–70.
25. Vlay SC. Innovations in the management of ischemic cardiomyopathy. Am Heart J 1994;127;235–242.
26. Marin-Neto JA, Maciel BC, Urbanetz LLT, et al. High output failure in patients with peripartum cardiomyopathy: A comparative study with dilated cardiomyopathy. Am Heart J 1991;121:134–140.
27. Goldman MR, Boucher CA. Value of radionuclide imaging techniques in assessing cardiomyopathy. Am J Cardiol 1980;46:1232–1236.
28. Johnson RA. Palacios I. Dilated cardiomyopathies of the adult. N Engl J Med 1982;307:1051–1058 (part I) and 1119–1126 (part 2).
29. Middlekauff HR, Stevenson WG, Woo MA, et al. Comparison of frequency of late potentials in idiopathic dilated car-

diomyopathy and ischemic cardiomyopathy with advanced congestive heart failure and their usefulness in predicting sudden death. Am J Cardiol 1990;66:1113–1117.
30. Maze SS, Adolph RJ. Myocarditis: Unresolved issues in diagnosis and treatment. Clin Cardiol 1990;13:69–79.
31. Rezkalla SH, Kloner RA. Management strategies in viral myocarditis. Am Heart J 1989;117:706–708.
32. Neumann DA, Burek CL, Baughman KL, et al. Circulating heart-reactive antibodies in patients with myocarditis or cardiomyopathy. J Am Coll Cardiol 1990;16:839–846.
33. Why HJ, Meany BT, Richardson PJ, et al. Clinical and prognostic significance of detection of enteroviral RNA in the myocardium of patients with myocarditis of dilated cardiomyopathy. Circulation 1994;89:2582–2589.
34. O'Connell JB, Mason JW. The applicability of results of streamlined trials to clinical practice: The myocarditis treatment trial. Stat Med 1990;9:193–197.
35. Mason JW, O'Connell JB, Herskowitz A, et al. A clinical trial of immunosuppressive therapy for myocarditis. N Engl J Med 1995;333:269–275.
36. Bristow MR. The beta-adrenergic receptor: Configuration, regulation, mechanism of action. Postgrad Med 1988;(Feb 29 Spec No):19–26.
37. Waagstein F, Caidahl K, Wallentin I, et al. Long-term beta-blockade in dilated cardiomyopathy. Effects of short- and long-term metoprolol treatment followed by withdrawal and readministration of metoprolol. Circulation 1989;80(3):551–563.
38. Waagstein F, Bristow MR, Swedberg K, et al. Beneficial effects of metoprolol in idiopathic dilated cardiomyopathy. Lancet 1993;342:1441–1446.
39. Doughty RN, MacMahon S, Sharpe N. Beta-blockers in heart failure: Promising or proved. J Am Coll Cardiol 1994;23:814–821.
40. Domanski MJ, Eichorn EJ. Beta blockade in congestive heart failure—the need for a definitive study. Am J Cardiol 1994;73:597–599.
41. Fisher ML, Gottlieb SS, Plotnick GD, et al. Beneficial effects of metoprolol in heart failure associated with coronary artery disease: A randomized trial. J Am Coll Cardiol 1994;23:943–950.
42. Brodde OE, Michel MC, Gordon EP, et al. Beta-adrenoceptor regulation in the human heart: Can it be monitored in circulating lymphocytes? Eur Heart J 1989;10(suppl B):2–10.
43. Gilbert EM, Anderson JL, Deitchman D, et al. Long-term β blocker vasodilator therapy improves cardiac function in idiopathic dilated cardiomyopathy: A double-blind, randomized study of bucindolol versus placebo. Am J Med 1990;88:223–229.
44. Pollock SG, Lytash J, Tedesco C, et al. Usefulness of bucindolol in congestive heart failure. Am J Cardiol 1990;66:603–607.
45. Das Gupta P, Lahiri A. Can intravenous beta blockade predict long-term haemodynamic benefit in chronic congestive heart failure secondary to ischaemic heart disease? A comparison between intravenous and oral carvedilol. Clin Investig 1992(suppl 1):S98–S104.
46. Olsen SL, Gilbert EM, Renlund DG, et al. Carvedilol improves left ventricular function and symptoms in chronic heart failure: A double-blind randomized study. J Am Coll Cardiol 1995;25:1225–1231.
47. Elkayam U, Shotan A, Mehra A, Ostrzega E. Calcium channel blockers in heart failure. J Am Coll Cardiol 1993;22(suppl A):139A–144A.
48. Garg R, Yusuf S. Current and ongoing randomized trilas in heart failure and left ventricular dysfunction. J Am Coll Cardiol 1993;22(suppl A):194A–207A.
49. Sonnenblick EH, Fein F, Capasso JM, Factor SM. Microvascular spasm as a cause of cardiomyopathies and the calcium-blocking agent verapamil as potent primary therapy. Am J Cardiol 1985;55:179B–184B.
50. Setaro JF, Schulman DS, Black HR, Soufer R. Usefulness of verapamil for congestive heart failure associated with abnormal left ventricular diastolic filling and normal left ventricular systolic performance. Am J Cardiol 1990;66:981–986.
51. Cohn JN. Nitrates are effective in the treatment of chronic congestive heart failure: The protagonist's view. Am J Cardiol 1990;66:444–446.
52. Packer M. Are nitrates effective in the treatment of chronic heart failure? Antagonist's viewpoint. Am J Cardiol 1990;66:458–461.
53. Sanders MR, Kostis JB, Frishman WH. The use of inotropic agents in acute and chronic heart failure. Med Clin N Am 1989;73(2):283–311.
54. Simonton CA, Daly PA, Kereiakes D, et al. Survival in severe left ventricular failure treated with the new nonglycoside, nonsympathomimetic oral inotrope agents. Chest 1987;92(1):118–123.
55. Yusuf S, Teo K. Intropic agents increase mortality in patients with congestive heart failure [abstract]. Circulation 1990;82(suppl III):III-673.
56. Feldman AM, Bristow MR, Parmley WW, et al. Effects of vesnarinone on morbidity in patients with heart failure. New Engl J Med 1993;329:149–155.
57. Podrid PJ, Wilson JS. Should asymptomatic ventricular arrhythmia in patients with congestive heart failure be treated? An antagonist's viewpoint. Am J Cardiol 1990;66:451–457.
58. Das SK, Morady F, DiCarlo L, et al. Prognostic usefulness of programmed ventricular stimulation in idiopathic dilated cardiomyopathy without symptomatic ventricular arrhythmias. Am J Cardiol 1986;58:998–1000.
59. Tamburro P, Wilbur D. Sudden death in idiopathic dilated cardiomyopathy. Am Heart J 1992;124:1035–1045.
60. Katz SD, Marantz PR, Biasucci L, et al. Low incidence of stroke in ambulatory patients with heart failure; a prospective study. Am Heart J 1993;126:141–146.
61. Falk RH. A plea for a clinical trial of anticoagulation in dilated cardiomyopathy. Am J Cardiol 1990;65:914–915.
62. Hochleitner M, Hortnagl H, Ng C, et al. Usefulness of physiologic dual-chamber pacing in drug-resistant idiopathic dilated cardiomyopathy. Am J Cardiol 1990;66:198–202.
63. Hill AB, Chiu RC. Dynamic cardiomyoplasty for treatment of heart failure. Clin Cardiol 1989;12:681–688.
64. Maron BJ, Bonow RO, Cannon RO, et al. Hypertrophic cardiomyopathy. Interrelations of clinical manifestations, pathophysiology and therapy. N Engl J Med 1987;316:780–789 (part 1) and 844–852 (part 2).
65. Maron BJ, Roberts WC. Hypertrophic cardiomyopathy, in Schlant RC, Alexander RW (eds): Hurst's the Heart, 8th ed. New York, McGraw-Hill, 1994, pp 1621–1635.

66. von Dohlen TW, Frank MJ. Current perspectives in hypertrophic cardiomyopathy: Diagnosis, clinical management, and prevention of disability and sudden cardiac death. Clin Cardiol 1990;13:247–252.
67. Watkins H, McKenna WJ, Thierfelder L, et al. Mutations in the genes for cardiac troponin T and α-tropomyosin in hypertrophic cardiomyopathy. N Engl J Med 1995;332:1058–1064.
68. Koga Y, Ogata M, Kihara K, et al. Sudden death in hypertrophic and dilated cardiomyopathy. Jpn Circ J 1989;53:1546–1556.
69. Martin AB, Garson A, Perry JC. Prolonged QT interval in hypertrophic and dilated cardiomyopathy in children. Am Heart J 1994;127:64–70.
70. Fay WP, Talierco CP, Ilstrup DM, et al. Natural history of hypertrophic cardiomyopathy in the elderly. J Am Coll Cardiol 1990;16:821–826.
71. Wagner JA, Sax FL, Weisman HF, et al. Calcium-antagonist receptors in the atrial tissue of patients with hypertrophic cardiomyopathy. N Engl J Med 1989;320:755–761.
72. Hopf R, Kaltenbach M. Management of hypertrophic cardiomyopathy. Ann Rev Med 1990;41:75–83.
73. Rosing DR, Idanpaan-Heikkla U, Maron BJ, et al. Use of calcium channel blocking drugs in hypertrophic cardiomyopathy. Am J Cardiol 1985;55:185B–195B.
74. Dimitrow PP, Dubiel JS. Effects on left ventricular function of pindolol added to verapamil in hypertrophic cardiomyopathy. Am J Cardiol 1993;71:313–316.
75. Fananapazir L, Leon MB, Bonow RO, et al. Sudden death during empiric amiodarone therapy in symptomatic hypertrophic cardiomyopathy. Am J Cardiol 1991;67:169–174.
76. Fananapazir L, Epstein SE. Value of electrophysiologic studies in hypertrophic cardiomyopathy treated with amiodarone. Am J Cardiol 1991;67:175–182.
77. Wilmhurst PT, Katritsis D. Restrictive cardiomyopathy. Br Heart J 1990;63:323–324.
78. Abelmann WH, Lorell BH. The challenge of cardiomyopathy. J Am Coll Cardiol 1989;13:1219–1239.
79. Shabetai R. Restrictive cardiomyopathy, in Schlant RC, Alexander RW (eds): Hurst's the Heart, 8th ed. New York, McGraw-Hill, 1994, pp 1637–1646.
80. Lewis AB. Clinical profile and outcome of restrictive cardiomyopathy in children. Am Heart J 1992;123:1589–1593.

Chapter 18

Cardiac Transplantation

Kathleen D. Lake, PharmD, BCPS, and Marc R. Pritzker, MD

Cardiac transplantation has emerged as a mainline therapeutic modality for selected patients with end-stage cardiac disease. The use of refined donor and recipient selection criteria, improved donor organ preservation, endomyocardial biopsy surveillance for rejection, improved diagnostic, prophylactic, and treatment strategies for infections in immunocompromised recipients, and the introduction of new immunosuppressive agents have all contributed to the dramatic improvements in survival. Actuarial survival rates following cardiac transplantation in excess of 82 and 77% at 1 and 2 years, respectively, point to the considerable progress made during the last two decades.[1] Long-term survival is now limited primarily by the development of late-stage problems including the particular graft atherosclerosis seen in transplanted organs and complications related to chronic maintenance immunosuppression (e.g., infections, hypertension, nephrotoxicity, malignancy).[2–4]

Historical Perspective (Table 18.1)

Although the idea of organ transplantation has intrigued scientists and writers since ancient times, the first serious investigations were conducted by Carrel and Guthrie in the early 1900s.[5] However, clinical cardiac transplantation as a potentially realistic therapeutic modality awaited the development of cardiopulmonary bypass and hypothermic preservation, which evolved in the middle decades of the twentieth century.

The first human-to-human heart transplant was carried out by Barnard of South Africa in 1967. This initial effort triggered a brief flurry of widespread transplantation activity at major centers around the world. However, the dismal results, owing to inadequate immunosuppression and subsequent acute rejection or infection, soon stifled the initial enthusiasm for the procedure, and all but two centers in the United States abandoned the procedure. During the subsequent fallow phase, the persevering efforts of Shumway at Stanford University and Lower at the University of Virginia were rewarded by the creation of immunosuppressive regimens that improved early survival while reducing the incidence of serious infections.[5]

The introduction of cyclosporin A (CsA) to these regimens in 1978 and the widespread adoption of CsA-based immunosuppressive regimens by 1983 resulted in a dramatic improvement in survival rates and reduced and altered the nature of the incidence of chronic complications.[6] In addition, CsA is credited with allowing the first successful heart–lung and single-lung transplantation in 1981 and 1983, respectively.[7,8]

Because of limited donor organ supply to meet the needs of potential transplant recipients, mechanical circulatory assistance with the idea of perfecting a chronically implantable mechanical device for the treatment of end-stage heart disease has remained attractive. Initial experience as a permanent implantation demonstrated the ability of the device to sustain bodily functions but it was plagued by an unacceptably high incidence of complications.[9] However, various forms of mechanical circulatory assistance were adopted as "bridges" to transplantation for patients with terminal cardiac failure for whom no donors were immediately available.[10] The overall survival rate following bridge-to-transplantation procedures (i.e., implantation through discharge from the hospital) utilizing mechanical devices has been approximately 50%.[11] The disappointing post-transplant survival rate following mechanical assistance has been largely due to its use in critically ill end-stage heart failure patients who go on to develop multisystem organ failure.[11] Thus, more restrictive selection criteria and improved risk stratification strategies are being evaluated. Clinical testing of two implantable chronic cardiac replacement systems is under way. The devices consist of a permanently implanted pump coupled to a rechargeable power supply. The Novacor wearable left ventricular assist system (LVAS) has been in use in Europe since 1994, for patients in and out of the hospital,[12] and is currently in clinical trials in the United States (Fig. 18.1). In 1995, the HeartMate implantable left ventricle assist device was approved by the FDA as a "bridge" to transplant[13] (Fig. 18.2).

With the improvement in survival rates, the number of cardiac transplant centers in the United States ballooned to more than 160 in the early 1990s, more than a 20-fold increase since 1981.[1] However, by 1994, that number had declined to 120 active centers reflecting changes caused by

TABLE 18.1. CARDIAC TRANSPLANTATION MILESTONES

1967	Dr. Christian Barnard performed the first heart transplant in the world.
1968	The Uniform Anatomical Gift Act formalized a consensus definition of brain death and paved the way for the legal donation of solid organs.
1968	Dr. Denton Cooley performed the first successful heart transplant in the United States at the Texas Heart Institute.
1973	Drs. Phillip Caves and Margaret Billingham developed the cardiac biopsy technique for monitoring rejection.
1981	Dr. Bruce Reitz performed the first heart–lung transplant at Stanford University.
1982	Dr. William DeVries performed the first Jarvik-7 total artificial heart implantation in Utah.
1983	Cyclosporine was approved by the FDA.
1984	Congress enacted the National Organ Transplant Act, establishing a national system to match donors and recipients.
1986	United Network for Organ Sharing (UNOS), Richmond, Virginia, was awarded the federal contract to ensure equitable access and allocation of organs. UNOS sets membership criteria and standards for transplant centers.
1987	Federal law began requiring hospitals to approach relatives of patients considered brain-dead about organ donation.
1987	Medicare began paying for heart transplantation at hospitals that meet survival and experience criteria set by the Health Care Financing Administration (HCFA).
1987	HCFA began certifying organ procurement agencies.
1994	Novacor wearable left ventricular assist system approved for commercial sale in Europe as a bridge and as an alternative to transplantation for patients in and out of the hospital.
1994	Tacrolimus was approved by the FDA.
1995	Mycophenolate mofetil was approved by the FDA.
1995	HeartMate left ventricular device FDA approved as a bridge to transplantation.

health care reform and the shortage of donor organs. The number of heart transplants performed in 1994 in the United States was 2298. Worldwide, more than 250 centers are currently performing heart transplant procedures. More than 26,700 heart and/or lung transplants had been performed as of 1994.[14]

Conditions Leading to the Need for Cardiac Transplantation

From a demographic perspective, it is estimated that there are 15,000 to 25,000 patients, 55 years of age and younger, with end-stage cardiac disease for whom the quality of life may be improved through cardiac transplantation[15] or through a perfected, permanent assistance device. This number increases to 40,000 if patients up to age 65 are included. In addition, this number is expected to grow as 400,000 new cases of heart failure are diagnosed each year.[16]

While demand for cardiac donors continues to grow, the number of potential organ donors, according to current brain death criteria, remains relatively fixed at 14,000 per year. Of these 14,000 patients, only 4500 become organ donors and, of these, only slightly more than 2000 are suitable cardiac donors. Currently, there are more than 4500 patients on the national organ network list awaiting donor availability for cardiothoracic transplantation.[1] Procurement of donor hearts with longer ischemic times, the use of older donors, and even the use of donors with borderline left ventricular function are being considered in an effort to increase donor supply.[17] This inequity between donor supply and recipient demand has resulted in a dramatic increase in waiting time from 6 weeks in 1988 to 6 months in 1990 to more than 1 year in 1993. Individual waiting times vary considerably based on recipient blood type, body size, clinical condition, and geographic location. As a result of this prolonged waiting time, one out of every five patients accepted for transplantation dies while awaiting donor organ availability.

Optimal recipient management in the pretransplantation period has been shown to reduce the morbidity and mortality associated with end-stage heart failure, but the timing for selection of the heart failure patient to become a transplant candidate is often difficult.[18] Optimal medical therapy includes the use of digoxin, angiotensin-converting enzyme (ACE) inhibitors, diuretics, potassium and magnesium supplements, and anticoagulants. Intermittent inotropic infusion therapy may also be required. Frequent patient follow-up (no less frequently than every 2 weeks) with careful attention to weight gain, nutrition, and electrolyte surveillance appears to reduce morbidity and the necessity for hospital admission. The high mortality rate of patients on the transplant waiting list will be altered only by improved methods of treating congestive heart failure or by alternatives to cardiac transplantation (e.g., cardiomyoplasty, mechanical devices, xenografts).[19]

The major etiologies of heart failure in potential recipients include idiopathic cardiomyopathy in 44% and ischemic heart disease in 47%.[14] Other less common etiologies include valvular disease, 4%; retransplantation for graft atherosclerosis or dysfunction, 2.3%; and congenital heart disease, 1.3%. Most recipients have been male between 30 and 55 years of age (mean 45 years).[20] However, the percentage of pediatric patients and patients greater than 55 years of age has continued to increase. Many centers are currently using modified criteria in which older patients with no secondary organ dysfunction may be transplanted.[21]

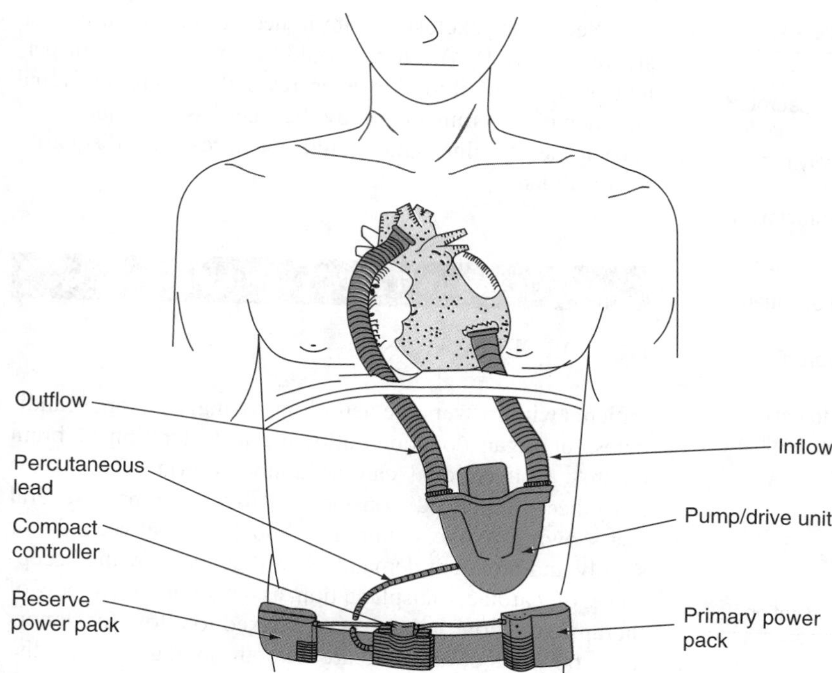

Figure 18.1. Wearable Novacor LVAS.

Historically, cardiac transplant candidates included those patients with end-stage heart failure who had New York Heart Association (NYHA) class III or IV symptoms, refractory to conventional medical management (Table 18.2), and who had a life expectancy of less than 1 year.

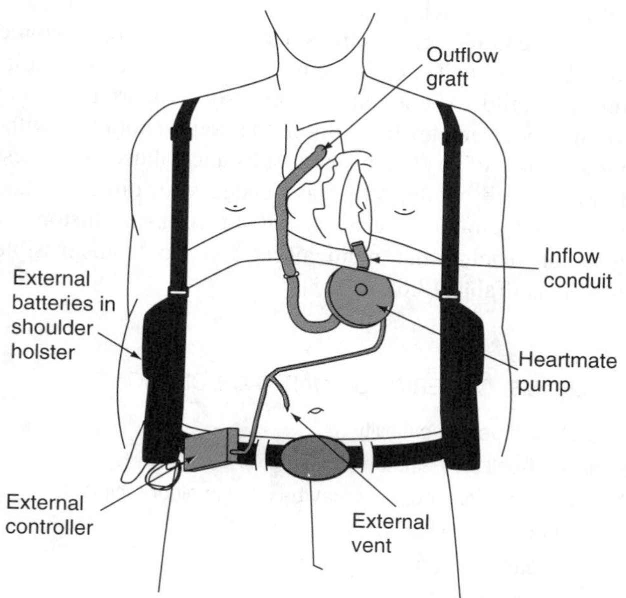

Figure 18.2. The vented electric HeartMate left ventricular assist device is battery powered and portable. Electrical wires and an air vent exit the skin to connect with the external controller. The pump also can be pneumatically actuated via the vent. *(From McCarthy PM, Sabik J. Implantable circulatory support devices as a bridge to heart transplantation. Semin Thorac Cardiovasc Surg 1994;6:174–180, with permission.)*

Based on the number of patients who currently meet these general criteria, more objective methods of identifying patients with the poorest prognosis are needed (Table 18.3).[18] Once maximal treatment has been instituted and maintained, peak V_{O_2} measured during maximal exercise testing provides an objective assessment of functional capacity and an indirect assessment of cardiovascular reserve; however, a variety of factors including age, gender, conditioning status, muscle mass and angina can limit peak V_{O_2}.[22]

Absolute contraindications to orthotopic cardiac transplantation include the presence of an active infection, the presence of other diseases that may limit survival (i.e., malignancy), or severe, irreversible pulmonary hypertension (PVR >6–8 Wood units or transpulmonary gradient >15 mm Hg), which could cause post-transplantation right ventricular failure. Candidates with borderline pulmonary pressures should be assessed to determine reversibility with agents such as nitroprusside, dobutamine, amrinone, milri-

TABLE 18.2. SELECTION AND EXCLUSION CRITERIA FOR HEART TRANSPLANTATION RECIPIENTS

Indications
Less than 65 years of age
End-stage cardiac disease (NYHA class III or IV), unlikely to benefit from conventional therapy or poor 6- to 12-month prognosis for survival
Normal function or reversible dysfunction of liver, kidneys, lungs, or CNS
Pulmonary vascular resistance <6 Wood units or pharmacologically reversible

TABLE 18.3. INDICATIONS FOR TRANSPLANTATION

I. Accepted Indications for Transplantation
1. Maximal Vo_2 <10 mL/kg/min with achievement of anaerobic metabolism
2. Severe ischemia consistently limiting routine activity not amenable to bypass surgery or angioplasty
3. Recurrent symptomatic ventricular arrhythmias refractory to all accepted therapeutic modalities

II. Probable Indications for Cardiac Transplantation
1. Maximal Vo_2 <14 mL/kg/min and major limitation of patient's daily activities
2. Recurrent unstable ischemia not amenable to bypass surgery or angioplasty
3. Instability of fluid balance/renal function not due to patient noncompliance with regimen of weight monitoring, flexible diuretic drugs, and salt restriction

III. Inadequate Indications for Transplantation
1. Ejection fraction <20%
2. History of class III or IV symptoms of heart failure
3. Previous ventricular arrhythmias
4. Maximal Vo_2 max >15 mL/kg/min without other indications

(From Ref. 18.)

none, PGE_1, or prostacyclin. A patient with a PVR >6 Wood units that decreases by 50% may be an acceptable candidate but the patient needs to be reassessed periodically to ensure suitability for transplant. Patients with elevated pulmonary artery resistance who do not respond to hemodynamic maneuvers may be candidates for heart–lung transplantation.

TABLE 18.4. SECONDARY EXCLUSION CRITERIA FOR HEART TRANSPLANTATION

Coexistent systemic illness with poor prognosis
Irreversible pulmonary parenchymal disease
Irreversible renal dysfunction with serum creatinine >2 mg/dL or creatinine clearance <50 mL/min
Irreversible hepatic dysfunction
Severe peripheral and cerebrovascular obstructive disease
Insulin-dependent diabetes with end-organ damage
Active infection
Coexisting neoplasm
Pulmonary hypertension with irreversibly high pulmonary vascular resistance (pulmonary vascular resistance >6 Wood units or 3.0 Wood units after treatment and vasodilators)
Acute pulmonary embolism or infarction
Active diverticulosis or diverticulitis
Active peptic ulcer disease
Myocardial infiltrative and inflammatory diseases
Severe obesity
Severe osteoporosis
Psychosocial instability or substance abuse, or both

(From Ref. 18).

Secondary exclusion criteria need to be carefully considered (Table 18.4). There should be no multiorgan or permanent system failure; however, reversible degrees of renal and hepatic dysfunction may be seen as a sequelae of chronic heart failure and should not necessarily disqualify the candidate.[18]

MECHANICS OF CARDIAC TRANSPLANTATION

DONOR SELECTION

Patients with irreversible neurologic damage become candidates for organ donation following a declaration of brain death.[23] Conventional cardiac donor criteria (Table 18.5) have been expanded considerably over the past several years owing to the continuing imbalance between donor supply and recipient demand as well as the growing acceptance of cardiac transplantation as an approved mode of therapy. Age criteria have been relaxed to allow for donors up to 60 years of age who are without obvious cardiac disease. Despite these changes, several principles remain standard in donor selection. There should be ABO blood group compatibility with the prospective heart recipient because mismatching in this system will result in a hyperacute rejection in most cases. Human leukocyte antigen (HLA) tissue matching of the donor organ and recipient is not performed routinely pretransplant unless the potential recipient is reactive against a panel of random donor antigens (i.e., positive cross-match), in which case a negative T-cell cross-match is required prior to transplantation. The donor should have a normal ECG and be hemodynamically stable, requiring only mild to moderate vasopressor support following volume replacement. In addition, the donor should be without a history of cardiac disease, substance abuse, and chest trauma severe enough to be associated with direct cardiac injury, and should have no active infections or history of behavior placing the recipient at risk for transmissible infections (Table 18.6).

TABLE 18.5. CRITERIA FOR CARDIAC DONATION

ABO blood type compatibility
Negative T-cell cross-match if PRA[a] ≥5%
Age ≤60 years (older organs may be used in older recipients)
Size within 30% of recipient
Negative cardiac history
Normal electrocardiogram
Normal echocardiogram
Minimal pressor support (e.g., <10 mcg/kg/min dopamine or equivalent)
Central venous pressure ≤12 mm Hg

[a]PRA, panel reactive antibody.

TABLE 18.6. ABSOLUTE AND RELATIVE CONTRAINDICATIONS TO CARDIAC DONATION

Absolute Contraindications Include:
1. HIV positivity (?, except in cases of HIV-positive recipients)
2. Death from carbon monoxide poisoning, with blood carboxyhemoglobin level >20%
3. Intractable ventricular arrhythmia
4. Inadequate oxygenation, with arterial saturation <80% on ventilatory support
5. Documented previous myocardial infarction
6. Clinically significant structural heart disease, intracardiac tumor, or severe global hypokinesia with ejection fraction <10% as determined by echocardiogram
7. Severe occlusive coronary artery disease on arteriography

Relative Contraindications Include:
1. Hepatitis B surface antigen positivity (?, except in cases of surface antigen-positive recipients)
2. Bacterial sepsis
3. Hepatitis C positivity
4. History of metastatic cancer
5. Extensive chest wall trauma with evidence of cardiac contusion by ECG or echocardiography
6. Prolonged hypotension, defined as a systolic blood pressure <60 mm Hg for >6 hours
7. Recurrent supraventricular arrhythmia
8. Prolonged need for inotropic support, defined as a dopamine dosage >20 μg/kg per min for >24 hours or comparable dosage of other β agonist or epinephrine, norepinephrine, or dobutamine for the same period
9. Prolonged resuscitation time after cardiopulmonary arrest, defined as attempted cardiopulmonary resuscitation for >30 min performed within 24 hours of organ harvest or multiple episodes of attempted cardiopulmonary resuscitation
10. Severe left ventricular hypertrophy on electrocardiogram or echocardiogram
11. Echocardiogram revealing moderate hypokinesia, which is typically segmental in brain injury, with shortening fraction 10–25%
12. Noncritical coronary disease on arteriogram
13. History of carbon monoxide inhalation, with blood carboxyhemoglobin <20%
14. History of intravenous drug abuse

(From Ref. 23.)

SURGICAL TECHNIQUE

Once a suitable donor has been identified, the first surgical priority is the coordination of the necessary logistical arrangements for donor organ transport and recipient preparation. The distant procurement radius is based on an optimal maximum total graft ischemia time of 4 hours, because it has been observed that early graft function and survival tend to be impaired with longer ischemic times. Donor organ preservation during transport is accomplished utilizing topical hypothermia and a variety of cardioplegic solutions.

Recipient preparation is based on a 3-hour time frame, which allows for antibiotic and immunosuppressive administration, presurgical preparation, initiation of hemodynamic monitoring, anesthesia induction, placement on cardiopulmonary bypass, and dissection of the recipient's heart. The diseased heart is removed, leaving behind a cuff of right atrium encompassing the superior and inferior venae cavae and a cuff of left atrium encompassing all of the pulmonary vein ostia.

The cardiac transplantation procedure is similar to that originally described by Lower and Shumway.[5] With the patient on total cardiopulmonary bypass and systemically cooled to 28°C, the left atrial anastomosis is performed first. Then the right atrial anastomosis, the aortic, and last, the pulmonary artery anastomosis are completed (Fig. 18.3).

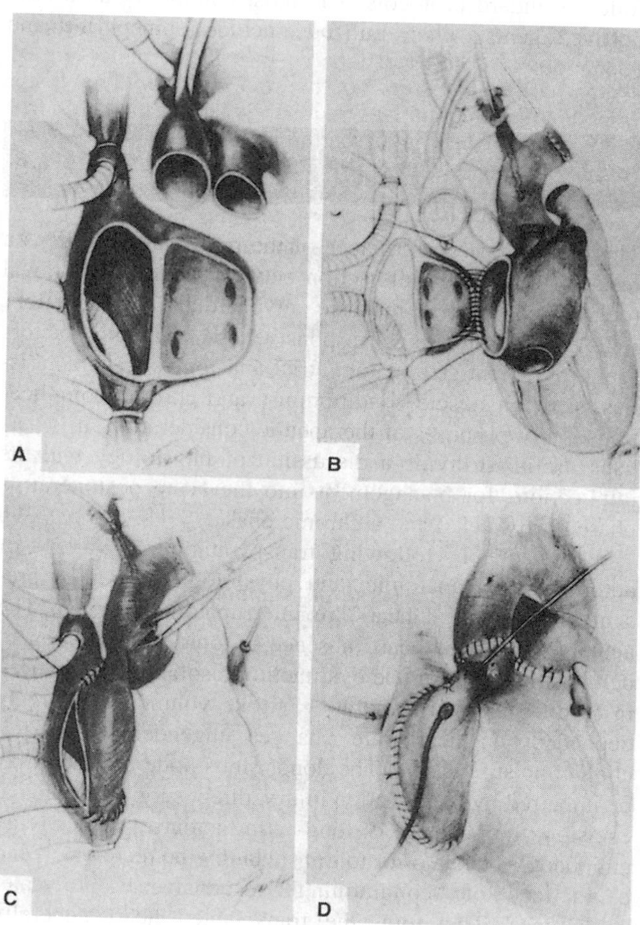

Figure 18.3. Heart transplantation procedure. (A) The recipient heart is excised, leaving behind a right and left atrial remnant. (B) The left atrial anastamosis is performed first. (C) The right atrial anastamosis is performed. (D) Finally, the aorta and pulmonary artery anastamoses are performed and an atrial-pacing electrode is placed. *(From Bolman RM, Molina EJ, Anderson R. Heart transplantation, in Najarian JS, Simmons RL, Ascher NL, et al [eds]: Manual of Vascular Access, Organ Donation, and Transplantation. New York, Springer-Verlag, 1984, pp 215, 216, 218, 222, with permission.)*

When the cross-clamp has been removed and rewarming is under way, the heart will often enter sinus rhythm spontaneously. Generation and maintenance of a hemodynamically optimal sinus rhythm is accomplished utilizing a combination of isoproterenol, temporary atrial pacing, and DC countershock. Lidocaine is used to suppress hemodynamically compromising ventricular arrhythmias. In the occasional patient who demonstrates prolonged asystole following bypass, metabolic parameters (electrolytes, acid–base status) are determined and corrected when necessary. Inotropic or vasopressive agents may also be necessary in this setting.

Hemodynamic goals following bypass include a systolic pressure between 90 and 140 mm Hg and a central venous pressure (CVP) of 8–18 cm H_2O. Inotropic and chronotropic agents are used to titrate systolic pressures and heart rate. Decannulation, heparin reversal, and closure follow standard protocols. The most commonly used supportive agents, when utilized, include epinephrine and dopamine.

Physiologic Consequences of Cardiac Transplantation

The physiologic performance of the transplanted heart is a result of a complex interaction between neural withdrawal (denervated heart), intrinsic myocardial autoregulatory reflexes, catecholamine responsiveness, anatomic factors (donor/recipient size match, atrial anastomosis characteristics, skeletal muscle conditioning), and chronic complications.[24] For purposes of therapeutic consideration, it is perhaps useful to divide a discussion of physiology with its implications for management into the acute postoperative phase (0–6 weeks) and a chronic phase.

Immediately following transplantation, a variety of autoregulatory, anatomic, and physiologic responses present in the normal heart are interrupted or blunted. The acutely denervated heart (absence of tonic vagal influence) demonstrates sinus node dysfunction insofar as the changes in cardiac output (heart rate × stroke volume) are largely dependent on heart rate changes engendered by catecholamine stimulation. The donor sinus node function may be impaired by preservation injury, direct surgical trauma at excision, the presence of long-acting antiarrhythmics (e.g., amiodarone) taken prior to transplant by the recipient,[25] and by a lack of "conditioning" responsiveness to catecholamines. Therefore, the transplanted heart generally requires chronotropic support with either isoproterenol or pacing in the early post-transplant period. Generally, either mode of heart rate manipulation is adjusted to maintain a heart rate of 90–110 beats/min and evidence of satisfactory hemodynamics (blood pressure, urine output, and tissue perfusion). Approximately 10% of transplant patients will have persistent chronotropic incompetence and require either extended (permanent) cardiac pacing or pharmacologic manipulation of the heart with isoproterenol or theophylline.[26]

In the early post-transplant period, anatomic variables may further compromise optimal hemodynamic function and complicate hemodynamic assessment of the patient. Atrial transport function, which normally contributes 15–20% to the cardiac output, is impaired following transplantation because the hybridized atria do not conduct the electrical activation signal across suture lines. Right ventricular function is frequently impaired, presumably as a result of "preservation" injury, and may demonstrate a "restrictive" hemodynamic pattern, which improves over 6 weeks following transplantation. Donor/recipient size mismatch may also contribute to early post-transplantation hemodynamic abnormalities characterized by increased heart rates and higher left ventricular end diastolic pressures.

The chronically transplanted heart has been studied extensively both at rest and in response to exercise, which may unmask physiologic abnormalities not seen in the resting state. In the resting state, left ventricular ejection fraction is well preserved but may not increase to the same degree with exercise when compared with normals. As pointed out previously, the chronically denervated heart is dependent on augmentation of cardiac output/ventricular function by stimulation of myocardial β-receptors. However, the denervated, exercising cardiac graft rarely achieves the maximum augmentation seen in normal hearts. In addition, persistent abnormalities of diastolic function are noted in the chronically transplanted heart such that intracardiac pressures increase in an exaggerated fashion with response to exercise and/or volume infusion. In the chronically transplanted heart, these abnormalities of diastolic function may be the result of acute rejection, scarring secondary to treated rejection, hypertension, coronary graft arteriopathy, or the abnormal neuroendocrine milieu in which the graft functions. Baroreceptor function is also abnormal in the transplanted heart, probably as a result of altered mechanoreceptor afferent impulses in the denervated heart, and may contribute to the observation of impaired hemodynamic responses to hypotension or exercise in the transplanted heart.

The peculiar physiology of the transplanted heart has several implications for pharmacologic therapy. Drugs such as digoxin and atropine, whose mechanisms of action are mediated by the sympathetic nervous system, will have little effect on the transplanted heart. Augmentation of cardiac output is primarily mediated via heart rate increases and to a lesser extent, inotropic responses. Thus, drugs such as epinephrine and isoproterenol with their marked β-adrenergic effect are particularly useful, while β-blocking agents may precipitate catastrophic cardiovascular collapse. The sinus node of the denervated heart is particularly sensitive to the negative chronotropic effects of acetylcholine or adenosine and caution must be used if these agents are administered. Wilson has suggested that reinnervation may occur in the previously denervated heart, thereby facilitating more normal physiologic and pharmacologic responses.[27] Supraventricular arrhythmias are not uncommon in the early post-transplant period. Chronic suppressive pharmacologic therapy with type IA or IC agents may be required but may depress sinus node or AV nodal function.

QUALITY OF LIFE AFTER TRANSPLANTATION

Quality of life indicators have been widely studied in cardiac transplantation recipients as researchers and society seek to objectify and justify the rewards of transplantation.[24] While cynics would maintain that heart transplantation involves the trading of one disease (heart failure) with a poor prognosis for another disease with a less dismal prognosis (post-transplantation status), most recipients self-assess themselves positively when compared with both their prior health status and in comparison to perceptions of normal.

CARE OF THE CARDIAC TRANSPLANT PATIENT

POSTOPERATIVE MANAGEMENT

Postoperative care is similar to that provided for other patients undergoing cardiac surgery. Patients are generally extubated on the first postoperative day, and early ambulation and vigorous pulmonary toilet are of considerable importance in minimizing complications. Chest tubes are usually removed within 48 hours. All central lines and catheters are removed within 24–48 hours. The uncomplicated patient is transferred out of the intensive care unit by 48–72 hours and discharged at 10–14 days.

Early postoperative complications in the heart transplant recipient can be avoided by carefully screening donors (Tables 18.5 and 18.6) and recipients (Table 18.4) prior to transplantation. Primary graft failure is usually evident in the operating room and, although frequently reversible, may necessitate mechanical assistance or re-transplantation. Right ventricular failure secondary to high pulmonary vascular resistance can be avoided by carefully screening recipients. On occasion, intra- or postoperative administration of prostaglandins, vasodilators, and inotropic agents may be necessary to treat right-sided failure in the transplant patient.

Following transplantation, myocardial depression may occur as a result of ischemia, pharmacologically induced myocardial catecholamine depletion, or elevated pulmonary artery resistances. Thus, vasopressor or inotropic support may be necessary in the early postoperative period; commonly used agents include dopamine and/or epinephrine. Early on, cardiac output in the transplanted heart is largely rate dependent and this chronotropic response may require "conditioning" with isoproterenol (0.005–0.01 mcg/kg/min) to maintain the heart rate in the range of 110–130 beats/min in order to optimize cardiac output. Cardiac function generally returns to normal within 3 to 4 days, during which time most patients can be weaned from chronotropic and inotropic support. While many patients require temporary pacing support for the first 3 to 7 days after transplantation, a few (2–10%) will require permanent pacemaker support because of chronotropic incompetency. Patients who received amiodarone preoperatively are at risk for prolonged bradycardia following transplantation.[25] Agents such as theophylline or terbutaline may enhance ventricular response and obviate the need for permanent pacing in these patients.[26]

Hypertension may occur following surgery and may be due to pain, hypothermia, stress, or the presence of preoperative hypertension. Systolic blood pressure is maintained at less than 140 mm Hg, utilizing afterload reduction with nitroprusside or nitroglycerin, thereby further augmenting cardiac function.

Because the incidence of acute rejection is highest during the first 6 months following transplantation, endomyocardial biopsies are performed empirically at regularly scheduled intervals following transplantation (e.g., every week first month, then every 2 weeks for 2–3 months, then every 4–6 weeks up to 6 months, and then every 3 months up to 1 year) and on an as-needed basis according to the clinical status of the patient.

IMMUNOSUPPRESSION PROTOCOLS

Preliminary work in the area of immunosuppression for cardiac transplantation evolved as an extension of experience gained from the treatment of cancer as well as from the partially successful control of rejection in renal transplant recipients. Early protocols included methotrexate, azathioprine, actinomycin D, and cyclophosphamide. The initial protocol used by Stanford in 1968 included azathioprine 2–3 mg/kg/d adjusted according to white blood count, prednisone 1.5 mg/kg/d tapered to a maintenance dose of 0.25–0.5 mg/kg/d by 6 months, and horse antilymphocyte globulin (ALG).[28] Initial 1-year survival rates increased from 28–50% with the substitution of six doses of rabbit antithymocyte globulin (RATG) for the ALG. By 1984, 1-year actuarial survival rates exceeded 67% with so-called "conventional" immunosuppression.[29]

CsA was introduced in the immunosuppressive protocol beginning in 1980. The initial protocol consisted of CsA 18 mg/kg/d, prednisone 1 mg/kg/d tapering to 0.2 mg/kg/d, and RATG 3 mg/kg/dose in the immediate postoperative period. The CsA-based regimen resulted in a marked reduction in the dosage of corticosteroids and an increase in early survival. Disadvantages of CsA therapy observed during these initial trials included the loss of the ECG as a sensitive and specific noninvasive test for the monitoring of rejection, hypertension, nephrotoxicity, and the occurrence of four lymphomas in the first 36 patients.[28] The implementation of triple-drug therapy regimens (CsA 6–12 mg/kg/d, azathioprine 2 mg/kg/d, and prednisone tapered from 1.5 to 0.2 mg/kg/d by the end of 3 months) by Bolman and associates in 1983 resulted in 1-year survival rates of 88% and reduced nephrotoxicity, infection, and hypertension.[30] This regimen remains the cornerstone of many immunosuppressive protocols in use today.[31]

Current preoperative regimens consist primarily of azathioprine (2–4 mg/kg orally or intravenously) and varying dosages of CsA (0–10 mg/kg) administered orally 4–6 hours prior to surgery. All patients receive methylprednisolone 500 mg intravenously immediately after discontinuing cardiopulmonary bypass, and 125 mg intravenously every 12 hours for the first 36 hours after surgery.

Postoperatively, the administration of CsA is either initiated on day 1 or delayed until day 3 or 4 to decrease potential nephrotoxicity in the immediate postoperative period. Based on the latter concern, the initial postoperative dosage of CsA varies from center to center (4–12 mg/kg/d). However, CsA is usually titrated to achieve whole blood levels as assayed by high-performance liquid chromatography in the range of 175–250 ng/mL, or plasma levels by radioimmunoassay of 180–250 ng/mL. Intravenous cyclosporine may be used in patients with absorption problems[32]; however, controversy exists as to what steady-state concentrations are desirable. Azathioprine is initiated at 2 mg/kg/d and is adjusted to maintain a peripheral white blood cell count of 3500–6000 cells/mm^3. Prednisone is tapered from an initial dose of 1.5 to 0.2 mg/kg/d by the end of 3 months and then tapered to approximately 0.1 mg/kg/d by 6–12 months.

Tacrolimus (formerly FK506) was approved in 1994, and has been used as an alternative agent for cyclosporine in double and triple drug regimens.[33] The drug is reviewed in greater detail in Chapter 9 (Overview of Transplantation). The usual starting dosage for tacrolimus, 0.1–0.2 mg/kg/d administered orally as a twice-daily dosage, or 0.025–0.075 mg/kg/d as a continuous intravenous infusion, is slightly lower in heart transplant patients based on the earlier experience gained with other organ recipients. Tacrolimus concentrations are titrated initially to achieve whole blood levels of 5–20 ng/mL or plasma levels of 0.5–2 ng/mL; however, lower concentrations are used after 6 months.[34,35] Drug concentrations need to be monitored whenever the patient's condition changes, toxicity is suspected, or when hepatically metabolized drugs are administered. The propensity for drug interactions for tacrolimus appears to be either similar or greater than CsA. Until clinical data document the contrary, drugs known to interact with CsA should be assumed to interact with tacrolimus (Table 18.7).[36] Because tacrolimus is a macrolide, it may also interact with other drugs (e.g., theophylline, terfenadine) known to interact with erythromycin.[37] Because of its very narrow therapeutic range, drug interactions may be even more problematic with tacrolimus than CsA. With mechanisms of action, pharmacokinetic profiles, analytical difficulties, and toxicity profiles similar to that of cyclosporine, tacrolimus' major advantages have been its efficacy as a (rescue) agent in patients with recalcitrant rejection, its steroid and azathioprine-sparing effects, and its lower propensity to cause hypertension.[36,38] However, the latter may be more related to its steroid-sparing effects,

TABLE 18.7. DRUG INTERACTIONS OF CSA AND TACROLIMUS

CsA Levels		Tacrolimus Levels	
Increase	**Decrease**	**Increase**	**Decrease**
Ketoconazole	Rifampicin	Ketoconazole	Rifampicin
Fluconazole	Phenytoin	Fluconazole	Dexamethasone
Itraconazole	Phenobarbital	Itraconazole	Phenytoin
Erythromycin	Carbamazepine	Erythromycin	
Diltiazem	Sulphadimine	Diltiazem	
Verapamil	Trimethoprim	Verapamil	
Danazol		Danazol	
Nicardipine		Cimetidine	
Metoclopramide		Clotrimazole	
Methylprednisolone		CsA	
Norethisterone			
Tacrolimus			

(From Ref. 36.)

because it appears to be equally or more nephrotoxic than CsA.[39]

Some centers use cytolytic agents (e.g., muromonab-CD3, OKT3, ALG, or ATG) as "induction" therapy during the first 7–14 postoperative days to minimize the adverse side effects observed with the other agents.[40–43] To date, pooled data series show no clear-cut survival advantages with induction therapy, though it appears that a higher percentage of patients may be weaned from prednisone, thereby reducing the incidence of steroid-associated complications. These protocols usually result in the discontinuation of prednisone by 3–6 months following transplantation. Controversy exists as to whether prophylactic therapy with these cytolytic agents confers any added benefit. In addition, cytolytic therapy is expensive, inconvenient to administer, possibly alters the incidence and character of infectious complications, and may result in a higher incidence of malignancy. These agents are best reserved for selective use in patients at high risk for toxicity from the other immunosuppressive agents and/or those who are more immunoreactive.

Mycophenolate mofetil (formerly RS61443) was approved for use in transplant patients in 1995, and is described in more detail in Chapter 9. This drug is an antiproliferative agent with similar but less toxicity than azathioprine. It has demonstrated efficacy both as maintenance immunosuppression and "rescue" therapy for rejection episodes.[44,45] Its exact role in cardiac transplant patients remains to be identified (clinical trials are still under way).

Complications After Heart Transplantation

Despite the improved survival, the major long-term complications reported today are virtually unchanged from the early 1980s. Post-transplant complications can be categorized as life-threatening (i.e., those related to either too much or too little immunosuppression) versus immunosuppressant-induced adverse effects (Table 18.8). The complications are reviewed extensively elsewhere in the literature.[2–4]

TABLE 18.8. POST-TRANSPLANT COMPLICATIONS

Immunosuppression-Related Life-Threatening Consequences	Immunosuppressant-Related Adverse Effects
Early	Nephrotoxicity
Acute rejection	Hypertension
Infection	Hyperlipidemia
Late	Osteoporosis
Allograft coronary artery disease	Obesity
Malignancy	Diabetes

MORTALITY

Mortality in the early post-transplant period (first 3 months) occurs as a result of either very early technical complications (failure of graft preservation, hemorrhage, postoperative pulmonary hypertension) or as a result of rejection or infection. Risk factors for death within the first postoperative year include prior transplantation, the use of a ventricular assist device or ventilator, very young or old recipient (<5 years or >60 years), older donor, female donor, and prolonged ischemic time.[14] Late mortality (>12 months) occurs as a result of chronic rejection (i.e., chronic graft atherosclerosis), malignancy, cerebrovascular accident, or renal and/or hepatic failure.

IMMUNOSUPPRESSION-RELATED COMPLICATIONS

Acute Rejection

Despite advances in immunosuppression and refinement of postoperative care, acute cardiac allograft rejection remains a major determinant of late survival following cardiac transplantation. Acute rejection continues to account for approximately 17% of all deaths.[46] The incidence of rejection is substantially higher during the early months following transplantation, with 90% of all rejections occurring within the first 6 months. In addition, the severity of rejection tends to be greater when it occurs early in the postoperative period. Although a minority of patients (37%) remain rejection free, most will experience at least one rejection episode during the first year (e.g., cumulative number of rejection episodes is 1.3 ± 0.7/patient).[46]

Clinical manifestations of rejection may include low-grade fever, malaise, heart failure (S3), or atrial arrhythmias; however, most patients remain entirely asymptomatic. In the pre-CsA era, ECG changes served as an indicator of rejection.[27] Besides a drop in voltage, other ECG changes seen with rejection included the onset of new atrial arrhythmias, a change in the axis, and the development of a conduction defect. With the introduction of CsA into immunosuppressive regimens, the reliability of ECG monitoring to detect rejection has diminished due to the subtle presentation of clinical findings. Currently, the gold standard for rejection detection is histologic confirmation using endomyocardial specimens obtained by transvenous biopsy. Biopsy specimens are examined for evidence of rejection and graded, based on histologic severity of the rejection.[47] Because endomyocardial biopsies are not only an invasive procedure but also are expensive and labor intensive, great efforts have been expended to identify an accurate and reproducible noninvasive method/marker to detect or predict acute rejection. Unfortunately, none of the methods studied thus far has the reliability of the endomyocardial biopsy.

The treatment of rejection is based on a number of factors including the type, histologic grade, clinical symptoms, hemodynamic changes, noninvasive findings, and time after transplantation.

Mild degrees of acute cellular rejection (grade 0–1) are not usually treated unless the patient is symptomatic, whereas the presence of moderate rejection (grades 2–4), with or without necrosis, generally mandates treatment. Acute rejection is usually treated with methylprednisolone 500–1000 mg intravenously daily for 3 days. Lower doses may be equally effective[48] and, in some situations, a prednisone taper (e.g., 1.5 mg/kg/d tapered to ≤0.15 mg/kg/d over 7–14 days) either alone or in addition to intravenous therapy may be used.[49] An endomyocardial biopsy is usually repeated within 7 days of augmented steroid therapy. If there is evidence of continuing or worsening rejection, the steroid therapy may be repeated and/or cytolytic therapy (ATG or OKT3) may be employed. Other innovative forms of therapy for persistent or intractable rejection have been investigated, including low-dose methotrexate,[50,51] mycophenolate mofetil (formerly RS61443),[44,45] tacrolimus (formerly FK506),[34,35] serolimus (formerly rapamycin),[52] total lymphoid irradiation,[53] and photopheresis.[54]

Infection

Both the severity and incidence of infections and deaths due to infections have decreased dramatically since the introduction in 1978 of cyclosporine, a more potent and selective T-cell immunosuppressant that also allowed for lower steroid dosages. Nonetheless, infection and rejection remain the most frequently encountered complications associated with immunosuppression in the first year post-transplant.[55] The overall risk of infection is directly related to the level of immunosuppression and is greatest during the first postoperative 3 months, as well as following treatment of rejection episodes.[56] During the months following transplantation, the patient is carefully observed for signs and symptoms of infection. Laboratory or clinical evidence of an evolving infectious process necessitates the institution of aggressive diagnostic and frequently empiric therapeutic strategies. Infections in the transplant recipient can be categorized as nosocomial (catheter or wound-related or pneumonia with staphylococcus or gram negatives), donor-related (toxoplasmosis, hepatitis, CMV), or opportunistic (CMV, pneumocystis, nocardia, fungal).[56–58] The infections usually present in a characteristic time course following transplant (Fig. 18.4).[57] The most common sites of infection include lung, blood, urine, gastrointestinal (GI) tract, and sternal wound.[2] The latter accounts for only 7% of infections but represents 25% of the deaths because mediastinitis in an immunosuppressed patient can be devastating.[55] A number of preventive strategies are employed routinely in the transplant recipient and include the use of trimethoprim–sulfamethoxazole (pneumocystis, toxoplasma, and nocardia prophylaxis), miconazole (candida), and antiviral agents (e.g., acyclovir, ganciclovir, immune globulin, CMV hyperimmune globulin) for CMV, herpes simplex virus (HSV), and Epstein–Barr virus (EBV).[58]

CMV infection can result in both direct (increased morbidity and mortality having an impact on the cost and success of transplantation) and indirect (stimulatory and inhibitory immune responses resulting in rejection, opportunistic infections, and possibly chronic rejection) consequences in the transplant recipient.[59] Based on the premise that preventing CMV infection is preferable to treating CMV disease, most centers have adopted some type of preventive regimen. The major limitation is that the anti-CMV agents appear to be most efficacious in preventing reactivation (secondary infection) but have had little impact on the incidence of primary infection in the highest risk group (seronegative recipients of seropositive allografts).[60,61] The added benefit of acyclovir and ganciclovir prophylaxis is that they have significant activity against the other herpes viruses including EBV, which may provide a protective effect against post-transplant lymphoproliferative disease. Based on the current literature, there is no one ideal regimen for CMV prevention. More aggressive strategies including intravenous ganciclovir ± CMV hyperimmune globulin followed by high-dose acyclovir or oral ganciclovir may be most appropriate for the highest risk patients (CMV-negative recipients of seropositive organs or those receiving antilymphocyte therapy with OKT3 or ATG), while selective preemptive therapy with ganciclovir (i.e., treating the infection once it manifests itself rather than administering prophylaxis to all patients) may be used in those seropositive recipients at risk for reactivation.[62]

Chronic Graft Atherosclerosis

Chronic graft atherosclerosis (CGAS), also referred to as transplant coronary artery disease, has been defined as the occurrence of an accelerated atherosclerosis in the coronary arteries of the graft. Numerous reports have suggested the average incidence of this disease is approximately 10% per year or approximately 40–50% of angiographically defined CGAS by year 5 following transplantation.[63,64] This entity is thought to be similar to the "chronic rejection" processes also seen in renal, lung (obliterative bronchiolitis), and liver (vanishing bile duct syndrome) allografts. Achieving an understanding of and treatment for CGAS remains the single major obstacle to improving long-term survival in cardiac transplant recipients.[65] Despite improvements in immunosuppression and consequently in overall survival, the incidence of the disease has not changed since the late 1970s.

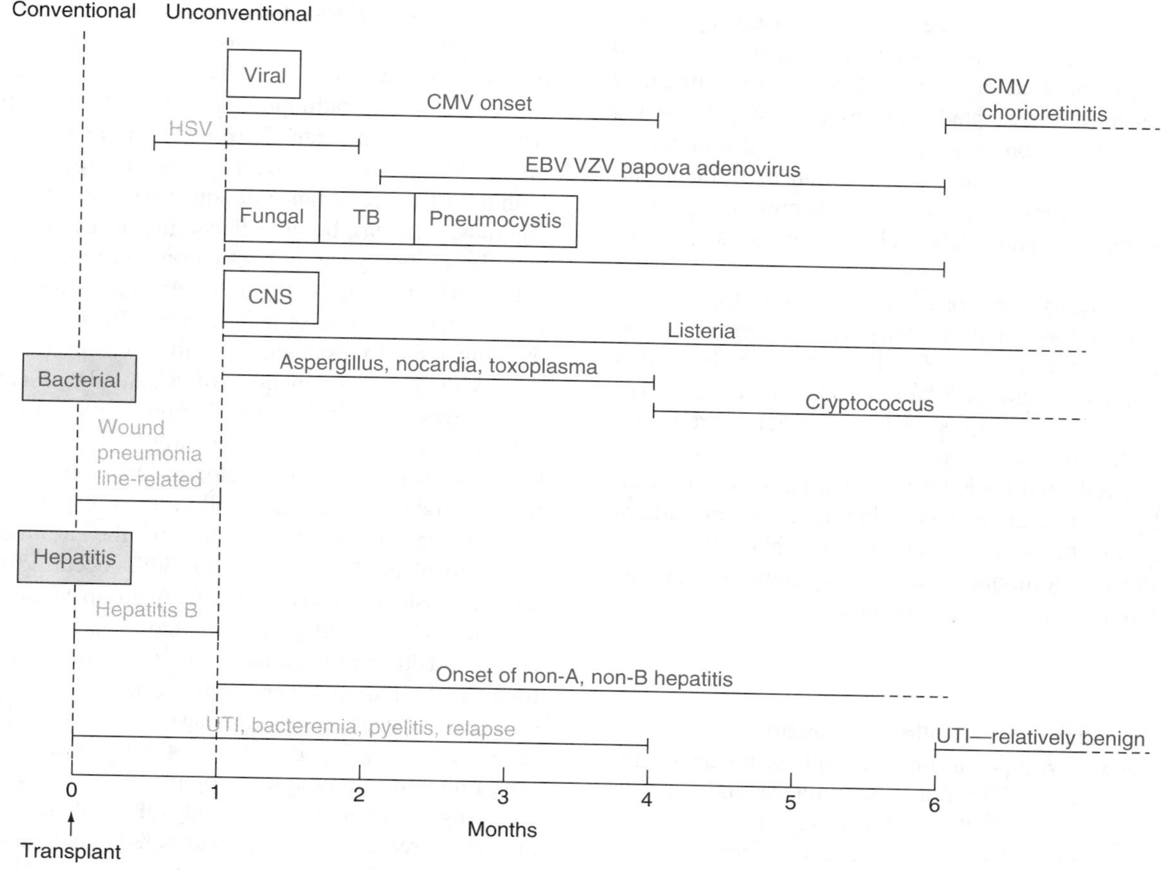

Figure 18.4. Timetable of infection for organ transplantation.

Manifestations of CGAS may include arrhythmias, impaired left ventricular function, congestive heart failure, acute myocardial infarction, and sudden cardiac death. Most heart transplant recipients with graft atherosclerosis do not experience "classic" angina because the allograft is denervated (i.e., true silent ischemia); however, angina should not be ignored because reinnervation has been reported.[27]

Accelerated graft atherosclerosis is characterized by a diffuse, concentric, intimal proliferation, which, in contrast to traditional atherosclerosis, is not usually focal but involves the entire vessel length, frequently resulting in obliteration of the small vessels of both epimyocardial and intramyocardial coronary branches. To aid in the diagnosis of CGAS, most centers perform annual cardiac evaluations including cardiac catheterization, thallium stress testing, and echocardiography. Because of the concentric, diffuse pattern of graft atherosclerosis, results of annual coronary angiography must be compared serially to appreciate the concentric reduction in luminal diameter or obliteration of second- and third-order vessels. By virtue of its diffuse nature, this type of graft atherosclerosis is rarely amenable to angioplasty or coronary artery bypass surgery.[66] Focal atherosclerotic involvement, as seen in nontransplant ischemic heart disease, may also be found in the transplanted allograft. This latter process tends to occur in the proximal portions of the extramural coronary vessels and may be amenable to percutaneous balloon dilation.

The pathogenesis of this problem has not yet been delineated, but the frequent observation of intimal thickening and a mononuclear cell inflammatory reaction within the thickened intima suggest that it may in part be due to chronic rejection, possibly as a result of a reaction to immunologic markers carried on vascular endothelial cells. CMV infection and subsequent rejection episodes are associated with the development of atherosclerosis in the transplanted heart.[67] It is possible the CMV contributes to an initial injury to the coronary endothelium, perhaps on an immunologic basis, that progresses to coronary artery disease. Another theory is that CMV expresses a protein that inhibits the beneficial function of a tumor suppression gene, thus promoting angiogenesis and accelerated atherosclerosis.[68] The potential long-term benefit of ganciclovir prophylaxis and treatment of CMV infections and its association with CGAS remain to be assessed.

Conventional preventive measures used to decrease the incidence of graft atherosclerosis in the transplant recipient include maintenance of ideal body weight, control of blood pressure, and implementation of dietary and drug therapy for lipid disorders.[69] The use of antiplatelet agents has become accepted preventive therapy following cardiac transplantation even though controlled clinical trials have not been conducted to demonstrate their efficacy.[70] Other therapies including angiopeptin, low molecular weight heparin, and calcium channel blockers are being studied.[2,71]

As previously mentioned, percutaneous transluminal coronary angioplasty and coronary bypass surgery are not usual options for treatment of diffuse graft atherosclerosis, leaving retransplantation as the only potential therapy once graft atherosclerosis has resulted in significant graft compromise. The prognosis following retransplantation is suboptimal, as reflected by a 1-year actuarial survival rate of 49%.[20] In addition, the extensive incidence of graft atherosclerosis potentially necessitating retransplantation introduces several additional ethical considerations regarding the allocation of scarce donor organs.

Malignancy

Successful maintenance of allograft function requires continuous therapy with potent immunosuppressive agents that interfere with normal immune surveillance and function. The biologic activity of these agents may engender diminished immune surveillance and direct carcinogenic or mutagenic action, chronic antigenic stimulation, or activation of oncogenic viruses resulting in an increased potential for tumor development.[72] Malignant neoplasms are an unfortunate consequence of chronic immunosuppression and may be an unavoidable complication of modifying the normal immune process.

The prevalence of cancers that occur most frequently in the general population (e.g., carcinomas of the lung, prostate, breast, and colon and invasive carcinomas of the uterine cervix) is not increased among transplant recipients. However, a variety of cancers that are uncommon in the general population often occur with a higher prevalence in transplant recipients: lymphomas (21% of cancers in transplant recipients are lymphomas, 93% of which are non–Hodgkin's or lymphoproliferative disorders), squamous-cell carcinomas of the lip and skin, Kaposi's sarcoma, other sarcomas, carcinomas of the vulva and perineum, carcinomas of the kidney, and hepatobiliary tumors.

The incidence of lymphoma appears to correlate with the intensity of immunosuppression. The use of more intensive immunosuppression in extrarenal transplant recipients is particularly common and is reflected in the higher incidence of lymphomas seen in cardiac recipients when compared to renal recipients.[73]

The incidence, time to occurrence, and features of the tumors appear to vary with use of various immunosuppressive agents.[74] Azathioprine-based immunosuppressive regimens have been associated with a high incidence (40% of all malignancies) of cutaneous malignancies. One possible mechanism to explain this unusually high incidence of skin cancer involves azathioprine's metabolite, nitroimidazole, which causes significant photosensitivity resulting in subsequent skin cancer.[75,76] Azathioprine therapy is associated with a 2 : 1 predominance of squamous over basal cell carcinomas, whereas basal cell carcinoma occurs more frequently in the general population. Azathioprine-induced cutaneous squamous cell carcinoma is also associated with more metastatic disease and accounts for 6% of all deaths in comparison to less than 1% with cyclosporine.[75]

With the introduction of CsA, the incidence of non–Hodgkin's lymphoma or lymphoproliferative disorder (LPD) increased to 29% as compared to 11% with regimens based on azathioprine or cyclophosphamide.[74] The tumors tended to occur earlier (15 months after transplantation in the CsA group versus 48 months in the azathioprine or cyclophosphamide group); and 32% occurred within 4 months postoperatively in the CsA group versus 11% for older non-CsA-based regimens. Among patients treated with OKT3 and other monoclonal antibodies, lymphomas account for 64% of all tumors. These lymphomas frequently develop soon after transplantation (average, 7 months).[74] In a recent report, LPD developed in 1.3% of patients receiving triple drug immunosuppression as compared to 11.4% in patients receiving the monoclonal antibody OKT3. A statistically significant increase in incidence was noted in patients receiving cumulative OKT3 dose of greater than 75 mg.[77] This report is in conflict with experiences of other centers.[78] Similarly, the use of ATG was found to increase the risk of LPD.[79]

T-cell-specific agents (e.g., CsA, OKT3, ATG) that directly impair T-cell function may produce a reduction in host response to viral infections, particularly EBV and CMV. EBV has been shown to have infectious as well as oncogenic properties and may play a causal role in the development of mononucleosis, Burkett's lymphoma, and nasal pharyngeal carcinoma. Reduction in immunosuppression intensity and concomitant therapy with acyclovir have resolved some forms of LPD.[80]

The clinical presentation of LPD may vary from a flu-like syndrome to multisystem organ failure.[80] A higher proportion of patients receiving conventional immunosuppression has extranodal involvement as compared with CsA-based regimens. Extranodal involvement occurs in 69% of cases in transplant recipients versus 24–48% in the general population. Central nervous system involvement occurs more frequently in patients with conventional immunosuppression (39%) as compared with CsA-based regimens (14%).

The diagnosis of LPD is made by a tissue biopsy. The histologic types of LPD are described elsewhere. Treatment depends on symptoms, presentation, and extent of involvement. In general, reduction of immunosuppression and concomitant therapy with acyclovir have been associated with resolution and remission of LPD.[80,81] Radiotherapy, chemotherapy, and surgical excision may be necessary in certain situations as palliative therapy but are rarely curative. Optimal preventive therapy is to avoid overimmunosuppression in transplant recipients. A 5-year mortality rate of 37% has been reported in patients with LPD.[81]

IMMUNOSUPPRESSANT-RELATED ADVERSE EFFECTS

Hypertension

Arterial hypertension is the most common post-transplantation medical problem, which, despite intensive investigation, is not well understood. The incidence of post-transplantation hypertension in cardiac recipients has increased from less than 20% in the conventional immunosuppression era to greater than 90% in the current era utilizing cyclosporine-based regimens.[82] In the conventional era, hypertension was believed to be a result of mineralocorticoid excess engendered by immunosuppressive regimens heavily based on prednisone. Paradoxically, with the introduction of cyclosporine-based regimens allowing for steroid dosage reduction or discontinuation, hypertension has become more prevalent.[82]

The primary mechanism of CsA-associated hypertension in heart transplant recipients may be related to the CsA-induced stimulation of intact renal sympathetic nerves and the absence of reflex cardiac inhibition of the sympathetic nervous system,[83] but a variety of other mechanisms have also been proposed.[84] In addition to CsA's propensity to cause peripheral vasoconstriction, it promotes sodium retention by increasing proximal tubular sodium retention, resulting in ECF volume expansion. Thus, diuretics and dietary sodium restriction are used routinely in heart transplant recipients. Because CsA and diuretics also induce renal magnesium wasting, hypomagnesemia may contribute to the hypertension because magnesium is purported to be a vasorelaxant. Magnesium supplementation is usually necessary in patients unless they have renal insufficiency.[84] Diuretics, while effective, may aggravate lipid abnormalities in these patients.

No single antihypertensive agent has been uniformly effective in controlling cyclosporine-associated hypertension. Currently, the use of calcium channel antagonists (e.g., diltiazem), inhibitors of central sympathetic outflow (e.g., clonidine), and, to a lesser extent, ACE inhibitors have been variably effective in the treatment of this form of hypertension. Calcium channel blockers, particularly diltiazem, are often considered drugs of choice because they have other purported benefits on the development of graft atherosclerosis[71] and may also be renal protective.[63,85] Polydrug regimens are often necessary. Additional hypertension control is seen as a salutary effect of current immunosuppressive protocols that eliminate prednisone after the third month following transplantation.[86]

Nephrotoxicity

One of the most common side effects observed in heart transplant recipients receiving maintenance cyclosporine therapy is nephrotoxicity.[87,88] Two types of toxicity occur: Acute nephrotoxicity is often seen early and is dose-dependent and reversible, while the more common type of toxicity is that of a chronic nephropathy. Clinical manifestations of cyclosporine nephrotoxicity include elevated serum creatinine and BUN, hyperkalemia, hyperuricemia, mild proteinuria, and a decreased fraction excretion of sodium.[89]

The predominant mechanism for cyclosporine nephrotoxicity is that of renal vasoconstriction, primarily of the afferent arteriole, resulting in increased renal vascular resistance, decreased renal blood flow by up to 40%, reduced glomerular filtration rate (GFR) by up to 30%, and increased proximal tubular sodium reabsorption with a reduction in urinary sodium and potassium excretion.[78] A number of other mechanisms have been implicated including changes in the renin–angiotensin–aldosterone system, prostaglandin synthesis, sympathetic nervous system activation, and alterations in calcium handling.[84]

Measures to reduce CsA nephrotoxicity include delaying its administration immediately postoperatively in patients at high risk for nephrotoxicity (i.e., using alternative induction protocols including OKT3 or ATG), monitoring CsA trough blood levels and reducing the cyclosporine dosage if the vasoconstrictive effects present, and cautiously using other nephrotoxins (e.g., aminoglycosides, amphotericin B, nonsteroidal anti-inflammatory agents). When using these agents, drug concentrations of CsA and that of the other drugs, if available, should be monitored closely. In addition, the concomitant administration of drugs (e.g., azole antifungals, especially ketoconazole and to a lesser extent fluconazole and itraconazole, the macrolide antibiotics—erythromycin, clarithromycin, tacrolimus—and the calcium antagonists—diltiazem, nicardipine, verapamil) known to elevate cyclosporine levels requires intentional dosage reductions to avoid unnecessary renal and other toxicity.[90–92] Other drugs may also increase CsA and tacrolimus concentrations (Table 18.7). Similar management strategies are useful when dealing with tacrolimus (FK-506) as it is equally or more nephrotoxic than CsA.[39]

Currently, no proven therapies consistently prevent or reverse the nephrotoxic effects of cyclosporine; however, a number of agents have been studied including prostaglandin analogues, pentoxyphylline, fish oils, and so on. Based on their effects on calcium flux and on endothelin production (i.e., vasoconstrictive substance), the calcium channel blockers appear to be the most promising.[85] Interestingly, calcium channel blockers have also been proposed to have a beneficial effect on chronic graft atherosclerosis in heart transplant patients.[63]

Hyperlipidemia

While hypercholesterolemia is a known risk factor for the development of coronary artery disease and reduction of serum cholesterol levels decreases coronary heart disease morbidity and mortality in the general population,[93] conflicting evidence exists regarding the relationship between the hyperlipidemia commonly seen in heart recipients and the development of CGAS.[70,94–96] A progressive rise in serum cholesterol and triglyceride occurs in a time-dependent fashion following cardiac transplantation. Both steroids and cyclosporine are known to increase serum cholesterol and triglyceride levels.[97] Other drugs including diuretics, β blockers, ethanol, and so on, may aggravate hyperlipidemia in transplant patients.[98] Drug therapy to reduce cholesterol and triglycerides may be used but dosage reduction of lovastatin and monitoring for myositis are necessary if it is used concomitantly with CsA.[96] The other "statins" (e.g., pravastatin, simvastatin, etc.) are preferred because of a lower interactive potential with CsA, and they may also have a salutary immunosuppressive effect.[99] Management of hyperlipidemia in the heart transplant recipient is reviewed extensively elsewhere.[100]

Future Prospects for Cardiac Transplantation and Treatment

A variety of factors, including refined selection criteria, improvements in immunosuppressive regimens, diagnostic techniques for rejection, donor organ preservation, and treatment of infectious complications, have contributed to the overall success of cardiothoracic transplantation. The majority of patients return to NYHA functional class I and are able to achieve a desirable quality of life following transplantation. Despite the tremendous progress made in cardiothoracic transplantation since the mid-1980s, much remains to be done.[18]

The therapeutic-to-toxic ratio of currently utilized immunosuppressive agents remains narrow, mandating lifelong monitoring of patients. The identification of more specific immunosuppressive agents, with a higher therapeutic-to-toxic index or one capable of inducing tolerance to the grafted organ, presently remains a desirable, although elusive, goal. Similarly, the development of noninvasive techniques for the diagnosis of graft rejection would substantially reduce the inconvenience, cost, and morbidity associated with long-term surveillance.

Chronic graft atherosclerosis remains to be understood and until the pathogenesis and appropriate treatment are defined, graft dysfunction secondary to this form of atherosclerosis will remain the leading impediment to long-term survival.

While ideally, legislative and public awareness programs will have an impact on resolving the chronic shortage of suitable donors, the rapidly increasing number of patients afflicted with congestive heart failure will necessitate developing alternative options for patients with end-stage disease. The roles of long-term mechanical circulatory assistance, xenotransplantation, and dynamic cardiomyoplasty remain to be defined. It is likely that the twenty-first century will witness enhanced therapeutic and laboratory research designed to evaluate and refine the clinical, immunologic, and socioeconomic impact of using these alternative options.

References

1. United Network for Organ Sharing, Richmond, Virginia.
2. Miller LW, Schlant RC, Kobashigawa T, et al. Task Force 5: Complications. JACC 1993;22(1):41–53.
3. Min DI, Monaco AP. Complications associated with immunosuppressive therapy and their management. Pharmacotherapy 1991;11:19S–25S.
4. Rossi SJ, Schroeder TJ, Hariharan S, First MR. Prevention and management of the adverse effects associated with immunosuppressive therapy. Drug Safety 1993;9(2):104–131.
5. Baldwin JC, Wolfgang TC, Shumway NE, Lower RR. Cardiac transplantation, in Flye MW (ed): Principles of Organ Transplantation. Philadelphia, PA, WB Saunders, 1989, pp 385–402.
6. Kahan BD. Cyclosporine. N Engl J Med 1989;321:1725–1738.
7. Reitz BA, Wallwork JL, Hunt SA, et al. Heart–lung transplantation: Successful therapy for patients with pulmonary vascular disease. N Engl J Med 1982;306(10):557–564.
8. Toronto Lung Transplant Group. Unilateral lung transplant for pulmonary fibrosis. N Engl J Med 1986;314:1140–1145.
9. DeVries WC, Anderson JL, Joyce LD, et al. Clinical use of the total artificial heart. N Engl J Med 1984;310(5):273–278.
10. Pennington DG, McBride LR, Kanter KR, et al. Bridging to heart transplantation with circulatory support devices. J Heart Transplant 1989;8:116–123.
11. Farrar DJ and Thoratec Ventricular Assist Device Principal Investigators. Preoperative predictors of survival in patients with thoratec ventricular assist devices as a bridge to heart transplantation. J Heart Lung Transplant 1994;13(1):93–101.
12. Vetter HO, Kaulbach HG, Schmitz C, et al. Experience with the Novacor left ventricular assist system as a bridge to cardiac transplantation, including the new wearable system. J Thorac Cardiovasc Surg 1995;109:74–80.
13. McCarthy PM. HeartMate implantable left ventricular assist device: Bridge to transplantation and future applications. Ann Thorac Surg 1995;59:S46–S51.
14. Hosenpud JD, Novick RJ, Breen TJ, Daily OP. The Registry of the International Society for Heart and Lung Transplantation: Eleventh official report—1994. J Heart Lung Transplant 1994;13(4):561–570.
15. Evans RW, Manninen DL, Dong F, et al. The National Cooperative Transplantation Study. Seattle, WA, Battelle Research Center, 1991.

16. O'Connell JB, Bristow MR. Economic impact of heart failure in the United States: Time for a different approach. J Heart Lung Transplant 1994;13:S107–S111.
17. O'Connell JB, Gunnar RM, Evans RW, et al. Task Force 1: Organization of heart transplantation in the U.S. J Am Coll Cardiol 1993;22(1):8–14.
18. Mudge GH, Goldstein S, Addonizio LJ, et al. Task Force 3: Recipient guidelines/prioritization. J Am Coll Cardiol 1993;22(1):21–31.
19. Costanzo-Nordin MR, Cooper DKC, Jessup M, et al. Task Force 6: Future developments. J Am Coll Cardiol 1993;22(1):54–64.
20. Kaye MP. The Registry of the International Society for Heart and Lung Transplantation: Tenth official report—1993. J Heart Transplant 1993;541–548.
21. Olivari MT, Antolick A, Kaye MP, et al. Heart transplantation in elderly patients. J Heart Transplant 1988;7:258–264.
22. Mancini DM, Eisen H, Kussmaul W, et al. Value of peak exercise oxygen consumption for optimal timing of cardiac transplantation in ambulatory patients with heart failure. Circulation 1991;83:778–786.
23. Baldwin JC, Anderson JL, Boucek MM, et al. Task Force 2: Donor guidelines. J Am Coll Cardiol 1993;22(1):15–20.
24. Young JB, Winters WL, Bourge R, Uretsky BF. Task Force 4: Function of the heart transplant recipient. J Am Coll Cardiol 1993;22(1):31–41.
25. Chelimsky-Fallick C, Middlekauff H, Stevenson W, et al. Amiodarone therapy does not compromise subsequent heart transplantation. J Am Coll Cardiol 1992;20(7):1556–1561.
26. Redmond JM et al. Use of theophylline for treatment of prolonged sinus node dysfunction in human orthotopic heart transplantation. J Heart Lung Transplant 1993;12(1):133–139.
27. Wilson RF, Christensen BV, Olivari MT, et al. Evidence for structural sympathetic reinnervation after orthotopic cardiac transplantation in humans. Circulation 1991;83(4):1210–1220.
28. Oyer PE, Stinson EB, Jamieson SW, et al. Cyclosporin A in cardiac allografting: A preliminary experience. Transplant Proc 1983;15:1247–1252.
29. Copeland JG, Mammana RB, Fuller JK, et al. Heart transplantation: Four year's experience with conventional immunosuppression. JAMA 1984;251:1563–1566.
30. Bolman RM, Elick B, Olivari MT, et al. Improved immunosuppression for heart transplantation. J Heart Transplant 1985;11:315–318.
31. Olivari MT, Kubo SH, Braunlin EA, et al. Five-year experience with triple-drug immunosuppression therapy in cardiac transplantation. Circulation 1990;82(5 suppl):IV276–IV280.
32. Schroeder TJ, Myre SA, Melvin DB, et al. Efficacy and safety of constant-rate intravenous cyclosporine infusion immediately after heart transplantation. J Heart Transplant 1989;8:5–10.
33. Peters D, Fitton A, Plosker G, Faulds D. Tacrolimus: A review of its pharmacology, and therapeutic potential in hepatic and renal transplantation. Drugs 1993;46(4):746–794.
34. Armitage JM, Kormos RL, Fung J, Starzl TE. The clinical trial of FK506 as primary and rescue immunosuppression in adult cardiac transplantation. Transplant Proc 1991;23(6):3054–3057.
35. Armitage JM, Kormos RL, Shigeki M, et al. Clinical trial of FK506 immunosuppression in adult cardiac transplantation. Ann Thorac Surg 1992;205–211.
36. Manez R, Jain A, Marino IR, Thomson AW. Comparative evaluation of tacrolimus (FK506) and cyclosporin A as immunosuppressive agents. Transplantation Reviews 1995;9(2):63–76.
37. Ludden TM. Pharmacokinetic interactions of the macrolide antibiotics. Clin Pharmacokinet 1985;10(1):63–79.
38. Dew MA, Harris RC, Simmons RG, et al. Quality-of-life advantages of FK506 vs conventional immunosuppressive drug therapy in cardiac transplantation. Transplant Proc 1991;23(6):3061–3064.
39. Porayko MK, Textor SC, Krom RA, et al. Nephrotoxic effects of primary immunosuppression with FK-506 and cyclosporine regimens after liver transplantation. Mayo Clinic Proc 1994;69(2):105–111.
40. Prieto M, Lake KD, Pritzker MR, et al. OKT3 induction and steroid-free maintenance immunosuppression for treatment of high-risk heart transplant recipients. J Heart Lung Transplant 1991;10:901–911.
41. Costanzo-Nordin MR, O'Sullivan JE, Johnson MR, et al. Prospective randomized trial of OKT3 versus horse antithymocyte globulin-based immunosuppressive prophylaxis in heart transplantation. J Heart Transplant 1990;9:306–315.
42. Kormos RL, Herlan DB, Armitage JM, et al. Monoclonal versus polyclonal therapy for prophylaxis against rejection after heart transplantation. J Heart Transplant 1990;9:1–10.
43. Renlund DG, O'Connell JB, Gilbert EM, et al. A prospective comparison of murine monoclonal CD3 (OKT3) antibody-based and equine antithymocyte globulin-based rejection prophylaxis in cardiac transplantation. Transplantation 1989;47:599–605.
44. Taylor DO, Ensley RD, Olsen SL, et al. Mycophenolate mofetil (RS-61443): Preclinical, clinical, and three-year experience in heart transplantation. J Heart Lung Transplant 1994;13(4):571–582.
45. Kirklin JK, Bourge RC, Naftel DC, et al. Treatment of recurrent heart rejection with mycophenolate mofetil (RS-61443): Initial clinical experience. J Heart Lung Transplant 1994;13:444–450.
46. Kobashigawa JA, Kirklin JK, Naftel DC, et al. Pre-transplantation risk factors for acute rejection after heart transplantation: A multi-institutional study. J Heart Lung Transplant 1993;12:355–366.
47. Billingham ME, Cary NRB, Hammond ME, et al. A working formulation for the standardization of nomenclature in the diagnosis of heart and lung rejection: Heart rejection study group. J Heart Transplant 1990;9(6):587–593.
48. Wahlers T, Heublein B, Cremer J, et al. Treatment of rejection after heart transplantation: What dosage of pulsed steroids is necessary? J Heart Transplant 1990;9:568–574.
49. Hosenpud JD, Norman DJ, Pantely GA. Low dose oral prednisone in the treatment of acute cardiac allograft rejection not associated with hemodynamic compromise. J Heart Transplant 1990;9(3 part 2):292–296.

50. Constanzo-Nordin MR, Grusk DB, Silver MA, et al. Reversal of recalcitrant cardiac allograft rejection with methotrexate. Circulation 1988;78(suppl III):III47–III57.
51. Olsen SL, O'Connell JB, Bristow MR, Renlund DG. Methotrexate as an adjunct in the treatment of persistent mild cardiac allograft rejection. Transplantation 1990;50:773–775.
52. Morris RE. New small molecule immunosuppressants for transplantation: Review of essential concepts. J Heart Lung Transplant 1993;12:S275–S286.
53. Salter MM, Kirklin JK, Bourge RC, et al. Total lymphoid irradiation in the treatment of early or recurrent heart rejection. J Heart Lung Transplant 1992;11:902–911.
54. Costanzo-Nordin MR, Hubbell EA, O'Sullivan EJ, et al. Reversal of heart transplant rejection with photochemotherapy. J Heart Lung Transplant 1992;11:746–750.
55. Miller LW, Naftel DC, Bourge RC, et al. and the Cardiac Transplant Research Database Group. Infection after heart transplantation: A multiinstitutional study. J Heart Lung Transplant 1994;13(3):381–393.
56. Dummer SJ. Infectious complications of transplantation. Cardiovasc Clin 1990;20:163–178.
57. Rubin RH, Young LS (eds). Clinical Approach to Infection in the Compromised Host, 2nd ed. New York, Plenum Medical Book Co, 1988, p 685.
58. Rubin RH, Tolkoff-Rubin NE. Antimicrobial strategies in the care of organ transplant recipients. Antimicrob Agents Chemother 1993;37:619–624.
59. McCarthy JM, Karim MA, Krueger H, et al. The cost impact of cytomegalovirus disease in renal transplant recipients. Transplantation 1993;55:1277–1282.
60. Glowacki LS, Smaill FM. Use of immune globulin to prevent symptomatic cytomegalovirus disease in trans-plant recipients—A meta-analysis. Clin Transplant 1994;8:10–18.
61. Merigan TC, Renlund DG, Keay S, et al. A controlled trial of ganciclovir to prevent cytomegalovirus disease after heart transplantation. N Engl J Med 1992;326:1182–1186.
62. Singh N, Yu VL, Mieles L, et al. High-dose acyclovir compared with short-course preemptive ganciclovir therapy to prevent cytomegalovirus in liver transplant recipients. Ann Intern Med 1994;120:375–381.
63. Schroeder JS, Gao S, Hunt SA, Stinson EB. Accelerated graft coronary artery disease: Diagnosis and prevention. J Heart Lung Transplant 1992;11:S258–S266.
64. Gao SZ, Schroeder JS, Alderman EL, et al. Prevalence of accelerated coronary artery disease in heart transplant survivors. Comparison of cyclosporine and azathioprine regimens. Circulation 1989;80(suppl III):III100–III105.
65. Libby P, Tanaka H. The pathogenesis of coronary arteriosclerosis ("chronic rejection") in transplanted hearts. Clin Transplant 1994;8(3 part 2):313–318.
66. Billingham ME. The postsurgical heart: The pathology of cardiac transplantation. Am J Cardiovasc Pathol 1988;1:319.
67. McDonald K, Rector TJ, Braunlin EA, et al. Association of coronary artery disease in cardiac transplant recipients with cytomegalovirus infection. Am J Cardiol 1989;64:359–362.
68. Speir E, Modali R, Huang E-S, et al. Potential role of human cytomegalovirus and p53 interaction in coronary restenosis. Science 1994;265:391–394.
69. Expert Panel on Detection, Evaluation, and Treatment of High Blood Cholesterol in Adults. Summary of the second report of the National Cholesterol Education Program (NCEP) Expert Panel on Detection, Evaluation, and Treatment of High Blood Cholesterol in Adults (Adult Treatment Panel II). JAMA 1993;269:3015–3023.
70. Griepp RB, Stinson EB, Bieber CP, et al. Control of graft arteriosclerosis in human heart transplant recipients. Surgery 1977;81:262–269.
71. Schroeder JS, Gao SZ, Alderman EL, et al. A preliminary study of diltiazem in the prevention of coronary artery disease in heart-transplant recipients. N Engl J Med 1993;328:164–170.
72. Penn I. Incidence and treatment of neoplasia after transplantation. J Heart Lung Transplant 1993;12(6 part 2):S328–S336.
73. Penn I. Tumors after renal and cardiac transplantation. Hematology-Oncology Clin N Am 1993;7(2):431–445.
74. Penn I. The changing patterns of post-transplant malignancies. Transplant Proc 1991;23(1):1101–1103.
75. Hemmens VJ, Moore D. Photochemical sensitization by azathioprine and its metabolites. II. Azathioprine and nitroimidazole metabolites. Photochem Photobiol 1986;43:257–262.
76. Edwards DI. Mechanisms of cytotoxicity of nitroimidazole drugs. Prog Med Chem 1981;18:87–116.
77. Swinnen LJ, Costanzo-Nordin MR, Fisher SG, et al. Increased incidence of lymphoproliferative disorder after immunosuppression with the monoclonal antibody OKT3 in cardiac transplant recipients. N Engl J Med 1990;323:1723–1728.
78. Emery RW, Lake KD. Post-transplantation lymphoproliferative disorder and OKT3 [letter]. N Engl J Med 1991;324(20):1437.
79. Brumbaugh J, Baldwin JC, Stinson EB, et al. Quantitative analysis of immunosuppression in cyclosporine-treated heart transplant patients with lymphoma. J Heart Transplant 1985;4:307–311.
80. Hanto DW, Frizzera G, Gajl-Peczalska KJ, et al. Epstein–Barr virus-induced B-cell lymphoma after renal transplantation: Acyclovir therapy and transition from polyclonal to monoclonal B-cell proliferation. N Engl J Med 1982;306:913–918.
81. Nalesnik MA, Locker J, Jaffe R, et al. Clonal characteristics of post-transplant lymphoproliferative disorders. Transplant Proc 1988;20(1 suppl 1):280–283.
82. Porter GA, Bennett WM, Sheps SG; on behalf of the National High Blood Pressure Education Program, National Heart, Lung, and Blood Institute, National Institutes of Health. Cyclosporine-associated hypertension. Arch Intern Med 1990;150:280–283.
83. Scherrer U, Vissing SF, Morgan BJ, et al. Cyclosporine-induced sympathetic activation and hypertension after heart transplantation. N Engl J Med 1990;323:693–699.
84. Sturrock ND, Struthers AD. Hormonal and other mechanisms involved in the pathogenesis of cyclosporin-induced nephrotoxicity and hypertension in man. Clin Sci 1994;86(1):1–9.
85. Epstein M. Calcium antagonists and the kidney. Implications for renal protection. Am J Hypertension 1993;6 (7 part 2):251S–259S.

86. Moore CK, Bristow MR, Renlund DG, et al. Long-term morbidity of cyclosporine with corticosteroid-free maintenance immunosuppression in cardiac transplantation. Transplant Proc 1990;22:25–29.
87. Myers BD, Sibley R, Newton L, et al. The long-term course of cyclosporine-associated chronic nephropathy. Kidney Int 1988;33:590–600.
88. Greenberg A, Thompson ME, Griffith BJ, et al. Cyclosporine nephrotoxicity in cardiac allograft patients—a seven-year follow-up. Transplantation 1990;50:589–593.
89. Weir MR, Klassen DK, Shen SY, et al. Acute effects of IV cyclosporine on renal function in healthy humans. Transplant Proc 1989;21(book 1):915–917.
90. Lake KD. Management of drug interactions with cyclosporine. Pharmacotherapy 1991;11:110S–118S.
91. Lake KD, Canafax DM. Important interactions of drugs with immunosuppressive agents used in transplant recipients. J Antimicrob Chemother 1995;36(Suppl B):11–22.
92. Lake KD. Drug interactions in transplant patients, in Emery RW, Miller L (eds): Handbook of Cardiac Transplantation. Philadelphia, PA, Hanley & Belfus, 1995.
93. Lipid Research Clinics. The Lipid Research Clinics coronary primary prevention trial results. I. Reduction in incidence of coronary heart disease. JAMA 1984;251:351–364.
94. Bilodeau M, Fitchett DH, Guerraty A, Sniderman AD. Dyslipoproteinemias after heart and heart-lung transplantation: Potential relation to accelerated graft arteriosclerosis. J Heart Transplant 1989;8(6):454–459.
95. Winters GL, Kendall TJ, Radio SJ, et al. Post-transplant obesity and hyperlipidemia: Major predictors of severity of coronary arteriopathy in failed human heart allografts. J Heart Transplant 1990;9:364–371.
96. Ballantyne CM, Radovancevic B, Farmer JA, et al. Hyperlipidemia after heart transplantation: Report of a 6-year experience, with treatment recommendations. J Am Coll Cardiol 1992;19(6):1315–1321.
97. Hricik DE, Mayes JT, Schulak JA. Independent effects of cyclosporine and prednisone on post-transplant hypercholesterolemia. Am J Kidney Dis 1991;18:353–358.
98. Henkin Y, Como JA, Oberman A. Secondary dyslipidemia inadvertent effects of drugs in clinical practice. JAMA 1992;267(7):961–968.
99. Katznelson S, Laks H, et al. Effect of pravastatin on outcomes after cardiac transplantation. N Engl J Med 1995;333:621–627.
100. Lake, KD. Management of post-transplant obesity and hyperlipidemia, in Emery RW, Miller L (eds): Handbook of Cardiac Transplantation. Philadelphia, PA, Hanley & Belfus, 1995.

Chapter 19

Thromboembolic Disorders

Sharon M. Erdman, PharmD, Keith A. Rodvold, PharmD, and William R. Friedenberg, MD

Venous thromboembolism, which includes both venous thrombosis and its most feared complication, pulmonary embolism, is a serious and potentially fatal disorder that can occur in bedridden hospitalized patients as well as in healthy ambulatory individuals. It is estimated that there are approximately 500,000 cases of pulmonary embolism in the United States each year, with about 10% (50,000) of these cases resulting in death.[1] In one-third of these patients, death can occur within the first few hours of onset, making rapid diagnosis and early, effective treatment critical determinants in patient outcome.[2]

A pulmonary embolism (PE) is a thrombus or foreign substance that arises from the systemic circulation and lodges in the pulmonary artery or one of its branches, causing complete or partial obstruction of pulmonary blood flow. It is estimated that greater than 95% of pulmonary emboli originate as thrombi in the deep-venous system of the lower extremities.[2,3] A deep vein thrombosis (DVT) is a thrombus composed of cellular material (red and white blood cells, and platelets) bound together with fibrin strands, which form in the venous portion of the vasculature.[3] Venous thrombosis can involve any vein in the body, but most often occurs in the lower limbs involving the superficial large veins, the deep veins of the calf, and the deep veins above the knee (including the popliteal and proximal veins). The larger leg veins (those above the knee) are the most common source of PE that reach clinical attention. Thrombi of the deep calf veins are often small in size and generally pose only a small risk of developing subsequent PE and long-term clinical disability.[1] In addition, a small number of patients develop PE secondary to pelvic, renal, or upper extremity vein thrombosis, or by the injection of a foreign substance (as in intravenous drug abusers).

Pulmonary embolism has often been called the "great masquerader" due to its multiple clinical presentations as well as the lack of specificity of associated signs and symptoms. In addition, the clinical diagnosis of venous thrombosis and PE is notoriously unreliable so that treatment is often initiated before a firm diagnosis has been made.

Etiology

A number of factors, either inherited or acquired, may place a patient at risk for the development of venous thromboembolism. Some acquired risk factors include immobility, heart disease, malignancy, surgery, and estrogen use. Inherited disorders such as antithrombin III deficiency and protein C deficiency may also play a role in the development of venous thromboembolism, and are also considered to be risk factors. Thrombosis may be due to resistance to activated protein C (APC resistance) in as many as 33% of patients who do not have an obvious predisposition to thromboembolic diseases.[4] A comprehensive list of risk factors is summarized in Table 19.1. It is not known if age itself is an independent risk factor for the development of venous thromboembolism but the prevalence of many risk factors increases with age.

The incidence or risk of developing venous thromboembolism also appears to differ depending on the surgical procedure being performed, the clinical situation (emergent versus elective), the duration of general anesthesia (increased risk with duration >30 minutes), and the age of the patient. In general, the overall incidence of a thrombotic event in patients who undergo major surgery is 30–35%. In addition, elective hip surgery patients are at a 0.3–1.7% risk of developing fatal PE, which increases to 4–7% in patients who undergo emergent hip surgery. Interestingly, new data suggest that the risk of postoperative PE continues for more than 1 month after surgery.[2]

Pathophysiology

Three primary components—venous stasis, vascular injury, and hypercoagulability (Virchow's triad)—play a role in the development of a thrombus.[1] In addition, the fibrinolytic state of the patient is also a key component. Venous stasis is characterized by altered or decreased blood flow in the deep veins of the lower limbs and is a critical determinant in the formation of thrombi in many patients. Ineffective

TABLE 19.1. RISK FACTORS PREDISPOSING TO THROMBOEMBOLISM

Inherited Risk Factors
Activated protein C resistance
Antithrombin III deficiency
Protein C deficiency
Protein S deficiency
Dysfibrinogenemia
Sickle cell anemia
Polycythemia
Acquired Risk Factors
Lupus anticoagulant
Malignancy (especially pancreatic, gastrointestinal, bronchogenic, genitourinary, breast)
Heart disease (congestive heart failure, atrial fibrillation, acute myocardial infarction, dilated cardiomyopathy)
Trauma/surgery of lower extremity, pelvis, hip
Immobility or paralysis
Estrogen use (oral contraceptives, hormonal replacement)
Peripartum period
Obesity
History of varicose veins
History DVT or PE
Inflammatory bowel disease
Antiphospholipid antibodies
Chronic lung disease
Chronic venous insufficiency
Renal transplantation
Splenectomy
Myeloproliferative disorders

(Adapted from JAMA 1986;256:744–749; JAMA 1992;268:1727–1733; and Semin Thromb Hemost 1991;17(3):250–253, with permission.)

venous emptying can lead to local endothelial damage to venous valves secondary to hypoxia, as well as the local concentration of activated clotting factors in the area of stasis. Venostasis may result from a number of conditions including immobility, prolonged bed rest, massive obesity, venous obstruction, congestive heart failure, hypovolemia, varicose veins, late-stage pregnancy, shock, or severe myocardial infarction.

Vascular wall injury or endothelial damage occurs secondary to mechanical or chemical trauma that evokes an inflammatory response (phlebitis), in addition to locally activating the coagulation cascade as a result of the exposure of collagen, leading to platelet aggregation to form an intraluminal thrombus. Mechanical injury to the intima of vessel walls may result from venipuncture, indwelling cannulas and catheters, fractured bones, and direct trauma as with surgery. Chemical irritation may result from the infusion or injection of agents such as potassium or hypertonic glucose.

The coagulation process is regulated by a number of feedback mechanisms that normally limit thrombus formation. However, there are circumstances (hypercoagulable states) when the activation of the coagulation cascade exceeds the ability of the body's natural fibrinolytic system to prevent thrombus formation, thus leading to the development of a thrombus. APC resistance, deficiencies of protein C, protein S, or antithrombin III, and certain types of malignancy are conditions in which there is an increased activation of the blood coagulation system above normal, which predisposes to the development of a thrombus.[4]

The coagulation process is activated by a number of factors including tissue or vascular trauma and inflammation, and it seems to be augmented by venous stasis due to the local concentration of activated clotting factors. The coagulation cascade can be triggered through either the intrinsic or extrinsic pathways (Fig. 19.1). The intrinsic pathway is activated by the contact of factor XII with exposed collagen from damaged subendothelial vessels, or by contact with a foreign substance such as a prosthetic surface. All of the clotting factors necessary for the activation of the intrinsic system are present in the circulating blood. The extrinsic pathway is activated by the exposure of blood to tissue thromboplastin, a tissue factor released after vascular wall damage, which combines with and activates factor VII to form a complex that activates factor X. It is at this point that the intrinsic and extrinsic pathways meet to continue along a common pathway ultimately leading to the activation of factor XII, which stabilizes the fibrin clot. In addition, tissue factor has been shown to activate factor IX, thus providing an alterative pathway of blood coagulation.[5] Tissue factor pathway inhibitor (TFPI) appears to play a role in regulating this alternative pathway.

NATURAL HISTORY OF DEEP VEIN THROMBOSIS AND PULMONARY EMBOLISM

Most venous thrombi involve the veins of the lower extremities where they develop behind venous valve cusps or at bifurcations in the intramuscular veins of the calf. The major consequences of DVT include venous valvular damage, which may lead to the postphlebitic syndrome; the compromise of venous blood flow to the lower extremity or chronic venous insufficiency, which can lead to tissue hypoxia; and embolization of the thrombus to the lungs or elsewhere. In most patients, venous thrombi and PE are broken up by the endogenous lytic system, with complete clot resolution occurring over several weeks. Subsequently, clinically apparent thrombotic disease is observed in patients in whom this mechanism fails.

As mentioned before, most pulmonary emboli originate as thrombi in the deep venous system, which dislodge and produce complete or partial interruption of blood flow to a portion of the lungs. It is estimated that 15–20% of proximal deep venous thrombi embolize to the lungs. Upper extremity thrombosis may lead to a PE, especially in the presence of a central indwelling catheter.

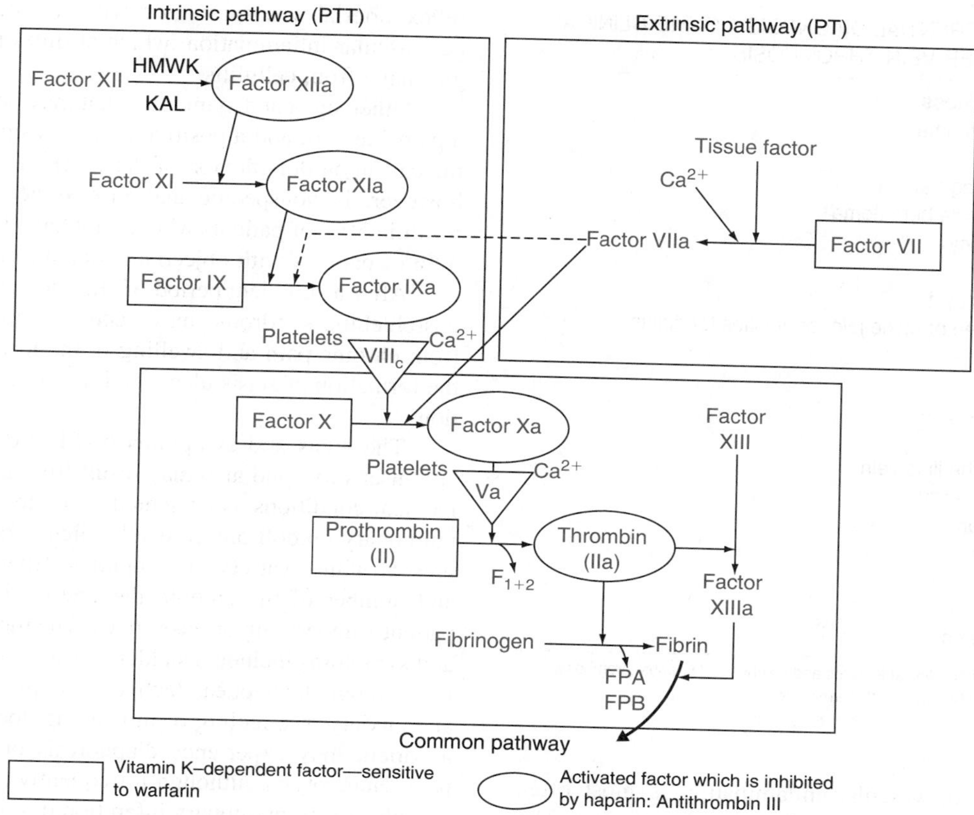

Figure 19.1. The coagulation cascade. **HMWK,** high molecular weight kininogen; **KAL,** kallikrein. *(From Stead RB: Clinical pharmacology, in Goldhaber SZ (ed). Pulmonary Embolism and Deep Venous Thrombosis. Philadelphia, PA, WB Saunders, 1985, p 100, with permission.)*

Pulmonary emboli may be generally classified into two groups: (1) submassive, in which less than 50% of the pulmonary vascular bed is occluded, and (2) massive, in which greater than 50% of the pulmonary vascular bed is occluded. The severity of the pulmonary and hemodynamic effects of a PE depends on several factors including the extent of anatomic obstruction and the underlying cardiopulmonary status of the patient.

The pulmonary effects of a PE may include the formation of an alveolar dead space (an area ventilated in excess of perfusion), pneumoconstriction (a decrease in the functional size of the area not being perfused), arterial hypoxemia; loss of pulmonary surfactant (which occurs after 24 hours) leading to atelectasis and transudation of alveolar fluid into alveolar spaces; and pulmonary infarction (<10%).[1]

Hemodynamically, a PE causes a decrease in the cross-sectional area of the pulmonary bed, which increases pulmonary vascular resistance and subsequently right ventricular afterload. If these changes become marked, they may lead to tricuspid regurgitation, pulmonary hypertension, right ventricular failure, and low cardiac output, especially in patients who have underlying cardiopulmonary disease.[1] In addition, chronic pulmonary hypertension and cor pulmonale may develop in a small number of patients who experience recurrent pulmonary emboli.

Clinical Presentation

Frequently, venous thrombi are clinically silent. Signs and symptoms develop as a consequence of venous outflow obstruction, inflammation of the vessel wall or perivascular tissue, or embolization of the thrombus to the pulmonary vascular bed. The signs and symptoms of venous thrombosis are relatively nonspecific and may result from a variety of other conditions, presented in Table 19.2. The most common clinical symptoms include pain, tenderness, swelling, and discoloration. The pain and tenderness are usually localized to the calf in patients with calf vein thrombosis, and tend to be more diffuse and intense in patients with proximal vein thrombosis. The severity of the pain and tenderness, however, does not appear to correlate with the size or extent of the thrombus. Edema secondary to proximal

TABLE 19.2. DIFFERENTIAL DIAGNOSIS OF THE CLINICAL FEATURES OF DEEP VEIN THROMBOSIS

Pain and/or Tenderness
- Muscle strain or trauma
- Muscle tear
- Direct muscle or leg trauma
- Spontaneous muscle hematoma
- Arterial insufficiency
- Neurogenic pain
- Ruptured Baker's cyst
- Arthritis of the knee or ankle joint or achilles tendinitis
- Varicose veins
- Pregnancy
- Oral contraceptive use

Leg Swelling
- Compression of the iliac vein
- Postphlebitic syndrome
- Leg immobilization
- Leg inflammation
- Lymphedema
- Lipedema
- Self-induced edema

(Adapted from Hirsh J et al. Clinical features and diagnosis of venous thrombosis. J Am Coll Cardiol 1986;8:114–127B, with permission.)

vein obstruction or vascular inflammation is most often responsible for the swelling and ranges in severity. The swelling is typically localized or unilateral and can occur with or without pain. Patients with DVT may exhibit a discolored lower extremity, which is manifested as cyanosis because of a large venous obstruction; pale secondary to reflex arterial vasospasm; or with a reddish color from perivascular inflammation, which at times may be indistinguishable from cellulitis.

Other signs and symptoms that may be present include a palpable cord and a positive Homan's sign (discomfort in the calf upon dorsiflexion of the foot).[6] The Homan's sign, however, is nonspecific and insensitive, with a positive result in 50% of patients who do not have DVT, and in only 30% of patients with objectively documented DVT.[3]

After a sufficient period of chronic venous obstruction, postphlebitic syndrome may occur. Symptoms may range from chronic pain and swelling in the lower extremities to the formation of stasis ulcers and the development of infection.

The signs and symptoms of PE are also nonspecific and insensitive and also may result from a number of other medical conditions as presented in Table 19.3. While most pulmonary emboli are clinically silent, some patients may present with a variety of symptoms depending on the size and number of the emboli, the arteries involved, and the patient's underlying disease states. The most common signs and symptoms include a sudden onset of unexplained dyspnea, cough, tachypnea, tachycardia, pleuritic chest pain, and anxiety or a feeling of impending doom. Occasionally, a patient may experience diaphoresis or substernal chest pain. Hemoptysis, although infrequently present, is usually an indicator of pulmonary infarction or congestive atelectasis. In addition, patients with massive PE often present with signs of circulatory collapse, such as syncope or shock, secondary to a reduced cardiac output, or with evidence of acute cor pulmonale or right ventricular failure.

TABLE 19.3. DIFFERENTIAL DIAGNOSIS OF THE CLINICAL FEATURES OF PULMONARY EMBOLISM

Dyspnea
- Atelectasis
- Pneumonia
- Pneumothorax
- Acute pulmonary edema
- Acute bronchitis
- Acute bronchiolitis
- Acute bronchial obstruction (asthma)
- Hyperventilation
- Metabolic acidosis

Pleuritic Chest Pain
- Pneumonia
- Pneumothorax
- Pericarditis
- Pulmonary neoplasm
- Bronchiectasis
- Subdiaphragmatic inflammation
- Myositis
- Muscle strain
- Rib fracture

Hemoptysis
- Pneumonia
- Bronchial neoplasm
- Bronchiectasis
- Acute bronchitis
- Mitral stenosis
- Tuberculosis

Acute Right Heart Failure
- Myocardial failure
- Myocarditis
- Cardiac tamponade
- Acute respiratory infection complicating chronic lung disease

Cardiovascular Collapse
- Myocardial infarction
- Acute massive hemorrhage
- Gram-negative hemorrhage
- Cardiac tamponade
- Spontaneous pneumothorax

(From Hirsh J et al. Diagnosis of pulmonary embolism. J Am Coll Cardiol 1986;8(suppl):130B, with permission.)

DIAGNOSIS

The diagnosis of DVT or PE should be suspected in any patient with suggestive clinical signs and symptoms. Because none of the signs or symptoms are specific for DVT or PE, the diagnosis cannot be made on the basis of clinical judgment alone, and objective testing methods are necessary to aid in the diagnosis.

In any patient suspected of having a DVT or PE, empiric therapy (e.g., heparin) is started to decrease the risk of further embolic events while waiting for the results of diagnostic tests. The initial steps in the evaluation of any patient with suspected thromboembolic disease should include a medical history, a medication history, and a thorough physical exam. All of these are important in identifying underlying risk factors that may have led to the development of the thrombus. As previously mentioned, objective testing is necessary for the diagnosis of either deep vein thrombosis or pulmonary embolism because of the nonspecificity of associated signs and symptoms. Diagnostic algorithms for DVT and PE are presented in Figs. 19.2 and 19.3, respectively.

Also, the use of new plasma markers, such as D-dimer, are currently being evaluated as negative predictors of DVT and PE.[7] D-dimer is an endogenous substance released upon fibrinolysis of a fibrin clot. In one study, quantitative plasma D-dimer concentrations less than 500 ng/mL were found to be strongly predictive of a normal pulmonary angiogram.[7] However, D-dimer concentrations greater than 500 ng/mL were noted in 42 of 45 patients with PE, and 96 of 128 patients without PE, making this a rather nonspecific finding. More studies are needed to determine if plasma D-dimer concentrations of less than 500 ng/mL may help a patient avoid angiography due to its negative predictor value of PE.

There are a number of invasive and noninvasive diagnostic techniques that may be useful for the detection of DVT.[5] Some techniques visualize the thrombus (contrast venography, ultrasound, magnetic resonance imaging); some measure obstructions to venous outflow (impedance plethysmography, Doppler ultrasound); and others detect the incorporation of radiolabeled proteins into the developing thrombus (^{125}I-fibrinogen scan, monoclonal antibodies). The clinical usefulness of any of these tests depends on whether the patient has clinically suspected DVT, or whether a high-risk patient is being screened for DVT.

The first of the noninvasive tests is ^{125}I-fibrinogen leg scanning, which can be used as a screening tool in high-risk patients or as an adjunctive test to impedance plethysmography in patients with suspected DVT. Radioiodine-labeled fibrinogen scanning depends on the incorporation of circulating labeled fibrinogen (which is injected into the patient) as fibrin into the thrombus, which is then detected by an isotope detector. This technique detects more than 90% of calf vein thrombi, but only 60–80% of proximal vein thrombi. This method should never be used as the only diagnostic tool in patients with suspected DVT because it fails to detect many high proximal vein thrombi.

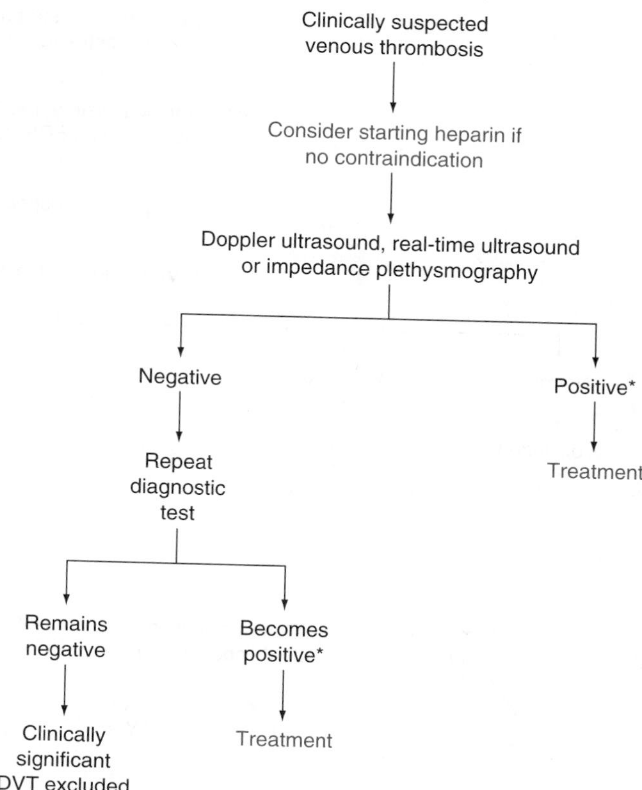

Figure 19.2. Diagnostic algorithm for patients with suspected deep vein thrombosis (DVT). *In the absence of clinical conditions known to produce false positive results. *(Adapted from Hirsh J et al. Clinical features and diagnosis of venous thrombosis. J Am Coll Cardiol 1986;8(suppl):124B, with permission.)*

Doppler ultrasonography is a noninvasive diagnostic test used for the evaluation of patients with suspected DVT. The Doppler flowmeter is a continuous-wave device that detects venous flow patterns. It uses a transducer in addition to an acoustic gel, which emits and then measures sound waves that are reflected from red blood cells. In a patient with DVT, an absence of spontaneous venous flow is observed. The Doppler is highly sensitive in detecting thrombi in proximal veins, but is less sensitive to thrombi that are nonocclusive or located in the calf veins. The accuracy of the device is also dependent on an experienced operator. The Doppler is almost as sensitive as impedance plethysmography in detecting symptomatic DVT, and the advantages over impedance plethysmography include its convenience, low cost, better sensitivity to calf vein throm-

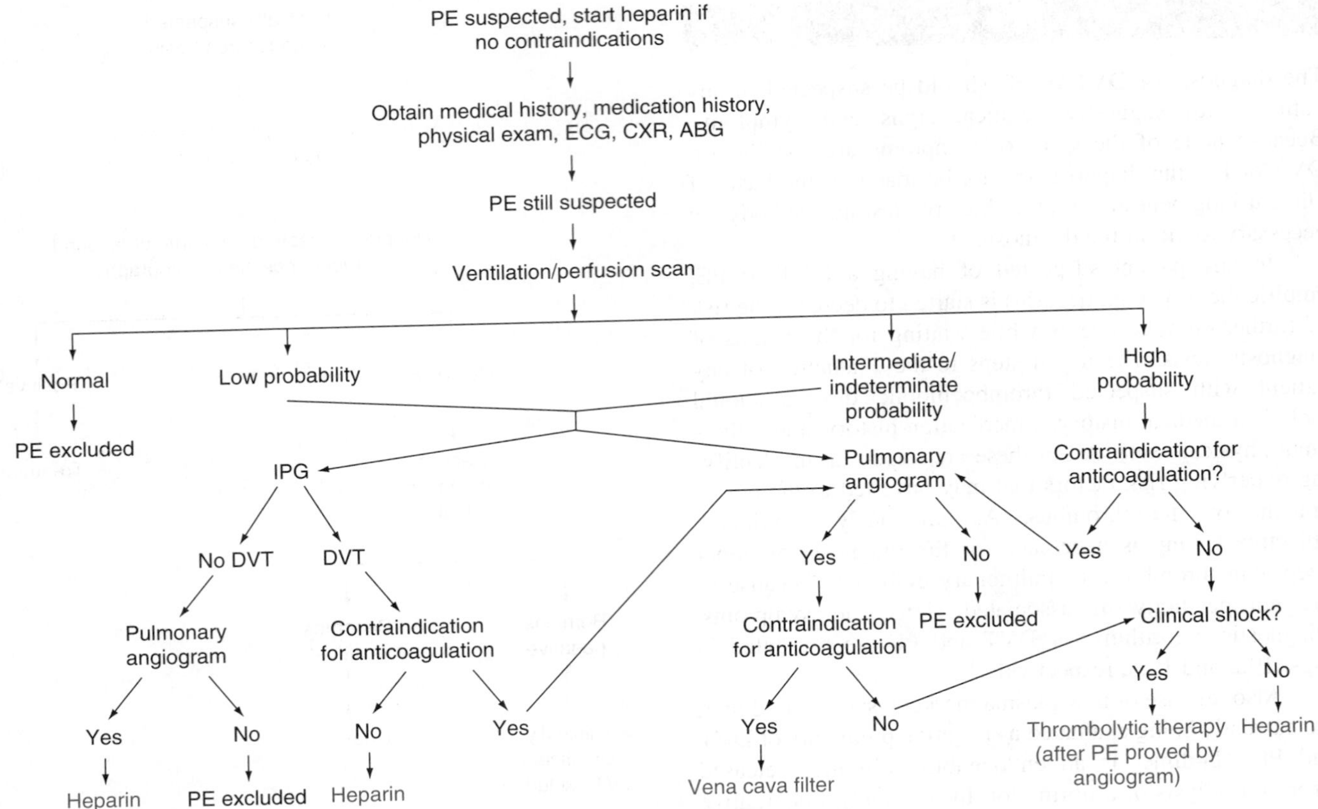

Figure 19.3. Diagnostic algorithm for patients with suspected pulmonary embolism (PE). V-Q, ventilation-perfusion; IPG, impedance plethysmography; DVT, deep vein thrombosis.

bosis, and applicability to patients with arterial insufficiency or plaster casts.

Impedance plethysmography (IPG) is also a noninvasive test for the diagnosis of DVT. It is based on the changes in electrical resistance that accompany changes in blood volume in the legs. A pneumatic cuff is applied to the midthigh and inflated to 50 mm Hg to occlude venous return. After a set period of time, the cuff is quickly deflated while changes in electrical resistance (impedance) from alterations in blood volume distal to the cuff are measured by calf electrodes. This method is sensitive and specific for thrombosis of the proximal veins, but is less sensitive for thrombosis of the calf veins and cannot distinguish between thrombotic and nonthrombotic obstruction to venous outflow. A normal result essentially excludes the diagnosis of proximal vein thrombosis, but not calf vein thrombosis.

Real-time ultrasonography is a commonly used ultrasound technique that provides a three-dimensional picture of the deep veins through the use of a transducer. It may be useful in detecting acute and chronic thrombi in the lower extremities. This method is often used in conjunction with Doppler ultrasound, and it is very accurate and sensitive in the diagnosis of proximal vein thrombosis, but is less accurate in detecting calf vein thrombi.

Doppler ultrasonography, IPG, and real-time ultrasonography all have the limitation in that they are insensitive to calf vein thrombosis, and need to be repeated serially if the initial test is negative. This is based on the observation that calf vein thrombosis is only clinically important when it extends into the proximal veins, at which point these noninvasive tests would be useful in detecting the thrombus. Serial exams are often obtained the day after the initial test, on day 5 to 7, and again on days 10 to 14. If the test becomes positive during the serial testing, the patient is diagnosed with DVT and anticoagulant therapy is initiated. A positive test in the presence of conditions known to produce false positives (i.e., congestive heart failure) should be confirmed by venography.

Venography is the accepted reference standard for the diagnosis of DVT to which all other tests are compared. Radiopaque contrast dye is injected into a dorsal foot vein or the femoral vein, which provides an outline of the deep venous system of the lower limbs. Ascending venography provides adequate visualization of the deep veins of the calf and several proximal veins. In patients who do not have adequate visualization of the external and common iliac veins with ascending venography, common femoral or iliac venography may be needed. The diagnosis of DVT is made based on the presence of intraluminal filling defects. Venography requires experienced personnel for both operation and interpretation, and is often used in patients in whom noninvasive techniques are inconclusive, or in whom ultrasonic techniques are not useful (morbidly obese, edema). Venography may be associated with immediate or delayed foot pain, superficial phlebitis, or hypersensitivity reactions to the contrast dye. If a patient with signs and symptoms suggestive of PE has a finding of proximal vein thrombosis of the legs, invasive studies that might be used to confirm the diagnosis of PE can be avoided since the same therapies would be employed. In contrast, PE cannot be excluded in patients with negative findings on leg examination so that further tests may be necessary to make the diagnosis in a patient with a compatible clinical picture.

In addition to the initial medical history and physical examination, an electrocardiogram (ECG), chest x-ray, and arterial blood gas should be obtained in any patient with suspected PE. Evidence of right heart strain caused by elevated pulmonary artery pressures may be seen on the ECG of patients with PE. Patterns may include nonspecific ST-segment elevations or depression, T-wave inversion, right axis deviation, new incomplete right bundle-branch block, or evidence of right ventricular hypertrophy.[2] The radiographic patterns in patients with PE may include effusions, infiltrates, enlargement of right descending pulmonary artery, Westermark's sign (avascular lung zones), and elevation of the diaphragm. An arterial blood gas may be useful in assessing the patient's degree of ventilation; however, approximately 10–20% of patients with PE have Po_2 values of >80 mm Hg. Although these tests are nonspecific for PE, they may be used to exclude other causes for the patient's condition, in addition to assisting in the interpretation of other diagnostic tests.

Ventilation–perfusion (V/Q) radionuclide scans are one of the objective testing methods used initially for the diagnosis of PE. The V/Q scan estimates the probability of PE in a given patient based on the anatomic patterns of injected and inhaled radioactive materials. Technetium-99-labeled macroaggregates of albumin are injected intravenously for the assessment of pulmonary perfusion. The distribution of these macroaggregates as they are trapped in the pulmonary capillary bed is detected radiographically and reflects the blood flow within the lungs. Because it cannot distinguish between pulmonary perfusion defects from PE and from other causes, it is nonspecific. Therefore, the assessment of ventilation is also used to help in the diagnosis. In the ventilation phase of the test, the patient inhales and exhales radioactive inert xenon, which permits imaging of the pattern of distribution of air in the alveolar gas-exchange units. Because an embolus obstructs arterial blood flow in one of the pulmonary arteries but does not affect ventilation, this scan can detect areas that are being ventilated but not perfused (a V/Q mismatch).

Results of this test are expressed in terms of the probability that a particular patient has a PE. A normal V/Q scan reliably excludes the diagnosis of PE, while a high probability V/Q scan supports the diagnosis of a PE.[8,9] If the results are interpreted as low or intermediate/indeterminate probabilities, diagnosing PE is more difficult. It is estimated that the prevalence of PE by pulmonary angiogram was 16% in patients with low probability lung scans, and 32% in patients with intermediate or indeterminate probability lung scans, although all of these emboli detected may not be clinically significant.[9] Therefore, in this subset of patients with inconclusive results from V/Q scans, further objective testing is necessary to confirm the diagnosis of PE.

As mentioned earlier, a number of patients with PE also have venographically detectable DVT, making IPG or Doppler ultrasonography possibly useful as a predictor of thromboembolism. It is estimated that approximately 70% of patients with angiographically proven PE have concurrent DVT by venography. If DVT is detected by venography testing, the patient should be treated with anticoagulant therapy, circumventing the need for pulmonary angiography. If the results of the above tests are negative or inconclusive, pulmonary angiography is then indicated to establish the diagnosis of PE.

Pulmonary angiography is the accepted diagnostic standard for PE to which all other tests are compared. In terms of diagnosing PE, it has the greatest diagnostic certainty, and can identify emboli as small as 0.5 mm. The procedure involves the injection of contrast media into the right and left pulmonary arteries, and radiographically detecting any filling defects on multiple magnification views. Some indications for pulmonary angiography include a nondiagnostic V/Q scan with or without a normal IPG in a patient with a picture suggestive of PE; a disagreement between V/Q scan interpretation and clinical impression; a contraindication to anticoagulation; and anticipation of thrombolytic therapy, inferior vena cava interruption, or embolectomy. Risks or complications of the pulmonary angiography include cardiac dysrhythmias, cardiac perforation, hypotension, and reaction to contrast media. Recently, modified pulmonary angiography techniques have improved diagnostic accuracy and reduced the risks of this procedure.[9]

Newer imaging techniques that are less invasive than pulmonary angiography are currently being investigated as diagnostic tools for PE. These techniques include magnetic resonance imaging (MRI); computed tomography (CT) with contrast; radiolabeled platelets; intravascular pulmonary ultrasound; fiberoptic pulmonary ultrasound; and digital subtraction angiography, which is simpler, faster, and does not require catheterization of the pulmonary artery.[1,2] Echocardiography is also emerging as an effective technique for the evaluation of patients with suspected PE.[2]

TREATMENT

The main objectives of treating venous thrombosis are (1) to prevent the development of pulmonary embolism, (2) to prevent the postphlebitic syndrome, (3) to reduce morbidity from the acute event, and (4) to achieve these objectives with a minimum of adverse effects and cost. Thus, successful treatment of DVT should prevent extension of the thrombus, prevent embolism to the lungs, and restore patency to the venous circulation while maintaining normal venous valve function. General management of DVT includes bed rest, with the heels elevated above the heart to enhance venous return, and administration of nonaspirin analgesics for pain. For PE, oxygen should be given and, if necessary, patients should be mechanically ventilated. Definitive management of acute DVT and PE includes anticoagulation, thrombolytic therapy, embolectomy, or inferior vena caval (IVC) interruption.

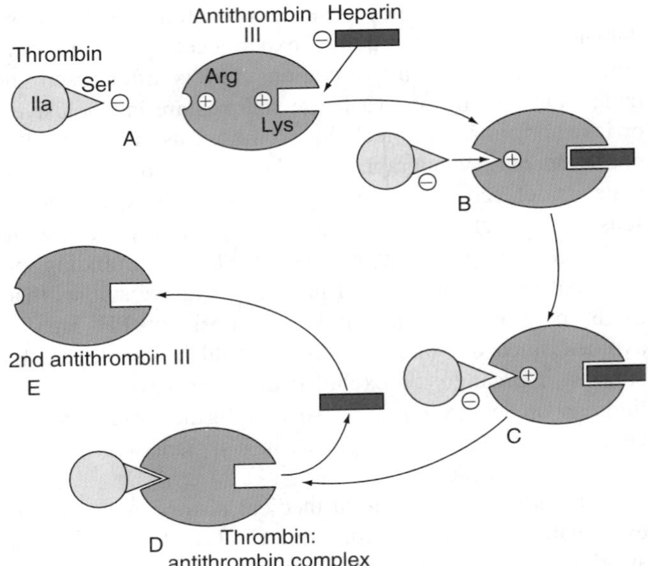

Figure 19.4. Mechanism of action of heparin. Heparin interacts with antithrombin III (A, B, C, E), which catalyzes the formation of thrombin:antithrombin complexes (D). Heparin and antithrombin also inactivate factors XIIa, XIa, and Xa by a similar mechanism. *(From Stead RB: Clinical pharmacology, in Goldhaber SZ (ed). Pulmonary Embolism and Deep Venous Thrombosis. Philadelphia, PA, WB Saunders, 1985, p 101, with permission.)*

HEPARIN

Heparin is the mainstay for the prevention and treatment of venous thromboembolism.[6,10] Heparin is a complex mucopolysaccharide that is extracted either from porcine gastrointestinal (GI) sources or from beef lung. Commercially available heparin is a heterogeneous mixture of polymers ranging from 3000–30,000 Da in molecular weight, with varying antithrombotic activity.[11] Apparently, a small and distinct fraction of the heparin molecule is responsible for most of its anticoagulant effect. Anticoagulant therapy with heparin is complicated by the chemical and pharmacologic heterogeneity of the product, which accounts for some of the inter- and intraindividual differences in its anticoagulant response.

The anticoagulant function of heparin is thought to depend on its ability to bind to and catalyze antithrombin III (ATIII) or heparin cofactor, a circulating anticoagulant that neutralizes the proteolytic activities of several clotting factors that have a serine residue at their enzymatically active site.[11] These activated factors include factors XII, XI, X, and IX, kallikrein, and thrombin (Fig. 19.4). Heparin halts further growth and propagation of the thrombus, allowing the patient's endogenous thrombolytic system to eradicate the existing clot. In addition, heparin may also promote thrombus resolution.[11]

The lack of a readily available direct chemical assay for heparin has limited pharmacokinetic data. Few carefully designed prospective evaluations of the disposition of heparin in patients are available. Data are not available on the rate and extent of absorption of heparin after oral administration. The total amount of heparin required to achieve the same degree of anticoagulant effect over the same time period does not appear to differ whether the agent is administered by intravenous, subcutaneous, or intrapulmonary routes.[12] Some studies have demonstrated significantly lower peak plasma heparin concentrations or decreased anticoagulant effects from the calcium salts; other investigators have failed to find significant differences between sodium and calcium salts.[12]

Heparin is distributed primarily throughout the vascular system, and the apparent volume of distribution (V_D) quantitatively resembles that of plasma or blood volume (mean $V_D = 60$ mL/kg; range: 40–100).[12] The V_D is directly related to body weight. However, there is no consensus as to whether ideal body weight or total body weight should be used when dosing heparin. The most recent data suggest that total body weight and estimations of blood volume should be used to dose heparin, especially in morbidly obese patients.[12]

The metabolism and excretion of heparin are complex, but involve primarily the metabolic processes of depolymerization and desulfation. Enzymes likely involved in heparin degradation include heparinases and desulfatases.[11,12]

The anticoagulant activity of heparin in plasma decreases exponentially with time after intravenous administration; however, the half-life increases with increasing dose. The biologic half-life of heparin in humans after a single intravenous injection has been reported to range from 0.4–2.5 hours.[12] Heparin clearance ranges from 0.25–2 mL/min/Kg, and has been found to be related to both total body weight and ideal body weight.[12] Up to a 10-fold range in heparin half-life has been reported within individual studies involving the administration of large doses. The interpatient variability in heparin clearance is reported to be 6- to 12-fold. The disappearance of the anticoagulant activity follows nonlinear pharmacokinetics, and has been described by a combination of a saturable and a linear mechanism.[12] The elimination of heparin is thought to be influenced by both renal and hepatic dysfunction.

Patients with PE have shorter heparin elimination half-lives and more rapid total clearances of heparin than patients treated for venous thrombosis.[12] This observation was supported by investigators who have recommended larger heparin doses for patients with pulmonary emboli. However, several other investigators have reported no significant differences in heparin dosage requirements between patients with PE and DVT.[12] White et al.[13] suggested that patients with verified thromboembolic diseases required significantly larger mean heparin doses (25 U/kg/h) than did patients without thromboembolic disease (15 U/kg/h). Cipolle et al.[14] found a correlation between the time delay from onset of symptoms to initiation of treatment and the heparin dosage requirements of 20 patients with thromboembolic disorders. These data indicate that patients with acute thromboembolic disorders have rapid clearance rates and require larger heparin doses to ensure adequate anticoagulant activity.

Therapeutic Indications

Anticoagulation with heparin is indicated in patients with a thrombus extending above the popliteal vein because of the high risk of PE and postphlebitic syndrome in these patients.[10,11] Patients with symptomatic calf vein thrombosis should receive heparin, because recent studies have shown a higher incidence of recurrent DVT in proximal veins in nonanticoagulated patients compared with anticoagulated patients. However, there are no definitive recommendations in patients with asymptomatic calf vein thrombosis detected by routine postoperative leg scanning. Patients with superficial thrombophlebitis should not receive anticoagulation. Heparin is clearly indicated for patients with documented PE. Heparin is also used for the prevention of venous thromboembolism.

Heparin therapy is contraindicated in patients who are hypersensitive to the drug, who are actively bleeding or who have hemophilia, thrombocytopenia, intracranial hemorrhage, bacterial endocarditis, active tuberculosis, ulcerative lesions of the GI tract, severe hypertension, threatened abortion, or visceral carcinoma. Heparin should be withheld during and after surgery of the brain, eye, or spinal cord, and should not be administered to patients undergoing lumbar puncture or regional anesthetic block. The drug should be used only when clearly indicated in pregnant women, despite its apparent lack of transfer across the placenta.[15]

Clinical Efficacy

The pharmacodynamic goals of heparin therapy are the prevention of thrombosis as well as hemorrhagic episodes, which may be caused by excessive anticoagulation. The evidence that heparin is effective as an anticoagulant is well documented.[10,11] In one evaluation of heparin for the treatment of PE in 114 patients, 5 out of the 19 control patients died as a result of the embolism and another 5 had a nonfatal recurrence of PE.[16] An 8% recurrence rate of PE was observed among patients given heparin. Several studies have documented a reduced mortality rate in patients with venous thromboembolic disease or PE when given heparin compared to patients in whom anticoagulants were withheld.[10,11]

Zero percent to 5% of patients treated with adequate doses of intravenous heparin develop clinical evidence of recurrence, and the likelihood of fatal embolism during treatment is very low.[10–12] Basu et al.[17] found that recurrence of venous thromboembolism, based on clinical diagnosis, was related to an activated partial thromboplastin time (APTT) less than 1.5 times the normal value on 2 or more consecutive days during continuous intravenous heparin therapy. In a study by Wilson et al.[18] using more objective diagnostic criteria, the same trend was observed in patients being monitored with coagulation tests. Raschke et al.[19] demonstrated that recurrent venous thromboembolism occurred less often (5% versus 25%) in patients who had achieved therapeutic APTT values with dosing by a weight-based heparin nomogram than patients receiving standard heparin doses (5000 U bolus followed by 1000 U/h). For both adjusted-dose subcutaneous heparin and continuous intravenous heparin therapy, several contemporary studies have demonstrated the relationship between clinical effectiveness and maintaining the APTT at least 1.5 times the control value.[10,11,19–21] In the future, heparin therapy will be monitored using heparin plasma concentrations rather than APTT.

Administration/Monitoring of Intravenous Heparin

Heparin has traditionally been initiated with an intravenous bolus injection (i.e., 5000 to 10,000 U) followed by either an intravenous continuous infusion (i.e., starting at 1000 U/h) or intermittent intravenous injections (i.e., 5000 U every 4–6 hours). Several issues regarding the optimal administration and monitoring of heparin continue to been reassessed: (1) What route of administration should be used to administer heparin: intravenous infusion, intermittent intravenous injection, or subcutaneous injection?

(2) Should the dose of heparin be adjusted using a coagulation test? (3) How should heparin be monitored? (4) What is the optimal duration of therapy for heparin administration? and (5) Should long-term anticoagulation therapy follow heparin therapy?[10,11]

The most efficient method for providing patients with rapid and effective heparin anticoagulation is for the clinician to consider individual heparin pharmacokinetic and pharmacodynamic data to determine initial dosages, systematically monitor anticoagulation tests, and make subsequent dosage adjustments as indicated. These points are exemplified in a study by Wheeler et al.[22] who identified the following five common practices that led to delays and/or less than adequate anticoagulation (APTT less than 1.5 times control) in patients treated with heparin. These practices are (1) failure to start heparin therapy at the time of clinical presentation, (2) suboptimal dosages, (3) delay in measuring APTT, (4) inadequate response to an APTT less than 1.5 times the control, and (5) excessive and prolonged reductions in heparin dosing when APTT is greater than 3 times the control.

Several standardized dosing techniques and predictive pharmacokinetic methods have been proposed to improve heparin dosing.[10,12,19,21] Figure 19.5 is an algorithm intended for the acute management of DVT or PE with heparin therapy as well as how to manage excessive anticoagulation. Doses should be based on total body weight: a loading dose of 70–100 U/kg followed by an initial infusion rate of 15–25 U/kg/h. Continuous intravenous infusion is the recommended route of administration for maintenance doses because it produces a more consistent degree of coagulation and may be associated with lower risk for bleeding.[10] Despite which route of heparin administration is used (intravenous or subcutaneous), the risk for recurrent venous thromboembolism is low as long as adequate doses of heparin are used.[10]

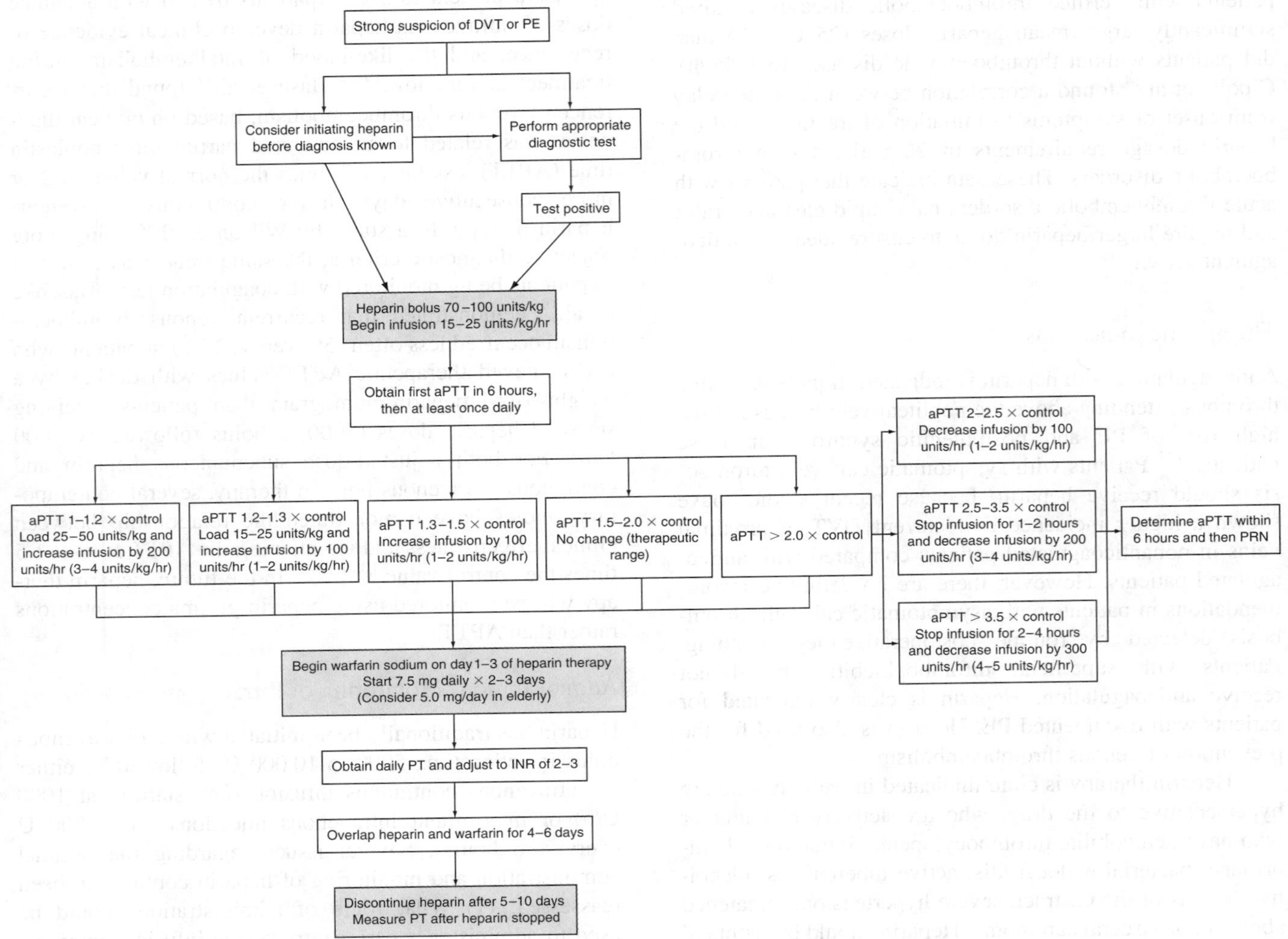

Figure 19.5. Algorithm for acute management of DVT or PE with heparin. *(Adapted from Carter BL. Therapy of acute thromboembolism with heparin and warfarin. Clin Pharm 1991;10:514, with permission.)*

A recent randomized controlled trial[19] evaluated the application of a weight-based dosing nomogram (initial dosing of 80 U/kg bolus followed by 18 U/kg/h; subsequent dosing based on APTT monitoring every 6 hours as needed, and a weight-based [U/kg for boluses and U/kg/h for infusion rates] nomogram) versus standard care dosing guidelines (initial dosing of 5000 U bolus followed by 1000 U/h; subsequent dosing based on APTT monitoring every 6 hours as needed, with bolus dose and infusion rates based on fixed amounts [U and U/h, respectively]). Compared to the standard care guidelines, weight-based heparin dosing resulted in a shorter period of time to achieve an APTT above (8.2 versus 20.2 hours) and within (14.1 versus 20.2 hours) the therapeutic range. In addition, weight-based dosing resulted in more patients with therapeutic APTT at 6 (86 versus 32%) and 24 hours (97 versus 77%) of initiating therapy than patients dosed with standard dosing guidelines. The standard care group had one major bleeding complication. Long-term follow-up demonstrated that recurrent venous thromboembolism occurred less often (5 versus 25%) in patients who received weight-based dosing. This study, as well as others, supports the use of weight-based nomograms or algorithms to provide effective and safe heparin therapy, and appears to avoid long periods of under- or overanticoagulation.

It is imperative that blood samples for coagulation tests (i.e., APTT) for monitoring heparin therapy be carefully timed. After beginning the heparin infusion or after any dosage change, the clinician should wait at least 6 hours to draw samples for coagulation tests to assess the effect of the heparin dose. Samples collected too early are often misleading, may result in inappropriate dosage alteration, and frequently start a costly cycle of "dosage change–coagulation test" in a clinically stable patient. It is often most efficient to wait until steady-state conditions exist to monitor the degree of anticoagulation and make dosage alterations. The risk of bleeding is minimal during the first 48 hours of heparin therapy (in patients without identified risk factors), and coagulation tests are helpful primarily to ensure adequate heparinization. In addition, a recent study found no association between APTT values considered above the therapeutic range during the first 4 days of therapy and bleeding complications.[21]

When a continuous infusion is not feasible, heparin can be administered by intravenous intermittent injections. The half-life of heparin ranges from 0.4–2.5 hours; therefore, an every-4-hours dosing interval is appropriate for most patients. Coagulation tests are best performed 3.5–4 hours after the heparin injection. It is imperative to schedule and document the times of heparin injections and blood sampling for coagulation tests. The heparin dosage is considered adequate when the coagulation test collected 3.5 hours after an intravenous injection is in the therapeutic range for the test (i.e., APTT 1.5–2.0 times baseline).

Once a heparin dose has been determined that produces the desired degree of anticoagulation, daily monitoring of coagulation tests is indicated for minor dosing adjustments. Laboratory monitoring should be performed at the same time of the day (i.e., every morning) to minimize the influence of circadian variation.[12] Large variations in subsequent coagulation tests necessitate investigation to ensure that the patient's condition has not dramatically changed (i.e., extension or recurrence of the thromboembolic event), that the prescribed heparin dose is being administered accurately, and that blood samples are being collected and assayed appropriately. If substantial changes in heparin dosage are made, the modified dosage regimen needs to be monitored in a manner similar to the initial heparin therapy.

The optimal duration of anticoagulation with heparin therapy for the treatment of thromboembolic diseases continues to be evaluated.[10] Several studies in patients with acute thromboembolic diseases have established the effectiveness and safety associated with a short course (4–5 days) of continuous intravenous heparin therapy (warfarin started on day 1 of heparin therapy) compared to the traditional 10-day course (warfarin started on day 5 of heparin therapy).[23–25] These studies demonstrated no significant difference between the groups in terms of rate of recurrence of venous thromboembolism (3.7 versus 4.6%), major bleeding complications (3.7 versus 3.2%), or fatal PE (0% for both groups). Mohiuddin et al.[25] showed that the length of hospital stay (8.62 versus 13.0 days), the cost of hospitalization ($10,485 versus $14,987), and the frequency of adverse reactions associated with heparin therapy (infusion phlebitis [2 versus 18%] and thrombocytopenia [0 versus 14%]) were significantly less for the short-course versus long-course groups. This approach seems appropriate for patients with uncomplicated and less extensive thromboembolic disorders. Patients with massive pulmonary embolism or ileofemoral thrombosis may require a more traditional duration of intravenous heparin therapy (i.e., 10 days), with oral anticoagulation being started on day 5 of heparin therapy to ensure a crossover period of 4–5 days.[10]

Coagulation tests should be performed prior to the initiation of heparin therapy to (1) establish the patient's baseline APTT value, which assists in determining the endpoint for heparin therapy, and (2) establish a baseline prothrombin time (PT and INR) as a guide for later oral anticoagulation with warfarin. Additional necessary baseline laboratory parameters include quantitative platelet count prior to heparinization, every 2 or 3 days during therapy, and after the discontinuation of therapy to monitor for heparin-associated thrombocytopenia. Hemoglobin and hematocrit measurements are indicated prior to heparinization and every 1–2 days while the patient is receiving heparin to identify the presence of bleeding. These laboratory parameters are especially useful in determining the existence of occult bleeding, such as retroperitoneal hemorrhage. The stool should be examined daily for the presence of blood.

Patients should be examined twice daily for signs of bleeding including intravenous catheter sites, hematomas, and ecchymosis. Intramuscular injections should be avoided in patients receiving therapeutic heparin.

Patients receiving heparin for DVT or PE should be monitored for signs and symptoms of pulmonary embolism every shift for 1–2 days, followed by daily monitoring for the incidence or changes in dyspnea, apprehension, cough, pleuritic chest pain, and hemoptysis. In addition, repeat arterial blood gases and lung scans and/or perfusion–ventilation studies may be indicated to assess progress of antithrombotic therapy in patients being treated for PE. Similarly, patients being treated for venous thrombosis should be initially monitored twice daily and then daily for changes in pain, limb circumference, swelling, and tenderness, as well as for signs of PE.

In addition to the laboratory and clinical monitoring parameters just mentioned, clinicians must be aware of other practical concerns in patients receiving heparin. Hattersley et al.[26] reported that the four most common errors associated with heparin therapy were (1) lack of precision of pumps being used to infuse heparin, (2) interruption in the continuous infusion, (3) errors in preparation of solution containing the heparin dose, and (4) errors in charting the dose administered. For the intravenous administration of continuous infusion heparin, reliable infusion pumps should be used. Every effort should be made not to interrupt the continuous infusions. During a 1-hour interruption, the APTT can fall from 60 seconds (therapeutic) to less than 40 seconds; hence, interruptions in the infusion longer than 60 minutes may require an additional bolus injection in addition to restarting the infusion (Fig. 19.5).

To interpret a coagulation test properly, it is essential to know the actual rate of heparin infusion. Failure to document and chart heparin infusion rates adequately can lead to potentially serious errors. The importance of this problem is exemplified by the Boston Collaborative Drug Surveillance Program, which involved 2656 heparinized patients. The actual heparin doses received could not be determined in 30% of the patients because of inadequate drug administration records.[27]

Administration/Monitoring of Dose-Adjusted Subcutaneous Heparin

Several randomized trials suggest that intermittent, adjusted-dose subcutaneous heparin is a safe and effective alternative route of therapy for the initial treatment of venous thrombosis.[10–12,20] In addition, this route of administration simplifies treatment and allows for outpatient therapy.

Initial heparin dosage guidelines should be 15,000–17,500 U or 250 U/kg total body weight administered subcutaneously every 12 hours.[11] The initial dose can be rapidly adjusted according to the APTT value drawn 4–6 hours after the first dose. A midinterval sample has been chosen because this predicts the maximal response of the APTT after subcutaneous injection and the sustained therapeutic response throughout the 12-hour dosing interval.

As with intravenous heparin therapy, adjusted-dose subcutaneous heparin must be administered to maintain APTT above 1.5 times the control value. The APTT should be performed (1) prior to the initiation of heparin therapy, (2) 4–6 hours after the first subcutaneous dose, and (3) once daily at the middle of the dosing interval. Failure to achieve an adequate anticoagulant response early in therapy is associated with an unacceptable recurrence rate of 20–25% of venous thromboembolism.[10] Major and minor bleeding complications have been similar to intravenous heparin administration.

Laboratory Monitoring

The APTT has become the most popular test for monitoring heparin therapy largely because of its routine use by clinical laboratories, the rapidity with which it can be performed, and its reproducibility.[28] The APTT is a global test that measures the resultant activity from the balance between activators and inhibitors of the intrinsic and common pathways of the coagulation system. Platelet-poor plasma is activated by contact agents in the presence of phospholipids and is then recalcified. The APTT uses the generation of a fibrin clot as its endpoint. The APTT reacts similarly with heparin derived from bovine lung and porcine mucosa. The three major disadvantages to using APTT to monitor heparin therapy are that (1) it is unable to distinguish between the anticoagulant activity of heparin and several clotting factor deficiencies, (2) the instrumentation used requires that the APTT be performed in a laboratory, and (3) the variability in heparin sensitivity of different commercial APTT reagents.[12,28,29] This latter point emphasizes the need for each clinical laboratory to use a standardized procedure in the reporting of APTT values.[29]

The goal of therapy is to balance the prevention of unwanted clotting and increased risk of hemorrhage by keeping the degree of anticoagulation within the therapeutic range (APTT between 1.5 and 2.5 times control or baseline).[10,11] Normal adult control values vary among laboratories and range from about 28–42 seconds. The association between subtherapeutic APTT values and recurrent thrombosis is firmly established.[10,17–19,21] However, in the absence of randomized studies, evidence of a correlation between elevated APTT and risk of hemorrhage is suggestive but not conclusive.[10,11]

A recent study has suggested that an antifactor Xa assay may be more useful for monitoring heparin therapy than APTT in patients who require large daily doses (e.g.,

>35,000 U/d).[30] Bleeding complications occurred in only 1 of 65 (1.5%) patients monitored by the antifactor Xa assay compared to 4 of 66 (6.1%) patients monitored by APTT values; recurrent thromboembolic complications were similar for the two groups (4.6 versus 6.1%, respectively). The antifactor Xa assay is not influenced by coagulation factors and is more specific for the effect of heparin to neutralize factor Xa or thrombin. In this select group of patients, the antifactor Xa assay avoids excessive heparin doses and the increased risk of bleeding complications encountered when the APTT is monitored.

Adverse Effects

Hemorrhage is the adverse effect of greatest concern with anticoagulant therapy. The risk of major bleeding (bleeding requiring blood transfusion and/or discontinuation of the anticoagulant) with therapeutic doses of heparin for the treatment of thromboembolic disease has been reported to range from 1–33%, although most studies have reported a frequency of 2–5%.[31–33] The frequency of fatal, major, and major plus minor bleeding during heparin therapy has been estimated to be 0.05, 0.8, and 2.0%, respectively.[33] These frequencies are approximately twice the expected values in patients not receiving heparin therapy.

The most common sites of bleeding with heparin therapy are from the GI tract, the urinary tract, soft tissues, and the oropharynx.[33] The most frequently encountered bleeding episodes include melena, hematomas, and hematuria, which occur in 2–3% of patients. Less common are ecchymosis, epistaxis, and hematemesis, which occur in 0.5–1.2% of patients.

The frequency of bleeding complications has been related to several treatment-related factors (i.e., dose, route, and duration of therapy) and patient-related factors (i.e., age, gender, past history of GI bleeding or peptic ulcer diseases, comorbid diseases, concurrent medications). Several studies have shown that the risk of bleeding greatly increases as the dose increases and with the administration of heparin by intermittent bolus as compared with continuous infusion. Exceeding the normal values of "therapeutic" coagulation tests has been suggested to be predictive of these hemorrhagic complications. However, Conti et al.[34] reported that 84.7% of patients experiencing major bleeding episodes had "therapeutic" activated coagulation times. Mant et al.[35] found that neither heparin dose nor APTT results could be related to bleeding complications.

In general, the risk of bleeding not only varies with the dose but also increases with the length of heparin therapy. The 7-day cumulative risk of bleeding during heparin therapy is 3.4–9.1%.[27,32] Also, this cumulative risk increases with the length of therapy, and by 3 weeks of continuous heparin therapy, bleeding occurs in nearly 20% of patients.

The risk of bleeding is also influenced by several patient-related factors. In an extensive review of 2656 patients, Walker and Jick[27] identified gender, age, dose, concurrent aspirin use, and heavy alcohol use as risk factors associated with both major and minor bleeding episodes in nonsurgical patients. Landefeld et al.[32] reported that the four predictors of major bleeding in hospitalized patients receiving anticoagulant (warfarin or heparin) therapy are (1) comorbid conditions such as heart, liver, or kidney failure, cancer, and severe anemia; (2) age greater than 60 years in patients receiving heparin; (3) the intensity of anticoagulation; and (4) liver failure that worsened during therapy. The risk of bleeding increased as the number of comorbid conditions increased, and was more likely in patients who received intravenous heparin than warfarin.

When bleeding occurs during heparin therapy, it is often related to preexisting hemostatic defects (uremia, drug-related defects in platelet aggregation, thrombocytopenia, liver disease), invasive procedures (venous cutdowns, arterial punctures, thoracentesis), or patient factors such as gender and age. Women have approximately a twofold greater risk of bleeding than males. This gender difference is further exaggerated when advanced age is examined as an additional risk factor. Overall, prophylactic low-dose heparin (5000 U subcutaneously every 12 hours) is not associated with an increased risk of major hemorrhage, and the risk of minor bleeding is also very low.

Minor bleeding from an excess of heparin can usually be controlled by discontinuing the drug. For major bleeding or the threat of significant hemorrhage, specific therapy is warranted. Blood transfusion will correct massive blood loss, but it is not a specific antidote. Protamine sulfate remains the drug of choice for reversal of heparin effect. Protamine combines quickly with heparin to form salts that are devoid of anticoagulant effect. One milligram of protamine sulfate neutralizes approximately 90 USP units of beef lung heparin or 115 USP units of porcine mucosal heparin. For patients receiving heparin as a continuous infusion, 1 mg of protamine should be administered for each 100 U of heparin delivered during the past 4 hours. Protamine should be administered by slow intravenous infusion (up to 50 mg over 10 minutes) to decrease the frequency and severity of adverse reactions (i.e., hypotension, vasodilation, bradycardia, and dyspnea). Excessive doses of protamine can also be associated with bleeding complications.

Other important adverse effects of heparin therapy are thrombocytopenia with thrombosis and osteoporosis. Although the reported incidence of thrombocytopenia has varied from less than 1–30%, the probable frequency is 1–5%.[36] Thrombocytopenia seems to be more frequent with beef lung heparin; however, switching to porcine mucosa heparin is not recommended because of the high incidence of cross-sensitivity between products. Two distinct platelet phenomena are associated with the administration of heparin, and can be seen in patients who receive therapeutic doses of heparin, as well as in patients who receive low-dose subcutaneous heparin and heparin flushes. An early, slight decrease in circulating platelets is almost universal. The effect is mild and transient, with platelet counts seldom dropping below 100,000/mm^3, and usually does not require discontinuation of heparin therapy. It is most likely due to a temporary sequestration of platelets, secondary to heparin's mild platelet aggregating effect. The patients are usually asymptomatic, and it appears to be of no clinical importance.

The second effect is a rare but severe thrombocytopenia that occurs between 5–14 days after the initiation of heparin therapy. The effect is independent of dose or route, and most likely has an immunologic basis, which increases platelet consumption. Platelet counts may fall below 100,000/mm^3, and will remain low until the heparin is discontinued. In addition, thromboembolic complications may occur in arteries (white clot) as well as veins (i.e., myocardial infarction, DVT, PE) with this type of thrombocytopenia. Careful monitoring of platelet counts (every 2–3 days) to evaluate the decline of platelet count (i.e., greater than 30%) as well as the absolute number (i.e., less than 100,000/mm^3) can minimize the risk of heparin-associated thrombocytopenia.[37]

A limited number of reports have described osteoporosis secondary to heparin therapy.[10,11] This adverse effect has been rarely reported and is generally found in patients receiving in excess of 20,000 U/d for 6 months or longer.

Other rare complications of heparin therapy include skin necrosis, local urticaria, hypoaldosteronism, and hypersensitivity reactions.

WARFARIN

The coumarin derivative warfarin was synthesized at the University of Wisconsin in 1948 (the name warfarin being derived from the Wisconsin Alumni Research Foundation). Warfarin is the most useful of the vitamin K antagonists because of its predictable clinical effects, including onset of action and long duration of effect. The indications for warfarin therapy include the treatment of venous thromboembolism, the prevention of recurrent venous thromboembolism, the prevention of thromboembolism in patients with prosthetic heart valves or chronic atrial fibrillation, the prophylaxis against venous thrombosis in patients undergoing moderate- to high-risk surgical procedures, or as an adjunct in the treatment of coronary artery occlusion.[38,39] Because the risk of recurrent thromboembolic disease is significant in the first 3 months after DVT or PE, and moderate for 6 months or greater, warfarin administration is indicated after the initial course of heparin therapy to prevent further thromboembolic complications.[10,39]

The pharmacologic effects of warfarin include anticoagulation and antithrombotic action. The mechanisms by which warfarin accomplishes these effects include prevention of the formation of γ-carboxyglutamic acid residues (by blocking the carboxylation system) and release of certain proteins that are deficient in γ-carboxyglutamic acid (Fig. 19.6). Six vitamin K-dependent proteins are involved in the coagulation system (factors II, VII, IX, X, and proteins C and S), whose synthesis is inhibited by warfarin.

The inhibition of coagulation factors and the indirect anticoagulation of warfarin occurs 12–24 hours after oral administration. This is at the same time that depression of protein C and factor VII occurs. In contrast, antithrombotic effects of warfarin may not occur until 2–7 days following

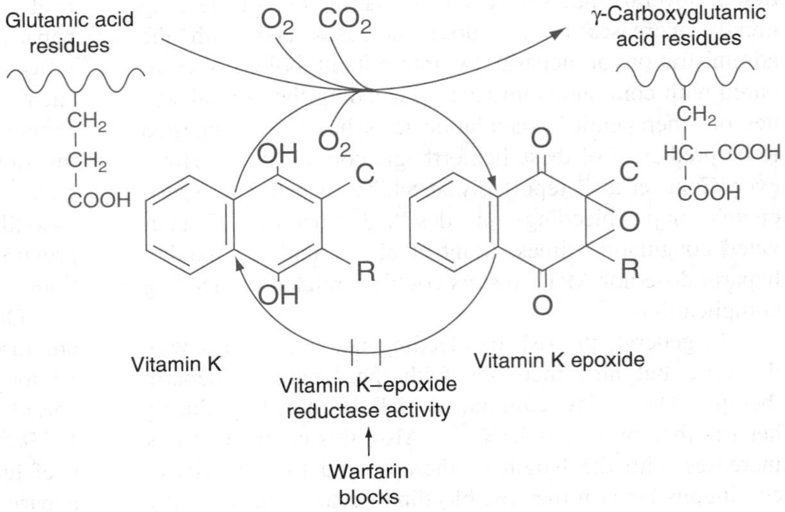

Figure 19.6. Interactions between vitamin K and warfarin. Warfarin and other vitamin K antagonists inhibit the reduction of vitamin K epoxide to vitamin K by the enzyme vitamin K–epoxide reductase. The oxidation–reduction cycle between the two forms of vitamin K is linked in some unknown way to the γ-carboxylation of glutamic acid residues on vitamin K-dependent coagulation factors II, VII, IX, and X. *(From Hirsh J, Genton E, Hull R (eds). Venous Thromboembolism. New York, Grune and Stratton, 1981, p 189, with permission.)*

the initiation of therapy. The *in vivo* antithrombotic effect occurs after a steady state has been achieved between the decrease in the rate of synthesis and the rate of disappearance of existing clotting factors in plasma. The average half-lives of the vitamin K-dependent clotting factors are 6, 24, 40, and 60 hours for factors VII, IX, X and II, respectively. Factor VII concentrations decrease first and account for the initial change in the PT.

Pharmacokinetics

Warfarin is commercially available as a racemic mixture of the enantiomers *R*- and *S*-warfarin that exhibit differing pharmacokinetic and pharmacodynamic characteristics.[38,40,41] After oral administration, warfarin is well absorbed, with peak plasma concentrations occurring from 0.3–8 hours (mean: 90 minutes) after a dose.[41] The bioavailability of warfarin is 100% with minimal differences among the various commercial warfarin products. However, difficulties may arise in controlling a patient's anticoagulant therapy when products are interchanged.

Warfarin is extensively protein bound (97.4–99.9%), principally to albumin, with the *R*-enantiomer having greater binding affinity than *S*-warfarin. When protein binding is taken into account, the *S*-enantiomer has an inherent potency approximately eight times greater than the *R*-enantiomer. Warfarin is stereoselectively oxidized by hepatic microsomal enzyme systems to hydroxy metabolites, and then reduced to alcohols that are renally excreted.

Warfarin is a capacity-limited binding-sensitive drug, which has a low intrinsic clearance and a low unbound fraction. Protein binding determines the unbound drug fraction available for metabolism and explains the linear relationship observed between total body clearance of warfarin and the unbound fraction in plasma. In addition, isomers of warfarin have different rates of elimination. Mean (range) half-lives for the *R*- and *S*-isomers are 45.4 (37.4–88.6) and 33 (21.2–42.6) hours, respectively. These differences in half-life of the isomers influence the contribution of the *R*-isomer to the anticoagulant effects of warfarin and have implications on drug interactions.

Plasma clearance of warfarin is increased in patients with renal insufficiency. More unbound fraction of warfarin is available for metabolism in patients with renal failure. In addition, there is the potential for the renally excreted active alcohol metabolites to accumulate. However, these alterations have not increased pharmacologic responsiveness of warfarin in patients with renal failure.

Therapeutic Indications/Clinical Efficacy

Warfarin effectively prevents recurrent thromboembolic events following the acute treatment of DVT or PE with heparin therapy. The rationale for warfarin after initial heparin therapy was derived from studies that showed a protective effect of anticoagulant therapy for the first 6 months after hospital discharge.[38–40,42] Beyond this time, the potential beneficial effects of anticoagulation must be weighed against the risk of bleeding complications. The incidence of serious bleeding complications while receiving warfarin ranges from 2.4–10% in most series.[31–33,43,44] The risk of recurrent thromboembolic disease is highest in those patients with previous episodes of the same phenomenon. Thus, warfarin administration is indicated for at least 3 months after an initial episode of DVT and indefinitely for long-term anticoagulation in patients with recurrent venous thromboembolism.[10,42]

Several studies have searched for a suitable alternative strategy for managing patients with long-term anticoagulation.[10,11,39] The clinical efficacy of fixed-low-dose subcutaneous heparin, dose-adjusted subcutaneous heparin, and "less intensive" warfarin therapy (prothrombin times ranging from 1.2–1.8 times control or baseline values) has been evaluated in patients initially treated with a continuous intravenous infusion of heparin for 10–14 days. These studies demonstrate that adjusted-dose heparin and less intense warfarin therapy are as effective as conventional warfarin therapy for treating proximal-vein thrombosis, with risk of hemorrhage significantly greater with conventional warfarin therapy. Fixed-low-dose heparin is not effective for treating proximal vein thrombosis. A cost-effectiveness analysis was performed for the various approaches to long-term treatment of proximal venous thrombosis. It was concluded that the less intense warfarin therapy was the most cost effective and that oral therapy was preferred by the majority of patients. However, dose-adjusted subcutaneous heparin is an acceptable alternative to warfarin therapy, particularly in patients who cannot take warfarin (i.e., pregnancy) and in those patients who cannot have their coagulation tests (PT) monitored on a continual basis.

All of the contraindications listed above for heparin apply to warfarin as well. Relative contraindications for warfarin therapy include severe hepatic or renal disease, vitamin K deficiency, chronic alcoholism, a requirement for intensive salicylate or nonsteroidal anti-inflammatory drug therapy, and the inability of the patient to comply with the regimen.

Laboratory Monitoring

The international normalized ratio (INR) is now considered the standard of practice for monitoring warfarin therapy.[10,38] The INR takes into account the sensitivity of the thromboplastin used in determining the PT for each specific laboratory.[45] The World Health Organization (WHO) has prepared a thromboplastin standard to promote standardization of oral anticoagulation therapy by allowing any commercial thromboplastin reagent to be calibrated against this reference standard.

The calculation of the INR is represented by the following equation demonstrating the relationship between the INR and the observed PT ratio:

$$\text{INR} = (\text{observed PT ratio})^{\text{ISI}}$$

where ISI is the international sensitivity index, which is calibrated based on the type of thromboplastin used. The sensitivity of the thromboplastin reagent can dramatically influence the INR value. For example, if a patient has a PT of 17 seconds using a more responsive thromboplastin with a low ISI value of 1.2, and the laboratory mean normal value for the PT is 12.6 seconds, the INR for this patient would be 1.43. However, the INR would be 1.99 in the same patient if the thromboplastin used was less sensitive and had an ISI value of 2.3. The different values in thromboplastin reagents illustrates the limitation of monitoring warfarin with only PT ratios, which have been associated with significant errors when monitoring warfarin therapy.[45,46]

The current recommendation for monitoring most indications of warfarin therapy is an INR of 2.0–3.0.[10,38] Patients with mechanical prosthetic heart values are the only exception, where an INR of 2.5–3.5 has been recommended. In addition, the use of standard PT ratios is no longer recommended for the "typical" North American thromboplastin (ISI = 2.3) since ISI values range from 1.3–2.8 with the various commercially available thromboplastins.[45]

It is important to recognize the effect that heparin has on the PT when heparin and warfarin therapies are "overlapped." It has been shown that heparin increases PT results. However, the effects are minimal and the PT will decrease once heparin therapy is discontinued, which may require further adjustment of warfarin maintenance doses.

Warfarin Administration/Monitoring

Warfarin can be initiated at any time during heparin treatment and should be initiated as soon as it becomes apparent that oral anticoagulation will be used. Initiation of warfarin should occur before intravenous heparin is discontinued to prevent a break in the level of anticoagulation. The "overlapping period" of heparin and warfarin should be 4–5 days because of the delayed onset of warfarin's effect and the hypercoagulable state occurring after heparin is discontinued.[10,22,38,39] Heparin can usually be discontinued once the INR is within the desired range for 2 consecutive days.

The risk of recurrent venous thromboembolism approaches 0% if warfarin therapy is initiated during a 5- to 14-day course of heparin therapy.[11] In addition, several studies have demonstrated that the number of hospitalization days, days of heparin therapy, adverse effects of heparin, and cost of hospitalization are decreased when warfarin is administered within the first 24–48 hours of heparin therapy.[23–25]

It must be emphasized that warfarin dosages must be individualized by monitoring the INR closely and examining the patient for signs of bleeding. The initiation of oral warfarin therapy with small doses of approximately 5–10 mg/d for 2–4 days is generally agreed to be less toxic than administration of large loading doses (i.e., 50–75 mg).[39,40] In elderly patients (i.e., age >65 years), initial doses may need to be lower (i.e., 1–3 mg/d) as well as laboratory monitoring intervals ≥1 week to allow steady-state effects to be achieved. Administration of a large loading dose places the patient at risk of hemorrhage and may precipitate the potentially serious dermatologic reaction (necrosis).[41]

The PT should be performed prior to the initiation of warfarin therapy for the following purposes: (1) as a screen for preexisting coagulation disorders; (2) to evaluate the effect, if any, that heparin therapy may have on the PT; and (3) to establish the patient's individual baseline value to determine the therapeutic endpoint of warfarin therapy from a laboratory standpoint (to calculate a PT ratio for determination of the INR). The INR should be monitored every 24–48 hours after warfarin therapy is initiated and until the INR results have stabilized (i.e., INRs that are similar for 2 or 3 consecutive days with the same warfarin dosage) or until a maintenance dose is determined. Alterations in warfarin dosage should be made in small increments to prevent excessive changes in the INR. A patient's discharge from the hospital need not be delayed due to an INR that has not stabilized because the patient can easily be monitored as an outpatient with frequent INR determinations.

The initial maintenance dosage requirements of a patient should not be considered as absolute requirements. Careful follow-up and weekly monitoring of the INR is required during the first 4 weeks of therapy after discharge from the hospital (Fig. 19.7). A number of "outpatient" factors including changes in diet, exercise, clinical state, social habits, and compliance frequently alter maintenance dose requirements. Once a stable therapeutic warfarin dose has been attained, the INR can be monitored less frequently (i.e., once monthly).

A number of specific factors may contribute to a patient's unusual response to warfarin.[39,41] These include (1) inaccurate laboratory monitoring, (2) failure to use the INR system appropriately, (3) alterations in the anticoagulant response because of drug–drug or drug–disease interactions, (4) fluctuations in nutritional status and/or dietary vitamin K intake, (5) altered receptor site sensitivity to warfarin (i.e., hereditary resistance), (6) alterations in drug administration or patient compliance, and (7) abnormal product performance or use of products from various manufacturers.

A number of pharmacokinetic equations, computer-assisted programs, and Bayesian forecasting programs intended to predict warfarin maintenance dose requirements have been evaluated.[41,47,48] These warfarin prediction meth-

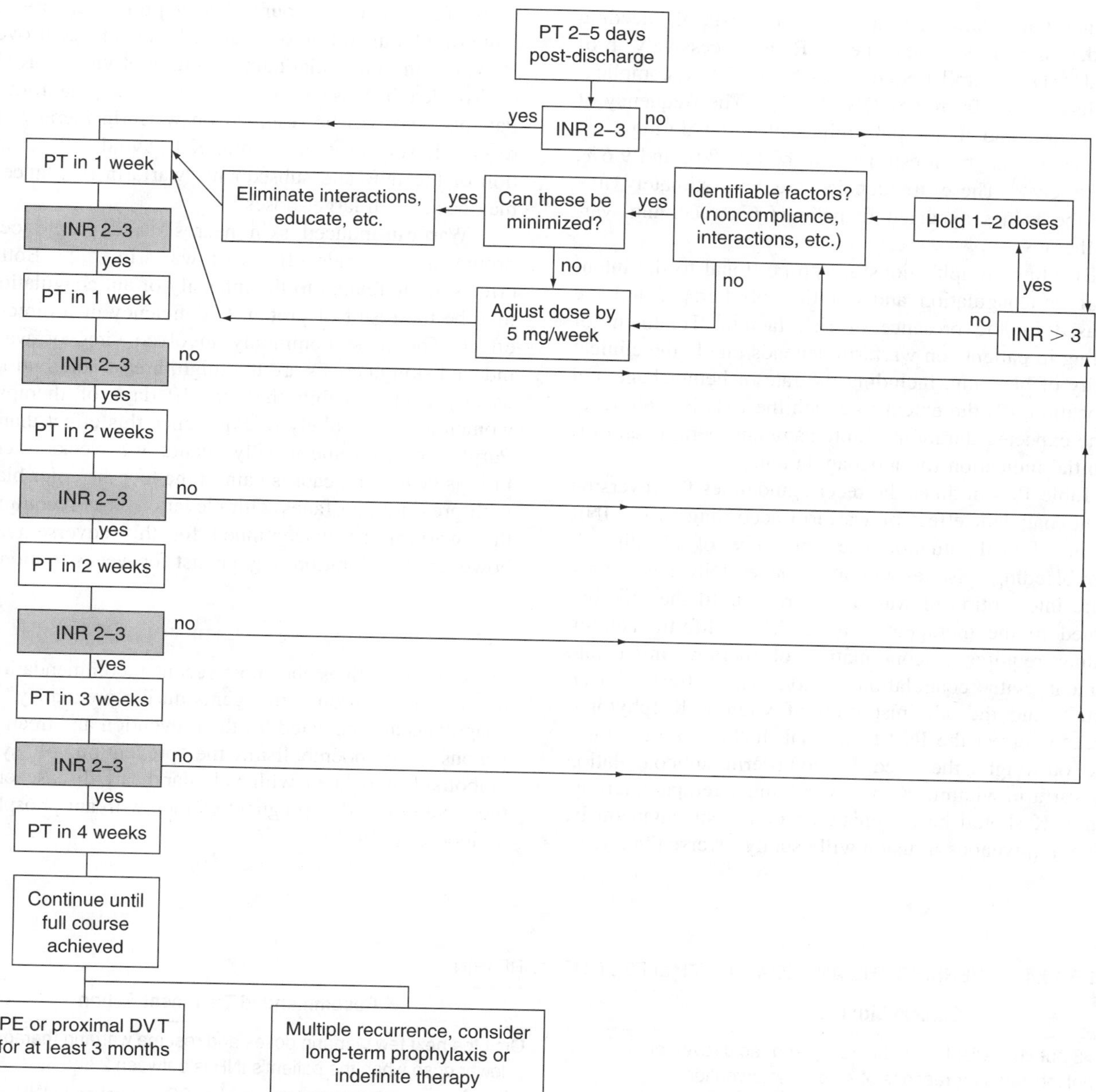

Figure 19.7. Algorithm for management of long-term warfarin therapy after hospital discharge. *(From Carter BL. Therapy of acute thromboembolism with heparin and warfarin. Clin Pharm 1991;10:514, with permission.)*

ods may not be clinically applicable because of interpatient variability, differences between laboratory techniques, and use of a therapeutic PT ratio of 1.5–2.5 making further evaluations necessary.

A guideline-based consultation service that uses specific practice guidelines (i.e., Antithrombotic Consensus Conference[10]) has been shown to be an effective method of decreasing major (from 13–4%) and minor (from 18–9%) bleeding episodes in medium- to high-risk hospitalized patients receiving heparin and warfarin therapy.[49] This type of service, as well as pharmacy-managed warfarin-monitoring services for inpatient and outpatient therapy,[40,50] provides an excellent way of (1) introducing standard of care guidelines, (2) evaluating risks and benefits of therapy, (3) assessing alternative treatments, (4) providing dosing recommendations, (5) monitoring efficacy and safety of therapy, and (6) improving patient compliance.

Adverse Effects

As with heparin, the major toxic effect of warfarin is hemorrhage. Bleeding during anticoagulation does not always correlate with the INR; however, the risk of bleeding episodes increases when the INR is excessively prolonged.[32] The overall frequency of hemorrhagic complications has ranged from 2.5–27%.[31–33,43,44] The frequency of fatal, major, and major plus minor bleeding during warfarin therapy has been estimated to be 0.6, 3.0, and 9.6%, respectively.[33] These frequencies are approximately five times the values expected in patients not receiving warfarin therapy.

Bleeding complications are proportional to the intensity of anticoagulation and duration of therapy, and are increased by the presence of risk factors. Treatment of bleeding in patients on warfarin depends on (1) the clinical severity of bleeding, including the rate of hemorrhage and the location; (2) the extent to which the INR is prolonged; (3) the expected duration of anticoagulant therapy; and (4) the initial indication for anticoagulation.

Table 19.4 outlines the recent guidelines for reversing the anticoagulant effect of warfarin according to the INR and the clinical situation (i.e., presence of bleeding).[45] Minor bleeding episodes with a prolonged INR may merely require interruption of warfarin therapy until the INR has returned to the therapeutic range. Major life-threatening bleeding requires discontinuation of therapy, immediate treatment with coagulation factors (i.e., fresh frozen plasma), and the administration of vitamin K (phytonadione) to correct the INR to normal. If the risk of hemorrhage outweighs the need for long-term anticoagulation with warfarin, vitamin K may be administered parenterally. Vitamin K should be administered orally, subcutaneously, or slow intravenous infusion will usually reverse the effects of warfarin in 6–12 hours. The appropriate dose and/or route of administration of vitamin K remains controversial. However, intramuscular administration of vitamin K should be avoided because of the risk of hematoma formation. Patients who will be resumed on warfarin therapy should receive lower doses of vitamin K to avoid full normalization of the INR and subsequent "warfarin resistance" that may occur with larger doses.

Warfarin-induced skin necrosis and purple-toe syndrome are rare side effects of warfarin.[39,40,51] Both side effects are unrelated to the intensity of anticoagulation and may be the result of protein C deficiency or a direct toxic effect. The most commonly involved sites of warfarin-induced skin necrosis are the thigh, breast, and buttocks. It usually occurs within the first 10 days of therapy, and women are more likely to experience this effect than men. Purple-toe syndrome usually occurs 3–8 weeks after warfarin is begun and causes pain in the toe; the color blanches with pressure and fades with elevation. It is recommended that warfarin be discontinued for this adverse reaction; however, discoloration may persist for weeks to months.

Anticoagulants During Pregnancy

Table 19.5 outlines the most recent recommendations for the use of antithrombotic agents during pregnancy.[15] Anticoagulants are indicated for the prevention and treatment of venous thromboembolism, the prevention of systemic embolism associated with valvular heart disease or prosthetic valves, and in pregnant women with antiphospholipid antibodies (APLA).

TABLE 19.4. REVERSING THE ANTICOAGULANT EFFECT OF WARFARIN

Clinical Situation	Recommended Treatment Action
INR >3 but <6, patient is not bleeding, and rapid reversal is not indicated for reasons of surgical intervention	Omit the next few warfarin doses and resume warfarin therapy at a lower dose when the patient's INR is between 2 and 3.
INR ≥6 but <10 and the patient is not bleeding, or more rapid reversal is required because the patient requires elective surgery	Administer vitamin K 0.5–1 mg, oral or SQ; reduction in INR will occur within 8 hours and many patients' INRs may be in the range of 2–3 in 24 hours. If the INR at 24 hours is still high, a second dose of vitamin K 0.5 mg SQ can be repeated. Warfarin can then be restarted at a lower dose.
INR ≥10 but <20 and the patient is not bleeding	Vitamin K 3–4 mg, oral or SQ, should be given with the INR reduced substantially at 6 hours. The INR should be checked every 6–12 hours, and vitamin K can be repeated as necessary.
Major warfarin overdose (e.g., INR >20) or a rapid reversal of an anticoagulant effect is required because of serious bleeding	Vitamin K 10 mg slow IV infusion (e.g., over 20–30 minutes) and the INR checked every 6 hours. Vitamin K may be repeated every 12 hours and supplemented with plasma transfusion or factor concentrate depending on the urgency of the situation.
Life-threatening bleeding or serious warfarin overdose	Replacement with factor concentrates as indicated supplemented with vitamin K 10 mg slow IV infusion (e.g., over 20–30 minutes). Vitamin K may be repeated as necessary depending on the INR.

(Adapted from Hirsh J, Poller L. The international normalized ratio: A guide to understanding and correcting its problems. Arch Intern Med 1994;154:282–288, with permission.)

TABLE 19.5. RECOMMENDATION OF ANTITHROMBOTIC AGENTS DURING PREGNANCY

Condition	Recommendation
Previous venous thrombosis or pulmonary embolism prior to current pregnancy	Heparin 5000 U subcutaneously q 12 hours throughout pregnancy.
Venous thrombosis or pulmonary embolism during current pregnancy	Heparin in full intravenous doses for 5–10 days, followed by q 12 hours subcutaneous injection to prolong 6-hour postinjection APTT to 1.5 times control until delivery. Warfarin can then be used postpartum.
Planning pregnancy in patients requiring long-term anticoagulation	Either heparin q 12 hours subcutaneously to prolong 6-hour postinjection APTT to 1.5 times control, or Frequent pregnancy tests and substitute heparin (as above) for warfarin when pregnancy achieved.
Mechanical prosthetic heart valves	Either heparin q 12 hours subcutaneously to prolong 6-hour postinjection APTT to 1.5 times control, or Adjusted dose subcutaneous heparin until the 13th week, warfarin until the middle of the third trimester, then adjusted dose subcutaneous heparin until delivery.
APLA and >1 previous pregnancy loss	Either aspirin plus prednisone, or heparin.
APLA and 0 or 1 previous pregnancy loss	Low-dose aspirin during the second and third trimester.
APLA and previous venous thrombosis	Heparin q 12 hours subcutaneously to prolong 6-hour postinjection APTT to 1.5–2.5 times control.
APLA without previous venous thrombosis	Either weekly or biweekly IPG or compression ultrasonography, or heparin 5000 U q 12 hours throughout pregnancy.

Key: APLA, antiphospholipid antibodies; IPG, impedance plethysmography. (Adapted from Ginsberg JS, Hirsh J. Use of antithrombotic agents during pregnancy. Chest 1992;102(suppl):385S–390S, with permission.)

Heparin is currently the anticoagulant of choice in pregnant females (FDA Pregnancy Category C) because it does not cross the placenta and does not cause fetal complications.[11,15] Maternal effects of anticoagulation include hemorrhage and osteoporosis. Hemorrhage is a possible adverse effect of treatment with heparin, and it must be used judiciously with careful monitoring. Long-term use of high doses of heparin (i.e., 20,000 U/day for greater than 5 months) during pregnancy has been associated with maternal osteoporosis.

Warfarin should be avoided in pregnant patients (FDA Pregnancy Category X) because it crosses the placenta and causes fetal malformation at *any* time during pregnancy.[15,39] During the first 6–12 weeks of pregnancy, "warfarin embryopathy" may occur, which is associated with skeletal abnormalities. Exposure after the first trimester carries the risk of central nervous system abnormalities. All women of child-bearing age should be counseled to use contraceptive methods to avoid becoming pregnant while on warfarin therapy. If the mother's condition requires anticoagulation, heparin should be used from at least the start of the sixth gestational week and until the end of the twelfth gestational week, and again at term to lessen the risks to the fetus.

During lactation, heparin is not secreted in breast milk and can be safely administered to nursing mothers. Warfarin has not been detected in breast milk and has not produced an anticoagulant effect in infants; however, further studies are needed before routine use of warfarin during lactation is recommended.

The use of low molecular weight heparin could also be considered. Enoxaparin is classified as FDA Pregnancy Category B. Enoxaparin does not cross the placenta, and has been used in a limited number of pregnant patients with no apparent adverse effects. Although dalteparin also appears not to cross the placenta, no data are currently available concerning its use in pregnancy or effects on the fetus. Further data are needed before the use of dalteparin in pregnancy can be recommended.

Food and Drug–Drug Interactions

There are more food and drug–drug interactions reported with warfarin than for any other drug.[39] Current use of warfarin with alcohol and prescription or over-the-counter medications must routinely be considered as a cause of increased or decreased anticoagulant effect. Mechanisms responsible for these interactions involve (1) altered vitamin K availability, (2) reduced warfarin absorption, (3) changes in warfarin protein binding, (4) effects on warfarin's metabolism, (5) changes in receptor affinity for warfarin, (6) reduction in vitamin K-dependent clotting factor levels, and (7) independent effect on hemostatic metabolism (Fig. 19.8). The clinician must be aware of the high probability of drug–drug and drug–food interactions.[52]

Each patient's response needs to be closely monitored and additional INR determinations may be indicated whenever other medications are initiated or discontinued, or an alternation in consumption of vitamin K-containing foods is noted.

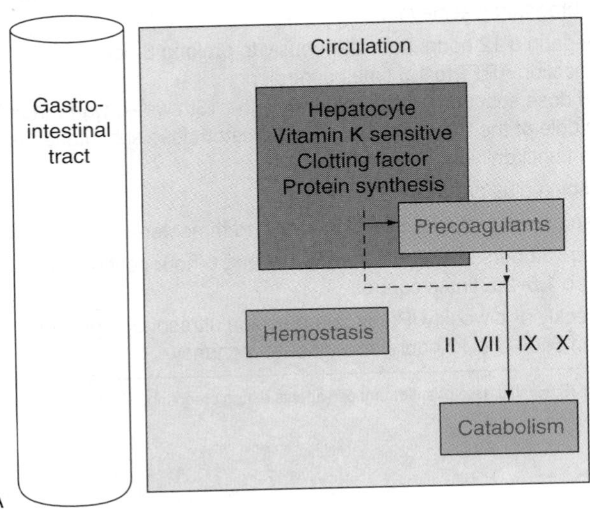

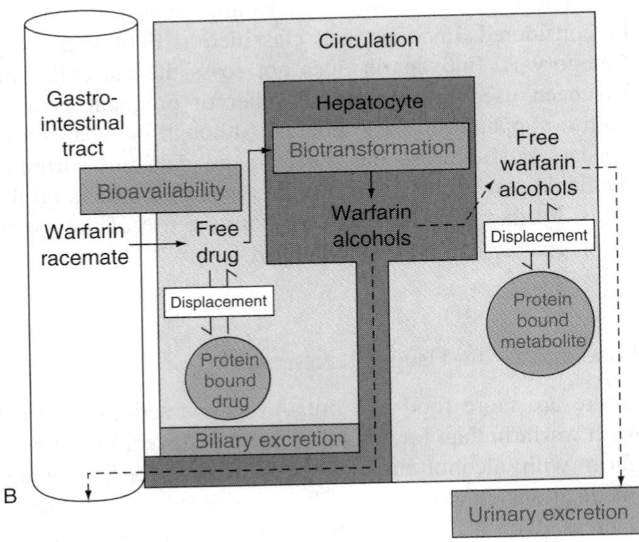

Figure 19.8. Pharmacodynamic and pharmacokinetic drug interactions with coumarin anticoagulants. (A) Mechanisms of pharmacodynamic interactions, i.e., pharmacologic actions of coumarins that may be altered by other drugs affecting clotting factor synthesis or the hemostatic process. (B) Mechanisms of pharmacokinetic interactions, i.e., interactions in which the absorption, biotransformation, or disposition of coumarin anticoagulants may be altered. *(From MacLeod SM, Seller EM. Pharmacodynamic and pharmacokinetic drug interactions with coumarin anticoagulants. Drugs 1976;11:463, with permission.)*

Patient Education

Safe and efficient warfarin therapy requires careful patient selection, cooperation of the patient, and patient education. Areas that need to be included in patient education are outlined in Table 19.6. It is also important that patients inform other health care professionals (i.e., physician, dentist, nurse) that they are taking warfarin. It may be useful for patients to carry an identification card or a MEDALERT bracelet stating that they are receiving warfarin.

THROMBOLYTIC THERAPY

The principal aim of thrombolytic therapy in the treatment of acute PE and DVT is to restore circulation through a previously occluded vessel by the rapid and complete removal of a pathologic intraluminal thrombus or embolus that has not been dissolved by the endogenous fibrinolytic system.[10,53–55] The potential benefits of thrombolytic therapy for the treatment of PE include prompt dissolution of physiologically compromising pulmonary emboli, faster recovery, prevention of recurrent thrombus formation, and rapid restoration of hemodynamic disturbances.[10,53,55–60] For DVT, lysis of thrombus can prevent PE and permanent pathologic changes such as venous valvular dysfunction and postphlebitic syndrome.[10,53,54,61–64] However, thrombolytic agents have not

TABLE 19.6. INFORMATION FOR THE PATIENT ON WARFARIN

1. *Need for strict compliance:* The importance of taking warfarin and other medications as directed and of following instructions regarding prothrombin times and follow-up office visits must be stressed.
2. *Side effects:* The sites and signs of bleeding as well as instructions on when and where to call if bleeding occurs should be reviewed.
3. *Dietary instruction:* The patient should be told that no major dietary restrictions are necessary; however, no abrupt changes in dietary habits should be made. Rarely, diets with excessive quantities of vitamin K have interfered with warfarin therapy.
4. *Frequent prothrombin times:* The patient needs to be aware of the required monitoring of prothrombin times and why this is necessary. Some patients question the need for continued monitoring of warfarin, and this issue is best addressed early in the course of treatment.
5. *Drug interactions:* The patient should be informed that other drugs can greatly influence the effect of warfarin and should be told not to start or stop medications without first asking the physician. It may be useful to make specific recommendations regarding the use of common nonprescription drugs, e.g., antacids, analgesics, and cold products.

(Adapted from Carter BL, Jones ME, Waickman LA. Pathophysiology and treatment of deep-vein thrombosis and pulmonary embolism. Clin Pharm 1985;4:292–293, with permission.)

been generally accepted as a standard form of therapy for DVT or PE because of the possible bleeding complications, the lack of mortality differences, and adequate long-term follow-up among studies performed, the amount of patient monitoring required once therapy is initiated, and the substantial cost of these agents.

Currently, four thrombolytic agents are available: streptokinase (SK), urokinase (UK), recombinant alteplase (rt-PA, recombinant human tissue-type plasminogen activator), and acylated plasminogen streptokinase activator complex (APSAC).[10,53] All thrombolytics are plasminogen activators and act either directly (UK, rt-PA) or indirectly (SK, APSAC) (Fig. 19.9). Plasminogen, an inactive proteolytic enzyme, is converted to plasmin, which has the ability to lyse fibrin, as well as to hydrolyze fibrinogen and other coagulation factors, leading to a systemic lytic state. The agents differ with respect to their mechanism of plasminogen activation, their specificity for fibrin, their half-lives, source, and cost (Table 19.7).

Streptokinase is a nonenzymatic protein derived from strains of β-hemolytic streptococci. It is an indirect plasminogen activator in that it must first form a complex with plasminogen, which then converts other plasminogen molecules to be activated to plasmin. Because streptokinase is a bacterial protein, it is antigenic and can lead to the production of antibodies as well as allergic reactions. Antibodies from previous streptococcus or streptokinase exposure can bind to streptokinase, rendering it biologically inactive. Part of the rationale for using a loading dose is to overcome the antibody binding and still achieve some therapeutic activity.

Urokinase is a direct plasminogen activator isolated from human fetal kidney cells grown in culture. The advantage of this agent is that it is nonantigenic; however, it is considerably more expensive than streptokinase, which limits its use. Neither urokinase nor streptokinase is specific for thrombi, making either agent prone to lysing any fresh platelet–fibrin hemostatic plug, which is thought to be responsible for the observed hemorrhagic complications. This led investigators to search for agents that were fibrin-specific in hopes of decreasing the incidence of bleeding complications while maintaining their effectiveness.

Alteplase (rt-PA) is a recombinant, second-generation thrombolytic agent that has relative fibrin specificity and is a direct activator of plasminogen. It is described as being more fibrin specific in that it activates plasminogen associated with thrombi or hemostatic plugs in preference to circulating plasminogen. It seems that systemic activation of the fibrinolytic system may be dependent on the dose and rate of administration of rt-PA. However, there is no evidence to date that this agent is associated with a lower incidence of bleeding.

APSAC is an equimolar complex of streptokinase and plasminogen, which can be given as an intravenous bolus

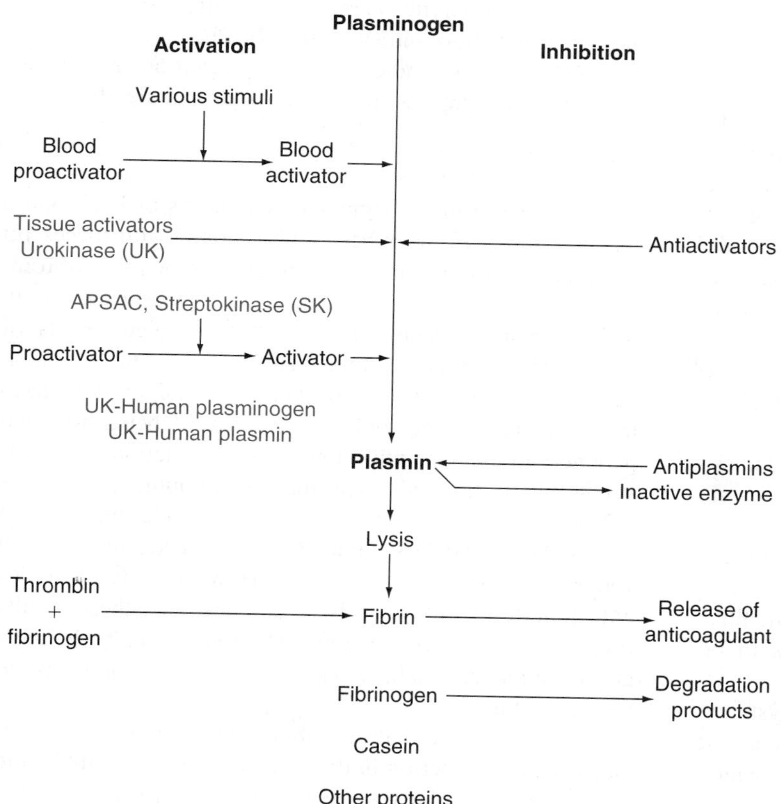

Figure 19.9. Fibrinolysis during thrombolytic therapy. Urokinase and streptokinase activate the fibrinolytic system and convert plasminogen to the active enzyme plasmin, which then lyses a fresh fibrin clot. *(From Sharma GVRK, Cella G, Parisi AF, Sasahara AA. Thrombolytic therapy. N Engl J Med 1982;306:1269, with permission.)*

TABLE 19.7. PROPERTIES OF THROMBOLYTIC AGENTS

	Streptokinase	Urokinase	rt-PA	APSAC
Source	Streptococcal culture	Heterologous mammalian tissue culture	Heterologous mammalian tissue culture	Streptococcal culture
Molecular weight	47,000	32,000–54,000	70,000	131,000
Type of agent	Bacterial proactivator	Tissue plasminogen activator	Tissue plasminogen activator	Bacterial proactivator
Plasma half-life (minutes)	12–18	15–20	2–6	40–60
Fibrinolytic activation	Systemic	Systemic	Systemic	Systemic
Antigenic	Yes	No	No	Yes
Cost[a]	$804 to 2260[b]	$5231[c]	$2641[d]	$2234[e]
Loading dose	250,000 U over 30 minutes	4400 U/kg over 30 minutes	100 mg over 2 hours	[f]
Maintenance dose	100,000 U/h	4400 U/kg/h	None	[f]
Duration of therapy	24–72 hours	12 hours	None	[f]

[a]Represents drug cost to the pharmacy, not actual cost to the patient.
[b]Based on a dosage of 250,000 U (bolus) and an infusion of 100,000 U/h for 24 hours.
[c]Based on a dosage for a 154-pound patient, bolus of 4400 U/kg and an infusion of 4400 U/kg/h for 12 hours.
[d]Based on 100-mg dose.
[e]A 30-unit dose.
[f]No approved dosage regimen for PE or DVT. (Adapted from Bell WR et al. Fibrinolytic therapy: Indications and management, in Hoffman R et al (eds): Hematology: Basic Principles and Practice. New York, Churchill Livingstone, 1991, p 1451, with permission.)

injection. It is chemically inert and relies on deacylation under physiologic conditions to become active. This agent has mainly been used for the treatment of evolving acute myocardial infarction.

Therapeutic Indications

Streptokinase is FDA approved for the treatment of acute PE and DVT; urokinase and rt-PA are FDA approved for the treatment of acute PE. All of the agents are approved for use in acute myocardial infarction. Although these agents have been investigated in numerous other thromboembolic disorders, the small number of patients studied does not permit any conclusions to be drawn, and therefore no clinical recommendation can be made.

The proposed indications for the use of thrombolytic therapy in patients with thromboembolic disease include massive/submassive PE with hemodynamic compromise, massive PE without hemodynamic compromise, submassive PE in patients who cannot tolerate further cardiopulmonary compromise, heparin treatment failures, and extensive proximal DVT. Presently, thrombolytic agents offer the greatest benefit to PE patients suffering from acute decompensation with hypotension and low cardiac output; their role in patients with less severe episodes remains to be defined.

Guidelines for selection of patients for systemic thrombolytic therapy should be based on the presence of clinical indications. This should include a documented diagnosis of thromboembolism and evidence that the thrombus is of recent origin (within the last 7 days). Recent origin of thrombus seems particularly important in the treatment of DVT. However, Goldhaber[55] suggests that effective thrombolytic therapy can administered up to 14 days after the signs and symptoms of PE.

Relative contraindications and precautions for the use of thrombolytic agents are summarized in Table 19.8.

Clinical Efficacy

A rapid decline in the signs and symptoms of DVT and a reduced risk of PE have been demonstrated with successful resolution of the thrombus. Streptokinase achieves thrombolysis 3.7 times more often than does heparin therapy in patients being treated for DVT.[54,56,61] Pooled results of short-term venographic studies suggest that either substantial or partial improvement occurs in 61% of streptokinase-treated patients compared to only 25% of heparin-treated patients. In studies with long-term evaluation of DVT, streptokinase resulted in normal venographic evaluations (57 versus 7%), less chronic post-thrombotic changes (43 versus 93%), and less clinically symptomatic patients (19 versus 75%) than heparin therapy. However, not all studies with long-term follow-up have demonstrated these results favoring thrombolytic therapy. Urokinase and rt-PA have also been reported to have results similar to streptokinase in the treatment of DVT.[54,62,64]

It is suggested that thrombolytic therapy may be associated with a reduction in the incidence of the postphlebitic syndrome, particularly if treatment is given soon after the

TABLE 19.8. CONTRAINDICATIONS TO THROMBOLYTIC THERAPY

Absolute Contraindications
- Active internal bleeding
- Cerebrovascular process, disease, or procedure within 2 months

Relative Contraindications
- Conditions requiring fibrin strands and plugs for normal hemostasis or healing (fibrinolysis is usually contraindicated within 10 days of onset of these conditions)
- Recent major surgery, organ biopsy, puncture of noncompressible blood vessel
- Postpartum period
- Cardiopulmonary resuscitation during presence of rib fractures
- Thoracentesis, paracentesis, lumbar puncture
- Recent serious trauma

Potentially Serious Bleeding
- Uncontrolled coagulation defects
- Uncontrolled severe hypertension
- Pregnancy
- Other conditions deemed potential bleeding risks

(From Sharma CVRK, Cella G, Parisi AF, Sasahara AA. Thrombolytic therapy. N Engl J Med 1982;306:1271, with permission.)

development of symptoms.[54,61,63,64] Successful clot resolution on venogram has been reported to occur in more than 65% of patients treated within 5 days of symptom onset, compared to 33% if treatment is initiated between 6–9 days and 0% if after 9 days.[54] In addition, predictive factors that appear to influence the effectiveness of streptokinase in patients treated for DVT include the following: (1) Nonocclusive clots are more easily lysed than occlusive clots; (2) among nonocclusive clots, proximal are more easily lysed than popliteal; and (3) long-term venous sequelae greater than 2 years occur less frequently when a normal phlebogram (compared residual occlusion) is observed at time of discharge.[63]

Successful resolution of pulmonary thromboemboli occurs in about 80–90% of patients with massive and submassive PE. Two controlled trials, one comparing urokinase with heparin[56] and a second comparing urokinase with streptokinase,[57] were performed to define the role of thrombolytic therapy in the treatment of PE. These two trials, in which 327 patients with angiographically confirmed pulmonary embolism were studied, showed that, compared with heparin, thrombolytic therapy produced (1) greater resolution of pulmonary emboli, (2) greater improvement of the abnormal hemodynamic status of the right heart and pulmonary circulation, (3) greater reperfusion of the original pulmonary perfusion defects, and (4) maximal clot resolution and general improvement in patients with the largest pulmonary emboli. However, in these studies there was no difference in the mortality rate among patients given heparin compared with those given thrombolytic therapy, and the incidence of bleeding complications was nearly double for those who received thrombolytic therapy.

A further potential advantage to the use of thrombolytic therapy is a reduction in the long-term effects of PE. Sharma et al.[58] have shown greater improvement in pulmonary capillary blood volume and perfusion at both 2 weeks and 1 year in a streptokinase-treated group when compared with a heparin-treated group. Follow-up of these patients at 7–10 years has continued to demonstrate a decrease in chronic pulmonary hypertension and functional impairment in the streptokinase-treated group.[53]

Several recent clinical studies have established the role of rt-PA in the treatment of PE.[55,59,60,65] Short-term hemodynamic and angiographic improvements have been demonstrated to occur more often with rt-PA and urokinase than heparin therapy. Major bleeding complications, including intracranial bleeding, occur more frequently with thrombolytic therapy.

Drug Administration

Safe and effective administration of thrombolytic agents is best accomplished with continuous intravenous infusion in a precise manner. The commonly recommended dosage schedules were derived from the large clinical trials for the treatment of PE and DVT.[10,53,54,56,57]

For streptokinase, the initial loading dose of 250,000 units in normal saline or 5% dextrose in water is administered over 30 minutes. Maintenance therapy consists of 100,000 U/h for 24–72 hours. For PE, results from the major studies favor 24 hours of administration. Infusions for DVT have been continued for up to 120 hours, but have not demonstrated additional benefit when continued beyond 72 hours. Intravenous administration of a bolus followed by intravenous infusion results in a systemic lytic state (decreased fibrinogen and increased fibrin degradation products) in more than 90% of patients.

Urokinase is given in a loading dose of 4400 U/kg of body weight in normal saline over 10 minutes. Maintenance therapy consists of 4400 U/kg/h for a total of 12 hours for PE. The total volume of fluid administered should not exceed 200 mL. In one study the drug was administered for 24 hours, but no additional benefit was demonstrated after 12 hours.[57]

The approved dose of rt-PA for treatment of PE is 100 mg administered by intravenous infusion over 2 hours. Other studies have been conducted that employ lower doses and/or shorter infusion rates of rt-PA and urokinase in the treatment of PE.[55,65] The most recent trials have included a reduced dose rt-PA as a short infusion (0.6 mg/kg infused over 15 minutes; maximum dose of 50 mg) compared to the traditional 2-hour infusion of 100 mg. No differences were observed in short-term efficacy or bleeding complications; however, death (5 versus 2) occurred more frequently with the 15-minute low-dose infusion group. Although these alternative delivery modalities are more convenient to administer and potentially less expensive, the frequency of therapeutic efficacy and bleeding complications have not changed compared to traditional dosing recommendations.

Thrombolytic therapy should not be considered as a substitute for anticoagulant therapy. Once thrombolytic therapy is discontinued and the thrombin time or APTT has fallen to less than twice the normal values (usually in 2–4 hours), continuous heparin should be given for 7–14 days.

Laboratory Monitoring/Treatment Guidelines

Laboratory monitoring of thrombolytic therapy is used simply to determine whether some degree of systemic fibrinolysis has been achieved.[66] As long as some degree of lysis is established, vigorous dissolution of clots can be expected, provided that the fibrin clots are fresh. Simple but adequate laboratory monitoring for safe and effective administration of thrombolytic therapy is outlined in Table 19.9.

The two most sensitive tests for fibrinolysis are whole-blood euglobulin lysis time and thrombin time. If they are unavailable, APTT and PT can be used. Whatever test is selected, it should be performed prior to the administration of thrombolytic therapy and 3–4 hours after the initiation of thrombolytic treatment. As long as the test values during thrombolytic infusion are prolonged beyond the control value (except the euglobulin lysis time, which should be shortened), it can be assumed that a systemic lytic state has been established.[10,66]

Treatment guidelines to minimize local and major hemorrhage of patients receiving thrombolytic therapy are summarized in Table 19.10.

TABLE 19.9. LABORATORY MONITORING FOR THROMBOLYTIC THERAPY

Tests
- Whole-blood euglobulin lysis time, or
- Thrombin time, or
- APTT and PT, or
- Fibrin(ogen) degradation products

Time of Testing

Before therapy
- Detect and correct coagulation defects (by means of thrombin time, APTT and PT)
- Determine baseline or control for fibrinolysis (any of the above tests; euglobulin lysis time or fibrin[ogen] degradation products if patient has been receiving heparin)

During therapy (3–4 h after start)
- Use same test(s) used for establishing baseline or control

After therapy
- Use APTT if heparin therapy is to begin

(From Sharma CVRK, Cella G, Parisi AF, Sasahara AA. Thrombolytic therapy. N Engl J Med 1982;306:1271, with permission.)

TABLE 19.10. CLINICAL GUIDELINES FOR PATIENT TREATMENT

1. Minimize physical handling of patient.
2. Discontinue parenteral (subcutaneous, intramuscular) medications.
3. Substitute appropriate oral medications.
4. Minimize invasive procedures, including needle punctures.
5. Apply compression bandages at sites of vessel puncture.
6. Avoid concurrent anticoagulation.
7. Avoid concurrent use of platelet-active drugs, aspirin-containing compounds (erosive), antiplatelet agents, and dextran.

(Adapted from Sharma CVRK, Cella G, Parisi AF, Sasahara AA. Thrombolytic therapy. N Engl J Med 1982;306:1274, with permission.)

Adverse Effects

Hemorrhage, allergy, and fever are the three major types of adverse reactions that have been reported with thrombolytic agents.[53,54,67] The most disturbing and common side effect is bleeding, causing thrombolytic therapy to be discontinued in 5–25% of patients. Thrombolytic therapy is associated with a 6–30% frequency of major bleeding complications in patients treated for DVT; and approximately 20% for patients being treated for PE. The relative risk of major bleeding during thrombolytic therapy is approximately threefold higher than with heparin therapy.

Sharma and Sasahara[68] reported their experience with almost 100 patients who were given thrombolytic agents for PE. Twenty-nine percent had minor oozing, 10% had major bleeding, and 4% required replacement transfusion. No deaths were attributable to bleeding. Their figures are considerably lower than those reported in the two trials sponsored by the NIH.[56,57] They believe that careful attention to local hemostasis, close patient observation, and avoidance of unnecessary invasive procedures were responsible for their low incidence of serious bleeding.

Minor bleeding or oozing at cutaneous puncture sites can be controlled locally with pressure dressings. In cases of serious bleeding, thrombolytic therapy should be quickly discontinued. Because of the very short half-life of these agents, the lytic activity stops promptly. If blood replacement is indicated, whole blood or blood products (packed red cells, fresh-frozen plasma, or cryoprecipitate) may be given and should rapidly reverse the hemostatic alterations. In situations where bleeding unresponsive to blood replacement therapy must be rapidly corrected, ε-aminocaproic acid (EACA) may be administered in 5-g doses.

A recent decision analysis evaluated the preference of patients based on possible outcomes (i.e., postphlebitic syndrome, PE, major bleeding, death) in choosing therapy of streptokinase plus heparin or heparin therapy alone for the treatment of DVT.[69] The preferred choice of all patients evaluated (n = 36) was heparin alone. Patients did not feel that the avoidance of the postphlebitic syndrome with thrombolytic therapy was worth the risk of death. This study emphasizes the need to consider the patient's preference in addition to the risks and benefits of thrombolytic therapy.

Allergic or hypersensitivity reactions associated with streptokinase include urticaria, itching, flushing, nausea, headache, and transient elevation or decrease of systolic blood pressure. Anaphylaxis (1.3–2.5%) has ranged in severity from minor breathing difficulties to bronchospasm, periorbital swelling, or angioneurotic edema. Although urokinase and rt-PA are considered to be nonantigenic, relatively mild allergic reactions have been reported (0.9–4.5%).

With streptokinase, the frequency of temperature increase greater than 1.5°F is 30%, but only 3.5% of patients have temperatures greater than 104°F. Fever, which is more common with streptokinase therapy, can also occur with the administration of rt-PA and urokinase (15%). Both allergic and febrile reactions may be treated with antihistamines at the time of detection, and acetaminophen is very effective for treating temperature increases. Corticosteroids have also been used for the prophylaxis of these adverse reactions.

Hypotension (10–20%) can occur with rapid infusions of streptokinase. Hypotensive reactions have also been reported for high-dose intravenous infusions of urokinase (14–24%) and rt-PA (10–16%). The hypotension can often be prevented by slowing the rate of administration.

Thrombocytopenia has been reported in approximately 10% of patients receiving rt-PA, and therapy should be discontinued if the platelet counts fall below 75,000/mm^3.

SURGICAL THERAPY

Surgical interventions are additional options usually reserved for situations in which anticoagulation and thrombolytic therapy have an absolute contraindication, cannot be safely administered, or have failed.[10] Surgical therapy for acute DVT remains controversial and thrombectomy is reserved for patients with severe limb ischemia (phlegmasia cerulea dolens).[3] Pulmonary embolectomy and venous interruption are the most common procedures considered for PE. The placement of percutaneous transvenous filters (i.e., Greenfield filter) and umbrellas (Mobin–Uddin) have replaced older surgical techniques to prevent recurrence of thromboembolism from the lower extremities. These procedures have replaced the use of caval ligation, a procedure only indicated for severe septic pelvic thrombophlebitis unresponsive to conventional therapy. In life-threatening situations, pulmonary embolectomy (Trendelenburg's procedure) can be considered; however, it is associated with an extremely high mortality rate.

Prevention of Venous Thromboembolism

The key to reducing the morbidity and mortality of venous thromboembolism is the prevention of DVT and subsequent PE.[3] The strategies for preventing DVT are aimed at preventing stasis and reversing coagulability changes, which allow thrombi to form in patients at risk for developing venous thromboembolism. The choice of a particular prophylactic drug or procedure for each patient will depend on the degree of risk of developing thromboembolism and/or bleeding complications from therapy.

Several patient populations have been identified as being at risk for developing DVT or PE and were discussed earlier in this chapter. All medical and surgical patients admitted to the hospital should be evaluated for the presence of these risk factors. Among surgical patients, those having procedures requiring general anesthesia for longer than 30 minutes, periods of prolonged immobility, or procedures involving injury/surgery to the lower extremities or the pelvis are at the highest risk of developing DVT or PE.[2,6] In addition, the period of risk of developing DVT for surgical patients extends from the time of operation to 30 days after surgery.[2] Because the risk for developing DVT or PE is longer than the immediate postoperative period, some patients may require prolonged prophylaxis after hospital discharge. Currently, there is debate as to exactly which patients require prolonged prophylaxis as well as how long they should receive it. It does appear, however, that a high risk for DVT or PE extends for at least 3–5 weeks after orthopedic surgery and that prolonged prophylaxis seems reasonable in these patients.[3,70]

Some general prophylactic guidelines have been developed through careful literature search and evaluation.[3,6] In conclusions made by the National Heart, Lung, and Blood Institute and the NIH Office of Medical Application of Research consensus panel, it was determined that none of the preventive measures is ideal, but most are relatively simple to use, complications are generally minor, and the need for laboratory monitoring is minimal. They also concluded that prophylactic therapy should be tailored to the patient's disease and degree of risk, and should be used more extensively to prevent DVT and PE in high-risk patients.

The prophylactic guidelines in Table 19.11 have been developed based on the age of the patient, his or her underlying risk factors for the development of thromboembolism, underlying characteristics of the patient, and the type of surgery or indication for prophylaxis. In addition, any patient who is at high risk of developing thromboembolism

TABLE 19.11. GUIDELINES FOR PROPHYLAXIS OF THROMBOEMBOLISM

Type of Surgery/Indication	Recommended Prophylaxis
General surgery	
Low-risk (minor surgery, <40 years old, no risk factors)	Early ambulation
Moderate-risk (major surgery, >40 years old, no risk factors)	GCS, LDH (every 12 hours), or IPC
High-risk (major surgery, >40 years old, some risk factors)	LDH (every 8 hours), or LMWH
Above characteristics but prone to wound complications (hematoma)	Above or IPC or dextran
Very high-risk (above with multiple risk factors)	LDH (every 8 hours), LMWH, or dextran with IPC, perioperative warfarin in some
Total hip replacement	Warfarin, LMWH, or dose-adjusted heparin
Hip fracture surgery	Warfarin or LMWH
Knee surgery	IPC (? LMWH)
Multiple trauma patients	IPC, warfarin, or LMWH
High-risk orthopedic and multiple trauma patients, other prophylaxis contraindicated	IVC filter
Neurosurgery, intracranial	IPC and/or GCS
Acute spinal cord injury	Dose-adjusted heparin, LMWH, IPC, or warfarin
Immobile general medicine patients	GCS, IPC, or LDH

Key: GCS, graduated compression stockings; IPC, intermittent pneumatic compression; LDH, low-dose subcutaneous heparin; LMWH, low molecular weight heparin; IVC, inferior vena cava.

should be monitored routinely for signs of DVT and/or PE through the use of careful clinical evaluation as well as objective tests such as impedance plethysmography or Doppler ultrasonography.

Because the pharmacologic agents used to prevent DVT and PE have serious potential side effects, many studies have been performed evaluating nonpharmacologic methods to decrease stasis and the incidence of thromboembolic disease, without the added risk or cost of pharmacologic therapy. Some nonpharmacologic techniques include early ambulation, leg elevation, leg exercises, elastic compression or thromboembolic deterrent stockings, intermittent calf compression, electrical stimulation of calf muscles during surgery, and inferior vena cava (IVC) interruption. Because these methods do not increase the risk of bleeding, they are especially useful in patients at increased risk of bleeding from anticoagulants.

One of the best nonpharmacologic techniques for the prevention of DVT in the postoperative period is early ambulation. However, because this may not be feasible in every patient, other techniques have been employed. Standard elastic compression stockings have a graduated pressure that is highest at the ankle and decreases as it approaches the thigh. These stockings decrease stasis by increasing blood flow to the proximal femoral vein. The stockings should be placed on the patient before surgery and worn until the patient is fully ambulatory. They have been shown to decrease moderately the incidence of DVT in general surgery patients and should not be used as sole prophylaxis in high-risk patients. If used, they must be properly fitted to achieve the greatest benefit of reducing stasis in the legs.

Intermittent pneumatic calf muscle compression employs an inflatable cuff placed around the calf of the patient to increase venous flow to the proximal femoral vein. It is especially useful in a patient who is at high risk of bleeding with heparin and in patients undergoing neurosurgery.[71] This technique prevents stasis by enhancing blood flow in the deep veins of the legs as well as activating the fibrinolytic system. This method is usually initiated at the time of surgery and is continued throughout the entire time of immobilization. Intermittent pneumatic compression has been shown to reduce the frequency of calf vein thrombosis in patients undergoing orthopedic procedures, but should not be considered as a sole prophylactic measure in this high-risk group since it is not as effective in preventing proximal vein thrombosis.[70]

Electrical stimulation of the calf muscles to induce muscle contractions has also been employed as a prophylactic agent and is mostly used during the surgical procedure. It has not gained patient acceptance because of the associated discomfort; therefore, its use is limited.

As mentioned earlier, a Greenfield filter can be placed in the IVC to prevent pulmonary embolism from deep vein thrombi. Inferior vena cava interruption is useful in patients in whom the use of anticoagulant therapy is contraindicated or in those patients who have failed previous anticoagulant therapy.[10] It is important to note that the IVC filter does not prevent the formation of DVT. In patients who received a filter secondary to anticoagulant treatment failure, anticoagulant therapy with heparin followed by warfarin should continue to prevent recurrence or extension of the thrombus in the leg, as well as thrombosis of the filter.

Pharmacologic approaches for prophylaxis for DVT include low-dose heparin, warfarin, dose-adjusted heparin, low molecular weight heparin (LMWH), and dextran.[6] In general, prophylaxis has conclusively been shown to decrease the risk of venous thromboembolism with an acceptably low risk of bleeding. Platelet inhibitors such as aspirin only affect thrombus formation that is dependent on prostaglandins such as thromboxane A_2 and have not been shown to be effective in preventing DVT.

The most widely applicable and carefully studied method of prophylaxis is low-dose heparin. Low doses of heparin given subcutaneously have been shown to be highly effective in reducing the incidence of postoperative DVT and fatal PE in general, abdominal, thoracic, urologic, and some orthopedic surgery patients,[3] bedridden patients after myocardial infarction and stroke, and immobilized medical patients.[3,6,72] A cost–benefit study of low-dose subcutaneous heparin as prophylaxis against postoperative venous thromboembolism has shown it to be cost effective by decreasing postoperative morbidity and mortality.[73] Low-dose heparin also has the added advantage of not requiring any laboratory monitoring. However, this regimen has been shown to be ineffective in preventing DVT in high-risk surgical patients (total hip replacement), so that other methods such as dose-adjusted heparin, LMWH, or warfarin should be employed.[3,6,74]

Low-dose heparin therapy involves the administration of 5000 U subcutaneously every 8–12 hours. The every-8-hours regimen (15,000 U/d) has not been shown to be more effective than the every-12-hours regimen and may be associated with a slightly higher rate of bleeding episodes. When heparin is used for prophylaxis in surgery patients, the heparin should be started 2 hours before the surgical procedure and then every 12 hours thereafter.

Dose-adjusted heparin therapy has also been used in high-risk patients in whom low-dose heparin is not effective or has limited effectiveness (i.e., hip surgery patients).[3,70] The heparin dose is adjusted to maintain the APTT in the high-normal range (i.e., 31.5–36 seconds). The APTT should be drawn 4–6 hours after the first dose, and at the midpoint of the dosing interval thereafter. Average daily doses are 15,000 to 17,500 U, and the dose is usually administered subcutaneously every 12 hours.

Warfarin has been used for the prophylaxis of DVT after major gynecologic, orthopedic (including joint replacement and hip fracture patients), thoracic, and abdominal surgeries.[2,3,6,75] It can be administered as either a fixed low dose (1–2 mg daily) or a dose adjusted to slightly prolong the prothrombin time (INR of 2–2.5; for hip surgery, INR of 2–3). Both methods usually require preoperative treatment and repeated laboratory monitoring. Although the risk of bleeding appears to be less than full anticoagulation, hemorrhagic episodes still occur so that warfarin is usually reserved for high-risk patients (previous thromboembolism, major orthopedic surgery).

Dextran is a partially hydrolyzed glucose polymer that has several antithrombotic effects, but most notably impairs platelet function and decreases their ability to aggregate.[6,72,75] It has shown limited efficacy as DVT prophylaxis in general surgery and hip surgery patients, and appears to be used only occasionally in patients who cannot receive heparin due to adverse effects or bleeding. In addition, several drawbacks have limited the use of dextran as a prophylactic agent such as (1) intravenous administration; (2) the risks of fluid overload, bleeding, and allergic reactions; and (3) cost.

LMWHs belong to a class of anticoagulants termed glycosaminoglycans to which standard heparin also belongs. LMWHs are derived from unfractionated heparin by various manufacturing methods to elaborate compounds with smaller, more standard average masses than unfractionated heparin, which is very heterogeneous.[76] Like unfractionated heparin, LMWHs bind to antithrombin III and produce a conformational change to expedite the natural function of antithrombin III. However, unlike standard heparin, LMWHs are less able to inhibit thrombin formation and exhibit a preferential inhibitory effect on factor Xa, with fewer effects on platelet activity.[76] It is thought that these characteristics should cause bleeding less often, while still retaining anticoagulant effects. Other favorable properties of LMWHs over standard heparin include greater bioavailability after subcutaneous administration, a longer duration of anti–factor Xa activity, linear pharmacokinetics, possibly fewer adverse effects, and lack of required routine laboratory monitoring (i.e., APTT).

Data from clinical trials have also suggested efficacy of LMWHs in terms of DVT prevention in general surgery, total knee replacement surgery, and abdominal surgery patients.[3,10,74,77–97] Several authors have evaluated the use of LMWHs as prophylaxis against DVT by meta-analysis for patients undergoing orthopedic[86–88] or general surgery.[87–97] In orthopedic surgery, LMWH significantly decreases the incidence of DVT over placebo in elective hip or knee replacement, tibial osteotomy, or femoral neck fracture repair patients[74]; and it significantly decreases the incidence of proximal vein thrombosis over standard heparin in total hip replacement patients.[86] A nonsignificant decrease in the mean incidence of DVT with LMWH was also seen when compared to (1) placebo and standard heparin in elective and acute hip surgery patients,[88] (2) standard heparin in elective hip replacement patients,[79,85] and (3) dextran in elective hip surgery patients.[88]

In general surgery patients, LMWH appears to be more effective at preventing DVT than placebo[88,89] or standard

TABLE 19.12. CLINICAL TRIALS EVALUATING THE EFFICACY OF ENOXAPARIN AS DVT PROPHYLAXIS

Reference	Type of Surgery	Regimens Compared	Number of Patients	Outcome (%)		Bleeding (%)		Comments
				DVT	PVT	Major	Minor	
77	Elective hip surgery	Enoxaparin 30 mg SubQ bid	50	12	4	2	2	• Therapy started 12–24 hours after surgery, continued until 14 days or until discharge
		Placebo	50	42[a]	20[b]	4		• No difference in transfusions
78	Tibial osteotomy or knee arthroplasty	Enoxaparin 30 mg SubQ bid	65	17	0	0	6	• Therapy started 12–24 hours after surgery, continued for 14 days or until discharge
		Placebo	64	58[c]	19[d]	2	6	• Enoxaparin more effective in knee arthroplasty
79	Elective hip replacement	Enoxaparin 10 mg SubQ qd	116 (A)	31	15	2.5	4.3	• Therapy started no later than postop day 1 and continued for 7 days
		Enoxapirin 40 mg SubQ qd	149 (B)	14	6	4.7	9.4	• DVT higher in group A vs B ($p = 0.003$) and C ($p = 0.002$)
		Enoxapirin 30 mg SubQ bid	143 (C)	11	6	7.7	11.2	• Two cases of PE in group B
80	Elective hip replacement	Enoxaparin 30 mg SubQ bid	333	17.1	4.8	3.3	1.8	• Therapy started 12–24 hours after surgery, continued for 14 days or until discharge
		Heparin 7500 U SubQ bid	332	19	5.4	5.7	3.6	• Two episodes each of PE and thrombocytopenia in heparin group • 42% risk reduction of bleeding in enoxaparin group
81	Elective hip replacement	Enoxaparin 40 mg SubQ qd	124	12.5	7.5	1.6	0.8	• Enoxaparin started 12 hours before surgery; heparin started 2 hours before surgery; both therapies continued for 12–15 days postop
		Heparin 5000 U SubQ tid	113	25[e]	18.5[f]		1.7	
82	Elective hip replacement	Enoxaparin 30 mg SubQ bid	194	2	2	4	8	• Therapy started within 24 hours postop and continued for 7 days
		Enoxaparin 40 mg SubQ qd	203	10	4	1	9	• PE in 4 heparin-treated patients
		Heparin 5000 U SubQ q8h	207	5	5	6	6	• Thrombocytopenia in 4% and 1% of patients who received enoxaparin 30 mg bid and 40 mg qd, respectively, and 2% of heparin-treated patients

83	Elective hip or knee implantation	Enoxaparin 75 U of factor Xa in U/kg SubQ qd	715	31.4	6.1		2.8	1.4	• Enoxaparin started 18–24 hours after surgery, both therapies continued for 14 days or until discharge
		Warfarin 10 mg day 1, then adjusted to INR of 2–3	721	37.4[g]	7.6		1.2[h]	1.9	• Increased rate of DVT and decreased hematoma rate in warfarin group • One patient in each group developed a PE
84	Elective hip replacement	Enoxaparin 40 mg SubQ qd	108	4.6	1.8			12.9	• Enoxaparin started 12 hours pre-op and continued for 7 days postop
		Dextran 60 mg/mL; 500 mL intraop, then 4–6 hours later, then days 1 and 3 postop	111	16.2	5.4			23.4	• If patient immobile, a fifth dose of dextran given on day 5 • Overall difference in phlebographic DVT was significant between the groups ($p = 0.013$) • Postop blood loss and transfusions were higher in dextran group
85	General surgery	Enoxaparin 60 mg SubQ qd	157	2.9					• Heparin therapy started 2 hours before surgery and then given 5000 U q8h SubQ for 7 days • Enoxaparin started 2 hours before surgery and given daily for 7 days • Patients included abdominal, gynecologic, urologic, and thoracic surgery patients
		Heparin	147	3.8					
		Enoxaparin 40 mg SubQ qd	124	2.8					
		Heparin	123	2.7					
		Enoxaparin 20 mg SubQ qd	167	3.8					
		Heparin	167	7.6					

Key: DVT, deep-vein thrombosis; PVT, proximal vein thrombosis; SubQ, subcutaneous administration; bid, twice daily; qd, once daily; U, units; PE, pulmonary embolism.

[a] $p = 0.0007$.
[b] $p = 0.014$.
[c] $p < 0.0001$.
[d] $p < 0.001$.
[e] $p = 0.03$.
[f] $p = 0.014$.
[g] $p = 0.03$.
[h] $p = 0.04$.

heparin.[87,88,97] An overall decrease in fatal PE has also been shown over standard heparin.[87] Overall, there was no significant difference in the rates of total, major, or minor bleeding.[86,87,92,94,96,97]

LMWHs have also proven effective in the treatment of DVT,[98,99] but are not currently FDA approved for this indication.

ENOXAPARIN

Enoxaparin (Lovenox, Rhone Poulenc Rorer) was the first LMWH to become commercially available in the United States. Currently, the only FDA-approved indication of enoxaparin is for the prevention of DVT following hip or knee replacement surgery.

Enoxaparin is derived from standard heparin by benzylation and alkaline depolymerization, and has an average mass of 3500–5000 Da. Following subcutaneous administration, the bioavailability is 91% and is linear within the dosage range of 20–80 mg.[90] The time to maximal anti–factor Xa activity is 3–5 hours after subcutaneous injection. The volume of distribution of enoxaparin in healthy volunteers is approximately 7 liters. In animals, the drug appears to accumulate in the liver, kidney, and spleen. Enoxaparin is excreted primarily as unchanged drug in the urine, mainly by glomerular filtration.[90] Following subcutaneous administration, the elimination half-life of enoxaparin is 4.5 hours and may be prolonged as much as twofold in patients with renal failure.[90]

One of the purposes of developing LMWHs was to maintain antithrombotic activity while decreasing the bleeding and thrombocytopenia that may occur during heparin therapy. However, the most common adverse effects of enoxaparin therapy are also bleeding and thrombocytopenia. Unfortunately, a decreased frequency of bleeding has not been convincingly shown in clinical trials, with a frequency as high as 4% being reported in one trial.[7] Bleeding episodes have been partially controlled with the administration of protamine sulfate.

The incidence of thrombocytopenia with enoxaparin therapy is less than 2%.[99,100] Because heparin-induced thrombocytopenia may be an immunogenic response to the secondary or tertiary structures of standard heparin, LMWHs may also produce this effect (but at a lower incidence). There are cases of both successful and unsuccessful use of enoxaparin in patients with heparin-induced thrombocytopenia. Other adverse effects with enoxaparin include elevations in serum transaminase levels, urticaria and pain, local irritation, and hematoma at the site of injection.

Numerous studies have evaluated enoxaparin for the prevention of DVT following orthopedic, general, gynecologic, urologic, and thoracic surgery (Table 19.12, see pages 426–427). When compared with placebo for elective hip replacement or knee arthroplasty, enoxaparin significantly decreased the incidence of both DVT and proximal vein thrombosis, without an increase in the incidence of adverse effects.[77,78] Trials comparing enoxaparin with heparin (each at varying doses) for the prevention of DVT have been conducted in patients undergoing elective hip replacement, abdominal, gynecologic, urologic, or thoracic surgery. An overall trend at preventing DVT was noted in favor of enoxaparin in all studies reviewed,[80–82,85] with one trial exhibiting a significant decrease in the rate of DVT and proximal vein thrombosis in elective hip replacement patients who received enoxaparin.[81] The frequency of major or minor bleeding and thrombocytopenia was not significantly different between the two groups.

When comparing enoxaparin with warfarin as prophylaxis in patients undergoing hip or knee replacement, a significant decrease in the incidence of DVT was noted with enoxaparin in knee replacement patients and with combined analysis (hip and knee replacement patients).[83] The incidence of DVT and proximal vein thrombosis was lower in hip replacement and knee replacement patients, respectively, who received enoxaparin, but this difference was not statistically significant. In addition, the incidence of major bleeding overall was significantly higher in the enoxaparin group.

Enoxaparin has been compared with dextran for the prophylaxis of DVT in hip replacement patients.[84] The overall difference in the incidence of DVT was significantly lower in the enoxaparin group. In addition, the amount of postoperative blood loss and number of transfusions were higher in the patients who received dextran.

In conclusion, although enoxaparin is currently only FDA-approved for prophylaxis of DVT in patients undergoing hip or knee replacement surgery, it appears to be effective prophylaxis in other surgical patients. It does not, however, appear to decrease significantly the risk of bleeding.

DALTEPARIN

Dalteparin (Fragmin, Pharmacia) has recently been approved by the FDA for the prevention of DVT in patients undergoing abdominal surgery who are at risk for thromboembolic complications.

Dalteparin is derived from standard heparin by nitrous acid depolymerization and has an average molecular weight of 5000 Da. After subcutaneous administration, dalteparin is almost completely absorbed with a bioavailability of 87%. Peak plasma anti–factor Xa activity occurs approximately 4 hours after subcutaneous injection. The volume of distribution ranges 40–60 mL/kg in healthy volunteers and seems to correlate with plasma volume. Dalteparin is excreted by primarily renal routes. Following subcutaneous administration, the average elimination half-life is 3.5 hours, which increases to 5.7 hours in patients with chronic renal insufficiency requiring dialysis.

Reported adverse effects with dalteparin therapy include hemorrhage, thrombocytopenia, hematoma, and pain at the site of injection. As with enoxaparin, a significant decrease in bleeding complications has not been definitely established with dalteparin as compared to standard heparin therapy. Hemorrhagic complications may be controlled by using slow infusions of protamine sulfate (1 mg of protamine for every 100 anti–factor Xa units of dalteparin given).

During clinical trials with dalteparin, the incidence of thrombocytopenia was less than 1%. Because heparin-induced thrombocytopenia may be due to an immunogenic response, extreme caution should be exercised when using dalteparin in these patients because LMWHs may also produce this effect. Other adverse effects associated with dalteparin therapy include pain and hematoma formation at the site of injection, allergic reactions, skin necrosis, and elevated transaminases.

There have been numerous prospective studies evaluating dalteparin for the prevention of DVT and PE in patients undergoing abdominal surgery. These studies are listed in Table 19.13. When compared to placebo,[89] dalteparin was significantly more effective in preventing the development of DVT. It also decreased the incidence of PE and displayed an insignificant increase in bleeding episodes. Once-daily dalteparin produced effects similar to that of twice-daily dalteparin, with a trend toward decreased bleeding episodes in the group given dalteparin once daily.[90] In studies using higher than recommended doses of dalteparin (5000–7500 IU/d),[92,93,97] similar efficacy in preventing thromboembolism was reported with significantly increased hemorrhagic complications noted in three studies[91,92,97] when compared to conventional heparin therapy. When dalteparin was used at the current recommended dosage (2500 IU daily),[94–96] comparable efficacy and toxicity to standard heparin therapy was noted.

Dalteparin (5000 IU/d) has also been compared to placebo and heparin as prophylaxis against thromboembolism in patients undergoing other surgical procedures such as total hip replacement and hip fracture surgery.[74] Studies have shown various results with a trend toward decreasing the incidence of DVT (significantly in several studies). One study demonstrated the use of more transfusions in the dalteparin-treated group when compared to those who received heparin, but no significant difference was noted in terms of operative blood loss, wound drain loss, or hemoglobin level. In addition, a significant decrease in the incidence of DVT was noted in acute stroke patients who received dalteparin prophylaxis when compared to placebo,[74] but the patients also experienced more bleeding episodes. Dalteparin has also been evaluated in several studies for the treatment of DVT with promising results. Results of these studies seem promising; however, further studies are needed before routine use in these areas can be recommended.

Evaluation of Therapeutic Outcomes

Venous thromboembolism is a potentially fatal disorder that employs either prophylactic therapy to prevent high-risk patients from developing a DVT or PE, or treatment of an existing thrombus. The overall pharmaceutical care plan, which includes the therapeutic goals, choice of a particular agent, and monitoring parameters, differs depending on whether prophylactic therapy or treatment against DVT or PE is being employed.

Because DVT and PE are potentially preventable diseases, health care professionals (including pharmacists) can play a major role in identifying which patients are at risk for developing venous thromboembolism, deciding which prophylactic modality would be most suitable based on the patient's degree of risk of developing DVT or PE and the potential for adverse effects from the therapy, and monitoring the patient for signs of DVT, PE, or adverse drug effects.

The therapeutic goals in the treatment of DVT or PE include (1) inhibiting the growth of the thrombus or embolus, (2) preventing recurrent embolic episodes, (3) restoring normal hemodynamics and oxygenation in the case of PE, and (4) minimizing the symptoms of the postphlebitic syndrome. The choice of a particular therapeutic agent will depend on the urgency of the case; the presence of contraindications to anticoagulants or thrombolytics; the relative safety, efficacy, and cost of the treatment; and the availability of resources necessary to carry out the treatment. Patients in this group should not only be monitored for adverse effects from treatment, but also for the resolution of symptoms, the development of recurrent thrombosis, and symptoms of the postphlebitic syndrome.

Conclusion

Venous thromboembolism continues to be the target of intensive clinical research. The disorder is an important source of morbidity and mortality owing to complicating pulmonary embolism in patients on both medical and surgical wards. A major problem in the care of these patients has always been diagnosis. Many patients are asymptomatic, and both false-positive and false-negative diagnoses are common. Significant progress has been made in recent years in diagnostic procedures, identification of high-risk groups, and therapeutic management, although studies are needed to better define the role of thrombolytic therapy in acute DVT and PE. Most clinicians agree, however, that management of venous thromboembolism is ideally achieved through prophylactic approaches rather than by allowing thromboembolism to occur.

TABLE 19.13. CLINICAL TRIALS EVALUATING THE EFFICACY OF DALTEPARIN PROPHYLAXIS IN PATIENTS UNDERGOING ABDOMINAL SURGERY

Reference	Regimens Compared	Number of Patients	Outcome (%)		Bleeding (%)		Comments
			DVT	PE	Major	Minor	
89	Dalteparin 2500 IU SubQ qd	95	4.2	0	4.2	6.3	• Therapy started 1–2 hours preop, and for 5–10 days postop
	Placebo	88	15.9	2.2	4.5	0	• Local injection site reaction in two dalteparin-treated patients
90	Dalteparin 2500 IU SubQ bid	112	2.6	0	8.9		• First dose given 1–2 hours preop, and for at least 7 days postop
	Dalteparin 2500 IU SubQ qd	94	7.4	1	4.2		• Difference between incidence of DVT and bleeding was insignificant
91	Dalteparin 5000 IU SubQ qd Heparin 5000 IU SubQ bid	190 192	6.8 4.6	0 0.5	11.6 4.6		• Therapy started 2 hours preop, and for 5–7 days postop • Bleeding % reported is overall % • More patients in dalteparin group had bleeding complications ($p = 0.047$) and required transfusions ($p = 0.02$)
92	Dalteparin 7500 IU SubQ qd	23	0		47		• First dose given 1 hour preop, and for at least 5 days postop
	Heparin 5000 IU SubQ bid	20	0		10		• Study prematurely stopped because of excessive bleeding complications
	Dalteparin 2500 IU SubQ qd Heparin 5000 IU SubQ bid	70 68	2.86 2.94	 1.47	14.9 15.3		• Bleeding % reported is overall % • In second study, patients in heparin group required more transfusions
93	Dalteparin 5000 IU SubQ qd	25	8	0	4		• Therapy started 2 hours preop and continued for 6 days postop
	Heparin 5000 IU SubQ bid	27	7.4	0	7.4		• Transfusion requirements similar in the 2 groups
94	Dalteparin 2500 IU SubQ qd Heparin 5000 IU SubQ bid	1894 1915	0.6 0.6	0.7 0.7	3.6 4.8	6.2 7.9	• Therapy started 1–4 hours preop and continued for at least 5 days postop • Incidence of injection site bruising was higher in heparin group ($p = 0.001$)
95	Dalteparin 2500 IU SubQ qd Heparin 5000 IU SubQ bid	190 195	3.1 3.7	0 0.5			• Therapy started 2 hours preop and continued for 7 days postop • Incidence of wound hematoma was 1.6% in dalteparin group and 2.1% in heparin group • Fall in hemoglobin levels was not significant between the 2 groups
97	Dalteparin 2500 IU SubQ qd Heparin 5000 IU SubQ bid	112 115	8 7.8	0.9 0.86	3.6 3.5		• Therapy started 2 hours preop and continued for 7 days postop • Bleeding % reported is overall % • Heparin group required significantly more transfusions
98	Dalteparin 5000 IU SubQ qd Heparin 5000 IU SubQ bid	405 421	5 9.2	0 1.2		6.7 2.7	• Dalteparin started the evening before surgery, heparin started 2 hours preop, both continued for 5–8 days postop • Significant difference in DVT incidence ($p = 0.02$)

Key: DVT, deep vein thrombosis; PE, pulmonary embolism; SubQ, subcutaneous administration; bid, twice daily; qd, once daily; IU, international units.

REFERENCES

1. Moser KM. Venous thromboembolism. Am Rev Resp Dis 1990;141:235–249.
2. Goldhaber SZ, Morpurgo M. Diagnosis, treatment, and prevention of pulmonary embolism. JAMA 1992;268:1727–1733.
3. Weinmann EE, Salzman EW. Deep-vein thrombosis. N Engl J Med 1994;331:1630–1641.
4. Dahlback B. Inherited thrombophilia: Resistance to activated protein C as a pathogenic factor of venous thromboembolism. Blood 1995;85:607–614.
5. Broze GJ. The role of tissue factor pathway inhibitor in a revised coagulation cascade. Semin Hematol 1992;29:159–169.
6. Clagett GP, Anderson FA, Levine MN, et al. Prevention of venous thromboembolism. Chest 1992;102(suppl):391S–407S.
7. Bounameaux H, Cirafici P, de Moerloose P, et al. Measurement of D-dimer in plasma as diagnostic aid in suspected pulmonary embolism. Lancet 1991;1:196–200.
8. Hull RD, Raskob GE, Coates G, Panju AA. Clinical validity of a normal perfusion lung scan in patients with suspected pulmonary embolism. Chest 1990;97:23–26.
9. PIOPED Investigators. Value of the ventilation/perfusion scan in acute pulmonary embolism: Results of the prospective investigation of pulmonary embolism diagnosis (PIOPED). JAMA 1990;263:2753–2759.
10. Hyers TM, Hull RD, Weg JG. Antithrombotic therapy for venous thromboembolis disease. Chest 1992;102(suppl):408S–425S.
11. Hirsh J, Fuster V. Guide to anticoagulant therapy part 1: Heparin. Circulation 1994;89:1449–1468.
12. Cipolle RJ, Rodvold KA. Heparin, in Evans WE, Schentag JJ, Jusko WJ (eds): Applied Pharmacokinetics, Principles of Therapeutic Drug Monitoring, 3rd ed. Vancouver, WA, Applied Therapeutics, 1992, pp 30:1–39.
13. White TM, Bernene JL, Marino AM. Continuous heparin infusion requirements: Diagnostic and therapeutic implications. JAMA 1979;241:2717–2720.
14. Cipolle RJ, Seifert RD, Neilan BA, et al. Heparin kinetics: Variables related to disposition and dosage. Clin Pharmacol Ther 1981;29:387–393.
15. Ginsberg JS, Hirsh J. Use of anticoagulants during pregnancy. Chest 1992;102(suppl):385S–390S.
16. Barritt DW, Jordan SC. Anticoagulant drugs in the treatment of pulmonary embolism: A controlled trial. Lancet 1960;1:1309–1312.
17. Basu D, Gallus A, Hirsh J, Cade J. A prospective study of the value of monitoring heparin treatment with the activated partial thromboplastin time. N Engl J Med 1972;287:324–327.
18. Wilson JE, Bynum LJ, Parkey RW. Heparin therapy in venous thromboembolism. Am J Med 1981;70:808–816.
19. Raschke RA, Reilly BM, Guidry JR, et al. The weight-based heparin dosing nomogram compared with a "standard care" nomogram: A randomized controlled trial. Ann Intern Med 1993;119:874–881.
20. Hommes DW, Bura A, Mazzolai L, et al. Subcutaneous heparin compared with continuous intravenous heparin administration in the initial treatment of deep vein thrombosis: A meta-analysis. Ann Intern Med 1992;116:279–284.
21. Hull RD, Raskob GE, Rosenbloom D, et al. Optimal therapeutic level of heparin therapy in patients with venous thrombosis. Arch Intern Med 1992;152:1589–1595.
22. Wheeler AP, Jaquiss RDB, Newman JH. Physician practices in the treatment of pulmonary embolism and deep venous thrombosis. Arch Intern Med 1988;148:1321–1325.
23. Hull RD, Raskob GE, Rosenbloom D, et al. Heparin for 5 days as compared with 10 days in the initial treatment of proximal venous thrombosis. N Engl J Med 1990;322:1260–1264.
24. Gallus A, Tillett J, Jackaman J, et al. Safety and efficacy of warfarin started early after submassive venous thrombosis or pulmonary embolism. Lancet 1986;2:1293–1296.
25. Mohiuddin SM, Hilleman DE, Destache CJ, et al. Efficacy and safety of early versus late initiation of warfarin during heparin therapy in acute thromboembolism. Am Heart J 1992;123:729–732.
26. Hattersley PG, Mitsouka JC, King JG. Sources of error in heparin therapy. Arch Intern Med 1980;140:1173–1175.
27. Walker AM, Jick H. Predictors of bleeding during heparin therapy. JAMA 1980;244:1209–1212.
28. Breddin HK, Radziwon P, Bocakowska-Radziwon B. Laboratory monitoring of new antithrombotic drugs. Clin Lab Med 1994;14:825–846.
29. Brill-Edwards P, Ginsberg JS, Johnston M, Hirsh J. Establishing a therapeutic range for heparin therapy. Ann Intern Med 1993;119:104–109.
30. Levine MN, Hirsh J, Gent M, et al. A randomized trial comparing activated thromboplastin time with heparin assay in patients with acute venous thromboembolism requiring large daily doses of heparin. Arch Intern Med 1994;154:49–56.
31. Levine MN, Hirsh J, Landefeld S, Raskob G. Hemorrhagic complications of anticoagulant treatment. Chest 1992;102(suppl):352S–63S.
32. Landefeld CS, Cook EF, Flatley M, et al. Identification and preliminary validation of predictors of major bleeding in hospitalized patients starting anticoagulant therapy. Am J Med 1987;82:703–713.
33. Landefeld CS, Beyth RJ. Anticoagulant-related bleeding: Clinical epidemiology, prediction, and prevention. Am J Med 1993;95:315–328.
34. Conti S, Daschbach M, Blaisdell FW. A comparison of high-dose versus conventional-dose heparin therapy for deep vein thrombosis. Surgery 1982;92:972–980.
35. Mant MJ, O'Brien BD, Thong KL, et al. Haemorrhagic complications of heparin therapy. Lancet 1977;1:1133–1135.
36. Schmitt BP, Adelman B. Heparin-associated thrombocytopenia: A critical review and pooled analysis. Am J Med Sci 1993;305:208–215.
37. Ramirez-Lassepas M, Cipolle RJ, Rodvold KA, et al. Heparin-induced thrombocytopenia in patients with cerebrovascular ischemic disease. Neurology 1984;34:736–740.

38. Hirsh J, Dalen JE, Deykin D, Poller L. Oral anticoagulants: Mechanism of action, clinical effectiveness, and optimal therapeutic range. Chest 1992;102(suppl):312S–326S.
39. Hirsh J, Fuster V. Guide to anticoagulant therapy part 2: Oral anticoagulants. Circulation 1994;89:1469–1480.
40. Ansell JE. Oral anticoagulant therapy: 50 years later. Arch Intern Med 1993;153:586–596.
41. Porter RS, Sawyer WT. Warfarin, in Evans WE, Schentag JJ, Jusko WJ (eds): Applied Pharmacokinetics, Principles of Therapeutic Drug Monitoring, 3rd ed. Vancouver, WA, Applied Therapeutics, 1992, pp 31:1–46.
42. Schulman S, Rhedin AS, Lindmarker P, et al. A comparison of six weeks with six months of oral anticoagulant therapy after a first episode of venous thromboembolism. N Engl J Med 1995;332:1661–1665.
43. Landefeld CS, Goldman L. Major bleeding in outpatients treated with warfarin: Incidence and prediction by factors known at start of outpatient therapy. Am J Med 1989;87:144–152.
44. Landefeld CS, Rosenblatt MW, Goldman L. Bleeding in outpatients treated with warfarin: Relation to the prothrombin time and important remediable lesions. Am J Med 1989;87:153–159.
45. Hirsh J, Poller L. The international normalized ratio: A guide to understanding and correcting its problems. Arch Intern Med 1994;154:282–288.
46. Bussey HI, Force RW, Bianco TM, Leonard AD. Reliance on prothrombin time ratios causes significant errors in anticoagulation therapy. Arch Intern Med 1992;152:278–282.
47. Fredriks DA, Coleman RW. Nomogram for dosing warfarin at steady-state. Clin Pharm 1991;10:923–927.
48. White RH, Mungall D. Outpatient management of warfarin therapy: Comparison of computer-predicted dosage adjustment to skilled professional care. Ther Drug Monitor 1991;13:46–50.
49. Landefeld CS, Anderson PA. Guideline-based consultation to prevent anticoagulant-related bleeding: A randomized, controlled trial in a teaching hospital. Ann Intern Med 1992;116:829–837.
50. Ellis RF, Stephens MA, Sharp GB. Evaluation of a pharmacy-managed warfarin-monitoring service to coordinate inpatient and outpatient therapy. Am J Hosp Pharm 1992;49:387–394.
51. Eby CS. Warfarin-induced skin necrosis. Hematol Oncol Clin N Am 1993;7:1291–1300.
52. Wells PS, Holbrook AM, Crowther NR, Hirsh J. Interactions of warfarin with drugs and food. Ann Intern Med 1994;121:676–683.
53. Sasahara AA, St. Martin CC, Henkin J, Barker WM. Approach to the patient with venous thromboembolism. Hematol Oncol Clin N Am 1992;6:1141–1159.
54. Francis CW, Marder VJ. Fibrinolytic therapy for venous thrombosis. Prog Cardiovasc Dis 1991;34:193–204.
55. Goldhaber SZ. Contemporary pulmonary embolism thrombolysis. Chest 1995;107(suppl):45S–51S.
56. A Cooperative Study. Urokinase-pulmonary embolism trial phase I results. JAMA 1970;214:2163–2172.
57. A Cooperative Study. Urokinase-streptokinase embolism trial phase 2 results. JAMA 1974;229:1606–1613.
58. Sharma GVRK, Burleson VA, Sasahara AA. Effect of thrombolytic therapy on pulmonary-capillary blood volume in patients with pulmonary embolism. N Engl J Med 1980;303:842–845.
59. Goldhaber SZ, Haire WD, Feldstein ML, et al. Alteplase versus heparin in acute pulmonary embolism: Randomized trial assessing right-ventricular function and pulmonary perfusion. Lancet 1993;341:507–511.
60. Dalla-Volta S, Palla A, Santolicandro A, et al. PAIMS 2: Alteplase combined with heparin versus heparin in the treatment of acute pulmonary embolism. Plasminogen activator Italian multicenter study 2. J Am Coll Cardiol 1992;20:520–526.
61. Rogers LQ, Lutcher CL. Streptokinase therapy for deep vein thrombosis: A comprehensive review of the English literature. Am J Med 1990;88:389–395.
62. Goldhaber SZ, Meyerovitz MF, Green D, et al. Randomized controlled trial of tissue plasminogen activator in proximal deep venous thrombosis. Am J Med 1990;88:235–240.
63. Thery C, Bauchart JJ, Lesenne, et al. Predictive factors of effectiveness of streptokinase in deep venous thrombosis. Am J Cardiol 1992;69:117–122.
64. Turpie AGG, Levine MN, Hirsh J, et al. Tissue plasminogen activator (rt-PA) vs heparin in deep vein thrombosis: Results of a randomized trial. Chest 1990;97(suppl):172S–175S.
65. Goldhaber SZ, Feldstein ML, Sors H. Two trials of reduced bolus alteplase in the treatment of pulmonary embolism: An overview. Chest 1994;106:725–726.
66. Bell WR. Laboratory monitoring of thrombolytic therapy. Clin Lab Med 1995;15:165–178.
67. Levine MN, Goldhaber SZ, Califf RM, et al. Hemorrhagic complications of thrombolytic therapy in the treatment of myocardial infarction and venous thromboembolism. Chest 1992;102(suppl):364S–373S.
68. Sharma GVRK, Sasahara AA. Thrombolytic therapy [letter]. N Engl J Med 1981;304:361.
69. O'Meara JJ, McNutt RA, Evans AT, et al. A decision analysis of streptokinase plus heparin as compared with heparin alone for deep-vein thrombosis. N Engl J Med 1994;330:1864–1869.
70. Merli GJ. Deep vein thrombosis and pulmonary embolism prophylaxis in orthopedic surgery. Med Clin N Am 1993;77:397–411.
71. Turpie AG, Hirsh J, Gent M, et al. Prevention of deep vein thrombosis in potential neurosurgical patients. Arch Intern Med 1989;149:679–681.
72. Collins R, Scrimgeour A, Yusuf S, Peto R. Reduction in fatal pulmonary embolism and venous thrombosis by perioperative administration of subcutaneous heparin: Overview of results of randomized trials in general, orthopedic, and urologic surgery. N Engl J Med 1988;318:1162–1172.
73. Hauch O, Khattar SC, Jorgensen LN. Cost–benefit analysis of prophylaxis against deep vein thrombosis in surgery. Semin Thromb Hemost 1991;17:280–283.
74. Green D, Hirsh J, Heit J, et al. Low molecular weight heparin: A critical analysis of clinical trials. Pharmacol Rev 1994;46:89–109.

75. Thromboembolic Risk Factors (THRIFT) Consensus Group. Risk of and prophylaxis for thromboembolism in hospital patients. Br Med J 1992;305:567–574.
76. Verstraete M. Pharmacotherapeutic aspects of unfractioned and low molecular weight heparin. Drugs 1990;40:498–530.
77. Turpie AG, Levine MN, Hirsh J, et al. A randomized controlled trial of a low-molecular-weight heparin (enoxaparin) to prevent deep-vein thrombosis in patients undergoing elective hip surgery. N Engl J Med 1986;315:925–929.
78. Leclerc JR, Geerts WH, Desjardins L, et al. Prevention of deep vein thrombosis after major knee surgery: A randomized double-blind trial comparing a low-molecular weight heparin fragment to placebo. Haemost 1992;67:417–423.
79. Spiro TE, Johnson GJ, Christie MJ, et al. Efficacy and safety of enoxaparin to prevent deep venous thrombosis after hip replacement surgery. Enoxaparin Clinical Trial Group. Ann Intern Med 1994;121:81–89.
80. Levine MN, Hirsh J, Gent M, et al. Prevention of deep vein thrombosis after elective hip surgery. Ann Intern Med 1991;114:545–551.
81. Planes A, Vochelle N, Fagola M, et al. Efficacy and safety of a perioperative enoxaparin regimen in total hip replacement under various anesthesia. Am J Surg 1991;161:525–531.
82. Colwell CW, Spiro TE, Trowbridge AA, et al. Use of enoxaparin, a low-molecular weight heparin, and unfractionated heparin for the prevention of deep venous thrombosis after elective hip replacement. J Bone Joint Surg 1994;76:3–14.
83. Hull R, Raskob G, Pineo G, et al. A comparison of subcutaneous low-molecular weight heparin with warfarin sodium for prophylaxis against deep-vein thrombosis after hip or knee implantation. N Engl J Med 1993;329:1370–1376.
84. Borris LC and The Danish Enoxaparin Study Group. Low-molecular-weight heparin (enoxaparin) vs. Dextran 70. Arch Intern Med 1991;151:1621–1624.
85. Combe S, Samama MM. Prevention of thromboembolic disease in general surgery with clexane (enoxaparin). Semin Thromb Hemost 1991;17:291–295.
86. Anderson DR, O'Brien BJ, Levine MN, et al. Efficacy and cost of low-molecular weight heparin compared with standard heparin for the prevention of deep vein thrombosis after total hip arthroplasty. Ann Intern Med 1993;119:1105–1112.
87. Nurmohamed MT, Rosendaal FR, Buller HR, et al. Low-molecular weight heparin versus standard heparin in general and orthopaedic surgery: A meta-analysis. Lancet 1992;340:152–156.
88. Lassen MR, Borris LC, Christiansen HM, et al. Clinical trials with low molecular weight heparins in the prevention of postoperative thromboembolic complications: A meta-analysis. Semin Thromb Hemost 1991;17:284–290.
89. Ockelford PA, Patterson J, Johns AS. A double-blind randomized placebo controlled trial of thromboprophylaxis in major elective general surgery using once daily injections of a low molecular weight heparin fragment (Fragmin). Thromb Haemost 1989;62:1046–1049.
90. Kakkar VV, Kakkar S, Sanderson RM, Peers CE. Efficacy and safety of two regimens of low molecular weight heparin fragment (Fragmin) in preventing postoperative venous thromboembolism. Haemostasis 1986;16(suppl 2):19–24.
91. Bergqvist D, Burmark US, Frisell J, et al. Prospective double blind comparison between Fragmin and conventional low-dose heparin: Thromboprophylactic effect and bleeding complications. Haemostasis 1986;16(suppl 2):11–18.
92. Koller M, Schoch U, Buchmann P, et al. Low molecular weight heparin (KABI 2165) as thromboprophylaxis in elective visceral surgery. Thromb Haemost 1986;56:243–245.
93. Onarheim H, Lund T, Heimdal A, Arnesjo B. A low molecular weight heparin (Kabi 2165) for prophylaxis of postoperative deep venous thrombosis. Acta Chir Scand 1986;152:593–596.
94. Kakkar VV, Cohen AT, Edmonson RA, et al. Low molecular weight versus standard heparin for prevention of venous thromboembolism after major abdominal surgery. Lancet 1993;341:259–265.
95. Caen JP. A randomized double-blind study between a low-molecular weight heparin (kabi 2165) and standard heparin in the prevention of deep vein thrombosis in general surgery. Thromb Haemost 1988;59:216–220.
96. Hartl P, Brucke P, Dienstl E, Vinazzer H. Prophylaxis of thromboembolism in general surgery: Comparison between standard heparin and Fragmin. Thromb Res 1990;57:577–584.
97. Bergqvist D, Matzsch T, Burmark US, et al. Low molecular weight heparin given the night before surgery compared with conventional low-dose heparin in prevention of thrombosis. Br J Surg 1988;75:888–891.
98. Cziraky MJ, Spinler SA. Low-molecular-weight heparins for the treatment of deep-vein thrombosis. Clin Pharm 1993;12:892–899.
99. Buckley MM, Sorkin EM. Enoxaparin: A review of its pharmacology and clinical applications in the prevention and treatment of thromboembolic disorders. Drugs 1992;44:465–497.
100. Warkentin TE, Levine MN, Hirsh J, et al. Heparin-induced thrombocytopenia in patients treated with low-molecular-weight heparin or unfractionated heparin. N Engl J Med 1995;332:1330–1335.

Chapter 20

Stroke

J. Chris Bradberry, PharmD

Stroke is a syndrome and is a major manifestation of cerebrovascular disease. Stroke refers to the sudden onset of a focal neurologic deficit. Cerebrovascular disease refers to any type of pathophysiologic vascular disease of the brain. This vascular pathology can include any abnormality of the vessel, blood flow, or quality of the blood. Abnormalities of the vessel include many processes such as developmental defects, arteritis, aneurysm, hypertensive disease, vasoconstriction, and atherosclerosis. Blood flow can be affected by disease of the vessel and also by thrombotic or embolic processes. The changes in the brain that these abnormalities can produce are either a decrease in blood flow, termed ischemia, or bleeding. Ischemia can be present with or without brain tissue infarction. When a stroke occurs, the neurologic manifestations produced are the result of the location of insult in the brain and the extent of ischemia, infarct, or hemorrhage. A stroke may show varied manifestations, reversible and irreversible, ranging from hemiplegia to sensory deficits. Hemiplegia may or may not be accompanied by other manifestations. It is a challenge for the clinician to accurately diagnose a particular lesion because of these variations in presentation; however, a good clinical examination can aid in locating a lesion as well as in helping to determine if the stroke is ischemic or hemorrhagic in nature. The advent of imaging studies such as computed tomography (CT) scan and magnetic resonance imaging (MRI) has been of tremendous importance in the diagnosis and assessment of stroke. Results of the CT scan must be known prior to therapy of certain stroke syndromes with anticoagulants or platelet antiaggregating agents. Although the causes of stroke are many, this chapter centers on the most common types of stroke, with further emphasis on ischemic cerebrovascular disease and pharmacotherapy and cardiogenic embolic stroke and pharmacotherapy. Hemorrhagic and other more unusual forms are deemphasized.

EPIDEMIOLOGY AND ETIOLOGY

Figure 20.1 outlines the causes of stroke. Since the 1940s, cerebrovascular disease death rates have declined in the United States.[1] In 1971, the American Heart Association (AHA) issued a special statement on risk factors.[2] At that time, major risk factors for ischemic stroke were identified as transient ischemic attacks, cerebral infarction, hypertension, cardiac abnormalities, and other consequences of atherosclerosis and diabetes mellitus.

Since that statement, mortality from stroke has continued to decline.[3,4] In fact, during the mid-1970s, the rate of decline in mortality from cerebrovascular disease was far greater than that from cardiovascular disease. The reasons for this decline are not clear, but evidence would suggest that this decline in mortality from cerebrovascular disease and ischemic stroke, in particular, may be related to more effective treatment of hypertension. Nevertheless, other factors have also undoubtedly contributed to this decline and, in 1984, the Stroke Council of the AHA issued an updated review of risk factors.[5]

General population studies show that atherothrombotic infarction is the most common type of stroke, representing almost 66% of the reported cases.[4,6] Therefore, the majority of strokes are caused by ischemia and infarction secondary to disease of the small and medium-sized arteries. Cerebral embolism causes stroke 5–14% of the time, although these data indicate cases for which there is a recognized embolic source. Hemorrhage into the brain tissue (cerebral hemorrhage) and subarachnoid hemorrhages account for 14–20% of all strokes. In 1992, the AHA estimated that in the United States more than 143,640 (1 of every 15 deaths) people died from a stroke, and that 3,080,000 people survived a stroke.[7] Stroke remains the third leading cause of death in the United States even though mortality is declining. It is estimated that 500,000 people per year have a new or recurrent stroke.

One of the major impacts of stroke is the resultant disability in up to 50% of patients hospitalized for cerebrovascular disease. The overall economic impact is estimated to be as high as $21.1 billion annually.[7] Obviously, with this impact, both economically and emotionally, stroke is one of the most devastating diseases in this country. Prevention is of primary importance and proper prevention requires correction of risk factors in persons at highest risk. As noted earlier, there is good evidence to show that improved treat-

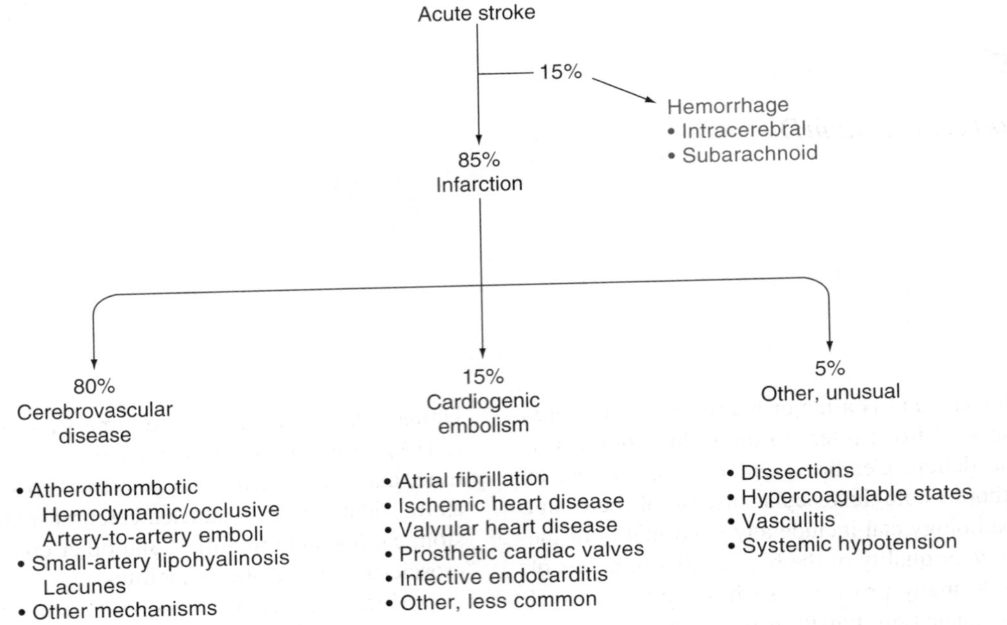

Figure 20.1. A general framework for conceptualizing the causes of stroke. The precise mechanisms are controversial. *(From Sherman DG, Dyken ML, Fisher M, et al: Cerebral embolism. Chest 1986;89(suppl 2):835, with permission.)*

ment, specifically of hypertension, may decrease death from stroke. The risk factors for stroke are shown in Table 20.1 and are divided into groups on the basis of their relationship to stroke.[5,7,8]

SINGLE RISK FACTORS

With regard to single risk factors, it is clear that stroke incidence is related to increasing age, with doubling of stroke rates each decade after 55.[7,9] Approximately 72% of stroke victims are 65 years or older.[7] Stroke generally has a 30% higher incidence in men than women. There is a higher death rate in blacks, Asian-Pacific Islanders, and Hispanics than whites. In blacks, this may be a result of the increased incidence of hypertension. Environmental factors, such as a high-sodium diet, may also play an important role in the increased stroke rate in blacks.[10] Diabetes mellitus contributes independently to atherothrombotic brain infarction and the risk is greater in women than men.[11] An individual with a prior stroke has a high risk of developing a recurrent stroke.[9] Carotid bruits are evidence of increased risk of stroke; however, asymptomatic carotid bruits have been a controversial topic with regard to treatment. In asymptomatic individuals, a carotid bruit is an indication of a generalized atherosclerotic disease and does not necessarily indicate that a cerebral infarction will occur in the cerebral territory supplied by the affected carotid.

Of the treatable single risk factors identified, hypertension is the major predisposing factor for stroke and is strongly related to atherothrombotic brain infarction as well as cerebral hemorrhage.[12] The Framingham study indicated that there is a direct relationship between elevation of blood pressure and stroke risk.[13] There does not seem to be a gender difference in the risk for hypertensive patients, and elevated blood pressure appears to be closely associated with stroke. The risk does not decrease with age; however, with effective treatment, the elderly have a reduction in stroke as great as or greater than that of the younger population. This was noted by the Hypertension Detection and Follow-up Program in 1982[14] and strongly suggested in the Framingham study. Impaired cardiac function is the next most important single treatable risk factor for stroke. Individuals with cardiac diseases such as coronary heart disease, congestive heart failure, left ventricular hypertrophy, and arrhythmias, and specifically atrial fibrillation, have more than twice the stroke risk compared with those with normal cardiac function.[8] The major controllable risk factor for coronary heart disease (CHD) must be addressed in order to reduce the risk of CHD and, in turn, stroke risk. Atrial fibrillation is strongly correlated with embolic stroke and those patients with nonrheumatic atrial fibrillation have a sixfold increase in stroke frequency over those without fibrillation.[15–17]

Transient ischemic attacks (TIAs) are defined as episodes of focal ischemic neurologic deficit lasting less than 24 hours. The neurologic deficit depends on the thrombotic or embolic activity in the particular arterial supply to the brain. TIAs precede an ischemic stroke in about 60% of cases, and 35% of untreated patients will develop a stroke within 5 years of a TIA. TIAs precede 10% of strokes from all causes. The greatest risk for stroke is early, within the

TABLE 20.1. RISK FACTORS IN STROKE

- Single risk factors
  - Well-documented risk factors
    - Treatment not feasible or value not established
      - Age and gender
      - Familial factors
      - Race
      - Diabetes mellitus
      - Prior stroke
      - Asymptomatic carotid bruits
    - Treatable
      - Hypertension
      - Cardiac disease
      - Transient ischemic attacks
      - Elevated hematocrit
      - Sickle cell disease
  - Less well-documented risk factors
    - Treatment not feasible or value not established
      - Geographic location
      - Season and climate
      - Socioeconomic factors
    - Treatable but value not established
      - Elevated blood cholesterol and lipids
      - Cigarette smoking
      - Alcohol consumption
      - Oral contraceptive use
      - Physical inactivity
      - Obesity
- Multiple risk factors
  - Framingham profile
    - Systolic blood pressure
    - Serum cholesterol
    - Glucose tolerance
    - Cigarette smoking
    - Electrocardiogram
    - Left ventricular hypertrophy
  - Paffenbarger and Williams criteria
    - Cigarette smoking
    - Systolic blood pressure
    - Low ponderal index
    - Body height
    - A parent dead
    - Not a varsity athlete

(From Dyken ML, Wolf PA, Barnett HJM, et al: Risk factors in stroke—a statement for physicians by the Subcommittee on Risk Factors and Stroke of the Stroke Council. Stroke 1984;15:1106, with permission.)

first few weeks of the TIA, with about 20% occurring within the first month after the TIA and 50% within the first year after the TIA.[18] The more frequently TIAs occur the higher the probability of stroke, and a previous stroke is a greater risk factor for subsequent stroke than a TIA alone.[19] TIAs as risk factors are also influenced by other stroke risk factors; therefore, treatment of other risk factors may influence the occurrence of stroke in patients with TIAs. Another treatable risk factor is elevated hematocrit. Several studies,[20–22] including data from the Framingham study,[23] point to the relationship between increased hematocrit and decreased cerebral blood flow and stroke. Stroke in patients with elevated hematocrits has been attributed to decreased collateral flow caused by increased blood viscosity.[24] Sickle cell disease patients also appear to have an increased incidence of stroke. One study[22] of hospitalized patients showed that 17% of sickle cell disease patients had one or more strokes. Those patients with sickle cell disease had a 1 in 20 rate of stroke and 4 of 227 with sickle cell trait developed stroke.[22] Stroke in middle-age men has been shown to correlate significantly with a maternal history of stroke.[25]

Risk factors that are less well documented but treatable are now briefly reviewed. Hyperlipidemia and hypercholesterolemia are risk factors for atherosclerosis and CHD related to stroke. It has been clearly established that lipoproteins play a primary role in atherogenesis and lowering plasma cholesterol concentration reduces arterial cholesterol accumulation.[26,27] In a recently published study, lowering cholesterol in patients with existing coronary heart disease also showed a very favorable risk reduction for stroke, thus emphasizing the importance of elevated cholesterol as a risk factor for stroke.[28] Cigarette smoking and alcohol consumption have been reported as having unclear contributions to stroke; however, recent reports indicate that cigarette smoking is indeed a major risk factor for ischemic stroke due to extracranial or intracranial vascular disease.[1,7,28,29] Alcohol intake was reviewed in 230 patients with stroke. It was found in men that heavy alcohol consumption (>300 g/week) is an independent risk factor but similar conclusions cannot be made for women on the basis of this study.[28] Twelve years of follow-up of the 7872 male subjects originally enrolled in the Honolulu Heart Program have shown that those who continued to smoke during follow-up had the highest risk of stroke.[28] Smokers had two to three times the risk of stroke compared with nonsmokers, and a fourfold to sixfold increase in stroke risk compared with those who had never smoked. It was also shown that cessation of smoking had significant benefits in reducing stroke risk. An association between the use of oral contraceptives as an independent risk factor and the incidence of stroke is not certain, and other risk factors for stroke such as coexisting hypertension, history of migraine, age greater than 35 years, cigarette smoking, diabetes, and hyperlipidemia are important.[5]

MULTIPLE RISK FACTORS

Data from two studies[8,30] have defined cerebrovascular risk profiles consisting of multiple risk factors. The Framingham study determined five factors: elevated systolic blood pressure, elevated serum cholesterol, glucose intolerance, cigarette smoking, and left ventricular hypertrophy by electrocardiogram (ECG). These factors, if present, can be used to identify the 10% of the population who will have one-third of the strokes. Individuals who have all of these factors require close supervision. Interestingly, various combinations of factors have been studied, including low ponderal index (height in inches/cube root of weight in pounds), and risk can vary fourfold to eightfold depending on the number of multiple risk factors present. The most important single factor, however, was found to be elevated blood pressure.

The treatable single risk factors should be vigorously addressed, and when risk factors occur in combination, therapy should be initiated aggressively, with particular emphasis on hypertension and lifestyle changes.

Pathophysiology of Acute Stroke

The vascular anatomy of the brain with blood flow from the heart is shown in Fig. 20.2. The reader may also refer to the diagrams of the brain territory supplied by the middle cerebral artery (Fig. 20.3), the anterior cerebral artery (Fig. 20.4), and the vertebral–basilar system (Fig. 20.5).

The large majority of acute strokes result either from ischemic infarction or from inadequate blood flow, while only 15% result from intracranial hemorrhage. Exact pathophysiologic mechanisms remain controversial. Figure 20.5 describes the anatomic basis of stroke. Using this schema, the pathophysiology of acute stroke is discussed.

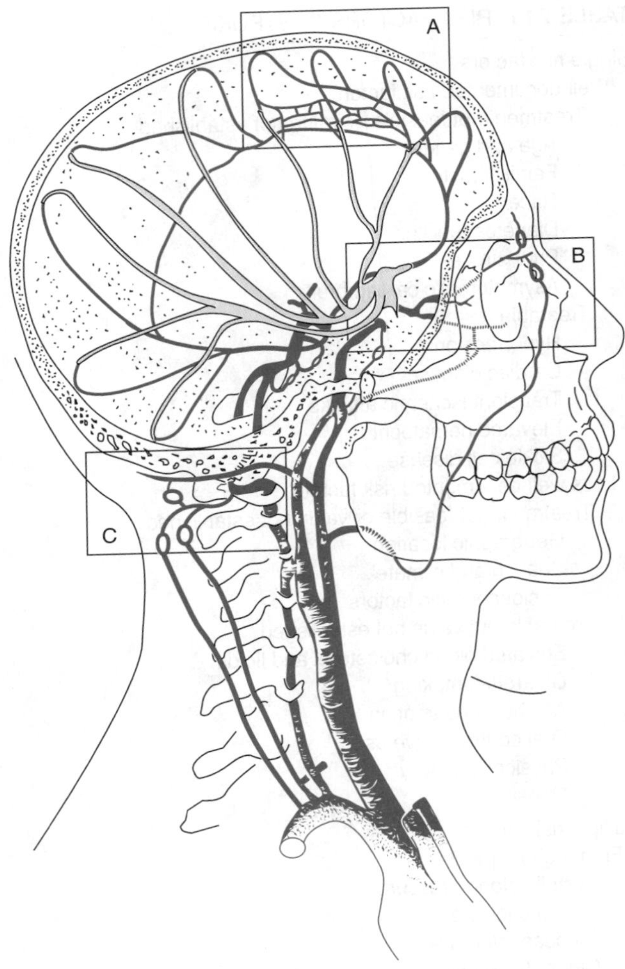

Figure 20.2. Arrangement of the major arteries of the right side carrying blood from the heart to the brain. Also shown are vessels of collateral circulation that may modify the effects of cerebral ischemia *(A–C)*. Not shown is the circle of Willis, which also provides a source for collateral circulation. *(A)* The anastomotic channels between the distal branches of the anterior and middle cerebral artery, termed *borderzone* or *watershed anastomotic channels.* Note that they also occur between the posterior and middle cerebral arteries and the anterior and posterior cerebral arteries. *(B)* Anastomotic channels occurring through the orbit between branches of the external carotid artery and the ophthalmic branch of the internal carotid artery. *(C)* Wholly extracranial anastomotic channels between the muscular branches of the ascending cervical arteries and the muscular branches of the occipital artery that anastomose with the distal vertebral artery. Note that the occipital artery arises from the external carotid artery, thereby allowing reconstitution of flow in the vertebral artery from the carotid circulation. *(From Braunwald E, Isselbacher KJ, et al (eds): Harrison's Principles of Internal Medicine, 11th ed. New York, McGraw-Hill, 1987, p 1931, with permission.)*

CEREBROVASCULAR DISEASE

Atherothrombotic Disease

Atherosclerosis of brain arteries is a process similar to that found in other extracranial vessels. It is generally held that the atherosclerotic process occurs in parallel fashion throughout the body, although the severity may be slightly less in arteries of the brain than in such arteries as the aorta, the arteries of the extremities, and the coronary arteries. Atherosclerosis and subsequent plaque formation result in arterial narrowing or occlusion and constitute the most common cause of aortacranial stenosis. Thrombosis is most likely to occur in areas where plaque has caused the greatest narrowing of the vessel. Formation of a blood clot superimposed on atherosclerotic plaque may cause significant stenosis of large extracranial arteries of the deep penetrating intracerebral arteries. Additional factors such as blood hypercoagulability and increased platelet counts and hematocrit may also contribute to clotting and sludging of blood flow. Embolism can produce a stroke when a clot, plaque, or platelet aggregate breaks off into the circulation and blocks an artery. When atherosclerotic plaque ulcerates and pieces embolize distally, the emboli are called artery-to-artery emboli. Other embolic phenomena are discussed in the section on Cardiogenic Embolism. Platelets play an important role in thrombosis and loss of integrity of the endothelial surface of the arterial wall, even if the defect is minor, and resultant platelet activation can lead to formation of a thrombus. This endothelial

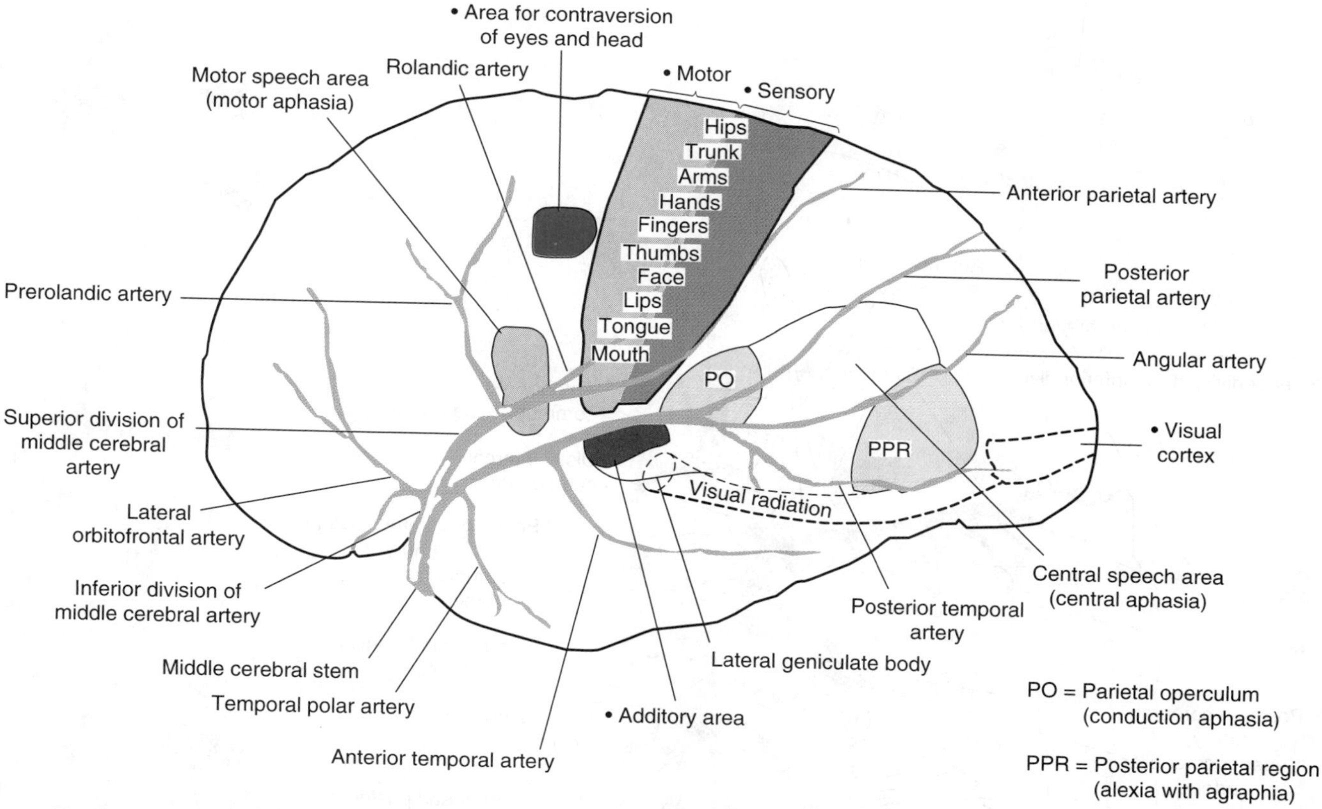

• Area for contraversion of eyes and head
Motor speech area (motor aphasia)
Rolandic artery
• Motor
• Sensory
Hips
Trunk
Arms
Hands
Fingers
Thumbs
Face
Lips
Tongue
Mouth
Anterior parietal artery
Posterior parietal artery
Prerolandic artery
Angular artery
PO
Superior division of middle cerebral artery
PPR
• Visual cortex
Visual radiation
Lateral orbitofrontal artery
Inferior division of middle cerebral artery
Central speech area (central aphasia)
Posterior temporal artery
Lateral geniculate body
Middle cerebral stem
Temporal polar artery
• Additory area
Anterior temporal artery
PO = Parietal operculum (conduction aphasia)
PPR = Posterior parietal region (alexia with agraphia)

Figure 20.3. Diagram of a cerebral hemisphere, lateral aspect, showing the branches and distribution of the middle cerebral artery and the principal regions of cerebral localization. Note the bifurcation of the middle cerebral artery into a superior and an inferior division. *(From Braunwald E, Isselbacher KJ, et al (eds): Harrison's Principles of Internal Medicine, 11th ed. New York, McGraw-Hill, 1987, p 1936, with permission.)*

Supplementary motor area
Motor area for foot, leg, and urinary bladder
Sensory area for foot and leg
Pericallosal artery
Callosomarginal artery
Artery of splenium
Frontopolar artery
Parietooccipital branch
Visual cortex with striate area along calcarine sulcus
Medial orbitofrontal artery
Anterior cerebral artery
Calcarine artery
Posterior cerebral artery
Posterior temporal artery
Anterior temporal artery

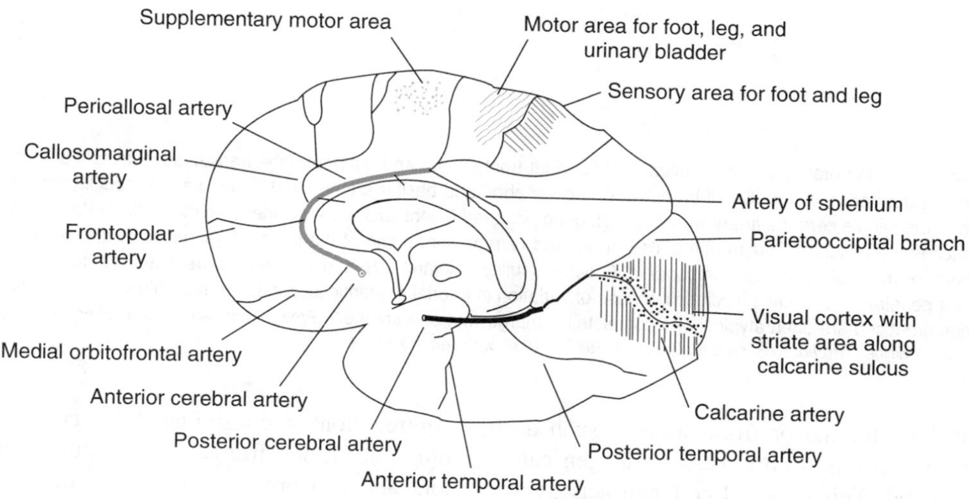

Figure 20.4. Diagram of a cerebral hemisphere, medial aspect, showing the branches and distribution of the anterior cerebral artery and the principal regions of cerebral localization. *(From Braunwald E, Isselbacher KJ, et al (eds): Harrison's Principles of Internal Medicine, 11th ed. New York, McGraw-Hill, 1987, p 1937, with permission.)*

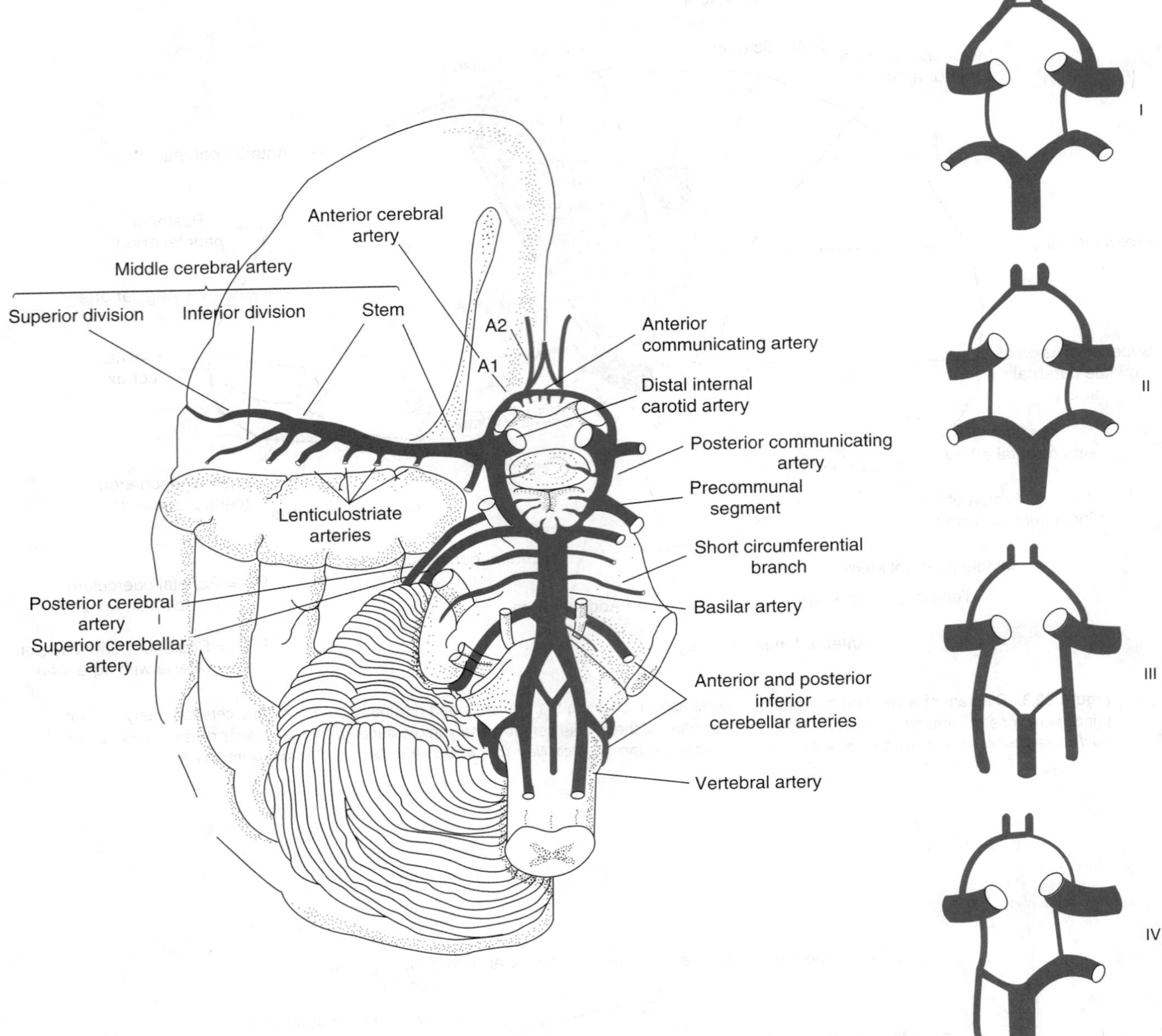

Figure 20.5. Diagram of the brain stem, cerebellum, inferior right frontal lobe, and temporal lobe transected. Principal branches of the vertebrobasilar arterial system are pictured. Small branches of the vertebral and basilar arteries that penetrate the medulla and pons are not pictured. The stem of the middle cerebral artery with its small, deep penetrating lenticulostriate arteries and the circle of Willis with its small, deep penetrating branches are pictured. Roman numerals I, II, III, and IV represent some of the possible variations of the circle of Willis resulting from atresia of one or more of its arterial components. Great variability in infarct size and location occurs when the basilar or vertebral arteries, or one of their penetrating branches, occlude because of variation in arterial anatomic location and available collateral circulation. Thus the stroke syndromes produced are often atypical or incomplete, or merge with one another. *(From Braunwald E, Isselbacher KJ et al. (eds): Harrison's Principles of Internal Medicine, 11th ed. New York, McGraw-Hill, 1987, p 1932, with permission.)*

damage can result from trauma or from diseases such as atherosclerosis and, when this occurs, vessel collagen can be exposed to the blood. This exposed collagen acts as a trigger mechanism to activate the platelets. This activation results in release of adenine diphosphate (ADP) from the platelets, which in turn causes platelets to aggregate. Aggregation is consolidated by coagulation factors, red blood cells, and formation of a fibrin network. Other factors are also produced including thromboxane A_2, which promotes platelet aggregation and vasoconstriction. This is balanced by the production of prostacyclin (PGI_2) by the vessel endothelium. Prostacyclin is a vasodilator and inhibitor of platelet aggregation. This thrombus may continue to increase in size until the entire lumen of the vessel is blocked, or pieces of the thrombus may break off and embolize into more distal areas. The process of atherosclerosis, as indicated previously, results in plaque formation, which stimulates platelet aggregation. Atherosclerosis itself is initially seen as a fatty streak on the vascular wall. This fatty streak starts as a deposition of lipids in the endothelial cells of the vessel wall. This process may regress, remain stable, or progress. If the process continues, yellow fatty, fibrous plaques are formed. Again, if there is progression, an atheromatous lesion may form and hemorrhage into the plaque, and subintimal necrosis, loss of intimal integrity, ulcer formation, or calcification may occur.[31–34] The atherosclerotic process is variable and the ischemic consequences resulting from this process depend on (1) adequacy of blood flow and collateral circulation and (2) embolism.[35] These factors determine the outcome of any individual ischemic event. To produce a low-blood-flow state leading to ischemia, the blood pressure must be reduced distal to the stenosis or occlusion and, usually, the carotid lumen must be reduced 75% in diameter.[36,37] Impaired collateral circulation to the affected area is also critical. The collateral circulation is composed of a network of arteries on the surface of the brain and those of the circle of Willis.

The most common sites for the atherosclerotic process to occur are at the bifurcation of the common carotid siphon, the origin of the common carotid artery from the aorta; at the bifurcation of the internal carotid artery into the anterior and middle cerebral arteries; and in the circle of Willis at the proximal segments of the anterior, middle, and posterior cerebral arteries (Fig. 20.6).[38]

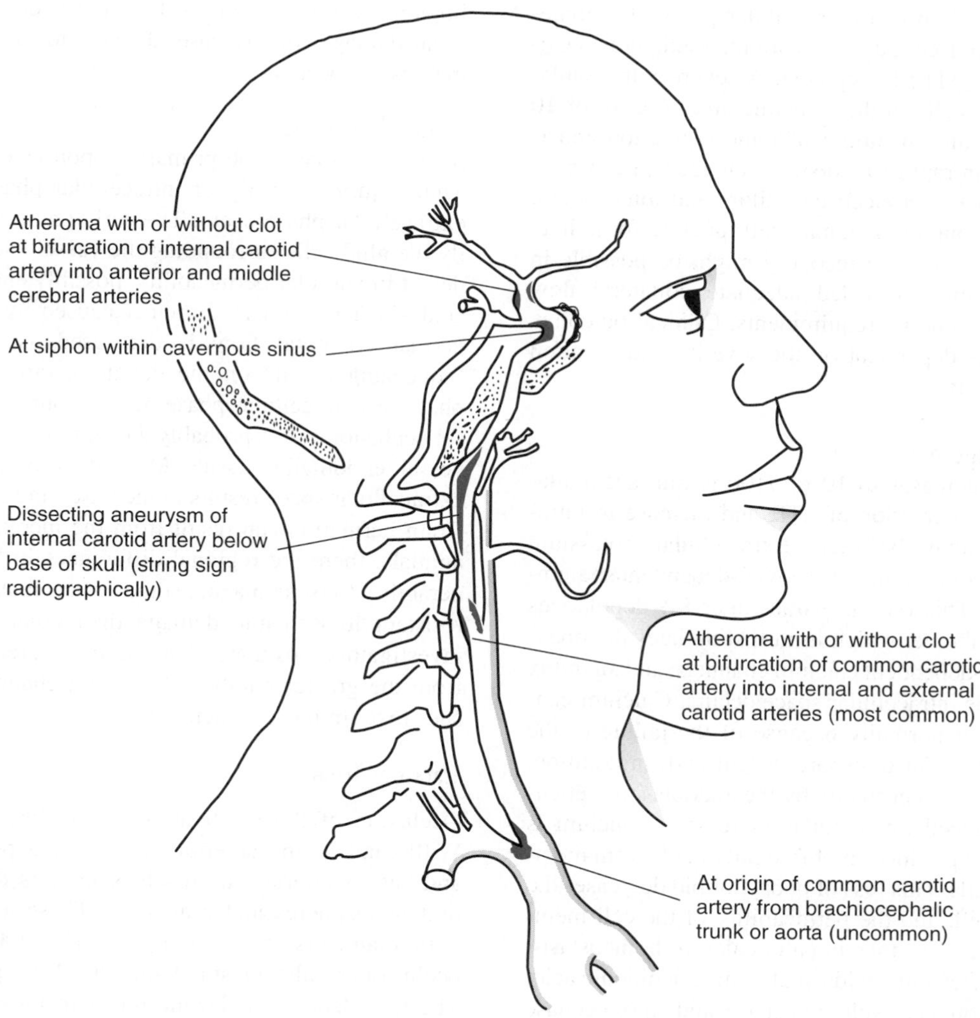

Figure 20.6. Common sites of atherosclerotic disease in the aortocranial circulation. *(From The Ciba Collection of Medical Illustrations. Ciba Foundaion, 1982, vol I pt II, p 55, with permission.)*

Cerebral Ischemia

Cerebral ischemia can be divided into focal and general (or global) ischemia. Global ischemia is associated with lack of collateral blood flow, and irreversible brain damage occurs in a short period of time (4–8 minutes).[39] In focal ischemia, however, there remains some degree of collateral circulation; therefore, this may allow for survival of brain cells and reversal of neuronal damage after periods of ischemia. Because of this potential for recovery, focal ischemia is considered treatable in some cases. The pathophysiologic characteristics of focal ischemia may be reviewed in terms of cerebral ischemia thresholds, metabolic derangements, and microcirculatory changes.[40]

Cerebral Ischemia Thresholds

Normal cerebral blood flow (CBF) in humans is about 53 mL per 100 g of brain tissue per minute. Reductions in CBF to the range 15–18 mL/100 g/min result in abnormal brain electrical activity. At a flow of 10 mL/100 g/min alterations in intracellular calcium and extracellular potassium homeostasis occur. Also, free fatty acids are released, and adenosine triphosphate (ATP) is depleted. A severe intracellular acidosis ensues in cells in the ischemic area. A CBF of 10 mL/100 g/min results in failure of ionic regulation and is thought to result in rapid irreversible damage to neurons.[40] The CBF range between electrical failure and ionic failure is thought to be enough to maintain cell function for a time, possibly up to 4 hours, and recovery might be possible in acute focal ischemia, provided adequate collateral flow could supply basic energy requirements. Clinical outcome, as noted earlier, is dependent on the severity and duration of the decreased CBF.

Metabolic Derangements

When the CBF decreases to 10 mL/100 g/min, accumulation of lactic acid, depletion of ATP, and increase in intracellular calcium may be seen. Extracellular potassium increases because of a failure of the ATP-dependent sodium-potassium pump. This rise in extracellular K+ depolarizes the neuronal membrane, which in turn stimulates the opening of the voltage-dependent calcium channels, and an influx of calcium into the intracellular space occurs. Calcium cannot be pumped out normally because of the failure of the ATP-dependent calcium transport system and, in addition, calcium is not taken up normally by the endoplasmic reticulum. This unbalanced intracellular increase in calcium is thought to result in production of free fatty acids from membrane phospholipids. This loss of phospholipid decreases the integrity of the cell, and the permeability of the cell membranes increases and further impairs calcium homeostasis. Accumulation of free fatty acids, including arachidonic acid, results in oxidation via cyclooxygenase and lipoxygenase pathways, producing prostaglandins, leukotrienes, and, possibly, free radicals.[40] Thromboxane A_2 is a potent vasoconstrictor, leukotrienes affect membrane permeability, and free radicals can attack cell membranes.[40] All of these actions can lead to further intracellular acidosis and increasingly impair cell function. Ischemia and the subsequent production of intracellular acidosis can have devastating effects on the brain cell. These effects include glial edema and denaturation of proteins. Focal ischemia is associated with preserved but marginal CBF, and continued glucose delivery in the face of ischemia promotes anaerobic glycolysis with production of lactic acidosis. This continues to worsen the intracellular acidosis.

Microcirculatory Changes and Edema

At the time of occlusion, blood viscosity and resistance to flow are increased,[41] and blood flow is further slowed as ischemia develops. Soon after this, an ischemia-induced arterial spasm occurs,[42] possibly as a result of the aforementioned increased extracellular potassium or increased intracellular calcium or both. It is not clear why vasospasm of the microcirculation occurs and it is also not clear if this impaired vascular filling is the primary determinant of neuronal damage. In any case, damage to the endothelium of the vessels occurs.

Ischemia Edema

Swelling is one of the primary responses of brain tissue to acute injury. An early or intracellular phase and a late or extracellular phase occur. The early phase involves primarily the glial cells surrounding the vessel itself, suggesting a defect in vascular permeability, possibly enhanced by lactic acidosis. The primary difficulty caused by the glial edema is that collateral flow is decreased as a result of the "squeezing down" on the collateral circulation. The late phase or extracellular phase occurs hours to days after vessel occlusion and is probably a result of ischemic damage to vessel endothelial tissue. Movement of plasma into the extracellular space results in increased intracranial pressure. Brain herniation can result from the increased pressure. In animals, there are regional differences in brain tissue vulnerability to ischemia and some tissues may be more or less resistant to ischemic damage than other tissues.[43] Some investigators postulate that these differences may result from the greater number of calcium channels in those tissues that are most vulnerable.[40]

Lacunar Infarcts

Occlusion of the small arterial branches of the circle of Willis and of the anterior, middle, and posterior cerebral and basilar arteries can result in infarcts deep in the cerebral hemispheres and brainstem. These are small arteries with diameters in the range of 100–400 μm and their occlusion results in small infarcts 2–15 μm in diameter. The term lacunar or lacune refers to the small cavity left after necrotic tissue has been removed. The pathophysiology of these infarcts is somewhat different from that of infarcts closer to the surface of the brain. About 10–20% of all strokes are a result of lacunar infarcts, which are the major risk factor for lacunar disease. Arterial hypertension is closely related to the occurrence of lacunar infarcts and is the major risk factor for lacunar disease. The pathophysiology of the small arteries has been described as being a degenerative process in the media of the artery (lipohyalinosis), leading to vessel occlusion.[44,45] The degenerative occlusive process may be, on occasion, histologically different in appearance compared with the atherosclerotic process affecting extracranial and other larger intracranial arteries and may, in fact, circumscribe portions of the involved artery. Microatheroma (plaque) may also be found in the proximal portions of the arterial branches. These different occlusive processes probably account for the multiple types of clinical presentations of lacunar infarcts. The patient's clinical presentation will reflect which small arterial branches are involved in the occlusive process. For example, the lenticulostriate artery is often involved and the most common lacunar syndrome results from an infarct in the internal capsule of the brain and a pure motor hemiparesis is seen.

Transient Ischemic Attacks

TIAs of cerebral origin are episodes of temporary focal cerebral dysfunction of vascular origin in which the onset is rapid, is of variable duration, and lasts from a few seconds up to 24 hours. The most common duration is a few seconds up to 5–10 minutes. Between attacks there may be no neurologic abnormality. The clinical manifestation reflects the territory of the artery involved and usually occurs in the carotid system or in the vertebrobasilar system or both. TIAs have greater significance in that they herald an impending stroke. Threatened stroke is a term used to describe any prestroke syndrome, such as TIAs, or patients who have had small or minor strokes or progressing or evolving stroke, and are at further risk for a major stroke.

The pathophysiology of TIAs involves the atherosclerotic process, thrombus formation, and low CBF. It is from the cerebral thrombus that small microemboli, in the form of platelet aggregates and cholesterol crystals, break off and travel to distal areas and lodge, producing the ischemic attack. Cerebral or cerebellar artery thrombosis is most commonly responsible for TIAs. Low flow will also result in a TIA when the CBF is sufficiently reduced in stenosed arteries. Other causes include emboli from the heart caused by valvular disease or endocardial damage and increased blood viscosity from conditions such as polycythemia. Polycythemia is an uncommon cause of TIA.

CEREBRAL EMBOLISM

Any region of the brain can be affected by embolism; however, the area or territory of the middle cerebral artery is commonly involved. Embolism may result from pieces or fragments of an arterial thrombus that have broken off or from a heart valve vegetation. Occasionally, an embolus may form from an ulcerated atheromatous plaque. Other forms of embolism such as air, fat, or tumor cells occur only rarely. Cerebral embolism from bacterial sepsis occurs frequently, but bacterial emboli large enough to produce a stroke are infrequent. After breaking off from a thrombus or heart valve vegetation, an embolism usually circulates until it is too large to traverse the arterial lumen. The point of occlusion may be at a bifurcation or other narrowed area. Both hemispheres of the brain appear to be equally affected. Hemorrhagic infarction frequently occurs in the embolic process because of the reperfusion of blood into the ischemic tissue, causing hemorrhage, and the area of the middle cerebral artery is often the involved site. The size of the embolus may vary from large to very small; in fact, the embolus may be so small that it produces no infarct or produces an infarct so small that it cannot be detected.

Cerebral embolism secondary to thrombotic disease usually has a rapid onset and it is not preceded by a TIA. This rapid onset is problematic because there is less time for collateral circulation to develop as in cerebral thrombosis. As a result, embolic strokes are often functionally devastating. Cerebral embolism may result from heart disease. It is currently recognized that cardiogenic embolism accounts for 6–23% of all ischemic strokes.[46,47] Embolism has been associated with many types of heart disease, and the following discussion focuses on the most common types (Table 20.2).

TABLE 20.2. MAJOR CAUSES OF CARDIOGENIC CEREBRAL EMBOLISM

Nonvalvular atrial fibrillation	50%
Coronary heart disease	20%
Myocardial infarction	
Rheumatic heart disease	15%
Mitral stenosis ± atrial fibrillation	
Prosthetic cardiac valves	10%
Other	5%
Cardiomyopathy	
Cardiac tumors	
Septic endocarditis	
Nonbacterial thrombotic endocarditis (marantic)	
Congenital heart disease	
Venous clots/intracardiac shunt (paradoxic emboli)	
Mitral annulus calcification	
Calcific aortic stenosis	
Mitral valve prolapse	

(From Easton JD, Hart RG, Sherman DG, et al: Diagnosis and management of ischemic stroke. Part 1. Threatened stroke and its management. Curr Prob Cardiol 1983;8:20, with permission.)

Cardiogenic Embolism

Atrial Fibrillation

Chronic atrial fibrillation (AF) is the most common cause of cardiogenic embolism and is the most common sustained dysrhythmia. The incidence of AF increases with age such that 2–5% of patients older than 60 years of age have AF, and more than half of AF-associated strokes occur in individuals older than 75 years.[15,16] Patients with nonvalvular atrial fibrillation have about the same stroke risk as patients who experience a TIA. Atrial fibrillation enhances the development of left atrial thrombi and arterial embolism. The most common site (75%) in which left atrial thrombi form in patients with nonvalvular AF (NVAF) is the atrial appendage rather than the atrial wall. Patients with AF and valvular disease have thrombi both on the atrial wall and on the appendage in equal incidence. Factors involved in the pathogenesis of atrial thrombus formation in patients with AF include increased left atrial pressure and outflow obstruction. Mitral valve obstruction can enhance left atrial stasis similar to that seen in AF alone. Enlargement of the left atrium occurs in AF and the incidence of thrombus formation increases with left atrial enlargement. Damage to the endothelial surface could also induce thrombus formation and initiate AF. Such disorders as rheumatic heart disease, myocardial infarction, and pericarditis can also initiate AF by involvement of the sinoatrial node and change the atrial endothelial surface such that thrombus formation is enhanced. The risk of stroke in patients with AF is high and 20–35% of all patients with AF will have an embolic stroke of clinical significance.[48] The risk of stroke in those with AF is five to six times that of the general population and average about 5% per year. Those at greatest risk are those patients with AF and rheumatic valvular disease. The risk for development of systemic embolism for these individuals is 17 times that of the general population.[49] The largest group of patients comprises those with NVAF; their rate of systemic embolism is around 35% and their stroke risk is six times that of the general population.[49,50] Predictors of stroke risk for AF during aspirin therapy are shown in Table 20.3. Major clinical risk factors for thromboembolism in NVAF are a history of hypertension and arterial thromboembolism, and recent (within 3 months) congestive heart failure and diabetes.[16,51] Electrocardiographic findings which correlate to embolic risk in AF are enlargements of the left atrium and impairment of left ventricular systolic function.[52] The clinical utility of this risk stratification will be discussed under treatment. Even those patients with idiopathic AF have an increased rate of embolism of 7% in the first year, and up to 14% at 5 years of AF.[53] The presence of carotid stenosis may also help to identify a subgroup of NVAF who are at higher risk of stroke.[54] Patients who develop AF have a high rate of embolus formation soon after the onset of AF. Recurrence of embolism is frequent. Up to 50% of patients who develop one embolus develop another.[18] In addition, changing the rhythm by cardioversion increases the rate of embolus occurrence, and about 2% of these patients may develop an embolus the first few days after cardioversion of AF to normal sinus rhythm.[55] Studies are necessary to establish the evidence for maintaining sinus rhythm after cardioversion in order to prevent strokes.

TABLE 20.3. STROKE RISK IN ATRIAL FIBRILLATION DURING ASPIRIN THERAPY

Risk Factors
Hypertension (SBP > 160 mm Hg)
Prior stroke/TIA
Age greater than 75 in women
Impaired left ventricular function (within previous 100 days)
Recent heart failure
Rate of stroke with a risk factor = 6.3%/yr
Rate of stroke without risk factors = 1.8%/yr

Ischemic heart disease and ischemic stroke share the same risk factors and most patients with TIAs and stroke die from myocardial infarction. In myocardial infarction the primary cause of emboli is mural thrombus formation in the left ventricle. Thrombus formation is thought to be started by platelet adherence to and deposition on the damaged (infarcted) akinetic or dyskinetic endocardial surface.[56] There is also an inflammatory white cell response in the damaged area secondary to the tissue infarction. Additionally, the infarcted area may develop into an aneurysmal region where fibrin accumulation can occur. Mural thrombus formation depends on the size and location of the infarct. Thrombus formation and the presence of apical akinesis or dyskinesis are seen almost exclusively in anterior myocardial infarctions. Aneurysms occur most frequently in the apex region of the heart. About 50–60% of patients with aneurysm formation in the left ventricle develop a mural thrombus.[56] Most of these mural thrombi develop within the first week of the acute myocardial infarction (AMI) and patients who have mural thrombi as evidenced by echocardiography after AMI are most probably those patients at risk for eventual embolization.[47,57] The overall incidence of systemic emboli in patients who suffer an AMI is around 5–6% and is similar to the incidence in those patients who develop a left ventricular aneurysm. Therefore, of the 50–60% of patients with an aneurysm who develop a mural thrombus only 5–6% develop a systemic embolus.

Valvular Heart Disease

Thromboembolism is commonly found in patients with valvular heart disease, such as rheumatic mitral disease, and in those with prosthetic heart valves. Thrombus formation in patients with valvular disease or prosthetic valves most often occurs in the left ventricle or on the prosthetic valve. Thrombi can also form, but with a lower incidence, in the left atrium. Mitral stenosis is also associated with an increased risk of thromboembolism.

In valvular heart disease, those patients with mitral stenosis and those with mitral stenosis combined with incompetence of the mitral valve have a thromboembolic event rate of 15–20%. Up to 16% of these events may be fatal.[58,59] Patients with only mitral incompetence are at less risk than those with mitral stenosis and the embolic rate is approximately 3%, although this rate may be higher in patients with a severe form of mitral incompetence. Prolapse of the mitral valve appears to carry a very low risk of embolism. The risk of embolism also appears to be low in patients with aortic valve disease. Additional factors that increase risk for systemic embolism in patients with valvular disease are atrial fibrillation, increased left atrial size, increased age, and history of a previous embolic event. Atrial fibrillation is the most important single risk factor and, as noted previously, thrombus formation is rare in patients with a normal sinus rhythm. Atrial fibrillation is closely associated with mitral valve disease and emboli may develop shortly after fibrillation develops. Enlargement of the left atrium usually occurs with mitral valve disease, and left atrial enlargement predisposes to atrial fibrillation; therefore, there is an indirect relationship between left atrial enlargement and embolism. Recurrent embolic events can occur in up to 20% of mitral stenosis patients with previous embolic history. The mortality rate is quite high in this group of patients and may reach 42%.[59]

Prosthetic Cardiac Valves

Thrombus formation on prosthetic cardiac valves (PCVs), whether aortic or mitral valves, is related to the production of turbulence in blood flow by the valve and the thrombogenic potential of the valve material. Patients who have had PCV replacement are at long-term risk of arterial thrombolism.[60] Examples of valves currently used are the Starr–Edwards ball valve, Bjork–Shiley disk valve, St. Jude Medical, and others. The early Starr–Edwards valve used in the 1960s may have a higher embolic rate than those used in recent years. This may be a result of improved operative procedures and valve factors, as well as less severe disease and better atrial and ventricular function. The embolism rate with the Bjork–Shiley valve is similar to that with the Starr–Edwards valve; however, a newer material, pyrolytic carbon in the disk of the valve is less thrombogenic and the embolism rate is lower. The bioprosthetic valves, such as the Hancock, Carpentier–Edwards, and Lonescu–Shiley, have a different design, a central flow design. This design produces less turbulence in blood flow, and the biologic material (i.e., porcine valve) is less thrombogenic. Thromboembolism occurs less frequently than with the other valves. Other risk factors include atrial fibrillation, large left atrium, inadequate anticoagulation, and a previous embolic event.[60] The overall risk of neurologic deficit with mechanical prosthetic valve-induced embolism is high. For instance, data from follow-up of the older Starr–Edwards ball valve show that 85% of systemic emboli entered the cerebral circulation and 50% of these emboli resulted in a neurologic deficit, with 10% of all embolic events being fatal.[61] Overall, the rate of embolism in anticoagulated patients with mechanical PCVs averages 3% per year for mitral valves and 1.5% per year for aortic valves. Embolic rates for nonanticoagulated patients with bioprosthetic valves are 2–4% per year. There is general agreement that all adults with any type of mechanical valve should be on long-term anticoagulation and that bioprosthetic valves also require treatment with short-term anticoagulation and optional long-term antiplatelet therapy.[62,63]

Infective Endocarditis

Emboli may result from bacterial vegetations that can form in infective endocarditis. Arterial emboli are one of the most frequent complications of this disease. Major cerebral emboli have been observed in nearly one-third of patients with endocarditis, with the middle cerebral artery and its branches being most frequently involved. The highest frequency of major embolic events occurs in association with infections on the left side of the heart that produce large, mobile vegetations from *Haemophilus parainfluenzae,* or slow-growing fastidious, gram-negative bacilli, fungi *(Aspergillus),* and *Streptococcus viridans.* Emboli from the right side of the heart, as seen in intravenous drug abusers, are often caused by staphylococcal organisms and can produce clinical manifestations of pulmonary emboli. There is another type of endocarditis, called marantic endocarditis, in which sterile thrombi are present on the valves. This condition is seen most often in patients with mucin-secreting adenocarcinomas. This process is nonbacterial and the vegetations are composed mainly of platelets and fibrin. The term *marantic* refers to old and debilitated; however, this thromboembolic process can occur in the young and non-debilitated.

Unusual and Other Causes of Infarction

There are a number of other causes of cerebral infarction, and these are listed in Table 20.4.

TABLE 20.4. UNUSUAL CAUSES OF INFARCTION

Venous thrombosis	Contraceptive steroid use
Systemic hypotension	Polycythemia
Arteriography	Idiopathic thrombocytosis
Carotid occlusion	Dissecting aortic aneurysm
Arteritis	Hypercoagulable states
Moyamoya disease	

TABLE 20.5. CAUSES OF INTRACRANIAL HEMORRHAGE

Hypertensive intracerebral hemorrhage
Lobar hemorrhage of undetermined cause and intracerebral hemorrhage associated with congophilic angiopathy (analyzed)
Ruptured saccular aneurysm, giant aneurysm, or mycotic aneurysm
Ruptured angioma
Hemorrhagic disorders: leukemia, aplastic anemia, thrombocytopenic purpura, liver disease, complication of anticoagulant therapy, hyperfibrinolysis, hypofibrinogenemia, hemophilia, Christmas disease
Trauma, including post-traumatic apoplexy
Hemorrhage into primary and secondary brain tissue
Hemorrhagic infarction, arterial or venous
Inflammatory disease of the arteries and veins
Miscellaneous rare types: after vasopressor drugs, upon exertion, during arteriography, during painful urologic examination, as a late complication of early-life carotid occlusion, complication of carotid–cavernous arteriovenous fistula, with anoxemia, migraine, teratomatous malformations (acute inclusion body encephalitis produces xanthochromia and up to 2000 red blood cells or more in the cerebrospinal fluid; acute necrotizing hemorrhagic encephalopathy may be associated with up to 100 red blood cells in the cerebrospinal fluid; tularemia and snake venom poisoning may cause bloody cerebrospinal fluid)

(From Braunwald E, Isselbacher KJ, et al (Eds): Harrison's Principles of Internal Medicine, 11th ed. New York, McGraw-Hill, 1987, p 1952, with permission.)

INTRACRANIAL HEMORRHAGE

Hemorrhage is the third most frequent cause of stroke. Approximately 15% of cases of stroke are due to intracranial hemorrhage. The more frequent causes of stroke from intracranial hemorrhage are hypertensive intracerebral hemorrhage, ruptured saccular aneurysms, hemorrhage associated with bleeding disorders, and arteriovenous malformations (AVMs).

Hypertensive intracerebral hemorrhage occurs generally when the blood pressure is significantly elevated. The bleeding occurs in the brain tissue as a result of the rupture of an artery. This allows for an extravasation of blood into the brain tissue, which forms a mass. This mass damages the tissue and continues to enlarge as bleeding continues. Brain tissue is pushed, displaced, and compressed and brain functions may be impaired. The larger the hemorrhage, the greater the displacement of tissue. Escape of blood into the ventricles of the brain can occur, and when this happens, the spinal fluid becomes bloody. The cerebrospinal fluid may remain clear if the hemorrhage is small or at a distance from the ventricular system. The extravascular blood undergoes changes such as phagocytosis, and the mass gradually shrinks; after 2–6 months, only discoloration is left at the site. Hemorrhagic infarcts, discussed earlier, are due primarily to the reflow or reperfusion of ischemic tissue, with resultant bleeding into the tissue. In hypertensive hemorrhage, the vessels most often involved are the penetrating arteries in the putamen and internal capsule and parts of the white matter, including the frontal lobe, thalamus, pons, and cerebellar hemisphere. Causes of intracranial hemorrhage are listed in Table 20.5.

CLINICAL PRESENTATION/DIAGNOSIS

ATHEROTHROMBOTIC DISEASE

Thrombosis of cerebral vessels produces variable clinical manifestations as compared with embolic disease or intracranial hemorrhage. In a large percentage of cases (>50%), the stroke is preceded by one or more transient ischemic attacks. If the evolving thrombosis involves the internal carotid and middle cerebral arteries, then such focal symptoms as mono- or hemiplegia, mono- or hemiparesthesia, blindness in one eye, and speech disturbance may occur. If the vertebrobasilar system is involved, such symptoms as dizziness, diplopia, numbness, impaired vision, and dysarthria may occur. Usually these attacks are short lived and resolve in less than 10 minutes. The stroke itself most often develops suddenly as a single attack, or it may show an intermittent or stuttering progression pattern over hours to days. Additionally, a patient may suffer a partial stroke, improve for several hours, then develop full paralysis of one or more parts of the body; other parts become paralyzed in a stepwise manner until the stroke is completed. When the thrombosis produces a developing involvement over hours, days, or weeks, it is called stroke in evolution or progressing stroke. Interestingly, the majority (60%) of cerebral thrombotic strokes occur at rest while sleeping or after arising.[18] Headache may occur, but is often absent; when present, it may occur several days prior to the other symptoms of the stroke.

Diagnosis consists of evaluation of the clinical presentation and laboratory findings. In addition to the clinical presentation just discussed, laboratory evaluation can include tests such as cerebral arteriography, imaging studies such as CAT and MRI, radioactive brain scan study (such as a technetium scan), x-rays of the head, electroencephalogram, ECG, transcranial Doppler studies, digital subtraction angiogram, and lumbar puncture (LP). The definitive test for arterial occlusion or narrowing is the arteriogram; however, the procedure carries a neurologic risk itself and should only be used if the diagnosis of vascular disease is not clear or if vascular surgery is a possibility, such as in carotid TIA patients. Complications from cerebral angiography occur in 2–12% of patients and consist primarily of aortic or carotid dissection and embolic stroke. Hydration may reduce these risks. Because of the risks of arteriography, brain imaging is the most important test after a stroke has occurred. When it is performed, transfemoral angiography is usually the procedure of choice as compared with the direct carotid puncture procedure.[18] The CT scan in cerebral thrombosis usually shows an area of decreased attenuation or hypodense lesion in the infarcted area. The CT scan is often normal, however, during the first 48 hours after the thrombotic infarction. The CT scan is extremely useful in excluding tumors and identifying intracranial hemorrhage, both of which dictate different treatment modalities. CT scans, however, may not show small ischemic strokes, especially on the cortical surface, and bone may cause difficulty in interpretation. MRI can adequately detect small infarcts in the cortical surface and elsewhere usually within 1 hour of occurrence. MRI is a noninvasive imaging technique that, unlike CT and PET, does not require x-rays or isotopes. MRI uses magnetic fields to generate images and it takes longer to perform than a CT scan.

Radioisotopic brain scans can be helpful and show infarcts earlier than CT scans. Skull x-rays are usually not helpful and the electroencephalogram and LP are of limited value, because they are usually normal. Noninvasive techniques like Doppler flow studies and Doppler scanning have been developed but have some disadvantages with consistent differentiation of stenosis from occlusion and detection of distal atherosclerosis.

Digital subtraction angiography (DSA) is a recent addition and it holds promise as a diagnostic tool. Arterial injection of contrast medium in DSA currently provides better imaging of the cerebral vasculature than does intravenous administration, which gives imperfect detail.

Other new diagnostic imaging techniques include transesophageal echocardiography, xenon blood flow, positron emission tomography (PET), which can give an image of dynamic physiology after injection of positron-emitting isotopes, and MRI angiography. These techniques are very promising advances and as they become more refined their place in diagnosis will become clear.[47]

Lacunar Infarcts

The clinical presentation varies depending on the perforating cerebral arteries involved. The most frequently occurring lacunar syndrome is pure motor hemiparesis, which is due to an infarct in the posterior portion of the internal capsule. This infarct results from occlusion of a middle or posterior cerebral perforating artery. The manifestations of the pure motor hemiparesis syndrome are hemiparesis or hemiplegia of the arm, leg, face, and trunk. In addition, a mild dysarthria occurs without sensory or consciousness alterations or visual field defects. The different parts of the body involved in the stroke display the same degree of weakness. This is in contrast to a stroke in the cortical region involving the middle or anterior cerebral artery where there is usually an unequal degree of weakness of the affected parts of the body.

Diagnosis is usually based on clinical evaluation of the patient after careful neurologic examination. A CT or MRI scan can provide evidence of the infarction if performed within about 7–10 days of the event; however, infarcts smaller than 2 mm may be missed. Treatment after lacunar strokes requires control of hypertension to help in the prevention of progression of the degenerative occlusive process.

Transient Ischemic Attacks

Most TIAs last 5–10 minutes, and those lasting one or more hours may be a result of embolism rather than ischemia or atherosclerosis. An ischemic event that lasts longer than 24 hours but completely resolves in a short period (up to 3 weeks) is termed a *reversible ischemic neurologic defect* (RIND). A TIA resulting from a carotid system lesion and anterior cerebral artery involvement manifests as weakness in the opposite leg and shoulder. If the anterior cortical branches of the middle cerebral artery are involved, a sensory and motor loss results in the contralateral face, arm, and hand. If the ischemia is in the dominant hemisphere, a nonfluent (Broca's) aphasia usually is present. Ischemia occurring in the posterior portions of the middle cerebral artery often produces contralateral sensory loss and homonymous hemianopia (defective vision or blindness affecting the right halves or the left halves of the visual fields of the two eyes). If there is posterior middle cerebral artery involvement in the dominant hemisphere, a fluent aphasia is likely to occur. Ischemia of the lenticulostriate arteries may result in findings that involve motor and sensory defects in the arms, legs, face, and trunk as noted in the discussion of lacunar infarcts. Clinical manifestations of TIAs arising from ischemia in the vertebrobasilar circulation are numerous. Vertigo and ataxia are seen in ischemia affecting cerebellar and vestibular areas. Bilateral weakness of the extremities indicates that the corticospinal nerve tracts are involved as they cross the brain stem.

Diagnosis of a TIA is difficult because the episode is usually over before the patient can be examined. Therefore, the diagnosis is really made on the basis of the patient's recollection of the symptoms. Table 20.6 shows the symp-

TABLE 20.6. SYMPTOMS OF TRANSIENT ISCHEMIC ATTACKS

Carotid system TIAs	
Unilateral weakness—usually hemiparesis	
Unilateral sensory complaints—numbness, paresthesia	
Aphasia—language comprehension, output or both	
Monocular visual loss (amaurosis fugax)	
Vertebrobasilar system TIAs	
Motor deficit—especially if bilateral	
Sensory complaints—especially if bilateral	
Simultaneous, bilateral visual complaints	
Diplopia	Only in combination, not as isolated symptoms
Vertigo	
Dysarthria[a]	
Ataxia without weakness	
Dysphagia	
Either carotid or vertebral TIAs	
Severe dysarthria[a]	
Homonymous visual complaints	
Isolated symptoms rarely resulting from TIAs	
Vertigo, dizziness	
Diplopia	
Loss of consciousness	
Confusion	
Bilateral leg weakness, falling spells	

[a]Often difficult to distinguish from nonfluent dysphasia on the basis of history. (From Easton JD, Hart RG, Sherman DG, et al: Diagnosis and management of ischemic stroke. Part 1. Threatened stroke and its management. Curr Prob Cardiol 1983;8:13, with permission.)

toms of TIAs. There are many singular symptoms or events that can be confused with TIAs and usually are not TIAs. Some of these events are fainting, convulsions, loss of consciousness, dizziness, spots before the eyes, dysarthria, imbalance and falling, and headache. Diagnostic studies may indicate the presence of vascular disease; however, history is the key to the diagnosis of a TIA. Proper attention to the history is important because treatment of TIAs is important in stroke prevention.

Laboratory studies in the diagnosis of TIA should rule out blood or other disorders that may produce decreased cerebral blood flow. Routine studies include erythrocyte sedimentation rate, complete blood count, platelet count, blood chemistry, urinalysis, coagulation profile, and syphilis (serology). To reveal systemic disease in selected patients, serum protein electrophoresis, antinuclear antibody titers, blood and plasma viscosities, plasma fibrinogen, and cerebrospinal fluid (CSF) examination may be performed. Embolism of cardiac origin should be a consideration in every patient with a single TIA. In these cases a 12-lead ECG should be performed to test for recent myocardial infarction and/or dysrhythmias such as atrial fibrillation. Other laboratory tests include a chest x-ray to exclude heart enlargement or disease of the valves. In patients suspected of having TIAs of embolic origin, echocardiography is an important diagnostic tool. Two-dimensional "echo" is indicated in patients with cerebral ischemia who have evidence of cardiac disease such as AF, enlarged heart, and mitral valve prolapse. The yield of thrombus detection in the hearts of these patients is 10–20%. The lower limit of clot size that is detected accurately by echocardiography is 2–3 mm. In addition, results from the Stroke Prevention in Atrial Fibrillation Investigators (SPAF) studies indicate that echocardiography in NVAF can serve as a clinical predictor of thromboembolism by detecting increased left atrial size and left ventricular dysfunctions.[50] Left atrial size and left ventricular size are strong independent predictors of later thromboembolism. Therefore, the echocardiogram can add to the clinical variables for risk stratification. As mentioned earlier, cerebral angiography should be performed only in selected patients, and patients who have had a carotid TIA should be studied with angiography as soon as reasonably possible because of the high risk of cerebral infarction in these patients.

CEREBRAL EMBOLISM/ CARDIOGENIC EMBOLISM

Cardiogenic brain embolism is the major cause of cerebral embolism and the brain is involved in approximately 70% of all emboli from the heart, whereas systemic or noncerebral nervous system emboli often go unrecognized. Cardiogenic brain embolism accounts for 6–23% of all ischemic strokes. The clinical diagnosis is based on a variety of findings as shown in Table 20.7. The onset is characteristically abrupt, often occurring in an awake patient.

A stuttering course may be seen in about 10% of patients. This represents a distal lodging of emboli. Most cardiogenic emboli that go to the brain lodge in the middle cerebral artery (MCA) or one of its branches. Vertebrobasilar or anterior cerebral artery emboli occur less frequently

TABLE 20.7. CLINICAL FEATURES SUGGESTIVE OF CARDIOGENIC BRAIN EMBOLISM

Primary Features
Abrupt onset of maximal deficit
Presence of a potential embolic source
Infarct involving the cerebral cortex or cerebellum
Previous ischemic events in other vascular territories
Secondary Evidence
Hemorrhagic infarct by CAT
Absence of occlusive cerebrovascular disease by cerebral angiography or reliable noninvasive imaging
Angiographic evidence of vanishing occlusions
Evidence of embolism to other organs
Cardiac thrombi demonstrated by echocardiography, catheterization, cardiac CAT or MRI

(From Sherman DG, Dyken ML, Fisher M, et al: Cerebral embolism. Chest 1986;89(suppl 2):845, Table 2, with permission.)

(<10%) than MCA emboli. Cardiogenic embolism may be suspected when there are multifocal neurologic findings. Seizure or headache at the onset of the stroke is not as useful an indicator as once thought. Cardiogenic embolism should be considered when the following conditions are present: age over 60, sudden onset of maximal neurologic deficit, prior cortical infarct, past history of valvular heart disease or left ventricular myocardial infarct, and atrial fibrillation or congestive heart failure. Laboratory studies in those with suspected cardiogenic brain embolism may include two-dimensional echocardiography (2-D echo) to assess the presence of left ventricular thrombi and mitral valve dysfunction and M-mode echo for the presence of left ventricular dysfunction. Echo does not reliably indicate atrial thrombi, although transesophogeal echo may be better at detection than 2-D echo. The ECG may indicate a dysrhythmia such as AF. MRI and CT are currently being evaluated for their clinical usefulness in detecting cardiogenic emboli.

INTRACRANIAL HEMORRHAGE

Usually the clinical manifestations of intracranial hemorrhage have an abrupt onset and changes generally occur over minutes to hours (up to 24 hours). This gradual evolution depends primarily on the bleeding rate and accounts for the time range for the neurologic deficit to become maximal. The neurologic physical findings vary with the site of bleeding and the size of the bleed. The majority of patients lose consciousness, and many die without recovering awareness.

Typically, the patient with spontaneous intracerebral hemorrhage may experience head pain and dizziness prior to losing consciousness. In the case of hypertension-related external capsule (putaminal) hemorrhage, the patient quickly develops signs of hemiplegia and loss of consciousness. Hypertensive intracerebral hemorrhages are most often associated with prolonged and sustained hypertension and frequently occur while the patient is awake.

Conjugate deviation of the eyes to the side opposite the affected limbs is commonly seen. If the lesion becomes larger, compression of the upper brainstem produces deepening coma and the patient has dilated and fixed pupils, Babinski signs, bilateral motor hypertonus, and irregular respirations.[63]

In the case of internal capsule (thalamic) hemorrhage, the onset is similar to that for putamenal hemorrhage; however, if the patient is still alert a homonymous hemianopia may be seen because of optic nerve involvement in the internal capsule. The location of this hemorrhage produces a variety of gaze disturbances including defective vertical and lateral gaze, fixed downward deviation of the eyes, and unequal pupils. The reader is referred to other sources for discussion of other types of intracranial hemorrhage.[63]

In the diagnosis of hypertensive intracerebral hemorrhage the sudden onset and quick evolution of the physical findings are important. Headache occurs at the onset in approximately 50% of the cases, whereas the occurrence of headaches in thromboembolism is less than 25%. Neck rigidity is common and the funduscopic examination of the eye may reveal periarteriolar hemorrhages and decreased arteriolar size. Ocular signs are very helpful in localizing hemorrhages of putaminal and thalamic origin. Convulsions are common as is vomiting, and a history of hypertension is an important clue. Generally, the immediate prognosis for intracerebral hemorrhage is extremely poor, with up to 70% of patients dying in a few days.[63]

Important laboratory findings include blood in the CSF and evidence of bleeding on the CT scan. CT is the diagnostic procedure of choice in assessing intracranial and subarachnoid hemorrhage. It is extremely sensitive in detection of blood in very small amounts and is extremely useful in the differential diagnosis of hemorrhage versus infarction.

TREATMENT

GENERAL THERAPEUTIC CONSIDERATIONS

The therapeutic approach to patients with cerebrovascular disease involves multiple phases, including preventive measures against stroke and vascular disease in general, supportive and medical management during the acute phase of a stroke, measures necessary to mitigate the pathologic or atherothrombotic process, and appropriate rehabilitative and physical therapy programs during the poststroke period.

Prevention of cerebrovascular disease is the most important aspect of therapeutic management, and elimination and/or management of the risk factors discussed earlier under the section on Epidemiology and Etiology are required. Control of hypertension, hyperlipidemia, obesity, cigarette smoking, and tobacco use as well as other risk factors for atherothrombotic disease is essential to the overall care of the patient with cerebrovascular disease. In the patient with hypertension who has atherosclerotic cerebrovascular disease or who has developed an ischemic infarction, care must be taken to avoid drug-induced or other hypotensive episodes. In general, preservation of the systemic circulation in acute stroke and avoidance of orthostatic changes are also advised.

SPECIFIC THERAPEUTIC CONSIDERATIONS

As indicated earlier, the focus of this chapter is on ischemic stroke, and the following discussion emphasizes this condition; however, therapeutic management of some of the other types of cerebrovascular disease covered in this chapter is discussed briefly.

Ischemic Cerebrovascular Disease

Anticoagulation Therapy

This mode of therapy was the first to gain acceptance in ischemic cerebrovascular disease, and because this therapy has been used for some time, some conclusions can be drawn about the usefulness of anticoagulation in various types of ischemic cerebrovascular disease. A number of studies have been performed with heparin and coumarin derivatives since the 1970s; however, criticisms of poor design, wrong diagnosis, and inadequate number of patients for comparative purposes have limited the acceptance of these studies.

The following is a brief review of anticoagulation therapy in TIA, progressing stroke, and completed stroke.

Transient Ischemic Attacks. Four randomized prospective studies comparing patients on anticoagulation therapy with control subjects showed no significant difference in the occurrence of stroke or death.[63] Only one of the four studies was a double-blind study; all had small numbers of patients and three studies had short follow-up periods. Although weak, data from these studies indicate that the rate of recurrence of TIAs is reduced. Definite conclusions regarding anticoagulation cannot be stated on the basis of these studies. Six nonrandomized studies have been reported and no reduction was shown in mortality; however, one study did show a decreased incidence of TIAs and one showed a decrease in recurrence of TIAs. It appears from the literature that anticoagulation does not decrease mortality in TIA patients, but it may reduce the rate of recurrence of TIAs and subsequent ischemic infarction.[63]

Progressing Stroke (Stroke-in-Evolution). Three randomized and three nonrandomized studies strongly suggest that anticoagulation is of benefit in this condition.[63] Although these studies are strongly suggestive, they are not conclusive because of flaws in study design. There were only slight differences in mortality in the treated groups (most patients were heparinized); however, there were favorable trends reported in the prevention of stroke progression. Other more recent data point out the variability of patient response to the heparin anticoagulation of acute brain ischemia and the problem of intracerebral hemorrhage in stroke patients.[64–67] It appears that although conclusive statements cannot be made since efficacy is unproven, heparin anticoagulation is still an anecdotal therapy and if it is to be used at all in the acute phase of a progressing stroke it must be made certain that cerebral hemorrhage has not occurred.

Completed Stroke. Seven randomized studies have addressed anticoagulation therapy in completed stroke.[63] These studies showed no difference between treatment and control groups in the incidence of recurrent stroke or death. There is also a risk of major bleeding in patients treated for several months with anticoagulation therapy. Therefore, the risk of anticoagulation therapy in completed stroke outweighs any benefits obtained, and based on the best studies to date, anticoagulation generally should not be used.

The risk of hemorrhage is highest in patients with ischemic cerebrovascular disease when anticoagulation therapy lasts longer than 4 weeks. Compared with other indications for anticoagulation, anticoagulation for stroke is associated with a greater risk of hemorrhagic complications.[63,68] Although intensity of therapy and type of reagents used in laboratory testing were the source of some of the differences in European and North American studies, hemorrhagic complications are still the major risk in anticoagulated patients with ischemic cerebrovascular disease.

Recommendations and Monitoring. It is recommended that anticoagulation not be routinely used in patients with TIAs and not be used at all in patients with completed stroke.[69] The use of anticoagulation in progressing stroke is still controversial; however, individual judgment must be used in this situation when intracerebral hemorrhage has been ruled out by CT scan. Short-term anticoagulation may be useful in TIA patients who refuse surgery for a surgically correctable lesion, who are not surgical candidates for whatever reason, or who are awaiting surgery. Patients who remain symptomatic with TIAs and on aspirin therapy who do not have surgical disease may be candidates for anticoagulation. If anticoagulation is used, careful monitoring is required and heparin should be administered acutely by continuous infusion to a target partial thromboplastin time of 1.5 times control value. In general, if warfarin is to be used to continue chronic anticoagulation, it should overlap with heparin for approximately 5 days to obtain warfarin antithrombotic activity. By maintaining an international normalized ratio of 2.0 to 3.0, a slightly less intensive anticoagulation effect is obtained with a decreased incidence of bleeding without a decrease in efficacy.[70] Continuous monitoring for minor and major bleeding is required.

Antiplatelet Therapy

Antiplatelet agents have been studied for use in ischemic cerebrovascular disease for a number of years; the proposed mechanism of action is an alteration in blood platelet aggregation, thus inhibiting the formation of thrombi in arterial vessels. Several antiplatelet agents have been used; however, aspirin and triclopidine are the only agents currently commercially available with convincing clinical effects.

Aspirin

Aspirin (acetylsalicylic acid) was found in the early 1970s to prevent amaurosis fugax (monocular visual loss); subsequently, in a retrospective study, aspirin was shown to decrease the number of TIAs without affecting the death rate.[71–73] The Aspirin in Transient Ischemic Attack Study was then initiated to study this potential beneficial effect on TIAs.[74] This multicenter study compared the use of 650 mg twice daily with placebo. Only patients with carotid system TIAs were enrolled in the study. In the analysis of the study, when deaths not caused by stroke were excluded, there was a significant difference in favor of the aspirin-treated group in preventing stroke. The study was small and short, and the definite conclusion that aspirin prevents stroke could not be made. The Canadian Cooperative Study Group was then formed and published its results in 1978.[75] This study involved treatment of 585 patients with one or more cerebral or retinal ischemic attacks. These patients were randomized to aspirin, sulfinpyrazone, and placebo. The average follow-up was 26 months and the aspirin dose was 325 mg four times daily and sulfinpyrazone 200 mg four times daily. For the overall study group, aspirin reduced the risk of TIA, stroke, or death by 19%. If only stroke or death was considered, aspirin reduced the risk of these by 31%. Interestingly, there was no significant benefit shown for women in this study, however this sex difference was not confirmed in later studies.[76] Sulfinpyrazone did not show any risk reduction for TIA. Other randomized trials have been done and all show statistically significant differences between aspirin and placebo for some ischemic events.[74,75]

The doses of aspirin used in ischemic cerebrovascular disease studies have ranged from ≤325 mg/d to 1.5 g/d. A controversy now exists over the appropriate dose of aspirin. Although low doses of aspirin (≤325 mg/d) have been shown to be effective in other conditions such as protection against myocardial infarction in unstable angina patients, prevention of coronary bypass shunt thrombosis, and prevention of thrombosis in arteriovenous shunts of chronic hemodialysis patients, the effectiveness of low doses in preventing stroke is just now being determined. One of the recent studies to address the low-dose issue is the United Kingdom Transient Ischemic Attack/Aspirin Trial (UKTIA).[77,78] This is the first large study to evaluate low dose versus high dose (300 mg/d versus 1200 mg/d). Between July 1979 and September 1985, 2435 patients were enrolled in the study. All patients had experienced at least one TIA or mild ischemic stroke within 3 months of entry. The mean age was 60, and 75% of patients were male. Patients were randomly assigned to three groups. One group received 600 mg aspirin twice daily, the second group received 300 mg daily, and the third group received placebo. The dose ranges were selected somewhat arbitrarily, and patients were followed an average of 4 years. Results that have been reported indicate that the incidence of stroke, myocardial infarction, or sudden death was the same in both aspirin-treated groups and 20% lower (statistically significant) than the incidence in the placebo-treated groups. The risk of cerebral infarction alone was 11% higher in the placebo group, although this was not statistically significant. When women were considered separately in the study, no significant differences were found between aspirin and placebo in risk for cerebral infarction or other major vascular event. The investigators note, significantly however, that the number of women in the study was small. Side effects were less frequent with the lower dose of aspirin (29%) as compared with the 1200-mg dose (39%) and were least frequent in the placebo group (24%). Therefore, the lower dose of aspirin in this study was just as effective as the higher dose but had fewer side effects. Although this study showed that aspirin had less effect on fatal events than on nonfatal events, antiplatelet treatment conclusively reduces the risk of nonfatal vascular events.

Another recent study to address the low-dose aspirin issue is the Dutch TIA Trial.[79] This study was a double-blind trial in patients with TIAs or nondisabling stroke. This particular study had a different twist in that two main hypotheses were tested; first is the question of the effectiveness of 30 mg aspirin per day versus 300 mg/d in preventing vascular death and disability, and secondly, is 50 mg of atenolol more effective versus placebo in preventing vascular death and disability? A double randomization technique was used to compare these two different therapeutic modalities. A total of 3131 patients were enrolled and follow-up was 2.6 years. It was found that 30 mg/d of aspirin is no less effective than 300 mg/d in the prevention of the composite outcome event of death from vascular causes, nonfatal stroke, or nonfatal myocardial infarction. There were also fewer adverse effects in the 30 mg/d group. Therefore, a dose of 30 mg/d of aspirin was effective in TIA prevention.

Meta-analysis of 29,000 patients with histories of TIAs, minor strokes, unstable angina, or myocardial infarction was reported by the Antiplatelet Trialists' Collaboration.[80,81] This analysis represented 25 trials. All antiplatelet agents and regimens were evaluated. Results of the analysis showed an overall 25% odds reduction (similar to relative risk reduction) for vascular events (stroke, myocardial infarction, or death from a vascular cause) and a 27% odds reduction in nonfatal stroke.[80] A second meta-analysis from this group evaluated more than 100,000 patients in 145 trials. A 25% overall odds reduction was shown for vascular events and 22% for patients with previous minor stroke or TIAs.[81]

The antiplatelet effects of aspirin are theoretically responsible for aspirin's beneficial antithrombotic effects in TIAs. Aspirin inhibits platelet aggregation by irreversible inactivation of the enzyme cyclooxygenase which, in platelets, prevents conversion of arachidonic acid to thromboxane A_2 (TXA_2), which is a powerful vasoconstrictor and stimulator of platelet aggregation. Platelets remain impaired for their life span (5–7 days) after exposure to aspirin. Aspirin also inhibits prostacyclin activity in the smooth muscle of vascular walls. PGI_2 inhibits platelet aggregation, and the vascular endothelium can synthesize prostacyclin such that the platelet antiaggregating effect is maintained. The suppression of PGI_2 production by aspirin has been found to be dose and duration related; the higher the dose, the longer the cyclooxygenase production is suppressed. Therefore, the lower the aspirin dose, the less effect on prostacyclin. The optimal dose of aspirin is still under study, but it should be the dose that inhibits TXA_2 with the least amount of prostacyclin inhibition. It has been shown that an aspirin dose of 325 mg/d will inhibit TXA_2, but will not significantly inhibit PGI_2 production.[77] There is probably a point at which lower doses of aspirin do not completely block TXA_2, and recent studies indicate the lowest effective dose may be in the range of 20–40 mg/d.[79,82] The effectiveness of doses lower than 300 mg/d for TIA or minor strokes of arterial origin is still not resolved and additional study is required to adequately answer the dose questions. Other potential mechanisms of antithrombotic action of aspirin are currently under investigation.

Pharmacodynamically, as aspirin is converted to salicylate during the normal metabolic process, the ratio of salicylate to aspirin may be important because salicylate may prevent aspirin inhibition of PGI_2. Excessive salicylate concentrations may displace or prevent aspirin from binding to platelets, thereby potentially minimizing the antiplatelet effect of aspirin. Whether or not this proves to be clinically relevant remains to be shown in clinical studies. The interaction can be minimized by using low doses and sustained-release preparations.

Dipyridamole

This drug has weak inhibiting properties *in vitro* on platelet aggregation and it also inhibits platelet phosphodiesterase. Clinical studies have not yielded supportive data for the use of this drug in ischemic cerebrovascular disease, and dipyridamole alone has no role in stroke prevention.[83–85]

Sulfinpyrazone

This agent has been studied in several trials for ischemic cerebrovascular disease. Sulfinpyrazone, like aspirin, produces an inhibition of cyclooxygenase; however, this inhibition is reversible, whereas the aspirin inhibition is not. The drug has metabolites that also have inhibitory effects on cyclooxygenase. Clinical studies have found no beneficial effect for sulfinpyrazone in the treatment of ischemic cerebrovascular disease.[86]

Ticlopidine

This recently approved agent has unique platelet antiaggregatory effects in that it is an inhibitor of the adenosine diphosphate pathway of platelet aggregation and inhibits known stimuli to platelet aggregation.[19,87,88] This effect causes an alteration of the platelet membrane and interference with the membrane–fibrinogenic interaction leading to a blocking of the platelet glycoprotein IIb/IIIa receptor.[89] A time lag of 8–11 days before the antiplatelet effect is maximal should be expected. The bleeding time is prolonged up to fivefold and will return to normal in 14 days after discontinuation. Ticlopidine has been evaluated in two large clinical trials and the results in stroke prevention have been beneficial in both men and women. In the TASS trial, the relative-risk reduction for fatal or nonfatal stroke at 3 years was 21% greater with ticlopidine as compared to aspirin. The CATS trial showed a 30% relative-risk reduction as compared to placebo. Ticlopidine does possess a significant side-effect profile and is costly. Side effects include suppression of bone marrow, rash and diarrhea, and elevation of serum cholesterol. Neutropenia may occur in up to 2% of patients but is reversible on discontinuation of therapy. Monitoring is required because of these side effects and it is recommended that patients have CBCs with differential every 2 weeks for 3 months. More than 50% of patients report at least one side effect with gastrointestinal complaints being the most common. Drug interactions may occur with digoxin, theophylline, and antacids and these efforts should be monitored. Ticlopidine's place in therapy will require further evaluation; however, ticlopidine (500 mg/d) in divided doses of 250 mg/d can be recommended as an alternative to aspirin in those patients who cannot tolerate aspirin or in whom aspirin treatment has not been effective.[19,90,91]

Recommendations and Monitoring

Clinical trials have shown the beneficial effects of aspirin in men in prevention of secondary TIAs as well as in producing a decrease in major vascular events. The National Conference on Antithrombotic Therapy in 1986 recommended an aspirin dose of 1 g/d for patients with TIAs.[69] With the more recent evidence a lower dose of aspirin is appropriate. A dose of 325–975 mg/d is recommended in preventing TIAs and stroke. An enteric-coated product may be better tolerated by some individuals and may be used if needed. Patients should be monitored for gastrointestinal bleeding since the risk for bleeding is slightly increased. Triclopidine is effective for the secondary prevention of stroke. It is superior to aspirin in patients with TIAs; however, ticlopidine is less tolerable and more costly than aspirin. Ticlopidine 250 mg twice daily should be used if aspirin has failed to decrease or eliminate TIAs or if the patient cannot tolerate or has an allergy to aspirin. Patients require careful monitoring while on ticlopidine as noted previously, particularly during the first 3 months of therapy.

Surgical Therapy

The purpose of surgery in ischemic cerebrovascular disease is to prevent the occurrence of cerebral infarctions and TIAs. Generally, the goal of a surgical procedure is to remove the source of occlusion and/or embolus and, hopefully, to increase cerebral blood flow to an ischemic area.

Carotid endarterectomy (CEA) is the most common surgical procedure used for occlusive cerebrovascular disease. This procedure has been popular since its introduction over 30 years ago. CEA involves exposing the carotid artery in the neck and removing the occlusive atheromatous plaque usually at the carotid bifurcation. The indications have generally been considered to be TIAs and mild completed stroke in the presence of ulcerated or highly stenotic (>75%) plaque.[18] Two recent ongoing multicenter studies of CEA in symptomatic carotid artery disease have been reported: the North American Symptomatic Carotid Endarterectomy Trial Collaborators (NASCET) and the European Carotid Surgery Trial (ECST). In both of these trials, interim analysis showed that for symptomatic patients with stenosis of 70% or greater, CEA was superior to medical treatment alone at 2–3 years. In both studies, surgery was not beneficial in patients with less than 70% stenosis. The rate of complications such as stroke or death of CEA for an institution should be equal to or better than NASCET (<5%) in order to have an acceptable risk-to-benefit ratio.[92,93] Other indications such as asymptomatic bruits and progressing stroke are controversial; however, results from the Asymptomatic Cartoid Atherosclerosis Study (ACAS) show that symptom-free patients with 60 to 99% carotid artery stenosis had a 55% relative risk reduction for ipsilateral stroke or any stroke or death after carotid endarectomy compared with medical therapy. This information may have significant future implications in asymptomatic patients.[94–96] CEA is not indicated in patients with permanent deficits from moderate to severe completed strokes. For patients with a complete occlusion of an extracranial vessel, CEA is usually unsuccessful, and these patients may be considered for an extracranial–intracranial (EC-IC) bypass procedure.[92] The most common EC-IC bypass procedure is anastomosis of the superficial temporal artery to a branch of the middle cerebral artery. This can augment blood flow to the brain by bypassing the stenotic or occluded artery. The clinical efficacy of this procedure has been disputed by a recent large international trial and the results indicate that this procedure does not prevent stroke.[19] However, an editorial review of that trial indicates that certain other subsets of patients may benefit from this procedure.[95,96] In any event, further well-controlled studies are needed to clarify this point.

Investigational Therapy

Investigational therapy for prevention of TIAs and stroke includes thromboxane synthetase inhibitors, such as imidazole and dazoxiben.[19,69] Therapy to improve or reverse the effects of an acute stroke is being actively pursued and includes prostacyclin and the calcium channel blocking agents nimodipine and nicardipine.[97–100] These agents are currently being tested in clinical trials; however, calcium channel blockers have not shown convincing evidence in reducing infarct size. Another agent, naloxone, has been studied in ischemic cerebrovascular disease; however, controlled trials have failed to show beneficial effects. Other therapies with steroids, vasoactive agents, and barbiturates have shown no benefit. Low molecular weight heparins and heparinoids are currently under study in ischemic stroke. They appear to have a decreased bleeding tendency and the potential of these compounds is promising.[101] The use of fibrinolysins such as tissue plasminogen activator has been promising in animal stroke studies and multicenter randomized trials in acute ischemic stroke are ongoing. Ancrod (pit viper venom extract) is still experimental. Research with glutamate receptor antagonists, such as the NMDA receptor subtype, is ongoing and there is promise that infarct size reduction can be attained.[19]

CEREBRAL EMBOLISM OF CARDIAC ORIGIN

In patients with cardiogenic brain embolism, immediate anticoagulation should be considered because approximately 12% of such patients have a second embolic stroke within 2 weeks.[46] In nonhypertensive patients with small to moderate stroke, heparin should be given 24 hours after stroke onset without a loading dose so that a less intensive anticoagulation effect is obtained. The partial thromboplastin time (PTT) should be no greater than 1.5 times the control value using rabbit brain thromboplastin. Before heparin is started, however, a CT scan should document the absence of spontaneous hemorrhagic transformation. Anticoagulation should be maintained with warfarin at an INR of 2.0 to 3.0. In patients who develop hemorrhagic transformation shortly after embolic stroke, anticoagulation should be postponed 8–10 days.

The role of platelet antiaggregating agents in this situation is not clear; however, antiplatelet agents are generally not recognized to have therapeutic value in those instances where red thrombi can develop, as in patients with cardiac mural thrombi, venous thrombosis, or large thrombi in any artery.[19] Anticoagulation with warfarin is recommended in these situations. Obviously, prevention of the embolic event is the best therapy, and those patients at high risk for cardiogenic embolism, such as patients with atrial fibrillation or mechanical or prosthetic valves, should be treated with prophylactic chronic anticoagulation with warfarin.[47] Six recent studies looking at preventative therapy in patients with nonvalvular atrial fibrillation (NVAF) have been completed. Five were primary intervention trials and one (EAFT) was for secondary intervention.[50]

The Copenhagen Atrial Fibrillation, Aspirin, Anticoagulation Study (AFASAK) evaluated 1007 older patients (median age = 74.2 years) treated with either warfarin (INR=2.8–4.2), aspirin (75 mg/d), or placebo. Patients were followed for an average of 11 months. The primary endpoints were ischemic stroke, transient cerebral ischemia, and systemic embolism. There was benefit to warfarin (although there was a large dropout rate in the warfarin group) but not to aspirin in preventing thromboembolic events.[102] In a recent report Petersen[103] performed an intention-to-treat analysis of all thromboembolic complications in those patients receiving treatment and in those who withdrew from the study. Using an efficacy analysis, total deaths and vascular death were significantly lower in the anticoagulant group; however, using the intention-to-treat analysis there was no difference in either total or vascular mortality. The Stroke Prevention in Atrial Fibrillation Study (SPAF 1) evaluated 1244 patients randomly assigned to one of two groups. Group 1 patients took warfarin (INR=1.7–4.6), aspirin (325 mg/d), or placebo. Group 2 patients took aspirin or placebo. Patients were followed for a mean of 1.3 years. The primary endpoints were ischemic stroke and systemic embolism. Although aspirin did not show benefit in patients over 75 years, the study was stopped early because of the beneficial effects of warfarin and aspirin in group 1 as compared to placebo.[52] The Canadian Atrial Fibrillation Anticoagulation Study (CAFA) evaluated 383 patients in a primary prevention trial with a warfarin target INR of 2.0–3.0 compared to placebo. The clinical outcomes were similar to those in the AFASAK trial except that TIAs were not included. Warfarin reduction of stroke and systemic embolism was statistically significant as compared to placebo. The Stroke Prevention in Nonrheumatic Atrial Fibrillation Study (SPINAF) was a primary prevention trial of 525 subjects with a warfarin target INR of 1.4–2.8 compared to placebo. The outcome measured was stroke rate. Results showed that warfarin significantly reduced the rate of stroke as compared to placebo.

The Boston Area Anticoagulation Trial for Atrial Fibrillation (BAATAF) studied 420 patients who were randomly assigned to warfarin (INR = 1.5–2.7) or control (no therapy). Aspirin, however, was taken by 46% of the patients in the control group. The follow-up was for 2.2 years and the primary endpoint was ischemic stroke. The follow-up methodology was done by phone and mail survey and was done infrequently. This issue raises concern about the validity of the data collected. The patients in the low-dose warfarin group had significantly lower death and stroke rates as compared to controls.[104] The European Atrial Fibrillation Trial (EAFT) was a secondary prevention study of warfarin and aspirin. Two groups were created in which 1007 patients participated. Group 1 compared warfarin to placebo and aspirin (325 mg/d) and group 2 compared aspirin and placebo. The primary endpoints were death from vascular disease, have failed stroke and MI, or systemic embolism. Target INR was 2.4–4.0 and the average duration was 2.3 years. Warfarin significantly reduced the risk of all strokes compared to placebo and aspirin. In summary, these studies indicate that patients with NVAF can be effectively and safely treated with either warfarin or aspirin. The overall reduction of the relative risk of stroke in AF patients treated with warfarin was 64% compared to placebo and aspirin was 22% compared to placebo.[105] In addition, warfarin may be the agent of choice in the stasis-related thromboembolism seen in patients with NVAF and heart failure.

Recommendations

Because of the potential of intracerebral hemorrhage in elderly patients and the probability of lifetime treatment with warfarin, identification of subgroups of AF patients with high and low rates of stroke has been studied in two large trials (SPAF I and SPAF II).[50] As shown in Table 20.3 AF patients with certain risk factors are more likely to develop stroke than those without these factors. Data from SPAF II indicate that the risk of thromboembolism in AF patients 75 years or younger given aspirin is low, less than 3%/year, and that younger low-risk AF patients can be treated with 325 mg/d aspirin for stroke prevention. High-risk patients in whom anticoagulation is judged to be safe can be treated with warfarin to an INR of 2.0–3.0. High-risk patients older than 75 years may be treated with lower intensity warfarin at an INR of 2.0. Aspirin is the alternative. In those AF patients who have had an ischemic stroke or TIA, anticoagulation will be necessary for most patients. Lone AF should be managed with aspirin.

Patients who have had prosthetic cardiac valve replacement have a clinically significant and long-term risk of thromboembolism. The pathophysiologic events that precede arterial thromboembolism actually begin as soon as the device is sewn in place and blood flows across the PCV. Generally, patients who have undergone aortic valve replacement are at a lower risk of thromboembolism than those with mitral PCV. Patients with both aortic and mitral valve replacement are usually considered to have the highest risk of thromboembolism. Other risk factors for thromboembolism include presence of atrial fibrillation, a large left atrium, previous thromboembolism, left ventricular dysfunction, and valve type and design.[19,47,59]

Treatment recommendations for patients with mechanical PCVs are based on prospective randomized trials of anticoagulant therapy with and without a platelet inhibitor.[59] These trials indicate that oral anticoagulation plus dipyridamole decreased the incidence of thromboembolism when compared to anticoagulation alone. Aspirin plus anticoagulation was found to produce excessive major bleeding (primarily gastrointestinal) when compared to warfarin plus dipyridamole. Oral anticoagulation plus dipyridamole for prevention of mechanical PCV induced thromboembolism in a now Food and Drug Administration (FDA)-approved therapy. Thromboembolism is less frequent after bioprosthetic valve replacement. Even though the thrombogenicity of bioprosthetic valves is lower than that of mechanical valves, specific therapy is still required. The current recommendations for antithrombotic therapy for PCV replacement are presented for mechanical and bioprosthetic valves.[62]

Mechanical PCVs

Therapy should begin with intravenous heparin 6 hours after surgery to maintain the activated partial thromboplastin time at 1.5 to 2 times control followed by subcutaneous heparin, 10,000 U every 12 hours after chest tube removal continuing until discharge. Warfarin should be started as soon as possible after operation and dosed to maintain the prothrombin time at an INR of 2.5–3.5. Aspirin 160 mg/d should be added to warfarin and may offer additional protection. Dipyridamole 5–6 mg/kg divided every 6 hours may be added to warfarin as as alternative to the warfarin–aspirin combination. For those patients who cannot take oral anticoagulants, dipyridamole plus sulfinpyrazone 800 mg/d may be tried empirically.

Bioprosthetic PCVs

Initial therapy with heparin is similar to mechanical PCVs as previously described. In those patients with aortic valve replacement who are in sinus rhythm, anticoagulation is optional. Aspirin 325 mg/d can be used empirically. For patients who have mitral valve replacement, initiate warfarin therapy as soon as possible after operation and for 3 months thereafter, at a less intense INR of 2.0–3.0. Aspirin 325 mg/d long term is optional. For patients who have atrial fibrillation, an enlarged left atrium or previous thromboembolism, warfarin should be continued indefinitely at an INR of 2.0 to 3.0.

INTRACRANIAL HEMORRHAGE

General medical management and supportive therapy are indicated in the patient with this condition. This condition, as noted earlier, has a generally poor prognosis. Preventive therapy of intracranial bleeding is possible in the case of hypertension, where blood pressure can be controlled by diet and/or medication. Surgical management in the acute or early stage of the event is removal of the clot by aspiration or evacuation; this treatment is usually beneficial only in those patients whose hemorrhage is near the surface of the brain and who are not comatose. Cerebellar hemorrhage, on the other hand, is often amenable to surgery within the first 2 days of onset.

Corticosteroids and, more recently, dexamethasone have been used in the treatment of cerebral edema resulting from primary intracerebral hemorrhage. A recent study has shown no beneficial effect; in fact, a harmful effect (infection and diabetic complications) was seen.[106] Therefore, the use of dexamethasone in this condition should be reconsidered. The use of mannitol and other osmotic agents to reduce edema around the hemorrhage is appropriate, provided systemic hypotensive and hypertensive episodes are avoided. The use of mannitol is well established and is guided by maintaining the serum osmolality and arterial pressure. Generally, 0.25–2 g/kg mannitol intravenously can be administered every 4–8 hours until the serum osmolality is raised between 300 and 310 mOsm/L. Cerebral edema is rarely a problem in ischemic stroke unless a very large MCA territory infarction occurs. Treatment is the same as noted above for intracranial hemorrhage. Cerebral vasospasm in subarachnoid hemorrhage can be severe and therapeutic efforts to prevent or treat the vasospasm have been disappointing. Reserpine, kanamycin, isoproterenol, aminophylline, and nitroprusside have all failed in this condition. Recently, dopamine (3–6 μg/kg/min) has been used, but there is a risk of rebleeding. Percutaneous intra-arterial angioplasty, although not recommended, may be considered when vasospasm persists in spite of optimal medical treatment. However, data from well-designed trials are lacking. Barbiturate coma has been used to reduce intracranial pressure resulting from intracerebral hemorrhage when pressure reduction with dopamine or mannitol has not been successful. Further research is needed in the treatment of cerebral vasospasm and the resulting increased intracranial pressure.[107–109]

REFERENCES

1. Abbott RD, Yin Y, Reed DM, et al. Risk of stroke in male cigarette smokers. N Engl J Med 1986;315:717–720.
2. Kannel WB, Blaisdell FW, Gifford R, et al. Risk factors in stroke. Stroke 1971;2:423.
3. Gillum RF. Cerebrovascular disease morbidity in the United States, 1970–1983—age, sex, region, and vascular surgery. Stroke 1986;17:656–661.
4. Garraway WM, Whisnant JP, Furlan AJ, et al. The declining incidence of stroke. N Engl J Med 1979;300:449.
5. Dyken ML, Wolf PA, Barnett HJM, et al. Risk factors in stroke—a statement for physicians by the Subcommittee on Risk Factors and Stroke of the Stroke Council. Stroke 1984;15:1105–1111.
6. Kurtzke JF. Epidemiology of cerebrovascular disease, in Cerebrovascular Survey Report for Joint Council Subcommittee on Cerebrovascular Disease. National Institute of Neurological and Communicative Disorders and Stroke and National Heart and Lung Institute (revised). Rochester, NY, Whiting Press, 1980, pp 135–176.
7. Anonymous. Heart and Stroke Facts: 1995 Statistical Supplement. Dallas, American Heart Association, 1994.
8. Wolf PA, Kannel WB, Verter J. Current status of risk factors for stroke. Neurol Clin 1983;1:317.
9. Robins M, Baum HM. The National Survey of Stroke Incidence. Stroke 1981;12(supp 1):1–45.
10. Heyman A, Karp HR, Heyden S, et al. Cerebrovascular disease in the biracial population of Evans County, Georgia. Arch Intern Med 1971;128:949.
11. Schoenberg BS, Schoenberg DS, Pritchard DA, et al. Differential risk factors for completed stroke and transient ischemic attacks (TIA): Study of vascular diseases (hypertension, cardiac disease, peripheral vascular disease) and diabetes mellitus, in Duvoisin RC (ed): Transactions of the American Neurological Association. New York, Springer, 1980, vol 105, p 165.

12. Wolf PA. Hypertension as a risk factor for stroke, in Whisnant JP, Sandok B (eds): Cerebral Vascular Diseases. New York, Grune and Stratton, 1975, pp 105–112.
13. Kannel WB, Wolf PA, Verter J, et al. Epidemiologic assessment of the role of blood pressure in stroke: The Framingham study. JAMA 1970;214:301.
14. Hypertension Detection and Follow-up Program Cooperative Group. Five year findings of the Hypertension Detection and Follow-up Program. III. Reduction in stroke incidence among persons with high blood pressure. JAMA 1982;247:633.
15. Wolf PA, Abbott RD, Kannel WB. Atrial fibrillation as an independent risk factor for stroke: The Framingham study. Stroke, 1991;22:983–988.
16. Hart RG, Halperin JL. Atrial fibrillation and stroke. Revisiting the dilemmas. Stroke 1994;25:1337–1341.
17. Chesebro JH, Fuster V, Halperin JL. Atrial fibrillation—risk marker for stroke. N Engl J Med 1990;323:1556–1558.
18. Easton JD, Hart RG, Sherman DG, et. al. Diagnosis and management of ischemic stroke. Part 1. Threatened stroke and its management. Curr Probl Cardiol 1983;8:1–80.
19. Anonymous. Stroke 1989. Recommendations on stroke prevention, diagnosis, and therapy. Report of the WHO Task Force on stroke and other cerebrovascular disorders. Stroke 1989;20:1407–1431.
20. Tohgi J, Yamanouchi H, Murakami M, et al. Importance of the hematocrit as a risk factor in cerebral infarction. Stroke 1978;9:369.
21. Thomas DJ, Marshall J, Russell RWR, et al. Effect of haematocrit on cerebral blood flow in man. Lancet 1977;2:941.
22. Portnoy BA, Herion JC. Neurological manifestations in sickle-cell disease, with a review of the literature and emphasis on the prevalence of hemiplegia. Ann Intern Med 1972;76:643.
23. Kannel WB, Gordon T, Wolf PA, et al. Hemoglobin and the risk of cerebral infarction: The Framingham study. Stroke 1972;3:409.
24. Harrison MJG, Pollock S, Kendall BE, et al. Effect of haematocrit on carotid stenosis and cerebral infarction. Lancet 1981;2:114.
25. Welin L, Svardsudd K, Wilhelmsen L, et al. Analysis of risk factors for stroke in a cohort of men born in 1913. N Engl J Med 1987;317:521–526.
26. Adult Treatment Panel II. National Cholesterol Education Program: Second report of the Expert Panel on Detection, Evaluation, and Treatment of High Blood Cholesterol in Adults. Circulation 1994;89;1333–1445.
27. Havel RJ. Biology of cholesterol, lipoproteins and atherosclerosis. Clin Exp Hypertens 1989;11:887–900.
28. Scandinavian Simvastatin Survival Study Group. Randomized trial of cholesterol lowering in 4444 patients with coronary heart disease: The Scandinavian Simvastatin Survival Study (4S). Lancet 1994;344:1383–1389.
29. Gill JS, Zezulka AV, Shipley MJ, et al. Stroke and alcohol consumption. N Engl J Med 1986;315:1042–1046.
30. Donnan GA, McNeil JJ, Adena MA, et al. Smoking as a risk factor for cerebral ischaemia. Lancet 1989;643–647.
31. Paffenbarger RS, Williams JL. Chronic disease in former college students. V. Early precursors of fatal stroke. Am J Public Health 1967;57:1290.
32. Grady PA. Pathophysiology of extracranial cerebral artery stenosis. A critical review. Stroke 1984;15:224–234.
33. Nerem RM. Arterial fluid dynamics and interactions with the vessel walls, in Schwartz CJ, Wertheisen NT, Wolf S (eds): Structure and Function of the Circulation. New York, Plenum, 1981, vol 2, pp 719–835.
34. Pessin MS, Hinton RC, Davis KR, et al. Mechanisms of acute carotid stroke. Ann Neurol 1979;5:152–157.
35. Gunning AJ, Pickering GW, Robb-Smith AHT, et al. Mural thrombosis of the carotid artery and subsequent embolism. Q J Med 1964;33:155–195.
36. Kistler JP, Ropper AH, Heros RC. Therapy of ischemic cerebral vascular disease due to atherothrombosis. N Engl J Med 1984;311:27–34.
37. DeWeese JA, May AG, Lipchick EO, et al. Anatomic and hemodynamic correlations in carotid artery stenosis. Stroke 1970;1:149–157.
38. Fisher M. Occlusion of the internal carotid artery. Arch Neurol Psychiatry 1951;65:346–377.
39. Tolle JF. Cerebrovascular Disorders, 3rd ed. New York, Raven, 1984, pp 214–230.
40. Ames A, Wright RL, Kowada M, et al. Cerebral ischemia. II. The no-reflow phenomenon. Am J Pathol 1968;52:437–453.
41. Meyer FB, Sundt TM, Yanagihara T, et al. Focal cerebral ischemia: Pathophysiologic mechanisms and rationale for future avenues of treatment. Mayo Clin Proc 1987;62:35–55.
42. Sundt TM, Davis DH. Reactions of cerebrovascular smooth muscle to blood and ischemia: Primary versus secondary vasospasm, in Wilkins RH (ed): Cerebral Arterial Spasm. Baltimore, MD, Williams and Wilkins, 1980, pp 244–250.
43. Sundt TM, Waltz AG. Cerebral ischemia and reactive hyperemia: Studies of cortical blood flow and microcirculation before, during, and after temporary occlusion of middle cerebral artery of squirrel monkeys. Circ Res 1971;28:426–433.
44. Matsumoto M, Hatakeyama T, Yanagihara T. Combination of cerebral blood flow measurement and immunohistochemical technique in cerebral ischemia [abstract]. Stroke 1986;17:137.
45. Mohr JP. Lacunes. Stroke 1982;13:3–11.
46. Fisher CM. Capsular infarcts. The underlying vascular lesions. Arch Neurol 1979;36:65–73.
47. Sherman DG, Dyken ML, Gent M, et al. Antithrombotic therapy for cerebrovascular disorders. An update. Chest 1995;108(supp):444S–456S.
48. Cerebral Embolism Task Force. Cardiogenic brain embolism. The second report of the Cerebral Embolism Task Force. Arch Neurol 1989;46:727–743.
49. Friedman GD, Loveland DB, Ehrlich SP. Relationship of stroke to other cardiovascular disease. Circulation 1968;38:533–541.
50. Nelson KM, Talbert RL. Preventing stroke in patients with nonrheumatic atrial fibrillation. Am J Hosp Pharm 1994;51:1175–1183.
51. Hinton RC, Kistler JP, Fallon JT, et al. Influence of etiology of atrial fibrillation on incidence of systemic embolism. Am J Cardiol 1977;40:509–513.
52. Stroke Prevention in Atrial Fibrillation Investigators. Predictors of thromboembolism in atrial fibrillation, I: Clinical features of patients at risk. Ann Intern Med 1992;116:1–5.

53. Bharucha NE, Wolf PA, Kannel WB, et al. Epidemiological study of cerebral embolism: The Framingham study [abstract]. Ann Neurol 1981;10:105.
54. Tegeler C. Carotid stenosis in atrial fibrillation [abstract]. Neurology 1989;39(suppl):159.
55. Bjerkelund CJ, Orning OM. The efficacy of anticoagulant therapy in preventing embolism related to D.C. electrical conversion of atrial fibrillation. Am J Cardiol 1969;23:208–216.
56. Chesebro JH, Ezekowitz M, Badimon L, et al. Intracardiac thrombi and systemic thromboembolism: Detection, incidence, and treatment. Ann Rev Med 1985;36:579–605.
57. Stroke Prevention in Atrial Fibrillation Investigators. Predictors of thromboembolism in atrial fibrillation, II: Echocardiographic features of patients at risk. Ann Intern Med 1992;116:6–12.
58. Abernathy WS, Willis PW. Thromboembolic complications of rheumatic heart disease. Cardiovasc Clin 1973;5:131.
59. Askey JM, Berstein S. The management of rheumatic heart disease in relation to systemic arterial embolism. Prog Cardiovasc Dis 1960;3:220.
60. Chesebro JH, Adams PC, Fuster V, et al. Antithrombotic therapy in patients with valvular heart disease and prosthetic heart valves. J Am Coll Cardiol 1986;8:41B–56B.
61. Fuster V, Pumphrey CW, McGoon MD, et al. Systemic thromboembolism in mitral and aortic Starr–Edwards prosthesis: A long term follow-up. Circulation 1982;66(suppl 1):1–157.
62. Barnett HJM. Cerebrovascular disease, in Wyngarden JB, Smith LD (eds): Cecil Textbook of Medicine, 18th ed. Philadelphia, WB Saunders, 1988, pp 2159–2180.
63. Stein PD, Alpert JS, Copeland J. et al. Antithrombotic therapy in patients with mechanical and prosthetic heart valves. Chest 1995;108(suppl):371S–379S.
64. Miller VT, Hart RG. Heparin anticoagulation in acute brain ischemia. Stroke 1988;19:403–406.
65. Slivka A, Levy D. Natural history of progressive ischemic stroke in a population treated with heparin. Stroke 1990;21:1657–1662.
66. Babikian VL, Kase CS, Pessin MS, et al. Intracerebral hemorrhage in stroke patients anticoagulated with heparin. Stroke 1989;20:1500–1503.
67. Estol CJ, Pessin MS. Anticoagulation: Is there still a role in atherothrombotic stroke? Stroke 1990;21:820–824.
68. Levine MN, Raskob G, Hirsh J. Risk of haemorrhage with long term anticoagulant therapy. Drugs 1985;30:444–460.
69. Dalen JE, Hirsh J. American College of Chest Physicians and the National Heart, Lung, and Blood Institute National Conference on Antithrombotic Therapy. Arch Intern Med 1986;146:462–472.
70. Hirsh J, Dalen JE, Deykin D, Poller L, Bussey H. Mechanism of action, clinical effectiveness, and optimal therapeutic range. Chest 1995;108(suppl):2315–2465.
71. Harrison MJG, Marshall J, Meadows JC, et al. Effect of aspirin in amaurosis fugax. Lancet 1971;2:743–745.
72. Mundall J, Quintero P, von Kaulla KN, et al. Transient monocular blindness and increased platelet aggregability treated with aspirin. Neurology 1972;22:280–285.
73. Dyken ML, Kolar OJ, Jones FH. Differences in the occurrence of carotid ischemic attack associated with antiplatelet aggregation therapy. Stroke 1973;4:732–736.
74. Fields WS, Lemak NA, Frankowski RF, et al. Controlled trial of aspirin in cerebral ischemia. Stroke 1977;8:301–306.
75. The Canadian Cooperative Study Group. A randomized trial of aspirin and sulfinpyrazone in threatened stroke. N Engl J Med 1978;299:53–59.
76. Kelton JG, Hirsh J, Carter CJ, et al. Sex differences in the antithrombotic effects of aspirin. Blood 1978;52:1073–1076.
77. Merz B. Multicenter study indicates one aspirin can do the job of four in preventing stroke. JAMA 1987;257:2134–2135.
78. UK–TIA Study Group. United Kingdom transient ischaemic attack (UK–TIA) aspirin trial: Interim results. Brit Med J 1988;296:316–320.
79. The Dutch TIA Study Group. The Dutch TIA trial: Protective effects of low-dose aspirin and atenolol in patients with transient ischemic attacks or nondisabling stroke. Stroke 1988;19:512–517.
80. Antiplatelet Trialists' Collaboration. Secondary prevention of vascular disease by prolonged antiplatelet treatment. BMJ 1988;296:320–331.
81. Antiplatelet Trialists' Collaboration. Collaborative overview of randomized trials of antiplatelet therapy. I. Prevention of death, myocardial infarction, and stroke by prolonged antiplatelet therapy in various categories of patients. BMJ 1994;308:81–106
82. Weksler BB, Tack-Goldman K, Subramanian A, et al. Cumulative inhibitory effect of low-dose aspirin on vascular prostacyclin and platelet thromboxane production in patients with atherosclerosis. Circulation 1985;71:332–340.
83. Merz B. Why a little aspirin is better than a lot. JAMA 1987;257:2135.
84. Acheson J, Danta G, Hutchinson EC. Controlled trial of dipyridamole in cerebral vascular disease. Br J Med 1969;1:614–615.
85. The American–Canadian Cooperative Study Group. Persantine aspirin trial in cerebral ischemia. Part II. Endpoint results. Stroke 1985;16:406–415.
86. Barnett HJM, Gent M, Sackett DL. The Canadian Cooperative Study Group: A randomized trial of aspirin and sulfinpyrazone in treated strokes. N Engl J Med 1978;299:53–59.
87. Gordon JL, Overview: Pharmacology of ticlopidine. Agents Action 1984;(suppl 15):108–115.
88. Hass WK, Easton D, Adams HP, et al. A randomized trial comparing ticlopidine hydrochloride with aspirin for the prevention of stroke in high-risk patients. N Engl J Med 1989;321:501–507.
89. Saltiel E, Ward A. Ticlopidine: A review of its pharmacodynamic and pharmacokinetic properties, and therapeutic efficacy in platelet-dependent disease states. Drugs 1987;34:222–262.
90. Gent M, Blakely JA, Easton JD, et al. The Canadian American Ticlopidine Study (CATS) in thromboembolic stroke. Design, organization, and baseline results. Stroke 1988;19:1203–1210.
91. Robert S. Miller AJ, Fagan SC. Ticlopidine: A new antiplatelet agent for cerebrovascular disease. Pharmacotherapy 1991;11(4):317–325.
92. North American Symptomatic Carotid Endarterectomy Trial Collaborators. Beneficial effect of carotid endarterectomy in symptomatic patients with high-grade carotid stenosis. N Engl J Med 1991;325:445–453.

93. European Carotid Surgery Trialists' Collaborative Group. MRC European Carotid Surgery Trial: Interim results for symptomatic patients with severe (70–99%) or with mild (0–29%) carotid stenosis. Lancet 1991;337:1235–1243.
94. Chambers BR, Norris JW. Outcome in patients with asymptomatic bruits. N Engl J Med 1986;315:860–865.
95. EC/IC Bypass Study Group. Failure of extracranial–intracranial arterial bypass to reduce the risk of ischemic stroke. Results of an international randomized trial. N Engl J Med 1985;313:1191–1200.
96. Executive Committee for the Asymptomatic Carotid Atherosclerosis Study. Endarterectomy for asymptomatic carotid artery stenosis. JAMA 1995;273:1421–1428.
97. Huczynski J, Kostha-Trabka E, Sotowska W, et al. Double blind controlled trial of the therapeutic effects of prostacyclin in patients with completed ischaemic stroke. Stroke 1985;16:810–814.
98. Philips JW, DeLong RE, Rowner JK. The effects of nifedipine and felodipine on cerebral blood flow during anoxic episodes. Stroke 1986;17:229–234.
99. Mabe H, Nagai H, Tukagi T, et al. Effect of nimodipine on cerebral functional and metabolic recovery following ischemia in the rat brain. Stroke 1986;17:501–505.
100. Gelmers HJ, Gorter K, DeWeerdt CJ, et al. A controlled trial of nimodipine in acute ischemic stroke. N Eng J Med 1988;318:203–207.
101. Massey EW, Biller J, Davis JN, et al. Large-dose infusion of heparinoid ORG 10172 in ischemic stroke. Stroke 1990;21:1289–1292.
102. Petersen P, Boysen G, Godtfredsen J, et al. Placebo controlled, randomized trial of warfarin and aspirin for prevention of thromboembolic complications in chronic atrial fibrillation: The Copenhagen AFASAK study. Lancet 1989;1:175–179.
103. Petersen P. Thromboembolic complications in atrial fibrillation. Stroke 1990;21:4–13.
104. The Boston Area Anticoagulation Trial for Atrial Fibrillation Investigators. The effect of low-dose warfarin on the risk of stroke in patients with non-rheumatic atrial fibrillation. N Engl J Med 1990;323:1505–1511.
105. Barnett HJM, Eliasziw M, Meldrum HE. Drugs and surgery in the prevention of ischemic stroke. N Engl J Med 1995;332:238–248.
106. Poungvarin N, Bhoopat W, Viriyavejakul A, et al. Effects of dexamethasone in primary supratentorial intracerebral hemorrhage. N Engl J Med 1987;316:1229–1233.
107. Aitkenhead A. Cerebral protection. Br J Hosp Med 1986;35(May):290–297.
108. Cook DA. The pharmacology of cerebral vasospasm. Pharmacology 1984;29:1–16.
109. Woster PS, LeBlanc KL. Management of elevated intracranial pressure. Clin Pharm 1990;9:762–772.

Chapter 21

Hyperlipidemia

Robert L. Talbert, PharmD, FCCP

Cholesterol, triglycerides, and phospholipids are the major lipids in the body and they are transported as complexes of lipid and specialized proteins (apolipoproteins) known as lipoproteins. Plasma lipoproteins are spherical particles with a surface that consists largely of phospholipid, free cholesterol, and protein, and a core that consists mostly of triglyceride and cholesterol ester (Fig. 21.1). Abnormalities of plasma lipoproteins can result in a predisposition of coronary artery disease, pancreatitis, xanthomas, or neurologic disease. Accumulating evidence over the last three decades had linked elevated total and low-density-lipoprotein cholesterol (LDL-C) and reduced high-density-lipoprotein cholesterol (HDL-C) to the development of coronary heart disease (CHD). Premature coronary atherosclerosis, leading to the manifestations of ischemic heart disease (see Chapter 14), is the most common and significant consequence of hyperlipidemia. In 1994, the National Cholesterol Education Program (NCEP) Adult Treatment Panel II (ATP II) published their second report summarizing these data and giving recommendations for the management of hypercholesterolemia in adults.[1]

Epidemiology

Total cholesterol and LDL-C increase throughout life in men and women, representing an atherogenic pattern characteristic of Westernized society (Fig. 21.2). Based on the National Health and Nutrition Examination Survey (1988–1991) and ATP II guidelines, 40% of all adults ages 20–74 years would require fasting lipoprotein analysis and 29% (52 million Americans) would be candidates for dietary therapy. Assuming that dietary intervention would reduce LDL-C by ~10%, then about 7% (approximately 12.7 million Americans) might be candidates for lipid-lowering drugs. This reflects about 4 million Americans with known CHD and about 8.7 million adults without established CHD. Of the latter group, up to 3.1 million are ages 65 years and older.[2] While these numbers seem staggering in their enormity, substantial progress has been made and the number of Americans with a desirable blood cholesterol level has risen to 49% from 45% from the earlier survey (1976–1980).

Data from the Framingham study and other studies demonstrate that the risk for developing cardiovascular disease is related to the degree of cholesterol and LDL-C elevation in a graded, continuous fashion.[3,4] Hypercholesterolemia is additive to the other nonlipid risk factors for CHD including cigarette smoking, hypertension, diabetes, and electrocardiographic abnormalities (Fig. 21.3). The presence of established CHD or prior myocardial infarction (MI) increases the risk of MI five to seven times that seen in men or women without CHD, and LDL-C is a significant predictor of subsequent morbidity and mortality.[1] Approximately 50% of all MIs and at least 70% of CHD deaths occur in patients with known CHD and, therefore, these patients should be a target for screening, identification, and treatment. Unfortunately, the identification of patients at high risk due to hypercholesterolemia or other lipid disorders is too frequently overlooked since blood lipid levels are not always evaluated in this population even after an event such as myocardial infarction.[5,6]

Comparison of the United States to other countries has shown similar relationships between total cholesterol, LDL-C, and an inverse relationship with HDL-C to coronary artery disease mortality (Fig. 21.4). On a positive note, the U.S. mortality rate is midway among the countries studied and this country has had the greatest decline in coronary artery disease mortality (35–40%) in men and women over the last 10 years compared with other countries.[7] A decline in the prevalence of hypercholesterolemia in certain segments of the U.S. population parallels these trends in mortality.[8] LDL-C and the ratio of LDL-C/HDL-C have also been used to assess risk but their use adds little information to total cholesterol alone unless HDL-C is abnormally high or low. HDL-C has been shown to be protective for the occurrence of coronary heart disease and an inverse relationship exists between CHD and HDL-C levels (Fig. 21.5).

Two fractions of HDL-C occur, HDL_2-C and HDL_3-C, and it is thought that HDL_2 is more important for prevention of cardiovascular disease. HDL transports cholesterol from lipid-ladened foam cells to the liver. In general, for every 1 mg/dL decline in HDL, CHD risk is increased 2–3%. Elevated triglycerides may cause pancreatitis but

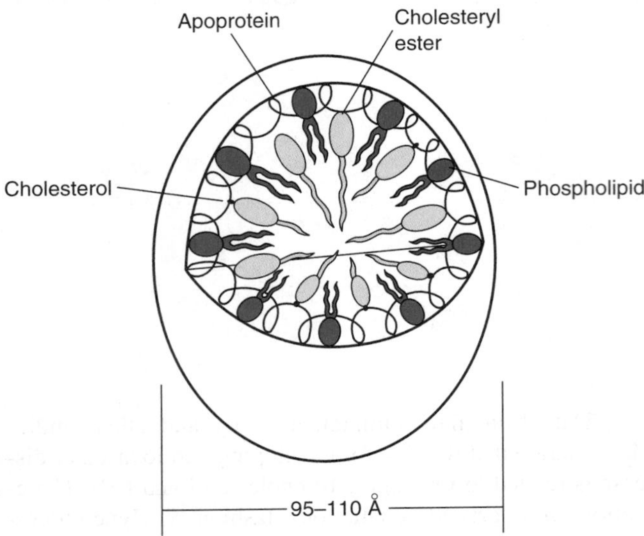

Figure 21.1. Schematic of a high-density-lipoprotein particle. The protein is represented as having a helical structure and forming the outer 110-Å shell of the particle. The polar head groups of phospholipids are shown interacting with the helices of the protein. Cholesteryl esters are drawn such that the cholesterol moiety interacts with the fatty acyl chains of the phospholipids. *(From Jackson RL, Morrisett JD, Gotto AM Jr. Lipoprotein structure and metabolism. Physiol Rev 1976;56:276, with permission.)*

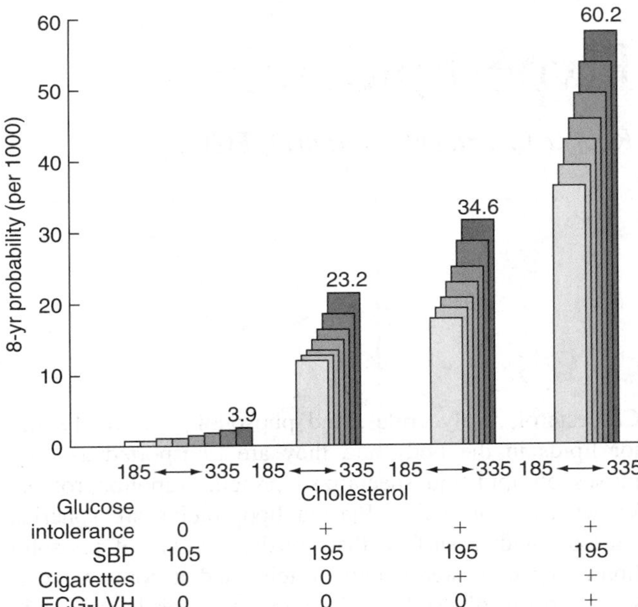

Figure 21.3. Risk of cardiovascular disease according to serum cholesterol at specified levels of other risk factors. ECG-LVH, electrocardiographic evidence of left ventricular hypertrophy; SBP, systolic blood pressure. *(From Kannel WB. High-density lipoproteins: Epidemiologic profile and risks of coronary artery disease. Am J Cardiol 1983;52:10B, with permission.)*

their relationship to coronary heart disease is much weaker than cholesterol, and studies of unselected patients have not found a significant relationship between triglycerides and the prevalence of CHD. Very-low-density lipoproteins (VLDL), which are enriched with cholesterol esters, are smaller, more dense, and more atherogenic than less dense VLDL.[1] Routine measurement of triglycerides cannot distinguish between the types of VLDL present in plasma. Elevation of triglyceride-rich lipoproteins is associated with low HDL and this ratio predicts increased risk. The Helsinki Heart Study has shown that the use of the LDL-C/HDL-C ratio along with serum triglyceride concentration can be used to predict high-risk patients and response to treatment.[8] The Stockholm Ischaemic Heart Disease Study using niacin and clofibrate found the greatest reduction in CHD in patients with elevated triglycerides.[9] Hypertriglyceridemia in certain instances, for example, diabetes mellitus, nephrotic syndrome, chronic renal disease, and perhaps in women, is associated with increased cardiovascular risk. This is thought to be due to the presence of atherogenic lipoproteins and hypertriglyceridemia being a marker for them as triglycerides are usually not independently predictive for CHD.[10]

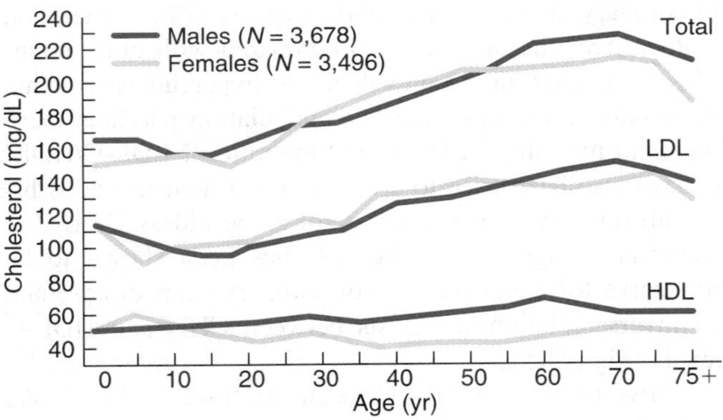

Figure 21.2. Mean plasma concentrations of total, low-density-lipoprotein (LDL) and high-density-lipoprotein (HDL) cholesterol by age and sex for whites (Lipid Research Clinics random sample). *(From Tyroler HA. An overview of Lipid Research Clinics (LRC) epidemiologic studies as background for the LRC Coronary Primary Prevention Trial. Am J Cardiol 1984;54:15C, with permission.)*

Lipoprotein Metabolism and Transport[11,12]

Cholesterol and triglycerides, as the major plasma lipids, are essential substrates for cell membrane formation and hormone synthesis, and they provide a source of free fatty acids. Hyperlipidemia is defined as an elevation of one or more of the following: cholesterol, cholesterol esters, phospholipids, or triglycerides. Lipids, being water immiscible, are not present in free form in the plasma but rather circulate as lipoproteins. Hyperlipoproteinemia describes an increased concentration of the lipoprotein macromolecules that transport lipids in the plasma. The density of plasma lipoproteins is determined by their relative content of pro-

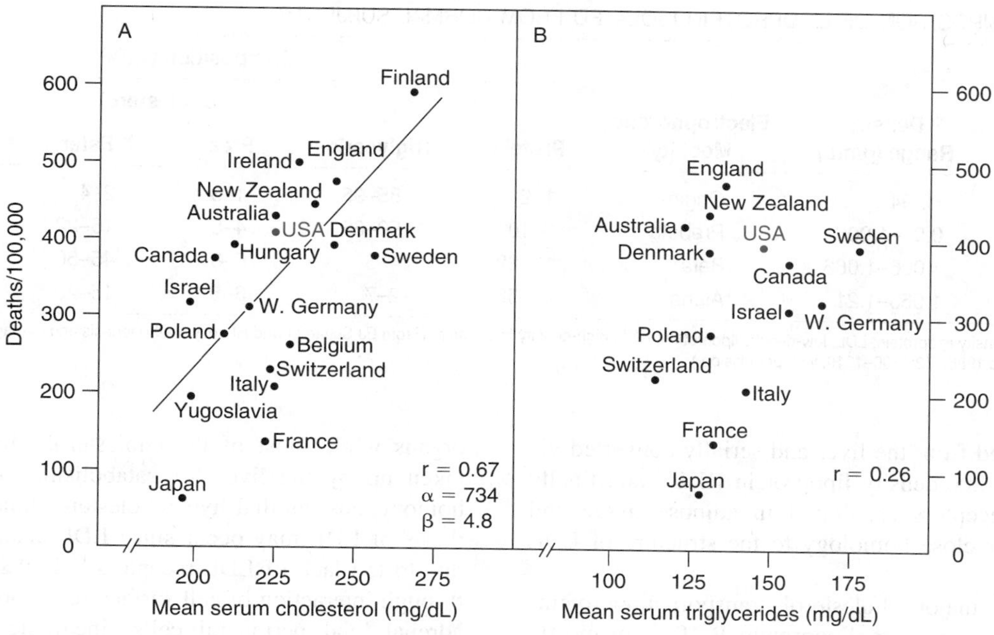

Figure 21.4. Coronary artery disease (A) mortality rate versus serum cholesterol and (B) triglyceride concentrations in men. NS, not significant; α, intercept; β, slope. *(From Simons LA. Interrelations of lipids and lipoproteins with coronary artery disease mortality in 19 countries. Am J Cardiol 1986;57:8G, with permission.)*

tein and lipid, and density, composition, and electrophoretic mobility have been used to divide lipoproteins into four classes (Table 21.1).

LDLs have been further divided into LDL_1, or intermediate-density lipoproteins (density of 1.006–1.019 g/mL) and LDL_2 (1.019–1.063 g/mL). LDL_2 is the major LDL component in plasma and it carries 60–70% of the total serum cholesterol. HDLs have been subfractionated into HDL_2 (density of 1.063–1.125 g/mL) and HDL_3 (1.125–1.21 g/mL). Fluctuations in HDLs are usually due to alterations

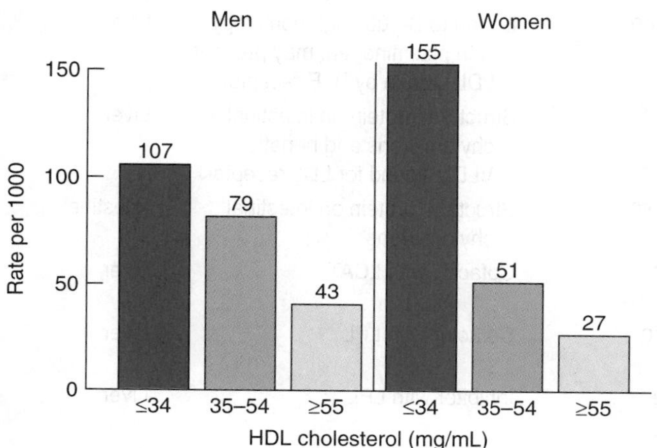

Figure 21.5. Incidence of coronary heart disease by HDL-C level. Framingham study, exam 11; men and women 50–79 years old. *(From Kannel WB. High-density lipoproteins: Epidemiologic profile and risks of coronary artery disease. Am J Cardiol 1983;52:10B, with permission.)*

in the levels of HDL_2. HDL normally carries about 20–30% of the total cholesterol. VLDL has also been subdivided into three classes and it carries about 10–15% of serum cholesterol and most of the triglyceride in the fasting state. VLDLs are the precursors for LDL, and VLDL remnants may also be atherogenic. The characteristics of the protein constituent of lipoproteins, known as apolipoproteins, are shown in Table 21.2.

Chylomicrons, large triglyceride-rich particles containing apolipoprotein B-48, B-100, and E, are formed from dietary fat solubilized by bile salts in intestinal mucosal cells. Chylomicrons are normally not present in the plasma after a fast of 12–14 hours and are catabolized by lipoprotein lipase (LPL), which is activated by apolipoprotein C-II and in the vascular endothelium and hepatic lipase to form chylomicron remnants. The remnants containing apolipoprotein E (Fig. 21.6) are taken up by the "remnant receptor," which may be a LDL receptor-related protein, in the liver. Free cholesterol is liberated intracellularly after attachment to the remnant receptor. Chylomicrons also function to deliver dietary triglyceride to skeletal muscle and adipose tissue. During the catabolism of nascent chylomicrons to remnants, triglyceride is converted to free fatty acids, and apolipoproteins A-I, A-II, A-IV (free in plasma), C-I, C-II, and C-III, and phospholipids are transferred to HDLs. Apolipoproteins E and C-II are transferred to chylomicrons from HDL and eventually back through these metabolic events. Hepatic VLDL synthesis is regulated in part by diet and hormones and is inhibited by uptake of chylomicron remnants in the liver.

TABLE 21.1. COMPOSITION OF LIPOPROTEIN ISOLATED FROM NORMAL SUBJECTS

Lipoprotein Class	Density Range (g/mL)	Electrophoretic Mobility	Composition (wt%) Protein	Triglyceride	Cholesterol Free	Cholesterol Ester	Phospholipid
Chylomicrons	<0.94	Origin	1–2	85–95	1–3	2–4	3–6
VLDL	0.94–1.006	Prebeta	6–10	50–65	4–8	16–22	15–20
LDL	1.006–1.063	Beta	18–22	4–8	6–8	45–50	18–24
HDL	1.063–1.21	Alpha	45–55	2–7	3–5	15–20	26–32

Key: VLDL, very-low-density lipoprotein; LDL, low-density lipoprotein; HDL, high-density lipoprotein. (From EJ Schaefer and RI Levy. Pathogenesis and management of lipoprotein disorders. *N Engl J Med* 1985;312:1300–1310, with permission.)

VLDL is secreted from the liver and serially converted via LPL to intermediate-density lipoprotein (IDL), and finally LDL. VLDL receptors are found in adipose tissue and muscle and bear close homology to the structure of LDL receptors.

LDLs, the major cholesterol transport lipoproteins that have virtually only apolipoprotein B-100, are mostly derived from VLDL catabolism and cellular synthesis. When fasted and on low fat intake in normals, most cholesterol is synthesized and utilized in the extrahepatic organs while most of the cholesterol carried by LDL is taken up by the liver for catabolism.[11] In patients with homozygous familial hypercholesterolemia, enhanced synthesis of LDL may occur since LDL clearance is reduced due to the lack of LDL receptors.[12] LDLs are catabolized through interaction of cell surface receptors found on liver, adrenal, and peripheral cells (including fibroblasts and smooth muscle cells). These cells recognize apolipoprotein B-100 on LDLs, and after binding to a receptor on the cell membrane, LDLs are internalized and degraded. In the

TABLE 21.2. CHARACTERISTICS AND FUNCTIONS OF APOLIPOPROTEINS

Apolipoprotein	Lipoprotein Density Class	Approximate Plasma Concentration (mg/dL)	Approximate Molecular Weight (kd)	Reported Functions	Major Site of Synthesis
A-I	Chylomicrons, HDL	120	28	Cofactor with LCAT, structural protein on HDL, ligand for HDL receptor	Liver, intestine
A-II	Chylomicrons, HDL	35	18	Structural protein for HDL, ligand for HDL receptor	Liver
A-IV	Chylomicrons, 1.21B	15	45	?	Intestine
ApoLp(a)	LDL, HDL	10	500±	Bound to B-100, high homology with plasminogen, may prevent LDL uptake by B, E receptor	Liver
B-100	VLDL, LDL	100	500	Structural protein on intestinal chylomicrons and hepatic VLDL, ligand for LDL receptor	Liver
B-48	Chylomicrons	Trace	250	Structural protein on intestinal chylomicrons	Intestine
C-I	Chylomicrons, VLDL, HDL	7	7	Cofactor with LCAT	Liver
C-II	Chylomicrons, VLDL, HDL	4	10	Cofactor with LPL	Liver
C-III	Chylomicrons, VLDL, HDL	13	9	Inhibitor with LPL	Liver
D	HDL	6	32	?	?
E2-E4	Chylomicrons, VLDL, HDL	5	34	Ligand for several cell receptors	Liver

Key: LCAT, lecithin-cholesterol acyltransferase; HL, hepatic lipase. Other abbreviations are given in Table 21.1.

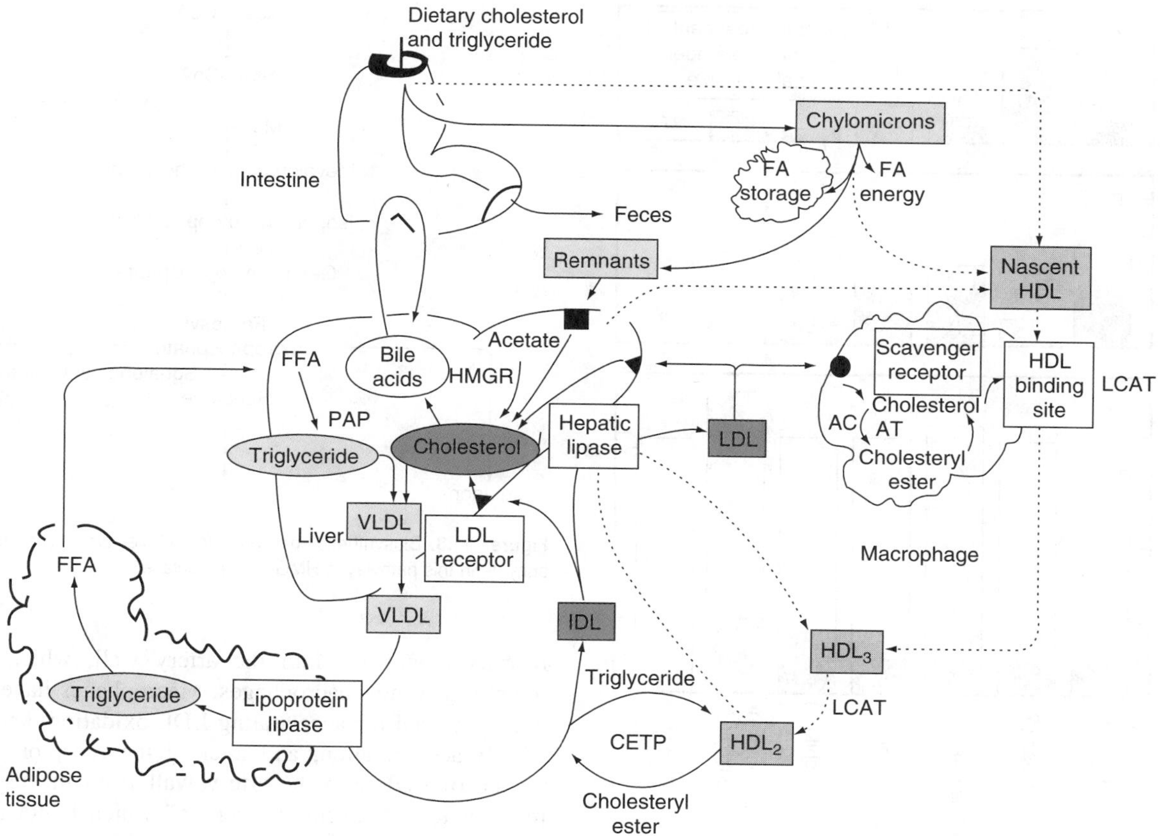

Figure 21.6. Overview of lipoprotein metabolism. ACAT, acyl CoA:cholesterol acyltransferase; LCAT, lecithin:cholesterol acyltransferase; HMGR, HMG CoA reductase; PAP, phosphatidic acid phosphatase; CETP, cholesteryl ester transfer protein; FFA, free fatty acid. *(From Shepherd J. Lipoprotein metabolism. An overview. Drugs 1984;(suppl 2):1–10, with permission.)*

normal fasting state, approximately 70% of LDL is cleared through a receptor-dependent mechanism although this is highly dependent on the availability and type of saturated and mono- or polyunsaturated fat from dietary sources. Ingestion of cholesterol and saturated fatty acids such as C12:0, 14:0, and 16:0 is associated with reduction in LDL receptor activity, increased LDL production rate, and elevation in LDL plasma concentration.[13] Receptor-independent mechanisms are also involved to a lesser extent in the catabolism of LDLs and these receptors are present in many tissues but are most active in animals in the adrenals and ovary (Fig. 21.7).[11] Increased intracellular cholesterol resulting from LDL catabolism inhibits the activity of 3-hydroxy-3-methylglutaryl coenzyme A (HMG-CoA) reductase, the rate-limiting enzyme for intracellular cholesterol biosynthesis (Fig. 21.8). Additional consequences of increased intracellular cholesterol include reduced synthesis of LDL receptors, which limits subsequent cholesterol uptake from the plasma, and accelerated activity of acyl coenzyme-A:cholesterol acyltransferase to facilitate cholesterol storage within cells. LDL cholesterol may also be excreted into bile and become part of the enterohepatic pool or be lost in the stool. Lp(a) is a cholesterol-rich lipoprotein similar to LDL in composition and density and it has been reported to be an important independent risk factor for the development of premature cardiovascular disease.[14]

Nascent HDLs are derived from liver and gut synthesis primarily in the form of apolipoprotein A-I phospholipid discs. Esterification of free cholesterol in nascent HDLs and from peripheral tissues to cholesteryl esters by lecithin:cholesterol acyltransferase (LCAT) results in the production of HDL_3. Further addition of tissue cholesterol to HDL_3 results in the formation of HDL_2. HDL_2 can also be formed from remodeling of chylomicrons and VLDL catabolism. HDL_2 may be converted back to HDL_3 by the action of hepatic lipase and the transfer of cholesteryl esters to the liver, LDL, and VLDL. Apolipoprotein A-I production is increased by estrogens, leading to higher HDL levels in women and in individuals receiving estrogen. Transfer of excess cholesterol from peripheral tissues by HDL is called *reverse cholesterol transport.* Putative HDL receptors in peripheral cells facilitate the uptake of cholesterol by HDL, which transfers cholesterol to either VLDL and LDL or to the liver for secretion into bile or conversion into bile acids. These processes serve to rid peripheral tissue (e.g., coro-

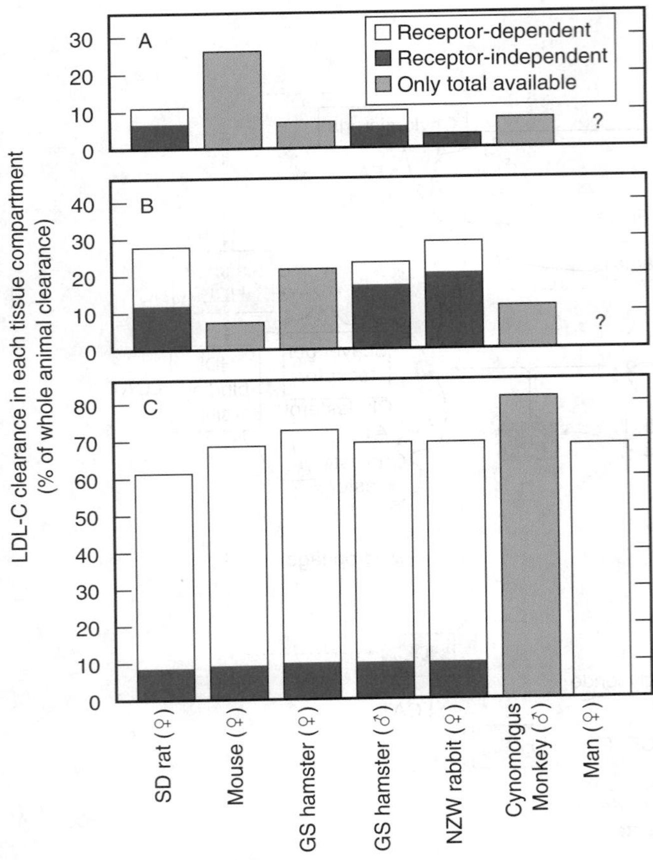

Figure 21.7. A is small intestine, B is extrahepatic tissues, and C is liver. LDL-C clearance from various tissues in several species via receptor-dependent and receptor-independent mechanisms. *(From Dietschy JM, Turley SD, Spady DK. Role of liver in the maintenance of cholesterol and low density lipoprotein homeostasis in different animal species, including humans. J Lipid Res 1993;34:1637–1659, with permission.)*

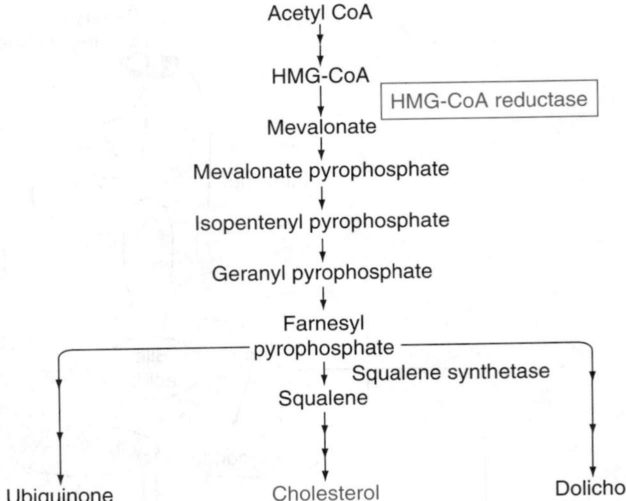

Figure 21.8. Biosynthetic pathway for cholesterol. The rate-limiting enzyme in this pathway is HMG-CoA reductase.

nary arteries) of excessive amounts of cholesterol and, thus, the protective effects noted with increasing HDL in women and other factors that elevate HDL levels. HDL has been further separated into subtypes HDL_{2a}, HDL_{2b}, HDL_{3a}, and HDL_{3c} and the importance of each subtype is being investigated.

The response-to-injury hypothesis states that risk factors such as oxidized LDL, mechanical injury to the endothelium (e.g., percutaneous transluminal angioplasty), excessive homocysteine, immunologic attack, or viral-induced changes in endothelial and intimal function lead to endothelial dysfunction and a series of cellular interactions that culminate in atherosclerosis.[15] The eventual outcomes of this cascade are clinical events such as angina and myocardial infarction. Atherosclerotic lesions are thought to arise from transport and retention of plasma LDL-C through the endothelial cell layer into the extracellular matrix of the subendothelial space. Once in the artery wall, LDL but not apolipoprotein B is oxidized by various oxidative products produced locally. Mildly oxidized LDL then recruits monocytes into the artery wall, which become transformed into macrophages. Macrophages have tremendous potential for accelerating LDL oxidation, apolipoprotein B accumulation, and altering the receptor mediated uptake of LDL into the artery wall from the usual LDL receptor to a "scavenger receptor," which is not regulated by cell content of cholesterol. Oxidized LDL increases plasminogen inhibitor levels (promotion of coagulation), induces the expression of endothelin (vasoconstrictive substance), inhibits the expression of nitric oxide (a vasodilator and platelet inhibitor) and is toxic to macrophages if highly oxidized. As oxidation of biologically active lipids proceeds, other lipids such as lysophosphatidylcholine and oxysterol are formed and continue the reaction within the tissue. These events lead to a massive accumulation of cholesterol and these cholesterol-laden cells are called *foam cells;* foam cells are the earliest recognized cell of the arterial fatty streak.[16]

Oxidized LDL provokes an inflammatory response which is mediated by a number of chemoattractants and cytokines. Examples of each which appear to be involved at different stages of lesion development include monocyte chemoattractant protein 1 (MCP-1), monocyte colony-stimulating factor (M-CSF), *gro,* vascular cell adhesion molecule (VCAM-1), E-selectin (ELAM-1), intercellular adhesion molecule (ICAM-1), platelet-derived growth factor (PDGF), vascular endothelial growth factor (VEGF), transforming growth factors (TGFa and TGFb), and interleukin-1 and interleukin-6 (IL-1 and IL-6). It appears that some of these factors, e.g., MCP-1 and M-CSF, participate early in the process of monocyte–macrophage attachment and transmigration across the endothelium while others such as PDGF and VCAM-1 promote later lesion growth.[15–17] The extent of oxidation and the inflammatory response are under genetic control of a major gene termed *Ath*-1 based on murine model studies.[18] Increased recognition of the role of these growth-regulatory molecules provides the possibility of future directions for antagonists to regulatory molecules such as PDGF, TGFb, and the interleukins.

Lipoprotein disorders have been classified into six categories and this categorization (Table 21.3) is commonly used today for the phenotypical description of hyperlipidemia. More recently, it has become apparent that specific genetic defects with disrupted protein, cell, and organ function give rise to several disorders within each family of lipoproteins (Table 21.4). In other words, an elevated cholesterol does not necessarily equate to familial hypercholesterolemia or type IIa, because cholesterol may also be elevated in other lipoprotein disorders and the lipoprotein pattern does not describe the underlying genetic defect. The preceding discussion has focused on primary or genetic hyperlipoproteinemia and it should be remembered that secondary forms exist and several drugs may also elevate lipid levels (Table 21.5). These secondary forms of hyperlipidemia should be initially managed by correcting the underlying abnormality, including modification of drug therapy when appropriate.

TABLE 21.3. FREDRICKSON–LEVY–LEES CLASSIFICATION OF HYPERLIPOPROTEINEMIA

Type	Lipoprotein Elevation	Approximate Mean Lipid Elevation: Cholesterol (mg/dL)	Approximate Mean Lipid Elevation: Triglycerides (mg/dL)
I	Chylomicrons	324	3316
IIa	LDL[a]	368	148
IIb	LDL + VLDL	354	135
III	IDL (LDL_1)	441	694
IV	VLDL	251	438
V	VLDL + chylomicrons	373	2071

[a]Heterozygotes for familial hypercholesterolemia. (Modified from Schafer EJ, Levy RI. Pathogenesis and management of lipoprotein disorders. N Engl J Med 1985;312:1302.)

Familial hypercholesterolemia is the best understood of the primary hyperlipoproteinemia disorders and this stems from the Nobel prize-winning work of Brown and Goldstein,[19] in their characterization of the LDL receptor (LDL-R) function and importance. It is characterized by (1)

TABLE 21.4. LIPOPROTEIN DISORDERS[a]

Increased Chylomicrons (Types I and V HLP)	Increased VLDL (Type IV HLP)	Increased Beta VLDL (Type III HLP)	Increased LDL (Type II HLP)	Abnormal LDL	Chylomicron, VLDL, and LDL Deficiency	HDL Deficiency
Familial hypertriglyceridemia[b]	Familial hypertriglyceridemia[b]	Apolipoprotein E2 phenotype[c]	Familial hypercholesterolemia[d]	Betasitosterolemia[b]	Abetalipoproteinemia[e]	Hypoalphalipoproteinemia[b]
Familial combined hyperlipidemia[b]	Familial combined hyperlipidemia[b]	Apolipoprotein E variants[c]	Familial combined hyperlipidemia[b]	Hyperapobetalipoproteinemia[b]	Hypobetalipoproteinemia[e]	Apolipoprotein A-I variants[c]
Lipoprotein lipase deficiency[f]	Apolipoprotein C-III DNA polymorphism[c]	Apolipoprotein E deficiency[e]		Cerebrotendinous xanthomatosis[f]	Normotriglyceridemic abetalipoproteinemia[e]	Tangier disease[c]
Lipoprotein lipase inhibitor[f]		Hepatic lipase deficiency[f]				HDL deficiency with planar xanthomas[b]
Apolipoprotein C-II deficiency[e]						Apolipoprotein A-I and C-III deficiency[e]
Abnormal apolipoprotein C-III sialylation[c]						LCAT deficiency[f]
Apoliprotein E4 phenotype[c]						Fish eye disease[b]

[a]HLP denotes hyperlipoproteinemia. Other abbreviations are explained in Tables 21.2 and 21.3.
[b]Unknown defect.
[c]Apolipoprotein abnormality.
[d]Receptor abnormality.
[e]Apolipoprotein deficiency.
[f]Enzyme abnormality. (From Schaefer EJ and Levy RI . Pathogenesis and management of liproprotein disorders. N Engl J Med 1985;312:1300–1310, with permission.)

TABLE 21.5. SECONDARY FORMS OF HYPERLIPOPROTEINEMIA

Disease-Induced	Drug-Induced
Endocrine/Metabolic	Alcohol
Diabetes mellitus	Progestins
von Gierke's disease	Thiazide diuretics
Lipodystrophies	β Blockers
Cushing's syndrome	Glucocorticoids
Sexual ateliotic dwarfism	
Acromegaly	
Hypothyroidism	
Anorexia nervosa	
Werner's syndrome	
Acute intermittent porphyria	
Renal	
Uremia	
Nephrotic syndrome	
Hepatic	
Primary biliary cirrhosis	
Acute hepatitis	
Hepatoma	
Immunologic	
Systemic lupus erythematosis	
Monoclonal gammapathies	
Stress-Induced	

a selective elevation in the plasma level of LDL; (2) deposition of LDL-derived cholesterol in tendons (xanthomas) and arteries (atheromas); and (3) inheritance as an autosomal dominant trait with homozygotes more severely affected than heterozygotes. Homozygotes (prevalence 1 in 1,000,000) have severe hypercholesterolemia (650–1000 mg/dL) with the early appearance of cutaneous xanthomas and fatal CHD generally before the age of 20. The primary defect in familial hypercholesterolemia is the inability to bind LDL to the LDL-R or, rarely, a defect of internalizing the LDL-R complex into the cell after normal binding. This leads to lack of LDL degradation by cells and unregulated biosynthesis of cholesterol, with total cholesterol and LDL-C being inversely proportional to the deficit in LDL receptors. Heterozygotes have only about one-half of the normal number of LDL receptors while homozygotes have essentially no functional LDL receptors. This is illustrated in Fig. 21.9, which relates the number of receptors to the fractional catabolic rate for LDL.

Familial lipoprotein lipase deficiency is characterized by a massive accumulation of chylomicrons and corresponding increase in plasma triglycerides or a type I lipoprotein pattern. VLDL concentration is normal. The presenting manifestations include repeated attacks of pancreatitis and abdominal pain, eruptive cutaneous xanthomatosis, and hepatosplenomegaly beginning in childhood. Symptom severity is proportional to dietary fat intake, and consequently to the elevation of chylomicrons. LPL is normally released from vascular endothelium or by heparin and hydrolyzes chylomicrons and VLDL (Fig. 21.6). Diagnosis is based on low or absent enzyme activity with normal human plasma or apolipoprotein C-II, a cofactor of the enzyme.[20] Accelerated atherosclerosis is not associated with this disease. Type V (VLDL + chylomicrons) is characterized by abdominal pain, pancreatitis, eruptive xanthomas, and peripheral polyneuropathy. Symptoms may occur in childhood but usually the disorder is expressed at a later age. The risk of atherosclerosis is increased with this disorder. These patients are commonly obese, hyperuricemic, and diabetic; alcohol intake, exogenous estrogens, and renal insufficiency tend to be exacerbating factors.

Patients with familial type III hyperlipoproteinemia (also called dysbetalipoproteinemia or beta VLDL) develop the following clinical features after age 20: xanthoma striata palmaris (yellow discolorations of the palmar and digital creases); tuberous or tuberoeruptive xanthomas (bulbous cutaneous xanthomas); and severe atherosclerosis involving the coronary arteries, internal carotids, and abdominal aorta. A defective structure of apolipoprotein E does not allow normal hepatic surface receptor binding of remnant

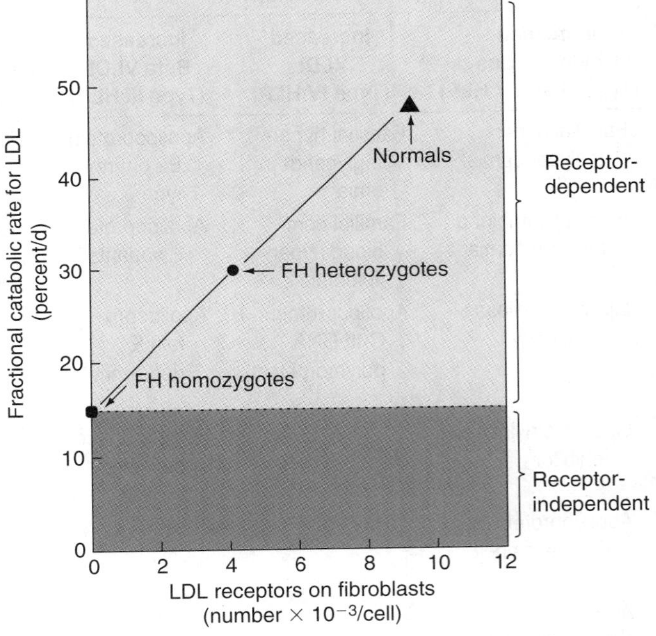

Figure 21.9. Relation between the fractional catabolic rate (FCR) for plasma LDL and the number of LDL receptors on fibroblasts in patients with familial hypercholesterolemia (FH). The values for the fractional catabolic rate were derived from studies of the turnover of ^{125}I-labeled apo-LDL in the plasma of 6 normal subjects, 6 FH heterozygotes, and 11 FH homozygotes. The number of LDL receptors per cell was calculated from experiments in which maximal ^{125}I-labeled LDL binding was measured at 4°C in actively growing fibroblasts deprived of LDL for 48 hours. *(From Stanbury JB, Wyngaarden JB, Fredrickson DS, et al [eds]. The Metabolic Basis of Inherited Disease, 5th ed. New York, McGraw-Hill, 1983, p 687, with permission.)*

particles derived from chylomicrons and VLDL (known as IDL). Although homozygosity for the defective allele is common (1 in 100), only 1 in 10,000 express the full-blown picture, and interaction with other genetic or environmental factors or both is needed to produce clinical disease.

Type IV hyperlipoproteinemia is common and occurs in adulthood primarily in patients who are obese, diabetic, and hyperuricemic and do not have xanthomas. It may be secondary to alcohol ingestion and can be aggravated by stress, progestins, oral contraceptives, thiazides, or β blockers. Two genetic patterns occur in type IV hyperlipoproteinemia: familial hypertriglyceridemia, which does not carry a great risk for premature coronary artery disease, and familial combined hyperlipidemia, which is associated with increased risk of cardiovascular disease.

Rare forms of lipoprotein disorders may include abnormal LDL or deficiencies in chylomicrons, VLDL, LDL, and HDL (Table 21.4). Most of these rare lipoprotein disorders do not result in premature atherosclerosis, with the exceptions of familial lecithin:cholesterol acyltransferase (LCAT) deficiency, cerebrotendinous xanthomatosis (CTX), and sitosterolemia with xanthomatosis. Their treatment consists of dietary restriction of plant sterols (sitosterolemia with xanthomatosis), chenodeoxycholic acid (CTX), or, potentially, blood transfusion (LCAT deficiency).

Patient Evaluation

Total cholesterol and HDL should be measured in all adults 20 years of age or older at least once every 5 years. Once hyperlipidemia is suspected, two major components of the evaluation are the history (including age, gender, and, if female, menstrual and estrogen replacement status) and physical examination and laboratory investigations. A complete history and physical exam should assess the following: (1) presence or absence of cardiovascular risk factors or definite cardiovascular disease in the individual; (2) family history of premature cardiovascular disease or lipid disorders; (3) presence or absence of secondary causes of hyperlipidemia, including concurrent medications (Table 21.5); and (4) presence or absence of xanthomas, abdominal pain, or history of pancreatitis, renal or liver disease, peripheral vascular disease, or cerebral vascular disease (carotid bruits, stroke or transient ischemic attack). This approach for a single patient is referred to as case finding or patient-based whereas large-scale screening and recommendations for the general populace, health care providers, and the food industry are called a population-based approach. Strategies for blood cholesterol reduction in the entire population have been described.[21]

Measurement of plasma cholesterol (which is about 3% lower than serum determinations), triglyceride, and HDL-C levels after a 12-hour or longer fast is important, because triglycerides may be elevated in nonfasted individuals; total cholesterol is only modestly affected by fasting. Analytic and biologic variability can have a major impact on the measurement and interpretation of cholesterol (or any other laboratory test). Analytic variability can be minimized through the use of adequate quality-control procedures including internal training, routine calibration and monitoring, and external proficiency testing. Even with these measures the coefficient of variability in the best procedures can acceptably be up to 5%, and when combined with average biologic variability, total variability may be as high as ±22%. Analytic variability with desk-top equipment generally is greater in the "finger stick" capillary blood methods (e.g., Reflotron, Vision, DT-60), usually yielding measurements less than those from a clinical laboratory, and this technology should be considered for use only as a screening method.[22,23] Reliance on desk-top methods can result in misclassification of 7–14% of patients if capillary blood is used. Two determinations, 1–8 weeks apart, with the patient on a stable diet and weight, and in the absence of acute illness, are recommended to minimize variability and to obtain a reliable baseline.[1] If the total cholesterol is greater than 200 mg/dL, a second determination is recommended and if the values are more than 30 mg/dL apart, the average of three values should be used. Familiarity with the method and quality-control procedures employed by local laboratories is essential for interpretation of reported values. If the physical examination and history are insufficient to diagnose a familial disorder, then agarose-gel lipoprotein electrophoresis is useful to determine which class of lipoproteins is affected. If the triglyceride levels are below 400 mg/dL and neither type III hyperlipidemia nor chylomicrons are detected by electrophoresis, then one can calculate VLDL-C and LDL-C concentrations: VLDL-C = triglyceride/5; LDL-C = total cholesterol − (VLDL-C + HDL-C). Initial testing utilizes total cholesterol for case finding but subsequent management decisions should be based on LDL-C.

Because total cholesterol is comprised of cholesterol derived from LDL, VLDL, and HDL, determination of HDL-C is useful when total plasma cholesterol is elevated. While HDL-C may be elevated by moderate alcohol ingestion (less than 2 drinks per day), physical exercise, smoking cessation, weight loss, oral contraceptives, phenytoin, and terbutaline, smoking, obesity, a sedentary lifestyle and drugs such as β blockers lower HDL. Of the former, only exercise and smoking cessation could be recommended as interventions for low HDL-C concentrations. The lipid lowering agents niacin and gemfibrozil also increase HDL concentrations but they are not Food and Drug Administration (FDA) approved for this use.

The range of lipid concentrations represents a population mean plus or minus two standard deviations and does not define the risk of disease. Reference values for plasma total, LDL, and HDL cholesterol concentrations from the

TABLE 21.6. TOTAL SERUM CHOLESTEROL (mg/dL) DISTRIBUTION IN THE U.S. POPULATION—NHANES III DATA 1988–1991

Race/Ethnicity, Sex, and Age	Mean	Percentile		
		50th	75th	90th
Men				
≤20 yr	205	201	231	260
20–34 yr	189	186	211	236
35–44 yr	207	205	231	258
45–54 yr	218	215	242	268
55–64 yr	221	221	245	274
65–74 yr	218	214	241	270
≥75 yr	205	202	232	257
Women				
≤20 yr	207	202	233	269
20–34 yr	185	182	204	229
35–44 yr	195	193	215	242
45–54 yr	217	212	240	279
55–64 yr	237	228	264	291
65–74 yr	234	232	261	290
≥75 yr	230	227	263	287
Mexican-Americans				
Men	202	199	225	257
Women	200	195	224	258
Non-Hispanic Blacks				
Men	199	195	224	252
Women	203	200	227	262
Non-Hispanic Whites				
Men	206	203	232	260
Women	208	202	234	271

National Health and Nutritional Survey (NHANES III) data are given in Tables 21.6, 21.7, and 21.8. Cholesterol and triglycerides increase throughout life until about the seventh decade for men and women. At that point, total and LDL plateau and fall slightly in men but continue to rise in women. HDL tends to fall slightly with time and more rapidly after menopause in women. Institution of a population-based approach for cholesterol reduction should shift the entire curve to the left and the potential reduction in cardiovascular mortality would be proportional to mean reductions at any cholesterol concentration.[21]

RECOMMENDATIONS FOR TREATMENT[1]

Based on a careful review of the experimental pathologic, genetic, and epidemiologic evidence relating to the relationship between blood cholesterol levels and CHD, the Adult Treatment Panel II of the NCEP has recommended that total cholesterol determinations and risk factor assessment be used in the initial classification of adults. If total cholesterol is less than 200 mg/dL, the patient has a *desirable blood cholesterol level* (Table 21.9). Cholesterol levels between 200 and 239 mg/dL are classified as *borderline high blood cholesterol* and assessment of risk factors (Table 21.10) is needed to more clearly define disease risk. Blood cholesterol levels of 240 mg/dL and above are classified as *high blood cholesterol levels.* If the total cholesterol is <200 mg/dL and the HDL is >35 mg/dL, no further follow-up is recommended for patients without known CHD and less than two risk factors. When the serum total cholesterol is ≥200 mg/dL, or when the HDL cholesterol is <35 mg/dL or at borderline-high levels with two or more risk factors, a lipoprotein analysis (two measurements 1–8 weeks apart) to measure total and HDL cholesterol and triglycerides so that LDL-C may be estimated is recommended. In patients with evidence of CHD or other clinical atherosclerotic disease the LDL goal is <100 mg/dL and most patients will require diet and/or drug intervention. Decisions regarding classification and management are based on the LDL-C levels as outlined in Table 21.11.

Screening of children and adolescents for elevated cholesterol remains a controversial issue; however, the Expert Panel on Children and Adolescents of the NCEP has recommended screening and dietary intervention in higher risk children.[24] The rationale, in part, for this approach is based on the recognition that atherosclerosis begins in the childhood and adolescent years as recently documented in the Pathobiological Determinants of Atherosclerosis in Youth (PDAY) studies.[25] Likewise, if children

TABLE 21.7. LOW-DENSITY CHOLESTEROL (mg/dL) DISTRIBUTION IN THE U.S. POPULATION—NHANES III DATA 1988–1991

Race/Ethnicity, Sex, and Age	Mean	Percentile		
		50th	75th	90th
Men				
≤20 yr	131	129	154	179
20–34 yr	120	121	139	165
35–44 yr	134	131	156	176
45–54 yr	138	136	163	187
55–64 yr	142	143	165	194
65–74 yr	141	134	163	185
≥75 yr	132	130	154	186
Women				
≤20 yr	126	122	150	175
20–34 yr	110	108	129	155
35–44 yr	117	116	138	155
45–54 yr	132	130	157	182
55–64 yr	145	145	170	189
65–74 yr	147	143	168	197
≥75 yr	147	143	168	197
Mexican-Americans				
Men	124	120	148	172
Women	122	118	144	166
Non-Hispanic Blacks				
Men	124	123	146	186
Women	122	124	147	174
Non-Hispanic Whites				
Men	132	129	154	179
Women	126	122	151	176

with high blood lipids or lipoprotein levels are identified, and the levels in the parents are not known, the parents should be screened as well because they are likely to be at high risk.[26] Racial and gender differences do exist in the determination of lipoprotein fractions and these factors should be considered in screening. Use of the serum cholesterol level alone may not be of sufficient specificity or sensitivity depending on the cut points used in screening, and other discretionary factors such as hypertension, smoking, obesity, high-fat diet, and use of cholesterol-raising medication may be needed to correctly identify children at risk.[27,28] These recommendations are presented in Table 21.12. Presently, children older than age 10 are candidates for drug therapy if a trial of diet (6 months to 1 year) proves to be inadequate and LDL-C remains above 190 mg/dL or above 160 mg/dL if two or more risk factors or CHD are present. Bile acid sequestrants are the recommended drugs for this population. The long-term consequences of drug therapy in this population are unknown. In special instances, familial hypercholesterolemia (particularly the homozygous form), or the existence of CHD or two or more risk factors in the child, would prompt the earlier institution of drug therapy after a trial of dietary intervention.

The goals of therapy expressed as LDL-C levels and the level of initiation of diet and drug therapy are provided in Tables 21.11 and 21.12 for adults and children, respectively. Ideally, dietary means should be used to attain even lower LDL-C, if possible, to achieve further reductions in CHD risk. Based on angiographic studies, aggressive reduction in total and LDL cholesterol is beneficial to prevent the development of atheromatous lesions in vascular beds and to induce the regression of existing lesions. Furthermore, data from trials of secondary and primary intervention also provide evidence that CHD morbidity and mortality as well as total mortality can be reduced with diet and drug therapy. The extent of lipid reduction is related to CHD risk reduction and the goals outlined in the tables should be considered as *minimal* goals. Hypertriglyceridemia is classified as normal, borderline, high, or very high as outlined in Table 21.9.

MANAGEMENT OF HYPERLIPIDEMIA

Many clinicians believe that reduction of elevated levels of cholesterol in patients with hypercholesterolemia should lessen the risk for CHD. Results from numerous epidemio-

TABLE 21.8. HIGH-DENSITY CHOLESTEROL (mg/dL) DISTRIBUTION IN THE U.S. POPULATION—NHANES III DATA 1988–1991

		Percentile		
Race/Ethnicity, Sex, and Age	**Mean**	**50th**	**75th**	**90th**
Men				
≤20 yr	46.5	44.1	53.1	64.0
20–34 yr	47.1	46.0	54.0	64.0
35–44 yr	46.3	44.0	53.0	63.0
45–54 yr	46.6	43.1	53.0	66.1
55–64 yr	45.6	43.0	53.0	62.0
65–74 yr	45.3	43.0	53.0	62.1
≥75 yr	47.2	45.0	54.0	67.0
Women				
≤20 yr	55.7	54.0	65.0	76.1
20–34 yr	55.7	54.0	64.1	75.1
35–44 yr	54.3	53.0	64.1	72.1
45–54 yr	56.7	56.0	65.0	77.1
55–64 yr	56.1	53.0	66.0	79.0
65–74 yr	55.7	54.0	65.1	78.0
≥75 yr	57.1	56.0	66.1	78.1
Mexican-Americans				
Men	46.9	45.0	54.0	64.0
Women	53.3	52.0	61.0	72.1
Non-Hispanic Blacks				
Men	53.3	51.0	62.0	75.1
Women	57.8	55.1	67.1	78.1
Non-Hispanic Whites				
Men	45.5	44.0	52.1	62.0
Women	55.7	54.0	65.1	77.0

logic studies are consistent with this concept. Without doubt, hypercholesterolemia increases the risk for CHD. However, proof of the lipid hypothesis (that reduction of elevated cholesterol would reduce risk) was lacking until the publication of the Lipid Research Clinics Coronary Primary Prevention Trial (LRC–CPPT) unequivocally demonstrated a reduction in CHD death and nonfatal myocardial infarction in a large number of asymptomatic men with primary hypercholesterolemia.[29,30] The investigators found that for every 1% reduction in cholesterol, approximately a 2% reduction in CHD was seen. More recently, the Scandinavian Simvastatin Survival Study (4S), a secondary intervention trial, demonstrated that intervention with diet and simvastatin reduces CHD mortality and total mortality compared to diet and placebo treatment.[31] Results from angiographic studies demonstrate halting of progression of established lesions, prevention of new lesion formation, and, to a lesser extent, regression of existing atherosclerotic plaques in coronary arteries. This has been shown in native vessels or venous bypass grafts in patients who have undergone coronary artery bypass grafting.[32,33] Of interest, these angiographic trials, which typically cause animalculine changes in luminal diameter (e.g., ~0.04-mm difference in change between placebo and active treatment), result in fewer clinical events such as myocardial infarction or the need for revascularization. This unexpected finding suggests that plaque size and luminal encroachment by plaque may be less important than the effects of cholesterol lower-

TABLE 21.9. INITIAL CLASSIFICATION OF TOTAL, LDL, AND HDL CHOLESTEROL AND TRIGLYCERIDES

Classification	**Total Cholesterol**	**LDL Cholesterol**	**HDL Cholesterol**	**Triglycerides**
Desirable/normal	<200 mg/dL	<130 mg/dL	—	<200 mg/dL
Borderline-high	200–239 mg/dL	130–159 mg/dL	—	200–400 mg/dL
High	≥240 mg/dL	>160 mg/dL	>60 mg/dL	400–1000 mg/dL
Very high	—	—	—	>1000 mg/dL
Low	—	—	<35 mg/dL	—

Key: HDL, high-density lipoproteins; LDL, low-density lipoproteins.

TABLE 21.10. RISK STATUS BASED ON PRESENCE OF CHD RISK FACTORS OTHER THAN LDL CHOLESTEROL

Positive Risk Factors
Men: ≥45 years
Women: ≥55 years or premature menopause without estrogen replacement therapy
Family history of premature CHD (definite myocardial infarction or sudden death before 55 years of age in father or other male first-degree relative, or before 65 years of age in mother or other female first-degree relative)
Current cigarette smoking
Hypertension (≥140/90 mm Hg or on antihypertensive medication).
Low HDL cholesterol (<35 mg/dL)
Diabetes mellitus
Negative Risk Factor[a]
High HDL cholesterol (≥60 mg/dL)

Key: CHD, coronary heart disease; LDL, low-density lipoproteins; HDL, high-density lipoproteins.
Note: High risk is defined as a net of two or more CHD risk factors or the presence of coronary or peripheral atherosclerosis.
[a]If the HDL cholesterol level is ≥60 mg/dL, subtract one risk factor since high HDL cholesterol levels decrease CHD risk.

TABLE 21.11. TREATMENT DECISIONS BASED ON LDL CHOLESTEROL

	Initiation Level	LDL Goal
Dietary therapy		
Without CHD and <2 risk factors	≥160 mg/dL	<160 mg/dL
Without CHD and ≥2 risk factors	≥130 mg/dL	<130 mg/dL
With CHD	>100 mg/dL	≤100 mg/dL
	Consideration Level	**LDL Goal**
Drug treatment		
Without CHD and <2 risk factors	≥190 mg/dL[a]	<160 mg/dL
Without CHD and ≥2 risk factors	≥160 mg/dL	<130 mg/dL
With CHD	≥130 mg/dL[b]	≤100 mg/dL

Key: LDL, low-density lipoproteins; CHD, coronary heart disease.
[a]In men less than 35 years old and premenopausal women with LDL cholesterol levels of 190–219 mg/dL, drug therapy should be delayed except in high-risk patients such as those with diabetes.
[b]In patients with CHD and LDL cholesterol levels of 100–129 mg/dL, the clinician should exercise clinical judgment in deciding whether to initiate drug treatment.

ing on the activity in the plaque and endothelial dysfunction.[34,35] These studies provide a strong rationale for attempting to lower plasma cholesterol and LDL in patients with hypercholesterolemia. Present evidence clearly demonstrates the benefit of cholesterol lowering in patients with known CHD and in patients with multiple risk factors. Many more patients without established CHD or risk factors must be treated to show a reduction in cardiovascular endpoints; however, the LRC–CPPT[29] and the West of Scotland[36] trials provide convincing evidence that primary intervention also is effective.

DIETARY THERAPY

The objectives of dietary therapy are to progressively decrease the intake of total fat, saturated fatty acids (i.e., saturated fat), and cholesterol and to achieve a desirable body weight. Typical American diets now include 13–20% of total calories from saturated fat and a cholesterol intake of 350–450 mg/d, both in excess of a "heart healthy" diet for normal Americans let alone patients with a lipid disorder. The targeted saturated fatty acids have carbon chain lengths of 12 (lauric acid), 14 (myritisc acid), and 16 (palmitic acid). The rationale for using a nutritionally balanced low-fat, low-cholesterol diet for the treatment of hypercholesterolemia is based on the following principles: (1) It represents a reasonable extension of the diet recommended for the general public; (2) it progressively decreases the major cholesterol-raising constituent of the diet; (3) it precludes large intakes of polyunsaturated fats; and (4) it facilitates weight reduction by removing foods of high caloric density.[1] Dietary modification, weight control,

TABLE 21.12. CLASSIFICATION OF TOTAL AND LOW-DENSITY LIPOPROTEIN CHOLESTEROL LEVELS IN CHILDREN AND ADOLESCENTS FROM FAMILIES WITH HYPERCHOLESTEROLEMIA OR PREMATURE CARDIOVASCULAR DISEASE[a]

Category	Total Cholesterol (mg/dL)	LDL Cholesterol (mg/dL)	Dietary Intervention
Acceptable	<170	<110	Recommended population eating pattern
Borderline	170–199	110–129	Step 1 diet prescribed and other risk factor intervention
High	≥200	≥130	Step 1 diet prescribed and then step 2 diet if necessary

[a]For use in children with a definite family history of premature (<50 yr in females; <60 yr in males) coronary heart disease including diagnostic coronary arteriography, angioplasty, coronary artery bypass grafting, myocardial infarction, angina pectoris, peripheral vascular disease, or cerebrovascular disease before age 55 yr. Screening should also be done in the offspring of a parent or sibling with blood cholesterol of ≥240 mg/dL or, in the absence of family history, the presence of other risk factors (corticosteroid use, juvenile diabetes mellitus, hypothyroidism or other renal, endocrine, or hepatic disease known to affect cholesterol level). (From Expert Panel. National Cholesterol Education Program. Report of the Expert Panel on blood cholesterol levels in children and adolescents. Pediatrics 1992;89(2 suppl):525–584.)

and increased physical activity are essential first steps in the treatment of most lipid disorders. The dietary approach recommended by the NCEP ATP II for treating high blood cholesterol is outlined in Table 21.13.

Many patients with hyperlipidemia may be managed with dietary therapy alone, obviating the need for drugs.[1] Diet is considered to be the cornerstone for most forms of hyperlipidemia and the use of a dietitian for patient counseling is recommended. Several cookbooks with recipes generally suitable for implementing an alternate diet as part of the stepped diet approach have been published. The basic rationale for reducing dietary cholesterol, saturated fat, and excessive calories is based on the overproduction of VLDL and, subsequently, LDL. Excessive dietary intake of cholesterol and saturated fatty acids leads to decreased hepatic clearance of LDL and deposition of LDL and oxidized LDL in peripheral tissues.[11] The predicted reduction in total serum cholesterol following institution of the step I diet would be reduction of 3–14% with average reductions of about 5–7% in men consuming 13–14% of their calories as saturated fat.[1] Progressing to step II diet therapy should provide an additional reduction of about 3–7%. Therefore, if the baseline cholesterol was 275 mg/dL, then cholesterol after dietary therapy could range from about 220–265 mg/dL in a compliant patient. Some individuals are more responsive to dietary therapy than others and deviation from the predictions mentioned can be expected. Assessment of response to dietary therapy can be done with a dietary assessment instrument as described in the NCEP report.[1] Depending on the response to diet, the patient may be advanced until the target total or LDL-C level is reached. Each phase of the diet should be maintained for a minimum of 4–6 weeks for the minimal goal; however, the optimal response may not be seen for 3–6 months or more. In general, drug therapy should not be instituted until the trial of diet has continued for 6 months in primary prevention. Exceptions to these suggestions include patients with severe forms of hyperlipidemia or the presence of two or more risk factors or definite CHD. Long-term counseling of the patient and his or her family to encourage diet compliance and education about the risks and benefits that can be derived from diet modification and lifestyle changes is important. Overall, reduction of cholesterol and saturated fat intake provides a reduction of CHD risk. This is true regardless of the time of intervention (primary versus secondary), and diet modification works adjunctively with other risk factor interventions, such as cessation of smoking and treating hypertension. Continuation of diet therapy is imperative if drug therapy is to be optimal.

Adherence to diet therapy may be improved by presenting the changes in diet in a positive perspective and making changes over a reasonable time frame. The entire family, including the preparer of meals, should be included in diet counseling, considering that the step I diet is recommended for all Americans. Realistic goals should be set and monitoring of response of diet intervention with feedback to the patient and family will improve compliance with diet therapy. A registered dietitian is an important member of the team and his or her expertise in providing a wide range of options and suggestions in preparation of food can make the difference between a good or an inadequate response to diet. Information concerning how one can eat out in a healthy fashion and advice about shopping are also important factors for success in diet therapy. For example, being aware of products with misleading labels such as coffee creamers which state they contain "no cholesterol" when they may contain hydrogenated (saturated) fats or oils (e.g., palmitic acid, palm kernel oil, or coconut oil), which makes them undesirable because of their saturated fat content. Variations in polyunsaturated and saturated fat and cholesterol intake influence the LDL concentration but the amount of cholesterol has been found by Fielding et al.[37] to have a greater effect than the proportion of poly- or saturated fat. In this small study there were also ethnic differences in elevation of LDL with high saturated fat diets being greater in Caucasians than other groups. The isomeric form of fatty acids is also important. Fatty acids with the *cis* configuration are the preferred substrate for the ACAT reaction and significantly increase hepatic LDL receptor clearance while reducing the LDL cholesterol production rate. The *trans*

TABLE 21.13. DIETARY THERAPY OF HIGH BLOOD CHOLESTEROL

Nutrient[a]	Step I Diet	Recommended Intake	Step II Diet
Total fat		≤30% of total calories	
Saturated fatty acids	8–10% of total calories		<7% of total calories
Polyunsaturated fatty acids		Up to 10% of total calories	
Monounsaturated fatty acids		Up to 15% of total calories	
Carbohydrates		≥55% of total calories	
Cholesterol	<300 mg/d		<200 mg/d
Total calories		To achieve and maintain desirable body weight	

[a]Calories from alcohol not included.

isomeric form cannot be utilized by ACAT and is biologically inactive with no effect on LDL concentration.[38] In addition to the commercial publications mentioned previously, the NCEP also has publications available to assist with diet therapy.

Other dietary interventions or diet supplements may be useful in certain patients with lipid disorders. Increased intake of soluble fiber in the form of oat bran, pectins, certain gums, and psyllium products can result in useful adjunctive reductions in total and LDL cholesterol but these dietary alterations or supplements should not be substituted for more active forms of treatment. Total daily fiber intake should be about 20–30 g/d with about 25% or 6 g/d being soluble fiber.[1] Studies with psyllium seeds in doses of 10–15 g/d have shown reductions in total and LDL cholesterol ranging from about 5–20%.[39] They have little or no effect on HDL-C or triglyceride concentrations. These products may also be useful in managing constipation associated with the bile acid sequestrants. Fish oil supplementation provides an increased amount of the omega-3 polyunsaturated fatty acids such as eicospentaenoic acid and docosahexaenoic acid. In epidemiologic studies from Scandinavia, ingestion of large amounts of cold water fish is associated with a reduction in CHD risk but it is unclear if the same advantage is conferred with commercially prepared fish oil products. Fish oil supplementation has a fairly large effect in reducing triglycerides and VLDL-C but it either has no effect on total and LDL cholesterol or may cause elevations in these fractions. Other actions of fish oil may account for their protective effects. These effects include quantitative and qualitative alterations in the synthesis of prostanoid substances, changes in immune function and cellular proliferation, and potential antioxidative actions.[40] Responses noted with fish oil are further discussed under drug therapy. Although much has been written about coffee, there appears to be little impact on any lipid level.

Fat substitutes such as Simplesse or Trailblazer may be useful in making diets more palatable but there is no evidence of lowering lipid concentrations or in weight reduction. Both products contain protein from egg whites and skim milk or whey and they are prepared by heating, agitation, and shearing to form spherical microparticles that taste and feel like fat. Both are unstable when heated, limiting their utility in cooking, and both carry some risk for allergic reactions in people allergic to milk products or egg protein.

Drug therapy is indicated following an adequate trial of diet therapy when LDL-C is greater than or equal to 190 mg/dL in patients without definite CHD or two other risk factors. In patients with CHD or two or more risk factors, drug therapy should be considered when LDL-C is greater than or equal to 160 mg/dL.[1] Drug therapy in patients with established CHD is indicated if LDL-C exceeds 130 mg/dL after dietary therapy (Table 21.11).

DRUG THERAPY

Several excellent reviews on the treatment of hyperlipidemia and the adverse effects of the drugs used have been published recently.[41–43] Although many efficacious lipid-lowering drugs exist, none is effective in all lipoprotein disorders, and all such agents are associated with some adverse effects.[44] Lipid-lowering drugs can be broadly divided into agents that decrease the synthesis of VLDLs and LDLs, agents that enhance VLDL clearance, agents that enhance LDL catabolism, agents that decrease cholesterol absorption, agents that elevate HDL, or some combination of these characteristics (Table 21.14). Recommended drugs of choice for each lipoprotein phenotype and alternate agents are given in Table 21.15. Available products and their doses are provided in Table 21.16.

Treatment of type I hyperlipoproteinemia is directed toward reduction of chylomicrons derived from dietary fat with the subsequent reduction in plasma triglycerides. Total daily fat intake should be no more than 10–25 g/d or approximately 15% of total calories. Secondary causes of hypertriglyceridemia (Table 21.15) should be excluded or, if present, the underlying disorder should be treated appropriately. Type V hyperlipoproteinemia also requires a stringent restriction of the fat component of dietary intake and, in addition, drug therapy is indicated, as outlined in Table 21.15, if the response to diet alone is inadequate. Medium-chain triglycerides, which are absorbed without chylomicron formation, may be used as a dietary supplement for caloric intake if needed for types I and V. Hepatic fibrosis has been reported with medium-chain triglycerides. Omega-3 fatty acids may be useful in lipoprotein lipase deficiency in some patients. In patients with apolipoprotein C-II deficiency, infusion of plasma may normalize plasma triglyceride levels.

Primary hypercholesterolemia (familial hypercholesterolemia, familial combined hyperlipidemia, type IIa hyperlipoproteinemia) is treated with the bile acid sequestrants, cholestyramine and colestipol. The primary action of both agents is to bind bile acids in the intestinal lumen, with a concurrent interruption of enterohepatic circulation of bile acids and a markedly increased excretion of acidic steroids in the feces. This decreases the bile acid pool size and stimulates hepatic synthesis of bile acids from cholesterol. Depletion of the hepatic pool of cholesterol results in an increase in cholesterol biosynthesis and an increase in the number of LDL-R on the hepatocyte membrane (Fig. 21.10). The increased number of LDL-Rs stimulates an enhanced rate of catabolism from plasma and lowers LDL levels.[43] Patients with homozygous familial hypercholesterolemia (FH) genetically lack the ability to increase synthesis of LDL-R, and bile acid resins are generally ineffective. The increase in hepatic cholesterol biosynthesis may be paralleled by increased hepatic VLDL production and, consequently, bile acid resins may aggravate hypertriglyceridemia in patients with combined hyperlipi-

TABLE 21.14. EFFECTS OF DRUG THERAPY ON LIPIDS AND LIPOPROTEINS

Drug	Mechanism of Action	Effects on Lipids	Effects on Lipoproteins	Comment
Cholestyramine and colestipol	↑ LDL catabolism Cholesterol absorption	↓ Cholesterol	↓ LDL ↑ VLDL	Problem with compliance; binds many coadministered drugs
Niacin	↓ LDL and VLDL synthesis	↓ Triglyceride and cholesterol	↓ VLDL, ↓ LDL, ↑ HDL	Problems with patient acceptance; good in combination with bile acid resins
Dextrothyroxine sodium	↑ LDL catabolism	↓ Cholesterol	↓ LDL	Caution in patients with heart disease
Clofibrate	↑ VLDL clearance	↓ Triglyceride and cholesterol	↓ VLDL and LDL. ↑ HDL	Possible long-term toxicity; only modest effects on cholesterol
Neomycin sulfate	↑ LDL catabolism ↓ Cholesterol absorption	↓ Cholesterol	↓ LDL	Potentially ototoxic and nephrotoxic
Probucol	↑ LDL clearance	↓ Cholesterol	↓ LDL and HDL	Lowers HDL; modest efficacy but inhibits LDL oxidation and facilitates reverse cholesterol transport
Gemfibrozil	↑ VLDL clearance ↓ VLDH synthesis	↓ Triglyceride and cholesterol	↓ VLDL, ↑↓ LDL, ↑ HDL	Similar to clofibrate; long-term toxicity may be less than clofibrate; raises HDL
Lovastatin, pravastatin, simvastatin	↑ LDL catabolism; inhibit LDL synthesis	↓ Cholesterol	↓ LDL	Highly effective in heterozygotous familial hypercholesterolemia and in combination with other agents

demia.[45] Gastrointestinal complaints of constipation, bloating, epigastric fullness, nausea, and flatulence are most commonly reported.[44] With intensive education, patients can learn to tolerate resins on a long-term basis as evidenced by adherence in clinical trials to active drug regimens but in routine clinical practice 40% or more of patients will discontinue therapy within 1 year.[46] These adverse effects can be managed by increasing the fluid intake, modifying the diet to increase bulk, and by use of stool softeners. The other major limiting complaint is the gritty texture and bulk; these prob-

TABLE 21.15. LIPOPROTEIN PHENOTYPE AND RECOMMENDED DRUG TREATMENT

Lipoprotein Type	Drug of Choice	Combination Therapy	Alternative Agents
I	Not indicated	—	—
IIa	Cholestyramine or colestipol HMG Co-ARI[a]	Niacin Neomycin	HMG Co-ARI Neomycin Probucol
IIb	Gemfibrozil Niacin	Cholestyramine or colestipol	Cholestyramine or colestipol HMG Co-ARI Clofibrate
III	Gemfibrozil Niacin	HMG Co-ARI	HMG Co-ARI Clofibrate Estrogen
IV	Gemfibrozil Niacin	Niacin Gemfibrozil	Clofibrate
V	Gemfibrozil Niacin		Clofibrate Oxandrolone Norethisterone Fish oils

[a]Not presently recommended as a first-line drug by the National Cholesterol Education Program. HMG Co-ARI, hydroxymethylglutaryl coenzyme-A reductase inhibitors; those available include lovastatin, pravastatin, and simvastatin.

TABLE 21.16. COMPARISON OF DRUGS USED IN THE TREATMENT OF HYPERLIPIDEMIA

Drug	Manufacturer	Dosage Forms	Usual Daily Dose	Maximum Daily Dose	Cost/Month[a] ($)
Cholestyramine (Questran)	Bristol-Myers Squibb	Bulk powder/4-g packets	8 g tid	32 g	66.27–238.23
Cholestyramine (Questran Light)	Bristol-Myers Squibb	Bulk powder/4-g packets			Same
Cholestyramine (Cholybar)	Parke-Davis	4-g resin per bar			97.20
Colestipol hydrochloride (Colestid)	Upjohn	Bulk powder/5-g packets	10 g bid	30 g	89.28–142.80
Niacin	Various	50-, 100-, 250-, and 500-mg tablets; 125-, 250-, and 500-mg capsules	2 g tid	9 g	10.44–338.76
Probucol (Lorelco)	Merrill Dow	250-mg tablets	500 mg bid	1 g	69.62
Dextrothyroxine sodium (Choloxin)	Boots	1-, 2-, and 4-mg tablets	6 mg qd	8 mg	91.55
Neomycin sulfate	Various	500-mg tablets	1 g bid	2 g	15.54–28.60
Clofibrate (Atromid-S)	Ayerst	500-mg capsules	1 g bid	2 g	101.52
Gemfibrozil (Lopid)	Parke-Davis	300-mg capsules	600 mg bid	1.5 g	65.74
Lovastatin (Mevacor)	MSD	20- and 40-mg tablets	20–40 mg	80 mg	62.40–112.50
Pravastatin (Pravachol)	Bristol-Myers Squibb	10- and 20-mg tablets	20–40 mg	40 mg	54.60–91.20
Simvastatin (Zocor)	MSD	5-, 10-, 20-, and 40-mg tablets	10–20 mg	40 mg	53.40–102.30
Fluvastatin (Lescol)	Sandoz	20- and 40-mg tablets	20–40 mg	40 mg	31.80–35.70

[a]Average wholesale cost based on 1995 Redbook for usual daily dose for treatment for 1 month.

lems may be minimized by mixing the powder with orange drink or juice.[47] Tablet forms of bile acid sequestrants should help in improving compliance with this form of therapy. Other potential adverse effects include impaired absorption of fat-soluble vitamins A, D, E, and K; hypernatremia and hyperchloremia; gastrointestinal obstruction; and reduced bioavailability of acidic drugs such as coumarin anticoagulants, digitoxin, nicotinic acid, thyroxine, acetaminophen, hydrocortisone, hydrochlorothiazide, loperamide, and possibly iron.[44] Hyperchloremic metabolic acidosis, hypernatremia, and gastrointestinal obstruction have been reported almost exclusively in children and malabsorption of fat-soluble vitamins is probably most common with high doses (e.g., 30 g/d of cholestyramine) of the bile acid resins. Drug

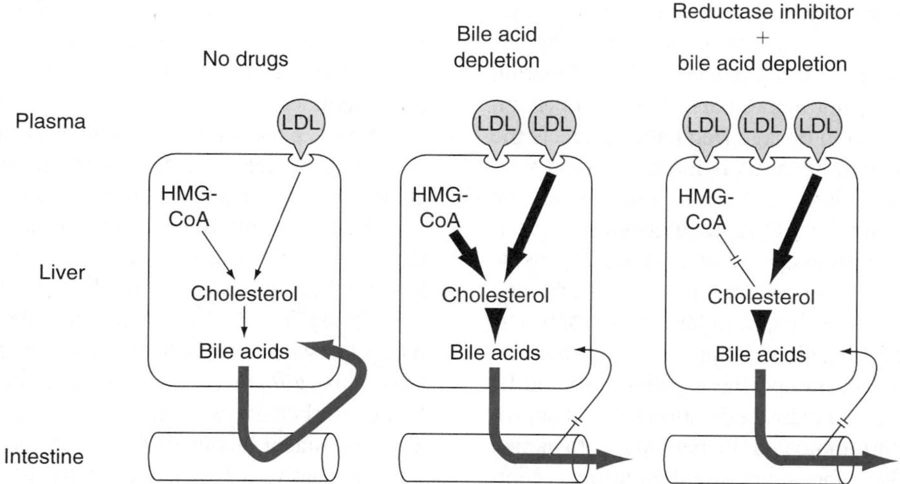

Figure 21.10. Function of the hepatic LDL-R with pharmacologic intervention, with the addition of a bile acid sequestrant, and with the combined use of bile acid sequestrant and an HMG-CoA reductase inhibitor. *(From Gotto AM Jr. Treatment of hyperlipidemia. Am J Cardiol 1986;57:14G, with permission.)*

interactions may be avoided by alternating administration times with an interval of 6 hours or greater between the bile acid resin and other drugs. Colestipol and cholestyramine have comparable side effects; however, colestipol may have better palatability since it is odorless and tasteless.

Niacin (nicotinic acid) may also be used in primary hypercholesterolemia in combination with bile acid sequestrants or as monotherapy for this disorder and others (Table 21.15). Niacin reduces the hepatic synthesis of VLDL, which in turn leads to a reduction in the synthesis of LDL. Factors responsible for decreased production of VLDL include inhibition of lipolysis with a decrease in free fatty acids in plasma, decreased hepatic esterification of triglycerides, and a possible direct effect on the hepatic production of apolipoprotein B. The complementary action of niacin and bile acid sequestrants to increase catabolism and decrease synthesis of LDL may account for the additive effects of this combination in hyperlipidemia.[48] Niacin also increases HDL by reducing its catabolism. The principal use of niacin is for mixed hyperlipemia or as a second-line agent in combination therapy for hypercholesterolemia. It is also considered to be the first-line agent or an alternative for the treatment of hypertriglyceridemia.[41]

Niacin has many adverse drug reactions that occur commonly; fortunately, most of the symptoms and biochemical abnormalities seen do not require discontinuation of therapy. Cutaneous flushing and itching appear to be prostaglandin mediated and can be reduced by aspirin 325 mg given shortly before niacin ingestion. Flushing seems to be related to rising plasma concentrations of niacin; taking the dose with meals and slowly titrating the dose upward may minimize these effects.[48] Gastrointestinal intolerance and flushing are common problems. Sustained-release products may minimize these complaints in some patients but controlled trials with regular release products do not demonstrate much of a difference between sustained- and regular-release products. Potentially important laboratory abnormalities occurring with niacin therapy include elevated liver function tests, hyperuricemia, and hyperglycemia. With less than 3 g/d the degree of liver function test elevation is generally not marked and is often transient, and a temporary reduction in dosage frequently corrects the problem. Niacin-associated hepatitis is more common with sustained-release preparations and their use should be restricted to patients intolerant of regular-release products.[49] Sustained-release products are often more expensive and given the lack of data for reduced adverse effects and increased incidence of hepatitis, regular-release products should always be used first. Preexisting gout and diabetes may be exacerbated by niacin and these patients should be monitored more closely and their medication titrated appropriately. Niacin is contraindicated in patients with active liver disease. Dry eyes and other ophthalmologic complaints are also occasionally noted. Concomitant alcohol and hot drinks may magnify flushing and pruritus with niacin and they should be avoided at the time of ingestion. Nicotinamide should not be used in the treatment of hyperlipidemia, because it does not effectively lower cholesterol or triglyceride levels.

Probucol, neomycin, and dextrothyroxine have also been used as alternative drugs for primary hypercholesterolemia; however, their utility is limited by detrimental changes in lipoproteins, adverse effects, and lack of efficacy. Fractional catabolism of LDL and increased biliary excretion of cholesterol reduce both LDL and HDL with probucol.[50] The decrease in HDL levels seen with probucol is due to a decreased synthesis of apolipoprotein A-I and decreased lipoprotein lipase activity.[43] VLDL levels are unaffected with probucol. Probucol reduces total and LDL cholesterol by 8–21% while *reducing* HDL concentrations by up to 26%.[44] Probucol inhibits the oxidation of LDL and it also facilitates reverse cholesterol transport. HDL levels may drop during reverse cholesterol transport and this may explain this lipoprotein change seen in probucol therapy.[51] The presumably undesirable effect of probucol on HDL, which may adversely affect CHD risk, as well as its propensity to increase the QT interval, relegates probucol to no more than a second-line drug.[44,52] Clinical trials to assess the potential for regression of atherosclerosis with probucol have been disappointing, and in the fall of 1995 the manufacturer announced that probucol would be removed from the market. Neomycin reduces the absorption of cholesterol from the small intestine and it is a second-line drug for use in patients with primary hypercholesterolemia who are unable to take bile acid sequestrants. Early in therapy 38–80% of patients experience increased stool frequency or diarrhea with neomycin but this usually resolves in 1–3 weeks of therapy. Although neomycin is ototoxic and small amounts are absorbed (3–5%), producing measurable plasma concentrations, at doses of 2 g/d or less for up to 3 years no toxicity has been reported. Neomycin may increase the absorption of digoxin, enhance the hypoprothrombinemic effects of warfarin, and interact synergistically with other nephrotoxic drugs and neuromuscular blocking agents. Dextrothyroxine can no longer be recommended for the treatment of hyperlipemia based on the CDP experience in which dextrothyroxine-treated patients experienced a higher mortality rate if ventricular ectopy was present at the initiation of therapy.[53]

Reductase inhibitors interrupt the conversion of HMG-CoA to mevalonate, the rate-limiting step in *de novo* cholesterol biosynthesis, by inhibiting HMG-CoA reductase (Fig. 21.8). The first product available was lovastatin (formerly known as mevinolin), a fermentation product derived from *Aspergillus terreus.* Currently, three other products are being marketed: pravastatin, simvastatin, and fluvastatin. The pharmacokinetics differ in that pravastatin and fluvastatin are active when given orally whereas lovastatin and simvastatin are prodrugs (lactone form), protein binding is extensive (95–98%) and liver excretion is high (70–95%)

with fluvastatin, lovastatin, and simvastatin but lower with pravastatin. The plasma half-lives for all the drugs have been reported to be short but since the principal site of action is the liver and a major first-pass effect is seen, the relevance of plasma half-life is unclear. Another potential difference is in tissue selectivity for inhibition of HMG-CoA reductase, but the clinical significance of this observation is unclear.[54] Simvastatin is more potent than lovastatin and pravastatin by a factor of approximately 1.5, and at higher doses, may be several times more potent than fluvastatin. Metabolic studies with lovastatin in normal volunteers and patients with hypercholesterolemia suggest reduced synthesis of LDL-C as well as enhanced catabolism of LDL mediated through LDL-R as the principal mechanisms for lipid-lowering effects.[1,43] Total and LDL cholesterol are reduced in a dose-related fashion by 30% or more on average when added to dietary therapy, with the effects being more pronounced in nonfamilial hypercholesterolemia than in FH. Combination therapy with bile acid sequestrants and lovastatin is rational as LDL-R numbers are increased, leading to greater degradation of LDL-C; intracellular synthesis of cholesterol is inhibited; and enterohe-patic recycling of bile acids is interrupted (Fig. 21.10). The addition of colestipol to lovastatin results in further reductions of total and LDL cholesterol of 28–46% compared with lovastatin alone.[55] In doses of 20 mg twice a day lovastatin produces reductions in total and LDL cholesterol of about 22–39%.[56] Twice-daily dosing appears to provide a greater reduction in lipid levels than once daily. In the Expanded Clinical Evaluation of Lovastatin (EXCEL) study of more than 8000 patients, lovastatin reduced LDL-C by 24–40% when given in doses ranging from 20 mg once daily to 40 mg twice daily.[57] Constipation in placebo-treated patients occurred in 4.7% of patients while lovastatin was associated with 4.2–7.7% (20 mg twice a day). Other adverse events related to lovastatin use were noted. Elevation of serum transaminase levels (primarily alanine aminotransferase) to above three times the upper limit of normal and associated muscle symptoms (myopathy) were most common at 40 mg given twice a day; 1.5% compared to placebo of 0.1%. Creatine kinase (CK) greater than 10 times the upper limit of normal and muscle symptoms occurred in 0% of the placebo group versus 0.2% of the lovastatin group, and any elevation of CK was highest at 40 mg given twice a day, 3.5% versus 1.6% for placebo. Lens opacities have been reported with lovastatin; however, in the age groups studied, these abnormalities are common and tend to wax and wane with time irrespective of drug therapy and no statistical association is known to exist. As a category of monotherapy, the HMG-CoA reductase inhibitors are the most potent total and LDL cholesterol lowering agents and among the best tolerated.[58–60]

Combined hyperlipoproteinemia (type IIb) may be treated with niacin or gemfibrozil to lower LDL cholesterol without elevating VLDL and triglycerides. Niacin is the most effective agent and may be combined with a bile acid sequestrant. Cholestyramine or colestipol alone in this disorder may elevate VLDL and triglycerides and their use as single agents for treating combined hyperlipoproteinemia should be avoided.[45] Gemfibrozil as a single agent is effective in reducing VLDL but a reciprocal rise in LDL may occur and total cholesterol values may remain relatively unchanged. Gemfibrozil reduces the synthesis of VLDL and, to a lesser extent, apolipoprotein B with a concurrent increase in the rate of removal of triglyceride-rich lipoproteins from plasma. Plasma HDL concentrations may rise 10–15% or more with gemfibrozil. As a fibric acid derivative of clofibrate, there has been concern that detrimental and adverse effects similar to those observed with clofibrate would occur; however, evidence from the Helsinki Heart Study has shown no significant differences between gemfibrozil and placebo.[44,61] Gastrointestinal complaints occur in 3–5% of patients, rash in 2%, dizziness in 2.4%, and transient elevations in transaminase levels and alkaline phosphatase in 4.5% and 1.3%, respectively. Similar to clofibrate, gemfibrozil may enhance the formation of gallstones associated with an increase in the lithogenic index; however, the rate is low (0.6%) and similar to that seen with placebo in the Helsinki Heart Study. Gemfibrozil may potentiate the effects of oral anticoagulants as seen with clofibrate, but this is not well documented.

Type III hyperlipoproteinemia may be treated with clofibrate, niacin, or gemfibrozil. Although clofibrate has been suggested as the drug of choice for this disorder, given the lack of data supporting its efficacy in altering cardiovascular mortality in the major studies on hypercholesterolemia and numerous, well-documented and serious adverse effects, it is reasonable to consider niacin or gemfibrozil prior to the use of clofibrate. Clofibrate increases the activity of lipoprotein lipase and reduces to a lesser extent the synthesis or secretion of VLDL from the liver into the plasma. Clofibrate is less effective than gemfibrozil or niacin in reducing VLDL production. The most disturbing aspects of clofibrate's adverse effects are its potential to induce gallstones (4.7%, clofibrate; 0.54%, placebo), promote ventricular ectopy, and potentially cause gastrointestinal malignancy causing a greater overall mortality than placebo alone.[44,62] A myositis syndrome of myalgia, weakness, stiffness, malaise, and elevations in creatinine phosphokinase and aspartate aminotransaminase is seen with clofibrate and it seems to be more common in patients with renal insufficiency. Enhanced hypoprothrombinemic and hypoglycemic effects are reported to occur when clofibrate is given to patients on coumarin anticoagulants and sulfonylurea compounds, but the mechanisms for these interactions are not well understood. Rifampin, an hepatic enzyme inducer of oxidative pathways, may induce the metabolism of clofibrate but the long-term consequences are unknown.

Two fibric acid derivatives (clofibrate and gemfibrozil) are approved in the United States; however, several others are under development or are being used in Europe. These include benzafibrate, fenofibrate, and ciprofibrate.[41] Fenofibrate is likely to be the next fibric acid analog available in this country. Diprofidrate and fenofibrate appear to be the most useful, with both reducing LDL-C by 20–25% in heterozygous FH.

As a potential alternative therapy for this phenotype, numerous epidemiologic and normal volunteer studies have found that diets high in omega-3 polyunsaturated fatty acids (from fish oil), most commonly eicosapentaenoic acid (EPA), reduce cholesterol, triglycerides, LDL-C, VLDL-C, and may elevate HDL-C.[63] The effects of fish oil on lipoprotein metabolism are mediated through a reduction in VLDL production and suppression of VLDL apolipoprotein B. In patients with hypertriglyceridemia, either phenotypes type IIb or type V, a diet high in omega-3 fatty acids given for 4 weeks reduced cholesterol 27 and 45% and triglyceride 64 and 79% in the type IIb and type V patients, respectively.[64] A diet high in EPA given to hyperlipidemic hemodialysis patients resulted in significant decreases in cholesterol and triglycerides for up to 13 weeks.[65] Fish oil supplementation may be most useful in patients with hypertriglyceridemia; however, its role in treatment is not well defined. Potential complications of fish oil supplementation such as thrombocytopenia and bleeding disorders have been noted especially with high doses (EPA, 15–30 g/d), and well-controlled trials are needed to determine if fish oils have safe and effective doses before their use may be broadly recommended.

Combination drug therapy may be considered after adequate trials of monotherapy and in patients documented as being compliant to the prescribed regimen. Two to three monthly lipoprotein determinations should confirm lack of response prior to initiation of combination therapy. Cholestyramine may be added in patients with fasting hypertriglyceridemia but it should not be used as the initial drug. Contraindications to and drug interactions with combined therapy should be carefully screened, as well as consideration of the extra cost of drug product and monitoring which may be required. Figure 21.11 summarizes the effects of combination therapy on LDL and HDL cholesterol concentrations. In general, an HMG-CoA reductase inhibitor and a bile acid sequestrant or niacin with a bile acid sequestrant provide the greatest reduction in total and LDL cholesterol. Regimens intended to increase HDL levels should include either gemfibrozil or niacin and it should be remembered that lovastatin combined with either of these drugs may result in a greater incidence of hepatoxicity or myositis. Familial combined hyperlipidemia may respond better to gemfibrozil and lovastatin than gemfibrozil and colestipol.[64]

Severe forms of hypercholesterolemia such as FH, familial defective apolipoprotein B-100, severe polygenic hypercholesterolemia, familial combined hyperlipidemia, and familial dysbetalipoproteinemia (Type III) may require more intensive therapy.[66] In particular, FH patients often require combination therapy (two to three drugs) and have been managed with surgical therapy (partial ileal bypass), plasmapheresis, and liver transplantation (to replace LDL-R).

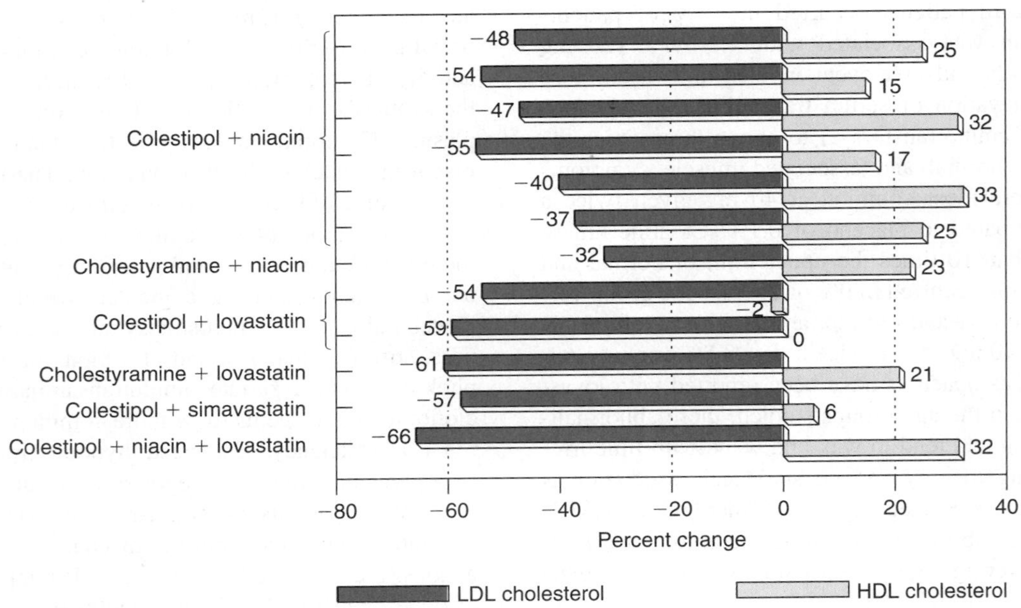

Figure 21.11. The effects of selected drug combinations on LDL and HDL cholesterol concentrations expressed as percent change from baseline. *(From Hoeg JM. Combination drug therapy, in Rifkind BM [ed]: Drug Treatment of Hyperlipidemia. New York, Marcel Dekker, 1991, p 220, with permission.)*

MANAGEMENT OF HYPERTRIGLYCERIDEMIA

It is important to remember that lipoprotein pattern types I, III, IV, and V are associated with hypertriglyceridemia and these primary lipoprotein disorders and underlying diseases should be excluded prior to implementing therapy. A positive family history of CHD is important in identifying patients at risk for premature atherosclerosis, and if a patient with CHD has elevated triglycerides, the associated abnormality is probably a contributing factor to CHD and should be treated.

High serum triglycerides (Table 21.9) should be treated by achieving desirable body weight, consumption of a low saturated and cholesterol diet, regular exercise, smoking cessation, and restriction of alcohol (in selected patients). In patients with borderline-high triglycerides but with accompanying risk factors of established CHD disease, family history of premature CHD, concomitant LDL elevation or low HDL, and genetic forms of hypertriglyceridemia associated with CHD (familial dysbetalipoproteinemia, familial combined hyperlipidemia), drug therapy with niacin should be considered. Niacin should not be used in diabetics because of the risk of worsening glycemic control. Alternative therapies include gemfibrozil and reductase inhibitors. Fibrates may increase LDL and their use in borderline-high triglyceridemia requires careful monitoring to detect this deleterious change in lipid profile. Reductase inhibitors may also be used since they provide modest reductions in triglycerides and modest elevations in HDL. The goal of therapy in this situation is to lower triglycerides and VLDL particles which may be atherogenic, increase HDL, and reduce LDL.

Very high triglycerides are associated with pancreatitis and other consequences of the chylomicron syndrome. At this level of elevation of triglycerides, a genetic form of hypertriglyceridemia often coexists with other causes of elevated triglycerides such as diabetes. Dietary fat restriction (10–20% of calories as fat), weight loss, alcohol restriction, and treatment of the coexisting disorder are the basic elements of management. Drugs useful in hypertriglyceridemia include gemfibrozil and niacin. Gemfibrozil is the preferred drug in diabetics due to the effect of niacin on glycemic control. Success in treatment is defined as a reduction in triglycerides below 500 mg/dL.[1]

SPECIAL CONSIDERATIONS

ELDERLY

Hypercholesterolemia is an independent risk factor for CHD in the elderly as it is in the younger patient. The attributable risk, which is the difference in absolute rates of CHD between segments of the population with higher or lower serum cholesterol levels, increases with age and older patients potentially benefit to a greater extent from cholesterol lowering than younger populations. Data from studies of elderly men in a variety of settings are consistent with a relative risk of at least 1.5 in the highest compared to lower quartile of cholesterol levels.[67] Treatment of hypercholesterolemia in the elderly may bring about a greater reduction in absolute risk than is obtained in younger persons.[1] The Framingham study suggests that elderly women are at higher risk due to high blood cholesterol levels but no other large studies have included women and their risks or benefits from cholesterol reduction are not well defined. Primary prevention in younger patients requires about 2 years before reduction in CHD risk is apparent and this lag time should be taken into consideration in patient selection for therapy. Nonlipid CHD risk factors do not decline in relative risk with aging, and aggressive management of the modifiable nonlipid risk factors is important in the older patient. Since most women with CHD are elderly and also at risk for osteoporosis, they are logical candidates for diet therapy with consideration of calcium intake consistent with osteoporosis prevention, exercise, and estrogen replacement therapy.

Step I diet can be recommended for most elderly patients with hypercholesterolemia but step II diets may not be advisable given potential malnutrition and concurrent disease in the elderly. Drug therapy in principle differs little from younger patients' and older patients' responses to lipid lowering drugs as well as younger patients based on the 4S trial and smaller studies.[31] Predicted reductions in CHD morbidity and mortality suggest that elderly patients with hypercholesterolemia should benefit from treatment; however, the gain in life expectancy may be small depending on the age at the start of treatment and the magnitude of cholesterol reduction.[68] Changes in body composition, renal function, and other physiologic changes of aging may make older patients more susceptible to adverse effects of lipid lowering drug therapy. In particular, older patients are more likely to have constipation (bile acid resins), skin and eye changes (niacin), gout (niacin), gallstones (fibric acid derivatives), conduction abnormalities (probucol), and bone/joint disorders (fibric acid derivatives, reductase inhibitors). Therapy should be started with lower doses and titrated up slowly to minimize adverse effects.

WOMEN/PREGNANCY

Cholesterol is an important determinant of CHD in women but the relationship is not as strong as that seen in men and HDL may be a more important predictor of disease in women.[69,70] LDL and HDL genetic regulation in women and men does not appear to be different. Based on the Nurses' Health Study, obesity is an important determinant of CHD in women with the relative risk being 3.3 in the highest Quetelet index (weight in kilograms divided by the square of the height in meters) compared to the lowest category (i.e., <21 versus ≥29); low HDL levels usually accompany obesity.[71] No major differences exist in the influence of exercise, alcohol ingestion, and smoking on lipid levels between men and women. Women in the highest tertile of cholesterol appear to be more responsive to dietary therapy than those in the lower tertiles and more responsive than formulas based on men predict.[72] Oral contraceptives adversely influence LDL and HDL and the products containing the lowest estrogen dose and the strongest antiestrogenic progestin produce the largest changes. Unopposed estrogen replacement for menopausal therapy increases HDL by 9–13% and decreases LDL by 4–10%, which is enough to influence CHD risk. Cyclic therapy with estrogen–progestin therapy may offset the beneficial effect of estrogen alone depending on the particular estrogen–progestin combination and the doses used. The Lipid Research Clinics study demonstrates the protective effect of estrogen in reducing CHD and suggests that lipid reduction with cholestyramine is beneficial in women.[73] Regression of coronary atherosclerosis in women can be induced with aggressive therapy and, based on one study, the mean percent change in area of stenosis was greater in women than men when LDL was reduced by about 38% and HDL was increased by 28%.[74]

Cholesterol and triglyceride levels rise progressively throughout pregnancy with an average increment in cholesterol of 30–40 mg/dL occurring around the 36th to 39th weeks. Triglyceride levels may go up by as much as 150 ng/dL. Drug therapy is not instituted nor is it usually continued during pregnancy. Dietary therapy is the mainstay of treatment with emphasis on maintaining a nutritionally balanced diet as per the needs of pregnancy.

CHILDREN

Drug therapy in children is not recommended until the age of 10 years or older and the guidelines for institution of therapy and the goals of therapy are different than those in adults (Table 21.12). Younger children are generally managed with dietary therapy following the NCEP step I and II diets after the age of 2 years. Bile acid sequestrants are used in children because they minimize the risks of systemic toxicity. Some literature does exist suggesting that resins are safe and effective in children. Severe forms of hypercholesterolemia (e.g., FH) may require more aggressive treatment.

CONCURRENT DISEASE STATES

Diabetes mellitus, nephrotic syndrome, end-stage renal disease, nephrotic syndrome, and hypertension compound the risk of dyslipemia and may present difficult-to-treat lipid abnormalities. Diabetic dyslipemia leads to threefold increased risk of CHD (women > men) and macrovascular complications which are associated with hyperinsulinemia and/or insulin resistance and may precede the onset of clinical diabetes during the prediabetic phase. Hyperinsulinemia may contribute to dyslipemia and hypertension and have direct atherogenic effects on the arterial wall (syndrome X); it is an independent predictor of future cardiovascular disease in a number of studies. Diabetics also have enhanced oxidation and glycation of LDL, making their LDL more atherogenic and have a pattern of smaller, more dense LDLs (pattern B) which are considered to be more atherogenic. The characteristic pattern in type II diabetes is hypertriglyceridemia, low HDL, and, less commonly, elevated total and LDL cholesterol. In the diabetic, hypertriglyceridemia is a stronger predictor of CHD risk than are cholesterol levels. Although the target LDL concentration in all diabetics is <130 mg/dL, because of the tremendous synergy between diabetes and the associated dyslipemic state, many feel that LDL cholesterol should be reduced to <100 mg/dL when possible. There are no trials currently to prove that more aggressive lipid lowering provides greater CHD risk reduction but this rationale is based on the interaction between diabetes and dyslipemia. Diet and weight reduction, if the patient is obese (particularly type II patients), and good glycemic control should be instituted prior to drug therapy. The availability of metformin should prove useful in dyslipemic diabetics since it induces weight loss and improves lipid levels slightly. Cholestyramine in diabetic patients may result in lower LDL levels but VLDL and triglyceride levels, which are commonly elevated in diabetes, may be further increased in this population. Resins may aggravate constipation, which is common in diabetics. Niacin is very effective in lowering total and LDL cholesterol and raising HDL concentrations but it is associated with worsened glycemic control.[75] Gemfibrozil principally lowers VLDL and triglycerides while increasing HDL with only modest lowering of total and LDL cholesterol; on occasion, fibric acid derivatives may increase LDL levels. Fibric acid derivatives tend to improve glucose tolerance in contrast to niacin and the greatest effect has been seen with bezafibrate. Data from the Helsinki Heart Study suggest that gemfibrozil should be an effective drug in diabetic patients because it corrects the common lipid defects that are seen.[8] HMG-CoA reductase inhibitors principally lower total and LDL cholesterol; they have modest effects on triglycerides and HDL.[76]

Abnormalities of lipoprotein metabolism in the nephrotic syndrome include elevated total and LDL cholesterol, elevated Lp (a), elevated VLDL and triglycerides. The apolipoprotein C-III/C-II ratio is elevated, consistent with greater lipoprotein lipase inhibitor activity, and the extent of hypoalbuminemia is correlated with dyslipemia. The basic abnormality appears to be one of overproduction rather than reduced clearance of LDL-C and related proteins.[77] Protein restriction and a "vegan" diet corrects lipid abnormalities to some extent. HMG-CoA reductase inhibitors have been shown to be effective in reducing elevated total and LDL cholesterol in the nephrotic syndrome, although the levels do not usually return to normal.[78,79] Combination therapy with resins and HMG-CoA reductase inhibitors may be useful, but this is untested. Clofibrate should not be used if renal insufficiency exists whereas the pharmacokinetics of gemfibrozil are apparently not altered by renal insufficiency and it is effective in lowering total cholesterol by about 15% for this disorder.[80]

Renal insufficiency without proteinuria leads to hypertriglyceridemia, slightly elevated total and LDL cholesterol (particularly with chronic ambulatory peritoneal dialysis), and low HDL levels (especially during hemodialysis). These abnormalities are thought to be due to a deficiency in apolipoprotein C-II, perhaps due to sustained use of heparin during hemodialysis and depletion of lipoprotein lipase, carbohydrate-induced obesity and hypertriglyceridemia, loss of carnitine during hemodialysis, use of acetate buffer (acetate is a precursor to fatty acid synthesis) during hemodialysis, and decreased lecithin–cholesterol acyltransferase (LCAT) activity during hemodialysis. Dialysis does not correct the lipid abnormalities. Renal transplantation may correct lipid abnormalities in some patients; however, in others the use of transplantation-related medications such as corticosteroids, cyclosporine, and certain antihypertensive agents (see Chapter 45 on renal transplantation and Chapter 12 on hypertension) may aggravate the lipid abnormalities. Cyclosporine interferes with the metabolism of reductase inhibitors and patients need to be observed closely for myositis and worsening renal function. Small, short-term studies have suggested that fluvastatin may be safer than other reductase inhibitors, but this needs to be validated in larger, long-term trials. Diet will modify lipoprotein levels, and polyunsaturated fatty acids may have a role in impeding the progression of renal disease as well as the cardiovascular complications. Clofibrate and neomycin should not be used in these patients due to the risks for toxicity. Bile acid sequestrants do not correct the lipid abnormalities seen in renal insufficiency. Lovastatin or its active metabolite may accumulate in renal insufficiency and lower doses of reductase inhibitors should be used to avoid adverse effects. Gemfibrozil may be used with caution as its pharmacokinetics are unchanged and it lowers triglycerides and increases HDL.[80] Both reductase inhibitors and fibric acid derivatives may increase the risk of severe myopathy and attention to symptoms of myositis is needed. Niacin may also be useful in nondiabetic patients with renal insufficiency.

Hypertensive patients have a greater than expected prevalence of high blood cholesterol levels, and, conversely, patients with hypercholesterolemia have a higher than expected prevalence of hypertension. Recommendations for the management of hypertension in patients with hypercholesterolemia include avoiding the use of drugs that elevate cholesterol such as diuretics and β blockers and using agents that are either lipid-neutral or may reduce cholesterol slightly (see Chapter 12, Hypertension).[81] Bile acid sequestrants may bind to thiazide diuretics and some β blockers and interfere with their absorption. This interaction may be avoided by giving the antihypertensive 1 hour before or 4 hours after the resin. Niacin may magnify the hypotensive effects of vasodilators.

COST-EFFECTIVENESS OF ANTIHYPERLIPEMIC THERAPY

The clinical benefits of lipid-lowering therapy are now well established based on the results of the LRC-CPPT, 4S, and other studies showing a reduction in CHD morbidity and mortality. The balance of benefits and costs has been examined in a few studies.[82–84] The cost per year of life saved has been estimated to range from about $17,000 to more than 1 million dollars depending on the age of the patient, the baseline level and reduction in cholesterol, the number of risk factors present, and assumptions made concerning the cost of treatment.[68,84] While this sounds like a lot of money, the cost per year of life saved is similar to that estimated for other common problems such as hypertension or renal dialysis, which are estimated to cost between $5000 and $50,000 per quality adjusted life year gained. Several studies suggest that niacin or an HMG-CoA reductase inhibitor would be more effective than cholestyramine based on the extent of cholesterol reduction or compliance.[83] Cost effectiveness is maximized by treating high-risk patients and those with established CHD.

OTHER THERAPIES

Partial ileal bypass has been used in severe heterozygous and homozygous FH; however, it is ineffective in the latter case. Ileal bypass removes the site of bile acid reabsorption, depleting the bile acid pool and increasing the catabolism of cholesterol. A randomized trial of diet versus surgery, Program on the Surgical Control of the Hyperlipidemias (POSCH), reported that total and LDL cholesterol were decreased (23.3% and 37.7%, respectively) and HDL increased (4.3%) in patients who had undergone ileal bypass for hypercholesterolemia.[85–87] Overall death was delayed by nearly 3 years ($p = 0.032$) and CHD mortality was delayed by nearly 4 years ($p = 0.046$) by surgery compared to the control group. Revascularization procedures were delayed by an average of 7 years ($p < 0.001$). Post-surgery diarrhea was more common in the surgical group as was the rate of kidney stones (4% versus 0.4%),[88] gallstones (10% versus 2%), and bowel obstruction (13.5% versus 3.6%).

Portacaval shunts have been used to decrease the formation of LDL-C and reductions of 10–20% have been reported. Plasma exchange combined with niacin was found to reduce plasma cholesterol levels by about 50% in homozygous FH over 5 years, and coronary atherosclerosis did not progress as documented by angiography. Combined liver and heart transplantation in a 6-year-old girl with homozygous FH reduced total and LDL cholesterol concentrations from 1079 and 988 mg/dL to 302 and 184 mg/dL, prior to and after surgery, respectively.[89] Liver transplantation replaced the missing LDL-R, enhanced catabolism, and reduced lipoprotein synthesis in this patient.

SUMMARY OF MAJOR STUDIES

Primary and secondary prevention diet and drug trials have been performed to determine if lowering of cholesterol will prevent CHD; these are summarized in Tables 21.17 and 21.18. A number of angiographic studies have also been performed (Table 21.19) that demonstrate that cholesterol reduction leads to regression of atherosclerosis. Most of the primary and secondary studies were double-blind, random, and placebo-controlled studies, lasting for 5 years or longer, and most had sufficient patient numbers to be meaningful. Exceptions to these qualifications were seen in the early studies such as Newcastle and Edinburgh trials which were small and the CDP using dextrothyroxine which was terminated early due to adverse effects on CHD mortality.[93,94] In the Edinburgh study,[94] 180 patients were also given warfarin and the patients remained blinded while the physicians were aware of the treatment group allocation. The Helsinki Heart Study, using gemfibrozil, resulted in a reduction in nonfatal myocardial infarction which was the primary contributor to reduced CHD incidence[9,126] (see Table 21.17).

Total and LDL cholesterol were reduced an average of 13.4% and 20.3%, respectively, by cholestyramine in the LRC–CPPT and the reduction of lipid levels was related to the amount of drug ingested[29,30] (e.g., one to two packets, 5.4% reduction in total cholesterol, versus five or more packets, 19.0% reduction). The prescribed dose of cholestyramine was 24 g or six packets per day. The cholestyramine group experienced a 19% reduction in risk ($p < 0.05$) of the primary endpoint—definite CHD death and/or definite nonfatal myocardial infarction—reflecting a 24% reduction in definite CHD death and a 19% reduction in nonfatal myocardial infarction. Other endpoints were reduced by 25, 20, and 21% for new positive exercise tests, angina, and coronary bypass surgery, respectively. Death from all causes was not significantly reduced by cholestyramine secondary to more accidents and violence in this group. The mean falls in total and LDL cholesterol in the cholestyramine group were 8% and 12% relative to levels in placebo-treated men, providing evidence that for every 1% reduction in cholesterol, a 2% decline in CHD mortality can be realized.

The cooperative trial sponsored by WHO used clofibrate 1.6 g/d in high-risk males (upper third of cholesterol distribution) compared to a similar high-risk group given placebo and a low-risk group (lower third of cholesterol distribution).[62] Cholesterol was reduced an average of 9% but

TABLE 21.17. PRIMARY PREVENTION TRIALS WITH LIPID LOWERING DRUGS

Trial	Treatment	No.	Baseline Cholesterol (mg/dL)	CHD Mortality (%)	Total Mortality (%)
Helsinki Heart Study[90]	Placebo	2030	298	1.13	2.07
	Gemfibrozil	2050	289	1.07	2.19
World Health Organization[62]	Placebo	5296	247	0.12	0.38
	Clofibrate	5331	249	0.13	0.49
LRC–CPPT[29,30]	Placebo	1900	292	2.3	3.7
	Cholesytramine	1906	292	1.7	3.6
WOSCOPS[36]	Placebo	3293	272	2.3	4.1
	Pravastatin	3302	272	1.6	3.2
ALLHAT[91]	Usual care	40,000+	NA	NA	NA
	Pravastatin				
WHI[91]	Usual care	63,000+	NA	NA	NA
	Diet, HRT				
AFCAPS/TexCAPS[91]	Placebo	7000+	NA	NA	NA
	Lovastatin				

Key: AFCAPS/TexCAPS, Air Force Coronary/Texas Atherosclerosis Prevention Study; ALLHAT, Antihypertensive and Lipid-Lowering Treatment to Prevent Heart Attack Trial; HRT, hormone replacement therapy; LRC–CPPT, Lipid Research Clinics–Coronary Primary Prevention Trial; NA, not available; WHI, Women's Health Initiative; WOSCOPS, West of Scotland Coronary Prevention Study.

TABLE 21.18. SECONDARY PREVENTION TRIALS WITH LIPID LOWERING DRUGS

Trial	Treatment	No.	CHD Mortality (%)	Total Mortality (%)
CDP[92]	Placebo	2789	22.7	25.4
	Clofibrate	1103	21.8	25.5
	Niacin	1119	21.3	24.4
Newcastle[93]	Placebo	253	NA	20.2
	Clofibrate	244		12.7
Edinburg[94]	Placebo	367	NA	11.7
	Clofibrate	350		12.3
Stockholm[9]	Placebo	276	27.2	29.7
	Clofibrate + niacin	279	19.4	21.9
4S[31]	Placebo	2223	9.3	11.5
	Simvastatin	2221	6.1	8.3
LIPID[95]	Placebo	9014	NA	NA
	Pravastatin			
CARE[96]	Placebo	4159	NA	NA
	Pravastatin			
GISSI prevention[91]	Usual care	6000	NA	NA
	Pravastatin			
BIP[91]	Placebo	3122	NA	NA
	Bezafibrate			
HIT[97]	Placebo	2500	NA	NA
	Gemfibrozil			

Key: BIP, Benzafibrate Infarction Prevention; CARE, Cholesterol and Recurrent Events; CDP, Coronary Drug Project; GISSI, Gruppo Italiano per lo Studio dell Sopravivenza nell'Infarto miocardico; HIT, High-density Lipoprotein Cholesterol Intervention Trial; LIPID, Long-term Intervention with Provastatin in Ischemic Disease; NA, not available; 4S, Scandinavian Simvastatin Survival Study.

ranged from 7–11% from the three study centers in the clofibrate-treated group. Clofibrate reduced nonfatal myocardial infarcts by 25% and CHD was reduced by 20%, primarily due to nonfatal MI reductions. Fatal MI was similar in the two high-cholesterol groups and all-cause mortality was higher (<0.05) in the clofibrate-treated group. Mortality from gastrointestinal malignancy was seen more commonly with clofibrate, and the cholecystectomy rate for gallstones was also significantly higher.

In the secondary intervention trials (Table 21.18), clofibrate (1.5 g/d) in the Newcastle study significantly reduced mortality (11.1% versus 19.0%) from sudden deaths (9 versus 21 patients in clofibrate and placebo groups, respectively) but not from myocardial infarction or congestive heart failure.[93] Nonfatal infarcts were 11.9% with clofibrate versus 18.2% in the placebo group (<0.055). Clofibrate (1.6–2 g/d) in the Edinburgh trial was less impressive with no significant effect on the occurrence of fatal or nonfatal myocardial infarction or overall mortality seen.[94]

Niacin in the CDP significantly reduced definite, nonfatal myocardial infarction compared to placebo (10.1% versus 13.9%) whereas clofibrate did not reduce death from any cause, or nonfatal or fatal myocardial infarction at the 5-year follow-up period.[92] Clofibrate did increase the rate of definite or suspected fatal or nonfatal pulmonary embolism or thrombophlebitis compared to placebo (5.8% versus 3.6%) after adjusting for baseline characteristics for total follow-up.[70] Other findings with clofibrate that occurred more frequently than with placebo included intermittent claudication, arrhythmias, palpable spleen, cholelithiasis (including cholecystectomy), and more frequent use of anticoagulants. Skin reactions, gastrointestinal complaints, and the use of gout medication were more common with niacin than with placebo. The 5-year total mortalities were 20.0% for clofibrate and 20.9% for placebo. The 5-year total mortality for niacin was 21.2%. Long-term follow-up of the CDP has shown a reduction in total mortality with niacin which occurred 9 years after the drug had been stopped.[108] The mechanism for this effect is unclear.

The most important study published in the last 5 years has been the 4S trial, which was a secondary intervention trial in a large number of patients.[31] Simvastatin, 20–40 mg/d, reduced LDL cholesterol by 35% and reduced the risk of death from any cause by 30%. Coronary deaths were also reduced with simvastatin (relative risk 0.58, CI 0.46–0.73). Therapy was also shown to be effective in women (18–19% of patients enrolled) and in the elderly (≥60 years). Indeed, the relative risk of death or major coronary event was reduced to a greater extent in the elderly than in younger patients. Death from noncardiovascular causes was similar for simvastatin and placebo (2.1% and 2.2%, respectively). The survival curves for simvastatin and

TABLE 21.19. ANGIOGRAPHIC TRIALS OF LIFESTYLE AND LIPID-LOWERING THERAPY TREATMENT/CONTROL OUTCOMES

Trial	Tx	No. Randomized	Baseline LDL (mg/dL)	% Reduction LDL	% Progression	% Regression	% Clinical Events
Lifestyle							
LHT[98]	Diet, other	53/43	149/164	36/3	14/32	41/32	5/5
Heidelberg[99]	Diet, exercise	50/56	164/165	9/0	20/42	30/4	13/8
STARS[100]	Diet	30/30	195/187	16/0	15/38	31/4	15/42
Resins							
NHLBI[32]	Ch	71/72	242/229	26/0	32/49	7/7	12/26
STARS[100]	Ch	30/30	201/187	34/4	4/38	21/4	4/42
Statins							
CCAIT[101]	L	165/166	172/171	30/2	33/50	10/7	12/14
MARS[102]	L	134/136	157/157	45/3	29/40	23/13	13/19
MAAS[103]	S	193/188	170/173	31/+1	23/32	19/12	14/20
ACAPS[104]	L	460/459	157/154	28/0	?	?	1/3
PLAC-II[104]	P		167/164	28/	?	?	5/13
REGRESS[104]	P	450/434	166/167	25/+2	45/55	17/9	16/24
Combinations							
CLAS[33]	C, N	94/94	171/169	43/5	33/55	19/7	4/7
FATS[105]	C, N	36/46	190/175	32/7	23/46	35/11	7/22
FATS[105]	C, L	38/46	196/175	45/7			
SCOR[48]	C, N, L	49/48	283/275	39/12	20/41	33/13	0/3
SCRIP[106]	C, N, G, L, P	145/155	158/156	23/4	50/50	20/10	32/37
HARP[107]	P, N, Ch, G	44/47	140/135	39/+2	35/38	10/13	10/10
Surgery							
POSCH[85]	Diet	421/417	178/176	42/6	38/65	13/5	38/72
All Trials		2023/1938	183/179	32/3	28/45	22/10	13/23

Key: Ch, cholestyramine; C, colestipol; N, niacin; L, lovastatin; G, gemfibrozil; P, probucol; HTN, hypertensive meds; PR, pravastatin; S, simvistatin. Events are defined in each study, but in general, they include cardiovascular events such as death, fatal and nonfatal MI, unstable angina, PTCA, and CABG. (Modified from Rossouw JE. Lipid-lowering interventions in angiographic trials. Am J Cardiol 1995;76:86C–92C.)

placebo began to separate at 1 year and became more divergent with additional follow-up. The 4S study clearly demonstrates the benefit in cholesterol lowering and placates long-held fears of death from non-CHD causes.

Regression of atherosclerosis and atheromatous plaques in various arterial systems has been demonstrated in numerous studies (Table 21.19). Intensive dietary and drug therapy has been used in these trials and the duration of therapy required for regression to be seen is about 2 years. Regression has been noted in native vessels as well as in grafted vessels in coronary artery bypass grafts and regression has been seen in the carotid as well as the coronary system. Presumably, regression can be induced in other vascular beds as well and these effects appear to be independent of the drug therapy used to induce regression. Based on meta-analysis and pooling project analysis of angiographic trial data, clinical outcomes such as MI and the need for interventions are reduced in a time frame not consistent with regression of plaque.[109–113] This interesting observation suggests that alteration in plaque activity, so-called "plaque stabilization," may play an important role favoring aggressive lipid lowering that has not been previously recognized.

Evaluation of Therapeutic Outcomes

Short-term evaluation of therapy for hyperlipidemia is based on response to diet and drug treatment as measured in the clinical laboratory by total cholesterol, LDL-C, HDL-C, and triglycerides for patients being treated for primary intervention as well as secondary intervention. Less commonly used laboratory measurements would include apolipoprotein B and Lp(a) levels. Since many patients being treated for primary have no symptoms and may not have any clinical manifestations of a genetic lipid disorder such as xanthomas or eruptions, then monitoring and outcome are solely laboratory based. In patients treated for secondary intervention, symptoms of atherosclerotic cardiovascular disease, such as angina or intermittent claudication, may improve over months to years. If patients have xanthomas or other external manifestations of hyperlipidemia, these lesions should regress with therapy. Lipid measurements should be obtained in the fasted state to minimize interference from chylomicrons and, once the patient is stable, monitoring is needed at intervals of 6 months to 1 year. The goals for LDL and HDL cholesterol are provided in Tables 21.11 and 21.12.

Patients with multiple risk factors and established CHD should also be monitored and evaluated for progress in managing their other risk factors such as hypertension, smoking cessation, exercise and weight control, and glycemic control if diabetic. The goals would be to maintain a blood pressure of <140/90 mm Hg, stop smoking, maintain an ideal body weight, exercise for at least 20 minutes three or more times per week, and keep plasma glucose below 140 mg/dL. Invasive evaluation such as cardiac catheterization is useful in patients with established CHD and is typically used for planning revascularization rather than monitoring of lipid-lowering therapy.

Evaluation of dietary therapy is part of the outcome evaluation for treating hyperlipidemia and the assistance of a dietitian is recommended. Use of diet diaries and recall survey instruments allow information about diet to be collected in a systemic fashion and may improve patient adherence to dietary recommendations.

Conclusion

Hypercholesterolemia is unequivocally linked to increased risk for CHD morbidity and mortality. Reductions in elevated total and LDL-C reduce CHD mortality and total mortality. Aggressive treatment of hypercholesterolemia results in fewer patients progressing to myocardial infarction, angina, and the need for interventions such as CABG and PTCA. Cholestyramine and niacin have been shown to decrease nonfatal myocardial infarction and CHD death. Niacin and simvastatin have been shown to reduce total mortality as well. Studies soon to be published may demonstrate a reduction in total mortality with other reductase inhibitors. Gemfibrozil has been shown to decrease the incidence of nonfatal CHD, especially in patients with reduced HDL and elevated LDL and triglycerides. Evidence for these beneficial effects with other lipid-lowering drugs is not currently available. Hypertriglyceridemia has not been conclusively associated with increased CHD; however, severely elevated triglyceride levels can produce pancreatitis. Hypertriglyceridemia and certain triglyceride-rich VLDL particles are associated with CHD and should be treated.

Initial therapy for any lipoprotein disorder is dietary restriction of fat and cholesterol and a modest increase in polyunsaturated fat intake along with a program of regular exercise. Hypercholesterolemia is best treated initially with a bile acid sequestrant, a reductase inhibitor, or niacin. Reductase inhibitors are the most potent form of monotherapy. Combinations of reductase inhibitors with resins are effective for hypercholesterolemia while reductase inhibitors may be used with caution with niacin or fibric acid derivatives in patients with mixed lipid disorders. Hypertriglyceridemia may be treated with niacin, gemfibrozil, or clofibrate and when considering the side-effect profile of each, gemfibrozil may be the best initial choice.

References

1. National Cholesterol Education Program: Second report of the National Cholesterol Education Program (NCEP) Expert Panel on detection, evaluation, and treatment of high blood cholesterol in adults (Adult Treatment Panel II). Circulation 1994;89:1329–1445.
2. Sempos CT, Cleeman JI, Carroll MD, et al. Prevalence of high blood cholesterol among US adults. An update based on guidelines from the second report of the National Cholesterol Education Program Adult Treatment Panel. JAMA 1993;269:3009–3014.
3. Kannel WB, Castelli WB, Gordon T. Cholesterol in the prediction of atherosclerotic disease. New perspectives based on the Framingham study. Ann Intern Med 1979;90:85–91.
4. Pooling Project Research Group. Relationship of blood pressure, serum cholesterol, relative weight and ECG abnormalities to incidence of major coronary events: Final report of the Pooling Project. J Chron Dis 1978;31:201–306.
5. Rossouw JE, Lewis B, Rifkind BM. The value of lowering cholesterol after myocardial infarction. N Engl J Med 1990;323:1112–1119.
6. Clinical Quality Improvement Network (CQIN) Investigators. Low incidence of assessment and modification of risk factors in acute care patients at high risk for cardiovascular events, particularly among females and the elderly. Am J Cardiol 1995;76:570–573.
7. Simons LA. Interrelations of lipids and lipoproteins with coronary artery disease mortality in 19 countries. Am J Cardiol 1986;57:5G–10G.
8. Manninen V, Tenkanen L, Koskenen P, et al. Joint effects of serum triglyceride and LDL cholesterol and HDL cholesterol concentrations on coronary heart disease risk in the Helsinki Heart Study. Implications for treatment. Circulation 1992;85:37–45.
9. Carlson LA, Rosenhamer G. Reduction of mortality in the Stockholm ischaemic heart disease secondary prevention study by combined treatment with clofibrate and nicotinic acid. Acta Med Scand 1988;223:405–418.
10. NIH Consensus Development Panel on triglyceride, high-density lipoprotein, and coronary heart disease. Triglyceride, high-density lipoprotein, and coronary heart disease. JAMA 1993;269:505–510.
11. Dietschy JM, Turley SD, Spady DK. Role of liver in the maintenance of cholesterol and low density lipoprotein homeostasis in different animal species, including humans. J Lipid Res 1993;34:1637–1659.
12. Shepherd J. Lipoprotein metabolism. Drugs 1994;47(suppl 2):1–10.
13. Wollett LA, Dietschy JM. Effect of long-chain fatty acids on low-density-lipoprotein-cholesterol metabolism. Am J Clin Nutr 1994;60(suppl):991S–996S.
14. Rosengren A, Wilhelmsen L, Eriksson E, et al. Lipoprotein(a) and coronary heart disease: A prospective case-con-

trol study in a general population sample of middle-aged men. Br Med J 1990;301:1248–1250.
15. Ross R. The pathogenesis of atherosclerosis: A perspective for the 1990's. Nature 1993;330:1431–1438.
16. Berliner JA, Navab M, Fogelman AM, et al. Atherosclerosis: Basic mechanisms. Oxidation, inflammation, and genetics. Circulation 1995;91:2488–2496.
17. Nagel T, Resnick N, Atkinson WJ, et al. Shear stress selectively upregulates intercellular adhesion molecule-1 expression in cultured human vascular endothelial cells. J Clin Invest 1994;94:885–891.
18. Liao F, Andalibi A, Qiao J-H, et al. Genetic evidence for a common pathway mediating oxidative stress, inflammatory gene induction, and aortic fatty streak formation in mice. J Clin Invest 1994;92:877–884.
19. Brown MS, Goldstein JL. Receptor-mediated control of cholesterol metabolism. Science 1976;191:150–154.
20. Santamarina-Fojo S, Brewer HB Jr. The familial hyperchylomicronemia syndrome. New insights into underlying genetic defects. JAMA 1991;265:904–908.
21. Carleton RA, Dwyer J, Finberg L, et al. Report of the Expert Panel on population strategies for blood cholesterol reduction. Circulation 1991;83:2154–2232.
22. Cooper GR, Smith SJ, Sampson EJ. Standardization of lipid, lipoprotein, and apolipoprotein measurements. Clin Chem 1988;34:B95–105.
23. Bachorik PS, Cloey TA, Finney CA, et al. Lipoprotein-cholesterol analysis during screening: Accuracy and reliability. Ann Intern Med 1991;114:741–747.
24. Expert Panel. National Cholesterol Education Program. Report of the Expert Panel on blood cholesterol levels in children and adolescents. Pediatrics 1992;89(suppl 2):525–584.
25. Wissler RW. New insights into the pathogenesis of atherosclerosis as revealed by PDAY, Pathobiological Determinants of Atherosclerosis in Youth. Atherosclerosis 1994;108(suppl):S3–S20.
26. Croft JB, Cresanta JL, Webber LS, et al. Cardiovascular risk in parents of children with extreme lipoproteins cholesterol levels: The Bogalusa Heart Study. South Med J 1988;81:341–349.
27. Meyers L, Coughlin SS, Webber LS, et al. Prediction of adult cardiovascular multifactorial risk status from childhood risk factor levels. The Bogalusa Heart Study. Am J Epdemiol 1995;142:918–924.
28. Diller PM, Huster GA, Leach AD, et al. Definition and application of the discretionary screening indicators according to the National Education Program for Children and Adolescents. J Pediatr 1994(Mar);126(3): 345–352.
29. Lipid Research Clinics Program. The Lipid Research Clinics coronary primary prevention trial results. I. Reduction in incidence of coronary heart disease. JAMA 1984;251:351–364.
30. Lipid Research Clinics Program. The Lipid Research Clinics coronary primary prevention trial results. II. The relationship of reduction in incidence of coronary heart disease to cholesterol lowering. JAMA 1984;251:365–374.
31. Scandinavian Simvastatin Survival Study Group. Randomized trial of cholesterol lowering in 4444 patients with coronary artery disease: The Scandinavian Simvastatin Survival Study (4S). Lancet 1994;344:1383–1389.
32. Brensike JF, Levy RI, Kelsey SF, et al. Effects of therapy with cholestyramine on progression of coronary arteriosclerosis: Results of the NHLBI type II Coronary Intervention Study. JAMA 1984;69:313–324.
33. Blankenhorn DH, Nessim SA, Johnson RL, et al. Beneficial effects of combined colestipol–niacin therapy on coronary atherosclerosis and coronary venous bypass grafts. JAMA 1987;257:3233–3240.
34. Anderson TJ, Meredith IT, Yeung AC, et al. The effect of cholesterol-lowering and antioxidant therapy on endothelium-dependent coronary vasomotion. N Engl J Med 1995;332:488–493.
35. Treasure CB, Klein JL, Weintraub WS, et al. Beneficial effects of cholesterol-lowering therapy on the coronary endothelium in patients with coronary artery disease. N Engl J Med 1995;332:481–487.
36. Shepherd J, Cobbe SM, Ford I, et al. Prevention of coronary heart disease with pravastatin in men with hypercholesterolemia. N Engl J Med 1995;333:1301–1307.
37. Fielding CJ, Havel RJ, Todd KM, et al. Effects of dietary cholesterol and fat saturation on plasma lipoprotein in an ethnically diverse population of healthy young men. J Clin Invest 1995;95:611–618.
38. Daumerie CM, Woollett LA, Dietschy JM. Fatty acids regulate hepatic low density lipoprotein receptor activity through redistribution of intracellular cholesterol pools. Proc Natl Acad Sci USA 1992;89:10797–10801.
39. Levin EG, Miller VT, Muesing RA, et al. Comparison of psyllium hydrophilic mucilloid and cellulose as adjuncts to a prudent diet in the treatment of mild to moderate hypercholesterolemia. Arch Intern Med 150;1990:1822–1827.
40. Schmidt EB, Dyerberg J. Omega-3 fatty acids. Current status in cardiovascular medicine. Drugs 1994;47:405–424.
41. Stein EA. Drug and alternative therapies for hyperlipidemia. Atherosclerosis 1994;108(suppl):S105–S116.
42. Jones PH. A clinical overview of dyslipidemias: Treatment strategies. Am J Med 1992;93:187–198.
43. Larsen ML, Illingworth DR. Drug treatment of dyslipoproteinemia. Med Clin North Am 1994;78:225–245.
44. Knodel LC, Talbert RL. Adverse effects of hypolipidaemic drugs. Med Toxicol 1987;2:10–32.
45. Crouse JR III. Hypertriglyceridemia: A contraindication to the use of bile acid-binding resins. Am J Med 1987;83:243–248.
46. Andrade SE, Walker AM, Gottlieb LK, et al. Discontinuation of antihyperlipidemic drugs—do rates reported in clinical trials reflect rates in primary care settings? N Engl J Med 1995;332:1125–1131.
47. Ito M, Morreale AP. Acceptability of cholestyramine and colestipol formulations in three common vehicles. Clin Pharm 1991;10:138–140.
48. Kane JP, Malloy MJ, Tun P, et al. Normalization of low-density-lipoprotein levels in heterozygous familial hypercholesterolemia with a combined drug regimen. N Engl J Med 1981;304: 251–258.
49. McKenney JM, Proctor JD, Harris S, Chinchili VM. A comparison of the efficacy and toxic effects of sustained-

vs immediate-release niacin in hypercholesterolemic patients. JAMA 1994(Mar 2);271(9):672–677.
50. Buckley MM, Goa KL, Price AH, et al. Probucol. A reappraisal of its pharmacological properties and therapeutic use in hypercholesterolemia. Drugs 1989; 37:761–800.
51. Franceschini G, Sirtori M, Vaccarino V, et al. Mechanisms of HDL reduction after probucol. Changes in HDL subfractions and increased reverse cholesteryl ester transfer. Arteriosclerosis 1989;9:462–469.
52. Dujovne CA, Atkins F, Wong B, et al. Electrocardiographic effects of probucol: A controlled perspective clinical trial. Eur J Clin Pharmacol 1984;26:735–739.
53. Coronary Drug Project Research Group. The Coronary Drug Project: Findings leading to further modifications of its protocol with respect to dextrothyroxine. JAMA 1972;220:996–1008.
54. Pan HY, DeVault AR, Wang-Iverson D, et al. Comparative pharmacokinetics and pharmacodynamics of pravastatin and lovastatin. J Clin Pharmacol 1990;30:1128–1135.
55. Illingworth DR. Mevinolin plus colestipol in therapy for severe heterozygous familial hypercholesterolemia. Ann Intern Med 1984;101:598–604.
56. Lovastatin Study Group II. Therapeutic response to lovastatin (mevinolin) in nonfamilial hypercholesterolemia. A multicenter study. JAMA 1986;256:2829–2834.
57. Bradford RH, Shear CI, Chremos AN, et al. Expanded clinical evaluation of lovastatin (EXCEL) study results. I. Efficacy in modifying plasma lipoproteins and adverse event profile in 8245 patients with moderate hypercholesterolemia. Arch Intern Med 1991;151:43–49.
58. Lovastatin Study Group II. A multicenter comparison of lovastatin and cholestyramine therapy for severe primary hypercholesterolemia. JAMA 1988;260:359–366.
59. Crepaldi G, Baggio G, Arca M, et al. Pravastatin vs gemfibrozil in the treatment of primary hypercholesterolemia. The Italian Multicenter Pravastatin Study I. Arch Intern Med 1990;151:146–152.
60. Tikkanen MJ, Helve E, Jaattela A, et al. Comparison between lovastatin and gemfibrozil in the treatment of primary hypercholesterolemia: The Finnish Multicenter Study. Am J Cardiol 1988;62:35J–43J.
61. Helsinki Heart Study Ethical Committee. Safety as a factor in lipid-regulating primary prevention trials: The Helsinki Heart Study Interim Report, in Wood C (ed): Further Progress with Gemfibrozil. International Congress and Symposium Series No. 87, Royal Society of Medicine Series Limited, 1986, pp 51–61.
62. Committee of Principal Investigators (WHO). A co-operative trial in the primary prevention of ischaemic heart disease using clofibrate. Br Heart J 1978;40:1069–1118.
63. Israel DH, Gorlin R. Fish oils in the prevention of atherosclerosis. J Am Coll Cardiol 1992;19:174–185.
64. Phillipson BE, Rothrock DW, Connor WE, et al. Reduction of plasma lipids, lipoproteins, and apoproteins by dietary fish oils in patients with hypertriglyceridemia. N Engl J Med 1985;312:1210–1216.
65. Hamazaki T, Nakazawa R, Tateno S, et al. Effects of fish oil rich in eicosapentaenoic acid on serum lipid hyperlipidemic haemodialysis patients. Kidney Int 1984;26:81–84.
66. East C, Bilheimer DW, Grundy SM. Combination drug therapy for familial combined hyperlipidemia. Ann Intern Med 1988;109:25–32.
67. Rubin SM, Sidney S, Black DM, et al. High blood cholesterol in elderly men and the excess risk for coronary heart disease. Ann Intern Med 1990;113:916–920.
68. Taylor WC, Pass TM, Shepard DS, et al. Cholesterol reduction and life expectancy: A model incorporating multiple risk factors. Ann Intern Med 1987;106:605–614.
69. Bush TL, Fried LP, Barrett-Connor E. Cholesterol, lipoproteins, and coronary heart disease in women. Clin Chem 1988;34:B60–B70.
70. Jacobs DR Jr, Mebane IL, Bangdiwala SI, et al. High density lipoprotein cholesterol as a predictor of cardiovascular disease mortality in men and women: The follow-up study of the Lipid Research Clinics Prevalence Study. Am J Epidemiol 1990;131:32–47.
71. Manson JE, Colditz GA, Stampfer MJ, et al. A prospective study of obesity and risk of coronary heart disease in women. N Engl J Med 1990;322:882–889.
72. Boyd NF, Cousin M, Berton M, et al. Quantitative changes in dietary fat intake and serum cholesterol in women: Results from a randomized, controlled trial. Am J Clin Nutr 1990;52:470–476.
73. Bush RL, Barrett-Connor E, Cowan LD, et al. Cardiovascular mortality and non-contraceptive estrogen use in women: Results from the Lipid Research Clinics Program Follow-Up Study. Circulation 1987;75:1102–1109.
74. Kane JP, Malloy MJ, Ports TA, et al. Regression of coronary atherosclerosis during treatment of familial hypercholesterolemia with combined drug regimens. JAMA 1990;264:3007–3012.
75. Garg A, Grundy SM. Nicotinic acid as therapy for dyslipidemia in non-insulin-dependent diabetes mellitus. JAMA 1990;264:723–726.
76. McKenney JM. Understanding and treating dyslipidemia associated with noninsulin-dependent diabetes mellitus and hypertension [review]. Pharmacotherapy 1993(Jul–Aug);13(4):340–352.
77. Joven J, Villabona C, Vilella E, et al. Abnormalities of lipoprotein metabolism in patients with the nephrotic syndrome. N Engl J Med 1990;323:579–584.
78. Vega GL, Grundy SM. Lovastatin therapy in nephrotic hyperlipidemia: Effects on lipoprotein metabolism. Kidney Int 1988;33:1160–1168.
79. Rabelink AJ, Erkelens DW, Hene RJ, et al. Effects of simvastatin and cholestyramine on lipoprotein profile in hyperlipidemia of nephrotic syndrome. Lancet 1988;2:1335–1338.
80. Evans JR, Falland SC, Cutler RE. The effect of renal function of the pharmacokinetics of gemfibrozil. J Clin Pharmacol 1987;27:994–1000.
81. Working Group on Management of Patients with Hypertension and High Blood Cholesterol. National Education Programs Working Group Report on the management of patients with hypertension and high blood cholesterol. Ann Intern Med 1991;114:224–237.
82. Schrott HG, Stein EA, Dujovne CA, Davidson MH. Enhanced low-density lipoprotein cholesterol reduction and cost-effectiveness by low-dose colestipol plus lova-

statin combination therapy. Am J Cardiol 1995;75:34–39.
83. Goldman L, Weinstein MC, Goldman PA, et al. Cost-effectiveness of HMG CoA reductase inhibition for primary and secondary prevention of coronary heart disease. JAMA 1991;265:1145–1151.
84. Hamilton VH, Racicot FE, Zowall H, Coupal L. The cost-effectiveness of HMG-CoA reductase inhibitors to prevent coronary heart disease. Estimating the benefits of increasing HDL-C. JAMA 1995;273:1032–1038.
85. Buchwald H, Varco RL, Matts JP, et al. Effect of partial ileal bypass surgery on mortality and morbidity from coronary heart disease in patients with hypercholesterolemia. Report of the Program on the Surgical Control of the Hyperlipidemias (POSCH). N Engl J Med 1990;323:946–955.
86. Buchwald H, Campos CT, Boen JR, et al. for the POSCH Group. Disease-free intervals after partial ileal bypass in patients with coronary heart disease and hypercholesterolemia: report from the Program on the Surgical Control of the Hyperlipidemias (POSCH). J Am Coll Cardiol 1995;26:351–357.
87. Buchwald H, Matts JP, Fitch LL, et al. for the Program on the Surgical Control of the Hyperlipidemias (POSCH) Group. Changes in sequential coronary arte--riograms and subsequent coronary events. JAMA 1992;268:1429–1433.
88. Obialo CI, Clayman RV, Matts JP, et al. Pathogenesis of nephrolithiasis postpartial ileal bypass surgery: Case-control study. The POSCH Group. Kidney Int 1991;39:1249–1254.
89. Bilheimer DW, Goldstein JL, Grundy SM, et al. Liver transplantation to provide low-density lipoprotein receptors and lower plasma cholesterol in a child with homozygous familial hypercholesterolemia. N Engl J Med 1984;311:1658–1664.
90. Frick MH, Helsinki Heart Study. Primary-prevention trial with gemfibrozil in middle-aged men with dyslipidemia. N Engl J Med 1987;317:1237–1245.
91. Simes RJ. Prospective meta-analysis of cholesterol-lowering studies: The Prospective Pravastatin Pooling (PPP) project and the Cholesterol Treatment Trialists (CTT) collaboration. AJC 1995;76:122C–126C.
92. Coronary Drug Project Research Group. Clofibrate and niacin in coronary heart disease. JAMA 1975;231:360–381.
93. Group of Physicians of the Newcastle upon Tyne Region. Trial of clofibrate in the treatment of ischaemic heart disease. Br Med J 1971;4:767–775.
94. Research Committee of the Scottish Society of Physicians. Ischaemic heart disease: A secondary prevention trial using clofibrate. Br Med J 1971;4:775–784.
95. LIPID Study Group. Design features and baseline characteristics of the LIPID (Long-term Intervention with Pravastatin in Ischemic Disease) Study: A randomized trial in patients with previous acute myocardial infarction and/or unstable angina pectoris. Am J Cardiol 1995;76:474–479.
96. Sacks FM, Rouleau J-L, Moye LA, et al. Baseline characteristics in the cholesterol and recurrent events (CARE) trial of secondary prevention in patients with average serum cholesterol levels. Am J Cardiol 1995;75:621–623.
97. Rubins HB, Robins SJ, Twane MK, Boden WE, et al. Rationale and design of the Department of Veterans Affairs High-density Lipoprotein Cholesterol Intervention Trial (HIT) for secondary prevention of coronary artery disease in men with low high-density lipoprotein cholesterol and desirable low-density lipoprotein cholesterol. Am J Cardiol 1993;71:45–52.
98. Ornish D, Brown SE, Scherwitz LW, Billings JH, et al. Can lifestyle changes reverse coronary heart disease? Lancet 1990;336:129–133.
99. Schuler G, Hambrecht R, Schlierf G, Niebauer J, et al. Regular physical exercise and low-fat diet. Effects on progression of coronary artery disease. Circulation 1992;86:1–11.
100. Watts GF, Lewis B, Brunt JN. Effects on coronary artery disease of lipid-lowering diet, or diet plus cholestyramine, in the St. Thomas Atherosclerosis Regression Study (STARS). Lancet 1992;339:563–569.
101. Waters D, Higginson L, Gladstone P, Kimball B, et al. Effects of monotherapy with an HMG-CoA reductase inhibitor on the progression of coronary atherosclerosis as assessed by serial quantitative arteriography. The Canadian Coronary Atherosclerosis Intervention Trial. Circulation 1994;89:959–968.
102. Blankenhorn DH, Azen SP, Kramsch DM, et al. Coronary angiographic changes with lovastatin therapy. The Monitored Atherosclerosis Regression Study (MARS). Ann Intern Med 1993;199:969–976.
103. MAAS Investigators. Effect of simvastatin on coronary atheroma: The Multicentre Anti-Atheroma Study (MAAS). Lancet 1994;344:633–638.
104. Jukema JW, Bruschke AVG, van Boven AJ, et al. Effects of lipid lowering by pravastatin on progression and regression of coronary artery disease in symptomatic men with normal to moderately elevated serum cholesterol levels. The Regression Growth Evaluation Statin Study (REGRESS). Circulation 1995;91:2528–2540.
105. Crouse JR III, Byington RP, Bond MG, et al. Pravastatin, lipids, and atherosclerosis in the carotid arteries (PLAC-II). Am J Cardiol 1995;75:455–459.
106. Brown BG, Albers JJ, Fisher LD. Regression of coronary artery disease as a result of intensive lipid-lowering therapy in men with high levels of apolipoprotein B. N Engl J Med 1990;323:1289–1298.
107. Haskell WL, Alderman EL, Fair JM, et al. Effects of intensive multiple risk factor reduction on coronary atherosclerosis and clinical cardiac events in men and women with coronary artery disease. The Stanford Coronary Risk Intervention Project (SCRIP). Circulation 1994;89:975–990.
108. Canner PL, Bierge KG, Wenger NK, et al. Fifteen year mortality in Coronary Drug Project patients: Long-term benefit with niacin. J Am Coll Cardiol 1986;8:1245–1255.
109. Sacks FM, Paternak RC, Gibson CM, et al. for the Harvard Atherosclerosis Reversibility Project (HARP)

Group. Effect on coronary atherosclerosis of decrease in plasma cholesterol concentrations in normocholesterolemic patients. Lancet 1994;344:1182–1186.

110. Gotto AM Jr. Lipid lowering regression, and coronary events. Circulation 1995;92:646–656.

111. Salonen R, Nyyssonen K, Porkkala E, et al. Kuopio Atherosclerosis Prevention Study (KAPS): A population-based primary preventive trial of the effect of LDL lowering on atherosclerosis progression in carotid and femoral arteries. Circulation 1995;92:1758–1764.

112. Pitt B, Mancini G, Ellis SG, et al. Pravastatin limitation of atherosclerosis in the coronary arteries (PLAC-I). J Am Coll Cardiol 1994;suppl IA:131A.

113. Furberg CD, Adams HP J, Applegate WB. Effect of lovastatin on early carotid artherosclerosis and cardiovascular events. Circulation 1994;90:1679–1687.

Chapter 22

Peripheral Vascular Disease

Robert L. Talbert, PharmD, FCCP

The term *peripheral vascular disease* (PVD), in its broadest sense, applies to disease of any of the blood vessels outside the heart and thoracic aorta and to disease of the lymph vessels. Although this term includes cerebrovascular and hypertensive vascular disease, these two topics are discussed in other chapters. The other major area included in this term is peripheral vascular disease of the extremities, which can be divided into two distinct systems: (1) venous disorders such as acute deep vein thrombosis and its complications of pulmonary embolism and post-thrombotic syndrome (Chapter 19), and (2) peripheral arterial disease resulting from occlusion and arterial vasospasm. This chapter focuses on peripheral vascular disease. Because there are several distinct peripheral vascular diseases, epidemiology, pathophysiology, clinical presentation, and treatment are oriented to the particular disease. A general review of the structure and function of the normal vascular system and its reactive changes is presented first to aid in the understanding of the specific peripheral vascular disorders.[1,2]

Structure/Function of the Normal Vascular System

The vascular system consists of varying histologic portions of five component parts: endothelium, basement membrane, elastic tissue, collagen, and smooth muscle.[2] The endothelium is the monolayer lining of the luminal surface of the entire vascular system and functions to regulate the flow of blood in and out of the vessel lumen. Endothelial cells have several important functions including the active transport of circulating substances through their cytoplasm. Endothelium-derived relaxing factor (EDRF), which is thought to be nitric oxide or a mixture of S-nitrosothiol and nitric oxide, is synthesized through three pathways by the endothelium from l-arginine in response to a host of neurochemical and mechanical stimuli including wall and shear stress, platelet activation, thrombin, serotonin, adenosine diphosphate (ADP), arachidonic acid, catecholamines, vasopressin, histamine, and acetylcholine.[3,4] EDRF diffuses from endothelial cells to adjacent smooth muscle cells and relaxes vascular smooth muscle. It also counteracts the action of numerous vasoconstrictor substances on smooth muscle as well as inhibiting platelet aggregation.[5] The effects of EDRF seem most pronounced in the basal state and contribute to dilator tone of the skin and extremities but less of an effect is seen during reflex sympathetic vasoconstriction.[4] Vasorelaxation and inhibition of platelet aggregation derived from the actions of EDRF stem from stimulation of the formation of cyclic guanosine monophosphate (cGMP) from guanosine triphosphate (GTP) and elevated cytosolic concentrations of cGMP, which stimulates intracellular binding of free calcium. Endothelin-1, the arachidonic acid metabolites prostacyclin H_2 and thromboxane A_2, and angiotensin II are vasconstricting substances derived from the endothelium which are counterbalanced by the vasodilating properties of nitric oxide when endothelial function is normal.[1] Loss of endothelium from atherosclerotic plaque formation, percutaneous transluminal angioplasty, or other means of disruption of this monolayer of cells such as smoking reduces synthesis of EDRF and the protective homeostatic function of this paracrine substance (Fig. 22.1). Disease states that facilitate this process or are worsened because of it include hypertension, diabetes mellitus, hypercholesterolemia, atherosclerosis, and coronary artery disease.[6,7]

Basement membrane is a dense sheath adjacent to the external surface of endothelial cells and serves as a transport barrier and support structure. The basement membrane contains a ground substance that is a mixture of mucopolysaccharides, protein–polysaccharide complexes, and glycoproteins, which retain large amounts of water and provide a gelatinous medium for transport of materials. Elastic tissue encircles the wall just outside the endothelium and basement membrane. It is also found in the media and adventitia of all vessels except the terminal arterioles, capillaries, and small venules, and allows for expansion of the vessel. The internal elastic lamella is prominently affected by nearly all pathologic changes that involve the vascular system.

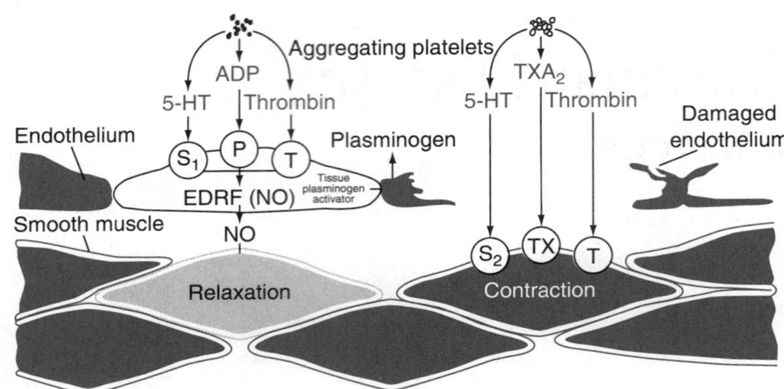

Figure 22.1. Mechanisms of vasospasm in atherosclerotic arteries. *Left:* Normal endothelium. If platelets were to aggregate and release 5-hydroxytryptamine (5-HT; serotonin) and ADP, these would act on specific receptors on the endothelial cells (S_1, serotoninergic receptor; P, purinergic receptor) to release EDRF. EDRF is nitric oxide (NO) or a nitrosothiol. Also, if any thrombin were formed, this would act on a specific receptor (T) to enhance the release of relaxing factor. Also, tissue plasminogen activator would be stimulated to form plasminogen. *Right:* If the endothelium is damaged, platelets aggregate because of the loss of the inhibitory action of NO and prostacyclin. The resultant release of 5-HT and thromboxane A_2 (TXA_2) and the formation of thrombin cause vasoconstriction or vasospasm by acting directly on receptors on the smooth muscle cells. Not shown is the fact that some of the 5-HT can be taken up by the sympathetic nerve endings and released again as a false transmitter to enhance the contraction. Also the resultant tissue hypoxia–anoxia releases a contracting factor from the vessel wall, which further aggravates and prolongs the vasospasm. *(From Shepherd JT, Katušić ZS: Hypertension 18(suppl 3):76–85, 1991. By permission of the American Heart Association, Inc.)*

Another important component of vessel walls is collagen. In normal vessels it is present in the media and adventitia and is involved in all reactions of vessels to injury. Collagen is highly resistant to stretching and functions to prevent overdistention of the vessels. The fifth component is smooth muscle, which is the actively contracting element of the vascular system. Arterial metabolism is dependent mainly on smooth muscle cells. These are the major connective tissue-forming cells of the vascular wall, producing elastic tissue, collagen, mucopolysaccharides, and myosin. Smooth muscle cells can metabolize glucose, synthesize fatty acids, cholesterol, phospholipids, and triglycerides, and facilitate the entry of lipoproteins into the cell. Several catabolic enzymes such as mixed-function oxidases, fibrinolysins, and lysosomal hydrolases are also present. This function and the proliferative nature of smooth muscle cells are important factors in the reaction of arterial walls to injury and atherogenesis.[7] In contrast to the differentiated, contractile type of smooth muscle cell usually seen in adults, smooth muscle cells lose their contractility and instead gain the ability to secrete extracellular matrix components and divide, which is thought to be an early step in the development of atherogenesis.[8]

The structural organization of the vessel wall consists of three well-defined layers: the intima, the media, and adventitia[2] (Fig. 22.2). The intima is a single continuous layer of endothelial cells and associated basement membrane. It is delineated on its outer surface by a perforated tube of elastic tissue, the internal elastic lamella. This structure is especially prominent in the large elastic arteries and medium-caliber muscular arteries, but is not seen in capillaries. The media consists of only one cell type, the smooth muscle cell. These cells are surrounded by small amounts of collagen and elastic tissue. The media is delineated on the luminal side by internal elastic lamina, and on the abluminal side by a less continuous sheet of elastic tissue, the external elastic lamella. The outer portion is nourished by small blood vessels (vasa vasorum) in the adventitia, and the inner layers receive nutrients from the lumen. The outer layer of the vascular wall is the adventitia. This layer contains a mixture of collagen, elastic fibers, smooth muscle fibers, and fibroblasts. This outer layer also contains nerve fibers, the vasa vasorum, and lymphatics that nourish the vessel wall and remove metabolic waste products.

The vascular system can be divided into elastic arteries, muscular arteries, arterioles, capillaries, veins, and lymphatics. Elastic arteries, such as the aorta and major pulmonary arteries, contain large amounts of elastic tissue. The walls of these arteries distend and increase their elastic tension with systole. During diastole, the elastic fibers recoil, which helps propel the blood distally and maintain flow (see Chapter 12, Hypertension).

Smooth muscle cells dominate in muscular arteries such as the renal, superior mesenteric, and femoral arteries. These arteries regulate peripheral flow and supply organs that require a specific blood supply based on the amount of work they are performing. These arteries can vary their caliber by contracting (vasoconstriction) and relaxing (vasodilation), so that a given cardiac output can be allocated to various tissues depending on their current needs. Thus, muscular arteries function as resistance vessels and are major regulators of systemic blood pressure.

Arterioles are branches of the muscular arteries that differ structurally and functionally from small arteries only by their size. Because of their large number, arterioles form

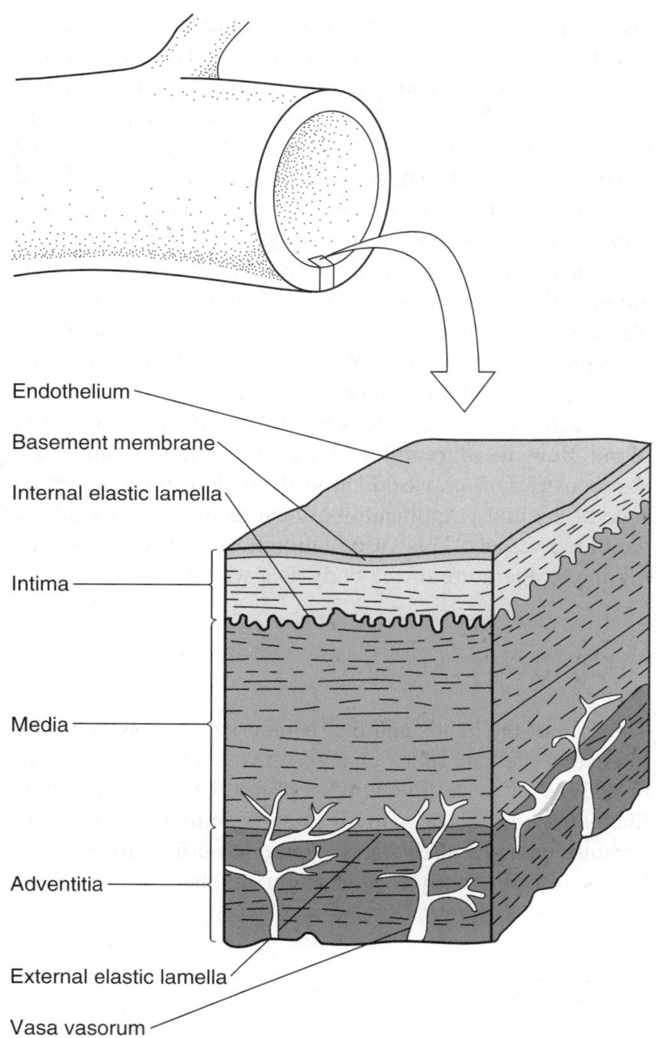

Figure 22.2. Schematic drawing of structural organization of the vascular wall. *(From Lie JR. The structure of the normal vascular system and its reactive changes, in Juergens JL, Spittell JA, Fairbairn JF [eds]: Peripheral Vascular Diseases. Philadelphia, WB Saunders, 1980, p 57, with permission.)*

the most important class of resistance channels in the vascular system. Capillaries are blood vessels that have a diameter similar to that of a red blood cell.

Veins are considerably larger than their associated arteries. Their structure reflects both the low pressure of this system and their reservoir function. The walls of the veins are thinner and the media contains fewer smooth muscle cells, collagen, and elastic fibers. Smooth muscle cells are responsible largely for the vasoconstrictive activity of the veins that is seen mainly in the small peripheral veins in the skin. The larger veins can actively constrict during acute changes in pressure, but they passively dilate with slow increases in pressure. The lymphatic channels are the simplest parts of the vascular system. The intima consists of endothelial cells and a few collagen and muscle fibers.

Reactive Changes of the Vascular System

The arteries are not static structures, but rather they change in response to various physical and chemical stimuli, react to injury, and undergo structural alterations throughout growth and aging.[2] The major change that occurs with normal aging is a slow, continuous symmetric increase in the intimal thickness, especially in the large elastic arteries. This process results from a gradual accumulation of smooth muscle cells (which presumably migrate from the media), diffuse connective tissue, and an accumulation of sphingomyelin and cholesterol. This diffuse age-related thickening is to be distinguished from discrete raised fibromuscular plaques, a characteristic feature of atherosclerosis. After the sixth decade, the intima also becomes more collagenized and there is a loss of cellular constituents and granular degranulation of elastic fibers. The rate of aortic intimal thickening is more prominent in men and accelerated in patients with hypertension. Structural changes in small arteries and arterioles differ somewhat from that in systemic vessels in that there is progressive fibrotic thickening of the adventitia and media, with little intimal change. These changes are closely linked to hypertension and diabetes mellitus.

In the normal arterial wall, lipid content, mainly cholesterol and phospholipid (especially sphingomyelin), also progressively increase with age. Phospholipid synthesis rises with age followed by a compensatory increase in all phospholipases except sphingomyelinase. Accumulations of cholesterol and low-density lipoprotein (LDL) appear to be derived from plasma. Functionally, these changes result in increased rigidity of arteries and loss of endothelial function. Endothelial dysfunction leads to vasoconstriction, thrombosis, and greater involvement of the inflammatory response, promoting atherosclerosis. The larger arteries may become dilated, elongated, and tortuous, and aneurysms may form in areas of degenerating arteriosclerotic plaques.

The veins also undergo age-related changes. Phlebosclerosis, also called hyperplastic phlebitis, refers to thickening of the veins. It appears to be age related and is particularly prominent in veins of the lower extremity that are subject to stasis and increased luminal pressure.

Physiology of Limb Blood Flow

Blood flow to the limbs is controlled by arterial blood pressure and resistance to flow, which is provided by the physical characteristics of blood vessels and of the blood itself. There are two major components to resistance: the viscosity of the blood and the tube factor or hindrance, based on size, shape, smoothness, branching, and other physical aspects of the wall. Poiseuille's law governs the flow of fluids through cylindrical tubes and it states that resistance to flow is proportional to the fourth power of the radius. Viscosity is usually fairly constant but exceptions to this would be the presence of abnormal or abnormally high numbers of red or white blood cells such as in chronic obstructive airways disease, sickle cell disease, or certain types of leukemia. Active changes in the radius of the resistance vessels in the limbs are caused by local and neurogenic mechanisms.[2]

LOCAL CONTROL

Local control of limb blood flow includes intrinsic, metabolic, humoral, and physical factors. The relative importance of each of these varies for different tissues and for different vessels within the same tissue. Intrinsic smooth muscle tone appears to be directly influenced by changes in wall tension, which in turn is determined by intravascular pressure. A decrease in intravascular pressure and wall tension would result in spontaneous activity of the smooth muscle cells, and an increase in intravascular pressure would have the opposite effect.

The intrinsic myogenic activity is modified by chemical changes in the resistance vessels, which adjust blood flow to the limbs (active hyperemia). Similar increases are seen after temporary arrest of circulation to the limbs (reactive hyperemia). Metabolic factors play an important role in controlling blood flow to skeletal muscles. The accumulation of metabolic products such as carbon dioxide, potassium, phosphate, and adenosine during exercise, an increase in the osmolality of venous effluent, or a change in pH causes direct vasodilation of peripheral vessels (Fig. 22.3). The humoral factors that cause dilation of skeletal muscle vessels include epinephrine, acetylcholine, histamine, prostaglandins, and serotonin. As described previously, many of the effects of these substances are mediated via the endothelial release of EDRF. Norepinephrine, angiotensin, and vasopressin cause vasoconstriction. In skin, epinephrine causes vasoconstriction because there is a preponderance of α adrenergic in cutaneous vessels, in contrast to skeletal muscle vessels, which have both α and β receptors. Epinephrine has a greater affinity for β_2 receptors in skeletal muscle resistance vessels, and thus causes vasodilation.

Such physical factors as local temperature also control blood flow to extremities. Low temperatures can cause vasoconstriction or vasodilation depending on the thermal state of the body. Application of heat to an extremity dilates the blood vessels. This vasodilation is enhanced by increasing the temperature of the body as a whole.

NEURAL CONTROL

The skin of the hands and feet is innervated by sympathetic fibers that mediate reflex changes in vessel tone. Alterations in activity of these fibers under central control cause large fluctuations in the flow to all fingers simultaneously. Temperature changes alter the sympathetic outflow to the skin. Exposure of the body to cold augments the vasoconstrictor

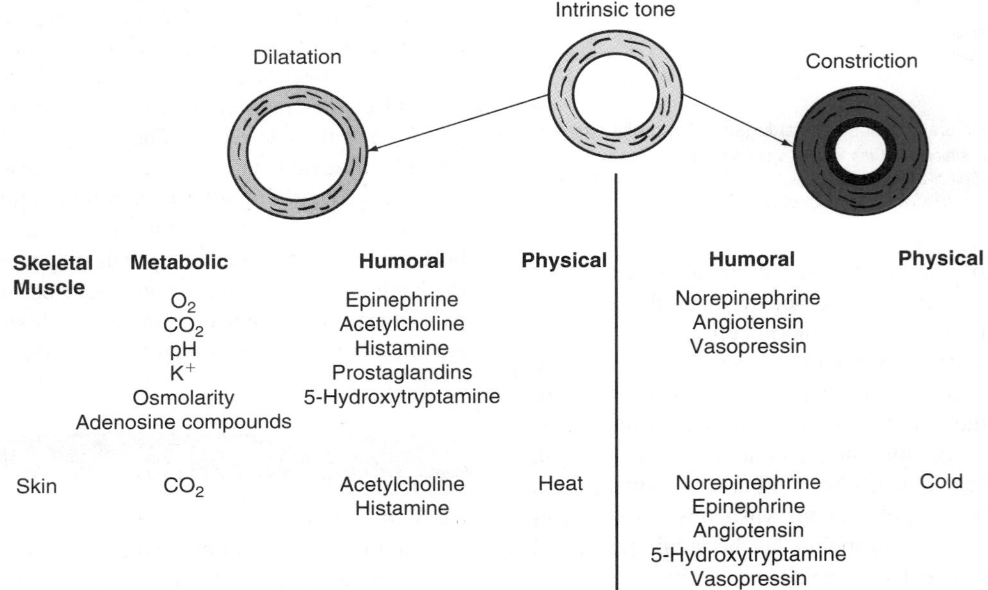

Figure 22.3. Active changes in vascular diameter are caused by local and nervous mechanisms. Local control includes intrinsic, metabolic, humoral, and physical factors, and the relative importance of each of these varies for different tissues and for different vessels within the same tissue. This figure identifies actions of local factors that can alter arterial diameter in skeletal muscle and skin. *(From McGrath MA, Verhaeghe RH, Shepherd JT. The physiology of limb blood flow, in Juergens JL, Spittell JA, Fairbairn JF [eds]: Peripheral Vascular Diseases. Philadelphia, WB Saunders, 1980, p 84, with permission).*

tone, whereas an increase in body temperature decreases tone. The circulation in the skin also plays an essential role in thermal homeostasis. Arteriovenous anastomoses, which are numerous in fingers and toes, favor heat dissipation. Sweat glands cause local production of bradykinin, and consequently vasodilation, when stimulated by sympathetic cholinergic nerves.

Changes in the diameter of resistance vessels in skeletal muscle are influenced by sympathetic adrenergic nerves, which are abundant in small arteries and arterioles. Sympathetic nerve fibers to muscle are of two types: vasoconstrictor fibers, whose activity is mediated by the release of norepinephrine, and vasodilator fibers, whose activity is mediated through the release of acetylcholine. Although vessels in both the skin and muscles are innervated by sympathetic fibers, the vasomotor centers controlling these vessels can function independently. In reflex control of body temperature, only the vessels to the skin are involved, whereas with alterations in position, the reflex changes are confined to the vessels in the muscles.

PERIPHERAL ARTERIAL DISORDERS

Peripheral vascular disease of the arteries can be generally classified as obstructive and vasospastic. Examples of an obstructive abnormality include arteriosclerosis obliterans and thromboangiitis obliterans (Buerger's disease). Raynaud's disease is the most common example of a vasospastic disorder.

ARTERIOSCLEROSIS OBLITERANS

Arteriosclerosis obliterans, also called atherosclerosis obliterans (ASO), is a chronic occlusive arterial disease of the aorta, particularly the terminal portion of the abdominal aorta and its major branches to the extremities. It is one of several types of chronic arterial occlusive disease (Table 22.1). This disease also involves the large- and medium-size arteries of the extremities, especially the iliofemoral and popliteal arteries and, in the lower leg, the posterior tibial artery at the ankle and the anterior tibial artery at its origin. Arteriosclerosis obliterans is considered a segmental disease, with significant variation in its extent. The clinical classification of the severity of peripheral vascular disease is based on exercise limitation and symptoms and is referred to as the Fontaine classification (Table 22.2).

TABLE 22.1. CAUSES OF CHRONIC ARTERIAL OCCLUSIVE DISEASE

Arteriosclerosis obliterans
Thromoboangiitis obliterans (Buerger's disease)
Arteritis
Trauma
Congenital arterial narrowing

Epidemiology

Arteriosclerosis obliterans occurs primarily in men between the ages of 50 and 70 years, and the reported incidence of symptomatic disease is about 1.5%; however, the incidence is age related.[1,9] In men aged 40–44 years, 50–54 years, and 60–64 years, the reported incidence is 0.9, 3.6, and 7.5%, respectively. The disease affects women less commonly, about 0.07%, usually after the age of 60 years, perhaps in part because of a menopausal loss of the protective effect of estrogens and an increased incidence of diabetes in women of this age. If noninvasive testing is performed, the incidence of large leg artery disease is 11.7% and small artery disease is 16% while only about 10% report symptoms.[10] As in the case of atherosclerosis, hypercholesterolemia plays an important role in the development of this disease. Arteriosclerotic lesions in the lower extremities are commonly associated with coronary and cerebrovascular disease as noted in the Coronary Artery Surgery Study and others.[11] Diabetes mellitus significantly increases the prevalence (11-fold) and severity of ASO (10 years earlier than if diabetes is not present). Other risk factors important for the pathogenesis of ASO include hypertension, hypercholesterolemia, and smoking.[9,12]

Pathophysiology

The primary lesion in ASO is an intimal plaque, which progressively narrows and, in many cases, leads to complete occlusion of these arteries. The histopathologic changes are essentially identical to those of arteriosclerotic occlusive disease of the visceral and cerebral arteries. The primary physiologic disturbance is obstruction of blood flow through large arteries and, therefore, ischemia of those tissues of the extremity supplied by these arteries. The degree of ischemia is proportional to (1) the proximal limit of the occluding process, (2) the patency of collateral blood vessels, and (3) the rapidity of occlusion development. The ischemia pro-

TABLE 22.2. FONTAINE CLASSIFICATION FOR CLAUDICATION

Stage	Symptoms
I	Asymptomatic
II	Intermittent claudication
IIa	Pain-free, claudication walking >200 m
IIb	Pain-free, claudication <200 m
III	Rest/nocturnal pain
IV	Necrosis/gangrene

duced by the obstruction may be increased by arteriolar constriction from any cause. If the occlusion is not too extensive, dilation may improve circulation. Obstruction of the large arteries decreases pressure and blood flow in smaller arteries distal to the obstruction, and thrombosis and gangrene may result. Peripheral occlusive arterial disease is often associated with increased blood viscosity, hyperfibrinogenemia, and a relatively high hematocrit.

Clinical Presentation

Unless there is an acute arterial occlusion such as a thrombosis, the signs and symptoms of ASO have a gradual onset. The most common is intermittent claudication, which is described as pain, cramping, numbness, or weakness in certain muscles that develops only during exercise. The distress is quickly relieved by rest without change in position. About one-third of patients do not have symptoms of intermittent claudication or any other ischemic symptoms. Intermittent claudication is caused by inadequate blood supply to muscles(s) stressed by exercise. The distance a person is able to walk before the pain develops varies with the extent and severity of arterial occlusion. It is usually unilateral at first, may become bilateral with time, and is often worse in one of the extremities if both are involved. The location of the involved muscle group may predict the most proximal level of occlusion. For example, claudication of the calf muscles suggests occlusion of the popliteal artery or higher; claudication of the hip indicates disease low in the aorta or in the iliac artery. Edema of disuse and dependency may occur if a limb is kept in the dependent position for long periods of time in an attempt to relieve symptoms.

Another important group of symptoms includes pain at rest, paresthesias, and numbness. These symptoms are usually the result of more severe ischemia of tissues and a more advanced form of the disease resulting from multiple levels of occlusion or obstruction of collateral vessels. It is usually felt in the digits but may be noted in the foot and lower leg as well. Ulceration and gangrene are common when the disease reaches this stage. Pain caused by ischemic neuropathy is another clinical feature of ASO, especially in diabetic patients. Peripheral nervous tissue has a low metabolism and requires very little blood to keep it healthy; this ischemic neuropathy, regardless of symptoms, is consistent with advanced disease. This pain may be continuous or paroxysmal and may be described as a series of sharp pains or the sensation of electrical shocks. A sensation of numbness, coldness, or burning may also occur. When diabetics with a neuropathy develop ulcers the lesions are often painless.

The physical findings in arteriosclerosis of the extremities are for the most part indistinguishable from those seen in other occlusive arterial diseases. Impairment of arterial pulsations, often noted by palpation, is the most important and consistent finding. Others include systolic bruits over the involved arteries, color (waxy, pale, and dry appearance) and temperature changes in the skin of the extremity, edema, and hypoesthesia and hyporeflexia in patients with severe neuropathy.

Diagnosis

The diagnosis of ASO is often made on the basis of a good history and physical examination. Sophisticated laboratory studies and diagnostic tests are rarely necessary to establish the diagnosis; however, routine laboratory tests such as blood chemistry, electrocardiogram, and x-ray studies may be needed to determine the extent of associated disease as well as prognosis and therapy. The magnitude of arterial occlusion can be assessed simply by measuring the extremity's blood pressure at rest and after exercise to the point of claudication. Another easily obtained measure of disease severity is the ankle/brachial index (ABI). This can be done using a Doppler ultrasonic probe or by a variety of plethysmographs. The ABI (sometimes called the arm/ankle index, AAI) is abnormal if the ratio of the arm (right or left) to dorsalis pedis (DP) or posterior tibial (PT) blood pressure is <0.8. If both DP and PT are abnormal the extent of disease is more severe and atherosclerosis is likely to be widespread.[13] ABI is inversely related to cardiovascular risk factor as well as subclinical and clinical cardiovascular disease in older adults. The lower the ABI, the greater the increase in CVD risk; even those with asymptomatic reductions in the ABI (0.8–1.0) appear to be at increased risk of cardiovascular disease.[14] Arteriography is rarely necessary to establish the diagnosis, but is usually used prior to surgery to precisely locate the disease. Traditional or digital subtraction arteriography are considered to be the "gold standard" diagnostic tests for peripheral vascular disease. Other techniques include vascular songraphy (standard and color Doppler), magnetic resonance imaging, computerized axial tomography, and angioscopy, which utilizes a thin, flexible fiberoptic scope to directly visualize the vessel lumen. After physical examination and ABI determination, the next diagnostic test is usually sonography.[12]

Noninvasive methods available for evaluating skin microcirculation include transcutaneous oxygen tension measurements ($tcPo_2$), laser Dopper fluxmetry (LDf), and vital capillaroscopy (VC).[1] These methods differ in the amount of skin area and depth of microcirculation which can be evaluated. They are all highly variable in assessing the blood flow. The clinical differentiation of ASO from other types of occlusive peripheral arterial diseases is given in Table 22.3.

Treatment

The goals of therapy in patients with ASO are to arrest progression of the disease, improve blood flow, relieve pain,

TABLE 22.3. FACTORS IN DIFFERENTIAL DIAGNOSIS OF PERIPHERAL VASCULAR DISEASE

Factor	Arteriosclerosis Obliterans	Thromboangiitis Obliterans	Raynaud's Phenomenon
Gender distribution	Predominantly male	98% male	90% female
Age at onset of symptoms	Usually over 50 yr Earlier in diabetes	<35 yr	Usually 11–45 yr
Symmetry	Often asymmetrical	Generally asymmetrical	Symmetrical
Onset	Insidious	Acute and preceded by migratory phlebitis (30–70%)	Often in cold climate and after stress
Intermittent claudication	Common	Common	Absent
Vasospasm	Not remarkable	Almost invariable in involved limb	Invariably symmetrical
Absent pulses	Infrequent in upper and common in lower extremities	Common in upper and lower extremities	Occurs only in late and extreme cases
Skin (if involved)	Thin, often hairless	Thin, atrophic, and red or cyanotic	Normal except during spasm
Ulcers (if any)	Dry and usually superficial	Moist, deep, inflamed, and invasive	Dry, fingertip
Plain radiograms	Calcification of artery	Normal	Often atrophy of phalanges
Cholesterol	High	Borderline	Normal
Presence of coronary or cerebral disease	Common	Rare early in disease	Coincidental

(Modified from McCombs PR, Horwitz O. Diseases of the arteries of extremities, in Horwitz O, McCombs PR, Roberts B (eds): Diseases of Blood Vessels. Philadelphia, Lea and Febiger, 1985, pp 210–211.)

and prevent and treat ulceration and gangrene. Progression of the disease may be prevented by control of hyperlipoproteinemia, control of any associated diseases such as diabetes and hypertension, and tobacco abstinence. Regression of atherosclerosis with lipid lowering is described in Chapter 21, Hyperlipidemia. Normalizing cholesterol serum levels in patients with peripheral atherosclerosis improves both endothelium-dependent and -independent relaxation in human peripheral small arteries. For patients who have severe ischemia manifested by rest pain, ulceration, and gangrene, rest of the extremity is an important adjunct of treatment. If the pain is severe, narcotics and other pain medications may be necessary. It is important to take meticulous care of the extremities and avoid even minor trauma because it may lead to ulceration. In these patients, ulceration is usually treated with local care, medical management, including antibiotics if necessary, and surgical amputation if required.

Another effective method of improving blood flow to the extremities is to increase collateral flow. This can be accomplished by a warm environmental temperature; avoidance of vasoconstriction caused by drugs, cold, and tobacco; elevation of the head of the bed 12–16 inches; and exercise. A daily exercise training program is very effective in patients with mild to moderate intermittent claudication. Important features of a successful program are (1) repetitive daily walks to 75% of the claudication distance with intermittent periods of rest (1–2 minutes); (2) weekly increase in walking time and distance; and (3) continuation of this program, as cessation results in loss of improvement. Controlled studies have shown a 25–30% increase in walking distance with an average of about 1000 feet, although 40% of patients may show increases of nearly a mile.[15] Compared to strength training, treadmill training provides more improvement in exercise time and maximum oxygen uptake.[16] A consistent exercise training program will prevent abrupt deterioration and the need for amputation and may reduce mortality compared to patients with claudication not on an exercise program.[17]

Various vasodilating drugs (e.g., tolazoline, nylidrin, isoxsuprine, niacin derivatives, cyclandelate, and papaverine) have been used in ASO, but none has been shown to be consistently effective. Ischemia is one of the most potent stimuli for vasodilation, and drug therapy does not augment the physiologic response to ischemia. Vasodilators may increase the caliber of nondiseased vessels creating a "steal" of flow from deficit areas to well-perfused areas or they may decrease systemic blood pressure and increase resistance further in diseased vessels. Therefore, vasodilators are of no value in treating ASO.[15]

Controversy surrounds the use of β-adrenergic blocking agents in PVD patients with concurrent coronary artery disease or hypertension. A number of case reports have been published indicating that these agents can cause or worsen intermittent claudication. By reducing systemic blood pressure, these agents could decrease blood flow through stenotic arteries or collateral vessels. A nonselective β blocker may attenuate epinephrine-induced vasodilation during exercise by blocking β_2 receptors in peripheral vessels. Controlled trials using both selective and nonselective agents have produced mixed results in patients with PVD. A few studies have demonstrated an increase in muscle blood flow and symptomatic improvement when β blockers were withdrawn.[18,19] Hiatt et al.,[20] however, demonstrated that calf blood flow was not affected by either propranolol or metoprolol compared with placebo in patients with mild to moderate occlusive PVD, and there was no difference in symptoms of claudication. In contrast, Roberts et al.,[21] in a 6-month randomized, double-blind study of captopril, atenolol, labetalol, and pindolol, found that all β blockers reduced pain-free walking distance and maximum walking distance as well as postexercise calf blood flow availability compared with captopril in hypertensive patients with intermittent claudication. β-Adrenergic blocking agents are probably best avoided in patients with intermittent claudication.[22]

Pentoxifylline (Trental®) has been shown to be of benefit in patients with chronic occlusive arterial disease. In a double-blind multicenter trial of 128 patients, pentoxifylline in doses up to 1200 mg/d was significantly more effective than placebo in increasing both the initial and the absolute claudication distances. The average increase in walking distance was about one-half of a city block. With regard to the subjective parameters, only incidences of paresthesias showed a significantly greater reduction in the pentoxifylline group compared with the placebo group.[23] Pentoxifylline has been shown to be effective in moderately severe chronic obstructive arterial disease if the resting AAI is less than 0.8 and if symptoms of intermittent claudication have been present for longer than 1 year.[24] Other studies with pentoxifylline have not shown objective benefit in treadmill exercise time.[15] Pentoxifylline increases red blood cell deformibility, decreases platelet adhesiveness, blood fibrinogen, and neutrophil elastase/α_1 proteinase inhibitor complex levels, which are thought to lead to a reduction in blood viscosity and improved blood flow.[25] Patients more likely to improve with pentoxifylline are those with moderately severe ischemia and without rest pain, ischemic ulcers, or severe claudication.[26] Pentoxifylline is also used to prevent postoperative rethrombosis after vascular surgery for arterial occlusive disease. This drug has been shown superior to the combination of acetylsalicylic acid and dipyridamole in maintaining vascular patency in these patients over a 6-month period.[27] Pentoxifylline may also be useful in aiding healing of diabetic foot ulcers but most of these studies are small and not well designed.[28] Some studies show that pentoxifylline is most effective early in therapy and may lose its effectiveness with time.[29] A cost-effectiveness analysis suggests that pentoxifylline may reduce the risk of vascular surgery while not increasing the total cost of PAD care.[30]

Antiplatelet therapy with aspirin and dipyridamole may decrease disease progression, whereas aspirin alone has less of an effect.[31] In earlier, smaller studies ticlopidine improved pain-free walking time, ABI ratios, and ulcer healing.[32,33] However, in the Swedish Ticlopidine Multicenter Study, a larger randomized, placebo-controlled trial lasting for 5 years, no significant improvement was noted with ticlopidine.[34] Prostaglandin E_1 (PGE_1) and I_2 (PGI_2, prostacyclin) are potent vasodilators and inhibitors of platelet aggregation that have been shown to improve claudication, relieve pain, and promote ulcer healing in short-term studies.[35] More recent studies have confirmed the earlier findings and suggest that the effects of infusions of PGE_1 and PGI_2 have persisting effects on blood flow and exercise capacity which may last for weeks to months after treatment.[36–40] The major drawback to prostaglandin therapy is the need for intravenous infusion of the drugs due to their short half-lives.[40] Other antiplatelet drugs undergoing clinical evaluation include trapidil, cilostazol, and picotamide.[41]

Short-term studies with calcium channel blockers have also shown some promise; however, interest recently has focused on the potential for antiatherosclerosis effects of calcium blockers.[42–44] This approach to therapy presently is only theoretical although there is some hope that calcium channel blockers may limit or delay the progression of atherosclerosis. Defibrotide, an investigational agent, has been shown in open label trials to improve symptoms and treadmill exercise time in about 50% of treated patients.[45] Defibrotide increases tissue plasminogen activator production and release and PGI_2 formation, and inhibits platelet activation.

Based on results from the Prevention of Atherosclerosis Complications with Ketanserin (PACK) trial, ketanserin has no significant effect in reducing the symptoms of intermittent claudication.[46] Another approach, based on improved muscle metabolism with L-carnitine (2 g twice a day for 3 weeks), was shown to improve walking distance.[47–49] Carnitine skeletal muscle stores are reduced in animal models and, when replenished, muscle performance is improved. At this point, an appropriate reminder would be that many trials in the treatment of PVD and intermittent claudication are either poorly controlled or have significant design flaws, and that an inverse correlation exists between the sample size and the number of studies reporting positive results.[50]

Low-dose regional catheter-directed thrombolytic therapy has been used as an alternative to surgical treatment in those patients considered poor surgical candidates. Ward et al.[51] used tissue plasminogen activator as either a bolus of 20 mg followed by continuous infusion of 1 mg/h or a continuous infusion of 1 mg/h only. More rapid dissolution of thrombus and greater angiographic and clinical success was noted with the bolus/infusion method; however, bleeding complications were also higher.[51] The short-term success rate ranges from 65–85% in appropriately selected patients and major complications have been reported to occur in 8–12% of patients.[12] Others have noted similar results but the exact method of delivering thrombolytics, the relative efficacy among available agents, optimal patients to be treated, and duration of response remain to be determined.[52,53] Another form of antithrombotic therapy, calcium heparin, has been found to be more effective than ticlopidine in trials lasting up to 3 months.[54]

When medical management with exercise, control of risk factors, and vasodilator or antithrombotic therapy is inadequate, interventional therapeutic technology is useful. The indications for revascularization are patients truly incapacitated by exercise limitations or critical limb ischemia. The types of technology which exist include atherectomy, atheroablation, balloon angioplasty and endovascular stents, angioscopy and laser angioplasty, and direct open arterial surgery utilizing endarterectomy, prosthetic bypass grafts, or vein-patch arterioplasty may be effective in bypassing or removing areas of stenosis but should be reserved for patients with severe and disabling symptoms (Fontaine class IIb and above).[12] Patients most likely to have complete relief of symptoms and normalization of pressure gradients are those with smaller, more focal segments involved (2–5 cm or so depending on the vascular bed), those without calcification, and those with less than total occlusion. Vein grafts are preferred because of a lower incidence of thrombosis compared with synthetic materials. For patients with venous insufficiency, sclerotherapy with hypertonic saline or dextrose of sodium morrhuate, sodium tetradecyl sulfate, or polidocanol and others may be useful in controlling telangiectasias and varicosities.

As with atherectomy, atheroablation and balloon angioplasty procedures for coronary revascularization, these revascularization procedures for peripheral artery occlusion are associated with primary failure and restenosis, hematomas at the site of device insertion, dissection, and pseudoaneurysms at the site of catheter entry.[55–58] Acute closure occurs in 1–4% of peripheral angioplasties and antithrombotic therapy with urokinase or other thrombolytics, and heparin may be used to reopen a vessel occluded with thrombus.[55,56] Spasm postprocedure is managed with nitroglycerin and calcium channel blockers. Longer term antithrombotic therapy may be continued with aspirin. Recently, Minar et al.[55] found aspirin 100 mg/d was as effective as 1000 mg/d to prevent restenosis; however, 30% of patients in either group still developed closure. Neither antiplatelet agents nor anticoagulation with warfarin have been shown to be very effective in preventing restenosis; however, omega-3 polyunsaturated fatty acid supplementation with fish oil shows some promise.[57] Longer term patency rates following angioplasty typically have ranged from about 60–75% at 1 year depending on the site of intervention and this rate compares favorably with surgery.

Lumbar sympathectomy may be useful in patients with mild ischemia rest pain but temporary sympathectomy with local anesthetics should be performed first to ensure benefit from the procedure. Sympathectomy does alter the long-term course of ASO.

THROMBOANGIITIS OBLITERANS (BUERGER'S OR VON WINIWERTER DISEASE)

Thromboangiitis obliterans (TAO) is a disease involving segmental inflammatory and proliferative nonartheromatous lesions of the medium and small arteries, veins, and nerves that usually occurs in young males and frequently leads to nonhealing ulcers and gangrene (see Table 22.2). The cause of thromboangiitis obliterans is unknown but virtually all patients are heavy smokers of cigarettes or use other forms of tobacco. Many patients show cutaneous sensitivity to tobacco and there is a high prevalence of the human leukocyte antigens (HLA)-A9 and HLA-B5 in affected persons, which suggests a genetic basis for the disease. Lymphocyte sensitivity to type I and III collagens has been shown for 77% of patients and about 50% have anti-collagen antibodies.[59]

Common presenting complaints include a superficial, migratory, nodular phlebitis, associated with cutaneous erythema, and tenderness. TAO may present with intermittent claudication, most commonly in the arch of the foot (relieved by rest), or less commonly in the calf and occasionally on both sides. Rest pain may present as a severe ache, or numb, gnawing pain that may worsen by elevation of the limb. Cold sensitivity of the hands occurs in about 50% of TAO patients. Pulsations in the posterior tibial and dorsalis pedis arteries may be impaired or absent and affected extremities may be abnormally red. Segmental thrombophlebitis occurs in about 40% of the patients.

Goals of therapy in TAO include arresting progression of the disease, producing vasodilation, relieving pain, and treating ulcers and gangrene. All patients with TAO should abstain completely and permanently from tobacco of any type. Failure to abstain from tobacco results in disease progression, severe rest pain, ulceration, and amputation. Other measures that have been suggested but do not work well include anticoagulants, sympathectomy, vascular surgery, and vasodilating drugs. None of these measures can be recommended. Patients should be advised to avoid cold exposure and vasoconstricting drugs.

RAYNAUD'S DISEASE[60–63]

In 1862 Maurice Raynaud described episodes of discoloration of the skin of the digits on exposure to cold and he thought this was due to increased sensitivity of the sympathetic nervous system. This condition, which is limited to the skin, usually accompanied by cyanosis, rubor, pain, or parethesias, and associated gangrene, came to be termed Raynaud's disease. More than a century later, the pathogenesis, diagnosis, and treatment are still unclear.[60] Raynaud's disease may be classified as primary, in which the cause is unknown, or secondary in which an associated condition exists (Table 22.4).

TABLE 22.4. CLASSIFICATION OF RAYNAUD'S PHENOMENON

I. Primary Raynaud's syndrome or phenomenon—no known association or contributing condition
   A. Raynaud's disease
II. Secondary Raynaud's phenomenon
   A. After trauma—pneumatic hammer, pianists, typists
   B. Neurogenic lesions—carpal tunnel syndrome, thoracic outlet syndrome
   C. Occlusive arterial disease—ASO, TAO, thrombotic arterial occlusion
   D. Miscellaneous diseases and conditions
      1. Common causes—connective tissue diseases
      2. Uncommon causes—cryoproteinemias, polycythemia, vinyl chloride, hepatitis B antigenemia, hypothyroidism, renal disease
   E. Drugs
      1. β-Adrenergic receptor blocking drugs
      2. Ergot preparations
      3. Methysergide
      4. Vinblastine and bleomycin
      5. Amphetamines (? cocaine)
      6. Imipramine
      7. Bromocriptine
      8. Clonidine
      9. Cyclosporin

(Modified from Coffman JD. Raynaud's phenomenon. An update. Hypertension 1991;17:593–602; and Spittell JA Jr. Raynaud's phenomenon and allied vasospastic disorders, in Juergens JL, Spittell JA, Fairbairn F (eds): Peripheral Vascular Diseases. Philadelphia, WB Saunders, 1980, pp 554–583.)

Epidemiology

The prevalence of Raynaud's disease in the general population is unknown, but the gender ratio is 4 or 5 to 1 female to male, and most cases occur prior to age 40 years (Table 22.3). Men with Raynaud's disease generally present at an older age, and have a much higher incidence of associated atherosclerosis, which accounts for their symptoms when compared with women.

One interesting group of patients with Raynaud's symptoms comprises those whose occupations involve routine use of vibratory equipment or frequent exposure to cold temperature. Forty percent to 90% of loggers and 50% of miners using vibratory equipment have been diagnosed with Raynaud's disease. Heredity may also play a role in the development of this disease.[61]

Pathophysiology

The two theories of the cause of digital artery vasospasm in primary Raynaud's disease are an increased activity of the sympathetic nervous system and a local fault in the digital arteries.[60] Although several lines of evidence favoring increased sympathetic activity exist, evidence against this mechanism includes lack of increased cutaneous nervous system activity, local cooling of one hand does not lead to reflex vasoconstriction in the opposite hand, and normal plasma and urinary catecholamine concentrations in primary Raynaud's disease. In contrast, the local fault theory is supported by the induction of vasospastic attacks in sympathetically denervated fingers, the induction of attacks in single fingers, an enhancement of reflex sympathetic vasoconstriction by local hand cooling, and a loss of digital systolic blood pressure with a local ischemia and cold stimulus. One of the mechanisms to explain these observations focuses on the activity of α_2-adrenergic receptors in patients with primary Raynaud's disease and the sensitivity of the receptor to cold exposure. Patients with primary Raynaud's disease have a greater sensitivity of the α_2 receptor with exposure to cold and specific agonists and antagonists for α_1 and α_2 receptors point to altered α_2 activity as one of the defects in this syndrome. Reflex sympathetic stimulation also leads to greater S_2-serotonergic receptor activity even in the presence of α_1 and α_2 blockade, suggesting a pathophysiologic role for serotonin (5-hydroxytryptamine) in vasospasm of Raynaud's disease. Coffman has recently studied Raynaud's patients and could not document a role for sertontin in these patients.[64] It is still possible that serotonin is produced at the local level and contributes to the disease but this remains to be further clarified. Young women with primary Raynaud's disease usually exhibit the purest form of vasospasm. These patients have lower digital, artery, and arteriolar systolic blood pressure than normal subjects.[61] Older male patients usually have secondary Raynaud's disease involving both a vasospastic and obstructive disease. In these patients a normal vasoconstrictive stimulus acting on an arterial bed with reduced intraluminal pressure is sufficient to cause arterial closure. Initially these patients may demonstrate pure vasospasm, but later they develop obstruction as underlying autoimmune processes cause damage to the arterial wall.

Additional factors that may contribute to the pathogenetic mechanisms of Raynaud's disease include increased blood viscosity, platelet abnormalities, abnormal secretion of prostacyclin and thromboxane B_2, and abnormal endothelial function. Evidence does exist of increased factor VIII/von Willebrand factor antigen and factor activity along with elevated fibrinogen levels that promote hyperviscosity (especially in connective tissue disorders) and thrombosis, but the importance of these factors as well as the others described remains to be determined.

Clinical Presentation

Digital color changes are a common manifestation of this disease. A classic attack begins with a sudden loss of arterial blood flow, causing blanching. Next, a small quantity of blood enters the capillary and venous system and desaturates, and the digits become cyanotic. The third phase of the attack involves vasodilation, causing rubor. Not all patients exhibit a triphasic color change; many demonstrate only pallor or cyanosis, during which the digits turn absolutely white. At first only the tips of the fingers of both hands are involved; later the more proximal parts of the fingers are affected. In the late stage the color change may extend back to involve the rest of the hands. Symptoms are worse in the cold season and less severe in warm weather. Pain is not a prominent symptom during the attack or in the interval between attacks. Paresthesias are common during the attack and consist of numbness, tingling, burning, or a feeling of tightness. Slight swelling of the involved fingers may occur, but only during attacks.

Diagnosis

Primary Raynaud's disease usually includes the following features:

1. Vasospastic attack induced by cold exposure
2. Bilateral involvement of the extremities
3. Absence of gangrene or involvement of only the skin of the fingertips
4. History of symptoms for at least 2 years
5. No evidence of underlying disease including absence of antinuclear antibodies, a normal erythrocyte sedimentation rate, and normal nailfold capillaroscopy and esophageal motility studies[60]

All patients should have a complete history and physical examination, with special emphasis on signs and symptoms of connective tissue disease. Routine laboratory tests should include a complete blood count, erythrocyte sedimentation rate, chemistry profile, antinuclear antibody, urinalysis, and hand radiography. Hand arteriography may sometimes be used in assessing the relative roles of vasospastic and occlusive disease, but is rarely used to establish a diagnosis. Digital plethysmography is often used to follow the course of the disease or to evaluate the response to therapy. Finger systolic blood pressure and its response to cold stress and ischemia has also been used to aid in diagnosis.

Treatment[60–62]

Conservative measures will suffice for the majority of patients with primary or secondary Raynaud's disease. General considerations for treatment include avoidance of cold temperatures, tobacco, emotional situations, and certain drugs (Table 22.4). These patients should dress warmly, wear lined gloves, and use Styrofoam coasters when handling iced drinks. Large meals and long periods of standing should be avoided as they both reduce peripheral circulation.

Therapy for Raynaud's disease is aimed at increasing digital blood flow and consists of behavioral therapy or biofeedback and drug therapy. Biofeedback is of benefit in some patients and it is used to lessen the severity of the attacks. The goal with these techniques is to self-regulate the nervous system and reduce vasoconstrictive autonomic tone. Biofeedback is accomplished with the use of a thermoprobe or thermistor attached to the person's finger or hand, which relays skin temperature information back to the patient. The patient can then concentrate further on raising the peripheral temperature. One of the more successful regimens has been immersing the hands in 43°C water while the body is exposed to 0°C temperatures. After 3 weeks of daily sessions, improvement has been noted for several months.[65] When attacks interfere with the patient's ability to function normally, drug therapy should be tried. Drug therapy is associated with significant adverse effects and objective changes in blood flow do not always correlate with symptom improvement. Only about two-thirds of patients can be expected to respond to drug therapy.

Drug therapy for Raynaud's disease is directed toward vasodilation and involves several classes of drugs toward this end, including sympatholytics, α-adrenergic antagonists, direct-acting vasodilators, calcium channel antagonists, serotonin receptor antagonists, angiotensin-converting enzyme inhibitors, prostaglandins, and thyroid hormones.

Sympatholytic Agents

Reserpine and other drugs have been used for years in the treatment of Raynaud's disease; unfortunately there are few controlled trials with these agents to suggest that any benefit is derived from their use. Reserpine in oral doses of 0.25–0.75 mg daily may increase capillary blood flow in short-term studies, but long-term improvement is doubtful. Reserpine in higher doses causes several unpleasant adverse effects including nasal congestion, bradycardia, postural hypotension, dyspepsia, fluid retention, lethargy, and depression. Intra-arterial reserpine has been shown to be no better than placebo. Guanethidine in doses of 10–50 mg daily produces postural hypotension, explosive diarrhea, fatigue, and impotence, and is generally not well tolerated. It may increase capillary blood flow during cooling in patients with Raynaud's disease resulting from scleroderma. Methyldopa has been shown to offer subjective improvement in uncontrolled studies but no objective benefit has been observed in comparisons with other drugs. Adverse effects seen with methyldopa include drowsiness, headache, dry mouth, postural hypotension, nasal congestion, edema, and diarrhea.

α-Adrenergic Antagonists

Prazosin is an α_1-adrenergic blocking agent, and studies of its use in Raynaud's disease are both positive and negative. Although prazosin produces about a 60% response rate, larger doses of prazosin lead to an unacceptable number of adverse effects and a dose of 1 mg three times a day is best tolerated and improves symptoms, finger skin blood flow, and temperature.[66] The early response to prazosin may dissipate in a few weeks, and an increase to the maximum tolerated doses leads to multiple adverse effects such as headache, dizziness, fatigue, edema, dyspnea, rash, or diarrhea.[67] Thymoxamine, an investigational α-adrenoceptor antagonist, blocks vasoconstriction in the vascular bed of

TABLE 22.5. EFFECT OF CALCIUM CHANNEL ANTAGONISTS IN THE TREATMENT OF RAYNAUD'S DISEASE

Reference	No. of Patients	Study Duration (wk)	Additional Assessment	Results
Nifedipine				
Aldoori et al. Cardiovasc Res 1986;20:446	30p + 10s	3	Digital blood flow	9/13 patients had improved clinical symptoms
Belcaro et al. Panmin Med 1987;29:223	34p	3	Digital blood flow	N improved digital blood flow
Challenor et al. Angiology 1989;40:122	22	3	Vibrotactile thresholds	40% reduction in mean number of attacks; better response at lower thresholds
Corbin et al. Eur Heart J 1986;7:165	23p	4	Digital blood pressure	N significantly reduced the number of attacks
Finch et al. Clin Rheum 1986;5:493	16s	4	Digital blood pressure	N produced "better" clinical results than placebo
Fisher et al. Zeit Kardiol 1985;74:298	6 PAH		Hemodynamic testing	Raynaud's patients more responsive to nifedipine than other PAH patients
Gjorup et al. Am Heart J 1986;3:742	19p	4		N significantly reduced frequency of attacks and attack severity
Gush et al. J Cardiovasc Pharmacol 1987;9:628	9p	5 d	Peripheral blood flow	Tendency for N to offer some protection against reductions in blood flow
Hawkins et al. Rhem Int 1986;6:85	20p + 37s	3	Mitogenic activity	Overall, N reduced both frequency and severity of attacks, but large individual variations in response. N inhibited mitogen-induced lymphocyte proliferation but only in patients who responded to the drug clinically
Kallenberg et al. J Rheum 1987;14:284	8p + 8s	4	Digital blood flow	N reduced frequency and severity of attacks and improved digital blood flow
Lewis et al. Eur Heart J 1987;8(suppl):83	20	OD	Radial artery blood flow	N prevented reduction in blood flow by cooling
Meyrick et al. Br J Derm 1987;117:237	10	6	Digital blood flow	Reduction in number and severity of attacks but no change in blood flow or red blood cell deformability or white blood cell CL
Nilsson et al. Acta Med Scand 1987;221:53	28p	2	Digital blood pressure	17 patients showed symptomatic improvement with N versus 5 with placebo; digital blood pressure improved significantly with N
Riccio et al. Clin Ther 1987;9:232	6p + 7s	5 d	Thermography	More marked increases of hand tissue temperature in patients with secondary disease (progressive systemic sclerosis) than primary disease
Sarkozi et al. J Rheum 1986;13:331	39p	10		N significantly reduced frequency and severity of attacks compared with placebo
Waller et al. Br J Clin Pharm 1986;22:449	34p	4	Rheology	N produced a 25% reduction in mean number of attacks; no difference versus placebo in red cell deformability
White et al. Am J Med 1986;80:623	6p + 5s	1	Digital skin temperature recovery time	9/11 patients reported symptomatic improvement; N significantly improved skin temperature recovery time
Wollersheim. J Clin Pharmacol 1987;27:907	16	4	Digital blood flow	Open label, no correlation between sublingual acute use and oral long term; lack of objective long-term benefit
Dompeling and Smit. Vasa Suppl 1992;34:34–37	14p	1d	Photoelectric plethysmography	Single-dose study; N better than placebo and a potassium channel opener, pinacidil
Diltiazem				
Da Costa, et al. J Rheumatol 1987;14:858–859	15s		Digital rheography	No significant effect on subjective or objective outcome measures

TABLE 22.5. EFFECT OF CALCIUM CHANNEL ANTAGONISTS IN THE TREATMENT OF RAYNAUD'S DISEASE *(Continued)*

Reference	No. of Patients	Study Duration (wk)	Additional Assessment	Results
Nicardipine		14d		
French Cooperative Multicenter Group Am Heart J 1991;122:352–355	69p		Symptomatic	Double-blind, placebo-controlled study; 21% symptomatic improvement; no improvement in cold-reactive hyperemia test
Ferri C, et al Clin Rheumatol 1992 Mar;11(1):76–80	21p + s	3	Peak flow after postischemic reactive hyperemia	18/21 completed study; subjective improvement noted with fewer episodes and improved hand disability score
Wollersheim H, et al. J Cardiovasc Pharmacol 1991;18:813–818	16p + 9s	3	Finger skin temperature and laser Doppler flux	Double-blind, placebo-controlled study; NS between nicardipine and placebo for number, duration, or severity of vasospastic attacks or for any of the microcirculatory parameters
Felodipine				
Kallenberg CG, et al. Eur J Clin Pharmacol 1991;40:313–315	10p	6	Symptomatic and finger plethysmography	Single blind; subjective improvement in the number and intensity of attacks; blood flow improved only at certain temperatures
Flunarizine				
Centonze V, et al. Clin Ter 1991;137:77–82	28		Symptomatic	Flunarizine caused NS clinical improvement; adverse effects were common

Key: p, primary Raynaud's disease; s, secondary Raynaud's disease; N, nifedipine; PAH, pulmonary arterial hypertension; CL, clearance; OD, one dose; NS, not significant.

the skin, but overall vascular resistance is unaffected.[68] The explanation for this effect may be related to its selectivity for α_1 receptors over α_2 receptors. Three controlled studies have shown that thymoxamine gives subjective relief of symptoms but also abolishes vasoconstriction after cold stimulus, and it appears to be well tolerated.[68]

Other nonselective α-adrenergic antagonists such as phentolamine and phenoxybenzamine provide inconsistent improvement in blood flow and symptoms. Their use is further limited by difficulties in oral dosing as well as frequent and bothersome adverse effects. Intra-arterial phentolamine infused at 50–150 g/min or as a single brachial artery injection of 0.05–10 mg improves finger blood flow, digital pulse volume amplitude, and forearm blood flow, and this route is useful for unrelenting vasospasm and ischemia when the sympathetic nervous system is the cause.[60]

Direct-Acting Vasodilators

Nitroglycerin, nitroprusside, niacin and its derivatives, papaverine, isoxsuprine, griseofulvin, cyclandelate, and hydralazine fall into this category. With the exception of nitroglycerin, none of these agents can be recommended because of the lack of controlled studies to support their use and the frequency of adverse effects.[60] Nitroglycerin ointment usually improves the symptoms and, at times, objective measures of effectiveness have been shown in patients with primary and secondary Raynaud's disease.[60,62] Headaches, dizziness, and postural hypotension are the most frequent reasons for failure with nitroglycerin.

Calcium Channel Antagonists

Numerous studies with calcium channel antagonists, particularly nifedipine, have been performed in patients with Raynaud's disease. As the name implies these drugs block the entry of calcium ions through the slow channel that reduces the availability of cytosolic calcium and decreases smooth muscle contractility. Additionally, they may inhibit vascular responses evoked by α_2-adrenergic receptors, which are activated predominantly during reflex sympathetic stimulation of body cooling.[15,61] Subjective and objective improvements have been demonstrated with drugs in this category. Table 22.5 summarizes clinical trials of calcium channel antagonists for Raynaud's disease. Nifedipine is more effective in primary Raynaud's disease and its effects are more pronounced early in therapy. Chronic therapy may result in loss of response as determined by objective measures as reported by Gush and Wollersheim (Table 22.5). Nifedipine may also be used as prophylactic therapy prior to cold exposure.

Diltiazem has been reported to reduce the number, severity, and duration of attacks in doses of 30–120 mg given three times a day.[61] Objective measures of effect have not demonstrated benefit with diltiazem. Verapamil has been reported to improve the symptoms in one small study, but diary data and objective measures did not confirm any beneficial effect.

Newer calcium blockers such as nicardipine, isradipine, and nisoldipine have also been used with varying degrees of success for Raynaud's disease. Nicardipine provides subjective improvement in about one-half of the patients receiving it, and the frequency and severity of attacks are significantly reduced with its use. It is more effective in primary Raynaud's disease than secondary, and subjective, symptomatic improvement is seen more often than objective improvement.[69,70] Other studies (also see Table 22.5) have shown no benefit, either subjective or objective, from nicardipine even though the drug was shown to inhibit platelet aggregation.[71] Isradipine, a calcium antagonist that is highly selective for peripheral vessels, in doses of 1.25 and 2.5 mg, has been shown to increase finger systolic blood pressure and improve symptoms during cold exposure and to have few adverse effects.[72] Nisoldipine, an investigational dihydropyridine, appears to be ineffective in primary Raynaud's disease.[73]

Serotonin Receptor Antagonists

Serotonin (5-hydroxytryptamine, 5-HT) has been shown to induce vasospasm and platelet aggregation in animals and humans through the 5-HT_2 receptor. Ketanserin is a selective antagonist of the 5-HT_2 receptor and it may also have some α_1-adrenoreceptor blocking activity. It increases finger blood flow with intra-arterial and intravenous injection during sympathetic vasoconstriction induced by body cooling, and its effects are evident in the presence of α blockade.[74] The largest study (N = 222) with oral use found that ketanserin (40 mg three times a day) decreased the duration and frequency of attacks (34% reduction versus 18%) and was preferred by both patients and investigators over placebo.[75] About 50–70% of the patients experienced subjective mild to moderate improvement. Ketanserin had no effect on total finger blood flow in warm or cold environments. There was no difference in response between primary and secondary Raynaud's disease. Headache, asthenia, dizziness, and gastrointestinal complaints were the most common symptoms seen with ketanserin; respiratory infections were also more common with ketanserin than placebo. Ketanserin may also prolong the QT interval and it should be used cautiously in patients with hypokalemia, second- or third-degree heart block, ventricular arrhythmias, prolonged QT interval at baseline, or in combination with potassium-losing diuretics or antiarrhythmics.[76] Part of the variability in response to ketanserin may be due to the frequency in dosing because some evidence exists that its effects on platelet aggregation are minimal at 12 hours after dosing.[77] When compared with other drugs such as nifedipine or pentoxiphylline, ketanserin may provide better subjective improvement and perhaps better objective improvement as illustrated in small studies to date.[78,79] Ketanserin may also be effective in combination therapy with prostacyclin derivatives.[80]

Angiotensin-Converting Enzyme Inhibitors[81]

The proposed mechanism for improvement of Raynaud's disease with angiotensin-converting enzyme (ACE) inhibitors is the inhibition of the breakdown of bradykinin and vasodilation resulting from its accumulation. Earlier studies showed improved blood flow and some improvement in symptoms. More recently, double-blind placebo-controlled trials have not documented any improvement with enalapril 20 mg/d.[82]

Prostanoids

Prostacyclin and prostaglandins E_1 and E_2 have been studied in Raynaud's disease because of their properties of vasodilation and inhibition of platelet aggregation. Iloprost, a synthetic analogue of prostacyclin, and PGE_1 infusions given for several hours over a few days have been shown to reduce the number and severity of attacks of Raynaud's disease, to induce healing of digital lesions, and in some instances to improve blood flow for periods of up to 6 weeks.[83–85] Because of the limitations of intravenous therapy, oral regimens with various prostanoid analogs have been performed. Belch et al.[86] gave iloprost 50–150 μg twice daily to 63 patients and found that symptoms, as assessed by diary cards, trended toward improvement but did not reach statistical significance. Other forms of prostanoids such as misoprostol have not been shown to have significant acute vasodilating properties.[87]

Thyroid Hormones

Triiodothyronine (T_3) 80 mcg/d has been shown in one small (N = 18), double-blind controlled crossover trial to reduce the frequency, duration, and severity of attacks as well as increase skin temperatures and promote ulcer healing.[88] The proposed mechanisms for this effect are activation of heat dissipating mechanisms and enhanced β_2-adrenoreceptor activity in vascular smooth muscle. T_3 significantly elevated T_3 and T_4 concentrations and reduced thyroid-stimulating hormone concentrations to less than 0.1 mIU/L in 14 of 18 patients. Palpitations, headaches, and weight loss were reported by about one-third of patients. The overall attack rate reduction was approximately 75%, somewhat higher than that reported for other types of treatment. The authors suggest follow-up studies using a lower dose of 60 μg/d of triiodothyronine to minimize adverse effects and chemical hyperthyroidism. Other case reports suggest similar findings.[89,90]

Other approaches to therapy have included β-adrenergic blocking agents and pentoxiphylline. Atenolol and propranolol have been reported to benefit some patients with Raynaud's disease based on diary data of attack frequency.[91] The premise for their use is that presynaptic blockade of β_2 receptors should prevent postsynaptic activation of adrenergic receptors; few data support this concept at the present time. Pentoxifylline, in a study of 11 patients, was reported to improve symptoms in 7 patients and to improve red cell filtration.[92] Improved skin temperatures to cold challenge have been noted with pentoxiphylline as well.[79]

Calcitonin gene-related peptide is an endogenous vasodilator which seems to be specific for skin blood flow and it may be deficient in Raynaud's disease. Trials giving this substance intravenously for up to 5 days have shown improved hand warming and skin temperature, improved hand and digital blood flow, and ulcer healing in small groups of patients and it seems to be better tolerated than prostacyclin.[93,94] Another drug with some promise is piracetam, an antiplatelet agent which also increases the synthesis of PGI_2.[95]

A cervicothoracic sympathectomy may produce temporary relief from symptoms but they usually return within 6 months to 2 years. Several complications may occur because of the surgery and the success rate is considered to be no better than conservative management.[60]

Evaluation of Therapeutic Outcomes

Drug therapy responses in peripheral vascular disease may be evaluated using patient symptoms, the presence or absence of peripheral pulses at various sites, the ABI index, exercise capacity, angiographic documentation of improved flow, and the need for subsequent procedures and surgery. Using the Fontaine classification system (Table 22.2) or other rating scales which are available,[57] semiquantitative assessments of symptomatic clinical improvement can be obtained. For example, a patient might move from class IIb to IIa or I as a measure of improvement following pharmacotherapeutic or interventional therapy. The ABI index provides an estimate of the restoration of blood flow to an extremity and this index can easily be obtained by measuring blood pressures at different points of the circulatory system. Exercise capacity can be evaluated using the Fontaine classification or through other estimates made by the patient or clinician of exercise duration or effort. This could be expressed as the time to cover a set distance, i.e., one block, or the total amount of distance covered without a time restriction. Angiographic studies to document improved blood flow are usually not necessary and are more often used for research purposes to objectively assess the outcome of some intervention. The need for a revascularization procedure as primary or secondary intervention or the need for vascular surgery after pharmacotherapy or interventional technologies could also be used as an outcome measure. This would be more important for groups of patients than individual patients but the need for revascularization certainly would suggest failure of the primary mode of therapy.

Symptom remission is the primary method of evaluating therapy for Raynaud's disease. Digital plethysmography and finger blood pressure would be used for a more objective method of assessment or for research purposes. Patients with TAO should be evaluated for symptom response but smoking cessation is important as well. This may be evaluated through history but a more objective means would be serum cotinine concentrations.

Conclusion

Peripheral vascular disease is a very common disorder affecting between 50 to 60 men or women per 10,000 after the age of 65 years. Patients with arteriosclerosis obliterans should begin a regular exercise program, control their other cardiovascular risk factors, and be given a trial of antithrombotic therapy (aspirin) and perhaps calcium channel blockers to limit disease progression and provide some vasodilation. An inadequate response to lifestyle modification and pharmacologic therapy may be managed by interventional therapy such as angioplasty or artherectomy. If these measures fail, open vascular surgery and reconstruction with grafts remains an option.

Raynaud's disease is a vasospastic disorder which is more common in women and responds moderately well to vasodilator therapy with calcium channel blockers and other vasodilators. Improved understanding of the etiology of this disorder may increase the number of therapeutic options for the future. TAO is a disease of smokers and smoking cessation is the primary intervention. Vasodilation may have a role but smoking cessation is much more important.

References

1. Clement DL, Shepherd JT (eds). Vascular Diseases in the Limbs. Mechanisms and Principles of Treatment. St. Louis, MO, Mosby Year Book, 1993.
2. Lie JR. The structure of the normal vascular system and its reactive changes, in Juergens JL, Spittell JA, Fairbairn JF (eds): Peripheral Vascular Diseases. Philadelphia, WB Saunders, 1980, pp 51–81.
3. Dusting GJ. Nitric oxide in cardiovascular disorders. J Vasc Res 1995;32:143–161.
4. Coffman JD. Effects of endothelium-derived nitric oxide on skin and digital blood flow in humans. Am J Physiol 1994;267(6 pt 2):H2087–2090.
5. Vane JR, Anggard EE, Botting RM. Regulatory functions of the vascular endothelium. N Engl J Med 1990;323:27–36.
6. Luscher TF, Vanhoutte PM. The endothelium: Modulator of cardiovascular function. Boca Raton, FL, CRC Press, 1990, pp 11–146.
7. Ross R. The pathogenesis of atherosclerosis: A perspective for the 1990's. Nature 1993;330:1431–1438.
8. Thyberg J, Hedin U, Sjolund M, et al. Regulation of differentiated properties and proliferation of arterial smooth muscle cells. Arteriosclerosis 1990;10:966–990.
9. Ouriel K (ed). Lower Extremity Vascular Disease. Philadelphia, WB Saunders Company, 1995.
10. Shepherd JT, Bergan JJ, Cohen RA, et al. Report of the Task Force on Vascular Medicine. Circulation 1994;89:532–535.

11. Rihal CS, Eagle KA, Mickel MC, Foster ED. Surgical therapy for coronary artery disease among patients with combined coronary artery and peripheral vascular disease. Circulation 1995;91:46–53.
12. Kerstein MD, White JV (eds). Alternatives to Open Vascular Surgery. Philadelphia, JB Lippincott Company, 1995.
13. Hiatt WR, Hoag S, Hamman RF. Effect of diagnostic criteria on the prevalence of peripheral arterial disease. The San Luis Valley Diabetes Study. Circulation 1995;91:1472–1479.
14. Newman AB, Siscovick DS, Manolio TA, et al. Ankle-arm index as a marker of atherosclerosis in the Cardiovascular Health Study. Cardiovascular Heart Study (CHS) Collaborative Research Group. Circulation 1993;88:837–845.
15. Coffman JD. New drug therapy in peripheral vascular disease. Med Clin North Am 1988;72:259–263.
16. Hiatt WR, Wolfel EE, Meier RH, Regensteiner JG. Superiority of treadmill walking exercise versus strength training for patients with peripheral arterial disease. Implications for the mechanism of the training response. Circulation 1994;90:1866–1874.
17. Hertzer NR. The natural history of peripheral vascular disease. Implications for its management. Circulation 1991;83(2 suppl):I12–19.
18. Ingram D, House A, Thompson G, et al. β-Adrenergic blockade and peripheral vascular disease. Med J Aust 1982;1:509–511.
19. Smith R, Warren D. Effect of β-blocking drugs on peripheral blood flow in intermittent claudication. J Cardiovasc Pharmacol 1982;4:2–4.
20. Hiatt WR, Stoll S, Nies AS. Effect of β-adrenergic blockade on the peripheral circulation in patients with peripheral vascular disease. Circulation 1985;72:1226–1231.
21. Roberts DH, McLoughlin GA, Tsao Y, et al. Placebo-controlled comparison of captopril, atenolol, labetalol, and pindolol in hypertension complicated by intermittent claudication. Lancet 1987;2:650–653.
22. Heintzen MP, Strauer BE. Peripheral vascular effects of beta-blockers. Eur Heart J 1994;15(suppl C):2–7.
23. Porter JM, Carter BS, Lee BY, et al. Pentoxifylline efficacy in the treatment of intermittent claudication: Multicenter controlled double-blind trial with objective assessment of chronic occlusive arterial disease patients. Am Heart J 1982;104:66–72.
24. Lindgarde F, Jelnes R, Bjorkman H, et al. Conservative drug treatment in patients with moderately severe chronic occlusive peripheral arterial disease. Scandinavian Study Group. Circulation 1989;80:1549–1556.
25. Currie MS, Simel DL, Christenson RH, et al. Anti-inflammatory effects of pentoxifylline in claudication. Am J Med Sci 1991;301:85–90.
26. AbuRahma AF, Woodruff BA. Effects and limitations of pentoxifylline therapy in various stages of peripheral vascular disease of the lower extremity. Am J Surg 1990;160:266–270.
27. Lucas MA. Prevention of postoperative thrombosis in peripheral arteriopathies. Pentoxifylline versus conventional antiaggregants. A 6-month randomized follow-up study. Angiology 1984;35:443–449.
28. Campbell RK. Clinical update on pentoxifylline therapy for diabetes-induced peripheral vascular disease. Ann Pharmacother 1993;27:1099–1105.
29. Ernst E, Kollar L, Resch KL. Does pentoxifylline prolong the walking distance in exercised claudicants? A placebo-controlled double-blind trial. Angiology 1992;43:121–125.
30. Stergachis A, Sheingold S, Luce BR, et al. Medical care and cost outcomes after pentoxifylline treatment for peripheral arterial disease. Arch Intern Med 1992;152:1220–1224.
31. Hess H, Mietaschk A, Deichsel G. Drug-induced inhibition of platelet function delays progression of peripheral occlusive arterial disease. A prospective double-blind arteriographically controlled trial. Lancet 1985;1:415–419.
32. Katsumura T, Mishima Y, Kamiya K, et al. Therapeutic effect of ticlopidine, a new inhibitor of platelet aggregation, on chronic arterial occlusive disease, a double-blind study versus placebo. Angiology 1982;33:357–367.
33. Balsano F, Coccheri S, Libretti A, et al. Ticlopidine in the treatment of intermittent claudication: A 21-month double-blind trial. J Lab Clin Med 1989;114:84–91.
34. Fagher B. Long-term effects of ticlopidine on lower limb blood flow, ankle/brachial index and symptoms in peripheral arteriosclerosis. A double-blind study. The STIMS Group in Lund. Swedish Ticlopidine Multicenter Study. Angiology 1994;45:777–788.
35. Grant SM, Goa KL. Iloprost. A review of its pharmacodynamic and pharmacokinetic properties, and therapeutic potential in peripheral vascular disease, myocardial ischaemia and extracorporeal circulation procedures. Drugs 1992;43:889–924.
36. Volteas N, Leon M, Labropoulos N, et al. The effect of iloprost in patients with rest pain. Eur J Vasc Surg 1993;7:654–658.
37. Loosemore TM, Chalmers TC, Dormandy JA. A meta-analysis of randomized placebo control trials in Fontaine stages III and IV peripheral occlusive arterial disease. Int Angiol 1994;13:133–142.
38. Altstaedt HO, Berzewski B, Breddin HK, et al. Treatment of patients with peripheral arterial occlusive disease Fontaine stage IV with intravenous iloprost and PGE1: A randomized open controlled study. Prostaglandins Leukot Essent Fatty Acids 1993;49:573–578.
39. Scheffler P, de la Hamette D, Gross J, et al. Intensive vascular training in stage IIb of peripheral arterial occlusive disease. The additive effects of intravenous prostaglandin E1 or intravenous pentoxifylline during training. Circulation 1994;90:818–822.
40. Wolf DL, Metzler CM, Froeschke MO, Luderer JR. Continuous intravenous dosing with ciprostene using a portable pump in ambulatory patients. J Clin Pharmacol 1993;33:150–153.
41. Balsano F, Violi F. Effect of picotamide on the clinical progression of peripheral vascular disease. A double-blind placebo-controlled study. The ADEP Group. Circulation 1993;87:1563–1569.
42. Fleckenstein-Grun G, Thimm F, Czirfuzs A, Matyas S. Experimental vasoprotection by calcium antagonists against calcium-mediated arteriosclerotic alterations. J Cardiovasc Pharmacol 1994;24(suppl 2):S75–84.
43. Frey M, Just H. Role of calcium antagonists in progression of arteriosclerosis. Evidence from animal experiments and clinical experience. Part I. Preventive effects of calcium antagonists in animal experiments. Basic Res Cardiol 1994;89(suppl 1):161–76.

44. Fleckenstein-Grun G, Frey M, Thimm F, et al. Calcium overload—an important cellular mechanism in hypertension and arteriosclerosis. Drugs 1992;44(suppl 1):23–30.
45. Ulutin ON. Clinical effectiveness of defibrotide in vaso-occlusive disorders and its mode of action. Sem Throm Hem 1988;14(suppl):58–63.
46. Prevention of Atherosclerosis Complications with Ketanserin (PACK) Investigators. Randomized placebo-controlled, double-blind trial of ketanserin in claudicants. Changes in claudication distance and ankle systolic pressure. Circulation 1989;80:1544–1548.
47. Brevetti G, Chiariello M, Ferulano G, et al. Increases in walking distance in patients with peripheral vascular disease treated with l-carnitine: A double-blind, crossover study. Circulation 1988;77:767–773.
48. Brevetti G, Angelini C, Rosa M, Carrozzo R, et al. Muscle carnitine deficiency in patients with severe peripheral vascular disease. Circulation 1991;84:1490–1495.
49. Corsico N, Nardone A, Lucreziotti MR, et al. Effect of propionyl-L-carnitine in a rat model of peripheral arteriopathy: A functional, histologic, and NMR spectroscopic study. Cardiovasc Drugs Ther 1993;7:241–251.
50. Cameron HA, Waller PC, Ramsay LE. Drug treatment of intermittent claudication: A critical analysis of the methods and findings of published clinical trials, 1965–1985. Br J Clin Pharmacol 1988;26:569–576.
51. Ward AS, Andaz SK, Bygrave S. Peripheral thrombolysis with tissue plasminogen activator. Results of two treatment regimens. Arch Surg 1994;129:861–865.
52. Smith CM, Yellin AE, Weaver FA, et al. Thrombolytic therapy for arterial occlusion: A mixed blessing. Am Surg 1994;60:371–375.
53. Comerota AJ, Cohen GS. Thrombolytic therapy in peripheral arterial occlusive disease: Mechanisms of action and drugs available. Can J Surg 1993;36:342–348.
54. Andreozzi GM, Signorelli SS, Cacciaguerra G, et al. Three-month therapy with calcium-heparin in comparison with ticlopidine in patients with peripheral arterial occlusive disease at Leriche-Fontaine IIb class. Angiology 1993;44:307–313.
55. Minar E, Ahmadi A, Koppensteiner R, et al. Comparison of effects of high-dose and low-dose aspirin on restenosis after femoropopliteal percutaneous transluminal angioplasty. Circulation 1995;91:2167–2173.
56. Lowe GD, Reid AW, Leiberman DP. Management of thrombosis in peripheral arterial disease. Br Med Bull 1994;50:923–935.
57. Pentecost MJ, Criqui MH, Dorros G, et al. Guidelines for peripheral percutaneous transluminal angioplasty of the abdominal aorta and lower extremity vessels. Councils on Cardiovascular Radiology, Arteriosclerosis, Cardio-Thoracic and Vascular Surgery, Clinical Cardiology, and Epidemiology and Prevention, American Heart Association. Circulation 1994;89:511–531.
58. Isner JM, Rosenfield K. Redefining the treatment of peripheral artery disease. Role of percutaneous revascularization. Circulation 1993;88:1534–1557.
59. Adar R, Papa MZ, Halpern Z, et al. Cellular sensitivity to collagen in thromboangiitis obliterans. N Engl J Med 1983;308:1113–1116.
60. Coffman JD. Raynaud's phenomenon. An update. Hypertension 1991;17:593–602.
61. Coffman JD. Raynaud's Phenomenon. New York, Oxford University Press, 1989.
62. Roath S. Management of Raynaud's phenomenon. Focus on newer treatments. Drugs 1989;37:700–712.
63. Coffman JD. The diagnosis of Raynaud's phenomenon. Clin Dermatol 1994;12:283–289.
64. Coffman JD, Cohen RA. Plasma levels of 5-hydroxytryptamine during sympathetic stimulation and in Raynaud's phenomenon. Clin Sci (Colch) 1994;86:269–273.
65. Jobe JB, Beetham WP, Roberts DE, et al. Induced vasodilation as a home treatment for Raynaud's disease. J Rheumatol 1985;12:953–956.
66. Wollersheim H, Thien T. Dose-response study of prazosin in Raynaud's phenomenon: Clinical effectiveness versus side effects. J Clin Pharmacol 1988;28:1089–1093.
67. Nielsen SL, Vitting K, Rasmussen K. Prazosin treatment of primary Raynaud's phenomenon. Eur J Clin Pharmacol 1983;24:421–423.
68. Cooke ED, Nicolaides AN. Raynaud's syndrome. Thymoxamine, iloprost, and ACE inhibitors are among the effective treatments now available. Br Med J 1990;300:553–555.
69. Rupp PAF, Mellinger S, Kohler J, et al. Nicardipine for the treatment of Raynaud's phenomena: A double-blind crossover trial of a new calcium entry blocker. J Rheumatol 1987;14:745–750.
70. van Heereveld H, Wollerhseim H, Gough K, et al. Intravenous nicardipine in Raynaud's phenomenon: A controlled trial. J Cardiovasc Pharmacol 1988;11:68–74.
71. Wigley FM, Wise RA, Malamet R, et al. Nicardipine in the treatment of Raynaud's phenomenon. Arthritis Rheum 1987;30:281–286.
72. Leppert J, Jonasson T, Nilsson, et al. The effect of isradipine, a new calcium-channel antagonist, in patients with primary Raynaud's phenomenon: A single-blind dose-response study. Cardiovasc Drugs Ther 1989;3:397–401.
73. Challenor VF, Waller DG, Francis, et al. Nisoldipine in primary Raynaud's phenomenon. Europ J Clin Pharmacol 1987;33:27–30.
74. Brouwer RML, Wenting GJ, Schalekamp ADH. Acute effects and mechanism of action of ketanserin in patients with primary Raynaud's phenomenon. J Cardiovasc Pharmacol 1990;15:868–876.
75. Coffman JD, Clement DL, Creager MA, et al. International study of ketanserin in Raynaud's phenomenon. Am J Med 1989;87:264–268.
76. Prevention of Atherosclerosis Complications with Ketanserin Trial Group. Prevention of atherosclerotic complications: Controlled trial of ketanserin. Br Med J 1989;298:424–430.
77. Marasini B, Biondi ML, Mollica R. Effect of chronic ketanserin treatment on serotonin-induced platelet aggregation in patients with Raynaud's phenomenon. Eur J Clin Pharmacol 1990;39:289–290.
78. Codella O, Caramaschi P, Olivieri O, et al. Controlled comparison of ketanserin and nifedipine in Raynaud's phenomenon. Angiology 1989;40:114–121.
79. Arosio E, Montesi G, Zannoni M, et al. Comparative efficacy of ketanserin and pentoxiphylline in treatment of Raynaud's phenomenon. Angiology 1989;40:633–638.
80. Pola P, Tondi P, Serricchio M, Favuzzi A, Gerardino L. New prospects for the treatment of Raynaud's phenomenon using

a serotoninergic S2 receptor antagonist (ketanserin) and stable derivatives of prostacyclin. Angiology 1993;44:123–128.

81. Challenor VF. Angiotensin converting enzyme inhibitors in Raynaud's phenomenon. Drugs 1994;48:864–867.
82. Challenor VF, Waller DG, Hayward RA, et al. Subjective and objective assessment of enalapril in primary Raynaud's phenomenon. Br J Clin Pharmacol 1991;31:477–480.
83. Wigley FM, Wise RA, Seibold JR, et al. Intravenous iloprost infusion in patients with Raynaud phenomenon secondary to systemic sclerosis. A multicenter, placebo-controlled, double-blind study. Ann Intern Med 1994(Feb 1);120(3):199–206.
84. Katoh K, Kawai T, Narita M, Uemura J, et al. Use of prostaglandin E1 (lipo-PGE1) to treat Raynaud's phenomenon associated with connective tissue disease: Thermographic and subjective assessment. J Pharm Pharmacol 1992;44:442–444.
85. Torley H, Madhok R, Capell HA, et al. A double blind, randomised, multicentre comparison of two doses of intravenous iloprost in the treatment of Raynaud's phenomenon secondary to connective tissue diseases. Ann Rheum Dis 1991;50:800–804.
86. Belch JJ, Capell HA, Cooke ED, et al. Oral iloprost as a treatment for Raynaud's syndrome: A double blind multicentre placebo controlled study. Ann Rheum Dis 1995;54:197–200.
87. Wise RA, Wigley F. Acute effects of misoprostol on digital circulation in patients with Raynaud's phenomenon. J Rheumatol 1994;21:80–83.
88. Dessein PH, Morrison RC, Lamparelli RD, et al. Triiodothyronine treatment for Raynaud's phenomenon: A controlled trial. J Rheumatol 1990;17:1025–1028.
89. Lateiwish AM, Feher J, Baraczka K, Racz K. Remission of Raynaud's phenomenon after L-thyroxine therapy in a patient with hypothyroidism. J Endocrinol Invest 1992;15:49–51.
90. Gledhill RF, Dessein PH, Van der Merwe CA. Treatment of Raynaud's phenomenon with triiodothyronine corrects coexistent autonomic dysfunction: Preliminary findings. Postgrad Med J 1992;68:263–267.
91. Brotzu G, Susanna F, Roberto M, et al. β-Blockers: A new therapeutic approach to Raynaud's disease. Microvas Res 1987;33:283–288.
92. Neirotti M, Longo F, Molaschi M, et al. Functional vascular disorders: Treatment with pentoxifylline. Angiology 1987;38:575–580.
93. Bunker CB, Reavley C, O'Shaughnessy DJ, Dowd PM. Calcitonin gene-related peptide in treatment of severe peripheral vascular insufficiency in Raynaud's phenomenon. Lancet 1993;342:80–83.
94. Shawket S, Dickerson C, Hazleman B, Brown MJ. Prolonged effect of CGRP in Raynaud's patients: A double-blind randomised comparison with prostacyclin. Br J Clin Pharmacol 1991;32:209–213.
95. Moriau M, Lavenne-Pardonge E, Crasborn L, et al. Treatment of the Raynaud's phenomenon with piracetam. Arzneimittelforschung 1993;43:526–535.

Chapter 23

Hypovolemic and Cardiogenic Shock

Edward Sypniewski, Jr., PharmD

In 1743, the word "shock" was first used medically by an English translator of Henri Francois Le Dran's *A Treatise of Reflections Drawn from Experience with Gunshot Wounds.*[1] Early observations in the nineteenth century described shock as a gradual decline in organ function following injury or surgery. Although Thomas Latta was the first to use intravenous saline in the treatment of hypovolemic shock,[1] George W. Crile, in 1899, was one of the first to publish experiments that formed the basis of our therapeutic approaches to both traumatic and hypovolemic shock. Using an animal model, he induced shock and then infused warmed saline, correlating increased venous return with improved myocardial contractility. During the following two decades, shock was thought to be due to either vasomotor exhaustion (resulting in venous pooling of blood) or vasoconstriction (diminished blood flow to vital organs).[1]

The next phase of research resulted from analyses of injuries to soldiers during World War I. In 1918, W. B. Cannon reported the correlation of low blood pressure (BP) with arterial blood acidosis while Keith correlated the degree of blood loss with severity of the shock syndrome the following year. W. B. Cannon and W. M. Bayliss organized the first shock team in 1923 and used the data from World War I to describe the phenomenon of shock. In the years that followed many researchers and clinicians confirmed blood loss as the major cause of the shock syndrome. Following World War II, Cournand et al. reported the first measurements of cardiac output (CO) in patients with shock. Invasive measurement of CO became a standard of care and, in 1970, Swan et al.[2] published their observations on assessment of intracardiac and intrapulmonary pressures using a flow-directed balloon-tipped catheter. The 1970s led to a better understanding of the hemodynamic alterations that accompany shock, as hypotension, tachycardia, low CO, and oliguria became hallmark signs and symptoms of hypovolemic and cardiogenic shock. Research during the last two decades has centered on the optimization of circulating blood volume and maintenance of organ perfusion. Regardless of which form of shock syndrome is present (e.g., cardiogenic, hypovolemic, septic), restoration of oxygen delivery to tissues and organs continues as the primary goal of therapy.

Although we have learned much about shock, this complex syndrome continues to be associated with a high level of mortality (40–90%). The rapid occurrence of cellular, tissue, and organ dysfunction secondary to hypoxia, coupled with our still limited understanding of the complex processes involved, impedes our ability to treat patients successfully even though this syndrome has been recognized for more than a century. The goal of this chapter is to provide the reader with a comprehensive summation of the underlying pathophysiology and clinical presentation of patients with hypovolemic and cardiogenic shock. Included are the monitoring parameters, empiric approaches, and treatment strategies for the management of hypovolemic and cardiogenic shock.

General Characteristics

PATHOPHYSIOLOGY

Pathophysiologic Alterations

The shock syndromes are often categorized based on clinical presentation, laboratory analysis, and changes in primary pathophysiology. The three categories consist of intravascular volume deficit (hypovolemic shock), peripheral vasodilation (septic, anaphylactic, neurogenic shock), or myocardial pump failure (cardiogenic shock).

A fall in BP due to either hypovolemia, vasodilation, or severely depressed CO is compensated by an increase in sympathetic outflow, activation of the renin–angiotensin system, and other humoral factors (vasopressin) that stimulate peripheral vasoconstriction in an attempt to restore BP and preserve cerebral and coronary perfusion. The increased sympathetic stimulation augments heart rate and myocardial contractility, which results in enhanced cardiac output unless there is damage to the myocardium (e.g., myocardial infarction) or profound hypovolemia. The reflex sympathetic stimulation may be successful in achieving a minimal systolic blood pressure (SBP) of 90 mm Hg, at least in the early stages of the shock syndrome. However, patients with a vasodilatory form of shock (anaphylactic, neurogenic, septic shock), or continued uncorrected intravascular volume losses (e.g., hypovolemia secondary to burns, hemorrhage from severe trauma, gastrointestinal bleeding) will often require immediate fluid resuscitation and pharmacologic intervention. The patient with cardiogenic shock (e.g., depressed cardiac output) may or may not achieve complete compensation by peripheral vasoconstriction to maintain blood pressure.

Compensatory vasoconstriction redistributes blood away from the extremities and kidneys, both of which may tolerate hypoxia to a greater degree, toward the vital organs (e.g., heart, brain) in an attempt to maintain oxygenation, nutrition, and organ function. The decreased rate of blood flow from cellular edema or local effects of humoral vasoactive substances causes sludging and microagglutination, ultimately resulting in microcirculatory failure, cell membrane injury, and tissue ischemia. A severe metabolic lactic acidosis often develops secondary to the tissue ischemia and causes localized vasodilation, which further exacerbates the impaired cardiovascular state. As shock progresses to this level, reversal of the syndrome is extremely difficult despite medical interventions because of the degree of end-organ damage that is occurring or has occurred. Death follows from multisystem organ failure (Fig. 23.1).

If circulation and oxygenation are restored in a timely manner, cellular, tissue, and organ function can be salvaged. The extent of damage and rehabilitation of the organ systems depend primarily on the severity and duration of the insult. The degree of cellular damage that results from generation of oxygen-derived free radicals (ODFRs) during tissue reperfusion is variable. Although postischemic myocardial damage occurs secondary to generation of ODFRs following successful coronary reperfusion in the setting of acute myocardial ischemia or restoration of coronary circulation following cardioplegia during open heart

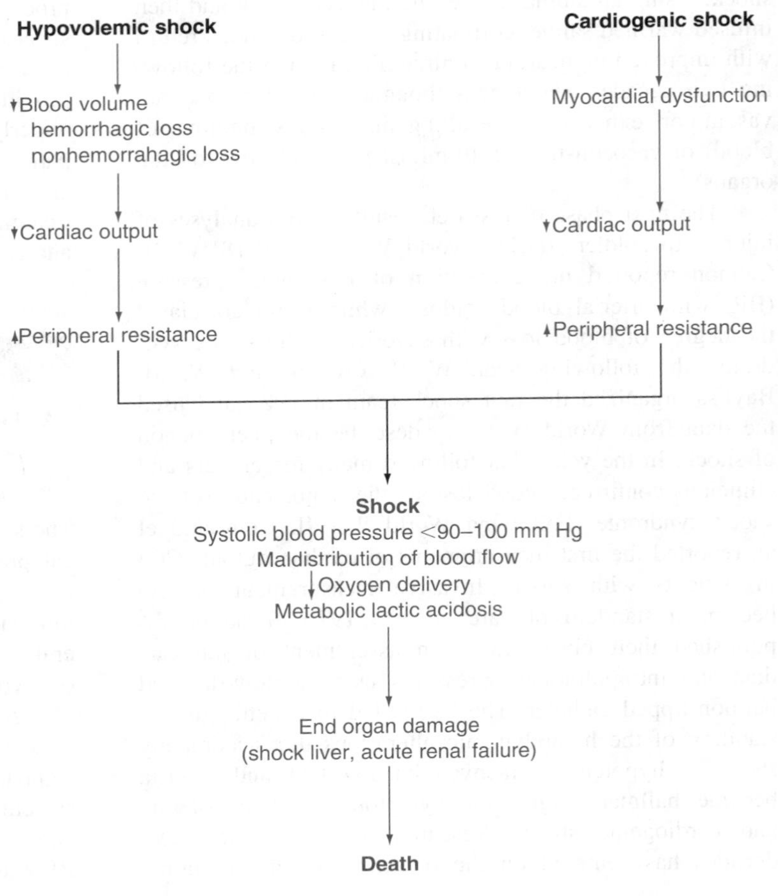

Figure 23.1. Pathophysiologic interrelationships between hypovolemic and cardiogenic shock.

surgery, the presence of this process at the microcirculatory level in the periphery during the shock states is still under investigation.

Oxygen Delivery

Both hypovolemic and cardiogenic shock result in failure of the circulatory system to deliver sufficient oxygen (O_2) to body tissues despite normal or reduced O_2 consumption.[3] The generation of a net deficit in O_2 supply is due to underdistribution of blood flow. The resultant tissue hypoxia causes a shift from aerobic to anaerobic metabolism, leading to the generation of metabolic acidosis (due to production of lactic acid). Organ dysfunction and death follow in a majority of patients despite aggressive medical care.

Oxygen delivery (Do_2), which normally ranges from 900–1100 mL/min, cannot be measured directly. However, it is dependent on two obtainable variables: CO and the arterial oxygen-carrying capacity (Cao_2) of the blood[4]:

$$Do_2 \text{ mL/min} = CO \times Cao_2 \quad (1)$$

Cardiac output is the product of heart rate (HR) and stroke volume (SV) and is measured directly by the Swan–Ganz catheter using the thermodilution method. Oxygen-carrying capacity (Cao_2) [Eq. (2)] is a function of hemoglobin (Hgb), the volume of O_2 carried per gram of hemoglobin (1.39) (at pH = 7.4 and temperature of 37°C), and arterial O_2 saturation (Sao_2) plus the product of plasma dissolved O_2 content ($0.0031 \times Pao_2$).

$$Cao_2 = (Hgb \times 1.39 \times Sao_2) + (0.0031 \times Pao_2) \quad (2)$$

The arterial blood gas (ABG) provides a measure of arterial pH, the partial pressure of O_2 (Pao_2), partial pressure of carbon dioxide ($Paco_2$), and oxygen saturation (Sao_2). Circulating Sao_2 can also be measured by an oximeter, which utilizes a sensor, attached to either the patient's earlobe or finger, that continuously relays the peripheral Sao_2 to a bedside monitor. Although some deviations from the standard ABG measurements have been identified, this device is fairly accurate and useful at the patient's bedside. However, one should always confirm the Sao_2 by direct ABG measurement before initiating any changes in therapy.

One can substitute Eq. (2) for Cao_2 into Eq. (1), thus yielding Eq. (3):

$$Do_2 \text{ mL/min} = CO \times [(Hgb \times 1.39 \times Sao_2) + (0.0031 \times Pao_2)] \quad (3)$$

Finally, if plasma-dissolved O_2 (i.e., $0.0031 \times Pao_2$) is deleted, because its contribution to the overall content of O_2 in the blood is essentially insignificant, and the number 10 (mL/min) is inserted as a conversion factor to arrive at the correct units of measure, the resultant equation defines the parameter of Do_2 as *the rate of O_2 delivery* to tissues:

$$Do_2 \text{ mL/min} = CO \times (Hgb \times 1.39 \times SaO_2) \times 10 \quad (4)$$

Oxygen delivery can be hindered if pH is altered despite adequate Hgb saturation and normal CO. Metabolic acidosis shifts the oxyhemoglobin dissociation curve to the right, whereas alkalosis shifts it to the left. A shift to the left is associated with poor unloading of O_2 from Hgb to the cells. Temperature also affects O_2 dissociation as hypothermia increases the affinity of Hgb for O_2, which results in suboptimum release of O_2 at the cellular level. Theoretically, a linear relationship exists between CO and Do_2 at varying concentrations of Hgb and Sao_2 (Fig. 23.2).[5] To achieve a normal O_2 delivery of 900 mL O_2/min in a patient with an Hgb of 15 g/dL and an Sao_2 of 95%, one must have a CO of about 4.5 L/min. Conversely, if the patient's Hgb was only 10 g/dL (similar Sao_2 = 95%), the CO would only be able to deliver approximately 600 mL O_2/min to the periphery. The 33% fall in Hgb would have to be met by a 44% increase in CO (to a total of 6.5 L/min) to achieve a normal level of O_2 delivery. Oxygen delivery is important since both improved patient survival and a reduction in organ system failure have been correlated with Do_2.[6,7] It appears that the critical level of Do_2 is about 600 mL/min or 8 mL/kg/min in a normal patient[6,8] and may increase to 15 mL/kg/min in those with septic shock[7] (Fig. 23.3).

The ideal setting in a patient with cardiogenic shock is to provide the optimal Do_2 at the lowest cardiac work; this would be consistent with maintaining the lowest adequate BP, with just enough preload to achieve the optimal CO at an HR between 60–100 beats/min with a minimal amount of inotropic and vasoactive drug support.

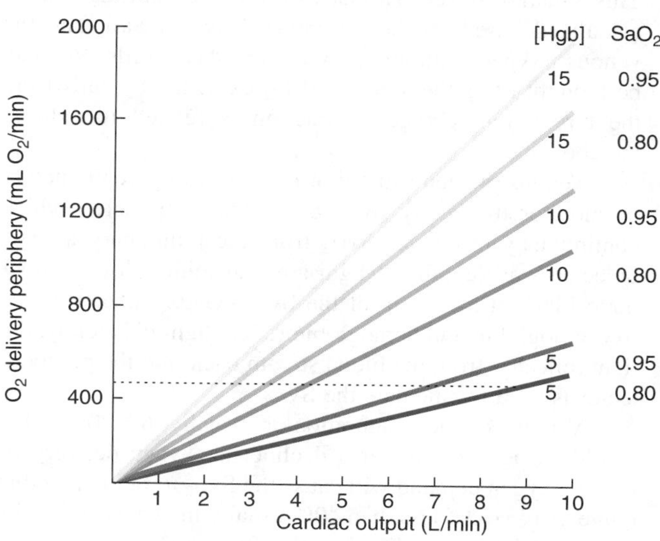

Figure 23.2. Theoretical oxygen delivery at varying hemoglobin concentrations and oxygen saturations. *(From Lyerly HK. Shock, in Lyerly HK [ed]: The Handbook of Surgical Intensive Care: Practices of the Surgery Residents at the Duke University Medical Center, 2nd ed. Chicago, Year Book Medical Publishers, 1989, pp 1–18, with permission.)*

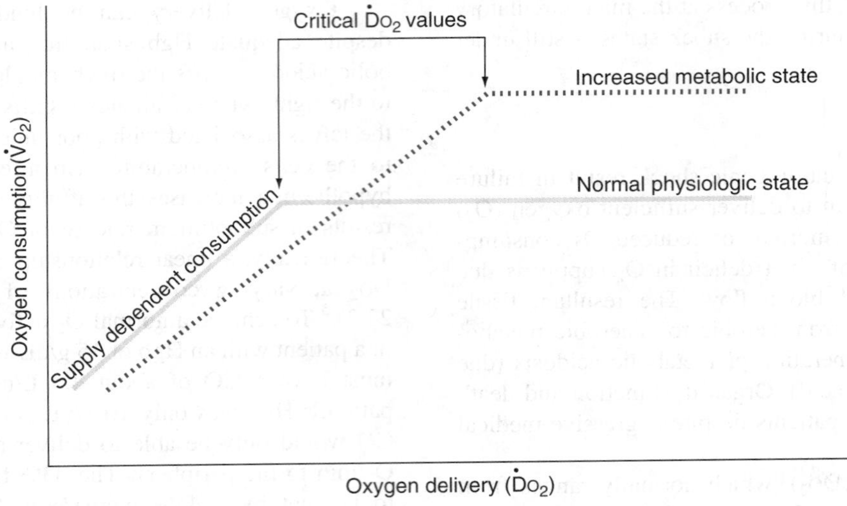

Figure 23.3. Conceptual representation of Vo_2 versus Do_2 in normal states and states of increased metabolism. *(From Tuchschmidt JA. Hemodynamic correlates of outcome, in Parrillo JE, Shoemaker WC, Tuchschmidt JA, Edwards JD [eds]: Acute Cardiac Dysfunction and Tissue Oxygen Debt in Septic Shock. New York, NCM Publishers, 1991, p 14, with permission.)*

Oxygen Consumption

Oxygen consumption (Vo_2) is approximately 225 mL/min (3.5 mL/kg/min) and is expressed by the following relationship[4]:

$$Vo_2 \text{ mL/min} = CO \times [Hb \times 1.39 \times (Sao_2 - Svo_2)] \times 10 \qquad (5)$$

This equation is very similar to Eq. (4), except that Vo_2 is calculated based on the difference between Sao_2 and the venous oxygen saturation (Svo_2). In other words, Vo_2 can be thought of as the amount of O_2 extracted by cells from the circulation. Oxygen extraction is related to cellular metabolism.

Venous oxygen saturation is obtained by venipuncture or monitored directly by a Swan–Ganz oximeter, which continuously calculates Svo_2 from the pulmonary artery.[9] Selected wavelengths of light are transmitted down a fiber optic filament to the tip of the Swan–Ganz catheter. Since oxyhemoglobin and hemoglobin reflect light differently, the light reflected from the blood stream back into the photodetector is used to calculate the Svo_2.

Venous oxygen saturation is usually 60–80%. One would suspect that either a decline in oxygen delivery or rise in oxygen demand will cause the Svo_2 to fall below this range. An Svo_2 of less than 40% usually indicates an inability to compensate and maintain sufficient Do_2. A low Hgb (anemia, hemorrhage), impaired Sao_2 (hypoxia, suctioning), or reduced CO (hypovolemia, cardiogenic shock, arrhythmias) may all depress Svo_2. In addition, an increase in O_2 demand and Vo_2 (hyperthermia, pain, shivering, seizures) can also reduce Svo_2. The Svo_2 can be elevated due to either an increase in O_2 delivery (e.g., high Fio_2, hyperoxia) or a decrease in O_2 demand (e.g., hypothermia, anesthesia, pharmacologic paralysis).

Normally, Vo_2 is *independent* of Do_2, unless there is significant impairment of Do_2, as depicted by the plateau phase of Do_2 in the normal physiologic state (solid line in Fig. 23.3). Initially, as Do_2 falls (moving right to left along solid plateau line in Fig. 23.3), Vo_2 is maintained by an increase in cellular oxygen extraction. Once Do_2 falls below the critical value, Vo_2 becomes *dependent* on Do_2 (sloping solid line, Fig. 23.3). Oxygen consumption is usually depressed in patients with decreased tissue O_2 utilization, diminished CO, decreased arterial O_2-carrying capacity, and intracardiac right to left shunting (desaturation of blood). Conversely, Vo_2 may be elevated in patients with increased O_2 utilization (sepsis, trauma), inappropriate elevation of CO, arteriovenous shunting, and altered oxyhemoglobin dissociation. If Do_2 does not meet the oxygen demands of the cell, aerobic metabolism shifts to anaerobic metabolism, thus generating lactic acid, which results in a metabolic acidosis.

CLINICAL PRESENTATION

The hallmark clinical signs and symptoms coupled with the patient's chief complaint, medical history, and laboratory values ultimately contribute to the definitive diagnosis of shock. The following discussion focuses on each of the organ systems involved.[10,11]

Cardiovascular

The cardiovascular system represents the initial and most critical organ system affected by the shock syndromes. Significant hypotension (SBP <90 mm Hg) with resultant reflex sinus tachycardia (>120–130 beats/min) is often observed in the hypovolemic patient. The reflex tachycardia represents the body's attempt to maintain CO and hence BP and DO_2 in spite of decreased circulating intravascular volume (preload), depressed vascular tone, or left ventricular (LV) dysfunction. Although sinus tachycardia may increase CO, an HR over 150 beats/min shortens diastolic filling time and reduces SV and CO. A maldistribution of blood flow occurs as the body compensates to maintain circulation to O_2 supply-dependent tissues (heart and brain) in lieu of supply-independent tissues (splanchnic bed, kidneys, skin, muscle). Clinically, the patient presents with extremities cool to the touch and a "thready pulse."

If BP does not rise via an increase in CO or humoral mechanisms, coronary perfusion will fall because it is directly related to the patient's aortic pressure minus the intraventricular pressure during diastole. A mean arterial pressure of <60 mm Hg will severely limit coronary filling, thereby straining the already limited aerobic metabolic capabilities of the myocardium. This leads to a further worsening of ventricular function since O_2 is in short supply. Cardiac arrhythmias may be observed if coronary hypoxia persists. Perpetuation of coronary hypoperfusion with declining myocardial contractility eventually leads to irreversible myocardial pump failure, pulmonary edema, and cardiovascular collapse.

Cardiac output may also be very low (2.5–3 L/min) in the patient with extensive myocardial damage because there often is not enough viable muscle remaining to eject ventricular volume adequately. A structural defect such as an incompetent valve or chemical mediators associated with septic shock also may adversely affect myocardial function. The patient's SvO_2 generally falls to about 70–75% because of the reduced CO. Auscultation of the chest may reveal heart sounds consistent with valvular heart disease (regurgitation, outflow obstruction) or significant ventricular dysfunction (S_3). A chest roentgenogram may detect a dissecting ascending aortic aneurysm (widened mediastinum) or cardiomegaly (large heart shadow). Normal autoregulatory responses may be inadequate in these instances and thus pharmacologic and/or mechanical support may be necessary.

Central Nervous System

One of the first signs/symptoms of shock may be an alteration of the patient's sensorium (i.e., the patient may be confused or combative). The brain is very adept at autoregulating central nervous system (CNS) perfusion pressure (mean arterial pressure [MAP] – intracranial pressure) despite wide swings in systemic BP. Although MAP is thought to play a significant role in CNS perfusion, patients with normal MAP and sepsis syndrome have been observed to have reduced cerebral blood flow. In general, however, prolonged and significant decreases in cerebral perfusion pressure based on an MAP of less than 60 mm Hg may induce coma.

Respiratory

Respiratory alkalosis secondary to hyperventilation is usually observed secondary to CNS stimulation of ventilatory centers as a result of trauma, sepsis, or shock. Tidal volume may be reduced secondary to hyperventilation and arterial blood gas determination will confirm a low $PaCO_2$ (25–35 mm Hg), normal bicarbonate, and alkaline pH. The PaO_2 remains in the normal range, at least during the initial stages of shock due to the tachypnea. Nevertheless, as the shock state continues, hypoxia will predominate, especially when extravascular lung water expands in the setting of cardiogenic shock. Auscultation of the lungs may reveal rales (pulmonary edema) or absence of breath sounds (pneumothorax, hemothorax). A chest roentgenogram can confirm early suspicions or disclose an undetected abnormality such as pneumonia (pulmonary infiltrates).

As shock progresses, there is a narrowing of the arterial–venous oxygen content (CaO_2–CvO_2) difference as oxygen delivery decreases due to microvascular low flow states or shunting of blood. Decreased tissue perfusion also causes accumulation of tissue carbon dioxide (PCO_2) secondary to altered clearance by low blood flow. This is accompanied by a widening of the arteriovenous pH gradient. Because of the arteriovenous variations, severely hemodynamically compromised patients should have both arterial and mixed venous blood gas samples drawn to assess acid–base status as tissue acidemia and hypercapnia will be better detected on the venous side of the circulation.

As the metabolic acidosis develops, compensatory respiratory alkalosis will be maintained through hyperventilation, unless there is alveolar obstruction or damage, significant pulmonary edema, or the patient is intubated and mechanically ventilated. Continued insult to the lungs may result in adult respiratory distress syndrome (ARDS) (see Chapter 27).

Renal

The kidneys are exquisitely sensitive to changes in perfusion pressures and moderate alterations can lead to significant changes in glomerular filtration rate (GFR) regardless of whether the precipitant is hypovolemic or cardiogenic in origin. Oliguria (urine output of <20 mL/h), progressing to anuria, occurs due to vasoconstriction of the afferent arterioles because of inadequate renal perfusion pressure from depressed CO, hypovolemia, or hypotension. The decrease in renal perfusion leads to increased proximal tubule reabsorption of solute (Na, blood urea nitrogen [BUN]) and the release of the mineralocorticoid, aldosterone; both result in Na retention and thus low sodium concentration in the urine (U_{Na}) (<30 mEq/L).

Renal function can be grossly assessed by hourly measurements of urine output. Creatinine clearance estimation (e.g., Cockroft and Gault formula), based on isolated serum creatinine values in critically ill patients, generally yields erroneous results. Trends, however, in serum creatinine and BUN are useful and should be followed. A rise in BUN may indicate increased proximal tubule reabsorption of solute due to depressed glomerular perfusion as mentioned above. Similarly, an increase in creatinine may be noted as GFR decreases. If the BUN to serum creatinine ratio is >20 : 1, a prerenal syndrome is suspected.

Because the creatinine clearance in the patient with fluctuating hemodynamics, and thus GFR, is ever changing, drug selection and dosing requires careful attention and should be appropriately modified (see Chapter 50).

Skin

The patient is often cool and will have severely slowed capillary refill of the digits as a result of the peripheral vasoconstriction. The skin may be pale or have cyanotic (bluish) color due to the presence of hypoxemia. Sympathetic stimulation accounts for sweating, giving the skin a moist, clammy feel. The patient's integument will undergo changes back to normal as peripheral and microcirculation is restored.

Metabolic

As the shock state progresses uncorrected, VO_2 increases due to hypercatabolism as the body attempts to repair cellular damage from either hypoperfusion or endotoxin from sepsis. Redistribution of blood flow induces peripheral O_2 debt as DO_2 is altered. This leads to a shift from aerobic to anaerobic metabolism to form adenosine triphosphate (ATP) as mentioned previously. Anaerobic conversion of glucose to pyruvate yields only 2 moles of ATP per mole of glucose rather than the 38 moles of ATP per mole of glucose generated via the aerobic Krebs cycle. This significant reduction of ATP energy adversely affects all cellular functions because the Na^+/K^+ plasma membrane pump is ATP dependent. Elevation in serum lactate, produced from pyruvate, has been implicated in increasing mortality in patients with circulatory shock.[12] The lactate is converted into lactic acid in the periphery, thereby causing the metabolic acidosis. Reversal of the metabolic acidosis, coupled with trends in decreasing serial serum lactate levels, is usually observed with overall clinical improvement of the patient and survival.

Gastrointestinal

Compensatory peripheral vasoconstriction from cardiogenic shock and/or hypovolemia results in a redistribution of blood flow away from the gastrointestinal (GI) tract and may cause stress gastritis, gut ischemia, and in some cases infarction, resulting in GI bleeding. If the integrity of the intestine is violated, translocation of bacteria and endotoxins may occur, further compounding the cardiovascular insult already under way by adding the potential of sepsis. Auscultation for bowel sounds and evaluation for stool and gas production determine the presence of ileus. If oral agents are to be given with expectations of being absorbed, GI motility must be present.

Hepatic

Hypovolemia and depressed CO accompanied by sympathetic vasoconstriction can reduce liver blood flow and thus alter the metabolism of endogenous compounds and drugs. Vasodilatory forms of shock may similarly diminish liver blood flow. Progressive liver damage (shock liver) manifests as a release of intracellular enzymes (aspartate aminotransferase [AST], alanine aminotransferase [ALT]) into the circulation; unconjugated bilirubin may also be elevated. Lastly, prothrombin time (PT), the international normalized ratio (INR) and the activated partial thromboplastin time (aPTT) may be increased above baseline as synthesis of clotting factors is impaired.

Summary

Shock presents with a diversity of signs and symptoms. Hypotension, tachycardia, confusion, and oliguria are key symptoms of the shock state. Myocardial and cerebral ischemia, pulmonary edema (cardiogenic shock), and multisystem organ failure will often follow. The astute clinician should recognize the early stages of shock and initiate immediate interventions in an attempt to prevent irreversible cellular, tissue, and organ damage that, if untreated, will ultimately lead to the patient's demise.

MONITORING

Information obtained from both noninvasive and invasive monitoring and an evaluation of the patient's past medical history, clinical presentation, and laboratory findings are key components in establishing the diagnosis, assessing the general mechanisms responsible for the shock state, and guiding therapy (Table 23.1). All instrumentation must be calibrated so that accurate values are recorded. Trends must be considered rather than isolated numbers because erroneous information and/or misinterpretation can result in an incorrect diagnosis, which may delay appropriate therapy. The noninvasive and invasive measures as well as calcu-

TABLE 23.1. COMPARATIVE HEMODYNAMIC PROFILES OF HYPOVOLEMIC AND CARDIOGENIC SHOCK

	MAP	RAP (CVP)	PCWP	HR	CO	SVR
Hypovolemic shock	↓↓	↓↓	↓↓	↑↑	↓–↓↓↓	↑–↑↑
Cardiogenic shock						
Left ventricular/biventricular failure	↔↓	↑–↑↑	↑↑	↓↔↑	↓↓	↑–↑↑
Right ventricular failure	↔↓	↑↑–↑↑↑	↓–↓↓	↓↔↑	↓↓	↑–↑↑

Key: MAP, mean arterial pressure; RAP, right atrial pressure; CVP, central venous pressure; HR, heart rate; CO, cardiac output; SVR, systemic vascular resistance; ↓, decrease; ↔, no change; ↑, increase. (Compiled from Sypniewski E, Ornato JP. Circulatory shock, in Ornato JP, Gonzalez ER (eds): Drug Therapy in Emergency Medicine. New York, Churchill Livingstone, 1990, p 55; and Kirby RR, Taylor RW, Civetta JM (eds). Shock in Handbook of Critical Care. Philadelphia, JB Lippincott, 1994, p 19, with permission.)

lated parameters from these measurements are listed in Table 23.2.

Blood Pressure

Noninvasive assessment of BP using the sphygmomanometer and stethoscope may be inaccurate in the presence of arrhythmias, low SV, profound peripheral vasodilation, or peripheral vascular disease, because all can cause an underestimation of BP due to inaudible Korotkoff sounds. Peripheral vasoconstriction in patients receiving α-adrenergic agonists (e.g., high-dose dopamine or epinephrine, norepinephrine, phenylephrine) also may invalidate cuff BP results because peripheral arterial pressures will be falsely elevated in relation to aortic pressures. The use of a Doppler device to amplify Korotkoff sounds in a hypotensive patient may improve the accuracy of BP measurements, especially if the SBP is less than 50–70 mm Hg, although reliability may still be questioned. Automated peripheral BP monitoring devices such as the Dynamapp suffer from the same limitations as the sphygmomanometer.

Because noninvasive cardiovascular monitoring provides information that may not be accurate, invasive hemodynamic monitoring is often utilized. Insertion of an indwelling catheter into the radial artery can supply reasonably accurate BP determinations, albeit they are dependent on the patient's arm position. In addition, this site serves as a port to readily obtain ABGs.

Cardiac and Pulmonary Pressures

A subclavian or internal jugular indwelling intravenous line in the superior vena cava can be used to measure central venous pressure (CVP) or right atrial pressure (RAP), thus providing an estimation of the filling pressure, or preload, of the right ventricle (RV). This measurement is useful in estimating intravascular volume status during acute changes and in the absence of other concomitant diseases such as pulmonary embolism or right-sided heart failure. However, the CVP is not always a reliable indicator of intravascular volume in intensive care unit (ICU) patients, probably due to physiologic changes in venous capacitance that is thought to occur over time in this patient population. However, it can be useful if trends in pressure changes are followed rather than absolute values. Volume expansion should lead to an increase in CVP. Conversely, venodilation following intravenous nitroglycerin infusion or intravascular volume loss secondary to bleeding will cause the CVP to fall.

A more complex instrument for invasive monitoring of central cardiovascular pressures is the flow-directed balloon-tipped catheter (Swan–Ganz).[2,13–15] Under aseptic conditions, the catheter is inserted via the subclavian or internal jugular vein and threaded through the superior vena cava, right atrium, and ventricle, into the pulmonary artery (Fig. 23.4). The pressure waveforms observed during passage of the Swan–Ganz catheter are depicted in Fig. 23.5. The pressure tracing in the right atrium is rather static because it measures the minor pressure changes indicative of CVP. The RAP and CVP are considered essentially the same because the right atria is an open chamber to both the inferior and superior vena cavas. This pressure reading (normally 0–10 mm Hg) provides an estimate of intravascular volume and RV preload as mentioned previously. Although a high CVP may suggest intravascular volume overload, right-sided heart failure, an incompetent tricuspid valve, pulmonary hypertension or embolism, and pericardial tamponade can all cause elevations. A further limitation of the CVP is that the pressure readings have not been found to correlate well with pulmonary capillary wedge pressure (PCWP), which is considered the preload to the left side of the heart.

The balloon at the tip of the catheter is inflated with air and the catheter is advanced into the RV. Wide variations in pressure are observed owing to ventricular diastole and systole, reaching a systolic pressure of 15–25 mm Hg and a diastolic pressure of 2–5 mm Hg (Fig. 23.5). Further advancement of the catheter into the pulmonary artery reveals the pulmonary artery systolic (PAS) and pulmonary artery diastolic (PAD) pressures. The PAS rises to about 15–30 mm Hg and the PAD falls to 5–15 mm Hg. These pressures may be elevated in patients with fluid overload, as well as in those with pulmonary hypertension, pulmonary embolus, severe obstructive lung disease, and left-sided ventricular failure. The pulmonary artery pressures may be depressed in hypovolemia and severe right-sided failure, the latter due to depressed CO from the RV.

The inflated balloon-tip will "wedge" in a pulmonary capillary artery at which time the PCWP can be determined

TABLE 23.2. KEY CARDIOVASCULAR AND RESPIRATORY PARAMETERS

Parameter	Abbreviation	Formula	Normal
Noninvasive			
Heart rate	HR	Direct measure	72–88 beats/min
Blood pressure (systolic/diastolic)	SBP/DBP	Direct measure cuff or arterial line	100–140/60–100 mm Hg
Mean arterial pressure	MAP	DBP + 1/3 (SBP – DBP) or arterial line	82–102 mm Hg
Pulse pressure	PP	SBP – DBP	40–80 mm Hg
Invasive: Swan–Ganz Determinations			
Central venous pressure (right atrial pressure)	CVP (RAP)	Direct measure	1–10 mm Hg
Pulmonary artery pressure (systolic/diastolic)	PAS/PAD	Direct measure	25–35 mm Hg/10–20 mm Hg
Mean pulmonary artery pressure	MPAP	Direct measure	11–15 mm Hg
Pulmonary capillary wedge pressure	PCWP	Direct measure	8–12 mm Hg
Cardiac output	CO	Thermodilution measure	4.5–6.5 L/min
Cardiac index	CI	CO/BSA	2.8–3.6 L/min/m^2
Calculated Parameters			
Rate pressure product	RPP	HR × SBP	12,000
Stroke volume	SV	CO/HR × 1000	60–90 mL
Stroke index	SI	CI/HR × 1000	30–50 mL/m^2
Left ventricular stroke work index	LVSWI	SI × MAP × 0.0136	44–68 g/m^2
Left cardiac work index	LCWI	CI × MAP × 0.0136	3–4.6 kg-m/m^2
Right ventricular stroke work index	RVSWI	SI × MPAP × 0.0136	4–8 g/m^2
Right cardiac work index	RCWI	CI × MPAP × 0.0136	0.4–0.6 kg-m/m^2
Systemic vascular resistance	SVR	[(MAP – CVP)/CO] × 79.9	900–1200 dynes-s/cm^5
Systemic vascular resistance index	SVRI	[(MAP – CVP)/CI] × 79.9	1760–2600 dynes-s/cm^5 × m^2
Pulmonary vascular resistance	PVR	[(MPAP – PCWP)/CO] × 79.9	75–400 dynes-s/cm^5 × m^2
Pulmonary vascular resistance index	PVRI	[(MPAP – PCWP)/CI] × 79.9	45–225 dynes-s/cm^5
Oxygen Transport			
Arterial pH	pH	Direct measure	7.36–7.44
Arterial oxygen tension	Pao_2	Direct measure	80–100 mm Hg
Arterial carbon dioxide tension	$Paco_2$	Direct measure	36–44 mm Hg (torr)
Arterial oxygen hemoglobin saturation	Sao_2	Direct measure	95–99%
Mixed venous oxygen tension	Pvo_2	Direct measure	33–53 mm Hg
Mixed venous oxygen saturation	Svo_2	Direct measure	60–80 mm Hg
Arterial oxygen content	Cao_2	Hb × Sao_2 × 1.39	20.1 vol%
Venous oxygen content	Cvo_2	Hb × Svo_2 × 1.39	15.5 vol%
Arterial–mixed venous content difference	$O_2C(a–v)O_2$	Cao_2 – Cvo_2	4–5.5 mL/dL
Oxygen delivery	Do_2	CO × Cao_2 × 10	900–1100 mL/min
Oxygen consumption	Vo_2	CO × Cvo_2 × 10	225–235 mL/min
Oxygen extraction	O_2 ext	(Cao_2 – Cvo_2)/Cao_2	22–30%

(Reprinted with modifications from Shoemaker WC. Shock states: Pathophysiology, monitoring, outcome prediction and therapy, in Shoemaker WC, Ayers S, Grenvik A, et al. (eds): Textbook of Critical Care, 2nd ed. Philadelphia, WB Saunders, 1989, p 979, with permission.)

(Fig. 23.4). The PCWP affords an estimate of the left ventricular end diastolic pressure (LVEDP) because there are no structural barriers through the lungs and left atrium into the LV except for the mitral valve. Also, the PCWP serves as an indicator of pulmonary congestion. The normal pressure range for the PCWP is 6–12 mm Hg.

Like the CVP, the PCWP is not an ideal index of intravascular volume status. One must remember that these readings are pressures, which are a function of not only plasma volume but the area inside the blood vessels (vascular tone), ventricular compliance, and CO. These pressures can be altered without change in plasma volume, by constriction or dilation of blood vessels, and changes in ventricular compliance. It is important to note that a nonlinear relationship between volume and pressure exists. As optimal intravascular volume is approached, the pressure rises at a disproportionate rate. It is therefore best to follow acute trends in PCWP rather than matching an isolated value to an estimated plasma volume.

A correlation between PCWP and PAD also exists in the absence of underlying structural heart or vascular lung disease. The PCWP will be about 1–3 mm Hg lower than the PAD. This is useful to know when there are difficulties in "wedging" the catheter.

Application of either positive end-expiratory pressure (PEEP) or continuous positive airway pressure (CPAP) will

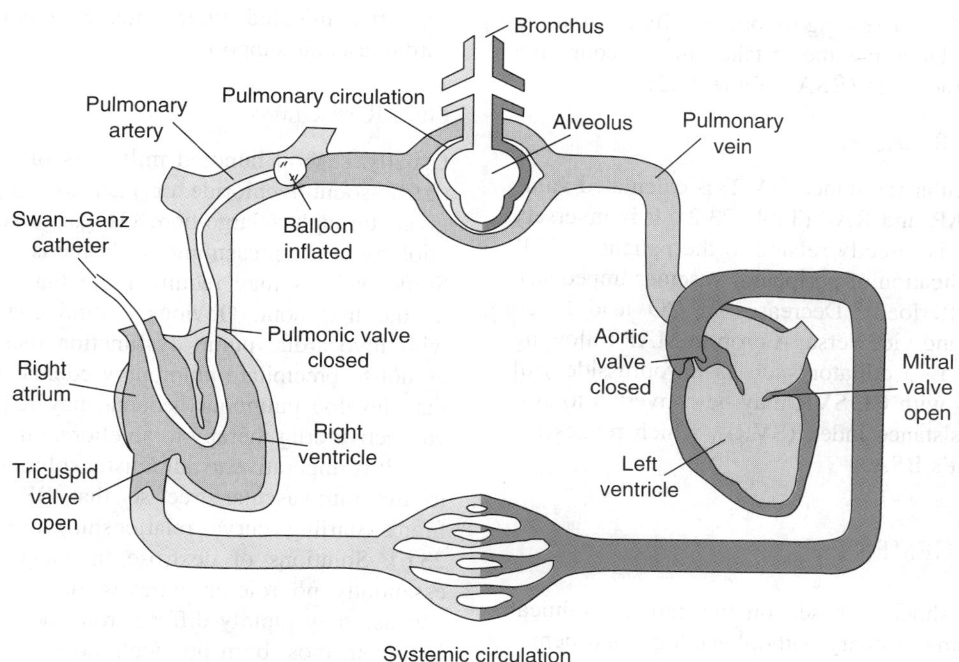

Figure 23.4. Insertion of the Swan–Ganz catheter. *(From Headley JM. Invasive Hemodynamic Monitoring: Physiological Principles and Clinical Applications. Santa Ana, CA, Edwards Critical Care Division, 1989, p 20, with permission.)*

result in false elevations of the PCWP. The extent of the deviation varies with the degree of lung compliance and transmission of airway pressure through the pulmonary vasculature. Generally, the PCWP will be falsely elevated by 1 mm Hg for every 5 cm H_2O increase in intrathoracic pressure from PEEP or CPAP. In addition, structural abnormalities such as atrial myxoma, mitral regurgitation, pericardial tamponade, or a noncompliant, stiff LV can cause a falsely elevated PCWP.

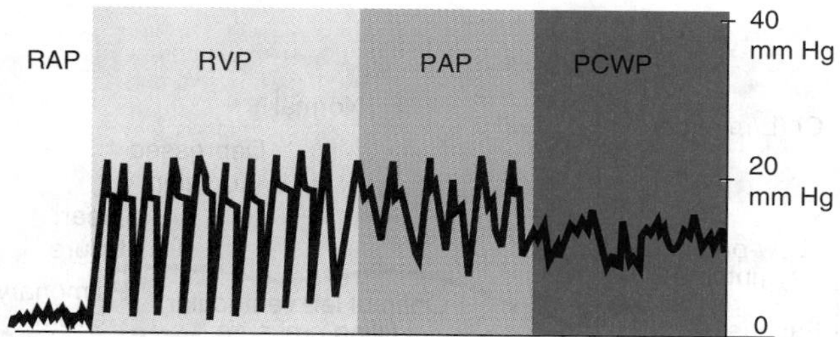

Figure 23.5. Swan–Ganz pressure waveforms during advancement and "wedging" of catheter. RAP, right atrial pressure (central venous pressure); RVP, right ventricular pressures; PAP, pulmonary artery pressures, PCWP, pulmonary capillary wedge pressure. *(From Anonymous. Understanding hemodynamic measurements made with the Swan–Ganz catheter. American Edwards Laboratories, 1984, p 6, with permission.)*

The Swan–Ganz catheter provides accurate readings when the catheter is calibrated and the exterior transducer is level with the patient's right atrium. Insertion of the Swan–Ganz catheter may trigger ventricular arrhythmias ranging from isolated premature ventricular contractions to rare transient ventricular tachycardia and fibrillation; therefore, lidocaine should be available at the bedside. Other complications of an indwelling Swan–Ganz catheter include thrombosis, infection (primarily *Staphylococcus* species), damage to either the tricuspid or pulmonary valve, pulmonary infarction, and rupture of the pulmonary artery.

Cardiac Output

Cardiac output is estimated using the thermodilution method.[16] An internal thermistor at the tip of the Swan–Ganz catheter determines the temperature of the blood in the pulmonary tree, compares that reading with the original temperature of the dextrose infusate, and calculates the CO based on the difference in temperature. Of note, the CO determined from this methodology is for the RV, not the LV. Because of the pathophysiology involved, we assume that the CO for the RV is equivalent to the LV. This assumption is not always true because structural abnormalities such as ventricular septal defect with left to right shunting of blood will elevate RV stoke volume over left, thus altering the CO from each ventricle.

Once the CO is known, SV can be calculated by dividing CO by HR. Many clinicians prefer to use cardiac index

(CI) rather than CO in assessing myocardial function at the bedside since the latter parameter takes into account the patient's body surface area (BSA) (Table 23.2).

Systemic Vascular Resistance

The systemic vascular resistance (SVR) is calculated value using the CO, MAP, and RAP (Table 23.2). It is inversely related to CO and is directly related to the patient's MAP. The SVR is an indication of peripheral vascular impedance to blood flow (afterload). Decreases in CO lead to an increase in SVR, and vice versa. A drop in MAP following administration of a vasodilator such as nitroprusside will decrease SVR. As with CI, SVR may be converted to systemic vascular resistance index (SVRI), which relates the SVR to the patient's BSA.

INITIAL MANAGEMENT

The diagnosis of shock is based on the patient's clinical signs and symptoms, primary pathophysiology, and hemodynamic profile. Hypotension (SBP < 90 mm Hg), depressed CI (<2.2 L/min/m^2), tachycardia (HR >100 beats/min), and low urine output (<20 mL/h) are consistent findings in both hypovolemic and cardiogenic shock. Although the severity of the initial event, degree of hypotension, duration of the shock state, associated disease states, and the patient's physiologic reserve are all important to survival, the key component to sustaining life appears to be the speed and appropriateness with which therapy is rendered.[17]

Empiric Therapy

The goal in the empiric management of shock is not to normalize each parameter since compensatory mechanisms such as sinus tachycardia are clearly necessary. Rather, the principal goal is to support the delivery of O_2 through the circulatory system by assuring effective intravascular plasma volume, optimal O_2-carrying capacity and adequate BP while a definitive diagnosis and strategy for therapy is being determined.[18]

Oxygen Therapy

The patient should receive supplemental oxygen at the earliest signs of shock, beginning with 4–6 L/min via nasal cannula or 6–10 L/min by face mask (with or without oxygen reservoir). Frank respiratory failure may not be evident during the initial stages of shock; however, it is likely that mechanical ventilatory support will eventually be necessary, especially for the patient with cardiogenic shock. Marginal gas exchange (hypoxemia), development of a mild metabolic acidosis, peripheral cyanosis, and mental obtundation all justify tracheal intubation and mechanical ventilation with pressure supported ventilation (PSV) and PEEP when necessary. Once the airway is secure and ventilatory support is initiated, future interventions can be directed at cardiovascular support.

Fluid Resuscitation

Usually, several hundred milliliters of isotonic crystalloid (0.9% sodium chloride or lactated Ringer's solution) is given through a large-bore (16-gauge) catheter while the etiology of the presenting syndrome is under investigation. Some patients may require more than 2 L of crystalloid in the first hour. Obviously, fluid challenge in patients with myocardial pump dysfunction must be tempered so as not to precipitate pulmonary edema. Likewise, patients that develop pulmonary edema may require diuretics and vasoactive drug therapy to ameliorate this situation.

It is imperative to administer solutions that will remain in the intravascular tree so that BP and CO (via the Frank–Starling curve relationship) are augmented (Fig. 23.6). Solutions of dextrose in water (e.g., D_5W) have essentially no role in intravascular volume resuscitation because they rapidly diffuse from the intravascular space. However, most burn protocols do recommend administration of dextrose in water solutions during the first 24–48 hours following major burns so that a hypertonic state does not develop.

An ongoing source of fluid or blood loss should be sought if substantial (>200 mL/h) fluid administration is associated with negligible changes in BP, CVP, and PCWP measurements. A similar effect can often be observed in the patient with septic shock due to profound peripheral vasodilation. Trends in cardiac filling pressures can be followed if the patient has an indwelling Swan–Ganz catheter. Successful fluid resuscitation should favorably increase SBP (>90 mm Hg), CI (>2.2 L/min/m^2), and urine output (0.5–1 mL/kg/h) while decreasing SVR to the normal range (900–1200 dynes-s/cm^5). It is essential that a MAP of greater than 60 mm Hg be achieved to ensure adequate cerebral and coronary perfusion pressure.

Colloid (5% plasmanate, 5% albumin, hydroxy ethyl starch), 250–500 mL, infused over several minutes may be

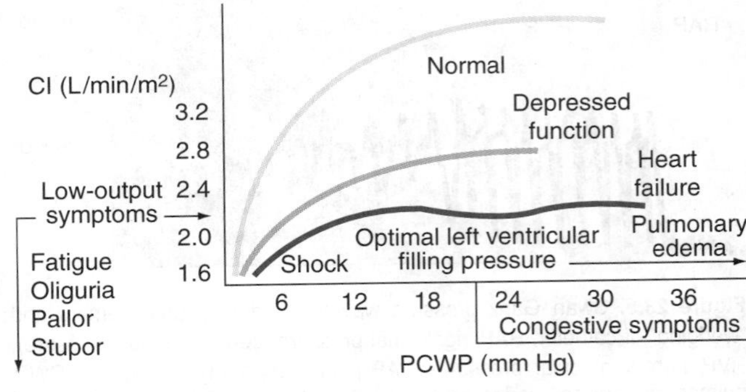

Figure 23.6. Idealized relationship between pulmonary capillary wedge pressure (PCWP) and cardiac index (CI).

preferred in the postoperative patient because the colloid will draw third-spaced interstitial fluid into the vascular tree. Burn patients, however, should not receive any colloid for the first 24 hours after burn injury, because the accompanying "leaky capillary" syndrome will result in interstitial colloid deposition, which may compromise lung gas exchange.

The patient's Hgb concentration must be monitored due to the dilutional effect of exogenous fluid administration. Blood products (whole blood, packed red blood cells) should be given, if necessary, to maintain the oxygen-carrying capacity of the circulation. Patients presenting with an Hgb of <10 g/dL should be evaluated for blood transfusion, especially if ongoing blood loss is detected and significant amounts of nonoxygen-carrying solutions will be used for volume resuscitation.

Pulmonary edema, the major consequence of fluid overload, should be avoided since further insult on the respiratory system, which is already under stress, will generally not be tolerated by the patient with compromised myocardial function.

Vasoactive Therapy

The intravascularly volume-depleted patient should respond to fluid challenge alone, provided that a sufficient volume of fluid is infused and the patient does not have an ongoing source of fluid loss (burns, hemorrhagic trauma). If fluid challenge is unsuccessful in achieving the desired endpoints, pharmacologic support is then necessary (Fig. 23.7). There is appreciable interpatient variability in dose and pharmacodynamic effect with most of the vasoactive agents; titration of dose will depend on both the desired and observed clinical outcomes, as well as the type of shock present (hypovolemic versus cardiogenic versus vasodilatory) (Table 23.3 on pages 522–523). One must also keep in mind that dosing recommendations of inotropic and vasoactive drugs are primarily based on patients that have little variability from normal or ideal body weight; hence, careful dose selection at initiation of therapy and during maintenance should be employed in obese individuals since the potential for overdose and subsequent sequelae may be significant. Finally, all vasoactive and inotropic medications must be infused using an infusion pump system to assure accuracy of dose and facilitate titration.

If the patient is believed to have a primary vascular component to the hypotension (secondary to vasodilation causing a relative hypovolemia such as in septic, neurogenic, or anaphylactic shock), the primary strategy is administration of vasopressors such as dopamine (Intropin) (5–20 μg/kg/min) or norepinephrine (Levophed) (0.5–30 μg/min) through a central intravenous line as outlined in the algorithm depicted in Fig. 23.7. Phenylephrine (Neosynephrine) (0.5 μg/kg/min) is a good first-line alternative in a patient that has accompanying ventricular ectopy since it only stimulates α_1 receptors and thus would be expected to have minimum adverse effects on the arrhythmia. Phenylephrine should also be infused via a central intravenous line. The catecholamines, in general, have very short half-lives (2 minutes), which affords quick onset and short duration of action, thus facilitating titration.

Alternatively, a patient that experiences significant myocardial dysfunction *without* signs or symptoms of shock, yet presents with mild to severe hypotension (SBP = 70–100 mm Hg), may optimally benefit from a β_1-adrenergic inotrope such as dobutamine (Dobutrex), in addition to modest intravascular volume expansion with crystalloid (Fig. 23.7). Because the Starling's curve response to volume administration is often limited in patients with myocardial dysfunction (Fig. 23.6), there is a high risk of developing pulmonary edema if too much volume is infused. Dobutamine primarily stimulates the β_1-adrenergic receptors of the heart to increase the force of contraction of viable muscle throughout the dosing range.[19] Dobutamine is usually initiated at a dose of 2–5 μg/kg/min through a peripheral (or central) intravenous line and titrated, at 1–2 μg/kg/min increments based on response, to a maximum of about 15–20 μg/kg/min. Although the drug also has combined α_1- and β_2-adrenergic stimulation,[20] at doses exceeding 10–15 μg/kg/min, the net effect on the pulmonary and peripheral vasculature is vasodilation.[19] Peripheral organ perfusion as evidenced by improvement in UO should be observed following the increase in CO.

If the patient with myocardial dysfunction presents with hypotension (SBP = 70–100 mm Hg) and accompanying signs and symptoms of shock/hypoperfusion (oliguria, pallor, cyanosis, etc.), dopamine may be the preferred agent in this setting (Fig. 23.7). At moderate doses (2.5–10 μg/kg/min), renal vascular dilation from dopaminergic receptor (DA_1) stimulation and β_1-adrenergic-mediated inotropy on the myocardium will be observed.[21] As dopamine is titrated beyond 10 μg/kg/min, stimulation of endogenous norepinephrine release,[22,23] along with direct α_1-adrenergic-mediated vasoconstriction[21] becomes prominent and BP should rise to a minimally acceptable level (SBP > 90–100 mm Hg). Although a rise in BP and resultant coronary filling pressure should improve myocardial function, the resultant increase in impedance to left ventricular outflow may be significant and thus depress CO. Unlike dobutamine, dopamine also increases pulmonary and ventricular filling pressures.[24,25]

Epinephrine is not usually used empirically because its strong inotropic and chronotropic effects may worsen the myocardial oxygen supply–demand mismatch, particularly if the patient has underlying ischemic heart disease or an ongoing ischemia process.[26] Systemic vascular resistance may already be elevated in an attempt to maintain BP as CO is depressed. Epinephrine is therefore reserved as a second- or third-line agent in spite of its superior inotropic effects. The usual dosage is 0.002 to 0.05 μg/kg/min, which

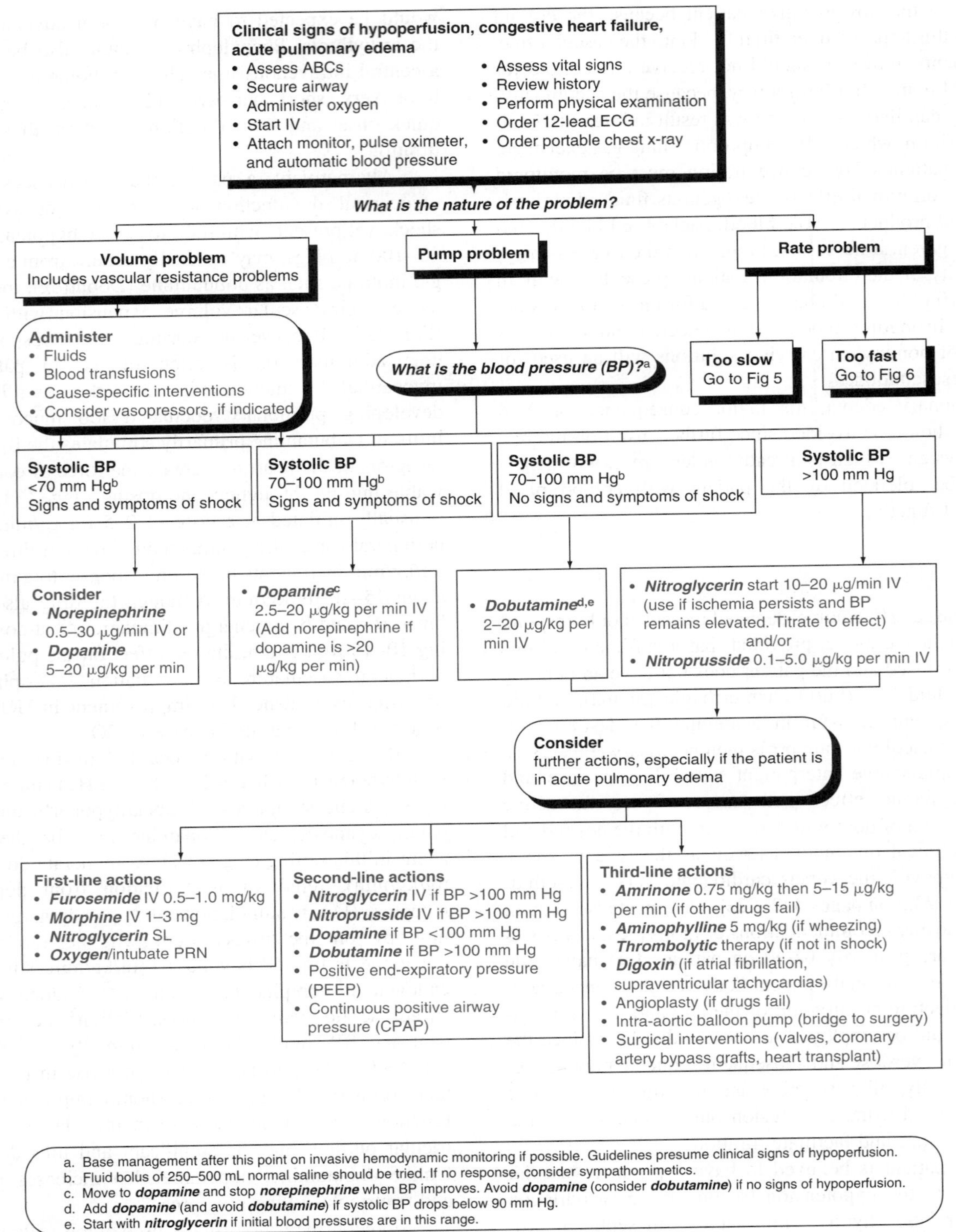

Figure 23.7. Acute pulmonary edema/hypotension/shock algorithm. *(From Cummins RO [ed]. Textbook of Advanced Cardiac Life Support, American Heart Association, 1994, pp 1–41, with permission.)*

primarily affects β_1 and β_2 receptors. As the dose is titrated upward, α_1-adrenergic stimulation produces a profound vasoconstriction. One advantage of using epinephrine in the setting of cardiac resuscitation or following a cardiac arrest is that despite significant increases in peripheral vascular tone, coronary and cerebral perfusion is maintained.[27]

Isoproterenol (Isuprel) has potent β_1- and β_2-adrenergic activity, which may benefit a select number of patients requiring a strong inotrope with afterload reduction. However, its chronotropic and arrhythmogenic effects preclude its use in most patients. In addition, the strong vasodilatory effects are not tolerated by hypovolemic patients or those with low to marginal BP (SBP ≤ 90 mm Hg). A fall in SVR, coupled with an increase in CO and HR, may precipitate ischemia in patients with ischemic heart disease.[28]

A third subset of patients with myocardial pump problems consists of those with a BP of >100 mm Hg systolic. The initial strategy in these patients is to initiate a vasodilator such as nitroglycerin (Tridil) (start at 10–20 μg/min) by constant infusion through either a peripheral or central line, either prior to initiation of inotropic therapy[29] or soon thereafter[30] (Fig. 23.7). Nitroglycerin causes venous dilation at lower doses (<100–150 μg/min) with the addition of arterial dilation at higher doses (>100–150 μg/min). It is also a coronary and collateral artery vasodilator and therefore the agent of choice in the setting of ongoing myocardial ischemia or in the patient with ischemic heart disease as the risk of coronary steal is minimized.[31,32] Nitroprusside provides a balanced arterial and venous dilation, however, it must be used with caution in patients with evolving myocardial infarction and high LVEDP, as discussed under the cardiogenic shock section of this chapter.[32,33] Nitroprusside is infused either peripherally or centrally starting at 0.1–0.5 μg/kg/min and titrated upward at 0.5 μg/kg/min increments at 10- to 15-minute intervals to a maximum of 8–10 μg/kg/min.

Patients who have myocardial dysfunction as a result of calcium-channel blocker administration or have hypocalcemia or severe hyperkalemia can be given calcium (either gluconate or chloride) 1 g by slow intravenous push to improve myocardial contractility. The chloride salt is used preferentially by many clinicians since it contributes approximately three times more elemental calcium than the gluconate salt; and the latter must undergo liver metabolism for calcium liberation. Rapid administration of the calcium salts can precipitate hypotension, bradycardia, or asystole.[34] Calcium can also induce vasoconstriction.[34] High doses of calcium have also been shown to attenuate the chronotropic effects of glucagon and the β-adrenergic effects of epinephrine.[35] Extreme care must be taken when administering calcium to a digitalized patient, especially if the patient is digoxin toxic based on levels and clinical presentation, due to the risk of ventricular arrhythmias or bradyasystole.

The phosphodiesterase III inhibitor amrinone (Inocor) has a tertiary role in the empiric management of the pump failure based on American Heart Association guidelines (Fig. 23.7). Amrinone has potent vasodilatory properties that accompany the indirect inotropic effect.[36,37] The long half-life of 3–5 hours does limit titration during acute management. Although the arrhythmia/tachycardia potential with amrinone may be less than that of the dobutamine, the hemodynamic effects are similar[38] and dobutamine is more easily titrated.

Acid–Base Management

The metabolic acidosis generated from lactic acid that accompanies shock can be prevented as long as ventilation is optimized and prolonged maldistribution of blood flow is prevented. Approximately 500–700 mEq of acid can be eliminated per hour in the form of CO_2 through ventilation of the lungs. However, patients in whom respiratory ventilation is compromised due to ventilation–perfusion mismatch (e.g., pulmonary embolus or edema, mucous plug, alveolar damage) or in those with a persistent source of acid load (e.g., continued hypoperfusion, ischemic limb, severe trauma), administration of sodium bicarbonate often may be required. Normalization of pH to at least 7.3 is essential because metabolic acidosis results in suboptimal hemodynamic response to both endogenous and exogenous catecholamines (e.g., dopamine, dobutamine, epinephrine).[39] It is not uncommon to observe a patient with virtually little or no response to high-dose dopamine, norepinephrine, or epinephrine in the presence of metabolic acidosis. A complete discussion of the pathophysiology and treatment of metabolic acidosis is presented in Chapter 52, Acid–Base Disorders.

Summary

Empiric therapeutic maneuvers should be undertaken while the underlying etiology of the shock syndrome is being established so that the most appropriate interventions can then be implemented. The pharmacist should review the patient's chart, the entire drug history, and medication administration record, as well as the events immediately preceding the development of shock. A complete battery of laboratory tests to include a multichannel chemistry panel, complete blood count (CBC) with differential, arterial, and venous blood gases, electrocardiogram, and chest roentgenogram may all be valuable in determining the cause of the shock syndrome and evaluating its present state.

Hypovolemic Shock

Hypovolemic shock is a hypotensive condition characterized by acute intravascular volume deficiency due to either external losses or internal redistribution of extracellular water. A relative hypovolemia leading to hypovolemic shock occurs during significant vasodilation, which accompanies anaphylaxis, sepsis, and neurogenic shock. Hemorrhage, burns, trauma, intestinal obstruction and dehydration from considerable insensible fluid loss, overaggressive loop-diuretic drug administration, and severe vomiting or diarrhea can precipitate hypovolemic shock. A fluid redistribution phenomenon can also be observed in patients with septic, neurogenic, and anaphylactic shock, as intravascular fluid shifts interstitially. Patients who receive intravenous morphine before intravascular volume status is corrected may develop hypotension secondary to morphine-induced venodilation in the setting of low circulating volume.

TABLE 23.3. PHARMACOLOGIC PROPERTIES AND CLINICAL EFFECTS OF SELECTED VASOACTIVE DRUGS

	Receptor Specificity					Pharmacologic Effect			
Drug/Usual Dose	α	β_1	β_2	**Dop**	**Sm Msc**	**VD**	**VC**	**INT**	**CHT**
Amrinone (Inocor)									
(750 mg/250 mL NS) (P,C)									
LD = 0.75 – 1.0 mg/kg									
MD = 5 – 15 μg/kg/min	—	—	—	—	++	++	—	+++	+++
Dobutamine (Dobutrex)									
(500 mg/250 mL D_5W or NS) (P,C)									
2–10 μg/kg/min	+	+++	++	—	—	+	+	+++	+
>10–20 μg/kg/min	++	++++	+++	—	—	++	+	++++	++
Dopamine (Intropin)									
(800 mg/250 mL D_5W or NS (C)									
1–3 μg/kg/min	—	+	—	++++	—	+	—	++	+
3–10 μg/kg/min	—	++++	++	++++	—	+	—	++++	++
>10–20 μg/kg/min	+++	++++	+	—	—	—	+++	+++	+++
Epinephrine (Adrenalin)									
(2 mg/250 mL D_5W or NS (C)									
0.01–0.05 μg/kg/min	+	++++	++	—	—	+	+	++++	++
>0.05 μg/kg/min	+++	+++	+	—	—	—	+++	+++	+++
Milrinone (Primacor)									
(50 mg/250 mL D_5W or NS) (P,C)									
LD = 50 μg/kg	—	—	—	—	++	++	—	+++	+++
MD = 0.375–0.75 μg/kg/min									
Norepinephrine (Levophed)									
(4 mg/250 mL D_5W or NS) (C)									
>2–20 μg/min	++++	++	—	—	—	—	++++	+	++
(0.02–1.0 μg/kg/min)									
Isoproterenol (Isuprel)									
(2 mg/250 mL D_5W or NS) (P,C)									
2–10 μg/min	—	++++	+++	—	—	+++	—	++++	++++
Phenylephrine (Neosynephrine)									
(50 mg/250 mL D_5W or NS) (C)									
0.5–5 μg/min	++++	—	—	—	—	—	++++	—	—
Nitroglycerin (Nitrol, Tridil)									
(50 mg/250 mL D_5W or NS) (P,C)									
5–300 μg/min	—	—	—	—	++++	++++ A<V	—	—	+
Nitroprusside (Nipride)									
(50 mg/250 mL D_5W or NS) (P,C)									
0.5–10 μg/kg/min	—	—	—	—	++++	++++ A=V	—	—	+

Key: α, alpha-adrenergic; β_1, beta-one adrenergic; β_2, beta-two adrenergic; Dop, dopaminergic; Sm Msc, smooth muscle; VD, vasodilation; VC, vasoconstriction; INT, inotropic; CHT, chronotropic; AP, arrhythmogenic potential; RBF, renal blood flow; MAP, mean arterial pressure; PCWP, pulmonary capillary wedge pressure; CO, cardiac output; SVR, systemic vascular resistance; UO, urine output; P, peripheral administration; C, central administration; LD, loading dose; MD, maintenance dose; A, arterial; V, venous; +, mild; ++, moderate; +++, high; ++++, maximal; —, no effect; ↑, increase; ↓, decrease; ↑↓, increase or decrease; ↔, no change. (Reprinted with modification from Gonzalez ER and Meyers DG. Assessment and management of cardiogenic shock, in Ornato JC (ed): Clinics in Emergency Medicine: Cardiovascular Emergencies. New York, Churchill Livingstone, 1986, p 125, with permission.)

Reduction of CO occurs simultaneously with loss of blood volume as preload falls. Peripheral vascular resistance (PVR) increases to maintain BP. The increase in PVR will be successful in maintaining BP provided blood losses are less than 15–20% of total circulating volume (Fig. 23.8). Once this amount of blood loss is exceeded, the degree to which vasoconstriction can maintain BP is surpassed, and both CO and BP fall. Hypotension and inadequate Do_2 result. The goal of treatment, therefore, is restoration of circulating volume to increase CO, BP, and tissue perfusion, normalize standard distribution of extracellular water, and achieve acceptable oxygen delivery.[40]

TABLE 23.3. PHARMACOLOGIC PROPERTIES AND CLINICAL EFFECTS OF SELECTED VASOACTIVE DRUGS *(Continued)*

	Hemodynamic Effect						
AP	**RBF**	**MAP**	**PCWP**	**CO**	**SVR**	**UO**	**Adverse Effects/Comments**
++	↑	↔↑↓	↓	↑	↓↓	↑	Thrombocytopenia, nausea flulike syndrome, hypotension, arrhythmias, dilute in saline only
+	↑	↑	↓	↑—	↔↓	↑	Hypotension, tachycardia, headache
++	↑	↔↑↓	↓	↑	↓	↑	
+	↑↑	↔	↔	↔	↔	↑↑	Tachyarrhythmias, painful extravasation, hypertension, decreased peripheral perfusion, angina, headache
++	↑↑	↑	↔↑	↑	↔↓	↑↑	
+++	↑↓	↑	↑	↑	↑	↑↓	
++	↑	↑	↔↓	↑↑	↔↓	↑	Hypertension, arrhythmias, decreased peripheral perfusion, angina, painful extravasation
+++	↑↓	↑↑	↑	↑↑	↑↑	↑↓	
++	↑	↔↑↓	↓	↑	↓↓	↑	Hypotension, possible increased incidence of tachyarrhythmias vs. amrinone, decreased incidence of thrombocytopenia vs. amrinone
++	↑↓	↑↑↑	↑↑	↔↑↓	↑↑↑	↑↓	Arrhythmias, angina, hypertension, decreased peripheral perfusion, painful extravasation
++++	↑	↓↓	↓↓	↑↑	↓↓↓	↑	Hypotension, arrhythmias, tachycardia
—	↑	↑	↑	↔↑↓	↑	↑	Reflex bradycardia, hypertension, painful extravasation
—	↑	↓	↓	↔↑↓	↔↓	↑	Headache, hypotension, reflex tachycardia, nausea
—	↑	↓↓	↓↓	↑	↓↓	↑	Headache, hypotension, nausea, tremor, confusion, reflex tachycardia, cyanide and thiocynate toxicity

PATHOPHYSIOLOGY

Water represents about 45–75% of total body weight. The anatomic water compartment, total body water (TBW), consists of intracellular water (ICW) (2/3 TBW), and extracellular water (ECW) (1/3 TBW). The ECW is further subdivided into the interstitial fluid/lymph (75%) and plasma (25%). Distribution of TBW between ICW and ECW is maintained by the balance of osmotic forces inside and outside the cell. The osmotic solutes governing ICW are potassium (primary), magnesium, protein, and organic phosphorus. The major osmotic solutes of the ECW are sodium and the anions, chloride and bicarbonate, which are relatively impermeable to the cell membrane and move intracellulary with great difficulty. Sodium is the primary ion contributing to the 285 mOsm/L found in the ECW. The following formula is useful in estimating serum osmolarity at the bedside:

$$\text{Serum mOsm} = 2 \times \text{Na (mEq/L)} + \frac{\text{Blood glucose}}{18} + \frac{\text{Blood urea nitrogen}}{2.8} \quad (6)$$

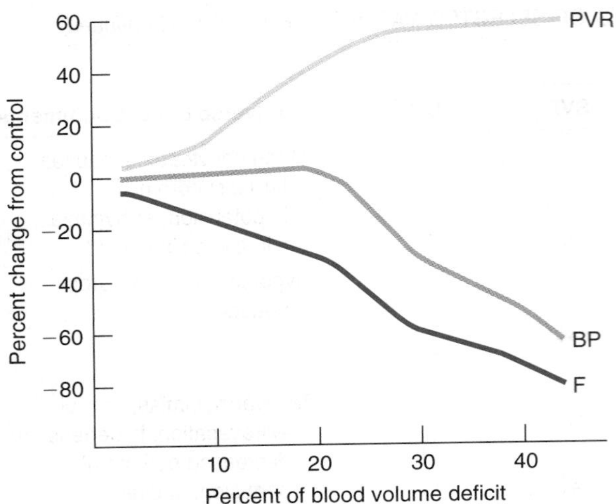

Figure 23.8. Relationship of blood pressure (BP) to cardiac output (F, flow) and peripheral vascular resistance (PVR) as blood volume is depleted. *(From Rackow EC, Falk JL. Colloid and crystalloid fluid resuscitation, in Shoemaker WC, Thompson WL, Holbrook PR [eds]: Textbook of Critical Care. Philadelphia, PA, WB Saunders, 1984, p 736, with permission.)*

The distribution of fluid within the body is best depicted by the following example. An 80-kg male with 48 L of total body water has 16 L of ECW and 32 L of ICW (Fig. 23.9). Of the 16 L in the ECW, 12 L (or 75%) is in the interstitial space and lymph, while 4 L (25%) is in the intravascular space. Addition of 3 L of D_5W shows a net increase of 250 mL of volume to the intravascular space, since this "free water" distributes readily throughout both the ECW and ICW. In comparison, infusion of 3 L of 0.9% sodium chloride or lactated Ringer's (LR) solution contributes 750 mL to the intravascular space since distribution is limited to the ECW, with no intracellular migration, because of the solute component (Na) of the administered solution(s).

Starling's Law of Fluid Movement

The maintenance of proper fluid distribution between the intravascular and extravascular space is necessary for homeostasis. *Starling's law of fluid movement* describes the major forces that maintain adequate plasma volume. Unlike osmolarity, which governs fluid movement into and out of the cells, hydrostatic pressure, protein oncotic pressure, and capillary permeability are key factors in fluid movement between the intravascular and extravascular spaces. These forces are dynamic yet remain controversial because some can only be measured experimentally and with little confidence. The Starling equation governing fluid movement is[41]

$$J_v = K_{F,c}\,[(P_c - P_T) - c\,(c - \pi_T)] \qquad (7)$$

where

J_v = rate of fluid movement into or out of capillary (mL/min/100 g)
$J_v > 0$ = fluid movement out of the capillary
$J_v < 0$ = fluid movement into the capillary
$K_{F,c}$ = capillary filtration coefficient (mL/mm Hg/min/100 g); normal = 0.1
P_c = capillary hydrostatic pressure (mm Hg); normal = 6
P_T = tissue fluid hydrostatic pressure (mm Hg); normal = −7
c = capillary membrane permeability reflection coefficient to proteins; range = 0–1
π_c = plasma oncotic pressure (colloid osmotic pressure) (mm Hg); normal = 26
π_T = tissue fluid oncotic pressure (tissue colloid osmotic pressure) (mm Hg); normal = 14.

Figure 23.10 details the normal values thought to exist on the arterial side of the human lung capillary. As blood flows through the capillary to the venous side, the hydrostatic pressure (P_c) drops from 7 to 4 mm Hg and the rate of fluid movement out of the capillary (J_v) decreases to below zero. Fluid movement shifts and now flow is *into* the capillary from the interstitial space.[42] The capillary filtration coefficient ($K_{F,c}$) is indicative of the capillary membrane's permeability to small solutes and water. Hence, this value depends on the porosity and surface area of the endothelium and varies depending on the organ system or disease state that is present. An increase in $K_{F,c}$ may occur during overexpansion of plasma volume, which could be associated with congestive heart failure.

Capillary hydrostatic pressure (P_c) is the outward driving force of fluid created by the SV of the heart. The P_c is the primary force that "pushes" fluid out of the capillaries. Clinically, the pulmonary P_c is approximated by the PCWP. The P_c values of various organs differ; for example, the lung P_c is 7 mm Hg,[43] skeletal muscle is 15–20 mm Hg,[44] and liver is 5–6 mm Hg.[44]

Plasma colloid osmotic pressure (π_c) is the inward pulling force of fluid exerted across the capillary membrane by the intravascular proteins as blood passes through to the venous side of the capillary. A more familiar term, colloid *oncotic* pressure, is synonymous with colloid *osmotic* pressure. The π_c is the only parameter in the Starling equation that can be measured directly in the clinical setting. All plasma proteins exert an oncotic pressure, and albumin, which represents about 50% of the total mass of serum protein, contributes 65–75% of the π_c.

Although albumin is found throughout the body, only 30–40% is located in the intravascular compartment. The remainder is found in extravascular sites such as the interstitial fluid of the skin, muscle, lungs, and lymph. Albumin moves from the vascular space of the capillaries to the

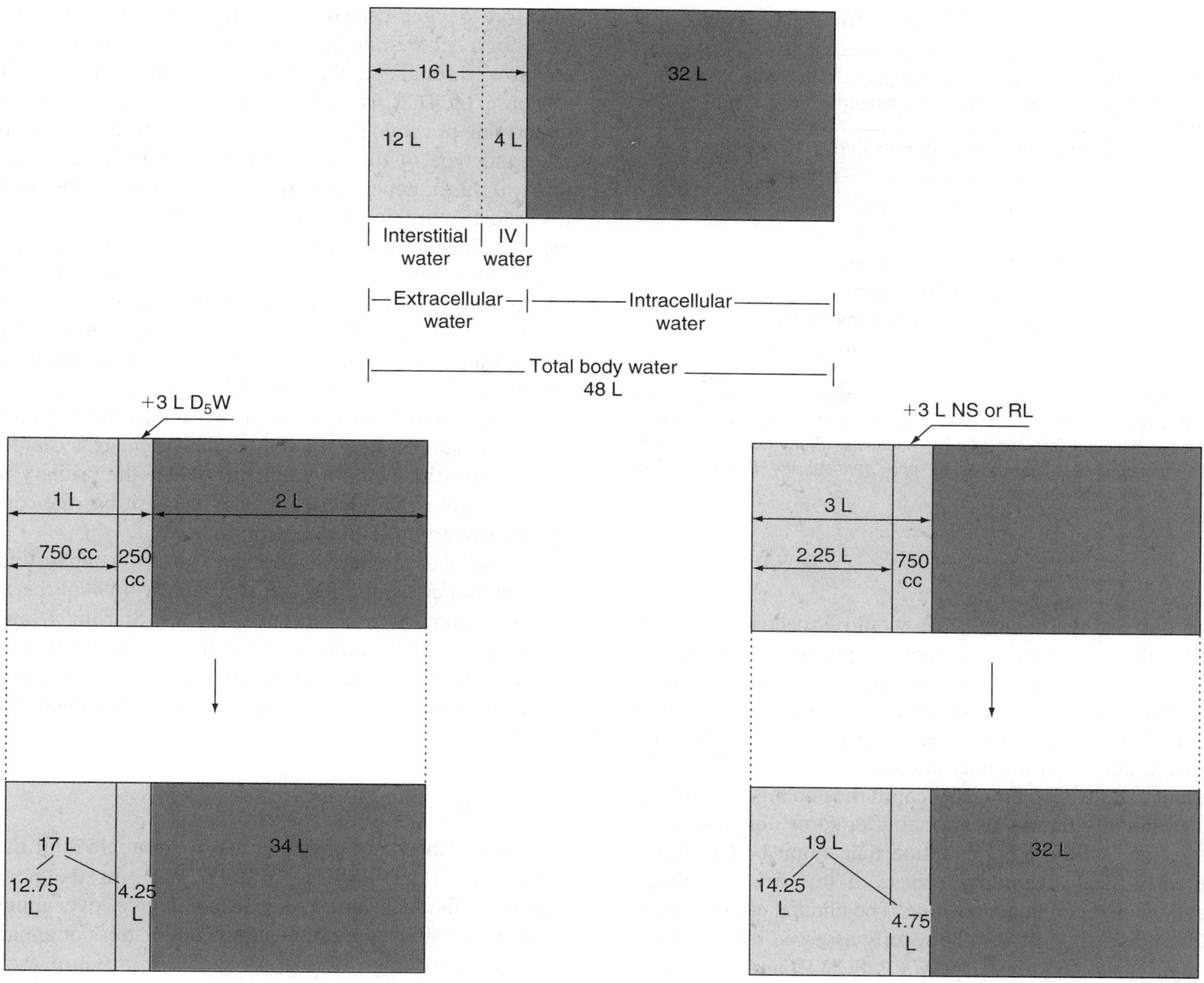

Figure 23.9. Distribution of fluid in an 80-kg man with total body water of 48 L following administration of dextrose in water 5% (D_5W) (left) and 0.9% sodium chloride (NS) or Ringer's lactate (RL) solution (right). IV, intravascular. *(From Rainey TG, English JF. Colloids and crystalloids, in Chernow B [ed]: Essentials of Critical Care Pharmacology (abridged). Baltimore, Williams and Wilkins, 1989, pp 132–133, with permission.)*

lymph and vice versa. The rate of movement may be altered by a change not only in σ (reflection coefficient) but also by variations in PV. Liver function and nutritional status play a vital role in maintaining albumin stores.

The normal π_c is 25–28 mm Hg and declines to 21 mm Hg in the recumbent position. This value is 1–2 mm Hg lower in older patients (>50 years) and 2 mm Hg lower in females.[45] As mentioned previously, oncotic pressure is the only variable that can be measured directly using the following formula where TPP is total plasma protein in g/dL[45]:

$$\pi_c = 2.1\ (\text{TPP}) + 0.16\ (\text{TPP})^2 + 0.009\ (\text{TPP})^3 \qquad (8)$$

Elevated temperature, changes in blood pH, liver disease, or administration of albumin can all affect the actual π_c; therefore, a good correlation between the calculated π_c and the actual π_c will not exist.

The reflection coefficient (σ) is the ability of capillary membranes to prevent plasma proteins and other molecules (>60,000 molecular weight) from crossing into the interstitium. The value of σ ranges from 1 (impermeable) to 0 (completely permeable) and differs among vascular beds. Although absolute values are not known, certain capillaries, such as those in the hepatic microcirculation, have a very low reflection coefficient (0.2), whereas the lung is higher (0.8) and skeletal muscle is essentially impermeable (1.0). The normal π_c–P_c pressure gradient is confounded when conditions such as sepsis increase permeability of the capillary membrane (from 0.8–0.4), allowing more protein to

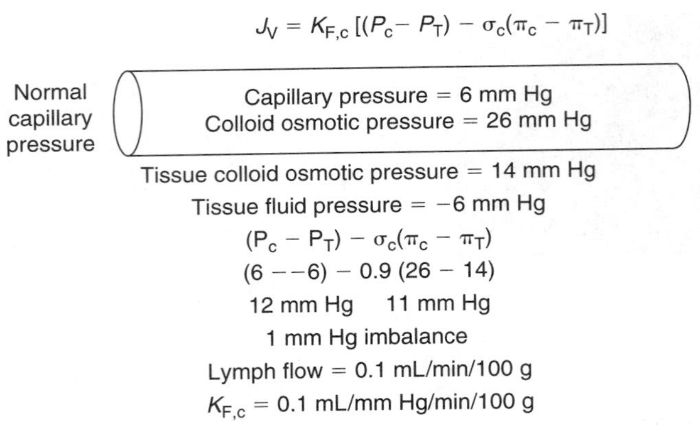

$$J_V = K_{F,c}\,[(P_c - P_T) - \sigma_c(\pi_c - \pi_T)]$$

Normal capillary pressure

Capillary pressure = 6 mm Hg
Colloid osmotic pressure = 26 mm Hg

Tissue colloid osmotic pressure = 14 mm Hg
Tissue fluid pressure = −6 mm Hg

$$(P_c - P_T) - \sigma_c(\pi_c - \pi_T)$$
$$(6 - -6) - 0.9\,(26 - 14)$$

12 mm Hg   11 mm Hg
1 mm Hg imbalance
Lymph flow = 0.1 mL/min/100 g
$K_{F,c}$ = 0.1 mL/mm Hg/min/100 g

Figure 23.10. Currently perceived normal values for the forces that govern fluid exchange across the pulmonary capillary. These approximate values can be substituted into the Starling equation. *(From Gabel JC, Drake RE. Pulmonary capillary pressure and permeability. Crit Care Med 1979;7:92–97, with permission.)*

leak out extravascularly. One would expect an albumin-containing solution to aggravate this phenomenon since the increased permeability of the capillary would facilitate albumin migration from the vasculature into the interstitial space. Consequently, the effective gradient to pull the necessary water out of the lung interstitium would no longer be present. The σ of pulmonary capillaries changes in ARDS, but eventually returns to normal after some unknown time. Therefore, colloid administration that might be harmful in the early "leaky capillary" phase of this disease process may be beneficial at a later time. The clinical effects of colloids and crystalloids can be readily assessed by measuring intravascular pressures (e.g., CVP, PCWP) and other parameters signifying adequate circulation (e.g., BP, HR, UO, CNS function).

The interstitium serves as a reservoir of fluid. It is composed primarily of hyaluronic acid, a mucopolysaccharide that has the ability to sequester fluid or release it into the plasma volume. The normal amount of water sequestered in the interstitium is two to three times the plasma volume and is the source of fluid for the transcapillary refill phenomenon seen after any fluid loss.

Hypovolemic shock, with the resultant reduction in plasma volume, is accompanied by a process called *transcapillary refill* (TCR). TCR is a physiologic process activated by pressure receptors in the atria, following reduction in volume and loss of oncotic pressure. The response to reduced pressure is an increase in ECW osmolarity and movement of protein and water from the interstitium into the capillary to maintain an adequate plasma volume. A drop in circulating hematocrit (Hct) concentration occurs because fluid with a 40% Hct is replaced by interstitial fluid absent of red blood cells (RBCs). The resultant hemodilution has two effects: (1) reduction of Hgb concentration and therefore oxygen-carrying capacity, and (2) the beneficial effect of a decrease in blood viscosity, which promotes better flow through small, vasoconstricted capillaries. The response of TCR is variable depending on the patient's underlying physiologic and hydration status and on amount, rate, and type of fluid loss. The rate of TCR varied from 40–100 mL/h, depending on the speed at which blood was lost and the time when the observations were made postbleed.[46] The TCR replacement rate was the greatest in the first 6 hours after rapid (20 minutes) blood loss. The TCR phenomenon is capable of meeting blood volume deficits of 10–15% (500–750 mL), equivalent to a class I hemorrhage.

Tissue hydrostatic pressure (P_T) of the interstitium is negative (−7 mm Hg) because of lymphatic drainage of the interstitium and fluid movement back into the capillaries. The lymphatic system serves as the drainage system for excess interstitial fluid. Lymphatic flow is the primary protection against pulmonary edema because it has the capacity to increase up to 20 times normal.[47,48]

Finally, tissue fluid oncotic pressure (π_T) approximates the albumin concentration and is normally 40% of the π_c.

In summary, one must realize that Starling's law of fluid movement is complex and still not completely understood. Its use in clinical situations is also hampered by the inability to measure directly the majority of parameters that are involved.

Fluid Loss

A class I hemorrhage involves loss of up to 15% of blood volume (750 mL or less) (Table 23.4). In the normal healthy individual, blood loss of this degree, over minutes to hours, is tolerated without significant distress or apparent physiologic damage. Complete recovery of intravascular volume, plasma proteins, and clotting factors takes only a few hours. Red cell replacement, however, takes several weeks. The TCR response depends in part on the previous hydration state, cardiovascular function, and general health status of the individual; older, sicker, dehydrated patients have difficulty compensating for even such mild losses.

Class II, III, and IV hemorrhages result in worsening clinical status, with volume of blood loss related to survival[49] (Table 23.4). Patients with class IV blood loss present in profound shock with the pulse only palpable in the carotid artery. This degree of intravascular volume depletion can quickly result in loss of arterial pressure and consciousness, pulselessness, and cardiovascular arrest. Cardiac arrest from exsanguination manifests as pulseless electrical activity (formerly known as electromechanical dissociation), which then progresses to asystole.

Not all intravascular fluid losses are due to bleeding outside the body. Blood or plasma can "third space" into various areas such as the chest, retroperitoneal areas, buttocks, shoulder girdle, or pelvis. Up to 6 L of extravascular volume may be sequestered in the abdomen with only a

TABLE 23.4. HYPOVOLEMIC CLASSES

Blood Loss	Blood Pressure	Vascular Response	Temperature	Color	Circulation (Blanching)	Endocrine Response	Metabolic Response	Signs and Symptoms
Class I (<15%) (750 mL)	Normal to 20%, ↓ BP	Contraction of great veins, ECF shift intravascularly	Cool	Pale	Normal, slight slowing	Slight	Slight	Mild thirst UO > 30 mL/h
Class II (20–25%) (1000–1250 mL)	↓ SBP, ↑ DBP, narrow pulse pressure	All of the above, mild tachycardia (>100 beats/min), ↓ CO, ↓ blood flow to all organs, shunting of blood flow to heart and brain	Cool	Pale	Definite slowing	↑ aldosterone, ADH, growth hormone and interleukin-1-β; some ↑ cortisol, catecholamines, clotting factors, no ↑ in insulin	↑ glycolysis, mild ↑ glucose, ↑ lipolysis/FFA, small ↑ lactate, respiratory alkalosis, ↑ O_2 consumption, ↓ U_{Na}	Thirst, orthostasis, hyperventilation, apprehension, weakness UO = 20–30 mL/h
Class III (30–35%) (1500–1750 mL)	Frank hypotension, ↓ BP 20–40%	As above, tachycardia (>120 beats/min), ↓↓ CO, ↓↓ blood flow to organs	Cold	Pale	Definite slowing	As above	As above	As above, confusion UO = 5–15 mL/h
Class IV (40–45%) (2000–2500 mL)	Very narrow pulse pressure, ↓↓ BP or nonrecordable	As above, CO < 50% tachycardia (>140 beats/min), increased shunting to heart and brain; bradycardia, asystole or ventricular fibrillation	Cold	Ashen, cyanotic (mottling)	Definite slowing	As above, marked ↑ in catecholamines	As above, ↑↑ lactic acidosis, mVo_2 20 mm Hg or less	As above, lethargic, comatose, anuria

Key: ↑, increase; ↓, decrease; BP, blood pressure; SBP, systolic blood pressure; DBP, diastolic blood pressure; ADH, antidiuretic hormone; FFA, free fatty acids; U_{Na}, urine sodium concentration; mVo_2, mixed venous oxygen; UO, urine output. (Compiled from Packman MI, Rackow EC. Optimum left heart filling pressure during fluid resuscitation of patients with hypovolemic and septic shock. Crit Care Med 1983;11:165–169; and Advanced Trauma Life Support Student Manual, American College of Surgeons Committee on Trauma, 1993, p 86, with permission.)

2-cm change in apparent length and radius. During peritonitis, fluid may accumulate in the abdomen for 24–48 hours and then return to the vascular space. This latter remobilization can increase urine output and lead the unsuspecting clinician to increase intravenous fluid administration to replace urine volume, thereby creating a vicious cycle.

The loss of hypotonic fluid from the body is different from that observed with hemorrhage. Hypotonic fluid loss involves not only the blood volume but also the ECW and ICW. A 4-L hypotonic loss, resulting from either diarrhea or osmotic diuresis, typically contains approximately 77 mEq of sodium per liter. This 4-L loss could be evaluated as 2 L of pure water from the TBW and 2 L of isotonic saline from ECW. The 2 L of isotonic saline loss reduces the PV by approximately 500 mL (PV = 0.25 × ECW 2 L), with another 160 mL decrease (PV = 0.08 × TBW 2 L) because of the 2-L pure water loss, for a total of 660 mL. A patient with a 4-L hypotonic loss would therefore be expected to present with hemodynamic effects similar to that of a class I hemorrhage.

TREATMENT

The primary goal of therapy is to restore circulating volume and assure adequate tissue perfusion, BP, CO, and Do_2. Initial fluid resuscitation consists of isotonic crystalloid (0.9% sodium chloride or lactated Ringer's solution), colloid (5% plasmanate or albumin, 6% hetastarch), or whole blood (Table 23.5).[40,50] Choice of solution is based on the patient's current oxygen-carrying capacity (e.g., hemoglobin, hematocrit), cause of the hypovolemic shock, accompanying disease states, degree of fluid loss (class I–IV), and speed of fluid delivery required. (A detailed discussion of colloid versus crystalloid fluid resuscitation is given in the next section.)

In most instances, crystalloid is administered at a rate of 500–2000 mL/h, depending on the severity of the deficit, degree of ongoing fluid loss, and tolerance to the volume infused. Usually 2–4 L of crystalloid should normalize intravascular volume. A "3 to 1" rule is employed by many clinicians, which translates to 300 mL of crystalloid administration for every 100 mL of blood loss. Patients may require blood products as part of the initial fluid resuscitation to assure maintenance of oxygen-carrying capacity, as well as clotting factors and platelets for blood hemostasis. If blood products are employed, the patient must be monitored for possible complications (Table 23.6).

Patients with class I or class II blood loss can usually be managed by crystalloid alone. Patients with class III or class IV blood loss require a combination of crystalloid and colloid because of the significant volume of fluid lost (>1500 mL), and hence oxygen-carrying capacity (Table 23.4).

As fluid resuscitation is under way, one must follow trends in HR and BP as well as cardiac filling pressures (CVP, PCWP) and CO, if available, to assess how intravascular volume expansion is affecting myocardial function. It is best to follow a trend rather than "shoot for" a specific CVP or PCWP number, because there is considerable variability in response depending on the status of the patient's vasculature and myocardium. Patients with a history of congestive heart failure or myocardial infarction and those in septic shock will have an atypical response to volume loading. The major side effect of excessive fluid resuscitation is intravascular volume overload characterized by high filling pressures (CVP > 12–15 mm Hg, PCWP > 20–24 mm Hg), and decreased CO (<3.5 L/min). Volume overload can degenerate to cardiogenic shock with emergence of pulmonary edema, the latter of which can be monitored by auscultation of the lungs with a stethoscope. If volume overload occurs, furosemide 20–40 mg slow intravenous push is effective in not only "unloading" the heart through venous dilation within minutes of injection, but also by diuresis of intravascular volume.[51]

Crystalloids

Crystalloids consist of electrolyte (e.g., Na^+, Cl^-, K^+) in water solutions, with or without dextrose (Table 23.5). The primary crystalloids used in fluid resuscitation include 0.9% sodium chloride (normal saline, NS), lactated Ringer's (LR), and rarely, hypertonic saline solutions (3% sodium chloride, or "hot salt"). Both NS and LR are essentially isotonic so distribution is limited to the ECW (Fig. 23.9). There is little clinical evidence to support the superiority of LR over NS in fluid resuscitation of patients.[52]

The advantages of crystalloids include the rapidity and ease of administration. Isotonic or hypotonic solutions can be administered peripherally, whereas hypertonic solutions should be infused through a central line. Because the isotonic solutions distribute fairly rapidly out of the intravascular space (1 liter of administered fluid results in about 250 mL of contribution to circulating volume), they may be safer to administer to patients who may not tolerate fluid challenges well (e.g., myocardial dysfunction). In addition, the degree of oncotic pull from outside the capillary is negligible because plasma colloid osmolarity remains unchanged. Therefore, use of these solutions is considered appropriate in patients with "leaky capillary syndrome." The solutions are compatible with most drugs, do not induce serum sickness, and are very inexpensive.

A disadvantage of crystalloids is the large volume necessary to replace or augment intravascular volume. Approximately 4 L of NS must be infused to replace 1 L of blood loss. In addition, dilution of colloid oncotic pressure leading to pulmonary edema can ensue following crystalloid resuscitation in comparison to colloid.[53,54] Lastly, administration of large volumes of NS is needed to reach hemodynamic end points seen with smaller volumes of colloids.

TABLE 23.5. CRYSTALLOID AND COLLOID PREPARATIONS

	0.9% NaCl (NS)	Lactated Ringer's	Plasma Protein Fraction 5%	Albumin 5%	Albumin 25%	Hetastarch 6% in NS
Sodium (mEq/L)	154	130	130–160	130–160	130–160	154
Chloride (mEq/L)	154	109	130–160	130–160	130–160	154
Other	—	Lactate 28 mEq/L, potassium 4 mEq/L, calcium 3 mEq/L	—	—	—	Hydroxyethyl starch average MW 450,000
Osmolality (mOsm)	308	273	290	300	1500	310
Albumin	—	—	≈44 g/L	≈50 g/L	≈250 g/L	—
Globulin	—	—	≈6 g/L	—	—	—
Colloid oncotic pressure (mm Hg)	—	—	20	20	100	30
Plasma volume expansion (per amount infused)	250 mL (per 1000 mL)	250 mL (per 1000 mL)	250–500 mL (per 250 mL)	250–500 mL (per 250 mL)	250 mL (per 50 mL)	500–750 mL (per 500 mL)
Distribution	ECW[a]	ECW[a]	Intravascular[b]	Intravascular[b]	Intravascular[b]	Intravascular[b]
Half-life of effect	Minutes	Minutes	5–6 hours	5–6 hours	5–6 hours	6–8 hours
Metabolism	—	Liver (lactate to bicarbonate)	Liver (amino acids)	Liver (amino acids)	Liver (amino acids)	40% urine unchanged, enzymatic degradation to smaller particles and glucose
Anaphylactoid reactions	—	—	0.019%[c]	0.019%	0.019%	0.085%
Life-threatening reactions	—	—	0.003%[c]	0.003%	0.003%	0.006%
Precautions	—	—	Dilutional effect on coagulation factors Relatively contraindicated during coagulopathy			Dilutional effect on coagulation factors, lowers factor VIII, do not exceed 1500 mL per 24 hours, do not administer to patients with history of coagulation or bleeding problems

[a] Will distribute into ICW if intracellular osmolarity > normal from dehydration.
[b] Will distribute into interstitial space if presence of "leaky capillary syndrome" associated with septic shock.
[c] Incidence slightly higher than 5% and 25% albumin due to presence of globulins. (Compiled from Ross AD, Angaran DM. Colloids vs. crystalloids: A continuing controversy. Drug Intell Clin Pharm 1984;18,108; and Gould SA, Sehgal LR, Sehgal HL, Moss GS. Hypovolemic shock. Crit Care Clin 1993;9:240, with permission.)

TABLE 23.6. BLOOD AND BLOOD PRODUCTS

Blood Product	Usual Package	Content	Complications
Whole blood	Unit	450 mL of blood; plasma (some clotting factors) RBCs, WBCs, platelets	Hepatitis, fever, chills, hemolytic/allergic reactions, hyperkalemia, hypocalcemia, intravascular overload, rare hemolytic reactions, CMV, HIV
Packed red blood cells (PRBCs)	Unit	220–300 mL of RBCs, includes WBCs and platelets	Same as with whole blood, except decreased risk, of intravascular overload
Platelets	Unit	5.5–10 × 10^{10} platelets in 30–50 mL plasma	Hepatitis, fever, chills, allergic reactions, development of antiplatelet antibodies, graft-versus-host disease, HIV
Fresh frozen plasma (FFP)	Unit	200–250 mL plasma; 200 units of all coagulation factors, 400 mg of fibrinogen, complement	Hepatitis, fever, chills, allergic reactions, HIV
Cryoprecipitate	Unit	80–120 units of factor VIII, 250 mg of fibrinogen 15–25 mL of plasma	Hepatitis, fever, chills, allergic reactions, hemolysis from anti-A or anti-B, HIV

(Compiled from Bojar RM. Manual of Perioperative Care in Cardiac and Thoracic Surgery, 2nd ed. Boston, Blackwell Scientific Publications, 1994, pp 93–97; and Kirby RR, Taylor RW, Civetta JM (eds). Handbook of Critical Care. Philadelphia, JB Lippincott, 1994, p 32, with permission.)

The hypertonicity of solutions with greater than 0.9% sodium chloride results in a greater degree of fluid retention in the vascular tree. In addition, free water will be pulled across the capillary membranes, thereby increasing the net intravascular volume expansion. Patients receiving hypertonic solutions usually require significantly less fluid than those receiving isotonic crystalloid.[55,56] Although a number of preliminary studies show these solutions to be beneficial with less risk of edema, precipitation of hypernatremia and metabolic hyperchloremic acidosis have been reported.[55] The role of the hypertonic solutions in hypovolemic shock remains unknown at this time.

Colloids

The colloids consist of natural protein solutions (e.g., albumin, plasmanate), synthetic complex sugars (e.g., dextran, hetastarch), and blood products; all exert oncotic pressure within the vascular tree. The ideal properties of a colloid are listed in Table 23.7. Unfortunately, no colloid with all of these properties is currently available. Blood products are discussed separately in the following section.

TABLE 23.7. IDEAL PROPERTIES OF A COLLOID

1. Osmotic pressure similar to plasma
2. Oxygen carrying and distribution properties
3. Reasonable duration of action
4. More than single route of metabolism and elimination
5. Lack of antigenicity, allergenicity, and pyretic properties
6. Easily manufactured and sterilized
7. Pharmacologically inert
8. Inexpensive

The natural protein solutions include albumin 5%, albumin 25%, and plasmanate 5%, all of which are effective in augmenting intravascular volume (Table 23.5). Early preparations of albumin contained high concentrations of sodium (300 mEq/L); however, reformulation following the Korean War has lead to the current product (130–160 mEq/L of sodium chloride), which was often referred to as "salt-poor" albumin prior to February 1978. Since then, the designation of "salt poor" has become obsolete.

Plasmanate is a combination of approximately 88% albumin and 12% globulins. It is thought that the globulins are responsible for a higher incidence of serum sickness (manifest as hypotension, fever) compared to pure albumin preparations. Plasmanate contains a similar amount of sodium chloride per volume.

Although dextran was the original synthetic plasma expander, its use today is limited, due to its relatively small molecular size and modest effects on oncotic pressure. Hetastarch (Hespan–DuPont Critical Care), a complex sugar (starch) with properties very similar to those of the protein colloids, has essentially replaced the use of dextran as a synthetic plasma volume expander. It has proven effects in terms of the resuscitation of patients with hypovolemia and shock.[57,58] The effects of hetastarch on the blood coagulation system have been of concern to many clinicians. When hydroxyethyl starch is infused in massive amounts to dogs (>25% of blood volume), overt bleeding is observed readily, with laboratory abnormalities in all aspects of hemostasis. Investigation in humans or animals after moderate replacement (hydroxyethyl starch volume <20 mL/kg/d or 1500 mL/d total volume) results in prolonged partial thromboplastin time (PTT) and prothrombin time (PT), which parallel those observed with albumin administration.[59] However, reduction in factor VIII levels have been reported following hetastarch administration.[60] Patients with a history of coagulation disorder or those with an ongoing coagulopathy should probably not receive hetastarch based on its reported effects on coagulation.

Albumin, plasmanate, and hetastarch must be administered through a large-bore central line because of the viscosity of the solutions. Plasma expansion following administration results in at a least a milliliter-for-milliliter increase in intravascular volume. The extent and duration of volume expansion achieved are a function of the dose, rate, volume status of the patient, baseline plasma oncotic pressure, cardiovascular function, renal function, and degree of capillary integrity (reflection coefficient). It is not uncommon to observe a "relative" 400- to 500-mL increase in intravascular volume following 250 mL of albumin 5% or hetastarch. Four-to-one volume expansion following administration of 25% albumin has been observed due to the strong oncotic forces as fluid is pulled into the vasculature across the capillary membranes. Both hetastarch and albumin are considered equivalent therapy for treatment of hypovolemic shock.[40,50,53,54] In fact, incidence of pulmonary edema has been shown to be lower in colloid-treated patients versus crystalloid provided capillary integrity is not violated.[54]

Advantages of the colloids include a long dwell time in the vasculature that ranges from several hours to days. Much less volume is required compared with the crystalloids because colloids stay in the intravascular space and draw in interstitial fluid as discussed previously. Hypovolemic patients with third-spaced fluid following surgery may benefit significantly from colloid administration, because small amounts of colloid (250–750 mL) will augment intravascular volume and aid in shifting fluid back into the vascular tree from the interstitium and "third-space" areas, for added volume support.

Disadvantages mirror the advantages, because long dwell times and large increases in intravascular volume can be detrimental to some patients with borderline hemodynamic status. Fluid overload is a more serious complication when compared with crystalloids, because diuretic administration will not affect circulating colloids. However, free intravascular water that may have shifted from the interstitium will be eliminated. Extreme care must be taken in the cardiovascular-compromised patient because colloids may precipitate congestive heart failure (CHF). Patients with "capillary leak" phenomenon may be at higher risk of developing pulmonary edema. Colloids leaking out of the vascular tree and into the interstitium exert oncotic pressure. Increased interstitial oncotic pressure causes increased interstitial fluid and pulmonary death. Finally, these agents are very expensive compared with crystalloids, and budget constraints may govern some of their use.

Crystalloids Versus Colloids

A meta-analysis to assess patient mortality following either crystalloid or colloid fluid administration for circulatory resuscitation has been performed.[61] The pooled data indicated a 5.7% lower mortality in those patients receiving crystalloid; however, the 95% confidence level was ±15.1%. Trauma patients (those patients in which capillary integrity may be altered) had a lower mortality with crystalloid (12.3%, 95% confidence of ±16.9%). However, in patients without trauma (those patients with expected intact capillary integrity or minor capillary leak), the difference in mortality shifted to those receiving colloids (7.8% lower, 95% confidence of ±11.2%). These data may support the theory that colloids may be less effective, and possibly detrimental by causing pulmonary edema when administered to patients with increased capillary permeability (i.e., leaky capillary syndrome).

In general, most clinicians agree that crystalloid administration (e.g., NS, LR) should be the initial therapy for intravascular volume replacement. The ease of administration, cost, and safety support this regimen. If volume resuscitation is suboptimal following several liters of crystalloid administration, colloids should be considered. Careful attention should be focused on the dilutional effects that these solutions may have on both Hgb and clotting factors in order to prevent further complications. The need for blood must be continually assessed during the resuscitative effort.

Blood Products

Blood is a colloid and the only carrier of oxygen in the circulation. Delivery of oxygen is based on CO and Cao_2 as described previously in this chapter. Although there is considerable debate with respect to blood transfusion, most clinicians will transfuse when the hematocrit is ≤20% (e.g., Hgb ≈ 7 g/dL) in stable patients.[40] Patients in shock should be more aggressively transfused, maintaining Hgb at a minimum of 10 g/dL since Hgb concentration plays a central role in Do_2. Blood should be fully cross-matched for ABO and Rh antigens to avoid serious reactions. If blood is required immediately, type O Rh-negative blood can be used.

Banked whole blood is often used; however, it lacks the labile clotting factors (V, VIII, IX) and platelets (Table 23.6). Fresh whole blood (<6 hours old) has intact clotting factors and platelets; however, it is obviously not as available as banked whole blood. The risk of hepatitis with blood administration is about 5%. In addition, transmission of cytomegalovirus (CMV) and human immunodeficiency virus (HIV) must be considered. An estimate by the American Association of Blood Banks in 1989 reported a 1 : 40,000 to 1 : 200,000 risk of incurring HIV via blood transfusion, but noted that the risk is very dependent on prevalence of HIV in the donor area.[62]

Hemolytic transfusion reactions are divided into two types, acute and delayed. The acute reaction is almost always associated with a clinical error resulting from mismatching of blood. Signs and symptoms vary from fever, chills, and flushing to dyspnea, chest pain, hypotension, shock, and generalized bleeding. Therapy consists of stopping the transfusion, hydrating the patient with crystalloid to treat hypotension and maintain urine output at >100 mL/h to prevent renal failure from hemoglobinuria. Should fluid therapy be insufficient to prevent or reverse hypotension, a vasopressor (dopamine, phenylephrine, norepinephrine) can be used. Some clinicians recommend loop diuretics or mannitol (25 g) to maintain renal blood flow and urine output.

The delayed hemolytic reaction occurs most often in patients who have been previously transfused or who are pregnant and have antibodies to antigens not screened in the ABO system. The signs and symptoms of the delayed reaction may be subtle or as apparent as in the acute reaction. These reactions occur 7–10 days after the transfusion and are rarely dangerous.

Transfusion of blood stored in either acid citrate dextrose (ACD) or citrate phosphate dextrose (CPD) is accompanied by a reduced P_{50} (affinity of hemoglobin for oxygen). The delivery of oxygen to the cells and its subsequent release from RBCs to tissue constitute a complex topic that involves RBC oxygen pressure, 2-diphosphoglycerate concentration, temperature, and pH. In addition, CPD sequesters calcium ion resulting in hypocalcemia, which may manifest as coagulation disorders, dysrhythmias, seizures, hyperactive reflexes, and tetany. The transfusion of one or two units of blood does not significantly alter calcium ion; however, further administration of blood products should be accompanied by administration of 4 mEq calcium per unit blood given. Hyperkalemia may be observed following blood administration due to RBC lysis that has occurred in the stored blood and does not usually require therapy. Metabolic alkalosis is the most common acid–base disturbance following blood administration as the citrate is metabolized to bicarbonate. Citrate toxicity is rare and administration of up to one unit every 5 minutes in adults is safe. Urticarial reactions are limited to the skin (hives, itching, erythema) and are not accompanied by fever. The transfusion may be continued and H_1 antihistamines (diphenhydramine) administered intravenously.

Coagulation problems are primarily associated with low levels of clotting factors in stored blood as well as dilution of endogenous clotting factors and platelets following administration of the blood. As a result, a coagulation panel (PT, INR, aPTT) should be checked in patients undergoing replacement of 50–100% or more of blood volume in 12–24 hours.

Blood is usually administered through a 170-μm filter to remove microaggregates. Blood administration is compatible with NS but incompatible with dextrose and LR solutions; coadministration of the latter in an IV line may cause clumping or hemolysis. Administration times are usually 1 unit over 1 hour; however, blood may be infused as rapidly as possible during an acute event. Administration times greater than 4 hours are not recommended because of bacterial proliferation and temperature-induced hemolysis. Usually, 1 unit of blood will raise the hemoglobin concentration by approximately 1 g/dL, provided there is no ongoing blood loss. Since blood is stored in the refrigerator, massive transfusions can also contribute to the hypothermia observed with hypovolemic shock.

Postoperative cardiothoracic surgery patients may receive their own blood collected from chest tubes. This autotransfused blood contains clotting factors and platelets, and obviously carries the least risk of viral inoculation of all the blood products available.

Packed red blood cells (PRBCs) consist of centrifuged cells minus plasma. This product is used in fluid-restricted patients, such as those with cardiovascular disease or renal failure or patients who have already undergone volume expansion. No clotting factors are present with PRBCs.

Platelets and fresh-frozen plasma (FFP) serve as the cornerstones of hemorrhage management. Typically, a unit of platelets will increase the platelet count by about 7000–10,000 mm^3. Since FFP contains clotting factors and fibrinogen, it is first-line therapy along with platelet administration in severe bleeding. Finally, for those patients with severe coagulopathy, cryoprecipitate provides the best source of factors I, VIII, and XIII as well as fibrinogen. Cryoprecipitate is prepared by centrifuging FFP and pooling the precipitated clotting factors with those of 9 or 10 other samples to provide a very concentrated solution. The pooling of samples significantly raises the risk of hepatitis over that of blood.

EVALUATION OF THERAPEUTIC OUTCOMES

Successful management of hypovolemic shock necessitates prompt identification, correct interpretation of the hypovolemia (absolute or relative) and appropriate management, especially in the setting of ongoing blood loss. Constant assessment of oxygen-carrying capacity, the need for blood, and clotting factors must be made. Patients who are not in the immediate postoperative stage should be resuscitated with crystalloid (0.9% NaCl or LR) to raise BP (SBP > 90–100 mm Hg, MAP > 60 mm Hg), decrease tachycardia (HR < 100 beats/min), and restore peripheral circulation (peripheral pulses, capillary refill, etc). Patients with a relative hypovolemia (secondary to peripheral vasodilation) usually require both fluids and vasopressors (dopamine, norepinephrine, etc.) to achieve desired outcomes as stated previously. Finally, postoperative patients are usually managed with colloids (blood, albumin 5%, hydroxyethylstarch). Care must be exercised so that endpoints are not "overshot" because pulmonary edema may occur.

CARDIOGENIC SHOCK

PATHOPHYSIOLOGY

Cardiogenic shock occurs as a result of direct insult to the heart muscle (acute myocardial infarction [AMI]) or other mechanical problem of the heart (valvular dysfunction) (Table 23.8), restriction of muscle function (tamponade, pericardotomy syndrome), or exacerbation of congestive heart failure due to drug or nondrug factors (Table 23.9). Hypoperfusion (cool extremities), impaired mental function, depressed myocardial function, pulmonary congestion, and oliguria are consistent with the findings of an arterial systolic blood pressure under 90 mm Hg, cardiac index less than 1.8 L/min/m^2, PCWP greater than 18–20 mm Hg, elevated SVR (>1300 dynes-s/cm^5), and urine output <20 mL/h.[63]

Electrocardiographic (ECG) monitoring, prompt recognition, and treatment of electrical complications have reduced the in-hospital mortality from AMI. Unfortunately, a similarly favorable trend has not been observed with AMI-associated pump failure despite advances in hemodynamic monitoring and newer strategies and methods of inotropic support. Failure to reperfuse the coronary arteries early in AMI with either thrombolytics, angioplasty, or surgical revascularization results in an incidence of cardiogenic shock equal to 7.5% of patients.[64] Mortality ranges from 70–95%.[64] Of the 10–30% of patients who survive, 40% die within the next 5 years, with prognosis related to the amount of functioning myocardium post-AMI. Mortality is also linked to the hemodynamic subset of the Forrester classification (Table 23.10).[65,66]

TABLE 23.8. ETIOLOGY OF CARDIOGENIC SHOCK

Acute Myocardial Infarction
Severely reduced left ventricular function
Ventricular septal rupture
Acute mitral regurgitation
Right ventricular infarction
Other Cardiac Entities
Dilated cardiomyopathy/severe myocarditis
End-stage valvular disease (aortic/mitral stenosis, aortic/mitral regurgitation)
Tachy- or bradyarrhythmias
Post cardiopulmonary bypass
Cardiac Obstruction or Compression
Pericardial tamponade or constriction
Pulmonary embolism
Severe pulmonary hypertension
Coarctation of the aorta
Myxoma
Severe hypertrophic cardiomyopathy
Tension pneumothorax

(Modified from Alpert JS, Becker RC. Mechanisms and management of cardiogenic shock. Crit Care Clin 1993;9:205–218.)

TABLE 23.9. MAJOR CAUSES OF LEFT VENTRICULAR FAILURE

Loss of Muscle
Acute myocardial infarction
Chronic coronary artery disease
Primary Muscle Disease (Cardiomyopathy)
Infection (viral)
Exposure to toxin (alcoholic)
Metabolic or other factors (idiopathic)
Mechanical Problems
Hypertension
Valvular stenosis and regurgitation
Rheumatic fever
Congenital heart disease
Pulmonary hypertension
Factors That Exacerbate CHF
Fever
Hot weather
Anemia
Atrioventricular fistula
Hyperthyroidism
Pulmonary embolism
Infection (pneumonia, bacteremia, endocarditis)
Arrhythmias
Salt and water retention
Pregnancy
Ventricular aneurysm
Drug-Induced CHF
Antiarrhythmics (quinidine, procainamide)—decrease contractility
Beta blockers—decrease contractility
Calcium-channel blockers (verapamil, diltiazem)—decrease contractility
Daunomycin—dose-dependent direct cardiotoxin
Diazoxide—sodium and water retention
Doxorubicin—dose-dependent direct cardiotoxin
Estrogens—sodium and water retention
Guanethidine—sodium and water retention
Licorice—sodium and water retention
Lithium carbonate—sodium and water retention
Methyldopa—sodium and water retention
Nonsteroidal anti-inflammatory agents—sodium and water retention
Salicylates (high doses)—sodium and water retention
Sodium content of drugs—sodium and water retention
Steroids—sodium and water retention
Tricyclic antidepressants—decrease contractility
Volume expanders (albumin, mannitol)—expand intravascular volume

(Reprinted from Donat WE, Weiner BH. Syndromes of left ventricular failure, in Rippe JM, Irwin RS, Alpert JS, Dalen JE (eds): Intensive Care Medicine. Boston, Little, Brown and Co, 1985, with permission.)

In the setting of AMI, about 35–40% of left ventricular mass must be damaged or destroyed before cardiogenic shock develops. Patients with AMI without history of congestive heart failure (CHF) who are predisposed to developing cardiogenic shock include elderly females, patients

TABLE 23.10. HEMODYNAMIC CLASSIFICATION AND RELATIONSHIP TO CLINICAL PRESENTATION AND PERCENT MORTALITY

	Subset I	**Subset II**
CI >2.2 L/min/m²	Normal hemodynamics Mortality ≈ 3%	Pulmonary congestion Rales present Mortality ≈ 9%
	Subset III	**Subset IV**
CI <2.2 L/min/m²	Peripheral hypoperfusion Rales absent Mortality ≈ 23% PCWP <18 mm Hg	Pulmonary congestion Rales present Peripheral hypoperfusion Mortality ≈ 51% PCWP > 18 mm Hg

Key: CI, cardiac index; PCWP, pulmonary capillary wedge pressure. (Compiled from Forrester JS, Waters DD. Hospital treatment of congestive heart failure: Management according to hemodynamic profile. Am J Med 1978;65:173).

with a history of vascular disease/complications (myocardial ischemia, peripheral vascular disease, stroke), hyperglycemia on admission, and patients that have greater than a fourfold increase over normal of lactic acid dehydrogenase (LDH).[67] Likewise, patients with underlying CHF are more susceptible to developing cardiogenic shock post-AMI since the myocardial contractility is already compromised to some degree. Rare complications of AMI include pericarditis; rupture of the myocardial wall, septum, or papillary muscle; or formation of a left ventricular aneurysm with mural thrombus and systemic embolization.

Patients with mitral valve disease often present with symptoms of CHF (dyspnea, orthopnea, fatigue, decreased exercise tolerance). Those with aortic valve disease present with symptoms of myocardial ischemia, in addition to CHF. The myocardial ischemia develops because of poor coronary filling during diastole, secondary to the incompetent aortic valve or inadequate forward flow as a result of aortic stenosis.

Drug-induced myocardial decompensation usually develops in patients with preexisting myocardial dysfunction. The negative inotropic effects of β-adrenergic blockers, selected calcium channel blockers, type I antiarrhythmics, tricyclic antidepressants, and certain antihypertensives have all been implicated. The antimetabolite drugs, such as daunomycin, are direct cardiotoxins (Table 23.9).

Overhydration with crystalloid or plasma volume expanders (e.g., hydroxyethyl starch, albumin, plasmanate) may also cause myocardial decompensation.

TREATMENT

The primary management of cardiogenic shock involves careful patient monitoring, insightful interpretation of both subjective and objective clinical data, and the logical selection of drug therapy, either individually or in combination.[63] Insertion of the Swan–Ganz catheter not only provides an initial cardiovascular assessment, but serves to guide therapy. Treatment centers on restoring pump function (CO) through manipulation of the inotropic state of the myocardium, systemic vascular tone, and cardiac filling pressures (CVP, PCWP). The intra-aortic balloon pump (IABP), the ventricular assist device (VAD), and extracorporeal membrane oxygenation (ECMO) provide options for patient management. In very severe instances, the aforementioned interventions may serve as a therapeutic bridge until the patient is able to undergo heart transplantation.

Acute Myocardial Infarction

Isolated Left Ventricular Failure/Biventricular Failure

The specific goals of medical management of cardiogenic shock associated with left ventricular infarction include (1) optimization of left ventricular filling pressure to maximize the Frank–Starling relationship, (2) afterload reduction to minimize the impedance to left ventricular outflow, and (3) maximization of myocardial contractility without excessive increases in myocardial oxygen demand. Therapeutic agent selection (Table 23.3) is based on the Forrester subset classification present (Table 23.10).[65,66]

Patients in subset I of the Forrester classification have a low incidence of mortality, optimum filling cardiac filling pressures and CI, and do not require treatment.

Treatment of subset II patients is directed at reducing PCWP by administering loop diuretics, such as furosemide (Lasix) 20–40 mg slow IV push. Two important effects result from furosemide administration: an immediate increase in venous capacitance, redistributing blood away from the lungs and decreasing pulmonary capillary pressures followed by diuresis, which eliminates some of the intravascular volume.[51] The combination of effects lowers pulmonary and ventricular filling pressures. Loop diuretics also produce renal vasodilation, which may increase their natriuretic effect.

Overzealous diuresis should be avoided because excessive reductions in left ventricular filling pressure may worsen cardiac output and further activate compensatory neurohumoral systems. To minimize the risk of suboptimal cardiac filling pressures as well as diuretic-induced electrolyte abnormalities, the smallest effective dose of the diuretic should be employed. The patient's hemodynamic parameters and urine output will guide subsequent diuretic administration. If diuretics are ineffective, intravenous nitroglycerin (titrated from 10–20 μg/min) should provide added preload reduction.

The finding of isolated peripheral hypoperfusion (subset III) is of major prognostic importance because of the high mortality associated with it. These patients present with hypovolemia and/or bradycardia. The goal of therapy is to improve the CI and to reverse the hypoperfusion while minimizing myocardial oxygen expenditure. Initial volume therapy should consist of 100–250 mL of 0.9% sodium chloride administered intravenously over 10–15 minutes to raise the PCWP to 15–18 mm Hg. If PCWP is increased and CI does not improve to ≥2.2 L/min/m^2, the patient will most likely progress to subset IV. Appropriate treatment should then be rendered as outlined below. A small group of patients in subset III have a normal SV but a slow HR. Temporary pacing may restore CO, but the increase in myocardial oxygen demand may outweigh the marginal increase in CO at paced rates beyond 90–100 beats/min.

Subset IV carries the highest mortality. The goal of therapy is the simultaneous improvement of CI and PCWP. The choice of therapy lies between inotropic agents and peripheral vasodilators. Vasodilators such as nitroglycerin (starting at 10–20 μg/min) are usually selected first because they minimize increases in myocardial oxygen demand[31,32]; however, when severe hypotension is present (SBP < 90 mm Hg), a positive inotropic agent may prevent further circulatory collapse. One must be aware that tolerance to nitroglycerin infusion can develop and that dose and effect must be evaluated on a daily basis. Nitroglycerin can also induce a hypotension-bradycardia syndrome, which responds to fluid administration and atropine.

An ideal inotropic agent must maintain or improve myocardial contractility while minimizing oxygen demand. Dobutamine has been found to be safe and effective in patients with AMI.[68] A starting dose of 2.5 μg/kg/min can be titrated upward with expected trends of increased CO, reduced PCWP, and an SBP of >90 mm Hg. Multiple drug therapy using various combinations has also been studied. The use of dobutamine in a mean dose of 7.7 μg/kg/min with nitroglycerin (average 267 μg/min) has been shown to be effective in both decreasing LV filling pressures and significantly improving cardiac index in patients with severe LV failure resulting from AMI.[30] In addition, dopamine (7.5 μg/kg/min) combined with dobutamine (7.5 μg/kg/min) administration results in substantial hemodynamic improvement when compared to doses of 15 μg/kg/min of either agent alone in patients with cardiogenic shock.[69] The combination of dobutamine (at 3, 6, and 9 μg/kg/min) and administration of amrinone (IV bolus of 1.5 mg/kg followed by second bolus of 0.75 mg/kg) produces a statistically significant increase in cardiac index and peak positive left ventricular pressure (DP/dt mm Hg/sec), with a commensurate decrease in systemic vascular resistance compared to dobutamine alone in patients with severe heart failure.[70] The latter additive effect is based on the direct increase in 3,5-cAMP levels from adenylate cyclase stimulation by the catecholamine and inhibition of 3,5-cAMP degredation by the phosphodiesterase III inhibitor.

If all of the preceding treatment approaches are without significant effect in decreasing pulmonary congestion and improving cardiac output, insertion of an IABP for counterpulsation, left VAD or biventricular assist device (BiVAD) should be considered.

Isolated Right Ventricular Failure

Right-sided failure should be suspected in patients with a history of inferior wall or anteroseptal AMI. The patient will exhibit jugular venous distention (JVD), and may have hepatojugular reflux, peripheral edema, and Kussmaul's sign (inspiratory JVD). The lungs are clear to percussion and auscultation. A high CVP and SVR accompanied by low pulmonary pressures, PCWP, and CO are all indicative of right-sided ventricular failure. Sine CO from the RV is depressed, suboptimal delivery of blood (preload) to the LV results. Left ventricular CO is therefore diminished because of low ventricular filling pressures (PCWP).

The strategy in managing patients with right ventricular infarction is to optimize CVP to maximize the Starling's curve response of myocardial contractility to intravascular volume.[71] One must remember that this response will be directly dependent on viable myocardial tissue. As one improves right-sided ventricular CO, filling pressures on the left side (PCWP) should rise, thereby enhancing left ventricular output. Further augmentation can be obtained by administration of an inotrope, such as dobutamine and/or amrinone (or milrinone), which does not increase pulmonary pressures (PAS/PAD) (e.g., right ventricular afterload). Dobutamine, is the easiest to use because it is readily titratable, and will increase stroke volume and CO while lowering cardiac filling pressures.[24,72] A modest (<10 beats/min) increase in HR is usually observed following dobutamine initiation, however, the magnitude of drug-induced tachycardia can vary significantly from patient to patient. The continuous infusion of 2.5–5 μg/kg/min can be titrated at 1–2 μg/kg/min increments at 10- to 15-minute intervals to a maximum of 15–20 μg/kg/min. One must be advised that tachyphylaxis to the inotropic effects of dobutamine have been reported with infusions greater than 72 hours in duration.[73]

Amrinone or milrinone may be the initial inotrope selected in this setting or, as in most instances, added to the dobutamine regimen for synergy. Amrinone and milrinone not only improve CO but also provide significant afterload reduction, which would be beneficial in this scenario. One must be careful that the peripheral vasodilation does not drop preload significantly since this would be extremely detrimental to the patient with RV failure. Regardless of which agent is used, a loading dose must be given because of the long half-lives of the phosphodiesterase inhibitors. Amrinone can be given as 0.75–1.5 mg/kg while the loading dose for milrinone is 50 μg/kg. This dose should be infused over 10–15 minutes, or longer if necessary, while the patient's BP is carefully monitored. If hypotension develops (SBP < 90 mm Hg) the infusion should be stopped and BP allowed to return to at least >90–100 mm Hg. Some patients may require administration of a vasoconstrictor, such as phenylephrine or norepinephrine if they remain hypotensive.

If significant benefit from the initial loading dose of amrinone or milrinone is not achieved within 30 minutes, a second load equivalent to the first can be administered. A maintenance infusion starting at 5 μg/kg/min of amrinone or 0.375 μg/kg/min of milrinone is instituted following completion of the loading dose, and can be increased by 2.5–5 μg/kg/min increments for amrinone and 0.125 μg/kg/min increments of milrinone to the maximum recommended dose (Table 23.3).

Dopamine and norepinephrine have essentially no role in the management of cardiogenic shock secondary to isolated RV failure because both agents will increase pulmonary vascular tone, thus impeding right ventricular outflow.[22,23] Isoproterenol can be used to improve CO and lower pulmonary pressures; however, extreme care must be exercised in patients with ischemic heart disease due to the risk of exacerbation of myocardial ischemia.[28] Administration of vasodilators, such as nitroglycerin or nitroprusside, or diuretics may decrease right ventricular preload and cause worsening of CO and hypotension if not given concurrently with an inotrope.

If all treatment strategies fail, insertion of an IABP or right VAD may provide support while the myocardium heals or serve as a bridge to transplantation.

Post–Cardiac Surgery

The myocardium is usually "stunned" during the first 24 hours following cardiopulmonary bypass surgery as a result of the patient undergoing heart stoppage (cardioplegia), hypothermia, and suffering postischemic myocardial damage.[74] The effects of low CI (<2.2 L/min/m^2) and decompensation to cardiogenic shock on the other organ systems is described in detail in the section on General Characteristics at the beginning of this chapter.

The SVR is usually elevated due to vasoconstriction as a result of both hypothermia and depressed CI. Intravascular volume is routinely low secondary to blood loss and third spacing of fluid. Intravascular volume replacement with colloids should improve CI and lower SVR.[75] As the patient warms, some degree of vasodilation will occur, further lowering the SVR and thus facilitating decreased impedance to left ventricular outflow and peripheral perfusion. If optimal filling pressures have been attained (CVP, 8–10 mm Hg; PCWP, 12–18 mm Hg) and CI has plateaued and remains suboptimal (CI < 2.2 L/min/m^2), pharmacologic interventions must be considered.

Pharmacotherapy is initiated with either afterload reduction with nitroprusside or inotropic support with dobutamine. The balanced arterial and venous dilation from nitroprusside can be titrated in increments of 0.5 μg/kg/min at 5- to 10-minute intervals from a starting dose of 0.5 μg/kg/min to a maximum of 8–10 μg/kg/min. A slow, deliberate titration is suggested to prevent "overshoot" hypotension. A sudden significant fall in BP may necessitate complete discontinuation of the infusion, with initiation at a lower dose once BP stabilizes. Hypotension with reflex tachycardia is more likely to occur in hypovolemic patients. Cyanide and thiocyanate toxicity are observed in patients with hepatic and renal dysfunction, respectively; most often occurring following doses >2–3 μg/kg/min for greater than 2–3 days.

If therapy is initiated with dobutamine, a starting dose of 2.5–5 μg/kg/min is utilized with incremental increases of 1–2 μg/kg/min at 10- to 15-minute intervals. Unlike dopamine, dobutamine enhances coronary blood flow and has a net positive effect on the myocardial oxygen supply and demand balance.[76–78] Should dobutamine fail to achieve a minimum CI of 2.2 L/min/m^2 then one may consider adding nitroprusside to further lower afterload and improve CO.

Although amrinone can also be used as initial therapy,[79–81] its long half-life, lack of rapid titratability, dose-related thrombocytopenia, and vasodilatory effects relegate its use as a second- or third-line agent unless the patient has pulmonary hypertension.[82] In most instances, amrinone[70,83,84] or milrinone is added to a catecholamine regimen for synergy to optimize CO. Some advantages of amrinone as compared to dobutamine include a lower increase in HR and myocardial oxygen demand following administration, fewer arrhythmias, and a lower incidence of perioperative infarction.[85] It is suggested that patients with postoperative low output syndrome may require a loading dose of 1–3 mg/kg of amrinone with a maintenance infusion of 10–20 μg/kg/min to attain optimal effects.[37] Milrinone is usually initiated as a 50 μg/kg bolus over 10–15 minutes followed by a 0.375–0.75 μg/kg/min infusion.[86,87] Milrinone has a much lower incidence of thrombocytopenia as compared to amrinone, but may be more arrhythmogenic. It is reasonable to consider amrinone or milrinone in patients that have a SBP of at least 90–100 mm Hg. Patients with marginal SBP (90–100 mm Hg) must be carefully monitored to evaluate BP tolerance to the amrinone or milrinone infusion.

Epinephrine can be used as an alternative to dopamine or dobutamine or in addition to either nitroprusside or amrinone. Epinephrine at low doses (<0.05 μg/kg/min) primarily stimulates β_1- and β_2-adrenergic receptors, resulting in significant positive inotropic effects with moderate peripheral vasodilation and bronchodilation. Epinephrine carries a risk of arrhythmogenicity and may induce tachycardia. In addition, the potent β_2-adrenergic stimulation transports potassium intracellularly[88] and inhibits insulin release from the pancreas[89] while simulating glycogenolysis by the liver.[90] A slight rise in blood glucose levels (<200 g/dL) occurs in many patients. An accentuated rise in serum glucose levels (500–700 g/dL) may be observed in the diabetic patient.

Although dopamine may adversely effect myocardial oxygen balance compared with dobutamine inotropic doses,[77] concurrent administration of low-dose dopamine (2–4 μg/kg/min) with other catecholamines may aid renal perfusion through dopaminergic (DA_1) dilation of the renal vasculature.[91,92]

Some patients with depressed CI and low BP (MAP < 60 mm Hg) may respond to slight increases in SVR. The increase in SVR should increase both BP and MAP. More importantly, coronary perfusion pressure (MAP–LVEDP), should rise, thus improving oxygen delivery to the myocardium. Low doses of norepinephrine (1–2 μg/min) increase vascular tone and improve coronary perfusion pressure. In addition, the β_1-adrenergic effects of norepinephrine may directly enhance CI. An alternative agent to use in this setting is low-dose phenylephrine 10–50 μg/min, a pure α-adrenergic agonist. This agent may be desirable in a patient who requires peripheral vasoconstriction but has either tachycardia or arrhythmias that preclude further β_1-adrenergic stimulation.

Lastly, IABP counterpulsation should be considered for support of ventricular function if the patient does not respond to adjustments in intravascular volume, and vasoactive and inotropic drug therapy.

Drug-Induced Ventricular Failure

Patients with left ventricular decompensation secondary to the drugs listed in Table 23.9 can best be managed by discontinuing the offending agent and administration of dobutamine or dopamine at β_1-adrenergic stimulating doses. Epinephrine or isoproterenol is usually reserved for severe cases such as the reversal of significant drug-induced β-adrenergic blockade. Dopamine or dobutamine can be infused at 5–10 μg/kg/min, epinephrine at 0.01–0.05 μg/kg/min, and isoproterenol at 2–10 μg/min.

If conventional therapy fails, glucagon 3- to 5- mg intravenous push should be given while maintaining the ongoing infusions.[93] A continuous infusion of glucagon (4 mg/min) is then started to maintain ventricular function while the effects of β-adrenergic blockade dissipate.[94] Left ventricular dysfunction induced by calcium channel blocker administration can be reversed by calcium (either gluconate or chloride) 1 g by slow intravenous push. This should improve myocardial contractility and also reverse hypotension if present.

Intra-Aortic Balloon Pump

The IABP is useful in augmenting CO when pharmacologic interventions are maximized and CO remains suboptimal.[95] Insertion of the IABP is performed under aseptic conditions, and the balloon catheter is threaded into the descending aorta via a femoral artery. The IABP is connected to the patient's electrocardiogram (ECG) monitor. Inflation and deflation of the balloon are directly activated by the patient's electrical conduction. The balloon deflates immediately prior to systole (just before or on the R wave) and inflates during diastole (peak of the T wave). The primary cardiovascular effect is one of a substantial decrease in afterload, which augments left ventricular stroke volume and results in a 10–20% increase in CO.[96] In addition, the condom-shaped balloon pushes blood back toward the heart when inflated, significantly improving coronary filling.

The IABP is usually employed for 24–72 hours; however, some patients may require several days to weeks of supportive intra-aortic counterpulsation, especially those awaiting heart transplant. There is a risk of thrombus formation around the catheter, which necessitates careful vigilance of lower extremity peripheral pulses. Dextran 40 at a rate of 10 mL/h is sometimes used to prevent thrombi by altering platelet aggregation. Other complications include infection, perforation or damage of the aortic wall, hemolysis, thrombocytopenia, and perforation of the balloon releasing helium gas, which is absorbed into the body without detrimental effects.

The IABP is weaned by adjusting the ratio of counterpulsations to heart beats. During initial therapy, the balloon inflates and deflates with every ventricular depolarization (1 : 1). Once the patient is stabilized, and a majority of vasoactive support has been discontinued, the IABP can be weaned to a 1 : 2 or 1 : 3 ratio (i.e., an inflation and deflation with every other or every third beat, respectively). The IABP can be removed once the patient's hemodynamic status stabilizes and vasoactive drugs have been weaned to low therapeutic doses or discontinued.

Extracorporeal Membrane Oxygenation

Extracorporeal membrane oxygenation (ECMO) is a device that provides blood gas exchange, while maintaining circulation of blood. In the setting of cardiogenic shock, ECMO has also been shown to lower intracardiac filling pressures, relieve pulmonary edema, and maintain peripheral perfusion.[97] Either the carotid or femoral artery is cannulated, blood is pumped out of the vascular tree, through the gas exchange canister, and back into the patient. The flow rate is governed by ABGs and is usually 80 mL/kg/min in adults. The patient must be fully anticoagulated with heparin during the course of therapy. Adverse effects are limited to bleeding secondary to the anticoagulation. The use of ECMO is reserved for patients with severe cardiac failure, in which pharmacologic and invasive (IABP) measures are futile, and either recovery or transplant is anticipated within a few days.

Ventricular Assist Devices

VADs, also known as circulatory assist devices, may be considered when there is an inability to wean the patient from cardiopulmonary bypass despite maximum pharmacologic support and use of an IABP. These devices can provide circulation while the myocardium has an opportunity to recover. In cases of severe myocardial damage, the VAD serves as a bridge to transplantation. Three devices are available, the left ventricular assist device (LVAD), right ventricular assist device (RVAD), and the biventricular assist device (BiVAD).[98] Anticoagulation with heparin is required for most devices. Inotropic support is usually withdrawn during ventricular assist. Recovery of myocardial function is assessed by periodic transesophageal echocardiography (TEE). Complications include mediastinal bleeding, mediastinitis, sepsis, stroke, renal failure, and respiratory failure.[99] Weaning from a ventricular assist device ranges from 35–50%, with about 25% of patients surviving to discharge.[100]

EVALUATION OF THERAPEUTIC OUTCOMES

The high mortality rate and the rapidity with which cardiogenic shock can progress to organ failure and death make prompt intervention absolutely critical. The primary focus in managing cardiogenic shock is to reverse the maldistribution of blood flow while restoring the Do_2 to the normal range (900–1100 mL/min). The Forrester classification system can serve as an assessment at initiation of therapy and guide further therapy, in patients with AMI, so that the patient eventually progresses into classification subset I (CI > 2.2 L/min/m^2, PCWP < 18 mm Hg). It is crucial to not only support the myocardium but also to prevent and reverse lung involvement so that pulmonary edema is managed if it occurs and oxygenation is restored and/or maintained. ABGs should be optimized so that values are in the normal ranges. Key goals should be attainment of acceptable blood pressure (SBP > 90–100 mm Hg, MAP > 60 mm Hg) and urine output (>0.5–1.0 mL/kg/h) and improvement in overall clinical status (peripheral perfusion, wakeable, oriented patient).

TAPER OF VASOACTIVE AND INOTROPIC DRUGS

Once the goals of therapy are attained and the patient has stabilized, a deliberate taper ("wean") of the vasoactive and inotropic medications should be undertaken. The selection of drug to be weaned and the rate at which weaning occurs are primarily dependent on the patient's current clinical and hemodynamic status, the number of medications that the patient is receiving, the doses, and the risk of potential adverse effects of the respective medications. In general, only one medication is weaned at a time, often starting with the vasoconstrictors, followed by the inotropes and/or vasodilators (or vice versa), depending on the patient's cardiovascular status. Small incremental decreases in dose are instituted at fixed intervals (e.g., every 15–60 minutes). Further weaning is guided by changes in hemodynamic parameters. Systolic blood pressure should be maintained at greater than 90 mm Hg, CI > 2.2 L/min/m^2, UO > 0.5 mL/kg/h, and other values within the accepted ranges. If the patient falls below the desired minimum endpoints, then weaning should be interrupted and the patient allowed to stabilize. Some patients may experience a disproportionate fall in hemodynamic parameters thus requiring an upward titration in the medication currently being weaned.

REFERENCES

1. MacLean LD. Shock: Causes and management of circulatory collapse, in Sabiston, DC Jr (ed): Textbook of Surgery, 11th ed. Philadelphia, WB Saunders, 1977, p 65.
2. Swan HJC, Forrester J, Markus H, et al. Catheterization of the heart in man with use of a flow-directed balloon-tipped catheter. N Engl J Med 1970;283:447–451.
3. Edwards JD. Practical application of oxygen transport principles. Crit Care Med 1990;18:S45–S48.
4. Naylor-Shepherd MF, Fuhs DW, Angaran DM. Oxygen homeostasis: Theory, measurement, and therapeutic implications. DICP Ann Pharmacother 1990;24:1195–1203.
5. Lyerly, HK. Shock, in Lyerly HK (ed): The Handbook of Surgical Intensive Care: Practices of the Surgery Residents at the Duke University Medical Center, 2nd ed. Chicago, Year Book Medical Publishers, 1989, pp 1–18.
6. Bland RD, Shoemaker WC, Abraham E, et al. Hemodynamic and oxygen transport patterns in surviving and nonsurviving postoperative patients. Crit Care Med 1985;13:85–90.
7. Tuchschmidt J, Fried J, Swinney R, et al. Early hemodynamic correlates of survival in patients with septic shock. Crit Care Med 1989;17:719–723.
8. Schlichting, R. O_2 uptake, critical O_2 delivery, and tissue wellness, in Pinsky MR, Dhainaut JA (eds). Pathophysiologic Foundations of Critical Care. Baltimore, Williams & Wilkins, 1993, pp 119–139.
9. Enger E. Understanding continuous mixed venous oxygen saturation (Svo_2) monitoring with the Swan–Ganz oximetry TD system. Santa Ana, CA, American Edwards Laboratories, 1987.
10. Bryan-Brown CW. Blood flow to organs: Parameters for function and survival in critical illness. Crit Care Med 1988;16(2):170–178.

11. Astiz ME, Rackow EC, Weil MH. Pathophysiology and treatment of circulatory shock. Crit Care Clin 1993;9:183–203.
12. Weil MH, Afifi AA. Experimental and clinical studies on lactate and pyruvate as indicators of the severity of acute circulatory failure (shock). Circulation 1970;41:989–1001.
13. Swan HJC, Ganz W. Use of balloon flotation catheters in critically ill patients. Surg Clin North Am 1975;55:501–509.
14. Headley JM. Invasive hemodynamic monitoring: Physiologic principles and clinical applications. Edwards Critical-Care Division, 1989.
15. Ermakor S, Hoyt JW. Pulmonary artery catheterization. Crit Care Clin 1994;8:773–806.
16. Ganz W, et al. A new technique for measurement of cardiac output by thermodilution in man. Am J Cardiol 1971;27:392–396.
17. Shoemaker WC. Shock states: Pathophysiology, monitoring, outcome prediction, and therapy, in Shoemaker WC, et al (eds): Textbook of Critical Care, 2nd ed. Philadelphia, WB Saunders, 1989, pp 977–993.
18. Shoemaker WC, Kram HB, Appel PL. Therapy of shock based on pathophysiology, monitoring, and outcome prediction. Crit Care Med 1990;18:S19–S25.
19. Williams RS, Bishop T. Selectivity of dobutamine for adrenergic receptors. J Clin Invest 1981;67:1703–1711.
20. Ruffolo RR Jr, Spradlin TA, Pollock GD, et al. α- and β-adrenergic effects of the stereoisomers of dobutamine. J Pharmacol Exp Ther 1981;219:447–452.
21. Murphy MB, Elliott WJ. Dopamine and dopamine receptor agonists in cardiovascular therapy. Crit Care Med 1990;18:S14–S18.
22. Goldberg LI. Dopamine—clinical uses of an endogenous catecholamine. N Engl J Med 1974;291:707–710.
23. Kawashima S, Combes J, Liang CS, et al. Contrasting effects of dopamine and dobutamine on myocardial release of norepinephrine during acute myocardial infarction. Jpn Heart J 1985;26:975–984.
24. Leier CV, Heban PT, Huss P, et al. Comparative systemic and regional hemodynamic effects of dopamine and dobutamine in patients with cardiomyopathic heart failure. Circulation 1978;58:466–475.
25. Vincent JL, Reuse C, Kahn RJ. Effects on right ventricular function of a change from dopamine to dobutamine in critically ill patients. Crit Care Med 1988;16(7):659–662.
26. Schechter E, Wilson MF, Kong Y-S. Physiologic responses to epinephrine infusion: The basis for a new stress test for coronary artery disease. Am Heart J 1983;105:554–560.
27. Holmes HR, Babbs CR, Voorhiss WE, et al. Influence of adrenergic drugs upon vital organ perfusion during CPR. Crit Care Med 1980;8:137–140.
28. Mueller HS, Ayers SM, Gregory JJ, et al. Hemodynamics, coronary blood flow and myocardial metabolism in coronary shock: Response to L-norepinephrine and isoproterenol. J Clin Invest 1970;49:1885–1902.
29. Mikulic E, Cohn JN, Fanciosa JA. Comparative hemodynamic effects of inotropic and vasodilator drugs in severe heart failure. Circulation 1977;56:528–533.
30. Awan NA, Evenson MK, Needham KE, et al. Effect of combined nitroglycerin and dobutamine infusion in left ventricular dysfunction. Am Heart J 1983;106:35–40.
31. Hill NS, Antman EM, Green LH, et al. Intravenous nitroglycerin: A review of pharmacology, indications, therapeutic effects, and complications. Chest 1981;79:69–76.
32. Chiariello M, Gold HK, Leinbach RC, et al. Comparison between the effects of nitroprusside and nitroglycerin on ischemic injury during acute myocardial infarction. Circulation 1976;54:766–773.
33. Passamani ER. Nitroprusside in myocardial infarction. N Engl J Med 1982;306:1168–1170.
34. Nerothin DD, Kaane PB. Calcium—vasodilator or vasoconstrictor [abstract]? Anesth Analg 1984;63:255.
35. Zaloga GP, Strickland RA, Butterworth JF, et al. Calcium attenuates epinephrine's β-adrenergic effects in postoperative heart surgery patients. Circulation 1989;81:196–200.
36. Mancini D, LeJemtel T, Sonnenblick E. Intravenous use of amrinone for the treatment of the failing heart. Am J Cardiol 1985;56:8B–15B.
37. Hines R. Clinical applications of amrinone. J Cardiothor Anesth 1989;3:24–32.
38. Klein N, Siskind S, Frishman W, et al. Hemodynamic comparison of intravenous amrinone and dobutamine in patients with chronic congestive heart failure. Am J Cardiol 1981;48:170–175.
39. Camilion de Hurtado M, Argel MI, Cingolani HE. Influence of acid–base alterations on myocardial sensitivity to catecholamines. Arch Pharmacol 1981;317:219–224.
40. Gould SA, Sehgal LR, Sehgal HL, Moss GS. Hypovolemic shock. Crit Care Clin 1993;9:239–259.
41. Civetta JM. A new look at the Starling equation. Crit Care Clin 1979;7:84–91.
42. Gabel JC, Drake RE. Pulmonary capillary pressure and permeability. Crit Care Med 1979;7:92–97.
43. Gaar KA, Taylor AE, Owens LJ, et al. Pulmonary capillary pressure and filtration coefficients in the isolated perfused lung. Am J Physiol 1967;23:910–914.
44. Landis EM. Capillary pressure and capillary permeability. Physiol Rev 1934;14:404–481.
45. Morisette MP. Colloid osmotic pressure: Its measurement and clinical value. Can Med Assoc J 1977;116:897–900.
46. Skillman JJ, Awwad HK, Moore FD. Plasma protein kinetics on the early transcapillary refill after hemorrhage in man. Surg Gynecol Obstet 1967;125:983–996.
47. Crandall ED, Staub NC, Goldberg HS, et al. UCLA conference: Recent developments in pulmonary edema. Ann Intern Med 1983;99:808–822.
48. Granger HJ. Role of interstitial matrix and lymphatic pump in regulation of transcapillary fluid balance. Microvasc Res 1979;18:209–216.
49. Knottenbelt JD. Low initial hemoglobin levels in trauma patients: An important indicator of ongoing hemorrhage. J Trauma 1991;31:1396–1399.
50. Imm A, Carlson RW. Fluid resuscitation in circulatory shock. Crit Care Clin 1993;9:313–333.
51. Biddle TL, Paul NY. Effect of furosemide on hemodynamic and lung water in acute pulmonary edema secondary to myocardial infarction. Am J Cardiol 1979;43:86–90.
52. Lowery BD, Cloutier CT, Carey LC. Electrolyte solutions in resuscitation in human hemorrhagic shock. Surg Gynecol Obstet 1971;133:273–284.

53. Haupt MT, Rackow EC. Colloid osmotic pressure and fluid resuscitation with hetastarch, albumin and saline solutions. Crit Care Med 1982;10:159–162.
54. Rackow EC, Falk JL, Fein IA, et al. Fluid resuscitation in circulatory shock: A comparison of the cardiorespiratory effects of albumin, hetastarch and saline solutions in patients with hypovolemic and septic shock. Crit Care Med 1983;11:839–850.
55. Maningas PA, Mattox KL, Pepe PE, et al. Hypertonic saline-dextran solutions for the prehospital management of traumatic hypotension. Am J Surg 1989;157:528–534.
56. Shackford SR, Sise JM, Friedlund PH, et al. Hypertonic sodium lactate versus lactated Ringer's solution for intravenous fluid therapy in operations on the abdominal aorta. Surgery 1983;94:41–51.
57. Puri VK, Paidipaty B, White L. Hydroxyethyl starch for resuscitation of patients with hypovolemia and shock. Crit Care Med 1981;9:833–837.
58. Shatney CH, Deepika K, Militello PR, et al. Efficacy of hetastarch in the resuscitation of patients with multisystem trauma and shock. Arch Surg 1983;118:804–809.
59. Kirklin JK, Lell WA, Kouchoukos NT. Hydroxyethyl starch versus albumin for colloid infusion following cardiopulmonary bypass in patients undergoing myocardial revascularization. Ann Thorac Surg 1994;37:40–46.
60. Stump DC, Strauss RG, Henriksen RA, et al. Effects of hydroxyethyl starch on blood coagulation, particularly factor VIII. Transfusion 1985;25:349–354.
61. Velanovich V. Crystalloid versus colloid fluid resuscitation: A meta-analysis of mortality. Surgery 1989;105:65–71.
62. American Association of Blood Banks. Blood Bank Week 1989;6(10):1.
63. Alpert JS, Becker RC. Mechanisms and management of cardiogenic shock. Crit Care Clin 1993;9:205–218.
64. Goldberg RJ, Gore JM, Alpert JS, et al. Cardiogenic shock after acute myocardial infarction. Incidence and mortality form a community-wide perspective, 1975 to 1988. N Engl J Med 1991;325(16):1117–1122.
65. Forrester JS, Diamond G, Chattrejee K, et al. Medical therapy of acute myocardial infarction by application of hemodynamic subsets (first of two parts). N Engl J Med 1976;295:1356–1362.
66. Forrester JS, Diamond G, Chatterjee K, et al. Medical therapy of acute myocardial infarction by application of hemodynamic subsets (second of two parts). N Engl J Med 1976;295:1404–1413.
67. Loer J, Golbourt U, Reicher-Reiss H, et al. Cardiogenic shock complicating acute myocardial infarction in patients without heart failure on admission: Incidence, risk factors and outcomes. SPRINT Study Group. Am J Med 1993;94:265–273.
68. Gillespie TA, Ambos HD, Sobel BE, et al. Effects of dobutamine in patients with acute myocardial infarction. Am J Cardiol 1977;39:588–594.
69. Richard C, Ricome JL, Rimailho A, et al. Combined hemodynamic effects of dopamine and dobutamine in cardiogenic shock. Circulation 1983;67:620–626.
70. Gage J, Rutman H, Lucido D, et al. Additive effects of dobutamine and amrinone on myocardial contractility and ventricular performance in patients with severe heart failure. Circulation 1986;74:367–373.
71. Lorell B, Leinbach RC, Pohost GM, et al. Right ventricular infarction. Am J Cardiol 1979;43:465–471.
72. Dell'Italia LJ, Starling MR, Blumhardt R, et al. Comparative effects of volume loading, dobutamine and nitroprusside in patients with predominant right ventricular infarction. Circulation 1985;72:1327–1335.
73. Unverferth DV, Blanford M, Kate RE, et al. Tolerance to dobutamine after a 72-hour continuous infusion. Am J Med 1980;69:262–266.
74. Briesblatt WM, Stein KL, Wolfe CJ et al. Acute myocardial dysfunction and recovery: A common occurrence after coronary bypass surgery. J AM Coll Cardiol 1990;15:1261–1269.
75. Kirklin JK, Lell WA, Kouchoukos NT. Hydroxyethyl starch versus albumin for colloid infusion following cardiopulmonary bypass in patients undergoing myocardial resuscitation. Ann Thor Surg 1984;37:40–46.
76. Schwenzer KJ, Kopel RF. Hemodynamic and metabolic effects of dobutamine in 18 patients after open heart surgery. Crit Care Med 1990;18:1107–1110.
77. Van Trigt PV, Spray TL, Pasque MK, et al. The comparative effects of dopamine and dobutamine on ventricular mechanics after coronary artery bypass grafting: A pressure dimension analysis. Circulation 1984;70(suppl I):112–117.
78. Fowler MB, Alderman EL, Oesterle SN, et al. Dobutamine and dopamine after cardiac surgery: Greater augmentation of myocardial blood flow with dobutamine. Circulation 1984;70(suppl I):103–111.
79. Goenen M, Pedemonte O, Baele P, et al. Amrinone in the management of low cardiac output after open heart surgery. Am J Cardiol 1985;56:33B–38B.
80. Gunnicker M, Hess W. Preliminary results with amrinone in perioperative low cardiac output syndromes. Thorac Cardiovasc Surg 1987;35:219–225.
81. Butterworth JF IV. Use of amrinone in cardiac surgery patients. J Cardiothorac Vasc Anesth 1993;7:1–7.
82. Hess W, Arnold B, Veit S. The hemodynamic effects of amrinone in patients with mitral stenosis and pulmonary hypertension. Eur Heart J 1986;7:800–807.
83. Uretsky BF, Lawless CE, Verbalis JG, et al. Combined therapy with dobutamine and amrinone in severe heart failure. Chest 1987;92:657–662.
84. Royster RL, Butterworth JF IV, Prielipp RC, et al. Combined inotropic effects of amrinone and epinephrine after cardiopulmonary bypass in humans. Anesth Analg 1993;77:662–672.
85. Dupuis JY, Bondy R, Cattran C, et al. Amrinone and dobutamine as primary treatment of low cardiac output syndrome following coronary artery surgery: A comparison of their effects on hemodynamics and outcome. J Cardiothorac Vasc Anesthesia 1992;6:542–553.
86. Feneck RO. The European Milrinone Multicenter Trial Group. Intravenous milrinone following cardiac surgery: 1. Effects of bolus infusion followed by variable dose maintenance infusion. J Cardiothorac Vasc Anesth 1992;6:554–562.
87. Copp MV, Hill AJ, Feneck RO. Overview of the effects of intravenous milrinone in acute heart failure following surgery. Eur J Anaesthesiol 1992;(suppl 5):35–41.
88. Brown MJ, Brown DC, Murphy MB. Hypokalemia from β_2-receptor stimulation by circulating epinephrine. N Engl J Med 1983;309:1414–1419.

89. Clutter WE, Bier DM, Shah SD, et al. Epinephrine plasma metabolic clearance rates and physiologic thresholds for metabolic and hemodynamic actions in man. J Clin Invest 1980;66:94–101.
90. Soman VR, Shamoon H, Sherwin RS. Effects of physiologic infusion of epinephrine in normal humans: Relationship between the metabolic response and β-adrenergic binding. J Clin Endocrinol Metab 1980;50:294–297.
91. Davis RF, Lappas DG, Kirklin JK, et al. Acute oliguria after cardiopulmonary bypass: Renal function improvement with low-dose dopamine infusion. Crit Care Med 1982:10;852–856.
92. El Allaf D, Cremers S, D'Orio V, et al. Combined hemodynamic effects of low doses of dopamine and dobutamine in patients with acute infarction and cardiac failure. Arch Int Physiol Biochem 1986;92:S49–S55.
93. Brogan E, Kozorris MC, Overy DC. Glucagon therapy in heart failure. Lancet 1969;1:482–484.
94. Vander Ark CR, Reynolds EW. Clinical evaluation of glucagon by continuous infusion in the treatment of low cardiac output states. Am Heart J 1970;79:481–487.
95. Maccioli GA, Lucas WJ, Norfleet EA. The intra-aortic balloon pump: A review. J Cardiothorac Vasc Anesth 1988;2:365–373.
96. Bregman D. Assessment of intra-aortic balloon counterpulsation in cardiogenic shock. Crit Care Med 1975;3:90–93.
97. Toomasian JM, Haiduc NJ, Zwischenberger JB, et al. Techniques for extracorporeal membrane oxygenation for cardiac failure. Proc Am Acad Cardiovasc Perf 1986;7:105.
98. Farrar DJ, Hill JD, Gray LA Jr, et al. Heterotopic prosthetic ventricles as a bridge to cardiac transplantation: A multicenter study in 29 patients. N Engl J Med 1988;318:333–340.
99. Bojar RM. Manual of Perioperative Care in Cardiac and Thoracic Surgery, 2nd ed. Boston, Blackwell Scientific Publications, 1994, p 162.
100. Bojar RM. Adult Cardiac Surgery. Boston, Blackwell Scientific Publications, 1992, pp 425–459.

Section 2
Respiratory Disorders

Chapter 24

Introduction to Pulmonary Function Testing

Shawn E. Wright, MD, Carlos A. Garza, MA, CRRT, CPFT, and Stephen G. Jenkinson, MD

Pulmonary function testing is an indispensable tool in the clinician's diagnostic armamentarium. Although most valuable in identifying and monitoring primary disorders of ventilation, pulmonary function testing can reveal dysfunction of cardiovascular, neurologic, and musculoskeletal systems responsible for respiratory symptoms. Many disease states may affect the lungs' capacity to exchange gas adequately; however, relatively few specific patterns of ventilatory abnormalities are described. Pulmonary function testing allows the clinician to form meaningful differential diagnostic categories, determine degree of impairment, and assess response to therapy. Pulmonary function testing is an increasingly complex technology. This chapter concentrates on the key aspects of pulmonary function interpretation required to diagnose and treat most patients with respiratory disorders.

Physiologic abnormalities that can be measured by pulmonary function testing include obstruction of airflow, restriction of lung size, and decrease in transfer of gases. Abnormal values of pulmonary function tests are those outside the range of values obtained from a group of normal individuals matched according to age, height, race, and sex. These normal "predicted values" are calculated from specific prediction equations. The equations give a mean value for the group of normals and usually a range defined by confidence limits that include 95% of the variation of the normal group. Before a pulmonary function test is labeled abnormal, the results should fall outside the range in which 95% of people the same age, height, and sex would be found. All lung volumes obtained by spirometry or gas dilution studies must be corrected to body temperature saturated with water vapor (BTPS) in order to produce uniformity of interpretation from one pulmonary function laboratory to another.

Obstructive Lung Disease

Obstructive ventilatory diseases are manifested by a reduction of airflow through the conducting airways due to a decrease in their diameter or loss of their integrity. This condition has a variety of causes, including bronchial smooth muscle contraction (asthma), airway collapse from loss of radial traction (emphysema), anatomic thickening of bronchial walls (chronic bronchitis), infiltration of the bronchial wall (tumor or granuloma), or aspiration of objects that mechanically obstruct bronchi (foreign bodies). The standard pulmonary function test used to measure airway obstruction is the forced expiratory spirogram. This test allows an assessment of the rate of change in volume that occurs as a function of time.

The forced expiratory spirogram can be analyzed several ways to decide whether obstructive lung disease is present. One of the simplest and most commonly used analyses is measurement of the forced expiratory volume exhaled after 1 second (FEV_1). A single value of this measurement can be compared with normal predicted values and different degrees of obstruction can be documented (Fig. 24.1).

The most widely used general classification for interpretation of obstructive lung dysfunction states that a decrease in FEV_1 to less than 75% of the predicted value is mild obstruction, less than 60% of the predicted value is moderate obstruction, and less than 40% of the predicted value is severe obstruction. Measurement of maximum expiratory flow rate, forced expiratory flow measured between 200 and 1200 mL of the FVC maneuver ($FEF_{0.2-1.2L}$), and maximum midexpiratory flow rate, flow between 25 and 75% of the forced expiratory volume ($FEF_{25-75\%}$) will also be abnormal in patients with obstructive airway disease. In general, neither of these two tests adds more information about an obstructed patient than the FEV_1 and both measurements are more variable. The $FEF_{25-75\%}$ has been of value in monitoring lung transplant patients for acute graft rejection.[1]

Although all patients with obstructive lung disease of any etiology have reduced flow rates on forced exhalation, the use of pulmonary function testing can sometimes be helpful in differentiating among the various causes. The different responses these patients show to selected pulmonary function tests are illustrated in Table 24.1. Patients with asthma usually exhibit increased airway resistance, a significant improvement in airflow in response to bronchodilators, and normal diffusing capacity for carbon monoxide (DLco) because asthma causes reversible bronchial obstruction. Patients with chronic bronchitis also have an increased airway resistance and a normal DLco, but they usually have only a slight increase in flow after bronchodilators. Patients with emphysema exhibit little increase in airway resistance, no response to bronchodilators, and a marked decrease in DLco because emphysema is a disease

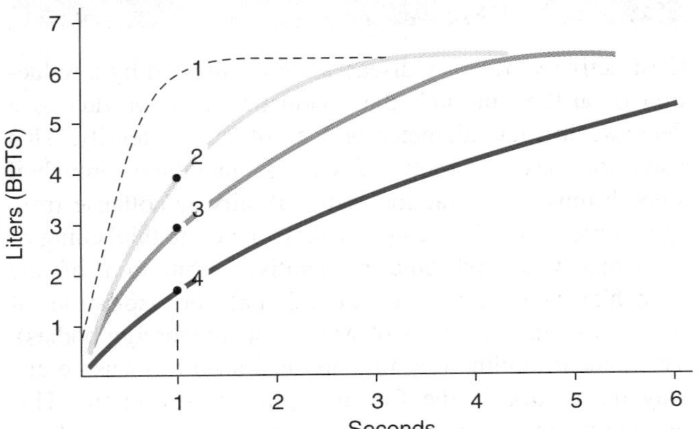

Figure 24.1. (1) The measurement of forced expiratory volume in 1 second (FEV_1) in a normal subject; (2) a patient with mild airway obstruction; (3) a patient with moderate airway obstruction; and (4) a patient with severe airway obstruction. BPTS, body temperature saturated with water vapor.

TABLE 24.1. SPECIFIC PULMONARY FUNCTION PATTERNS IN PATIENTS WITH CHRONIC OBSTRUCTIVE PULMONARY DISEASE (COPD)

	Causes of COPD		
	Asthma	Chronic Bronchitis	Emphysema
Decreased FEV_1	++++	++++	++++
Decreased FEV_1/FVC ratio	++++	++++	++++
Increased airway resistance	++++	++++	+
Decreased DLco	–	–	++++
Response to bronchodilators	++++	+	–

Key: FEV_1, forced expiratory volume expired after 1 second; FVC, forced vital capacity; DLco, diffusing capacity for carbon monoxide.

of the terminal respiratory units characterized by loss of alveoli. A near-normal specific resistance in the face of decreased forced expiratory flow is characteristic of emphysema, as airway resistance is measured in the absence of dynamic airway compression. The use of these pulmonary function tests combined with the clinical assessment of a patient can often reveal the prevalent cause of obstructive lung disease in a given subject.

FEV_1 measured as a percent of predicted normal value cannot be used to assess airway obstruction if a patient also has restrictive lung disease because all lung volumes are reduced. A better measurement in these patients is the percentage of FVC exhaled in the first second (FEV_1/FVC%). A normal FEV_1/FVC% is 75%. (The ratio is age dependent and lower values may be normal in older patients.) This ratio remains accurate even in the presence of severe restrictive lung disease. Measurement of FEV_1/FVC% is very useful at the bedside because it can be interpreted rapidly without having to consult a table of normal values. There is some decline of these ratios with increasing age, but even in the elderly the decline is very modest. Mild obstruction is represented by an FEV_1/FVC% ratio between 75 and 60%. Moderate obstruction produces an FEV_1/FVC% ratio between 60 and 40%; and severe obstruction produces an FEV_1/FVC% ratio of $<40\%$. The predicted percentage FEV_1 and the FEV_1/FVC% ratio are usually similar in a given patient. When, in a single patient, they are found to differ (e.g., FEV_1 equals 55% of predicted and the FEV_1/FVC% ratio equals 64%), then the FEV_1/FVC% ratio measurement should be used for the interpretation because FEV_1 can be decreased by concomitant restrictive disease.

Forced expiratory flow can also be measured by plotting instantaneous airflow against lung volume during a maximum forced expiration. This is called a maximum expiratory flow volume (MEFV) curve (Fig. 24.2). The early portion of this maneuver is effort dependent and flow will increase in proportion to the intensity of effort. The latter portion is effort independent and flow depends on the resistance of the peripheral bronchi and the recoil pressure of the lung in the midvital capacity range. Computerized pulmonary function equipment is capable of extracting and reporting the FEV_1 and FVC from this curve.

UPPER AIRWAY OBSTRUCTION

Obstructing lesions of the upper airway can go unrecognized and misdiagnosed if pulmonary function test results are not interpreted properly. These patients have physiologic derangements similar to patients with asthma or chronic obstructive pulmonary diseases (COPD). Upper airway obstruction in these patients can be either fixed or variable.[2] Fixed lesions do not allow the airway to change cross-sectional area regardless of the changes in transmural pressure. With variable lesions, however, the size of the airway can respond to changes in transmural pressure. Variable lesions are subclassified as intrathoracic or extrathoracic because of their location and response to changes in transmural pressure.[3] Pulmonary function testing can usually distinguish among the various types of upper airway obstruction. Note, however, that in patients with bilateral obstruction of both main bronchi, a plateau in the inspiratory limb of a flow-volume loop, similar to patients with intrathoracic upper airway obstruction, may be seen.

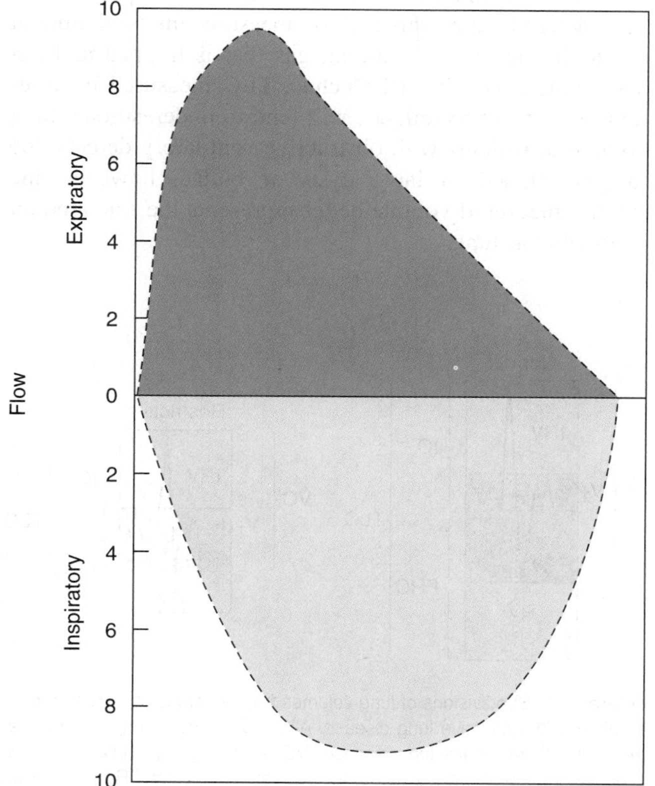

Figure 24.2. Maximum expiratory flow volume curve in a normal subject.

Pulmonary function tests used to diagnose and classify upper airway obstruction include spirometry and MEFV curves. MEFV curves are the pulmonary function tests of choice in diagnosing upper airway obstruction because they define the site of obstruction as well as document its presence. The various changes in MEFV curves from upper airway obstruction can be seen in Fig. 24.3. With fixed obstruction, the plateau and limitation of flow is seen during both inspiration and expiration. Variable extrathoracic obstruction produces flow limitation and a plateau only on inspiration for the reasons mentioned previously. Variable intrathoracic obstruction causes flow limitation and a plateau only on expiration because the pressure outside the lumen (pleural pressure) becomes much greater than intraluminal pressure. Spirometry can sometimes be misleading in patients with variable extrathoracic obstruction. With this lesion, intraluminal pressure during expiration is much higher than extraluminal pressure. This actually causes the airway to dilate in the area of the obstruction during an expiratory maneuver.

Rotman et al.[4] have defined spirometric variables that can be used to distinguish patients with upper airway obstruction from those with COPD or asthma. With spirometry alone, the $FEV_1/FVC_{0.5}$ (forced expiratory volume in 1 second/forced expiratory volume in 0.5 seconds) ratio in patients with upper airway obstruction is greater than or equal to 1.5. This is because $FEV_{0.5}$ is proportionately more reduced by obstruction of the upper airway because forced expiration measured at 0.5 seconds ($FEV_{0.5}$) occurs at higher lung volumes than at 1.0 seconds (FEV_1). The abnormality seen with upper airway obstruction has been referred to as "straightening" of the curve during the early portion of expiration.

REVERSIBILITY OF OBSTRUCTION

Patients with obstructive ventilatory defects should be evaluated for their response to bronchodilators. If a patient improves after the use of a bronchodilator at the time of their pulmonary function testing, they are more likely to benefit from long-term administration of these drugs.[5] The interpretation of bronchodilator studies is often difficult because even small changes in reversibility of airway obstruction could be significant in a given patient if the obstruction is very severe.

Studies in which bronchodilators were administered to normal persons have shown a mean increase in FEV_1 of 2.5% with a standard deviation of 3.9%.[3] If a posi-

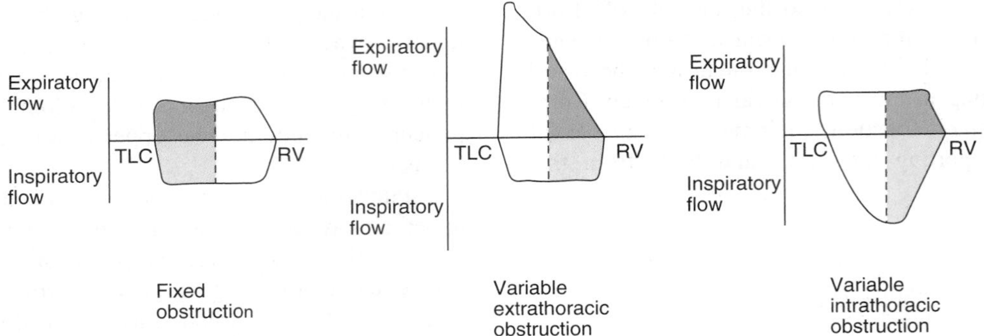

Figure 24.3. Maximum expiratory flow volume curves from patients with fixed obstruction, variable extrathoracic obstruction, and variable intrathoracic obstruction. TLC, total lung capacity; RV, residual volume.

tive response to bronchodilators is defined as a response of at least two standard deviations (SDs) above the mean response in normal individuals, then the FEV_1 must improve by at least 10% with bronchodilators to be considered significant. Other spirometric parameters, such as the FVC or $FEF_{25-75\%}$, have also been used by some to detect reversibility, but FEV_1 remains the best test for evaluating bronchodilator response. This is because increases in FEV_1, although not large, have a very small variability, which makes it a good discriminating test.[6] Several issues complicate the interpretation of bronchodilator responses in obstructive lung disease. Failure to respond significantly to a single bronchodilator exposure should not be construed as *a priori* evidence of irreversible obstruction. For example, use of bronchodilating agents prior to the pulmonary function test may reduce the observed improvement in the test by "predilating" the airways. Delayed improvement has been reported in some patients with "irreversible" airway obstruction after prolonged corticosteroid therapy. Finally, there are no well-established criteria for a significant response in acutely ill patients due to the variable severity of bronchospasm in these patients.

Restrictive Lung Disease

Restrictive lung disease results in decreased lung volumes without reduction of airflow. This abnormality can be measured using static lung volumes. In Fig. 24.4, the subdivisions of lung volumes are seen for a normal patient and a patient with restrictive lung disease. Restrictive disease reduces all the various subdivisions of lung volume. These patients have normal airway resistance, and their FEV_1 is greater than 75% of their forced vital capacity (FEV_1/FVC greater than 75%).

Total lung capacity (TLC) is the total volume of gas in the lungs and airways after a maximum inspiration. A reduction in TLC is the most accurate measurement of restrictive lung function. The degree of restrictive ventilatory defect is determined by grouping patients with reduced TLC into mild (TLC less than 80%), moderate (TLC less than 60%), or severe (TLC less than 40%) categories.[7] TLC can be measured by closed-circuit helium dilution, open-circuit nitrogen washout, or body plethysmography. All of these methods determine functional residual capacity (FRC) and TLC is calculated from this value. When the body plethysmograph is used to determine TLC, the volume measured is termed the thoracic gas volume (V_T) and usually equals FRC. TLC is then calculated as the sum of V_T and the inspiratory capacity (IC). TLC determined by this method measures the total amount of gas in the chest, including gas that is trapped and not communicating with a bronchus. TLC measured by dilution or washout techniques will tend to underestimate lung volume in patients with obstructive ventilatory defects due to gas trapped in large cysts or bullae, however, the smaller measured volume better represents the true amount of functional lung.

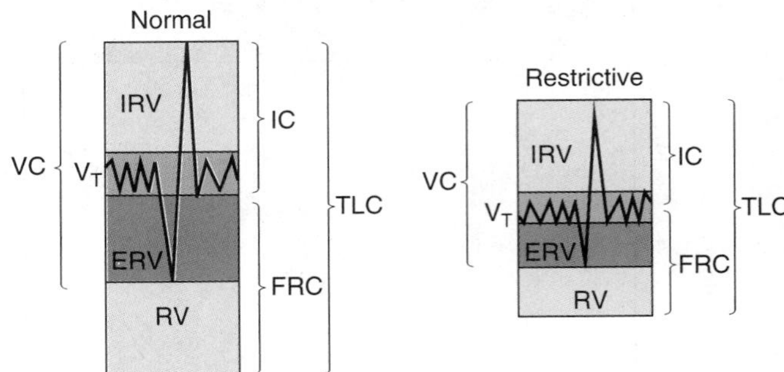

Figure 24.4. Subdivisions of lung volumes from a normal subject and from a patient with restrictive lung disease. All subdivisions of lung volume are reduced with restrictive lung disease. VC, vital capacity; TLC, total lung capacity; V_T, thoracic gas volume; IC, inspiratory capacity; FRC, functional residual capacity; IRV, inspiratory reserve volume; ERV, expiratory reserve volume; RV, residual volume.

The diagnosis of restrictive ventilatory dysfunction in patients who also exhibit airway obstruction should always be confirmed by measurement of TLC. In addition, race must also be considered in the diagnosis of restrictive lung disease because black subjects have been shown to have a VC approximately 12% lower than that of whites of the same age and height.[8] This is thought to be due to differences in chest wall configuration.

Restriction of lung function can be produced by diseases that affect the lungs themselves or by decreases in the ability of the chest to perform as a bellows. A list of the common causes of restrictive lung disease is given in Table 24.2.

RESTRICTIVE PARENCHYMAL DISEASES

Intrinsic restriction of lung function associated with diseased lung parenchyma can usually be differentiated from processes causing mechanical restriction due to chest bellows malfunction. Restrictive parenchymal diseases are associated with a reduction in alveolar volume or an increase in lung elastic recoil. Pulmonary function testing reveals decreased lung volumes, decreased static compliance, increased lung elastic recoil, and decreased DLco (Table 24.3). The measurement of static lung compliance is the single best test for determining whether restriction is caused by parenchymal disease.[9] In addition, these patients exhibit mild resting hypoxemia that worsens with exercise. Monitoring gas exchange during exercise is the most sensitive test for detecting worsening interstitial disease in patients with restrictive parenchymal diseases.[10] DLco can also be abnormal in patients with restrictive parenchymal disease, even with a normal chest radiograph.

Rarely, patients with pulmonary fibrosis may also have evidence of obstructive airway disease caused by peribronchiolar fibrosis. More sensitive tests of small airway function, such as frequency dependence of dynamic lung compliance, slope of phase III on the single-breath nitrogen washout test, and closing volume (CV) expressed as a percentage of the VC, are often abnormal in patients with obstructive forms of pulmonary fibrosis or sarcoidosis. Other tests of obstructive airway disease, such as the absolute value of FEV_1, the FEV_1/FVC ratio, and airway resistance, are usually normal in these patients. A summary of changes observed in restrictive pulmonary dysfunction caused by parenchymal disease is given in Table 24.4.

TABLE 24.2. CAUSES OF RESTRICTIVE LUNG DISEASE

- Interstitial lung diseases
  - Collagen vascular disease
  - Interstitial pneumonitis
  - Hypersensitivity pneumonitis
  - Pneumoconiosis
  - Pulmonary fibrosis
  - Pulmonary edema
- Infiltrative lung diseases
  - Granulomatosis
  - Tumor
- Pleural diseases
  - Fibrothorax
  - Pleural effusion
  - Pneumothorax
- Chest wall diseases
  - Kyphoscoliosis
  - Ankylosing spondylitis
  - Neuromuscular disease
- Miscellaneous causes
  - Obesity
  - Paralyzed diaphragm
  - Ascites
  - Pregnancy
  - Flail chest
  - Resectional surgery

TABLE 24.3. PULMONARY FUNCTIONS IN A 28-YEAR-OLD MAN WITH IDIOPATHIC PULMONARY FIBROSIS

Function	Observed	Predicted (%)
FEV_1	3.0 L	64
FVC	3.2 L	66
TLC	4.6 L	64
RV	1.5 L	70
RV/TLC	32%	104
MVV	150 L/min	96
DLco	14 mL/min/mm Hg	58

Key: FEV_1, forced expiratory volume exhaled after 1 second; FVC, forced vital capacity; TLC, total lung capacity; RV, residual volume; MVV, maximum voluntary ventilation; DLco, diffusing capacity for carbon monoxide.

CHEST BELLOWS DYSFUNCTION

Diseases that mechanically inhibit the chest bellows mechanism may cause restricted ventilation. Clinical syndromes of bellows dysfunction involve deformity of the chest wall and skeleton, loss of neuromuscular function to perform inspiration, fibrosis of the pleural space, and abdominal overdistention causing upward displacement of the diaphragm and decreased diaphragm movement. The lung parenchyma itself remains normal in these disorders. The most common pulmonary function pattern seen with mechanically deforming diseases is a decrease in TLC and VC with only a slight decrease in RV. This situation produces an increased ratio of RV to TLC. RV is maintained in these diseases because lung compliance remains normal.

The specific diffusing capacity (DLco corrected for lung volume) is also normal because no intrinsic lung disease exists. With chest wall deformities, ventilation can usually be increased in these patients by increasing the respiratory rate; therefore, the measurement of maximum vol-

TABLE 24.4. RESTRICTIVE LUNG DISEASE

Restrictive Parenchymal Disease	Restrictive Chest Bellows Disease
Decreased lung volumes	Decreased lung volumes
$FEV_1/FVC \geq 75\%$	$FEV_1/FVC \geq 75\%$
Normal airway resistance	Normal airway resistance
Decreased static compliance	Increased RV/TLC ratio
Decreased diffusing capacity	Normal compliance
	Normal diffusing capacity

See Table 24.3 for explanation of abbreviations.

untary ventilation (MVV) is not affected unless the restrictive dysfunction is extremely severe (Table 24.5).[9]

Clinical conditions that inhibit proper function of the chest bellows mechanism may produce subtle differences in pulmonary function testing suggesting a particular diagnosis. Obesity and abdominal distention from pregnancy or ascitic fluid produce a decrease in both functional residual capacity (FRC) and the expiratory reserve volume (ERV). (Doubling a patient's predictive body weight decreases FRC by 25% and ERV by 40%.) The closing capacity (CC) can rise above FRC in these patients and airway closure will consequently occur, resulting in hypoxemia. With massive obesity, chest wall compliance also decreases and MVV falls, probably because of the increase in oxygen demand required per unit of work done by the respiratory muscles. Deforming skeletal abnormalities, such as kyphoscoliosis, cause a reduction in VC and TLC in proportion to the degree of the physical defect. FRC and RV, however, remain essentially normal, resulting in a diagnostically useful increased ratio of RV to TLC. Ankylosing spondylitis also produces a decrease in VC and TLC, but FRC and RV are increased above normal values. This increase is caused by a decrease in chest wall compliance.

Neuromuscular diseases produce decreases in VC, TLC, and MVV, and increases in RV as chest wall compliance falls. Flow rates during the early part of a forced expiration (effort-dependent flows) are reduced because these patients cannot generate the amount of force necessary to greatly distend the lung beyond its mechanical resting point.

TABLE 24.5. PULMONARY FUNCTION IN A 62-YEAR-OLD MAN WITH ANKYLOSING SPONDYLITIS

Function	Observed	Predicted (%)
FEV_1	2.5 L	67
FVC	3.1 L	67
TLC	4.6 L	69
RV	1.8 L	94
RV/TLC	37%	146
MVV	140 L/min	92
DLco	24 mL/min/mm Hg	92

See Table 24.3 for explanation of abbreviations.

Abnormal Gas Transfer

Measurement of diffusing capacity permits evaluation of the alveolar endothelial-pulmonary vascular bed interface. A reduction in diffusing capacity occurs with loss of alveolar surface area, thickening of alveolar endothelium, loss of pulmonary capillary bed, increases in ventilation/perfusion (V/Q) mismatch, or decreases in the amount of circulating hemoglobin. Single-breath diffusing capacity for carbon monoxide (DLco) is the most common measurement of diffusing capacity performed in pulmonary function laboratories. When the measurement of diffusing capacity is corrected for alveolar volume, it is referred to as the "specific" DLco ($DLco/V_A$). A decrease in DLco is most commonly seen with emphysema, loss of parenchymal tissue from surgery, interstitial lung disease, or pulmonary vascular disease. DLco should be less than 80% of predicted value to be considered abnormal because of the marked variability of the test.

Increased DLco can also occur in patients with polycythemia, high-altitude dwellers, patients with intracardiac shunts, patients with congestive heart failure, and in some patients with asthma (thought to be caused by redistribution of perfusion). Increased DLco is normally seen during exercise because of an increase in blood flow into the lung. This same mechanism causes a slight increase in DLco when one assumes the supine position. All of the changes that cause an increase in DLco do so by increasing the amount of blood available in the pulmonary capillaries to take up carbon monoxide.

Misinterpretation of Pulmonary Function Tests

The information obtained from pulmonary function tests must be carefully assessed to avoid any misinterpretation of a patient's functional status. Data generated from pulmonary function tests can be misleading if the tests are not performed properly. Flow–volume curves provide graphic representation of data gathered during a test and must be examined to obtain a meaningful interpretation of the results. Abnormalities such as coughing, inconsistent effort, or mechanical malfunctions can be identified easily by direct examination of the tracings.

Other potential errors of interpretation include changes in function caused by variability in patients themselves. A normal diurnal rhythm exists that produces the worst pulmonary function in the early morning, improves during the day, and again falls during the evening.[11] Large variations can also occur on a day-to-day basis in a single patient, especially with significant reversible obstructive airway disease. Patients may also inadvertently cause changes in their test results by doing such things as smoking immediately before the tests or using bronchodilator medications prior to arrival at the laboratory. This information must be made available to the physician interpreting the pulmonary function tests before a test result is deemed abnormal or a patient labeled as unresponsive to bronchodilators.

Finally, repetitive testing is essential to confirm an abnormal test result. A lack of response to inhaled bronchodilators should be repeatedly documented prior to recommending that a patient with obstructive lung disease refrain from using these drugs.

The performance of pulmonary function tests requires the interaction of a machine, a technician, a patient, and the physician.[11] On a given day, problems pertaining to any of these four components can arise and produce data that do not represent a patient's pulmonary functional status. To avoid any problems with misinterpretation, the following rules should be applied:

1. Pulmonary function equipment should be calibrated regularly.
2. Volumes should be corrected for BTPS.
3. Patients should be instructed not to smoke or use inhaled bronchodilators within 4 hours of testing, or use oral bronchodilators within 12 hours of testing.
4. Testing should be performed according to strict protocol.
5. Repeat tests should be performed at the same time of day.
6. Patient effort should be recorded as good or poor.
7. Copies of pulmonary function tracings should be provided to the interpreter along with the computerized data printout sheets.

Adherence to these guidelines will assist in reducing interpretive errors. The medical, psychological, financial, and legal implications of misinterpreting pulmonary function tests can be significant. Results that are not clearly abnormal should be repeated and scrutinized before a final interpretation is made.

Cardiopulmonary Exercise Testing

Integrative cardiopulmonary exercise testing permits the clinician to simultaneously assess several key components of gas exchange. While routine pulmonary function testing is capable of demonstrating ventilatory abnormalities (obstructive versus restrictive lung defects, etc.), cardiopulmonary exercise testing better defines the physiologic responses to exercise and characterizes the disease processes responsible for the observed ventilatory abnormalities.[12] In addition, many disease states result in discordance between symptoms and routine spirometric findings; cardiopulmonary exercise testing allows more in-depth evaluation of these individuals' symptoms and their ability to respond to cardiopulmonary stress.[12]

The fundamentals of exercise testing rely on an accurate assessment of the cardiovascular and respiratory systems' ability to efficiently consume oxygen and produce carbon dioxide (and water) during the metabolism of energy-containing substrate. At the cellular level, hydrolysis of adenosine triphosphate (ATP) releases stored energy, which will ultimately be used by muscle to perform work. Oxidative phosphorylation is required to maintain cellular energy levels to sustain this work. This phosphorylation sequence utilizes oxygen intermediaries to accomplish the mitochondrial transfer of electrons from donor to acceptor via the NAD(P)-cytochrome chain. Consumption of molecular oxygen results in the formation of high-energy phosphate bonds available for energy transfer to muscle. Altered cellular metabolism of oxygen may manifest at the organ level as abnormal changes in molecular gas consumption and production. Thus, a primary physiologic goal of exercise testing is determination of the balance between oxygen uptake (V_{O_2}) and carbon dioxide output (V_{CO_2}) under a given workload (Fig. 24.5). Exercise testing attempts to characterize these biophysiologic events on the whole-body level in an effort to recognize patterns of disease.

Although a wide spectrum of clinical disorders is encompassed by derangements of gas exchange, several criteria may be used to determine when cardiopulmonary exercise will likely be of most value[13]:

1. Clarification of dyspnea or exercise limitation of unclear etiology (Patients with lung disease are often limited by dyspnea, a complex subjective symptom reflecting the balance of ventilatory capacity and demand.)
2. Evaluation of the degree of cardiopulmonary disability
3. Evaluation of drug therapy or rehabilitation capacity on exercise as indirect measures of treatment success
4. As additional, and possibly more accurate information on ability of an individual to withstand cardiopulmonary stress (i.e., preoperative evaluation)

Most complications of exercise testing are cardiovascular in origin. Relative contraindications to exercise testing include active heart disease (e.g., angina, arrhythmias, severe hypertension, congestive heart failure, etc.), significant asthma, hypoxemia, or uncontrolled metabolic disturbances (e.g., acidosis, thyrotoxicosis, etc.).[14]

Successful application of exercise testing depends on accurate determination of V_{O_2}, V_{CO_2}, and other important measures of cardiopulmonary function; most often, a proto-

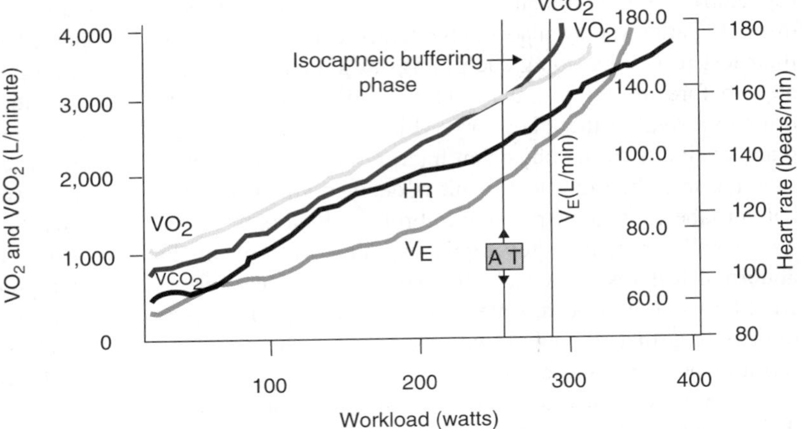

Figure 24.5. Graphic representation of the relationship between fundamental variables of gas exchange in a normal subject during cardiopulmonary exercise testing. O_2, oxygen consumption; VCO_2, carbon dioxide production; V_E, minute ventilation; AT, anaerobic threshold; HR, heart rate.

col of progressively increasing work rate testing is used to obtain these values. Patients are typically exercised by walking or cycling "against" an incremental load to a maximum or symptom-limited end. Steady-state protocols work a patient at a constant level for a predetermined time and are most useful when specific variables (e.g., cardiac output) are to be measured. Clinical signs and symptoms that may limit or terminate the test (e.g., dyspnea, chest pain, arrhythmias, wheezing, oxygen desaturation, etc.) are monitored. Electrocardiographic monitoring of at least one lead (12 leads are used when evaluating patients with ischemic heart disease) permits an indirect assessment of oxygen availability and requirements for myocardial work. Physiologically, the cardiovascular and ventilatory responses to exercise are interrelated, however, for purposes of discussion they are dealt with somewhat independently.

Normally, the fundamental ventilatory response to exercise is an increase in rate and tidal volume. During a cardiopulmonary exercise test, ventilation is determined by measuring total expired minute ventilation (V_E) in L/min BTPS using a mouthpiece connected to a volume measuring device. Analysis of expired gas allows measurement of VO_2 and VCO_2:

$$VO_2 = (V_I \times F_IO_2) - (V_E \times F_EO_2) \quad (1)$$

$$VCO_2 = V_E \times F_ECO_2 \quad (2)$$

where F_IO_2 = fraction of inspired oxygen; F_EO_2 = fraction of expired oxygen; and F_ECO_2 = fraction of expired carbon dioxide.

The level above which the body cannot increase VO_2 despite increases in work rate is termed the maximal oxygen uptake (VO_{2max}). This maximal aerobic power is rarely achieved. More commonly, a normal individual attains his or her own peak oxygen uptake (VO_{2peak}), which is slightly below VO_{2max}. Individuals with exercise limitation of any sort (including poor effort) will have a much lower VO_{2peak} for a given work rate. Determination of VO_{2peak} establishes whether a patient has approached maximal aerobic function and should be among the first values examined in an exercise test.

Ventilatory limitation of exercise may be assessed by measurement of a patient's ability to increase ventilation when maximally exercised. Termed the breathing reserve (BR), which is the patient's maximal voluntary ventilation at rest (L/min) − V_E (L/min) at maximum exercise, this value is reduced in patients who are limited primarily by pulmonary disease and elevated in those limited by cardiovascular disease.

Coupling VO_2 and VCO_2 with minute ventilation is another useful method of assessing abnormal ventilation. Patients with pulmonary disease often have an increased V_E/VCO_2 response to exercise indicating significant ventilation–perfusion imbalance due to either vascular or parenchymal disease or both. In normal, maximally exercised individuals, both V_E/VCO_2 and V_E/VO_2 initially decrease, with V_E/VO_2 reaching its nadir when exercise-induced metabolic acidosis (anaerobic threshold) occurs (Fig. 24.6). V_E/VCO_2 reaches its nadir when respiratory compensation (RC) begins in response to an anaerobic threshold (Fig. 24.6). The anaerobic threshold is defined as the exercise VO_2 above which there is a net increase in lactate production due to increased anaerobic metabolism.[15] Determination of the anaerobic threshold assists in discriminating patients with oxygen delivery deficiencies from patients limited primarily by parenchymal diseases. Patients with impaired cardiac pump function, pulmonary vascular disease, and systemic vascular disease demonstrate a reduced anaerobic threshold reflecting impaired oxygen delivery to tissue (Table 24.6). The anaerobic threshold can be determined invasively by measuring blood lactate levels. For most studies, however, noninvasive methods using the point where the VCO_2 and VO_2 slopes intersect (Fig. 24.5), or by observing V_E/VO_2 increasing out of proportion to V_E/VCO_2 (Fig. 24.6) are usually sufficient for determining the anaerobic threshold.[12]

Cardiovascular disease-related exercise intolerance is characterized by several altered physiologic responses. Because the primary role of the cardiovascular system is

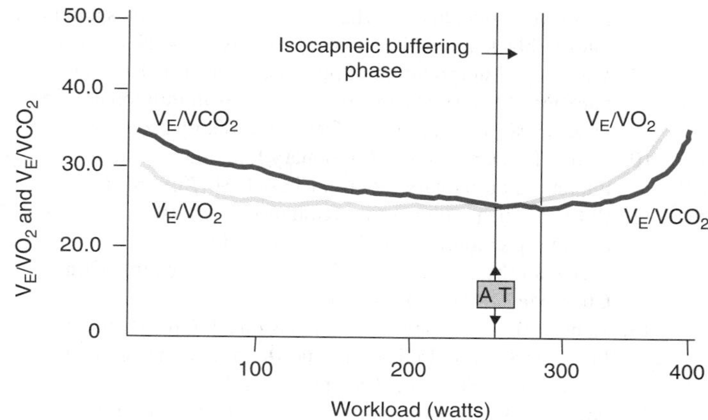

Figure 24.6. Line graph showing the relationship between the ventilatory equivalents of oxygen consumption (V_E/V_{O_2}) and carbon dioxide production (V_E/V_{CO_2}) with increasing workloads. Lactate produced by anerobiasis is buffered without an increase in Pa_{CO_2} or net hydrogen ion concentration during the isocapneic buffering phase.

ultimately oxygen transport, the major cardiovascular abnormalities associated with exercise include impaired V_{O_2}, V_{CO_2}, and heart rate response. The fundamental cardiovascular response to exercise is an increase in cardiac output (the volume of blood pumped by the heart per minute) and is expressed as the product of heart rate and stroke volume. Low cardiac output is characteristic of poor cardiac status. The normal myocardial response to increasing work is a linear increase in cardiac output and heart rate (HR), the latter to an age-dependent maximum:

$$HR_{max}\text{ (beats/min)} = 210 - 0.65 \times \text{Age (years) (95\% CI} \pm 20\text{ beats/min)}$$

Measurement of the heart rate reserve (HRR) gives an indication of cardiovascular reserve:

$$\text{HRR (beats/min)} = \text{Predicted maximum HR} - \text{HR at maximum exercise}$$

Normally the HRR is small (less than 15 beats/min), however, in patients who have intrinsic heart disease, systemic vascular disease, or ischemic heart disease may prematurely discontinue exercising giving rise to an increased HRR (Table 24.6). In addition, abnormalities of the ECG, presence of hypertension, and symptoms of coronary ischemia suggest cardiovascular limitation of exercise.

Interpretation of cardiopulmonary exercise tests can be complex. Many of the so-called "normal" values differ significantly depending on the protocols and formulas used to derive the data. The use of established algorithms facilitates interpretation by permitting pattern recognition of certain disease states.[15] Some of the most common patterns of cardiopulmonary exercise responses in different clinical settings are described in Table 24.6.

TABLE 24.6. PATTERNS OF RESPONSES TO CARDIOPULMONARY EXERCISE TESTING

Cardiovascular Disease	Deconditioning	COPD
Decreased $V_{O_{2peak}}$	Decreased $V_{O_{2peak}}$	Decrease $V_{O_{2peak}}$
Decreased AT (<40% pred.)	Low-normal AT	Variable AT
Variable HRR	No HRR	Increased HRR
Normal BR	Normal BR	Decreased BRR
Normal Pa_{O_2}	Normal Pa_{O_2}	Decreased Pa_{O_2} (usually)
Abnormal ECG, angina	Difficult to distinguish from mild cardiovascular diseases	Increased P(A-a) O_2 gradient; Pa_{CO_2} variable

Interstitial Lung Disease	Pulmonary Vascular Disease
Decreased $V_{O_{2peak}}$	Decreased $V_{O_{2peak}}$
Variable HRR	Decreased AT (< 40% pred.)
Decreased BRR	Decreased HRR
Decreased Pa_{O_2}	Normal BR
Increased P(A-a) O_2 gradient	Decreased Pa_{O_2}
Increased V_E/V_{CO_2}	Increased P(A-a) O_2 gradient
Increased V_D/V_T	Increased V_D/V_T

REFERENCES

1. Tillis W, Levine SM, Anzueto A, et al. Clinical predictors of graft dysfunction following single lung transplantation. Chest 1992;102(2):73S.
2. Acres JC, Kryger MH. Upper airway obstruction. Chest 1981;80:207–211.
3. Lazarus A. Pulmonary function tests in upper airway obstruction. Basics of RD 1980;8:1.
4. Rotman HH, Liss HP, Weg JG. Diagnosis of upper airway obstruction by pulmonary function testing. Chest 1975;68:796–799.
5. Light RW. Use of the pulmonary function laboratory in the treatment of obstructive airway disease. Adv Asthma Allergy 1978;5:10.
6. Light RW, Conrad SA, George RB. The one best test for evaluating the effects of bronchodilator therapy. Chest 1977;72:512–516.
7. Scheinhorn DJ, Emory WB. Putting spirometry to use in your practice. J Resp Dis 1981;2(8):8.
8. Lapp NL, Amandus HE, Hall R, et al. Lung volumes and flow rates in black and white subjects. Thorax 1974;29:185–188.
9. Wanner A. Interpretation of pulmonary function tests, in Sackner MA (ed): Diagnostic Techniques in Pulmonary Disease. New York, Marcel Dekker, 1980, pp 353–426.
10. Keogh BA, Crystal RG. Pulmonary function testing in interstitial pulmonary disease. Chest 1980;78:856–865.
11. Butler J. The pulmonary function test, cautious overinterpretation. Chest 1981;79:498–500.
12. Weisman IM, Zeballos RJ. Clinical exercise testing. Clin Chest Med 1994;15:173–450.
13. Hansen JE. Exercise testing, in Wilson AF (ed): Pulmonary Function Testing: Indications and Interpretations. Orlando, FL, Grune & Stratton, 1985, pp 175–199.
14. American College of Sports Medicine, Guidelines for Exercise Testing and Prescription, 4th ed. Philadelphia, Lea & Febiger, 1991.
15. Wasserman K, Hansen JE, Sue DY, Whipp BJ. Principles of Exercise Testing and Interpretation. Philadelphia, Lea & Febiger, 1987.

Chapter 25

Asthma

H. William Kelly, PharmD, and Alan K. Kamada, PharmD

Bronchial asthma is a common disease of children and adults. Although the clinical manifestations of asthma have been known since antiquity, it is a disease that still defies precise definition. The word *asthma* is of Greek origin and means "panting." More than 2000 years ago, Hippocrates used the word *asthma* to describe episodic shortness of breath; however, the first detailed clinical description of the asthmatic patient was made by Aretaeus in the second century.[1] Since that time asthma has been used to describe any disorder with episodic shortness of breath or dyspnea; thus, the terms *cardiac asthma* and *bronchial asthma* have been used to delineate the etiologies of the dyspnea. These terms are now obsolete and asthma refers to a disorder of the respiratory system characterized by episodes of difficulty in breathing. An Expert Panel of the National Institutes of Health National Asthma Education Program (NAEP)[2] has defined asthma as a lung disease characterized by "1) airway obstruction that is reversible (but not completely so in some patients) either spontaneously or with treatment; 2) airway inflammation; and 3) increased airway responsiveness to a variety of stimuli." This descriptive definition for asthma is attributed to our lack of knowledge of the precise pathogenic defect that results in the clinical syndrome we recognize as asthma. The current definition does allow for the important heterogeneity of the clinical presentation of asthma. New technologies have added substantially to our understanding of the interrelationships of immunology, biochemistry, and physiology to the clinical presentation of asthma, and further research may yet uncover a specific genetic defect in asthma. Until such time, asthma will continue to defy exact definition.

Epidemiology

An estimated 10 million persons in the United States have asthma (about 5% of the population). The reported prevalence has increased 29% from 1980 to 1987 to 40.1 per 1000 population.[2] African-Americans have a 19% higher incidence of asthma than whites and are twice as likely to be hospitalized.[2] The estimated cost of asthma in the United States in 1990 was $6.2 billion.[3] The largest single direct medical expenditure was inpatient hospital services (emergency care), reaching almost $1.5 billion, followed by prescription medications ($1.1 billion). The costs of medication increased 54% between 1985 and 1990. In total, 43% of the economic impact was associated with emergency room use, hospitalization, and death. Asthma accounted for 1% of all ambulatory care visits according to the National Ambulatory Medical Care Survey and results in more than 450,000 hospitalizations per year.[2]

Asthma continues to be a significant cause of missed school days in children, with more than 10 million school days missed in 1990. This resulted in an estimated cost of $900 million dollars lost to parents to stay home and care for their children.[3] In a national cohort of reported asthma in 6- to 24-year-olds, approximately 50% reported the onset of asthma by 4 years of age with the age of reported onset highly dependent on the age at which patients are asked.[4] The 6- to 14-year-old age group reported onset less than 2 years in 45.2 versus 34.1% for 15- to 24-year-olds. This suggests a significant bias in data retrieved from large retrospective questionnaires. A comparison of surveys from Aberdeen, Scotland, 25 years apart showed doubling of the prevalence of asthma from 4.1 to 10.2% from 1964 to 1989.[5] While there has been some speculation that the increasing prevalence of asthma worldwide has been a result of improved diagnosis these questionnaires also showed doubling rises in respiratory symptoms (wheeze and episodes of shortness of breath) suggestive of asthma, indicating a true rise in the prevalence in the United States and worldwide. Although the precise reason for this increase is unknown, early exposure to allergens and airway irritants such as tobacco smoke in infancy increases the risk of developing asthma. Worsening air quality has also been promoted as a cause of the increased asthma prevalence.

Natural History

The natural history of asthma is still not well defined. Most of the studies are retrospective and either clinic or hospital based, leading to possible bias in patient selection. Between

30 and 70% of children with asthma will markedly improve or become symptom free by early adulthood; chronic disease persists in about 30% of patients. Although asthmatic patients who develop the disease in childhood are more likely to have remissions, patients who present at an early age have a poorer prognosis. A recent study reported that ongoing airway obstruction may persist undetected in asthmatic children who are clinically well if objective measures are not made.[6] Weiss et al.[7] reported that females developing asthma by age 7 could expect a 7% reduction in lung function by age 15. These studies raise the question of whether ongoing asthma may produce fixed airways obstructions and whether therapy may be able to change the natural history of childhood asthma. Approximately 60% of patients who are symptom free as adults continue to exhibit bronchial hyperreactivity to inhaled histamine challenges. In general, subjects with less frequent attacks and normal pulmonary function on initial assessment have higher remission rates, while smokers have the lowest remission and highest relapse rates.

Evidence exists that morbidity and mortality from asthma are increasing. Although death from asthma is still relatively rare, among 5- to 34-year-olds the death rate increased 6.2% per annum in the 1980s in the United States with 4580 deaths in 1988.[8] This is consistent with the increase in death rates found worldwide. African-Americans have two to three times the death rate from asthma as whites. This discrepancy is even more evident in children, for which the death rate for African-Americans was three to nine times higher than for whites in children 10–14 years old.[2] Analysis of hospitalization rates over the same time period from the National Hospital Discharge Survey would indicate that asthma morbidity is also increasing.[9] Hospitalizations for asthma among children 0–17 years increased 4.5% per annum while total hospitalizations for all causes actually decreased. The increase for African-Americans was 1.8 times that of whites. In a study in New York City, the highest annual rate of hospitalizations for asthma was in Hispanics (62.9 per 10,000) followed by blacks at 59.9 per 10,000 and non-Hispanic whites at 12.2 per 10,000.[10]

Studies of the cause and prevention of death from asthma have presented disturbing results. They indicate that 80–90% of the deaths are preventable.[2] Most deaths from asthma occur outside of the hospital and death is rare after hospitalization. The most common cause of death from asthma is inadequate assessment of the severity of airway obstruction by the patient or physician and inadequate therapy. Because poor, inner-city, minority populations have a disproportionate share of deaths from asthma,[9] inadequate access to the health care system is felt to play a significant role.[10,11] The most common cause of death in the hospitalized patient is also inadequate or inappropriate therapy. Thus, the key to prevention of death from asthma as advocated by the NAEP is education.[2] This includes education of the patients as well as the clinicians caring for them.

PATHOPHYSIOLOGY

BRONCHIAL HYPERREACTIVITY

Although a single underlying cellular defect has not yet been discovered, new technologies have substantially advanced our understanding of the pathogenesis of asthma. Hyperreactivity of the airways to physical, chemical, and pharmacologic stimuli is the hallmark of asthma.[11,12] Bronchial hyperreactivity also occurs in some patients with chronic bronchitis and allergic rhinitis, although to a lesser degree.[11,12] Normal healthy subjects may also develop a transient increased bronchial reactivity after viral respiratory infections or exposure to ozone.[12] However, the degree of reactivity is quantitatively greater in asthmatic patients than in other groups who demonstrate hyperreactivity. Bronchial reactivity of the general population fits a unimodal distribution that is skewed toward increased reactivity.[7] Patients with clinical asthma represent the extreme end of the distribution. The degree of bronchial hyperreactivity with asthmatics correlates with the clinical course of their disease and medication requirement necessary to control symptoms.[12] Patients with mild symptoms or in remission demonstrate lower levels of reactivity, although still greater than the normal population. Much of the recent research on the pathogenesis of asthma has focused on explaining airway hyperreactivity. A number of excellent reviews and symposia have highlighted new discoveries and summarized the current state of knowledge of this expanding area of research.[11,12]

Our current understanding recognizes that the increased bronchial responsiveness seen in asthma is at least in part due to an inflammatory response within the airway.[11] The intact lungs of patients at autopsy are hyperinflated because of air trapping from widespread mucus plugging. The histologic examination is characterized by three findings: (1) marked hypertrophy and hyperplasia of the airway smooth muscle, (2) increased airway wall thickness caused by an exudative inflammatory reaction and edema, and (3) mucous gland hypertrophy and mucus hypersecretion[12] (Fig. 25.1). Although the precise link is not known, bronchial hyperresponsiveness is thought to be related to the extent of inflammation in the airways.

HISTOLOGIC CHANGES IN THE LINING OF THE AIRWAYS

Histologic studies performed on patients with mild–intermittent to moderate–chronic asthma have shown marked inflammatory changes within the airway along with extensive epithelial damage.[11] Similar but more severe changes have also been seen in patients who have died from acute asthma attacks.[11,12] The correlation between the degree of

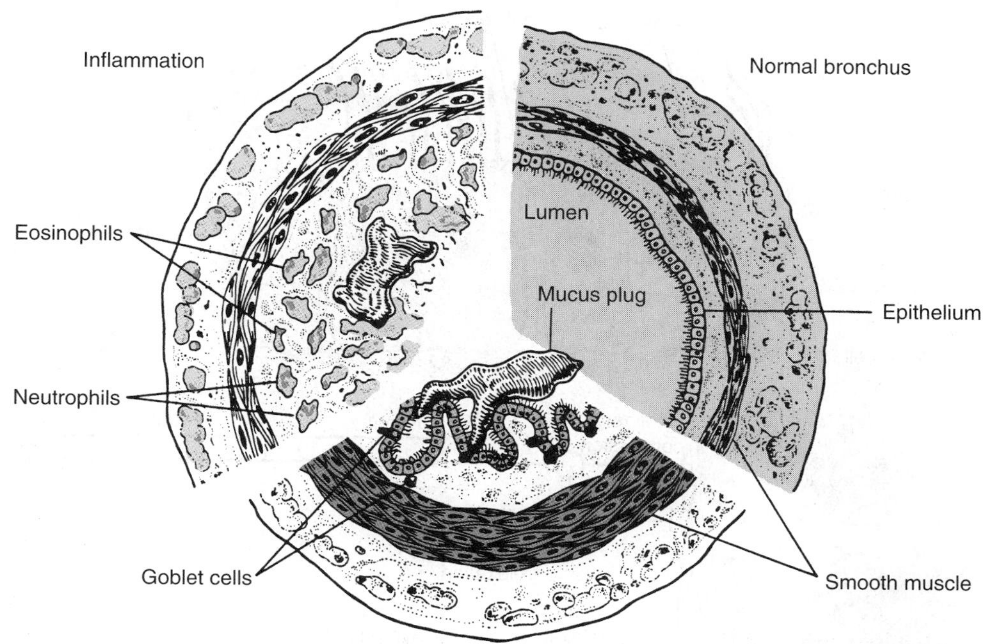

Figure 25.1. Representative illustration of the pathology found in the asthmatic bronchus compared with a normal bronchus (upper right). Each section demonstrates how the lumen is narrowed. Edema of the basement membrane, mucus plugging, smooth muscle hypertrophy, and constriction contribute (lower section). Inflammatory cells producing epithelial desquammation fill the airway lumen with cellular debris and expose the airway smooth muscle to other mediators (upper left).

epithelial denudation and airways reactivity suggests that patients with the most reactive airways have the least amount of normal bronchial epithelium.[13] Subepithelial fibrosis has also been described in the bronchi of patients with mild asthma.[11] This finding is not surprising considering that fibrosis occurs as a result of other chronic inflammatory diseases. It is not known whether the epithelial damage precedes the development of reactive airways or if these features occur simultaneously. It is also not known whether epithelial damage is a universal feature in all patients. The presence of subepithelial fibrosis is of most concern because it remains to be determined whether this type of fibrosis represents a reversible or transient process, or can have more serious sequelae such as the development of chronic obstructive pulmonary disease.

Cellular and Biochemical Features

INFLAMMATORY PROCESSES

The inflammatory reaction appears to be the key mechanism to explain the pathologic changes seen in asthma. In addition, inflammation of the airways and the release of mediators of inflammation appears to be necessary for the development and maintenance of bronchial hyperreactivity.[11] Inflammation of the airways is associated with epithelial cell damage and increased mucosal permeability.[12] This improves access of noxious stimuli from the lumen to the airway smooth muscle, submucosal mast cells, and the cholinergic irritant receptors located in the junction between cells (Fig. 25.2).[11,12] The epithelial damage and turnover leads to the hypertrophy of the basement membrane.[12]

Inflammation can also account for mucus hypersecretion.[12] Therefore, recent research on the pathogenesis of bronchial hyperreactivity has focused on inflammation and the mediators of the inflammatory process.[13] Figure 25.3 lists a number of identified mediators, their origin, and pathophysiologic processes with which they are associated.[12] While our understanding of the complex interactions involved in the inflammatory process is still incomplete, the central role of inflammation in producing or increasing bronchial hyperreactivity appears clear. With the increased awareness of the role of inflammation in the pathogenesis of asthma, it has become apparent that therapy directed solely at bronchospasm is incomplete. Attempting to minimize inflammation is an important aspect of asthma therapy.

Inflammatory Cells

Numerous types of leukocytes are present in the circulation, lung tissues, and lumen of airways. The involvement of

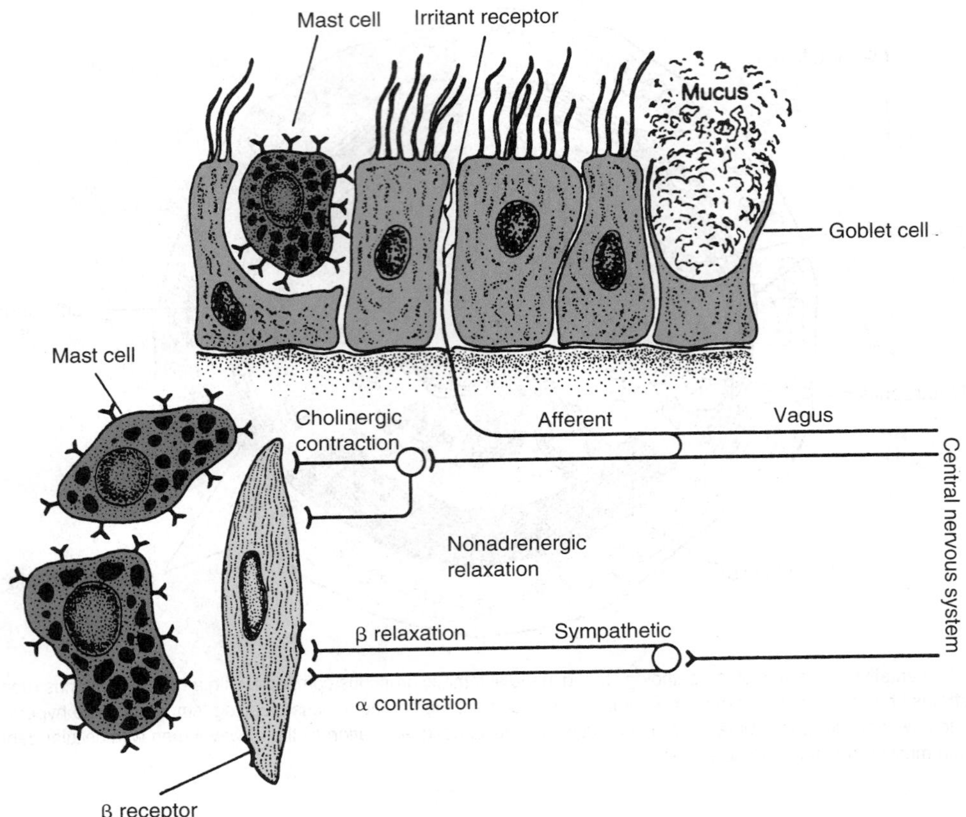

Figure 25.2. Innervation of the airways by the sympathetic, cholinergic, and nonadrenergic inhibitory systems. Mast cell concentration increases from the epithelial lumen to the submucosa.

mast cells, eosinophils, neutrophils, alveolar macrophages, and lymphocytes within the airways and surrounding tissues are important in asthma. The contributions of these cell types to asthma are important in terms of pathogenesis and for understanding how therapy may alter cellular presence and function. Future therapeutic strategies aimed specifically at decreasing the number of inflammatory cells or removing their effect on asthma pathogenesis are being developed.

Mast Cells

The mast cell degranulation is important in the initiation of immediate responses following exposure to allergens. Mast cells are found throughout the walls of the respiratory tract, and increased numbers of these cells (threefold to fivefold) have been described in the airways of asthmatics with an allergic component.[12] Once binding of allergen to cell-bound immunoglobulin E (IgE) occurs, mediators such as histamine; eosinophil and neutrophil chemotatic factors; leukotrienes C_4, D_4, and E_4; prostaglandins; platelet-activating factor; and others are released from mast cells (Fig. 25.3). Histologic examination has revealed decreased numbers of granulated mast cells in the airways of patients who have died from acute asthma attacks, suggesting that mast cell degranulation is a contributing factor in the progression of the disease.[12] Mast cell degranulation is felt to be an integral cause of exercise-induced bronchospasm following either drying or cooling of the airways.[14]

Eosinophils

Eosinophils have long been linked to asthma, primarily due to the association between asthma and peripheral blood eosinophilia.[15] The degree of bronchial reactivity has been related to the number of eosinophils in peripheral blood and bronchoalveolar lavage fluid.[15] Major basic protein (MBP), a constituent of the granules present in the eosinophil, is responsible for damage to airway epithelium and has been found in very high quantities in the sputum of patients with asthma.[15] The damage to airway epithelium and the subsequent disruption of normal physiology may contribute to development of the airway hyperreactivity characteristic of asthma.[15]

Alveolar Macrophages

The role of alveolar macrophages in the pathogenesis of asthma is becoming clearer.[11] The primary function of these cells in the normal airway is to serve as "scavengers," engulfing and digesting bacteria and other foreign materi-

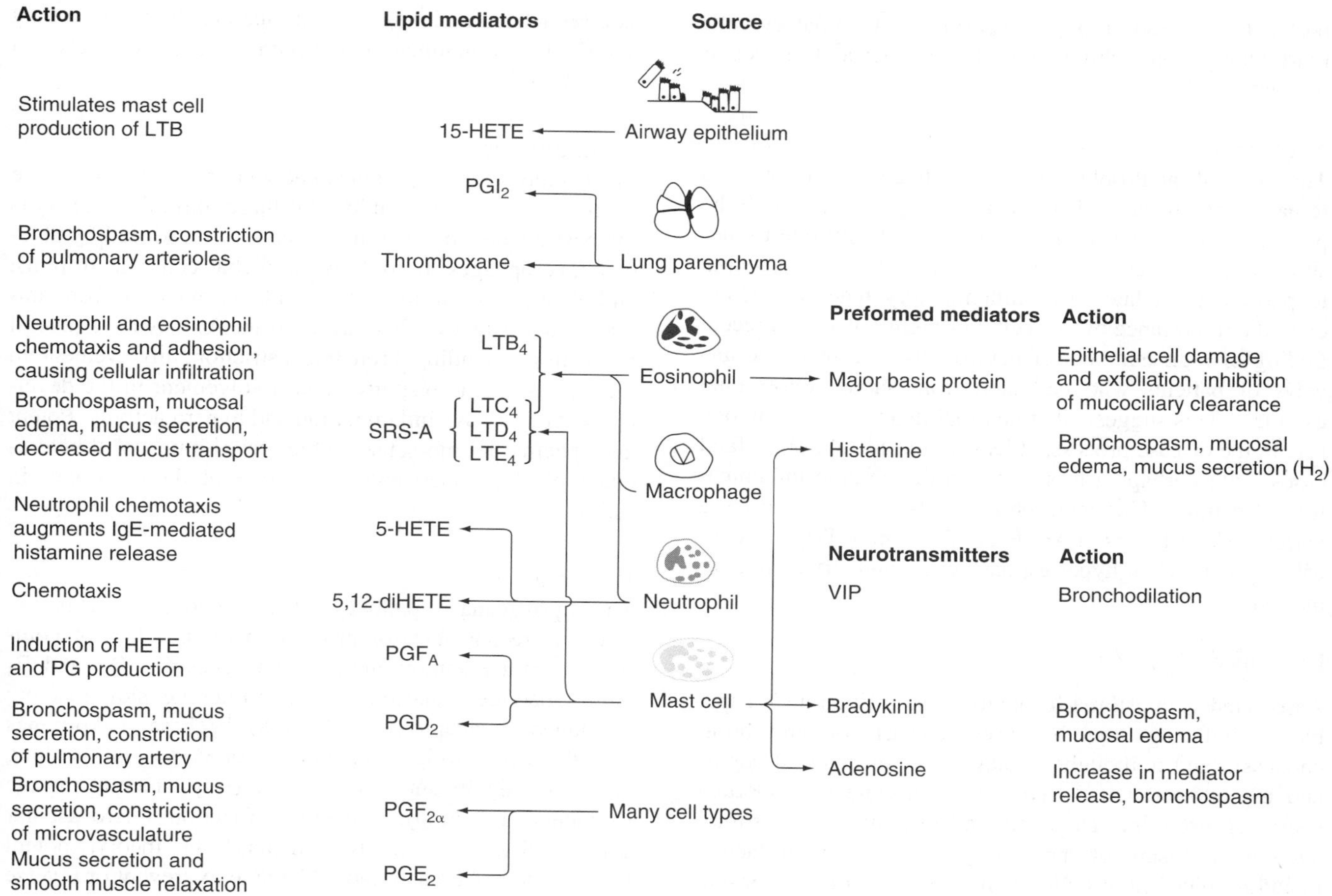

Figure 25.3. Diagrammatic presentation of the source, variety, and pathogenetic effects of lipid and preformed mediators as well as neurotransmitters involved in asthma. See text for details. HETE, hydroxyeicosatetaraenoic acid; PG, prostaglandin; LT, leukotriene; SRS-A, slow-reacting substance of anaphylaxis; VIP, vasoactive intestinal polypeptide.

als. They are found in large and small airways, ideally located for affecting the asthmatic response. A number of mediators produced and released by macrophages have been identified and their roles in initiating and amplifying inflammation in allergic asthma have been determined.[16] A partial list of mediators produced by these cells includes platelet-activating factor, leukotriene B_4, leukotriene C_4, and leukotriene D_4. Additionally, alveolar macrophages are able to produce neutrophil chemotactic factor and eosinophil chemotactic factor.[12] These substances attract neutrophils and eosinophils, which in turn further facilitate the inflammatory process.

T Lymphocytes

In recent years much emphasis has been placed on the role of T lymphocytes in the pathogenesis of asthma, specifically the regulation of inflammation. Several studies have demonstrated increased numbers of T lymphocytes in bronchoalveolar lavage fluid and airway biopsy specimens of asthmatics,[17,18] even in mild and newly diagnosed cases.[19] In addition, the presence of T lymphocytes has been correlated to bronchial hyperresponsiveness.[17] The T_{H2} subset of T lymphocytes has received particular attention due to the profile of cytokines produced and released by these cells, which includes interleukin (IL)-4, IL-5, IL-6, and IL-10, but not IL-2 and interferon gamma (IFN-γ). Conversely, T_{H1} cells secrete IL-2, IFN-γ, and tumor necrosis factor beta (TNF-β), with both T_{H1} and T_{H2} cells producing IL-3, granulocyte-macrophage colony-stimulating factor (GM-CSF), and IFN-α.[20] Evidence for the importance of T_{H2}-like cells in the pathogenesis of allergic inflammation includes their requirement for IgE production by B cells, induction of their proliferation by allergens, production of IL-4 and IL-5 by cells from atopic individuals, and accumulation of cells expressing messenger ribonucleic acid (mRNA) for IL-4 and IL-5 in the airways of atopic asthmatics.[20] Cytokines liberated by T_{H2} cells appear to be intimately involved in inflammation, thus these cells are thought to orchestrate the inflammatory process, particularly microvascular changes, up-regulation of adhesion molecules, migration and activation of inflammatory cells (particularly eosinophils), and other cellular and molecular interactions.[20]

Neutrophils

The role of neutrophils in the pathogenesis of asthma remains somewhat unclear, because they may normally be present in the airways and usually do not infiltrate tissues showing chronic allergic inflammation despite the potential to participate in late-phase inflammatory reactions. However, the importance of this cell was highlighted by a recent finding of high numbers of neutrophils present in the airways of patients who had died from sudden-onset fatal asthma.[21] This suggests that neutrophils may play a pivotal role in the disease process, at least in the sudden-onset fatal cases, with perhaps a lesser role in the chronic inflammation of asthma. The neutrophil can also be a source for a variety of mediators (PAF, PGs, Txs, and LTs) that contribute to bronchial hyperresponsiveness and airway inflammation.

Preformed Mediators

Associated with asthma for many years, histamine is capable of inducing smooth muscle constriction and bronchospasm and is thought to play a role in mucosal edema and mucus secretion.[12] Lung mast cells are an important source of histamine. The release of histamine can be stimulated by exposure of the airway to a variety of factors including physical stimuli (such as exercise) and exposure to relevant allergens.[12]

Membrane-Derived Lipid Mediators

Chemical substances known as phospholipids are found in rich supply in the membranes of most cells involved with inflammation. Several classes of important mediators, including arachidonic acid and its metabolites, prostaglandins, leukotrienes, and platelet-activating factor, are derived from these membrane phospholipids (Fig. 25.3).

Prostaglandins

Once arachidonic acid is released it can be broken down by the enzyme cyclooxygenase to form the prostaglandins. A further breakdown product, prostaglandin D_2, has been well characterized and is a potent bronchoconstricting agent.[12] It is unlikely that prostaglandin D_2 can produce sustained effects on airway function or inflammation; however, its role in asthma remains to be determined. Similarly, prostaglandin $F_{2\alpha}$ is a potent bronchoconstrictor in patients with asthma and can enhance the effects of histamine.[12] It is not clear whether this substance has any other pathophysiologic effects and its specific origin from within the lung is also unknown. Another cyclooxygenase product, prostacyclin (prostaglandin I_2) is known to be produced in the lung. It is unclear whether prostaglandin I_2 is important as a bronchoconstricting agent in humans; however, it may contribute to inflammation and edema due to its effects as a vasodilator.[12]

Thromboxanes

The cyclooxygenase products known as thromboxanes have received increasing attention. Of these, thromboxane A_2 is the best understood. Thromboxane A_2 is produced by alveolar macrophages, fibroblasts, epithelial cells, neutrophils, and platelets within the lung.[12] Indirect evidence from animal models suggests that thromboxane A_2 may have several properties, including bronchoconstriction, involvement in the late asthmatic response, and involvement in the development of airways inflammation and hyperreactivity. Potent and specific thromboxane synthetase inhibitors will be crucial tools for understanding the role of thromboxanes in asthma.

Leukotrienes

The lipoxygenase pathway of arachidonic acid breakdown is responsible for production of the class of compounds called leukotrienes. Leukotrienes C_4, D_4, and E_4 (sulfidopeptide leukotrienes) constitute the slow-reacting substance of anaphylaxis (SRS-A).[11] These leukotrienes are liberated during inflammatory processes in the lung and have significant effects on airway smooth muscle (bronchoconstriction), mucociliary function, microvascular permeability, and airways edema.[11] In theory, potent leukotriene antagonists should be able to prevent or reverse some of the pathologic features of asthma. Specific leukotriene antagonists and 5-lipoxygenase inhibitors are undergoing clinical trials at this time. Zileuton a 5-lipoxygenase inhibitor recently gained approval from an FDA advisory panel for the treatment of asthma.

Platelet-Activating Factor

Thought to be produced by macrophages, eosinophils, and neutrophils within the lung, platelet-activating factor (PAF) is involved in the mediation of many of the important steps in the development of the asthmatic response. These steps include immediate bronchoconstriction and sustained induction of airway hyperreactivity, edema formation, and cellular changes associated with generalized inflammatory responses, including chemotaxis of eosinophils.[12] PAF is the only mediator known to produce a sustained increase in bronchial reactivity.[12] As selective and potent PAF-receptor antagonists are developed and clinical trials are completed, the relative importance of PAF as a mediator in asthma will be more completely understood.

Adhesion Molecules

An important step in the inflammatory process is the adhesion of the various cells to each other and the tissue matrix to facilitate infiltration and migration of these cells to the site of inflammation. To promote this, cell membranes express a number of glycoproteins, or adhesion molecules. Adhesion molecules have additional functions involved in the inflammatory process aside from promoting cell adhesion, including activation of cells and cell-to-cell communication, and promoting cellular migration and infiltration.[22,23] The many adhesion molecules are divided into families on the basis of their chemical structure. These families are the integrins, cadherins, immunoglobulin supergene family, selectins, vascular adressins, and carbohydrate ligands. Those thought to be important in inflammation include the integrins, immunoglobulin supergene family, selectins, and carbohydrate ligands.[23]

Adhesion molecules are found on a variety of cells, such as neutrophils, monocytes, lymphocytes, basophils, eosinophils, granulocytes, platelets, endothelial cells, and epithelial cells[23] and can be expressed or activated by the many inflammatory mediators present in asthma.[22] Thus, complex interactions occur whereby mediators affect expression of adhesion molecules, and adhesion molecules can produce mediators. In addition to these interactions, a major role of adhesion molecules is in the recruitment of leukocytes from the vascular lumen to tissues. The initial step involved in this leukocyte–endothelial cell adhesion cascade is transient, and reversible binding of the adhesion molecule to specific ligands on endothelial cells results in slowing or rolling of the circulating leukocyte along the surface of the vasculature. Activation of the leukocyte or endothelial cell follows in response to a mediator or the initial adhesion event. Finally, firm adhesion, or anchoring, of the leukocyte to the endothelial cell surface allows for diapedesis between endothelial cells and migration of the leukocyte into the extracellular matrix.[23]

While the role of adhesion molecules in the pathogenesis of asthma remains undefined, studies have begun to address the mechanisms of leukocyte infiltration into the airways. The availability of monoclonal antibodies to the functional epitopes of adhesion molecules will facilitate our understanding of their role in inflammation. In addition, specific blocking of adhesion molecules by monoclonal antibodies appears promising as a novel therapeutic approach or compliment to existing anti-inflammatory therapy.

MUCUS PRODUCTION

The mucociliary system is the lung's primary defense mechanism against irritants and infectious agents. Mucus is composed of 95% water and 5% glycoproteins and is produced by bronchial epithelial glands and goblet cells.[24] The lining of the airway consists of a continuous aqueous layer controlled by active ion transport across the epithelium where water moves toward the lumen along the concentration gradient. Catecholamines and vagal stimulation enhance the ion transport and fluid movement.[24] Mucus transport is dependent on the viscoelastic properties of the mucus. Mucus that is either too watery or too viscous will not be optimally transported. The exudative inflammatory process and sloughing of epithelial cells into the airway lumen impairs mucociliary transport. The bronchial glands are increased in size and the goblet cells are increased in size and number in asthma, suggesting an increased production of mucus.[24]

Expectorated mucus from patients with asthma tends to have a high viscosity. The mucous plugs in the airways of patients who died in status asthmaticus are tenacious and tend to be connected by mucous strands to the goblet cells.[24] Asthmatic airways may also become plugged with casts consisting of epithelial and inflammatory cells. While it is tempting to speculate that death from asthma attacks is a result of the mucus plugging resulting in irreversible obstruction, there is no direct evidence for this. Autopsies of asthmatics who died from other causes have shown similar pathology.[12] In addition, some subjects who have died of sudden severe asthma did not show the characteristic mucus plugging on necropsy.[12,24]

AIRWAYS SMOOTH MUSCLE

The smooth muscle of the airways does not form a uniform coat around the airways but is wrapped around in a connecting network best described as a spiral arrangement.[12,24] The muscle contraction displays a sphincteric action that is capable of completely occluding the airway lumen. The airway smooth muscle extends from the trachea through the respiratory bronchioles. When expressed as percent of wall thickness, the smooth muscle represents 5% of the large central airways and up to 20% of the wall thickness in the bronchioles.[12] Total smooth muscle mass decreases rapidly past the terminal bronchioles to the alveoli so the contribution of smooth muscle tone to airway diameter in this region is relatively small.[12] In the large airways of asthmatics, smooth muscle may account for 11% of the wall thickness.[12] Airway smooth muscle contraction *in vivo* is measured indirectly by determining the flow of air into and out of the patient. The difficulties in using changes in airflow as a measurement of smooth muscle contraction have been delineated elsewhere.[12] The relationship between airway diameter and flow is dictated by Poiseuille's law[12]:

$$\Delta P = \frac{8nl}{\pi r^4}$$

where n = viscosity of the air, l = length of the tube, r = radius of the tube, and ΔP = drop in pressure. Because resistance is equal to P divided by airflow, a twofold change in airway diameter would produce a 16-fold change in airflow resistance. It is possible that the increased smooth muscle mass of the asthmatic airways is important in magnifying and maintaining bronchial hyperreactivity in chronic asthma.[12,24] However, it appears that the hypertrophy and hyperplasia are secondary processes caused by chronic stimulation and are not the primary cause of bronchial hyperreactivity.[12,24]

NERVOUS SYSTEM

The airway is innervated by parasympathetic, sympathetic, and nonadrenergic inhibitory nerves (Fig. 25.2). Parasympathetic innervation of the smooth muscle consists of efferent motor fibers contained in the vagus nerves and sensory afferent fibers in the vagus and other nerves.[12] The normal resting tone of human airway smooth muscle is maintained by vagal efferent activity.[12] Maximum bronchoconstriction mediated by vagal stimulation occurs in the small bronchi and is absent in the small bronchioles.[12] The nonmyelinated C fibers of the afferent system lie immediately beneath the tight junctions between epithelial cells lining the airway lumen.[12] These endings probably represent the irritant receptors of the airways. Stimulation of these irritant receptors by mechanical stimulation, chemical and particulate irritants, and pharmacologic agents such as histamine produces reflex bronchoconstriction.[12] The sympathetic innervation of the airway smooth muscle is sparse and does not directly control airway smooth muscle tone.[12] All airway smooth muscle contains noninnervated β_2-adrenergic receptors that produce bronchodilation.[12] Circulating catecholamines play an important role in regulating bronchial tone. There is some evidence for α-adrenergic receptors in the major resistant airways. Stimulation of these receptors produces bronchoconstriction that is enhanced by pretreatment with histamine.[24] The importance of these receptors in asthma is unknown; however, specific α-adrenergic blockers have minimal effect on asthma.[12] One theory on the pathogenesis of bronchial hyperreactivity is that asthma represents a relative β-adrenergic blockade. The demonstration of a β-adrenergic defect in asthmatic patients has been inconsistent, and the production of β blockade in normal subjects is insufficient, by itself, to cause bronchial hyperreactivity. Recent studies have suggested the existence of a nonadrenergic, noncholinergic (NANC) nervous system in the trachea and bronchi. The importance of this system is still unknown largely because the exact neurotransmitters are unknown. It has recently been postulated that a defect in the nonadrenergic inhibitory system exists in asthma, as a result of the lack of significant amounts of the neurotransmitter vasoactive intestinal peptide (VIP).[12] NANC excitatory neuropeptides such as substance P and neurokinin A are released by C-fiber sensory nerve endings.[12] The NANC system may play an important role in amplifying inflammation in asthma.

CLINICAL PRESENTATION

The heterogeneity of asthma appears most obvious when listing the diverse triggers of bronchospasm in asthmatic subjects (Table 25.1). In the past, a good deal of the confusion concerning the definition and etiology of asthma centered on the inclusion of the various triggering events as the etiology. Thus, asthma has been variously defined as an allergic, emotional, and infectious disease. However, it has become clear that asthma is first a lung disease, and specific triggering events have relative degrees of importance from patient to patient. Epidemiologic studies support the concept of a genetic predisposition to the development of asthma.[25] Studies of occupational asthma and the induction of hyperreactivity in healthy individuals emphasize the effect of environment on the development of asthma.[24,25] Asthma is still frequently classified according to its predominant trigger; however, it should be emphasized that this method of classification is at best arbitrary and many patients respond to a number of stimuli. Indeed it is the uniform increased responsiveness to challenge with the nonspecific stimuli methacholine, histamine, and exercise that is often used to define and diagnose asthma.

CHRONIC ASTHMA

Classic asthma is characterized by episodic dyspnea associated with wheezing; however, the clinical presentation of asthma is as diverse as the number of triggering events.[11,26] Although wheezing is the characteristic symptom of asthma, the medical literature is replete with the warning that "not all that wheezes is asthma." A wheeze is a high-pitched, whistling sound created by turbulent airflow through an obstructed airway so that any condition that produces significant obstruction can result in wheezing as a symptom. In addition, "all of asthma does not wheeze" is an equally justifiable warning. Patients may present with a chronic persistent cough as their only symptom.[11]

The diagnosis of asthma is based primarily on a good history of recurrent episodes of dyspnea and/or wheezing.[2,27] The patient may complain of a feeling of tightness in the chest or sometimes a burning sensation. The patient may have a family history of allergy or asthma or have symptoms of allergic rhinitis.[27] A history of exercise or cold air precipitating the dyspnea or an association of increased symptoms during specific allergen seasons would also point to asthma.

Asthma has a widely variable presentation from chronic daily symptoms to only intermittent symptoms. The intervals between symptoms could be weeks, months, or years. It is a disease characterized by recurrent exacerbations and remissions. The next variable is severity. The intermittent and/or chronic nature of symptoms does not necessarily determine the severity of symptoms during exacerbations. The severity is primarily determined by the

TABLE 25.1. REPRESENTATIVE LIST OF AGENTS AND EVENTS TRIGGERING ASTHMA

Trigger	Mechanism
Respiratory infection Respiratory syncytial virus (RSV), rhinovirus, influenza, parainfluenza, *Mycoplasma* pneumonia	Inflammation and epithelial damage sensitizing cholinergic irritant receptors; virus-induced relative β-blockade possibly contributes
Allergens Airborne pollens (grasses, trees, weeds), house dust, animal danders, dust mites, insect parts, fungal spores, food	IgE-mediated mast cell mediator release
Exercise	Hyperventilation with loss of water and cooling of the airways and mast cell mediator release
Occupational stimuli Animal handlers; antibiotic drug manufacturing; bakers (flour dust); spice and enzyme workers; printers (arabic gum); chemical workers (azo dyes, anthraquinone, ethylenediamine, toluene diisocyanates, meat wrappers heated polyvinyl chloride); plastics, rubber, and wood workers (formaldehyde, western red cedar, dimethylethanolamine, anhydrides)	IgE-mediated mast cell release Airway epithelial damage, increased permeability and sensitization of irritant receptors
Environment Cold air, ozone, sulfur dioxide, nitrogen dioxide	Unknown (irritation?); epithelial damage and neutrophil infiltration
Emotions Anxiety, fatigue, stress, laughter	Parasympathetic stimulation; augments preexisting event, generally not a primary event
Drugs	See text for discussion

number of medications required to adequately control patients' symptoms. Patients can present with mild intermittent symptoms that require no medications or only occasional use of inhaled bronchodilators to severe chronic asthma symptoms despite receiving multiple medications.

Chronic Severe Asthma

Chronic severe asthma is defined by the requirement of continuous or frequent intermittent glucocorticoids for control of symptoms. These patients frequently demonstrate significant residual pulmonary function abnormalities and require chronic bronchodilator therapy for control of symptoms. These patients can be frustrating for the general practitioner and specialist alike, and therefore it is fortunate that they comprise a relatively small percentage of all asthmatics. Short lapses in compliance with the treatment regimen can lead to hospitalization with life-threatening asthma attacks. The most severe patients may infrequently require hospitalization for acute attacks of asthma despite compliance with maximum dosages of chronic medications. In this sense, they are not unlike the "brittle diabetics" who need only a small insult to tip the balance. These patients are in the greatest danger of death from asthma and present the greatest challenge to the clinicians caring for them. The clinician is frequently forced to assess the risk/benefit ratio of the therapeutic plan because it is frequently necessary to use a number of drugs including daily long-term oral glucocorticoids at their maximum recommended dosages.

ACUTE SEVERE ASTHMA

Uncontrolled asthma, with its inherent variability, can progress to an acute state where inflammation, airways edema, excessive accumulation of mucus, and severe bronchospasm result in a profound airways narrowing, which is poorly responsive to usual bronchodilator therapy. This clinical situation is a common circumstance necessitating emergency department care. In many cases, emergency department visits for acute severe asthma represent the failure of an adequate therapeutic regimen for chronic asthma. Patients present with severe dyspnea, inspiratory as well as expiratory wheezing, anxiety, tachypnea, tachycardia, and in severe cases cyanosis. They exhibit supraclavicular and intercostal retractions, a hyperinflated chest, and coughing. In severe obstruction, air movement in and out of the lungs is substantially decreased so that wheezing may actually decrease.

ASTHMA TRIGGERS

ALLERGIC ASTHMA

An allergic component can be demonstrated in 35–55% of asthmatic patients, and this may be higher in childhood asthma.[2,11,26] The allergens (Table 25.1) that provoke asthma are airborne and evoke the asthmatic response through the classical allergic pathway, depicted in Fig. 25.4.

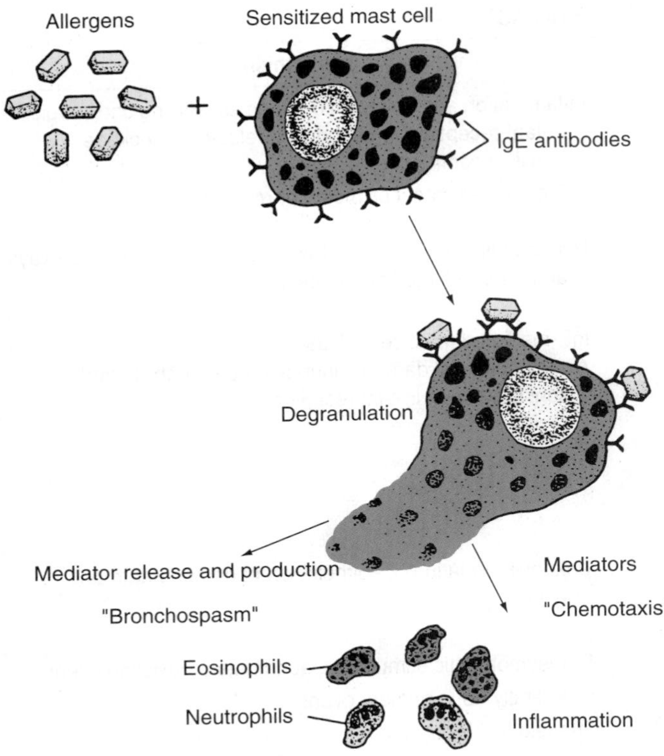

Figure 25.4. IgE-mediated allergic response. Allergens produce steric changes in a mast cell, leading to the spillage of granules with preformed mediators as well as initiating production of other mediators of anaphylaxis through the lipoxygenase pathway.

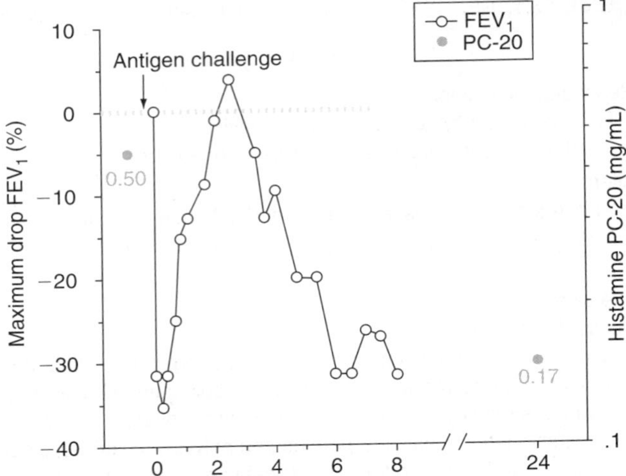

Figure 25.5. Biphasic response to allergen exposure in a sensitive patient with asthma. The immediate response occurs within 10–30 minutes following exposure and may revert to baseline without intervention. The late asthmatic response occurs within 2–8 hours following exposure. The provocative concentration of inhaled histamine, which produces a 20% decrease in forced expiratory volume in 1 second (FEV_1) (PC-20), an index of airways reactivity, also shows a marked decrease following development of a late asthmatic response. This is suggestive of an increase in the propensity of the airways to constrict to nonspecific stimuli.

The role of allergy in the etiology of asthma has been controversial and asthma has been considered an allergic disease by many.[27,28] Although the allergic reaction plays an important role in the atopic asthmatic patient, atopy is not necessary for the development of asthma and not all atopic individuals develop asthma.[11] Many patients with hay fever will develop some airway hyperreactivity (although less than asthmatics) during their allergen season.

When allergic asthmatics are given an inhalational challenge with an allergen to which they are sensitized, the patients demonstrate an immediate asthmatic reaction (EAR) (Fig. 25.5). The reaction is characterized by a drop in pulmonary function that reaches maximum intensity in 10–20 minutes and reverses spontaneously by 60–120 minutes.[25] In addition, many subjects experience a late asthmatic reaction (Fig. 25.5) that begins 4 hours after the challenge, reaches maximum intensity in 6–8 hours, is often more severe than the immediate response, and may last as long as 24 hours. The late asthmatic reaction (LAR) may be the pathogenetic mechanism for inducing and maintaining bronchial hyperreactivity in atopic asthmatics.[25] Patients who experience an LAR demonstrate increased responsiveness to methacholine, histamine, and exercise that may last up to 6 weeks, while subjects who only experience the immediate response demonstrate no increased bronchial reactivity.[25] The degree of hyperresponsiveness and its duration correlate with the intensity of the LAR. The LAR is associated with increased serum concentrations of neutrophil and eosinophil chemotactic factors and the influx of neutrophils and eosinophils into the tissue as well as the degranulation of mast cells.[25] The LAR is associated with greater degrees of obstruction in small airways and air trapping than occur with the immediate response. The immediate response, due to the degranulation of mast cells and preformed mediator (histamine) release, is easily blocked or reversed with inhaled β_2 agonists.[29] Theophylline, anticholinergics, and oral β_2 agonists blunt the response but are inconsistently effective.[30] The LAR is not prevented by pretreatment with any of these bronchodilators, although the bronchospastic component may be attenuated if therapeutic doses are administered at the time of the LAR. Glucocorticoid pretreatment does not alter the EAR but prevents the LAR, whereas pretreatment with cromolyn sodium or nedocromil blocks both responses.[30] Long-term treatment with glucocorticoids can attenuate the immediate response by decreasing overall bronchial hyperresponsiveness.[30]

Clinically, allergic asthmatics develop increased bronchial hyperreactivity with increased exposure to allergens during a pollen season.[28] Avoidance of the pollen or prophylaxis with cromolyn sodium prevents the increased bronchial hyperreactivity.[26,28] Studies have shown that long-term therapy with both cromolyn sodium and glucocorticoids reduces bronchial hyperreactivity.[30] In contrast, long-term therapy with β_2 agonists and theophylline has not been associated with similar decreases in bronchial hyperreactivity.[26,30]

EXERCISE-INDUCED ASTHMA

During vigorous exercise, pulmonary function in asthmatic patients (as measured by forced expiratory maneuvers) increases during the first few minutes but then begins to decrease after 6–8 minutes (Fig. 25.6). Exercise-induced asthma (EIA) is defined as a drop in forced expiratory volume in 1 second (FEV_1) of greater than 15–20% of baseline (preexercise value).[2,14] Most studies suggest that 70–90% of all asthmatics experience EIA.[2] The exact pathogenesis of EIA is unknown; however, heat loss and or water loss from the central airways appears to play an important role.[14] EIA is more easily provoked in cold, dry air, and warm, humid air can blunt or block it.[14]

Studies using isocapnic hyperventilation of cold air and inhalation of hypertonic saline have demonstrated sim-ilar degrees of bronchospasm as seen in EIA.[14] A number of studies have demonstrated increased plasma histamine and tryptase concentrations during EIA, suggesting a role for mast cell degranulation. In addition, pretreatment with cro-molyn sodium, a drug that stabilizes mast cells, inhibits EIA and inhibits the associated rise in neutrophil chemotactic factor.[14] A small number of patients with EIA will have a late response similar to the LAR and associated with a secondary rise in neutrophil chemotactic factor.[14]

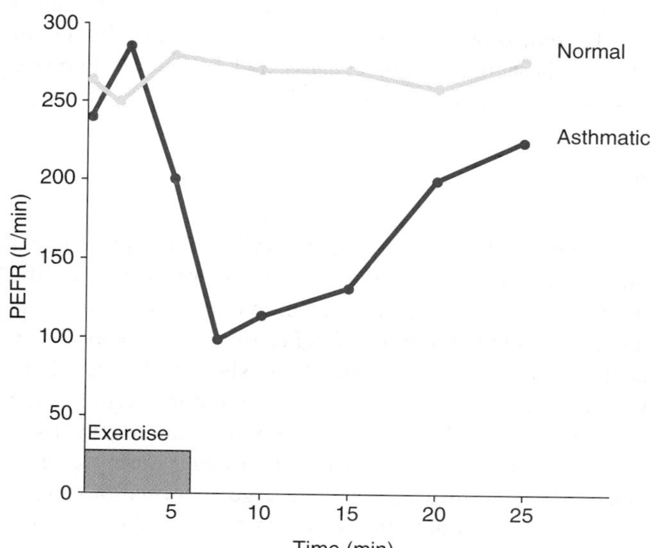

Figure 25.6. Typical responses to exercise in a normal subject and an asthmatic subject. Note the initial bronchodilation. PEFR, peak expiratory flow rate.

A refractory period with EIA lasts up to 3 hours after exercise. During this period, repeat exercise of the same intensity either produces no decrease in pulmonary functions or a drop of less than 50% of the initial response.[14,24] The refractory period is thought to be caused by an acute depletion of mast cell mediators and time required for their repletion. Patients with known refractoriness to exercise will still respond to histamine so that acute hyporesponsiveness of airway smooth muscle does not appear to be a factor.[14,24]

EIA is believed to be a reflection of the increased hyperreactivity of asthmatics. A correlation, though not perfect, exists between EIA and reactivity to histamine and methacholine.[24] Other patient groups with increased airway reactivity (postviral infection, cystic fibrosis, hay fever) show bronchoconstriction after exercise to a lesser degree (5–10%) than asthmatics (20–40%).[14] Asthmatics will not always demonstrate the same sensitivity. During periods of remission, they often have a decreased sensitivity to the same degree of exercise. Finally, a number of children and adults with EIA are otherwise normal, without symptoms or abnormal pulmonary function.

NOCTURNAL ASTHMA

Worsening of asthma during sleep is referred to as nocturnal asthma. Patients with nocturnal asthma exhibit significant falls in pulmonary function between bedtime and awakening.[31] Although the pathogenesis of this phenomenon is unknown, it has been associated with diurnal patterns of endogenous cortisol secretion and circulating epinephrine.[31] Direct evidence for an inflammatory component to nocturnal asthma includes increased circulating histamine and activated eosinophils at night associated with increased hyperresponsiveness to methacholine.[32] It has been postulated that the decrease in endogenous hormones results in enhanced pulmonary T-cell release of proinflammatory cytokines, which then activates the airway inflammatory cells at night.[31]

Numerous other factors that may affect nocturnal worsening of asthma, including allergies and improper environmental control, gastroesophageal reflux, and sinusitis, must also be considered when evaluating these patients.[33] Some experts consider nocturnal asthma to be a separate entity and advocate therapy with long-acting bronchodilators,[32] while others consider it a symptom of inadequately treated chronic asthma and advocate increased anti-inflammatory therapy.[24]

MISCELLANEOUS FACTORS

Viral Infections

Viral upper respiratory infections are associated with exacerbations of asthma. Well-controlled investigations have convincingly demonstrated that viral infections and not bacteria are primarily responsible for exacerbations of asthma.[2,34] Viral upper respiratory tract infections are a major precipitant of acute asthma in children, being involved in up to 20–40% of acute episodes.[34] The viruses isolated most frequently are respiratory syncytial virus (RSV), parainfluenza virus, coronavirus, rhinovirus, and influenza viruses.[34] Although the exact mechanism is unknown, the inflammatory response to viral infection is thought to be directly associated with the increasing bronchial hyperresponsiveness. Certain viruses (RSV and parainfluenza) are capable of inducing specific IgE antibodies, and viral infections increase the incidence of LAR responses to specific allergen exposure.[34] The increase in asthma symptoms and bronchial hyperresponsiveness that occurs may last for days or weeks following resolution of the symptoms of the viral infection.

Environmental and Occupational Factors

Agents and events and the mechanisms that are known to trigger asthma are listed in Table 25.1. The general mechanisms are unknown, but it is presumably caused by epithelial damage and inflammation in the airway mucosa. Ozone and sulfur dioxide, common components of air pollution, have been used to induce airways hyperreactivity in animals. Exposure to ozone 0.2 ppm for 2 to 3 hours can induce bronchoconstriction and increase bronchial reactivity in asthmatics.[24] Sulfur dioxide in the ambient atmosphere is highly irritating, but it is not known how it induces bronchoconstriction. Pretreatment with cromolyn sodium will block the obstruction, implicating mast cell or irritant receptor involvement.[24] Asthma produced by repeated prolonged exposure to industrial inhalants is a significant health problem. It has been estimated that occupational asthma accounts for 2% of all asthmatic persons.[2] Persons with occupational asthma have the typical symptoms of asthma with cough, dyspnea, and wheeze. Typically, the symptoms are related to work with improvement on weekends and vacations.[24] In some instances, symptoms may persist even after termination of exposure.[2]

Psychologic Factors

Emotions and stress rarely precipitate attacks of asthma, but more commonly worsen an attack in progress.[2] Bronchoconstriction from psychologic factors appears to be primarily mediated through excess parasympathetic input.[24] Atropine has been shown to block experimental psychogenic bronchoconstriction.[24] It is most important to emphasize to patients and to parents of asthmatic children that asthma is not an emotional disease; however, calming influences and relaxation techniques may benefit the patient who becomes severely emotionally distraught during asthma attacks.

Sinusitis/Rhinitis

Disorders of the upper respiratory tract, particularly sinusitis and rhinitis, have been linked with asthma for many years. As many as 40–50% of asthmatics have abnormal sinus radiographs.[33] Studies have shown that asthma symptoms improve with treatment of sinusitis.[33] The mechanism by which sinusitis aggravates asthma is unknown. Transport of mucus chemotactic factors, and inflammatory mediators from nasal passages into the lung may accentuate bronchial hyperresponsiveness.

OTHER FACTORS

Gastroesophageal reflux has been associated with asthma for many years. Reflux of acidic gastric contents into the esophagus is thought to initiate a vagally mediated reflex bronchoconstriction.[33] Also of concern is that most medications that decrease airways smooth muscle tone have a relaxant effect on gastroesophageal sphincter tone as well. The therapeutic approach most commonly taken for patients with gastroesophageal reflux and asthma is to initiate standard antireflux therapy and observe the asthma symptoms.

Premenstrual worsening of asthma has been reported in as many as 33% of women in some studies.[33] While other studies have not confirmed these results, others have noted worsening of pulmonary functions associated with menstruation even in women not aware of worsening of symptoms.[33] This and asthma in pregnancy have been a poorly studied phenomenon. Studies would indicate that, in general, bronchial responsiveness and symptoms improve in asthmatics during pregnancy.[24]

BLOOD GAS MEASUREMENT

Gas exchange at the alveoli–capillary interface is dependent on ventilation (V_a), or the mechanical properties of the lung, perfusion (Q), the flow of blood, and diffusion of the gases across the membrane. Studies of diffusion capacity in acute asthma indicate that it is slightly increased or unchanged.[24] Arterial hypoxia is common during acute asthma attacks and is caused by significant derangements in V_a/Q relationships.[24] The airway narrowing during asthma attacks, though diffuse, results in large abnormalities in the distribution of ventilation. The perfusion abnormalities appear to be secondary to changes in ventilation. The normal response to alveolar hypoxia is active vasoconstriction to shunt blood flow to better ventilated areas.[24] Unfortunately, the V_a and Q are not perfectly matched in acute asthma. This may in part be caused by the increased vascu-

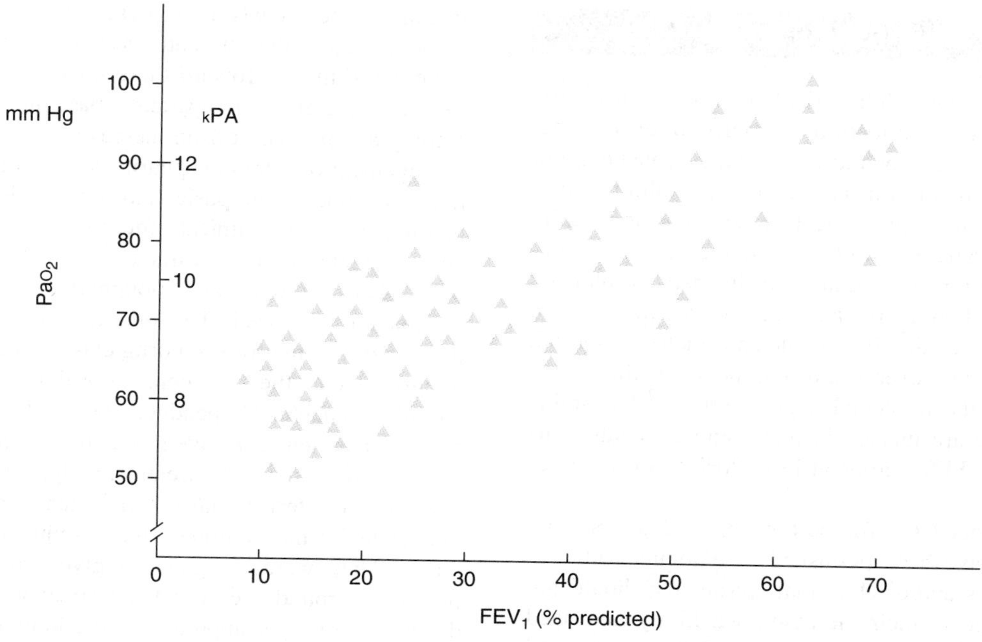

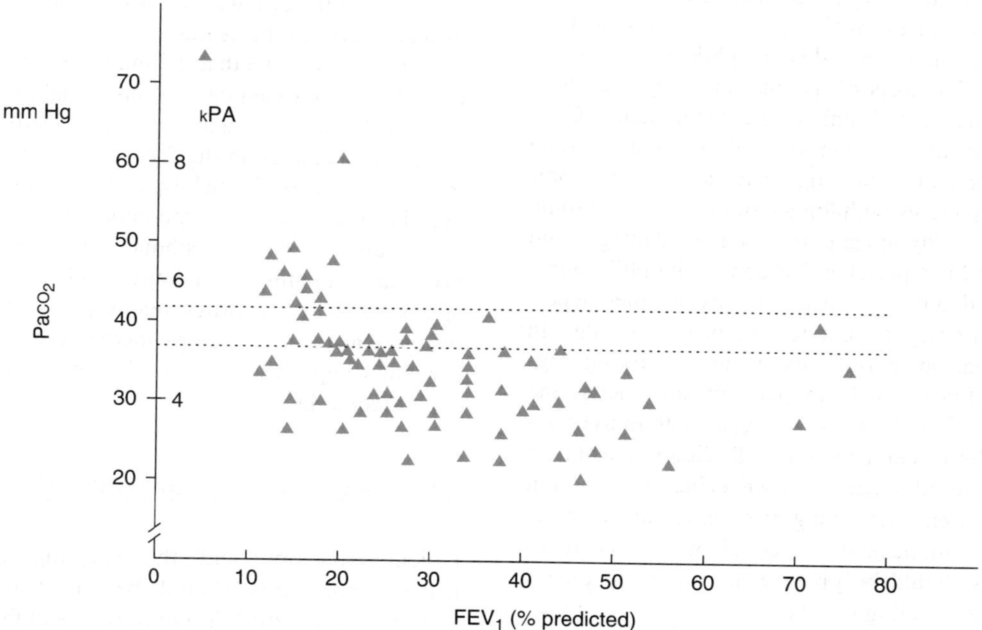

Figure 25.7. Effect of increasing airway obstruction on arterial (A) PaO_2 and (B) PaCO_2. The dashed lines show the normal range of PaCO_2. *(From McFadden ER Jr, Lyons HA. Arterial blood gas tension in asthma. N Engl J Med 1968;278:1029, with permission.)*

lar resistance produced by lung hyperinflation.[24] Figure 25.7 demonstrates the effect of increasing airway obstruction on arterial blood gases. When lungs initially become obstructed, patients demonstrate a marked respiratory drive thought to be caused by the stimulation of the irritant receptors because it is not obliterated by correcting the hypoxemia.[24] As a result, the asthmatic tends to "blow off" carbon dioxide and the arterial carbon dioxide concentration decreases (Fig. 25.7). Unfortunately, the patient is forced to breathe at higher lung volumes because of air trapping. This requires the use of accessory respiratory muscles. When the respiratory muscles begin to fatigue, the patient will retain carbon dioxide, and this may signal impending respiratory failure.

Diagnostic Tests

In the older child and adult patient in whom spirometric evaluations can be performed, abnormal pulmonary functions that improve 15% or more following bronchodilator administration help confirm the diagnosis.[2] Failure of pulmonary functions to improve acutely does not necessarily rule out asthma. Patients with long-standing disease or substantial inflammation may require an intensive prolonged course of bronchodilators and glucocorticoids before reversibility is detected.[24] If baseline spirometry is normal, challenge testing with exercise, histamine, or methacholine can be used to elicit bronchial hyperreactivity.[2] Histamine and methacholine are inhaled in increasing concentrations until the patient's FEV_1 drops at least 20% from the baseline.[13,26]

Standard procedures for performing and interpreting challenge tests have been published.[2,24] Patients with significant symptoms and/or abnormal spirometry should not be challenged due to their increased sensitivity and need not be challenged for diagnostic purposes.[24] Spirometry and bronchoprovocation have been shown to be more reliable indicators of bronchial hyperreactivity than history of wheezing and physical exam.[24] Studies for atopy such as serum IgE and sputum and blood eosinophils are not necessary to make the diagnosis of asthma, but they may help differentiate asthma from chronic bronchitis in adults. Clinically, this distinction is often difficult to make. Some patients with chronic bronchitis may have a reversible component and some patients with long-standing severe chronic asthma may have significant irreversible damage and obstruction. Very high peripheral blood eosinophil counts may point to the diagnosis of aspergillosis or other hypereosinophilic syndromes.[33] Skin testing is of no value in diagnosing asthma, but may be useful in identifying triggers. In small infants unable to perform spirometry, the diagnosis is more difficult. They may demonstrate hyperinflation on the chest roentgenogram. Radiologic exam is helpful in ruling out other causes of wheezing (e.g., foreign body aspiration, parenchymal lung disease, cardiac disease, and congenital anomalies).[2] In place of pulmonary functions, the parents should be given a diary card to record symptoms and precipitating events.

Treatment

The NAEP has provided the following goals for asthma management: "1) Maintain normal activity levels (including exercise); 2) Maintain (near) "normal" pulmonary function rates; 3) Prevent chronic and troublesome symptoms (e.g., coughing or breathlessness in the night, in the early morning, or after exertion); 4) Prevent recurrent exacerbations of asthma; 5) Avoid adverse effects from asthma medication."[2] These goals are represented in expanded form in Appendix 25.1 (the International Consensus Report's treatment algorithm).[27] Toward these goals, every effort should be made to decrease the patient's baseline airways hyperreactivity and prevent it from increasing. The mainstay of the management of asthma is pharmacologic therapy. There are numerous books, symposia, and reviews detailing the basic pharmacology and clinical efficacy of the various pharmacologic agents used in asthma.[2,11,24,26,35–38] In this section both pharmacologic and nonpharmacologic therapy of asthma are reviewed. The pharmacology relevant to the therapy of asthma for each drug class will be discussed and integrated into the treatment algorithms illustrated at the end of the chapter (Appendixes 25.1 and 25.2). In addition, current treatment controversies and experimental therapies will be addressed. The treatment algorithms were developed by the International Asthma Management Project and published by the National Heart, Lung, and Blood Institute.[27] They were designed to give primary health care providers around the world a framework from which to develop the proper approach to the individualized therapy of patients and are not to be used as practice standards. The heterogeneity of asthma demands an individualized approach to therapy with the four basic goals of therapy as primary outcome measures.[2]

The knowledge that inflammation plays a primary role in both the increased chronic bronchial hyperreactivity and the development of acute severe exacerbations in asthma has led to a change in the focus of therapy from the symptomatic relief of bronchospasm to preventing and suppressing the underlying inflammation.[2,11,26,27] Thus current therapeutic options in asthma consist of rescue, prophylaxis, and suppressive therapy.[2,27] The currently accepted approach is to use drugs that suppress the inflammatory response as primary therapy thereby reducing the degree of bronchial hyperreactivity and improving long-term control and outcome in asthma.

NONPHARMACOLOGIC MANAGEMENT

Patient education and the teaching of patient self-management skills should be the cornerstone of any treatment program.[2] There are a number of published self-management programs for children and adults available through local American Lung Association chapters and asthma treatment centers and nationally through the National Heart, Lung, and Blood Institute and the Asthma and Allergy Foundation of America.[24,39] Asthma self-management programs have been shown to improve patient adherence to medication regimens, improve self-management skills, and improve utilization of health care services.[39] The object of these programs is to develop a partnership relationship between the patient and the health care provider.

Self-management programs instruct patients in the pathogenesis of asthma and the appropriate use of their medications, but they focus principally on teaching patients to recognize triggers for their asthma and how to recognize early signs of deterioration. Use of objective measurements of airflow obstruction with a home peak flow meter is integral to many of the programs.[39] However, a recent study would suggest that routine peak flow monitoring in and of itself does not improve patient outcomes.[40] Patient education has proven successful regardless of the health professional who provided the information (physician, nurse, or pharmacist).

The NAEP Expert Panel has advocated the use of objective pulmonary function monitoring at home with portable peak expiratory flow meters as a means of improving the care of asthmatics.[2] They have recommended a system based on a traffic light scenario: green zone equal to 80–100% of normal or personal best; yellow zone equal to 50–80% of normal; and red zone less than 50% of normal peak flows. The yellow zone is cautionary and requires increasing bronchodilation as needed and either increasing the anti-inflammatory dose or beginning prednisone if not improved. The red zone warrants contacting the patient's health care provider.[2] This may be of particular importance for the chronic severe asthmatic who may not be able to detect deterioration of lung function. It can also assist the health professional to determine the next level of therapy for a specific patient. The provision of written treatment plans enhances the success of education and peak flow monitoring.[39,40]

In patients with known allergenic triggers for their asthma, allergen avoidance has resulted in an improvement in symptoms, a reduction in medications, and a decrease in bronchial hyperreactivity.[28] Relatively simple environmental controls for patients allergic to house dust such as removing carpeting from bedrooms and using plastic pillow and mattress covers can reduce symptoms and need for medications.[28] Therefore, obvious environmental triggers (i.e., animals) should be avoided; however, there is very little evidence that extensive environmental controls (i.e., home air filtering systems) are of any value. Patients who smoke should be encouraged to stop. Numerous studies have shown that asthmatic children of smoking parents do worse than children of nonsmoking parents.[26]

The role of immunotherapy (i.e., allergy shots) in asthma, although a proven and accepted therapy for allergic rhinitis, is still controversial.[26,28] Some studies have shown that immunotherapy of patients with a very specific allergy reduces the number of late asthmatic responses and decreases bronchial sensitivity to the allergen while others have shown no effect.[26] A recent meta-analysis of immunotherapy trials suggested a positive benefit for specific immunotherapy against known allergens, however, the benefit was small in comparison to placebo.[41] Further studies comparing immunotherapy to pharmacotherapy are warranted to determine the role for immunotherapy in asthma treatment.[28]

Oxygen therapy is indicated in patients requiring emergency therapy for acute severe asthma.[2,24,38] Oxygen reverses bronchial hyperreactivity induced by hypoxemia, as well as the hemoglobin desaturation produced by V_a/Q mismatching. Patients hospitalized with acute severe asthma should be given adequate maintenance hydration in order to mobilize secretions; however, excessive hydration should be avoided to prevent excessive lung fluid at a time when patients have inflammation and bronchial edema.[24]

PHARMACOLOGIC MANAGEMENT

β_2 Agonists

The β_2 agonists are the most effective bronchodilators available. β_2-Adrenergic receptor stimulation activates adenyl cyclase, which produces an increase in intracellular cyclic AMP.[35] This increase results in a decrease in unbound intracellular calcium, producing smooth muscle relaxation, mast cell membrane stabilization, and skeletal muscle stimulation.[24,35] β_2-Adrenergic stimulation also activates Na^+/K^+-ATPase, produces gluconeogenesis, and enhances insulin secretion. These three effects combine to produce a mild to moderate decrease in serum potassium concentration by driving potassium intracellularly.[35] The chronotropic response to β_2 agonists is mediated in part by baroreceptor reflex mechanisms as a result of the drop in blood pressure from vascular smooth muscle relaxation, as well as by direct stimulation of cardiac β_2 receptors and some β_1 stimulation at high concentrations.[24,35] Table 25.2 lists the pharmacologic effects of adrenergic receptor stimulation. Because the excessive cardiac stimulation produces cardiac arrhythmias and the inotropic effect enhancing myocardial oxygen consumption leads to myocardial necrosis, there is no rationale for using non-β_2-selective agonists in the treatment of asthma.[24,37]

Table 25.3 compares the various β-adrenergic agonists in terms of selectivity, potency, oral activity, and duration of action. The β_2 agonists are functional or physiologic antagonists in that they relax airway smooth muscle regardless of the mechanism for constriction.[24,35] When administered in equipotent doses, all the drugs will produce the same intensity of response; the only differences will be in duration of action and cardiac toxicity. All of the β agonists are more bronchoselective when administered by the aerosol route.[24,35] Differences in myocardial effects are discernible between selective and nonselective agents even when administered as aerosols, particularly at the higher doses used for acute severe asthma.

The aerosol administration of β_2 agonists not only enhances bronchoselectivity but provides a more rapid response and a greater degree of protection against provo-

TABLE 25.2. PHARMACOLOGIC RESPONSES TO SYMPATHOMIMETIC STIMULATION

Tissue	Receptor Type	Response
Airways	β_2	Bronchodilation, increased ciliary beat, increased mucus production, and inhibition of histamine release from mast cells
	α	Bronchoconstriction?
Heart	β_1	Chronotropic, inotropic
	β_2	Chronotropic
Vasculature	β_2	Vasodilatation
	α	Vasoconstriction
Skeletal	β_2	Increased neuromuscular transmission muscle (tremor, increased strength of contraction)
Uterus	β_2	Relaxation (tocolysis)
Metabolic	α, β_1	Glycogenolysis, lipolysis
	β_2	Gluconeogenesis, lactic acidemia, hypokalemia
Mast cells	α	Augment mediator release
	β_2	Inhibit mediator

cations that induce bronchospasm, such as exercise and allergen challenges, than does systemic administration. Currently, the only disadvantage to aerosol administration of β_2 agonists is the relative complexity of administration. The two new long-acting β_2 agonists, formoterol and the newly FDA-approved salmeterol, provide long-lasting protection (12 or more hours) when administered as aerosols.[42] Salmeterol is more β_2 selective than albuterol.[43] However, it is more bronchoselective by virtue of its property of remaining in the lung, which produces its longer duration.[42,43] Because aerosol administration is so important to the use of β_2 agonists and other antiasthmatics, we discuss the various aerosol delivery techniques at the end of this section.

The dose–response relationship for β_2-agonist-induced bronchodilation has been extensively studied and two aspects have significant clinical relevance. Both the intensity and duration of response are dose dependent, and more important, the dose–response is a dynamic relationship. At increasing levels of baseline bronchoconstriction (irrespective of the stimulus), the dose–response curve is shifted to the right and the duration of bronchodilation is decreased.[24,35] This is reflected in the need for higher, more frequent doses in acute asthma exacerbations and why the duration of protection against significant provocation is much less than the duration of bronchodilation in chronic stable asthma (Table 25.3). The ability to increase the dose of the short-acting aerosolized β_2 agonists by as much as 5-fold to 10-fold over those doses producing adequate bronchodilation in chronic stable asthmatics is what contributes to their efficacy in reversing the bronchospasm of acute severe asthma.[38]

Despite the fact that β_2 agonists are potent inhibitors of mast cell degranulation they do not inhibit the late asthmatic response to allergen challenge or the subsequent bronchial hyperresponsiveness.[12,24] Initial studies suggested that the long-acting β_2 agonists formoterol and salmeterol inhibited the LAR to allergen challenge and prevented the rise in bronchial hyperresponsiveness.[42] However, this effect most likely represents only functional antagonism of the bronchospastic portion of the LAR and not an anti-inflammatory effect. Long-term administration of β_2 agonists does not reduce bronchial hyperreactivity confirming a lack of significant anti-inflammatory activity.[42]

Chronic administration of β_2 agonists can lead to down-regulation (decreased number of β_2 receptors) and a decreased binding affinity for these receptors.[35,37] Glucocorticoid therapy can both prevent and reverse this phenomenon.[12,35] Studies of β_2 receptors *in vivo* as well as β_2-

TABLE 25.3. RELATIVE SELECTIVITY, POTENCY, AND DURATION OF ACTION OF THE β-ADRENERGIC AGONISTS

	Selectivity			*Duration of Action*		
Agent	β_1	β_2	β_2 Potency[a]	Bronchodilation (h)	Protection[b] (h)	Oral Activity
Isoproterenol	++++	++++	1	0.5–2	0.5–1.0	No
Metaproterenol	+++	+++	15	3–4	1–2	Yes
Isoetharine	++	+++	6	0.5–2	0.5–1.0	No
Albuterol	+	++++	2	4–8	2–4	Yes
Bitolterol	+	++++	5	4–8	2–4	No
Pirbuterol	+	++++	5	4–8	2–4	Yes
Terbutaline	+	++++	4	4–8	2–4	Yes
Formoterol	+	++++	0.24	>12	>12	Yes
Salmeterol	+	++++	0.50	>12	>12	UK[c]

[a]Relative molar potency: 1 = most potent.
[b]Protection refers to the duration of time that bronchoconstriction may be prevented.
[c]UK, unknown. (Compiled from Refs. 24, 35, 36, and 40.)

receptor end-organ responses have indicated that a significantly greater tolerance develops in all other β_2 receptors in comparison with respiratory smooth muscle β_2 receptors.[24] Thus, the development of tolerance to the extrapulmonary effects (cardiac stimulation and hypokalemia) may account for a lack of significant cardiac effects with retention of the bronchodilator response despite chronic inhaled β_2-agonist therapy, whereas tolerance to mast cell stabilization may be a drawback to chronic use.[24,35] The body of literature suggests that chronic β_2-agonist administration may produce a small degree of tolerance of minimal clinical significance that is easily overcome by increasing the dose or by administering glucocorticoids. Tolerance also develops to the long-acting β_2 agonists when assessed with bronchoprovocation as would be expected from a receptor phenomenon.[43,44]

The β_2-Agonist Controversy

The potential for chronic use of inhaled β_2 agonists to worsen asthma and for excessive use to increase the risk of dying from asthma has gained a great deal of attention recently.[44,45] The concern has existed for more than 20 years since the first publication of the association between increased asthma deaths and isoproterenol metered-dose inhalers (MDIs), and the more recent studies have been extensively reviewed in a monograph.[37] A complete review is beyond the scope of this chapter. Briefly, two studies that have been extensively analyzed have brought the issue to the forefront.[45]

In a double-blind crossover trial of regular versus as-needed fenoterol, it was reported that 70% of the patients had better control on as-needed therapy.[44] However, a later publication of the actual measurements of asthma control failed to demonstrate a significant difference in number of asthma exacerbations or bronchial hyperreactivity.[45] A more recent double-blind crossover trial of regular versus as-needed albuterol in 341 patients failed to show worsening and actually demonstrated better control in asthma symptoms during regular treatment.[45] Long-term studies of bronchial hyperreactivity have failed to document an adverse effect of chronic inhaled β_2-agonist use.[44]

A case-control epidemiologic study suggested an increased risk of asthma death associated with excessive use of both fenoterol and albuterol by MDI that correlated with the number of canisters used.[44] They also found a risk of death was similar between albuterol by MDI and theophylline. The authors' follow-up cohort analysis that attempted to control for severity of illness confirmed the initial findings. It demonstrated that the increased risk of death occurred primarily after usage exceeded 2 canisters per month, which was in excess of recommended limits.[45] However, case-control epidemiologic studies purporting to show that inhaled β_2 agonists increase the risk of death from asthma are all confounded by the fact that the indication for treatment is inextricably related to the outcome.[45] The assumption that confounding by the indication can be adequately controlled is erroneous unless assignment to therapy is randomized. Thus, the increased risk is as likely a result of inappropriate therapy with bronchodilators in severe asthma because the anti-inflammatory drugs did not show an increased risk of death.[44] Others have implied cardiac deaths as a possibility because fenoterol is not as β_2 selective as albuterol, terbutaline, or pirbuterol.[35,37] A follow-up meta-analysis of all case-control trials evaluating the role of inhaled β_2 agonists and asthma deaths demonstrated only a weak association with nebulized β_2 agonists.[44] As the more severe patients receive home nebulizers, this again suggests that asthma severity is the strongest link to death from asthma.[44,45]

Clinical Use

Inhaled short-acting selective β_2 agonists are indicated for the treatment of intermittent episodes of bronchospasm and are the bronchodilator as well as the first treatment of choice for acute severe asthma.[24,38] In acute severe asthma, β_2 agonists should be given in high doses by jet nebulization in frequent intervals or alternatively via MDI plus a spacer device by trained personnel (Table 25.4).[38] Initially, the patient should receive dosages every 20 minutes for the first 1 or 2 hours, and then the dosage should be adjusted based on response (see treatment algorithms). During the recovery phase, the dose is generally lowered first and then the dosing interval is extended.

The inhaled selective β_2 agonists are the treatment of choice for EIA.[14,24] They inhibit EIA in a dose-dependent fashion and provide complete protection for a 2-hour period following inhalation with varying levels of patient-dependent protection over 4 hours while the new long-acting agents provide significant protection for 8–12 hours.[14,42] The inhaled route is significantly more effective than the oral route of administration, which provides a moderate blocking effect similar to that seen for oral theophylline.[24]

The duration of the short-acting inhaled β_2 agonists limits their usefulness in those patients who require chronic maintenance bronchodilators to prevent and control symptoms, particularly for those patients suffering from nocturnal asthma.[24,30] These patients can be treated with long-acting inhaled β_2 agonists,[31,42] oral sustained-release β_2 agonists, or sustained-release theophylline.[24] The need for chronic bronchodilator therapy may be an indicator of inadequate anti-inflammatory treatment and a dosage adjustment of these agents should be considered.

The exact role of long-acting inhaled β_2 agonists in the therapy of chronic asthma has yet to be definitively determined. The International Consensus Report (Appendix 25.1) places them for chronic maintenance in patients with symptoms who are already on standard doses of anti-inflammatories prior to advancing to high-dose inhaled corticosteroids.[27] A recent study suggests that twice daily inhaled salmeterol will improve peak flows and symptom

TABLE 25.4. DOSAGES OF MEDICATIONS FOR ACUTE SEVERE ASTHMA

Medication	Dosage: Pediatric	Dosage: Adult	Comment
Sympathomimetics			For optimal delivery, dilute aerosols to minimum of 4 mL, maximum 6 mL; gas flow at 6–12 L/min
Isoetharine	0.1–1.0% 0.1–0.2 mg/kg every 20 min for 3 doses, then every 1–2 h as needed	3–10 mg every 20 min for 3 doses then every 1–2 h as needed	Not recommended due to low potency and short duration
Metaproterenol 5% (50 mg/mL), 15-µg unit dose	0.25–0.5 mg/kg every 2–4 h as needed, maximum 15 mg	15 mg every 20 min for 3 doses, then 15–30 mg every 2–4 h as needed	Do not exceed maximum; not recommended in high dose due to lack of β_2 selectivity
Terbutaline Injection (1 mg/mL) Nebulizer solution (10 mg/mL)	0.1–0.3 mg/kg every 20 min or 3 doses, then every 2–4 h as needed	10 mg every 20 min then 10 mg every 2–4 h as needed	Currently not approved for this mode of administration; no advantage over albuterol so not recommended
Albuterol (5 mg/mL)	0.05–0.15 mg/kg every 20 min for 3 doses, then 0.15–0.3 mg/kg up to 10 mg every 2–4 h as needed, or 0.5 mg/kg/h by continuous nebulization	5–10 mg every 20 min for 3 doses every 2–4 h as needed, or 10–15 mg/h by continuous nebulization	May continue every 20 min for 2–4 h in severe cases
Systemic			No proven advantage of systemic therapy over aerosol in patients capable of moving air
Epinephrine 1:1000 (1 mg/mL)	0.01 mg/kg up to 0.5 mg every 20 min for 3 doses SQ	0.3–0.5 mg every 20 min for 3 doses	
Sustained-action susphrine 1:200 (5 mg/mL)	0.005–0.01 mL/kg every 6–10 h as needed SQ	0.5–0.75 mg every 6–10 h as needed	
Terbutaline (1 mg/mL)	0.01 mg/kg every 20 min for 3 doses, then every 2–6 h as needed SQ	0.25–0.5 mg every 20 min for 3 doses, then every 2–6 h as needed	
	10 µg/kg over 10 min intravenously followed by 0.4 µg/kg/min. Increase as necessary by 0.2 µg/kg/min up to 3–6 µg/kg/min	Not recommended	Due to cardiac toxicity high dose inhaled agonists preferred
Anticholinergics			
Aerosol Atropine sulfate	0.5–0.075 mg/kg every 4–6 h as needed	0.025 mg/kg or 2.5–5 mg every 4–5 h as needed	Due to excellent absorption atropine sulfate not recommended
Ipratropium bromide 0.025%	250 µg every 4–6 h as needed	250–500 µg every 4–6 h as needed	
Glycopyrrolate (Robinul) 0.2 mg/mL injection	0.025–0.05 mg/kg nebulized every 4–6 h	2 mg nebulized every 2–6 h as needed	
Glucocorticoids			
Methylprednisolone	1–2 mg/kg every 6 h for 24–48 h or severe symptoms abate, then reduce to 1–2 mg/kg/d every 12 h	80–200 mg/d in 2–4 divided doses	Duration of steroid therapy is dependent on response; continue full dose until patient at least 70–75% of normal predicted FEV_1; hydrocortisone produces greater sodium retention; no advantage over parenteral therapy
Hydrocortisone	4 mg/kg every 4–6 h for 24–48 h, then reduce	200–400 mg/d 2–4 divided doses	
Prednisone	1–2 mg/kg/d in 2–3 doses for outpatient use for 3–5 days. Inpatient same as for methylprednisolone	40–160 mg/d in 2–4 divided doses	
Methylxanthines	See Fig. 25.6		Monitor theophylline serum concentration

control in moderate to severe patients already receiving inhaled corticosteroid therapy and improves sleep quality as well as airflow obstruction in nocturnal asthma more effectively than doubling the dose of inhaled corticosteroids.[46] However, the FDA-approved use for salmeterol is for the chronic maintenance therapy of asthma (i.e., not qualified by severity), and it has proven efficacious as primary therapy for chronic asthma whether or not administered with inhaled corticosteroids.[43] Patients should be warned that salmeterol is ineffective for acute severe asthma because it can take up to 20 minutes for onset and 1–4 hours for maximum bronchodilation following inhalation. Patients need to be counseled to continue to use their short-acting inhaled β_2 agonists for acute exacerbations.

Methylxanthines

Methylxanthines have been used for asthma therapy for 50 years. Theophylline is the primary methylxanthine of interest, although others such as caffeine, dyphylline, and enprofylline also produce bronchodilation.[24,35] Caffeine and dyphylline are less potent than theophylline, while enprofylline, which is available in Europe, has greater bronchodilator potency.[35] Like the β_2 agonists, the methylxanthines are functional antagonists; however, their clinical potency is limited by their low therapeutic index.[24,35] Methylxanthines are ineffective by aerosol and therefore must be taken systemically. Theophylline as a sustained-release product is the preferred oral preparation, whereas its complex with ethylenediamine (aminophylline) is the preferred injectable product.

The mechanism by which theophylline produces bronchodilation is unknown but may involve inhibition of the release of intracellular calcium.[24,35] Theophylline is a competitive antagonist of the bronchoconstrictor adenosine; however, this property is not shared by enprofylline, a more potent bronchodilator than theophylline.[35] Theophylline also stimulates endogenous catecholamine release.[35] These latter two effects are important determinants of toxic symptoms of excess theophylline. Renewed attention has been placed on theophylline's potential for inhibition of phosphodiesterases (PDEs).[47,48] Inhibition of PDEs results in increased cyclic AMP and cyclic GMP concentrations. The PDE isoenzymes currently thought to be important in asthma are PDE III, predominant in airway smooth muscle, and PDE IV, important in inflammatory cell regulation such as mast cells, eosinophils, and T lymphocytes.[48] PDE inhibition is consistent with various nonbronchodilator activities that may be relevant to asthma including decreased mast cell mediator release, decreased eosinophil basic protein release, decreased T-lymphocyte proliferation, decreased T-cell cytokine release, and decreased plasma exudation.[47,48] Selective PDE isoenzyme inhibitors are currently being developed for possible treatment of asthma. Theophylline is a nonselective PDE inhibitor.[48] Although these properties indicate a potential for theophylline to provide anti-inflammatory activity in asthma, to date clinical trials have not borne this out.[24,35]

Both bronchodilation and protection against bronchoprovocation challenges are concentration dependent. Theophylline produces linear increases in bronchodilation with logarithmic increments in serum drug concentrations.[35,47] The majority of chronic stable asthmatics will obtain significant bronchodilation when the serum theophylline concentration reaches 5 μg/mL, and most patients will have no toxic symptoms with serum concentrations less than 15 μg/mL.[35] The percentage of patients experiencing adverse effects is approximately 18% at serum concentrations between 15 and 20 μg/mL.[35] This increases sharply to 60% at concentrations between 20 and 30 μg/mL, and 80% at concentrations greater than 30 μg/mL.[35]

As with the β_2 agonists, the dose–response curves for smooth muscle relaxation by theophylline are dynamic and shifted to the right in the face of increasing contractile stimuli.[35] This probably explains theophylline's relative lack of bronchodilatory effect in acute severe asthma.[38,49,50] The severity of theophylline's toxicity precludes even doubling the usual dosage.

Theophylline has other effects that may be important to its antiasthmatic action. Theophylline inhibits pulmonary edema by decreasing vascular permeability, enhances mucociliary clearance, and strengthens contraction of a fatigued diaphragm.[35] *In vitro* theophylline inhibits the release of histamine in sensitized human lung fragments but has provided inconsistent protection against the early asthmatic response to allergen.[35] When present in therapeutic concentrations, theophylline and enprofylline attenuate the bronchospasm of the late asthmatic response,[35] but have no apparent effect on the inflammation and subsequent increase in bronchial hyperresponsiveness.[24] Long-term administration does not reduce bronchial hyperreactivity.[24]

Other Effects

Theophylline stimulates the central nervous system through its adenosine antagonism and produces cerebral vasoconstriction.[35] Both effects contribute to the neurotoxicities seen with theophylline. Theophylline acts as a respiratory stimulant by enhancing the hypoxic ventilatory drive, it decreases the lower esophageal sphincter pressure and increases gastric acid secretion, and has both inotropic and chronotropic cardiac effects.[24] Acutely theophylline acts as a diuretic but tolerance develops rapidly.

Pharmacokinetics

An understanding of the pharmacokinetics combined with routine monitoring of serum concentrations is essential for the safe and effective use of theophylline.[47] Theophylline is primarily eliminated by metabolism via the hepatic cytochrome P-450 mixed-function oxidase microsomal enzymes (primarily the CYP1A2 isozyme) with 10% or less excreted unchanged in the kidney.[51] Each of the major metabolic pathways for theophylline is saturable within the usual therapeutic concentration so that theophylline frequently, although not always, exhibits nonlinear pharmacokinetics.[35,51] This may partially explain the relatively large intrapatient variability in theophylline clearance (often as great as 30%) over time.[51] Part of the intrapatient variability in clearance is age dependent with 1- to 9-year-olds having the greatest clearance rates and therefore requiring the largest dosages for theophylline. However, even within the same age groups theophylline clearance can vary twofold to threefold so that no patient should be treated with theophylline without routine monitoring of serum theophylline concentrations. Figures 25.8 and 25.9 give recommended dosages, monitoring schedules, and dosage adjustments for theophylline.

The hepatic P-450 enzymes are susceptible to induction and inhibition by various environmental factors and drugs, as listed in Table 25.5. Only those drugs or diseases that produce a 20% or greater inhibition or 50% or greater induction of theophylline metabolism are likely to result in clinically significant interactions. Also, there is a significant interpatient susceptibility to developing an interaction even with potent P-450 inhibitors such as cimetidine. However, the clinician needs to be aware of drugs that have been proven to alter theophylline metabolism, or could potentially do so, in order to provide appropriate alternatives and monitor the patient appropriately.

Due to the relatively short elimination half-life of theophylline (3–5 hours in children and 6–12 hours in adults), sustained-release oral preparations are favored for outpatient therapy.[47] These preparations can be administered every 8–24 hours in patients and maintain relatively constant therapeutic serum concentrations, and the decreased dosing frequency improves compliance.[47] The degree of serum theophylline concentration fluctuation over the dosing interval is dependent on the release characteristics of the products as well as the elimination rate characteristics of the patients.[47] Thus, patients with rapid clearances for theophylline will experience greater fluctuations than patients with slow clearances, given the same product over the same dosing interval.[47] Neither an optimal nor an acceptable maximum fluctuation has been absolutely established for theophylline serum concentrations but it seems reasonable that it should not exceed the usual therapeutic range. That is, it should not exceed 100% for twice daily dosing or 150% for once daily dosing where

$$\%\ \text{fluctuation} = Cp_{\text{max}} - Cp_{\text{min}}/Cp_{\text{min}}$$

Each of the sustained-release theophylline products has different release characteristics and the products are variably susceptible to altered absorption from food or gastric pH changes.[47] Preparations with slower release characteristically exhibit a significant diurnal variation in absorption with the rate significantly slower at night in the recumbent patient.[51] As a result of these differences, it is best not to consider the sustained-release preparations to be interchangeable. In general, preparations unaffected by food that can be administered a minimum of every 12 hours in most patients are preferable.

Clinical Use

In the 1970s and 1980s, theophylline was a primary drug for the treatment of both acute and chronic asthma in the United States. However, the availability of safer more effective inhaled β_2 agonists and anti-inflammatory agents (cromolyn and topically active inhaled glucocorticoids), coupled with a better understanding of the pathogenesis of asthma and bronchial hyperreactivity, has curtailed the use of theophylline.

A series of investigations in the 1980s evaluating the therapy of acute asthma in the emergency room demonstrated that theophylline did not add to the efficacy of aerosolized β_2 agonists but frequently increased toxicity.[2,24] A number of recent double-blind, placebo-controlled trials of aminophylline for hospitalized adult and child asthmatics failed to detect any benefit of adding aminophylline to optimal inhaled β_2 agonists and oral glucocorticoids.[49,50]

In the outpatient setting, chronic theophylline administration can reduce asthma symptoms, reduce the amount of as-needed inhaled β_2 agonists used, and reduce the oral steroid requirement in steroid-dependent asthmatics.[24,47] Sustained-release theophylline once nightly is effective for nocturnal asthma.[47] Comparative studies between sustained-release theophylline and oral sustained-release β_2 agonists have not shown any advantage for theophylline.[52] Significant disadvantages to chronic theophylline therapy include theophylline's lack of effect on underlying bronchial hyperreactivity and the dangers inherent in giving a drug that can produce severe neurologic toxicity, including seizures, permanent neurologic deficit, and death at serum concentrations only twofold greater than optimal therapeutic concentrations. Death has occurred in children receiving their usual doses of theophylline during acute systemic viral illnesses.[35] Studies comparing cromolyn and theophylline as first-line therapy for chronic asthma have failed to demonstrate an advantage for theophylline over cromolyn.[53]

Serum theophylline concentrations must be routinely monitored for the safe and effective use of theophylline. The usually accepted therapeutic range of 10–20 μg/mL is not an absolute but a statistical concept.[51] Many patients will respond to lower concentrations. A range of 5–15 μg/mL has been recommended by the NAEP[2] and others[27] as an effective and safer range of steady-state concentrations for most patients. Due to the log–linear nature of the concentration–response curve, there is little to gain in terms of bronchodilation by going from 15 to 20 μg/mL.[35] Patients whose theophylline concentrations are maintained near 20 μg/mL are more susceptible to developing serious

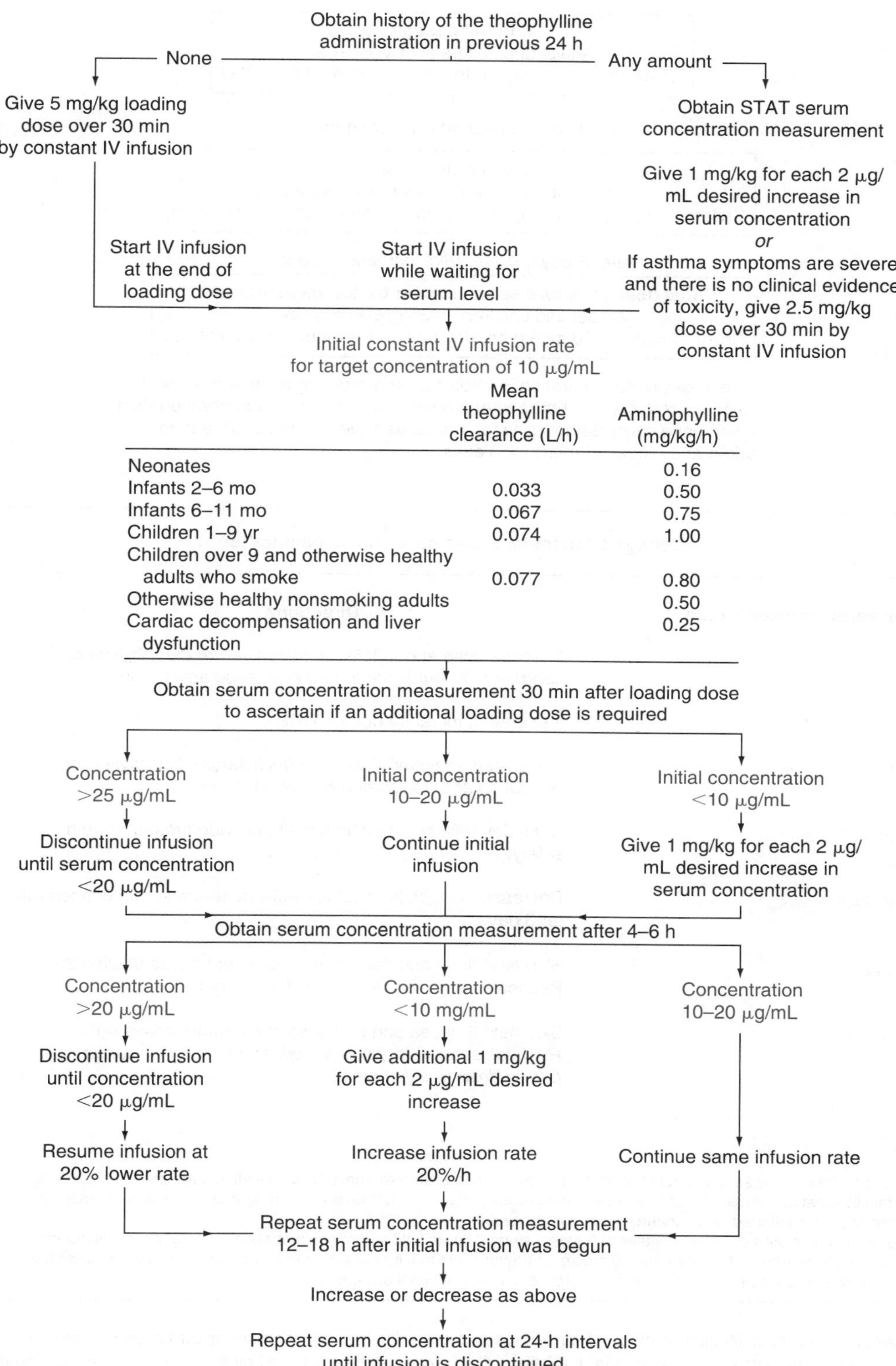

	Mean theophylline clearance (L/h)	Aminophylline (mg/kg/h)
Neonates		0.16
Infants 2–6 mo	0.033	0.50
Infants 6–11 mo	0.067	0.75
Children 1–9 yr	0.074	1.00
Children over 9 and otherwise healthy adults who smoke	0.077	0.80
Otherwise healthy nonsmoking adults		0.50
Cardiac decompensation and liver dysfunction		0.25

Figure 25.8. Algorithm for the use of theophylline to relieve acute symptoms of asthma. Aminophylline = 80% theophylline. *(From Jenne JW, Murphy S (eds). Drug Therapy for Asthma: Research and Clinical Practice. New York, Marcel Dekker, 1987, with permission.)*

Initial dosage
Adults and children >1 yr of age:
12–14 mg/kg per day up to a maximum of 300 mg/day

↓

After 3 days, *if tolerated*, increase dose to:

Incremental increase
Adults and children ≥45 kg: 400 mg/day
Children <45 kg: 16 mg/kg per day up to a maximum of 400 mg/day

↓

After 3 days, *if tolerated*, increase dose to:

Final dosage before serum concentration measurement
Adults and children ≥45 kg: 600 mg/day
Children <45 kg: 20 mg/kg per day up to a maximum of 600 mg/day

↓

Check serum concentration ~4 hours after a morning dose of most slow-release products or 8 hours after a dose of a very slowly absorbed product given once every 24 hours, when no doses have been missed, added, or taken at unequal intervals for 3 days.

↓

Dosage adjustment based on serum concentration

Peak serum concentration	Directions
<7.5 μg/mL	Increase dose about 25%. *Recheck serum theophylline concentration for guidance in further dosage adjustment.*
7.5 to 9.9 μg/mL	If tolerated, increase dose ~25%.
10 to 14.9 μg/mL	If tolerated, maintain dose. *Recheck serum theophylline concentration at 6- to 12-month intervals.**
15 to 19.9 μg/mL	Consider 10% decrease in dose to provide greater margin of safety.*
20 to 24.9 μg/mL	Decrease dose 10% to 25%. Recheck serum serum concentration after 3 days.
25 to 30 μg/mL	Skip next dose and decrease subsequent doses at least 25%. Recheck serum concentration after 3 days.
>30 μg/mL	Skip next 2 doses and decrease subsequent doses 50%. *Recheck serum theophylline concentration for guidance in further dosage adjustment.†*

*Dosage reduction or serum concentration measurement is indicated whenever adverse effects are present, physiologic abnormalities that can reduce theophylline clearance occur (e.g., persistent fever), or a drug that interacts with theophylline is added or discontinued (e.g., erythromycin, carbamazepine).

†Administer activated charcoal in water, 0.5 gm/kg every 2 hours until serum concentration <20 μg/mL. Consider intravenously administered phenobarbital, 20 mg/kg, to prevent seizures if excessive serum concentration has resulted from multiple doses. Consult a regional poison control center for additional advice.

Figure 25.9. Algorithm for slow titration of theophylline dosage and guide for final dosage adjustment based on serum theophylline concentration measurement. For infants <1 year of age, the initial daily dosage can be calculated by the following regression equation: Dose = (mg/kg) = (0.2)(age in weeks) + 5.0. Whenever side effects occur, dosage should be reduced to a previously tolerated lower dose. *(From Ref. 49 with permission.)*

TABLE 25.5. FACTORS AFFECTING THEOPHYLLINE CLEARANCE

Decreased Clearance	Decrease in Clearance[a] (%)	Increased Clearance	Increase in Clearance[a] (%)
Cimetidine	−35 to −60	Rifampin	+53
Troleandomycin	−25 to −50	Carbamazepine	+50
Erythromycin	−25	Phenobarbital	+34
Allopurinol	−20		
Propranolol	−30	Phenytoin	+70
Oral contraceptives	−10 to −30	Smoking	+40
Enoxacin	−65	High-protein diet	+25
Ciprofloxacin	−25 to −30	Charcoal broiled meat	+30
Norfloxacin	−10	Intravenous isoproterenol	
Ofloxacin	−26	Sulphinpyrazone	+22
Systemic viral illness	−50		
Thiabendazole	−65		

[a]Approximate means reported across studies. (From Refs. 24, 35, 49, and 55.)

adverse effects when confronted with an environmental exposure that inhibits theophylline metabolism. Due to its high risk/benefit ratio, theophylline should be considered as a second- or third-line drug in the therapy of asthma. Current recommendations place theophylline as an alternative to the long-acting inhaled β_2 agonists for patients still symptomatic despite standard or high-dose anti-inflammatory therapy (Appendix 25.1).[27]

Anticholinergics

The anticholinergic agents have been used for centuries in the form of stramonium herbal treatments for asthma.[35] However, their systemic effects, particularly involving the central nervous system, limited their usefulness. The introduction of quaternary ammonium derivatives such as ipratropium bromide has renewed interest in these compounds.[24] Anticholinergic bronchodilators are competitive inhibitors of muscarinic receptors.[35] Unlike β_2 agonists and theophylline, they are not functional antagonists; they only produce bronchodilation in cholinergic-mediated bronchoconstriction. Normal bronchial tone is maintained through parasympathetic innervation of the airways via the vagus nerve. A number of the triggers and mediators of asthma (i.e., histamine, prostaglandins, sulfur dioxide, exercise, allergens) produce bronchoconstriction in part through vagal reflex mechanisms.[24,35] Studies of asthmatics consistently demonstrate that anticholinergics are effective bronchodilators though not as potent as β_2 agonists. Anticholinergics attenuate but do not block allergen- or exercise-induced asthma in a dose-dependent fashion and have no effect on the late asthmatic response.[35] Anticholinergics consistently produce bronchodilation in acute severe asthma. Most studies suggest that anticholinergics can be expected to produce a further 20–25% improvement in FEV_1 over β_2 agonists alone.[54] However, a significant interpatient variability exists with some patients obtaining significantly greater (40–80%) improvements, and others minimal improvement.

Currently available anticholinergics are nonselective muscarinic receptor blockers, and blockade of inhibitory muscarinic receptors could theoretically result in an increased release of acetylcholine and overcome the block on the smooth muscle receptors (M3).[35] This mechanism may explain why some patients have experienced paradoxical bronchoconstriction from nebulized anticholinergics. All anticholinergics are somewhat selective in that bronchodilation occurs at a lower dose than is required to dry secretions or produce tachycardia.[35] The bronchoselectivity is enhanced by aerosol administration.

Atropine sulfate is a tertiary ammonium compound that is completely absorbed from the lungs and gastrointestinal tract.[24,35] It has an elimination half-life of 3–4 hours in young adults, which is prolonged in young children and the elderly who may accumulate toxic concentrations with continued dosing.[35] The quaternary ammonium derivatives (ipratropium bromide, atropine methonitrate, oxitropium, and glycopyrrolate) have the advantage of poor absorption across mucosae and the blood–brain barrier. This results in negligible systemic effects with a prolonged local effect (i.e., bronchodilation). In addition, the quaternary compounds appear not to produce the decrease in mucociliary clearance seen with the tertiary compounds (atropine and hyoscine).[35] Table 25.6 compares the anticholinergic agents.

The quaternary anticholinergics have a duration of action of 4–8 hours. Both intensity and duration of action are dose dependent. Time to reach maximum bronchodilation from aerosolized anticholinergics is considerably slower than from aerosolized short-acting β_2 agonists (2

TABLE 25.6. COMPARISON OF ANTICHOLINERGICS[a]

Agent	Availability	Relative Potency[b]	Duration (h)	Dosages	
				Pediatrics	Adults
Atropine methonitrate	Investigational only	1	5–6	ND[c]	1.5 mg nebulized q 6 h
Ipratropium bromide (Atrovent)	MDI[d] 18 μg/actuation; 300 actuations; 0.025% (0.25 mg/mL) nebulizer solution	Unknown 0.5	5–6	2 inhalations q 6 h nebulized 250 μg nebulized q 4–6 h for acute asthma	2–4 inhalations q 6 h or 500 μg nebulized q 6 h for acute asthma
Glycopyrrolate (Robinul)	0.2 mg/mL injectable solution	1	6–12	0.025–0.05 mg/kg nebulized q 6 h	2 mg nebulized q 6 h
Oxitropium bromide	Investigational	Unknown	8	ND[c]	500 μg

[a]At the current time there are no anticholinergics approved by the FDA for use in asthma.
[b]Dose required to produce equivalent bronchodilation.
[c]ND, not determined.
[d]MDI, metered-dose inhaler. (Compiled from Refs. 24, 35, and 36.)

hours versus 30 minutes). However, this is of little clinical consequence because some bronchodilation is seen within 30 seconds, 50% of maximum response occurs within 3 minutes, and 80% of maximum is reached within 30 minutes.[35,54]

Clinical Use

The role of anticholinergics in the treatment of asthma is limited. Due to potential toxicities and availability of quaternary compounds, there is no rationale for using atropine sulfate. Studies in chronic bronchitis, a disease in which increased parasympathetic action is the predominant reversible component, show that anticholinergics produce similar bronchodilation to β_2 agonists with fewer side effects. However, anticholinergics are unable to produce maximum bronchodilation in asthma and in the usual recommended doses are significantly less effective than the β_2 agonists.[10] Although they produce additive bronchodilation to β_2 agonists and/or theophylline in chronic asthma, the significance of this is unknown. A recent 2.5-year placebo-controlled trial of the addition of ipratropium to chronic inhaled terbutaline in asthmatics and chronic bronchitics failed to demonstrate an improved outcome in association with the increased cost of therapy.[55]

Significant tolerance is not produced with prolonged administration nor is there any effect on bronchial hyperreactivity.[24] Both the β_2 agonists and cromolyn provide superior protection against EIA.[24,31] Anticholinergics produce additive bronchodilation with β_2 agonists in acute severe asthma.[54] However, the effect is inconsistent and, even in those studies demonstrating significant further bronchodilation, the overall outcome of the patients (i.e., number admitted to hospital or length of hospital stay) was not altered.[54] Despite these results, anticholinergics represent a safer and more effective additional bronchodilator than theophylline in this setting. Anticholinergics appear to be as effective as β_2 agonists for reversing the bronchospastic component of acute exacerbations of chronic bronchitis.[24,35]

Cromolyn Sodium and Nedocromil Sodium

Cromolyn sodium has been available for the prophylactic treatment of asthma for almost 20 years, while nedocromil sodium, a pyranoquinoline dicarboxylic acid that is pharmacologically similar, has just recently been released in the United States. The exact mechanism of action for these agents is still unknown. While minor differences in activity do exist, the principal difference appears to be potency with 4 mg of nedocromil by MDI equivalent to 20 mg of cromolyn sodium by Spinhaler.[36] Initially, it was thought that all of cromolyn's activity was a result of mast cell membrane stabilization. As such, it inhibits the EAR to allergen challenge as well as EIA.[53] Unlike the β_2 agonists and other experimental mast cell membrane stabilizers, cromolyn and nedocromil also inhibit the LAR and prevent the subsequent increased bronchial hyperreactivity.[24,36] Long-term prophylaxis with cromolyn prevents the usual rise in bronchial hyperreactivity associated with specific pollen seasons and may produce a modest decrease in baseline bronchial hyperreactivity.[53] Both cromolyn and nedocromil inhibit *in vitro* activation of human neutrophils, macrophages, and eosinophils.[24,36] Each agent also inhibits neurally mediated bronchoconstriction through C-fiber sensory nerve stimulation in the airways.[56] Neither drug has a bronchodilatory effect.

Cromolyn and nedocromil are only effective by inhalation and are available as MDIs, while cromolyn also comes as a nebulizer solution and Spinhaler. The pharmacokinetics of both drugs are also very similar. They are not bioavailable orally but the portion of the dose that reaches the lung is completely absorbed.[24,36] Absorption from the airway is significantly slower than elimination (hours versus minutes). Both the intensity and duration of protection against various challenges is dose dependent.[24,56] Higher doses produce greater and more prolonged protection.

Both drugs are remarkably nontoxic. No evidence of mutagenesis or teratogenesis has been found for cromolyn and less than 0.1% of an intravenous dose crosses the placenta or enters breast milk.[53] Cough and wheeze has also been reported following inhalation of the dry powder inhaler of cromolyn and bad taste and headache following nedocromil. Cromolyn is the least toxic drug used to treat asthma with significant adverse effects occurring in less than 1 in 10,000 patients.[53] Tolerance to cromolyn or nedocromil has not been demonstrated.

Approximately 60–75% of patients (adults and children) with mild to moderate chronic asthma will be adequately controlled with cromolyn.[53] Comparative studies between cromolyn and theophylline do not demonstrate a significant advantage for either agent in controlling symptoms of asthma or improving baseline pulmonary functions.[57] However, cromolyn produced a significant decrease in bronchial hyperreactivity and theophylline did not, and theophylline therapy produced more side effects and required more patient visits for monitoring.

Clinical Use

Cromolyn and nedocromil are indicated for the prophylaxis of chronic mild to moderate asthma in both children and adults regardless of etiology. They are particularly effective for the allergic asthmatics on a seasonal basis or just prior to an acute exposure (i.e., animals or mowing the lawn).[36] Cromolyn is the second drug of choice for the prevention of EIA and may be used in conjunction with a β_2 agonist in more severe cases not completely responding to either agent alone.[14] In those patients with a history of a LAR following exercise, cromolyn would be the first choice.[53] The NAEP and International Consensus have suggested that cromolyn and nedocromil be the anti-inflammatories of first choice for childhood asthma due to their efficacy and safety.[2,27] Nedocromil therapy may be able to produce a decrease in inhaled steroid dosage.[56]

The efficacy of each drug is directly related to its degree of deposition in the lung so when beginning therapy, it is important that the airways are patent. A short course of systemic glucocorticoids and around-the-clock inhaled β_2 agonists may initially be required in patients with significant obstruction. Most patients will experience an improvement in 1–2 weeks but it may take longer to achieve maximum benefit. Patients should initially receive cromolyn or nedocromil four times daily and then only after stabilization of symptoms may the frequency be reduced to two or three times daily. It is not necessary to maintain the regular use of concomitant β_2 agonists after the patient becomes stable; they can be reduced as needed.

GLUCOCORTICOID THERAPY

General Characteristics

Evidence that inhaled corticosteroids can alter the level of hyperreactivity has reestablished the utility of glucocorticoid therapy for asthma.[2,11,57] The mechanism of action and use of glucocorticoids in asthma have been reviewed.[57,58] Actions useful in treating asthma include (1) increasing the number of β_2-adrenergic receptors and improving the receptor responsiveness to β_2-adrenergic stimulation (glucocorticoids also restore and prevent tolerance induced with chronic administration of β_2 agonists); (2) reducing mucus production and hypersecretion; and (3) inhibiting the inflammatory response at all levels.[57] Glucocorticoids constrict the microvasculature inhibiting fluid and protein influx, and inhibit migration of neutrophils and eosinophils into tissues as well as inhibiting their function.[57] Glucocorticoids inhibit the synthesis but not release of histamine from mast cells. Glucocorticoids inhibit the production of prostaglandins and leukotrienes by inhibiting phospholipase release of arachidonic acid from membrane phospholipids.[57]

Cortisol and its synthetic derivatives such as prednisolone, methylprednisolone, triamcinolone, dexamethasone, and betamethasone all have beneficial effects in the treatment of asthma related to the prevention or suppression of airway inflammation.[12,35,57] The major cellular and biochemical activity of the glucocorticoids includes decreasing synthesis and release of several proinflammatory cytokines such as IL-1, GM-CSF, IL-3, IL-4, IL-5, IL-6, and IL-8; reducing inflammatory cell activation, recruitment, and infiltration; and decreasing vascular permeability.[58] Suppressing the ongoing airways inflammation results in prevention or inhibition of mucus secretion, decreased edema of airway mucosa, and perhaps decreased airway epithelial denudation, leading to a reduction in airways reactivity.[57] Airway epithelium appears to regenerate toward normal with ongoing therapy with inhaled glucocorticoids.[58]

Time Course of Response

The anti-inflammatory effects of glucocorticoids are mediated through the production of lipocortin; therefore, the time required to see the particular effect is dependent on the time required for lipocortin synthesis, decreased formation of the particular mediator, and resolution of the response.[57] Generally, the cellular and biochemical effects are immediate, but varying amounts of time are required to produce a clinical response. β-Receptor density increases within 4 hours of glucocorticoid administration.[57] Improved responsiveness to β_2 agonists occurs within 2 hours.[35] In acute severe asthma (status asthmaticus), 4–12 hours may be required before any clinical response is noted, most likely due to the time required to produce sufficient lipocortin.[58] Reversal of seasonal increased bronchial hyperreactivity requires at least 1 week of therapy.[57] Reactivity to EIA decreases after 4 weeks of therapy.[14] Although single doses do not inhibit the immediate asthmatic response to antigen challenge, continued therapy for 1 week partially suppresses the response. These latter two effects are likely a result of a reduction in the number of mucosal mast cells.[58]

The response to inhaled glucocorticoids is somewhat delayed. Most patients' symptoms will improve in the first 1–2 weeks of therapy and reach maximum improvement in 4–8 weeks. However, the improvement in bronchial hyperreactivity may take up to 3 months and may continue to show improvement over 12 months of therapy.[58] No evidence exists that the use of glucocorticoids in the moderate asthmatic will induce a state of steroid dependence. In fact, most of the evidence demonstrating a decrease in bronchial hyperreactivity with steroid therapy implies just the opposite.

Systemic Glucocorticoid Therapy

Acute severe asthma, status asthmaticus, is treated with high-dose systemic glucocorticoids combined with frequent administration of inhaled β_2 agonists.[24,59] Glucocorticoids can be administered by the parenteral route (methylprednisolone sodium succinate, hydrocortisone sodium succinate) or alternatively by the oral route (prednisone, methylprednisolone), which provide a rapid onset of action and a systemic effect.[59] The glucocorticoids used in asthma are compared in Table 25.7. Systemic steroids should be administered in a dose approximately equivalent to methylprednisolone 0.5–1 mg/kg intravenously or orally every 6–8 hours.[59,60] There is no difference in response to intravenous and oral administration. The duration of action of steroids in acute asthma has been poorly studied, but existing evidence suggests that divided doses should be used.[59,60] Following resolution of severe obstruction (achievement of 50% of predicted normal FEV_1, which generally occurs in the first 48–72 hours), the steroid dose is reduced to 1 mg/kg/d in children or 60 mg/d in adults as one or two doses administered by the oral route.[59,60] The duration of treatment is dependent on the patient's response and past history. The usual practice of tapering the steroid dosage after hospitalization does not affect outcome in terms of recovery or reexacerbation rate and, therefore, is unnecessary.[61]

Glucocorticoids are also recommended for the treatment of impending episodes of severe asthma unresponsive to bronchodilator therapy.[2,27] Prednisone, approximately 1–2 mg/kg/d (up to 30–40 mg/dose), is administered orally in two divided doses for 3–7 days.[59] If an adequate response is not achieved, administration of prednisone three times daily may be worthwhile. Once again, the dose and duration of treatment is based on the patient's response and past history. The effects of glucocorticoids in asthma are dose and duration dependent. This is true as well for the adverse effects of systemic steroids (Table 25.8). The clinician is continually forced to balance the toxicity of chronic systemic glucocorticoid therapy versus control of asthma symptoms. Because short-term (1–2 weeks) high-dose steroids (1–2 mg/kg/d methylprednisolone) do not produce serious toxicities, the ideal use is to administer the glucocorticoids for a short course or "burst" and then maintain the patient on bronchodilators, inhaled corticosteroids,

TABLE 25.7. GLUCOCORTICOID COMPARISON CHART

Systemic	Relative Anti-Inflammatory Potency	Relative Sodium-Retaining Potency	Duration Biologic Activity (h)	Plasma Elimination Half-Life (h)	Equivalent Dose (mg)
Hydrocortisone	1	1	8–12	1.5–2	20
Prednisone	4	0.8	12–36	2.5–3.5	5
Prednisolone	4	0.8	12–36	2.5–3.6	5
Methylprednisolone	5	0.5	12–36	3.3	4
Triamcinolone	5	0	12–36	2.5–3.3	4
Betamethasone	25	0	36–54	5–7	0.75
Dexamethosone	25	0	36–54	3.4–4	0.75

Aerosol	Relative Topical Potency	Systemic Bioavailability (%)	Dosage per Inhalation (μg)	Plasma Elimination Half-Life (h)
Beclomethasone-16, 17-dipropionate (Forte)	0.3–0.5	<5	42 (250)	15
Budesonide[a]	1.0	10	50	2–2.8
Flunisolide	0.05	20	250	1.6
Triamcinolone-16,17-acetonide	0.2	Unknown	100	Unknown
Fluticasone dipropionate[a]	2.0	Unknown	—	3.0

[a]Investigational.

TABLE 25.8. ADVERSE EFFECTS OF CHRONIC SYSTEMIC GLUCOCORTICOID ADMINISTRATION

Hypothalamic–pituitary–adrenal suppression
Growth retardation
Skeletal muscle myopathy
Osteoporosis fractures
Aseptic necrosis of bone
Pancreatitis
Pseudotumor cerebri
Psychiatric disturbances
Sodium and water retention
Hypokalemia alkalosis
Hypertension
Skin striae
Impaired wound healing
Inhibition of leukocyte and monocyte function
Subcutaneous tissue atrophy
Glaucoma
Posterior subcapsular cataracts
Moon facies
Central redistribution of fat

and/or cromolyn with long periods between systemic glucocorticoid treatment.[59] In general, glucocorticoid therapy for more than 5 days at doses that exceed the usual physiologic endogenous cortisol production will cause temporary aberration in adrenal cortisol release. However, in studies this hypothalamic–pituitary–adrenal (HPA) axis suppression is short lived (1–3 days) and readily reversible following short bursts (10 days or less) of pharmacologic doses of glucocorticoids.[59] There is probably a maximum number of short bursts a patient can receive after which chronic steroid side effects occur. Patients receiving at least eight bursts were shown to have a decrease in trabecular bone density similar to those patients on daily or alternate day steroids over 1 year.[59] Children who received four or more bursts of prednisone exhibited a subnormal response to hypoglycemic stress or adrenocorticotropic hormone (ACTH) administration.[59] Very short courses of glucocorticoids (3–5 days) have been effective in reducing hospitalization from acute exacerbations. Short-burst steroid therapy is often effective in reducing hospitalizations in moderate asthmatics.[59,60]

In patients who require chronic systemic glucocorticoids for control of asthma, the lowest possible dose required to control symptoms is the goal of therapy. Physicians will often sacrifice complete control of the patient's symptoms to avoid toxicity. Two methods of decreasing the toxicities of systemic glucocorticoid therapy is to use alternate-day therapy or the topical inhaled glucocorticoids. In patients with poorly controlled chronic asthma, oral glucocorticoids may be administered in a dosing schedule similar to that previously described, to maximize pulmonary function. Once this goal is achieved, the prednisone dose is tapered and may be supplemented and eventually replaced by inhaled glucocorticoids.[35,57]

Inhaled Glucocorticoids

The inhaled glucocorticoids are becoming more popular in the United States as first-line therapy for chronic asthma. This is because the contribution of inflammation to the pathogenesis of asthma is becoming better understood and the inhaled glucocorticoids allow the application of potent topical anti-inflammatory agents to the relevant site of action within the airways.[57] The glucocorticoids currently available for inhaled use are beclomethasone diproprionate, triamcinolone acetonide, and flunisolide (Table 25.7). Fluticasone diproprionate and budesonide are undergoing clinical trials for asthma in the United States.

Few studies of the bioequivalence between the inhaled glucocorticoids or between inhaled and systemic glucocorticoids have been performed. In one such study, inhaled budesonide was compared to prednisone to establish the dose required to control moderate to severe asthma and measure the relative degree of systemic effects (suppression of serum cortisol and serum eosinophils). It was found that a budesonide dose (2.0 mg) that produced an antiasthmatic effect equivalent to prednisone 60 mg/d produced systemic effects equivalent to only 15 mg/d of prednisone.[57] These results indicate that inhaled glucocorticoids demonstrate a favorable topical/systemic potency ratio, but should not be considered benign. The "ideal" glucocorticoid for inhaled use should have a higher degree of topical potency, minimal systemic absorption of active drug, and minimal local or systemic side effects. None of the available inhaled glucocorticoids are considered ideal and ongoing investigation into topical/systemic potency ratios will reveal important and much needed information. The bronchoselectivity of the inhaled glucocorticoids is primarily a result of metabolism to less active substances following absorption from the lung. Beclomethasone dipropionate, triamcinolone acetonide, and flunisolide appear to have relatively similar topical/systemic potency ratios, whereas budesonide and fluticasone have improved bronchoselectivity[58]; however, more clinical studies are needed to clarify issues of comparative efficacy and toxicity.[24,58]

As with systemic glucocorticoid therapy, the lowest dose required to control symptoms is the appropriate dose. The inhaled glucocorticoids have varying binding affinities for human lung glucocorticoid receptors and demonstrate differing potencies for producing skin blanching (Table 25.7).[58] Skin blanching potency is a standard bioassay for anti-inflammatory activity. The relationship between skin blanching and inhibition of the inflammatory process in asthmatic airways has not been clearly delineated. In addition, insufficient clinical trials comparing the relative efficacy of the available inhaled glucocorticoids in asthma have been performed to warrant an absolute confidence in dose equivalency. As a result, the current guidelines (Appendix 25.1) assume the same relative potency for all of the available inhaled glucocorticoids despite the documented differences *in vitro* (Table 25.7); thus, they lump all the inhaled glucocorticoids in terms of daily microgram dosage.[2,27] Comparisons between beclomethasone and budesonide generally confirm this approach,[58] whereas an initial comparison between beclomethasone 2 mg daily and fluticasone 1 mg daily would indicate fluticasone to be both more potent and have greater bronchoselectivity.[62]

The inhaled glucocorticoids produce dose-dependent suppression of the adrenal cortex, but much less than systemic glucocorticoids.[57] Patients derive increased antiasthmatic benefits from increasing the dose of inhaled glucocorticoids from 400 to 2000 μg daily.[58] Measurable suppression of basal serum cortisol occurs consistently at dosages greater than 1500 μg daily in adults and ≥800 μg daily in children.[57,58] Dosages between 1000 and 1500 μg in adults and 400 and 800 μg daily in children have been inconsistent, with only a few reports suggesting a suppressive effect though the basal morning cortisol concentration remained in the normal range.[58] Some of these studies were confounded by systemic glucocorticoid administration. As with efficacy, the paucity of comparative studies between inhaled glucocorticoids precludes definitive comparisons of toxicity potential. However, initial evaluations would suggest that both budesonide and fluticasone produce less cortisol suppression.[58,62]

Glucocorticoids can have profound effects on bone metabolism including decreasing calcium deposition and enhancing calcium resorption, thereby predisposing adults to osteoporosis.[58] In addition, chronic glucocorticoid administration can result in growth retardation in prepubertal children.[58] The adverse effects of glucocorticoids on bone metabolism and growth can occur at dosages that do not affect cortisol secretion. Studies utilizing bone densitometry measurements have demonstrated decreased bone mineralization in adult patients receiving on average 600 μg of beclomethasone daily.[58] Growth suppression has been reported to occur with as little as 400 μg daily beclomethasone but not at 200–400 μg daily of budesonide.[58] However, it has also been reported that uncontrolled moderate to severe asthma may produce deceleration of growth velocity.[58] Long-term, well-controlled trials assessing the effect of inhaled glucocorticoid on bone metabolism and growth are still lacking.

Local adverse effects of inhaled steroids include oropharyngeal candidiasis and dysphonia that are dose dependent. The dysphonia appears to be due to a local steroid-induced myopathy of the vocal chords. The use of a spacer device can decrease oropharyngeal deposition and decrease the incidence and severity of local side effects.[57] Oropharyngeal candidiasis is due to local immunosuppression and can be reduced with less frequent administration and rinsing of the oropharynx as well as use of a spacer device.[57]

Optimal dosing of inhaled steroids has not been thoroughly investigated. A number of patients may be controlled with bid dosing; however, investigations have demonstrated an improved asthma response with decreased systemic effects by giving the same total daily dose four times daily as opposed to twice daily.[57] So although twice-daily dosing may improve adherence, it may be at the cost of decreased efficacy and increased toxicity. Daily aerosol glucocorticoid administration often produces greater control than alternate-day systemic glucocorticoids.[11,35] The combination can be used for further improvement; in addition, inhaled steroids may allow the systemic dose to be lowered in the severe steroid-dependent asthmatic. Regardless of the type of glucocorticoid therapy, bronchodilator therapy should be considered in conjunction to allow a decrease in the glucocorticoid dose required to control symptoms. There is no evidence that the use of glucocorticoids in the moderate asthmatic will induce a state of steroid dependence. In fact, most of the evidence demonstrating a decrease in bronchial hyperreactivity with steroid therapy implies just the opposite.

At the present time, product information is clear regarding maximum dosing guidelines for adults and children with the available inhaled glucocorticoids. The maximum recommended dose for adults is equivalent to 1600 and 2000 μg daily. It is recommended that patients requiring greater than 1000 μg daily be seen by a specialist in asthma care.[27] These patients should be periodically monitored for adverse systemic effects, particularly if they periodically require oral steroid bursts. The maximum dosing guidelines are even lower for children. Needless to say, more studies are needed in both adults and children to establish safety for doses that exceed the product recommendations.

Spacer Devices and Inhaled Glucocorticoids

The bioavailability of the inhaled glucocorticoids is influenced by the method of delivery, systemic absorption from the gastrointestinal tract and lung, and general factors affecting elimination of the drug. Deposition to the site of drug action within the airways can be substantially increased by application of spacer devices available from various manufacturers. This enhanced deposition will decrease asthma symptoms and improve spirometry in patients with moderate to severe asthma.[57] Coincident with the improvement in asthma is the decrease in frequency of colonization of the oropharynx with candida.

MISCELLANEOUS THERAPIES

Antihistamines

Antihistamines have had a controversial role in asthma therapy. Early studies demonstrating the role of histamine release in bronchoconstriction suggested a potential benefit of antihistamine therapy; however, studies in chronic and acute asthma did not support the initial enthusiasm.[24] The pendulum then swung in the opposite direction on the theoretical (but unproven) grounds that antihistamines through their anticholinergic and mucus-drying effect could be harmful in asthma. This concern has now been refuted and should be finally put to rest.[24] Thus, while antihistamines are generally not indicated for asthma, they are not contraindicated. Indeed, most studies of chronic and acute administration of antihistamines in asthma have demonstrated small improvement of symptoms and pulmonary functions or no effect.[24] Some of the newer agents—terfenadine, cetirizine, loratidine, and azelastine—have demonstrated other anti-inflammatory effects or bronchodilation (azelastine) that may enhance their efficacy in asthma.[24] Currently, antihistamines are useful adjunctive therapy for the patient with allergic rhinitis and asthma.

Methotrexate

Low-dose methotrexate (5–25 mg/week) has been approved for the treatment of the inflammatory diseases psoriatic and rheumatoid arthritis and polymyositis. Initial trials of this agent in the treatment of severe steroid-dependent asthma allowed the reduction of systemic steroid dose in some patients.[24] Although its primary mechanism of action is not understood, methotrexate may be acting as an anti-inflammatory agent.[24] Methotrexate may also have immunomodulatory effects at very low and relevant concentrations because it inhibits chemotaxis of neutrophils, inhibits leukotriene B_4-induced adherence to endothelium, and inhibits the proinflammatory activity of IL-1.[24] Low-dose weekly methotrexate is not without hazard. Hepatotoxicity, opportunistic infections, and pulmonary fibrosis have been reported in patients receiving similar therapy for psoriasis and rheumatoid arthritis.[24] At least one double-blind placebo-controlled trial failed to detect any benefit from methotrexate and had one subject expired from *Pneumocystis carinii* pneumonia.[24] At best, methotrexate therapy results in a moderate reduction in systemic steroid dosage (14–35%) in patients with severe steroid-dependent asthma and does not induce a remission in the disease.[23] Methotrexate should still be considered experimental and reserved for only severe steroid-dependent asthmatics. Patients require careful monitoring including periodic liver biopsies.[24]

The potential beneficial effects of methotrexate have raised questions about whether other anti-inflammatory or immunosuppressant agents might be effective in the treatment of asthma. Thus, many of the drugs active in rheumatoid arthritis such as hydroxychloroquine, dapsone, and gold have been studied in severe steroid-dependent asthma with mixed results.[23,24]

Gold Therapy

Because of its anti-inflammatory properties, gold therapy has been used as a standard therapy in Japan for the past 50 years.[24] However, these studies have been poorly controlled and better well-controlled trials are essential prior to subjecting patients to the potential serious toxicities associated with gold therapy. Similar to the findings with methotrexate, early studies with gold suggest its usefulness in the treatment of steroid-dependent patients. Trials with injectable gold demonstrated improvement in asthmatic symptoms, reduction in glucocorticoid requirements, and diminished airways reactivity.[24] A long-term open trial with oral gold conducted in a population of severe asthmatics demonstrated a small reduction in glucocorticoid use and decreased airways reactivity in about half of the patients evaluated, but 10% of patients were forced to discontinue gold due to side effects.[24] The relatively slow and incremental response observed and significant side effects do not support recommendation of its use.

Macrolides

The macrolide antibiotics troleandomycin (TAO) and erythromycin produce a steroid sparing effect.[23,24] This was initially thought to be primarily due to their ability to inhibit methylprednisolone metabolism. However, the macrolides inhibit activation and chemotaxis of neutrophils and reduce asthmatic bronchial hyperreactivity in trials.[24] Three open trials and two double-blind, crossover trials of TAO in a total of 125 patients have documented a positive steroid sparing effect and/or improvement in symptoms.[24] The potential for hepatotoxicity limits their usefulness. They also inhibit the metabolism of a number of drugs used by asthmatics—most notably theophylline, terfenadine, and astemizole, producing life-threatening cardiac arrhythmias (torsades de pointes) with the latter two drugs and life-threatening seizures with theophylline.[24]

Other Agents

The nonsteroidal anti-inflammatory drugs (NSAIDs) will be dealt with in detail elsewhere. Most asthmatics are unaffected by these agents but up to 25% may have their asthma aggravated; however, a few (less than 1%) benefit from these agents. Currently, there is no method of predicting which patients may benefit. Intravenous gamma globulin (2 gm/kg over 2 consecutive days every 4 weeks for 6 months) has been used in eight children in an open trial and was reported to reduce symptoms and oral corticosteroid dosage.[63] Cyclosporine inhibits T-lymphocyte function and has provided a modest steroid-sparing effect in a small number of patients.[64] Cyclosporine's nephrotoxicity limits its usefulness. Inhaled heparin through its inactivation of histamine and other mast cell mediators and inhaled furosemide by possibly blocking specific chloride channels inhibit EIA.[24,64] Furosemide also inhibits allergen, adenosine, and metabisulfite challenges but is not active orally.[64]

The use of expectorants has not been demonstrated to be beneficial in asthma, although mucolytic therapy to assist removal of impacted mucus plugs in a large bronchus has been life saving in a few instances. Adequate hydration is usually all that is required. In acute asthma, the large negative intrathoracic pressures coupled with mediator-induced capillary permeability may predispose to pulmonary edema that will worsen oxygenation so that excessive hydration should be avoided.[24]

Therapies for Recalcitrant Acute Severe Asthma

Intravenous magnesium sulfate ($MgSO_4$) has been advocated for patients with acute severe asthma who exhibit a suboptimal response to inhaled β_2 agonists.[24] However, the initial trials often used inadequate doses of inhaled β_2 agonists and the bronchodilation from the $MgSO_4$ was modest and did not exceed the β_2-agonist response. Two recent placebo-controlled trials of intravenous $MgSO_4$ in emergency department patients failed to detect any significant bronchodilation or outcome difference from $MgSO_4$ added to optimal inhaled β_2 agonists.[65,66] Numerous other therapies have been reported on an anecdotal basis only; these include ketamine infusion, halothane and isoflurane anesthesia, and ventilation of patients with a helium/oxygen mixture.[24]

Future Therapies

Lipoxygenase System

A number of compounds that either inhibit the production of leukotrienes or antagonize their receptors are undergoing clinical trials in asthma.[23,24,64] Zileuton, an orally active 5-lipoxygenase inhibitor, abolishes aspirin-induced asthma and inhibits allergen-induced asthma and EIA.[64] Zileuton 600 mg four times daily produced significant bronchodilation and improvement in symptoms compared to placebo in mild to moderate adult asthmatics.[67] Zileuton received a positive recommendation for approval for marketing by the FDA Pulmonary and Allergy Drugs Advisory Committee in April 1995. There is some concern about liver enzyme elevations in a small number of patients that was reversible upon discontinuation of the drug. The exact role of zileuton in the therapy of asthma remains to be defined. Early studies of LTD_4 receptor antagonists MK-571 and SKF-104,353 demonstrated inhibition of both EAR and LAR following allergen challenge.[24]

Other Immunomodulators

Much research has focused on evaluating ways of inhibiting the airways inflammatory response. Thus, selective phosphodiesterase inhibitors may have anti-inflammatory activity. Investigations of monoclonal antibodies to specific cytokines and intercellular adhesion molecules (ICAM-1) are in preclinical investigation as well as PAF and neurokinin antagonists.[24,64]

AEROSOL THERAPY FOR ASTHMA

Aerosol delivery of drugs for asthma has the advantages of being site-specific, which enhances the therapeutic ratio. In addition, inhalation of β_2 agonists provides more rapid bronchodilation than either parenteral or oral administration as well as a greater degree of protection against EIA and other challenges.[14,24] Inhalation of glucocorticoids appears to have a greater effect on bronchial hyperreactivity than systemic administration,[57] and finally the newer prophylactic agents, salmeterol and nedocromil, are only effective by inhalation. Therefore, an understanding of aerosol drug delivery is essential to optimal asthma therapy. Table 25.9

TABLE 25.9. FACTORS DETERMINING LUNG DEPOSITION OF AEROSOLS

Device	Device Factors	Patient Factors
Metered-dose inhaler	Canister held inverted Formulation (solution versus micronized suspension) Actuator cleanliness Addition of large volume spacer	Rate of inhalation (slow inspiration) Breathholding Coordinating actuation and inhalation Shaking device
Jet nebulizer	Volume fill (4–6 mL) Gas flow rate (6–12 L/min) Open versus closed system Dead space volume Thumb activating valve	Inhalation rate (slow, deep inspiration) Breathholding Tapping nebulizer
Ultrasonic nebulizer	Volume fill	Inhalation rate (slow, deep inspiration) Breathholding Tapping nebulizer
Dry powder inhaler	Actuator cleanliness	Inhalation rate (rapid, deep inspiration) Breathholding Tilting head back

lists the factors determining lung deposition of therapeutic aerosols. They are divided into device and patient factors.

The various devices used to generate therapeutic aerosols include jet nebulizers, ultrasonic nebulizers, MDIs, and dry powder inhalers (DPIs). The single most important device factor determining the site of aerosol deposition is droplet size.[68] Devices for delivering therapeutic aerosols generate particles with aerodynamic diameters from 0.5–35 μm in diameter.[68] Particles greater than 10 μm deposit in the oropharynx, particles between 5 and 10 μm deposit in the trachea and large bronchi, particles 1 to 5 μm reach the lower airways, and particles smaller than 0.5 μm act as a gas and are exhaled. Respirable particles are deposited in the airway by three mechanisms: (1) inertial impaction, (2) gravitational sedimentation, and (3) Brownian diffusion.[68] The first two are the most important for therapeutic aerosols and are probably the only factors that can be manipulated by patients.

The most important patient factor determining aerosol deposition is inspiratory rate. High inspiratory flow rates increase the degree of deposition due to impaction of all sized particles, thereby increasing deposition centrally (i.e., large airways) and decreasing peripheral deposition.

Besides the two major factors, a number of other factors can be altered to improve delivery and efficacy of clinical aerosols. Most of these factors tend to be device specific and will be discussed under the individual device. Patient factors that cannot be controlled include interpatient variability in airway geometry (particularly the differences between children and adults), the effect of bronchospasm edema, and mucus hypersecretion. Studies indicate that mild obstruction actually increases aerosol deposition[35]; however, severe obstruction probably leads to increased central deposition from impaction.[68]

Metered-Dose Inhalers

Metered-dose inhalers are the most popular form of aerosol delivery due to their convenience (easy portability) and efficacy. They consist of a pressurized canister with a metering valve containing active drug, low vapor pressure chlorofluorocarbon (CFC) propellants, cosolvents, and/or surfactants.[36] The drug is either in solution or a suspended micronized powder. To disperse the suspension for accurate delivery, the canister must be shaken. The metering chamber measures a liquid volume and therefore the device must be held with the valve stem downward so that the chamber is covered with liquid.[35,36] The canister is placed inverted in an actuator and, when pressed, the device releases the propellant and drug in a forceful spray whose particles are large, a mass median aerodynamic diameter (MMAD) of 45 μm with an initial velocity of 100 mph.[35] As evaporation occurs, the particle size is reduced to a final MMAD of 2.8–5.5 μm, depending on the MDI. The aerosol cloud extends at least 10 inches beyond the MDI at the lowest MMAD.[36] Although CFCs can produce cardiac arrhythmias at high doses, investigations have failed to detect adverse effects from the dose delivered via MDIs in recommended dosages. As a result of the Montreal Accord, which phases out the production and use of CFCs by 1996, newer propellants are being developed.[49] Despite a 2-year exemption for medical devices, most manufacturers are in the process of developing alternative aerosol delivery systems. Surfactants, particularly oleates, can produce lung irritation and coughing at excessive doses.[35,36]

Appropriate technique is required to achieve optimal drug delivery and therapeutic effect from an MDI (Table 25.9). Even with optimal technique, only about 10% (5–15%) of the metered dose is deposited in the lung. Approximately 80% impacts on the oropharynx due to the initial high velocity and this portion is then swallowed; the rest is either left in the actuator or exhaled.[68] It is important for actuation to occur during inhalation although the time during inspiration is unimportant provided the inspiratory rate is slow (30 L/min or 5–10 seconds for entire inspiration).[68] A number of authors advocate holding the actuator 2–3 cm in front of an open mouth to allow more evaporation and less impaction. Although radiolabel studies indicate improved delivery, physiologic studies with bronchodilators have failed to document an advantage for this method.[24,35] A large number of studies have shown that many patients do not use their MDIs optimally and also that patient instruction with demonstration is the most effective means of improving inhaler technique.[39,68] Even with instruction, up to 30% of patients, particularly young children and the elderly, cannot master the use of an MDI. For these patients the attachment of auxiliary devices or spacers to the MDI or use of a breath-activated MDI can significantly improve efficacy.[49,68]

Holding Chamber/Spacer Devices

Advantages to the use of spacers with an MDI are decreased oropharyngeal deposition and enhanced lung delivery.[69,70] However, not all spacer devices produce similar effects. The design of spacers varies from simple open-ended tubes that maintain the MDI away from the mouth to holding chambers with one-way valves that open during inhalation. The purpose of a spacer is to allow evaporation of the propellant prior to inhalation. This allows inhalation after actuation of the device, obviating the need for good hand–lung coordination and for a greater number of drug particles to achieve a respirable droplet size.[68] Additionally, most of the large particles that would normally deposit in the oropharynx rain out in the spacer.[68] All of the available spacers significantly reduce oropharyngeal deposition of aerosols from various MDIs.[69] This is an important factor in reducing local adverse effects (hoarseness, thrush) and may decrease HPA-axis suppression from inhaled glucocorticoids,[58,70] and may have clinical importance for bronchodilators delivered by MDI in acute severe asthma.[38] The use of spacers significantly enhances the clinical effect from bronchodilators in ambulatory patients with poor hand–lung coordination but offers no advantage in those patients who can optimally use an MDI alone, despite the fact that radiolabeled studies show increased lung deposition.[49,68] Either the increased amount of bronchodilator drug deposited in the lung is clinically insignificant or these patients reside at the top of the dose–response curve. The inconsistent result may also be due to the utilization of different spacers. Only the large-volume spacers such as the Nebuhaler and InspirEase consistently increase aerosol lung delivery.[69] The increased delivery produced by the use of large-volume spacers appears to be more clinically significant for inhaled glucocorticoids, but may also be important for bronchodilators during acute severe asthma.[58,70]

Breath-Actuated MDIs

Breath-actuated MDIs include the Autohaler and E-Z-V devices. After cocking a lever to "load" the dose of medication, a baffle is opened by inspiratory pressure and the dose is expelled from the canister metering chamber. The E-Z-V device also has a button for manual actuation. While the need for hand–lung coordination for proper actuation is significantly reduced with breath-actuated MDI, these devices do not allow the use of a spacer and they still utilize CFC propellants (although the Autohaler releases 60% less than conventional MDIs).[36] Also, use of these devices improves pulmonary drug deposition only in patients unable to adequately coordinate the use of conventional MDIs.[71] These devices may be particularly helpful in the elderly who have difficulty actuating conventional MDIs.[72]

Jet Nebulizers

Jet nebulizers are primarily used to deliver aerosols to hospitalized patients or patients with acute asthma exacerbations presenting to the clinic or emergency room. They have the advantage of not requiring significant patient coordination or cooperation other than tidal breathing. Jet nebulizers produce an aerosol from a liquid solution placed in a cup. A tube connected to a stream of compressed air or oxygen flows up through the bottom and draws the liquid up an adjacent open-ended tube. The air and liquid strike a baffle creating a droplet cloud that is then inhaled.[35,36] Large droplets adhere to the sides of the nebulizer and baffles, coalesce, and drip to the bottom to be renebulized. The aerosol output and lung delivery vary between the commercially available nebulizers even when operated in the same manner.[68] This is due to differing dead-space volumes and baffle systems. Altering the operating parameters can also significantly effect lung delivery. Because dead space (i.e., the volume left behind after nebulization stops) remains constant, increasing the fill volume will increase total amount of drug delivered; however, it will also take longer to nebulize the dose.[68] A total fill volume of 4–6 mL is considered optimal but will take 10–15 minutes to complete.[35,36] While this may be an inconvenience to the outpatient, the slower nebulization is probably an advantage in the patient experiencing an acute exacerbation. Tapping the side of the nebulizer during operation induces the droplets on the sides to fall back into the reservoir, minimizing loss.[68] The MMAD of the droplets is directly related to the gas flow rate with flow rates of 5–12 L/min, providing an aerosol cloud with MMAD of 4–8 µm for most nebulizers.[68] Putting a hole in the gas supply tube so nebulization will only occur during inhalation when the patients close their thumb over the hole also decreases aerosol loss. Quiet tidal breathing through a mouthpiece or face mask is the usual method of aerosol delivery from a nebulizer; however, slow deep inhalation and breathholding will also improve delivery from this device as well as from an MDI.

Approximately 10% (5–15%) of the dose placed in a nebulizer is delivered to the patient's lung with 60–80% lost in the apparatus, up to 20% exhaled, and 2% deposited in the mouth under usual operating conditions.[35,36,68] Ultrasonic nebulizers that produce an aerosol by vibrating liquid lying above a transducer at speeds of about 1 mHz produce similar degrees of lung deposition as jet nebulizers.[68] It is easy to see why patients not responding to multiple doses of bronchodilator via MDI during acute attacks respond to the usual doses administered via nebulizer. For example, 2.5 mg of albuterol via a nebulizer should deliver approximately 0.25 mg into the airways whereas 10 puffs from an MDI would only be expected to deliver 0.1 mg to the airways. This is without the increased risk of poor MDI technique during the attack. However, this should not be interpreted as meaning that jet nebulizers are superior to MDIs, for even in acute asthma when β_2 agonists are given in the same dosage by MDI plus spacer or nebulizer over the same time period, they have been shown to be equally effective.[24,38] A number of studies have now shown that the administration of β_2 agonists by MDI plus a spacer with the assistance of trained personnel is as effective as nebulization.

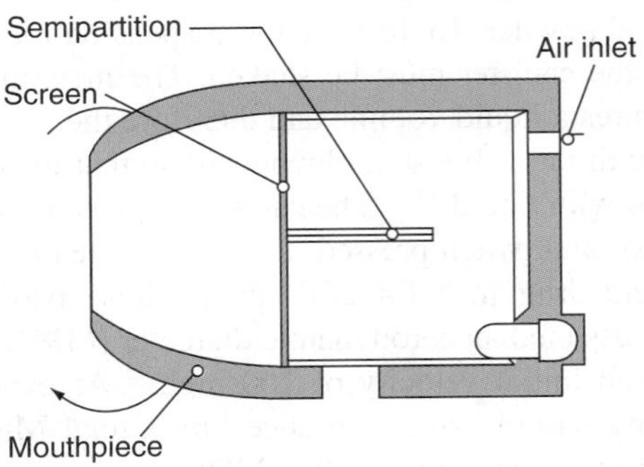

Figure 25.10. Rotahaler (Glaxo).

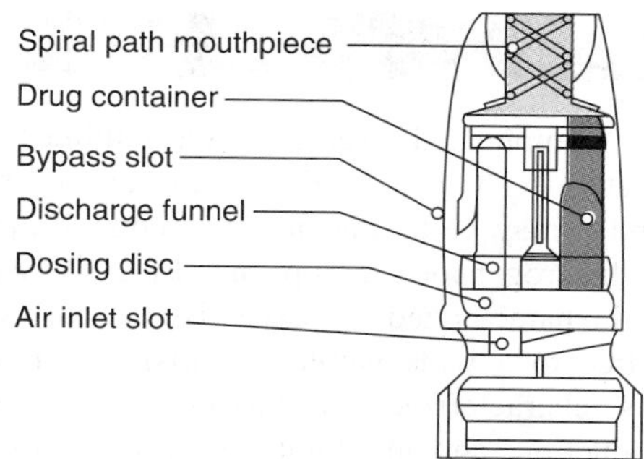

Figure 25.11. Turbuhaler (Draco).

Dry Powder Inhalers

Dry micronized powders can be inhaled directly into the lung. Cromolyn was first introduced for administration in this fashion via a Spinhaler. Due to the impending ban on CFC propellants (scheduled for January 1, 1998, with the 2-year exemption for MDIs), a number of other DPI devices have been developed.[49] These include the *Rotahaler* (Fig. 25.10), *Turbuhaler* (Fig. 25.11), and *Diskhaler* (Fig. 25.12), with other devices undergoing development. The Rotahaler requires that a capsule of medication be placed in the back of the device. Then the device is twisted to break open the capsule and release the medication for inhalation.[73] The Turbuhaler and Diskhaler are multidose devices which require "loading" a dose prior to inhalation by twisting the grip and puncturing a blister of medication, respectively.[49]

An advantage of DPIs is that they are breath actuated and require minimal hand–lung coordination.[24,49] DPIs require higher inspiratory flows (≥60 L/min) and a change in inhalation technique (deep, forceful inspiration) for optimal actuation as compared to conventional MDI, which in turn increases the amount of drug impacted into the oropharynx.[49] Thus, mouth rinsing following treatment with glucocorticoids will be important to minimize absorption and the risk of systemic adverse effects. The higher inspiratory flows required and the inherent inhaler resistance of DPIs have increased concern that patients in acute distress will be unable to adequately actuate the devices for symptomatic relief. However, preliminary studies in acutely obstructed asthmatics have shown that adequate (equivalent to or better than with conventional MDIs) relief can be achieved when bronchodilator medications are administered via DPIs.[49] The Turbuhaler only requires an inspiratory flow of 20 L/min, however, children less than 4 years may not be able to generate a sufficient inspiratory flow for optimal delivery.[74,75] Another concern is that the powder may be irritating and may produce cough, but this has not been widely reported.[24] Finally, the Turbuhaler device is thought to facilitate twice the pulmonary and systemic drug availability as compared to conventional MDI.[49] This is of particular importance with inhaled glucocorticoids because this can influence not only the efficacy of the medication, but its safety profile.[49]

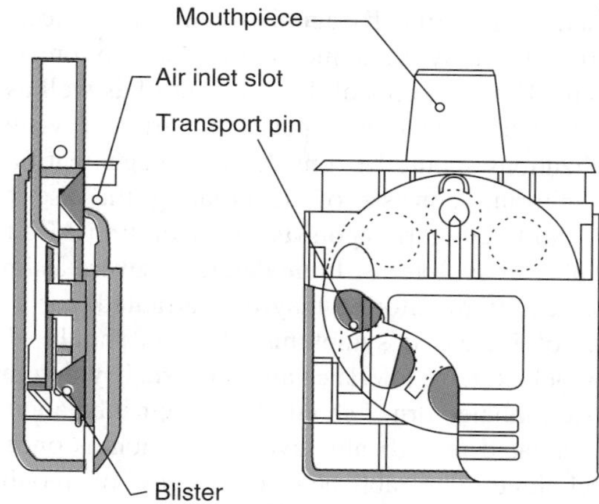

Figure 25.12. Diskhaler (Glaxo).

Alternative Propellants

The impending ban on CFCs has also prompted research into alternative propellants for MDIs. The characteristics of alternative propellants should include allowing solubility of the surfactant, formation of homogeneous suspension (no density gradients), atomization and evaporation characteristics similar to CFCs, no degradation or other effects on metering valve seals, no crystal growth with long-term storage, stability of the drug, and finally, safety to the patient. Two promising alternative propellants currently in development are HFA-134a and HFA-227.[49] Neither, however, possesses all of the ideal features necessary, and the availability of an alternative to CFCs is not expected until 1998 at the earliest. More likely estimates place availability after the end of the century.

MONITORING OF THERAPEUTIC OUTCOMES

CHRONIC ASTHMA

The desired outcomes of successful asthma management are defined by the ICR (Appendix 25.1).[27] Control of asthma is defined as achieving a minimal need for as-needed short-acting β_2 agonists (ideally none), no acute episodes, no limitation of activity, no emergency visits, no nocturnal symptoms, normal peak flows, a peak flow diurnal variation of <20%, and minimal or no adverse effects from medicine. Depending on the severity of the patient's asthma the desired outcome is either control of asthma or the best possible results. For instance, in a severe chronic asthmatic, systemic steroid toxicity is an acceptable alternative to severe morbidity or death from asthma, or in a moderate asthmatic once- or twice-daily administration of as-needed short-acting β_2 agonists may be an acceptable alternative to daily systemic steroid use to prevent all symptoms. Both in terms of disease control as well as cost-effective management, emergency department visits and hospitalizations should be considered management failures.

Monitoring consists of quantitating the use of as-needed short-acting β_2 agonists, days of limited activity, and number of symptoms. In moderate to severe asthmatics daily peak flow monitoring may be warranted, particularly at times of increased symptoms. Patients should also be asked about exercise tolerance and nocturnal symptoms. All patients on inhaled drugs should have their inhalation technique evaluated periodically, every 3–6 months once optimal technique is established. Frequency of monitoring depends on the clinical condition, with severe patients or patients who present as adherence problems seen monthly and mild to moderate patients evaluated every 3–6 months.

Following initiation of anti-inflammatory therapy or a change in dosage, most patients should begin experiencing a decrease in symptoms within 1–2 weeks and achieve maximum symptomatic improvement within 4–8 weeks. Improvement in baseline FEV_1 or PEF should follow a similar time frame, however a decrease in bronchial hyperreactivity as measured by diurnal variation in PEF and exercise tolerance may take longer and slowly improve over 1–3 months and continue to improve from 6 months to 1 year.[2,27]

ACUTE SEVERE ASTHMA

If a patient has an acute severe asthma exacerbation, the goals of therapy are to:

- Relieve airway obstruction as quickly as possible (within minutes).
- Relieve hypoxemia.
- Restore lung function to normal as soon as possible (within hours).
- Plan avoidance of future relapses.
- Develop a written action plan in case of further exacerbations.

Patients who are at risk for acute severe exacerbations should monitor peak flows twice daily at home during periods of increased symptoms or acute exacerbations and continue to monitor peak flows until both the evening and morning PEFs are in the green zone (80% of normal or personal best). If in the yellow zone (50–80% of normal), patients should intensify bronchodilator and possibly anti-inflammatory therapy until they improve into the green zone or contact their physician or begin their home action plan if not improved in 1–2 days. Patients who fall below 50% of normal PEF should contact their physician as soon as possible and seek urgent medical care. In children unable to perform PEFs, supraclavicular retractions and increased respiratory rate and heart rates correlate with severe obstruction.

CONCLUSION

Asthma is a complicated disease with a multitude of clinical presentations. The exact defect in asthma has not been defined, and it may be that asthma is a common presentation of a heterogeneous group of diseases. Asthma is defined and characterized by excessive reactivity of the bronchial tree to a wide variety of noxious stimuli. The reaction is characterized by bronchospasm, excessive mucus production, and inflammation. The central role of inflammation in inducing and maintaining bronchial hyperreactivity is now becoming widely appreciated and studied. The goal of asthma therapy is to normalize, as much as possible, the patient's life and prevent chronic irreversible lung changes. Drugs are the mainstay of asthma therapy. The goal of drug therapy is to use the minimum amount possible to completely control the disease. In chronic asthma, therapy should be aimed at both bronchospasm and inflammation in order to produce the best results. Patients should be diligently followed and monitored for toxicities. Although death from asthma is a rare event, the most common cause of death is underassessment of the severity of obstruction either by the patient or clinician; the next most common is undertreatment. A cornerstone of any therapy is education and the realization that most asthma exacerbations requiring emergency care utilization, hospitalization, and deaths are avoidable.

REFERENCES

1. Rosenblatt MB. History of bronchial asthma, in Weiss EB, Segal MS, Stein M (eds): Bronchial Asthma: Mechanisms and Therapeutics, 2nd ed. Boston, Little, Brown, 1976, pp 5–17.
2. NHLBI, National Asthma Education Program, Expert Panel Report. Guidelines for the diagnosis and management of asthma. Publication No. 91-3042. Bethesda, MD, U.S. Department of Health and Human Services, 1991.
3. Weiss KB, Gergen PJ, Hodgson TA. An economic evaluation of asthma in the United States. N Engl J Med 1992;326:862–866.
4. Gergen PJ, Turkeltaub PC, Kramer RA. Age of onset in childhood asthma: Data from a national cohort. Ann Allergy 1992;68:507–514.
5. Ninan TK, Russell G. Respiratory symptoms and atopy in Aberdeen school children: Evidence from two surveys 25 years apart. Br Med J 1992;304:873–875.
6. Bye MR, Kerstein D, Barsh E. The importance of spirometry in the assessment of childhood asthma. Am J Dis Child 1992;146:977–978.
7. Weiss ST, Tosteson TD, Segal MR, et al. Effects of asthma on pulmonary function in children. A longitudinal population-based study. Am Rev Respir Dis 1992;145:58–64.
8. Weiss KB, Wagener DK. Changing patterns of asthma mortality: Identifying target populations at risk. JAMA 1990;264:1683–1687.

9. Gergen PJ, Weiss KB. Changing patterns of asthma hospitalization among children: 1979 to 1987. JAMA 1990;264:1688–1692.
10. Coultas DB, Gong H Jr, Grad R, et al. Respiratory diseases in minorities of the United States. Am J Respir Crit Care Med 1993;149:S93–S131.
11. McFadden ER, Gilbert IA. Asthma. N Engl J Med 1992;327:1928–1937.
12. Kaliner MA, Barnes PJ, Persson CGA (eds). Asthma: Its Pathology and Treatment. New York, Marcel Dekker, 1991.
13. Murphy S, Kelly HW. Asthma, inflammation, and airway hyperresponsiveness in children. Curr Opin Pediatr 1993;5:255–265.
14. McFadden ER, Gilbert IA. Exercise-induced asthma. N Engl J Med 1994;330:1362–1367.
15. Gleich GJ. The eosinophil and bronchial asthma: Current understanding. J Allergy Clin Immunol 1990;85:422–436.
16. Rankin JA. The contribution of alveolar macrophages to hyperreactive airway disease. J Allergy Clin Immunol 1989;83:722–729.
17. Smith H. Asthma, inflammation, eosinophils and bronchial hyperresponsiveness. Clin Exp Allergy 1992;22:187–197.
18. Kay AB. Asthma and inflammation. J Allergy Clin Immunol 1991;87:893–910.
19. Laitinen LA, Laitinen A, Haahtela T. Airway mucosal inflammation even in patients with newly diagnosed asthma. Am Rev Respir Dis 1993;147:697–704.
20. Ricci M, Rossi O, Bertoni M, Matucci A. The importance of T_{H2}-like cells in the pathogenesis of airway allergic inflammation. Clin Exp Allergy 1993;23:360–369.
21. Sur S, Crotty TB, Kephart GM, et al. Sudden-onset fatal asthma. A distinct entity with few eosinophils and relatively more neutrophils in the airway submucosa? Am Rev Respir Dis 1993;148:713–719.
22. Calderón E, Lockey RF. A possible role for adhesion molecules in asthma. J Allergy Clin Immunol 1992;90:852–865.
23. Corrigan CJ. Immunological aspects of asthma: Implications for future treatment. Clin Immunother 1994;1:31–42.
24. Weiss EB, Stein M (eds). Bronchial Asthma: Mechanisms and Therapeutics, 3rd ed. Boston, Little, Brown, 1993.
25. Morgan WJ, Martinez FD. Risk factors for developing wheezing and asthma in childhood. Pediatr Clin North Am 1992;39:1185–1203.
26. Larsen GL. Asthma in children. N Engl J Med 1992;326:1540–1545.
27. International Asthma Management Project. International consensus report on diagnosis and management of asthma. Publication No. 92-3091. Bethesda, MD, U.S. Department of Health and Human Services, 1992.
28. Duff AL, Platts-Mills TAE. Allergens and asthma. Pediatr Clin North Am 1992;39:1277–1291.
29. Hill M, Szefler SJ, Larson GL. Asthma pathogenesis and the implications for therapy in children. Pediatr Clin North Am 1992;39:1205–1223.
30. Stempel DA, Szefler SJ. Management of chronic asthma. Pediatr Clin North Am 1992;39:1293–1310.
31. Martin RJ (ed). Nocturnal Asthma: Mechanisms and Treatment. Mount Cisco, NY, Futura Publishing Co, 1993.
32. Postma DS, Oosterhoff Y, van Aalderen WMC, et al. Inflammation in nocturnal asthma? Am J Respir Crit Care Med 1994;150(suppl):S83–S86.
33. Reid MJ. Complicating features of asthma. Pediatr Clin North Am 1992;39:1327–1341.
34. Cypcar D, Stark J, Lemanske, RF Jr. The impact of respiratory infections on asthma. Pediatr Clin North Am 1992;39:1259–1276.
35. Jenne JS, Murphy SA (eds). Drug Therapy for Asthma: Research and Clinical Practice. New York, Marcel Dekker, 1987.
36. D'Arcy PF, McElnay JC (eds). The Pharmacy and Pharmacotherapy of Asthma. Chichester, England, Ellis Horwood, 1989.
37. Beasley R, Pearce NE (eds). The Role of Beta Receptor Agonist Therapy in Asthma Mortality. Boca Raton, FL, CRC Press, 1993.
38. Kelly HW, Murphy S. Beta-adrenergic agonists for acute, severe asthma. Ann Pharmacother 1992;26:81–91.
39. Howell JH, Flaim T, Lum Lung C. Patient education. Pediatr Clin North Am 1992;39:1343–1361.
40. Drummond N, Abdalla M, Buckingham JK, et al. Integrated care for asthma: A clinical, social, and economic evaluation: Grampian Asthma Study of Integrated Care (GRASSIC). Br Med J 1994;308:559–571.
41. Abramson MJ, Puy RM, Weiner JM. Is allergen immunotherapy effective in asthma? A meta-analysis of randomized controlled trials. Am J Respir Crit Care Med 1995;151:969–974.
42. Boulet LP. Long- versus short-acting β_2-agonists: Implications for drug therapy. Drugs 1994;47:207–222.
43. Meyer JM, Wenzel CL, Kradjan WA. Salmeterol: A novel, long-acting $beta_2$-agonist. Ann Pharmacother 1993;27:1478–1487.
44. Barrett TE, Strom BL. Inhaled beta-adrenergic receptor agonists in asthma: More harm than good? Am J Respir Crit Care Med 1995;151:574–577.
45. McFadden ER Jr. Perspectives in β_2-agonist therapy: Vox clamantis in deserto vel lux in tenebris? J Allergy Clin Immunol 1995;95:641–651.
46. Greening AP, Ind PW, Northfield M, et al. Added salmeterol versus higher-dose corticosteroid in asthma patients with symptoms on existing inhaled corticosteroid. Lancet 1994;344:219–224.
47. Hendeles L, Weinberger M, Szefler S, Ellis E. Safety and efficacy of theophylline in children with asthma. J Pediatr 1992;120:177–183.
48. Barnes PJ. Theophylline in the management of asthma: Time for a reappraisal? Eur Respir J 1994;7:579–591.
49. Kamada AK. Therapeutics controversies in the treatment of asthma. Ann Pharmacother 1994;28:904–914.
50. Strauss RE, Wertheim DL, Bonagura VR, Valacer DJ. Aminophylline therapy does not improve outcome and increases adverse effects in children hospitalized with acute asthmatic exacerbations. Pediatrics 1994;93:205–210.
51. Edwards D, Zarowitz BJ, Slaughter RL. Theophylline, in Evans WE, Schentag JJ, Jusko WJ (eds). Applied Pharmacokinetics: Principles of Therapeutic Drug Monitoring, 3rd ed. Vancouver, Applied Therapeutics, 1992, pp 13-1–13-38.

52. Pierson WE, LaForce CF, Bell TD, et al. Long-term, double-blind comparison of controlled-release albuterol versus sustained-release theophylline in adolescents and adults with asthma. J Allergy Clin Immunol 1990;85:618–626.
53. Murphy S, Kelly HW. Cromolyn sodium: A review of mechanisms and clinical use in asthma. Drug Intell Clin Pharm 1987;21:22–35.
54. Kelly HW, Murphy S. Should anticholinergics be used in acute severe asthma? DICP Ann Pharmacother 1990;24:409–416.
55. Rutten-van Molken MPMH, van Doorslaer EKA, Jansen MCC, et al. Costs and effects of inhaled corticosteroids and bronchodilators in asthma and chronic obstructive pulmonary disease. Am J Respir Crit Care Med 1995;151:975–982.
56. Wasserman SI (ed). Nedocromil sodium: A pyranoquinolone antiinflammatory agent for the treatment of asthma. J Allergy Clin Immunol 1993;92(suppl):143–216.
57. Sertl K, Clark T, Kaliner M (eds). Corticosteroids: Their biologic mechanisms and application to the treatment of asthma. Am Rev Respir Dis 1990;141(suppl):S1–S96.
58. Barnes PJ, Pedersen S. Efficacy and safety of inhaled corticosteroids in asthma. Am Rev Respir Dis 1993;148(suppl):S1–S26.
59. Kelly HW, Murphy S. Corticosteroids for acute severe asthma. DICP Ann Pharmacother 1991;25:72–79.
60. McFadden ER Jr. Dosages of corticosteroids in asthma. Am Rev Respir Dis 1993;147:1306–1310.
61. O'Driscoll BR, Kalra S, Wilson M, et al. Double-blind trial of steroid tapering in acute asthma. Lancet 1993;341:324–327.
62. Barnes NC, Marone G, Di Maria GU, et al. A comparison of fluticasone propionate, 1 mg daily, with beclomethasone dipropionate, 2 mg daily, in the treatment of severe asthma. Eur Respir J 1993;6:877–884.
63. Mazer BD, Gelfand EW. An open-label study of high-dose intravenous immunoglobulin in severe childhood asthma. J Allergy Clin Immunol 1991;87:976–983.
64. Barnes PJ. New drugs for asthma. Eur Respir J 1992;1126–1136.
65. Tiffany BR, Berk WA, Todd IK, White SR. Magnesium bolus or infusion fails to improve expiratory flow in acute asthma exacerbations. Chest 1993;104:831–834.
66. Green SM, Rothrock SG. Intravenous magnesium for acute asthma: Failure to decrease emergency treatment duration or need for hospitalization. Ann Emerg Med 1992;21:260–265.
67. Israel E, Rubin P, Kemp JP, et al. The effect of inhibition of 5-lipoxygenase by zileuton in mild-to-moderate asthma. Ann Intern Med 1993;119:1059–1066.
68. Newman SP. Aerosol deposition considerations in inhalation therapy. Chest 1985;88(suppl):152–160.
69. Kim CS, Eldridge MA, Sackner MA. Oropharyngeal deposition and delivery aspects of metered-dose inhaler aerosols. Am Rev Respir Dis 1987;135:157–164.
70. Brown PH, Blundell G, Greening AP, et al. Do large-volume spacer devices reduce the systemic effects of high-dose inhaled corticosteroids? Thorax 1990;45:736–739.
71. Newman SP, Weisz AWB, Talaee N, Clarke SW. Improvement of drug delivery with a breath actuated pressurized aerosol for patients with poor inhaler technique. Thorax 1991;46:712–716.
72. Chapman KR, Love L, Brubaker H. A comparison of breath-actuated and conventional metered-dose inhaler inhalation techniques in elderly subjects. Chest 1993;104:1332–1337.
73. Pedersen S. How to use a rotahaler. Arch Dis Child 1986;61:11–14.
74. Pedersen S, Hansen OR, Fuglsang G. Influence of inspiratory flow rate upon the effect of a Turbuhaler. Arch Dis Child 1990;65:308–319.
75. Goren A, Noviski N, Avital A, et al. Assessment of the ability of young children to use a powder inhaler device (Turbuhaler). Pediatr Pulmonol 1994;18:77–80.

Chronic Management of Asthma: Stepwise Approach to Asthma Therapy

Step-up: Progression to the next higher step is indicated when control cannot be achieved at the current step and there is assurance that medication is used correctly. If PEFR ≤60% predicted or personal best, consider a burst of oral corticosteroids and then proceed.

Step-down: Reduction in therapy is considered when the outcome for therapy has been achieved and sustained for several weeks or even months at the current step. Reduction in therapy is also needed to identify the minimum therapy required to maintain control.

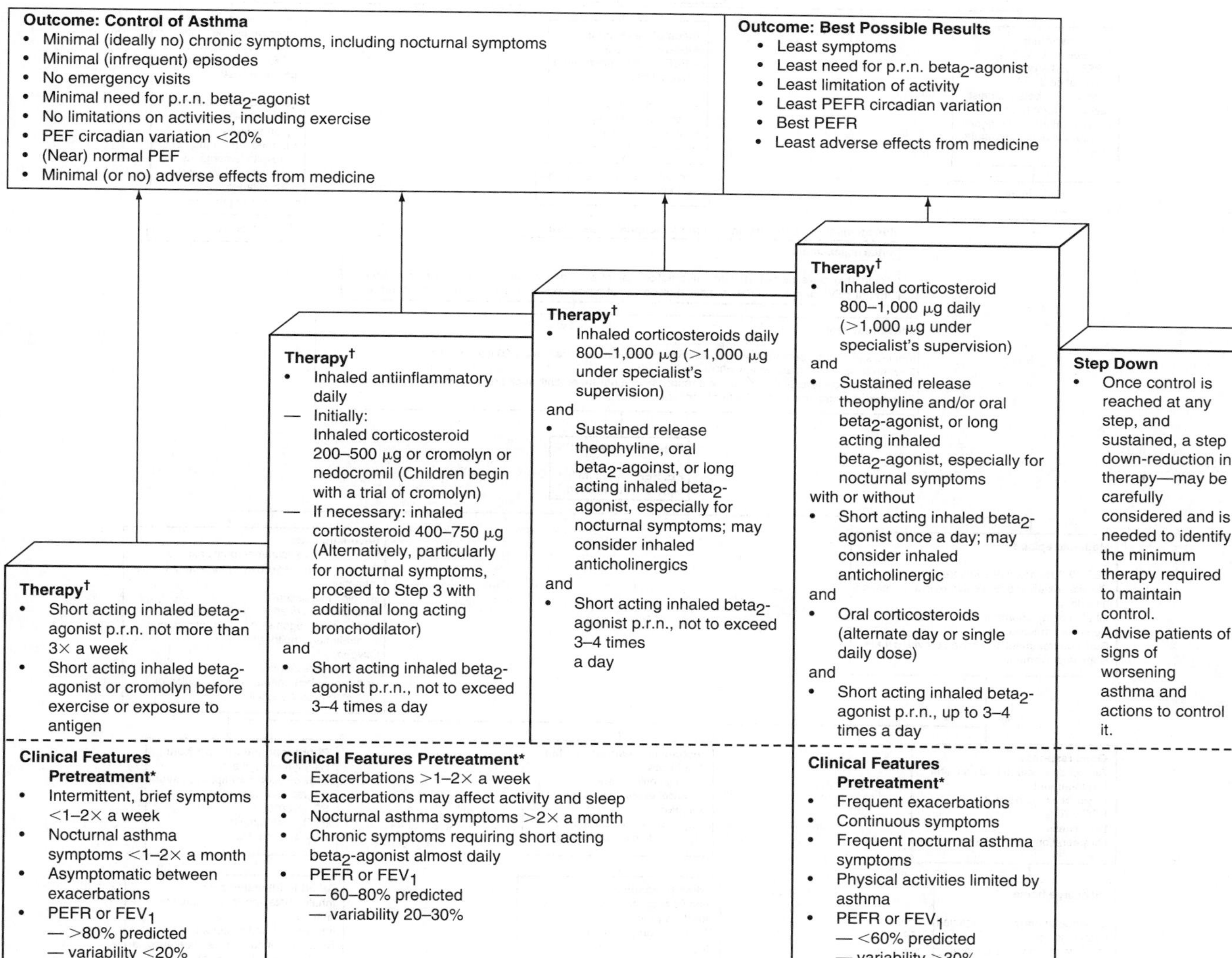

*One or more features may be present to be assigned a grade of severity; an individual should usually be assigned to the most severe grade in which any feature occurs.

†All therapy must include patient education about prevention (including environmental control where appropriate) as well as control of symptoms.

From *International Consensus Report on Diagnosis and Management of Asthma*, March 1992.

Management of Exacerbation of Asthma: Home Treatment

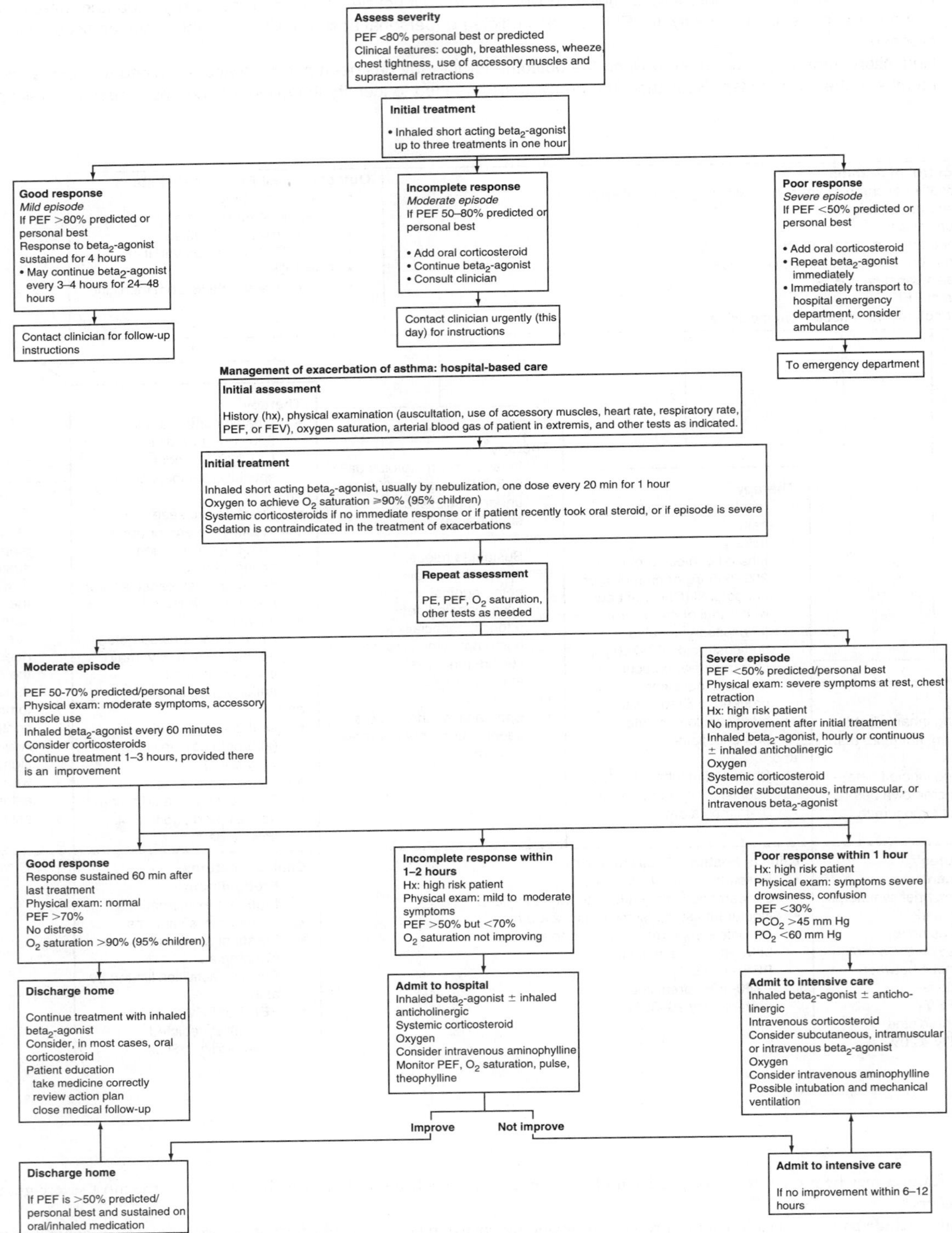

From *International Consensus Report on Diagnosis and Management of Asthma,* March 1992.

Chapter 26

Chronic Obstructive Lung Disease

Margaret A. Noyes, PharmD, BCPS,
and Mark A. Stratton, PharmD, BCPS, FASHP

Chronic obstructive lung disease (COLD) is a term used to describe a pulmonary disorder characterized by abnormal results of tests of expiratory flow that do not change markedly over a several-months' period of observation. Patients with this disease may show some improvement in pulmonary function with bronchodilators. At autopsy, however, they exhibit characteristic changes in their airways and alveoli. While the term COLD initially evolved in the 1950s and 1960s, a uniform definition was elusive due to inconsistencies in descriptions used in the United States and Great Britain. The definition provided here is the one adopted by the American Thoracic Society and serves to distinguish COLD from asthma or other potentially reversible causes of lung dysfunction such as tuberculosis or tumors.[1] The terms chronic obstructive airway disease (COAD) and chronic obstructive pulmonary disease (COPD) are synonymous with COLD.

COLD has conventionally included the subsets of chronic bronchitis and emphysema, although one should note that COLD may exist before evidence of airflow obstruction is demonstrated.[2] Recently, two additional subsets have been made, one from a pathologic perspective, peripheral airway disease, and the other from a clinical perspective, asthmatic bronchitis. Although the pathology and clinical characteristics of these subsets differ, most patients with COLD show characteristics of most of these subsets.

Chronic bronchitis, as reaffirmed by the American Thoracic Society in 1986, is a condition with chronic or recurrent excess mucus secretion into the bronchial tree that occurs on most days during a period of at least 3 months of the year for at least 2 consecutive years.[1] Patients with predominant chronic bronchitis may have an associated asthmatic bronchitis, which implies some degree of reversibility to their disorder. Emphysema classically was defined on histologic examination at autopsy. Since this definition is of no clinical value, it has been defined as a condition of the lung characterized by abnormal, permanent enlargement of the airspaces distal to the terminal bronchiole, accompanied by destruction of their walls, yet without obvious fibrosis. Peripheral airway disease is a condition that includes inflammation of the terminal and respiratory bronchioles, fibrosis with narrowing of airway walls, and goblet cell metaplasia of the bronchiolar epithelium.[1] These changes appear before clinically detectable emphysema is present and are consistent with the pathology traditionally associated with chronic bronchitis.

Epidemiology

Approximately 15 million Americans have COLD.[3,4] It is the fourth most common cause of death in the United States. This is notable because COLD is the only leading cause of death other than congestive heart failure that is increasing in prevalence.[4] The group with the highest increase in deaths from COLD most recently has been white women. Data from the National Center for Health Statistics indicate that in a 13-year period, the age-adjusted mortality rate from COLD increased approximately 5.8% in men and 100% in women (Fig. 26.1).[3,4] Rates of death from COLD increase with age, and are 1.8 times higher in males than females and 2.8 times higher in whites than in blacks. In 1986, 71,099 people in the United States died from COLD. This represented a 33% increase in COLD mortality since 1979 even though the prevalence of smoking has decreased since 1965 (Fig. 26.2). This probably reflects the long latency period between smoking exposure and death from COLD. Cigarette smoking is clearly recognized as the principal risk factor for the development of COLD and is implicated in 90% of cases.[5]

According to the National Health Interview Survey, in 1985, nearly 5.5 million Americans 55 years of age and over were estimated to have COLD. This same survey revealed that, from the period 1979–1985, prevalence rates for COLD for the age group 65 to 74 years were 136/1000 for men and 118/1000 for women.[6] This striking increase from earlier data may reflect a broadening acceptance of the definition of COLD rather than an increased incidence of the disease.

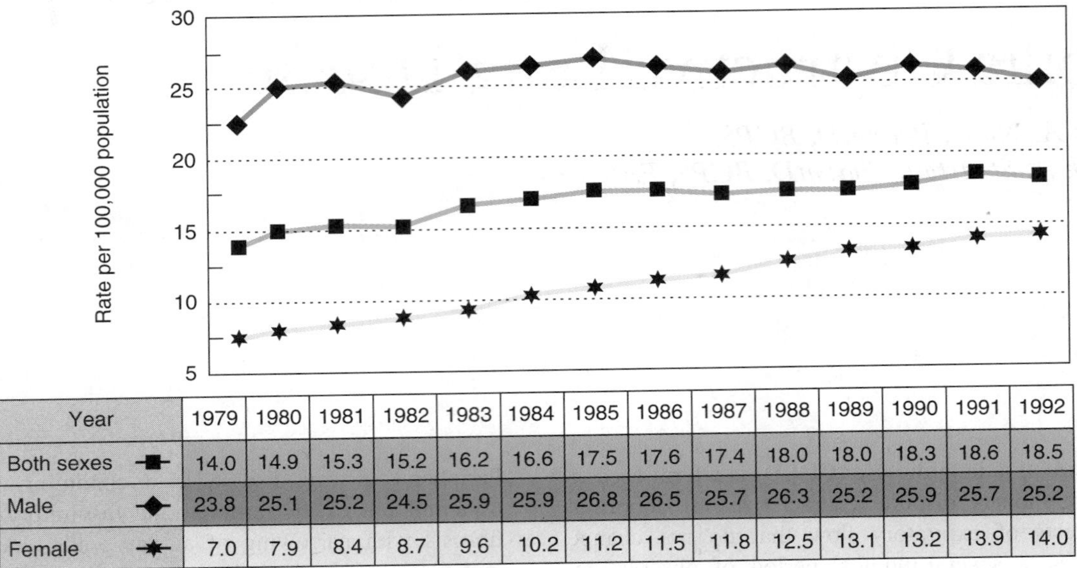

Year	1979	1980	1981	1982	1983	1984	1985	1986	1987	1988	1989	1990	1991	1992
Both sexes	14.0	14.9	15.3	15.2	16.2	16.6	17.5	17.6	17.4	18.0	18.0	18.3	18.6	18.5
Male	23.8	25.1	25.2	24.5	25.9	25.9	26.8	26.5	25.7	26.3	25.2	25.9	25.7	25.2
Female	7.0	7.9	8.4	8.7	9.6	10.2	11.2	11.5	11.8	12.5	13.1	13.2	13.9	14.0

Figure 26.1. COPD death rate, 1979–1992, age-adjusted by sex. *(From NCHS, Annual Summary of Vital Statistics, 1979–1992.)* This figure refers exclusively to data on chronic bronchitis and emphysema. Data on asthma are not included.

While the mortality associated with COLD is impressive, the disability associated with it is also of concern. COLD is the second leading cause of disability in the United States.[7] The prevalence rate of chronic bronchitis and emphysema increases with age and is higher in men than women and in whites than nonwhites[3,4] (Figs. 26.3 through 26.6). However, the ratio of men to women is higher for emphysema than for chronic bronchitis. The prevalence rate of chronic bronchitis increased from 1982–1992 from 33.9 per 1000 to 53.7 per 1000 persons.[3,4] In 1992, the prevalence rate of emphysema was 7.6 per 1000 persons, a 25% decrease over that reported in 1982.[3,4]

Assessing the use of medical resources can provide an estimate of the impact of COLD on society. Data indicate that from 1979–1985, physician office visits for COLD increased 15% for men and 8% for women. In addition, individuals with COLD have approximately double the number of hospital stays, days of restricted activity, and days of being confined to bed than do individuals without COLD.[2]

Of the numerous risk factors (Table 26.1) associated with the development of chronic bronchitis and emphysema, clearly cigarette smoking is the most common. The median risk ratio for smokers versus nonsmokers to develop chronic bronchitis is 5.3 for men and 4.2 for women. Of concern is that the incidence of women with chronic bronchitis or emphysema has increased because of the increased number of women smokers.

Only 15% of smokers go on to develop COLD.[8] Note, however, that in 1986, 82% of COLD mortality was due to smoking.[9] Although the risk is lower in pipe and cigar smokers, it is still higher than for nonsmokers. Not all smokers who have equivalent smoking histories develop

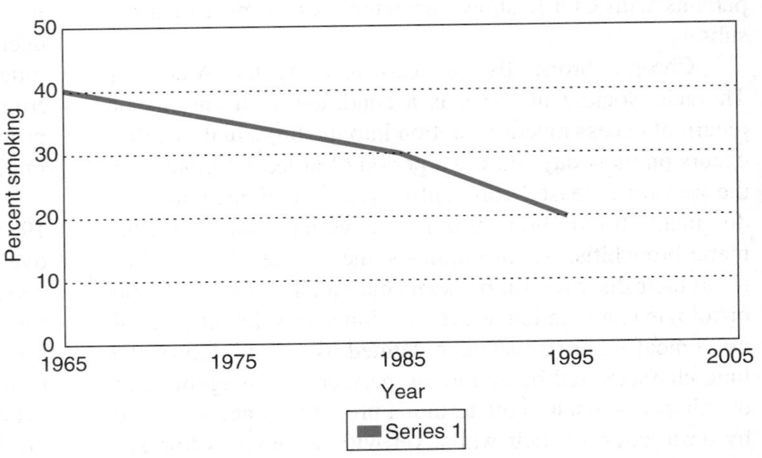

Figure 26.2. Smoking prevalence.

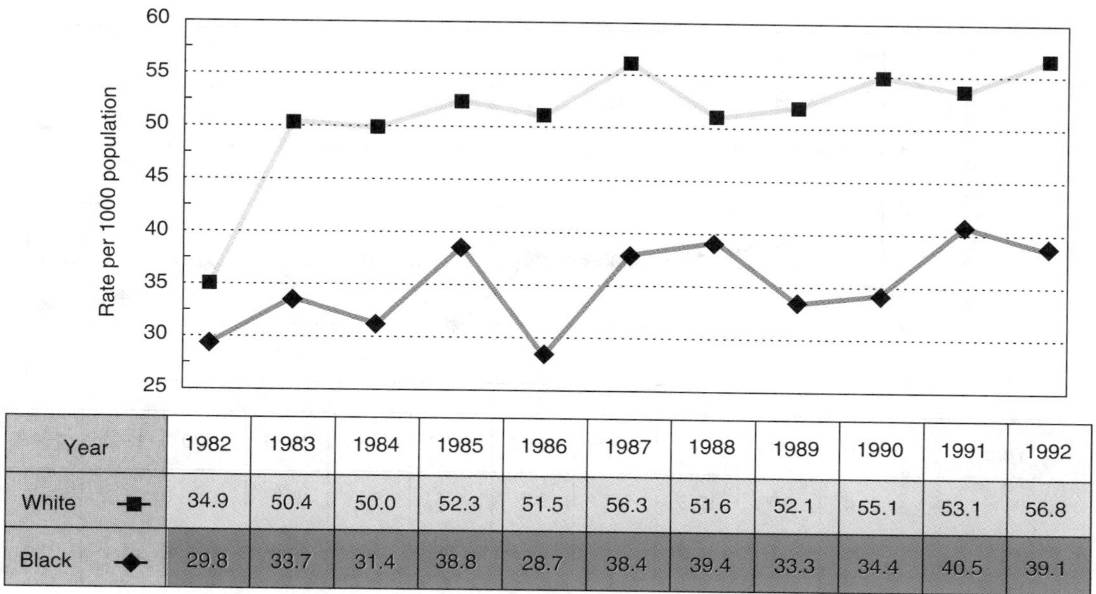

Year	1982	1983	1984	1985	1986	1987	1988	1989	1990	1991	1992
White ■	34.9	50.4	50.0	52.3	51.5	56.3	51.6	52.1	55.1	53.1	56.8
Black ◆	29.8	33.7	31.4	38.8	28.7	38.4	39.4	33.3	34.4	40.5	39.1

Figure 26.3. Chronic bronchitis prevalence, 1982–1992, by race (all ages). *(From NCHS, National Health Interview Survey, 1982–1992.)*

the same degree of pulmonary impairment, suggesting that other physiologic or environmental factors contribute to the degree of lung dysfunction in smokers.[10,11] Children and spouses of smokers are also at increased risk of developing significant pulmonary dysfunction.

Increasing age, male gender, and existing impaired lung function have also been identified as risk factors for the development of COLD. Individuals with existing impairment experience a greater decline in lung function over time than their counterparts with normal pulmonary function. Other increasingly identified familial factors are genetic and environmental.

Occupational hazards are difficult to identify, as they primarily affect blue-collar workers who also have a higher

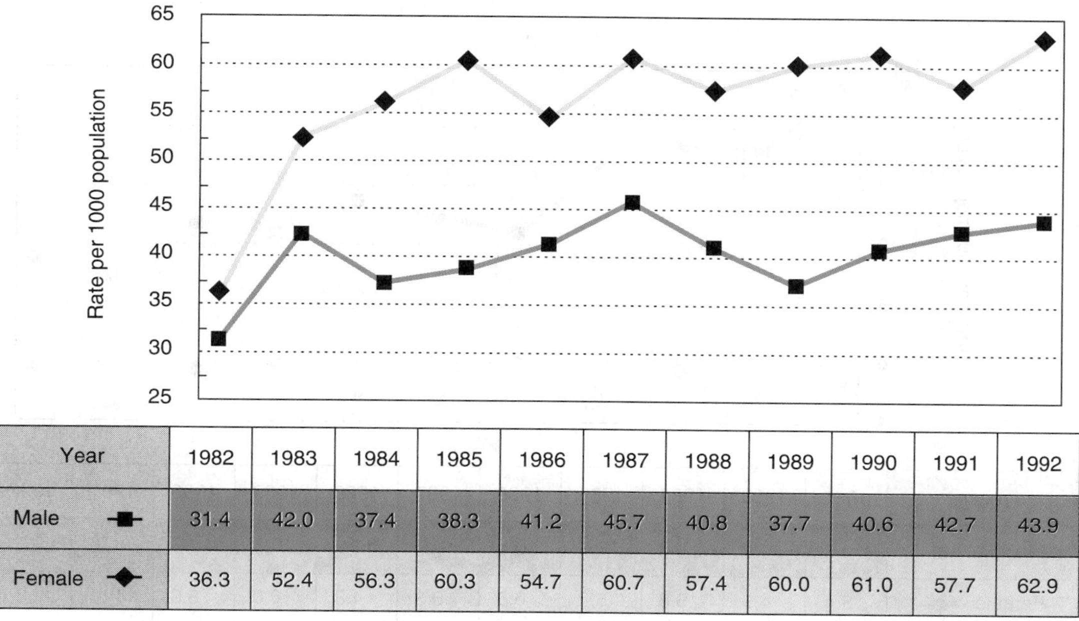

Year	1982	1983	1984	1985	1986	1987	1988	1989	1990	1991	1992
Male ■	31.4	42.0	37.4	38.3	41.2	45.7	40.8	37.7	40.6	42.7	43.9
Female ◆	36.3	52.4	56.3	60.3	54.7	60.7	57.4	60.0	61.0	57.7	62.9

Figure 26.4. Chronic bronchitis prevalence, 1982–1992, by sex. *(From NCHS, National Health Interview Survey, 1982–1992.)*

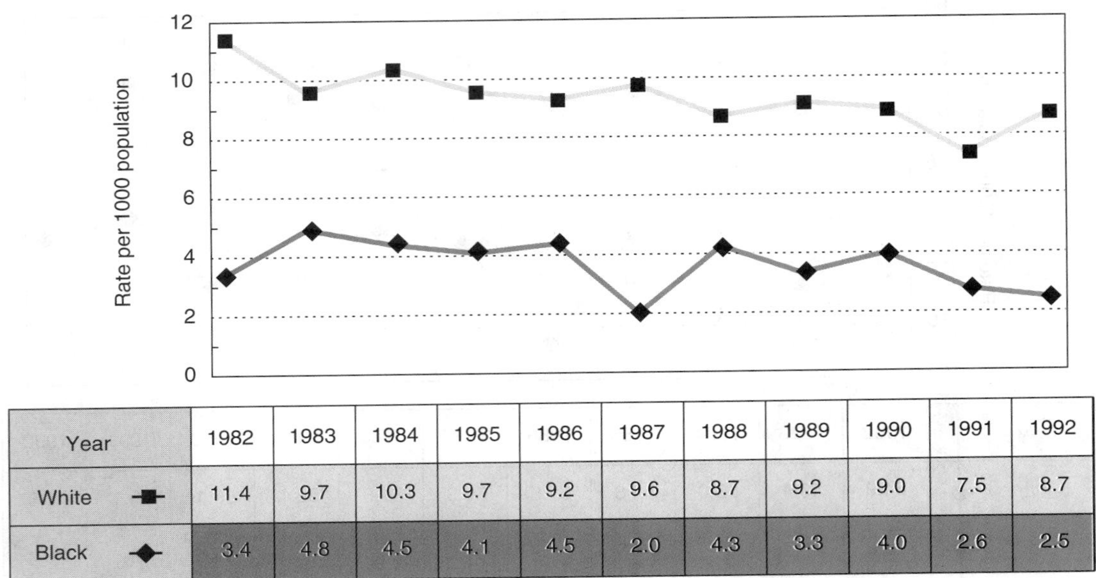

Year	1982	1983	1984	1985	1986	1987	1988	1989	1990	1991	1992
White	11.4	9.7	10.3	9.7	9.2	9.6	8.7	9.2	9.0	7.5	8.7
Black	3.4	4.8	4.5	4.1	4.5	2.0	4.3	3.3	4.0	2.6	2.5

Figure 26.5. Emphysema prevalence, 1982–1992, by race (all ages). *(From NCHS, National Health Interview Survey, 1982–1992.)*

incidence of cigarette smoking and may live in areas of higher air pollution. Reduced lung function and deaths from COLD are higher for individuals engaged in numerous occupations such as gold and coal mining, working in glass or ceramic industries with exposure to silica dust, and in jobs that expose workers to cotton dust or grain dust, toluene diisocyanate, or asbestos. Cigarette smokers have a higher incidence of pulmonary dysfunction than their nonsmoking counterpart in jobs with this type of exposure.[11,12] Numerous other possible occupational risk factors also exist.

It is unclear whether or not air pollution alone is a significant risk factor for the development of COLD. However, in individuals with existing pulmonary dysfunction, significant air pollution worsens symptoms. Studies have shown an association between intensity of air pollution and number of emergency room admissions for COLD.[13] There are as yet insufficient data to suggest that air pollution con-

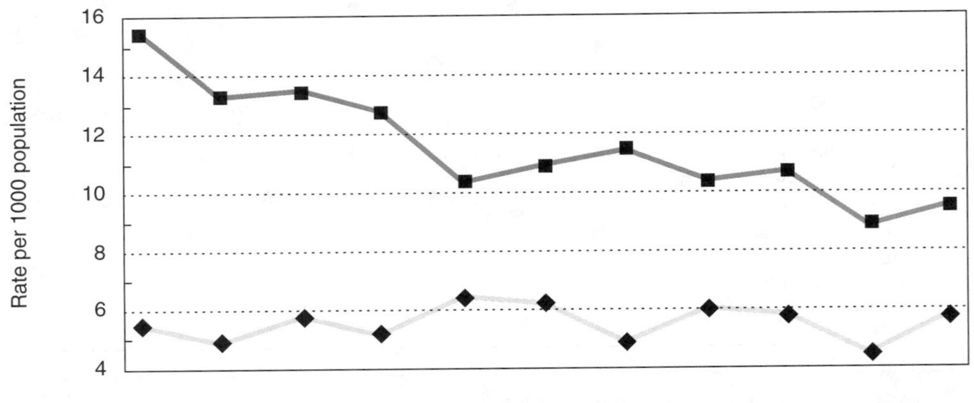

Year	1982	1983	1984	1985	1986	1987	1988	1989	1990	1991	1992
Male	15.4	13.2	13.3	12.8	10.5	10.9	11.2	10.5	10.7	8.8	9.5
Female	5.4	4.9	5.8	5.2	6.5	6.3	4.8	6.0	5.9	4.6	5.8

Figure 26.6. Emphysema prevalence, 1982–1992, by sex. *(From NCHS, National Health Interview Survey, 1982–1992.)*

TABLE 26.1. RISK FACTORS FOR THE DEVELOPMENT OF COLD

Major	Minor
Smoking	Air pollution
Age	Alcohol
Male gender	Race
Existing impaired lung function	Nutritional status
Occupation	Family history
α_1-Antitrypsin deficiency	Socioeconomic status
	Respiratory tract infections
	Bronchial reactivity

tributes to the development of COLD in individuals with normal pulmonary function, whether smokers or not.

α_1-Antitrypsin deficiency has been clearly defined as a genetic factor that contributes significantly to the risk of developing COLD, specifically emphysema. α_1-Antitrypsin is a protease inhibitor that normally inhibits trypsin and other proteases from destroying normal lung tissue. The protease inhibitor (Pi) phenotypes with the highest incidence of COLD are the homozygous PiZ (because they have the lowest level of α_1-antitrypsin) and, to a lesser extent, the heterozygous PiMZ individuals.

PATHOPHYSIOLOGY

The pathophysiology of COLD can best be understood by examining chronic bronchitis and emphysema separately. Peripheral airway disease is a major component of both conditions contributing to obstruction. In the majority of patients, evidence of each condition is present.

CHRONIC BRONCHITIS

As described earlier, chronic bronchitis is characterized by excessive tracheobronchial mucous secretion with cough. This excessive production of mucus results from hyperplasia and hypertrophy of mucus-producing glands and goblet cells due to continued bronchial irritation. Additional morphologic changes occur in the bronchi, including increased smooth muscle, cartilage atrophy, inflammation characterized by neutrophil and lymphocyte infiltration, and loss of cilia. These bronchial changes do not contribute significantly to obstruction.[15]

In the COLD patient with predominant chronic bronchitis, changes in the peripheral airways contribute most to obstruction. Inflammation exists with mucus production and narrowing of the lumen in the more distal noncartilagenous or membranous bronchioles. In addition, there is fibrosis, tortuosity, and irregularity of these smaller airways. Autopsies have shown that individuals with chronic bronchitis have more airways smaller than 0.4 mm in diameter when compared with nonbronchitic patients. This is thought to be a result of the previously described morphologic changes.

Many chronic bronchitis patients will show minimal improvement with bronchodilators. Some display much more improvement in obstruction after bronchodilator therapy and would be more appropriately referred to as patients with asthmatic bronchitis. There may be a significant component of atopy in these patients.[15] Ventilatory impairment is unrelated to atopic status in individuals without a history of asthma, according to a recent study,[16] further supporting the theory that nonallergic inflammation is important in the pathogenesis of chronic airflow obstruction.

The lung damage produced by smoking or exposure to other chronic irritants has long been considered to begin in the small airways. Airways less than 2 mm in diameter contribute only 10–20% of normal resistance to airflow, because their total cross-sectional diameter is much greater than that of larger airways. By the time obstruction is detected by pulmonary function tests, extensive damage has occurred. The best predictor of moderate disease has been suggested to be the presence of diminished breath sounds on physical examination, especially when combined with a clinical history consistent with COLD.[17] As chronic bronchitis progresses over several years, the changes in small airways begin to impair ventilation (V), while perfusion (Q) remains fairly adequate, resulting in a V/Q imbalance and hypoxemia. The hypoxemia leads to pulmonary hypertension with subsequent right ventricular failure (cor pulmonale). Autopsy data indicate that patients with pulmonary hypertension have markedly increased percentages of the intima and media in the musculature of the pulmonary arteries, specifically the larger vessels. These alterations do not, however, correlate with either the severity of the pulmonary hypertension nor the ability of the vasculature to respond to oxygen.[18] The persistent hypoxemia stimulates erythropoiesis with resultant secondary polycythemia and increased blood viscosity, with its attendant complications of mental confusion and thrombotic stroke.

An additional component of chronic bronchitis is repeated respiratory infections. Patients are predisposed to repeated infections due to mucus stagnation and plugging as well as lack of cilia or ciliary movement to clear mucus. The signs of infection usually consist of sputum changes; such as an increase in volume, thickening, and a change in color. Fever or other objective evidence of infection need not be present. Repeated respiratory infections in the chronic bronchitis patient can cause severe acute exacerbations in pulmonary status and can contribute significantly to accelerating the decline in pulmonary function tests due to the inflammation-induced fibrosis of bronchi and bronchioles. The most frequent respiratory pathogens are viral, although bacterial infection may follow a viral infection. The respiratory syncytial virus is considered the most common overall pathogen, while *Streptococcus pneumoniae* and *Haemophilus influenzae* are the most common bacterial pathogens. Because these are not the only bacteria that act as pathogens, the host's condition and environment must be considered when searching for a pathogen in a patient with chronic bronchitis with a suspected respiratory infection.

EMPHYSEMA

Emphysema refers specifically to involvement of the acinus, which is the unit of the lung responsible for gas exchange. It consists of three levels—respiratory bronchioles, alveolar ducts, and alveolar sacs—proceeding distally. In a simplistic sense, emphysema is a condition in which there is destruction of walls within the acinus such that the surface area for gas exchange is diminished. Data indicate it is intrinsic damage to the small airways that is the major cause of airflow limitation and not emphysema.[19]

Several types of emphysema have been described and deserve comment:

1. *Proximal acinar emphysema:* This type includes the centrilobular emphysema (i.e., central lobes of the acinus) characteristically seen in cigarette smokers, especially in the upper lobes, and simple pneumoconiosis of coal workers. This type of emphysema is confined largely to the proximal portion of the acinus, with the respiratory bronchioles being particularly affected (Fig. 26.7).
2. *Panacinar emphysema:* The entire acinus is involved in this type. It is found in those genetically susceptible individuals who possess the homozygous PiZ phenotype (i.e., 1–2% of all emphysema patients). These patients have a deficiency of protease inhibitors (α_1-antitrypsin) such that proteases are allowed to destroy the alveolar walls of the acinus. This type usually involves the entire lung field (Fig. 26.7).
3. *Distal (paraseptal) emphysema:* As the term suggests, this type of emphysema is associated with the distal portion of the acinus. It is seen as a consequence of spontaneous pneumothorax in young adults.
4. *Irregular emphysema:* This type of emphysema is produced as a consequence of trauma to lung tissue.

Our understanding of the pathogenesis of centrilobular emphysema (the most common type) extends from an understanding of the panacinar emphysema associated with protease inhibitor deficiency states. In centrilobular emphysema specifically caused by smoking, an imbalance develops between the protective protein inhibitors and proteases from activated neutrophils and mast cells. Women are less likely to experience this imbalance, possibly because of a protective effect of estrogens that may stimulate synthesis of protease inhibitors. Damage occurs because cigarette smoke causes a macrophage alveolitis and a respiratory bronchiolitis. These macrophages are chemotactic for neutrophils. Both the macrophages and neutrophils release a greater amount of elastase (which breaks down elastin, a protein integral to the structural integrity of alveolar walls) in response to smoke in smokers than in nonsmokers. Cigarette smoke is also thought to impair the synthesis of elastin.[20] Alveolar inflammatory cells in smokers with emphysema have been shown to spontaneously inactivate α_1-proteinase inhibitor, suggesting that the progressive lung damage is related to an ongoing inflammation in peripheral airways.[21] Protease inhibitor (Pi) phenotype M patients are particularly susceptible to these effects of cigarette smoke.[9]

The destruction of the surface area for gas exchange within the acinus results in a loss of elastic recoil. This loss permits compression of distal airways during expiration, contributing to the significant obstructive pattern that is seen in pulmonary function tests. The exact changes in pulmonary function are described later in this chapter. In cigarette smokers with centrilobular emphysema, the respiratory bronchiolitis leads to narrowing of the terminal bronchioles.[22]

In addition to a reduction in elastic recoil, loss of alveolar walls results in a loss of the capillary network essential to adequate perfusion. This results in not only a decrease in

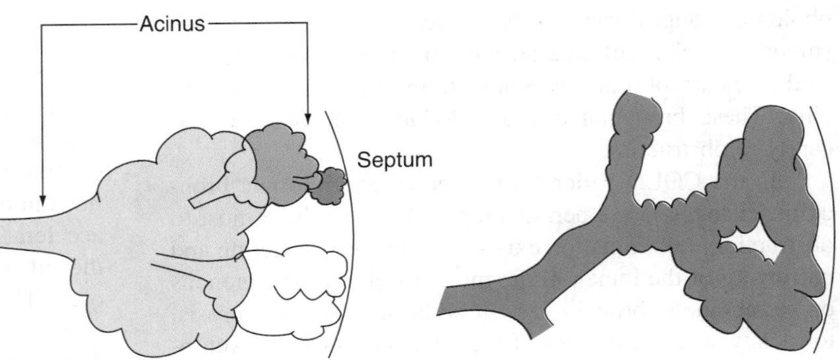

Figure 26.7. In centrilobular emphysema the terminal bronchioles are involved, whereas in panacinar emphysema the entire acinus is involved.

ventilation (V) but also a loss in perfusion (Q), thus, the V/Q ratio is maintained better than in chronic bronchitis.[23] Therefore, while predominant emphysematous patients experience greater dyspnea than predominant chronic bronchitis patients, the former are better able to preserve gas exchange because their respiratory centers are more responsive to hypoxia. The net result of this on other physiologic systems is less cor pulmonale and less polycythemia than seen in the predominant chronic bronchitic.

CLINICAL PRESENTATION

By the time a patient presents with obstructive airway disease, the diagnosis can be rapidly made often by simply observing the patient's breathing pattern. The clinical features are presented in Table 26.2. As described previously, while the majority of patients with COLD will have components of both chronic bronchitis and emphysema, it is best to describe the physical examination of each predominant constituent condition separately.

CHRONIC BRONCHITIS

The patient presenting with predominant chronic bronchitis is often overweight and has an impressive history of productive cough and increasing dyspnea on exertion. By history the cough has been increasing in frequency and duration. Predominant chronic bronchitis patients are referred to classically as "blue bloaters" (type B) as they tend to retain carbon dioxide because of a decreased responsiveness of the respiratory center to hypoxemia and ultimately hypercarbia. They will commonly have peripheral edema from cor pulmonale and usually have a normal or only slightly increased respiratory rate at rest. With advanced disease, the anteroposterior diameter of the chest is often increased resulting in the classical "barrel chest" appearance. This does not always indicate advanced disease, because it is also a normal part of the aging process. Percussion of the chest is resonant, and the breath sounds are distant on auscultation. Rhonchi and wheezes are frequently heard and change in location as the patient breathes deeply or coughs. A rapid assessment of obstruction can be done by placing the stethoscope over the trachea and instructing the patient to forcefully expire. Forced expiration lasting greater than 4 seconds correlates with obstruction in pulmonary function tests. The use of the scalene or sternocleidomastoid muscles of the neck to assist respiration may not be apparent unless severe obstruction is present.

As the degree of obstruction worsens and the arterial oxygen tension ($Pa{O_2}$) continues to drop, pulmonary hypertension from vasoconstriction ensues. This leads to right ventricular strain and ultimately cor pulmonale. On physical examination this is manifested by jugular venous distention, hepatomegaly, hepatojugular reflux, and peripheral edema. Conventional cardiac examination may be difficult if a barrel chest is present; however, by palpating the epigastric area, a heave may be felt or even seen in thin patients and auscultation of the area may reveal a gallop rhythm suggestive of right ventricular hypertrophy.

In the face of chronic hypoxemia, cyanosis of the lips, mucous membranes, or extremities may be seen. The cyanosis worsens during the night, frequently because of

TABLE 26.2. CLINICAL FEATURES OF COLD

	Predominant Emphysema	Predominant Chronic Bronchitis
Age (yr)	60±	50±
Dyspnea	Severe	Mild
Cough	After dyspnea starts	Before dyspnea starts
Sputum	Scanty, mucoid	Copious, purulent
Bronchial infection	Less frequent	More frequent
Respiratory insufficiency episode	Often terminal	Repeated
Chest film	Increased diameter Flattened diaphragms	Increased bronchovascular markings, large heart
$Pa{CO_2}$ (mm Hg)	35–40	50–60
$Pa{O_2}$ (mm Hg)	65–75	45–60
Hematocrit (%)	35–45	50–60
Pulmonary hypertension		
Rest	None to mild	Moderate to severe
Exercise	Moderate	Worsens
Cor pulmonale	Rare	Common
Diffusion capacity	Decreased	None to slightly decreased

(Adapted from Ref. 29.)

chronic oxygen desaturation secondary to sleep apnea. Clubbing of the fingers is rarely seen in chronic bronchitis. Sleep apnea has recently become an area of increasing study in patients with COLD and may play a much greater role than previously understood in the pathogenesis of disease, especially with respect to cor pulmonale. Recent data indicate that individuals with sleep apnea are at greater risk for developing respiratory insufficiency and cor pulmonale than expected.[24]

EMPHYSEMA

The patient presenting with predominant emphysema is characteristically older than the chronic bronchitis patient. The chief complaint is often increasing dyspnea, even at rest, with minimal cough. These patients have been classically termed "pink puffers" (type A) because of their obvious tachypnea and flushed appearance, which is due to their respiratory centers being quite responsive to hypoxemia as a stimulus to breathe.

These patients are frequently thin in physical stature and will present with "pursed lip" breathing. This maneuver compensates for loss of elastic recoil so that exhalation of a larger volume of air is possible. They also are tachypneic at rest and often sit with their chests forward and hands resting on their knees; this position requires the least energy for breathing. Frequently, the patient uses accessory muscles of the chest and neck to assist in the work of breathing. Percussion of the chest is hyperresonant and auscultation reveals diminished breath sounds with rhonchi and minimal wheezes. Excursion of the diaphragms is limited because of persistent hyperinflation of the lungs.

Hypoxemia is not a significant problem in the predominant emphysema patient until late in the disease state. As a result, cor pulmonale is not as common a problem as seen in the predominant chronic bronchitic until the terminal stages.

Diagnostic Tests

PULMONARY FUNCTION TESTS

Measurements of pulmonary function by objective means are considered essential in any patient with COLD to determine the severity of the disease, responsiveness to therapeutic agents, and prognosis. Several tests of small airway function are available, including the single-breath nitrogen test and mid- and end-expiratory flows from spirometry. Spirometry has been extensively used and is preferred due to its cost, technical ease, and clinical applicability.[25]

In the predominant chronic bronchitic, the vital capacity (VC) is decreased, the residual volume (RV) is increased, and the total lung capacity (TLC) is often normal. The VC is decreased while the RV is increased in the emphysematous patient as compared with the chronic bronchitic, and the TLC is usually increased.

In patients with chronic bronchitis and/or emphysema leading to COLD there are reductions in forced expiratory volume after 1 second (FEV_1), forced vital capacity (FVC), FEV_1/FVC%, and forced expiratory flow ($FEF_{25-75\%}$). The FVC is used in conjunction with the FEV_1. The FEV_1/FVC ratio expressed as a percentage is helpful in determining the degree of obstruction. If it is less than 80%, obstruction is present. The forced expiratory flow over the middle 50% of the expiratory curve (MMFR, $FEF_{25-75\%}$, or $FEF_{50\%}$) is helpful specifically in the predominant emphysema patient because it represents the elastic recoil of the lung. In predominant chronic bronchitis, flow rates are decreased. It is now understood that in addition to loss of elastic recoil (i.e., elasticity of the lung parenchyma) in the emphysema patient, there is also a significant component of peripheral airway disease, also referred to as bronchiolitis, which contributes to the obstructive picture.

The majority of patients with mixed disease will usually experience exertional dyspnea when the FEV_1 is less than 50% of predicted and will have dyspnea at rest when the FEV_1 is less than 25% of predicted. Patients with predominant chronic bronchitis experience carbon dioxide retention and cor pulmonale when the FEV_1 is greater than 25% of predicted values, but the predominantly emphysematous patient does not experience these complications until the FEV_1 is less than 25% of predicted.

Measurement of diffusion capacity using carbon monoxide (DCO) can help distinguish predominant bronchitis from emphysema. In emphysema, the diffusion capacity is diminished because of loss of surface area available for gas diffusion. In bronchitis the diffusion capacity is normal or only slightly decreased.

ARTERIAL BLOOD GASES

Just as pulmonary function tests are essential for determining the severity and prognosis of patients with COLD, so are arterial blood gases. Arterial blood gases should be determined at rest and after exercise. The predominant chronic bronchitis patient is characterized as having a low arterial oxygen tension (Pao_2 = 45–60 mm Hg) and an elevated arterial carbon dioxide tension ($Paco_2$ = 50–60 mm Hg). The predominantly emphysematous patient has by comparison a higher Pao_2 and usually normal $Paco_2$ with similar degrees of pulmonary dysfunction. In the predominant chronic bronchitis patient the initial abnormality is a decrease in the Pao_2. The major cause of this hypoxemia is an underventilation (V) of acini relative to the perfusion (Q) of the area. This low V/Q ratio will progress over a period of several years resulting in a consistent decline in the Pao_2. For reasons that are not entirely understood, the predominant chronic bronchitic loses the ability to increase the rate or depth of respiration in response to persistent hypoxemia. This decreased ventilatory drive may have its origin in either abnormal peripheral or central respiratory receptors. This relative hypoventilation subsequently leads to hypercapnia. The respiratory centers again do not respond to the persistently increasing $Paco_2$.

These changes in Pao_2 and $Paco_2$ are subtle and progress over a period of many years; as a result the pH is usually near normal because the kidneys compensate by retaining bicarbonate. If an acute change occurs such as might be seen in an acute pneumonia with impending respiratory failure, the $Paco_2$ may rise sharply, temporarily resulting in a primary respiratory acidosis until the kidneys can compensate (24–72 hours later) or the acid–base defect is corrected by mechanical ventilation.

The persistent hypoxemia leads to pulmonary vascular constriction and cor pulmonale. The hypoxemia and hypercarbia leads to an increase in 2,3-diphosphoglyceric acid (2,3-DPG) and a shift of the oxyhemoglobin dissociation curve to the right. This results in a decrease in the affinity of hemoglobin for oxygen, allowing more oxygen to be released to tissues in which the Po_2 is lowest. Hypoxemia also stimulates erythropoiesis, which leads to the secondary polycythemia common in the predominant chronic bronchitic.

Compared with the predominant chronic bronchitic, the predominant emphysematous patient can maintain a near-normal Pao_2 in the face of declining pulmonary function, until the terminal stages, because ventilation and perfusion decrease proportionately. These individuals have normal or excess responsiveness of peripheral and central respiratory receptors to hypoxemia or hypercarbia. This explains why the predominant emphysematous patient does not develop cor pulmonale, cyanosis, or polycythemia until the end stages of the disease process.

CHEST ROENTGENOGRAM

A chest roentgenogram (posteroanterior and lateral views) is most useful in the diagnosis of the predominant emphysema patient. Characteristic findings include flattened diaphragms that move less than 3 cm between inspiration and expiration, loss of peripheral vascular markings, bullous lesions, and increased retrosternal air space (Fig. 26.8). All these findings indicate extensive air trapping consistent with severe emphysema. Whether or not the dimensions of the thoracic cage itself are truly increased is a matter of controversy; it may be that the cage appears large because of the loss of physical mass in the rest of the body. In the

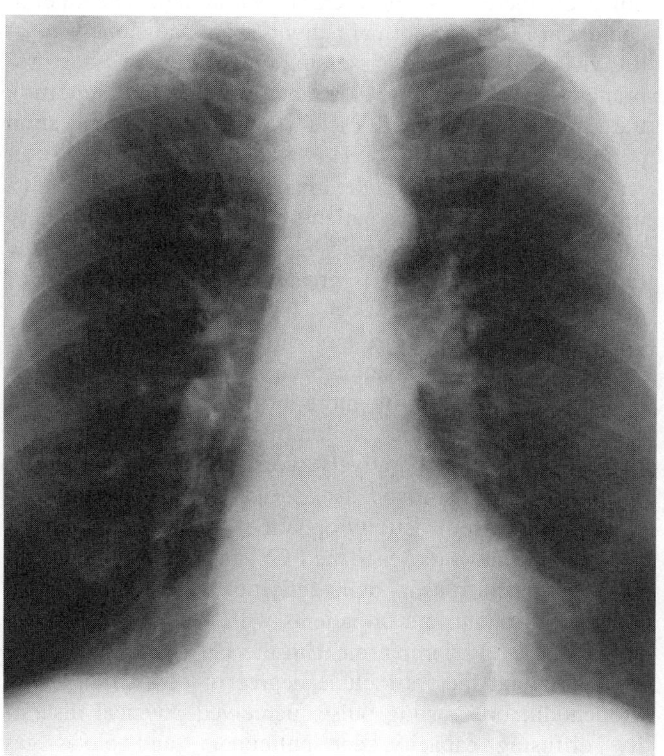

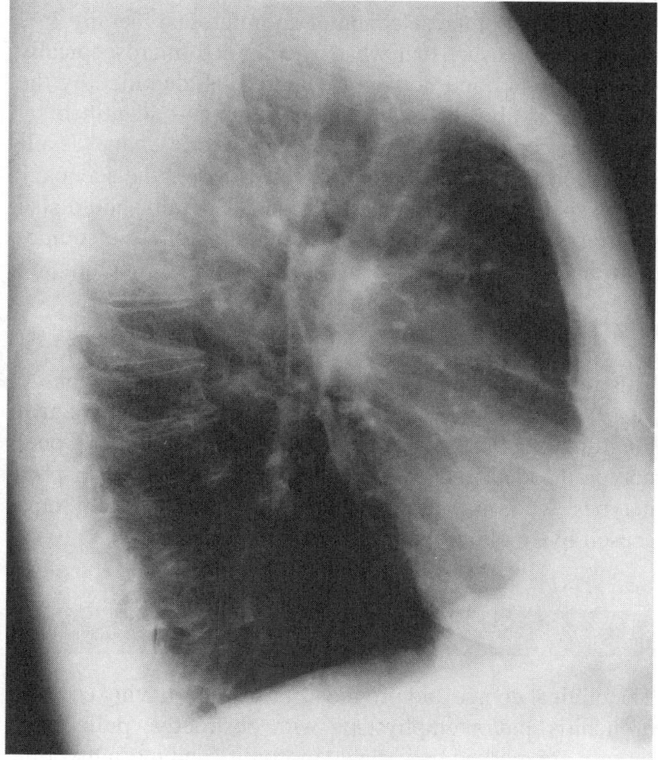

Figure 26.8. Characteristic emphysematous lungs. Note flattened diaphragms, loss of peripheral vascular markings, and a bullous lesion in the right lower lobe on the posteroanterior view (left), and the increased retrosternal air space on the lateral view (right).

predominant chronic bronchitic, the only changes are increased bronchovascular markings in the lower lung field and an increased cardiac silhouette in the presence of right ventricular failure with prominent pulmonary arteries.

ELECTROCARDIOGRAM

The electrocardiogram is helpful in COLD patients only when cor pulmonale develops. Common findings are right-axis deviation, prominent R waves in V1 and V2, S wave in V5 or V6 ≥ 7 mm, and tall peaked P waves in lead II.

OTHER LABORATORY TESTS

Hematology

In the predominant chronic bronchitic patient, the hemoglobin and hematocrit will be elevated secondary to erythropoiesis caused by hypoxemia. In exacerbations of chronic bronchitis, the white cell count may or may not rise and a left shift may or may not be present.

Sputum

Examination of sputum (e.g., Gram stain) is helpful in exacerbations of chronic bronchitis to identify potential bacterial pathogens that may have precipitated the exacerbation and aid in the selection of antimicrobial therapy. It is important to ensure that what is examined microscopically is truly sputum and not saliva. Sputum is identified by the presence of alveolar macrophages; saliva is identified by squamous epithelial cells. Many laboratories have developed scoring systems to help clinicians assess the adequacy of the sputum sample being examined. Sputum should also be examined for eosinophils to rule out an allergic component that would be consistent with asthmatic bronchitis.

α_1-Antitrypsin Assay

This test is particularly useful in patients younger than 40 years of age who present with emphysema and obstructive lung disease. Markedly low levels may indicate a PiZ phenotype. Moderately low levels may indicate other Pi phenotypes who may be more predisposed to emphysema caused by smoking than the general population.

COURSE/PROGNOSIS

The clinical course and prognosis of patients having chronic bronchitis and/or emphysema with obstructive pulmonary disease are marked by variable morbidity and mortality. Little is known of the early natural history of COLD, but it is probably characterized by slowly deteriorating pulmonary function for several years before clinical illness is appreciated by patients. Much more is known of the prognosis and clinical course once symptomology has become evident.

The predominant emphysema patient's pattern is characterized by progressive dyspnea without exacerbations precipitated by increased sputum production, as is characteristic of the predominant chronic bronchitic patient. The predominant emphysema patient's terminal event is often characterized by rapidly progressive cor pulmonale and intractable hypercapnia leading to respiratory arrest. The usual course of a patient with predominant bronchitis is characterized by increasing frequency of exacerbations of acute pulmonary insufficiency precipitated by bronchitis. This is accompanied by progressive decline in pulmonary function, with the chronic complications (previously described) of cor pulmonale, hypercapnia, and polycythemia. Exacerbations of bronchitis are characterized by increased mucopurulent sputum and frequently lead to acute respiratory failure from which the patient rapidly recovers with appropriate antibiotics and other therapies. These episodes tend to increase in severity and frequency until intractable cor pulmonale and hypercapnia occur.

Mean rate of decline of FEV_1 appears to be the most useful objective tool to assess the course of COLD. The rates of decline in prospective follow-up studies of patients with initially abnormal FEV_1s or FEV_1/FVC ratios followed for 3 to 16 years revealed a decline in the FEV_1 of 44–75 mL/yr; however, there was considerable variability. The rate of decline in FEV_1 for normal patients from age alone was 24 mL/yr.[26–28] In any study assessing rate of decline, an appropriate observation period is essential. In the study reporting the rate of decline in FEV_1 of 44 mL/yr, the observation period was only 3 years.[26] This may be too short to project rate of decline throughout the life of the patient, because during the first year many patients improve their pulmonary function with pharmacologic agents. In longer studies the rate of decline of FEV_1 is greater and linear.[27,28] Rate of decline of blood gases has not been shown to be a useful parameter to assess progression of the disease.

In terms of functional capacity, the predominant bronchitic patient will show more physical impairment at a higher FEV_1 than the predominant emphysema patient because of the comparatively worse arterial blood gases. Most people with mixed disease are not able to perform extremely vigorous activity once the FEV_1 falls below 1.5 L, but they can work. Once the FEV_1 falls below 1.0 L their ability to perform usual daily activities becomes impaired.

The survival rate in patients with COLD is related to the initial level of impairment in the FEV_1 and age. Other less important factors include degree of reversibility with bronchodilators, resting pulse, perceived physical disability, diffusing capacity, cor pulmonale, and blood gas abnormalities.[29]

A rapid decline in pulmonary function tests indicates a poor prognosis. People living at high altitudes also have a reduced survival rate.[28] Median survival is approximately 10 years when the FEV_1 is 1.4 L, 4 years when the FEV_1 is 1.0 L, and about 2 years when the FEV_1 is 0.5 L.[28]

As of yet, it is not clear that treatment with pharmacologic agents improves survival; however, they do improve the quality of life, probably reduce hospitalizations, and may prevent some premature deaths. The only intervention shown to improve survival rate is oxygen therapy.[28] Smoking cessation leads to decreased symptomology and slows the rate of decline of pulmonary function even after significant abnormality in pulmonary function tests have been detected (FEV_1/FVC less than 60%).[27]

ACUTE RESPIRATORY FAILURE IN COLD

The diagnosis of acute respiratory failure in COLD is definitively made on the basis of an acute change in the arterial blood gases. Defining acute respiratory failure as a PaO_2 of less than 50 mm Hg or a $PaCO_2$ of greater than 50 mm Hg may often be incorrect and inadequate because these values may not represent a significant change from a patient's baseline values. A more precise definition is an acute drop in PaO_2 of 10 to 15 mm Hg or any acute increase in $PaCO_2$ that decreases the serum pH to 7.30 or less.[30] Additional acute clinical manifestations of respiratory failure include restlessness, confusion, tachycardia, diaphoresis, cyanosis, hypotension, irregular breathing, miosis, and unconsciousness.[31]

The most common cause of acute respiratory failure in COLD is acute exacerbation of bronchitis with an increase in the volume and viscosity of sputum. This serves to worsen obstruction and further impair alveolar ventilation, resulting in worsening hypoxemia and hypercapnea. Additional causes of acute respiratory failure in COLD are pneumonia, pulmonary embolism, left ventricular failure, pneumothorax, and central nervous system depressants.

TREATMENT

Therapy of the patient with COLD is multifaceted. The goals of therapy are presented in Table 26.3. The importance of smoking cessation cannot be overemphasized—it is the obvious and first step in the secondary prevention plan. Smoking cessation will slow the rate of decline in pulmonary function tests, decrease symptoms,[32] and improve the patient's quality of life. The use of nicotine gum, patch, or clonidine may be helpful in assisting the smoker to quit. Behavioral modification techniques or other forms of psychotherapy may also be helpful. Programs that address the many issues associated with smoking (i.e., learned behaviors, environmental influences, chemical dependence) using a team approach are more likely to be successful.[33]

There was a long-standing opinion that COLD was associated with irreversible obstruction. This reasoning allowed pharmacotherapy to be chosen empirically. This opinion, however, has been challenged by the Intermittent Positive Pressure Breathing Group.[34] The data reported from their studies suggest that many individuals with COLD do obtain some degree of improvement in their obstruction from bronchodilators. This group may include many patients who would now be described as having asthmatic bronchitis. In addition, COLD patients with the greatest bronchodilatory response have the lowest annual decline in FEV_1 and the greatest 5-year survival.[2] It also appears that a single test of reversibility using an inhaled sympathomimetic followed by pulmonary function tests is not adequate to assess whether patients with COLD will benefit from bronchodilators. Even if a positive response is not detected, these patients deserve an adequate therapeutic trial of pharmacologic agents for the following reasons: (1) While objective tests may not reveal a response, possibly because of sensitivity of equipment, a subjective improvement may occur; (2) some patients may respond to inhaled sympathomimetics on one occasion and not on another; (3) the response to bronchodilators may require prolonged administration; (4) patients may respond to pharmacologic agents via mechanisms besides bronchodilation; (5) patients not responding in initial tests with sympathomimetics may respond to anticholinergics or methylxanthines; and (6) some parameters may be improved (e.g., exercise capacity) while others are not (e.g., FEV_1). The hypothesis that regular bronchodilation may slow the deterioration of lung function is being studied.[2]

TABLE 26.3. GOALS OF THERAPY

Smoking cessation
Improvement of the chronic obstructive state
Treatment and prevention of acute exacerbations
Reduction of the rate of progression of the disease
Improvement of physical and psychologic well-being of the patient so that daily activities can be resumed or maintained
Reduction in days lost from work
Reduction in hospitalizations
Reduction in mortality

There is no clear answer to the question of which bronchodilator class to initiate first. The decision should be based on patient compliance, response, and side effects. For the purposes of this chapter, agents will be presented in the sequence in which trends in therapy currently seem to indicate. These are anticholinergics, sympathomimetics, methylxanthines, and corticosteroids.

ANTICHOLINERGICS

During the past decade, the use of anticholinergic agents has increased in this country. These drugs have emerged as first-line therapy for the stable COLD patient; sympathomimetics remain the bronchodilators of choice for acute exacerbations. The only agents currently available in the United States are atropine and ipratropium bromide. When given by inhalation, anticholinergics produce bronchodilation by competitively inhibiting cholinergic receptors in bronchial smooth muscle. This activity blocks acetylcholine, with the net effect being a reduction in cyclic guanosine monophosphate (GMP), which normally acts to constrict bronchial smooth muscle. These agents maintain their effectiveness during years of regular continuous use.[33–35]

The effects of anticholinergics on mucociliary clearance are at this time unclear. Two studies that have addressed this question reached opposite conclusions.[36,37] However, ipratropium bromide has been shown to decrease the effectiveness of voluntary cough on clearing mucus from the airways, which may affect its role in the treatment of patients who have excessive mucus production.[38] The clinical significance of this effect is unknown.

Several studies have demonstrated the effectiveness of inhaled anticholinergics in patients with COLD.[39–42] Anticholinergic agents have been compared with an inhaled sympathomimetic and in all of the studies the anticholinergic agent was found to produce greater improvement in pulmonary function tests than the sympathomimetic agents. These studies point out the relative importance of the cholinergic system as a mediator of bronchial tone in COLD patients.

Atropine can be administered via either a hand-held or a jet nebulizer using the parenteral or ophthalmic solution, which is diluted with 2–4 mL of saline for administration. The dose of atropine is initiated at 0.025–0.05 mg/kg. The duration of effect is approximately 4 hours. Systemic absorption may be substantial, therefore patients should be monitored for signs of toxicity after several doses.[43] An alternative to atropine with less systemic side effects (due to its quaternary structure) is glycopyrrolate.

Ipratropium bromide is available as a metered dose inhaler and a solution for inhalation. It is three to five times more potent on muscarinic receptors than atropine.[44] It provides a peak effect in 1.5–2 hours and has a duration of 4–6 hours.[45] Systemic absorption is minimal since it has a quaternary structure.[45] While the recommended dose is two puffs 4 times a day, many clinicians prescribe two to three times that dose to produce maximal bronchodilation.[46] Oxitropium bromide and Ba679Br are long-acting agents being studied in Europe that appear to be even more potent.[47]

The objective in therapy with inhaled bronchodilators is to provide relatively small doses to the affected airways and to achieve the desired pharmacologic effect with minimal systemic toxicity. The remaining issue is to determine which method of inhaling bronchodilators best achieves this objective: (1) use of a metered-dose inhaler (MDI); (2) use of a MDI with a spacer; or (3) use of a powered nebulizer to deliver the medication. Regardless of which method is used, the most critical factor is proper technique. Although usual doses and dosing intervals may be obtained from several sources, a patient's dose and frequency should be adjusted based on their needs and tolerance.

MDIs are convenient for the mobile patient and are quite adequate when used appropriately. (A description of appropriate administration technique is provided in Chapter 25, Asthma). The greatest problems are inappropriate technique and overuse, therefore patient education and reinforcement are critical. Spacer devices improve aerosol delivery from MDIs in patients who are unable to adequately coordinate MDI actuation with inhalation (e.g., elderly COLD patients). The wet nebulization method should be reserved for those with the most debilitated lung function. This method of delivery has been considered superior to the MDI, but it may be equivalent to a MDI with a spacer.[48] When a wet nebulizer is used, the bronchodilator is diluted with 2–3 mL of normal saline or water, which is sufficient to provide a treatment for approximately 10 minutes. A T-tube is necessary to prevent excessive loss of drug and diluent. As when using the MDI, inspiration must be slow and deep. The patient should try to hold each inspiration for 3–5 seconds. Exhalation should be through the nose. It may be desirable to use more diluent to further moisten secretions and promote their expectoration, but this will alter the delivered dose because the dead volume (the volume of liquid left in the nebulizer following treatment) remains the same but will contain less drug.

SYMPATHOMIMETICS

Sympathomimetics have traditionally been the cornerstone of pharmacotherapy for COLD, but have now fallen behind anticholinergics as preferred therapy. Numerous sympathomimetics are currently available in the U.S. market, however it is more desirable to use the newer agents with greater β_2 selectivity and longer duration of action. These agents include albuterol, bitolterol, salmeterol, and terbutaline. β_2-selective sympathomimetics cause bronchodilation by stimulating the enzyme adenyl cyclase to increase the formation of adenosine 3′, 5′ monophosphate (3′,5′-cAMP). In addition, they are thought to improve mucociliary clearance. Although shorter-acting and less selective β agonists are still widely used (i.e., metaproterenol, isoetharine, isoproterenol), it is difficult to advocate their continued use because of the shorter duration of action and increased cardiostimulatory effects. Note that salmeterol is used for chronic, not acute, therapy. Regular use of long-acting β agonists has been suggested to be potentially deleterious,[2] however this referred to patients with bronchial asthma and has not been determined to occur in patients with COLD. The reader is referred to Chapter 25, Asthma, for a comparative table of these agents.

The preferred route of administration of the selective β_2 agonist is an issue that has prompted considerable research in the past several years. This decision is based on comparative efficacy and toxicity of the parenteral, oral, or inhalation route. The accumulated data suggest that the inhalation route is preferred in terms of both efficacy and toxicity.[44,49,50] Inhalation is equal, if not superior, to the parenteral route and unquestionably superior to the oral route in bronchodilating effect. The inhalation route consistently has shown fewer cardiostimulatory and other systemic effects (e.g., hand tremor) than either the parenteral or oral routes. This route minimizes the intracellular shift of potassium and resultant hypokalemia, which is augmented by theophylline.[35] In-depth reviews on these newer agents and routes of administration are available.[51,52]

All patients with COLD deserve a trial of inhaled β_2 agonist even if their FEV_1 is not changed because mechanisms other than bronchodilation may be helpful (e.g., increase in mucociliary clearance). It is still unclear if COLD patients with extremely poor inspiratory effort on aerosolized β_2 agonists receive additional benefit or simply greater toxicity by the addition of an oral β_2 agonist. An individual's perceived benefit from these agents may significantly affect their usefulness.[53] The dose of the β_2 agonist can be increased in an acute exacerbation, although the limiting factor is an excessive increase in heart rate.

COMBINATION ANTICHOLINERGICS AND SYMPATHOMIMETICS

The body of evidence indicates that combination inhaled anticholinergic and sympathomimetic regimens are more effective than either as monotherapy.[33,54,55] Before the combination is used, the dose of the anticholinergic should first be titrated. When used together, the most recent recommendation is to use the anticholinergic 2 hours prior to using the sympathomimetic. Combination MDIs that contain both a β agonist and an anticholinergic agent (available outside of the United States) have been shown to be more effective than using either agent alone.[54–56]

METHYLXANTHINES

The role of methylxanthines in the treatment of COLD is controversial. Data indicate that theophylline, the most common methylxanthine used in clinical practice, appears to be an effective bronchodilator in patients with chronic, stable disease. Early studies suggested methylxanthines produce bronchodilation through inhibition of phosphodiesterase, thus preventing the enzymatic breakdown of 3′,5′-cAMP. This proposed mechanism is no longer generally accepted because this effect requires concentrations of methylxanthines much higher than those obtainable in clinical practice.[51] Numerous other mechanisms have been proposed to explain bronchodilation and other respiratory effects, including (1) inhibition of calcium ion influx into smooth muscle, (2) prostaglandin antagonism, (3) stimulation of endogenous catecholamines, (4) adenosine receptor antagonism, and (5) inhibition of release of mediators from mast cells and leukocytes.[51,57,58] Beneficial respiratory effects other than bronchodilation that have been attributed to methylxanthines in COLD patients include (1) improved diaphragmatic strength and reduction of fatigue, (2) stimulation of mucociliary clearance, and (3) improved central respiratory response to hypoxemia (especially helpful in patients with a significant sleep apnea component to their disease).[51,57,58] The data to support these effects are varied, because many of the studies are not standardized or have methodological flaws. In addition, the objective measurements used as endpoints (e.g., pulmonary function tests) may not correlate with clinical improvement or quality of life benefits to the patient. However, the majority of studies do indicate that theophylline as chronic therapy is of therapeutic benefit.[59] The reader is referred to a review by Vaz Fragoso and Miller[59] for a thorough discussion of the topic.

Numerous reliably absorbed sustained-release theophylline (1,3-dimethylxanthine) preparations are currently available. These have the advantages of improving patient compliance and achieving more consistent serum concentrations over rapid-release theophylline and aminophylline preparations; however, caution must be used in switching from one sustained-release preparation to another, because there are considerable variations in sustained-release characteristics.[51] Aside from aminophylline, there is no need to use any of the various other theophylline complexes. There is no indication for rectal suppositories of theophylline or aminophylline or intramuscular administration of these drugs. Dissolution from rectal suppositories is inconsistent, absorption from intramuscular injections is unreliable, and the injections are painful.

Aminophylline, USP is the complex of ethylenediamine and theophylline dihydrate (containing 80% anhydrous theophylline). Aminophylline has increased water solubility over theophylline, which is why it is commonly used for parenteral administration. Parenteral administration is indicated for severe acute decompensation or if the patient is unable to take oral medications. Note that Rice et al.[60] were unable to document any objective improvement in pulmonary function tests or arterial blood gases when intravenous aminophylline was added to a regimen of metaproterenol and methylprednisolone in patients suffering acute exacerbations of their COLD symptoms. However, a recent double-blind placebo-controlled study demonstrated that administering relatively low doses of aminophylline in the emergency room to COLD patients with acute exacerbations decreased hospital admissions.[61]

Because aminophylline is still widely used in clinical practice, pharmacists should apply an appropriate knowledge base to the objective use of this drug. During acute exacerbations, loading doses of intravenous aminophylline should be administered to patients in order to achieve therapeutic serum theophylline concentrations rapidly. Without a loading dose, COLD patients would require 40–60 hours (5 half-lives, using the usual elimination half-life of 8–12 hours) before steady-state serum concentrations would be reached with maintenance dosing only.[57] The loading dose is based on actual body weight.[56] Recommended loading doses of intravenous aminophylline are 6–9 mg/kg for patients who have not taken any theophylline in the previous 24 hours, or 3 mg/kg if they have taken sustained-release theophylline within the past 24 hours or rapid-release theophylline within the past 12 hours.

If serum concentration measurements are readily available, one may use the average distribution volume (V_D) of 0.5 L/kg for theophylline in adults to estimate the loading dose required to produce the desired increment in serum theophylline concentration:

$$\text{Loading dose}/V_D = \text{Serum level increment}$$

or

$$\frac{1\ \text{mg/kg}}{0.5\ \text{L/kg}} = 2\ \text{mg/L}$$

The administration rate should not exceed 25 mg/min to avoid cardiac arrhythmias or cardiovascular collapse. A controlling device is recommended when infusing aminophylline.

The desired therapeutic range is 10–20 mcg/mL. Because most COLD patients are elderly and often have a rapidly changing clinical picture that may affect theophylline clearance, it is prudent to aim for levels in the range of 10–15 mcg/mL in order to minimize the likelihood of toxicity. The initial intravenous maintenance dose recommendation (based on ideal body weight) for acute exacerbations of COLD with pneumonia or ventricular failure is 0.45–0.7 mg/kg/h of aminophylline. One may wish to initiate therapy at the upper end of this range if the patient is a smoker because of the increased clearance induced by smoking. Factors in COLD patients that decrease theophylline clearance leading to reduced maintenance dose requirements include advanced age, bacterial or viral pneumonia, left or right ventricular failure, liver dysfunction, hypoxemia from the acute decompensation, and use of drugs such as cimetidine, erythromycin, and ciprofloxacin. Maintenance dose recommendations for these conditions have been proposed (Table 26.4). These recommendations should be considered as starting points, as serum theophylline concentrations must be obtained to guide and individualize further therapy. The conditions described are dynamic and as they fluctuate so will the clearance of theophylline.

Serum concentrations should be obtained 12–24 hours after the initiation of therapy, with adjustments made accordingly. The reason for evaluating concentrations early is that, should the patient have a clearance much lower than anticipated, the dose can be reduced before the patient becomes toxic, and should the clearance be much higher than anticipated, modest elevations in dose can be made. The serum concentration should be obtained every 24 hours thereafter until the patient is stable.

TABLE 26.4. MAINTENANCE DOSES OF PARENTERAL AMINOPHYLLINE IN EXACERBATIONS OF COLD

Age (>50 yr)	0.6–0.7 mg/kg/h
Bacterial or viral pneumonia	0.45–0.7 mg/kg/h
Heart failure (left or right)	0.45–0.7 mg/kg/h
Liver disease (total bilirubin >1.5 mg/dL)	0.2–0.25 mg/kg/h

Attempting to make adjustments in dose to attain a desired concentration using first-order pharmacokinetic equations is fraught with error. Theophylline is metabolized by microsomal enzymes to three major metabolites: 1,3-dimethyluric acid, 1-methyluric acid, and 3-methylxanthine.[56] Each metabolic pathway is potentially saturable. This results in the nonlinear kinetics of theophylline that are witnessed in acute overdoses. Apparent nonlinearity may occur because of physiologic changes that happen during therapy of acute exacerbations. For example, diminished hemodynamics due to either right or left ventricular failure may result in hepatic congestion, which affects theophylline clearance. Each patient's physiologic character should be carefully monitored, with serum theophylline concentrations obtained if any significant changes are noted. Since there are other pharmacologic interventions for COLD, it is unnecessary to push the theophylline dose to toxicity.

Serum theophylline concentrations above 20 mcg/mL are associated with nausea and vomiting and those above 35–40 mcg/mL with arrhythmias and seizures. In the elderly with exacerbations of COLD, these values should not be used to judge the likelihood of toxicity, because this population exhibits these catastrophic side effects at lower serum concentrations. Nausea is a common complication in elderly patients with concentrations greater than 15 mcg/mL, and seizures and atrial tachyarrhythmias have been reported with serum concentrations of 20–30 mcg/mL. These seizures and arrhythmias are quite refractory to conventional treatment.

Once the patient is stabilized and serum concentrations are reasonably consistent, one can switch to oral therapy. The oral sustained-release preparation can be initiated at the time the intravenous solution is stopped. The oral dose is calculated from the 24-hour intravenous theophylline dose. The total 24-hour dose may then be divided in thirds or in halves depending on the desired interval and strength of preparation available. Follow-up trough serum concentrations should be obtained several days after initiation of therapy to ensure the appropriateness of the dose and dosing interval for the selected product. Once a dose is established, it should not be necessary to routinely monitor serum concentrations unless the patient's disease worsens or toxicity is suspected.

Another regimen that is used clinically is to administer long-acting theophylline preparations at bedtime. This has been demonstrated to reduce overnight declines in FEV_1 and morning respiratory symptoms.[62]

There has been considerable debate as to the relative risk/benefit ratio of methylxanthines in COLD patients.[2] Data indicate that adding theophylline may not result in improvement of a patient's symptoms.[63] Because of the uncertainty regarding their role, they are now placed after anticholinergics and sympathomimetics when listing preferred therapies. Should a COLD patient not receive optimal benefit from anticholinergics and sympathomimetics, a judicious trial of a sustained-release theophylline preparation would be warranted. The evidence supporting an additive bronchodilatory effect of a methylxanthine with a sympathomimetic or ipratropium bromide is convincing.[63–65] When methylxanthines are used to treat COLD patients, parameters other than objective measurements, such as FEV_1, should be monitored to assess efficacy. Subjective parameters, such as perceived exercise tolerance, become increasingly important in assessing the acceptability of methylxanthines for the COLD patient. Note that although objective improvement may be minimal, clinical benefit to the individual may be meaningful.

CORTICOSTEROIDS

The use of corticosteroids in either acute exacerbations of COLD or as chronic treatment had been an issue of considerable controversy until 1980, when a study published by Albert et al.[66] established the efficacy of corticosteroids in COLD patients with acute exacerbations. The patients, who were on standard therapy of methylxanthines and sympathomimetics, were randomly allocated to receive either placebo or methylprednisolone 0.5 mg/kg every 6 hours intravenously for 72 hours. The steroid-treated group showed greater improvement in pulmonary function tests than the placebo group.

The role of steroids in chronic stable COLD patients was clarified in a review by Callahan et al.[67] In this meta-analysis, 33 original studies of oral steroids in COLD published since 1951 were evaluated. The authors concluded that COLD patients treated with steroids showed clinically significant improvement in baseline FEV_1 (increase of 20%) 10% more often than similar patients who received placebo. It therefore appears that the number of stable COLD patients who will benefit from steroids is modest. Attempts to determine patient characteristics that may be helpful in assessing which patients would most likely benefit from steroid administration appear to show that either a significant eosinophilia (>300/mm^3), eosinophils on sputum examination, or significant response on pulmonary function tests to sympathomimetics are the best predictors. A 25% or greater response of the FEV_1 has been reported to be the best predictor of responsiveness.[2]

Corticosteroids produce significant side effects; therefore, many clinicians follow the axiom that as soon as a decision is made to initiate therapy, a similar plan should be made to discontinue therapy as soon as is feasibly possible. Objective parameters should be followed to substantiate drug use. The anti-inflammatory mechanisms whereby corticosteroids exert their beneficial effect in COLD include (1) reduction in capillary permeability to decrease mucus, (2) inhibition of release of proteolytic enzymes from leukocytes, and (3) inhibition of prostaglandins. These desired effects occur because of the ability of steroids to be transported into the nucleus of the cell and stimulate RNA synthesis.

The decision to use corticosteroids is usually initiated during an acute exacerbation when the patient is deteriorating or not improving as expected despite adequate anticholinergic and/or sympathomimetic therapy and possibly methylxanthines. Patients taking chronic oral steroids who present in acute distress should be immediately started on parenteral steroids. Therapy is initiated with methylprednisolone or its equivalent 0.5–1.0 mg/kg intravenously every 6 hours. It generally requires 3–6 hours or longer for a beneficial pharmacologic effect to be observed.

As soon as the patient's symptoms have stabilized, he or she may be switched to 40–60 mg of prednisone daily. The oral dose is largely empiric. A short- to intermediate-acting corticosteroid is preferred to minimize suppression of the hypothalamic-pituitary-adrenal (HPA) axis. If possible, steroids should be stopped in 7–14 days, since extending beyond 2–4 weeks with supraphysiologic doses suppresses the HPA axis. If therapy needs to be prolonged, the ideal is to achieve the lowest possible effective dose with a minimal likelihood of HPA axis suppression (e.g., prednisone 7.5 mg/d). The dose should be given once per day in the morning to mimic the normal diurnal variation of endogenous cortisol secretion. If possible, the patient should be moved to an alternate-day schedule, shown by Blair and Light[68] to be just as effective as daily therapy in COLD patients. This is accomplished by raising one day's dose, while decreasing the alternate day's dose. If a patient requires continuous steroid therapy, giving short bursts of higher doses of oral prednisone during periods of worsening clinical status may be effective at decreasing hospitalizations.

The role of inhaled corticosteroids is controversial. Previously, they were thought to be of no benefit in patients with COLD. Recent studies, including a prospective 4-year trial from Europe, indicate that inhaled corticosteroids have a positive effect on the annual decline of FEV_1.[69–72] In the prospective study by Dompeling et al.,[69] adding inhaled beclomethasone to bronchodilator therapy was found to slow the unfavorable course of COLD, but the effect was not as positive as that exhibited by the asthmatic patients who were studied. The results of another multicenter trial indicate that while younger, nonsmoking individuals had the greatest response when inhaled corticosteroids were added to maintenance regimens of β agonists, all groups showed benefit from the combination in terms of reduction in morbidity, hyperresponsiveness, and airway obstruction.[71] Evidence from these and other studies gives strength to the use of inhaled corticosteroids in COLD; however, the data indicate that asthmatic patients gain greater benefit from these agents than do COLD patients.

LONG-TERM OXYGEN

While long-term oxygen has been used for many years in patients with advanced COLD, it was not until 1980 that data became available documenting its benefits. At that time, the Nocturnal Oxygen Therapy Trial Group published their data comparing nocturnal oxygen therapy (NOT) (12 hours per day) with continuous oxygen therapy (COT) (average of 20 hours per day).[73] The patients were followed for at least 12 months. The results revealed a mortality rate in the NOT group nearly double that of the COT group, 41/80 versus 23/87. Statistical estimates of the COT group suggest that COT may have added 3.25 years to a COLD patient's life.[74] The decline in mortality with oxygen therapy was further substantiated in 1981 in a study by the British Medical Research Council, which compared 15 hours per day of oxygen versus no supplemental oxygen in COLD patients.[75] Additional data from the Nocturnal Oxygen Therapy Trial Group revealed that COT patients had fewer (but statistically insignificant) hospitalizations, improved quality of life and neuropsychologic function, reduced hematocrits, and decreased pulmonary vascular resistance. Recent analyses have shown that long-term oxygen therapy provides even more benefit in terms of survival after at least 5 years of use, and it improves the quality of life of these patients by increasing walking distance, neuropsychological condition, and reducing time spent in the hospital.[76] Whether oxygen therapy consistently improves exercise tolerance or sleep remains controversial.

Before patients are considered for long-term oxygen therapy, they should be stabilized in the outpatient setting for one month and pharmacotherapy should be optimized. Once this is accomplished, long-term oxygen therapy should be instituted if either of two conditions exists:

1. A resting Pa_{O_2} of less than 55 mm Hg
2. Evidence of right heart failure, polycythemia, or impaired neuropsychiatric function with a Pa_{O_2} of less than 60 mm Hg.

Oxygen therapy may also be used during exercise in those patients who show serious hypoxemia during episodes of increased activity, and during the night in individuals who have nocturnal hypoxemia. The possible benefits of long-term oxygen in borderline hypoxemic patients is currently under study in a large multicenter trial.[77]

The most practical means of administering long-term oxygen is with the nasal cannula, which provides 24–28% oxygen. The goal is to raise the Pa_{O_2} above 60 mm Hg. Patients known to retain carbon dioxide should be cautioned to not raise the Pa_{O_2} so high that they depress their respiratory drive. Patient education about flow rates and avoidance of flames is of the utmost importance.

Currently, there are three different oxygen delivery systems. While the conventional liquid oxygen and compressed oxygen are quite bulky, smaller, portable tanks are available to permit the patient more mobility. The newest method of oxygen delivery is with an oxygen concentrator; these devices separate the nitrogen from room air and concentrate the oxygen. These may prove the most convenient and ultimately the least expensive method of oxygen delivery. Disadvantages of these devices are that they currently require a continuous electrical supply, thus necessitating a backup system, and are somewhat noisy.

The cost of oxygen therapy may be substantial. The use of an oxygen concentrator may cost between $200 and $400 per month. Portable oxygen tanks may cost $300 per month. It is therefore important to discuss the economic issues of therapy with the patient and family before initiating oxygen.

ANTIBIOTICS

Antibiotics are reasonable therapy in COLD patients who exhibit signs suggestive of bronchial infection, such as increased sputum, increased viscosity of sputum, and/or change in sputum color. Sputum Gram's stain may be helpful in determining the need for oral antibiotic therapy; however, given the difficulty of obtaining an appropriate sputum in the outpatient setting, this may not always be practical. Early in the stage of infectious exacerbations patients do not always have fever, chills, or a leukocytosis. Sputum cultures, initially, are of little practical value and were shown to be of less benefit at identifying the organism than Gram's stain.[77]

While as many as one-third of infections are viral, bacterial infection may follow the initial viral infection. Therapy should be initiated within 24 hours of symptoms to prevent unnecessary hospitalization. It is also important to prevent an accelerated rate of decline in pulmonary function from irritation and mucus plugging due to the infectious process. In a recent large double-blind placebo-controlled study, higher success rates were shown with antibiotic therapy, but it should be noted that those patients with less severe exacerbations did not show benefit.[78]

The bacterial organisms usually responsible for exacerbations are *Streptococcus pneumoniae* and *Haemophilus influenzae.* Oral ampicillin and amoxicillin are considered the agents of choice in patients not allergic to penicillins. Other acceptable oral alternatives include tetracyclines, cephalosporins, and cotrimoxazole. If bacterial resistance to the penicillins through β-lactamase is suspected, a β-lactamase inhibitor such as clavulanate may be an appropriate choice (e.g., Augmentin). Therapy should generally be continued for at least 7–10 days. Certain regimens of shorter duration are as effective (e.g., azithromycin 3- or 5-day regimens).[78] If the patient deteriorates or does not improve as anticipated, hospitalization may be necessary and more aggressive attempts should be made to identify potential pathogens responsible for the exacerbation. Parenteral antibiotics may be required.

IMMUNOTHERAPY

An empiric recommendation has been that all patients with COLD should receive one dose of pneumococcal vaccine. This recommendation has been questioned in articles by Williams and Moser[79] and Davis et al.[80] The argument for continued use of the vaccine, however, is that the current vaccine has 23 antigens and now provides coverage for 87% of pneumococcal disease. Currently, administering the vaccine remains the standard of practice and is recommended by the Centers for Disease Control and Prevention and the American Lung Association. Repeated vaccination with the 23 valent product is not recommended but is controversial. However, individuals who received the original 18 valent product should receive the 23 valent vaccine. COLD patients should also receive a yearly influenza vaccination. If a patient has been exposed to influenza before vaccination, a course of amantadine or rimantadine may be considered. These antivirals are only effective against influenza A. Their dose should be decreased from 100 mg twice daily to 100 mg once daily in those older than 65 years of age.

RESPIRATORY STIMULANTS

The role of acetazolamide and progesterone in COLD patients has been investigated for the past 25 years. Acetazolamide, a carbonic anhydrase inhibitor, may exert a beneficial effect by increasing cerebral blood flow, decreasing cerebrospinal fluid bicarbonate, and increasing the responsiveness of central respiratory centers to hypoxemia and hypercarbia.[51] It may be especially useful in COLD patients who are alkalemic as a result of diuretic therapy, as alkalosis depresses the respiratory drive. Acetazolamide does not work when the arterial pH is less than 7.35. Its exact role has not been determined nor has the dose or duration of therapy been established.

Progesterone shares an equally unclear role in patients with COLD and its effectiveness is controversial.[51] Originally, this agent was promoted to be of benefit as a respiratory stimulant in patients with Pickwickian syndrome with sleep apnea. However, progesterone more consistently shows benefit in awake patients than in those who are asleep.[51]

The newest agent that has shown considerable promise as a "respiratory stimulant" is almitrine bimesylate. This peripheral chemoreceptor agonist, not currently available in the United States, has consistently been shown to increase Pa_{O_2} during wakefulness and even more strikingly during sleep.[81] Recent data indicate that low-dose oral therapy (75 mg daily) results in sustained elevation of arterial oxygen tension in hypoxemic patients.[82] Its potential to impair peripheral motor nerve function has been documented and may limit its usefulness.[82] Protriptyline has also been shown in one study to improve diurnal and nocturnal hypoxemia.[83] However, nortriptyline has been reported to depress ventilatory control, although exercise tolerance increased.[84] Further work with these agents may establish their role in COLD more definitively.

CHOICE OF THERAPY

An algorithm to provide guidance in the choice of therapy for a patient with COLD is shown in Fig. 26.9. It cannot be stressed enough that individualized treatment regimens are necessary in order to optimize outcome because patients differ in their compliance with medication, technique in using inhalers and equipment, and values in terms of quality of life.

COMPLICATIONS

COR PULMONALE

Diuretics have been the mainstay of therapy for cor pulmonale. The greatest concern with using diuretics is hypokalemic metabolic alkalosis. The hypokalemia may be exacerbated by concomitant use of β agonists or corticosteroids. Therefore, the decision to use diuretics must be based on a risk/benefit ratio. If only peripheral edema exists without hepatic congestion, the risk of diuretics may exceed potential benefit. If hepatic congestion is evident, judicious use of diuretics is certainly indicated because other modes of therapy may be compromised by the congestion. Digitalis glycosides have no role in the treatment of cor pulmonale.

Recently, research into the treatment of cor pulmonale has been directed at reducing the force against which the right ventricle has to work by dilating the pulmonary vasculature. One method of doing this is to remove a primary

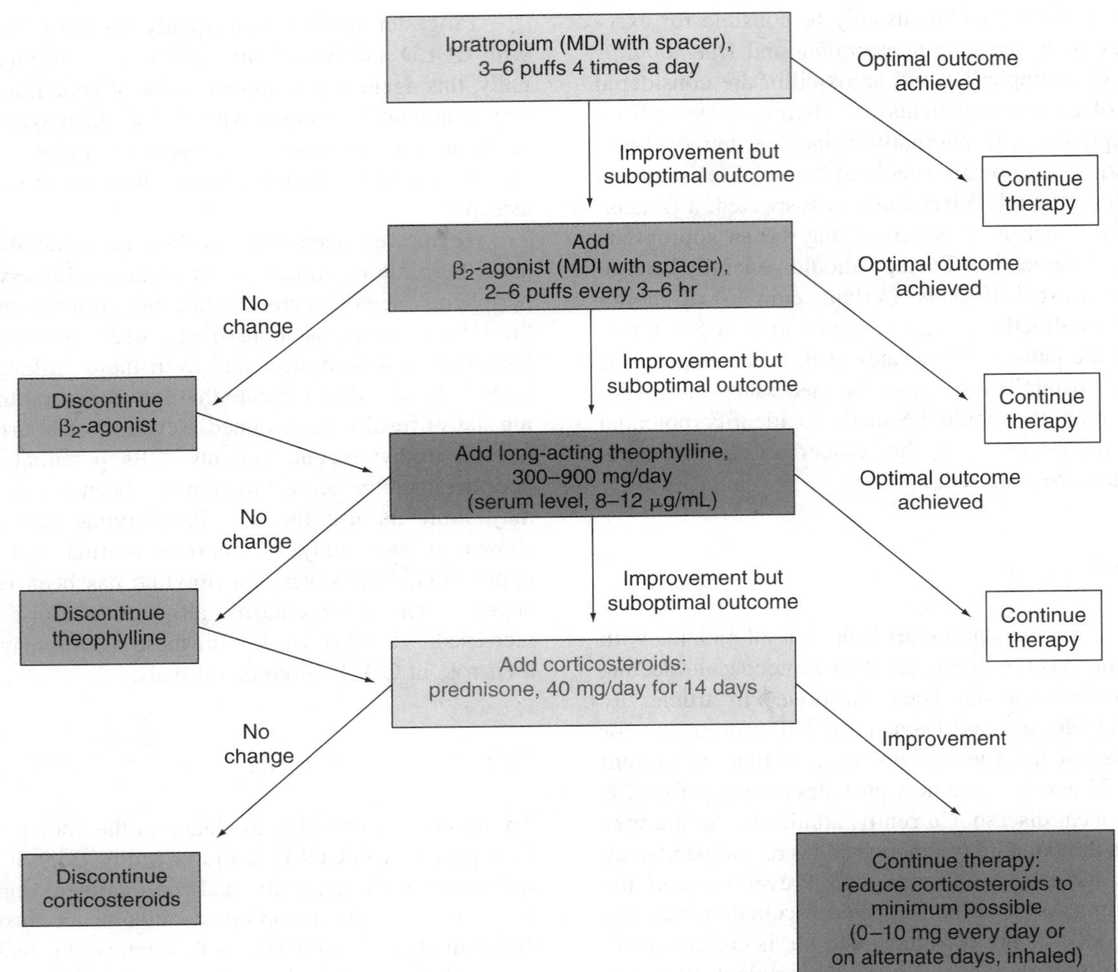

Figure 26.9. Typical treatment algorithm for patients with COLD. Outcome is measured in terms of improvement in the FEV_1:FVC and peak flow; improvement in the distance covered in a 6- or 12-minute walk; and objectively observed reduction in dyspnea, medication use, and nocturnal symptoms. MDI, metered dose inhaler. *(Reprinted by permission of The New England Journal of Medicine, vol 328, pp 1017–1022, 1993.)*

cause of pulmonary hypertension (e.g., hypoxia). This can be improved by raising the PaO_2 higher than 60 mm Hg. Hydralazine and nifedipine have been the most extensively examined pharmacologic agents, although other calcium antagonists (e.g., felodipine) have also shown promise.[85] Data are currently insufficient to offer guidelines for the role of these agents on COLD patients with cor pulmonale. The investigational α_1 blocker, urapadil, has shown limited promise in improving gas exchange and pulmonary hemodynamics.[86]

POLYCYTHEMIA

Polycythemia secondary to chronic hypoxemia in COLD patients can be improved by either oxygen therapy or by periodic phlebotomy if oxygen is not sufficient. Continuous oxygen therapy was shown by the Nocturnal Oxygen Therapy Trial Group to reduce hematocrits.[73] Acute phlebotomy is indicated if the hematocrit is above 55–60% and the patient is experiencing central nervous system effects suggestive of sludging from high blood viscosity. Long-term oxygen can then be used to maintain a lower hematocrit.

α_1-PROTEINASE INHIBITOR (α_1-ANTITRYPSIN)

This genetically engineered compound is indicated for those patients with panacinar emphysema who have the PiZ phenotype. Its use should not be considered in patients with emphysema who are other Pi phenotypes. The therapeutic objective is to maintain α_1-antitrypsin serum concentrations higher than 80 mg/dL in order to have sufficient antielastase activity in the lung epithelial lining fluid. The recommended dosing regimen is 60 mg/kg administered intravenously once a week, at a rate of 0.08 mL/kg/min (adjusted to patient tolerance). It has been estimated that this form of augmentation therapy will have an annual cost of $20,000 to $30,000 per patient.[87]

ACUTE RESPIRATORY FAILURE

Acute respiratory failure is an emergency situation. When it occurs in a patient with COLD, all pharmacologic maneuvers should be optimized initially and low-flow oxygen delivered. If these agents fail to stabilize or improve the patient's condition, intubation and mechanical ventilation must be considered. This is an extremely difficult decision. Ideally, all severe COLD patients should be involved in the decision to intubate. Preferably, this decision should be made before an acute event occurs. If a decision is made to mechanically ventilate because of impending respiratory failure, it is important that ventilator settings not be adjusted to return the patient to normal values; rather, settings should be adjusted to achieve the patient's baseline values in a stable state. This will facilitate weaning from the ventilator. Maintaining the physical strength and nutritional status of the patient is vital in aiding the weaning procedure. Recent data indicate that a systematic multiparameter approach to assessing nutritional status is critical for COLD patients requiring mechanical ventilation, as malnutrition is common and has a deleterious effect on the weaning process.[88] Physical therapy and a nutritional intake of 3000 kcal/d with a relatively high proportion of protein are advised. If mechanical ventilation persists beyond 5–7 days, the patient should be switched to a tracheostomy to prevent tracheal erosion and to facilitate feeding.

Extubation can be considered if the patient's arterial blood gases have reached baseline and are maintained on an FiO_2 of 40% or less and a tidal volume of 400 mL or less. Once this is achieved, the following parameters can be measured to allow a reasonable prediction of successful extubation: a minute ventilation of less than 10 L/min and the ability to double this on command; a low spontaneous respiratory rate of 20 per minute or less; and the ability to achieve an inspiratory force of greater than –20 cm of water. At this point with the patient alert and willing to comply, a T-tube should be used for 30 minutes with 40% oxygen while the patient is observed for excessive fatigue. Blood gases, respiratory rate, pulse, and general appearance are evaluated. If this is successful, extubation may be attempted. The patient should be closely observed on oxygen via nasal canula or mask, with blood gases, respiratory rate, pulse, and general appearance again being monitored. Intermittent mandatory ventilation (IMV) is another method of weaning before extubation. The reader is referred to a more in-depth discussion of this topic by Petty.[31]

CONTROVERSIES

EXPECTORANTS AND MUCOLYTICS

Water has been, and continues to be, the expectorant of choice in COLD patients. Adequate hydration is safe and effective when compared with saturated solution of potassium iodide, ammonium chloride, or guaifenesin. Although these agents may promote expectoration, the doses required are so large that they are frequently associated with undesirable side effects.

Use of the mucolytic agent acetylcysteine to aid the clearance of mucus has been a matter of controversy for some time. There is no question that it is effective as a mucolytic. However, it causes irritation when administered via the inhaled route, which may cause further narrowing of the airways. For this reason, use of inhaled acetylcysteine has fallen into disfavor. It should always be preceded by an inhaled sympathomimetic if this route is chosen. Attention has recently been focused on the oral and intravenous routes of administration.[51] Although these routes appear to provide a beneficial mucolytic effect, there have not been sufficient studies to determine their place in therapy.

Another mucolytic, iodinated glycerol, was compared with placebo at a dose of 60 mg four times a day and was found to be superior in terms of cough frequency, cough severity, and chest discomfort but no improvement in blood oxygenation or pulmonary function was reported.[89] Data are still insufficient to recommend this agent but it may become a useful adjunct in selected patients.

INTERMITTENT POSITIVE PRESSURE BREATHING

Intermittent positive pressure breathing (IPPB) has, for more than 30 years, been a method of delivery of aerosolized medications to patients with COLD. While some patients experience subjective benefit, IPPB is not without risk, especially for patients with predominant emphysema. It may produce bronchospasm and also cause pneumothorax when used improperly. As a means of delivering bronchodilators, it is no more effective than compressor-driven nebulizers.[90] If IPPB is to be used at all, it should be in patients whose FEV_1 values are less than 750 mL and who are too weak to comply with other measures to promote bronchial drainage.[51]

OTHER ASPECTS OF MANAGEMENT

The standard of practice for many years was to avoid administering narcotics and benzodiazepines to patients with COLD. These drugs can further depress respiration, especially when given parenterally. Recent work in this area suggests that this issue is not yet settled. The current debate is over the risk of loss of sleep versus the risk of sedatives. As yet, there is no clear resolution to this issue. Some have found diphenhydramine useful as an anxiolytic or sedative, but there has not been an objective analysis of its effectiveness or safety in patients with COLD. Opiates have been used to increase exercise tolerance in individuals in whom dyspnea is severely disabling.[46]

The importance of psychological variables cannot be ignored in determining the functional status of the patient with COLD. Recent studies indicate that exercise capacity and depression are the best predictors of functional status.[91]

A substantial number of COLD patients have nutritional abnormalities. The association between weight loss and COLD, especially emphysema, is well established. Weight loss adversely impacts the progression of COLD; however, whether it is a marker for more severe disease or represents the pathogenesis of deterioration of pulmonary function is unclear. Recent data indicate that BMI (body mass index) is a simple and accurate indicator of nutritional status that correlates with several pulmonary function tests.[92]

While these topics are beyond the scope of this chapter, the role of chest physiotherapy, breathing retraining, and nutrition cannot be overlooked. The reader is referred to discussions by Hodgkin et al.,[93] Miller and Geumei,[51] and Lewis and Belman[94] for in-depth information.

CONCLUSION

Chronic obstructive lung disease is indeed a multifaceted disease process. The obstructive process is a result of the progression of chronic bronchitis and emphysema. Most people with COLD have both processes. The most common cause is cigarette smoking. Primary prevention is essential if the incidence of this disease is to decrease. Education is vital to prevent people from starting to smoke and to stop those who do smoke.

The therapeutic management involves numerous medications, oxygen, and physiotherapy. Unfortunately, pharmacologic management is still largely empiric, with anticholinergics, sympathomimetics, methylxanthines, and corticosteroids forming the foundation of therapy. These agents, especially methylxanthines and corticosteroids, are not without considerable risk of toxicity. Therefore, embarking on a pharmacologic plan requires weighing the risk/benefit ratio carefully and having a comprehensive plan to assess subjectively and objectively the efficacy and toxicity of the chosen therapy.

ADDENDUM

An official statement of the American Thoracic Society regarding the standards for the diagnosis and care of patients with chronic obstructive lung disease has recently been published after the text of this chapter was approved and finalized. This official statement is the first from ATS regarding COLD since 1987. The reader is referred to this reference for the most up-to-date information regarding the following information for COLD and its management; definitions, epidemiology, pathophysiology, diagnosis, staging, outpatient management, inpatient management, surgical evaluation for COLD patients, sleep, nutrition, and ethical issues.[95]

REFERENCES

1. American Thoracic Society. Standards for the diagnosis and care of patients with chronic obstructive pulmonary disease (COPD) and asthma. Am Rev Respir Dis 1987;136: 225–244.
2. Edelman NH, et al. Chronic obstructive pulmonary disease. Chest 1992;102(suppl 3):243–256.
3. National Center for Health Statistics, Current Estimates from the National Health Interview Survey, United States, Selected Years 1971–1994.
4. National Center for Health Statistics, Advanced Report of Final Mortality Statistics, 1973–1994.
5. Anonymous. Deaths from chronic obstructive pulmonary disease in the United States, 1987. Stat Bull 1990;July–Sept:20–26.
6. Feinlieb M, et al. Trends in COPD morbidity and mortality in the United States. Am Rev Respir Dis 1989;140:S9–S18.
7. Murray JF, Nadel JA. Textbook of Respiratory Medicine. Philadelphia, WB Saunders, 1988, pp 1001–1003.
8. Pauwels RA, et al. European Respiratory Society study on chronic obstructive pulmonary disease (EUROSCOP): Hypothesis and design. Eur Respir J 1992;5:1254–1261.
9. Chronic Disease Reports. Chronic obstructive pulmonary disease mortality—United States, 1986. MMWR 1989;38:549–552.
10. Higgens M. Epidemiology of COPD: State of the art. Chest 1984;85:3S–8S.
11. Tackman MS, Knoury MS, Cohen BH. The epidemiology of COPD, in Petty TL (ed): Chronic Obstructive Pulmonary Disease. New York, Marcel Dekker, 1985, pp 43–92.
12. Oxman AD, et al. Occupational dust exposure and chronic obstructive pulmonary disease. A systemic overview of the evidence. Am Rev Resp Dis 1993;148:38–48.
13. Sunyer J, et al. Air pollution and emergency room admissions for chronic obstructive pulmonary disease: A 5-year study. Am J Epidemiol 1993;137:701–705.
14. Snider GL. Chronic obstructive pulmonary disease: Risk factors, pathophysiology and pathogenesis. Ann Rev Med 1989;40:411–429.

15. Petty TL. Definitions in chronic obstructive pulmonary disease. Clin Chest Med 1990;11:363–373.
16. O'Connor GT, Sparrow D, Segal M, Weiss ST. Risk factors for ventilatory impairment among middle-aged and elderly men. Chest 1993;103:376–382.
17. Badgett RG, et al. Can moderate chronic obstructive pulmonary disease be diagnosed by historical and physical findings alone? Am J Med 1993;94:188–195.
18. Wright JL, Petty T, Thurlbeck WM. Analysis of the structure of the muscular pulmonary arteries in patients with pulmonary hypertension and COPD: National Institutes of Health Nocturnal Oxygen Therapy Trial. Lung 1992;170:109–124.
19. Gelb AF, et al. Limited contribution of emphysema in advanced chronic obstructive pulmonary disease. Am Rev Resp Dis 1993;147:1157–1161.
20. Kimbel P. Proteolytic damage and emphysema pathogenesis, in Petty TL (ed): Chronic Obstructive Pulmonary Disease. New York, Marcel Dekker, 1985, pp 105–127.
21. Wallaert B, et al. Inactivation of α_1-proteinase inhibitor by alveolar inflammatory cells from smoking patients with or without emphysema. Am Rev Resp Dis 1993; 147:1537–1543.
22. Robins AG. Pathophysiology of emphysema. Clin Chest Med 1983;4:413–420.
23. Macklem PT. The pathophysiology of chronic bronchitis and emphysema. Med Clin North Am 1973;57:669–679.
24. Weitzenblum E, et al. Chronic obstructive pulmonary disease and sleep apnea syndrome. Sleep 1992;15:S33–S35.
25. Hayes GB, Christiani DC. Measures of small airways disease as predictors of chronic obstructive pulmonary disease. Occup Med State Art Rev 1993;8(2):375–395.
26. Anthonisen NR, Wright SC, Hodgkin JE. Prognosis in chronic obstructive pulmonary disease. Am Rev Respir Dis 1986;133:14–20.
27. Petty TL, Good JT, White DP. Long-term follow-up of a random population observed for the prevalence and outcome of COPD, in Petty TL (ed): Chronic Obstructive Pulmonary Diseases. New York, Marcel Dekker, 1985, pp 93–103.
28. Burrows B. Cause and prognosis in advanced disease, in Petty TL (ed): Chronic Obstructive Pulmonary Disease. New York, Marcel Dekker, 1985, pp 31–42.
29. Anthonisen NR. Prognosis in chronic obstructive pulmonary disease: Results from multicenter clinical trials. Am Rev Respir Dis 1989;140:S95–S99.
30. Ingram RH. Chronic bronchitis, emphysema, and airway obstruction, in Wilson JD, Braunwald E, Isselbacher KJ, et al. (eds): Harrison's Textbook of Internal Medicine. New York, McGraw-Hill, 1991, pp 1074–1082.
31. Petty TL. Acute respiratory failure in COPD, in Petty TL (ed): Chronic Obstructive Pulmonary Disease. New York, Marcel Dekker, 1985, pp 389–410.
32. Leader WG, Wolf KM, Cooper TM, Chandler MHH. Symptomatology, pulmonary function and response, and T lymphocyte B2-receptors during smoking cessation in patients with chronic obstructive pulmonary disease. Pharmacotherapy 1994;14(2):162–172.
33. Chapman KR. Therapeutic algorithm for chronic obstructive pulmonary disease. Am J Med 1991; 91(suppl 4A):17–23.
34. Gross NJ. Ipratropium bromide. N Engl J Med 1989;319:486–494.
35. Skorodin MS. Pharmacotherapy for asthma and chronic obstructive pulmonary disease. Arch Intern Med 1993;153:814–828.
36. Pavia D, Bateman JR, Sheahan NF, et al. Clearance of lung secretions in patients with chronic bronchitis: Effect of terbutaline and ipratropium bromide aerosols. Eur J Respir Dis 1980;61:245–253.
37. Matthys H, Hundenborn J, Daikeler, et al. Influence of 0.2 mg ipratropium bromide on mucociliary clearance in patients with chronic bronchitis. Respiration 1985;48:329–339.
38. Bennett WD, Chapman WF, Mascarella JM. The acute effect of ipratropium bromide bronchodilator therapy on cough clearance in COPD. Chest 1993;103:488–495.
39. Gross NJ, Skorodin MS. Role of the parasympathetic system in airway obstruction due to emphysema. N Engl J Med 1984;311:421–425.
40. Passamonte PM, Martinez AJ. Effect of inhaled atropine or metaproterenol in patients with chronic airway obstruction and therapeutic serum theophylline levels. Chest 1984;85:610–615.
41. Marini JJ, Lakshminarayan S, Kradjan WA. Atropine and terbutaline aerosols in chronic bronchitis. Chest 1981;80:285–291.
42. Ashutosh K, Lang H. Comparison between long-term treatment of chronic bronchitic airway obstruction with ipratropium bromide and metaproterenol. Ann Allergy 1984;53:401–406.
43. Kradjan WA, Smallridge RC, Davis R, et al. Atropine serum concentrations after multiple inhaled doses of atropine sulfate. Clin Pharmacol Ther 1985;38:12–15.
44. Shim CS, Williams MH. Bronchodilator response to oral aminophylline and terbutaline versus aerosol albuterol in patients with chronic obstructive pulmonary disease. Am J Med 1983;75:697–701.
45. Massey KL, Gotz VP. Ipratropium bromide. Drug Intell Clin Pharm 1985;19:5–12.
46. Ferguson GT, Cherniack RM. Management of chronic obstructive pulmonary disease. N Engl J Med 1993;328:1017–1022.
47. Maesen FPV, et al. Ba 679 Br, a new long-acting antimuscarinic bronchodilator: a pilot dose-escalation study in COPD. Eur Resp J 1993;6:1031–1036.
48. Berry RB, Shinto RA, Wong FH, et al. Nebulizer versus spacer for bronchodilator delivery in patients hospitalized for acute exacerbations of COPD. Chest 1989;96:1241–1246.
49. Larsson S, Svedmyr N. Bronchodilating effect and side effects of β_2 adrenoceptor stimulants by different modes of administration. Am Rev Respir Dis 1977;116:861–869.
50. Shim C, Williams MH. Bronchial response to oral versus aerosol metaproterenol in asthma. Ann Intern Med 1980;93:428–431.
51. Miller WF, Geumei AM. Respiratory and pharmacological therapy in COPD, in Petty TL (ed): Chronic Obstructive Pulmonary Disease. New York, Marcel Dekker, 1985, pp 205–338.
52. Kelly HW. New β_2-adrenergic agonist aerosols. Clin Pharm 1985;4:393–404.

53. Noseda A, Schmerber J, Prigogine T, Yernault JC. Perceived effect on shortness of breath of an acute inhalation of saline or terbutaline: Variability and sensitivity of a visual analogue scale in patients with asthma or COPD. Eur Resp J 1992;5:1043–1053.
54. Imhof E, Elsasser S, Karrer W, et al. Comparison of bronchodilator effects of fenoterol/ipratropium bromide and salbutamol in patients with chronic obstructive pulmonary lung disease. Respiration 1993;60:84–88.
55. Wesseling G, Mostert R, Wouters EFM. A comparison of the effects of anticholinergic and β_2-agonist and combination therapy on respiratory impedance in COPD. Chest 1992;101:166–173.
56. Combivent Inhalation Aerosol Study Group. In chronic obstructive pulmonary disease, a combination of ipratropium and albuterol is more effective than either agent alone. Chest 1994;105:1411–1419.
57. Bukowskyj M, Nakatsu K, Munt PW. Theophylline reassessed. Ann Intern Med 1984;101:63–73.
58. Hill NS. The use of theophylline in "irreversible" chronic obstructive pulmonary disease. Arch Intern Med 1988;148:2579–2584.
59. Vaz Fragoso CA, Miller MA. Review of the clinical efficacy of theophylline in the treatment of chronic obstructive pulmonary disease. Am Rev Resp Dis 1993;147:S40–S47.
60. Rice KL, Leatherman JW, Duane PG, et al. Aminophylline for acute exacerbations of chronic obstructive pulmonary disease. Ann Intern Med 1987;107:305–309.
61. Wrenn K, Slovis CM, Murphy F, Greenberg RS. Aminophylline therapy for acute bronchospastic disease in the emergency room. Ann Intern Med 1991;115:241–247.
62. Nesse RE. COPD pharmacotherapy. Postgrad Med 1992;91(1):76–84.
63. Nishimura K, Koyama H, Ikeda A, Izumi T. Is oral theophylline effective in combination with both inhaled anticholinergic agent and inhaled β_2-agonist in the treatment of stable COPD? Chest 1993;104:179–184.
64. Georgopoulos A, Wong D, Anthonisen NR. Interactive effects of systematically administered salbutamol and aminophylline in chronic obstructive pulmonary disease. Am Rev Respir Dis 1988;138:1499–1503.
65. Taylor DR, Buick B, Kinney F. The efficacy of orally administered theophylline, inhaled salbutamol, and a combination of the two as chronic therapy in the management of chronic bronchitis with reversible air-flow obstruction. Am Rev Respir Dis 1985;131:747–751.
66. Albert RK, Marten TR, Lewis SW. Controlled clinical trial of methylprednisolone in patients with chronic bronchitis and acute respiratory insufficiency. Ann Intern Med 1980;92:753–758.
67. Callahan CM, Dittus RS, Katz BP. Oral corticosteroid therapy for patients with stable chronic obstructive pulmonary disease. Ann Intern Med 1991;114:216–223.
68. Blair GP, Light RW. Treatment of chronic obstructive pulmonary disease with corticosteroids. Chest 1984;86:525–528.
69. Dompeling E, et al. Slowing the deterioration of asthma and chronic obstructive pulmonary disease observed during bronchodilator therapy by adding inhaled corticosteroids. Ann Intern Med 1993;118:770–778.
70. Thompson AB, et al. Aerosolized beclomethasone in chronic bronchitis. Am Rev Resp Dis 1992;146:389–395.
71. Kerstjens HAM, et al. A comparison of bronchodilator therapy with or without inhaled corticosteroid therapy for obstructive airways disease. N Engl J Med 1992;327:1413–1419.
72. Weir DC, Burge PS. Effects of high dose inhaled beclomethasone dipropionate, 750 mcg and 1500 mcg twice daily, and 40 mg per day oral prednisolone on lung function, symptoms, and bronchial hyperresponsiveness in patients with non-asthmatic chronic airflow obstruction. Thorax 1993;48:309–316.
73. Nocturnal Oxygen Therapy Trial Group. Continuous or nocturnal oxygen therapy in hypoxemic chronic obstructive lung disease. Ann Intern Med 1980;93:391–398.
74. Petty TL. Long-term outpatient oxygen therapy, in Petty TL (ed): Chronic Obstructive Pulmonary Disease. New York, Marcel Dekker, 1985, pp 375–388.
75. Medical Research Council Working Party. Long-term domiciliary oxygen therapy in chronic hypoxic cor pulmonale complicating chronic bronchitis and emphysema. Lancet 1981;1:681–685.
76. Weitzenblum E, Apprill M, Oswald M. Benefit from long-term O_2 therapy in chronic obstructive pulmonary disease patients. Respiration 1992:59(suppl 1):14–17.
77. Mitlehner W. Effects of long-term oxygen therapy due to portable liquid oxygen tanks in disabled malnourished chronic obstructive pulmonary disease patients with borderline hypoxemia. Respiration 1992;24(suppl 2):40–45.
78. Staley H, McDade HB, Paes D. Is an objective assessment of antibiotic therapy in exacerbations of chronic bronchitis possible? J Antimicrob Chemother 1993;31:193–197.
79. Williams JH, Moser KN. Pneumococcal vaccine and patients with chronic lung disease. Ann Intern Med 1986;104:106–109.
80. Davis AL, Aranda CP, Schiffman G, et al. Pneumococcal infection and immunologic response to pneumococcal vaccine in chronic obstructive pulmonary disease. Chest 1987;92:204–212.
81. Gothe B, Cherniack NS, Bachand RT, et al. Long-term effects of amiltrine bimesylate on oxygenation during wakefulness and sleep in chronic obstructive pulmonary disease. Am J Med 1988;84:436–444.
82. Winkelmann BR, Kullmer TH, Kneissl DG, Trenk D, Kronenberger H. Low-dose almitrine bismesylate in the treatment of hypoxemia due to chronic obstructive pulmonary disease. Chest 1994;105:1383–1391.
83. Series F, Cormier Y. Effects of protriptyline on diurnal and nocturnal oxygenation in patients with chronic obstructive pulmonary disease. Ann Intern Med 1990;113:507–511.
84. Greenberg HE, Scharf SM, Green H. Nortriptyline-induced depression of ventilatory control in a patient with chronic obstructive pulmonary disease. Am Rev Respir Dis 1993;147:1303–1305.
85. Sajkov D, et al. Felodipine improves pulmonary hemodynamics in chronic obstructive pulmonary disease. Chest 1993;103:1354–1361.

86. Adnot S, Andrivet P, Piguet J, et al. The effects of urapadil therapy on hemodynamics and gas exchange in exercising patients with chronic obstructive pulmonary disease and pulmonary hypertension. Am Rev Respir Dis 1988;137:1068–1074.
87. MacDonald JL, Johnson CE. Pathophysiology and treatment of α_1-antitrypsin deficiency. Am J Health-Syst Pharm 1995;52:481–489.
88. Laaban J-P, et al. Nutritional status of patients with chronic obstructive pulmonary disease and acute respiratory failure. Chest 1993;103:1362–1368.
89. Morgan EJ, Petty TL. Summary of the national mucolytic study. Chest 1990;97:24S–27S.
90. The Intermittent Positive Pressure Breathing Trial Group. Intermittent positive pressure breathing therapy of chronic obstructive pulmonary disease. Ann Intern Med 1983;99:612–620.
91. Weaver TE, Narsavage GL. Physiological and psychological variables related to functional status in chronic obstructive pulmonary disease. Nursing Research 1992;41(5):286–291.
92. Sahebjami H, Doers JT, Render ML, Bond TL. Anthropometric and pulmonary function test profiles of outpatients with stable chronic obstructive pulmonary disease. Am J Med 1993;94:469–474.
93. Hodgkin JE, et al (eds). Chronic Obstructive Pulmonary Disease: Current Concepts in Diagnosis and Comprehensive Care. Park Ridge, IL, American College of Chest Physicians, 1979, p 10.
94. Lewis MI, Belman MJ. Nutrition and the respiratory muscles. Clin Chest Med 1988;9:337–348.
95. American Thoracic Society. Standards for the diagnosis and care of patients with chronic obstructive pulmonary disease. Am J Respir Crit Car Med 1995;152:s77–s120.

Chapter 27

Respiratory Distress Syndrome

Peter Gal, PharmD, FCCP, BCPS,
and Sharon M. Watling, PharmD, BCPS

This chapter addresses the problems of acute respiratory distress syndromes in neonates, children, and adults. The first half is dedicated to neonatal RDS and is followed by a discussion of acute respiratory distress syndrome in adults and children.

Respiratory Distress Syndrome

Respiratory distress syndromes (RDSs) in the neonate are a major source of neonatal morbidity and mortality. Acute forms of RDS include hyaline membrane disease (HMD) and transient tachypnea of the newborn (TTN). Chronic forms of RDS include chronic pulmonary insufficiency of prematurity (CPIP), bronchopulmonary dysplasia (BPD), and Wilson–Mikity syndrome. This discussion is limited to surfactant-deficiency respiratory distress syndrome, often referred to as hyaline membrane disease.

PHYSIOLOGY AND PATHOPHYSIOLOGY

Hyaline membrane disease, perhaps more appropriately called surfactant-deficiency respiratory distress syndrome, is common in neonates less than 36 weeks' gestation; the incidence increases as the gestational age decreases (Fig. 27.1).[1]

Pulmonary surfactant, containing phospholipids, functions to stabilize the air-filled alveolus against the collapsing forces of surface tension at the air/liquid interface.[1] Thus surfactant deficiency results in atelectasis and impaired gas exchange. Alveolar transudation of protein-rich fluids forms a hyaline membrane, giving rise to the name hyaline membrane disease.[1] Surfactant is secreted primarily by type II alveolar cells, which are sufficiently abundant and differentiated by 35 weeks' gestation to make HMD unlikely. Before 35 weeks' gestation, the risk of HMD and the severity of the disease increase as a consequence of (1) the immaturity of the alveolar lining cells, (2) impaired surfactant production, (3) impaired release of surface-active phospholipids, and (4) death of many cells responsible for surfactant production.[1–3]

Several problems associated with acute fetal or intrapartum stress worsen the severity of HMD, possibly as a consequence of further compromising the limited pulmonary blood supply and causing the death of an already limited number of type II alveolar cells. Chronic intrauterine stress, on the contrary, lowers the risk of HMD by promoting lung maturation, perhaps by increasing endogenous glucocorticoid concentrations. The factors influencing the incidence and severity of HMD are summarized in Table 27.1.

Once HMD has occurred and ventilatory assistance is required, morbidity and mortality are substantial. Those with a gestation of 30 to 35 weeks typically have improved pulmonary function and spontaneous diuresis 3–4 days after birth. The more immature newborns often have a more complicated course due to secondary lung damage and complications of immaturity such as intrapulmonary and intraventricular or periventricular hemorrhage and patent ductus arteriosus (PDA). Complications from ventilator and oxygen therapy may result in a prolonged, complex clinical course.[1–5] These complications, which include bronchopulmonary dysplasia, retinopathy of prematurity, and developmental delays, may persist into adulthood.[5–6]

CLINICAL PRESENTATION

Clinically, a premature infant with HMD may appear normal at birth, although often evidence of intrapartum depression or asphyxia is present. During the first few hours after birth, these newborns develop early signs of respiratory failure (i.e., forceful intercostal retractions, the use of accessory neck muscles, expiratory grunting, paradoxical seesaw respirations, gradually increasing oxygen requirements, and tachycardia). Pallor or cyanosis may also develop. Fluid retention, edema, and oliguria are common in the first 48 hours.

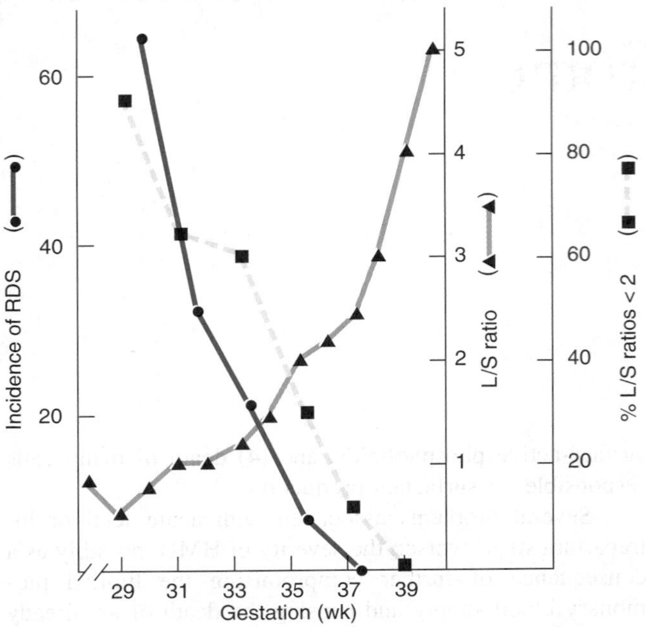

Figure 27.1. Comparison of the frequency of RDS with lecithin/sphingomyelin (L/S) ratio in amniotic fluid and with gestational age. *(From Farrell PM, Avery ME. Hyaline membrane disease. Am Rev Resp Dis 1975;111–657, with permission.)*

A characteristic chest x-ray film (Fig. 27.2) shows a reticulogranular (ground glass) pattern to the peripheral lung fields, along with clearly defined large airways (air bronchograms) resulting from the presence of air in the large airways and the collapse of small air spaces around the large airways.[1]

A number of neonatal disorders may clinically mimic and be indistinguishable from HMD (Table 27.2). By far the most important disorder is sepsis due to group B β-hemolytic streptococcus, pneumococcus, or gram-negative bacilli. Sepsis accounted for 8% of consecutively admitted infants with RDS during a 1-year study.[2] All neonates with suspected HMD should be evaluated for sepsis. Antibiotics should be used until sepsis can be ruled out or a full therapeutic course is completed.

TABLE 27.1. FACTORS WORSENING THE SEVERITY AND INCREASING THE INCIDENCE OF RESPIRATORY DISTRESS SYNDROME

Perinatal asphyxia or hypoxia
Cold stress
Prematurity
Failure of closure of the patent ductus arteriosus
Diabetes mellitus in mother
Acidosis

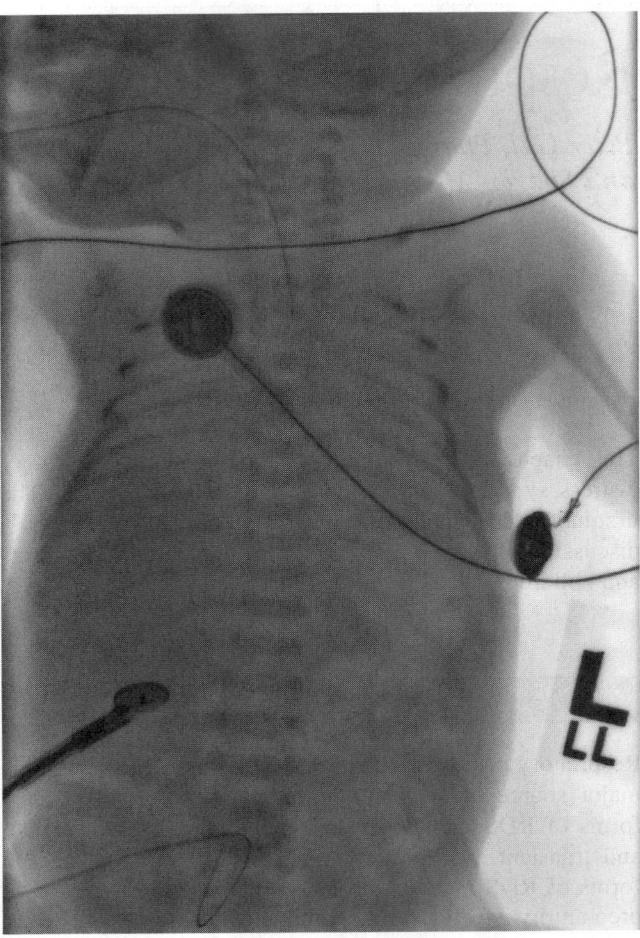

Figure 27.2. Chest x-ray demonstrating hyaline membrane disease with ground glass appearance and air bronchograms.

THERAPY

Prevention of, or minimizing the severity of, HMD is the most important goal of therapy. Several interventions can provide substantial benefit to the newborn. These can be divided into the four categories listed in Table 27.3.

Management of the premature infant during labor and delivery to prevent hypoxia and hypothermia is critical to limiting the severity of RDS. This involves preventing or minimizing maternal hypotension and hemorrhage, supply-

TABLE 27.2. DIFFERENTIAL DIAGNOSIS OF HYALINE MEMBRANE DISEASE

Pneumonia, especially group B streptococcus
Spontaneous pneumothorax
Transient tachypnea of the newborn
Congenital cyanotic heart disease
Hypoplastic lungs
Diaphragmatic hernia

TABLE 27.3. METHODS OF PREVENTING OR MINIMIZING THE SEVERITY OF HYALINE MEMBRANE DISEASE

Initiate maternal and neonatal care during labor and delivery to minimize hypoxia and optimize the time for delivery
Delay premature delivery to allow more lung maturation (e.g., with tocolytics)
Promote lung development and surfactant formation (e.g., with prenatal steroids)
Provide exogenous surfactant

TABLE 27.4. DRUGS USED FOR INHIBITING PRETERM LABOR

β-Adrenergic agonists (ritodrine, terbutaline)
Magnesium sulfate
Isoxsuprine hydrochloride
Calcium channel blockers
Ethanol
NSAIDs[a] (indomethacin, ibuprofen)

[a]Nonsteroid anti-inflammatory drugs.

ing adequate warmth to the newborn at delivery to maintain normal body temperature, and providing supplemental oxygen as needed to maintain adequate oxygenation.[1]

In some cases, particularly with premature infants, delaying delivery to allow time for lung maturation should be considered. To assist with this decision, measurement of the lecithin/sphingomyelin (L/S) ratio in amniotic fluid is valuable (Fig. 27.1). An L/S ratio higher than 2 is generally considered compatible with relatively mature lung function.[1] L/S values less than 2 are associated with a risk of RDS of approximately 50%, compared with a risk less than 1% when L/S ratios are greater than 2. However, L/S ratios are often falsely elevated for select high-risk populations (e.g., diabetics, chronic toxemia of pregnancy, hypertensives from cardiovascular or renal origin, sickle-cell disease, narcotic addiction). In these situations other markers are used as adjuncts to evaluate lung maturity. Other phospholipids including desaturated lecithin and phosphatidylglycerol (PG) determined in amniotic fluid are also predictive of lung maturation.[3,7] PG concentrations in amniotic fluid are 3% or greater if lung maturation is sufficient to avoid RDS.[7]

In cases where the L/S ratio is less than 2 or PG is negative, tocolytic agents (agents inhibiting labor) can reduce the risk of RDS. Although several tocolytics are available and have been used clinically (Table 27.4), the β sympathomimetics are the best studied and should be considered the agents of choice. Promising results have also been noted with the calcium channel blockers but are accompanied by some concerns about decreased uterine blood flow and fetal hypoxemia.[8] Since different β agonists are equally effective provided comparable doses are used, drug selection should be based on the convenience of the dosing schedule and cost. Most patients are started in the hospital on an intravenous regimen, then converted to oral therapy once labor is stopped. Tocolytics are generally not used at less than 20 weeks' gestation since usually they delay delivery by a few weeks and viability in most centers is about 24 weeks.[8] Therapy is continued until the etiology for preterm labor (e.g., urinary tract infection) is resolved or until the fetus is sufficiently mature to be safely delivered (e.g., L/S ratio becomes greater than 2 or positive PG).

Tocolytics are generally started when frequent contractions are noted, although preterm labor may be overdiagnosed in up to 70% of cases using this approach. Ideally, the diagnosis of premature labor should only be made when regular contractions are accompanied by progressive cervical dilatation and/or effacement. However, waiting for cervical changes will reduce the likelihood of successful inhibition of labor and thus compromise the fetus.[8,9]

Corticosteroids (e.g., betamethasone 12 mg daily for two doses or dexamethasone 5 mg every 12 hours for four doses) given at least 24 hours prenatally to a pregnant mother under 32 weeks' gestation to accelerate lung maturation and prevent RDS in the infant, have been used since 1972.[10,11] Two mechanisms by which lung maturation is enhanced by corticosteroids are increased production of surfactant[10–12] and acceleration of the normal rise in the antioxidant enzymes, for example, superoxide dismutase, catalase, and glutathione peroxidase, which protect lungs against damage from O_2 free radicals.[10–12] Several studies have observed a reduction in RDS with the use of antenatal corticosteroids.[10–14] However, some studies have noted that the benefits may be limited to a small population (i.e., infants 30 to 32 weeks' gestation, white, and female).[13] Overt toxicity from antenatal steroids appears to be minimal, prompting some authors to speculate that use of corticosteroids to prevent RDS is warranted for all mothers with pregnancies less than 34 weeks.[14] Others have argued that the relative benefits are inadequate to justify routine antenatal corticosteroid use.[15] This issue was resolved in a recent NIH consensus conference,[11] which indicated that with few exceptions, women with preterm labor should be treated with corticosteroids. The odds ratio (95% confidence interval) for developing RDS is reduced to 0.49 (0.41–0.6) if steroids are started 24 hours to 7 days before delivery. Even if treatment is started before 24 hours or >7 days from delivery, risk is reduced OR 0.69 (CI 0.50–0.94). Antenatal steroids also reduce the risk of intraventricular hemorrhage (OR 0.5, CI 0.3–0.9) and neonatal mortality (OR 0.6, CI 0.5–0.8).[11] One additional consideration favoring corticosteroid use antenatally is the apparent additive effects with surfactant treatment of RDS,[12] again supporting a liberal policy for prenatal corticosteroid use.

TREATMENT

Treatment of RDS can involve the use of surfactant, the use of mechanical ventilation, management of acidosis, and diuresis. These treatment considerations are discussed in the following sections.

Surfactant Therapy

Administration of lung surfactant to neonates with surfactant deficiency RDS is now widely recognized as the most physiologic and cost-effective approach.[16–18] Both natural and synthetic surfactants have been shown to modify the severity and duration of RDS, reduce multisystem morbidity (e.g., bronchopulmonary dysplasia), and decrease mortality from RDS by 40–60%.[16–18] This decreased mortality due to surfactant treatment of RDS is thought to account for over half of the 6% reduction in neonatal mortality observed from 1989 to 1990.[17] Surfactant use was also cost effective, because inflation-adjusted resource use declined by $5800 for survivors and $4400 for infants who died, subsequent to introduction of surfactant into clinical practice.[17]

Numerous surfactant preparations have been used in clinical trials with favorable outcomes. The surfactants are generally separated into natural or synthetic products, which contain different components of surfactant proteins and lipids (Table 27.5).[19]

Natural human surfactant is composed of phospholipids (85%), neutral lipids (10%), and surfactant proteins (SP) or apolipoproteins (5%). Animal surfactants have similar protein and lipid content. Most exogenous surfactants incorporate dipalmitoyl phosphatidylcholine (DPPC), which constitutes 45–70% of endogenous lung surfactant and is the major factor causing the low surface tension of surfactant. Other phospholipids, mainly phosphatidyl ethanolamine, phosphatidyl glycerol, phosphatidylinositol, and sphingomyelin are responsible for adsorbing to the air/liquid interface. Four surfactant proteins (SP), SP-A, SP-B, SP-C, and SP-D, are known and have different functions. SP-A and SP-D have immunomodulatory properties, while SP-B and SP-C improve surface adsorption of phospholipids, thus lowering surface tension. SP-A also serves to enhance the effects of SP-B and SP-C to facilitate lipid adsorption, and it regulates surfactant reuptake and secretion of phospholipids and proteins by type II pneumocytes. SP-B and SP-C may also enhance surfactant reuptake by type II pneumocytes. Different ingredients and quantities appear in different surfactants, accounting for some of the observed pharmacodynamic differences among exogenous surfactants. For practical purposes, only two surfactants are currently marketed in the United States, the synthetic surfactant, Exosurf, and the modified natural surfactant, Survanta. The natural surfactant extracts, Infasurf and Curosurf, are expected to be marketed in the near future.

Several questions about exogenously administered surfactants remain partially resolved or unresolved: (1) What is the optimum method of administration? (2) Should surfactant be administered "prophylactically" before RDS or as "res-

TABLE 27.5. EXOGENOUS SURFACTANTS USED FOR THE TREATMENT OF NEONATES WITH RESPIRATORY DISTRESS SYNDROME

	Source	Components	Concentration (g/L)	Initial Dose (mg/kg)
Artificial Surfactants				
ALEC (Pumactant)	Synthetic	DPPC, unsaturatedphosphatidylglycerol	100	100
Colfosceril palmitate (Exosurf)	Synthetic	DPPC, hexadecanol, tyloxapol	13.5	67.5
Human Surfactants				
Human	Amniotic fluid	Surfactant lipids, SP-A, SP-B, SP-C, SP-D	20	60–70
Animal Surfactants				
Infasurf	Lipid extract of calf lung lavage	Surfactant lipids, SP-B, SP-C	25	100
CLSE	Lipid extract of calf lung lavage		30	90
Alveofact	Lipid extract of cow lung lavage	Surfactant lipids, SP-B, SP-C	45	50
Curosurf	Organic solvent of pig lung purified by chromatography	Lung phospholipids, SP-B, SP-C	80	200
Surfactant-TA (Surfacten)	Lipid extract of cow lung + added synthetic lipids	Lung lipids + DPPC, tripalmitin, palmitic acid	30	100
Survanta	Lipid extract of cow lung + synthetic lipids	Lung lipids + DPPC, tripalmitin, palmitic acid, SP-B, SP-C	25	100

Key: ALEC, artificial lung expanding compound; CLSE, calf lung surfactant extract; DPPC, dipalmitoyl phosphatidylcholine; SP-A, surfactant protein A; SP-B, surfactant protein B; SP-C, surfactant protein C. (Adapted with permission from Hallman M, Merritt TA, Bry K. The fate of exogenous surfactant in neonates with respiratory distress syndrome. Clin Pharmacokinet 1994;26(3):215–232.)

cue therapy" after the onset of disease? (3) What is the optimum dose and how many doses should be administered? (4) Which surfactant preparation is best? (5) Should surfactant treatment be repeated if RDS recurs or causes of treatment failure resolve? (6) Can toxicities associated with exogenous surfactant be reduced? These issues are addressed as follows.

Surfactant administration technique differed in clinical trials for Exosurf and Survanta. Exosurf was administered via the side port of an endotracheal tube adapter with each inspiratory cycle of the ventilator, which allowed the maintenance of positive pressure during instillation.[18] Survanta was administered in most clinical trials via a feeding tube measured to deliver drug to the distal end of the endotracheal tube in four aliquots. Manual ventilation and positioning are used to disperse the drug.[18] The basis for dividing Survanta administration into four parts appears to be empiric. A recent clinical trial[20] compared Survanta administration by three methods: (1) the standard method requiring removal from the ventilator, dividing the dose into four fractional doses, and hand-bagging the dose into the lungs at 45° tilts upward or downward and angled to the right then left sides; (2) the same technique in two fractional doses at 45° upward tilt angled to the right then left; and (3) via a catheter placed through the suction valve of the endotracheal tube without removing the patient from the ventilator and administering two fractional doses at a 45° upward tilt angled to the right then left. All three doses were equal for response and administration-related problems. Recent animal studies support these clinical findings.[21–24] The use of two, rather than the usual four, positions to administer bolus doses of Survanta was demonstrated to deliver and distribute surfactant evenly and equally well.[21] Slow infusion technique was shown to deliver surfactant primarily to the upper lobes[21] and nebulized surfactant tended to concentrate in select pockets of each lobe of the lung resulting in areas of hypo- or hyperinflation.[22] Relative delivery was only one-twentieth of the instilled dose.[23] Thus, instilled surfactant doses in two to four divided doses seem most efficient.

The timing of treatment initiation is also controversial. Overall, delivery room prophylaxis seems unnecessary as a window of at least 2 hours after birth appears to exist where outcome is not compromised by delayed delivery.[16,18] This allows time for stabilization of the patient and confirmation of the need for surfactant. Delayed administration beyond 2 hours of age has been associated with increased complications of RDS although this information remains to be confirmed.[18] Early instillation of exogenous surfactant as rescue therapy appears to be the best medical management at this time. Prophylaxis should be reserved for patients at particularly high risk for RDS (e.g., those known to have immature L/S ratio or absence of PG or preterm infants of ≤26 weeks' gestation).[18]

The optimal dose of exogenous surfactant is uncertain. Controlled trials comparing single and multiple doses of surfactant have shown significant reductions in pneumothorax and neonatal mortality with multiple doses relative to single doses.[16,18] This makes some physiologic sense since animal studies suggest that much of the initial surfactant dose is inhibited by soluble proteins and other factors in the small airways and alveoli. Multiple doses may overcome this initial inactivation. While many clinicians use up to four doses of surfactant over 24–48 hours, an Exosurf study comparing two doses versus two to four doses depending on clinical need failed to show advantages to more than two doses.[24] A summary of the clinical trials comparing surfactant doses is given in Table 27.6.[25–31] Nevertheless, the

TABLE 27.6. DOSING COMPARISON STUDIES FOR DIFFERENT SURFACTANTS

			Effects of Higher Doses Compared to Lower Doses	
Ref.	**Surfactant**	**Doses**	**Short-Term**	**Long-Term**
27	Exosurf	5 mL/kg ≤4 vs ≤ 2 doses	Not stated	*28 days:* no differences
28	Exosurf	2.5 vs 5 mL 2.5 vs 7.5 mL 5 vs 7.5 mL	↓ Fio_2, ↓ vent (MAP) ↓ Fio_2, ↓ vent (MAP) No difference	*14 days:* no differences
25	Infasurf	100 mg/kg 1 vs ≤ 4 doses	↓ Fio_2, ↓ vent (PIP × IMV)	*28 days:* ↓ O_2 suppl (0 vs 8.3%) ↓ pneumothorax (11.1 vs 16.7%)
26	Surfactant TA	30 mg/mL 2 vs 4 mL/kg	↓ Fio_2	*30 days:* ↓ O_2 suppl (13 vs 43.5%) ↓ vent (4.3 vs 30.4%)
29	Curosurf	200 mg/kg × 1 vs 200 mg/kg × 1 + 100 mg/kg ($x \le 2$)	↓ Fio_2, ↓ vent (MAP)	*28 days:* ↓ death (13 vs 21%) ↓ pneumothorax (9 vs 18%)
30	Curosurf	100 mg/kg ($x \le 3$) vs 200 mg/kg + 100 mg/kg ($x \le 4$)	↓ Fio_2	*28 days:* no differences
31	Alveofact	100 mg/kg vs 50 mg/kg (repeat doses to max 200 mg/kg)	↓ Fio_2	*28 days:* ↓ pulmonary air leak (14 vs 33%)

question of optimum doses is not fully resolved. Currently, it appears that repetitive dosing based on clinical necessity is reasonable up to at least four doses of Survanta. A recent study[32] associated requiring four doses of Survanta with a subsequent increased requirement for oxygen, beginning on about day 10, and a predisposition to bronchopulmonary dysplasia (BPD). Thus, the need for a fourth Survanta dose may be of prognostic importance.

Comparing different sufactants requires documentation of short- and long-term risks and benefits and the number of doses needed and costs to administer surfactant. Endpoints reported by various investigators include acute changes in supplemental oxygen and ventilator pressures, the incidence of PDA, intraventricular hemorrhage (IVH), pulmonary hemorrhage, pneumothorax, BPD, and death. In individual studies, surfactant has not been reported to reduce PDA, IVH, BPD, or pulmonary hemorrhage. Using meta-analysis, both natural and synthetic surfactants have been shown to reduce only the risk of pneumothorax and death[16,33] (Table 27.7). Based on these meta-analyses and animal studies,[21–23] early oxygen requirements and the incidence of pneumothorax would be the most likely differences.

Studies in humans are limited. A meta-analysis of three abstracts published in 1993 compared the relative risks of several outcomes in neonates treated with Exosurf versus Survanta.[34] The projected difference for relative risk of pneumothorax and death for the Exosurf group increased by 3.3 and 2.7%, respectively. It was projected that 9000 patients would need to be studied to show this difference in death rates with a $p = .05$ and 90% power. Also it was projected that for preferential use of Survanta to benefit one patient would require treatment of 30 patients to prevent pneumothorax and 37 patients to prevent death. Thus, while a recently published study comparing outcomes in 617 newborns treated with Exosurf or Survanta failed to show statistically significant differences, the study could only detect differences of 38.5% for death and 50% for BPD.[36] Thus, although pneumothorax occurred in 13% of Exosurf-treated neonates and 9% of Survanta-treated neonates (risk ratio 1.51, 95% CI 0.95–2.39), a statistically significant greater benefit for Survanta could not be shown. A recent comparison of Curosurf and Survanta in 75 neonates showed both drugs to provide rapid improvement in oxygenation and ventilator pressure requirements.[35] Curosurf, however, had greater effects as well as a reduction in pneumothorax (6 versus 12.5%), grades 3–4 intraventricular hemorrhage (IVH) (3 versus 12.5%), and death (3 versus 12.5%). None of these differences reached statistical significance and the small population studied precludes attributing any differences between these products.

As more surfactant products become available, selection will depend largely on clinical efficacy for prevention of short- and long-term sequelae, adverse effects, and cost. The trend toward reduction in early oxygen and ventilator requirements, and pneumothorax, favors natural over synthetic surfactants.[37–39] Differentiating natural surfactants will be based primarily on cost, unless sufficiently large studies are performed to show differences.

Despite the overwhelming success of surfactant to improve the outcome of neonatal RDS, 20% of neonates fail to respond to treatment.[16,33] Factors associated with poor response include sepsis or pneumonia, PDA, congenital heart disease, and pulmonary hypoplasia.[33] It remains unclear if treatment with surfactant is appropriate once the cause of failure resolves or if a patient initially responding to surfactant appears to have recurrent RDS. Most centers do not currently use surfactant in this situation and such expensive therapy should not routinely be undertaken without supporting trials.

While surfactant appears to be generally well tolerated, some toxicities are observed. Pulmonary hemorrhage is perhaps the most common problem. This is primarily a problem with Exosurf (odds ratio 2.32, 95% CI 1.32–4.06), and may not be a real risk with natural surfactant (odds

TABLE 27.7. RELATIVE RISKS FOR POTENTIAL BENEFICIAL AND ADVERSE EFFECTS OF SYNTHETIC AND NATURAL SURFACTANTS

	Synthetic Surfactant				Natural Surfactant			
Outcome	**No.**	**Prophylaxis**	**No.**	**Rescue**	**No.**	**Prophylaxis**	**No.**	**Rescue**
Pneumothorax	5	0.64 (0.49–0.89)	3	0.52 (0.42–0.65)	9	0.31 (0.22–0.44)	12	0.34 (0.27–0.44)
BPD	5	1.09 (0.80–1.47)	3	0.68 (0.46–0.99)	7	0.88 (0.67–1.17)	10	1.01 (0.81–1.27)
Death	7	0.67 (0.52–0.88)	3	0.47 (0.30–0.74)	9	0.60 (0.42–0.85)	11	0.59 (0.47–0.74)
Death + BPD	3	0.82 (0.63–1.08)	2	0.65 (0.50–0.82)	7	0.64 (0.49–0.84)	10	0.66 (0.53–0.82)
All IVH	4	0.94 (0.73–1.21)	2	0.77 (0.62–0.97)	8	0.95 (0.73–1.24)	10	0.94 (0.76–1.15)
Severe IVH						1.05 (0.86–1.18)		0.91 (0.72–1.14)
PDA	5	1.27 (1.03–1.57)	3	0.73 (0.60–0.88)	9	1.16 (0.89–1.50)	12	0.96 (0.79–1.18)
Pulmonary bleed	4	3.12 (1.54–6.32)	3	1.49 (0.57–3.79)	2	0.73 (0.31–1.69)	2	1.25 (0.74–2.13)

Key: BPD, bronchopulmonary dysplasia; IVH, intraventricular hemorrhage; PDA, patent ductus arteriosus; #, number of studies reporting each outcome.
Based on meta-analysis of controlled clinical trials.
Numbers expressed as adjusted odds ratio (95% confidence interval). (Data summarized from information in Refs. 16, 33, and 36.)

ratio 1.09, 95% CI 0.69–1.72).[36] Massive pulmonary hemorrhage was described in 10–45% of neonates with RDS before the introduction of surfactant and may still primarily be the consequence of disease. Physiologically, the marked reduction in pulmonary pressure is believed to promote a significantly larger shunting of blood through the PDA. Therefore, surfactant treatment appears to increase the likelihood of clinically significant PDA. Furthermore, the consequent pulmonary edema from this increased PDA shunting is thought to cause a hemorrhagic pulmonary edema rather than a serious pulmonary hemorrhage.[18] Early closure of the PDA should minimize this complication as well as improve surfactant response rates. Some studies have also shown increased rates of IVH among surfactant-treated neonates. This is not a consistent finding and some reports show a reduction in IVH incidence with surfactant therapy. Cerebral blood flow velocity has been shown to be altered in some studies.[18] It is possible that changes in arterial and cerebral blood flow are associated with PDA shunting.[18] Since IVH prophylaxis with indomethacin has been shown to be beneficial, it is possible that such therapy would be particularly useful in surfactant-treated neonates to prevent both IVH and hemorrhagic pulmonary edema in newborns. Sufficient research to make this a standard of practice is currently lacking.

Synthetic surfactant manufacturers have highlighted the allergenic risks of natural surfactants in marketing their products.[40] While this may prove important for adults and children receiving surfactant for ARDS, it appears of little consequence in neonates, since they do not produce antibodies to Survanta.[41]

Ventilator Management of the Newborn

Once RDS has occurred, mechanical ventilation is necessary for maintaining adequate oxygenation and ventilation, and delivery of exogenous surfactant. A comprehensive review of mechanical ventilation is beyond the scope of this chapter but can be found in other reviews.[42] In general, the goal is to maintain arterial partial pressure of oxygen $Pa{O_2}$ of 50–70 mm Hg and a pH of 7.28–7.40. A glossary of terms used with standard pressure ventilation is given in Table 27.8 and typical ventilator responses based on arterial blood gases are described in Table 27.9. Use of oxygen monitoring devices (e.g., pulse oximetry) can reduce the frequency of arterial blood gas collection and allow clinicians to be more responsive to the rapidly changing pulmonary status noted with surfactant use. This is important and pulmonary overdistention due to increased lung compliance and hyperoxia due to improved alveolar function can result in air leak syndromes and oxygen toxicity to lungs and eyes. Other ventilator maneuvers that require further study but have positive results in experimental animal models of RDS include high-frequency jet ventilation (HFV)[43] and perfluorocarbons to provide liquid ventilation.[44] These may play important roles in the future.

Other maneuvers important during management of RDS include maintaining adequate blood pressure, sedation to prevent ventilator fighting, use of alkali to correct metabolic acidosis, and diuretics to treat pulmonary edema.

Hypotension is commonly observed in neonates with RDS. This is considered important when systolic blood pressure is less than 35 mm Hg or higher values if markers of organ perfusion (e.g., urine output or capillary refill) appear compromised. Since fluid is usually restricted, only a limited challenge with colloids is reasonable. Once pressors are needed, dopamine has been shown to be superior to dobutamine[45] and should be the first agent tried.

Use of Sedatives and Muscle Relaxants

Prevention of ventilator complications secondary to barotrauma involves using the lowest possible airway pressure and can often be minimized by use of sedatives or muscle relaxants. For example, pneumothorax, a common

TABLE 27.8. GLOSSARY OF TERMS FOR VENTILATOR MANAGEMENT

Term	Definition
Et	Expiratory time; in the ventilatory cycle, the amount of time devoted to exhalation.
It	Inspiratory time; in the ventilatory cycle, the amount of time devoted to inspiration.
I : E	Ratio of inspiratory time to expiratory time; in a normal, spontaneously breathing patient this is 1 : 1.5 $Pa{CO_2}$, partial pressure of carbon dioxide present in arterial blood; normal is 35–45 mm Hg, but higher $Pa{CO_2}$ is acceptable to minimize ventilator support.
$Pa{O_2}$	Partial pressure of oxygen present in arterial blood; normal level for adults is 80–100 mm Hg; normal level for premature babies is 50–70 mm Hg.
PEEP	Positive end expiratory pressure; positive pressure at the end of exhalation; designed to prevent alveoli from collapsing during expiration.
PIP	Peak inspiratory pressure; the maximum level of pressure achieved by the ventilator during inspiration.
IMV	Intermittent mandatory ventilation; a mode of ventilation designed to deliver a present inspiratory rate; continuous flow of gas is available for patient's spontaneous breaths.
$Fi{O_2}$	Fraction (percentage) of inspired oxygen.

(Prepared by Rene Mize, BS, RRT, Assistant Director, Department of Respiratory Therapy, The Moses H. Cone Memorial Hospital, Greensboro, NC.)

TABLE 27.9. VENTILATOR MANEUVERS FOR NEONATES ON A POSITIVE-PRESSURE VENTILATOR IN RESPONSE TO ARTERIAL BLOOD GAS RESULTS

pH	Pao_2	$Paco_2$	Ventilator Maneuvers	Possible Complications
Normal, high, or low	Low (<50 mm Hg)	Normal	↑ Fio_2	Oxygen toxicity
		Normal to high	↑ PIP	Barotrauma, overdistention, ↓ cardiac output
		Normal	↑ PEEP	Barotrauma, ↑ $Paco_2$, ↓ cardiac output
		Normal	↑ It	Barotrauma, ↑ $Paco_2$, ↓ cardiac output
	High (>80 mm Hg)	Normal to high	↓ Fio_2	Hypoxemia ↑ $Paco_2$, atelectasis
		Normal to high	↓ PIP	Hypoxemia, atelectasis
		Normal to high	↓ PEEP	Hypoxemia
		Normal to high	↓ It	
Low (<7.25)	Low to normal	High (>45 mm Hg)	↑ PIP	Barotrauma, overdistention, ↓ $Paco_2$
	Low, normal, high		↓ PEEP	Hypoxemia, atelectasis
	Normal to high		↓ It	
	Low, normal, high		↑ IMV	Hypoxemia $Paco_2$ (secondary ↓ Et)
	Normal	Low	↓ PIP	
	Normal		↓ IMV	Hypoxemia, atelectasis ↑ $Paco_2$

Assume that there are no other causes for abnormality (i.e., misplaced or obstructed endotracheal tube). (Prepared by Rene Mize, BS, RRT, Assistant Director, Department of Respiratory Therapy, The Moses H. Cone Memorial Hospital, Greensboro, NC.)

complication of ventilator support, is strongly associated with breathing against the ventilator.[46] Capturing the infant's own respiratory rate is helpful and this usually requires at least 50 breaths per minute. However, sedation or paralysis is usually needed to allow optimal ventilator manipulation without neonatal resistance. The selection of a sedative or muscle relaxant is very controversial as each treatment has important clinical benefits and toxicities. Approaches differ in each center based on individual clinicians' experiences with the various options and their interpretation of the literature. The approach discussed in the following section represents the authors' and may differ from that in many centers. In general, only intravenous (IV) drugs are recommended until proper gastrointestinal (GI) function is established. The advantages and disadvantages for each option are discussed as follows, and dosing recommendations are described in Table 27.10.

TABLE 27.10. GUIDELINES FOR SEDATION AND MUSCLE RELAXATION IN NEONATES REQUIRING MECHANICAL VENTILATION

Drug	Dose	Comments
Phenobarbital	20 mg/kg IV for four doses then 5–10 mg/kg/d	Keep plasma concentration above 60 μg/mL; avoid hypotension by administering doses slowly, i.e., ≥15 min
Lorazepam	0.1–0.4 mg/kg IV every 2–6 h PRN	Short duration of effects; low toxicity risk
Diazepam	0.1–1.0 mg/kg IV every 6 h PRN	Risk excess accumulation in neonates due to long half-life; may cause phlebitis. Use as adjunct to phenobarbital
Morphine	0.1–0.2 mg/kg IV every 3–6 h PRN	May be preferred for short postoperative therapy because it also produces analgesia; monitor blood pressure for hypotension and decrease dose if it occurs
Fentanyl	Loading dose 1–2 μg/kg IV may repeat every 5–10 min to total 8 μg/kg IV; maintenance dose = 1–8 μg/kg/h; continuous infusion or every 2 h dosing may be used	Short pharmacologic effect; high addiction potential; rate-related wooden chest syndrome; may use clonidine 1–2 μg/kg every 6 h as an adjunct to assist tapering doses by blunting abstinence syndrome
Pancuronium	0.01–0.03 mg/kg IV PRN	Dosing requirements gradually increase with continuous therapy. Monitor closely for sudden drop in Pao_2 within minutes of a dose—either increase PIP or D/C Pavulon if this occurs. Must administer phenobarbital to a concentration of 40 μg/mL to minimize the risk of undetected seizures and provide sedation
Chloral hydrate	25–50 μg/kg PO every 4–6 h PRN	Only oral form available. May cause GI irritability, vasodilation, hypotension, respiratory depression, and direct hyperbilirubinemia

Pancuronium

Several studies have used pancuronium (Pavulon) paralysis to reduce ventilator fighting and the consequent complications. These studies have demonstrated a reduction in the duration of oxygen support needed for babies with HMD,[47] reduced periods of hypoxia and hyperoxia,[48] lower incidence of pneumothorax,[49] which was not confirmed in other studies,[47] and reduced intracranial pressure and cerebral blood flow associated with a decreased incidence of intraventricular hemorrhage.[49,50] While these findings are encouraging, they are not consistent across studies.[49,51] In addition, the toxicities and hazards of treatment with pancuronium are substantial. These include acute hypoventilation (19 of 35 neonates with HMD),[49,52] increased ventilator pressure support needs,[50] and increased massive intracranial hemorrhage,[52] perhaps precipitated by acute increases in blood pressure and heart rate.[53] Excessive edema and fluid and electrolyte problems occur in all paralyzed neonates.

Another consideration is the risk of masking seizure activity,[54,55] thus allowing it to go untreated. Neonates receiving pancuronium should be given concurrent prophylactic phenobarbital as electroencephalographic seizure activity has been noted in 13 of 16 paralyzed neonates[54] without clinically noticeable symptoms. Twitching, which may be misinterpreted as seizures, often occurs when the pancuronium dose is tapered or discontinued. Some authors feel the risks outweigh any possible benefits while others are strong proponents. One issue not discussed in neonatal literature, but commonly known for adults, is the need for adjunctive sedatives in paralyzed patients. It is likely that the feeling of paralysis is stressful and terrifying in the neonate. The only patients in whom the risk/benefit ratio currently favors pancuronium is the 15% of prematures with HMD where an elevated intracranial pressure is documented. Other less hazardous agents that can provide adequate sedation and avoid the need for paralysis, such as phenobarbital, lorazepam, or fentanyl, may suffice even in this situation.[51,56]

Phenobarbital

Phenobarbital, alone or in combination with a benzodiazepine, provides sedation as well as several other possible beneficial, but controversial, actions. Beneficial actions include reduced intracranial pressure[57] and possibly lower incidence of intraventricular hemorrhage,[58] and a reduction in the central nervous system sequelae from asphyxia,[59,60] which is common in this population. Sedation is rarely achieved unless plasma concentrations exceed 60 μg/mL.[60]

The concerns with this regimen are the potential hazards to brain growth[61] and the prolonged half-life, which results in persistent high plasma concentrations for several days after the drug is stopped. Concerns about the cardiovascular toxicity of phenobarbital appear ill founded and probably reflect the effects of propylene glycol when the product is administered by rapid intravenous push.[60] No cardiovascular toxicity is seen when 20 mg/kg doses are given over 5 minutes.[62]

Narcotics

Morphine has been used in some circumstances for sedation and respiratory depression in ventilated neonates.[63] While it appears effective, the risks of hypotension, decreased GI motility, and physiologic dependency with prolonged use are important risks that relegate morphine to a second- or third-line drug in our nursery except in neonates who also have a component of pain (e.g., postsurgery). One advantage of morphine is its rapid reversibility with narcotic antagonists.

Fentanyl has been used increasingly in the neonatal intensive care unit population. Its main benefit is in larger neonates with persistent pulmonary hypertension as it blocks the sympathetic response to stress[50] and ablation of pulmonary vascular responsiveness.[64] While it is clinically effective, addiction potential appears to be high, occurring in 4–5 days of treatment, and tolerance to sedative effects may develop.[64]

Benzodiazepines

Diazepam has been used by some clinicians to sedate neonates although literature supporting its use in neonates is lacking. While the therapeutic index is wide, accumulation of diazepam and its active metabolite, *N*-desmethyldiazepam, may occur with repeated doses and result in severe hypotonia.[65] An additional disadvantage of intravenous diazepam is the propensity for producing phlebitis, which can be reduced but not eliminated by slow administration.

Lorazepam is the preferred agent due to its lower risk for accumulation than diazepam as its half-life is shorter (28–65 hours for lorazepam[66] versus 40–400 hours for diazepam metabolites). Although the available literature about neonatal lorazepam use is limited,[66] our experience in more than 150 patients has been that it is a safe, effective sedative, which clinically lasts 2–4 hours. Doses used clinically range from 0.1–0.4 mg/kg every 2–6 hours depending on clinical response and desired level of sedation.[67]

Chloral Hydrate

Chloral hydrate has been an effective, relatively safe sedative in children and has been used by some clinicians for neonates. It is metabolized in the liver to the active metabolite tricholethanol, which has an average half-life of 37 hours. However, doses of 25–50 mg/kg result in only 1 or 2 hours of sedation. The major disadvantages of chloral hydrate are that it must be given orally and it can cause GI irritation. Other reported toxicities include vasodilation, hypotension, respiratory depression, cardiac arrhythmias,[68] and direct hyperbilirubinemia.[69]

Acidosis

Acidosis is associated with a number of physiologic effects that increase the severity of RDS, including increased pulmonary vascular resistance, impaired synthesis of surfactant, reduced cardiac output, and depressed ventilation. Consequently, measures that reduce the risk of acidosis, such as prevention of hypoxemia, hypotension, excessive blood loss through venipuncture or bleeding, and minimizing oxygen consumption through careful temperature control, are critical. Correction of metabolic acidosis with sodium bicarbonate or 0.3 *M* tromethamine (THAM) is recommended when blood pH falls below 7.25. Alkali is needed fairly often in neonates. The trade-off for increasing ventilator settings to correct for acidosis is pulmonary and ocular toxicity; thus, increased ventilator support creates considerable toxicity. Because available scientific data do not clearly identify a "safe" ventilator setting in neonates, the decision on whether increased ventilator support should be provided or alkali should be given is empiric and clinician dependent.

Diuretics

Pulmonary edema is a prominent feature of RDS. Clinically, the severity of RDS is correlated to the presence of factors that cause pulmonary edema. This is not unexpected since excess fluid in the alveolar and interstitial spaces impairs pulmonary gas exchange, lowers lung compliance, and reduces functional residual capacity. Prevention of fluid overload and pulmonary edema is critical to minimize the risk of opening the ductus arteriosus and creating a need for high ventilator pressures and oxygen requirements due to stiff lungs.[70] Pulmonary edema can be benefited by positive end expiratory pressure (PEEP) because it redistributes fluid from air spaces to interstitial tissue and improves respiratory gas exchange. It does not, however, reduce lung water content.[70] Oliguria is well recognized during the early stages of RDS. An abrupt diuresis occurs during the recovery phase of RDS. Heaf et al.[71] showed that pulmonary function improved immediately after the onset of diuresis. This diuretic phase was thought to represent the removal of alveolar or interstitial lung water. The association of diuresis with improvement in RDS prompted several investigators to study furosemide for mobilizing lung edema and improving RDS. In general, studies have not justified the routine use of furosemide for treatment of infants with RDS.[72,73] However, all the studies have serious limitations, including inadequate definition of RDS (leading to a nonuniform patient population); the timing of doses often coincides with the time for expected spontaneous diuresis and improved lung functions; and selection of too low furosemide doses (1 mg/kg) by most researchers, as 2 mg/kg appears necessary for most RDS cases.[71,74] The potential but uncertain benefits of furosemide must be weighed against its risks. These risks include the promotion of prostaglandin synthesis, which may cause an increased incidence of PDA that could worsen the RDS. Also, if neonates have inadequate right atrial venous return, diuresis may be detrimental. Electrolyte imbalance may also result from furosemide-induced diuresis.[70,71,73] More studies need to be done to determine the potential value of diuretics.

CONCLUSION

Advances in prevention and reversal of RDS have had considerable impact on morbidity and mortality from RDS. Nevertheless, chronic lung disease, although less severe, continues to occur in about 35–45% of neonates. The challenge for the future is to manage effectively the 20% of neonates with RDS responding poorly to surfactant and to add therapies that will further reduce long-term pulmonary sequelae associated with RDS. This is a valuable area for future research.

ACUTE RESPIRATORY DISTRESS SYNDROME

Acute respiratory distress syndrome (ARDS) was first described by Ashbaugh and colleagues in 1967.[75] They describe a syndrome including diffuse bilateral lung infiltrates on chest x ray, a high oxygen requirement, high ventilatory inflation pressures, and an improvement in oxygenation after the addition of PEEP. In all cases, the syndrome occurred 1–96 hours after an acute insult such as trauma, pancreatitis, pneumonia, or drug overdose. Although described more than 20 years ago, tremendous work continues in an effort to elicit the causes and treatment of this often fatal disease. Because data regarding treatment and causality are limited, nomenclature, diagnosis, and therapy are highly controversial.

PATHOPHYSIOLOGY

The incidence and mortality of ARDS is controversial secondary to nomenclature and definition issues. A recent consensus conference recommends use of "acute" rather than the previously used "adult" terminology. Some divide the lung injury into acute lung injury (ALI) describing the initial clinical findings, and ARDS, describing the severe, sustained lung injury with or without multisystem organ damage. The American-European Consensus Conference on ARDS agreed on the criteria listed in Table 27.11 to define ARDS/ALI which includes chest x-ray findings, pulmonary artery catheter pressures, and onset.[76]

Because of the controversies, understanding the pathophysiology of ARDS is important in order to evaluate ther-

TABLE 27.11. AMERICAN-EUROPEAN CONSENSUS CRITERIA DEFINING ARDS

Timing	Oxygenation	Chest Radiograph	Pulmonary Artery Wedge Pressure
Acute onset	$Pao_2/Fio_2 \leq 200$ mm Hg (ALI ≤ 300 mm Hg)	Bilateral infiltrates	≤18 mm Hg (without pulmonary hypertension)

Note: Acute lung injury (ALI) criteria differ only by allowing $Pao_2/Fio_2 \leq 300$ mm Hg) (From Ref. 76.)

apeutic modalities. This requires discussing the Starling equation of fluid movement across cellular membranes:

$$Q_T = K_f[(P_{mv} - P_{is}) - \sigma(\pi_{mv} - \pi_{is})] \qquad (1)$$

where Q_T is amount of fluid filtered per unit time; K_f is the vessel permeability to fluid; $(P_{mv} - P_{is})$ is the hydrostatic pressure gradient across the membrane separating the pulmonary microvasculature (mv) from the interstitium (is); $(\pi_{mv} - \pi_{is})$ is the osmotic gradient between the pulmonary microvasculature (mv) and interstitium (is); and σ is the membrane permeability to protein.

ARDS describes the situation in which σ approaches zero, that is, the membrane allows protein and fluid to cross freely into the pulmonary interstitium. Many clinicians call this "leak." This differs from congestive heart failure (CHF) in which σ is normal (approximately one) and the membrane is relatively impermeable to fluid and protein movement. In CHF the hydrostatic pressure increases, forcing fluid across the membrane. Because formation of lung edema differs, the therapeutic endpoints of ARDS and CHF differ (Table 27.12).[77]

Clinically, lung injury allowing σ to approach zero occurs after a variety of insults including trauma, sepsis, pancreatitis, and other diseases causing tissue inflammation. This lung injury (altered membrane permeability) causes an increase in lung water. Increased lung water increases shunt fraction, which is a ventilation/perfusion mismatch where areas of lung are being perfused, but not ventilated. This ventilation/perfusion mismatch leads to the clinical hallmark of ARDS, severe hypoxemia.[78] A fall in pulmonary compliance ensues, all with normal microvascular pressure (P_{mv}) and normal pulmonary capillary wedge pressures (PCWPs). The clinical vernacular describing decreased compliance is "stiff lung." The increase in lung water appears on chest x ray as bilateral symmetrical infiltrates.

TABLE 27.12. DIFFERENCES BETWEEN CARDIOGENIC AND NONCARDIOGENIC (ARDS) CAUSES OF PULMONARY EDEMA

Cause Parameter	Cardiogenic Hydrostatic Gradient ($P_{mv} - P_{is}$)	ARDS Membrane Permeability (σ)
Protein in fluid	↓	↑
Resolution	Fast	Slow
Pulmonary capillary wedge pressure	↑	↓
Left ventricular dysfunction	Yes	No

EPIDEMIOLOGY

The definition controversy clouds the issue of incidence. A reasonable estimate is 1.5 cases/100,000 with 70% mortality.[79] ARDS has been associated with sepsis, aspiration, multiple emergency transfusions, pulmonary contusion, multiple fractures, surgery involving cardiopulmonary bypass, burns, disseminated intravascular coagulation (DIC), and pneumonia requiring an ICU admission. Notice that all of these illnesses can cause an acute inflammatory response. Organisms causing ARDS include gram-negative bacilli, gram-positive cocci, and atypical organisms such as fungi, viruses, *Pneumocystis carinii,* and *Legionella* species. Most commonly an abdominal infection is the source that causes ARDS secondary to sepsis. Sepsis occurring after an initial episode of ARDS is usually due to a pulmonary source.[80]

The survival of ARDS is dependent on the occurrence of concomitant end-organ damage and infection. Uninfected patients and patients with an identifiable source survive more often than their counterparts.[81] The incidence of end-organ failure increases with infection.

TREATMENT

No effective therapy is available to treat the underlying cause of ARDS. Therapy is primarily supportive.[82] The clinical goals are to improve cardiopulmonary status with the goal of delivering adequate oxygen to the tissues (i.e., perfusion). Equally important is the prevention of ARDS-associated complications (end-organ disease and infection) while the underlying lung injury heals.

Monitoring Parameters

Rather than following single therapeutic endpoints, monitoring the critically ill ARDS patient requires synthesis of all endpoints in order to make rational therapeutic decisions. Ventilatory and hemodynamic endpoints are discussed in detail elsewhere in this text. In addition, drug therapy, end-organ function, and drug effects on end-organ function require careful monitoring to treat the ARDS patient appropriately.

Monitoring of ventilatory parameters, arterial blood gases, and oxygen saturation assists in the determination of severity of illness and also provides rudimentary endpoints of perfusion. For example, most clinicians agree that maintaining an oxygen saturation (Sao_2) ≥ 90 is an important endpoint.

Although some centers try to manage ARDS patients without a pulmonary artery catheter, very few patients with severe ARDS are managed this way. The diagnosis of ARDS depends on measuring PCWP, which can only be obtained by a pulmonary artery catheter. Radiographically, noncardiogenic pulmonary edema (ARDS) cannot be distinguished from cardiogenic pulmonary edema.[83] In addition, high-pressure ventilation interferes with cardiac function, which must be measured and managed to improve perfusion. Unfortunately, these ventilatory pressures also interfere with measurements obtained with central venous catheters (e.g., central venous pressure, PCWP). To assist with these problems, many centers use pulmonary artery catheters, which include an oxygen saturation monitor to measure oxygen saturation directly and mixed venous oxygenation (mVo_2). This catheter obviates the need for pulse oximetry, which may not be accurate in poorly perfused patients. In the truly ill ARDS patient, monitoring of oxygen saturation, cardiac output, and PCWP (and, in some institutions, other endpoints) is essential to determine whether specific therapeutic interventions improve perfusion.

Finally, adequate perfusion supplies necessary nutrients (oxygen, glucose, and electrolytes) and also disposes of metabolic by-products. Monitoring perfusion consists of two basic approaches. The first follows end-organ function, such as central nervous or renal function. ARDS patients are usually sedated; therefore, central nervous function is difficult to assess. Urine output as a marker of renal function rapidly becomes the most available measure of perfusion.

The second approach equates adequate oxygen delivery with perfusion. Therapy is based on optimizing oxygen delivery. Remember, hypoxemia is the predominant effect of ARDS; therefore, this latter approach addresses the most abnormal aspect of organ perfusion. Oxygen saturation, mixed venous oxygenation, and arterial blood gas oxygen (Pao_2) are usually followed. Lactate levels aid oxygen delivery assessment. Lactate production occurs during anaerobic metabolism. Monitoring serum lactate is less than ideal because lactate clearance is abnormal in renal and hepatic dysfunction and lactate metabolism is altered by endotoxin.[84] Monitoring mixed venous oxygen saturation also follows oxygen delivery. Maintaining a mixed venous saturation (mVo_2) in the normal range (65–75%) assumes adequate delivery if oxygen extraction is not deranged by sepsis. Table 27.13 lists monitoring parameters to be followed.

Hemodynamic Management

Theoretically, improving the oxygen supply should improve oxygen delivery to the tissues. A classic and often cited study in ARDS patients showed a linear relationship between oxygen supply and uptake.[85] Unfortunately, this study suffers from methodologic flaws. The methods used to calculate supply and uptake both incorporate cardiac output. Because altering cardiac output was the method used to increase oxygen supply, a linear relationship is to be expected. The inherent variability in these measures could also describe the relationship.

The most rigorous evaluation of oxygen supply and utilization refutes the linear relationship.[86] Oxygen uptake was measured by respiratory gas analysis and oxygen delivery altered using blood transfusions. Using these methods, oxygen consumption was independent of delivery.

Regardless, most clinicians optimize cardiac output in ARDS patients to assure adequate perfusion by using fluids, red cell transfusions, inotropic agents, and afterload reducing agents. Arterial oxygen (Pao_2), urine output, blood pressure, PCWP, cardiac output, oxygen saturation, and hemoglobin must be monitored to determine which agent is most appropriate to improve perfusion. Oxygen saturation ≥90%, hemoglobin ≥10 g/dL are the only numbers generally agreed on across the United States. Specific

TABLE 27.13. MONITORING PARAMETERS IN ARDS

Hemodynamic	Ventilator Status	Infection	End-Organ Damage
PCWP	Fio_2	White blood cells/differential	BUN
Cardiac output/index	Pao_2	Chest x-ray findings	Creatinine
Oxygen saturation (Sao_2)	Sao_2	Temperature	Urine output
Mixed venous oxygenation (mVo_2)	mVo_2	Cultures	Liver function tests
Hemoglogin/hematocrit	Plateau pressure	Change in color/quantity sputum	PT/PTT
Urine output	Respiratory effort/rate	New onset hypotension	
		Abdominal examination	
		Number of central catheter days	

numbers for the other monitoring parameters actually depend on the overall perfusion of the patient, rather than a specific number. One reason arterial oxygen (and saturation) are particularly important is that inotropic agents and vasodilators may increase shunt by decreasing blood transport time in the vasculature adjacent to alveoli flooded with edema fluid. This could worsen oxygenation. In most cases, increased shunt is overcome by an increased mixed venous oxygen, which allows a higher percentage of tissue oxygen transport. The net effect is usually an increase in Pa_{O_2} and improved organ perfusion, but both should be monitored.[64]

Fluid Management

Fluid management is an important component of hemodynamic monitoring. Two hotly debated fluid management strategies exist. The "dry" theorists lower PCWP, keeping it just high enough to maintain perfusion.[87] Often this approach requires vasopressors and inotropic agents to maintain blood pressure. Theoretically, although all fluid leaks across the pulmonary membranes, the amount of leak will be minimized. The "dry" method requires extreme vigilance to avoid acute renal failure, which often causes death in ARDS patients.

The other strategy argues that most patients die from end-organ disease, not from hypoxemia, therefore, maintaining organ perfusion is the only way to improve survival. The amount of leak cannot be altered until the membrane returns to normal[88]; therefore, fluid restriction is futile. Defenders of this theory discuss data showing only 16% of deaths due to an inability to oxygenate the patient.[89] The remaining deaths were due to sepsis and severe organ dysfunction.

Data support both viewpoints. Many clinicians blend both views when caring for patients and limit fluids whenever adequacy of perfusion permits. As discussed previously, this requires monitoring of cardiac output, PCWP, urine output, hemoglobin, blood pressure, BUN, and creatinine.

Hypoxia

As described previously, careful hemodynamic monitoring can improve oxygenation of tissues and perfusion. Additional modalities are also useful to improve hypoxia.

Ventilator Management

Optimizing mechanical ventilation is another therapeutic goal. Mechanical ventilation can be lifesaving, yet details are critical to avoiding and managing the life-threatening complications caused by mechanical ventilation. Mechanical ventilation may also effect drug disposition.[90] Clinicians caring for the critically ill must have a rudimentary understanding of the technical aspects of mechanical ventilation to optimize drug therapy. A recent review is available.[91]

Endpoints include an oxygen saturation ≥90% on the lowest fraction inspired oxygen (Fi_{O_2}) possible. Oxygen therapy can lead to lung injury including fibrosis, although how, when, and at what level this occurs is debated. Most clinicians try to use the least amount of Fi_{O_2} possible.

Patients requiring mechanical ventilation usually receive inhaled β agonists by metered dose inhaler to combat ARDS associated increased airway resistance.[92] The increase in resistance is not clearly associated with hyperreactivity. Mechanically ventilated patients require at least twice the usual dose due to drug delivery problems associated with ventilator tubing and, therefore, the dose should be adjusted to decrease airway resistance.[93] No particular β agonist is preferred.

Positive End Expiratory Pressure

One method used to limit Fi_{O_2} is application of positive end expiratory pressure (PEEP). PEEP is a pressure applied by the ventilator that prevents complete lung emptying at end expiration, thereby increasing lung volume. The therapeutic goal is to keep alveoli from collapsing, thus improving gas exchange. Lung water is not decreased but redistributed, reducing shunt. In most, both processes reduce hypoxemia by reducing shunt (unventilated lung areas that are perfused).[78] Early PEEP does not decrease atelectasis, pneumonia, barotrauma, or mortality.[94] ARDS-induced lung injury is not consistent throughout the lung, but patchy; therefore, PEEP has variable effects on gas exchange. PEEP reaching only normal lung regions causes overdistention. Overdistention can send blood from normal to abnormal areas, worsening shunt and hypoxemia; therefore, the effects of PEEP on arterial oxygen (Pa_{O_2}) saturation and mixed venous oxygen are monitored closely.[78] PEEP can decrease cardiac output primarily by decreasing venous return. Because of this, hemodynamic parameters such as cardiac output and PCWP are monitored to assess and correct any problems induced by high levels of PEEP. The overall goal is to find the amount of PEEP (referred to as "best PEEP") that improves oxygenation without causing major hemodynamic compromise.

Barotrauma

High-pressure ventilation associated lung injury is referred to as barotrauma. The most life-threatening complication of this lung injury is hemodynamic compromise in which patients acutely lower their blood pressure and decrease perfusion. Historically, to avoid barotrauma, goals included low peak airway pressures, modest amounts of PEEP, and volume ventilation modes. Recently, barotrauma has taken on new meaning. Besides pneumomediastinum and pneumothorax, mechanical ventilation-induced alveolar damage may occur. This realization occurred concurrent with an appreciation of the inhomogeneous nature of ARDS. On computed tomography (CT) scans, relatively normal lung is interspersed with damaged lung. High pressures or volumes may overdistend normal alveoli, perhaps worsening lung injury. This led to ventilator modes designed to minimize alveolar overdistention.[95] Overdistention is best measured by alveolar pressure, which is directly related to alveolar volume. Alveolar pressure is measured by stopping flow at end inspiration, allowing pressure equilibration throughout the system. Under these circumstances, the airway opening pressure measured by the ventilator during the end inspiratory occlusion (plateau pressure) is equal to alveolar pressure. Guidelines suggest alveolar (plateau) pressure should not exceed 35 cm water, the pressure associated with overdistention in normal lungs.[76] Nonphysiologic ventilatory methods used to accomplish this involve pressure control ventilation, permissive hypercapnia, and inverse ratio ventilation.[96] Pressure control ventilation differs from volume ventilation by discontinuing airflow at a specific pressure rather than delivering a specific tidal volume. This allows maintenance of low intra-alveolar pressures. In addition, patients can be underventilated (permissive hypercapnia). This causes a rise in $Paco_2$, which is thought to be relatively harmless in the ventilated ICU patient. Arterial pH is maintained at approximately 7.4 using intravenous sodium bicarbonate. Inverse ratio is a type of pressure control that prolongs the inspiratory time in relation to the expiratory time (usual physiology is longer expiratory time) on the theory that oxygenation will be improved. The effect of these ventilatory modes on reducing lung injury is unproven; however, these modes are rapidly being adopted in critical care settings.

Limiting Oxygen Utilization

Standard ARDS management includes limiting oxygen utilization by aggressively managing fever, seizures, respiratory drive, and other causes of increased metabolism. Sedation is critical to patient survival because increased oxygen usage can be detrimental. Nonphysiologic ventilatory modes such as inverse ratio cannot be tolerated by patients with an intact respiratory drive and, therefore, patients must be heavily sedated.

Obliteration of respiratory drive is often a goal and a variety of methods are available. Typically, patients receive a benzodiazepine/opiate combination. Neuromuscular blockade use is undergoing heated debate,[97] but single doses are often needed to gain acute control during titration of other sedatives. Continuous infusion neuromuscular blockade is fraught with danger, and attempts should be made to optimize other sedative regimens.[98]

SURFACTANT

Surfactant is secreted by the type II alveolar cells lining the alveolar surface. The detergent action of surfactant stabilizes alveoli, helps keep the alveolus dry, and reduces the work of breathing, promoting gas exchange.[99]

Theoretically in ARDS, proteins leaking into the alveolar–capillary junction inactivate surfactant causing further leakage. Unlike neonatal respiratory distress syndromes due to a primary surfactant deficiency, the injury associated with ARDS is much more complex. Malfunction of the surfactant system is probably a secondary effect of the underlying disease process. A recently published multicentered, double-blind, placebo-controlled, randomized pilot study showed no difference between placebo and treated groups; however, the study lacked significant power to detect a difference between the two groups.[100] In the end, surfactant therapy may play a minor supportive therapeutic role. Currently, its use is considered experimental and further work is necessary before it can be recommended for widespread use.[99]

AVOIDING ARDS COMPLICATIONS

Multisystem Organ Failure

Multisystem organ failure is a leading cause of mortality in ICU patients. Mortality approaches 100% when three or more organs fail.[101] Patients with multisystem organ failure are also more likely to be infected.[81] End-organ function, as well as drug effects on end-organ function, should be monitored closely.

Stress Ulcerations

Stress-induced GI bleeding complicates ARDS therapy. Sepsis, mechanical ventilation, and coagulopathy increase the risk of stress ulceration. ICU stress ulcer prophylaxis is undergoing debate; however, ARDS patients should receive therapy. Studies suggesting fewer nosocomial pneumonias with sucralfate are widely criticized; therefore, drug choice is based on patient-specific factors rather than advantages of a particular agent.[102]

Nosocomial Infection

Nosocomial pneumonia in ARDS patients causes mortality in 67 versus 23% of patients without pneumonia.[81] Prevention and early treatment is critical to decreasing ARDS mortality. Concurrently, bacterial resistance is increasingly prevalent among hospitalized patients. Each ICU must develop a strategy for diagnosis and treatment of nosocomial pneumonia, while limiting the incidence of resistance.

Some ICUs use selective gut decontamination in an attempt to decrease the incidence of nosocomial pneumonia. To date, selective gut decontamination has not been shown to decrease mortality.[103] Historically, such approaches increased bacterial resistance. Further studies are needed before recommending widespread usage in ARDS patients.

Catheter-Related Infections

ARDS patients have multiple central venous catheters to measure hemodynamic parameters and deliver intravenous medications. The major life-threatening complication associated with central venous catheters is bacteremia.[104] Attention to aseptic placement and follow-up care is extremely important to avoid infection. Some centers use antibiotic impregnated lines or dressings in hope of reducing the infection rate. Diagnosis of catheter-related infections is relatively difficult, although most clinicians agree that semiquantitative cultures of the removed catheters are the most helpful. Organisms are usually gram positive, with methicillin-resistant *Staphylococcus* being relatively common in ICU patients. Catheter removal and antimicrobial therapy are cornerstones of therapy.

NUTRITIONAL SUPPORT

Although not clearly shown to affect outcome and survival of ARDS patients, most clinicians pay particular attention to achieving nutritional goals. Parenteral nutrition may be necessary in seriously ill ARDS patients because blood flow to the GI tract can be compromised. Enteral nutrition is preferred if the patient can tolerate enteral feedings, even in small amounts. Enteral feedings are advantageous because infectious complications from central access are decreased. Enteral feeding increases in GI blood flow, perhaps decreasing the risk of bacterial transport across the gut and the risk of stress ulceration. Lipid administration in ARDS is controversial, although withholding lipids from ARDS patients is not clearly supported or recommended in the literature. Hypercarbia solely due to excessive calorie and/or dextrose administration should be avoided. Excellent reviews on the subject of critical care nutrition are available.[105]

NONSTEROIDAL ANTI-INFLAMMATORY AGENTS

In animal models, nonsteroidal anti-inflammatory agents (NSAIDs) alter the late phases of lung injury.[82] In blocking the sepsis-induced activated arachidonic acid pathway, NSAIDs decrease inflammatory processes in the lung. To date, there is no human evidence in a large trial showing efficacy.

CORTICOSTEROIDS

Part of the pathogenesis of ARDS is an acute inflammatory lung process. Corticosteroid anti-inflammatory effects were initially thought to ameliorate this process. A multicentered trial showed that corticosteroid treatment of ARDS patients did not affect outcome.[76] Furthermore, early corticosteroid administration in septic patients did not prevent ARDS development. In fact, the time to ARDS resolution was shorter in the placebo group.[106]

Two uncontrolled, open label studies have investigated corticosteroid use in patients with persistent ARDS. This group progresses from acute inflammation to fibrosis. Corticosteroids improved lung injury scores. Until a controlled trial is completed, use of corticosteroids to prevent the fibroproliferative stage of ARDS is extremely controversial and not recommended.[106]

ANTIOXIDANTS

Oxygen radical scavengers such as vitamins C and E reduce lung injury. ARDS patients have been shown to have lower vitamin E concentrations than patients without ARDS. Conversely, higher concentrations of both agents have been shown to induce free-radical-mediated damage. Increased mortality in smokers receiving vitamin E in comparison to smokers receiving placebo is also of concern. Trials are currently under way to determine dosage and place in therapy.[82]

NITRIC OXIDE

As ARDS progresses to fibrosis, pulmonary vascular resistance increases and hypoxemia worsens. Systemic vasodilators decrease pulmonary vascular resistance and increase perfusion to ventilated areas. Unfortunately, most patients with ARDS cannot tolerate the hypotension associated with systemic vasodilatation. Inhaled nitric oxide offers a means to vasodilate the ventilated lung areas, yet not worsen shunt while minimizing systemic effects.[107–110]

Animal studies of hypoxic vasoconstriction and bilateral lung lavage induced ARDS have shown vasodilatory effects, decreased shunt and decreased hypoxemia.[108,109] Neither model closely mimics ARDS lung injury, therefore, the findings are suggestive but not conclusive for ARDS treatment.

A small open label inhaled nitric oxide clinical trial showed decreased shunt, decreased pulmonary artery pressure, and improved oxygenation.[107] Major study limitations include size and homogeneity of the population. Several patients received extracorporeal membrane oxygenation therapy (ECMO), which is not standard therapy in the United States.

Nitric oxide toxicity is worth mention. Few animal or human safety studies are currently available. Nitric oxide mixes with oxygen to create nitric acid, whose effects are unknown in humans.[110] It also causes methemoglobinemia from reaction with oxyhemoglobin. Nitric oxide may worsen "leak" by increasing intracellular pore size.[107] Nitric oxide has been shown to increase alveolar septal injuries in an animal model.[111] A controlled, multicentered trial is currently under way and, until completed, routine nitric oxide use cannot be recommended.

MONOCLONAL ANTIBODIES

Mediators of sepsis are associated with the protein and fluid leak across the alveolar-vascular membrane in ARDS. Blocking the sepsis mediators should decrease the incidence and mortality of ARDS. Unfortunately, monoclonal antibody studies did not improve the outcome of sepsis.[112] In fact, our worst fears were realized because some patients with less severe illness actually had an increased mortality rate when treated with active drug in comparison to placebo. Attenuating the inflammatory process may actually be harmful rather than helpful to patients with sepsis and ARDS. Research regarding mechanisms, timing, and dosing requires completion before these agents find a place in ARDS treatment.

PROGNOSIS/OUTCOME

ARDS mortality is approximately 70%.[79,113] Median survival time is 13 days. Acidemic and uremic patients are less likely to survive.[114]

In ARDS survivors, respiratory impairment, measured by pulmonary function tests, occurs in 67% of patients when measured a year or more after their illness.[115] Smoking status did not impact the degree of impairment, but severity of ARDS did. Functional improvement as measured by pulmonary function tests and perceived improvement of self-health status occurs up to 3 months after extubation.[116] Improvement after 3 months is minimal.

CONCLUSION

ARDS-related mortality plagues the modern ICU. Therapy is supportive with vigilant attention to detail perhaps providing the only means to decrease mortality. In particular, the search for and avoidance of nosocomial infection is critical to survival. Improving perfusion and avoiding end-organ damage is also critical. Research is ongoing for pharmacologic therapy directed at the underlying disease process.

REFERENCES

1. Farrell PM, Avery ME. Hyaline membrane disease. Am Rev Resp Dis 1975;111:657–668.
2. Boyle RJ, Oh W. Respiratory distress syndrome. Clin Perinatol 1978;5:287–297.
3. Reynolds MS, Wallander KA. Use of surfactant in the prevention and treatment of neonatal respiratory distress syndrome. Clin Pharm 1989;8:559–576.
4. Wiseman LR, Bryson HM. Porcine-derived lung surfactant: A review of the therapeutic efficacy and clinical tolerability of a natural surfactant preparation (Curosurf) in neonatal respiratory distress syndrome. Drugs 1994;48:386–403.
5. Northway WH, Moss RB, Carlisle KB, et al. Late pulmonary sequelae of bronchopulmonary dysplasia. N Engl J Med 1990;323:1793–1799.
6. Bregman J, Kimberlin LVS. Developmental outcome in extremely premature infants. Pediatr Clin North Am 1993;40:937–953.
7. Maberry MC. Methods to diagnose fetal lung maturity. Semin Perinatol 1993;17:241–246.
8. Leonardi MR, Hankins GDV. What's new in tocolytics. Clin Perinatol 1992;19:367–384.
9. Caritis SN. Treatment of preterm labour. A review of options. Drugs 1983;26:243–261.
10. Liggins GC, Howie RN. A controlled trial of antepartum glucocorticoid treatment of prevention of the respiratory distress syndrome in premature infants. Pediatrics 1972;515.
11. NIH Consensus Panel. Effect of corticosteroids for fetal maturation on perinatal outcomes. JAMA 1995;273:413–418.
12. Yeomans ER. Prenatal corticosteroid therapy to prevent respiratory distress syndrome. Semin Perinatol 1993;17:253–259.
13. Sepkowitz S. Prenatal corticosteroid therapy to prevent respiratory distress syndrome. J Pediatr 1984;105:338–339.
14. Avery ME. The argument for prenatal administration of dexamethasone to prevent respiratory distress syndrome. J Pediatr 1984;104:240.
15. Levy DL. Maternal administration of dexamethasone to prevent RDS. J Pediatr 1984;105:339–340.
16. Jobe AH. Pulmonary surfactant therapy. N Engl J Med 1993;328:861–868.
17. Schwartz RM, Luby AM, Scanlon JW, et al. Effect of surfactant on morbidity, mortality, and resource use in newborn infants weighing 500 to 1500 g. N Engl J Med 1994;330:1476–1480.
18. Pramanik AK, Holtzman RB, Merritt TA. Surfactant replacement therapy for pulmonary diseases. Pediatr Clin North Am 1993;40:913–936.
19. Hallman M, Merritt TA, Bry K. The fate of exogenous surfactant in neonates with respiratory distress syndrome. Clin Pharmacokinet 1994;26:215–232.
20. Zola EM, Gunkel JH, Chan RK, et al. Comparison of three dosing procedures for administration of bovine surfactant to neonates with respiratory distress syndrome. J Pediatr 1993;122:453–459.
21. Veda T, Ikegami M, Rider ED, Jobe AH. Distribution of surfactant and ventilation in surfactant-treated preterm lambs. J Appl Physio 1994;76:45–55.
22. Lewis JF, Tabor B, Ikegami M, et al. Lung function and surfactant distribution in saline-lavaged sheep given instilled vs. nebulized surfactant. J Appl Physiol 1993;74:1256–1264.

23. Lewis JF, Ikegami M, Jobe AH, Tabor B. Aerosolized surfactant treatment of preterm lambs. J Appl Physiol 1991;70:869–876.
24. Fujiwara T, Adams FH. Surfactant for hyaline membrane disease. Pediatrics 1980;66:795–798.
25. Dunn MS, Shennan AT, Possmayer F. Single- versus multiple-dose surfactant replacement therapy in neonates of 30 to 36 weeks gestation with respiratory distress syndrome. Pediatrics 1990;86:564–570.
26. Konishi M, Fujiwara T, Naito T, et al. Surfactant replacement therapy in neonatal respiratory distress syndrome. A multicentre randomized clinical trial: Comparison of high- versus low-dose of surfactant-TA. Eur J Pediatr 1988;147:20–25.
27. OSIRIS. Early v. delayed neonatal administration of a synthetic surfactant—the judgement of OSIRIS. Lancet 1992;340:1363–1369.
28. Berry DD, Pramanik AK, Phillips JB, et al. Comparison of the effect of three doses of a synthetic surfactant on the alveolar-arterial oxygen gradient in infants weighing ≥1250 grams with respiratory distress syndrome. J Pediatr 1994;124:294–301.
29. Speer CP, Robertson B, Curstedt T, et al. Randomized European Multicenter Trial of Surfactant Replacement Therapy for Severe Neonatal Respiratory Distress Syndrome: Single versus multiple doses of Curosurf. Pediatrics 1992;89:13–20.
30. Halliday HL, Tarnow-Mordi WO, Corcoran JD, Paterson CC. Multicentre randomized trial comparing high and low dose surfactant regimens for the treatment of respiratory distress syndrome (the Curosurf 4 trial). Arch Dis Child 1993;69:276–280.
31. Gortner L, Pohlandt F, Bartmann P, et al. High-dose versus low-dose bovine surfactant treatment in very premature infants. Acta Pediatr 1994;83:135–141.
32. Sobel BB, Carroll A. Postsurfactant slump: Early prediction of neonatal chronic lung disease? J Perinatol 1994;268–274.
33. Merritt TA, Soll RF, Hallman M. Overview of exogenous surfactant replacement. J Intensive Care Med 1993;8:205–228.
34. Tarnow-Mardi WO, Soll RF. Artificial versus natural surfactant—Can we base clinical practice on a firm scientific footing? Eur J Pediatr 1994;153(suppl):17–21.
35. Speer CP, Gofeller O, Groneck P, et al. Randomized clinical trial of two treatment regimens of natural surfactant preparations in neonatal respiratory distress syndrome. Arch Dis Child 1995;72:8–13.
36. Rajo TNK, Langenberg P. Pulmonary hemorrhage and exogenous surfactant therapy: A metaanalysis. J Pediatr 1995;123:603–610.
37. Harbor JD, Wright LL, Sol RF, et al. A multicenter randomized trial comparing two surfactants for the treatment of neonatal respiratory distress syndrome. J Pediatr 1993;123:757–766.
38. Modanlou HD, Beharry K, Norris K, et al. Comparative efficacy of survanta (Surv) and exosurf (Exo) on early clinical course of respiratory distress syndrome (RDS). Pediatr Res 1994;35(4 PT 2):345A.
39. Bloom BT, Delmore P, Kattwinkel J, et al. Randomized double blind multicenter trial of survanta (SURV) and infasurf (IS). Pediatr Res 1994;35(4 PT 2):326A.
40. Long W. Synthetic surfactant. Semin Perinatol 1994;17:275–284.
41. Spafford PS, Kendig JW, Maniscalco WM. Use of natural surfactants to prevent and treat respiratory distress syndrome. Semin Perinatol 1993;17:285–294.
42. Kirby RR, Smith RA, Desautels DA (eds). Mechanical Ventilation. New York, Churchill Livingstone, 1985, pp 1–475.
43. Venegas JG, Fredberg JJ. Understanding the pressure cost of ventilation: Why does high-frequency ventilation work? Crit Care Med 1994;22:S49–S57.
44. Jacobs HC, Mercurio MR. Perfluorocarbons in the treatment of respiratory distress syndrome. Semin Perinatol 1993;17:295–302.
45. Klarr JM, Faix RG, Pryce CJE, Bhatt-Mehta V. A randomized, blinded trial of dopamine versus dobutamine for treatment of hypotension in preterm infants with respiratory distress syndrome. J Pediatr 1994;125:117–122.
46. Greenough A, Morely C, Davis J. Interaction of spontaneous respiration with artificial ventilation in preterm babies. J Pediatr 1983;103:769–773.
47. Pollitzer MJ, Reynolds EO, Shaw DG, et al. Pancuronium during mechanical ventilation speeds recovery of lungs of infants with hyaline membrane disease. Lancet 1981;1:346–348.
48. Finer NN, Tomney PM. Controlled evaluation of muscle relaxation in the ventilated neonate. Pediatrics 1981;67:641–646.
49. Greenough A, Woods S, Morely CH, et al. Pancuronium prevents pneumothoraces in ventilated premature babies who actively expire against positive pressure inflation. Lancet 1984;1:1–3.
50. Perlman JM, Goodman S, Kreusser KL, et al. Reduction in intraventricular hemorrhage by elimination of fluctuating cerebral blood-flow velocity in preterm infants with respiratory distress syndrome. N Engl J Med 1985;312:1353–1357.
51. Ment LR. Prevention of neonatal intraventricular hemorrhage. N Engl J Med 1985;312:1385–1387.
52. Runkle B, Bancalari E. Acute cardiopulmonary effects of pancuronium bromide in mechanically ventilated newborn infants. J Pediatr 1984;104:614–617.
53. Cabal LA, Siassi B, Artal R, et al. Cardiovascular and catecholamine changes after administration of pancuronium in distressed neonates. Pediatrics 1982;69:583–586.
54. Goldberg RN, Goldman SL, Ramsay ER, et al. Detection of seizure activity in the paralyzed neonates using continuous monitoring. Pediatrics 1982;69:583–586.
55. Coen RW, McCutchen CB, Wermer D, et al. Continuous monitoring of the electroencephalogram following perinatal asphyxia. J Pediatr 1982;100:628–630.
56. Kilchevsky ES, Wung JT. Pancuronium risks [letter]. Pediatrics 1985;76:653.
57. Wimberly PD, Lou HC, Pederson H, et al. Hypertensive peaks in the pathogenesis of intraventricular hemorrhage in the newborn: Abolition by phenobarbitone sedation. Acta Paediatr Scand 1982;71:537–542.
58. Donn SM, Roloff DW, Goldstein GW. Prevention of intraventricular haemorrhage in preterm infants by phenobarbitone. Lancet 1981;1:215–217.

59. Svenningsen NW, Blennow G, Lindroth M, et al. Brain-oriented intensive care treatment in severe neonatal asphyxia. Arch Dis Child 1982;57:176–183.
60. Pippenger CE, Rosen TS. Phenobarbital plasma levels in neonates. Clin Perinatol 1975;111–115.
61. Diaz J, Schain RJ, Bailey BG. Phenobarbital-induced brain growth retardation in artificially reared rat pups. Biol Neonate 1977;32:77–88.
62. Donn SM, Goldstein GW, Roloff DW. Prevention of intraventricular hemorrhage with phenobarbital therapy: Now what? Pediatrics 1986;77:779–781.
63. Maguire DP, Maloney P. A comparison of fentanyl and morphine use in neonates. Neonatal Netw 1988;7:27–32.
64. Arnold JH, Truog RD, Orav EJ, et al. Tolerance and dependence in neonates sedated with fentanyl during extracorporeal membrane oxygenation. Anesthesiol 1990;73:1136–1140.
65. Langslet A, Meberg A, Bredesen JE, et al. Plasma concentrations of diazepam and *N*-desmethyldiazepam in newborn infants after intravenous, intramuscular, rectal, and oral administration. Acta Paediatr Scand 1978;67:699–703.
66. Desmulch A, Wittert W, Schnitzler E, et al. Lorazepam in the treatment of refractory neonatal seizures. Am J Dis Child 1986;140:1042–1044.
67. Mololey P, Gal P, Mize R, et al. Lorazepam dosing in neonates: Application of objective sedation scores. DICP Ann Pharmacother 1990;24:326–327.
68. Laptook AR, Rosenfeld CR. Chloral hydrate toxicity in a preterm infant. Pediatr Pharmacol 1984;4:161–165.
69. Muraskas J, Lambert GH, Ayuste O, et al. Neonatal direct hyperbilirubinemia associated with chloral hydrate dosage. Pediatr Res 1987;2:239.
70. Bland RD. Edema formation in the newborn lung. Clin Perinatol 1982;9:593–611.
71. Heaf DP, Belik J, Spitzer AR, et al. Changes in pulmonary function during the diuretic phase of respiratory distress syndrome. J Pediatr 1982;101:103–107.
72. Green T. The use of diuretics in infants with respiratory distress syndrome. Semin Perinatol 1982;6:172–180.
73. Yeh TF, Raval D, John E, et al. Renal response to furosemide in preterm infants with respiratory distress syndrome during the first three postnatal days. Arch Dis Child 1985;60:621–626.
74. Yeh TF, Shibli A, Lev ST, et al. Early furosemide therapy in premature infants (<2000 gm) with respiratory distress syndrome: A randomized controlled trial. J Pediatr 1984;105:603–609.
75. Ashbaugh DG, Bigelow DB, Petty TL, and Levine B. Acute respiratory distress in adults. Lancet 1967;2:319–323.
76. Bernard GR, Artigas A, Brigham KL, et al. and the Consensus Committee. The American-European Consensus Conference on ARDS. Am J Respir Crit Care Med 1994;149:818–824.
77. Wood LD, Prewitt RM. Cardiovascular management in acute hypoxemic respiratory failure. Am J Cardiol 1981;47:963–972.
78. Dantzker DR. Gas exchange in the adult respiratory distress syndrome. Clin Chest Med 1982;3:57–67.
79. Villar J, Slutsky AS. The incidence of the adult respiratory distress syndrome. Am Rev Respir Dis 1989;140:814–816.
80. Seidenfeld JJ, Pohl DF, Bell RC, et al. Incidence, site, and outcome of infections in patients with the adult respiratory distress syndrome. Am Rev Respir Dis 1986;134:12–16.
81. Bell R, Coalson JJ, Smith JD, Johanson WG. Multiple organ system failure and infection in adult respiratory distress syndrome. Ann Intern Med 1983;99:293–298.
82. Messent M, Griffiths M. Pharmacotherapy in lung injury. Thorax 1992;47:651–656.
83. Aberle DR, Wiener-Kronish JP, Webb WR, Matthay MA. Hydrostatic versus increased permeability pulmonary edema: Diagnosis based on radiographic criteria in critically ill patients. Radiology 1988;168:73–79.
84. Curtis S, Cain S. Regional and systemic oxygen delivery/uptake relations and lactate flux in hyperdynamic endotoxin-treated dogs. Am Rev Respir Dis 1992;145:348–354.
85. Danek SJ, Lynch JP, Weg JG, Dantzker DR. The dependence of oxygen uptake on oxygen delivery in the adult respiratory distress syndrome. Am Rev Respir Dis 1980;122:387–395.
86. Ronco JJ, Phlang T, Walley KR, et al. Oxygen consumption is independent of changes in oxygen delivery in severe adult respiratory distress syndrome. Am Rev Respir Dis 1991;143:1267–1273.
87. Simmons RS, Berdine GG, Seidenfeld JJ, et al. Fluid balance and the adult respiratory distress syndrome. Am Rev Respir Dis 1987;135:924–929.
88. Matthay MA, Wiener-Kronish JP. Intact epithelial barrier function is critical for the resolution of alveolar edema in humans. Am Rev Respir Dis 1990;142:1250–1257.
89. Montgomery AB, Stager MA, Carrico CJ, Hudson LD. Causes of mortality in patients with the adult respiratory distress syndrome. Am Rev Respir Dis 1985;132:485–489.
90. Perkins MW, Dasta JF, DeHaven B. Physiologic implications of mechanical ventilation on pharmacokinetics. Ann Pharmacother 1989;23:316–323.
91. Tobin MJ. Mechanical ventilation. N Engl J Med 1994;330:1056–1061.
92. Wright PE, Bernard GR. The role of airflow resistance in patients with the adult respiratory distress syndrome. Am Rev Respir Dis 1989;139:1169–1174.
93. Htan E, Shalansky KF, Mouat B. Use of metered-dose inhalers in mechanically ventilated patients. Ann Pharmacother 1992;26:1247–1248.
94. Pepe PE, Hudson LD, Carrico CJ. Early application of positive end-expiratory pressure in patients at risk for the adult respiratory distress syndrome. N Engl J Med 1984;311:281–286.
95. Marini JJ, Kelsen SG. Re-targeting ventilatory objectives in adult respiratory distress syndrome. Am Rev Respir Dis 1992;146:2–3.
96. Abraham E, Yoshihara G. Cardiorespiratory effects of pressure controlled ventilation in severe respiratory failure. Chest 1990;98:1445–1449.
97. Watling SM, Dasta JF. Prolonged paralysis in intensive care unit patients after the use of neuromuscular blocking agents: A review of the literature. Crit Care Med 1994;22:884–893.
98. Wheeler AP. Sedation, analgesia, and paralysis in the intensive care unit. Chest 1993;104:566–577.

99. Lewis JF, Jobe AH. Surfactant and the adult respiratory distress syndrome. Am Rev Respir Dis 1993;147:218–233.
100. Weg JG, Balk RA, Tharratt RS, et al. and the Exosurf ARDS Sepsis Study Group. Safety and potential efficacy of an aerosolized surfactant in human sepsis induced adult respiratory distress syndrome. JAMA 1994;272:1433–1448.
101. Knaus WA, Wagner DP. Multiple systems organ failure: Epidemiology and prognosis. Crit Care Clin 1989;5:221–232.
102. Smythe MA, Zarowitz BJ. Changing perspectives of stress gastritis prophylaxis. Ann Pharmacother 1994;28:1073–1085.
103. Gomez EC, Markowsky SJ, Rotschafer JC. Selective decontamination of the digestive tract in intensive care patients: A review and commentary. Ann Pharmacother 1992;26:963–976.
104. Mermel LA, Maki DG. Infectious complications of Swan-Ganz pulmonary artery catheters. Am Rev Respir Crit Care Med 1994;149:1020–1036.
105. Berger R, Adams L. Nutritional support in the critical care setting (part 1). Chest 1989;96:139–150.
106. Putterman C. Use of corticosteroids in the adult respiratory distress syndrome: A clinical review. J Crit Care 1990;5:241–251.
107. Rossaint R, Falke KJ, Lopez F, et al. Inhaled nitric oxide for the adult respiratory distress syndrome. N Engl J Med 1993;328:399–405.
108. Pison U, Lopez FA, Heidelmeyer, et al. Inhaled nitric oxide reverses hypoxic pulmonary vasoconstriction without impairing gas exchange. J Appl Physiol 1993;74:1287–1292.
109. Rovira I, Chen T, Winkler M, et al. Effects of inhaled nitric oxide on pulmonary hemodynamics and gas exchange in an ovine model of ARDS. J Appl Physiol 1994;76:345–355.
110. Zapol WM, Rimar S, Gillis N, et al. Nitric oxide and the lung. Am Rev Respir Crit Care Med 1994;149:1375–1380.
111. Mercer RR, Costa DL, Crapo JD. Alveolar septal injury from low level exposures to nitric oxide and nitrogen dioxide. Am Rev Respir Dis 1993;1477(4):A385.
112. McCloskey RV, Straube RC, Sanders C, et al. and the CHESS Trial Study Group. Treatment of septic shock with human monoclonal antibody HA-1A. Ann Intern Med 1994;121:1–5.
113. Fowler AA, Hamman RF, Good JT, et al. Adult respiratory distress syndrome: Risk with common predispositions. Ann Intern Med 1983;98:593–597.
114. Fowler AA, Hamman RF, Zerbe GO, et al. Adult respiratory distress syndrome: Prognosis after onset. Am Rev Respir Dis 1985;98:472–478.
115. Ghio AJ, Elliott G, Crapo RO, et al. Impairment after adult respiratory distress syndrome. Am Rev Respir Dis 1989;139:1158–1162.
116. McHugh LG, Milberg JA, Whitcomb ME, et al. Recovery of function in survivors of the acute respiratory distress syndrome. Am J Respir Crit Care Med 1994;150:90–94.

Chapter 28

Drug-Induced Pulmonary Diseases

H. William Kelly, PharmD

The manifestations of drug-induced pulmonary diseases span the entire spectrum of pathophysiologic conditions of the respiratory tract. As with most drug-induced diseases, the pathologic changes are nonspecific. Therefore, the diagnosis is often difficult and in most cases is based on exclusion of all other possible causes. In addition, the true incidence of specific drug-induced pulmonary disease is difficult to assess as a result of the pathologic nonspecificity and the interaction between the underlying disease state and the drugs.

Considering the physiologic and metabolic capacity of the lung, it is surprising that drug-induced pulmonary disease is not more common. The lung is the only organ of the body that receives the entire circulation. In addition, the lung contains a heterogeneous population of cells capable of various metabolic functions, including *N*-alkylation, *N*-dialkylation, *N*-oxidation, reduction of *N*-oxides, and *C*-hydroxylation.

Evaluation of epidemiologic studies on adverse drug reactions provides a perspective of the importance of drug-induced pulmonary disease in the general population. In a 2-year prospective survey of a community-based general practice, 41% of 817 patients experienced adverse drug reactions.[1] Four patients, or 0.5% of the total respondents, experienced adverse respiratory symptoms. Respiratory symptoms occurred in 1.2% of patients experiencing adverse drug reactions. A more recent surveillance study of 3181 general pediatric outpatients receiving 4244 courses of drug therapy reported adverse reactions in 473 (11.1%) of the courses.[2] Of these, only 200 were considered definite or probable. Gastrointestinal symptoms, skin reactions, and central nervous system (CNS) symptoms made up 96.5% of the reactions with respiratory symptoms included with all other reactions.

Adverse pulmonary reactions would appear to be uncommon in the general population, but they are among the most serious reactions, often requiring intervention. This is illustrated by studies of adverse reactions requiring hospitalization. In a study of 270 adverse reactions leading to hospitalization from two populations, 3.0% were respiratory in nature.[3] Of the reactions considered to be life-threatening, 12.3% were respiratory. An early report on death caused by drug reactions from the Boston Collaborative Drug Surveillance Program indicated that 7 of 27 drug-induced deaths were respiratory in nature.[4] This was confirmed in a follow-up study in which 6 of 24 drug-induced deaths were respiratory in nature.[5]

This chapter is arranged according to the clinical presentation of the respiratory illness. The pathophysiologic mechanism and usual clinical presentation of the most important agents in each disease group are discussed. Tables listing all the agents that have been associated with each disease and their relative frequency complement the discussions. Secondary literature references (i.e., review articles, book chapters) are used to expedite referencing and to provide the student with a bibliography of reviews on the subject. The interested student is encouraged to seek out the reviews and the primary literature on this interesting and complex subject.

Apnea

Apnea may be induced by CNS depression or respiratory neuromuscular blockade (Table 28.1). Patients with chronic obstructive airways disease, alveolar hypoventilation, and chronic carbon dioxide retention have an exaggerated respiratory depressant response to narcotic analgesics and sedatives. In addition, the injudicious administration of oxygen in patients with carbon dioxide retention can remove their hypoxic ventilatory drive, producing apnea.[6] Although the benzodiazepines are touted as causing less respiratory depression than barbiturates, they may produce a profound additive or synergistic effect when taken in combination with other respiratory depressants. Combining intravenous diazepam with phenobarbital to stop seizures in patients in an emergency department frequently results in admissions to an intensive care unit (ICU) for a short period of assisted mechanical ventilation, regardless of administration rate.

TABLE 28.1. DRUGS THAT INDUCE APNEA

Central Nervous System Depression	
Narcotic analgesics	F[a]
Barbiturates	F
Benzodiazepines	F
Other sedative and hypnotics	I
Tricyclic antidepressants	R
Phenothiazines	R
Ketamine	R
Promazine	R
Anesthetics	R
Antihistamines	R
Alcohol	I
Fenfluramine	R
L-Dopa	R
Oxygen	R
Respiratory Muscle Dysfunction	
Aminoglycoside antibiotics	I
Polymyxin antibiotics	I
Neuromuscular blockers	I
Quinine	R
Digitalis	R
Myopathy	
Corticosteroids	F
Diuretics	I
Aminocaproic acid	R
Clofibrate	R

[a]Relative frequency of reactions: F, frequent; I, infrequent; R, rare.

Too rapid intravenous administration of any of the benzodiazepines, even without coadministration of other respiratory depressants, will result in apnea. The risk appears to be the same for all of the available agents (i.e., diazepam, lorazepam, midazolam). Respiratory depression and arrests resulting in death and hypoxic encephalopathy have occurred following rapid intravenous administration of midazolam for conscious sedation prior to medical procedures. This has been reported more commonly in the elderly and the chronically debilitated or in combination with opioid analgesics.

Prolonged apnea may follow the administration of any of the neuromuscular blocking agents following surgery, particularly in patients with hepatic or renal dysfunction. In addition, persistent neuromuscular blockade and muscle weakness has been reported in a number of critically ill patients receiving neuromuscular blockers continuously for more than 2 days to facilitate mechanical ventilation.[7] This has resulted in delayed weaning from mechanical ventilation and prolonged ICU stays. The prolonged neuromuscular blockade has been principally confined to pancuronium and vecuronium in patients with renal disease. Both agents have pharmacologic active metabolites that are renally excreted. The persistent muscular weakness is less well defined but appears to represent an acute myopathy.[7] High-dose corticosteroids appear to produce a synergistic effect supported by animal studies showing that corticosteroids at dosages greater than or equal to 2 mg/kg/d prednisone produce atrophy in denervated muscle. The fluorinated corticosteroids (i.e., triamcinolone) appear to be more myopathic. More recently, dose-dependent respiratory muscle weakness has been reported in COPD and asthma patients receiving repeated short courses of oral prednisone in the previous 6 months.

Respiratory failure has been known to occur following local spinal anesthesia. Apnea from respiratory paralysis and rapid respiratory muscle fatigue has followed the administration of polymyxin and aminoglycoside antibiotics.[6] The mechanism appears to be related to the complexation of calcium and its depletion at the myoneural junction. Intravenous calcium chloride has been variably effective in reversing the paralysis.[6] The aminoglycosides competitively block neuromuscular junctions. This has resulted in life-threatening apnea when neomycin, gentamicin, streptomycin, or bacitracin have been administered in the peritoneal and pleural cavities.[6] The aminoglycosides will produce an additive blockade and ventilatory paralysis with curare or succinylcholine and in patients with myasthenia gravis or myasthenic syndromes.[6] Intravenous administration of aminoglycosides has resulted in respiratory failure in babies with infantile botulism. The treatment consists of ventilatory support and administration of an anticholinesterase (neostigmine or edrophonium).[6]

ASTHMA

Bronchoconstriction is the most common drug-induced respiratory problem. Bronchospasm can be induced by a wide variety of drugs through a number of disparate pathophysiologic mechanisms (Table 28.2). Regardless of the pathophysiologic mechanism, drug-induced bronchospasm is almost exclusively a problem of patients with preexisting bronchial hyperreactivity (i.e., asthma, chronic obstructive lung disease).[8] By definition, all patients with nonspecific bronchial hyperreactivity will experience bronchospasm if given sufficiently high doses of cholinergic or anticholinesterase agents. Severe asthmatics with a high degree of bronchial reactivity may wheeze following the inhalation of a number of particulate substances, such as the lactose in cromolyn (by Spinhaler) or corticosteroids, presumably through direct stimulation of the central airway irritant receptors. Other pharmacologic mechanisms for inducing bronchospasm include β_2-receptor blockade and nonimmunologic histamine release from mast cells and basophils.[8] A wide variety of agents are capable of producing bronchospasm through IgE-mediated reactions.[8] These drugs can become a significant occupational hazard for pharmacists, nurses, and pharmaceutical industry workers.[8]

TABLE 28.2. DRUGS THAT INDUCE BRONCHOSPASM

Drug	Frequency	Drug	Frequency
Anaphylaxis (IgE-Mediated)		**Anaphylactoid Mast Cell Degranulation**	
Penicillins	F[a]	Narcotic analgesics	I
Sulfonamides	F	Ethylenediamine	R
Serum	F	Iodinated-radiocontrast media	F
Cephalosporins	F	Platinum	R
Bromelin	R	Local Anesthetics	I
Cimetidine	R	Steroidal anesthetics	I
Papain	F	Iron–dextran complex	I
Pancreatic extract	I	Pancuronium bromide	R
Psyllium	I	Benzalkonium chloride	I
Subtilase	I	**Pharmacologic Effect**	
Tetracyclines	I	β-Adrenergic receptor blockers	I–F
Allergen extracts	I	Cholinergic stimulants	I
L-Aspariginase	F	Anticholinesterases	R
Pyrazolone analgesics	I	α-Adrenergic agonists	R
Direct Airway Irritation		Ethylenediamine tetraacetic acid (EDTA)	R
Acetate	R	**Unknown Mechanisms**	
Bisulfite	F	ACE inhibitors	I
Cromolyn	R	Anticholinergics	R
Smoke	F	Hydrocortisone	R
N-Acetylcysteine	F	Isoproterenol	R
Inhaled steroids	I	Monosodium glutamate	I
Precipitating IgG Antibodies		Piperazine	R
α-Methyl dopa	R	Tartrazine	R
Carbamazepine	R	Sulfinpyrazone	R
Spiramycin	R	Zinostatin	R
Cyclooxygenase Inhibition			
Aspirin/NSAIDs	F		
Phenylbutazone	I		
Acetaminophen	R		

[a]Relative frequency of reactions: F, frequent; I, infrequent; R, rare.

ASPIRIN

Epidemiology

Aspirin-induced asthma was first recognized in 1902 shortly after the introduction of aspirin. Aspirin sensitivity or intolerance occurs in 4–20% of all asthmatics.[9] The frequency of aspirin-induced bronchospasm increases with age. Patients older than 40 years have a frequency approximately four times that of patients younger than 20 years.[9] The frequency increases to 14–23% in patients with nasal polyps.[9]

Clinical Presentation

The classic description of the aspirin-intolerant asthmatic includes the triad of severe asthma, nasal polyps, and aspirin intolerance. The typical patient experiences intense vasomotor rhinitis, which may or may not be associated with aspirin exposure, beginning during the third or fourth decade of life.[10] Over a period of months, nasal polyps begin to appear followed by severe asthma exacerbated by aspirin. Bronchospasm typically begins within minutes to hours following ingestion of aspirin and is associated with rhinnorhea, flushing of the head and neck, and conjunctivitis.[10] The reactions are severe and often life threatening.

All aspirin-sensitive asthmatics do not fit the classic "aspirin triad" picture and not all patients with asthma and nasal polyps develop sensitivity to aspirin.[11] In most cases, aspirin-sensitive asthmatics are indistinguishable clinically from the general population of asthmatics except for their intolerance to aspirin and other nonsteroidal anti-inflammatory drugs (NSAIDs). Women predominate over men, and there is no evidence for a genetic or familial predisposition.[11]

Pathogenesis

Aspirin-induced asthma is correctly classified as an idiosyncratic reaction in that the pathogenesis is still unknown. Patients with aspirin intolerance have increased plasma histamine concentrations after ingestion of aspirin and elevated peripheral eosinophil counts.[10,11] All attempts to define an immunologic mechanism have been unsuccessful.

Chemically similar drugs such as salicylamide and choline salicylate do not cross-react whereas a large number of chemically dissimilar NSAIDs do produce reactions.[10,11] Table 28.3 lists the analgesics that do and do not cross-react with aspirin.

The currently accepted hypothesis is that aspirin intolerance is integrally related to inhibition of cyclooxygenase. This is supported by the following evidence: (1) All NSAIDs that inhibit cyclooxygenase produce reactions; (2) the degree of cross-reactivity is proportional to the potency of cyclooxygenase inhibition; and (3) each patient with aspirin sensitivity has a threshold dose for precipitating bronchospasm that is specific for the degree of cyclooxygenase inhibition produced and, once established, the dose of another cyclooxygenase inhibitor needed to induce bronchospasm can be estimated.[10]

The mechanism by which cyclooxygenase inhibition produces bronchospasm in susceptible individuals is unknown. Recent evidence suggests that arachidonic acid metabolism through the 5-lipoxygenase pathway leading to the excess production of leukotrienes (LTs) C_4 and D_4 plays a pivotal role.[12] LTC_4, LTD_4, and LTE_4 produce bronchospasm and promote histamine release from mast cells,[10] while the administration of leukotriene receptor antagonists and 5-lipoxygenase inhibitors ablate the pulmonary and nonpulmonary responses to aspirin in aspirin-sensitive asthmatics.[12] The precise mechanism by which augmented leukotriene excretion occurs is unknown and available hypotheses do not explain why only a small number of asthmatic patients react to aspirin and NSAIDs.

TABLE 28.3. TOLERANCE OF ANTI-INFLAMMATORY/ ANALGESIC DRUGS IN ASPIRIN-INDUCED ASTHMA

Cross-Reactive Drugs	Drugs with No Cross-Reactivity
Diclofenac	Acetaminophen[a]
Diflunisal	Benzydamine
Fenoprofen	Chloroquine
Flufenamic acid	Choline salicylate
Flurbiprofen	Corticosteroids
Hydrocortisone hemisuccinate	Dextropropoxyphene
	Phenacetin[a]
Ibuprofen	Salicylamide
Indomethacin	Sodium salicylate
Ketoprofen	
Mefenamic acid	
Naproxen	
Noramidopyrine	
Oxyphenbutazone	
Phenylbutazone	
Piroxicam	
Sulindac	
Sulphinpyrazone	
Tartrazine	
Tolmetin	

[a]A very small percentage (5%) of aspirin-sensitive patients react to acetaminophen and phenacetin.

Desensitization

Patients with aspirin sensitivity can be desensitized. The ease of desensitization correlates with the sensitivity of the patient.[11] Highly sensitive patients who initially react to less than 100 mg of aspirin require multiple rechallenges to produce desensitization.[11] Desensitization usually persists for 2–5 days following discontinuance, with full sensitivity reestablished within 7 days.[11] Cross-desensitization has been established between aspirin and all NSAIDs tested to date. Because patients may experience life-threatening reactions, desensitization should only be attempted in a controlled environment by personnel with expertise in handling these patients. In addition, there have been reports of patients who have failed to maintain a desensitized state despite continued aspirin administration.[11] The chronic asthma symptoms have markedly improved in a number of aspirin-sensitive asthmatics who have undergone desensitization.[11] The explanation for this is not clear.

Food and Drug Additives

It has been reported that up to 80% of aspirin-sensitive asthmatics will have an adverse reaction to the yellow azo dye tartrazine (FD&C Yellow No. 5), which is widely used for coloring foods, drinks, drugs, and cosmetics.[9] However, those studies reporting high cross-reactivity were poorly controlled and often used only subjective criteria.[9,13] In double-blind placebo-controlled trials using pulmonary-function testing, sensitivity to tartrazine has proven to be a rare event.[13] Tartrazine sensitivity appears to occur only in aspirin-intolerant patients at a prevalence of 2%.[13]

Reactions to other azo dyes, monosodium glutamate (MSG), parabens, and non–azo dyes have been reported much less frequently than reactions to tartrazine and have been equally difficult to confirm with controlled challenges.[13] Positive reactions to sodium benzoate, a food preservative, have been reported in as many as 23% of aspirin-sensitive individuals.[9] Acetaminophen is a weak inhibitor of cyclooxygenase. As such, a small number of aspirin-sensitive asthmatics, approximately 5%, will experience reactions to acetaminophen.[9] Most aspirin-sensitive asthmatics can use acetaminophen as a safe alternative to aspirin. Sporadic cases of worsening bronchospasm and anaphylaxis have been reported in aspirin-sensitive asthmatics receiving intravenous hydrocortisone succinate but have not been reported with the use of other corticosteroids.[10] It is not known whether it is the hydrocortisone or the succinate that is the problem.

Treatment

Therapy of aspirin-sensitive asthmatics takes one of two general approaches: desensitization or avoidance. Avoidance of triggering substances seldom alters the clinical course of patients' asthma. The therapy of patients' asthma has been nonspecific, however, the availability of 5-lipoxygenase inhibitors such as zileuton or leukotriene antagonists should provide specific therapy. Many of these patients require chronic steroid therapy to control the asthma. The respiratory symptoms can be decreased but not prevented by pretreatment with antihistamines and cromolyn.[11]

β Blockers

β-Adrenergic receptor blockers comprise the other large class of drugs that can be hazardous to the asthmatic. Even the more cardioselective agents such as acebutolol, atenolol, and metoprolol have been reported to cause asthma attacks.[8] Asthmatics may take nonselective and β_1-selective blockers without incident for long periods; however, the occasional reports of fatal asthma attacks resistant to therapy with β agonists should provide ample warning of the dangers inherent in β-blocker therapy.[8]

If a patient with bronchial hyperreactivity requires β-blocker therapy, one of the relatively selective β_1 blockers (acebutol, atenolol, metoprolol, or pindolol) should be used at the lowest possible dose. Two newer agents, celiprolol and betaxolol, appear to possess greater cardioselectivity than currently marketed drugs.[14] Fatal status asthmaticus has occurred with the topical administration of the nonselective timolol maleate ophthalmic solution for the treatment of open-angle glaucoma.[15] Early investigations with ophthalmic betaxolol suggest that it is well tolerated even in timolol-sensitive asthmatics.[16]

SULFITES

Epidemiology

Severe, life-threatening asthmatic reactions following restaurant meals and wine have occurred secondary to ingestion of the food preservative potassium metabisulfite.[13] Sulfites have been used for centuries as preservatives in wine and food. As antioxidants, they prevent fermentation of wine and discoloration of fruits and vegetables due to contaminating bacteria.[17] Previously sulfites had been given generally-recognized-as-safe (GRAS) status by the Food and Drug Administration (FDA). Sensitive patients react to concentrations ranging from 5–100 mg, amounts that are routinely consumed by anyone eating in restaurants. Consumption of sulfites in U.S. diets is estimated to be 2–3 mg/d in the home with 5–10 mg per 30 mL of beer or wine consumed.[13] Anaphylactic or anaphylactoid reactions to sulfites in nonasthmatics is extremely rare. In the general asthmatic population, reactions to sulfites are uncommon. Approximately 5% of steroid-dependent asthmatics demonstrate a sensitivity to sulfiting agents, but the prevalence is only around 1% in non-steroid-dependent asthmatic patients.[17]

Mechanism

The mechanism by which sulfites induce asthma is still unknown. The inhalation of 1–5 ppm sulfur dioxide produces bronchoconstriction in all asthmatics through direct stimulation of afferent parasympathetic irritant receptors.[17] When SO_2 comes in contact with water, it forms H_2SO_3, which dissociates to H^+ and HSO_3^-. It is unknown whether SO_2 or HSO_3^- is the asthmagenic stimulus. Upon oral ingestion of metabisulfites, less than 10% of all asthmatics will develop bronchospasm. It has therefore been postulated that sulfite-sensitive asthmatics have an inability to clear a sulfite load normally and therefore the sulfite accumulates.[13,17] At the air–fluid surface of the bronchial mucosa, HSO_3^- ions associate with water to form H_2SO_3 and SO_2. A reduced concentration of sulfite oxidase enzyme (the enzyme that catalyzes oxidation of sulfites to sulfates) compared with normals has been demonstrated in a group of sulfite-sensitive asthmatics.[13] There has been no correlation between sulfite sensitivity and sensitivity to cyclooxygenase inhibitors.

A number of pharmacologic agents contain sulfites as preservatives and antioxidants. The FDA now requires warning labels on drugs containing sulfites. Most manufacturers of drugs for the treatment of asthma have discontinued the use of sulfites. In addition, labeling is required on packaged foods that contain sulfites at 10 ppm or more, and sulfiting agents are no longer allowed on fresh fruits and vegetables (excluding potatoes) intended for sale.

Pretreatment with cromolyn, anticholinergics, and cyanocobalamin have protected sulfite-sensitive patients.[18] Presumably, pharmacologic doses of vitamin B_{12} catalyze the nonenzymatic oxidation of sulfite to sulfate.

Other Preservatives

Both ethylenediamine tetraacetic acid (EDTA) and benzalkonium chloride used as bacteriostatic and stabilizing agents, respectively, can produce bronchoconstriction.[19] In addition to producing bronchoconstriction, EDTA potentiates the bronchial responsiveness to histamine.[19] These effects are presumably mediated through calcium chelation by EDTA. Benzalkonium chloride is more potent than EDTA and its mechanism appears to be a result of mast cell degranulation and stimulation of irritant C fibers in the airways.[19]

The bronchoconstriction from benzalkonium chloride can be blocked by cromolyn but not the anticholinergic ipratropium bromide.[20] Benzalkonium chloride is found in the commercial multiple-dose nebulizer preparations of ipratropium bromide and beclomethasone diproprionate found in the United Kingdom and Europe and is presumed to be in part responsible for paradoxical wheezing following administration of these agents.[19,20] Benzalkonium chloride is also found in albuterol nebulizer solutions marketed in the United States and has been implicated as a possible cause of paradoxical wheezing in infants receiving this preparation.[19] However, β_2 agonists are potent mast cell stabilizers and the anecdotal reports have not yet been confirmed with controlled investigations.[19,20]

Contrast Media

Iodinated-radiocontrast materials are the most common cause of anaphylactoid reactions producing bronchospasm occurring in 2–8% of all contrast-media infusions. The risk appears to be similar for both ionic and nonionic agents. Fatalities occur as frequently as 1 in 3000 procedures for cholangiography.[21] These reactions are associated with increased plasma histamine concentrations, although the mechanism of the histamine release is unknown. Patients with previous reactions have an increased incidence on second exposure (35–60%). Pretreatment with prednisone and antihistamines reduces the rate of recurrence to 9%.[21]

ANGIOTENSIN-CONVERTING ENZYME INHIBITORS

Epidemiology

In recent years cough has become a well-recognized side effect of angiotensin-converting enzyme (ACE) inhibitor therapy. Studies utilizing spontaneous reporting by patients estimate that it occurs in 1–10% of patients receiving ACE inhibitors with a preponderance of females. Studies specifically evaluating cough due to ACE inhibitors have reported prevalences of 19–25%.[22,23] Patients receiving ACE inhibitors had a 2.3 times greater likelihood of developing cough than a similar group of patients receiving diuretics.[22] Patients with hyperreactive airways do not appear to be at greater risk.[24] It occurs with all ACE inhibitors.[24]

Clinical Presentation

The cough typically is dry and nonproductive, it is persistent and not paroxysmal.[24] The cough can begin within 3 days or have a delayed onset of up to 12 months following initiation of ACE inhibitor therapy.[24] The cough remits within 1–4 days of discontinuing therapy but rarely can last up to 4 weeks and recurs with rechallenge.[24] The chest x-ray is normal as are pulmonary function tests (spirometry and diffusing capacity). Bronchial hyperreactivity, as measured by histamine and methacholine provocation, may be worsened in patients with underlying bronchial hyperreactivity such as asthma and chronic bronchitis. However, bronchial hyperreactivity is not induced in others.[24,25] The cough reflex to capsaicin is enhanced but not to nebulized distilled water or citric acid.[24]

Pathogenesis and Treatment

The mechanism of ACE inhibitor-induced cough is still unknown. ACE is a nonspecific enzyme that also catalyzes the hydrolysis of bradykinin and substance P (see Chapter 25, Asthma) that produce or facilitate inflammation and stimulate lung irritant receptors.[24] ACE inhibitors may also induce cyclooxygenase to induce the production of prostaglandins. NSAIDs suppress or inhibit ACE inhibitor-induced cough.[24] The cough has generally not proven responsive to cough suppressants or bronchodilator therapy. It is recommended that patients be given a 4-day withdrawal to determine if the cough is ACE inhibitor-induced. The preferred therapy is withdrawal of the ACE inhibitor and replacement with an alternative antihypertensive agent. The use of NSAIDs is not generally recommended.[24]

PULMONARY EDEMA

Pulmonary edema may result from the failure of any of a number of homeostatic mechanisms. The most common cause of pulmonary edema is an increase in capillary hydrostatic pressure because of left ventricular failure. Excessive fluid administration in compromised and noncompromised cardiovascular patients is the most frequent cause of iatrogenic pulmonary edema. Besides hydrostatic forces, other homeostatic mechanisms that may be disrupted include the osmotic and oncotic pressures in the vasculature, the integrity of alveolar epithelium, interstitial pulmonary pressure, and the interstitial lymph flow.[6] The edema fluid in cardiogenic pulmonary edema contains a low amount of protein, whereas noncardiogenic pulmonary edema fluid has a high protein concentration.[6] This indicates that noncardiogenic pulmonary edema results primarily from disruption of the alveolar epithelium.

The clinical presentation of pulmonary edema includes persistent cough, tachypnea, dyspnea, tachycardia, rales on auscultation, hypoxemia from ventilation perfusion imbalance and intrapulmonary shunting, widespread fluffy infiltrates on chest roentgenogram, and decreased lung compliance (stiff lungs). Noncardiogenic pulmonary edema may progress to hemorrhage; cellular debris collects in the alveoli followed by hyperplasia and fibrosis with a residual restrictive mechanical defect.[6]

NARCOTICS

The most common drug-induced noncardiogenic pulmonary edema is produced by the narcotic analgesics

(Table 28.4).[6] Narcotic-induced pulmonary edema is most commonly associated with intravenous heroin use but has also occurred with morphine, methadone, meperidine, and propoxyphene use.[6,26] There have also been two reported cases associated with the use of the opiate agonist naloxone.[26] The mechanism is unknown but may be related to hypoxemia similar to the neurogenic pulmonary edema associated with cerebral tumors or trauma, or a direct toxic effect on the alveolar capillary membrane.[26] Initially thought to occur only with overdoses, most evidence now supports the theory that narcotic-induced pulmonary edema is an idiosyncratic reaction to moderate as well as high doses.[26]

Symptoms

Patients may be comatose with depressed respirations or dyspneic and tachypneic. They may or may not have other signs of narcotic overdose. Symptomology varies from cough and mild crepitations on auscultation with characteristic radiological findings to severe cyanosis and hypoxemia even with supplemental oxygen. Symptoms may appear within minutes of intravenous administration, but may take up to 2 hours particularly following oral methadone.[26] Hemodynamic studies in the first 24 hours have demonstrated normal pulmonary capillary wedge pressures in the presence of pulmonary edema.

Clinical symptoms generally improve within 24–48 hours and radiologic clearing occurs in 2–5 days, but abnormalities in pulmonary-function tests may persist for 10–12 weeks. Therapy consists of naloxone administration, supplemental oxygen, and ventilatory support if required. Mortality is less than 1%.[26]

TABLE 28.4. DRUGS THAT INDUCE PULMONARY EDEMA

Cardiogenic Pulmonary Edema	
Excessive intravenous fluids	F[a]
Blood and plasma transfusions	F
Corticosteroids	F
Phenylbutazone	R
Sodium diatrizoate	R
Hypertonic intrathecal saline	R
β_2-Adrenergic agonists	I
Noncardiogenic Pulmonary Edema	
Heroin	F
Methadone	I
Morphine	I
Oxygen	I
Propoxyphene	R
Ethchlorvynol	R
Chlordiazepoxide	R
Salicylate	R
Hydrochlorothiazide	R
Triamterene + hydrochlorothiazide	R
Leukoagglutinin reactions	R
Iron dextran	R
Methotrexate	R
Cytosine arabinoside	R
Nitrofurantoin	R
Dextran 40	R
Fluorescein	R
Amitriptyline	R
Colchicine	R
Nitrogen mustard	R
Epinephrine	R
Metaraminol	R
Bleomycin	R
Iodide	R
Cyclophosphamide	R
VM-26	R

[a]Relative frequency of reactions: F, frequent; I, infrequent; R, rare.

OTHER DRUGS

Noncardiogenic pulmonary edema has also been associated with the oral and intravenous administration of ethchlorvynol.[26] A parodoxical pulmonary edema has been reported in a few patients following hydrochlorothiazide ingestion but not any other benzothiazide diuretic.[6] Acute pulmonary edema has rarely followed the injection of high concentrations of contrast medium into the pulmonary circulation during angiocardiography.[6] Rare occurrences of pulmonary edema have followed the intravenous administration of bleomycin, cyclophosphamide, and vinblastine.[6]

The selective β_2-adrenergic agonists terbutaline and ritodrine have been reported to induce pulmonary edema when used as tocolytics.[6] This has never occurred with their use in asthma patients, even in inadvertent overdosage. This reaction may result from excess fluid administration used to prevent the hypotension from β_2-mediated vasodilation or the particular hemodynamics of pregnancy.

Pulmonary edema has occasionally occurred with salicylate overdoses. The serum salicylate concentrations are often greater than 45 mg/dL and the patients have other signs of toxicity, although some cases have been associated with concentrations in the usual therapeutic range.[26]

PULMONARY EOSINOPHILIA

Pulmonary infiltrates with eosinophilia (Loeffler's syndrome) have been associated with nitrofurantoin, paraaminosalicylic acid, methotrexate, sulfonamides, tetracycline, chlorpropamide, phenytoin, NSAIDs, and imipramine (Table 28.5).[6,27] The disorder is characterized by fever, nonproductive cough, dyspnea, cyanosis, bilateral pulmonary infiltrates, and eosinophilia in the blood.[6] Lung biopsy has revealed perivasculitis with infiltration of eosinophils, macrophages, and proteinaceous edema fluid in the alveoli. The symptoms and eosinophilia generally respond rapidly to withdrawal of the offending drug.

TABLE 28.5. DRUGS THAT INDUCE PULMONARY INFILTRATES WITH EOSINOPHILIA (LOEFFLER'S SYNDROME)

Nitrofurantoin	F[a]	Tetracycline	R
para-Aminosalicylic acid	F	Procarbazine	R
Sulfonamides	I	Cromolyn	R
Penicillins	I	Niridazole	R
Methotrexate	I	Gold salts	R
Imipramine	I	Chlorpromazine	R
Chlorpropamide	R	Naproxen	R
Carbamazepine	R	Sulindac	R
Phenytoin	R	Ibuprofen	R
Mephenesin	R		

[a]Relative frequency of reactions: F, frequent; I, infrequent; R, rare.

Sulfonamides were first reported as causative agents in users of sulfanilamide vaginal cream.[6] Para-aminosalicylic acid frequently produced the syndrome in tuberculosis patients being treated with this agent.[6] There have been nine reported cases associated with sulfasalazine use in inflammatory bowel disease.[26] The drug most frequently associated with this syndrome is nitrofurantoin.[6,26] Nitrofurantoin-induced lung disorders appear to be more common in postmenopausal women.[26] Lung reactions made up 43% of 921 adverse reactions to nitrofurantoin reported to the Swedish Adverse Drug Reaction Committee between 1966 and 1976.[27] No apparent correlation exists between duration of drug exposure and severity or reversibility of the reaction.[27] Most cases occur within 1 month of therapy. Typical symptoms include fever, tachypnea, dyspnea, dry cough, and less commonly pleuritic chest pain. Radiographic findings include bilateral interstitial infiltrates, predominant in the bases and pleural effusions 25% of the time. Although there are anecdotal reports that steroids are beneficial, the usual rapid improvement following discontinuation of the drug brings their utility into question. Complete recovery usually occurs within 15 days of withdrawal.

A few cases of pulmonary eosinophilia have been reported in asthmatics treated with cromolyn.[6,27] The significance of this is unknown in light of the occasional spontaneous occurrence of pulmonary eosinophilia in asthmatic patients. Cases of acute pneumonitis and eosinophilia have been reported to occur with phenytoin and carbamazepine therapy.[27] Patients have had other symptoms of hypersensitivity including fever and rashes. The symptoms of dyspnea and cough subside following discontinuation of the drug.

OXYGEN TOXICITY

Because of the similarity to pulmonary fibrosis, oxygen-induced lung toxicity are briefly reviewed. More extensive reviews on this topic have been published.[28,29]

Pathophysiology

Oxygen-induced lung damage has been systematically characterized. These are generally separated into the acute exudative phase and the subacute or chronic proliferative phase. The acute phase consists of perivascular, peribronchiolar, interstitial, and alveolar edema with alveolar hemorrhage and necrosis of pulmonary endothelium and type I epithelial cells.[28] The proliferative phase consists of resorption of the exudates and hyperplasia of interstitial and type II alveolar lining cells. Collagen and elastin deposition in the interstitium of alveolar walls then leads to thickening of the gas exchange area and the fibrosis.[28]

Etiology

The fractional concentration of inspired oxygen (FIO_2) and duration of exposure are both important determinants of the severity of damage. Normal human volunteers can tolerate 100% oxygen at sea level for 24–48 hours with minimal to no damage.[28] Oxygen concentrations of less than 50% are well tolerated even for extended periods. Inspired oxygen concentrations between 50% and 100% carry a substantial risk of lung damage and the duration required is inversely proportional to the FIO_2.[27] Underlying disease states may alter this relationship.

Symptoms

The earliest manifestation of oxygen toxicity is substernal pleuritic pain from tracheobronchitis.[29] The onset of toxicity follows an asymptomatic period and presents as cough, chest pain, and dyspnea. Early symptoms are usually masked in ventilator-dependent patients. The first noted physiologic change is a decrease in pulmonary compliance caused by reversible atelectasis. Then decreases in vital capacity occur, followed by progressive abnormalities in carbon monoxide-diffusing capacity (DLCO).[29] Decreased inspiratory flow rates, reflected in the need for high inspiratory pressures in ventilator-dependent patients, occur as the FIO_2 requirement increases. The lungs become progressively stiffer as the ability to oxygenate becomes more compromised.

Mechanism

The biochemical mechanism of the tissue damage during hyperoxia is the increased production of highly reactive, partially reduced oxygen metabolites (Fig. 28.1).[29] These oxidants are normally produced in small quantities during cellular respiration and include the superoxide anion (O_2^-), hydrogen peroxide (H_2O_2), the hydroxyl radical (OH), singlet oxygen ($^1O_2$), and hypochlorous acid (HOCl).[29] Oxygen-free radicals are normally formed in phagocytic cells in order to kill invading microorganisms, but they are also toxic to normal cell components. The oxidants produce toxicity through destructive redox reactions with protein sulfhydryl groups, membrane lipids, and nucleic acids.[29]

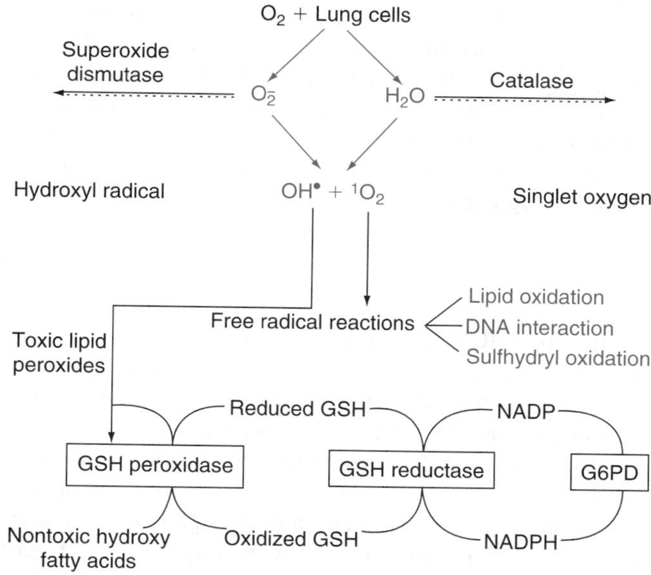

Figure 28.1. Schematic of the interaction of oxygen radicals and the antioxidant system. GSH, glutathione; G6PD, glucose-6-phosphate dehydrogenase.

The oxidants are products of normal cellular respiration that are normally counterbalanced by an antioxidant defense system that prevents tissue destruction. The antioxidants include superoxide dismutase, catalase, glutathione peroxidase, ceruloplasmin, and alphatocopherol (vitamin E). Antioxidants are ubiquitous in the body. Hyperoxia produces toxicity by overwhelming the antioxidant system. There is experimental evidence that a number of drugs and chemicals produce lung toxicity through increasing production of oxidants (e.g., bleomycin, cyclophosphamide, nitrofurantoin, paraquat) and/or by inhibiting the antioxidant system (e.g., carmustine, cyclophosphamide, nitrofurantoin).[30,31]

PULMONARY FIBROSIS

A large variety of drugs have been associated with chronic pulmonary fibrosis with or without a preceding acute pneumonitis (Table 28.6). The cancer chemotherapeutic agents make up the largest group and have been the subject of numerous reviews.[30,31] Although the mechanisms by which all of the drugs produce pneumonitis and/or fibrosis are not known, the clinical syndrome, pulmonary-function abnormalities, and histopathology present a relatively homogeneous pattern.[30] The histopathologic picture closely resembles oxidant lung damage and in some experimental cases oxygen enhances the pulmonary injury.[30]

The lung damage following ingestion of the contact herbicide paraquat classically resembles hyperoxic lung damage. Hyperoxia accelerates the lung damage induced by paraquat. Lung toxicity from paraquat occurs following oral administration in man and aerosol administration and inhalation in experimental animals.[31] The pulmonary specificity of paraquat results in part from its active uptake into lung tissue. Paraquat readily accepts an electron from NADPH and is then rapidly reoxidized, forming superoxide and other oxygen radicals.[31] The toxicity may be a result of NADPH depletion (Fig. 28.1) and/or excess oxygen-free radical generation with lipid peroxidation. Treatment with exogenous superoxide dismutase has had limited and conflicting results.[31]

A number of furans have been shown to produce oxidant injury to lungs.[31] Occasionally, patients with acute nitrofurantoin lung toxicity will progress to a chronic reaction leading to fibrosis and rarely a patient may develop

TABLE 28.6. DRUGS THAT INDUCE PNEUMONITIS AND/OR FIBROSIS

Oxygen	F[a]
Radiation	F
Bleomycin	F
Busulfan	F
Carmustine	F
Hexamethonium	F
Paraquat	F
Amiodarone	F
Mecamylamine	I
Pentolinium	I
Cyclophosphamide	I
Practolol	I
Methotrexate	I
Mitomycin	I
Nitrofurantoin	I
Methysergide	I
Azathioprine, 6-mercaptopurine	R
Chlorambucil	R
Melphalan	R
Lomustine and semustine	R
Zinostatin	R
Procarbazine	R
Teniposide	R
Sulphasalazine	R
Phenytoin	R
Gold salts	R
Pindolol	R
Imipramine	R
Penicillamine	R
Phenylbutazone	R
Chlorphentermine	R
Fenfluramine	R

[a]Relative frequency of reactions: F, frequent; I, infrequent; R, rare.

chronic toxicity without an antecedent acute reaction. Like paraquat, nitrofurantoin undergoes cyclic reduction and reoxidation that may produce superoxide radicals or deplete NADPH. In addition, nitrofurantoin inhibits glutathione reductase, an enzyme involved in the glutathione antioxidant system (Fig. 28.1). Table 28.7 provides a list of possible causes of pulmonary fibrosis, drug and nondrug.

ANTINEOPLASTICS

A number of cancer chemotherapeutic agents produce pulmonary fibrosis. In an excellent review, Cooper et al.[30] listed six predisposing factors for the development of cytotoxic drug-induced pulmonary disease: (1) cumulative dose, (2) increased age, (3) concurrent or previous radiotherapy, (4) oxygen therapy, (5) other cytotoxic drug therapy, and (6) preexisting pulmonary disease. Drugs that are directly toxic to the lung would be expected to show a dose–response relationship. Dose–response relationships have been established for bleomycin, busulfan, and carmustine (BCNU).[30] Bleomycin and busulfan exhibit threshold-cumulative doses below which a very small percentage of patients exhibit toxicity, but carmustine shows a more linear relationship.[31] Older patients appear to be more susceptible, possibly as a result of a decrease in the antioxidant defense system.

Excessive irradiation produces a pneumonitis and fibrosis thought to be caused by oxygen-radical formation.[30] Evidence for synergistic toxicity with radiation exists for bleomycin, busulfan, and mitomycin.[30] Hyperoxia has shown synergistic toxicity with bleomycin, cyclophosphamide, and mitomycin.[30] Carmustine, mitomycin, cyclophosphamide, bleomycin, and methotrexate all appear to show increased lung toxicity when they are part of multiple-drug regimens.

TABLE 28.7. POSSIBLE CAUSES OF PULMONARY FIBROSIS

Idiopathic pulmonary fibrosis (fibrosing alveolitis)
Pneumoconiosis (asbestosis, silicosis, coal dust, talc berylliosis)
Hypersensitivity pneumonitis (molds, bacteria, animal proteins, toluene diisocyanate, epoxy resins)
Smoking
Sarcoidosis
Tuberculosis
Lipoid pneumonia
Systemic lupus erythematosus
Rheumatoid arthritis
Systemic sclerosis
Polymyositis/dermatomyositis
Sjögren's syndrome
Polyarteritis nodosa
Wegener's granuloma
Byssinosis (cotton workers)
Siderosis (arc welders' lung)
Radiation
Oxygen
Chemicals (thioureas, trialkylphosphorothioates, furans)
Drugs (see Tables 28.5, 28.6, and 28.8)

NITROSOUREAS

Carmustine (BCNU) is associated with the highest incidence of pulmonary toxicity (20–30%).[30] The lung pathology generally resembles that produced by bleomycin and busulfan. Unique to carmustine is the finding of fibrosis in the absence of inflammatory infiltrates. Carmustine preferentially inhibits glutathione reductase, the enzyme required to regenerate glutathione, thus reducing glutathione tissue stores.[30,31] The patients present with dyspnea, tachypnea, and nonproductive cough that may begin within a month of initiation of therapy but may not develop for as long as 3 years.[30] A more recent report suggested that most patients receiving carmustine develop fibrosis that may remain asymptomatic or become symptomatic anytime up to 17 years after therapy.[32] The cumulative dose has ranged from 580–2100 mg/m^2.[28] The disease is usually slowly progressive with a mortality rate from 15% to greater than 90% depending on the study and period of follow-up. Rapid progression and death within a few days occur in a small percentage of patients.[30] Corticosteroids do not appear to be effective in reducing damage.[30] Other nitrosoureas, lomustine and semustine, have also been reported to produce lung damage in patients receiving unusually high doses.[30]

BLEOMYCIN

Bleomycin is the best studied cytotoxic pulmonary toxin. Because of its lack of bone marrow suppression, pulmonary toxicity is the dose-limiting toxicity of bleomycin therapy. The cumulative dose above which the incidence of toxicity significantly increases is 450–500 units.[30] However, rapidly fatal pulmonary toxicity has occurred with doses as low as 100 units.[30]

Experimentally bleomycin generates superoxide anions, and the lung toxicity is increased by radiation and hyperoxia.[30] Pretreatment with superoxide dismutase and catalase reduces toxicity in experimental animals.[30] Bleomycin also oxidizes arachidonic acid, which may account for the marked inflammation. Bleomycin may also affect collagen deposition by its stimulation of fibroblast growth.[30] Combination of bleomycin with other cytotoxic agents, particularly regimens containing cyclophosphamide, may predispose patients to pulmonary damage.

There are two distinct clinical patterns of bleomycin pulmonary toxicity. Chronic progressive fibrosis is the most common; acute hypersensitivity reactions occur infrequently. Patients present with cough and dyspnea. The first physiologic abnormality seen is a decreased carbon monoxide-diffusing capacity.[30] Chest radiographs show a bibasilar reticular pattern, and gallium scans show marked uptake in the involved lung.[30] Chest radiographic changes lag behind pulmonary-function abnormalities. Spirometry tests before each bleomycin dose are not predictive of toxicity. The DLCO is the most sensitive indicator of bleomycin-induced lung disease. Although it is not absolutely predictive, a drop of 20% or greater in the DLCO is an indication for using alternative therapies.[30] Corticosteroid therapy appears to be helpful in patients with acute pneumonitis, although there have been no controlled trials. Patients with chronic fibrosis would be less likely to respond. Although corticosteroids have been used for a number of drug-induced pulmonary problems, a study in mice showing a potential for worsening of lung damage when administered early during the repair stage should sound a word of caution against their indiscriminate use.[33]

Mitomycin is an alkylating antibiotic that produces pulmonary fibrosis at a frequency of 3–12%.[30] The mechanism is unknown, but oxygen and radiation therapy appear to enhance the development of toxicity.[30] The clinical presentation and symptoms are the same as for bleomycin. The mortality rate is about 50%. Early withdrawal of the drug and administration of corticosteroids appear to significantly improve the outcome.

ALKYLATING AGENTS

A number of alkylating agents have been associated with pulmonary fibrosis (Table 28.5). In 1961, busulfan, the first cytotoxic agent reported to do so, was found to cause pulmonary fibrosis.[30] The incidence of clinical toxicity is around 4%, although subclinical damage is apparent in up to 46% of patients at autopsy. The mechanism of toxicity is unknown; however, epithelial cell damage that triggers the arachidonic acid inflammatory cascade may be the initiating event.[30] The clinical presentation is insidious, with 4 years being the average duration of therapy before the onset of symptoms.[30] Patients present with low-grade fever, weight loss, weakness, dyspnea, cough, and rales.[30] Pulmonary-function tests initially show abnormal diffusion capacity followed by a restrictive pattern (low vital capacity). The histopathologic findings are nonspecific. The prognosis is one of slow progression with a mean survival of 5 months following diagnosis.[30] Although there is no direct dose-dependent correlation, patients receiving less than 500 mg do not develop the syndrome without concomitant radiation or use of other pulmonary-toxic chemotherapeutic agents.[30] There are anecdotal reports of beneficial responses to corticosteroids, but no controlled studies have been done.

Cyclophosphamide infrequently produces pulmonary toxicity. More than 20 well-documented cases have been reported to date. In animal models cyclophosphamide produces reactive oxygen radicals. High oxygen concentrations produce synergistic toxicity with cyclophosphamide. The duration of therapy before the onset of symptoms is highly variable, and there may be a delay of several months between the onset of symptoms and discontinuation of drugs.[30] Cyclophosphamide may potentiate carmustine lung toxicity.[30] Clinical symptoms usually consist of dyspnea on exertion, cough, and fever. Inspiratory crackles and the bibasilar reticular pattern typical of cytotoxic drug-induced radiographic changes are present. Histopathologic changes are also nonspecific. Approximately 60% of patients recover. Corticosteroid therapy has been reported to be beneficial; however, death despite corticosteroid administration has also been reported.

Chlorambucil, melphalan, and uracil mustard have also been associated with pulmonary fibrosis. Of the alkylating agents, only nitrogen mustard and thiotepa have not been reported to cause fibrotic pulmonary toxicity.[30]

ANTIMETABOLITES

Methotrexate was first reported to induce pulmonary toxicity in 1969.[30] The pulmonary toxicity to methotrexate is unique in that discontinuation is not always necessary and reinstitution of the drug may not produce recurrence of symptoms.[6] Methotrexate pulmonary toxicity most commonly appears to result from hypersensitivity.[27] Pulmonary edema and eosinophilia are common and fibrosis occurs in only 10% of the patients who develop acute pneumonitis.[30] Systemic symptoms of chills, fever, and malaise are common before the onset of dyspnea, cough, and acute pleuritic chest pain. Methotrexate has also been associated with granuloma formation.[30]

The prognosis of methotrexate-induced pulmonary toxicity is good with a 1% or less mortality rate.[27] Pulmonary toxicity has followed intrathecal as well as oral administration, and has occurred after single doses as well as long-term daily and intermittent administration.[30] Pneumonitis has been reported to occur up to 4 weeks following discontinuation of therapy.[30] Numerous anecdotal reports have claimed dramatic benefit from corticosteroid therapy. It is unknown whether intermittent dosing as is done for rheumatoid arthritis decreases the risk of methotrexate-induced pulmonary toxicity, and pneumonitis has occurred with this form of dosing.

Rarely azathioprine and its major metabolite 6-mercaptopurine have been reported to produce an acute restrictive lung disease. Procarbazine, a methylhydrazine more commonly associated with Loeffler's syndrome, has rarely been associated with pulmonary fibrosis.[27] The vinca alkaloids, vinblastine and vindesine, have been reported to produce severe respiratory toxicity in association with mitomycin. The incidence with the combination is 39% and may represent a true synergistic effect between these agents.[30]

NONCYTOTOXIC DRUGS

Pulmonary fibrosis associated with the ganglionic-blocking agent hexamethonium was first reported in 1954 (Table 28.6).[6] Patients developed extreme dyspnea after several months on the drug. Pathologic findings were consistent with bronchiectasis, bronchiolectasis, and fibrosis.[6] This phenomenon has occasionally occurred with the use of the other ganglionic blockers, mecamylamine and pentolinium.[6]

In 1959 radiographic changes characteristic of diffuse pulmonary fibrosis were reported in 87% of 31 patients who had taken phenytoin for 2 years or more.[26] Since then studies have been conflicting. If phenytoin does produce chronic fibrosis, it would appear to be a relatively rare event.

Gold salts (sodium aurothiomalate) used in the treatment of rheumatoid arthritis have produced pulmonary fibrosis with cough, dyspnea, and pleuritic pain 5–16 weeks following institution of therapy.[26] Pulmonary function tests show a restrictive defect and patients generally have an eosinophilia. The reactions improve on discontinuation of the gold therapy and promptly recur on reexposure. The pulmonary deficit may not completely improve.

AMIODARONE

Amiodarone, a benzofuran derivative, produces pulmonary fibrosis when used for supraventricular and ventricular arrhythmias (Table 28.6).[34] The duration of amiodarone therapy before the onset of symptoms has ranged from 4 weeks to 6 years.[26,34] The estimated incidence is 1 in 1000 to 2000 treated patients per year. The clinical course is variable, ranging from acute onset of dyspnea with rapid progression into severe respiratory failure and death caused by slowly developing exertional dyspnea over a few months. Patients generally improve upon discontinuation of the drug.[34] The majority of patients develop reactions while taking maintenance doses greater than 400 mg daily.[34] Routine spirometry does not appear to be predictive for identifying patients at risk.[35] Carbon monoxide diffusing capacity studies are sensitive indicators of amiodarone pulmonary toxicity but have only a 21% positive predictive value.[35] Clinical findings include exertional dyspnea, nonproductive cough, weight loss, and occasionally low-grade fever.[26,34] Radiographic changes are nondiagnostic and consist of diffuse bilateral interstitial changes consistent with a pneumonitis. Pulmonary function abnormalities include hypoxia, restrictive changes, and diffusion abnormalities.

The mechanism of amiodarone-induced pulmonary toxicity is unknown. Amiodarone is an amphiphilic molecule that contains both a highly apolar aromatic ring system and a polar side chain with a positively charged nitrogen atom.[34] Amphiphilic drugs characteristically produce a phospholipid storage disorder in the lungs of experimental animals and man.[31] Chlorphentermine, an anorectic, is the prototype amphiphilic compound. The mechanism is currently believed to be the inhibition of lysosomal phospholipases.[31] The inflammation and fibrosis is thought to be a late finding resulting from nonspecific inflammation following the breakdown of phospholipid-laden macrophages.[34]

In a review of 39 cases, 9 patients died and the remaining 30 patients had resolution of abnormalities after withdrawal of the drug.[34] Some patients have had resolution with lowering of the dosage, and therapy has been reinstituted at lower doses without problems in others. Of the patients who died, one-half received corticosteroids. There have been reports of a protective effect with prophylactic corticosteroids and other reports of patients developing amiodarone lung toxicity while on corticosteroids.[24] At this time any benefit of corticosteroids is unclear because most patients improve upon stopping the drug.

MISCELLANEOUS PULMONARY TOXICITY

A number of drugs may produce serious pulmonary toxicity as part of a more generalized disorder. The pleural thickening, effusions, and fibrosis that occur as an extension of the retroperitoneal fibrotic reactions of methysergide and practolol or as part of a drug-induced lupus syndrome are the most common examples (Table 28.8).

Methysergide therapy for prophylaxis of poorly controlled migraine headache occasionally results in pulmonary toxicity associated with pleural effusions. The patients develop pleural pain, dyspnea, and fever. Chest radiography reveals a uniform hazy shadowing over the lower lung fields and a loud pleural rub is heard on auscultation.[6] The mechanism is unknown and most patients improve with discontinuation of the drug. Pleural and pulmonary fibrosis has been reported in one patient taking pindolol, a β blocker, structurally similar to practolol, an agent known to produce fibrosis.[26] Acute pleuritis with pleural effusions and fibrosis is a prominent manifestation of drug-induced lupus syndrome. Procainamide is associated with the largest number of pulmonary reactions, with 46% of patients with the lupus syndrome developing pulmonary complications.[6] Symptoms include pleuritic pain and fever with muscle and joint pain. Chest radiographs show bilateral pleural effusions and linear atelectasis. Patients have a positive antinuclear antibody (ANA) test. Symptoms usually resolve within 6 weeks of drug withdrawal.[6]

TABLE 28.8. DRUGS THAT MAY INDUCE PLEURAL EFFUSIONS AND FIBROSIS

Idiopathic	
Methysergide	F[a]
Practolol	F
Pindolol	R
Methotrexate	R
Nitrofurantoin	R
Due to Drug-Induced Lupus Syndrome	
Procainamide	F
Hydralazine	F
Isoniazid	R
Phenytoin	R
Mephenytoin	R
Griseofulvin	R
Trimethadione	R
Sulfonamides	R
Phenylbutazone	R
Streptomycin	R
Ethosuximide	R
Tetracycline	R
Pseudolymphoma Syndrome	
Cyclosporine	R
Phenytoin	R

[a]Relative frequency of reactions: F, frequent; I, infrequent; R, rare.

Hydralazine is the next most common cause of lupus syndrome. Most patients who develop pleuropulmonary manifestations have antecedent symptoms of generalized lupus.[6] Other drugs that produce the lupus syndrome include isoniazid and phenytoin. Phenytoin can also produce hilar lymphadenopathy as part of a generalized pseudolymphoma or lymphadenopathy syndrome.[6]

Monitoring Therapeutic Outcomes

Monitoring for drug-induced pulmonary diseases consists primarily of having a high index of suspicion that a particular syndrome may be drug induced. Most hypersensitivity or allergic reactions (bronchospasm) occur rapidly, within the first 2 weeks of therapy with the offending agent and reverse rapidly with appropriate therapy (i.e., withdrawal of the offending agent, administration of corticosteroids and bronchodilators). Loeffler's syndrome and acute pulmonary edema syndromes also improve rapidly in 1–2 days for the dyspnea. However, some residual defect in diffusion capacity and roentgenogram may persist for a few weeks. It is probably unnecessary to do follow-up spirometry or diffusion capacity in these patients unless there is some concern that the syndrome will progress to pulmonary fibrosis (i.e., through use of bleomycin or nitrofurantoin).

The routine monitoring of patients receiving known pulmonary toxins with dose-dependent toxicity such as amiodarone, bleomycin, or carmustine is still controversial. For chronic fibrosis the DLCO is the most sensitive test and may be useful in patients receiving bleomycin for detecting and preventing further deterioration of lung function with continued administration. Carmustine lung toxicity may be delayed up to 10 years following administration and routine monitoring has not proven preventive. Monitoring patients every 4–6 months receiving amiodarone in doses greater than 400 mg daily may prove useful in detecting early disease that requires lowering the amiodarone dose or stopping the drug. Because there is no evidence of a cumulative dose effect once it has been established that the patient can tolerate the elevated dose, continued routine monitoring past the first year is unnecessary.

References

1. Martys CR. Adverse reactions to drugs in general practice. Br Med J 1979;2:1194–1197.
2. Kramer MS, Hutchinson TA, Flegel KM, et al. Adverse drug reactions in general pediatric outpatients. J Pediatr 1985;106:305–310.
3. Levy M, Kewitz H, Altwein W, et al. Hospital admissions due to adverse drug reactions: A comparative study from Jerusalem and Berlin. Eur J Clin Pharmacol 1980;17:25–31.
4. Shapiro S, Slone D, Lewis GP, et al. Fatal drug reactions among medical inpatients. JAMA 1971;216:467–472.
5. Porter J, Jick H. Drug-related deaths among medical inpatients. JAMA 1977;237:879–881.
6. Brewis RAL. Respiratory disorders, in Davies DM (ed): Textbook of Adverse Drug Reactions, 2nd ed. New York, Oxford University Press, 1981, pp 154–178.
7. Hansen-Flaschen J, Cowen J, Raps EC. Neuromuscular blockade in the intensive care unit: More than we bargained for. Am Rev Respir Dis 1993;147:234–236.
8. Fisher HK. Drug-induced asthma syndromes, in Weiss EB, Segal MS, Stein M (eds): Bronchial Asthma: Mechanisms and Therapeutics, 2nd ed. Boston, Little, Brown, 1985, pp 938–949.
9. Settipane GA. Aspirin and allergic diseases: A review. Am J Med 1983;74(suppl 6a):102–109.
10. Szczeklik A, Gryglewski RJ. Asthma and antiinflammatory drugs: Mechanisms and clinical patterns. Drugs 1983;25:533–543.
11. Stevenson DD. Diagnosis, prevention, and treatment of adverse reactions to aspirin and nonsteroidal antiinflammatory drugs. J Allergy Clin Immunol 1984;74:617–622.
12. Lee TH. Mechanism of bronchospasm in aspirin-sensitive asthma. Am Rev Respir Dis 1993;148:1442–1443.
13. Mathison DA, Stevenson DD, Simon RA. Precipitating factors in asthma: Aspirin, sulfites, and other drugs and chemicals. Chest 1985;87(suppl):50–54.
14. Riddell JG, Shanks RG. Effects of betaxolol, propranolol, and atenolol on isoproterenol-induced β-adrenoceptor responses. Clin Pharmacol Ther 1985;38:554–559.
15. Fraunfeder FT, Barker AF. Respiratory effects of timolol. N Engl J Med 1984;311:1441.
16. Dunn TL, Gerber MJ, Shen AS, et al. The effect of topical ophthalmic instillation of timolol and betaxolol on lung

function in asthmatic subjects. Am Rev Respir Dis 1986;133:264–268.
17. Bush RK, Taylor SL, Busse W. A critical evaluation of clinical trials in reactions to sulfites. J Allergy Clin Immunol 1986;78:191–202.
18. Anibarro B, Caballero T, Garcia-Ara C, et al. Asthma with sulfite intolerance in children: A blocking study with cyanocobalamin. J Allergy Clin Immunol 1992;90:103–109.
19. Beasley R, Rafferty P, Holgate ST. Adverse reactions to the nondrug constituents of nebulizer solutions. Br J Clin Pharmacol 1988;25:283–287.
20. Zhang YG, Wright WJ, Tam WK, et al. Effect of inhaled preservatives on asthmatic subjects II. Benzalkonium chloride. Am Rev Respir Dis 1990;141:1405–1408.
21. Greenberger PA. Contrast media reactions. J Allergy Clin Immunol 1984;74:600–605.
22. Sebastian JL, McKinney WP, Kaufman J, et al. Angiotensin-converting enzyme inhibitors and cough: Prevalence in an outpatient medical clinic population. Chest 1991;99:36–39.
23. Simon SR, Black HR, Moser M, Berland WE. Cough and ACE inhibitors. Arch Intern Med 1992;152:1698–1700.
24. Israili ZH, Hall WD. Cough and angioneurotic edema associated with angiotensin-converting enzyme inhibitor therapy: A review of the literature and pathophysiology. Ann Intern Med 1992;117:234–242.
25. Kaufman J, Casanova JE, Riendl P, et al. Bronchial hyperreactivity and cough due to angiotensin-converting enzyme inhibitors. Chest 1989;95:544–548.
26. Cooper JAD, White DA, Matthay RA. Drug-induced pulmonary disease. Part 2: Noncytotoxic drugs. Am Rev Respir Dis 1986;133:488–505.
27. Obermiller T, Lakshminarayan S. Drug-induced hypersensitivity reactions in the lung. Immunol Allergy Clin North Am 1991;11:575–594.
28. Frank L, Massaro D. Oxygen toxicity. Am J Med 1980;69:117–126.
29. Jackson RM. Pulmonary oxygen toxicity. Chest 1985;88:900–905.
30. Cooper JAD, White DA, Matthay RA. State of the art: Drug-induced pulmonary disease. Part 1: Cytotoxic drugs. Am Rev Respir Dis 1986;133:321–340.
31. Kehrer JP, Kacew S. Systematically applied chemicals that damage lung tissue. Toxicology 1985;35:251–293.
32. O'Driscoll BR, Hasleton PS, Taylor PM, et al. Active lung fibrosis up to 17 years after chemotherapy with carmustine (BCNU) in childhood. N Engl J Med 1990;323:378–382.
33. Kehrer JP, Klein-Szanto AJP, Sorensen EMB, et al. Enhanced acute lung damage following corticosteroid treatment. Am Rev Respir Dis 1984;130:256–261.
34. Rakita L, Sobol SM, Mostow N, et al. Amiodarone pulmonary toxicity. Am Heart J 1983;106:906–914.
35. Gleadhill IC, Wise RA, Schonfeld SA, et al. Serial lung-function testing in patients treated with amiodarone: A prospective study. Am J Med 1989;86:4–10.

Chapter 29

Cystic Fibrosis

John A. Bosso, PharmD, FCCP

Cystic fibrosis is the most common lethal, genetically inherited disease affecting the Caucasian population. While considered a pediatric disease since it was first described by Anderson in 1938,[1] early diagnosis and more effective therapy now enable many patients to survive into adulthood. It is a disease mainly involving the exocrine glands and thus affects a number of organs or organ systems (Table 29.1). The more common manifestations of the disease involve the gastrointestinal (GI) and pulmonary systems with most of the observed morbidity and mortality associated with the latter. Most pathology is due to production of viscous secretions. The underlying disorder leading to this pathophysiology is a chloride transport channel defect at the secretory epithelial cell level. The protean nature of the disease dictates that care be multidisciplinary with a wide variety of therapeutic interventions.

INCIDENCE AND EPIDEMIOLOGY

Cystic fibrosis is inherited through an autosomal (Mendelian) recessive genetic mode. This implies that each parent must be at least a carrier (heterozygous) for the trait and, with such a couple, each child would have a one-in-four chance of having the disease, a one-in-two chance of being a carrier, and a one-in-four chance of being normal (having neither the disease nor the trait). The incidence of cystic fibrosis is greatest in the Caucasian population, with a rate of 1 in 2000 live births in the United States.[2] The incidence of the trait (carrier state) in this group is about 5%. The frequency of the disease is considerably less in other races, occurring at a rate of 1 in 17,000 Blacks and about 1 in 90,000 Asians.[3] After years of intensive research, the cystic fibrosis gene was discovered, cloned, and was described in the literature in 1989.[4–6] The protein (cystic fibrosis transmembrane regulator, or CFTR) encoded by this gene, which is on the long arm of chromosome 7, is a membrane protein that represents a channel involved in the transport of electrolytes and water. The most common genetic mutation associated with cystic fibrosis involves a specific base pair deletion at position 508,[4–6] but more than 200 cystic fibrosis-associated mutations within the gene have been described. The common mutation is referred to as the Δf_{508} allele and is present in about 70% of patients. The possible mutations have been divided into four classes: (I) defective protein production, (II) defective protein processing, (III) defective regulation, and (IV) defective conduction.[7] Patients who are homozygous for the ΔF_{508} mutation, which falls into class II, tend to be diagnosed at an earlier age, due to earlier onset of airway disease, and have a greater frequency of pancreatic insufficiency (99 versus 72% in heterozygotes and 36% in patients with other genotypes).[8,9]

PATHOPHYSIOLOGY

Cystic fibrosis is basically a disease of secretory epithelial cells or tissues. Such tissues are involved with the transport of chloride, sodium, and water in and out of the blood. In the normal state, there is a net chloride transport out of blood with sodium and water following this flux. This net secretion is activated or affected by hormones or neurotransmitters such as protein kinases and further involves intracellular second messengers such as adenosine 3′,5′-monophosphate (cAMP) or calcium.[10] It is an apical membrane chloride channel where activity is apparently affected in cystic fibrosis, leading to a decrease in secretion of chloride, sodium, and water. ΔF_{508} homozygous individuals have this abnormal chloride channel in the cells of several exocrine organs including pancreatic and hepatobiliary ducts, microvilli of the GI tract, and the lungs. In pulmonary epithelial cells, there also appears to be excessive absorption of sodium. These phenomena then lead to the thick, dehydrated mucus. This mucus can block pancreatic and hepatobiliary exocrine outflow and also accumulate in and obstruct the airways.

GASTROINTESTINAL TRACT

Involvement of the GI tract in cystic fibrosis is due to both the increased viscosity of mucus secretions and a relative

TABLE 29.1. ORGAN INVOLVEMENT IN CYSTIC FIBROSIS

Organ System/Organ	Abnormality	Consequence
Gastrointestinal		
Pancreas	Digestive enzyme deficiency	Maldigestion, malnutrition
	Insulin deficiency	Glucose intolerance
Intestines	Viscous secretions	Obstruction
Liver	Biliary cirrhosis/fatty infiltration	Portal hypertension/esophageal varices
Pulmonary	Viscous secretions	Chronic obstructive disease, hypoxia, cor pulmonale
	Infection	Endobronchial infection
Sweat glands	Failure to reabsorb sodium	Hyponatremia
Reproductive	Obstruction of epididymus, vas deferens, and seminal vesicles	Aspermia
	Viscous cervical mucus	Decreased fertility
Hematologic	Chronic disease?	Anemia
Bone and joint	Unknown	Arthritis, osteopenia

deficiency of pancreatic digestive enzymes. In 10–16% of cystic fibrosis patients, the first GI manifestation of the disease is an intestinal obstruction evident shortly after birth and known as meconium ileus. Again, the basic electrolyte transport defect is involved, and this complication is caused by an inability to evacuate the abnormally viscid meconium in these patients. A similar condition, known as distal intestinal obstruction syndrome (formerly referred to as meconium ileus equivalent), occurs in older cystic fibrosis patients; it is also thought to result from abnormally viscous GI secretions and fecal impaction. Other intestinal complications include intussusception, volvulus, atresia, perforation, giant cystic meconium peritonitis, and rectal prolapse.

A deficiency of pancreatic digestive enzymes, also known as pancreatic achylia, is present with most genotypes and, thus, 85% of cystic fibrosis patients. Pancreatic lesions include fibrosis, fatty replacement, and cyst formation and are secondary to obstruction of small pancreatic ducts by thickened secretions and cellular debris. Inspissated eosinophilic material is also present in acini and ductules. As a result, pancreatic secretions (as reflected by duodenal aspirates) are viscous and low in volume and in concentrations of pancreatic enzymes and bicarbonate. Affected enzyme levels include trypsin, chymotrypsin, carboxypeptidase, amylase, and lipase. This leads to a maldigestion of ingested nutrients including fats and protein.

Because of the lipase deficiency, fat-soluble vitamin (A, D, E, and K) deficiencies sometimes occur. Whether lipase is involved in fat-soluble vitamin absorption directly (e.g., micelle formation) or indirectly, with continuing steatorrhea resulting in abnormally high losses of these nutrients in the feces, is unclear. While pancreatic involvement is predominantly exocrine in nature, insulin deficiency has been described in many older cystic fibrosis patients. The carbohydrate intolerance observed is characterized by low insulin concentrations and enhanced peripheral sensitivity to insulin. This complication involves an increase in the number of insulin receptors with decreased affinity for insulin. Despite a concomitantly increased tissue affinity for insulin, 8% of cystic fibrosis children older than 12 years of age require insulin therapy. Whether this endocrine dysfunction is actually caused by the exocrine disease or results independently through a common pathogenic process is unclear.[11]

The liver is sometimes involved in cystic fibrosis. Biliary cirrhosis secondary to bile duct obstruction occurs in as many as 18% of patients, while fatty infiltration may occur in about 30% of patients in a pattern unrelated to nutritional status. Bile duct obstruction occurs with inspissated mucus and may lead to focal or multilobar cirrhosis.[12] Such hepatic involvement, which can occur at any age, is more common as the cystic fibrosis life span increases and can lead to portal hypertension and thus bleeding esophageal varices and hypersplenism. The most common laboratory abnormality associated with hepatic involvement is elevated serum alkaline phosphatase (hepatic isoenzyme).

PULMONARY SYSTEM

Involvement of the respiratory tract accounts for the vast majority of morbidity and mortality associated with cystic fibrosis. Manifestations within this organ system result from the accumulation of viscous mucus in the small airways. There are two important consequences of this pulmonary condition: obstruction and infection/inflammation.

Obstruction of both small and large airways by thick mucus results in air trapping, bronchiectasis, and atelectasis, resulting in a COPD phenomenon not unlike emphysema in presentation (although little alveolar septal destruction occurs). Hyperinflation or dilation of the air spaces is the common lesion. Further, the persistence of this same mucus is an excellent growth medium for microorganisms, and pulmonary infections are commonplace despite normal host defense mechanisms. While bacterial infection is thought to be the major factor in this aspect of the respiratory disease, it is clear that viruses and other nonbacterial pathogens play an important pathologic role as well.[13–15] Environmental factors, such as exposure to tobacco smoke, also contribute.[16] The three most common bacterial pathogens isolated from the respiratory secretions (sputum) of cystic fibrosis patients are *Staphylococcus aureus, Pseudomonas aeruginosa,* and *Haemophilus influenzae,* with *P. aeruginosa* predominating throughout life. *Proteus* and *Klebsiella* species are observed much less frequently. The mucoid strains (alginate producers) of *P. aeruginosa* commonly observed in cystic fibrosis have been reported by some to be particularly resistant to antibiotics,[17] as are nonmotile forms. The isolation of *Burkholderia cepacia* from the sputum of cystic fibrosis patients has become more common at some cystic fibrosis centers. The significance of the presence of this highly contagious organism varies from one patient to the next. Three fairly distinct syndromes associated with this *B. cepacia* have been described: asymptomatic colonization, chronic deterioration with intermittent fever and weight loss, and rapid, usually fatal deterioration.[18] The nature of the initially cultured oropharyngeal flora in patients less than 2 years of age has prognostic significance. The finding of *P. aeruginosa* or *P. aeruginosa* plus *S. aureus* in initial cultures appears to be related to increased morbidity and mortality, respectively.[19]

It is believed that the presence of the above bacteria is responsible for a portion of the destructive changes to the lungs in cystic fibrosis due to both direct damage from bacterial toxins and the body's immune reaction to the presence of these same bacteria. For example, it has been shown that *P. aeruginosa,* which elaborates a number of extracellular toxins, proteases, hemolysins, and exopolysaccharides that may be responsible for direct or indirect pulmonary damage, increases mucin production in respiratory epithelium and stimulates the production of immune complexes (IgG and IgM), which may also contribute to local damage. Elevated levels of such mediators as granulocyte elastase, tumor necrosis factor-alpha, interleukin 1 and 2, and related complexes with associated inhibitors have been well documented in cystic fibrosis patients. The inflammatory reaction in response to the inability to clear the lower airways of bacterial pathogens tends to be excessive. One inflammatory mediator that clearly contributes to pulmonary pathophysiology is neutrophil elastase.[20] Present in excess, it overwhelms and neutralizes native antiproteases (α_1 antitrypsin and secretory leukocyte protease inhibitor), destroys structural fibers, and inhibits complement mediated phagocytosis and antipseudomonal antibodies. Combined with other inflammatory mediators, a self-sustaining, vicious cycle leading to progressive and often permanent tissue damage is established. The neutrophil influx that is part of this cycle results in release of neutrophil-derived DNA, which is thought to contribute to sputum viscosity. The occasional presence of *Aspergillus fumagatus* in the sputum of these patients may also contribute to the pulmonary pathology.

The major consequence of these pulmonary processes is a decrease in gas exchange by the lungs. The challenge of moving air into and out of such congested airways often requires the use of accessory muscles resulting in an increased anterior-posterior chest diameter (also referred to as "barrel chest"), a flattened diaphragm, and pulmonary hypertension. Pneumothorax occurs, as does right-sided heart failure (cor pulmonale), secondary to the pulmonary hypertension. While seldom overt clinically, findings such as right ventricular hypertrophy, increased heart weight, and right atrial and right ventricular chamber dilation are usually present at autopsy.[21] Digital clubbing, a common finding in cystic fibrosis as well as other chronic pulmonary conditions, is thought to be related to chronic hypoxia.

The upper respiratory tract is also involved; sinusitis and nasal polyposis occur in 90 and 50% of patients, respectively.[22] Sinusitis is chronic in character and acute symptoms are unusual. While its etiology is not entirely clear, sinusitis may result from obstruction of the sinus ducts, preventing drainage, and is apparently not related to the underlying lung disease.[23] The bacteria generally isolated in these cases of sinusitis include *P. aeruginosa, H. influenzae,* streptococci, and anaerobes. Usually, the same strain of *P. aeruginosa* found in the lungs is present in the upper airways (nasopharynx, sinuses) and may represent a reservoir for the pathogen. Symptomatic patients are often treated medically or surgically.

SWEAT GLANDS

The abnormally high concentrations of both sodium and chloride in the sweat of cystic fibrosis patients due to defective salt reabsorption can result in the need for supplementary dietary intake of these electrolytes and forms the basis for the diagnosis of the disease. Sodium and chloride are not excreted in abnormally high concentrations by the sweat glands. Instead, there is a failure of the sweat ducts to reabsorb these electrolytes in a normal fashion, apparently because of a chloride impermeability in the sweat ducts. Similar abnormalities are seen in the excretions of the salivary glands.

REPRODUCTIVE SYSTEM

Of males with cystic fibrosis, 95% are sterile because of abnormal development or obstruction of the epididymis, vas deferens, and seminal vesicles, with resulting aspermia. There is late maturation of the reproductive system in both sexes. Females also have less than normal fertility due to the production of abnormal cervical mucus. Nonetheless, due to greater life expectancy in these patients, increasing numbers are becoming mothers. In these individuals, the course and tolerance of pregnancy are related to pregravid nutritional and pulmonary status.[24]

HEMATOLOGIC SYSTEM

Anemia is observed in some cystic fibrosis patients despite chronic hypoxia. The apparent deficient erythroid response occurs, at least in part, from disturbances in erythropoietin regulation and iron availability (impaired GI absorption). Despite the chronic hypoxia characteristic of cystic fibrosis, erythropoietin concentrations are normal or low. The condition is characterized by decreased hematocrit, and serum ferritin, increased carboxyhemoglobin and normal or low hemoglobin. Vitamin E concentrations are usually normal. Many patients have documentable iron deficiency the causes of which appear to include decreased dietary intake, malabsorption, and blood loss.

BONE AND JOINT

Arthritis occurs in cystic fibrosis patients and can take one of several forms.[25] This arthritis may be either mono- or polyarticular and is usually nondestructive. An episodic form is most common and may be due to immune complexes formed in response to the chronic pulmonary infections. Hypertrophic osteoarthropathy occurs in cystic fibrosis as it does in association with other pulmonary diseases. The incidence of arthritis may be increasing as median survival age increases. Osteopenia and osteoporosis also occur with abnormally high frequency in adult cystic fibrosis patients. The causes of the resultant bone demineralization are mutifactorial and include vitamin D malabsorption and decreased vitamin conversion (via sunlight), delayed puberty and endocrine development, poor nutrition, limited physical activity, and chronic acidosis.

DIAGNOSIS

Cystic fibrosis is normally diagnosed on the basis of an abnormal sweat test. In such a test, a sample of sweat is collected (usually with the use of pilocarpine iontophoresis) and the concentration of chloride is determined. A chloride concentration of 60 mEq/L or more is considered diagnostic, although values up to 80 may be observed in noncystic fibrosis adults. A number of other disorders, such as adrenal insufficiency and hypothyroidism, may be inconsistently associated with elevated sweat chloride concentrations but do not generally present a problem in the differential diagnosis of cystic fibrosis. Ninety-eight percent of cystic fibrosis patients will have a sweat chloride concentration 60 mEq/L or greater. The remaining 2% will have sweat chloride concentrations between 50 and 60 mEq/L and the test may have to be repeated one or more times to obtain definitive results. Nonetheless, the results of a sweat test are not necessarily proof-positive of the presence or absence of cystic fibrosis. The presence of chronic obstructive respiratory disease, exocrine pancreatic insufficiency, and/or a positive family history of the disease help to confirm the diagnosis. Genetic analysis is now also possible and may be used to diagnose the disease *in utero* or to detect heterozygotes (carriers) with obvious implications for genetic counseling.

CLINICAL PRESENTATION AND COURSE

The clinical signs and symptoms of cystic fibrosis occur as direct consequences of the pathophysiologic processes previously described. Thus, the clinical findings can be conveniently subdivided by organ system.

GASTROINTESTINAL SYSTEM

Intestinal symptomatology is secondary to obstruction and maldigestion of nutrients. Obstruction, manifested as meconium ileus or distal intestinal obstruction syndrome, causes symptoms such as vomiting of bile-stained material, abdominal distention, and pain. Pain may be an especially prominent feature when obstruction results in intussusception.

The more frequent GI clinical presentation is due to maldigestion of ingested food resulting in steatorrhea and malnutrition. Stools are characterized by their foul smell, bulky, greasy nature, and abnormally high number per day and may precipitate rectal prolapse. The stool's high fat content results from the relative lipase deficiency. Perhaps the most significant consequence of maldigestion is malnutrition. Cystic fibrosis children characteristically fall below age-related norms for both weight and height.

PULMONARY SYSTEM

The respiratory symptoms of cystic fibrosis are those of obstructive disease and pneumonia. Hypoxia with resultant cyanosis and digital clubbing are common. Likewise, labored breathing with retractions and resultant increased anterior-posterior chest diameter, flattened diaphragm, and overaeration observed on chest roentgenogram are frequent findings.

Acutely, a patient's respiratory status follows a cyclical pattern, from a state of relative well-being to one of acute pulmonary deterioration theoretically paralleling the course of the infectious process. Marked declines in pulmonary status (presumably secondary to infection) are referred to as acute respiratory exacerbations and are generally associated with symptoms of acute bacterial endobronchial infection. Thus, fever, increased coughing, increased sputum production, change in sputum character (e.g., thicker, change in color), increased respiratory rate, dyspnea on exertion, increased oxygen requirements, and decreased exercise tolerance are commonly described. Symptoms of chronic sinusitis and nasal polyposis may include rhinorrhea, nasal obstruction, pain over affected sinuses, and disturbances of smell.

Concomitantly, laboratory tests of peripheral blood reveal an increased white blood count with increased polymorphonuclear leukocytes and immature forms consistent with acute infection. Tests of pulmonary function often demonstrate both acute and long-term changes in forced vital capacity, forced expiratory volume, and residual volume. Tests reflective of small airway function are more markedly affected as the pulmonary disease progresses. Arterial blood gases typically reveal hypoxia and hypercapnia.

OTHER SIGNS AND SYMPTOMS

The relative insulin deficiency observed in older cystic fibrosis patients is often asymptomatic and only detected on laboratory analysis of serum performed for other reasons. Symptomatic patients present as untreated cases of diabetes mellitus type II. Cases of cor pulmonale are not usually clinically evident until signs of left-sided heart failure ensue. An enlargement of cardiac size is often noted on routine chest roentgenogram prior to that time, however. Signs and symptoms of anemia and arthritis with cystic fibrosis patients do not differ from those in other patients.

While the abnormal loss of sodium and chloride in the sweat of cystic fibrosis patients seldom results in profound symptoms such as those of heat prostration, this phenomenon has formed the basis of some large-scale public awareness/screening programs due to the resultant "salty" taste on the skin of affected patients.

COURSE OF DISEASE

Cystic fibrosis is a heterogeneous disease in terms of initial presentation, organ involvement, and clinical course. Most patients are not diagnosed at birth. Only 16% of affected patients have meconium ileus, few neonatal screening programs are in place, and prenatal diagnosis is early in its implementation. Therefore, the average patient is diagnosed later in life based on a history of recurrent respiratory infections, steatorrhea, and/or failure to thrive. The median age at diagnosis is 7 months and most are diagnosed by 12 years of age.[26]

The course of the disease after diagnosis varies markedly from one patient to the next, perhaps based on genotype, as discussed previously. Some patients have a rapid downhill course based on pulmonary involvement, while others suffer only from GI complaints for many years. While the expected life span of cystic fibrosis patients has increased to 25–30 years of age in the last two decades, some patients still die early in life secondary to a fulminant pulmonary process. Some, however, due to minimal involvement and mild course, are not diagnosed until their second decade of life. The increased longevity now realized with early diagnosis and aggressive treatment has led to an increase in formerly unusual complications, such as diabetes and hepatic disease. Two-year mortality rates higher than 50% are associated with FEV_1 less than 30% of predicted, Pa_{O_2} less than 50 mm Hg or P_{CO_2} greater than 50 mm Hg.[27]

TREATMENT

GASTROINTESTINAL SYSTEM

The treatment of GI involvement is ultimately aimed at correcting the nutritional deficit present in so many patients. In addition to the pancreatic enzyme replacement and other drug therapy described in the following section, nutritional supplementation is frequently employed. Nutritional interventions range from behavioral modification to nocturnal feedings via gastrostomies.[28,29]

Pancreatic Enzyme Supplementation

The backbone of GI therapy in cystic fibrosis is pancreatic enzyme replacement or supplementation. The preferred products are microencapsulated, although powders are marketed and useful in patients who are unable to swallow capsules or to otherwise use the microencapsulated beads they contain. Microencapsulated products protect the contained enzymes from destruction by gastric acid and may be given in much lower doses than their predecessors, which were susceptible to acid breakdown. The most contemporary enzyme replacement products vary mainly in enzyme content per capsule, with lipase content being the chief variable. Whether such variations from one product or brand to the next make a difference clinically is often a matter for speculation as scant data exist to support the superiority of one over another. Representative products and their contents are presented in Table 29.2.

Before the introduction of microencapsulated enzyme products, various maneuvers were utilized to circumvent or overcome the problem of acid breakdown. The most obvious of these was to administer large quantities of

TABLE 29.2. PANCREATIC ENZYME PRODUCTS

Trade Name	Manufacturer	Enzyme Content (units)			Form[a]
		Lipase	Protease	Amylase	
Cotazym	Organon	8000	30,000	30,000	C
Cotazym-S		5000	20,000	20,000	ECM
Creon	Reid-Rowell	8000	13,000	30,000	ECM
Ilozyme	Adria	11,000	30,000	30,000	T
Pancrease	McNeil	4000	25,000	20,000	ECM
Pancrease MT4		4000	12,000	12,000	ECM
Pancrease MT10		10,000	30,000	30,000	ECM
Pancrease MT16		16,000	48,000	48,000	ECM
Ultrase MT12	Scandipharm	12,000	39,000	39,000	ECM
Ultrase MT20		20,000	65,000	66,000	ECM
Ultrase MT24		24,000	78,000	78,000	ECM
Viokase	Robins	s8000	30,000	30,000	T
Viokase		16,800	70,000	70,000	P[b]
Zymase	Organon	12,000	24,000	24,000	ECM

[a]Dosage form: C, capsule; ECM, enteric coated microspheres or beads; T, tablet; P, powder.
[b]Viokase powder, units of enzymes per 700 mg.

enzyme product. Enteric coated (microencapsulated) have largely solved this problem. The occasional patient may yet require large quantities of even the microencapsulated enzyme product. Whether such difficulties are due to residual acid breakdown or perhaps low pH in the upper small intestine (secondary to deficient bicarbonate excretion by the pancreas), resulting in a failure to dissolve the coating of the microencapsulated beads, is unknown. Defective enteric coating on some generic brands has also been described and led to FDA reclassification of these products as prescription drugs, requiring bioequivalence data. Histamine H_2-receptor antagonists have been used to reduce the enzyme dose when residual acid breakdown is suspected. Omeprazole, which decreases gastric acid by inhibiting parietal cell H^+/K^+-ATPase, has been shown to be an effective adjunct in patients with some residual pancreatic function but steatorrhea despite high-dose enzyme supplementation.

For patients who are unable to swallow capsules, the contents may be emptied into applesauce, jelly, or some other vehicle provided that the patient does not chew the microencapsulated beads. Side effects of pancreatic enzyme products are unusual. Perianal irritation resembling diaper rash may occur in infants fed excess quantities of enzyme powders. Hyperuricosuria has also been reported to occur secondary to pancreatic enzyme use, apparently related to their high purine content. A dose-related side effect of lipase consisting of colonic strictures, termed *fibrosing colonopathy,* has been described in patients receiving per meal lipase doses in excess of 6000 units/kg, leading to dosage recommendations below this threshold.[30]

Vitamin Supplementation

While clinically evident fat-soluble vitamin deficiencies are unusual in those patients taking adequate pancreatic enzymes and receiving a balanced diet, obvious vitamin K deficiency, manifested as bleeding diathesis, has been reported.[31] Demineralization of bone has also been described,[32] and vitamin E deficiency has been related to neurologic dysfunction.[33] Further, appropriate laboratory tests (serum carotene, vitamin E, and cholecalciferol concentrations) often will help document other deficiencies, leading to recommendations for additional supplementation of these vitamins. Water-miscibilized vitamin A, 4000 IU/d, vitamin E, 50 mg (50 IU *dl*-alpha-tocopherol acetate) per day, and vitamin K, 5 mg orally twice a week, have each been recommended. To put these doses in perspective, it should be noted that the adult recommended daily allowances (RDA) for vitamins A and E are 1000 IU and 8–10 mg, respectively. It should also be noted that appropriately adjusted doses of fat-soluble preparations may be more cost effective than their water-miscible counterparts (e.g., 800 IU fat-soluble vitamin E versus 200 IU water miscible vitamin E).[34]

Treating Meconium Ileus

The treatment of meconium ileus or distal intestinal obstruction syndrome can sometimes be limited to the use of enemas with contrast materials such as Gastrografin (Squibb) or Hypaque (Winthrop–Breon).[35] Unfortunately, surgery (bowel resection and primary anastomosis) is more often necessary to treat this condition and prevent its complications.[36]

Prevention and Treatment of Cirrhosis

Ursodeoxycholic acid, a bile acid with choleretic properties, has been shown to produce morphologic and functional improvement in affected patients with long-term treatment.[37] The effects are dose-related and 20 mg/kg/d has been recommended.[38] The potential of administering this agent prophylactically to patients at risk for liver disease, if feasible, has been speculatively proposed.[39]

CARDIOVASCULAR SYSTEM

Various modalities have been used in attempts to treat the pulmonary hypertension and secondary cor pulmonale of cystic fibrosis. These treatments, which include the use of vasodilators, inotropic agents, and diuretics, have all resulted in limited and transient effects. This is most likely due to the fact that none of these modes of therapy addresses the underlying cause of the cor pulmonale, hypoxia. Likewise, supplemental (often nocturnal) oxygen treatment has also failed to affect mortality rates or disease progression, although it does appear to prevent exercise-induced oxygen desaturation as well as that occurring with sleep.

PULMONARY SYSTEM

Management of the pulmonary component of cystic fibrosis can be broken down into two areas: respiratory therapy, including anti-inflammatory therapy, and anti-infective therapy.

Respiratory Therapy

The cornerstone of pulmonary therapy is percussion and postural drainage, which aids in the clearance of pulmonary mucus and is performed as often as five times daily or more during an acute pulmonary exacerbation. Note that the benefits of percussion and postural drainage are acute in nature, that data demonstrating long-term benefit are scant, and that exercise alone, in capable patients, may be just as effective in helping to clear mucus from the airways.[40] New flutter devices also appear promising in this regard. Percussion is often preceded by nebulizer therapy during which nebulized sterile water or 0.9% sodium chloride solution is breathed to liquefy pulmonary secretions. Bronchodilators and/or mucolytic agents (e.g., *N*-acetylcysteine) may be added to the nebulizer solution to prevent bronchospasm and further liquefy pulmonary secretions, respectively. While the effects of bronchodilators administered by inhalation are readily demonstrated with pulmonary function tests, those of mucolytic agents are not as obvious and a number of attempts to demonstrate the effects of inhaled *N*-acetylcysteine (Mucomyst, Mead Johnson) have been unsuccessful. Moreover, many patients prefer not to use *N*-acetylcysteine because of its unpleasant taste and odor and because it often induces bronchospasm. Normal saline and sodium bicarbonate solution are also commonly administered by aerosol as aids to sputum expectoration, but again documentation of efficacy is elusive.

Recently, recombinant human DNase has been approved for use in cystic fibrosis. When given by inhalation (2.5 mg once or twice daily), rhDNase reduces the viscosity of cystic fibrosis sputum and leads to statistically significant, although modest, improvement in indices of pulmonary function.[41] The cost of this therapy may not be justified for the majority of cystic fibrosis patients because the average improvement in pulmonary function is small.

In attempts to block the consequence of the inflammatory component of the disease, corticosteroid therapy has been evaluated. While early results were encouraging,[42] a large, multicenter, placebo-controlled trial found alternate-day prednisone treatment to be neither effective nor safe.[43] The efficacy of short-term corticosteroid use as well as that of less toxic agents, such as ibuprofen, will continue to be evaluated. While data concerning inhaled corticosteroids are lacking, a recently reported long-term trial of oral ibuprofen indicates a positive effect in slowing pulmonary deterioration.[44]

Because many cystic fibrosis patients have a reactive airways component to their pulmonary disease, systemic bronchodilators such as theophylline and β agonists may be of benefit. Responsiveness to such agents should be documented, however, before a protracted course is begun. Normal antiasthmatic doses of most bronchodilators should be appropriate for cystic fibrosis patients. However, theophylline clearance may be different in cystic fibrosis patients,[45,46] and bioavailability of some products may be decreased,[46] sometimes necessitating the use of higher than usual doses. The determination of a theophylline dose in a specific cystic fibrosis patient should be based on that individual's dose/serum concentration relationship (i.e., individual pharmacokinetic values). Because cystic fibrosis patients are at high risk to develop the complications of influenza, influenza vaccine should be administered on a yearly basis and amantadine prophylaxis or treatment may be indicated as well. Approximately 20% of patients with chronic sinusitis will eventually require surgical intervention.

Antibiotic Therapy

The use of antibiotics in cystic fibrosis patients is somewhat controversial and certainly challenging. Controversy exists because of the observation that during treatment for an acute pulmonary exacerbation, clinical improvement occurs despite failure to eradicate bacterial pathogens from the sputum. This suggests to some that the bacteria present are colonizers rather than pathogens, which would argue against the use of antibiotics. The results of one published study comparing antibiotic to placebo suggested antibiotics may not always contribute to recovery from an acute exacerbation.[47] However, this small study only evaluated patients with mild to moderate disease and therefore is not convincing. At the same time, these results do emphasize the fact that not all exacerbations of pulmonary disease in cystic fibrosis are due to bacteria. It is logical that other factors such as viral infection and air pollutants could at least contribute to such episodes. Clearly, bacteria such as *P. aeruginosa* are pathogenic both by virtue of inherent properties such as exotoxin release and the body's immune response to their presence and products. Moreover, it is apparent that sublethal effects of antibiotics on *P. aeruginosa* (e.g., decreased exoenzyme production) contribute to clinical improvement.[48] Therefore, the routine presence of known bacterial pathogens dictates antibiotic use and most if not all clinicians caring for cystic fibrosis patients regularly employ antibiotic therapy.

Once one is committed to antibiotic therapy, a number of other important, and sometimes perplexing, issues emerge. These include the selection of the best antibiotic(s), for the individual patient, the best dosage and dosage regimen, given altered pharmacokinetics, the optimal route of administration, emergence of antibiotic resistant bacteria, and identification of appropriate endpoints of therapy.

Selection of Antibiotic

Specific therapy is directed at proven or likely pathogens such as *P. aeruginosa* and *S. aureus,* and usually includes an aminoglycoside and an extended-spectrum penicillin. Single-agent therapy with newer antibiotics, especially on an outpatient basis, is frequently employed at some centers where significant resistance to these agents has not yet emerged. Such agents would include ceftazidime, aztreonam, and ciprofloxacin (Cipro, Miles). However, the evidence supporting the clinical superiority of two-drug combinations over single-agent therapy leads many clinicians to treat only with combinations.[49–52] The fact that such combinations are sometimes synergistic *in vitro* and the possibility that they may act to suppress or delay the emergence of resistance[53,54] provide attractive rationales for their use. Further, *in vitro* synergism has been reported to persist even in the face of resistance to one of the single agents in a given combination.[55] Lastly, monodrug therapy has been met with rapid emergence of resistance.[56]

Unlike other cases of lower respiratory tract infection, organism-specific drug treatment may be based on results from sputum cultures in cystic fibrosis patients because good agreement between sputum and thoracotomy cultures has been demonstrated.[57] Typically, such results will lead one to prescribe or recommend aminoglycoside/extended-spectrum penicillin combinations although newer antibiotics such as ciprofloxacin and older agents such as colistin may also play a role. While the complete eradication of *S. aureus* and *H. influenzae* are practical goals or endpoints of antibiotic therapy, the total eradication of *Pseudomonas* species is infrequent and transient. Similarly, the complete resolution of pulmonary signs and symptoms becomes less and less likely as the disease progresses.

Selection of Dose—Altered Pharmacokinetics

While altered pharmacokinetics in cystic fibrosis is not limited to antibiotics (Table 29.3), this drug class has been the most extensively studied. As is true for theophylline, many cystic fibrosis patients have increased total body clearance for many antibiotics, including the aminoglycosides, some of the beta-lactams and trimethoprim/sulfamethoxazole. Thus, higher doses of these agents may be necessary to produce therapeutic concentrations (Table 29.4). Unfortunately, these alterations in pharmacokinetics are neither consistent nor predictable. Why the pharmacokinetics of these antibiotics are different in cystic fibrosis patients is unknown. It appears that for many beta-lactam antibiotics, increased total body clearance could be accounted for by increased renal clearance. It should also be pointed out that renal function, as reflected by glomerular filtration rate and renal blood flow, is not different in cystic fibrosis patients as compared to non-cystic fibrosis controls.[75] Moreover, a concomitant increase in renal clearance does not completely explain the increase in total body clearance of aminoglycosides, leading some to speculate about extrarenal pathways for elimination.[69] In any event, increased total body clearance dictates higher doses in many, but not all, patients. However, a range of dosage requirements should be expected consistent with a range in the variation of pharmacokinetics in these patients. For example, experience with netilmicin revealed a dosage requirement range of 7–17 mg/kg/d to achieve peak concentrations (0.5 hour after the end of a drug infusion) of 8 μg/mL or greater.[71] The mean dosage requirement in this study was approximately 12 mg/kg/d. Peak concentrations of this magnitude are believed to be necessary to adequately treat pneumonia caused by gram-negative bacteria.[76,77]

While the pharmacokinetics of antibiotics may correlate with the severity of pulmonary disease,[78,79] it is not possible to predict changes in antibiotic pharmacokinetics in cystic fibrosis patients based on markers of clinical status or disease progression. Attempts to correlate antibiotic pharmacokinetics with Shwachman score (a gross method for quantitation of disease status) have been unsuccessful.[59,80] Therefore, attempts to guide aminoglycoside dosing are often based on measured serum concentrations during a course of therapy. However, this method may also meet with mixed success due to the changing pharmacokinetics of this family of antibiotics during an acute pulmonary exacerbation.[81] This observation should not deter one from attempts to adjust doses to desirable concentrations based on serum concentration determinations and subsequent pharmacokinetic calculations.

Alternate Routes of Administration

An additional form of antibiotic administration that is intuitively attractive in patients with cystic fibrosis is by inhala-

TABLE 29.3. CHANGES IN PHARMACOKINETICS IN CYSTIC FIBROSIS

Agent	$\beta t_{1/2}$	V_d	CL_B	CL_R	Ref.
Antibiotics					
Methicillin	NC	I	I	I	58
Cloxacillin	D	I	I	I	59
Dicloxacillin	I	NR	NR	I	60
Azlocillin	D	I	I	NR	61
Piperacillin	D	I	I	NR	62
Ticarcillin	D	NC	I	I	63
Aztreonam	D	I	I	I	64
Ceftazidime	D	I	I	I	65
Imipenem	NC	I	I	NR	66
Trimethoprim/sulfamethoxazole	D/D	NC/NC	I/I	I/NC	67
Gentamicin	NC	I	I	NR	68
Tobramycin	NC	I	I	NC	69
Amikacin	NC	I	I	I	70
Netilmicin	NC	I	I	NR	71
Fleroxacin	D	D	I	D	72
Other					
Theophylline	D	I	I	I	45
Furosemide	NC	NC	I	NC	73
Acetaminophen	NC	NR	I	NR	74

Key: $\beta t_{1/2}$, elimination half-life; V_d, apparent volume of distribution; CL_B, total body clearance; CL_R, renal clearance; D, decreased; I, increased; NC, no change; NR, not reported.

tion of aerosolized solution. Such a route of administration should, theoretically, deliver the drug to the actual site of infection and perhaps avoid systemic toxicity. Certainly, many classes of antibiotics including beta-lactams, aminoglycosides, and polymyxins have been administered to cystic fibrosis patients in this fashion, often in conjunction with systemic antibiotics. However, until recently no clear effect or advantage had been consistently demonstrated. Earlier studies suffered from lack of controls, small sample size, and a failure to ensure that the respiratory equipment used would, in fact, guarantee that the drug is delivered to the small airways. In a recent, placebo-controlled, multicenter trial, 600 mg tobramycin administered by aerosol three times daily was found to produce a small but statistically significant improvement in FEV_1, FVC, $FEF_{25-75\%}$, *P. aeruginosa* density in sputum, and peripheral white blood cell count.[82] This being recognized, appropriate clinical circumstances for this form (type and condition of patient), length, and frequency of therapy remain to be clarified. Last, if such doses are to be used, preservative-free antibiotic preparations should be utilized. The efficacy of smaller doses of inhaled aminoglycosides remains unproven.

Bacterial Resistance

As already noted, emergence of antimicrobial resistance seems to follow the introduction and use of new antibiotics.[56] *P. aeruginosa* can exhibit many resistance mechanisms revealed as resistance to quinolones (altered DNA gyrase target site), β-lactams (production of Bush group 1 β-lactamase), aminoglycosides (decreased permeability and modifying enzymes), and carbapenems (decreased permeability). *B. cepacia* is inherently resistant to most antibiotics. Methicillin-resistant staphylococci are increasingly common in institutional settings and will become a more pervasive problem in cystic fibrosis populations. These phenomena require close attention to susceptibility reports in selecting therapy and the avoidance of unnecessary or unnecessarily protracted courses of antibiotic therapy.

Recommendations for Antibiotic Therapy

Despite these inherent difficulties, a number of recommendations regarding the use of systemic antibiotics in cystic fibrosis can be made. The selection of antibiotics should be based on specific culture and susceptibility results. Aminoglycosides should be initially dosed at the upper end of the normal dosage range (e.g., 6–7.5 mg/kg/d for tobramycin) and serum concentrations should be determined frequently so that dosage can be appropriately adjusted to achieve peak concentrations of at least 8 but not exceeding 12 μg/mL. Keep in mind that aminoglycoside serum half-lives may lengthen during the course of treatment so that a constant relationship between dose and serum concentration may not exist. Upward adjustments in dosage should therefore be made with some degree of caution and should be followed with further determination of serum concentrations. Once-

TABLE 29.4. ANTIBIOTIC DOSES IN CYSTIC FIBROSIS

Antibiotic	Dose (mg/kg/d)	Regimen	Adult Maximum Dose (g/d)
Parenteral Antibiotics			
Tobramycin,[a] Gentamicin,[a] or Netilmicin[a]	6–9	q 6–8 h	NA
Amikacin[a]	20–30	q 6–8 h	NA
Azlocillin	400–600	q 4–6 h	24
Aztreonam	200	q 6 h	8
Carbenicillin	400–600	q 4–6 h	40
Ceftazidime	150	q 8 h	6
Colistin	6–8	q 6–8 h	NA
Imipenem	45–100	q 6 h	4
Nafcillin	100	q 4–6 h	6
Ticarcillin	400–600	q 4–6 h	18
Ticarcillin/clavulanate	400–600	q 4–6 h	18
Piperacillin	400–600	q 4–6 h	18
Oral Antibiotics			
Ciprofloxacin[b]	1500 mg/d	q 12 h	1.5
Cephalexin	50–100	q 6–8 h	6
Dicloxacillin	80–100	q 6 h	6
Trimethoprim/sulfamethoxazole	10–15[c]	q 12 h	0.64[c]
Inhaled Antibiotics			
Colistin	150 mg/d	q 6–12 h	NA
Gentamicin or Tobramycin	60–1800 mg/d	q 6–12 h	NA
Polymixin B	250 mg/d	q 6–12 h	NA

[a]Starting doses; adjust to desired serum concentrations based on dose/serum concentration relationship.
[b]Adult dose.
[c]Based on trimethoprim.

daily administration of aminoglycosides is gaining popularity in other settings. Obviously, such a dosing practice would result in much larger peak concentrations than those previously mentioned. Efficacy of such dosing regimens in cystic fibrosis patients has not yet been determined, but this practice is likely to be increasingly employed as cystic fibrosis-specific data are generated.

Beta-lactam antibiotics such as extended-spectrum penicillins should be prescribed with aminoglycosides to take advantage of their frequent synergy and prevent the emergence of resistance. These agents should be prescribed in large doses to delay stepwise resistance. Ticarcillin, azlocillin, and piperacillin should be prescribed in a dose of at least 350 mg/kg/d divided into 4–6 doses. For patients with *P. aeruginosa* and *S. aureus,* the combination of an aminoglycoside and ticarcillin/clavulanate or piperacillin/tazobactam would be expected to be as effective as an aminoglycoside, and extended-spectrum penicillin and nafcillin. Selection among these agents should be based on local susceptibility patterns and cost considerations. The possible increased incidence of fever and exanthema with the newer pencillins should be kept in mind.[83] Aztreonam would be a safe and effective β-lactam to use in patients experiencing these serum sickness-like reactions to the penicillins.[84] In older patients with *P. aeruginosa* isolates with broad resistance patterns, the clinician should work closely with the microbiology laboratory to identify effective agents or combinations. The potential use of older agents with unique mechanisms of action, such as colistin, should not be overlooked.

Oral antibiotics should be prescribed in symptomatic outpatients with susceptible pathogens in their sputum. Agents with activity against common pathogens such as *S. aureus* and *H. influenzae* are useful in this setting. These typically include such antibiotics as first-generation cephalosporins, trimethoprim/sulfamethoxazole, and amoxicillin/clavulanic acid. The use of such agents on a "prophylactic" basis is discouraged because the presently available data suggesting a beneficial effect does not outweigh the risk of development of resistance among the common bacterial pathogens of cystic fibrosis.[85] The 4-fluoroquinolone antibiotic, ciprofloxacin, possesses potent activity against most cystic fibrosis pathogens and has been evaluated in adult patients undergoing pulmonary exacerbations. While not conclusive because of shortcomings in the studies, available data suggest that this oral agent is as effective as standard intravenous therapy.[86] The availability of a potent, oral antipseudomonal agent poses a number of potential uses in the cystic fibrosis population. However, keep in mind that repeated or long-term use will likely lead to resistance and that antibiotics only play a supportive role in the treatment of these patients. Thus, oral antibiotic therapy, regardless of efficacy, does not negate the need for other forms of therapy that are often best administered in the hospital setting. It should also be pointed out that while ciprofloxacin appears to be safe in patients less than 18 years of age with little evidence of joint or cartilage toxicity, the drug is yet to be approved for use in children by the FDA.[87] In the meantime, this agent should be used with caution in the younger population.

MONITORING DRUG THERAPY

GASTROINTESTINAL SYSTEM

The ultimate goal of pharmacotherapy for the GI involvement of cystic fibrosis is to affect optimal nutrition. Therefore, the patient's nutritional status should be closely monitored on both short- and long-term bases. Height and weight should be followed with time and anthropometric measure to give more precise information. From a specific drug standpoint, the adequacy of pancreatic enzyme replacement can be grossly assessed by following stool patterns with the goal of normal number per day and normal consistency. Any evidence of steatorrhea indicates suboptimal enzyme therapy. A more precise method would involve assessment of fat quantities in the stool. Vitamin status can be assessed though serum monitoring of fat-soluble vitamin concentrations.

PULMONARY SYSTEM

Pulmonary status can be monitored by a combination of clinical observation and examination and a variety of laboratory tests. Physical examination should focus on signs and symptoms of upper and lower respiratory tract infection. In addition, exercise tolerance, recent character of sputum production, and oxygen requirements are key to long-term and short-term assessment. With antibiotic and bronchodilator treatment of acute respiratory exacerbations, a return to pre-exacerbation clinical status, based on physical examination or pulmonary function testing, becomes a practical endpoint for antimicrobial treatment. While the goal of bacterial eradication is desirable, other attainable endpoints may be more reasonable, as discussed earlier. Bacterial density in sputum as well as sputum DNA and protein content have also been shown to be useful monitoring parameters.[88] Plasma inflammatory markers such as C-reactive protein may also be useful in this regard.[89] However, it should be noted that, of objective parameters, pulmonary function tests correlate best with clinical observations and scoring systems.[90] Response to intravenous antibiotics and aggressive chest physiotherapy, as measured by FEV_1 at the end of 1 week of treatment, has been used to predict total necessary length of therapy. In patients whose FEV_1 had recovered more than 40% at the end of 1 week, a total of 2 weeks of therapy was generally sufficient.[91] Little has been done by way of pharmacodynamic studies in treating cystic fibrosis. Therefore, symptomatic improvement is largely relied on to assess the relative success of antibiotic therapy. Oral antibiotic therapy should also be limited in length with specific endpoints, such as decreased cough and/or improved pulmonary function, identified as treatment commences.

NEW DIRECTIONS IN THERAPY

Now that the gene and gene product of cystic fibrosis have been identified, gene therapy becomes an obvious potential of treatment. Research to date has centered on introduction of the correct gene into affected tissues. Viral vectors, chiefly adenovirus, have been studied in animal models[92] and human trials are under way.[93] Liposomes may represent another useful delivery mode to introduce the correct gene.[94]

Other, novel approaches to therapy are currently being investigated. Protease inhibitors hold potential in this condition for reasons cited earlier. α_1-Antitrypsin administered by aerosol shows promise[95] as does secretory leukocyte protease inhibitor (SLPI). Further attempts to aid the body's host-defense mechanisms, as with intravenously administered immune globulin,[96] will also receive additional evaluation. In an attempt to approach directly the cellular defect in cystic fibrosis, the diuretic amiloride has been shown to possess positive activity in improving respiratory secretion rheology and clearance,[97] presumably by blocking excessive sodium reabsorption, and it is being further evaluated in a large-scale, controlled trial. At a similar level, the secretagogues, adenosine and uridine triphosphate (ATP and UTP), have been shown to increase chloride excretion in the epithelial cells of cystic fibrosis patients.[98]

It is hoped that some, if not all, of these approaches will provide viable additions to our pharmacologic armamentarium for this disease. For older, more severely affected patients who may not be able to benefit from such advances, organ transplants (single lung, double lung, heart/lung) are becoming more widely available. Although intraoperative mortality is high, overall results are positive.[99,100]

PROGNOSIS AND CONCLUSIONS

The prognosis for cystic fibrosis patients has improved substantially in the last few decades due to early diagnosis, aggressive management, and improved antibiotic therapy. Nonetheless the average life span of these patients has only risen into the third decade of life. Presumably because of the heterogeneous nature of the clinical presentation and course of the disease, there are still early deaths and substantial morbidity throughout life.

Pharmacotherapeutic intervention plays an important role in the management of these patients but is complex. The clinician is, as yet, faced with many unresolved issues in attempting to apply sound therapeutic principles in this population. While close attention should be paid to pharmacologic treatment, the approach to these patients should be multifaceted and multidisciplinary in character. In addition to the involvement of such pediatric subspecialties as pulmonology, gastroenterology, pharmacology, and infectious diseases, contributions from such areas as nutrition support and social work should be a regular and ongoing part of the management effort.

References

1. Anderson DH. Cystic fibrosis of the pancreas and its relation to celiac disease. Am J Dis Child 1938;56:344–399.
2. Steinberg AG, Brown DC. On the incidence of cystic fibrosis of the pancreas. Am J Hum Genet 1960;12:416–424.
3. Wright SE, Morton NE. Genetic studies on cystic fibrosis in Hawaii. Am J Hum Genet 1968;20:157–169.
4. Rommens JM, Iannuzzi MC, Kerem B, et al. Identification of the cystic fibrosis gene: Chromosome walking and jumping. Science 1989;245:1059–1065.
5. Riordan JR, Rommens JM, Kerem B, et al. Identification of the cystic fibrosis gene: Cloning and characterization of complementary DNA. Science 1989;245:1066–1073.
6. Kerem B, Rommens JM, Buchanan JA, et al. Identification of the cystic fibrosis gene: Genetic analysis. Science 1989; 245:1073–1080.
7. Welsh MJ, Smith AE. Molecular mechanisms of CFTR chloride channel dysfunction in cystic fibrosis. Cell 1993;73:1251–1254.
8. Kerem E, Corey M, Kerem B, et al. The relationship between genotype and phenotype in cystic fibrosis—analysis of the most common mutation (ΔF_{508}). N Engl J Med 1991;323:1517–1522.
9. Mohon RT, Wagener JS, Abman SH, et al. Relationship of genotype to early pulmonary function in infants with cystic fibrosis identified through neonatal screening. J Pediatr 1993;122:550–555.
10. Collins FC. Cystic fibrosis: Molecular biology and therapeutic implications. Science 1992;256:774–779.
11. Moran A, Diem P, Klein DJ, et al. Pancreatic endocrine function in cystic fibrosis. J Pediatr 1991;118:715–723.
12. Feigelson J, Anagnostopoulos C, Poquet M, et al. Liver cirrhosis—therapeutic implications and long term follow up. Arch Dis Child 1993;68:653–657.
13. Wang EEL, Prober CG, Manson B, et al. Association of respiratory viral infections with pulmonary deterioration in patients with cystic fibrosis. N Engl J Med 1984;311:1653–1658.
14. Abman SH, Ogle JW, Butler-Simon N, et al. Role of respiratory syncytial virus in early hospitalizations for respiratory distress of young infants with cystic fibrosis. J Pediatr 1988;113:826–830.
15. Pribble CG, Black PG, Bosso JA, et al. Clinical manifestations of exacerbations of cystic fibrosis associated with nonbacterial infections. J Pediatr 1990;117:200–204.
16. Campbell PW, Parker RA, Roberts BT, et al. Association of poor clinical status and heavy exposure to tobacco smoke in patients with cystic fibrosis who are homozygous for the F_{508} deletion. J Pediatr 1992;120:261–264.
17. May TB, Shinabarger D, Maharaj R, et al. Alginate synthesis by *Pseudomonas aeruginosa:* A key pathogenic factor in chronic pulmonary infections of cystic fibrosis patients. Clin Microbiol Rev 1991;4:191–206.
18. Isles A, Maclusky I, Corey M, et al. *Pseudomonas cepacia* infection in cystic fibrosis: An emerging problem. J Pediatr 1984;104:206–210.
19. Hudson VL, Wielinski CL, Regelmann WE. Prognostic implications of initial oropharyngeal bacterial flora in patients with cystic fibrosis diagnosed before the age of two years. J Pediatr 1993;122:854–860.
20. Davis PB. Cystic fibrosis from bench to bedside. N Engl J Med 1991;325:575–577.
21. Royce SW. Cor pulmonale in infancy and early childhood: Report of 34 patients with special reference to the occurrence of pulmonary disease in cystic fibrosis of the pancreas. Pediatrics 1951;8:255–274.
22. Triglia JM, Belus JF, Dessi P, et al. Rhinonasal manifestations of cystic fibrosis. Ann Otolaryngol Chir Cervicofac 1993;110:98–102.
23. Ledesma-Medina J, Osman MZ, Dirdany BR. Abnormal paranasal sinuses in patients with cystic fibrosis of the pancreas. Pediatr Radiol 1980;9:61–64.
24. Palmer J, Dillon-Baker C, Tecklin JS, et al. Pregnancy in patients with cystic fibrosis. Ann Int Med 1983;99:596–600.
25. Lawrence JM, Moore TL, Madson KL, et al. Arthropathies of cystic fibrosis: Case reports and review of the literature. J Rheumatol 1993;20(suppl 38):12–15.
26. FitzSimmons SC. The changing epidemiology of cystic fibrosis. J Pediatr 1993;122:1–9.
27. Kerem E, Reisman J, Corey M, et al. Prediction of mortality in patients with cystic fibrosis. N Engl J Med 1992;326:1187–1191.
28. Passero MA, Mulvihill MM, Hovell M. Increasing calorie consumption in children with cystic fibrosis: Replication with 2-year follow-up. J Appl Behav Anal 1993;26:435–450.
29. Steinkamp G, von der Hardt L. Improvement of nutritional status and lung function after long-term nocturnal gastrostomy feedings in cystic fibrosis. J Pediatr 1994;124:244–249.
30. Borowitz DS, Grand RJ, Durie PR. Use of pancreatic enzyme supplements for patients with cystic fibrosis in the context of fibrosing colonopathy. J Pediatr 1995;127:681–684.
31. Walters TR, Koch HF. Hemorrhagic diathesis and cystic fibrosis in infancy. Am J Dis Child 1972;124:641–642.
32. Mischler EH, Chesney J, Chesney RW, et al. Demineralization in cystic fibrosis. Am J Dis Child 1979;133:632–635.
33. Cynamon HA, Milov DE, Valenstein E, et al. Effect of vitamin E deficiency on neurologic function in patients with cystic fibrosis. J Pediatr 1988;113:637–640.

34. Nasr SZ, O'Leary MH, Hillerman C. Correction of vitamin E deficiency with fat-soluble versus water-miscible preparations of vitamin E in patients with cystic fibrosis. J Pediatr 1993;122:810–812.
35. Wagget J, Johnson DG, Borns P, et al. The nonoperative treatment of meconium ileus by Gastrografin enema. J Pediatr 1970;77:407–411.
36. Rescorla FJ, Grosfeld JL. Contemporary management of meconium ileus. World J Surg 1993;17:318–325.
37. Columbo C, Castellani MR, Balistreri WF, et al. Scintigraphic documentation of an improvement in hepatobiliary excretory function after treatment with ursodeoxycholic acid in patients with cystic fibrosis and associated liver disease. Hepatology 1992;15:677–684.
38. Columbo C, Crosignani A, Assaisso M, et al. Ursodeoxycholic acid therapy in cystic fibrosis—associated liver disease: A dose response study. Hepatology 1992;16:924–930.
39. Columbo C, Grazia M, Ferrari M, et al. Analysis of risk factors for the development of liver disease associated with cystic fibrosis. J Pediatr 1994;124:393–399.
40. Zach MS, Purrer B, Oberwaldner B. Effect of swimming on forced expiration and sputum clearance in cystic fibrosis. Lancet 1981;2:1201–1203.
41. Fuchs HJ et al, Borwitz DS, Christainsen DH, et al. Effect of aerosolized recombinant human DNase on exacerbations of respiratory symptoms and on pulmonary function in patients with cystic fibrosis. N Engl J Med 1994;331:637–642.
42. Auerbach HS, Williams M, Kirkpatrick JA, et al. Alternate-day prednisone reduces morbidity and improves pulmonary function in cystic fibrosis. Lancet 1985;2:686–688.
43. Rosenstein BJ, Eigen H. Risks of alternate-day prednisone in patients with cystic fibrosis. Pediatrics 1991;87:245–246.
44. Konstan MW, Byard PJ, Hoppel CL, et al. Effect of high-dose ibuprofen in patients with cystic fibrosis. N Engl J Med 1995;332:848–854.
45. Knoppert DC, Spino M, Beck R, et al. Cystic fibrosis: Enhanced theophylline metabolism may be linked to the disease. Clin Pharmacol Ther 1988;44:254–264.
46. Valet SB, Schwartz RH, Brooks JG. Pharmacokinetics of theophylline and bioavailability of sustained release theophylline preparation in patients with cystic fibrosis. Ann Allergy 1983;50:161–165.
47. Gold R, Carpenter S, Heurter H, et al. Randomized trial of ceftazidime versus placebo in the management of acute respiratory exacerbations in patients with cystic fibrosis. J Pediatr 1987;111:907–913.
48. Grimwood K, Semple RA, Rabin HR, et al. Elevated exoenzyme expression by *Pseudomonas aeruginosa* is correlated with exacerbations of lung disease in cystic fibrosis. Pediatr Pulmonol 1993;15:135–139.
49. Parry MF, Neu HC, Merlino M, et al. Treatment of pulmonary infections in patients with cystic fibrosis: A comparative study of ticarcillin and gentamicin. J Pediatr 1977;90:144–148.
50. Møller NE, Høiby N. Antibiotic treatment of chronic *Pseudomonas aeruginosa* infection in cystic fibrosis patients. Scand J Infect Dis 1981;24(suppl):87–91.
51. Friis B. Chemotherapy of chronic infections with mucoid *Pseudomonas aeruginosa* in lower airways of patients with cystic fibrosis. Scand J Infect Dis 1979;11:211–217.
52. Krause PJ, Young LS, Cherry JD, et al. The treatment of exacerbations of pulmonary disease in cystic fibrosis: Netilmicin compared with netilmicin and carbenicillin. Curr Ther Res 1979;25:609–617.
53. Gerber AU, Vastola AP, Brandel J, et al. Selection of aminoglycoside-resistant variants of *Pseudomonas aeruginosa* in an in vivo model. J Infect Dis 1982;146:691–697.
54. Gerber AU, Craig WA. Aminoglycoside-selected subpopulations of *Pseudomonas aeruginosa.* J Lab Clin Med 1982;100:671–681.
55. Aronoff SC, Klinger JD. In vitro activities of aztreonam, piperacillin and ticarcillin combined with amikacin against amikacin-resistant *Pseudomonas aeruginosa* and *P. cepacia* isolates from children with cystic fibrosis. Antimicrob Agents Chemother 1984;25:279–280.
56. Bosso JA, Allen JE, Matsen JM. Changing susceptibility of *Pseudomonas aeruginosa* isolates from cystic fibrosis patients with the clinical use of newer antibiotics. Antimicrob Agents Chemother 1989;33:526–528.
57. Thomassen MJ, Klinger JD, Badger SJ, et al. Cultures of thoracotomy specimens confirm usefulness of sputum cultures in cystic fibrosis. J Pediatr 1984;104:352–356.
58. Yaffe SJ, Gerbracht LM, Mosovich LL, et al. Pharmacokinetics of methicillin in patients with cystic fibrosis. J Infect Dis 1977;135:828–831.
59. Spino M, Chai RP, Isles AF, et al. Cloxacillin absorption and disposition in cystic fibrosis. J Pediatr 1984;105:829–835.
60. Jusko WJ, Mosovich LL, Gerbracht LM, et al. Enhanced renal excretion of dicloxacillin in patients with cystic fibrosis. Pediatrics 1975;56:1038–1044.
61. Woolf RA, Koup JR, Smith AL, et al. Pharmacokinetics of high-dose azlocillin sodium in patients with cystic fibrosis. Clin Pharm 1985;4:664–669.
62. Prince AS, Neu HC. Use of piperacillin, a semisynthetic penicillin, in the therapy of acute exacerbations of pulmonary disease in patients with cystic fibrosis. J Pediatr 1980;97:148–151.
63. deGroot R, Hack BD, Weber A, et al. Pharmacokinetics of ticarcillin in patients with cystic fibrosis: A controlled prospective study. Clin Pharmacol Ther 1990;47:73–78.
64. Reed MD, Aronoff SC, Stern RC, et al. Single-dose pharmacokinetics of aztreonam in children with cystic fibrosis. Pediatr Pulmonol 1986;2:282–286.
65. Leeder JS, Spino M, Isles AF, et al. Ceftazidime disposition in acute and stable cystic fibrosis. Clin Pharmacol Ther 1984;36:355–362.
66. Reed MD, Stern RC, O'Brien CA, et al. Pharmacokinetics of imipenem and cilistatin in patients with cystic fibrosis. Antimicrob Agents Chemother 1985;27:583–588.
67. Hutabarat RM, Unadkat JD, Sahauwalla C, et al. Disposition of drugs in cystic fibrosis. I. Sulfamethoxazole and trimethoprim. Clin Pharmcol Ther 91;49:402–409.
68. Kearns GL, Hilman BA, Wilson JT. Dosing implications of altered gentamicin disposition in patients with cystic fibrosis. J Pediatr 1982;100:312–318.

69. Levy J, Smith AL, Koup JR, et al. Disposition of tobramycin in patients with cystic fibrosis: A prospective controlled study. J Pediatr 1984;105:117–124.
70. Finkelstein E, Hall K. Aminoglycoside clearance in patients with cystic fibrosis. J Pediatr 1979;94:163–164.
71. Bosso JA, Townsend PL, Herbst JJ, et al. Pharmacokinetics and dosage requirements of netilmicin in cystic fibrosis patients. Antimicrob Agents Chemother 1985;28:829–831.
72. Mimeault J, Vallée F, Seelman R, et al. Altered disposition of fleroxacin in patients with cystic fibrosis. Clin Pharmacol Ther 1990;47:618–628.
73. Alván G, Beerman B, Hjelte L, et al. Increased nonrenal clearance and increased diuretic efficiency of furosemide in cystic fibrosis. Clin Pharmacol Ther 1988;44:436–441.
74. Hutabarat RM, Unadkat JD, Kushmerick P, et al. Disposition of drugs in cystic fibrosis. III. Acetaminophen. Clin Pharmacol Ther 1991;50:695–701.
75. Spino M, Chai RP, Isles AF, et al. Assessment of glomerular filtration rate and effective renal plasma flow in cystic fibrosis. J Pediatr 1985;107:64–70.
76. Moore RD, Smith CR, Lietman PS. Association of aminoglycoside plasma levels with therapeutic outcome in gram-negative pneumonia. Am J Med 1984;77:657–662.
77. Noone P, Parsons MC, Pattison JR, et al. Experience in monitoring gentamicin therapy during treatment of serious gram negative sepsis. Br J Med 1974;1:477–481.
78. MacDonald NE, Anas NG, Peterson RG, et al. Renal clearance of gentamicin in cystic fibrosis. J Pediatr 1983;103: 985–990.
79. Nahata MC, Lubion AH, Visconti JA. Cephalexin pharmacokinetics in patients with cystic fibrosis. Dev Pharmacol Ther 1984;7:221–228.
80. Jacobs RF, Trang JM, Kearns GL, et al. Ticarcillin/clavulanic acid pharmacokinetics in children and young adults with cystic fibrosis. J Pediatr 1985;106:1001–1007.
81. Bosso JA, Relling MV, Townsend PL, et al. Intrapatient variations in aminoglycoside disposition in cystic fibrosis. Clin Pharm 1987;6:54–58.
82. Ramsey BW, Dorkin HL, Eisenberg JD, et al. Efficacy of aerosolized tobramycin in patients with cystic fibrosis. N Engl J Med 1993;328:1740–1746.
83. Møller NE, Eriksen KR, Feddersen C, et al. Chemotherapy against *Pseudomonas aeruginosa* in cystic fibrosis. A study of carbenicillin, azlocillin or piperacillin in combination with tobramycin. Eur J Respir Dis 1982;63:130–139.
84. Jensen T, Koch C, Pedersen SS, et al. Aztreonam for cystic fibrosis patients who are hypersensitive to other betalactams. Lancet 1987;1:1319–1320.
85. Beardsmore CS, Thompson JR, Williams A, et al. Pulmonary function in infants with cystic fibrosis. Arch Dis Child 1994;71:133–137.
86. Bosso JA. Use of ciprofloxacin in cystic fibrosis patients. Am J Med 1989;87(suppl 5A):123S–127S.
87. Høiby N, Pedersen SS, Jensen T, et al. Fluoroquinolones in the treatment of cystic fibrosis. Drugs 1993;45(suppl 3):98–101.
88. Smith AL, Redding G, Doershuk C, et al. Sputum changes associated with therapy for endobronchial exacerbation in cystic fibrosis. J Pediatr 1988;112:547–554.
89. Rayner RJ, Wiseman MS, Cordon SM, et al. Inflammatory markers in cystic fibrosis. Resp Med 1991;85:139–145.
90. Bosso JA, Walker KB. Lack of correlation between objective indicators and clinical-response scores during antimicrobial therapy for acute pulmonary exacerbations of cystic fibrosis. Clin Pharm 1988;7:897–901.
91. Rosenberg SM, Schramm CM. Predictive value of pulmonary function testing during pulmonary exacerbations in cystic fibrosis. Pediatr Pulmonol 1993;16:227–235.
92. Rosenfeld MA, Yoshimura K, et al. In vivo transfer of the human cystic fibrosis transmembrane conductance regulator gene to the airway epithelium. Cell 1992;68:143–155.
93. Zabner J, Couture LA, Gregory RJ, et al. Adenovirus-mediated gene transfer transiently corrects the chloride transport defect in nasal epithelia of patients with cystic fibrosis. Cell 1993;75:1–10.
94. Hyde SC, Gill DR, Higgins CF, et al. Correction of the ion transport defect in cystic fibrosis transgenic mice by gene therapy. Nature 1993;362:250–255.
95. McElvaney NG, Hubbard RC, Birrer P, et al. Aerosol α_1-antitrypsin treatment for cystic fibrosis. Lancet 1991;337: 392–394.
96. Winnie GB, Cowan RG, Wade NA. Intravenous immune globulin treatment of pulmonary exacerbations in cystic fibrosis. J Pediatr 1989;114:309–314.
97. Knowles MR, Church NL, Waltner WE, et al. A pilot study of aerosolized amiloride for the treatment of lung disease in cystic fibrosis. N Engl J Med 1990;322:1189–1194.
98. Knowles MR, Clarke LL, Boucher RC. Activation by extracellular nucleotides of chloride secretion in the airway epithelia of patients with cystic fibrosis. N Engl J Med 1991;325:533–538.
99. Ramirez JC, Patterson GA, Winton TL, et al. Bilateral lung transplantation for cystic fibrosis. J Thorac Cardiovasc Surg 1992;103:287–294.
100. Shennib H, Noirclerc M, Ernst P, et al. Double-lung transplantation for cystic fibrosis. Ann Thorac Surg 1992;54: 27–32.

Section 3
Gastrointestinal Disorders

Chapter 30

Evaluation of the Gastrointestinal Tract

Marie A. Chisholm, PharmD, and Mark W. Jackson, MD

The gastrointestinal (GI) system encompasses organs and tissues that have richly diverse forms and functions. It includes the esophagus, stomach, small intestine, large intestine, colon, rectum, gallbladder, biliary tract, liver, and pancreas. Abnormalities in digestive function and structure can lead to severe consequences, and identification of the specific abnormality is of vital importance for prevention and effective therapeutic management. Despite the rapid proliferation of technology for the diagnosis of digestive diseases, the patient history and physical examination still play an important role. Combined with patient history and physical examination, diagnostic procedures are extremely useful in the evaluation of GI disorders. This chapter describes the most commonly used tools available to evaluate patients with GI diseases.

Patient History

A comprehensive patient history is paramount when approaching patients with digestive complaints. A clear, chronological account of the patient's problems should include the onset of the problem, the setting in which it developed, and its manifestations. Identification of factors that alleviate or exacerbate patient's symptoms is helpful. Ask questions that address the potential etiologic possibilities including motility disorders, structural diseases, malignancies, infections, psychosocial factors, dietary factors, and travel-associated diseases.[1,2] Past history detailing illnesses, surgeries, injuries, habits, and family illnesses is valuable. Because many drugs have been reported to cause GI injury, a patient's medication history is vital (Table 30.1).

Physical Examination

A complete physical examination is necessary to evaluate patients with GI complaints.[3] The general appearances and vital signs of patients may suggest clues to their overall condition and stability. Inspection of the abdomen may disclose signs of abdominal inflammation, scars, abdominal bulges, or hernias. Abdominal auscultation permits an appraisal of bowel sounds and other noises such as abdominal bruits. The liver and spleen are measured and air in the stomach and bowel is identified by abdominal percussion. Marked tenderness, involuntary rigidity, or muscle spasm detected by palpating the abdomen may indicate peritoneal inflammation. Digital rectal examinations are used to detect rectal cancers and other lesions.[1,3] The hemoccult slide is a fecal occult blood test that is used to screen for colon cancer.

Laboratory and Microbiologic Tests

Nonspecific laboratory serum blood tests that measure sodium, chloride, potassium, blood urea nitrogen, serum creatinine, bicarbonate, albumin, and glucose serve as

TABLE 30.1. DRUGS THAT COMMONLY CAUSE GASTROINTESTINAL INJURY

Gastrointestinal Mucosal Injury	**Liver Damage (continued)**
Aspirin	Ethanol
Chemotherapeutic agents	Glyburide
Corticosteroids	Isoniazid
Ethacrynic acid	Ketoconazole
Ethanol	Methotrexate
Gentian violet	Methyldopa
Isoproterenol	Monamine oxidase inhibitors
Nonsteroidal anti-inflammatory agents	Niacin
Pancreatin	Nifedipine
Potassium chloride	Nitrofurantoin
Reserpine	Phenytoin
Warfarin	Propylthiouracil
Jaundice	Pyridium
Acetohexamide	Rifampin
Androgens	Salicylates
Chlorpropamide	Sulfonamides
Corticosteroids	Tetracycline
Erythromycin	Verapamil
Estrogens	Warfarin
Ethanol	Zidovudine
Gold salts	**Pancreatitis**
Nitrofurantoin	Azathioprine
Phenothiazines	Corticosteroids
Warfarin	Estrogens
Liver Damage	Ethacrynic acid
Acetaminophen	Ethanol
Allopurinol	Furosemide
Aminosalicylic acid	Opiates
Dapsone	Sulfonamides
Erythromycin	Thiazides

indicators for electrolyte depletion, renal function, nutritional status, hypoglycemia, and hyperglycemia. The complete blood count is an important indicator of infection, malignancy, bone marrow suppression, anemia, and blood loss. Increases in liver enzymes such as aspartate transaminase (AST), alanine transaminase (ALT), and alkaline phosphatase suggest liver disorders, while amylase and lipase are generally elevated with pancreatitis.[4,5] Microbiologic studies may be necessary to evaluate patients with unexplained diarrhea, abdominal pain, and suspected GI infections. Microbiologic studies of GI tissues are performed to determine the presence of specific pathogens, and microscopic examinations of stools are performed to detect leukocytes, bacteria, and parasites. Common pathogens that can cause GI infections include bacteria such as *Shigella, Salmonella, Helicobacter pylori, Escherichia coli, gonococcus, Chlamydia, Clostridium difficle, tuberculosis,* and *Yersinia;* viruses such as *cytomegalovirus;* and parasites such as *Entamoeba histolytica* and *Giardia lambia.*[6]

DIAGNOSTIC TESTS AND PROCEDURES

The patient history, physical examination, and routine laboratory tests are surprisingly accurate in establishing a GI diagnosis, but frequently a more specific study is required to confirm or deny a clinical suspicion. The most appropriate diagnostic test depends on the anatomic region involved, the suspected abnormality, patient preferences, and clinical manifestation of the patient. The following sections outline the most frequently used diagnostic studies and procedures and their role in evaluating the GI tract.

RADIOLOGY

Radiologic procedures rely on the differential absorption of radiation between adjacent tissues to highlight anatomy and pathology. Radiologic procedures including plain radiography, upper GI series, lower GI series, and enteroclysis are important in evaluating the GI tract.[7,8]

Plain Radiography of Gastrointestinal System

Radiographic evaluation of the GI tract often starts with "plain films" of the abdomen that are straightforward, uncontrasted radiographs.[8] Specific abdominal organ structures that may be identified include the kidney, ureters, and bladder (KUB), esophagus, stomach, intestine, stones, and vessels. Plain films are often used to evaluate abdominal pain.[9] Clinicians frequently employ plain radiographic fluoroscopy to guide and position other instruments used to evaluate and treat GI disorders, for example, the manipulation of dilation devices to treat esophageal strictures. Bowel obstruction and free perforation are especially well identified by this technique.

Contrast Agents

Many different types of contrast agents are available. Two types of contrast agents commonly used to enhance visualization of the GI tract are barium sulfate and iodinated aqueous compounds. Barium sulfate is the contrast agent of choice for studying the esophagus, stomach, and intestine except in special clinical situations.[8] Barium sulfate is not generally absorbed and constipation is the most frequent adverse effect reported with its use. Two widely used iodinated contrast agents for visualizing the GI tract are diatrizoate meglumine and diatrizoate sodium (Gastrografin®) and diatrizoate sodium (Hypaque Sodium®). Unlike barium, these agents are relatively nontoxic if inadvertently introduced into the peritoneal cavity; therefore, the main indications for iodinated agents in GI radiologic films are for suspected bowel perforations. Since iodinated contrast agents are hyperosmolar, they possess the potential to cause severe diarrhea, dehydration, and electrolyte imbalances.

Nephrotoxicity associated with iodinated contrast agents may occur and is generally self-limited.[8,10] Allergies and hypersensitivity reactions such as rashes associated with contrast agents are possible and should be monitored and treated accordingly.

Upper Gastrointestinal Series

The upper GI series refers to the radiographic visualization of the esophagus, stomach, and small intestine. Patient preparation for an upper GI usually consists of instructing patients to refrain from eating or drinking 8–12 hours prior to testing, allowing the upper GI tract to empty. A contrast agent such as barium sulfate is administered to the patient at the beginning of the study. The observed swallowing of the contrast agent permits visualization and monitoring of esophageal structural and motor functions. This phase of the procedure is most often referred to as a "barium swallow." As the contrast medium flows into the stomach and small intestine, several regional radiographic films are taken in order to inspect these areas. This tracking of contrast agents through the small intestine is referred to as the "small bowel follow-through." The upper GI series with the small bowel follow-through includes the examination of the esophagus to the end of the small intestine and is useful to evaluate and detect obstructions, tumors, ulcers, and abnormal intestinal loops.[11,12] The upper GI series with small bowel follow-through commonly uncovers gastric cancer, peptic ulcer disease, esophagitis, gastric outlet obstruction, and Crohn's disease (Fig. 30.1).

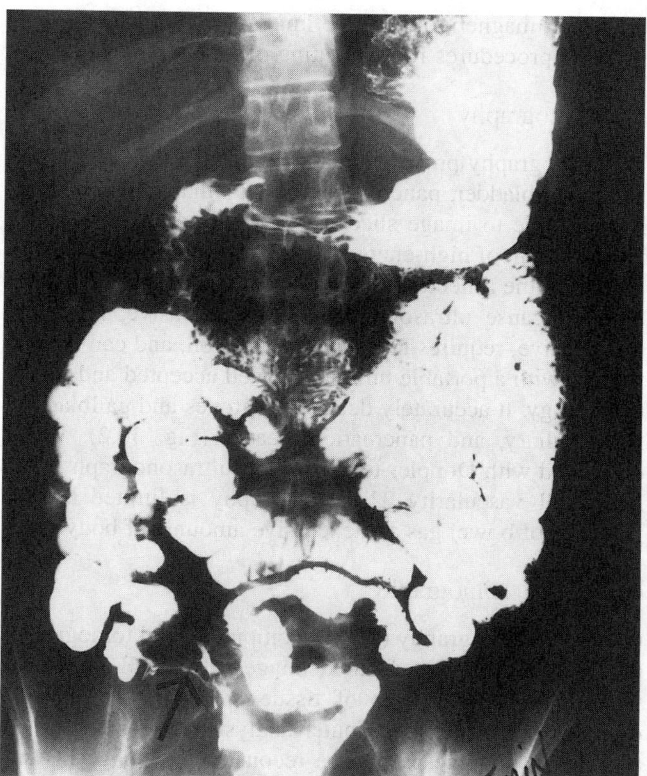

Figure 30.1. Upper GI series with small bowel follow-through demonstrating narrowed distal terminal ileum and separation of small bowel loops. These findings are consistent with Crohn's disease.

Lower Gastrointestinal Series

Patients complaining of lower abdominal pain, constipation, or diarrhea are often referred for a lower GI series. Before the procedure the colon is prepared by instructing the patient to refrain from eating or drinking 8–12 hours before the procedure and by administering bowel cleansing agents such as magnesium citrate and bisacodyl (Table 30.2). During a lower GI series a barium sulfate enema is given to contrast the terminal large intestine and rectum. The lower GI series is useful to detect and evaluate enterocolitis, obstructions, volvulus, and mucosal and structural lesions.[8] The lower GI series is commonly used to diagnose Crohn's disease, ulcerative colitis, colon cancers, and diverticulitis.

Small Bowel Enteroclysis

Enteroclysis or small bowel enema refers to the technique of direct small bowel introduction of a contrast agent through a tube inserted through the patient's mouth or nose. Intermittent radiographic films are taken of the small bowel as the contrast agent flows distally.[8] Because enteroclysis provides detailed imaging, it is the most accurate method for evaluating the small bowel and detects small mucosal lesions that have been missed on the traditional small bowel follow-through.[13,14] Adding methylcellulose to the barium enhances the detail of the small intestine in enteroclysis. Patient preparation for this procedure involves instructing patients to refrain from eating or drinking 8–12 hours before testing and administering bowel cleansing agents. The most frequent disorder evaluated by enteroclysis is obscure GI bleeding.

GASTROINTESTINAL IMAGING STUDIES

Through computer-assisted techniques, it is possible to generate cross-sectional radiographic images through the body. Ultrasonography, computed tomography, radionuclide scan-

TABLE 30.2. COMMONLY USED BOWEL CLEANSING AGENTS

Bisacodyl
Magnesium citrate
Magnesium hydroxide
Polyethylene glycol–electrolyte solution
Sodium bisphosphate and sodium phosphate

ning, and magnetic resonance imaging are frequently used imaging procedures for evaluating digestive disorders.[15–18]

Ultrasonography

Ultrasonography provides images of deeper structures such as the gallbladder, pancreas, and abdominal wall. The clinician is able to image slices of the GI tract by directing a narrow beam of high-energy sound waves into the body and recording the reflections from the various organs and structures. Because ultrasonography is noninvasive, relatively inexpensive, requires no ionizing radiation, and can be performed with a portable unit, it is a well accepted and useful technology. It accurately detects gallstones and gallbladder, hepatobiliary, and pancreatic diseases (Fig. 30.2). When combined with Doppler technologies, ultrasonography may image GI vascularity. Ultrasonography is limited by the presence of bowel gas and excessive amounts of body fat.[18]

Computed Tomography

Computed tomography (CT) or computed axial tomography (CAT) scans provide detailed images of the GI system in which transverse planes of tissue are swept by a radiographic beam and a computer analysis of the variance in absorption produces a precise reconstructed image of that area.[7,18] Contrast agents may be added in a CT procedure to illuminate specific hollow structures and vascularity of the GI tract. The abdominal CT displays organs from the diaphragm down to the pelvic brim and is especially valuable for detecting GI diseases of the liver, pancreas, spleen, and colon. Patient preparation for CT includes refraining from eating or drinking for a minimum of 4 hours before the test. The remarkable detail that CT offers in imaging organs and tissues adds to its popularity for evaluation of the GI system. CT is useful in the identification of liver cancer, pancreatitis, pancreatic cancer, intra-abdominal abscesses, and cysts[18] (Fig. 30.3). Unlike ultrasonography, patient body size or the presence of gas does not limit the quality of imaging with CT.

Radionuclide Imaging

Radionuclide imaging involves intravenous injections of a radiopharmaceutical imaging agent and the use of a computerized detection camera to gather images. Choice of a radiopharmaceutical agent depends on the specific organ or function being studied; however, the most commonly used agent is technetium (Tc-99*m*) tagged to a carrier molecule. Radiographic imaging is useful to visualize the liver and spleen ("liver-spleen scan"), bile ducts, gallbladder ("HIDA scan"), and gut ("bleeding scan").[17,18] Cysts, abscesses, tumors, and obstructions are detected and displayed as areas of differential uptake of radioactivity[7] (Fig. 30.4). Radionuclide bleeding scans may detect hemorrhages and assist in localization.

MAGNETIC RESONANCE IMAGING

Magnetic resonance imaging (MRI) places the patient in close proximity to a high-strength magnetic field through which pulses of radio-frequency irradiation are projected, thereby exciting the nuclei of hydrogen, phosphorus, oxygen, and other elements. The radio-frequency signals are manipu-

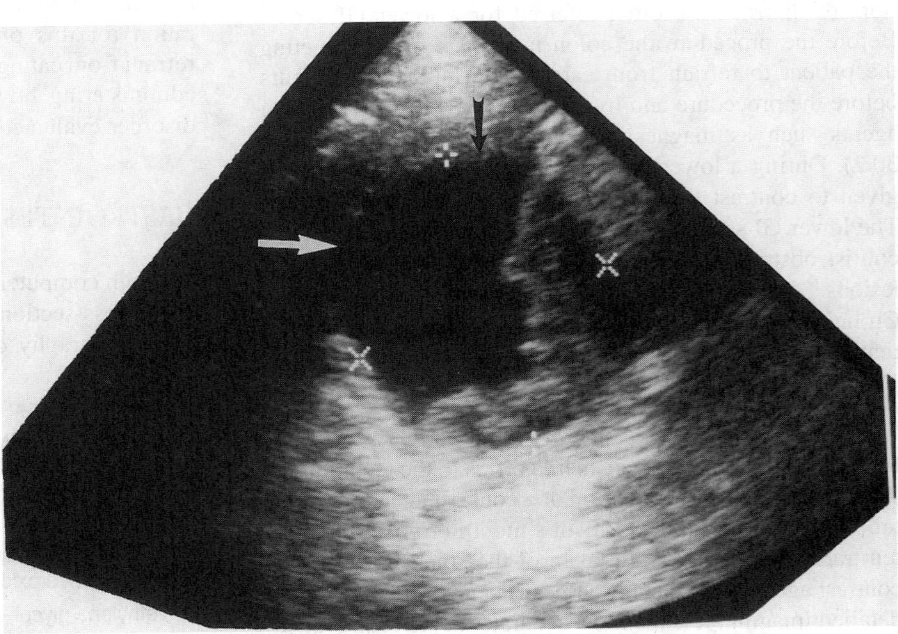

Figure 30.2. Abdominal ultrasound demonstrating a chronic pancreatic pseudocyst *(arrows)*.

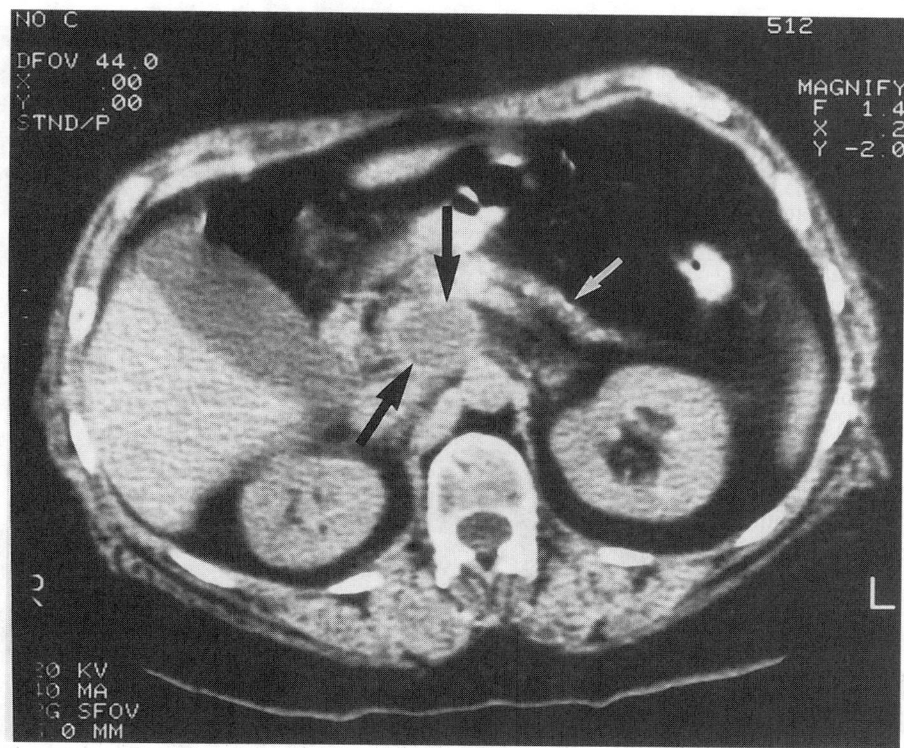

Figure 30.3. CT scan of the abdomen showing pancreatitis with calcification *(white arrow)* and pancreatic pseudocyst *(black arrows).*

lated and recorded by computer and a two-dimensional picture representing a section of the patient is produced.[7,18] MRI has greater sensitivity to identify liver tumors than ultrasonography, CT, or radionuclide imaging. Although the current use of MRI is not as popular as other imaging techniques due to limited availability, expense, slow scanning time, and problems associated with the use of powerful magnetic fields, its use is predicted to increase in the future.[19]

ARTERIOGRAPHY

Arteriography of the gut defines the configuration of visceral blood vessels after administration of a contrast media intravenously. Arteriography may be employed for detecting tumors and bleeding lesions and therapeutic applications including embolization of bleeding vessels, fistulas, and inoperable tumors.[16,18]

GASTROINTESTINAL ENDOSCOPY

Refinement in optical engineering and fiber optics has made possible the development of the endoscope, which has revolutionized the management of GI disorders. An endoscope is an illuminated optical instrument designed to inspect the interior of the GI tract. Endoscopes allow the practitioner to inspect intraluminal mucosal lesions and obtain biopsies

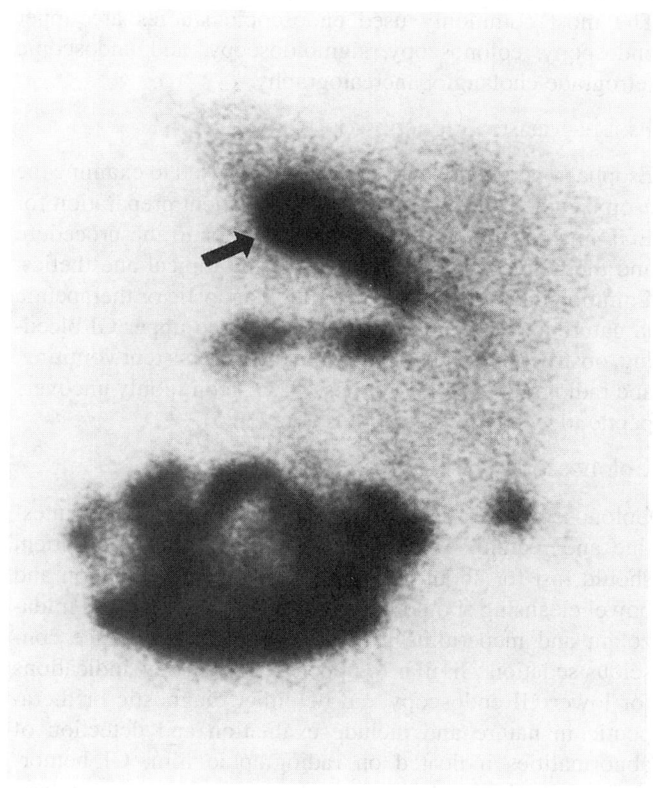

Figure 30.4. HIDA scan demonstrating normal gallbladder *(arrow).*

and washings for cytology studies. The upper GI tract endoscopy by esophagogastroduodenoscopy is capable of inspecting the esophagus, stomach, and proximal small bowel. The lower GI tract endoscopy of the rectum and colon may be accomplished by colonoscopy or sigmoidoscopy.

Preparation for endoscopic examinations includes instructing patients to refrain from eating or drinking 8–12 hours prior to the endoscopic procedures. Bowel cleansing is necessary for colonoscopy and sigmoidoscopy. Topical pharyngeal anesthetics such as viscous lidocaine or benzocaine usually improve patient acceptance of the upper endoscopic tube. Intravenous sedating agents such as meperidine hydrochloride, diazepam, lorazepam, and midazolam hydrochloride are among the agents used to induce "conscious sedation" minutes prior to the endoscopy; they improve patient acceptance and ease of procedure. With the development of flumazenil, a benzodiazepine antagonist, the popularity of benzodiazepines for mild sedation with GI procedures has increased. In addition, antimuscuranic agents such as atropine sulfate are used occasionally for their cardiovascular effects such as increasing a patient's heart rate or its antispasmodic effects such as reducing duodenal and colonic motility. Glucagon is also effective at reducing bowel motility and is often used. Endoscopy is contraindicated for patients with severe respiratory or cardiac failure, and patients with suspected perforated viscera. The most commonly used endoscopic studies are upper endoscopy, colonoscopy, sigmoidoscopy, and endoscopic retrograde cholangiopancreatography.[16]

Esophagogastroduodenoscopy

Esophagogastroduodenoscopy (EGD) is used to examine the esophagus, stomach, and duodenum. Patient preparation for EGD includes fasting for 6–8 hours prior to the procedure and the administration of sedatives and topical anesthetics. Common indications may be either diagnostic or therapeutic in nature and include evaluating suspected upper GI bleeding, obstructions, upper abdominal pain, persistent vomiting, and radiographic abnormalities.[20] EGD commonly uncovers peptic ulcers and other lesions (Fig. 30.5).

Colonoscopy

Colonoscopy permits direct examination of the large intestine and rectum. To prepare for colonoscopy, the patient should fast for about 8 hours prior to the examination and bowel cleansing should be completed. Agents such as midazolam and meperidine are usually given to produce conscious sedation. Similar to upper GI endoscopy, indications for lower GI endoscopy can be either diagnostic or therapeutic in nature and include evaluation and detection of abnormalities indicated on radiographic film, GI hemorrhaging, colonic lesions, volvulus, ulcerative colitis, Crohn's disease, diverticulitis, and excision of colonic polyps.[21]

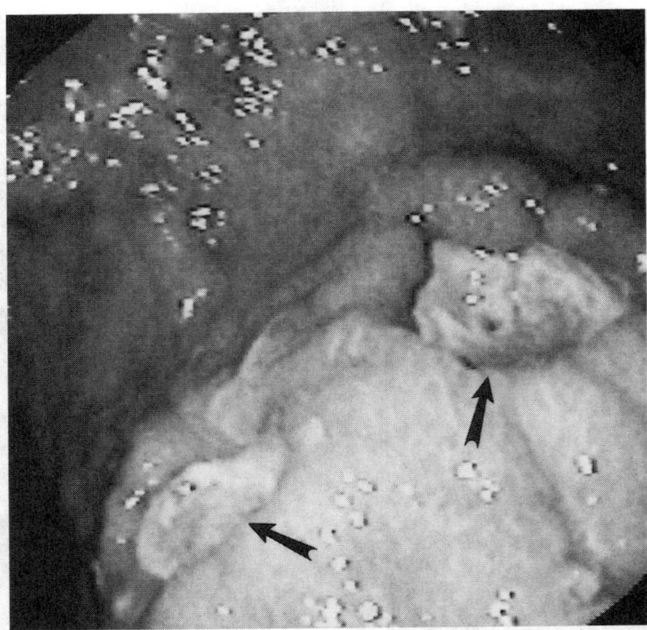

Figure 30.5. Deep "punched out" gastric ulcers *(arrows)* seen by EGD.

Sigmoidoscopy

Sigmoidoscopy is used to evaluate the sigmoid colon and rectum. Flexible sigmoidoscopy has virtually replaced the rigid sigmoidoscopy because of increased patient comfort and superior examining.[22,23] The major indication for this examination is to evaluate symptoms related to the colon or rectum and to conduct screening of asymptomatic patients for colon polyps or cancer. Patient preparation involves instructing patients to refrain from eating or drinking 8–12 hours prior to the procedure and administering bowel cleansing agents. Anoscopy is especially useful in evaluating the anus. The major indications for the anoscopic examination include symptoms related to the anus and rectum such as bleeding, protrusions or swelling, pain, and severe itching. Patients undergoing sigmoidoscopy or anoscopy generally do not require sedation.

Endoscopic Retrograde Cholangiopancreatography

Endoscopic retrograde cholangiopancreatography (ERCP) is an important procedure used to evaluate and treat diseases of the biliary tree and pancreas. By injecting contrast agents through a catheter placed in the pancreaticobiliary ducts during ERCP, abnormalities such as obstructions, calculi, and strictures can be examined. Preparation for ERCP consists of conscious sedation and glucagon to relax gut motility. Common reasons for ERCP include detection and evaluation of pancreatic malignancy, pancreatitis, biliary obstruction, bile duct stones, jaundice, and patients whose clinical presentation suggests biliary disease[24] (Fig. 30.6).

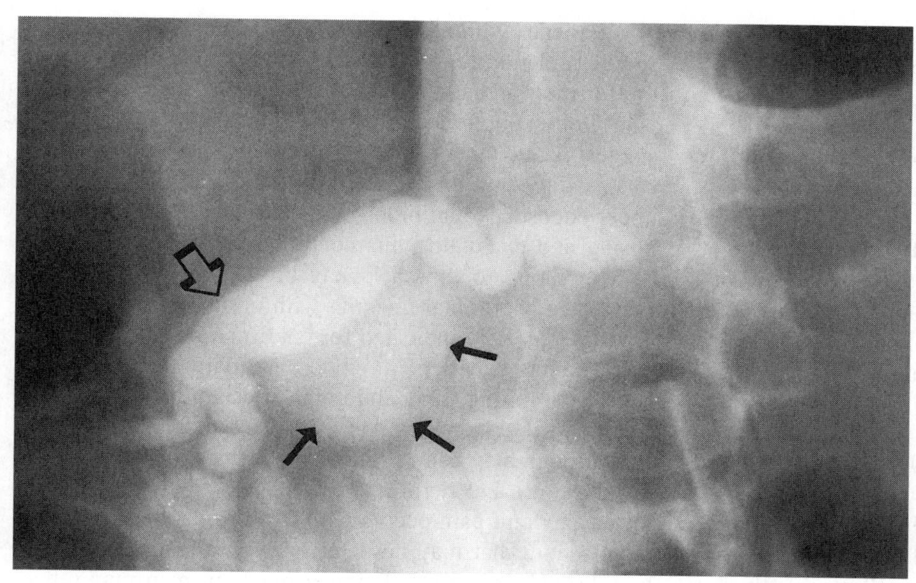

Figure 30.6. ERCP demonstrating a dilated, irregular pancreatic duct with areas of stricturing *(large arrow)*. A pancreatic pseudocyst is visible immediately adjacent to the spine *(small arrows)*.

MISCELLANEOUS TESTS

Esophageal Manometry

Esophageal manometry is used to evaluate esophageal motor functions. Common indications for this procedure include dysphagia and obscure chest pain. A special catheter equipped with pressure transducers is placed into the esophagus to measure esophageal pressures and peristalsis. Provocative testing with pharmacologic agents such as edrophonium chloride, a cholinergic muscle stimulant, may be used to precipitate esophageal pain during this procedure.[25] Typical reasons for esophageal manometry include evaluating esophageal dysmotility, nonobstructive dysphagia, obscure chest pain, scleroderma, intestinal pseudo-obstruction, achalasia, and aiding in positioning instruments such as pH probes.[16]

Ambulatory pH Monitoring

Gastric fluid pH monitoring in patients who complain of gastroesophageal reflux may be necessary. Indications for pH monitoring include evaluating atypical chest pain and severe or unusual reflux disorders. Ambulatory 24-hour pH monitoring is an elegant way to link esophageal acid exposure, as defined by a probe in the esophagus, with patient's symptoms. The pH probe is placed approximately 5 cm above the distal esophagus. Since intra-esophageal pH is normally higher (pH $\geq$ 6) than that of the stomach (pH approximately 1–3), the pH probe will record a decrease in pH if gastroesophageal reflux occurs.[26,27]

The Bernstein test, another procedure used to measure gastric fluid pH, is less expensive than ambulatory pH monitoring. This procedure requires inserting a nasogastric (NG) tube and administrating alternating dripped solutions of normal saline and 0.1 N hydrochloric acid (HCl) into the esophagus via the NG tube. If patient symptoms are reproduced by the acid perfusion and not the saline, the study is considered abnormal and indicative of acid hypersensitivity.[28,29]

LAPAROSCOPY

Laparoscopy uses a tubelike device with an elaborate optical system that permits distinct visualization of the peritoneal cavity. General anesthesia is often done and a surgical incision is made in the abdomen to allow the passage of the laparoscopic instrument. The exterior of the liver, gallbladder, spleen, peritoneum, diaphragm, and pelvic organs may be clearly examined during the laparoscopic examination. Similar to the other endoscopic techniques mentioned, biopsies and therapeutic interventions may occur during the laparoscopy. Reasons for doing laparoscopy include evaluating patients with ascites, abdominal masses, chronic abdominal pain, abnormalities indicated on liver–spleen scan, liver diseases, obstructive jaundice, and hepatic malignancy.[30]

CLINICAL APPLICATIONS OF GASTOINTESTINAL STUDIES

Putting to effective use the litany of available diagnostic studies is a regular challenge confronting today's clinicians managing patients with GI disorders. Numerous tests and procedures are available to evaluate the GI tract. Therefore, it is the responsibility of the practitioner to conduct efficient, direct, and comprehensive strategies of GI evaluation with the ultimate goal of achieving a reasonable degree of diagnostic certainty about the disease process in order to permit rational and effective therapy.

GI evaluations are largely driven by patient's dominant symptoms. Therefore, a brief evaluation overview is given for some common symptom complexes. The most common GI symptoms can be classified in the following sections: (1) heartburn, dysphagia, and odynophagia; (2) abdominal pain and dyspepsia; (3) nausea and vomiting; (4) diarrhea and constipation; (5) malabsorption; (6) gastrointestinal bleeding; and (7) hepatitis and jaundice.

HEARTBURN, DYSPHAGIA, AND ODYNOPHAGIA

The patient's history is especially useful in evaluating esophageal disease. Cardinal symptoms of the esophagus are heartburn, dysphagia (difficulty in swallowing), and odynophagia (painful swallowing). Heartburn is the most common esophageal complaint and when present is often sufficient to make the diagnosis of gastroesophageal reflux disease (GERD). The ambulatory 24-hour pH study may convincingly link the patient's symptom to an acid event. The role of endoscopy in reflux disease is to evaluate severe or atypical cases and to uncover complications of reflux including esophageal stricture, bleeding, ulcers, and Barrett's esophagus. Dysphagia prompts concern for structural diseases that may be either benign such as peptic strictures or malignant such as esophageal carcinomas. When dysphagia is the dominant symptom, the patient is appropriately referred for a barium swallow. Upper endoscopy offers the ability to inspect the mucosa of the esophagus and take biopsies.

Esophageal manometry may prove useful in documenting abnormal motility as a basis for dysphagia in those patients who lack evidence for structural disease. Achalasia, also diagnosed with manometry, is an unusual cause of dysphagia due to absent peristalsis in the esophagus. Odynophagia often results from infection and requires biopsy for confirmation.

ABDOMINAL PAIN AND DYSPEPSIA

Abdominal pain is a common reason for patients to seek medical care. A rapid onset of acute pain accompanied by signs of peritonitis, fever, and leukocytosis suggests the possibility of a severe intra-abdominal infection or inflammation. An upright abdominal film may reveal evidence of free peritoneal air under the diaphragm, suggesting a perforated bowel. A serum amylase confirms or denies the possibility of acute pancreatitis. The evaluation may include ultrasonography or CT scans that may be helpful in demonstrating inflammatory or structural diseases such as appendicitis, cholecystitis, diverticulitis, abscesses, or aneurysm.

Patients with long-standing, chronic abdominal pain should undergo a more deliberate evaluation depending on the location and the temporal patterns of their abdominal pain. For example nocturnal pain relieved by antacids may suggest peptic ulcer disease. A patient with abdominal pain, early satiety, and weight loss may have gastric cancer, and upper endoscopy and biopsy are particularly useful in diagnosing and evaluating this condition. Persistent attacks of pain radiating to the back may be due to pancreatic diseases, and abdominal imaging with ultrasonography or CT scans is generally indicated for confirmation.

Patients experiencing abdominal pain associated with nausea, vomiting, and abdominal distention may have a small bowel obstruction. An upper GI with small bowel follow-through may demonstrate a mechanical obstruction due to adhesions and hernias. Postprandial bloating and right lower quadrant pain occurs with Crohn's disease of the terminal ileum that may be detected with a small bowel follow-through as well. Left lower quadrant pain may reflect diverticulitis; although not always necessary, this may be detected by flexible sigmoidoscopy or barium enema. Patients with an iron deficiency of anemia or GI blood loss should undergo an evaluation by colonoscopy.

Dyspepsia generally refers to a variety of symptoms associated with the ingestion of food and can include such symptoms as belching, burning, epigastric pain, and bloating. Dyspepsia may be the presenting symptom for a variety of disorders including gastric and pancreatic carcinoma, cholelithiasis, intestinal obstruction, and functional disorders. An upper endoscopy can provide visual and histologic information that greatly aids in the differential diagnosis of patients with dyspepsia. An upper GI tract barium series is reasonably accurate in making a diagnosis although it is unable to define mucosal disease. Recently, tests have become available to detect *Helicobacter pylori,* which is the etiologic organism in many cases of gastritis and ulcers. Urease-based tissue tests, urea breath tests, or serology studies can be used to detect the presence of *H. pylori.*

NAUSEA AND VOMITING

As usual, evaluation of nausea and vomiting begins with a careful history. Is the patient pregnant? Is the patient undergoing chemotherapy? Does the patient have an obvious central nervous system disease? Is the patient experiencing an adverse or toxic effect from a drug such as theophylline, digoxin, or an antibiotic? After "ruling out" the more common causes for persistent nausea and vomiting such as food-borne or viral gastroenteritis, it is advantageous to consider "working up" the patient to detect bowel obstructions. A plain abdominal film may detect bowel obstruction. An upper GI series or an upper endoscopy may show structural lesions or obstructions of the GI tract as well. If an obstruction is not found, serum amylase and lipase should be measured to evaluate the diagnosis of acute pancreatitis. Timing of vomiting relative to meals provides important information. Nausea and vomiting on awakening suggest alcoholic gastritis; vomiting after meals suggests peptic ulcer disease and gastric cancer; and vomiting 3–8 hours after meals suggests an obstruction in the upper gastrointestinal tract.

DIARRHEA AND CONSTIPATION

Patient history may be useful in identifying diarrhea associated with recent travel, male homosexuality, antibiotics, or food-borne gastroenteritis. It is helpful to quantify the average number of stools per day, presence of blood and mucus, and color. Many patients experience mild abdominal discomfort and diarrhea when taking antibiotics. Other patients may continue to have diarrhea after discontinuing the antibiotics and experience fever and abdominal tenderness, suggesting antibiotic-associated colitis. This diagnosis can be achieved through sigmoidoscopy by observing yellow adherent plaques or "pseudo membranes" (Fig. 30.7). A stool sample may also be examined to detect *Clostridium difficile* toxins. A patient with acute diarrhea who appears feverish and dehydrated or has bloody diarrhea may have an infection and should undergo stool cultures to detect *C. difficile,* ova, and parasites. In addition, evaluation of diarrhea for leukocytes is useful to determine if inflammation is present.

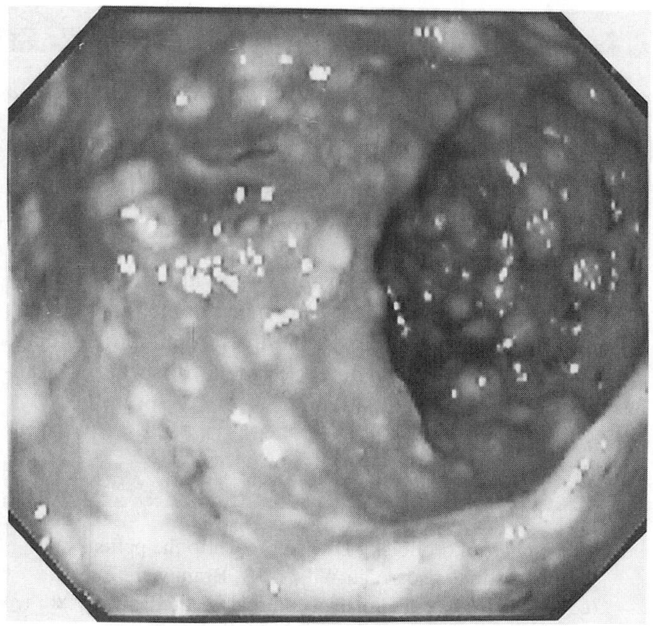

Figure 30.7. Sigmoidoscopic photograph revealing the light raised lesions of antibiotic-associated pseudomembranous colitis.

The history and physical examination may provide important clues to direct evaluation of chronic diarrhea. Sigmoidoscopy is reliable for excluding colitis and obstruction due to cancer or diverticula. A patient with a normal sigmoidoscopy may have the remainder of his or her colon evaluated with an air contrast barium enema to "rule out" inflammatory bowel disease or obstruction. A patient with a negative evaluation probably has irritable bowel syndrome ("spastic colon").

Constipation is an imprecise term that implies either infrequent or difficult defecation. It is important for clinicians to obtain a detailed dietary, laxative, and medication history since these may play a role. Appropriate laboratory tests should be performed to exclude metabolic disorders such as hypothyroidism, hypokalemia, hypocalcemia, and hypomagnesemia. If a metabolic disorder cannot be found, an underlying structural abnormality should be sought. Sigmoidoscopy and an air contrast barium enema are usually the best approaches for evaluation.

MALABSORPTION

Malabsorption is classically manifested by steatorrhea (fat in the stool) and weight loss. Steatorrhea is evaluated by first examining the stool for the presence of fat and, once established, tests are performed to differentiate pancreatic insufficiency from small bowel disease. The D-xylose test is a measure of small bowel absorption that is nearly always abnormal in small bowel malabsorption. A 5-g dose of D-xylose is taken orally by the patient and should normally be absorbed and secreted in the urine. A patient with a normal D-xylose test and steatorrhea probably has pancreatic insufficiency. However, a patient with an abnormal D-xylose test and steatorrhea favors small bowel disease. An upper GI with small bowel follow-through or small bowel biopsies may prove useful to show the presence of celiac sprue, Whipple disease, lymphoma, or other lesions.

GASTROINTESTINAL BLEEDING

GI bleeding may occur as a life-threatening emergency marked by hematemesis (bloody vomit), hematochezia (bloody stool), or melena (black, tarry stool due to upper GI bleeding), or, at the other extreme, may be chronic or occult and discovered in the course of evaluating anemia. The goal in evaluating a bleeding patient is to ascertain the site of bleeding (upper versus lower GI tract) and the nature of the bleeding lesion. After the patient is stabilized, endoscopy can be performed to identify bleeding ulcers, erosive gastritis, and esophageal varices. Endoscopy accurately determines the nature of the bleeding lesion in more than 90% of presenting patients and is often the vehicle for the delivery of therapy (sclerosis injections or cautery). In cases where endoscopy has technically failed to identify or treat the source of the bleeding or in cases of rapid bleeding, arteriography (angiography) may be advisable. Under these circumstances, arteriography can be used to localize the bleeding site and afford treatment of the bleeding vessel. Barium studies have no role in the management of acute GI bleeding.

HEPATITIS AND JAUNDICE

When the history and physical examination identify active or chronic liver disease, a detailed medication history is critical since numerous agents are known to induce these disorders. When transaminases are 10 times normal, viral hepatitis or acute cholangitis is considered and should prompt further specific diagnostic efforts including viral markers. Milder elevation of the transaminases is a nonspecific finding and considerations should include alcohol liver disease. In a symptomatic patient with hepatomegaly or clinical signs of liver disease, liver ultrasonography or CT scans may help exclude cancer. The function of the liver may be measured indirectly by measuring serum albumin and performing coagulation studies.

When hepatocellular disease is suspected, ultrasonography or CT scans of the liver are performed to exclude focal defects such as tumors, abscesses, and vascular lesions prior to performing a percutaneous liver biopsy (Fig. 30.8). Often a liver biopsy is the best way to resolve questions as to the reason for underlying hepatocellular injury. When alkaline phosphatase is elevated, especially in conjunction with transaminases, one considers cholestatic liver diseases. In suspected biliary disease, an abdominal ultrasound is usually done with special attention to the interhepatic ducts. If the ducts are dilated, one considers an obstructive pancreas, bile duct cancer, bile duct strictures, or common bile duct stones. "Cholestatic" patients without dilated bile ducts may have primary biliary cirrhosis, diagnosed by liver biopsy, or primary sclerosing cholangitis, diagnosed by characteristic bile duct changes on ERCP. Cholestasis may occur with or without jaundice.

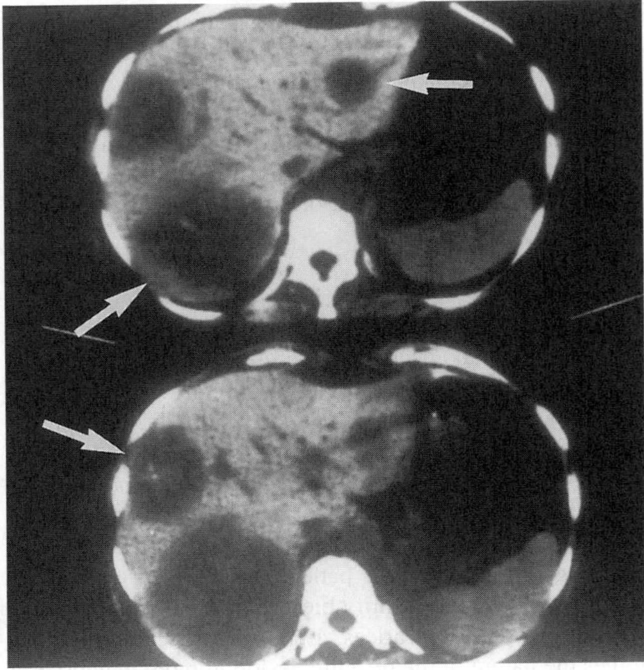

Figure 30.8. CT scans of the abdomen showing metastatic cancer of the liver *(arrows)*.

Jaundice often, but not always, reflects underlying liver disease. The clinician is commonly faced with the question as to whether the patient's jaundice is due to an extrahepatic process or an intrahepatic parenchymal liver disease. An extrahepatic lesion is suggested by a disproportionate elevation in alkaline phosphatase and may be confirmed by observing dilated intrahepatic ducts on ultrasonography or CT scan. Often an ERCP is necessary to visualize the biliary tree and pancreatic ducts to identify the precise location and character of the obstructing lesion. Liver biopsy plays a role in determining the parenchymal role in the cholestatic process.

Hepatomegaly found on physical exam suggests chronic disease. Hepatitis might be the culprit under these circumstances and is easily detected by measurement of serum transaminases. Ultrasonography or CT scans are used to determine if there is focal or diffuse liver disease and obstruction of the biliary tree. A patient with abdominal pain and an enlarged liver may have an abscess, hematoma, or tumor that may be best demonstrated by a CT scan.

CONCLUSION

A comprehensive history and physical examination play a pivotal role in evaluating patients with digestive diseases. Laboratory and microbiologic tests, radiography, ultrasonography, computed tomography, radionuclide scanning, magnetic resonance imaging, arteriography, endoscopy, esophageal manometry, pH monitoring, and laparoscopy have definite roles in diagnosing and evaluating GI disorders. These tests should be used in combination with the patient's history and physical examination to facilitate diagnosis and effective management of the GI disorder at nominal cost and risk to the patient.

REFERENCES

1. Isselbacher KJ, Podolsky DK. Approach to the patient with gastrointestinal disease, in Wilson JD, Braunwald E, et al (eds): Harrison's Principles of Internal Medicine. New York, McGraw-Hill, 1991, pp 1213–1216.
2. Janowitz HD. Approach to the patient with gastrointestinal symptoms, in Sachar DB, Waye JD, et al (eds): Pocket Guide

to Gastroenterology. Baltimore, Williams & Wilkins, 1989, pp 1–7.

3. Bates B. A Guide to Physical Examination. Philadelphia, JB Lippincott, 1979.
4. Ravel R. Clinical Laboratory Medicine: Clinical Applications of Laboratory Data. Chicago, Year Book Medical Publishers, 1984.
5. Wallach J. Interpretation of Diagnostic Tests. Boston, Little, Brown and Company, 1986.
6. Guerrant RL. Principles and syndromes of enteric infection, in Mandell GL, Douglas RG, et al (eds): Principles and Practice of Infectious Diseases. New York, Churchill Livingstone, 1990, pp 837–851.
7. Squire LF, Novelline RA. Fundamentals of Radiology. Cambridge, Harvard University Press, 1988.
8. Federle MP, Goldberg HJ. Convential radiography of the alimentary tract, in Sleisenger MH, Fordtran JS (eds): Gastrointestinal Diseases: Pathophysiology, Diagnosis, Management. Philadelphia, WB Saunders, 1983, pp 1634–1667.
9. Eisenberg RL, Heineken P, Hedgcock MW, et al. Evaluation of plain abdominal radiographs in the diagnosis of abdominal pain. Ann Intern Med 1982;97:257–261.
10. Smith CR, Petty BG. Specific complications of medical management, in Harvey AM, Johns RT, et al (eds): The Principles and Practice of Medicine. Norwalk, CT, Appleton & Lange, 1988, pp 1155–1162.
11. Laufer I. Assessment of the accuracy of double-contrast gastroduodenal radiology. Gastroenterology 1976;71:874–878.
12. Maruyama M. Early gastric cancer, in Laufer I (ed): Double Contrast Gastrointestinal Radiology. Philadelphia, WB Saunders, 1979, pp 241–287.
13. Miller RE, Sellink JL. Enteroclysis: The small bowel enema. How to succeed and how to fail. Gastrointest Radiol 1979;4:269–283.
14. Herlinger H. Small bowel, in Laufer I (ed): Double Contrast Gastrointestinal Radiology. Philadelphia, WB Saunders, 1979, pp 423–494.
15. Laing FC, Jeffrey RB. Echography of the abdomen, in Sleidenger MH, Fordtran JS (eds): Gastrointestinal Disease: Pathophysiology, Diagnosis, Management. Philadelphia, WB Saunders, 1983, pp 1688–1707.
16. Spiro HM. Clinical Gastroenterology. New York, Macmillan Publishing, 1977.
17. Hattner RS, Englestad BL. Diagnostic imaging and quantitating physiologic function using radionuclide techniques in gastrointestinal disease, in Sleisenger MH, Fordtran JS (eds): Gastrointestinal Diseases: Pathophysiology, Diagnosis, Management. Philadelphia, WB Saunders, 1983, pp 1667–1688.
18. Friedman LS, Needleman L. Hepatobiliary imaging, in Wilson JD, Braunwald E, et al (eds): Harrison's Principles of Internal Medicine. New York, McGraw-Hill, 1991, pp 1303–1308.
19. Berk RN. Diagnostic imaging procedures in gastroenterology, in Wyngaarden JB, Smith LH (eds): Cecil Textbook of Medicine. Philadelphia, WB Saunders, 1985, pp 650–658.
20. Sartor RB. Upper gastrointestinal endoscopy, in Drossman DA (ed): Manual of Gastroenterologic Procedures. New York, Raven Press, 1987, pp 90–97.
21. Shinya H, Wolf WI. Colonoscopy. Surg Ann 1976;8:257–295.
22. Hogan WJ. Flexible sigmoidoscopy versus colonoscopy—when to use which instrument. Gastrointest Endosc 1983;29:126–128.
23. Winawer SJ, Cummins R, Baldwin MP, Ptak A. A new flexible sigmoidoscope for the generalist. Gastrointest Endosc 1982;28:233–236.
24. Geenen JE. New diagnostic and treatment modalities involving endoscopic retrograde cholangiopancreatography and esophagastroduodenostromy. Scand J Gastroenterol 1982;77:93–106.
25. Benjamin SB, Richter JE, Cordova CM, et al. Prospective manometric evaluation with pharmacologic provocation of patients with suspected esophageal motility dysfunction. Gastroenterology 1983;84:893–901.
26. Tuttle SG, Bettarello A, Grossman MI. Esophageal acid perfusion test and a gastroesophageal reflux test in patients with esophagitis. Gastroenterology 1960;38:861–872.
27. Orlando RC. pH probe for reflux (tuttle test), in Drossman DA (ed): Manual of Gastroenterologic Procedures. New York, Raven Press, 1987, pp 51–54.
28. Sandler RS. Bernstein (acid perfusion) test, in Drossman DA (ed): Manual of Gastroenterologic Procedures. New York, Raven Press, 1987, pp 55–58.
29. Bernstein LM, Baker LA. A clinical test for esophagitis. Gastroenterology 1958;34:760–781.
30. Boyer TD. Laparoscopy, in Sleisenger MH, Fordtran JS (eds): Gastrointestinal Disease: Pathophysiology, Diagnosis, Management. Philadelphia, WB Saunders, 1983, pp 1627–1633.

Chapter 31

Gastroesophageal Reflux Disease

Dianne B. Williams, PharmD, and Lynda S. Welage, PharmD

Gastroesophageal reflux disease (GERD) is a common medical disorder seen by health care practitioners of all specialties. It is generally chronic in nature, and long-term therapy may be required. While the mortality associated with GERD is very low (1 death per 100,000 patients), the quality of life experienced by the patient can be greatly diminished.[1]

GERD refers to any symptomatic clinical condition or histologic alteration that results from episodes of gastroesophageal reflux. Gastroesophageal reflux refers to the retrograde movement of gastric contents from the stomach into the esophagus. Many people experience some degree of reflux, especially after eating, which may be considered a benign physiologic process. When the esophagus is repeatedly exposed to refluxed material for prolonged periods of time, inflammation of the esophagus (i.e., reflux esophagitis) can occur.[2] It is important to realize that, by definition, gastroesophageal reflux must precede the development of GERD or reflux esophagitis. In severe cases, reflux may lead to a multitude of serious complications including esophageal strictures, esophageal ulcers, motility disorders, perforation, hemorrhage, aspiration, and Barrett's esophagus.[3,4] While mild disease is often managed with lifestyle changes and antacids, more intensive therapeutic intervention with histamine (H_2) antagonists, sucralfate, prokinetic agents, or proton pump inhibitors is generally required for patients with more severe disease. In general, response to pharmacologic intervention is dependent on the efficacy of the agent, dosage regimen employed, duration of therapy, and severity of the disease. Following discontinuation of therapy, relapse is common and long-term maintenance therapy may be required. Historically, surgical intervention has been reserved for patients who fail conventional treatment modalities. However, the recent development of laparoscopic antireflux surgical procedures has led to a reevaluation of the role of surgery in the long-term management of GERD.[5,6] Some clinicians have suggested that laparoscopic antireflux surgery may be a cost-effective alternative to long-term maintenance therapy in young patients.[7,8] However, long-term comparative trials evaluating the cost effectiveness of the various treatment modalities are warranted.

The pathogenesis of gastroesophageal reflux is related to the complex balance between defense mechanisms and aggressive factors.[9] Understanding both the normal protective mechanisms and the aggressive factors that may contribute to or promote gastroesophageal reflux helps one to design rational therapeutic treatment regimens. Gastric acid, pepsin, bile acids, and pancreatic enzymes are considered aggressive factors and may promote esophageal damage upon reflux into the esophagus. Thus, the composition (potency) and volume of the refluxate are aggressive factors that may lead to esophageal injury. Conversely, normal protective mechanisms include anatomic factors, lower esophageal sphincter pressure, esophageal clearing, mucosal resistance, and gastric emptying. Rational therapeutic regimens in the treatment of gastroesophageal reflux are designed to maximize normal defense mechanisms and/or attenuate the aggressive factors.

EPIDEMIOLOGY

Gastroesophageal reflux disease occurs in both adults and children. The true prevalence and incidence of GERD is difficult to assess due to several factors: (1) many patients do not seek medical treatment, (2) symptoms do not always correlate well with severity of disease, and (3) there is no standardized definition or universal gold standard method for diagnosing the disease.[1]

The prevalence of GERD is dependent on the geographic region and is noted to be highest in Western countries.[1] In general, the prevalence increases in adults over the age of 40 years.[10] Except for pregnant women, there does not appear to be a major difference in incidence between men and women. Heartburn is a common complaint during pregnancy with as many as 25% of women experiencing heartburn on a daily basis.[11] While gender does not play a major role in the development of GERD, it is an important factor in the development of Barrett's esophagus, a complication of GERD, which occurs when normal squamous epithelium is replaced with columnar epithelium. Spechler et al.[12] found that Barrett's esophagus affected males more than women by a ratio of 6:1.

A national survey estimated that approximately 44% of adult Americans experience heartburn at least once every month and that 13% of the adult population take medications for indigestion at least a couple of times per week.[13] Similarly, Nebel et al.[11] found that 36% of 335 hospital employees experienced heartburn at least once a month, and 7% experienced reflux symptoms on a daily basis. It is well recognized that most patients with gastroesophageal reflux disease do not seek medical help from a physician. A smaller group of patients who have persistent symptoms occasionally may seek medical attention. Individuals with chronic severe symptoms and/or complications of GERD are often seen by a physician. This phenomenon has been referred to as the "iceberg of gastroesophageal reflux disease."[14] Factors that may cause an individual to seek medical attention include worsening symptoms, decreased tolerance to symptoms, fear of cancer, increased time to dwell on the symptoms, etc.[15] Many patients who do not seek medical help from a physician self-treat with over-the-counter (OTC) medications. Therefore, a pharmacist may be the primary health care professional encountered by these patients.

Even in symptomatic patients who seek medical treatment, symptoms do not always correlate well with the presence of esophageal inflammation or erosion. This makes it extremely difficult to identify which patients will have severe esophageal damage as opposed to those with merely symptoms. The overall prevalence of esophagitis in the general population is approximately 2–4%.[1,16,17] However, of the 20–40% of patients who experience heartburn, approximately 30–79% of these patients will have evidence of esophagitis.[17] Less than 15% of patients suffer severe esophagitis, indicating that most patients only suffer from mild to moderate degrees of esophagitis. Many patients with esophageal damage may not experience symptoms or they may present with atypical symptoms, such as chest pain.[2] For example, only 65% of patients with esophageal inflammation were found to complain of frequent heartburn.[18]

Another problem in assessing epidemiological data is the lack of a standardized definition and a universal gold standard method for diagnosing the disease. Behar et al.[19] evaluated 77 patients with chronic heartburn and regurgitation using endoscopy, basal lower esophageal sphincter pressure measurements, acid perfusion test, and esophageal biopsy. The prevalence of GERD varied from 61–94% depending on the diagnostic test used. The significance a patient places on their symptoms is very subjective and, therefore, difficult to evaluate objectively. Since reflux occurs to some degree in almost everyone, it is difficult to assess how many reflux episodes are considered normal.

The number of new cases that develop in a given population followed over time (incidence) is even harder to estimate than prevalence. The annual incidence of severe esophagitis was found to be 4.5 per 100,000 based on a study that used endoscopy of 443,000 people from northeast Scotland.[10] However, when a similar population was evaluated using barium swallows, the annual incidence based on radiographic evidence of gastroesophageal reflux was estimated to be 86 per 100,000.[10]

PATHOPHYSIOLOGY

The body of the esophagus lies within the negative pressure thoracic cavity, while the abdominal cavity has a positive pressure gradient. Without normal defense mechanisms the pressure gradients would favor continual reflux of gastric material into the esophagus.

ANATOMIC FACTORS

In the 1940s and 1950s anatomic factors were considered of primary importance in the prevention of gastroesophageal reflux. Proposed anatomic factors can be categorized into valvular mechanisms, extrinsic compression, intra-abdominal esophageal segment, mucosal choke, and spiral stretch mechanisms. Disruptions of the normal anatomic barriers, such as a sliding hiatal hernia, were considered the primary etiology of gastroesophageal reflux and esophagitis; however, it was later found that numerous patients with esophageal reflux did not have hiatal hernias.[9,20] Several studies have demonstrated that the presence or absence of hiatal hernia does not always correlate well with symptoms.[21–23] In a series of 1,011 patients, 786 patients were found to have a hiatal hernia, while only 23.9% had esophagitis and 4.3% had esophageal strictures.[21] Hiatal hernia was present in only 45.8% of 413 patients who were found to have esophagitis. A more important factor related to the presence or absence of symptoms is the lower esophageal sphincter pressure. Sloan et al.[24] demonstrated that patients with hypotensive lower esophageal sphincter pressures and large hiatal hernias are more likely to experience gastroesophageal reflux following abrupt increases in intra-abdominal pressure as compared to patients with hypotensive lower esophageal sphincter and no hiatal hernia. The presence of a hiatal hernia may impair esophageal clearance and predispose a patient to GERD.[22] However, patients with gastroesophageal reflux do not always have a herniated stomach and, conversely, individuals with hiatal hernias do not always have gastroesophageal reflux symptoms.[21–23] Anatomic factors are still considered by some to be of major importance in the prevention of reflux, but the diagnosis of hiatal hernia is currently considered a separate entity with which gastroesophageal reflux may or may not simultaneously occur.

LOWER ESOPHAGEAL SPHINCTER PRESSURE

The lower esophageal sphincter is a manometrically defined zone of high resting pressure.[25] This physiologic sphincter had been hypothesized since 1822, and supported by observations that food tends to be held up in the lower esophagus.[20] The lower esophageal sphincter, however, was not demonstrated until the development of pressure-recording devices. In the 1950s, Sanchez et al.[26] demonstrated the presence of the lower esophageal sphincter in humans. In the 1960s and 1970s an incompetent lower esophageal sphincter was considered the primary mechanism of gastroesophageal reflux.[27]

Physiologic control of the lower esophageal sphincter has been extensively studied but remains controversial. Sphincter control appears to be a complex system related to the intrinsic smooth musculature, autonomic innervation, and gastrointestinal hormones.[25] Both the vagus nerves (parasympathetic) and the thoracic greater splanchic nerve (sympathetic) innervate the lower esophageal sphincter.[28] Numerous hormones, pharmacologic agents, and interventions may increase or decrease lower esophageal sphincter pressure (Table 31.1).[25] The sphincter is normally in a tonic state, preventing the reflux of gastric material from the stomach, but relaxes on swallowing to permit the free passage of food into the stomach.[25] Resting pressures of the lower esophageal sphincter range from 15–35 mm Hg above gastric baseline pressure and vary with manometric methodology.[3,4] Patients with gastroesophageal reflux usually have decreased basal lower esophageal sphincter pressures, frequently less than 10 mm Hg and often less than 6 mm Hg.[3] Typically, patients with more severe gastroesophageal disease have resting lower esophageal sphincter pressures below 5 mm Hg. Although a correlation exists between lower esophageal sphincter pressures and the propensity to reflux, there is significant overlap between pressure values of normal healthy individuals and those of patients with gastroesophageal reflux.[27,29]

Mechanisms by which gastroesophageal reflux may occur are threefold.[30,31] First, and probably most important, reflux may occur following spontaneous transient lower esophageal sphincter relaxations that are not associated with swallowing.[4,30,31] The exact mechanism by which transient decreases in sphincter tone develop is unclear, but swallowing, esophageal distention, vomiting, belching, and retching have been shown to cause relaxation of the lower esophageal sphincter. A transient decrease in sphincter pressure is not always associated

TABLE 31.1. FACTORS THAT AFFECT LOWER ESOPHAGEAL SPHINCTER PRESSURES

Decrease Lower Esophageal Sphincter	Increase Lower Esophageal Sphincter
Foods	
Carminatives (peppermint, spearmint)	Protein meal
Chocolate	
Fatty meal	
Drugs	
Atropine	Bethanechol
Barbiturates	Cisapride
Calcium channel blockers	Edrophonium
Diazepam	Methacholine
Dopamine	Metoclopramide
Estrogen	Norepinephrine
Ethanol	Pentagastrin
Isoproterenol	Phenylephrine
Meperidine	
Morphine	
Nicotine (smoking)	
Phentolamine	
Progesterone	
Theophylline	
Hormones/Physiologic Factors	
Cholecytokinin	Gastric alkalinization
Estrogen	Gastrin
Gastric acidification	Prostaglandin F_2
Glucagon	
Progesterone	
Prostaglandins (E_1, E_2, A_2)	
Secretin	
Vasoactive intestinal peptide (VIP)	

(Adapted, with permission, from Castell DO. The lower esophageal sphincter. Physiologic and clinical aspects. *Ann Intern Med* 1975;83:396.)

with gastroesophageal reflux. However, in general, almost all episodes of reflux in normal subjects are results of transient decreases in sphincter pressure. Furthermore, transient decreases in sphincter pressure are responsible for approximately 65% of the reflux episodes in patients with GERD.[30] The propensity to develop gastroesophageal reflux secondary to transient decreases in lower esophageal sphincter pressure is probably dependent on numerous factors including degree of sphincter relaxation, efficacy of esophageal clearance, patient position, gastric volume, and intragastric pressure.[4] Second, reflux may also occur following transient increases in intra-abdominal pressure (stress reflux).[30,31] An increase in intra-abdominal pressure such as that occurring during straining, bending over, coughing, eating, or a Valsalva maneuver may overcome a weak lower esophageal sphincter, and thus may lead to reflux. Third, the lower esophageal sphincter may be atonic thus permitting free reflux.[4,30]

A decrease in lower esophageal sphincter pressure resulting from any of the previously mentioned causes is not always associated with gastroesophageal reflux. It has also been shown that individuals who experience decreases in sphincter pressures and subsequently reflux do not always develop GERD. The other natural defense mechanisms (esophageal clearance, mucosal resistance, and gastric factors) must be evoked to explain this phenomenon.

ESOPHAGEAL CLEARANCE

In many patients with GERD, the problem is not that they produce too much acid, but that the acid produced spends too much time in contact with the esophageal mucosa. The symptoms and/or severity of damage produced by gastroesophageal reflux are partially dependent on the duration of contact between the gastric contents and the esophageal mucosa.[32] This contact time is in turn dependent on the rate at which the esophagus clears the noxious material and the frequency of reflux. The esophagus is cleared by primary peristalsis in response to swallowing, secondary peristalsis in response to esophageal distention, and gravitational effects. Swallowing may also contribute to esophageal clearance by increasing salivary flow. Saliva buffers the residual gastric material on the surface of the esophagus. Saliva production decreases with increasing age, making it more difficult to maintain a neutral intraesophageal pH. Therefore, esophageal damage due to reflux occurs more often in the elderly and, similarly, in those patients with Sjögren's syndrome.[33]

Decreased esophageal clearance has been observed in some patients who have symptomatic gastroesophageal reflux. This decrease in esophageal clearance is marked by a defect in esophageal emptying and/or a decrease in the amplitude of esophageal peristalsis.[9,32] Gastroesophageal reflux may contribute to decreased clearing and decreased lower esophageal sphincter pressures, both of which can potentiate further reflux. Defective esophageal clearance may be both a primary event and a secondary consequence in gastroesophageal reflux.

When a patient is in an upright position, gravity facilitates esophageal clearance. Individuals who have symptomatic reflux while upright experience excessive acid exposure secondary to an increased frequency of reflux episodes.[34] Because esophageal clearance is impaired during sleep, excessive acid exposure in symptomatic patients in the supine position is primarily due to an increase in the duration of the reflux episodes (decreased clearance). The patient's awareness of heartburn during sleep may be impaired and this may contribute to the extended duration of acid exposure while recumbent.[34,35]

MUCOSAL RESISTANCE

Within the esophageal mucosa and submucosa there are mucus-secreting glands. The mucus secreted by these glands may contribute to the protection of the esophagus.[36] Bicarbonate moving from the blood to the lumen can neutralize acidic refluxate in the esophagus. In theory, mucosal resistance may be related not only to esophageal mucus, but also to tight epithelial junctions, epithelial cell turnover, nitrogen balance, mucosal blood flow, tissue prostaglandins, and the acid–base status of the tissue.[4,9,20,35,36]

COMPOSITION OF REFLUXATE

As previously discussed the tendency to reflux depends on a complex balance of natural defense mechanisms and aggressive mechanisms. The composition and volume of the refluxate are the most important aggressive factors in determining the consequences of gastroesophageal reflux. In animals it has been shown that acid has two primary effects when it is refluxed into the esophagus. First, if the pH of the refluxate is less than 2.0, esophagitis may develop secondary to protein denaturation. In addition, pepsin is activated at this pH and may also cause esophagitis. Alkaline esophagitis refers to esophagitis induced by the reflux of bilious and pancreatic fluid.[4] The term *alkaline esophagitis* may be a misnomer in that the refluxate may be either weakly alkaline or acidic in nature. Bile acids have both a direct irritant effect on the esophageal mucosa and an indirect effect of increasing hydrogen ion permeability of the mucosa.[37] Pure alkaline reflux is relatively rare.[38] The combination of acid, pepsin, and bile has been shown to be a potent refluxate in producing esophageal damage.[4,37] Esophageal pH monitoring has demonstrated that severity of disease is related to degree of esophageal acid exposure. Specifically, the percentage of time esophageal pH is <4.0 is greater for patients with severe disease as compared to patients with mild disease.[39,40]

GASTRIC EMPTYING

Delayed gastric emptying can also contribute to gastroesophageal reflux. An increase in gastric volume may increase both the frequency of reflux and the amount of gastric fluid available to be refluxed.[4] Gastric volume is related to the volume of material ingested, rate of gastric secretion, rate of gastric emptying, and amount and frequency of duodenal reflux into the stomach.[4] Patients with Barrett's esophagus may have a hypersecretory condition that is unresponsive to standard doses of H_2 antagonists. Factors that increase gastric volume and/or decrease gastric emptying are often associated with gastroesophageal reflux. This in part explains the prevalence of postprandial gastroesophageal reflux. Fatty foods may increase postprandial gastroesophageal reflux by increasing gastric volume, delaying the gastric emptying rate, and decreasing the lower esophageal sphincter pressure. Delayed gastric emptying of liquid-solid meals has been shown to occur in approximately 41% of patients with symptoms of gastroesophageal reflux.[41] It is theorized that patients with gastroesophageal reflux have a defect in antral motility.[42] This is commonly seen in infants. The delay in emptying may promote regurgitation of feedings, which may in turn contribute to the development of the two most common complications of gastroesophageal reflux disease in infants (e.g., failure to thrive and pulmonary aspiration).[43]

The pathophysiology of gastroesophageal reflux is a complex, cyclic process (Fig. 31.1).[9] It is difficult, if not impossible, to determine which event occurred first in a given patient. Did gastroesophageal reflux lead to the noted changes or did the noted changes produce reflux? Understanding the factors associated with the development of GERD provides insight into the treatment modalities currently used to manage a patient who suffers from this disease. Overall, treatment is designed to minimize gastroesophageal reflux and thus its consequences.

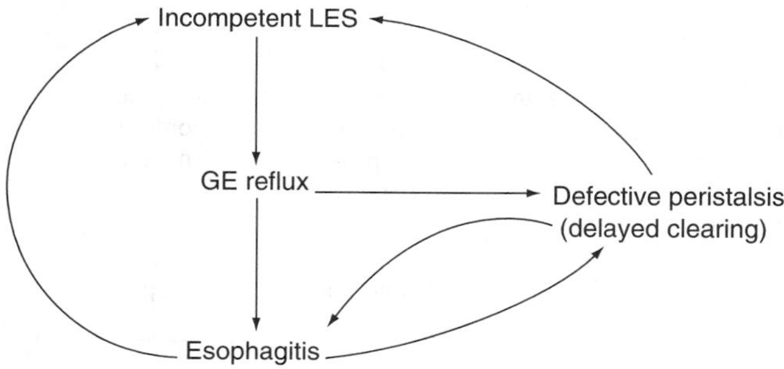

Figure 31.1. Schematic representation of classical concept of the pathogenesis of gastroesophageal (GE) reflux disease and various cyclic mechanisms of potential importance. LES, lower esophageal sphincter. *(Reproduced with permission from Richter JE, Castell DO. Gastroesophageal reflux. Pathogenesis, diagnosis, and therapy. Ann Intern Med 1982;97:94.)*

CLINICAL PRESENTATION

The hallmark symptom of gastroesophageal reflux and esophagitis is heartburn or pyrosis. It is classically described as a substernal sensation of warmth or burning that may radiate to the neck. It is waxing and waning in character, and is often aggravated by activities that potentiate gastroesophageal reflux (i.e., supine position, bending over). Heartburn is a common complaint of both healthy individuals and patients. It most commonly occurs when the gastric pH falls below 4.

Other symptoms that may occur in patients with GERD include regurgitation, water brash (hypersalivation), dysphagia (difficulty swallowing), odynophagia (pain on swallowing), and hemorrhage.[29] These symptoms are less specific and may occur in other esophageal disorders such as esophageal diverticulum, achalasia, obstruction, esophageal spasm, esophageal infections, scleroderma, and malignancy.[44] Regurgitation is the effortless movement of food or liquid from the esophagus into the mouth; it is frequently associated with gastroesophageal reflux (especially in infants). In contrast, dysphagia and odynophagia are less common and usually signify more severe disease. Chest pain may be present and must be distinguished from chest pain that is cardiac in nature. Other symptoms that are more atypical of GERD include pulmonary symptoms, cough, hoarseness, and hiccups. The severity of the symptoms of gastroesophageal reflux does not usually correlate with the degree of esophagitis, but it does correlate with the duration of reflux.[29]

Numerous factors and conditions have been associated with the potentiation of reflux and its symptomology. Factors that decrease lower esophageal sphincter pressure (Table 31.1) predispose patients to gastroesophageal reflux. Various foods aggravate esophageal reflux. Some of these foods cause a decrease in lower esophageal sphincter pressure; other foods such as spicy foods, orange juice, tomato juice, and coffee may precipitate symptomatic reflux by direct mucosal irritation.[11] Pregnancy, achalasia, and scleroderma are conditions in which reflux is common. There are many postulated reasons for the increased incidence of heartburn during pregnancy including hormonal effects on esophageal muscle, lower esophageal sphincter tone, and physical factors (increased intra-abdominal pressure) resulting from an enlarging uterus.[7]

Gastroesophageal reflux may lead to many severe complications, including esophageal ulceration, stricture formation, esophageal perforation, pharyngeal/oral disturbances, hemorrhage, and Barrett's esophagus.[45] Strictures are common in the distal esophagus and are generally 1–2 cm in length. The use of nonsteroidal anti-inflammatory drugs (NSAIDs) or aspirin has been implicated as an additional risk factor that may contribute to the development or worsening of esophageal strictures. In one study, 31% of patients undergoing initial dilation for benign esophageal strictures used NSAIDs compared with only 14% in controlled subjects.[46] Pulmonary complications including aspiration, recurrent pneumonia, and bronchospasm occur quite frequently in patients with GERD. Pulmonary symptoms are thought to result from either direct irritation of the vagus nerve by the refluxate, yielding bronchospasm or aspiration of the refluxate into the lungs, which causes chemical irritation.[45,47,48] Although GERD may lead to esophageal bleeding, the blood loss is usually chronic and low grade in nature and may lead to anemia. In some patients the reparative process leads to the replacement of the squamous epithelial lining of the esophagus by columnar-type epithelium. This condition, known as Barrett's esophagus, is found in 4.5–12.4% of patients undergoing endoscopy for reflux symptoms.[45] Barrett's esophagus is associated with a 5–10% incidence of adenocarcinoma and a 30–80% incidence of esophageal stricture formation.[45]

DIAGNOSIS

The most useful tool in the diagnosis of gastroesophageal reflux is the clinical history, including both presenting symptomology and associated risk factors. Patients presenting with classic symptoms of reflux do not usually require invasive esophageal evaluation; however, esophageal studies should be used as a tool to guide the diagnosis of gastroesophageal reflux when (1) the diagnosis is uncertain or the presentation is atypical; (2) the patient fails to respond to treatment; (3) the possibility of associated disease exists (i.e., peptic ulcer disease); or (4) the symptomology includes dysphagia, odynophagia, or bleeding.[49] Patients presenting with weight loss or anemia should also be thoroughly evaluated to determine cause.[33]

The numerous diagnostic tests used to diagnose GERD can be categorized on the basis of their ability to detect (1) potential for esophageal reflux, such as the presence of a hiatal hernia or decreased lower esophageal sphincter pressure; (2) esophageal damage, such as the acid perfusion test, endoscopy, mucosal biopsy, or barium esophagram; and (3) presence of reflux, such as barium esophagram, standard acid reflux test, gastrointestinal scintiscanning, or pH monitoring. Each of the tests currently available has some limitation associated with it; some lack specificity or sensitivity, some are difficult to perform, some are invasive, and some are expensive. Figure 31.2 depicts an algorithm that can be used to direct the selection of diagnostic tests based on the patient's clinical presentation.[50]

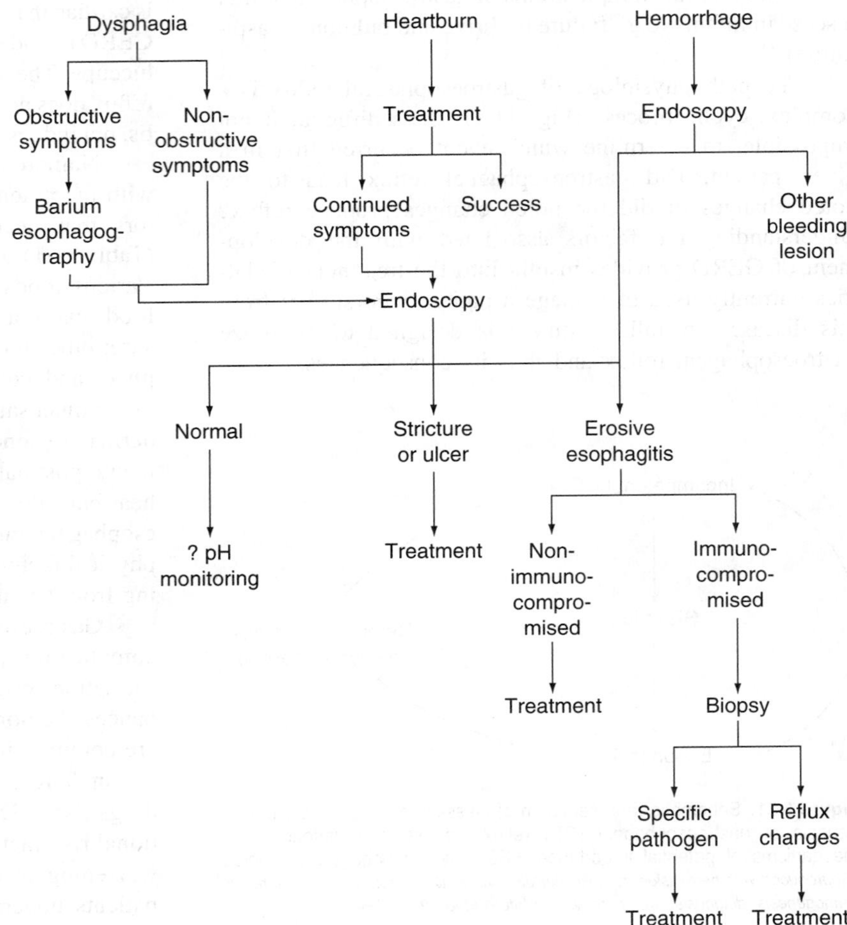

Figure 31.2. An algorithm to direct the selection of diagnostic tests based on the patient's clinical presentation. *(From Pope CE. Acid-reflux disorders. New Engl J Med 1994;331[10]: 656–660. Reprinted by permission of The New England Journal of Medicine, Copyright 1994, Massachusetts Medical Society.)*

Endoscopy allows visualization and biopsy of the esophageal mucosa, which permits assessment of the severity of esophageal injury. Several systems have been used to classify severity of disease; a common grading scale is depicted in Table 31.2.[51] While endoscopy is a highly specific test, it is not extremely sensitive. In mild cases of GERD the esophageal mucosa may appear relatively normal. The diagnostic yield may be increased by obtaining mucosal biopsies.[52] Noninflammatory GERD and major motor disorders may be missed by endoscopy. In these cases, 24-hour ambulatory pH monitoring or manometry may be useful to determine the degree of acid reflux or presence of a major motor disorder, respectively.

Twenty-four hour ambulatory pH monitoring, considered the gold standard by many, documents the percentage of time the intraesophageal pH is low.[33] It is very effective at determining the frequency and severity of reflux. Continuous pH monitoring can be performed by passing a small electrode pH probe intranasally and placing it approximately 5 cm above the lower esophageal sphincter.[33] Patients keep a diary of symptoms and these can be correlated with the pH measurement corresponding to the time the symptom was reported. It is useful in those patients with uncertain diagnosis, presence of noncardiac chest pain or other atypical symptoms, symptoms refractory to standard treatment, or in patients who are candidates for antireflux surgery.[53] Problems with esophageal pH monitoring arise when different methods are used to perform the test or a patient's baseline differs significantly from the standard.

Esophageal manometry is useful in excluding motility disorders and should be performed in any patient who is a candidate for antireflux surgery.[33] A multilumen tube is passed in the stomach and the pressures are measured as the tube is pulled back across the lower esophageal sphincter, the esophagus, and the pharynx.

The use or lack of use of the other diagnostic procedures, such as acid perfusion (Bernstein) test, barium esophagram, and gastrointestinal scintiscanning, is dependent on the patient's symptoms and the diagnostic facilities available.

Patients who present with atypical chest pain often require both cardiac and esophageal evaluations. The diagnosis is complicated because esophageal pain may cause electrocardiographic disorders, and both esophageal and cardiac disorders may occur simultaneously. In establishing a diagnosis of esophageal disease in these patients, it is crucial to document production of chest pain simultaneously with an esophageal abnormality.[54]

TABLE 31.2. ENDOSCOPIC CLASSIFICATION OF ESOPHAGITIS

Grade 0	Normal esophageal mucosa
Grade 1	Erythema or diffusely red mucosa, edema causing accentuated folds
Grade 2	Isolated round or linear erosions extending from the gastroesophageal junction upwards, not involving entire circumference
Grade 3	Confluent erosions extending around entire circumference or superficial ulceration without stenosis
Grade 4	Complicated cases; erosions as above plus deep ulcerations, stricture, or columnar epithelium-lined esophagus

(Adapted from Savary M, Miller G. The esophagus. Handbook and Atlas of Endoscopy. Solothurn, Gassman, 1978, with permission.)

TREATMENT

Therapeutic modalities utilized in the treatment of gastroesophageal reflux are targeted at reversing the various pathophysiologic abnormalities. The multifold goals of treatments are to (1) alleviate/eliminate the patient's symptoms, (2) decrease the frequency and duration of gastroesophageal reflux, (3) promote healing of the injured mucosa, and (4) prevent the development of complications. Therapy is directed at augmenting defense mechanisms that may prevent reflux and/or decreasing the aggressive factors that potentiate reflux or mucosal damage (Fig. 31.3). Specifically, therapy is directed at (1) increasing lower esophageal sphincter pressure, (2) enhancing esophageal acid clearance, (3) improving gastric emptying, (4) protecting the esophageal mucosa, (5) decreasing the acidity of the refluxate, and (6) decreasing the gastric volume available to be refluxed.[55] Treatment is categorized into the following modalities: lifestyle changes, pharmacologic interventions, and surgical interventions.

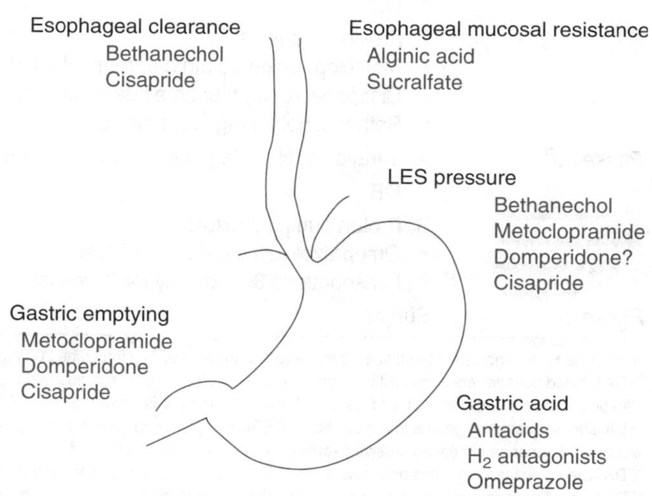

Figure 31.3. Therapeutic interventions in the management of gastroesophageal reflux disease. Pharmacologic interventions are targeted at improving defense mechanisms or decreasing aggressive factors. LES, lower esophageal sphincter.

The initial therapeutic modality used is in part dependent on the patient's condition (degree of esophagitis, presence of complications, etc.).[56] However, historically a stepwise approach has been used starting with noninvasive lifestyle modifications (Table 31.3).[2,9,53,56,57]

With the multitude of pharmacologic agents available to treat GERD, it becomes quite easy to relegate lifestyle modifications to historical therapy. However, lifestyle modifications are effective and are frequently used by patients with gastroesophageal reflux, many of whom have not sought medical attention (Table 31.4).[2,58,59] Patients not responding to lifestyle changes alone are generally started on a treatment regimen consisting of either antacids, H_2 antagonists, prokinetic agents, mucosal protectants, or proton pump inhibitors. Modifications of standard treatment regimens have been used in those patients who have failed traditional regimens. These modifications include increasing standard doses of H_2 antagonists to 2–4× the normal dose, administering combination therapy, or administering more potent acid-suppressive agents, such as omeprazole or lansoprazole.[60]

ANTACIDS AND ANTACID–ALGINIC ACID PRODUCTS

Antacids are commonly used in the treatment of gastroesophageal reflux because of their acid-neutralizing ability. Maintenance of the intragastric pH above 4 decreases the activation of pepsin from pepsinogen. Also, neutralization of gastric fluid leads to an increased lower esophageal sphincter pressure. Originally, the ability to increase lower esophageal sphincter pressure was thought to be gastrin mediated; however, serum gastrin levels were not altered by gastric alkalinization.[61]

While antacids are commonly used to treat gastroesophageal reflux and esophagitis, documentation of their efficacy in placebo-controlled clinical trials is lacking. One double-blind study compared the efficacy of liquid antacid (80 mEq per dose) taken seven times a day with placebo in 32 patients.[62] After 5 weeks of therapy, both treatment groups showed significant improvement in heartburn frequency and severity and degree of esophagitis, when compared with baseline. There was no significant difference in

TABLE 31.3. THERAPEUTIC APPROACH TO GASTROESOPHAGEAL REFLUX DISEASE

Phase I	Lifestyle changes/antacids/OTC H_2 antagonists[a]
Phase IIa	A. Standard doses of H_2 antagonists for 8–12 weeks (usually first-line therapy after phase I). • Cimetidine 400 mg four times daily or 800 mg twice daily[b] • Ranitidine 150 mg twice daily[c] • Famotidine 20 mg twice daily[d] • Nizatidine 150 mg twice daily[e] **OR** B. Mucosal protective agents (alternative to H_2 antagonist) Sucralfate 1 g after meals and at bedtime **OR** C. Prokinetic agents[f,g] • Metoclopramide 10 mg before meals and at bedtime (up to 15 mg four times daily) • Cisapride 10 mg four times daily (up to 20 mg four times daily) • Bethanechol 25 mg four times daily
Phase IIb[h]	A. Titration of H_2 antagonists to 1.5–2× standard dose **OR** B. Proton pump inhibitors • Omeprazole 20 mg daily for 8 weeks[i] • Lansoprazole 30 mg daily for 8 weeks[i]
Phase III	Surgery

[a]Low-dose H_2 antagonists: famotidine 10 mg taken up to twice daily; cimetidine 200 mg taken up to twice daily. (See Table 31.4).
[b]FDA labeled dosage regimens and indications: erosive esophagitis, cimetidine 800 mg twice daily or 400 mg four times daily for up to 12 weeks. Cimetidine 400 mg twice daily may also be effective in patients with mild disease, however, this dose is lower than the FDA approved dose.
[c]FDA labeled dosage regimens and indications: GERD symptoms, ranitidine 150 mg twice daily for up to 6 weeks; erosive esophagitis, ranitidine 150 mg four times daily for up to 12 weeks; maintenance of healing erosive esophagitis, ranitidine 150 mg twice daily.
[d]FDA labeled dosage regimens and indications: GERD symptoms, famotidine 20 mg twice daily for up to 6 weeks; esophagitis, famotidine 20–40 mg twice daily for up to 12 weeks.
[e]FDA labeled dosage regimen and indication: esophagitis, nizatidine 150 mg twice daily for up to 12 weeks.
[f]Concurrent use of an H_2 antagonist + prokinetic agent may be considered in those patients refractory to single-agent therapy or in those patients who have multifactoral problems contributing to their disease state. (e.g., esophagitis + motor dysfunction).
[g]Use in the presence of motor dysfunction, such as decreased lower esophageal sphincter pressure or decreased gastric emptying.
[h]Phase IIb therapy is often reserved for those patients who fail on phase I or IIa therapy or in those patients who present with even more severe disease (grade 3 or 4 esophagitis).
[i]Higher dosage regimens or longer durations of therapy may be used in refractory patients. (From Refs. 2, 9, 53, 56, and 57.)

TABLE 31.4. PHASE I TREATMENT MODALITIES

- Elevate the head of the bed (increases esophageal clearance)[58]
  - Use 6–8 1-inch blocks or 1 6- to 8-inch block under the head of the bed
  - Sleep on a foam wedge
- Dietary changes
  - Avoid foods that may decrease lower esophageal sphincter pressure (fats, chocolate, alcohol, peppermint, and spearmint)
  - Avoid foods that have a direct irritant effect on the esophageal mucosa (spicy foods, orange juice, tomato juice, and coffee)[2,59]
  - Include protein-rich meals in diet (augments lower esophageal sphincter pressure)
  - Eat small meals and avoid eating immediately prior to sleeping (decreases gastric volume)
  - Weight reduction (reduces symptoms)
- Stop smoking (decreases spontaneous esophageal sphincter relaxation)
- Avoid alcohol (increases amplitude of the lower esophageal sphincter, peristaltic waves, and frequency of contraction)
- Avoid tight-fitting clothes
- Discontinue drugs that may promote reflux, if possible
- Take drugs that have a direct irritant effect on the esophageal mucosa with plenty of liquid if they cannot be avoided (tetracyclines, quinidine, KCL, iron salts, aspirin, NSAIDs)
- Take antacids or over-the-counter H_2 antagonists as directed to relieve symptoms

(From Refs. 2, 58, and 59.)

response between placebo and antacid-treated patients. In contrast, two additional trials have demonstrated that antacids are superior to placebo in providing symptomatic relief.[63,64] Although, the literature is somewhat controversial on the superiority of antacids as compared with placebo, physicians and patients clearly consider antacids to be effective for symptomatic relief.

The dosage recommendations for antacids in the management of GERD are somewhat difficult to derive from the literature. Clinical trials have used various dosage schedules ranging from hourly antacid administration while awake to antacid regimens that are only taken on an as-needed basis.[61–65] Interestingly, low-dose antacids (30 mmol/tablet given four times a day) have been found to be superior to placebo in providing symptomatic relief.[64] In general, antacids have a short duration of action, which necessitates frequent administration throughout the day to provide continuous neutralization of acid. Night-time acid suppression cannot be maintained with bedtime doses of antacids.

An antacid combination product, containing alginic acid, sodium bicarbonate, aluminum hydroxide, and magnesium trisilicate (Gaviscon), is frequently used in the treatment of GERD. Unlike antacids, this product is not a potent neutralizing agent and does not enhance lower esophageal sphincter pressure. The alginic acid component forms a highly viscous solution that floats on the surface of the gastric contents. This viscous solution may act by mechanically impairing reflux, or by coating the esophagus, thus preventing mucosal contact of the irritants in refluxate.[66] Antacid–alginic acid tablets significantly decrease the number of reflux episodes and the percentage of time in which esophageal pH is less than 4.[67] In contrast, Johnson and DeMeester[58] found that the antacid–alginic acid product did not decrease esophageal acid exposure.

Several studies have compared the efficacy of the combination product (antacid–alginic acid) with that of antacids alone.[66,68,69] Overall, these studies demonstrate that the combination product (Gaviscon) usually relieves symptoms associated with reflux. Efficacy data indicating endoscopic healing are lacking.

Antacid and/or antacid combination products may cause gastrointestinal adverse effects (diarrhea or constipation, depending on the product), alterations in mineral metabolism, and possible acid–base disturbances. Aluminum-containing antacids may bind to phosphate in the gut and lead to bone damage. In addition, antacids interact with a variety of drugs by altering gastric pH, increasing urinary pH, absorbing medications to their surfaces, providing a physical barrier to absorption, or forming insoluble complexes with other medications.[70] Clinically significant antacid–drug interactions include tetracycline, ferrous sulfate, isoniazid, and quinolone antibiotics. Antacid–drug interactions are influenced by composition, dose, and dosage schedule of the antacid, as well as the formulation of the drug.

Antacids and/or antacid combination products are frequently used in the treatment of gastroesophageal reflux without complications. Antacids are generally used to provide symptomatic relief in patients who have mild to moderate intermittent symptoms. Patients with significant symptoms and/or severe disease often require more aggressive pharmacologic intervention with H_2 antagonists, prokinetic agents, mucosal protectants, or proton pump inhibitors. However, antacids are sometimes employed as adjunctive therapy to provide symptomatic relief.

H_2 ANTAGONISTS: CIMETIDINE, RANITIDINE, FAMOTIDINE, AND NIZATIDINE

The H_2 antagonists have historically been the mainstay in the treatment of GERD. These agents decrease gastric acid secretion by competitively and reversibly inhibiting the stimulation of the parietal cell by histamine. Decreasing the gastric acid secretion results in a less irritating refluxant. In addition, inhibition of gastric acid secretion results in a lower volume of gastric fluid available to be refluxed.

Extensive literature exists regarding the efficacy of the H_2 antagonists in the treatment of GERD.[15,57,60,71–85]

Indeed, all of the currently marketed H_2 antagonists (cimetidine, ranitidine, nizatidine, and famotidine) are approved for the management of GERD. Numerous placebo-controlled studies have demonstrated that H_2 antagonists are superior to placebo in the treatment of GERD.[15,57,60] The majority of the trials assessing the efficacy of standard dosage regimens of H_2 antagonists indicate that symptomatic improvement is achieved. However, healing rates are lower than those seen in duodenal ulcer disease and are far less than ideal. In general, endoscopic evidence of improvement in the degree of esophagitis is observed in approximately 45–80% of patients receiving standard doses of H_2 antagonists.[15,57,60] However, importantly, endoscopic healing rates tend to be lower.

Four major studies have compared the efficacy of H_2 antagonists with antacid therapy and have yielded conflicting results.[63,71–73] Two trials demonstrated that H_2 antagonists provided superior symptomatic and/or endoscopic healing rates compared to antacids.[71,72] In contrast, two other studies found no significant difference between the two agents.[63,73]

The clinical trials clearly indicate that the efficacy of H_2 antagonists in the management of GERD is extremely variable and is frequently lower than desired. Response to the H_2 antagonists appears to be dependent on the (1) severity of disease, (2) duration of therapy, and (3) dosage regimen used. These factors are important to keep in mind when comparing various clinical trials and/or assessing a patient's response to therapy.

Severity of Disease

The severity of esophagitis at baseline has a profound impact on a patient's response to H_2 antagonists. Tytgat et al.[74] demonstrated that patients with severe esophagitis (grade 3) had dramatically lower healing rates compared to those with less severe disease independent of the dosage regimen used. Following 12 weeks of cimetidine therapy (400 mg four times daily), endoscopic healing was observed in 80% of patients with mild esophagitis (grade 1) and only 46% of patients with severe disease (grade 3). Clearly, the more severe the esophageal damage, the poorer the response to H_2 antagonists.

Duration of Therapy

Unlike duodenal ulcer disease, in which the duration of therapy is relatively short (e.g., 4–6 weeks), prolonged courses of H_2 antagonists are frequently required in the treatment of GERD.[74,75] In an open-label trial of famotidine 40 mg daily, endoscopic healing increased as the duration of therapy increased.[75] After 4 weeks of therapy, healing was observed in 50% of patients. The healing rate increased with continued therapy, to yield healing rates of 75, 82, and 83% after 4, 12, and 16 weeks of therapy, respectively. Similar results were observed with cimetidine.[74] Based on the contribution of duration of therapy to the efficacy of H_2 antagonists, prolonged therapy (8 weeks or more) is frequently used when treating patients with GERD.

Dosage Regimen Used

The efficacy of numerous H_2 antagonist dosage regimens has been evaluated in the treatment of GERD. Low-dose H_2 antagonists have been shown to be effective in treating intermittent heartburn and in preventing meal-provoked heartburn.[76,77] Simon et al.[76] demonstrated the superiority of famotidine 5, 10, and 20 mg and antacids in relieving episodes of heartburn as compared to placebo. Patients were instructed to ingest the study medication on an as-needed basis at the onset of a heartburn episode. Overall, 41, 59, 70, 69, and 62% of the heartburn episodes were relieved following treatment with placebo, famotidine 5 mg, 10 mg, 20 mg, or antacids, respectively. Although the majority of patients enrolled in the study had mild disease without evidence of esophagitis at study entry, evaluation of the subset of patients with esophagitis (usually grade 1 or grade 2) revealed that famotidine 10 and 20 mg was superior to placebo in providing heartburn relief. However, no significant difference was detected between famotidine 5 mg, antacids, and placebo in this subset of patients. This further stresses the impact of severity of disease on response. Recently, low-dose famotidine (10 mg used up to twice daily) and cimetidine (200 mg used up to twice daily) gained FDA approval as OTC medications to prevent heartburn and acid indigestion. Based on their similar mechanism of action, one would anticipate that low-dose ranitidine and nizatidine will also be effective in relieving heartburn and, therefore, their manufacturers may also seek FDA approval for OTC usage. With the availability of OTC H_2 antagonists, it is imperative that pharmacists have a thorough understanding of GERD and be willing to educate the consumer.

As previously stated standard-dose H_2 antagonists are effective in providing symptomatic relief and endoscopic healing in patients with GERD. In general, standard-dose H_2 antagonists provide improvement in the degree of esophagitis in 45–80% of patients.[15,57,60] In one study assessing the efficacy of various cimetidine regimens, response was primarily dependent on the severity of disease and not the dosage regimen employed.[74] Healing rates ranging from 47–84% and 49–79% were achieved with cimetidine 800 mg at bedtime and cimetidine 400 mg four times daily, respectively. Although the results of Tytgat et al.[74] suggest that as low as 800 mg of cimetidine may be effective in healing esophagitis, usual doses have been 1–1.6 g daily.

Due to the somewhat disappointing healing rates observed with standard dosages of H_2 antagonists, many recent studies have evaluated the efficacy of higher doses.[78–83,85] One study demonstrated that high-dose ranitidine (300 mg four times daily) provided a higher healing rate than that achieved with a standard dose (150 mg twice daily) regimen, with healing rates of 75 and 54%, respectively.[78] Similarly, Euler et al.[80] demonstrated that ranitidine 150 mg four times daily and ranitidine 300 mg four times daily was more effective than placebo in healing esophagitis and relieving symptoms in patients with erosive esophagitis. Healing rates following 12 weeks of therapy were 79, 74, and 40% for patients receiving 150 mg three times daily, 300 mg four times daily, or placebo, respectively.

Famotidine dosage regimens used in various trials have ranged from 40 mg at bedtime to 40 mg three times daily.[81–83] Endoscopic healing was shown to be superior following famotidine 40 mg twice daily as compared to famotidine 20 mg twice daily; with healing rates of 58% versus 43% at 6 weeks and 76% versus 67% at 12 weeks, respectively.[82]

The efficacy of once, twice, and three times a day regimens of nizatidine have been evaluated.[84,85] Although Cloud et al.[84] demonstrated that standard-dose nizatidine (150 mg twice daily) was more effective than placebo in healing esophagitis, nizatidine 300 mg given at bedtime was not effective. Higher dosage regimens of nizatidine have been shown to provide higher healing rates.[85] Specifically, endoscopic healing rates of 81.3, 79.2, and 67% have been reported for patients receiving nizatidine 150 mg three times daily, 150 mg + 150 mg + 300 mg, or 300 mg twice daily, respectively.[85] Both of the three-times-daily regimens were superior to the twice-daily regimen, $P < 0.005$. Because H_2 antagonists may not adequately block acid suppression in those patients who have an increased stimulus to secrete acid, dosage adjustments should be made according to patient response.

Although high-dose H_2 antagonists may provide higher symptomatic and endoscopic healing rates, it is important to realize that limited information exists regarding the safety of high-dose regimens. Based on the lack of safety information regarding high-dose H_2 antagonist therapy, it is prudent to recommend starting a patient on standard doses (cimetidine 400 mg four times a day or 800 mg twice daily, ranitidine 150 mg twice daily, famotidine 20 mg twice daily, or nizatidine 150 mg twice daily). If the patient fails to respond to standard regimens or if the patient has severe disease, higher dose regimens may be recommended.

Although data identifying the ideal H_2-antagonist dosage regimen to be used in the treatment of GERD are lacking, it is theorized that profound acid suppression may lead to increased healing rates. This theory is based on five observations. First, gastroesophageal reflux occurs during both daytime and night-time hours. Thus, acid suppression for only part of the day may not be sufficient to prevent the refluxate from injuring the esophageal mucosa, especially postprandially and during the night-time hours. H_2 antagonists do not easily overcome the stimulus for acid secretion following a meal and, thus, postprandial acid secretion may be inadequately suppressed.[40] Dividing the H_2-antagonist dose may provide coverage for both daytime and night-time acid reflux and may theoretically improve symptom control and esophageal healing. However, studies have yielded conflicting results.[40,84] Second, high-dose ranitidine (>300 mg daily) provides a greater degree of acid suppression compared with the standard-dose regimen of 300 mg daily and is also associated with higher healing rates.[78] Third, the profound acid suppression achieved with omeprazole results in dramatically increased response rates.[86] Fourth, a subset of patients with GERD has been reported to have hypersecretion of gastric acid and may, therefore, require higher doses of antisecretory agents.[87] Finally, Bell et al.[40] demonstrated a relationship between the 8-week healing rate of esophagitis and the time duration that gastric pH is > 4.0. Similarly, an inverse relationship between healing rate and esophageal acid exposure was also found. Based on Bell's findings one may be able to predict responses to antisecretory regimens based on their ability to maintain intragastric pH> 4.0.

Since all of the H_2 antagonists are efficacious, selection of the specific agent to be used in the management of GERD should be based on other factors such as differences in pharmacokinetics and safety profiles, as well as cost. In general, these agents are extremely safe. However, agents decrease gastric acid secretion and therefore may lead to a decrease in absorption of weak bases, such as ketoconazole.[70] In addition, cimetidine inhibits the metabolism of several drugs and concomitant therapy may need to be closely monitored or adjusted. Ranitidine also binds to the cytochrome P-450 system, but it does so less avidly than cimetidine. The pharmacokinetic profile, as well as cost of the individual agents, may in part impact this decision, and the reader is referred to two excellent reviews comparing agents.[88,89]

PROKINETIC AGENTS: BETHANECHOL, METOCLOPRAMIDE, AND CISAPRIDE

The efficacy of bethanechol, metoclopramide, and cisapride has been evaluated in the treatment of GERD. All of these agents have been shown to increase lower esophageal sphincter pressure and thereby may minimize the number of reflux episodes.[90–93] Bethanechol and cisapride have also been shown to improve esophageal clearance.[90,93] Metoclopramide and cisapride promote gastric emptying and thus may be of benefit in patients with GERD, many of whom have delayed gastric emptying.[93,94] Bethanechol does not improve gastric emptying.[90]

Bethanechol

Although bethanechol has been shown to increase lower esophageal sphincter pressure, improve esophageal clearance, and provide similar symptomatic and endoscopic healing compared with cimetidine 300 mg four times a day, its side-effect profile severely limits its use.[95,96] Oral bethanechol may cause abdominal cramps, urinary frequency, malaise, blurred vision, and diarrhea. In addition, bethanechol may increase gastric acid secretion. Because bethanechol is a cholinergic agonist, relative contraindications for its use include asthma, chronic obstructive pulmonary disease, and peptic ulcer disease.

Metoclopramide

Metoclopramide, a dopamine antagonist, increases lower esophageal sphincter pressure in a dose-related manner and has also been shown to accelerate gastric emptying in gastroesophageal reflux patients.[42,94] Ten milligrams of oral metoclopramide significantly increased gastric emptying of a solid-liquid meal in reflux patients with delayed gastric emptying as well as in patients with normal gastric emptying rates.[94] Another study found that antral contractility is reduced in patients with esophagitis and both antral contractility and gastric emptying are significantly improved after a single 15-mg dose of metoclopramide.[42]

Based on metoclopramide's ability to increase lower esophageal sphincter pressure and improve gastric emptying, it may be useful in the treatment of gastroesophageal reflux. However, there was no significant difference between placebo and metoclopramide (10 mg four times daily) in symptomatic response rates reported in one study.[97] Conversely, in two studies[98,99] metoclopramide 10 mg four times daily was superior to placebo in providing symptomatic relief; however, metoclopramide did not provide significant endoscopic and histologic improvement as compared to placebo.[99]

A double-blind trial comparing cimetidine 300 mg four times daily and metoclopramide 10 mg four times daily with placebo showed that metoclopramide and cimetidine significantly improved symptomatic response rates, but not endoscopic response rates, compared with placebo.[100] Ranitidine 150 mg twice daily was found to be superior to metoclopramide 10 mg three times daily in promoting improvement in the endoscopic appearance of esophagitis.[101]

A limiting factor with metoclopramide therapy may be the high incidence of adverse effects. The safety of this agent was evaluated in 269 gastroesophageal reflux patients who received doses ranging from 10–50 mg daily.[102] Forty-eight percent of the participants experienced adverse effects and 17% of the population withdrew from the study because of adverse reactions. Most commonly reported adverse reactions were somnolence (9%), nervousness (9%), fatigue (8%), dizziness (5%), weakness (3%), depression (2%), diarrhea (2%), and rash (2%). Other possible adverse reactions include anxiety, insomnia, and extrapyramidal reactions.[9] Metoclopramide elevates serum prolactin concentrations and may lead to gynecomastia, galactorrhea, or menstrual irregularity. The risk of adverse effects is much greater in patients with renal dysfunction since the drug is primarily eliminated by the kidneys. Because metoclopramide is a dopamine antagonist, its activity may undermine the treatment of Parkinson's disease. Additional contraindications to metoclopramide use include mechanical obstruction, concomitant use of other dopamine antagonists, anticholingeric agents, pheochromocytoma, and Parkinson's disease.

Overall, metoclopramide improves gastric emptying and increases lower esophageal sphincter pressure. Although studies suggest that metoclopramide provides symptomatic improvement for patients with gastroesophageal reflux disease, substantial data indicating that metoclopramide provides endoscopic healing are currently lacking. In addition, metoclopramide's side-effect profile often limits its use.

Cisapride

Cisapride is a synthetic, substituted piperidinyl benzamide chemically related to metoclopramide.[93] It is indicated for the symptomatic treatment of patients with nocturnal heartburn due to gastroesophageal reflux disease. Cisapride is thought to increase lower esophageal sphincter pressure and accelerate gastric emptying through the facilitation of acetylcholine release at the myenteric plexus.[93] Cisapride also increases the amplitude of esophageal contractions and is effective in improving esophageal clearance in some select patient populations.[93]

Cisapride 10 mg four times daily has been shown to be superior to placebo in providing both symptomatic relief and endoscopic healing in patients with gastroesophageal reflux disease.[103,104] The endoscopic healing rate observed in these studies ranged from 63–73%. The efficacy of cisapride 10 mg four times daily in the treatment of GERD has been shown to be similar to that of cimetidine 400 mg four times daily and ranitidine 150 mg twice daily.[105,106] Cisapride 10 mg twice daily or 20 mg four times daily was compared with cimetidine 400 mg twice daily or 400 mg four times daily.[107] All patients showed improvement in severity of diurnal and nocturnal heartburn and regurgitation. Endoscopic healing rates were similar with 69, 64, 55, and 55% for cisapride 10 mg twice daily, 20 mg four times daily, cimetidine 400 mg twice daily, and 400 mg four times daily showing healing rates, respectively. In another study, a greater percentage of patients treated with cisapride 10 mg three times daily for 4 weeks were asymptomatic compared with patients receiving metoclopramide 10 mg three times daily, although the difference was not statistically significant.[108] In addition, cisapride was better tolerated.

Cisapride appears to be a potential agent for the treatment of infants with gastroesophageal reflux. One study demonstrated the superiority of cisapride (0.15–0.3 mg/kg given three times daily) as compared with placebo in the management of GERD in infants.[109]

Unlike metoclopramide, this newer prokinetic agent is devoid of antidopaminergic effects and, therefore, does not cause extrapyramidal side effects or prolactin secretion.[90] The most commonly reported adverse effects following cisapride administration are gastrointestinal in nature and include transient abdominal cramping, borborygmi, diarrhea, and loose stools. Cisapride is extensively metabolized via oxidative *N*-dealkylation and hydroxylation pathways. Recent reports indicate that patients taking cisapride concurrently with ketoconazole, miconazole, itraconazole, or troleandomycin may lead to prolongation of the QT interval leading to ventricular arrhythmias. For this reason, the concurrent use of cisapride with these agents is contraindicated.

While many of the studies performed in other countries have shown promising results, some of the U.S. studies evaluating cisapride 10 mg three times daily have not consistently shown benefits over placebo.[110] However, doses of 10–20 mg four times daily may be more effective in attaining therapeutic effect.[93] More studies are needed to assess the effectiveness in more severe disease (grade 2 and 3), as well as the effectiveness of long-term use, possibly as maintenance therapy for patients with GERD. In addition, studies comparing cisapride to omeprazole are needed.

MUCOSAL PROTECTANTS: SUCRALFATE

Sucralfate is a nonabsorbable aluminum salt of sucrose octasulfate that is effective in the treatment of duodenal ulcer disease.[111] While the precise mechanism of action is unclear, local mucosal protection is achieved. On the basis of mucosal protective properties, sucralfate may be effective in the treatment of gastroesophageal reflux. One study demonstrated endoscopic improvement in 7 of 18 patients following 12 weeks of treatment with sucralfate granulate 1 g four times daily.[112] In contrast, a multicenter, double-blind placebo-controlled trial found that sucralfate suspension (1 g after meals and 2 g at bedtime) yielded healing rates similar to those seen with placebo.[113] Following 8 weeks of therapy, 36% of patients who received sucralfate and 35% of those who received placebo were completely healed. Although neither endoscopic healing nor symptomatic relief were different among the two groups, more patients tended to improve on sucralfate (81%) as compared with placebo (49%), $P = 0.07$.

Limited comparative trials are available assessing the efficacy of sucralfate as compared with standard therapy in the treatment of GERD.[114–122] Sucralfate was found to provide similar healing rates as compared with antacid–alginic acid therapy in patients with endoscopically proven esophagitis.[114,115] Sucralfate has comparable healing rates with H_2 antagonists for patients with less severe disease.[116–122] Healing rates of 64 and 68% were demonstrated for sucralfate-treated patients (1 g suspension four times daily) or ranitidine 150 mg twice daily, respectively.[116] Similarly, in a multicenter trial, endoscopic improvement was seen in 67% of patients receiving cimetidine 400 mg four times daily as compared with 53% of those receiving sucralfate suspension 1 g four times daily.[117] Although endoscopic improvement was noted in the majority of patients regardless of treatment, endoscopic healing rates were rather low. Thirty-one percent of patients demonstrated endoscopic healing following 8 weeks of sucralfate, as compared with 14% for those receiving cimetidine. Another study failed to show comparable efficacy of sucralfate to high-dose famotidine in patients with refractory esophagitis.[123]

Overall, the efficacy of sucralfate varies greatly among the studies. The wide range of response rates may in part be related to (1) patient population, (2) baseline degree of esophagitis, (3) duration of treatment, (4) dose used, or (5) sucralfate formulation used. A suspension formulation of sucralfate was used in many of the trials. Theoretically, a suspension may more effectively coat the esophagus as it is swallowed and/or act as a barrier on reflux than a tablet. A commercially available suspension makes giving this dosage form more convenient than previously possible.

Sucralfate is generally well tolerated; however, constipation, dry mouth, nausea, and abdominal discomfort may occur. Caution should be used when sucralfate is administered to a patient with renal dysfunction, because the aluminum may accumulate. Sucralfate may also lead to hypophosphatemia, presumably due to binding with phosphate in the gut. Sucralfate may also interact with several drugs leading to a decrease in drug absorption.[70]

In general, sucralfate appears effective in some patients and may therefore be a suitable alternative to standard-dose H_2 antagonists or antacid–alginic acid therapy for treating mild esophagitis. Additional trials are needed to further elucidate the precise role of sucralfate in the management of GERD.

PROTON PUMP INHIBITORS: OMEPRAZOLE AND LANSOPRAZOLE

Omeprazole and lansoprazole belong to the class of drugs commonly referred to as proton pump inhibitors. These agents inhibit gastric acid secretion by inhibiting gastric H^+/K^+-adenosine triphosphatase.[86,124–126] The net result is profound long-lasting inhibition of acid secretion.

Because gastric acid secretion is the major aggressive factor responsible for esophageal damage in patients with gastroesophageal reflux disease, it appears logical that potent inhibitors of gastric acid secretion, such as the proton pump inhibitors omeprazole and lansoprazole, may have a prominent role in our armamentarium. Studies document the superior efficacy of both lansoprazole and omeprazole as compared with placebo in the treatment of patients with GERD.[86,124–128] Omeprazole dose-finding (20 mg versus 40 mg daily versus placebo) studies revealed that both 20 and 40 mg given once daily were superior to placebo in healing esophagitis.[127,128] In a U.S. multicenter trial, healing rates of 73.5, 74.7, and 14% were observed for patients treated with omeprazole 20 mg daily, 40 mg daily, and placebo, respectively.[128] Similarly, dose-ranging studies with lansoprazole have revealed that lansoprazole 15, 30, and 60 mg daily is more effective than placebo in healing esophagitis.[125,126] Furthermore, lansoprazole regimens of 30 and 60 mg daily have been shown to be superior to lansoprazole 15 mg daily.

The comparative efficacy of proton pump inhibitors (omeprazole or lansoprazole) with either ranitidine or cimetidine has been assessed in several randomized, controlled trials.[86,124–126,129–132] Studies demonstrate esophageal healing in 57–85% of patients after 4 weeks of omeprazole (20–60 mg daily) therapy as compared with healing rates of 27–45% during ranitidine or cimetidine therapy.[86] Meta-analysis of these trials revealed a significant therapeutic advantage, as measured by both symptom relief and endoscopic healing, for omeprazole as compared with ranitidine after both 4 and 8 weeks of therapy. In addition, the benefit of omeprazole as compared to ranitidine was more evident in patients with severe disease. Lansoprazole 30 and 60 mg daily were also shown to provide superior symptom relief and healing rates as compared with ranitidine 150 mg twice daily.[130–132] Comparative trials have reported healing rates ranging from 91–92% following 8 weeks of therapy with lansoprazole 30 mg daily as compared with 53–70% following ranitidine therapy.[130–132]

Two studies have compared the efficacy of lansoprazole and omeprazole.[133,134] The results from these studies indicate that the healing rates after 8 weeks of treatment with lansoprazole 30 mg daily are similar to those observed following 8 weeks of omeprazole therapy (20 mg daily). In one study, following 4 weeks of therapy, symptomatic relief was greater for patients treated with lansoprazole as compared to those receiving omeprazole.[134] However, following 8 weeks of treatment no significant difference in symptom relief was noted between the two regimens.

Omeprazole and lansoprazole have also been shown to be efficacious in patients who are refractory to standard doses of H_2 antagonists[135–137] and in those with gastroesophageal reflux complications, such as Barrett's esophagitis.[138–140] The efficacy of omeprazole 40 mg daily was compared with high-dose ranitidine (600 mg daily) in patients who were refractory to standard-dose H_2 antagonist regimens.[135] After 12 weeks of therapy significantly more patients were healed with the omeprazole regimen (90%) as compared with those who received ranitidine (47%), $P < 0.0001$. Similarly, Feldman et al.[137] assessed the efficacy of lansoprazole (30 mg daily) and ranitidine (150 mg twice daily) for the treatment erosive esophagitis that was resistant to H_2 antagonists. Following 8 weeks of treatment, the healing rate was significantly higher for patients receiving lansoprazole compared with those receiving ranitidine (i.e., 89 and 38%, respectively). Preliminary reports indicate that omeprazole 40–60 mg daily and lansoprazole 30–60 mg daily are effective in healing esophagitis and esophageal ulcers in patients with Barrett's esophagus.[138–140]

Clinical trials clearly indicate that omeprazole and lansoprazole are effective in providing symptomatic relief and esophageal healing in a significant percentage of patients with severe GERD. Both lansoprazole and omeprazole have an FDA-approved indication for the treatment of erosive esophagitis. Omeprazole also has an FDA-approved indication for the treatment of poorly responsive symptomatic GERD. Because both omeprazole and lansoprazole degrade in acidic environments, these agents have been formulated as delayed release capsules that contain enteric coated (pH-sensitive) granules.

Omeprazole and lansoprazole are usually well tolerated; however, potential adverse effects include headache, dizziness, somnolence, diarrhea, constipation, and nausea.[86,124–126] The frequency of adverse events with omeprazole or lansoprazole appears to be similar to that seen with the H_2 antagonists. Concern and controversy regarding the safety of therapy with a proton pump inhibitor are based on their ability to produce hypergastrinemia and gastric carcinoid tumors in rats. Importantly neither omeprazole nor lansoprazole has been shown to produce tumors in humans and an excellent review of this controversy is available.[86]

COMBINATION THERAPY

Combination therapy would seem to be a logical choice in treating patients with GERD given the multifactorial nature of the disease, particularly in light of the disappointing results seen to date with many single-agent regimens. Unfortunately, sufficient data to support use of combination therapy are limited. Most of the information available suggests that combination therapy offers only modest improvements over standard-dose H_2 antagonists alone. Therefore, until more data are available, combination therapy should be reserved for those patients failing to respond to traditional single-agent therapy or for those patients who obviously have multifactorial problems contributing to their disease (e.g., esophagitis + motor dysfunction).

The most frequently used combinations include H_2 antagonists with prokinetic agents. Cimetidine 1200 mg daily plus metoclopramide 40 mg daily or cimetidine plus placebo were compared in 25 patients with persistent heartburn and endoscopic evidence of disease, despite 1 month of treatment with lifestyle changes, antacids, and cimetidine 1200 mg daily.[141] After 8 weeks, 25% of patients treated with single-drug therapy versus 75% of patients treated with combination therapy had improvement of symptoms, $P < 0.05$. Side effects were more common in the patients receiving combination therapy, primarily related to the use of metoclopramide. This may have been a source of bias in this study. Another study compared cimetidine 1 g daily plus cisapride 40 mg daily with cimetidine plus placebo in 47 patients with endoscopically diagnosed severe reflux esophagitis.[142] After 12 weeks, 46% of patients treated with single-drug therapy versus 70% of patients treated with combination therapy were healed. Symptomatic improvement was also significantly better in patients receiving the combination regimen compared with the single-dose regimen, $P < 0.05$.

Although some reports of H_2 antagonist plus a prokinetic agent have shown promising results, others have not been as convincing.[143] Data on famotidine or nizatidine in combination with a prokinetic agent are insufficient to recommend their use.

Data with other drug combinations for the treatment of GERD are even more limited. One study demonstrated the benefit from the combination of cimetidine 300 mg four times daily plus sucralfate (1 g after meals and 2 g at bedtime) as compared with cimetidine alone.[144] While patients receiving combination therapy showed greater endoscopic improvement of esophagitis when compared with those patients receiving single-drug therapy, healing rates were not significantly different. No added benefit was found when sucralfate 1 g three times daily plus cimetidine 400 mg at night was compared with sucralfate 1 g four times daily alone.[145] Until studies show a true benefit resulting from an H_2 antagonist combined with sucralfate, this combination cannot be recommended.

MAINTENANCE THERAPY

Although healing and/or symptomatic improvement may be achieved via many different therapeutic modalities, a large percentage of patients with gastroesophageal reflux will relapse following discontinuation of therapy. Follow-up studies indicate that 70–90% of patients will relapse within 1 year of discontinuation of therapy.[127] Due to the high rate of relapse, several maintenance regimens have been used. The primary goal of maintenance therapy is to keep the patient in remission using lower dosages than those routinely used therapeutically. More studies are needed to determine which dosage regimen is most beneficial and if maintenance therapy should consist of standard doses or lower doses to prevent relapse of gastroesophageal reflux disease.

Maintenance therapy with the H_2 antagonists is extremely effective in preventing duodenal ulcer recurrence; however, their efficacy in maintaining GERD patients in remission is somewhat disappointing. Neither cimetidine 300 mg twice daily nor cimetidine 400 mg at bedtime was significantly superior to placebo in preventing recurrence over the 12-month study period.[146] There was a slight tendency for the twice-daily regimen to be more effective than the once-daily regimen, suggesting that higher doses may be required. In a similar study comparing ranitidine 150 mg twice daily and ranitidine 150 mg at bedtime with placebo in preventing recurrence there was a trend for the twice-daily regimen to be more effective; however, no significant differences were seen between the active treatments and placebo.[147] In contrast Euler et al.[148] demonstrated that recurrence rates of esophagitis were significantly less in patients receiving ranitidine 150 mg twice daily as compared to placebo. Similarly, one study demonstrated that ranitidine 150 mg twice daily was superior to placebo in preventing the recurrence of symptoms.[149] Ranitidine 150 mg twice daily has an FDA approved indication for maintenance of healing of erosive esophagitis.

Emerging data suggest that cisapride may be effective in preventing relapse in certain patients. One hundred and thirty-eight patients with endoscopically diagnosed reflux esophagitis received cisapride 10 mg four times daily for 8–16 weeks (phase I).[150] Healing was seen in 69% and symptoms decreased by 67%. Eighty patients from phase I who were healed on cisapride (10 mg four times daily) received cisapride 10 mg twice daily or placebo as maintenance therapy. Patients in the cisapride group had a 20% relapse rate compared with 39% in the placebo group, $P < 0.06$. Patients with less severe disease remained in remission longer than patients with more severe disease. Cisapride 20 mg at bedtime, cisapride 10 mg twice daily, or placebo were evaluated for preventing relapse in 443 patients whose reflux esophagitis was previously healed with an antisecretory agent.[151] Maintenance therapy was continued for 12 months or until there was endoscopic evidence of relapse. Both cisapride regimens were significantly better than placebo in preventing relapse, $P = 0.012$. Fifty-one percent of patients showed relapse at 12 months in the placebo group compared with 32 and 34% in the cisapride 20 mg at bedtime and cisapride 10 mg twice daily groups, respectively, $P = 0.02$. Patients whose disease was more severe before treatment tended to relapse faster than those with less severe disease. The severity of esophagitis before treatment appears to be a prognostic marker suggestive of a greater risk of relapse during maintenance therapy.

The efficacy of omeprazole 20 mg daily was compared with that of ranitidine 150 mg twice daily in preventing recurrence.[152] Only 25% of patients receiving omeprazole relapsed during the year-long study, as compared with the greater than 80% of patients receiving ranitidine. In a similar study, the efficacy of omeprazole 20 mg daily, omeprazole 20 mg daily taken only on weekends (Friday, Saturday, Sunday), and ranitidine 150 mg twice daily in preventing recurrence was assessed.[153] The standard omeprazole regimen (20 mg daily) was effective; however, the alternative regimens did not appear to be beneficial. The efficacy of a lower dose of omeprazole (10 mg daily) as compared with the omeprazole weekend regimen (20 mg daily) was also assessed.[154] The 10 mg daily regimen prevented relapse in 79% of the patients. The weekend regimen was significantly inferior to the 10 mg daily regimen. The use of omeprazole for maintenance therapy in GERD was recently approved by the FDA.

SURGERY

Surgical intervention is indicated when (1) the patient fails to respond to conservative and pharmacologic treatment modalities, (2) strictures are present, (3) major bleeding occurs, and (4) pulmonary complications exist.[29] Surgical procedures include Nissen, Belsey Mark IV, and Hill operations. Recently laparoscopic surgical procedures have been introduced.[5,6] Due to diminished surgical complications with these newer procedures the role of surgery in the long-term management of GERD has become controversial.[5–8] In general, these surgical techniques increase resting pressure of the lower esophageal sphincter.[9,29] Successful surgery does not guarantee that GERD will not recur. Historically, because the long-term results of surgery have been somewhat disappointing, many clinicians opt for more aggressive pharmacologic therapy.

INVESTIGATIONAL AGENTS

Several investigational agents have been evaluated in the treatment of GERD. These include the prokinetic agents clebopride and domperidone, and a proton pump inhibitor, pantoprazole.[155–160] New H_2 antagonists under development include etintidine and roxatidine.

Domperidone is a new prokinetic agent currently undergoing clinical investigations. It is similar to metoclopramide in that it is a specific dopamine antagonist; however, because it works more peripherally, it does not readily penetrate the central nervous system and therefore rarely causes extrapyramidal reactions.[155] Like metoclopramide and cisapride, domperidone has been shown to accelerate gastric emptying. Oral domperidone has not shown effect on lower esophageal sphincter pressure.

The efficacy of oral domperidone in the treatment of GERD has been assessed in a limited number of clinical trials with somewhat conflicting reports.[156–158] The comparative efficacy of domperidone 20 mg four times daily, metoclopramide 10 mg four times daily, and placebo were assessed in a double-blind crossover trial involving 23 patients with gastroesophageal reflux.[158] All three treatment regimens were associated with symptomatic improvement as compared with baseline; however, no difference was detected among the treatment regimens. Although preliminary studies suggest that domperidone may be effective in the treatment of GERD and is associated with less adverse reactions than metoclopramide, delineation of the role of this agent in the treatment of GERD awaits additional trials.

These newer agents will be a welcomed addition to our armamentarium of drugs used in the management of GERD. As more studies are done on these agents, their true niche in the management of GERD will be delineated.

EVALUATION OF THERAPEUTIC OUTCOMES

Evaluation of the long-term benefits of treatment are difficult to assess due to limited information known about the epidemiology and natural history of GERD. Therefore, successful outcomes are generally measured in terms of symptomatic relief. Healing of the esophageal mucosa should be considered a separate endpoint.

The short-term goal of therapy is to relieve symptoms, such as heartburn and regurgitation, to the point where they do not impair the patient's quality of life. Pharmacists should take an active role in educating the patient about potential adverse effects and drug interactions that may occur with drug therapy. The frequency and severity of symptoms should be monitored; and patients should be counseled on symptoms that may suggest the presence of complications requiring immediate medical attention, such as dysphagia or odynophagia. Patients with persistent dysphagia should be evaluated for the presence of strictures or other complications. Long-term treatment is indicated in patients who have strictures because they commonly recur if esophagitis is not treated.[161]

Patient compliance is another factor that will affect the outcome of drug therapy. Drug regimens that are easily managed will improve compliance and therefore outcome for the patient. This can especially be a problem in patients who require high-dose therapy with H_2 antagonists. Not only are they required to take the drug more often in higher doses, but there is also an increased expense associated with such regimens. The patient may be unable to afford the drug. Choosing a drug that is the least expensive and provides the greatest benefit related to dosing interval and number of tablets taken is the optimal regimen. Studies comparing the cost effectiveness of the various treatment strategies for GERD are limited.[162,163] Hillman et al.[162] utilized decision analysis to evaluate the cost effectiveness of phase I therapy, or phase I therapy combined with omeprazole 20 mg daily or ranitidine 150 mg twice daily for patients with persistent symptomatic gastroesophageal reflux disease who had failed phase I therapy. A complex model that evaluated the influence of empiric versus definitive therapy, compliance, and efficacy of the three treatment regimens was employed. Although the retail cost of omeprazole was the highest among the treatments evaluated, it was the most effective strategy and was associated with the lowest overall cost. Additional studies evaluating the cost effectiveness of various treatment regimens as well as studies assessing the impact of these treatments on quality of life issues are needed.

The long-term goal is to decrease the risk of complications (esophagitis, strictures, Barrett's esophagus) and prevent recurrence associated with GERD. A small subset of patients may continue to fail treatment, despite therapy with higher doses of H_2 antagonists or omeprazole. Maintenance therapy with standard to higher doses of antisecretory agents may be indicated in these acid hypersecretors since severe esophagitis that is not adequately treated may lead to Barrett's esophagitis and its associated risk of adenocarcinoma. Unfortunately, data are lacking that show effective treatment of esophagitis decreases the risk of developing adenocarcinoma in patients with Barrett's esophagitis.

Pharmacists must have a clear understanding about the pathophysiology and management of GERD in order to develop an appropriate pharmaceutical care plan for the patient.

CONCLUSION

Gastroesophageal reflux disease is a common entity that classically presents as heartburn. The pathophysiology of reflux is complex, involving both aggressive factors (acid, pepsin, bile acids, pancreatic enzymes, prostaglandins) and defense mechanisms (anatomic factors, lower esophageal sphincter pressure, esophageal clearance, gastric emptying); however, an understanding of the pathophysiology allows the design of rational treatment regimens. Therapeutic modalities (Fig. 31.3) are designed to minimize aggressive factors and/or augment defense mechanisms. The treatment of GERD often involves a multidisciplinary stepwise approach. Patients with mild esophagitis may be satisfactorily treated with lifestyle modifications and antacids or OTC H_2 antagonists. Pharmacologic therapy should be instituted in patients in whom lifestyle modifications have not provided satisfactory results. The H_2 antagonists have been the mainstay of treatment; however, a significant portion of patients fail to respond to standard doses of H_2 antagonists. Proton pump inhibitors or high-dose H_2 antagonists are often reserved for patients who are refractory to standard treatment or have severe disease. Potent antisecretory agents are, however, also effective in treating patients with lower grades of esophagitis. For example, endoscopic healing has been observed in 90% of patients with grade I esophagitis treated with 4 weeks of omeprazole 40 mg daily as compared with 55% of the patients receiving ranitidine 150 mg twice daily for 4 weeks.[164] Further studies evaluating the efficacy of lower doses of proton pump inhibitors in the treatment of patients with mild to moderate GERD are warranted. In addition, studies assessing quality of life issues and the cost effectiveness of various treatment strategies are needed to further elucidate their place in therapy. Other pharmacologic agents such as bethanechol, metoclopramide, cisapride, or sucralfate are alternative agents that may be used in the management of GERD. These agents are sometimes used as either adjunctive therapy or in patients who have an identifiable abnormality that the drug may correct (e.g., decreased lower esophageal sphincter pressure, delayed esophageal clearance or delayed gastric emptying, etc.).

Although patients may respond to pharmacologic therapy, a significant percentage of patients will relapse following discontinuation. Maintenance therapy to prevent relapses of GERD needs to be more clearly elucidated. Surgical intervention is usually reserved for patients who fail to respond to conservative and pharmacologic therapy or for those who develop severe complications as a result of the disease. In conclusion, GERD is a complex entity in which treatment may be approached from several angles. To design appropriate regimens, a detailed understanding of the pathophysiology of the disease is required.

REFERENCES

1. Spechler SJ. Epidemiology and natural history of gastro-oesophageal reflux disease. Digestion 1992;51(suppl 1):24–29.
2. Kitchin LI, Castell DO. Rationale and efficacy of conservative therapy for gastroesophageal reflux disease. Arch Intern Med 1991;151:448–454.
3. Navab F, Texter EC. Gastroesophageal reflux. Pathophysiologic concepts. Arch Intern Med 1985;145:329–333.
4. Dodds WJ, Hogan WJ, Helm JF, et al. Pathogenesis of reflux esophagitis. Gastroenterology 1981;81:376–394.
5. McKernan JB. Laparoscopic repair of gastroesophageal reflux disease: Toupet partial fundoplication versus Nissen fundoplication. Surg Endosc 1994;8:851–856.
6. Aye RW, Hill LD, Kaemer SJM, Snopkowski P. Early results with the laparoscopic Hill repair. Am J Surg 1994;167:542–546.
7. Castell DO. Long-term management of GERD: The pill, the knife or the endoscope? Gastrointestinal Endoscopy 1994;40(2):252–253.
8. Coley CM, Barry MJ, Spechler SJ, et al. Initial medical v. surgical therapy for complicated or chronic gastroesophageal reflux disease (GERD): A cost-effective analysis [abstract]. Gastroenterology 1993;104:A4.
9. Richter JE, Castell DO. Gastroesophageal reflux. Pathogenesis, diagnosis and therapy. Ann Intern Med 1982;97:93–103.
10. Brunnen PL, Karmody AM, Needham CD. Severe peptic oesophagitis. Gut 1969;10:831–837.

11. Nebel OT, Fornes MF, Castell DO. Symptomatic gastroesophageal reflux: Incidence and precipitating factors. Dig Dis 1976;21:953–956.
12. Spechler SJ, Goyal RK. Barrett's esophagus. N Engl J Med 1986;315:362–371.
13. Heartburn across America: A Gallup Organization National Survey, Princeton, NJ, The Gallup Organization, Inc., 1988.
14. Castell DO. Introduction to pathophysiology of gastroesophageal reflux, in Castell DO, Wu WC, Ott DJ (eds): Gastroesophageal Reflux Disease. Mount Kisco, NY, Futura Publishing Co., 1985, pp 3–9.
15. Sontag SJ. The medical management of reflux esophagitis: Role of antacids and acid inhibition. Gastroenterol Clin North Am 1990;19(3):683–712.
16. Wienbeck M, Barnert J. Epidemiology of reflux disease and reflux esophagitis. Scand J Gastroenterology 1989;24 (suppl 156):7–13.
17. Richter JE. Severe reflux esophagitis. Gastrointestinal Endoscopy Clin North Am 1994;4(4):677–698.
18. Knill-Jones RP, Card WI, Crean CP, James WB, Spiegelhalter DJ. The symptoms of gastro-oesophageal reflux and oesophagitis. Scand J Gastroenterol 1984;19 (suppl 106):72–76.
19. Behar J, Biancani P, Sheahan DG. Evaluation of esophageal tests in the diagnosis of reflux esophagitis. Gastroenterology 1976;71:9–15.
20. Jamieson GG, Duranceau AC. The defense mechanisms of the esophagus. Surg Clin North Am 1983;63:787–799.
21. Palmer ED. The hiatus hernia esophagitis-esophageal stricture complex. Am J Med 1968;44:566–579.
22. DeMeester TR, Lafontaine E, Joelsson BE, et al. Relationship of a hiatal hernia to the function of the body of the esophagus and the gastroesophageal junction. J Thorac Cardiovasc Surg 1989;82:547–558.
23. Berstad A, Weberg R, Larsen I, et al. Relationship of hiatus hernia to reflux oesophagitis. Scand J Gastroenterol 1986;21:55–58.
24. Sloan S, Rademaker AW, Kahrilas PJ. Determinants of gastroesophageal junction incompetence: Hiatal hernia, lower esophageal sphincter or both? Ann Intern Med 1992;117:977–982.
25. Castell DO. The lower esophageal sphincter. Physiologic and clinical aspects. Ann Intern Med 1975; 83:390–401.
26. Sanchez GC, Kramer P, Ingelfinger FJ. Motor mechanisms of the esophagus, particularly of its distal portion. Gastroenterology 1953;25:321–332.
27. Robinson MG. Management of reflux esophageal disease. Am J Med 1984;77 (suppl 5B):106–110.
28. Goyal RK, Rattan S. Neurohumoral, hormonal and drug receptors for the lower esophageal sphincter. Gastroenterology 1978;74:598–619.
29. Hogan WJ, Dodds WJ. Gastroesophageal reflux disease (reflux esophagitis), in Sleisinger MH, Fordtran JS (eds): Gastrointestinal Disease: Pathophysiology, Diagnosis, Management, 4th ed. Philadelphia, WB Saunders, 1989, pp 594–618.
30. Dodds WJ, Dent J, Hogan WJ, et al. Mechanisms of gastroesophageal reflux in patients with reflux esophagitis. N Engl J Med 1982;307:1547–1552.
31. Holloway RH, Dent J. Pathophysiology of gastroesophageal reflux: Lower esophageal sphincter dysfunction in gastroesophageal reflux disease. Gastroenterol Clin North Am 1990;19:517–535.
32. Kahrilas PJ. Esophageal motor activity and acid clearance. Gastroenterol Clin North Am 1990;19:537–550.
33. Bozymski EM. Pathophysiology and diagnosis of gastroesophageal reflux disease. Am J Hosp Pharm 1993;50 (suppl 1):S4–S6.
34. DeMeester TR, Johnson LF, Joseph GL, et al. Patterns of gastroesophageal reflux in health and disease. Ann Surg 1976;184(4):459–470.
35. Orr WC, Robinson MG, Johnson LF. Acid clearance during sleep in the pathogenesis of reflux esophagitis. Dig Dis Sci 1981;26:423–427.
36. Goldstein JL, Schlesinger PK, Mozwecz HL, et al. Esophageal mucosal resistance: A factor in esophagitis. Gastroenterol Clin North Am 1990;19:565–585.
37. Safaie-Shirazi S, DenBesten L, Zike WL. Effect of bile salts on the ionic permeability of the esophageal mucosa and their role in the production of esophagitis. Gastroenterology 1975;68:728–733.
38. Fiorucci S, Santucci L, Chiucchiu S, Morelli A. Gastric acidity and gastroesophageal reflux patterns in patients with esophagitis. Gastroenterology 1992;103:855–861.
39. Dent J. Roles of gastric acid and pH in the pathogenesis of gastro-oesophageal reflux disease. Scand J Gastroenterol 1994; 29 (suppl 201):55–61.
40. Bell NJV, Burger D, Howden CW, Wilkinson J, Hunt RH. Appropriate acid suppression for the management of gastro-oesophageal reflux disease. Digestion 1992;51 (suppl 1):59–67.
41. McCallum RW, Berkowitz DM, Lerner E. Gastric emptying in patients with gastroesophageal reflux. Gastroenterology 1981;80:285–291.
42. Behar J, Ramsby G. Gastric emptying and antral motility in reflux esophagitis: Effect of oral metoclopramide. Gastroenterology 1978;74:253–256.
43. McCallum RW. Gastric emptying in gastroesophageal reflux and the therapeutic role of prokinetic agents. Gastroenterol Clin North Am 1990;19:551–564.
44. Goff JS. Diagnosis and evaluation of esophageal disorders. Ear Nose Throat J 1984;63:19–26.
45. Kozarek RA. Complications of reflux esophagitis and their medical management. Gastroenterol Clin North Am 1990;19:713–731.
46. Orenstein SR. Gastroesophageal reflux disease. Sem Gastrointestinal Dis 1994;5(1):2–14.
47. Simpson WG. Gastroesophageal reflux disease and asthma. Diagnosis and management. Arch Intern Med 1995;155:798–803.
48. Heller SR, Fellows IW, Ogilvie AL, Atkinson M. Non-steroidal anti-inflammatory drugs and benign oesophageal stricture. BMJ 1982;2:425–454.
49. Whelan G. Management of gastroesophageal reflux. Aust NZ J Med 1982;12:90–96.
50. Pope CE. Acid-reflux disorders. New Engl J Med 1994;331(10):656–660.
51. Savary M, Miller G. The Esophagus. Handbook and Atlas of Endoscopy. Solothurn, Gassman, 1978.

52. Holloway RH, McCallum RW. A practical approach to gastroesophageal reflux. Drug Ther 1983;13:151–160.
53. Morton LS, Fromkes JJ. Gastroesophageal reflux disease: Diagnosis and medical therapy. Geriatrics 1993;48(3):60–66.
54. Castell DO. Esophageal chest pain. Am J Gastroenterol 1984;79:969–971.
55. Tytgat GNJ, Nio CY, Schotborgh RH. Reflux esophagitis. Scand J Gastroenterol 1990;25 (suppl 175):1–12.
56. Hogan WJ. Gastroesophageal reflux disease: An update on management. J Clin Gastroenterol 1990;12 (suppl 2):S21–S28.
57. Hixson LJ, Kelley CL, Jones WN, Tuohy CD. Current trends in the pharmacotherapy for gastroesophageal reflux disease. Arch Intern Med 1992;152:717–723.
58. Johnson LF, DeMeester TR. Evaluation of elevation of the head of the bed, bethanechol and antacid foam tablets on gastroesophageal reflux. Dig Dis Sci 1981;26:673–680.
59. Richter JE, Castell DO. Drugs, foods and other substances in the cause and treatment of reflux esophagitis. Med Clin North Am 1981;65:1223–1234.
60. Johnson DA. Medical therapy for gastroesophageal reflux disease. Am J Med 1992;92 (suppl 5A):88S–97S.
61. Higgs RH, Smyth RD, Castell DO. Gastric alkalinization: Effect on lower esophageal-sphincter pressure and serum gastrin. N Engl J Med 1974;291:486–490.
62. Graham DY, Patterson DJ. Double-blind comparison of liquid antacid and placebo in the treatment of symptomatic reflux esophagitis. Dig Dis Sci 1983;28:559–563.
63. Grove O, Bekker C, Jeppe-Hansen MG, et al. Ranitidine and high-dose antacid in reflux oesophagitis. Scand J Gastroenterol 1985;20:457–461.
64. Weberg R, Berstad A. Symptomatic effect of a low-dose antacid regimen in reflux oesophagitis. Scand J Gastroenterol 1989;24:401–406.
65. Thanik KD, Chey WY, Shah AN, et al. Reflux esophagitis: Effect of oral bethanechol on symptoms and endoscopic findings. Ann Intern Med 1980;93:805–808.
66. Bamardo DE, Lancaster-Smith M, Strickland ID, et al. A double-blind controlled trial of "Gaviscon" in patients with symptomatic gastro-oesophageal reflux. Curr Med Res Opin 1975;3:388–391.
67. Stanciu C, Bennett JR. Alginate/antacid in the reduction of gastro-oesophageal reflux. Lancet 1974;1:109–111.
68. Chevrel B. A comparative crossover study on the treatment of heartburn and epigastric pain: Liquid Gaviscon and a magnesium-aluminum antacid gel. J Int Med Res 1980;8:300–302.
69. Graham DY, Lanza F, Dorsch ER. Symptomatic reflux esophagitis: A double-blind controlled comparison of antacids and alginate. Curr Ther Res 1977;22:653–658.
70. Welage LS, Berardi RB. Drug interactions with antiulcer agents: Considerations in the treatment of acid-peptic disease. J Pharm Prac 1994;VII(4):177–195.
71. Petrokubi RJ, Jeffries GH. Cimetidine versus antacid in scleroderma with reflux esophagitis: A randomized double-blind controlled study. Gastroenterology 1979;77:691–695.
72. Furman D, Mensh R, Winan G, et al. A double-blind trial comparing high-dose liquid antacid to placebo and cimetidine in improving symptoms and objective parameters in gastroesophageal reflux. Gastroenterology 1982;5 (part 2):1062.
73. Farup PG, Weberg R, Berstad A, et al. Low-dose antacids versus 40 mg cimetidine twice daily for reflux oesophagitis. Scand J Gastroenterol 1990;25:315–320.
74. Tytgat GNJ, Nicolai JJ, Reman FC. Efficacy of different doses of cimetidine in the treatment of reflux esophagitis. Gastroenterology 1990;99:629–634.
75. Sekiguchi T, Nishioka T, Kogure M, et al. Once-daily administration of famotidine for reflux esophagitis. Scand J Gastroenterol 1987;22 (suppl 134):51–54.
76. Simon TJ, Berlin RG, Gardner AH, et al. Self-directed treatment of intermittent heartburn: A randomized, multicenter, double-blind, placebo-controlled evaluation of antacid and low doses of an H_2-receptor antagonist (famotidine). Am J Therap 1995;2:304–313.
77. Gottlieb S, Decktor DL, Eckert JM, et al. Efficacy and tolerability of famotidine in preventing heartburn and related symptoms of upper gastrointestinal discomfort. Am J Therap 1995;2:314–319.
78. Johnson NJ, Boyd EJS, Mills JG, et al. Acute treatment of reflux oesophagitis: A multicentre trial to compare 150 mg ranitidine b.d. with 300 mg ranitidine q.d.s. Aliment Pharmacol Ther 1989;3:259–266.
79. Castell DO. Rationale for high-dose H_2 blockade in the treatment of gastroesophageal reflux disease. Aliment Pharmacol Therap 1991;5 (suppl):59–67.
80. Euler AR, Murdock RH, Wilson TH, et al. Ranitidine is effective therapy for erosive esophagitis. Am J Gastroenterol 1993;88(4):520–524.
81. Edge DP. High-dose famotidine in ranitidine-resistant severe oesophagitis: A pilot study. NA Med J 1990;103:150–152.
82. Wesdorp ICE, Dekker W, Festen HPM. Efficacy of famotidine 20 mg twice a day versus 40 mg twice a day in the treatment of erosive or ulcerative reflux esophagitis. Dig Dis Sci 1993;38(12):2287–2293.
83. Festen HPM, Wesdorp ICE, Dekker W. The efficacy of famotidine 20 mg bid vs 40 mg bid in the treatment of erosive/ulcerative esophagitis: Significance of severity of esophagitis and duration of therapy. Gastroenterology 1991;100(5)(part 2, suppl):A63.
84. Cloud ML, Offen WW, Robinson M. Nizatidine versus placebo in gastroesophageal reflux disease: A 12 week, multicenter, randomized, double-blind study. Am J Gastroenterol 1991;86:1735–1742.
85. Baldi F, Longanesi A, Ferrarini F, et al. Nizatidine in gastroesophageal reflux disease: A review. Gastrointest Res 1991;20:5–6.
86. Maton PN. Drug therapy: Omeprazole. N Engl J Med 1991;324:965–975.
87. Collen MJ, Johnson DA, Sheridan MJ. Basal acid output and gastric acid hypersecretion in gastroesophageal reflux disease. Dig Dis Sci 1994;39(2):410–417.
88. Feldman M, Burton ME. $Histamine_2$ receptor antagonists: Standard therapy for acid peptic diseases (first of 2 parts). N Engl J Med 1990;323:1672.
89. Feldman M, Burton ME. $Histamine_2$ receptor antagonists: Standard therapy for acid peptic diseases (second of 2 parts). N Engl J Med 1990;323:1749.

90. Reynolds JC. Prokinetic agents: A key in the future of gastroenterology. Gastroenterol Clin North Am 1989;18(2):437–456.
91. Stanciu C, Bennett JR. Metoclopramide in gastroesophageal reflux. Gut 1973;14:275–279.
92. McCallum RW, Kline MM, Curry N, et al. Comparative effects of metoclopramide and bethanechol on lower esophageal sphincter pressure in reflux patients. Gastroenterology 1975;68:1114–1118.
93. McCallum RW. Cisapride: A new class of prokinetic agent. Am J Gastroenterol 1991;86(2):135–149.
94. Fink SM, Lange RC, McCallum RW. Effect of metoclopramide on normal and delayed gastric emptying in gastroesophageal reflux patients. Dig Dis Sci 1983;28:1057–1061.
95. Farrell RL, Roling GT, Castell DO. Cholinergic therapy of chronic heartburn: A controlled trial. Ann Intern Med 1974;8:573–576.
96. Thanik K, Chey WY, Shak A, et al. Bethanechol or cimetidine in the treatment of symptomatic reflux esophagitis: A double-blind control study. Arch Intern Med 1982;142:1479–1481.
97. Paull A, Grant A. A controlled trial of metoclopramide in reflux oesophagitis. Med J Aust 1974;2:627–629.
98. McCallum RW, Ippoliti AF, Cooney C, et al. A controlled trial of metoclopramide in symptomatic gastroesophageal reflux. N Engl J Med 1977;296:354–357.
99. McCallum RW, Fink SM, Winnan GR, et al. Metoclopramide in gastroesophageal reflux disease: Rationale for its use and results of a double-blind trial. Am J Gastroenterol 1984;79:165–172.
100. Bright-Asare P, El-Bassoussi M. Cimetidine, metoclopramide, or placebo in the treatment of symptomatic gastroesophageal reflux. J Clin Gastroenterol 1980;2:149–156.
101. Guslandi M, Testoni PA, Passaretti S, et al. Ranitidine versus metodopramide in the medical treatment of reflux esophagitis. Hepato-enterol 1983;30:96–98.
102. Taylor DM. Evaluation of the safety of metoclopramide in patients with gastroesophageal reflux disease. Clin Ther 1984;7:28–32.
103. Lepoutre L, Van Der Spek P, Vanderlinden I, et al. Healing of grade II and III oesophagitis through motility stimulation with cisapride. Digestion 1990;45:109–114.
104. Baldi F, Bianchi Porro GP, Dobrilla G, et al. Cisapride versus placebo in reflux esophagitis. A multicenter double-blind trial. J Clin Gastroenterol 1988;10(6):614–618.
105. Galmiche JP, Fraitag B, Filoche B, et al. Double-blind comparison of cisapride and cimetidine in treatment of reflux esophagitis. Dig Dis Sci 1990;35:649–655.
106. Janisch HD, Huttemann W, Bouzo MH. Cisapride versus ranitidine in the treatment of reflux esophagitis. Hepatogastroenterology 1988;35:125–127.
107. Maleev A, Mendizova A, Popov P, et al. Cisapride and cimetidine in the treatment of erosive esophagitis. Hepatogastroenterology 1990;37:403–407.
108. Manousos ON, Apostolos M, Michailidis D. Treatment of reflux symptoms in esophagitis patients: Comparative trial of cisapride and metoclopramide. Curr Ther Res 1987;42:807–813.
109. Cucchiara S, Staiano A, Boccieri A, et al. Effects of cisapride on parameters of oesophageal motility and on the prolonged intraoesophageal pH test in infants with gastro-oesophageal reflux disease. Gut 1990;31:21–25.
110. Barone JA, Jessen LM, Colaizzi JL, et al. Cisapride: A gastrointestinal prokinetic agent. Ann Pharmacother 1994;28:488–500.
111. Siepler JK, Mahakain K, Trudeau WT. Current concepts in clinical therapeutics: Peptic ulcer disease. Clin Pharm 1986;5:128–142.
112. Elsborg L, Beck B, Stubgaard M. Effect of sucralfate on gastroesophageal reflux in esophagitis. Hepatogastroenterology 1985;32:181–184.
113. Williams RM, Orlando RC, Bozymski EM, et al. Multicenter trial of sucralfate suspension for the treatment of reflux esophagitis. Am J Med 1987;83 (suppl 3B):61–66.
114. Evreux M. Sucralfate versus alginate/antacid in the treatment of peptic esophagitis. Am J Med 1987;83 (suppl 3B):48–50.
115. Laitinen S, Stahlberg M, Kairaluoma MI, et al. Sucralfate and alginate/antacid in reflux esophagitis. Scand J Gastroenterol 1985;20:229–232.
116. Simon B, Dammann HG, Muller P. Sucralfate in the treatment of reflux esophagitis in adults: An update. Scand J Gastroenterol 1989;24 (suppl 156):37–41.
117. Hameeteman W, Boomgaard DMvd, Dekker W, et al. Sucralfate versus cimetidine in reflux esophagitis. J Clin Gastroenterol 1987;9:390–394.
118. Tytgat GNJ. Clinical efficacy of sucralfate in reflux esophagitis: Comparison with cimetidine. Am J Med 1987;83(suppl 3B):38–42.
119. Ross E, Toledo-Pimentel V, Bordas JM, et al. Healing of erosive esophagitis with sucralfate and cimetidine: Influence of pretreatment lower esophageal sphincter pressure and serum pepsinogen I levels. Am J Med 1991;91 (suppl 2A):107S–113S.
120. Bremner CG, Marks IN, Segal I, Simjee A. Reflux esophagitis therapy: Sucralfate versus ranitidine in a double-blind multicenter trial. Am J Med 1991;91 (suppl 2A):119S–122S.
121. Elsborg L, Jorgensen F. Sucralfate vs. cimetidine in reflux esophagitis: A double-blind clinical study. Scand J Gastroenterol 1991;26:146–150.
122. Jorgensen F, Elsborg L. Sucralfate vs. cimetidine in treatment of reflux esophagitis with special reference to the esophageal motor function. Am J Med 1991;91 (suppl 2A):114–117.
123. Pace F, Lazzaroni M, Bianchi-Porro G. Failure of sucralfate in the treatment of refractory esophagitis vs. high dose famotidine: An endoscopic study. Scand J Gastroenterol 1991;26:491–494.
124. Berardi RR, Dunn-Kucharski VA. Omeprazole: Defining its role in gastroesophageal reflux disease. Hosp Formul 1995;30:216–225.
125. Barradell LB, Faulds D, McTavish D. Lansoprazole: A review of its pharmacodynamic and pharmacokinetic properties and its therapeutic efficacy in acid related disorders. Drugs 1992;44:225–250.
126. Spencer CM, Faulds D. Lansoprazole: A reappraisal of its pharmacodynamic and pharmacokinetic properties, and its

therapeutic efficacy in acid related disorders. Drugs 1994;48:404–430.

127. Hetzel DJ, Dent J, Reed WD, et al. Healing and relapse of severe peptic esophagitis after treatment with omeprazole. Gastroenterology 1988;95:903–912.

128. Sontag SJ, Hirschowitz BL, Holt S, et al. Two doses of omeprazole versus placebo in symptomatic erosive esophagitis: The U.S. multicenter study. Gastroenterology 1992;102:109–118.

129. Dehn TCB, Shepherd HA, Colin-Jones D, et al. Double-blind comparison of omeprazole (40 mg od) versus cimetidine (400 mg qd) in the treatment of symptomatic erosive reflux oesophagitis, assessed endoscopically, histologically and by 24-h pH monitoring. Gut 1990;31:509–513.

130. Bardhan KD, Long R, Hawkey CJ, et al. Lansoprazole, a new proton pump inhibitor vs ranitidine in the treatment of reflux erosive esophagitis [abstract]. Gastroenterology 1991;100:A30.

131. Benhaim MC, Evreux M, Salduccci J, et al. Lansoprazole and ranitidine in treatment of reflux oesophagitis: Double blind comparative trial [abstract]. Gastroenterology 1990;A20.

132. Robinson M, Kogut D, Jennings D, et al. Lansoprazole heals erosive reflux esophagitis better than ranitidine [abstract]. Meeting of American Gastroenterological Association. San Francisco, May 9–14, 1992.

133. Corallo J, Vicari F, Forestier S, et al. Lansoprazole in acute treatment of reflux esophagitis [abstract]. Gastroenterology 1003;104 (suppl):A58.

134. Hatlebakk JG, Berstad A, Carling L, et al. Lansoprazole versus omeprazole in short-term treatment of reflux oesophagitis. Results of a Scandinavian multicentre trial. Scand J Gastroenterol 1993;28:224–228.

135. Lundell L, Westin IH, Sandmark S, et al. Omeprazole or high-dose ranitidine in the treatment of patients with reflux esophagitis not responding to standard doses of H_2-receptor antagonists [abstract]. Gastroenterology 1989;96(5):310.

136. Klinkenberg-Knol EC, Jansen JBMJ, Lamers CBHW, et al. Use of omeprazole in the management of reflux esophagitis resistant to H_2-receptor antagonists. Scand J Gastroenterol 1989;24 (suppl 166):88–93.

137. Feldman M, Harford WV, Fisher RS, et al. Treatment of reflux esophagitis resistant to H_2 receptor antagonists with lansoprazole, a new H^+/K^+-ATPase inhibitor: A controlled, double-blind study. Am J Gastroenterol 1993;88:1212–1217.

138. Deviere J, Buset M, Dumonceau JM, et al. Regression of Barrett's epithelium with omeprazole. N Engl Med J 1989;320(22):1497–1498.

139. Hameeteman W, Tytgat GN. Healing of chronic Barrett ulcers with omeprazole. Am J Gastroenterol 1986;81(9):764–766.

140. Sampliner RE. Effect of up to 3 years of high dose lansoprazole on Barrett's esophagus. Am J Gastroenterol 1994;89:1844–1848.

141. Lieberman DA, Keeffe EB. Treatment of severe reflux esophagitis with cimetidine and metoclopramide. Ann Intern Med 1986;104:21–26.

142. Galmiche JP, Brandstatter G, Evreux M, et al. Combined therapy with cisapride and cimetidine in severe reflux oesophagitis: A double blind controlled trial. Gut 1988;29:675–681.

143. Temple JG, Bradby GV, O'Connor F, et al. Cimetidine and metoclopramide in oesophageal reflux disease. Br Med J 1983;286:1863–1864.

144. Herrera IL, Shay SS, McCabe M, et al. Sucralfate used as adjunctive therapy in patients with severe erosive peptic esophagitis resulting from gastroesophageal reflux. Am J Gastroenterol 1990;85:1335–1338.

145. Schotborgh RH, Hameeteman W, Dekker W, et al. Combination therapy of sucralfate and cimetidine, compared with sucralfate monotherapy, in patients with peptic reflux esophagitis. Am J Med 1989;86 (suppl 6A):77–80.

146. Bright-Asare P, Behar J, Brand DL, et al. Effects of long-term maintenance cimetidine (CIM) therapy on gastroesophageal reflux disease (GERD). Gastroenterology 1985;82(5)(part 2):1025.

147. Sontag S, Vlahcevic R, Orr W, et al. Ranitidine versus placebo in long-term treatment of gastroesophageal reflux. Gastroenterology 1985;88(5)(part 2):1595.

148. Euler AR, Murdock RH, Brotherton BJ, et al. Ranitidine 150mg b.i.d. prevents erosive esophagitis [abstract]. Gastroenterology 1992;102:A65.

149. McCallum RW, Sontag SJ, Vlahcevic ZR, et al. Ranitidine versus placebo in long-term treatment of gastroesophageal reflux (GERD). Am J Gastroenterol 1985;80:864.

150. Toussaint J, Gossuin A, Deruyttere M, et al. Healing and prevention of relapse of reflux oesophagitis by cisapride. Gut 1991;32:1280–1285.

151. Blum AL, Adami B, Bouzo MH, et al. Effect of cisapride on relapse of esophagitis. Dig Dis Sci 1993;38(3):551–560.

152. Lundell L, Backman L, Ekstrom P, et al. Prevention of relapse of esophagitis after endoscopic healing: The efficacy of omeprazole (OME) compared with ranitidine (RAN). Gastroenterology 1990;98(5)(part 2):82.

153. Dent J, Mackinnon M, Reed W, et al. Omeprazole prevents relapse of peptic oesophagitis. World Congress, 1990.

154. Isal JP, Zeitoun P, Barbier P, et al. Comparison of two dosage regimens of omeprazole—10 mg once daily and 20 mg weekends. Gastroenterology 1990;98:A63.

155. Brogden RN, Carmine AA, Heel RC, et al. Domperidone: A review of its pharmacologic activity, pharmacokinetics and therapeutic efficacy in the symptomatic treatment of chronic dyspepsia and as an antiemetic. Drugs 1982;24:360–400.

156. Blackwell JN, Heading RC, Fettes MR. Effects of domperidone on lower esophageal sphincter pressure and gastroesophageal reflux in patients with peptic esophagitis, in Towse G (ed): Progress with Domperidone, a Gastrokinetic and Antiemetic Agent. London, Royal Society of Medicine International Congress and Symposia Series no 36, 1981, pp 57–65.

157. Masci E, Testoni PA, Passaretti S, et al. Comparison of ranitidine, domperidone maleate and ranitidine and domperidone maleate in the short-term treatment of reflux esophagitis. Drugs Exp Clin Res 1985;10:1–6.

158. Maddern GJ, Kiroff GK, Leppard PI, et al. Domperidone, metoclopramide, and placebo: All give symptomatic improvement in gastroesophageal reflux. J Clin Gastroenterol 1986;8:135–140.

159. Koop H, Schepp W, Dammann HG, et al. Comparative trial of pantoprazole and ranitidine in the treatment of reflux esophagitis: Results of a German multicenter study. J Clin Gastroenterol 1995;20:192–195.
160. Bader JP, Delchier JC. Clinical efficacy of pantoprazole compared with ranitidine. Aliment Pharmacol Ther 1994;8 (suppl 1):47–52.
161. Dent J. Long-term aims of treatment of reflux disease, and the role of non-drug measures. Digestion 1992;51 (suppl 1):30–34.
162. Hillman AL, Bloom BS, Fendrick AM, et al. Cost and quality effects of alternative treatments for persistent gastroesophageal reflux disease. Arch Intern Med 1992;152:1467–1472.
163. Marks RD, Richter JE, Rizzo J, et al. Omeprazole versus H_2 receptor antagonists in treating patients with peptic stricture and esophagitis. Gastroenterology 1994;106:907–915.
164. Havelund T, Laursen LS, Lauritsen K. Efficacy of omeprazole in lower grades of gastro-oesophageal reflux disease. Scand J Gastroenterol 1994;29 (suppl 201):69–73.

Chapter 32

Peptic Ulcer Disease and Zollinger–Ellison Syndrome

Rosemary R. Berardi, PharmD, FASHP

Peptic ulcer disease (PUD) refers to a group of ulcerative disorders of the upper gastrointestinal (GI) tract that require acid and pepsin for their formation. Ulcers differ from superficial mucosal erosions in that they extend deeper into the muscularis mucosa. In light of recent data, there are three common forms of peptic ulcer: *Helicobacter pylori* (HP)-associated, nonsteroidal anti-inflammatory drug (NSAID)-associated, and stress ulcers.[1] Stress ulcers develop in critically ill patients and are discussed elsewhere. Chronic ulcers (HP- and NSAID-associated) differ from acute ulcers (stress ulcers) by their depth, etiology, clinical presentation, and tendency to recur. Duodenal ulcer (DU) and gastric ulcer (GU) occur most often, but occasionally ulcers develop in the esophagus, jejunum, or ileum. Uncommon ulcers are associated with Zollinger–Ellison syndrome (ZES), radiation, chemotherapy, and vascular insufficiency.[1]

EPIDEMIOLOGY

Approximately 10% of Americans will develop PUD during their lifetime.[1] The incidence varies with ulcer type, age, gender, and geographic location. Racial, occupational, and societal variables require reevaluation in light of differences in HP infection rates.[1] In the United States, the overall prevalence of PUD has shifted from predominance in men to nearly comparable prevalence of DU and GU in men and women, although DU emerges 20 years earlier than GU in men.[1] These recent trends suggest a declining rate for younger men and an increasing rate for older women. Factors that may have influenced these trends include the increasing prevalence of HP infection with age, NSAID-induced ulcers in the elderly, and declining smoking rates, especially in younger men. Stress associated with increased social, occupational, and family responsibilities may also be related to recent changes observed in the male-to-female ratio.[1]

A number of genetic, environmental, and therapeutic factors have been implicated in the changing patterns of PUD over time. Since 1960, ulcer-related hospitalizations, operations, and deaths in the United States have declined, suggesting a decrease in the incidence of PUD.[1] The decline in hospitalizations has resulted primarily from a reduction in hospital admissions for uncomplicated DU, with a less dramatic decrease in GU. It is uncertain whether this decline reflects an actual decrease in the incidence of PUD or the combined influences of changes in diagnostic practices, more effective treatment, hospitalization criteria, and the shift to ambulatory care. Mortality from PUD has declined among persons of all ages, but declining death rates for men are in contrast to increasing rates for women.[1] Despite these changes, PUD is one of the most common GI diseases resulting in work loss, disability, and high-cost medical care.

GASTRIC PHYSIOLOGY

ACID SECRETION

Parietal Cell Function

The parietal, or oxyntic, cells are located in the mucosa of the fundus and body of the stomach. When stimulated, they secrete acid into the gastric lumen through the secretory canaliculi. In the resting state, the parietal cell secretes intrinsic factor, which serves as a carrier protein for vitamin B_{12}.

Stimulants

Three major endogenous substances, acetylcholine, histamine, and gastrin, stimulate specific receptors on the parietal cell to secrete acid (Fig. 32.1). The neurocrine pathway delivers acetylcholine released from postganglionic vagal neurons in the stomach. Although five muscarinic subtypes have been identified, acid stimulation is mediated through the M_3 receptor.[2] The paracrine pathway delivers histamine released by mucosal mast or enterochromaffin-like (ECL) cells. Recent data suggest that ECL cells may be primarily

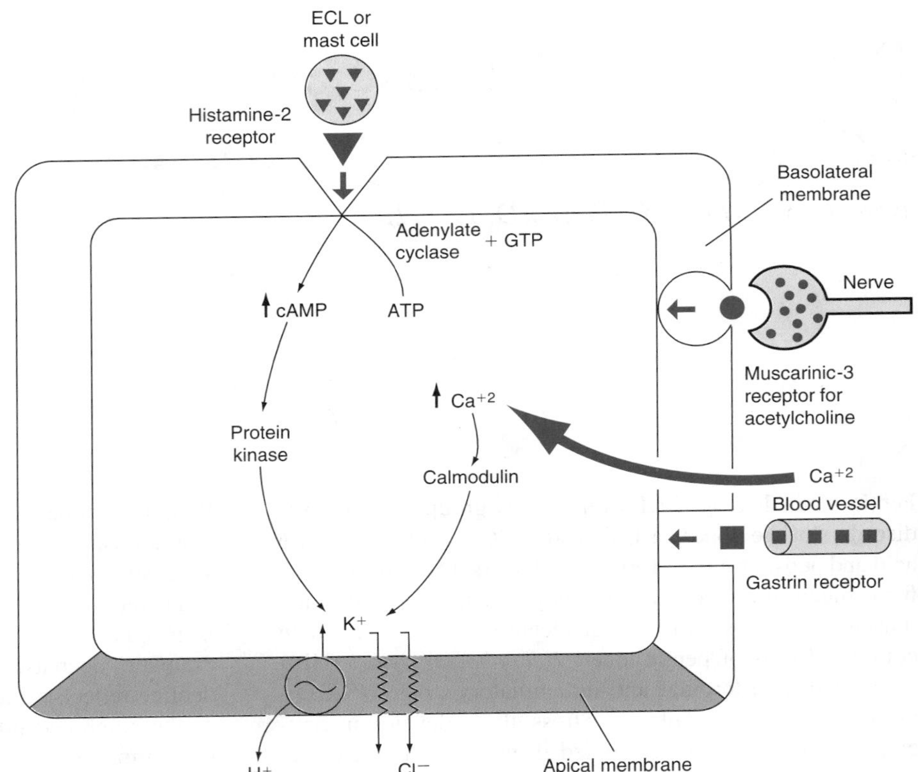

Figure 32.1. Model for receptors and pathways regulating acid secretion. Histamine from mast cells or enterochromaffin-like (ECL) cells activates the proton pump on the apical membrane of the cell by increasing intracellular cyclic adenosine monophosphate (cAMP). Acetylcholi from nerves and gastrin from the blood act by increasing intracellular calcium. *(From Goldschmiedt M, Feldman M. Gastric secretion in health and disease, in Sleisenger MH, Fordtran JS (eds): Gastrointestinal Disease: Pathophysiology/Diagnosis/Management, 5th ed. (Vol 1). Philadelphia, WB Saunders, 1993, p 526, with permission.)*

responsible for the postprandial release of histamine.[2,3] The endocrine pathway delivers gastrin from antral and duodenal G cells. Gastrin acts directly on the parietal cell receptor or stimulates histamine from ECL cells.

Intracellular Second Messengers

Once an agonist binds to a specific parietal cell receptor, two second messengers within the parietal cell, cyclic AMP and free calcium, mediate acid secretion.[2,3] Histamine stimulates cyclic AMP by activating the enzyme adenylate cyclase, which converts adenosine triphosphate (ATP) to cyclic AMP. Gastrin and acetylcholine release calcium from intracellular stores, although increases in intracellular calcium may arise from extracellular sources (Fig. 32.1). The complex arrangement of receptors and pathways culminates in activation of hydrogen/potassium adenosine triphosphatase (H^+/K^+-ATPase), the gastric proton pump.

Gastric Proton Pump

Acid is secreted by the parietal cell into the gastric lumen against a concentration gradient and requires an active energy-dependent process. Through a series of intracellular events, the actions of cyclic AMP and calcium converge on H^+/K^+-ATPase, the proton pump located in the apical membrane of the parietal cell. H^+/K^+-ATPase catalyzes a one-to-one exchange of intracellular hydrogen ions for luminal potassium ions, the terminal step in acid secretion (Fig. 32.1).[2,3]

Inhibitors

Low intragastric pH (<3.0) suppresses antral gastrin stimulation of acid by a negative feedback mechanism. Prostaglandins (PGs) of the E_2 type (PGE_2) inhibit histamine-stimulated acid secretion by acting on a parietal cell membrane receptor that prevents histamine from activating adenylate cyclase. Although acid suppression results from the release of a number of endogenous peptides, somatostatin and secretin are the most important.[2,3]

Acid Secretory Capacity

Basal, maximal, and meal-stimulated acid secretion varies according to time of day, psychological state, age, gender, and health status. Parietal cell mass and acid secretory rates are often lower in women. Decreased acid secretion (hypochlorhydria) or an absence of acid secretion (achlorhydria) has been reported in the elderly. Hypersecretion of acid occurs in subsets of patients with DU, gastrinoma, or mastocytosis.[2]

Basal Acid Secretion

Basal acid output (BAO) reflects continuous fasting gastric acid secretion in the absence of avoidable stimuli.

BAO is variable and follows a circadian rhythm. Higher secretory rates occur in the afternoon and evening (between 2 and 11 PM), while lower rates occur in the morning (between 5 and 11 AM).[2] The BAO in healthy individuals is usually between 2 to 10 mEq/h, with higher rates reported in men than in women.

Maximal Secretory Capacity

The maximal secretory capacity can be estimated by the maximum acid output (MAO), following an injection of pentagastrin, betazole, or histamine. The MAO represents the sum of four 15-minute acid output measurements and is an indirect estimate of parietal cell mass (total number of gastric parietal cells). Peak acid output (PAO) represents the sum of the two highest stimulated acid outputs multiplied by two. Normal MAO is usually 20 to 40 mEq/h. The ratio of BAO/MAO or PAO represents the fraction of the parietal cell mass that is functional under basal conditions. An increase in the BAO/MAO ratio often suggests a basal hypersecretory state such as ZES.

Meal-Stimulated Acid Secretion

Meal-stimulated acid secretion can be divided into three phases: cephalic, gastric, and intestinal. Each phase has different mechanisms of stimulation and inhibition. The cephalic phase is initiated by the sight, smell, and taste of food and is mediated primarily by the vagal pathway; hormonal stimulation by gastrin plays only a small role. The gastric phase is activated by stimuli within the stomach. Gastric distention activates vagal nerves in the gastric wall and the chemical constituents of food (amino acids and peptides) stimulate gastrin release. The increased acid response provides a negative feedback mechanism that suppresses gastrin output. The intestinal phase of acid secretion has both stimulatory and inhibitory components. Stimulation results from the intraluminal effect of amino acids on the parietal cell or the effect of circulating amino acids in the blood. Intraluminal acid, fat, and hyperosmolar solutions inhibit acid secretion. Secretin is released upon acidification of the duodenal mucosa and inhibits gastrin-stimulated acid secretion. Fats inhibit acid secretion through the release of various gut peptides, including cholecystokinin (CCK) and gastric inhibitory peptide (GIP).

PEPSIN AND PEPSINOGEN SECRETION

Gastric mucosal cells secrete two distinct types of proteolytic proenzymes, pepsinogen group I (PGI) and pepsinogen group II (PGII). PGI is produced in the chief and mucus neck cells of the acid-secreting mucosa; PGII is produced in the mucus cells of the gastric and duodenal mucosa. Pepsin is activated by acid pH (optimal pH of 1.8–3.5), inactivated reversibly at pH 4 and irreversibly destroyed at pH 7. PGI secretion is directly proportional to the rate of acid secretion. Hypergastrinemia and HP infection are associated with increased serum PGI concentrations, although HP itself may induce hypergastrinemia.[1]

MUCOSAL PROTECTION

Several mechanisms protect the GI mucosa from endogenous and exogenous noxious substances. These defensive mechanisms include mucus secretion, bicarbonate secretion, mucosal blood flow, and epithelial cell restitution, growth, and wound healing after injury. The maintenance of mucosal integrity, by mechanisms independent of acid inhibition, is mediated by the production of endogenous PGs.[4,5] The term *cytoprotection* is used to describe this process although it is semantically incorrect. The terms *mucosal defense* or *mucosal protection* are more accurate because PGs prevent deep mucosal injury and not superficial damage to individual cells. *Adaptive cytoprotection,* the short-term adaptation of mucosal cells to mild topical irritants, is characterized by gastric hyperemia and increased PG synthesis.[4] This phenomenon allows the stomach to withstand initially the damaging effects of stronger irritants.

Mucus Secretion

Mucus is secreted continuously onto the surface of the mucosa and is thought to have several major functions. Mucus protects underlying cells and acts as a lubricant layer between the mucosa and its contents. It also forms a mucus–gel or "unstirred" layer that impedes hydrogen ion back-diffusion (the permeability of hydrogen ions from the stomach lumen into the gastric mucosa). The extent to which mucus alters the susceptibility of individuals to ulceration is unknown.

Bicarbonate Secretion

Bicarbonate is secreted by gastric and duodenal surface epithelial cells, the pancreas, and the biliary system. Most gastric bicarbonate remains trapped within the mucus–gel layer, where a pH gradient is established between the mucosal epithelial cells and the lumen. The surface of the gel facing the gastric lumen approaches pH 2, whereas that in contact with the mucosal surface is about pH 7. Luminal hydrogen ions are neutralized by mucosal bicarbonate as they diffuse through the mucus–gel layer. Pepsin activity also declines as it diffuses toward the mucosa. Some secreted bicarbonate reaches the lumen where it is neutralized by hydrogen ions. Pancreatic bicarbonate is secreted into the proximal duodenum when the duodenum is exposed to acid or chyme.

Mucosal Blood Flow

Gastric and duodenal blood flow is essential in maintaining mucosal integrity. Vascular insufficiency, resulting in local ischemia, has been linked to the pathogenesis of stress ulcers. It is unclear how alterations in mucosal blood flow contribute to the pathogenesis of PUD.

Epithelial Restitution, Cell Growth, and Wound Healing

GI surface epithelial cells have a rapid turnover rate, and when injured, migrating gastric pit cells are immediately available to restore the damaged surface epithelium. Growth factors, particularly epidermal growth factor (EGF), appear to stimulate growth of various cell types and also play an important role in mucosal protection and wound healing.[4]

Prostaglandins

Prostaglandins have numerous effects on the GI tract. Endogenous PGE_2, produced in gastric and duodenal mucosal cells, stimulate mucus and bicarbonate secretion, maintain mucosal blood flow, and participate in epithelial restitution and cell growth.[4,5]

Etiology and Pathogenesis

Most peptic ulcers occur in the presence of acid and pepsin when HP, NSAIDs, or other possible factors disrupt normal mucosal defense and healing mechanisms. Hypersecretion of acid is the primary pathogenic mechanism in hypersecretory states such as ZES (Fig. 32.2).[1,6,7] The pathogenesis of DU and GU is multifactorial and most likely reflects a combination of pathophysiologic abnormalities, environmental, and genetic factors. Ulcer location appears to be related to a number of etiologic factors. Most DUs occur in the first part of the duodenum (duodenal bulb). Benign GUs can occur anywhere in the stomach, although most are located on the lesser curvature, just distal to the junction of the antral and acid-secreting mucosa.

Association with *Helicobacter pylori*

A strong association exists between *Helicobacter pylori* (HP) (formerly *Campylobacter pylori*) and PUD (Fig. 32.3).[1,6–8] Virtually all patients with DU and GU who are not taking NSAIDs have evidence of HP infection and antral gastritis. Although a causal relationship between HP and chronic superficial antral gastritis is well established, a similar relationship between HP and PUD is difficult to confirm, in part because only a small number of individuals infected with HP actually develop an ulcer. It is likely that unidentified host-specific cofactors or strain variability also play an important role in the pathogenesis of PUD. Never-

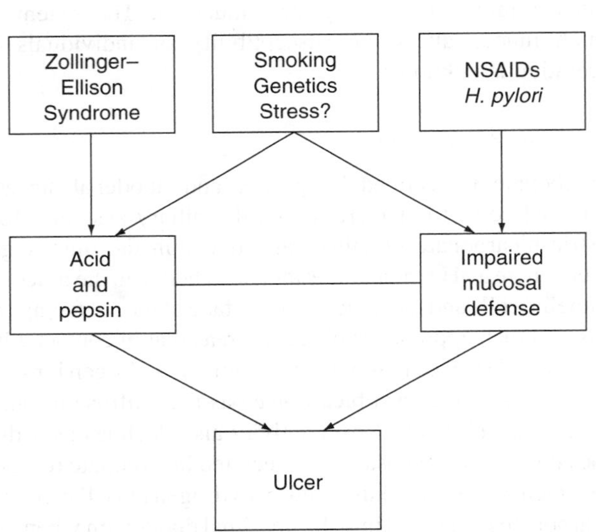

Figure 32.2. Proposed model for the pathophysiology of peptic ulcer. Acid and pepsin cause ulcers when mucosal defense mechanisms are impaired by NSAIDs or *H. pylori*. Smoking, genetic factors, and psychological stress probably modulate the secretion of acid and/or impair mucosal defense. Hypersecretion of gastric acid causes ulcers in ZES. *(Modified and reprinted, by permission of The New England Journal of Medicine, (vol 322; p 910, 1990.)*

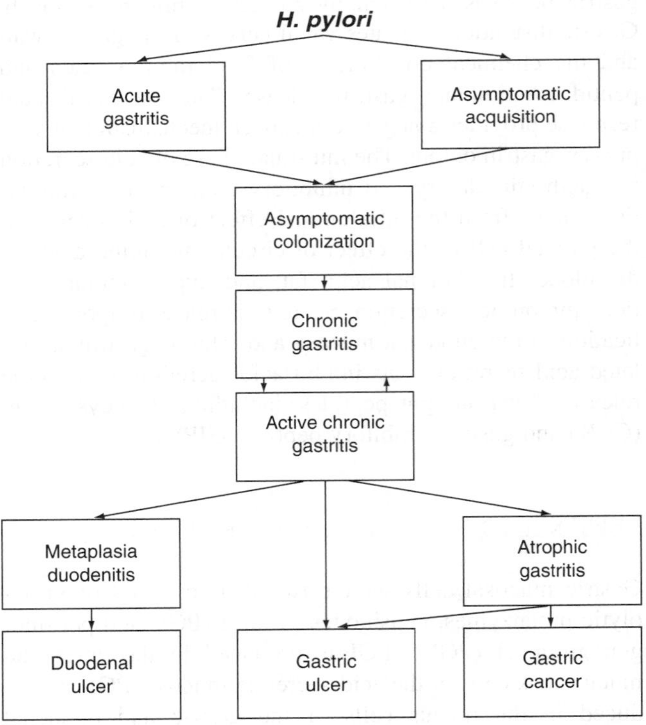

Figure 32.3. The natural history of *H. pylori* infection and its role in the pathogenesis of gastric and duodenal ulcer. *(From Wyle FA. J Clin Gastroenterol 1991;13(suppl 1): S114–S124, with permission.)*

theless, it is noteworthy that nearly all patients with PUD not taking NSAIDs have HP gastritis. In addition, there is a marked decrease in DU and GU recurrence rates following eradication of HP infection.[6–8]

HP is an acid-labile, spiral-shaped gram-negative rod that resides between the mucus layer and surface epithelial cells in the stomach or any location where gastric epithelium is found.[7,9] Antral organisms colonize gastric metaplasia in the duodenum, which is thought to arise secondary to changes in acid or bicarbonate secretion, products of HP, or host inflammatory responses.[1,6] The shape and motility of the bacterium permit penetration of the mucus layer where the local pH is less acid. Before HP enters the mucus, it produces large amounts of urease, which breaks down urea in gastric juice and converts it to ammonia and carbon dioxide. This metabolic process continues after HP reaches the "safe haven" of the mucus. The neutralizing effect of ammonia forms a microenvironment that protects the organism from the lethal effect of acid. HP attaches to epithelial surfaces by adhesions or pedestals specific for gastric-type epithelium.[9,10]

The specific pathophysiologic mechanism(s) by which HP causes ulcers is controversial and remains unknown; however, several theories have been proposed.[10,11] The "leaking roof" theory suggests that HP impairs mucosal defense by the elaboration of toxins, potentially toxic enzymes and inflammation. Candidates include lipopolysaccharide, vacuolizing cytotoxin, urease, and ammonia, as well as macrophage and neutrophil activation. The role of the immune system in HP infection requires further study. The "gastrin-link" theory hypothesizes that HP increases antral gastrin release, which leads to increased acidity and ultimately gastroduodenal damage. Although chronic HP infections have been shown to induce a chronic hypergastrinemia, increased gastrin does not appear to be a critical factor.[10]

Transmission of the organism in Western countries is thought to be person to person via the fecal–oral and oral–oral routes as humans are the only reservoir of infection.[1,7–9] Most infections are passed from parents to their children.[9,12] It is also possible to transmit HP via infected instruments such as endoscopes. The overall prevalence of HP is much higher in underdeveloped countries where people become infected much earlier. It appears that HP infection rates correlate with lower socioeconomic status and health standards. In the asymptomatic population of the United States, the prevalence of HP is age dependent with a rate of 60% occurring in individuals over the age of 60 years compared to 10% in children. Differences exist among ethnic groups with infection more common in African Americans and Hispanics than in whites.[1,7] HP infection rates do not differ with gender or smoking status. There is an epidemiologic association between HP and gastric cancer, although whether a causal relationship exists remains unknown.[1,6,7,13]

ABNORMALITIES IN ACID SECRETION AND MOTILITY

Most people with DU have normal acid secretory rates; however, a subgroup are acid hypersecretors. Factors responsible for acid hypersecretion include increased parietal cell mass, increased basal secretory drive (high BAO/MAO ratio), and increased postprandial secretory drive. Mechanisms that underlie basal and postprandial hypersecretion include enhanced sensitivity of the parietal cell to secretogogues or vagal stimulation as well as impaired acid inhibitory mechanisms. Sustained hypergastrinemia in ZES patients increases parietal cell mass. The implications of HP-induced hypergastrinemia on acid secretion and its potential pathogenic role in PUD are controversial and require further investigation. In contrast to DU, patients with GU have normal or reduced rates of acid secretion.

Gastric motility determines the rate of delivery of stomach contents to the duodenum, whereas duodenal motility affects the clearance of gastric, biliary, and pancreatic secretions from the duodenal bulb. In a subset of DU patients, accelerated gastric emptying may contribute to a relative increase in the acidity of the proximal duodenum. Abnormal antral-pylorus-duodenal motility patterns permit duodenal contents containing bile salts and pancreatic enzymes to reflux into the stomach. Delayed gastric emptying increases exposure of the stomach to acid, pepsin, and refluxed duodenal contents. It is possible that in a subset of patients, gastric stasis and duodenal reflux may influence the severity of gastric injury induced by HP or NSAIDs.[1]

ASSOCIATION WITH NSAIDS

There is overwhelming evidence linking chronic NSAID (including aspirin) use and gastroduodenal ulcers.[1,5] In patients receiving NSAIDs, ulcers occur more frequently in the stomach than in the duodenum. Hospitalizations, complications, and mortality are increased in chronic NSAID users and are, in part, related to ulcer bleeding and perforation. Several factors, including a history of PUD, NSAID dose, duration of exposure, and disability, may predispose people to ulcers and complications.[1,14–16] There is no evidence that cigarette smoking or ethanol ingestion serve as independent risk factors for NSAID-induced ulcers. The high incidence of NSAID-related ulcer complications in the elderly and the increased risk of ulcers in older women are probably related to increased consumption.[1,15] Although patients with NSAID-induced ulcers may have HP, NSAIDs appear to induce ulcers through a mechanism that does not require HP.[14] Conversely, NSAID-induced ulcers do not seem to increase susceptibility to HP infection. Ulcers have been reported with low doses of aspirin or nonaspirin NSAIDs and complications have occurred following a few days of treatment.[1,16] Acute low-dose NSAID-induced lesions, however, usually undergo adaptive mucosal cytoprotection and have the capacity for rapid, spontaneous healing.

Chronic NSAID therapy produces gastroduodenal injury by two mechanisms: a direct action on the mucosa and a systemic effect whereby endogenous PG synthesis is inhibited (Fig. 32.4).[1,5] NSAID inhibition of cyclooxygenase not only decreases protective PGs, but also generates oxygen-derived free radicals and makes available more arachidonic acid for metabolism via the lipoxygenase pathway. Leukotrienes, products of lipoxygenase metabolism, are inflammatory substances that may contribute to mucosal injury. Although most nonaspirin NSAIDs have topical irritative effects, aspirin appears to be the most ulcerogenic. Even though prodrugs, enteric-coated aspirin tablets or capsules, salicylate derivatives, and parenteral or rectal preparations may not cause as many superficial gastric erosions, they can cause GU and DU and related life-threatening complications.

ADRENOCORTICOSTEROIDS

The association between adrenocorticosteroids and PUD remains controversial. Although it is likely that adrenocorticosteroids induce ulcers because of their ability to increase gastric acid secretion and inhibit PG production, sufficient evidence is lacking to support a causal relationship. Discrepant findings among earlier retrospective studies may have been due, in part, to differences in the use of NSAIDs among study participants. A recent study suggests that elderly patients on concurrent oral adrenocorticosteroids and NSAIDs are at a much higher risk for PUD than those receiving either of these agents alone, and that ulcer risk is related to adrenocorticosteroid dose and duration of therapy.[17] It is possible that adrenocorticosteroids either delay or inhibit the healing of ulcers caused by aspirin and other NSAIDs. Patients receiving adrenocorticosteroids and NSAIDs should be considered high risk for PUD.

UNCOMMON FORMS OF PEPTIC ULCER

DU and GU have been reported in individuals using crack cocaine and in patients with viral infections, receiving radiation, or undergoing chemotherapy administration through an hepatic artery pump. The infusion of 5-fluorouracil, mitomycin C, doxorubicin, or cisplatin probably causes ulcers by a direct toxic effect.[1]

POTENTIAL RISK FACTORS

Cigarette Smoking

There is strong epidemiologic evidence that links cigarette smoking to PUD. Cigarette smoking increases the risk for the development and recurrence of DU and GU and the risk appears to be proportional to the amount smoked. The threshold for measurable risk appears to be about one-half pack (10 cigarettes) per day. The adverse relationship of cigarette smoking to PUD is supported by the fact that smokers are more likely than nonsmokers to develop ulcers and that relapse occurs sooner and more frequently in smokers than in nonsmokers. In addition, smoking may impair ulcer healing as evidenced by the need for longer treatment periods or higher antisecretory doses. Smoking also increases the likelihood of complications and the need for surgery. Death rates are higher among patients who smoke than among nonsmokers, although it is not known whether this apparent increase in mortality reflects PUD or the cardiac and pulmonary sequelae of smoking.[1]

The specific reasons why cigarette smoking influences ulcer incidence, recurrence, healing, and complications

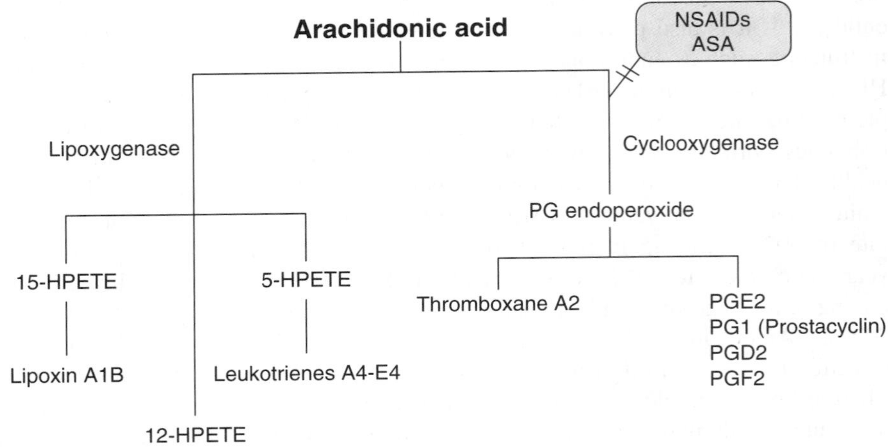

Figure 32.4. The arachidonic acid cascade; postulated mechanism whereby NSAIDs exert gastroduodenal injury. NSAIDs act by both a direct action on the mucosa and by systemic inhibition of cyclooxygenase. ASA, acetylsalicylic acid; HPETE, hydroperoxyeicosatetraenoic acid; NSAIDs, nonsteroidal anti-inflammatory drugs; PG, prostaglandins.

remains unclear. Possible mechanisms include accelerated gastric emptying of liquids, inhibition of pancreatic bicarbonate secretion, promotion of duodenogastric reflux, and reduction in mucosal PG production. It is uncertain whether nicotine is the component of smoke responsible for these physiologic alterations. Although smoking has been reported to increase gastric acid, it appears to have no consistent effect on acid secretion. There are no satisfactory data on whether smoking cigars or pipes is also associated with PUD.

Genetic Factors

A number of genetic factors have been proposed to explain familial aggregation of PUD. However, recent data suggest that HP, and its association with hypergastrinemia and hyperpepsinogenemia I, offers a more plausible explanation for family clustering than inherited autosomal dominance.[1] Whether the gene for blood group O is associated with an increased incidence in DU requires studies to confirm its independence of HP. Conversely, genetic syndromes such as multiple endocrine neoplasia (MEN) type I, systemic mastocytosis, and amyloidosis type IV maintain their association with peptic ulcers.[1]

Psychological Stress

The importance of psychological factors in the genesis of PUD is controversial. Although clinical observation supports the belief that ulcer patients are adversely affected by stressful life events, controlled studies have failed to document a cause-and-effect relationship. Alternatively, psychological factors may predispose selected patients to PUD or alter the degree of pain or disability that results from an ulcer. It is possible that stressors induce behavioral risks such as smoking and the use of NSAIDs or alter the inflammatory response or resistance to HP infection. Because of the difficulty in quantitating and assessing the response to stress, its role in ulcer pathogenesis is uncertain.[1]

Dietary Factors

The role of diet and nutrition in PUD is uncertain, but may explain regional variations. Coffee, tea, cola beverages, beer, milk, and spices may cause dyspepsia, but do not increase the risk for PUD. In addition, beverage restrictions and bland diets do not alter the frequency of ulcer recurrence. Although caffeine is a gastric acid stimulant, other constituents in decaffeinated coffee/tea, caffeine-free carbonated beverages, beer, and wine are responsible for increasing gastric acid. Ethanol, in high concentrations, is associated with acute gastric mucosal damage and upper GI bleeding; however, there is insufficient evidence to confirm that ethanol causes ulcers. An association between high salt intake and GU as well as low dietary fiber and DU has been hypothesized, but not substantiated.[1]

DISEASES ASSOCIATED WITH PEPTIC ULCER

A few diseases have been associated with peptic ulcer, although some of these associations have been based on inconclusive evidence. Duodenal ulcer is commonly associated with reflux esophagitis and Barrett's esophagus. In patients with chronic pulmonary disease and cancer of the lung, cigarette smoking appears to fully account for the association. The increased incidence of ulcers in patients with rheumatoid arthritis is thought to be related to the use of aspirin, NSAIDs, and adrenocorticosteroids. The incidence and prevalence of DU and GU appear to be increased in cirrhosis, but a relationship has not been confirmed. The association between PUD and renal failure in patients on hemodialysis and after transplant is controversial. A negative association exists in patients with pernicious anemia and atrophic gastritis, Addison's disease, autoimmune thyroid disease, and hypoparathyroidism.[1]

CLINICAL PRESENTATION

Patients with PUD usually present with dyspeptic symptoms such as nausea, vomiting, belching, and bloating in addition to heartburn or epigastric pain. When patients with dyspepsia are found not to have ulcers, they are diagnosed as having "nonulcer" dyspepsia. Although it is important to distinguish between nonulcer dyspepsia and PUD, there is no reliable way to make this distinction based on symptoms. Information obtained from the medical history often leads to suspicion of an ulcer, but direct visualization of the crater is required to confirm the diagnosis. Occasionally, patients present with complications such as bleeding, obstruction, or perforation without dyspeptic symptoms.

SYMPTOMS AND SIGNS

Epigastric pain is the classic and most frequent symptom of DU and GU. The pain is often described as burning but can present as a vague discomfort, abdominal fullness, or cramping (Table 32.1). Many patients with DU describe a typical nocturnal pain that awakens them at night. Ulcer-related pain in DU often occurs 1–3 hours after meals and is usually relieved by food, but this is variable. In GU, food may precipitate or accentuate ulcer pain. Antacid ingestion usually provides immediate pain relief in most patients with either DU or GU. Pain usually diminishes or disappears during treatment; recurrence of pain after healing usually indicates a recurrent ulcer.

The severity of symptoms varies from patient to patient and, in some patients, symptoms may be seasonal, occurring more frequently in the spring or fall. Episodes of discomfort usually occur in clusters lasting up to a few

TABLE 32.1. CLINICAL FEATURES OF GASTRIC AND DUODENAL ULCER[a]

Feature	Gastric Ulcer	Duodenal Ulcer
Pain	++++	++++
Epigastric	+++	++++
Frequently severe	+++	+++
Radiation to back	++	++
Episodic (clusters)	+	+++
Nocturnal	+++	++++
Within 30 minutes of food	++	+
Food relief	++	+++
Relieved by antacids	++++	++++
Anorexia	+++	++
Weight loss	+++	++
Nausea	++++	+++
Vomiting	++++	+++
Heartburn	+	+++
Bloating	+++	+++
Belching	+++	+++
Ulcer recurrence	+++	++++

[a]Frequencies represent estimates and are categorized as being consistent (++++), frequent (+++), infrequent (++), or rare (+). None of the features is always present or always absent.

weeks followed by a symptom-free period or remission lasting from weeks to years. Pain does not always correlate with the presence or absence of acid or ulcer craters. Asymptomatic patients may have an ulcer at endoscopy and patients with endoscopically proven healed ulcers may have persistent symptoms. Changes in the character of the pain or failure to respond to antacids suggest the presence of complications. Persons consuming NSAIDs and the elderly are often symptom free (silent ulcer) prior to bleeding or perforation. The reasons for this are unclear, but may relate to differences in which the elderly perceive pain or result from the analgesic effect of the NSAID. Nausea, vomiting, anorexia, and weight loss are more common in patients with GU (Table 32.1).

PHYSICAL EXAMINATION

The physical examination generally reveals epigastric tenderness, which usually occurs between the umbilicus and the xiphoid process and less commonly radiates to the back. Although pain is a common finding, it is insensitive and nonspecific. The development of complications associated with PUD (obstruction, perforation, penetration, or bleeding) may be present on physical examination. Unusual findings may be present when ulcers are associated with hypersecretory states such as ZES (see the section on Zollinger–Ellison Syndrome).

DIAGNOSTIC TESTS AND PROCEDURES

LABORATORY TESTS

Routine laboratory tests are not helpful in establishing a diagnosis of uncomplicated PUD. Acid secretory studies and a fasting serum gastrin concentration are only recommended in patients unresponsive to therapy or for cases in which hypersecretory diseases are suspected. The hematocrit, hemoglobin, and stool hemoccult tests are used to detect bleeding. An elevated serum PGI may provide indirect evidence of HP, but its clinical utility is questionable and the test is not widely available.

HELICOBACTER PYLORI TESTS

The diagnosis of HP can be made using invasive or noninvasive tests (Table 32.2).[6,7,18] The invasive methods require upper GI endoscopy with a mucosal biopsy taken for histology, culture, gram stain, or detection of urease activity. Histologic identification has a sensitivity and specificity of >95%. Although culture has a specificity of 100%, it lacks sensitivity for HP. The sensitivity and specificity of the biopsy urease test, which detects HP urease enzyme activity, is >90%. The ^{13}C and ^{14}C urea breath tests require that patients ingest radiolabeled urea, which, in the presence of urease, forms ammonia and radiolabeled bicarbonate. The absorbed bicarbonate is excreted in the breath and detected by a scintillation counter (^{13}C) or mass spectography (^{14}C). With the exception of serology, all of the diagnostic tests for HP may produce false-negative results if antibiotics were used within the previous 4 weeks. Serologic tests can detect antibodies produced against high molecular weight HP cell proteins; however, a positive test indicates both active as well as past infections. Until inexpensive and accurate noninvasive tests are available, the routine monitoring of HP eradication for relapse, reinfection, or treatment failure cannot be recommended.

ENDOSCOPIC/RADIOGRAPHIC EXAMINATION

The diagnosis of PUD depends on visualizing the ulcer crater. DU should be distinguished from other acid-peptic diseases, and benign GU must be distinguished from those that are malignant. The clinical presentation of these disorders does not allow differentiation on the basis of symptoms and physical examination. Therefore, the diagnosis depends on radiologic or endoscopic findings. Routine single barium contrast techniques can detect 30% of peptic ulcers, whereas it is possible to detect 60–80% of ulcers using optimal double-contrast radiography. Fiber optic endoscopy detects more than 90% of peptic ulcers

TABLE 32.2. TESTS FOR DETECTION OF *HELICOBACTER PYLORI*

Test	Sensitivity[a]	Specificity[a]	Endoscopy	Cost[b]	Comments
Histology	+++	+++	Yes	+++	At least two biopsies from antrum
Culture	++	+++	Yes	+++	Reserved for cases of antibiotic resistance
Biopsy/gram stain	++	++	Yes	+++	Rapid microbiologic detection
Biopsy/urease	+++	+++	Yes	+++	Quick, often endoscopic method of choice
Breath/urease (^{13}C/^{14}C)	+++	+++	No	++	May be used to monitor antimicrobial therapy
Serology	++	++	No	+	Does not differentiate active versus previous infection

[a]Categorized as very good (+++), good (++), or poor (+).

[b]Represents cost estimates: most expensive (+++), expensive (++), or least expensive (+). Includes cost of endoscopy, when appropriate. (Modified from Loffeld RJLF, Stobberingh E, Arends JW. A review of diagnostic techniques for *Helicobacter pylori* infection. Dig Dis 1993;11:177.)

and permits direct inspection, biopsy, visualization of superficial erosions, and sites of active bleeding. Because of its lower cost, greater availability, and perhaps greater safety, many physicians believe that radiography should remain the initial diagnostic procedure in evaluating patients with suspected uncomplicated peptic ulcer; however, if complications are thought to exist or if an accurate diagnosis of PUD is warranted, endoscopy is the diagnostic procedure of choice. If a GU is found on radiography, malignancy should be excluded by direct endoscopic visualization and biopsy for histologic examination.

Clinical Course and Prognosis

The natural history of PUD is characterized by periods of exacerbations and remissions. Ulcer pain is usually recognizable and episodic, but symptoms are variable, especially in the elderly and in patients taking NSAIDs. Untreated patients with uncomplicated ulcers often become asymptomatic within several weeks of the diagnosis. Most ulcers will eventually heal on their own, but the healing process is accelerated with treatment. Conventional drug therapy accelerates ulcer healing and alleviates symptoms in most patients; however, rapid and frequent ulcer recurrence can be expected following initial healing of both GU and DU. Low-dose maintenance therapy with conventional antiulcer medications decreases the rate of ulcer recurrence. Two-thirds of patients with DU can expect to have their disease subside over a 10- to 15-year period. About 20% of all patients will experience complications from their ulcer disease. Mortality in patients with GU is slightly higher than in patients with DU and the general population. Eradication of HP infection cures the disease, dramatically reduces ulcer recurrence, and may prevent future complications. The epidemiologic association between HP and gastric carcinoma requires further definition. Although conventional antiulcer medications heal and prevent ulcers, they do not affect the natural history of the disease. Anti-HP therapy offers the possibility of altering the natural history of PUD rather than temporary control of the diathesis.[6,7]

Treatment

The treatment of PUD is traditionally aimed at relieving ulcer pain, accelerating ulcer healing, minimizing ulcer recurrence, and reducing ulcer-related complications. The discovery that HP is responsible for nearly all DU and most GU has had important therapeutic implications. Treatment strategies have been modified to reflect new information on the efficacy of anti-HP drug regimens. Peptic ulcer disease, however, remains a multifactorial disease and a number of factors continue to influence ulcer healing.

FACTORS THAT INFLUENCE ULCER HEALING

The natural history of PUD varies from spontaneous ulcer healing to refractory ulcerations despite drug therapy. In the United States, DU placebo healing rates range from 20% to about 60% over 2–6 weeks, respectively. Drug therapy with standard doses of the H_2-receptor antagonists (H_2RAs), antacids, or sucralfate increases the rate of active ulcer healing. Approximately 70%, 80%, or 90% of DUs heal by 4, 6, or 8 weeks, respectively. Increasing the degree of acid suppression with proton pump inhibitors or higher doses of H_2RAs accelerates DU healing so that comparable rates are seen over a 2- to 4-week period. In contrast, GU healing does not correlate as strongly with acid suppression. A longer duration of treatment is often required to heal GUs, because the average ulcer size is larger than a DU. Once full-dose antiulcer medication is stopped, 50–90% of patients develop a recurrent ulcer within 1 year. Effective maintenance therapy reduces the recurrence rate of symptomatic DU to 20–40%.

Cigarette smoking is a risk factor for PUD and ulcer-related complications. There is strong evidence that smoking impairs healing and promotes recurrence and that the risk is increased with 10 or more cigarettes/day. NSAID (including aspirin) consumption causes "virgin" ulcers and delays ulcer healing. Although certain foods and beverages may cause dyspepsia, there is no evidence that they alter ulcer healing or recurrence. Psychosocial factors may influence the perception of ulcer symptoms and ulcer healing.

H_2-RECEPTOR ANTAGONISTS

The H_2RAs (cimetidine, famotidine, nizatidine, and ranitidine) competitively and reversibly bind H_2 receptors on the parietal cell, diminishing cytosolic cyclic AMP production and the secretion of histamine-stimulated gastric acid. An interaction between the cyclic AMP and calcium pathways also results in partial inhibition of acetylcholine- and gastrin-stimulated acid secretion (Fig. 32.1).

Structure/Antisecretory Potency

The chemical structures of the H_2RAs differ in that cimetidine, famotidine, and ranitidine contain an imidazole, thiazole, and furan ring, respectively. Nizatidine combines the thiazole ring of famotidine and the side chain of ranitidine. The relative antisecretory potencies of the H_2RAs vary from the least potent, cimetidine, to the most potent, famotidine; however, increased potency does not confer greater efficacy if these agents are administered in similar antisecretory doses. The recommended oral ulcer-healing doses tend to minimize differences in antisecretory potency (Table 32.3).[19,20] The pharmacokinetics of the H_2RAs are similar and are discussed elsewhere.[19,21,22]

Efficacy

Cimetidine, famotidine, nizatidine, and ranitidine, when used in recommended oral doses (Table 32.3), have similar DU and GU healing rates.[20,23] In most patients, DU and GU healing is comparable with multiple daily doses or a single full dose given after dinner or at bedtime. Similar DU healing rates have been achieved by giving the full daily dose in the morning.[1] Twice-daily administration suppresses daytime acid and benefits patients with daytime ulcer pain. Treatment duration for most patients with an uncomplicated DU is 6–8 weeks; however, a small number may remain symptomatic and unhealed.[20] An additional 2–4 weeks is sometimes recommended in the elderly and smokers, as longer treatment is more likely to heal the ulcer and possibly reduce ulcer recurrence. Data are conflicting regarding a dose-response for healing.[1] On-demand therapy (treatment until pain is symptomatically controlled) may be similar to conventional therapy in controlling DU pain, but ulcer healing is slower and complications may occur more often.[24] Although H_2RAs are effective in healing benign GU, their ability to relieve symptoms and prevent complications is less convincing than in DU. In patients with GU, H_2RAs are usually given for 8 weeks; however, ulcers greater than 1 cm may require up to 12 weeks for complete healing. Endoscopy is often recommended to confirm GU healing and to assure that the ulcer is not malignant. A reduction in H_2RA daily dose is recommended in patients with moderate-to-severe renal failure (Table 32.4).

TABLE 32.3. ORAL ANTIULCER DRUG TREATMENT REGIMENS[a]

Drug	DU Healing (mg/dose)	GU Healing (mg/dose)	DU Maintenance (mg/dose)	GU Maintenance (mg/dose)
H_2-Receptor Antagonists				
Cimetidine	300 qid 400 bid 800 hs	300 qid 800 hs	400 hs	400 hs
Famotidine	20 bid 40 hs	20 bid[a] 40 hs	20 hs	20 hs[a]
Nizatidine	150 bid 300 hs	150 bid 300 hs	150 hs	150 hs[a]
Ranitidine	150 bid 300 hs	150 bid 300 hs[a]	150 hs	150 hs[a]
Proton Pump Inhibitors				—
Omeprazole	20 qd	20 qd[a]		
Lansoprazole	15 qd	15 qd		
Enhances Mucosal Defense				
Sucralfate[b]	1 qid 2 bid[a]	1 qid[a] 2 bid[a]	1 bid	1 bid[a]

[a]Not a Food and Drug Administration (FDA)-approved indication/dose regimen.
[b]Dose = (g/dose).

TABLE 32.4. PRACTICAL GUIDELINES FOR ADJUSTING THE ORAL DOSE OF ANTIULCER DRUGS IN RENAL IMPAIRMENT[a]

Drug	Creatinine Clearance (mL/min)			
	>50	**20–50**	**10–20**	**<10**
Cimetidine	800–1200	800–1000	600–800	300–400
Famotidine	40	40	20–40	20–20[b]
Nizatidine	300	150	150–150[b]	150[b]
Ranitidine	300	150	150–150[b]	150[b]
Omeprazole	20	20	20	20–20[b]
Lansoprazole	15	15	15	15–15[b]
Sucralfate[c]	4	4	4	2–4

[a]Estimated daily dose (mg) required to heal a duodenal or gastric ulcer.
[b]Give dose every other day.
[c]Dose = (g).

Safety

In general, H_2RAs are safe and well tolerated. When used in recommended therapeutic doses for the treatment of PUD, their short- and long-term safety profiles are quite similar.[1,20] GI disturbances occur most frequently. Central nervous system (CNS) effects, particularly drowsiness and headache, occur most often in ambulatory patients and have been reported with all of the H_2RAs. The H_2RAs are associated with a rare incidence of reversible adverse hematologic reactions; thrombocytopenia is the most common, regardless of the H_2RA implicated. Gynecomastia and impotence can occur in men receiving prolonged, high doses of cimetidine and is thought to be a dose-related antiandrogen effect of the drug.[1] The cardiovascular effects and changes in gastric emptying associated with the oral H_2RAs are probably of minimal clinical consequence in most patients. Cimetidine and, to a lesser extent, ranitidine interfere with the renal tubular secretion of creatinine; however, increases in serum creatinine do not represent renal toxicity.[20]

The potential for drug interactions exists with all of the H_2RAs and is reviewed extensively elsewhere.[25] H_2RAs may interact with drugs by several mechanisms (Table 32.5); they may (1) alter the bioavailability of orally administered drugs as a consequence of increasing intragastric pH; (2) bind reversibly to hepatic cytochromes P-450 and decrease the hepatic clearance of drugs that undergo phase I metabolism; (3) inhibit gastric mucosal alcohol dehydrogenase (ADH), thereby influencing the mucosal metabolism of ethanol; and (4) decrease the renal clearance of drugs by inhibiting their renal tubular secretion.[25] None of the H_2RAs has a clinically important effect on hepatic blood flow. Numerous drug interactions have been reported, especially with cimetidine, but the majority do not lead to pharmacodynamic effects.[20,25] Important drug interactions do exist, however, particularly with drugs that have a narrow therapeutic index (e.g., theophylline, phenytoin, and warfarin). Metabolic interactions with cimetidine may be dose dependent. The clinical relevance of the H_2RA–ethanol interaction remains uncertain.

TABLE 32.5. MECHANISMS OF DRUG INTERACTIONS WITH ANTIULCER AGENTS[a]

Drug	Absorption		Metabolism		
	pH Effect	**Adsorption**	**Hepatic P-450**	**Gastric ADH**	**Elimination**
Antacids	+	+	–	–	+[b]
Cimetidine	+	–	++	+	++[c]
Famotidine	+	–	–	–	–
Nizatidine	+	–	–	+	–
Ranitidine	+	–	+	+	+[c]
Misoprostol	+	–	–	–	–
Omeprazole	++	–	+	–	?
Lansoprazole	++	–	+	–	?
Sucralfate	–	+	–	?	–

[a]Estimates are categorized as predominant effect (++), an effect (+), no effect (–), or unknown (?).
[b]Elevates urinary pH.
[c]Inhibits renal tubular secretion. (Modified from Welage LS, Berardi RR. Drug interactions with antiulcer agents: Considerations in the treatment of acid-peptic disease. J Pharm Prac 1994;7:190.)

PROTON PUMP INHIBITORS

The proton pump inhibitors (PPIs), omeprazole and lansoprazole (a benzimidazole derivative structurally similar to omeprazole), dose-dependently inhibit basal and stimulated gastric acid secretion. Under acidic conditions in the parietal cell, the parent compounds are protonated and converted to active metabolites, which react covalently with H+/K+-ATPase. A sulfhydryl bond is formed that noncompetitively and irreversibly inhibits activity of the enzyme (Fig. 32.1). PPIs produce a profound, long-acting, but reversible acid suppression that persists for several days after stopping the drug. Resumption of acid secretion requires the synthesis of new H+/K+-ATPase. Rebound hypersecretion does not usually occur.[26–30]

Omeprazole and lansoprazole are inactivated by gastric acid; therefore, the drugs are administered orally in a capsule that contains pH-sensitive granules that release the drug when the pH is higher than 6. Upon dissolution of the capsule in the stomach, the granules pass into the duodenum where the drug is released and absorbed. In patients who are unable to swallow, the capsule may be opened but the granules should be administered in an acidic juice (e.g., orange, apple, or cranberry juice) to avoid dissolution of the protective coating.[1,26] Although omeprazole and lansoprazole have an elimination half-life of about 1 hour, their prolonged antisecretory effects enable once-a-day dosing, usually in the morning. Higher daily doses should be divided in order to enhance 24-hour control of acid secretion. Both drugs are most effective when taken shortly before meals.[1] The pharmacokinetics of these agents are similar and are reviewed elsewhere.[27–30]

Efficacy

Omeprazole and lansoprazole are effective in healing DU and GU (Table 32.3). Duodenal ulcer healing rates at 4 weeks, with omeprazole 20 mg/d or lansoprazole 15 mg/d, are similar and more effective than H_2RA antiulcer regimens.[26–31] Although PPIs accelerate DU healing, healing rates vary with cigarette smoking, NSAID use, and the size or severity of the ulcer. Gastric ulcer healing rates are only slightly higher than those observed with the H_2RAs.[26–30] When compared with conventional H_2RA doses, PPIs usually provide a more rapid resolution of symptoms. Initial treatment should be limited to 4 weeks; however, an additional 2–4 weeks may be needed in some patients. Patients with resistant DU or GU and those refractory to H_2RA treatment may benefit from omeprazole 40 mg/d or lansoprazole 30 mg/d. The daily dose of both drugs should be reduced in patients with severe hepatic failure, but a reduction is not necessary in renal failure or in the elderly.

Safety

Adverse effects related to the short-term (<12 weeks) use of PPIs are well established and similar to those observed with the H_2RAs (e.g., diarrhea, nausea, constipation, headache, and skin rash[26,30,32,33]). Within the last few years isolated cases of gynecomastia,[34] hemolytic anemia,[35] peripheral neuropathy,[36] acute interstitial nephritis,[37] fulminant hepatic failure,[38] and male sexual dysfunction[39] have been reported with omeprazole. In general, the adverse effects observed with long-term (>12 weeks) PPI treatment are similar to those reported with short-term use.[32,33] The potential long-term consequences of hypergastrinemia are discussed elsewhere (see section on Consequences of Hypochlorhydria). Gastric polyposis has been reported after 12 months of treatment with omeprazole.[40] A dose-dependent decrease in protein-bound cyanocobalamin absorption has been observed in patients receiving long-term omeprazole therapy.[41] Omeprazole and lansoprazole selectively inhibit isoenzymes of the hepatic cytochrome P-450 subfamily IIC. Interactions may occur with omeprazole and either warfarin, phenytoin, or diazepam or with lansoprazole and theophylline. (Table 32.5).[25,30]

ANTACIDS

High and frequent antacid doses (100–144 mEq of acid neutralizing capacity 1 and 3 hours after meals and at bedtime) heal DU more effectively than placebo and are comparable to the H_2RAs and sucralfate. Low-dose aluminum/magnesium-containing liquid or tablet regimens are also effective in healing DU and GU; however, the lower limits of the ulcer-healing dosage regimens are unknown.[1,42,43] Recent data support the argument that antacids heal ulcers by acid-independent mechanisms in addition to their acid-neutralizing effects. Antacids inactive pepsin and bind bile salts; aluminum-mediated complexes suppress HP, enhance mucosal defense, and may deliver EGF to the injured mucosa.[1] Although antacids heal ulcers, they are primarily used in combination with other antiulcer drugs when needed for the relief of ulcer pain or dyspepsia, in part, because of their adverse effects and frequent administration. Antacids, taken in the fasted state, have a neutralizing effect of 15 to 30 minutes. When taken 1 hour after meals, the meal provides a buffering effect for about 1 hour; gastric emptying is delayed and prolongs the antacid-neutralizing effects for an additional 2 hours.

Preparations/Formulations

Magnesium/aluminum-containing antacids are most widely used in PUD. Sodium-containing salts are not used long term because they can lead to systemic alkalosis. Magnesium hydroxide has a more prolonged neutralizing effect than either sodium bicarbonate or calcium carbonate; however, the effects of magnesium oxide and carbonate are similar to those of magnesium hydroxide. Magnesium trisilicate is considered a weak antacid. Aluminum hydroxide possesses a relatively low neutralizing capacity; aluminum phosphate has very little antacid activity. Magaldrate (hydroxymagnesium aluminate) is transformed to magnesium and aluminum ions in the presence of hydrochloric acid. Its effects resemble those of other magnesium/aluminum-containing antacids, but it contains less magnesium per unit of weight. Simethicone may reduce flatulence and bloating, but does not have antiulcer properties. Antacid tablets should be chewed prior to swallowing. Compliance can be increased by selecting a high-potency antacid and by determining the patient's taste preference.

Safety

GI effects occur most frequently with antacid use. Magnesium salts cause a dose-dependent osmotic diarrhea, whereas constipation occurs with aluminum salts. Diarrhea predominates with magnesium/aluminum-containing antacids. These effects can be minimized by lowering the dose or alternating magnesium/aluminum with aluminum-containing antacids. Antacids that are similar in potency, but contain less magnesium, may cause less diarrhea. Aluminum-containing antacids (except aluminum phosphate) form insoluble salts with dietary phosphorus and block phosphorus absorption. Hypophosphotemia may develop especially in patients with low dietary phosphate intake (e.g., malnutrition, alcoholism). Combined treatment with sucralfate can also potentially amplify the hypophosphotemia.[1]

Aluminum elimination may be impaired in patients with renal failure (see section on Sucralfate). Magnesium-containing antacids should not be used in patients with a creatinine clearance of <30 mL/min, because magnesium excretion is impaired. Although calcium stimulates gastrin, acid rebound is questionable.[42] Patients with normal renal function taking >20 g/d of calcium carbonate and those with impaired renal function taking >4 g/d may develop hypercalcemia. Most antacids have been reformulated to contain insignificant amounts of sodium. The milk-alkali syndrome occurs with high calcium intake in patients with systemic alkalosis. The alkalosis may be produced by absorbable antacids (sodium bicarbonate) or by prolonged vomiting. The main features of the syndrome include hypercalcemia, alkalosis, renal stones, and elevated blood urea nitrogen and creatinine concentrations.

Antacids can alter the absorption and excretion of drugs when administered concomitantly (Table 32.5).[25] The magnitude of the interaction depends on antacid dose, salt, and the ability to separate the antacid from other oral drugs. Antacids interact by elevating intragastric pH, adsorption, chelation, or by increasing urinary pH. Most interactions can be avoided by separating the antacid from the oral drug by 2 hours. If possible, it is advisable to avoid coadministering antacids with other oral medications. Clinically important interactions can occur when antacids are administered with tetracycline, warfarin, digoxin, quinidine, isoniazid, ketoconazole, or the fluoroquinolones.[25]

SUCRALFATE

Sucralfate is an aluminum salt of a sulfated disaccharide that is only minimally absorbed (3–5%) from the GI tract. When exposed to acid, sucralfate forms a viscous adhesive that binds electrostatically to positively charged protein molecules in the ulcer crater, forming a protective barrier that inhibits back-diffusion of hydrogen ions, pepsin, and bile salts.[44,45] Although the drug has a greater affinity for damaged mucosa, binding to normal mucosa does occur; attachment to the ulcer crater lasts for up to 6 hours following oral administration. Sucralfate inhibits pepsin, adsorbs bile salts, stimulates endogenous PGs and EGF, and may suppress HP.[45] Although aluminum appears to mediate some of these actions, the sucrose moiety may also play a role in ulcer healing. Sucralfate does not have an important effect on acid secretion. The majority of the dose is excreted unchanged in the feces with only a small amount of the absorbed drug excreted in the urine. Aluminum excretion is decreased in uremia.[44] Although a liquid form of the drug is available, a suspension can be prepared by dispersing the tablet in 20–30 mL of water.

Efficacy

Sucralfate is effective in the short-term treatment of DU and is comparable to the H_2RAs. Although the recommended dosing regimen is 1 g four times per day 1 hour before meals and at bedtime, a regimen of 2 g twice per day appears to be as effective (Table 32.3).[44] Treatment should be continued for 6–8 weeks. Sucralfate should be taken on an empty stomach to prevent binding to dietary protein and phosphate. Fewer studies indicate that sucralfate is effective in healing GU.[44] Combined sucralfate and H_2RA regimens permit two different mechanisms of action, but appear to offer no advantage over either agent alone. Sucralfate may overcome the negative effect of smoking on DU healing and recurrence.

Safety

Adverse effects to sucralfate are usually minor and occur in less than 5% of patients. Constipation is most common and develops in about 2% of patients.[44] Elderly patients, who are sensitive to alterations in bowel function, may not tolerate the drug. Nausea, indigestion, dry mouth, dizziness, and a metallic taste occur infrequently. Seizures resulting from aluminum accumulation have occurred in dialysis patients who were also receiving aluminum-containing antacids. It is best to avoid combining these agents in chronic renal failure. Simultaneous consumption of citric acid has been reported to significantly enhance aluminum absorption and probably should be avoided as well.[1] Hypophosphotemia may develop in patients on prolonged sucralfate therapy (see section on Antacids). Gastric bezoar formation has been reported.[44]

The concomitant administration of sucralfate with phenytoin, digoxin, theophylline, quinidine, amitriptyline, warfarin, ketoconazole, fluoroquinolones, and L-thyroxine may reduce their bioavailability and effectiveness (Table 32.5).[25,46] In most instances, the interaction can be minimized by separating the drug and the sucralfate dose by 2 hours. The sequence of administration can profoundly influence the magnitude of the fluoroquinolone interaction; therefore, the fluoroquinolone should be given at least 2 hours before sucralfate.[25] Alternative antiulcer therapy may be warranted in some patients.

PROSTAGLANDINS

Prostaglandins (PGs) are produced by the GI mucosa and play an important role in maintaining mucosal resistance to injury (see section on Gastric Physiology). The synthetic PGE analogues also inhibit acid secretion by binding to a PG receptor on the parietal cell. Although structurally similar, there are subtle differences in the actions of the PGEs with regard to their antisecretory effects and actions on the uterus. A number of PGE analogues (misoprostol, enprostil, arbaprostil, rioprostil) are in various stages of clinical development in the United States; however, only misoprostol is indicated for the prevention of NSAID-induced GU.

Misoprostol

Misoprostol, a synthetic PGE_1 analogue, moderately inhibits acid secretion and enhances mucosal defense. Antisecretory effects are dose dependent over the range of 50 to 200 μg; cytoprotective effects occur in humans at doses of at least 200 μg.[1] Misoprostol heals uncomplicated DU and GU in a dose-dependent fashion. Thus, the ability of misoprostol to heal ulcers appears to be related primarily to its antisecretory effect. Because protective effects occur at higher ulcer-healing doses, it is difficult to establish the protective effect independent of antisecretory action. Although not recommended for the treatment of PUD in the United States, a dose of 200 μg four times daily or 400 μg twice daily heals DU and GU comparable to conventional H_2RA or sucralfate regimens. Misoprostol, 200 μg four times per day, also effectively protects against NSAID-induced GU and DU (see section on NSAID-Induced Ulcers).[47,48] Lower doses of 200 mcg three times a day or twice daily provide adequate protection in most patients. A reduction in dose is not necessary in renal or hepatic impairment.

The most frequent adverse effects reported with misoprostol are crampy abdominal pain and diarrhea. The diarrhea is dose dependent and is due to stimulation of intestinal smooth muscle as well as fluid and electrolyte secretion. Diarrhea is reported to develop within 1–2 weeks of initiating therapy in about 40% of patients on NSAIDs receiving 800 μg/d and in 25% of patients receiving 400 μg/d; however, the incidence of diarrhea in clinical studies is variable and reflects differences in definition and study design.[1,47,48] Life-threatening diarrhea has been reported in a patient with inflammatory bowel disease.[49] Nausea, flatulence, headache, dyspepsia, vomiting, and constipation occur frequently. Because misoprostol does not relieve GI pain associated with NSAIDs, antacids (other than magnesium-containing antacids) may be used as needed for abdominal discomfort. Taking the drug with or after meals and at bedtime may minimize diarrhea. Misoprostol is uterotrophic and produces contractions that may endanger pregnancy; therefore, the drug is contraindicated in pregnant women. If misoprostol is prescribed to women in their childbearing years, use of adequate contraceptive measures should be confirmed and a negative serum pregnancy test should be documented within 2 weeks of starting the drug. Patients should be advised about the potential GI effects and the need to avoid magnesium-containing antacids, and younger women should be warned about the importance of adequate contraception. In patients with rheumatoid arthritis, misoprostol does not interfere with the beneficial effects of NSAIDs.

BISMUTH PREPARATIONS

Bismuth preparations have been used for many years to treat acid-peptic disorders. The most commonly used salts are bismuth subsalicylate (BSS or Pepto-Bismol™), available in the United States, and colloidal bismuth subcitrate (CBS) and tripotassium dicitrato bismuthate (TDB, DeNol), available in Europe. Ranitidine bismuth citrate has recently become available in the United States. Bismuth subsalicylate is an insoluble complex that, at a pH <3.5, reacts with acid to form bismuth oxide and salicylic acid, which is readily absorbed.[1,50] In the colon, bismuth oxide reacts with hydrogen sulfide to form bismuth sulfide, which blackens the stool. Although the precise method by which bismuth acts to heal ulcers remains uncertain, possible mechanisms include its local gastroprotective effect, its ability to stimulate endogenous PGs, and its ability to suppress HP.[1,51,52] Bismuth does not inhibit or neutralize acid. Both CBS and TDB are effective in healing DU and GU; healing rates are similar to conventional doses of the H_2RAs and sucralfate.[51,52] Ulcer recurrence rates following short-term treatment with CBS or TDB are lower than those with other antiulcer medications. Various BSS regimens, including 525 mg (305 mg elemental bismuth) four times daily, are being investigated; however, preliminary data suggest that BSS may not have the same antiulcer effects as CBS or TDB when used as a single agent.

Bismuth absorption varies with the specific salt; however, absorption is greater with other bismuth salts than with BSS.[1] A decrease in intragastric acidity has been reported to enhance CBS absorption, but not that of BSS.[53] Although prolonged treatment with bismuth subgallate has been associated with neurologic toxicity, clinical trials with intermittent use of CBS, TDB, and BSS have not reported significant neurologic effects.[51,52] Renal failure decreases bismuth elimination and may result in an increased bismuth load. BSS should be used with caution in the elderly or patients with renal failure, salicylate sensitivity, bleeding disorders, and in combination with high-dose salicylate therapy. Patients should be advised that bismuth preparations may impart a black color to their stool.

ERADICATION OF *HELICOBACTER PYLORI*

In the 1990s, a growing body of knowledge has convincingly shown the important role that HP plays in the pathogenesis and recurrence of PUD. Recent studies indicate that eradication of HP infection heals ulcers, alters the natural history of PUD, and reduces the risk of recurrence to <10% in 1 year.[6,8,54–56] In addition, eradication of HP may heal ulcers refractory to conventional antiulcer regimens. The aim of anti-HP drug therapy is to eradicate the organism, rapidly ameliorate symptoms, cure the infection, heal the ulcer, and prevent recurrence. Failure to detect HP after a course of antimicrobial therapy does not confirm that the organism is eradicated. In some instances, HP may have only been suppressed and will ultimately emerge again. Therefore, eradication of HP is defined as absence of the organism at least 4 weeks after cessation of therapy. The disease is successfully cured when eradication is permanent.

Numerous clinical trials of multiple drugs, drug combinations, and dosage regimens have been conducted in an attempt to eradicate HP and cure PUD.[8,54–61] In general, drug combinations are more effective than single agents; however, combinations tend to cause more adverse effects. An increasing concern is the emergence of resistant strains. Resistance to antimicrobials, in particular to metronidazole and clarithromycin, is a cause for treatment failure.[8,62] Although the optimal drug regimen has yet to be identified, acceptable results can be obtained by using a number of different approaches to treatment. When multiple drugs are administered at various times, patient compliance may become an important factor in determining efficacy.[62] The selection of a particular therapeutic regimen should take into account efficacy, resistance, safety, cost, and compliance. HP eradication for DU appears to be more cost-effective than conventional anti-ulcer treatment.

Single Agents

None of the conventional antiulcer agents (including ranitidine bismuth citrate) has any meaningful effect on HP (Table 32.6). When given alone, bismuth eradication rates range from 5–35% after 4–6 weeks of therapy.[55,57] Although many antimicrobials have been investigated, including amoxicillin, metronidazole, tetracycline, erythromycin, furazolidone, and the fluoroquinolones, monotherapy with most is ineffective.[55,57] A discrepancy between high *in vitro* and low *in vivo* efficacy may be explained, in part, by the degradation of the antimicrobial in the acidic environment of the stomach or by insufficient penetration through the gastric mucus.[62,63] The reduced effect may also be caused by HP resistance, although resistance with amoxicillin or tetracycline has not been reported. The most promising antimicrobial, given as monotherapy, is clarithromycin (Table 32.6). Because of the poor results with monotherapy and the emergence of resistance to selected antimicrobials, a remarkable number of combined drug regimens has been investigated. The methodologies and results of these studies can be found elsewhere; only the most important are discussed in this chapter.[6–8,54–61,64]

Bismuth/Antimicrobial Regimens

Numerous clinical trials have confirmed the superiority of bismuth plus metronidazole and either amoxicillin or tetracycline in eradicating HP (Tables 32.6 and 32.7).[8,55,57] Use of amoxicillin is generally associated with lower eradication rates compared with tetracycline-containing regimens.[6,54,55,57] Therapy with bismuth plus two antimicrobials is begun concurrently and continued for 2 weeks. An H_2RA is usually added to the initial regimen and continued for 4–6 weeks. DU healing may be modestly accelerated with the addition of an H_2RA. Similar regimens have been associated with a 30% incidence of diarrhea, occasional antibiotic-associated colitis, and other numerous adverse effects.[8,62,64] Medication noncompliance is also a significant problem. An HP eradication rate of 69% was reported in patients who took less than 60% of their medications.[62]

Because of these and other problems, new and shorter regimens have been investigated. Clinical trials using bismuth, higher doses of metronidazole plus tetracycline or amoxicillin and a proton pump inhibitor yield excellent eradication rates after 1 week of treatment, but adverse effects occur in up to 20% of patients (Tables 32.6 and 32.7).[57,64] Whether these regimens lead to better compli-

TABLE 32.6. *HELICOBACTER PYLORI* **ERADICATION RATES WITH SINGLE AGENTS AND COMBINATION THERAPY**

Regimen	Eradication Rate (%)[a]
Monotherapy	
Bismuth subsalicylate, antibiotics (most), ciprofloxacin, or H_2-receptor antagonists (H_2RA), proton pump inhibitors alone	0–10
Colloidal bismuth subcitrate, amoxicillin, erythromycin base, or furazolidone alone	10–40
Clarithromycin	40–60
One Antimicrobial Plus an Antisecretory Agent	
Amoxicillin + PPI	30–90
Clarithromycin + PPI	70–90
Two Antimicrobials Plus an Antisecretory Agent	
Bismuth + amoxicillin + H_2RA	30–60
Bismuth + metronidazole + H_2RA	30–75
Metronidazole + amoxicillin + H_2RA	55–90
Metronidazole + clarithromycin + PPI	90–95
Metronidazole + amoxicillin + PPI	90–95
Three Antimicrobials Plus an Antisecretory Agent	
Bismuth + metronidazole + tetracycline + H_2RA	90–95
Bismuth + metronidazole + amoxicillin + H_2RA	80–90
Bismuth + metronidazole + tetracycline + PPI	>95

[a]Eradication rates are dependent on individual drug doses and duration of therapy. (Compiled from Refs. 6, 54, 55, and 57–59.)

ance remains unknown. A one-day, high-dose regimen using bismuth, amoxicillin, metronidazole, and omeprazole was effective in eradicating HP in 72% of patients with PUD.[60] When bismuth is combined with either amoxicillin or metronidazole the results are disappointing.

TABLE 32.7. DRUG REGIMENS FREQUENTLY USED IN THE TREATMENT OF *HELICOBACTER PYLORI*-ASSOCIATED PEPTIC ULCER DISEASE[a]

Regimen	Drug
1.	Bismuth subsalicylate 525 mg qid × 2 weeks Metronidazole 250 mg tid/qid × 2 weeks Tetracycline/Amoxicillin 500 mg qid × 2 weeks H_2RA (e.g., ranitidine 300 mg/d) × 4–6 weeks
2.	Bismuth subsalicylate 525 mg qid × 2 weeks Metronidazole 500 mg qid × 1 week Tetracycline/Amoxicillin 500 mg qid × 1 week PPI (e.g., omeprazole 20 mg bid × 1 week)
3.	Metronidazole 500 mg bid × 1 week Omeprazole 20 mg bid × 1 week Clarithromycin 250–500 mg bid × 1 week Metronidazole 500 mg tid × 12–14 days H_2RA (e.g., ranitidine 300 mg/d) × 6–10 weeks
4.	Omeprazole 20 mg bid × 2 weeks then 20 mg/day × 2 weeks Amoxicillin 1 g bid or 500 mg qid × 2 weeks
5.	Omeprazole 20 mg bid × 2 weeks; then 20 mg/day × 2 weeks Clarithromycin 1000–1500 mg/d × 2 weeks
6.	Metronidazole 500 mg bid × 1 week Omeprazole 20 mg bid × 1 week Amoxicillin 250–500 mg bid × 1 week

[a]Selection of a specific treatment regimen should take into account drug efficacy/resistance, compliance, adverse effects, and cost.

The observation that omeprazole might be associated with a decrease in HP led to the exploration of studies using omeprazole and various antimicrobials.

Regimens that combine omeprazole with amoxicillin are associated with variable efficacy (Tables 32.6 and 32.7).[6,8,26,57,59,64] These regimens involve the coadministration of omeprazole 20 mg twice daily preprandially for 2–4 weeks and amoxicillin 2 g/d (either 1 g twice daily or 500 mg four times daily) after meals for 2 weeks. Explanations as to why omeprazole enhances the efficacy of amoxicillin include possible omeprazole-induced suppression of HP; better activity or stability of amoxicillin in the hypoacidic stomach; a higher topical antibiotic concentration due to decreased gastric secretions; prolonged amoxicillin after postprandial administration; and a number of host factors such as prolonged action of immunoglobulins and increased neutrophil function.[59,64] Immediate pretreatment with omeprazole lowers the effectiveness of the omeprazole-amoxicillin regimen.[6,59] Favorable results have been obtained by administering omeprazole with varying doses of clarithromycin (Tables 32.6 and 32.7).[26,64] Regimens recently approved for use in the United States include: 1) omeprazole 40 mg once daily with clarithromycin 500 mg three times daily for 2 weeks, followed by omeprazole 20 mg daily for 2 weeks, and 2) ranitidine bismuth citrate 400 mg twice daily for 4 weeks with clarithromycin 500 mg three times daily. One advantage of these combinations is that they can be used in penicillin-allergic individuals. The major disadvantage is that HP resistance to clarithromycin may develop. Limited data indicate that lansoprazole-antimicrobial anti-HP regimens provide results similar to that of omeprazole.

Numerous other anti-HP regimens have been investigated.[8,57,58,61] The combination of metronidazole, clarithromycin, and omeprazole, or metronidazole, amoxicillin, and omeprazole for 1 to 2 weeks results in an eradication rate of more than 90%.[8] In most instances, HP eradication does not appear to be significantly enhanced with the 2 week regimen. (Tables 32.6 and 32.7).[58] Combined treatment with furazolidone, amoxicillin, and metronidazole for 5 days eradicated HP and abolished DU relapse.[61]

OTHER ANTIULCER AGENTS

A number of other agents have been used to treat PUD. The anticholinergics have been replaced by more potent antisecretory drugs with fewer adverse effects. Pirenzepine and telenzepine, antimuscarinic drugs that inhibit cholinergic-mediated acid secretion by selectively blocking specific muscarinic receptors, are associated with a lower incidence of anticholinergic side effects, but dry mouth and visual disturbances have been reported with ulcer-healing doses. The mechanisms by which tricyclic antidepressants, such as doxepin and trimipramine, act in PUD are complex but most likely include H_2-receptor blockade and an anticholinergic effect. Although these agents may be effective in PUD, anticholinergic and cardiac side effects limit their use. Metoclopramide, domperidone, and cisapride accelerate gastric emptying and may be of value in treating GU. Proglumide, a gastrin antagonist, inhibits gastrin stimulation of the parietal cell. Somatostatin may heal ulcers by way of its inhibitory effects on acid, pepsin, and gastrin release. Zinc salts have been reported to be effective in the treatment of PUD.[65]

MAINTENANCE THERAPY

Peptic ulcer disease (PUD) is a chronic disorder characterized by frequent ulcer recurrence. Approximately 50–90% of ulcers recur within 1 year of initial ulcer healing with conventional antiulcer regimens.[20,23] Recurrence following treatment with colloidal bismuth subcitrate is less common than after treatment with the H_2RAs, PPIs, or sucralfate. A number of factors influence the tendency for ulcers to recur. These include the presence of HP, cigarette smoking, NSAID use, gastric acid hypersecretion, patient noncompliance, incomplete ulcer healing, a long duration of PUD, and a history of complications.[1,23,66] The cause of ulcer recurrence, like that of the initial ulcer, is probably multifactorial. Maintenance therapy reduces symptomatic recurrence to about 20–40% within a year. Prevention lasts only as long as treatment is continued; up to 90% of ulcers recur after the drug is withdrawn.

In the United States, the H_2RAs (cimetidine, famotidine, nizatidine, and ranitidine) and sucralfate are recommended as DU maintenance therapy; however, only ranitidine is approved for GU maintenance. When the H_2RAs are given in a reduced dose at bedtime (Table 32.3), all four agents are effective and comparable in preventing DU recurrence.[20,23,66] Although ranitidine 150 mg may be superior to cimetidine 400 mg, the differences observed in comparative maintenance trials is of questionable clinical importance in most patients. A bedtime dose of cimetidine 300 mg/d is often prescribed, but there are no controlled clinical trials to support this dose. Although it appears that H_2RA maintenance regimens are effective in preventing GU recurrence, a subset of GU patients may require continuation of the full ulcer-healing dose. In addition, full-dose H_2RA maintenance therapy may be warranted in DU or GU patients who are heavy smokers, take NSAIDs, or have a history of refractory ulcers or complications. Long-term maintenance therapy (beyond 10 years) with cimetidine or ranitidine appears to be safe and effective; results with nizatidine and famotidine will probably be similar.

Maintenance therapy with either 10 or 20 mg/d of omeprazole is superior to placebo, and symptomatic recurrence rates are generally similar to those achieved with low-dose H_2RAs or sucralfate.[20,26–29] However, the antisecretory response to 10 mg/d is widely variable.[67] Intermittent dosage schedules, such as weekend therapy (20 mg daily on Friday, Saturday, and Sunday), or 20 mg every other day, appear promising.[20,67] Neither of these regimens is associated with clinically important changes in fasting serum gastrin concentrations. Patients with severe DU have been maintained ulcer-free for as long as 6 years while receiving omeprazole 20 to 40 mg/d.[20] However, PPIs should not be used routinely as maintenance therapy in PUD until studies document the lowest effective dose (see section on Consequences of Hypochlorhydria). Clinical trials evaluating the efficacy and safety of lansoprazole maintenance therapy are currently under way, but similar results are expected.

DU recurrence rates with sucralfate 1 g twice daily are similar to those reported with maintenance doses of the H_2RAs. Long-term maintenance therapy with sucralfate should probably be avoided in patients with chronic renal failure. The efficacy of sucralfate in preventing GU recurrence remains to be established. Maintenance trials with antacids and prostaglandins are inconclusive. The future of maintenance therapy in PUD is uncertain given the ability of anti-HP regimens to cure ulcers.

CONSEQUENCES OF HYPOCHLORHYDRIA

Most antisecretory agents increase fasting and postprandial serum gastrin concentrations as a function of their acid-inhibitory effect. Low intragastric pH serves as a feedback mechanism to inhibit gastrin secretion from the antral G cells. Sustained hypo- or achlorhydria induces a release of gastrin into the circulation that is directly proportional to the degree of gastric acid inhibition. Usually small, but variable, increases in serum gastrin have been observed following several weeks of treatment with conventional doses of the H_2RAs. In most patients, these increases are within the normal range and return to baseline within a few days of discontinuing therapy.[20] Hypergastrinemia has been reported with high-dose H_2RAs.[68]

Treatment with the more potent PPIs (omeprazole and lansoprazole) produces greater increases in fasting and postprandial serum gastrin.[1,28,30,33] The effects are dose and time dependent.[28,30,68–70] Although drug-induced hypergastrinemia may be of no direct clinical concern, an important consequence is its trophic effect on ECL cells in the gastric epithelium (Figure 32.5). ECL cell hyperplasia has led to the development of gastric carcinoid tumors in female rats receiving long-term omeprazole and in patients with pernicious anemia or gastrinoma.[68–70] There is no evidence, however, to indicate that hypergastrinemia and the subsequent development of ECL hyperplasia has led to dysplastic lesions in patients receiving omeprazole for as long as 8 years.[70] The degree and duration of hypergastrinemia needed to produce ECL hyperplasia or carcinoid formation in humans is unknown. It is possible that, in humans, progression of ECL hyperplasia to carcinoid tumor requires the presence of unknown factors in addition to hypergastrinemia.[1,68–70] Alternatively, ECL hyperplasia may be related to an underlying HP gastritis rather than to the drug. In any case, periodic determinations (every 6–12 months) of fasting serum gastrin may be warranted in patients receiving long-term (>12 weeks) PPI therapy. If marked elevations are present (>300 pg/mL), a dosage reduction.

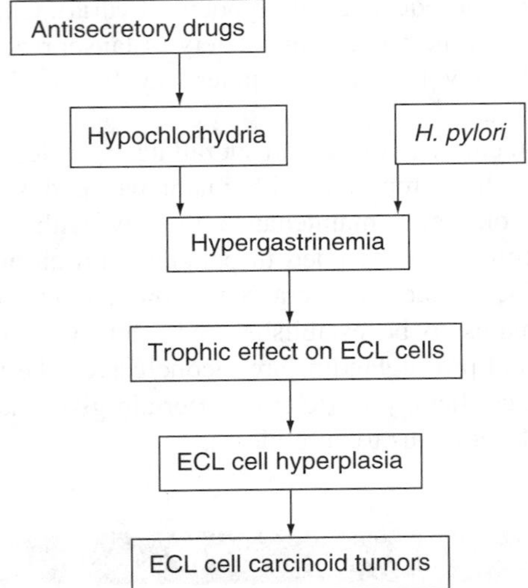

Figure 32.5. The gastrin hypothesis suggests that prolonged hypergastrinemia results in hyperplasia of the enterochromaffin-like (ECL) cells of the gastric fundus. The trophic influence of gastrin may be a risk factor for ECL cell carcinoid tumor formation.

Bacterial overgrowth occurs in the stomach as a consequence of hypochlorhydria and may lead to the formation of carcinogenic *N*-nitroso compounds in animals. There is no evidence, however, that a causal association exists in humans.[1,70] Alternatively, descriptive epidemiologic studies indicate that gastric cancer occurs more frequently in patients with long-standing HP infection.[6,13] Although HP is not known to produce direct carcinogens, it may promote the development of gastric cancer indirectly. The relationship among chronic HP infections, hypergastrinemia, and gastric cancer remains unclear.

NSAID-Induced Ulcers

NSAIDs (including aspirin) cause *de novo* ulcers and exacerbate the underlying ulcer diathesis in patients with a history of PUD. However, controversy exists as to whether there are important differences between NSAIDs and their propensity to cause ulcers. Endoscopic studies confirm that NSAID-induced GUs occur more commonly than DU. Elderly patients, patients with a history of PUD recurrence and complications, patients with a coagulopathy or underlying cardiovascular disease, and those taking high-dose NSAIDs, NSAID combinations, or NSAIDs and adrenocorticosteroids appear to be at greatest risk of developing NSAID-related complications and death. High-risk patients should probably stop or reduce smoking and ethanol use. If possible, NSAIDs should be withdrawn and alternative agents such as acetaminophen or nonacetylated salicylates (e.g., salsalate) should be used for analgesia. In those patients in whom NSAIDs cannot be discontinued, a lower NSAID dose or the use of a less damaging agent, coadministered with food or antacids, may minimize dyspepsia or direct mucosal damage.

Treatment

When a NSAID-induced ulcer is confirmed, the NSAID should be discontinued or the dose reduced. If the NSAID is stopped, full-dose therapy with either an H_2RA, PPI, or sucralfate will heal most ulcers. Large GUs or DUs may require prolonged therapy or treatment with higher antisecretory doses. If the NSAID is continued, treatment with a conventional H_2RA or PPI antiulcer regimen will promote healing, but ulcers tend to heal at a slower rate.[1,47,71] Therefore, a longer duration of antiulcer therapy may be indicated in these patients. Alternatively, higher doses of a PPI (e.g., omeprazole 40 mg/d) may be preferred in patients with GUs who continue to take NSAIDs.[1,26,47] Data are limited regarding the ulcer-healing efficacy of sucralfate or misoprostol in the setting of continued NSAID use.

Prevention

Misoprostol is the drug of choice for preventing GU and DU in chronic NSAID users; however, the drug has not been approved in the United States for prophylaxis of DU.[47,48] Data are limited with regard to the cost effectiveness of such treatment. Coadministration of misoprostol (200 μg four times per day) with NSAIDs is indicated for high-risk patients, although the definition of "high risk" remains elusive. The use of a lower misoprostol dose (200 μg two to three times per day) is better tolerated, but efficacy in preventing endoscopic ulcers may be somewhat diminished.[48] No data support the efficacy of the H_2RAs, sucralfate, or PPIs in preventing NSAID-induced GU.[1,47,72] H_2RAs and PPIs appear to reduce chronic NSAID-induced DU, but dosage guidelines have not been established.[1,47] No data support the use of low-dose maintenance therapy with either the H_2RAs or PPIs.

Recommendations

INITIAL TREATMENT

Recent advances in the pathogenesis of PUD have altered therapeutic goals and long-standing strategies for management. Treatment, at present, poses several unique challenges because it is not entirely clear who should undergo HP eradication and what is optimal therapy. Clinicians have been slow to embrace HP treatment because of the complexity and inconvenience of the regimens, as well as the possibilities for increased adverse effects and antimicrobial resistance. Although excellent eradication rates are achieved with bismuth-metronidazole-tetracycline or bismuth-metronidazole-amoxicillin plus an H_2RA, or PPI the search continues for regimens that combine simplicity, safety, and efficacy. A 2-week course of clarithromycin and either a PPI or ranitidine bismuth citrate permits almost all DU to heal and affords a cure of about 80%. A one-week course of metronidazole, clarithromycin or amoxicillin and a PPI also provides excellent eradication rates and ulcer healing (Table 32.7).

The H_2RAs (cimetidine, famotidine, nizatidine, and ranitidine), PPIs (omeprazole and lansoprazole), sucralfate, and antacids are all effective in healing peptic ulcers but do not alter the underlying ulcer diathesis. The convenience of a single nighttime dose and a remarkable safety profile explains why the H_2RAs have become the preferred agents for most patients with an initial ulcer. In patients with daytime ulcer pain, a twice-daily regimen may be necessary. The use of either famotidine or nizatidine spares interactions with drugs metabolized by hepatic P-450 enzymes. PPIs heal DU and possibly GU more rapidly than conventional antiulcer doses of the H_2RAs. When used for short-term treatment of PUD, the adverse effects profile of the PPIs is similar to that observed with the H_2RAs. Long-term studies with omeprazole reveal a safety profile not unlike short-term therapy. Although omeprazole and lansoprazole may interact with drugs metabolized by selected hepatic P-450 isoenzymes, they are more likely to alter the bioavailability of other drugs whose absorption is pH dependent.

The efficacy of sucralfate is well established in DU, but is less so in GU. Deterrents to its use include a multiple-dosing regimen, large tablet size, and the need to separate the drug from meals and other potentially interacting medications. In addition, sucralfate should be used with caution in patients on dialysis, especially when they are receiving other aluminum-containing medications. Because the drug is not extensively absorbed, it may be the drug of choice in pregnancy. Antacids are not used to heal ulcers; however, they are often used in combination with other antiulcer agents to provide rapid relief of ulcer pain and dyspepsia. When given after meals, their neutralizing effect can be prolonged for several hours.

A reasonable approach to the initial treatment of non–NSAID-induced DU or GU is presented in Fig. 32.6. If possible, the patient should stop or reduce smoking. In patients with uncomplicated DU, treatment can be initiated. with either an H_2RA, sucralfate, or a PPI. Therapy with an H_2RA or sucralfate is usually continued for 6–8 weeks, while therapy with a PPI is usually continued for 4 weeks. If the patient is asymptomatic, ulcer healing is assumed and treatment is discontinued. Visual confirmation of the healed ulcer is not necessary. In patients with GU, treatment with an H_2RA (8 weeks) or PPI (4 weeks), should be initiated. The patient should undergo endoscopy to confirm ulcer healing. If the ulcer is healed, therapy is stopped. However, if either a DU or GU remains unhealed, it is reasonable to continue treatment with the same dose and the same drug for an additional 4 weeks or switch from an H_2RA to a PPI. Anti-HP treatment should be instituted in HP-positive patients. Because ulcer healing is time dependent, nearly all ulcers will heal with any of the agents if therapy is continued for 12 weeks.

There is a strong belief among most gastroenterologists that all patients with non–NSAID-induced DU or GU should be initially treated with one of the more effective anti-HP regimens, although the optimal regimen has not been identified (Table 32.7). It is their belief that all patients should receive treatment regardless of whether they are suffering from the first symptomatic presentation of the disease or from a recurrence. Although this strategy offers a relatively simple way to cure the disease or dramatically reduce ulcer recurrence, there is no inexpensive and accurate noninvasive method to routinely monitor the absence of HP. It also remains unclear as to whether all patients with symptomatic DU and GU should receive eradication therapy without confirmation of HP-positivity. Ultimately, the

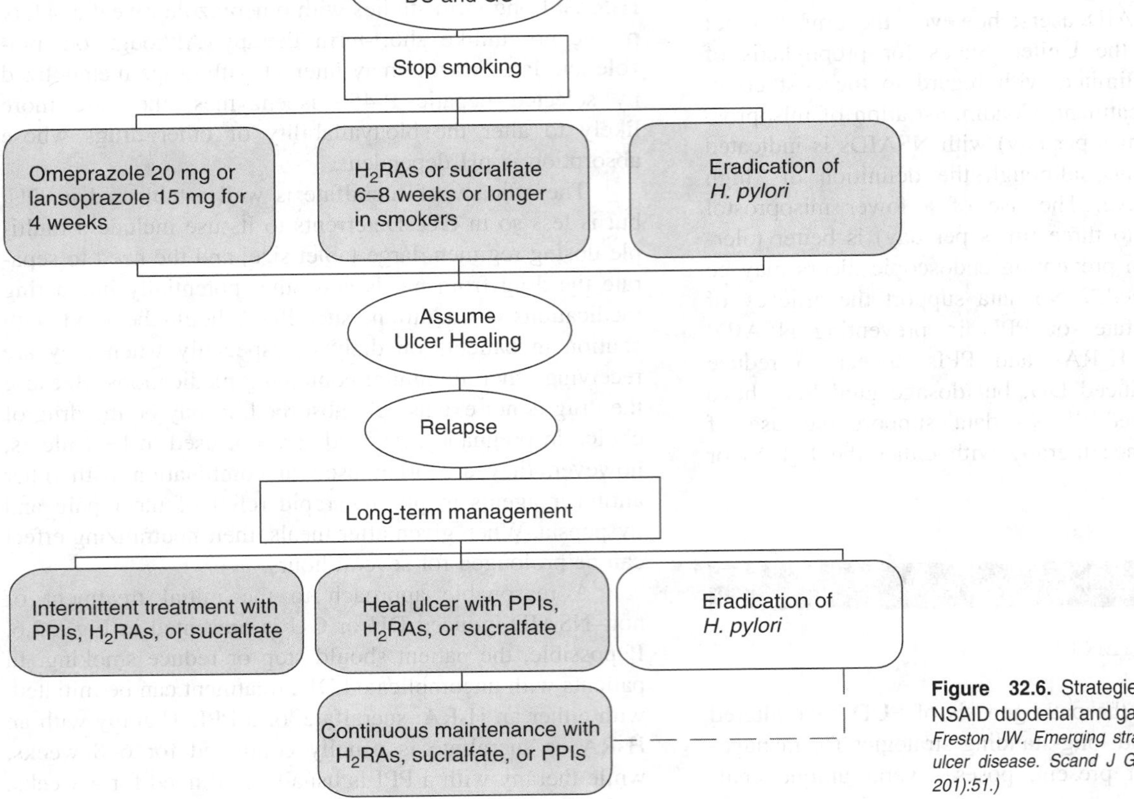

Figure 32.6. Strategies for managing non-NSAID duodenal and gastric ulcers. *(Modified from Freston JW. Emerging strategies for managing peptic ulcer disease. Scand J Gastroenterol 1994;29:(suppl 201):51.)*

choice of a specific ulcer-healing regimen should be individualized and based on efficacy, safety, compliance, and cost. The cost effectiveness of anti-HP therapy requires further evaluation and comparison with other treatment options.

There are several groups of patients who may not warrant HP eradication therapy. These include patients with very mild disease, those who are old or might not tolerate the antimicrobial regimens, HP patients with a history of bleeding or perforation, individuals with HP-free NSAID-induced ulcers, and patients with ZES. There are no data to support HP eradication in patients with asymptomatic HP, nonulcer dyspepsia, or to prevent gastric cancer.

LONG-TERM STRATEGIES

Long-term strategies for managing ulcer recurrence are currently undergoing revision in light of the fact that recurrence of PUD is infrequent after HP eradication and ulcer healing (Figure 32.6). If symptoms persist or recur after initial treatment (regardless of the initial ulcer-healing regimen), a second course of antiulcer therapy should be instituted. Diagnostic reevaluation may favor the use of an anti-HP regimen. Alternatively, most patients with a single episode of an uncomplicated recurrent ulcer, who have few if any risk factors, can be managed with another course of intermittent full-dose therapy (6–8 weeks) with an H_2RA, PPI, or sucralfate. On-demand treatment (full-dose therapy until symptoms are relieved) is generally not advocated because it has been associated with increased ulcer-related complications. High-risk patients who relapse early (within 3–6 months of ulcer healing) or frequently (two or more relapses per year) after ulcer healing, and those with a history of ulcer complications or multiple risk factors, may be placed on continuous maintenance therapy. Low-dose therapy with an H_2RA, sucralfate, or possibly a PPI keeps a majority of ulcers healed and patients symptom free. Ulcer recurrence, while on maintenance therapy, suggests smoking, noncompliance, NSAIDs, persistent HP infection, or ZES.

REFRACTORY ULCERS

Ulcers are usually considered refractory to therapy when symptoms, ulcers, or both persist beyond 12 weeks despite conventional treatment or when several courses of HP eradication fail. Poor patient compliance, antimicrobial resistance, cigarette smoking, the use of NSAID, or a gastrinoma, may contribute to refractory PUD. The exact role of HP infection is uncertain; however, in patients not previously treated with an anti-HP regimen, eradication therapy is appropriate. A number of patients will respond to markedly suppressed gastric acid, which possibly destroys pepsin.[1] An omeprazole dose of 40 mg/d successfully heals the majority of ulcers proven refractory to omeprazole 20 mg/d as well as conventional or high-dose H_2RAs.[26] However, ulcers usually recur when therapy is discontinued or reduced to lower levels. Switching from one H_2RA or PPI to another is not beneficial. Combination therapy with an H_2RA or a PPI and sucralfate or misoprostol may appear rational because of the different mechanisms by which these drugs act, but it is without established benefit. Repeat endoscopy is required to determine ulcer healing. Combined treatment with an H_2RA is irrational. Patients with refractory GU will usually have surgery because of the fear of malignancy.

NSAID-INDUCED ULCERS

Treatment with conventional full-dose H_2RAs, PPIs, or sucralfate will heal most ulcers if NSAIDs are discontinued. Larger ulcers may require prolonged therapy at higher doses. Most therapeutic regimens will also heal ulcers despite continued NSAID use, but a longer duration of therapy or higher doses are usually required. A proton pump inhibitor (e.g., omeprazole 40 mg/d is probably the treatment of choice in patients who continue to take NSAIDs. High-risk patients with healed ulcers who continue to take NSAIDs should receive cotherapy with misoprostol. The initial dose may be 200 μg four times daily, but 200-μg dose given two or three times per day may be used in patients unable to tolerate the higher regimen. Antacids (other than magnesium-containing) may be taken with misoprostol when needed for abdominal discomfort. Conventional doses of the H_2RAs and PPIs prevent NSAID-induced DU, but not GU. The possibility of curing NSAID-induced ulcers by eradicating HP has not been adequately investigated.

Evaluation of Therapeutic Outcomes

Patients should be monitored for symptomatic relief of ulcer pain as well as potential adverse effects and drug interactions related to drug therapy. Most patients with uncomplicated PUD will be rendered symptom-free after appropriate treatment with any one of the recommended antiulcer regimens. Symptoms, however, cannot be used to guide therapeutic decisions in patients taking NSAIDs. Patient noncompliance, antimicrobial resistance, continued smoking, or NSAID use can compromise the efficacy of therapeutic regimens. Follow-up endoscopy to determine if ulcers or HP are present can be justified in patients with frequent symptomatic recurrence, refractory disease, complications, or suspected hypersecretory states. Alternatively, the urea breath test can be performed to confirm eradication of HP. A second course of therapy should be considered in patients with recurrent disease.

Complications

BLEEDING

GI bleeding may be the first manifestation of chronic PUD and occurs in approximately 15–20% of patients.[73] Bleeding is caused by erosion of the ulcer into an artery. Recurrence of bleeding after the bleeding has stopped or after ulcer healing is common. Bleeding may be insidious or may present as melena or hematemesis. In about 90% of patients, bleeding responds satisfactorily to gastric lavage and supportive therapy. In most controlled trials, treatment with drugs, such as the H_2RAs, sucralfate, antacids, PPIs and somatostatin, or drug combinations, appears to be ineffective in stopping bleeding. Although controversial, initial eradication of HP may lead to a reduction in ulcer complications and bleeding.[74]

PERFORATION AND PENETRATION

Perforation of a peptic ulcer into the peritoneal cavity occurs in 5–10% of ulcer patients.[73] Most perforations are preceded by ulcer symptoms that intensify before the perforation. The pain of perforation is usually sudden and severe, with mortality higher for GU than DU. Penetration occurs when an ulcer burrows into an adjacent structure rather than opening freely into a cavity. Duodenal ulcers may penetrate the pancreas, biliary tract, or liver. Bleeding occurs in one-third of patients.

GASTRIC OUTLET OBSTRUCTION

Gastric outlet obstruction occurs in less than 5% of hospitalized patients with peptic ulcer.[73] Mechanical obstruction is caused by scarring or edema of the duodenal bulb or pyloric channel and can lead to delayed gastric emptying. Symptoms usually occur over several months and include nausea, vomiting, and weight loss.

INTRACTABILITY

Intractability implies that all forms of drug therapy have failed. Medical therapy has improved so dramatically over the last few years that even the most virulent hypersecretory states can be managed medically.[73] Intractability is now an infrequent manifestation of PUD and an infrequent indication for surgery.

SURGERY

Advances in the medical management of PUD has led to a steady decline in operations.[75] However, a subset of patients will require emergency surgery for bleeding, perforation, or obstruction. Confirmation that HP eradication cures most HP-positive ulcers and alters the natural history of the disease should have a dramatic effect on the need for future surgery. Classically, surgical procedures performed for PUD include vagotomy with pyloroplasty or vagotomy with antrectomy.[75] Vagotomy inhibits vagal stimulation of gastric acid and may be of three types: truncal, selective, or parietal cell. A truncal or selective vagotomy frequently results in postoperative gastric dysfunction and requires a pyloroplasty or antrectomy to facilitate gastric drainage. When an antrectomy is performed, the remaining stomach is anastomosed with the duodenum (Billroth I) or with the jejunum (Billroth II). A vagotomy is not necessary when an antrectory is performed for GU. Although surgery for PUD is effective, postoperative consequences (e.g., recurrent ulceration, postvagotomy diarrhea, dumping syndrome, and anemia) occur and alter quality of life.

ZOLLINGER–ELLISON SYNDROME

Zollinger–Ellison syndrome (ZES) is characterized by gastric acid hypersecretion and recurrent peptic ulceration that results from a gastrin-producing tumor (gastrinoma). In the United States, ZES is found in approximately 0.1% of patients with DU. At surgery, more than 90% of the gastrinomas are located in the region of the pancreas known as the "gastrinoma triangle." Although most gastrinomas were thought to occur in the pancreas, recent studies indicate that as many as two-thirds of patients have extrapancreatic gastrinomas, the most common site being duodenum. Gastrinomas have also been found in the liver, spleen, kidney, and rarely the ovaries. Malignant gastrinomas occur in about 30–50% of patients with metastases to distant sites including regional lymph nodes, liver, spleen, bone, and skin. About 25–60% of cases are associated with MEN type I.[76,77]

PATHOGENESIS

Gastrin is normally secreted by antral G cells located in the stomach. In ZES, ectopic production of gastrin occurs within the gastrinoma, which results in potent stimulation of gastric acid secretion by the parietal cell. The trophic effect of gastrin leads to an increase in parietal cell mass, which provides further enhancement of acid secretion; thus, the normal feedback mechanism whereby acidification of the antrum inhibits gastrin release is lost. Despite its importance in ZES, hypergastrinemia is not specific for the diagnosis.

CLINICAL PRESENTATION

The most frequent clinical manifestation of ZES is severe and recurrent peptic ulceration typically accompanied by abdominal pain and often associated with complications such as bleeding or perforation. Ulcers occur most often in the duodenum, but may involve the stomach or jejunum. In some patients, reflux esophagitis is the prominent feature and the major complaint is heartburn. Diarrhea occurs in 30–50% of patients and may precede ulcer symptoms by several years. The diarrhea appears to result from high concentrations of gastric acid that overwhelm the duodenum's buffering capacity and damage the mucosa. Enormous amounts of intraluminal acid in the duodenum also causes steatorrhea by inactivating pancreatic lipase and precipitating bile acids. Vitamin B_{12} malabsorption may result from reduced intrinsic factor activity. Patients with MEN I may have other symptoms when the parathyroid, pituitary, thyroid, or adrenal glands are involved. Hypercalcemia related to hyperparathyroidism appears to be most common.

DIAGNOSIS

ZES should be suspected in those individuals with a compatible clinical history and evidence of gastric acid hypersecretion. The diagnosis can be established in patients with a BAO greater than 15 mEq/h (without prior gastric surgery) or in patients with a BAO greater than 5 mEq/h (with prior acid-reducing surgery) when the fasting serum gastrin is higher than 1000 pg/mL. In healthy individuals and some patients with DU, fasting serum gastrin concentrations usually do not exceed 150 pg/mL. Patients with a fasting serum gastrin in the intermediate range (200 to 1000 pg/mL) may require a provocative test to confirm the diagnosis. Although several provocative tests (secretin, calcium, and test meals) are available, the secretin test is most widely used. A positive test, consistent with a gastrinoma, is defined as an absolute increase in the gastrin level of greater than 200 pg/mL over baseline. A BAO/MAO ratio in excess of 0.6 helps reinforce the diagnosis. Tumor localization and staging must be undertaken to determine metastatic, unresectable disease from those with solitary or localized tumors. Diagnostic techniques include computed tomography (CT), magnetic resonance imaging (MRI), selective venous sampling of serum gastrin from portal venous tributaries, and abdominal ultrasonography. Location of the gastrinoma is essential in patients with localized disease as surgical resection is curative.[76]

TREATMENT

The medical approach to treating ZES is based on the presence or absence of peptic ulcers, esophagitis, diarrhea, and a gastrinoma, which may be malignant. The major threat to life is not complications from ulcer disease, but potential malignant invasion by the tumor. Surgical resection of the gastrinoma is the optimal treatment, but is not always possible. In the past, large H_2RA doses of up to 14.2 g of cimetidine, 9.6 g of ranitidine, and 0.8 g of famotidine were used to control symptoms related to acid hypersecretion. Frequently, an anticholinergic agent was added to the regimen to potentiate antisecretory effects. Because of the need for large doses, as well as the cost and inconvenience of therapy, most ZES patients on oral H_2RAs have been switched to a PPI. Occasionally, patients will require parenteral antisecretory therapy. Continuous infusion of either famotidine or ranitidine is highly effective in controlling gastric acid hypersecretion, without any significant dose-related adverse effects.

The high potency and prolonged antisecretory effect of the PPIs makes them the drugs of choice for managing acid hypersecretory states. The specific dose cannot be predicted, but may be determined by titrating the BAO to less than 10 mEq/h (or less than 5 mEq/h if the patient has severe esophagitis or prior gastric surgery) in the hour preceding the next dose of the drug. The recommended initial oral dose of omeprazole is 60 mg/d and should be adjusted to individual patient response. Dividing the daily dose and giving the drug every 8–12 hours appears to be most effective in controlling acid output and relieving symptoms. Although doses as high as 360 mg/d have been administered, an average omeprazole dose of 60 to 80 mg/d has been reported to reduce basal acid output to target levels.[26,28,76,77] In a subset of patients, acid hypersecretion can be adequately controlled with 20 to 40 mg/d.[78] Omeprazole appears safe and effective when administered by IV bolus every 12 hours, but the parenteral dosage form is not approved for use in the United States.[79] An average dose of 60 to 90 mg/d of lansoprazole appears to provide adequate control of acid secretion in most patients with ZES.[80] In general, the PPIs appear to be safe and well tolerated. ZES patients have been treated with omeprazole for as long as 10 years.

Octreotide, the long-acting somatostatin analogue, decreases acid secretion both by reducing the serum concentration of gastrin and by a direct inhibitory effect on the parietal cell. A subcutaneous dose of 100 to 250 μg three times per day has been reported to reduce serum gastrin and acid secretion substantially.[76] In theory, octreotide may also reduce the formation of gastric carcinoid by reducing the serum gastrin concentration. The use of misoprostol, sucralfate, or anti-HP regimens in patients with ZES has not been established.

Total gastrectomy, as a means to control acid, is considered in those few patients who do not respond to drug treatment; however, there is no evidence that this procedure provides protection from tumor growth or metastasis. Patients with metastatic gastrinoma require tumor resection or treatment with chemotherapeutic agents. Drugs such as streptozotocin, 5-fluorouracil, and doxorubicin have been reported to be effective in some patients. Most patients with unresectable gastrinoma avoid antisecretory surgery and are managed with PPIs.

CONCLUSION

The discovery of HP has had a profound effect on the pathogenesis and treatment of PUD. This new knowledge has revolutionized the way in which ulcers are treated and, for the most part, cured. Although much is known, numerous questions remain and many issues are still unresolved. One certainly is why some HP-infected individuals develop an ulcer or gastric cancer and why others do not. Fundamental questions about the organism, including methods of transmission, virulence, and specific pathogenic mechanisms, need to be answered. Issues related to who should be treated and what constitutes optimal drug therapy need to be further delineated. Future research may provide us with less complicated and safer antimicrobial regimens that provide novel ways of attacking the organism, including vaccines. Finally, pharmacoeconomic studies will have to confirm the cost effectiveness of HP therapy. Until many of these questions are addressed, drug treatment of PUD should be individualized using any one of the effective and safe options available. It seems reasonable, however, to treat all proven HP-positive patients with the simplest effective antimicrobial regimen.

REFERENCES

1. Soll AH. Gastric, duodenal, and stress ulcer, in Sleisenger MH, Fordtran JS (eds): Gastrointestinal Disease: Pathophysiology, Diagnosis, Management, 5th ed. Philadelphia, WB Saunders, 1993, p 580.
2. Goldschmiedt M, Feldman M. Gastric secretion in health and disease, in Sleisenger MH, Fordtran JS (eds): Gastrointestinal Disease: Pathophysiology, Diagnosis, Management, 5th ed. Philadelphia, WB Saunders, 1993, p 524.
3. Shamburek RD, Schubert ML. Control of gastric acid secretion. Gastroenterol Clin North Am 1993;21:527–550.

4. Konturek SJ, Konturek JW. Gastric adaptation: Basic and clinical aspects. Digestion 1994;55:131–138.
5. Wallace JL. Prostaglandins, NSAIDs, and cytoprotection. Gastroenterol Clin North Am 1992;21:631–641.
6. NIH Consensus Development Panel on *Helicobacter pylori* in Peptic Ulcer Disease. *Helicobacter pylori* in peptic ulcer disease. JAMA 1994;272:65–69.
7. Fennerty MB. *Helicobacter pylori.* Arch Intern Med 1994; 154:721–727.
8. Walsh JH, Peterson WL. The treatment of *Helicobacter pylori* infection in the management of peptic ulcer disease. N Engl J Med 1995;33:984–991.
9. Lee A. The microbiology and epidemiology of *Helicobacter pylori* infection. Scand J Gastroenterol 1994;29(suppl 201): 2–6.
10. Dunn BE. Pathogenic mechanisms of *Helicobacter pylori.* Gastroenterol Clin North Am 1993;22:43–57.
11. Dixon MF. Pathophysiology of *Helicobacter pylori* infection. Scand J Gastroenterol 1994;29(suppl 201):7–10.
12. Malaty HM, Engstrand L, Pedersen NL, Graham DY. *Helicobacter pylori* infection: Genetic and environmental influences: A study of twins. Ann Intern Med 1994;120: 982–986.
13. Sipponen P. Gastric cancer—a long term consequence of *Helicobacter pylori* infection. Scand J Gastroenterol 1994;29 (suppl 201):24–27.
14. Janssen M, Dijkmans AC, Lamers CBHL, et al. A gastroscopic study of the predictive value of risk factors for nonsteroidal anti-inflammatory drug-associated ulcer disease in rheumatoid arthritis patients. Br J Rheumatol 1994;33: 449–454.
15. Griffin MR, Piper JM, Daugherty JR, et al. Nonsteroidal anti-inflammatory drug use and increased risk for peptic ulcer disease in elderly persons. Ann Intern Med 1991;114: 257–263.
16. Kaufman DW, Kelly JP, Sheehan JE, et al. Nonsteroidal anti-inflammatory drug use in relation to major upper gastrointestinal bleeding. Clin Pharmacol Ther 1993;53:485–494.
17. Piper JM, Ray WA, Daugherty JR, et al. Corticosteroid use and peptic ulcer disease: Role of nonsteroidal anti-inflammatory drugs. Ann Intern Med 1991;114:735–740.
18. Loffeld RJLF, Stobberingh E, Arends JW. A review of diagnostic techniques for *Helicobacter pylori* infection. Dig Dis 1993;11:173–180.
19. Feldman M, Burton ME. Histamine$_2$-receptor antagonists: Standard therapy for acid-peptic diseases. Part I. N Engl J Med 1990;323:1672–1680.
20. Feldman M, Burton ME. Histamine$_2$-receptor antagonists: Standard therapy for acid-peptic diseases. Part II. N Engl J Med 1990;323:1749–1755.
21. Lauritsen K, Laursen LS, Rask-Madsen J. Clinical pharmacokinetics of drugs used in the treatment of gastrointestinal diseases. Part I. Clin Pharmacokinet 1990;19:11–31.
22. Lauritsen K, Laursen LS, Rask-Madsen J. Clinical pharmacokinetics of drugs used in the treatment of gastrointestinal diseases. Part II. Clin Pharmacokinet 1990;19:94–125.
23. Brooks WS. Short- and long-term management of peptic ulcer disease: Current role of H$_2$-antagonists. Hepato-Gastroenterology 1992;39:47–52.
24. Thorat VK, Misra SP, Anand BS, et al. Conventional versus on-demand therapy for duodenal ulcer: Results of a controlled therapeutic trial. Am J Gastroenterol 1990; 85:243–248.
25. Welage LS, Berardi RR. Drug interactions with antiulcer agents: Considerations in the treatment of peptic ulcer disease. J Pharm Prac 1994;7:177–195.
26. Berardi RR, Welage RR. Current status of proton pump inhibitors in the treatment of acid-peptic disease. J Pharm Prac 1994;7:165–176.
27. Wilde MI, McTavish D. Omeprazole: An update of its pharmacology and therapeutic use in acid-related disorders. Drugs 1994;48:91–132.
28. Maton PN. Omeprazole. N Engl J Med 1991;324:965–975.
29. Massoomi F, Savage J, Destache CJ. Omeprazole: A comprehensive review. Pharmacotherapy 1993;13:46–59.
30. Spencer CM, Faulds D. Lansoprazole: A reappraisal of its pharmacodynamic and pharmacokinetic properties, and its therapeutic efficacy in acid-related disorders. Drugs 1994;48: 404–430.
31. Morgan DG, Burget DW, Howden CW, et al. Rates of duodenal ulcer (DU) healing by drug class: A meta-analysis [abstract]. Gastroenterology 1993;104:A150.
32. Joelson S, Joelson IB, Lundbort P, et al. Safety experience from long-term treatment with omeprazole. Digestion 1992; 51(suppl 1):93–101.
33. Conlin-Jones DG. Safety of lansoprazole. Aliment Pharmacol Ther 1993;7(suppl 1):56–60.
34. Santucci L, Garroni F, Fiorucci S, et al. Gynecomastia dur ing omeprazole therapy [letter]. N Engl J Med 1991;324: 635.
35. Marks DR, Joy JV, Bonheim NA. Hemolytic anemia associated with the use of omeprazole. Am J Gastroenterol 1991; 86:217–218.
36. Sellapah S. An unusual side effect of omeprazole: Case report [letter]. Br J Gen Pract 1990;40:389.
37. Kuiper JJ. Omeprazole-induced acute interstitial nephritis [letter]. Am J Med 1993;95:248.
38. Jochem V, Kirkpatrick R, Greenson J, et al. Fulminant hepatic failure related to omeprazole. Am J Gastroenterol 1992;87: 523–525.
39. Nasser K, Irshad M, Howden CW. Prevalence of male sexual dysfunction during treatment with omeprazole [abstract]. Gastroenterology 1992;102:A133.
40. Graham JR. Omeprazole and gastric polyposis in humans [letter]. Gastroenterology 1993;104:1584.
41. Marcuard SP, Albernaz L, Khazanie PG. Omeprazole therapy causes malabsorption of cyanocobalamin (vitamin B$_{12}$). Ann Intern Med 1994;120:211–215.
42. Texter EC. A critical look at the clinical use of antacids in acid-peptic disease and gastric acid rebound. Am J Gastroenterol 1989;84:97–108.
43. Sewing KF. Efficacy of low-dose antacids in the treatment of peptic ulcers: Pharmacological explanation? J Clin Gastroenterol 1991;13 (suppl 1):S134–S138.
44. McCarthy DM. Sucralfate. N Engl J Med 1991;325: 1017–1025.
45. Jensen SL, Jensen PF. Role of sucralfate in peptic disease. Dig Dis 1992;10:153–161.

46. Sherman SI, Tielens ET, Ladeson PW. Sucralfate causes malabsorption of L-thyroxine. Am J Med 1994;96:531–535.
47. Ballinger A. Cytoprotection with misoprostol: Use in the treatment and prevention of ulcers. Dig Dis 1994;12:37–45.
48. Raskin JB, White RH, Jackson JE, et al. Misoprostil dosage in the prevention of nonsteroidal anti-inflammatory drug-induced gastric and duodenal ulcers: a comparison of three regimens. Ann Intern Med 1995;123:344–350.
49. Kornbluth A. Life-threatening diarrhea after short-term misoprostol use in a patient with Crohn's ileocolitis. Ann Intern Med 1990;113:474–475.
50. Bierer DWS. Bismuth subsalicylate: History, chemistry, and safety. Rev Infect Dis 1990;12:S3–S8.
51. Gorbach SL. Bismuth therapy in gastrointestinal diseases. Gastroenterology 1990;99:863–875.
52. Marshall BJ. The use of bismuth in gastroenterology. Am J Gastroenterol 1991;86:16–25.
53. Nwokolo CU, Prewett EJ, Sawyer AF, et al. The effect of histamine H_2-receptor blockade on bismuth absorption from three ulcer-healing compounds. Gastroenterology 1991;101: 889–894.
54. Ateshkadi A, Lam NP, Johnson CA. *Helicobacter pylori* and peptic ulcer disease. Clin Pharm 1993;12:32–48.
55. Tytgat GNJ, Noach LA, Rauws EAJ. *Helicobacter pylori* infection and duodenal ulcer disease. Gastroenterol Clin North Am 1993;22:127–139.
56. Graham DY, Lew GM, Klein PD, et al. Effect of treatment of *Helicobacter pylori* infection on the long-term recurrence of gastric or duodenal ulcer: A randomized, controlled study. Ann Intern Med 1992;116:705–708.
57. Marshall BJ. *Helicobacter pylori.* Am J Gastroenterol 1994;89:S116–S128.
58. Hentschel E, Brandstatter G, Dragosics B, et al. Effect of ranitidine and amoxicillin plus metronidazole on the eradication of *Helicobacter pylori* and the recurrence of duodenal ulcer. N Engl J Med 1993;328:308–312.
59. Graham KS, Malaty H, El-Zimaity HMT, et al. Variability with omeprazole-amoxicillin combinations for treatment of *Helicobacter pylori* infection. Am J Gastroenterol 1995;90: 1415–1417.
60. Tucci A, Corinaldesi R, Stanghellini V, et al. One-day therapy for treatment of *Helicobacter pylori* infection. Dig Dis Sci 1993;38:1670–1673.
61. Vaz Coelho LG, Passos MCF, Chausson Y, et al. Five-day bismuth-free triple therapy for the eradication of *Helicobacter pylori* and reduction of duodenal ulcer relapse. Am J Gastroenterol 1991;86:971–975.
62. Malfertheiner P. Compliance, adverse events and antibiotic resistance in *Helicobacter pylori* treatment. Scand J Gastroenterol 1993;28(suppl 196):34–37.
63. Freston JW. Emerging strategies for managing peptic ulcer disease. Scand J Gastroenterol 1994;29(suppl 201):49–54.
64. Axon ATR. The role of acid inhibition in the treatment of *Helicobacter pylori* infection. Scand J Gastroenterol 1994; 29(suppl 201):16–23.
65. Jimenez E, Bosch F, Galmes JL, Banol JE. Meta-analysis of efficacy of zinc acexamate in peptic ulcer. Digestion 1992; 51:18–26.
66. Kohn A, Annibale B, Delle Fave G, Levenstein S. Maintenance treatment with H_2-receptor antagonists for duodenal ulcer disease: Toward a rational use. Dig Dis 1993;11: 228–238.
67. Savarino V, Mela GS, Zentilin P, et al. Antisecretory effects of three omeprazole regimens for maintenance treatment in duodenal ulcer. Dig Dis Sci 1994;39:1473–1482.
68. Lamberts R, Creutzfeldt W, Struber HG, et al. Long-term omeprazole therapy in peptic ulcer disease: Gastrin, endocrine cell growth, and gastritis. Gastroenterology 1993;104:1456–1470.
69. Solcia E, Villani L, Luinetti O, et al. Proton pump inhibitors, enterochromaffin-like cell growth and *Helicobacter pylori* gastritis. Aliment Pharmacol Ther 1993;7(suppl 1): 25–28.
70. McCloy RF, Arnold R, Bardhan KD, et al. Pathophysiological effects of long-term acid suppression in man. Dig Dis Sci 1995;40(Suppl):96S–120S.
71. Hawkey CJ, Hudson N. Healing and prevention of NSAID-induced peptic ulcers. Scand J Gastroenterol 1994;29(suppl 201):42–44.
72. Agrawal NM, Roth S, Graham DY, et al. Misoprostol compared with sucralfate in the prevention of nonsteroidal anti-inflammatory drug-induced gastric ulcer. Ann Intern Med 1991;115:195–200.
73. Graham DY. Ulcer complications and their nonoperative treatment, in Sleisenger MH, Fordtran JS (eds): Gastrointestinal Disease: Pathophysiology, Diagnosis, Management, 5th ed. Philadelphia, WB Saunders, 1993, p 698.
74. Labenz J, Borsch G. Role of *Helicobacter pylori* eradication in the prevention of peptic ulcer bleeding relapse. Digestion 1994;55:19–23.
75. Matthews JB, Silen W. Operations for peptic ulcer disease and early postoperative complications, in Sleisenger MN, Fordtran JS (eds): Gastrointestinal Disease: Pathophysiology, Diagnosis, Management, 5th ed. Philadelphia, WB Saunders, 1993, p 713.
76. McGuigan JE. Zollinger–Ellison syndrome and other hypersecretory states, in Sleisenger MN, Fordtran JS (eds): Gastrointestinal Disease: Pathophysiology, Diagnosis, Management, 5th ed. Philadelphia, WB Saunders, 1993, p 679.
77. Jensen RT, Fraker DL. Zollinger–Ellison syndrome: Advances in treatment of gastric hypersecretion and the gastrinoma. JAMA 1994;271:1429–1435.
78. Metz DC, Pisegna JR, Fishbeyn VA, et al. Currently used doses of omeprazole in Zollinger–Ellison syndrome are too high. Gastroenterology 1992;103:1498–1508.
79. Vinayek R, Frucht H, London JF, et al. Intravenous omeprazole in patients with Zollinger–Ellison syndrome undergoing surgery. Gastroenterology 1990;99:10–16.
80. Jensen RT, Metz DC, Koviak PD, et al. Prospective study of the long-term efficacy and safety of lansoprazole in patients with Zollinger–Ellison syndrome. Aliment Pharmacol Ther 1993;7(suppl 1):41–50.

Chapter 33

Upper Gastrointestinal Bleeding

John K. Siepler, PharmD, BCNSD, and Robert M. Mowers, PharmD, BCPS

Upper gastrointestinal bleeding (UGIB) is a condition resulting from a bleeding lesion located in the esophagus, stomach, or duodenum. UGIB is most often a result of esophageal varices, stress ulceration, or a complication of peptic ulcer disease (PUD). UGIB resulting from a complication of PUD is usually caused by an ulcer eroding into a blood vessel in the gastric or duodenal mucosa. This vessel then bleeds into the lumen of the digestive tract. Stress-related mucosal lesions (stress gastritis) may also cause UGIB. Patients susceptible to stress ulcers generally include those who are critically ill and in intensive care units. Esophageal varices can bleed in patients with liver disease associated with portal hypertension.

Other causes of UGIB include erosions from feeding or nasogastric (NG) tubes and Mallory–Weiss tears (a longitudinal tear of the esophagus that results from retching). Patients with NG tube-related bleeding are usually treated by removal of the tube. Most (95%) of Mallory–Weiss tears stop bleeding without intervention. This chapter focuses on the treatment of UGIB that occurs as a complication of PUD, bleeding esophageal varices, and stress-related bleeding.

EPIDEMIOLOGY

In one study severe, *active* UGIB was seen in only 32 of 174 PUD-related admissions for over 3 years, suggesting that active UGIB as a severe complication of PUD is not a common occurrence.[1] The mortality for massive hemorrhage from peptic ulcer is about 10%. This complication occurs in about 25% of patients presenting with UGIB and is the most common cause of mortality in this group.[2] Another study evaluated 100 patients with iron deficiency anemia of unknown cause. After performing both upper and lower endoscopy, 28% of the patients were found to have upper GI lesions consistent with a bleeding site sufficient to cause the anemia.[3] We also know that a significant number of patients who present with UGIB have been ingesting aspirin or other nonsteroidal anti-inflammatory drugs (NSAIDs).

The severity of stress ulcers varies from superficial erosions of the stomach and duodenum to deep ulcers that produce life-threatening hemorrhage. Mucosal lesions occur almost immediately upon initiation of stress. Whereas early reports suggest a frequency of about 10%, lesions can occur in up to 90% of severely stressed patients. Burn patients, patients with head injuries, those with medical conditions serious enough to warrant admission to an intensive care unit, patients receiving mechanical ventilation, those with coagulopathy, and patients who have survived major surgery are all at risk for development of stress ulcers.[4] The incidence of severe bleeding in these patients may be much lower. Some suggest that less than 10% of these stressed patients will have serious bleeding episodes.[5,6]

PATHOPHYSIOLOGY

ESOPHAGEAL VARICES

Patients with severe liver disease often have portal hypertension. The portal vein receives its blood supply from the GI tract, and the only outlet is through hepatic tissue. In advanced cirrhosis with fibrosis of the liver, an increased resistance to blood flow in the portal system develops, which causes increased pressures. When significant portal hypertension develops, the blood bypasses the liver through collateral vessels, including the esophageal veins, which become engorged with blood. These engorged veins located in the lower part of the esophagus are called *esophageal varices.* The presence of esophageal varices in a patient with liver disease is consistent with a diagnosis of portal hypertension. Variceal bleeding occurs when these veins bleed into the GI tract.

PEPTIC ULCER DISEASE-RELATED BLEEDING EPISODES

Bleeding can occur in patients with PUD when an ulcer erodes into a blood vessel or when generalized gastritis is so severe that oozing of blood occurs. A small amount of bleeding (5 to 30 mL) may only be evident by heme-positive stools. Larger amounts (30 to 50 mL) may cause the stools to turn black. Severe bleeding (greater than 50 mL) may cause emesis.

Bleeding peptic ulcers can be classified as Forrest class I, II, or III.[7] Forrest class I lesions are actively bleeding lesions. These lesions are classified further into lesions that are spurting or oozing blood. In a Forrest class II lesion, a blood vessel is visible at the base of the ulcer crater when viewed by an endoscope. This type is called a *visible vessel.* The remaining lesions are grouped as Forrest class III. Patients with Forrest class I and II lesions have a higher frequency of rebleeding compared to those with class III lesions.

The specific reason why one patient with PUD develops a bleeding episode and another does not is unknown; however, it is thought that the peptic ulcer patient whose disease is more severe is at greater risk. Often bleeding occurs in association with the ingestion of aspirin or other NSAIDs. Lesions in 35% of the patients admitted for UGIB were associated with ingestion of drugs of this class.[8–11] Another study reported that 80% of patients admitted for UGIB had evidence of prior aspirin or NSAID use compared with 34.3% of a control group.[12] All evidence suggests that aspirin and NSAID ingestion is a major cause of UGIB. We also know that patients with a prior UGIB incident are at an increased risk for another bleeding episode compared to the general population of patients with PUD.[13]

Clinical Presentation

The clinical presentation of the patient with UGIB is similar regardless of etiology. In severe cases, the chief complaint will be a history of bright red or coffee-ground–appearing emesis. In less severe cases, the patient may complain of weakness and is generally found to have a heme-positive stool. The source of bleeding cannot be determined by history alone without further diagnostic intervention. The patient with a severe UGIB may be hypotensive from blood loss and will usually be nontender on abdominal palpation. Many patients who bleed from a peptic ulcer will usually be otherwise asymptomatic. Some patients notice a dark, tarry, or black stool as the first hint of bleeding. If the bleeding is a slow ooze or trickle, weakness and anemia can be the first symptoms of UGIB.[3]

Stabilization and Diagnosis

STABILIZATION

Many patients with severe UGIB are hemodynamically unstable when they present for diagnosis and treatment. Thus, it is often necessary to stabilize the patient before diagnosis can take place. When a patient presents with severe UGIB, a large-bore intravenous line is inserted, appropriate laboratory samples are drawn, and the patient is typed and cross-matched for several units of blood. Intravenous normal saline (0.9% sodium chloride injection) is given at a rapid rate until vital signs are stable. If the patient does not respond, intravenous pressors may be used. In addition, a large-bore nasogastric tube is placed, and the stomach is lavaged with large amounts of water or saline to allow the endoscopist a better view of the stomach and duodenum. Attempts to use iced saline or addition of pressors to the irrigation fluid to cut down blood flow to the mucosa and decrease bleeding have not proven more effective than saline. Sterile saline is not necessary for gastric lavage. When the return from the nasogastric tube becomes clear, the tube is removed, the patient sedated, and an endoscopy performed for diagnosis of the cause of the bleeding episode.

DIAGNOSIS

When the patient with UGIB is admitted to the emergency room or clinic, an adequate history must be taken. The pharmacist must pay particular attention to the drug history and focus specifically on alcohol and ulcerogenic medications. The patient may not consider aspirin or over-the-counter (OTC) NSAIDs as drugs and may not mention taking them in a conventional drug history. Other important contributing factors include previous bleeding episodes or a history of PUD or alcoholic liver disease. Of note, only half of alcoholic patients who present with an UGIB bleed from esophageal varices.[1]

A physical examination should be performed as soon as possible. Particular attention must be given to the patients's pulse rate, rhythm, the presence or absence of neck vein distention, and the presence of cutaneous vasoconstriction (cool to cold, clammy skin). Further attention in the examination must be placed on the abdomen. The presence of ascites, spider nevi, or hepatosplenomegaly is often an indication of long-standing alcoholic liver disease. When examining the rectum, tarry stools may suggest chronic bleeding that preexisted this acute episode. Bright red blood without obvious cause (e.g., hemorrhoids) may result from colonic lesions or massive UGIB and rapid transit through the alimentary canal.

Endoscopic examination is the most accurate way to determine the bleeding site in a patient presenting with UGIB. The diagnostic accuracy of early endoscopy is greater than 90% and considered crucial to progressing to the next step of therapy.[14] Once the patient's vital signs are stable, endoscopy may be performed. Several studies have shown that a significant proportion of alcoholic patients who are suspected of bleeding from esophageal varices are actually bleeding from a peptic ulcer lesion.[1,9] The recommended treatment and diagnostic scheme is shown in Table 33.1.

TABLE 33.1. TREATMENT AND DIAGNOSTIC SCHEME IN UPPER GASTROINTESTINAL BLEEDING

1. Stabilize patient hemodynamically. Stabilize blood pressure. Start an intravenous line (lactated Ringers with 5% dextrose or 0.9% sodium chloride). Use vasopressors (e.g., vasopressin) if necessary.
2. Insert large-bore nasogastric tube (large enough to lavage with water or saline). Lavage until clear (to aid diagnosis with endoscope).
3. Obtain medical and drug history. Identify any previous bleeding episodes and possible causes.
4. Conduct physical examination.
5. Perform endoscopy.
6. Treatment initiation depends on diagnosis.

Endoscopy is performed specifically to determine the source of bleeding. The presence or absence of esophageal varices is noted. The endoscopist also notes if the varices or peptic ulcer lesions are bleeding, because the presence of nonbleeding varices is not uncommon in a patient who is bleeding from a peptic ulcer. The endoscopist should continue to examine the stomach and duodenum even if bleeding varices are seen. The entire stomach should be examined including inspection for gastric varices (extension of esophageal varices into the stomach). Next, the duodenum should be entered and inspected for a duodenal ulcer. Therapeutic endoscopy using bipolar electrocautery, laser photocoagulation, or heater probe may be performed at the initial endoscopic examination.

TREATMENT

The proper mode of treatment involves specific treatment of the bleeding lesion. The goal of this specific treatment is to stop the acute bleeding episode. The patient with bleeding esophageal varices demands a different treatment scheme than the patient who presents with bleeding peptic ulcers. The treatment methods are summarized in the following paragraphs.

ESOPHAGEAL VARICES

When esophageal varices are the source of bleeding, treatment is centered on two principles: (1) local injection of the varices (sclerotherapy to attempt to stop bleeding), and (2) reduction of portal pressure. The following sections discuss the effectiveness of these treatment methods to stop acute bleeding.

Sclerotherapy

Development of the flexible fiber optic endoscope and long-needle injectors that fit down one of the channels of the scope has allowed sclerotherapy to become widely used. Esophageal sclerotherapy is performed by direct injection of a varix with a sclerosant to obliterate the varix and stop acute bleeding. The solutions most often used in the United States have been limited to sodium tetradecyl sulfate (Sotradecol®), ethanolamine oleate (Ethamolin®), and sodium morrhuate. Among single-drug agents, comparative studies indicate a similar efficacy for sodium morrhuate and sodium tetradecyl sulfate. Sodium morrhuate appears to form superficial ulcers at the injection site more often than sodium tetradecyl sulfate.[15] No comparative data exist for ethanolamine oleate. In animal experiments, combinations of agents have been found more effective than the solutions alone. The most popular combination agent is a mixture of 50% dextrose, cephalothin, and alcohol. A trial in humans has yet to show the superiority of combination solutions to a single agent.

The selection of patients for injection sclerotherapy is critical. To date, no trial shows that life expectancy is prolonged in patients that receive injection sclerotherapy. However, sclerotherapy remains an effective means of stopping *acute* bleeding episodes. Patients who receive injection sclerotherapy on an emergent basis (immediately upon stabilization), rather than an urgent basis (within 24 hours), have lower transfusion requirements and better chances of survival.[9]

While injection sclerotherapy has received acceptance in acute hemostasis of bleeding esophageal varices, proving this premise has been difficult. A large multicenter study found that mortality and rebleeding rates were greater among patients randomly selected to receive sclerotherapy than in those who did not have sclerotherapy. The investigators delayed as long as 24 hours after initial presentation to enter a patient into the trial. This practice may have excluded many of the most critically ill patients who expired before entry into the trial. Also, unequal numbers of patients were entered into each group of the study by different institutions. Some hospitals had larger samples of nonsclerotherapy patients, and other hospitals had larger samples of sclerotherapy patients. This tended to skew the data regarding survival, favoring the nonsclerotherapy group.[16]

A meta-analysis suggested that endoscopic sclerotherapy is effective at stopping acute variceal bleeding.[17,18] Other forms of endoscopic therapy for variceal bleeding have also been proposed. Endoscopic ligation has also recently been demonstrated to be effective.[19]

The efficacy of injection sclerotherapy for *prevention of recurrent variceal bleeding* remains controversial. Several researchers have attempted to use sclerotherapy to obliterate varices in patients who were not actively bleeding. The success of this practice depends on the assumption that the obliterated varix will be less likely to bleed than one not injected. Also, many patients who receive repeated endoscopic sclerotherapy develop esophageal stricture, thus this practice cannot be recommended. Injection sclerotherapy cannot be recommended for *prophylaxis* of bleeding in patients with esophageal varices.

Vasopressin

The antidiuretic hormone vasopressin (Pitressin®) has been used for treatment of esophageal variceal bleeding for more than 20 years. Early researchers used intermittent, intravenous doses of vasopressin in an effort to lower portal pressure to stop bleeding of varices.[20]

In the mid-1970s, investigators found that intravenous vasopressin was as effective in lowering portal pressure as intra-arterial vasopressin. By the late 1970s, intravenous vasopressin had become the most common therapy for esophageal varices. Intravenous vasopressin therapy is initiated with an infusion of 30 to 40 units over 30 to 40 minutes and is followed by a 0.4 unit/min infusion. The infusion is continued until 24 hours after bleeding stops. The infusion dose is then decreased by half for 12 hours and then the dose is halved again for another 12 hours. A multicenter study randomized trial compared patients that received vasopressin or placebo.[21] There were no significant differences in the amount of blood transfused or survival rates between the two groups. This study was plagued by the same problem that limited the sclerotherapy study mentioned earlier. The effort to allow all patients to sign a consent form meant that the mean time between arrival in the emergency room and entry into the study was about 1.5 days. As a result, the most critically ill patients (and those most likely to benefit from vasopressin) may have died within that 36-hour period. Despite the negative nature of this study, vasopressin remains a common treatment for patients with bleeding esophageal varices.

Octreotide

In addition to inhibiting the release of several GI hormones, somatostatin and its longer acting analogue, octreotide, are also strong inhibitors of pancreatic and gastric secretions and increase splanchnic arteriolar resistance. This increase in splanchnic arteriolar resistance is associated with a decrease in hepatic blood flow, portal pressure, and intravariceal pressure. The inhibition of gastric secretions produces an increase of intragastric pH, maintaining an adequate medium for facilitating blood coagulation.[22] Studies suggest that octreotide at a dose of 25–50 mcg/h may be of benefit in patients who continue to bleed after sclerotherapy.[23,24] However, further controlled trials are necessary to evaluate not only the activity of octreotide in controlling hemorrhage, but also efficacy in reducing mortality.

Nonpharmacologic Treatment

One of the nonpharmacologic treatments is the Sengstaken–Blakemore or Minnesota tube. These tubes are designed to compress the varices mechanically and stop bleeding. This form of treatment has received insufficient scientific evaluation and is prone to such complications as spontaneous bacterial peritonitis, perforation of the esophagus, and esophageal stricture. Therefore, use of these tubes cannot be recommended.

Surgery is another form of therapy for bleeding esophageal varices. Various operations have been designed to lower the portal pressure by shunting blood around the liver. These operations are long and difficult to perform, especially in patients that are often unstable. Thus, the best candidates are those who are stable and are not acutely bleeding, which is often not the case with these patients. Postoperative follow-up of these patients reveals that they often suffer from hepatic encephalopathy. Nevertheless, such surgical procedures may prolong life in certain patients with portal hypertension who *are* stable and considered good risks.

A newer radiologic approach for managing variceal hemorrhage, transjugular intrahepatic portosystemic stent shunt (TIPPS), has been developed with promising initial results. In this technique, the portal system is decompressed with the creation of an intrahepatic shunt from the hepatic to portal veins, using a percutaneous transjugular approach. One hundred patients underwent TIPPS for variceal bleeding, ascites, hepatorenal syndrome, and preoperative portal decompression.[25] Shunts were completed in 96 patients. Acute variceal bleeding was controlled in 29 of 30 patients and recurrent variceal bleeding was seen in only 9 of 95 patients because of either shunt stenosis or occlusion. TIPPS is an effective method for lowering portal pressure and controlling variceal bleeding.

BLEEDING PEPTIC ULCERS

Therapeutic trials designed to determine the effectiveness of drug treatment for acute bleeding from PUD concentrate on drugs that lower gastric acid. Acid secretory suppression with H_2-receptor antagonists (H_2RAs), proton pump inhibitors (PPIs), and buffering with antacids are the primary drugs used and are also used in patients with UGIB as a result of PUD. The two desirable clinical outcomes in patients with bleeding peptic ulcers are (1) cessation of the acute bleeding episode, and (2) prevention of rebleeding. Endoscopic therapy is also used for UGIB from PUD. In addition, these drugs are used for prophylaxis against UGIB from stress-related lesions in critically ill patients.

Endoscopic Therapy

Hemostasis in an acute bleeding episode is often effectively accomplished with endoscopic therapy. This consists of the endoscopic use of laser photocoagulation, heater probe, monopolar and bipolar electrocautery, and/or injection of epinephrine. This form of therapy is designed to promote the formation of a clot at the bleeding site. Although it is not possible to stop all acute bleeding episodes with endoscopic therapy, an experienced endoscopist will be able to stop the bleeding in many patients.

Acid Suppressive Therapy

When an acute bleeding episode is stopped, a clot forms at the bleeding point in the ulcer crater that eroded into the bleeding vessel. This leaves the clot in direct contact with the acidic gastric contents. It has been shown that clots are more stable in gastric juice that is titrated to a pH of 7 than at a lower pH.[26] This is the basis of the use of acid-reducing agents in the treatment of acute bleeding episodes and is responsible for the trend to attempt to achieve maximal gastric acid suppression in this class of patients.

Reducing gastric acid is achieved by several pharmacologic mechanisms. Antacids buffer the acid produced in the stomach, histamine H_2RAs prevent acid from being produced by the parietal cells,[27] and PPIs prevent the transport of acid across the parietal cell membrane. Conventional schemes of dosing require that antacids and H_2RAs be given on an intermittent basis, with antacids administered orally or via NG tube 8–24 times daily (every 1–3 hours). Cimetidine, ranitidine, and famotidine are generally administered intravenously up to four times daily. Omeprazole is only available in an oral form (capsule) in the United States and is not applicable to acute UGIB.

These dosing regimens produce periods of good acid secretory control (right after the dose is given) and periods of poor acid secretory control (right before the next dose is given). Because current concepts of treatment require acid secretory suppression to a level of pH 7 in an effort to stabilize the clot formed and prevent a rebleeding episode, the intermittent regimens may be at a disadvantage. If the goal of treatment is a constant gastric pH of 7, alternatives to conventional dose regimens that produce a more consistent acid secretion control by constant infusions may be more effective.

Four regimens are available that control acid secretion and thus treat this type of bleeding: (1) oral antacids given at frequent dosing intervals (as often as hourly); (2) H_2RAs administered in conventional intermittent intravenous regimens every 6–8 hours (cimetidine and ranitidine) or every 12 hours (famotidine); (3) H_2RAs administered via constant intravenous infusion; and (4) oral PPIs (only possible in patients who are able to take oral medications).

Titration of intragastric pH with antacids was introduced by Czaja and colleagues.[4] Hourly administration of antacids with intragastric pH determinations made before each scheduled dose is designed to follow the effect of antacids on pH. If the pH is less than 7, the antacid dose is doubled and monitoring is continued hourly. Since that time, other investigators have used antacid titration with lower pH goals.

In the mid-1970s, the development of histamine H_2RAs was a significant pharmacologic achievement.[27] In most patients, intravenous cimetidine (300 mg) and ranitidine (50 mg) are quite effective at reducing gastric acid for 4–5 hours after an intravenous dose.[28,29] Intravenous famotidine will reduce gastric acid for approximately 8–11 hours after a 20-mg dose.[30,31]

These pharmacodynamic properties explain the apparent failure of H_2RAs to control intragastric pH better than antacids. If the intragastric pH testing is done near the time the next dose is due, the serum drug concentration is very low, and the intragastric fluid is often acidic. Thus, frequent intragastric pH testing (at least every 3–4 hours) is essential to ensure that the patient responds effectively to the drug therapy.

Alternatives to intermittent H_2RAs have been used for many years. In 1975, constant-infusion metiamide was used to demonstrate effective acid control in a patient who had Zollinger–Ellison syndrome.[32] Others have compared the intragastric pH response of duodenal ulcer patients to intermittent and constant-infusion cimetidine. In contrast to the peaks and valleys of acid control produced by intermittent dosing, a bolus of cimetidine 300 mg followed by a 37.5 mg/h—50 mg/h intravenous infusion of cimetidine produced an intragastric pH that remained in the 4–5 range. Doses of 100 mg/h plus antacids were necessary to achieve a pH response that was uniformly higher than 7.[17,33]

Others have found similar intragastric pH responses with ranitidine at continuous infusions of 6.25 mg/h—12.5 mg/h.[34,35] A comparison of the effect of constant-infusion cimetidine and ranitidine found a similar intragastric pH response.[31] Famotidine at a constant intravenous dose of 1.67 mg/h has also been found to provide consistent acid secretory suppression in critically ill patients.[30,31] Others have used famotidine at higher doses (3.2 mg/h—4 mg/h) with good pH control.[31]

Clinical studies using these regimens in patients with UGIB from peptic ulcers to stop acute bleeding and prevent rebleeding have been published.[36–41] Controlled, comparative studies of intravenous cimetidine reveal that it offers no significant advantage over placebo with regard to cessation of acute bleeding, prevention of rebleeding, or need for surgery[41,42]; however, a slight but statistically significant reduction in mortality has been noted subsequent to cimetidine therapy in patients with gastric ulcers.[37] The trend toward clinical improvement among patients with gastric ulcers was also noted in studies of intravenous ranitidine therapy.[41] Comparisons of cimetidine and ranitidine in acute UGIB have revealed no significant differences.[40,41]

Fullarton and associates[42] compared famotidine 10-mg bolus followed by 3.2 mg/h constant infusion (80 mg/d) with placebo to treat bleeding PUD. Intragastric pH was monitored with the median values in the famotidine group (n = 10) ranging from 6.8 to 7.1. This was significantly higher than the placebo group (n = 10), whose median pH was 1.6. Four patients rebled in the placebo group and none in the famotidine group. The significance of this study is limited by a small patient population (n = 20) and the short follow-up period (22 hours). Walt and associates[43] studied 1005 patients who received either famotidine at the dose previously given or placebo. The rebleed rate, mortality, and need for surgery were not significantly different, suggesting that aggressive pH control is not effective at preventing rebleeding or reducing mortality or the rate of surgery in patients who bleed from acute peptic ulcers. This study included a large number of patients with minor UGIB episodes, so their results may not apply to the more critical patient.

Omeprazole is a H^+/K^+-ATPase inhibitor that produces a profound inhibition of acid secretion. Brunner and Chang[44] studied 39 critically ill patients with actively bleeding peptic ulcers. Patients were randomized to either ranitidine (50-mg load followed by continuous infusion of 400 mg/d) or omeprazole (80-mg intravenous bolus then 40 mg intravenous every 12 hours) for 5 days of therapy. Therapeutic endoscopy was not performed. Treatment failure (inability to control bleeding or rebleeding) occurred in 85% of the ranitidine patients and 16% of the omeprazole patients. Intravenous omeprazole is not available in the United States and the results should be considered preliminary.

Stress Ulcer Prophylaxis

Many patients who experience trauma, burns, major surgery, or sepsis will develop mucosal ulcers, or erosions in the stomach and duodenum. In 5–20% of these patients, clinically important bleeding from these mucosal lesions will develop within 3–7 days after the initial insult.[45] Clinically important bleeding is usually defined as overt blood or coffee-ground emesis on return from a nasogastric (NG) tube. Occult bleeding, such as "guiac positive" NG return is not considered significant bleeding, because there is no evidence that this predisposes a patient to a more severe bleeding episode. Critically ill patients who are ventilator dependent or have a coagulopathy are also at risk for clinically important bleeding.[6] Although many of the bleeding lesions may be stress gastritis, a significant number of bleeding episodes are actually from bleeding gastric or duodenal ulcers.[46] Presumably, these are preexisting lesions that bleed in critically ill patients.

The pathogenesis of stress ulcers and stress-related bleeding does not generally involve gastric hypersecretion. Factors that may be pathogenetic include reduced mucosal blood flow and oxygenation, disruption of the integrity of the mucosal barrier, and the presence of high local mucosal concentration of gastric acid. The contribution of *Helicobacter pylori* to this syndrome is just now being investigated. A combination of these factors predisposes the critically ill patient to potentially life-threatening gastric mucosal erosions and resultant bleeding.

Despite the fact that gastric hypersecretion is not common in patients at risk for stress-related bleeding, the neutralization of gastric acid remains the main form of prophylaxis. One exception to this principle is sucralfate, which has a mechanism that remains a mystery. Raising intragastric pH to values higher than 3.5–4 appears to reduce the incidence of stress gastritis and stress-related bleeding. Titration of gastric acidity using intragastric pH determinations has been used in an attempt to prevent stress ulcers. McAlhaney et al.[47] gave antacids on an hourly basis to burn patients in increasing doses titrating their intragastric pH to 7. Only 4% of the antacid-treated patients required transfusions compared with 25% of the control group. The antacid regimen also prevented the development of stress ulcers. Their method of hourly administration is time consuming and can cause adverse effects (usually diarrhea) in more than 50% of patients. Others have used pH endpoints for antacid titration that are less aggressive (3.5–4).[40,41,48]

Numerous comparisons of the efficacy of H_2RAs and antacids have been performed. Zuckerman et al.[38] reviewed 16 prospective trials comparing intravenous cimetidine (given intermittently) or antacids to prevent overt bleeding in patients in intensive care units. There was no significant difference in the prophylaxis of UGIB between cimetidine and antacids. Compilation of data revealed that 11 of 402 patients receiving cimetidine (2.7%) and 25 of 458 patients receiving antacids (3.3%) bled, concluding that cimetidine and antacids are equally effective in preventing bleeding. Antacids used alone are effective, but are labor intensive and produce a significant number of side effects.

Lamothe et al.[49] compared the ability of cimetidine (300 mg intravenously every 6 hours), famotidine (20 mg intravenously every 12 hours), or ranitidine (50 mg intravenously every 8 hours) to prevent stress-related mucosal bleeding in patients undergoing cardiac surgery. There was no clinical difference between any of the agents in preventing overt bleeding from stress ulceration. Mean gastric pH was better controlled (pH higher than 4.5) with famotidine and ranitidine than with cimetidine. The clinical relevance of the study is debatable because no overt bleeding was observed in any group.

A constant infusion of H_2RAs will maintain the intragastric pH higher than 4 on a more consistent basis than intermittent bolus doses.[26,31,33,41,50] In a double-blind, randomized, controlled trial, intravenous cimetidine (50 mg/h after a 300-mg bolus dose) was compared with placebo.[51] Of the 54 patients treated with cimetidine, overt bleeding developed in 1 patient (1.9%) compared with 7 of the 33 patients (21.2%) receiving placebo.

The constant-infusion regimen provides a more consistent effect on gastric pH. To date, no large, randomized, double-blind, controlled trial comparing the three intravenous H_2RAs has been conducted. Based on available data, one would expect all of them to be equally effective.

Despite the fact that it does not affect gastric acidity, sucralfate given at a dose of 1 g every 4–6 hours via the NG tube has been shown to be effective at preventing stress-related bleeding in numerous studies. Tryba[52] compared sucralfate to antacids, finding equal efficacy at preventing stress bleeding. He also found the sucralfate group to have a lower incidence of nosocomial pneumonia than the antacid group. He postulated that the increased gastric pH allowed bacteria to grow in the stomach and as patients aspirated this content, pneumonia developed. Driks et al.[53] conducted a randomized study in 130 patients who were receiving mechanical ventilation in an intensive care unit. There were two treatment groups, the first received sucralfate (1 g every 6 hours) and the second received antacids, H_2RAs, or both. Overt bleeding was observed in one patient (1.4%) in the antacid plus H_2RA group and in two patients in the sucralfate group (3.3%). These rates of bleeding were not statistically different.

Driks et al.[53] also discussed the concern that the elevation of the intragastric pH by antacids or H_2RAs may lead to gastric colonization with gram-negative bacteria and predispose the patient to nosocomial pneumonia. Thus, he suggests that agents that prevent the development of stress ulcers without altering the intragastric pH may be preferential. Seven of 61 patients (11.5%) receiving sucralfate, 1 patient of 17 (5.9%) receiving an H_2RA alone, 6 of 13 (46.2%) patients receiving the antacid–H_2RA combination, and 9 of 39 (23.1%) patients receiving antacids alone developed nosocomial pneumonia. It appears that the volume of antacids given may be a greater risk factor for aspiration than an increase in pH for overgrowth. Other studies examining this problem have produced conflicting results. Some investigators have found that there appears to be no significant difference in the incidence of nosocomial pneumonia in critically ill patients treated with H_2RA compared with those treated with sucralfate. Recently, a study from Switzerland comparing the incidence of development of pneumonia in patients who received ranitidine, antacids, or sucralfate found that the incidence of pneumonia was higher (p = 0.065) in the two groups who received antacids or ranitidine than the sucralfate group.[54] Also, recent reviews of the literature suggest there is evidence that patients with elevated intragastric pH are at greater risk for development of nosocomial pneumonia.[55,56] Research continues to unravel the complex relationships involved. There is no proven advantage to combining sucralfate with H_2RAs.

CONCLUSION

Esophageal variceal bleeding is a catastrophic event that has a high mortality. Patients who do not expire from bleeding often die from the many other complications of alcoholic liver disease. Patients who present with acute variceal bleeding should be stabilized, and, after diagnosis, acute hemostasis may be achieved by using sclerotherapy if physicians are available who are experienced in that form of therapy. If no experienced endoscopist is available, it is advisable to use an agent to lower the portal pressure (e.g., vasopressin or octreotide) and wait for the bleeding to stop. Patients who stop bleeding are usually admitted to an intensive care unit for observation for at least several days. Rebleeding usually occurs within 3 days in 75% of patients who present with UGIB. Recurrent bleeding episodes can be treated with additional sclerotherapy, octreotide, or vasopressin. Vasopressin is not indicated in patients whose bleeding stops with sclerotherapy. Sclerotherapy is not indicated to prevent recurrent bleeding episodes. Other treatment options are surgery or transjugular intrahepatic portosystemic shunt.

Studies of UGIB have included several slightly different subpopulations of patients who present with UGIB from peptic ulcer. While no study conclusively shows the efficacy of acid secretory suppression in the treatment of UGIB, conventional therapy continues to employ aggressive acid suppression in the form of one of the three H_2RAs. After stabilization, hemostasis may be achieved by endoscopic therapy. To prevent a rebleeding episode, acid secretory suppression continues to be the conventional method of treatment. This can be achieved by using intermittent or constant-infusion H_2RAs. If constant infusions are chosen, a loading dose of cimetidine (300 mg), ranitidine (50 mg), or famotidine (20 mg) is given followed by a constant infusion that is titrated (with the addition of antacids if necessary) to produce an intragastric pH as near 7 as possible. The initial infusion dose currently recommended is cimetidine 50 mg/h, ranitidine 8 mg/h, or famotidine 1.67 mg/h. If the intragastric pH is not controlled with the starting dose, the dose can be doubled and pH monitoring continued. Treatment should continue for at least 3 days. If the patient rebleeds during this period, alternative therapy such as surgery or endoscopic therapy may be considered.

The maintenance of intragastric pH in a range of 3.5–4 decreases the frequency of stress-related mucosal lesions and resultant bleeding in critically ill patients. Most complications of stress ulcers are related to bleeding. However, bleeding is often rare (less than 5%). Intravenous H_2RAs given by intermittent bolus or continuous infusions, antacids, or sucralfate are effective in preventing clinically overt bleeding. If H_2RAs are used, a constant-infusion regimen in doses previously described offers a consistent effect on gastric pH. Antacids are rarely used alone for prophylaxis because their required frequent administration is difficult in these complicated intensive care patients. Sucralfate appears to be efficacious when given in a dose of 1 g every 4–6 hours. Data using omeprazole for prophylaxis are not available, and thus it cannot be recommended at this time. There are no data to suggest that any one of these agents is clinically superior to any other in prevention of bleeding. A combination of these agents has never been shown to improve the efficacy over a single agent.

The effect of prophylaxis on outcome of the critically ill patient remains controversial. The risk of nosocomial pneumonia may be higher in patients receiving acid suppression regimens. The impact of this complication has yet to be shown to be significant in patient outcome, but must be considered when choosing a prophylaxis regimen. A reevaluation of the need for stress-related bleeding prophylaxis using outcome parameters should be performed to allow a full evaluation of the clinical need for this therapy.

References

1. Krejs GJ, Little KH, Westergaard H, et al. Laser photocoagulation for the treatment of acute peptic ulcer bleeding. N Engl J Med 1987;316:1618–1621.
2. Crohn BB. The need for aggressive therapy in massive upper gastrointestinal hemorrhage. JAMA 1954;151:626–627.
3. Rockey DC, Cello JP. Evaluation of the gastrointestinal tract in patients with iron-deficiency anemia. N Engl J Med 1993;329:1691–1695.
4. Czaja AJ, McAlheny JC, Pruitt BA. Gastric acid secretion and acute gastroduodenal disease after burns. Arch Surg 1976;111:243–246.
5. Day SB, MacMillan BF, Altheimer WA. Curlings Ulcer: An Experiment of Nature. Springfield, IL, Charles C Thomas, 1972, pp 183–184.
6. Cook DJ, Fuller HD, Guyatt GH, et al. Risk factors for gastrointestinal bleeding in critically ill patients. N Engl J Med 1994;330:377–381.
7. Forrest JAH, Finlayson NDC, Shearman DJC. Endoscopy in gastrointestinal bleeding. Lancet 1974;2:394–397.
8. Siepler JK. A dosage alternative for H_2-receptor antagonists. Clin Ther 1986;8 (suppl A) :24–33.
9. Spiro H. Complications of peptic ulcer disease, in Clinical Gastroenterology, 3rd ed. New York, Macmillan, 1983.
10. Silverstein FE, Kimmey MB, Saunders DR, Levine DS. Gastric protection by misoprostol against 1,300 mg aspirin. Dig Dis Sci 1986;31:137S–142S.
11. Levy M. Aspirin use in patients with major upper gastrointestinal bleeding and peptic ulcer disease. N Engl J Med 1974;290:1158–1162.
12. Lanas A, Sekar MC, Hirschowitz BI. Objective evidence of aspirin use in both ulcer and nonulcer upper and lower gastrointestinal bleeding. Gastroenterology 1992;103:862–869.
13. Jensen DM, Cheng S, Kovacs TO, et al. A controlled study of ranitidine for the prevention of recurrent hemorrhage from duodenal ulcer. N Engl J Med 1994;330:382–386.
14. Jones FA, King WE. A study of acute gastric ulcers causing hemorrhage. Aust Ann Med 1953;2:179–182.
15. Prindiville T, Trudeau W. A comparison of immediate versus delayed endoscopic injection sclerosis of bleeding esophageal varices. Gastroenterol Endosc 1986;32:385–388.
16. Larson AW, Cohen H, Zweiban B, et al. Acute esophageal variceal sclerotherapy: Results of a randomized trial. JAMA 1986;255:497–500.
17. Henry D, Cook D. Meta-analysis workshop in upper GI bleeding. Gastroenterology 1991;100:1481–1482.
18. Pagliaro L, Burroughs AK, Sorensen IPA, et al. Therapeutic controversies and randomized controlled trials: Prevention of rebleeding in cirrhosis. Gastroenterol Int 1989;2:71–84.
19. Laine L, el-Newihi HM, Migikovsky B, et al. Endoscopic ligation compared with sclerotherapy for the treatment of bleeding esophageal varicies. Ann Intern Med 1993;119:1–7.
20. Siepler JK. Esophageal variceal bleeding. US Pharmacist 1979;24:H8–H11.
21. Choskier M, Grossman RJ, et al. A controlled comparison of intra-arterial and intravenous vasopressin [abstract]. Gastroenterology 1979;77:540.
22. Cello JP, Chan MF. Octreotide therapy for variceal hemorrhage. Digestion 1993;54:20–26.
23. McKee R. A study of octreotide in esophageal varices. Digestion 1990;45:60–65.
24. Sung JJ, Chung SC, Lai CW, et al. Octreotide infusion and emergency sclerotherapy for variceal haemorrhage. Lancet 1993;342:637–641.
25. LaBerge JM, Ring EJ, Gordon RL, et al. Creation of transjugular intrahepatic portosystemic shunts with the Wallstent endoprothesis: Results in 100 patients. Radiology 1993;87:413–420.
26. Peterson WL, Richardson CT. Sustained fasting achlorhydria: A comparison of two medical regimens. Gastroenterology 1985;88:666–669.
27. Black JW, Duncan WAM, Durant GJ, et al. Definition and antagonism of histamine H_2-receptors. Nature 1972;236:385–390.
28. Berner BD, Conner C, Sawyer D, et al. Ranitidine: A new H_2-receptor antagonist. Clin Pharm 1982;1:499–509.
29. Frank WO, Peace KE, Watson M, et al. The effect of single intravenous doses of cimetidine and ranitidine on gastric secretion. Clin Pharmacol Ther 1987;40:665–672.
30. Cicale M. Stress ulcer bleeding: Prophylaxis in the ICU. Hosp Formulary 1992;27:584–594.
31. Siepler JK, Trudeau W, Petty DE, et al. Use of continuous infusion of histamine H_2-receptor antagonists in critically ill patients. Drug Intell Clin Pharm 1989;23:S40–S43.
32. Siepler JK, Donahue P, Campagna K, Bombeck CT, Zollinger–Ellison syndrome. Ill Med J 1978;153:282–284.
33. Ostro MJ, Russell JA, Soldin SJ, et al. Control of gastric pH with cimetidine: Boluses versus primed infusions. Gastroenterology 1985;89:532–537.
34. Rigaud D, Chastre J, Accary JP, et al. Intragastric pH profile during acute respiratory failure in patients with chronic obstructive pulmonary disease. Chest 1986;90:58–63.
35. Ballesteros MA, Hogan DL, Koss MA, Isenberg JI. Bolus or intravenous, infusion of ranitidine: Effects on gastric pH and acid secretion. Ann Intern Med 1990;112:334–339.
36. Bauer H. Cimetidine in the preoperative treatment of acute bleeding gastroduodenal lesions. Munch Med Wochenschr 1979;121:1085–1089.
37. Barer D, Oglivie A, Henry D, et al. Cimetidine and tranexaminic acid in the treatment of upper gastrointestinal bleeding. N Engl J Med 1983;308:1571–1575.
38. Zuckerman G, Welch R, Douglas S, et al. Controlled trial of medical therapy for active gastrointestinal bleeding and prevention of rebleeding. Am J Med 1984;76:361–366.
39. Nowak A, Saldinski C, Gorka Z, et al. Ranitidine in the treatment of acute upper gastrointestinal haemorrhage. Hepatogastroenterology 1981;28:267–269.

40. Falk A, Darle N, Haglund U, Tornqvist A. Histamine H_2-receptor antagonists in gastroduodenal hemorrhage. Scand J Gastroenterol 1985;20(suppl 110):95–100.
41. Thomson AB, Maguire T, Wensel RH, et al. Ranitidine versus cimetidine in the management of acute gastrointestinal tract bleeding. J Clin Gastroenterol 1984;6:295–299.
42. Fullarton GM, MacDonald AM, Mann SG, McColl KE. Controlled study of the effects of intravenous famotidine on intragastric pH in bleeding ulcers. Aliment Pharmacol Ther 1991:77–84.
43. Walt RP, Cottrell J, Mann SG, et al. Continuous intravenous famotidine for hemorrhage from peptic ulcer. Lancet 1992;340:1058–1062.
44. Brunner G, Chang J. Intravenous therapy and high doses of ranitidine and omeprazole in critically ill patients with bleeding peptic ulceration of the upper intestinal tract: An open randomized trial. Digestion 1990;45:217–225.
45. Peura DA. Stress-related mucosal damage: An overview. Am J Med 1987;83 (suppl 6A) :3–7.
46. Davidson JS, Trudeau WL, Prindiville T. Emergence of acute ulcers as a major cause of significant gastrointestinal hemorrhage in critically ill patients [abstract]. Am J Gastroenterol 1987;97:1277.
47. McAlhany JC Jr, Colmic L, Czaja AJ, Pruitt BA Jr. Antacid control of complications from acute gastroduodenal disease after burn. J Trauma 1976;16:645–648.
48. Shuman RB, Schuster DP, Zuckerman GR. Prophylactic therapy for stress ulcers bleeding: A reappraisal. Ann Intern Med 1987;106:562–567.
49. Lamothe PH, Rao E, Serra AJ, et al. Comparative efficacy of cimetidine, famotidine, ranitidine, and mylanta in postoperative stress ulcers. Gastroenterology 1991;100:1515–1520.
50. Santucci L, Fiorucci S, Pelli MA, et al. Control of gastric pH with ranitidine in critically ill patients. Dig Dis Sci 1991;36:583–587.
51. Karlstadt RG, Iberti TJ, Silverstein J, et al. Comparison of cimetidine and placebo for the prophylaxis of upper gastrointestinal bleeding due to stress-related mucosal damage in the intensive care unit. J Intensive Care Med 1990;5:26–32.
52. Tryba M. Risk of acute stress bleeding and nosocomial pneumonia in ventilated patients: Sucralfate versus antacids. Am J Med 1987;83:117–124.
53. Driks MR, Craven DE, Celli B, et al. Nosocomial pneumonia in intubated patients given sucralfate as compared with antacids or histamine type 2 blockers. N Engl J Med 1987;317:1376–1382.
54. Prod'hom G, Leuenberger P, Koerfer J, et al. Nosocomial pneumonia in mechanically ventilated patients receiving ranitidine, sucralfate, or antacids for stress ulcer. Ann Intern Med 1994;120:653–662.
55. Scheld WM, Mandell GL. Nosocomial pneumonia: Pathogenesis and recent advances in diagnosis and therapy. Rev Infect Dis 1994;13 (suppl 9) :S743–S751.
56. Simms HH, DeMaria E, McDonald L, et al. Role of gastric colonization in the development of pneumonia in critically ill trauma patients: Results of a randomized prospective trial. J Trauma 1991;31:531–537.

Chapter 34

Inflammatory Bowel Disease

Joseph T. DiPiro, PharmD, FCCP, and Talmadge A. Bowden, Jr., MD

Two forms of idiopathic inflammatory bowel disease (IBD) are of primary concern to the pharmacy clinician: ulcerative colitis, a mucosal inflammatory condition confined to the rectum and colon, and Crohn's disease, a transmural inflammation of gastrointestinal (GI) mucosa that may occur in any part of the GI tract. The etiologies of both conditions are unknown, but they may have a common pathogenetic mechanism.

In this chapter, these conditions are discussed separately but compared and contrasted when appropriate. Antibiotic-associated colitis (covered in a later chapter) and other forms of drug- or chemical-induced inflammatory GI diseases are not discussed here.

Ulcerative colitis was first identified in 1875[1] and was for many years thought to be a condition of North Americans and Europeans. Today its reported incidence is rising in many parts of the world, with increasing recognition of the disorder as distinct from infectious diarrhea. Crohn's disease, described initially in 1932,[2] was originally thought to be a disease of the ileum. Experience has taught that the disease, sometimes incorrectly called regional enteritis, may occur in any portion of the GI tract.

The patterns of clinical presentation of IBD can vary widely. Patients may have a single acute episode that resolves and does not recur, but most patients experience acute exacerbations after periods of remission. With more severe disease, prolonged illness may occur.

Although IBD is expressed primarily in the GI tract, it should be recognized as a systemic disease. IBD may be associated with arthritis, uveitis, liver disease, and other complications.

The cause of IBD is not known; therefore, effective therapy has been difficult to define. For Crohn's disease, no true cure exists, whereas for ulcerative colitis a true cure is achieved by proctocolectomy. Treatment for IBD has changed little over the past 25 years. Sulfasalazine was first used in the early 1940s and steroids were introduced in 1948. Over the past few years the introduction of other mesalamine derivatives has expended therapeutic options. Immunosuppressive agents, antibiotics, and nutritional support offer help in the management of complications, but the natural progression of these diseases has remained unchanged.

EPIDEMIOLOGY

At least 1 million Americans are believed to have IBD, with 15,000 to 30,000 new cases diagnosed annually.[3] Two key studies, one in Baltimore, Maryland,[4] and the other in Rochester, Minnesota,[5] established a generally accepted incidence (new cases per year) for ulcerative colitis of 3 to 6 per 100,000 and a prevalence (number of cases at any point in time) of 35 to 70 cases per 100,000 Americans. Crohn's disease has a reported incidence of 4.3 to 6.8 and a prevalence of 20 to 40 per 100,000 people.[6] The increase is believed to be real, not just increased awareness or better diagnosis.[3]

Both sexes are affected equally,[3,6] although some studies have shown slightly greater numbers of women with the disease.[7] Ulcerative colitis and Crohn's disease have bimodal distributions in age of initial presentation. The peak incidence occurs in the second or third decade of life, but infants and the elderly may present with either disorder. Significantly increased incidence (four to five times normal) has been observed in Ashkenazi Jews, while blacks and Orientals have a relatively low incidence of occurrence.[6]

ETIOLOGY

Although the exact etiology of ulcerative colitis and Crohn's disease is unknown, similar factors are believed responsible for each condition (Table 34.1). The major theories of the cause of IBD involve infectious or immunologic causes. The infectious theory assumes that the body is reacting normally to an unrecognized pathogen, whereas the immunologic theory assumes that the immune system is acting inappropriately to antigens to which most people are exposed.[8]

INFECTIOUS THEORIES

A number of different microorganisms have been suspected of being involved in the pathogenesis of IBD, including

TABLE 34.1. PROPOSED ETIOLOGIES FOR INFLAMMATORY BOWEL DISEASE

Infectious Agents
- Viruses
- L-forms of bacteria
- *Mycobacteria*
- *Chlamydia*

Genetics
- Metabolic defects
- Connective tissue disorders

Environmental Factors
- Diet

Immune Defects
- Altered host susceptibility
- Immune-mediated mucosal damage

Psychologic Factors
- Stress
- Emotional or physical trauma
- Occupation

viruses, protozoans, mycoplasmas, and other bacteria.[9] However, no definitive infectious cause of IBD has been found even though the presentation is similar to that caused by some invasive microbial pathogens. Also, certain strains of bacteria produce toxins (necrotoxins, hemolysins, and enterotoxins) that cause mucosal damage. Bacteria also elaborate peptides (e.g., formyl-methionyl-leucyl-phenylalanine [FMLP]) that have chemotactic properties and cause an influx of inflammatory cells with subsequent release of inflammatory mediators and tissue destruction. In addition, microbes may elaborate super antigens, which are capable of global T lymphocyte stimulation and subsequent inflammatory response.[9]

Investigators have examined the difference in bowel flora of IBD patients and normal individuals.[10] In up to one-third of patients with Crohn's disease abnormal flora (increased anaerobes) were observed in the upper small bowel. However, it is recognized that diarrhea alone can cause changes in bowel flora.

GENETIC FACTORS

Genetic factors are believed to predispose patients to both ulcerative colitis and Crohn's disease.[11,12] In studies of monozygotic twins, there has been a high concordance rate, with both individuals of the pair having an IBD (particularly Crohn's disease). Also, first-degree relatives of patients with IBDs had a 10-fold increase in the risk of disease. Other investigators have observed genetic markers that are found more frequently in those with IBDs (particularly human leukocyte antigens [HLA]). A number of genes have been associated with IBDs; however, the nature of the gene products has not been established.

IMMUNOLOGIC MECHANISMS

The immunologic basis of IBD is supported by a number of observations.[8] First is the pathology of the lesions. With Crohn's disease, the bowel wall has been observed to be infiltrated with lymphocytes, plasma cells, mast cells, macrophages, and neutrophils. Similar infiltration has been observed in the mucosal layer of the colon in patients with ulcerative colitis. Second, many of the systemic manifestations of IBD have an immunologic etiology (e.g., arthritis or uveitis). Finally, IBD is responsive to immunosuppressive drugs (e.g., corticosteroids and azathioprine).

As previously stated, the immune theory of IBD assumes that IBD is caused by an "inappropriate" reaction of the immune system. This may involve an immunodeficiency, such as a defect in cell-mediated immunity or of macrophages or neutrophils. Autoimmunity may be involved.

Potential immunologic mechanisms include both autoimmune and nonautoimmune phenomena.[9,13] Autoimmunity may be directed against mucosal epithelial cells or against neutrophil cytoplasmic elements. Some patients with IBD have abnormal structural features for colonic epithelial cells even in the absence of active disease. Autoantibodies to these structures have been reported. Also, up to 70% of patients with ulcerative colitis are reported to have an antineutrophil cytoplasmic antibody. It is not clear if autoimmune mechanisms are responsible for these diseases.

A number of nonautoimmune phenomena have been reported with IBDs. Patients with IBDs have increased numbers of IgG bearing cells and altered production of IgG subtypes. Mucosal injury with IBD may result from mucosal T cell activation. These cells may have cytotoxic effects directly or through the actions of cytokines. Inflammatory cytokines such as interleukin-1 and interleukin-6 are reported to be increased with IBDs. Also, inflammatory products such as leukotriene B_4 are related to disease activity.

PSYCHOLOGIC FACTORS

Mental health changes appear to correlate with remissions and exacerbations, especially of ulcerative colitis, but psychologic factors overall are not thought to be a major etiologic factor. Most rigorous studies have concluded that no connection can be made between stress-inducing events and disease symptoms.[7,9]

DIET AND SMOKING

Changes in diet by people in industrialized countries where Crohn's disease is more common have not been consistently associated with the disease. Studies of increased intake of refined sugars or chemical food additives and reduced fiber intake have been conflicting regarding risk for Crohn's disease.

Smoking is believed to play an important but contrasting role in ulcerative colitis and Crohn's disease. The incidence of ulcerative colitis is inversely associated with smoking.[12,14] Clinical relapses have been associated with smoking cessation, and nicotine transdermal administration has been effective in improving symptoms in patients with ulcerative colitis.[15] In contrast, Crohn's disease has been directly associated with smoking.[12]

PATHOPHYSIOLOGY

Ulcerative colitis and Crohn's disease differ in two general respects: anatomic sites and depth of involvement within the bowel wall. There is, however, overlap between the two conditions, with a small fraction of patients showing features of both diseases. Confusion can occur, particularly when the inflammatory process is limited to the colon. Table 34.2 compares pathologic and clinical findings of the two diseases.

ULCERATIVE COLITIS

Ulcerative colitis is confined to the colon and rectum, and affects primarily the mucosa and the submucosa. In some instances, a short segment of terminal ileum may be inflamed; this is referred to as "backwash ileitis." The histopathology of ulcerative colitis is similar to that of other inflammations of the colon such as that caused by infectious agents. Unlike Crohn's disease, the deeper longitudinal muscular layers, serosa, and regional lymph nodes are not usually involved.[7] Because inflammation is usually confined to the mucosa and submucosa, fistulas, perforation, or obstruction is uncommon.

The primary lesion occurs in the crypts of the mucosa (crypts of Lieberkuhn) in the form of a crypt abscess. Here, frank necrosis of the epithelium occurs; it is usually visible

TABLE 34.2. COMPARISON OF THE CLINICAL AND PATHOLOGIC FEATURES OF CROHN'S GRANULOMATOUS COLITIS AND ULCERATIVE COLITIS

Feature	Crohn's Colitis	Ulcerative Colitis
Intestinal		
Malaise, fever	Common	Uncommon
Rectal bleeding	Intermittent about 50%	Common
Abdominal tenderness	Common	May be present
Abdominal mass	Very common (especially with ileocolitis)	Not present
Abdominal pain	Very common	Unusual
Abdominal wall and internal fistulas	Very common	Rare
Endoscopic		
Rectal disease	About 20%	Almost 100%
Diffuse, continuous symmetric involvement	Uncommon	Very common
Aphthous or linear ulcers	Common	Rare
Friability	Rare	Rare
Radiologic		
Continuous disease	Rare	Very common
Ileal involvement	Very common	Rare
Asymmetry	Very common	Rare
Strictures	Common	Rare
Fistulas	Very common	Rare
Pathologic		
Discontinuity	Common	Rare
Rectal involvement	Rare	Common
Intense vascularity	Rare	Common
Ileal involvement	Common	Nonexistent
Transmural involvement	Common	Rare
Lymphoid aggregates	Common	Uncommon
Crypt abscesses	Rare	Very common
Granulomas	Common	Rare
Linear clefts	Common	Rare
Surgical treatment	Subtotal or total colectomy, rectum frequently preserved	Proctocolectomy with ileostomy

(Adapted from Ramming KP. Diseases of the rectum and colon, in Sabiston DC (ed): Essentials of Surgery. Philadelphia, WB Saunders, 1987, p 483, with permission.)

only with microscopy but may be seen grossly when coalescence of ulcers occurs. Extension and coalescence ulcers may surround areas of uninvolved mucosa. These islands of mucosa are called *pseudopolyps*. Other typical ulceration patterns include a "collar-button ulcer," which results from extensive submucosal undermining at the ulcer edge.[7,16] The extensive mucosal damage seen in ulcerative colitis can result in significant diarrhea and bleeding, although a small percent of patients experience constipation.

Ulcerative colitis can be accompanied by complications that may be local (involving the colon) or systemic (not directly associated with the colon). With either type the complications may be mild, serious, or even life-threatening.

Local complications occur in the majority of ulcerative colitis patients. Relatively minor complications include hemorrhoids, anal fissures, or perirectal abscesses. These complications are more likely to be present during active colitis. Enteroenteric fistulas are rare.

A major complication is toxic megacolon, a severe condition that occurs in 1–3% of patients with ulcerative colitis or Crohn's disease. With toxic megacolon, ulceration extends below the submucosa, sometimes even reaching the serosa. Vasculitis, swelling of the vascular endothelium, and thrombosis of small arteries occur; involvement of the muscularis propria causes loss of colonic tone, which leads to dilatation and potential perforation.[7] Colonic perforation, however, may occur with or without toxic megacolon and is a greater risk with the first attack.

Another major local complication is massive colonic hemorrhage. Although rectal bleeding is common, massive hemorrhage occurs infrequently. Colonic stricture, sometimes with clinical obstruction, may also complicate ulcerative colitis. Finally, the risk of colonic carcinoma is much greater in patients with ulcerative colitis as compared with the general population. The risk of colon cancer begins to increase 10–15 years after the diagnosis of ulcerative colitis. The absolute risk may be as high as 30% 35 years after diagnosis and 49% for patients who were less than 15 years of age at the time of diagnosis.[13]

The inflammatory response seen in IBD has also been blamed for the "systemic" complications seen in both Crohn's disease and ulcerative colitis. The systemic complications of ulcerative colitis are summarized in the following section.

Hepatobiliary Complications

Approximately 11% of patients with ulcerative colitis have been reported to have hepatobiliary complications.[17] However, the reported frequency ranges from 5–95% in IBD patients overall.[18] Hepatic complications include fatty liver, pericholangitis, chronic active hepatitis, and cirrhosis. Biliary complications include sclerosing cholangitis, cholangiocarcinoma, and gallstones.

Fatty infiltration of the liver may be due to malabsorption, protein-losing enteropathy, or concomitant steroid use. The most common hepatic complication is pericholangitis (acute inflammation surrounding the intrahepatic portal venules, bile ducts, and lymphatics). Chronic active hepatitis occurs in up to 1% of patients with ulcerative colitis but not with Crohn's disease. Cirrhosis may be a sequela of cholangitis or chronic active hepatitis. Often the severity of hepatic disease does not correlate with GI disease.

Gallstones occur more commonly in patients with Crohn's disease (particularly with terminal ileal disease) and may be related to bile salt malabsorption. Also, cholangiocarcinoma occurs 10–20 times more frequently in IBD patients compared with the general population.[17]

Joint Complications

Arthritis was found to be present in 4.9% of patients.[17] Arthritis is typically migratory and involves one or a few joints. The joints most often affected, in decreasing frequency, are the knees, hips, ankles, wrists, and elbows. Arthritis associated with ulcerative colitis is generally related to the severity of colonic disease, and resolution without recurrence is seen with proctocolectomy. Also, arthritis in this setting is different from rheumatoid arthritis in that rheumatoid factors are generally not detected.

Another potential joint complication is ankylosing spondylitis, which is often unresponsive to treatment. The incidence of ankylosing spondylitis in patients with ulcerative colitis is 30 times that of the general population.

Ocular Complications

Ocular complications, including iritis, uveitis, episcleritis, or conjunctivitis, occur in about 10% of patients with IBDs.[18] The most commonly reported symptoms include blurred vision, headaches, eye pain, and photophobia. These complications often do not parallel the severity of intestinal disease although recurrence after colectomy with ulcerative colitis is uncommon.

Dermatologic and Mucosal Complications

A number of different skin and mucosal lesions are associated with IBDs, including erythema nodosum, pyoderma gangrenosum, and aphthalous ulceration. Overall, most studies report 5–10% of IBD patients experience dermatologic or mucosal complications.[19]

Erythema nodosum is manifested by raised, red, tender nodules that vary in size from one to several centimeters. They are typically found on the tibial surfaces of the legs and arms. These lesions are more commonly observed in Crohn's disease patients and are noted to correlate with disease severity.

Pyoderma gangrenosum occurs more commonly in patients with ulcerative colitis (1–5% incidence) and is noted by discrete skin ulcerations that have a necrotic center and a violaceous color of the surrounding skin.[19] They can be seen on any part of the body but are more commonly found on the lower extremities.

Oral lesions are found in 6–20% of patients with Crohn's disease and 8% of patients with ulcerative colitis.[19] The most common lesion is aphthous stomatitis, which is most often seen with Crohn's disease. The severity of these lesions tends to parallel GI disease.

CROHN'S DISEASE

Crohn's disease is best characterized as a transmural inflammatory process. The terminal ileum is the most common site of the disorder (14–30%), but it may occur in any part of the GI tract. About two-thirds of patients have some colonic involvement, and 15–25% of patients have only colonic disease.[9] Patients often have normal bowel separating segments of diseased bowel; that is, the disease is often discontinuous.

Regardless of the site, bowel wall destruction is extensive and the intestinal lumen is often narrowed. The mesentery becomes first thickened and edematous and then fibrotic. Ulcers tend to be deep and elongated and extend along the longitudinal axis of the bowel, at least into the submucosa. The "cobblestone" appearance of the bowel wall results from deep mucosal ulceration intermingled with nodular submucosal thickening.

Complications of Crohn's disease may involve the intestinal tract or organs unrelated to it. Small bowel stricture and subsequent obstruction is a complication that may require surgery. Fistula formation is common and occurs much more frequently than with ulcerative colitis.[9,20] Fistulas often occur in the areas of worst inflammation where loops of bowel have become matted together by fibrous adhesions. Fistulas may connect a segment of the GI tract to skin (enterocutaneous fistula), two segments of the GI tract (enteroenteric fistula), or the intestinal tract with the bladder (enterovesicular fistula). Crohn's disease fistulas almost always require surgical treatment.

Bleeding with Crohn's disease is usually not as severe as with ulcerative colitis, although patients with Crohn's disease may have hypochromic anemia. Also, as with ulcerative colitis, the risk of carcinoma is increased but not as great as with ulcerative colitis.

Systemic complications of Crohn's disease are common, and similar to those found with ulcerative colitis. Arthritis, iritis, skin lesions, and liver disease often accompany Crohn's disease.

CLINICAL PRESENTATION

ULCERATIVE COLITIS

Although a typical clinical picture of ulcerative colitis can be described, there is a very wide range of presentation. Symptoms may range from mild abdominal cramping with frequent small-volume bowel movements to profuse diarrhea. Most patients with ulcerative colitis experience intermittent bouts of illness after varying intervals with no symptoms. Only a small percentage of patients have continuous unremitting symptoms or have a single acute attack with no subsequent symptoms.

Complex disease classifications are generally not used in clinical practice for ulcerative colitis. The arbitrarily determined distinctions of "mild," "moderate," and "severe" disease are generally used, and these are determined largely by clinical signs and symptoms. Mild disease has been defined as less than four stools daily without anemia, tachycardia, weight loss, or hypoalbuminemia, and severe disease as greater than six stools daily with the signs just listed (Table 34.3).[7]

Two-thirds of patients with ulcerative colitis have mild disease.[21] Occasionally, the mild form may progress to severe or fulminant disease. Systemic signs and symptoms of the disease (e.g., arthritis, uveitis, pyoderma gangreno-

TABLE 34.3. SEVERITY CRITERIA FOR ULCERATIVE COLITIS

Variables	Mild	Severe	Fulminant
Bowel frequency	<4/day	>6/day	>10/day
Blood in stool	+/–	++	Continuous
Fever	Normal	>37.5°C	>37.5°C
Pulse	Normal	>90/mm	<90/mm
Hemoglobin	Normal	<75% normal	Transfusion required
ESR	<30 mm/h	>30 mm/h	>30 mm/h
Colon		Colonic air	Dilated colon
Radiography		Edematous wall, thumbprinting	
Clinical sign		Abdominal tenderness	Abdominal distension + tenderness

(From Hanauer SB. Medical therapy of ulcerative colitis. Lancet 1993;342:412–417.)

sum) may be present in these patients and, in fact, may be the reason the patient seeks medical attention. Patients with mild disease are believed to be at lower risk of colon cancer. Moderate disease is observed in one-fourth of patients.[21] These patients have more prominent abdominal discomfort and usually present with diarrhea as the major complaint. They may be noted to have a low-grade fever.

With severe disease the patient is usually found to be in acute distress, has profuse bloody diarrhea, and often has a high fever with leukocytosis and hypoalbuminemia. Often the patient is dehydrated and therefore may be tachycardic and hypotensive. This presentation may have a sudden onset with rapid progression.

The diagnosis of ulcerative colitis is made on clinical suspicion and confirmed by biopsy, stool examinations, sigmoidoscopy or colonoscopy, and barium radiographic contrast studies. The presence of extracolonic manifestations such as arthritis, uveitis, and pyoderma gangrenosum may also aid in establishing the diagnosis.

CROHN'S DISEASE

As with ulcerative colitis, the presentation of Crohn's disease is highly variable. A single episode may not be followed by further episodes, or the patient may experience continuous, unremitting disease. Because the symptoms can be confusing, an average of 3 years between the onset of complaints and the initial diagnosis has been reported. The patient typically presents with diarrhea and abdominal pain. Hematochezia occurs in about one-half of the patients with colonic involvement and much less frequently when there is no colonic involvement. Commonly, a patient may first present with a perirectal or perianal lesion. The diagnosis should be suspected in children with growth retardation.

The course of Crohn's disease is characterized by periods of remission and exacerbation. Some patients may be free of symptoms for years, while others experience chronic problems in spite of medical therapy. Nearly all patients have a recurrence of Crohn's disease within 10 years of the initial episode.[12] As in ulcerative colitis the diagnosis of Crohn's disease involves a thorough evaluation using laboratory, endoscopic, and radiologic testing to detect the characteristic features of the disease. Because of similarities that may exist between ulcerative colitis and Crohn's disease, a definitive diagnosis cannot be made in up to 15% of cases, even with pathologic specimens in hand.

TREATMENT

Treatment of IBD centers on agents used to lessen the inflammatory process. Salicylates, corticosteroids, antimicrobials, and immunosuppressive agents such as azathioprine and 6-mercaptopurine are commonly used to treat active disease and, for some agents, to lengthen remission from disease.

In addition to the use of drugs, surgical procedures are sometimes performed when active disease is not adequately controlled or when the required drug dosages pose an unacceptable risk of adverse effects. For most patients with IBD, nutritional considerations are also very important because these patients are often malnourished. Finally, a variety of therapies may be used to address complications or symptoms of IBD. For example, antidiarrheals may be used in some patients, although these are generally to be avoided in ulcerative colitis because they may contribute to the development of toxic colonic dilatation. Antimicrobial agents may be used in conjunction with drainage when abscesses are present. Iron may be required, particularly with ulcerative colitis where blood loss from the colon can be significant.

GOALS

To treat IBD properly, the clinician must have a clear concept of realistic therapeutic goals for each patient. These goals may relate to resolution of acute inflammatory processes, to resolution of attendant complications (e.g., fistulas, abscesses), to alleviation of systemic manifestations (e.g., arthritis), to maintenance of remission from acute inflammation, or to surgical palliation or cure. The approach to the therapeutic regimen differs considerably with varying goals as well as with the two diseases, ulcerative colitis and Crohn's disease.

In determining goals of therapy and selecting therapeutic regimens it is important to understand the natural history of IBD when untreated.[22] This knowledge is necessary to estimate the value of therapeutic regimens. Admittedly, there is relatively little information on the natural history in IBD, and most of it is derived from placebo-controlled trials. Since the first recognition of these clinical syndromes, virtually all patients have received some therapeutic measures.

Some types of acute ulcerative colitis are self-limited. With mild to moderate acute colitis, without systemic symptoms, 20% of patients may experience improvement in their disease within a few weeks; however, a small percentage of patients may go on to experience more serious disease. With severe colitis, improvement without treatment cannot be expected. For instance, the response to medical management of toxic megacolon is poor and colectomy is usually required. When remission of ulcerative colitis is achieved, it is likely to last at least 1 year with medical therapy. In the absence of medical therapy, one-half to two-thirds of patients are likely to relapse within 9 months.[22] In some reports, remission rates with placebo have approached those with active treatment.

A considerable number of patients with active Crohn's disease may achieve at least temporary remission without drug therapy. In two large trials, 26% and 42% of ambulatory patients on placebo achieved remission.[23,24] Once remission is achieved, two-thirds to three-fourths of patients remain in remission up to 2 years without drug therapy.[22] The implication of these data is that up to 40% of patients with active Crohn's disease improve in 3 to 4 months with observation alone, and that most patients remain in remission for prolonged periods without medical intervention. These observations apply more to mild or moderate disease than to severe disease.

NUTRITIONAL SUPPORT

Proper nutritional support is an important aspect of the treatment of patients with IBD, not because specific types of diets are useful in alleviating the inflammatory conditions but because patients with moderate to severe disease are often malnourished. The patient with IBD may be malnourished because of decreased nutrient intake (anorexia or when eating causes exacerbation of symptoms), because the inflammatory process results in significant malabsorption, or because of the catabolic effects of the disease process. Malabsorption may occur in the patient with Crohn's disease with inflammatory involvement of the small bowel where many nutrients are absorbed, and also in patients who have undergone multiple small bowel resections with subsequent reduction in absorptive surface ("short gut").

A number of specific diets have been tried in attempts to improve the condition of patients with IBD, but none has gained widespread acceptance. With each individual it is helpful to eliminate specific foods that exacerbate symptoms. This elimination process must be conducted cautiously, as patients have been known to exclude a wide range of nutritious products without adequate justification. Many patients with IBD, although not the majority, have lactase deficiency; therefore, diarrhea may be associated with milk intake. In these patients, avoidance of milk or supplementation with lactase generally improves the patient's symptoms.

Dietary supplementation with fish oil has been proposed to treat IBDs. In one placebo-controlled trial, patients with active ulcerative colitis were treated with fish oil supplementation for 4 months and had significant improvements in histologic findings and weight gain.[25] Fish oil contains eicosapentaenoic acid, which is metabolized by lipoxygenase and cyclooxygenase (similar to arachidonic acid), and results in lower production of leukotriene B_4 and prostaglandin E_2, which are believed to be important mediators in IBDs.

The nutritional needs of the majority of patients can be adequately addressed with enteral supplementation. Patients who have severe disease may require a course of parenteral nutrition to attain a reasonable nutritional status or in preparation for surgery. In one report of patients with severe acute ulcerative colitis, enteral nutrition resulted in significantly greater increase in serum albumin, fewer adverse effects related to the nutritional regimen, and fewer postoperative infections, compared with isocaloric, isonitrogenous parenteral nutrition. The regimens were similar with regard to remission rate and the need for colectomy.[26] Consideration should be given to lipid administration, not only for caloric value but also in recognition of depleted peripheral fat stores in many IBD patients and the greater potential for fatty acid deficiency.

Parenteral nutrition is an important component of the treatment of severe Crohn's disease or ulcerative colitis. The use of parenteral nutrition allows complete bowel rest in patients with severe ulcerative colitis, which may alter the need for proctocolectomy. Parenteral nutrition has also been valuable in Crohn's disease because remission may be achieved with parenteral nutrition in about one-half of patients.[27] In some patients, the disease may worsen when parenteral nutrition is stopped. Patients with enterocutaneous fistulas of various etiologies have been reported to benefit from parenteral nutrition.[27] Parenteral nutrition may also be valuable in children or adolescents with growth retardation associated with Crohn's disease, but surgery is usually necessary with severe disease. Finally, when possible, home parenteral institution should be used for patients requiring long-term therapy, particularly with "short gut."

SURGERY

Surgical procedures have an established place in the treatment of IBD. Although surgery (proctocolectomy) is curative for ulcerative colitis, this is not the case for Crohn's disease. Surgical procedures involve resection of segments of intestine that are affected, as well as correction of complications (e.g., fistulas) or drainage of abscesses.

For ulcerative colitis, colectomy may be performed when the patient has disease uncontrolled by maximum medical therapy or when there are complications of the disease such as colonic perforation, toxic dilatation (megacolon), uncontrolled colonic hemorrhage, or colonic strictures. Colectomy may be indicated in patients with long-standing disease (greater than 8–10 years), as a prophylactic measure against the development of cancer, and in patients with premalignant changes (severe dysplasia) on surveillance mucosal biopsies. The most common surgical procedures include proctocolectomy, after which the patient is left with a permanent ileostomy, and abdominal colectomy, with removal of the mucosa of the rectum and anastomosis of an ileal pouch to the anus. The risk from surgery in these patients is relatively low if the operations are performed on a nonemergency basis.

The indications for surgery with Crohn's disease are not as well established as they are for ulcerative colitis, and surgery is usually reserved for the complications of the disease. A recognized problem with intestinal resection for Crohn's disease is the high recurrence rate. Surgery may be appropriate in well-selected patients who are documented to continue to have severe or incapacitating disease in spite of aggressive medical management. The surgical procedures performed include resections of the major intestinal areas of involvement. In some patients with severe rectal or perineal disease, diversion of the fecal stream is performed with a colostomy. Other indications for surgery include the finding of colon cancer, inflammatory mass, or intestinal perforations.

DRUG THERAPY

Drug therapy plays an integral part in the overall treatment of IBD. It is important to emphasize that none of the drugs used for IBD is curative; at best they serve to control the disease process. Therefore, a reasonable goal of drug therapy is resolution of disease symptoms such that the patient can carry on normal daily functions. The major types of drug therapy used in IBD include aminosalicylates, corticosteroids, immunosuppressives (azathioprine, mercaptopurine, cyclosporin A), antimicrobials (metronidazole), and other agents used investigationally, such as immune enhancers (e.g., levamisole or bacillus Calmette-Guérin, BCG) and mast cell stabilizers (cromolyn sodium).

Sulfasalazine, an agent that combines a sulfonamide (sulfapyridine) antibiotic and 5-aminosalicylic acid (5-ASA, mesalamine) in the same molecule, has been used for many years to treat IBD. The agent has a unique route of disposition in the body that relates to its effectiveness in treating IBD. When administered orally, sulfasalazine is absorbed intact from the small bowel. Most of the drug is then excreted unchanged in the bile where it then progresses to the colon. In the colon, sulfasalazine is cleaved by gut bacteria to sulfapyridine (which is mostly reabsorbed and excreted in the urine) and 5-ASA (which mostly remains in the colon and is excreted in stool). When given by mouth, however, both sulfapyridine and 5-ASA are absorbed in the small bowel and excreted primarily in the urine.

The active component of sulfasalazine is 5-ASA (mesalamine), which has a local anti-inflammatory effect on the lumen of the intestine; however, other mechanisms are still considered.[28] One theory holds that mesalamine's main beneficial effect is inhibition of prostaglandin synthetase and 5-lipoxygenase.[13] Alternative theories suggest that mesalamine inhibits the migration of inflammatory cells into the bowel wall[29] or that it acts as a superoxide-free radical scavenger.[30] As the mechanism of action of sulfasalazine is not related to the sulfapyridine component and as sulfapyridine is believed responsible for many of the adverse reactions to sulfasalazine, new 5-aminosalicylate derivatives have been developed. Mesalamine (5-aminosalicylate) has been used topically as an enema for the treatment of proctitis. Oral derivatives of 5-aminosalicylate have also been developed. Olsalazine is a dimer of two 5-aminosalicylate molecules linked by an azo bond. With this product there is minimal GI absorption. Mesalamine is released in the colon after olsalazine is acted on by bacteria. Other products have used inert, pH-dependent coatings to delay 5-aminosalicylate release until the tablet reaches the small bowel (Table 34.4).

Corticosteroids and adrenocorticotropic hormone (ACTH) have been widely used for the treatment of ulcerative colitis and Crohn's disease. There has been a long-standing controversy as to the relative merits of corticosteroids versus ACTH; however, most clinicians currently prefer corticosteroids.[31] ACTH may be more effective in patients who have not previously received steroids.[32–34] Although ACTH is administered parenterally, corticosteroids may be given parenterally, orally, and/or rectally. The exact mechanism of action of corticosteroids is not

TABLE 34.4. MESALAMINE DERIVATIVES FOR TREATMENT OF INFLAMMATORY BOWEL DISEASE

Product	Trade Name(s)	Formulation	Dose/Day	Site of Action
Sulfasalazine	Azulfidine	Tablet	1–4 g	Colon
Mesalamine	Rowasa, Salofalk, Claversal, Pentasa	Enema	1–4 g	Rectum, terminal colon
	Rowasa	Suppository	1 g	Rectum
	Asacol	5-ASA coated with Eudragit-S (delayed release acrylic resin)	2.4 g	Distal ileum and colon
	Claversal (Salofalk)	5-ASA coated with Eudragit-L (delayed release acrylic resin)	1–4 g	Ileum and colon
	Pentasa	5-ASA encapsulated in ethylcellulose microgranules (oral tablet)	1–4 g	Small bowel and colon
Olsalazine	Dipentum	Dimer of 5-ASA oral capsule	1–3 g	Colon
Balsalazide	Colazide	Capsule	2.16 g	Colon

known but is believed to involve modulation of the immune system.

Immunosuppressive agents such as azathioprine and 6-mercaptopurine (a metabolite of azathioprine) are sometimes used for the treatment of IBDs. These agents are generally reserved for cases that are refractory to steroids and may be associated with serious adverse effects such as lymphomas, pancreatitis, or nephrotoxicity. The agents are usually used in conjunction with mesalamine derivatives and/or steroids and must be used for long periods of time (up to 6 months) before benefits may be observed.[35] The proper role for these agents in the treatment of ulcerative colitis has not been determined.

Antimicrobial agents, particularly metronidazole, are frequently used in attempts to control Crohn's disease. Metronidazole has been demonstrated to be of value in some patients with active Crohn's disease, particularly that involving the perineal area or fistulas.[36] The mechanism of metronidazole's effect on Crohn's disease has not been determined but is theorized to relate to interruption of a bacterial role in the inflammatory process. Although other antimicrobial agents have been studied, none has gained as much attention as metronidazole.

Other agents that have been investigated for treatment of IBD include mast cell stabilizers, such as cromolyn sodium, bile salt sequestrants, such as cholestyramine, and sucralfate. These agents have not resulted in consistent improvement in patients with IBD and cannot be recommended for routine use.

Drug treatment is differentiated by the type of IBD, as well as by the extent of disease, principal site of inflammation, and degree of severity. The data employed to support the use of an agent in one type of disease, or even in a subset of a specific type of IBD, should not be used to justify use under other conditions.

Ulcerative Colitis

Mild to Moderate Disease

The majority of patients with active ulcerative colitis are considered to have mild to moderate disease. These patients do not require parenteral medications. The first line of drug therapy for the patient with mild to moderate colitis is oral sulfasalazine or an oral mesalamine derivative. For proctitis the preferred therapy is rectally administered steroids or mesalamine. The value of sulfasalazine for treatment of ulcerative colitis has been documented in early studies that compared the agent with placebo.[37,38] From these reports and others it has been recognized that usually 4 g/d, and up to 8 g/d, of sulfasalazine is required to attain control of active inflammation. There does not appear to be an increased rate of response with increased dosage over 4 g/d. Even with the use of adequate doses, patient improvement usually takes 2 to 3 weeks and sometimes up to 4 weeks. The dosage of sulfasalazine that can be given is usually limited by the patient's tolerance of the agent; most adverse effects of sulfasalazine are dose related.[39] Sulfasalazine therapy should be instituted at 500 mg/d and increased every few days up to 4 g or the maximum tolerated (up to 8 g/d).

Oral mesalamine derivatives (such as those listed in Table 34.4) are reasonable alternatives to sulfasalazine for treatment of ulcerative colitis. Most of these agents have been demonstrated to be effective for ulcerative colitis but no more effective than sulfasalazine.[40] A major reason for the use of one of these agents is intolerance to sulfasalazine. The majority of patients intolerant to sulfasalazine should tolerate one of the other oral mesalamine derivatives.

Olsalazine (a dimer of 5-ASA, given orally) has been demonstrated effective for treatment of mild to moderate ulcerative colitis. Of patients taking olsalazine, however, 15–25% experience severe diarrhea, often necessitating discontinuation of the drug. In some patients, combined use of oral sulfasalazine or olsalazine and rectal steroids or rectal 5-ASA may provide advantages.

Steroids have a place in the treatment of moderate to severe ulcerative colitis. Oral steroids (usually up to 1 mg/kg/d of prednisone equivalent) may be used for patients who do not have an adequate response to sulfasalazine. Prednisone dosages in the range of 40–60 mg/d have been superior to regimens of 20 mg/d in producing remission.[41] Overall, steroids and sulfasalazine appear to be equally efficacious; however, the response to steroids may be evident sooner.[42,43] The use of oral steroids as initial therapy for mild to moderate ulcerative colitis should be avoided, mainly because of the known risks of steroid use. If steroids are used to attain remission, tapered drug withdrawal should be accomplished to minimize steroid exposure.

Rectally administered steroids or mesalamine can be used as initial therapy for ulcerative proctitis or distal colitis. With these agents, local actions are believed to be responsible for drug effects. In a trial of 86 patients with mild to moderate colitis who received rectal hydrocortisone or 5-ASA, the latter agent was found superior (93% remission rate).[44]

The choice of rectally administered steroid has been a subject of debate as there is varying potential for systemic steroid absorption with different products. Although many steroids have been administered rectally, certain agents such as betamethasone-17-valerate, beclomethasone dipropionate, prednisolone metasulfobenzoate, prednisolone-21-phosphate, and budesonide have been used in attempts to reduce systemic steroid effects. Betamethasone-17-valerate appears to result in less adrenal suppression compared with prednisolone-21-phosphate.[45] Systemic side effects may be the least severe with beclomethasone dipropionate because this agent is rapidly metabolized by the gut wall and liver.[46,47] With whatever product is used rectally, the systemic effects are less severe than those of oral steroids of the same equivalent dose. Most patients do not experience adrenal suppression from rectal steroids. The use of rectal steroids may often result in reduction of the required oral dose.

A number of investigational drug therapies have been studied for ulcerative colitis. Cyclosporine (usually given as an enema) has gained increasing attention for the treatment of ulcerative colitis. To date, relatively small studies have demonstrated a beneficial effect of cyclosporine enemas for distal colitis.[48] One of the potential benefits of cyclosporine is a more rapid onset of action (usually within 1 to 2 weeks) compared with azathioprine or 6-mercaptopurine. Nicotine has been proposed as a treatment for ulcerative colitis (but not Crohn's disease) since the observation of onset of ulcerative colitis after smoking cessation in some individuals. Transdermal nicotine has been shown to improve symptoms of patients with active ulcerative colitis (when given along with mesalamine).[15]

Severe or Intractable Disease

Patients with uncontrolled severe colitis or incapacitating symptoms require hospitalization for effective management. Under these conditions, patients generally receive nothing by mouth to put the bowel at rest; however, one study has demonstrated the benefit of enteral nutrition in these patients.[26] Most medication is given by the parenteral route. With severe colitis, there is a much greater reliance on parenteral steroids and surgical procedures. Sulfasalazine or mesalamine derivatives have not been proven beneficial for treatment of severe colitis. The reason for this may relate to rapid elimination of these agents from the colon with diarrhea, thereby not allowing sufficient time for gut bacteria to cleave the molecules.[49] Overall, it is very difficult to evaluate drugs in this setting, because patients with severe disease almost always receive additional medications including steroids. In one trial, sulfasalazine did not demonstrate added benefit when combined with steroids.[50]

Steroids have been valuable in the treatment of severe disease because the use of these agents may allow some patients to avoid colectomy. A trial of steroids is warranted in most patients before proceeding to colectomy, unless the condition is grave or rapidly deteriorating. In one trial of 87 patients with severe colitis, the use of intravenous steroids and parenteral nutrition resulted in remission in 60% of patients, with only 5% of those requiring colectomy after 6 weeks.[51] The dose of steroid generally used is 1 mg/kg of prednisone equivalent daily, although some patients may require much less or much more for satisfactory control. With higher doses, however, steroid side effects may limit drug benefits. The length of the medical trial before consideration of surgery is open to debate. When steroids must be used, it is well recognized that they may mask such complications as intra-abdominal sepsis. Steroids also increase surgical risk, particularly infectious risk, if an operation is required later. After a colectomy is performed, steroids should no longer be required for the disease; however, they must be withdrawn gradually (usually over 3 to 4 weeks) to avoid hypoadrenal crisis from adrenal suppression. Adler and Korelitz[52] recently reported that 6-mercaptopurine was effective in reducing steroid dosage in 61% of patients with refractory ulcerative colitis.

A major development in the treatment of severe ulcerative colitis refractory to steroids has been intravenous cyclosporine.[53] Continuous intravenous infusion of cyclosporine (4 mg/kg/d) was rapidly effective in steroid-resistant ulcerative colitis and reduced the need for colectomy.[54] Intravenous cyclosporine has been recommended for all patients with active ulcerative colitis refractory to steroids.[55]

Maintenance of Remission

Once remission from active disease has been achieved, the goal of therapy is to maintain remission. The major agents used for maintenance of remission are sulfasalazine and the mesalamine derivatives; steroids usually do not have a role. The value of sulfasalazine in preventing recurrences has been documented in placebo-controlled trials. Misiewicz and associates[56] found that one-fourth of patients taking sulfasalazine (2 g/d) had a relapse within 1 year, while three-fourths of patients taking placebo had a relapse.

Olsalazine, Pentasa (a slow-release oral form of mesalamine), and mesalamine enema have also been demonstrated effective for maintaining remission in patients with ulcerative colitis. In one trial of 164 patients, olsalazine given 500 mg twice daily and sulfasalazine given 1 g twice daily had 6-month relapse rates of 19.5% and 12.2%, respectively (not significant).[57] Pentasa, given 500 mg three times daily, was as effective as sulfasalazine, given 1 g three times daily, in maintaining remission (54% versus 46% in remission at 12 months, respectively).[58] Mesalamine coated with Eudragit-S (Asacol), 1.2 g daily, was found not as effective as olsalazine, 1 g daily, for prevention of relapses over a 12-month period.[59]

A major question about the use of sulfasalazine for maintenance of remission with ulcerative colitis is the duration of the preventive regimen. In one trial, the rate of recurrence of acute colitis was the same with placebo or sulfasalazine after 1 year.[60] In another trial, the rate of recurrence was much greater with placebo compared with sulfasalazine for periods of 6 months to 3 years after a year of remission.[61] The efficacy of sulfasalazine appears to be related to dose administered, up to a point. In a trial to assess the effect of daily dosage on recurrence, patients received 1, 2, or 4 g of sulfasalazine per day. The recurrence rates were 33%, 14%, and 9%, respectively. The 4 g/d regimen resulted in intolerable side effects in about one-fourth of patients.

Steroids do not have a role in the maintenance of remission with ulcerative colitis because they have been demonstrated to be ineffective.[35,62] Steroids should be gradually withdrawn after remission is induced (over 3 to 4 weeks). If they are continued, the patient will be exposed to steroid side effects without likelihood of benefits. For patients who require chronic steroid use (>20 mg/d), there is a strong justification for colectomy. Azathioprine has been demonstrated effective in preventing relapse of ulcerative colitis for periods of up to 2 years.[63] However, 3 to 6 months may be required for beneficial effect.

Crohn's Disease

Management of Crohn's disease often proves more difficult than that of ulcerative colitis, partly because of the greater complexity of presentation with Crohn's disease. The disease may be found to involve any segment of the GI tract, from mouth to anus, and may involve other visceral structures and soft tissues through fistulization. There is a greater reliance on drug therapy with Crohn's disease, because resection of all involved intestine may not be possible and recurrence after surgery is possible. Also, it is more difficult to evaluate the published literature with this disease because there is a large diversity in presentation and trial groups may involve widely differing patients.

Active Crohn's Disease

The goal of treatment for active Crohn's disease is to achieve remission; however, in many patients, reduction of symptoms so that the patient may carry out normal activities or reduction of the steroid dose required for control is a significant accomplishment. In the majority of patients, active Crohn's disease is treated with sulfasalazine, mesalamine derivatives, or steroids, although azathioprine, 6-mercaptopurine, or metronidazole are frequently used.

The role of sulfasalazine in the treatment of active Crohn's disease is accepted but not as well established as its role in the treatment of ulcerative colitis. It appears that sulfasalazine is more effective when Crohn's disease involves the colon[23] and in patients who have not undergone surgery for their disease.[64] In these circumstances, sulfasalazine has been reported to be as effective as prednisone.[23,65] There is limited information also suggesting the benefit of sulfasalazine in ileal Crohn's disease.[66] Other mesalamine derivatives (such as Pentasa or Asacol) that release mesalamine in the small bowel may be more effective than sulfasalazine for ileal involvement. In a trial of 310 patients with active Crohn's disease, Pentasa alone was more effective than placebo in achieving remission in a 16-week trial (43% versus 18%, respectively).[67] This beneficial effect was dose dependent and greatest with a dose of 4 g/d. The regimen was well tolerated by most patients. It appears reasonable to initiate a trial of sulfasalazine or oral mesalamine derivative in patients with mild to moderate Crohn's disease, particularly when the colon is involved. A course of steroids would be appropriate in patients who then cannot be controlled. When a patient is maintained on steroids, however, there appears to be no benefit from the addition of sulfasalazine.[50]

Steroids are frequently used for the treatment of active Crohn's disease, particularly with more severe presentations. In the National Cooperative Crohn's Disease Study[23] prednisone was documented to be significantly more effective than placebo in achieving remission. In this trial, the prednisone doses were 0.25 mg/kg/d for mild disease, 0.5 mg/kg/d for moderate disease, and 0.75 mg/kg/d for severe disease. Prednisone was found to be effective for disease limited to the small bowel. The major limitation of steroids is the risk of adverse effects with long-term use.

The European Cooperative Crohn's Disease Study Group examined the effectiveness of 6-methylprednisolone and/or sulfasalazine.[24] They reported that the steroid provided a better overall response than sulfasalazine for treatment of active disease. The combination of steroid and sulfasalazine was more effective in previously untreated patients or in those with disease localized to the colon.

Steroids are preferred for treatment of severe Crohn's disease, mainly because these agents can be given parenterally and response to therapy may occur sooner. Once remission is achieved, however, it may prove difficult to reduce steroid dosage without reintroduction of active disease.

Metronidazole may be useful in some patients with Crohn's disease, particularly in patients with colonic involvement or those with perineal disease. In most patients, metronidazole would be added to sulfasalazine, a mesalamine derivative, or steroid therapy when those agents alone are not effective. In one trial, metronidazole was not significantly different from placebo in terms of clinical response scores; however, about one-half of patients on metronidazole had significant improvement.[68] In a comparative trial with sulfasalazine, metronidazole was found to be as effective overall, and more effective in patients with colonic disease. Metronidazole has also been reported effective in noncomparative trials for treatment of Crohn's disease with perineal involvement.[69] The role for metronidazole is not fully defined. It may deserve a trial as adjunctive therapy for patients with colonic or perineal disease, where satisfactory control is not gained with first-line agents, or in attempts to reduce steroid dosage.

The immunosuppressive agents (azathioprine and 6-mercaptopurine) are generally limited to use in patients not achieving adequate response to standard medical therapy, or to reduce steroid doses when toxic doses are required. Azathioprine has been determined effective for active disease when added to a steroid regimen.[70] When administered 2.5 mg/kg/d for 4 months the frequency of remission was significantly increased. The major benefits of azathioprine may be in allowing reduction of the steroid dosage.[71,72] Also, treatment with azathioprine may need to be continued for up to 6 months to observe a response.[35] 6-Mercaptopurine may have advantages over azathioprine for adjunctive treatment of Crohn's disease.[73] In one trial of patients already receiving sulfasalazine or prednisone, 6-mercaptopurine was compared with placebo.[74] Significant improvements were noted in the 6-mercaptopurine group, mainly in decreasing steroid requirement and in healing fistulas. One problem noted with 6-mercaptopurine was that more than 3 months was required to observe a response in 32% of patients. In a report of 20 years of experience with 148 patients, 6-mercaptopurine (50 mg/d for mean 34 months) was judged effective for reduction of steroid dosage or elimination of the need for steroids, healing of fistulas and abscesses, and healing of Crohn's disease of the stomach and duodenum.[75] Some investigators have suggested that azathioprine or 6-mercaptopurine should be started earlier in the course of treatment than has been traditional.

Cyclosporine has also demonstrated benefit in active Crohn's disease.[53] In a placebo-controlled trial improvement was noted with cyclosporine in patients who were resistant or intolerant to corticosteroids.[76] It appears that the dose of cyclosporine is important in determining efficacy. An oral dose of 5 mg/kg/d was not effective,[77] whereas 7.9 mg/kg/d was effective.[76] However, toxic effects limit application of the higher dosage. At present, the therapeutic blood or plasma concentration range for cyclosporine has not been established. When using cyclosporine, however, clinicians should recognize the accompanying risk of renal toxicity.

Maintenance of Remission

Prevention of recurrence of disease is clearly more difficult with Crohn's disease than with ulcerative colitis. In the past few years there has been increasing evidence that some agents, particularly sulfasalazine and oral mesalamine derivatives are effective in preventing acute recurrences in quiescent Crohn's disease.[77] The support for sulfasalazine has been largely anecdotal[78]; however, a trial of 232 patients demonstrated a lower relapse rate compared with placebo for up to 2 years when given 3 g/d.[79]

There is greater support for the use of oral mesalamine derivatives for maintenance of symptomatic remission. On average, oral mesalamine derivatives decrease recurrence rates by 40% compared with placebo in long-term studies.[77] In one trial of 161 patients in remission 2 g/d of mesalamine as Pentasa for 2 years resulted in a significantly reduced relapse rate when begun within 3 months of achieving remission.[80] In another trial of mesalamine as Asacol, 125 patients received 2.4 g/d or placebo for 12 months resulting in a significantly reduced relapse rate with Asacol.[81] Steroids also have no place in the prevention of recurrence of Crohn's disease; these agents do not appear to alter the long-term course of the disease.[82]

Azathioprine has been studied as an adjunctive agent for the treatment and prevention of Crohn's disease.[71,72] Although the published data are not consistent, there is evidence to suggest that azathioprine and 6-mercaptopurine are effective in maintaining remission in Crohn's disease.[83] This agent should be reserved for patients who cannot tolerate dosages of steroids required to control their disease and who are not good surgical candidates.

SELECTED COMPLICATIONS

TOXIC MEGACOLON

Toxic megacolon or "toxic colonic dilatation" is a serious complication of IBD that occurs in about 1% or 2% of patients with IBDs, particularly ulcerative colitis. As previously described, the patient with toxic megacolon is usually severely ill with fever, abdominal pain and distention, decreased bowel sounds, and is often dehydrated. Immediate and aggressive measures are required to minimize mortality.

The treatment required for toxic megacolon includes general supportive measures to maintain vital functions, consideration for early surgical intervention, and drugs (steroids and antimicrobials). Aggressive fluid and electrolyte management is required for dehydration. Fluids and electrolytes may be lost through vomiting, diarrhea, and nasogastric intubation, as well as through fluid accumulation in the bowel. When the patient has lost significant amounts of blood (through the rectum), blood replacement is also necessary. Opiates and anticholinergics should be discontinued because these agents enhance colonic dilatation, thereby increasing the risk of bowel perforation.

Steroids in high dosages should be administered intravenously to reduce acute inflammation. Doses as high as 2 mg/kg/d of prednisone equivalent have been recommended (generally administered as hydrocortisone).[7] The duration of steroid administration is not certain; however, most clinicians continue the high-dose steroids for up to 2 weeks after improvement is observed and then reduce the dosages (approximately 0.5 to 1 mg/kg/d) for a few additional weeks. Antimicrobial regimens that are effective against enteric aerobes and anaerobes (e.g., aminoglycoside with clindamycin or metronidazole, imipenem, or extended-spectrum penicillin with a β-lactamase inhibitor) should be administered from the time of diagnosis and continued until patient improvement is assured. The duration of the antimicrobial regimen (often 2 to 3 weeks) should be determined with consideration that there may be significant intra-abdominal contamination with signs and symptoms hidden by steroid effects.

Surgical intervention, mainly an abdominal colectomy with formation of an ileostomy, is an important consideration in patients with toxic megacolon and prevents death in some patients. Early surgical intervention in these patients may result in a reduced mortality rate. In most cases in which colectomy is performed in the face of toxic megacolon, there is a significant risk of operative complications, including postoperative infection.

SYSTEMIC MANIFESTATIONS

The common systemic manifestations of IBD include arthritis, anemia, skin manifestations such as erythema nodosum and pyoderma gangrenosum, uveitis, and liver disease. Certain of these problems may be related to the inflammatory process. For some of these manifestations, specific therapies can be instituted, while for others, treatment that is used for the GI inflammatory process also addresses the systemic manifestations.

Anemia may be a common problem where there is significant blood loss from the GI tract. When the patient can consume oral medication, ferrous sulfate should be administered. If the patient is not able to take oral medication and the patient's hematocrit is sufficiently low, blood transfusions may be required. Anemia may also be related to malabsorption of vitamin B_{12} or folic acid, so these may also be required.

There are no consistently recommended therapies for liver disease, skin manifestations, or uveitis associated with IBD. Some reports suggest that these manifestations are worse during exacerbations of the intestinal disease and that measures improving intestinal disease will improve these systemic manifestations. Unfortunately, this association has not been demonstrated consistently. Liver transplantation is being used more frequently for definitive treatment of sclerosing cholangitis. For arthritis associated with IBD, aspirin or other NSAID may be beneficial as would be steroids.

SPECIAL CONSIDERATIONS

PREGNANCY

Pregnancy, either the occurrence or consideration of, may cause significant concerns in the patient with IBD. Questions arise as to fertility in patients with IBD, the effect of pregnancy on the disease course, the effect of the disease on the outcome of pregnancy, and the effects of the drugs used in IBD on the fetus.[84]

It does not appear that patients with IBD are less fertile than women in general.[7,85] The rate of normal childbirth is similar to that for healthy populations. Some studies have noted, however, a greater rate of spontaneous abortions in patients with IBD. It does not appear that pregnancy affects the course of IBD. Patients who are pregnant experience recurrence rates similar to those of nonpregnant females. Also, there is no justification for therapeutic abortion with IBD because termination of the pregnancy has not been observed to improve the disease.

Steroids and sulfasalazine should be administered during pregnancy with the same guidelines that would be applied to the nonpregnant patient.[7,85] Steroids given systemically do not appear to be detrimental to the fetus. Sulfasalazine is generally well tolerated; however, there has been suggestion of increased frequency of congenital abnormalities when it is given during pregnancy.[86] Interestingly, sulfasalazine has also been reported to cause decreased sperm counts in males.[87] This effect is reversible on discontinuation of the drug. Immunosuppressive drugs (azathioprine and 6-mercaptopurine) may be associated with fetal deformities in humans; however, they have been used without detriment in some patients.[85]

Overall, drug therapy for IBD is not a contraindication for pregnancy, and most pregnancies are well managed in patients with these diseases. The indications for medical and surgical treatment are similar to those in the nonpregnant patient. If a patient has an initial bout of IBD during pregnancy, a standard approach to treatment should be initiated.

ADVERSE DRUG REACTIONS TO AGENTS USED FOR TREATMENT OF IBD

Drug intolerance often limits the usefulness of agents used to treat IBD. Many patients receiving sulfasalazine, corticosteroids, metronidazole, azathioprine, or 6-mercaptopurine experience some undesired effects. In some cases, these adverse effects can be significant and require discontinuation of the therapy. Knowledge of the common or important adverse reactions will assist in avoiding or minimizing their effects.

Sulfasalazine is often associated with adverse drug effects and these effects may be classified as either dose related or idiosyncratic. Dose-related side effects usually include GI disturbances such as nausea, vomiting, diarrhea, or anorexia, but may also include headache and arthralgia.[49,88] These adverse reactions tend to occur more commonly on initiation of therapy and decrease in frequency as therapy is continued. Patients may experience these adverse effects at the commonly used dosages. One approach to the management of these reactions is to discontinue the agent for a short period and then reinstitute therapy at a reduced dosage. Some have suggested that the rate of adverse effects may be related to the concentration of free sulfapyridine in serum, suggesting that the sulfa portion of the molecule is responsible for the adverse effects.[89]

Non–dose-related adverse effects include rash, fever, or hepatotoxicity most commonly (20–50% of patients), as well as relatively uncommon but serious reactions such as agranulocytosis, pancreatitis, thrombocytopenia, and toxic epidermal necrolysis.[90] For most patients with idiosyncratic reactions, sulfasalazine must be discontinued. In some patients who have experienced allergic reactions to sulfasalazine, a desensitization procedure can be instituted. By gradually increasing sulfasalazine dosage over weeks to months, patient tolerance has been improved.[91] Most of the idiosyncratic reactions observed with sulfasalazine are similar to those with the class of sulfonamides in general.

Oral mesalamine derivatives may impose a lower frequency of adverse effects compared with sulfasalazine. Many patients who are intolerant to sulfasalazine will tolerate oral mesalamine derivatives.[92] Olsalazine, however, may frequently (up to 25%) cause watery diarrhea, sometimes requiring drug discontinuation.[93,94]

Adverse reactions to corticosteroids have been well recognized and may occur when corticosteroids are used for any indication. There is a greater potential for adverse effects when corticosteroids are used for the treatment of IBD, however, because high doses must often be used for extended periods. In the National Cooperative Crohn's Disease Study, 50% of patients receiving high-dose steroid therapy experienced side effects as did one-third of the patients on the lower dose regimens for prophylaxis.[49] The well-appreciated adverse effects of corticosteroids include hyperglycemia, hypertension, osteoporosis, fluid retention and electrolyte disturbances, myopathies, psychosis, and reduced resistance to infection. In addition, corticosteroid use may cause adrenocortical suppression. Specific regimens for withdrawal of corticosteroid therapy have been suggested.[95] To minimize corticosteroid effects, clinicians have used alternate-day steroid therapy; however, some patients do not do well on the days when no steroid is given. For most patients, a single daily corticosteroid dose suffices, and divided daily doses are unnecessary.

Immunosuppressants such as azathioprine and 6-mercaptopurine have a significant potential for adverse reactions. Azathioprine causes bone marrow suppression and has been associated with lymphomas (in renal transplant patients) and pancreatitis. 6-Mercaptopurine causes adverse reactions similar to azathioprine; however, there are fewer reports of lymphomas with this agent. With 6-mercaptopurine, pancreatitis usually occurs within 1 month of initiating therapy and recurs if the patient is rechallenged.[96] In one trial, 10% of patients that received azathioprine or 6-mercaptopurine required discontinuation of treatment due to adverse effects.[97]

Most patients receiving metronidazole for Crohn's disease tolerate the agent fairly well; however, mild adverse effects occur frequently. They commonly include paresthesias and reversible peripheral neuropathy, metallic taste, urticaria, and glossitis.[36,98] Other effects include a disulfiram-like reaction if alcohol is ingested in conjunction.

Assessment of Therapeutic Outcomes

The success of therapeutic regimens to treat IBDs can be measured by patient-reported complaints, signs, and symptoms, direct physician examination (including endoscopy), history and physical examination, selected laboratory tests, and quality of life measures. Evaluation of IBD severity is difficult since much of the assessment is subjective. To create more objective measures, disease rating scales or indices have been created. The Crohn's Disease Activity Index (CDAI) is a commonly used scale, particularly for evaluation of patients during clinical trials.[99] The scale incorporates eight elements: (1) number of stools in the past 7 days, (2) sum of abdominal pain ratings from the past 7 days, (3) rating of general well-being in the past 7 days, (4) use of antidiarrheals, (5) body weight, (6) hematocrit, (7) finding of abdominal mass, and (8) a sum of symptoms present in the past week. Elements of this index provide a guide for those measures that may be useful in assessing the effectiveness of treatment regimens.

Standardized assessment tools have also been constructed for ulcerative colitis.[15,48] Elements in these scales include (1) stool frequency, (2) presence of blood in the stool, (3) mucosal appearance (from endoscopy), and (4) physician's global assessment based on physical examination, endoscopy, and laboratory data.

Additional studies that are often useful include direct endoscopic examination of affected areas and/or radiocontrast studies. For patients with acute disease, assessment of fluid and electrolyte status is important since these may be lost during diarrheal episodes. Other laboratory tests such as serum albumin, transferrin, or other markers of visceral protein status as well as markers of inflammation (e.g., the erythrocyte sedimentation rate) may be used.

Assessment of the IBD patient must include consideration for adverse drug effects. Given that many of the agents used have a relatively high probability of causing adverse effects, particularly corticosteroids and other immunosuppressive agents, patient assessment should include collection of history and physical and laboratory data that are necessary to prevent or recognize adverse drug effects.

Finally, a patient quality of life assessment should be performed regularly. Agents that appear clinically equivalent may differ substantially in resulting quality of life. Inquiry should be made regarding general well-being, emotional function, and social function. The latter may include assessment of the ability to perform routine daily functions, maintain occupational activities, sexual function, and recreation.

References

1. Wilks S, Moxon W. Lectures on Pathological Anatomy, 2nd ed. London, J and A Churchill, 1875.
2. Crohn BB. Granulomatous diseases of the large and small bowel. A historical survey. Gastroenterology 1967;52:767.
3. Kraft SC. Modern clinical aspects of inflammatory bowel disease. Radiol Clin North Am 1987;25:213–224.
4. Monk M, Mendeloff AI, Siegel CI, et al. An epidemiological study of ulcerative colitis and regional enteritis among adults in Baltimore: II. Social and demographic factors. Gastroenterology 1969;56:847–857.
5. Sedlack RE, Nobrega FT, Karland LT, et al. Inflammatory colon disease in Rochester, Minnesota, 1935–1964. Gastroenterology 1972;62:935–941.
6. Whelan G. Epidemiology of inflammatory bowel disease. Med Clin North Am 1990;74:1–12.
7. Cello JP. Ulcerative colitis, in Sleisenger MH, Fordtran JS (eds): Gastrointestinal Disease. Philadelphia, WB Saunders, 1983, pp 1122–1168.
8. Elson CO. The immunology of inflammatory bowel disease, in Kirsner JB, Shorter RG (eds): Inflammatory Bowel Disease. Philadelphia, Lea & Febiger, 1988, pp 97–164.
9. Shanahan F. Pathogenesis of ulcerative colitis. Lancet 1993;342:407–411.
10. Gorbach SI. Intestinal microflora in inflammatory bowel disease—implications for etiology, in Kirsner JB, Shorter RG (eds): Inflammatory Bowel Disease. Philadelphia, Lea & Febiger, 1988, pp 51–64.
11. Hellers G, Bernell O. Genetic aspects of inflammatory bowel disease. Med Clin North Am 1990;74:13–19.
12. Podolsky DK. Inflammatory bowel disease. First of two parts. N Engl J Med 1991;325:928–937.
13. Podolsky DK. Inflammatory bowel disease. Second of two parts. N Engl J Med 1991;325:1008–1015.
14. Boyko ES, Koesell TD, Perera DR, Inui TS. Risk of ulcerative colitis among former and current cigarette smokers. N Engl J Med 1987;316:707–710.
15. Pullan RD, Rhodes J, Ganesh S, et al. Transdermal nicotine for active ulcerative colitis. N Engl J Med 1994;330:811–815.
16. Lichenstein JE. Radiologic-pathologic correlation of inflammatory bowel disease. Radiol Clin North Am 1987;25:3–24.
17. Monsen V, Sorstad J, Hellers G, et al. Extracolonic diagnosis in ulcerative colitis: An epidemiologic study. Am J Gastroenterol 1990;85:711–716.
18. Mayer L, Janowitz H. Extraintestinal manifestations of inflammatory bowel disease, in Kirsner JB, Shorter RG (eds): Inflammatory Bowel Disease. Philadelphia, Lea & Febiger, 1988, pp 299–317.
19. Rankin GB. Extraintestinal and systemic manifestations of inflammatory bowel disease. Med Clin North Am 1990;74:39–50.
20. Glick SN. Crohn's disease of the small intestine. Radiol Clin North Am 1987;25:25–45.
21. Edwards FC, Truelove SC. The cause and prognosis of ulcerative colitis. I. Short-term prognosis. Gut 1964;4:299.
22. Janowicz HD. The "natural history" of inflammatory bowel disease and therapeutic decisions. Am J Gastroenterol 1987;82:498–503.
23. Summers RW, Switz DM, Sessions JT, et al. National Cooperative Crohn's Disease Study: Results of drug treatment. Gastroenterology 1979;77:847–869.
24. Malchow H, Ewe K, Brandes JW, et al. European Cooperative Crohn's Disease Study (ECCDS): Results of drug treatment. Gastroenterology 1984;86:249–266.
25. Stenson WF, Cort D, Rogers J, et al. Dietary supplementation with fish oil in ulcerative colitis. Ann Intern Med 1992;116:609–614.
26. Gonzalez-Huix F, Fernandez-Banares F, Esteve-Comas M, et al. Am J Gastroenterol 1993;88:227–232.
27. Clouse RE, Rosenberg IH. Intensive nutritional support, in Sleisenger MH, Fordtran JS (eds): Gastrointestinal Disease. Philadelphia, WB Saunders, 1983, pp 1831–1850.
28. Klotz U, Maier K, Fischer C, et al. Therapeutic efficacy of sulfasalazine and its metabolites in patients with ulcerative colitis and Crohn's disease. N Engl J Med 1980;303:1499–1502.
29. Sack DM, Peppercorn MA. Drug therapy of inflammatory bowel disease. Pharmacotherapy 1983;3:158–176.
30. Ruderman WB. Newer pharmacologic agents for therapy of inflammatory bowel disease. Med Clin North Am 1990;74:133–153.
31. Peppercorn MA. Role of corticotropin therapy in ulcerative colitis: The controversy continues. Gastroenterology 1983;85:472–475.
32. Meyers S, Sachar DB, Goldberg JD, Janowitz HD. Corticotropin versus hydrocortisone in the intravenous treatment of ulcerative colitis. A prospective, randomized, double-blind trial. Gastroenterology 1983;85:351–357.
33. Kaplan HP, Portnoy B, Binder HJ, et al. A controlled evaluation of intravenous adrenocorticotropic hormone and hydrocortisone in the treatment of acute colitis. Gastroenterology 1975;69:91–95.
34. Powell-Tuck J, Buckness NA, Lennard-Jones JE. A controlled comparison of corticotropin and hydrocortisone in the treatment of severe proctocolitis. Scand J Gastroenterol 1977;12:971–975.
35. Ginsburg AL. The azathioprine controversy. Dig Dis Sci 1981;26:364–371.
36. Jakobovits J, Schuster MM. Metronidazole therapy for Crohn's disease and associated fistulae. Am J Gastroenterol 1984;79:533–540.
37. Baron JH, Connell AM, Lennard-Jones JE, et al. Sulfasalazine and salicylazosulphadimidine in ulcerative colitis. Lancet 1962;1:1094–1096.
38. Dick AP, Grayson MJ, Carpenter RG, et al. Controlled trial of sulfasalazine in the treatment of ulcerative colitis. Gut 1964;5:437–441.
39. Das KM. Pharmacotherapy of inflammatory bowel disease. Part 1. Sulfasalazine. Postgrad Med 1983;74:141–151.
40. Sutherland LR, May GR, Shaffer EA. Sulfasalazine revisited: A meta-analysis of 5-aminosalicylic acid in the treatment of ulcerative colitis. Ann Intern Med 1993;118:540–549.
41. Powell-Tuck J, Brown RL, Lennard-Jones JE. A comparison of oral prednisone given as single or multiple daily doses for active proctocolitis. Scand J Gastroenterol 1975;13:833–837.

42. Lennard-Jones JE, Longmore AJ, Newell AC, et al. Assessment of prednisone, salazopyrin, and topical hydrocortisone hemisuccinate used as outpatient treatment for ulcerative colitis. Gut 1960;1:217–222.
43. Truelove SC, Watkinson G, Draper G. Comparison of corticosteroid and sulphasalazine therapy in ulcerative colitis. Br Med J 1962;2:1708–1711.
44. Campieri M, Lanfranchi GA, Bazzocchi G, et al. Treatment of ulcerative colitis with high-dose 5-aminosalicyclic acid enemas. Lancet 1981;2:270–271.
45. Anonymous. Multicentre trial. Betamethasone-17-valerate and prednisolone-21-phosphate retention enemata in proctocolitis. Br Med J 1971;3:84–86.
46. Kumana CR, Seaton T, Meghi M, et al. Beclomethasone dipropionate enemas for treating bowel disease without producing Cushing's syndrome or hypothalamic-pituitary suppression. Lancet 1982;1:579–582.
47. Bansky G, Buhler H, Stamm B, et al. Treatment of distal ulcerative colitis with beclomethasone enemas: High therapeutic efficacy without endocrine side effects. Dis Colon Rectum 1987;30:288–292.
48. Sandborn WJ, Tremaine WJ, Schroeder KW, et al. Cyclosporine enemas for treatment-resistant, mildly to moderately active, left sided ulcerative colitis. Am J Gastroenterol 1993;88:640–645.
49. Azad Khan AK, Truelove SC. Circulating levels of sulphasalazine and its metabolites and their relation to the clinical efficacy of the drug in ulcerative colitis. Gut 1980;21:706–710.
50. Singleton JW, Law DH, Kelley ML, et al. National Cooperative Crohn's Disease Study: Adverse reactions to study drugs. Gastroenterology 1979;77:870–882.
51. Truelove SC, Willoughby CP, Lee EG, et al. Further experience in the treatment of severe attacks of ulcerative colitis. Lancet 1978;2:1086–1088.
52. Adler DJ, Korelitz BI. The therapeutic efficacy of 6-mercaptopurine in refractory ulcerative colitis. Am J Gastroenterol 1990;85:717–721.
53. Sandborn WJ, Tremaine WJ. Cyclosporine treatment of inflammatory bowel disease. Mayo Clin Proc 1992;67:981–990.
54. Lichtiger S, Present DH, Kornbluth A, et al. Cyclosporine in severe ulcerative colitis refractory to steroid therapy. N Engl J Med 1994;330:1841–1845.
55. Present DH. Cyclosporine and other immunosuppressive agents: Current and future role in the treatment of inflammatory bowel disease. Am J Gastroenterol 1993;88:627–630.
56. Misiewicz JJ, Lennard-Jones JE, Connell AM, et al. Controlled trial of sulphasalazine in maintenance therapy for ulcerative colitis. Lancet 1965;1:185–188.
57. Ireland A, Mason CH, Jewell DP. Controlled trial comparing olsalazine and sulfasalazine for maintenance treatment of ulcerative colitis. Gut 1988; 29:835–837.
58. Mulder CJ, Tytgat GNJ, Weterman IT, et al. Double-blind comparison of slow-release 5-aminosalicylate and sulfasalazine in remission maintenance in ulcerative colitis. Gastroenterology 1988;95:1449–1453.
59. Courtney MG, Nunes DP, Bergin CF, et al. Randomized comparison of olsalazine and mesalamine in prevention of relapses in ulcerative colitis. Lancet 1992;339:1279–1281.
60. Riis P, Anthonisen P, Wulff HR, et al. The prophylactic effect of salazosulphapyridine in ulcerative colitis during long-term treatment: A double-blind trial on patients symptomatic for 1 year. Scand J Gastroenterol 1973;8:71–75.
61. Dissanayake PS, Truelove SC. A controlled therapeutic trial of long-term maintenance treatment of ulcerative colitis with sulphasalazine (salazopyrin). Gut 1973;14:923–926.
62. Lennard-Jones JE, Misiewicz JJ, Connell AM, et al. Prednisone as maintenance treatment for ulcerative colitis in remission. Lancet 1965;1:199–209.
63. Hawthorne AB, Logan RFA, Hawkey CJ. Randomized controlled trial of azathioprine withdrawal in ulcerative colitis. Br Med J 1992;305:20–22.
64. Anthonisen P, Baraby F, Folkenborg O, et al. The clinical effect of salazosulphapyridine (salazopyrin) in Crohn's disease. Scand J Gastroenterol 1974;9:549–554.
65. Van Hees PA, Van Lier HJ, Van Elteren PH, et al. Effect of sulphasalazine in patients with active Crohn's disease: A controlled double-blind study. Gut 1981;22:404–409.
66. Goldstein F, Farquhar S, Thornton JJ, et al. Favorable effects of sulfasalazine on small-bowel Crohn's disease. A long-term study. Am J Gastroenterol 1987;82:848–853.
67. Singleton JW, Hanauer SB, Gitnick GL, et al. Mesalamine capsules for the treatment of active Crohn's disease: Results of a 16-week trial. Gastroenterology 1993;104:1293–1301.
68. Blichfeldt PER, Blomhoff JP, Myhre E, et al. Metronidazole in Crohn's disease: A double-blind cross-over trial. Scand J Gastroenterol 1978;13:123–127.
69. Bernstein LH, Frank MS, Brandt LJ, et al. Healing of perineal Crohn's disease with metronidazole. Gastroenterology 1980;79:357–365.
70. Ewe K, Press AG, Singe CC, et al. Azathioprine combined with prednisolone or monotherapy with prednisolone in active Crohn's disease. Gastroenterology 1993;105:367–372.
71. Willoughby JMT, Kumar Praveen J, Beckett J, et al. Controlled trial of azathioprine in Crohn's disease. Lancet 1971;2:294.
72. Rosenberg JL, Levin B, Wall AJ, et al. A controlled trial of azathioprine in Crohn's disease. Dig Dis Sci 1975;20:721.
73. Korelitz BI. Pharmacotherapy of inflammatory bowel disease. Part 3. 6-Mercaptopurine. Postgrad Med 1983;74:165–172.
74. Present DH, Korelitz BI, Wisch N, et al. Treatment of Crohn's disease with 6-mercaptopurine: A long-term, randomized, double-blind study. N Engl J Med 1980;302:981–987.
75. Korelitz BI, Adler DJ, Mendelsohn RA, Sacknoff AL. Long-term experience with 6-mercaptopurine in the treatment of Crohn's disease. Am J Gastroenterol 1993;88:1198–1205.
76. Brynskov J, Freund L, Rasmussen SN, et al. A placebo-controlled, double-blind, randomized trial of cyclosporine therapy in active chronic Crohn's disease. N Engl J Med 1989;321:845–850.
77. Stark ME, Tremaine WJ. Maintenance of symptomatic remission in patients with Crohn's disease. Mayo Clin Proc 1993;68:1183–1190.

78. Goldstein F. Maintenance treatment for Crohn's disease: Has the time arrived? Am J Gastroenterol 1992;87:551–556.
79. Ewe K, Herfarth C, Malchow H, Jesdinsky HJ. Postoperative recurrence of Crohn's disease in relation to radicality of operation and sulfasalazine prophylaxis: A multicenter trial. Digestion 1989;42:224–232.
80. Gendre JP, Mary JY, Florent C, et al. Oral mesalamine (Pentasa) as maintenance treatment in Crohn's disease: A multicenter placebo-controlled study. Gastroenterology 1993;104:435–439.
81. Prantera C, Pallone F, Brunetti G, et al. Oral 5-aminosalicylic acid (Asacol) in the maintenance treatment of Crohn's disease. Gastroenterology 1992;103:363–368.
82. Allen R, Steinberg DM, Williams JA, et al. Crohn's disease involving the colon: An audit of clinical management. Gastroenterology 1977;73:723–732.
83. Present DH. 6-Mercaptopurine and other immunosuppressive agents in the treatment of Crohn's disease and ulcerative colitis. Gastroenterol Clin North Am 1989;18:57–71.
84. Donaldson RM. Management of medical problems in pregnancy—inflammatory bowel disease. N Engl J Med 1986;312:1616–1619.
85. Baiocco P. Pregnancy and inflammatory bowel disease, in Korelitz BI, Sohn N (eds): Inflammatory Bowel Disease. Orlando, FL, Harcourt Brace Jovanovich, 1985, pp 91–95.
86. Willoughby JMT, Truelove SC. Ulcerative colitis and pregnancy. Gut 1980;21:469.
87. Toovey S, Hudson E, Hendry WF, et al. Sulfasalazine and male infertility: Reversibility and possible mechanism. Gut 1981;22:445–451.
88. Taffet SL, Das KM. Sulfasalazine: Adverse effects and desensitization. Dig Dis Sci 1983;28:833–842.
89. Das KM, Eastwood MA, McManus JPA, et al. Adverse reactions during salicylazosulfapyridine therapy and the relation with drug metabolism and acetylator phenotype. N Engl J Med 1973;289:491–495.
90. Goldman P, Peppercorn MA. Sulfasalazine. N Engl J Med 1975;293:20–23.
91. Korelitz BI, Present DH, Rubin PH, et al. Desensitization to sulfasalazine after hypersensitivity reactions in patients with inflammatory bowel disease. J Clin Gastroenterol 1984;6:27–31.
92. Linn FV, Peppercorn MA. Drug therapy for inflammatory bowel disease: Part I. Am J Surg 1992;164:85–89.
93. Feurle GE, Theuer D, Velasco S, et al. Olsalazine versus placebo in the treatment of mild to moderate ulcerative colitis: A randomized double-blind trial. Gut 1989;30:1354–1361.
94. Zinberg J, Molinas S, Das KM. Double-blind placebo-controlled study of olsalazine in the treatment of ulcerative colitis. Am J Gastroenterol 1990;85:562–566.
95. Byyny RL. Withdrawal from glucocorticoid therapy. N Engl J Med 1976;295:30–32.
96. Haber CJ, Meltzer SJ, Present DH, et al. Nature and course of pancreatitis caused by 6-mercaptopurine in the treatment of inflammatory bowel disease. Gastroenterology 1986;91:982–986.
97. O'Brien JJ, Bayless TM, Bayless JA. Use of azathioprine or 6-mercaptopurine in the treatment of Crohn's disease. Gastroenterology 1991;101:39–46.
98. Duffy LF, Daum F, Fisher SE, et al. Peripheral neuropathy in Crohn's disease patients treated with metronidazole. Gastroenterology 1984;88:681–684.
99. Best WR, Becktel JM, Singleton JW, et al. Development of a Crohn's disease activity index. Gastroenterology 1976;70:439–444.

Chapter 35

Nausea and Vomiting

A. Thomas Taylor, PharmD, and Eileen G. Holland, PharmD

Nausea and vomiting are common complaints among most individuals with gastrointestinal (GI) disorders. However, because of the variable etiologies of these problems, management may be quite simple or detailed and complex, essentially innocuous or associated with therapy-induced adverse reactions. This chapter provides an overview of nausea and vomiting, two multifaceted subjects.

Etiology

Nausea is usually defined as the inclination to vomit or as a feeling in the throat or epigastric region alerting an individual that vomiting is imminent. Vomiting is defined as the ejection or expulsion of gastric contents through the mouth, often requiring a forceful event. Both of these conditions may occur transiently with no other associated signs or symptoms; however, these conditions also may be only part of a more complex clinical presentation.

Nausea and vomiting may be associated with a variety of clinical presentations. In addition to numerous GI diseases, either or both may accompany cardiovascular, infectious, neurologic, or metabolic disease processes. Nausea and/or vomiting may be a feature of such conditions as pregnancy or may follow operative procedures or administration of certain medications such as those used in cancer chemotherapy. Psychogenic etiologies of these symptoms may be present, especially in young women with an underlying emotional disturbance. Anticipatory etiologies may be involved, such as in patients who have previously received cytotoxic chemotherapy. Specific etiologies associated with nausea and vomiting are presented in Table 35.1.[1]

In addition to identifying general areas associated with nausea and vomiting, it is important to address specific related medical problems. For example, nausea and/or vomiting may occur in as many as 70% of patients with inferior myocardial infarction or diabetic ketoacidosis. As many as 80–90% of patients with an Addisonian crisis, acute pancreatitis, or acute appendicitis may present with nausea and vomiting.

Drug-induced nausea and vomiting have been of particular interest, especially when caused by cytotoxic agents. The reasons for this awareness include the increasing number of patients receiving cytotoxic treatment and the number of agents implicated. Included in Table 35.2 are specific cytotoxic agents categorized by their emetogenic potential. Although some agents may have greater emetogenic potential than others, combinations of agents, high doses, clinical settings, psychologic conditions, prior treatment experiences, and unusual stimuli to sight, smell, or taste may alter a patient's response to a drug treatment. Not only are nausea and vomiting unpredictable, but also they may be unavoidable and potentially devastating to the continued delivery of care. Indeed, some patients may experience these problems so intensely that chemotherapy may be postponed or discontinued. In addition to the emetogenic potential of various cytotoxic regimens, a variety of other common etiologies have been proposed for the development of nausea and vomiting in cancer patients. These are presented in Table 35.3.[2]

The etiology of nausea and vomiting may vary with the age of the patient. For example, vomiting in the newborn during the first day of life suggests upper digestive tract obstruction or an increase in intracranial pressure. Other illnesses associated with vomiting in children include pyloric stenosis, duodenal ulcer, stress ulcer, adrenal insufficiency, septicemia, or diseases of the pancreas, liver, or biliary tree. Also, the hepatocellular failure seen in Reye's syndrome may lead to profound cerebral edema followed by persistent emesis. One of the most common etiologies of vomiting in children, however, is viral gastroenteritis caused by rotavirus. Vomiting in infants may also be associated with something as simple as overfeeding, rapid feeding, inadequate burping, or lying down too soon after feeding. It should be recognized that these types of vomiting are usually indicative of minor problems and may be altered by changing the approach to feeding.

Pathophysiology

The three consecutive phases of emesis include nausea, retching, and vomiting. Nausea, the imminent need to vomit, is associated with gastric stasis and may be considered a separate and singular symptom. Retching is the

TABLE 35.1. SPECIFIC ETIOLOGIES OF NAUSEA AND VOMITING

Gastrointestinal Mechanisms
- Mechanical gastric outlet obstruction
  - Peptic ulcer disease
  - Gastric carcinoma
  - Pancreatic disease
- Motility disorders
  - Gastroparesis
  - Drug-induced gastric stasis
  - Chronic intestinal pseudo-obstruction
  - Postviral gastroenteritis
  - Irritable bowel syndrome
  - Postgastric surgery
  - Idiopathic gastric stasis
  - Anorexia nervosa
- Intra-abdominal emergencies
  - Intestinal obstruction
  - Acute pancreatitis
  - Acute pyelonephritis
  - Acute cholecystitis
  - Acute cholangitis
  - Acute viral hepatitis
- Acute gastroenteritis
  - Viral gastroenteritis
  - Salmonellosis
  - Shigellosis
  - Staphylococcal gastroenteritis (enterotoxins)

Cardiovascular Diseases
- Acute myocardial infarction
- Congestive heart failure
- Shock and circulatory collapse

Neurologic Processes
- Midline cerebellar hemorrhage
- Increased intracranial pressure
- Migraine headache
- Vestibular disorders
- Head trauma

Metabolic Disorders
- Diabetes mellitus (diabetic ketoacidosis)
- Addison's disease
- Renal disease (uremia)

Psychogenic Causes
- Self-induced
- Anticipatory

Therapy-Induced Causes
- Cytotoxic chemotherapy
- Radiation therapy
- Theophylline preparations (intolerance, toxic)
- Anticonvulsant preparations (toxic)
- Digitalis preparations (toxic)
- Opiates
- Amphotericin
- Antibiotics

Drug Withdrawal
- Opiates
- Benzodiazepines

Miscellaneous Causes
- Pregnancy
- Any swallowed irritant (foods, drugs)
- Noxious odors
- Operative procedures

(Partially adapted from Hanson JS, McCallum RW. The diagnosis and management of nausea and vomiting: A review. Am J Gastroenterol 1985;80:210–218, with permission.)

TABLE 35.2. EMETOGENIC POTENTIAL OF CYTOTOXIC CHEMOTHERAPY

Most Emetogenic	Moderate	Least Emetogenic
Amsacrine	Azacytidine	Asparaginase
Cisplatin	Etoposide	Bleomycin
Cyclophosphamide	Mitomycin C	Busulfan
Dacarbazine	Procarbazine	Chlorambucil
Dactinomycin	Thiotepa	Cytarabine
Daunorubicin		Diaziquone
Doxorubicin		Estramustine
Hexamethylmethamine		Floxuridine
Mechlorethamine		Fluorouracil
Mitoxantrone		Hydroxyurea
Nitrosoureas		Melphalan
Streptozocin		Mercaptopurine
		Methotrexate
		Teniposide
		Thioguanine
		Vinca alkaloids

TABLE 35.3. NONCHEMOTHERAPY ETIOLOGIES OF NAUSEA AND VOMITING IN CANCER PATIENTS

Fluid and electrolyte abnormalities
- Hypercalcemia
- Volume depletion
- Water intoxication
- Adrenocortical insufficiency

Drug induced
- Opiates
- Antibiotics

Gastrointestinal obstruction
Increased intracranial pressure
Peritonitis
Metastases
- Brain
- Meninges
- Hepatic

Uremia
Infections (septicemia, local)
Radiation therapy

(Adapted from Frytak S, Moertel CG. Management of nausea and vomiting in the cancer patient. JAMA 1981;245:393–396, with permission. Copyright 1981, American Medical Association.)

labored movement of abdominal and thoracic muscles before vomiting. The final phase of emesis is vomiting, the forceful expulsion of gastric contents due to GI retroperistalsis. The act of vomiting requires the coordinated contractions of the abdominal muscles, pylorus, and antrum, a raised gastric cardia, diminished lower esophageal sphincter pressure, and esophageal dilatation.[3] Vomiting should not be confused with regurgitation, an act in which the gastric or esophageal contents rise to the pharynx because of pressure differences due to, for example, an incompetent lower esophageal sphincter. Accompanying autonomic symptoms of pallor, tachycardia, and diaphoresis account for many of the distressing feelings associated with emesis.

Vomiting is triggered by afferent impulses to the vomiting center, a nucleus of cells in the medulla. Impulses are received from sensory centers, such as the chemoreceptor trigger zone (CTZ), cerebral cortex, and visceral afferents from the pharynx and GI tract. When excited, afferent impulses are integrated by the vomiting center, resulting in efferent impulses to the salivation center, respiratory center, and the pharyngeal, GI, and abdominal muscles, leading to vomiting.

The CTZ, located in the area postrema of the fourth ventricle of the brain, is a major chemosensory organ for emesis and is usually associated with chemically induced vomiting. Due to its location, blood-borne and cerebrospinal fluid toxins have easy access to the CTZ. Therefore, cytotoxic agents stimulate primarily this area rather than the cerebral cortex and visceral afferents. Similarly, pregnancy-associated vomiting probably occurs through stimulation of the CTZ.

Numerous neurotransmitter receptors are located in the vomiting center, CTZ, and GI tract. Examples of such receptors include cholinergic and histaminic, dopaminergic, opiate, serotonin, and benzodiazepine receptors. It is theorized that chemotherapeutic agents, their metabolites, or other emetic compounds trigger the process of emesis through stimulation of one or more of these receptors. Effective antiemetics are able to antagonize or block the emetogenic receptors.

Anticipatory nausea and vomiting may be elicited either by specific stimuli associated with the administration of noxious, often cytotoxic, agents or by the anxiety associated with such treatments. Many patients demonstrate both types. The most often accepted theory for this pattern of conditioning is that by repeated pairing of chemotherapy and its aftereffects, previously neutral stimuli such as odors, sounds, and settings acquire the ability to elicit nausea and vomiting.[4,5] These types of stimuli should be expected to be most troublesome in patients receiving agents with the greatest inherent emetogenic potential.

CLINICAL PRESENTATION

Included in the GI etiologies of nausea and vomiting are a variety of specific disorders associated with mechanical obstruction, motility changes, and infectious diseases of the vital organs within the abdominal cavity. Although each of these conditions may vary in onset, duration, and severity of symptoms, each is nevertheless a potential source of nausea and vomiting that may need to be addressed. In this regard, attention to simultaneous signs and symptoms is helpful in making an accurate diagnosis and evaluation of a specific patient. Additional knowledge of a patient's GI history, with particular emphasis on the presence of abdominal pain or discomfort, diarrhea, and blood from the upper or lower GI tract, should always be sought. Knowledge of the patient's tolerance of food is important. Also, the timing of these symptoms in relation to meals as well as the consistency, content, odor, and frequency of the vomitus may be characteristic findings in certain conditions. Further information that may be helpful in understanding a specific clinical presentation includes concomitant findings such as fever or weight loss, a description of precipitating factors, a complete history of recent medication use, and the history or presence of myalgias, behavioral or visual changes, headache, or pain outside the abdomen.

Because it is impossible to discuss all clinical settings in which the presence of nausea and vomiting might be a pertinent finding, these processes are presented as they might occur together and also as *simple* or *complex* in presentation. Defined here, the term *simple* applies to those episodes of nausea and/or vomiting described by one of the following criteria: (1) occur occasionally and are self-limiting or relieved by the minimal use of antiemetic methods or medications; (2) account for little patient deterioration such as fluid–electrolyte imbalances, pain, or noncompliance with prescribed therapies; or (3) are not related to the administration of or exposure to noxious agents. Conversely, the term *complex* is used when describing a patient's clinical course as including symptoms that (1) are not adequately or readily relieved by the administration of a single antiemetic method or medication; (2) lead to progressive patient deterioration secondary to fluid–electrolyte imbalances, pain, or noncompliance with prescribed therapies; or (3) are caused by noxious agents or psychogenic events. Psychogenic vomiting is often related to sexual or marital disturbances, health problems of friends or family members, or deeper emotional strains. Pertinent features of this condition may include a positive family history of this condition. Episodes may be induced by meals, are recurrent, generally not accompanied by nausea, and may be suppressed by the patient. Often these events are not noted to be important by the patient. Unless associated with anorexia nervosa, appetite is usually normal. Many of these conditions subside with reductions in stress.

TREATMENT

Most episodes of nausea and vomiting decrease in frequency, duration, and severity as the underlying process resolves. However, during the recovery period, it may be desirable to combat the specific symptoms of nausea and vomiting. Most cases of nausea and vomiting are self-limiting, resolve spontaneously, and only require symptomatic therapy. Antiemetic therapy is indicated in patients with electrolyte disturbances secondary to vomiting, severe anorexia or weight loss, or progression of disease either due to refusal of continued therapy or poor nutritional status.

Although many approaches to the treatment of nausea and vomiting have been suggested, antiemetic drugs (over-the-counter [OTC] and prescription) are most often recommended. These agents represent a variety of pharmacologic and chemical classes as well as dosage regimens and routes of administration. With so many treatment possibilities available, factors that enable the clinician to discriminate among various choices must be recognized. These factors include (1) the suspected etiology of the symptoms; (2) the frequency, duration, and severity of the episodes; (3) the ability of the patient to use oral, rectal, injectable, or transdermal topical medications; and (4) the success of previous antiemetic medications. For example, many antiemetics are commercially available as oral agents. Provided a patient can and will adhere to oral dosing, a suitable and effective agent can often be selected; however, for certain other patients, oral medications may be inappropriate because of their inability to retain any appreciable oral ingestions. In these patients, rectal or injectable routes of administration might be preferred. Information concerning commonly available antiemetic preparations is compiled in Table 35.4.

Often an individual initially experiences nausea and vomiting at home or outside formal medical settings. For these symptoms, patients may choose from a lengthy list of OTC products. While suitable for occasional simple nausea and vomiting, OTC agents are often abandoned by the patient as symptoms continue or become progressively worse. As the patient's condition warrants, prescription medications may be chosen, either as single-agent therapy or in combination. For most conditions, a single-agent antiemetic is preferred; however, for those patients not responding to such therapy and those receiving highly emetogenic chemotherapy, multiple-agent regimens are usually recommended. Numerous combinations have been employed through clinical investigation and practice.

The treatment of simple nausea and vomiting usually requires minimal therapy. Products available for self-medication include antacids; antihistamine–anticholinergic agents such as cyclizine, dimenhydrinate, diphenhydramine, and meclizine; and phosphorated carbohydrate solutions. Agents requiring physician prescription include some antihistaminic–anticholinergic drugs and phenothiazine agents. These latter agents include benzquinamide, buclizine, parenteral dimenhydrinate and diphenhydramine, hydroxyzine, prochlorperazine, promethazine, and trimethobenzamide. Both OTC and prescription drugs useful in the treatment of simple nausea and vomiting are usually effective in small, infrequently administered doses. Side effects and toxic effects in these settings are also usually minimal.

The management of complex nausea and vomiting may require aggressive drug therapy, possibly with more than one antiemetic agent. For patients with complex symptoms, effective combinations may include two of the following drugs: benzquinamide, chlorpromazine, dimenhydrinate, droperidol, hydroxyzine, prochlorperazine, promethazine, thiethylperazine, or trimethobenzamide. In combination, each of these drugs is prescribed in small to moderate dosages, achieving symptomatic control through different pharmacologic mechanisms while avoiding the untoward effects caused by high doses. For patients receiving highly emetogenic chemotherapy, antiemetic regimens may include one or more of the following agents: prochlorperazine, metoclopramide, ondansetron, granisetron, dexamethasone, or lorazepam (see section on Chemotherapy-Induced Nausea and Vomiting).

ANTIEMETIC AGENTS

In general, the clinician should evaluate the patient's condition and determine the need for antiemetic treatment of an existing condition or prophylactic therapy to prevent or lessen anticipated nausea and vomiting episodes, as is seen in patients requiring cytotoxic drugs or operative procedures. Once this decision has been made, along with the complete and overall medical evaluation, the antiemetic selection process may proceed. Common antiemetic preparations are presented in Table 35.4.

Various antacids may be sought by patients experiencing simple nausea and vomiting. In this setting, single or combination OTC antacid products, especially those containing magnesium hydroxide, aluminum hydroxide, and/or calcium carbonate, may provide sufficient relief, primarily through gastric acid neutralization. Patients responding to small and occasional doses of antacids probably do not have significant pathology; however, it is not uncommon for patients with significant GI disease to self-medicate with larger and more frequent doses of antacids.

Common antacid dosage regimens for the relief of nausea and vomiting include one or more small doses of single- or multiple-agent products. Although antacid therapy may be aggressively applied for the treatment of known ulcer disease, OTC products sought by patients are usually taken in response to acute and sporadic episodes of nausea and vomiting. Depending on dose, common commercial products usually supply sufficient ingredients to allow a range of approximately 40–180 mEq of acid-neutralizing capacity.[6–8] Potential adverse effects from antacids are usually related to the presence of magnesium, aluminum, or calcium salts. Specifically, osmotic diarrhea from magnesium and constipation from aluminum or calcium salts may be of concern to patients, particularly those self-medicating or using high or frequently administered antacid doses. Generally, however, when used occasionally for acute episodic relief of nausea and vomiting, antacids do not produce serious toxicities.

Antiemetic drugs from the antihistaminic–anticholinergic category appear to interrupt various visceral afferent pathways that stimulate nausea and vomiting and may be appropriate in the treatment of simple symptomology. However, when used alone, each provides little efficacy in patients with more complex complaints such as those caused by cytotoxic chemotherapy. Adverse reactions that may be apparent with the use of the antihistaminic–anticholinergic agents primarily include drowsiness or confusion, blurred vision, dry mouth, urinary retention, and possibly tachycardia, particularly in elderly patients. Also, as doses are increased or are more frequently administered, patients with narrow-angle glaucoma, prostatic hyperplasia, or asthma are at greater risk of complications from the anticholinergic effects of these drugs.

Historically, phenothiazines have been the most widely prescribed antiemetic agents. These agents appear to block dopamine receptors, most likely in the CTZ. Some investigators have found phenothiazines to demonstrate greatest efficacy when compared with placebo and less efficacy when compared with other more potent antiemetics.[9–11] Phenothiazines are marketed in an array of dosage forms, none of which appears to be more efficacious than another; however, there are perhaps some important generalizations concerning their use in overall clinical practice. These agents may be most practical for long-term treatment and are inexpensive in comparison with newer drugs, with the exception of slow-release products that may be too costly and of no established clinical advantage. Little distinguishing information is available in the present literature concerning the efficacy of rectal preparations. Rectal administration is most preferred in patients in whom parenteral administration is impractical or oral medications cannot be retained and are therefore ineffective. In many patients, low doses of phenothiazine drugs may not be effective, while larger doses may produce unacceptable risks.[2] Phenothiazines are most useful in patients with simple nausea and vomiting or in those receiving mildly emetogenic doses of chemotherapy. Problems associated with these drugs include troublesome and potentially dangerous side effects, including extrapyramidal reactions, hypersensitivity reactions with possible liver dysfunction, marrow aplasia, and excessive sedation.

Two butyrophenone compounds have antiemetic activity, haloperidol and its congener droperidol. Each agent blocks dopaminergic stimulation of the CTZ. Although each agent is effective in relieving nausea and vomiting, droperidol has been used most often. Depending on its specific indication, the optimal dosage range may vary considerably. For example, preoperative doses may range from 2.5–10 mg, while dosage regimens during cytotoxic chemotherapy have been documented as low as 0.5–2.5 mg by intermittent injection to as great as 1.0–1.5 mg/h by intravenous infusion.[12–15] Adverse reactions resulting from the use of the butyrophenone compounds include primarily sedation and the possibility of dystonic reactions. Although dystonia may occur after the initial dose, some patients may experience this problem later in therapy. Injectable diphenhydramine usually rapidly resolves these extrapyramidal reactions.[13]

Corticosteroids have been used successfully in the management of chemotherapy-induced nausea and vomiting with few problems. However, reported adverse effects have included mood changes ranging from anxiety to euphoria as well as headache, metallic taste, abdominal discomfort, hyperglycemia, and itchy throat.[16] For patients with simple nausea and vomiting, steroids are not indicated and may be associated with unacceptable risks. As with other conditions, steroids should be employed only when the benefit-to-risk ratio is sufficient to warrant a medication with such complex and potentially deleterious effects. Metoclopramide, procainamide's congener, has been studied for its antiemetic effects. Its ability to block the dopaminergic receptors centrally in the CTZ as well as peripherally makes it an agent with documented and

TABLE 35.4. COMMON ANTIEMETIC PREPARATIONS AND ADULT DOSAGE REGIMENS

Drug (Brand Name)	Adult Dosage Regimen	Dosage Form/Route	Availability
Antacids			
Antacids (various)	15–30 mL every 2–4 h prn	Liquid	OTC
Antihistaminic–Anticholinergic Agents			
Benzquinamide (Emete-Con)	25–50 mg every 3–4 h prn	IM, IV	Rx
Buclizine (Bucladin-S)	50 mg twice daily	Tab	Rx
Cyclizine (Marezine)	50 mg every 4–6 h prn	Tab, IM	Rx/OTC
Dimenhydrinate (Dramamine)	50–100 mg every 4–6 h prn	Tab, chew tab, cap, liquid, IM, IV	Rx/OTC
Diphenhydramine (Benadryl)	10–50 mg every 4–6 h prn	Tab, cap, liquid, IM, IV	Rx/OTC
Hydroxyzine (Vistaril, Atarax)	25–100 mg every 6 h prn	Tab, cap, liquid, IM	Rx
Meclizine (Bonine, Antivert)	25–50 mg every 24 h prn	Tab, chew tab, cap	Rx/OTC
Promethazine (Phenergan)	12.5–25 mg every 4–6 h prn	Tab, liquid, IM, IV, supp	Rx
Pyrilamine (Nisaval)	25–50 mg three to four times daily	Tab	Rx/OTC
Scopolamine (Transderm Scop)	0.5 mg every 72 h prn	Transdermal patch	Rx
Trimethobenzamide (Tigan)	200–250 mg three to four times daily prn	Cap, IM, supp	Rx
Phenothiazines			
Chlorpromazine (Thorazine)	10–25 mg every 4–6 h prn	SR cap, tab, liquid, IM, IV	Rx
	50–100 mg every 6–8 h prn	Supp	Rx
Fluphenazine (Prolixin)	1.25–2.5 mg every 6–8 h prn	Tab, liquid, IM	Rx
Perphenazine (Trilafon)	8–30 mg/d divided prn	Tab, liquid, IM, IV	Rx
Prochlorperazine (Compazine)	5–10 mg three to four times daily prn	SR cap, tab, liquid, IM, IV	Rx
	25 mg twice daily prn	Supp	Rx
Promazine (Sparine)	25–50 mg every 4–6 h prn	Tab, IM	Rx
Thiethylperazine (Torecan)	10 mg three times daily	Tab, IM, supp	Rx
Cannabinoids			
Dronabinol (Marinol)	5–7.5 mg/m^2 every 2–4 h prn	Cap	Rx (C-II)
Nabilone (Cesamet)	1–2 mg two to three times daily prn	Cap	Rx (C-II)
Butyrophenones			
Droperidol (Inapsine)	2.5–5.0 mg every 4–6 h prn	IM, IV	Rx
Haloperidol (Haldol)	1–5 mg every 12 h prn	Tab, liquid, IM, IV	Rx

promising efficacy. Peripherally, metoclopramide increases lower esophageal sphincter tone, aids gastric emptying, and accelerates transit through the small bowel, possibly through the release of acetylcholine. Because the adverse reactions to metoclopramide include extrapyramidal effects, intravenous diphenhydramine 25–50 mg should be prophylactically administered or provided on-call for its anticipated need. Other adverse effects produced by metoclopramide include restlessness, drowsiness, fatigue, nausea, and diarrhea.[17,18]

Serotonin-receptor antagonists have become increasingly important to antiemetic therapy in recent years, particularly in the management of chemotherapy-induced and postoperative nausea and vomiting. Issues involved in the use of ondansetron and granisetron are reviewed in detail in the sections that follow.

A final group of antiemetic preparations available to patients complaining of nausea and vomiting necessitates some mention. First, the phosphorated carbohydrate solutions (mixtures of fructose, dextrose, and phosphoric acid) are available OTC and may be administered in 15- to 30-mL doses as often as every 3 hours or as needed. As one might predict from quick assessment of the ingredients, this mixture is intended only for mild and infrequent symptoms. Because of the inability of these agents to relieve significant symptoms, the solution should not be used in patients with complex problems, especially those receiving chemotherapy. However, this combination is safe and effective in patients with morning sickness. Adverse reactions to these solutions are most often noted as abdominal pain or diarrhea as a consequence of large doses of fructose or as lack of control in diabetic patients because of the

TABLE 35.4. (Continued)

Drug (Brand Name)	Adult Dosage Regimen	Dosage Form/Route	Availability
Corticosteroids			
Dexamethasone (Decadron)	10 mg prior to chemotherapy, repeat with 4–8 mg every 6 h for total of four doses	IV	Rx
Methylprednisolone (Solu-Medrol)	125–500 mg every 6 h for total of four doses	IV	Rx
Benzodiazepines			
Diazepam (Valium)	2–5 mg every 3 h	Tab	Rx (C-IV)
Lorazepam (Ativan)	0.5–4.0 mg prior to chemotherapy	IV	Rx (C-IV)
Selective Serotonin Antagonists			
Granisetron (Kytril), for CINV diluted, give over 5 min	10 mcg/kg prior to chemotherapy	IV	Rx
Ondansetron (Zofran), for CINV, IV diluted, give over 15 min	32 mg prior to chemotherapy as a single dose, or 0.15 mg/kg prior to chemotherapy, repeat at 4 and 8 h	IV	Rx
Ondansetron (Zofran), for CINV, oral	8 mg 30 min prior to chemotherapy, repeat at 4 and 8 h and every 8 h for 1–2 days after chemotherapy completion	Tab	Rx
Ondansetron (Zofran), for PONV, IV undiluted, give over 2–5 min	4 mg prior to induction of anesthesia or postoperatively	IV	Rx
Miscellaneous Agents			
Dextrose, fructose, phosphoric acid (Emetrol)	15–30 mL every 1–3 h prn	Liquid	OTC
Diphenidol (Vontrol)	25–50 mg every 4 h prn	Tab	Rx
Metoclopramide (Reglan)	1–2 mg/kg every 2 h × 2, then every 3 h × 3	IV	Rx

Key: Rx, prescription; OTC, over the counter; cap, capsule; chew tab, chewable tablet; IM, intramuscular; IV, intravenous; liquid, oral syrup, concentrate, suspension; SR cap, sustained-release capsule; supp, rectal suppository; tab, tablet; CINV, chemotherapy-induced nausea and vomiting; PONV, postoperative nausea and vomiting.

dextrose included in the formulations; however, with the use of small doses, most patients experience little benefit or adversity.

An agent that has received comparatively little attention in the antiemetic literature is diphenidol. Although this agent inhibits the CTZ as well as conduction in vestibular–cerebellar pathways and is indicated in most references for the management of nausea and vomiting associated with surgery, malignant neoplasms, antineoplastic chemotherapy, radiation sickness, infectious diseases, and labyrinthine disturbances, it should be used extremely cautiously. Diphenidol should be used only when there is a clear and unquestionable benefit potential. Even though it is an oral agent, this product should be utilized only in a hospital or under comparable conditions. The primary reason for these measures required for the use of diphenidol is its adverse reaction profile. Auditory and visual hallucinations, disorientation, and confusion have been reported and are the usual warnings against its use. These problems may be even more pronounced in elderly patients or those with declining renal function, because approximately 90% of diphenidol is excreted in the urine. Lastly, diphenidol should be avoided during pregnancy or lactation and in children weighing less than 50 pounds.

Pyridoxine has also been cited as an antiemetic agent; however, its efficacy has not been accepted beyond that of a placebo and probably has little place in the approach to simple or complex symptoms. In patients in whom it may offer benefit, its beneficial mechanism has been suggested to be restoration of depleted pyridoxine body stores.

CHEMOTHERAPY-INDUCED NAUSEA AND VOMITING

Information concerning antiemetic drug selection for patients with chemotherapy-induced nausea and vomiting is changing rapidly, and although newer agents may be readily acceptable in clinical practice, older agents may be appropriately prescribed. For example, prior to the use of metoclopramide, phenothiazine antiemetics were frequently chosen in patients with chemotherapy-induced nausea and vomiting. Even with newer therapies, if relief of symptoms is provided and side effects are absent or acceptable, these drugs may be continued. Conversely, failure to achieve adequate antiemetic efficacy during the first course of chemotherapy should prompt the clinician to search for more acceptable agents, possibly combination therapies.[10,11,19]

Droperidol, usually given intravenously, has been documented as safe and effective, even in ambulatory cancer patients.[12,20–22] Although the optimal antiemetic dose of droperidol for patients receiving chemotherapy is not well established, many patients benefit from small doses, particularly when combined with other antiemetic drugs.

Corticosteroids have demonstrated antiemetic efficacy since the initial recognition that patients receiving prednisone as part of their Hodgkin's disease protocol appeared to develop less nausea and vomiting than those treated with protocols excluding this agent. This is of particular interest because the alkylating agents often employed in such protocols rank high in emetogenicity, especially mechlorethamine and cyclophosphamide. Other corticosteroids that have shown efficacy include methylprednisolone and dexamethasone. The exact mechanism by which corticosteroids provide antiemetic activity is unknown; however, the inhibition of prostaglandin synthesis has been postulated and questioned.[16,23] Such mechanism theories are most appealing in light of the known high emetogenic potential of prostaglandins themselves; however, because of their numerous metabolic effects, a single site of steroid antiemetic activity may be difficult to locate or assess. In addition to the antiemetic benefits of corticosteroids, other desirable effects include increased appetite and an elevation of mood or feelings of well-being. Depending on the patient and the drug regimen, these effects may be the primary considerations for corticosteroid preferences.

A variety of study protocols have been employed in corticosteroid antiemetic clinical trials. Variations in drug, dosage regimen, and route of administration plague the unraveling of the clinical literature. Although studies utilizing steroids in both single- and multiple-agent protocols have demonstrated acceptable efficacy, their exact ranking among antiemetic alternatives is not clear for patients receiving cytotoxic chemotherapy.

Benefits from corticosteroids have been quite variable. Of the corticosteroids studied, the use of dexamethasone has been best defined. In clinical trials, dexamethasone has been compared with metoclopramide and prochlorperazine.[24–26] During therapy with mildly to moderately emetogenic agents, dexamethasone appeared to be comparable to metoclopramide and superior to prochlorperazine when each was used alone; however, metoclopramide has shown greater efficacy when studied in patients receiving highly emetogenic regimens, especially those including cisplatin. Methylprednisolone has been compared with metoclopramide and thiethylperazine. Benefit appeared to be greater for methylprednisolone than thiethylperazine and comparable to typical metoclopramide doses of less than 2 mg/kg.[27–30] Dosage regimens vary widely among steroid antiemetic protocols. When used alone, dexamethasone has often been administered parenterally as a single dose of 8–20 mg prior to chemotherapy, followed by oral doses of 4–12 mg up to 24 hours after completion of chemotherapy. There is less variation in the dosage regimens of other steroids. Usually, methylprednisolone has been administered prior to chemotherapy in a dose of 250 mg. After chemotherapy, up to four subsequent doses have been given.

Metoclopramide is most often prescribed for the prevention and treatment of complex nausea and vomiting in response to chemotherapy administration, particularly cisplatin. For such patients, it has been employed in multiagent combination protocols; however, it has shown efficacy as a single therapy. Alone or in combination, metoclopramide has demonstrated significant efficacy in high doses (1–2 mg/kg intravenously), with one dose administered approximately 30 minutes prior to chemotherapy. Up to four subsequent doses are given at 2-hour intervals after chemotherapy. Although cisapride, an agent similar to metoclopramide, may provide relief in select patients with nausea and vomiting this agent is at present indicated primarily for the management of acid-reflux disorders.[31]

Several selective 5-HT_3 serotonin antagonists, including ondansetron, granisetron, and tropisetron, have been evaluated and clinically accepted in the management of chemotherapy-induced nausea and vomiting. Ondansetron, the first of these agents, and granisetron are safe and effective in the treatment of nausea and vomiting associated with cytotoxic chemotherapy and radiation therapy.[32] By blocking serotonin receptors located in the area postrema and possibly vagal afferent fibers in the upper GI tract, these agents inhibit emesis.[33] Although potentially important agents for cancer patients, 5-HT_3 serotonin receptor antagonists have provided no beneficial effects in reducing motion sickness when compared with placebo.[34]

Ondansetron is usually administered intravenously 30 minutes prior to chemotherapy at a dose of 0.15 mg/kg over 15 minutes. Similar subsequent doses are given 4 and 8 hours after the first dose. Investigated in both oral and parenteral forms, ondansetron is generally well tolerated. Reported side effects include headache, diarrhea, and transient elevations in hepatic aminotransferases. Because ondansetron does not affect dopamine receptors, it is not associated with akathisia or acute dystonia.[35–37]

In adults and children at least 2 years of age, granisetron should be intravenously infused in a dose of 10 mcg/kg over 5 minutes, beginning within 30 minutes before the initiation of chemotherapy, only on the day(s) chemotherapy is given. Children under the age of 2 years have not been adequately studied. Reported side effects of granisetron include headache, asthenia, somnolence, diarrhea, and constipation.

Although the availability of serotonin antagonists has made a significant impact on the management of patients receiving cytotoxic chemotherapy, two issues may hamper their overall usefulness. The first issue in most institutions is that of cost since these medications may be quite expensive compared to other agents. However, the overall costs of using each medication and not just the medication costs must be compared. Included in this type of comparison must be consideration of the overall expectations from the antiemetic chosen for individual patient variables. These variables include the patient's age, prior adverse reactions that may have been experienced, the effects of anticipatory nausea and vomiting, and certainly the costs associated with an increased duration of hospitalization due to clinically important nausea and vomiting. In addition to cost considerations, serotonin antagonists have not been adequately effective in controlling delayed emesis in some studies. Furthermore, some patients have experienced a reduction of efficacy with multiple-day chemotherapy or after several cycles of chemotherapy.[38] In this latter situation, some clinicians recommend the addition of a corticosteroid to the regimen to increase the response rate.

The cannabinoids are effective antiemetic agents, even in patients in whom other regimens have failed.[39,40] Dronabinol, Δ-9-tetrahydrocannabinol (THC), is the major psychoactive substance present in marijuana. Cannabinoids are only indicated for nausea and vomiting associated with cancer chemotherapy. The mechanism of action is unknown; however, it may be related to effects on opiate receptors and the cortical and vomiting centers of the brain and probably does not involve the CTZ.[39–41] Cannabinoids have been associated with potentially undesirable features and are not equally effective against all stimuli or all doses of the same stimuli. As expected, a number of transient central nervous system (CNS) effects are common, including mood changes, anxiety, memory loss, fear, confusion, motor incoordination, time distortion, hallucinations, euphoria, relaxation, and hunger. Depending on the severity of these effects, doses should be lowered or discontinued. However, there is a strong correlation between a subjective "high" and antiemetic efficacy. Nabilone has been associated with less euphoric effects than dronabinol. Other potential side effects of the cannabinoids include sedation, blurred vision, hypotension, tachycardia, and paranoid ideation. Tolerance usually develops to most of the side effects, but not to the antiemetic activity.[42,43] Both increased effectiveness and improved tolerance of the cannabinoids may be observed in younger patients. Administration of the cannabinoids should be initiated the night before chemotherapy because failure to achieve adequate blood concentrations will likely result in vomiting.

Anticipatory nausea and vomiting is a somewhat unique problem sometimes associated with cytotoxic chemotherapy. As many as one in four cancer patients may experience this condition during repeated courses of therapy. According to one study, patients with four or more of the following characteristics may be more likely to develop anticipatory symptoms by their fourth chemotherapy treatment: nausea and/or vomiting experienced after first treatment; nausea after treatment described as "moderate, severe, or intolerable"; vomiting after treatment described as "moderate, severe, or intolerable"; less than 50 years of age; a susceptibility to motion sickness; feeling warm or hot all over after treatment; sweating following treatment; or feelings of generalized weakness following treatment.[44]

Benzodiazepines represent the best of the therapeutic alternatives in the treatment of anticipatory nausea and vomiting. The most often prescribed agent in this pharmacologic class is lorazepam, usually administered intravenously for its amnestic effects. Dosage regimens include one dose before and multiple doses after each treatment with cytotoxic chemotherapy. Although some patients appreciate their lack of recall of having received chemotherapy, others find it uncomfortable and unacceptable. The latter patients may refuse lorazepam for subsequent treatments; however, acceptability of this feature of one's care may be highly dependent on the overall severity of symptoms. Maher has reported the use of lorazepam and a phenothiazine with improvement in anticipatory and chemotherapy-induced symptoms.[45] Others believe this combination requires additional study because of the increased risk of respiratory and CNS depression. Similar to other benzodiazepines, lorazepam may display an array of pharmacologic activities including sedation, hypnosis, anxiolysis, and muscle relaxation in doses of 0.5–4.0 mg, with little change in a patient's respiratory or cardiovascular function; however, other effects on the CNS such as disorientation, hallucinations, incontinence, and amnesia appear directly related to dose escalation.[46,47]

Because of the complexities of chemotherapy-induced nausea and vomiting and the variable patient response, many patients require two or more antiemetic agents, particularly when the cytotoxic regimen includes high-dose cisplatin. Considerations for the use of multiple antiemetic drugs are provided later in the section on Combination Antiemetic Protocols.

POSTOPERATIVE NAUSEA AND VOMITING

Nausea and vomiting associated with operative procedures are common problems for some patients. However, not all operative procedures produce such problems to the same degree. Specifically, procedures of the abdomen, eye, ear, nose, and throat are generally associated with higher incidences of nausea and vomiting than other procedures. Women, perhaps related to high gonadotropin levels, appear more susceptible to such postoperative problems and experience a threefold higher incidence of nausea and vomiting compared to men, independent of the type of operation or anesthetic.[48] Children are about twice as susceptible as adults.[49] Other risk factors that may be associated with an increase in postoperative symptoms include patient variables such as obesity, increased age, a history of motion sickness or prior postoperative emesis, as well as drug therapy variables such as the choice of premedication or general anesthetic agent. For example, inhalational anesthetics such as cyclopropane, an older agent, and nitrous oxide are particularly emetogenic, whereas agents such as isoflurane, enflurane, and halothane cause less, but still significant, postoperative nausea and vomiting. Of the intravenous anesthetics, propofol may be less emetogenic than some agents previously used.[49]

Most patients do not require preoperative prophylactic antiemetic therapy. In 70–90% of cases, patients either do not experience these symptoms or may have incomplete resolution when they occur. Also, simple premedication with atropine may decrease the potential occurrence of these symptoms in some patients. Other anticholinergic agents that may be effective include promethazine, scopolamine, cyclizine, and possibly glycopyrrolate. Although each of these agents has been effective in the prevention of nausea and vomiting in some clinical settings, sedation, dry mouth, and disorientation may limit their usefulness. Few patients will require the administration of additional preoperatively administered therapy.

The use of antiemetic therapy immediately following an operative procedure has been much more aggressively evaluated and applied, either as prophylaxis for potential postoperative symptoms or as acute management of actual nausea and vomiting. A variety of pharmacologic approaches are available and should be prescribed as single or combination therapy in their minimally effective dosage regimens. In doing so, patients will experience fewer adverse effects, some of which may otherwise be very troublesome for the overall recovery of the patient. Among the commonly prescribed antiemetic therapies in the postoperative setting, droperidol has been effective, particularly in patients undergoing obstetric and gynecologic procedures. Limiting effects, however, may include sedation, hypotension, and extrapyramidal signs.

Studies of metoclopramide have provided conflicting results, with some clinical trials documenting control of symptoms and others having concluded little value. Such findings perhaps have been due to metoclopramide's short duration of action, particularly when compared in settings in which patients had received morphine, a known emetogenic analgesic. Adverse effects of metoclopramide include sedation and infrequently extrapyramidal signs. Although possible, extrapyramidal effects appear to be much less likely with the low doses most often prescribed in this setting.

Selective serotonin antagonists have been evaluated in the prevention of postoperative nausea and vomiting. To date, ondansetron has generally provided favorable outcomes when compared to placebo, metoclopramide, and droperidol. Similar agents, including granisetron, may provide similar results. The most often cited reason for selecting a serotonin antagonist in the postoperative period appears to be a probable reduction in the occurrence of extrapyramidal signs noted with these agents compared particularly to droperidol and metoclopramide. Even so, the true role of serotonin antagonists is presently unknown, with many clinicians preferring the use of older, more traditional and less expensive antiemetic therapy. With the unpredictable occurrence and severity of nausea and vomiting for many patients, perhaps newer therapies are best reserved for patients who have failed to respond to traditional therapy, or for patients in whom drug allergies or other specific risk factors exist.

Other antiemetic medications with value in the management of postoperative nausea and vomiting include promethazine, prochlorperazine, scopolamine, diphenhydramine, lorazepam, and ephedrine. These latter medications may be prescribed in doses similar to those used in other settings and produce similar beneficial and adverse effects. With or without antiemetic therapy, certain nonpharmacologic methods may be effective in reducing the potential for emesis and should be universally applied. These include assisting patients with movement and providing particularly close attention to adequate hydration and pain management.

DISORDERS OF BALANCE

A variety of clinical conditions may be associated with vertigo and dizziness. The etiology of these complaints may include diseases that are infectious, postinfectious, demyelinative, vascular, neoplastic, degenerative, traumatic, toxic, psychogenic, or idiopathic. Therefore, symptoms of imbalance or perceived imbalance by the patient present a particular clinical challenge. Whether associated with a minor or complex disorder, motion sickness may be associated with nausea and vomiting.

Although much progress has been made in the management of other illnesses associated with emesis, motion sickness represents an area in which newer agents have provided little benefit. Studies of serotonin antagonists in motion sickness suggest that the 5-HT$_3$ receptor is not involved in the neural pathways that bring about motion sickness.[50] Interestingly, vertigo has been documented among the adverse reactions of these agents. Therefore, beneficial therapy for patients in this setting can most reliably be found among the antihistaminic–anticholinergic agents.[51] However, their precise mechanisms of action are unknown to date. Neither the antihistaminic nor the anticholinergic potency appears to correlate well with the ability of these agents to prevent or treat the nausea and vomiting associated with motion sickness.

When used for their depressant effects on labyrinth excitability, these agents have been shown to produce variable efficacy and safety profiles. The most useful antiemetic agent for motion sickness prophylaxis appears to be scopolamine, particularly when used 1 to 2 hours prior to symptom-producing exposures.[52] Typical regimens of antihistaminic–anticholinergic agents include the oral administration of small to moderate doses one to several times each day.

COMBINATION ANTIEMETIC PROTOCOLS

The management of nausea and vomiting may include various combinations of known antiemetic drugs. Most often these combination protocols are reserved for patients whose symptoms are complex, especially those receiving cytotoxic chemotherapy. Such combinations may include as few as two or as many as five antiemetic agents, each in moderate to high doses. These multiagent regimens should be carefully administered by experienced personnel in a hospital or specialty clinic setting. Although oral agents may be used, most regimens are administered intravenously and require fairly continuous patient assessment and feedback for evaluation of efficacy and side effects. Because an increasing number of patients may require such regimens, careful monitoring should be developed and employed to eliminate possibly severe adverse reactions.

The primary goal of combination antiemetic regimens is to select beneficial agents that have different pharmacologic mechanisms as well as toxic effects that are not considered additive or synergistic. These protocols may affect the vomiting center, the CTZ, the cerebral cortex, and/or the peripheral mechanisms that mediate nausea and vomiting.[53] Combinations often include metoclopramide, diphenhydramine, and dexamethasone. Other agents that may be added to the regimen include droperidol, diazepam, thiethylperazine, secobarbital, pentobarbital, chlorpromazine, or prochlorperazine. Dexamethasone may be combined with ondansetron or granisetron. From this list of possible combinations, it should be apparent that the ideal multiagent antiemetic protocol has not been well defined. Nevertheless, protocols utilizing injectable metoclopramide or a setotonin antagonist appear to have a high degree of efficacy in preventing nausea and vomiting, even in patients receiving cisplatin.[53–55]

ANTIEMETIC USE DURING PREGNANCY

More than one-half of pregnant women experience nausea and vomiting or hyperemesis gravidarum.[56] Because drugs may influence embryonic development most during the first 2 months of pregnancy, there has been much interest in the potential maternal and fetal benefits and risks of the antiemetic agents during this early phase.[57] Included in the list of agents that have commonly been prescribed are the phenothiazines (prochlorperazine and promethazine), the antihistaminic–anticholinergic agents (dimenhydrinate, diphenhydramine, meclizine, and scopolamine), metoclopramide, pyridoxine, and Bendectin. Once the most commonly prescribed antiemetic therapy in pregnancy, Bendectin, a combination of doxylamine succinate and pyridoxine hydrochloride, is no longer commercially available. Although not reviewed here, this combination has been included in other reference material.[58] By its removal, the most studied antiemetic during pregnancy is no longer a part of the treatment for this commonly troublesome condition.

Although many women experience nausea and vomiting during pregnancy, the etiology of hyperemesis gravidarum is not well understood. Numerous mechanisms have been proposed. In addition, the severity of symptoms may vary greatly. In its most severe state, hyperemesis gravidarum may result in volume contraction, starvation, and electrolyte abnormalities; however, as a mild condition, it may be self-limiting and intermittent and may respond favorably to placebo. The efficacy of antiemetics has been questioned while the importance of specific management plans has been addressed. These plans have included emphasis on fluid and electrolyte management, vitamin supplements, and efforts aimed at reducing psychosomatic complaints.[59,60]

Evaluation of teratogenicity of products administered during the first trimester of pregnancy is of great importance, particularly in patients with a condition with such variability in its presentation; however, proof of teratogenicity varies among animals and humans. In animals, tests of this nature are performed in the laboratory, may vary with animal strain and breed, and may not be good predictors of human experience. Conversely, the clinical laboratory of patient care is the testing ground for agents used in humans. From this setting, case reports and often retrospective epidemiologic reports document the outcome of these human experiences.

Teratogenicity is a major consideration for the use of antiemetic drugs during pregnancy and is the primary factor that dictates this condition's drug of choice. Therefore, both the benefit and side effect profiles for the mother as well as potential fetal risks are important. Of the agents commonly used, those that have demonstrated teratogenicity in animals include diphenhydramine, meclizine, prochlorperazine, and thiethylperazine[61–63]; however, in humans meclizine has not been shown to have these same effects. Most authors currently do not recommend metoclopramide because its use during pregnancy requires further study. Also, its primary benefit in nonpregnant patients with nausea and vomiting has been in association with cancer, chemotherapy, and high intravenous doses. In addition, serotonin antagonists cannot be recommended in this setting, even though animal studies to date have revealed no harm. Presently, cyclizine and meclizine are considered the drugs of choice for the treatment of nausea and vomiting during pregnancy.[64] Promethazine should be considered as a third choice and prescribed only if symptoms are severe and cannot be controlled by adequate trials of one of the first two agents.

ANTIEMETIC USE IN CHILDREN

In general, most studies of antiemetic drugs have included primarily adult patients; however, nausea and vomiting in children present unique problems that deserve mention. There are perhaps more uncertainties concerning drug and dosage selection as well as the appropriateness of combination regimens for use in children. One apparent finding is that children may not require or tolerate the same milligram-per-kilogram (mg/kg) doses of drugs commonly used in adults. Striking examples of this finding include the use of metoclopramide. During the 1960s and 1970s this drug was given as an antiemetic to European children with gastroenteritis. From these populations came numerous reports citing extrapyramidal reactions at cumulative daily doses less than 2.0 mg/kg.[65,66] It is now appreciated that these side effects should be anticipated in children and may occur at intravenous doses as low as 0.5 mg/kg given as repeated doses four times per day. Also, it is interesting that differences in drug disposition, including plasma metoclopramide concentrations, probably do not explain the occurrence of dystonia.[67]

Dosage regimens and anticipated outcome of other antiemetic drugs in children are also quite interesting compared with adults. Phenothiazines appear more likely to produce neuromuscular reactions, particularly dystonias, in this age group than in adults, especially when administered during acute viral illnesses such as chicken pox, measles, and gastroenteritis. Therefore, phenothiazines should be reserved for patients with prolonged vomiting in whom the benefit-to-risk ratio has been examined carefully. Promethazine may be the best agent in this class because its activity is most like that of the antihistamines rather than the phenothiazines.

The antihistaminic–anticholinergic agents also present some difficulty in selection depending on the exact age of the child. For example, the use of benzquinamide, buclizine, cyclizine, and scopolamine is not recommended in children under the age of 12 years. Dimenhydrinate, however, has been used in children at doses that differ by age for those less than 2 years, those 2 to 6 years, and children 6 to 12 years. Interestingly, trimethobenzamide may be used in children orally or rectally but is not recommended for injection. When chosen, it should be prescribed according to weight. Trimethobenzamide is also not recommended by any route for premature or newborn infants. The butyrophenones, haloperidol and droperidol, have been used in children but not usually in those younger than 2 to 3 years. In children older than 3 years of age, most patients studied have received droperidol in the preoperative setting as an adjunct to general anesthesia. Fewer children, comparatively, have received droperidol during chemotherapy. Diphenidol, an agent associated with significant adverse effects, is usually not prescribed in children and is not recommended in patients weighing less than 50 pounds. Parenteral lorazepam, although perhaps useful in adults, is not generally recommended for patients younger than 18 years. Likewise, dronabinol is not indicated for children because it has been studied most in patients older than 12 years. Corticosteroids are often included in the anticancer regimens received by children but are not generally utilized as antiemetics in this age group. Finally, serotonin antagonists have been evaluated in children of various ages and have been shown to be both safe and effective, particularly in patients receiving cytotoxic chemotherapy or those in the postoperative period. These agents have been shown to provide a significant reduction in nausea and vomiting in the absence of extrapyramidal effects.[68–70] However, dosage information is primarily available for children 4 to 18 years of age. Comparatively little information is available for children 3 years of age and younger.

NONPHARMACOLOGIC MANAGEMENT

Nonpharmacologic management of nausea and vomiting may include a variety of dietary, physical, or psychologic changes consistent with the etiology of symptoms. For patients with simple complaints, perhaps resulting from excessive or disagreeable food or beverage consumption, avoidance or moderation in dietary intake may be preferable. Patients suffering symptoms of systemic illness may improve dramatically as their underlying condition resolves. Finally, patients in whom these symptoms result from labyrinthine changes produced by motion may benefit quickly by assuming a stable physical position.

The variables associated with the development of anticipatory nausea and vomiting have been studied. These variables include the use of cisplatin, the severity of postchemotherapy vomiting, and the duration of the patient's worst nausea.[71] Although many clinicians believe antiemetic and antianxiety agents are most successful in treating these patients, others have been disappointed. Various techniques involving relaxation have been reported.

These techniques include hypnosis, behavior modification, and guided mental imagery.[72–74] Presently, the efficacy of such nonpharmacologic approaches remains inadequately tested and requires further evaluation. Nevertheless, it is apparent that prevention of these symptoms is extremely important. This may be accomplished through supportive care coupled with potent prophylactic antiemetic regimens prior to chemotherapy treatment.

The management of psychogenic vomiting is greatly dependent on nonpharmacologic methods. Pharmacologic approaches, although not well studied in this setting, may exhibit only minimal benefit, if any. Surgery, such as gastroenterostomy, is of no value. The most likely beneficial interventions are psychologic; however, even these therapies may require in-depth follow-up as the ultimate problems are complex and intertwined in the relationships of the patient and individuals with whom he or she often associates.

Evaluation of Therapeutic Outcomes

With the increasing use of highly emetogenic chemotherapeutic agents, numerous single- and multiple-agent antiemetic clinical trials have been reported in the medical and pharmaceutical literature. However, these studies have used different methods of evaluation. Variables affecting the assessment of antiemetic trials have been addressed.[75] In broad terms, there may be variability in patients, emetic stimuli, antiemetic drugs, and study design. More specifically, in evaluating such studies, close attention should be paid to pretreatment variables as well as to the types of patients studied. The onset, duration, and frequency of symptoms should be compared as should the various etiologic situations. Anticipatory nausea and vomiting require careful evaluation because this condition may often be refractory to antiemetic drugs.[71,76] Another patient factor that should be considered is age. Age-related responsiveness has been noted particularly in studies in which the greatest efficacy of Δ-9-tetrahydrocannabinol (THC) was reported among younger patients.[77–79]

Another variable that affects patient response to antiemetic therapy, and therefore influences the overall interpretation of study results, is the setting in which nausea and vomiting occurs. For example, hospital inpatients may tolerate chemotherapy better than outpatients, perhaps because of more security in the inpatient environment. In addition, the presence of stress or depression as well as the lack of social support may adversely affect patient response.[80,81] Dosage, schedule, and route of administration of each antiemetic agent may greatly influence beneficial as well as toxic effects. Unfortunately, many clinical trials to date have not adequately addressed the pharmacodynamic issues of these drugs. Therefore, efficacy is difficult to compare because of the wide variety of study protocols.

The etiology of a patient's nausea and vomiting determines the expected outcome of antiemetic therapy. Depending on the patient's ability to tolerate antiemetics, symptomatic relief is often unattainable until definitive therapy can be instituted (i.e., delivery of fetus, GI surgery, correction of metabolic disorders, or removal of emetogenic agents). If nausea and vomiting persist despite maximal and frequent dosing of an antiemetic agent, an agent with a different mechanism of action may be administered. In addition, the patient should be examined closely to elicit any signs of volume contraction and assess the need for aggressive fluid replacement.

In accordance with the above information concerning age and clinical condition, individualized therapy may be possible through drug selection and dosage adjustment. Monitoring criteria for drug therapy should include the subjective assessment of the patient's severity of nausea as well as objective parameters such as the number of vomiting episodes each day, the volume of vomitus lost, and evaluation of fluid, acid–base balance, and electrolyte status, with particular attention to serum sodium, potassium, and chloride concentrations. In addition, evaluation of renal function may become important, particularly in patients with volume contraction and progressive electrolyte disturbances. Specific parameters include daily urine volume, urine specific gravity, and urine electrolyte concentrations. Physical assessment of patients should include evaluation of mucous membranes and skin turgor, since dryness of these tissues may be indicative of significant volume loss.

Conclusion

The approach to the diagnosis and management of nausea and vomiting depends on the clinical setting in which these problems occur. Only with a clear understanding of these settings can therapeutic plans involving nonpharmacologic as well as pharmacologic approaches be adequately developed. In treating an individual patient, a systematic approach should be initially prescribed; alterations should be based on follow-up assessments. These initial and follow-up management protocols should always take into consideration the uniqueness of the patient, with attention to the specific details of the prescribed regimen as well as the unique clinical setting in which it occurs.

References

1. Hanson JS, McCallum RW. The diagnosis and management of nausea and vomiting: A review. Am J Gastroenterol 1985;80:210–218.
2. Frytak S, Moertel CG. Management of nausea and vomiting in the cancer patient. JAMA 1981;245:393–396.
3. Feldman M. Nausea and vomiting, in Sleisenger MH, Fordtran JS (eds): Gastrointestinal Disease. Philadelphia, WB Saunders, 1983, pp 160–177.

4. Redd WH. Control of nausea and vomiting in chemotherapy patients: Four effective behavioral methods. Postgrad Med 1984;75:105–113.
5. Eyre HJ, Ward JH. Control of cancer chemotherapy-induced nausea and vomiting. Cancer 1984;54:2642–2648.
6. Dutro MP, Ammerson AB. Comparison of liquid antacids. N Engl J Med 1980;302:967.
7. Fordtran JS, Morawski S, Richardson C. *In vitro* and *in vivo* evaluation of antacids. N Engl J Med 1973;288:923.
8. Seipler JK, Mahakian K, Trudeau WT. Current concepts in clinical therapeutics: Peptic ulcer disease. Clin Pharm 1986;5:128–142.
9. Edmunds SJ, Prys RC. Pharmacology of drugs used in neuroleptanalgesia. Br J Anaesthesia 1970;42:207–216.
10. Wampler G. The pharmacology and clinical effectiveness of phenothiazines and related drugs for managing chemotherapy-induced emesis. Drugs 1983;25(suppl):35–51.
11. Lucas VS. Phenothiazines as antiemetics, in Lazlo J (ed): Antiemetics and Cancer Chemotherapy. Baltimore, Williams & Wilkins, 1983, pp 93–107.
12. Jacobs AJ, Deppe G, Cohen CJ. A comparison of the antiemetic effects of droperidol and prochlorperazine in chemotherapy with *cis*-platinum. Gynecol Oncol 1980;10:55–57.
13. Cersosimo RJ, Bromer R, Hoffer S, et al. The antiemetic activity of droperidol administered by intramuscular injection during cisplatin chemotherapy: A pilot study. Drug Intell Clin Pharm 1985;19:118–121.
14. Paladine W, Price L, Sokol G, et al. Antiemetic trial of droperidol. Proc Am Soc Clin Oncol 1980;21:381.
15. Brown RE, Gregg RE, Hood JC. Droperidol treatment of streptozotocin-induced nausea and vomiting. Drug Intell Clin Pharm 1982;16:775–776.
16. Cersosimo RJ, Karp DD. Adrenal corticosteroids as antiemetics during cancer chemotherapy. Pharmacotherapy 1986;6:118–127.
17. Gralla RJ. Metoclopramide: A review of antiemetic trials. Drugs 1983;25(suppl):63–73.
18. Schyulze-Delriev K. Metoclopramide. Gastroenterology 1979;77:768–779.
19. Stoudemire A, Cotanch P, Lazlo J. Recent advances in the pharmacologic and behavioral management of chemotherapy-induced emesis. Arch Intern Med 1984;144:1029–1033.
20. Grossman B, Lessin LS, Cohen P. Droperidol prevents nausea and vomiting from *cis*-platinum. N Engl J Med 1979;301:147.
21. Mehrota S, Rosenthal CJ, Barile B, et al. A comparison between droperidol and prochlorperazine in combination with trimethobenzamide as antiemetics for antineoplastic combination chemotherapy [abstract]. Proc Am Assoc Cancer Res/Am Soc Clin Oncol 1981;22:417.
22. Wilson J, Weltz D, Solimando D, et al. Continuous infusion droperidol. Antiemetic therapy for *cis*-platinum toxicity [abstract]. Proc Am Assoc Cancer Res/Am Soc Clin Oncol 1981;22:421.
23. Curry SL, Rine J, Whitney CW, et al. The role of prostaglandins in the excessive nausea and vomiting after intravascular *cis*-platinum therapy. Gynecol Oncol 1981;12:89–91.
24. Cognetti F, Pinnaro P, Carlini P, et al. Randomized open crossover trial between metoclopramide and dexamethasone for the prevention of cisplatin-induced nausea and vomiting. Eur J Cancer Clin Oncol 1984;20:183–187.
25. Aapro MS, Plezia PM, Albert DS, et al. Double-blind crossover study of the antiemetic efficacy of high-dose dexamethasone versus high-dose metoclopramide. J Clin Oncol 1984;2:466–471.
26. Markman M, Sheidler V, Ettinger DS, et al. Antiemetic efficacy of dexamethasone. Randomized, double-blind, crossover study with prochlorperazine in patients receiving cancer chemotherapy. N Engl J Med 1984;311:549–552.
27. Kolaric K, Roth A. Methylprednisolone as an antiemetic in patients on *cis*-platinum chemotherapy. Results of a controlled randomized study. Tumori 1983;69:43–46.
28. Giaconne G, Donadio M, Musella R, et al. Comparison of methylprednisolone and metoclopramide in the prophylactic treatment of cisplatin-induced nausea and vomiting. Tumori 1984;70:237–241.
29. Schallier D, Van Belle S, De Greve J, et al. Methylprednisolone as an antiemetic drug. A randomized double-blind study. Cancer Chemother Pharmacol 1985;14:235–237.
30. Ell C, Konig HJ, Brockmann P, et al. Antiemetic efficacy of moderately high-dose metoclopramide in patients receiving varying doses of cisplatin. Controlled comparison with combination of methylprednisolone and metoclopramide. Oncology 1985;42:354–357.
31. Pope CE II. Acid-reflux disorders. N Engl J Med 1994;331:656–660.
32. Marty M, Pouillart P, Scholl S, et al. Comparison of the 5-hydroxytryptamine$_3$ (serotonin) antagonist ondansetron (GR 38032F) with high-dose metoclopramide in the control of cisplatin-induced emesis. N Engl J Med 1990;322:816–821.
33. Tyers MB, Bunce KT, Humphrey PPA. Pharmacological and antiemetic properties of ondansetron. Eur J Cancer Clin Oncol 1989;25(suppl):S15–S19.
34. Stott JR, Barnes GR, Wright RJ, et al. The effect on motion sickness and oculomotor function of GR 38032F, a 5-HT$_3$-receptor antagonist with antiemetic properties. Br J Clin Pharmacol 1989;27:147–157.
35. Bryson JC, Finn AL, Plagge PB, et al. The safety profile of IV ondansetron from clinical trials [abstract]. Proc ASCL 1990;9:328.
36. Smith RN. Safety of ondansetron. Eur J Cancer Clin Oncol 1989;25(suppl):S47–S50.
37. Chaffee BJ, Tankanow RM. Ondansetron—the first of a new class of antiemetic agents. Clin Pharm 1991;10:430–446.
38. Aapro MS. Review of experience with ondansetron and granisetron. Ann Oncol 1993;4(suppl 3):S9–S14.
39. Lazlo J, Lucas VS. Synthetic cannabinoids, in Lazlo J (ed): Antiemetics and Cancer Chemotherapy. Baltimore, Williams & Wilkins, 1983, pp 116–128.
40. Herman TS, Einhorn LH, Jones SE, et al. Superiority of nabilone over prochlorperazine as an antiemetic in patients receiving cancer chemotherapy. N Engl J Med 1979;300:1295–1297.
41. Tortorice PV, O'Connell MB. Management of chemotherapy-induced nausea and vomiting. Pharmacotherapy 1990;10:129–145.

42. Anderson PO, McGuire GG. Δ-9-Tetrahydrocannabinol as an antiemetic. Am J Hosp Pharm 1981;38:639–646.
43. Neidhart JA, Gagen M. Experimental antiemetic agents (other than cannabinoids and metoclopramide), in Lazlo J (ed): Antiemetics and Cancer Chemotherapy. Baltimore, Williams & Wilkins, 1983, pp 142–163.
44. Morrow FR, Lindke J, Black PM. Predicting development of anticipatory nausea in cancer patients: Prospective examination of eight clinical characteristics. J Pain Symptom Manage 1991;6:215–223.
45. Maher J. Intravenous lorazepam to prevent nausea and vomiting associated with cancer chemotherapy. Lancet 1981;1:91–92.
46. Lazlo J. Oral lorazepam to improve tolerance of cytotoxic therapy. Lancet 1981;1:1316–1317.
47. Meyer M, Long AM, Natale RB, et al. Phase I, II and III trials of a new antiemetic agent—lorazepam. Proc Am Soc Clin Oncol 1983;2:88.
48. Mitchelson F. Pharmacological agents affecting emesis: A review. Drugs 1992;43:443–463.
49. Kenny GN. Risk factors for postoperative nausea and vomiting. Anaesthesia 1994;49(suppl):6–10.
50. Scott JR, Barnes GR, Wright RJ, Ruddock CJ. The effect on motion sickness and oculomotor function of GR 38032F, a 5-HT_3-receptor antagonist with anti-emetic properties. Br J Clin Pharmacol 1989;27:147–157.
51. Maule WF, Parry MC. Management of chemotherapy-induced nausea and emesis. Am Fam Physician 1983;27:226–234.
52. Wood CD. Antimotion sickness and antiemetic drugs. Drugs 1979;17:471–479.
53. Strum SB, McDermed JE, Lauer D, et al. Control of acute-onset and delayed-onset chemotherapy-induced nausea and emesis with metoclopramide-based regimens. Intern Med Specialist 1985;6:104–112.
54. Fortner CL, Finley RS, Grove WR. Combination antiemetic therapy in the control of chemotherapy-induced emesis. Drug Intell Clin Pharm 1985;19:21–24.
55. Plezia PM, Alberts DS, Kessler J, et al. Immediate termination of intractable vomiting induced by cisplatin combination chemotherapy using an intensive five-drug antiemetic regimen. Cancer Treat Rep 1984;68:1493–1495.
56. Jarnfelt-Samsioe A, Samsioe G, Velinder GM. Nausea and vomiting in pregnancy—A contribution to its epidemiology. Gynecol Obstet Invest 1983;16:221–229.
57. Tuchmann-Duplessis H. Drugs and xenobiotics as teratogens. Pharmacol Ther 1984;26:273–344.
58. Leathem AM. Safety and efficacy of antiemetics used to treat nausea and vomiting in pregnancy. Clin Pharm 1986;5:660–668.
59. Fairweather DV. Nausea and vomiting during pregnancy. Obstet Gynecol Annu 1978;7:91–105.
60. Mellencamp E, Wang RI. The patient with nausea. III. Cancer, pregnancy, or surgery. Drug Ther 1977;7:49–54.
61. Schardein JL. Drugs as Teratogens. Cleveland, OH, CRC Press, 1976, pp 5, 130.
62. Shepard TH. Catalog of Teratogenic Agents, 4th ed. Baltimore, The Johns Hopkins University Press, 1983.
63. Nishimura H, Tanimura T. Clinical Aspects of Teratogenicity of Drugs. New York, Elsevier, 1976, pp 212, 241.
64. American Medical Association Department of Drugs. AMA Drug Evaluations Annual. Chicago, AMA, 1993, pp 428–429.
65. Low LCK, Goel KM. Metoclopramide poisoning in children. Arch Dis Child 1980;55:310–312.
66. Casteels-Van Daele M, Jaeken J, Van Der Schueren P, et al. Dystonic reactions in children caused by metoclopramide. Arch Dis Child 1970;45:130–133.
67. Bateman DN, Craft AW, Nicholson E, et al. Dystonic reactions and the pharmacokinetics of metoclopramide in children. Br J Clin Pharmacol 1983;15:557–559.
68. Furst SR, Rodarte A, Demars P. Ondansetron reduces postoperative vomiting in children undergoing tonsillectomy [abstract]. Anesthesiology 1993;79:A1197.
69. Lawhorn CD, Brown RE, Jr., Schmitz ML, et al. Prevention of postoperative vomiting in pediatric outpatient strabismus surgery [abstract]. Anesthesiology 1993;79:A1196.
70. Stevens RF. The role of ondansetron in paediatric patients: A review of three studies. European J Cancer 1991;27(suppl 1):S20–S22.
71. Morrow GR. Prevalence and correlation of anticipatory nausea and vomiting in chemotherapy patients. J Natl Cancer Inst 1982;68:585–588.
72. Lyles JN, Burish TG, Knozely MG, et al. Efficacy of relaxation training and guided imagery in reducing the aversiveness of cancer chemotherapy. J Consult Clin Psychol 1982;50:509–524.
73. Morrow GR, Morrell C. Behavioral treatment for the anticipatory nausea and vomiting induced by cancer chemotherapy. N Engl J Med 1982;307:1476–1480.
74. Redd WH, Andresen GV, Minagawa RY. Hypnotic control of anticipatory emesis in patients receiving cancer chemotherapy. J Consult Clin Psychol 1982;50:14–19.
75. Olver IN, Simon RM, Aisner J. Antiemetic studies: A methodological discussion. Cancer Treat Rep 1986;70:555–563.
76. Moher D, Arthur AZ, Peter JL. Anticipatory nausea and/or vomiting. Cancer Treat Rev 1984;11:257–264.
77. Sallan SE, Zinberg NE, Frei E III. Antiemetic effect of Δ-9-tetrahydrocannabinol in patients receiving cancer chemotherapy. N Engl J Med 1975;293:795–797.
78. Sallan SE, Cronin C, Zelen M, et al. Antiemetics in patients receiving chemotherapy for cancer: A randomized comparison of Δ-9-tetrahydrocannabinol and prochlorperazine. N Engl J Med 1980;302:135–138.
79. Chang AE, Shilling DJ, Stillman RC, et al. Δ-9-Tetrahydrocannabinol as an antiemetic in cancer patients receiving high dose methotrexate: A prospective randomized evaluation. Ann Intern Med 1979;91:819–824.
80. Carey MP, Burish TG, Brenner DE. Δ-9-Tetrahydrocannabinol in cancer chemotherapy: Research problems and issues. Ann Intern Med 1983;99:106–114.
81. Broadhead WE, Kaplan BH, James SA, et al. The epidemiologic evidence for a relationship between social support and health. Am J Epidemiol 1983;117:521.

Chapter 36

Diarrhea and Constipation

R. Leon Longe, PharmD, and Joseph T. DiPiro, PharmD, FCCP

DIARRHEA

In the United States, diarrhea is a troublesome discomfort that is sometimes fatal. Usually, diarrheal episodes begin abruptly and subside within 1 or 2 days without treatment. This review focuses primarily on noninfectious diarrhea, with only minor reference to infectious diarrhea (see later chapter). Diarrhea is often a symptom of a systemic disease and not all possible causes are covered. This chapter presents a basic understanding of management.

To understand diarrhea, one must have a reasonable definition of the condition, but the literature is extremely variable on this. Simply, diarrhea is abnormal frequency and liquidity of fecal discharge compared with the patient's normal stools. Frequency and consistency are variable within and between individuals. For example, some individuals defecate as many as three times per day, while others defecate only two or three times per week. A Western diet usually produces a daily stool weighing between 100 and 300 g, depending on nonabsorbable materials (mainly carbohydrates). Patients with serious diarrhea have a stool of more than 300 g/d; however, a subset of cases have frequent small, watery passages. Another exception is the vegetable fiber-rich diet (e.g., some Eastern cultures such as African), which normally produces stools weighing more than 300 g/d.

Diarrhea may be associated with a specific disease of the intestines or secondary to a disease outside the intestines. For instance, bacillary dysentery directly affects the gut; diabetes mellitus causes neuropathic diarrheal episodes. Furthermore, diarrhea is divided into acute or chronic. Infectious diarrhea is often acute; diabetic diarrhea is chronic. Whether acute or chronic, diarrhea shares some common pathophysiologic causes that help identification of specific treatments.

EPIDEMIOLOGY

The epidemiology of diarrhea is different in developed (e.g., United States) versus underdeveloped countries (e.g., Tanzania).[1] In the United States, diarrheal illnesses usually are not reported to the Centers for Disease Control and Prevention (CDC) unless associated with an outbreak or an unusual organism or condition. For example, acquired immune deficiency syndrome (AIDS) has been identified with protracted diarrheal illness. Some populations are particularly affected and generate a public health concern. Diarrhea is a major problem in day care centers and nursing homes, probably because early childhood and senescence plus environmental conditions are risk factors. However, an exact epidemiologic profile in the United States is not available through the CDC or published literature.

In the United States viral and bacterial organisms account for most of the infectious diarrhea. Common bacterial organisms are *Shigella, Salmonella, Campylobacter, Staphylococcus,* and *Escherichia coli.* Acute viral infections are attributed mostly to Norwalk and rotavirus groups.

In developing cultures, acute diarrhea kills 5 million children annually.[2] The World Health Organization (WHO) estimates that 744 million to 1 billion diarrheal attacks occur annually in the world's children. These findings are associated with poor sanitation, poor nutrition, and age less than 5 years, especially infancy. The leading cause is invasion by infectious organisms (e.g., parasites, cholera).

PATHOPHYSIOLOGY

In the fasting state, 9 L of intestinal fluid enters the proximal small intestine each day.[3] Of this fluid, 2 L are ingested with the diet; the remainder comes from internal secretions. Because of meal content, duodenal chyme is usually hypertonic. When chyme reaches the ileum, osmolality adjusts to equal that of plasma, with most dietary fat, carbohydrate, and protein absorbed. Ileal chyme reduces to about 1 L/d entering the colon. The electrolyte profile of ileal chyme per liter is normally sodium 140 mEq, potassium 8 mEq, chloride 60 mEq, and bicarbonate 70 mEq. In the normal state, the colon absorbs 900 mL, reducing chyme to 100 mL water loss daily. Fecal electrolyte content (mEq/L) is sodium 40, chloride 15, potassium 90, and bicarbonate 30.

From the preceding description, one visualizes diarrhea as an imbalance in absorption and secretion of water and electrolytes. In normal volunteers, small intestine water has a maximum rate of absorption. If the small intestine absorption capacity is exceeded, chyme overloads the colon, resulting in diarrhea. In humans, the colon absorptive capacity is about 5 L daily.[3] Colonic fluid transport is critical to water and electrolyte balance. In simplistic terms, diarrhea is a seesaw with absorption on one end and secretion on the other. If these processes are equally weighed, one has a normal bowel movement. If absorption decreases or secretion increases beyond normal, diarrhea results. Normally, the absorption of water and electrolytes exceeds secretory fluxes. One should understand the mechanisms at work controlling water, electrolyte, and glucose movements.

Water passively moves across the gut after the movement of solutes such as sodium.[4] The intestinal mucosa is semipermeable and allows selective solute and solvent movements. For instance, the proximal intestine rapidly makes meal content isosmotic. In the small intestine, absorption occurs in the villous cells and secretion in the cryptic cells. In the colon, chyme may be hypertonic; this is partly explained by bacterial metabolism of carbohydrates into absorbable solutes. Unabsorbed carbohydrates metabolize into volatile fatty acids and absorb across the colon.

Electrolyte transport, like water transport, is handled by villi (absorption) and crypt (secretion) cells. Sodium is the principal ion absorbed and chloride is the primary ion secreted. In both absorption and secretion, an active sodium-potassium–activated ATPase pump secretes sodium into the blood in exchange for potassium. Because of membrane lipophilic properties, specific carrier proteins transport sodium and chloride. A cotransporter carries both sodium and chloride from the extracellular fluid into enterocytes. Also, animal studies show a one-to-one exchange of Na^+ for H^+ and a one-to-one exchange of Cl^- for either OH^- or HCO_3^- as another NaCl absorption mechanism. Chloride channels opened by cyclic adenosine monophosphate (AMP) permit movement of chloride into the intestinal lumen.[5]

Paracellular pathways are another major route of ion movement. As ions, monosaccharides, and amino acids are actively transported, they create an osmotic pressure, drawing water and electrolytes across the intestinal wall. This pathway accounts for very large amounts of ion transport, especially sodium. Glucose plays an important role in stimulating sodium absorption.

Gut motility influences absorption and secretion.[6] Time in which luminal content is in contact with epithelium is under neural and hormonal control. Neurohormonal substances and neurotransmitters also regulate ion transport.[7] Some are circulating hormones like angiotensin, vasopressin, glucocorticoids, and aldosterone. For instance, glucocorticoids improve sodium absorption and sodium-coupled chloride absorption. Angiotensin has absorptive effect.

Four general pathophysiologic mechanisms disrupt water and electrolyte balance, leading to diarrhea. These four mechanisms are the basis of diagnosis and therapy: (1) a change in active ion transport by either decreased sodium absorption or increased chloride secretion, (2) change in intestinal motility, (3) increase in luminal osmolarity, and (4) increase in tissue hydrostatic pressure. These mechanisms have been related to four broad clinical diarrheal groups: secretory, osmotic, exudative, and altered intestinal transit.

Secretory diarrhea occurs when a stimulating substance either increases secretion or decreases absorption of large amounts of water and electrolytes. Substances that cause excess secretion include vasoactive intestinal peptide (VIP) from a pancreatic tumor, unabsorbed dietary fat in steatorrhea, laxatives, hormones (e.g., secretin), bacterial toxins, and excessive bile salts. Many of these agents stimulate intracellular cyclic AMP and inhibit Na^+/K^+-ATPase, leading to increased secretion. Also, many of these mediators inhibit ion absorption simultaneously. Clinically, secretory diarrhea is recognized by large stool volumes (>1 L/d) with normal ionic contents and osmolality about equal to plasma. Fasting does not change the stool volume.

Poorly absorbed substances retain intestinal fluids, making osmotic diarrhea. This mechanism occurs with malabsorption, lactose intolerance, divalent ions (e.g., antacids), or poorly soluble carbohydrate (e.g., lactulose). As a poorly soluble solute is transported, the gut adjusts the osmolality to plasma; in so doing, water and electrolytes flux into the lumen. The loss of sodium and water is less than with some diarrheal mechanisms. Clinically, osmotic diarrhea is distinguishable from other types because it stops when the patient fasts.

Inflammatory gut diseases discharge mucus, serum proteins, and blood into the gut. Sometimes bowel movements consist only of mucus, exudate, and blood. Exudative diarrhea probably affects other absorptive, secretory, or motility functions to account for the large stool volume.

Changed intestinal motility causes diarrhea by three mechanisms: reduction of contact time in the small intestine, premature emptying of the colon, and bacterial overgrowth. Chyme must be exposed long enough for normal absorption and secretion. If contact time decreases, diarrhea occurs. Intestinal resection or bypass surgery and drugs (e.g., metoclopramide) cause this type of diarrhea. Increased exposure time also allows fecal bacteria overgrowth. A characteristic small intestine diarrheal pattern is rapid, small, coupling bursts of waves. These waves are inefficient, do not allow absorption, and rapidly dump chyme into the colon. Once in the colon, chyme exceeds the colonic capabilities to absorb water or a diseased colon does not function properly.

CLINICAL PRESENTATION

Diarrhea is divided into acute and chronic diarrheal disorders. Usually, acute diarrheal episodes subside with 72 hours of onset. Chronic diarrhea involves frequent attacks over two to three extended periods. If diarrhea persists or gross blood is present, an extensive study is needed.

History/Physical Examination

Onset and duration differentiate acute and chronic diarrhea. With acute diarrhea, the patient complains of abrupt onset of frequent, watery, loose stools, flatulence, malaise, and abdominal pain. Pain is evaluated for duration, location, and character. Intermittent periumbilical or lower right quadrant pain with cramps and audible bowel sounds is characteristic of small intestinal disease. When pain is present in large intestinal diarrhea, it is a gripping, aching sensation with tenesmus (straining ineffective and painful stooling). Pain localizes to the hypogastric region, right or left lower quadrant, or sacral region. Depending on the specific etiology, the patient complains of fever, vomiting, and muscle aches. In chronic diarrhea, previous bouts, weight loss, anorexia, and chronic weakness are important findings. Certain diarrheal diseases are associated with specific ages. For example, diarrhea from colon cancer is common with advancing age while diarrhea from viral gastroenteritis is largely a childhood condition.

Americans traveling abroad recently may have traveler's or parasitic diarrhea. Environmental conditions such as the recent ingestion of bacteria-contaminated foods identifies "food poisoning" as a possible etiology. An attentive dietary history identifies offending foods (e.g., dairy products with lactose intolerance). With AIDS, a history that focuses on high-risk situations cannot be overlooked. Recent gastrointestinal (GI) surgery may cause a "dumping syndrome."

TABLE 36.1. DRUG-INDUCED DIARRHEA

- Laxatives
- Antacids (magnesium-containing)
- Antibiotics
  - Clindamycin
  - Tetracyclines
  - Sulfonamides
  - Any broad-spectrum antibiotic
- Antihypertensives
  - Reserpine
  - Guanethidine
  - Methyldopa
  - Guanabenz
  - Guanadrel
- Cholinergics
  - Bethanechol
  - Metaclopramide
  - Neostigmine
- Cardiac agents
  - Quinidine
  - Digitalis
  - Digoxin

A medication history is extremely important in identifying drug-induced diarrhea (Table 36.1). For example, many agents, including antibiotics and other drugs, cause pseudomembranous colitis. Self-inflicted laxative abuse for weight loss is popular. Neurotic or psychotic behavior leads to laxative abuse. Drug side effects (e.g., quinidine) often present as diarrhea.

Stool characteristics are important. A description of the frequency, volume, consistency, and color provides diagnostic clues. For instance, diarrhea starting in the small intestine produces copious, watery or fatty (greasy), and foul-smelling stool; contains undigested food particles; and is usually free from gross blood. Colonic diarrhea appears as small, pasty, and sometimes bloody or mucoid movements. Rectal tenesmus with flatus accompanies large intestine diarrhea.

In diarrhea, physical examination of the abdomen shows hyperperistalsis with borborygmi (growling stomach sounds) and generalized or local tenderness. A rectal examination detects masses or possibly fecal impaction, a common cause of diarrhea in the elderly. Hydration is assessed by checking skin turgor and mouth mucosal moisture. Physical signs of systemic disease (e.g., diabetic neuropathy) should be identified. If the patient has hypotension, tachycardia, absent radial pulse, or stupor, severe dehydration is present. Fever strongly suggests an infectious cause.

Laboratory and Endoscopic Tests

Special tests are used for diagnosing unexplained diarrhea, especially in chronic situations.[8,9] Stool studies include examination for parasites and ova, blood, mucus, fat, osmolality, pH, electrolyte analysis, and cultures. Total daily stool volume is also determined. Besides stool studies, direct endoscopic visualization and biopsy are used to diagnose certain conditions such as colitis. Radiographic studies are helpful in neoplastic and inflammatory conditions.

Prognosis

Most diarrhea is self-limiting, subsiding within 72 hours. However, infants, young children, the elderly, and debilitated persons are at risk for morbid and mortal events in prolonged or voluminous diarrhea. These groups are at risk for water, electrolyte, and acid–base disturbances, and potentially cardiovascular collapse and death.

PREVENTION

Acute diarrheal illness often occurs in day care centers and nursing homes.[10] Isolation techniques prevent spread among these populations and health care workers. Hidden dietary sources, such as sorbitol in dietetic products or "Chinese food dumping" syndrome, should be identified and avoided; milk allergy is also a cause.[11] If diarrhea is secondary to another illness, controlling the primary condition is necessary. Antibiotics and bismuth subsalicylate are advocated for preventing traveler's diarrhea, plus special care with drinking water and fresh vegetables.

TREATMENT

If prevention is not successful and diarrhea occurs, the therapeutic goals are (1) to prevent excessive water, electrolyte, and acid–base disturbances; (2) to provide symptomatic relief; (3) to treat curable causes; and (4) to manage secondary disorders causing diarrhea (Figs. 36.1 and 36.2). Clinicians must clearly understand that diarrhea, like a cough, may be a body defense mechanism for ridding itself of harmful substances or pathogens. The correct therapeutic response is not necessarily to stop diarrhea at all costs!

Management of the diet is a first priority. Most clinicians recommend stopping solid foods for 24 hours and avoiding dairy products. In osmotic diarrhea these maneuvers control the problem. If the mechanism is secretory, the diarrhea persists. When nausea or vomiting is mild, digestible low-residue diet is administered for 24 hours. If vomiting is present and uncontrollable with antiemetics (see Chapter 35), nothing is taken by mouth. As bowel movements decrease, a bland diet is begun. Research shows that feeding should continue in children with acute bacterial diarrhea.[12] Fed children have less morbidity and mortality, whether or not they receive oral rehydration fluids. Studies are not available in the elderly or other risk groups to determine the value of continued feeding in bacterial diarrhea.

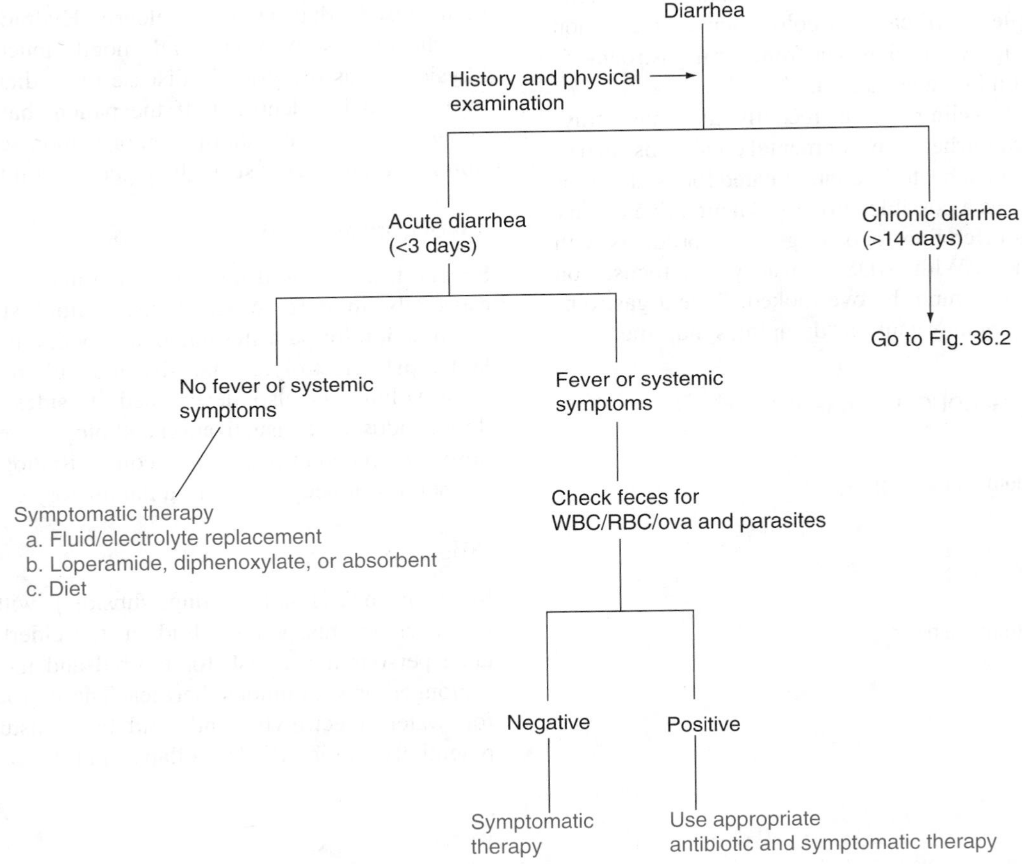

Figure 36.1. Recommendations for treating acute diarrhea. Follow these steps: (1) Perform a complete history and physical examination. (2) Is the diarrhea acute or chronic? If chronic diarrhea, go to Fig. 36.2. (3) If acute diarrhea, check for fever and/or systemic signs and symptoms (i.e., toxic patient). If systemic illness (fever, anorexia, volume depletion), check for infectious source. If positive for infectious diarrhea, use appropriate antibiotic/anthelminthic drug, and symptomatic therapy. If negative for infectious cause, use only symptomatic treatment. (4) If no systemic findings, then use symptomatic therapy, based on severity of volume depletion, oral or parenteral fluid/electrolytes (see Chapter 51, Body Electrolyte Homeostasis), antidiarrheal agents (see Table 36.3), and diet.

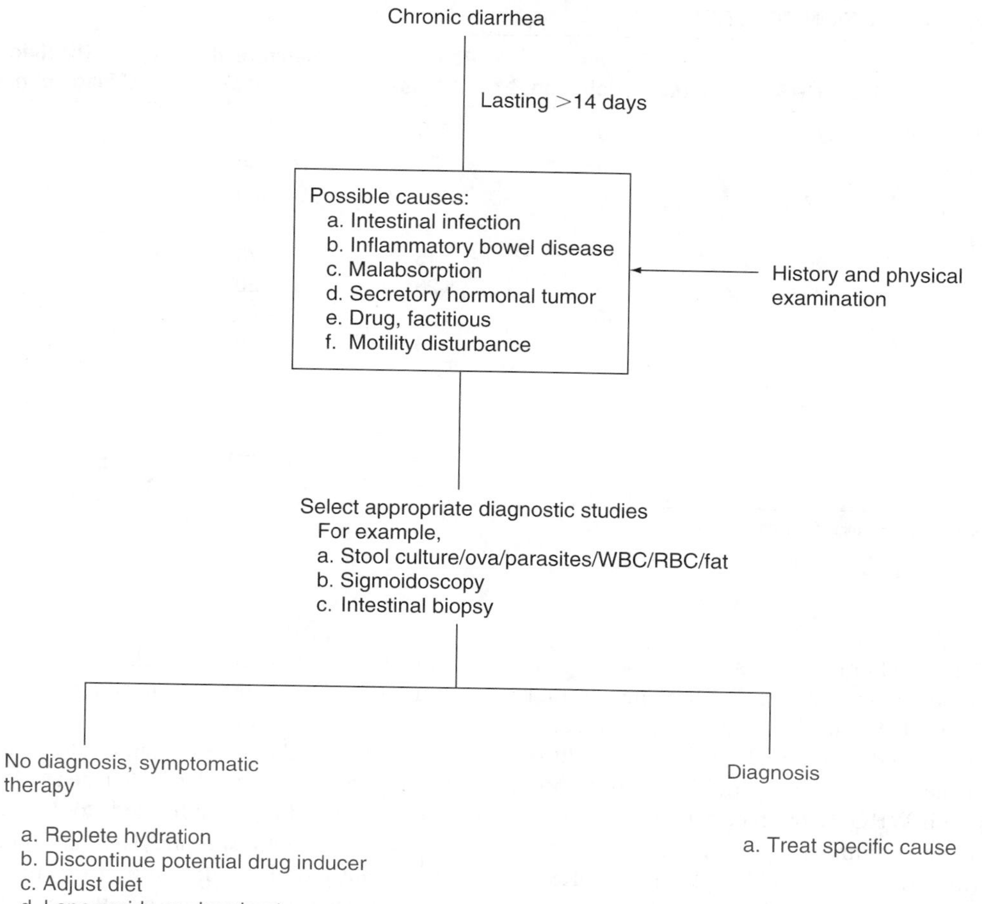

Figure 36.2. Recommendations for treating chronic diarrhea. Follow these steps: (1) Perform a careful history and physical examination. (2) The possible causes of chronic diarrhea are many. These can be classified into intestinal infections (bacterial, protozoal), inflammatory (Crohn's disease, ulcerative colitis), malabsorption (lactose intolerance), secretory hormonal tumor (intestinal carcinoid tumor, VIPoma), drug (antacid), factitious (laxative abuse), or motility disturbance (diabetes mellitus, irritable bowel syndrome, hyperthyroidism). (3) If the diagnosis is uncertain, selected appropriate diagnostic studies should be ordered. (4) Once diagnosed, treatment is planned for the underlying cause with symptomatic antidiarrheal therapy. (5) If no specific cause can be identified, symptomatic therapy is prescribed.

Iatrogenic and surreptitious causes should be sought. Overzealous laxative use in the elderly, whether self- or physician-prescribed, is a common cause of diarrhea and must be identified and stopped.[13] In the nursing home, four to six laxatives are commonly prescribed on an as-needed basis, leading to diarrhea. Community practitioners often encounter elderly patients who falsely believe a daily bowel movement is essential for good health. Besides antibiotics and laxatives, many other drugs induce diarrhea and should be stopped or the dosage reduced.[14]

Repletion and maintenance of water and electrolytes are the primary goals until the diarrheal episode ends. Parenteral and enteral routes supply water and electrolytes. If vomiting and dehydration are not severe, enteral feeding is the less costly and preferred method. In the United States many commercial oral rehydration preparations are available (Table 36.2). These products have been criticized as worsening diarrhea by drawing water into the gut by hypertonicity.[15] However, U.S. physicians continue to hospitalize and intravenously correct these deficits for severe dehydration. Avery and Snyder[16] urge American physicians to use the oral solutions. In developing countries, the World Health Organization Oral Rehydration Solution (WHO–ORS) saves the lives of millions of children (Table 36.2).

During diarrhea, the small intestine retains its ability to actively transport monosaccharides such as glucose. Glu-

TABLE 36.2. ORAL REHYDRATION SOLUTIONS

	WHO–ORS[a]	Lytren (Mead Johnson)	Pedialyte (Ross)	Rehydralyte (Ross)	Ricelyte (Mead Johnson)	Resol (Wyeth)
Osmolality (mOsm/L)	333	220	249	304	200	269
Carbohydrates[b](g/L)	20	20	25	25	30[c]	20
Calories (cal/L)	77	85	100	100	126	80
Electrolytes (mEq/L)						
Sodium	90	50	45	75	50	50
Potassium	20	25	20	20	25	20
Chloride	80	45	35	65	45	50
Citrate	—	30	30	30	34	34
Bicarbonate	30	—	—	—	—	—
Calcium	—	—	—	—	—	4
Magnesium	—	—	—	—	—	4
Sulfate	—	—	—	—	—	—
Phosphate	—	—	—	—	—	5

[a]World Health Organization Oral Rehydration Solution.
[b]Carbohydrate is glucose.
[c]Rice syrup solids is carbohydrate source.

cose actively carries sodium with water and other electrolytes passively. Because the WHO–ORS has a high sodium concentration, U.S. physicians have been reluctant to use it in well-nourished children. This attitude could be changing as controlled comparative studies describe more favorable results with WHO–ORS than parenteral fluids.[17] Amino acids promote sodium transport and act as an antisecretory agent. Researchers have added glycine to ORS in an attempt to create a "super–ORS." Reports, however, are disappointing because glycine causes an osmotic diarrhea and diuresis in experimental concentrations.[18] Rice-based oral solution is an hyposmotically active substrate. Rice supplies long-chain molecules and elutes glucose without increasing stool or urine outflow. Pizarro et al.[19] reported effective rehydration of infants with acute diarrhea using a rice-based solution. They also reported decreased stool output and greater absorption and retention of fluid and electrolytes. These starch solutions reach 5%, a concentration possibly causing an osmotic diarrhea.

Various drugs have been used to treat diarrheal attacks (Table 36.3). These drugs are grouped into several categories: antimotility, adsorbents, antisecretory compounds, antibiotics, enzymes, and intestinal microflora. Usually, these drugs are not curative but palliative.

Opiates and opioid derivatives (1) delay the transit of intraluminal content or (2) increase gut capacity, prolonging contact and absorption. Enkephalins, endogenous opioid substances, regulate fluid movement across the mucosa by stimulating absorptive processes. Most opiates act through peripheral and central mechanisms, except loperamide, which acts peripherally.[20] Loperamide is antisecretory; it inhibits the calcium-binding protein calmodulin, controlling chloride secretion.[21,22] Although many studies support this mechanism, Schiller et al.[23] questioned loperamide's antisecretory mechanism as the important antidiarrheal control.

Loperamide was comparable to bismuth subsalicylate for treatment of traveler's diarrhea.[24] People taking loperamide passed fewer unformed stools compared with those receiving bismuth subsalicylate, and shigellosis was not significantly prolonged. The limits of the opiates are addiction potential (a real concern with long-term use) and worsening of diarrhea in selected infectious diarrhea.

Adsorbents are used for symptomatic relief (Table 36.3). These products, many not needing a prescription, are nontoxic but their effectiveness remains unproven. Adsorbents are nonspecific in their action; they adsorb nutrients, toxins, drugs, and digestive juices. Coadministration with other drugs reduces their bioavailability. Portnoy and associates[25] compared kaolin and pectin suspension and diphenoxylate liquid in acute childhood diarrhea, and did not show relief. The Food and Drug Administration over-the-counter (FDA OTC) review panel recommends only polycarbophil as an effective adsorbent. Polycarbophil absorbs 60 times its weight in water and treats both diarrhea and constipation.

Lactobacillus preparations replace colonic microflora secondary to antibiotic action. A controversial treatment is seeding the gut with this organism. This supposedly restores intestinal functions and suppresses the growth of pathogenic microorganisms. However, a dairy product diet containing 200–400 g of lactose or dextrin is equally effective in recolonization. Again, clinical studies are lacking.

Anticholinergic drugs, such as atropine, block vagal tone and prolong gut transit time (Table 36.3). They are available in combination in many nonprescription products

TABLE 36.3. SELECTED ANTIDIARRHEAL PREPARATIONS

	Dose Form	Adult Dose
Antimotility		
Diphenoxylate	2.5 mg/tablet 2.5 mg/5 mL	5 mg QID; do not exceed 20 mg/d
Loperamide	2 mg/capsule 1 mg/5 mL	Initially 4 mg, then 2 mg after each loose stool; do not exceed 16 mg/d
Paregoric	2 mg/5 mL (morphine)	5–10 mL 1–4 times daily
Opium tincture	5 mg/mL (morphine)	0.6 mL QID
Atropine	0.3, 0.4, 0.6 mg/tablet	0.4–0.6 mg every 4–6 h
Adsorbents		
Kaolin–pectin mixture	0.98 g kaolin + 21.7 mg pectin per 5 mL	30–120 mL after each loose stool
Polycarbophil	500 mg/tablet	Chew 2 tablets QID or after each loose stool; do not exceed 12 tablets a day
Antisecretory (bismuth subsalicylate)	300/mg tablet 525 mg/30 mL	Two tablets or 30 mL every 30 min as needed up to 8 doses per day
Enzymes (lactase)	1250 neutral lactase units per 4 drops 3300 FCC lactase units per tablet	3–4 drops taken with milk or dairy product 1 or 2 tablets as above
Bacterial replacement (*Lactobacillus acidophilus, L. bulgaricus*)		2 tablets or 1 granule packet 3 to 4 times daily; give with milk, juice, or water

and as single entities. Their value in controlling diarrhea is questionable and limited by side effects. To stop diarrhea, clinicians have been falsely taught to dose anticholinergics until they decrease salivary and sweat secretion. Despite anticholinergic side effects in 54% of test subjects, Reves et al.[26] did not prove the effectiveness of mepenzolate bromide in acute infectious diarrhea. Angle closure glaucoma, selected heart diseases, and obstructive uropathies are relative contraindications to use of anticholinergic agents.

Many acute diarrheas are caused by infectious agents, which have a strong secretory component. Agents blocking copious fluid flow are highly desirable in secretory diarrheas, so bismuth subsalicylate suspension has been studied. When 30 mL of this suspension was given every 30 minutes for eight doses, unformed stools decreased in the first 24 hours in active infection.[27] Bismuth subsalicylate has also been studied to prevent traveler's diarrhea. Bismuth subsalicylate tablets (1.05 or 2.1 g versus placebo twice daily) reduced the incidence of diarrhea in 231 volunteers and caused only minor undesirable complaints (taste, constipation, nausea).[28]

Bismuth subsalicylate contains multiple components that might be toxic if given excessively to prevent or treat diarrhea. For instance, the active ingredient is salicylate, which may interact with anticoagulants or cause effects of salicylism (tinnitus, nausea, and vomiting). Bismuth toxicity is another potential problem at excessive doses, but clinical problems are rarely encountered. Despite these potential problems, bismuth subsalicylate can be effective and safe in treatment and prevention of traveler's diarrhea with proper dosing.

The role of antibiotics is controversial. Antibiotics are curative if the organism is susceptible, but most infectious diarrheas are self-limiting and treated with supportive therapy. In traveler's diarrhea, antibiotic prophylaxis (e.g., with tetracycline and cotrimoxazole) is effective but antibiotic resistance is possible.

Octreotide (Sandostatin™), a synthetic octapeptide analogue of endogenous somatostatin, is prescribed for the symptomatic treatment of carcinoid tumors and vasoactive intestinal peptide-secreting tumors (VIPomas).[29,30] Metastatic intestinal carcinoid tumors secrete excessive amounts of vasoactive substances, including histamine, bradykinin, serotonin, and prostaglandins. Primary carcinoid tumors are located throughout the GI tract with most in the ileum. The predominant clinical signs and symptoms are attributable to excessive 5-hydroxytryptophan and serotonin. The collection of their clinical effects is termed the *carcinoid syndrome.* Carcinoid syndrome is characterized by paroxysmal vasomotor attacks, most notably sudden red to purple flushing of the face and neck. These attacks are often precipitated by emotional outbursts or by ingestion of food or alcohol. Some patients have a violent, watery diarrhea with cramping. Initially diarrhea might be managed with various agents such as codeine, diphenoxylate, cyproheptadine, methysergide, phenoxybenzamine, or methyldopa. Octreotide, a parenteral drug, is used in selected patients. Octreotide blocks the release of serotonin and other active peptides and has been effective in controlling diarrhea and flushing. Dosage range is 100–600 mcg/d in two to four divided doses subcutaneously. Nongastrin-secreting adenomas of the pancreas are tumors associated with profuse watery diarrhea. This condition is termed by various names including "Verner–Morrison syndrome," "WDHA syndrome" (watery diarrhea, hypokalemia, achlorhydria), "pancreatic cholera," "watery diarrhea syndrome," and "VIPoma." Excessive secretion of VIP from a retroperitoneal or pancreatic tumor is believed to cause most of the clinical features. Excessive VIP is isolated in about half of patients along with numerous other peptide hormones (peptide histidine methionine [PHM], serotonin, somatostatin, gastrin, glucagon). Surgical tumor dissection is the treatment of choice. In nonsurgical candidates, however, the profuse watery diarrhea is managed with octreotide. The dosage range is 200–300 mcg/d in two to four divided doses. The adverse reactions most often reported are GI (nausea, cramping, diarrhea) and injection site pain.

EVALUATION OF THERAPEUTIC OUTCOMES

Acute Diarrhea

Most patients have mild to moderate distress with acute diarrhea. Without moderate to severe dehydration, high fever, and blood or mucus in their stool, the illness is usually self-limiting within 3 to 7 days. Mild to moderate acute diarrhea is usually managed without hospitalization using oral rehydration, symptomatic treatment, and diet. Elderly persons with chronic illness and infants may need hospitalization for parenteral rehydration and close monitoring.

With the urgency/emergency situation, evaluation of the patient's volume status is the most important outcome. Toxic patients (fever, dehydration, hematochezia, hypotensive) require hospitalization; they need intravenous electrolyte solutions and empiric antibiotics while awaiting cultures. With quick management, they usually recover within a few days.

Therapeutic outcomes are directed to key symptoms, signs, and laboratory studies. The constitutional symptoms usually improve within 24 to 72 hours. One should check the frequency and character of bowel movements each day along with the vital signs and improving appetite. Also, the clinician needs to monitor body weight, serum osmolality, serum electrolytes, complete blood cell count, urinalysis, and cultures (if appropriate).

Chronic Diarrhea

Chronic diarrhea has myriad causes and the prognosis is extremely variable. Antidiarrheal drugs are prescribed for symptomatic control, as are antibiotics and anthelmintic drugs when appropriate. The therapeutic outcome depends on diagnosing and correcting the underlying disease. Short-term management goals are similar to those with acute diarrhea.

CONTROVERSIES IN DRUG MANAGEMENT

Many experimental drugs have been used to control diarrhea. Phenothiazines, β blockers, nonsteroidal anti-inflammatory drugs (NSAIDs), calcium channel blockers, somatostatin, and α-adrenergic agonists are only a few agents under investigation in either animals or humans.

Nifalatide is an enkephalin analogue that delays the onset of castor oil-induced diarrhea and decreases stool frequency. Dizziness and dry mouth are frequent side effects.[31] Enkephalinase inhibitors (e.g., acetorphan) offer another therapeutic choice.[32] In the search for proabsorption/antisecretory drugs, lidamidine, a prototype α_2-adrenergic agonist, was compared with loperamide and found to counter diarrhea by either promoting absorption or preventing secretion.[31] With lidamidine, a clonidine analogue, hypotension is a limiting dose-related problem. Prostaglandin inhibitors, aspirin and its analogues, and indomethacin are safe and effective in childhood gastroenteritis; studies in animals support indomethacin in enteropathogen secretory states such as with *Vibrio cholerae.*[33–35]

Vaccines are a new therapeutic frontier in controlling infectious diarrheas, especially in developing countries.[2] Cholera vaccine yields some protection but is not totally effective and does not prevent transmission. Oral *Shigella* vaccine was effective under field conditions, but calls for five doses with repeat booster doses, limiting its practicality in developing nations. With about 1500 serotypes for *Salmonella,* a vaccine still is not available. In the United States, rotavirus vaccine would protect many infants and children, and a vaccine is under development.

SUMMARY

In the United States, diarrhea is most often a minor discomfort, not life threatening and usually self-limited. Children and the elderly are groups at high risk for severe complications of acute diarrhea. Usually, a diagnosis is based on the history and physical examination, with extensive diagnostic tests reserved for chronic diarrhea.

Management focuses on preventing excessive water and electrolyte losses, relieving symptoms, treating curable causes, and treating secondary disorders. Acute diarrhea is usually self-limiting and managed with supportive therapy. Chronic diarrhea is managed by identifying (if possible) and treating the cause or at least supportively managing each diarrheal episode.

CONSTIPATION

Constipation is a very common problem as evidenced by the tremendous dollar volumes spent on laxatives and the prominence they have gained in the advertising media and on the shelves of retail outlets. Currently, more than 125 laxative products are available OTC[36] and a few are available by prescription.

Most treatments for constipation are initiated by the patient, often without consultation from a health professional. One reason constipation continues to be a frequent problem in the United States is the inadequate diets of many people. Another unfortunate problem is that many people have misconceptions about normal bowel function, thinking that daily bowel movements are required for health and well-being. Others believe that the lack of a daily bowel movement contributes to the accumulation of toxic substances or is associated with various somatic complaints. These misconceptions lead to the inappropriate use of laxatives by the general public.

Constipation does not have one consistently used definition. When using the term *constipation,* the lay public or health care professional may be referring to several difficult-to-quantify variables: bowel movement frequency, stool size or consistency, and such symptoms as a feeling of incomplete defecation. Stool frequency is most often used to describe constipation. The frequency of bowel movements used to define constipation is not well established, but it has been determined that normal subjects pass at least three stools per week. In one study of more than 1400 people in Great Britain, 99% of subjects had a bowel movement more than twice weekly but not more than 3 times daily.[37] In an older population, 95% of men and 90% of women had a bowel movement from once every 2 days to twice daily.[38] A study of 115 healthy men showed mean (±SD) stool frequency to be 27.6 ± 9.5 hours.[39]

A number of other definitions have been used in clinical studies. Some of the definitions used include (1) less than three stools per week for women and five for men despite a high residue diet, or a period of greater than 3 days without a bowel movement, (2) straining at stool greater than 25% of the time and/or two or fewer stools per week, or (3) straining at defecation and less than one stool daily with minimal effort. These varying definitions demonstrate the difficulty in characterizing this problem.

Constipation may be caused by a wide range of diseases (e.g., diseases of the GI tract, endocrine or metabolic derangements), drugs, or improper diets. Evaluation of the patient complaining of constipation requires a thorough history to determine the nature and frequency of bowel movements and dietary habits, and may include physical and laboratory assessments to evaluate the possibility of underlying diseases. The proper treatment of constipation requires alteration of diet to include a greater quantity of fiber, correction of diseases that may be responsible, and elimination (if possible) of drugs that may cause constipation. Once these factors have been considered, judicious use of selected laxative products is sometimes required.

Constipation requires treatment (not necessarily with drug therapy), mainly because it is usually uncomfortable for the patient, and also because it may be associated with more serious diseases. Constipation associated with inadequate dietary fiber may worsen hemorrhoidal disease by the passage of infrequent, relatively hard stool. With some causes of constipation the loops of bowel may become dangerously dilated, with risk of perforation or infarction. Also, some studies have shown that constipation is associated with a greater risk of colon and rectal cancer, particularly in women, although this relationship is not well accepted.[40–42]

ETIOLOGY

Constipation is not a disease but a symptom of an underlying disease or problem. Approaches to treatment of constipation should begin with attempts to determine its cause. Disorders of the GI tract (e.g., irritable bowel syndrome or diverticulitis), metabolic disorders (e.g., diabetes), or endocrine disorders (e.g., hypothyroidism) may be involved. Constipation commonly results from a diet low in fiber or from use of constipating drugs such as opiates. Finally, it is believed that constipation may sometimes be psychogenic in origin. Each of these causes is discussed.

Constipation is a frequent problem in the elderly, probably the result of improper diets (low in fiber and liquids), diminished abdominal wall muscular strength, and possibly diminished physical activity. In addition, diseases that may cause constipation, such as colon cancers and diverticulitis, are more common with increasing age.

Gastrointestinal Disorders

GI disorders are a common cause of constipation. The most frequent GI causes of constipation are disorders of the large bowel, but diseases of the upper GI tract (e.g., gastroduodenal obstruction from ulceration or cancer) may also be responsible. The most common colonic disorders causing constipation are irritable bowel syndrome and diverticulitis. Irritable bowel syndrome may be associated with constipation, diarrhea, or both. In these patients, objective findings of disease are often absent, but colonic motility is usually abnormal.

Anal and rectal diseases associated with pain on defecation may cause constipation. Hemorrhoids, anal fissures, or ulcerative proctitis may all result in painful elimination and inhibition of the urge to defecate. The result may be a decreased frequency of bowel movements.

Constipation may be an indication of obstruction of the colon. The colon may become obstructed from tumors that originate in the lumen of the colon or from organs or structures adjacent to the colon. Also, constipation may result from hernias, volvulus of the bowel (torsion or twisting of a loop of intestine), or a variety of diseases (syphilis, tuberculosis, helminthic infections, or lymphogranuloma venereum), all of which may cause stricture of the lumen of the colon.

Neurologic disorders of the GI tract also may be a cause of constipation. The most prominent neurologic disorder of the GI tract resulting in constipation is Hirschsprung's disease, also called aganglionosis. With this disorder there is a congenital absence of neurons to the terminal segments of the bowel. The disorder is usually diagnosed by rectal biopsy and manometric studies of the rectum.

Metabolic and Endocrine Disorders

Many metabolic and endocrine disorders affect bowel function. Examples include diabetes mellitus with associated neuropathy, which may affect multiple segments of the GI tract and result in an atonic colon, uremia, and hypokalemia. Hypothyroidism and panhypopituitarism may result in inhibited bowel function. In fact, for some cases of hypothyroidism the presenting symptom is constipation or bowel obstruction. Other disorders such as pheochromocytoma may cause constipation, because catecholamines inhibit GI smooth muscle activity. Hypercalcemia (from any cause) and enteric glucagon excess may also result in inhibited bowel function.

Pregnancy

Constipation is a frequent problem during pregnancy, possibly resulting from complex factors that include depressed gut motility, increased fluid absorption from the colon, decreased physical activity, and dietary changes.[43] Predisposing dietary factors include inadequate fluid intake, low dietary fiber, and the use of iron salts.

Neurogenic Constipation

In addition to peripheral neurologic disorders that may cause constipation, central nervous system (CNS) disorders also may be responsible. The CNS is an important component in GI regulation, either through GI reflexes or through coordination of other organs of the body. In addition, the CNS modifies GI function in response to conscious effort or emotional stimuli. Many diseases of the CNS can therefore affect GI function. Trauma to the brain (particularly the medulla) or spinal cord may result in inhibited bowel function as may CNS tumors. Also, cerebrovascular accidents and Parkinson's disease may cause inhibited bowel function.

Psychogenic Constipation

The term *psychogenic constipation* has variable acceptance among experts in the field because objective evidence for its existence is slim; however, it has been recognized that bowel habits, particularly those developed early in life, may relate to chronic constipation. Ignoring or postponing the urge to defecate may cause blunting of the colonic and rectal response and may possibly lead to prolonged retention of stool. People in certain occupations, such as truck drivers, may be particularly predisposed to this problem. Finally, patients with psychiatric diseases often have constipation. In many instances, improvement in constipation is observed with the onset of psychotherapy.

Drug-Induced Constipation

Drugs that inhibit the neurologic or muscular function of the GI tract, particularly the colon, may result in constipation. A large number of drugs have such properties (Table 36.4). The majority of cases of drug-induced constipation are caused by opiates, various agents with anticholinergic properties, and antacids containing aluminum or calcium. With most of the agents listed, the inhibitory bowel effects are dose dependent, with larger doses clearly causing constipation more frequently.

Opiates have been known for their GI inhibitory effects at least as long as they have been known as analgesics. Clearly, opiates used to treat diarrhea have considerable antimotility effects. Opiates have effects on all segments of the bowel, but effects are most pronounced on the colon. The major mechanism of opiate action has been proposed to be prolongation of intestinal transit time by causing spastic, nonpropulsive contractions.[44] An additional, contributory mechanism of action may be an increase in electrolyte absorption.[45]

All opiate derivatives are associated with constipation, but the degree of intestinal inhibitory effects seems to differ between agents. Orally administered opiates appear to have

TABLE 36.4. DRUGS CAUSING CONSTIPATION

- Analgesics
  - Inhibitors of prostaglandin synthesis
  - Opiates
- Anticholinergics
  - Antihistamines
  - Antiparkinsonian agents (e.g., benztropine or trihexaphenidyl)
  - Phenothiazines
  - Tricyclic antidepressants
- Antacids containing calcium carbonate or aluminum hydroxide
- Barium sulfate
- Clonidine
- Diuretics (non–potassium sparing)
- Ganglionic blockers
- Iron preparations
- Muscle blockers (*d*-tubocurarine, succinylcholine)
- Polystyrene sodium sulfonate

greater inhibitory effect than parenterally administered agents; oral codeine is well known as a potent antimotility agent. Orally administered enkephalins (endogenous opiatelike polypeptides) are recognized to have antimotility properties.

Agents with anticholinergic properties inhibit bowel function by parasympatholytic actions on innervation to many regions of the GI tract, particularly the colon and rectum. Many types of drugs possess anticholinergic action (Table 36.4), and these agents are used commonly in hospitalized and nonhospitalized patients. One recent study demonstrated that amitriptylline, diphenhydramine, and thioridazine were associated with laxative use in 800 nursing home patients.[46]

A prospective study included 3166 people over the age of 65 in a Florida community.[47] Twenty-six percent of women and 15.8% of men reported recurrent constipation. Factors found to correlate with self-reported constipation were age, sex (higher frequency in females), total number of drugs taken, abdominal pain, and hemorrhoids. Drugs correlated with constipation were anticholinergics, aspirin, furosemide, nitroglycerin, and amitriptylline. Serum chloride and aspartate aminotransferase, as well as alcohol consumption, were found to be negatively related to constipation. The most important predictors of constipation were age and the total number of medications taken.

CLINICAL PRESENTATION

The patient presenting with constipation (usually with abdominal discomfort and distention) should be questioned and examined; constipation may vary in implication from minor discomfort in the otherwise healthy adult to a symptom of colon cancer or other serious diseases. A basis for evaluation and treatment should be a thorough history including questions about the nature of the "constipation." It is important to ascertain whether the patient perceives the problem as infrequent bowel movements, stools of insufficient size, a feeling of fullness, or difficulty and pain on passing stool. The patient should be asked about the frequency of bowel movements and the chronicity of constipation. Constipation occurring recently in an adult may indicate significant colon pathology such as malignancy; constipation present since early infancy may be indicative of neurologic disorders. The patient also should be carefully questioned about usual diet and laxative regimens. Does the patient have a diet consistently deficient in high-fiber items and containing mainly highly refined foods? What laxatives or cathartics has the patient used to attempt relief of constipation? It should be noted that laxative abusers frequently deny laxative use. Finally, the patient should be questioned about other concurrent medications, with interest toward agents that might cause constipation.

For most patients complaining of constipation, a thorough physical examination is not required once it is established that constipation (1) is not a chronic problem, (2) is not accompanied by signs of significant GI disease (e.g., rectal bleeding), and (3) does not cause severe discomfort. In these circumstances the patient may be referred directly to the first-line therapies for constipation described under the Treatment section (mainly bulk-forming laxatives and dietary fiber with occasional use of saline or stimulant laxatives). Certain patients, however, require a full examination by a physician to determine the cause of constipation. Patients may then have a series of examinations, proctoscopy, sigmoidoscopy, colonoscopy, or barium enema to determine the presence of colorectal pathology. Also, tests such as thyroid function studies may be performed to determine the presence of metabolic or endocrine disorders.

Chronic constipation can result in a more complex picture. Patients may have long-standing complaints of GI irregularities with a variety of symptoms. The laxative abuser may present with contradictory findings, sometimes diarrhea or weight loss. Laxative abusers may also have vomiting, abdominal pain, lassitude, thirst, edema, and bone pain (due to osteomalacia). With prolonged abuse patients may have fluid and electrolyte imbalances (most commonly hypokalemia), protein losing gastroenteropathy with hypoalbuminemia, and syndromes resembling colitis.

TREATMENT

The proper management of constipation requires a number of different modalities; however, the basis for therapy should be dietary modification. The major dietary change should be an increase in the amount of fiber consumed daily. In addition to dietary management, patients should be encouraged to alter other aspects of their lifestyle to some extent if necessary and where possible. Important considerations would be to encourage the patients to exercise (achieved even by brisk walking after dinner) and to adjust bowel habits so that a regular and adequate time is made to respond to the urge to defecate. Another general measure is to increase fluid intake. This is generally recommended and believed beneficial, although there is little objective evidence of benefit.

If an underlying disease is recognized as the cause of constipation, attempts should be made to correct it. GI malignancies may be removed through a surgical resection. Endocrine and metabolic derangements should be corrected by the appropriate methods. For example, when hypothyroidism is the cause of constipation, cautious institution of thyroid-replacement therapy is the most important treatment measure.

As discussed earlier, many drug substances may cause constipation. After determination of a patient's prescription and nonprescription drug therapy, potential drug causes of constipation should be identified. If the patient is consuming medications well known to cause constipation, consideration should be given to alternative agents. For some medications (e.g., antacids), nonconstipating alternatives exist. If no reasonable alternatives exist to the medication thought to be responsible for constipation, consideration should be given to lowering the dose. If a patient must remain on constipating medications, then more attention must be paid to general measures for prevention of constipation, as discussed next.

Dietary Modification and Bulk-Forming Agents

The most important aspect of the therapy for constipation for the majority of patients is dietary modification to increase the amount of fiber consumed. Fiber, the portion of vegetable matter not digested in the human GI tract, increases stool bulk, retention of stool water, and rate of transit of stool through the intestine.[48] The result of fiber therapy is an increased frequency of defecation. Also, fiber has been shown to decrease intraluminal pressures in the colon and rectum, which is thought to be beneficial for diverticular disease and irritable bowel syndrome. The specific physiologic effects of fiber are not well understood.

Patients should be advised to include at least 14 g of crude fiber in their daily diets.[49] Fruits, vegetables, and cereals have the highest fiber content. Bran, a by-product of milling of wheat, is often added to foods to increase fiber content. Raw bran is generally 40% fiber. Medicinal products, often called "bulk-forming agents," such as psyllium hydrophillic colloids (e.g., Effersyllium), methylcellulose (e.g., Cologel), or polycarbophil (e.g., Mitrolan) have properties similar to those of dietary fiber and may be taken as tablets, powders, or granules (Table 36.5).

A trial of dietary modification with high-fiber content should be continued for at least 1 month before effects on bowel function are determined. Most patients begin to notice effects on bowel function 3 to 5 days after beginning a high-fiber diet, but some patients may require a considerably longer time. When beginning fiber therapies, the patient should be cautioned that abdominal distention and flatus may be particularly troublesome in the first few weeks, particularly with high bran consumption.[50] In most patients, these problems resolve with continued use.

Bulk-forming laxatives have few side effects and minimal systemic effects. The only major caution in the use of bulk-forming laxatives is that obstruction of the esophagus, stomach, small intestine, and colon has been reported when the agents have been consumed without fluid, so these products should not be used without adequate fluids or in patients with intestinal stenosis.

TABLE 36.5. DOSAGE RECOMMENDATIONS FOR LAXATIVES AND CATHARTICS

Agent	Recommended Dose
Agents That Cause Softening of Feces in 1–3 d	
Bulk-forming agents	
Methylcellulose	4–6 g/d
Polycarbophil	4–6 g/d
Psyllium	Varies with product
Emollients	
Docusate sodium	50–360 mg/d
Docusate calcium	50–360 mg/d
Docusate potassium	100–300 mg/d
Lactulose	15–30 mL orally
Sorbitol	30–50 g/d orally
Mineral oil	15–30 mL orally
Agents That Result in Soft or Semifluid Stool in 6–12 h	
Bisacodyl (oral)	5–15 mg orally
Phenolphthalein	30–270 mg orally
Cascara sagrada	Dose varies with formulation
Senna	Dose varies with formulation
Magnesium sulfate (low dose)	<10 g orally
Agents That Cause Watery Evacuation in 1–6 h	
Magnesium citrate	18 g in 300 mL water
Magnesium hydroxide	2.4–4.8 g orally
Magnesium sulfate (high dose)	10–30 g orally
Sodium phosphates	Varies with salt used
Bisacodyl	10 mg rectally
Polyethylene glycol–electrolyte preparations	4 L

Surgery

In a small percentage of patients presenting with complaints of constipation, surgical procedures are necessary. Surgery is usually necessary with most colonic malignancies and with GI obstruction from a number of causes. In each case, the involved segment of intestine may be resected or revised to allow flow of GI contents through an enterostomy or through the anus. Surgery may be required in some endocrine disorders causing constipation, such as pheochromocytoma, which requires removal of a tumor.

Drug Therapy

The traditional classification system for laxatives and cathartics, by suspected mode of action, has not been very useful; the mode of action of many products is not clearly understood.[51,52] In general, most agents work by promoting some of the mechanisms involved in diarrhea, including active electrolyte secretion, decreased water and electrolyte absorption, increased intraluminal osmolarity, and increased hydrostatic pressure in the gut. Laxatives convert the intestine from primarily an organ that absorbs water and electrolytes to an organ that secretes water and electrolytes.[52] The various types of laxatives are discussed in this section. The agents are divided into three general classifications: (1) those causing softening of feces in 1 to 3 days (bulk-forming laxatives, docusates, and lactulose); (2) those that result in soft or semifluid stool in 6 to 12 hours (diphenylmethane derivatives and anthraquinone derivatives); and (3) those causing water evacuation in 1 to 6 hours (saline cathartics, castor oil, and polyethylene glycol–electrolyte lavage solution).[53]

Emollient Laxatives

These surfactant agents, docusate in its various salts, work by facilitating mixing of aqueous and fatty materials within the intestinal tract. They may increase water and electrolyte secretion in the small and large bowel.[54] These products are generally given orally, although docusate potassium has also been used rectally. These products result in a softening of stools within 1 to 3 days.

Emollient laxatives are not effective in treating constipation but are used mainly to prevent constipation. They may be helpful in situations where straining at stool should be avoided, such as after recovery from myocardial infarction, with acute perianal disease, or after rectal surgery. It is unlikely that these agents would be very effective in preventing constipation if major causative factors (e.g., heavy opiate use, uncorrected pathology, inadequate dietary fiber) are not concurrently addressed.

Although docusates are generally safe, a few adverse effects have been noted. They may increase the intestinal absorption of agents administered concurrently and alter toxic potential. Danthron, a laxative previously used in combination with docusates, has been noted to be hepatotoxic when there is increased absorption.[55,56]

Lubricants

Mineral oil is the only lubricant laxative in routine use. This agent, obtained from petroleum refining, acts by coating stool and allowing easier passage. It inhibits colonic absorption of water, thereby increasing stool weight and decreasing stool transit time. Mineral oil may be given orally or rectally in a dose of 15 to 45 mL. Generally, the effect on bowel function is noted after 2 or 3 days of use.

Mineral oil is helpful in situations similar to those suggested for docusates: to maintain a soft stool and avoid straining for relatively short periods of time (a few days to 2 weeks); however, it possesses a much greater potential for adverse effects and its routine use should be discouraged. Mineral oil may be absorbed systemically and cause a foreign-body reaction in lymphoid tissue. Also, in debilitated or recumbent patients, mineral oil may be aspirated causing lipoid pneumonia.[57,58] For this reason it should not be used just before bedtime or when a patient is recumbent. Mineral oil has been reported to decrease the absorption of fat-soluble vitamins (A, D, E, and K) with chronic use by causing retention in the GI tract. Finally, even when given orally, mineral oil may leak from the anal sphincter, causing pruritus and soiling of clothing.

Lactulose and Sorbitol

Lactulose is a disaccharide used orally or rectally. It is metabolized by colonic bacteria to low molecular weight acids, resulting in an osmotic effect whereby fluid is retained in the colon. The fluid retained in the colon lowers the pH and increases colonic peristalsis. Lactulose is generally not recommended as a first-line agent for the treatment of constipation because it is costly and not necessarily more effective than such agents as milk of magnesia.[59] It may be justified as an alternative for acute constipation and has been found useful particularly in elderly patients. Occasionally, the use of lactulose may result in flatulence, cramps, diarrhea, and electrolyte imbalances.[60] Sorbitol, a monosaccharide, is occasionally used as a laxative, exerting its effect by osmotic action. It is as effective as lactulose and much less expensive.[61]

Diphenylmethane Derivatives

The two commonly used agents in this class are bisacodyl and phenolphthalein. The actions of these agents are believed to be primarily on the colon. Bisacodyl stimulates the mucosal nerve plexus of the colon; the mechanism of action of phenolphthalein is poorly understood (possibly it inhibits active glucose absorption and sodium absorption, resulting in fluid accumulation in the colon by osmotic action). The dose of these agents effective in various individuals appears to vary greatly. A dose that causes no effects in one patient may result in excessive cramping and fluid evacuation in others. With phenolphthalein, a small portion of the dose undergoes enterohepatic recirculation, which may result in a prolonged laxative action.

These agents are not recommended for daily use on a regular basis. Their use is acceptable intermittently (every few weeks) to treat constipation or as a bowel preparation before diagnostic procedures in which cleansing of the colon is necessary. These agents may sometimes cause severe abdominal cramping as well as significant fluid and electrolyte imbalances with chronic use. These agents should not be used for patients in whom appendicitis is a possibility (perforation of the appendix may result) or during pregnancy or lactation. Finally, the patient taking phenolphthalein-containing laxatives should be cautioned that it may turn urine pink.

Anthraquinone Derivatives

The agents in this class are cascara sagrada, sennosides, and casanthrol. These agents are metabolized by gut bacteria to their active compounds, but the exact mechanisms of action are not understood. Effects are limited to the colon, and stimulation of Auerbach's plexus may be involved. Recommendations for the use of these agents are similar to those for the diphenylmethane derivatives. In most cases, intermittent use is acceptable; daily use should be strongly discouraged.

Most of the concerns with the use of diphenylmethane derivatives (bisacodyl and phenolphthalein) apply to the anthraquinone derivatives. In addition, the anthraquinone derivatives may cause melanosis coli, an accumulation of dark pigment, mainly in the cecum and rectum, that is evident after 4 to 13 months of use. A pathologic effect of melanosis coli has not been demonstrated, and it appears reversible after anthraquinones have been discontinued for 3 to 6 months.

Saline Cathartics

Saline cathartics are composed of relatively poorly absorbed ions such as magnesium, sulfate, phosphate, and citrate, which produce their effects primarily by osmotic action to retain fluid in the GI tract. Magnesium has been shown to stimulate the secretion of cholecystokinin, a hormone that causes stimulation of bowel motility and fluid secretion. These agents may be given orally or rectally. A bowel movement may result within a few hours after oral doses and in 1 hour or less after rectal administration.

These agents should be used primarily for acute evacuation of the bowel, which may be necessary before diagnostic examinations, after poisonings, and in conjunction with some anthelmintics to eliminate parasites. Such agents as milk of magnesia (an 8% suspension of magnesium hydroxide) may be used occasionally (every few weeks) to treat constipation in otherwise healthy adults. Saline cathartics should not be used on a routine basis to treat constipation. With fecal impactions the enema formulations of these agents may be helpful.

As with most laxatives, these agents may cause fluid and electrolyte depletion. Also, magnesium or sodium accumulation may occur when magnesium-containing cathartics are used in patients with renal dysfunction or when sodium phosphate is used in patients with congestive heart failure.

Castor Oil

Castor oil is metabolized in the GI tract to an active compound, ricinoleic acid, which stimulates secretory processes, decreases glucose absorption, and promotes intestinal motility, primarily in the small intestine. Castor oil usually results in a bowel movement within 1 to 3 hours of administration. Because the agent has such a strong purgative action it should not be used for the routine treatment of constipation.

Glycerin

This agent is usually administered as a 3-g suppository and exerts its effect by osmotic action in the rectum. As with most agents given as suppositories, the onset of action is usually less than 30 minutes. Glycerin is considered a very safe laxative, although it may occasionally cause rectal irritation. Its use is acceptable on an intermittent basis for constipation, particularly in children.

Polyethylene Glycol–Electrolyte Lavage Solution

Whole-bowel irrigation with polyethylene glycol–electrolyte lavage solution (PEG–ELS) has become popular for colon cleansing before diagnostic procedures or colorectal operations.[62] Four liters of this solution is administered over 3 hours to obtain complete evacuation of the GI tract. The solution is not recommended for the routine treatment of constipation and its use should be avoided in patients with intestinal obstruction.

Other Agents

Tap-water enemas may be used to treat simple constipation. The administration of 200 mL of water by enema to an adult often results in a bowel movement within one-half an hour. Soapsuds are no longer recommended for use in enemas because their use may result in proctitis or colitis.

Cisapride is a GI prokinetic agent that is used in GI motility disorders. It has been demonstrated to be effective in relieving acute constipation in both adults and children.[63] The agent is considerably more expensive than most alternatives.

Recommendations

Treatment and prevention of constipation should consist of bulk-forming agents in addition to dietary modifications that increase dietary fiber.[64] A variety of products are available that provide adequate bulk. Whichever agent is chosen, it should be used daily and continued indefinitely in most patients, particularly those with chronic constipation. Some bulk-forming agents are available in combination with diphenylmethane or anthraquinone derivatives. Generally, these combinations should be avoided because the added agents should not be used routinely.

For most nonhospitalized persons with acute constipation, the infrequent use (less than every few weeks) of most laxative products is acceptable; however, before more potent laxative/cathartics are used, relatively simple measures may be tried. For example, acute constipation may be relieved by the use of a tap-water enema or a glycerin suppository; if neither is effective, the use of low doses of diphenylmethane or anthraquinone derivatives or saline laxatives (e.g., milk of magnesia) may provide relief. If laxative treatment is required for longer than 1 week, the person should be advised to consult a physician to determine if there is an underlying cause of constipation that requires treatment with agents other than laxatives.

For some bedridden or geriatric patients, or others with chronic constipation, bulk-forming laxatives remain the first line of treatment, but the use of more potent laxatives may be required relatively frequently. When other than bulk-forming laxatives are used, they should be administered in the lowest effective dose and as infrequently as possible to maintain regular bowel function (more than three stools per week). Agents that may be used in these situations include diphenylmethane and anthraquinone derivatives, milk of magnesia, and lactulose. Mineral oil should be avoided, particularly in bedridden patients, because of the risk of aspiration and lipoid pneumonia. Some patients with chronic constipation may present with fecal impactions. Before vigorous oral laxatives can be used, the impaction needs to be removed using mechanical methods, including tap-water or saline enemas and digital extraction.

In the hospitalized patient without GI disease, constipation may be related to the use of general anesthesia and/or opiate substances. Most orally or rectally administered laxatives may be used. For prompt initiation of a bowel movement, a tap-water enema or glycerin suppository is recommended, or milk of magnesia.

With infants and children, constipation may occur commonly. The approach to the treatment of constipation in young persons should consider neurologic, metabolic, or anatomic abnormalities when constipation is a persistent problem. When not related to an underlying disease, the approach to constipation is similar to that in an adult. Dietary modification should be considered emphasizing high-fiber food. For acute constipation in most age groups, a tap-water enema or glycerin suppository may be helpful. Occasional use of milk of magnesia or anthraquinone derivatives in low doses is justified for acute constipation.

Patients with chronic, intractable constipation were commonly found to have slow GI transit, pelvic floor dysfunction, both of the above, or irritable bowel syndrome.[65] With failure of medical management, surgery may be indicated in patients with slow transit. Behavioral treatments such as biofeedback are successful in about 70% of patients with pelvic floor dysfunction.

PREVENTION

For certain groups of patients, such as those recovering from myocardial infarction or rectal surgery, straining at defecation is to be avoided. For these patients, the basis of preventive therapy should be the use of bulk-forming laxatives. In addition to these products, the use of docusate has become popular, although its effectiveness is debated. In pregnant patients, constipation may result because of alterations in anatomy or iron supplementation. As described earlier, bulk-forming laxatives and docusates should be the first line of prevention.

LAXATIVE ABUSE SYNDROME

Misconceptions about normal bowel patterns and the effect of laxatives have contributed to a syndrome of laxative abuse that is relatively common in the United States. The availability of laxatives as chocolates or gums conveys to the public that the use of these agents is without adverse consequences. Abuse of laxatives has occurred traditionally in persons trying to maintain daily bowel function, but more recently has extended to others who use laxatives for the purpose of controlling weight. In either case, the consistent abuse of strong laxatives and cathartics may lead to serious illness.

Laxative abuse for the purpose of maintaining daily bowel function begins with misconceptions about the frequency, quantity, or consistency of stools. With the use of strong purgatives, the colon may be so thoroughly cleansed that a bowel movement may not occur normally until a few days later. This delay reinforces the need for more purgatives and the cycle of laxative dependence is begun. Eventually the patient may require daily laxatives to maintain bowel function.

The laxative abuser may present with contradictory findings of diarrhea and weight loss.[66,67] In addition, long-term abusers of laxatives tend to have vomiting, abdominal pain, lassitude and weakness, thirst, edema, and bone pain (caused by osteomalacia). With prolonged use of laxatives a number of serious illnesses may arise. These include fluid and electrolyte imbalances (including acid–base imbalances and hypokalemia), protein-losing gastroenteropathy with hypoalbuminemia, and syndromes resembling colitis.

The determination of laxative abuse syndrome can be difficult because many laxative abusers vigorously deny laxative use. Middle-age women tend to be the most common laxative abusers. The chronic laxative abuse problem should be addressed by a combination of measures, including psychiatric evaluation, dietary modification with reliance on bulk-forming laxatives, and specific guidelines to the patient for the withdrawal of stimulant laxatives.

A variation of laxative abuse is seen in persons who use them as a method of weight loss.[68] It appears from the medical literature and daily news sources that this type of abuse is on the increase. Treatment of patients who abuse laxatives in this way has proven very difficult.

SUMMARY

Constipation is a very common problem in our society mostly because the average person's diet has inadequate fiber. Although improper diet is the major cause of constipation, various underlying diseases, such as GI cancers, neurologic or metabolic disorders, or use of constipating drugs, are important and relatively frequent causes of constipation.

The primary treatment of constipation should be to correct underlying disease, if present, and to increase dietary fiber. Dietary fiber can be increased by consumption of high-fiber-content foods or by use of bulk-forming laxatives. Stronger laxatives (diphenylmethane and anthraquinone derivatives, and saline laxatives) should be reserved for infrequent use in constipation more difficult to treat. Unlike many of the diseases described in this text, new drugs are not being developed to treat constipation, because new agents would not be expected to change the approach to the treatment of constipation.

References

1. Nelson JD. Etiology and epidemiology of diarrheal diseases in the United States. Am J Med 1985;78(suppl 6B):78–80.
2. Rohde JE. Selective primary health care: Strategies for control of disease in the developing world. XV. Acute diarrhea. Rev Infect Dis 1984;6:840–854.
3. Ooms L. Alterations in intestinal fluid movement. Scand J Gastroenterol 1983;84(suppl):65–77.
4. Keusch GT, Donowitz M. Pathophysiological mechanisms of diarrhoeal diseases: Diverse aetiologies and common mechanisms. Scand J Gastroenterol 1983;84(suppl):33–43.
5. Field M, Ras MC, Chang EB. Intestinal electrolyte transport and diarrheal disease. N Engl J Med 1989;321:879–883.
6. Read NW. Speculations of the role of motility in the pathogenesis and treatment of diarrhoea. Scand J Gastroenterol 1983;84(suppl):45–63.
7. Gyr K. Infectious diarrhoea and gastrointestinal hormones: Potential therapeutic implications. Scand J Gastroenterol 1983;84(suppl):135–140.
8. Johnson DA, Cattau EL. Stool chemistries in patients with unexplained diarrhea. Am Fam Physician 1986;33:131–134.
9. Shiau YF, Feldman GM, Resnick MA, et al. Stool electrolyte and osmolality measurements in the evaluation of diarrheal disorders. Ann Intern Med 1985;102:773–775.
10. Haskins R, Kotch J. Day care and illness: Evidence, costs and public policy. Pediatrics 1986;77(suppl):951–958.
11. Babb RR. Coffee, sugars, and chronic diarrhea. Tx-Diet 1984;75:82–87.
12. Anonymous. Feeding during diarrhea. Nutr Rev 1986;44:102.
13. Slugg PH, Carey WD. Clinical features and follow-up of surreptitious laxative users. Cleve Clin Q 1984;51:167–171.
14. George WL. Antimicrobial agent-associated colitis and diarrhea: Historical background and clinical aspects. Rev Infect Dis 1984;6(suppl 1):S208–S213.
15. Brown JD. Oral rehydration therapy for diarrhea. Milit Med 1985;150:577–581.
16. Avery ME, Snyder JD. Oral therapy for acute diarrhea. N Eng J Med 1990;323:891–894.
17. Santosham M, Burns B, Nadkarni V, et al. Oral rehydration therapy for acute diarrhea in ambulatory children in the United States: A double-blind comparison of four different solutions. Pediatrics 1985;76:159–166.
18. Vesikari T, Isolauri E. Glycine supplemented oral rehydration solutions for diarrhoea. Arch Dis Child 1986;61:372–376.
19. Pizarro D, Posada G, Sandi L, et al. Rice-based electrolyte solutions for the management of infantile diarrhea. N Engl J Med 1991;324:518–521.
20. Turnberg LA. Antisecretory activity of opiates *in vitro* and *in vivo* in man. Scand J Gastroenterol 1983;84:79–83.
21. Sandu BK, Milla PJ, Harries JT. Mechanisms of action of loperamide. Scand J Gastroenterol 1983;84:85–92.
22. Merritt JE, Brown BL, Tomlinson S. Loperamide and calmodulin [letter]. Lancet 1982;283.
23. Schiller LR, Santa CA, Morawski SG, et al. Mechanism of the antidiarrheal effect of loperamide. Gastroenterology 1984;86:1475–1480.
24. Johnson PC, Ericsson CD, DuPont HL, et al. Comparison of loperamide with bismuth subsalicylate for the treatment of acute travelers' diarrhea. JAMA 1986;255:757–760.
25. Portnoy BL, DuPont HL, Pruitt D, et al. Antidiarrheal agents in the treatment of acute diarrhea in children. JAMA 1976;236:844–846.
26. Reves R, Bass P, DuPont HL, et al. Failure to demonstrate effectiveness of an anticholinergic drug in the symptomatic treatment of acute travelers' diarrhea. J Clin Gastroenterol 1983;5:223–227.
27. DuPont HL, Sullivan P, Pickering LK, et al. Symptomatic treatment of diarrhea with bismuth subsalicylate among students attending a Mexican university. Gastroenterology 1977;73:715–718.
28. Steffen R, DuPont HL, Heusser R, et al. Prevention of traveler's diarrhea by the tablet form of bismuth subsalicylate. Antimicrob Agents Chemother 1986;29:625–627.
29. Gordon P, Comi RJ, Maton PN, et al. NIH conference: Somatostatin and somatostain analogue (SMS 201-995) in treatment of hormone-secreting tumors of the pituitary and gastrointestinal tract and non-neoplastic diseases of the gut. Ann Intern Med 1989;110:35–50.
30. Grosman I, Simon D. Potential gastrointestinal uses of somatostatin and its synthetic analogue octreotide. Am J Gastroenterol 1990;85:1061–1072.
31. Ryan J, Leighton J, Kirksey D, et al. Evaluation of an enkephalin analog in men with castor oil-induced diarrhea. Clin Pharmacol Ther 1986;39:40–42.
32. Lecomte JM, Costentin J, Vlaiculescu A, et al. Pharmacological properties of acetorphan, a parenterally active "enkephalinase" inhibitor. J Pharmacol Exp Ther 1986;237:937–944.
33. Sninsky CA, Davis RH, Clench MH, et al. Effect of lidamidine hydrochloride and loperamide on gastric emptying and transit of the small intestine. Gastroenterology 1986;90:68–73.
34. Gots RE, Formal SB, Giannella RA. Indomethacin inhibition of *Salmonella typhimurium, Shigella flexneri,* and cholera-mediated rabbit ileal secretion. J Infect Dis 1974;130:280–284.

35. Burke V, Gracey M. Reduction by aspirin of intestinal fluid-loss in acute childhood gastroenteritis. Lancet 1980;i:1329–1330.
36. Curry CE. Laxative products, in Handbook of Nonprescription Drugs, 10th ed. Washington, DC, American Pharmaceutical Association, 1993.
37. Connell AM, Hilton C, Irvine G, et al. Variation of bowel habits in two population samples. Br Med J 1965;2:1095–1099.
38. Milne JS, Williamson J. Bowel habits in older people. Gerontol Clin 1972;14:56–60.
39. Rendtorff RC, Kashgarian M. Stool patterns of healthy adult males. Dis Colon Rectum 1969;10:222–228.
40. Bjelke E. Epidemiologic studies of cancer of the stomach, colon and rectum. Scand J Gastroenterol 1974;9 (suppl):31.
41. Wynder EL, Shigematsu T. Environmental factors of cancer of the colon. Cancer 1967;20:1520.
42. Sonnenberg A, Muller AD. Constipation and cathartics as risk factors for colorectal cancer: A meta-analysis. Pharmacology 1993;47 (suppl 1):224–233.
43. Anderson AS. Dietary factors in the aetiology and treatment of constipation during pregnancy. Br J Obstet Gynaecol 1986;93:245–249.
44. Sandgren JE, McPhee MS, Greenberger NJ. Narcotic bowel syndrome treated with clonidine. Ann Intern Med 1984;101:331–334.
45. Schiller LR, Davis GR, Santa Ana CA, et al. Mechanism of antidiarrheal action of codeine. Gastroenterology 1981;80:1275.
46. Monane M, Avorn J, Beers MH, Everitt DE. Anticholinergic drug use and bowel function in nursing home patients. Arch Intern Med 1993;153:633–638.
47. Stewart RB, Moore MT, Marks RG, Hale WE. Correlates of constipation in an ambulatory elderly population. Am J Gastroenterol 1992;87:859–864.
48. Dwyer JT, Goldin B, Gorbach S, et al. Drug therapy reviews: Dietary fiber and fiber supplements in the therapy of gastrointestinal disorders. Am J Hosp Pharm 1978;35:278–287.
49. DeVroede G. Constipation: Mechanisms and management, in Sleisenger MH, Fordtran JS (eds): Gastrointestinal Disease, 2nd ed. Philadelphia, WB Saunders, 1983, pp 288–308.
50. Almy TP, Howell DA. Diverticular disease of the colon. N Engl J Med 1980;302:324–331.
51. Donowitz M. Current concepts of laxative action: Mechanisms by which laxatives increase stool water. Clin Gastroenterol 1979;1:77–84.
52. Binder HJ, Donowitz M. A new look at laxative action. Gastroenterology 1975;69:1001–1005.
53. Brunton LL. Laxatives, in Goodman LS, Gilman AG (eds): The Pharmacologic Basis of Therapeutics, 7th ed. New York, Macmillan, 1985, pp 994–1003.
54. Moriarity KJ, Kelly MJ, Beetham R, et al. Studies on the mechanism of action of dioctyl sodium sulphosuccinate in the human jejunum. Gut 1985;26:1008–1013.
55. Tolman KG, Hammar S, Sannella JJ. Possible hepatotoxicity of doxidan. Ann Intern Med 1976;84:290–292.
56. Anonymous. Safety of stool softeners. Med Lett 1977;19:45–46.
57. Forbes G, Bradley A. Liquid paraffin as a cause of oil aspiration pneumonia. Br Med J 1958;2:1566–1568.
58. Schneider L. Pulmonary hazard of the ingestion of mineral oil in the apparently healthy adult: A clinicoroentgenologic study. N Engl J Med 1949;240:284–291.
59. Anonymous. Lactulose for constipation. Med Lett 1980;22:2–4.
60. Gattuso JM, Kamm A. Adverse effects of drugs used in the management of constipation and diarrhea. Drug Safety 1994;10:47–65.
61. Lederle FA, Busch DL, Mattox KM, et al. Cost-effective treatment of constipation in the elderly: A randomized double-blind comparison of sorbitol and lactulose. Am J Med 1990;89:597–601.
62. Michael KA, DiPiro JT, Bowden TA, et al. Whole-bowel irrigation for mechanical colon cleansing. Clin Pharm 1985;4:414–424.
63. Staiano A, Cucchiara S, Andreotti MR, et al. Effect of cisapride on chronic idiopathic constipation in children. Dig Dis Sci 1991;36:733–736.
64. Tedesco FJ, DiPiro JT. Laxative use in constipation. Am J Gastroenterol 1985;80:303–309.
65. Camilleri M, Thompson G, Fleshman JW, Pemberton JH. Clinical management of intractable constipation. Ann Intern Med 1994;121:520–528.
66. Scully RE, Mark EJ, McNeely BU. Case records of the Massachusetts General Hospital. N Engl J Med 1985;313:1341–1346.
67. Oster JR, Materson BJ, Rogers A. Laxative abuse syndrome. Am J Gastroenterol 1980;74:451–458.
68. Beumont PJV, George GCW, Smart DE. "Dieters" and "vomiters and purgers" in anorexia nervosa. Psychological Med 1976;6:617–622.

Chapter 37

Alcoholic Liver Disease

Mark A. Gill, PharmD, and William R. Kirchain, PharmD

Alcoholic liver disease (ALD) is one of the most prevalent drug-induced liver diseases seen by clinicians worldwide. The health costs of ALD range in the millions of dollars. The trend in the United States, however, during the 1980s was a decrease in mortality (25% decline) and rate of hospitalization (44% decline) from chronic liver disease (all causes), associated with a decline in alcohol consumption.[1] Death from chronic liver disease (which is predominantly secondary to alcoholism in the United States) was the ninth leading cause of death in 1989.[2] The following year, chronic liver disease dropped to the eleventh most frequent cause of death with a decrease of 3.5%.[3] It has been estimated that 90% of deaths from cirrhosis would be preventable if alcohol use were to be eliminated. It is an ancient disease; in fact, some of the earliest descriptions of cirrhosis resulted from the observations of the livers of alcoholics.[4] However, the earliest recognition that alcoholism led to liver disease was in 1793 by Matthew Baille.[5]

PATHOPHYSIOLOGY

ALD is associated with chronic ingestion of 60–80 g of ethanol daily for long periods of time (e.g., over 10 years).[6] The type of ethanol does not appear to be important. An individual's susceptibility is dependent on individual host factors leading to a 1 in 12 risk of cirrhosis from chronic ethanol abuse. Other factors related to the risk of developing ALD include nutritional status and female sex.[7] The increased risk for female alcoholics seems to derive from differences in first-pass metabolism of ethanol by alcohol dehydrogenase in gastric mucosal cells. Even accounting for weight, females have higher blood ethanol concentrations than males. This disparity can be accounted for by the decreased enzyme activity in females and even lower activity in female alcoholics.[8]

Although some controversy still remains, ALD can be viewed as a progressive, chronic condition with four basic stages (Fig. 37.1). The initial lesion, steatosis or fatty metamorphosis, may begin as early as the first drink.[9,10] If the pattern of heavy alcohol use is continued, these lesions become necrotic, inducing a mild inflammatory reaction called alcoholic hepatitis or steatonecrosis.[10,11] In some cases, these lesions lead to a third stage involving fibrotic changes of cirrhosis.[11] The endpoint of the disease is hepatic failure and death.

Many theories have been put forth to explain the toxic effect of alcohol on the liver. Originally, a great deal of attention was paid to possible adulterants or contaminants in the alcohol consumed by those with liver disease.[12] Another popular theory held that ALD is primarily a nutritional deficit.[9] Most alcoholics do have serious nutritional deficits and the treatment of ALD often includes nutritional replacement/supplementation. It has been postulated that virtually 100% of patients with ALD have malnutrition.[13] Estimates of typical patients with chronic liver disease suggest an intake of 47 g protein and 1320 kcal daily,[14] compared with roughly 50 g of protein and 1800 kcal for an average healthy adult. A nutritional deficit does not predict the development of ALD. Yet patients with a nutritional deficit do suffer the highest mortality rate.[15]

The best explanation of ALD comes from an understanding of how alcohol is metabolized in the liver. When alcohol is ingested, it is metabolized in the liver, intestinal lumen, and pancreas via alcohol dehydrogenase to acetaldehyde, which in turn is, via the mixed-function oxidase system, broken down to acetic acid.[16] This simple reaction series has tremendous cellular consequences. Both the conversion of alcohol to acetaldehyde and the mixed-function oxidase system require NADH-NAD^+or NADPH-$NADP^+$conversions. This increases the ratio of NADH to NAD^+, which increases fatty acid synthesis and triglyceride accumulation within the cell.[16] Concurrently, the production of lactic acid increases, which can lead to increased collagen production. The increase in lactic acid can also decrease the pH slightly, decreasing uric acid excretion.[16]

The cellular toxicity of alcohol can be separated into the intrinsic and idiosyncratic mechanisms. The idiosyncratic mechanisms of genetics, sex, nutrition, and other hepatotoxins may predispose individuals to the uncommon development of alcoholic hepatitis despite the chronic abuse of excessive amounts of alcohol. Continued use of alcohol appears to induce the mixed-function oxidase sys-

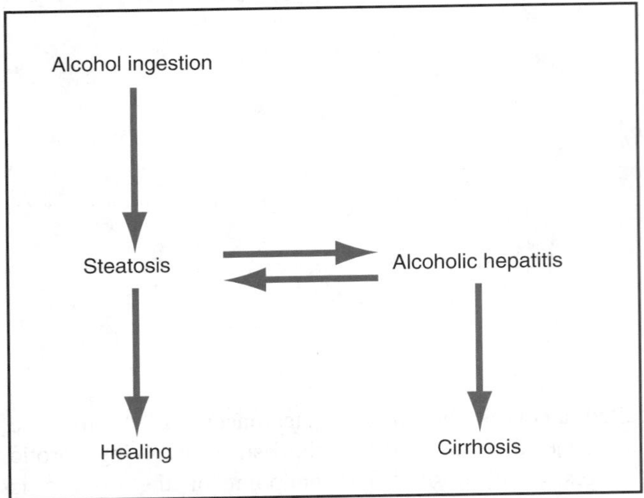

Figure 37.1. Progression of alcoholic liver disease.

tem. This increase in lipid synthesis, along with a decrease in oxidation of fatty acids perhaps caused by acetaldehyde, leads directly to steatosis, the first lesion of ALD.[11]

Steatosis is a lesion characteristic of, although not exclusive to, ALD. When seen at biopsy, the hepatocytes are filled with large lipid-containing vesicles.[4] The pattern of steatosis induced by alcohol is largely centrilobular (now often referred to as perivenular—the lobule immediately surrounding the central vein).[11] This pathologic change is easily reversed by abstinence from alcohol, and little functional impairment is usually encountered.[9]

The next major pathologic event in the progression of ALD is steatonecrosis or alcoholic hepatitis. Lysis and necrosis of the fat-filled hepatocytes provoke an immune response. In susceptible persons, there is an apparent alteration of cell-mediated immunity, leading to an increased rate of damage.[17] The most obvious changes of alcoholic hepatitis seen histologically occur in zone 3 of the hepatic acinus. This is the part furthest from oxygenated blood entering the liver. Alcohol may lead to cell necrosis by increasing the metabolic rate of cells that are already relatively hypoxic. Alcoholic hepatitis is also marked by the development of the alcoholic hyaline or Mallory bodies. These are intracellular eosinophilic perinuclear inclusion bodies. Although not diagnostic, Mallory bodies portend a more severe form of alcoholic hepatitis.[18] Besides alcohol, griseofulvin and amiodarone may induce Mallory bodies. The fibrosis that occurs in alcoholic hepatitis often obliterates the central veins, leading to portal vein hypertension even before the patient has progressed to cirrhosis. Even at the alcoholic hepatitis stage of the disease, many patients can avoid the eventual sequelae by abstinence, although the cellular structure may never return to normal.[19] Surprisingly, 18% of patients at this stage of ALD will continue to develop cirrhosis despite abstinence from alcohol.[20] If there is no continued insult to the liver, a resolution of symptoms can be anticipated in 3 to 8 months. The 7-year survival rate for abstainers is 80%, whereas for those continuing to drink the rate is only 50%.[21]

Cirrhosis leading to hepatic failure and its complications is the terminal event in ALD. Cirrhosis is primarily the result of fibrotic changes that distort the architectural integrity of the liver. This is generally accompanied by a loss of parenchymal mass and a concurrent loss of liver function. It is these changes in structure and decreases in function that result in the signs and symptoms of alcoholic cirrhosis, such as portal hypertension or bleeding abnormalities. The fibrosis may compress the hepatic veins, decreasing hepatic outflow and thus leading to portal hypertension.[21]

CLINICAL PRESENTATION

Patients typically present with scleral icterus, spider angiomata generally observed on the trunk, and palmar erythema. Spider angiomata are star-shaped vascular defects observed on the skin. The liver is usually distended, measured in finger breadths below the right costal margin. Typically the spleen is palpable because of increased pressures from the portal hypertension. Gynecomastia is common in males because of the testicular atrophy induced by alcohol.

LABORATORY

A valuable laboratory test to evaluate several aspects of liver function is the serum bilirubin. Bilirubin is a breakdown product of hemoglobin. This breakdown occurs in the spleen and bone marrow. The bilirubin released is an insoluble form of bilirubin (called indirect bilirubin) that is bound to plasma proteins and delivered to the liver parenchymal cells, which conjugate bilirubin; this is measured as direct bilirubin. Most of the bilirubin glucuronide is excreted into the bile and then converted by gut bacteria to urobilinogen, which gives stool its characteristic brown color. With advancing liver disease less bilirubin gets conjugated leading to increases in indirect bilirubin. Liver cell death leads to release of conjugated bilirubin from the liver into the systemic circulation, which then leads to increases in direct bilirubin. Excess conjugated bilirubin may be filtered by the kidneys giving urine the characteristic "cola" color. Excess bilirubin leads to accumulation in the epidermis and sclera. Termed jaundice or icterus, it is characterized by a yellow tinge to the skin or eye that is noticeable when total bilirubin levels exceed 3 to 5 mg%. Another useful test is the alkaline phosphatase concentration in serum. This enzyme is made in cells lining the biliary tract and in bone tissue. In processes that disrupt bile flow, alkaline phosphatase will increase in the blood.

Once jaundice is evident, it is helpful to analyze the relative incremental increases in serum bilirubin versus alkaline phosphatase. In alcoholic liver disease the ratio of patient to normal bilirubin is much greater than that ratio for alkaline phosphatase. The transaminase tests are also valuable in assessing liver damage from alcohol. The transaminases are the alanine aminotransferase (ALT) and aspartate aminotransferase (AST), with a typical normal range of 5–40 IU/dL. Typically, the AST increases beyond the ALT (about twofold difference). The highest increase in AST or ALT is seen with alcoholic hepatitis and may reach into the hundreds. As the liver disease progresses into cirrhosis, the transaminases may actually fall despite worsening liver function. Another enzyme that may be useful is the γ-glutamyltranspeptidase (GGTP), with a typical normal range of 0–65 IU/dL. GGTP is a biliary excretory enzyme that is more specific for liver disease than alkaline phosphatase (i.e., the former will not be elevated in bone disease while the latter may). Generally, GGTP and alkaline phosphatase rise in concert with cholestasis; however, with ALD a disproportionate increase in GGTP can be expected and is a useful diagnostic clue. An elevation in GGTP in ALD may reflect microsomal enzyme induction rather than cellular toxicity.[22] Whereas in viral hepatitis the enzyme elevation correlates with the extent of cellular destruction, this is not the case in ALD. As liver damage progresses, protein synthesis decreases, which will affect plasma protein concentrations of albumin and clotting factors. Combined with the malnutrition of ALD patients, the decreased hepatic protein synthesis results in serious abnormalities in serum oncotic pressure and hemostasis. Prolongation of clotting tests such as prothrombin time and activated partial thromboplastin time can be expected. The serum albumin may fall as low as 2 g/dL (normal 4.5–5.5 g/dL). The value of monitoring all of these lab tests has been questioned. Several of these tests used individually (GGTP, AST, or ALT) had no prognostic value in relative risk estimates of 1 year mortality from ALD.[23] However, albumin, serum bilirubin, hemoglobin, or prothrombin time had very significant predictive ability.

A classification system for the severity of liver disease has been developed that incorporates several laboratory tests. The Child–Pugh classification is frequently used to stratify patients into categories for selection of various therapies. The system may be useful in monitoring the response to therapies. Patients are labeled grade A for point scores of 5–6, grade B for scores of 7–9, and grade C with scores above 10 using the point system given in Table 37.1.[24]

COMPLICATIONS

PORTAL HYPERTENSION AND ASCITES

Portal hypertension in ALD is the direct result of increased mechanical resistance to blood flow through the liver.[25] In individuals with no cirrhosis, the normal liver blood flow is roughly 1–1.5 L/min at a pressure of only 4–6 mm Hg.[25] As the flow is inhibited by the distorted liver architecture in cirrhotic patients, the pressure rises not only in the liver but also along the gastrointestinal (GI) tract and in the spleen as well. The manifestations then of portal hypertension are primarily the result of low-pressure vessels handling high-pressure loads. To cope with this pressure, blood is diverted into a large number of minor small collateral vessels. This collateral flow is very prominent in the azygous and subclavian veins through the lower esophagus, the abdominal wall, and between the spleen and the left renal vein. Esophageal and abdominal varices often develop; these can rupture and sometimes lead to life-threatening hemorrhage. It is believed that the portal pressure correlates poorly with the risk of variceal bleeding. There is a minimum pressure of 12 mm Hg that appears to be necessary for varices to form, then bleed.[26] Splenomegaly is also a common feature, occasionally requiring splenectomy.

Another significant complication of portal hypertension is ascites (Fig. 37.2). Ascites results from the higher pressures of portal hypertension coupled with an increased porosity in the liver sinusoids, and an increase in intrahepatic interstitial fluid.[25] The lymphatic system of the liver is able to handle a great deal of excess fluid, but some leakage into the peritoneal cavity still occurs. The amount of fluid leaked into the peritoneal cavity can become quite large over time, leading to mechanical problems with many body systems. The increased intra-abdominal pressure acting on the diaphragm can, by affecting thoracic pressure, decrease

TABLE 37.1. CHILD–PUGH GRADING OF LIVER DISEASE

Clinical and Biochemical Measurements	Points Scored for Increasing Abnormality		
	1	2	3
Encephalopathy (grade)	None	1 and 2	3 and 4
Ascites	Absent	Slight	Moderate
Bilirubin (mg/dL)	1–2	2–3	>3
Albumin (g/dL)	3.5	2.8–3.5	<2.8
Prothrombin time (increased seconds)	1–4	4–6	>6

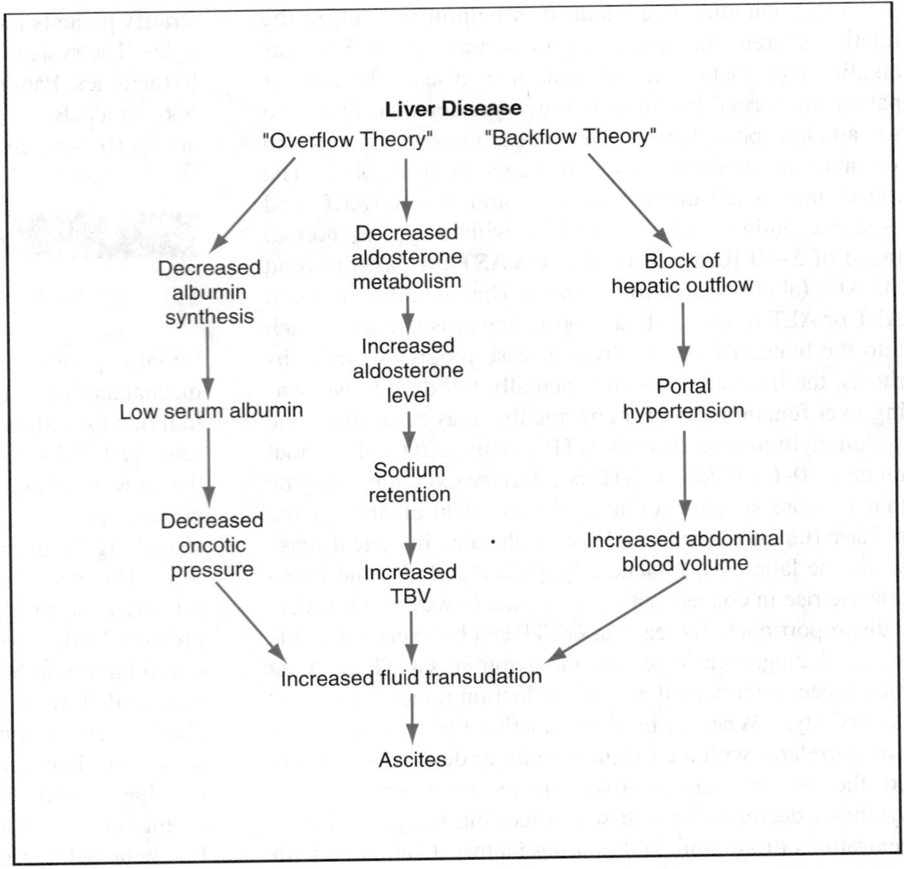

Figure 37.2. Theories for developing ascites.

transmural filling pressure of the heart, increase right atrial pressure, and decrease venous return to the right ventricle.[27] The increased pooling of blood associated with portal hypertension leads to a sequestration of blood in the spleen, which, along with the sequestration of fluid in the peritoneum, leads to a relative decrease in renal arteriolar perfusion. This induces the release of renin, which may lead to the increased ability of cirrhotics to reabsorb sodium (and water). Renin levels are higher in cirrhotic patients. Because cirrhosis is often accompanied by a decrease in the hepatic production of albumin, the serum oncotic pressure is also decreased, thus reducing the ability of the body to retain fluid in the vascular space.

ESOPHAGEAL AND GASTRIC VARICES

Portal hypertension causes pooling of blood in both the spleen and the mesenteric veins and arteries. This causes engorgement of the small capillaries along the entire GI tract. These overfilled blood vessels are much easier to rupture than normal vessels. Concurrently there is a breakdown in the gastric mucosa, leading to increased damage from acid and pepsin in the stomach and esophagus caused by an apparent direct toxic effect of alcohol on the mucosal surface.

DECREASED LIVER FUNCTION

Along with the effects of the mechanical problems of cirrhosis there is a progressive loss of basic hepatocyte function because of an overall loss of parenchymal mass. There is generally a decrease in protein synthesis and utilization of available substrates. A loss of enzymes leads to a decrease in the liver's ability to handle both drugs and endogenous toxins, which begin to accumulate. A decrease in serum albumin leads to a decrease in the protein binding of certain drugs and a decrease in the serum oncotic pressure. Vitamin K-dependent coagulation factors (II, VII, IX, X) synthesized by the liver slowly diminish, resulting in an increased frequency of bleeding problems. The ability of the hepatic transaminases to detoxify ammonia is decreased. Ammonia, octopamine, mercaptans, phenols, methanethiols, and other by-products of metabolism begin to accumulate.[28] There is some evidence that benzodiazepine-receptor reactivity is increased and that an endogenous benzodiazepine-receptor ligand accumulates in liver disease.[29] This ligand is known to be produced in very small amounts by plants.

Along with this decrease in transamination there is an apparent increase in ammonia production in the gut.[30] The catabolism induced by the decrease in albumin leads to an increase in aromatic amino acids (AAAs) at a rate 24 times the production of branched-chain amino acids (BCAAs).[31]

HEPATIC ENCEPHALOPATHY

Hepatic encephalopathy (HE) is a syndrome of altered mental status associated with liver impairment characterized by impaired cognitive skills, worsened motor abilities, and steadily depressed levels of consciousness beginning with somnolence and ending with coma. The spectrum of impairment is broad and may be classified in stages as the syndrome progresses (Table 37.2). Alternative scales are in use. One, summarized in Table 37.3 may be useful in assessing the progression of the disease or response to therapies. The incidence of hepatic encephalopathy may be much greater than generally perceived. In one study only 15% of patients with chronic liver disease but without a diagnosis of encephalopathy could pass standardized psychometric tests.[32] The cause of HE is not known; several factors, such as increased blood levels of ammonia and aromatic amino acids, have been associated with the development of HE (Table 37.4). Elevated ammonia levels have long been associated with HE. It is unclear if this elevation is the actual cause of the encephalopathic symptomatology. Ammonia metabolites (glutamine, α-ketoglutaramate) rather than ammonia in cerebrospinal fluid (CSF) correlate well with the grade of encephalopathy.[33] Mechanisms for the accumulation of ammonia and other nitrogenous compounds include reduced metabolic clearance of ammonia by the liver and bypass of the liver via collateral blood vessels because of intrahepatic outflow blockade.

As stated earlier, there is also a tremendous change in the relative levels of aromatic amino acids in the encephalopathic patient. Increased levels of blood glucagon and/or insulin in liver impairment lead to muscle breakdown of BCAAs, gluconeogenesis, and possibly hyperammonemia. The BCAA normally compete for central nervous system (CNS) entry with AAAs. Thus, the abnormal ratio of BCAA:AAA in liver disease allows for enhanced CNS entry of tryptophan, tyrosine, and phenylalanine. Free fatty acids have been implicated in HE. Long-chain fatty acids are elevated in cirrhotic patients secondary to decreased hepatic oxidation and increased absorption. They are thought to displace neuroactive chemicals from serum albumin (e.g., tryptophan, benzodiazepines). There is evidence of increased brain concentrations of 1,4-benzodiazepines in

TABLE 37.2. SCALE FOR ASSESSING THE DEPTH OF HEPATIC ENCEPHALOPATHY

Grade	Cognitive/Motor	Behavior
1	Mild tremor, altered handwriting	Anxiety, insomnia, mild confusion
2	Dysarthria, ataxia asterixis	Lethargy, disorientation
3	Seizures, muscle twitching	Delirium, bizarre behavior
4	Posturing	Coma

(From Barber JR, Teasley KM. Nutritional support of patients with severe hepatic failure. Clin Pharm 1984;3:245–253, with permission.)

TABLE 37.3. HEPATIC ENCEPHALOPATHY SCORES

I. Verbal Response	1. None
	2. Incomprehensible
	3. Confused
	4. Normal
II. Eye Opening	1. None
	2. Noxious stimuli only
	3. Verbal stimuli
	4. Spontaneous
III. Pupils	1. Nonreactive
	2. Sluggish
	3. Brisk
IV. Oculocephalic/ Oculovestibular	1. No reaction
	2. Partial or dysconjugate
	3. Full
	4. Normal
V. Best Motor Response	1. None
	2. Abnormal extensor
	3. Abnormal flexor
	4. Withdrawal or localizes
	5. Obeys commands
VI. Respiration	1. Nil on ventilator
	2. Irregular
	3. Regular >22/min
	4. Regular <22/min

(From Berk PD, Hopper H. Fulminant hepatic failure. Am J Gastroenterol 1978;69:349–400, with permission.)

TABLE 37.4. THEORIES FOR THE DEVELOPMENT OF HEPATIC ENCEPHALOPATHY

Toxin	Description
Ammonia	Direct neurotoxin
Multiple synergistic neurotoxins	Mercaptans (produced by dietary methionine), elevated free fatty acids
False neurotransmitters	Elevated aromatic amino acids lead to increased serotonin, octopamine, and phenylethylamine (depressants) while decreasing dopamine and noradrenaline (stimulants)
γ-Aminobutyric acid neurotransmission	Endogenous and/or exogenous benzodiazepine-like compounds

some patients with hepatic encephalopathy due to fulminant hepatic failure.[34] γ-Aminobutyric acid is a product of intestinal flora and intestinal mucosa. With hepatic failure, blood and CNS levels rise allowing for its CNS depression. Evident are decreased catabolism of GABA by the impaired liver and lowered blood–brain barrier to GABA.

PHARMACOKINETIC/ PHARMACODYNAMIC CHANGES ASSOCIATED WITH LIVER FAILURE

There is currently no exact mathematical approach to adjusting drug doses during liver failure. Drugs that are primarily excreted by the liver or extensively metabolized before renal excretion are the most affected by changes in hepatic function. As stated earlier, liver disease is a complex process that involves changes in blood flow, blood pressure, metabolic capacity, and protein binding. These changes will occur at different rates and to varying degrees, depending on the patient. The most important pharmacokinetic parameter when adjusting drug doses for liver impairment is the clinical response. Frequent close observation of an individual's response to a dose is the best way to meet the needs of the liver disabled patient. There is value in pharmacokinetic assessment of the patient as well, but it is difficult to be exact with these assessments. Table 37.5 lists a few drugs and the known pharmacokinetic changes associated with liver impairment. Note that one of the most important considerations is the extraction ratio of a drug.[35] Highly extracted drugs tend to be affected more by changes in hepatic blood flow than by changes in metabolic rate. The opposite is true of low extraction ratio drugs. Cirrhosis would then have a greater impact on a drug such as labetalol than would an inflammatory process such as hepatitis. Beyond the observed changes in clearance, half-life, and volume of distribution, it is important to note the impact of disease and extraction ratio. Drugs with a high extraction ratio are more affected by changes in hepatic blood flow than drugs with low extraction ratios. Changes during acute hepatitis are often transitory and new changes in drug dosage must be made as the disease subsides.

Another important factor in considering the pharmacokinetic changes associated with liver failure is protein binding. There is a slow but steady decrease in serum albumin that occurs with decreasing liver function. Highly protein-bound drugs experience increases in their free fractions during this period. This increase in free fraction can cause an increase in the observed clinical action of the drug, usually seen as increased toxicity. An increased free fraction also means that there is more drug available to be metabolized by the still functioning hepatic enzymes. Thus until these enzymes become saturated, the clearance of a highly protein-bound drug during liver impairment can increase and the half-life can shorten. Patients with high GGTP and alkaline phosphatase levels may experience a decrease in biliary excretion. Drugs that are excreted through the bile will accumulate in these patients.

The third spacing associated with chronic liver disease may also alter pharmacokinetics/dynamics. Dramatic shifts in fluid can be expected in the pancreatitis of ALD thus increasing the distribution volume of drugs with low protein binding. The fluid shift into the peritoneum from ascites has also been shown to increase the distribution volume of drugs such as the aminoglycosides, oftentimes necessitating larger drug dosages.[36]

The clinical components of liver disease also can change the dose–response relationships of drugs. Encephalopathic patients will be much more sensitive to CNS depressants. Varices, particularly bleeding varices, may increase the absorption of drugs that would normally exhibit poor absorption. Diarrhea associated with hepatitis will decrease the absorption of many drugs. Besides the hepatic components most end-stage liver disease patients have some mild to moderate renal impairment that will further decrease drug elimination.

TABLE 37.5. SELECTED EXAMPLES OF PHARMACOKINETIC CHANGES DURING LIVER FAILURE

Drug	Extraction	Disease	Plasma Clearance	Volume of Distribution	Terminal Half-Life
Diazepam	Low	Cirrhosis	Decreases 30–50%	May increase slightly	Increases 40–50%
Diazepam	Low	Acute hepatitis	Decreases	May increase slightly	Increases 20–40%
Oxazepam	Low	Cirrhosis	Increases slightly	Increases 10–20%	Increases slightly
Phenobarbital	Low	Cirrhosis			Increases 10–30%
Phenobarbital	Low	Acute hepatitis			Increases 10–40%
Propranolol	High	Cirrhosis	Decreases 33–50%	Increases 50%	Increases 100–200%
Labetolol	High	Cirrhosis	Decreases 25–60%	Decreases 20–40%	Increases slightly
Lidocaine	High	Cirrhosis	Decreases 35–40%		
Clindamycin	Low	Cirrhosis	Decreases 60%	Decreases 40%	Increases slightly
Theophylline	High	Cirrhosis	Decreases 33–50%	Increases 30–40%	Increases 100–300%

Once the individual factors are accounted for, it is important when dosing drugs in the hepatically impaired patient to account for the multiorgan system nature of liver disease. One bedside method for assessing the extent of liver disease is Pugh's score. Originally developed for comparing the survival of mild versus severely diseased patients after surgical procedures this system allows one to estimate total hepatic function.[37] Encephalopathy, ascites, bilirubin levels, serum albumin, and the prothrombin time combine to give a score that increases with increasing disease. As seen in Table 37.1, this technique accounts for the differing presentations of liver impairment by allowing each element to increase the score. Scores of 6 or less are associated with highly survivable liver disease. Scores between 7 to 9 suggest moderate disease and loss of function and scores greater than 10 represent end-stage disease. The use of this system can give clues to the extent that drug dosage should be changed or monitored more closely. Antipyrine and other hepatic function markers such as indocyanine green can also be used to assess hepatic function. The administration of these agents in the clinical setting of severe liver disease is uncommon. Preprandial and postprandial bile acid levels with galactose clearance studies have also been used to assess liver function. Caffeine is also used for the study of hepatic function because of its widespread acceptance as a benign agent in low doses. Caffeine clearance studies, however, have difficulty differentiating patients at or near the end stages of the disease.[38,39]

TREATMENT

The most important treatment for drug-induced liver disease is the discontinuance of drug exposure. It cannot be overemphasized that patients with alcoholic liver disease (ALD) must stop drinking. With discontinuation of alcohol exposure, many patients improve dramatically. Steatosis often resolves within weeks, and alcohol hepatitis within a few months, of the last drink.[19]

ALCOHOLIC HEPATITIS

After the discontinuation of alcohol, the therapy for ALD is primarily symptomatic. In alcoholic hepatitis, glucocorticoids are sometimes used during the acute phase; the rationale is to decrease the inflammatory response to the alcoholic hyaline and other antigenic substances present. There appears to be increased class 1 major histocompatibility complex antigens that have been found on the plasma membrane of hepatocytes in patients with alcoholic hepatitis. Subsequently effector T cells attack the liver cells. Glucocorticoids may act by decreasing T-cell-mediated cytotoxicity.[40] There is conflicting evidence regarding glucocorticoid effect on reducing the overall morbidity of alcoholic hepatitis patients (Table 37.6). Most recently, dramatic improvement in short-term mortality was demonstrated with methylprednisolone in very sick patients. The steroid reduced mortality from 35% seen with placebo to 6%.[41] Prior studies with negative results may not have randomized subjects who were ill enough. To circumvent the latter problem, meta-analysis has been employed. When studies have been combined, the positive effects of glucocorticoids become more apparent.[48] The analysis revealed a particular benefit in those patients with hepatic encephalopathy. Another meta-analysis also showed a reduction in mortality with corticosteroids.[49] This analysis also found that encephalopathy was a predictor for success and additionally that the presence of GI bleeding would reverse the positive effects of glucocorticoids. Generally, prednisolone or methylprednisolone are the preferred steroids since they do not require liver metabolism to an active compound such as prednisone does. The long-term prognosis with glucocorticoids still remains uncertain particularly if alcohol is still

TABLE 37.6. STUDIES OF STEROID THERAPY FOR ALCOHOLIC HEPATITIS

Reference	Agent	Dosage	Total Duration (d)	Mortality (%) Placebo Group	Mortality (%) Steroid Group
41	MePr[a]	32 mg	28	35	6
42	MePr	1 g	3	57	63
43	Pred[a]	40 mg	28	100	11
44	MePr	80 mg	4–7	47	50
45	Pred	40 mg	30	100	29
46	Pred	0.5 mg/kg for 3 wks then 0.25 mg/kg for 3 wks	42	35	36
47	MePr	40 mg	14	78	55

[a]MePr, methylprednisolone; Pred, prednisone.

ingested. Regardless of treatment, many patients do not survive severe bouts of the disease (survival rate 22–45%). Those who do survive often develop cirrhosis in 3 to 5 years (Figure 37.3).

CIRRHOSIS

The treatment of cirrhosis is again symptomatic, directed at the particular manifestations in the particular patient. If the patient shows signs of nutritional deficiency, it should be corrected. Deficiencies in folate, thiamine, and vitamin C are very common and often severe.[50] In addition, potassium, phosphorus, magnesium, and iron can be quite low in these patients.[50] Replacement of iron should be done with particular caution in cirrhotic patients, because liver iron stores are often higher than normal despite low serum concentrations, and hemochromatosis can develop.[11] Vitamin K injections can sometimes help regenerate clotting factors, but as cirrhosis worsens the response to vitamin K lessens. Treatment of the coagulopathy may require fresh whole blood or fresh frozen plasma transfusions. Replenishment of serum protein can be very difficult in cirrhotic patients who often require protein restriction, but adequate calories should be given.

Liver transplantation is a consideration for end-stage liver disease. Alcoholics have not been viewed as optimal candidates because the high rates of recidivism and poor compliance to immunosuppressive agents might result in unacceptably high rejection rates. However, in a series of 73 alcoholic patients receiving liver transplants, 71% were alive after a mean of 25 months, which was felt to be comparable to a nonalcoholic population receiving transplants.[51]

An experimental treatment for ALD with propylthiouracil (PTU) has been shown to reduce mortality compared to placebo.[52] Response to PTU was dependent on a reduced intake of alcohol. PTU may reduce the hypoxic conditions in the liver produced by alcohol. PTU was given in a dose of 150 mg bid with changes in thyroid function tests but no clinical hypothyroidism. These results, however, need confirmation before PTU can be recommended for alcoholics.

ASCITES

Ascites is primarily an accumulation of fluid; therefore, the objective in treating ascites should be removal of fluid. In practice, this is often not an easy task.

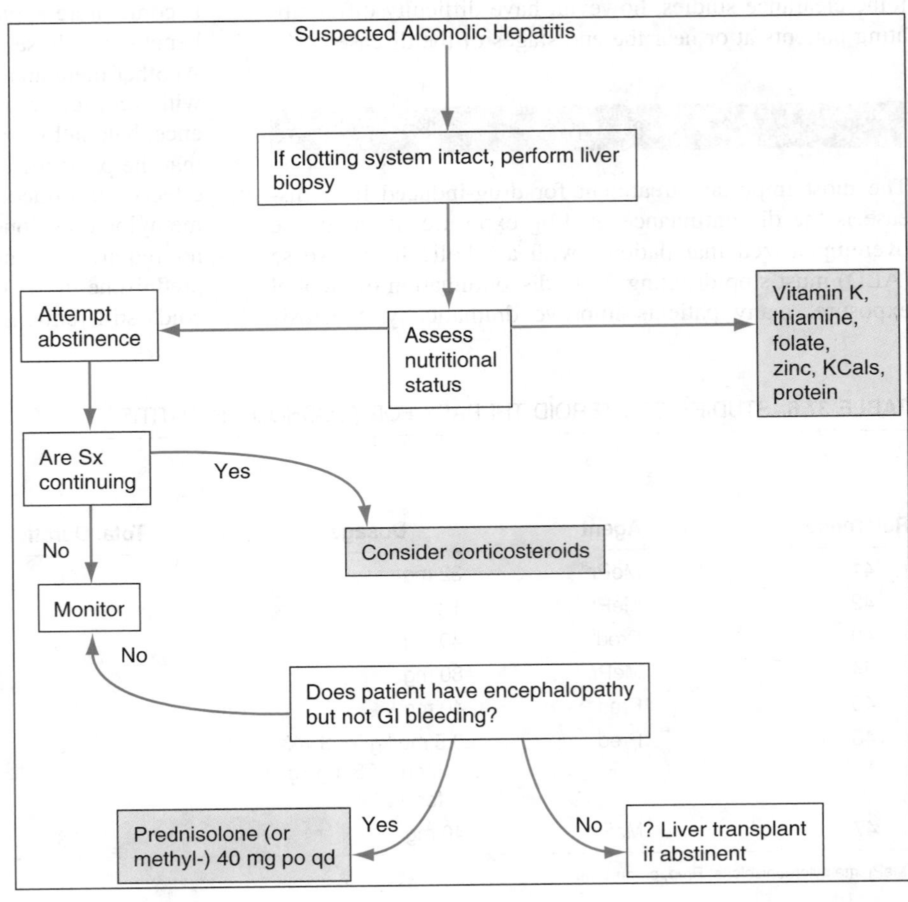

Figure 37.3. Treatment algorithm for a patient with alcoholic hepatitis.

Table 37.7 summarizes the stepwise treatment of ascites. The increase in fluid in the peritoneal cavity causes a relative decrease in intravascular volume. The kidney responds by retaining sodium; sodium restriction is then the first step in treating ascites.[53] Most patients with ascites can tolerate 1 g of sodium per day, which essentially means no added salt and no salted foods. The diuresis observed from this approach though is very slow, often taking as long as 30 days for obvious loss of ascites volume.[54] Salt restriction is generally accompanied by a concurrent restriction of fluid intake to a few hundred milliliters per day. Patients who are not hospitalized generally find this a difficult regimen. As the ascites begins to resolve, the amount of sodium can sometimes be increased to a more tolerable 2 to 3 g, and the amount of fluid intake increased upward to a liter per day. The overall fluid loss per day should not exceed 1–2 L.[55] Patients with peripheral edema seem to tolerate faster mobilization of ascites than patients who have no edema. Nonedematous patients transfer water from the peritoneal cavity to the vascular space at a rate of 200–400 mL/d and should not be diuresed beyond a weight loss of about 0.5 kg/d. Because maximal ascitic fluid mobilization occurs at a rate of only 1–2 L/d, diuresis that is too brisk can lead to problems of relative dehydration and a potentially fatal hepatorenal syndrome. Hepatorenal syndrome is a progressive, fatal loss of renal function in the face of severe hepatic dysfunction. The onset of hepatorenal syndrome is insidious and often unrecognized. A slow but continuous rise in serum creatinine and blood urea nitrogen eventually progresses to complete failure of the kidneys. The patient must then deal not only with a failed liver but also with all the problems associated with acute renal failure. Drug dosing can become extremely difficult in these patients, often requiring extensive use of blood levels and sophisticated pharmacokinetic methods. Ultimately, however, hepatorenal syndrome is almost uniformly fatal.

TABLE 37.7. TREATMENT ALGORITHM FOR ASCITES

Therapy	Goal
Sodium and water restriction	Loss = 1–2 L/d (weight loss = 1–2 kg)
If inadequate response after 3–5 d, add	
Mild diuretic (spironolactone 100–400 mg/d)	As above
If inadequate response after 4–7 d, add	
Loop diuretic (furosemide 40–120 mg/d)	As above
If inadequate response after 30–60 d, add	
Peritoneal dialysis with reinfusion	As above
or	
Peritoneovenous shunt	As above

Paracentesis or diuretic therapy can be used to deplete the volume of ascites when sodium and fluid restriction fail to produce adequate diuresis. Paracentesis as a palliative measure designed to relieve pressure, respiratory insufficiency from a displaced diaphragm, and/or umbilical hernia has been employed for centuries. It is said that the composer Beethoven was "tapped" toward the end of his life. The result was reported to be a loss of 25 pounds worth of fluid and that he was symptomatically improved.[56] Paracentesis of large volumes of fluid usually results in immediate resorption of water from the vascular space into the peritoneal space that may be complete in as little as 4 days.[55] This rapid shift may lead to vascular volume depletion. To avoid these shifts, recent studies employed simultaneous administration of parenteral albumin in order to increase plasma oncotic pressure and prevent movement of substantial volumes of fluid. Paracentesis without albumin was reported to produce hyponatremia, increased plasma renin activity, and renal insufficiency more frequently than paracentesis with albumin.[57] In a randomized trial of paracentesis/albumin versus spironolactone/furosemide, diuretics were more likely to cause hyponatremia, encephalopathy, and renal impairment.[58] In addition, a satisfactory response to treatment was more common for paracentesis/albumin, 96.5%, than for diuretics, 72.8%. Perhaps more startling was the shorter hospital stay and lower mortality rate observed for the paracentesis group.

Many patients who continue to develop ascites and those who do not respond to diuretics or paracentesis may be eligible to receive a LeVeen or peritoneovenous shunt (Fig. 37.4). Even this does not always prevent ascites from recurring; 30% of patients with a LeVeen shunt in place may develop ascites again later.[59] In addition, one trial revealed that after 3 months, 40% of shunts were no longer patent.[60] However, a large-scale trial in veterans demonstrated delayed recurrence, shorter hospital stays, and faster ascites removal with shunting as opposed to medical treatment.[61] Encephalopathy was more common with medical treatment in certain subgroups of patients. Shunts may lead to postoperative disseminated intravascular coagulopathy, presumably from deficiency of circulating fibrinogen and platelets induced by the infusion of ascitic fluid through the shunt. Soluble collagen present in ascitic fluid causes intravascular platelet agglutination. In addition, peritoneal tissues secrete tissue plasminogen activator, which when it enters the bloodstream through the shunt may cause fibrinolysis. Approaches to reduce the risk of coagulopathy include completely draining the ascites at the time the shunt is placed, preoperative aspirin, heparin, or EACA.[62] Nonetheless, mortality rate is not improved with shunts relative to medical treatment.

Diuretic therapy for ascites is effective in most patients yet the process is slow. Patients may require as long as 35–40 days of continuous therapy before the ascites has resolved.[53] The drugs most frequently used are the

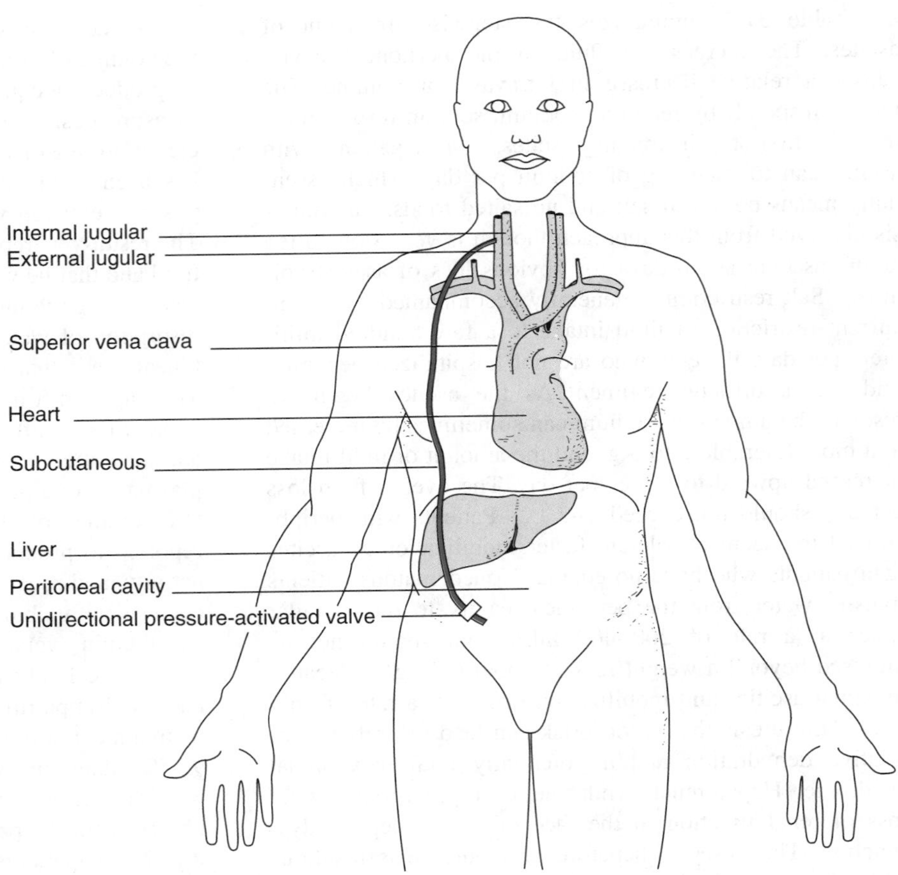

Figure 37.4. Anatomical representation of the placement of a peritoneovenous or LeVeen shunt.

potassium-sparing diuretics, because of the ability of spironolactone, in particular, to inhibit the action of aldosterone in the kidney tubule. It is believed that ascites causes a relative decrease in intravascular volume that stimulates the aldosterone-mediated retention of sodium and water in the kidney.[63] The dose of spironolactone required ranges from 100–800 mg/d and is usually not effective without concurrent sodium and water restriction.[63] The half-life of spironolactone and its active metabolites is prolonged in patients with liver disease. Thus, one expert has recommended single daily doses to improve compliance.[64] The onset of the diuretic effect with spironolactone is slow, 3–5 days in some cases, and loop diuretics such as furosemide are sometimes added to increase the rate of weight loss. Spironolactone is a competitive inhibitor of aldosterone in the distal segment of the renal tubule. Aldosterone causes the reabsorption of sodium from the peritubular fluid and the concurrent excretion of potassium. The amount normally presented to the distal tubule is small and inhibiting this reabsorption produces only a mild increase in sodium and water excretion. Again, the rate of weight loss should not exceed 1–2 kg/d. The relative efficacy of diuretics has been examined and revealed that spironolactone produces a positive response more often than furosemide.[65] Regardless of the diuretic selected, serum electrolytes must be monitored carefully during therapy and signs of dehydration (orthostatic blood pressure changes, changes in heart rate, decreased urine output) must be carefully monitored.

PORTAL HYPERTENSION

The therapy for portal hypertension is directed at reducing flow to the portal bed. Operative procedures such as splenectomy or portacaval shunts attempt to do this mechanically.[25] Drug therapy with propranolol has also been used with some success (see a summary of studies in Table 37.8). In one study, propranolol was shown superior to placebo in preventing rebleeding in patients with esophageal varices. The propranolol dose used was the dose sufficient to decrease the blood pressure by 25 mm Hg.[75] In another trial of propranolol versus placebo, the dose was adjusted to reduce the heart rate by 20–25%.[66]

Propranolol reduced the incidence of first rebleeding and lowered the mortality rate relative to placebo. Selective beta blockade (with atenolol) that is given in a fixed dose may not be as effective as pharmacodynamically adjusted

TABLE 37.8. STUDIES OF THERAPY FOR ESOPHAGEAL VARICES

Reference	Agent	Dosage (mg)[a]	Indication	Class[b]	Bleeding (%)		
					Placebo Group	β Blocker Group	Sclerotherapy
66	Propranolol	40–320	1° prevention	A,B,C	61	26[c]	—
67	Propranolol	60–320	2° prevention	A,B,C	—	29[d]	28
68	Propranolol/ atenolol	Up to 160p/ 100a	2° prevention	A,B	51[c]	24p/31a	—
69	Propranolol	40–360	2° prevention	A,B	—	62[c]	29
70	Propranolol	160	2° prevention	A,B,C	75	25[c]	—
71	Propranolol	160	2° prevention	A,B,C	73	15[c]	—
72	Propranolol	20–240	2° prevention	A,B,C	30	27[d]	—
73	Propranolol	160	2° prevention	A,B,C	31	50	E,F
74	Propranolol	20–360	2° prevention	A,B,C	40	10	G

[a]Single doses indicate fixed regimens; dose ranges indicate adjustment toward a physiologic goal, e.g., pulse or pressure reduction.
[b]Child–Pugh classification.
[c]$p < 0.05$.
[d]$p > 0.05$.

propranolol in preventing rebleeding.[68] However, propranolol produces desirable (decreased portal vein pressure) and undesirable effects (decreased liver blood flow). A selective β_1 blocker (metoprolol) may reduce portal hypertension without reducing hepatic blood flow like the nonselective β blocker propranolol.[76] One result of the reduced hepatic blood flow has been the demonstration that propranolol increases arterial blood ammonia and may precipitate hepatic encephalopathy.[77]

Sclerotherapy is the direct application of a chemical with necroinflammatory or thrombotic properties. Sclerosants are typically introduced via a fiber optic endoscope and injected into the bleeding varix. Ethanolamine, sodium tetradecyl sulfate, and sodium morrhuate have been used to treat esophageal varices. Sclerosants may be used to manage the acute bleeding episode and, when used prophylactically, to prevent relapse. Ulcers that develop after therapy are a serious complication of this procedure.[25] In addition, esophageal perforation, strictures, and pleural effusions may result from sclerotherapy. There is no consensus regarding the sclerosant of choice. Efficacy varies from 70–100% in stopping blood loss from varices depending on the agent, site of injection, dose, and frequency.[78] (For additional information on management of bleeding see Chapter 33 on GI bleeding.)

Medical therapy with propranolol has been compared with sclerotherapy with some studies showing no difference[79] while others favor sclerotherapy.[69] One factor to consider in favor of repeated sclerotherapy is the potential for noncompliance with propranolol. Some authors avoid this compliance risk by only using sustained-release β blockers.[73] There may be an advantage to using propranolol for secondary prevention after initial treatment of the bleeding with sclerotherapy. Alternatively, an intravenous infusion of vasopressin at 0.2–0.6 unit per minute can be used to treat acutely bleeding varices.[25] Vasopressin increases the contractility of smooth muscles, particularly the small arterioles of the splanchnic, coronary, pancreatic, and mesenteric beds. Patients must then be monitored for adverse effects resulting from the decreased perfusion of these areas. Coronary and venous thrombosis can occur along with arrhythmias secondary to ischemia. Increases in blood pressure are possible as are severe vascular headaches and angina. It is prudent to have any patient treated with vasopressin monitored by electrocardiogram. Nitroglycerin has been advocated as an adjunct to vasopressin to limit the coronary vasospasm. In addition, vasopressin and nitroglycerin appear to be additive in their effects on the portal bed.[80] Vasopressin can also be administered intra-arterially into the superior mesenteric artery. This technique is usually reserved for varices that do not respond to intravenous infusions. Ice water lavage can also be used to slow bleeding; surgery is often required in severe cases.[25] Portocaval shunting has been compared to sclerotherapy for acute variceal bleeding. Initially sclerotherapy looked superior with shorter hospital stays, fewer transfusions, and equivalent survival compared to surgery. Yet, follow-up revealed that sclerotherapy had more frequent rebleeding episodes, more rehospitalizations, and higher use of transfusions than surgery. Overall mortality and therapy costs were similar for both treatments. At this time, sclerotherapy is recommended as the initial treatment with shunt surgery indicated for failures to sclerosants.[81]

HEPATIC ENCEPHALOPATHY

> Methinks sometime I have no more wit than a Christian or an ordinary man has; but I am a great eater of beef, and I believe that does harm to my wit.
>
> Sir Andrew in "Twelfth Night," Act 1, Scene 3—Shakespeare (1603)

There are a variety of precipitating events for HE that may be preventable or reversible (Table 37.9). Most patients with HE respond to some type of protein restriction. Care must be exercised since nearly all patients with ALD have varying degrees of protein malnutrition and would require at least 60 g of protein daily to maintain positive nitrogen balance.[82] To further complicate the issue, much of the elevations in aromatic amino acids present in liver failure derive from endogenous protein breakdown rather than exogenous intake. Fully 5–12 times as much of the former compared to the latter suggests that dietary restriction would not be as effective as suppressing protein catabolism.[83] The source and types of amino acids in the diet may also be important, because AAAs, already higher than normal cirrhotics, can be utilized in the CNS to produce false neurotransmitters.[50] This ratio of AAAs to BCAAs can be reversed by the use of feedings high in BCAAs.[84] Vegetable sources of protein that are high in BCAAs can often aid in this therapy by increasing the amount of fiber in the diet. This increase in fiber can also decrease total urea production in the colon and increase fecal urea excretion.[85] Further, dairy products are less likely to precipitate HE than meat protein.[86] The classic management has been to restrict intake to about 20 g of protein per day; this was increased as the patient's symptoms improved. This approach is refuted by the false neurotransmitter theory for HE that suggests quality of protein rather than quantity especially in light of protein malnutrition and anorexia present in this population.

Specialized Protein Diet

The variable effectiveness of BCAA solutions has been the rule for the management of HE. Many of the trials producing equivocal results suffer from small sample sizes and limited power. It is useful to consider HE in acute, chronic, latent (i.e., subclinical), and fulminant phases. In latent HE, oral BCAA improves psychomotor disturbances and automobile driving capacity compared to placebo.[87] The status of BCAA in *acute* HE is more uncertain. In addition, most studies do *not* show deterioration of HE despite standard parenteral amino acid solutions or even lipid solutions. Meta-analysis did not reveal a preference for parenteral nutrition in HE.[88] In contrast, oral BCAA has improved some measures in *chronic* HE including liver function tests (increased serum albumin), nutritional measures (amino acid profile, nitrogen balance), and in some studies mortality. Given the years of anticipated treatment, oral BCAA for chronic use may be cost prohibitive for widespread use. Overall, to prevent negative nitrogen balance, stable cirrhotic patients may require 0.5–1 g/kg of protein. However, catabolic states such as alcoholic hepatitis require intakes of 1.0 g/kg of protein.

Antiammonia

Therapies that reduce the blood ammonia level appear to be effective in the management of HE that does not respond to protein restriction alone (Fig. 37.5). Cirrhotic patients have a higher rate of urea breakdown in the GI tract than do normal individuals. Lactulose, a nonabsorbed disaccharide, decreases this rate of urea breakdown and thus decreases the

TABLE 37.9. PRECIPITATING CAUSES OF HEPATIC ENCEPHALOPATHY

Cause	Mechanism	Management
Infection	Increased tissue catabolism leads to more nitrogen load; hypotension-induced azotemia	Treat infection
Constipation	Increased production and absorption of ammonia from longer contact time for bacteria and substrates	Prophylactic use of stool softeners or laxatives
Metabolic alkalosis	Leads to diffusion of un-ionized ammonia across blood–brain barrier	KCl treatment in moderate cases; 0.1 N HCl infusion in severe cases
Excess dietary protein	Substrate for bacterial production of ammonia or other nitrogenous toxins	Limit total protein intake or restrict red meat protein
Gastrointestinal bleeding	Hypovolemia may decrease perfusion to liver/brain/kidneys; blood provides 15–20 g protein/100 ml as ammonia substrate	Evacuate bowel
Drugs: sedative/hypnotics; opiates	Direct CNS depression	Avoid use; otherwise select short-acting nonliver metabolized or adjust dose
Azotemia	Sedative effect of uremia	Use diuretics gently

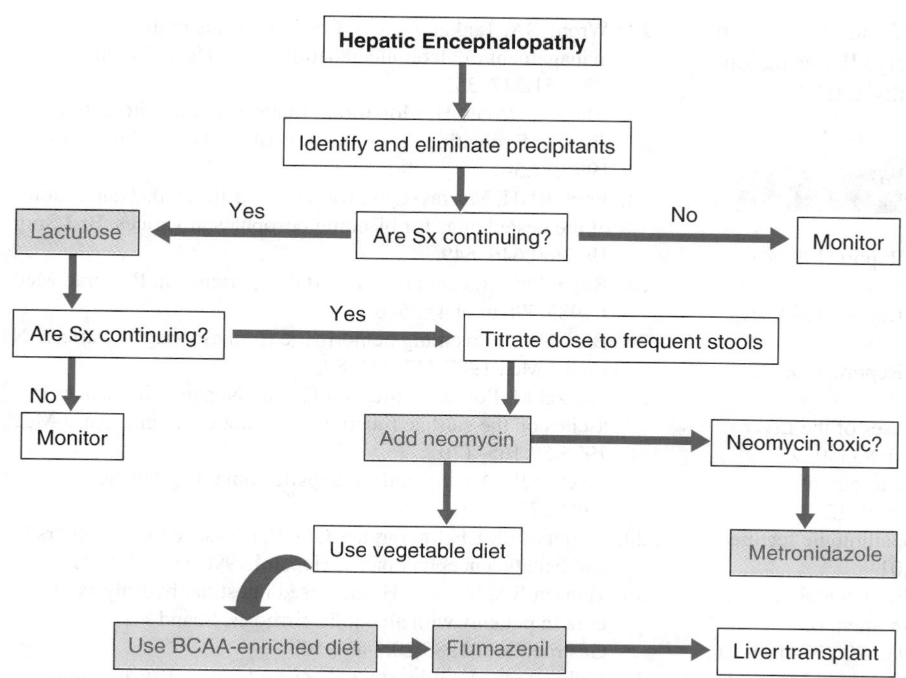

Figure 37.5. Treatment algorithm for the management of hepatic encephalopathy.

ammonia in the blood derived from the gut.[32] The exact mechanism is unclear, but an increased frequency of stools per day appears to be necessary for efficacy and may rely on less contact time of protein with gut bacteria for breakdown into ammonia. Unfortunately, use of lactulose has not been shown to increase overall fecal ammonia discharge. Rather, lactulose may increase ammonia incorporation into colonic bacteria. Optimally, the lactulose dose should be titrated to produce two to three stools per day. Lactulose is broken down in the colon to acetic, lactic, and formic acids and to carbon dioxide.[32] It has been shown to increase relative concentrations of *Lactobacillus* and other fermentative bacteria in the colon and to inhibit the proteolytic enzymes of many bacteria. By decreasing the pH in the colon, lactulose also reduces the ability of ammonia to diffuse across the gut wall. Another mechanism may well be to reduce bacterial production and systemic absorption of GABA. Lactulose should be started at 50 mL every hour until catharsis occurs. The dose is then titrated to maintain two to three stools per day.

Neomycin given orally is also used to change colonic flora and decrease blood ammonia. Another mechanism may well be to reduce bacterial production and systemic absorption of GABA. The optimal dosing regimen is not known; however, a starting dose of 0.5 g four times daily may be used up to 4–6 g/d. The disadvantage with neomycin is that it is partially absorbed, causing ototoxicity and nephrotoxicity. If either agent alone does not work, neomycin and lactulose may be given together with additive effects.[89] Neomycin was first released in 1957. Despite decades of neomycin use for HE, there is some question concerning the product's efficacy. A recent double-blinded trial versus placebo did not reveal a statistical difference in regression to grade zero symptoms between neomycin and placebo for the acute management of hospitalized subjects.[90]

Flumazenil

Small numbers of patients have been treated with the benzodiazepine antagonist, flumazenil. On occasion, rapid and startling clinical response has been seen with doses of 0.2–15 mg IV in uncontrolled studies. Controlled studies versus placebo show improvement in 40–70% treated with flumazenil and no response to placebo.[91] Thus flumazenil may be an alternative when conventional treatment of HE has failed. The parenteral route and short half-life of flumazenil (about 4 hours) precludes its use in chronic HE.

The endpoint of therapies directed at HE is an overall increase in the cognitive ability of the patient from baseline. If the patient is comatose, a return to consciousness is the goal. It is sometimes difficult in patients with milder forms of HE to detect changes resulting from therapy. In these patients, improvements in the mental status exam, electroencephalogram, and asterixis are sometimes used.[92] Simple bedside psychomotor exams, such as serial signatures, nine-number connection tests, or drawing a familiar simple figure (a star, a house), can also be of assistance.

Conclusion

ALD is often a frustrating disease for the clinician. There are few direct therapies, and symptomatic treatment often does not work or works poorly. The overall success of therapy depends ultimately on the patient. If the patient can stop drinking, there is a chance of recovery. If the patient does not stop drinking, the disease is usually fatal.

References

1. Anonymous. Morbidity Mortality Weekly Report. 1992;41, no. 7, Feb. 21:123–124.
2. Anonymous. Morbidity Mortality Weekly Report. 1993;41, no. 52–53, Jan. 8:969–973.
3. Anonymous. Morbidity Mortality Weekly Report. 1993;42, no. 46, Nov. 26:897.
4. Conn HO. Cirrhosis, in Schiff L (ed): Diseases of the Liver, 4th ed. Philadelphia, JB Lippincott, 1975, pp 833–939.
5. Grant BF, Dufour MC, Harford TC. Epidemiology of alcoholic liver disease. Semin Liver Dis 1988;8:12–25.
6. Maddrey WC. Alcoholic hepatitis: Clinicopathologic features and therapy. Semin Liver Dis 1988;8:91–101.
7. Johnson RD, Williams R. Genetic and environmental factors in the individual susceptibility to the development of alcoholic liver disease. Alcohol Alcohol 1985;20:137–160.
8. Frezza M, di Padova C, Pozzato G, et al. High blood alcohol levels in women. The role of decreased gastric alcohol dehydrogenase activity and first-pass metabolism. N Engl J Med 1990;322:95–99.
9. Klatskin G. Alcohol and its relationship to the liver. Gastroenterology 1961;41:443–451.
10. Iseri OA, Lieber CS, Gottlieb LS. The ultrastructure of the fatty liver induced by prolonged ethanol ingestion. Am J Pathol 1966;48:535–538.
11. Zimmermann HJ. Hepatotoxicity, in The Adverse Effects of Drugs and Other Chemicals on the Liver. New York, Appleton-Century-Crofts, 1978, pp 122–144.
12. Mallory FB. Phosphorous poisoning and alcoholic cirrhosis. Am J Pathol 1933;9:551–560.
13. Marsano L, McClain CJ. Nutrition and alcoholic liver disease. J Parenter Enteral Nutr 1991;15:337–344.
14. Silk DBA, O'Keefe SJD, Wicks C. Nutritional support in liver disease. Gut Supplement 1991;Sept:29–33.
15. Cabre E, Gonzalez-Huix F, Abad-Lacruz A, et al. Effect of total enteral nutrition on the short term outcome of severely malnourished cirrhotics. A randomized controlled trial. Gastroenterology 1990;98:715–720.
16. Steinmetz PR, Balko C. Liver adaptation and injury in alcoholism. N Engl J Med 1973;288:356–362.
17. Sorrell MF, Leevy CM. Lymphocyte transformation and alcoholic liver injury. Gastroenterology 1972;63:1020–1025.
18. Harinasuta U, Zimmermann HJ. Alcoholic steatonecrosis: Relationship between severity of hepatic disease and presence of Mallory bodies in the liver. Gastroenterology 1967;60:1036–1045.
19. Galambos JT. Natural history of alcoholic hepatitis. Gastroenterology 1972;63:1026–1035.
20. Ezzell JH, Werkman RF, Dean P. Treatment of alcoholic hepatitis. Am J Gastroenterol 1989;84:1217–1221.
21. Lieber CS, Guadagnini KS. The spectrum of alcoholic liver disease. Hosp Pract 1990;25:51–69.
22. Wrona SA, Tankanow RM. Corticosteroids in the management of alcoholic hepatitis. Am J Hosp Pharm 1994;51:347–353.
23. Blake J, Orrgeo H. Monitoring treatment of alcoholic liver disease: Evaluation of various severity indices. Clin Chem 1991;37:5–13.
24. Pugh RNH, Murray-Lyon IM, Dawson JL, et al. Transection of the oesophagus for bleeding oesophageal varices. Br J Surg 1973;60:646–649.
25. Reynolds TB, Campra TL. Portal hypertension. Postgrad Med J 1983;59(suppl 4):55–63.
26. Bass NM. Preventing hemorrhage from esophageal varices. N Engl J Med 1987;317:893–895.
27. Guazzi M, Polese A, Magrini F, et al. Negative influences of ascites on the cardiac function of cirrhotic patients. Am J Med 1975;59:165–170.
28. Fischer JE. Amino acids in hepatic coma. Dig Dis Sci 1982;27:97–101.
29. Butterworth RF, Layrargues GO. Benzodiazepine receptors and hepatic encephalopathy. Hepatol 1990;11:499–501.
30. Hansen BA, Vilstrup H. Increased intestinal hydrolysis of urea in patients with alcoholic cirrhosis. Scand J Gastroenterol 1985;20:346–350.
31. Gilberstadt SJ, Gilberstadt H, Zieve L, et al. Psychomotor performance defects in cirrhotic patients without overt encephalopathy. Arch Intern Med 1980;140:519–521.
32. Crossley IR, Williams R. Progress in the treatment of chronic portasystemic encephalopathy. Gut 1984;25:85–98.
33. Hourani BT, Hamlin EM, Reynolds TB. Cerebrospinal fluid glutamine as a measure of hepatic encephalopathy. Arch Intern Med 1971;127:1033–1036.
34. Basile AS, Hughes RD, Harrison PM, et al. Elevated brain concentrations of 1,4-benzodiazepines in fulminant hepatic failure. N Engl J Med 1991;325:473–478.
35. Williams RL, Mamelok RD. Hepatic disease and drug pharmacokinetics. Clin Pharmacokinetics 1980;5:528–547.
36. Gill MA, Kern JW. Altered gentamicin distribution in ascitic patients. Am J Hosp Pharm 1979;36:1704–1706.
37. Goode HF, Kellelher J, Walker BE. Relation between zinc status and hepatic functional reserve in patients with liver disease. Gut 1990;31:694–697.
38. Scott NR, Stambuck D, Chakraborty J, et al. The pharmacokinetics of caffeine in patients with chronic liver disease. Br J Clin Pharmacol 1989;27:205–213.
39. Juhl RP, Van Thiel DH, Dittert LW, et al. Alprazolam pharmacokinetics in alcoholic liver disease. J Clin Pharmacol 1984;24:113–119.
40. Black M, Tavill AS. Corticosteroids in severe alcoholic hepatitis. Ann Intern Med 1989;110:677–680.
41. Carithers RL, Herlong HF, Diehl AM, et al. Methylprednisolone therapy in patients with severe alcoholic hepatitis. A randomized multicenter trial. Ann Intern Med 1989;110:685–690.
42. Theodossi A, Eddleston ALWF, Williams R. Controlled trial of methylprednisolone therapy in severe acute alcoholic hepatitis. Gut 1982;23:75–79.
43. Helman RA, Temko MH, Nye SW, et al. Alcoholic hepatitis natural history and evaluation of prednisone therapy. Ann Intern Med 1971;74:311–321.

44. Shumaker JB, Resnik RH, Galambos JT, et al. A controlled trial of 6-methylprednisolone in acute alcoholic hepatitis. Am J Gastroenterol 1978;69:443–449.
45. Lesesne HR, Bozymski EM, Fallon HJ. Treatment of alcoholic hepatitis with encephalopathy, comparison of prednisone with caloric supplements. Gastroenterology 1978;74:169–173.
46. Campra JL, Hamlin EM, Kirshbaum RJ, et al. Prednisone therapy of acute alcoholic hepatitis, report of a controlled trial. Ann Intern Med 1973;79:625–631.
47. Porter HP, Simon FR, Pope CE, et al. Corticosteroid therapy in severe alcoholic hepatitis. N Engl J Med 1971;284:1350–1355.
48. Reynolds TB, Benhamou JP, Blake J, et al. Treatment of acute alcoholic hepatitis. Gastroenterol Int 1989;2:208–216.
49. Imperiale TF, McCullough AJ. Do corticosteroids reduce mortality from alcoholic hepatitis? A meta-analysis of the randomized trials. Ann Intern Med 1990;113:299–307.
50. Mills PR, Shenkin A, Anthony RS, et al. Assessment of nutritional status and *in vivo* immune responses in alcoholic liver disease. Am J Clin Nutr 1983;38:849–859.
51. Kumar S, Stauber RE, Gavaler JS, et al. Orthotopic liver transplantation for alcoholic liver disease. Hepatol 1990;11:159–164.
52. Orrego H, Blake JE, Blendis LM, et al. Long-term treatment of alcoholic liver disease with propylthiouracil. N Engl J Med 1987;317:1421–1427.
53. Quintero E, Arroyo V, Bory F, et al. Paracentesis versus diuretics in the treatment of cirrhotics with tense ascites. Lancet 1985;2:611–612.
54. Gauthier A, Levy VG, Quinton A, et al. Salt or no salt in the treatment of cirrhotic ascites. Gut 1986;27:705–709.
55. Shear L, Ching S, Gabuzda GJ. Compartmentalization of ascites and edema in patients with hepatic cirrhosis. N Engl J Med 1970;282:1391–1396.
56. Correia JP, Conn HO. Spontaneous bacterial peritonitis in cirrhosis: Endemic or epidemic? Med Clin North Am 1975;59:963–981.
57. Gines P, Arroyo V, Quintero E, et al. Comparison of paracentesis and diuretics in the treatment of cirrhotics with tense ascites. Gastroenterology 1987;93:234–241.
58. Gines P, Tito L, Arroyo V, et al. Randomized comparative study of therapeutic paracentesis with and without intravenous albumin in cirrhosis. Gastroenterology 1988;94:1493–1502.
59. Smadja C, Franco D. The LeVeen shunt in the elective treatment of intractable ascites in cirrhosis. Ann Surg 1985;201:488–493.
60. Ring-Larsen H, Siemssen O, Krintel JJ, et al. Denver shunt in the treatment of refractory ascites in cirrhosis: A randomized controlled trial [abstract] . J Hepatol 1989;9(suppl 1):S77.
61. Stanley MM, Ochi S, Lee KK, et al. Peritoneovenous shunting as compared with medical treatment in patients with alcoholic cirrhosis and massive ascites. N Engl J Med 1989;321:1632–1638.
62. LeVeen HH, Ahmed N, Hiutto RB, et al. Coagulopathy post peritoneovenous shunt. Ann Surg 1987;205:305–311.
63. Sherlock S. Ascites formation in cirrhosis and its management. Scand J Gastroenterol 1970;5(suppl 7):9–15.
64. Sungaila I, Bartle WR, Walker SE, et al. Spironolactone pharmacokinetics and pharmacodynamics in patients with cirrhotic ascites. Gastroenterology 1992;102:1680–1685.
65. Perez-Ayuso RM, Arroyo V, Planas R, et al. Randomized comparative study of efficacy of furosemide versus spironolactone in nonazotemic cirrhosis with ascites. Gastroenterology 1983;84:961–968.
66. Pascal JP, Cales P, and a multicenter study group. Propranolol in the prevention of first upper gastrointestinal tract hemorrhage in patients with cirrhosis of the liver and esophageal varices. N Engl J Med 1987;317:856–861.
67. Fleig WE, Stange EF, Hunecke R, et al. Prevention of recurrent bleeding in cirrhotics with recent variceal hemorrhage: Prospective, randomized comparison of propranolol and sclerotherapy. Hepatol 1987;7:355–361.
68. Colombo M, Franchis RD, Tommasini M, et al. Beta-blockade prevents recurrent gastrointestinal bleeding in well-compensated patients with alcoholic cirrhosis: A multicenter randomized controlled trial. Hepatol 1989;9:433–438.
69. Alexandrino PT, Alves MM, Correia JP. Propranolol or endoscopic sclerotherapy in the prevention of recurrence of variceal bleeding: A prospective, randomized controlled trial. J Hepatol 1988;7:175–185.
70. Jensen LS, Krarup N. Propranolol in prevention of rebleeding from oesophageal varices during the course of endoscopic sclerotherapy. Scand J Gastroenterol 1989;24:339–345.
71. Jensen LS, Krarup N. Propranolol may prevent recurrence of oesophageal varices after obliteration by endoscopic sclerotherapy. Scand J Gastroenterol 1990;25:352–356.
72. Westaby D, Hegarty J, Gimson AES, et al. Use of propranolol to reduce the rebleeding rate during injection sclerotherapy prior to variceal obliteration. Hepatol 1986;6:673–675.
73. Garden OJ, Mills PR, Birnie GG, et al. Propranolol in the prevention of recurrent variceal hemorrhage in cirrhotic patients: A controlled trial. Gastroenterology 1990;98:185–190.
74. O'Connor KW, Lehman G, Yune H, et al. Comparison of three nonsurgical treatments for bleeding esophageal varices. Gastroenterology 1989;96:899–906.
75. Lebrec D, Poynard T, Hillon P, et al. Propranolol for prevention of recurrent gastrointestinal bleeding in patients with cirrhosis. N Engl J Med 1981;305:1371–1374.
76. Westaby D, Bihari DJ, Gimson AES, et al: Selective and non-selective beta receptor blockade in the reduction of portal pressure in patients with cirrhosis and portal hypertension. Gut 1984;25:121–124.
77. Snady H, Lieber CS. Venous, arterial, and arterialized-venous blood ammonia levels and their relationship to hepatic encephalopathy after propranolol. Am J Gastroenterol 1988;83:249–255.
78. Sarin SK, Kumar A. Sclerosants for variceal sclerotherapy: A critical appraisal. Am J Gastroenterol 1990;85:641–649.
79. Westaby D, Polson RJ, Gimson AE, et al. A controlled trial of oral propranolol compared with injection sclerotherapy for the long term management of variceal bleeding. Hepatol 1990;11:353–359.
80. Terblanch J, Burroughs AK, Hobbs KEF. Controversies in the management of bleeding esophageal varices. N Engl J Med 1989;320:1393–1398.

81. Cello JP, Grendell JH, Crass RA, et al. Endoscopic sclerotherapy versus portacaval shunt in patients with severe cirrhosis and acute variceal hemorrhage. N Engl J Med 1987;316:11–15.
82. Marsano L, McClain CJ. Nutrition and alcoholic liver disease. J Parenter Enteral Nutr 1991;15:337–344.
83. Silk DBA, O'Keefe SJD, Wicks C. Nutritional support in liver disease. Gut Supplement 1991;Sept:S29–S33.
84. Fischer JE. Amino acids in hepatic coma. Dig Dis Sci 1982;27:97–101.
85. Weber FL, Minco D, Fresard KM, et al. Effects of vegetable diets on nitrogen metabolism in cirrhotic subjects. Gastroenterology 1985;89:538–544.
86. Mullen KD, Weber FL. Role of nutrition in hepatic encephalopathy. Semin Liv Dis 1991;11:292–304.
87. Plauth M, Egberts EH, Hamster W, et al. Long-term treatment of latent portosystemic encephalopathy with branched-chain amino acids. A double-blind placebo controlled crossover study. J Hepatol 1993;17:308–314.
88. Ericksson LS, Conn HO. Branched chain amino acids in the management of hepatic encephalopathy: An analysis of varient. Hepatol 1989;10:228–246.
89. Pirotte J, Guffens JM, Devos J. Comparative study of basal arterial ammonemia and of orally-induced hyperammonemia in chronic portal systemic encephalopathy, treated with neomycin, lactulose, and an association of neomycin and lactulose. Digestion 1974;10:435–444.
90. Strauss E, Tramote R, Silva EPS, et al. Double-blinded randomized clinical trial comparing neomycin and placebo in the treatment of exogenous hepatic encephalopathy. Hepatogastroenterol 1992;39:542–545.
91. Pomier-Layrargues G, Giguere JF, Lavoie J, et al. Flumazenil in cirrhotic patients in hepatic coma: A randomized double-blind placebo-controlled crossover trial. Hepatol 1994;19:32–37.
92. Atterbury CE, Maddrey WC, Conn HO. Neomycin-sorbital and lactulose in the treatment of acute portal-systemic encephalopathy: A controlled, double-blind clinical trial. Am J Dig Dis 1978;23:398–406.

Chapter 38

Drug-Induced Liver Disease

William R. Kirchain, PharmD, and Mark A. Gill, PharmD

The number of drugs associated with adverse reactions involving the liver is extensive. The National Library of Medicine lists more than 1000 case reports of drug-induced liver injury. The overall incidence of human liver injury from most drugs is fortunately very low. Chronic liver disease and cirrhosis collectively account for approximately 1% of annual mortality in the United States (about 26,000 of 2,150,000 deaths/year). Alcohol-induced liver disease accounts for most of these deaths.[1] Drug-related symptoms are the reason for about 1% of liver biopsies done each year.[2] Still, for an individual patient, liver disease is usually a profound, life-changing disease. The liver's function affects almost every other organ system in the body. It is important for a person providing pharmaceutical care to know basic patterns of drug-related pathology and toxicity to assess adverse reactions when they occur. It is also important to understand how and when to monitor for these reactions in day-to-day patient care and clinical research situations.

Hepatic Physiology and Function

For most drugs taken orally, the liver is the entrance to the systemic circulation. Blood laden with newly absorbed chemicals flows via the superior mesenteric vein into the liver's portal vein (Fig. 38.1).[3] Once in the sinusoidal portions of the liver, these chemicals are either actively or passively taken up by the hepatocytes. This "first-pass" effect causes the liver to be the first organ exposed to potentially toxic substances. In addition, any drug undergoing enterohepatic recirculation will first pass through the liver.

For most metabolized compounds, the hepatocytes that absorb these drugs are the primary site of biotransformation. These cells have a tremendous capacity for metabolizing substrates. One cubic centimeter of tissue in the average liver contains an estimated 20 m^2 of rough endoplasmic reticulum. This also predisposes the cells to damage from compounds that become more, not less, toxic following the phase I reactions of biotransformation (Fig. 38.2). These bioactivated compounds are often directly toxic to the organelles of the hepatocytes, leading to cell damage.[4] For example, valproic acid becomes toxic to the hepatocyte only after it is converted to Δ-4-valproic acid by cytochrome P-450.[5]

Along with its metabolic role, the liver serves as a primary storage organ for many substrates. Apparently, certain toxins are concentrated in the liver, leading to selective adverse reactions.[3,6] Over time, vitamin A stored in the space of Disse can, in high doses, lead to marked liver hypertrophy and fibrosis. Similarly, amiodarone that has a very long residence time in the liver can induce phospholipidosis within the lysosomal lamellar bodies of the hepatocyte. Besides their metabolic role, the hepatocytes connect to the bile canalicular system and produce bile. Drugs excreted via this system may cause a decrease in bile production or bile flow through the system.[4,7,8] Estrogens, for example, can reduce bile-salt–dependent flow, thus decreasing the excretion of bile and causing congestion. This congestion in turn leads to the formation of cholestatic lesions in the liver. Cholestatic lesions are often characterized by bile plugs within the biliary capillaries seen at biopsy.

There are anatomic and physiologic divisions in the liver that control the development of the different patterns of hepatic damage. Hepatocytes are in constant contact with other hepatocytes, the perisinusoidal space, and a biliary capillary (Fig. 38.3).[4] The hepatocytes develop around an axis consisting of a central vein, portal venule, bile ductule, and lymph vessels that grow outward from a small triangular field called an acinus. This arrangement can be divided physiologically into three zones. Moving from the central vein toward the portal vein, the function of the hepatocyte shifts from respiration to biotransformation and storage.[3,6] The hepatocytes in zone 1, the best oxygenated zone, tend to have higher concentrations of the enzymes of respiration, particularly glucose-6-phosphatase and the Kreb's cycle enzymes. These cells tend to be more resistant to nutritional and circulatory disease. The hepatocytes in zone 3 tend to have higher concentrations of NAD and NADP, and a higher rate of fatty acid production and glycogen stores.[3]

Necrotic lesions then develop in patterns correlating with both the type of toxic compound and the position of the most sensitive hepatocytes. For example, a bioactivated compound that requires a specific enzyme, such as isoni-

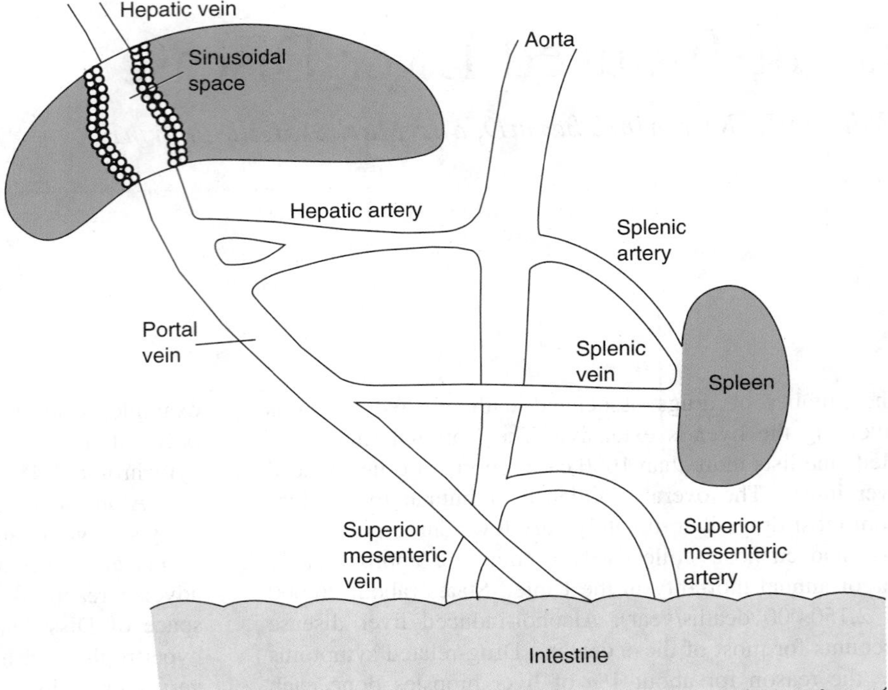

Figure 38.1. Diagram of hepatic blood flow. The interconnections of the hepatic circulatory system are important in understanding the physiology and pathology of the liver. All substances taken orally pass through the liver via the superior mesenteric vein and hepatic artery. These are low-pressure, low-speed systems that allow for the extraction of substrates from the blood by the hepatocytes.

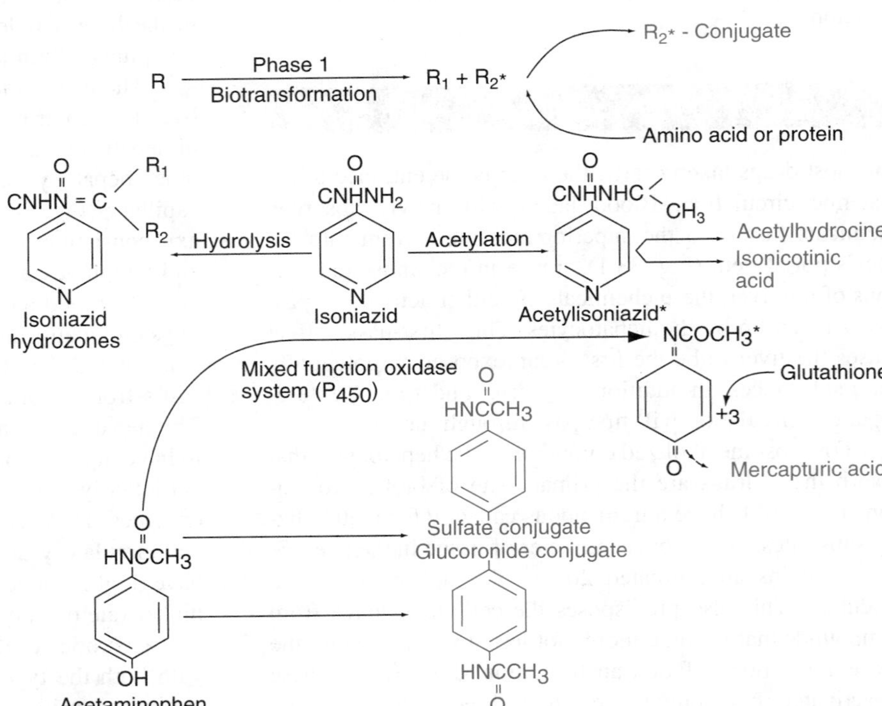

Figure 38.2. Bioactivation. Usually during a phase I reaction, a drug *(R)* is converted to an intermediate compound that is intrinsically toxic to the hepatocyte or the canaliculi. Isoniazid is thought to be bioactivated by acetylation, acetaminophen by the mixed-function oxidase system (cytochrome P-450).

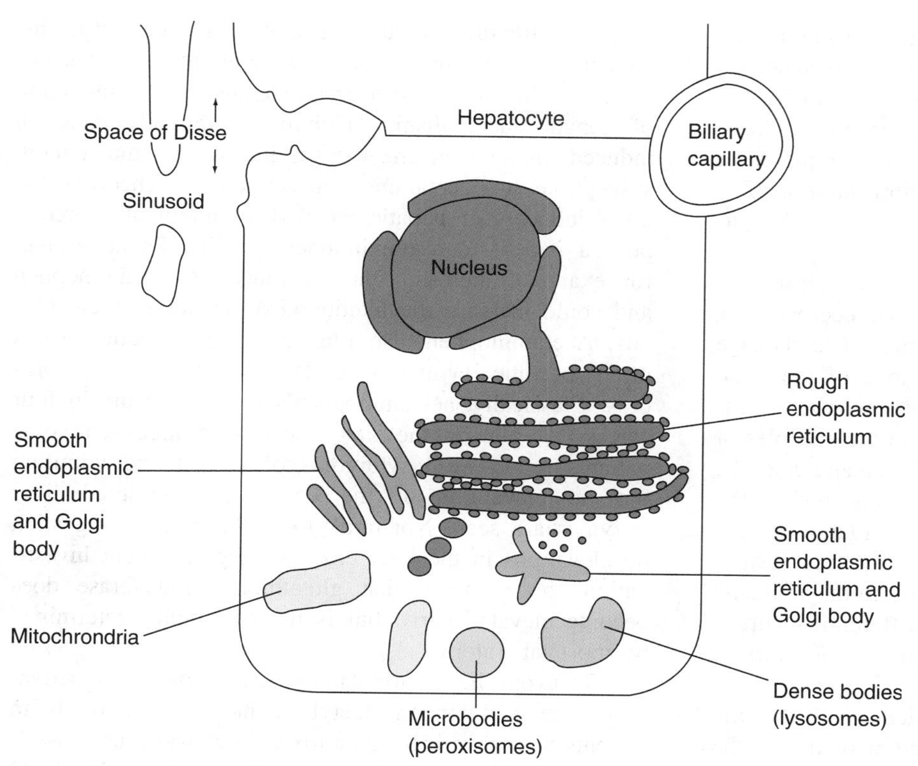

Figure 38.3. A typical hepatocyte is in constant contact with the hepatic blood, another hepatocyte, and a biliary capillary. There are always large amounts of endoplasmic reticulum, along with many mitochondria and microbodies, in each hepatocyte.

azid, will tend to produce lesions in areas of the liver where acetylation is a predominant function.[9] The lesions associated with acetaminophen overdose tend to occur in zone 3 where there is a higher rate of redox reactions.[10]

If the liver parenchyma is continually exposed to periods of acute cell damage and necrosis, nonfunctional fibrous tissue will begin to replace functional hepatocytes.[3] Because of the liver's tremendous capacity, small fibrotic changes can usually be tolerated without significant reduction in function. As these changes continue, the architectural integrity of the organ is lost; when these changes are accompanied by nodular regeneration, cirrhosis follows. The cirrhotic liver can take many forms depending on the rate of nodular regeneration and the extent of the initial necrotic process.[4] The terms used to describe the results of a liver biopsy reflect this process. The size of the nodules of collagen are indicated by the terms *micro*nodular or *macro*nodular. Congestive cirrhosis describes a large backflow of blood in the tissue secondary to scarring. Disease restricted to the bile canalicular system is termed biliary cirrhosis. Cirrhosis can develop after only one exposure to a drug, but usually results from months to years of exposure.[11,12]

As the normal liver ages, hepatic blood flow decreases as much as 30% by age 65.[13] This decrease in liver blood flow increases the bioavailability of highly extracted drugs, such as labetolol, propranolol, lidocaine, and chlormethiazole. The risk of hepatotoxicity is apparently greater in persons 70 years old or older, according to data from the United Kingdom. There >5% of all adverse reactions in persons 70 years old or older occur in the liver, while only 2% of all adverse reactions in children (0–14 years old) occur in the liver.[14] The potential mortality from hepatoxic reactions is also higher in the elderly, who often have concurrent decreases in renal or cardiac function. Neoplastic disease and hepatocellular carcinomas are also more common in the elderly than in younger patients.[14]

Patterns of Drug-Induced Liver Disease

The two primary types of drug-induced liver disease are predictable reactions and idiosyncratic or unpredictable reactions. Predictable reactions usually can be explained by a toxic dose–response relationship. For some drugs, there also must coexist a genetic or acquired abnormality in a particular metabolic pathway for a predictable reaction to take place. Predictable reactions occur in greater than 2% of persons taking the drug. Predictable reactions have a very well-defined slow onset and long duration, usually manifesting after a few weeks to months of therapy. These reactions are typically associated with a drug concentration and often respond to simply lowering the dose of the offending drug. Idiosyncratic reactions, however, tend to occur without association to particular blood concentrations or specifically identified metabolic abnormalities. Idiosyncratic reactions are rare and are sometimes described as a type of liver hypersensitivity to a drug. These reactions occur within the first days to weeks of therapy with a rapid onset and, although severe in nature, have a short duration. The offending drug must be discontinued before an idiosyncratic reaction can resolve.

Predictable and idiosyncratic reactions can cause similar patterns of liver damage. Centrolobular necrosis is a pattern of acute cell death and disruption. The damage spreads outward from the middle of a lobe of the liver. Steatonecrosis is a specialized type of acute necrosis resulting from the accumulation of fatty acids in the vacuoles of the hepatocyte. If no cells have yet burst open and died, the pattern of damage is termed steatosis. Steatonecrosis is the primary lesion in alcoholic hepatitis. When a large number of liver cells become damaged acutely, hepatitis ensues. Hepatitis is an immune reaction in the liver to the antigenic proteins within the hepatocyte. To differentiate drug-induced hepatitis from other types the term *toxic hepatitis* is sometimes used.

Hepatitis also can be induced by damage to the bile canalicular system. Typically in this pattern of illness the flow of bile is decreased, causing accumulation in the biliary capillaries. If enough accumulation occurs, cells lining the biliary capillary will die. Another rarer pattern of disease in the liver involves the loss of cell membrane integrity. These are the liver vascular disorders and are marked by numerous blood-filled sacks found throughout the organ. With each insult to the liver—regardless of type—healthy tissue is lost and replaced with functionless scar tissue. If enough scar tissue has built up in the right places cirrhosis is the result. Based on the pattern of the scar tissue laid down, cirrhosis can be classified as either micronodular, macronodular, congestive, or biliary cirrhosis.

CENTROLOBULAR NECROSIS

Centrolobular necrosis is often a dose-related, predictable reaction secondary to drugs such as acetaminophen; however, it also can be associated with idiosyncratic reactions, such as those caused by halothane.[15] Also called *direct* or *metabolite-related hepatotoxicity,* centrolobular necrosis is usually the result of the production of a toxic metabolite. The process by which a nontoxic parent compound converts into a toxic metabolite is termed *bioactivation.* Bioactivation of a hepatically cleared compound is a very important concept. Drugs cleared by the cytochrome P-450 system are often associated with a bioactivated toxic process.

Acetaminophen, when taken in overdose, becomes bioactivated to a toxic intermediate (Fig. 38.2). When the liver's glutathione stores are depleted and there are no longer sulfhydral groups available to detoxify this metabolite, it begins to react directly with the hepatocyte.[16,17] This process can be accelerated by the induction of hepatic metabolism. Alcoholics commonly have an induced microsomal enzyme system and are much more susceptible to acetaminophen toxicity.[18] Theoretically, other inducers of hepatic metabolism might also predispose a patient to acetaminophen toxicity. Phenobarbital, for example, increases the clearance of acetaminophen and could increase the likelihood of acetaminophen toxicity. Acetaminophen also illustrates how hepatic lesions often become symptomatic late in the disease process. Classically, acetaminophen's toxicity occurs in four stages.[16,17] During the first hours after ingestion some patients report mild symptoms of nausea and vomiting but no elevations of the commonly measured liver enzymes are seen. Not until 40–50 hours after ingestion do elevations in the liver enzymes begin. Recent investigations have shown that glutathione-*S*-transferase does become elevated early, but is not commonly determined by most laboratories.[15–17]

To avoid the hepatic damage caused by the bioactivation of acetaminophen, acetylcysteine is given orally to patients who have ingested a toxic dose. The usual dose is 140 mg/kg of body weight given every 4–6 hours for 48–72 hours. Although acetylcysteine does not reverse damage that has already occurred, it provides additional sulfhydral groups replacing the spent stores of glutathione. These sulfhydral groups are then available to conjugate the toxic metabolite being produced by the cytochrome P-450 system.[16,17] It is interesting to note that known cytochrome P-450 inhibitors, such as cimetidine, have not proven useful in treating acetaminophen overdose.

Halothane may produce centrolobular necrosis in patients who have been exposed to the drug more than once. There is no dose–response relationship associated with halothane exposure, but there is a correlation between the extent of liver damage and the number of times the patient has been anesthetized with halothane.[19] The frequency of halothane-induced hepatic disease is one in several thousand.[20] Halothane is metabolized by both oxidative and reductive pathways. Trifluoroacetic acid is its major oxidative metabolite, while the products of reduction include several chloronated ethylenes and trifluorocarbene.[21] With these compounds several intermediates also may be produced including a reactive metabolite that can bind to macromolecules in the hepatocyte and disrupt the normal metabolic processes.[22]

Patients suffering from centrolobular necrosis tend to present in one of two ways, depending on the extent of necrosis. Mild drug reactions, involving only small amounts of parenchymal tissue, may be detected as asymptomatic elevations in the serum transaminases. If the reaction is diagnosed at this stage, most of these patients will recover with minimal cirrhosis and thus minimal chronic liver impairment. More severe forms of centrolobular necrosis are accompanied by nausea, vomiting, upper abdominal pain, and jaundice. These patients can progress rapidly into both complete hepatic and renal failure and require intensive supportive care.[17] Those who survive this initial period often go on to develop chronic liver failure secondary to cirrhosis.

STEATONECROSIS

Steatonecrosis is the accumulation of large amounts of microvesicular fat within the hepatocyte. Drugs or their metabolites that cause steatonecrosis do so by affecting fatty-acid oxidation within the mitochondria of the hepatocyte. Hepatic vesicles become engorged with fatty acids, eventually disrupting the homeostasis of the hepatocyte. Alcohol is the most common drug that produces steatonecrotic changes in the liver. When alcohol converts into acetaldehyde the synthesis of fatty acids is increased.[23] When the hepatocyte has become completely engorged with microvesicular fat, it often breaks open spilling its contents into the blood. If enough hepatocytes break open, an inflammatory response begins. If the offending agent is withdrawn before significant numbers of hepatocytes become necrotic the process is completely reversible without long-term sequelae.[24] Steatonecrotic reactions are the most reversible of all drug-induced liver diseases.

Steatonecrosis is often a drug or toxin concentration-related phenomena. Tetracycline has produced steatonecrosis and steatosis.[25] The lesions are characterized by large vesicles of fat found diffused throughout the liver. This is typical of most steatonecrotic drug reactions in the liver. The development of this reaction is related to the high concentrations achieved when tetracycline is given intravenously and in doses greater than 1.5 g/d.[26] The first reports of this reaction related the fatal outcome of several patients given tetracycline intravenously to treat pelvic inflammatory disease. The mortality of tetracycline steatonecrosis is very high (70–80%) and those that do survive often develop cirrhosis.

Valproate also can produce steatonecrosis through the process of bioactivation. Cytochrome P-450 converts valproate to Δ-4-valproic acid. Δ-4-Valproate is a potent inducer of microvesicular fat accumulation.[5] Estimates of the frequency of this reaction range from 1 in 500 to 1 in 50,000, depending on age and concomitant therapy.[27,28] As stated earlier, phenobarbital can induce the cytochrome P-450 system and increase Δ-4-valproic acid production.[5] Caution is therefore appropriate when the two drugs are given together to control epilepsy.

Patients experiencing steatonecrosis may present with abdominal fullness or pain as their only complaint. This is particularly true in cases of mild steatonecrosis. Patients with more severe steatonecrosis will present with all the symptoms characteristic of alcoholic hepatitis such as nausea, vomiting, steatorrhea, abdominal pain, pruritis, and fatigue. With the discontinuance of the offending agent most of these patients will heal with only moderate cirrhosis.

Phospholipidosis is similar to steatonecrosis except that it is the accumulation of phospholipids instead of fatty acids. The phospholipids usually engorge the lysosomal bodies of the hepatocyte.[29] Amiodarone has been documented to cause this reaction. It has been argued that this phenomenon is not the mechanism of amiodarone toxicity but simply the normal storage pattern of the drug. This argument is based on the fact that all patients given the drug have some degree of phospholipidosis. Patients treated with amiodarone that develop overt hepatic disease tend to have received higher doses of the drug. These patients also have higher amiodarone to *N*-desethyl-amiodarone ratios indicating a greater accumulation of the parent compound. Amiodarone and its major metabolite *N*-desethyl-amiodarone remain in the liver of all patients for several months after therapy is stopped. Usually the phospholipidosis develops in patients treated for more than a year. The patient can present with either elevated transaminases or hepatomegaly; jaundice is rare.[25,30,31]

REYE'S SYNDROME

Reye's syndrome is an aggressive form of hepatocellular disease often associated with aspirin use in children. Valproate toxicity can also present in this pattern. Early in the process of Reye's syndrome mitochondrial dysfunction leads to the depletion of acyl coenzyme A (CoA) and carnitine. Fatty acids accumulate and gluconeogenesis is impaired, resulting in hypoglycemia. A concurrent disruption of the urea cycle leading to decrease in the removal of ammonia and a slowing of protein utilization occurs. A threefold or greater rise in the blood ammonia level and an increase in the prothrombin time are common findings. In advanced stages of Reye's syndrome many patients develop intracranial hypertension that can be life-threatening and refractory to therapy.[32]

TOXIC HEPATITIS

Drug-induced or toxic hepatitis resembles acute viral hepatitis. The onset of symptoms is usually delayed, as much as a week or more after exposure to toxin. Bioactivation is often important for toxic hepatitis to develop, but may not be the immediate cause of damage. Many drugs that have been associated with toxic hepatitis produce metabolites that are not inherently toxic to the liver. Instead they act as haptens, binding to specific cell proteins and inducing an autoimmune reaction.[33] Halothane produces centrolobular necrosis in some patients as described earlier and toxic hepatitis in others. Eosinophilia and fever are commonly present in these patients.[34,35] Methyldopa has also been known to cause toxic hepatitis through the production of a methyldopa-antigen complex. Methyldopa can also induce a lupus-like autoimmune reaction that develops into chronic active hepatitis. These antiorganelle antibodies have been identified for many drugs associated with toxic hepatitis, including nitrofurantoin.[33]

Isoniazid produces a pattern of hepatocellular necrosis in affected patients that is almost identical with viral hepatitis.[9,36] The long-term administration of isoniazid can lead to hepatic dysfunction in 10–20% of those receiving the drug. Yet severe toxic hepatitis develops in only 1% or less of this population.[37,38] Although the exact mechanism is still controversial, patients who are rapid acetylators have a greater susceptibility. Isoniazid is metabolized by several pathways, acetylation being the major pathway. It is acetylated to acetylisoniazid, which is, in turn, hydrolyzed to acetylhydrazine. The acetylhydrazine and, to a lesser extent, the acetylisoniazid are directly toxic to the cellular proteins in the hepatocyte.[37] The role of acetylator phenotype is even more complex; studies have shown that rapid acetylators also detoxify acetylhydrazine very rapidly converting it to diacetylhydrazine. It may be the relative rates of reaction and affinities of the various pathways that determine susceptibility to hepatotoxicity.

Acetylator phenotype can be determined before the initiation of therapy, but this is seldom done in clinical practice due to the amount of time required and the costs involved. Most methods require the administration of a small dose of another acetylated compound and the determination of serial blood levels. Sulfadimidine is given in doses of 1 g, and urine is then collected over an 8-hour period. This method was first introduced in 1939 and is still used in studies of acetylator phenotype today.[39,40] Another method involves the administration of dapsone 5 mg/kg to fasting subjects; blood samples are then drawn at 0, 2, 3, 4, and 5 hours and a half-life is calculated from the data. Rapid acetylators tend to have a half-life of less than 2 hours.[41] Alternatively a blood sample taken 3 hours after a dose of 100 mg dapsone can be assayed for the content of both dapsone and monoacetyldapsone in the blood. Rapid acetylators should have a calculated ratio of monoacetylated dapsone to dapsone greater than or equal to 70%, while slow acetylators will have values less than or equal to 26%.[42] These methods are contraindicated in persons with hypersensitivity to sulfonamides or sulfones.

Aspirin has also been reported to cause toxic hepatitis in adults taking high doses of the drug. The incidence of this reaction in patients taking more than 2 g of aspirin daily is high. Elevated transaminases are noted in 20–60% of patients in this group. Severe hepatoxicity is rare and may have some relationship to serum concentrations greater than 25 mg/dL.[43,44] These patients may go on to develop chronic active hepatitis after the initial insult.

Ketoconazole produces toxic hepatitis or milder forms of hepatic dysfunction in 1–2% of patients treated for fungal infections.[45] This reaction has been reported to be fatal in many patients. The onset is usually early in therapy although it can be delayed until several months into therapy. Because the relative risk from most fungal infections is low in persons with good immune function, the hepatotoxic potential of ketoconazole has relegated it to the level of secondary therapy. In immune-compromised patients where ketoconazole is used for long periods of time, special care should be taken to watch for changes in liver function.

Chronic active hepatitis is a sequela to the development of toxic hepatitis.[46] It is a progressive necroinflammatory disease that carries a very high mortality rate if not aggressively treated. Methyldopa, isoniazid, nitrofurantoin, and dantrolene have all been associated with its development.[46–48] It is more common in females than males and is characterized by high levels of autoimmune antibodies.[46] Treatment includes the use of immunosuppressants such as prednisone and azathioprine, usually given in low doses for several months.[46,48]

HYPERSENSITIVITY REACTIONS

Allergic reactions in the liver can be manifested by either hepatocellular or cholestatic patterns of injury. In addition, patients may present with a mixed pattern with both cholestatic and hepatocellular lesions. The sulfonamides, including trimethoprin-sulfamethoxazole, induce a reaction typical of hepatic hypersensitivity in a few patients.[49–52] The reaction usually develops within 4 weeks of the start of therapy. It is marked by fever, rash, eosinophilia, arthritis, and hemolytic anemia. The formation of granulomas within the liver is often seen on biopsy.[52] The reaction reverses with discontinued therapy and reappears upon rechallenge. Many other anti-infectives, penicillin, cloxacillin, oxacillin, and amoxicillin-clavulinic acid have been associated with this type of reaction.[52–54] The incidence of an allergic liver reaction is low, but fatal in some cases.[52]

Erythromycin and troleandomycin are associated with a classic idiosyncratic hypersensitivity reaction marked by a diffuse rash, pruritis, abdominal pain, and eosinophilia. Granulomas are often seen on liver biopsy. The incidence of this reaction has been estimated to be 1–2% of patients treated with erythromycin.[55] The two macrolide antibiotics produce nitrosoalkanes when metabolized by cytochrome P-450. Nitrosoalkanes react readily with sulfhydral groups within the hepatocyte. It is theorized that when enough hepatocytes are damaged by this reaction there is a release of hepatic intracellular protein that stimulates an allergic reaction within the liver.[55]

Allopurinol also has been associated with a number of reports of hypersensitivity reactions involving the liver. The onset of symptoms is 1–6 weeks after initiation of therapy.[56,57] The incidence, like all the allergic liver reactions is low, estimated at less than 1%. The clinical presentation includes eosinophilia, fever, rash, and arthritis as previously mentioned. The biopsy may show a pattern of fibrin-ring granulomas similar to those seen in Q-fever.[56,57] The bulk of reported idiosyncratic liver damage associated with antibiotic use also follows this pattern.

CHOLESTATIC JAUNDICE

Cholestatic jaundice or cholestasis can be histologically classified by the area of the bile canalicular or ductal system that is impaired. Canalicular cholestasis is very often associated with long-term estrogen therapy. A significant decrease in bile flow without secondary inflammation is usually seen.[58,59] The actual incidence is very low and is decreasing as the estrogen doses in oral contraceptives decrease. Clinically, these patients are often asymptomatic and present with mild to moderate elevations of serum bilirubin. At times, androgens are also associated with canalicular cholestasis. α-Tocopherol acetate, an intravenous form of vitamin E, was noted to cause cholestatic jaundice, primarily involving the canaliculi, in premature infants. The children were being treated with the drug to avoid hemolytic anemia secondary to the vitamin E deficiency often seen in premature infants.[60] The incidence of this reaction in this group was very high (greater than 10%) and the mortality even higher (greater than 50%). The drug was withdrawn from the market because of this problem.

Hepatocellular cholestasis is a much more serious form of cholestatic jaundice that involves both the parenchyma and bile canalicular cells. Chlorpromazine is the most cited example of heptocellular cholestatic jaundice. The reaction occurs in about 1% of patients treated with the drug.[61] Chlorpromazine can precipitate bile salts and decrease total bile flow. The reaction typically begins in the first 4 weeks of therapy, but may be delayed for months.[61,62] The administration of total parenteral nutrition induces cholestatic changes and nonspecific enzyme elevations in as many as 80% of patients treated, although the exact incidence is probably only around 25%.[63] Patients with low serum albumin concentrations may be at greater risk than patients with normal serum albumin concentrations.[64] It also has been suggested that aluminum deposition may play a role.[65] This reaction also has been reported to occur rarely with sulfonamides, sulfonylureas, erythromycin estolate and ethylsuccinate, captopril, and other phenothiazines.[66–71] Ductular cholestasis is the least reported form of cholestatic jaundice. This reaction is similar to canalicular cholestasis in that no inflammation is usually seen. The bile ducts and, to a lesser degree, the canaliculi become plugged with very dense bile casts. The anti-inflammatory agents are associated with the development of ductular cholestasis, but only in rare cases.[72]

LIVER VASCULAR DISORDERS

Focal lesions in hepatic venules, sinusoids, and portal veins occur with various drugs. The most commonly associated drugs are the cytotoxic agents used to treat cancer, the pyrrolizidine alkaloids, and the sex hormones.[73–75] Veno-occlusive disease is a phlebitis of the central veins in the liver. A centralized necrosis often follows and can result in cirrhosis, usually with a significant amount of concurrent congestion.[73,76] Azathioprine and herbal teas that contain comfrey (a source of pyrrolizidine alkaloids) have been reported in association with the development of veno-occlusive disease. The exact incidence is rare and may be, for the pyrrolizidine alkaloids, dose related.[73,74]

Peliosis hepatitis is an unusual type of hepatic vascular lesion that can be seen as both an acute and a chronic disease. The liver develops large, blood-filled lacunae within the parenchyma.[75,77] Rupture of the lacunae can lead to severe peritoneal hemorrhage. Peliosis hepatitis has been associated with exposure of the liver to androgens, estrogens, tamoxifen, azathioprine, and danazol.[73,78,79] Androgens with a 17, α-testosterone structure are the most frequently reported agents to cause peliosis hepatitis, usually after at least 6 months of therapy. The actual incidence of this reaction is rare, with less than 40 cases reported in the literature in the last 40 years.[80]

CIRRHOSIS

The deposition of fibrotic tissue and the secondary development of cirrhosis are usually sequelae to a primarily necrotic or cholestatic lesion, but sometimes can be the dominant presenting feature of a hepatotoxic reaction. Methotrexate causes periportal fibrosis in most patients. The lesion results from the action of a bioactivated metabolite produced by cytochrome P-450.[81] This process has most commonly been noted in patients treated for psoriasis.[81–83] The extent of damage can be reduced or controlled by increasing the dosage interval to once weekly. The addition of leucovorin to the regimen also decreases the rate of fibrosis.[82,83] Leucovorin is a completely reduced form of folic acid. It can act in metabolic reactions without being first reduced by dihydroreductase, the enzyme inhibited by methotrexate. Cells treated with leucovorin may be more resistant to the deteriorating effect of methotrexate. Vitamin A, which is normally stored in the space of Disse, specifically in Ito cells, can cause significant hypertrophy and fibrosis when taken for long periods in high doses. Hepatomegaly is a common finding along with other signs of advanced liver disease including ascites and portal hypertension. In patients with vitamin A toxicity, gingivitis and dry skin are also very common.[84] Tragically, patients who develop this hepatotoxic reaction are often extremely interested in their health and have taken megavitamins to become healthier.

NEOPLASTIC DISEASE

A large body of the current literature on adverse reactions and the liver addresses the development of neoplasms following drug therapy. Both carcinoma- and sarcoma-like lesions have been identified. Fortunately, hepatic tumors associated with drug therapy are usually benign and remit when drug therapy is discontinued. Except in rare instances, these lesions are associated with long-term exposure to the offending agent.[4,80] Androgens, estrogens, and other hormonal-related agents are the most frequently associated causes of neoplastic disease.

IDENTIFYING HEPATOTOXICITY

The best and most important technique for assessing and monitoring for drug-induced liver disease is the medication history. Questions addressing the patient's drug usage along with a thorough review of systems are essential. It is also good to try to determine nondrug hepatic disease risk. Here one is looking for a history of exposure to known environmental toxins. Arsenic, for example, is known to induce both acute and chronic hepatic reactions. Arsenic in low concentrations is found in most rot- and insect-resistant lumber. Persons working with what is sometimes referred to as pressure-treated lumber may predispose themselves to liver damage from other agents. Following Occupational Safety and Health Agency (OSHA) guidelines should decrease this danger, but not eliminate it. Even if exposure to an environmental toxin in and of itself does not produce a hepatic reaction, it may predispose a patient to a drug-induced hepatic reaction when the drug is added. Table 38.1 lists some of the more common hepatic toxins that can add to a patient's risk for developing a hepatic lesion. All potential drug reactions should be judged as to the timing of the reaction versus drug administration, pharmacokinetic considerations, the literature records of previous reactions, the inclusion of alternative nondrug causes, and close clinical observation when the drug in question is stopped.

Often there is no good clinical test available to determine the type of hepatic lesion exactly, short of biopsy. There are, still, certain patterns of enzyme elevation that have been identified and can be helpful (Table 38.2).[85] These enzymes are also useful in monitoring patients on certain potentially hepatotoxic drugs. The specificity of any serum enzyme depends on the distribution of that enzyme in the body. Alkaline phosphatase is usually found in the bile duct epithelium, but it is also found in bone and intestinal and kidney cells. Alkaline phosphatase, therefore, although indicative of cholestatic disease, is not absolutely specific for cholestatic disease.[86] 5′-Nucleotidase is more specific for hepatic disease than alkaline phosphatase, because most of the body's store of 5′-nucleotidase is in the liver. This rule of specificity also holds true within the liver.

TABLE 38.1. ENVIRONMENTAL HEPATIC TOXINS[a]

Toxin	Group or Use Associated with Exposure
Arsenic	Chemical, construction, agricultural workers
Copper	Use of copper utensils, copper plumbing
Dimethylformanide	Chemical workers
Fluorine	Chemical workers
Pyrrizolidine alkaloids	Users of herbal teas
Toluene	Chemical and agricultural workers
Trichloroethylene	Printers, dye workers, cleaners
Vinyl chloride	Chemical workers

[a]A partial list of environmental toxins that can cause liver injury. At lower exposure rates, these compounds may also predispose the patient to liver injury from a drug.

Glutamate dehydrogenase is a very good indicator of centrolobular necrosis because it is found primarily in centrolobularly located mitochondria. The sensitivity of serum enzymes, as indicators of organ damage, depends on the relative concentration and rate of production of the enzyme within the cell. Most hepatic cells have extremely high concentrations of transaminases. Aspartamine transferase (AST or SGOT) and alanine transferase (ALT or SGPT) are commonly measured. Because of their high concentrations and easy liberation from the hepatocyte cytoplasm, AST and ALT are very sensitive indicators of necrotic lesions within the liver. Once an acute hepatic lesion is established it may take weeks for these concentrations to return to normal. An abrupt fall in concentration suggests the total destruction of the hepatic parenchyma.

Liver enzymes commonly available to the clinician often have little prognostic value. Serum bilirubin concentration is an exception, having some prognostic value when dramatically elevated.[86] Patients with halothane hepatitis have an increased mortality rate when the serum bilirubin concentration is greater than 10 mg/dL.[85,86] The breakdown product of porphyrin, myoglobin, and various cytochromes, bilirubin is actively taken into the hepatic cells, conjugated with glucuronic acid, and excreted into the bile. In the intestine, bilirubin is converted to several compounds through the action of bacteria. These urobilinogens are then reabsorbed and excreted via the kidney. When the hepatic production of conjugated bilirubin decreases, a proportional decrease occurs in the amount of urobilinogen excreted in the urine. Antibiotics, however, can also cause decreased urine urobilinogen.[86]

The relative amounts of conjugated (direct) versus unconjugated (indirect) bilirubin are at times useful in differentiating a cholestatic hepatic lesion from an extrahepatic disease or a parenchymal hepatic lesion. The direct (conjugated) bilirubin would be expected to increase when-

TABLE 38.2. RELATIVE PATTERNS OF HEPATIC ENZYME ELEVATION VERSUS TYPE OF HEPATIC LESION

Enzyme	Abbreviation	Necrotic	Cholestatic	Chronic
Alkaline phosphatase	Alk Phos	+	+++	+
5′-Nucleotidase	5NC	+	+++	+
γ-Glutamyltransferase	GGTP	+	+++	++
Leucine aminopeptidase	LAP	+	+++	+
Aspartamine transferase	AST	+++	+	++
Alanine transferase	ALT	+++	+	++
Malate dehydrogenase	MDH	+++	+	+
Lactate dehydrogenase	LDH	+++	+	+

Key: + = minimal elevation above normal, ++ = median elevation above normal, +++ = significant elevation above normal.

ever there is a decrease in bile flow. The total bilirubin would be expected to increase whenever there is a large decrease in the ability of the liver to process bilirubin.

Bilirubin concentrations and serum enzyme elevations give a static picture of the liver's condition. They do not indicate hepatic function. Readily available tests to predict hepatic function are serum protein measurement and prothrombin time. As hepatic parenchymal function decreases, serum protein concentrations in the body decrease at a rate determined by each protein's own elimination rate. Overhydration and starvation can also decrease serum protein concentrations. In addition, serum protein concentrations give only a rough estimate of the degree of hepatic dysfunction. The coagulation factors II, VII, IX, and X are produced in the liver and are dependent on the utilization of vitamin K by liver carboxylase. The function of this enzyme–vitamin system is indicated by the prothrombin time. The prothrombin time increases in a fashion similar to the decrease in serum proteins during hepatic dysfunction. The changes in the prothrombin time often occur earlier than the changes in albumin or transferrin. The response of the prothrombin time to the administration of parenteral 10 mg vitamin K is often used to test between hepatic and extrahepatic disease and to estimate the residual metabolic capacity of the liver.

One of the common problems associated with a decrease in liver function is the lack of a good clinical determinant of this change. A good compound for a liver function test would theoretically match the following criteria: (1) It should be nontoxic, lacking any pharmacologic effect. (2) It should be either rapidly and completely absorbed orally or easily administered via a peripheral vein. (3) It must be eliminated only by the liver. (4) The drug and its metabolite should be easily measured in blood, saliva, or urine.[87]

Several tests are used in research settings and in liver transplant patients to indicate liver function. The breath test uses ^{14}C-labeled aminopyrine to measure the capacity of the mixed-function oxidase system via the production of $^{14}CO_2$. Because this test requires sophisticated radiation detection equipment it has not become a widely available clinical test for mixed-function oxidase activity.[88] The more traditional tests of hepatic function, such as sulfobromophthalein excretion or indocyanine green excretion, measure less exact qualities of hepatic clearance. Sulfobromophthalein is injected intravenously, absorbed by parenchymal cells, conjugated to glutathione, and then excreted in the bile. A blood sample taken 45 minutes after the injection is reported as a percentage of dye retained in the blood. Sulfobromophthalein is very irritating at the injection site and has rarely been associated with anaphylactic reactions. Indocyanine green follows a similar pathway except for conjugation and is also measured as percentage of dye retained. Indocyanine green clearance is used in comparative studies of highly extracted hepatically cleared drugs to measure changes in hepatic blood flow.[89]

There are also a few drugs that have been used to test liver function. Most of these drugs do continue to have pharmacologic activity when used for this purpose. Sorbitol is administered by intravenous infusion 50 mg/min over a period of 3 hours. Blood samples taken at 0, 135, and 180 minutes are used to determine hepatic blood flow. Sorbitol's advantage over indocyanine green is a much lower incidence of allergic reactions. It is unfortunately partially cleared by the kidney, and urine levels must also be determined during the test. In diabetics, where sorbitol levels are higher than nondiabetics, the results may be suspect.[87,90] Oxpurinol production as the result of allopurinol administration can be used to determine purine metabolism and hepatic blood flow. This reaction can occur in other tissues outside of the liver and does not test other enzyme systems.[91] The conversion of lidocaine to its metabolite monoethylglycinexyline (MEGX) is used first before and then after liver transplantation as an indicator of liver blood flow.[92] Caffeine can be given in very low doses to reduce its cardiac and central nervous system effects to measure demethylation and hepatic blood flow. Either blood or saliva concentrations can be used to determine clearance. Caffeine is very good at differentiating patients with mild to moderate disease as rated by Pugh's score (see Chapter 37, Alcoholic Liver Disease), but has trouble differentiating between patients with Pugh's scores much above 10.[93] The administration of various benzodiazepines has also been studied. The appeal here is for patients with alcoholic liver disease. Many of these patients require benzodiazepines for the treatment of the symptoms of delirium tremors while hospitalized for alcoholic hepatitis. A good estimate of hepatic clearance can be obtained by serial blood levels of these drugs if an assay is locally available.[94,95]

Ultrasound pictures and computed tomography (CT) scans can be used on a periodic basis to monitor for the development of fibrosis or vascular lesion in the liver and for hepatocellular carcinomas. Significant loss of total liver volume documented by serial CT scans has been associated with an increased death rate in patients in fulminant liver failure.[96] Recent advances in magnetic resonance imaging are also promising for research studies of the liver. Hepatobiliary scanning using Tc-99*m*-labeled carriers also can be useful in quantifying the location and extent of obstruction or damage.[86] The use of a more sensitive assay such as glutathione-*S*-transferase has also been advocated in particular cases when sensitive early markers of intrinsic damage are needed.[15] In cases of idiosyncratic hypersensitivity reactions, a macrophage inhibition test can be useful in predicting which drug may have caused the reaction in question.[97]

Classifying Hepatotoxicity

As patient records become computerized there will be increasing pressure to classify diseases by commonly accepted terms. The following system for drug-induced liver disease proposed in 1990 by the Council for International Organizations of Medical Science is useful for many clinical situations.[98] First and foremost, the patient must have symptoms associated with liver injury. If the patient is not experiencing jaundice, ascites, abdominal pain, pruritus, nausea, vomiting, or other symptoms then there is no liver injury. Liver disease may be indicated by elevated laboratory values, but there is no liver injury. Liver disease may precede liver injury and it is not to be discounted, but it also must not be overinterpreted. Elevations in laboratory values are important and are considered abnormal, but not an absolute marker of liver injury.

If there is a liver biopsy available, the injury should be classified by the histological findings. If there is no biopsy, then it is best to avoid using the terms "cirrhosis," "hepatic necrosis," or "hepatitis." These terms indicate specific patterns of cell damage, which cannot be directly related to a specific clinical presentation. In cases where there is no biopsy but the patient is symptomatic, the pattern of liver enzyme elevation is sometimes used to estimate the type of injury. Hepatocellular injuries are marked by profound elevations in transaminase—at least two times normal. If the alkaline phosphatase is also elevated, then a hepatocellular lesion is still suspected when elevation of ALT is significantly higher than the elevation of alkaline phosphatase. If the magnitude of elevation is nearly equal between ALT and alkaline phosphatase, then the lesion is likely cholestatic.

A liver injury is acute if the symptoms and enzyme elevations last less than 3 months. It is considered a chronic lesion after 3 months of consistent symptoms or enzyme elevation. A liver injury is severe if the patient has marked jaundice. It is more severe if the prothrombin time does not improve by more than 50% after the administration of vitamin K or if hepatic encephalopathy is detectable. If an acute liver injury progresses from normal to severe in a matter of a few days or weeks it is considered fulminant.[98]

Monitoring for Hepatotoxicity

When selecting which tests to use in monitoring a patient placed on a hepatotoxic drug it is important to distinguish the predictable hepatotoxic reaction from the idiosyncratic reaction. Predictable reactions have a high incidence of occurrence and are usually dose related (Table 38.3). Methotrexate and chlorpromazine are examples of predictable hepatotoxic reactions with somewhat high incidences of occurrence. Methotrexate, a drug that induces acute parenchymal damage and fibrosis, is best monitored by using those measures of acute hepatocellular damage. The serum transaminases, AST and ALT (SGOT and SGPT), are the most commonly used in the clinical setting. Concentrations of these enzymes should be obtained about every 4 weeks depending on the reported characteristics of the reaction in question. Methotrexate should be monitored every 4 weeks, because toxicity usually develops over a period of several weeks to months.[82,83] In addition, some recommend that sulfobromophthalein or indocyanine green excretion studies be performed on a regular basis and that patients treated for very long periods of time should have a liver biopsy performed every 12 months.[83]

Chlorpromazine, which produces cholestatic lesions, is best monitored with a serum bilirubin concentration and regular determinations of the serum enzymes usually found in high concentrations in the canalicular system. As the onset of action reported for this reaction is within the first 4 weeks of therapy, determinations of the bilirubin concentration, alkaline phosphatase, and γ-glutamyltransferase should be obtained every 2 weeks for the first month of therapy then at monthly intervals for the first 6 months of therapy to pick up the few cases that may be delayed.[61,62] This pattern of decreasing incidence with increasing length of therapy is true for most drugs that cause liver disease. The important exceptions to this rule include any drug associated with the development of hepatocellular carcinomas or veno-occlusive disease. Oral contraceptives are associated with a higher risk of hepatocellular carcinoma after 15 to 20 years of use.

If a person is in a higher risk group for the development of a particular reaction, the intervals between serum

TABLE 38.3. GENERAL RECOMMENDATIONS FOR MONITORING OF DRUGS WITH LIVER INJURY RISK

Routine AST, ALT, LDH[a] Determinations Are Useful in the General Population
Cytidine analogues[b]
Interleukins
Folic acid analogues[b]
Anthracendiones
Amiodarone[b]
Sodium valproate
Megadose vitamin A[b]
Retenoic acid and derivatives
Inhaled anesthetics[c]
Routine AST, ALT, LDH Determinations May Be Helpful in High-Risk Populations
Quinolone antibiotics
Nonsteroidal anti-inflammatory agents[b,d]
Estrogen agonist/antagonists[e]
Acetaminophen[f]
Bis-triazole antifungals
Iron salts[f]
Hetastarch[g]
Routine GGTP, Alk Phos,[a] Bilirubin Determinations Are Useful in the General Population
L-asparaginase
Carmustine
Alkylating agents
Purine antimetabolites[h]
Gold sodium thiomalate
Flutamide, gosseralin
Fluosol-DA 20%
Routine GGTP, Alk Phos, Bilirubin Determinations May Be Helpful in High-Risk Populations
Tetracyclines[b]
Griseofulvin
Heavy metal chemotherapeutics
Testosterone and derivatives
Clozapine
Phenothiazines
Thioxanthenes
Butyrophenones
Megadose α-tocopherol

[a]AST, aspartate transaminase; ALT, alanine transaminase; LDH, lactate dehydrogenase; GGTP, γ-glutamyltransferase; Alk Phos, alkaline phosphotase.
[b]Dose-related, risk increases with increasing doses and, in some cases, with length of therapy.
[c]Risk increases with repeated exposures within the class.
[d]Aspirin, one of the NSAIDs, also is associated with Reye's syndrome.
[e]Estrogens, estrogen antagonists, testosterone, and its derivatives are all associated with an increased risk for rare hepatocellular cancers; this risk increases with high doses and long periods of use.
[f]Most commonly seen after accidental or intentional overdose.
[g]In patients with renal insufficiency that causes secondary hepatic accumulation.
[h]Usually associated with high doses (>1.5 g/d) given intravenously.

enzyme determination should be shortened. Isoniazid, for example, carries a greater risk for patients older than 35 years. Young patients less than 14 years old also may need more intensive monitoring.[38] Isoniazid-induced hepatotoxicity is not a predictable reaction and would not be routinely monitored on a monthly basis, except in these populations. Valproate toxicity is also much more common in patients less than 20 years of age.[28] Patients with preexisting liver or kidney disease, in whom even a mild hepatotoxic reaction would have profound negative consequences, also should be more intensely monitored. In patients who are not in high-risk groups or have no preexisting disease, routine monitoring for idiosyncratic reactions is of little value.

REFERENCES

1. National Center for Health Statistics. Advance report of final mortality statistics 1990. U.S. Department of Health and Human Services, Monthly Vital Statistics Report 1993;41(7).
2. Olmos M, Guma C, Colombato LO, et al. Hepatic lesions induced by drugs. Report of 26 cases. Acta Gastroenterol Latinoam 1987;17:105–111.
3. Rapport AM. Anatomic considerations, in Schiff L (ed): Diseases of the Liver. Philadelphia, JB Lippincott, 1975, pp 1–43.
4. Zimmerman HJ. General considerations, in Zimmerman HJ (ed): Hepatotoxicity, the Adverse Effects of Drugs and Other Chemicals on the Liver. New York, Appleton-Century-Croft, 1978, pp 3–164.
5. Rettie AE, Rettenmeier AW, Howald WN, et al. Cytochrome P-450-catalyzed formation of Δ-4-VPA, a toxic metabolite of valproic acid. Science 1987;235:890–893.
6. Recknagel RO, Glende EA, Jr. Carbon tetrachloride hepatoxicity: An example of lethal clevage. CRC Critical Review Toxicol 1973;2:263–297.
7. Forker EL. Mechanisms of hepatic bile formation. Ann Rev Physiol 1977;39:323–347.
8. Kelsey WM, Scharyj M. Fatal hepatitis probably due to indomethacin. JAMA 1967;199:154–155.
9. Mitchell JR, Zimmerman HJ, Ishak KG, et al. NIH conference—Isoniazid liver injury: Clinical spectrum, pathology, and possible pathogenesis. Ann Intern Med 1976;84:181–192.
10. Black M. Acetaminophen hepatotoxicity. Gastroenterology 1980;78:382–392.
11. Comfort MW, Weir JF. Toxic cirrhosis caused by cincophen. Arch Intern Med 1933;52:685–724.
12. Maddrey WC, Boitnott JK. Drug-induced chronic liver disease. Gastroenterology 1977;72:1348–1353.
13. James OFW. Gastrointestinal and liver function in old age. Clin Gastoenterol 1983;12:671–691.
14. James OFW. Drugs and the aging liver. J Hepatol 1985;1:431–435.
15. Beckett GJ, Chapman BJ, Dyson EH, et al. Plasma glutathione-*S*-transferase measurements after paracetamol overdose: Evidence for early hepatocellular damage. Gut 1985;26:26–31.

16. Mitchell JR, Thorgiersson SS, Potter WR, et al. Acetaminophen-induced hepatic injury: Protective role of glutathione in man and rationale for therapy. Clin Pharmacol Ther 1974;16:676–684.
17. Beckett GJ, Foster GR, Hussey AJ, et al. Plasma glutathione-*S*-transferase and F protein are more sensitive than alanine aminotransferase as markers of paracetamol (acetaminophen)-induced liver damage. Clin Chem 1989;35:2186–2189.
18. Seeff LB, Cuccherini BA, Zimmerman HJ, et al. Acetaminophen hepatotoxicity in alcoholics, a therapeutic misadventure. Ann Intern Med 1986;104:399–404.
19. Rosenal D, Halevy A, Orda R. Halothane and liver damage. Postgrad Med J 1989;65:129–135.
20. Timbrell JA. Drug hepatotoxicity. Br J Clin Pharmacol 1983;15:3–14.
21. Maiorino RM, Sipes IG, Gandolf AJ, et al. Quantative analysis of volatile halothane metabolites in biological tissues by gas chromatography. J Chromatogr 1979;164:63–72.
22. DeGroot H, Noll TL. Halothane hepatotoxicity: Relation between metabolic activation, hypoxia, covalent binding, lipid peroxidation, and liver cell damage. Hepatology 1983;3:601–606.
23. Rubin E, Cederbaum AT. Organelle pathology of alcohol-induced hepatic injury, in Fischer MM, Rankin JG (eds): Alcohol and the Liver. New York, Plenum Press, 1977, pp 167–193.
24. Galambos JT. Alcoholic hepatitis, in Schaffner F, Sherlock S, Leevy CM (eds): The Liver and Its Diseases. New York, Intercontinental Medical Book, 1974, pp 225–267.
25. Guigul B, Perrot S, Berry JP, et al. Amiodarone-induced hepatic phospholipidosis: A morphological alteration independent of pseudoalcoholic liver disease. Hepatology 1988;8:1063–1068.
26. Breen KJ, Schenker S, Heimberg M. Fatty liver induced by tetracycline in the rat: Dose–response relationship and effect of sex. Gastroenterology 1975;69:714–723.
27. Itoh S, Yamaba Y, Matuso S, et al. Sodium valproate-induced liver injury. Am J Gastroenterol 1982;77:875–879.
28. Dreifuss FE, Langer DH, Moline KA, et al. Valproic acid hepatic fatalities. II. US experience since 1984. Neurology 1989;39:201–207.
29. Lullman H, Lullman R, Wasserman O. Drug-induced phospholipidosis II. Tissue distribution of the amphiphilic drug chlorphentermine. CRC Crit Drug Rev Toxicol 1975;4:185–218.
30. Pollak PT, Sharma AD, Carruthers SG. Relation of amiodarone hepatic and pulmonary toxicity to serum drug concentrations and superoxide dismutase activity. Am J Cardiol 1990;65:1185–1191.
31. Pourcell S, Ireton J, Valencia-Mayoral P, et al. Amiodarone-associated phospholipidosis of the liver: Light, immunohistochemical and electron microscopic studies. Gastroenterology 1984;86:926–936.
32. Glasgow JFT. Clinical features and prognosis of Reye's syndrome. Arch Dis Child 1984;59:230–235.
33. Neuberger J, Kenna JG, NouriAria K, et al. Antibody-mediated hepatocyte injury in methyldopa-induced hepatotoxicity. Gut 1985;26:1233–1239.
34. Brown BR, Jr. Halothane hepatitis revisited. N Engl J Med 1985;313:1347–1348.
35. Zarday Z, Rosenthal WS, Wolff FW. Severe liver toxicity after methyldopa. NY State J Med 1967;67:1897–1899.
36. Black M, Mitchell JR, Zimmerman HJ. Drug-induced chronic liver disease. Gastroenterology 1977;72:1348–1353.
37. Maddrey WC. Isoniazid-induced liver disease. Semin Liver Dis 1981;1:129–131.
38. Tsagaropoou-Stinga H, Mataki-Emmanouilidon T, Karida-Kavalioti S, et al. Hepatotoxic reactions in children with severe tuberculosis treated with isoniazid-rifampin. Pediatr Infect Dis 1985;4:270–273.
39. Bratton AC, Marshall EK, Jr. A new coupling component for sulfadimidine determination. J Biol Chem 1939;128:537–550.
40. Ylitalo P, Rousteenoja R, LesKinen O, et al. Significance of acetylator phenotype in pharmacokinetics and adverse effects of procainamide. Eur J Clin Pharm 1983;25:791–795.
41. Kergueris MF, Bourin M, Larousse C. Pharmacokinetics of isoniazid: Influence of age. Eur J Clin Pharm 1986;30:335–340.
42. Reidenberg MM, Drayer DE, Levy M, et al. Polymorphic acetylation of procainamide in man. Clin Pharmacol Ther 1975;17:722–730.
43. Miller JJ, Weissman DB. Correlations between transaminase concentrations and serum salicylate concentrations in juvenile rheumatoid arthritis. Arthritis Rheum 1976;19:115–118.
44. Zimmerman HJ. Effects of aspirin and acetaminophen on the liver. Arch Intern Med 1981;141:333–342.
45. Lake-Bakaar G, Scheuer PJ, Sherlock S. Hepatic reactions associated with ketoconazole in the United Kingdom. Br Med J 1987;294:419–422.
46. Zimmerman HJ. Drug-induced chronic active hepatic disease. Med Clin North Am 1979;63:567–582.
47. Reynolds TB, Peters RL, Yamada S. Chronic active and lupoid hepatitis caused by a laxative, oxphenisatin. N Engl J Med 1971;285:813–820.
48. Maddrey WC, Boitwott JK. Drug-induced chronic liver disease. Gastroenterology 1977;72:1348–1353.
49. Nair SS, Kaplan JM, Levine LH, et al. Trimethoprin-sulfamethoxazole-induced intrahepatic cholestasis. Ann Intern Med 1980;92:511–512.
50. Dujovne CA, Chan CH, Zimmerman HJ. Sulfonamide hepatic injury. N Engl J Med 1967;277:785–788.
51. Alberti-Flor JJ, Hernandez ME, Ferrer JP, et al. Fulminant liver failure and pancreatitis associated with the use of sulfamethoxazole-trimethoprim. Am J Gastroenterol 1989;84:1577–1579.
52. Verhamme M, Ramboer C, Van de Bruaene P, et al. Cholestatic hepatitis due to an amoxycillin/clavulinic acid preparation. J Hepatol 1989;9:260–264.
53. Valdiva-Barriga V, Feldman A, Orellana J. Generalized hypersensitivity with hepatitis and jaundice after the use of penicillin and streptomicin. Gastroenterology 1963;45:114–117.
54. Keeffe EB, Reis TC, Berland JE. Hepatotoxicity to both erythromycin estolate and erythromycin ethylsuccinate. Dig Dis Sci 1982;27:701–704.

55. Pessayre D, Larrey D, Funck-Bretano A, et al. Drug interactions and hepatitis produced by some macrolide antibiotics. J Antimicrob Chemother 1985;16:181–192.
56. Vanderstigel M, Zafrani ES, Deyone JL, et al. Allopurinol hypersensitivity syndrome as a cause of hepatic fibrin ring granulomas. Gastroenterology 1986;90:188–190.
57. Al-Kawas FH, Seeff LB, Berendson RA, et al. Allopurinol hepatotoxicity. Report of two cases and review of the literature. Ann Intern Med 1981;95:588–590.
58. Foitl DR, Hyman G, Leflowitch JH. Jaundice and intrahepatic cholestasis following high-dose megestrol acetate for breast cancer. Cancer 1989;63:438–439.
59. Boelsterli UA, Rakhit G, Balazas T. Modulation of *S*-adenosyl-*L*-methionate, hepatic Na+,K+-ATPase, membrane fluidity and bile flow in rats with ethinyl estradiol-induced cholestasis. Hepatology 1983;3:12–17.
60. Lorch V, Murphy D, Hoersten L, et al. Unusual syndrome among premature infants: Associated with a new intravenous vitamin E product. Pediatrics 1985;75:598–601.
61. Ishak KG, Irey NS. Hepatic injury associated with the phenothiazines. Clinicopathological follow-up study of 36 patients. Arch Pathol 1972;93:283–304.
62. Carey MC, Hiram PC, Small DM. A study of physiochemical interactions between biliary lipids and chlorpromazine-HCl. Biochem J 1976;153:519–531.
63. Bowyer BA, Fleming CR, Ludwig J, et al. Does long-term home parenteral nutrition in adult patients cause chronic liver disease? J Parenter Enter Nutr 1985;9:11.
64. Nanji AA, Anderson FH. Relationship between serum albumin and parenteral nutrition-associated cholestasis. J Parenter Enter Nutr 1984;8:438.
65. Klein GL, Berquist WE, Ament ME, et al. Hepatic aluminum accumulation in children on total parenteral nutrition. J Pediatr Gastroenterol Nutr 1984;3:740.
66. Reichel J, Goldberg SB, Ellenberg M, et al. Intrahepatic cholestasis following administration of chlorpropamide. Report of a case with electron microscopic observations. Am J Med 1960;28:654–660.
67. Gilbert FI. Cholestatic hepatitis caused by esters of erythromycin and oleandomycin. JAMA 1962;182:1048–1050.
68. Bachman BA, Boyd WP, Brady PG. Erythromycin ethylsuccinate-induced cholestasis. Am J Gastroenterol 1982;77:397–400.
69. Johnson DF, Hall WH. Allergic hepatitis caused by the propionyl erythromycin ester of lauryl sulfate. N Engl J Med 1961;265:1200–1202.
70. Rahmat J, Gelfand RL, Gelfand MC, et al. Captopril-associated cholestatic jaundice. Ann Intern Med 1985;102:56–58.
71. Reichel J, Goldberg SB, Ellenberg M, et al. Intrahepatic cholestasis following administration of chlorpropamide. Am J Med 1960;28:654–660.
72. Taggart HMA, Alderdice JM. Fatal cholestatic jaundice in elderly patients taking benoxaprofen. Br Med J 1982;284:1372.
73. Larrey D, Fr'eneaux E, Berson A, et al. Peliosis hepatitis induced by 6-thioguanine administration. Gut 1988;29:1265–1269.
74. Kumara CR, Ng M, Lin JH, et al. Herbal tea-induced hepatic veno-oclusive disease: Quantification of toxic alkaloid exposure in adults. Case report. Gut 1985;26:101–104.
75. Bagheri SA, Boyer JL. Peliosis hepatitis associated with androgenic anabolic steroid therapy. Ann Intern Med 1974;81:610–618.
76. Fajard OLF, Colby JV. Pathogenesis of veno-occlusive liver disease. Arch Pathol Lab Med 1980;104:584–588.
77. Schomberg LA. Peliosis hepatitis and oral contraceptives. J Reprod Med 1982;27:753–756.
78. Nescher G, Dollberg L, Ziman A, et al. Hepatosplenic peliosis after danazol and glucocorticoids for ITP. N Engl J Med 1985;312:242.
79. Loomus GN, Aneja P, Bota RA, et al. A case of peliosis hepatitis in association with tamoxifen therapy. Am J Clin Pathol 1983;80:881–883.
80. Haupt HA, Rovere GD. Anabolic steroids: A review of the literature. Am J Sports Med 1984;12:469–479.
81. Bjorkman DJ, Hammond EH, Lee RG, et al. Hepatic ultrastructure after methotrexate therapy for rheumatoid arthritis. Arthritis Rheum 1988;31:1465–1472.
82. Zachariae H, Bjerring P. Methotrexate in psoriasis with and without leukovorin: Effect of different dosage schedules on acute liver toxicity. Acta Derm Venereol (Stockh) 1982;62:446–448.
83. Leonard PA, Clegg DO, Carson CC, et al. Low-dose pulse methotrexate in rheumatoid arthritis: An 8-year experience with hepatotoxicity. Clin Rheumatol 1987;6:575–582.
84. Sarles J, Scheiner C, Sarran M, et al. Hepatic hypervitaminosis A: A familial observation. J Pediatr Gastroenterol Nutr 1990;10:71–76.
85. Zimmerman HJ. Chemical hepatic injury and its detection, in Plaa GG, Hewitt WR (eds): Toxicology of the Liver, Target Organ Series. Philadelphia, Raven Press, 1981, pp 1–46.
86. Choppa S, Griffin PH. Laboratory tests and diagnostic procedures in evaluation of liver disease. Am J Med 1985;79:221–230.
87. Barstow L, Smith RE. Liver function assessment by drug metabolism. Pharmacotherapy 1990;10:280–288.
88. Williams CN, McCauley D, Malatjalian DA, et al. The aminopyrine breath test, an inadequate early indicator of methotrexate-induced liver disease in patients with psoriasis. Clin Invest Med 1987;10:54–58.
89. Caesar J, Shaldon S, Chiandussi L, et al. The use of indocyanine green in the measurement of hepatic blood flow and as a test of hepatic function. Clin Sci 1961;21:43–57.
90. Zeeh J, Lange H, Bosch J, et al. Steady-state extrarenal sorbitol clearance as a measure of hepatic plasma flow. Gastroenterology 1988;95:749–759.
91. VanWaeg G, Groth T, Nikiasson F, et al. Allopurinol kientics in humans as a means to assess liver function: Comparison of different models. Am J Physiol 1987;253:R352–R360.
92. Potter JM, Hickman PE, Lynch SV, et al. Use of monethylglycinexyline as a liver function test in liver transplant recipient. Transplant 1993;56:1385–1388.
93. Scott NR, Stambuk D, Chakraborty J, et al. The pharmacokinetics of caffeine and its dimethylxanthine metabolites in patients with chronic liver disease. Br J Clin Pharmacol 1989;27:205–213.

94. Crom WR, Webster SL, Bobo L, et al. Simultaneous administration of multiple-model substrates to assess hepatic drug clearance. Clin Pharm Ther 1987;41:645–650.
95. Juhl RP, VanThiel DH, Dittert LW. Alprazolam pharmacokinetics in alcoholic liver disease. J Clin Pharmacol 1984;24:113–119.
96. Sekiyama K, Yoshiba M, Inoue K, et al. Prognostic value of hepatic volumetry in fulminant hepatic failure. Dig Dis Sci 1994;39:240–244.
97. Enat R, Pollack S, Ben-Arieh Y, et al. Cholestatic jaundice caused by cloxacillin: Macrophage inhibition factor test in preventing rechallenge with hepatic drugs. Br Med J 1980;280:982–983.
98. Report of an International Consensus Meeting. Standardization of definitions and criteria of causality assessment of adverse drug reactions, drug-induced liver disorders: Report of an international consensus meeting. Int J Clin Pharmacol Ther Toxicol 1990;28:317–322.

Chapter 39

Pancreatitis

Rosemary R. Berardi, PharmD, FASHP, and Lisa M. Henderson, PharmD

Inflammatory disease of the pancreas may be defined as either acute or chronic. These terms do not describe the onset or resolution of symptoms, but rather the reversibility of functional and morphologic changes in the pancreas. Acute pancreatitis (AP) is characterized by a discrete episode of symptoms, with restoration of normal exocrine and endocrine function when the cause is removed. The attack may be mild or severe and may occur as an initial single or recurrent event. The occurrence of local and systemic complications accompany the more severe forms of the disease. Although exocrine and endocrine function may remain impaired for variable periods after the attack, the disease rarely progresses to chronic pancreatitis.[1,2]

Chronic pancreatitis (CP) results in functional and structural damage to the pancreas that persists after the causative factor is eliminated. The disease is often progressive and loss of pancreatic function is irreversible. Improvement may occur in a subset of patients with obstructive CP when obstruction of the main pancreatic duct is relieved. In the acutely ill, symptomatic exacerbations closely resemble attacks of AP and may not be distinguishable. Patients with CP suffer from many of the same complications associated with AP.[3,4]

The prevalence of pancreatitis varies in different geographic areas and depends primarily on etiologic factors. The incidence of AP in the United States is less than 1%, while the number of patients with CP is largely undefined. The overall male-to-female ratio appears to be nearly equal; however, there is an increased incidence of alcoholic pancreatitis in younger men and of gallstone-related disease in older women.[1,2]

Physiology of Exocrine Pancreatic Secretion

The pancreas is a lobulated organ that possesses both endocrine and exocrine functions. Interspersed between the lobules are the islets of Langerhans, which contain the cells of the endocrine pancreas, which secrete insulin, glucagon, somatostatin, and other polypeptide hormones. The exocrine pancreas consists of lobular subunits composed of acini. Each acinus contains pyramidal and centroacinar cells and is drained by a ductule. The acinar ductules join intralobular ducts and eventually form the duct of Wirsong, the main pancreatic duct, which enters the duodenum at the ampulla of Vater, after joining the common bile duct.[1,2] The final common channel, as well as the common bile and pancreatic ducts independently, are encased by the muscular sphincter of Oddi, which controls entry of pancreatic juice and bile into the duodenum. The exocrine pancreas secretes about 1 to 2 L/d of alkaline pancreatic juice, which contains water, electrolytes, and enzymes necessary for digestion.

COMPOSITION OF PANCREATIC JUICE

Water and Electrolytes

The acinar cells of the pancreas secrete an isotonic fluid that contains sodium, potassium, chloride, calcium, and traces of magnesium, zinc, phosphate, and sulfate. The major cations, sodium and potassium, are secreted at a fixed concentration similar to their extracellular concentrations. Bicarbonate is secreted primarily by the centroacinar (ductular) cells and is the principal ion of physiologic importance. The pH of pancreatic juice is about 8.3.[5] Water enters the juice passively along osmotic gradients established by the active secretion of the electrolytes. The alkaline pancreatic juice neutralizes gastric acid in the duodenum and provides an appropriate pH for maintaining the activity of pancreatic enzymes.

Enzymes

Pancreatic juice contains less than 10% protein; more than 90% of the protein consists of enzymes or proenzymes secreted by the pancreatic acinar cells.[5] The four major enzyme groups are identified in Table 39.1. The proteolytic enzymes are secreted as inactive proenzymes, which are activated in the lumen of the duodenum. Enterokinase, an enzyme secreted by the duodenal mucosa, converts trypsinogen to trypsin, which then activates all other pro-teolytic

TABLE 39.1. DIGESTIVE ENZYMES IN THE PANCREATIC ACINAR CELL

Proteolytic Enzymes	**Lipolytic Enzymes**
Trypsinogen	Lipase
Chymotrypsinogen	Prophospholipase A_2
Proelastase	Caroboxylesterase lipase
Procarboxypeptidase A	**Nucleases**
Procarboxypeptidase B	Deoxyribonuclease (DNAse)
Amylolytic Enzymes	Ribonuclease (RNAse)
Amylase	**Others**
	Procolipase
	Trypsin inhibitor

(From Pandol SJ. Pancreatic physiology, in Sleisenger MH, Fordtran JS (eds): Gastrointestinal Disease: Pathophysiology/Diagnosis/Management, 5th ed. Philadelphia, WB Saunders, 1993, p 1587, with permission.)

proenzymes in a cascade fashion. Two important mechanisms protect the pancreas from the potential degradative action of its own digestive enzymes. The synthesis of proteolytic enzymes as proenzymes requires extrapancreatic trigger enzymes for activation. In addition, pancreatic juice contains a low concentration of trypsin inhibitor, which inactivates trypsin and partially inhibits chymotrypsin. Proteolytic activity in the intestinal lumen is not inhibited because the concentration is minimal. The proteolytic enzymes, lipase, amylase, and ribonuclease are secreted in their active form by the acinar cells. Colipase, another constituent of pancreatic secretion, binds to the bile salt–lipid surface and facilitates the action of lipase. It also enhances lipase activity by lowering the optimum pH of lipase from 8.5 to 6.5, the normal luminal pH in the duodenum.[5]

REGULATION OF PANCREATIC SECRETION

The regulation of exocrine pancreatic secretion is complex and depends on stimulatory and inhibitory factors exerted through hormonal and neuronal mechanisms. Two hormones, secretin (SC) and cholecystokinin (CCK), play an important role in mediating pancreatic secretions and have synergistic effects: SC primarily stimulates ductular cells to increase water and bicarbonate; CCK stimulates acinar cells to secrete a juice that is low in volume and bicarbonate, but rich in enzyme content. The release of SC from the intestinal mucosa is pH dependent and occurs when the duodenal pH is approximately 4.5. Below this pH, titratable acid in the duodenum governs pancreatic bicarbonate output. Although the postprandial release of SC is small, nonacid factors such as products of fat digestion and bile can also stimulate SC release. The release of CCK from the small intestine is largely dependent on the presence of fatty acids and amino acids in the duodenum. Vasoactive intestinal polypeptide (VIP) is structurally similar to SC and exhibits weak secretin-like effects on exocrine pancreatic secretion. Other peptides (bombesin and gastrin) have been shown to stimulate pancreatic enzyme secretion, but their role in regulating pancreatic secretion remains unclear. Much less is known about the mechanisms that inhibit pancreatic enzyme secretion. Gastrointestinal (GI) peptides such as somatostatin, enkephalin, glucagon, pancreatic polypeptide (PP), neuropeptide Y, and pancreastatin inhibit pancreatic enzyme secretion, in part, by modulating cholinergic transmission.[5]

Pancreatic exocrine secretion is divided into four phases: basal, cephalic, gastric, and intestinal. In the fasted state, basal pancreatic secretion occurs at a low rate; output fluctuates in cycles with the interdigestive migrating myoelectric complex (IMMC) so that peak secretions occur during phase III of the IMMC.[5] The cephalic phase is stimulated by the sight and smell of food and is thought to be mediated by vagal pathways. Gastric distention and the rate of gastric emptying stimulate an increase in enzyme-rich pancreatic fluid. In the intestinal phase, chyme and acid stimulate pancreatic secretion, largely through the release of SC and CCK. Because the pancreas normally secretes more enzymes than are actually needed for digestion, maldigestion or malabsorption does not usually occur until postprandial secretions fall below 15% of normal. A comprehensive discussion of pancreatic physiology and the role of pancreatic enzymes in digestion can be found elsewhere.[5]

ACUTE PANCREATITIS

AP is an inflammatory disorder of the pancreas resulting from premature activation of proteolytic enzymes within the pancreas. The spectrum of the disease varies from mild, which is usually self-limiting, to severe, in which the severity of the attack correlates with the degree of the pancreatic involvement and complications. The morphologic appearance of the pancreas and surrounding tissue represents a spectrum of severity ranging from the early stages, characterized as *edematous,* to necrosis of surrounding fatty tissue, termed *necrotizing.* The rupture of blood vessels within or around the pancreas may lead to a collection of blood in the retroperitoneal spaces and is referred to as *hemorrhagic* pancreatitis.

ETIOLOGY

The etiologic factors associated with AP are presented in Table 39.2. Ethanol abuse and gallstone-associated biliary tract disease (choledocholithiasis) together account for 60–80% of all cases; however, the frequency varies depending on the patient population and geographic location. Because of the great functional reserve of the pancreas and the insidious loss of pancreatic function, it is possible that many patients who experience attacks of ethanol-related AP have CP. About 10–15% of acute attacks are

TABLE 39.2. ETIOLOGIC FACTORS IN ACUTE PANCREATITIS

Obstruction	**Trauma**
Choledocholithiasis	Accidental abdominal trauma
Pancreatic tumors	Abdominal surgery
Infection	ERCP[a]
Mumps/rubella	**Metabolic Abnormalities**
Hepatitis	Hypertriglyceridemia
Human immunodeficiency virus	Hypercalcemia
Mycoplasma	**Vascular Abnormalities**
Mycobacterium tuberculosis	Vasculitis
Toxins	Ischemia postcardiac surgery
Ethanol	**Miscellaneous**
Scorpion venom	Crohn's disease
Organophosphorous insecticides	Cystic fibrosis
Medications	**Idiopathic Causes**

[a]ERCP, endoscopic retrograde cholangiopancreatography. (Modified from Steinberg WS, Tenner S. Acute pancreatitis. N Engl J Med 1994;330:1198–1210.)

associated with a variety of other causes (Table 39.2). The remaining 10–15% have *idiopathic* pancreatitis, as a cause cannot be determined.[1,2] Pregnancy is not considered a cause of AP because most pregnant women develop AP as a result of coincident processes, most commonly cholelithiasis.

Drug-Induced Pancreatitis

A number of medications have been implicated in AP, but a causal association is difficult to confirm because ethical and practical considerations prevent rechallenge with the suspected agent.[1,2,6,7] Table 39.3 lists drugs according to their certainty to cause AP. A "definite" association is based on the temporal relationship of drug administration to abdominal pain and hyperamylasemia or on a positive response to rechallenge with the offending agent. Suggestive evidence exists for drugs with a "probable" association, while evidence is inadequate or contradictory for drugs having a "questionable" association.

The pathogenesis of drug-induced pancreatitis does not appear to differ from other causes of AP. The method by which medications induce pancreatitis is unknown, but probably involves both direct and indirect mechanisms. Postulated mechanisms include immune-mediated inflammatory response, direct cellular toxicity, pancreatic duct constriction, arteriolar thrombosis and metabolic effects; however, none of these mechanisms has been confirmed.[6,7] Allergic reactions (e.g., urticaria) usually do not accompany drug-induced pancreatic disease. Pancreatitis is an infrequent complication of drug therapy; however, when there appears to be an association between a drug and AP, it is prudent to withdraw the drug. A more in-depth discussion of the specific medications associated with AP can be found elsewhere.[6,7]

TABLE 39.3. DRUGS ASSOCIATED WITH ACUTE PANCREATITIS

Definite Association	
5-Aminosalicylic acid	Metronidazole
Azathioprine	Pentamidine
Didanosine	Sulfonamides
Estrogens	Sulindac
Furosemide	Tetracycline
6-Mercaptopurine	Thiazide diuretics
Methyldopa	Valproic acid
Probable Association	
Ampicillin	Corticosteroids
Asparaginase	Cytarbine
Bumetamide	Ethacrynic acid
Calcium	Phenformin
Cimetidine	Piroxicam
Chlorthalidone	Procainamide
Cisplatin	Salicylates
Clozapine	Zalcitabine
Colaspase	
Questionable Association	
Acetaminophen	Isotretinoin
β-Adrenergic blockers	Ketoprofen
Amiodarone	Lipid emulsions
Amoxapine	Lisinopril
Carbamazepine	Mefenamic acid
Cholestyramine	Metolazone
Clonidine	Nitrofunantoin
Cyclosporine	Octreotide
Cyproheptadine	Opiates
Danazol	Oxyphenbutazone
Diazoxide	Phenolphthalein
Diphenoxylate	Potassium permanganate
Enalapril	Propoxyphene
Ergotamine	Rifampicin
Erythromycin	Ranitidine
Gold therapy	Roxithromycin
Ibuprofen	Sodium stibogluconate
Indomethacin	Ticarcillin/clavulanic acid
Interleukin-2	L-Tryptophan
Isoniazid	Warfarin

(Compiled from Refs. 1, 2, 6, and 7.)

PATHOPHYSIOLOGY

The pathophysiology of AP is related to autodigestion of the pancreas as a result of premature intrapancreatic activation of proteases (Fig. 39.1). Several mechanisms may initiate enzymatic activation within the pancreas, including reflux of duodenal contents containing enterokinase, activated pancreatic enzymes, and bile salts into the pancreatic duct; disruption of the pancreatic ducts and extravasation of juice as a result of gallstone-induced ductal hypertension; and intracellular activation of proteases by lysosomal enzymes such as cathepsin B.[1,2,8] Activation of trypsin digests cell membranes and leads to the activation of other

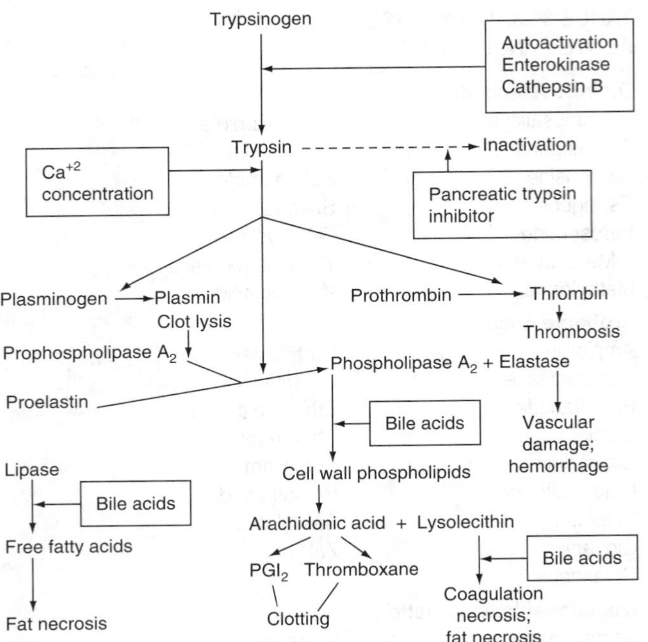

Figure 39.1. Hypothesis for pathophysiology of pancreatic autodigestion. *(From Soergel KH. Acute pancreatitis, in Sleisenger MH, Fordtran JS (eds): Gastrointestinal Disease: Pathophysiology/Diagnosis/Management, 5th ed. Philadelphia, WB Saunders, 1993, p 1631, with permission.)*

pancreatic enzymes within the pancreas. Elastase dissolves vascular wall connective tissue and contributes to hemorrhage. Coagulation is altered by the activation of thrombolytic and thrombotic factors. Lysolecithin formed from phospholipase induces pancreatic necrosis. Bile salts may activate lipase and enhance the cytotoxic effects of phopholipase. The manifestations of these events on the pancreas include inflammation, edema, and ischemia, which combine to produce a local and regional necrosis. When digestive enzymes enter the systemic circulation, widespread necrosis of extra-abdominal organs occurs. Vasoactive substances (histamine, prostaglandins, kinins) are released from the inflamed pancreas into the circulation causing increased vascular permeability, vasodilation, and edema.[1,2,8] Release of these substances also contributes to local and systemic complications.

CLINICAL PRESENTATION

The clinical presentation of AP varies depending on the severity of the inflammatory process and whether damage is confined to the pancreas or involves contiguous organs. Typical signs and symptoms are listed in Table 39.4. The initial presentation ranges from mild abdominal discomfort to excruciating pain, shock, and respiratory distress. Abdominal pain, the major symptom of nearly all patients, is usually epigastric, often radiating to either of the upper quadrants or the back. The onset is usually sudden and the intensity is often described as "knifelike" or "boring." Generally, the pain of AP tends to be steady and usually persists for several days. Partial relief of pain can be obtained by repositioning the patient so that the knees are flexed against the chest. Nausea and vomiting usually follow the onset of pain. Marked epigastric tenderness, abdominal distention, hypotension, and low-grade fever are often observed with widespread pancreatic inflammation and necrosis. In severe disease, bowel sounds are usually diminished or absent; dyspnea and tachypnea are signs of acute respiratory complications.[1]

TABLE 39.4. CLINICAL FINDINGS IN ACUTE PANCREATITIS

Observation	Incidence (%)
Abdominal pain	95
Radiation of pain to back	50
Abdominal distention	75
Nausea and vomiting	80
Low-grade fever	75
Hypotension	30
Mental aberrations	25
Jaundice	20

DIAGNOSIS

The "gold standard" for diagnosis of AP is surgical examination of the pancreas or pancreatic histology. In the absence of these procedures, the diagnosis depends on the recognition of an etiologic factor, the clinical signs and symptoms, abnormal laboratory tests, and imaging techniques that predict the severity and course of the disease.

Laboratory Tests

Acute pancreatitis and its complications may be associated with leukocytosis, hyperglycemia, hypoalbuminemia, and mild hyperbilirubinemia; elevations in serum alkaline phosphatase and liver transaminases are common. Dehydration may lead to hemoconcentration with elevated hemoglobin, hematocrit, blood urea nitrogen (BUN), and serum creatinine concentration. The total serum calcium is usually normal initially, but hypocalcemia out of proportion to the hypoalbuminemia may develop. Marked hypocalcemia is an indication of severe necrosis and a poor prognostic sign. Some patients with severe pancreatitis develop thrombocytopenia and a prolongation in the prothrombin time.

Pancreatic Enzymes

A number of laboratory tests are used to detect pancreatic enzymes in the blood and urine. Many of these tests do not provide sufficiently reliable information to be of clinical value. The serum amylase concentration usually rises within 24 hours of the onset of symptoms and returns to normal over the next 3–5 days. Persistent elevations suggest extensive pancreatic necrosis and/or related complications; however, serum amylase elevations do not correlate with either the etiology or severity of the disease. In addition, many nonpancreatic diseases may be associated with hyperamylasemia, including salivary, renal, hepatobiliary, metabolic, female reproductive tract, and neoplastic diseases.[1,9,10] Pancreatic isoamylase studies assist in determining the origin of elevated serum amylase concentrations, but have not proven useful for the diagnosis of AP because the diseases that simulate pancreatitis cause pancreatic rather than nonpancreatic amylase concentration to rise.

Serum lipase is specific to the pancreas and concentrations are usually elevated in AP. Serum lipase persists longer than serum amylase elevations and can be detected in the serum after the amylase has returned to normal. Urine amylase is increased in AP and may be elevated for 7–10 days after serum values have returned to normal. Urinary amylase concentrations are of little value, because they reflect the hydration and renal status of the patient. The amylase-to-creatinine clearance ratio is not widely used because it is associated with high false-negative and false-positive rates. In many cases, the diagnosis of AP is based on the clinical presentation and an elevated serum amylase or lipase.[9,10]

Imaging Techniques

A number of radiologic imaging techniques reveal pancreatic abnormalities during the disease course. None, however, provides a positive diagnosis of AP. The plain film of the abdomen radiograph often suggests AP. Ultrasonography is indicated in patients with suspected biliary involvement. Contrast-enhanced computed tomography (CECT) is useful in demonstrating the severity of the inflammatory process.

CLINICAL COURSE AND PROGNOSIS

The majority of patients with AP recover uneventfully. Mortality rates appear to be influenced by the etiology of the disease and whether the acute attack is an initial or recurrent episode. Patients with ethanol-related AP appear to have a decreased mortality rate when compared to patients with pancreatitis from other causes.[1,2] Mortality is higher during the first attack of pancreatitis than during recurrent acute attacks. The severity of an acute attack may be predicted using criteria (Table 39.5) obtained upon admission and during the initial 48 hours of hospitalization.[1,2,9,10] Patients with less than three criteria have a mortality rate of less than 1%, while those with six or more criteria have a 100% mortality rate.[2] Early recognition of severe pancreatitis requires aggressive clinical monitoring and therapy. The Acute Physiology and Chronic Health Enquiry (APACHE-II) score, however, is more sensitive and specific than Ranson's criteria and can be calculated on admission.[11] Death during the first few days or weeks often results from systemic complications. When death occurs after this period, it is usually associated with local complications.

COMPLICATIONS

Local complications, including phlegmon (mass of inflamed pancreas containing patchy areas of necrosis), pseudocyst (fluid collections of necrotic debris, blood, and pancreatic enzymes without an epithelial lining), hemorrhage, abscess, and ascites, usually occur within 2–4 weeks

TABLE 39.5. PROGNOSTIC FACTORS IN SEVERE ACUTE PANCREATITIS—RANSON'S CRITERIA

	Nongallstone Pancreatitis	Gallstone Pancreatitis
On Admission		
Age (yr)	>55	>70
White-cell count/mm^3	>16,000	>18,000
Glucose (mg/dL)	>200	>220
Lactic dehydrogenase (IU/L)	>350	>400
Aspartate aminotransferase (U/L)	>250	>250
Within 48 Hours		
Decrease in hematocrit (% points)	>10	>10
Increase in blood urea nitrogen (mg/dL)	>5	>2
Calcium (mg/dL)	<8	<8
Partial pressure of oxygen (mm Hg)	<60	<60
Base deficit (mmol/L)	>4	>5
Fluid deficit (L)	>6	>4

(Modified from Steinberg WS, Tenner S. Acute pancreatitis. N Engl J Med 1994;330:1198–1210.)

after the initial attack.[1] Gastrointestinal bleeding may occur secondary to numerous causes including rupture of a pseudocyst. Mortality after a pseudocyst rupture may be as high as 50%.[1] Pancreatic abscess is usually a secondary infection of necrotic tissue or pseudocysts and appears to correlate with the severity of the pancreatitis. Pancreatic ascites occurs when pancreatic secretions spread throughout the peritoneal cavity.

Systemic complications include pulmonary, cardiovascular, hematologic, renal, metabolic, and central nervous system abnormalities.[1] Of the early complications, shock is the main cause of death. Hypotension results from hypovolemia, hypoalbuminemia, the release of kinins, and sepsis. Renal complications are usually caused by hypovolemia. Pulmonary complications develop in approximately 10–20% of patients. Of the respiratory complications, hypoxia occurs in more than 50% of patients; pleural effusions occur more frequently on the left. The most serious respiratory complication is acute respiratory distress syndrome (ARDS), which usually occurs within a week after the onset of AP. Approximately 50% of patients who have hypoxemia and pulmonary infiltrates die.[1] Additional information on the complications of AP can be found elsewhere.[1,2]

TREATMENT

The overall treatment of AP varies depending on the severity of the attack. Initial treatment should be aimed at relieving pain, minimizing complications, and preventing subsequent episodes. In most patients, the disease is self-limiting and subsides spontaneously within 2–7 days of the initiation of supportive care and the reduction of pancreatic secretions; however, the disease takes a fulminant course in about 10–15% of patients. Because acute mild pancreatitis can progress to the severe form, all patients should be treated aggressively and monitored closely.

General Measures

In the early phase of the attack, most patients are treated by withholding food or liquids in order to minimize exocrine stimulation of the pancreas. The use of nasogastric (NG) aspiration offers no clear advantage in patients with mild AP; however, it is beneficial in patients with profound pain, severe disease, paralytic ileus, and intractable vomiting.[1]

A primary goal of therapy is to replace fluid and electrolyte losses that result from a "chemical burn" induced by the pancreatic exudate. The prognosis of the patient depends, to a great extent, on the rapidity and adequacy of volume restoration. In severe disease, large quantities of fluid are sequestered within the peritoneal and retroperitoneal spaces. Vomiting and NG suction contribute to fluid and electrolyte losses. Intravenous colloids may be required to maintain intravascular volume and blood pressure in severe pancreatitis, because fluid losses are rich in protein. A high priority should be placed on the frequent monitoring of physical findings and vital signs. Patients with severe AP will require intensive treatment of cardiovascular, respiratory, renal, and metabolic complications. Intravenous potassium, calcium, and magnesium should be used to correct deficiency states. Insulin may be needed to treat hyperglycemia. Parenteral nutrition is indicated in patients with severe, protracted pancreatitis who are unable to tolerate enteral feedings. Local complications resolve as the inflammatory process subsides; however, secondary infections require the use of antibiotics and surgical intervention.[1]

Analgesics

Analgesics should be administered to reduce the severity of abdominal pain. The administration of narcotics has been associated with mild and transient increases in serum amylase and lipase; however, because these effects do not appear to be deleterious to the patient, it is not necessary to delay or curtail their use. A traditional approach is to begin therapy with parenteral meperidine (50–100 mg) at regular intervals, because theoretically it causes less spasm of the sphincter of Oddi than other narcotic medications.[1,12] Although increased pancreatic duct pressure may correlate with the severity of pain, the difference in the degree of spasm produced by meperidine and equipotent doses of morphine is of questionable clinical significance. The primary basis for drug selection should be analgesic efficacy. Morphine may be warranted in patients whose pain is severe or unresponsive to meperidine.

Unproven Therapies

Specific medical therapy is aimed at directly or indirectly reducing pancreatic secretions or inhibiting the action of proteolytic enzymes. Although numerous therapeutic approaches have been proposed, their ability to interrupt the process of autodigestion that is central to AP has not been proven by well-designed and controlled studies (Table 39.6).

In patients with mild to moderate AP, the inhibition of gastric acid secretion by antisecretory drugs does not appear to be more effective than NG suction or withholding food when these modalities are used to diminish the pain associated with pancreatic exocrine secretion.[1,16] Alternatively, an H_2-receptor antagonist (H_2RA) is often used to prevent stress-bleeding in the critically ill patient. Conflicting data exist regarding the efficacy of prophylactic antibiotics, corticosteroids, glucagon somatostatin, calcitonin, and pancreatic enzymes.[1,13–16] Studies have failed to confirm the value of fresh frozen plasma, parenteral nutrition, aprotinin, snake antivenom, ε-aminocaproic acid, propylthiouracil, xylocaine, and acetazolamide.[1,13,16] The administration of vasopressin, low molecular weight dextran, and other vasoactive drugs may decrease the severity of experimental AP, but their efficacy in patients is uncertain.[1,13,16]

TABLE 39.6. UNPROVEN THERAPIES FOR ACUTE PANCREATITIS

Drugs	
Acetazolamide	Glucagon
ε-Aminocaproic acid	H_2 blockers
Antacids	Heparin
Antibiotics	Indomethacin
Anticholinergics	Octreotide
Aprotinin	Pancreatic enzymes
Calcitonin	Propylthiouracil
Calcium/sodium EDTA[a]	Prostaglandins
Corticosteroids	Snake antivenom
Chlorophyll	Xylocaine
Dextran	Vasopressin
Gabexate meslilate	
Procedures	
Hypothermia	Peritoneal lavage
Nasogastric suction	Thoracic duct drainage
Pancreatic irradiation	
Other	
Fresh frozen plasma	Parenteral nutrition

[a]Ethylenediamine-tetraacetic acid. (Compiled from Refs. 1, 2, 11, and 13–15.)

Antibiotics

The use of prophylactic antibiotics does not offer any therapeutic advantage in patients with mild to moderate ethanol-induced AP.[1,16] Controlled trials also fail to demonstrate the benefit of early antibiotic therapy in severe disease; however, the empiric use of appropriate antibiotics may be warranted in patients with biliary or pancreatic duct obstruction, and in those with pancreatic abscess or severe necrotizing pancreatitis. The selection of an empiric antibiotic regimen should be based on the premise that enteric aerobic gram-negative bacilli and anaerobic microorganisms are often the cause of pancreatic infections. Adjustments in the antibiotic regimen should be made once the results of culture and sensitivity tests are known.

Somatostatin and Octreotide

Somatostatin and its analogue octreotide inhibit pancreatic enzyme secretion and may have a cytoprotective effect on pancreatic acinus cells. Experimental animal models, however, indicate that basal and stimulated pancreatic secretion is reduced in AP.[15] It appears that after an acute attack, the secreting capacity of the pancreas becomes temporarily impaired. In patients with transplant pancreatitis, exocrine function has been shown to be dependent on the severity of the pancreatitis. To date, there is no conclusive support for or against the use of these agents in the treatment of AP. The results of large randomized controlled trials currently under way will provide information that should clarify the use of these agents in the treatment of AP.

Biliary Tract Disease

There is considerable controversy as to the role of surgery or endoscopy in the early phase of gallstone-induced AP.[1,11] Once a patient with choledocholithiasis recovers from an episode of AP, removal of the underlying biliary tract stone should reduce the risk of recurrent pancreatitis.

Peritoneal Lavage

Lavage of the peritoneal cavity is associated with numerous risks and is of questionable value.[1,13] Although removal of toxic pancreatic exudate may assist in the treatment of early cardiovascular and respiratory complications, it does not appear to prevent necrosis or late abscess formation.

Recommendations

A first priority of treatment is to discontinue medications listed in Table 39.3, whenever possible. Administer intravenous fluids to maintain intravascular volume and analgesics to control pain. Measures to reduce pancreatic secretions should be initiated. Nasogastric aspiration is indicated if pain is severe and if ileus or intractable vomiting are present. Patients with a prolonged course of severe AP should be treated with NG suction and parenteral nutrition. Antisecretory agents do not appear to be of benefit, but may be used to prevent stress-bleeding. Antibiotics should not be used in the absence of signs of infection except in patients with choledocholithiasis or when pancreatic necrosis or abscess is likely. Octreotide or glucagon may be tried, but their efficacy remains unproven. Patients with life-threatening complications require additional intensive medical therapy or surgery.

CHRONIC PANCREATITIS

Chronic pancreatitis results in functional and structural damage to the pancreas that persists after the causative factor is eliminated. In contrast to ethanol-induced CP, structural and functional changes may improve in obstructive CP when the obstruction is removed. In most individuals, CP is progressive and loss of pancreatic function is irreversible. Permanent destruction of pancreatic tissue usually leads to exocrine and endocrine insufficiency. Cystic fibrosis, a cause of pancreatic exocrine insufficiency in children, is discussed in Chapter 29.

ETIOLOGY AND PATHOGENESIS

Prolonged ethanol consumption is the main cause of CP in the United States, accounting for approximately 70% of all cases, while half of the remaining 30% of nonethanol cases are idiopathic.[3] Infrequent causes of CP include hyperparathyroidism (and other chronic hypercalcemic states), protein-calorie malnutrition, heredity, trauma, pancreatic divisum, and obstruction of the main pancreatic duct by tumors, scars, stenosis, and pseudocysts. Although cholelithiasis may coexist with CP, gallstones rarely lead to chronic disease.

The pathophysiology of ethanol-induced CP is related to ethanol-induced changes in the composition of pancreatic secretion, which leads to the precipitation of protein within the pancreatic ducts.[3,8] The precipitates form "protein plugs," which occlude the secondary pancreatic ducts causing duct dilation, inflammation, acinar cell atrophy, fibrosis, scarring, and eventual calcification. It is also possible that chronic ethanol ingestion initiates conditions conducive to autodigestion. The end result is varying degrees of pancreatic destruction and insufficiency.

CLINICAL PRESENTATION

The main features of CP are abdominal pain, malabsorption, weight loss, and diabetes. Prolonged jaundice occurs in about 10% of patients and is usually due to extrahepatic biliary tract obstruction secondary to fibrosis of the head of the pancreas and stenosis of the common bile duct. Complications such as pancreatic pseudocysts, pleural effusions, or ascites may be detected on physical examination.

Pain

Abdominal pain is the most prominent clinical feature of CP and is classically described by many patients as dull, constant, epigastric, and radiating to the back. Characteristically, the pain is deep-seated, positional, and unresponsive to medication. The intensity of the pain varies from mild to severe and does not usually correlate directly with the inflammatory process or other physical findings. Severe attacks usually last from several days to several weeks and may be aggravated by eating. Up to 50% of alcoholic patients have chronic pain, while the remainder have intermittent attacks or a painless pancreatitis. Nausea, vomiting, and weight loss may accompany the episodes of pain. Although the pathogenesis of the pain is unclear, its cause is multifactorial and related to increased intraductal pressure secondary to continued pancreatic secretion and possibly to pancreatic ischemia.[3,17] Abstinence from ethanol may provide relief from pain, but does not prevent continuous exocrine dysfunction. The course of pain is unpredictable, but frequently lessens as pancreatic insufficiency progresses.

Malabsorption

Permanent destruction of the pancreas and obstruction of the pancreatic ducts leads to a decrease in the amount of pancreatic enzymes that reach the proximal duodenum. Although the secretion of digestive enzymes decreases early in the course of the disease, protein and fat are not malabsorbed until at least 90% of the secretory capacity of the pancreas is lost.[3,4] Steatorrhea (excessive loss of fat in the feces) and azotorrhea (excessive loss of protein in the feces) are seen in the majority of patients once significant pancreatic destruction occurs. Because lipase secretion decreases more rapidly than secretion of proteolytic enzymes, steatorrhea is an earlier and more severe problem than azotorrhea.[3] Diarrhea may occur secondary to fat malabsorption. Severe CP may also affect gastric emptying, intraluminal duodenal pH, and bile acids. Abnormally low duodenal pH values reported postprandially in severe pancreatic insufficiency may affect the efficacy of exogenous pancreatic enzymes.[3,4] At least 50% of patients with advanced pancreatic insufficiency present with vitamin B_{12} malabsorption.

Weight Loss

Nausea, vomiting, anorexia, and weight loss are often seen in CP patients. Weight loss occurs primarily from avoidance of food due to fear of a painful response to eating. Malabsorption and uncontrolled diabetes may contribute to a reduction in weight.

Pancreatic Diabetes

Pancreatic diabetes is usually a late manifestation commonly associated with pancreatic calcification. Neuropathy is common and may result from the additive effects of alcohol abuse and malnutrition. Ketoacidosis, vascular complications, and nephropathy are uncommon with this form of diabetes.

DIAGNOSIS

Numerous tests have been introduced into clinical practice; however, the classic triad of calcification, steatorrhea, and diabetes usually confirms the diagnosis of CP. Total serum amylase and the amylase-to-creatinine clearance ratio are not useful in diagnosing and monitoring the course of CP. The quantitative fecal fat test is of value in assessing the efficacy of pancreatic enzyme treatment.

Direct tests of pancreatic exocrine function involve the collection of pancreatic juice after stimulation with exogenous hormones such as secretin or cholecystokinin and serve as the best indicators for detecting CP. Because these tests are complicated and require intubation and special collection techniques, they are performed infrequently. Indirect tests of pancreatic secretory capacity (bentiromide test, dual-label Schilling test) are not as difficult to perform, but are less sensitive (especially in patients with mild disease) and produce a significant number of false-positives.[3] Imaging techniques are helpful in detecting calcification of the pancreas, other causes of pain (ductal obstruction secondary to stones, strictures, or pancreatic pseudocysts), and in differentiating CP from pancreatic cancer. ERCP may assist in the diagnosis and permits the identification of surgically correctable lesions.

CLINICAL COURSE/COMPLICATIONS

Patients with alcoholic CP usually present with an initial acute attack followed by successive attacks that are slower to resolve. Continued ethanol use leads to chronic abdominal pain and progressive exocrine and endocrine insufficiency. In 50% of the patients, the pain diminishes in about 5–10 years after the onset of symptoms.[3] Steatorrhea, calcification, and diabetes usually develop after 10–20 years of heavy ethanol ingestion.

Most patients with CP are affected by varying degrees of pain, malnutrition, and glucose intolerance. Complications frequently occur as a consequence of ethanol and narcotic abuse. A minority of patients will develop pancreatic pseudocyst, ascites, or abscess; common bile duct obstruction leading to cholangitis or secondary biliary cirrhosis; or GI bleeding resulting from multiple sources, including gastritis, peptic ulcer, and splenic/portal vein thrombosis. Most deaths are due to hepatic, cardiovascular, or malignant disease and rarely are directly related to pancreatitis or its complications.[3]

TREATMENT

The treatment of uncomplicated CP is directed at the control of chronic pain and the correction of malabsorption.[3,4,16–23]

Chronic Pain

Nonsurgical treatment modalities have been advocated for abdominal pain relief, but none is completely effective. In some patients, pain may be associated with pseudocysts, peptic ulcer, cholelithiasis, biliary or duodenal obstruction, or pancreatic cancer and, if detected, may be amenable to other forms of treatment. If all nonsurgical measures fail and severe pain continues, surgery is indicated.

Diet

In patients with ethanol-induced CP, abstinence is the most important factor in the prevention of chronic pain in the early stages of the disease. Small and frequent meals (six meals per day) and a diet restricted in fat (50–75 g/d) is recommended to minimize postprandial pancreatic secretion and resulting pain.

Analgesics

Nonnarcotic analgesics such as aspirin or acetaminophen should be tried initially, preferably before meals to prevent postprandial exacerbation of pain.[3,16–18] Treatment should be individualized and should begin with the lowest effective dose. The dosage regimen should be maximized before switching to narcotic alternatives. Analgesics should be prescribed around-the-clock because they may be more effective and the total amount of medication required over 24 hours may be less. Frequently, severe pain relief necessitates the use of opiate analgesics. Narcotics should not be withheld because of the risk of inducing addiction. Oral agents (e.g., codeine derivatives) should be added to the nonnarcotic drug regimen before parenteral narcotics are administered. Exogenous pancreatic enzymes may be attempted prior to narcotics.

Enzyme Therapy

The administration of large doses of pancreatic enzymes early in the course of the disease may afford pain relief by suppressing pancreatic enzyme secretion through a negative feedback mechanism involving proteases present in the duodenum.[3,17–21] Beneficial effects seem to occur primarily in patients with mild to moderate disease (without steatorrhea) and treatment appears to be especially useful in patients with a nonethanol etiology. Possible reasons for the symptomatic failure of enzyme therapy include insufficient concentrations of trypsin content within the pancreatic enzyme preparation and a delayed release of trypsin from pH-dependent dosage forms.[19,20] If enzymes are ineffective in reducing pain after 1–2 months, the addition of an H_2RA may enhance their efficacy.

Nonsurgical Modalities

If systemic drug therapy is unsuccessful, a percutaneous corticosteroid injection into the celiac ganglion (celiac plexus block) may be attempted. Unfortunately, pain relief obtained by this procedure may last for only 3–6 months and repeated treatments are usually not as effective. A number of new endoscopic procedures (sphincterotomy, pancreatic duct stenting, and lithotriptic destruction of pancreatic calculi) are available, but are of questionable benefit to the patient.[3,11] As a last resort, the epidural administration of opiates via an epidural catheter may provide pain control.

Malabsorption

The clinical manifestation of exocrine pancreatic insufficiency related to CP is malabsorption. Steatorrhea (greater than 7 g of fat in the feces per 24 hours while on a 100 g/day of fat diet), due to maldigestion of fats, does not occur until the pancreatic secretory capacity is less than 10% of normal.[3,4] Malabsorption requires treatment when steatorrhea is documented and persistent weight loss occurs in spite of efforts to correct it. Because steatorrhea is often the first sign of malabsorption, treatment efficacy is commonly expressed as a reduction in the degree of steatorrhea. The standard therapy for malabsorption resulting from exocrine pancreatic insufficiency is the use of pancreatic enzyme supplements that contain lipase.[3,4,16,23] The combination of enzyme supplementation and a reduction in dietary fat (to less than 25 g per meal) enhances the patient's nutritional status, reduces (but does not totally correct) steatorrhea, and may alleviate other symptoms.

Principles of Enzyme Replacement

The success of pancreatic enzyme supplementation requires the understanding of important physiologic factors. First, lipase is rapidly and irreversibly inactivated at a pH <4, whereas trypsin is more resistant to acid.[3,4,22,23] Second, a critical amount of enzymes must be delivered to the duodenum in sufficient concentrations in order for digestion to occur. The maximal delivery of pancreatic lipase following a meal is approximately 140,000 IU/h for 4 hours.[3,4,16,23] Malabsorption is minimized if the concentration of enzymes delivered to the duodenum is at least 5% of normal maximal enzyme output. This requires that approximately 30,000 IU of lipase and 10,000 IU of trypsin be delivered during a 4-hour postprandial period.[3,4,16,23] Third, gastric and duodenal pH may vary depending on age, etiology of the disease, and disease severity.[3,4,23] These factors help to explain why steatorrhea is not as readily corrected as azotorrhea and why there is such a variable response to pancreatic enzyme therapy.

Pancreatic Enzyme Supplements

Oral pancreatic enzyme supplements are available as powders, uncoated or coated tablets, capsules, enteric-coated spheres (ECS) and microspheres (ECMS), or enteric-coated microtablets (ECMT) encased in a cellulose capsule (Table 39.7). Most of the available preparations in the United States contain pancrealipase, which has about 12 times the lipolytic activity, 4 times the amylolytic activity, and 4 times the proteolytic activity of pancreatin. These products differ in enzyme content and activity, bioavailability, clinical efficacy, patient acceptance, and cost. Of importance is the relatively low potency and variable nature of lipase, usually requiring that several tablets or capsules be taken per meal. If a commercially available product contains 8000 IU/tablet of lipase, at least four tablets must be taken per meal.

Controversy exists over the optimal dosage schedule, although the consensus is that tablets/capsules should be taken with meals.[3,4] Dividing the total mealtime dose and administering a portion of the dose before, with, and after meals, or hourly, may further decrease steatorrhea in certain patients. The frequency of the dosage regimen, however, must be weighed against the ability of the patient to comply with this schedule. Because of the number of tablets/capsules required per dose, the need to take them with each meal or snack, and the cost of pan-

TABLE 39.7. ENZYME CONTENT OF SELECTED PANCREATIC ENZYME PREPARATIONS

Product	Dosage Form[b]	Enzyme Content (Units)[a]		
		Lipase	Amylase	Protease
Cotazym	C	8000	30,000	30,000
Cotazym-S	ECS	5000	20,000	20,000
Creon-5	ECMS	5000	16,600	18,750
Creon-10	ECMS	10,000	33,200	37,500
Creon-20	ECMS	20,000	66,400	75,000
Ku-Zyme HP	C	8000	30,000	30,000
Pancrease	ECMS	4000	20,000	25,000
Pancrease MT-4	ECMT	4000	12,000	12,000
Pancrease MT-10	ECMT	10,000	30,000	30,000
Pancrease MT-16	ECMT	16,000	48,000	48,000
Pancrease MT-20	ECMT	20,000	56,000	44,000
Ultrase MT-6	ECMT	6000	19,500	19,500
Ultrase MT-12	ECMT	12,000	39,000	39,000
Ultrase MT-18	ECMT	18,000	58,500	58,500
Ultrase MT-20	ECMT	20,000	65,000	65,000
Viokase	UCT	8000	30,000	30,000
Viokase[c]	P	16,800	70,000	70,000
Zymase	ECS	12,000	24,000	24,000

[a]All listed products contain pancrealipase. Pancrealipase contains not less than 24 USP units of lipase activity, not less than 100 USP units of amylase activity, and not less than 100 USP units of protease activity per mg.

[b]C, powder encased in a cellulose capsule; ECS, enteric-coated sphere encased in a cellulose capsule; ECMS, enteric-coated microspheres encased in a cellulose capsule; ECMT, enteric-coated microtablets encased in a cellulose capsule; UCT, uncoated tablet; P, powder.

[c]Units of 0.7 g of powder.

creatic enzyme therapy, compliance (especially among alcoholics) is often poor. Consideration should be given to selecting a product that contains higher lipase activity (Table 39.7).

Gastric inactivation of pancreatic enzymes and the inability to correct steatorrhea has led to the development of dosage formulations that consist of a cellulose capsule that contains pancreatic enzyme granules within an acid-resistant ECS, ECMS, or ECMT.[4,16,22,23] The polymer used to coat each granule is pH dependent and dissolves in the duodenum (pH >5) where the enzymes are released.[4,16,22] An intragastric pH >5 may liberate the enzymes in the stomach and later inactivate them when the intragastric pH is <4. If a low (<4) gastric pH prevails, the enteric-coating should remain intact and the enzymes will be released in the upper portion of the small intestine. A low (<5) duodenal pH may prolong dissolution of the enteric-coating and release of the enzymes. Microencapsulated enteric-coated products do not appear to be superior to standard doses of conventional nonenteric-coated pancreatic enzyme preparations such as Viokase.[4,16] Perhaps this is related to the fact that a lesser quantity of lipase is often administered when an ECS, ECMS, or ECMT is prescribed. The quantity of active lipase delivered to the duodenum appears to be a more important determinant in pancreatic replacement therapy than the actual dosage form.[4,16,23] Factors other than the intragastric destruction of lipase may play a role in the failure of enzymes to normalize fat absorption in pancreatic insufficiency. Large enteric-coated tablets do not empty with partially digested stomach contents and usually are ineffective in treating pancreatic enzyme insufficiency.

Adjuncts to Enzyme Therapy

The use of antacids or H_2RAs as an adjunct to pancreatic enzyme supplementation does not unequivocally improve their efficacy.[3,4,16,23] Theoretically, the use of these agents in conjunction with oral pancreatic enzymes should maintain luminal gastric and duodenal pH >4 and enhance lipase activity. Increased duodenal pH also prevents bile acid precipitation and thus increases fatty acid solubility. In most studies, antacids appear to have little or no added effect on reducing steatorrhea. Sodium bicarbonate and aluminum hydroxide may be more effective than calcium- and magnesium-containing antacids and do not cause diarrhea.[3,4,16] The beneficial effects of an H_2RA result from both an increase in pH and a decrease in intragastric volume. Divergent results reported with the use of H_2RAs in pancreatic steatorrhea may result from differences in the acid secretory status of subjects.[4,16,23] Symptomatic patients whose steatorrhea is not corrected by enzyme replacement therapy and who have a low duodenal pH, may benefit from the addition of an H_2RA. The additional cost of therapy and the potential for adverse effects should be considered. Adjunct therapy with omeprazole has been reported to reduce fecal fat in cystic fibrosis patients with steatorrhea.[24]

Adverse Effects

Pancreatic enzymes contain nucleic acids and, when given in high therapeutic doses, have been associated with hyperuricosuria, hyperuricemia, and kidney stones.[3,16] Impaired folic acid absorption by oral pancreatic enzymes may lead to folic acid deficiency.[3,16] Serum uric acid and folic acid concentrations should be monitored periodically in patients prone to hyperuricemia or folic acid deficiency. GI side effects appear to be dose-related, but occur less frequently with the enteric-coated products. Reports of colonic strictures in cystic fibrosis patients taking high-dose pancreatic enzymes (>20,000 units lipase/capsule) has lead to their withdrawal from the market.[25,26] Sensitization and allergic reactions are uncommon but may occur in patients taking the powder.

Recommendations

Abdominal pain is the most prominent and challenging clinical feature in alcoholic CP and may cease with abstinence. Pain management should begin with simple analgesics such as aspirin or acetaminophen. If pain persists, the response to exogenous pancreatic enzymes should be evaluated in patients with mild to moderate nonalcoholic pancreatitis. If these measures fail, the addition of an oral narcotic should be considered. Parenteral narcotics should be reserved for those patients with severe pain unresponsive to oral analgesics. In each case, the lowest effective analgesic dose should be used and administered around-the-clock. In some patients, a celiac ganglion nerve block may be recommended for pain management. When all medical measures fail, surgery is indicated (Fig. 39.2).

Most patients placed on a reduced fat diet and an adequate dose of conventional pancreatic enzyme supplements usually achieve a satisfactory nutritional status and become relatively asymptomatic. An initial prandial dose of 30,000 IU of lipase should be given with each meal; however, the lipase dose should be titrated to a reduction in steatorrhea. A further reduction in dietary fat may be necessary in some patients. In those patients who do not respond adequately, the use of microencapsulated enteric-coated dosage forms may be indicated. These products offer greater patient acceptance because fewer capsules are needed to produce an adequate response and they are associated with fewer GI side effects. When cost is based on the number of tablets/capsules per day, the high potency ECS, ECMS, or ECMT preparations are usually similar in price to the conventional dosage forms. Addition of an H_2RA should be reserved for those occasional patients resistant to enzyme therapy (Fig. 39.3). If all of these measures are ineffective, documentation of the diagnosis and exclusion of other diseases must be undertaken.

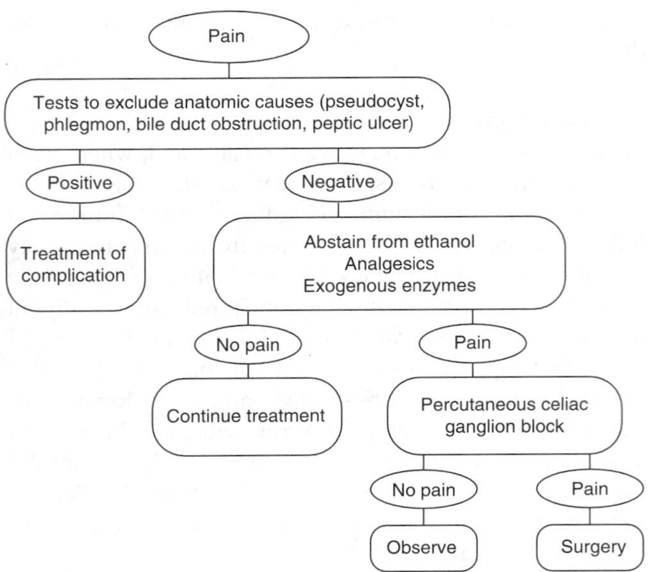

Figure 39.2. Algorithm for treatment of pain. *(Modified from DiMagno EP, Layer P, Clain JE. Chronic pancreatitis, in Go VLW, Gardner JD, Brooks FP, et al (eds): The Pancreas: Biology, Pathobiology, and Diseases, 2nd ed. New York, Raven Press, 1993, p 676, with permission.)*

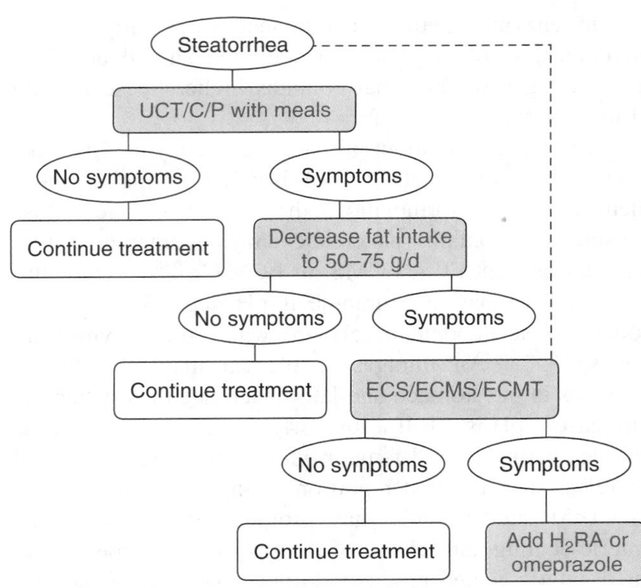

Figure 39.3. Algorithm for treatment of malabsorption. UCT, uncoated tablet; C, capsule; P, powder; ECS, enteric-coated sphere; ECMS, enteric-coated microsphere; ECMT, enteric-coated microtablet; H_2RA, H_2-receptor antagonist *(Modified from DiMagno EP, Layer P, Clain JE. Chronic pancreatitis, in Go VLW, Gardner JD, Brooks FP, et al (eds): The Pancreas: Biology, Pathobiology, and Diseases, 2nd ed. New York, Raven Press, 1993, p 684, with permission.)*

Nutritional Support in Pancreatic Disease

Nutritional deficits develop rapidly in patients with AP complicated by tissue necrosis, organ failure, and surgery. In addition, a number of factors including ileus may preclude oral feeding for prolonged periods of time. Nutritional support should be implemented in patients with AP before protein and calorie depletion becomes advanced. Although parenteral nutrition as a primary therapeutic modality does not alter the course of AP, it should be regarded as a useful adjunct in restoring and maintaining nutritional status.[27] Parenteral or enteral nutrition (elemental diets) may be necessary in patients with CP, especially if the patient is chronically debilitated. The intravenous administration of amino acids and lipids does not significantly stimulate pancreatic secretion. When weight loss is refractory to diet and exogenous enzymes, supplementation with medium-chain triglycerides (MCTs) should be considered.

Surgical Treatment of Pancreatitis

Surgery may be necessary in AP to treat pseudocyst or abscess or to drain the pancreatic bed if hemorrhagic or necrotic pancreatitis is present. Surgical correction of biliary tract disease may reduce the risk of recurrent episodes of AP. The most common indication for surgery in CP is abdominal pain refractory to medical therapy. Although the pain may "burn out" as the gland deteriorates, it is unreasonable that a patient wait years for spontaneous relief. Surgical procedures that alleviate pain include a subtotal or total pancreatectomy, drainage of the pancreatic duct, or interruption of the splanchnic nerves.

Conclusion

Despite modern medical knowledge, much of what we know about the pathophysiologic mechanisms, diagnosis, and treatment of AP and CP remains incomplete. In the future, answers to the many questions surrounding the mysteries of these diseases will become known. Until then, our role as pharmacists is largely supportive, but should include the provision of information to patients and the public regarding the complications and consequences of ethanol-related diseases such as pancreatitis.

References

1. Soergel KH. Acute pancreatitis, in Sleisenger MH, Fordtran JS (eds): Gastrointestinal Disease: Pathophysiology, Diagnosis, Management, 5th ed. Philadelphia, WB Saunders, 1993, p 1628.
2. Steinberg W, Tenner S. Acute pancreatitis. N Engl J Med 1994;330:1198–1210.
3. Grendell JH, Cello JP. Chronic pancreatitis, in Sleisenger MH, Fordtran JS (eds): Gastrointestinal Disease: Pathophysiology, Diagnosis, Management, 5th ed. Philadelphia, WB Saunders, 1993, p 1654.

4. DiMagno EP, Layer P, Clain JE. Chronic pancreatitis, in Go VLW, Gardner JD, Brooks FP, et al. (eds): The Pancreas: Biology, Pathobiology, and Diseases, 2nd ed. New York, Raven Press, 1993, p 665.
5. Pandol SJ. Pancreatic physiology, in Sleisenger MH, Fordtran JS (eds): Gastrointestinal Disease: Pathophysiology, Diagnosis, Management, 5th ed. Philadelphia, WB Saunders, 1993, p 1585.
6. Underwood TW, Frye CB. Drug-induced pancreatitis. Clin Pharm 1993;12:440–448.
7. Frick TW, Speiser DE, Bimmier D, Largiader F. Drug-induced acute pancreatitis: Further criticism. Dig Dis 1993;11:113–132.
8. Kloppel G, Maillet B. Pathology of acute and chronic pancreatitis. Pancreas 1993;8:659–670.
9. Ventrucci M. Update on laboratory diagnosis and prognosis of acute pancreatitis. Dig Dis 1993;11:189–196.
10. Calleja GA, Barkin JS. Acute pancreatitis. Med Clin North Am 1993;77:1037–1056.
11. Irani SK. Endoscopic management of pancreatic disorders. Gastroenterol Clin North Am 1990;19:975–997.
12. Steinberg WM. Sphincter of Oddi dysfunction: A clinical controversy. Gastroenterology 1988;95:1409–1515.
13. Marshall SB. Acute pancreatitis: Review with an emphasis on new developments. Arch Intern Med 1993;153:1185–1198.
14. McMahon MJ. Acute pancreatitis: When is enzyme treatment indicated? Digestion 1993;54(suppl 2):40–42.
15. Buchler MW, Binder M, Friess H, Malfertheimer P. Potential role of somatostatin and octreotide in the management of acute pancreatitis. Digestion 1994;44(suppl 1):16–19.
16. Tenner S, Levine RS, Steinberg WM. Drug treatment of acute and chronic pancreatitis, in Lewis JH (ed): A Pharmacologic Approach to Gastrointestinal Disorders. Baltimore, Williams & Wilkins, 1994, p 311.
17. Ihse I, Anderson R, Axelson J. Pancreatic pain: Is there a medical alternative to surgery? Digestion 1993; 54(suppl 2):30–34.
18. Malfertheiner P, Dominguez-Munoz JE, Buchler MW. Chronic pancreatitis: Management of pain. Digestion 1994;55(suppl 1):29–34.
19. Mossner J. Is there a place for pancreatic enzymes in the treatment of pain in chronic pancreatitis? Digestion 1993;54(suppl 2):35–39.
20. Mossner J, Secknus R, Meyer J, et al. Treatment of pain with pancreatic extracts in chronic pancreatitis: Results of a prospective placebo-controlled multicenter trial. Digestion 1992;53:54–66.
21. Malfertheiner P, Dominguez-Munoz JE. Effect of exogenous pancreatic enzymes on gastrointestinal and pancreatic hormone release and gastrointestinal motility. Digestion 1993;54(suppl 2):15–20.
22. Layer P, Groger G. Fate of pancreatic enzymes in the human intestinal lumen in health and pancreatic insufficiency. Digestion 1993;54(suppl 2):10–14.
23. Lankisch PG. Enzyme treatment of exocrine pancreatic insufficiency in chronic pancreatitis. Digestion 1993; 54(suppl 2):21–29.
24. Heijerman HG, Lamers CB, Bakker W. Omeprazole enhances the efficacy of pancreatin (Pancrease) in cystic fibrosis. Ann Intern Med 1991;114:200–201.
25. FDC Report. High-dose pancreatic enzymes may require clinical trials to return to market following removal due to safety concerns: Cystic fibrosis patient registry suggested. The Pink Sheet. 1994(Feb 21):13–14.
26. Smyth RL, van Velzen D, Smyth AR, et al. Strictures of ascending colon in cystic fibrosis and high-strength pancreatic enzymes. Lancet 1994;343:85–86.
27. Pisters PWT, Ranson JH. Nutritional support for acute pancreatitis. Surg Gynecol Obstet 1992;175:275–284.

Chapter 40

Viral Hepatitis

Marsha A. Raebel, PharmD, FCCP, BCPS

Viral hepatitis is a major cause of morbidity and mortality in the United States.[1] Several distinct viruses are responsible for the 56,000 cases of hepatitis reported yearly.[2] Reporting is incomplete, however, and the actual number of patients infected is closer to 600,000.[3] Hepatitis A causes an estimated 300,000 infections, while hepatitis B is responsible for 120,000 to 200,000 cases.[1] Six to 10% of all patients infected with hepatitis B develop chronic hepatitis, while chronic disease develops in more than 50% of patients infected with hepatitis C. Many of these patients ultimately die of complications of chronic hepatitis such as cirrhosis or hepatocellular carcinoma (HCC).

Outside the United States, viral hepatitis is a major health problem. More than 300 million people are infected with hepatitis B worldwide. The World Health Organization (WHO) lists hepatitis B as the ninth leading cause of death in the world.

Viral hepatitis refers to the clinically important hepatotrophic viruses responsible for hepatitis A (HAV), hepatitis B (HBV), delta hepatitis (HDV), hepatitis C (HCV), and hepatitis E (HEV). Those viruses that cause hepatitis as part of a generalized illness, such as Epstein–Barr virus, herpes simplex virus, measles virus, and cytomegalovirus, are not discussed in this chapter.

Viral hepatitis has several clinical forms (acute, fulminant, chronic), defined by duration or severity of infection. The clinical, biochemical, immunoserologic, and histologic features of viral hepatitis follow similar patterns despite the virus responsible for the patient's illness. The hepatocellular response to injury and the resulting physical signs and symptoms are all nonspecific in nature.[4]

Acute Viral Hepatitis

Acute viral hepatitis is a systemic viral infection of up to but not exceeding 6 months in duration producing inflammatory necrosis of the liver. The natural history of the infection is divided into three stages based on viral serologic markers: incubation, acute hepatitis, and convalescence. Clinical severity of illness varies widely from asymptomatic, anicteric hepatitis to fulminant hepatitis, a rapidly fatal disease.[4]

The incubation stage begins shortly after parenteral or oral inoculation with the virus. Once access is gained to the circulation, the infective virions accumulate in hepatic sinusoids and are internalized by the hepatocytes. The internalized viral particles replicate within either the cytoplasm or the nucleus with the assistance of the host cellular apparatus. Infective viral particles are shed into blood, bile, and other body secretions during the later phases of the incubation stage. Complete virions and/or viral antigens are found in body fluids and tissues. The duration of the incubation stage is virus specific and varies (Table 40.1).[5,6] The host is essentially asymptomatic during the incubation stage of the infection.[4]

The hepatotrophic viruses cause hepatic injury either because of the host immune response or from direct viral damage to hepatocytes. For example, the acute hepatitis stage in hepatitis B begins once the host recognizes the virus and initiates an active immune response against the invading virions. The resulting cellular and humoral immune response is directed against viral antigens found on the host hepatocyte membranes and/or circulating within the vascular compartment.[7] The severity of the inflammatory response and resulting liver cell damage is variable. Under conditions of viral antigen excess, antigen–antibody complexes form within the vascular compartment and may produce immune complex-related phenomena and symptoms such as arthritis, skin rash, and urticaria.[4]

This acute hepatitis stage begins with a preicteric phase (before the onset of jaundice), which parallels initiation of the host immune response and occurs before significant liver cell injury. The preicteric phase is frequently associated with nonspecific influenza-like symptoms consisting of anorexia, nausea, fatigue, and malaise.[4]

Most patients with acute viral hepatitis develop only a few, mild symptoms and minimal hepatocyte damage. This mild disease is called *acute anicteric hepatitis.* The minimal degree of liver cell damage is reflected by mild elevations of serum bilirubin, gamma globulin, and hepatic

TABLE 40.1. IMPORTANT FEATURES OF HAV, HBV, HCV, HDV AND HEV

	Hepatitis A	Hepatitis B	Hepatitis C	Hepatitis D	Hepatitis E
Virus	HAV	HBV	HCV	HDV	HEV
Family	Picornavirus	Hepadnavirus	Flavivirus	Satellite	Calcivirus
Size (nm)	27	42	30–60	40	32
Genome	ssRNA	dsDNA	ssRNA	ssRNA	ssRNA
Incubation (days)	14–45	40–180	35–84	40–180 coinf[a] 14–45 superinf[b]	14–42
Transmission	Fecal-oral	Parenteral Sexual Perinatal	Parenteral Sexual (?)	Parenteral Sexual (?)	Fecal-oral
Serologic markers					
Antigens	HAVAg[c]	HbsAg HBcAg HBeAg	HCVAg	HDVAg	HEVAg
Antibodies	Anti-HAV	Anti-HBs Anti-HBc Anti-HBe	Anti-HCV	Anti-HDV	Anti-HEV
Viral markers	HAV RNA	HBV DNA DNA polymerase	HCV RNA	HDV RNA	Viruslike particles
Clinical illness					
Children	Anicteric	Anicteric 70%	Anicteric 75%	Not known	High % anicteric
Adults	Icteric	Icteric 30%	Most icteric	Icteric 25%	Not known
Acute mortality (%)	0.2	0.2–1	0.2	2–20	0.2 (pregnancy)
Chronicity	No	2–7% Neonates 90%	50–70%	2–70%	No
HCC[d]	No	Yes	Yes	Yes	No

[a]coinf, coinfection.
[b]superinf, superinfection.
[c]Ag, antigen.
[d]HCC, hepatocellular carcinoma. (Adapted with permission from Seminars in Liver Disease, vol 11, p 74, 1991, Thieme Medical Publishers, Inc.)

transaminase (ALT, AST) values to about twice normal. A subset of patients experiences enough hepatocyte destruction to produce significant liver function derangement characterized by interruption of bilirubin metabolism and flow. This results in clinical jaundice. The icteric phase is generally accompanied by fever, right upper quadrant abdominal pain, nausea, vomiting, dark urine, acholic stools, and worsening of systemic symptoms. Clinical symptoms are accompanied by moderate to marked elevations of the serum bilirubin, gamma globulin, and hepatic transaminases (4–10 times normal). Viral serologic markers and host antibodies are detectable during this stage of the illness.[4]

Most patients with either acute anicteric or icteric hepatitis go through the convalescence stage to complete recovery without developing complications or chronic sequelae. The duration of disease stages and the risk for developing chronic sequelae are virus-specific phenomena (Table 40.1).[4]

HEPATITIS A VIRUS (HAV)

Hepatitis A is the primary etiologic agent of worldwide hepatitis epidemics throughout recorded history.[5,8] HAV, an RNA virus, remains a significant cause of clinical hepatitis worldwide, although HEV plays a role in many epidemics.

Epidemiology

HAV is well suited to produce epidemics given its fecal-to-oral route of transmission and its ability to resist both gastric acid and the digestive enzymes of the upper gastrointestinal (GI) tract.[8] HAV infection also occurs sporadically. Both patterns of occurrence are related to overcrowded conditions and person-to-person or fecal-to-oral spread; thus, the incidence of HAV correlates directly with poor sanitary conditions and hygienic practices.[2] In most developing countries, almost all children are infected by 10 years of age. As hygienic standards improve, the frequency of HAV infection decreases in all age groups.[8]

In the United States, HAV infection occurs primarily in communitywide outbreaks, in lower socioeconomic groups, or in sporadic common-source outbreaks (outbreaks where all infected patients contract the infection from a single person or source). Children aged 5–14 years are more likely to be involved in communitywide outbreaks, whereas common-source outbreaks primarily involve young adults. Both children and young adults can be infected from common-source outbreaks at day care centers.[2]

The incubation period of HAV is 14–45 days, with a median of 28 days. The dose of infective inoculum alters the length of the incubation period but not the severity of clinical illness, which is host dependent.[28]

Pathogenesis

Hepatitis A viral replication occurs in the liver. Viral antigens are found in the hepatocyte cytoplasm during the incubation stage. They are subsequently shed into bile and feces. The largest concentration of viral particles is found in stool specimens during the 1–2 weeks preceding clinical illness. Viral shedding declines as clinical symptoms appear. Viremia is extremely short lived, thus explaining the rare occurrence of blood-borne transmission of hepatitis A.[5,9] Cases of HAV associated with parenteral drug abuse are increasing. Liver injury is immune mediated with cytolytic T cells the most likely effector cells.[7,8] Death of hepatocytes results in viral elimination and eventual resolution of the clinical illness.

The host serologic response to HAV initially appears as the viral particles begin to disappear from stool. Two classes of anti-HAV antibodies can be detected, immunoglobulin (Ig) M and IgG. Like most host antibody responses, antibodies of the IgM class appear first and imply recent infection. After 2–6 months, the IgM antibodies are replaced with IgG antibodies, whose presence indicates immunity to HAV. IgG antibodies can be detected for many years following infection.[8]

Clinical Features

Clinical symptoms are age dependent, with children less than 6 years old generally displaying a mild, influenza-like illness without clinical jaundice. In contrast, infected adults display the characteristic clinical syndrome of acute hepatitis with elevated hepatic transaminase levels and jaundice.[8]

HAV infection usually produces a mild, self-limited illness, although rarely HAV results in fulminant hepatitis or death. Alternatively, a minority of patients exhibits a cholestatic illness with predominant elevations of alkaline phosphatase, gamma-glutamyl transferase and total bilirubin that last several months. Pruritus may be the primary complaint of this latter patient group.[9] No cases of a chronic carrier state or chronic hepatitis have been reported. However, up to 20% of patients relapse with acute hepatitis 2–8 weeks after the initial illness. Recurrent symptoms tend to be milder than the initial episode.[8] Rarely, a relapse is associated with cryoglobulinemia, arthritis, and vasculitis.[9]

Diagnosis

The diagnosis of acute HAV infection depends on clinical suspicion, characteristic symptoms (if present), elevated aminotransferases and bilirubin, and a positive anti-HAV IgM (Table 40.1). Without characteristic symptoms, clinical suspicion of HAV is extremely important.[8] Patients who receive gamma globulin will have low titers of anti-HAV for several weeks after inoculation.[6] Patients who receive hepatitis A vaccine will also have anti-HAV.[6]

HEPATITIS B VIRUS (HBV)

The existence of a parenterally transmitted form of viral hepatitis was proposed in the late 1800s. However, such transmission was not confirmed until the 1930s when vaccinations for yellow fever (containing human convalescent serum) produced clinical jaundice. Despite extensive research, an infectious agent was not identified until 1965. In that year, Blumberg and colleagues[10] isolated an antibody from multitransfused patients that reacted with the serum of an Australian aborigine. Thus, the term *Australia antigen* came into use. In 1970, when David Dane and colleagues described the 42-nm particles ("Dane particles") that are the hepatitis B virions, the term "Australia antigen" was replaced with *hepatitis B surface antigen (HBsAg)* to denote its association with the envelope of HBV.[3]

Unlike HAV, HBV is a DNA virus of the Hepadnaviridae family (Table 40.1). As the family name implies (Hepadnaviridae are *hepa*totrophic *DNA vir*uses), these DNA viruses undergo primary replication in the liver. The Hepadnaviridae viruses cause chronic infection resulting in chronic liver injury. These viruses also have a propensity for integration into the host genome with associated oncogenesis.[2,11] The HBV produces complete virions and 22-nm spherotubules composed of the viral coat known serologically as HBsAg.[2,11] These forms are found in the plasma of patients with acute HBV infection, chronic carrier state, or chronic HBV infection. The hepatitis B virus is extremely hardy, remaining infective in human blood products frozen for up to 1 month. This complicates human blood banking.[2,11]

Epidemiology

HBV infection is a public health problem worldwide because of the chronic liver disease and primary HCC produced. There are more than 1 million chronic carriers of HBV in the United States alone.[12] HBV infection has extreme geographic variation in endemicity. In highly endemic areas (China, Southeast Asia, the Middle East, and parts of Africa and South America) HBV spread is predominantly by mother-to-infant perinatal transmission and child-to-child transmission.[9] High rates of chronic viral carriage and virus-associated primary HCC are seen in such areas. In parts of the world where the endemicity of HBV is relatively low (North America, Australia, Western Europe, and temperate South America) the chronic viral carriage rate is correspondingly low and mother-to-infant transmission is relatively uncommon. Rather, HBV transmission occurs either through intimate contact or by the parenteral route. High-risk groups in these areas include intravenous drug abusers, multitransfused patients, health care providers, male homosexuals, heterosexual partners of HBV-infected people, and heterosexual partners of human immunodeficiency virus (HIV)-infected individuals.[2] Transmission of HBV in the United States occurs predominantly through contact with infected blood products or body secretions (e.g., saliva, vaginal fluids, semen). The routine practice of screening blood donors for HBsAg has essentially eliminated hepatitis B as a cause of post-transfusion hepatitis. However, products or concentrates of blood such as clotting factors can remain infective despite prescreening for HBsAg. Excluding cases resulting from clotting factor concentrates, most blood-borne HBV transmissions are due to accidental inoculation by health care workers and to the sharing of needles by intravenous drug abusers (percutaneous exposure).[2]

The chief obstacles to eradication of hepatitis B include the carrier state and infections *in utero,* which are not preventable.

Pathogenesis

Although the HBV has been completely characterized and much is known about the biologic features of HBV infection, little is known about the mechanisms responsible for virus hepatocyte uptake, induction of viral replication, hepatocyte injury, persistent infection, or HBV-associated oncogenesis.[11]

Once the HBV gains access to the vascular compartment, the virus "homes in" to the liver, where primary replication occurs. HBV has a much longer incubation period than HAV (1–6 months).[2,11] HBV replication occurs in liver cell nuclei with HBsAg produced in the cell cytoplasm and expressed on the cell surface. During acute infection, usually only a small number of hepatocytes express viral antigens.[11,13] HBV is not cytopathic. The liver injury (like HAV infection) is immune related and T lymphocytes are important for both the host cellular and humoral responses.[7,13]

Antibody to HBsAg (anti-HBs) is initially detected in plasma as the concentration of HBsAg in plasma wanes. However, identification of HBsAg/anti-HBs immune complexes suggests that the surface antibody response occurs much earlier than detected by standard serologic assays. The presence of circulating immune complexes in antigen excess (generally in the prodromal stage) is associated with extrahepatic manifestations, including arthritis, urticaria, vasculitis, and glomerulonephritis.[11,13]

Additional antibodies directed against other HBV antigens are found in plasma of individuals with acute HBV infection. Anti-HBc, the antibody directed against the inner core viral antigen present in hepatocyte nuclei, is first detected shortly after the onset of acute cellular injury. Anti-HBc is initially of the IgM class and, when detectable, signifies acute HBV infection. IgG-class anti-HBc antibodies become detectable several months following the acute HBV infection and persist along with HBs antibody for life. Therefore, the presence of plasma anti-HBc IgG class antibodies signifies prior infection.[11]

A third antigen–antibody system of HBV is comprised of e antigen (HBeAg) and e antibody (anti-HBe). HBe antigen is a protein subunit of the viral core detected in plasma immediately prior to or at the onset of hepatocyte injury. Its presence correlates with a high degree of infectivity, presumably due to concomitantly circulating Dane particles. In contrast, the presence of HBe antibody correlates with a very low degree of infectivity and portends a complete recovery. The HBe antibody becomes detectable either immediately after the peak of liver injury or in early convalescence.[11]

Clinical Features

The clinical course of HBV infection and the associated clinical features cannot be differentiated from other types of viral hepatitis based on symptoms. A wide range of disease expression from asymptomatic infection to fulminant hepatitis occurs. In the typical case of acute HBV infection, the incubation period is followed by a symptomatic prodromal phase consisting of malaise, fatigue, weakness, anorexia, myalgias, and arthralgias. Jaundice develops in about one-third of patients as liver cell destruction increases. Jaundice may persist for several weeks.[2,11]

Clinical manifestations of HBV infection are age dependent. For example, newborns infected with HBV are generally asymptomatic, while about one-third of adult patients with acute HBV infection have symptoms. Of the approximately 65% of adults with subclinical infection, most recover completely. Twenty-five percent have symptomatic illness with jaundice and 1% develop fulminant hepatic failure during the acute illness. Approximately 10% of adult patients develop chronic or persistent infection. Chronicity is more likely to occur in patients with mild, anicteric forms of acute hepatitis, and is much more likely to occur when the infection is acquired as a newborn or infant.[2,11] Over a period of years, about 25% of adults with chronic HBV infection develop chronic active hepatitis

(CAH), and a smaller percentage progress to cirrhosis.[9] Immunosuppression with HIV results in more severe clinical disease with HBV infection, a higher incidence of both chronic HBV carriers and chronic hepatitis B and reactivation of HBV in late stages of HIV.[14]

Extrahepatic manifestations such as neuropathies, glomerulonephritis, pancreatitis, and hematopoietic stem cell suppression (aplastic anemia, thrombocytopenia) are occasionally seen. In chronic hepatitis B, essential mixed cryoglobulinemia (presence of abnormal plasma proteins of different types that precipitate or crystallize when cooled), polyarteritis nodosa (inflammation and necrosis of segments of medium-sized or small arteries), and other vasculitis-like lesions have been described.[15] Formerly it was thought that extrahepatic disease was mediated by circulating immune complexes. However, there is evidence now that these clinical symptoms are a direct consequence of the HBV infection.[16] In addition, hemolytic uremic syndrome, thrombotic thrombocytopenic purpura, Raynaud syndrome, Schonlein–Henoch purpura (an eruption of hemorrhaging into the skin that is nonthrombocytopenic; associated with joint pains or swelling and bleeding from the GI tract, as well as other manifestations), infantile papular acrodermatitis (an inflammatory papular eruption of the skin of the extremities of infants), Guillain–Barré syndrome, meningitis, myelitis, and meningoencephalomyelitis have all been reported.

Diagnosis

HBV has four potential gene regions: the nucleocapsid region (HBcAg and HBeAg), the envelope region (HBsAg), the P region (DNA polymerase), and the poorly understood X region.[6] In typical acute HBV infection, serologic markers proceed in sequence from the development of HBsAg followed by HBeAg (30–60 days prior to onset of clinical symptoms) through to the appearance of anti-HBs in late convalescence. The presence of anti-HBs without HBsAg usually indicates protective immunity. Occasionally HBsAg and anti-HBs will be present in the serum of a patient. This coexpression results from the presence of heterotypic antibody (i.e., the presence of more than one of the eight subtypes of HBV that have been defined by various combinations of epitopes in the surface antigen). It is important to remember that HBsAg is present in chronic infection as well as in acute HBV infection.

Acute HBV infection is diagnosed by the presence of anti-HBc IgM. There are periods during the course of HBV infection when specific serologic markers are absent; the lack of such markers complicates diagnosis of the acute infection. These serologic "window" periods can be seen in the early incubation phase when HBsAg and HBeAg are not detectable despite the presence of ongoing viral replication, and early in convalescence when these two antigens are cleared prior to the appearance of anti-HBs antibody. Markers of HBV replication (HBV DNA and DNA polymerase) are sensitive indicators. Soluble or dot-blot hybridization assays for HBV DNA are commercially available from several reference laboratories. Less sensitive modified Western blot assays are also available and useful. Fortunately, anti-HBc IgM can almost always be detected in acute hepatitis and serves to identify "HBsAg-negative" cases of acute HBV infection.[11,13]

Three new markers of HBV infection include pre-S1, pre-S2 for the envelope, and the functional X protein.[17] When monitored, presence of the pre-S1 antigen (pre-S1 Ag) correlates with viral replication. Pre-S1 Ag, HBV DNA, and anti-HBc IgM help guide interferon (IFN) therapy.

Anti-HBc IgG confirms current (or implies previous) HBV infection. The finding of anti-HBc IgG, without other HBV markers, indicates one of four things: (1) the patient is in the window phase of acute HBV infection; (2) the duration of anti-HBc exceeds that of anti-HBs in a resolved infection; (3) the patient has chronic HBV infection in which HBsAg is produced at levels below the detectable limit; or (4) it is falsely positive.[9]

Two types of HBV variants have been identified. In the first, a point mutation in the precore region of the HBV genome precludes the production of HBeAg. This variant is associated with active liver disease, IFN treatment is less effective, and HCC development and mortality are higher than in those infected with wild-type HBV. This HBV mutant has been linked to epidemics of fulminant HBV.[18,19] The second HBV variant has mutations in the pre-S and S genes and has significant subtype variation. This variant is associated with nonresponse to HBV vaccination. Clinical cases that present with atypical serologies may be caused by infection with HBV variants.

HEPATITIS C VIRUS (HCV)

HCV is a single-stranded RNA virus that accounts for most cases of what was previously termed non-A, non-B hepatitis (NANBH). HCV is a member of the Flaviviridae family, which includes the viruses that cause human diseases such as dengue and yellow fever and animal diseases including hog cholera and bovine viral diarrhea. In addition to the structural components of the virus (core and envelope), the virion also has several nonstructural proteins (Ns).[20,21] The functions of these Ns are not well understood. There are several HCV strains with considerable genetic and immunogenic variability.

Epidemiology

HCV is found worldwide. Patients at risk for HCV infection in the United States include those who receive blood products, intravenous drug users, and health care workers.

Together these three groups account for approximately 41–62% of cases of HCV.[9] HCV antibodies are detected in 85–90% of patients with post-transfusion hepatitis, 70% of patients with a history of intravenous drug abuse and who test positive for HIV, 30–50% of patients with sporadic NANBH, 20% of patients undergoing hemodialysis, and up to 75% of patients with primary HCC.[22] Up to 40% of all cases of hepatitis C report no known risk factors, and the mechanism(s) of transmission for these sporadically occurring cases is poorly understood. Permucosal, sexual, and maternal–neonatal transmission rates of HCV are low.[9,23] Sexual transmission rates are much less for HCV than for HBV or HIV.[24] Sexual transmission is facilitated by HIV coinfection.[9] Spouses of patients with HCV infection and chronic liver disease are at increased risk of acquiring HCV. The risk is proportional to the length of the marriage, but is low.[25]

Antibody to HCV has been reported in groups of patients with chronic liver disease, such as alcoholics, and in patients with classic (type 1) autoimmune hepatitis. However, many of the positives in these groups are false-positives, based on, for example, high gamma globulin levels of the patients. HCV virus may play a role in alcoholics with chronic liver disease and in certain patients with some forms of autoimmune liver disease, however.[9,24]

Pathogenesis

In contrast to HBV where the liver cell damage is primarily immunologically mediated, the liver injury with HCV infection most closely resembles that of a cytopathic virus. For example, the general histologic picture of chronic hepatitis C is predominant lobular hepatitis with scarce periportal piecemeal necrosis. There may be immune-mediated features as well.[25]

HCV persists in the majority of infected patients. The mechanism by which this occurs is unknown, although the simultaneous presence of multiple variant genomes appears to play a role.[25]

Clinical Features

Acute hepatitis C is clinically indistinguishable from other types of viral hepatitis. The incubation period for HCV is usually 5–12 weeks, although the range is 2–26 weeks.[2,22] The clinical course is generally mild with less than 25% of patients developing jaundice. Major complaints are frequently limited to fatigue and malaise.[12] Similar to other types of viral hepatitis, the hepatic transaminase values in HCV hepatitis vary from mildly to markedly elevated. Unlike the other types, HCV infections characteristically demonstrate a pattern of widely fluctuating enzyme values over the course of the infection.[22] It is not yet clear whether fulminant hepatocellular failure can be a consequence of infection with hepatitis C. Infection with HIV results in more severe clinical disease with HCV infection.

An important feature of this form of hepatitis is that 60–70% of cases progress to chronic infection. Within 5 years, 30–35% develop CAH and 20–33% progress to cirrhosis.[9,26] Others who eventually develop cirrhosis and hepatic failure do so after up to 20 years of indolent, asymptomatic infection. Chronic HCV infection-related cirrhosis is an etiologic factor in the development of HCC.[22]

In general, the extent of liver damage evident on liver biopsy is far greater than the degree of elevation of serum enzymes would lead one to believe. The disease progresses insidiously with continuing damage to the liver in those patients who develop chronic infection with the virus.

Extrahepatic manifestations occasionally occur with hepatitis C. They include the following: erythema multiforme, thrombocytopenia, serum sickness, rash, blood dyscrasias, cryoglobulinemia with cutaneous vasculitis, arthralgia, and glomerulonephritis.[27]

Diagnosis

HCV RNA is detectable by PCR as early as 1 week after infection.[9] This test is still primarily a research tool and diagnosis of acute HCV depends on clinical symptoms and sequential monitoring of liver transaminase levels until the HCV antibody becomes positive.[26] Seroconversion to anti-HCV appears from 3–6 months following initial exposure and, in rare instances, can take up to 12 months. This lag time is a major limitation in testing for hepatitis C.

Serologic testing for HCV has progressed rapidly since the introduction of the first antibody test in 1990. The first-generation enzyme-linked immunosorbent assay (ELISA I) test for HCV detects only the antibody to a recombinant HCV protein known as c100-3 (from a nonstructural region of the HCV genome) and is plagued by false-positive and false-negative results. However, use of the first-generation test markedly reduced the risk and incidence of post-transfusion hepatitis due to HCV. The second-generation assay (ELISA II, Ortho Diagnostics, Raritan, NJ) is both more sensitive and more specific. It detects the antibody to a recombinant hybrid antigen (c100-3 and c33c nonstructural regions and c22 core region). Second-generation ELISAs require confirmation by supplement assays, but the biggest limitation remains the delayed appearance of anti-HCV after acute infection.[17] The recombinant immunoblot assay (RIBA II) is used as a supplemental test to confirm ELISA II results because of its high specificity and positive predictive value.[9,24] Even the second-generation tests, however, are not 100% accurate confirmatory tests for HCV.

Viral RNA remains positive and histologic progression continues in those who develop chronic infection with HCV. However, serum aminotransferase levels can fluctuate, or even normalize, confounding the diagnosis of chronic HCV infection. To assess chronic HCV, liver biopsy is the only reliable indicator of disease progression.

It is not uncommon for a patient to present to physician with cirrhosis or portal hypertension secondary to HCV infection years to decades prior, yet to have had few or no clinical signs or symptoms during the intervening years.

DELTA HEPATITIS VIRUS

The hepatitis delta virus (HDV), first identified in 1977, is a defective RNA virus that requires the presence of HBV to cause infection. Infection with HDV usually worsens the course of the HBV-infected patient. HDV is composed of a single strand of RNA, an internal protein (the delta antigen), and an outer coat of HBsAg. Serologic tests for detection of serum antibodies to the delta antigen (anti-HDV) are useful in diagnosing acute hepatitis and chronic infection.[2,28]

Epidemiology

HDV parallels the transmission patterns and areas of endemicity of HBV, with only a few differences. These differences include lower endemicity rates of HDV in East and Southeast Asia and lower incidence rates in homosexual males. Three forms of HDV infection have been identified and are designated acute HDV–HBV coinfection, acute HDV superinfection, and HDV chronic infection. Coinfection describes simultaneous infection with both HBV and HDV while superinfection occurs when HDV is transmitted after the patient has been exposed to HBV.[2,28,29] Chronic infection and liver disease result from acute HDV–HBV coinfection in approximately 5% of cases.[9]

HDV infection in the United States is strongly associated with intravenous drug abuse, exposure to infected blood, and/or fulminant hepatitis. Epidemics among drug abusers have been reported and usually involve coinfection with HBV.[2,28]

Clinical Features

Because of the dependence of HDV on HBV for its infectivity, the natural course of HDV coinfection and superinfection differ significantly. In coinfection, the acute delta hepatitis is almost always self-limited, owing to the transient hepatitis B surface antigenemia, and follows the usual course of HBV infection. Similar to HBV, replication of the delta virus occurs in the liver. Unlike the typical HBV infection, a biphasic rise in liver transaminase levels may be seen, the first peak attributable to HBV and the second to HDV. The disappearance of HBsAg from serum heralds resolution of both infections and development of specific antibodies to both agents. Lasting immunity to both viruses is provided by the antibodies to HBsAg.[28,29]

In HDV superinfection, delta viral replication occurs rapidly due to the persistent HBV infection, providing a ready supply of HBsAg. Liver injury and clinical symptoms appear quickly and may be severe, leading to a fulminant course. Rapid clinical decompensation in a previously stable HBV carrier should raise the possibility of HDV superinfection. Many of these patients develop chronic liver disease and some develop HCC.[28,29]

Diagnosis

The diagnosis of HDV infection depends on clinical suspicion, elevated hepatic aminotransferases, and serologic evidence of HBV and HDV infection. In acute superinfection of a chronic HBV carrier, markers for acute HBV are negative. HBsAg, HDVAg, and anti-HDV IgM are usually present. In acute coinfection, HDVAg, anti-HDV IgM, and markers for acute HBV are usually present. Anti-HDV IgG follows. Currently, only a test for total anti-HDV is commercially available.[2]

Prognosis

The mortality rate in acute delta hepatitis is 2–20%. Cirrhosis develops in ≥70% of patients with chronic delta hepatitis.[30]

HEPATITIS E VIRUS

During the past century, enterically transmitted, waterborne hepatitis caused major epidemics throughout the Third World. These epidemics, originally attributed to HAV, were later found to be serologically unrelated to HAV infection. In the 1980s, a 27- to 34-nm, spherical RNA virus of the Caliciviridae family was isolated from fecal samples of infected patients and produced hepatitis in human volunteers, thus supporting its role as a cause of enterically transmitted hepatitis.[22,31] This agent was designated hepatitis E virus (HEV), in part to identify it as the agent responsible for enterically transmitted hepatitis epidemics (enterically transmitted non-A, non-B hepatitis [NANBH]).[2,22,31]

HEV is endemic in Africa, Southeast and Central Asia, Mexico, and Central and South America. Many sporadic cases of acute hepatitis in areas endemic for HEV are also attributed to HEV. To date, Western travelers to endemic areas provide the reported cases of HEV in developed countries.[2,22,31] HEV accounts for a portion of acute NANBH in Americans with no travel history.[9]

Although serologically distinct, HEV infection is similar to HAV infection. The similar features include enteric transmission, ability to cause epidemics, existence of areas of endemicity relating to poor sanitary conditions, occurrence of primary viral replication in hepatocyte cytoplasm, heavy shedding of viral particles into bile and feces, similarity of incubation period and clinical course, and lack of demonstrated chronic persistent viral infection.[22,31]

Infection with HEV follows a benign course, except in pregnant women; women who contract HEV during the third trimester are at considerable risk for developing fulminant hepatitis.[22,31]

The diagnosis is made on clinical grounds in conjunction with exclusion of other viruses. A convenient serologic test for HEV is not yet available. Until diagnostic studies become available, questions concerning specific epidemiologic characteristics, incidence and prevalence rates, host response to infection, and protective immunity cannot be answered.[22,31]

VIRUS VARIANTS

Variants of hepatitis viruses—especially HBV variants—have been acknowledged for years. They have gained new attention because of the association of these mutants with fulminant hepatitis and escape from hepatitis B vaccination response. These variants can also be useful, however. For example, genetic variants of HAV that have lost their virulence and that are adapted to efficient growth in cell culture are the bases for inactivated and live attenuated hepatitis A vaccines. Recently, variants among HCV have also been documented.

In summary, at least five hepatotrophic viruses are responsible for the clinical entity known as acute viral hepatitis. Accurate diagnosis is frequently complicated by the similar patterns of the clinical, biochemical, and histologic features produced by the different viral agents. For the purpose of diagnosing acute hepatitis, four tests should be done initially: anti HAV-IgM, anti-HBc IgM, HBsAg, and anti-HCV.[6] If HBsAg is present, anti-HDV should be checked.

TREATMENT OF ACUTE VIRAL HEPATITIS

Management of acute viral hepatitis is primarily supportive. General measures include a healthy diet, rest, maintaining fluid balance, and avoiding hepatotoxic drugs and alcohol. The patient should avoid becoming fatigued; bed rest may be required during the acute phase of the illness. Management includes monitoring for development of chronic liver disease and preventing disease spread.[32]

Treatments that offer no benefit include special diets, corticosteroids, and antiemetics. Vitamin K is recommended only if the patient has a prolonged prothrombin time. Hospitalization is necessary only for those who have prolonged vomiting, coagulation defects, or fulminant hepatitis.[32]

Preliminary trials and case reports of the use of IFN-α and IFN-β as therapy in acute HBV and HCV infections report promising results.[33,34] Because not all studies have demonstrated IFN to be useful, further studies are ongoing to define the place of IFN in acute hepatitis treatment. If results from these studies demonstrate that a lower rate of chronicity results when treatment is initiated during the acute phase of infection, early identification and treatment will become the primary focus. The role of antiviral agents is undefined.

FULMINANT HEPATITIS

Liver injury that results in fulminant hepatic necrosis and hepatic failure is relatively rare. When it occurs, death results in a few days or weeks in nearly 80% of cases. Any potential hepatotoxic agent can be responsible, although the most frequent cause is viral hepatitis (70%), especially HBV.[35] In the United States, fulminant hepatitis is mainly due to HBV, and occasionally, HCV. Acute hepatitis B leads to acute liver failure in 1% of patients.[36]

Although patients with acute HBV usually are viremic for weeks, many of those who develop liver failure become seronegative for HBsAg within a few days.[36] This rapid viral clearance is secondary to a massive immune response by the infected patient. Patients with fulminant hepatic necrosis typically develop signs and symptoms of viral hepatitis, then rapidly develop evidence of hepatic failure. The clinical syndrome is usually a 1- to 3-week course of hepatic failure and encephalopathy with coma developing within a few weeks of the onset of acute hepatitis. Hyperexcitability, insomnia, somnolence, irritability, and impaired mental status are evidence of impending hepatic failure in patients with acute hepatitis.[15] Particularly ominous signs include a rapid decrease in liver size, a rapid decline in aminotransferase levels, prolonged prothrombin time, and hypoglycemia.[15] Manifestations of hepatic failure include metabolic encephalopathy, coma, coagulation defects, ascites, and edema. In fulminant liver failure, complications include GI hemorrhage, sepsis, cerebral edema, renal failure, lactic acidosis, and disseminated coagulopathy, with death resulting from bleeding, cerebral edema, hypoglycemia, infection, and/or multisystem organ failure.[15,35]

There is no specific treatment for fulminant hepatic failure. Management of fulminant hepatitis focuses on recognition, prevention of complications, and aggressive management of complications. Measures that improve survival of patients include intensive supportive care plus early referral for liver transplantation.[37,38] Fresh frozen plasma should be administered for bleeding, H_2-blocker therapy given to prevent GI bleeding, and aggressive antibiotic therapy should be used for infections. Cerebral edema occurs in the majority of cases that progress to grade IV encephalopathy, and it is the leading cause of death in these patients.[36] Management includes intracranial-pressure monitoring and administration of mannitol (0.3–0.4 g/kg body weight as a 20% solution).[15,36] Dexamethasone and hyperventilation are of little value in cerebral edema related to acute liver failure.[36] Pentobarbital will lower intracranial pressure, but often lowers systemic blood pressure, too.[36]

For further information on therapy and dosing of these drugs, the reader is referred to the corresponding topics in appropriate chapters of this book.

Urgent liver transplantation is the therapy of choice for patients with fulminant hepatic failure. Patients who could potentially be candidates for liver transplantation should be transferred at the first sign of altered mentation, because these patients can worsen very rapidly. Survival rates with liver transplantation for fulminant hepatitis approach 55–75%.[15] Prognosis is improved if transplantation is done prior to development of dense coma, the diagnosis is acute HAV infection, there are no comorbid conditions, the patient is between 11 and 40 years of age, the patient was jaundiced for less than 7 days before encephalopathy occurred, the prothrombin time was less than 50 seconds, and the serum bilirubin was less than 17.6 mg/dL.[15]

Patients do not benefit from administration of corticosteroids, heparin, insulin, or glucagon.[36] The role of antiviral therapy is not clear.[37] Agents such as foscarnet have been tried in uncontrolled studies with apparent improvement in survival. Antiviral therapy would not be expected to help, however, because viral replication in fulminant hepatitis is low (or has ceased) by the time the patient is admitted to hospital. Other treatments that do not improve survival (if liver transplantation is not done) include plasmapheresis, peritoneal dialysis, cross-circulation with nonhuman primate livers, extracorporeal liver perfusion, plasma perfusion over sorbents, and total body washout.[15] Experimental treatments with prostaglandins show potential benefit.[15]

Chronic Viral Hepatitis

Chronic viral hepatitis describes prolongation or continuation of the hepatic necroinflammatory process 6 months or more beyond the onset of the acute illness. Chronic hepatitis was first described in 1941 as a sequela of acute viral hepatitis. Drugs, metabolic conditions, and autoimmune disorders may also produce chronic hepatic inflammatory injury; such injury often leads to cirrhosis.[39]

The clinical findings, course, and histologic features are similar in all patients with chronic hepatitis regardless of the etiologic agent.[39] HAV and HEV, however, do not produce a persistent infection in humans. Further, the delta virus cannot produce chronic infection without HBV assistance. Thus, HBV and HCV are the primary hepatitis viruses capable of producing chronic hepatitis.[4] Sixty to 80% of all cases are related to HBV or HCV infection.[12] Worldwide, chronic infection with hepatitis B is the most important, while in the United States, most cases of chronic hepatitis are due to chronic HCV infection. The principal reservoir of HBV for infection of others is the chronically infected individual.

Complications of chronic hepatitis include cirrhosis, hepatic failure, and HCC. Both chronic HBV and chronic HCV infection are associated with HCC. For example, HBV carriers have a relative risk of acquiring HCC that is more than 100-fold that of noncarriers. Furthermore, 40% of male HBV carriers die of causes related to their liver disease. HBV and HCV infections are thus convincing causes of human cancer as well as important causes of chronic liver damage.[3]

HBV causes chronic infection in up to 90% of infected neonates, 20–50% of infected children under 6 years of age, and 6–10% of infected adults.[1] Persistent HBsAg is much more common in males and neonates.[11,39,40] The Centers for Disease Control and Prevention (CDC) estimates that 5000 people die yearly in the United States as a consequence of acute and chronic HBV infections.[1]

Failure to clear viral antigen from the serum within 6 months of acute infection indicates ongoing viral replication, persistent infection, and inflammation with resulting liver cell injury. In hepatitis B infection, subsequent clearance of serum HBsAg may occur, but at a rate of only 1% per year.

Clinical Features

The spectrum of clinical symptoms, course, and histologic features is broad in chronic hepatitis B. "Healthy" carriers exhibit no symptoms, have normal or near normal liver transaminase values, and minimal nonspecific histologic abnormalities. The majority of these carriers are found to be HBeAg negative and anti-HBe positive and do not appear to develop chronic active hepatitis or cirrhosis.[11,40]

In contrast to the healthy carriers, chronic HBsAg carriers with markers of ongoing viral replication (HBcAb–IgM, HBeAg, and HBV DNA) display persistent hepatic injury. Chronicity is more likely to occur in individuals with antecedent episodes of mild, anicteric acute hepatitis, suggesting that viral clearance is the ultimate result of significant hepatic necrosis. This has been repeatedly demonstrated in patients with acute fulminant hepatitis. If the patient with fulminant hepatitis survives, complete recovery without development of chronic sequelae generally occurs. Another important factor in determining chronicity is host immune competence. Persistent infection is much more common in immunologically compromised individuals such as patients with the acquired immune deficiency syndrome (AIDS), cancer, or renal failure; those on chemotherapeutic and immunosuppressive treatments; and newborns.[11,40]

Although there is considerable variability in the clinical features of chronic hepatitis B, males predominate in most series (80%). The mean age at presentation is greater than 30 years. Unlike acute hepatitis, physical symptoms do not correlate well with the severity of liver injury. Many patients are asymptomatic and therefore are diagnosed only after elevated serum liver transaminases and/or HBsAg are found in patients' serum upon routine testing. An additional group of patients presents with a complication of their chronic hepatitis/cirrhosis such as ascites or esophageal variceal bleeding.[39,40]

In either chronic HBV or chronic HCV, if the patient is symptomatic, fatigue, malaise, anorexia, and weight loss are common. Many patients have a history of jaundice. On physical examination, hepatomegaly is usually present, but the stigmata of chronic liver disease (spider nevi, splenomegaly, palmar erythema, testicular atrophy, caput medusa, female escutcheon) are generally absent until late in the disease course. Mild but persistent elevations of the serum aminotransferases, bilirubin, and gamma globulin levels are most commonly seen.[39] Both chronic HBV and chronic HCV are associated with extrahepatic syndromes. These include mixed cryoglobulinemia, polyarteritis nodosa, and a sicca-like syndrome that resembles Sjogren's syndrome. HBV infection is also occasionally associated with renal failure. Whether this is also true for HCV is not known.

In chronic hepatitis C, there is frequently little clinical evidence that the disease process is progressing. The patient is asymptomatic, yet liver biopsy would demonstrate ongoing liver injury and progressive histologic changes. Serum enzymes can be normal or only mildly elevated; unfortunately, the patient is on an insidious course that progresses to complications after a period of 15–20 years. Thus, extra vigilance is important in the patient with hepatitis C to assess whether "silent" progression is occurring.

Pathogenesis

The host immune response appears responsible for the persistence of HBV infection in healthy carriers and the hepatocyte damage in CAH. A weak cell-mediated immune response has been demonstrated in these patients. In healthy carriers an absent or poor cell-mediated response results in persistent viral replication but only minimal liver damage. As previously stated, viral clearance is dependent on destruction and elimination of infected hepatocytes. Thus, a poor host immune response ensures persistent viral replication. Therefore, it is not surprising that healthy carriers have high titers of serum HBsAg and correspondingly high HBsAg concentrations within infected hepatocytes.[7,13,39,40]

Patients with chronic HBV infection are deficient in producing, or responding to, IFN, which is needed to stimulate production of HLA class I protein.[12] This lack of HLA class I protein expression on the hepatocyte membrane results in incomplete direction of the lymphocyte to the target infected cell.[12]

A poor immune response may also produce a smoldering inflammatory form of hepatic injury as seen in chronic active hepatitis (CAH). While the host immune response is capable of destroying some infected hepatocytes, such a response is incapable of eliminating the virus entirely. The result is persistent viral replication and continued stimulation of the host immune system.[7,13,39,40]

If persistent viral replication and subsequent hepatocyte inflammatory destruction continue unabated, the number of functioning hepatocytes gradually decreases over time, and fibrosis resulting from cellular repair mechanisms distorts the basic cellular architecture. Hepatic nodules are thus formed. When widespread, the hepatic fibrosis with nodule formation is termed cirrhosis. The consequences of cirrhosis do not differ with regard to initial etiologies and can produce portal hypertension and ascites.[13]

In addition to cirrhosis, another long-term complication of chronic HBV infection is primary hepatocellular carcinoma. The exact mechanism of HBV in the development of HCC is not clear. Worldwide, HBV is the most important etiologic factor in the development of HCC, although it does appear that the presence of cofactors (toxins and carcinogens) and cirrhosis (premalignant condition) play a role.[11,13,40] HCV and delta hepatitis are also associated with HCC in patients with chronic infections.[22,29]

More than 50% of patients who are infected with HCV will progress to chronic disease, and more than 20% of those with chronic hepatitis C will have a low-grade, smoldering progression to cirrhosis.[12] The mechanism of liver injury in chronic HCV infection is not well understood, however, in contrast to HBV, HCV is considered a cytopathic virus.

Diagnosis

The natural histories and treatments of the various types of chronic hepatitis differ significantly. Thus, it is important to establish an accurate etiology. The diagnostic tests previously discussed are excellent in differentiating a specific viral cause of chronic hepatitis from an autoimmune, metabolic, drug, or other etiology. The duration of inflammation coupled with assessment of extent of histologic injury (liver biopsy), will further define the expected course and treatment plan.

Aminotransferase levels in patients with chronic HBV infection can be minimally elevated or normal. The extent of elevation correlates roughly with the extent of active inflammation. When a relatively asymptomatic carrier of HBV experiences an acute exacerbation of hepatitis, then superinfection with another virus, spontaneous reactivation of hepatitis B, or clearance of the hepatitis B e antigen all must be considered. In chronic hepatitis B, markers include HBsAg, HBV DNA, pre-S1 Ag, pre-S2 Ag, and anti-HBx. HBeAg can be positive or negative, depending on the virus variant. HBeAg is lost spontaneously at the rate of 7–20% per year.

In a patient with a history of blood transfusion, chronically elevated aminotransferase levels, a positive ELISA II for anti-HCV and CAH on liver biopsy, the diagnosis of chronic HCV is easily made. For patients without risk factors, other potential causes must be ruled out before making the diagnosis of chronic HCV. Serum aminotransferase levels correlate poorly with the histologic extent of disease, and liver biopsy provides diagnostic and prognostic information.

Prognosis

In patients with chronic viral hepatitis, the presence of ongoing viral replication is the most important factor in evaluating disease progression.[12] However, the prognosis for a patient with chronic viral hepatitis is indicated by the degree of liver damage noted on liver biopsy. The typical histologic features are the presence of chronic inflammatory cells within portal triads, hepatocellular necrosis, and a variable degree of fibrosis. The severity of these histologic features varies within regions of the involved liver and among individual patients.

In an attempt to standardize the histologic features and to provide prognostic information based on these features, a classification scheme was developed. This scheme divides chronic hepatitis into two categories: chronic persistent hepatitis (CPH, good prognosis) and chronic active hepatitis (CAH), which can proceed to further hepatic damage and eventually cirrhosis. CAH is divided into mild and severe forms. A third category, chronic lobular hepatitis, describes the histologic picture of persistent acute hepatitis of greater than 3 months duration and, like CPH, this histologic diagnosis carries a good prognosis.

Although there are limitations to use of this schema, long-term prognosis of patients with chronic HBV infection correlates as follows: 97% of those with CPH are alive at 5 years compared with 86% of those with CAH without cirrhosis and 55% of those with CAH and cirrhosis.[9] Age greater than 40, the presence of spider nevi, bilirubin greater than 1.5 mg/dL, and ascites correlates with a worse prognosis. Patients with evidence of end-stage liver disease have a much lower 5-year survival rate.[41]

Prognosis in chronic HCV correlates with histologic findings. Recently, investigations into HCV genotype have suggested that genotype may have important implications for benign or severe disease.

TREATMENT OF CHRONIC VIRAL HEPATITIS

General therapeutic measures in patients with compensated chronic hepatitis include exercise as tolerated, avoidance of potentially hepatotoxic drugs and chemicals (i.e., alcohol), and a healthy diet. Patients should not donate blood and serum monitoring for exacerbations of disease or spontaneous seroconversion should be done periodically. Sexual partners and children of patients with chronic HBV should be vaccinated against hepatitis B.

Effective treatment of chronic viral hepatitis should decrease morbidity and mortality and prevent infected patients from serving as reservoirs of infection.[42] Ideal treatment of chronic hepatitis would permanently inhibit viral replication, prevent cirrhosis, avert incorporation of the viral genome, stop progression of disease, and eliminate the virus entirely (Table 40.2).[42,43]

The decision to treat patients with chronic hepatitis should not be made based on the presence or absence of symptoms or the degree of abnormality of biochemical tests. The activity and extent of the liver disease do not correlate with the level of serum aminotransferases or the patient's symptoms. Rather, a systematic approach to the treatment should be made, such as the management approach shown in the algorithm in Fig. 40.1.[44]

Interferons

Inhibition of replication of HBV by adenine arabinoside (ara-A) and interferon (IFN) was first reported in 1976.[45] Early clinical study of IFN was impeded by short supply, and undefined dose and duration of therapy,[45] but improved

TABLE 40.2. GOALS OF THERAPY IN PATIENTS WITH CHRONIC HEPATITIS B AND CHRONIC HEPATITIS C

Goal	Chronic Hepatitis B	Chronic Hepatitis C
Loss of HBV DNA (loss of ability of HBV to replicate)	X	
Loss of HBeAg (loss of infectious potential)	X	
Loss of HBsAg (eradication of HBV)	X	
Loss of HCV RNA (loss of ability of HCV to replicate)		X
Loss of HCVAg (loss of infectious potential)		X
Normalization of aminotransferases (cessation of hepatic inflammation)	X	X
Improve symptoms	X	X
Decreased progression of liver disease	X	X
Reduce risk of cirrhosis	X	X
Reduce risk of hepatocellular carcinoma	X	X
Increase survival	X	X

(Compiled, in part, from Ref. 12.)

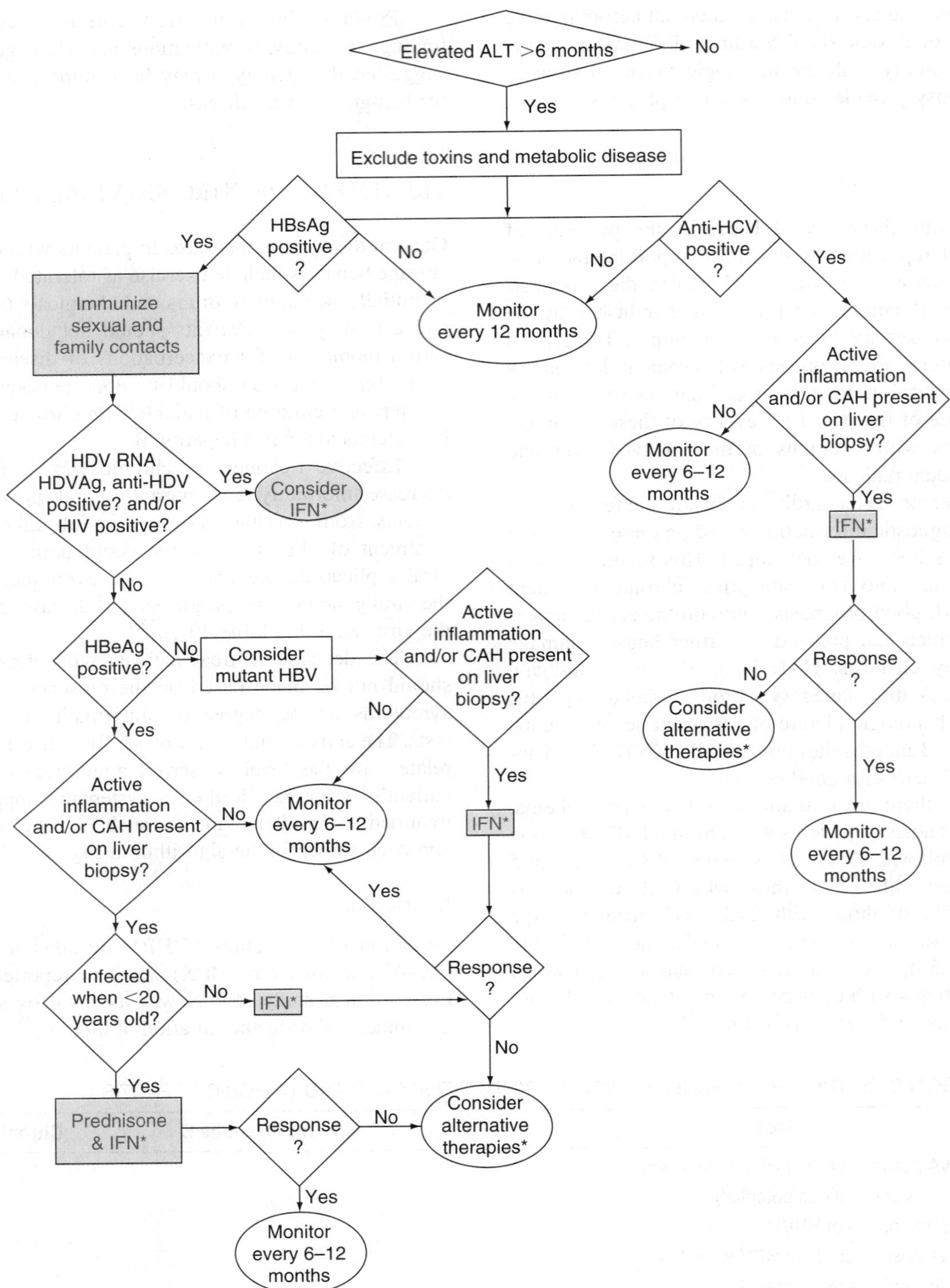

Figure 40.1. Algorithm for the management of chronic viral hepatitis. *See text for IFN dosing and alternative therapies. *(Adapted, in part, from Ref. 44.)*

availability of IFN due to recombinant DNA techniques has fostered an increased number of clinical trials. IFN is now the treatment of choice for patients with chronic HBV, HCV, and HDV infection. Unfortunately, IFN therapy has limitations in management of chronic hepatitis: Only a proportion of patients respond favorably; considerably fewer have lasting response; very few are cured. There remains a need for more effective, more widely applicable, and less costly therapy for chronic hepatitis.

The IFNs are a family of endogenous proteins grouped together on the basis of their biological effects. IFN-α and IFN-β act through a common receptor and have more pronounced antiviral effects, while IFN-γ acts through a separate receptor and has more pronounced immunological actions. IFN-α is the most extensively studied of the IFNs in chronic hepatitis. IFN-α exerts its action in chronic hepatitis partly through induction of transcription of cellular genes that encode proteins that cause an antiviral state, and partly via its immunomodulatory actions (Fig. 40.2).[46,47] IFNs bind to specific cell receptors causing the release of a group of intracellular enzymes such as 2′,5′-oligoadenylate synthetase and double-stranded RNA-dependent protein kinases. Activation of these enzymes leads to a chain of reactions resulting in destruction of viral mRNA and phosphorylation of cellular proteins within infected cells.[12] IFNs also increase expression of cell surface membrane proteins, including HLA class I proteins, increase natural killer cell activity, and enhance maturation of cytotoxic T cells.[12] Which of the multiple actions of IFN-α account for its effectiveness in chronic viral hepatitis is unclear.

Recombinant IFNs (alfa-2A, Roferon A, Hoffmann-LaRoche; α-2B, Intron A, Schering) and lymphoblastoid IFN (α-n1, Wellferon, Burroughs Wellcome) are effective in relieving symptoms and halting progression of chronic hepatitis B in one-third to one-half of immunocompetent patients from Western countries.[42,47–49] Remissions are marked by loss of HBV DNA, HBeAg, normalization of serum aminotransferases, and improvement in liver histology. The typical biochemical response to IFN-α in a patient with chronic HBV infection is shown in Fig. 40.3.[50] More than half of the responders subsequently lose HBsAg and develop anti-HBs. Termination of the HBV carrier state occurs in the majority of individuals who lose HBsAg.[51]

Effective dosing regimens of IFN in clinically stable patients with chronic HBV are 5 million units daily (MU) or 10 MU subcutaneously three times weekly for 4–6 months. One specific regimen (FDA-approved) for IFN-α 2b: 5 MU 5 days per week or 10 MU every other day for 16 weeks. Therapy should be started as early as possible after diagnosis.[48] Mildly or moderately decompensated patients should receive only 2 MU daily or 2–5 MU three times weekly, if IFN is used at all.[52]

Predictors of good response (sustained loss of HBeAg and HBV DNA) in chronic HBV include age greater than 20 years when acquiring the disease, high pretreatment aminotransferases (ALT and AST), no coinfection with HIV, female sex, low serum titer of HBV–DNA, and active liver disease prior to therapy.[42,48,49] A transient increase in ALT is often seen in responders during the second or third month of therapy.[42] Response is usually sustained when therapy is stopped. Patients infected with HBV mutants that prevent HBeAg expression may be less likely to respond to IFN therapy and/or have a high rate of relapse upon discontinuation of IFN.[51]

It is important to measure the markers of chronic HBV infection (HBeAg and HBV DNA) immediately prior to initiating treatment because a few patients with chronic HBV infection spontaneously lose HBV DNA and seroconvert each year without treatment.[42] Laboratory monitoring parameters during treatment include the aminotransferases, HBeAg, and HBV DNA. Clinical vigilance for decompensation is essential.

The long-term effect of therapy is not well defined, however, evidence is accumulating that liver disease progression is delayed or halted and HBsAg positivity and HBV DNA are lost in responders.[53] In a study of 23 patients who had responded to therapy with a loss of HBsAg and improvement in serum aminotransferases, only three patients relapsed in 3–7 years of follow-up.[53] All the relapsing patients did so within the first year after discontinuing therapy. A meta-analysis of randomized, controlled trials indicated a loss of HBV DNA in 37% and a loss of HBsAg in 7.8% of IFN-treated patients.[54] Thus, termination of the HBV carrier state is possible in some patients. Further study is needed to define whether long-term protection from cirrhosis or HCC occurs.[42,43]

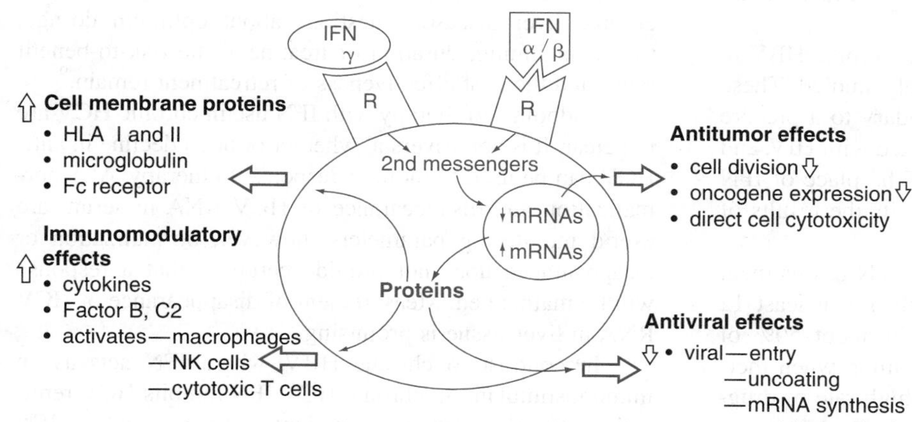

Figure 40.2. The mechanisms of action of interferons. *(Reprinted with permission from Seminars in Liver Disease, vol 9, p 235, 1989, Thieme Medical Publishers, Inc.)*

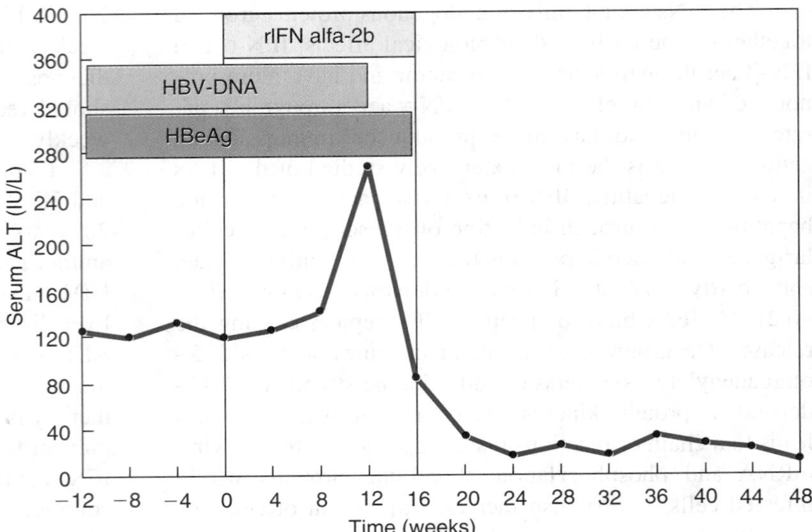

Figure 40.3. Typical biochemical response to IFN-α in a patient with chronic hepatitis B. *(Adapted from Lambiase L, Davis GL. Treatment of chronic hepatitis. Gastroenterol Clin North Am 1992;21:659–677, with permission.)*

Use of IFN in patients with cirrhosis is controversial. These patients appear to respond to IFN at rates similar to those with less advanced disease, however, IFN side effects are more common and severe—even life-threatening.[52] Extreme caution must be used in treating patients with cirrhosis with IFN and should be attempted only in those patients with mild or early decompensation. Therapy should be closely supervised.

Interestingly, IFN therapy alone has little benefit in most Chinese patients with HBV infection.[55] This is related to immunologic tolerance to HBV induced by exposure to the virus early in life.[55]

Patients with HBV in whom IFN should not be used include those whose liver disease has progressed to end stage (very low serum albumin, prolonged prothrombin time, elevated bilirubin, leukopenia, thrombocytopenia, bleeding esophageal varices, ascites, encephalopathy, and/or progressive jaundice), those with liver disease of other causes, patients on immunosuppressive therapy, patients actively abusing drugs, those with significant psychiatric illness, and those with significant other medical illnesses such as cardiac, renal, or thyroid disease that are not successfully treated.[54]

There are several patient groups with chronic HBV in whom IFN therapy has not been adequately studied. These include patients whose infection is secondary to a precore mutant virus, children, individuals coinfected with HIV, and those with decompensated liver disease. The place of IFN in therapy of these groups of patients awaits the results of clinical trials.

In chronic delta hepatitis high-dose IFN-α treatment (5 MU daily or 9 MU three times weekly for at least 12 months) produces disease improvement in about 50% of patients.[30,56] Unfortunately, relapse is common when therapy is stopped and these patients have a high rate of drug-related adverse effects necessitating dosage reduction or termination of therapy.[42] Prolonged IFN therapy may be necessary to achieve a sustained response. IFN has not been specifically approved for use in chronic HDV. Use of IFN should be limited to those patients who have elevated aminotransferases, HBsAg and anti-HDV in serum, HDVAg in liver, and either CAH or active cirrhosis.[30]

The long-term effectiveness of IFNs in chronic hepatitis C is unclear, but recent reports suggest that IFN-α therapy can lead to complete eradication of HCV infection in long-term responders.[57] IFN-α-2b at a dose of 3 MU three times weekly for 24 weeks is approved for treatment of chronic hepatitis C. One-third to one-half of treated patients improve (aminotransferase levels normalize, hepatic inflammation improves, HCV RNA becomes undetectable), but approximately 50% of responders relapse within 6 months when therapy is discontinued.[58–61] Longer treatment periods do not lower relapse rates. Relapse correlates with a return of HCV RNA. The time course of response to IFN-α in chronic HCV is given in Fig. 40.4.[50] Retreatment of initial responders who relapse after discontinuing therapy will usually result in response. IFN is most effective in those patients without clinically advanced chronic liver disease. Questions about optimum dosage, treatment timing, duration of treatment, the risk-to-benefit ratio, and the cost effectiveness of retreatment remain.[9]

Endpoints of therapy with IFN use in chronic HCV are not clear. It is controversial whether or not a decline in anti-HCV can be used to monitor response to therapy. ALT normalization and disappearance of HCV RNA in serum are useful monitoring parameters, however, normalization or disappearance does not provide certainty that a response will be maintained. Measurement of disappearance of HCV RNA in liver tissue is promising.

In contrast to chronic HBV, where IFN acts as an immunostimulant, in chronic HCV IFN inhibits HCV replication directly.[9] Typically, patients who respond to IFN

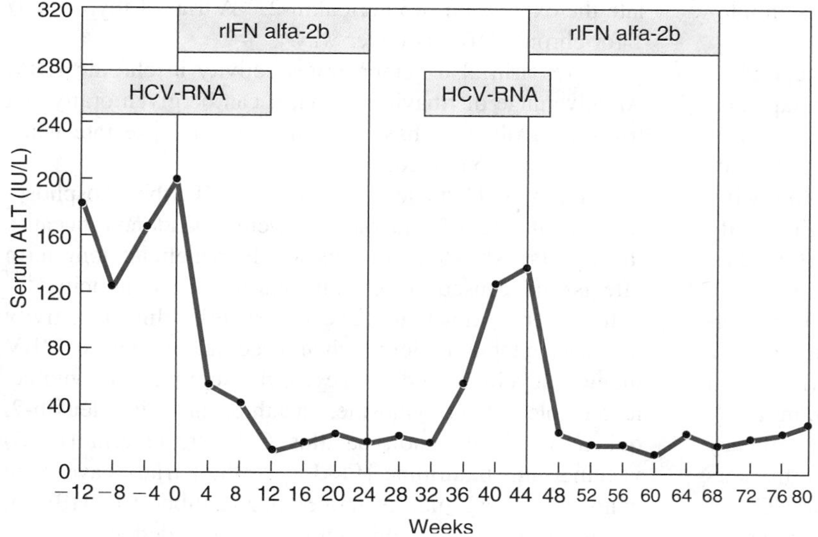

Figure 40.4. Typical biochemical response to IFN-α in a patient with chronic hepatitis C. *(From Lambiase L, Davis GL. Treatment of chronic hepatitis. Gastroenterol Clin North Am 1992;21:659–677, with permission.)*

treatment have a rapid decrease in ALT levels. In chronic HBV, IFN responders have a transient increase in ALT during the second to third month of therapy (Figs. 40.3 and 40.4).[50] Also in contrast to chronic HBV, little has been clarified regarding predictors of response to IFN therapy in chronic HCV. One study suggests that low pretreatment gamma glutamyltransferase activity, absence of obesity, and absence of cirrhosis are predictive of response.[61] Another suggests that intermittent IFN administration after daily IFN and chronic persistent or mild chronic aggressive hepatitis on liver biopsy prior to treatment correlate with response to IFN.[62] An intriguing research area is that genotypic variability and/or genomic hypervariability of HCV contributes to different response rates to IFN.[9]

There are many patient groups with chronic HCV in whom IFN has not yet been studied. These include patients with clinically unstable disease, children, those with decompensated liver disease, and the immunosuppressed. For the present time, IFN therapy for chronic HCV should be offered at least to those in whom disease symptoms are disabling, those in whom the disease is histologically advanced, patients with rapidly progressive disease and those with markedly elevated aminotransferase levels. IFN should not be used in patients with evidence of hepatic decompensation (hepatic encephalopathy, variceal bleeding, ascites, serum bilirubin concentration >3 mg/dL, low serum albumin, prolonged prothrombin time, leukopenia, and thrombocytopenia).

The cost of a 6-month course of IFN-α-2b 3 MU three times weekly is $1900 (based on average wholesale price).[63] This cost must be balanced against the risk, the chance of response, and the expected consequences of untreated chronic hepatitis along with the fact that the optimal dose, duration, and combination of therapy are poorly defined. Recent cost–benefit analyses of IFN in chronic HCV suggests that, if IFN can reduce the costs of disease progression by 30% or more, it is cost effective based on medical costs alone.[64,65]

The side effects of IFN are frequent enough that the patient should be informed about them before treatment begins. Early side effects include fatigue, malaise, muscle aches, headaches, changes in appetite, fever, chills, nausea, and sleep disturbance.[49,66] Premedication with acetaminophen will ameliorate the flu-like symptoms. Severity decreases with subsequent injections.[66] Late adverse reactions include those previously mentioned plus mild myelosuppression, bacterial infection, weight loss, loss of libido, thyroiditis, alopecia, IFN-induced autoimmune hepatitis (very rarely), exacerbation of other autoimmune phenomena, development of a variety of autoantibodies (e.g., antinuclear antibody, smooth muscle antibody, or antibody to thyroid microsomal antigen), irritability, anxiety, depression, attention span deficits, seizures, psychosis, delirium, and, most commonly, fatigue.[12] Thrombocytopenia and granulocytopenia are more common in those patients with cirrhosis and hypersplenism. IFN therapy induces the formation of IFN antibody, but the clinical significance is controversial. Patients with a preexisting autoimmune disorder should be treated with IFN with extreme caution because IFN can exacerbate the autoimmune disease. The psychiatric complications are especially severe in those with severe liver disease, occur in up to 20% of patients, and are the most common dose-limiting side effects.[47,66] IFN should be discontinued if serious complications occur. Reassuring the patient and family that these are therapy related and will disappear when therapy is stopped is important.

Several drugs can potentially interact with IFN. Examples include theophylline (increased theophylline concentration), zidovudine (enhanced hematologic toxicity), vidarabine (vidarabine-induced neurotoxicity), and cytotoxic agents (increased myelosuppression). Careful review of, and evaluation for, drug interactions with IFN is an integral part of monitoring IFN therapy.

Ongoing monitoring of IFN toxicity includes complete blood counts weekly during the first 2 weeks of therapy and monthly thereafter. Patients should be asked about level of performance, mood changes, and symptoms. The dose of IFN should be decreased by 50% if any of the following develop: fatigue that interferes with the daily routine, daily nausea with occasional vomiting, granulocytopenia (less than 750/mm^3), and/or thrombocytopenia (less than 50,000/mm^3). IFN should be immediately discontinued if any of the following develop: fatigue that requires bed rest, vomiting more than twice daily, profound granulocytopenia (less than 500/mm^3), or thrombocytopenia (less than 30,000/mm^3).[51]

Pre- and post-therapy monitoring for IFN efficacy includes liver biopsy, concentrations of serum markers (HCV RNA and anti-HCV in treatment of chronic HCV or HBeAG, HBsAg, HBV DNA, and anti-HBs in treatment of chronic HBV), and serum thyrotropin. Serum markers can also be followed during therapy. Other laboratory monitoring includes aminotransferases, prothrombin time, alkaline phosphatase, albumin, and bilirubin concentrations before therapy, monthly for the first 3 months of therapy, and then every 2 months.

Corticosteroids, Antiviral Agents, and Immunostimulants

Corticosteroids were initially studied in chronic HBV infection because such therapy had proven beneficial in autoimmune hepatitis.[47] However, controlled trials show corticosteroids to be harmful in most patients with chronic hepatitis B.[67,68] Corticosteroids lead to reduced hepatic inflammation, but also result in dramatic increases in viral replication. In addition, withdrawal of the steroids causes a flare in hepatitis disease activity. Thus, corticosteroids can cause further decompensation and death in patients with clinically unstable disease. Corticosteroid treatment can also worsen disease activity in patients with cirrhosis secondary to HBV and should not be used in such patients.[37]

Certain patients (Chinese patients and those patients with mild disease and low levels of HBV DNA) can be exceptions to the above relative contraindication. These "exception" patients can be tried on a 4- to 8-week tapering course of prednisone (e.g., decreasing daily doses of 60, 40, and 20 mg, each for 2 weeks) followed by IFN-α 3 to 5 MU daily for 16 weeks.[48,49] This short course of prednisone acts as an "immunologic conditioner" in such patients.[49]

Corticosteroids have not been used successfully in chronic hepatitis C or delta hepatitis.[69]

Many other therapies have been studied for chronic viral hepatitis (see Table 40.3). Both thymosin and AM-3, a biologic response modifier, have activity in chronic HBV.[9] Thymosins are hormone-like polypeptides that regulate the maturation of T cells, modulate IFN production, and stimulate the expression of interleukin-2.[70] A trial of thymosin α 1 for chronic HBV is under way.

Ribavirin also demonstrates activity in chronic HBV. An advantage of ribavirin is that it can be given orally. All trials with ribavirin have shown a high relapse rate when therapy is discontinued.[71]

Trials with vidarabine and ara-AMP (the phosphorylated analogue of vidarabine) were abandoned because the agents exhibited no consistently beneficial long-term effects and caused significant neuromuscular toxicity.[42,47] Other agents shown to have either little clinical activity or unacceptable toxicity when used alone against HBV include acyclovir, 6-deoxyacyclovir, suramin, zidovudine, levamisole, dideoxyinosine, azathioprine, interleukin-2, quinacrine, cyanidanol, bacillus Calmette–Guérin (BCG) vaccine, and fialuridine (FIAU).[9,42] Pilot trials have been conducted using murine monoclonal antibody to HBsAg, but the usefulness of this antibody is not defined.

Antiviral agents have, in general, not been useful alone in chronic hepatitis C. Short-term treatment with ribavirin induces a decrease in serum aminotransferases, but response persists only until therapy is discontinued. Studies with thymosin are under way. The greatest potential use for these agents may be in combination therapy with IFN. Combination therapy could potentially allow reduction of IFN dose and decrease IFN side effects.

Combination Therapy

In chronic HBV, regimens involving combination antiviral chemotherapy or combinations of antiviral plus immunomodulating agents (e.g., prednisone and IFN, as previously discussed) have been studied with the hope that synergistic or additive effects would be seen (Table 40.3).[42] Cyclooxygenase inhibitors have also been studied in combination with IFN to boost the arachidonic acid pathway-mediated effects of IFN.[9]

Many combinations of therapeutic agents show promise for the treatment of chronic HBV. This is not true for all combinations, however. Levamisole plus lymphoblastoid IFN is associated with a lower rate of response than IFN alone.[70] Nevertheless, combining therapeutic agents to treat chronic HBV is one of the most promising areas of therapy.

In chronic HCV, the possible role of IFN plus ribavirin or other antiviral agents has not been defined. Preliminary evidence suggests that prednisolone pretreatment reduces cumulative relapse rate with IFN treatment.[70] These results require confirmation.

Liver Transplantation

Liver transplantation is an option for patients with end-stage chronic liver disease secondary to viral infection. Recurrent viral hepatitis B infection in the transplanted liver almost always occurs.[38] The primary strategy to protect the

TABLE 40.3. DRUG THERAPY FOR CHRONIC HBV INFECTION

Agent	Status
Immunologic	
IFN-α	Therapy of choice; approved
IFN-β, -γ	Possibly effective if started within 4 years of infection
Corticosteroids	Little to no role in primary therapy (see text)
Thymosin	Undergoing evaluation; preliminary data promising
Levamisole	Conflicting data
Transfer factor	No role in therapy
Autolymphocyte therapy	Phase I trials in progress
Interleukin-2	Undergoing evaluation; preliminary data promising
Antiviral	
Acyclovir	Partially effective
Adenine arabinoside monophosphate (ara-AMP)	Toxicity outweighs clinical benefit
Suramin	Toxicity outweighs clinical benefit
Vidarabine	Toxicity outweighs clinical benefit
Fialuridine	Toxicity outweighs clinical benefit
Ribavirin	Somewhat effective; less effective than IFN
Foscarnet	Little data
Ganciclovir	Little data
Zidovudine	Little data
Lamivudine	Little data
Quinacrine	Little data
(+) -cyanidanol-3	Little data
Dideoxynucleosides	Little data
Erythromycin 9-0 methyloxime	Little data
Combination Therapy	
IFN + ara-A	Little added benefit over IFN alone; increased toxicity
IFN + ara-AMP	Toxicity outweighs clinical benefit
IFN-α + IFN-γ	Little data
Prednisone + ara-A	Toxicity outweighs clinical benefit
Prednisone + ara-AMP	Toxicity outweighs clinical benefit
Prednisone + IFN	Useful in selected patients (see text)
Prednisolone + ara-A + IFN	Little data
Acyclovir + IFN; deoxyacyclovir + IFN	Little added benefit over IFN alone
Prednisone + acyclovir	Little data
Levamisole + IFN	Little data

(Compiled from Refs. 53 and 69.)

graft from reinfection is to transplant HBV DNA negative patients and then treat them for life with HBIG.[72] Further trials are necessary to confirm the effectiveness of this approach. IFN is of little value. Transplanting HBV DNA and/or HBeAg positive patients is not routine because these patients have a more aggressive postoperative course and a lower 1-year survival rate.[54] This area is controversial, and some believe that liver transplant in HBV patients should only be done in the context of prospective clinical studies.[72] Hepatitis B reinfection in the graft results in a characteristic histologic lesion known as fibrosing cholestatic hepatitis.[9] Why HBV infection is so devastating in liver transplant recipients is an active area of research.

In liver transplantation for end-stage chronic HCV disease, HCV–RNA persists in the great majority of patients with pretransplant RNA positivity.[9] However, data on the clinical impact of HCV infection in the transplanted liver are limited, and patients with chronic hepatitis C and liver decompensation are considered candidates for liver transplantation.

Hepatitis D infection recurs in the majority of patients who receive liver transplant.

Prevention of Viral Hepatitis

The mainstays of hepatitis prevention are risk reduction, education, passive immunization with immune globulins, and, for hepatitis B, active immunization through vaccination programs.[73] The spread of HAV can be controlled by cautious handling of fomites contaminated with feces coupled with good handwashing techniques. Universal precautions are used to prevent hepatitis spread within the hospital setting. HBV and HCV spread are reduced, but not eliminated, through screening of blood donors and testing for HBsAg and anti-HCV.

HEPATITIS A PREVENTION

Prevention of HAV has traditionally focused on avoiding exposure as well as preexposure and postexposure prophylaxis with immune globulin (IG). The importance of avoiding exposure through good handwashing and good personal hygienic practices cannot be overemphasized. IG is effective in modifying the course and preventing the spread of HAV.[2] IG contains antibodies against the hepatitis A virus (anti-HAV) and the HBsAg (anti-HBs). International travelers are the major group receiving preexposure prophylaxis with IG.[2] The risk of hepatitis varies with the incidence of hepatitis A from country to country, living conditions, and length of stay. IG is recommended for all susceptible persons traveling to developing countries. The CDC publication, *Health Information for International Travel,* should be consulted for specific recommendations. Travelers can minimize risk by avoiding uncooked shellfish, uncooked fruits and vegetables, and by avoiding drinking water (and other beverages with ice) of unknown purity.

A single dose of IG of 0.02 mL/kg intramuscularly (IM) is recommended if travel is for less than 3 months. For lengthy stays, 0.06 mL/kg IM should be given every 3 to 5 months. Dosing is the same for adults and children. Screening for total anti-HAV prior to travel is useful to eliminate unnecessary doses of IG for immune individuals who would otherwise require repeated IG prophylaxis. People who need repeat doses while overseas should use products that meet the U.S. standards for purity.

The postexposure prophylactic benefit from IG is greatest early in the incubation period and is of no benefit more than 2 weeks after exposure.[2] Serologic screening of contacts for anti-HAV is not recommended before IG administration because such screening is costly and delays prophylaxis.

A single IG dose of 0.02 mL/kg IM is used for postexposure prophylaxis of hepatitis A. Some groups recommended to receive postexposure prophylaxis are listed in Table 40.4.[2]

Unfortunately, the use of IG has had little impact on the incidence of hepatitis A in the United States.[1] For this reason, data are awaited on the short- and long-term clinical impact of the hepatitis A vaccine.

An inactivated HAV vaccine, Havrix (SmithKline Beecham), was marketed in early 1995. This vaccine demonstrates protective efficacy in at least 94% of vaccines within 1 month after vaccination.[74–77] Live, attenuated vaccines have also been developed, but their efficacy has not been fully defined.[75] Havrix is indicated for immunization of individuals 2 years of age or greater who are at increased risk of hepatitis A infection.[78] Much controversy surrounds who should receive this vaccine. Current recommendations include that the vaccination should be offered to individuals in high-risk groups. Groups considered at increased risk of infection with hepatitis A are listed in Table 40.5.[78] Sewage workers could possibly be added to these increased risk groups.

TABLE 40.4. GROUPS RECOMMENDED FOR POSTEXPOSURE PROPHYLAXIS OF HEPATITIS A

Household or sexual contacts
Staff and children in day care centers where cases of hepatitis A are diagnosed (or identified in households of children attending the center)
Members of households that have children in diapers attending a day care center where cases of hepatitis A are identified
Residents and staff of prisons and facilities for developmentally disabled
Hospital personnel exposed to feces of infected patients
Food handlers and patrons of restaurants if the (1) infected food handler is directly involved in handling foods, without gloves, that will not be cooked; (2) source has deficient hygienic practices; and (3) exposed patrons can be identified and treated within 2 weeks of exposure

(Modified from Ref. 2.)

Approved dosing for hepatitis A vaccine in adults is a single dose of 1440 enzyme-linked immunosorbent assay units (ELU)/mL injected intramuscularly into the deltoid muscle followed by a booster dose 6 to 12 months after the primary immunization to prolong protection. The primary immunization should be given at least 2 weeks prior to expected exposure to HAV. For children, the primary immunization is two doses, each containing 360 ELU/0.5 mL, given 1 month apart. A booster dose is given 6 to 12 months later. The vaccine can be given at the same time as a wide variety of other vaccines without interfering with the immune responses. Each vaccine should be given with a different syringe and at a different injection site. Havrix can be given concomitantly with IG; however, the antibody titer ultimately obtained is likely to be lower than when the vaccine is given alone.

The inactivated vaccine has generally mild side effects. These include local reactions at the injection site (soreness, induration, redness, and swelling), headache, fatigue, fever, and GI upset.[77]

Many questions remain about where and when hepatitis A vaccination should be used. For example: (1) Young children generally have a clinically insignificant illness when infected with hepatitis A (yet children with asymptomatic hepatitis A serve as reservoirs for infecting others). (2) The incidence of hepatitis A in the United States is low (thus, should the vaccine even be offered to some of the

TABLE 40.5. PEOPLE AT INCREASED RISK OF HEPATITIS A INFECTION

Persons traveling to areas of high endemicity for hepatitis A[a]
Residents of a community experiencing an outbreak of hepatitis A
Military personnel
Persons engaging in high-risk sexual activity (including bisexual and homosexual males)
Native peoples of Alaska and the Americas
Users of illicit injectable drugs
Institutional workers, such as caretakers for the developmentally disabled
Employees of child day care centers
Laboratory workers who handle live hepatitis A virus
Handlers of primate animals that may be harboring HAV
People living in, or relocating to, areas of high endemicity

[a]Africa, Asia (except Japan), the Mediterranean basin, Eastern Europe, the Middle East, Central and South America, Mexico, and parts of the Caribbean. (From Ref. 78.)

high-risk groups, such as day care providers, in the absence of a hepatitis A outbreak?). (3) For some groups it is more cost effective to screen for antibodies to hepatitis A before administering the vaccine (the vaccine cost is approximately $40 per dose).

At Kaiser Permanente of Colorado, Aurora, guidelines for the prevention of hepatitis A in travelers have been developed and implemented.[79] The guidelines have received the most widespread use within the International Travel Clinic. These guidelines include recommendations to screen for prior exposure to hepatitis A in those individuals 40 years of age or greater, in individuals born in a country of high endemicity for hepatitis A, and in frequent travelers. The incidence of protective antibodies against hepatitis A in our patient population is such that screening is cost effective in these groups of individuals. For a patient who is traveling within 2 weeks of initially contacting the Travel Clinic, it is recommended that he or she receive IG, and the patient is counseled to contact the Travel Clinic with more advanced notice before future travel. If the traveler contacts us within 2 weeks of travel and will be traveling for more than 3 months, the patient is offered both IG and the first dose of hepatitis A vaccine. In all cases, it is important to counsel the patient about receiving the booster dose 6 to 12 months after the primary series, as well as to talk with the patient about food and water precautions.

Questions also remain about whether long-term (several decades) immunity is induced by the vaccine. It is unknown whether protective immunity persists into adulthood when an individual is immunized as a child. Other questions include whether vaccination should simply be universally recommended (especially if long-term data continue to document the safety of the vaccine) or whether use should be encouraged only for high-risk groups (Table 40.5). In addition, the place of the vaccine in postexposure prophylaxis has yet to be determined.

To lower substantially the incidence of hepatitis A in the United States, immunization of infants and young children would be necessary. However, the currently licensed vaccine is approved for use only in people 2 years of age or older. For people less than 2 years of age, the only option is passive immunization with IG. The very young can therefore continue to serve as reservoirs of infection. Initial vaccination efforts focus on selective preexposure immunization of "high-risk" groups.[74] Cost-effectiveness analyses are necessary to determine the final place of the vaccine in prevention of HAV.

HEPATITIS B PREVENTION

Two products are available for prevention of hepatitis B infection: hepatitis B vaccine, which provides active immunity, and HBIG, which provides temporary passive immunity.[2]

The goals of immunization against viral hepatitis include prevention of (1) the short-term viremia that can lead to transmission of infection, (2) clinical disease, and (3) chronic HBV infection.[80,81] Vaccination remains the most effective method for reaching these goals. The vaccine is used in preexposure prophylaxis in risk groups, and in postexposure prophylaxis in combination with HBIG.[32]

HBIG

HBIG is used only in postexposure prophylaxis. Postexposure prophylaxis for HBV is recommended for perinatal exposure of infants of HBV-carrier mothers, sexual exposure to HBsAg-positive persons, accidental percutaneous or permucosal exposure to HBsAg-positive blood, and exposure of an infant to a caregiver who has acute hepatitis B.[2] HBIG should be given to immunocompromised patients for the same indications and in the same doses as immunocompetent individuals.[82] The recommended dose is 0.06 mL/kg administered intramuscularly. Guidelines for use are listed in Tables 40.6 and 40.7.[2,83]

Use of IG for prophylaxis of HBV infection is only recommended when HBIG is not available. IG contains anti-HBs in titers of 1:100 to 1:1000, in comparison to the 1:100,000 or greater anti-HBs titer found in HBIG.[84] IG and HBIG available in the United States do not transmit HBV, HIV, or other viruses.

Hepatitis B Vaccine

In 1982 a plasma-derived vaccine against HBV was licensed in the United States. This vaccine has since been replaced by two recombinant vaccines: Recombivax HB (Merck Sharp & Dohme) and Engerix-B (SmithKline Beecham). The immune responses and safety profiles of the vaccines are comparable,[2] although higher antibody levels

TABLE 40.6. RECOMMENDED SCHEDULE OF IMMUNOPROPHYLAXIS TO PREVENT PERINATAL OR SEXUAL TRANSMISSION OF HBV INFECTION

Vaccine Recipient	Immunoprophylaxis	Timing
Infant born to HBsAg-positive mother	Vaccine dose 1	Within 12 hours of birth
	HBIG[a]	Within 12 hours of birth
	Vaccine doses 2 and 3[b]	Usual schedule
Infant born to mother not screened for HBsAg	Vaccine dose 1[c]	Within 12 hours of birth
	HBIG	If mother is found to be HBsAg-positive, administer dose to infant as soon as possible, but no later than 1 week after birth
	Vaccine doses 2 and 3[b]	Usual schedule
Sexual exposure	HBIG[d]	Single dose within 14 days of sexual contact
	Vaccine dose 1	At time of HBIG treatment[e]

[a]0.5 ml, intramuscularly, at a site different from that used for the vaccine.
[b]The four-dose schedule for Engerix-B can also be used.
[c]The first dose of vaccine is the same as that for the infant of an HBsAg-positive mother. If the mother is found to be HBsAg-positive, that dose is continued. If the mother is found to be HBsAg-negative, the remaining vaccine doses are those appropriate for other infants and children.
[d]0.06 mL/kg intramuscularly.
[e]The first dose can be given at the same time as the HBIG dose but in a different site; subsequent doses should be given as recommended in Table 40.8. (Adapted, in part, from Refs. 2 and 82.)

are obtained with Engerix-B in people over 40 years of age. Hepatitis B vaccines contain 5–40 g HBsAg protein per mL adsorbed onto aluminum per mL of vaccine, with thimerosal added as preservative.[2] Side effects of the vaccine are soreness at the injection site, headache, fatigue, and fever. The number of patients experiencing these adverse reactions decreases with each vaccine dose, and adverse reactions are less common in infants and children than in adults. A possible association between Guillain–Barré syndrome and the plasma-derived vaccine was found in adults. This has not been found with the recombinant vaccine. The hepatitis B vaccine is contraindicated in patients with anaphylaxis to common baker's yeast. The vaccine does not transmit HIV.[85]

The dose of HBsAg to induce the desired antibody response/protective effect varies between the two available

TABLE 40.7. RECOMMENDATIONS FOR HEPATITIS B PROPHYLAXIS FOLLOWING PERCUTANEOUS OR PERMUCOSAL EXPOSURE

	Treatment When Source Is Found to Be:		
Exposed Person	HBsAg-Positive	HBsAg-Negative	Source Not Tested or Unknown
Unvaccinated	HBIG × 1[a] and initiate HB vaccine[b]	Initiate HB vaccine[b]	Initiate HB vaccine[b]
Previously vaccinated			
Known responder	Test exposed for anti-HBs 1. If adequate,[c] no treatment 2. If inadequate, HB vaccine booster dose	No treatment	No treatment
Known nonresponder	HBIG × 2 or HBIG × 1 plus 1 dose HB vaccine	No treatment	If known high-risk source, may treat as if source were HBsAg-positive
Response unknown	Test exposed for anti-HBs 1. If inadequate,[c] HBIG × 1 plus HB vaccine booster dose 2. If adequate, no treatment	No treatment	Test exposed for anti-HBs 1. If inadequate,[c] HB vaccine booster dose 2. If adequate, no treatment

[a]HBIG dose 0.06 mL/kg IM.
[b]HB vaccine dose; see Table 40.8.
[c]Adequate anti-HBs is ≥10 sample ratio units by radioimmunoassay or enzyme immunoassay. (Modified from Ref. 2.)

TABLE 40.8. RECOMMENDED DOSES AND SCHEDULES OF CURRENTLY LICENSED HB VACCINES

Group	Vaccine	
	Recombivax HB[a] dose, μg (mL)	**Engerix-B[a,b] dose, μg (mL)**
Infants of HBsAg-positive mothers	Adult formulation: 5 (0.5) Pediatric formulation: 5 (1)[c]	10 (0.5)
Other infants and children <11 years	Adult formulation: 2.5 (0.25) Pediatric formulation: 2.5 (0.5)[c]	10 (0.5)
Children and adolescents 11–19 years	5 (0.5)	20 (1.0)
Adults >19 years	10 (1.0)	20 (1.0)
Dialysis patients and other immunocompromised persons	40 (1.0)[d]	40 (2.0)[e,f]

[a]Usual schedules: three doses given at 0, 1, and 6 months or, for infants, with other routine immunizations at 2, 4, and 6 months.
[b]Alternative schedule: four doses at 0, 1, 2, and 12 months.
[c]A special pediatric formulation of Recombivax HB is available that contains 5 μg/ml.
[d]Special formulation for dialysis patients.
[e]Two 1.0-mL doses given at different sites.
[f]Four-dose schedule recommended at 0, 1, 2, and 6 months. (Modified from Ref. 82.)

vaccines (Table 40.8).[83] HBV vaccine is given as a series of three IM doses into the deltoid (anterolateral thigh in infants), given over a period of months. A pediatric formulation is available that contains 5 μg/mL. Specific dosing guidelines for all age groups are listed in Tables 40.8 and 40.9.[83] An alternate four-dose schedule is approved for Engerix-B (0, 1, 2, 12 months). All dosing schedules (birth, 1, 6 months; birth, 1, 2 months; birth, 2, 4 months; birth, 2, 6 months; 2, 4, 6 months) give excellent seroconversion rates, although the postvaccination titer is higher with longer intervals between the second and third dose.[86] In addition, the vaccine can be given with doses administered at even longer intervals with equal protection attained, and the vaccination process need not be restarted because of missed doses.[2] Dosing guidelines for infants born to HBsAg-positive mothers and mothers whose HBsAg status is unknown are given in Table 40.6.[83] Premature infants born to a HBsAg-positive mothers should receive hepatitis B vaccine and HBIG beginning at or shortly after birth. Premature infants of HBsAg-negative mothers should be immunized at the same chronologic age as term infants. Partial protection is achieved after the second dose.[1] The vaccination series can be started with one vaccine type and completed with another.[87]

Hepatitis B vaccines are inactivated and can be simultaneously administered with other vaccines.[2] Breastfed infants can be vaccinated with hepatitis B vaccine, as can immunocompromised infants and children.[82,87] The three-dose vaccination series induces an adequate anti-HBs response in more than 90% of healthy adults and more than 95% of infants and children.[2] An adequate response is defined as anti-HBs of 10 mIU/mL or greater, which is approximately equal to 10 sample ratio units (SRU), measured 1 to 6 months after completion of the vaccine series.[2] Low responders (10–100 mIU/mL), as well as those with good response (greater than or equal to 100 mIU/mL) have complete protection against clinical infection with the virus.

Persistence of anti-HBs is directly related to the height of the antibody response.[80] The level of circulating antibody declines dramatically during the first year after vaccination.[81] Up to 50% of responders lose detectable antibody within 7 years, but immunologic memory and protection against viremia and clinical illness persist for at least 10 years in immunocompetent individuals.[88,89]

Host factors, immunization factors, and the characteristics of the vaccine itself affect the immunogenicity of hepatitis B vaccines.[1,2,81,85] Factors that diminish vaccine immunogenicity include smoking, increased age, and increased body mass.

Postvaccination testing for immunity is not routinely done. It is recommended for those whose management depends on their immune status and those in whom a suboptimal response is expected.[1,2] Examples include

TABLE 40.9. RECOMMENDED SCHEDULE FOR ROUTINE HEPATITIS B VACCINATION OF INFANTS AND CHILDREN

Hepatitis B Vaccination[a]	At Birth (Before Hospital Discharge)	1–2 Months	4 Months	6–18 Months
Option 1[b]	X	X		X
Option 2[b]		X	X	X

[a]For use among infants born to HBsAg-negative mothers. The first dose should be administered during the newborn period, no later than age 2 months. Premature infants of HBsAg-negative mothers should receive the first dose of the hepatitis B vaccine series at the time of hospital discharge or when the other routine childhood vaccines are initiated. (All infants born to HBsAg-positive mothers should receive immunoprophylaxis for hepatitis B as soon as possible after birth.)
[b] Hepatitis B vaccine can be administered simultaneously at the same visit with DTP (or DTaP), OPV, Hib, and/or MMR. (Modified from Ref. 82.)

hemodialysis patients, HIV-infected patients, certain public safety personnel, smokers, the extremely obese, and those who receive intradermal vaccine administration.[2,90] Testing for peak anti-HBs should be conducted 1 to 3 months after completion of the vaccine series to determine if a response occurred and to evaluate the need for booster dose(s).[85]

Healthy nonresponders are not at increased risk of becoming chronic carriers when infected with HBV. Such individuals have a normal reaction after infection.

Timing and need for booster doses are controversial. It is clear that nonresponders and inadequate responders should be immediately revaccinated with one or two injections of vaccine (Table 40.10).[2,81] Up to 50% of nonresponders will develop anti-HBs after two additional doses of vaccine,[2,91] although the level of antibody achieved is low. Inadequate responders should receive at least one booster 1 to 2 years after the basic immunization,[81] and low responders should receive boosters every 1 to 2 years.[85]

The extent of long-term protection in vaccine responders remains controversial.[81] On average, 35% of healthy adults who initially respond to the vaccine have antibody levels of less than 10 mIU/mL (the level below which protection against HBV is uncertain) by 5 years after vaccination.[88,89,92] However, these persons promptly respond to booster doses.[81,92] The few vaccine responders who develop serologic evidence of HBV infection do not have detectable HBsAg or clinical hepatitis.[2,85,88] In addition, cohort- and population-based studies demonstrate that persons immunized against HBV retain protective immune response for up to 10 years, even if antibody is undetectable.[75] Additional data are necessary to define recommendations for appropriate booster dosing in vaccine responders.[2,93] It is not yet known whether an initial infant hepatitis B immunization series confers lifelong immunity, however, data from long-term studies indicate that the vast majority of vaccine responders continue to be protected from both symptomatic and chronic HBV infection.[94]

Immunocompromised adults can receive hepatitis B vaccine when indicated. Hemodialysis patients have decreased seroconversion rates, decreased antibody titers to surface antigens, and a faster rate of loss of antibody after HBV vaccination.[85] These patients require higher vaccine doses or an increased number of doses.[82] A special formulation of Recombivax HB (40 µg/mL) is available for these patients. A more rapid rise in antibody concentration is observed with a 0-, 1-, 2-, and 6-month vaccination schedule in these patients, although overall conversion rate is similar whether the final (fourth) dose is given 6 or 12 months after the series begins.[95] Protection in this group is maintained only as long as the anti-HBs level remains above 10 mIU.[1] Routine anti-HBs testing (at 12-month intervals) and booster doses to maintain adequate anti-HBs are recommended in hemodialysis patients.[2] Patients with renal disease who will likely need dialysis or transplantation should also receive hepatitis B vaccination.

Vaccine response is reduced to less than 70% in males infected with HIV,[96] even in those in early stages of the infection.[85,97] Nonresponders and inadequate responders are unlikely to respond to revaccination.[96] HIV-infected patients are prone to have an impaired response to HBV infection and are more likely to become chronic carriers.[73,96] Testing for antibody response is recommended, with notification of nonresponders of the potential consequences (infection, carrier state, delta virus superinfection).[96]

Other immunosuppressed groups with decreased response to HBV vaccine include alcoholics with clinical liver disease and patients with hematologic malignancies, organ transplants, diabetes, or hemophilia.[85]

The vaccine is safe in chronic carriers, but ineffective in eliminating HBsAg.[88] Antibody acquired from HBIG or IG administration or via the placenta will not interfere with development of active immunity[2]; for example, HBIG can be administered concomitantly with the first dose of vaccine.[85]

Groups Recommended for Preexposure Vaccination

The primary eradication strategy for hepatitis B is routine infant vaccination, which, over several decades, could eliminate transmission of the virus. There is little immediate impact on the incidence of clinical hepatitis B. That effect will become apparent only when those vaccinated as infants become adolescents and young adults. However, this vaccination strategy almost immediately has an impact on the number of new HBV carriers and reduces the chance for chronic liver disease.

TABLE 40.10. GUIDELINES FOR BOOSTER DOSE INOCULATIONS FOLLOWING HEPATITIS B IMMUNIZATION

Type of Response	Anti-HBs Level (IU/L)	Booster Dose Recommendations
Nonresponse	Negative	Immediate
Inadequate response	<10	Immediate
Low response	10–100	1–2 years
Good or adequate response	>100	5–10 years or none

(From Hollinger FB. Immunogenicity of a yeast-derived hepatitis B vaccine in hemodialysis patients. Am J Med 1989;87 (suppl 3A):38S, with permission.)

Routine infant vaccination raises issues relative to vaccine cost. At the current cost of the vaccine ($22 to $40 per infant vaccination series; about $100 per adult vaccination series), hepatitis B could be eventually eliminated from the United States at a cost of about $120 million per year, compared with an estimated annual cost of $750 million for treating persons who contract the disease.[98] This is the cost justification used as the basis for the CDC recommendation of routine infant vaccination. Others, on the basis of a cost-effectiveness analysis, recommend a strategy of screening pregnant women for active HBV infection and vaccinating babies born to mothers with positive screening tests combined with routine vaccination of 10-year-old children.[99] Both approaches are currently used (and debated) in the United States.

In countries such as the United States, where the risk of hepatitis B is relatively low, determination of whom to vaccinate prior to exposure depends on the risk of infection in that group and the relative cost of pretesting versus the cost of vaccination.[2,85] Cost–benefit analyses favor vaccination for high-risk groups.[2] The groups currently recommended for preexposure vaccination are listed in Table 40.11.[2] Everyone in high-risk, low-prevalence groups (such as health professionals in training) can be vaccinated without screening.[2,85] To comply with federal guidelines, health care workers with potential exposure to blood are offered hepatitis B vaccination at no cost by their employers.

For vaccination to have an impact on the incidence of hepatitis B in the United States, the vaccine must be provided to patients before they are placed at increased risk of acquiring the virus.[2] Unfortunately, selective adult immunization (the strategy used during the first several years of vaccine availability) failed to lower the rate of infection. This led to the comprehensive vaccination strategy now in place, which targets interruption of transmission at all age groups through routine infant immunization, continued vaccination of high-risk adolescents and adults, and routine screening of pregnant women for HBsAg.

TABLE 40.11. HIGH-RISK GROUPS RECOMMENDED FOR PREEXPOSURE HEPATITIS B VACCINATION[a]

Health care and public safety workers who have occupational exposure to blood
Parenteral drug abusers
Individuals with multiple sexual partners (homosexual, bisexual, or heterosexual)
Hemodialysis patients
Recipients of certain blood products, i.e., uninfected patients with hemophilia and other clotting disorders
Clients and staff of institutions for the developmentally disabled
Household and sexual contacts of HBV carriers
Adoptees from countries where HBV is highly endemic
Populations where HBV is highly endemic (e.g., Alaskan Eskimos)
Inmates of long-term correctional facilities
International travelers to highly endemic HBV regions for >6 months
Unvaccinated infants under 12 months of age exposed to acute HBV infection through primary caregiver
Household contacts with blood exposure to a patient with acute HBV infection

[a]CDC recommendations are that all newborns be vaccinated against hepatitis B. (Compiled from Refs. 1, 2, 86, and 98.)

Postexposure Prophylaxis for Hepatitis B

If a patient is infected with HBV within 72 hours of receiving the vaccine and the person responds to the vaccine, symptoms of the infection either are absent or less severe.[88] This forms the basis for vaccination plus HBIG treatment as postexposure prophylaxis.[85] In addition, the antibody response to the vaccine is not attenuated by administration of HBIG.[32] Hepatitis B vaccination is recommended for any person not previously vaccinated who is exposed to blood potentially containing HBsAg. The source should be tested for HBsAg. If positive, the exposed person should receive HBIG.[1] Specific recommendations are in Tables 40.6 and 40.7.

One dose of HBIG prevents hepatitis B in 75% of people with sexual exposure to HBV, if given within 2 weeks of exposure.[2] Testing of sexual partners for susceptibility is recommended before treatment.[2] All sexual partners of persons with acute HBV infections or hepatitis B carriers should receive one dose of HBIG. Hepatitis B vaccination should be started if ongoing sexual contact with the infected person will occur.[2]

Perinatal transmission of HBV occurs in 70–90% of cases and depends on the hepatitis B e antigen status of the mother.[2] Even with administration of three doses of HBIG, 25% of infants exposed to HBV will become carriers.[85] With one dose of HBIG given within 24 hours of birth plus the hepatitis B vaccine series started within 1 week of birth, only 5–15% of infants develop the carrier state.[1,2,85] Current recommendations therefore include administration of both HBIG and HBV vaccine to neonates with HBV exposure,[100] although vaccination without HBIG may be effective.[85] Unfortunately, those 5–15% of infants infected *in utero* cannot be helped with treatment.[85]

Because infants experience substantial morbidity from this infection—and die of the complications at a rate of 20–30%[101]—routine HBsAg screening of pregnant women with the at-risk infant receiving HBIG and hepatitis B vaccine shortly after birth is routine.[2] If the HBV status of a woman is unknown at the time she presents for delivery, HBsAg testing is done then, and the baby receives appropriate prophylaxis. Infants born to HBsAg-positive mothers should begin prophylaxis within 12 hours of birth, or as soon as possible, using the schedule in Table 40.6. These infants should be tested for HBsAg and anti-HBs at 12–15 months of age. Testing for anti-HBs is not useful, because the maternal antibody can persist longer than 1 year.[2] Routine childhood vaccinations can be given.

Future Strategies for Prevention of Hepatitis B

Research is ongoing combining hepatitis B vaccine with DTP and Hib conjugate vaccines. Other possible combinations include hepatitis B vaccine with inactivated polio vaccine or hepatitis A vaccine. Such combinations would reduce the number of injections infants and children need at each visit.

Research in hepatitis B vaccines centers on vaccines that solve the problem of the nonresponder and are inexpensive to manufacture.[85] Vaccines in various stages of research include polypeptide HBsAg vaccines containing pre-S2 plus S polypeptides and/or the HBcAg.[1] The pre-S region elicits a stronger antibody response than does the S region. Nonresponders to the current vaccine might respond to a hepatitis B vaccine containing the pre-S regions or may generate an immune response to a different part of the virus, such as the core protein.[1] Other research is with recombinant HBsAg vaccines produced in mammalian or virus cells; and anti-idiotype vaccines.[1,85] The clinical role of these vaccines is not defined.

The delta virus depends on HBV for replication, and thus prevention of HBV infection will prevent HDV.[2] Exposure to HBV and HDV should be treated as an exposure to HBV alone.[2] No products are available to help prevent HDV infection in HBsAg carriers.

HEPATITIS C PREVENTION

Screening blood donors only has a modest effect on the magnitude of the hepatitis C problem because only a small percentage of cases of acute hepatitis C are a result of blood transfusion. It is obvious that much remains to be learned about the hepatitis C virus. Necessary strategies in preventing hepatitis C include defining the mechanism of sporadic spread and delineating the immunopathogenesis of the HCV. A reliable and readily available marker of the infection is needed, as is a vaccine.

Vaccine development for HCV is difficult for many of the same reasons that have made vaccine development difficult for HIV. HCV is a rapidly mutating virus with no readily defined or constant neutralizing epitopes.[24] In addition, because anti-HCV is not a protective antibody, hyperimmune globulin for passive immunoprophylaxis is not promising.[24]

Data on the use of IG for passive immunization are conflicting. For persons with percutaneous exposure to blood from a person with hepatitis C, or for newborns of anti-HCV-positive mothers, it may be useful to give IG (0.06 mL/kg). For other pre- and postexposure situations, no clear guidelines exist.[2]

HEPATITIS E PREVENTION

The best prevention method for hepatitis E is avoidance of potentially contaminated food or water and maintenance of good sanitary practices.[2] There is no evidence that IG or HBIG will prevent hepatitis E, and it is unlikely that immunoglobulins prepared in the United States would have high concentrations of antibody to hepatitis E, because the disease is rare in the United States. It is likely that a vaccine for HEV will be developed before the year 2000.

CONCLUSION

Despite breakthroughs in diagnosis and management in the last few years, acute and chronic viral hepatitis infections remain a worldwide health problem. Up to 5% of community-acquired viral hepatitis and 10% of transfusion-associated hepatitis are still not identified as any known virus. Knowledge is rapidly expanding, but unfortunately, limitations in diagnostic and therapeutic options continue to contribute to morbidity and mortality.

Further clarification of the role of IFN in chronic HCV and HBV (dosing, evaluation parameters, optimal population for use, etc.) is needed. Additional therapeutic options and therapeutic combinations are desirable for management of both chronic HCV and HBV infections. Finally, health care professionals must be informed about the HCV, the disease it causes, and the potential impact on society. Education and recognition about all viral hepatitis infections and their complications is important.

More widespread use of currently available and future vaccines provides the best weapon against viral hepatitis. Prospects for control of viral hepatitis by immunoprophylaxis are encouraging—if the vaccines reach the populations in need of them. Immunoprophylaxis of viral diseases is one of the most cost effective of medical strategies—far less costly than managing end-stage liver disease, cirrhosis, and HCC.

REFERENCES

1. Hadler SC. Vaccines to prevent hepatitis B and hepatitis A infections. Infect Dis Clin North Am 1990;4:29–46.
2. Centers for Disease Control and Prevention (CDC). Protection against viral hepatitis: Recommendations of the Immunization Practices Advisory Committee (ACIP). MMWR 1990;39(RR-2):1–26.
3. Purcell RH. The discovery of the hepatitis viruses. Gastroenterology 1993;104:955–963.
4. Losowsky MS. The clinical course of viral hepatitis. Clin Gastroenterol 1980;91:3–21.

5. Cohen JI. Hepatitis A virus: Insights from molecular biology. Hepatology 1989;9:889–895.
6. Hoofnagle JH, DiBisceglie AM. Serologic diagnosis of acute and chronic viral hepatitis. Seminars Liver Dis 1991;11:73–83.
7. Vento S, Eddleston A. Autoimmunity and liver diseases. Prog Liver Dis 1990;9:335–343.
8. Gust ID, Feinstone SM. Hepatitis A. Prog Liver Dis 1990;9:371–378.
9. Kiyasu PK, Caldwell SH. Diagnosis and treatment of the major hepatotropic viruses. Am J Med Sci 1993;306(4):248–261.
10. Blumberg BS, Alter HJ, Visnick S. A "new" antigen in leukemia sera. JAMA 1965;191:541–546.
11. Hoofnagle JH, Schafer DF. Serologic markers of hepatitis B virus infection. Semin Liver Dis 1986;6:1–10.
12. Maddrey WC. Chronic hepatitis. Dis Mon 1993;39(2):53–125.
13. Thomas HC, Jacyna M, Waters J, et al. Virus–host interaction in chronic hepatitis B virus infection. Semin Liver Dis 1988;8:342–349.
14. Bernstein BM, Gill JC. Natural history and therapy of hepatitis B and C in patients with HIV disease. AIDS Clin Rev 1993–94;129–143.
15. Carey WD, Patel G. Viral hepatitis in the 1990s, part I: Current principles of management. Cleve Clin J Med 1992;59:317–325.
16. Yoffe B, Noonan CA. Hepatitis B virus. Digest Dis Sci 1992;37:1–9.
17. Trepo C, Zoulim F, Alonso C, et al. Diagnostic markers of viral hepatitis B and C. Gut 1993;34(suppl):S20–S25.
18. Oren I, Hershow RC, Ben-Porath E, et al. A common-source outbreak of fulminant hepatitis B in a hospital. Ann Intern Med 1989;110:691–698.
19. Liang TJ, Hasegawa K, Rimon N, et al. A hepatitis B virus mutant associated with an epidemic of fulminant hepatitis. N Engl J Med 1991;324:1705–1709.
20. Sherlock S, Dusheiko G. Hepatitis C virus updated. Gut 1991;32:965–967.
21. Weiland O, Schvarcz R. Hepatitis C: Virology, epidemiology, clinical course and treatment. Scand J Gastroenterol 1992;27:337–342.
22. Alter MJ. Non-A, non-B hepatitis: Sorting through a diagnosis of exclusion. Ann Intern Med 1989;110:583–585.
23. Ohto H, Terazawa S, Sasaki N, et al. Transmission of hepatitis C virus from mothers to infants. N Engl J Med 1994;330:744–750.
24. Esteban JI, Genesca J, Alter HJ. Hepatitis C: Molecular biology, pathogenesis, epidemiology, clinical features, and prevention. Prog Liver Dis 1992;10:253–282.
25. Akahane Y, Kojima M, Sugai Y, et al. Hepatitis C virus infection in spouses of patients with type C chronic liver disease. Ann Intern Med 1994;120:748–752.
26. Alter HJ, Purcell RH, Shih JW, et al. Detection of antibody of hepatitis C virus in prospectively followed transfusion recipients with acute and chronic non-A, non-B hepatitis. N Engl J Med 1989;321:1494–1500.
27. Weintrub PS. Hepatitis. Adv Pediatr Infect Dis 1993;8:67–89.
28. Bonino F, Smedile A. Delta agent (type D) hepatitis. Semin Liver Dis 1986;6:28–33.
29. Rizzetto M, Bonino F, Verme G. Hepatitis delta virus infection of the liver: Progress in virology, pathobiology, and diagnosis. Semin Liver Dis 1988;8:350–356.
30. Hoofnagle JH, DiBisceglie AM. Therapy of chronic delta hepatitis: Overview. Prog Clin Biol Res 1993;382:337–343.
31. Purcell RH. Enterically transmitted non-A, non-B hepatitis, in Popper H, Schaffner F (eds): Progress in Liver Diseases, Vol 9. New York, Grune and Stratton, 1990, pp 371–378.
32. Balistreri WF. Viral hepatitis. Pediatr Clin North Am 1988;35:637–639.
33. Omata M, et al. Resolution of acute hepatitis C after therapy with natural beta interferon. Lancet 1991;338:914–915.
34. Halevy J, Achiron A, Spiegel D, et al. Recombinant αIFN may be efficacious in acute hepatitis B. Am J Gastroenterol 1990;85:210–212.
35. Katelaris PH, Jones DB. Fulminant hepatic failure. Med Clin North Am 1989;73:955–970.
36. Lee WM. Acute liver failure. N Engl J Med 1993;329;1862–1872.
37. DiBisceglie AM. IFN therapy of complicated hepatitis B virus infection. Semin Liver Dis 1989;9:254–258.
38. Starzl TE, Demetris AJ, Van Thiel D. Liver transplantation. N Engl J Med 1989;321:1014–1022, 1092–1099.
39. Wright R. Type B hepatitis: Progression to chronic hepatitis. Clin Gastroenterol 1980;9:97–115.
40. Hoofnagle JH, Shafritz DA, Popper H. Chronic type B hepatitis and the "healthy" HBsAg carrier state. Hepatology 1987;7:758–763.
41. Weissberg JI, Andres LL, Smith CI, et al. Survival in chronic hepatitis B: An analysis of 397 patients. Ann Intern Med 1984;101:613–616.
42. Perrillo RP. Treatment of chronic hepatitis B with IFN: Experience in Western countries. Semin Liver Dis 1989;9:240–248.
43. Alexander GJ, Williams R. Natural history and therapy of chronic hepatitis B virus infection. Am J Med 1988;85(suppl 2A):143–146.
44. Main J, Jacyna MR, Thomas HC. The diagnosis and management of viral hepatitis. Communicable Dis Rep 1992;2:R117–R120.
45. Greenberg HB, Pollard RB, Lutwick LI, et al. Effect of human leukocyte IFN on hepatitis B virus infection in patients with chronic active hepatitis. N Engl J Med 1976;295:517–522.
46. Peters M. Mechanisms of action of interferons. Semin Liver Dis 1989;9:235–239.
47. Hoofnagle JH, Jones EA. Therapy of chronic viral hepatitis: Past, present, and future. Semin Liver Dis 1989;9:231–234.
48. Perrillo RP, Schiff ER, Davis GL, et al. A randomized, controlled trial of IFNα2b alone and after prednisone withdrawal for the treatment of chronic hepatitis B. N Engl J Med 1990;323:295–301.
49. Perrillo RP, Regenstein FG, Peters MG, et al. Prednisone withdrawal followed by recombinant alpha IFN in the treatment of chronic type B hepatitis. A randomized, controlled trial. Ann Intern Med 1988;109:95–100.
50. Lambiase L, Davis GL. Treatment of chronic hepatitis. Gastroenterol Clin North Am 1992;21:659–677.

51. Perrillo RP. Interferon in the management of chronic hepatitis B. Digest Dis Sci 1993;38:577–593.
52. Hoofnagle JH, DiBisceglie AM, Waggoner JG, Park Y. Interferon alfa for patients with clinically apparent cirrhosis due to chronic hepatitis B. Gastroenterology 1993;104:1116–1121.
53. Korenman J, Baker B, Waggoner J, et al. Long-term remission of chronic hepatitis B after alpha-IFN therapy. Ann Intern Med 1991;114:629–634.
54. Wright TL, Lau JYN. Clinical aspects of hepatitis B virus infection. Lancet 1993;342:1340–1344.
55. Lok AS, Lai CL, Wu PC, et al. Treatment of chronic hepatitis B with IFN: Experience in Asian patients. Semin Liver Dis 1989;9:249–253.
56. Farci P, Mandas A, Coiana A, et al. Treatment of chronic hepatitis D with interferon alfa-2a. N Engl J Med 1994;330:88–94.
57. Romeo R, Pol S, Berthelot P, Brechot C. Eradication of hepatitis C virus RNA after alpha-IFN therapy. Ann Intern Med 1994;121:276–277.
58. Jacyna MR, Brooks MG, Loke RH, et al. Randomised controlled trial of IFN alfa (lymphoblastoid IFN) in chronic non-A, non-B hepatitis. Br Med J 1989;298:80–82.
59. DiBisceglie AM, Martin P, Kassianides C, et al. Recombinant IFN alfa therapy for chronic hepatitis C. A randomized, double-blind, placebo-controlled trial. N Engl J Med 1989;321:1506–1510.
60. Davis GL, Balart LA, Schiff ER, et al. Treatment of chronic hepatitis C with recombinant IFN alfa. A multicenter randomized, controlled trial. Hepatitis International Therapy Group. N Engl J Med 1989;321:1501–1506.
61. Camps J, Crisostomo S, Garcia-Granero M, et al. Prediction of the response of chronic hepatitis C to IFNα: A statistical analysis of pretreatment variables. Gut 1993;34:1714–1717.
62. Tsubota A, Chayama K, Arase Y, et al. Factors useful in predicting the response to interferon therapy in chronic hepatitis C. J Gastroenterol Hepatol 1993;8:535–539.
63. 1993 Red Book. Montvale, NJ, Medical Economics Data, 1993, p 489.
64. Davis GL. Recombinant α-interferon treatment of non-A, non-B (type C) hepatitis: Review of studies and recommendations for treatment. J Hepatol 1990;11:S72–S77.
65. Garcia de Ancos JL, Roberts JA, Dusheiko GM. An economic evaluation of the costs of α-interferon treatment of chronic active hepatitis due to hepatitis B or C virus. J Hepatol 1990;11:S11–S18.
66. Renault PF, Hoofnagle JH. Side effects of alpha IFN. Semin Liver Dis 1989;9:273–277.
67. Hoofnagle JH, Davis GL, Pappas SC, et al. A short course of prednisolone in chronic type B hepatitis. Report of a randomized double-blind, placebo controlled trial. Ann Intern Med 1986;104:12–17.
68. A trial group of the European Association for the Study of the Liver. Steroids in chronic B-hepatitis. A randomized, double-blind, multinational trial on the effect of low-dose, long-term treatment on survival. Liver 1986;6:227–232.
69. Dienstag JL, Alter HJ. Non-A, non-B hepatitis: Evolving epidemiologic and clinical perspective. Semin Liver Dis 1986;6:67–81.
70. Perillo RP. Antiviral agents in the treatment of chronic viral hepatitis. Prog Liver Dis 1992;10:283–309.
71. DiBisceglie AM, Shindo M, Fong TL, et al. A pilot study of ribavirin therapy for chronic hepatitis C. Hepatology 1992;16:649–654.
72. Shorrock C, Neuberger J. The changing face of liver transplantation. Gut 1993;34:295–298.
73. Goilav C, Piot T. Vaccination against hepatitis B in homosexual men. Am J Med 1989;87(suppl 3A):21S–25S.
74. Werzberger A, Mensch B, Kuter B, et al. A controlled trial of a formalin-inactivated hepatitis A vaccine in healthy children. N Engl J Med 1992;327:453–457.
75. Margolis HS. Prevention of acute and chronic liver disease through immunization: Hepatitis B and beyond. J Infect Dis 1993;168:9–14.
76. Innis BL, Snitbhan R, Kunasol P, et al. Protection against hepatitis A by an inactivated vaccine. JAMA 1994;271:1328–1334.
77. Lee SD, Lo KJ, Chan CY, et al. Immunogenicity of inactivated hepatitis A vaccine in children. Gastroenterology 1993;104:1129–1132.
78. Olin BR (ed). Hepatitis A vaccine, inactivated, in Facts and Comparisons. St. Louis, MO, Facts and Comparisons, Inc. May 1995, pp 467f–467h.
79. Guidelines for the prevention of hepatitis A in travelers. Kaiser Permanente of Colorado. May 1995, pp 1–2 (unpublished).
80. Ambrosch F, Courouce AM, Coursaget P, et al. Immunisation against hepatitis B. Lancet 1988;1(8590):875–876.
81. Hollinger FB. Factors influencing the immune response to hepatitis B vaccine, booster dose guidelines, and vaccine protocol recommendations. Am J Med 1989;87(suppl 3A):36S–40S.
82. CDC. Recommendations of the Advisory Committee on Immunization Practices (ACIP): Use of vaccines and immune globulins in persons with altered immunocompetence. MMWR 1993;42(RR-4):1–18.
83. CDC. Hepatitis B virus: A comprehensive strategy for eliminating transmission in the United States through universal childhood vaccination. MMWR 1991;40(RR-13):1–25.
84. Tabor E. Etiology, diagnosis, and treatment of viral hepatitis in children. Adv Pediatr Infect Dis 1988;3:19–46.
85. Troisi CL, Hollinger FB. Hepatitis B vaccines. Prog Liver Dis 1990;405–442.
86. West DJ, Margolis HS. Prevention of hepatitis B virus infection in the United States: A pediatric perspective. Pediatr Infect Dis J 1992;11:866–874.
87. CDC. General recommendations on immunization: Recommendations of the Advisory Committee on Immunization Practices (ACIP). MMWR 1994;43 (RR-1):1–38.
88. Hadler SC. Are booster doses of hepatitis B vaccine necessary? Ann Intern Med 1988;108:457–458.
89. Hadler SC, Francis DP, Maynard JE, et al. Long-term immunogenicity and efficacy of hepatitis B vaccine in homosexual men. N Engl J Med 1986;315:209–214.

90. Roome AJ, Walsh SJ, Carter ML, Hadler JL. Hepatitis B vaccine responsiveness in Connecticut public safety personnel. JAMA 1993;270:2931–2934.
91. Craven DE, Awdeh ZL, Kunches LM, et al. Nonresponsiveness to hepatitis B vaccine in health care workers. Results of revaccination and genetic typings. Ann Intern Med 1986;105:356–360.
92. Horowitz MM, Ershler WB, McKinney WP, et al. Duration of immunity after hepatitis B vaccination: Efficacy of low-dose booster vaccine. Ann Intern Med 1988;108:185–189.
93. International Advisory Group. Immunization against hepatitis B. Lancet 1988;1:875–876.
94. Greenberg DP. Pediatric experience with recombinant hepatitis B vaccines and relevant safety and immunogenicity studies. Pediatr Infect Dis J 1993;12:438–445.
95. Bruguera M, Cremades M, Rodicio JL, et al. Immunogenicity of a yeast-derived hepatitis B vaccine in hemodialysis patients. Am J Med 1989;87(suppl 3A):30S–32S.
96. Hadler SC. Hepatitis B prevention and human immunodeficiency virus (HIV) infection [editorial]. Ann Intern Med 1988;109:92–94.
97. Collier AC, Corey L, Murphy VL, et al. Antibody to human immunodeficiency virus (HIV) and suboptimal response to hepatitis B vaccination. Ann Intern Med 1988;109:101–105.
98. CDC. Recommendations of the International Task Force for Disease Eradication. MMWR 1993;42(RR-16):1–38.
99. Bloom BS, Hillman AL, Fendrick AM, Schwartz JS. A reappraisal of hepatitis B virus vaccination strategies using cost-effectiveness analysis. Ann Intern Med 1993;118:298–306.
100. Tong MJ. Hepatitis B vaccination of neonates and children. Am J Med 1989;87(suppl 3A):33S–35S.
101. Arevalo JA, Washington AE. Cost-effectiveness of prenatal screening and immunization for hepatitis B virus. JAMA 1988;259:365–369.

Chapter 41

Liver Transplantation

Gilbert J. Burckart, PharmD, FCCP,
and Raman Venkataramanan, PhD, FCP

Liver transplantation is a lifesaving procedure for many patients with severe hepatic disease who have no other medical option. From 1981 to 1994, the number of liver transplant operations in the United States increased from approximately 100 to more than 3500 procedures per year. In spite of this increase in the number of liver transplantation procedures, more than 5000 patients are now on the waiting list for a liver in the United States. Through this large number of transplants, knowledge has been gained not only about the liver transplant procedure, but also about the role of the liver in metabolic diseases that affect the liver.

The concept of whole liver transplantation in animals was first mentioned in a publication in 1955 by Welch.[1] Welch envisioned that auxiliary liver transplants (the original liver was left in place, and a donor liver graft was added) would provide a therapeutic option for patients with liver disease, but all such attempts in patients failed with rare exceptions. In 1958, research using an orthotopic (donor liver replaces recipient liver in the same position) liver transplantation (OLTx) model in dogs was initiated in Chicago by Dr. Thomas Starzl and by a research team in Boston. In 1965, Starzl reported the first long-term survival (4 months) of liver-transplanted dogs receiving azathioprine for immunosuppression. The first patient to survive 1 year after OLTx was operated on in 1967, but the 5-year survival of the first 111 patients who underwent the procedure from 1963 to 1976 was under 20% in spite of triple drug therapy with azathioprine, prednisone, and antilymphocytic globulin (ALG). The 5-year survival rate improved only minimally over the period of 1976 to 1980, when cyclosporine (CyA) was introduced in OLTx patients. Eleven of the 12 patients who underwent the transplant operation in 1980 and received CyA survived for at least 1 year. This striking improvement in survival following liver transplantation with CyA led to a major expansion of the operative procedure to the point where approximately 117 transplant centers in the United States now perform the operation. Current 1-year and 3-year patient survival data for liver transplantation yield 79% and 72% survivals, respectively, in the United States.[2]

The diseases leading to hepatic dysfunction that warrant the liver transplantation procedure are varied. The principal indications for transplantation in adults have been postnecrotic cirrhosis and primary biliary cirrhosis, but other common indications have included alcoholic cirrhosis, primary sclerosing cholangitis, acute hepatic failure, primary liver cancer, and inborn errors of metabolism (Table 41.1).[3] Pediatric liver transplantation has been performed primarily for biliary atresia and inborn errors of metabolism. Postnecrotic cirrhosis, biliary atresia, and primary biliary cirrhosis make up almost 60% of all OLTx indications. The postnecrotic cirrhosis caused by hepatic parenchymal disease is most commonly caused by alcohol use or hepatitis B or C.

Some relative contraindications to liver transplantation do exist. The patient should have a reasonable life expectancy after transplantation. The results following surgery for primary liver cancer have been discouraging in that patients develop recurrent malignancy, but work with selected cancer patient populations and with neoadjuvant chemotherapy continues at some transplant centers. With careful selection of patients with Laënnec's cirrhosis, alcoholism has recurred in less than 10% of OLTx patients and the long-term survival has paralleled other patient populations. Age does not appear to be a barrier to liver transplantation with good 5-year survival rates in patients older than 50 years. Patients who have had multiple abdominal surgical procedures previously are more difficult to operate on due to adhesions, but management techniques for these patients are improving. Patients who have a major systemic infection or who have a disease that is expected to recur are generally excluded from liver transplantation. Patients who have a positive screening test for the acquired immune deficiency (AIDS) virus have not uniformly died of AIDS after transplantation, but would be excluded at some centers.

Hepatitis B has a high rate of recurrence in OLTx patients, and liver transplantation for chronic hepatitis B virus (HBV) is still controversial. Recurrence rates of up to 83% have been reported in specific patient populations. A recent European consensus report[4] recommends that chronic HBV carriers without evidence of hepatitis D virus (HDV) infection who are seropositive for either the HBe antigen or

TABLE 41.1. INDICATIONS FOR LIVER TRANSPLANTATION

Indication	Number of Patients		Percentage
	Pediatric	Adult	
Acute hepatic failure	23	48	4.8
Postnecrotic cirrhosis	44	361	27.6
Alcoholic cirrhosis		113	7.7
Biliary atresia	236	5	16.4
Inborn errors of metabolism	75	52	8.6
Primary biliary cirrhosis		210	14.3
Primary sclerosing cholangitis	4	99	7.0
Primary liver cancer	8	59	4.6
Other	48	84	9.0
Total	438	1031	100

(From Starzl TE, Demetris AJ. Liver Transplantation: A 31-Year Perspective. Chicago, Year Book Medical Publishers, 1990, with permission.)

HBV–DNA constitute a risk group of patients who should not be transplanted. The use of hyperimmune globulin (HBIG) may be useful in reducing graft infection with the HBV in patients with acute liver failure, and transplantation should be considered in this group. Patients who have HDV infection superimposed on chronic HBV infection also have a low graft reinfection rate and should be considered as candidates for liver transplantation. Other pharmacologic means for controlling HBV recurrence include recombinant interferon-α, which has not been found to be useful in post-transplantation HBV recurrence in OLTx patients, combination antiviral therapy with ganciclovir and foscarnet, and investigational approaches such as prostaglandin E (PGE) administration. Therefore, select populations with HBV may be candidates for OLTx, and new drug therapy regimens may improve the outlook for this group of patients.

The inborn errors of metabolism that have been treated by OLTx are a heterogeneous group of disorders, and correction of the metabolic defect has not always occurred. α_1-Antitrypsin deficiency; Wilson's disease; tyrosinemia; types I, III, and IV glycogen storage diseases; type I hyperoxaluria; and hemophilia A and B have been corrected through liver transplantation. Correction has been incomplete in other disorders such as familial hypercholesterolemia. Timing is critical for correction of the metabolic disease in order to prevent irreversible damage to the end organ (e.g., central nervous system in ornithine transcarbamylase deficiency) or to prevent hepatocellular carcinoma (e.g., tyrosinemia).

The Liver Transplantation Procedure

Liver transplantation is the most technically demanding of the surgical transplant procedures. This difficulty has produced a slow increase in the number of successful centers performing liver transplant procedures. Figure 41.1 depicts the anatomical structures critical to liver transplantation.

The first critical step in liver transplantation is the proper procurement of the donor organ. In approximately one-third of human donors, arterial abnormalities in the liver will be encountered that would make the organ useless without special techniques. Preservation of the donor organ is critical and has been discussed in Chapter 9. New preservation solutions have extended the 6- to 8-hour maximal preservation period previously used for livers to up to 24 hours. This extension in preservation has dramatically affected liver procurement practices and the availability of viable organs.

No uniform method of assessing the adequacy of the donor liver and predicting primary graft dysfunction have been found. One widely published method is to administer lidocaine to the donor or recipient and document the formation of the metabolite monoethylglycinexylidide (MEGX).[5] Other methods of assessment that have been advocated include administration of indocyanine green (ICG), galactose, and caffeine to the recipient with subsequent clearance measurements. A combination of the ICG clearance test and MEGX test appears to be superior to conventional liver function tests and a Pugh score in assessing short-term prognosis in cirrhotic patients.[6] These methods involve some added expense, timed sampling and interpretation, and therefore have been widely ignored by clinicians in favor of monitoring transaminase activity, bile production, and hemostasis.

The recipient operation is roughly conducted in three phases: removal of recipient liver, donor graft revascularization, and biliary reconstruction. The venous hypertension produced by clamping of the inferior vena cava and portal vein during the anhepatic phase can cause edema of the intestinal mucosa, and has been circumvented in adult patients through the use of the venovenous bypass. Graft revascularization involves performing anastomosis of the vena cava above and below the liver (Fig. 41.1a) followed by the portal venous anastomosis (Fig. 41.1b). Biliary reconstruction can be accomplished in several ways: by end-to-end anastomosis of the donor and recipient common bile ducts over a T-tube stent, by side-to-side choledochostomy after closure of the donor and recipient duct ends, or by anastomosing the graft's common duct to a defunctionalized limb of jejunum (Roux limb, Fig. 41.1c). The complete procedure takes many hours, often requires several teams of surgeons, and is frequently accomplished with the replacement of multiple blood volumes for the patient.

One of the most difficult problems in pediatric transplantation is the availability of size-matched allografts. A donor liver allograft has to be within about 20% of the recipient's size; it can impair breathing or closure of the abdomen if too large and may not be adequate for survival if too small. Because of this problem, reduced-size liver transplantation has evolved as a technique where the donor liver is surgically reduced in size to meet the needs of the recipient. This technique has been most commonly used in split-liver transplantation where a donor graft provides livers for two recipients, and in living-related donor operations where a portion of the left lobe of the healthy liver is taken for the donor graft from the parent. The University of Chicago performed 69 living-related donor grafts for 62 infants and young children between 1989 and 1994.[7] Fifty-nine of the 66 (89%) recipients are alive and 53 of the 69 grafts are functioning well (77%). Although some donor morbidity has resulted, there have been no cases of donor mortality. Immunosuppressive therapy is similar to a cadaveric donor graft, but episodes of rejection that are resistant to corticosteroids appear to be less common in the recipient of a living-related donor liver allograft. Living-related donor operations may become more common at other centers as the shortage of donor organs continues.

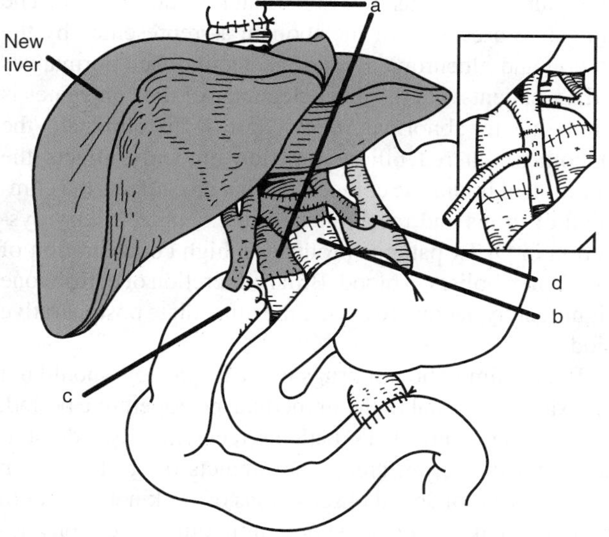

Figure 41.1. Orthotopic liver transplantation with (a) suprahepatic and intrahepatic inferior vena cava anastomosis, (b) portal venous anastomosis, (c) choledochojejunostomy, and (d) hepatic arterial anastomosis.

Failure of the newly transplanted liver occurs in 10–15% of cases and can result through several different mechanisms. Early graft failure can result from preexisting disease in the donor, and even coagulation defects have been transmitted through donor organs. The technical complexity of the operation can produce flaws in revascularization that also lead to graft nonfunction; portal vein thrombosis, hepatic artery thrombosis, and bile duct leaks are all technical problems that have been encountered. Ischemic injury to the donor liver through preservation is difficult to predict, but can produce early graft dysfunction. Perioperative immune events rarely lead to the classic picture of hyperacute rejection in liver transplantation, but graft failure in the first 2 weeks postoperatively may still indicate antibody-mediated graft destruction.

Endotoxemia has been recognized as a potential cause of early graft failure following liver transplantation. Animal studies have demonstrated large increases in plasma endotoxin concentrations during the anhepatic phase of liver transplantation, and patients with early graft failure and no positive cytotoxic cross-matches have been found to have elevated plasma concentrations of endotoxin. A recent study of selective decontamination of the bowel using oral amphotericin, polymixin E, and tobramycin in liver transplant patients demonstrated that this approach may reduce pulmonary infections but has no effect on endotoxemia or the development of organ failure.[8] Selective decontamination is expensive and is not presently being practiced at the University of Pittsburgh liver transplant program, and the importance of reducing the endotoxin load following liver transplantation remains unclear.

The shortage of donor organs has stimulated work in the area of hepatocyte transplantation and in the development of artificial liver support. Hepatocyte transplantation, where the cells are implanted into the liver or the spleen, may be considered as a temporary bridge to provide liver function in patients with end-stage liver failure until a donor becomes available. Cellular transplantation with hepatocytes is potentially a simpler, less expensive, and less invasive procedure when compared to liver transplantation.[9] Hepatocyte transplantation can involve the use of (1) heterologous cells being transplanted into an immunosuppressed recipient or (2) partial hepatectomy of the recipient with an *in vitro* genetic correction with a recombinant vector to reverse the genetic defect, followed by retransplantation of the autologous cells into a nonimmunocompromised recipient. Studies in animals and some preliminary human data indicate that the transplanted hepatocytes seed and proliferate in organs such as the spleen and liver over an entire life span.

The bioartificial liver consists of an implantable system or an extracorporeal liver support device that contains human hepatocytes.[10] A hollow fiber hepatocyte bioreactor appears to be a promising support system. Such systems will not only serve as temporary support but may provide an opportunity for the recipient's liver to regenerate after an acute insult. Bioartificial livers are currently entering clinical trials.

Physiologic and Pharmacologic Consequences of Liver Transplantation

The physiologic consequences of liver transplantation are complex, but an oversimplification can be made by combining models of rapidly changing hepatic function, postoperative patients with ileus and biliary tract dysfunction, catabolic patients on high doses of steroids, and immunocompromised patients. The OLTx patient represents each of these models with each intricate component interacting with the other models in an individualized manner. The transition from poor hepatic function to normal liver processes is one that involves changes in both metabolic and synthetic function. The postoperative patient will have fluid, electrolyte, and nutritional abnormalities that will be combined with biliary tract dysfunction with its subsequent gastrointestinal (GI) implications. Disruption of bile flow through removal of the gallbladder and, in some cases, temporary placement of a drainage tube (T tube) in the bile duct will alter the absorption of fats and fat-soluble drugs. Corticosteroids and the other immunosuppressive drugs have metabolic consequences that affect both endogenous and exogenous substrates. As an immunosuppressed patient, the OLTx patient will have the attendant risk of infection and requirement for the use of multiple anti-infective drugs.

The physiologic changes that the patient is undergoing result in alterations in the biopharmaceutic profile in an OLTx patient, and these changes have been reviewed previously.[11] Changes in drug absorption are quite dramatic in OLTx patients. After a successful liver transplant operation, the absorption of lipid-soluble compounds such as CyA, vitamin A, and vitamin E are considerably improved. The poor absorption of the lipid-soluble drug CyA improves after successful liver transplantation and reestablishment of bile flow. Vitamin E deficiency and the neurologic complications associated with it are reversed after successful liver transplantation in pediatric patients. In stable adult OLTx patients, the concentrations of retinol and tocopherol are similar to that seen in normal healthy subjects, indicating recovery of the ability of the transplanted liver to produce and excrete the bile salts needed for fat-soluble vitamin absorption.

The protein binding of drugs in OLTx patients is affected both by the synthetic capacity of the liver and by the pathophysiologic changes associated with the postoperative state. The serum concentration of albumin in OLTx patients is frequently lower than that observed in normal subjects for months following surgery, resulting in a lower protein-bound fraction for drugs binding to albumin. When compared with patients with chronic liver disease, the binding of both diazepam and salicylic acid is greater in OLTx patients due to the removal of endogenous binding inhibitors. Studies in OLTx patients indicate that the concentration of α_1-acid glycoprotein (AAG) increases after surgery and stays at an elevated level for at least 45 days. Correspondingly, the unbound fraction of lidocaine in plasma obtained from stable OLTx patients was lower than the free fraction values observed in plasma from normal volunteers. Propranolol also binds to AAG, but no significant difference was observed in the unbound fraction of propranolol in stable OLTx patients when compared with normal subjects. An increase in propranolol binding due to an increase in AAG concentration is offset by a reduction in albumin concentration because albumin also contributes significantly to the binding of propranolol.

Liver metabolism is altered by a combination of factors relating to physiologic changes (preservation injury or decreased effective hepatic blood flow initially), stimulation of hepatic microsomes by some immunosuppressant agents, and inhibition of microsomal drug transformation by other immunosuppressant agents. The oxidative metabolizing capacity of the liver as determined by antipyrine kinetics is similar in clinically stable OLTx patients to that observed in normal subjects. First-pass metabolism is expected to be altered during the transition to normal hepatic function. The conjugative processes of metabolism as represented by the sulfation and glucuronidation of acetaminophen normalizes in OLTx patients, but the renal clearance of the conjugates is altered due to abnormal renal capacity to eliminate the metabolites. Altered biliary function not only affects the absorption of lipophilic compounds, but also affects the elimination of drugs and metabolites. For example, biliary dysfunction in OLTx patients produces a high concentration of the CyA metabolites in blood. Biliary excretion of ceftriaxone is significantly decreased during the immediate postoperative period.

Renal elimination of drugs in OLTx patients should not be considered normal in the immediate postoperative period. Earlier studies with OLTx patients receiving CyA demonstrated that the serum creatinine predicts drug elimination that is in excess of actual observations of the kinetics of both gentamicin and the cephalosporin antibiotics. These physiologic alterations in an OLTx patient must be considered when developing individualized drug regimens.

CARE OF THE LIVER TRANSPLANT PATIENT

Table 41.2 lists the routine postoperative ICU medication orders for an adult liver transplant patient in June 1995. Immunosuppressive and management protocols vary tremendously among centers and within a center over time. For example, the University of Pittsburgh protocol has previously contained antacids in addition to the H_2 blocker, routine acyclovir prophylaxis for cytomegalovirus for all patients, antithrombotic therapy including dextran infusions, aspirin and dipyridamole, and PGE_1 infusions. Immunosuppressive protocols at other centers may include CyA instead of tacrolimus and may include an antiproliferative agent such as azathioprine or mycophenolate mofetil. So-called "induction" protocols may include 5–14 days of initial antithymocytic or antilymphocytic globulin or muromonab-CD3, after which the CyA or tacrolimus therapy would be initiated.

An intensive laboratory assessment program is used to monitor the patient following liver transplantation. Table 41.3 lists the monitoring parameters and their use in following an OLTx patient. No one single test can be interpreted independently; an adequate assessment comes only after considering the clinical, radiologic, and laboratory examinations as a composite representation of the patient's condition. This is particularly true when attempting to assess whether an adverse event is due to drug therapy, to an infection, to rejection, or due to some technical complication of the transplant surgery.

The use of prostaglandins or the use of thromboxane receptor antagonists in patients receiving CyA or tacrolimus has been of particular interest since these mediators may have an impact on the nephrotoxicity of these drugs. Some centers do administer PGE_1 in the postoperative period and/or misoprostil orally, but no studies to date have documented the cost effectiveness of this therapy. The administration of PGE may have additional beneficial effects relating to its immunomodulating properties and hepatoprotective properties.

Neurologic complications are common after the OLTx procedure and occur in as many as 47% of patients. Four primary immunosuppressants have been associated with adverse neurologic symptoms ranging from ataxia to seizures, psychosis, visual hallucinations, and meningoencephalitis: CyA, tacrolimus, muromonab-CD3, and corticosteroids. Drug-induced adverse effects must therefore always be considered as a possible cause when a neurologic anomaly is observed.

Many women with liver disease have menstrual irregularities and reproductive problems, and these problems are corrected by liver transplantation. Healthy infants have been delivered by mothers receiving CyA or receiving tacrolimus, but couples should be counseled about the possible hypertension and graft dysfunction that can accompany pregnancy in a mother with a liver transplant. These discussions are particularly important since estrogen-containing hormonal birth control is generally withheld from OLTx patients due to the interaction with CyA or tacrolimus.

TABLE 41.2. ROUTINE INTENSIVE CARE UNIT MEDICATION ORDERS FOR AN ADULT POSTOPERATIVE LIVER TRANSPLANT PATIENT AT THE UNIVERSITY OF PITTSBURGH IN JUNE 1995

- Fentanyl 50–100 mcg IV every 2 hours as needed
- Dopamine 2–3 mcg/kg/min IV infusion
- Famotidine 20 mg IV (or 40 mg per NG) every 12 hours
- Cefotaxime 1.0 gram every 8 hours for 3 days and ampicillin 1.0 gram every 6 hours for 3 days
- Nystatin suspension 15 mL swish and swallow four times daily once the NG tube is out (and one vaginal suppository daily for female patients)
- Trimethoprim-sulfamethoxazole single-strength tablet or suspension Monday–Wednesday–Friday
- Tacrolimus (see dosage discussion in text) IV to run continuously
- Methylprednisolone 50 mg IV every 6 hours × 4; then 40 mg IV every 6 hours × 4; then 30 mg IV every 6 hours × 4; then 20 mg IV every 6 hours × 4; then 20 mg every 12 hours × 2; then 20 mg IV once daily
- Furosemide and albumin as required
- Antihypertensives as required with sublingual nifedipine for acute hypertension

IMMUNOSUPPRESSIVE MEASURES

The liver appears to be less immunogenic and more likely to promote immunologic tolerance than the other vascularized organs. Hyperacute rejection rarely occurs in patients receiving a liver transplant. The liver's special status for transplantation is not fully understood, but local release of cytokines may alter the immunologic reaction taking place in the liver. One recent investigator identified a massive local release of interleukin-10 (IL-10) that appears to accompany liver transplantation, and IL-10 is considered to be an endogenous immunosuppressive cytokine.[12]

The specific immunosuppressive measures chosen for an OLTx patient are largely specific for the protocol at an individual transplant center, and are empiric due to our inability to distinguish small differences in several effective drug regimens. The ability to perform cooperative studies on immunosuppressive protocols for OLTx patients has therefore been limited.

The University of Pittsburgh liver transplant program and Dr. Thomas Starzl have performed over 4000 OLTx

TABLE 41.3. MONITORING PARAMETERS IN A PATIENT FOLLOWING LIVER TRANSPLANTATION

Measurement	Application
Serum bilirubin and liver enzymes	Assess the functional status of the liver. These tests should improve rapidly unless there is delayed graft function or primary nonfunction. An increase in these values may indicate a technical complication or rejection.
Serum creatinine and blood urea nitrogen (BUN)	Assess renal function. The BUN/creatinine ratio is normally increased in an OLTx patient. These values should stabilize to the high normal range in an OLTx patient; rapid increases may indicate drug toxicity or a change in the hydration status of the patient.
Serum electrolytes	Hypomagnesemia requiring supplementation has been observed. Hyperkalemia requiring fludrocortisone therapy is common. Other abnormalities related to intensive diuretic therapy are also common.
Serum prothrombin time, INR	Assess functional capacity of liver to make coagulation factors. Also is important in the event of bleeding episodes due to technical complications.
Blood pressure, weight, vital signs	Prevents hypertensive encephalopathy and the other complications of hypertension. Monitors fluid status and temperature elevations that may accompany infection or graft rejection.
Leukocyte cytomegalovirus (CMV) antigenemia	Assess CMV status through identification of pp65 marker on cells. Allows preemptive antiviral therapy when the level of antigenemia increases.
Physical examination	Assess graft tenderness, neurologic status, sites of infection on skin incisions or body cavities.
Serum albumin	Assess plasma oncotic pressure and hepatic synthetic function. Albumin supplementation is occasionally prescribed to improve diuretic efficiency until synthesis can restore normal plasma proteins.
Complete blood count	Assess white cell number and differential to monitor for infection. Follow hematocrit to observe for bleeding episodes that may indicate technical complications with the graft.

procedures between 1980 and 1994. During this period, the prophylactic immunosuppressive regimen has changed from an earlier protocol of CyA and corticosteroids to a triple drug regimen of CyA, azathioprine, and corticosteroids and then finally to the tacrolimus and steroid protocol that is in use in 1995.

The earlier high-dose oral CyA regimen (17.5 mg/kg/d) was effective in OLTx patients, but frequently resulted in complications of severe hypertension and renal dysfunction. The judicious dosing of CyA and the monitoring of CyA blood concentrations could avoid some early increases in serum creatinine, but long-term changes in renal function were consistently unrelated to blood or plasma concentrations. The contribution of CyA assays and monitoring to appropriate CyA dosing was critical for the OLTx patient due to the changing status of the graft function, biliary duct obstruction, bile fistulas, and the presence or absence of T-tube bile drainage. Original concerns about the CyA monitoring by blood or plasma or by specific chromatographic means versus immunoassay did not significantly affect monitoring programs for the OLTx patient. The addition of azathioprine to CyA and steroids did allow the CyA dosage to be reduced to the currently used range of 6–14 mg/kg/d with similar efficacy. The long-term reductions in CyA dosage to less than 4 mg/kg/d may have contributed to problems with chronic rejection, and is not a common practice at the present time.

An important characteristic of CyA for OLTx patients that was identified in early animal studies was the ability of CyA to promote the regeneration of hepatocytes following hepatectomy. The transplanted liver goes through a period of volume adjustment to conform to the space provided in the recipient, and the hepatotrophic growth factors involved in liver regeneration are incompletely understood. CyA, tacrolimus (FK-506), and insulin are recognized as positive hepatotrophic factors.

An open-label randomized multicenter trial comparing CyA and tacrolimus in liver transplantation in the United States found that the actuarial survival rates for patients and grafts were similar between the two groups.[13] The tacrolimus group did have significantly lower incidences of acute rejection and corticosteroid-resistant rejection. Nephrotoxicity and neurotoxicity required that more patients be withdrawn from tacrolimus therapy than from CyA therapy. A European trial found similar results in that survival and adverse effects were similar with CyA and tacrolimus in OLTx patients, but that the incidence of acute, refractory, and chronic rejection was lower in the tacrolimus group.[14] One of the primary uses for tacrolimus in centers that use CyA as their primary immunosuppressant drug is as rescue therapy. Patient survival rates exceeding 80% have been reported in OLTx patients who were converted from CyA to tacrolimus due to failure of the conventional immunosuppressive therapy; this percentage is considered an outstanding response rate.

Tacrolimus is now used as the primary immunosuppressant for OLTx patients at the University of Pittsburgh in conjunction with corticosteroids. Many long-term patients have been weaned from corticosteroids and are being maintained on tacrolimus alone. The incidence of hypertension resulting from the immunosuppressive therapy has decreased with tacrolimus therapy in the Pittsburgh experience.

DRUG DOSING CONSIDERATIONS

The intravenous administration of medications is considered essential in the immediate postoperative period for the OLTx patient. While methylprednisolone and azathioprine are administered preoperatively or intraoperatively, CyA and tacrolimus are usually withheld for postoperative administration. Intravenous therapy with CyA or tacrolimus must be monitored carefully in the immediate postoperative period because of considerable patient variation in liver function and drug metabolism, and continuous drug infusion can assist in the accurate determination of changes in drug metabolizing or eliminating capabilities. Oral therapy with CyA or tacrolimus can usually be initiated on day 2 to 4 postoperatively, and CyA often is given in increasing daily oral increments as the intravenous therapy is weaned while monitoring CyA blood or plasma concentrations. This CyA dosing schedule has been used to protect the patient who malabsorbs CyA during this critical period. With tacrolimus, the intravenous therapy is discontinued and oral therapy is initiated with the next dose.

Intravenous and oral CyA and tacrolimus therapy are adjusted to provide concentrations within an accepted range for each transplant center. The ranges vary widely for CyA and are dependent on whether blood or plasma is used, and whether a specific (high-performance liquid chromatography [HPLC], monoclonal radioimmunoassay [RIA], or fluorescence polarization immunoassay [FPIA]) or nonspecific laboratory test is used. For oral therapy, morning trough drug concentrations are used by tradition but some reports support the use of a time point (often 5–8 hours post oral dose), which is more representative of the total concentration–time exposure. Once the patient is stabilized, concentration monitoring at twice-weekly intervals is sufficient for the first month unless acute patient changes (rejection, removal of the T tube) warrant closer monitoring.

The most recent protocols using tacrolimus as the primary immunosuppressant in OLTx administer 0.1 mg/kg/d intravenously as an infusion over 24 hours beginning 4–6 hours after revascularization of the graft. Oral dosing of tacrolimus begins at 0.15 mg/kg every 12 hours and is usually initiated 8–12 hours after the intravenous infusion has been stopped. The target 12-hour trough blood concentration of tacrolimus is between 5 and 15 ng/mL using the microparticle enzyme immunoassay (MEIA).

Distinct differences in CyA and tacrolimus dosing in relation to hepatic and biliary function are notable. With CyA, diminished hepatic and/or biliary function results in poor CyA absorption with relatively small changes in CyA clearance. Therefore, the oral dosage of CyA must be increased significantly to maintain CyA blood or plasma concentrations, and doses of more than 70 mg/kg/d have been administered to a few patients. Reinitiation of intravenous CyA must be considered an alternative for the OLTx patient with continued hepatic or biliary dysfunction. An opposite effect is observed when the patient's T tube is clamped and all bile drainage is diverted into the GI tract; CyA oral dosage must be significantly reduced to maintain stable blood or plasma concentrations. With tacrolimus, drug absorption does not appear to be affected by the presence of bile, and presystemic first-pass metabolism may be diminished with hepatic dysfunction. The oral dosage of tacrolimus must therefore be decreased significantly during periods of diminished hepatic function. Clamping the patient's T tube has no effect on the oral dosage requirements of tacrolimus.

Because CyA absorption appears to be a process that occurs slowly in the small bowel, the length of the small bowel to which CyA is exposed affects cumulative drug absorption. Drug administration through a small bowel feeding tube reduces the total CyA absorbed in comparison with oral absorption, and connection of the biliary system at a distal rather than a proximal small bowel site may also reduce drug absorption.

COMPLICATIONS FOLLOWING LIVER TRANSPLANATION

GRAFT DYSFUNCTION

Early graft dysfunction is treated with supportive care and retransplantation if possible. An immunologic explanation for graft dysfunction becomes more probable as time passes in a patient with an initially functioning liver graft. Initial episodes of acute cellular rejection often occur between 6 days and 6 weeks post-transplantation, but can also occur earlier or later. Other reasons for delayed graft dysfunction include defects in bile duct reconstruction, opportunistic infections, toxicity from parenteral nutrition, sepsis, or drug-induced hepatotoxicity. The clinical signs of acute cellular rejection are fever, lethargy, graft tenderness, leukocytosis, and a change in the color or quantity of bile. An increased serum bilirubin and increases in hepatic enzymes are the most common biochemical parameters monitored and are sensitive markers of rejection. The liver biopsy is used as definitive evidence of the diagnosis of rejection, but response to antirejection medication has also been used in differentiating rejection from other causes of hepatic dysfunction in an OLTx patient.

The treatment of acute cellular rejection varies widely from center to center, but generally involves the concepts of (1) optimizing the present immunosuppressive therapy, (2) initially giving high-dose corticosteroids, and (3) the use of OKT3 monoclonal antibody or antilymphocyte (ALG)/antithymocyte (ATG) globulin for a 7- to 14-day course. Increasing the dosage of CyA can be effective in mild cases of rejection, but is infrequently used because of concerns of nephrotoxicity with the drug. The tacrolimus dosage is increased in patients for mild rejection and is effective in some OLTx patients. The administration of corticosteroids for rejection can be done as a "pulse" of one to three large doses of methylprednisolone, or can be achieved as a "recycle" of an increased dosage of methylprednisolone, prednisolone, or prednisone for 5–10 days. The dosages of other immunosuppressant drugs are often decreased while administering corticosteroids, OKT3, or ALG/ATG therapy. Patients who are deemed "steroid resistant" are treated with a 7- to 14-day course of OKT3, ALG, or ATG. Repeated courses of immunosuppressant agents for rejection will put the patient at an increased risk for infection, which is always a concern in immunocompromised patients, and at risk for the development of post-transplant lymphoproliferative disease (PTLD).

Chronic rejection of the liver is characterized by an obliterative arteriopathy and the loss of bile ducts, which has been referred to as the vanishing bile duct syndrome. These patients experience an asymptomatic rise in the canalicular liver enzymes (alkaline phosphatase and γ-glutamyl transpeptidase) and become jaundiced. These changes can be seen in patients who have not responded adequately to therapy for acute rejection, and are considered the result of immunologic and ischemic injury. The changes of chronic rejection are not reversible, and CMV infection has been implicated in the initiation of the process in some OLTx patients.

INFECTION

The balance between immunosuppression and infection control is critical in the OLTx patient because of the constant exposure of the graft to intestinal flora. In the presence of rejection, the liver can become an open portal for entry of bacterial organisms from the GI tract. Bacterial or fungal invasion can result in local abscess formation or in general sepsis, both of which represent life-threatening infectious complications of transplantation and immunosuppression.

OLTx patients have an increased incidence of symptomatic CMV infection in comparison with renal transplant patients (32% versus 8%, respectively).[15] These infections are most frequently observed from 3–8 weeks following transplantation or after an intensive treatment course for rejection. As with other transplants, liver recipients who are seronegative for CMV prior to transplantation are at increased risk for symptomatic CMV infections (88% of infections) in comparison with liver recipients who were preoperatively seropositive (32% of symptomatic infections). While prophylactic therapy with ganciclovir or acyclovir is used in some centers, a newer approach is to follow the patient's CMV leukocyte antigen concentration and to treat the patient aggressively when the antigen concentration increases.[16] The antigen level can then also be used as a measure of response to therapy in patients undergoing treatment with intravenous ganciclovir. The place of oral ganciclovir in the prophylaxis against CMV disease has not been determined in OLTx patients. Other significant viral diseases in OLTx patients include herpes simplex types 1 and 2, HBV, adenoviral hepatitis, and Epstein–Barr viral diseases ranging from an infectious mononucleosis syndrome to life-threatening lymphoproliferative disease. An expanded discussion of the PTLD seen in transplant patients can be seen in Chapter 18 on cardiac transplantation.

CONCLUSION

Improved organ preservation techniques have made liver transplantation a more widely available and accepted technique for an expanding list of congenital, autoimmune, and metabolic diseases. New agents such as tacrolimus have improved the immunosuppressive management of OLTx patients, but the absence of subtle immunologic monitoring techniques means that infection and rejection are persistent clinical problems in these patients. Drug therapy in the OLTx patients is complicated by rapidly changing hepatic function and the need for intense immunosuppression. Their drug regimen is initially complex and requires intensive monitoring to optimize therapy in the presence of drug interactions and changing drug absorption, distribution, metabolism, and elimination. The pharmacotherapist can make significant contributions to the care of OLTx patients through knowledge of the physiologic changes that affect the biopharmaceutic properties of drugs in these patients.

REFERENCES

1. Welch CS. A note on transplantation of the whole liver in dogs. Transplant Bull 1955;2:54–55.
2. UNOS Scientific Registry as of July 29, 1994. United Network for Organ Sharing, Richmond, VA.
3. Starzl TE, Demetris AJ. Liver Transplantation: A 31-Year Perspective. Chicago, Year Book Medical Publishers, 1990, p 120.
4. Muller R, Samuel D, Fassati LR, et al. 'EUROHEP' consensus report on the management of liver transplantation for hepatitis B virus infection. J Hepatol 1994;21: 1140–1143.
5. Potter JM, Hickman PE, Lynch SV, et al. Use of monoethylglycinexylidide as a liver function test in the liver transplant recipients. Transplantation 1993;56: 1385–1388.
6. Ollerich M, Burdelski M, Lautz HU, et al. Assessment of pretransplant prognosis with cirrhosis. Transplantation 1991;51:801–806.
7. Whitington PF, Alonso EM, Piper JB. Pediatric liver transplantation. Semin Liver Dis 1994;14:303–317.
8. Bion JF, Badger I, Crosby HA, et al. Selective decontamination of the digestive tract reduces gram-negative pulmonary colonization but not systemic endotoxemia in patients undergoing elective liver transplantation. Crit Care Med 1994;22:40–49.
9. Mito M, Kusano M. Hepatocyte transplantation in man. Cell Transplantation 1993;2:65–74.
10. Dixit V. Development of bioartificial liver using isolated hepatocytes. Artif Organs 1994;18:371–384.
11. Venkataramanan R, Habucky K, Burckart GJ, et al. Clinical pharmacokinetics in organ transplant patients. Clin Pharmacokinet 1989;16:134–161.
12. LeMoine O, Marchant A, Durand F, et al. Systemic release of IL-10 during orthotopic liver transplantation. Hepatology 1994;20:889–892.
13. The U.S. Multicenter Tacrolimus Liver Study Group. A comparison of tacrolimus (FK-506) and cyclosporine for immunosuppression in liver transplantation. N Engl J Med 1994;331(17):1110–1115.
14. European Tacrolimus Multicenter Liver Study Group. Randomized trial comparing tacrolimus (FK-506) and cyclosporine in prevention of liver allograft rejection. Lancet 1994;344(8920):423–428.
15. Dummer JS. Cytomegalovirus infection after liver transplantation: Clinical manifestations and strategies for prevention. J Infect Dis 1990;12(suppl 7):S767–S775.
16. Halwachs G, Zach R, Pogglitsch H, et al. A rapid immunocytochemical assay for CMV detection in peripheral blood of organ-transplanted patients in clinical practice. Transplantation 1993;56:338–342.

Section 4
Renal Disorders

Chapter 42
Quantification of Renal Function

Thomas J. Comstock, PharmD

Renal function includes the processes of filtration, secretion, and reabsorption, as well as endocrine and metabolic functions. Alterations of all five renal functions, whether declining or improving, have been associated primarily with glomerular filtration rate (GFR).[1] This chapter discusses the predominant methods currently available to quantify renal function, with emphasis on GFR, renal plasma and blood flow, as well as tubular function indices (Table 42.1).

Renal Function

ENDOCRINE

Secretion of renin by the cells of the juxtaglomerular apparatus, production and metabolism of prostaglandins and kinins, and the production and secretion of erythropoietin by the interstitial cells in response to decreased oxygen tension in the blood are among the kidney's endocrine functions.[2] Since these functions are related to renal mass, decreased endocrine activity has been associated with the loss of viable cells. Hematocrit, for example, declines as a function of decreasing GFR, primarily due to a loss of erythropoietin production, leading to the complications associated with anemia, which include fatigue, dyspnea, anorexia, and the development of, or increased, angina.[3,4]

METABOLIC

The kidneys are capable of a wide variety of metabolic activities, including the activation of vitamin D_3, gluconeogenesis, and metabolism of endogenous compounds such as insulin and steroids, as well as xenobiotics. Impaired renal function results in decreased formation of activated vitamin D_3 and decreased insulin metabolism. It is common for patients with diabetes and chronic renal failure to have reduced requirements for exogenous insulin,[5,6] and supplemental therapy with activated vitamin D_3 (calcitriol) is often necessary in the management of renal osteodystrophy.[7] Numerous enzymes have been identified in the kidneys, primarily the cortex. These include cytochrome P-450, *N*-acetyltransferase, glutathione transferase, renal peptidases, and others.[8,9] Reversible metabolism may also be affected by renal disease when normal enzyme function is disrupted. This has been observed with clofibrate[10] and may apply to other compounds eliminated by the same route, such as ketoprofen.[11]

EXCRETORY

Although endocrine and metabolic functions are important aspects of the kidney, it is the excretory function that is often perceived as the "kidney function." Through the combined processes of glomerular filtration, tubular secretion, and tubular reabsorption, the nephron, as the functional unit of the kidney, maintains balance between input and output of water and solutes from the body. This is represented as:

$$\text{Rate of excretion} = \text{Rate of filtration} + \text{Rate of secretion} - \text{Rate of reabsorption}$$

Glomerular filtration occurs by passive diffusion of water and small molecular weight ions and molecules across the

TABLE 42.1. MARKERS OF RENAL FUNCTION

Renal plasma/ blood flow	*p*-Aminohippurate (PAH) ^{125}I- or ^{131}I-orthoiodohippurate (^{125}I-OIH or ^{131}I-OIH) 5-Hydroxyindoleacetic acid (5-HIAA)
Glomerular filtration rate	Inulin Iothalamate, Iohexol ^{99m}Tc-DTPA ^{169}Yb-DTPA ^{125}I-Iothalamate Creatinine Cystatin C
Tubular function	PAH, 5-HIAA *N*-1-Methylnicotinamide (NMN) Tetraethyl ammonium (TEA) β_2-Microglobulin Retinol-binding protein (RBP) Protein HC (α_1-Microglobulin) *N*-Acetylglucosaminidase (NAG) Alanine aminopeptidase (AAP) Adenosine binding protein (ABP)

glomerular-capillary membrane into Bowman's capsule and the proximal tubule. Since most proteins are too large to be filtered, compounds presented to the glomerulus in the bound state are not filtered and enter the peritubular circulation. Secretion occurs primarily along the proximal tubule and facilitates elimination of compounds through active transport from the plasma into the tubular lumen. Anionic and cationic transport systems have been characterized and are involved in the transport of many endogenous and exogenous substances. Examples include probenecid, *p*-aminohippurate (PAH), and penicillin as anions, and creatinine, cimetidine, and procainamide as cations.[12] These systems are not mutually exclusive, because probenecid has been observed to compete with the tubular secretion of cimetidine.[13] Reabsorption of water and solutes occurs throughout the nephron, while drug reabsorption occurs predominantly along the distal tubule and collecting tubules. These processes are influenced by urine flow rate and physicochemical characteristics of the molecule. Highly ionized compounds are not reabsorbed unless pH changes within the urine alter the fraction unionized, whereby reabsorption may be facilitated.[14]

The homeostasis afforded by the kidneys is affected by catecholamines, prostaglandins, renin, antidiuretic hormone, natriuretic hormone, and the number of functioning nephrons. The "intact nephron hypothesis" of Bricker[15,16] proposes that whole kidney function is the net result of a reduced number of appropriately functioning nephrons. As the number of nephrons is reduced from the initial complement of 2 million, those unaffected will compensate for those damaged by disease or toxic insult. The cornerstone of this hypothesis is that glomerulotubule balance is maintained, such that those nephrons capable of functioning will continue to perform in an appropriate fashion. As GFR declines, tubular reabsorption must decrease in order to allow for elimination of the solute load. Single nephron GFR increases in the remnant nephrons, whereas the whole kidney GFR represents the sum of the remaining functional nephrons. Based on this, one would presume that a measure of one component of nephron function could be used as an estimate of all renal functions. This indeed has been and remains our clinical approach.

Measurement of GFR, however, may not be appropriate to assess how a drug will be handled that undergoes active tubular secretion, or reabsorption. As an example, Hori et al.[17,18] demonstrated that the postfiltration renal handling of ampicillin, which is secreted, and cephalexin, which is secreted and reabsorbed, remained normal in patients with renal failure due to glomerulonephritis, but was reduced in patients with renal failure and tubular dysfunction. They concluded that dosage adjustment based on creatinine clearance is not appropriate for drugs eliminated by tubular secretion. Maiza and Daley-Yates[19] have also observed glomerulotubule imbalance in experimentally induced renal failure in rats based on differential effects on inulin (GFR), PAH (an index of anionic secretion), and *N*-1-methylnicotinamide clearance (an index of cationic secretion). Using an experimental nephrotoxic (uranyl nitrate) acute renal failure model in rats, Lin and Lin[20] and Gloff and Benet[21] demonstrated differential handling of tetraethylammonium bromide (TEAB) and PAH, with greater impairment of tubular secretion than GFR. Lin and Lin[20] further studied an ischemic acute renal failure model (glycerol) and showed a parallel decline of secretion and GFR for TEAB, whereas secretion of PAH decreased at a greater rate than GFR. These results support the differential pathways for elimination of compounds, which may be dependent on the mode of injury as well as the chemical characteristics of the compound itself. Thus, the kidney should not be considered as a single homogeneously functioning organ, but one with several different, discrete functions. It is thus analogous to the liver in which the multiple metabolic pathways may be impaired to variable degrees dependent on the type of injury or disease.[22]

Quantification of renal function is not only an important diagnostic index, but it also serves as an important parameter for monitoring therapy directed at the etiology of the diminished function itself, thereby allowing for objective measurement of the success or failure of treatment.[23–25] Measurement of renal function also serves as a useful indicator of the ability of the kidneys to eliminate drugs from the body[26,27] (see Chapter 50). Furthermore, alterations of drug distribution[28,29] and metabolism[30–32] have also been associated with the degree of renal function. Although several indices have been used for the quantification of renal function in the research setting, GFR and, more specifically, creatinine clearance has been the primary marker of renal function in the clinical arena.

Measurement of Renal Plasma and Blood Flow

Renal blood and plasma flow are not common clinical measures of renal function, but may provide insight into hemodynamic changes related to disease or drug therapy. The kidneys receive approximately 20% of cardiac output and representative values of renal blood flow in men and women of 1209 ± 256 and 982 ± 184 mL/min/1.73 m^2 have been reported, respectively.[33] Renal plasma flow (RPF) is estimated to be 60% of blood flow if one assumes the average hematocrit is 40%, and it can be measured by the use of model compounds that are eliminated from the plasma compartment on a single pass through the kidneys. Since only 20% of the plasma is filtered at the glomerulus, the compound must undergo active tubular secretion and minimal to no reabsorption in order to be completely eliminated. To accurately reflect RPF, the extraction through the kidney must be nearly 100%. Aminohippurate sodium (PAH or sodium *p*-aminohippurate) is an organic anion that has been used extensively for the quantitation of renal plasma flow. PAH is bound approximately 83% to plasma proteins and is eliminated extensively by active tubular secretion. Since PAH elimination is active, saturation of the transport processes should be anticipated. Indeed, concentrations of PAH in plasma should not exceed 20 mg/L. Furthermore, PAH is metabolized, possibly within the kidney to *N*-acetyl-PAH, and the renal clearance of PAH alone has been noted by Prescott et al.[34] to decrease with decreasing plasma concentrations while the clearance of the acetyl metabolite increases. Total PAH clearance remained unchanged. Further studies are necessary to evaluate the mechanisms and significance of these findings. The extraction ratio for PAH is 70–90% at plasma concentrations of 10–20 mg/L, hence the term "effective" renal plasma flow (ERPF) has been used when the clearance of PAH is not corrected for the extraction ratio or if it is assumed to be one.[12] Normal values are 654 ± 163 mL/min for men and 592 ± 153 mL/min for women.[33] Children will reach normalized adult values by 3 years of age, and ERPF will begin to decline as a function of age after 30 years. The method for calculation of RPF is based on the relationship between organ clearance, extraction ratio, and flow:

$$CL_{r,\,PAH} = Q_{r,\,p} \times E \qquad \text{or} \qquad Q_{r,\,p} = CL_{r,\,PAH}/E$$

where CL_r = renal clearance of PAH, $Q_{r,p}$ = renal plasma flow, and E = extraction ratio of PAH by the kidneys. Effective renal blood flow ($Q_{r,b}$) can be estimated from ERPF assuming the extraction ratio is one and correcting for the red blood cell volume of the blood (hematocrit):

$$Q_{r,\,b} = Q_{r,\,p}/(1 - \text{Hct})$$

where Hct is the patient's hematocrit at the time of the study.

ERPF can also be measured using the radioisotopes ^{125}I- or ^{131}I-orthoiodohippurate (^{125}I-OIH or ^{131}I-OIH). One important advantage of this method is the ability to measure ERPF in total or for each kidney independently. Taylor et al.[35] compared four methods of calculating the RPF following injection of a single dose of ^{125}I-OIH in patients with various degrees of renal function. A two-compartment model, fitted to blood samples obtained during the 6 hours after injection, yielded the most accurate measurement. Other methods using fewer observations and a shorter time period resulted in overestimation of the ERPF by as much as 70% in patients with reduced renal function. These data support the biexponential approach to calculating ERPF following a single injection of ^{125}I-OIH.

Hannedouche et al.[36] have evaluated plasma 5-hydroxyindoleacetic acid (5-HIAA) as an endogenous marker of RPF. It is a metabolite of serotonin and eliminated by glomerular filtration and tubular secretion. Plasma 5-HIAA can, however, be affected by changes in dietary serotonin intake, and ethanol ingestion will impair the formation of 5-HIAA from serotonin. Furthermore, the analytic method to determine plasma 5-HIAA concentrations is high-pressure liquid chromatography (HPLC), with electrochemical detection, a procedure that is often delicate. Thus, although this method may minimize the need for administration of exogenous compounds to assess RPF, it is not likely to be widely available clinically. The study of 27 samples resulted in a correlation of $CL_{5\text{-HIAA}} = 1.15\ CL_{PAH} - 16$ mL/min, r = 0.76.

Measurement of Glomerular Filtration Rate

The single best measure or index of renal function is the GFR. Normally there are approximately 1 million nephrons per kidney, and each nephron functions independently with regard to filtration. The net effect, or the total GFR, is a representation of the functional renal mass. As renal mass declines, due to normal physiologic loss of nephrons secondary to the aging process or due to disease, there is a progressive decline in GFR. As such, the total filtration rate represents the functional status of the kidneys.[37,38]

GFR is the volume of plasma filtered across the glomerulus per unit time. Considering a normal RBF of approximately 1.0 L/min, plasma volume 60% of blood volume, and filtration fraction across the glomerulus of 20%, the normal GFR would then be approximately 120 mL/min/1.73 m^2.[2]

Accurate measurement of the GFR requires a compound that has unrestricted diffusion across the glomerulus and into Bowman's capsule without additional contribution by tubular secretion nor loss by reabsorption. Furthermore, the solute should not undergo metabolism by renal tubular cells or alter renal function. Given these conditions, the

GFR would be equivalent to the renal clearance of the solute marker:

$$GFR = CL_r = (A_e)/AUC_{0-t}$$

where CL_r is renal clearance of the marker, A_e is the amount of marker excreted in a specified period of time, t, and AUC_{0-t} is the area under the plasma concentration time curve of the marker. Under steady-state conditions, the expression simplifies to

$$GFR = CL_r = (A_e)/[(C_{ss}) \times t]$$

where C_{ss} is the steady-state plasma concentration of the marker. Several solutes have been utilized for the measurement of GFR and include both exogenous and endogenous compounds. Those administered as exogenous agents, such as inulin, iothalamate, or radioisotopes, require specialized administration techniques and detection methods for the quantitation of function, but generally provide a more accurate measure of GFR. Methods that employ endogenous compounds, such as creatinine, require less technical expertise, but produce results with greater variability.[1] The compound of choice will depend on the purpose of the test, as research protocols will generally utilize a more accurate test than one used in the clinical setting (Table 42.2).

INULIN CLEARANCE

Inulin is a relatively large molecule (5200 daltons) compared to most drugs, and has the necessary characteristics to serve as a marker for the measurement of GFR. Inulin is a fructose polysaccharide, obtained from plant tubers of the Jerusalem artichoke, dahlia, and chicory plants. It is not bound to plasma proteins, is freely filtered at the glomerulus, is not secreted or reabsorbed, and is not metabolized by the kidney.[1] The apparent volume of distribution for inulin is approximately extracellular volume, or 20% of ideal body weight. Since it is eliminated by glomerular filtration, its elimination half-life is dependent on renal function, and is approximately 1.3 hr in subjects with normal renal function. For a subject with a GFR of 10 mL/min, the elimination half-life increases to approximately 16 hr. Therefore, a loading dose is essential when using the steady-state approach for estimation of GFR.

TABLE 42.2. SENSITIVITY AND CLINICAL UTILITY OF RENAL FUNCTION TESTS

	Accuracy	Clinical Utility
Inulin clearance	++++	+
Radiolabeled markers	+++	+
Nonisotopic contrast agents	+++	++
Creatinine clearance	++	+++
Serum creatinine	+	++++

+, least acceptable.
++, adequate.
+++, better.
++++, best.

The most common technique for determination of GFR with inulin involves bolus administration followed by a continuous infusion of inulin.[38,39] The infusion dose must be adjusted in patients with diminished renal function due to the dependence of inulin elimination on GFR. A typical loading dose of 40 mg/kg is administered followed by a maintenance infusion of 25 mg/min/1.73 m^2 × RF, where RF is the estimated fraction of normal renal function. For such situations, the maintenance infusion is reduced to the fraction of expected GFR based on an estimated creatinine clearance. Following a 60-min equilibration period, sequential measurements of inulin clearance are made over a period of 30 min for three intervals. Urine is collected, and blood samples bracket each collection period. Because GFR may be dependent on renal blood flow, it is necessary to maintain adequate hydration during the test for the purposes of adequate filtration as well as urine production. A relatively constant urine flow will decrease the variability among repeated measurements and should be within the range of 1–10 mL/min. An initial water load of 10–15 mL/kg body weight will usually initiate a diuresis, and additional water equal to the output of each interval should be given for each collection period.[39]

Inulin clearance has also been estimated following a single-dose intravenous injection via multiple sampling of blood to estimate area under the curve and calculation of clearance from the disappearance curve. Rosenbaum et al.[40] collected blood samples over 90 and 120 min and calculated plasma inulin clearance; correlations were 0.87 and 0.92, respectively, compared with the standard inulin infusion technique. Rose[41] employed a continuous infusion of inulin following a bolus injection and determined plasma clearance from a single plasma concentration. Approximately 4 hr were needed to achieve steady state, and the results were similar to those obtained using the traditional urine collection method. Florijn et al.[42] compared the infusion and single-shot techniques for both total body and urinary clearance in 14 patients with autosomal-dominant polycystic kidney disease. Variability was lower using total body clearance, but it overestimated the renal clearance by 10–20%. The authors provide a regression equation to account for the overestimation, however, measurement of renal clearance will avoid the need to introduce additional variability into the assessment of renal function.

Measurement of plasma and urine inulin concentrations can be performed using a colorimetric reaction to detect fructose following acid hydrolysis of inulin, or enzymatically.[43] Glucose cross-reacts with the colorimetric measurement; therefore, it is necessary to correct samples with a "blank" obtained prior to infusion of the inulin. Individuals with elevated plasma glucose concentrations that change during the evaluation will show increased variability in their results.[1]

The majority of variability in the inulin clearance can be attributed to body size and is reduced if corrected to body surface area. The normal range will decrease with increasing age, at a rate of approximately 10 mL/min/1.73 m^2 for each decade over 30 years. Gender and differences in renal function, due to physiologic conditions and/or disease state, may also contribute to the observed variability in the test. Normal inulin clearance is approximately 120 mL/min/1.73 m^2, slightly higher for men and lower for women.[1]

IOTHALAMATE CLEARANCE

Alternatives have been sought for inulin as a marker for GFR due to the problems of intermittent availability, high cost, invasiveness, sample preparation, and assay variability. Iothalamate has been commonly used in radiocontrast studies, but is also available in an unlabeled form. This agent is handled in a manner similar to that of inulin. It appears to be freely filtered at the glomerulus, and does not undergo substantial tubular secretion or reabsorption.[44] Iothalamate has most commonly been employed in its radiolabeled form, ^{125}I-iothalamate, but recently has been used as a nonisotopic probe. Plasma and urine iothalamate concentrations have been measured using HPLC methods,[45,46] and can be analyzed simultaneously with PAH.[47] Protein binding in humans was found to be less than 1%, and iothalamate renal clearance would appear to be an excellent alternative to inulin for the measurement of GFR.

Iohexol, a nonionic, low osmolar, iodinated contrast agent, has also been used for the determination of GFR. It is eliminated almost entirely by glomerular filtration and plasma and renal clearance values are similar.[48] Brown and O'Reilly[49] performed simultaneous renal clearance studies of inulin and iohexol in 30 patients with various degrees of renal function. Clearance values were very similar, $CL_{iohexol} = 0.998\ CL_{inulin} - 2.309$ mL/min, $r = 0.986$. Detection of iohexol in plasma and urine samples was based on x-ray fluorescence analysis.

LABELED MARKERS

The GFR has also been evaluated using radiolabeled markers,[50,51] the most common including ^{125}I-iothalamate (614 daltons, radioactive half-life of 60 days),[52,53] ^{99m}Tc-diethylenetriamine penta-acetic acid (DTPA, 393 daltons, radioactive half-life of 6.03 hr),[54,55] and ^{51}Cr-ethylenediaminetetraacetic acid (EDTA, 292 daltons, radioactive half-life of 27 days).[56] They are all relatively small molecules that are minimally bound to plasma proteins and do not undergo tubular secretion or reabsorption to any significant degree.[1,50] ^{125}I-Iothalamate and ^{99m}Tc-DTPA are used in the United States, whereas ^{51}Cr-EDTA is used extensively in Europe. Various protocols exist for the administration of the marker and subsequent determination of renal clearance. These protocols center around the issue of plasma clearance versus renal clearance and the collection of urine during the evaluation period. The primary concern is whether the marker is cleared solely by filtration in the kidneys or by other routes of elimination. Measurement of radioactivity in blood samples and standard pharmacokinetic approaches using either a single point estimation based on a constant[57] or a slope and intercept method[58] results in plasma clearance, which will overestimate GFR if elimination occurs by routes other than the kidneys. A more accurate approach would necessitate the measurement of urine excretion rates and activity in the blood.

Tepe et al.[59] studied the relationship of various methods of GFR determination to inulin clearance using ^{131}I-diatrizoate administered as an intravenous injection. The single-sample method was found to be superior to the slope/intercept methods, which employ at least two post-dose plasma measurements. Generally, the single-sample method produced a lower value than the slope/intercept technique and resulted in values closer to a simultaneously determined inulin clearance, $R^2 = 0.994$. Nevertheless, both methods for the calculation of clearance resulted in values similar to the observed inulin clearance. Of note, the range of inulin clearance was approximately 40–160 mL/min in the patients evaluated. In contrast, LaFrance et al.[54] reported that the plasma clearance of ^{99m}Tc-DTPA correlated poorly with its renal clearance in 64 clearance determinations in 22 patients with severe renal insufficiency (iothalamate renal clearance <35 mL/min, $R^2 = 0.48$). The same patients showed a good correlation between renal ^{99m}Tc-DTPA and ^{125}I-iothalamate clearance. ^{125}I-Iothalamate has also been compared with inulin in this same population and indicated a good correlation with the inulin measurement of renal clearance. These data strongly suggest the use of renal clearance protocols for patients with impaired kidney function.

Perrone et al.,[55] as part of the multicenter Modification of Diet in Renal Disease Study, simultaneously evaluated three radiolabeled markers of GFR using renal clearance, compared to inulin. These included ^{125}I-iothalamate, ^{169}Yb-DTPA, and ^{99m}Tc-DTPA. All radiolabeled markers overestimated inulin clearance in normal subjects by approximately 5–10%. Patients with renal impairment showed a small but significant overestimation of their inulin clearance when measured using ^{125}I-iothalamate or ^{169}Yb-DTPA. Clearance of creatinine overestimated the GFR at all levels of kidney function. Based on their results, the authors suggested the radioisotopic filtration markers would be suitable alternatives to inulin for measurement of GFR.

^{51}Cr-EDTA also yields estimates of GFR similar to inulin and in some cases slightly lower. This may be due to plasma protein binding or tubular reabsorption. As with ^{125}I-iothalamate and ^{99m}Tc-DTPA, ^{51}Cr-EDTA plasma clearance is greater than renal clearance, probably due to nonrenal routes of elimination.[54]

Rodman et al.[60] evaluated ^{99m}Tc-DTPA serum clearance as a predictor of GFR in 17 children with cancer, 3–17 years of age. Using unbound ^{99m}Tc-DTPA as the reference, a limited sampling schedule using three samples was shown to overestimate the reference method, but the application of a correction factor of 0.8 produced nearly identical results.

Labeled markers have also been used for real-time monitoring of GFR during critical care of patients. Rabito et al.[61] studied 20 patients in an intensive care unit using an external radionuclide counting system to measure the rate of disappearance of ^{99m}Tc-DTPA from the extracellular space. Comparisons were made with short-term creatinine clearance measurements, and the rate constant for the ^{99m}Tc-DTPA disappearance predicted the renal function status in 94% of the patients. Patient outcomes were not assessed and further studies are needed to determine its utility in the early detection of acute renal dysfunction.

CREATININE CLEARANCE

The most common clinical test for the assessment of renal function is the serum creatinine concentration. Creatinine is a product of creatine metabolism from muscle, therefore its production is directly dependent on muscle mass.[62] At steady state, the "normal" serum creatinine concentration is approximately 0.5–1.5 mg/dL, although numerous factors, such as age, body mass, and gender, will affect the concentration, making its interpretation alone difficult at best.[1,62–64] Creatinine is eliminated primarily by glomerular filtration, and as GFR declines, the serum creatinine concentration will rise (Fig. 42.1).

Several methods are used for the determination of the serum creatinine concentration, most of which are based on the nonspecific method using the Jaffé reaction: a colorimetric method based on the reaction of creatinine with alkaline picrate. This nonspecific method also reacts with noncreatinine chromogens in the serum, which may result in a falsely increased serum creatinine concentration.[62] Other substances that also react with this procedure in the serum include glucose, protein, pyruvate, acetoacetate, fructose, uric acid, and ascorbic acid[62,63,65] (Table 42.3). The chromogens are not present in the urine. The impact of this interference is seen with the clearance calculation:

$$CL_{Cr} = (U_{cr} \times V)/(S_{cr} \times t)$$

where U_{cr} = urine creatinine concentration, V = urine volume, S_{cr} = serum creatinine concentration, and t = time. The extent of the interference is to increase the serum creatinine

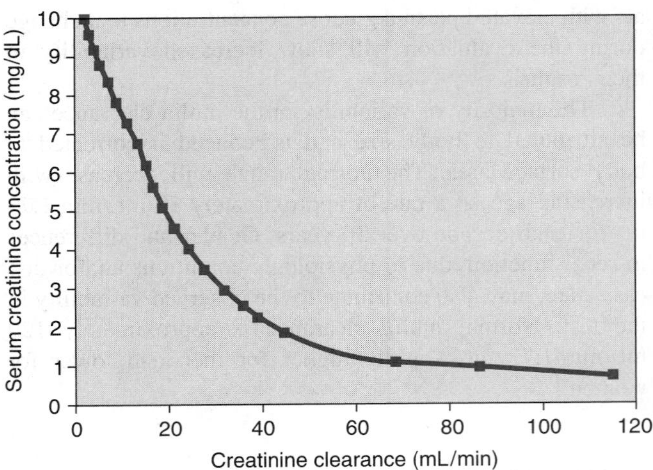

Figure 42.1. Relationship between serum creatinine concentration and creatinine clearance.

concentration approximately 10% and thereby the creatinine clearance would underestimate the GFR by 10%. In subjects with normal renal function, this tends to counterbalance the effect of the contribution of tubular secretion of creatinine, which increases urine creatinine by nearly 10%. Thus, CL_{cr} may serve as a good measure of GFR in subjects with normal renal function. However, this false increase in serum creatinine becomes less noticeable as the true creatinine concentration rises due to the increasing contribution of tubular secretion to the renal clearance of creatinine.[1,63,66,67]

Diabetic ketoacidosis may produce increased concentrations of acetoacetate, which serves as a chromophore in the Jaffé reaction, thereby increasing the serum creatinine concentration.[68] In addition, some cephalosporin antibiotics have been associated with a false increase in the serum creatinine concentration, including cephalothin, cefazolin, cephalexin, cefoxitin, cefaclor, and cephra-

TABLE 42.3. FACTORS THAT MAY ALTER CREATININE CLEARANCE DETERMINATIONS

Analytic	Physiologic
Glucose	Age, weight, gender
Protein	Exercise
Pyruvate	Diurnal variation
Acetoacetate	Diet
Fructose	Drugs (cimetidine, trimethoprim, probenecid)
Uric acid	
Ascorbic acid	
Cephalosporins (cephalothin, cefazolin, cephalexin, cefoxitin, cefaclor, cephradine)	
5-Flucytosine	

dine,[69] while other antibiotics, such as the fluoroquinolones (ciprofloxacin, fleroxacin, lomafloxacin, ofloxacin, 1-ofloxacin, sparfloxacin, and temafloxacin) have been shown not to interact.[70] The degree of interference is dependent on the serum concentration of the antibiotic, so blood samples for creatinine should be obtained when the antibiotic concentration is lowest (i.e., at the end of a dosing interval). These interferences are not observed when the serum creatinine is measured using an enzymatic technique. The antifungal agent, 5-flucytosine, causes an increase in the serum creatinine when measured using the Ektachem system, but does not interact with the Jaffé method.[71] The Ektachem system has also been observed by Apple et al.[72] to yield serum creatinine concentrations 0.2–0.3 mg/dL higher than with nonenzymatic methods. These differences emphasize the need to standardize a method within the research or clinic setting.

Other compounds are known to interfere with the serum creatinine concentration, through inhibition of the active tubular secretion of creatinine. Among these are cimetidine[73] and trimethoprim,[74] which compete for creatinine secretion at the cationic transport system. Cibenzoline,[46] an antiarrhythmic agent and organic base that also undergoes tubular secretion, failed to show any effect on the CL_{cr} when given at doses of 130 mg orally every 12 hr. Competition with creatinine for tubular secretion appears to be dose dependent, and the cibenzoline dose may have been inadequate to compete for creatinine secretion. Both trimethoprim and cimetidine have demonstrated dose dependency with respect to competition with creatinine for secretion.[46]

The serum creatinine concentration is dependent on the "input" function, or formation rate, and "output" function, or elimination rate. Its formation rate depends on the zero-order production from creatine metabolism as well as input from other sources, such as dietary intake.[62] Creatine metabolism is directly proportional to muscle mass, therefore individuals with larger amounts of muscle will have a higher serum creatinine concentration at any given degree of kidney function than one with less muscle mass. Exercise has been associated with an increase of approximately 10% in the serum creatinine concentration.[75] Cachectic patients, as the result of minimal muscle mass, will have very low serum creatinine concentrations, as do those with spinal cord injuries.[76] Elderly patients and those with poor nutrition may also have low serum creatinine concentrations (<1.0 mg/dL) secondary to decreased muscle mass. Other factors that influence the serum creatinine concentration include the dietary intake of creatinine. During the cooking of meat, some creatine is converted to creatinine, which is rapidly absorbed following ingestion. Serum creatinine concentrations may rise as much as 50% within 2 hr of a meat meal and remain elevated for as long as 8–24 hr as shown in Fig. 42.2.[77] This presents a problem only when a single serum creatinine concentration is used to represent the entire 24-hr collection period. An alternative is to obtain multiple samples and calculate the area under the serum concentration time curve and divide by the collection time interval to obtain the average plasma creatinine concentration. This is rarely done in clinical practice, but points out the need to question patients regarding dietary intake for the 24 hr preceding the measurement.

Diurnal variation in serum creatinine concentration may also affect the accuracy of the CL_{cr} determination. Although the fluctuation is minimal, the observed peak plasma creatinine concentration generally occurs at approximately 7:00 PM while the nadir is in the morning.[78] To minimize this effect, the CL_{cr} is usually performed over a 24-hr period with the plasma creatinine obtained in the morning, as long as the patient has stable kidney function. Collection of urine remains a limiting factor in the 24-hour CL_{cr} due to variability likely caused by incomplete collections. Although Forbes et al.[79] reported day-to-day variability can be further reduced by collecting urine over 3 days, urine collection intervals of less than 24 hr have been advocated by most. Bingham et al.[80] used *para*-amino benzoic acid as

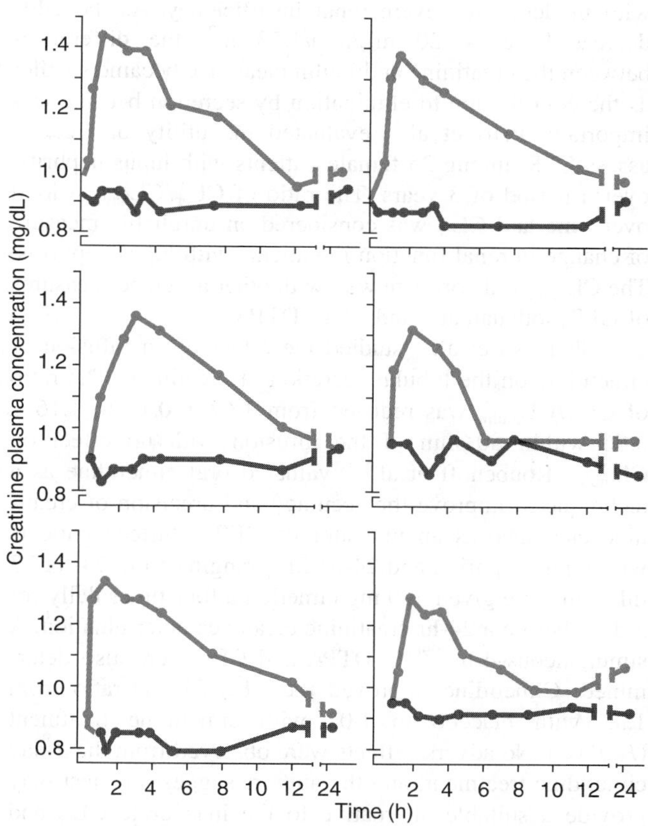

Figure 42.2. Creatinine plasma concentration as a function of time following a control breakfast devoid of meat protein (●) and following experimental breakfast of cooked meat protein (●). *(From Br J Clin Pharmaco 1983;15:228, with permission.)*

an oral marker to assess the completeness of 24-hr urine collections in 63 hospital outpatients. Twenty-nine percent were judged incomplete. Fuller and Elia[81] identified an additional complicating factor—the interconversion between creatinine and creatine that can occur if the urine is not maintained at a pH <6.

Creatinine is eliminated by both glomerular filtration and tubular secretion. Tubular secretion augments the filtered creatinine by about 10% in subjects with normal kidney function. This, however, increases to as much as 100% in patients with renal insufficiency.[63,64] As renal impairment develops, the remaining nephrons hypertrophy, and the degree of tubular secretion increases disproportionately to the increase in filtration. The result is an overestimation of creatinine clearance as a function of GFR as assessed using inulin clearance (Fig. 42.3). Bauer et al.[63] assessed creatinine clearance as a function of inulin clearance in 123 subjects with various degrees of kidney function. Using a specific assay for the measurement of creatinine, the ratio of CL_{cr} exceeded CL_{inulin} by 14%, thus suggesting 14% of the creatinine was eliminated by secretion. The CL_{cr}/CL_{inulin} ratio in subjects with mild impairment was 1.20; for moderate impairment 1.87; and severe impairment 2.32. Thus, creatinine clearance is a poor indicator of GFR in patients with moderate to severe renal insufficiency. As the GFR decreased below 20 mL/min/1.73 m^2, the differences between the creatinine and inulin clearance became smaller as the contribution to elimination by secretion became less important. Petri et al.[82] evaluated the utility of CL_{cr} to assess GFR among 25 female patients with lupus nephritis over a period of 3 years. The ratio of CL_{cr}/CL_{inulin} varied over time and CL_{cr} was considered an unreliable measure of change in renal function in patients with lupus nephritis. The CL_{inulin} did correlate well with other accepted measures of GFR, iothalamate, and ^{99m}Tc-DTPA.

Shemesh et al.[83] studied the effect of an infusion of cimetidine on the tubular secretion of creatinine. The ratio of CL_{cr}/CL_{inulin} was reduced from 1.67 ± 0.10 to 1.16 ± 0.06 within 80 min of the infusion with no effect on CL_{inulin}. Roubenoff et al.[84] evaluated oral cimetidine as a technique to improve the accuracy and precision of creatinine clearance as an indicator of GFR. Thirteen patients with lupus nephritis and 24-hr CL_{cr} ranging from 24–115.3 mL/min were given 400 mg cimetidine four times daily for 2 days before a 24-hr creatinine clearance determination. A simultaneous 4-hr ^{99m}Tc-DTPA and CL_{cr} were also determined. Cimetidine improved the CL_{cr}/CL_{DTPA} ratio from 1.33 with placebo to 1.07 with cimetidine treatment (P<0.05). No adverse effects were observed from the 2-day cimetidine treatment, and the authors suggest this test may provide a suitable alternative to the inaccurate CL_{cr} and expensive CL_{DTPA} tests to estimate GFR. Hilbrands et al.[85] and Van Acker et al.[86] have confirmed these results although the latter group noted a dose-dependency effect of cimetidine; subjects with higher renal cimetidine clearance

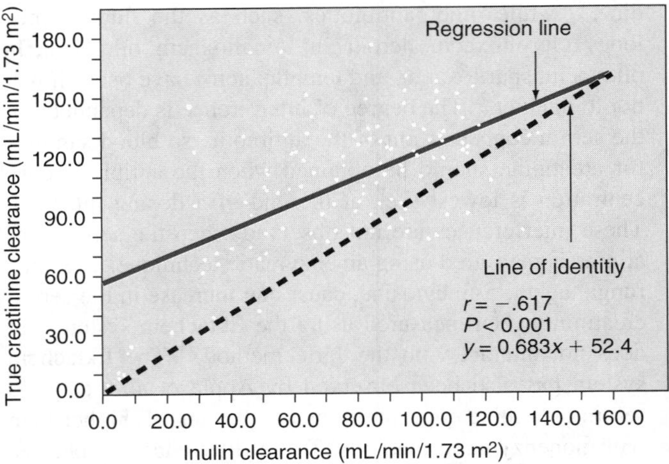

Figure 42.3. Relationship between true creatinine clearance, using a specific assay for creatinine, and inulin clearance (duplicate points have been omitted for clarity). *(From Am J Kidney Dis 1982;2:341, with permission.)*

required larger cimetidine doses for complete blockade of creatinine tubular secretion.

Despite the common use of CL_{cr} to estimate GFR, it is a controversial measurement. Lemann et al.[24] have shown that CL_{cr} correlates very well with iothalamate clearance performed using the single injection technique. In a multicenter study designed to evaluate the effects of angiotensin-converting enzyme inhibition in 136 patients with type I diabetic nephropathy, GFR was assessed using duplicate serum creatinine and 24-hr CL_{cr} and four iothalamate clearance periods by single injection technique during water diuresis with simultaneous CL_{cr}. Creatinine clearance was also estimated for each patient using the Cockcroft–Gault method,[87] corrected for weight and gender. The simultaneous $CL_{iothalamate}$ and CL_{cr} were 78 ± 35 and 86 ± 35 mL/min while the separate 24-hr CL_{cr} was 75 ± 33 mL/min. The Cockcroft–Gault estimate was 79 ± 29 mL/min. Compared to $CL_{iothalamate}$ as the standard, the R^2 values for the simultaneous CL_{cr}, 24-hr CL_{cr}, and Cockcroft–Gault CL_{cr} were 0.81, 0.49, and 0.67, indicating increased variability with the 24-hr clearance determinations. It was not stated whether the 24-hr CL_{cr} measurements were performed as inpatient or ambulatory procedures. For a group of 110 mainly healthy men—comprised of normals, kidney stone patients, and one nephritic—the mean CL_{inulin} was 117 ± 18 mL/min compared to 129 ± 20 mL/min for measured CL_{cr} and 108 ± 19 for estimated CL_{cr} using the Cockcroft–Gault method. The range of inulin clearance was approximately 80–160 mL/min except for a single patient with a clearance of 51 mL/min. The relationship between the 24-hr CL_{cr} and CL_{inulin} showed an R^2 of 0.74, whereas the Cockcroft–Gault CL_{cr} was 0.41. Measurement of a 4-hr CL_{cr} during water diuresis provided the best estimate of the GFR as determined by the $CL_{iothalamate}$, and the ratio of $CL_{cr}/CL_{iothalamate}$ did not appear to increase as the GFR decreased (Fig. 42.4). These data suggest that a shorter collection period with a water diuresis may be the best method for determination of GFR when using creatinine clearance.

Estimation of Creatinine Clearance

Another approach to the clinical estimation of GFR is estimation of CL_{cr}, which incorporates the variables responsible for differences in the serum creatinine among individuals. Cockcroft and Gault (CG)[87] identified age and body mass as factors to incorporate in an equation to estimate CL_{cr}. Their relationship was based on 249 male patients with stable kidney function. Creatinine clearance ranged from 11 mL/min to normal for a 24-hr collection and creatinine excretion was greater than 10 mg/kg, except for 23 patients who were included when their 24-hr urine volume was greater than 500 mL. The relation between creatinine excretion and age reveals a significant decrease with increasing age (Fig. 42.5). Based on the usual CL_{cr} formula and the regression line obtained, the empiric formula to estimate CL_{cr} was derived and expressed as:

$$CL_{cr}\ (\text{mL/min}) = [(140 - \text{Age}) \times \text{IBW}]\ /(S_{cr} \times 72)$$

where age is expressed in years, S_{cr} is the serum creatinine in mg/dL, and IBW is ideal body weight in kg. For females, the result is multiplied by 0.85. It should be recognized that this expression yields an individualized CL_{cr} and that a standardized CL_{cr} is expressed as

$$CL_{cr}\ (\text{mL/min/72kg}) = (140 - \text{Age})/S_{cr}$$

Luke et al.[88] have evaluated the ability of the CG method and four other methods to predict renal function with inulin clearance being considered the standard. Simultaneous inulin and creatinine clearances, and a 24-hr ambulatory CL_{cr}, were conducted in 109 patients. The CL_{cr} was also estimated using five different methods as listed in Table 42.4. The simultaneously determined inulin and creatinine clearances correlated best, $R^2 = 0.85$, and the CL_{inulin} was overestimated by approximately 15% due to tubular secretion of creatinine. The 24-hr ambulatory CL_{cr} R^2 was 0.71. For the five calculated clearances, CG and Mawer et al.[89] correlated the best with inulin clearance. The CG method showed a linear relationship with CL_{inulin} = 1.121

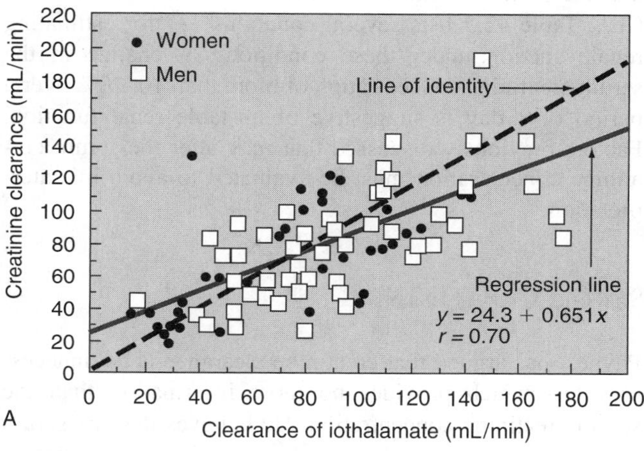

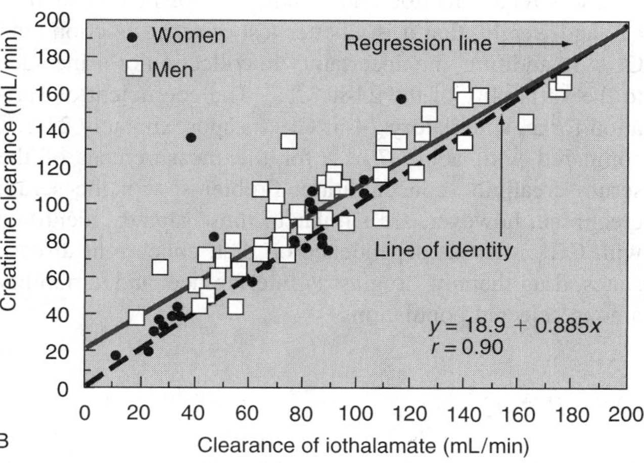

Figure 42.4. Relationships among patients with diabetic nephropathy between creatinine clearances, based on 24-hour urine collection (A) and four 30-minute urine collections (B). The solid line shows the mean regression relationships; the dashed line shows the line of identity. *(From Am J Kidney Dis 1990;16:238, with permission.)*

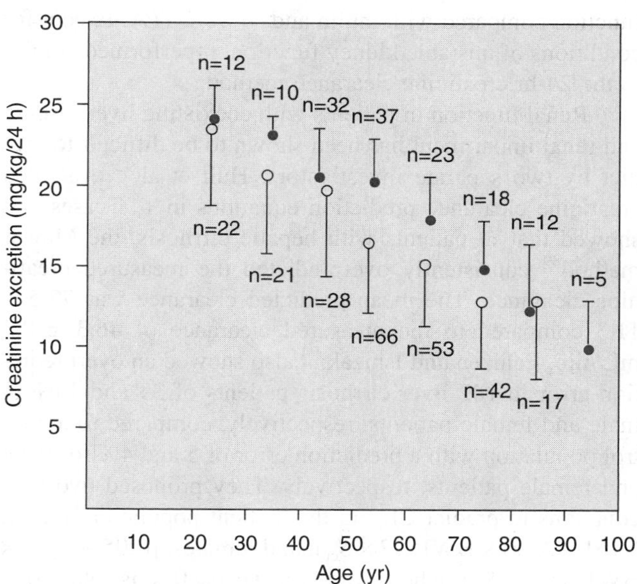

Figure 42.5. Creatinine excretion as a function of age. Solid circles, 149 males, age 20–99 years; open circles, 249 males, age 18–92 years. *(From Nephron 1976;16:34, with permission.)*

TABLE 42.4. EQUATIONS FOR THE ESTIMATION OF CREATININE CLEARANCE IN ADULTS WITH STABLE RENAL FUNCTION

1. Cockroft and Gault[87]	Men: CL_{cr} = (140 – Age) IBW / (S_{cr} × 72) Women: CL_{cr} × 0.85
2. Jelliffe[90]	Men: CL_{cr} = (100/S_{cr}) – 12 Women: CL_{cr} = (80/S_{cr}) – 7
3. Jelliffe[91]	Men: CL_{cr} = 98 – [0.8 (Age – 20)]/S_{cr} Women: CL_{cr} × 0.9
4. Mawer et al.[89]	Men: IBW [29.3 – (0.203 × Age)] [1 – (0.03 × S_{cr})]/(14.4 × S_{cr}) Women: IBW [25.3 – (0.175 × Age)] [1 – (0.03 × S_{cr})]/(14.4 × S_{cr})
5. Hull et al.[92]	Men: CL_{cr} = [(145 – Age)/S_{cr}] – 3 Women: CL_{cr} × 0.85

(CL_{cr}) + 20.6, R^2 = 0.66, whereas for Mawer the relationship was CL_{inulin} = 1.051 (CL_{cr}) + 18.3, R^2 = 0.66. The calculated CL_{cr} values from CG and Mawer both appeared to correlate well with the ambulatory and 4-hr CL_{cr}, but the regressions were not reported. Based on their findings, Luke et al.[88] propose continued use of the CG or Mawer method for rapid estimation of CL_{cr} in patients with stable kidney function. The other methods of Jelliffe[90,91] and Hull et al.[92] consistently underestimated the CL_{cr}. As kidney function declined, there was an increase in the fraction of creatinine eliminated by secretion as measured by the CL_{cr}/CL_{inulin} ratio, consistent with earlier reports. This limitation should be taken into consideration when attempting to use CL_{cr} for the estimation of renal function and the individualization of drug dosage regimens. Gault et al.[93] also evaluated the performance of the CG estimator of renal function compared with inulin and ^{99m}Tc-DTPA. Except for conditions of unstable kidney function, it performed similar to the 24-hr creatinine clearance method.

Renal function in patients with coexisting liver disease and renal impairment has been shown to be difficult to predict by two separate investigators. Hull et al.[92] evaluated creatinine clearance prediction equations in 144 cases and showed that in patients with hepatic cirrhosis, the Mawer method[89] consistently overpredicted the measured creatinine clearance. The mean predicted clearance was 73.5 ± 11.3 compared to the measured clearance of 46.3 ± 8.3 mL/min. Echizen and Ishizaki[94] also showed an overprediction error in 142 liver cirrhosis patients of 35 and 14% in male and female patients, respectively, compared to a control population with a prediction error of 5 and 4% for male and female patients, respectively. They proposed two new equations to predict CL_{cr} in this patient population: males, [(161 – Age) × BW]/(97 × S_{cr}); and females, [(205 – Age) × BW]/(152 × S_{cr}), where Age is in years, BW is total body weight in kg, and S_{cr} is serum creatinine concentration in mg/dL. In a prospective evaluation of the new equations, the investigators showed a prediction error of 2 and –7% for males and females, respectively. The proposed mechanism for these observations is based on a decreased excretion rate of creatinine compared to controls, increased extrahepatic creatinine metabolism or decreased synthesis of creatine in the liver, and subsequent decreased storage in the muscle and therefore, lowered production of creatinine. These data illustrate the inherent limitations of nomogram approaches to the estimation of renal function.

Renal function assessment during pregnancy is usually performed using a 24-hr creatinine clearance determination. Quadri and colleagues[95] evaluated the CG formula to estimate renal function in 34 pregnant women during each trimester, compared with the measured 24-hr creatinine clearance. Prepregnancy weights were used throughout the study for the CG estimate, and results correlated well with those for the measured clearance (R^2 = 0.76). Peak clearance occurred during the second trimester for both methods.

Patients with unstable kidney function present a unique situation since the serum creatinine is changing and the rate of change must be considered in the estimation of CL_{cr}. Table 42.5 lists several equations[96–98] for estimating renal function under these conditions. A change in the serum creatinine concentration of more than 10–20% over a period of 1 day is suggestive of unstable renal function. Factors previously discussed that may alter the serum creatinine concentration must be evaluated to avoid misinterpretation.

SERUM CREATININE

Payne[66] has argued that creatinine clearance is an unnecessary test which provides no more information than the serum creatinine concentration. He believes that the serum creatinine concentration alone gives sufficient information to assess renal function and, if adjusted for factors such as age and weight, that it is a better test of renal function than CL_{cr}. In addition, the uncertainty in collection of urine adds to the variability of the 24-hr CL_{cr}. The coefficient of variation for an ambulatory 24-hr CL_{cr} is approximately 27%,[99] compared with about 7%[100] for the measurement of the serum creatinine concentration. Problems with the serum creatinine, however, are similar to those already identified with CL_{cr}, such as dependence on diet, concurrent disease states, drug therapy, drug assay interference, and variability among selected populations.

CYSTATIN C

A relatively new marker for renal function has been identified and evaluated in small populations for its utility as a tool to assess changes in GFR. Cystatin C is a nonglycosylated 13-kDa basic protein of the cystatin superfamily of inhibitors of cysteine proteases.[48,101–103] It is produced by

TABLE 42.5. EQUATIONS FOR THE ESTIMATION OF CREATININE CLEARANCE IN ADULTS WITH UNSTABLE RENAL FUNCTION

Reference	Units	Equations: Males	Equations: Females
Jelliffe and Jelliffe[96]	mL/min/1.73 m²	$E^{ss} = \text{IBW}\,[29.3 - 0.203\,(\text{Age})]$ $E^{ss}_{corr} = E^{ss}\,[1.035 - 0.0337\,(Scr)]$ $E = E^{ss}_{corr} - \dfrac{[4\,\text{IBW}\,(Scr_2 - Scr_1)]}{\Delta t\ \text{day}}$ $\text{CL}_{cr} = \dfrac{E}{14.4\,(Scr)}$	$E^{ss} = \text{IBW}\,[25.1 - 0.175\,(\text{Age})]$ $E^{ss}_{corr} = E^{ss}[1.035 - 0.0337\,(Scr)]$ $E = E^{ss}_{corr} - \dfrac{[4\,\text{IBW}\,(Scr_2 - Scr_1)]}{\Delta t\ \text{day}}$ $\text{CL}_{cr} = \dfrac{E}{14.4(Scr)}$
Chiou et al.[97]	mL/min	$V_d = 0.6\ \text{L (IBW)}$ $\text{CL}_{cr} = \dfrac{2\,\text{IBW}\,[28 - 0.2\,(\text{Age})]}{14.4(Scr_1 + Scr_2)} + \dfrac{2\,[V_d\text{IBW}\,(Scr_1 - Scr_2)]}{(Scr_1 + Scr_2)\Delta t\ \text{min}} - [\text{CL}^{NR}_{cr} \times \text{IBW}]$	$V_d = 0.6\text{L (IBW)}$ $\text{CL}_{cr} = \dfrac{2\,\text{IBW}\,[22.4 - 0.16\,(\text{Age})]}{14.4(Scr_1 + Scr_2)} + \dfrac{2\,[V_d\text{IBW}\,(Scr_1 - Scr_2)]}{(Scr_1 + Scr_2)\Delta t\ \text{min}} - [\text{CL}^{NR}_{cr} \times \text{IBW}]$
Brater[98]	mL/min/70 kg	$\text{CL}_{cr} = [293 - 2.03(\text{Age})] \times [1.035 - 0.01685\,(Scr_1 + Scr_2)] + \dfrac{49\,(Scr_1 - Scr_2)}{(Scr_1 + Scr_2)\,\Delta t\ \text{day}}$	$\text{CL}_{cr} = \text{Male value} \times 0.86$

E^{ss}, steady state urinary creatinine excretion; Δt day, time in days between $Scr_1 + Scr_2$; Δt min, time in minutes between Scr_1 and Scr_2; CL^{NR}_{cr}, nonrenal clearance of creatinine = 0.048 ml/min/kg.

nucleated cells of the body and is present in stable concentrations, apparently not affected by infection or malignancy. It was initially recommended as a test of kidney function in 1985,[104] and shown to correlate with GFR as well as creatinine. The recent development of an automated immunoassay technique by Newman et al.[101] and their validation of the test as a more sensitive indicator of reduced renal function than creatinine suggest it may have future clinical utility in the assessment of renal function. Comparison of Cr-labeled EDTA with 1/cystatin C and 1/creatinine for 106 measurements resulted in $r = 0.81$ and 0.50, respectively.

MEASUREMENT OF TUBULAR FUNCTION

While GFR is perhaps the best overall indicator of renal function, it may not be reflective of tubular function, either secretory capacity[17,105] or cellular damage.[106–110] Tubular function is best assessed by measurement of ERPF, where PAH serves as the prototype marker of the organic anion secretory system.[111] *N*-1-methylnicotinamide (NMN) and tetraethyl ammonium (TEA) are prototype compounds secreted by the cationic transport system and may be used as markers of cationic secretory capacity.[12,112] Edwards et al.[113] demonstrated delayed recovery of NMN clearance among patients with psoriasis treated with low-dose cyclosporine, compared with the recovery of GFR and renal blood flow. Earlier studies with NMN have suggested its use to assess the effects of selected renal diseases on drug handling by the kidneys.[114] It should be recognized, however, that these transport systems are not mutually exclusive. Indeed probenecid that is secreted by the anionic pathway has been shown to inhibit the secretion of cationic compounds. Quantitative measures of tubular transport capacity are currently limited primarily to the research setting.

Other measures of tubular function are less specific and are regarded primarily as indices of damage within the nephron.[115] Schentag and Plaut[110] demonstrated a delay in the increase of serum creatinine following aminoglycoside toxicity when compared to markers for tubular damage such as the low molecular weight protein β_2-microglobulin (11.8 kDa) and urinary enzymes. The rise in β_2-microglobulin is related to an early functional defect in the proximal tubular cell. This is followed by a rise in the excretion of enzymes released due to structural damage of the cells and finally the formation and excretion of cellular casts. Other low-molecular-weight proteins that have been used as markers of tubular function include retinol-binding protein[116,117] (21 kDa) and protein HC (also known as α_1-microglobulin, 27 kDa).[103,106,115] These proteins are normally freely filtered at the glomerulus, then completely reabsorbed by the proximal tubule. Increases in their excretion are thus suggestive of tubular dysfunction but are not diagnostic, as an increased production rate or GFR less than 30 mL/min may lead to increased excretion. In both cases, the maximal reabsorptive capacity may be exceeded, leading to net excretion of the protein. β_2-Microglobulin has been studied most commonly among the proteins, however, it is unstable at pH <5.5 at room temperature or pH <6.0 at body temperature.[107] Retinol-binding protein and protein HC have also been shown to be elevated with tubular damage and may be more appropriate markers than β_2-microglobulin.[106]

Numerous urinary enzymes such as *N*-acetylglucosaminidase (NAG), alanine aminopeptidase (AAP), alkaline phosphatase (AP), γ-glutamyltransferase (GGT), pyruvate kinase, glutathione transferase, lysozyme, and pancreatic ribonuclease have been used as diagnostic markers for renal disease.[106] Jung et al.[118] compared the ability of five enzymes (NAG, AAP, AP, GGT, and lysozyme) to detect early rejection episodes in kidney transplant patients. Only NAG and AAP were early predictors of rejection. NAG is an enzyme contained within the lysosome of the tubular cell and is released by damage to the lysosome, whereas AAP is an enzyme of the brush border. Both markers were increased approximately 2 days earlier than standard methods in patients with transplant rejection.

The kidney tissue protein, adenosine-binding protein (ABP), is a large, 120-kDa protein bound to the brush border of the proximal tubule and shed during damage to the tubule. It has been shown by Thompson et al.[119] to be significantly elevated in patients with acute tubular necrosis but remained near normal in patients with glomerular lesions. It has also been shown to be elevated in the urine of kidney transplant patients during acute rejection episodes. This increase often preceded elevations of the serum creatinine by 1–7 days. Flynn[106] has suggested that the battery of tests available for evaluation of urinary proteins and enzymes may be useful in identifying the location of injury in the kidneys and may some day provide an alternative to the renal biopsy for identification of the renal pathology.

Clinical Issues

PEDIATRICS

Kidney function in the neonate is difficult to assess due to difficulty in urine and blood collection, the frequent presence of a nonsteady-state serum creatinine, and apparent disparity between development of glomerular and tubular function.[120–123] Inulin clearance performed in infants during the first 4 days of life was 10.8 ± 1.0 mL/min/m^2 and increased twofold at 14 days.[120] There was no relationship between inulin clearance and gestational age. PAH clearance was 30.8 ± 3.8 mL/min/m^2 and increased to a similar degree during the same time period. The value of PAH as a measure of plasma flow is difficult to assess because the extraction ratio of PAH is decreased in newborn infants. Creatinine clearance has also been evaluated in infants less than 1 week of age and values of 17.8 mL/min/1.73 m^2 on day 1 increased to 36.4 mL/min/1.73 m^2 by day 6.[121] Preterm infants demonstrate significantly reduced GFR prior to 34 weeks, then rapidly increase to be similar to term infants during the first week of life.[124] The degree of creatinine excretion through tubular secretion is unknown. However, the results are similar to those observed with inulin.

Due to difficulty in assessing GFR, Clark et al.[123] suggested monitoring the excretion ratio of retinol-binding protein/creatinine as an indicator of early tubular damage. Small molecular weight proteins (<30,000 Da) such as β_2-microglobulin and retinol-binding protein are normally reabsorbed through the proximal tubule following glomerular filtration. Excretion of this protein into the urine is an indication of a tubular functional defect, which usually precedes a reduction in glomerular filtration. Retinol-binding protein is more stable in an acid urine, therefore it may be a preferred marker for tubular function. Clark et al.[123] demonstrated decreased retinol-binding protein/creatinine ratio with increasing gestational age, without changes in creatinine, suggesting it may be a more sensitive indicator of tubular function. It was also related to the severity of illness, whereas there were no differences for plasma creatinine alone. Kidney function expressed as GFR standardized to body surface area increases with age and stabilizes at approximately 1 year.[125,126] Individual studies in older children are best assessed using standard measurement techniques for GFR. Table 42.6 lists formulas for estimating renal function in children.[127–129]

GERIATRICS

Cross-sectional studies have demonstrated decreased GFR as a function of age when GFR was measured as inulin, iothalamate, or creatinine clearance.[87,130] The Baltimore Longitudinal Study on Aging[131] has shown in an evaluation of 254 normal healthy subjects a decrease in creatinine clearance at the rate of approximately 0.75 mL/min/1.73 m^2/yr beginning at the fourth decade of life. These subjects were evaluated prospectively for up to 23 years. Interestingly, approximately one-third of the subjects showed no change in renal function from their baseline value, and a small number showed an increased clearance. These changes may be due to normal physiologic changes or subclinical insults to the kidneys initiating the events leading to chronic progressive loss of renal function.

Interpretation of the serum creatinine concentration alone is difficult in the elderly patient due to the decreased

TABLE 42.6. EQUATIONS FOR THE ESTIMATION OF CREATININE CLEARANCE (ML/MIN/1.73 M^2) IN CHILDREN WITH STABLE RENAL FUNCTION

Ref. No.	Equation	Age
127	$CL_{cr} = (0.45 \times Ht)/S_{cr}$	(Birth–1 year)
128	$CL_{cr} = (0.55 \times Ht)/S_{cr}$	1–20 years
129	$CL_{cr} = (0.48\ Ht/S_{cr}) \times (Wt/70)^{0.7}$	1–20 years

Height in cm and weight in kg.

muscle mass and lower production rate of creatinine. As a result, the body load of creatinine is reduced, yet the fewer functional nephrons tend to maintain the serum creatinine within the normal range. As renal function declines, a larger fraction of creatinine is excreted by the kidneys. This perpetuates the "normal" serum creatinine. A reasonable approach to interpretation of the plasma creatinine is use of the Cockcroft–Gault formula[87] to estimate the patient's CL_{cr}. Durakovic[132] utilized this method to estimate the CL_{cr} in a group of 53 patients at least 70 years old who were admitted to the intensive care unit. The correlation between the estimated and measured CL_{cr} was 0.46, however the units of measure were not the same and may have accounted for some of the variability. Smythe et al.[133] estimated CL_{cr} in 23 patients >60 years of age using seven different methods, and compared the results to a measured 24-hr CL_{cr} determination. Estimations were performed with the actual serum creatinine concentration and also with the serum creatinine rounded to 1.0 mg/dL if the actual value was <1.0 mg/dL. Rounding the serum creatinine to 1.0 mg/dL resulted in a significantly lower (bias 28.8 mL/min) estimate of GFR compared with the actual clearance than when the unadjusted creatinine (bias 2.3 mL/min) was used. These data strongly suggest that one should not arbitrarily adjust the serum creatinine concentration in elderly patients. An alternative to the estimation of GFR or a 24-hr clearance determination is a 4-hr clearance performed during water diuresis.[24] This correlates with the inulin clearance as well as the inpatient 24-hr collection, although one must be aware of the potential risk of hyponatremia in the geriatric patient unable to tolerate an oral water load. O'Connell et al.[134] assessed the accuracy of 2- and 8-hr urine collections compared with 24-hr creatinine clearance determinations in 45 hospitalized patients ≥65 years old with indwelling urethral catheters. Single, timed urine collections for CL_{cr} showed minimal bias with the 8-hr collection compared with the 24-hr value, whereas the 2-hr determination was both biased and imprecise. Unfortunately, urinary residual was not determined, the bladder not rinsed at each collection period, and the mean urine flow was low at 1.23 mL/min; all of these factors may have affected the results of the 2-hr collection.

ASSESSMENT OF PROGRESSION

It has long been recognized that chronic progressive kidney disease will eventually lead to end-stage renal disease (ESRD), necessitating dialysis or transplantation for survival. Attempts to slow the rate of progression, through dietary and blood pressure control,[135] angiotensin-converting enzyme inhibitor therapy,[136] and improved glucose control in patients with Type I diabetes mellitus[137] have recently proven successful. As a result, therapeutic intervention can now successfully decrease the incidence of ESRD. The efficacy of these interventions must be assessed with an accurate and sensitive tool to measure changes in renal function.

A linear decline in the reciprocal of the serum creatinine concentration as a function of time has been used as a simple technique to evaluate the rate of progression of renal disease and to predict the time when dialysis is necessary.[25,138–140] Fundamentally, the serum creatinine concentration is a function of input from the breakdown of creatine derived from muscle or dietary sources and its elimination, predominantly through glomerular filtration and tubular secretion. Under steady-state conditions, the formation rate equals the elimination rate:

$$S_{cr} = R/CL_{cr}$$

where R is the elimination rate of creatinine. For a constant input and reduced output (i.e., decreased GFR), the reciprocal of the serum creatinine concentration will increase as a linear function of the creatinine clearance:

$$1/S_{cr} = 1/R \times CL_{cr}$$

This is depicted in Fig. 42.6, and the slope of the relationship is the reciprocal of the elimination rate. For a constant input, there is a direct, linear relationship between $1/S_{cr}$ and CL_{cr}. Under conditions of progressively decreasing kidney function, this relationship assumes that filtration clearance and secretion clearance decrease proportionately as well as any nonrenal elimination of creatinine. In addition, the rate of input is assumed constant. Based on these assumptions, clinicians can use the reciprocal serum creatinine plotted as a function of time as a prognostic tool regarding the need for dialysis or as a marker for evaluating the success of treatment interventions in the prevention of progressive renal impairment. If these assumptions change over time, then the linearity of the relationship will also change. Several factors such as changes in dietary intake of creatine and decreased muscle mass with associated reduction in the production of creatinine may alter the utility of the relationship. Furthermore, if tubular secretion increases in response to nephron hypertrophy, disproportionately to filtration, or nonrenal routes of elimination of creatinine, such as metabolism by intestinal bacteria become more important, then changes in the slope of the reciprocal creatinine versus time relationship may be altered.[25]

Walser et al.[141] evaluated the relationship between the renal clearance of ^{99m}Tc-DTPA and creatinine clearance and serum creatinine on 22 occasions in 17 patients with moderate to severe chronic renal failure (GFR 4–23 mL/min) over time periods ranging from 6–33 months. Radioisotope GFR was measured bimonthly and 24-hour CL_{cr} at monthly intervals. The 24-hour CL_{cr} and serum creatinine gave misleading impressions of the rate of progression in 9 and 10 of the 22 studies, respectively. Some cases showed apparent improvement in renal function while others showed a more severe rate of progression when using the creatinine data.

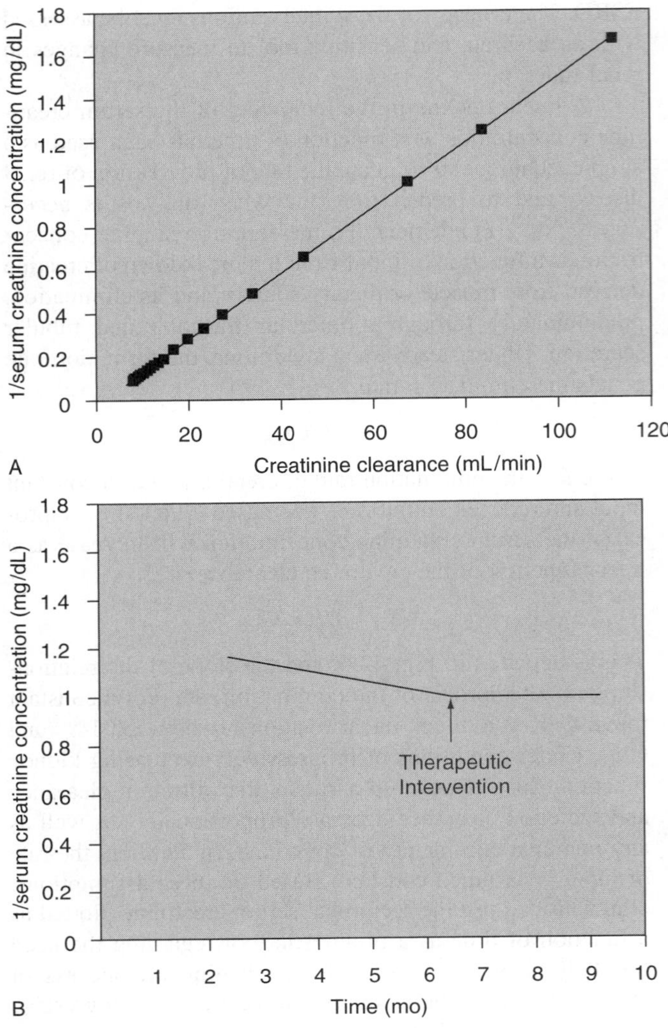

Figure 42.6. Linear relationship between 1/serum creatinine concentration and creatinine clearance (A) and 1/serum creatinine concentration as a function of time in a hypothetical patient with progressive renal impairment (B). The arrow indicates a change in the rate of progression which may be related to a therapeutic intervention.

Walser et al.[141] conclude that serum creatinine measurements of renal function to monitor patients with chronic renal failure should be replaced, when possible, with radioisotope or inulin clearance. Levey, in comprehensive reviews,[1,23] suggests that the variability in measurement of CL_{cr} as an index of GFR is a major limitation to accurate assessment of the decline in renal function over time. It is most important to be aware of the limitations of serum creatinine measurement, and to realize that it is not an adequate test to detect early chronic renal disease or to precisely estimate the disease's rate of progression.

Although not a quantitative measure of renal function, urinary microalbuminuria has been used as an early marker of renal disease in patients with diabetic nephropathy.[142,143] Recently developed guidelines indicate that a urine albumin/creatinine ratio of >30 mg/g places the patient at increased risk of developing diabetic nephropathy and is an indication for the initiation of pharmacotherapeutic intervention.[144] Microalbuminuria has also been suggested as a risk factor for renal dysfunction among patients with essential hypertension.[145] A recent NIDDK Workshop[146] has reported recommendations for management of the progression of chronic renal disease, and identifies microalbuminuria as the best early marker of nephropathy in patients with insulin-dependent diabetes mellitus (IDDM). Annual evaluations should be performed in patients with a 5- to 10-year history of IDDM. Patients with microalbuminuria (30–300 mg/day) on at least two or three occasions or overt albuminuria (>300 mg/day) should begin to receive pharmacotherapy. For children, microalbuminuria is considered present at >15 μg/kg/h, and overt albuminuria at >4 mg/kg/d.

Regarding the quantification of kidney function, the NIDDK report[146] recommends the measurement of GFR with inulin or iothalamate. Creatinine clearance was noted to overestimate the GFR consistently by an average of 30% among whites, and numerous factors, noted earlier, interfere with the renal handling of creatinine.

Conclusion

The glomerular filtration rate is the single best test to assess overall renal function, yet it is nonspecific regarding the site of injury. Measurement of the GFR is ideally performed using inulin or iothalamate as the test marker, or radioisotope techniques such as ^{99m}Tc-DTPA, when renal clearance is measured. Creatinine clearance is the most commonly performed test of renal function, whether measured in the ambulatory or inpatient setting, or estimated using the serum creatinine along with the patient's age, gender, and weight. The best measure of GFR can be obtained if the creatinine clearance is determined during a 4-hr water-induced diuresis. Although creatinine is secreted, the variability associated with inadequate urine collection is eliminated by the use of this short, defined time period. The pretreatment of patients with cimetidine prior to the creatinine clearance determination should enhance the accuracy of the GFR measurement, especially in patients with severe renal dysfunction.

Caution should be exercised when interpreting the serum creatinine concentration as the sole measure of kidney function. Many factors influence the creatinine concentration, only one of which is the GFR. Consideration should be given to patient age, lean body mass, gender, diet, concomitant diseases and drug therapy, circadian rhythm, stability of kidney function, tubular secretion, and analytic method. Use of the reciprocal creatinine as a measure of

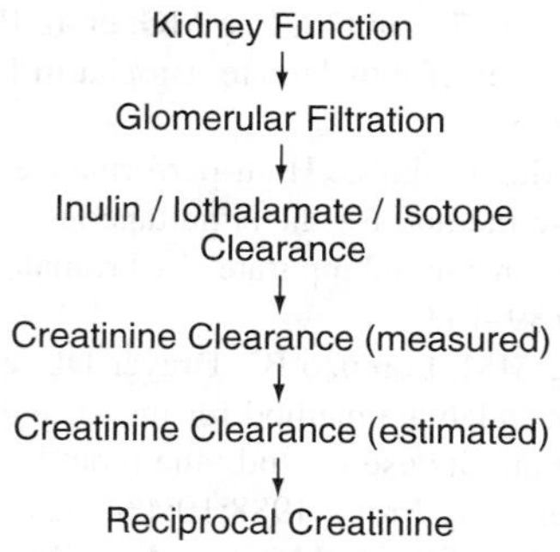

Kidney Function
↓
Glomerular Filtration
↓
Inulin / Iothalamate / Isotope Clearance
↓
Creatinine Clearance (measured)
↓
Creatinine Clearance (estimated)
↓
Reciprocal Creatinine

Figure 42.7. Representation of various measures of kidney function and how removed they are from the "true" value.

progression of kidney disease is not an acceptable alternative to the measurement of GFR. Its use in clinical practice should be limited to those settings where more specific methods are unavailable (Fig. 42.7).

Markers of tubular function such as *N*-1-methylnicotinamide and *p*-aminohippuric acid may provide quantitative insight to secretory processes within the nephron. Other measures, including measures of urinary proteins, enzymes, and kidney tissue proteins, may prove useful to the clinician in identifying sites of drug-induced kidney damage, onset of rejection episodes in kidney transplantation, and monitoring of therapeutic interventions in specific kidney diseases.

The role of pharmacists continues to evolve, creating new opportunities for patient care. Their responsibility as related to monitoring of renal function extends beyond the institutional setting into the ambulatory and extended care environments. Specific functions for pharmacists now include the development of monitoring protocols for potential nephrotoxins, the evaluation of therapeutic interventions on progression of renal disease, and the development of guidelines for dosage regimen adjustment in patients with renal dysfunction.

References

1. Levey AS, Madaio MP, Perrone RD. Laboratory assessment of renal disease: Clearance, urinalysis, and renal biopsy, in Brenner BM, Rector FC (eds): The Kidney, 4th ed. Philadelphia, WB Saunders, 1991, pp 919–968.
2. Vander AJ. Renal Physiology, 5th ed. New York, McGraw-Hill, 1995.
3. Radtke HW, Claussner A, Erbes PM, et al. Serum erythropoietin concentration in chronic renal failure: Relationship to degree of anaemia and excretory function. Blood 1979;54:877–884.
4. Eschbach JW. The anemia of chronic renal failure: Pathophysiology and the effect of recombinant EPO. Kidney Int 1989;35:134.
5. Rabkin R, Simon NM, Steiner S, et al. Effect of renal disease on renal uptake and excretion of insulin in man. New Engl J Med 1970;282:182–187.
6. Hostetter TH. Diabetic nephropathy, in Brenner BM, Rector FC (eds): The Kidney, 4th ed. Philadelphia, WB Saunders, 1991, pp 1695–1727.
7. Coburn JW, Slatopolsky E. Vitamin D, parathyroid hormone, and the renal osteodystrophies, in Brenner BM, Rector FC (eds): The Kidney, 4th ed. Philadelphia, WB Saunders, 1991, pp 2036–2120.
8. Anders MW. Metabolism of drugs by the kidney. Kidney Int 1980;18:636–647.
9. Hook JB, Hewitt WR. Development of mechanisms for drug excretion. Am J Med 1977;62:497–506.
10. Meffin PJ, Zilm DM, Veenendaal JR. Reduced clofibric acid clearance in renal dysfunction is due to a futile cycle. J Pharmacol Exp Therap 1983;227:732–738.
11. Verbeeck RK, Wallace SM, Loewen GR. Reduced elimination of ketoprofen in the elderly is not necessarily due to impairment of glucuronidation. Br J Clin Pharmacol 1984;17:783–784.
12. Grantham JJ, Chonko AM. Renal handling of organic anions and cations: Excretion of uric acid, in Brenner BM, Rector FC (eds): The Kidney, 4th ed. Philadelphia, WB Saunders, 1991, pp 483–509.
13. Poe-Hirr H, Gisclon LG, Hui AC, Giacomini KM. Interactions of organic anions with the organic cation transporter in renal BBMV. Am J Physiol 1988;254:F56–F61.
14. Rowland M, Tozer TN. Clinical Pharmacokinetics: Concepts and Applications, 3rd ed. Baltimore, Williams & Wilkins, 1995, pp 172–173.
15. Bricker NS. On the meaning of the intact nephron hypothesis. Am J Med 1969;46:1–11.
16. Meyer TW, Scholey JW, Brenner BM. Nephron adaptation to renal injury, in Brenner BM, Rector FC (eds): The Kidney, 4th ed. Philadelphia, WB Saunders, 1991, p 1872.
17. Hori R, Okumura K, Kamiya A, et al. Ampicillin and cephalexin in renal insufficiency. Clin Pharmacol Ther 1983;34:792–798.
18. Hori R, Okumura K, Nihira H. A new dosing regimen in renal insufficiency: Application to cephalexin. Clin Pharmacol Therap 1985;38:290–295.
19. Maiza A, Daley-Yates PT. The clearance of drugs in different types of renal disease [abstract]. Renal Failure 1988;11:67.
20. Lin JH, Lin T. Renal handling of drugs in renal failure I. Differential effects of uranyl nitrate- and glycerol-induced acute renal failure on renal excretion of TEAB and PAH in rats. J Pharmacol Exp Therap 1988;246:896–901.
21. Gloff CA, Benet LZ: Differential effects of the degree of renal damage on *p*-aminohippuric acid and inulin clearances in rats. J Pharmacokinet Biopharm 1989;17:169–177.
22. Brouwer KLR, Dukes GE, Powell JR. Influence of liver function on drug disposition, in Evans WE, Schentag JJ, Jusko WJ, (eds): Applied Pharmacokinetics, Principles of Therapeutic Drug Monitoring, 3rd ed. Vancouver, WA, Applied Therapeutics, 1992, pp 6/1–6/59.
23. Levey AS. Assessing the effectiveness of therapy to prevent the progression of renal disease. Am J Kidney Dis 1993;22:207–214.

24. Lemann J, Bidani AK, Bain RP, et al. Use of the serum creatinine to estimate glomerular filtration rate in health and early diabetic nephropathy. Am J Kidney Dis 1990;16:236–243.
25. Hunsicker LG. Studies of therapy of progressive renal failure in humans. Semin Nephrol 1989;9:380–394.
26. Schrier RW, Gambertoglio JG. Handbook of Drug Therapy in Liver and Kidney Disease. Boston, Little, Brown, 1991.
27. Matzke GR, Millikin SP. Influence of renal function and dialysis on drug disposition, in Evans WE, Schentag JJ, Jusko WJ (eds): Applied Pharmacokinetics, Principles of Therapeutic Drug Monitoring, 3rd ed. Vancouver, WA, Applied Therapeutics, 1992, pp 8/1–8/49.
28. Zini R, Riant P, Barre J, et al. Disease-induced variations in plasma protein levels: Implications for drug dosage regimens (Part I). Clin Pharmacokinet 1990;19:147–159.
29. Zini R, Riant P, Barre J, et al. Disease-induced variations in plasma protein levels: Implications for drug dosage regimens (Part II). Clin Pharmacokinet 1990;19:218–222.
30. Gibson TP. Renal disease and drug metabolism: An overview. Am J Kidney Dis 1986;8:7–17.
31. Verbeeck RK. Glucuronidation and disposition of drug glucuronides in patients with renal failure. A review. Drug Metab Dispos 1982;10:87–89.
32. Simon P, Meyrier A, Brissot P. Uremia and the liver. II. Drugs and the liver in the uremic patient. Nephron 1981;29:7–13.
33. Dworkin LD, Brenner BM. The renal circulations, in Brenner BM, Rector FC (eds): The Kidney, 4th ed. Philadelphia, WB Saunders, 1991, p 182.
34. Prescott LF, Freestone S, McAuslane JAN: The concentration-dependent disposition of intravenous *p*-aminohippurate in subjects with normal and impaired renal function. Br J Clin Pharmacol 1993;35:20–29.
35. Taylor DJ, Griffiths P, Swainson CP, et al. Calculation of effective renal plasma flow using ^{125}I-orthoiodohippuran: Comparison of four methods. Clin Nephrol 1985;23:169–172.
36. Hannedouche T, Laude D, Déchaux M, et al. Plasma 5-hydroxyindoleacetic acid as an endogenous index of renal plasma flow. Kidney Int 1989;35:95–98.
37. Levey AS. Measurement of renal function in chronic renal disease. Kidney Int 1990;38:167–184.
38. Maack T. Renal clearance and isolated kidney perfusion techniques. Kidney Int 1986;30:142–151.
39. Levey AS. Use of glomerular filtration rate measurements to assess the progression of renal disease. Semin Nephrol 1989;9:370–379.
40. Rosenbaum JL, Kramer MS, Raja RM, et al. Determination of inulin and *p*-aminohippurate clearances without urine collections. Nephron 1973;10:347–354.
41. Rose GA. Measurement of glomerular filtration rate by inulin clearance without urine collection. Br Med J 1969;2:91–93.
42. Florijn KW, Barendregt JNM, Lentjes EGWM, et al. Glomerular filtration rate measurement by "single-shot" injection of inulin. Kidney Int 1994;46:252–259.
43. Degenaar CP, Frenken LAM, van Hoof JP. Enzymatic method for determination of inulin. Clin Chem 1987;33:1070–1071.
44. Prueksaritanont T, Lui CY, Lee MG, et al. Renal and nonrenal clearances of iothalamate. Biopharm Drug Disp 1986;7:347–355.
45. Boschi S, Marchesini B. High-performance liquid chromatographic method for the simultaneous determination of iothalamate an *o*-iodohippurate. J Chromatogr Biomed Appl 1981;224:139–143.
46. Reidenberg MM, Lorenzo BJ, Drayer DE, et al. A nonradioactive iothalamate method for measuring glomerular filtration rate and its use to study the renal handling of cibenzoline. Ther Drug Monit 1988;10:434–437.
47. Prueksaritanont T, Chen M, Chiou WL. Simple and micro high-performance liquid chromatographic method for simultaneous determination of *p*-aminohippuric acid and iothalamate in biological fluids. J Chromatogr Biomed Appl 1984;306:89–97.
48. Nilsson-Ehle P, Grubb A. New markers for the determination of GFR: Iohexol clearance and cystatin C serum concentration. Kidney Int 1994;46(suppl 47):S17–S19.
49. Brown SCW, O'Reilly PH. Iohexol clearance for the determination of glomerular filtration rate in clinical practice: Evidence for a new gold standard. J Urol 1991;146:675–679.
50. Taylor A. Radionuclide evaluation of renal function. CRC Crit Rev Diagn Imaging 1991;32:1–36.
51. O'Malley JP, Ziessman HA. Quantitation of renal function using radioisotopic techniques. Clin Lab Med 1993;13:53–68.
52. Ott NT, Wilson DM. A simple technique for estimating glomerular filtration rate with subcutaneous injection of [^{125}I] iothalamate. Mayo Clin Proc 1975;50:664–668.
53. Evans JR, Cutler RE, Forland SC. Pharmacokinetics of iothalamate in end stage renal disease. J Clin Pharmacol 1988;28:826–830.
54. LaFrance ND, Drew HH, Walser M. Radioisotopic measurement of glomerular filtration rate in severe chronic renal failure. J Nucl Med 1988;29:1927–1930.
55. Perrone RD, Steinman TI, Beck GJ, et al. Utility of radioisotopic filtration markers in chronic renal insufficiency: Simultaneous comparison of ^{125}I-iothalamate, ^{169}Yb-DTPA, ^{99m}Tc-DTPA, and inulin. Am J Kidney Dis 1990;16:224–235.
56. Rehling M, Moller ML, Thamdrup B, et al. Simultaneous measurement of renal clearance and plasma clearance of ^{99m}Tc-labelled diethylenetriaminepenta-acetate, ^{51}Cr-labelled ethylenediaminetetra-acetate and inulin in man. Clin Sci 1984;66:613–619.
57. Tauxe WN. Determination of glomerular filtration rate by single sample technique following injection of radioiodinated diatrizoate. J Nucl Med 1986;27:45–50.
58. Farmer CD, Tauxe WN, Maher FT, et al. Measurement of renal function with radioiodinate diatrizoate and *o*-iodohippurate. Am J Clin Pathol 1967;467:9–16.
59. Tepe PG, Tauxe WN, Bagchi A, et al. Comparison of measurement of glomerular filtration rate by single sample, plasma disappearance slope/intercept and other methods. Eur J Nucl Med 1987;13:28–31.
60. Rodman JH, Maneval DC, Magill HL, et al. Measurement of Tc-99*m* DTPA serum clearance for stimating glomerular

filtration rate in children with cancer. Pharmacotherapy 1993;13:10–16.
61. Rabito CA, Panico F, Rubin R, et al. Noninvasive, real-time monitoring of renal function during critical care. J Am Soc Nephrol 1994;4:1421–1428.
62. Narayanan S, Appleton HD. Creatinine: A review. Clin Chem 1980;26:1119–1126.
63. Bauer JH, Brooks CS, Burch RN. Clinical appraisal of creatinine clearance as a measurement of glomerular filtration rate. Am J Kidney Dis 1982;2:337–346.
64. Bauer JH, Brooks CS, Burch RN. Renal function studies in man with advanced renal insufficiency. Am J Kidney Dis 1982;2:30–35.
65. Murther RS. Drug interference with renal function tests. Am J Kidney Dis 1983;3:118–120.
66. Payne RB. Creatinine clearance: A redundant clinical investigation. Ann Clin Biochem 1986;23:243–250.
67. Sjostrom P, Odlind B, Wolgast M. Extensive tubular secretion and reabsorption of creatinine in humans. Scand J Urol Nephrol 1988;22:129–131.
68. Molitch ME, Rodman E, Hirsch CA, et al. Spurious serum creatinine elevations in ketoacidosis. Ann Intern Med 1980;93:280–281.
69. Green AJE, Halloran SP, Mould GP, et al. Interference by newer cephalosporins in current methods for measuring creatinine. Clin Chem 1990;36:2139–2140.
70. Massoomi F, Matthews III HG, Destache CJ. Effect of seven fluoroquinolones on the determination of serum creatinine by the picric acid and enzymatic methods. Ann Pharmacother 1993;27:586–588.
71. Herrington D, Drusano GL, Smalls U, Standiford H. False elevation in serum creatinine levels [letter]. JAMA 1984;252:2962.
72. Apple FS, Benson P, Abraham PA, et al. Assessment of renal function by inulin clearance: Comparison with creatinine clearance as determined by enzymatic methods. Clin Chem 1989;35:312–314.
73. Burgess E, Blair A, Krichman K, et al. Inhibition of renal creatinine secretion by cimetidine in humans. Renal Physiol Basel 1982;5:27–30.
74. Roy MT, First MR, Myre SA, et al. Effect of co-trimoxazole and sulfamethoxazole on serum creatinine in normal subjects. Ther Drug Monit 1982;4:77–79.
75. Statland BE, Winkel P, Bokelund H. Factors contributing to intra-individual variation of serum constituents: 2. Effects of exercise and diet on variation of serum constituents in healthy subjects. Clin Chem 1973;19:1380–1383.
76. Mirahmadi MK, Byrne C, Barton C, et al. Prediction of creatinine clearance from serum creatinine in spinal cord injury patients. Paraplegia 1983;21:23–29.
77. Mayersohn M, Conrad KA, Achari R. The influence of a cooked meat meal on creatinine plasma concentration and creatinine clearance. Br J Clin Pharmacol 1983;15:227–230.
78. Pasternack A, Kuhlbäck B. Diurnal variations of serum and urine creatine and creatinine. Scand J Clin Lab Invest 1971;27:1–7.
79. Forbes GG, Bruining GS. Urinary creatinine excretion and lean body mass. Am J Clin Nutr 1978;29:1359.
80. Bingham SA, Murphy J, Waller E, et al. Para-amino benzoic acid in the assessment of completeness of 24-hour urine collections from hospital outpatients and the effect of impaired renal function. Eur J Clin Nutr 1992;46:131–135.
81. Fuller NJ, Elia M. Factors influencing the production of creatinine: Implications for the determination and interpretation of urinary creatine and creatinine in man. Clin Chim Acta 1988;175:199.
82. Petri M, Bockenstedt L, Colman J, et al. Serial assessment of glomerular filtration rate in lupus nephropathy. Kidney Int 1988;34:832–839.
83. Shemesh O, Golbetz H, Kriss JP, et al. Limitations of creatinine as a filtration marker in glomerulopathic patients. Kidney Int 1985;28:830–838.
84. Roubenoff R, Drew H, Moyer M, et al. Oral cimetidine improves the accuracy and precision of creatinine clearance in lupus nephritis. Ann Intern Med 1990;113:501–506.
85. Hilbrands LB, Artz MA, Wetzels JFM, et al. Cimetidine improves the reliability of creatinine as a marker of glomerular filtration. Kidney Int 1991;40:1171–1176.
86. Van Acker BAC, Koomen GCM, Koopman MG, et al. Creatinine clearance during cimetidine administration for measurement of glomerular filtration rate. Lancet 1992;340:1326–1329.
87. Cockroft, DW, Gault MH. Prediction of creatinine clearance from serum creatinine. Nephron 1976;16:31–41.
88. Luke DR, Halstenson CE, Opsahl JA, et al. Validity of creatinine clearance estimates in the assessment of renal function. Clin Pharmacol Ther 1990;48:503–508.
89. Mawer CE, Knowles BR, Lucas SB, et al. Computer-assisted prescribing of kanamycin for patients with renal insufficiency. Lancet 1972;1:12–15.
90. Jelliffe RW. Estimation of creatinine clearance when urine cannot be collected. Lancet 1971;1:975–976.
91. Jelliffe RW. Creatinine clearance: Bedside estimate. Ann Intern Med 1973;79:604–605.
92. Hull JH, Hak LJ, Koch GC, et al. Influence of range of renal function and liver disease on predictability of creatinine clearance. Clin Pharmacol Ther 1981;29:516–521.
93. Gault MH, Longerich LL, Harnett JD, et al. Predicting glomerular function from adjusted serum creatinine. Nephron 1992;62:249–256.
94. Echizen H, Ishizaki T. Superiority of disease-specific over conventional formula in predicting creatinine clearance from serum creatinine in patients with liver cirrhosis. Ther Drug Monit 1988;10:369–375.
95. Quadri KHM, Bernardini J, Greenberg A, et al. Assessment of renal function during pregnancy using a random urine protein to creatinine ratio and Cockcroft-Gault formula. Am J Kidney Dis 1994;24:416–420.
96. Jeliffe RW, Jeliffe SM. A computer program for estimation of creatinine clearance from unstable serum creatinine concentration. Math Biosci 1972;14:17–24.
97. Chiou WL, Hsu FH. A new simple rapid method to monitor renal function based on pharmacokinetic considerations of endogenous creatinine. Res Comm Chem Path Pharmacl 1975;10:15.
98. Brater DC. Drug Use in Renal Disease. Balgowlah, Australia, ADIS Health Science Press, 1983, pp 22–56.
99. Brochner-Mortensen I, Rodbro P. Selection of routine method for determination of glomerular filtration rate in adult patients. Scand J Clin Lab Invest 1976;36:35–43.

100. Rosano TG, Brown HH. Analytical and biological variability of serum creatinine and creatinine clearance: Implications for clinical interpretation [letter]. Clin Chem 1982;28:2330–2331.
101. Newman DJ, Thakkar H, Edwards RG, et al. Serum cystatin C measured by automated immunoassay: A more sensitive marker of changes in GFR than serum creatinine. Kidney Int 1995;47:312–318.
102. Pergande M, Jung K. Sandwich enzyme immunoassay of cystatin C in serum with commercially available antibodies. Clin Chem 1993;39:1885–1890.
103. Grubb A. Diagnostic value of analysis of cystatin C and protein HC in biological fluids. Clin Nephrol 1992;38(suppl 1):S20–S27.
104. Simonsen O, Grubb A, Thysell H. The blood serum concentration of cystatin C (γ-trace) as a measure of the glomerular filtration rate. Scand J Clin Lab Invest 1985;45:97–101.
105. Dubovsky EV, Russell CD. Quantitation of renal function with glomerular and tubular agents. Semin Nucl Med 1982;12:308–329.
106. Flynn FV. Assessment of renal function: Selected developments. Clin Biochem 1990;23:49–54.
107. Schardijn GHC, Statius van Eps LW. β_2-microglobulin: Its significance in the evaluation of renal function. Kidney Int 1987;32:635–641.
108. Floege J, Wilks MF, Soose M, et al. Renal elimination of beta-2-microglobulin and myoglobin in patients with normal and impaired renal function. Nephron 1990;55:361–367.
109. Sherman RL, Drayer DE, Leyland-Jones BR, et al. N-acetyl-β-glucosaminidase and β_2-microglobulin: Their urinary excretion in patients with renal parenchymal disease. Arch Intern Med 1983;143:1183–1185.
110. Schentag JJ, Plaut ME. Patterns of urinary β_2-microglobulin excretion by patients treated with aminoglycosides. Kidney Int 1980;17:654–661.
111. Gloff CA, Benet LZ. Differential effects of the degree of renal damage on *p*-aminohippuric acid and inulin clearances in rats. J Pharmacokinet Biopharm 1989;17:169–177.
112. Nassseri K, Daley-Yates PT. A comparison of N-1-methylnicotinamide clearance with 5 other markers of renal function in models of acute and chronic renal failure. Toxicol Letters 1990;53:243–245.
113. Edwards BD, Maiza A, Daley-Yates PT, et al. Altered clearance of N-1 methylnicotinamide associated with the use of low doses of cyclosporine. Am J Kidney Dis 1994;23:23–30.
114. Maiza A, Daley-Yates PT. Estimation of the renal clearance of drugs using endogenous N-1-methylnicotinamide. Toxicol Lett 190;53:231–235.
115. Jung K. Urinary enzymes and low molecular weight proteins as markers of tubular dysfunction. Kidney Int 1994;46(suppl 47):S29–S33.
116. Ayatse JOI, Kwan JTC. Relative sensitivity of serum and urinary retinol binding protein and alpha-1 microglobulin in the assessment of renal function. Ann Clin Biochem 1991;28:514–516.
117. Verplanke AJW, Heber RFM, de Wit R, et al. Comparison of renal function parameters in the assessment of cis-platin induced nephrotoxicity. Nephron 1994;66:267–272.
118. Jung K, Diego J, Strobelt V, et al. Diagnostic significance of some urinary enzymes for detecting acute rejection crises in renal transplant recipients: Alanine aminopeptidase, alkaline phosphatase, gamma-glutamyl transferase, *N*-acetyl-beta-glucosaminidase, and lysozyme. Clin Chem 1986;32:1807–1811.
119. Thompson RE, Piper DJ, Galberg C, et al. Adenosine deaminase binding protein, a new diagnostic marker for kidney disease. Clin Chem 1985;31:679–683.
120. Guignard JP, Torrado A, Da Cunha O, et al. Glomerular filtration rate in the first three weeks of life. J Pediatr 1975;87:268–272.
121. Sertel H, Scopes J. Rates of creatinine clearance in babies less than one week of age. Arch Dis Child 1973;48:717–720.
122. Rudd PT, Hughes EA, Placzek MM, et al. Reference ranges for plasma creatinine during the first month of life. Arch Dis Child 1983;58:212–215.
123. Clark PMR, Bryant TN, Hal MA, et al. Neonatal renal function assessment. Arch Dis Child 1989;64:1264–1269.
124. Arant BS Jr. Developmental patterns of renal functional maturation compared in the human neonate. J Pediatr 1978;92:705–712.
125. Rose BD. Clinical assessment of renal function, in Rose BD (ed): Pathophysiology of Renal Disease, 2nd ed. New York, McGraw-Hill, 1987, p 5.
126. Hurley RM. Assessment of renal function in the young. Special considerations. Clin Lab Med 1993;13:257–267.
127. Schwartz GJ et al. A simple estimate of glomerular filtration rate in full-term infants during the first year of life. J Pediatr 1984;104:849–854.
128. Schwartz GJ et al. A simple estimate of glomerular filtration rate in children derived from body length and plasma creatinine. Pediatrics 1976;58:259–263.
129. Traub SL, Johnson CE: Comparison of methods of estimating creatinine clearance in children. Am J Hosp Pharm 1980;37:195–201.
130. Lindeman RD. Assessment of renal function in the old. Clin Lab Med 1993;13:269–277.
131. Lindeman RD, Tobin J, Shrock NW. Longitudinal studies on the rate of decline in renal function with age. J Am Geriatr Soc 1985;33:278–281.
132. Durakovic Z. Creatinine clearance in the elderly: A comparison of direct measurement and calculation from serum creatinine. Nephron 1986;44:66–69.
133. Smythe M, Hoffman J, Kizy K, et al. Estimating creatinine clearance in elderly patients with low serum creatinine concentrations. Am J Hosp Pharm 1994;51:198–204.
134. O'Connell MB, Wong MO, Bannick-Mohrland SD, et al. Accuracy of 2- and 8-hour urine collections for measuring creatinine clearance in the hospitalized elderly. Pharmacotherapy 1993;13:135–142.
135. Klahr S, Levey A, Beck G, et al. and the MDRD Study Group. The effects of dietary protein restriction and blood pressure control on the progression of chronic renal disease. New Engl J Med 1994;330:877–884.
136. Lewis E, Hunsicker L, Bain R, et al. The effect of angitensin-converting-enzyme inhibition on diabetic nephropathy. New Engl J Med 1993;329:1456–1462.
137. DCCT Research Group. The effect of intensive treatment on the development and progression of long-term complications

in insulin-dependent diabetes mellitus. New Engl J Med 1993;329:977–986.
138. Mitch WE, Walser M, Buffington GA, et al. A simple method of estimating progression of chronic renal failure. Lancet 1976;2:1326–1328.
139. Rutherford WE, Blondin J, Miller JP, et al. Chronic progressive renal disease: Rate of change of serum creatinine concentration. Kidney Int 1977;11:62–70.
140. Kirschbaum BB. Analysis of reciprocal creatinine plots in renal failure. Am J Med Sci 1986;291:401–404.
141. Walser M, Drew HH, LaFrance ND. Creatinine measurements often yield false estimates of progression in chronic renal failure. Kidney Int 1988;34:412–418.
142. Rossing P, Astrup A-S, Smidt UM, et al. Monitoring kidney function in diabetic nephropathy. Diabetologia 1994;37:708–712.
143. Mogensen CE, Hansen KW, Nielson S, et al. Monitoring diabetic nephropathy: Glomerular filtration rate and abnormal albuminuria in diabetic renal disease-reproducibility, progression, and efficacy of antihyptensive intervention. Am J Kidney Dis 1993;22:174–187.
144. Bennett PH, Haffner S, Kasiske BL, et al. Screening and management of microalbuminuria in patients with diabetes mellitus: Recommendations to the scientific advisory board of the National Kidney Foundation from an ad hoc committee of the council on diabetes mellitus of the National Kidney Foundation. Am J Kidney Dis 1995;25:107–112.
145. Mimran A, Ribstein J, DuCailar G. Is microalbuminuria a marker of early intrarenal vascular dysfunction in essential hypertensin? Hypertension 1994;23:1018–1021.
146. Striker G. Report on a workshop to develop management recommendations for the prevention of progression in chronic renal disease. J Am Soc Nephrol 1995;5:1537–1540.

Chapter 43

Acute Renal Failure

Bruce A. Mueller, PharmD, BCPS, and William L. Macias, MD, PhD

Acute renal failure is an abrupt decline in renal function characterized by the inability of the kidney to excrete metabolic waste products (nitrogenous wastes and water) and maintain acid–base balance. An elevation in nitrogenous waste products (e.g., creatinine and urea nitrogen) is referred to as azotemia. Uremia, characterized by anorexia, nausea, vomiting, and mental status changes, is the clinical syndrome resulting from azotemia. An increase in the serum creatinine concentration of 0.5 mg/dL when the baseline creatinine is less than 3.0 mg/dL or an increase of 1.0 mg/dL if the baseline is equal to or greater than 3.0 mg/dL has been the most commonly used definition of acute renal failure.[1]

The use of the serum creatinine to define renal failure, although probably appropriate in chronic renal disease, may by itself be inadequate to define renal failure in a significant number of individuals who develop acute renal failure. This inadequacy stems from the fact that a large percentage of individuals who develop acute renal failure are critically ill and highly catabolic. Consequently, these individuals frequently accumulate noncreatinine waste products (e.g., urea nitrogen and water) out of proportion to the increase in serum creatinine. Therefore, the diagnosis of acute renal failure in critically ill patients should be made whenever the kidneys are unable to maintain acceptable control of body volume, acid–base balance, and the levels of nitrogenous waste products, regardless of whether the serum creatinine concentration has risen significantly. By employing this broadened definition, a more realistic estimate of patient outcome, anticipation of possible complications, and an increased awareness of the need for early intervention with renal replacement therapies can be made.

Epidemiology

With few exceptions (i.e., glomerulonephritis, obstruction, renal vasculitis), the development of acute renal failure is primarily a phenomenon of hospitalized patients with the diagnosis appearing in their discharge or death summaries and not in their admitting history.[2] Community-acquired acute renal failure occurs in only 1% of hospital admissions.[3] Risk factors for the development of acute renal failure in the intensive care unit include sepsis, bleeding, volume depletion, chronic liver disease, mechanical ventilation, and surgery.[4] However, because of the difficulties in defining acute renal failure, the exact incidence and prevalence of acute renal failure are difficult to quantify.

Conceptually, one can achieve a better understanding of the magnitude of the problem by dividing the patient population into those individuals who develop acute renal failure but never require renal replacement therapy, those who develop acute renal failure but do require renal replacement therapy, and those who develop acute renal failure in association with established multiple organ failure. The exact incidence of acute renal failure (as defined by an increase in the serum creatinine) not requiring renal replacement therapy is unknown, largely because this syndrome frequently is not recognized as acute renal failure and even more frequently not recorded as a discharge diagnosis. Almost by definition the prognosis for this group of patients is excellent since they have had a recovery of renal function, which usually heralds recovery from the underlying condition.

The incidence, in hospitalized patients, of acute renal failure requiring renal replacement therapy is better documented and ranges from <1% to ≈5% depending on whether the hospital is a primary care facility or a tertiary care referral institution.[2,5] Multiple investigators have attempted to identify those clinical and demographic factors that are associated with survival.[6–10] Unfortunately, most analyses have been unduly complex and not extremely useful for the nonstatistically inclined clinician. However, certain trends that are useful in predicting outcome have been documented. For individuals with acute renal failure requiring renal replacement therapy and having no other major organ system failure, the mortality rate ranges from 10–25%.[11,12] As the number of failed organ systems increases, so does the mortality rate such that for individuals with multiple organ failure (≥3 failed organ systems) the mortality rate currently exceeds 80%.[6] This mortality rate is a slight improvement from the rate described for these patients just 10 years ago.[13] This improvement in survival may relate to the recognition of the need for increased attention to the nutritional status of the patient,[14] earlier intervention with renal replacement therapy, the choice of renal replacement therapy (continuous versus intermittent),[15] and possibly the choice of hemodialysis membrane.[16]

Lastly, the incidence of acute renal failure as a consequence of preexisting multiple organ failure is, fortunately, relatively low (<1% of hospitalized patients in tertiary referral centers). However, their prognosis is extremely dismal.[9] Aggressive attempts at providing renal replacement therapy usually result in futile care at exorbitant expense.

CLASSIFICATION

The classification of acute renal failure into broad categories based on precipitating factors facilitates the diagnosis and management of patients presenting with this disorder (Table 43.1). Traditionally, the scheme most frequently utilized has categorized the causes of acute renal failure into prerenal azotemia (resulting from decreased renal perfusion), acute intrinsic renal failure (resulting from structural damage to the kidney), and postrenal obstruction (resulting from the obstruction of urine flow from the kidney out of the body). The addition of the category "functional acute renal failure" aids in the understanding of the pathophysiology of acute renal failure resulting from hemodynamic changes at the level of the glomerulus without decreased perfusion of the kidney or structural damage to it.

PRERENAL AZOTEMIA

Prerenal acute renal failure results from hypoperfusion of the renal parenchyma, with or without systemic arterial hypotension. Renal hypoperfusion with systemic arterial hypotension may be caused by a decline in intravascular volume (e.g., hemorrhage, dehydration) or a decline in effective blood volume (i.e., the blood volume perceived by the arterial baroreceptors). Examples of disease states in which there is a decline in effective blood volume without a decrease in intravascular volume include congestive heart failure and liver failure. Since the kidney is undamaged, at least early on, the urinalysis will be normal. The fractional excretion of sodium will be low, reflecting an increase in the concentrations of the sodium-retentive hormones: renin, angiotensin, and aldosterone. Urinary solute will be concentrated as a result of the increased circulating levels of antidiuretic hormone, which is released in response to the diminished arterial blood pressure.

Renal hypoperfusion without systemic hypotension most commonly results from bilateral renal artery occlusion, or unilateral occlusion in a patient with a single functioning kidney. In these conditions, the sodium-retentive hormones are activated by the decline in renal parenchymal perfusion. However, systemic arterial blood pressure is usually elevated, leading to an inhibition of antidiuretic release. Consequently, the urinary indices will reflect enhanced sodium reabsorption (i.e., a low fractional excretion of sodium), but the urinary solute may not be maximally concentrated.

FUNCTIONAL ACUTE RENAL FAILURE

Functional acute renal failure refers to those entities that result in a decline in glomerular ultrafiltrate production secondary to a reduced glomerular hydrostatic pressure without damage to the kidney itself. The decline in glomerular hydrostatic pressure is a direct consequence of changes in glomerular afferent (vasoconstriction) and efferent (vasodilation) arteriolar circumference (Fig. 43.1). These clinical conditions most commonly occur in individuals who have reduced effective blood volume (e.g., congestive heart failure, cirrhosis, severe pulmonary disease, hypoalbuminemia) or renovascular disease (e.g., renal artery stenosis) and cannot compensate for changes in afferent or efferent arteriolar tone. Examples of disorders that result in afferent arteriolar vasoconstriction (and an increase in afferent arteriolar resistance) include hypercalcemia and the administration of certain medications (e.g., cyclosporin A and nonsteroidal anti-inflammatory drugs). A decrease in efferent arteriolar resistance usually results from the administration of an angiotensin converting enzyme inhibitor. With correction of the underlying pathologic process or discontinuation of the responsible medication, renal function rapidly returns to baseline. The hepatorenal syndrome is included in this classification scheme since the kidney itself is not damaged and there is intense afferent arteriolar vasoconstriction (possibly mediated by endothelin[17]) leading to a decline in glomerular filtration. In all of the previously mentioned conditions, the urinalysis is not different from its baseline state and the urinary indices suggest prerenal azotemia. The urinary solute concentration may be variable depending on circulating levels of antidiuretic hormone.

This syndrome of functional acute renal failure is very common in individuals with congestive heart failure who receive an angiotensin converting enzyme inhibitor in an attempt to improve left ventricular function. Unfortunately, the improvement in left ventricular function resulting from the administration of an angiotensin converting enzyme inhibitor may take weeks to be clinically significant.[18] However, the decline in efferent arteriolar resistance resulting from the inhibition of angiotensin II occurs rapidly.[19] Therefore, if the dose of the angiotensin converting enzyme inhibitor is increased too rapidly, a decline in glomerular ultrafiltrate production will occur with a concomitant rise in the serum creatinine, leading to functional acute renal fail-

TABLE 43.1. CLASSIFICATION OF ACUTE RENAL FAILURE

Category	Classification of Acute Renal Failure	Differential Diagnosis
Prerenal renal failure	With hypotension	Intravascular volume depletion dehydration hemorrhage
	Without hypotension	Bilateral renal artery stenosis (unilateral renal artery stenosis in solitary kidney) Emboli cholesterol thrombotic
Functional acute renal failure		Medications Cyclosporin A ACE inhibitors NSAIDs Hypercalcemia Hepatorenal syndrome
Acute intrinsic renal failure	Vascular	Vasculitis polyarteritis nodosa hemolytic uremic syndrome Emboli cholesterol thrombotic
	Glomerular	Systemic lupus erythematosus Poststreptococcal glomerulonephritis Antiglomerular basement membrane disease
	Acute tubular necrosis	Ischemic hypotension vasoconstriction Exogenous toxins contrast dye heavy metals drugs (amphotericin B, aminoglycosides, etc.) Endogenous toxins myoglobin hemoglobin
	Acute interstitial nephritis	Drugs penicillins ciprofloxacin sulfonamides Infection streptococcal
Postrenal renal failure (obstruction)	Bladder outlet obstruction	Prostatic hypertrophy Improperly placed bladder catheter
	Ureteral (bilateral or unilateral with solitary functioning kidney)	Cervical cancer Retroperitoneal fibrosis
	Renal pelvis or tubules	Crystal deposition oxalate sulfonamides tumor lysis syndrome

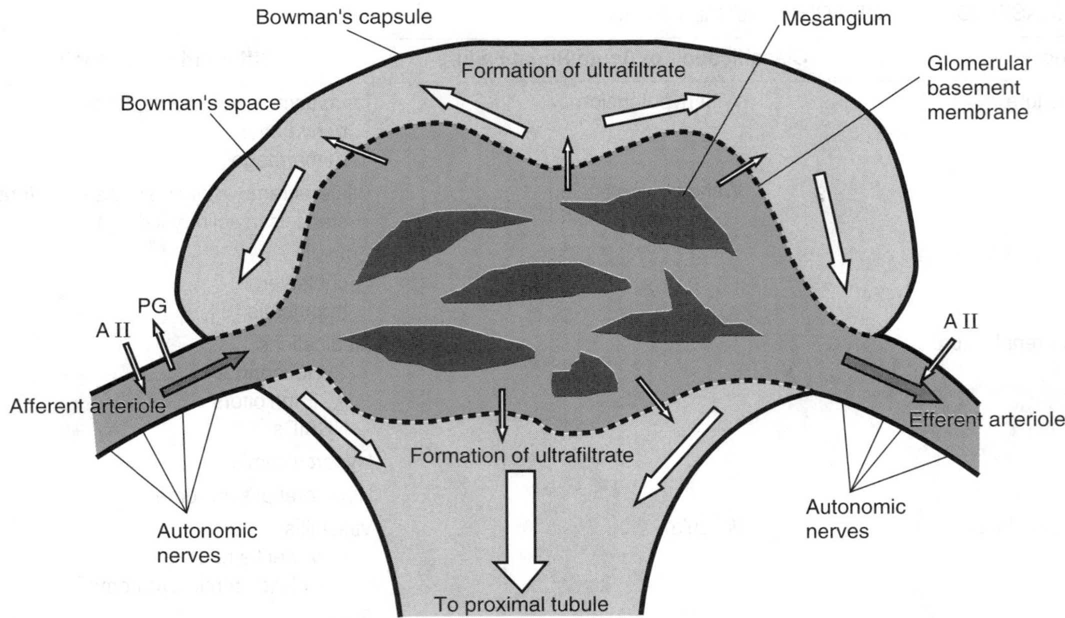

Figure 43.1. The formation of glomerular ultrafiltrate is dependent on the surface area of the glomerular capillaries, their permeability, and the net hydrostatic pressure across the capillary wall. As the glomerular capillary surface area increases, secondary to mesangial cell relaxation, the formation of glomerular ultrafiltrate is increased. An increase or decrease in glomerular hydrostatic pressure results in either an increase or decrease in glomerular ultrafiltrate production. Afferent arteriolar vasoconstriction (which is primarily mediated by angiotensin II) or vasodilation (which is primarily mediated by prostaglandins) can result in a decrease or increase, respectively, in hydrostatic pressure across the capillary. Efferent arteriolar vasoconstriction (which is primarily mediated by angiotensin II) results in an increase in glomerular hydrostatic pressure. Under conditions where renal blood flow is diminished, the kidney maintains glomerular ultrafiltration by vasodilating the afferent and vasoconstricting the efferent arterioles. Medications that may interfere with these processes might result in an abrupt decline in glomerular filtration.

ure. If the increase in the serum creatinine is not too severe (usually <1 mg/dL), the medication can be continued. Renal function should gradually improve as renal parenchymal perfusion pressure increases with improvement in left ventricular function.

ACUTE INTRINSIC RENAL FAILURE

Acute intrinsic renal failure results from damage to the kidney itself. Conceptually, acute intrinsic renal failure can best be organized by the structures within the kidney; the small blood vessels, glomeruli, renal tubules, and interstitium (Table 43.1). Renal failure secondary to small vessel vasculitis (e.g., polyarteritis nodosa, hemolytic uremic syndrome, malignant hypertension) or cholesterol emboli can present with a relatively normal urinary sediment since the glomerulus and tubules, at least initially, are not damaged. When renal failure results from a small vessel vasculitis, the vasculitic process is rarely confined solely to the kidney. A careful search for diagnostic clues suggesting other organ system involvement usually provides evidence of the diffuse nature of these disease processes (see section on Approach to the Patient with Acute Renal Failure).

Acute glomerular inflammation (acute glomerulonephritis) can result from a variety of precipitating causes (systemic lupus erythematosus, antiglomerular basement membrane disease, etc.). In these disorders, the urinalysis usually reveals the presence of heavy proteinuria (>3 grams urinary protein per 24-hour collection period) and hemoglobinuria. Microscopic analysis of the urinary sediment frequently shows numerous red blood cells and red blood cell casts, the latter being considered diagnostic for glomerulonephritis. In the early stages of the illness, the fractional excretion of sodium is less than 1 because tubular function is still intact. However, as renal failure becomes more established, the fractional excretion of sodium may increase.

The renal tubules are susceptible to a variety of insults. The tubules contained within the medulla of the kidney are particularly at risk from ischemic injury because this portion of the kidney is very metabolically active and thereby has a high oxygen requirement. Severe hypotension or the administration of vasoconstricting drugs preferentially affects the tubules more than any other portion of the kidney.[20] In addition, exogenous toxic substances (e.g., contrast agents, heavy metals, and pharmacological agents such as aminoglycosides, amphotericin B, foscarnet) and endogenous toxins (e.g., myoglobin, hemoglobin, uric acid) may cause tubular injury. Regardless of the etiology, tubular injury leads to a loss of urine concentrating ability, defective distal sodium reabsorption, and a reduction in the glomerular filtration rate. The etiology of acute intrinsic renal failure secondary to tubular injury (referred to as acute tubular necrosis) is usually discernible by reviewing the patient's history and medication list. The urinalysis suggests tubular injury by the presence of coarse "dirty brown" casts. Red blood cells and red blood cell casts are only rarely seen. The urinary indices suggest intrinsic renal dysfunction (i.e., high fractional excretion of sodium, isosthenuria [urine osmolality equal to plasma osmolality], and a low urine creatinine to serum creatinine ratio).

The interstitium of the kidney is also susceptible to injury from a variety of causes. Although acute interstitial nephritis is caused most commonly by medications (see Chapter 47), infections (e.g., streptococcal, Leptospirosis, Hantavirus, and HIV infections) also may produce a similar syndrome. The presence in the urine of white blood cells, white blood cell casts, and coarse granular casts, all suggest interstitial inflammation. The presence of eosinophilia and eosinophiluria also strongly suggest the presence of an interstitial nephritis. Interestingly, acute interstitial nephritis resulting from the administration of nonsteroidal anti-inflammatory drugs is not associated with eosinophilia and eosinophiluria. This clinical syndrome is frequently accompanied by an acute glomerulonephritis. As a consequence, the urinalysis has characteristics of both acute interstitial nephritis (i.e., white blood cells, white blood cell casts) and an acute glomerulonephritis (i.e., proteinuria, red blood cells, red blood cell casts).

POSTRENAL OBSTRUCTION

Acute renal failure resulting from obstruction may occur at any level within the urinary system from renal tubule to urethra. However, to cause acute renal failure, the obstructing process must involve both kidneys or one kidney in a patient with a single functioning kidney. Bladder outlet obstruction is the most common cause of obstructive uropathy. Crystal deposition within the tubules (e.g., secondary to uric acid, sulfonamide, or oxalate) and ureteral obstruction (e.g., secondary to shed renal papilla or calculi) are infrequent causes of obstructive acute renal failure. The onset of acute anuria, in the absence of a catastrophic event, should suggest acute urinary tract obstruction. However, the development of acute renal failure in a hospitalized patient who was admitted with normal renal function is rarely secondary to obstruction unless an indwelling urinary catheter has been misplaced. When the obstructing process (e.g., prostatic hypertrophy, cervical cancer) is gradual and incomplete, the patient may present with complaints of a decreased force of the urinary stream and polyuria.

Physiology and Pathophysiology of Renal Function

A basic knowledge of renal function facilitates the understanding of how acute renal failure manifests itself clinically. The most logical approach to understanding renal function is to divide the kidney into its four basic component parts: the vasculature, the glomeruli, the tubules, and the interstitium surrounding the other three component parts.

RENAL VASCULATURE

Blood flows to each kidney via a main renal artery, which divides in two just prior to entering the renal parenchyma. These two main branches divide into approximately five segmental branches, each of which is the sole provider of blood flow to its respective section. Consequently, arterial occlusion at the level of the segmental branch will result in complete ischemia of that portion of the kidney. In the setting of renal artery occlusion, the creatinine may or may not rise depending on the number of segmental arteries involved. If only a few segmental arteries are occluded, the serum creatinine will remain unchanged and the urinalysis will be normal. With significant renal infarction, the urinalysis will show hematuria and proteinuria, and the urine indices will show an inability to concentrate urinary solutes.

Each segmental renal artery divides into a series of smaller arteries leading to the afferent arterioles of the glomeruli. Lesions at this level of the arterial tree (e.g., cholesterol emboli, vasculitic lesions, platelet plugs) will present as isolated decreased perfusion of the glomeruli. The serum creatinine frequently is increased since the lesions are usually diffuse. However, the urinalysis most commonly will be normal since the kidney itself is not ischemic and the glomeruli are not involved. The urine indices suggest prerenal azotemia (i.e., a low urine sodium concentration and a low fractional excretion of sodium) in the absence of systemic hypotension or a decrease in effective blood volume. The urine volume may or may not be diminished. However, the onset of oliguria secondary to diffuse arterial lesions within the kidney, such as that which occurs with hemolytic uremic syndrome, denotes a poor chance for salvage of renal function.

GLOMERULUS

The glomerulus consists of an enlargement of the proximal end of the renal tubule to incorporate a vascular tuft connecting the afferent and efferent arterioles (see Fig. 43.1). Surrounding the vascular tuft is the mesangial region consisting of mesangial cells and the mesangial matrix. The production of glomerular ultrafiltrate is predominantly dependent on the transcapillary hydrostatic pressure (dictated by the afferent and efferent arteriolar resistance) and the glomerular surface area (primarily governed by the contraction and relaxation of mesangial cells that open and close glomerular capillaries). Afferent arteriolar tone is determined predominantly by the local levels of angiotensin II (which induces vasoconstriction) and prostaglandins (which induce vasodilation). Efferent arteriolar tone is predominantly determined by the local concentration of angiotensin II.

Pathophysiologic processes and medications that result in alterations of the afferent and efferent arteriolar tone (i.e., systemic hypotension, hypercalcemia, angiotensin converting enzyme inhibitors, and nonsteroidal anti-inflammatory drugs) reduce glomerular ultrafiltrate production as a result of a decrease in glomerular hydrostatic pressure. Under these conditions, the serum creatinine will rise, the urine sediment will be normal, and the urine indices will suggest prerenal azotemia. However, the urinary solutes may or may not be maximally concentrated depending on the circulating level of antidiuretic hormone that is necessary to maximally concentrate the urine. Damage to the glomerular capillary tuft (e.g., acute glomerulonephritis) results in a decline in the glomerular ultrafiltrate production as a result of a decrease in glomerular capillary surface area. Under these conditions the serum creatinine rises. The urinalysis is significant for hematuria and proteinuria because of the increased permeability of the damaged glomerular capillaries. Red cell casts are found often and are considered diagnostic of glomerular capillary injury. The urine indices may suggest prerenal azotemia because the renal tubules are intact. The urinary solutes may or may not be maximally concentrated.

RENAL TUBULES

Under normal conditions, approximately 180 liters of glomerular ultrafiltrate are produced per day, the vast majority of which must be reabsorbed by the renal tubules to maintain homeostasis. Clinically, the renal tubule can be divided into three major sections: the proximal tubule, Henle's loop, and the distal nephron, which includes the distal tubule, the cortical collecting tubule, and the medullary collecting ducts (Fig. 43.2). In the proximal tubule, approximately 60–70% of the filtered load of water and solute is isovolemically reabsorbed as well as the vast

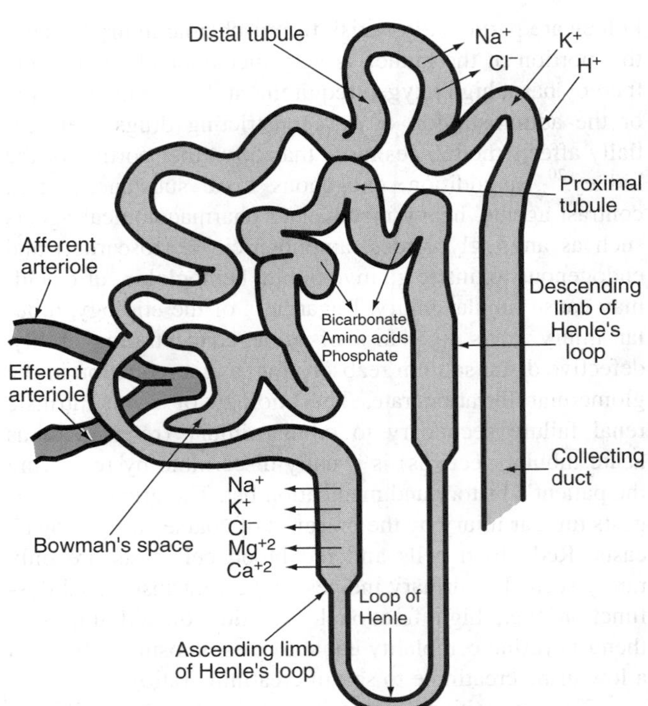

Figure 43.2. Schematic diagram of the renal tubule. As indicated by the arrows, different portions of the renal tubule modify the glomerular ultrafiltrate. Damage to a specific portion of the renal tubule may manifest itself by characteristic changes in the urinary composition. For example, proximal tubular damage secondary to multiple myeloma proteins results in renal failure and the abnormal presence of glucose and amino acids in the urine.

majority of filtered amino acids, glucose, and bicarbonate. Isolated injury to the proximal tubule (e.g., as occurs with heavy metal poisoning or paraproteinemia) results in significant aminoaciduria, glucosuria, and bicarbonaturia. The serum creatinine may rise because of intratubular obstruction, damage to the tubular epithelial cells, or the back leak of glomerular ultrafiltrate across the renal tubule.

In addition to its other functions, Henle's loop is responsible for a significant portion of the total reabsorption of potassium, calcium, and magnesium as well as for generating the osmotic gradient within the kidney necessary for the concentration of urinary solutes. Damage to this portion of the nephron results in wasting of potassium and magnesium by the kidney and an inability of the kidney to concentrate the urine. The medullary portions of Henle's loop are very sensitive to ischemia secondary to hypoperfusion. Consequently, in severe prerenal azotemia with renal hypoperfusion, there may be a loss of urinary concentrating ability despite the continued presence of a low urinary sodium concentration and a low fractional excretion of sodium.

Major functions of the distal nephron include the regeneration of bicarbonate, the excretion of acid (hydrogen ion), the secretion of potassium, and the reabsorption of water. Damage to this portion of the nephron may present as significant acidemia and either hypo- or hyperkalemia, depending on the mechanism of injury. For example, amphotericin B produces small pores in the lumenal membrane of distal tubular cells. These pores allow small molecules such as potassium to leak out; the molecules are then wasted in the urine.[21] Consequently, amphotericin B nephrotoxicity is characterized by hypokalemia secondary to renal potassium wasting. Hyperkalemia may occur if the damage to the distal nephron is severe enough to cause oliguria or if the damage disrupts the renin–aldosterone axis. Defects in urine concentrating ability also are fre-quent. In addition to the previously mentioned findings, acute tubular necrosis as a cause of acute renal failure is associated with a urinary sediment characterized by the presence of tubular cells, coarse granular casts, and rarely red blood cell casts.

INTERSTITIUM

The interstitium of the kidney provides the structural support for the kidney and serves to provide the environment in which concentrating gradients can be established. In addition, the interstitium of the kidney plays a major role in urinary ammonia handling. To facilitate the regeneration of bicarbonate and the excretion of acid by the distal nephron, the kidney utilizes ammonia as a urinary buffer. When the interstitium of the kidney is damaged (e.g., in acute allergic interstitial nephritis), the concentrating gradient within the kidney may be dissipated and ammonia handling disrupted. Consequently, patients presenting with acute interstitial nephritis frequently are not able to concentrate the urinary solute. They also may have a metabolic acidosis with hyperkalemia, the degree of which is out of proportion to the rise in serum creatinine. The urinalysis may show mild proteinuria and hematuria. However, the striking finding on microscopic examination of the sediment is the presence of numerous white blood cells and white blood cell casts.

APPROACH TO THE PATIENT WITH ACUTE RENAL FAILURE

Rapid determination of the etiology of acute renal failure is essential. Nearly 90% of patients presenting to the hospital with community-acquired acute renal failure have a potentially reversible cause.[22] The most common cause of acute renal failure in hospitalized patients is prerenal azotemia, which may be attenuated with prompt treatment of the renal hypoperfusion. A delay in the diagnosis of the etiology of acute renal failure may result in a more severe nephrologic injury.

HISTORY

The diagnostic approach to the patient with acute renal failure differs depending on the clinical setting in which the kidneys fail. For patients who present to the outpatient clinic or hospital with an elevated serum creatinine, the first objective is to determine if the renal failure is acute or chronic. A past medical history of renal disease, previous laboratory data documenting the presence of proteinuria or an elevated serum creatinine, and the finding of bilaterally small kidneys on renal ultrasonography suggest the presence of chronic renal failure. The finding of an elevated parathyroid hormone concentration or evidence of renal osteodystrophy on radiographic bone survey also suggest chronicity.

For patients who do not have these findings, their renal failure should be considered acute until proven otherwise. In these individuals, a careful review of their recent medications, including over-the-counter medications and vitamins, is mandatory. The patient's recent history can usually provide an indication of when the onset of renal dysfunction began. Frequently, patients may notice a change in their voiding habits with an increase in urinary frequency or nocturia, both suggesting a urinary concentrating defect. A decrease in the force of the urinary stream may suggest an obstructive process. The presence of cola-colored urine, indicating the presence of blood in the urine, is common in acute glomerulonephritis. If the accompanying proteinuria is heavy, the patient may note excessive foaming of the urine in the toilet. The onset of bilateral flank pain may suggest swelling of the kidneys secondary to either acute glomerulonephritis or acute interstitial nephritis. The onset of severe headaches may suggest the development of hypertension as a result of acute renal failure. A recent increase in the patient's weight secondary to salt and water retention also may be helpful in defining the onset of renal failure.

For patients who develop acute renal failure while hospitalized, a review of the laboratory data is usually sufficient to define the onset of acute renal failure. However, significant renal injury can occur prior to an increase in the serum creatinine. Consequently, clinicians must pay careful attention to subtle changes in the patient's weight, blood pressure, and urine output if they are to diagnose the onset of acute renal failure. Urine output is one of the easiest parameters to measure and is one of the most useful. In the absence of obstruction, urine output directly correlates with glomerular filtration rate in patients with acute renal failure.[23] Changes in urine output may be helpful in diagnosing the type of renal dysfunction that is present. Acute anuria (<50 mL urine production/24 hours) is either secondary to complete urinary obstruction or a catastrophic event (e.g., shock, hemolytic uremic syndrome, acute cortical necrosis). Oliguria (≤400 mL urine production/24 hours) suggests either prerenal azotemia, functional acute renal failure, or acute intrinsic renal failure. Nonoliguric renal failure (>400 mL urine production/24 hours) usually results from acute intrinsic renal failure or incomplete urinary obstruction. As with outpatients who present with acute renal failure, a careful review of the administered medications is also mandatory for individuals who develop acute renal failure while hospitalized.

PHYSICAL EXAMINATION AND URINALYSIS

A physical examination, including assessment of the patient's volume and hemodynamic status, is the next step in evaluating individuals with acute renal failure. Common physical findings in patients with acute renal failure are listed in Table 43.2. The urinalysis is an extremely important component of the physical examination when the clinician is attempting to classify the cause of renal failure as prerenal azotemia, functional acute renal failure, acute intrinsic renal failure, or obstruction. The finding of a high urinary specific gravity, in the absence of glucosuria or mannitol administration, suggests an intact urinary concentrating mechanism and prerenal azotemia or functional acute renal failure. The presence of proteinuria and hematuria indicates a glomerular injury. Glucosuria, aminoaciduria, and phosphaturia are associated with acute proximal tubular dysfunction. As noted earlier, the microscopic examination can provide helpful cues regarding the cause of acute renal failure. A benign urine sediment suggests either prerenal azotemia, functional acute renal failure, or urinary obstruction. The presence of red blood cells and red blood cell casts indicates a glomerular injury. The finding of white blood cells and white blood cell casts results from interstitial inflammation (i.e., interstitial nephritis), which can be secondary to an allergic, granulomatous, or infectious process.

LABORATORY DATA

Simultaneous measurement of serum and urinary chemistries is often helpful in determining the etiology of acute renal failure (Table 43.3). Calculation of the fractional excretion of sodium from urinary and plasma creatinine and sodium concentrations can yield important information about the patient with acute renal failure. The equation for the calculation of the fractional excretion of sodium is:

$$FE_{Na} = (\text{excreted Na/filtered Na}) \times 100$$
$$= [(U_{vol} \times U_{Na})/(GFR \times P_{Na})] \times 100$$

where $GFR = U_{vol} \times U_{Cr}/P_{Cr} \times \text{time}$. Thus,

$$FE_{Na} = (U_{Na} \times P_{Cr} \times 100)/(U_{Cr} \times P_{Na})$$

where U_{vol} = urine volume, U_{Cr} = urine creatinine, U_{Na} = urine sodium, P_{Cr} = plasma creatinine, P_{Na} = plasma sodium, and time = the time period over which the urine is collected.

The fractional excretion of sodium has clinical utility in differentiating prerenal azotemia and functional acute renal failure from acute intrinsic renal failure. A low urinary sodium concentration and low fractional excretion of sodium (<1%) in a patient with oliguria suggest that there is stimulation of the sodium-retentive mechanisms in the kidney and that tubular function is intact. These findings are most characteristic of prerenal azotemia or functional acute renal failure. Similarly, a fractional excretion of sodium exceeding 1–2% suggests acute intrinsic renal failure. However, a number of the causes of acute intrinsic renal failure are, at least early on, associated with a low fractional excretion of sodium (e.g., contrast nephropathy, myoglobinuria, interstitial nephritis). Diuretic use can limit the diagnostic utility of the fractional excretion of sodium calculation by increasing natriuresis even in hypovolemic patients.

A highly concentrated urine (>500 mOsm/L) suggests stimulation of antidiuretic hormone, indicating prerenal azotemia secondary to either hypovolemia or a decrease in effective blood volume. Under these conditions, the urine creatinine to serum creatinine ratio usually exceeds 40. On occasion, some patients may develop an extremely high blood urea nitrogen (BUN) concentration while the serum creatinine remains only mildly elevated. In these instances, measurement of the urinary urea nitrogen will allow the clinician to determine if the elevated BUN concentration is secondary to the underexcretion of urea nitrogen or the overproduction of urea nitrogen. A critically ill patient will produce approximately 18–19 grams of urea nitrogen per day. Excretion of a urinary urea nitrogen load substantially less than that suggests acute renal failure. Excretion of substantially more than that suggests overproduction of urea as the cause for the increased BUN concentration, such as might occur with gastrointestinal (GI) tract bleeding or excessive protein administration.

DIAGNOSTIC PROCEDURES

Although frequently ordered by physicians, a renal ultrasound is rarely helpful in determining the cause of acute renal failure in a hospitalized patient who previously had normal renal function. Insertion of a urinary catheter into the patient's bladder is usually adequate to exclude postrenal obstruction as the cause of acute renal failure. However, for the outpatient who presents with renal failure, the renal ultrasound is instrumental in determining whether the renal failure is acute or chronic and whether obstruction is present. A plain film radiograph of the abdomen will document the presence of two kidneys and also provide a check for renal stones. If the possibility of renal artery obstruction exists, a radioisotope scan or renal angiography may be required. Intravenous pyelography is rarely used in the diagnostic workup of acute renal failure. Cystoscopy with

TABLE 43.2. PHYSICAL EXAM FINDINGS IN ACUTE RENAL FAILURE[a]

Physical Examination Finding	Clinical Implication If Present	Possible Diagnoses	Category of Acute Renal Failure	Possible Confounding Factors
Vital Signs				
Orthostatic hypotension	Intravascular volume status	Volume depletion	Prerenal azotemia	Antihypertensive therapy Neuropathies (diabetes mellitus)
Skin				
Tenting	Volume status	Volume depletion	Prerenal azotemia	Advanced age
Rash	Allergic reaction	Hypersensitivity reaction	Acute interstitial nephritis	Contact dermatitis
Petechiae	Platelet dysfunction	Thrombotic thrombocytopenic purpura Hemolytic uremic syndrome Sepsis	Acute intrinsic renal failure—vasculitis	Bone marrow suppression Antiplatelet drugs
Splinter hemorrhages Janeway lesions Osler's nodes	Embolic phenomenon	Endocarditis	Acute intrinsic renal failure—acute Glomerulonephritis	Small vessel vasculitis
Edema	Volume status	Total body volume overload	Suggests prerenal azotemia unlikely	Right heart failure, deep venous thrombosis
HEENT				
Hollenhorst plaque	Embolic phenomenon	Cholesterol emboli	Acute intrinsic renal failure—vascular	Plaque must be in aorta to affect kidney
Roth spots	Embolic phenomenon	Endocarditis	Acute intrinsic renal failure—acute Glomerulonephritis	Other systemic infection
Heart				
S_3 heart sound	Left ventricular dysfunction	Congestive heart failure	Prerenal azotemia	Preexisting compensated congestive heart failure
New murmur (particularly diastolic murmurs)	Valvular dysfunction	Endocarditis	Acute intrinsic renal failure—acute Glomerulonephritis	Preexisting valvular disease Hyperdynamic state
Lung				
Rales	Pulmonary congestion	Pulmonary edema with volume overload or left ventricular dysfunction	Prerenal azotemia	Compensated CHF
Abdomen				
Renal artery bruit	Arterial integrity	Renal artery stenosis	Prerenal azotemia	Generalized atherosclerosis
Ascites	Elevated venous pressure	Liver failure or right heart failure	Prerenal azotemia Hepatorenal syndrome	Peritoneal membrane disorder (tumor)
Bladder distention	Bladder capacity	Bladder outlet obstruction	Postobstruction renal failure	
GU				
Prostatic enlargement	Prostate enlargement	Prostatic hypertrophy or cancer	Postobstruction renal failure	Nonenlarged prostate does not exclude obstruction
GYN				
Abnormal bimanual exam	Uterine size Cervical status	Possible bilateral ureteral obstruction or cervical cancer	Postobstruction renal failure	

[a]A variety of physical examination findings may be found in patients with acute renal failure. The first column lists the physical finding, while the second column is the clinical implications if these abnormal findings are present. Columns 3 and 4 list the possible diagnoses and category of acute renal failure that is likely to be present. Possible confounding factors that could also explain the physical examination findings are listed in the final column.

retrograde pyelography may be helpful if the possibility of obstruction exists. This last procedure may be necessary in a patient with the history of a single functioning kidney even if the ultrasound does not demonstrate hydronephrosis. If, despite a careful history, physical examination, and the above diagnostic tests, the etiology of the acute renal failure is unclear, a percutaneous renal biopsy may be indicated. When renal biopsies are performed to determine the cause of acute renal failure, the majority of cases demonstrate acute tubular necrosis.

Clinical Course and Prognosis

The clinical course and prognosis for patients with acute renal failure depends on a number of clinical variables including (1) the definition of acute renal failure employed, (2) the etiology of acute renal failure, (3) the presence or absence of oliguria, (4) the patient's nutritional status, (5) the presence of comorbidities, and (6) whether the patient requires renal replacement therapy. Many texts divide the clinical course of acute tubular necrosis into an initial, oliguric, and recovery phase. The utility of this approach is questionable because recovery from acute tubular necrosis does not begin at a defined time from onset of renal failure. Rather, recovery from acute tubular necrosis occurs 10–14 days after the last insult to the kidney. Critically ill patients with acute renal failure often have recurring episodes of hypoxia and hypotension and are treated with many ongoing doses of nephrotoxins, which may delay the recovery process.[24] Furthermore, the autoregulation of renal blood flow is deranged in acute renal failure.[25] Renal vasoconstriction results in continued reduced blood flow to the nephron even after the insult to the kidneys is removed and the tubules begin recovering from acute tubular necrosis. Actual improvements in glomerular filtration rate will not be manifested until tubular cell necrosis is repaired and renal blood flow is normalized.[25]

TABLE 43.3. DIAGNOSTIC PARAMETERS FOR DIFFERENTIATING CAUSES OF ACUTE RENAL FAILURE[a]

Lab Test	Prerenal Azotemia	Acute Intrinsic Renal Failure	Postrenal Obstruction
Urine sediment	Normal	Casts, cellular debris	Cellular debris
Urinary RBC	None	2–4+	Variable
Urinary WBC	None	2–4+	1+
Urine sodium	<20	>40	>40
FE Na (%)	<1	>1–2	Variable
Urine osmolality / Serum osmolality	>1.5	<1.3	<1.5
Urine creatinine / Plasma creatinine	>40:1	<20:1	<20:1
BUN/SCr	>20	15	15

[a]Common laboratory tests are listed that are used to classify the cause of acute renal failure. Functional acute renal failure, which is not included in this table, would have laboratory values similar to that seen in prerenal azotemia. However, the urine osmolality to plasma osmolality ratios may not exceed 1.5 depending on the circulating levels of antidiuretic hormone. The laboratory results listed under acute intrinsic renal failure are those seen in acute tubular necrosis, the most common cause of acute intrinsic renal failure.

Retrospective analyses suggest that patients with mildly increased serum creatinine concentrations have increased risk of mortality compared to those patients that do not have an increase in their creatinine during their hospitalization. However, whether this is a cause-and-effect phenomenon or a selection bias is unclear. In fact, patients who have a mild increase in their serum creatinine concentration have an excellent renal prognosis. Their eventual outcome is almost entirely dependent on their associated illnesses[11] and procedures performed on them (e.g., cardiac catheterization).

The etiology of acute renal failure has a major influence on the eventual outcome for patients with acute renal failure. Hospitalized patients who develop acute renal failure secondary to obstruction (e.g., an improperly placed urinary catheter) tend to have a rapid recovery of renal function following relief of the obstruction. Patients with prerenal azotemia resulting from renal hypoperfusion also have rapid recovery of function following an improvement in perfusion pressure. Individuals who develop functional acute renal failure generally recover renal function once the effects of the offending agents resolve. In each of these three clinical conditions, the patient's prognosis is largely dependent on his or her comorbid conditions. However, for those patients who develop intrinsic renal failure, the disruption in their internal milieu and the associated systemic effects of their uremia may adversely affect their preexisting illnesses and adversely influence their outcome.

The presence or absence of oliguria has been suggested to be an independent predictor of eventual patient outcome. In multiple reports of mortality in acute renal failure, individuals with nonoliguria have a significantly higher survival rate than individuals who develop oliguria or anuria.[5,26] A portion of this perceived improvement in outcome may relate to selection bias, in that patients developing nonoliguric renal failure frequently have more reversible renal insults such as obstruction or prerenal azotemia. However, the continued ability of the kidney to control volume homeostasis, even in the absence of solute control, may delay the need for renal replacement therapy and its associated risks.

Individuals who require renal replacement therapy for their acute renal failure have a more complicated clinical course and a higher mortality rate. The use of renal replacement therapy may delay the recovery of renal function[27]; activate endogenous inflammatory mediators, which may promote catabolism and enhance organ injury[16]; and expose the patient to the risks related to the renal replacement therapy itself.

THERAPEUTIC MANAGEMENT OF ACUTE RENAL FAILURE

PREVENTION OF ACUTE RENAL FAILURE

Acute renal failure frequently is iatrogenic, resulting from drug therapy, surgical procedures, and diagnostic tests. Ideally, preventative therapy should be instituted in patients who are at risk for developing acute renal failure and are about to receive known nephrotoxins or procedures likely to induce nephrotoxicity. Risk factors for the development of acute renal failure have been identified for many different patient populations. Suggested preoperative risk factors for the development of postoperative acute renal failure include preexisting renal insufficiency, advanced age, left ventricular dysfunction, male sex, and either hypertension or hypotension.[28] Risk factors for the development of aminoglycoside nephrotoxicity include high cumulative aminoglycoside doses, renal hypoperfusion, concomitant nephrotoxins, advanced age, and hypokalemia.[24] Risk factors for the development of contrast media-induced nephrotoxicity include the use of ionic contrast agents, the concomitant administration of nephrotoxins, a history of diabetes mellitus, hepatic disease, advanced age, or preexisting renal insufficiency.[24] The latter risk factor is the most significant indicator of those patients at risk for contrast dye nephrotoxicity. However, the overall risk of developing clinically significant renal failure from intravenous contrast dye is less than 0.01% for all patients undergoing intravascular contrast examinations.[29] The exclusive use of nonionic contrast agents would add an estimated $1.2 billion to the cost of health care in the United States, suggesting that the use of these agents be restricted to patients predisposed to nephrotoxicity.[30]

Hydration

Once the patient at risk for the development of acute renal failure has been identified prospectively, a few preventive maneuvers can be instituted. These preventive therapies include hydration, sodium loading, and the use of medications. The simplest and most effective method of acute renal failure prevention is to ensure that the patient is adequately hydrated prior to the nephrotoxic event. Adequate hydration improves renal perfusion and lowers tubular workload by reducing the need for urinary concentration. Reduced tubular work results in lower medullary oxygen requirements. Vigorous hydration will also dilute the nephrotoxin concentration within the tubule, possibly reducing the chances of developing nephrotoxicity.[24] Usually 0.45% or 0.9% NaCl is used to hydrate these patients in order to maintain a high intravascular volume. Care must be taken not to overhydrate, particularly in patients with preexisting liver or left ventricular dysfunction.

Clinical examples where aggressive hydration would be useful in flushing tubules and diluting possible nephrotoxins include tumor lysis syndrome and rhabdomyolysis. In both of these instances, cellular contents (i.e., phosphate and nucleic acids that are converted to uric acid) are released into the bloodstream due to tissue destruction. Some of this cellular debris is nephrotoxic. Aggressive hydration will help to flush these substances from the tubules. In the case of tumor lysis syndrome, alkalinization of the urine to a pH of >6 is attempted in order to prevent uric acid crystals from forming in the kidneys. The value of urinary alkalinization and diuretic therapy for the prevention and treatment of acute renal failure secondary to rhabdomyolysis is equivocal.[31]

Sodium Loading

A related means to prevent acute renal failure from occurring is to sodium load the patient prior to the scheduled nephrotoxic event in order to inhibit the tubular glomerular reflex. When the tubule senses high volume flow or an increased delivery of sodium chloride resulting from tubular damage or high sodium chloride administration, the reflex results in a decrease in renal blood flow, glomerular filtration rate and tubular flow, and ultimately conservation of solutes and fluid.

Amphotericin B nephrotoxicity may be prevented by mediation of this feedback mechanism. Sodium loading prior to the initiation of amphotericin B therapy enhances the tubular glomerular reflex, and the resultant reduction in the glomerular filtration rate may minimize or prevent amphotericin B-induced tubular damage since the amount of amphotericin B delivered to the distal nephron will be reduced. Dietary sodium liberalization was shown to improve renal function during amphotericin B therapy in a small case series of patients who had already developed nephrotoxicity.[32] Whether sodium loading prior to the initiation of therapy will prevent the development of amphotericin B nephrotoxicity is unknown.

Pharmacologic Interventions

In theory, the beneficial effects of diuretic therapy should include some of the benefits seen with hydration therapy as well as some additional benefits. Tubular obstruction from cellular debris is often associated with vasoconstriction and a reduced glomerular filtration rate, which may exacerbate acute renal failure.[25] Diuretics increase tubule fluid flow and, therefore, may prevent tubular obstruction. Loop diuretics increase renal blood flow via their vasodilating effects, which may be beneficial in the prevention of acute renal failure. Furosemide may also be useful in preventing acute renal failure since it inhibits tubuloglomerular feedback. This reflex may be harmful in acute renal failure because reductions in glomerular filtration rate may worsen tubular damage. Mannitol, an osmotic diuretic, may also have some utility in preventing acute renal failure. Mannitol theoretically may reduce tubular cell damage by acting as an impermeable solute that reduces cell swelling. Although these espoused theoretical benefits of diuretic therapy appear reasonable, actual documentation of their value in controlled studies is nearly nonexistent.

Diuretic therapy has potential benefits but the overwhelming majority of carefully controlled and blinded studies find no benefit to these treatments. Some studies have found that "preventive" diuretic therapy may worsen the incidence of acute renal failure.[33] Vigorous hydration and intravenous furosemide 1.5 mg/kg given 30 minutes before administration of radiocontrast dye was associated with a significant increase in serum creatinine compared to a control group that did not receive diuretics.[34] In contrast, a later study found that hydration plus either furosemide or mannitol resulted in a higher rate of radiocontrast dye-induced nephropathy compared to hydration alone.[35] Diuretics given prior to or during amphotericin B therapy increase the risk of developing amphotericin B nephrotoxicity, probably due to sodium depletion associated with diuretic therapy.[36]

Despite the majority of evidence that diuretic therapy does not prevent acute renal failure, small numbers of retrospective reports and case series have suggested a benefit. Consequently, many clinicians continue to utilize these agents in an attempt to prevent acute renal failure in settings where nephrotoxicity is likely. Caution should be exercised when diuretic therapy is attempted to prevent acute renal failure. Overaggressive "preventive" diuresis with any diuretic can result in hypovolemia and may induce or worsen acute renal failure. Adequate hydration and tissue perfusion is probably of more value than diuretic use in this setting.

Resistance to diuretic therapy is a common problem in acute renal failure. Many different mechanisms are thought to be responsible for diuretic resistance in this setting (Table 43.4).[37] Identification of the cause of diuretic resistance in an individual patient will allow the clinician to develop therapeutic strategies to obviate the problem. Sometimes the solution is as simple as changing to a parenteral route of administration to avoid poor oral bioavailability.[38] Other times it requires the use of a continuous infusion of loop diuretics[39] or the addition of low-dose dopamine to the diuretic therapy.

Combination therapy of loop diuretics and a diuretic from a different pharmacologic class and a different mechanism of action can be an effective tool in the setting of acute renal failure. Loop diuretics increase the delivery of sodium chloride to the distal convoluted tubule and collecting duct. With time, these areas of the kidney attempt to compensate for the activity of the loop diuretic and increase sodium and chloride reabsorption. In animals, this compensation can begin after a week of continuous furosemide infusion.[37] Whether this compensation can occur in humans with acute renal failure is unclear. Diuretics that work at the distal convoluted tubule (thiazides) or the collecting duct (amiloride, triamterene, and spironolactone) may have a synergistic effect when administered with loop diuretics by blocking the compensatory increase in sodium and chloride reabsorption. Metolazone is a thiazide diuretic commonly used in combination with loop diuretics because, unlike other thiazides, it produces effective diuresis at glomerular filtration rates below 20 mL/min. The combination of loop diuretics and usual doses of thiazide diuretics may be effective in renal disease despite the accumulation of endogenous organic acids, which blocks the transport of loop diuretics into the lumen.[40] Larger doses of loop diuretics may also be necessary to overcome this reduced transport.

Excessive sodium intake is the most likely cause of diuretic resistance in an outpatient setting. However, in the institutional setting, unrecognized sodium intake may occur in enteral and parenteral nutrition formulas, maintenance intravenous fluids, and from drug therapy. Restriction of sodium intake to <100 mmol/d should eliminate this cause of diuretic resistance.

TABLE 43.4. COMMON CAUSES OF DIURETIC RESISTANCE IN PATIENTS WITH ACUTE RENAL FAILURE

Excessive sodium intake
Inadequate diuretic dose or inappropriate regimen
Reduced oral bioavailability
Reduced delivery of diuretic to urine in renal failure
Nephrotic syndrome (diuretic protein binding in tubule lumen)
Reduced renal blood flow
Drugs (NSAID, ACE inhibitors, vasodilators)
Hypotension
Intravascular depletion
Increased sodium reabsorption
Nephron adaptation to chronic diuretic therapy
NSAID
CHF
Cirrhosis

(Adapted from Ref. 37.)

Theoretically, pharmacologic prevention of acute renal failure with low doses of dopamine may be of some benefit. Low doses of dopamine (1–3 μg/kg/min) selectively increase renal blood flow, while higher doses result in renal vasoconstriction. Exploitation of this salutary finding should allow for optimization of renal blood flow without as much concern for fluid overload, as is seen with vigorous hydration. However, the application of this pharmacologic finding has not translated into documented evidence of acute renal failure prevention. Pretreatment with dopamine (2 μg/kg/min) did not prevent radiocontrast-induced nephropathy in patients with chronic renal insufficiency despite a documented increase in renal blood flow prior to receiving ionic radiocontrast dye.[41] Indeed, in this study, the patients with the highest increase in renal blood flow were the patients who subsequently developed radiocontrast-induced nephropathy. This study suggests that dopamine-induced renal vasodilation alone is insufficient to prevent acute renal failure.

Calcium channel blockers may prevent the development of acute renal failure since they inhibit the vasoconstrictive response of the afferent arterioles of the kidney to vasoconstrictive agonists.[42] A subsequent increase in glomerular filtration is noted because the efferent arterioles are relatively resistant to the vasodilating effects of the calcium antagonists. These agents also may interfere with the damaging role of intracellular calcium in the mitochondria and tubules in the presence of hypoxia.[43] The elevated uptake of calcium by the mitochondria in the hypoxic state ultimately is responsible for cell death. It has been suggested that calcium channel blocker administration prior to the nephrotoxic insult may be a promising prophylactic therapy.[44]

Although calcium channel blockers have been shown to prevent acute renal failure in experimental models, few human studies have been conducted. Two studies have documented the efficacy of nitrendipine[45] and nifedipine[46] in the prevention of radiocontrast-induced nephropathy. Other positive findings are found in the renal transplant literature. Diltiazem-perfused kidneys, which are transplanted into patients who are also receiving diltiazem, have a lower incidence of acute tubular necrosis.[47] Similar findings have been reported with verapamil. In a randomized trial, verapamil 20 mg or placebo was administered to brain-dead kidney donors prior to organ harvest.[48] Urine output was significantly higher and serum creatinine significantly lower on the first day post-transplant in the verapamil group. This effect was lost by day seven post-transplant, suggesting that verapamil was efficacious in the prevention of oliguric acute renal failure post-transplant, possibly by preventing intracellular calcium accumulation. Larger studies in different clinical situations will help determine the role of calcium antagonists in the prevention of acute renal failure.

Investigational agents for the prevention of acute renal failure have shown some promise in animal models and in a few limited trials in humans. Endothelin and platelet activating factor (PAF) are vasoactive substances that have been identified from damaged kidneys. These substances are thought to mediate the compromised renal blood flow and glomerular filtration rate in acute renal failure. Antiendothelin and PAF antagonist[49] therapies may hold promise in the prevention and treatment of acute renal failure. Atrial natriuretic peptide (ANP) administration is associated with an increase in the glomerular filtration rate, natriuresis, and systemic hypotension. ANP causes the dilation of the afferent arterioles and a constriction of the efferent arterioles, possibly due to blockage of the tubuloglomerular feedback mechanism. These investigational therapies have been reviewed extensively elsewhere.[44]

PHARMACOLOGIC TREATMENT OF ACUTE RENAL FAILURE

Once acute renal failure is established, supportive treatments, some of which are pharmacologic, have been the primary options. The initial treatment of acute renal failure should be to alleviate the underlying cause, when possible. The most common cause of acute renal failure in the hospital setting is acute tubular necrosis from renal hypoxia. Therefore, immediate attention should be given to improving renal oxygenation and perfusion through the use of oxygen and hydration. Once fluid repletion has been accomplished, sodium and fluid restriction may be necessary to avoid fluid overload in oliguric patients. Sources of excess exogenous fluids that can be reduced include minimizing the volume of fluid used to administer intravenous medications, reassessing the need for and rate of "keep-open" intravenous solutions, and using concentrated sources of enteral and parenteral feedings. Identifiable nephrotoxins such as amphotericin B and the aminoglycosides should be avoided in these patients if possible; however, a risk–benefit analysis of therapy may indicate that no alternative is available. Other important supportive therapies include adequate nutrition and renal replacement therapy.

Once supportive measures are in place, active intervention with pharmacotherapy may be instituted, usually with the same agents that may have been utilized to try to prevent acute renal failure. Nonoliguric acute renal failure has a significantly better prognosis than oliguric acute renal failure.[26] Whether patients with nonoliguric acute renal failure have less extensive damage to their kidneys than their oliguric counterparts or if something is intrinsically therapeutic about having increased urine flow is unclear. Advantages of nonoliguric renal failure include easier management of fluid and electrolyte balance, the ability to administer adequate nutrition, reduced risk of developing pulmonary edema, and the reduced need for renal replacement therapies. Diuretic therapy is the most commonly used therapy to change the patient's status from oliguria to nonoliguria. The rationale for diuretic use to treat acute renal failure is similar to that of their use in preventing acute renal failure. However, like the findings for diuretics in the prevention of acute renal failure, most studies examining the effects of diuretic therapy in established acute renal failure find that diuretics do not improve patient outcome. Secondary considerations such as increased urine output and reduced need for renal replacement therapy, however, have been improved by diuretic use in most studies.[50] A clinical situation where diuretic use has been postulated to improve survival is in patients with "early" acute renal failure. In this small window of time, acute renal failure remains reversible before intrinsic renal failure establishes itself. Although early acute renal failure is difficult to define clinically, trials utilizing mannitol or loop diuretic therapy in early acute renal failure have demonstrated benefit. Unfortunately, most of these studies were not adequately controlled. In a crude meta-analysis of these reports of diuretic use in early acute renal failure, a significant improvement in survival rate was found in patients who increased their urine flow in response to diuretics compared to those who remained oliguric (76% versus 58%).[50] Whether this difference corresponds to an actual improvement due to diuretics or simply demonstrates that those with less severe disease are able to respond to diuretic therapy is not clear.

Furosemide, bumetanide, and torsemide are the three parenteral loop diuretics available to the practitioner, but nearly all studies in acute renal failure have been conducted with furosemide. Torsemide and bumetanide have better oral bioavailability compared to furosemide, and torsemide has a longer duration of action.[51] However, when given parenterally in equipotent doses, it does not appear that there is a difference in efficacy in patients with acute renal failure.[52] Interestingly, the equipotency ratio of parenteral bumetanide:torsemide:furosemide in patients with normal renal function is 1:20:40 but in renal failure this ratio changes to 1:11:11.[52] Most clinicians routinely choose furosemide in the treatment of acute renal failure for reasons of familiarity and cost.

An initial dose of intravenous furosemide 80–320 mg or mannitol 12.5–25 g can be used in the treatment of acute renal failure[50] (Table 43.5). Patient response to this initial dose will determine the utility of future dosing. Response to an initial dose of furosemide should be followed with subsequent intermittent dosing or the institution of a continuous infusion. Continuous infusion of loop diuretics is a relatively new dosing approach, but may result in an improved, titratable, diuretic response.[53]

Occasionally, low dose dopamine infusions combined with diuretics will increase urine output in poor responders, but this combination has not been documented to improve survival in patients with acute renal failure. Low-dose dopamine (200 μg/min) monotherapy increases urine output without improving measured creatinine clearance in critically ill patients without acute renal failure.[54] In contrast, low doses of the positive inotrope, dobutamine (175 μg/min), have been documented to elevate creatinine clearance significantly without increasing urine output in this same population.[54] It is unclear if these findings will apply to patients with acute renal failure and whether combination dobutamine and dopamine therapy will have additive salutary effects.[55]

Clinical trials utilizing calcium channel blockers in the treatment of established acute renal failure have shown promise. Much of the kidney damage in early acute renal failure has been attributed to the influx of calcium into the cell, which eventually causes cell death. As described earlier, calcium channel blockers appear to be beneficial in preventing acute renal failure if given prior to a nephrotoxic insult. Based on these findings, investigators have attempted to administer calcium antagonists early in the course of acute renal failure in an attempt to prevent mitochondrial changes and cell death.

One difficulty of using systemic calcium antagonists in critically ill patients with acute renal failure is that the hypotensive effects of the calcium channel blockers are not well tolerated. Often patients with acute renal failure are already hypotensive and require vasopressor therapies. To obviate this undesirable effect of the calcium channel blockers, some investigators have attempted to administer these agents directly into the kidney via an infusion into the renal artery. Six patients with acute renal failure caused by malaria or leptospirosis received 3 hours of intrarenal verapamil and intravenous furosemide for 24 hours and were compared to six others who received furosemide alone.[56] Patients receiving verapamil plus furosemide had a significantly improved glomerular filtration rate and had a significantly shorter duration of acute renal failure than did the furosemide alone group. Similar findings were reported by this research group with another calcium antagonist, gallopamil.[57] Intrarenal catheterization for the purposes of administering medications is not a common practice at most institutions. Studies of calcium channel blockers in the treatment of acute renal failure using more conventional routes of administration are necessary.

Increased endogenous ANP concentrations have been identified in patients with acute renal failure, possibly as an adaptive biological response to the fluid overload associated with acute renal failure.[58] Based on these findings, exogenous ANP has been administered to patients with established acute renal failure to determine whether pharmacologic intervention improves patient outcome or hastens recovery of renal function. ANP infusion added to mannitol or furosemide therapy was compared to conven-

TABLE 43.5. AGENTS USED IN THE TREATMENT OF ACUTE RENAL FAILURE

Agent	Adult Dosage	Special Considerations
Furosemide	100 mg IV, if no response within 1 hour, give 240 mg IV; if urine output follows, give 5–50 mg/h continuous infusion or 500–1500 mg/d in divided doses to maintain urine output	Other IV loop diuretics probably offer no additional benefit. Monitor urine output and serum electrolytes. Infuse ≤4 mg/min to avoid ototoxicity.
Metolazone	10 mg PO Q12h can be given in along with loop diuretic therapy to increase urine output	If patient cannot take oral meds, IV chlorothiazide 500 mg Q12h can be used. Same monitoring as for furosemide.
Mannitol (20%)	12.5–25 g IV over 3–5 min, may repeat in 1 hour if no response; if urine output follows, give 20 mL/h mannitol 20% along with furosemide	Monitor patient's fluid status, urine output, and serum electrolytes. Serum osmolality >310 mOsm/L is contraindication for mannitol therapy.
Dopamine	1–5 μg/kg/min IV	Monitor urine output, blood pressure, IV site for extravasation.

tional therapy with or without diuretics in patients with established acute renal failure.[59] The ANP-treated group experienced a significant improvement in creatinine clearance and a reduced need for dialysis treatments, although a significant difference in mortality was not found.

ANP causes systemic hypotension, prompting an interest in combination therapy with low-dose dopamine. This combination may be useful because dopamine could mitigate the hypotensive effects of ANP while increasing renal blood flow. Results of studies using this promising combination in humans have not yet been published. Another experimental approach to the treatment of established acute renal failure is therapy directed toward enhancing renal cell repair. Epidermal growth factor, insulin growth factor I, and hepatocyte growth factor may help the tubular cells to regenerate faster, but these therapies remain experimental for the treatment of acute renal failure.[60]

Complications of Acute Renal Failure

HYPERKALEMIA

The most common and life-threatening electrolyte disorder of acute renal failure is hyperkalemia. Patients with acute renal failure lose the ability to eliminate the potassium ion via the kidneys. More important, comorbid conditions such as diabetes mellitus often induce hyperkalemia via shifting intracellular potassium ions into the serum. Hyperkalemia is defined as a serum potassium concentration of >5.5 mEq/L. Clinical symptoms of hyperkalemia include paresthesias and weakness. Paralysis leading to respiratory demise may follow but usually the cardiac manifestations of hyperkalemia cause death before paralysis occurs. The electrocardiogram manifestations of hyperkalemia are depicted in Figure 43.3. The earliest electrocardiologic sign of hyperkalemia is the peaking of the T waves, which usually occurs at potassium concentrations of 5.5–6.0 mEq/L. As the serum potassium rises, the PR interval lengthens and the QRS complex widens (6.0–7.0 mEq/L). Further elevation in serum concentrations results in a disappearance of the P wave and a merging of the QRS complex into the T wave, resulting in a characteristic sine wave. Unless treatment is instituted rapidly, ventricular fibrillation and asystole will ensue. This is particularly true in acute renal failure because acute elevations in serum potassium are not tolerated as well as the chronic elevation in serum potassium seen in patients with chronic renal failure.

The treatment of hyperkalemia in acute renal failure results from a working knowledge of potassium physiology. Although potassium is predominantly an intracellular ion, serum potassium concentration measures only extracellular potassium. Hyperkalemia, therefore, can result from an elevated total body load of potassium or a shifting of intracellular potassium ions outside of the cells. Extensive tissue breakdown (as seen in rhabdomyolysis, tumor lysis syndrome, or crush injuries) results in large quantities of potassium entering the extracellular compartment. Because these patients frequently have a concurrent respiratory or metabolic acidosis, the serum potassium concentration will be further exaggerated. Acidotic states result in increased hydrogen ion concentrations, which subsequently enter the cells of the body. For cells to maintain electroneutrality, intracellular potassium ions shift extracellularly, raising the serum potassium concentration. No matter what the cause of the hyperkalemia, the effect on myocardial muscle is the same and a serum concentration above 5.5 mEq/L may cause toxicity. Hyperkalemia therapy is directed at either removing potassium ions from the body or shifting the extracellular potassium ions into cells. Typical pharmacologic regimens used to treat hyperkalemia are listed in Table 43.6. All therapies must work rapidly to lower serum concentrations if they are to prevent and reverse cardiac manifestations.

Only two of the therapies in Table 43.6 actually remove potassium from the body: sodium polystyrene sulfonate and renal replacement therapy (usually dialysis). Diuretics will also remove potassium but they are often ineffective in acute renal failure because of reduced urine output. Sodium polystyrene sulfonate is a cation exchange resin that exchanges sodium ion for potassium. This agent may be given orally or as a retention enema, with the oral route preferred because of increased contact time with the GI tract. Sorbitol is given with the oral and rectal administration of sodium polystyrene sulfonate to prevent constipation. Colonic necrosis has been reported when sodium polystyrene sulfonate along with sorbitol was given as a retention enema and may be due to the sorbitol in this combination.[61,62] Thus care should be taken when sodium polystyrene sulfonate is given to patients with acute renal failure, especially in those patients that may have preexisting bowel ischemia. Oral administration yields an exchange of approximately 1 mEq of potassium for every gram of sodium polystyrene sulfonate. Rectal administration usually results in an exchange of only 0.5 mEq for each gram because of reduced GI contact time compared to oral administration. The onset of action of sodium polystyrene sulfonate is slow and therefore it should not be used as monotherapy for patients with hyperkalemia who already exhibit EKG changes.

Dialytic therapies are effective in rapidly removing extracellular potassium. Hemodialysate potassium concentrations can be lowered to more rapidly eliminate serum potassium. Peritoneal dialysis may be used; however, more frequent exchanges of dialysate are necessary to remove adequate amounts of potassium at a clinically useful rate.

Serum concentrations above 6.0 mEq/L or the presence of EKG changes warrant immediate treatment. If dialysis is not imminent, therapy should be directed toward

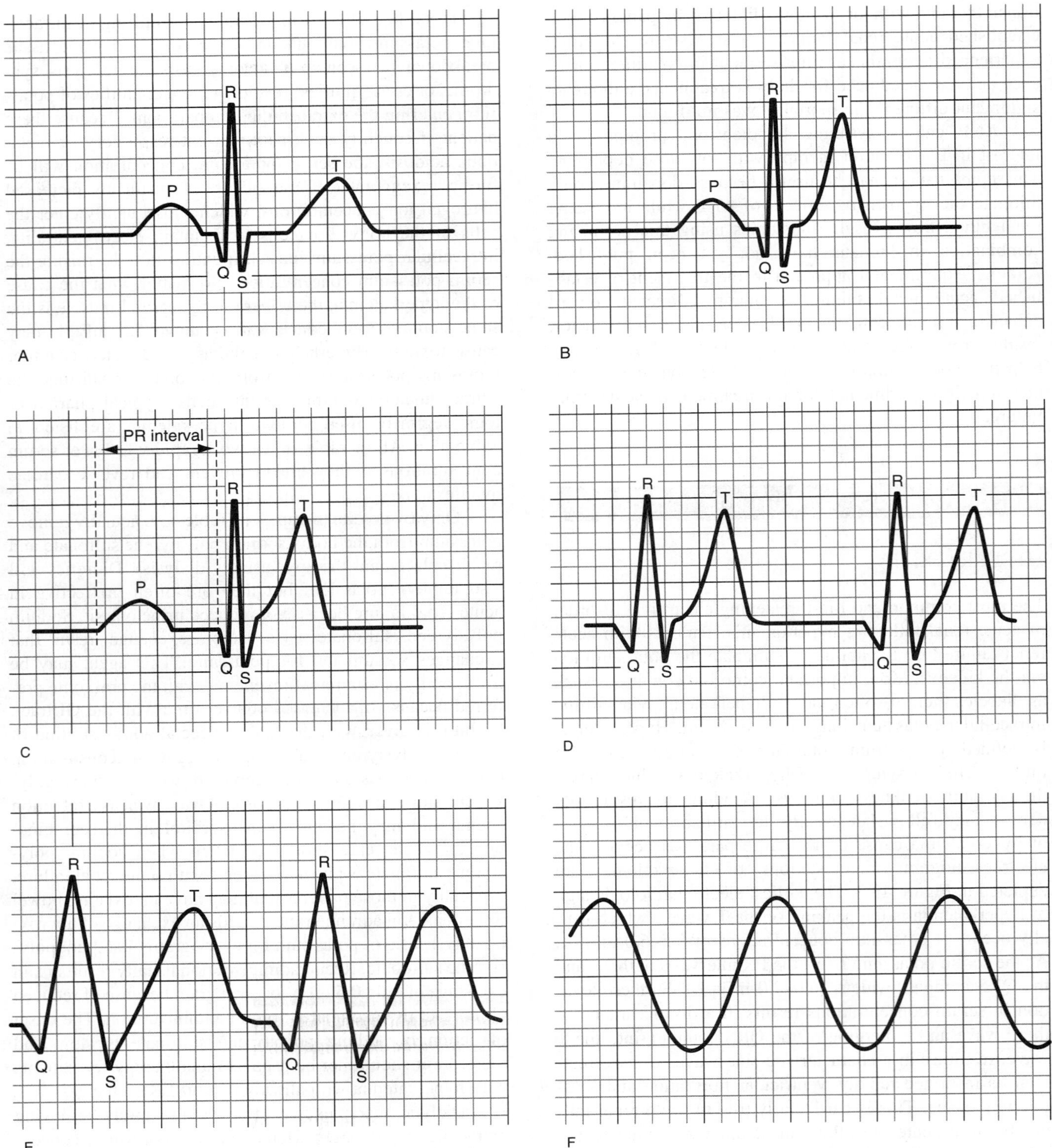

Figure 43.3. The earliest electrocardiogram (EKG) manifestation of hyperkalemia is an increase in the rate of ventricular repolarization, which results in a "peaking" of the T wave at serum potassium concentration of ≈5.5–6.0 mEq/L (B), relative to the normal EKG presentation (A). Further increases in the serum potassium concentration above 6 mEq/L result in conduction delays through the His–Purkinje system, the atrial myocardium, and the ventricular myocardium. The EKG manifestations of these conduction delays and the sequence in which they occur are a widening of the PR interval (C, delay through the His–Purkinje system), a loss of the P wave (D, delay through the atrial myocardium), and a widening of the QRS complex (E, delay through the ventricular myocardium). Finally, (F) there is a merging of the QRS complex with the T wave, which results in a sine-wave appearance to the tracing.

TABLE 43.6. TREATMENT OF HYPERKALEMIA

Treatment	Adult Dosage	Onset	Duration of Effect	Clinical Considerations
Calcium gluconate (10%)	10–20 mL IV at 1–3 mL/min	Immediate	5–20 minutes	Calcium and bicarbonate incompatible, monitor EKG
Sodium bicarbonate	50 mEq IV over 1–5 min	30–60 minutes	0.5–3 hours	Large sodium load
Regular insulin and glucose	10 units IV and 50 mL $D_{50}W$ bolus or 500 mL $D_{10}W$ over 1 hour	30–60 minutes	3–4 hours	Glucose monitoring necessary
Albuterol	10–20 mg nebulized or 0.5 mg IV over 15 minutes	<30 minutes	2–6 hours	Tachycardia, tremor
Sodium polystyrene sulfonate and sorbitol	25–50 g PO or PR as retention enema	2–3 hours	Irreversibly binds K^+	Constipation, large sodium load
Dialysis	—	Hours	Dependent on patient status and diet	Requires dialysis access

reducing extracellular potassium concentrations and increasing conduction velocity in the myocardium. Calcium infusion has an almost immediate onset of action and will reverse the membrane effects of potassium. Calcium does not reduce extracellular potassium concentrations, so after calcium is infused, other therapies directed at lowering potassium levels must be instituted. Decreasing the serum potassium concentration by redistribution of potassium into cells may be accomplished by intravenous administration of bicarbonate. Alternatively, an insulin infusion will also stimulate the cellular uptake of potassium. Glucose should be administered along with the insulin, and blood sugar concentrations should be monitored frequently to prevent hypoglycemia.

Inhaled or intravenous β-adrenergic agonist therapy also will reduce serum potassium concentrations. Beta agonists stimulate the ATPase pump by the activation of cyclic AMP thereby shifting potassium into the intracellular compartment. Intravenous albuterol increases plasma insulin concentrations, which may be an additional hypokalemic mechanism.[63] In one study of adult hemodialysis patients, nebulized albuterol 10–20 mg maximally reduced mean serum potassium concentrations by 0.62–0.98 mEq/L with an onset of activity of 30 minutes.[64] In a similar study in 11 children with chronic renal failure, nebulized albuterol 2.5–5 mg has been documented to lower mean serum potassium concentrations by 1.2 mEq/L for at least 5 hours after administration.[65] This noninvasive therapy may be useful in hyperkalemic patients when intravenous access is unavailable.

Hyperkalemic patients often need combination therapy to control serum potassium concentrations. In severe hyperkalemia, therapy often begins with calcium infusion followed by another modality until dialysis can be instituted. One combination that has been documented to be beneficial is insulin and glucose therapy combined with albuterol. Intravenous albuterol added to glucose and insulin therapy results in a significantly greater hypokalemic effect than glucose and insulin therapy alone.[66]

INFECTION

The most common cause of death in patients with acute renal failure is infection.[67] Interestingly, sepsis itself is a very common cause of acute renal failure.[11] Acute renal failure contributes somewhat to the high infection rate by altering leukocyte function and cell-mediated immunity. Other aspects in the care of the patient with acute renal failure can lead to infection. Renal replacement therapy usually necessitates indwelling vascular or peritoneal access, which can serve as a locus of infection. Peritoneal and vascular access site erythema or purulent drainage should be monitored routinely. Indwelling urinary catheters also predispose patients with acute renal failure to infection. Urinary catheters should be used for no longer than necessary, but in many instances their use cannot be avoided. Frequent evaluation of urine for signs of infection is warranted.

The comorbidities found in patients with acute renal failure may play a more important role in the development of infection. Critically ill patients with acute renal failure often have failures of other organ systems. These failures predispose them to infection. Concomitant cardiopulmonary failure necessitating mechanical ventilation increases the risk of pneumonia. High-dose vasopressor therapy results in reduced blood flow to the GI tract, which may cause ischemia and introduction of gut flora to the bloodstream. The management of a patient with acute renal failure requires (1) prevention of infection where possible, (2) a high index of suspicion in the recognition of infection, and (3) aggressive antibiotic therapy that has been adjusted appropriately for renal disease and renal replacement therapy.

CARDIOVASCULAR

Patients with acute renal failure often manifest cardiovascular abnormalities. Hypertension, hypotension, heart failure, pericarditis, arrhythmias, and pulmonary edema all may be associated with acute renal failure. The causes of cardiovascular complications in these patients include electrolyte disturbances, impaired acid–base balance, uremia, and volume overload. Volume overload may cause hypertension, which may be best treated with diuretics and renal replacement therapy. Aggressive renal replacement therapy can also alleviate uremic pericarditis and electrolyte and acid–base disorders. Swan–Ganz pressure and clinical monitoring will give an accurate assessment of the patient's volume status, which can be helpful in determining fluid replacement needs.

GASTROINTESTINAL

Critically ill patients with acute renal failure have long been recognized to be at increased risk for GI bleeding.[68,69] Hypotension, the use of vasoconstrictive agents, and the high catabolic state seen in acute renal failure can contribute to stress ulceration in these patients. The uremic state also may induce bleeding by causing a defect in platelet function. Patients with acute renal failure and additional risk factors for stress-related hemorrhage (e.g., respiratory failure or high-dose corticosteroid use) are at an even higher risk for bleeding.[70] Other common GI complaints in patients with acute renal failure include nausea and vomiting associated with uremia and electrolyte imbalances.

NEUROLOGIC

Uremia more commonly affects patients with chronic renal failure than acute renal failure. Nonetheless, the neurologic sequelae associated with uremia, altered mentation myoclonus, and lethargy can occur in the setting of acute renal failure. Other causes of neurologic symptoms must be examined in the patient with acute renal failure before attributing them to uremia. Electrolyte disturbances are common in acute renal failure[71] and frequently cause neurologic changes. Calcium, phosphate, and sodium disorders must be ruled out in these patients. Adverse effects from improperly dosed renally eliminated drugs can also manifest as neurologic abnormalities like seizures or somnolence. Because acute renal failure often has a sudden onset, electrolyte imbalance and drug accumulation can occur rapidly in these patients. Diligent monitoring of laboratory results, renal replacement schedules, and drug dosing can help to prevent these neurologic sequelae.

RENAL REPLACEMENT THERAPIES IN ACUTE RENAL FAILURE

Renal replacement therapy is often required to treat acute renal failure. The decision as to when to implement renal replacement therapy and which renal replacement therapy to use is patient specific. Table 43.7 lists the accepted indications for instituting renal replacement therapy in patients with acute renal failure. The most common reasons to begin renal replacement therapy in acute renal failure are for azotemic control, hyperkalemia, and fluid overload. Renal replacement options for acute renal failure can be divided into two main categories: intermittent and continuous therapies. The most commonly used intermittent and continuous renal replacement therapies are listed in Table 43.8. Historically, intermittent therapies, usually hemodialysis, have been the most commonly chosen modality. The advantages of these therapies are that they are technically simple, the hardware for instituting treatment is available at most institutions, and clinicians usually have expertise using them. Hemodialysis is effective for azotemic control in acute renal failure, providing that it is done frequently enough. In order to achieve azotemic control similar to that achieved by some continuous therapies, hemodialysis must be performed 5–6 times per week.[72] Larger patients with acute renal failure may require even more frequent or prolonged hemodialysis sessions to control azotemia.[73] However, hypotensive critically ill patients with acute renal failure frequently cannot tolerate hemodialysis, especially when aggressive attempts are made to remove excess volume.

Peritoneal dialysis is a continuous renal replacement therapy, which is usually used for ambulatory patients with chronic renal failure but can also be used in acute renal failure. Glucose-containing dialysate solutions are instilled into the patient's peritoneum. The patient's own peritoneal membrane acts as the dialysis membrane. An advantage of peritoneal dialysis in acute renal failure is that it is rela-

TABLE 43.7. THE A, E, I, O AND U'S THAT DESCRIBE THE CLINICAL INDICATIONS FOR RENAL REPLACEMENT THERAPY

	Indications for Renal Replacement Therapy	Clinical Setting
A	***A***cid-base abnormalities	Metabolic acidosis resulting from the accumulation of organic and inorganic acids
E	***E***lectrolyte imbalance	Hyperkalemia, hypermagnesemia
I	***I***ntoxications	Salicylates, lithium, methanol, ethylene glycol, theophylline, phenobarbital
O	fluid ***O***verload	Postoperative fluid gain
U	***U***remia	High catabolism of acute renal failure

TABLE 43.8. ADVANTAGES AND DISADVANTAGES OF COMMON RENAL REPLACEMENT THERAPIES FOR ACUTE RENAL FAILURE

	Intermittent Hemodialysis	Intermittent Hemofiltration	Perionteal Dialysis	Slow Continuous Ultrafiltration (SCUF)	Continuous Arteriovenous Hemofiltration (CAVH)	Continuous Venovenous Hemofiltration (CVVH)	Continuous Arteriovenous Hemodiafiltration (CAVHD)	Continuous Venovenous Hemodiafiltration (CVVHD)
Solute control	Usually adequate	Inadequate	Inadequate	Inadequate	Inadequate	Adequate	Adequate	Adequate
Volume control	Variable	Adequate	Adequate	Adequate	Adequate	Adequate	Adequate	Adequate
Hemodynamic stability	Variable	Well tolerated	Well tolerated	Well tolerated	Well tolerated	Well tolerated	Well tolerated	Well tolerated
Access	Venous	Venous	Peritoneal	Arterial and venous	Arterial and venous	Venous	Arterial and venous	Venous
Anticoagulation	Short duration	Short duration	None	Continuous high dose	Continuous low dose	Continuous high dose	Continuous low dose	Continuous
Technical complexity	High	High	Low	Low	Low	Moderate	Moderate	High
Workload	Intermittent	Intermittent	Low	Low	Low	Moderate	Moderate	High
Drug dosing ease	Many published recommendations	Difficult	Difficult	Negligible drug removal	Difficult	Many published recommendations	Difficult	Difficult
Convective clearance (small and middle molecules)	Mixed	Minimal	Moderate	Moderate	Large	Large	Large	Large
Dialytic clearance (small molecules)	Large	None	Large	None	None	None	Large	Large
Common complications	Hypotension	Hypotension	Hyperglycemia, atelectasis, peritonitis	Arterial bleeding, hypotension	Arterial bleeding, filter clotting	Hypotension	Arterial bleeding, ↑ serum lactate	↑ Serum lactate, hypotension

tively easy to perform once the dialysis catheter is placed into the patient's peritoneum. A disadvantage of peritoneal dialysis is that it is not very efficient for volume and solute removal and can provide a large glucose load to the patient. Patients with acute renal failure receiving rapid (30- to 90-minute dwell times) exchanges of peritoneal dialysate containing 4.25% dextrose absorbed an average of 1922 kcal/d of glucose from the dialysate, resulting in significant overfeeding.[74] Whatever renal replacement therapy is chosen, the goals of therapy remain the same: to provide adequate metabolic (azotemic), electrolyte, and fluid control.

The most commonly used continuous therapies in acute renal failure—continuous hemofiltration and hemodiafiltration—are more technically difficult thereby requiring more nursing time to perform. However, the advantages of continuous therapies are improved fluid and metabolic control, especially in patients unable to tolerate hemodialysis. Continuous therapies are generally better tolerated because the fluid and electrolyte shifts are more gradual than with the intermittent therapies.

Solute removal from the body by dialysis occurs as molecules diffuse across the dialysis membrane in an attempt to achieve equal concentrations in the blood and the dialysate. Smaller molecules, such as electrolytes and urea, cross the dialysis membrane easily and therefore are removed efficiently by dialysis. In contrast, hemofiltration employs no dialysate. Solutes dissolved in the plasma water that are small enough to pass through the hemofilter pores are removed as the plasma water they are dissolved in traverses through the hemofilter. This plasma water solution is called *ultrafiltrate,* and this type of solute removal is called *convection.* Because no diffusion occurs with convective solute removal, the molecular weight of removed substances will be as large as the hemofilter sieve allows, often as high as 5000–10,000 Daltons (Da). Consequently, hemofiltration is more effective that dialytic therapies in the removal of large molecular weight substances. Convective removal of larger molecular weight substances may be desirable in patients with diseases such as septic shock. Since many of the mediators of septic shock have molecular weights of 600–30,000 Da, continuous hemofiltration has been proposed as an adjunctive therapy for septic shock.[75]

The most common types of hemofiltration, continuous arteriovenous hemofiltration (CAVH) and continuous venovenous hemofiltration (CVVH), and the most common method of hemodiafiltration, continuous venovenous hemodiafiltration (CVVHD), are depicted in Figures 43.4, 43.5, and 43.6, respectively. Ultrafiltrate production in CAVH is dependent on the patient's cardiovascular status. This frequently yields adequate volume control but inadequate solute removal in critically ill patients with acute renal failure. However, no special machinery is needed to

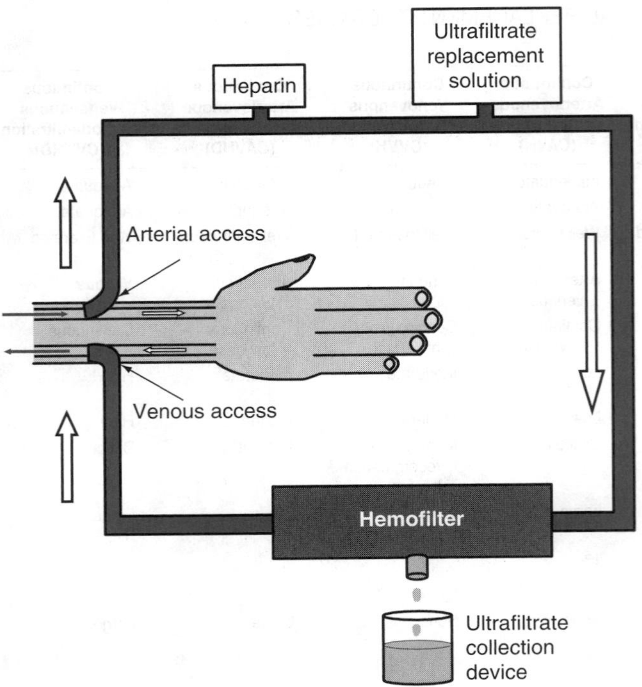

Figure 43.4. Schematic of continuous arteriovenous hemofiltration (CAVH). Blood enters the extracorporeal circuit from an arterial catheter and returns via a separate venous catheter. The hydrostatic force for making ultrafiltrate is provided by the patient's arterial pressure. Blood flow through the circuit and ultrafiltrate production rates are a function of the patient's cardiovascular status. Generally higher heparin doses are required to prevent hemofilter clotting in CAVH versus CVVH because of the slower blood flow through the hemofilter in CAVH.

conduct CAVH, making it a widely used renal replacement modality.[76] CVVH does not require arterial access but uses pumps to move blood through the circuit and to regulate ultrafiltrate production.[77] This increase in complexity compared to CAVH is balanced by more effective volume and solute control in the patient with acute renal failure. In hemodiafiltration modalities such as CVVHD, dialysate solution bathes the hemofilter membranes, yielding both diffusive and convective solute removal. Although this renal replacement modality provides the most solute removal of any of the continuous therapies, it does so at the expense of requiring more complex machinery and increased training for intensive care unit personnel. Clinician expertise and availability of resources are probably the most important determinants in choosing one of the continuous therapies for a patient with acute renal failure.[76]

The dialyzer or hemofilter used in these renal replacement therapies may affect the outcome of patients with acute renal failure. As blood comes into contact with the materials used in some of these membranes, many biochemical changes occur, including complement activation, cytokine generation, and clotting cascade activation.[78] Membranes that activate these systems are considered to be "bioincompatible" because it is postulated that these effects may be responsible for the slow recovery of renal function in acute renal failure. New synthetic, "biocompatible" membranes have been developed that do not activate these systems as much. Use of these biocompatible membranes for hemodialysis may confer an improved recovery of renal function and mortality rate in patients with acute renal failure compared to bioincompatible dialysis membranes.[16]

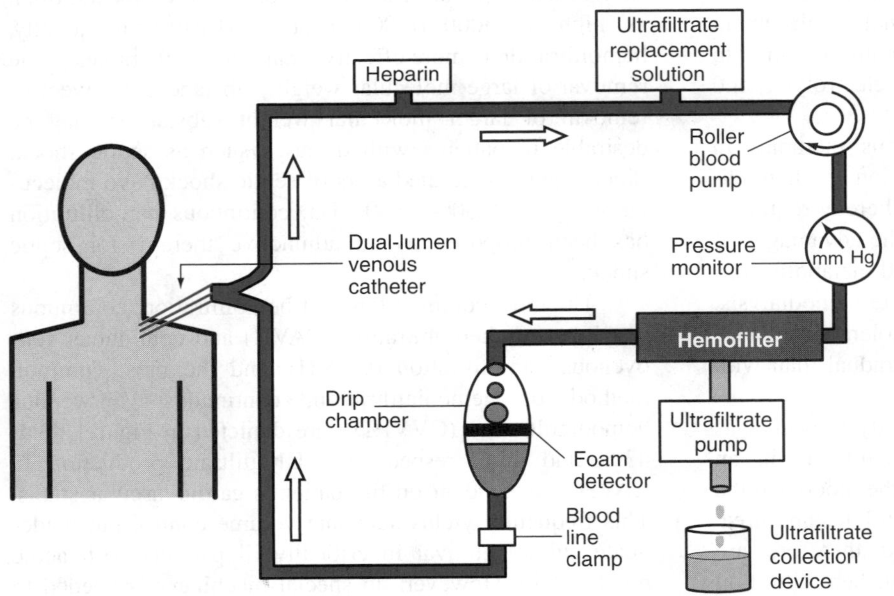

Figure 43.5. Schematic of continuous venovenous hemofiltration (CVVH). Blood is pulled into the extracorporeal circuit from a dual-lumen central venous catheter by a roller blood pump. The blood pump is responsible for the hydrostatic force that forms the ultrafiltrate. Blood is anticoagulated prior to the hemofilter to prevent clotting of the hemofilter. Ultrafiltrate is formed at a constant rate because it is regulated by an ultrafiltrate pump. A drip chamber and bubble-foam detector are safety features that prevent accidental air embolization. Blood returns to the patient via the other port of the venous catheter. This is the basic system used by the authors at the Indiana University Medical Center for critically ill patients with acute renal failure.[77]

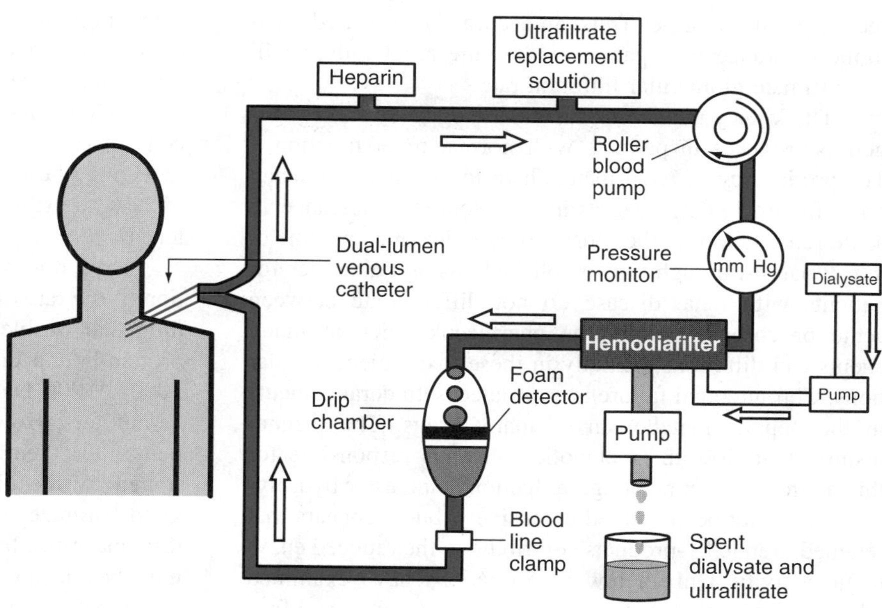

Figure 43.6. Schematic of continuous venovenous hemodiafiltration (CVVHD). CVVHD (occasionally called SCUF-D for slow continuous ultrafiltration and dialysis) incorporates a dialytic component to the extracorporeal CVVH circuit. The hemofiltration part of the circuit provides convective solute removal as it does in CVVH, usually at a rate of 500 mL/h. A premixed dialysate solution, usually a lactate-based peritoneal dialysate, is infused on the dialysate side of the hemodiafilter, at a rate of ~1,000 mL/h. The addition of dialysate to the system increases the small molecule clearance. CVVHD provides the highest amount of solute removal of all of the continuous therapies, but it does so at the cost of having the most complicated system for health care workers to operate and the highest daily cost.

CLINICAL CONSIDERATIONS IN ACUTE RENAL FAILURE

PHARMACOKINETIC ALTERATIONS IN ACUTE RENAL FAILURE

Distribution

Drug therapy in patients with acute renal failure may be complicated by pharmacokinetic changes that are specific to acute renal failure. Critically ill patients with acute renal failure frequently have substantial fluid overload, which may increase a drug's volume of distribution. Another important determinant of distribution volume is the reduction in protein binding that can occur in acute or chronic renal failure with highly albumin-bound acidic drugs like phenytoin. This alteration in protein binding is described in more depth in Chapter 50 on drug dosing of patients with renal disease.

Clearance

Assessing drug clearance in the patient with acute renal failure can be problematic. Total drug clearance is a function of residual renal clearance, nonrenal clearance, and the clearance of the renal replacement therapy used to treat the acute renal failure. Each of these factors can be difficult to quantitate, yet all are essential when designing pharmacotherapeutic regimens. Most patients with acute renal failure are not anuric and therefore may have some renal drug clearance. Estimation of glomerular filtration rate in the patient with acute renal failure is difficult because this patient population is usually not in a "steady-state" situation. Most clinically utilized methods (Cockcroft–Gault, Jelliffe, etc.) of estimating the glomerular filtration rate and creatinine clearance from serum creatinine determinations assume the patient has stable renal function. Acute renal failure violates this assumption. Laboratory values like serum creatinine concentration continually rise as creatinine is produced but is no longer eliminated by the kidneys. Furthermore, creatinine production in critically ill patients may no longer be constant because of the concomitant disease states in the patient with acute renal failure.[79] Creatinine clearance can be estimated in nonsteady-state patients with acute renal failure using equations specially designed for nonsteady-state conditions[80,81] (see Table 39.5). The predictive performance of these nonsteady-state equations is adequate for the clinical setting.[82]

The most accurate method to predict glomerular filtration rate from creatinine clearance is to actually measure the amount of creatinine that appears in a timed urine collection, although this technique can overestimate glomerular filtration rate if precise measurements of urine volume are not made. Urine collection over 24 hours in the intensive care unit can be cumbersome, but shortened collection periods can lead to increased error in glomerular filtration rate estimation.[79] Incomplete urine collection will result in a spuriously low creatinine clearance, while a falsely elevated creatinine clearance will be calculated if the bladder is not emptied prior to collection. Although creatinine secretion accounts for a small amount (<10%) of creatinine elimination at high glomerular filtration rates, at low glomerular filtration rates, creatinine secretion can contribute substantially (>50%) to the amount of creatinine recovered in the urine. Thus, an accurately measured creatinine clearance in a patient with acute renal failure will overestimate glomerular filtration rate.

The kidney metabolizes many endogenous and exogenous substances in patients with normal renal function.[83] The proficiency of renal metabolism in patients with acute renal failure has not been studied. Nonrenal clearance in acute renal failure is the most difficult clearance parameter to estimate. Although most published dosing guidelines for patients with renal disease do not differentiate between acute or chronic failure, the pharmacokinetics of many agents can differ substantially in these two patient populations. Chronic renal failure is associated with derangements in the hepatic metabolism of many drugs. The mechanism(s) that slow the metabolic pathways responsible for this nonrenal clearance (e.g., reduction[84] and ester hydrolysis[85]) have not been studied extensively, but it appears that retained uremic by-products contribute to the reduced enzymatic activity. Only a few investigations have examined whether nonrenal clearance in patients with acute renal failure approximates normal values or values reported in patients with chronic renal failure. The nonrenal clearance of vancomycin and imipenem in adults with acute renal failure lies somewhere between the normal (40 and 130 mL/min, respectively) and chronic renal failure values (6 and 50 mL/min).[86,87] In theory, this may occur because uremic by-products may not have had time to accumulate and affect hepatic function. Indirect evidence from vancomycin indicates that in early acute renal failure, the nonrenal clearance is preserved but declines for 1 to 2 weeks until the nonrenal clearance approaches the values observed in patients with chronic renal failure.[86] Further studies are needed to confirm these findings and evaluate whether this pattern of change is evident with other medications. If nonrenal clearance of antibiotics in early acute renal failure is greater than anticipated, the resultant serum concentrations would be lower. This could contribute to the fact that the primary cause of death in acute renal failure is usually infection. Clearly, frequent therapeutic drug monitoring is needed in these patients to assess whether nonrenal clearance changes with time. Because most of the published dosing guidelines in renal failure were generated from patients with chronic renal failure, future dosing guidelines for drugs with significant nonrenal clearance may need to differentiate between acute or chronic renal failure.

DRUG CLEARANCE BY THE RENAL REPLACEMENT THERAPY

The final source of drug clearance in the patient with acute renal failure is from renal replacement therapy. Drug clearance will differ substantially in the diffusion-based therapies (conventional hemodialysis) compared to the convective therapies (hemofiltration). Useful dosing recommendations for replacement of drug loss by diffusion and convection have been published; however, newer renal replacement therapies (e.g., continuous hemodiafiltration, high-flux hemodialysis, etc.) combine both diffusive and convective drug loss, complicating the dosing in patients receiving these therapies.[88] A more complete discussion of how to estimate clearance by dialysis appears in Chapter 50.

Drug removal by continuous hemofiltration is a function of the rate of ultrafiltrate production and the amount of drug that is able to cross the hemofilter membrane. Non-protein-bound drugs with molecular weights of less than 5000–10,000 Da usually can be removed by conventional hemofilters. However, only unbound drugs can cross the hemofilter; therefore, the unbound fraction of the drug multiplied by the ultrafiltrate production rate will provide a good estimate of the hemofiltration clearance rate. Once drug clearance by the hemofiltration system is calculated, it must be added to the patient's nonrenal clearance and residual renal clearance before a dosing regimen can be designed. Several excellent reviews delineate drug dosing recommendations for continuous hemofiltration[89] and other continuous renal replacement therapies.[90] However, none of these recommendations accounts for the preservation of nonrenal clearance that could occur in acute renal failure. Frequent therapeutic drug monitoring in patients with acute renal failure receiving continuous therapies is essential. A "steady-state" condition rarely occurs in these patients because their renal function may improve or worsen, their nonrenal drug clearance rates may change, and their renal replacement therapies may be modified as their clinical situation changes.

NUTRITIONAL CONSIDERATIONS IN ACUTE RENAL FAILURE

Patients with acute renal failure have special nutritional needs compared to patients with chronic renal failure. Profound catabolism is a hallmark of acute renal failure, with protein catabolic rates of 150–200 g/d.[91] Higher protein catabolic rates in patients with acute renal failure are associated with skeletal muscle wasting, amino acid oxidation, and impairment of immunologic and wound healing functions. Surprisingly, the protein catabolism is not linked with an overall increase in energy expenditure unless sepsis is also present.[92] The elevated protein catabolic rate frequently generates higher nitrogenous waste product concentrations than many renal replacement therapies can remove, thus worsening azotemic control. Higher protein administration rates can improve the net nitrogen balance but at the risk of further increasing azotemia.[93] Historically, protein administration recommendations in acute renal failure were based on patients receiving older, less efficient forms of renal replacement.

Consequently, low protein administration rates were suggested in an effort to reduce the degree of azotemia. Similarly, energy administration often was constrained by fluid restrictions imposed to reduce the need for frequent dialysis. The newer, more efficient renal replacement therapies such as CVVH and CVVHD remove more fluid and nitrogenous wastes, allowing the administration of protein and energy limited only by the patient's ability to utilize these nutrients.

The renal replacement therapy itself thus can influence the nutritional regimen of a patient with acute renal failure. As previously stated, more efficient continuous renal replacement therapies such as CVVH or CVVHD remove the constraints on fluid and nitrogen administration that were imposed by older, less efficient therapies. However, renal replacement therapies remove more than simply fluids, drugs, and nitrogenous wastes. Water soluble vitamins are also cleared efficiently and must be replaced in patients receiving renal replacement therapies. Nutritional considerations in patients with multisystem organ failure are discussed in Chapter 136.

EVALUATION OF THERAPEUTIC OUTCOMES

Much of the treatment of acute renal failure is a "wait and see" proposition. Clinicians can maximize the chances of the kidney to recover function by instituting supportive measures and trying some therapeutic measures, but every patient's course is different. Renal function may recover quickly, within a few months, or never. Close monitoring of the patient's status during the recovery period is essential.

Data derived from the physical exam can be very helpful in evaluating these patients. Gross measurements of daily weight and fluid intake versus fluid output will help discern the day-to-day recovery of the patient. These measurements are especially important in patients receiving continuous hemofiltration and hemodiafiltration because the ultrafiltrate replacement solution volumes are partially dependent on them. Urine output may be the best single test to assess recovery from acute renal failure. Fluid status should be assessed by checking lung sounds and looking for edema. Critically ill patients with acute renal failure frequently receive continuous hemodynamic monitoring via a Swan–Ganz catheter. These values can be helpful in assessing fluid status. Azotemic control can be assessed in the physical exam by looking for signs of uremia. The sound of a friction rub on chest exam can be a sign of a pericardial effusion due to uremia. Rales can be indicative of pulmonary edema secondary to fluid overload.

Laboratory values should be monitored closely, especially in the patient with changing renal function. Urine collection and measurement of urinary creatinine may be beneficial to assess changes in renal function. Urinalysis also can help discern the cause of acute renal failure, so attention should be given to the presence of urinary sediment, specific gravity, and sodium concentration in order to decide on a therapy to treat the cause of the acute renal failure. Blood urea nitrogen and creatinine measurements are useful but one must remember that creatinine clearance calculations may be unreliable in a nonsteady-state patient with changing serum creatinine values. Furthermore, any renal replacement therapy will reduce these values, so reliance on these indices alone to assess renal function can be misleading. Therapeutic drug monitoring should be performed frequently, not only because these patients are not at steady state, but also because of the paucity of data regarding drug disposition in acute renal failure. Serum electrolytes should be monitored daily with particular attention given to potassium, phosphorus, and calcium in early acute renal failure. Arterial blood gas determinations can help determine the respiratory status of a critically ill patient with acute renal failure and whether the kidney is able to compensate for any acid–base disturbances.

REFERENCES

1. Rose BD. Acute renal failure–prerenal disease versus acute tubular necrosis, in Rose BD (ed): Pathophysiology of Renal Disease, 2nd ed. New York, McGraw-Hill, 1987, pp 63–117.
2. Kjellstrand CM, Solez K. Treatment of acute renal failure, in Schrier RW, Gottschalk CW (eds): Diseases of the Kidney, 5th ed. Boston, Little, Brown and Company, 1992, pp 1371–1404.
3. Kaufman J, Dhakal M, Patel B, Hamburger R. Community acquired renal failure. Am J Kidney Dis 1991;17:191–198.
4. Jochimsen F, Schäfer JH, Maurer A, Distler A. Impairment of renal function in medical intensive care: Predictability of acute renal failure. Crit Care Med 1990;18:480–485.
5. Hou SH, Bushinsky DA, Wish JB, et al. Hospital-acquired renal insufficiency: A prospective study. Am J Med 1983;74:243–248.
6. Lohr JW, McFarlane MJ, Grantham JJ. A clinical index to predict survival in acute renal failure patients requiring dialysis. Am J Kidney Dis 1988;11:254–259.
7. Corwin HL, Bonventre JV. Factors influencing survival in acute renal failure. Semin Dial 1989;4:220–225.
8. Liano F, Garcia-Martin F, Gallego A, et al. Easy and early prognosis in acute tubular necrosis: A forward analysis of 228 cases. Nephron 1989;51:307–313.
9. Smithies MN, Cameron JS. Can we predict outcome in acute renal failure? Nephron 1989;51:297–300.
10. Liano F, Gallego A, Pascual J, et al. Prognosis of acute tubular necrosis: An extended prospectively contrasted study. Nephron 1993;63:21–31.
11. McMurray DS, Luft FC, Maxwell DR, et al. Prevailing patterns and predictor variables in patients with acute tubular necrosis. Arch Intern Med 1978;138:950–955.

12. Turney JH, Marshall DH, Brownjohn AM, et al. The evolution of acute renal failure: 1956–1988. Q J Med 1990;74:83–104.
13. Barton IK, Hilton PJ, Taub NA, et al. Acute renal failure treated by haemofiltration: Factors affecting outcome. Q J Med 1993;86:81–90.
14. Macias W, Alaka K, Clark W, et al. Nutritional status may predict outcome for critically ill patients undergoing continuous hemofiltration [abstract]. J Am Soc Nephrol 1994;5:497.
15. Kierdorf H. Continuous versus intermittent treatment: Clinical results in acute renal failure. Contrib Nephrol 1991;93:1–12.
16. Hakim R, Wingard RL, Parker RA. Effect of the dialysis membrane in the treatment of patients with acute renal failure. N Engl J Med 1994;331:1338–1342.
17. Moore K, Wendon J, Frazer M, et al. Plasma endothelin immunoreactivity in liver disease and the hepatorenal syndrome. N Engl J Med 1992;327:1774–1778.
18. Parmley WW. Pathophysiology and current therapy of congestive heart failure. J Am Coll Cardiol 1989;13:771–785.
19. Dunnick NR, Sfakianakis GN. Screening for renovascular hypertension. Radiol Clin N Am 1991;29:497–510.
20. Brezis M, Rosen S, Silva P, Epstein FH. Selective vulnerability of the medullary thick ascending limb to anoxia in the isolated perfused rat kidney. J Clin Invest 1984;73:182–190.
21. Finkelstein A, Holz R. Aqueous pores created in thin lipid membranes by the polyene antibiotics nystatin and amphotericin B, in Eisenman G (ed): Membranes: Lipid Bilayers and Antibiotics, Vol. 2. New York, Marcel Dekker, 1973, pp 377–408.
22. Kaufman J, Dhakal M, Patel B, Hamburger R. Community-acquired acute renal failure. Am J Kidney Dis 1991;17:191–198.
23. Rahman SN, Conger JD. Glomerular and tubular factors in urine flow rates of acute renal failure. Am J Kidney Dis 1994;23:788–793.
24. Agmon Y, Brezis M. Acute renal failure: A multifactorial syndrome, in Bourke E, Mallik NP, Pollak VE (eds): Moving Points in Nephrology, Contributions in Nephrology, Vol. 102. Basel, Karger, 1993, pp 23–36.
25. Paller MS. Pathophysiology of acute renal failure, in Greenberg A (ed): Primer on Kidney Diseases, 1st ed. San Diego, Academic Press, 1994, pp 126–133.
26. Corwin HL, Teplick RS, Schreiber MJ, et al. Prediction of outcome in acute renal failure. Am J Nephrol 1987;7:8–12.
27. Conger JD. Does hemodialysis delay recovery from acute renal failure? Semin Dial 1990;3:146–148.
28. Novis BK, Roizen MF, Aronson S, Thisted RA. Association of preoperative risk factors with postoperative acute renal failure. Anesth Analg 1994;78:143–149.
29. Conlon PJ, Schwab SJ. Time to abandon nonionic contrast? J Am Soc Nephrol 1994;5:123–124.
30. Steinberg EP, Moore RD, Powe N, et al. Safety and cost effectiveness of high-osmolality compared to low-osmolality contrast material in patients undergoing cardiac angiography. N Engl J Med 1992;326:425–430.
31. Farmer JC. Rhabdomyolysis, in Civetta JM, Taylor RW, Kirby RR (eds): Critical Care. Philadelphia, JB Lippincott, 1988, pp 1569–1573.
32. Heidemann HT, Gerkens JF, Spickard WA, et al. Amphotericin B nephrotoxicity in humans decreased by salt repletion. Am J Med 1983;75:476–481.
33. Gubern JM, Sancho JJ, Simo J, Sitges-Serra A. A randomized trial on the effect of mannitol on postoperative renal function in patients with obstructive jaundice. Surgery 1988;103:39–44.
34. Weinstein JM, Heyman S, Brezis M. Potential deleterious effect of furosemide in radiocontrast nephropathy. Nephron 1992;62:413–415.
35. Solomon R, Werner C, Mann D, et al. Effects of saline, mannitol, and furosemide on acute decreases in renal function induced by radiocontrast agents. N Engl J Med 1994;331:1416–1420.
36. Fisher MA, Talbot GH, Maislin G, et al. Risk factors for amphotericin B-associated nephrotoxicity. Am J Med 1989;87:547–552.
37. Ellison DH. The physiologic basis of diuretic synergism: Its role in treating diuretic resistance. Ann Intern Med 1991;114:886–894.
38. Vasko MR, Brown-Cartwright DB, Knochel JP, et al. Furosemide absorption altered in decompensated congestive heart failure. Ann Intern Med 1985;102:314–318.
39. Krasna MJ, Scott GE, Scholz PM, et al. Postoperative enhancement of urinary output in patients with acute renal failure using continuous furosemide therapy. Chest 1986;89:294–295.
40. Wollam G, Tarazi RC, Bravo EL, Dustan HP. Diuretic potency of combined hydrochlorothiazide and furosemide therapy in patients with azotemia. Am J Med 1982;72:929–938.
41. Weisberg LS, Kurnik PB, Kurnik BRC. Dopamine and renal blood flow in radiocontrast-induced nephropathy in humans. Renal Failure 1993;15:61–68.
42. Epstein M. Calcium antagonists and the kidney: Future therapeutic perspectives. Am J Kidney Dis 1993;21(suppl):16–25.
43. Schrier RW. Role of calcium channel blockers in protection against experimental injury. Am J Med 1991;90(suppl 5A):21S–26S.
44. Fischereder M, Trick W, Nath KA. Therapeutic strategies in the prevention of acute renal failure. Semin Nephrol 1994;14:41–52.
45. Neumayer HH, Junge W, Kufner A, Wenning A. Prevention of radiocontrast–media-induced nephrotoxicity by the calcium channel blocker nitrendipine: A prospective randomized clinical trial. Nephrol Dial Transplant 1989;4:1030–1036.
46. Russo D, Testa A, Della Volpe L, Sansone G. Randomized prospective study on renal effects of two different contrast media in humans: Protective role of calcium channel blocker. Nephron 1990;55:254–257.
47. Neumayer HH, Kunzendorf U. Renal protection with the calcium antagonists. J Cardio Pharm 1991;18:S11–S18.
48. Duggan KA, Macdonald GJ, Charlesworth JA, Pussell BA. Verapamil prevents post-traumatic oliguric renal failure. Clin Nephrol 1985;24:289–291.
49. Grino JM. BN 52021: A platelet activating factor antagonist for preventing post-transplant renal failure. Ann Intern Med 1994;121:345–347.

50. Levinsky NG, Bernard DB. Mannitol and loop diuretics in acute renal failure, in Brenner BM, Lazarus JM (eds): Acute Renal Failure, 2nd ed. New York, Churchill-Livingstone, 1988, pp 841–856.
51. Brater DC. Clinical pharmacology of loop diuretics. Drugs 1991;41(suppl 3):14–22.
52. Risler T, Krämer B, Müller GA. The efficacy of diuretics in acute or chronic failure. Drugs 1991;41(suppl 3):69–79.
53. Martin SJ, Danziger LH. Continuous infusion of loop diuretics in the critically ill: A review of the literature. Crit Care Med 1994;22:1323–1329.
54. Duke GJ, Briedis JH, Weaver RA. Renal support in critically ill patients: Low-dose dopamine or low-dose dobutamine? Crit Care Med 1994;22:1919–1925.
55. Vendegna TR, Anderson RJ. Are dopamine and/or dopamine renoprotective in intensive care unit patients? Crit Care Med 1994;22:1893–1894.
56. Lumlertgul D, Hutdagoon P, Sirivanichai C, et al. Beneficial effect of intrarenal verapamil in human acute renal failure. Renal Failure 1989–1990;11:201–208.
57. Lumlertgul D, Wongmekiat O, Sirivanichai C, et al. Intrarenal infusion of gallopamil in acute renal failure. Drugs 1991;42(suppl 1):44–50.
58. Kanfer A, Dussaule JC, Czekalski S, et al. Physiological significance of increased endogenous atrial natriuretic factor in human acute renal failure. Clin Nephrol 1989;32:51–56.
59. Rahman SN, Kim GE, Mathew AS, et al. Effects of atrial natriuretic peptide in clinical acute renal failure. Kidney Int 1994;45:1731–1738.
60. Lake EW, Humes HD. Acute renal failure: Directed therapy to enhance renal tubular regeneration. Semin Nephrol 1994;14:83–97.
61. Lillemoe KD, Romolo JL, Hamilton SR, et al. Intestinal necrosis due to sodium polystyrene (Kayexelate) in sorbitol enemas: Clinical and experimental support for the hypothesis. Surgery 1987;101:266–272.
62. Wootton FT, Rhodes DF, Lee WM, Fitts CT. Colonic necrosis with Kayexelate-sorbitol enemas after renal transplantation. Ann Intern Med 1989;111:947–949.
63. Montoliu J, Lens XM, Revert L. Potassium-lowering effect of albuterol for hyperkalemia in renal failure. Arch Intern Med 1987;147:713–717.
64. Allon M, Dunlay R, Copkney C. Nebulized albuterol for acute hyperkalemia in patients on hemodialysis. Ann Intern Med 1989;110:426–429.
65. McClure RJ, Prasad VK, Brocklebank JT. Treatment of hyperkalemia using intravenous and nebulised salbutamol. Arch Dis Child 1994;70:126–128.
66. Lens XM, Montoliu J, Cases A, et al. Treatment of hyperkalaemia in renal failure: Salbutamol v. insulin. Nephrol Dial Transplant 1989;4:228–232.
67. Woodrow G, Turney JH. Cause of death in acute renal failure. Nephrol Dial Transplant 1992;7:230–234.
68. Fischer RP, Stremble JF. Stress ulcers in post-traumatic renal insufficiency in patients from Vietnam. Surg Gynecol Obstet 1972;134:790–794.
69. Priebe HJ, Skillman JJ, Bushnell LS, et al. Antacid versus cimetidine in preventing acute gastrointestinal bleeding. N Engl J Med 1980;302:426–430.
70. Ben-Menachem T, Fogel R, Patel RV, et al. Prophylaxis for stress-related gastric hemorrhage in the medical intensive care unit. Ann Intern Med 1994;121:568–575.
71. Dolson GM. Electrolyte abnormalities before and after the onset of acute renal failure. Miner Electrolyte Metab 1991;17:133–140.
72. Clark WR, Mueller BA, Alaka KJ, Macias WL. A comparison of metabolic control by continuous and intermittent therapies in acute renal failure. J Am Soc Nephrol 1994;4:1413–1420.
73. Clark W, Kraus M, Alaka K, et al. Prediction of therapy requirements in CVVH [abstract]. Am J Kidney Dis 1993;22:A2.
74. Manji N, Shikora S, McMahon M, et al. Peritoneal dialysis for acute renal failure: Overfeeding resulting from dextrose absorbed during dialysis. Crit Care Med 1990;18:29–31.
75. Grootendorst AF. The potential role of hemofiltration in the treatment of patients with septic shock and multiple organ dysfunction syndrome. Adv Renal Replacement Ther 1994;1:176–184.
76. Paganini EP. General application of continuous therapeutic techniques, in Henrich WL (ed): Principles and Practice of Dialysis, 1st ed. Baltimore, Williams & Wilkins, 1994, pp 98–110.
77. Macias WL, Mueller BA, Scarim SK, et al. Continuous venovenous hemofiltration: An alternative to continuous arteriovenous hemofiltration and hemodiafiltration in acute renal failure. Am J Kidney Dis 1991;18:451–458.
78. Schulman G, Hakim R. Hemodialysis membrane biocompatibility in acute renal failure. Adv Renal Replacement Ther 1994;1:75–82.
79. Robert S, Zarowitz BJ. Is there a reliable index of glomerular filtration rate in critically ill patients? Drug Intell Clin Pharm 1991;25:169–178.
80. Jelliffe RW, Jelliffe SM. A computer program for estimation of creatinine clearance from unstable serum creatinine levels, age, sex, and weight. Math Biosci 1972;14:17–24.
81. Chiou WL, Hsu FH. A new simple and rapid method to monitor the renal function based on pharmacokinetic consideration of endogenous creatinine. Res Commun Chem Pathol Pharmacol 1975;10:315–330.
82. Chow MSS, Schweizer R. Estimation of renal creatinine clearance in patients with unstable serum creatinine concentrations: Comparison of multiple methods. Drug Intell Clin Pharm 1985;19:385–390.
83. Gibson TP. Renal disease and drug metabolism: An overview. Am J Kidney Dis1986;8:7–17.
84. Reidenberg MM. The biotransformation of drugs in renal failure. Am J Med 1977;62:482–485.
85. Reidenberg MM, James M, Dring LG. The rate of procaine hydrolysis in serum of normal subjects and diseased patients. Clin Pharmacol Ther 1972;13:279–284.
86. Macias WL, Mueller BA, Scarim SK. Vancomycin pharmacokinetics in acute renal failure: Preservation of nonrenal clearance. Clin Pharmacol Ther 1991;50:688–694.
87. Mueller BA, Scarim SK, Macias WL. Comparison of imipenem pharmacokinetics in patients with acute or chronic renal failure treated with continuous hemofiltration. Am J Kidney Dis 1993;21:172–179.

88. Matzke GR. Pharmacotherapeutic consequences of recent advances in hemodialysis therapy. Ann Pharmacother 1994;28:512–514.
89. Bressolle F, Kinowski JM, de la Coussaye JE, et al. Clinical pharmacokinetics during continuous hemofiltration. Clin Pharmacokinet 1994;26:457–471.
90. Reetze-Bonorden P, Böhler J, Keller E. Drug dosage in patients during continuous renal replacement therapy. Clin Pharmacokinet 1993;24:362–379.
91. Feinstein EI, Blumenkrantz MJ, Healy M, et al. Clinical and metabolic responses to parenteral nutrition in acute renal failure. Medicine 1981;60:124–137.
92. Schneeweiss B, Graninger W, Stockenhuber F, et al. Energy metabolism in acute and chronic renal failure. Am J Clin Nutr 1990;52:596–601.
93. Murphy MH, Alaka KJ, Miller ME, Macias WL. Assessment of urea appearance rates and net nitrogen deficits in patients with acute renal failure receiving continuous venovenous hemofiltration. J Ren Nutr 1993;3:67–74.

Chapter 44

Chronic Renal Failure and End-Stage Renal Disease

Wendy L. St. Peter, PharmD, BCPS, Scott W. Mihalovic, PharmD, BCPS, Marigel Vargas-Ruiz, RPh, MS, and Lawrence J. Lambrecht, PharmD, BCPS

Normal human kidneys contain approximately 2 million functionally integrated glomerulotubular units called nephrons. Under normal conditions these nephrons work in a highly organized fashion to filter, reabsorb, and excrete various solutes and fluid. In addition, the kidney plays an important role in the metabolism of various peptide hormones and in the production of renin, ammonia, erythropoietin, and 1,25-dihydroxyvitamin D_3.

Renal disease is characterized by disturbances in many of these normal functions. Evidence suggests that even as renal disease develops and adaptations take place, functioning (remnant) nephrons continue to function in a highly organized fashion. Although total kidney glomerular filtration rate (GFR) falls, the GFR of remnant nephrons rises. This adaptation blunts the drop in whole kidney GFR that would occur in the absence of compensatory changes. Unfortunately, this adaptive hyperfiltration process ultimately results in glomerular hypertension, which plays a significant role in glomerular injury. Indeed, in most instances, when serum creatinine rises above 3 mg/dL or creatinine clearance (Cr Cl) falls to approximately 25 mL/min, the injury process will progress to end-stage renal failure regardless of the initial etiology of kidney disease.[1]

Solute balance is maintained in chronic renal failure by increases in the fractional excretion of solutes such as sodium, potassium, creatinine, blood urea nitrogen (BUN), and phosphorus by remnant nephrons, although the adaptive mechanisms differ in each case. The urinary excretion of any substance is dependent on the amount of solute filtered at the glomerulus plus the net contribution of tubular secretion and tubular reabsorption (Fig. 44.1).

There are several ways in which remnant nephrons can adapt to maintain solute balance. Plasma concentrations of solutes that undergo minimal tubular secretion or reabsorption, such as creatinine and BUN, rise predictably as renal function declines. This results in an increase in the filtered load presented to each tubule, which allows remnant nephrons to increase excretion proportionally. Serum creatinine rises in proportion to the decline in GFR and can be used clinically to estimate renal function (see Chapter 42). Renal tubular reabsorption is the predominant mechanism of regulation of excretion for sodium and phosphorus; therefore, in chronic renal failure, tubular reabsorption of these solutes decreases in order to prevent or minimize the increase in plasma concentrations. Potassium balance, normally maintained by distal tubular potassium secretion, is maintained via further increases in tubular secretion. Thus the plasma concentrations of some solutes rise while the plasma concentrations of others remain relatively constant until residual renal function is quite low. These adaptations, which appear to be solute specific, are discussed in detail later in this chapter.

There may be "trade-offs" to many of these adaptations that actually contribute to the uremic state and its complications.[2] An understanding of these renal adaptations is crucial to an understanding of the conservative management of chronic renal failure since many therapeutic interventions follow logically from the disordered physiology.

Definitions

For practical purposes the clinical course of progressive renal disease is best divided into four stages. The accompanying signs and symptoms and laboratory parameters of each stage is described in Fig. 44.2.

Decreased Renal Reserve (Cr Cl: 60–90 mL/min)

The glomerular filtration rate, as measured by the Cr Cl, may decrease by as much as 50% before the plasma concentrations of creatinine or urea nitrogen rise above the normal range. Adaptive increases in solute excretion in remaining nephrons compensate for the decline in functioning kidney mass.

$$\text{Excretion} = \text{filtered load} + \text{tubular secretion} - \text{tubular reabsorption}$$

$$\text{Filtered load} = \text{glomerular filtration rate} \times \text{plasma concentration}$$

$$\text{Fraction excretion} = \frac{\text{amount excreted}}{\text{filtered load}}$$

Figure 44.1 Determinants of renal excretion.

Renal Insufficiency (Cr Cl: 30–60 mL/min)

A thorough evaluation to determine the etiology of the renal impairment is especially critical at this point since the underlying disease process may reverse or stabilize with appropriate treatment.

Chronic Renal Failure (Cr Cl: 15–30 mL/min)

In general, patients with this degree of renal dysfunction will progress to end-stage renal disease albeit at individual rates of decline. Nephrologists often use a plot of 1/Scr versus time to evaluate disease progression in individual patients. Unfortunately, the relationship between GFR and 1/Scr is not constant over time; changes in tubular secretion, extrarenal elimination, and rate of generation of creatinine in patients with renal failure can alter the 1/Scr slope without a change in GFR. Therefore, misinterpretation of the rate of decline in renal function can occur if this is the only method used to estimate renal function[3] (see Chapter 42).

Uremia (Cr Cl: <15 mL/min)

Uremia is a clinical syndrome that develops insidiously as renal function declines. It begins with nonspecific symptoms, which become progressively worse as the creatinine clearance drops below 10 mL/min. It is at this stage (preferably before the full syndrome develops) that dialysis is indicated to remove the by-products of protein metabolism, such as urea, thought to be largely responsible for this symptom complex. The patient requiring chronic dialysis or renal transplantation for relief of uremic symptoms is said to have *end-stage renal disease* (ESRD).

Prevalence, Incidence, and Etiology of End-Stage Renal Disease

Many diseases of the kidney, either idiopathic or secondary to systemic illness, can ultimately result in ESRD. More than 242,000 Americans were treated for ESRD in 1992.[4] Black individuals have approximately a fourfold greater incidence of renal failure (per 1 million population) than white individuals. The average life expectancy of a 20- and 60-year-old ESRD patient in the United States is only 12 and 4 years, respectively, compared to 50–60 and 16–23 years, respectively, for an adult without renal disease.[4]

Overall, the increase in incidence of patients starting ESRD therapy has increased 8.8% annually with the largest increase in the 65- to 74-year-old population[4] (Fig. 44.3).

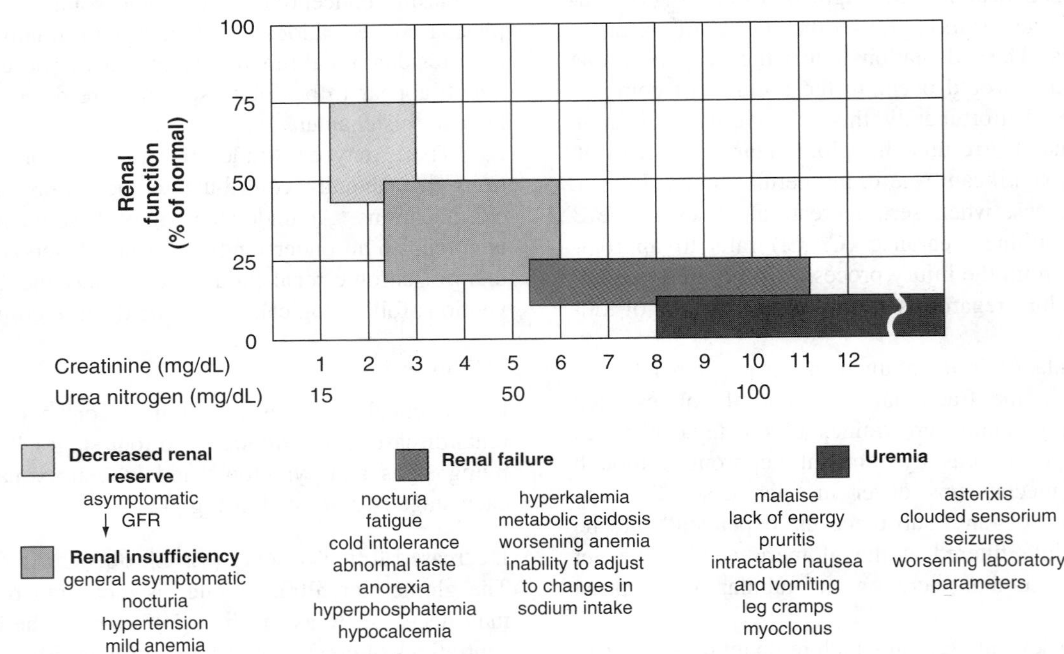

Figure 44.2. Staging of chronic renal disease. *(Adapted from Knochel JP. The pathophysiology of uremia. Hospital Pract 1981;16(11):67, with permission. Illustration by Albert Miller.)*

The largest increase in treated ESRD incidence by race has been in Native Americans and Asian/Pacific Islanders. The incidence rates for the five major causes of ESRD are shown in Fig. 44.4. Diabetes is the most common cause of renal failure in the United States. Sixty-four percent of Native Americans and 36% of Caucasians with ESRD developed the disease as a direct result of diabetes mellitus.[4] In 1992, the annual cost to treat an individual with ESRD on dialytic therapy was approximately $47,000, with 82% of the cost borne by the federal government. This translated into total expenditures of more than 9.5 billion dollars in 1992 for the U.S. ESRD program.[4]

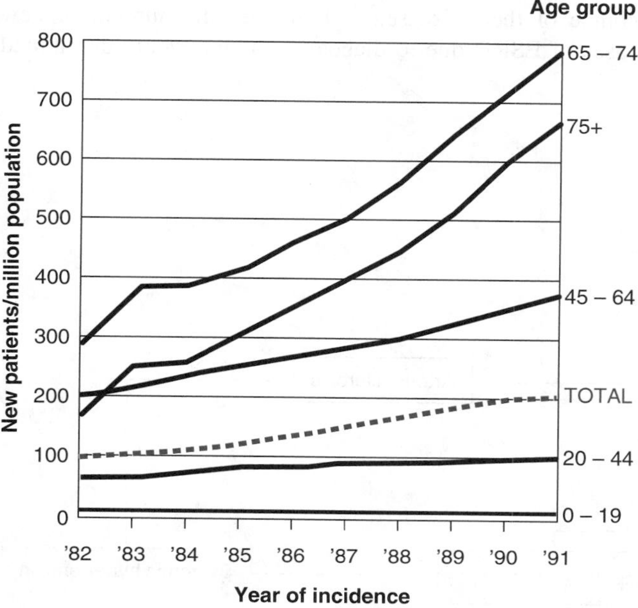

Figure 44.3. Incidence rates of treated ESRD per million population, by age group, 1982–1991. Rates are unadjusted. Rates do not include patients from Puerto Rico or U.S. territories. Medicare patients only. *(From U.S. Renal Data System, USRDS 1995 Annual Data Report, National Institutes of Health, National Institute of Diabetes and Digestive and Kidney Diseases, Bethesda, MD April 1995.)*

PROGRESSIVE NATURE OF RENAL DISEASE

PATHOPHYSIOLOGY

The exact mechanisms involved in the pathogenesis of progressive renal failure have not been completely identified, but most individuals with creatinine clearance of 25 mL/min or less progress to ESRD regardless of the underlying etiology.[1] Based on experimental animal models, hemodynamic changes at the glomerulus have been shown to exert a major influence on and/or regulate the rate of progression of renal disease.[5] Increased glomerular capillary plasma flow and glomerular capillary hydraulic pressure lead to glomerular hyperfiltration. Glomerular hyperfiltration and hypertension lead to progressive glomerular sclerosis and development of overt proteinuria.[5] In addition, glomerular capillary hypertension plays a key role in declining function of remaining intact nephrons. In experimental renal disease, pharmacologic or dietary interventions that decrease glomerular capillary pressure limit the rate and extent of overt proteinuria and glomerulosclerosis.[1] The presence of systemic hypertension is not required for the development of glomerular hyperfiltration and hypertension but, when present, may

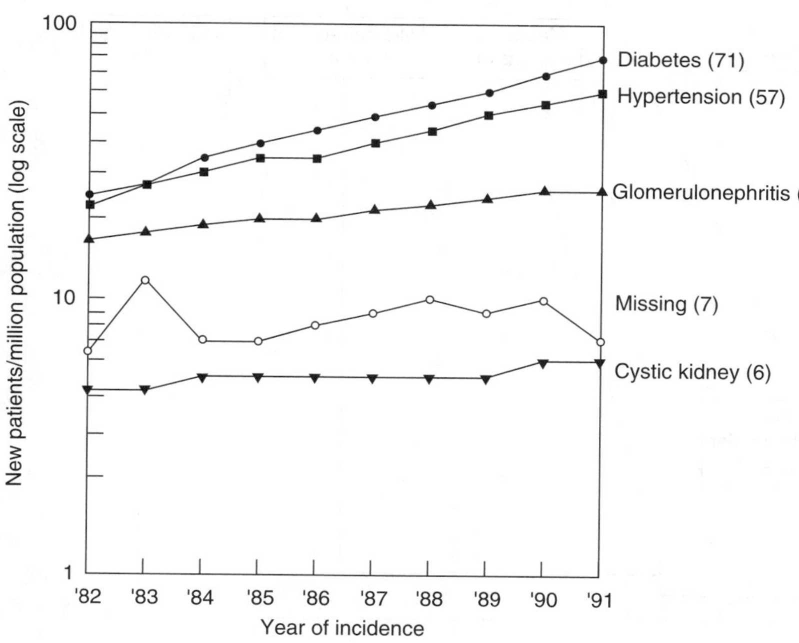

Figure 44.4 Incidence rates of treated ESRD per million population, by selected primary disease groups, 1982–1991. Rates are unadjusted. Semi-log scale used to show smaller rates. Rates do not include patients from Puerto Rico or U.S. territories. Medicare patients only. *(From U.S. Renal Data System, USRDS 1995 Annual Data Report, National Institutes of Health, National Institute of Diabetes and Digestive and Kidney Diseases, Bethesda, MD April 1995.)*

amplify the pathologic effects of these intrarenal changes.[6] Other risk factors considered important in the pathogenesis of progressive renal failure are summarized in Fig. 44.5. A reduction of filtration area secondary to glomerular cell injury can lead to hemodynamic changes that increase glomerular capillary pressure, flow, and volume, which causes functional and structural changes to the glomerulus. These pathologic processes lead to glomerulosclerosis, causing an elevation of systemic blood pressure, which may elicit further renal structure damage and consequent worsening of blood pressure control.[6–8]

In the United States, diabetes and hypertension are the most common causes of ESRD (Fig. 44.4). Approximately 30–40% of insulin-dependent diabetes mellitus (IDDM) patients and 5–10% of noninsulin-dependent diabetes mellitus (NIDDM) develop diabetic nephropathy during the course of their disease.[9–11] However, the number of new cases of ESRD due to diabetes is about evenly distributed

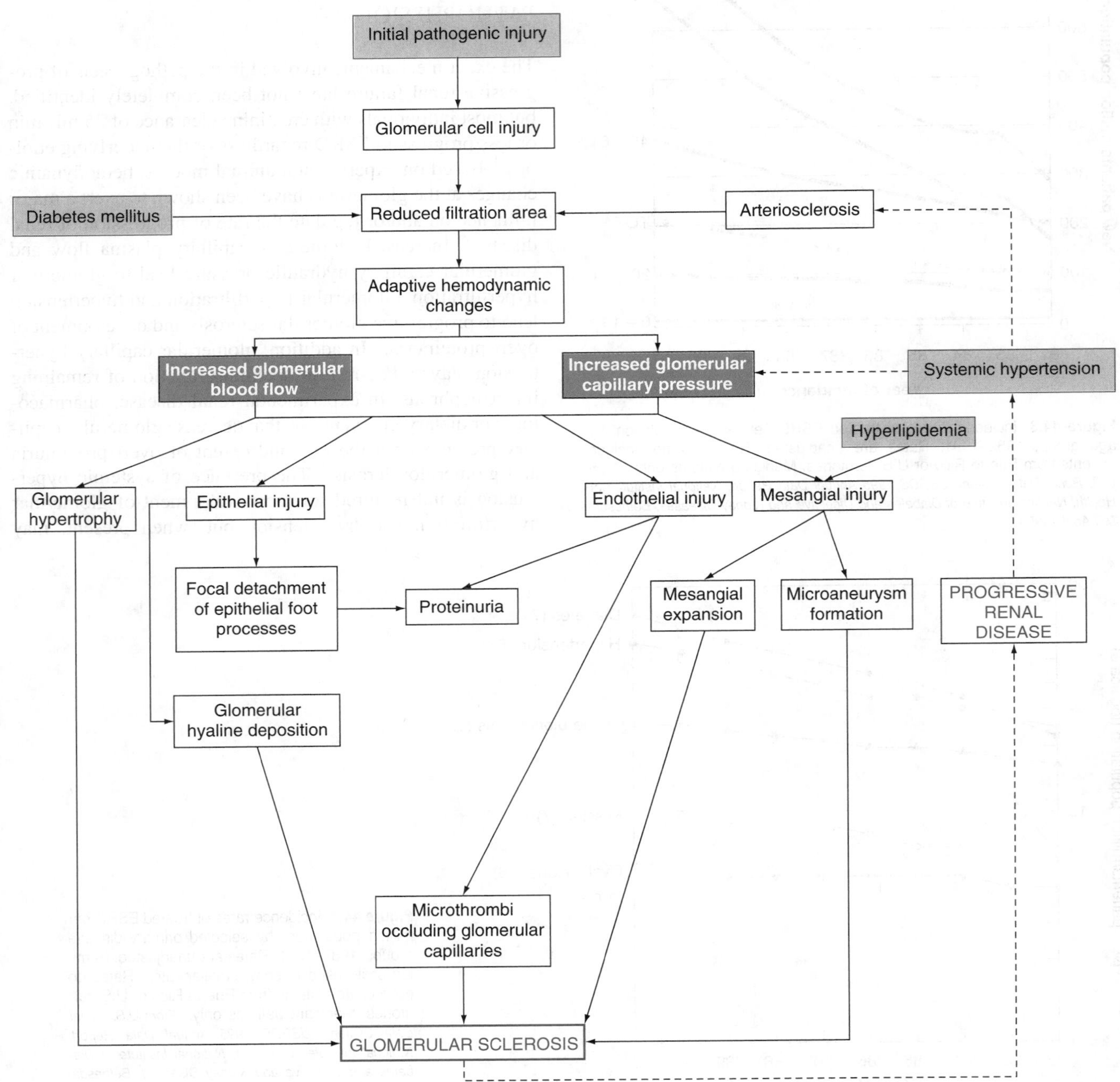

Figure 44.5. Proposed mechanisms of progressive glomerular sclerosis in chronic renal failure.

between IDDM and NIDDM patients probably due to the high prevalence of NIDDM patients. Diabetic nephropathy is characterized by persistent albuminuria (>300 mg/24 h), an increase in blood pressure, and decline in GFR, causing progression of renal disease to ESRD.[9] Diabetic nephropathy is clinically diagnosed if persistent proteinuria, defined as a total protein excretion exceeding 0.5 g/24 h (equivalent to a urinary albumin excretion rate [UAE] of 300 mg/24 h), is present in two out of three consecutive urine samples. If the UAE ranges between 30–300 mg/24 h, the patient is classified as having persistent microalbuminuria.[10] Clinical studies in diabetic patients have demonstrated that persistent microalbuminuria is highly predictive of progression of renal disease and is one of the best available early predictors of diabetic nephropathy.[10]

Approximately 25–28% of ESRD patients develop ESRD secondary to hypertension.[4] ESRD secondary to essential hypertension has continued to increase despite decreases in cardiovascular and stroke mortality.[12] The exact mechanisms involved in the development of ESRD among hypertensive individuals remains controversial. However, some of the major mechanisms include ischemia in the renal tubule, causing reduction of renal mass and increased glomerular capillary pressure.[1,13] Microalbuminuria occurs in approximately 30% of hypertensive patients, which significantly increases overall mortality rate.[14] The increased UAE in hypertension may be induced by renal hemodynamic changes, glomerular filter permeability changes, and glomerular structural changes due to nephrosclerosis (Fig. 44.5).

Hyperlipidemia is a major risk factor associated with progression of renal disease[15] (Fig. 44.5). Experimental studies in rats have demonstrated accelerated glomerulosclerosis when dietary cholesterol supplementation is given in the presence of various renal diseases, whereas pharmacologic therapy or low-fat diets have been shown to limit the progression of renal disease.[1] Lipid metabolism abnormalities alone in patients with normal renal function have not been shown to promote glomerular injury.[16] In IDDM and NIDDM patients with chronic renal insufficiency, low-density–lipoprotein (LDL cholesterol) concentrations appear to be predictive of the rate of decline of glomerular function.[17]

CLINICAL CONSEQUENCES

The incidence and prevalence of ESRD continue to rise.[4] The availability of chronic dialysis and renal transplantation is limited and expensive for ESRD patients. In addition, these treatments are associated with early morbidity and mortality and less than optimal quality of life.[18] Recent clinical trials have focused on the use of pharmacologic and nonpharmacologic treatment interventions during the early stages of renal disease when some reversibility or delay of ESRD may be possible. Treatment and prevention programs focusing on major risk factors, such as diabetes and hypertension, that promote progression of renal disease will hopefully reduce the incidence and prevalence of ESRD.

THERAPEUTIC MANAGEMENT

Diabetics

Screening Microalbuminuria

Early hyperfiltration is followed by persistent microalbuminuria.[19] Diabetic patients (IDDM) with elevated UAE are at high risk to develop overt nephropathy within 10–14 years.[10] Therefore, the early detection of microalbuminuria in the diabetic patient facilitates therapeutic intervention that can slow the progression of renal disease and other vascular complications.[20] Accurate assays that can detect UAE between 30–300 mg/24 h have been developed.[9] Routine dipstick urinalysis does not measure UAE less than 150 mg/d and should not be used to screen for microalbuminuria. Another acceptable alternative method is measurement of the albumin-to-creatinine ratio in the first morning urine sample. A urinary albumin-to-creatinine ratio greater than or equal to 30 mg/g and less than 300 mg/g can identify patients at high risk to develop diabetic nephropathy.[21] All diabetic patients older than 12 years of age should have their urine checked annually for microalbuminuria.[21]

Intensive Blood Glucose Control

Intensive blood glucose control in IDDM patients has been reported to reduce the frequency, decrease the severity, and delay the development or progression of diabetic complications including nephropathy in several randomized clinical trials.[22] Although most of these studies included small numbers of subjects (less than 100), and short duration of follow-up (less than 5 years), a meta-analysis of 16 clinical trials demonstrated a statistically significant effect of long-term intensive insulin therapy on reducing the risk of nephropathy progression.[22]

The Diabetes Control and Complications Trial (DCCT) was a multicenter (1441 patients), randomized study designed with sufficient statistical power to compare intensive versus standard diabetes therapy with regard to effects on the development and progression of diabetic nephropathy, retinopathy, and neuropathy.[23,24] Intensive therapy either by the administration of insulin three or more times daily by injection or by external pump reduced the incidence of microalbuminuria and albuminuria when compared to conventional therapy in both a primary prevention (n = 726) and a secondary prevention (n = 715) group.[24] Unfortunately, long-term rigid glycemic control with insulin was associated with a higher incidence of hypoglycemic reactions.[24] However, decreased diabetic complications in the intensive therapy group outweighed the increased risk of hypoglycemia.[25] A longer follow-up period is needed to evaluate the degree by which intensive glucose control will prevent or delay the development of diabetic nephropathy.[25]

Antihypertensive Agents

The prevalence of hypertension is high in diabetic nephropathy. Elevated blood pressure is observed more often in IDDM patients with persistent microalbuminuria when compared to normoalbuminuric IDDM patients. Blood pressure continues to rise at the onset of diabetic nephropathy and with the progression of renal failure (Fig. 44.5).

Many studies have demonstrated that adequate blood pressure control can reduce the rate of decline in GFR and albuminuria in hypertensive patients with either IDDM or NIDDM.[1] A long-term study in IDDM patients with microalbuminuria demonstrated that blood pressure control with β-blocker and diuretic therapy decreased UAE.[26] Animal models of diabetic nephropathy have demonstrated that decreasing glomerular capillary pressure and volume preserve renal function.[27] Angiotensin-converting enzyme inhibitors (ACEI) reduce both of these parameters.[28] In contrast, calcium channel blockers mainly dilate the afferent arteriole with no change or increase in glomerular capillary pressure. Nevertheless, calcium channel blockers decrease glomerular injury without changing renal hemodynamics.[28] The postulated mechanisms for this decrease in renal injury include suppression of glomerular hypertrophy, inhibition of platelet aggregation, and decreased salt accumulation.[28] Combination therapy with ACEI and calcium channel blockers resulted in a larger reduction of albuminuria than with either agent given alone in one small human study.[29]

A recent metaregression analysis of 100 controlled and uncontrolled clinical studies assessed the relative effect of different antihypertensive agents on proteinuria and renal function in IDDM and NIDDM patients.[30] None of the antihypertensive agents or classes analyzed had a greater effect on blood pressure reduction than any other agent or class. However, only ACEI decreased proteinuria and preserved GFR independently of blood pressure changes.

Given the preliminary evidence for the potential benefit of ACEI in diabetic nephropathy, a multicenter controlled clinical trial was designed to determine if long-term administration of captopril in IDDM patients with nephropathy ($n = 409$) would reduce the progression of renal failure independent of its blood pressure lowering effect.[31,32] The outcomes measured included the time elapsed to double the patient's baseline serum creatinine and the time to reach ESRD or death. Patients with the highest baseline serum creatinine had a greater risk reduction for doubling serum creatinine or for reaching ESRD than subjects with lower baseline values. However, a longer follow-up study may demonstrate similar benefits for patients with lower serum creatinine. Captopril also delayed the progression of renal disease independent of blood pressure control.

A long-term (5-year) double-blind trial of enalapril 10 mg/d or placebo in normotensive NIDDM patients with microalbuminuria resulted in stabilization of plasma creatinine concentrations and decreased albuminuria in the enalapril group as compared to the placebo group. Unfortunately, blood pressure was not as well controlled in the placebo group and the investigators monitored renal function using 1/Scr, which is a relatively crude way to measure GFR. Therefore, firm conclusions on the efficacy of enalapril above that of blood pressure control alone in NIDDM patients cannot be reached.[33]

Antilipidemic Agents

In animal models, use of lipid-lowering agents decreases the extent of glomerular injury when both underlying renal disease and hyperlipidemia are present.[15,17] Therefore, the correction of lipid abnormalities in patients with renal damage may be important in retarding the progression of renal disease (see section on Hyperlipidemia).

Nondiabetics

Renal disease secondary to causes other than diabetes (nondiabetic nephropathy) includes glomerular and tubulointerstitial disease, nephrosclerosis, and polycystic kidney disease. These etiologies are frequently grouped in large clinical trials due to the lower number of subjects with each disease. It is likely that each of these disease states progresses to ESRD and responds to therapeutic interventions differently. Therefore, it is difficult to extrapolate data from each trial to define a single optimal treatment pathway for patients with nondiabetic nephropathy.

Nutritional Management

The effect of dietary protein on the progression of chronic renal disease has been reported in animal and human studies.[34–37] A meta-analysis of six randomized clinical trials concluded that patients with mild to severe renal disease who followed a low-protein diet could delay the onset of ESRD.[38] Deficiencies of these clinical trials included inappropriate randomization procedures, methods of assessing renal function, lack of control groups, and poor documentation of patient's compliance to dietary regimens. One of the complications of decreasing protein intake is malnutrition. Some of these clinical trials failed to document if adequate nutrition and quality of life were maintained in these patients on low-protein diets.

The Modification of Diet in Renal Disease (MDRD) multicenter study was a well-designed trial. It evaluated the influence of dietary restriction of protein and phosphorus on the progression of renal function in nondiabetic patients.[39–42] Results from a pilot study revealed a high correlation between decreased renal function and increased mean blood pressure. Consequently, the full-scale study added blood pressure control as a second independent intervention.

The full-scale MDRD study (n = 840 patients) divided the subjects into moderate (n = 585) and severe (n = 255) renal dysfunction classifications based on GFR. Subjects in the moderate renal function group (GFR = 25–55 mL/min/1.73 m^2) were randomized into one of four groups: usual or a low-protein diet (1.3 versus 0.58 g/kg/d) with a usual or low mean arterial pressure (MAP) goal (107 versus 92 mm Hg). Subjects with severe renal dysfunction (GFR = 13–24 mL/min/1.73 m^2) were randomized to one of four groups: a low- or very low-protein diet (0.28 g/kg/d) with a usual or low MAP goal as previously described. Patients with moderate renal dysfunction who were in the low-protein diet or low blood pressure groups had a more rapid decline in renal function during the first 4 months of treatment than the baseline period. However, from 4 months to 3 years, the mean rate of decline was reduced in the patients receiving the low-protein diet albeit not significantly from the baseline period. In patients with severe renal dysfunction, a very low-protein diet did not significantly slow the progression of renal disease when compared to the low-protein diet group. In conclusion, no significant benefit of protein restriction was demonstrated in this study at the end of the follow-up period in either renal disease group when all the patients with different renal disease etiologies were considered together.

Antihypertensive Agents

Based on the results of multiple controlled and uncontrolled studies in diabetic patients, ACEI decrease proteinuria and preserve glomerular function.[30] The question of whether pharmacologic treatment of hypertension in nondiabetic patients delays the progression of renal disease has been addressed in various epidemiologic and clinical studies.[43] Thirty-five short-term (<12 months) and 17 long-term (>12 months) clinical trials evaluated the effect of ACEI inhibitors on renal hemodynamics in nondiabetic patients.[43] Renal function remained stable during the short-term ACEI therapy in the majority of studies. Results from two small long-term studies (follow-up to 2 years) demonstrated reduction in the rate of progression of renal disease with ACEI therapy. Therefore, it is not clear whether observed short-term hemodynamic effects will persist during long-term therapy. Large controlled randomized prospective studies are needed to determine what degree of blood pressure control is most effective in delaying renal disease and which hypertensive agents or combination of agents provides the greatest advantage. All hypertensive agents do not preserve renal function to the same degree despite equal blood pressure control. The effects of antihypertensive agents on renal hemodynamics are summarized in Table 44.1.[44,45] Regardless of the treat-

TABLE 44.1. EFFECTS OF ANTIHYPERTENSIVE AGENTS ON RENAL BLOOD FLOW (RBF) AND GLOMERULAR FILTRATION RATE (GRF)

Antihypertensive Agent	Mechanism of Action	Effects on Renal Hemodynamics
Diuretics	Sodium and volume depletion	⇓ in GFR and RBF
	⇑ vasodilatory prostaglandin levels [intravenous (IV) loop diuretics]	⇑ in RBF
	Renal vasoconstriction (IV thiazide)	⇓ in GFR and RBF
β-Adrenergic blockers	⇓ cardiac output	⇓ in GFR and RBF
	⇑ renal vascular resistance (nonselective agents)	⇓ in GFR and RBF
	⇓ renal vascular resistance (β_1-selective agents)	No change in GFR and RBF ⇓ or no change microalbuminuria
Centrally acting antiadrenergic drugs	⇓ renal vascular resistance (α-methyldopa)	No change in GFR and RBF
	⇓ renal perfusion pressure (clonidine, α_2-adrenergic agonist)	GFR and RBF are preserved
Peripherally acting antiadrenergic drugs	Direct vasodilation (postsynaptic α_1-adrenoreceptor blocking agents)	No adverse effect on GFR and RBF
Direct vasodilator agents	⇓ renal vascular resistance (hydralazine, minoxidil)	⇑ in RBF and no effect on GFR
Direct vasodilator agents	Arterial vasodilation plus dilatation of venous capacitance vessels (nitroprusside) (diazoxide-less venous dilatation)	⇓ in GFR and RBF (acute effect)
ACEI	Dilation of the efferent arteriole	⇑ in RBF and GFR (only in patients with hypertension, renal insufficiency, and ⇑ renin states)
	Dilatation of the efferent arteriole plus inhibition of angiotensin II concentration	⇓ glomerular capillary pressure
Calcium channel blockers	⇓ renal vascular resistance by vasodilation of afferent arterioles (hypertensive patients)	⇑ in RBF ⇑/no change on GFR
	⇓ renal vasoconstriction (isolated perfused kidney)	⇑ in RBF and GFR

ment regimen, hypertension should be controlled in the presence of underlying renal disease (see section on Hypertension). If proteinuria is present, the use of ACEI and calcium channel blockers may be superior to conventional treatment in decreasing proteinuria and glomerular hypertension.

EVALUATION OF THERAPEUTIC OUTCOMES

Diabetics

Based on the available clinical and experimental data, pharmacologic intervention can attenuate hemodynamic adaptations associated with progression of renal disease in diabetic patients. Overall recommendations for the prevention of progression of renal disease in this population are summarized in Fig. 44.6.[46] All patients with IDDM for more than 5–10 years, and/or a family history of renal disease or hypertension should be screened every year for microalbuminuria (annual UAE or urinary albumin-to-creatinine ratio). Blood glucose should be maintained within or close to normal range either by frequent insulin injections or use of an insulin pump while minimizing the risk of hypoglycemia with frequent blood glucose monitoring. If there are no contraindications, ACEI therapy should be initiated in normotensive or hypertensive IDDM patients with persistent microalbuminuria or overt albuminuria (>300 mg/d).[21] ACEI should be titrated every 1 to 3 months to achieve a maximal effect on UAE. Within 1 week of initiating or increasing a dose of an ACEI, serum

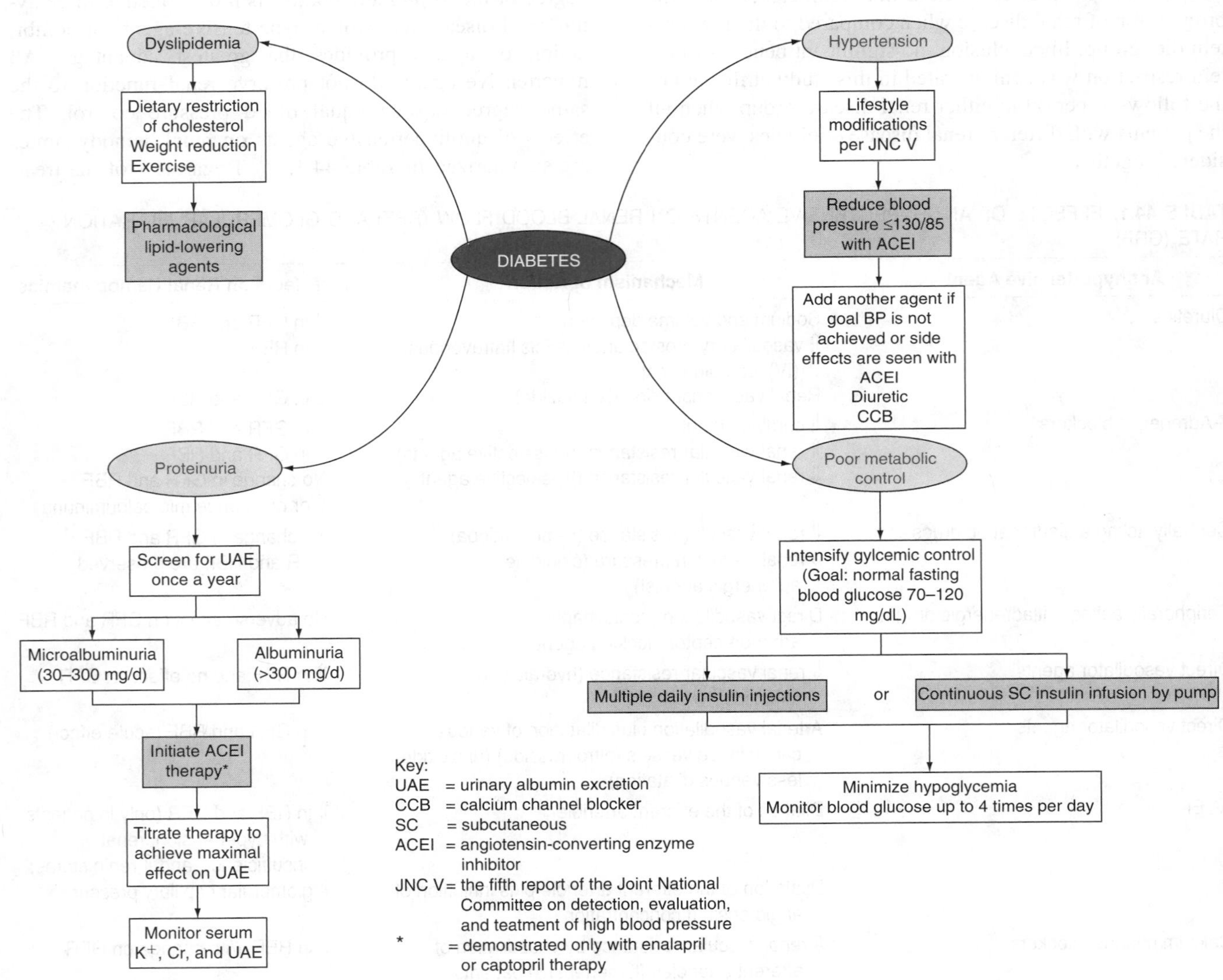

Figure 44.6. Therapeutic strategies to prevent progression of renal disease in diabetic individuals.

creatinine and potassium should be evaluated to detect abrupt reductions in GFR or development of hyperkalemia. Currently, data are limited on benefits of ACEI in slowing the rate of renal impairment in NIDDM patients who are normotensive and have microalbuminuria. However, until further data are available, ACEI may be considered in NIDDM patients with hypertension and/or in those who demonstrate persistent albuminuria (>300 mg/d).[46] Calcium channel blockers may be an effective alternative in hypertensive diabetic patients with advanced renal disease and/or proteinuria.

Experimental data indicate that hyperlipidemia may interact with concomitant risk factors such as hypertension, diabetes, and preexisting renal damage to accelerate progression of glomerular injury. The use of a low-fat diet and/or addition of antilipidemic agents to the therapeutic regimen may be beneficial in diabetic and nondiabetic patients with renal disease and lipid abnormalities (see section on Hyperlipidemia).

Nondiabetics

Therapeutic interventions for nondiabetic patients with renal insufficiency are summarized in Fig. 44.7. Nutritional management should be monitored frequently, regardless of the amount of protein intake prescribed, to avoid complications from malnutrition. Nutrition goals include maintenance of serum albumin >4 g/dL and transferrin >200 mg/dL. Based on the results of the MDRD study, a low-protein diet is of questionable benefit in patients with moderate renal function (GFR = 25–55 mL/min/1.73 m^2). Therefore, a standard protein diet (>0.8 g/kg/d) should be followed unless the patient develops rapid progression of renal failure and/or uremic symptoms. For patients with severe renal function (GFR = 13–24 mL/min/1.73 m^2), a low-protein diet of 0.6 g/kg/d may reduce the rate of decline in renal function, time to reach ESRD, and onset of uremic symptoms.[46]

Blood pressure control should target normotensive levels (130/80–85 mm Hg).[47] If proteinuria >1 g/d is present, providing there are no contraindications, blood pressure should be reduced further (125/75 mm Hg). But, if patient has proteinuria >3 g/d and chronic renal failure, ACEI and perhaps calcium channel blockers should be considered as first-line therapy.[46]

The Uremic State

PATHOPHYSIOLOGY

Despite multiple investigations, the exact toxin or toxins responsible for the manifestations of the uremic syndrome have not been determined. No single toxin is responsible for all of the abnormalities observed in patients with uremia, and the clinical picture likely results from an interplay of multiple factors.

Several mechanisms could contribute to the presence of uremic toxins as chronic renal failure progresses. Most likely, the uremic syndrome results from elevations in blood concentrations of various molecules. A number of organic compounds are known to accumulate in uremia (Table 44.2). Accumulation could result from several potential mechanisms including:

1. Decreased excretion; this would be most typical of the metabolic by-products of protein metabolism that accumulate as the whole kidney GFR decreases.
2. Increased secretion of biologically active substances such as parathyroid hormone and atrial natriuretic peptide, which are overproduced as part of the adaptation to the loss of renal mass.
3. Decreased clearance of endogenous substances normally metabolized by the kidney, including parathyroid hormone, gastrin, growth hormone, glucagon, somatostatin, prolactin, calcitonin, and insulin.

The ability of uremic toxins to produce clinical manifestations results in large part from their effects at the cellular level. The uremic syndrome is characterized by prominent alterations in transmembrane transport as well as cellular water and electrolyte content.[48] It seems most likely that the uremic syndrome is due to the retention of by-products of protein metabolism, because many manifestations of the uremic syndrome can be improved markedly with protein restriction. The role of other potential toxins has been much more difficult to determine.

CLINICAL PRESENTATION

Cardiovascular System

Sodium retention leads to volume expansion, which can result in volume overload and pulmonary edema. Hypertension induced by volume expansion and increased systemic vascular resistance increases myocardial work and results in left ventricular hypertrophy. In addition, hypertension represents a major risk factor for cardiovascular disease, and complications of atherosclerosis are common in these patients. Hyperlipidemia may enhance atherogenesis, while some uremic toxins decrease myocardial contractility. Uremic toxins can also induce uremic pericarditis, a potentially fatal complication of chronic renal failure. The high cardiac output state induced by anemia may be poorly tolerated in the face of underlying heart disease. Therapeutic measures for treating sodium and fluid retention along with hypertension are detailed later in this chapter.

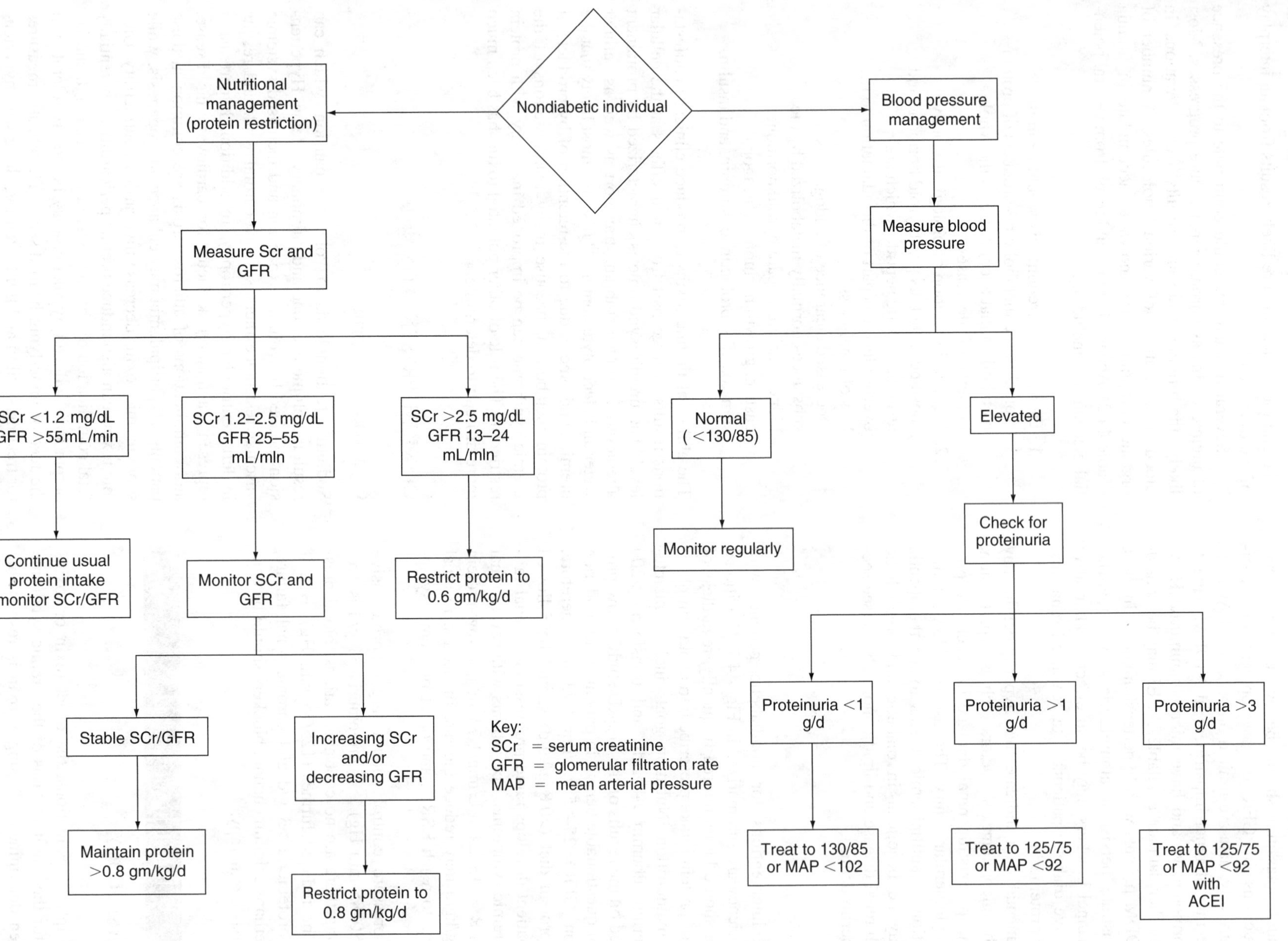

Figure 44.7. Therapeutic strategies to prevent progression of renal disease in nondiabetic individuals.

TABLE 44.2. POTENTIAL TOXINS IN UREMIA

2,3-Butylene	Indoles
Acetoin	Insulin
Aliphatic amines	Lipochromes
α_2-Glucoprotein	Lysozyme
Amino acids	Mannitol
Aromatic amines	Methylguanidine
Atrial natriuretic peptide	Middle molecules
β_1-Microglobulin	Myoinositol
β_2-Microglobulin	Natriuretic hormone
Calcitonin	Other guanidines
Creatinine	Oxalic acid
Cyanate	Parathyroid hormone
Cyclic AMP	Phenols
Gastric inhibitory peptide	Prolactin
Gastrin	Pyridine derivatives
Glucagon	Renin
Glucuronic acid	Retinol-binding protein
Growth hormone	Ribonuclease
Guanidinosuccinic acid	Urea
Human pancreatic polypeptide	Uric acid

Pulmonary System

The combination of volume overload and uremic toxin-induced increases in capillary permeability can result in noncardiogenic pulmonary edema.

Gastrointestinal System

Anorexia, hiccups, and a metallic taste in the mouth are common in chronic renal failure. In uremia, nausea, vomiting, diarrhea, or abdominal distention may occur. Gastric and colonic mucosal ulcerations and telangiectasias with resultant gastrointestinal (GI) bleeding are common.

Nervous System

Uremic toxins may increase neuromuscular irritability and result in leg cramps, restless leg syndrome, and reversal of the sleep–wake cycle. Uremic toxins can induce a peripheral neuropathy. The clinical manifestations of uremic encephalopathy include clouded sensorium, coma, seizures, myoclonic jerks, and asterixis. Dialysis dementia can result from aluminum intoxication in chronic dialysis patients.

Hematologic System

A normochromic, normocytic anemia secondary to decreased erythropoietin production and shortened erythrocyte survival is common. A prolongation in the bleeding time and a bleeding diathesis can result from platelet dysfunction. Gastrointestinal bleeding is common in ESRD, which contributes to anemia. In addition, vitamin and iron deficiency can lead to mixed anemia patterns in this population. The pathophysiology and treatment of anemia and uremic bleeding in patients with chronic renal failure is discussed later in the chapter.

Musculoskeletal System

Renal osteodystrophy (bone disease) is a common manifestation of chronic renal disease. Calcification of blood vessels or soft tissues may occur. These manifestations of renal disease are discussed in detail later.

Endocrine System

Various endocrine and metabolic abnormalities are common in ESRD.[49] The hypothalamus is "reset" as seen in other acute illnesses. Most patients are symptomatic as if hypothyroid (i.e., low energy, cold intolerance, constipation), but typically the levothyroxine (T_4) concentration is low, and the thyroid-stimulating hormone concentration is normal. Hypothermia is common; body temperatures are approximately 1°F lower as compared to individuals with normal renal function. Hyperglycemia secondary to peripheral resistance to insulin can occur. Diabetic patients with chronic renal failure often present with more frequent hypoglycemic episodes because the kidney is responsible, in large part, for the degradation of insulin. Insulin doses must be adjusted downward as renal failure progresses. Primary hypogonadism as well as hypothalamic abnormalities contribute to sexual dysfunction and sterility.

Dermatologic System

Dry, flaking skin and generalized pruritus (discussed later) are common manifestations of uremia.

Immune System

Infectious diseases are common and result in significant morbidity and mortality in patients with chronic renal failure/ESRD. Although multiple abnormalities in host defenses and an increased susceptibility to infection have been described, the causal link between these observations remains speculative.[50] Absolute lymphopenia and impaired cell-mediated immunity are common in uremic patients and may be due to the presence of uremic toxins or protein-calorie malnutrition. A variable mild defect in immunoglobulin production has been described. Macrophage-mediated F_c-receptor-dependent clearance is impaired and may contribute to the increased risk of infection observed in patients with ESRD.[51]

GENERAL THERAPEUTIC MANAGEMENT

The therapeutic management of the patient with chronic renal failure hinges on several important principles. First, those treatments known to slow the rate of progression of renal disease progression should be applied. Second, patients must receive dietary instruction to limit protein, potassium, and phosphorus intake and maintain adequate caloric intake (see Chapter 136). Phosphate-binding medications and/or calcium supplementation should be used to control serum phosphorus and calcium concentrations in order to suppress parathyroid hormone secretion and prevent renal bone disease. Therapy with alkalinizing agents should be administered to patients with systemic acidosis. Third, renal function must be monitored closely.

If a patient's renal function is deteriorating more rapidly than predicted, a vigorous search for reversible causes is warranted. Potential reasons for acceleration in the rate of decline of renal function in a patient with chronic renal failure include:

1. Volume depletion secondary to vomiting, diarrhea, or inappropriate salt restriction or diuretic therapy
2. Uncontrolled hypertension
3. Impaired renal perfusion secondary to hypotension, reduced cardiac output, or renovascular disease
4. Pyelonephritis
5. Urinary tract obstruction (i.e., prostatic hypertrophy, papillary necrosis, nephrolithiasis)
6. Drug-related effects

As renal function declines below 20 mL/min and treatable problems have been identified and addressed, the patient should be prepared for the eventuality of dialysis therapy. Hemodialysis and peritoneal dialysis options need to be discussed (see Chapter 46). In addition, if the patient is an appropriate candidate, they should be given information about renal transplantation (see Chapter 45).

Indications for the Initiation of Dialytic Therapy

In general, patients are managed conservatively until uremic symptoms become prominent (most commonly seen when creatinine clearance drops below 10 mL/min). Criteria for the initiation of dialysis in chronic renal failure patients are largely clinical and include:

1. Intractable nausea and vomiting
2. Uremic encephalopathy—confusion, asterixis, seizures
3. Myoclonus
4. Uremic pericarditis
5. Development of peripheral neuropathy
6. Development of pruritus
7. Prophylactically before major surgery

Once dialysis therapy is initiated, patients need further dietary instruction since dietary protein intake can be liberalized. Adequate caloric intake and dietary phosphate restriction remain important goals of dietary management. A no–added-salt diet and fluid restriction to approximately 1000 mL/d will minimize interdialysis weight gains and hyponatremia. Vitamin D therapy is commonly prescribed to prevent renal osteodystrophy along with epoetin and iron therapy for treatment of anemia. Aggressive antihypertensive therapy remains important since blood pressure elevation before each dialysis treatment is a strong predictor of future cardiovascular and cerebrovascular mortality.

Pathophysiology and Therapeutic Management of the ESRD Patient

SODIUM AND WATER HOMEOSTASIS

Pathophysiology

In normal subjects sodium balance is maintained with sodium intake of 120–150 mEq/d. The fractional excretion of sodium (FE_{Na}) is approximately 1%. Water balance is also maintained with a normal range of urinary osmolality of 50–1200 mOsm/L. In patients with chronic renal failure sodium balance is maintained but in a mildly volume expanded state. FE_{Na} increases to as high as 10–20%. The exact mechanism whereby FE_{Na} increases is unknown but may be the result of increased concentrations of atrial natriuretic peptide (ANP). The increased secretion of ANP is probably triggered by increased intravascular volume and atrial pressure.

Volume expansion results in hypertension. Increased levels of ANP may interfere with sodium and calcium transport in vascular smooth muscle resulting in increased resting muscle tone. The resultant increase in peripheral vascular resistance probably contributes to hypertension. Elevated levels of ANP may inhibit sodium and potassium ATPase-dependent pumps in many cells of the body, resulting in altered cellular electrolyte content and membrane potentials that may contribute to the uremic state.

Water balance is generally maintained but within a limited range. Since the fractional reabsorption of sodium is decreased secondary to ANP, free water generation by the kidney is impaired. An osmotic diuresis due to a large solute load per remnant nephron results in obligatory water losses. The ability to dilute or concentrate the urine is impaired and urine becomes isosthenuric (urinary osmolality fixed at that of plasma or approximately 300 mOsm/L).

Clinical Consequences

The ability of the kidney to adjust to abrupt changes in sodium intake is greatly diminished. Sodium restriction beyond a no–added-salt diet should not be recommended except in the face of hypertension or edema. Although it has been taught that patients with chronic renal failure are frequently "salt wasters" (i.e., develop volume depletion secondary to negative sodium balance when sodium intake is restricted), this is untrue in most cases. In fact, the kidney maintains the ability to lower urinary sodium content to essentially zero, but this can only be accomplished by very gradual sodium restriction over a prolonged time period.[52] Nocturia is present relatively early in the course of renal disease secondary to the defect in urinary concentrating ability.

Therapeutic Management

Under most circumstances, the inappropriate natriuresis and weight loss seen with sodium restriction in patients with chronic renal failure is a direct result of the sluggishness of the deadaptation process rather than "salt wasting." Hospitalized patients, therefore, should not routinely be sodium restricted since they have adapted to their outpatient intake. Negative sodium balance and its resultant volume contraction can result in decreased renal perfusion and subsequent further decline in GFR. Saline-containing intravenous solutions should be used cautiously in patients with chronic renal failure since the kidney's ability to excrete a salt load is impaired and such patients are prone to volume overload. Sodium retention and volume expansion contribute to hypertension in many patients with chronic renal failure and diuretic therapy may be necessary for control of edema or blood pressure.

Fluid restriction is generally not necessary provided sodium intake is controlled. An intact thirst mechanism maintains total body water and effective plasma osmolality near normal. Since urine volume is relatively fixed at approximately 2 L/d, fluid restriction below this amount should be avoided. Large amounts of free water administered orally or as intravenous fluid may induce hyponatremia and volume overload.

POTASSIUM HOMEOSTASIS

Pathophysiology

Potassium balance is maintained by renal and extrarenal mechanisms. The kidneys normally excrete 90–95% of a daily potassium dietary load, predominantly through distal tubular secretion. The fractional renal excretion of potassium (FE_K) is approximately 25%. Normally only 5–10% of ingested potassium is excreted through the gut. Potassium homeostasis is also maintained by shifting extracellular potassium to intracellular spaces, acutely, following ingestion of a potassium load.[53] In chronic renal failure, potassium balance is maintained by an increase in distal tubular potassium secretion in which aldosterone plays an important role. FE_K can increase to as high as 125%. The serum potassium concentration is usually maintained in the normal range until the patient reaches ESRD (GFR < 10 mL/min). A significant increase in potassium secretion by the colon contributes to the maintenance of external balance. Although aldosterone receptors are found in the colon, it is unclear whether they play a significant role in the upregulation of colonic potassium secretion in ESRD patients.[54]

Clinical Consequences

Although restriction of dietary intake is usually unnecessary, patients with chronic renal failure tolerate potassium loads poorly. Potassium-sparing diuretics are relatively contraindicated in chronic renal failure patients because of the high risk of hyperkalemia. Beta blockers, predominantly via β_2-antagonistic effects, interfere with the extrarenal translocation of potassium into cells and may result in a further impairment in potassium handling and life-threatening hyperkalemia. ACEI should be monitored closely in patients with chronic renal failure since they may provoke hyperkalemia by reducing aldosterone production.

Therapeutic Management

The management of hyperkalemia in ESRD can be divided into chronic (Fig. 44.8) and acute treatment.[53,54] The majority of patients can be chronically managed with dietary potassium restriction and alterations in dialysate potassium concentrations. Constipation in dialysis patients can interfere with colonic potassium excretion, therefore a good bowel regimen is important. Extrarenal handling of potassium is important in ESRD, therefore discontinuing ACEI and β blockers may be necessary in some. Pharmacologic treatment is rarely necessary during chronic management of hyperkalemia. Sodium polystyrene sulfonate, a potassium–sodium exchange resin, can be given between dialysis sessions to increase potassium excretion in the ileum and colon. Mineralocorticoids may enhance secretion of potassium into the gut by stimulating aldosterone receptors, although no clinical trials exist to support this. Finally, a short-term study showed that diltiazem lessened the rate of increase in plasma potassium between dialysis sessions.[55]

The definitive treatment of severe hyperkalemia in ESRD is hemodialysis. In reality there is often a delay between diagnosis of hyperkalemia and institution of dialysis, which necessitates the use of other temporizing measures such as intravenous calcium gluconate, insulin and glucose, nebulized albuterol, and sodium polystyrene sulfonate (see Chapter 43, Acute Renal Failure). Unfortunately, shifting potassium into the intracellular fluid compartment with insulin and glucose or with albuterol then makes dialysis removal of potassium more difficult. Multiple dialysis sessions may be necessary following potassium redistribution to the extracellular space. Lastly, sodium bicarbonate therapy is no longer advocated in the treatment

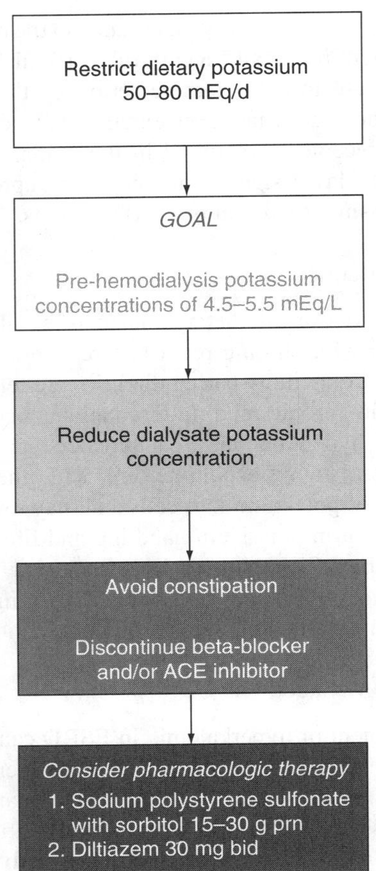

Figure 44.8. Chronic management of hyperkalemia in ESRD patients.

of ESRD hyperkalemia unless severe metabolic acidosis is also present because the potassium-lowering effect is not reliable.[53]

METABOLIC ACIDOSIS

Pathophysiology

A constant body fluid pH is maintained through the buffering of hydrogen ion by proteins, hemoglobin, phosphate, and especially bicarbonate. In normal renal function enough hydrogen ion is generated by the kidney to reclaim all filtered bicarbonate and secrete approximately 1 mEq/kg/d of hydrogen ions, which are generated from the metabolism of dietary proteins. Renal ammoniagenesis and phosphate excretion provide urinary buffer that facilitates acid excretion. In chronic renal failure all filtered bicarbonate is reclaimed, but the ability of the kidneys to synthesize ammonia is impaired.[56] This decrease in urinary buffer results in decreased net acid excretion and continuous positive hydrogen ion balance, thus metabolic acidosis develops. A clinically significant metabolic acidosis is uncommonly seen before the glomerular filtration rate drops below 20 mL/min. The plasma bicarbonate concentration tends to stabilize at 10 to 20 mEq/L.

Clinical Consequences

Metabolic acidosis, through unknown mechanisms, contributes to renal bone disease.[57] Dietary phosphate restriction or treatment with phosphate binders will decrease urinary phosphate excretion and can further impair renal hydrogen ion excretion. The presence of metabolic acidosis may contribute to hyperkalemia as well as fatigue and decreased exercise tolerance in patients with chronic renal failure. Finally, metabolic acidosis appears to stimulate protein catabolism, which can worsen uremia and contribute to a negative nitrogen balance.[58]

Therapeutic Management

The prevention and treatment of severe metabolic acidosis in patients with chronic renal failure (CRF) may be important for the prevention of the sequelae of the chronic acidotic state such as bone demineralization,[57] reduced cardiac contractility, increased ventricular irritability, potential for hyperkalemia, and growth retardation in children. Generally, treatment should be instituted when plasma bicarbonate has fallen below 20 mEq/L.

In patients with residual renal function, the use of alkalinizing salts such as sodium bicarbonate or citrate/citric acid preparations are useful to replenish depleted body bicarbonate stores. Citrate is metabolized in the liver to bicarbonate and citric acid is metabolized to CO_2 and water. Sodium bicarbonate tablets are manufactured in 325- and 650-mg strengths (a 650-mg tablet contains 7.7 mEq sodium and 7.7 mEq bicarbonate). Shohl's Solution® and Bicitra® contain sodium citrate and citric acid. Each milliliter contains 1 mEq sodium and the equivalent of 1 mEq bicarbonate. Polycitra®, which contains potassium citrate, should not be used in patients with severe CRF because hyperkalemia may result. Each milliliter of this product contains 1 mEq of sodium and potassium and 2 mEq of bicarbonate. Alkali therapy should be initiated at 0.5 mEq/kg/d in divided doses. Doses are subsequently titrated to produce plasma bicarbonate concentrations of 20 mEq/L or greater. Fluid balance should be monitored carefully because of the sodium content of these agents. Citrate-containing solutions should not be used in combination with aluminum-containing compounds because they can enhance aluminum absorption and increase the risk of aluminum intoxication. Excessive doses of alkalinizing agents may cause metabolic alkalosis as well as lethargy or cardiac depression secondary to a decrease in ionized serum calcium concentration. Gastrointestinal distress characterized by gastric distention and flatulence is relatively common with high doses of oral sodium bicarbonate. Patients with renal tubular acidosis (RTA) may require higher doses of these agents. Recommended initial doses of sodium bicarbonate for distal (type 1) and proximal (type 2) RTA of 0.5–2.0 mEq/kg/d and 4–10 mEq/kg/d, respectively, have been suggested.[59] Metabolic acidosis in patients undergoing hemodialysis can almost always be managed solely by dialysis. Measures used include dialysis against acetate (a bicarbonate precursor) or bicarbonate dialysate baths.[60]

RENAL OSTEODYSTROPHY AND SECONDARY HYPERPARATHYROIDISM

Metabolic bone disease is a major cause of morbidity and mortality in patients undergoing chronic dialysis treatment. Three types of bone lesions can be detected on bone biopsy in patients on dialysis.[61,62] When dialysis therapy was first available in the 1960s, a high-turnover bone disease called osteitis fibrosa cystica was detected. This bone lesion is characterized histologically by areas of peritrabecular fibrosis. Dynamic measurements show a high bone formation rate, which results from high circulating concentrations of parathyroid hormone (PTH). In that era, aluminum-containing phosphate binders were often initiated because the nephrology community was not aware that aluminum could be absorbed intestinally. In the 1970s a new bone lesion, osteomalacia, was observed. Osteomalacia is characterized by a high volume of osteoid tissue. After several years, aluminum toxicity was implicated as the main cause when histological stains revealed high levels of aluminum in patients with dialysis-associated osteomalacia. In the 1980s, a third abnormality, an aplastic lesion, was characterized. Histologically, this lesion shows low amounts of fibrosis or osteoid tissue. Characteristically, bone formation rates are low with this form of bone disease. Initially, aplastic bone disease was also linked to aluminum toxicity as many patients exhibited high amounts of stainable aluminum in bone biopsies. Today, aluminum-containing phosphate binders are not routinely used. However, the incidence of this lesion has increased dramatically over the last 10 years, and may be seen in up to 50% of unselected dialysis patients.[62] Multiple factors including aluminum toxicity, peritoneal dialysis utilizing high concentrations of dialysate calcium along with high doses of calcium-containing phosphate binders, aggressive management with vitamin D therapy, diabetes, and advanced age may also increase one's risk of developing this type of bone disease.[61] Management of phosphorus and calcium balance and minimizing patient exposure to aluminum are important in preventing the development of secondary hyperparathyroidism and slowing or preventing the progression of renal osteodystrophy.

Pathophysiology

Calcium and phosphorus balance is mediated through a complex interplay of hormones and their effects on bone, GI tract, kidney, and parathyroid gland. Phosphate retention inhibits renal activation (C_1-α hydroxylation) of vitamin D, which in turn reduces gut absorption of calcium. Phosphorus retention directly decreases blood ionized (free) calcium through a physiochemical interaction. Low blood calcium concentrations provide a major stimulus for parathyroid hormone (PTH) secretion. PTH decreases proximal tubular phosphate reabsorption and restores phosphate balance until the GFR falls below 30 mL/min at which time blood phosphorus concentrations are often noted to rise.

As seen in Fig. 44.9, the parathyroid glands release PTH in a physiologic attempt to restore normal blood calcium and phosphorus concentrations. However, as functional renal mass declines, serum calcium balance can only be maintained at the expense of increased bone resorption. Decreased production of 1,25 dihydroxyvitamin D_3 (calcitriol) results in impaired intestinal absorption of calcium, provides a stimulus for PTH release, and may contribute to defective bone mineralization.

Secondary hyperparathyroidism, a common manifestation in ESRD, can result in osteitis fibrosa cystica if left untreated. Underlying mechanisms are complex and somewhat controversial, but include continued phosphorus retention and subsequent development of hypocalcemia (Fig. 44.9), which provides a stimulus for PTH secretion. Although not clearly established, high phosphorus concentrations may also directly increase secretion of PTH. Parathyroid hyperplasia (nodular or diffuse) is another characteristic feature of secondary hyperparathyroidism. Nodular tissue demonstrates more rapid growth potential and appears to have lower numbers of calcitriol receptors than diffusely hyperplastic tissue.[63] Nodular hyperplasia along with low concentrations of circulating calcitriol is thought to result in an increased set point (the concentration of calcium causing half-maximal inhibition of PTH secretion).[64,65] Unfortunately, hypercalcemia may develop in the pharmacologic attempt to achieve suppression of PTH release.

Clinical Consequences

Development of secondary hyperparathyroidism and subsequent high circulating concentrations of PTH promote progression of osteitis fibrosa cystica and may adversely affect lipid metabolism, myocardial and skeletal muscle, and neurologic function.[66] Common signs and symptoms of secondary hyperparathyroidism include fatigue and musculoskeletal and GI complaints. Uncontrolled hyperphosphatemia can also result in metastatic calcification of joints, vessels, and soft tissue when the calcium (mg/dL)–phosphorus (mg/dL) product exceeds 70.[67]

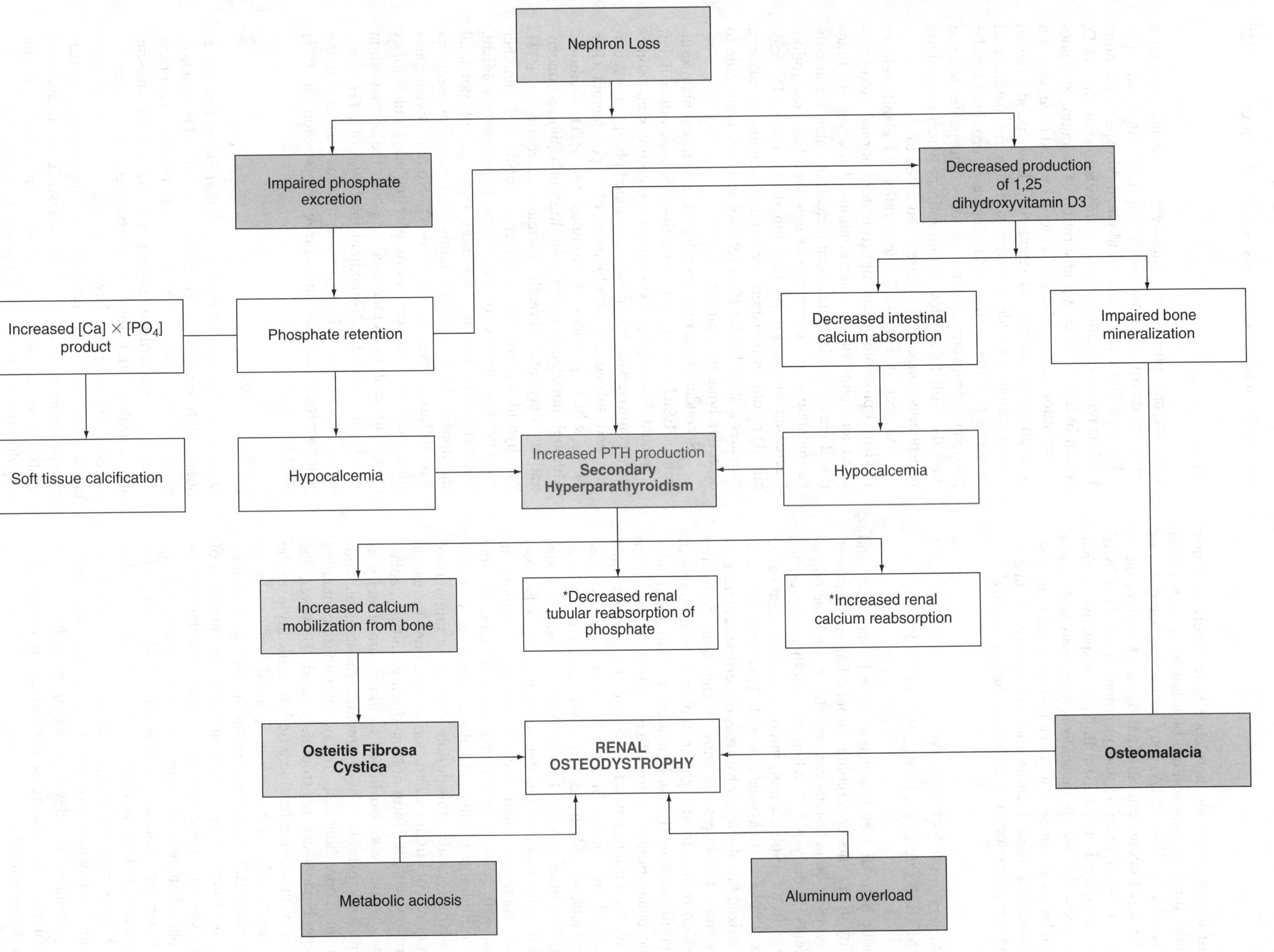

* These adaptations are lost as renal failure progresses.

Figure 44.9. Pathogenesis of secondary hyperparathyroidism and renal osteodystrophy in patients with chronic renal failure.

Clinical bone symptoms are rare in patients with mild to moderate renal impairment, although target organs (bone, kidney, and intestine) are affected. Intestinal calcium absorption can be decreased even at a GFR of 75 mL/min/1.73 m^2.[68] Hyperparathyroidism has been observed in patients with a GFR of 60–90 mL/min,[69] and 50% of patients with GFR less than 50 mL/min have abnormal bone histology.[68] Renal osteodystrophy progresses insidiously for several years before patients become symptomatic. When symptoms such as bone pain and skeletal fractures occur, the disease is not easily amenable to treatment. Bone marrow fibrosis and decreased hematopoiesis are also consequences of severe osteitis fibrosa. Therefore, preventive measures should be initiated in patients with mild to moderate degrees of renal failure.[68]

Because renal osteodystrophy is heterogenic, knowledge of the underlying bone abnormality is essential to guide therapy. Transiliac bone biopsy is the only technology that clearly differentiates between different etiologies and thus is the gold standard for evaluation of renal osteodystrophy. Tetracycline administration prior to bone biopsy provides dynamic information about bone turnover.[65] Bone mineral densitometry studies are mainly useful to follow progress after therapeutic intervention.[65] High-resolution x-ray techniques can aid in scoring the severity of bone disease and have been significantly correlated with serum PTH concentrations.[65] Serum calcium, phosphorous, PTH, alkaline phosphatase, and osteocalcin are serum biochemical markers that are used in the diagnostic workup and follow-up of renal osteodystrophy. New double antibody assays for measurement of serum intact-PTH, the biologically active molecule, are more sensitive in distinguishing between histologic patterns of renal osteodystrophy than older midregion and carboxy terminal PTH assays.[65,70] Alkaline phosphatase is a nonspecific marker of ongoing bone disease. Osteocalcin, a protein synthesized by osteoblasts, is a marker for bone formation.[65] A recent study found that the combination of *N*-terminal PTH, a deferoxamine stimulation test for aluminum toxicity, and bone biopsy provided a more specific means of diagnosis of renal osteodystrophy than total serum calcium, phosphorous, and alkaline phosphatase concentrations. High calcium concentrations were significantly associated with total body aluminum excess.[71] Calculation of the calcium set point following a modified calcium infusion test may be a time-intensive noninvasive method to monitor progression of hyperparathyroidism.[72]

Therapeutic Management

The goal of therapy across the spectrum of renal dysfunction is to prevent secondary hyperparathyroidism and renal osteodystrophy. Initially, dietary phosphorus restriction (6.5–12.0 mg/kg/d) should be initiated in patients with Cr Cl <50 mL/min to prevent early renal osteodystrophy and perhaps slow progression of renal disease.[73] This amount of phosphorus restriction is usually achievable with 0.6–0.8 g of protein per kilogram body weight. PTH concentrations should be monitored annually and should be maintained in the normal range. In addition, the fractional reabsorption of phosphorus (FR_{phos}, normally 80–95%) should also be monitored (Fig. 44.10). Elevations in PTH concentrations and a declining FR_{phos} will indicate the need for further phosphorus restriction. As the number of functioning nephrons declines, dietary restriction alone is usually inadequate to control serum phosphorous, and phosphate-binding agents are instituted. Dietary phosphorus can be liberalized to 800–1200 mg/d (10–17 mg/kg/d) once dialysis is initiated because a single hemodialysis or daily peritoneal dialysis treatment can remove up to 500–700 or 300 mg of phosphorus, respectively.[73] After control of serum phosphorus has been achieved, the goal shifts to optimizing serum calcium concentrations. By the time ESRD develops, most patients will require a combination of phosphate-binding medication, calcium supplements, and/or vitamin D therapy to prevent the development of secondary hyperparathyroidism, renal osteodystrophy, and metastatic calcification.

Phosphate-Binding Agents

Currently, the ideal phosphate-binding agent does not exist. A variety of calcium, aluminum, and magnesium containing phosphate-binding medications are available (Table 44.3). Phosphate-binding agents retard phosphorus absorption from the gut. These agents should be administered with meals to maximize the phosphate-binding effect. The dose in ESRD should be titrated to achieve normal to slightly high (4.5–6.0 mg/dL) serum phosphorus concentrations. Hypophosphatemia secondary to excessive binder use should be avoided in order to reduce the risk of osteomalacia. Unfortunately, many phosphate binders are marketed as antacids or calcium supplements and many dialysis patients do not know the indicated use,[74] which can lead to noncompliance.

Aluminum salts were once widely used as phosphate-binding agents because of their high-binding potency. However, aluminum binders can no longer be recommended as first-line therapy due to the toxicities previously discussed. Aluminum binders should be reserved for cases of severe hyperphosphatemia in conjunction with high serum calcium

$$FR_{phos} = \left(1 - \frac{U_{phos} \times P_{cr}}{P_{phos} \times U_{cr}}\right) \times 100$$

U_{phos} = urine phosphorus concentration
P_{cr} = plasma creatinine concentration
P_{phos} = plasma phosphorus concentration
U_{cr} = urine creatinine concentration

Figure 44.10. Fractional reabsorption of phosphorus (FR_{phos}).

TABLE 44.3. PHOSPHATE-BINDING AGENTS USED IN THE TREATMENT OF HYPERPHOSPHATEMIA OF RENAL FAILURE

Agents	Calcium, Aluminum, or Magnesium Content	Dosage Form	Starting Doses	Comments
Calcium Carbonate (40% calcium)			0.5–1 g (elemental calcium) tid with meals	Dissolution characteristics and phosphate binding effect may vary from product to product. Usual maintenance dosage ranges from 2.4–5.6 g (elemental calcium) or 6–14 g (calcium carbonate) per day.
Os-Cal 500	500 mg	Tablet		
Caltrate 600	600 mg	Tablet		
Nephro-Calci	600 mg	Tablet		
CalCarb HD	2400 mg/packet	Powder		To be mixed with food.
Calci-Mix	500 mg	Capsule		To be mixed with food.
Calci-Chew	500 mg	Tablet		Chewable.
Tums	200, 300, 400 mg	Tablet		Chewable.
Calcium carbonate	500 mg/5 ml	Suspension		
Many other trade names and generic brands available.				
Content represents amount of elemental calcium in product.				
Calcium Acetate (25% calcium)			2 tablets tid with meals	Comparable efficacy to calcium carbonate with half the dose of elemental calcium.
Phos-Lo	169 mg	Tablet		
Content represents amount of elemental calcium in product.				
Calcium Citrate (21% calcium)			0.5–1 g (elemental calcium) tid with meals	Citrate enhances absorption of aluminum. Should not be administered concurrently with aluminum binders, antacids, or sulcralfate.
Citracal	200 mg 500 mg	Tablet Effervescent tablet		Contains aspartame.
Content represents amount of aluminum carbonate in product.				
Aluminum Carbonate			400–500 mg tid with meals	Second line agent after calcium binders. Do not use concurrently with citrate-containing products.
Basaljel	500 mg 400 mg/5 mL	Tablet, capsule Suspension		
Content represents amount of elemental calcium in product.				
Aluminum Hydroxide			300–600 mg tid with meals	Second line agent after calcium binders. Do not use concurrently with citrate-containing products.
Amphogel	300, 600 mg 320 mg/5 mL	Tablet Suspension		
AlternaGel	600 mg/5 mL	Suspension		
Many other trade names and generic brands available.				
Content represents amount of aluminum hydroxide in product.				
Magnesium Hydroxide			300–400 mg tid with meals	Magnesium concentration in dialysate needs to be reduced to avoid hypermagnesemia. Serum magnesium concentration should be routinely monitored and kept within the normal range. Diarrhea is a common side effect.
Milk of Magnesia	300, 600 mg 400 mg/5 ml 800 mg/5 ml	Tablet Suspension Suspension		
Content represents amount of magnesium hydroxide in product.				

concentrations when the patient is at risk for metastatic calcification. Sucralfate, an aluminum-containing compound, has been shown to be an effective phosphate binder. However, aluminum contained in sucralfate may be more readily absorbed than with aluminum hydroxide,[75] and therefore should be avoided. Thus, oral calcium compounds have emerged as first-line agents for controlling both serum phosphorus and calcium concentrations.

Calcium carbonate, calcium citrate, and calcium acetate therapy have the potential advantage of partially correcting metabolic acidosis and increasing ionized calcium concentrations, thereby decreasing PTH secretion.[76] Bone mineral content may decrease less rapidly when patients are given calcium binders as compared to aluminum binders.[77] Prevention of phosphate retention by calcium binders also allows normal synthesis of calcitriol until low levels of renal function are reached.[78] However, maintaining a high positive calcium balance may predispose patients to metastatic calcification.[68] Multiple studies have demonstrated that calcium carbonate alone can successfully normalize phosphate concentrations in a high percentage of dialysis patients[78,79]; however, large doses (average 6–14 g/d of calcium carbonate) may be required.[79,80] Calcium carbonate is marketed in a variety of dosage forms (Table 44.3) and is relatively inexpensive. Unfortunately, many calcium carbonate products fall under the category of food supplements and are not required by law to meet USP disintegration and dissolution requirements. Intact calcium carbonate tablets have been detected in the stool of hemodialysis patients.[81] In general, nationally advertised brands meet USP quality standards for disintegration and dissolution, but it is difficult to determine whether private label or house brands conform to these same standards.[82] A home test for determining the quality of calcium carbonate tablets has been described.[81]

Single meal GI balance experiments and short-term human trials have shown that calcium acetate binds approximately twice as much phosphorus as calcium carbonate at comparable doses of elemental calcium.[83–85] Increased binding potency limits GI calcium absorption. However, calcium acetate is more soluble and therefore better absorbed than calcium carbonate in an alkaline pH, which may explain the similar incidence of hypercalcemia when equivalent phosphorus concentrations are achieved.[83,84] Hypercalcemia associated with the use of calcium-containing phosphate binders may be related to the presence of adynamic bone disease and not necessarily to dietary calcium intake or absorption,[86] although one short-term crossover study demonstrated a higher incidence of hypercalcemia and better PTH suppression with calcium acetate as compared to calcium carbonate.[87] Unfortunately, calcium acetate also causes more nausea and diarrhea than does calcium carbonate, which resulted in poorer medication compliance.[87] A long-term pharmacoeconomic study comparing the cost effectiveness of calcium acetate versus calcium carbonate on suppression of secondary hyperparathyroidism, bone mass, and metastatic calcification is needed to definitively support calcium carbonate or acetate as the superior phosphate-binding agent.

Although the chloride and citrate salts of calcium may be used as phosphate binders, these agents exhibit several disadvantages compared to the carbonate and acetate salts. The chloride salt is very astringent and unpalatable and absorbed chloride may contribute to systemic acidosis. The citrate salt binds phosphate poorly *in vitro,* markedly increases intestinal aluminum absorption due to the formation of soluble aluminum citrate complexes, and may contribute to aluminum intoxication.[88,89] Thus, citrate-containing compounds should not be combined with aluminum-containing compounds. In contrast, calcium acetate does not appear to influence the intestinal absorption of aluminum.[88] In most cases when calcium binders are used as the primary phosphate binder, a low-calcium dialysate (2.25–2.75 mEq/L) should be used concomitantly to reduce the potential for frank hypercalcemia and metastatic calcification.

Magnesium-containing antacids are also fairly effective phosphate binders. Several investigators have shown that magnesium-containing phosphate binders can lessen the amount of aluminum-containing binders necessary for optimal phosphorus control,[90] although serum potassium concentrations may rise and diarrhea is a problem.[91] Dialysate magnesium concentrations must be reduced to avoid hypermagnesemia when magnesium-binding agents are used.[90] Magnesium carbonate is less well absorbed and better tolerated than magnesium hydroxide; however, it is not available commercially in the United States in tablet or liquid form except in fixed combinations with aluminum hydroxide. Magnesium and potassium serum concentrations must be closely monitored to avoid hypermagnesemia or hyperkalemia.

In summary, patients should be initiated on calcium-containing phosphate binders. If necessary, magnesium- or aluminum-containing phosphate binders can be added to optimize phosphorus control. If magnesium-containing binders are used, a reduction in dialysate magnesium is necessary to prevent hypermagnesemia. If aluminum-containing binders are used, then serum aluminum concentrations should be monitored periodically to prevent aluminum toxicity.

Calcium Supplementation

Once normophosphatemia has been achieved, normocalcemia should be sought using both dietary and pharmacologic means. Before calcium-containing phosphate binders were routinely used, calcium supplements were often given between meals to optimize total corrected serum calcium concentration at high-normal limits (i.e., 10–10.5 mg/dL) to reduce the stimulus for PTH secretion. Although dietary calcium intake is often subnormal in renal failure patients due to the reduced intake of phosphate-containing dairy products, administration of calcium-containing phosphate binders should ensure a positive calcium balance. Therefore, calcium supplementation is no longer necessary in the majority of patients above that provided by the phosphate-lowering regimen.

Vitamin D Therapy

Vitamin D therapy should be added in patients who do not achieve normocalcemia or those with biochemical features of progressive bone disease (elevated PTH and alkaline phosphatase concentrations) by means of calcium-containing binders alone (Fig. 44.11). Many vitamin D analogues are available; however, all but dihydrotachysterol 1,25-dihydroxyvitamin D_3 (calcitriol) and 1-α hydroxyvitamin D_3 (alfacalcidiol, not yet available in the United States) require hydroxylation in the kidney to produce the physiologically active hormone. Although biochemical, radiologic, and histologic improvements in renal osteodystrophy have been noted in patients receiving massive doses of vitamins D_2 or D_3,[92] use of these sterols has been rendered

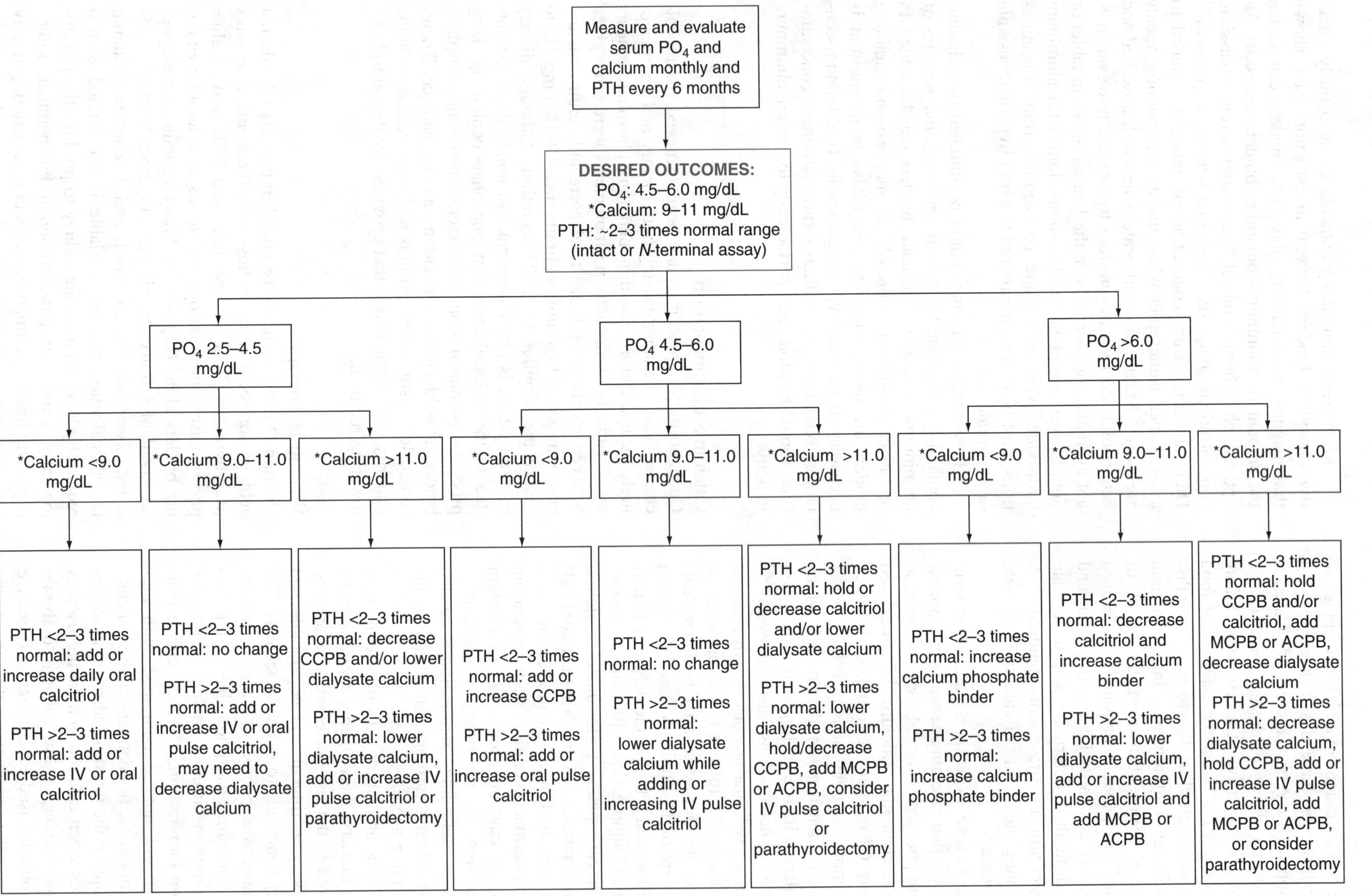

Key:
*Corrected calcium = [(4.0 − albumin) × 0.8] + serum calcium
CCPB = calcium containing phosphate binder
MCPB = magnesium containing phosphate binder
ACPB = aluminum containing phosphate binder

Figure 44.11. Approach to prevention and treatment of secondary hyperparathyroidism and renal osteodystrophy in ESRD patients.

obsolete by more physiologically active analogues with shorter half-lives. Calcitriol has largely replaced dihydrotachysterol in the management of renal osteodystrophy in the United States because calcitriol inhibits PTH secretion directly in addition to stimulating intestinal absorption of calcium.

Recent reviews[93,94] point out that calcitriol treatment has been shown to reduce bone pain, muscle weakness, and impaired growth in children. Calcitriol can suppress PTH secretion by increasing serum calcium concentrations through enhanced gut absorption of calcium as well as by directly decreasing PTH synthesis by parathyroid cells.[94] Calcitriol can be administered orally as well as by intravenous injection (Table 44.4). Controversy exists regarding the most effective route of administration, the optimal dose, and the dosage interval.

It appears that calcitriol directly suppresses PTH secretion by decreasing the set point for calcium-regulated PTH production.[95] Thus, the high plasma levels of this sterol achievable following intermittent intravenous dosing two or three times weekly may more effectively suppress PTH secretion than daily doses of oral calcitriol. In fact, intravenous calcitriol has been safely used in the treatment of patients with hyperparathyroid bone disease in whom hypercalcemia developed during oral therapy with the same agent.[96,97] Other small, uncontrolled clinical investigations indicate that oral pulse doses of calcitriol can suppress PTH concentrations effectively in patients with severe hyperparathyroidism[98,99] and may be able to reduce parathyroid hyperplasia.[100]

Oral and intravenous pulse doses of calcitriol (1–2 mcg three times weekly) were compared in a prospective crossover study lasting 8 months in 11 hemodialysis patients. Similar efficacy and rates of hypercalcemia were reported in both groups with no reduction in parathyroid gland size.[101] In the most well-designed study to date, Quarles and colleagues[102] studied 19 hemodialysis patients with severe hyperparathyroidism (mean intact PTH >900 pg/mL). Intravenous and oral calcitriol pulse doses (mean doses of 2.5 and 2.4 mcg, respectively, three times weekly) were evaluated in a randomized, double-blind, placebo-controlled fashion over 36 weeks. Oral and intravenous administration of calcitriol resulted in similar decreases in PTH, but neither therapy decreased parathyroid gland size or altered sensitivity to calcium loading. In summary, oral pulse doses of calcitriol appear to be as effective as intravenous pulse doses of calcitriol in suppression of PTH. However, insufficient power (small sample sizes) may limit the ability of these comparative studies to detect small differences in PTH suppression. The discrepancies between studies that have evaluated parathyroid gland size and calcium set-point changes probably can be explained by major differences in study population such as length of dialytic therapy, dose of calcitriol, use of aluminum versus calcium binders, presence or absence of aluminum bone disease, nodular versus diffuse parathyroid hyperplasia, and dialysate calcium concentration.

Unfortunately, use of calcitriol enhances phosphorus absorption from the gut and frequently leads to hypercalcemia.[96,101] Conventional daily oral doses of calcitriol (0.25 mcg) may be more frequently associated with hypercalcemia and hyperphosphatemia since calcitriol receptors are located in intestinal mucosa where direct stimulation can occur. Strategies to minimize hypercalcemia while maximizing PTH suppression have included use of oral or intravenous pulse doses of calcitriol and calcitriol administration at bedtime or between meals when gut calcium/phosphorus content is lowest.[99,103] Calcitriol pharmacokinetic and dosing information can be found in Table 44.4. Vitamin D analogues, such as 22-oxacalcitriol, which result in less calcium absorption from the gut but retain the positive physiologic action on bone and parathyroid tissue, are under investigation.[104]

Whether vitamin D analogues should be used as prophylactic agents in CRF patients with no evidence of renal osteodystrophy is unclear. Although such therapy may retard the development of renal osteodystrophy, there is some risk that drug-induced hypercalcemia and hyperphosphatemia may accelerate deterioration in renal function.[105,106] However, several investigators have documented biochemical and histologic improvement in renal bone disease with no alteration in the rate of decline of renal function provided that hypercalcemia and hyperphosphatemia are avoided.[107–109]

TABLE 44.4. COMPARISON OF VITAMIN D ANALOGUES COMMONLY USED IN THE TREATMENT OF RENAL OSTEODYSTROPHY

	Alfacalcidiol[a] [1α(OH)D_3]	Calcitriol [1,25$(OH)_2D_3$]
Physiologic dose (μg/d)	1	0.5
Pharmacologic dose (μg/d)	0.25–2.0	0.25–2.0[b,c]
Pharmacologic half-life (d)	3–5	1–3
Onset of maximal effects (d)	5–10	2–5
Time for reversal of toxic effects (d)	3–10	1–5

[a]Not available in the United States.
[b]Pulse (intermittent) doses of 2–5 mcg orally or IV two to three times weekly can be used.
[c]For treatment of renal osteodystrophy.

Other Pharmacologic Measures

Preliminary investigations with biphosphonates that block osteoclastic bone reabsorption (etidronate also inhibits bone mineralization) have shown conflicting results, thus, along with calcitonin, their place in therapy is currently confined to the acute treatment of hypercalcemia resulting from hyperparathyroidism.[79]

Parathyroidectomy

Parathyroidectomy should be undertaken as the last therapeutic option for patients with secondary hyperparathyroidism. Criteria for surgery include (1) persistent hypercalcemia (serum calcium >11.5 mg/dL) provided aluminum toxicity has been ruled out[93]; (2) a persistently elevated calcium–phosphorus product above 70 and progressive soft-tissue calcification that persists despite vigorous dietary phosphate restriction and phosphate binder use; (3) progressive radiographic lesions of secondary hyperparathyroidism, particularly when associated with severe or debilitating symptoms; (4) intractable pruritus recalcitrant to other therapy; and (5) syndrome of calciphylaxis (a rare syndrome characterized by ischemic necrosis of the skin, muscles, and/or subcutaneous fat caused by vascular calcification).

Total parathyroidectomy is not recommended because the presence of PTH appears to be necessary for bone remodeling. Generally, surgical approaches include either subtotal parathyroidectomy or total parathyroidectomy with transplantation of parathyroid tissue to an accessible site such as the forearm.[110] Postoperative hypocalcemia, hypophosphatemia, and hypomagnesemia may occur because of a marked increase in bone production in relation to bone absorption ("hungry bone syndrome"). The severity of the hypocalcemia depends on the degree of osteitis fibrosa, and preoperative treatment with calcitriol may prevent or minimize the risk. Treatment with supplemental calcium and calcitriol may be necessary for weeks or months. After surgery, continual efforts to prevent hyperphosphatemia and the recurrence of secondary hyperparathyroidism are necessary.

Evaluation of Therapeutic Outcomes

The therapeutic goals for treatment with phosphate-binding agents and vitamin D therapy are to prevent secondary hyperparathyroidism, vitamin D deficiency, and subsequent renal osteodystrophy without inducing adynamic bone disease from oversuppression of PTH. Figure 44.11 outlines an algorithm approach for the treatment and evaluation of the ESRD patient on dialysis using clinically available noninvasive markers (total serum calcium, serum phosphorus, and intact PTH). Intact or *N*-terminal PTH concentrations of 2.0–3.0 times normal, total calcium concentrations (corrected for albumin) of 9–11 mg/dL, and serum phosphorus concentrations of 4.5–6.0 mg/dL are the goals. A calcium (mg/dL) times phosphorus product (mg/dL) >70 should be avoided to lessen the risk of metastatic calcification. Aluminum toxicity should be suspected in a patient with a past or current history of aluminum binder use, low PTH, and development of hypercalcemia within weeks to months of starting calcitriol therapy.[93] In this case a deferoxamine (DFO) challenge and/or bone biopsy should be performed and, if positive, maintenance deferoxamine therapy begun (see section on Aluminum Toxicity). If the patient develops hypercalcemia after many months of calcitriol therapy, this may indicate healing of osteitis fibrosa cystica.[93]

ALUMINUM TOXICITY

Pathophysiology and Clinical Consequences

Although once a major problem, aluminum toxicity occurs less frequently due to use of deionizers and reverse osmosis filters for dialysate water purification and decreased use of aluminum phosphate binders.[111] Aluminum-associated toxicity has recently been reviewed in detail and therefore is briefly discussed here.[111] Aluminum toxicity can contribute to renal osteodystrophy (Fig. 44.9) and result in decreased hematopoiesis and encephalopathy. Impaired bone mineralization and altered bone cell proliferation from aluminum excess results in an osteomalacic or adynamic bone histologic pattern.[112] Aluminum appears to disrupt cellular iron metabolism causing an iron-deficiency–like pattern and decreased erythropoiesis (i.e., microcytic anemia) in the presence of normal iron balance.[112,113] Interestingly, patients with low serum iron may be predisposed to aluminum toxicity since aluminum binds to transferrin, the major transport protein for iron.[112,113] Aluminum neurotoxicity can occur insidiously with speech disturbances and can progress to asterixis, myoclonus, visual and auditory hallucinations, seizures, and ultimately death. Rapid manifestations of aluminum toxicity can occur under three circumstances: (1) high concentrations of aluminum in dialysate, (2) concurrent use of aluminum and citrate containing products, and (3) acute elevations in plasma and cerebrospinal fluid aluminum concentrations secondary to DFO administration.[114,115]

Therapeutic Management

The most important aspect of aluminum intoxication in ESRD is prevention. Prevention is accomplished by (1) using water purified by deionization or reverse osmosis such that dialysate aluminum concentrations are less than 10 mcg/L and (2) minimizing the use of aluminum-containing phosphate binders or medications and aluminum-containing drinks and foods (especially in the presence of citrate). Maintaining adequate iron balance may also lessen the risk for aluminum toxicity.

The gold standard for diagnosis of aluminum-related bone disease is by transiliac bone biopsy. Indirect, less invasive methods such as elevated plasma aluminum, low PTH concentrations, and positive DFO infusion test are also used to identify patients with aluminum overload, but these methods are less specific and sensitive. The DFO infusion test is based on the concept that the amount of aluminum mobilized following a single dose of DFO is representative of the total body burden of aluminum. The DFO test consists of an intravenous infusion of 5–40 mg/kg of DFO administered preferably after a dialysis session to minimize DFO loss through the dialyzer. Blood samples for aluminum content should be drawn before the hemodialysis session at which DFO was given and before the subsequent dialysis session.[111] The change in serum aluminum concentration is the key factor on which therapeutic decisions are made. Although the DFO infusion test is not entirely reliable in identifying patients with aluminum overload, it continues to be widely used. A combination of a negative DFO infusion test plus high PTH concentration may be useful to rule out aluminum toxicity.[116] Although the optimal way to evaluate aluminum toxicity is controversial, a recent consensus paper outlines a detailed approach to diagnosis and treatment (Figs. 44.12 and 44.13).[111]

All patients with symptoms of organ dysfunction from aluminum overload should receive DFO therapy. Hemodialysis alone does not significantly remove aluminum because it is highly bound to the plasma protein transferrin. However, hemodialysis can remove substantial amounts of aluminum–DFO complex. High-flux dialysis (utilizing membranes with high middle molecule clearances) and hemofiltration are particularly effective in removing the complex.[117]

Evaluation of Therapeutic Outcomes

Figure 44.13 outlines a therapeutic approach for treatment of aluminum overload with DFO. The use of DFO carries some risk of hypotension and ocular toxicity and has been linked to unusual systemic infections such as mucormycosis.[118,119] Cerebrospinal fluid aluminum concentrations have been shown to rise after DFO administration,[114] and plasma concentrations greater than 500 mcg/L following DFO administration have been associated with acute encephalopathy.[120] In an effort to minimize adverse reactions, once-weekly, low-dose (5 mg/kg) DFO administration has been recommended.[111] The prophylactic use of DFO also remains an unresolved issue since not all patients develop aluminum intoxication while taking aluminum-containing phosphate binders.

ANEMIA OF CHRONIC RENAL FAILURE

Pathophysiology

The primary cause of anemia in patients with chronic renal failure and ESRD is a relative erythropoietin (EPO) deficiency, for which therapy with recombinant human erythropoietin (epoetin) is now available. In adults, the kidneys synthesize about 90% of circulating EPO, the remainder is synthesized by the liver. EPO is a glycoprotein of approximately 30,000 Da, which is secreted in response to hypoxia.[121,122] Plasma concentrations of EPO increase to approximately 1000 mU/mL when the hematocrit drops to 20% in individuals with normal renal function. In contrast, anemic dialysis patients have serum EPO concentrations of about 20 mU/mL or less.[123] EPO stimulates the proliferation and differentiation of erythroid progenitor cells.[121] Anemia begins to develop when the GFR drops to less than 20–30 mL/min/1.73 m^2. It is of interest that patients with ESRD secondary to polycystic kidney disease can often maintain a normal hematocrit without exogenous administration of EPO. Other factors such as blood loss; iron, folic acid, or vitamin B_{12} deficiency; severe osteitis fibrosa; systemic infection or inflammatory illness; aluminum toxicity; or hypersplenism may also contribute to the anemia of ESRD.[124] Blood loss commonly occurs due to routine laboratory monitoring, dialyzer clotting, and bleeding from hemodialysis needle puncture sites. In addition, dialysis patients are prone to GI bleeding.[125] Iron deficiency is now commonly seen due mainly to aggressive use of recombinant human erythropoietin (epoetin).[126] Prior to epoetin availability, many patients were dependent on intermittent packed red blood cell (RBC) transfusions. Figure 44.14 shows the percentage of hemodialysis patients receiving outpatient blood transfusions before and following the introduction of epoetin in July 1989. Currently, the majority of eligible U.S. dialysis patients are receiving epoetin.[127]

Clinical Consequences

Signs and symptoms of fatigue, exertional dyspnea, dizziness, headache, and pallor are commonly seen even though some adaptation to a decreased hematocrit (HCT) occurs during the slow progression of ESRD anemia. Prior to availability of epoetin, HCTs commonly ranged from 18–25% in patients on hemodialysis. Although ESRD anemia is typically a hypoproliferative disorder in which normochromic and normocytic cells are seen on peripheral blood smear, iron deficiency secondary to blood loss or exogenous erythropoietin administration can result in a microcytic, hypochromic pattern. Vitamin B_{12} or folate deficiency can lead to a macrocytic anemia. Since the etiology of anemia in this population is often multifactorial, the workup of an ESRD patient with anemia should be approached in an economical stepwise fashion (Fig. 44.15).

Prior to epoetin availability, many patients were dependent on RBC transfusions, which increased patient risk for transfusion reactions and viral infections such as hepatitis and the acquired immunodeficiency syndrome. In addition, the development of iron overload and hemosiderosis was fairly common in patients receiving massive numbers of blood transfusions.

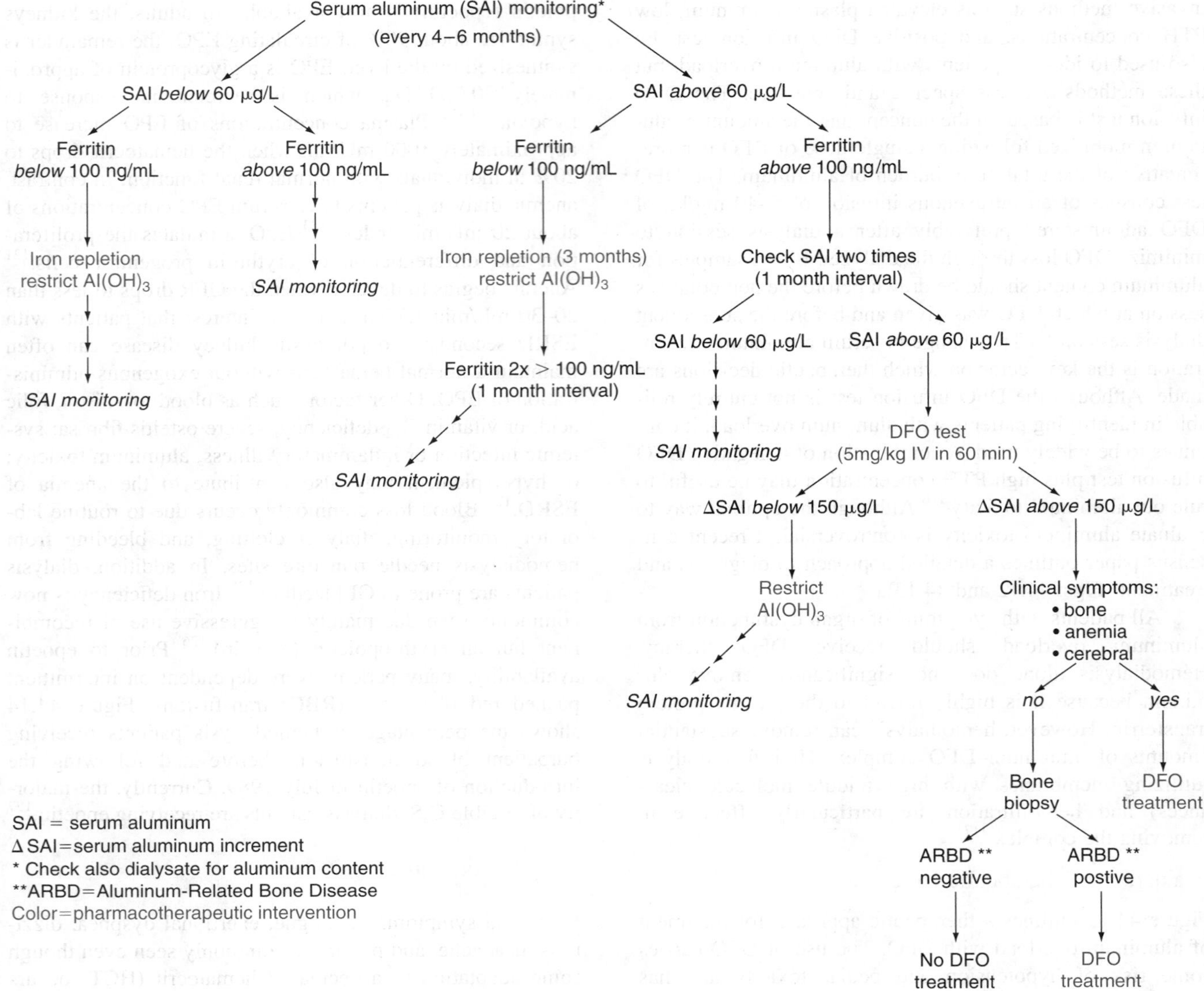

Figure 44.12. Diagnosis of aluminum overload. *(From Consensus conference. Diagnosis and treatment of aluminum overload in end-stage renal failure patients. Nephrol Dial Transplant 1993;8(suppl 1):3, by permission of Oxford University Press.)*

Therapeutic Management

RBC transfusions and androgen therapy are currently second-line treatment options. RBC transfusions carry many undesirable risks and therefore should be utilized in three situations: (1) acute management of symptomatic anemia, (2) after significant acute blood loss, and (3) prior to surgical procedures that carry a high risk of blood loss. Androgen therapy was also used extensively before epoetin availability, but hemopoietic response was suboptimal in the majority of patients.[128] However, androgen therapy may potentiate the effects of epoetin by increasing the sensitivity of erythroid precursors. Although *in vitro* results have been encouraging, small human trials testing androgen effects on erythropoiesis have yielded conflicting results.[128,129] In addition, side effects such as liver toxicity, malignancy, virilization, and hypertriglyceridemia limit the usefulness of this approach.

Currently, epoetin is the therapy of choice for long-term correction and maintenance of HCT levels in predialysis and dialysis patients. It is reasonable to begin epoetin therapy in CRF patients with hematocrits that fall to less than 30%. Epoetin therapy results in dose-dependent increases in effective erythropoiesis in both predialysis and

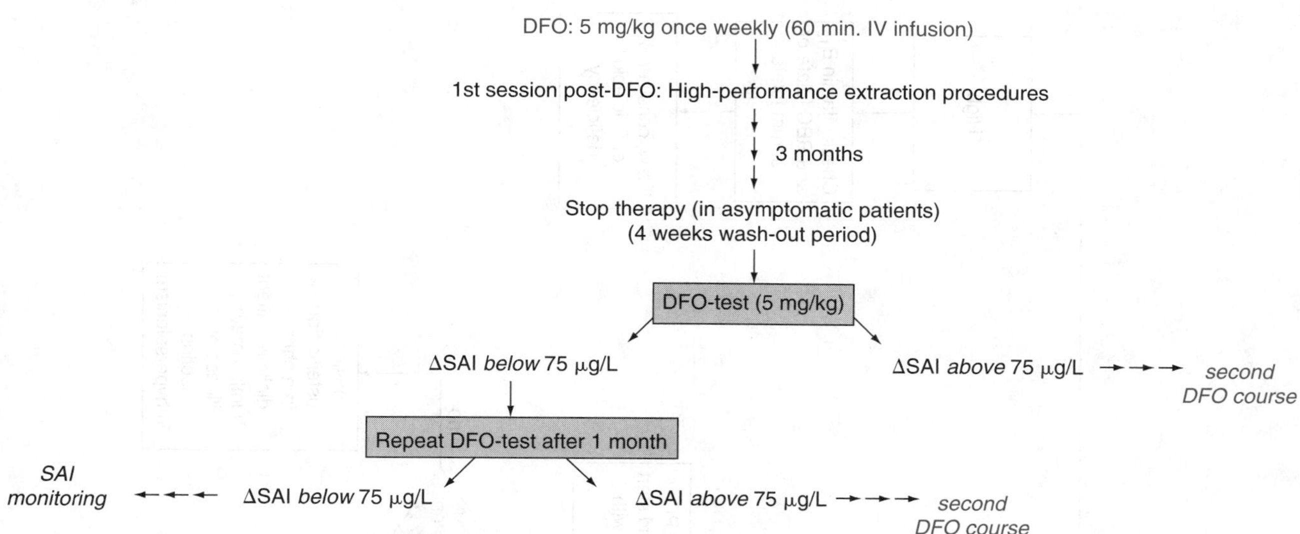

Figure 44.13. Treatment of aluminum overload. *(From Consensus conference. Diagnosis and treatment of aluminum overload in end-stage renal failure patients. Nephrol Dial Transplant 1993;8(suppl 1):3, by permission of Oxford University Press.)*

dialysis patients. Prior to initiation of epoetin, iron balance should be assessed because iron deficiency is the most common cause of suboptimal response to epoetin.

Iron Assessment

Iron status is usually assessed by monitoring serum iron, ferritin, total iron-binding capacity (TIBC), and transferrin saturation (serum iron divided by TIBC). Plasma ferritin values usually correlate with body stores of iron located in the liver, bone marrow, and spleen. Unfortunately, ferritin is an acute phase reactant and serum ferritin values can rise independently of body stores in response to an inflammatory state, in liver disease, malignancy, and infection. Circulating iron is highly bound to a protein called transferrin. Transferrin-bound iron is readily utilizable by the bone marrow for erythropoiesis. To prevent an absolute (low body stores) or functional (low amount of readily utilizable iron) iron deficiency in CRF patients receiving

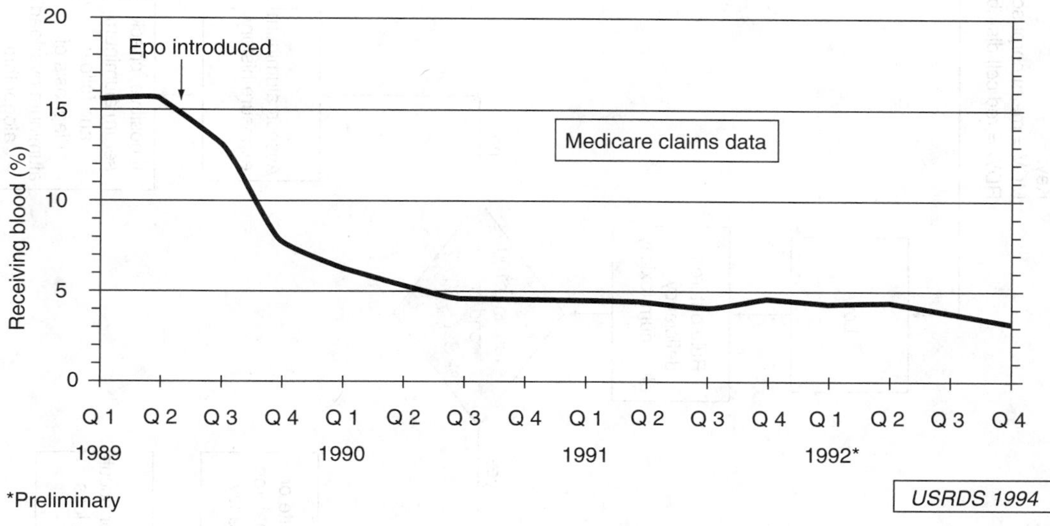

Figure 44.14. Hemodialysis patients receiving outpatient blood transfusions by quarter, 1989–1992. *(From U.S. Renal Data System, USRDS 1995 Annual Data Report, National Institutes of Health, National Institute of Diabetes and Digestive and Kidney Diseases, Bethesda, MD April 1995.)*

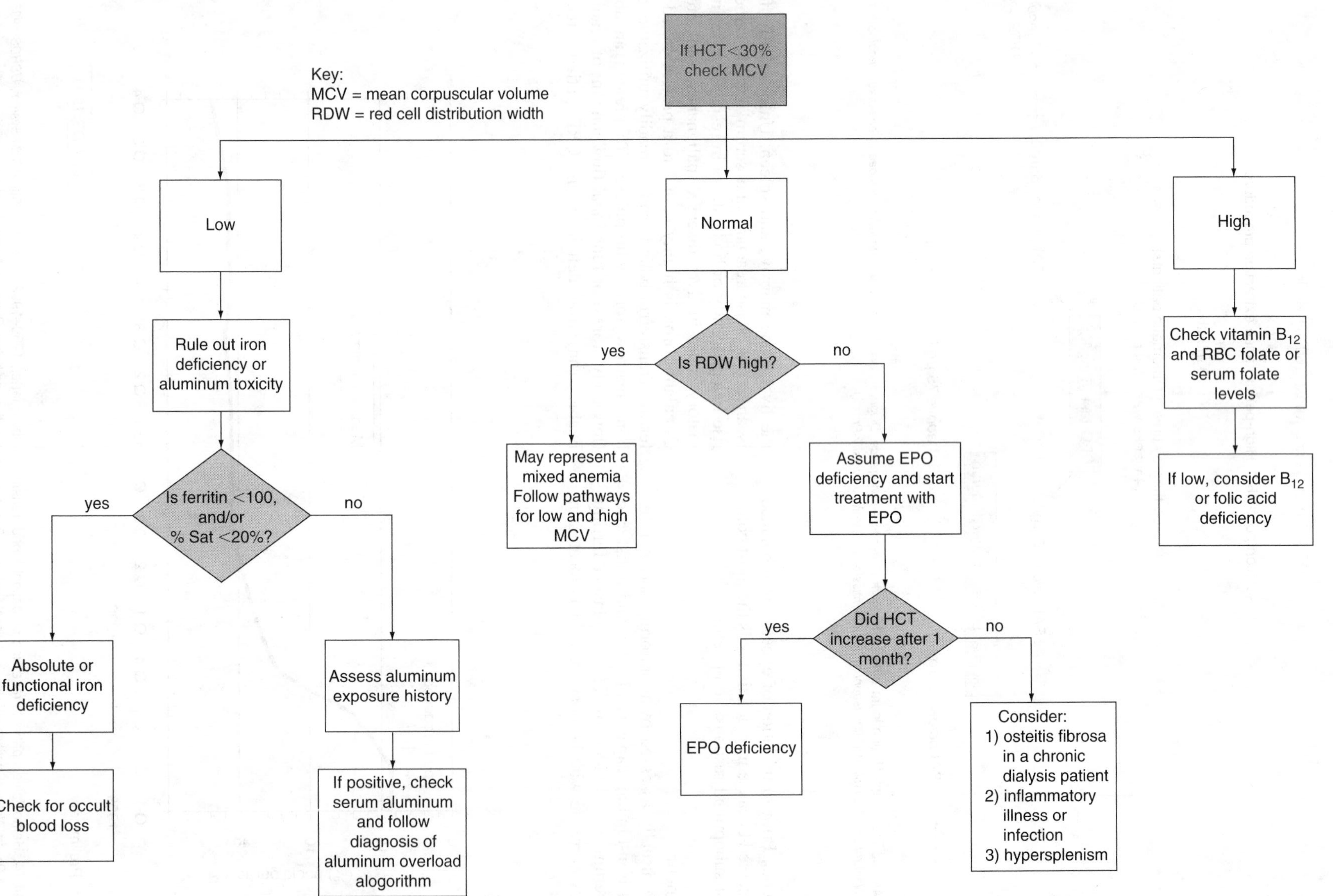

Figure 44.15. Diagnostic workup of anemia in ESRD.

epoetin, it is suggested that ferritin and transferrin saturation values of at least 100 ng/mL and 20%, respectively, be maintained.[130] Prior to epoetin therapy, an evaluation is necessary to determine whether current iron stores can meet future iron needs. Ideally, iron deficiency should be corrected before epoetin therapy is initiated, which can be accomplished slowly with oral iron or rapidly with intravenous iron. Several investigators have suggested methods to calculate iron needs.[131–133] However, a prospective evaluation needs to be conducted to determine if any method is superior to the others.

Oral Iron

Oral iron management should begin with agents that have relatively high bioavailability and low cost.[134] Initially, ferrous salts (sulfate, gluconate, and fumarate) should be prescribed to provide approximately 200 mg of elemental iron per day. Patients should be given divided daily doses of iron and instructed to take iron on an empty stomach to maximize absorption. If patients have GI complaints (nausea, vomiting, constipation, diarrhea), they can take oral iron with a small snack or try another dosage form or product such as ferrous sulfate solution, iron-polysaccharide complex, or a sustained-release preparation. However, the two latter compounds are more expensive and bioavailability is a problem. Administration with meals reduces iron absorption due to the interactions among iron, food, and phosphate binders. Some clinicians suggest giving vitamin C concomitantly with oral iron to enhance absorption. Unfortunately, serum oxalate concentrations have been shown to rise in dialysis patients who receive more than 250 mg a day of vitamin C,[135] therefore this maneuver is not recommended. Aggressive oral iron replacement therapy may reduce the amounts of intravenous (IV) iron dextran needed, which can minimize costs of iron therapy.

Intravenous Iron

Iron dextran is not immediately available to the bone marrow for heme synthesis, but must be processed by the reticuloendothelial system (RES) before being released to transferrin or stored within the RES in bone marrow, splenic, or hepatic tissue.[136] The incorporation of iron into hemoglobin occurs over weeks, with a plasma disappearance half-time that is dose-dependent.[136,137] Serum iron, TIBC, and ferritin values should be evaluated at least 4 weeks after iron dextran has been administered to avoid errors in serum iron determination from circulating iron dextran. Controversy exists over the best method to dose iron dextran. Some dialysis centers administer iron dextran as total dose infusions (500–2000 mg IV at one time), while others give 100 mg (2 mL) with each dialysis session until the calculated needs have been met, or more commonly, until 1 gram has been administered. Large dose infusions are more practical in peritoneal dialysis patients or in patients where IV access is limited. To date, no method has demonstrated superiority; however, total dose infusions have been associated with more delayed side effects such as arthralgias, myalgias, and serum-sickness–like symptoms.[138] However, some investigators have reported a low incidence of problems with doses equal to or less than 500 mg.[139] A 25-mg test dose should be administered IV before the first course of therapy to detect the small risk (<0.3%) of anaphylaxis. Aggressive use of intravenous iron dextran can enhance erythropoiesis, but may increase the risk of iron overload and development of hemosiderosis over time. Iron dextran should not be administered to patients with a serum ferritin level of >1000 ng/mL.[140]

Pharmacokinetic and Pharmacodynamic Properties of Epoetin

The pharmacokinetic profile of epoetin has been compared in healthy and uremic subjects after IV and subcutaneous injection.[141] Uremic patients have reduced subcutaneous bioavailability (23.7 versus 38.5%), and prolonged half-life ($t_{1/2}$) after IV administration (8.3 versus 4.92 hours).[141] However, understanding the pharmacodynamic profile of epoetin is more important than the pharmacokinetics of this agent. Unlike many drugs where pharmacodynamic action can be related to peak or trough concentrations or $t_{1/2}$ can be used to predict the duration of action or attainment of steady state, epoetin action must be evaluated on the basis of changes in RBC production rate and the individual's RBC life span.[142] An understanding of the pharmacodynamic action of epoetin can lead to appropriate dosing adjustments and diminish fluctuations in HCT levels.

Uremic patients have a shortened RBC life span, which averages 64 days[142] in contrast to 120 days in normal subjects. The HCT response to the pharmacodynamic effect of epoetin (i.e., increase in HCT) is illustrated in Fig. 44.16. Prior to starting epoetin, the baseline HCT is constant, demonstrating that RBC production is at steady state (i.e., the rate at which RBCs are being produced equals the rate at which they are dying). Although the HCT may begin to rise shortly following epoetin initiation as the result of demargination of reticulocytes, it takes approximately 10 days before erythrocyte progenitor cells mature and begin to be continuously released into the circulation at an increased rate. Gradually HCT rises as the RBC production rate exceeds daily RBC death. The HCT will continue to increase until the life span of the cells stimulated by epoetin is reached (range 1–4 months) and a new steady state is achieved. Clinical trials have shown successful treatment of ESRD anemia with doses of 50–100 U/kg IV three times a week.[143–146]

Epoetin can be administered by either the IV or subcutaneous route. Subcutaneous administration is preferable in chronic ambulatory peritoneal dialysis and prehemodialysis patients because these patients usually do not have permanent IV access. Although subcutaneous administration

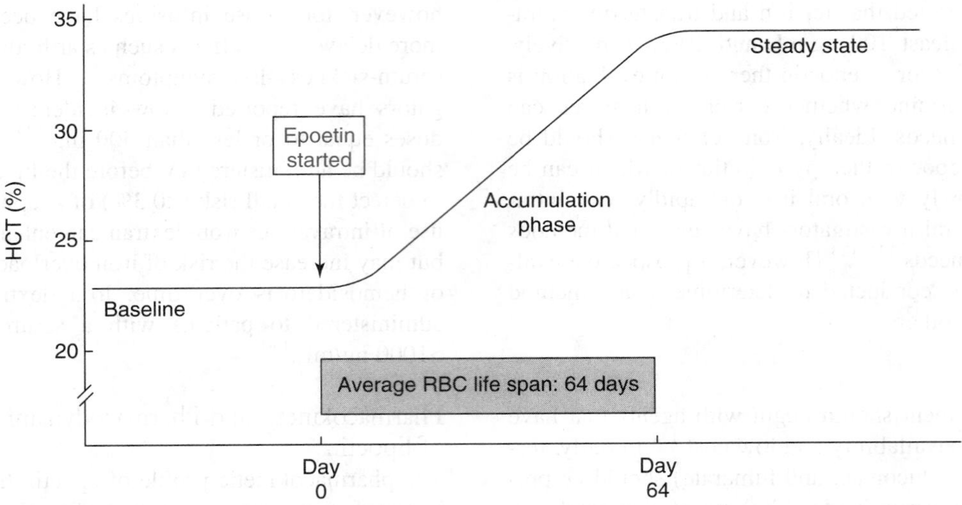

Figure 44.16. Pharmacodynamic effect of epoetin on hematocrit response.

results in poor bioavailability (approximately 25%), low peak serum concentrations, and a prolonged $t_{1/2}$ (approximately 22 hours), HCT response is at least as good or better than IV administration.[141,147,148] This enhanced efficacy is presumed to be due to a more prolonged, physiologic stimulation of erythroid precursors. A recent review points out that even though many of these comparative studies suffer from design flaws, the preponderance of data supports the use of subcutaneous epoetin in many clinical settings.[147] Once-a-week, twice-a-week, and three-times-a-week subcutaneous dosing have all been shown to be effective.

Resistance to Epoetin

Real or pseudoresistance to epoetin therapy can stem from multiple factors. Iron deficiency is the most common cause of resistance to epoetin and is routinely seen during epoetin therapy.[126] Evaluation and treatment should proceed as previously outlined for predialysis patients. Inflammation (localized or systemic infection, active inflammatory disease, surgical trauma) is associated with defective iron utilization known as reticuloendothelial (RE) block. RE block is characterized by a reduction in iron delivery from body stores to the bone marrow and is generally refractory to iron therapy. Malignancy and autoimmune diseases can cause resistance to epoetin by decreasing endogenous erythropoietin production, RE block, and reduced bone marrow responsiveness.[134] Cancer cells can also invade the bone marrow, while radiation and chemotherapy can damage erythroid progenitor cells. Epoetin therapy can be continued in the infected or postoperative patient, although increased amounts are often required to maintain or slow the rate of decline in hematocrit.

Hyperparathyroidism is known to cause resistance to epoetin. Erythropoietic response to epoetin therapy in patients with hyperparathyroidism appears to be linked to the severity of bone marrow fibrosis.[134] Aluminum toxicity, which was discussed earlier in this chapter, can reduce iron transport. Aluminum also inhibits key enzymes necessary in heme synthesis. Recognition of aluminum toxicity and appropriate chelation therapy with DFO are key steps in improving bone marrow response to epoetin. Unfortunately, DFO also chelates iron, making therapeutic management of anemia more difficult.

Finally, pseudoresistance can occur with occult bleeding or hemolysis. In this case, bone marrow response to epoetin is normal, but the rate of rise in hematocrit with epoetin is negatively offset by blood loss or hemolysis. Therefore, a workup of apparent epoetin resistance should always include an evaluation of potential sources of blood loss or hemolysis.

Evaluation of Therapeutic Outcomes

Figure 44.17 outlines an algorithm approach to patient evaluation and treatment with epoetin and iron therapy. Several studies have found improvements in various quality of life measurements such as physical energy, exercise capacity, cognitive function, peripheral perfusion, and nutrition with epoetin therapy. In addition, decreases in left-ventricular diastolic diameter and decreases in angina and ischemic EKG changes have been noted.[149] Improvements in quality of life parameters during a multicenter phase III clinical trial were more striking than interim data from a multicenter phase IV clinical trial. The mean hematocrit levels obtained during these two clinical trials were 34.6 and 30.4%, respectively, which could account for the differences. Interestingly, less than 10% of patients on maintenance hemodialysis have achieved steady hematocrit levels of 35%.[149] This suggests that epoetin and iron therapy can be further optimized in a large percentage of dialysis patients.

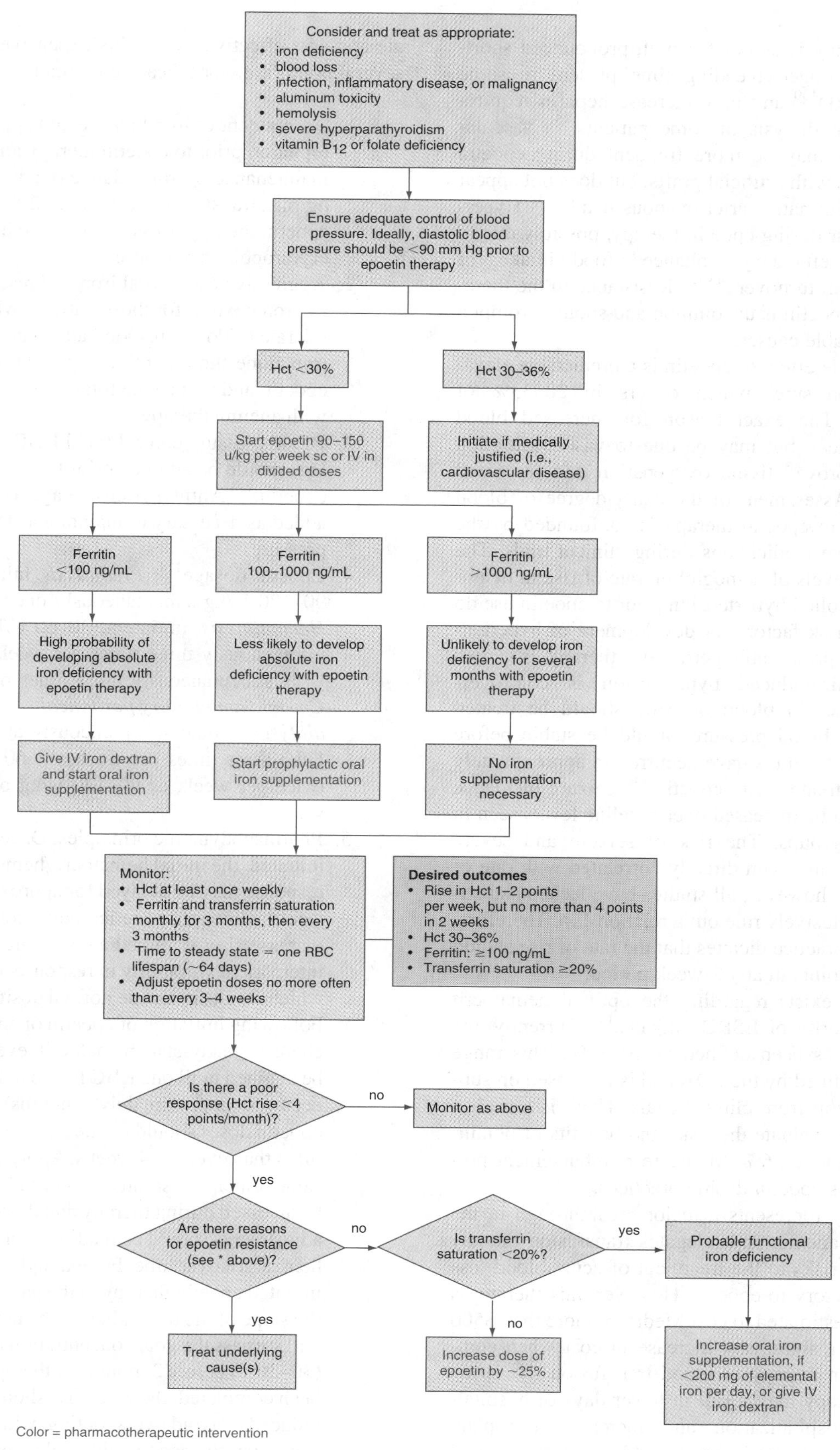

Figure 44.17. Algorithm approach to epoetin and iron therapy in the treatment of ESRD anemia.

Epoetin therapy is associated with pronounced shortening of the prolonged bleeding time present in some patients with ESRD[150] and may increase heparin requirements during hemodialysis in some patients.[151] Vascular access thrombosis may be more frequent during epoetin therapy in patients with artificial grafts, but does not appear to be increased with native arteriovenous fistula.[152] Hyperkalemia may occur during epoetin therapy, possibly due to reduced dialysis efficiency, enhanced food intake, or increased blood cell turnover.[144,153] Resistance to the therapeutic effects of epoetin is uncommon and should prompt a search for correctable causes.

The major side effect of epoetin is a predictable elevation in blood pressure, which occurs in 20–33% of patients.[146,154,155] The exact reason for increased blood pressure is not clear, but may be due to vasoconstriction secondary to improved tissue oxygenation and increased blood viscosity. Assessment of the exact degree of blood pressure increase to epoetin therapy is confounded by the use of hypertensive medications during clinical trials. The baseline or final levels of hemoglobin, rate of rise in hemoglobin, or uncontrolled hypertension prior to epoetin use do not appear to be risk factors for development of hypertension.[154] Whether prior antihypertensive therapy is a risk factor for epoetin-induced hypertension is controversial.[154,155] Increases in blood pressure should be treated aggressively, and blood pressure should be stable before epoetin initiation. Seizures have occurred in approximately 2.5% of patients treated with epoetin.[146] Seizure incidence does not appear to be increased over baseline levels seen in placebo control groups. The risk of seizure and severe hypertension have not been directly correlated with rate of rise in hematocrit; however, all studies have lacked statistical power to conclusively rule out a relationship. Therefore, standard clinical practice dictates that the rate of rise should not exceed four points in any 2-week period.

Controversy exists regarding the optimal hematocrit level for the majority of ESRD patients.[152] Currently, the goal hematocrit has been defined as 30–36%. This range was arbitrarily defined by the FDA and is not based on substantive information from clinical trials. There is a trial in progress that will evaluate the risks and benefits of obtaining hematocrits above 36%. Medicare reimbursement policy also influences epoetin dosing practices.

Epoetin truly represents a major breakthrough in the therapy of renal anemia and relegates transfusion therapy and its attendant risks to the treatment of acute blood loss and anemia refractory to epoetin. However, this therapy is expensive and is estimated to cost Medicare more than $500 million in 1994, a significant increase in cost when compared to androgen therapy or blood transfusions.[156] However, epoetin therapy may result in fewer days of hospitalization and rehospitalization and increased transplant success.[157,158] The economical use of this agent is essential in the face of limited health care dollars. To assure appropriate and cost-effective use of this expensive biologic agent, several points are worth bearing in mind:

1. Assessment of iron balance and appropriate repletion prior to epoetin therapy and maintenance of iron balance (ferritin, >100 ng/mL; transferrin saturation, >20%) during epoetin therapy is essential to maximize erythropoietic response.
2. Aggressive use of oral iron and reservation of IV iron dextran for those patients who cannot tolerate or do not respond adequately to oral iron alone should optimize patient response to epoetin and reduce the total cost associated with anemia therapy.
3. Blood pressure control (goal DBP <90 mm Hg) should be attained prior to starting epoetin.[124] Antihypertensive agents should be added as necessary to maintain a stable blood pressure.
4. Epoetin dosage[124]: *Predialysis,* initiate at 90–120 U/kg subcutaneously once per week; *Hemodialysis,* initiate at 30–60 U/kg intravenously three times per week or 30–45 U/kg subcutaneously three times per week; *Chronic ambulatory peritoneal dialysis,* initiate subcutaneously at 30–45 U/kg three times per week, 45–60 U/kg twice per week, or 90–120 U/kg once per week.
5. Pharmacodynamic principles: Once epoetin is initiated, the initial hematocrit/hemoglobin response may be delayed for approximately 2 weeks, although the reticulocyte count will increase almost immediately. There is a large interpatient variability in response to epoetin, which results in a wide normal dosing range. Following initiation of epoetin or any dose change, steady-state hematocrit levels will not be attained until one RBC life span has occurred (approximately 2 months). Therefore, epoetin doses should not be adjusted more often than every 3–4 weeks. Applying these same principles, serial hematocrit levels should be assessed during therapy and dosage adjustments should be made on trends in hematocrit over time. For example, if a patient initiated epoetin therapy in the past month and the slope of the line indicates the hematocrit will surpass the goal concentration range (30–36%) before 2 months of therapy have been completed, then the dose should be reduced to avoid overshooting, which could subsequently lead to holding the dose and "bouncing" hematocrit levels.

6. The rate of rise in hematocrit should not exceed four points in any 2-week period. Dosage should be adjusted downward if this occurs.
7. Goal hematocrit is 30–36%. Hematocrit levels should be drawn prior to hemodialysis, or anytime in peritoneal dialysis patients. For consistency, hematocrit levels should be drawn on the same day each week.
8. If the rate of rise in hematocrit is less than optimal (i.e., less than four points in 1 month), causes for epoetin resistance should be investigated. If no obvious reasons exist, then the dosage can be increased by approximately 25%.

If these simple guidelines are followed, the management of anemia in ESRD may be improved.

UREMIC BLEEDING

Pathophysiology

Renal failure is associated with a tendency to bleed. Bleeding complications are usually mild, but can result in major hemorrhagic events. The etiology of uremic bleeding is multifactorial (Table 44.5). The primary mechanisms underlying the hemostatic problem are platelet biochemical abnormalities and alterations in platelet–blood vessel wall interactions. Decreased platelet aggregation and adhesiveness have been shown in a number of studies.[159] In addition, there is a decreased plasma concentration and defective binding of the large multimer of von Willebrand factor, which results in abnormal platelet–blood vessel wall interactions. Normally platelets flow in a skimming pattern close to the vessel wall while RBCs occupy the center of the vessel, a situation that is ideal for platelet–vessel wall interaction. Anemia results in dispersion of platelets and RBCs during flow through vessels, which makes it difficult for primary hemostasis to occur.[160] Heparinization during dialysis procedures also increases risk of bleeding. In addition, dialysis patients often receive systemic anticoagulation (i.e., warfarin) or antiplatelet therapy (aspirin or ticlopidine) for prevention of access clotting or other cardiovascular problems.

TABLE 44.5. ETIOLOGY OF UREMIC BLEEDING

Platelet Defect
Circulating toxins
Imbalance in prostacyclin/thromboxane A_2
Decrease in ADP and serotonin
Increase in parathyroid hormone
Questionable abnormal vWF
Decreased platelet factor III
Increased platelet-derived levels of β-thromboglobulin
Anemia
Relative deficiency in erythropoietin
Shortened RBC life span
Blood loss
Iron, vitamin B_{12}, or folate deficiency
Antithrombotic Therapy
Heparinization during hemodialysis
Anticoagulant therapy for access clotting or other thrombotic disorder
Antiplatelet therapy for access clotting or other cardiovascular disorder

Clinical Consequences

Uremic patients commonly experience purpura, ecchymoses, epistaxis, and prolonged bleeding from hemodialysis venipuncture sites. Gastrointestinal bleeding occurs less commonly, but can be severe and is often related to GI telangiectasias. Other severe hemorrhagic complications such as spontaneous retroperitoneal bleeding, hemorrhagic pericarditis or pleural effusion occur less frequently.[125] Subdural hematoma, which may occur in up to 3% of hemodialysis patients,[125] should be suspected with symptoms of headache, vomiting, seizures, somnolence, confusion, or coma. Risk factors for subdural bleeding include head trauma or hypertension. The bleeding time is the clinical test that is most often prolonged in uremia. This test measures the time required for bleeding from a small standardized skin puncture site to cease. Filter paper is used to wipe off the blood from the incision every 30 seconds.[123] This test reflects primary hemostatic function and measures interaction between platelets and the vessel wall following injury. The normal bleeding time averages 4–5 minutes (range 2–9 minutes).[123] Unfortunately, this test has not been found to be useful in predicting the risk of bleeding in individual patients.[161]

Therapeutic Management

A number of studies have shown that dialysis therapy shortens the bleeding time, but the effect is short lived (1–2 days) and usually only partial.[160] Marked improvement in bleeding times have been found in patients whose hematocrit was corrected to above 30% with epoetin and iron therapy. The proposed mechanism is enhanced interaction between platelets and the blood vessel wall. Patients receiving warfarin anticoagulation need to be followed closely for clinical signs of bleeding; the international normalized ratio (INR) should be routinely evaluated. Patients receiving antibiotics (a common scenario in ESRD) need intensified monitoring for early detection of antibiotic-associated increases in INR.

Swartz and Port described a system to classify risk of hemorrhage in dialysis patients.[162] Patients at high risk for bleeding can undergo alternative dialysis procedures rather than traditional hemodialysis with systemic heparinization. Dialytic techniques with less risk of bleeding include peritoneal dialysis; hemodialysis with minimal heparinization, regional heparinization, or regional citrate anticoagulation; or hemodialysis without heparinization. A recent review describes each procedure in detail.[125]

Several nondialytic adjunctive therapies are available that may temporarily shorten the increased bleeding time observed in patients with renal failure.[125,159,160,163] Cryoprecipitate is rich in factor VIII, fibrinogen, and fibronectin, and it has been shown to shorten bleeding time in CRF patients. Based on positive results with cryoprecipitate, IV infusions of 1-deamino-8-*D*-arginine vasopressin (DDAVP) were evaluated. DDAVP has minimal vasoconstrictive effects compared to vasopressin, but effectively releases autologous factor VIII (von Willebrand factor, vWF) from the endothelial lining of vessel walls. Again a consistent lowering of bleeding time was noted. A drawback to the use of DDAVP is tachyphylaxis with repeated doses; response may return after 3–4 days. This effect is felt to be due to depletion of vWF stores following the first dose. Side effects of DDAVP are minimal and include mild flushing, headache, or hyponatremia. Based on the observation that women with von Willebrand disease improved during pregnancy, estrogens were evaluated and been shown to reduce bleeding time in uremic subjects.[164] The mechanism of action is unknown. Five daily IV infusions of conjugated estrogens have been demonstrated to have a prolonged effect on bleeding time. Oral conjugated estrogens have also been shown to be successful. Side effects, which are uncommon and usually mild, include hot flashes, nausea, vomiting, hypertension, gynecomastia, and loss of libido. An increased risk of thromboembolism may result from estrogen therapy especially with chronic use. Indications and dosage of each agent can be found in Table 44.6.

Evaluation of Therapeutic Outcomes

Each agent previously discussed has a place in the therapeutic management of uremic bleeding. The onset of action, maximal response, and duration of action of each therapeutic entity is found in Table 44.6. Preoperative and high-risk patients with uremia should have their bleeding times and other measures of coagulation (INR, aPTT, and platelet counts) assessed. Abnormal bleeding times should be corrected with DDAVP and cryoprecipitate if a rapid effect is desired, and estrogens should be used in situations where prolonged bleeding risk is a consideration. Alternative dialytic procedures can be performed in patients with high bleeding risk.

HYPERLIPIDEMIA

Pathophysiology

Chronic renal failure with or without nephrotic syndrome is frequently accompanied by abnormalities in lipoprotein metabolism. In chronic renal failure without nephrotic syndrome, type IV hyperlipidemia with hypertriglyceridemia (plasma concentrations 200–600 mg/dL) secondary to increased plasma concentrations of very low-density lipoprotein (VLDL) is commonly seen. In addition, normal to modest increases in total cholesterol (TC) and low-density lipoprotein (LDL) and reductions in high-density lipoprotein (HDL) concentrations and variable affects on apoproteins (reduction in apo A-I, A-II, and E and elevations in apo B and lipoprotein [a]) may accompany hypertriglyceridemia.[165] In part, lipid abnormalities in ESRD may result from reduced plasma clearance of triglyceride-rich lipoproteins secondary to inhibition of peripheral lipoprotein lipase and hepatic triglyceride lipase activity.[166] Peripheral insulin resistance, carnitine deficiency, and

TABLE 44.6. MANAGEMENT OF UREMIC BLEEDING

Indication	Agent	Effect: Start	Maximum	End	Dosage
Long-term management	Adequate dialysis	—	—	—	—
	Epoetin	10 days	2–3 months	—	See section on Anemia of Chronic Renal Failure. Goal: Hct >30%
Acute bleeding episodes	Packed RBC transfusion	Immediate	—	—	Goal: Hct >30%
	DDAVP	1–2 hours	2–4 hours	6–8 hours	0.3 μg/kg IV
	Conjugated estrogens	6 hours	5–7 days	21–30 days	0.6 mg/kg IV each day × 5 days
Life-threatening bleeding	Cryoprecipitate	1 hour	4–12 hours	24–36 hours	10 "bags" IV
Chronic treatment of telangiectasias	Estrogen/progestin combinations	6 hours	5–7 days	—	Various products and dosages used in studies
Management of chronic bleeding tendency	Conjugated estrogens	6 hours	5–7 days	—	50 mg orally each day; only studied short term (<2 weeks)

hyperparathyroidism may also contribute to lipid abnormalities.[166]

In the nephrotic syndrome, the major lipid abnormalities are elevation of plasma total and LDL cholesterol with variable changes in HDL cholesterol.[167,168] The proposed mechanisms involved in dyslipidemia of the nephrotic syndrome are outlined in Fig. 44.18.[168]

Clinical Consequences

Clearly, patients with chronic renal failure are at increased risk from cardiovascular mortality. "Myocardial infarction" and "other cardiac causes" are the most commonly reported causes of death in the ESRD population.[4] Whether hypertriglyceridemia or other lipoprotein changes per se contribute to the high incidence of cardiovascular disease in these patients is controversial. Clearly, other concomitant risk factors such as diabetes, smoking, hypertension, and left ventricular enlargement are often present before patients initiate dialysis therapies. In addition, hypertriglyceridemia alone has not been shown to be a strong independent risk factor for coronary heart disease in patients with normal renal function following multivariate analysis of several studies.[169,170] However, high triglyceride concentrations are known to raise the concentrations of other lipoproteins that do promote atherogenesis, including chylomicron remnants, VLDL remnants, intermediate-density lipoproteins, and small, dense LDL.[171] Finally, hypertriglyceridemia may reduce levels of "protective" HDL, which is now classified as a major risk factor for coronary heart disease.[169] Thus, while hypertriglyceridemia per se may not be atherogenic, it may increase coronary risk through its effects on other lipoproteins.

Although several reports claim that patients with nephrotic syndrome are at increased risk for coronary artery disease, conflicting data also exist.[168] Unfortunately, no prospective randomized human clinical trials have been designed to evaluate cardiovascular outcome following therapeutic interventions for hyperlipidemia in nephrotic syndrome. Thus, the extent to which hyperlipidemia contributes to cardiovascular disease in patients with the nephrotic syndrome remains unknown.

Therapeutic Management

Dietary restriction of carbohydrate and cholesterol combined with an increase in the polyunsaturated to saturated fat ratio can reduce plasma triglycerides in some patients.[172] Unfortunately, most patients with chronic renal insufficiency and those receiving dialysis have already been advised to adhere to difficult dietary regimens, which may include protein, phosphorus, sodium, potassium, and fluid restrictions as well as diabetic exchanges. Although diet therapy is a reasonable first step approach, it is unlikely to be successful in a majority of renal disease patients due to noncompliance.

Many nephrologists find dietary modification or use of triglyceride-lowering agents difficult to justify in hypertriglyceridemic chronic renal failure patients because (1) the specific contribution of hypertriglyceridemia to increased coronary artery disease risk in this condition is unknown, (2) a beneficial effect of drugs for reducing coronary artery disease risk in this condition has not been demonstrated, and (3) long-term drug safety has not been proven. However, it also has not been proven that patients with renal disease are more or less prone to the atherogenic effects of abnormal lipoprotein patterns. In the absence of solid data in this population, it seems prudent to follow the guidelines set forth by the National Cholesterol Education Program Expert Panel[169] (Chapter 21). The panel recommends nonpharmacologic treatment (weight reduction, alcohol restriction, and increased exercise) for all patients with elevated triglycerides. Drug therapy is probably indicated for triglyceride concentrations greater than 1000

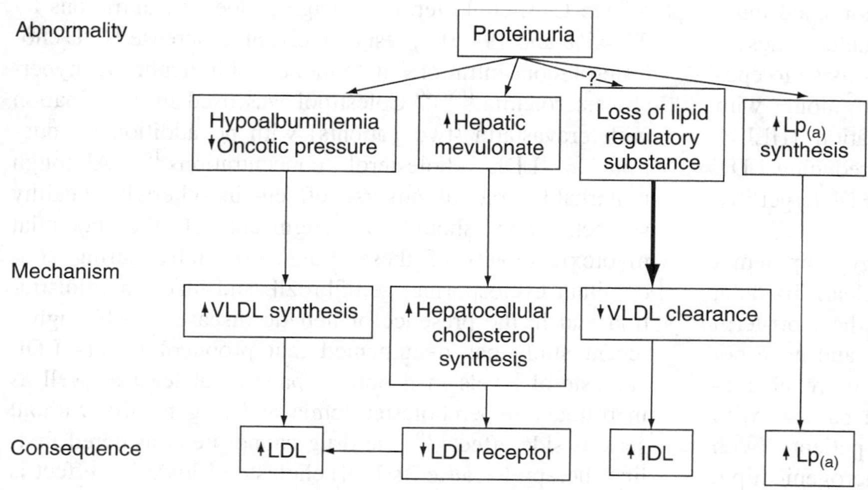

Figure 44.18. Potential effects of proteinuria on hyperlipidemia in the nephrotic syndrome. *(From Keane WF, St. Peter JV, Kasiske BL. Is the aggressive management of hyperlipidemia in nephrotic syndrome mandatory? Kidney Int 1992;42(suppl 38):S136, with permission.)*

mg/dL to prevent pancreatitis. For patients with "atherogenic" lipoprotein abnormalities, drug therapy may also be indicated.

Several studies have documented the triglyceride-lowering effect of clofibrate and gemfibrozil in chronic renal failure patients.[165,173–175] However, myositis and myalgias along with increased serum creatine phosphokinase (CPK) have been reported in renal failure patients using clofibrate.[176] Determining the optimal dose of clofibrate in this patient population is difficult because plasma protein-binding changes markedly affect free concentrations of the active metabolite, clofibric acid, which has a prolonged half-life in renal failure.[177] Gemfibrozil may be a safer alternative because the half-life is not altered in renal dysfunction.[178] However, some investigators have reported significant increases in CPK concentrations following usual doses of gemfibrozil in dialysis patients,[174,175] which has led some authors to suggest lower doses of 300 mg bid with close monitoring of CPK levels.[173,174]

The safety and efficacy of 3-hydroxy-3-methylglutaryl-coenzyme A reductase inhibitors (HMG-CoA) have been shown in hemodialysis and chronic ambulatory peritoneal dialysis with elevated total cholesterol levels and moderately elevated triglyceride levels.[179–181]Both lovastatin and simvastatin in usual doses effectively lowered LDL cholesterol by 30–41% and triglycerides by 5.5–29% and increased HDL cholesterol by 8–31.3% without significant side effects.

Large doses of omega-3 polyunsaturated fatty acids (fish oils) have been shown to lower triglyceride levels in hemodialysis patients[165,182] but they may interfere with platelet function, predisposing to bleeding. In addition, the high doses necessary to lower triglycerides makes noncompliance more likely. The effect of L-carnitine supplementation on abnormal lipid metabolism in dialysis patients has been assessed in several trials, however, the results have been contradictory. Although L-carnitine supplementation cannot be advocated at this time for hyperlipidemia treatment, carnitine may prove useful for dialysis-related muscle cramps or hypotension, lack of energy, skeletal muscle weakness, cardiomyopathy, or anemia unresponsive to epoetin.[183] Interestingly, reverse flux filtration along with heparin-induced extracorpeal LDL precipitation (HELP) during hemodialysis has been successful in reducing LDL cholesterol in hemodialysis patients with type IIb hyperlipidemia.[184]

The best approach to the treatment of hyperlipidemia in patients with nephrotic syndrome is unclear. To date, clinical trials have been designed to evaluate the short-term efficacy and safety of diet and drug therapy and have not been designed to define effects on cardiac or renal endpoints.[168] However, if clinical experience in patients with hyperlipidemia can be extrapolated to patients with nephrotic syndrome, then patients with atherogenic lipid profiles should be treated. Reductions of 20–25% in total and LDL cholesterol have been reported with strict soy-based vegetarian low cholesterol and fat diets[185] but short-term use of the American Heart Association step 1 diet has only minimal effects.[168,186] Step II diet therapy as recommended by the National Cholesterol Education Program Expert Panel may be a reasonable first step in management[169]; however, if LDL cholesterol reduction is suboptimal after 6 months of intensive diet therapy, lipid-lowering drugs should be added.

Five drug classes may prove useful as hypocholesterolemic therapies in nephrotic syndrome: the bile acid sequestrants, nicotinic acid, HMG-CoA reductase inhibitors, fibric acids, and probucol. Bile acid sequestrants are able to lower LDL cholesterol concentrations in patients with nephrotic syndrome, with decreases usually in the range of 19–32%.[168] However, absolute LDL cholesterol concentrations remained markedly elevated even with high doses of the resins, and triglyceride concentrations tend to rise. The nonselective binding activity of these agents may reduce absorption of corticosteroids, digoxin, thiazide diuretics, warfarin, and other commonly used medications. Bile acid sequestrants as monotherapy in nephrotic syndrome hyperlipidemia appear to be inadequate, however, they may be useful in combination with other agents.

Gemfibrozil (fibric acid derivative) has been evaluated alone and in combination with bile acid sequestrants in nephrotic hyperlipidemia.[168] Marginal lowering of total and LDL cholesterol was demonstrated with gemfibrozil alone. Colestipol in combination (three patients) produced further reductions in LDL cholesterol, but negated the positive effect on HDL cholesterol and reduced the triglyceride lowering effect. Although nicotinic acid has theoretical advantages for nephrotic patients, the drug has not been systematically studied for this purpose. It also exhibits a variety of adverse effects that may mitigate its usefulness.

Recent studies have suggested that HMG-CoA reductase inhibitors (lovastatin, simvastatin, and pravastatin) can reduce LDL cholesterol and triglyceride concentrations by 27–45% and 19–40%, respectively, and increase HDL cholesterol concentrations in patients with nephrotic hypercholesterolemia.[168,186] Colestipol was used in combination with pravastatin (two patients) with no additional reduction in LDL cholesterol concentrations.[186] Although remarkably free of adverse effects in otherwise healthy subjects, one should be cognizant of the potential myotoxic effects of these drugs, especially during concomitant cyclosporine, gemfibrozil, and niacin administration and in the presence of hepatic disease.[187] Although a recent study has documented that probucol lowers LDL cholesterol levels in nephrotic patients at least as well as in primary hypercholesterolemia and is generally without serious side effects,[168] the drug cannot be considered first-line therapy because its LDL cholesterol-lowering effect is modest at best.

Combined drug therapy has provided enhanced efficacy in primary dyslipidemia but has not been studied systematically in nephrotic hypercholesterolemia. Bile acid sequestrants combined with nicotinic acid (often poorly tolerated), gemfibrozil, or HMG-CoA reductase inhibitors may be useful in these patients. Probucol plus HMG-CoA reductase inhibitor therapy may be a third-line alternative combination.

Evaluation of Therapeutic Outcomes

Clearly, large-scale placebo-controlled prospective clinical trials of diet and antihyperlipidemic drug therapy are necessary in patients with nephrotic syndrome to determine if long-term treatment affects coronary artery disease risk and morbidity in this patient population. Clinical trials that evaluate the risk of hypertriglyceridemia as a primary risk factor for coronary heart disease need to be completed in the general adult population. Until these types of data are available, the following recommendations seem prudent. Nonpharmacologic treatment (weight reduction, alcohol restriction, and increased exercise) should be initiated for all patients with hypertriglyceridemia alone. Patients with triglyceride concentrations >1000 mg/dL after 3–6 months of nonpharmacologic treatment should begin gemfibrozil 300 mg bid with dose titration upward if necessary (CPK concentrations permitting) to prevent pancreatitis. Nonnephrotic patients with atherogenic concentrations of LDL cholesterol and other risk factors for coronary artery disease should be initiated on HMG-CoA reductase inhibitors. Dosages should be titrated per National Cholesterol Education Program (NCEP) Panel guidelines for LDL cholesterol concentrations.[169] Nephrotic patients with elevated LDL cholesterol should be initiated on a step II diet and/or drug therapy based on NCEP Panel guidelines.[169] HMG-CoA reductase inhibitors appear to be a good first choice, with addition of fibric acid derivatives, bile resins, or niacin as appropriate.

HYPERTENSION IN CHRONIC RENAL FAILURE AND END-STAGE RENAL DISEASE

In sharp contrast to the decrease in prevalence of stroke and coronary heart disease during the last two decades, ESRD prevalence appears to be increasing.[18] Hypertension was thought to be the underlying cause of ESRD in more than one-fourth of new cases from 1989–1992,[4] although the diagnosis of hypertensive ESRD is one of exclusion and no pathologic data corroborate this classification. In one multivariate analysis, poorly controlled hypertension, black race, and lack of health insurance were independently associated with the incidence of hypertensive ESRD.[18] Treatment and/or prevention of risk factors, including hypertension, may impact the prevalence and enormous cost of ESRD treatment. The pathogenesis and treatment of hypertension are reviewed in detail in another section of this text, therefore the present discussion focuses on pathogenesis and therapeutic management of hypertension in patients with chronic renal failure and ESRD.

Pathogenesis

The kidney has a dual role in hypertension. It can be a cause or a consequence of renal insufficiency. High blood pressure may also promote renal damage independently of the underlying mechanism of renal disease. The major pressor mechanisms are inappropriate activation of the renin–angiotensin system and an abnormal pressure–natriuresis relationship.[188] Several morphologic changes, collectively termed hypertensive nephrosclerosis, have been noted in kidneys of patients with essential hypertension. Seventy-five to 90% of patients initiating dialysis for ESRD are hypertensive. The pathogenesis is multifactorial but the majority of hypertensive dialysis patients have a volume component to blood pressure elevation (i.e., fluid retention promotes high blood pressure).[189] In addition to the pathogenic factors previously listed for chronic renal insufficiency, erythropoietin use and structural changes in the arteries (e.g., metastatic calcification) may contribute to hypertension in the ESRD patient.

Clinical Consequences

High blood pressure can accelerate the rate of decline in renal function (see section on Progressive Nature of Renal Disease) and cause other end-organ damage.[12] In addition, hypertension is a risk factor for the severe atherosclerosis and cardiovascular disease noted in ESRD.[190] Unfortunately, hypertension may not be adequately controlled in a significant number of ESRD patients.[191]

Therapeutic Management

Chronic Renal Failure

Unresolved issues in the management of hypertension in chronic renal failure patients include the degree of reduction in blood pressure that is necessary to benefit the kidney and whether reduction of blood pressure to values within the normal range would be helpful. In addition, the issues of control of systemic versus intraglomerular pressure and the potential benefit of specific agents remain to be answered. In 1991, the National High Blood Pressure Education Program provided a consensus document on the treatment of blood pressure in CRF.[192] Special attention should be paid to hypertensive black patients, those with CRF or diabetes, and the elderly—groups who are at the highest risk of progression to ESRD if left untreated. Blood pressure control was defined as less than 140/90; further reductions to <130/85 in patients with renal insufficiency may be beneficial.[192]

It is important to realize that precipitous falls in blood pressure to normotensive levels may be acutely deleterious to renal function in patients with impaired renal function. This may be especially problematic in the patient treated for hypertensive crisis. Target blood pressure[12] should be achieved reasonably slowly so as to allow adaptation to reduced perfusion pressures. In addition, it is preferable to use antihypertensive agents that maintain renal blood flow and thus do not contribute to declining renal function. Table 44.1 outlines the effects of various antihypertensive agents on renal blood flow and glomerular filtration rate.[44]

Diuretics are commonly used to treat fluid overload and hypertension in patients with impaired renal function. They may be particularly suited for treatment of the renally compromised older patient who tends to have salt-sensitive blood pressure.[193] Diuretic therapy is clearly indicated in the patient with volume overload or in patients with fluid retention secondary to other antihypertensive agents. As creatinine clearance falls below 20 to 30 mL/min, the thiazide-like diuretics lose their saluretic action but still maintain a modest antihypertensive effect, possibly because of vasodilation.[194] Saluresis in these patients can be maintained through the use of potent loop diuretics such as furosemide, torsemide, or bumetanide. As creatinine clearance declines further, these agents may become ineffective saliuretics as well. In such patients, a combination of a loop diuretic plus a thiazide diuretic or metolazone may prove beneficial,[195] although close clinical and laboratory monitoring should be undertaken to prevent the profound dehydration and metabolic derangements that may ensue.[195,196] Potassium-sparing diuretics such as spironolactone, triamterene, and amiloride should be used with extreme caution or not at all in patients with renal impairment because of the risk of hyperkalemia. Triamterene should probably be avoided in renally impaired patients also receiving nonsteroidal anti-inflammatory drugs (NSAIDs) because of the potential risk of precipitating more severe renal impairment.[197]

Extensive experience with ACEI in hypertensive patients with chronic renal failure has been documented recently (see section on Progressive Nature of Renal Disease). These drugs effectively lower blood pressure and may reduce proteinuria and/or slow the rate of decline in renal function in many patients with chronic renal failure. However, hyperkalemia can complicate their use especially in diabetics and/or those concurrently using nonsteroidal anti-inflammatory agents.[12] With the exception of fosinopril, the half-lives of all ACEI (or active metabolites) are prolonged in renal failure and lower doses may suffice.[198]

The calcium channel blocking agents are also effective in the treatment of hypertension in patients with chronic renal failure.[47] As with the ACEI, there is some experimental data that suggest that this class of drugs may slow the rate of decline of renal function in chronic renal failure (see section on Progressive Nature of Renal Disease). Dosage alterations are unnecessary in renal insufficiency.

Oral and transdermal clonidine has been used with some success in patients with renal insufficiency.[199] Although the bioavailability of the transdermal system has not been evaluated in CRF, plasma concentrations are comparable to that achieved with oral dosing.[199] Patients who respond to oral clonidine should maintain blood pressure control when switched to equivalent dosages of the transdermal patch. There are no data available to determine if clonidine is useful in retarding renal failure progression.

Alpha-1-adrenoceptor antagonists (prazosin, terazosin, doxazosin) are well tolerated and reduce blood pressure in short-term clinical trials in patients with renal insufficiency.[200] Again, currently no data are available on usefulness in preventing renal failure progression.

Although advocated as first- or second-line therapy in the treatment of essential hypertension,[12] β-blocking agents, with the exception of nadolol and labetolol,[201,202] may reduce renal blood flow secondary to a reduction in cardiac output in patients with renal failure although a deterioration in the GFR is uncommon. Hydrophilic β blockers such as nadolol, acebutolol, and atenolol are mainly eliminated via urinary excretion of unchanged drug and may require significant dosage adjustment with progressive renal failure.

Minoxidil with concurrent β-adrenoceptor-blocking agents and diuretics (to control tachycardia and fluid retention, respectively) have been shown to effectively lower blood pressure long term in antihypertensive resistant patients with renal insufficiency.[203] However, it is unclear if minoxidil reduces the rate of decline in renal function.

End-Stage Renal Disease

Achievement of an individual's "dry weight" and control of total body sodium through the dialytic process results in normalization of blood pressure in 50–60% of dialysis patients.[189] The percentage of dialysis patients considered to have dialysis-resistant hypertension requiring antihypertensive medications varies considerably depending on the approach of the specific dialysis unit or physician, demographic differences, differences in the definition of hypertension in dialysis patients, and the patient's primary disease. In general, antihypertensive medications will control elevated blood pressure in the vast majority of these individuals, with bilateral nephrectomy rarely being employed today.

The major initial effort in treating hypertension in ESRD is to restrict salt (2–3 grams per day) and water intake to reduce fluid volume accumulation between dialysis sessions. Massive doses of loop diuretics are generally ineffective in promoting diuresis and expose the patient to risks of ototoxicity, GI upset, muscle cramps, and hyperglycemia.

Patients in whom salt and water restriction and aggressive dialysis therapy fail to control high blood pressure may benefit from treatment with ACE inhibition in light of the important role of the renin–angiotensin axis in the etiology of dialysis-resistant hypertension. Since the elimination half-lives of the parent compound (captopril, lisinopril) or active metabolite (enalapril, benazepril, ramipril) are prolonged in ESRD patients, downward adjustment of doses is usually necessary.[189,198] Bone marrow depression has been noted in up to 10% of renal failure subjects receiving captopril, especially those with autoimmune diseases.[189] If captopril therapy is initiated in the dialysis patient, close monitoring of white blood cell counts should be undertaken and drug doses kept as low as possible. Other ACEI, which lack the sulfhydryl group of captopril, may be less likely to cause bone marrow depression and are probably the ACEI of choice in these patients.

Calcium channel blockers, particularly the dihydropyridines, which selectively lower systemic vascular resistance, also appear to be effective in the treatment of hypertension in the ESRD patient. In one study, nitrendipine lowered blood pressure effectively in hemodialysis patients with large interdialytic weight gains.[204] This is similar to the observation that a high sodium intake enhances the blood pressure response to calcium channel blockade in essential hypertension. Thus, either ACE inhibition or calcium channel blocker therapy would be appropriate first-line therapy in the hypertensive ESRD patient in whom achievement of their goal postdialysis weight (i.e., dry weight) is inadequate to control blood pressure.

A number of other antihypertensive drugs may also be effective in patients with ESRD, including drugs that interfere with renin release such as the β blockers or the combined α- and β-blocker labetolol. The choice of β blocker in dialysis patients should take into account the alterations in drug pharmacokinetics with ESRD and the effect of the dialysis procedure. Agents such as esmolol, timolol, pindolol, metoprolol, or labetalol, which are metabolized and not significantly dialyzable, may be easier to dose titrate than agents that are both dialyzable and extensively eliminated unchanged by the kidney (atenolol, nadolol, or acebutolol).[190]

Sympathetic nervous system active agents such as prazosin, terazosin, doxazosin, clonidine, guanabenz, or guanfacine may be required in patients unresponsive to dialytic therapy plus ACEI, calcium channel blocker, or β-blocker therapy. Central α_2 agonists such as clonidine appear to be the safest of these agents to use in the dialysis population. Transdermal clonidine in doses up to 1.2 mg/d (four 0.3-mg patches) has demonstrated success as monotherapy in one short-term study of hypertensive dialysis patients.[205] Postsynaptic α blockers (e.g., prazosin) have been associated with postural hypotension following hemodialysis.[206] Guanethidine and methyldopa should also be avoided because of potential complications including severe postural hypotension, severe dialysis-related hypotension, and impotence.[189]

The addition of vasodilators such as minoxidil or hydralazine may prove useful in patients resistant to combinations of the previously mentioned agents. Hydralazine is often effective as first-line therapy for hypertension and is generally well tolerated. In addition, monotherapy with the drug is well tolerated in diabetic patients because of the underlying autonomic neuropathy that prevents reflex tachycardia. The incidence of drug-induced systemic lupus erythematosus (SLE) does not appear to be increased by the presence of ESRD. Minoxidil therapy may be associated with a profound reflex tachycardia and most patients should receive a β blocker or a central α adenoreceptor agonist to suppress this.

Therapeutic Outcomes

A treatment algorithm for chronic renal insufficiency and ESRD patients with hypertension can be found in Figure 44.19. Other guidelines for antihypertensive therapy selection based on other patient characteristics can be found in the Joint National Committee (JNC) V report.[12] Gradual achievement of normotension in patients with chronic renal insufficiency may delay the progression of renal disease and ultimately reduce the prevalence of hypertensive patients who require dialytic therapy. The relative safety of ACEI and their ability to slow the rate of decline in renal function in diabetic patients with micro- or macro-proteinuria makes them the primary option for control of hypertension in diabetic chronic renal insufficiency patients. Prolonged antihypertensive therapy with a combination of β blockers, ACEI, and calcium channel blockers has clearly been shown to cause regression of left ventricular hypertrophy in hypertensive ESRD patients.[207] They also may be useful in patients with connective tissue diseases.[208]

Other considerations in selection of antihypertensive therapy in CRF and ESRD should include patient compliance and economic factors. In general, most ESRD patients are prescribed an average of 10 medications. Choosing agents that can be administered once or twice daily may improve patient compliance. In addition, there are now many selections within some antihypertensive classes such as calcium channel blockers (dihydropyridine structure), ACEI, and β blockers. In most cases, no clear therapeutic advantage has been demonstrated with any particular agent within a class. Therefore, selecting the least costly agent that can be administered once or twice daily should have a favorable economic impact over the lifetime of the patient.

MISCELLANEOUS THERAPEUTIC CONSIDERATIONS

Pruritus

Despite advances in dialysis treatment, pruritus (itching) remains a vexing problem that occurs in up to 86% of ESRD patients. Uremic pruritus is a manifestation of chronic but not acute renal failure.[209] The pathogenesis of

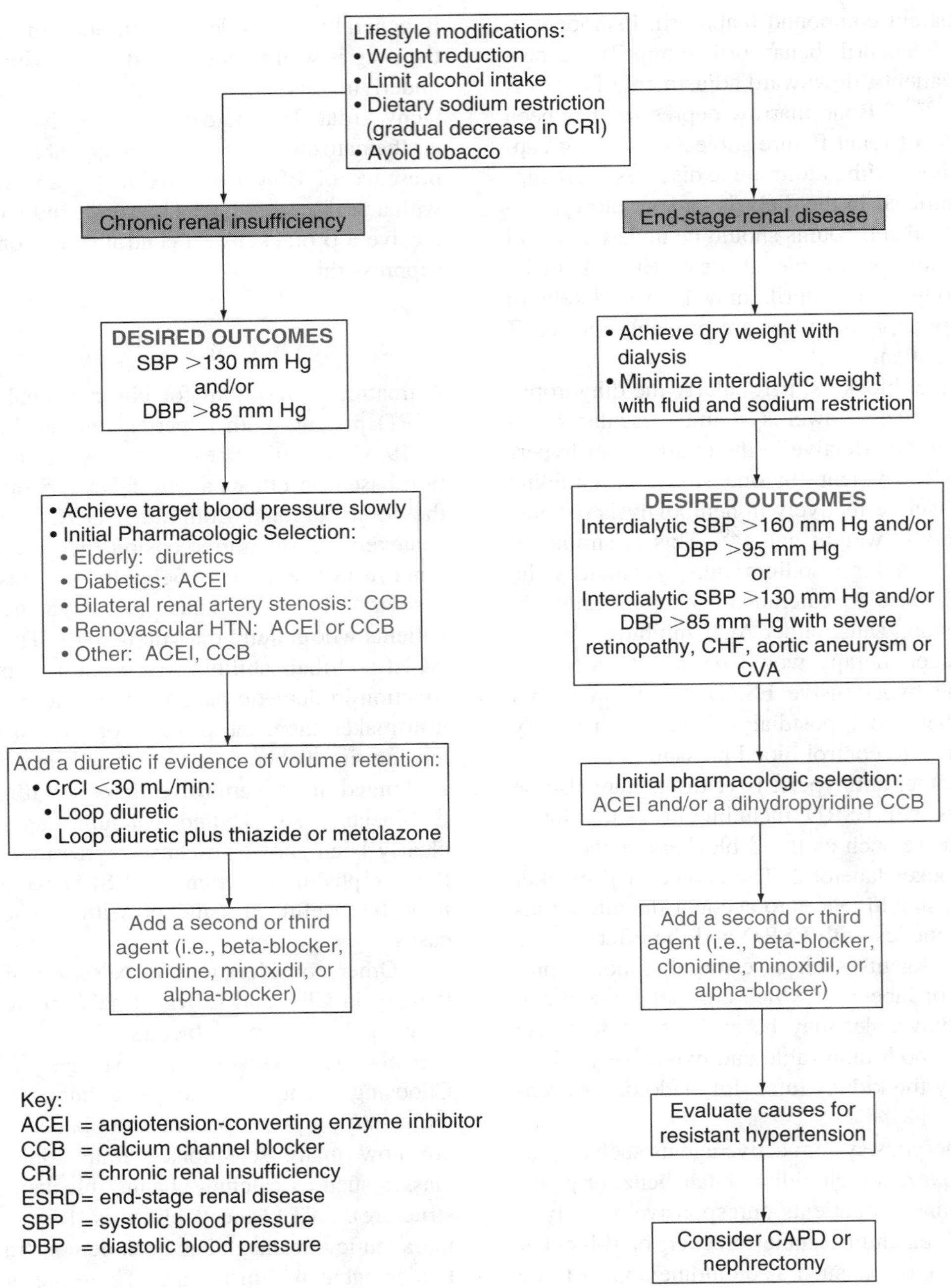

Figure 44.19. Treatment algorithm for chronic renal insufficiency and ESRD patients with hypertension.

uremic pruritus is poorly understood, but has been attributed to multiple factors such as skin dryness, secondary hyperparathyroidism, increased vitamin A and histamine plasma concentrations, and increased sensitivity to histamine.[209] A small study in hemodialysis and peritoneal dialysis patients showed that patients with pruritus demonstrated higher numbers of degranulated mass cells compared to patients without pruritus. In addition, higher concentrations of histamine, PTH, and middle molecular weight substances and lower serum iron concentrations were seen in patients with pruritus.[210] Uremic patients with pruritus experience exaggerated itching sensation to exogenous administration of histamine as compared with uremic patients with no pruritus or control patients.[209]

Therapy for pruritus is largely empirical. Strategies have included antihistamines, lidocaine, heparin, cholestyramine, parathyroidectomy, and ultraviolet phototherapy. Even though elevated plasma histamine concentrations and exaggerated responses to histamine have been noted in uremic patients with pruritus, antihistamine treatment often fails to reduce symptoms. In fact, no single therapy has proven more effective than another in individual patients. Interestingly, epoetin therapy significantly reduced pruritus as compared to placebo in a small well-designed clinical trial.[211] Some specific strategies are outlined in Table 44.7.[210,212]

Vitamin Replacement

Vitamin requirements for ESRD patients receiving dialysis are different from that of a healthy person due to dietary modifications, renal dysfunction, and dialytic therapy.[135,213] Both vitamins A and E have been shown to be elevated in ESRD. Hypervitaminosis of vitamin A has been correlated with anemia and hypercalcemia (increased bone resorption) in hemodialysis patients. Vitamin K supplementation is probably unnecessary in most dialysis patients except for those with an elevated INR during or after a course of antibiotics. Vitamin D plays a major role in bone metabolism in uremia; the dose of 1,25-dihydroxyvitamin D_3 (calcitriol) needs to be individualized (see sections on Renal Osteodystrophy and Secondary Hyperparathyroidism). The water-soluble vitamins (B_1, B_2, B_6, B_{12}, niacin, pantothenic acid, folic acid, biotin, and vitamin C) have been shown to be low or deficient in the average Western diet. Some of the water-soluble vitamins are dialyzable, others such as vitamins C and B complex may be destroyed or the amounts reduced with cooking methods used by dialysis patients to leach out potassium. Vitamins B_6 (pyridoxine) and C (ascorbic acid) as well as folic acid are the three vitamins that have consistently been reported to be deficient in dialysis patients. Vitamin C is necessary for the normal production of oxalic acid. Higher concentrations of oxalate have been reported in hemodialysis patients receiving greater than 250 mg of vitamin C per day. Increased plasma concentrations of oxalate may lead to deposition in soft tissues, muscles, vessels, and organs. The goal for vitamin supplementation in this population should be to prevent subclinical and frank deficiency and to avoid pathology from overdosage. Table 44.8 outlines recommended allowances for ESRD patients.[213] Special vitamin supplements have been formulated for the dialysis patient, but these preparations are fairly costly. Lower cost vitamin B with C formulations are available, although additional folic acid supplementation is then necessary.

TABLE 44.7. MANAGEMENT OF UREMIC PRURITUS

- Antihistamine therapy
- Lidocaine 200 mg IV over 20 minutes during hemodialysis
- Activated charcoal orally 6 g/d
- Cholestryramine orally 5 g twice daily
- High-flux hemodialysis with polyacrylonitrile membrane
- Ultraviolet phototherapy
- Parathyroidectomy

TABLE 44.8. RECOMMENDED DAILY ALLOWANCE OF VITAMINS IN ESRD PATIENTS

Vitamin	Recommended Amounts
A	0
E	0
K	0
D	Individualized
B_1	1.5 mg
B_2	1.7 mg
B_6	10 mg
B_{12}	6 μg
Biotin	300 μg
Pantothenic acid	10 mg
Niacinamide	20 mg
Folic acid	0.8–1 mg
C	60 mg

References

1. Rennke HG, Anderson S, Brenner BM. The progression of renal disease: Structural and functional correlations, in Tisher CC, Brenner BM (eds): Renal Pathology: With Clinical and Functional Correlations. Philadelphia, JB Lippincott, 1994, pp 116–139.
2. Bricker NS, Fine LG. The trade-off hypothesis: Current status. Kidney Int 1978;13(suppl 8):S5–S8.
3. Levey AS. Measurement of renal function in chronic renal disease. Kidney Int 1990;38:167–184.
4. U.S. Renal Data System. USRDS 1995 Annual Report, NIH Publication No. 94–3176. Bethesda, MD, USRDS Coordinating Center, by the Renal Research Program of the Urban Institute, 1994.
5. Neuringer JR, Brenner BM. Hemodynamic theory of progressive renal disease: A 10-year update in brief review. Am J Kidney Dis 1993;22:98–104.
6. Hostetter TH. Mechanisms of diabetic nephropathy. Am J Kidney Dis 1994;23:188–192.
7. Inomata S. Renal hypertrophy as a prognostic index for the progression of diabetic renal disease in non–insulin-dependent diabetes mellitus. J Diab Comp 1993;7:28–33.
8. Nath KA. Tubulointerstitial changes as a major determinant in the progression of renal damage. Am J Kidney Dis 1992;20:1–17.

9. Mathiesen ER. Prevention of diabetic nephropathy—Microalbuminuria and perspectives for intervention in insulin-dependent diabetes. Dan Med Bull 1993;40:273–285.
10. Carella MJ, Gossain VV, Rovner DR. Early diabetic nephropathy—Emerging treatment options. Arch Intern Med 1994;154:625–630.
11. Breyer JA. Diabetic nephropathy in insulin-dependent patients. Am J Kidney Dis 1992;20:533–547.
12. The fifth report of the Joint National Committee on detection, evaluation and treatment of high blood pressure (JNC V). Arch Intern Med 1993;153:154–183.
13. Brown TER, Carter BL. Hypertension and end stage renal disease. Ann Pharmacother 1994;28:359–366.
14. Erley CM, Haefele U, Heyne N, et al. Microalbuminuria in essential hypertension—Reduction by different antihypertensive drugs. Hypertension 1993;21:810–815.
15. Scanferla F, Landini S, Fracasso A, et al. Risk factors for the progression of diabetic nephropathy: Role of hyperlipidemia and its correction. Acta Diabetol 1992;29:268–272.
16. Keane WF, Mulcahy WS, Kasiske BL, et al. Hyperlipidemia and progressive renal disease. Kidney Int 1991;39(suppl 31):S-41–S-48.
17. Walker WG. Relation of lipid abnormalities to progression of renal damage in essential hypertension, insulin-dependent and non–insulin-dependent diabetes mellitus. Miner Electrolyte Metab 1993;19:137–143.
18. Whelton PK, Perneger TV, Brancati FL, Klag MJ. Epidemiology and prevention of blood pressure-related renal disease. J Hypertens 1992;10(suppl 7):S77–S84.
19. Neuringer JR, Levey AS. Strategies to slow the progression of renal disease. Semin Nephrol 1994;14:261–273.
20. Borch-Johnsen K, Wenzel H, Viberti GC, Mogensen CE. Is screening and intervention for microalbuminuria worthwhile in patients with insulin dependent diabetes? BMJ 1993;306:1722–1725.
21. Bennett PH, Haffner S, Kasiske BL, et al. Screening and management of microalbuminuria in patients with diabetes mellitus: Recommendations to the Scientific Advisory Board of the National Kidney Foundation from an Ad Hoc Committee of the Council on Diabetes Mellitus of the National Kidney Foundation. Am J Kidney Dis 1995;25:107–112.
22. Wang PH, Lau J, Chalmers TC. Meta-analysis of effects of intensive blood-glucose control on late complications of type I diabetes. Lancet 1993;341:1306–1309.
23. Skyler JS. Awaiting the DCCT. Int Diab Monit 1993;5:1–4.
24. The Diabetes Control and Complications Trial Research Group. The effect of intensive treatment of diabetes on the development and progression of long-term complications in insulin-dependent diabetes mellitus. N Engl J Med 1993;329:977–986.
25. Santiago JV. Perspectives in diabetes—Lessons from the Diabetes Control and Complications Trial. Diabetes 1993;42:1549–1554.
26. Parving H-H. Impact of blood pressure and antihypertensive treatment on incipient and overt nephropathy, retinopathy and endothelial permability in diabetes mellitus. Diabetes Care 1991;14:260–269.
27. Hoelscher D. Bakris G. Antihypertensive therapy and progression of diabetic renal disease. J Cardiovasc Pharmacol 1994;23(suppl 1):S34–S38.
28. Dworkin LD, Benstein JA, Parker M, et al. Calcium antagonists and converting enzyme inhibitors reduce renal injury by different mechanisms. Kidney Int 1993;43:808–814.
29. Brown SA, Walton CL, Crawford P, et al. Long term effects of antihypertensive regimens on renal hemodynamics and proteinuria. Kidney Int 1992;43:1210–1218.
30. Kasiske BL, Kalil RSN, Ma JZ, et al. Effect of antihypertensive therapy on the kidney in patients with diabetes: A meta-regression analysis. Ann Intern Med 1993;118:129–138.
31. Lewis EJ, Hunsicker LG, Bain RP, Rohde RD. The effect of angiotensin-converting enzyme inhibition on diabetic nephropathy. N Engl J Med 1993;329:1456–1462.
32. Pohl MA. Changing the course of diabetic nephropathy: Angiotensin-converting enzyme inhibition in type I diabetic renal disease. Cleve Clin J Med 1994;61:38–42.
33. Ravid M, Savin H, Jutrin I, et al. Long-term stabilizing effect of angiotensin-converting enzyme inhibition on plasma creatinine and on proteinuria in normotensive Type II diabetic patients. Ann Intern Med 1993;118:577–581.
34. Ihle BU, Becker GJ, Whitworth JA, et al. The effect of protein restriction on the progression of renal insufficiency. N Engl J Med 1989;321:1773–1777.
35. Locatelli F, Alberti D, Graziani G, et al: Prospective, randomized, multicentre trial of effect of protein restriction on progression of chronic renal insufficiency. Lancet 1991;337:1299–1304.
36. Rosman JB, Langer K, Brandl M, et al: Protein-restricted diets in chronic renal failure: A four year follow-up shows limited indications. Kidney Int 1989:36(suppl 27): S96–S102.
37. Zeller K, Whittaker E, Sullivan L, et al. Effect of restricting dietary protein on the progression of renal failure in patients with insulin-dependent diabetes mellitus. N Engl J Med 1991;324:78–84.
38. Fouque D, Laville M, Boissel JP, et al. Controlled low protein diets in chronic renal insufficiency: Meta-analysis. BMJ 1992;304:216–220.
39. Modification of Diet in Renal Disease Study Group. The modification of diet in renal disease study: Design, methods, and results from the feasibility study. Am J Kidney Dis 1992;20:18–33.
40. Klahr S, Levey AS, Beck GJ, et al. The effects of dietary protein restriction and blood-pressure control on the progression of chronic renal disease. N Engl J Med 1994;330:877–884.
41. Klahr S. The modification of diet in renal disease study. N Engl J Med 1989;320:864–866.
42. Greene T, Bourgoignie J, Habwe V, et al. Baseline characteristics in the modification of diet in renal disease study. J Am Soc Nephrol 1993;3:1819–1834.
43. ter Wee PM, Epstein M. Angiotensin-converting enzyme inhibitors and progression of nondiabetic chronic renal disease. Arch Intern Med 1993;153:1749–1759.
44. Schlueter WA, Batlle DC. Renal effects of antihypertensive drugs. Drugs 1989;37:900–925.

45. Risler T, Krämer B, Müller GA. The efficacy of diuretics in acute and chronic renal failure: Focus on torasemide. Drugs 1991;41(suppl 3):69–79.
46. Jacobson HR, Striker GE. Report on a workshop to develop management recommendations for the prevention of progression in chronic renal disease. Am J Kidney Dis 1995;25:103–106.
47. Moreira J, Barata JD, Olias J. Antihypertensive action of calcium blockade in hypertensive patients with chronic renal disease. Nephron 1985;41:314–319.
48. Mitch WE, Wilcox CS. Disorders of body fluids, sodium and potassium in chronic renal failure. Am J Med 1982;72:536–550.
49. Emmanouel DS, Lindheimer MD, Katz AI. Pathogenesis of endocrine abnormalities in uremia. Endocr Rev 1980;1:28–44.
50. Moran J, Blumenstein M, Gurland HJ. Immunodeficiencies in chronic renal failure. Contrib Nephrol 1990;86:91–110.
51. Ruiz P, Gomez F, Schreiber AD. Impaired function of macrophage Fc_y receptors in end-stage renal disease. N Engl J Med 1990;322:717–722.
52. Danovitch GM, Bourgoignie J, Bricker NS. Reversibility of the "salt-losing" tendency of chronic renal failure. N Engl J Med 1977;296:14–19.
53. Allon M. Treatment and prevention of hyperkalemia in end-stage renal disease. Kidney Int 1993;43:1197–1209.
54. Salem MM, Rosa RM, Batlle DC. Extrarenal potassium tolerance in chronic renal failure: Implications for the treatment of acute hyperkalemia. Am J Kidney Dis 1991;18:421–440.
55. Solomon R, Dubey A. Diltiazem enhances potassium disposal in subjects with end-stage renal disease. Am J Kidney Dis 1992;19:420–426.
56. Giovannetti S, Cupisti A, Barsotti G. The metabolic acidosis of chronic renal failure: Pathophysiology and treatment. Contrib Nephrol 1992;100:48–57.
57. Kraut JA. The role of metabolic acidosis in the pathogenesis of renal osteodystrophy. Adv Renal Replacement Ther 1995;2:40–51.
58. Reaich D, Channon SM, Schrimgeour CM, et al. Correction of acidosis in humans with CRF decreases protein degradation and amino acid oxidation. Am J Physiol 1993;265(2 Pt 1):E230–E235.
59. Batlle D. Renal tubular acidosis. Med Clin North Am 1983;67:859–878.
60. Gennari JF. Acid–base balance in dialysis patients. Kidney Int 1985;28:678–688.
61. Sherrard DJ. Aplastic bone: A nondisease of medical progress. Adv Renal Replacement Ther 1995;2:20–23.
62. Sherrard DJ, Hercz G, Pei Y, et al. The spectrum of bone disease in end-stage renal failure—An evolving disorder. Kidney Int 1993;43:436–442.
63. Akizawa T, Fukagawa M, Koshikawa S, Kurokawa K. Recent progress in management of secondary hyperparathyroidism of chronic renal failure. Curr Opin Nephrol Hypertens 1993;2:558–565.
64. Slatopolsky E, Delmez JA. Pathogenesis of secondary hyperparathyroidism. Am J Kidney Dis 1994;23:229–236.
65. Coen G, Mazzaferro S. Bone metabolism and its assessment in renal failure. Nephron 1994;67:383–401.
66. Akmal M, Kasim SE, Soliman AR, Massry SG. Excess parathyroid hormone adversely affects lipid metabolism in chronic renal failure. Kidney Int 1990;37:854–858.
67. Parfitt AM. Soft-tissue calcification in uremia. Arch Intern Med 1969;124:544–556.
68. Malluche HH, Monier-Faugere M-C. Uremic bone disease: Current knowledge, controversial issues and new horizons. Miner Electrolyte Metab 1991;17:281–296.
69. Reichel H, Deibert B, Schmidt-Gayk H, Ritz E. Calcium metabolism in early chronic renal failure: Implications for the pathogenesis of hyperparathyroidism. Nephrol Dial Transplant 1991;6:162–169.
70. Solal M-EC, Sebert J-L, Boudailliez B, et al. Comparison of intact, midregion, and carboxy terminal assays of parathyroid hormone for the diagnosis of bone disease in hemodialyzed patients. J Clin Endocrinol Metab 1991;73:516–524.
71. DeVita MV, Rasenas LL, Bansal M, et al. Assessment of renal osteodystrophy in hemodialysis patients. Medicine 1992;71:284–290.
72. Ali AA, Varghese Z, Moorhead JF, et al. Calcium set point progressively worsens in hemodialysis patients despite conventional oral 1-α hydroxycholecalciferol supplementation. Clin Nephrol 1993;39:205–209.
73. Brookhyser J, Pahre SN. Dietary and pharmacotherapeutic considerations in the management of renal osteodystrophy. Adv Renal Replacement Ther 1995;2:5–13.
74. Cleary DJ, Matzke GM, Alexander AM, Joy MS. Medication knowledge and compliance among patients receiving long-term dialysis. Am J Health-Syst Pharm 1995;52:1895–1900.
75. Roxe DM, Mistovich M, Barch DH. Phosphate-binding effects of sulcralfate in patients with chronic renal failure. Am J Kidney Dis 1989;13:194–199.
76. Rudnicki M, Frolich A, Haaber A, et al. Serum ionized calcium, parathyroid hormone and phosphate in uremic patients during and between hemodialysis. Clin Nephrol 1993;40:225–229.
77. Jespersen B, Jensen JD, Nielsen HK, et al. Comparison of calcium carbonate and aluminum hydroxide as phosphate binders on biochemical bone markers, PTH(1-84), and bone mineral content in dialysis patients. Nephrol Dial Transplant 1991;6:98–104.
78. Fournier A, Morinière P, Hamida FB, et al. Use of alkaline calcium salts as phosphate binder in uremic patients. Kidney Int 1992;42(suppl 38):S-50–S-61.
79. Fournier A, Drüeke T, Morinière P, et al. The new treatments of hyperparathyroidism secondary to renal insufficiency. Adv Nephrol 1992;21:237–306.
80. Slatopolsky E, Weerts C, Lopez-Hilker S, et al. Calcium carbonate as a phosphate binder in patients with chronic renal failure undergoing dialysis. N Engl J Med 1986;315:157–161.
81. Kobrin SM, Goldstein SJ, Shangraw RF, Raja RM. Variable efficacy of calcium carbonate tablets. Am J Kidney Dis 1989;14:461–465.
82. Carr CJ, Shangraw RF. Nutritional and pharmaceutical aspects of calcium supplementation. Am Pharm 1987;NS27:49–57.

83. Schaefer K, Scheer J, Asmus G, et al. The treatment of uraemic hyperphosphataemia with calcium acetate and calcium carbonate: A comparative study. Nephrol Dial Transplant 1991;6:170–175.
84. Morinière P, Djerad M, Boudailliez B, et al. Control of predialytic hyperphosphatemia by oral calcium acetate and calcium carbonate. Nephron 1992;60:6–11.
85. Mai ML, Emmett M, Sheikh MS, et al. Calcium acetate, an effective phosphorus binder in patients with renal failure. Kidney Int 1989;36:690–695.
86. Meric F, Yap P, Bia MJ. Etiology of hypercalcemia in hemodialysis patients on calcium carbonate therapy. Am J Kidney Dis 1990;16:459–464.
87. Pflanz S, Henderson IS, McElduff N, Jones MC. Calcium acetate versus calcium carbonate as phosphate-binding agents in chronic haemodialysis. Nephrol Dial Transplant 1994;9:1121–1124.
88. Nolan CR, Califano JR, Butzin CA. Influence of calcium acetate or calcium citrate on intestinal aluminum absorption. Kidney Int 1990;38:937–941.
89. Molitoris BA, Froment DH, Mackenzie TA, et al. Citrate: A major factor in the toxicity of orally administered aluminum compounds. Kidney Int 1989;36:949–953.
90. Delmez JA, Slatopolsky E. Hyperphosphatemia: Its consequences and treatment in patients with chronic renal disease. Am J Kidney Dis 1992;19:303–317.
91. Oe PL, Lips P, van der Meulen J, et al. Long-term use of magnesium hydroxide as a phosphate binder in patients on hemodialysis. Clin Nephrol 1987;28:180–185.
92. Eastwood JB, Bordier PJ, Clarkson EM, et al. The contrasting effects on bone histology of vitamin D and of calcium carbonate in the osteomalacia of chronic renal failure. Clin Sci 1974;47:23–42.
93. Sakhaee K. Management of renal osteodystrophy. Semin Nephrol 1992;12:101–108.
94. Silver J, Naveh-Many T. Regulation of parathyroid hormone synthesis and secretion. Semin Nephrol 1994;14:175–194.
95. Felsenfeld AJ, Llach F. Parathyroid gland function in chronic renal disease. Kidney Int 1993;43:771–789.
96. Malberti F, Surian M, Cosci P. Effect of chronic intravenous calcitriol on parathyroid function and set point of calcium in dialysis patients with refractory secondary hyperparathyroidism. Nephrol Dial Transplant 1992;7:822–828.
97. Andress DL, Norris KC, Coburn JW, et al. Intravenous calcitriol in the treatment of refractory osteitis fibrosa of chronic renal failure. N Engl J Med 1989;321:274–279.
98. Tsukamoto Y, Nomura M, Takahashi Y, et al. The "oral 1,25-dihydroxyvitamin D_3 pulse therapy" in hemodialysis patients with severe secondary hyperparathyroidism. Nephron 1991;57:23–28.
99. Muramoto H, Haruki K, Yoshimura A, et al. Treatment of refractory hyperparathyroidism in patients on hemodialysis by intermittent oral administration of $1,25(OH)_2$ vitamin D_3. Nephron 1991;58:288–294.
100. Hyodo T, Ono K, Koumi T, et al. Can oral $1,25(OH)_2D_3$ pulse therapy reduce parathyroid hyperplasia? Nephron 1991;59:171–172.
101. Fischer ER, Harris DCH. Comparison of intermittent oral and intravenous calcitriol in hemodialysis patients with secondary hyperparathyroidism. Clin Nephrol 1993;40:216–220.
102. Quarles LD, Yohay DA, Carroll BA, et al. Prospective trial of pulse oral versus intravenous calcitriol treatment of hyperparathyroidism in ESRD. Kidney Int 1994;45:1710–1721.
103. Schaefer K, Umlauf E, von Herrath D. Reduced risk of hypercalcemia for hemodialysis patients by administering calcitriol at night. Am J Kidney Dis 1992;19:460–464.
104. Brown AJ, Dusso A, Slatopolsky E. Selective vitamin D analogs and their therapeutic applications. Semin Nephrol 1994;14:156–174.
105. Christiansen C, Rodbro P, Christensen MS, et al. Deterioration of renal function during treatment of chronic renal failure with 1,25-dihydroxycholecalciferol. Lancet 1978;2:700–703.
106. Chan JCM, Young RB, Alon U, Mamunes P. Hypercalcemia in children with disorders of calcium and phosphate metabolism during long-term treatment with 1,25-dihydroxyvitamin D_3. Pediatrics 1983;72:225–233.
107. Mazur AT, Norman ME. Effects of 25-OHD_3 on renal function in pediatric patients with chronic renal failure. Miner Electrolyte Metab 1984;10:351–358.
108. Hymes LC, Warshaw BL. Vitamin D replacement therapy and renal function. Am J Dis Child 1984;138:1125–1128.
109. Baker LRI, Abrams SML, Roe CJ, et al. $1,25(OH)_2D_3$ administration in moderate renal failure: A prospective double-blind trial. Kidney Int 1989;35:661–669.
110. Mallette LE, Eisenberg KL, Schwaitzberg SD, et al. Total parathyroidectomy and autogenous parathyroid graft replacement for treatment of hyperparathyroidism due to chronic renal failure. Am J Surg 1983;146:727–733.
111. Consensus Conference. Diagnosis and treatment of aluminium overload in end-stage renal failure patients. Nephrol Dial Transplant 1993;8(suppl 1):1–54.
112. Drüeke TB. Adynamic bone disease, anaemia, resistance to erythropoietin and iron-aluminium interaction. Nephrol Dial Transplant 1993;8(suppl 1):12–16.
113. Abreo K, Glass J. Cellular, biochemical, and molecular mechanisms of aluminum toxicity. Nephrol Dial Transplant 1993;8(suppl 1):5–11.
114. Ellenberg R, King AL, Sica DA, et al. Cerebrospinal fluid aluminium levels following deferoxamine. Am J Kidney Dis 1990;16:157–159.
115. Alfrey AC. Aluminum toxicity in patients with chronic renal failure. Ther Drug Monit 1993;15:593–597.
116. Mazzaferro S, Coen G, Ballanti P, et al. Deferoxamine test and PTH serum levels are useful not to recognize but to exclude aluminum-related bone disease. Nephron 1992;61:151–157.
117. Day JP, Ackrill P. The chemistry of desferrioxamine chelation for aluminum overload in renal dialysis patients. Ther Drug Monit 1993;15:598–601.
118. Bentur Y, McGuigan M, Koren G. Deferoxamine (desferrioxamine) new toxicities for an old drug. Drug Saf 1991;6:37–46.

119. Boelaert JR, de Locht M. Side-effects of desferrioxamine in dialysis patients. Nephrol Dial Transplant 1993;8(suppl 1):43–46.
120. McCarthy JT, Milliner DS, Johnson WJ. Clinical experience with desferrioxamine in dialysis patients with aluminum toxicity. Q J Med 1990;74:257–276.
121. Jelkmann W. Erythropoietin: Structure, control of production, and function. Physiol Rev 1992;72:449–489.
122. Koury ST, Koury MJ. Erythropoietin production by the kidney. Semin Nephrol 1993;13:78–86.
123. Paganini EP. Hematologic abnormalities, in Daugirdas JT, Ing TS (eds): Handbook of Dialysis. Boston, Little, Brown and Company, 1994, pp 445–468.
124. Paganini EP. Overview of anemia associated with chronic renal disease: Primary and secondary mechanisms. Semin Nephrol 1989;9(suppl 1):3–8.
125. Lohr JW, Schwab SJ. Minimizing hemorrhagic complications in dialysis patients. J Am Soc Nephrol 1991;2:961–975.
126. St. Peter WL, Mihalovic SM. Efficacy and utilization of erythropoietin before and after intravenous iron dextran availability [abstract]. Pharmacotherapy 1993;13:681.
127. Powe NR, Eggers PW, Johnson CB. Early adoption of cyclosporine and recombinant human erythropoietin: Clinical, economic, and policy issues with emergence of high-cost drugs. Am J Kidney Dis 1994;24:33–41.
128. Ballal SH, Domoto DT, Polack DC, et al. Androgens potentiate the effects of erythropoietin in the treatment of anemia of end-stage renal disease. Am J Kidney Dis 1991;17:29–33.
129. Berns JS, Rudnick MR, Cohen RM. A controlled trial of recombinant human erythropoietin and nandrolone decanoate in the treatment of anemia in patients on chronic hemodialysis. Clin Nephrol 1992;37:264–267.
130. Van Wyck DB. Iron management during recombinant human erythropoietin therapy. Am J Kidney Dis 1989;14(suppl 1): 9–13.
131. Alexander ACM, Matzke GR, Nespor C, Rault R. Clinical utility of three methods of iron needs assessment [abstract]. Pharmacotherapy 1994;14:366.
132. Van Wyck DB. Iron deficiency in patients with dialysis-associated anemia during erythropoietin replacement therapy: Strategies for assessment and management. Semin Nephrol 1989;9(suppl 2):21–24.
133. Anastassiades EG, Howarth D, Howarth J, et al. Monitoring of iron requirements in renal patients on erythropoietin. Nephrol Dial Transplant 1993;8:846–853.
134. Kleiner MJ, Van Wyck DB, Kaupke CJ, Kirlin LF. The role of iron and other factors in patients unresponsive to erythropoietin therapy. Semin Dialysis 1995;8:29–34.
135. Makoff R. Water-soluble vitamin status in patients with renal disease treated with hemodialysis or peritoneal dialysis. J Renal Nutrition 1991;1:56–73.
136. Henderson PA, Hillman RS. Characteristics of iron dextran utilization in man. Blood 1969;34:357–375.
137. Wood JK, Milner PFA, Pathak UN. The metabolism of iron-dextran given as a total-dose infusion to iron deficient Jamaican subjects. Brit J Haematol 1968;14:119–129.
138. Watson A. Iron management during treatment with recombinant human erythropoietin in chronic renal failure. J Clin Pharmacol 1993;33:1134–1138.
139. Rault R, Nespor S, Holley J. Safety and efficacy of 500 mg of iron-dextran as a single IV infusion in patients on chronic dialysis [abstract]. ASAIO Trans 1994;23:74.
140. Rao KV, Anderson WR. Hemosiderosis and hemochromatosis in renal transplant recipients. Clinical and pathological features, diagnostic correlations, predisposing factors and treatment. Am J Nephrol 1985;5:419–430.
141. Jensen JD, Madsen JK, Jensen LW, Pedersen EB. Reduced production, absorption, and elimination of erythropoietin in uremia compared with healthy volunteers. J Am Soc Nephrol 1994;5:177–185.
142. Uehlinger DE, Gotch FA, Sheiner LB. A pharmacodynamic model of erythropoietin therapy for uremic anemia. Clin Pharmacol Ther 1992;51:76–89.
143. Watson AJ, Gimenez LF, Cotton S, et al. Treatment of anemia of chronic renal failure with subcutaneous recombinant human erythropoietin. Am J Med 1990;89:432–435.
144. Eschbach JW, Kelley MR, Haley NR, et al. Treatment of the anemia of progressive renal failure with recombinant human erythropoietin. N Engl J Med 1989;321:158–163.
145. Winearls CG, Oliver DO, Pippard MJ, et al. Effect of human erythropoietin derived from recombinant DNA on the anemia of patients maintained by chronic hemodialysis. Lancet 1986;2:1175–1177.
146. Eschbach JW, Egrie JC, Downing MR, et al. Correction of the anemia of end-stage renal disease with recombinant human erythropoietin. N Engl J Med 1987;316:73–78.
147. Ashai NI, Paganini EP, Wilson JM. Intravenous versus subcutaneous dosing of epoetin: A review of the literature. Am J Kidney Dis 1993;22(suppl 1):23–31.
148. Besarab A. Optimizing epoetin therapy in end-stage renal disease: the case for subcutaneous administration. Am J Kidney Dis 1993;22(suppl 1):13–22.
149. Paganini EP. In search of an optimal hematocrit level in dialysis patients: Rehabilitation and quality-of-life implications. Am J Kidney Dis 1994;24:S10–S16.
150. Moia M, Mannucci PM, Vizzotto L, et al. Improvement in the hemostatic defect of uremia after treatment with recombinant human erythropoietin. Lancet 1987;2:1227–1229.
151. Bommer J, Alexiou C, Müller-Bühl U, et al. Recombinant human erythropoietin therapy in hemodialysis patients—Dose determination and clinical experience. Nephrol Dial Transplant 1987;2:238–242.
152. Eschbach JW. Erythropoietin: The promise and the facts. Kidney Int 1994;45(suppl 44):S70–S76.
153. Zehnder C, Glück Z, Descoeudres C, et al. Human recombinant erythropoietin in anemia patients on maintenance hemodialysis. Secondary effects of the increase of hemoglobin. Nephrol Dial Transplant 1988;3:657–660.
154. Abraham PA, Macres MG. Blood pressure in hemodialysis patients during amelioration of anemia with erythropoietin. J Am Soc Nephrol 1991;2:927–936.
155. Canadian Erythropoietin Study Group. Effect of recombinant human erythropoietin therapy on blood

pressure in hemodialysis patients. Am J Nephrol 1991;11:23–26.
156. Powe NR, Griffiths RI, Bass EB. Cost implications to Medicare of recombinant erythropoietin therapy for the anemia of end-stage renal disease. J Am Soc Nephrol 1993;3:1660–1671.
157. Sheingold S, Churchill D, Muirhead N, et al. The impact of recombinant human erythropoietin on medical care costs for hemodialysis patients in Canada. Soc Sci Med 1992;34:983–991.
158. Powe NR, Griffiths RI, Watson AJ, et al. Effect of recombinant erythropoietin on hospital admissions, readmissions, length of stay, and costs of dialysis patients. J Am Soc Nephrol 1994;4:1455–1465.
159. Remuzzi G. Bleeding disorders in uremia: Pathophysiology and treatment. Adv Nephrol 1989;18:171–186.
160. Eberst ME, Berkowitz LR. Hemostasis in renal disease: Pathophysiology and management. Am J Med 1994;96:168–179.
161. George JN, Shattil SJ. The clinical importance of acquired abnormalities of platelet function. N Engl J Med 1991;324:27–39.
162. Swartz RD, Port FK. Preventing hemorrhage in high-risk hemodialysis: Regional versus low-dose heparin. Kidney Int 1979;16:513–518.
163. Watson AJ, Gimenez LF. The bleeding diathesis of uremia. Semin Dialysis 1991;4:86–93.
164. McCarthy ML, Stoukides CA. Estrogen therapy of uremic bleeding. Ann Pharmacother 1994;28:60–61.
165. Beccari M. Must we treat uremic dyslipidemia? Int J Artif Organs 1993;16:235–244.
166. Wanner C, Frommherz K, Hörl WH. Hyperlipoproteinemia in chronic renal failure: Pathophysiological and therapeutic aspects. Cardiology 1991;78:202–217.
167. Olbricht CJ, Koch KM. Treatment of hyperlipidemia in nephrotic syndrome: Time for a change? Nephron 1992;62:125–129.
168. Keane WF, St. Peter JV, Kasiske BL. Is the aggressive management of hyperlipidemia in nephrotic syndrome mandatory? Kidney Int 1992;42(suppl 38):S134–S141.
169. Expert Panel on Detection, and Treatment of High Blood Cholesterol in Adults. Summary of the second report of the National Cholesterol Education Program expert panel on detection, evaluation and treatment of high blood cholesterol in adults (Adult Treatment Panel II). JAMA 1993;269:3015–3023.
170. NIH Consensus Development Conference. Triglyceride, high density lipoprotein, and coronary heart disease. Sponsored by the National Heart, Lung and Blood Institute and the Office of Medical Applications of Research of the National Institutes of Health, 1992.
171. Richards EG, Grundy SM, Cooper K. Influence of plasma triglycerides on lipoprotein patterns in normal subjects and in patients with coronary artery disease. Am J Cardiol 1969;63:1214–1220.
172. D'Amico G, Gentile MG. Treatment of hyperlipidemia in human renal disease. Miner Electrolyte Metab 1993;19:196–204.
173. Elisaf MS, Dardamanis MA, Papagalanis ND, Siamopoulos KC. Lipid abnormalities in chronic uremic patients—Reponse to treatment with gemfibrozil. Scand J Urol Nephrol 1993;27:101–108.
174. Chan MK. Gemfibrozil improves abnormalities of lipid metabolism in patients on continuous ambulatory peritoneal dialysis: The role of postheparin lipases in the metabolism of high-density lipoprotein subfractions. Metabolism 1989;38:939–945.
175. Pasternack A, Vanttinen T, Solakivi T, et al. Normalization of lipoprotein lipase and hepatic lipase by gemfibrozil results in correction of lipoprotein abnormalities in chronic renal failure. Clin Nephrol 1987;27:163–168.
176. Sherrard DJ, Goldberg AB, Haas LB, Brunzell JD. Chronic clofibrate therapy in maintenance hemodialysis patients. Nephron 1980;25:219–221.
177. Merk W, Graben N, Hartmann H, et al. Serum levels of free non-protein bound clofibrinic acid after single dosing to patients with impaired renal function of various degrees—A multicenter study. Int J Clin Pharmacol Ther Toxicol 1987;25:59–62.
178. Evans JR, Forland SC, Cutler RE. The effect of renal function on the pharmacokinetics of gemfibrozil. J Clin Pharmacol 1987;27:994–1000.
179. Di Paolo B, Del Rosso G, Catucci G, et al. Therapeutic effects of simvastatin on hyperlipidemia in CAPD patients. ASAIO Trans 1990;36:M578–M580.
180. Li PKT, Mak TWL, Chiu K, et al. Effect of lovastatin on serum lipid profile in the treatment of dyslipoproteinaemia in uraemic patients on continuous ambulatory peritoneal dialysis. Aust NZ J Med 1993;23:252–257.
181. Wanner C, Hörl WH, Luley CH, Wieland H. Effects of HMG-CoA reductase inhibitors in hypercholesterolemic patients on hemodialysis. Kidney Int 1991;39:754–760.
182. Azar R, Dequiedt F, Awada J, et al. Effects of fish oil rich in polyunsaturated fatty acids on hyperlipidemia of hemodialysis patients. Kidney Int 1989;36(suppl 27):S239–S242.
183. AAKP Carnitine Renal Dialysis Consensus Group. Role of L-carnitine in treating renal dialysis patients. Dial Transplant 1994;23:177–181.
184. Bosch T, Samtleben W, Thiery J, et al. Reverse flux filtration: A new mode of therapy improving the efficacy of heparin-induced extracorporeal LDL precipitation in hyperlipidemic hemodialysis patients. Int J Artif Organs 1993;16:75–85.
185. D'Amico G, Gentile MG. Influence of diet on lipid abnormalities in human renal disease. Am J Kidney Dis 1993;22:151–157.
186. Spitalewitz S, Porush JG, Cattran D, Wright N. Treatment of hyperlipidemia in the nephrotic syndrome: The effects of pravastatin therapy. Am J Kidney Dis 1993;22:143–150.
187. Grundy SM. HMG-CoA reductase inhibitors for treatment of hypercholesterolemia. N Engl J Med 1988;319:24–33.
188. Ritz E, Fliser D. Hypertension and the kidney—An overview. Am J Kidney Dis 1993;21(suppl 3):3–9.
189. Campese VM, Chervu I. Hypertension in dialysis subjects, in Henrich WL (ed): Principles and Practice of Dialysis. Baltimore, Williams & Wilkins, 1994, pp 148–169.
190. Ritz E, Koch M. Hypertension as risk factor for renal patients—Morbidity and mortality due to hypertension in

patients with renal failure. Am J Kidney Dis 1993;21(suppl 2):113–118.

191. Cheigh JS, Milite C, Sullivan JF, et al. Hypertension is not adequately controlled in hemodialysis patients. Am J Kidney Dis 1992;19:453–459.
192. National High Blood Pressure Education Program. National High Blood Pressure Education Program working group report on hypertension and chronic renal failure. Arch Intern Med 1991;151:1280–1287.
193. Weder AB. The renally compromised older hypertensive: Therapeutic considerations. Geriatrics 1991;46:36–48.
194. Jones B, Nanra RS. Double-blind trial of antihypertensive effect of chlorothiazide in severe renal failure. Lancet 1979;2:1258–1260.
195. Wollam GL, Tarazi RC, Bravo EL, Dustan HP. Diuretic potency of combined hydrochlorothiazide and furosemide therapy in patients with azotemia. Am J Med 1982;72:929–938.
196. Oster JR, Epstein M, Smoller S. Combined therapy with thiazide-type and loop diuretic agents for resistant sodium retention. Ann Intern Med 1983;99:405–406.
197. Favre L, Glasson P, Vallotton MB. Reversible acute renal failure from combined triamterene and indomethacin: A study in healthy subjects. Ann Intern Med 1982;96:317–320.
198. Sica DA, Gehr TWB. The pharmacokinetics of angiotensin-converting enzyme inhibitors in end-stage renal disease. Semin Dialysis 1994;7:205–213.
199. Lowenthal DT, Saris SD, Paran E, Cristal N. The use of transdermal clonidine in the hypertensive patient with chronic renal failure. Clin Nephrol 1993;39:37–43.
200. Miura Y, Watanabe M, Yoshinaga K. An evaluation of the efficacy and safety of doxazosin in hypertension associated with renal dysfunction. Am Heart J 1991;121:381–388.
201. Innes A, Gemmell HG, Smith FW, et al. The short term effects of oral labetalol in patients with chronic renal disease and hypertension. J Hum Hypertens 1992;6:211–214.
202. Waal-Manning HJ, Hobson CH. Renal function in patients with essential hypertension receiving nadolol. Br Med J 1980;281:423–424.
203. Pontremoli R, Robaudo C, Gaiter A, et al. Long-term minoxidil treatment in refractory hypertension and renal failure. Clin Nephrol 1991;35:39–43.
204. London GM, Marchais SJ, Guerin AP, et al. Salt and water retention and calcium blockade in uremia. Circulation 1990;82:105–113.
205. Rosansky SJ, Johnson KL, McConnell J. Use of transdermal clonidine in chronic hemodialysis patients. Clin Nephrol 1993;39:32–36.
206. Harter HR, Delmez JA. Effects of prazosin in the control of blood pressure in hypertensive dialysis patients. J Cardiovasc Pharmacol 1979;1(suppl):S43–S55.
207. Cannella G, Paoletti E, Delfino R, et al. Regression of left ventricular hypertrophy in hypertensive dialyzed uremic patients on long-term antihypertensive therapy. Kidney Int 1993;44:881–886.
208. Asher JP, Murray KM. Use of angiotensin-converting-enzyme inhibitors in the management of renal disease. Clin Pharm 1991;10:25–31.
209. Stahle-Bäckdahl M. Pruritis in hemodialysis patients. Skin Pharmacol 1992;5:14–20.
210. Dimkovic N, Djukanovic L, Radmilovic A, et al. Uremic pruritis and skin mast cells. Nephron 1992;61:5–9.
211. DeMarchi S, Cecchin E, Villalta D, et al. Relief of pruritus and decreases in plasma histamine concentrations during erythropoietin therapy in patients with uremia. N Engl J Med 1992;326:969–974.
212. Lorette G, Vaillant L. Pruritus—Current concepts in pathogenesis and treatment. Drugs 1990;39:218–223.
213. Makoff R. Vitamin supplementation in persons with renal disease. EDTNA ERCA Journal 1992;18:11–14.

Chapter 45

Renal Transplantation

Richard J. Ptachcinski, PharmD, FCCP, and Karen Heim-Duthoy, PharmD, FCCP

Conditions Leading to Renal Transplantation

Each year the number of new patients diagnosed with end-stage renal disease (ESRD) increases by approximately 50,000. The primary therapeutic options for these individuals are hemodialysis, peritoneal dialysis, and/or renal transplantation. Hemodialysis (HD) and continuous ambulatory peritoneal dialysis (CAPD) remain options for patients with chronic, irreversible renal failure who choose not to be transplanted or for patients awaiting a suitable donor. Renal transplantation is the preferred long-term therapeutic option for most patients with ESRD because it provides patients with the greatest opportunity to improve their overall quality of life.

Currently there are more than 250,000 patients with ESRD in the United States.[1,2] In spite of efforts to increase public awareness about organ donation, the waiting list continues to grow, and reached 27,498 by the end of 1994 (Fig. 45.1).[1] The largest increase in patients waiting for kidneys was in patients over the age 64 years. In 1990, the median waiting time for an organ was 465 days and 935 patients died waiting for organs. In 1993, kidneys were retrieved from 4610 donors, which corresponds to a procurement rate of 17 per million population, which represents only 35–50% of potentially available kidneys. The reported causes of ESRD leading to transplantation include insulin-dependent diabetes mellitus (33.8%), hypertension (28.3%), chronic glomerulonephritis by all causes (12.6%), polycystic kidney disease (3%), interstitial nephritis (3%), and a number of minor causes.[2]

Renal transplantation has several advantages over dialysis. Vascular access problems are minimized, frequent (two to three times per week) dialysis treatments are avoided, dietary restrictions are less stringent and the problem of peritonitis associated with CAPD is avoided. While the analysis of quality of life is quite complex, patients generally report improved quality of life following transplantation as compared to patients on maintenance dialysis.[3]

Patient and graft survival rates following renal transplantation have improved steadily over the past 30 years due to advances in drug therapy, surgical techniques, organ preservation techniques, and the postoperative management of patients. One-year patient and graft survival rates prior to the availability of cyclosporine (prior to 1979) ranged from 85–95% and 60–80%, respectively.[1] While success rates vary among transplant centers, 1-year patient survival rates range from 96–98% for living related transplants (LRT) and 92–94% for cadaveric renal transplants (CRT). The 1-year graft survival rates for LRTs and CRTs range from 89–95% and 66–80%, respectively. Five-year graft survival rates currently range from 50–60% in most transplant centers.

While transplantation is a less costly method than dialysis for treating patients with chronic renal failure over the long term, the 5-year patient survival rate for each treatment is similar. The net cost benefit (or "breakeven point") to Medicare from transplantation has been estimated at 3 years in patients with a functioning graft.[4]

Several factors have been identified that are associated with decreased success rates for renal transplants.[5] These factors include early graft dysfunction, more than one transplantation, age under 15 and over 50 years, race (blacks have lower graft survival than whites), immunologic sensitization, or the presence of preformed anti-HLA antibodies. HLA matching continues to be an important factor influencing the success of renal transplantation. It is estimated that the half-life of HLA-matched grafts is 17.3 years as compared to 7.8 years for mismatched kidneys.[6]

Because of its continuously improving success, cost effectiveness, and ability to improve quality of life, renal transplantation is the treatment option that provides the patient with renal failure the best chance of survival and a return to a normal or near-normal lifestyle. However, patients with medical conditions where the risk of surgery or chronic immunosuppression would be greater than the risks associated with chronic dialysis are excluded from renal transplantation. The most frequent reason for patient exclusion is unstable cardiac disease or a recently diagnosed malignancy. Some transplant centers will also exclude patients that are human immunodeficiency virus antibody positive, and patients with a history of drug abuse or noncompliance with medical regimens.

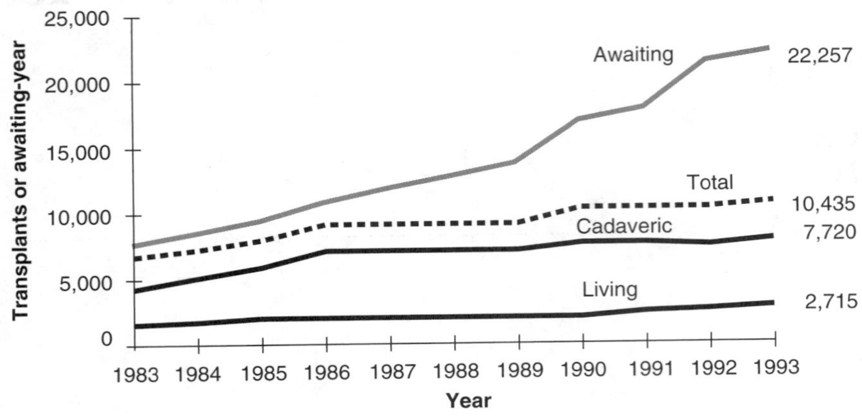

Figure 45.1. Kidney transplants by donor type and patients awaiting a transplant by year, 1983–1993. *(From U.S. Renal Data System, 1995 Annual Report. Am J Kid Dis 1995;26:S56.)*

The pharmacotherapy required for the management of patients following renal transplantation, including immunosuppression, antibiotic therapy, and other treatments, is discussed in the remainder of this chapter.

Renal Transplantation: Surgery and Perioperative Management

The immunologic cascade regulating a host response to a transplanted kidney is presented in Chapter 9. Allograft rejection depends on the activation of alloreactive T cells and antigen presenting cells such as B lymphocytes, macrophages, and dendritic cells. Acute allograft rejection is primarily caused by the infiltration of T cells into the allograft, which triggers the inflammatory and cytotoxic effects on the graft. Complex interactions between the allograft and cellular cytokines, cell-to-cell interactions, CD4+ and CD8+ T cells, and B cells ultimately lead to chronic rejection and ultimately graft loss if adequate immunosuppression is not maintained.[5]

Prior to surgery, patients receive antibiotic prophylaxis. The antibiotic chosen is usually a first-generation cephalosporin or vancomycin in a penicillin-allergic patient. Bowel cleansing with enemas is also indicated prior to surgery. Most transplant centers start immunosuppression prior to surgery but some withhold cyclosporine until postoperative diuresis has occurred.

Following the removal of the kidney from the donor, blood is flushed from the kidney and the core is cooled with a 4° Euro-Collins or University of Wisconsin (UW) solution for preservation (see Table 9.4).[7] While preservation of kidneys in UW solution allows for storage for up to 48 hours, it is preferable to transplant the kidney within 24 hours of harvesting from the donor.

The renal graft is placed extraperitoneally in either the right or left lower quadrant of the abdomen, just above the inguinal ligament (iliac fossa) in adults, and is placed retroperitoneally through a midline incision in small children. The usual vascular anastomoses are as follows: the end of the donor renal artery to the end of the recipient's hypogastric artery or side of the common iliac artery, the end of the renal vein to the iliac vein (in adults) or the inferior vena cava (in children).[8]

Following the completion of the revascularization, the urinary tract is then established. The donor ureter is inserted by creating a submucosal tunnel in the recipient's bladder. The shortest length of donor ureter is used in the procedure to decrease the risk of anastomotic leak or loss of ureteral integrity secondary to ischemic necrosis.

Physiologic Consequences of Renal Transplantation

Based on a rapid fall in serum creatinine, the glomerular filtration rate of a successfully transplanted kidney may be near normal almost immediately after transplantation. However, in some patients, the concentrations of standard biochemical indicators of renal function, such as serum creatinine and blood urea nitrogen (BUN), may remain elevated for several days. Therefore, standard formulas used to predict drug dosing, which rely on a stable serum creatinine, may be inaccurate immediately following transplantation.

Although the allograft is able to remove uremic toxins from the body, it may take several weeks for the other physiologic complications of chronic renal failure, such as anemia, calcium and phosphate imbalance, and altered lipid profiles, to show improvement. The renal production of erythropoietin and 1-hydroxylation of vitamin D may occur in the early postoperative period, but because their effects may be delayed, some continuation of pretransplant therapy with erythropoietin, calcium supplements, and/or phosphate binders may be indicated.

Primary nonfunction of a renal allograft may result in postoperative anuria. The primary cause is acute tubular necrosis (ATN). A number of circumstances related to the donor may cause, worsen, or prolong ATN. The incidence of ATN increases when kidneys have been harvested from donors following cardiac arrest, from donors who have been hypotensive or on vasopressors, or from older donors. Prolonged periods of warm and cold ischemia, greater than 40 minutes and 48 hours, respectively, have been recognized to increase a patient's risk of developing ATN. The management of patients with ATN becomes quite difficult since serum creatinine, which is a major parameter used to monitor for acute rejection, remains elevated. Therapy with cyclosporine either in high doses or via the intravenous route has been implicated as a cause of ATN, although a clear cause-and-effect relationship has not been established.

Acute allograft rejection continues to be a major management problem in the perioperative period. The immunologic mechanisms of transplant rejection are discussed in detail in Chapter 9. An episode of acute rejection occurs in 30–40% of patients undergoing a first transplant. While acute rejection can occur at any time in the postoperative period, first rejection episodes typically occur between 5–15 days following surgery. Chronic rejection, which is generally thought to be secondary to humoral injury, rarely occurs in the first 3 months following transplantation. It is usually responsible for a slow deterioration of renal function at any time from 6 months to years after transplantation.

Immunosuppressive Pharmacotherapy in the Renal Transplant Patient

Transplant immunosuppression must be balanced in terms of graft and patient survival (i.e., the prevention of rejection versus the risk of adverse effects associated with therapy including life-threatening infection or malignancy). A multidrug approach is rational from the immunomechanistic viewpoint since the agents have overlapping and potentially synergistic mechanisms. Furthermore, multidrug immunosuppression may allow for the use of lower doses of individual agents, which is generally associated with fewer or less severe adverse effects.

The goals of immunosuppression vary depending on the time interval since the transplant surgery. Immediately following surgery, the primary goal of therapy is to prevent hyperacute and acute graft rejection. The high doses of immunosuppressants required to achieve this goal may result in serious complications (e.g., infection, thrombocytopenia, and steroid-induced diabetes).

During the first 1–3 months following transplantation, acute graft rejection is common. It has been determined that acute rejection is the single strongest determinant of long-term renal graft survival.[9] Therefore, the doses of immunosuppressants are usually kept high to prevent rejection during this high-risk period. The doses of immunosuppressants are generally reduced if the patient develops serious adverse effects such as opportunistic infections, nephrotoxicity, or hepatotoxicity. The goal of maintenance immunosuppression is to prevent acute and chronic rejection while minimizing drug-related toxicity. In the long-term management of the transplant patient, the doses of immunosuppressants are gradually (over 6–12 months) reduced in an effort to minimize adverse effects. Many institutions may completely withdraw specific immunosuppressives, in select patients, to reduce long-term toxicity as well as cost. It is important to recognize that even though the goals of transplant immunosuppression are universal, protocols for induction, maintenance, and rejection therapy vary greatly between institutions. Table 45.1 includes the immunosuppressive options for induction, maintenance, and the management of acute rejection. This discussion of immunosuppression includes the rationale for the most commonly used regimens and success rates generally achieved with the most popular regimens.

INDUCTION THERAPY

Induction therapy often involves the use of sequential immunosuppression. This form of immunosuppression incorporates induction with a polyclonal or monoclonal antilymphocyte (ALG)/antithymocyte (ATG) antibody preparation along with azathioprine (AZA) and/or glucocorticoid, followed by the delayed administration of cyclosporine (CSA). CSA may be delayed until postoperative diuresis has been established or for a standard time frame (e.g., 5 days). Induction therapy using this combination with delayed initiation of CSA has been based on the following rationale: (1) The newly transplanted kidney is

TABLE 45.1. OPTIONS FOR IMMUNOSUPPRESSION DURING INDUCTION, MAINTENANCE, AND REJECTION THERAPY

Type of Therapy	Options
Induction therapy	1. Sequential, quadruple, or triple therapy: ALG/ATG or OKT3, azathioprine and/or glucocorticoid, cyclosporine 2. Other induction
Maintenance therapy	1. Monotherapy: immunosuppression with one drug, usually cyclosporine 2. Dual therapy: immunosuppression with two drugs 3. Triple therapy: immunosuppression with three drugs, usually a glucocorticoid plus azathioprine and cyclosporine
Rejection therapy	1. Glucocorticoid 2. OKT3 3. ALG/ATG 4. Radiation

very susceptible to nephrotoxic injury from CSA; (2) CSA dosage adjustment is difficult in the early post-transplant period; and (3) a theoretical immunologic benefit from initial, more intensive immunosuppression is achieved with the use of the ALG/ATG preparation.[10]

The presence of nephrotoxic drugs such as CSA, tacrolimus, or aminoglycosides may exacerbate damage to the transplanted kidney that results from prolonged cold and/or warm ischemia or the cellular damage caused by the release of oxygen free radicals that results upon reperfusion of the kidney with oxygenated blood. Therefore, immunosuppressive regimens that eliminate or use only low doses of CSA in the early postoperative period are frequently used. In addition to the nephrotoxic potential, CSA trough plasma/blood levels are difficult to adjust because of gastrointestinal (GI) dysfunction (i.e., postoperative ileus), which is common in the early post-transplant period. The microemulsion formulation of CSA may minimize these early absorption problems. However, during this initial stabilization period, while CSA dosage is adjusted to achieve the desired trough concentrations, patients still should be adequately immunosuppressed with other agents.

More intense immunosuppression is often indicated in the immediate post-transplant period when the risk for organ rejection is highest. This acts to decrease the overall incidence of acute rejection as well as to delay onset of early rejection. This may ultimately improve long-term graft survival. The prophylactic use of antibody preparations (ALG/ATG and muromonab CD-3 [OKT3]) during induction therapy is controversial. Some studies report higher graft survival with antibody prophylaxis,[11–14] whereas others report no significant improvement.[15–17] However, immunosuppressive regimens that include induction therapy are frequently preferred. Although the majority of literature on polyclonal antibody preparations was based on results with the investigational agent, Minnesota ALG, this product is no longer available. Because of their differences in antibody composition, potency, and preparation procedures, it is inappropriate to extrapolate results with the use of Minnesota ALG to other polyclonal antibody preparations. Further evaluation of these products is needed to define their specific role with induction therapy.

Induction therapy incorporating ALG, CSA, and steroids has been compared to conventional therapy utilizing CSA and steroids. Graft survival at 3 years post-transplant was significantly greater for the ALG group (89%) versus the conventional group (73%), $p = 0.041$.[12] Similarly, OKT3 induction with azathioprine, steroids, and delayed CSA has been compared to conventional therapy (azathioprine, steroids, and CSA).[11–14] OKT3 use was associated with significantly fewer rejection episodes (51% versus 66%) and a longer time to initial rejection (46 days versus 8 days).[14] Furthermore, the prophylactic use of OKT3 has resulted in improved graft survival at 18 months post-transplant (92% with OKT3 versus 79% with conventional therapy)[11] and at 5 years post-transplant (73% with OKT3 versus 64% with conventional therapy).[14]

The efficacy of induction therapy with polyclonal antibody preparations and OKT3 has been shown to be similar.[18–21] Light et al.[21] compared sequential therapy with delayed CSA initiation utilizing perioperative Minnesota ALG to OKT3. The ALG and OKT3 groups had similar 3-year graft (83% versus 87%, respectively) and patient (96% versus 94%, respectively) survival rates. The incidence of rejection in the first-year post-transplantation was similar in both groups (<40%).[21]

In contrast, other studies have reported no benefit from the use of induction therapy.[15–17] However, Belitsky et al.[16] utilized intravenous CSA during induction and Michael et al.[15] evaluated induction therapy in patients that had been diagnosed with delayed graft function. These factors may have contributed to the lack of outcome improvement with induction therapy.

Although there are no data indicating that sequential induction immunosuppression should be abandoned, some believe that it may be associated with an increased incidence of viral infection and malignancy. ALG/ATG doses commonly utilized for induction are 10–30 mg/kg/d for 5–14 days. Disadvantages for the use of either polyclonal antibody product include nonstandardized preparations (MALG), dose-limiting side effects, and cost. Daily pharmacy cost for antithymocyte globulin (ATGAM) (Upjohn Co., Kalamazoo, MI) for a 70-kg patient (20 mg/kg) is approximately $1300. ALG/ATG administration may be problematic secondary to the use of a central line, lengthy duration of infusion, and significant quantity of infusion volume. Anaphylactic reactions may occur with ALG/ATG products, therefore, the use of a test dose prior to the initial infusion is a common practice. Fever and chills often accompany the first few doses of ALG/ATG; acetaminophen, diphenhydramine, and glucocorticoid can be used as premedications. ALG and ATG are bone marrow suppressive, commonly causing leukopenia and thrombocytopenia.

The OKT3 dosage for induction is 5 mg/d for 5–14 days. Its rapid intravenous administration is an advantage over ALG/ATG infusions. OKT3 administration is associated with significant first-dose adverse effects and high cost (average wholesale price $535/5 mg). A first-dose reaction to OKT3, which may include fever, chills, rigors, pruritus, and alterations in blood pressure, may occur with the first several doses; methylprednisolone, acetaminophen, diphenhydramine, and pentoxifylline may be used as premedications. Pulmonary edema has been associated with OKT3 use in transplant patients that are significantly fluid overloaded; therefore, patients may need to be dialyzed prior to administration. Aseptic meningitis may result as a complication of OKT3 therapy. If encephalitic symptoms develop,

OKT3 should be discontinued and appropriate care initiated. Finally, due to the potential development of host antibodies and possible inability to reuse it as an effective rejection therapy, previous concern existed regarding its use for induction. However, it has been demonstrated that OKT3 can be safely and successfully used as rejection therapy in patients that have undergone previous OKT3 induction.[14,22,23] Specifically, these studies have confirmed that the presence of low anti-OKT3 antibody titers (≤1:100) does not preclude successful retreatment with OKT3 for rejection.

High-risk patients (e.g., those with poor HLA matching, or with high preformed antibody titers) who received a graft with a long cold ischemia time and therefore are more susceptible to CSA toxicity, or retransplants) may benefit from induction therapy. Further investigation, however, will be required to identify those patients that would benefit most from induction therapy.

MAINTENANCE THERAPY

Maintenance therapy can involve combinations of the various available immunosuppressives. Transplant type (cadaveric versus living related), the degree of HLA mismatch, time post-transplant, post-transplant complications including the number of acute rejection(s), previous immunosuppressive adverse reactions, compliance, and financial considerations are among the patient-specific factors considered in individualizing maintenance immunosuppression. CSA is generally a central component in most maintenance regimens, however, it is unknown whether tacrolimus will ultimately replace CSA in most renal transplant regimens. Renal transplant patients may receive mono-, dual, or triple therapy during the maintenance phase. In the early post-transplant period (up to 6 months following transplantation) most cadaveric renal transplant recipients will be maintained on triple drug therapy (CSA, azathioprine, and prednisone).[24] In contrast, recipients of living-related grafts may receive only dual therapy, such as azathioprine and prednisone. As patients progress through the post-transplant course, acute rejection becomes less of a risk; therefore, maintenance immunosuppression is commonly tapered and, in some cases, certain agents may be discontinued.

Azathioprine and Glucocorticoids

The efficacy of azathioprine (AZA) and glucocorticoids in renal transplantation has been recognized for more than 30 years.[25,26] They remained the two most important maintenance drugs until CSA was introduced for clinical use in 1983. Although most protocols today include CSA, dual therapy with azathioprine and glucocorticoid may be appropriate in instances such as HLA-identical renal transplants, significant CSA nephrotoxicity unresponsive to CSA dose reduction, and financial inability to pay for CSA.

Azathioprine, a prodrug for 6-mercaptopurine, is commonly used following renal transplantation. The immunosuppressive activity of azathioprine is correlated with its reduction in white blood cells (WBCs). Initial doses of 3–5 mg/kg/d are given with subsequent individualization (1–3 mg/kg/d) to maintain a stable serum creatinine and a WBC count of 5 to 7×10^3 cells/mm^3. Dose-limiting adverse effects of azathioprine are often hematologic in origin (Table 45.2). Leukopenia, anemia, and thrombocytopenia are common adverse effects and can be managed by dose reduction or discontinuation of azathioprine. Hepatic toxicity and pancreatitis are less common adverse effects of azathioprine; they are generally reversible upon dose adjustment or discontinuation. Azathioprine is also associated with an increased risk of malignancy, especially skin cancer. Transplant patients should be properly counseled about the risks of malignancy, the importance of sun-blocking preparations, and avoidance of sun exposure. In addition, careful screening for the detection of malignancy should be completed on a routine basis. Pelvic exams with cervical smears as well as breast and rectal exams should be completed at annual visits. Any change in bowel function or uterine/vaginal bleeding as well as the presence of melena, hematuria, or suspicious lesions should be aggressively evaluated.

An intravenous glucocorticoid, commonly high-dose (125–1000 mg/d) methylprednisolone, is given perioperatively, immediately following, and for several days post-transplant. The dose of methylprednisolone is rapidly tapered and discontinued as oral prednisone is initiated. Prednisone doses are tapered progressively over time to a baseline dose of 15 mg/d by the sixth month post-transplant. At 1-year post-transplantation, maintenance prednisone doses may be less than 10 mg/d in some patients. Prednisone doses may be reduced even lower with concurrent tacrolimus administration. As doses are tapered, it is preferable to administer steroids every other day and between 7 and 8 AM to mimic the body's diurnal release of

TABLE 45.2. AZATHIOPRINE: ADVERSE EFFECTS AND MANAGEMENT IN THE RENAL TRANSPLANT PATIENT

Adverse Effect	Management
Bone marrow suppression	Patient education; monitor WBC, RBC, and platelets; adjust dose or discontinue as needed
Hepatic abnormalities and pancreatitis	Monitor enzymes monthly; adjust dose or discontinue as needed
Malignancy	Patient education regarding prevention, signs, and symptoms; routine screening on annual exams

cortisol. Although conversion to alternate-day regimens or complete withdrawal of prednisone in patients with stable post-transplant courses has been used with success in some transplant centers,[27–29] steroids are often continued for the entire life of the functional graft. However, long-term steroid use and its associated deleterious effects are well recognized and particularly troublesome in transplant patients.[30–33] Specific adverse effects of glucocorticoids that are commonly encountered in transplant patients are summarized in Table 45.3.

Cyclosporine

The introduction of CSA has significantly improved the outcomes of renal transplantation. Patient and graft survival rates have improved secondary to a lower incidence of acute rejection episodes and severe infectious complications.[34–36] Despite these improvements in survival, concerns regarding its long-term usage include long-term survival, incidence of late-rejection episodes, frequency of hypertension, drug cost, and quality of kidney function. CSA maintenance regimens vary between transplant centers secondary to different institutional strategies. Mono-, dual, and triple therapy with CSA are all employed during maintenance immunosuppression although dual and triple therapy are most common.

A 5-year experience with CSA monotherapy as primary immunosuppression in renal transplant recipients was recently reported.[37] Actuarial patient and graft survival rates at 5 years were 89.7% and 80.0%, respectively. Sixty-four percent of patients experienced rejection episodes within the first 6 months and only 3.9% of patients experienced first rejection after the first post-transplant year. The avoidance of long-term steroids is the primary advantage with CSA monotherapy, whereas the primary disadvantage is its high incidence of rejection. Although CSA monotherapy may not jeopardize graft function, the effect of acute rejection on long-term graft survival is controversial and a subject of debate. Maintenance glucocorticoid may be necessary in those patients initiated on CSA monotherapy who experience recurrent rejection episodes.[38,39]

CSA dual therapy usually includes a combination of CSA and a glucocorticoid. Dual therapy with CSA and prednisone has been compared to AZA and prednisone.[40,41] With a follow-up period ranging from 3–6 years, Ghoneim et al.[40] demonstrated no significant difference in the overall frequency of acute rejection episodes or graft survival between the two living-related transplant groups; however, the number of patients experiencing two or more rejection episodes was greater in the azathioprine/prednisone group. In contrast, Amend et al.[41] observed significant differences in graft survival between CSA/prednisone and azathioprine/prednisone-treated cadaveric renal transplant patients; a significantly greater graft survival for all study periods during the 5-year follow-up was demonstrated for both diabetics (20–22%) and nondiabetics (35–40%) in the CSA/prednisone group. The different outcomes of these two studies could be attributed to the difference in study subjects and the source of the kidney, cadaveric versus living related, since survival rates are improved following living-related transplants.

CSA triple therapy usually consists of CSA, glucocorticoid, and azathioprine. Eventual tapering and/or elimination of glucocorticoid or CSA is attempted in many patients. CSA dual therapy (CSA/prednisone and CSA/AZA) has been compared to CSA triple therapy (CSA, prednisone, and AZA) in cadaveric renal transplant patients. Although the CSA/AZA group had more frequent early rejection, no significant differences in 1-year patient or graft survival, morbidity, and mortality were identified.[42] The long-term (4-year follow-up) effects of CSA dual versus CSA triple immunosuppression have been evaluated.[43,44] Both studies reported no differences in graft and patient survival. However, Isoniemi et al.[44] demonstrated other parameters of follow-up including graft function and "chronic allograft damage index" from renal biopsy to be

TABLE 45.3. GLUCOCORTICOIDS: ADVERSE EFFECTS AND MANAGEMENT IN THE RENAL TRANSPLANT PATIENT

Adverse Effect	Management
Adrenal suppression	If reduced or discontinued, taper slowly; identification card to be carried
Glucose alterations	Monitor glucose; begin or adjust oral hypoglycemic or insulin therapy as needed
Weight gain	Patient education; dietary intervention
Fluid and electrolyte alterations	Diuretic therapy with careful monitoring and adjustment of electrolytes
Hypertension	Monitor blood pressure; sodium restriction and antihypertensive therapy as needed
Hyperlipidemia	Patient education; dietary intervention and lipid-lowering agents as needed
Personality changes	Patient and family education
Epithelial changes	Patient education, especially with diabetics
Acne	Topical agents
Gastrointestinal bleeding	Prophylaxis with antacid or H_2 blocker therapy during high dose steroid use
Osteoporosis and aseptic necrosis	Regular bone examinations; if severe, surgical intervention
Cataracts and glaucoma	Regular eye examinations

significantly better in the triple therapy group, whereas Lindholm et al.[43] reported no difference in renal function determined by serum creatinine between groups.

The impact of CSA on long-term (≥5 years) renal allograft function has been analyzed. Although patient survival did not differ between treatment groups,[45,46] Monaco[46] demonstrated a significantly greater 5-year graft survival in CSA-treated patients (triple therapy). A retrospective study evaluated 5-year graft survival in patients who had received either (1) azathioprine and steroids or (2) CSA mono-, dual, or triple therapy.[47] The 5-year actual graft survival rate was not different between the azathioprine and CSA groups (88% versus 90%, respectively). In fact, 5-year graft survival after the development of chronic graft dysfunction was 34% in AZA patients and 53% in CSA patients. Similarly, Slaton et al.[48] compared 1- and 5-year patient and graft survival in cadaveric renal transplant recipients treated with either azathioprine or CSA as the primary immunosuppressive agent. Although patient survival rates did not differ between groups, the 5-year graft survival rate was greater in the CSA than AZA group (61% versus 29%); the mean serum creatinine level at 5 years was significantly greater in the CSA group (CSA 1.79 versus azathioprine 1.30 mg/dL, p <0.05). The results of a meta-analysis evaluating chronic immunosuppression in renal transplant patients refute these reports.[49] One- and 5-year graft and patient survival, rejection rate per patient, and infection rate were analyzed; no statistical differences between CSA triple therapy over dual therapy (CSA/prednisone) were detected. As the literature indicates, the optimal immunosuppressive regimen is not always clear-cut; further study in terms of longer follow-up may help determine which maintenance regimen(s) should be employed.

The results of a multicenter, long-term efficacy and safety of CSA evaluation in renal transplant patients was reported by Burke et al.[50] Graft survival was 78% after a median follow-up of 36 months. In the 1663 patients evaluated, there were 279 grafts lost. The leading cause of graft loss was acute rejection (68 patients) and chronic graft dysfunction (125 patients).

Dosing

Initiation of oral CSA therapy generally begins with a dose of 8–18 mg/kg/d divided into two daily doses. Higher CSA doses are more commonly used in dual therapy regimens, while lower doses are part of triple therapy regimens. Doses are adjusted on the basis of whole blood concentrations of the drug and the clinical response of the patient. The desired blood concentration range is dependent on the assay methodology utilized and individual risk factors for rejection such as time post-transplant. As the risk for acute rejection becomes less with time, oral CSA doses are reduced and may be as low as 3 mg/kg/d or less during maintenance therapy.[50] If oral administration is not possible, CSA may be administered intravenously at one-third the oral dosage.

Therapeutic Drug Monitoring

The absorption, distribution, and metabolism of CSA is highly variable; many factors contribute to this intrapatient and interpatient variability.[50–52] These factors are discussed in detail in Chapter 9. As these factors change in the post-transplant course, CSA pharmacokinetic parameters change.[53] Therefore, CSA blood concentrations are routinely measured in an attempt to optimize therapy (i.e., to minimize the adverse effects of the drug as well as acute rejection episodes in transplant patients).[54]

Radioimmunoassay and fluorescence polarization immunoassay are the most commonly utilized methods; however, high-performance liquid chromatography is recognized as the reference procedure.[55] It is important to determine which assay methodology the laboratory is using since target ranges vary between specific (which quantitates parent CSA) and nonspecific assays (which quantitates parent plus metabolite concentration) (Table 45.4). In addition, it is extremely important to interpret CSA concentrations not only in relation to goal ranges, but also in the context of relevant clinical and laboratory data.

The most common and practical method of CSA monitoring is the measurement of trough blood concentrations.[54,56] CSA trough concentrations are measured frequently (daily or three times per week) following the initiation of the drug and during the stabilization period after transplantation. Although CSA trough concentrations may document patient compliance, they are widely variable.

An alternative to the assessment of CSA trough concentrations is the characterization of the individual's CSA pharmacokinetic profile.[57–59] Theoretically, a pharmacokinetic profile consisting of serial samples collected throughout a CSA dosage interval is more reflective of overall CSA exposure than are individual trough concentrations. Sequential CSA profiles provide a more comprehensive pharmacokinetic characterization and AUC has been suggested to correlate with graft outcome.[60] However, due to the intrapatient variability in the pharmacokinetics of CSA the usefulness of a single pharmacokinetic profile to predict long-term dosing strategies is controversial. Unlike the ease

TABLE 45.4. THERAPEUTIC CYCLOSPORINE LEVELS AS MEASURED BY VARIOUS ASSAYS

Assay	Whole Blood	Serum
High-pressure liquid chromatography (HPLC)	100–300 ng/mL	—
Fluorescence polarization immunoassay (FPIA/TDx)	250–1000 ng/mL	100–300 ng/mL
Radioimmunoassay (polyclonal antibody)	200–800 ng/mL	100–250 ng/mL
Radioimmunoassay (specific monoclonal antibody)	150–400 ng/mL	50–125 ng/mL

(From Ref. 55.)

and convenience of obtaining CSA trough concentrations, measurement of CSA pharmacokinetic profiles is a more complicated procedure. The cost of additional blood samples and practicality of using these profiles for therapeutic monitoring at individual institutions must be considered. Finally, the optimal sampling strategy for CSA pharmacokinetic profiles remains to be determined and compared to CSA trough monitoring in a prospective, randomized study to simplify sampling routines.

CSA concentrations may be markedly increased as the result of drug interactions. Diltiazem[61] and ketoconazole[62] inhibit the hepatic elimination of CSA and thus can be used to achieve desired concentrations of CSA with lower drug doses. A complete discussion of CSA drug interactions and their implications related to CSA monitoring is found in Chapter 9.

Adverse Effects

A summary of CSA adverse effects and management in the renal transplant patient is presented in Table 45.5. The clinician is frequently required to differentiate between allograft rejection and CSA nephrotoxicity, which is generally a diagnosis of exclusion. Typically, nephrotoxicity is defined as an increase in serum creatinine of 25% over several days, that reverses following a CSA dose reduction. Patients are usually afebrile, have nontender grafts, and frequently maintain a good urine output. In contrast, patients experiencing renal allograft rejection frequently present with a sudden, rapid rise in serum creatinine, often associated with fever, graft edema, and tenderness, diminished urine output, and decreased renal blood flow on renal scan.[63] Because the clinical features of acute allograft rejection and CSA nephrotoxicity may overlap considerably, a renal biopsy continues to be the differential diagnosis gold standard. Acute cellular rejection is associated with an interstitial infiltrate of lymphocytes, whereas histologic findings in CSA nephrotoxicity include interstitial fibrosis, tubular atrophy, glomerular thrombosis, and arterial inflammation.[63,64] Differentiating between CSA nephrotoxicity and chronic rejection is also difficult, because the clinical signs and symptoms may be similar. Since biopsy findings are similar in patients with CSA nephrotoxicity and chronic rejection, this is a much more difficult differential diagnosis.

TABLE 45.5. CYCLOSPORINE: ADVERSE EFFECTS AND MANAGEMENT IN THE RENAL TRANSPLANT PATIENT

Adverse Effect	Management
Nephrotoxicity	Monitor creatinine; therapeutic drug monitoring with concurrent evaluation of concomitant therapy; adjust dose and discontinue as needed
Hyperkalemia	Monitor potassium; avoid concomitant agents causing hyperkalemia; initiate diuretic and sodium polystyrene sulfonate therapy as needed
Hypertension	Monitor blood pressure; antihypertensive therapy as needed
Hyperuricemia	Monitor uric acid; begin drug therapy as needed (caution: allopurinol/azathioprine drug interaction)
Hepatic toxicity	Monitor liver enzymes; adjust dose and discontinue as needed
Tremor, numbness	Adjust dose as needed
Hair growth and gingival hyperplasia	Patient education; cosmetic treatment; appropriate dental hygiene

CSA discontinuation in renal transplant patients may be considered in some cases of chronic nephrotoxicity, or uncontrolled hypertension. In these patients, immunosuppression is generally maintained with prednisone and azathioprine or by the addition of tacrolimus. Improved renal function may result from such a change in therapy, but it may take several weeks for the beneficial effects to be fully realized. However, CSA discontinuation may precipitate an episode of acute graft rejection and should, therefore, be completed in conjunction with careful monitoring. The financial impact of additional monitoring during the conversion period and the potential adverse effects of tacrolimus including hyperkalemia and neurologic effects must also be considered.

Tacrolimus (FK-506)

Tacrolimus, formerly called FK-506 is a potent immunosuppressant, which was approved by the FDA in 1994 for patients undergoing orthotopic liver transplantation. Tacrolimus has been used since 1989 as a primary immunosuppressant and in an attempt to rescue failing kidneys.[65] Most of the published reports describing the use of tacrolimus are from the University of Pittsburgh, although there are also reports of uncontrolled studies from other transplant centers.[65–68]

The early experience using tacrolimus in renal transplant patients was derived from a small randomized trial comparing tacrolimus with cyclosporine, and a larger group of patients undergoing retransplantation and individuals who had failed conventional immunosuppressive regimens. One-year actuarial patient survival for individuals receiving tacrolimus ($n = 240$) was 90% as compared to 94% for patients receiving cyclosporine ($n = 196$), while the 1-year graft survival for both groups was also similar: 74% for tacrolimus and 77% for CSA. Forty-four percent (105) of tacrolimus-treated patients were able to have steroids withdrawn as compared to no patients treated with cyclosporine, although this difference was not statistically significant. Hypertension was less of a problem in patients treated with tacrolimus as evidenced by the fact that there were more patients maintained without hypertensive therapy in the tacrolimus-treated patients, 43%, compared to 25% in the CSA group. Finally, the mean serum cholesterol in tacrolimus-treated patients was significantly lower (187 ± 51 mg/dL) than the serum cholesterol in cyclosporine patients (236 ± 59) (p <0.0001).[66] These results are similar to the preliminary results of the Japanese multicenter kidney transplant study, which indicated a 3-month patient survival rate of 95.7% and a 3-month graft survival rate of 94.2%.[67]

Once it was established that tacrolimus was as effective as CSA in the prevention of rejection following renal transplantation, additional studies were initiated to optimize its use. A study was initiated to compare immunosuppression with tacrolimus and prednisone to tacrolimus, prednisone, and azathioprine. There was no difference in the 2-year actuarial patient and graft survival between the groups. The 2-year actuarial patient survival was 95% for the two-drug combination and 90% for the three-drug combination. Graft survival was 86% and 79% for the double and triple therapy, respectively. There were also no differences between the study groups with regard to steroid withdrawal, antihypertensive therapy, or serum cholesterol.[66]

Adverse Effects

The adverse effects associated with tacrolimus in renal transplant patients include neurologic toxicity, nephrotoxicity, and electrolyte alterations.[66] The neurotoxicity, which was more common in patients treated with high doses of the drug in early trials, may include coma, tremor, headaches, and insomnia. Nephrotoxicity associated with tacrolimus has been reported in renal transplant patients. The incidence and severity of nephrotoxicity appears to be less than that seen with CSA, although because the differential diagnosis between nephrotoxicity and rejection is so difficult in renal transplant patients, a direct comparison of these two therapies in this population would be difficult to complete. Infections following renal transplantation appear to occur at a rate similar to that observed in patients receiving CSA. Other adverse effects related to tacrolimus include post-transplant lymphoproliferative disease, hyperkalemia, hypomagnesemia, rash, and itching. As observed with CSA, most adverse effects related to tacrolimus improve with dosage reduction or discontinuation of the drug.

Early experience and clinical trials indicate that tacrolimus is effective in preventing rejection in patients following renal transplantation. Additional studies, however, will be required to determine whether the preliminary observations of lower steroid and antihypertensive requirements and less hypercholesterolemia can be verified.

Mycophenolate Mofetil

Mycophenolate mofetil (MMF) is the morpholineoethyl ester of the immunosuppressant mycophenolic acid (MPA). Following oral administration, MMF is rapidly and completely converted into MPA. MPA exerts its immunosuppressive activity through noncompetitive binding to inosine monophosphate dehydrogenase, ultimately leading to a decrease in guanosine nucleotide synthesis.[69] Preliminary dose ranging and open-label trials suggested that MMF was a safe and effective agent for use in transplant recipients.[70] In addition, some preliminary animal studies suggest that MPA may prevent or slow the progression of chronic rejection.[71,72]

MMF has primarily been studied in regimens that include CSA and corticosteroids. Two large, double blind trials have compared MMF (plus CSA and steroids) to regimens that include either placebo or AZA. In the MMF European Trial,[73] significantly fewer patients had biopsy-proven rejection or treatment failure during the first 6 months after transplantation with MMF 2 g/d (30.3%) or MMF 3 g/d (38.8%), than with placebo (56.0%). The frequency of adverse effects among the groups was similar, although gastrointestinal disturbances, neutropenia, and opportunistic infections were more common in MMF-treated patients. Similar results were reported in the MMF U.S. Trial.[74] Biopsy-proven acute rejection or treatment failure occurred in 47.6% of patients in the AZA group compared with 31.1 and 31.3% of patients in the MMF 2 g/d and 3 g/d treatment groups, respectively. Adverse effects in the groups were similar, although diarrhea, gastrointestinal dysfunction, neutropenia, and tissue invasive CMV disease occurred more frequently during MMF therapy. The annual cost of MMF is 10- to 12-fold higher than AZA. Thus, the potential long-term therapeutic benefits must be balanced with the cost of this new agent.

IMMUNOSUPPRESSIVE THERAPY SWITCHES

Steroid Withdrawal

Withdrawal of corticosteroids following renal transplantation was not a realistic therapeutic option prior to the availability of CSA. Since CSA and tacrolimus have been available, steroid withdrawal protocols are a part of routine practice. However, they must be initiated and completed with caution. There is evidence suggesting that the avoidance or discontinuation of steroids is beneficial in transplant patients receiving CSA-based immunosuppression. Six-year actual graft survival was 69% in patients withdrawn from steroids at 6 months and maintained on cyclosporine monotherapy; reinstitution of steroids was necessary in 25% of patients secondary to rejection or graft dysfunction.[27] Hricik et al.[28] demonstrated late steroid withdrawal (≥6 months post-transplant) to be successful in 79% of patients. Furthermore, a meta-analysis indicated that patient and graft survival were not adversely compromised with the avoidance or withdrawal of steroids; however, the risk of acute allograft rejection was increased.[21] These results are in contrast with previous reports.[75] The actuarial 5-year graft survival rates were 73% and 85%, respectively ($p = 0.03$), among patients who received placebo to low-dose prednisone given on alternate days. The actuarial 5-year patient survival rates, however, were not significantly different (≥92%).[55] Additional prospective, randomized trials are needed to further evaluate the long-term effects of steroid withdrawal in renal transplant patients, specifically addressing issues of time and protocol of steroid withdrawal.

Special concerns exist regarding the long-term use of corticosteroids in children.[30,31] Growth rates in children receiving corticosteroid therapy are often not much better than growth rates of children with chronic renal, hepatic, or cardiac disease. Some transplant centers withhold prednisone therapy in children until a first rejection episode occurs. Alternate-day steroids may improve growth rates in patients who require corticosteroids to maintain allograft function.[22] Steroid withdrawal has been demonstrated to be beneficial by reducing blood pressure and lipids while improving growth in transplant children maintained on CSA with or without azathioprine; however, acute rejection episodes following withdrawal may occur in a high percentage of patients.[32,33] Although, multidrug immunosuppression regimens have resulted in improved graft and patient survival, the optimal utilization of corticosteroids remains unclear.

CSA Conversion

Ongoing concerns about chronic CSA nephrotoxic effects and the high cost of prolonged therapy have led to a large number of investigations examining different strategies for electively withdrawing CSA. Unfortunately, there have been major differences in the designs, results, and conclusions of these studies. In a meta-analysis evaluating elective CSA withdrawal in renal transplant patients, there was a greater combined rate of acute rejection in patients undergoing CSA withdrawal compared with control patients who continued to receive CSA, no matter when or how the CSA was withdrawn.[76] Although there was no evidence that the higher incidence of acute rejection following CSA withdrawal led to increased graft loss or patient mortality, it is possible that the duration of follow-up was too brief to have allowed the detection of significant differences in graft or patient survival. Conversion from CSA may be considered for patients because of the high cost of CSA therapy. When considering a conversion for economic reasons, the cost of additional monitoring and the treatment of potential rejection following conversion must be included in the analysis. Well-designed randomized controlled clinical trials are needed to compare the effects of CSA withdrawal versus continued CSA therapy on long-term graft and patient survival. Any long-term negative consequences from an increased incidence of acute rejection episodes following CSA withdrawal will need to be weighed against both the increased cost and the risk of long-term toxic effects of CSA associated with continued CSA therapy.

ACUTE REJECTION THERAPY

There is no standard protocol for the management of transplant rejection. Rejection therapy should be individualized for each patient. A specific histologic diagnosis should be made since treatment is often individualized based on histology. Hypertension often worsens during a rejection episode while sodium and fluid retention and azotemia may also develop. Appropriate adjustments in pharmacotherapy are therefore warranted if such circumstances occur. Prophylactic agents such as mycostatin, trimethoprim/sulfamethoxazole (TMP/SMX), ranitidine, and/or antacids may be used during the course of antirejection therapy.[77,78]

Acute cellular rejection is the only type of rejection that responds well to antirejection therapy. High-dose steroids continue to be the first-line therapy for acute cellular rejection. Specific protocols vary between transplant centers; however, the general practice is to increase the steroid dose for 3–7 days and then taper to the maintenance level or prerejection dose, whichever is higher. One approach is to use 250–1000 mg/d intravenous methylprednisolone for 3 days. A common alternative is to use an "oral recycle" of steroids consisting of 200 mg oral prednisone, which is decreased by 40 mg each day until a maintenance dose of 20 mg per day is achieved. Although no corticosteroid regimen has been shown to be superior to another, oral steroid cycles are less costly and easier to administer than intravenous therapy.

OKT3 therapy may also be used as a first-line treatment of acute cellular rejection. The reversal rate for acute rejection in patients treated with OKT3 is more than 80%.[79] This reversal rate compares to a reversal rate of 65–75% achieved with high-dose steroids.[80] In addition, it has been suggested that long-term graft survival may be higher where OKT3 is used as primary treatment for first episodes of rejection.[81] Factors that must be considered with OKT3 use are the added potential for infectious and/or CNS toxicity and increased cost when compared to high-dose steroids. As a result of these factors and the responsiveness of acute cellular rejections to steroid treatment, OKT3 is often reserved as a second-line agent.[82]

FACTORS AFFECTING TRANSPLANT OUTCOMES

A number of factors will influence the long- and short-term success of renal transplantation. These factors include early graft function, more than one transplant, age under 15 or over 50 years, or the presence of preformed anti-HLA antibodies.

HLA antigen matching is a major factor influencing the short- and long-term success of renal transplants. The

1-year graft survival rate was 94% in recipients of HLA-identical kidneys for two haplotypes, and 89% and 90%, respectively, when a parent or sibling matched for one haplotype was the donor. Long term, the estimated half-lives for kidneys is estimated to be 26.9 years for HLA identical grafts and 12.2 and 10.8 years, respectively, for grafts from a sibling or parent that are one-haplotype matches. One-year survival for cadaveric kidneys was 88% for HLA matched kidneys and 79% for mismatched kidneys. The estimated half-life for HLA matched grafts was 17.3 years and 7.8 years for mismatched kidneys.[1]

In some patients there is a delay of several days to several weeks before sufficient kidney function is established. During this period of delayed graft function (generally secondary to ATN), the patient must be maintained on chronic dialysis. Factors contributing to ATN following renal transplantation include cold and warm ischemic damage, reperfusion injury, perioperative hypotension, and acute CSA-induced nephrotoxicity. Urinary complications such as ureteral obstruction, thrombosis or leak, or vascular complications including arterial or venous stenosis or thrombosis may also result in early graft dysfunction. The presence of delayed graft function is a poor prognostic factor for the success of a renal transplant.

The management of patients with delayed graft function is often difficult since the traditional markers of graft rejection including BUN and serum creatinine remain elevated post-transplantation. Patients with delayed graft function may receive ALG/ATG or OKT3, azathioprine, and glucocorticoid as initial therapy. The initiation of CSA may be delayed until kidney function has been established because the severity and duration of delayed graft function may be worsened by CSA and difficult to differentiate from potential CSA nephrotoxicity. Induction therapy using this strategy of delayed CSA initiation was discussed earlier in more detail in the Induction Therapy section.

Pharmacotherapy of Infectious Complications

Infectious complications following transplantation are generally classified according to the causative organism, site of the infection, and time of appearance following surgery. Bacterial infections occur most frequently within the first month post-transplantation and generally affect the urinary tract, respiratory tract, wound, or vascular access sites. Viral infections are most commonly caused by herpes simplex (early post-transplant), herpes zoster (late post-transplant), or cytomegalovirus. Infections due to nocardia, fungi, or protozoa occur rarely in renal transplant recipients.[83]

The treatment of infection in the immunocompromised host is discussed in Chapter 113. Special considerations of therapy in renal transplant patients for cytomegalovirus, herpes, and *Pneumocystis carinii* infections are described in the following sections.

Cytomegalovirus Infections

Cytomegalovirus (CMV) is the most important viral pathogen affecting transplant patients; 50–60% of the patients have been infected with the virus.[84] In individuals with a normal immune system, CMV rarely produces symptoms. However, in patients with a suppressed immune system due to drug therapy or an underlying disease state, CMV is usually symptomatic, can be quite serious, and may be fatal. Following transplantation, patients may develop symptomatic primary or secondary CMV infections. A previously CMV-seronegative patient who receives an organ or blood product from a CMV-positive donor is considered to have a primary CMV infection. A secondary infection occurs in previously seropositive patients either due to reactivation of the latent virus or reinfection. Patients with primary infections are generally more symptomatic than patients with secondary infections.

A typical patient with a CMV infection will present between 4–10 weeks following transplantation with general malaise, gastritis, and abnormal liver function studies as well as fever, leukopenia, thrombocytopenia, and atypical lymphocytes on a WBC differential. Patients with CMV infection may develop retinitis leading to a permanent reduction in visual acuity. Deterioration in renal function may also be observed in patients with CMV. CMV gastritis is a common complication in transplant patients. The leading cause of death associated with CMV infection is pneumonia.

The incidence and severity of symptomatic CMV infections in transplant recipients is related to the intensity of immunosuppression required to prevent graft rejection. Patients treated on multiple occasions with high-dose steroids or patients receiving one or more courses of OKT3 or ALG/ATG are at high risk for developing symptomatic CMV infections.[84,85]

Because many transplant patients have primary CMV infections or reinfections, it would be ideal to limit the transplantation of CMV-positive organs. This option is not practical given the high prevalence of CMV in most donor pools. Therefore, multiple strategies have been utilized for the prevention of CMV. These strategies have included both prophylactic (to prevent disease) and preemptive (to prevent disease when it is likely to occur based on the detection of CMV infection without the presence of symptoms) interventions. However, because no large, well-controlled comparative studies have been completed, there is controversy as to which agent(s), if any, should be used in renal transplant recipients.

Prophylaxis of CMV Infections

High-dose acyclovir has been reported to reduce the incidence and severity of CMV disease in renal allograft recipients.[86] This widely quoted study was a prospective, double-blind, 12-week evaluation of 104 kidney transplant patients. Patients were randomized to receive either placebo or high-dose oral acyclovir (800 mg qid with dose adjustment based on renal function) for 12 weeks post-transplantation. There was a significant reduction in CMV isolation from blood (11% versus 41%) and disease requiring ganciclovir therapy (4% versus 13%) in patients receiving acyclovir versus placebo. Furthermore, the greatest benefit of acyclovir was demonstrated in seronegative recipients receiving seropositive donor kidneys; however, there were only 13 patients in this subgroup.[86]

Subsequent studies however, have failed to produce similar results.[86–89] The failure of acyclovir, in these subsequent reports, is consistent with *in vitro* data suggesting that CMV is unlikely to be inhibited by levels of acyclovir that are achievable *in vivo*.

Acyclovir therapy, if used, is given for the first 12 weeks following transplantation since the risk for developing CMV is greatest during this period. Because acyclovir is primarily excreted unchanged via the kidney, the dose of acyclovir should be individualized based on renal function (see Chapter 50). Oral acyclovir is well tolerated, with headache and nausea being the most commonly reported adverse effects. With high-dose therapy, adverse effects appear to be more common and include nausea, severe headaches, and neurologic toxicity, such as tremor and paresthesias, which improve with dose reduction. High-dose oral acyclovir (800 mg qid), may cost \$300 to \$400 per month, which needs to be considered along with clinical factors before acyclovir is used routinely in renal transplant patients.

Ganciclovir triphosphate, the active metabolite of ganciclovir, is a potent inhibitor of the replication of human herpes viruses including CMV. Therefore, the effect of prophylactic ganciclovir on CMV in renal transplant recipients has been evaluated.[90] Intravenous ganciclovir 5 mg/kg was initiated on day 14 post-transplantation in seronegative patients receiving seropositive grafts. Although there was no difference in incidence of CMV infection or disease between ganciclovir and control patients, ganciclovir use was associated with a delayed onset and decreased severity of CMV.

Future studies of monotherapy as well as combination strategies will be needed to determine the optimal dose and duration for preventative therapy as well as the long-term toxicity of ganciclovir.

The major side effects of ganciclovir include neutropenia and thrombocytopenia. Neutropenia may occur in up to 50% of patients treated with ganciclovir. Unfortunately, neutropenia is frequently observed in patients with CMV as a consequence of the disease, making the differentiation between causes of neutropenia in these patients difficult. Thrombocytopenia occurs less frequently (20%) and, in general, the adverse hematologic effects of ganciclovir are reversible within 3–7 days following discontinuation of therapy. Other less common toxicities associated with ganciclovir therapy include central nervous system toxicity (headache, tremor, confusion, seizures, and hallucinations). Fever, rash, and alterations in liver function have also been reported in patients receiving ganciclovir therapy, but these side effects are uncommon and a definite cause-and-effect relationship has been difficult to establish.

The utility of foscarnet for CMV prevention in the transplant setting has not been defined. Foscarnet prophylaxis is not advocated in renal transplant patients because of the potential additive nephrotoxicity that may occur when it is concurrently administered with agents such as CSA and amphotericin B.

Immunoglobulins, including polyclonal IVIG and CMV hyperimmune (CMVIG) immunoglobulin, have demonstrated variable efficacy for preventing CMV disease. Polyclonal immunoglobulin preparations are not standardized with regard to CMV-antibody content.[91] As a result, high doses of polyclonal immunoglobulin preparations are generally required to deliver an effective amount of CMV antibodies. The large volumes may be especially difficult in renal transplant patients who may not be in fluid balance. Furthermore, IVIG's high cost and significant patient inconvenience combined with a yet-to-be-proven benefit in the transplant setting are major limitations of its use.

The safety and efficacy of preventive CMVIG was evaluated in a prospective, controlled, randomized, multicenter trial in seronegative renal transplant patients receiving seropositive grafts.[92] Patients received 550 mg/kg over a 16-week period and were followed for up to 1 year. Patients who received CMVIG had significantly less confirmed CMV syndromes, marked leukopenia, and fungal and protozoal infections compared to controls. Furthermore, the incidence of serious CMV disease was reduced in the CMVIG group. These results have been confirmed by other investigators.[93] Adverse effects associated with CMVIG are rare but include flushing, anxiety, nausea, a metallic taste, headache, shortness of breath, palpitations, backache, and muscle cramps. Combination strategies using CMVIG and antiviral agents for CMV prevention need to be evaluated and may be more effective than monotherapy, especially in high-risk patients.

Treatment of CMV Infections

Ganciclovir is currently the therapy of choice for the treatment of CMV infections in renal transplant patients despite the fact that there is limited clinical experience in this population.[94,95] Hrebinko et al.[94] reported their experience in 36 renal transplant patients. Clinical improvement occurred in all patients following the initial course of treatment (2.5 mg/kg every 12 hours, for a minimum of 7 days, mean 12.2 ± 3.5 days). Seven patients had persistent asymptomatic viuria and two had recurrent invasive disease, which was eradicated with a second course of therapy. Neutropenia occurred in seven patients, thrombocytopenia occurred in two patients, and rash in one patient. Cure rates in renal transplant patients ranged from 89.2–100%, with recurrent CMV infection occurring in 5–21.2% of patients. Adverse effects reported in renal transplant patients include neutropenia, thrombocytopenia, and GI effects, which have been observed in other populations requiring the drug. Sixty-four patients in the study of Dunn et al.[95] had undergone renal transplantation. Improvement at 30 days following treatment with ganciclovir was seen in 58/64 (90.6%) patients. Retreatment was required in 16 of these patients. Toxicity (neutropenia or thrombocytopenia) was reported in four of the patients, which resolved when the drug was held for 1–2 days or a dosage reduction was made.[95] Recently, the oral dosage form of ganciclovir has become available. There are no clinical trials describing the use of this formulation in renal transplant patients. Studies evaluating its efficacy as primary treatment or as follow-up to shorten a course of IV therapy are warranted.

Foscarnet is generally reserved for the treatment of CMV infections that are unresponsive to therapy with ganciclovir. Only limited experience using the drug in renal transplant patients has been published.[96,97] Andersson et al.[96] used foscarnet as a continuous IV infusion (0.15 mg/kg/min) in eight renal transplant recipients. Seven of the patients were CMV virus culture negative 1 week after starting the foscarnet. Side effects included an increase in serum creatinine (5/8 patients), hypocalcemia (4/8 patients), and confusion (1/8 patients). All side effects were reversible after dosage reduction or discontinuation of the drug. Favorable clinical responses were noted in two of three renal transplant patients described by Klintmalm et al.[97] A rise in serum creatinine was noted in all patients, which may have been secondary to foscarnet or other clinical factors. For the present, foscarnet may be used cautiously in patients unresponsive or intolerant to therapy with ganciclovir.

CMVIG is effective in preventing CMV disease in high-risk renal transplant recipients. However, the use of CMVIG to treat CMV infections in renal transplant patients has not been evaluated. The combination of CMVIG and ganciclovir was compared to ganciclovir alone in a limited number of patients following liver transplantation.[98] No difference in clinical outcomes was noted between the two study groups. There are no available studies evaluating the use of CMVIG in renal transplant patients. Because of the high cost of the medication and follow-up, until well-controlled studies of CMVIG in the treatment of CMV disease in renal transplant patients are completed, its use for this purpose is not justified.

HERPES VIRUS INFECTIONS

Herpes simplex virus (HSV) infections in renal transplant patients are most commonly the result of reactivation of a previous infection. Symptomatic HSV infection usually presents with labial or oral lesions in the first 1–3 months post-transplantation. Prophylactic therapy with low-dose acyclovir has been shown to delay the development of HSV infections in patients following renal transplantation.[99] However, patients may still develop active HSV infections after discontinuation of therapy. The use of high-dose acyclovir therapy has been shown to prevent HSV infections.[68,77] As described in Chapter 113, intravenous acyclovir therapy is indicated in patients who develop disseminated HSV infections.

PNEUMOCYSTIS CARINII PNEUMONIA

The cumulative incidence of patients who develop *Pneumocystis carinii* pneumonia (PCP) within the first-year post-transplantation has been reported to be 3–5%.[100–102] PCP is a serious complication of immunosuppression in these patients. In the early 1980s, TMP/SMX was reported to be effective in the prevention of *Pneumocystis* infections.[100,103] As a result, many transplant centers choose to treat prophylactically all transplant patients with low-dose (one single strength tablet daily) TMP/SMX. After 3 months of therapy, it is frequently possible to change therapy from once daily to three times per week.[103] TMP/SMX is highly effective, relatively inexpensive, and offers protection against other susceptible bacterial pathogens.

Aerosolized pentamidine (300 mg every month) may be used prophylactically as an alternative to TMP/SMX in patients with allergies or intolerable adverse effects to sulfonamides.[104,105] Although it is generally well tolerated, the prophylactic use of aerosolized pentamidine is expensive and offers no systemic benefits. In addition, its aerosolized administration is associated with two concerns: (1) The sensitivity of induced sputum and bronchoalveolar lavage is reduced and, therefore, the diagnosis of breakthrough PCP is more difficult to establish[106,107]; and (2) patients cough secondary to the irritating effects and thereby the risk of spreading transmissible agents is increased.[108] Dapsone may also be used as an alternative for PCP prophylaxis. Its use has been evaluated in patients with HIV and appears to be promising.[109,110] However, further study of dapsone in the setting of renal transplantation is needed to substantiate its role.

The duration of *Pneumocystis* prophylaxis is unclear. The risk of infection caused by *P. carinii* is likely to decrease as immunosuppression is reduced; therefore, prophylaxis is generally discontinued within 6–12 months following transplantation. However, some centers maintain lifelong PCP prophylaxis.

The therapy of choice for the treatment of PCP continues to be TMP/SMX. The use of TMP/SMX as well as alternative agents for PCP treatment is described in Chapter 113.

PHARMACOTHERAPY OF NONINFECTIOUS COMPLICATIONS

Following renal transplantation, patients may develop other diseases unrelated to their transplant or other complications related to their transplant. In addition, the treatment of some preexisting medical problems may require modifications due to the transplant or medications required to maintain the transplant.

HYPERTENSION

Hypertension may have been present prior to transplantation or may develop as a result of the immunosuppressive medications required in the postoperative period. Impaired graft function following transplantation, corticosteroids, CSA, and tacrolimus may cause post-transplant hypertension. The treatment of hypertension is generally approached according to the guidelines established by the Joint National Committee on the Detection, Evaluation, and Treatment of High Blood Pressure.[111] However, some special precautions are required in this patient population.[112–115]

The treatment of hypertension following renal transplantation is most often achieved using a diuretic alone or in combination with another agent. Because of impaired renal function, thiazide diuretics may be ineffective, necessitating the use of a loop diuretic. Calcium channel blocking drugs, especially those of the dihydropiridine subclass, are highly effective in treating postoperative hypertension.[115] These agents are generally well tolerated at normal maintenance doses, with headache and edema more common at high doses. These agents may also have an additional benefit of improving renal blood flow and glomerular filtration in transplant patients. Verapamil and diltiazem may inhibit the hepatic metabolism of CSA and should be used with caution in these patients.[61] While several case reports describing interactions between CSA and the dihydropyridine calcium channel blockers are available, these interactions appear to be of little clinical significance.

Centrally acting agents (e.g., clonidine, guanabenz) and peripheral alpha blockers (e.g., prazosin, doxazosin, terazosin) are also effective in treating hypertension in these patients. Sedation, anticholinergic effects, and first-dose hypotension, respectively, which can occur in any patient receiving these agents must be considered. Beta-adrenergic blockers may be effective in some patients. However, since the leading cause of renal failure resulting in transplantation is diabetes mellitus, concerns related to impaired responses to hypoglycemia and effects on the peripheral vasculature in diabetics must be considered. In addition, decreased renal blood flow caused by β-adrenergic blockers may be undesirable in renal transplant patients. Direct-acting vasodilators may be required in some patients to control post-transplant hypertension. They are most often used in the early postoperative period. Since other agents are so effective, vasodilators are rarely required as maintenance therapy following transplantation.

Angiotensin-converting enzyme (ACE) inhibitors, which are frequently used in diabetics to slow the progression of renal disease, may be effective post renal transplantation. However, the combination of efferent arteriolar vasodilation caused by the ACE inhibitor and afferent vasoconstriction caused by CSA or tacrolimus may result in a decrease in glomerular filtration when these combinations are used. In addition, the hyperkalemia caused by CSA and/or tacrolimus is frequently worsened by concomitant therapy with an ACE inhibitor. If ACE inhibitor therapy is used in patients post-transplantation, close monitoring of serum creatinine and potassium is required.

HYPERLIPIDEMIA

Many renal transplant patients had elevated cholesterol prior to transplantation or developed it as a result of postoperative medications. Therapy with CSA, corticosteroids, diuretics, and β-adrenergic blockers can have a detrimental effect on serum lipids. The management of hyperlipidemia in these patients should follow the guidelines established by the National Cholesterol Education Program for diet and medication use.[116] Some special therapeutic issues must be considered in the management of hyperlipidemia in transplant patients.

Niacin is highly effective in improving lipid profiles in nontransplant patients. Niacin may be used in renal transplant patients; however, since transplant patients may require other hepatotoxic medications, liver function tests should be closely monitored. While gemfibrozil is most effective in lowering serum triglyceride concentrations, a recent study of renal transplant patients reported decreases in total cholesterol, triglycerides, and LDL-cholesterol following gemfibrizol therapy.[117]

Bile acid binding resins may be used to lower cholesterol in renal transplant patients. Since the absorption of CSA is dependent on the presence of bile in the GI tract, patients should be instructed to separate dosing of bile acid binding resins and CSA. Because the absorption of tacrolimus is not dependent on bile, this interaction is not of significance in patients immunosuppressed with tacrolimus.

HMG-CoA reductase inhibitors are highly effective in the treatment of hyperlipidemia in renal transplant patients.[118] These agents should be used with caution because of several reports of rhabdomyolysis resulting in renal failure when lovastatin was used in combination with CSA. In addition, because of the potential for hepatotoxicity from HMG-CoA reductase inhibitors, close monitoring of liver function is indicated. It is currently unknown whether HMG-CoA reductase inhibitors other than lovastatin interact with CSA or whether similar interactions would occur in patients receiving tacrolimus. Until additional information is available, the use of HMG-CoA reductase inhibitors should be used with caution in transplant patients. Patients should be informed of the signs and symptoms of rhabdomyolysis. Baseline and follow-up CPK measurements (every 6 months) have been used to identify patients who develop subclinical rhabdomyolysis when cholesterol lowering therapy is used.

GASTROINTESTINAL ULCER PROPHYLAXIS

Patients following renal transplantation are at high risk for gastrointestinal bleeding either due to their preexisting renal failure or as the result of chronic corticosteroid therapy. No studies have demonstrated a benefit to GI ulcer prophylaxis in renal transplant patients. However, patients frequently receive H_2-blocker therapy for ulcer prophylaxis. When utilized, H_2 blockers should be prescribed at the doses appropriate for prophylaxis based on renal function. Sucralfate, at prophylactic doses (1.0 g PO, BID), may also be used for ulcer prophylaxis. The use of combination antiulcer therapy, omeprazole or misoprostil, plus an H_2 blocker for post-transplant GI ulcer prophylaxis is not indicated.

LIVER DISEASE

Liver disease is a common cause of morbidity and mortality in renal transplant recipients, with abnormalities in liver function occurring in 7 to 24% of patients in the early post-transplant period.[119] Many factors have been implicated in the etiology of post-transplantation liver disease, including drug toxicity and viral infection. The management of cyclosporine- or azathioprine-induced hepatotoxicity usually responds to dosage reductions (see Chapter 38). However, discontinuation of the offending agent with a switch to another immunosuppressant (e.g., tacrolimus, MMF) may be warranted. Although hepatitis B virus was thought to play an important role, the incidence of post-transplantation chronic liver disease remained high after the exclusion of organ and blood donors who were hepatitis B surface antigen positive.

Transplant recipients are potentially at risk of developing hepatitis C virus (HCV) due to reactivation of pretransplantation HCV infection, infection acquired from blood products received at the time of transplantation, or HVC-infected organ donors. The prevalence of anti-hepatitis C virus antibodies varies from 2.4 to 5.1% among cadaveric organ donors.[120] In comparison, the prevalence of anti-HCV among healthy blood donors in the United States is only 0.6%. The higher prevalence among cadaver organ donors may reflect an increased incidence of risk factors associated with the spread of viral infections, such as unsuspected intravenous drug use or sexual promiscuity.

Recent studies suggest that the natural history of HCV infection and the host response to the virus in transplant recipients[121] are different from that observed in healthy individuals with post-transfusion hepatitis C.[122] A large proportion of nontransplanted patients with HCV infection have no evidence of liver disease. Possible explanations for this finding include the criteria used to define liver disease, extrahepatic sites of viral replication, a healthy carrier state, or indolent liver disease. Approximately 50% of patients with post-transfusion non-A, non-B hepatitis progress to chronic liver disease; in contrast, a majority of patients with post-transplantation liver disease progress to chronic hepatitis or develop subfulminant liver failure, and none clear the virus from the serum. The immunosuppressive therapy in transplant recipients could play an important role in preventing clearing of virus and recovery from liver disease. Finally, immunosuppression impairs the anti-HCV response in transplant recipients with HCV.

In otherwise healthy adults, acute HCV infection resolves in about 50%, while the rest progress to chronic liver disease, including chronic persistent hepatitis, chronic active hepatitis, and cirrhosis. Treatment is not generally recommended for acute hepatitis or chronic persistent hepatitis. However, interferon-α has been used with considerable success in nontransplant patients with chronic active hepatitis due to HCV.[123] Unfortunately, these results cannot necessarily be extrapolated to transplant recipients with chronic liver disease due to HCV. Interferon-α has pleiotropic effects that include antiviral, antiproliferative, and immunomodulatory properties. In particular, this agent can induce cytokine gene expression, increase cell surface expression of HLA antigens, and enhance the function of natural killer cells, cytotoxic T cells, and monocytes. As a result, therapy with interferon-α carries the risk of inducing or facilitating rejection in the allograft.[124] Thus, the risk of rejection in transplantation recipients must be weighed against the potential benefits of slowing or preventing the progression of chronic liver disease.

PATIENT OUTCOMES

Renal transplantation remains the therapy of choice for most patients with chronic renal failure. The development of new immunosuppressive agents and improved immunologic monitoring methods has reduced complications and prolonged graft survival. The application of studies of antigen-specific tolerance in the clinical setting make the future of renal transplantation even brighter. The importance of pharmacotherapy in the successful management of renal transplant patients has created an opportunity for pharmacists to enhance patient outcomes. Pharmacists are involved in the management of renal transplant patients along the continuum of care. Pharmacists can assist in the management of blood pressure, diabetes mellitus, anemia (e.g., erythropoietin, iron), and hyperlipidemia, and provide patient medication counseling for pretransplant patients in the dialysis unit or pretransplant renal clinic. In the perioperative period, pharmacists consult on operating room teams, and assist in the early postoperative management of fluids, electrolytes, hypertension, diabetes, immunosuppression, and general drug dosing in these patients with continuously changing renal function. Long term, pharmacists manage many of the complications experienced by these patients, including hypertension, diabetes, hyperlipidemia, infection, and GI disease. Pharmacists provide patient and family medication education and compliance monitoring, and are frequently an invaluable source of information regarding payment and reimbursement for medication. Although there may be a direct link between these activities and improved patient outcomes, documentation is limited.

References

1. United Network for Organ Sharing, 1995.
2. U.S. Renal Data System, 1995 Annual Report. Am J Kid Dis 1995;26:S1–S186.
3. Christensen AJ, Holman JM, Turner CW, Slaughter JR. Quality of life in end stage renal disease. Influence of renal transplantation. Clin Transplantation 1989;3:46–53.
4. Effers PW. Effect of transplantation on the Medicare end-stage renal disease program. N Engl J Med 1988;318:223–229.
5. Suthanthiran M, Strom TB. Renal transplantation. N Engl J Med 1994;331:365–376.
6. Opelz G, Wujciak T, Mytilineos J, Scherer S. Revisiting HLA matching for kidney transplantation. Transplant Proc 1993;25:173–175.
7. Wahlberg JA, Love R, Langford L, et al. Seventy-two hour preservation of canine pancreas. Transplantation 1987;43:5–8.
8. Lee HM. Surgical techniques for renal transplantation, in Morris PJ (ed): Kidney Transplantation, 3rd ed. Philadelphia, WB Saunders, 1988, pp 215–234.
9. Lindholm A, Ohlman S, Albrechtsen D, et al. The impact of acute rejection episodes of long-term graft function and outcome in 1347 primary renal transplants treated by 3 cyclosporine regimens. Transplantation 1993;56:307–315.
10. Bertolatus JA. Clinical immunosuppressive regimens and clinical results in renal transplantation. Semin Nephrol 1992;12:332–342.
11. Goldman M, Abramowicz D, De Pauw L, et al. Beneficial effects of prophylactic OKT3 in cadaver kidney transplantation: Comparison with cyclosporin A in a single-center prospective randomized study. Transplant Proc 1991;23:1046–1047.
12. Griño JM, Alsina J, Sabater R, et al. Antilymphoblast globulin, cyclosporine, and steroids in cadaveric renal transplantation. Transplantation 1990;49:1114–1117.
13. Cecka JM, Gjertson D, Terasaki PI. Do prophylactic antilymphocyte globulins (ALG and OKT3) improve renal transplant survival in recipient and donor high-risk groups? Transplant Proc 1993;25:548–549.
14. Norman DJ, Kahana L, Stuart FP, Jr., et al. A randomized clinical trial of induction therapy with OKT3 in kidney transplantation. Transplantation 1993;55:44–50.
15. Michael HJ, Francos GC, Burke JF, et al. A comparison of the effects of cyclosporine versus antilymphocyte globulin on delayed graft function in cadaver renal transplant recipients. Transplantation 1989;48:805–808.
16. Belitsky P, MacDonald AS, Cohen AD, et al. Comparison of antilymphocyte globulin and continuous IV cyclosporine A as induction immunosuppression for cadaver kidney transplants: A prospective randomized study. Transplant Proc 1991;23:999–1000.
17. Slakey DP, Johnson CP, Callaluce RD, et al. A prospective randomized comparison of quadruple versus triple therapy for first cadaver transplants with immediate function. Transplantation 1993;56:827–831.
18. Steinmuller DR, Hayes JM, Novick AC, et al. Comparison of OKT3 with ALG for prophylaxis for patients with acute renal failure after cadaveric renal transplantation. Transplantation 1991;52:67–71.
19. Hanto DW, Jendrisak MD, McCullough CS, et al. A prospective randomized comparison of prophylactic ALG and OKT3 in cadaver kidney allograft recipients. Transplant Proc 1991;23:1050–1051.
20. Frey DJ, Matas AJ, Gillingham KJ, et al. MALG and OKT3 following renal transplantation: A randomized prospective trial. Transplant Proc 1991;23:1048–1049.
21. Light JA, Jonsson J, Khawand N, et al. Sequential immunosuppression: Three years' experience in 240 cadaveric renal transplants. Transplant Proc 1991;23:1032–1035.
22. Shield CF, III. Consequences of anti-OKT3 antibody development: OKT3 reuse and long-term graft survival. Transplant Proc 1993;25(suppl 1):81–82.
23. Mayes JT, Thistlethwaite JR, Stuart JK, et al. Reexposure to OKT3 in renal allograft recipients. Transplantation 1988;45:349–353.
24. Walker AM, ed. Transplant Protocols. Chestnut Hill, MA, Epidemiology Resources Inc., 1990.
25. Murray JE, Merrill JP, Harrison JH, et al. Prolonged survival of human kidney homografts by immunosuppressive drug therapy. N Engl J Med 1963;268:1315–1323.
26. Starzl TE, Marchioro TL, Waddell WR. The reversal of rejection in human renal homografts with subsequent development of homograft tolerance. Surg Gynecol Obstet 1963;117:385–395.
27. Hillebrand G, Schneeberger H, Schleibner S, et al. Ten years' experience with cyclosporine monotherapy after renal transplantation. Transplant Proc 1993;25:513–514.
28. Hricik DE, Whalen CC, Lautman J, et al. Withdrawal of steroids after renal transplantation—clinical predictors of outcome. Transplantation 1992;53:41–45.
29. Hricik DE, O'Toole MA, Schulak JA, Herson J. Steroid-free immunosuppression in cyclosporine-treated renal transplant recipients: A meta-analysis. J Am Soc Nephrol 1993;4:1300–1305.
30. Ettenger RB, Blifeld C, Prince H, et al. The pediatric nephrologist's dilemma: Growth after renal transplantation

and its interaction with age as a possible immunologic variable. J Pediatr 1987;111:1022–1025.
31. Tejani A, Butt KMH, Rajpoot D, et al. Strategies for optimizing growth in children with kidney transplants. Transplantation 1989;47:229–233.
32. Walker RG, Jones CL, Powell HR, et al. Steroid withdrawal in paediatric renal transplant patients receiving cyclosporine and azathioprine. Transplant Proc 1993;25:2883–2885.
33. Ingulli E, Tejani A, Markell M. The beneficial effects of steroid withdrawal on blood pressure and lipid profile in children posttransplantation in the cyclosporine era. Transplantation 1993;55:1029–1033.
34. Canadian Multicentre Transplant Study Group. A randomized clinical trial of cyclosporine in cadaveric renal transplantation. N Engl J Med 1983;309:809–815.
35. European Multicentre Trial Group. Cyclosporin in cadaveric renal transplantation: One-year follow-up of a multicentre trial. Lancet 1983;2:986–989.
36. Najarian JS, Fryd DS, Strand M, et al. A single institution, randomized, prospective trial of cyclosporine versus azathioprine-antilymphocyte globulin for immunosuppression in renal allograft recipients. Ann Surg 1985;201:142–157.
37. Andreu J, Campistol JM, Oppenheimer F, et al. Cyclosporine monotherapy as primary immunosuppression in renal transplantation—five-year experience. Transplant Proc 1994;26:337–340.
38. Griffin PJA, Gomes Da Costa CA, Salaman JR. A controlled trial of steroids in cyclosporine-treated renal transplant recipients. Transplantation 1987;43:505–508.
39. Tarantino A, Aroldi A, Stucchi L, et al. A randomized prospective trial comparing cyclosporine monotherapy with triple-drug therapy in renal transplantation. Transplantation 1991;52:53–57.
40. Ghoneim MA, Sobh MA, Shokeir AA, et al. Prospective randomized study of azathioprine versus cyclosporin in live-donor kidney transplantation. Am J Nephrol 1993;13:437–441.
41. Amend W, Soskin T, Vincenti F, et al. Long-term experience in primary cadaver renal transplants using cyclosporine. Clin Transplantation 1990;4:341–346.
42. Hardie IR, Tiller DJ, Mahony JF, et al. Optimal combination of immunosuppressive agents for renal transplantation: First report of a multicentre, randomized trial comparing cyclosporine+prednisolone with cyclosporine+azathioprine and with triple therapy in cadaver renal transplantation. Transplant Proc 1993;25:583–584.
43. Lindholm A, Albrechtsen D, Tufveson G, et al. A randomized trial of cyclosporine and prednisone versus cyclosporine, azathioprine, and prednisolone in primary cadaveric renal transplantation. Transplantation 1992;54:624–631.
44. Isoniemi H, Ahonen J, Tikkanen MJ, et al. Long-term consequences of different immunosuppressive regimens for renal allografts. Transplantation 1993;55:494–499.
45. Ghoneim MA, Sobh MA, Shokeir AA, et al. Prospective randomized study of triple vs conventional immunosuppression in living donor kidney transplantation. Transplant Proc 1993;25:2243–2245.
46. Monaco AP, Sahyoun AI, Madras PN, et al. Cyclosporine in multi-drug therapy in living-related kidney transplantation. Clin Transplantation 1990;4:347–356.
47. Montagnino G, Colturi C, Tarantino A, et al. The impact of azathioprine and cyclosporine on long-term function in kidney transplantation. Transplantation 1991;51:772–776.
48. Slaton JW, Kropp KA, Jhunjhunwala JS, Selman SH. Cyclosporine versus azathioprine: A 5-year follow-up of 200 consecutive cadaver renal transplant recipients. J Urol 1994;151:582–585.
49. Helderman JH, Van Buren DH, Amend WJC, Jr, Pirsch JD. Chronic immunosuppression of the renal transplant patient. J Am Soc Nephrol 1994;4(suppl 1):S2–S9.
50. Burke JF, Pirsh JD, Ramos EL, et al. Long-term efficacy and safety of cyclosporine in renal-transplant recipients. N Engl J Med 1994;331:358–363.
51. Lindholm A, Welsh M, Alton C, Kahan BD. Demographic factors influencing cyclosporine pharmacokinetic parameters in patients with uremia: Racial differences in bioavailability. Clin Pharmacol Ther 1992;52:359–371.
52. Ohlman S, Lindholm A, Hägglund H, et al. On the intraindividual variability and chronobiology of cyclosporine pharmacokinetics in renal transplantation. Eur J Clin Pharmacol 1993;44:265–269.
53. Awni WM, Kasiske BL, Heim-Duthoy KL, Rao KV. Long-term cyclosporine pharmacokinetic changes in renal transplant recipients: Effects of binding and metabolism. Clin Pharmacol Ther 1989;45:41–48.
54. Kahan BD, Shaw LM, Holt D, et al. Consensus document: Hawk's Cay meeting on therapeutic drug monitoring of cyclosporine. Clin Chem 1990;36:1510–1516.
55. Kivisto KT. A review of assay methods for cyclosporin. Clinical implications. Clin Pharmacokinet 1992;23:173–190.
56. Rodighiero V. Therapeutic drug monitoring of cyclosporin—practical applications and limitations. Clin Pharmacokinet 1989;16:27–37.
57. Grevel J, Welsh MS, Kahan BD. Cyclosporine monitoring in renal transplantation: Area under the curve monitoring is superior to trough-level monitoring. Ther Drug Monit 1989;11:246–248.
58. Awni WM, Heim-Duthoy K, Kasiske BL. Monitoring of cyclosporine by serial posttransplant pharmacokinetic studies in renal transplant patients. Transplant Proc 1990;22:1343–1344.
59. Grevel J, Kahan BD. Abbreviated kinetic profiles in area-under-the-curve monitoring of cyclosporine therapy. Clin Chem 1991;37:1905–1908.
60. Lindholm A, Kahan BD. Influence of cyclosporine pharmacokinetics, trough concentrations, and AUC monitoring on outcome after kidney transplantation. Clin Pharmacol Ther 1993;54:205–218.
61. McDonald P, Keough A, Connell J, et al. Diltiazem co-administration reduces cyclosporine toxicity after heart transplantation: A prospective randomized study. Transplant Proc 1992;24:2259–2262.
62. Keough A, Spratt P, McCosker C, et al. Ketoconazole to reduce the need for cyclosporine after cardiac transplantation. N Engl J Med 1995;333:628–633.
63. Alexopoulos E, Leontsini M, Daniilidis M, et al. Differentiation between renal allograft rejection and cyclosporine

toxicity: A clinicopathological study. Am J Kidney Dis 1991;18:108–115.

64. Palestine AG, Austin HA, III, Balow JE, et al. Renal histopathologic alterations in patients treated with cyclosporine for uveitis. N Engl J Med 1986;314:1293–1298.
65. Starzl RE, Fung J, Jordan M, et al., Kidney transplantation under FK 506. JAMA 1990;264:63–67.
66. Shapiro R, Jordan M, Scantlebury VP, et al. Renal transplantation at the University of Pittsburgh: Impact of FK 506, in Terasaki PI, Cecka JM (eds): Clinical Transplants, 1994. Los Angeles, UCLA Tissue Typing Laboratory, 1995, pp 229–236.
67. Japanese FK 506 Study Group. Japanese study of FK 506 on kidney transplantation: Results of late phase II study. Transplant Proc 1993;25:649–654.
68. Mayer D, Buist L, Erhard J, et al. A European, pilot, multicenter, randomized study to compare the efficacy and safety of FK 506 with that of cyclosporin in patients undergoing primary renal transplantation: 6-week results[abstract 142]. 6th Congress European Society for Organ Transplantation, 1993.
69. Young CJ, Sollinger HW. Mycophenolate mofetil (RS-61443), in Kupiec-Weglinski JW (ed): New Immunosuppressive Modalities in Organ Transplantation. Austin, TX, R.G. Landes Co., 1994.
70. Sollinger HW, Deierhol MH, Belzer FO, et al. RS-61443-A phase I clinical trial and pilot rescue study. Transplantation 1992;53:428–432.
71. Morris RE, Wang J, Blum JR, et al. Immunosuppressive effects of the morpholineoethyl ester of mycophenolic acid (RS-61443) in rat and nonhuman primate recipients of heart allografts. Transplant Proc 1991;23(suppl 2):19.
72. Steele DM, Hullett DA, Bechstein WO, et al. Effects of immunosuppressive therapy on the rat aortic allograft model. Transplant Proc 1993;25:754.
73. European Mycophenolate Mofetil Cooperative Study Group. Placebo-controlled study of mycophenolate mofetil combined with cyclosporin and corticosteroids for the prevention of acute rejection. Lancet 1995;345:1321–1325.
74. Sollinger HW for the U.S. Renal Transplant Mycophenolate Mofetil Study Group. Mycophenolate mofetil for the prevention of acute rejection in primary cadaveric renal allograft recipients. Transplantation 1995;60:225–232.
75. St. Sinclair NR. Low-dose steroid therapy in cyclosporine-treated renal transplant recipients with well-functioning grafts. Can Med Assoc J 1992;147:645–655.
76. Kasiske BL, Heim-Duthoy KL, Ma JZ. Elective cyclosporine withdrawal after renal transplantation: A meta-analysis. JAMA 1993;269:395–400.
77. Rao KV. Mechanism, pathophysiology, diagnosis, and management of renal transplant rejection. Med Clin North Am 1990;74:1039–1057.
78. Gray D, Daar A, Shepherd H, et al. Oral versus intravenous high-dose steroid treatment of renal allograft rejection. The big shot or not? Lancet 1978;1:117–118.
79. Ortho Multicenter Transplant Study Group. A randomized clinical trial of OKT3 monoclonal antibody for acute rejection of cadaveric renal transplants. N Engl J Med 1985;313:337–342.
80. Deierhoi MH, Barber WH, Curtis JJ, et al. A comparison of OKT3 monoclonal antibody and corticosteroids in the treatment of acute renal allograft rejection. Am J Kidney Dis 1988;11:86–89.
81. Tesi RJ, Elkhammas EA, Henry ML, Ferguson RM. OKT3 for primary therapy of the first rejection episode in kidney transplants. Transplantation 1993;55:1023–1029.
82. Oh C-S, Stratta RJ, Fox BC, et al. Increased infections associated with the use of OKT3 for treatment of steroid-resistant rejection in renal transplantation. Transplantation 1988;45:68–73.
83. Rubin RH, Wolfson JA, Cosimi AB, Tolkoff-Rubin NE. Infection in the renal transplant recipient. Am J Med 1981;70:405–411.
84. Farrugia E, Schwab TR. Management and prevention of cytomegalovirus infection after renal transplantation. Mayo Clin Proc 1992;67:879–890.
85. Snydman DR, Rubin RH, Werner BG. New developments in cytomegalovirus prevention and management. Am J Kidney Dis 1993;21:217–228.
86. Balfour HH, Jr, Chace BA, Stapleton JT, et al. A randomized, placebo-controlled trial of oral acyclovir for the prevention of cytomegalovirus disease in recipients of renal allografts. N Engl J Med 1989;320:1381–1387.
87. Bailey TC, Ettinger NA, Storch GA, et al. Failure of high-dose oral acyclovir with or without immune globulin to prevent primary cytomegalovirus disease in recipients of solid organ transplants. Am J Med 1993;95:273–278.
88. Vasquez EM, Sanchez J, Pollak R, et al. High-dose oral acyclovir prophylaxis for primary cytomegalovirus infection in seronegative renal allograft recipients. Transplantation 1993;55:448–450.
89. Chitwood KK, Heim-Duthoy KL, Ney AL, Kasiske BL. Questionable benefit of prophylactic acyclovir in renal transplant recipients at high risk for cytomegalovirus disease. Clin Transplantation 1993;7:320–324.
90. Rondeau E, Bourgeon B, Peraldi MN, et al. Effect of prophylactic ganciclovir on cytomegalovirus infection in renal transplant recipients. Nephrol Dial Transplant 1993;8:858–862.
91. Roy DM, Grundy JE. Evaluation of neutralizing antibody titers against human cytomegalovirus in intravenous gamma globulin preparations. Transplantation 1992;54:1109–1110.
92. Snydman DR, Werner BG, Heinze-Lacey B, et al. Use of cytomegalovirus immune globulin to prevent cytomegalovirus disease in renal transplant recipients. N Engl J Med 1987;317:1049–1054.
93. Werner BG, Snydman DR, Freeman R, et al. Cytomegalovirus immune globulin for the prevention of primary CMV disease in renal transplant patients: Analysis of usage under treatment IND status. Transplant Proc 1993;25:1441–1443.
94. Hrebinko R, Jordan ML, Dummer JS, et al. Ganciclovir for invasive cytomegalovirus infection in renal allograft recipients. Transplant Proc 1991;23:1346–1347.
95. Dunn DL, Mayoral JL, Gillingham KJ, et al. Treatment of invasive cytomegalovirus disease in solid organ transplant patients with ganciclovir. Transplantation 1991;51:98–106.
96. Andersson J, Akesson-Johansson A, Brattstrom C. Evaluation by immune scanning electron microscopy of foscarnet

treatment of cytomegalovirus infection in patients with renal transplants. Scand J Inf Dis 1989;21:605–610.

97. Klintmalm G, Lonnqvist B, Oberg B, et al. Intravenous foscarnet for the treatment of severe cytomegalovirus infection in allograft recipients. Scand J Inf Dis 1985;17:157–163.
98. George MJ, Snydman DR, Werner BG, et al. Use of ganciclovir plus cytomegalovirus immune globulin to treat CMV pneumonia in orthotopic liver transplant recipients. Transplant Proc 1993;25:2(suppl 4):22–24.
99. Seale L, Jones CJ, Kathpalia S, et al. Prevention of herpes virus infections in renal allograft recipients by low-dose oral acyclovir. JAMA 1985;254:3435–3438.
100. Hardy AM, Wajszcsuk CP, Suffredini AF, et al. *Pneumocystis carinii* pneumonia in renal-transplant recipients treated with cyclosporine and steroids. J Infect Dis 1984;149:143–147.
101. Higgins RM, Bloom SL, Hopkin JM, Morris PJ. The risks and benefits of low-dose cotrimoxazole prophylaxis for *pneumocystis* pneumonia in renal transplantation. Transplantation 1989;47:558–560.
102. Santiago-Delpín EA, Mora E, González ZA, et al. Factors in an outbreak of *pneumocystis carinii* in a transplant unit. Transplant Proc 1988;20:462–465.
103. Hughes WT, Rivera GK, Schell MJ, et al. Successful intermittent chemoprophylaxis for *pneumocystis carinii* pneumonitis. N Engl J Med 1987;316:1627–1632.
104. Hirschel B, Lazzarin A, Chopard P, et al. A controlled study of inhaled pentamidine for primary prevention of *pneumocystis carinii* pneumonia. N Engl J Med 1991;324:1079–1083.
105. Hardy WD, Feinberg J, Finkelstein DM, et al. A controlled trial of trimethoprim-sulfamethoxazole for aerosolized pentamidine for secondary prophylaxis of *pneumocystis carinii* pneumonia in patients with the acquired immunodeficiency syndrome. N Engl J Med 1992;327:1842–1848.
106. Jules-Elysee KM, Stover DE, Zaman MB, et al. Aerosolized pentamidine: Effect on diagnosis and presentation of *pneumocystis carinii* pneumonia. Ann Intern Med 1990;112:750–757.
107. Levine SJ, Masur H, Gill VJ, et al. Effect of aerosolized pentamidine prophylaxis on the diagnosis of *pneumocystis carinii* pneumonia by induced sputum examination in patients infected with the human immunodeficiency virus. Am Rev Respir Dis 1991;144:760–764.
108. U.S. Department of Health and Human Services/Public Health Service. Nosocomial transmission of multidrug-resistant tuberculosis among HIV-infected persons—Florida and New York, 1988–1991. MMWR 1991;40:585–591.
109. Hughes WT, Kennedy W, Dugdale M, et al. Prevention of *pneumocystis carinii* pneumonitis in AIDS patients with weekly dapsone. Lancet 1990;2:1066.
110. Kemper CA, Tucker RM, Lang OS, et al. Low-dose dapsone prophylaxis of *pneumocystis carinii* pneumonia in AIDS and AIDS-related complex. AIDS 1990;4:1145–1148.
111. The Fifth Report of the Joint National Committee on the Detection, Evaluation and Treatment of High Blood Pressure (JNC V). Arch Int Med 1993;153;154–183.
112. Curtis JJ. Hypertension following kidney transplantation. Am J Kidney Dis 1994;23:471–475.
113. First RJ, Neylan JF, Rocher LL, Tejani A. Hypertension after renal transplantation. J Am Soc Nephrol 1994;4(suppl);S30–S36.
114. Curtis JJ. Management of hypertension after renal transplantation. Kidney Int 1993;44:S45–S49.
115. van der Schaaf MR, Hene RJ, Floor M, et al. Hypertension after renal transplantation. Hypertension 1995;25:77–81.
116. Summary of the Second Report of the National Cholesterol Education Program (NCEP) Expert Panel on Detection, Evaluation and Treatment of High Blood Cholesterol in Adults (Adult Treatment Panel II). JAMA 1993;269:3015–3023.
117. Chan M, Cheng KP, Tam CF. Hyperlipidemia after renal transplantation: Treatment with gemfibrozil. Nephron 1994;67:317–324.
118. Kirk JK, Dupuis RE. Approaches to the treatment of hyperlipidemia in the solid organ transplant recipient. Ann Pharmacother 1995;29:879–891.
119. Weir MR, Kirkman RL, Strom TB, Tilney NL. Liver disease in recipients of long-surviving renal allografts. Kidney Int 1985;28:839.
120. Pereira BJ, Wright TL, Schmid CH, et al. Screening and confirmatory testing of cadaver donors for hepatitis C virus infection: A U.S. National Collaborative Study. Kidney Int 1994;46:886.
121. Aeder MI, Shield CF, Tegtmeier GE, et al. The incidence and clinical impact of hepatitis C virus (HCV) positive donors in cadaveric transplantation. Transplant Proc 1993;25:1469.
122. Kortez RL, Stone O, Mousa M, Gitnick GL. Non-A, non-B post-transfusion hepatitis—a decade later. Gastroenterology 1985;88:1251.
123. Black M. Alpha-interferon treatment of chronic hepatitis C: Need for accurate diagnosis in selecting patients. Ann Intern Med 1992;116:86.
124. Kovarik J, Mayer G, Pohanak E, et al. Adverse effects of low-dose prophylactic human recombinant leukocyte interferon-alpha treatment in renal transplant recipients. Transplantation 1988;45:402.

Chapter 46

Principles and Practice of Chronic Renal Replacement Therapy

Gary R. Matzke, PharmD, FCP, FCCP, and George R. Bailie, MSc, PharmD, PhD, FCCP

Hemodialysis and peritoneal dialysis are the major treatment options for patients with end-stage renal disease (ESRD). Globally the dialysis population is estimated to number more than 650,000 patients, and the United States contributes almost 30% to this population. Japan and Europe contribute about 23 and 22% each, respectively.[1] The global growth of hemodialysis (HD) is estimated to be about 8.2% per year, whereas it is about 12% per year for peritoneal dialysis (PD). Thus, worldwide, there are now about 550,000 HD patients and 100,000 PD patients. The ratio of hemodialysis to peritoneal dialysis patients varies enormously among countries.[2] The percentage of dialysis patients treated by PD in 1992 was Japan, 5.0%; Germany, 6.0%; Australia, 31.0%; Canada, 34.0%; United Kingdom, 49.0%; and the United States, 14.0%.[2] There are several reasons for these differences, including the difference in costs between PD and HD, availability of equipment and trained personnel, political pressures, and physician and patient preferences.[3]

In the United States, estimates by the Health Care Financing Administration suggest that the number of dialysis patients will increase from 130,000 in 1990 to about 338,000 by the year 2000, a growth rate of about 10% per year.[4] The increase in the growth of PD is currently greater than for hemodialysis in the United States—about 17% of dialysis patients (29,300 in 1993) were treated by PD. The number of kidney transplants performed each year has remained relatively static over the last 5–10 years at about 8000 to 10,000, while the number of patients with end-stage renal disease awaiting transplants has increased sharply from 10,000 in 1986 to more than 27,000 in 1994.[5] The limited availability of transplantation as a treatment option for patients with ESRD has thus compounded the demand for chronic renal replacement therapy.

A number of studies have compared the mortality rates of peritoneal versus hemodialysis patients.[6–11] A recent study examined the mortality rate and causes of death in 42,372 dialysis patients over 170,700 years at risk.[10] Bloembergen et al.[10,11] found that there was a 19% increase in the relative risk of death with peritoneal dialysis compared to hemodialysis, and that peritoneal dialysis patients had more deaths as a result of infections, acute myocardial infarctions, and other cardiac causes, and as a result of cerebrovascular diseases. Other studies indicate that elderly nondiabetic patients and younger diabetic patients have an increased risk of death on hemodialysis, while older diabetic patients have an increased risk on PD.[6,8] The 1-year patient survival from 1991 data was 69.6 and 65.7% for diabetic hemodialysis and continuous ambulatory peritoneal dialysis (CAPD) patients, and 78.6 and 78.3% for nondiabetic hemodialysis and CAPD patients.[6] It is difficult to interpret accurately some of the U.S. Renal Data System (USRDS) data, however, since it remains unclear whether the older diabetic patients also had an increased cardiac disease severity. Causes of death with both treatment modalities are similar (Fig. 46.1).[12] Cardiovascular events account for 25–40% of all deaths, while peritonitis is the second most common cause of mortality among peritoneal dialysis patients. Of patients leaving PD, the major reasons are death or transfer to hemodialysis because of frequent episodes of peritonitis.[13]

Irrespective of the mode of chronic renal replacement therapy, patient survival remains poor. According to the USRDS, age- and sex-matched ESRD patients have about 20–25% of the expected remaining lifetime of the general population (Fig. 46.2).[14] Age-adjusted mortality rates for U.S. dialysis patients are about 15–30% higher than patients in Western Europe or Japan (Fig. 46.3).[15] Possible reasons for this include the increased age and number of comorbid conditions including cardiovascular diseases, diabetes, and malnutrition among U.S. patients. Other variables that may contribute to this phenomenon are the increasing use of PD[2] and the decreased duration of hemodialysis sessions,[16] both of which may be responsible for an inadequate delivery of dialysis to the patient. The later issue is currently under study by the National Institute

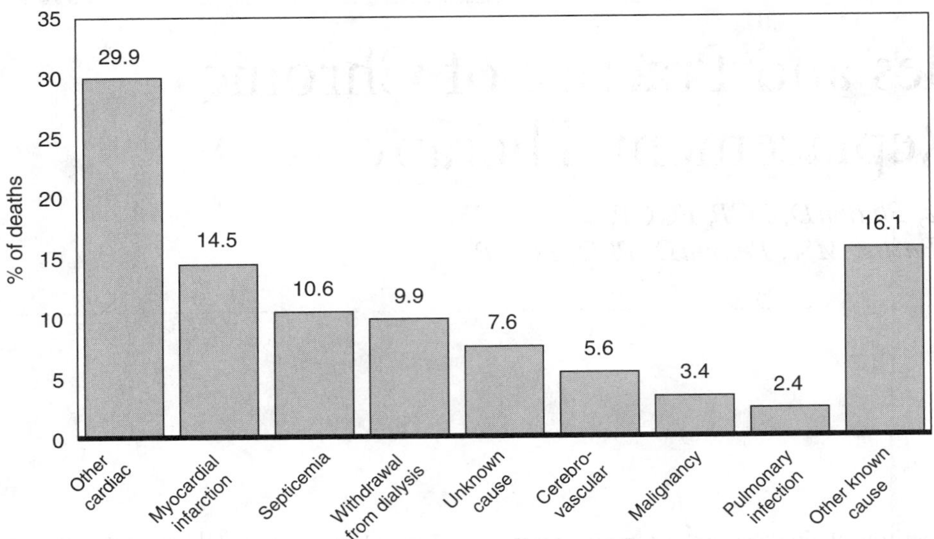

Figure 46.1. Predominant causes of death for ESRD patients between 45 and 64 years of age who died in 1989–1991. *(Adapted from Ref. 2.)*

of Diabetes and Digestive and Kidney Diseases for hemodialysis patients in the United States.

Morbidity can be grossly assessed by the number of hospitalizations per patient-year, the number of days hospitalized, or the incidence of certain complications such as cardiovascular events.[17,18] Early comparative studies demonstrated more hospitalized days with PD, but the policy at that time was for inpatient treatment of peritonitis. If one excludes peritonitis, there may not be much of a difference in hospitalization risk for PD patients compared to hemodialysis patients. If peritonitis is included in the comparison, the number of hospitalization days for PD patients is significantly greater than for HD patients (21.9 versus 17.3 per year).[18] Hospitalizations are more frequent in Caucasians than blacks and increase with age in both groups. Vascular access problems and cardiovascular complications are the most common reasons for hospital admission.[14] Cardiovascular morbidity is significantly reduced with PD, especially for arrhythmias and hypotensive episodes and cardiac performance appears to be improved as evidenced by decreases in intraventricular septum and left ventricular mass index and the lower incidence of pericarditis.[9]

The provision of pharmaceutical care to patients with ESRD is extremely complicated due to the multiplicity of concomitant diseases they have, as well as the complications they develop while receiving dialytic therapy. Although the average hemodialysis and peritoneal dialysis patient is prescribed an extensive number of pharmaceuti-

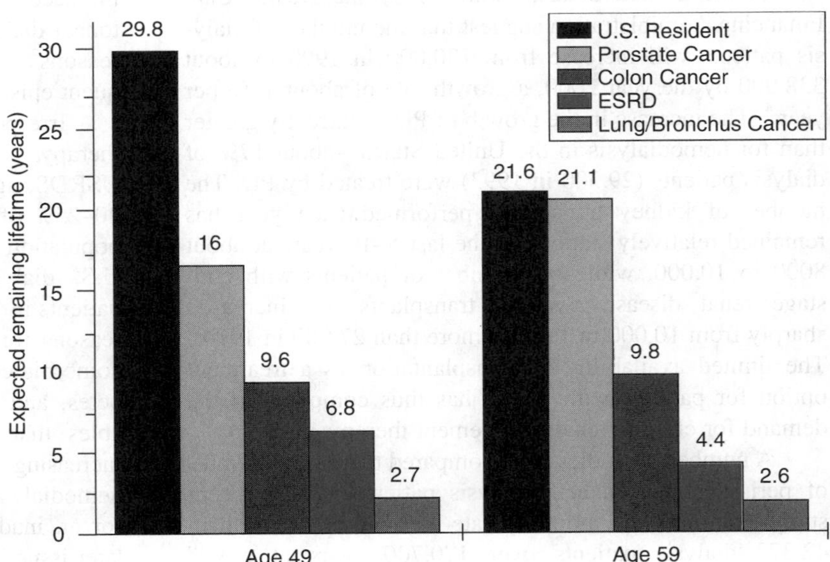

Figure 46.2. Life expectancy at age 49 and 59 years for patients with ESRD, the general population, and patients with various oncologic diseases. *(Adapted from Ref. 12.)*

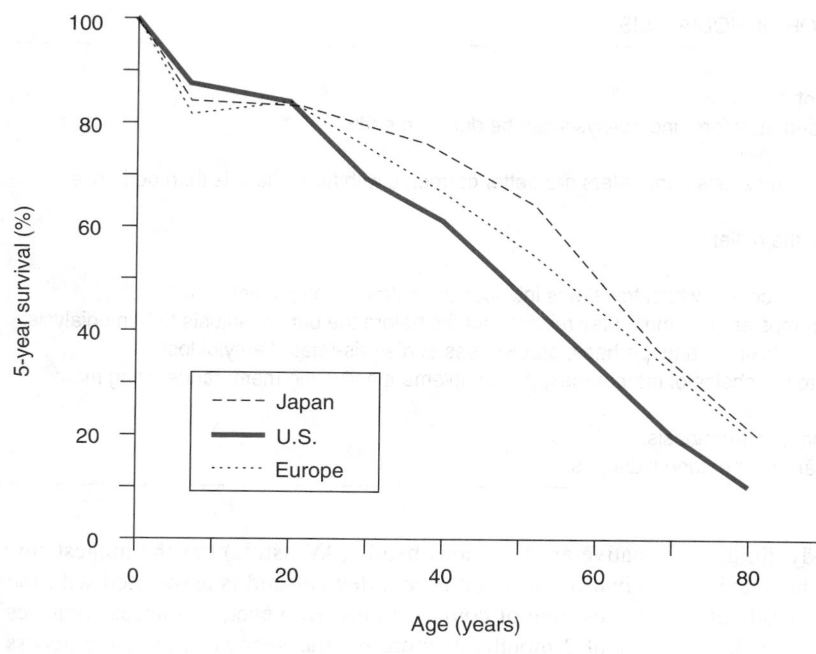

Figure 46.3. Five-year survival for ESRD patients in the United States, Europe, and Japan during 1982–1987. *(Adapted from Ref. 15 with permission.)*

cals,[19] the efficacy of these agents may be limited by inappropriate duplications[20] and lack of understanding by the patient of why, when, and how they should take their medication.[19–21] In the last decade, several models of pharmaceutical care have been developed to meet the needs of this population of patients in the institutional and ambulatory environment.[22–25]

It is our goal in this chapter to provide a primer on the principles of chronic renal replacement therapy, discuss the multiple types of catheters and procedures used as access for HD and PD, and differentiate between the various types of HD and PD since dialysis by either route is not a generic procedure. The "optimal" dose of dialysis for each patient population is reviewed and methodologies to quantitate what dose of dialysis an individual patient receives are described. Finally, the complications of both dialytic therapies are presented along with pertinent pharmacotherapy management plans.

Indications for Dialysis

Dialysis should be initiated electively rather than urgently in patients with chronic renal disease (see Chapter 44, Chronic Renal Failure and End-Stage Renal Disease). Because of the progressive nature of the disease, the need for dialysis should begin to be planned for once the serum creatinine or blood urea nitrogen (BUN) rises above a certain upper limit such as 8–10 or 100 mg/dL, respectively.[26] Although many patients may be symptom free with serum chemistries in this range, it is difficult to maintain values in this range without initiating severe dietary protein restrictions, which may result in malnutrition. Beginning the preparation process at this point should allow adequate time for proper education of the patient and their family and for the creation of a suitable vascular or peritoneal access. The advantages and disadvantages of hemodialysis are listed in Table 46.1, while those for peritoneal dialysis are delineated in Table 46.2. These factors along with the patients' concomitant diseases, preferences, and support environments are the principle determinants of the dialysis mode they will receive.[27] Finally, the initiation of dialysis in the ambulatory setting before the onset of severe complications such as pericarditis, encephalopathy, or pulmonary edema will also result in significant cost savings compared with the initiation in an acute care environment.

Principles of Hemodialysis

The basic principles of hemodialysis and peritoneal dialysis have remained unchanged since the clinical introduction of these modes of therapy almost 30 years ago.[28] Fundamentally, hemodialysis consists of the perfusion of heparinized blood and physiologic salt solution on opposite sides of a semipermeable membrane. The waste products such as urea and creatinine move from the blood into the dialysate by passive diffusion along concentration gradients. Inversely, if a substance is in the physiologic salt solution (i.e., dialysate) in a higher concentration than that in the blood, this solute will diffuse from the dialysate into the systemic circulation. The rate of diffusion depends on the difference between the concentrations of solute in blood and dialysate, solute characteristics, the dialysis filter composition and blood and dialysate flow rates. The second process that occurs during dialysis is ultrafiltration or convection. This

TABLE 46.1. ADVANTAGES AND DISADVANTAGES OF HEMODIALYSIS

Advantages

1. Higher solute clearance allows intermittent treatment.
2. Parameters of adequacy of dialysis better defined and therefore underdialysis can be detected early.
3. Technique failure rate is low.
4. Even though intermittent heparinization is required, hemostasis parameters are better corrected with hemodialysis than peritoneal dialysis.
5. In-center hemodialysis enables closer monitoring of the patient.

Disadvantages

1. Requires multiple visits each week to the hemodialysis center, which translates into loss of control by the patient.
2. Disequilibrium, dialysis hypotension, and muscle cramps are common. May require months before the patient adjusts to hemodialysis.
3. Bioincompatibility causes activation of complement, cytokines, and, perhaps, predisposes to dialysis-related amyloidosis.
4. Infections in hemodialysis patients may be related to the choice of membranes, the complement activating membranes being more deleterious.
5. Vascular access frequently associated with infection and thrombosis.
6. Decline of residual renal function more rapid compared to peritoneal dialysis.

is the primary mode for removal of excess body fluids. Ultrafiltration (expressed as mL/h/mm Hg) can be maximized by increasing the hydrostatic pressure gradient across the dialysis membrane. Those solutes that are dissolved in plasma water will be removed along with water if the size of the pores in the filter are large enough to allow it to pass. These two processes can be controlled independently and thus a patient's hemodialysis prescription can be individualized to attain the desired degree of solute (urea) removal and fluid balance.

VASCULAR ACCESS

Permanent access to the bloodstream for hemodialysis may be accomplished by several techniques[29,30] (Fig. 46.4). The native arteriovenous fistula (AV fistula) has the longest survival of all blood access devices and is associated with the lowest rate of complications. However, this access requires about 2 months or more for the venous limb of the access to "mature," that is, to dilate as the result of the increased pressure, before it can be utilized. This type of access is now used less frequently especially in diabetic patients (26% in 1990 versus 45% in 1986) because of poor vascular anatomy and indiscriminate use of the peripheral veins.[31]

Synthetic vascular grafts are the method of choice for access creation in most patients who have poor peripheral vasculature. Although these grafts can be made from multiple materials, polytetrafluorethylene (PTFE) has become the agent of choice and is now utilized as the initial access in 43–59% of patients.[31] PTFE grafts require only 2–3 weeks to endothelialize before they can be routinely uti-

TABLE 46.2. ADVANTAGES AND DISADVANTAGES OF PERITONEAL DIALYSIS

Advantages

1. Little risk of disequilibrium due to slow solute removal rate.
2. CAPD becomes more effective than HD as the solute size increases, which may explain good clinical state of the patient in spite of lower urea clearance.
3. Hypotension less frequent.
4. Better control of blood pressure.
5. Better preservation of residual renal function.
6. Convenient intraperitoneal route of administration of drugs such as antibiotics and insulin.
7. Can be done in elderly and the very young—age groups who may not tolerate HD well.
8. Freedom from the "machine" gives the patient a sense of independence.

Disadvantages

1. Protein losses through peritoneum and reduced appetite due to continuous glucose load and sense of abdominal fullness predispose to malnutrition.
2. Risk of peritonitis.
3. Catheter malfunction, exit site, and tunnel infection.
4. Inadequate ultrafiltration.
5. Patient burnout and high rate of technique failure.
6. Risk of obesity with excessive glucose absorption.
7. Mechanical problems such as hernias, dialysate leaks, hemorrhoids, or back pain may occur.
8. Extensive abdominal surgery may preclude peritoneal dialysis.

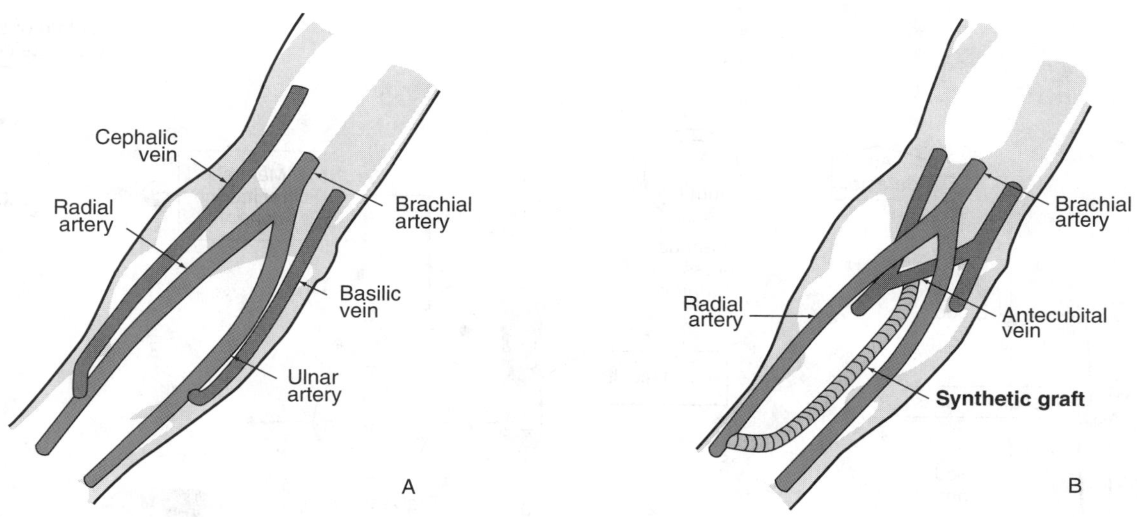

Figure 46.4. The predominant types of vascular access for chronic dialysis patients are (A) the arteriovenous fistula and (B) the synthetic arteriovenous forearm graft. The anteriovenous fistula is usually created by the surgical anastomosis of the end of the cephalic vein with the side of the radial artery. The anastomosis of the basilic vein to the ulnar artery is the primary alternative site.

lized. The primary disadvantages of this type of access are the shorter survival life and the fact that they have higher rates of infection and thrombosis than native AV fistulas.

The choice of vascular access type is dependent not only on the adequacy of the patients' vasculature but also how soon the patient will require hemodialysis. Acute dialysis access can be achieved by the insertion of a dual lumen catheter into the internal jugular, subclavian, or femoral vein or via the creation of an external AV fistula (i.e., a Scribner shunt). Once placed these devices can be used immediately and for up to several months as the bridge between permanent access for patients with ESRD. The primary complications associated with all vascular accesses are infection, thrombosis, and stenosis.[29,32]

HEMODIALYSIS PROCEDURES

Since the introduction of hemodialysis into clinical practice in the 1960s, some components have remained constant while others have changed dramatically.[28,33] Hemodialysis in all its variants still consists of an external vascular circuit through which the patient's blood is transferred in sterile polyethylene tubing to the dialysis filter (dialyzer) via a mechanical pump (Fig. 46.5). The patient's blood then passes through the dialyzer on one side of the semipermeable membrane material and is returned to the patient. The dialysate solution, which consists of purified water and electrolytes, is pumped through the dialyzer countercurrent to the flow of blood on the other side of the semipermeable membrane. The dialysate circuit, unlike the vascular circuit, is not sterile and is a potential source of infection for the patient particularly if the membrane were to rupture.

Conventional or standard hemodialysis is currently the predominant therapeutic modality prescribed in the United States.[34] However, the utilization of rapid high-efficiency dialysis (RHED) and high-flux dialysis (HFD) has gained increased acceptance since the first clinical reports almost 10 years ago.[35,36] These variants of hemodialysis were developed for a multiplicity of reasons including (1) a desire to improve patient acceptance by decreasing dialysis time while maintaining the dose of dialysis that could be administered; (2) to enhance patient survival and decrease morbidity by utilizing filters that remove higher molecular weight solutes; and (3) economic realities in which reimbursement per procedure was capitated and in order to be fiscally responsible dialysis units needed to find a way to deliver the desired dose of dialysis more efficiently. The higher efficiency of these two therapeutic variants has resulted in a shortening of the duration of dialysis therapy from approximately 4–5 hours three times per week to 2–3 hours three times per week.[37–39]

In conventional or standard hemodialysis, low-permeability (low-flux) membranes (Table 46.3) are used and diffusion is the primary mechanism by which uremic waste products such as urea are removed from the patient (Fig. 46.5). The rate of blood flow through the dialyzer ranges from 200–350 mL/min, and the dialysate flow rate is generally fixed at 400–500 mL/min. Under this set of clinical conditions, the clearance of urea by the dialyzer rarely exceeds 200 mL/min, and the duration of therapy required to deliver the desired amount of dialysis is usually 4 to 5 hours per session.

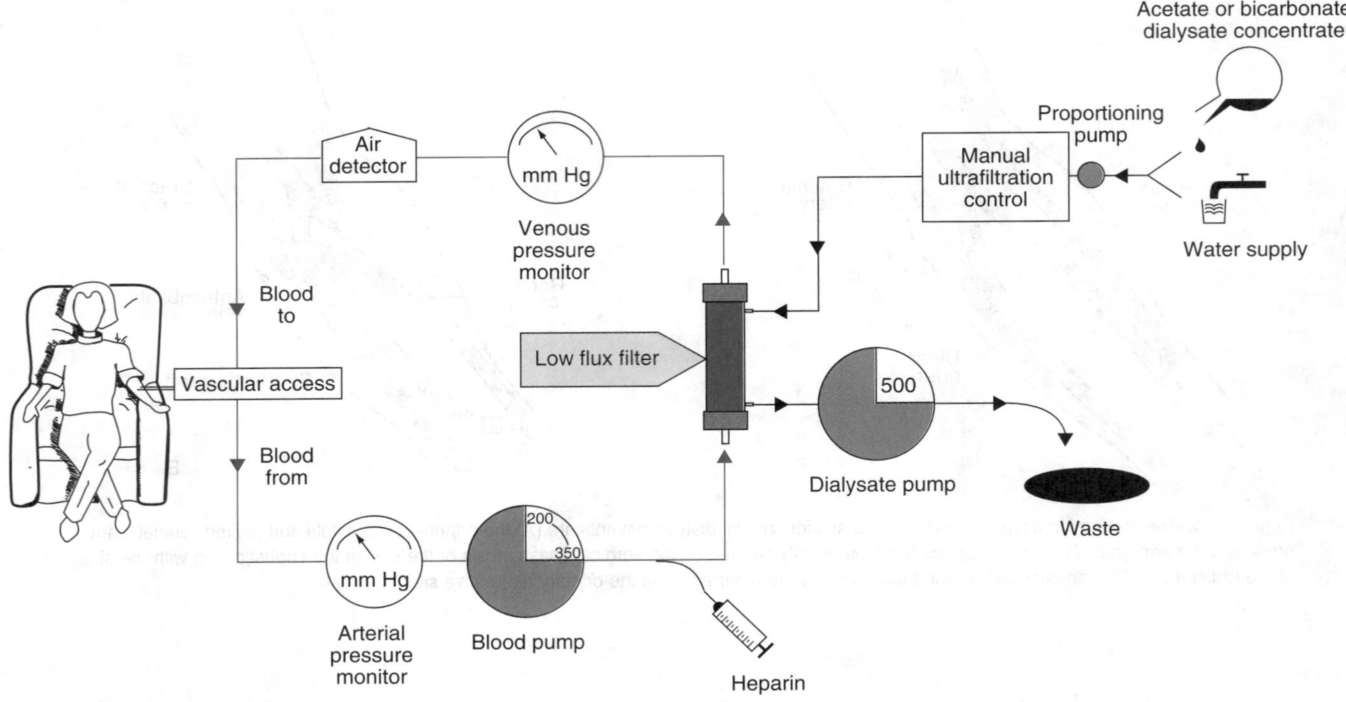

Figure 46.5. In conventional hemodialysis, the patient's blood is pumped to the dialyzer at the rate of 200–350 mL/min. Heparin is administered to prevent clotting in the dialyzer. The predominant dialyzers are small (0.8–1.5 m^2), low flux filters made of cellulose acetate, cuprophane, or hemophan. The dialysate, which may be acetate or bicarbonate buffered, is pumped at a rate of 500 mL/min through the dialyzer countercurrent to the flow of blood. The rate of fluid removal from the patient is manually controlled by adjusting the pressure in the dialysate compartment.

Although a myriad of names have been used to describe RHED and HFD, the common features of these treatments are procedure times usually under 3 hours, blood flow rates greater than 400 mL/min, dialysate flow rates greater than 500 mL/min, urea clearances that are usually in excess of 220 mL/min, and the utilization of strict controls on the rate of fluid removal. RHED (Fig. 46.6) differs from HFD (Fig. 46.7) in several ways. The primary difference is that cellulose-based membranes such as cuprophane, hemophan, cellulose acetate, and cuproammonium are used in RHED. These dialyzers are larger versions of the filters used in conventional dialysis and also have moderate ultrafiltration coefficients (K_{uf}) of 8–20 mL/h/mm Hg of transmembrane pressure (Table 46.3). The clearance of low molecular weight solutes such as urea is increased dramatically in RHED as the result of the contribution of convective transfer of the solute dissolved in the ultrafiltrate. However, middle and high molecular weight solutes including many drugs will not be cleared at a higher rate since the major limitation to their removal is the small pore size of this type of dialyzer membrane.[33,40]

HFD also combines diffusion and convection; however, in contrast to RHED the membranes are much more open, that is, the pore sizes are larger and the K_{uf} is generally in the range of 20–60 mL/h/mm Hg. Typically, these dialyzers, which are composed of polysulfone (PS), polymethylmethacrylate (PMMA), polyamide (PA), cellulose triacetate (CTA), and polyacrylonitrile (PAN), have higher middle molecule clearances than are attainable with RHED or standard hemodialysis.[41] The other major difference between RHED and HFD is that volumetric ultrafiltration control is required due to the high K_{uf} of these filters (Fig. 46.7).

There are currently more than 500 dialyzers available in the United States. They differ in regard to the composition of the membrane and ultrafiltration coefficient as described above as well as in structural design (hollow fiber versus flat plate), membrane surface area, degree of biocompatibility, and sterilization method. Despite numerous choices, almost 75% of the patients are dialyzed with one of the filters listed in Table 46.3.[34] In fact, most dialysis centers select the optimal dialysis filter for an individual patient from a small formulary of 5–10 filters. Although little attention has been focused on patient selection criteria for RHED or HFD versus standard hemodialysis, the best candidates for these new therapies are those with a vascular access that can deliver at least 400 mL/min, absence of severe cerebrovascular or cardiovascular disease, and weight gains of less than 5 kg between dialysis.[38,39] In addition to patient factors, the economics of the individual dial-

TABLE 46.3. CHARACTERISTICS OF THE DIALYZERS MOST FREQUENTLY USED IN THE UNITED STATES

Manufacturer	Membrane[a]	Surface Area (m^2)	K_{uf} (mL/h/mm Hg)	KOA	Urea Clearance Q_B (mL/min) 200	300	400	Vitamin B_{12} Clearance Q_B (mL/min) 200
Low Flux								
Baxter CF1511	CU	1.1	4.2	526	165	201	222	34
CF2308	CU	1.3	4.7	635	181	227	—[b]	46
CA90	CA	0.9	4.3	484	169	208	231	42
CA110	CA	1.1	5.3	562	176	221	248	52
NMC FoCus 90	CU	0.9	3.5	506	169	116	42	42
FoCus 120	CU	1.2	4.8	599	179	227	256	46
Terumo TAF10	CR	1.0	4.8	—	170	210	233	54
TAF12	CR	1.2	6.1	—	180	229	258	61
Medium Flux								
Baxter CA170	CA	1.7	8.3	1005	187	244	279	70
CA210	CA	2.1	10.1	911	192	258	299	79
Terumo T220	CR	2.2	11.1	1103	195	268	317	94
T175	CR	1.75	8.8	916	198	276	328	86
High Flux								
Fresenius F60	PS	1.2	40	709	187	244	279	134
F80	PS	1.8	60	986	193	259	301	160
Baxter CT110G	CTA	1.1	22	—	185	239	272	126
CT190G	CTA	1.9	36	—	192	257	297	157

[a] CU = cuprophane, CA = cellulose acetate, CR = cuparammonium rayon, PS = polysulfone, and CTA = cellulose triacetate.
[b] —, no data.

ysis unit enter into the selection process. High-flux filters are three to four times as expensive as low- or medium-flux filters, plus new dialysis machines that have more precise ultrafiltration controllers are usually required and, finally, a dialyzer reprocessing system to utilize these expensive filters multiple times will usually be needed if this treatment modality is going to be made available. RHED, however, can be performed on standard dialysis machines and, because the filters are not nearly as costly, reprocessing is not mandatory.

THE HEMODIALYSIS PRESCRIPTION

Hemodialysis in its multiple types has been available for 10–25 years, but there is still no clear agreement as to the dose of dialysis that should be prescribed.[42–44] Although even a small dose will sustain life longer than no dialysis, the goal is to prescribe and deliver the "optimal" dose of dialysis for each individual patient, that is, the amount of therapy above which there is no cost-effective increment in the patient's quality adjusted life expectancy.[45] Unfortunately, many nephrologists still prescribe dialysis by specifying a dialyzer manufacturer, size of the dialyzer, blood and dialysate flow rate, and the amount of weight to be removed within a certain time period with no clear understanding of the amount (dose) of dialysis being delivered (Table 46.4).[43]

In the last 5 years, the annual mortality rate of U.S. dialysis patients has ranged between 22.6–25.2%, a value 30–50% higher than their counterparts in Europe and Japan.[15,46] Although multiple factors such as patient age, concomitant disease states, and compliance may contribute to this difference, one factor that was evident is that European patients receive approximately 30% more dialysis than U.S. patients.[44] During this same period, multiple studies, mostly retrospective analyses, have reported that U.S. patient survival is improved when the dose of dialysis is increased.[44,47–53] The critical role of the dialysis dose is evident from the data of Hakim et al.[51] In this prospective trial, as the dose of dialysis was increased by 62% over a 3-year period the annual mortality rate declined from 22.8% in 1988 to 9.1% in 1991 and the number of hospital days per patient per year decreased from 15.2 to 10.3. The key question that remains is what is the optimal amount of dialysis that patients should receive.

Multiple methods have been developed to quantify the delivered dose of dialysis. The two predominant methods in use today are the urea reduction ratio (URR), which is the predialysis BUN minus the postdialysis BUN divided by predialysis BUN,[54] and the "Kt/V," which is the ratio of the dialyzer clearance of urea (K) in L/h multiplied by the dura-

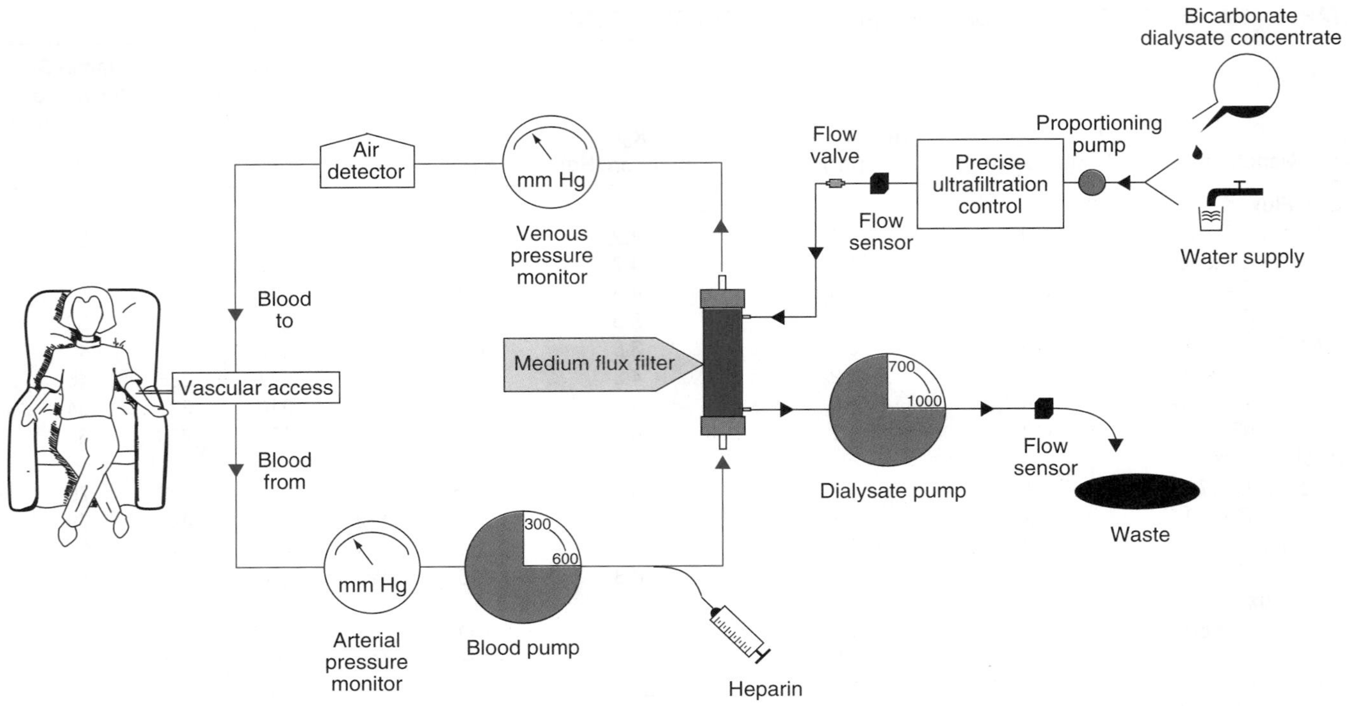

Figure 46.6. Rapid high-efficiency hemodialysis differs from conventional hemodialysis with regard to blood and dialysate flow rates, size of the dialyzer, and dialysate delivery system. The blood and dialysate flow rates range from 300–600 and 700–1000 mL/min, respectively. The dialyzer is often made of the same material but the size is larger, 1.5–2.1 m^2, and the filters are usually medium flux, that is, the rate of fluid removal is 8–20 mL/h/mm Hg. Bicarbonate buffered dialysate is usually used and more precise ultrafiltration control via adjustments of the rates of two dialysate pumps may be needed, especially if a medium-flux dialyzer is used.

tion of dialysis *(t)* in hours divided by the urea distribution volume of the patient *(V)* in liters.[55] *Kt/V* is a unitless parameter that quantitates the fraction of the patient's total body water which is cleared of urea during a dialysis session. This term was developed from the only prospective national cooperative dialysis study (NCDS), which characterized the relationship between the delivered dialysis dose (as the time-averaged urea concentration) and patient morbidity and mortality.[56,57] The only accurate way to determine *Kt/V* requires the collection of BUN concentrations prior to, during, or after the dialysis session and the application of a nomographic[58] or computerized urea kinetic modeling approach.[59] Although urea kinetic modeling *(Kt/V)* has been challenged, no other method has proven to be superior.[60]

On the basis of the NCDS study, a *Kt/V* of 0.9 to 1.3 was deemed to be sufficient and the implication in the mid-1980s through the early 1990s was that dialysis beyond that level would not likely improve patient survival. However, we now know that patient mortality decreases as the *Kt/V* is increased within this range and above.[49–51] The mortality risk appears to be reduced by 7% for every 0.1 increase in *Kt/V.*[44] This translates into a 21% decrease in mortality if the *Kt/V* was increased from 1.0 to 1.3 or, in other words, 17 rather than 22 deaths per 100 patient years. Indeed many nephrologists now recommend a target *Kt/V* of at least 1.3 for nondiabetic patients receiving standard dialysis and 1.4 to 1.5 or greater for diabetics and/or patients receiving RHED or HFD therapy.[39,43,53] The ultimate answer to this "optimal" question will hopefully be rigorously addressed and answered once the NIH sponsored morbidity and mortality in hemodialysis trial is completed near the turn of the century.[61] In the interim, the attainment of these new target *Kt/V*'s will not be easy. In the late 1980s when the target values were 1.0 to 1.2 several studies indicated that about 50% of patients had prescribed values less than 1.0 and more than 70% had delivered values less than 1.0.[43]

Clinical Assessment of the Delivered Dialysis Dose

Urea kinetic modeling of measured BUN levels is the optimal means to determine the delivered dose of dialysis.[60] Although simplified single-compartment models have been used and may still be applicable for patients receiving standard dialysis with the introduction of RHED

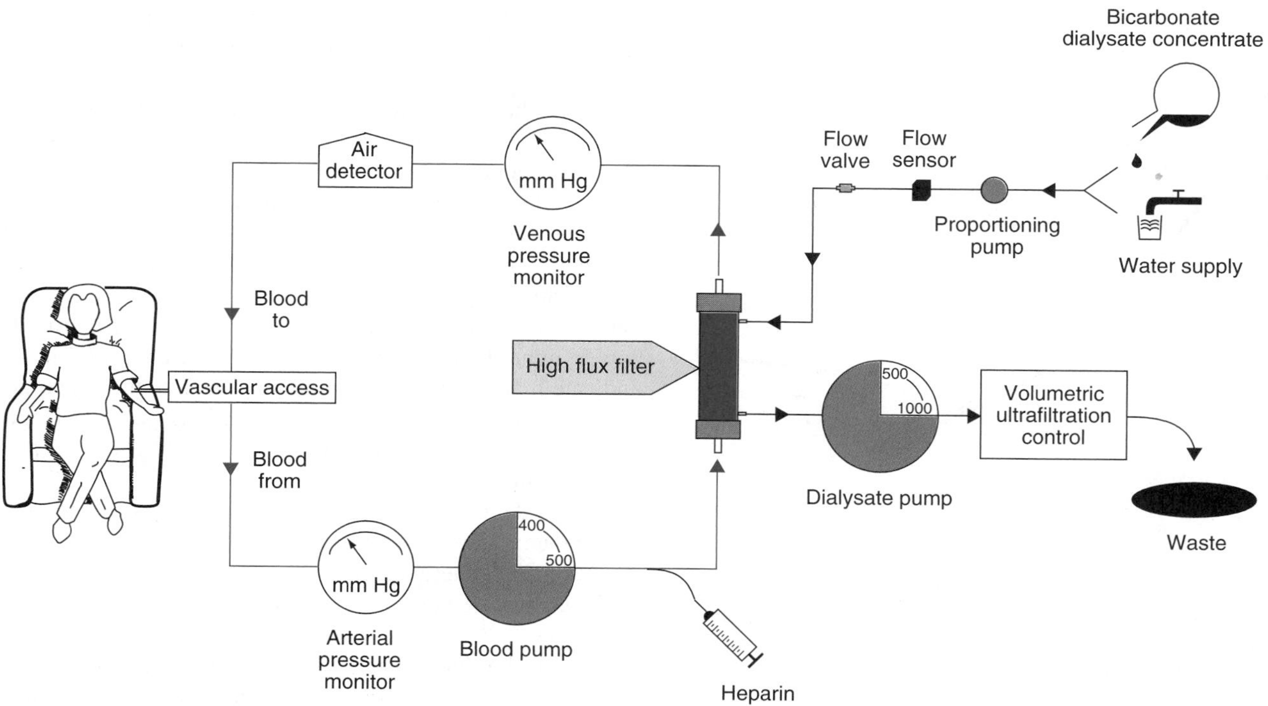

Figure 46.7. High-flux hemodialysis systems incorporate a synthetic dialyzer made of polysulfone, polyacrylonitrile, polymethylmethacrylate, etc., or a high-flux cellulosic based filter, e.g., cellulose triacetate of variable size (0.65–2.1 m^2). The blood flow rates are generally between 400–500 mL/min while dialysate flow rates may range from 500–1000 mL/min. Due to the high ultrafiltration coefficients of these dialyzers, volumetric ultrafiltration control and bicarbonate buffered dialysate are required.

TABLE 46.4. CONSIDERATIONS IN DESIGN OF THE HEMODIALYSIS PRESCRIPTION

Patient Variables
- Urea distribution volume
- Urea generation rate from protein catabolism
- Residual (native kidney) urea clearance
- Fluid accumulation

Procedure Variables
- Dialyzer clearance
  - Model of dialyzer
  - Blood flow rate
  - Dialysate flow rate
- Duration of dialysis
- Frequency of dialysis
- Desired adequacy index

and HFD, we now see the limitation of this simplified approach.[59,62–63] When the urea clearance of the dialyzer exceeds 180 mL/min and/or blood sampling is rigorous, one can clearly see that urea kinetics are best characterized by a two-compartment model with a central compartment volume that increases during the interdialytic period (Fig. 46.8). As the result of this kinetic behavior, a marked rebound in urea concentrations is seen after dialysis as has been described for many drugs (see Chapter 50, Drug Therapy Individualization for Patients with Renal Insufficiency).

The easiest way to assess the dose of dialysis actually administered to the patient is to determine the ratio of [BUN] post to [BUN] pre and from it, the *Kt/V.* Several formulas have been described by Daugirdas[58,64] to estimate *Kt/V* from the post/pre [BUN] ratio *(R)* (Table 46.5). The formula $Kt/V = -\ln(R - 0.008t) + [(4 - 3.5\,R) \times \text{UF/Wt}]$, gives an excellent approximation to the kinetically modeled *Kt/V.* This equation takes into consideration the effect of the efficiency of the treatment as a function of the treatment time, and the convective removal of urea in the ultrafiltrate (UF/Wt). Alternatively, urea kinetic modeling can be used to calculate the *Kt/V,* using a two-compartment model.

Because of the two-compartment behavior of urea, the timing of the post-treatment BUN sample is critical. If the sample is obtained immediately after the end of the treatment, equilibration between the two compartments is not complete and the sample will overestimate the magnitude of the treatment administered. The only "true" sample is the one obtained after the two compartments have reached equilibrium. In the majority of cases an almost complete equilibration between compartments would have been reached by 15–30 minutes after the end of the treatment. At this time, the sample truly represents the concentration of BUN in the body water. It is possible to obtain a sample

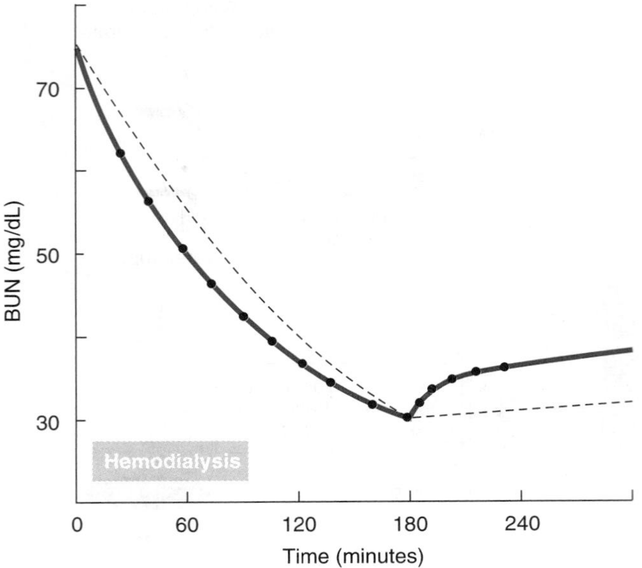

Figure 46.8. A two-compartment model (solid line) predicts the measured BUN value (solid dots) during and following high-flux hemodialysis. A single-compartment variable-volume model (dotted line) overestimates BUN removal during dialysis and fails to predict the rebound postdialysis.

immediately after the treatment if appropriate corrections are made to transform that sample into an equilibrated one (that is, the one obtained after 15–30 minutes). This correction must take into consideration the clearance used during the treatment because the magnitude of the rebound is proportional to the efficiency of the treatment. For example, if the treatment length was 240 minutes or greater, the urea reduction ratio goal should be 60–65%; 65–70% if the treatment is 180 minutes or greater; and 70–75% if the treatment was 120 minutes or less.[42] These are among the multiple situations that may contribute to variances between the prescribed and delivered dose of dialysis (Table 46.6).

Once the dialysis prescription has been determined, the ability of dialysis facilities to deliver the prescribed dose becomes critical. Unfortunately, multiple factors may result in the patient receiving less dialysis than was prescribed (Table 46.6). Sargent[65] reported several years ago that the average facility was not able to deliver the prescribed dose in more than one-third of the dialyses. The average "underdelivery" was 15%, but some treatments were up to 40% less than prescribed. USRDS data from the mid-1980s suggested that the mean delivered *Kt/V* was only 72% of the prescribed value of 1.0, which is grossly low in light of current data.[43] Although these reports clearly indicate that the dialysis community has a long way to go, the data from Collins[39] indicates that it is possible to get there since they delivered *Kt/V*'s of 87–89% of the prescribed values of 1.40–1.43.

The deficiency in delivered hemodialysis therapy is also related to patient compliance with their dialysis prescription.[66,67] Sherman et al.[66] reported that 50% of the patients they reviewed had either missed or ended their treatment early in the 3-month study period. Since compliance with the dialysis prescription is important for patient survival, different behavioral compliance styles will need to be devised and evaluated.

Lastly, the effect of other components of the dialysis prescription such as reuse of the dialyzer,[68] heparin dosage,[69] and elevations in hematocrit secondary to erythropoietin administration may alter the delivered dose of dialysis.[70] The number of dialysis facilities reusing dialyzers varies from 73.6% who use low-flux filters, to about 95% who use medium- to high-flux filters.[34] Since the effective volume of the dialyzer may decrease due to the clotting of the individual fibers, most centers that do reuse filters discard them if the volume loss exceeds 20%. Despite the application of this guidance, Sherman et al.[68] recently observed a significant decline in *Kt/V* when high-reuse dialyzers (mean number of uses = 13.8) were compared with low-reuse dialyzers (mean number of uses = 3.8). Optimal anticoagulation via heparin modeling appears to improve

TABLE 46.5. SIMPLIFIED APPROACHES FOR THE CALCULATION OF DELIVERED DIALYSIS DOSE

Kt/V	URR (%)		Formula[a]
0.8	50		
0.9	54	**Good**	$Kt/V = 2.2 - [3.3 \bullet (R - 0.03) - UF/Wt]$
1.0	58		
1.1	62	**Better**	$Kt/V = -\ln [(R - 0.03) - (0.75 \bullet UF/Wt)]$
1.2	65		
1.3	68	**Best**	$Kt/V = -\ln (R - 0.008\ h) + [(4 - 3.5\ R)\ UF/Wt]$
1.4	70		
1.5	72		

[a]*R* = post BUN/pre BUN; UF = ultrafiltration volume removed in liters (this is approximated as preweight minus postweight in kg); h = dialysis time in hours. *Note:* The first method underestimates K_t/V at low URR and overestimates at high URR. The second method will be adequate in most situations while the third is best when the URR is greater than 72.

TABLE 46.6. SITUATIONS IN WHICH DELIVERED *Kt/V* MAY VARY FROM PRESCRIBED

Less Than Prescribed

- True blood flow less than marked on blood pump
- Blood flow lowered during dialysis
- Recirculation of blood in the patient's vascular access
- Postdialysis BUN drawn late (>5 minutes post) and not adjusted for equilibration
- Time on dialysis reduced
- Patient's urea distribution volume larger than expected

Greater Than Prescribed

- Postdialysis BUN artifactually low (drawn too early or from dialyzer outflow line)
- Patient's urea distribution volume is lower than expected
- Patient stayed on dialysis longer than prescribed (unusual)
- Dialyzer clearance of urea is greater than expected (unusual)

the urea clearance of polysulfone dialyzers (213–240 mL/min) and increase the delivered *Kt/V* (0.99 to 1.10) despite extensive reuse of the filters (average use: 13 to 17 with a maximum of 50).[69] Thus, dialyzer urea clearance may be preserved and patient care improved if anticoagulation is rigorously monitored.

The impact of elevations in hematocrit secondary to the initiation of erythropoietin therapy on dialyzer clearance and *Kt/V* has been evaluated by more than 10 investigators.[70] These studies have uniformly reported that urea, as well as creatinine, potassium, and phosphate clearances were reduced by approximately 5, 15, 13, and 15%, respectively, when the hematocrit was increased from 20 to 36%. Although the decrement in *Kt/V*, a reflection of reduced urea clearance, was not large, the impact of an increasing hematocrit may necessitate a change in the patient's dialysis prescription to maintain the desired potassium and phosphate levels.

COMPLICATIONS OF HEMODIALYSIS

Patients with ESRD develop several sequelae as the result of the reduction in functioning nephron mass. The pathophysiology and management of complications such as anemia, acid–base and electrolyte disorders, aluminum overload, uremic bleeding, and hyperparathyroidism are discussed in Chapter 44 (Chronic Renal Failure and End-Stage Renal Disease). In addition to these new disorders, the primary pathology responsible for the patient's development of ESRD such as hypertension, diabetes mellitus, or hyperlipidemia may progress and contribute significantly to the patient's morbidity and risk of death.[61,71–76]

Intradialytic complications such as hypotension, acute hemorrhage due to dialyzer rupture, hemolysis, cardiac arrhythmia, muscle cramps, nausea and vomiting, air embolism, chest or back pain, and pruritus are relatively frequently reported in patients receiving RHED, HFD, or standard hemodialysis (Table 46.7).[77–82] Despite the use of higher blood flow rates and dialyzers with increased K_{uf}, the incidence of almost all of these complications is 30–40% lower in patients receiving RHED or HFD compared to standard hemodialysis.[35,39,80] The replacement of acetate with bicarbonate as the dialysate buffer has been a major reason for the decrease in hypotension and nausea and vomiting. The utilization of volumetric ultrafiltration controllers during RHED and HFD, as well as individualized dialysate sodium levels has likely also contributed to the lower incidence of these symptoms.[39] The incidence of pruritis and headache appear to be similar among the three types of hemodialysis. The etiology and predisposing factors, as well as initial management for the six most commonly observed intradialytic complications, are delineated in Table 46.7.

Dialyzer reactions encompass a broad range of clinical symptoms that include anaphylactic (Type A) and nonspecific (Type B) events.[83] In the past, these two types of reactions were considered to be part of the "first-use" syndrome because they presented much more frequently when new as opposed to reprocessed dialyzers were used. Although reprocessing may reduce the incidence of Type B events it has little to no benefit for patients who have experienced a Type A reaction.[84] The symptom complex associated with Type A reactions is similar to a drug-induced anaphylactic reaction and may be due to hypersensitivity to ethylene oxide (a common dialyzer sterilant), heparin, formaldehyde, or glutaraldehyde (common reuse sterilants). This type of reaction has also been associated with activation of the bradykinin system by some dialyzer membranes (especially the AN69), particularly in patients receiving angiotensin-converting enzyme (ACE) inhibitors since these agents block bradykinin inactivation.[85] The dialysis procedure should be stopped immediately for those patients who experience this type of reaction. The blood in the dialyzer should not be returned to them and resuscitative therapy with epinephrine, antihistamines, and steroids will likely be required.

Type B reactions are more common than Type A but less severe. Chest and back pain are the most frequently reported symptoms and they may be noted within minutes or delayed (up to 1–2 hours). Complement activation and subsequent anaphylatoxin formation has been associated to some degree with all dialysis membranes. Synthetic high-flux membranes have the least potential to produce this syndrome followed by modified cellulose membranes, such as hemophan and cellulose triacetate, while cuprophane and cellulose acetate membranes, particularly those in the Dow dialyzers, have the greatest potential to produce this syndrome.[86] Although no specific treatment is warranted and the patient can continue with their dialysis treatment, they

TABLE 46.7. COMMON COMPLICATIONS DURING HEMODIALYSIS

	Incidence	Etiology/Predisposing Factors	Management
Hypotension	20–30%	Excessive ultrafiltration Target weight too low Acetate dialysate→vasodilation Autonomic neuropathy Patient unable to compensatorily increase cardiac output	Place in Trendelenburg position 100–200 mL bolus of normal saline Decrease ultrafiltration rate 10–20 ml of 23.4% hypertonic saline over 5 minutes[79]
Cramps	5–20%	Hypotension Dehydration Sodium level in dialysate too low	100–200 mL bolus of normal saline 10–20 ml of 23.4% hypertonic saline over 5 minutes[79] Give oxazepam 5–10 mg 2 h before dialysis Prophylaxis with carnitine 20 mg/kg IV TIW[80]
Nausea and vomiting	5–15%	Hypotension May be an early sign of disequilibrium syndrome	Treat hypotension Prochlorperazine 10 mg PO or 2.5 mg IV
Headache	5%	For most, mechanism unknown Acute caffeine withdrawal due to dialytic removal Vasodilatation secondary to acetate dialysate solution	Acetaminophen 650 mg PO (PRN)
Chest or back pain	2.5%	Underlying cardiac disease Type B dialyzer reaction	Change dialyzer or start reuse program Nasal oxygen
Itching	5%	Uremic toxins Elevated calcium-phosphorus product Dry skin Allergy to heparin, plasticizers in dialysis tubing, sterilizer used or any other medication	Activated charcoal 6 g daily Reduce hyperphosphatemia Topical emollients Topical capsaicum cream 0.025% Diphenhydramine 25–50 mg PO Switch from ethylene oxide to gamma-ray-sterilized dialyzer

should be switched to a more biocompatible dialyzer and/or put on a reprocessing program since this may minimize the occurrence of this reaction in the future. Biocompatible dialyzers utilize a synthetic membrane of polysulfone, polyacrylonitrile, polymethylmethacrylate, etc., and may have a low, medium, or high ultrafiltration coefficient. In addition to their minimal activation of the complement system, these dialyzers also have minimal effects on the immune system, cytokine release, production of β_2 microglobulin and have been associated with a reduced risk of morbidity and mortality.[86,87]

Complications associated with hemodialysis therapy that began after and/or persist include immune system dysfunction,[87–89] disequilibrium syndrome,[90] and β_2 microglobulin amyloidosis.[91–93] ESRD patients demonstrate several abnormalities of immune function, some of which are aggravated by the mode of dialysis therapy they receive. For example, granulocyte phagocytic ability, natural killer cell functions, and lymphocyte interleukin 2 receptor density was impaired to a greater extent when dialysis was performed using bioincompatible filters relative to certain biocompatible synthetic filters.[89] Furthermore, Hornberger and colleagues[94] reported a significant reduction (almost 50%) in mortality and infection-related hospital admissions for patients treated with a high-flux biocompatible membrane, compared to patients treated with standard hemodialysis.

Disequilibrium syndrome is characterized by a set of systemic and neurologic symptoms, as well as EEG changes that may occur during but generally soon (hours) after the end of dialysis.[90] It has been reported in the acute and chronic setting and may be caused by an acute increase in brain water content. In mild cases, one may only observe nonspecific symptoms such as nausea, vomiting, headache, or restlessness. Severe disequilibrium is characterized by the development of seizures, obtundation, or coma. Prevention is the key to the management of this syndrome. The incidence of the syndrome can be minimized by the adjustment of dialysate sodium (at least 140 mEq/L) and glucose (at least 200 mg/dL) levels, a reduction in ultrafiltration rate and the target urea reduction ratio.

Dialysis-related amyloidosis is commonly seen in ESRD patients who have received dialysis for more than 8–10 years secondary to the accumulation of β_2 microglobulin.[91,95] The first and most prominent clinical manifestation of this syndrome is carpal tunnel syndrome. Approximately 20–25% of dialysis patients develop it after 5 years while the incidence increases to around 80% after 10 years.[95] Other clinical manifestations include shoulder, knee, ankle, elbow, and hip pain and stiffness with soft-tissue swelling. Radiologic lesions are usually evident before the onset of pain.

Serum β_2 microglobulin levels are significantly elevated in the presence of renal insufficiency; however, serum levels do not continuously rise, a finding that is compatible with its deposition in tissues.[93] Although the role of the dialyzer membrane is controversial, cuprophan and cellulose acetate membranes stimulate β_2 microglobulin production and because of their small pores the clearance of this compound is negligible.[87] In contrast, high-flux biocompatible membranes produce little to no stimulus of β_2 microglobulin production. Furthermore, due to their high porosity and the absorption of β_2 microglobulin to some of the membranes, postdialysis levels may be 50% lower than those prior to dialysis. Despite these beneficial effects, no progressive decrease in predialysis levels has been reported. This may be the result of the short-term nature of some of the evaluations and the massive tissue stores that would need to be removed before one could see progressive declines.[92] At present, there is no adequate definitive treatment for this syndrome. Treatment with nonsteroidal anti-inflammatory agents, systemic corticosteroids, therapeutic ultrasound, and physical therapy may be of benefit for some patients.[95] The utilization of biocompatible dialyzers may be beneficial and warrants further study.

Peritoneal Dialysis

Although the first use of peritoneal dialysis was described in 1923, this mode of therapy was used only intermittently in humans until the early 1970s.[28] The first patients treated with continuous ambulatory peritoneal dialysis (CAPD) were described in 1975 and the number of patients receiving this form of dialytic therapy increased at a slow rate until the early 1980s.[96] A number of mechanical and clinical improvements to the delivery system, such as improved intraperitoneal catheters and the replacement of glass dialysate containers by flexible plastic bags, has led to a rapid increase in the use of CAPD as a viable alternative to hemodialysis for the treatment of ESRD in the last decade.

Principles of Peritoneal Dialysis

The three basic components of any dialytic system, namely, a blood-filled compartment separated from a dialysate-filled compartment by a semipermeable membrane, are also utilized for the performance of peritoneal dialysis. In peritoneal dialysis, the dialysate-filled compartment is the peritoneal cavity, into which dialysate is instilled via a permanent peritoneal catheter that traverses the abdominal wall.[97] The peritoneal cavity is surrounded by the contiguous peritoneal membrane. The cavity normally contains about 100 mL of lipid-rich fluid, which has lubricating qualities and also has the ability to expand to a capacity of several liters. The peritoneal membrane that lines the cavity functions as the semipermeable membrane, across which dialysis occurs. The peritoneal membrane is classically described as a monocellular layer of mesothelial cells. However, in reality, the dialyzing membrane is also comprised of the basement membrane and underlying connective and interstitial tissue. The peritoneal membrane is termed parietal (that part which underlies the abdominal wall) or visceral (which overlies the abdominal organs) and its total area approximates body surface area (about 1.73 m^2). Blood vessels supplying and draining the abdominal viscera, musculature, and mesentery constitute the blood-filled compartment.

Solutes and water to be removed from blood during PD are not in intimate contact with the dialyzing membrane as they are in hemodialysis and must therefore travel a considerable distance to the dialysate-filled compartment.[98] There are several resistances to the movement of solutes and water by diffusion, represented by the basement membrane and endothelium of the blood vessels, the thickness of the interstitial tissue surrounding the vessels, the peritoneal mesothelial cells, the peritoneal basement membrane, and a stagnant layer of dialysate fluid in contact with the peritoneal membrane. Unlike hemodialysis, there is no easy method to regulate blood flow to the dialyzing surface, nor is there a countercurrent flow of blood and dialysate to increase diffusion and convective flow via changes in hydrostatic pressure. For these reasons, PD is a much less efficient process for dialysis per unit time compared with hemodialysis, and must therefore be a more frequent or virtually continuous procedure.

During peritoneal dialysis, therefore, there is a different solute profile compared to hemodialysis (Fig. 46.9).[98] In intermittent hemodialysis or peritoneal dialysis, there is a "sawtooth" pattern of solute concentration over time. Since CAPD is essentially continuous, conditions similar to a steady state occur, and solute profiles are almost level over time. The argument has been proposed that CAPD, therefore, represents a more physiologic process that is similar to endogenous renal function. Furthermore, the massive swings in body water content and high peak concentrations of uremic toxins in hemodialysis patients are less than optimal. There is also some evidence that CAPD may be more beneficial for patients with cardiovascular instability.[7–9]

The peritoneal membrane has different transport characteristics than conventional low-flux (cuprophane) or high-flux (cellulose triacetate) hemodialysis membranes

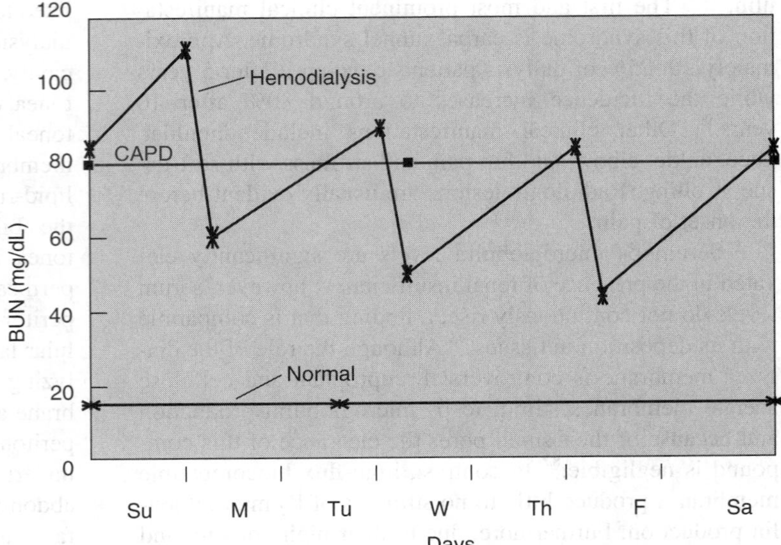

Figure 46.9. BUN concentration time profile in a patient with normal renal function, one maintained on CAPD, and one treated with intermittent hemodialysis. *(Reproduced from Ref. 98, p. 1141, with permission from Harvey Whitney Books Company. Cincinnati, OH.)*

(Table 46.8).[99] The peritoneal membrane permits the passage of larger molecular weight solutes than the older, low-flux conventional type of hemodialysis membranes. However, this difference is less marked for newer, high-flux membranes. These differences are important for understanding not only the relative efficiency of each system in the removal of endogenous solutes, but also the dialyzability of exogenously administered drugs.

The relative advantages of CAPD include steady-state hemostasis, hemodynamic tolerance, peptide and middle molecule removal, simplicity, relative independence, and no systemic heparinization (Table 46.2). Potential disadvantages of CAPD compared to hemodialysis include the requirement of continuous aseptic technique, possible injury to the peritoneum, infectious complications, excessive systemic glucose loading, protein loss, and body image issues (Table 46.2).

PERITONEAL ACCESS

Access to the peritoneal cavity is via the placement of an indwelling catheter. There are many styles of such catheters available,[97] and a typical sample is shown in Fig. 46.10. Catheters are manufactured from a silastic material, which is soft, flexible, and biocompatible. A typical adult catheter is about 40–45 cm long, 20–22 cm of which are inside the peritoneal cavity. Placement of the catheter is such that the distal end lies low in a pelvic gutter. The center section of the catheter has one or two cuffs, made of a porous material. This section is tunneled inside the anterior abdominal wall so that the cuffs provide mechanical support and stability to the catheter. The cuffs are placed at different sites surrounding the abdominal rectus muscle. The remainder of the central section of the catheter is tunneled subcutaneously before exiting the abdominal surface, usually midway between the umbilicus and pubis, offset to one side by a few centimeters.[98]

In addition to provision of support to the catheter, the cuffs and tunnel provide a mechanical barrier to skin organisms and prevent their migration down the catheter to the peritoneal cavity. The placement of the exit site of the catheter is one of the key factors to the development or prevention of exit-site infections and peritonitis, and many studies describe the development of new catheters and the surgical techniques for catheter placement. A recent exam-

TABLE 46.8. COMPARISON OF WEEKLY CLEARANCES OF SOLUTES BY PERITONEAL AND HEMODIALYSIS MEMBRANES

Solute	MW	Peritoneal Membrane[a] (L/wk)	Cuprophane[b] (L/wk)	Cellulose Triacetate[c] (L/wk)
Urea	60	64	119	139
Creatinine	113	57	96	126
Vitamin B_{12}	1355	37	27	86
Inulin	5200	17	14	51
Beta-2 microglobulin	11800	8	0	38

[a]Based on 4 • 2 liter exchanges daily.
[b]Based on 3 • 3 hour dialyses per week.
[c]Based on 3 • 3 hour dialyses per week. (Adapted from Ref. 99.)

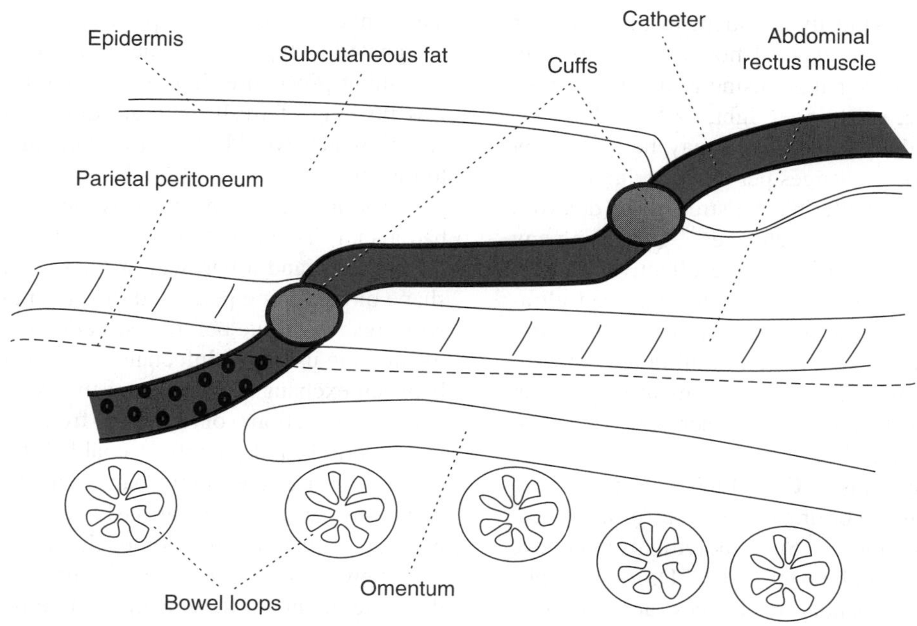

Figure 46.10. Schematic diagram of the placement of a peritoneal dialysis catheter through the abdominal wall into the peritoneal cavity. *(Reproduced from Ref. 24, p. 126, with permission from WB Saunders Company, Orlando, FL.)*

ple is the swan-neck presternal peritoneal catheter, which may have three or more cuffs.[100] These catheters are tunneled from the abdominal surface, along the surface of the thorax, and exit from the anterior chest wall. The external section of most peritoneal catheters ends with a Luer-lock, which can be connected to a variety of administration sets.[101] These catheters can be utilized immediately, if necessary, provided small initial volumes are instilled, however, a maturation period of 2–6 weeks is preferred.

PERITONEAL DIALYSIS PROCEDURES

There are several types of peritoneal dialysis, of which continuous ambulatory peritoneal dialysis (CAPD) is the most common. Others include continuous cycling (CCPD), daily ambulatory (DAPD), and nightly intermittent (NIPD).[102] All variants of PD require the placement of a dialysis solution in the peritoneal cavity, allowing it to remain *in situ* for a period (called the dwell time), removing the spent dialysate, and then repeating the process. All forms use the same dialysate, which is commercially available in volumes of 1 to 3 L presented in a flexible polyvinyl chloride plastic bag. The osmotic load is provided by dextrose, in concentrations ranging from 1.5–4.25%, which provides osmolarities of 350–480 mOsm/L, compared to that of serum, which is 280 mOsm/L. Other osmotic agents have been used, including mannitol, glycerol, glucose polymers such as icodextrin, and amino acids, but are not widespread because of expense or difficulty in manufacture.[103] It should be recognized that dextrose is not the ideal osmotic agent for dialysate, since these solutions are not biocompatible with peritoneal mesothelial cells or with peritoneal leukocytes.[104] These effects are mediated by both the osmolar load and by the low pH of the solutions. Other problems may arise from a plasticizer-induced peritoneal sclerosis.[105]

The other constituents of commercial PD solutions include sodium 132 mEq/L (132 mmol/L), chloride 102 mEq/L (102 mmol/L), lactate 35 mEq/L, and magnesium 1.5 mEq/L (0.75 mmol/L). Solutions have traditionally contained calcium 3.5 mEq/L (1.75 mmol/L), although there is a current trend to use low-calcium-containing solutions of 2.5 mEq/L (1.25 mmol/L), to reduce the risk of hypercalcemia, aluminum bone disease, or metastatic calcification.[106]

In a basic CAPD system, dialysate is permitted to flow into the peritoneal cavity under gravity. The inflow occurs over a period of about 15 minutes, and the dialysate is preheated to body temperature. A typical dwell period for daytime exchanges in CAPD is about 4 hours, using one of the lower dextrose concentration dialysate solutions. At the end of the prescribed dwell period, the empty dialysate bag is placed in a dependent position, the administration set is unclamped, and the dialysate is permitted to flow out of the peritoneal cavity via the catheter and administration set into the original container. The bag containing the spent fluid is detached and discarded. A new bag of dialysate is attached, and the process repeated. The process of outflow, aseptic manipulation of the administration set and catheter, and inflow requires a total time of about 30 minutes. Thus, actual dialysis occurs for about 3.5 hours out of the prescribed 4-hour period. Typically a patient instills a 2-liter exchange of dialysate about every 4 hours during the day and then a single 2-liter exchange, using a higher dextrose concentration dialysate, for an overnight, 12-hour dwell.

The quantity of dialysis delivered may be altered by changing the number of exchanges per day, altering the volume of each exchange, or altering the strength of dextrose in the dialysate for some or all exchanges.[98] Increasing any one of these variables will increase the effective osmotic gradient across the peritoneum, leading to increased ultrafiltration. Eventually an equilibrium will be reached after which time there will be no further ultrafiltration. Indeed, after a critical period, reverse water movement may occur. Solute movement by diffusion will also increase by increasing any of the above variables.

Alternative PD systems to CAPD have been designed for patients who are unable or unwilling to perform the necessary aseptic manipulations.[102] Such individuals may have poor visual acuity or manual dexterity. CCPD, for example, removes the need for manual exchanges and provides instead an automated cycler that performs these functions. The device is set up in the evening, and the patient attaches the peritoneal catheter to it at bedtime. The machine performs several short-dwell exchanges during the night and this permits a long cycle-free daytime dwell of up to 12–14 hours. Thus, CCPD provides an exchange profile in reverse of that of CAPD. NIPD has a similar theme, except that the peritoneal cavity tends to be dialysate-free during the day. A number of variants exist, and depend largely on equipment availability, patient and prescriber preference, and whether the patient retains any residual renal function, which influences the quantity of dialysis prescribed.

One of the paramount factors that influences the rate of peritonitis in PD patients is the type of administration set and method of its connection to the peritoneal catheter. In the late 1970s and early 1980s, a simple spike method was used to connect these sections. However, the rate of peritonitis was excessive and resulted from a breakdown of aseptic technique by patients, leading to touch contamination of the catheter. During the last decade, significant steps have been made to minimize this risk.[101] There have been approximately seven major types of connection systems introduced during the last 15 years, each one of which has had several variants. There is, thus, a confusing variety of systems available today. The relative success and acceptability of the systems is dependent on their ease of use, reliability, cost, aesthetics, and ability to prevent peritonitis. A system, for example, may be user friendly for the patient in that it requires few steps, but may carry an unacceptable risk for peritonitis.

The initial dialysate delivery system used dialysate in glass bottles with a long, disposable transfer set. This system required 44 steps per day and had a risk of biofilm formation inside the catheter.[107] The first significant improvement was the production of a wearable bag, which reduced the number of steps to 12 per day. However all steps were designated as high risk because they were not protected by a flushing procedure; indeed the first step after connection was flushing of fresh dialysate directly into the peritoneal cavity, which would deposit any contaminating organisms to that site.

The next development was the Perugia system, which had a short Y-shaped transfer set connected permanently to the catheter, and a bag with a long downflow tube.[101] The shape of the tubing permitted the patient to flush the system with fresh dialysate before instillation to the peritoneal cavity, and the use of disinfectant to fill the end of the catheter between exchanges. Variants of the Perugia system permitted disconnections of the bag from the catheter during dwell periods and, therefore, enabled the patient to dispose of, or to reuse, the empty bags. These variants remain in common use, and are variously termed O-sets or Y-sets, because of the configuration of the tubing.

Newer systems have the Y tubing on the bag side of the system. One of these is the double-bag system, and permits both a flush-before-fill procedure and disconnection during the dwell. Although the number of steps is reduced (20 per day), the risks of biofilm formation and peritonitis remain high.[107] The translation connection device, the nondisconnect Y, and the double-bag plus T-set are all new variants of the Y on the bag side. These systems sacrifice cost for the benefit of decreased infection risk.

ADEQUACY OF PERITONEAL DIALYSIS

Peritoneal dialysis patients have numerous metabolic and nutritional abnormalities, such as sustained uremia, accumulation of "middle molecule" toxins, amino acid and albumin loss into the dialysate, glucose absorption from the dialysate, loss of muscle mass and increased adipose tissue, and poor appetite.[108–112] Many studies indicate that although the nutritional status of CAPD patients improves for up to 1 year following the initiation of CAPD, long term they experience a deterioration in nutritional status, as measured by serum albumin, plasma amino acid concentrations, and anthropometric parameters. Poor nutritional status appears to correlate with poor clinical outcome.[108–110] Many PD patients may be malnourished as they start PD, due to the practice of placing patients on a low-protein diet as a means of slowing the progression of renal failure, together with the general loss of appetite that accompanies ESRD.[111,112] Many progressive renal diseases are treated using corticosteroids, which may increase net protein catabolism, and there may be a substantial loss of albumin (5–15 g/d) in the dialysate. The recommended daily protein intake for CAPD patients is >1.2 g/kg body weight/d, which exceeds that for normal individuals (0.75–1.0 g/kg/d). The BUN concentration is therefore a net result of both a patient's nutritional status (in terms of dietary protein intake and protein catabolic rate) and the quantity of dialysis the patient has received. For these reasons, the assessment of the adequacy of dialysis requires more than a simple examination of the BUN profile. The most common methods for assessment of the adequacy of PD are the peritoneal equilibration test (PET), *Kt/V,* and creatinine clearance.[99,113]

PERITONEAL EQUILIBRATION TEST

The PET is a diagnostic test designed to determine an individual PD patient's peritoneal membrane clearance and ultrafiltration characteristics.[113] It quantitates the ability with which solutes and water can transfer across the membrane. Since the peritoneal membrane permits movement of solutes in both directions, the PET simultaneously determines the passage of creatinine from blood to dialysate, glucose from dialysate to blood, and free water transfer. The objective of the PET is to determine which variant of PD is appropriate for an individual patient and to quantitate the daily dialysis requirement. Solute transport is defined as high, high average, low average, or low, and ultrafiltration rates as poor, adequate, good, or excellent (Table 46.9). To perform a PET, a patient receives a standardized exchange, and simultaneous blood and dialysate samples are obtained before the exchange (time 0), and at 1, 2, 3, and 4 hours into the exchange. Dialysate to plasma ratios of creatinine are plotted at each time point, and the rate and magnitude of the increase over 4 hours predicts the permeability of the membrane (Fig. 46.11). The ratio of glucose concentration in the dialysate at each time point *(D)* to the glucose concentration at time 0 (D_0) is calculated. The ratio therefore drops from a value of 1.0 over the following 4 hours (Fig. 46.11). A highly permeable membrane will allow easy passage of both creatinine and glucose. Since the glucose concentration in the dialysate is the primary force that results in ultrafiltration, it therefore follows that patients who have a high solute transport rate (in other words, a high dialysis clearance of creatinine) will also have a poor ultrafiltration rate. The prognostic interpretation of the PET results is depicted in Table 46.9 where APD is automated PD performed every night for 8–12 hours using 10–20 liters of dialysate. DAPD is daily ambulatory PD performed using 3–4 exchanges during the daytime only. Standard dose PD is CAPD with 7.5–9 liters of dialysate per 24 hours or standard CCPD with 6–8 liters overnight and 2 liters during the day. High dose is CAPD with >9 liters dialysate per 24 hours or CCPD with >8 liters of dialysate overnight and >2 liters of dialysate during the day.

Kt/V

The *Kt/V* test is based on urea kinetic modeling,[55] and for PD patients has been derived from data obtained from hemodialysis patients. In hemodialysis, the minimum acceptable value of *Kt/V* is 1.3 although some authors believe the optimal value is 1.4–1.5 per treatment.[39,43,53] In CAPD patients, *Kt/V* values usually exceed 1.9 per week. This is explained by the peak concentration and time-average concentration hypotheses, which have endeavored to correlate urea concentration parameters to patient outcome. As in hemodialysis, a *Kt/V* is a unitless value that correlates the patient's peritoneal membrane urea clearance *(K)* with the duration of dialysis *(t)* and the volume of distribution *(V)* of urea.

Calculation of *Kt/V* for PD requires that the total volume of drained effluent per day be determined (this value is the volume instilled plus volume of water ultrafiltered). A dialysate to plasma (D/P) urea concentration is determined, and *Kt* is estimated as:

$$Kt = \text{D/P} \times \text{volume drained (L/day)}$$

An estimate of *V* is determined from a nomogram based on height, weight, age, and gender.[58] The *Kt/V* calculated in this way is a value per day, and must be multiplied by 7 and divided by 3 to produce a value equivalent to that of intermittent, thrice-weekly hemodialysis. In this manner, appropriate *Kt/V*s for hemodialysis per treatment might be 1.2–1.4; and for PD (HD equivalent treatment), *Kt/V* might be 0.5–0.6. The exact requirements of *Kt/V* for PD patients remain unknown because of the lack of definitive published data.[114,115] A large, multicenter study is currently under way, in centers in the United States and Canada (the CANUSA study) that has this as its main objective.

One problem associated with the determination of *Kt/V* for PD patients is the impracticality of 24-hour collections of dialysis effluent. Recently, abbreviated collection periods have been used, demonstrating that calculations based on the first morning exchange after an overnight dwell correlated well ($r = 0.92$) with a 24-hour collection.[116,117]

TABLE 46.9. PROGNOSTIC VALUE OF PET RESULTS

Creatinine or Dextrose Transport	Ultrafiltration Rate	Predicted Solute Clearance	Preferred Type[a]
High	Poor	Adequate	APD, DAPD
High average	Adequate	Adequate	Standard dose PD
Low average	Good	Adequate/inadequate	Standard to high dose PD
Low	Excellent	Inadequate	High dose PD, hemodialysis

[a]See text for discussion of terms. (Reproduced from Ref. 113, p. 102, with permission from S. Karger AG, Basel, Switzerland.)

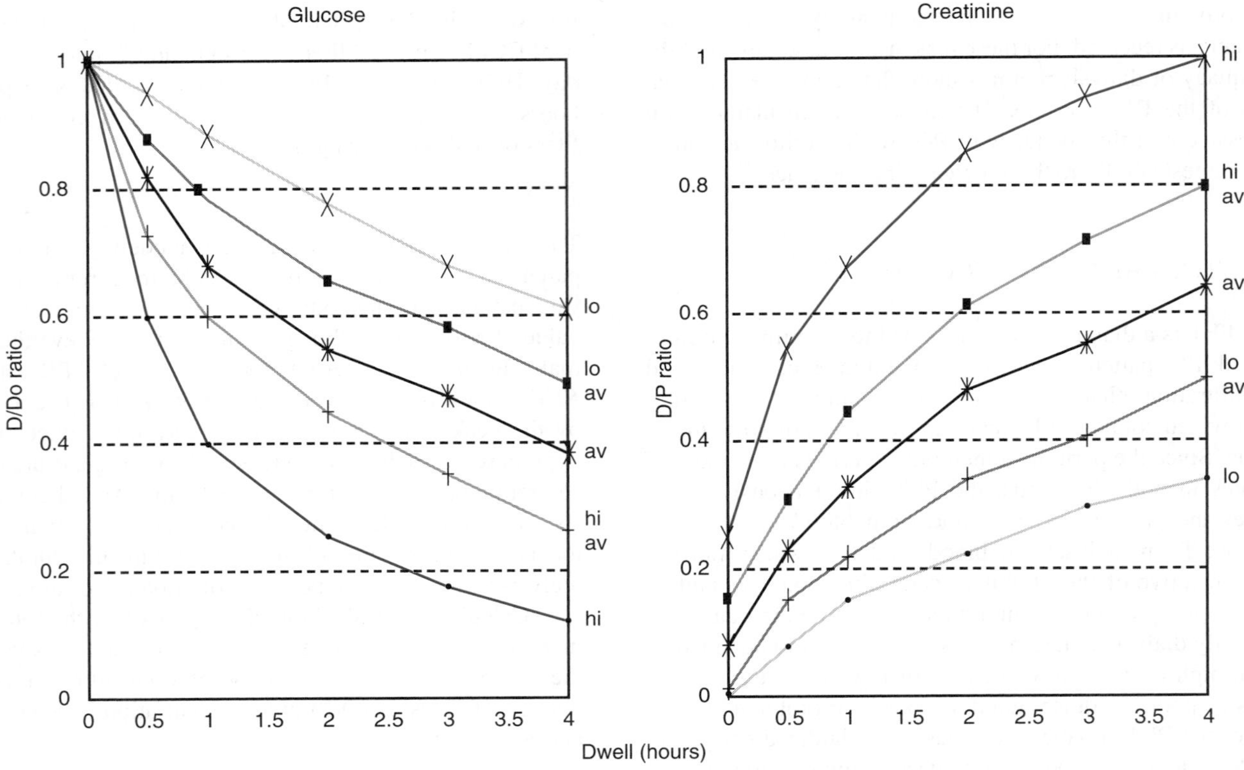

Figure 46.11. Glucose and creatinine ratio nomograms for interpretation of the peritoneal equilibration test. *(Reproduced from Ref. 113, p. 100, with permission from S Karger AG, Basel, Switzerland.)*

Creatinine Clearance

The determination of weekly creatinine clearance can also be used to assess the adequacy of peritoneal dialysis.[118,119] There is a reasonable correlation ($r = 0.71$) between weekly creatinine clearance, standardized to 1.73 m^2 body surface area, and *Kt/V*. A minimum weekly clearance of 40 liters has been recommended, while a weekly *Kt/V* of 2.0 represents a creatinine clearance of about 50–60 L/wk.[119] Such a value is the sum of both peritoneal and residual renal clearance and is influenced by body muscle mass. However this method may also overestimate the amount of dialysis delivered, since creatinine is eliminated by active tubular secretion as well as by glomerular filtration.

Complications of Peritoneal Dialysis

Mechanical, medical, and infectious problems complicate peritoneal dialysis therapy.[96,98,102] Mechanical complications include those that are effected by technical issues, such as kinking of the catheter and inflow and outflow obstruction. Most of these issues are solved by manipulation of the catheter, or prevented by careful initial placement of the catheter. Other mechanical problems include excessive catheter motion at the exit site leading to induration and possible infection and aggravation of tissues; pain from impingement of the catheter tip on the viscera; or inflow pain resulting from a jet-effect of too rapid dialysate inflow.

Numerous medical complications may arise (Table 46.10). An average PD patient will absorb up to 60% of each load of dextrose placed in the peritoneal cavity (Fig. 46.11). This continuous supply of calories leads to increased adipose tissue deposition and altered requirements for insulin in diabetic patients.

Infectious complications of PD are a major cause of morbidity and mortality, and are the leading cause of technique failure and transfer from PD to hemodialysis.[13,120] The two predominant infectious complications are peritonitis and catheter-related infections, which include both exit-site and tunnel infections. Although 40–60% of patients develop their first episode of peritonitis within 1 year of starting PD, the range reported is influenced by the type of connector technology the patient was using.[120] The use of Y-set systems was associated with the lowest incidence of peritonitis (40%). Peritonitis is a major cause of catheter loss in PD patients. In one series, peritonitis was responsible for the loss of 17% of all catheters lost in PD patients younger than 50 years, and for 25% of all

TABLE 46.10. MEDICAL COMPLICATIONS OF PERITONEAL DIALYSIS

Glucose load	Exacerbation of diabetes mellitus
Fluid overload	Exacerbation of CHF
	Edema
	Pulmonary congestion
Electrolyte abnormalities	Hyper- and hypocalcemia
Chemical peritonitis	
Malnutrition	Albumin loss
	Loss of amino acids
	Muscle wasting
	Increased adipose tissue
Fibrin formation in dialysate	

catheters lost in patients older than 60 years of age.[121] Together, catheter-related infections plus peritonitis were the most common cause of catheter loss in this population, responsible for 61 and 60% of catheters lost in the <50 and >60 year age groups, respectively.

A statistically significant correlation between infectious complications and death rates has been reported.[7] Fifty percent of patients who had more than 1 peritonitis episode per year, 0.5 to 1 episode per year, or less than 0.5 episode per year, died after 3, 4, and 5 years of therapy, respectively. It is important to note that these relationships are not necessarily cause and effect, since many of these patients succumb to cardiovascular events.

PERITONITIS

The reported incidence of peritonitis is influenced by connector technology and by at-risk patient populations, including the elderly and diabetic individuals.[120,121] Thus, the incidence of peritonitis in the literature varies from as frequent as one episode every 5 to 6 patient-months, to as infrequent as one episode every 5 to 6 patient-years. The mean incidence for most dialysis centers in the United States is about one episode every 12 to 24 patient-months.

The typical signs and symptoms of peritonitis are shown in Table 46.11. Peritonitis is defined in a variety of ways, but most would agree on a diagnosis based on the presentation of a patient with any two of the following: abdominal pain, cloudy effluent, or >100 WBCs per milliliter of dialysate. Inherent in this definition will be a number of false-positive and false-negative diagnoses, since 5% of patients with culture-proven peritonitis will have clear dialysate,[122] and some patients, such as menstruating females, may have cloudy PD effluent without clinical infection.

Sterile culture peritonitis remains problematic. It is defined as an episode where there is clinical evidence of peritonitis (abdominal pain, cloudy effluent, etc.), but where the culture of the dialysate reveals no organism. There are several postulates for the high incidence (up to 20% of episodes) of culture-negative peritonitis. Many peritonitis-producing organisms are slime producers.[107] These organisms may adhere to the peritoneal membrane or to the catheter surface and be protected from exogenous antibiotics. Sufficient numbers of these bacteria may proliferate to cause peritoneal membrane inflammation and clinical peritonitis, but an inadequate number may seed into the peritoneal cavity to be recovered by conventional microbiological techniques. In addition, planktonic bacteria may be rapidly phagocytosed by peritoneal WBCs, which would render them unavailable for culture.

TABLE 46.11. SIGNS AND SYMPTOMS OF PERITONITIS

	% Patients
Symptoms	
Cloudy effluent	98
Abdominal pain	78
Fever	38
Nausea, vomiting	25–30
Chills	18
Signs	
Abdominal tenderness	76
Fever >37°C	28

Clinical peritonitis is a relatively "dilute" infection, with as few as 10^4 organisms per milliliter of dialysate. Removal of a small volume of dialysate from the bag may thus result in too few organisms to culture. Contemporary methods have increased the recovery rate of organisms and decreased the culture-negative rate.[123] These methods all utilize some type of concentrating technique. Centrifugation is commonly employed, where a large volume of dialysate (100 mL) is centrifuged, and the resultant pellet may be cultured on agar plates or in broth. Filtration of a large volume through a 0.44-μm filter can be used for clear effluent, which contains few WBCs or fibrin that would otherwise clog the filter. The filter can subsequently be divided and cultured as above. Other methods that have been used for very cloudy effluent include attempts to lyse WBC to release bacteria trapped within them. Distilled water, surfactants, and ultrasound lysis are in widespread use, and have substantially increased the yield of positive peritonitis cultures. Blood-culturing methods (e.g., Bactec) also decrease the sterile culture rate.

The primary organisms responsible for causing peritonitis are listed in Table 46.12. The majority of infections (40–65%) are caused by gram-positive bacteria, of which *S. epidermidis* is the predominant organism.[124] There is no single predominant gram-negative organism. Together, gram-positive and gram-negative organisms account for 65–90% of all episodes of peritonitis, and thus are the spectrum against which initial empiric therapy is directed.

TABLE 46.12. ORGANISMS CAUSING PERITONITIS

Organisms	% Episodes
Gram positive	40–65
S. epidermidis	30–45
S. aureus	10–20
Streptococci	10–15
Enterococci	3–5
Diphtheroids	<5
Gram negative	20–35
E. coli	5–12
P. aeruginosa	5–8
Enterobacter	2–3
Acinetobacter	2–3
Klebsiella	2–3
Proteus	2–3
Mixed gram positive and negative	10–15
Fungi	5–10
Sterile culture, presumed bacterial	5–20
Other	5

Prophylaxis of Peritonitis

Attempts to prevent peritonitis and catheter-related infections have included technological developments of connector systems and the use of prophylactic antibiotic regimens[125–127] and vaccines.[128,129] In one study, 64 CAPD patients were randomized to either no treatment or to intermittent rifampin, 300 mg orally twice a day for 5 days, repeated every 3 months.[125] A number of outcomes were measured, including the incidence of peritonitis and catheter-related infections, and the percent of nasal and exit-site cultures positive for *S. aureus.* There was no significant change in the incidence of peritonitis: 0.84 episode per patient-year for the control group and 0.52 episode per patient-year for the rifampin-treated group. However, there was a significant decrease in the onset and number of catheter-related infections. There was a decrease ($p < 0.001$) in the infection rate (0.65 versus 0.22 episode per patient-year for control and treated groups), and a delay ($p = 0.015$) in the onset of the first catheter-related infection in the treated group. The authors also noted an early decrease in the positive culture rate of *S. aureus* from both the nares and exit site, but these returned to baseline within about a month during continued rifampin administration, which suggests that colonization is not the sole risk factor. There were few problems of patient intolerance of rifampin, and resistant organisms did not appear until 6 months. This same regimen of rifampin was recently compared to daily application of mupirocin to the exit site.[126] Although peritonitis was not measured as an outcome, both rifampin and mupirocin were demonstrated to reduce the incidence of *S. aureus* catheter infections.

In a randomized study, 56 CAPD patients treated with 160 mg trimethoprim/800 mg sulfamethoxazole once daily for 1 year were compared to 49 patients treated with placebo.[127] There was no difference in the time to the development of first peritonitis: at 6 months, 64.1% of co-trimoxazole and 62.5% of placebo patients were peritonitis-free; at 12 months 41.9% of cotrimoxazole and 35% of placebo patients were peritonitis-free. Sixteen patients required removal of the peritoneal catheter due to peritonitis, seven from the cotrimoxazole group and nine from the control group. Seventeen patients withdrew from the cotrimoxazole group because of adverse effects. The authors concluded that prophylactic cotrimoxazole was ineffective in the prevention of peritonitis.

Another approach to the prevention of peritonitis and catheter-related infections has been the use of staphylococcal vaccines.[128] In one multicenter study, 124 CAPD patients were randomly assigned to receive a control injection of normal saline, or a vaccine of combined staphylococcus toxoid and whole killed staphylococci. The vaccine did not alter the incidence of peritonitis or exit-site infections, nor did it change the rate of nasal carriage of *S. aureus.* However, the vaccine did increase serum anti-alpha hemolysin and dialysate levels of specific antibodies against *S. aureus.* Although vaccination was not successful against staphylococci, this approach is still being considered for gram-negative organisms such as *E. coli* or *Pseudomonas.*[129] Thus, the literature to date suggests ambivalent results using antibiotics or vaccines to prevent peritonitis, but that reductions in catheter-related infections may be possible.

Treatment of Peritonitis

The latest recommendations from the Ad Hoc Advisory Committee on Peritonitis Management include a series of algorithms that provide excellent guidelines for diagnosis and pharmacotherapy of peritoneal dialysis associated infections.[123] These guidelines are currently undergoing revision and should be available in 1996. Initial empiric therapy for peritonitis, in the situation where either organisms are not identified on a Gram stain or where such a stain was not performed, should include agents effective against both gram-positive and gram-negative organisms. Intraperitoneal (IP) administration is favored over the intravenous route, and combinations of vancomycin with either an aminoglycoside or ceftazidime are recommended. For vancomycin, pharmacokinetic and efficacy studies demonstrate that a single IP dose of 2 grams or 30 mg/kg vancomycin in one 6-hour exchange every 7 days, for a total of two doses, is adequate.[130–132] An alternative approach is the instillation of 25–50 mg/L of vancomycin into each dialysate exchange.[123] Once-weekly administration results in about 65–75% of the vancomycin being absorbed into the systemic circulation over the duration of the exchange, prevents transient high peak serum concentrations observed after intravenous administration, is convenient for a patient to use at home, and is as effective as intravenous therapy (about 90%).[131–133]

In the late 1980s and early 1990s, a series of case reports suggested an association between the administration of large doses of IP vancomycin and onset of peritonitis-like signs and symptoms, such as cloudy effluent and elevated dialysate leukocyte and polymorphonuclear cell counts.[134] The exact etiology of this phenomenon remains unknown and the number of published reports has abruptly declined over the last several years. The incidence is unknown, but is probably rare, and appears not to be brand specific.

For aminoglycosides, the latest recommendation is the use of once-daily IP administration.[123,135,136] When these guidelines were published, there were no clinical efficacy studies to demonstrate the effectiveness of this regimen. The recommendation was extrapolated from the use of once-daily aminoglycosides in other severe systemic infections in nondialysis patients, and knowledge of the disposition of aminoglycosides in PD.[136] For gentamicin, tobramycin, and netilmicin, recommended dosing is an IP loading dose of 1–2 mg/kg, in one 2-liter bag of dialysate, followed by 0.6 mg/kg IP into one 6-hour exchange daily.[123]

Two studies have recently been published that indicate the efficacy of once-daily IP gentamicin may be less than optimal.[132,137] The first prospective, randomized study compared once-daily versus multiple-dose gentamicin for the treatment of CAPD peritonitis. The regimens were 40 mg/2 L in the overnight exchange for the once-daily dose, and 10 mg/2 L in each of four exchanges per day for the multiple-dose regimen. Although the authors did not separately assess the differences in outcome between gram-negative and gram-positive organisms, 4 of 16 (25%) gram negative infections treated with multiple dosing resulted in treatment failure, compared with 3 of 19 (16%) treated with once-daily dosing.[137] Furthermore, 4 of the failures (2 in each group) resulted in relapsing infections.

Bailie et al.[132] treated all CAPD patients presenting with gram-negative infections with 0.6 mg/kg IP gentamicin in a 6-hour dwell. Of the 9 episodes of peritonitis caused by 10 gram-negative species, 6 (67%) were cured and 3 (4 organisms) were treatment failures. These limited efficacy data suggest that the clinical outcomes with once-daily dosing may be unsatisfactory.

The concept behind once-daily IP gentamicin was to employ the ideal antimicrobial characteristics of aminoglycosides, namely concentration-dependent killing, the postantibiotic effect, and saturable uptake by sensitive mammalian tissue. Thus, for peritonitis, once-daily IP dosing should ideally produce dialysate concentrations at least 10 times the minimum inhibitory concentration (MIC) of susceptible bacteria, and minimize the sustained, elevated serum aminoglycoside concentrations that predispose patients to ototoxicity or nephrotoxicity (in those PD patients who have residual renal function).

Unfortunately, the pharmacokinetic disposition of gentamicin following once-daily IP administration does not produce favorable serum and dialysate concentrations in many patients.[138] Mean concentrations at the end of the second, third, and fourth dwells, all of which have no added gentamicin, are approximately 0.5 to 1.0 mg/L and 0.2 to 0.7 mg/L for serum and dialysate, respectively. In addition, there may be prolonged periods of many hours during which dialysate concentrations are below the MIC of susceptible organisms. Furthermore, patients who are not yet anuric may attain even lower dialysate concentrations because of continued renal clearance.

On confirmation, by culture results, of the infecting organism, the appropriate antibiotic may be continued as monotherapy for a total treatment duration of 10–14 days and the other agent discontinued. If *S. aureus* is cultured and no clinical improvement is observed in 4–5 days, rifampin 600 mg PO daily should be added to the vancomycin.[123] Culture of enterococci should lead to a continued use of both vancomycin and an aminoglycoside. Culture-negative episodes of peritonitis require continued combination therapy. If there is clinical improvement within 4–5 days, the aminoglycoside may be discontinued and the patient should receive one additional dose of vancomycin on day 7, on the assumption that the organism was gram positive.

Single gram-negative species may be treated with aminoglycoside monotherapy, as long as sensitivity data support this. However, isolation of *Pseudomonas* or *Xanthomonas* should dictate the use of two concurrent agents with activity against these organisms.[139] An extensive list of appropriate antibiotics together with recommended dosing regimens derived from the report of the peritonitis advisory committee is provided in Table 50.9.[123]

Fungal peritonitis is associated with a poor prognosis, high morbidity, and high mortality.[133,140,141] One problem with prospective assessment of antifungal regimens is the relative infrequency with which these infections occur. It is therefore difficult to design and implement comparative studies. Most literature about antifungal treatment is therefore retrospective or a report of local experience.[140–143] There is controversy as to whether the PD catheter should be removed once fungal organisms are identified, and the patient transferred to hemodialysis. Based on retrospective analysis of data, the Ad Hoc Advisory Committee recommendations are to treat with oral flucytosine (2 gram loading dose then 1000 mg daily) plus fluconazole 150 mg IP every 2 days.[123] Treatment should be continued for 4–6 weeks if the patient is responding, but the catheter should be removed in 4–7 days if there is inadequate clinical response.

The recent trend of using oral fluoroquinolones for the treatment of peritonitis is no longer recommended. The propensity of chelation drug interactions with divalent and trivalent metal ions,[144] the relatively small margin between dialysate concentrations and MICs,[145] and reports of high incidences of relapsing and recurrent peritonitis suggest that other regimens may be preferred.[146,147]

CATHETER-RELATED INFECTIONS

The incidence of exit-site infections is about 0.8–1.2 episodes per patient-year.[148] There is a decreased incidence in older (>60 years) versus younger (<50 years) patients.[121] Causative organisms are different that those causing peritonitis—the most common is *S. aureus* (about 40–45% of episodes), followed by *S. epidermidis, P. aeruginosa,* and other enteric gram-negative bacilli (about 15–20% each).[124,149,150] The definitions of these infections are also vague, but generally include the presence of purulent drainage and erythema.[151] There appears to be an association between an increased risk of exit-site infections in patients who are nasal carriers of *S. aureus.* [152–154] Carriers of *S. aureus* had a significantly higher ($p = 0.012$) rate of exit-site infection (0.4 episode per patient year) than noncarriers (0.1).[154]

The use of topical antibiotics and disinfectants to treat catheter-related infections is controversial.[126,155] There are few adequately controlled studies to determine the effectiveness of systemic antibiotics. However, current recommendations for gram-positive infections are that oral cephalexin or cephradine or IP vancomycin be used.[123] Gram-negative organisms should be treated with ciprofloxacin 500 mg PO twice daily. Treatment should be continued for 2–3 weeks.

INTRAPERITONEAL DRUG THERAPY

In recent years, sound pharmacokinetic information has become available for antibiotics and other drugs in CAPD patients.[156–159] Indeed, the use of IP antibiotics for systemic infections has recently been reported.[160] Potential benefits of the IP versus IV route for the management of systemic infections include use of an already existent access for administration, ability to treat infections as outpatients, avoidance of costs for intravenous lines, possible avoidance of intravenous drug-related toxicities, and improved patient acceptance.

The IP route is frequently used for the administration of soluble insulin for maintenance of diabetic patients.[161] Possible advantages of the IP versus the subcutaneous route include the avoidance of erratic absorption (both rate and extent of absorption), convenience, avoidance of subcutaneous injection-site-related complications, and prevention of peripheral hyperinsulinemia. Insulin appears to be cleared into the systemic compartment by an active transport process, or via the peritoneal lymphatics. A number of studies have demonstrated the bioavailability of IP insulin to be about 25–30%, although none clearly compares the clinical effectiveness of IP versus subcutaneous insulin in diabetes control. Insulin requirements for PD patients may be greater than hemodialysis patients because of the continued absorption of dextrose from the peritoneal cavity. Further, because of adsorption of insulin to the PVC bag and administration set, the IP dose of insulin often needs to be two to three times the subcutaneous maintenance dose.

Many PD patients secrete large quantities of fibrinogen into the peritoneal cavity, which results in fibrin formation. This can lead to intraperitoneal adhesions and outflow obstruction. The instillation of heparin 500 U/L to each exchange may prevent this complication due to its local antifibrin effect.[162] Since standard heparin has a molecular weight of 12,000–15,000 Da, it is minimally absorbed and thereby has limited systemic effects.

Other drugs that have been administered by the IP route include calcitriol for the treatment of secondary hyperparathyroidism,[163] deferoxamine for the treatment of aluminum bone disease and hyperaluminumism,[164,165] erythromycin for the treatment of diabetic gastroparesis,[166] lithium for treatment of bipolar affective disorder,[167] streptokinase and urokinase for the treatment of recurrent peritonitis,[168,169] and amino acids for nutritional disorders.[170] The absorption of IP erythropoietin has also been studied,[171] and although its bioavailability is low ($F = 0.11$ into a dry peritoneum), its use has been suggested as an alternative for some but not all patients.[172]

NUTRITION AND PERITONEAL DIALYSIS

A recent, international study demonstrated that 41% of 224 CAPD patients were protein malnourished, on the basis of biochemical, anthropometric, and subjective measurements.[109] Some 8% of the study group were defined as severely malnourished and diabetic patients were disproportionally represented. Other studies have demonstrated similar findings with a range of 20–70% of PD patients being malnourished.[173–175] Malnutrition in these patients, thus, has a significant impact on patient outcome. One study in 51 CAPD patients conducted over 5 years showed that there was a 3.5-fold increase in mortality in those patients who had a serum albumin of less than 3.5 g/dL.[175] Serum albumin concentrations were determined to be the strongest single predictor of decreased survival.[174,176] Other investigators also demonstrated correlations between protein malnutrition and other morbidities, such as increased incidence of peritonitis and hospitalization. There is a strong interrelationship between nutritional status and adequacy of dialysis.[50,55] As *Kt/V* increases, serum albumin increases and mortality and morbidity decrease.[51] One technique for ensuring an adequate protein supply while minimizing phosphate delivery has been the use of IP amino acids (IPAA).[170,177] Short-term studies, over periods of up to 8 weeks, have shown that IPAA do improve nutritional status. One study examined the use of a 1% IPAA solution in seven nondiabetic CAPD patients over 8 weeks.[170] In each case, two of the four daily dextrose-containing exchanges were replaced by IPAA. It was noted that mean 24-hour concentrations of plasma total and essential amino acids, and branched chain amino acids (leucine, isoleucine, and valine), were higher following IPAA. Serum albumin increased over 4 weeks but fell to baseline again by 8 weeks. All other indices remained normal except for the development of metabolic acidosis due to a decreased plasma bicarbonate concentration.

In another study, 15 CAPD patients were treated with 1 or 2.7% IPAA and compared with normal exchanges containing 1.36 or 3.86% dextrose, in a single 6-hour dwell.[177] Plasma amino acid concentrations increased substantially (valine and methionine increased 800 and 1100%, respectively) following IPAA, but other solutes (creatinine, urea, glucose, albumin, beta-2 microglobulin, and total protein) showed no difference between regimens. Ultrafiltration was decreased with IPAA.

Few studies have exceeded 6 months, and all appear to be in small groups of less than 10 patients. However, these pilot data suggest that IPAAs are absorbed into the systemic correlation where they may positively influence nutritional parameters. In addition, higher concentrations of IPAAs may produce an adequate ultrafiltration. The results of long-term studies on patient outcome, however, should be awaited before the use of IPAA is generally accepted.

Patient Outcomes

During the past two decades, the renal community has focused much of their attention on technologically advancing the dialysis procedure, devising methods to quantitate the dose of dialysis they delivered, and assessing the impact of the therapy on the morbidity and mortality of the patients. During this time frame, the demographics of the U.S. dialysis population has changed dramatically. The median age of ESRD patients has increased from 55 to 61 years since 1980, and currently the United States has the oldest dialysis population of any industrialized nation.[178] These older patients have a larger number of coexistent medical conditions many of which independently are associated with marked morbidity and mortality and, thereby, significantly contribute to the higher mortality seen in U.S. ESRD patients.[71] The nutritional status of the patients at the time of dialysis initiation has also been shown to be a strong predictor of mortality.[173]

The optimal success of medical care has traditionally been defined as "curing" the disease. Recently, the paradigm has shifted in many settings to the prevention of a disease. In light of the persistent increase in the incidence of ESRD, these should remain avid avenues of research for the foreseeable future. For the patient with ESRD, however, the ultimate outcome may not be attainable, that is, decreasing annual mortality must surely have a finite limit based on the patient's concomitant disease states and lifestyle. Thus, a focus on quality of life (QOL)[72,178] and rehabilitation[179,180] may be a valuable and viable avenue toward which the nephrology community should redirect its research resources.

Some efforts in these fields have been initiated recently but much remains to be done. Pharmacists along with others on the health care team need to become involved with the development, validation, and use of QOL assessments,[181,182] so that they can quantitate the contributions of their innovative interventions.[20,22–25]

References

1. Baxter Survey Data. Deerfield, IL, Baxter Healthcare Corporation, 1994.
2. US Renal Data System 1995 Annual Data Report. Bethesda, MD, The National Institutes of Diabetes and Digestive and Kidney Diseases, July 1995, p 167.
3. Ismail N, Hakin RM, Oreopoulos DG, Patrikarea A. Renal replacement therapies in the elderly: Part 1. Hemodialysis and chronic peritoneal dialysis. In-depth review. Am J Kidney Dis 1993;22:759–782.
4. Ozminkowski RJ, Hasod A, Firkusny I, et al. Estimating increases in outpatient dialysis costs resulting from scientific and technologic advancement. Adv Renal Replace Ther 1995;2:127–142.
5. US Renal Data System 1995 Annual Data Report. Bethesda, MD, The National Institutes of Diabetes and Digestive and Kidney Diseases, July 1995, p 44.
6. US Renal Data System 1991 Annual Data Report. Bethesda, MD, The National Institutes of Health and National Institute of Diabetes and Digestive and Kidney Diseases, August 1991.
7. Maiorca R, Giovanni CC, Giulio B, et al. Morbidity and mortality of CAPD and hemodialysis. Kidney Int 1993;43(suppl 40):S4–S15.
8. Held PJ, Port FK, Turenne MN, et al. Continuous ambulatory peritoneal dialysis and hemodialysis: Comparison of patient mortality with adjustment for comorbid conditions. Kidney Int 1994;45:1163–1169.
9. Churchill DN. Comparative morbidity among hemodialysis and continuous ambulatory peritoneal dialysis patients. Kidney Int 1993;43(suppl 40):S16–S22.
10. Bloembergen WE, Port FK, Mauger EA, Wolfe RA. A comparison of mortality between patients treated with hemodialysis and peritoneal dialysis. J Am Soc Nephrol 1995;6:177–183.

11. Bloembergen WE, Port FK, Mauger EA, Wolfe RA. A comparison of cause of death between patients treated with hemodialysis and peritoneal dialysis. J Am Soc Nephrol 1995;6:184–191.
12. US Renal Data System 1994 Annual Data Report. Bethesda, MD, The National Institutes of Diabetes and Digestive and Kidney Diseases, July 1994, p 52.
13. de Fijter CWH, Oe LP, Nauta JJP, et al. Clinical efficacy and morbidity associated with continuous cyclic compared with continuous ambulatory peritoneal dialysis. Ann Intern Med 1994;120:264–271.
14. US Renal Data System 1993 Annual Data Report. Bethesda, MD, The National Institutes of Diabetes and Digestive and Kidney Diseases, July 1993, p 13.
15. Held PJ, Brunner F, Odaka M, et al. Five year survival for end-stage renal disease patients in the United States, Europe and Japan. Am J Kidney Dis 1990;15:451–457.
16. Held PJ, Levin NW, Boubjerg RR, et al. Mortality and duration of hemodialysis treatment. JAMA 1991;265:871–875.
17. Burton PR, Walls J. Selection-adjusted comparison of hospitalization on continuous ambulatory peritoneal dialysis and haemodialysis. J Clin Epidemiol 1989;42:531–539.
18. Habach G, Bloembergen WE, Mauger EA, et al. Hospitalization among United States dialysis patients: Hemodialysis versus peritoneal dialysis. J Am Soc Nephrol 1995;5:1940–1948.
19. Cleary DJ, Matzke GR, Alexander ACM, Joy MS. Medication knowledge and prescription drug taking behavior of patients receiving chronic dialysis. Am J Health-Sys Pharm 1995;52:1895–1900.
20. Kaplan B, Mason NA, Shimp LA, Ascion FJ. Chronic hemodialysis patients. Part I: Characterization and drug-related problems. Ann Pharmacother 1994;28:316–319.
21. Blanchard R, Berger W, Bailie GR, et al. Knowledge of hemodialysis and CAPD patients about their prescribed medicine. Clin Nephrol 1990;34:173–178.
22. St Peter WL. Clinical pharmacy nephrology consultation and documentation: A comprehensive approach. J Pharm Prac 1993;6:140–147.
23. Norwood CE, Pahre SN. Clinical pharmacy nephrology practice in the outpatient dialysis center. J Pharm Prac 1993;6:140–147.
24. Bailie GR. Clinical pharmacy care in continuous ambulatory peritoneal dialysis patients. J Pharm Prac 1993;6:123–132.
25. Tang I, Vrahnos D, Hatoum H, Lau A. Effectiveness of clinical pharmacists interventions in a hemodialysis unit. Clin Ther 1993;15:459–464.
26. Zawada ET. Indications for dialysis, in Daugirdas JT, Ing TS (eds): Handbook of Dialysis, 2nd ed. Boston, Little Brown and Company, 1994, pp 3–9.
27. Agarwal R, Levi M. Selection of therapy for patients with end-stage renal disease, in Henrich WE (ed): Principles and Practice of Dialysis. Baltimore, Williams & Wilkins, 1994, pp 261–276.
28. Drukker W. Hemodialysis: a historical review, in Maher JF (ed): Replacement of Renal Function by Dialysis, 3rd ed. Dordecht, Holland, Kluwer Academic Publishers, 1989, pp 21–86.
29. Fan PY, Schwab SJ. Hemodialysis vascular access, in Henrich WL (ed): Principles and Practice of Dialysis. Baltimore, Williams & Wilkins, 1994, pp 22–37.
30. Raja RM. Vascular access for hemodialysis, in Daugirdas JT, Ing TS (eds): Handbook of Dialysis, 2nd ed. Boston, Little Brown and Company, 1994, pp 53–77.
31. US Renal Data System 1995 Annual Data Report. Bethesda, MD, The National Institutes of Diabetes and Digestive and Kidney Diseases. April 1995, p 55.
32. Kaufman JL, Berman JA, Rhee SW, Friedman P. Major complications from vascular access for chronic hemodialysis, in Nissenson AR, Fine RN (eds): Dialysis Therapy, 2nd ed. Philadelphia, Hanley & Belfus, 1993, pp 15–19.
33. Matzke GR. Pharmacotherapeutic consequences of recent advances in hemodialysis therapy. Ann Pharmacother 1994;28:512–514.
34. US Renal Data System 1994 Annual Data Report. Bethesda, MD, The National Institutes of Diabetes and Digestive and Kidney Diseases. July 1994, p S66.
35. Keshaviah P, Collins A. Rapid high-efficiency bicarbonate hemodialysis. Trans Am Soc Artif Intern Organs 1986;32:17.
36. Von Albertini B, Miller J, Garder P, Shinaberger J. High flux hemodiafiltration: Under six hours/week treatment. Trans Am Soc Artif Intern Organs 1984;30:227.
37. Collins AJ. High-efficiency treatments using conventional equipment, in Bosch JP (ed): Contemporary Issues in Nephrology: Hemodialysis High-Efficiency Treatments, vol 27. New York, Churchill Livingstone, 1993, pp 91–104.
38. Acchiardo SR. High-flux hemodialysis, in Bosch JP (ed): Contemporary Issues in Nephrology: Hemodialysis High-Efficiency Treatments, vol 27. New York, Churchill Livingstone, 1993, pp 105–117.
39. Collins AJ. High-flux, high-efficiency procedures, in Henrich WE (ed): Principles and Practice of Dialysis. Baltimore, Williams & Wilkins, 1994, pp 22–37.
40. Golper TA, Vincent HH, Gleason JR, Vos MC. Drug removal during high-efficiency and high-flux hemodialysis, in Bosch JP (ed): Contemporary Issues in Nephrology: Hemodialysis High-Efficiency Treatments, vol 27. New York, Churchill Livingstone, 1993, pp 175–208.
41. Konstantin P. Newer membranes: Cuprophane versus polysulfone versus polyacrylonitrile, in Bosch JP (ed): Contemporary Issues in Nephrology: Hemodialysis High-Efficiency Treatments, vol 27. New York, Churchill Livingstone, 1993, pp 63–77.
42. Bosch JP. The prescriptions of hemodialysis. Adv Renal Repl Ther 1994;1:281–287.
43. Parker T. Hemodialysis adequacy, in Henrich WL (ed): Principles of Practice of Dialysis. Baltimore, Williams & Wilkins, 1994, pp 63–75.
44. Held PJ, Carroll CE, Liska DW, et al. Hemodialysis therapy in the United States: What is the dose and does it matter? Am J Kidney Dis 1994;24:974–980.
45. Hornberger JC. The hemodialysis prescription and cost effectiveness. J Am Soc Nephrol 1993;4:1021–1027.
46. US Renal Data System. USRDS 1994 Annual Data Report. Bethesda, MD. July, 1994, pp 171–177.
47. Kopple JD, Hakim RM, Held PJ, et al. Recommendations for reducing the high morbidity and mortality of United

States maintenance dialysis patients. Am J Kidney Dis 1994;24:968–973.
48. Parker TF III. Role of dialysis dose on morbidity and mortality in maintenance hemodialysis patients. Am J Kidney Dis 1994;24:981–989.
49. Collins AJ, Ma JZ, Umen A, et al. Urea index and other predictors of hemodialysis patient survival. Am J Kidney Dis 1994;23:272–282.
50. Owen WFJ, Lew NL, Liu Y, et al. The urea reduction ratio and serum albumin concentration as predictors of mortality in patients undergoing hemodialysis. N Engl J Med 1993;329:1001–1006.
51. Hakim RM, Breyer J, Ismail N, et al. Effects of dose of dialysis on morbidity and mortality. Am J Kidney Dis 1994;23:661–669.
52. Lowrie EG, Lew NL. Death risk in hemodialysis patients: The predictive value of commonly measured variables and an evaluation of death rate differences between facilities. Am J Kidney Dis 1990;15:458–482.
53. Charra B, Calemard E, Ruffet M, et al. Survival as an index of adequacy of dialysis. Kidney Int 1992;4:1286–1291.
54. Lowrie EG, Lew NL. The urea reduction ratio (URR): A simple method for evaluating hemodialysis treatment. Contemp Dial Nephrol 1991;12:11–20.
55. Gotch FA, Sargent JA. A mechanistic analysis of the National Cooperative Dialysis Study (NCDS). Kidney Int 1985;28:526–534.
56. Lowrie EG, Laird NM, Parker TF III, et al. Effect of the hemodialysis on patient morbidity: Report from the National Cooperative Dialysis Study. N Engl J Med 1981;305:1176–1181.
57. Hakim RM, Depner TA, Parker TF III. Adequacy of hemodialysis. Am J Kidney Dis 1992;20:107–123.
58. Daugirdas JT, Depner TA. A nomogram approach to hemodialysis urea modeling. Am J Kidney Dis 1994;23:33–40.
59. Depner TA. Approach to hemodialysis urea modeling, in Henrich WL (ed): Principles of Practice of Dialysis. Baltimore, Williams & Wilkins, 1994, pp 47–62.
60. Delmez JA, Windus DW, St. Louis Nephrology Study Group. Hemodialysis prescription and delivery in a metropolitan community. Kidney Int 1992;41:1023–1028.
61. Port FK. Morbidity and mortality in dialysis patients. Kidney Int 1994;46:1728–1737.
62. Abramson F, Gibson S, Barlee V, et al. Urea kinetic modeling at high urea clearances: Implications for clinical practice. Adv Renal Repl Ther 1994;1:5–14.
63. Pearson P, Lew S, Abramson F, Bosch J. Measurement of kinetic parameters for urea in end-stage renal disease patients using a two compartment model. J Am Soc Nephrol 1994;4:1869–1873.
64. Daugirdas JT. Chronic hemodialysis prescription: A urea kinetic approach, in Daugirdas JT, Ing TS (eds): Handbook of Dialysis, 2nd ed. Boston, Little, Brown and Company, 1994, pp 92–120.
65. Sargent J. Short falls in the delivery of dialysis. Am J Kidney Dis 1990;15:500–510.
66. Sherman RA, Cody RP, Matera JJ, et al. Deficiencies in delivered hemodialysis therapy due to missed and shortened treatments. Am J Kidney Dis 1994;24:921–923.
67. Kimmel PL, Peterson RA, Weihs KL, et al. Behavioral compliance with dialysis prescription in hemodialysis patients. J Am Soc Nephrol 1995;5:1826–1834.
68. Sherman RA, Cody RP, Rogers ME, Solanchick JC. The effect of dialyzer reuse on dialysis delivery. Am J Kidney Dis 1994;24:924–926.
69. Wei SS, Ellis PW, Magnusson MO, Paganini EP. Effect of heparin modeling on delivered hemodialysis therapy. Am J Kidney Dis 1994;23:389–393.
70. Morcos AWB, Nissenson AR. Erythropoietin and high-efficiency dialysis, in Bosch JP (ed): Contemporary Issues in Nephrology: Hemodialysis High-Efficiency Treatments, vol 27. New York, Churchill Livingstone, 1993, pp 151–174.
71. Keane WF, Collins AJ. Influence of co-morbidity on mortality and morbidity in patients treated with hemodialysis. Am J Kidney Dis 1994;24:1010–1018.
72. Consensus Development Conference Panel. Morbidity and mortality or renal dialysis: NIH Consensus Conference Statement. Ann Intern Med 1994;121:62–70.
73. Khanna R. Dialysis considerations for diabetic patients. Kidney Int 1993;43(suppl 40):S58–S64.
74. Wizemann V, Timio M, Alpert MA, et al. Options in dialysis therapy: Significance of cardiovascular findings. Kidney Int 1993;43(suppl 40):S85–S91.
75. Ritz E, Deppisch R, Stier E, et al. Atherogenesis and cardiac death: Are they related to dialysis procedure and biocompatibility? Nephrol Dial Transplant 1994;9(suppl 2):165–172.
76. Cheung AK, Wu LL, Kablitz C, et al. Atherogenic lipids and lipoproteins in hemodialysis patients. Am J Kidney Dis 1993;22:271–276.
77. Bregman H, Daugirdas JT, Ing TS. Complications during hemodialysis, in Daugirdas JT, Ing TS (eds): Handbook of Dialysis, 2nd ed. Boston, Little, Brown and Company, 1994, pp 149–168.
78. Rutsky E. Arrhythmias in hemodialysis patients, in Nissenson AR, Fine RN (eds): Dialysis Therapy, 2nd ed. Philadelphia, Hanley & Belfus, 1993, pp 116–123.
79. Kaufman AM, Polaschegg HD, Levin N. Common clinical problems during hemodialysis, in Nissenson AR, Fine RN (eds): Dialysis Therapy, 2nd ed. Philadelphia, Hanley & Belfus, 1993, pp 109–112.
80. Levin NW, Kupin WL, Zasuwa G, Venkat KK. Complications during hemodialysis, in Nissenson AR, Fine RN, Gentile DE (eds): Clinical Dialysis, 2nd ed. Norwalk, CT, Appleton & Lange, 1990, pp 172–201.
81. Gong R, Lindberg J, Abrams J, et al. Comparison of hypertonic saline solutions and dextran in dialysis-induced hypotension. J Am Soc Nephrol 1993;3:1808–1812.
82. Anonomyous. Role of 1-carnitine in treating renal dialysis patients. Dialysis Transplant 1994;23:177–179, 181.
83. Salem M, Ivanovich PT, Ing TS, et al. Adverse effects of dialyzers manifesting during the dialysis session. Nephrol Dial Transplant 1994;9(suppl 2):127–137.
84. Kaufman AM, Godmere RO, Levin NW. Dialyzer reuse, in Daugirdas JT, Ing TS (eds): Handbook of Dialysis, 2nd ed. Boston, Little, Brown and Company, 1994.
85. Lemke HD, Fink E. Accumulation of bradykinine formed by the AN69—or PAN 17DX—membrane is due to the

presence of an ACE-inhibitor in vitro [abstract]. J Am Soc Nephrol 1992;3:376.
86. Henderson LW. Biocompatibility issues in high-efficiency treatments, in Bosch JP (ed): Contemporary Issues in Nephrology: Hemodialysis High-Efficiency Treatments, vol 27. New York, Churchill Livingstone, 1993, pp 225–240.
87. Lazarus JM, Owen WF. Role of biocompatibility in dialysis morbidity and mortality. Am J Kidney Dis 1994;24:1019–1032.
88. Keane WF, Maddy MM. Host defenses and infectious complications in hemodialysis patients, in Maher JF (ed): Replacement of Renal Function by Dialysis, 3rd ed. Norwell, MA, Kluwer Academic Publishers, 1989, pp 840–850.
89. Descamps-Latscha B, Herbelin A. Long-term dialysis and cellular immunity: A critical survey. Kidney Int 1993;43(suppl 41):S135–S142.
90. Arieff AI. Dialysis disequilibrium syndrome: Current concepts on pathogenesis and prevention. Kidney Int 1994;45:629–635.
91. Gejyo F, Homma N, Arakawa M. Long-term complications of dialysis: Pathogenic factors with special reference to amyloidosis. Kidney Int 1993;43(suppl 41):S78–S82.
92. van Ypersele de Strehow C, Floege J, Jadoul M, Koch KM. Amyloidosis and its relationship to different dialyzers. Nephrol Dial Transplant 1994;9(suppl 2):156–161.
93. Fariyike B, Levin NW. Amyloid and β-microglobulin: Metabolism and kinetics, in Bosch JP (ed): Contemporary Issues in Nephrology: Hemodialysis High-Efficiency Treatments, vol 27. New York, Churchill Livingstone, 1993, pp 283–294.
94. Hornberger JC, Chernew M, Peterson J, Garber AM. A multioariate analysis of mortality and hospital admissions with high-flux dialysis. J Am Soc Nephrol 1992;3:1227–1237.
95. Acchiardo S. Dialysis amyloidosis, in Nissenson AR, Fine RN (eds): Dialysis Therapy, 2nd ed. Philadelphia, Hanley & Belfus, 1993, pp 313–315.
96. Moncrief JW, Popovich RP, Nolph KD. The history and current status of continuous ambulatory peritoneal dialysis. Am J Kidney Dis 1990;16:579–584.
97. Twardowski ZJ. Peritoneal catheter development: Currently used catheters—advantages/disadvantages/complications and catheter tunnel morphology in humans. ASAIO Trans 1988;34:937–940.
98. Bailie GR, Eisele G. Continuous ambulatory peritoneal dialysis: A review of its mechanics, advantages, complications, and areas of controversy. Ann Pharmacother 1992;26:1409–1420.
99. Keshaviah P. Urea kinetic and middle molecule approaches to assessing the adequacy of hemodialysis and CAPD. Kidney Int 1993;43(suppl 40):S28–S38.
100. Twardowski ZJ, Nichols WK, Nolph KD, Khanna R. Swan neck presternal peritoneal dialysis catheter. Perit Dial Int 1993;13(suppl 2):S130–S132.
101. Buoncristiani U. Continuous ambulatory peritoneal dialysis connection systems. Perit Dial Int 1993;13(suppl 2):S139–S145.
102. Diaz-Buxo JA, Suki WN. Automated peritoneal dialysis, in Gokal R, Nolph KD (eds): The Textbook of Peritoneal Dialysis. Boston, Kluwer Academic Publishers, 1994, pp 399–418.
103. Gokal R, Mistry CD, Peers E. A United Kingdom multicenter study of icodextrin in continuous ambulatory peritoneal dialysis. Perit Dial Int 1994;14(suppl 2):S22–S27.
104. Holmes CJ. Biocompatibility of peritoneal dialysis solutions [editorial]. Perit Dial Int 1993;13:88–94.
105. Fracasso A, Calo L, Landini S, et al. Peritoneal sclerosis: The role of plasticizers in stimulating interleukin-1 production. Perit Dial Int 1993;13(suppl 2):S517–S519.
106. Piraino B. A review of clinical trials with 2.5 mEq/L calcium dialysate. Perit Dial Int 1993;13(suppl 2):S464–S466.
107. Dasgupta MX, Ward K, Noble PA, et al. Development of bacterial biofilms on silastic catheter materials in peritoneal dialysis fluid. Am J Kidney Dis 1994;23:709–716.
108. Lindholm B, Bergstrom J. Nutritional aspects on peritoneal dialysis. Kidney Int 1992;42(suppl 38):S165–S171.
109. Young GA, Kopple JD, Lindholm B, et al. Nutritional assessment of CAPD patients: An international study. Am J Kidney 1991;17:462–471.
110. Struijk DG, Krediet RT, Koomen GCM, et al. Analysis of factors determining patient survival during CAPD [abstract]. Perit Dial Int 1993;13(suppl 1):S61.
111. Marckmann P. Nutritional status and mortality of patients in regular dialysis therapy. J Intern Med 1989;226:429–432.
112. Bergstrom J, Lindholm B. Nutrition and adequacy of dialysis. How do hemodialysis and CAPD compare? Kidney Int 1993;43(suppl 40):S39–S50.
113. Twardowski ZJ. Clinical value of standardized equilibration tests in CAPD patients. Blood Purif 1989;7:95–108.
114. Arkouche W, Delawari E, Laville M, et al. Which quantity of CAPD for a good clinical outcome? [abstract]. Perit Dial Int 1993;13(suppl 1):S76.
115. Schreiber M, Kawabe M, Cosentino F. KT/V in CAPD and APD [abstract]. J Am Soc Nephrol 1993;4:417.
116. Dumler F, Schmidt R, Cruz C. Abbreviated method for urea kinetic modeling in continuous ambulatory peritoneal dialysis patients. Perit Dial Int 1993;13(suppl 2):S50–S52.
117. Spinowitz B, Gupta B, Kulogowski J, et al. A new dialysate sampling method for determination of dialysis adequacy in CAPD patients [abstract]. J Am Soc Nephrol 1993;4:417.
118. Keshaviah P. Adequacy of CAPD: A quantitative approach. Kidney Int 1992;42(suppl 38):S160–S164.
119. Tzamoloukas AH, Murata GH, Sena P. Assessing the adequacy of peritoneal dialysis. Perit Dial Int 1993;13:236–237.
120. Port FK. Risk of peritonitis and technique failure by CAPD connection technique. A national study. Kidney Int 1992;42:967–974.
121. Holley JL, Bernardini J, Perlmutter JA, Piraino B. A comparison of infection rates among older and younger patients on continuous peritoneal dialysis. Perit Dial Int 1994;14:66–69.
122. Bunke M, Brier ME, Golper TA. CAPD peritonitis with low PD cell counts: Network #9 peritonitis study. [abstract]. Perit Dial Int 1994;14(suppl 1):S26.
123. Keane WF, Everett ED, Golper TA, et al. The Ad Hoc Advisory Committee on Peritonitis Management. Peritoneal dialysis-related peritonitis treatment recommendations: 1993 update. Perit Dial Int 1993;13:14–28.

124. Vas SI. The diagnosis of peritonitis in patients on continuous ambulatory peritoneal dialysis. Sem Dial 1995;8(4):232–237.
125. Zimmerman SW, Ahrens E, Johnson CA, et al. Randomized controlled trial of prophylactic rifampin for peritoneal dialysis-related infections. Am J Kidney Dis 1991;18:225–231.
126. Piraino B, Bernardini J, Lutes R, et al. Randomized trial of mupirocin at exit-site vs oral rifampin to prevent *S. aureus* catheter infections [abstract]. Perit Dial Int 1994;14(suppl 1):S27.
127. Churchill DN, Taylor DW, Vas SI, et al. Peritonitis in CAPD patients: A randomized clinical trial of cotrimoxazole prophylaxis. Perit Dial Int 1988;8:125–128.
128. Poole-Warren LA, Hallett MD, Hone PW, et al. Vaccination for prevention of CAPD associated staphylococcal infection: Results of a prospective multicentre clinical trial. Clin Nephrol 1991;35:198–206.
129. Poole-Warren LA, Farrell PC. The role of vaccination in the prevention of staphylococcal peritonitis in continuous ambulatory peritoneal dialysis. Perit Dial Int 1993;13:176–177.
130. Morse GD, Farolino DF, Apicella MA, Walshe JJ. Comparative study of intraperitoneal and intravenous vancomycin pharmacokinetics during continuous ambulatory peritoneal dialysis. Antimicrob Agents Chemother 1987;31:171–177.
131. Bailie GR, Eisele G, Venezia RA, et al. Prediction of serum vancomycin concentrations following intraperitoneal loading doses in continuous ambulatory peritoneal dialysis patients with peritonitis. Clin Pharmacokinet 1992;22:298–307.
132. Bailie GR, Haqqie SS, Eisele G, et al. Effectiveness of once-weekly vancomycin and once-daily gentamicin, intraperitoneally, for CAPD peritonitis. Perit Dial Int 1995;15(6):269–271.
133. Millikin SP, Matzke GR, Keane WF. Antimicrobial treatment of peritonitis associated with continuous ambulatory peritoneal dialysis. Perit Dial Int 1991;11:252–260.
134. Johnson CA. Intraperitoneal vancomycin administration [editorial]. Perit Dial Int 1991;11:9–11.
135. Vas SI. Single daily dose of aminoglycosides in the treatment of continuous ambulatory peritoneal dialysis peritonitis. Perit Dial Int 1993;13(suppl 2):S355–S356.
136. Bailie GR, Eisele G. Pharmacokinetic issues in the treatment of continuous ambulatory peritoneal dialysis-associated peritonitis. J Antimicrob Chemother 1995;35:563–567.
137. Lye WC, Wong PL, van der Straaten JC, et al. A prospective randomized comparison of single versus multidose gentamicin in the treatment of CAPD peritonitis. Adv Perit Dial 1995;11:179–181.
138. Low CL, Bailie GR, Evans A, Eisele G, Venezia RA. Pharmacokinetics of once-daily intraperitoneal gentamicin in CAPD patients. Unpublished data.
139. Taber TE, Hegeman TF, York SM, et al. Treatment of *Pseudomonas* infections in peritoneal dialysis patients. Perit Dial Int 1991;11:213–216.
140. Nagappan R, Collins JF, Lee WT. Fungal peritonitis in continuous ambulatory peritoneal dialysis—the Auckland experience. Am J Kidney Dis 1992;20:492–496.
141. Cheng IKP, Fang G-X, Chan T-M, et al. Fungal peritonitis complicating peritoneal dialysis: Report of 27 cases and review of treatment. Q J Med 1987;71:407–416.
142. Amici G, Grandesso S, Mottola A, et al. Fungal peritonitis in peritoneal dialysis: critical review of 6 cases [abstract]. Perit Dial Int 1994;14(suppl 1):S91.
143. Chart TN, Chan CY, Cheung SW, et al. Treatment of fungal peritonitis complicating continuous ambulatory peritoneal dialysis with oral fluconazole: A series of 21 patients. Nephrol Dial Transplant 1994;9:539–542.
144. Lomaestro BM, Bailie GR. Quinolone-cation interactions: A review. DICP Ann Pharmacother 1991;25:1249–1259.
145. Kowalsky SF, Echols M, Schwartz MT, et al. Pharmacokinetics of ciprofloxacin in subjects with varying degrees of renal function and undergoing hemodialysis or CAPD. Clin Nephrol 1993;39:53–58.
146. Janknegt R. CAPD peritonitis and fluoroquinolones: A review. Perit Dial Int 1991;11:48, 53–58.
147. Nikolaidis P. Newer quinolones in the treatment of CAPD related infections. Perit Dial Int 1990;10:127–133.
148. Flanagan MJ, Hochstetler LA, Langholdt D, Lim VS. Continuous ambulatory peritoneal dialysis catheter infections: Diagnosis and management. Perit Dial Int 1995;14:248–254.
149. Piraino B. A review of *Staphylococcus aureus* exit-site and tunnel infections in peritoneal dialysis patients. Am J Kidney Dis 1990;16:89–95.
150. Kazmi HR, Raffone FD, Kliger AS, Finkelstein FO. *Pseudomonas* exit-site infections in continuous ambulatory peritoneal dialysis patients. J Am Soc Nephrol 1992;2:1498–1501.
151. Ahlmen J, Schonborg C. Grading of exit-sites cannot predict peritonitis in patients on CAPD. Adv Perit Dial 1991;7:117–119.
152. Luzar MA, Coles GA, Faller B, et al. *Staphylococcus aureus* nasal carriage and infection in patients on continuous ambulatory peritoneal dialysis. N Engl J Med 1990;322:505–509.
153. Herwaldt LA. *Staphylococcus aureus* nasal carriage: Role in continuous ambulatory peritoneal dialysis-associated infections. Perit Dial Int 1993;13(suppl 2):S301–S305.
154. Piraino B, Perlmutter JA, Holley JL, Bernardini J. *Staphylococcus aureus* peritonitis is associated with *Staphylococcus aureus* nasal carriage in peritoneal dialysis patients. Perit Dial Int 1993;13(suppl 2):S332–S334.
155. Hasbargen BJ, Rodgers DJ, Hasbargen JA, et al. Exit site care—is it time for a change? Perit Dial Int 1993;12(suppl 2):S313–S315.
156. O'Brien M, Mason NA. Systemic absorption of intraperitoneal antimicrobials in continuous ambulatory peritoneal dialysis. Clin Pharm 1992;11:246–254.
157. Keller E, Reetze P, Schollmeyer P. Drug therapy in patients undergoing continuous ambulatory peritoneal dialysis. Clinical pharmacokinetic considerations. Clin Pharmacokinet 1990;18:104–117.
158. Lameire N, Belpaire F. Pharmacokinetics of antibiotics against gram-negative infections in continuous ambulatory peritoneal dialysis patients. Perit Dial Int 1993;12(suppl 2):S371–S376.
159. Bailie GR, Kane MP. Stability of drug additives to peritoneal dialysate: A review. Perit Dial Int 1995;15(8):328–325.

160. Gorman T, Eisele G, Bailie GR. Intraperitoneal antibiotics effectively treat non-dialysis-related infections. Perit Dial Int 1995;15:283–284.
161. Chan E, Montgomery PA. Administration of insulin via continuous ambulatory peritoneal dialysis. Pharmacother 1993;13:455–460.
162. Tabata T, Shimada H, Emoto M, et al. Inhibitory effect of heparin and/or antithrombin III on intraperitoneal fibrin formation in continuous ambulatory peritoneal dialysis. Nephron 1990;56:391–395.
163. Salusky IB, Goodman WG, Horst R, et al. Pharmacokinetics of calcitriol in continuous ambulatory and cycling peritoneal dialysis. Am J Kidney Dis 1990;16:126–132.
164. Hercz G, Salusky IB, Norris KC, et al. Aluminum removal by peritoneal dialysis: Intravenous vs intraperitoneal deferoxamine. Kidney Int 1986;30:944–948.
165. Andreoli SP, Cohen M. Intraperitoneal deferoxamine therapy for iron overload in children undergoing CAPD. Kidney Int 1989;35:1330–1335.
166. Galler P, Vigil A, Oliet A, Ortega O, Guijo G. Intraperitoneal erythromycin for diabetic gastroparesis in CAPD. Perit Dial Int 1992;12:265–266.
167. Flynn CT, Chandran PKG, Taylor MJ, Shadur CA. Intraperitoneal lithium administration for bipolar affective disorder in a patient on continuous ambulatory peritoneal dialysis. Int J Artif Organs 1987;10:105–107.
168. Everett ED. Relapsing peritonitis: Augmentation therapy with enzymes. Perit Dial Int 1990;10:9.
169. Nankirell BJ, Lake N, Gillies A. Intracatheter streptokinase for recurrent peritonitis in CAPD. Clin Nephrol 1991;35:20–23.
170. Arfeen S, Goodship THJ, Kirkwood A, Ward MK. The nutritional/metabolic and hormonal effects of 8 weeks of continuous ambulatory peritoneal dialysis with a 1% amino acid solution. Clin Nephrol 1990;33:192–199.
171. Ateshkadi A, Johnson CA, Oxton LL, et al. Pharmacokinetics of intraperitoneal, intravenous, and subcutaneous recombinant human erythropoietin in patients on continuous ambulatory peritoneal dialysis. Am J Kidney Dis 1993;21:635–642.
172. Zachee P. Controversies in selection of Epoetin doses. Drugs 1995;49:536–547.
173. Kopple JD. Effect of nutrition on morbidity and mortality in maintenance dialysis patients. Am J Kidney Dis 1994;24:1002–1009.
174. Spiegel DM, Anderson M, Campbell U, et al. Serum albumin: A marker for morbidity in peritoneal dialysis patients. Am J Kidney Dis 1993;21:26–30.
175. Teehan BP, Schleifer CR, Brown JM, et al. Urea kinetic analysis and clinical outcome on CAPD. A 5-year longitudinal study. Adv Perit Dial 1990;6:181–185.
176. Dabbagh S, Fassinger N, Clement K, Fleischmann LE. The effect of aggressive nutrition on infection rates in patients maintained on peritoneal dialysis. Adv Perit Dial 1991;7:161–164.
177. Park MS, Heimburger O, Bergstrom J, et al. Peritoneal transport during dialysis with amino acid-based solutions. Perit Dial Int 1993;13:280–288.
178. Kurtin P, Nissenson AR. Variation in end-stage renal disease patient outcomes: What we know, what should we know, and how do we find it out? J Am Soc Nephrol 1993;3:1738–1747.
179. Holley JL, Nespor S. An analysis of factors affecting employment of chronic dialysis patients. Am J Kidney Dis 1994;23:681–685.
180. Proceedings from renal rehabilitation and health care reform: Strategies for a changing era. Am J Kidney Dis 1994;24(suppl 1):S1–S32.
181. Hays RD, Kallich JD, Mapes DL, et al. Development of the kidney disease quality of life (KDQOL) instrument. Qual Life Res 1994;3:329–338.
182. Chapman MM, Meyer KB. Assessing health status in a dialysis clinic. Am J Health-Syst Pharm 1995;52(suppl 3):S31–S32.

Chapter 47

Drug-Induced Renal Disease

Mario Zarama, MD, and Paul A. Abraham, MD

Drug-induced renal disease occurs frequently in patients treated with diagnostic and therapeutic agents. The disease can be manifested as alterations or a decline in renal function. In addition, fluid, electrolyte, and acid–base disorders may result (see Chapters 51 and 52). These renal effects occur by many different mechanisms in association with a variety of risk factors.

Drug nephrotoxicity is seen in both the inpatient and outpatient settings and presents differently depending on the drug and clinical setting. Loss of renal function is often reversible on discontinuation of therapy, but may occasionally lead to end-stage renal failure. The ongoing development of more potent and specific drugs provides the potential for more nephropathy by an increasing variety of agents and mechanisms. Analyses of these effects can further our understanding of the mechanisms of renal disease and potentially result in new therapeutic approaches, as demonstrated by the recent application of angiotensin-converting enzyme (ACE) inhibitors to slow the loss of renal function in progressive renal disease.[1,2]

Incidence

Drug toxicity in hospitalized patients is a frequent adverse event with nephrotoxicity accounting for nearly 7% of all drug toxicity.[3] Drug nephrotoxicity was identified in one analysis as the cause of one-fifth of all cases of hospital-acquired acute renal failure, with a mortality of 8%.[4] Aminoglycosides, radiographic contrast media, and cisplatin were most commonly implicated.[4] In a more recent analysis, drugs contributed to 29% of all acute renal failure in hospitalized patients with antibiotics (aminoglycosides, pentamidine, and a cephalosporin), nonsteroidal anti-inflammatory drugs (NSAIDs), ACE inhibitors, and diuretics most commonly implicated.[5] The introduction of newer NSAIDs, antihypertensives, and antibiotics and their changed usage, coupled with the decline in use of aminoglycosides, has changed the spectrum of commonly implicated drugs.[6] In particular, NSAIDs and ACE inhibitors, used alone or in combination, are more predominant.[6,7]

The incidence and characteristics of drug nephropathy in the ambulatory care setting are less well understood, particularly since mild toxicity is often unrecognized and only more severe reactions requiring hospital care may be reported. As many as 3–6% of hospital admissions have been attributed to adverse drug effects.[8] The pharmacoepidemiology of these effects has become more important as care increasingly shifts to the outpatient setting with the potential use of more toxic agents in these patients. ACE inhibitors have contributed to transient acute renal failure.[9] Similarly, over-the-counter (OTC) availability of ibuprofen has contributed to cases of acute renal failure, but overall safety has been favorable in comparison to alternative analgesics.[10] This experience has resulted in recent approval of naproxen for OTC use in the United States. Other agents, particularly combination analgesics and cyclosporin, have resulted in end-stage renal failure during chronic outpatient use. Fortunately, with these agents early recognition of renal dysfunction and discontinuation of therapy may allow stabilization or recovery of renal function.

Risk Factors

Drug nephrotoxicity develops as a result of such a wide range of mechanisms, from idiosyncratic hypersensitivity reactions to direct cumulative toxicity, and spans the full spectrum of age, from the newborn[11] to the very elderly, that no generalizable risk factors are applicable to all drug classes and patient situations. An exception is hemodynamically mediated acute renal failure due to NSAIDs and ACE inhibitors. Their toxicity is frequently preventable by recognizing risk factors including preexisting renal insufficiency and decreased effective renal blood flow from volume depletion, heart failure, or liver disease. The elderly arthritic patient with hypertension or heart failure may be especially sensitive to the combined use of ACE inhibitors and NSAIDs.[7]

Recognition and Assessment of Renal Toxicity

The onset of acute renal failure associated with drug use in hospitalized acutely ill patients is most often recognized quickly by routine laboratory monitoring of serum creatinine or blood urea nitrogen (BUN) concentrations. Decreased urine output may also be the initial sign of toxicity, particularly with radiographic contrast media, NSAIDs, and ACE inhibitors. In the outpatient setting, nephrotoxicity is often recognized only with advanced renal dysfunction causing symptoms of uremia (malaise, anorexia, and vomiting) or volume overload (shortness of breath or edema). Serum creatinine or BUN concentrations identify the renal insult, whereas a urine collection for creatinine clearance quantifies the loss of glomerular filtration.

Nephrotoxity may also selectively alter renal tubular function, particularly early in toxicity, without loss of glomerular filtration. In these cases, indicators of proximal tubular injury include metabolic acidosis with bicarbonaturia, glycosuria in the absence of hyperglycemia, and hypophosphatemia and hypouricemia due to increased urinary losses of phosphorus and uric acid. Indicators of distal tubular injury include polyuria from failure to maximally concentrate urine, metabolic acidosis from impaired urinary acidification, and hyperkalemia from impaired potassium excretion. Urinary excretion of enzymes and low molecular weight proteins, including N-acetyl-β-D-glucosaminidase[12] and β_2 microglobulin,[13] respectively, have been used to detect early tubular injury, particularly during aminoglycoside therapy. However, these indicators have been too sensitive to be useful clinically since drug administration can increase their excretion without causing clinically important toxicity.

Classification of Drug-Induced Renal Disease

Drug nephropathy is highly heterogeneous with respect to the drugs involved and lesions produced. No system of classification has been satisfactory. For the student, classification based on mechanisms of toxicity is preferred but has been inadequate due to insufficient knowledge. Alternative classifications used include presenting the renal manifestations (e.g., acute or chronic renal failure, hematuria, pyuria, or proteinuria) to facilitate clinical diagnosis of nephrotoxicity; indexing of drugs by their therapeutic use and the various types of nephropathies they may produce (Table 47.1) to facilitate use as a reference; and finally by the renal structural and functional alterations they induce (Table 47.2) to emphasize current knowledge of mechanisms of drug nephrotoxicity. The latter classification is used in this discussion.

Overview of Mechanisms for Renal Susceptibility to Drug Toxicity

The kidneys appear more sensitive than other organs to drug toxicity. Both immunologic and nonimmunologic mechanisms appear to contribute. Immune-mediated drug nephropathies include glomerulonephritides and allergic interstitial nephritis, either with or without the nephrotic syndrome. Mechanisms for immune susceptibility are not clear, but could include the large vascular surface area with exposure to circulating immune mediators as well as an intrinsic immune function of glomerular mesangial cells and renal cytokine activation.[14–16] Nonimmunologic mechanisms of drug nephropathy relate to several specialized characteristics of normal renal physiology (Fig. 47.1).

HIGH BLOOD FLOW AND SPECIALIZED HEMODYNAMICS

While the kidneys constitute only 0.4% of body weight, they receive 20–25% of resting cardiac output, enhancing exposure to circulating drugs. Within the kidney, blood flow is distributed to superficial and deep nephron populations as well as the medulla and the papillae. Within each nephron unit, blood flow and pressure are regulated between glomerular afferent and efferent arterioles to maintain capillary hydrostatic pressure and glomerular filtration. This specialized blood flow is precisely regulated by mechanisms including interrelations between renal prostaglandins, vasoactive peptides, the sympathetic nervous system, the endocrine and autocrine renin-angiotensin systems, and the macula densa response to distal tubular solute delivery. In this unique vascular setting, beta blockers may reduce total renal blood flow,[17] radiographic contrast media may shunt intrarenal blood flow away from superficial nephrons,[18] mannitol osmotic diuresis may reduce glomerular blood flow due to tubuloglomerular feedback,[19] and ACE inhibitors may dilate glomerular efferent arterioles leading to a decrease in glomerular filtration pressure in the presence of ischemic renal vascular disease.[1]

TUBULAR EPITHELIAL CELL ABSORPTIVE AND SECRETORY FUNCTIONS

Drugs or their metabolites can accumulate in renal tubular epithelial cells, particularly in the proximal tubule, by active tubular transport processes involving secretion and absorption of organic acids and bases. This process can be prevented by inhibitors of tubular transport such as probenecid. They may also accumulate passively through lipid permeability. Toxic drugs or metabolites that accu-

TABLE 47.1. CLASSIFICATION OF NEPHROTOXIC DRUGS BY THEIR THERAPEUTIC USE

Cardiovascular
Angiotensin-converting enzyme inhibitors (H)
Calcium channel blockers (H)
Captopril (G, H,[a] I)
Hydralazine (G)
Mannitol (T, H)
Methyldopa (I)
Propranolol (H)
Thiazide and loop diuretics (I)
Triamterene (H, I, N[a])
Thromboclytics (V)
Warfarin sodium (I, V)
Antimicrobial
Acyclovir (O)
Aminoglycosides (T,[a] I)
Amphotericin B (T)
Aztreonam (I)
Cephalosporins (I,[a] T)
Ciprofloxacin (I)
Erythromycin (I)
Penicillins (I)
Pentamidine (T)
Rifampin (I,[a] G)
Sulfadiazine (O)
Sulfonamides (I,[a] O)
Tetracyclines (P, T, I)
Trimethoprim (P)
Vancomycin (I)
Rheumatologic
Acetaminophen (T, PN)
Acetylsalicylic acid (H)
Allopurinol (I,[a] N)
d-Penicillamine (G)
Nonsteroidal anti-inflammatory drugs (G, H,[a] I, T, PN)
Gold (G,[a] I)
Neuropsychiatric
Amoxapine (T)
Carbamazepine (I)
Lithium (G, I)
Phenobarbital (I)
Phenytoin (I)
Valproic acid (I)
Gastrointestinal
Cimetidine (I, P[a])
Magnesium antacids (N)
Phosphate enemas (O)
Ranitidine (I)
Vasopressin (O)
Cancer Chemotherapy
Carboplatinum (T)
Cisplatin (T,[a] V)
Interleukin 2
Methotrexate (O)
Mithramycin (T)
Mitomycin C (V)
Nitrosoureas (methyl CCNU) (I)
Streptozotocin (T)
Immunosuppressive
Corticosteroids (P)
Cyclosporine (H,[a] I,[a] T, V)
FK-506 (H, I)
Leukocyte A interferon (G, I)
OKT3 (H)
Drugs of Abuse
Amphetamine (V)
Cocaine (O)
Heroin (G, O)
Phencyclidine (O)
Miscellaneous
Ascorbic acid (O)
Glyburide (I)
Lovastatin (O)
Methoxyflurane anesthesia (T, O)
Radiographic contrast agents (H, T)

Key: I, interstitial nephritis; H, hemodynamically mediated; N, nephrolithiasis; G, glomerulopathy; T, tubular necrosis; O, intratubular obstruction; P, pseudo renal failure; V, vasculopathy; PN, papillary necrosis.
[a]Most common of multiple mechanisms.

mulate intracellularly may cause cell injury by mechanisms including impairment of mitochondrial function and decreased adenosine triphosphate (ATP) synthesis, increased oxidative stress, depletion of reduced glutathione and other antioxidants, inhibition of phospholipid metabolism, and disruption of protein synthesis. Intracellular accumulation of nephrotoxic agents is a lesser mechanism in immature animals with undeveloped tubular transport mechanisms. Aminoglycosides and cyclosporin are agents that appear to mediate nephrotoxicity through intracellular accumulation.[20,21]

TABLE 47.2. DRUG-INDUCED RENAL STRUCTURAL–FUNCTIONAL ALTERATIONS

Pseudo renal failure	Interstitial nephritis
Hemodynamically mediated renal failure	Acute allergic
Vascular alterations	Chronic
Glomerulopathy	Papillary necrosis
Nephrotic syndrome	Obstructive nephropathy
Glomerulonephritis	Intratubular
Tubular necrosis	Lower urinary tract
	Nephrolithiasis

DRUG METABOLISM TO TOXIC SPECIES

Multiple renal enzymes contribute to drug metabolism. These include cytochrome P-450 and mixed function oxidases with activity in proximal tubular epithelial cells similar to activity in the liver. In contrast, prostaglandin endoperoxide synthetase activity is more localized to the renal papilla and medulla. The kidney may thus transform a

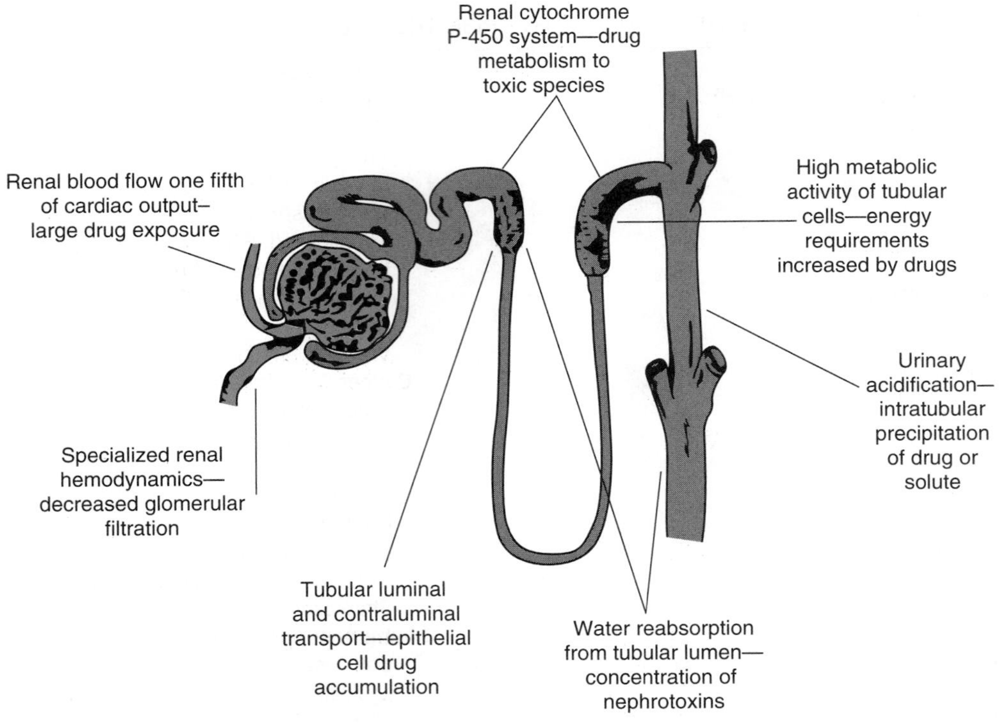

Figure 47.1. Mechanisms of renal susceptibility to drug toxicity. See text for discussion. CRF, chronic renal failure.

drug to an inactive or active metabolite, which may be nephrotoxic. As an example, acetaminophen can be oxidized to reactive species that contribute to acute tubular necrosis following acute acetaminophen overdose and likely contribute to analgesic nephropathy with chronic consumption.[20–22]

HIGH ENERGY REQUIREMENT BY RENAL TUBULAR CELLS

Renal tubular epithelial cells have high energy requirements that are necessary for active tubular transport and ongoing metabolic processes. Of relevance to nephrotoxicity, these energy needs are precariously supplied to medullary tubular epithelial cells, which function in a state of chronic hypoxia due to their perfusion with venous blood returning from the deep medulla. As a consequence these medullary tubular epithelial cells are especially sensitive to drugs, which accentuate this hypoxia by increasing energy demands or by decreasing energy production or oxygen delivery. An example is amphotericin B-induced medullary tubular cell damage, which appears to result from an imbalance between increased cellular energy requirements and inadequate oxygen delivery.[20,21,23]

CONCENTRATION OF SOLUTE IN THE TUBULAR LUMEN

Ninety-nine percent of the water filtered by the glomerulus is reabsorbed. Normally, 50–85% of water reabsorption occurs in the proximal tubule while the remainder occurs in the descending loop of Henle and collecting duct. Systemic volume depletion increases the percent of water reabsorption in the proximal tubule. As water reabsorption increases, the rate of tubular flow decreases and the concentration of solutes and toxins increases within the tubular lumen. Thus, the lumenal surfaces of cells, particularly in the proximal tubule, can be exposed to higher concentrations of potential toxins and for a longer time than most other tissues in the body. This enhances binding of drugs to tubular epithelial cells and promotes active and passive transport into cells. The enhancement of aminoglycoside nephrotoxicity by systemic volume depletion is an example.[24]

URINE ACIDIFICATION

Urine pH decreases to approximately 4.5 during maximal stimulation of renal tubular hydrogen ion secretion. Certain solutes can precipitate and obstruct the tubular lumen at this acid pH, particularly when urine is concentrated. Thus, a maximally acid urine can contribute to acute uric acid nephropathy as a potential complication of chemotherapy-induced tumor lysis.[25]

INCREASED FUNCTION OF INDIVIDUAL NEPHRONS IN ADAPTATION TO CHRONIC RENAL INSUFFICIENCY

Chronic renal insufficiency is associated with injury to some glomerular and tubular units while others remain relatively intact. The remaining functional nephron units have hyperfiltering glomeruli and hyperfunctioning tubules, which compensate for the loss of other nephrons. These residual nephrons are more susceptible to nephrotoxic injury due to their increased workload and accentuation of the previously described physiologic mechanisms. The nephrotoxicity of radiographic contrast media in patients with chronic renal insufficiency is such an example.[26]

PRINCIPLES FOR PREVENTION OF DRUG NEPHROPATHY

The basic principle for prevention of drug-induced renal disease is to avoid the use of potentially nephrotoxic agents in patients at increased risk for toxicity. However, when exposure to these drugs cannot be avoided, specific techniques may be used to reduce potential nephrotoxicity (Table 47.3).

Certain approaches to reduce drug toxicity are prudent and generally effective. These include careful and adequate hydration to establish high renal tubular flow rates and thereby permit more aggressive drug administration to maximize efficacy while minimizing toxicity. However, other measures to reduce drug toxicity are still theoretical and investigational. Thus, administration of oral prostaglandin analogues may reduce NSAID toxicity,[27] while calcium channel blockers reduce amphotericin B toxicity in animals.[28]

DRUG-INDUCED RENAL STRUCTURAL–FUNCTIONAL ALTERATIONS

Specific drug-induced renal structural–functional alterations constitute the remainder of this discussion under the eight broad headings listed in Table 47.2. The general orientation of these topics is from the systemic, hemodynamic, and renal vascular effects on renal function, through the glomerulus, the filtering surface of the kidney vasculature, into the renal tubules and surrounding interstitial support tissue of the kidney and finally into the urinary collecting system of the kidney and lower urinary tract. Mechanisms of nephrotoxicity will be emphasized in addition to clinical findings, prevention, and management.

PSEUDO RENAL FAILURE

BUN or creatinine concentrations may increase during drug therapy without a decrease in the glomerular filtration rate. This "pseudo" renal failure is most common during therapy with corticosteroids or tetracyclines, drugs that increase protein catabolism. These drugs can increase the BUN level while the serum creatinine concentration remains unchanged. The glomerular filtration rate is accurately indicated by the serum creatinine concentration or creatinine clearance.

Alternatively, pseudo renal failure may be characterized by a rise in the serum creatinine concentration while the BUN concentration remains unchanged. This can occur during trimethoprim, pyrimethamine, or cimetidine therapy because these drugs competitively inhibit proximal tubular creatinine secretion into the tubular lumen.[29,30] This effect is minimal in patients with normal renal function in whom the serum creatinine concentration usually remains in the normal range.[31] In contrast, in renal-insufficient patients, the rise in serum creatinine is greater since tubular secretion of creatinine contributes a proportionately greater amount to urinary creatinine excretion.[32] Ranitidine and other H_2-receptor antagonists that are more potent than cimetidine on a molar basis and therefore have a lower molar concentration in the blood are less likely to raise the serum creatinine concentration.[31] Competitive inhibition of creatinine secretion has been considered clinically useful in the evaluation of renal function. Thus, administration of large doses of cimetidine during urine collections gives a measure of creatinine clearance that closely approximates the true glomerular filtration rate.[33,34]

Pseudo renal failure also occurs with several drugs (see Table 47.4), particularly cefoxitin and other cephalosporin antibiotics, which can increase the serum creatinine concentration by direct interference with the enzymatic measurement of creatinine by the Jaffe method.[29] This effect is most pronounced in patients with decreased renal function. These drugs that directly interfere with creatinine measurement and increase serum creatinine concentrations also alter the creatinine clearance so it does not reflect the glomerular filtration rate. In this setting, renal function can only be determined accurately by nonenzymatic determination of creatinine concentration, inulin clearance, or another non-creatinine measure of renal function.

HEMODYNAMICALLY MEDIATED RENAL FAILURE

Reduced Glomerular Capillary Hydrostatic Pressure

Experience with ACE inhibitors has uncovered a new mechanism of hemodynamically mediated nephropathy caused by inhibition of the renin-angiotensin system (RAS) within the kidney. The RAS can operate as both an endocrine (circulating) and an autocrine/paracrine (tissue)

TABLE 47.3. MECHANISMS AND PRINCIPLES FOR PREVENTION OF DRUG NEPHROPATHY

Mechanisms of Renal Susceptibility	Principles for Prevention	Example
A. Large drug exposure due to high renal blood flow	1. Avoid systemic drug administration	1. Intraperitoneal administration of cisplatin for localized intraperitoneal tumor[95]
	2. Limit total drug dose	2. Monitor aminoglycoside levels to maintain in therapeutic range[120]; substitute nontoxic antibiotic based on microbial sensitivities
B. Specialized renal hemodynamics regulated by vasoactive substances	Avoid drugs that inhibit prostaglandin synthesis	Substitute acetaminophen or nonacetylated salicylates and sulindac for other NSAIDs[49]
C. Tubular epithelial cell drug accumulation due to luminal and contraluminal transport	1. Inhibit drug absorption from the luminal membrane	1. Hydration with chloride anions during cisplatin therapy[95]; calcium supplementation during aminoglycoside therapy[120]
	2. Inhibit drug absorption from the contraluminal membrane	2. Cilastatin inhibition of imipenem toxicity[230]
D. Renal metabolism of drugs to toxic species	Use drugs with nontoxic renal metabolites	Renal metabolism of active sulindac sulfide to inactive sulindac sulfoxide[53]
E. Cellular dysfunction due to drug-induced increased energy requirements	Decrease cell energy needs by reducing cell membrane transport activity	Furosemide use during amphotericin therapy to reduce ischemia and toxicity to the medullary thick ascending loop of Henle[23]
F. Water reabsorption and concentration of nephrotoxins within the tubular lumen promoting increased epithelial cell membrane contact and transport into cells	1. Prevent dehydration	1. NaCl repletion to prevent amphotericin toxicity[156]
	2. Use of osmotic diuresis to increase luminal water concentration and tubular flow rate	2. Possible reduction of contrast nephropathy by mannitol diuresis[134]
G. Urinary acidification with intratubular precipitation of drug or solute	Alkalinize urine	Urinary alkalinization to prevent uric acid and methotrexate nephropathy[206]
H. In chronic renal failure, increased toxin exposure per residual viable nephron due to nephron hyperfunction	Avoid drug use or reduce drug dose in renal failure patients	Choose alternatives to radiographic contrast agents for renal imaging: ultrasonography, computerized tomography without contrast use, radionuclide studies, magnetic resonance imaging

system. The endocrine RAS is involved with acute circulatory homeostasis, whereas the tissue RAS participates in the tonic regulation of cardiovascular function and structure.[35] In the kidney these components of the RAS have hemodynamic and nonhemodynamic effects that help balance glomerular afferent and efferent arteriolar pressures to maintain the glomerular filtration rate, influence renal tubular sodium reabsorption, regulate renal sympathetic nervous system activity, modify mesangial cell function, promote growth, and maintain endothelial cell function.[36]

TABLE 47.4. DRUGS THAT INTERFERE WITH THE JAFFE MEASUREMENT OF CREATININE AND CAN FALSELY INCREASE THE SERUM CREATININE CONCENTRATION

Cefoxitin
Cephalothin
Cefazolin
Cefotaxime
Flucytosine
Methyldopa

ACE inhibitor therapy can acutely deteriorate the glomerular filtration rate of kidneys perfused by stenotic renal arteries.[1] This reverses on discontinuation of therapy. The rise in serum creatinine is usually minimal if only one renal artery is stenotic. However, patients with bilateral renal artery stenosis or a single kidney with renovascular disease are at significant risk to develop severe renal failure. The diagnosis can be suspected by a rise in the serum creatinine concentration as well as reversible alterations in the radionuclide renogram of the involved kidney.[1,37] ACE inhibitor nephropathy may also occur in the absence of renal artery stenosis when renal blood flow is reduced by a systemic disease, such as congestive heart failure, or an intrarenal vascular process, such as small vessel afferent arteriolar narrowing due to severe hypertension. Of interest, the fetal kidney is also sensitive to ACE inhibitors and anuria has been observed in the newborn following maternal ACE inhibitor therapy late in pregnancy.[11]

The pathogenesis of ACE inhibitor nephropathy is a decrease in glomerular capillary hydrostatic pressure sufficient to reduce glomerular ultrafiltration[1] (Fig. 47.2). This occurs in settings where glomerular afferent arteriolar blood flow is reduced and the efferent arteriole is vasoconstricted by angiotensin II to maintain glomerular capillary hydrostatic pressure for ultrafiltration. ACE inhibitor therapy reduces angiotensin II production, thereby dilating the efferent arteriole, reducing glomerular capillary hydrostatic pressure, and decreasing glomerular ultrafiltration. Renal function must be monitored carefully during initiation of ACE inhibitor therapy in conditions where glomerular filtration pressure is dependent on the presence of angiotensin II through the RAS.

The pathophysiologic principles of ACE inhibitor nephropathy have now been extensively investigated and applied to diagnostic and therapeutic benefits. Diagnostically, the captopril renogram is now the most sensitive and specific screening test for the diagnosis of renovascular hypertension.[1,37] This test involves radionuclide imaging of the kidneys before and after a single dose of captopril. In the presence of hemodynamically significant renal artery stenosis, the involved kidney will show a reversible decrease in function after captopril compared to without captopril. This functional renal insufficiency induced by captopril is highly sensitive and specific for renal artery stenosis that may benefit by treatment. Therapeutically, captopril in a dose of 25 mg three times daily has received FDA approval to reduce proteinuria and slow the progressive deterioration of renal function in patients with diabetic nephropathy.[2]

Inhibition of Prostaglandin-Dependent Renal Blood Flow

NSAIDs inhibit cyclooxygenase and can impair renal function by decreasing synthesis of vasodilatory prostaglandins from arachidonic acid. Renal prostaglandins are synthesized in the renal cortex and medulla by vascular endothelial and glomerular mesangial cells. Their effects are primarily local renal vasodilation (particularly prostacyclin and PGE_2). They have limited activity in states of normal renal blood flow, but in states of decreased renal blood flow their synthesis is increased and they protect against renal ischemia and hypoxia by antagonizing renal vasoconstriction due to angiotensin II, norepinephrine, endothelin, and vasopressin.[38,39] Administration of NSAIDs in the setting of renal ischemia and compensatory increased prostaglandin

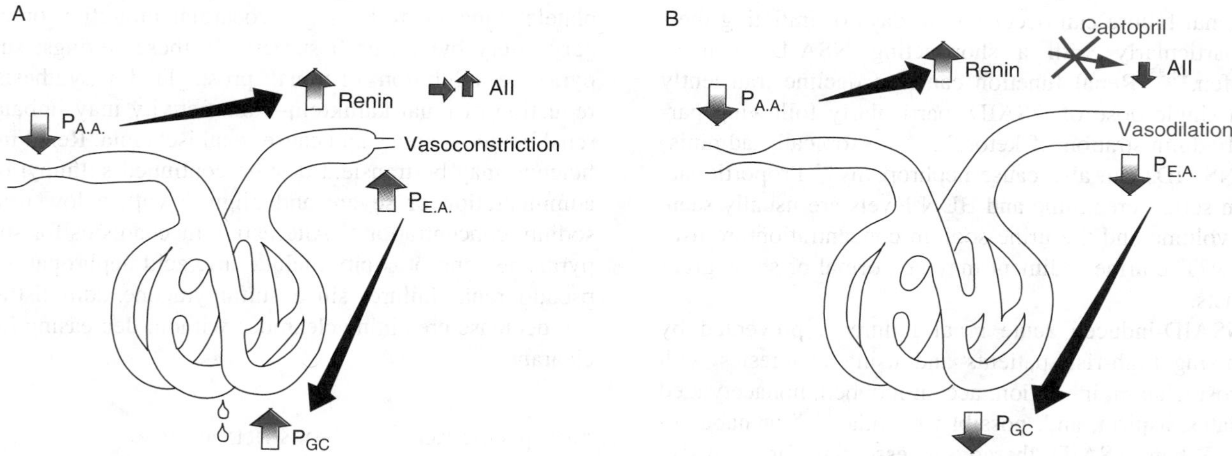

Figure 47.2. ACE inhibitor nephropathy occurs in the setting of reduced blood flow (involving large or small artery) to the glomerulus. In this setting (A), pressure in the afferent arterioles (P_{AA}) is reduced, causing the juxtaglomerular apparatus to increase renin secretion. Increased plasma renin activity converts angiotensinogen to angiotensin I, which is converted to angiotensin II (AII) by angiotensin-converting enzyme. Increased angiotensin II constricts the efferent arteriole increasing pressure in the efferent arteriole (P_{EA}) and thereby increases hydrostatic pressure in the glomerular capillaries (P_{GC}) to maintain glomerular filtration. When ACE inhibitor (captopril) therapy is initiated (B) the synthesis of angiotensin II is decreased, thereby dilating the efferent arteriole. This reduces outflow resistance from the glomerulus and decreases hydrostatic pressure in the glomerular capillaries which alters Starling's forces across the glomerular capillaries to decrease glomerular filtration. P_{AA}, afferent arteriole pressure; P_{EA}, efferent arteriole pressure; P_{GC}, glomerular capillary pressure; AII, angiotensin II.

activity may thus alter the balance of activity between renal vasoconstrictors and vasodilators. This leaves the activity of renal vasoconstrictors unopposed and promotes renal ischemia with loss of glomerular filtration. This hemodynamically mediated acute renal failure is the most common adverse renal effect of NSAIDs, but other renal effects can occur (Table 47.1).[38,39]

NSAIDs have an overall favorable safety profile resulting in OTC availability of ibuprofen and naproxen for short-term therapy. While the potential for adverse renal effects from OTC NSAIDs has been a concern,[10] activity of vasodilatory prostaglandins is not necessary to maintain renal function in the absence of renal ischemia or excess renal vasoconstrictor activity. NSAIDs are therefore unlikely to impair renal function in patients with normal kidneys. However, NSAIDs have been reported to cause small reductions in glomerular filtration rate even in normal subjects, as shown during short[40] and sustained[41] indomethacin therapy.

Persons at greatest risk for NSAID nephropathy generally have preexisting renal insufficiency, medical problems associated with high plasma renin activity (hepatic disease with ascites, decompensated congestive heart failure, or intravascular volume depletion), or systemic lupus erythematosus.[38,39] Additional risk factors continue to be clarified for otherwise healthy patients, but include age over 60 years, atherosclerotic cardiovascular disease, and diuretic therapy.[38,39,42] Combined NSAID and ACE inhibitor or cyclosporine therapy is also reason for concern.[7,39,43] Fetal and newborn kidneys also appear sensitive to the effects of NSAIDs administered late in pregnancy to prevent premature labor or shortly after birth to close a patent ductus arteriosus.[11]

Renal failure can occur within days of initiating therapy, particularly with a short-acting NSAID such as ibuprofen.[44,45] Renal function can also decline transiently after a single dose of NSAID, particularly following parenteral administration of ketorolac.[46,47] Topically administered NSAIDs can also cause nephropathy.[48] Proportionate rises in serum creatinine and BUN levels are usually seen. Urine volume and the urine sodium concentration are usually low. The urine sediment may be normal or show granular casts.

NSAID-induced acute renal failure is prevented by recognizing high-risk patients and using analgesics with less prostaglandin inhibition: acetaminophen, nonacetylated salicylates, aspirin, and, possibly, sulindac[49,50] or nabumetone.[51] When NSAID therapy is essential for high-risk patients, management of predisposing medical problems should be optimized and renal function monitored from the initial days of therapy. The use and pharmacology of sulindac is of particular interest in high-risk patients since it is a potent NSAID that may have lesser effects on renal prostaglandin synthesis and function.[39,50,52] The mechanism of renal prostaglandin sparing is unclear, but may involve intrarenal metabolism of the active drug, sulindac sulfide, by cytochrome P-450-dependent mixed-function oxidases to an inactive metabolite, sulindac sulfoxide.[53] However, this favorable effect of sulindac has not been consistently observed, especially at higher therapeutic doses, in patients with hepatic disease, or during prolonged therapy.[6,39,45,54] Finally, the oral prostaglandin E analogue, misoprostol, may be useful to prevent NSAID nephropathy.[27] Future NSAIDs, possibly including nabumetome,[51] may selectively inhibit an isozyme of prostaglandin synthase mediating tissue inflammation while maintaining activity of an isozyme for prostaglandin synthase in the kidney.[55]

Acute renal failure due to NSAIDs is treated by discontinuation of therapy and supportive care. Renal failure may be severe, but recovery is usually rapid and dialysis is rarely necessary. Occasionally the hemodynamic insult is sufficiently severe to cause frank tubular necrosis, which can prolong recovery. The differential diagnosis of NSAID hemodynamically mediated acute renal failure must include NSAID-induced acute interstitial nephritis, with or without the nephrotic syndrome, since steroid therapy may benefit this lesion.[56]

The renal hemodynamic effects of NSAIDs have been applied therapeutically to reduce proteinuria in patients with nephrotic syndrome.[57] The efficacy of various NSAIDs for this purpose is directly proportional to their ability to inhibit renal prostaglandin synthesis. Renal function declines, but the decrease in proteinuria is proportionately greater than the decline in renal function.

Sulfinpyrazone, a uricosuric congener of phenylbutazone, can also cause hemodynamically mediated acute renal failure.[58] Sulfinpyrazone has been used to impair platelet function following myocardial infarction or coronary artery bypass graft surgery. In these settings, sulfinpyrazone inhibition of renal prostaglandin synthesis or reduction of renal kallikrein–kinin activity may imbalance renal hemodynamics and cause renal ischemia. Renal insufficiency may be transient despite continued sulfinpyrazone administration or severe and oliguric with a low urinary sodium concentration.[58] Alternative mechanisms for sulfinpyrazone nephrotoxicity include uric acid nephropathy and pseudo renal failure, since sulfinpyrazone administration can decrease creatinine clearance without decreasing inulin clearance.[59]

Nonspecific Renal Vasoconstriction

Triamterene, a potassium-sparing diuretic, has been associated with transient decreases in creatinine clearance and abnormal urinary sediment in normal subjects and hypertensive patients.[60] In combination with hydrochlorothiazide, triamterene has caused reversible acute renal failure in elderly patients. In combination with indomethacin, triamterene has induced acute renal failure in normal subjects and patients at risk for NSAID nephropathy. A hemodynamic mechanism is most likely as suggested by the apparent increased risk for nephrotoxicity during combined triamterene and indomethacin therapy. Presumably, triamterene causes renal vasoconstriction that is counterbalanced by increased renal synthesis of vasodilatory prostaglandins. Concomitant NSAID therapy may induce renal ischemia by preventing the compensatory increase in renal prostaglandin synthesis. The implications of these observations are unclear because triamterene and NSAIDs are frequently used together without apparent nephrotoxicity.

Propranolol, a nonselective β-adrenergic receptor blocker, reduces renal blood flow 10–20% in hypertensive patients.[17] The glomerular filtration rate is less consistently reduced.[17] In contrast, nadolol, another nonselective β blocker, increases renal blood flow while other β blockers do not appear to alter renal hemodynamics.[61] The mechanism of the propranolol-induced decrease in renal blood flow is unknown. Since renal function does not decrease with other β blockers the effect is unlikely to result from blockade of β receptors or decreased cardiac output. Other postulated mechanisms include renal vasoconstriction due to unopposed alpha-adrenergic activity or inhibition of renal vasodilator activity, possibly mediated by the kallikrein–kinin system.[17] The clinical significance of these effects is unknown. However, it may be prudent to avoid propranolol therapy in patients with renal insufficiency.

Cyclosporine, a potent lipophilic immunosuppressive agent, has dramatically enhanced the survival of transplanted organs, including kidneys.[62] The mechanism of action is predominantly inhibition of lymphokine production by T lymphocytes. Acute hemodynamically mediated renal failure is the predominant adverse renal effect early in therapy. This can lead to interstitial fibrosis and progress to chronic failure.[62,63] The pathophysiology of cyclosporine nephrotoxicity has been difficult to assess in renal transplant patients because of changes due to concomitant graft rejection. Adverse renal effects have been quantified best in heart and liver transplant patients,[64–66] where up to 10% of patients progressed to chronic renal failure using higher dose regimens. Variable severity of nephrotoxicity developed in 21–25% of patients during immunosuppression for autoimmune diseases such as rheumatoid arthritis, uveitis, psoriasis, and diabetes mellitus despite lower cyclosporine doses.[67–69] Risk factors included increased age and higher initial cyclosporine doses.

Historically, renal function deteriorated acutely, and usually reversibly, in approximately 80% of transplant patients during the first 6 months of cyclosporine therapy. This high incidence of acute renal insufficiency with potential progression to chronic nephropathy has decreased with the advent of lower dose therapy,[66,70] but concern remains for a dose-dependent decline in the glomerular filtration rate, which may not progress to chronic renal failure.[62–64,66] Decreased renal function may occur within days of initiating therapy and may be accentuated by concurrent illness, including renal graft rejection, hypotension, infection, and therapy with other nephrotoxic drugs such as aminoglycosides, amphotericin B, acyclovir, NSAIDs, and radiocontrast agents, as well as drugs that inhibit cyclosporine hepatic metabolism.[62] Clinically, no consistent urine sediment abnormalities are seen. Urinary enzyme excretions are not reliable indicators of cyclosporine nephrotoxicity. Hypertension, hyperkalemia, sodium avidity, and hypomagnesemia may occur. Renal biopsy distinguishes cyclosporine nephrotoxicity from acute renal allograft rejection[62] and reveals thickening of arterioles, mild focal glomerular sclerosis, proximal tubular epithelial cell vacuolization and atrophy, and progressive interstitial fibrosis.[63] This contrasts with the cellular interstitial infiltrate seen in acute transplant rejection. However, renal biopsy may not distinguish chronic cyclosporine toxicity from chronic rejection.

A hemodynamic pathogenesis is suggested for cyclosporine nephrotoxicity during the initial months of therapy by the usually rapid improvement of renal function following dose reduction. Reversible vasoconstriction and injury to preglomerular arterioles may be involved as a consequence of decreased prostacyclin synthesis or, more likely, increased thromboxane synthesis,[62,63] possibly potentiated by increased endothelin vasoconstrictor activity.[71] Activity of the endothelial vasodilator, nitric oxide, may also be diminished.[72] Neither activation of the sympathetic nervous system nor the systemic renin–angiotensin system appears to contribute to human toxicity.[62,63] Functional evidence for vasoconstrictor-mediated renal failure by cyclosporine is supported by improved renal blood flow, glomerular filtration rate, and fractional excretion of sodium during infusion of renal vasodilatory doses of dopamine.[73] Direct proximal tubule damage by cyclosporine may add to hemodynamic effects.[63]

Therapy is limited to dose reduction and treatment of concomitant illness. Renal function usually recovers after dose reduction or discontinuation of cyclosporine.[62,63] Since irreversible chronic renal failure can occur with prolonged use,[64] (see section on Chronic Interstitial Nephritis) the benefits of short- and long-term therapy continue to be compared.[74] Most favor continued long-term therapy. Therefore, prevention of cyclosporine nephrotoxicity continues to be an important objective. Since toxicity appears to be dose related, measuring drug concentrations, pharmacokinetics including the area under the curve, and pharmacodynamic evaluations have been used to reduce toxicity.[75–77] However, neither therapeutic nor low cyclosporine levels can exclude a diagnosis of cyclosporine nephrotoxicity.[62] Lower dose cyclosporine therapy in various combinations with prednisone, az athioprine, and antilymphocyte globulin continues to be a practical approach to balance nephrotoxicity and graft rejection.[62,70,78] Prophylaxis with misoprostol during combined cyclosporine and prednisone immunosuppression improved renal allograft function, but did not prevent cyclosporine nephrotoxicity.[79] Suppression of thromboxane production using oral thromboxane synthase inhibitors has shown favorable acute,[80] but not long-term,[81] effects with regard to reversal of renal dysfunction in cyclosporine-treated renal allograft recipients. Calcium channel blockers may enhance,[80] while ACE inhibitors may prevent,[82] the favorable effects of thromboxane synthase inhibitors on cyclosporine renal dysfunction. Immunosuppression with FK-506, an agent also affecting T lymphocytes, appears to cause nephrotoxicity similar to that of cyclosporine.[83,84]

Mannitol, an osmotic diuretic used to reduce intracranial pressure, treat glaucoma, and prevent acute ischemic or nephrotoxic renal failure, may cause acute oligoanuric renal failure.[19] Potential mechanisms include accentuated osmotic diuresis with increased solute delivery to the macula densa causing a tubuloglomerular feedback response and vasoconstriction of the glomerular afferent arteriole, direct renal vasoconstriction, or proximal tubular "osmotic nephrosis" with tubular obstruction due to epithelial cell swelling.[19] Risk factors include excessive doses, preexistent renal insufficiency, and concomitant diuretic therapy.[19,85] Nephrotoxicity may be prevented by limiting the dose and avoiding dehydration and concomitant diuretic therapy. Serum mannitol concentration should be maintained at less than 1000 mg/dL (osmolal gap <55 mOsm/kg water), although an osmolal gap of 20 mOsm/kg water is usually therapeutic.[19] Urine flow and renal function generally recover when elevated mannitol concentrations decrease following drug withdrawal or hemodialysis.[85] In addition, massive mannitol dosing in an oliguric renal transplant patient treated with cyclosporine caused severe tubular damage with graft swelling and kidney rupture.[86] Mannitol-induced osmotic diuresis and volume depletion could increase the nephrotoxicity of other drugs, particularly NSAIDs and ACE inhibitors.

Increases in Vascular Permeability

OKT3 therapy, effective for the prevention and treatment of acute renal and cardiac allograft rejection, is accompanied by a rise in the serum creatinine concentration and return to near baseline after 3–5 days.[87] Renal biopsy findings of mild interstitial edema or no abnormalities suggest the mechanism is increased vascular permeability due to a renal capillary leak. This renal dysfunction is believed to be part of a cytokine syndrome associated with OKT3 therapy.[88] OKT3 causes lymphocyte activation and release of cytokines, particularly tumor necrosis factor-alpha, interferon gamma, and interleukin-2. Renal function improves spontaneously despite continued OKT3 therapy.

Increases in Colloid Oncotic Pressure and Blood Viscosity

Drugs that alter blood rheology may have renal hemodynamic effects. Thus, intravenous dextran-40 in sufficient quantities to increase plasma oncotic pressure above plasma hydrostatic pressure may reversibly imbalance Starling's forces in the glomerular capillaries and reduce glomerular filtration.[89] Alternatively, renal insufficiency could be due to "osmotic nephrosis" with tubular obstruction from epithelial cell swelling. Dialysis and plasmapheresis can remove dextran, resulting in rapid recovery of renal function.

Exogenous erythropoietin therapy in an animal model of progressive renal failure accelerated the rate of loss of renal function, possibly due to increased blood viscosity from an inappropriately increased red cell mass.[90] The proposed mechanism is increased blood viscosity, which exacerbates systemic hypertension and raises glomerular efferent arteriolar resistance leading to increased glomerular capillary pressure and renal damage.[90] Renal function, however, has not declined more rapidly than expected in humans during erythropoietin therapy when systemic blood pressure is controlled and the hematocrit does not rise above normal.[91]

RENAL VASCULAR ALTERATIONS

Systemic polyarteritis nodosa with involvement of small- and medium-sized renal arteries has been described following methamphetamine abuse.[92] Patients may have hematuria, proteinuria, renal insufficiency, and hypertension. Renal and visceral vascular aneurysms can be demonstrated by angiography. The pathogenesis may be a toxic reaction to methamphetamine or the result of associated hepatitis B infection. Penicillin and sulfonamide therapies have also been considered as causes of polyarteritis nodosa, although these associations have been less clear.[92]

Thrombotic microangiopathy (hemolytic-uremic syndrome, thrombotic thrombocytopenic purpura) resulting in thrombus formation in the renal vasculature has been described with various drugs, including oral contraceptive agents,[93] cyclosporine,[94] mitomycin C,[95,96] cisplatin,[97] and quinine.[98] The association with mitomycin C is of particular interest since the pathogenesis appears to be a direct toxic effect with a predictable incidence: 1.6% in patients receiving less than 50 mg/m^2 and 27.8% in patients receiving more than 70 mg/m^2.[95,96] Nephrotoxicity has occurred following long-term chemotherapy with mitomycin C alone and in combination with 5-fluorouracil, cisplatin, bleomycin, and a Vinca alkaloid.[95,99] Microangiopathic hemolytic anemia and thrombocytopenia are usually present. Renal failure can be severe and irreversible, although corticosteroids, antiplatelet agents, vincristine sulfate, plasma exchange, plasmapheresis, and high-dose intravenous IgG therapies have each induced clinical improvement.

Cholesterol emboli from large atherosclerotic arteries to small renal arteries and arterioles can induce an inflammatory obliterative vascular lesion with renal failure due to ischemia. This most commonly occurs following invasive angiographic procedures, but may also occur after thrombolytic or anticoagulant therapies, which remove or prevent thrombus formation over ulcerative atherosclerotic plaques.[100]

GLOMERULAR ALTERATIONS: NEPHROTIC SYNDROME AND GLOMERULONEPHRITIS

Drug-induced glomerular disease is uncommon, although a variety of agents have been implicated.[101] The mechanisms are mostly immunologic rather than direct toxic effects. The nephrotic syndrome, defined as proteinuria greater than 3.5 g/d, with or without renal insufficiency is the usual manifestation of glomerular damage. Several lesions have been described.

Minimal change nephrotic syndrome is characterized by normal glomeruli by light microscopy. Drug-induced minimal change nephropathy is frequently accompanied by interstitial nephritis and is most common during NSAID therapy. Ampicillin, rifampin, hydantoin anticonvulsants, and lithium have also been implicated.[102] The pathogenesis is unknown, but nephrotic range proteinuria due to NSAID therapy is frequently associated with a T-lymphocytic interstitial infiltrate suggesting disordered cell-mediated immunity.[103] These cells may release lymphokines that increase glomerular capillary permeability to proteins.[56] Proteinuria usually resolves rapidly after discontinuation of the offending drug. Prednisone therapy, in doses ranging from 0.5–1 mg/kg body weight for 2–4 weeks, may help resolve the lesion.[56] NSAID glomerulopathy may also mimick lupus nephritis.[104]

Focal segmental glomerulosclerosis is characterized by areas of sclerosis in some glomeruli along with renal interstitial inflammation and fibrosis. Chronic heroin abuse is the most common drug cause of this lesion.[105] The specific pathogenesis is unknown but may include direct toxicity by heroin or adulterants as well as injury from bacterial or viral infections accompanying intravenous drug use. End-stage renal failure develops in most cases. No specific therapy is available, although discontinuation of heroin use may prevent progression.[105] Focal segmental glomerulosclerosis is the predominant renal lesion in acquired immunodeficiency syndrome (AIDS) patients and may result from human immunodeficiency virus (HIV) or heroin abuse.[105,106] Glomerulosclerosis due to HIV infection may be distinguished from heroin nephropathy by tubuloreticular structures in endothelial cells on electron microscopy and, clinically, by a more rapid course and poorer prognosis. Focal segmental sclerosis has been attributed to lithium therapy.[107]

Membranous nephropathy, the most common drug-induced glomerular lesion,[108] is an immune-mediated disorder characterized by immune complex deposition along glomerular capillary loops. Parenteral gold is the most common cause, with an incidence of 1–10% in patients treated for rheumatoid arthritis.[109] Oral gold therapy has a lesser incidence. The pathogenesis may involve damage to proximal tubule epithelium with antigen release, antibody formation, and glomerular immune complex deposition. Gold has been identified in proximal tubular cells, but not in the glomerular deposits. Genetic factors appear to be important since patients with human leucocyte antigens (HLAs) DR3 or B8 have increased susceptibility. Renal function is preserved and proteinuria resolves within 6–39 months of discontinuing gold therapy.[109] Mercury found in diuretics, topical skin preparations, and industrial vapors as well as penicillamine cause membranous nephropathy.[108] The pathogenesis for both also appears to be immune mediated.[108]

Membranoproliferative glomerulonephritis is a rare consequence of drug therapy that is most commonly associated with hydralazine-induced systemic lupus erythematosus.[110] Other reported drug-induced glomerular lesions include rapidly progressive or crescentic glomerulonephritis due to penicillamine therapy[108,111] and combined interleukin-2 and interferon-alpha therapy,[112] proliferative glomerulonephritis due to chlorpropamide,[113] and crescentic IgA glomerulonephritis following recombinant interleukin-2 therapy.[114] Glomerular amyloidosis has been associated with heroin abuse, particularly in users who inject subcutaneously.[105] The pathogenesis may be immune stimulation from chronic skin inflammation.

ACUTE TUBULAR NECROSIS

Acute necrosis of renal tubular epithelium is one of the most common mechanisms responsible for drug-induced renal insufficiency. Proximal tubular cells appear to be quite susceptible to pharmacologic injury and multiple drugs have been implicated (Table 47.5). Aminoglycosides, radiographic contrast media, cisplatin, and amphotericin, however, are most important. Subclinical manifestations of toxicity include tubular proteinuria and enzymuria.[12,13] Clinical toxicity becomes apparent as a rise in serum creatinine and BUN concentrations, a decline in creatinine clearance, and disturbances of renal tubular electrolyte and water handling. Repetitive therapy causing recurrent subclinical toxicity can have cumulative effects resulting in chronic tubulointerstitial disease.[95]

TABLE 47.5. DRUGS THAT CAUSE TUBULAR NECROSIS

Higher Incidence	Lower Incidence
Acetaminophen (overdose)	Amoxapine
Aminoglycosides	Carboplatin
Amphotericin B	Cyclosporine
Cisplatin	Low-molecular-weight dextran
Radiographic contrast agents	Mannitol
Streptozocin	Methoxyflurane anesthesia
	NSAIDs
	Tetracycline

The mechanism of renal failure in acute tubular necrosis is unclear. The glomerular filtration rate decreases proportionately more than renal blood flow decreases, suggesting that renal ischemia is not the primary mechanism.[115,116] Other mechanisms include a shunt of blood away from the glomerulus, reduction of glomerular capillary filtration pressure, decreased permeability of the glomerular filtration surface, obstruction of tubular flow by damaged epithelial cells and cellular debris, and backleak of the glomerular filtrate across damaged tubular epithelia into the systemic circulation.[115,116] The relative role of each mechanism may depend on the specific nephrotoxic drug.

Aminoglycoside Nephrotoxicity

Clinically significant reductions in glomerular filtration have been reported in 5–25% of patients during a continued course of aminoglycoside therapy, making these agents an important cause of hospital-acquired renal disease.[4,5,117] Nephrotoxicity continues to contribute to the overall cost of aminoglycoside therapy.[118]

The initial manifestation of aminoglycoside toxicity is increased renal tubular proteinuria (β_2 microglobulin) and brush border enzymuria.[13,117] After 5–7 days of therapy the serum creatinine concentration rises gradually and the creatinine clearance decreases. Oliguria (urine volume less than 500 mL/d) is uncommon. Renal magnesium and potassium wasting can occur. Renal failure is usually mild if aminoglycoside therapy is stopped, but renal dialysis therapy is occasionally required. Renal function usually recovers, even when dialysis is necessary. Occurrences of aminoglycoside nephropathy must be evaluated carefully since not all renal failure during a course of therapy is due to aminoglycosides. Dehydration, sepsis, and concomitant drug therapy can contribute.

The pathogenesis of aminoglycoside nephrotoxicity is predominantly the result of tubular epithelial cell damage with obstruction of the tubular lumen and backleak of the glomerular filtrate.[117] Direct glomerular damage by aminoglycosides is unlikely,[117] but tubuloglomerular feedback from nephrotoxic tubular injury may contribute to reduced glomerular filtration.[119] The toxicity of various aminoglycosides is directly proportional to the number of their cationic charges.[120] Neomycin with six cationic amino groups is the most nephrotoxic while streptomycin with three groups is least toxic. Gentamicin and tobramycin with five aminogroups have similar and intermediate toxicity, while amikacin with four amino groups and netilmicin, with three amino groups, may be the least toxic of the commonly used aminoglycosides. Cationic charges facilitate binding of filtered aminoglycosides to renal tubular epithelial cell luminal membranes. This is followed by intracellular transport and concentration in lysosomes.[24,117,120] Phospholipidosis results, apparently by aminoglycoside interaction with negatively charged phospholipids (phosphatidylinositol), which inhibits phospholipase activity and causes accumulation of phospholipids. This can be seen histopathologically as abnormal lysosomal structures (myeloid bodies) within renal tubular epithelial cells. The membrane function of other cell organelles (e.g., mitochondria) is also affected.[117,120] Cellular dysfunction and death may result from release of lysosomal enzymes into the cytosol, altered cellular metabolism, and alterations in cell membrane fluidity leading to reduced activity of membrane-bound enzymes, including Na^+/K^+-ATPase, dipeptidyl peptidase IV, and neutral aminopeptidase.[20,21,117,120] Experimentally, administration of polyaspartic acid, a polyanionic peptide, forms electrostatic complexes with aminoglycosides that reduces their interaction with anionic phospholipids and decreases cell injury.[20,21,24]

Multiple potential risk factors for aminoglycoside nephrotoxicity have been identified and related to aminoglycoside dosing, synergistic effects of aminoglycosides in combination with other drugs, and predisposing conditions in the patient (Table 47.6). Certain of these risk factors have been variably identified as risks by different analyses and the reader is referred to the references for in-depth review.[24,117,120–123] While combined vancomycin and aminoglycoside therapy has been considered especially nephrotoxic, recent meta-analysis suggests only a 1–7% greater risk of nephrotoxicity with combination therapy compared to aminoglycoside therapy alone with the greater toxicity associated with more prolonged therapy.[123]

Nephrotoxicity can be prevented by switching to alternative antibiotics as soon as microbial sensitivities are known.[124] Toxicity may be reduced by avoiding volume depletion, limiting the total dose administered, and avoiding concomitant therapy with other nephrotoxic drugs. The role of therapeutic drug monitoring and pharmacokinetic modeling to prevent nephrotoxicity has shown benefit in uncontrolled studies,[125] but has not consistently prevented nephrotoxicity and therefore remains controversial.[126] The primary value of measuring drug levels may be to improve antimicrobial efficacy. Association between elevated trough aminoglycoside levels and nephrotoxicity may be the result, rather than a cause, of toxicity. The specific aminoglycoside used does not appear to affect significantly the

TABLE 47.6. POTENTIAL RISK FACTORS FOR AMINOGLYCOSIDE NEPHROTOXICITY

A. Related to aminoglycoside dosing:
- Large total cumulative dose
- Prolonged therapy
- High 1-hour postdose concentration
- Trough concentration exceeding 2 mg/L
- Recent previous aminoglycoside therapy

B. Related to synergistic nephrotoxicity. Aminoglycosides in combination with:
- Cyclosporine
- Amphotericin B
- Vancomycin
- Diuretics

C. Related to predisposing conditions in the patient:
- Preexisting renal insufficiency
- Increased age
- Poor nutrition
- Shock
- Gram-negative bacteremia
- Liver disease
- Hypoalbuminemia
- Obstructive jaundice
- Dehydration
- Potassium or magnesium deficiencies

risk of nephrotoxicity and therapy should be selected to optimize antimicrobial effects.[117] Once-daily dosing of aminoglycosides[127–129] may preserve efficacy and reduce nephrotoxicity, particularly for gentamicin, but this continues to be controversial[130] and remains to be established.[24,131] With once-daily dosing, transient high serum aminoglycoside levels may be less nephrotoxic because they are accompanied by low levels during a greater proportion of the dosing interval. Investigational use of calcium supplementation during aminoglycoside therapy has decreased nephrotoxicity, apparently by inhibiting aminoglycoside binding to luminal membranes of renal tubular epithelial cells and preventing uptake into cells.[117] Strategies using calcium channel blockers, pyridoxal phosphate, and ACE inhibitors are being evaluated.[132]

Radiographic Contrast Media Nephrotoxicity

Intravenous administration of radiographic contrast media is a common cause of hospital-acquired acute renal failure.[4,5] Toxicity ranges from transient tubular enzymuria to irreversible oliguric renal failure requiring dialysis therapy.[133,134] Toxicity is usually mild and rapidly reversible. Severe toxicity is most frequent in diabetic patients with preexistent severe renal insufficiency. The typical course is an initial transient osmotic diuresis followed by tubular proteinuria and enzymuria. The serum creatinine rises and peaks between 2 and 5 days after exposure with recovery after 4–10 days. Oliguria is present in about 50% of cases. No laboratory test is diagnostic and urinalysis reveals only hyaline and granular casts. The urine sodium concentration and fractional excretion of sodium are frequently low.[133,134] A decrease in renal function following contrast administration may not always reflect contrast toxicity since concomitant medical illness and dehydration due to fluid restriction and cathartics used for study preparation may also contribute.[134]

The major risk factor for contrast nephropathy is preexistent renal insufficiency.[133,134] Hospitalized patients with a serum creatinine concentration greater than 1.5 mg/dL have up to a 30–40% incidence, while those with serum creatinine concentrations greater than 5 mg/dL may have a 70% incidence of renal dysfunction after intravenous or intra-arterial contrast injection. Diabetic patients with renal insufficiency have a greater risk of nephropathy than nondiabetic patients with renal insufficiency.[134–136] Conditions associated with decreased renal blood flow, including congestive heart failure and dehydration, also confer risk. The presence of multiple myeloma has been considered a relative contraindication for contrast use, but this risk appears to be that of concomitant dehydration, renal insufficiency, or hypercalcemia. The risk of contrast nephropathy in multiple myeloma is minimal if renal function is normal and patients are well hydrated.[137]

The pathogenesis of contrast nephropathy includes both direct tubular toxicity and renal ischemia.[18,133,134] Direct tubular toxicity is suggested by renal tubular enzymuria and biopsy findings of proximal tubular epithelial cell vacuolization and acute tubular necrosis. In addition to the direct toxic effects of contrast media, the nonselective proteinuria induced by contrast media may indirectly damage tubular epithelial cells. In contrast to these findings, both the low urine sodium concentration and low fractional excretion of sodium frequently observed with contrast nephropathy indicate good tubular function and suggest that renal ischemia may participate more than tubular toxicity. Renal ischemia results from systemic hypotension associated with contrast injection as well as selective direct renal vasoconstriction. Renal ischemia may also result from dehydration due to the osmotic diuresis that accompanies use of hyperosmolar agents (900–1780 mOsm/kg) and increased blood viscosity due to red blood cell crenation and aggregation.

Contrast nephropathy can be prevented by using alternative imaging procedures in high-risk patients and thereby avoiding use of radiographic contrast media. If contrast media must be used, the smallest adequate dose should be administered. Dose reduction proportional to the level of renal insufficiency may be protective,[138] but could limit the adequacy of imaging in some patients.

The utility of newer lower osmolar nonionic (iohexol and iopamidol) and ionic (ioxaglate) contrast agents to prevent nephrotoxicity remains unclear. Early studies suggested that these newer agents had little renal protective effect, but few truly high-risk patients were studied.[139,140]

Subsequent larger prospective controlled trials[141,142] and a meta-analysis[143] indicated reduced nephrotoxicity with lower osmolar, mostly nonionic, agents in patients with preexisting renal insufficiency. Of these, a large prospective trial of 1196 patients compared the lower osmolar nonionic iohexol to the higher osmolar ionic diatrizoate.[142] This trial revealed that a 0.5 mg/dL or greater rise in plasma creatinine occurred 55% less often in patients with preexisting renal insufficiency and 30% less often in patients with diabetic nephropathy using iohexol compared to diatrizoate. However, these newer agents have not eliminated nephrotoxicity and caution must be continued with their use. Since lower osmolar agents are considerably more expensive than higher osmolar ionic agents and have an unclear cost–benefit profile, their most appropriate use remains controversial (Table 47.7). A cost-effective strategy may be to use newer lower osmolar contrast agents in patients with preexisting renal insufficiency, particularly those with diabetic nephropathy, and older higher osmolar constrast agents in patients with normal renal function. Additionally, the newer agents cause less histamine release and may be advantageous for hemodynamically unstable patients or those with a history of a hypersensitivity response to contrast media.[144]

Dehydration should be corrected before contrast agent administration, other nephrotoxic drugs should be discontinued, and subsequent contrast studies should be appropriately delayed to avoid cumulative toxicity. Aggressive hydration and mannitol administration before contrast exposure have been advocated to promote diuresis and renal vasodilation and help prevent nephropathy in high-risk patients.[133,134] More recently, neither mannitol nor furosemide were found helpful in preventing nephrotoxicity.[145] Investigationally, calcium channel blockers[134] and intravenous theophylline[146] may be protective while intravenous mannitol, dopamine, or atrial natriuretic peptide may ameliorate contrast toxicity by renal vasodilation in nondiabetic, but not diabetic, patients with renal insufficiency.[136]

Cisplatin Nephrotoxicity

Cisplatin, an important chemotherapeutic agent, may cause renal tubular damage due, in part, to the heavy metal, platinum.[95,147] During early investigations with multiple-course cisplatin therapy, the incidence of nephrotoxicity was 50–100%. Subsequently, the incidence of toxicity decreased to 6–13% by limiting the total drug dose and reducing the rate of administration. Risk factors include increased age, renal irradiation, and alcohol abuse.[148] Nephrotoxicity is usually reversible and manifests early during therapy by transient proximal tubular cell brush border and lysosomal enzymuria.[95,148] Peak serum creatinine concentrations occur approximately 10–12 days after initiation of therapy with recovery by 21 days. However, renal damage can be cumulative and the serum creatinine concentration may continue to rise with subsequent cycles of therapy.[95] Chronic renal insufficiency may result.[149] Renal magnesium wasting is also common and can be accompanied by hypocalcemia.[95,148] Hypomagnesemia may be severe, causing seizures, neuromuscular irritability, or personality changes, and persist long after chemotherapy has ended.

The mechanism of cisplatin toxicity involves impairment of cell energy production by binding of platinum to proximal tubular cell sulphydryl groups, with disruption of cell enzyme activity and uncoupling of oxidative phosphorylation.[147] Renal biopsies show sparing of glomeruli with necrosis of both proximal and distal tubules and collecting ducts.[147] Toxicity may be prevented by dose reduction and decreased frequency of administration. These are usually accomplished by using cisplatin in combination with other chemotherapeutic agents. Vigorous saline hydration is important, but roles for furosemide or mannitol diuresis are less clear.[147,148] Investigational techniques, which have decreased toxicity, include the use of hypertonic saline to reduce tubular cisplatin uptake,[95,147,148] and reduction of renal exposure for therapy of localized peritoneal tumors by intraperitoneal administration in conjunction with systemic administration of sodium thiosulfate, a cisplatin neutralizer.[95,148] Treatment with probenecid and glutathione may also have renal protective effects.[148] Carboplatin and ormaplatin, second-generation platinum analogues, appear to have less nephrotoxicity, but still induce dose-dependent azotemia and salt wasting.[95,147] Saline hydration also appears useful to reduce nephrotoxicity with these cisplatin analogs.[147]

Hypomagnesemia results from renal magnesium wasting due to tubular damage as well as magnesuric effects of saline hydration and diuretic therapy to prevent tubular toxicity. Anorexia and diarrhea also contribute. The incidence of hypomagnesemia increases with recurrent cycles of cisplatin and combination chemotherapy. Management requires frequent monitoring of serum magnesium concentrations and repletion with magnesium chloride.

TABLE 47.7. CONSIDERATIONS FOR USE OF NEWER, LOWER OSMOLAR RADIOCONTRAST AGENTS COMPARED TO OLDER, HIGHER OSMOLAR IONIC RADIOCONTRAST AGENTS

Advantages:
Less histamine release with fewer allergic or hemodynamic adverse effects.[144]
Less nephrotoxicity (30–50% decreased incidence in patients with preexisting nondiabetic or diabetic renal insufficiency).[142,143]
Disadvantage:
Greater than 10-fold higher cost.

Amphotericin B Nephrotoxicity

The frequency of fungal infections has increased during the last decade due to modern therapeutic interventions leading to more immunocompromised patients. Amphotericin B remains the antifungal drug of choice for most systemic infections, but dose-dependent nephrotoxicity occurs to varying degrees in almost all patients receiving the drug.[150,151] Toxicity may be manifest as a decrease in renal blood flow and glomerular filtration rate with a rise in the serum creatinine concentration, distal renal tubular acidosis due to a leak of hydrogen ions back out of the tubular lumen, impaired renal ability to concentrate urine, and renal tubular potassium, sodium, and magnesium wasting into urine.[152] Toxicity may occur with doses as low as 300–400 mg,[153] and reaches a prevalence of 80% with cumulative doses approaching 4 g.[150] Risk factors include higher average daily doses, diuretic use and volume depletion, and abnormal baseline renal function.[153,154]

Renal pathologic findings include focal vacuolization of small arterial and arteriolar smooth muscle cells as well as proximal and distal tubular epithelial cell damage.[155] The mechanisms of nephrotoxicity include cell membrane effects, which increase tubular permeability and cause arterial vasoconstriction.[151] Renal vasoconstriction occurs as either a direct effect of amphotericin or as a reflex effect mediated through tubuloglomerular feedback when the proximal tubule is damaged and sodium delivery is increased to the macula densa.[156] Tubular membrane permeability appears to increase when amphotericin binds to membranes and acts as an ionophore increasing permeability to solutes such as sodium and potassium.[156] These effects combine to increase cell energy requirements due to altered membrane permeability and reduce oxygen delivery due to vasoconstriction, which may damage renal medullary tubular epithelial cells.[23,151]

Nephrotoxicity may be minimized by limiting the dose, but this results in loss of efficacy. Volume repletion and administration of amphotericin with an intravenous saline load appear to reduce toxicity in humans.[156,157] Mannitol infusion to induce an osmotic diuresis has not been protective.[151] Rapid amphotericin infusion does not appear to enhance or prevent nephrotoxicity.[158] A new preparation of the drug, liposomal amphotericin B, appears useful in minimizing nephrotoxicity[159,160] as does administration with intravenous lipids.[161] Pretreatment with a calcium channel blocker may also prove useful.[28,162] Amphotericin nephrotoxicity is best treated by discontinuation of therapy. Renal tubular dysfunction and the glomerular filtration will improve to some degree in most patients, although damage may be irreversible in others.

Pentamidine Nephrotoxicity

Pentamidine therapy for *Pneumocystis carinii* infections is also limited by nephrotoxicity.[163,165] Prospective studies have shown azotemia in 60–90% of treated patients.[163,164] Hyperkalemia, metabolic acidosis, hypomagnesemia, and hypocalcemia may also occur.[164,166] Toxicity is more frequent in patients with AIDS than patients without this immune deficiency and may be accentuated by concomitant amphotericin B therapy.[167] The mechanism of toxicity is unknown, but tubular degeneration has been seen histopathologically. The primary alternative therapy for *P. carinii,* trimethoprim-sulfamethoxazole, may also cause renal dysfunction due to allergic interstitial nephritis and inhibition of tubular secretion of creatinine, but the incidence is lower than with pentamidine.[163]

Foscarnet, an antiviral pyrophosphate analogue used in AIDS and other immunosuppressed patients to treat cytomegalovirus (CMV) retinitis and life-threatening CMV infections, appears to be highly nephrotoxic.[168] As many as 65% of patients treated with foscarnet develop renal insufficiency[168] or electrolyte disturbances including hypokalemia, hypocalcemia, hypomagnesemia, and hypo- or hyperphosphatemia.[169] The mechanism appears to be renal tubular necrosis.[168] Vigorous isotonic saline hydration throughout the course of therapy may prevent nephrotoxicity.[168]

TUBULOINTERSTITIAL DISEASE

Acute Allergic Interstitial Nephritis

Acute allergic interstitial nephritis is common and the underlying cause for 3–14% of all cases of acute renal failure.[6,170,171] Multiple drugs have been implicated and the list continues to increase (Table 47.8). Methicillin allergic interstitial nephritis has been best characterized.[172] Clinical signs occurred about 17 days (range 2-44 days) after initiation of therapy and included (with their approximate incidence):[171–173] fever (75%), maculopapular rash (25%), eosinophilia (80%), pyuria and hematuria (90%), low-level proteinuria (90%), and oliguria (18%). Eosinophiluria, when present, has been considered an important marker of allergic interstitial nephritis from drug causes. However, the incidence is variable,[170,174] possibly due to instability of eosinophils in urine and inadequate laboratory methodology.[174,175] Anemia, leukocytosis, and elevated IgE levels, as well as tubular dysfunction, including renal tubular acidosis, hyperkalemia, salt wasting, and concentrating defects, may also occur.[170,174]

Allergic interstitial nephritis due to NSAID therapy has a different clinical presentation.[56] Older patients appear to be affected more frequently. The onset of nephropathy is delayed, a mean of 5.4 months from initiation of therapy. Manifestations of a systemic hypersensitivity response are infrequent, occurring in only 19% of the cases. A concomitant nil lesion nephrotic syndrome is characteristic.

Cytokine therapy induces a unique nephropathy usually considered to be hemodynamically mediated due to a systemic capillary leak syndrome.[88,95] However, acute interstitial nephritis has occurred during leukocyte A inter-

TABLE 47.8. COMMONLY USED DRUGS THAT CAUSE ALLERGIC INTERSTITIAL NEPHRITIS

Antibiotics	Amiloride
Acyclovir	Chlorthalidone
Aminoglycosides	Furosemide
Amphotericin B	Triamterene
Aztreonam	Thiazides
Cephalosporins	**Miscellaneous**
Ciprofloxacin	Acetaminophen
Erythromycin	Allopurinol
Ethambutol	Interferon-α
Penicillins	Aspirin
Polymyxin B	Captopril
Rifampin	Cimetidine
Sulfonamides	Clofibrate
Tetracyclines	Cyclosporine
Trimethoprim-sulfamethoxazole	Glyburide
Vancomycin	Gold
Neuropsychiatric	Methyldopa
Carbamazepine	*p*-Aminosalicylic acid
Lithium	Phenylpropanolamine
Phenobarbital	Propylthiouracil
Nonsteroidal anti-inflammatory drugs	Radiographic contrast media
Phenytoin	Ranitidine
Valproic acid	Sulfinpyrazone
Diuretics	Warfarin sodium
Acetazolamide	

feron therapy for mycosis fungoides[176] and also during adoptive cancer immunotherapy with interleukin-2 (IL-2) and lymphokine-activated killer (LAK) cells, causing a predominantly T-lymphocytic renal interstitial infiltrate.[177] Combined therapy with alpha human interferon and human granulocyte colony stimulating factor (rhG-CSF) has also been associated with acute renal failure and a course consistent with allergic interstitial nephritis.[178]

The renal pathology of allergic interstitial nephritis is a diffuse or focal interstitial infiltrate of lymphocytes, plasma cells, eosinophils, and occasional polymorphonuclear neutrophils.[170,174] Granulomas may also occur.[179] Patchy peritubular inflammation and epithelial cell atrophy with tubular necrosis is also present.[171,173] The pathogenesis is an allergic hypersensitivity response.[15,170,173] In certain cases a humoral, antibody-mediated mechanism may be involved as indicated by the occasional presence of circulating antibody to a drug hapten-tubular basement membrane complex, low serum complement levels, and tubular basement membrane deposition of IgG and complement. More commonly, a cell-mediated immune mechanism is suggested by the absence of these findings and the presence of a predominantly T-lymphocyte infiltrate with an increased helper to suppressor cell ratio. The pathogenesis of NSAID interstitial nephritis also involves T lymphocytes, possibly in response to altered prostaglandin synthesis.[56] Patients who are slow acetylators may be predisposed to idiosyncratic sulfonamide hypersensitivity, including nephritis.[180]

Prompt and accurate diagnosis of allergic interstitial nephritis is important since failure to stop the offending drug can result in chronic renal insufficiency. The presence of fever, rash, eosinophilia, and eosinophiluria suggests the diagnosis, but these findings are not reliable because one or more of them are frequently absent. When possible, a renal biopsy is recommended as the most specific and direct method for diagnosis.[15,170] Alternatively, gallium[67] renal imaging is a sensitive but nonspecific diagnostic technique.[170] Other interstitial and glomerular lesions including pyelonephritis, nil lesion nephrotic syndrome, and cholesterol embolization can give positive scans limiting the usefulness of this test. Treatment with corticosteroids in a dose of 0.5–1 mg/kg body weight for 1–4 weeks may shorten the duration and improve the extent of renal function recovery,[170,174] although no prospective comparative studies have been reported.

Chronic Interstitial Nephritis

Lithium and cyclosporine are two of the few drugs that have been considered to cause this usually progressive and irreversible nephropathy. Streptozotocin and other antineoplastic nitrosoureas can also cause dose-dependent chronic tubulointerstitial disease.[95]

Lithium therapy has been associated with several renal tubular lesions, including chronic tubulointerstitial nephritis,[181] impaired ability to concentrate urine (nephrogenic diabetes insipidus) in approximately 20–70% of patients,[181,182] incomplete distal renal tubular acidosis,[181] and acute renal failure.[183] Impaired ability to concentrate urine is due to a dose-related decrease in collecting duct response to antidiuretic hormone. This results from impaired formation of cellular cAMP in response to antidiuretic hormone and can frequently be reversed by discontinuation of lithium therapy or ameliorated with amiloride during continued lithium therapy.[184] Lithium-induced acute renal failure occurs during episodes of lithium intoxication.[183] The pathogenesis includes dehydration secondary to nephrogenic diabetes insipidus as well as direct proximal and distal tubular cell toxicity. Severe renal insufficiency has been reported and can be reversible with supportive care, including dialysis therapy to reduce toxic serum lithium concentrations.

Mild renal insufficiency occurs in as many as 10% of patients undergoing long-term lithium therapy.[181,185] Patients have rarely developed end-stage renal failure. The renal lesion includes interstitial fibrosis with focal tubular atrophy and glomerular sclerosis.[186,187] The role of lithium in this loss of renal function is debated. The duration of lithium therapy has correlated with the decline in the glomerular filtration rate suggesting the pathogenesis may involve direct lithium toxicity.[188] However, chronic renal insufficiency has not been convincingly demonstrated when lithium concentrations have been maintained within the therapeutic range. Furthermore, in prospective studies renal function has not declined during short-term lithium therapy.[189,190] Alternative mechanisms of nephrotoxicity associated with lithium therapy could include the cumulative effects of acute episodes of lithium toxicity,[186] use of concomitant drugs such as neuroleptic agents[187] or ACE inhibitors,[191] and concurrent renal tubulointerstitial disease.

Preventive measures include maintenance of lithium serum concentrations in the therapeutic range, avoidance of dehydration, and close monitoring of renal function including urinary concentrating ability. It is unknown whether progression to severe renal failure can be prevented by discontinuing lithium therapy when mild renal insufficiency is first recognized.

Cyclosporine can also cause interstitial fibrosis and chronic irreversible renal insufficiency after approximately 6–12 months of therapy.[62,63] This has been a major limitation to therapy since as many as 10% of cardiac transplant patients developed end-stage renal failure with prolonged higher dose therapy.[64] The pathogenesis appears to involve sustained renal endothelial cell injury and ischemia or direct tubular toxicity (see section on Hemodynamically Mediated Renal Failure). Cyclosporine-induced interstitial matrix synthesis and accumulation, apparently due to increased activity of cytokines, peptide growth factors, or thromboxane, may also contribute.[63] The risk of chronic interstitial renal disease appears to be lessened with the current lower dose therapy.[70]

Papillary Necrosis

Chronic excessive consumption of combination analgesics containing phenacetin can cause chronic renal tubulointerstitial disease with papillary necrosis and lead to increased hypertension and atherosclerotic cardiovascular disease.[192,193] In addition, high-dose dapsone therapy, used more frequently recently for *P. carinii* infections during the HIV epidemic, may also cause papillary necrosis.[194]

Analgesic or "phenacetin" nephropathy was initially reported from Switzerland in 1953 and was subsequently recognized as a worldwide public health concern.[195] It has been responsible for as much as 36% of all cases of end-stage renal failure in certain areas of the world, although the incidence is much lower in North America.[193,195] In addition, the incidence of lower urinary tract transitional cell carcinoma is increased in patients with a history of heavy phenacetin use.[196]

Analgesic nephropathy evolves insidiously over years with clinical expression following a cumulative phenacetin ingestion of 3 kg or more.[195,197] Women have been affected more frequently than men. Upper gastrointestinal irritation from analgesics with blood loss leading to anemia has been characteristic. Early renal manifestations include impaired maximal urinary concentration, sterile pyuria, microscopic hematuria, proteinuria, and hypertension. Creatinine clearance declines slowly. The diagnosis is confirmed by intravenous pyelography with the demonstration of papillary necrosis or by computed tomography (CT) scan, which shows decreased renal mass and bumpy contours or papillary calcifications. Frequently, however, urography only demonstrates "chronic pyelonephritis"—small kidneys with thin renal cortices and blunted calyces. Renal biopsy reveals nonspecific chronic interstitial inflammation and scarring.

The epidemiology of analgesic use and risk for analgesic nephropathy continues to evolve.[193,197] The classic concept is that risk for end-stage renal disease increases with cumulative consumption of combination analgesics[195,198] and that ingestion of single analgesics[198] and, particularly, acetylsalicylic acid alone[195] does not cause end-stage renal failure. In contrast, recent epidemiologic studies have suggested that phenacetin alone can cause chronic nephropathy.[192] Evidence is also accumulating that ingestion of high-dose acetaminophen alone, a phenacetin metabolite, may be a risk for renal disease.[22,199] In addition, chronic interstitial disease and papillary necrosis may occur with use of NSAIDs alone, particularly in males.[193,200]

The pathogenesis of analgesic nephropathy remains unclear and has been difficult to study since the evolving lesion is not easily recognized in humans because of the lack of diagnostic markers and since appropriate animal models have been difficult to establish.[201] Conceptualization of "classic analgesic nephropathy" is based on increased risk with combination analgesics containing phenacetin or acetaminophen and salicylates or NSAIDs. Evidence for nephrotoxicity from chronic ingestion of phenacetin or acetaminophen alone challenges these concepts. The renal lesion begins in the papillary tip as a result of accumulated toxic metabolites, decreased blood flow, and impaired cellular energy production.[197,201,202] The biochemical mechanisms appear to involve metabolism of phenacetin to acetaminophen, which is then oxidized to toxic free radicals that are concentrated in the papilla during urinary concentration.[197,202] The ability of the kidney to oxidize acetaminophen has been questioned because of an apparent lack of renal cytochrome P-450. However, co-oxidation of acetaminophen may occur with renal prostaglandin synthesis.[197,203] Papillary ischemia results from the ability of both salicylate and acetaminophen to inhibit renal medullary synthesis of vasodilatory prostaglandins. Impaired cellular energy production results from the ability of salicylate to uncouple mitochondrial oxidative phosphorylation.[202]

Prevention has depended primarily on public health efforts to restrict the sale of phenacetin and combination analgesics.[193] However, OTC combination analgesics containing aspirin, acetaminophen, and caffeine remain available in the United States and throughout the world. Caffeine appears to contribute to nephrotoxicity in this analgesic mixture.[200] While the withdrawal of phenacetin-containing analgesics has decreased the incidence of analgesic nephropathy,[193,204] the continued extensive use of acetaminophen, aspirin, and NSAIDs, frequently together, constitutes a potential health problem.

Individuals requiring chronic analgesic therapy may reduce their risk by limiting the total dose, avoiding the combined use of two or more analgesics, and maintaining adequate hydration to prevent renal ischemia and decrease the papillary concentration of toxic substances. Treatment of established nephrotoxicity requires cessation of analgesic consumption, which can prevent progression and may improve renal function. Persistent surreptitious analgesic abuse should be considered if renal function continues to decline.[205] Patients should also be evaluated carefully for associated transitional cell carcinoma of the renal pelvis, calyces, ureters, and bladder.[196] Carcinoma may present years after analgesic nephropathy is diagnosed.

OBSTRUCTIVE NEPHROPATHY

Renal Tubular Obstruction

Drug-induced acute renal failure due to renal tubular obstruction can be caused by intratubular precipitation of tissue degradation products as well as by drugs or their metabolites. Acute uric acid nephropathy following chemotherapy, usually for hematologic malignancies, is the most common cause of renal failure due to obstruction by tissue degradation products.[206] Acute oliguric or anuric renal failure develops rapidly. The diagnosis is supported by a urine uric acid to creatinine ratio greater than one.[206] Uric acid precipitation can be prevented by pretreatment hydration, urinary alkalinization to pH 7.0, and administration of allopurinol. Uric acid nephropathy was also observed at the initiation of therapy with ticrynafen, a uricosuric diuretic, and suprofen,[207] a uricosuric NSAID, both of which shared similar chemical structures and are no longer available in the United States.

Drug-induced muscle necrosis, nontraumatic rhabdomyolysis, is an important cause of acute renal failure due, in part, to intratubular precipitation of myoglobin. Drug-induced rhabdomyolysis may result from pressure necrosis during stupor or coma following alcohol or heroin abuse,[208] extreme neuromuscular stimulation and metabolic demands with abuse of phencyclidine[209] or therapy with adrenergic agents, including terbutaline,[210] and vasoconstriction and muscle ischemia due to abuse of cocaine[211] or therapeutic vasopressin infusion.[212] Rhabdomyolysis has also occurred during lovastatin therapy for hypercholesterolemia,[213] particularly in a dose-dependent association with cyclosporine therapy, but also with use of erythromycin, gemfibrozil, or niacin. One mechanism of toxicity appears to be accumulation of myotoxic levels of lovastatin due to competitive inhibition by cyclosporin for metabolism through the cytochrome P-450 system.[213]

Precipitation of drugs or their metabolites in concentrated acidic urine has been an important cause of acute renal failure, particularly with previous generations of sulfonamides. While this problem has been rare with the currently used more soluble sulfonamides, it may occur during acetazolamide therapy[214] and has become more frequent with the resurgence of sulfadiazine therapy for toxoplasmosis in AIDS patients.[215] Methotrexate and its less soluble metabolite, 7-hydroxymethotrexate, have also precipitated in acid urine and caused oligoanuric renal failure during high-dose chemotherapy.[95] Intravenous[216] and high-dose oral[217] acyclovir therapy for acute herpes zoster has caused renal insufficiency, possibly by intratubular precipitation in dehydrated oliguric patients. Massive administration of ascorbic acid can also result in obstruction of renal tubules with calcium oxalate crystals.[218] Oxalate, a poorly soluble ascorbic acid metabolite, can also precipitate and worsen renal function when ascorbic acid is administered to patients with acute renal failure or the congenital nephrotic syndrome.[218] Oxalate precipitation may also contribute to renal failure induced by methoxyfluorane, although proximal tubular necrosis due to fluoride toxicity is predominant in the pathogenesis.[219] Low molecular weight dextran therapy for volume expansion and rheological effects has also caused renal failure, possibly by intratubular precipitation of filtered dextran.[220] Triamterene may also precipitate in renal tubules and cause renal failure.[221] Renal failure due to intratubular precipitation of tissue degradation products or drugs and their metabolites can be largely prevented and possibly treated by maintaining a high urine volume and urinary alkalinization.[95,206]

Therapeutic agents not intended for systemic administration can cause renal failure in rare cases, apparently by intratubular or intrarenal precipitation. Severe hyperphosphatemia following administration of a hypertonic phosphate enema further reduced renal function in a renal-insufficient patient, possibly by intratubular precipitation of calcium phosphate.[222] Hypermagnesemia due to renacidin irrigation of the renal collecting system caused end-stage renal failure in a patient with preexistent renal insufficiency.[223] This may have involved intrarenal precipitation of magnesium whitlockite.

Extrarenal Urinary Tract Obstruction

Drug therapy may also cause renal insufficiency due to lower urinary tract obstruction. Ureteral obstruction can be caused by calculi (see Chapter 48, Nephrolithiasis, and below) or retroperitoneal fibrosis due to analgesics, methysergide, or radiation therapy.[224] Bladder dysfunction with urinary outflow obstruction can result, particularly in males with prostatic hypertrophy, from anticholinergic drugs, including tricyclic antidepressants. In particular, disopyramide phosphate, an antiarrhythmic with anticholinergic effects, has caused acute renal failure due to urinary retention.[225] Bladder outlet and ureteral obstruction may result from bladder fibrosis following hemorrhagic cystitis with cyclophosphamide or ifosfamide therapy.[95] Mesna cotherapy can prevent cystitis and this complication.

NEPHROLITHIASIS

Renal calculus formation, distinct from intratubular precipitation of crystalline material, is a rare complication of drug therapy. Historically, calculus formation occurred in 6% of patients during long-term therapy with sulfdiazine, a poorly soluble sulfonamide, for meningitis and endocarditis. Currently, triamterene appears to be the most frequent cause of calculus formation with an incidence approximating 1/1500 users of triamterene-hydrochlorothiazide.[60] However, it is unclear whether triamterene or its metabolites actually cause stone formation or are passively absorbed onto the organic matrix of calculi. Uricosuric agents, such as streptozotocin,[226] may cause uric acid stones and renal failure due to urinary obstruction. Allopurinal may rarely cause xanthine, hypoxanthine, and oxypurinol stones during therapy for conditions having excess uric acid production: such as Lesch–Nyhan syndrome and chemotherapy of lymphosarcoma.[227] Allopurinol inhibits xanthine oxidase and increases the urinary excretion of poorly soluble xanthine, hypoxanthine, and oxypurinol. Massive ingestion of magnesium trisilicate-aluminum hydroxide for gastric symptoms has been associated with magnesium ammonium phosphate (struvite) stone formation, possibly due to hypermagnesuria and increased urinary pH.[228] Laxative abuse may lead to the unusual formation of ammonium urate stones, possibly due to increased urinary pH and ammonium concentration.[229]

PATIENT OUTCOMES

Drug-induced renal disease is an important clinical problem that limits the optimal utilization of pharmacologic agents for diagnosis and therapy. In particular, new pharmacologic agents continue to demonstrate nephrotoxicity. Much research is necessary to increase our understanding of the pathogenesis of this heterogeneous group of disorders to turn apparent adverse effects to diagnostic and therapeutic advantage. In this regard, recent experience with captopril and other ACE inhibitors is a clear example of how understanding mechanisms of pathophysiology can lead to future benefits. Clinicians who remain observant and strive to understand mechanisms of disease and pharmacology will expand the horizons of pharmacotherapy and thereby enhance patient outcomes.

For management of individual patients, several guidelines can help maximize efficacy and safety:

- Know the potential nephrotoxicity of diagnostic and therapeutic pharmacologic agents used.
- Compare the potential risks and expected benefits for each course of treatment.
- Consider alternative diagnostic and therapeutic approaches.
- Use the lowest dose and shortest course of therapy that is efficacious.
- Monitor appropriately for potential toxicity.
- Modify therapy if toxicity occurs.

REFERENCES

1. Hricik DE, Dunn MJ. Angiotensin-converting enzyme inhibitor-induced renal failure: Causes, consequences and diagnostic uses. J Am Soc Nephrol 1991;1:845–858.
2. Lewis EJ, Hunsicker LG, Bain RP, et al. The effect of angiotensin-converting-enzyme inhibition on diabetic nephropathy. N Engl J Med 1993;329:1456–1462.
3. Leape LL, Brennan TA, Laird N, et al. The nature of adverse events in hospitalized patients. Results of the Harvard medical practice study II. N Engl J Med 1991;324:377–384.
4. Hou SH, Bushinsky DA, Wish JB, et al. Hospital-acquired renal insufficiency: A prospective study. Am J Med 1983;74:243–248.
5. Davidman M, Olson P, Kohen J, et al. Iatrogenic renal disease. Arch Intern Med 1991;151:1809–1812.
6. Hoitsma AJ, Welzels JFM, Koene AP. Drug induced nephrotoxicity. Aetiology, clinical features and management. Drug Safety 1991;6:131–147.
7. Sturrock NDC, Struthers AD. Non-steroidal anti-inflammatory drugs and angiotensin converting enzyme inhibitors: A commonly prescribed combination with variable effects on renal function. Br J Clin Pharmac 1993;35:343–348.
8. Strom BL, Tugwell P. Pharmacoepidemiology: Current status, prospects, and problems. Ann Intern Med 1990;113:179–181.
9. Kaufman J, Dhakal M, Patel B, Hamburger R. Community-acquired acute renal failure. Am J Kidney Dis 1991;17:191–198.
10. Mann JFE, Goerig M, Brune K, Luft FC. Ibuprofen as an over-the-counter drug: Is there a risk for renal injury? Clin Nephrol 1993;39:1–6.
11. Guignard J-P. Effect of drugs on the immature kidney. Adv Nephrol Necker Hosp 1993;22:193–211.
12. Price RG. The role of NAG (N-acetyl-beta-D-glucosaminidase) in the diagnosis of kidney disease including the monitoring of nephrotoxicity. Clin Nephrol 1992;38(suppl 1):S14–S19.
13. Schardijn GHC, Statius Van Eps LW. β_2-microglobulin: Its significance in the evaluation of renal function. Kidney Int 1987;32:635–641.
14. Couser WG. Mediation of immune glomerular injury. J Am Soc Nephrol 1990;1:13–29.

15. Neilson EG. Pathogenesis and therapy of interstitial nephritis. Kidney Int 1989;35:1257–1270.
16. Floege J, Johnson RJ. Cytokines in renal inflammation. Curr Opinion Nephrol Hypertens 1993;2:449–457.
17. Epstein M, Oster JR. Beta blockers and renal function: A reappraisal. J Clin Hypertens 1985;1:85–99.
18. Porter GA. Effects of contrast agents on renal function. Invest Radiol 1993;28(suppl 5):S1–S5.
19. Dorman HR, Sondheimer JH, Cadnapaphornchai P. Mannitol-induced acute renal failure. Medicine 1990;69:153–159.
20. Walker RJ, Fawcett JP. Drug nephrotoxicity—the significance of cellular mechanisms. Prog Drug Res 1993;41:51–94.
21. Weinberg JM. The cellular basis of nephrotoxicity, in Schrier RW, Gottschalk CW (eds): Diseases of the Kidney, 5th ed. Boston, Little, Brown and Company, 1993, pp 1031–1097.
22. Perneger TV, Whelton PK, Klag MJ. Risk of kidney failure associated with the use of acetaminophen, aspirin, and nonsteroidal antiinflammatory drugs. N Engl J Med 1994;331:1675–1679.
23. Brezis M, Rosen S. Hypoxia of the renal medulla—its implications for disease. N Engl J Med 1995;332:647–655.
24. Walker R. Aminoglycoside nephrotoxicity: Recent developments. NZ Med J 1994;107:54–55.
25. Patterson WP, Reams GP. Renal toxicities of chemotherapy. Semin Oncol 1992;19:521–528.
26. Berns AS. Nephrotoxicity of contrast media. Kidney Int 1989;36:730–740.
27. Antillon M, Cominelli F, Lo S, et al. Effects of oral prostaglandins on indomethacin-induced renal failure in patients with cirrhosis and ascites. J Rheumatol 1990;7(suppl 20):46–49.
28. Tolins JP, Raij L. Chronic amphotericin B nephrotoxicity in the rat: Protective effect of calcium channel blockade. J Am Soc Nephrol 1991;2:98–102.
29. Muther RS. Drug interference with renal function tests. Am J Kidney Dis 1983;3:118–120.
30. Opravil M, Keusch G, Luthy R. Pyrimethamine inhibits renal secretion of creatinine. Antimicrob Agents Chemother 1993;37:1056–1060.
31. Collen MJ, Howard JM, McArthur KE, et al. Comparison of ranitidine and cimetidine in the treatment of gastric hypersecretion. Ann Intern Med 1984;100:52–58.
32. Shemesh O, Golbetz H, Kriss JP, Myers BD. Limitations of creatinine as a filtration marker in glomerulopathic patients. Kidney Int 1985;28:830–838.
33. Roubenoff R, Drew H, Moyer M, et al. Oral cimetidine improves the accuracy and precision of creatinine clearance in lupus nephritis. Ann Intern Med 1990;113:501–506.
34. Van Acker BAC, Koomen GCM, Koopman MG, et al. Creatinine clearance during cimetidine administration for measurement of glomerular filtration rate. Lancet 1992;340:1326–1329.
35. Rosenthal J. Role of renal and extrarenal renin-angiotensin system in the mechanism of arterial hypertension and its sequelae. Steroids 1993;58:556–572.
36. Johnston CI, Fabris B, Jandeleit K. Intrarenal renin-angiotensin system in renal physiology and pathophysiology. Kidney Int 1993;44(suppl 42):S59–S63.
37. Davidson RA, Wilcox CS. Newer tests for the diagnosis of renovascular disease. JAMA 1992;268:3353–3358.
38. Clive DM, Stoff JS. Renal syndromes associated with nonsteroidal anti-inflammatory drugs. N Engl J Med 1984;310:563–572.
39. Schlondorff D. Renal complications of nonsteroidal anti-inflammatory drugs. Kidney Int 1993;44:643–653.
40. Bergamo RR, Cominelli F, Kopple JD, Zipser RD. Comparative acute effects of aspirin, diflunisal, ibuprofen and indomethacin on renal function in healthy man. Am J Nephrol 1989;9:460–463.
41. Ruilope LM, Robles RG, Paya C, et al. Effects of long-term treatment with indomethacin on renal function. Hypertension 1986;8:677–684.
42. Gurwitz JH, Avorn J, Ross-Degnan D, Lipsitz LA. Nonsteroidal anti-inflammatory drug-associated azotemia in the very old. JAMA 1990;264:471–475.
43. Seelig CB, Maloley PA, Campbell JR. Nephrotoxicity associated with concomitant ACE inhibitor and NSAID therapy. South Med J 1990;83:1144–1148.
44. Murray MD, Brater DC, Tierney WM, et al. Ibuprofen-associated renal impairment in a large general internal medicine practice. Am J Med Sci 1990;299:222–229.
45. Whelton A, Stout RL, Spilman PS, Klassen DK. Renal effects of ibuprofen, piroxicam, and sulindac in patients with asymptomatic renal failure: A prospective, randomized, crossover comparison. Ann Intern Med 1990;112:568–576.
46. Schoch PH, Ranno A, North DS. Acute renal failure in an elderly woman following intramuscular ketorolac administration. Ann Pharmacother 1992;26:1233–1236.
47. Boras-Uber LA, Brackett NC, Jr. Ketorolac-induced acute renal failure. Am J Med 1992;92:450–452.
48. O'Callaghan CA, Andrews PA, Ogg CS. Renal disease and use of topical non-steroidal anti-inflammatory drugs. BMJ 1994;308:110–111.
49. Stillman MT, Schlesinger PA. Nonsteroidal anti-inflammatory drug nephrotoxicity. Arch Intern Med 1990;150:268–270.
50. Ciabattoni G, Cinotti GA, Pierucci A, et al. Effects of sulindac and ibuprofen in patients with chronic glomerular disease. Evidence for the dependence of renal function on prostacyclin. N Engl J Med 1984;310:279–283.
51. Aronoff GR. Therapeutic implications associated with renal studies of nabumetone. J Rheumol 1992;19(suppl 36):25–31.
52. Eriksson LO, Sturfelt G, Thysell H, Wollheim FA. Effects of sulindac and naproxen on prostaglandin excretion in patients with impaired renal function and rheumatoid arthritis. Am J Med 1990;89:313–321.
53. Dibona GF. Prostaglandins and nonsteroidal anti-inflammatory drugs. Effects on renal hemodynamics. Am J Med 1986;80(suppl 1A):12–21.
54. Klassen DK, Stout RL, Spilman PS, Whelton A. Sulindac kinetics and effects on renal function and prostaglandin excretion in renal insufficiency. J Clin Pharmacol 1989;29:1037–1042.
55. DeWitt DL, Meade EA, Smith WL. PGH synthase isoenzyme selectivity: The potential for safer nonsteroidal antiinflammatory drugs. Am J Med 1993;95(suppl 2A):40S–44S.

56. Abraham PA, Keane WF. Glomerular and interstitial disease induced by nonsteroidal anti-inflammatory drugs. Am J Nephrol 1984;4:1–6.
57. Dunn MJ. The roles of angiotensin II and prostaglandins in the regulation of the glomerular filtration of albumin. J Hypertens 1990;8(suppl 1):S47–S52.
58. Boelaert J, Lijnen P, Robbens E, et al. Impairment of renal function due to sulphinpyrazone after coronary artery bypass surgery: A prospective double-blind study. J Cardiovasc Pharmacol 1986;8:386–391.
59. Rosenkranz B, Fejes-Tóth G, Diener U, Frölich JG. Effects of sulfinpyrazone on renal function and prostaglandin formation in man. Nephron 1985;39:237–243.
60. Sica DA, Gehr TWB. Triamterene and the kidney. Nephron 1989;51:454–461.
61. Danesh BJZ, Brunton J, Sumner DJ. Comparison between short-term renal hemodynamic effects of propranolol and nadolol in essential hypertension: A cross-over study. Clin Sci 1984;67:243–248.
62. Kahan BD. Cyclosporine. N Engl J Med 1989;321:1725–1738.
63. Kopp JB, Klotman PE. Cellular and molecular mechanisms of cyclosporine nephrotoxicity. J Am Soc Nephrol 1990;1:162–179.
64. Myers BD, Newton L. Cyclosporine-induced chronic nephropathy: An obliterative microvascular renal injury. J Am Soc Nephrol 1991;2:S45–S52.
65. Puschett JB, Greenberg A, Holley J, McCauley J. The spectrum of cyclosporin nephrotoxicity. Am J Nephrol 1990;10:296–309.
66. Ruggenenti P, Perico N, Amuchastegui CS, et al. Following an initial decline, glomerular filtration rate stabilizes in heart transplant patients on chronic cyclosporine. Am J Kidney Dis 1994;24:549–553.
67. Messana JM, Johnson KJ, Mihatsch MJ. Renal structure and function effects after low dose cyclosporine in psoriasis patients: A preliminary report. Clin Nephrol 1995;43:150–153.
68. Feutren G, Mihatsch MJ, for the International Kidney Biopsy Registry of Cyclosporine in Autoimmune Diseases. Risk factors for cyclosporine-induced nephropathy in patients with autoimmune diseases. N Engl J Med 1992;326:1654–1660.
69. Cohen DJ, Appel GB. Cyclosporine: Nephrotoxic effects and guidelines for safe use in patients with rheumatoid arthritis. Semin Arthritis Rheum 1992;21(suppl 3):43–48.
70. Burke, Jr. JF, Pirsch JD, Ramos EL, et al. Long-term efficacy and safety of cyclosporine in renal-transplant recipients. N Engl J Med 1994;331:358–363.
71. Brooks DP, Ohlstein EH, Contino LC, et al. Effects of nifedipine on cyclosporine A-induced nephrotoxicity, urinary endothelin excretion and renal endothelin receptor number. Eur J Pharmacol 1991;194:115–117.
72. De Nicola L, Thomson SC, Wead LM, et al. Arginine feeding modifies cyclosporine nephrotoxicity in rats. J Clin Invest 1993;92:1859–1865.
73. Conte G, Dal Canton A, Sabbatini M, et al. Acute cyclosporine renal dysfunction reversed by dopamine infusion in healthy subjects. Kidney Int 1989;36:1086–1092.
74. Kasiske BL, Heim-Duthoy K, Ma JZ. Elective cyclosporine withdrawal after renal transplantation. A meta-analysis. JAMA 1993;269:395–400.
75. Kahan BD. Development of synergistic immunosuppressive drug regimens based upon cyclosporine. Kidney Int 1993;44(suppl 43):S12–S15.
76. Meyer MM, Munar M, Udeaja J, Bennett W. Efficacy of area under the curve cyclosporine monitoring in renal transplantation. J Am Soc Nephrol 1993;4:1306–1315.
77. Awni WM. Pharmacodynamic monitoring of cyclosporin. Clin Pharmacokinet 1992;23:428–448.
78. Wrenshall LE, Matas AJ, Canafax DM, et al. An increased incidence of late acute rejection episodes in cadaver renal allograft recipients given azathioprine, cyclosporine, and prednisone. Transplantation 1990;50:233–237.
79. Moran M, Mozes MF, Maddux MS, et al. Prevention of acute graft rejection by the prostaglandin E_1 analogue misoprostol in renal-transplant recipients treated with cyclosporine and prednisone. N Engl J Med 1990;322:1183–1188.
80. Smith SR, Creech EA, Schaffer AV, et al. Effects of thromboxane synthase inhibition with CGS 13080 in human cyclosporine nephrotoxicity. Kidney Int 1992;41:199–205.
81. Smith SR, Kubacki VB, Rakhit A, et al. Chronic thromboxane synthase inhibition with CGS 12970 in human cyclosporine nephrotoxicity. Transplantation 1993;56:1422–1426.
82. Grieve EM, Hawksworth GM, Simpson JG, Whiting PH. Effect of thromboxane synthetase inhibition and angiotensin converting enzyme inhibition on acute cyclosporin A nephrotoxicity. Biochem Pharmacol 1990;40:2323–2329.
83. Porayko MK, Textor SC, Krom RAF, et al. Nephrotoxic effects of primary immunosuppression with FK-506 and cyclosporine regimens after liver transplantation. Mayo Clin Proc 1994;69:105–111.
84. Randhawa PS, Shapiro R, Jordan ML, et al. The histopathological changes associated with allograft rejection and drug toxicity in renal transplant recipients maintained on FK506. Clinical significance and comparison with cyclosporine. Am J Surg Pathol 1993;17:60–68.
85. Horgan KJ, Ottaviano YL, Watson AJ. Acute renal failure due to mannitol intoxication. Am J Nephrol 1989;9:106–109.
86. Biesenbach G, Zazgornik J, Kaiser W, et al. Severe tubulopathy and kidney graft rupture after coadministration of mannitol and cyclosporin. Nephron 1992;62:93–96.
87. Baiuk TD, Bennett WM, Norman DJ. Cytokine nephropathy during antilymphocyte therapy. Transplantation Proc 1993;2(suppl 1):27–30.
88. First MR, Schroeder TJ, Hariharan S. OKT3-induced cytokine-release syndrome: Renal effects (cytokine nephropathy). Transplantation Proc 1993;2(suppl 1):25–26.
89. Moran M, Kapsner C. Acute renal failure associated with elevated plasma oncotic pressure. N Engl J Med 1987;317:150–153.
90. Garcia DL, Anderson S, Rennke HG, et al. Anemia lessens and its prevention with recombinant human erythropoietin worsens glomerular injury and hypertension in rats with reduced renal mass. Proc Natl Acad Sci USA 1988;85:6142–6146.

91. Abraham PA, Opsahl JA, Rachael KM, et al. Renal function during erythropoietin therapy for anemia in predialysis chronic renal failure patients. Am J Nephrol 1990;10:128–136.
92. Porter GA, Bennett WM. Nephrotoxin-induced acute renal failure, in Brenner BM, Stein JH (eds): Contemporary Issues in Nephrology. New York, Churchill Livingstone, 1980, vol 6, pp 123–162.
93. Ridolfi RL, Bell WF. Thrombotic thrombocytopenic purpura. Report of 25 cases and review of the literature. Medicine 1981;60:413–427.
94. Hochstetler LS, Flanigan MJ, Lager DJ. Transplant-associated thrombotic microangiopathy: The role of IgG administration as initial therapy. Am J Kidney Dis 1994;23:444–450.
95. Narins RG, Carley M, Bloom EJ, Harrison DS. The nephrotoxicity of chemotherapeutic agents. Semin Nephrol 1990;10:556–564.
96. Valavaara R, Nordman E. Renal complications of mitomycin C therapy with special reference to the total dose. Cancer 1985;55:47–50.
97. Khansur T, Kennedy A. Case report: Cisplatin-induced hemolytic uremic syndrome. Am J Med Sci 1991;301:390–392.
98. Hagley MT, Hosney IA, Hulisz DT, Davis HH. Hemolytic-uremic syndrome associated with ingestion of quinine. Am J Nephrol 1992;12:192–195.
99. Jackson AM, Rose BD, Graff LG, et al. Thrombotic microangiography and renal failure associated with antineoplastic chemotherapy. Ann Intern Med 1984;101:41–44.
100. Lye WC, Cheah JS, Sinniah R. Renal cholesterol embolic disease. Case report and review of the literature. Am J Nephrol 1993;13:489–493.
101. Fillastre J-P, Mery J-P, Druet P. Drug-induced glomerulonephritis, in Solez K, Whelton A (eds): Acute Renal Failure. Correlations Between Morphology and Function. New York, Marcel Dekker, 1984, pp 389–407.
102. Baum M, Peil CF, Goodman JR. Antibiotic-associated interstitial nephritis and nephrotic syndrome. Am J Nephrol 1986;6:149–151.
103. Finkelstein A, Fraley DS, Stachura I, et al. Fenoprofen nephropathy: Lipoid nephrosis and interstitial nephritis. A possible T-lymphocyte disorder. Am J Med 1982;72:81–87.
104. Ling BN, Bourke E, Campbell Jr WG, Delaney VB. Naproxen-induced nephropathy in systemic lupus erythematosus. Nephron 1990;54:249–255.
105. Barbiano di Belgiojoso G, Genderini A, Scorza D, Landriani N. Renal damage in drug abusers. Contrib Nephrol 1990;77:142–156.
106. Rao TKS, Friedman EA, Nicastri AD. The types of renal disease in the acquired immunodeficiency syndrome. N Engl J Med 1987;316:1062–1068.
107. Santella RN, Rimmer JH, MacPherson BR. Focal segmental glomerulosclerosis in patients receiving lithium carbonate. Am J Med 1988;84:951–954.
108. Fillastre J-P, Druet P, Méry J-P. Proteinuric nephropathies associated with drugs and substances of abuse, in Cameron JS, Glassock RJ (eds): The Nephrotic Syndrome. New York, Marcel Dekker, 1988, pp 697–744.
109. Hall CL. Gold nephropathy. Nephron 1988;50:265–272.
110. Cush JJ, Goldings EA. Southwestern internal medicine conference: Drug-induced lupus: Clinical spectrum and pathogenesis. Am J Med Sci 1985;290:36–44.
111. Almirall J, Alcorta I, Botey A, Revert L. Penicillamine-induced rapidly progressive glomerulonephritis in a patient with rheumatoid arthritis. Am J Nephrol 1993;13:286–288.
112. Parker MG, Atkins MB, Ucci AA, Levey AS. Rapidly progressive glomerulonephritis after immunotherapy for cancer. J Am Soc Nephrol 1995;5:1740–1744.
113. Appel GB, D'Agati V, Bergman M, Pirani CL. Nephrotic syndrome and immune complex glomerulonephritis associated with chlorpropamide therapy. Am J Med 1983;74:337–342.
114. Chan TM, Cheng IKP, Wong KL, et al. Crescentic IgA glomerulonephritis following interleukin-2 therapy for hepatocellular carcinoma of the liver. Am J Nephrol 1991;11:493–496.
115. Oken DE. Hemodynamic basis for human acute renal failure (vasomotor nephropathy). Am J Med 1984;76:702–710.
116. Myers BD, Moran SM. Hemodynamically mediated acute renal failure. N Engl J Med 1986;314:97–105.
117. Humes HD. Aminoglycoside nephrotoxicity. Kidney Int 1988;33:900–911.
118. Eisenberg JM, Koffer H, Glick HA, et al. What is the cost of nephrotoxicity associated with aminoglycosides? Ann Int Med 1987;107:900–909.
119. Peterson OW, Gabbai FB, Myers RR, et al. A single nephron model of acute tubular injury: role of tubuloglomerular feedback. Kidney Int 1989;36:1037–1044.
120. Humes HD, Weinberg JM, Krauss TC. Clinical and pathophysiologic aspects of aminoglycoside nephrotoxicity. Am J Kidney Dis 1982;2:5–29.
121. Smith CR, Moore RD, Lietman PS. Studies of risk factors for aminoglycoside nephrotoxicity. Am J Kidney Dis 1986;8:308–313.
122. Bertino Jr JS, Booker LA, Franck PA, et al. Incidence of and significant risk factors for aminoglycoside associated nephrotoxicity in patients dosed by using individualized pharmacokinetic monitoring. J Infect Dis 1993;167:173–179.
123. Goetz MB, Sayers J. Nephrotoxicity of vancomycin and aminoglycoside therapy separately and in combination. J Antimicrob Chemother 1993;32:325–334.
124. Bailey RR, Lynn KL, Robson RA, et al. Comparison of ciprofloxacin with netilmicin for the treatment of acute pyelonephritis. NZ Med J 1992;105:102–103.
125. Bertino JS, Rodvold KA, Destache CJ. Cost considerations in therapeutic drug monitoring of aminoglycosides. Clin Pharmacokinet 1994;26:71–81.
126. Leehey DJ, Braun BI, Tholl DA, et al. Can pharmacokinetic dosing decrease nephrotoxicity associated with aminoglycoside therapy? J Am Soc Nephrol 1993;4:81–90.
127. Prins JM, Büller HR, Kuijper EJ, et al. Once versus thrice daily gentamicin in patients with serious infections. Lancet 1993;341:335–339.
128. Gilbert DN. Once-daily aminoglycoside therapy. Antimicrob Agents Chemother 1991;35:399–405.
129. Levison ME. New dosing regimens for aminoglycoside antibiotics. Ann Int Med 1992;117:693–694.

130. Rotschafer JC, Rybak MJ. Single dosing of aminoglycosides: A commentary. Ann Pharmacother 1994;28:797–801.
131. McLean AJ, Bastone EB, Ioannides-Demos LL, Spicer WJ. Bactericidal effect of gentamicin trough concentration provides a rationale for administration of bolus doses and maintenance of trough levels. J Antimicrob Chemother 1994;33:99–1004.
132. Ali BH, Bashir AA. Comparative modulating effects of captopril, diltiazem, dietary calcium and pyridoxal-5′phosphate on gentamicin-induced nephrotoxicity in the rat. Gen Pharmacol 1993;24:1279–1283.
133. Cronin RE. Southwestern internal medicine conference: Renal failure following radiologic procedures. Am J Med Sci 1989;298:342–356.
134. Barrett BJ. Contrast nephrotoxicity. J Am Soc Nephrol 1994;5:125–137.
135. Parfrey PS, Griffiths SM, Barrett BJ, et al. Contrast material–induced renal failure in patients with diabetes mellitus, renal insufficiency, or both: A prospective controlled study. N Engl J Med 1989;320:143–149.
136. Weisberg LS, Kurnik PB, Kurnik BRC. Risk of radiocontrast nephropathy in patients with and without diabetes mellitus. Kidney Int 1994;45:259–265.
137. McCarthy CS, Becker JS. Multiple myeloma and contrast media. Radiology 1992;183:519–521.
138. Cigarroa RG, Lange RA, Williams RH, Hillis LD. Dosing of contrast material to prevent contrast nephropathy in patients with renal disease. Am J Med 1989;86:649–652.
139. Schwab SJ, Hlatky MA, Pieper KS, et al. Contrast nephrotoxicity: A randomized controlled trial of a nonionic and an ionic radiographic contrast agent. N Engl J Med 1989;320:149–153.
140. Taliercio CP, Vlietstra RE, Ilstrup DM, et al. A randomized comparison of the nephrotoxicity of iopamidol and diatrizoate in high risk patients undergoing cardiac angiography. J Am Coll Cardiol 1991;17:384–390.
141. Katholi RE, Taylor GJ, Woods WT, et al. Nephrotoxicity of nonionic low-osmolality versus ionic high-osmolality contrast media: A prospective double-blind randomized comparison in human beings. Radiology 1993;186:183–187.
142. Rudnick MR, Goldfarb S, Wexler L, et al. Nephrotoxicity of ionic and nonionic contrast media in 1196 patients: A randomized trial. Kidney Int 1995;47:254–261.
143. Barrett BJ, Carlisle EJ. Metaanalysis of the relative nephrotoxicity of high- and low-osmolality iodinated contrast media. Radiology 1993;188:171–178.
144. Salem DN, Findlay SR, Isner JM, et al. Comparison of histamine release effects of ionic and non-ionic radiographic contrast media. Am J Med 1986;80:382–384.
145. Solomon R, Werner C, Mann D, et al. Effects of saline, mannitol, and furosemide on acute decreases in renal function induced by radiocontrast agents. N Engl J Med 1994;331:1416–1420.
146. Erley CM, Duda SH, Schlepckow S, et al. Adenosine antagonist theophylline prevents the reduction of glomerular filtration rate after contrast media application. Kidney Int 1994;45:1425–1431.
147. Cornelison TL, Reed E. Nephrotoxicity and hydration management for cisplatin, carboplatin, and ormaplatin. Gynecol Oncol 1992;50:147–158.
148. Anand AJ, Bashey B. Newer insights into cisplatin nephrotoxicity. Ann Pharmacother 1993;27:1519–1525.
149. Brillet G, Deray G, Jacquiaud C, et al. Long-term renal effect of cisplatin in man. Am J Nephrol 1994;14:81–84.
150. Butler WT, Bennett JE, Alling DW, et al. Nephrotoxicity of amphotericin B: Early and late effects in 81 patients. Ann Intern Med 1964;61:175–187.
151. Hoeprich PD. Clinical use of amphotericin B and derivatives: Lore, mystique, and fact. Clin Infect Dis 1992;14(suppl 1):S114–S119.
152. Burgess JL, Birchall R. Nephrotoxicity of amphotericin B, with emphasis on changes in tubular function. Am J Med 1972;53:77–84.
153. Fisher MA, Talbot GH, Maislin G, et al. Risk factors for amphotericin B-associated nephrotoxicity. Am J Med 1989;87:547–552.
154. Sabra R, Branch RA. Amphotericin B nephrotoxicity. Drug Saf 1990;5:94–108.
155. Bhathena DB, Bullock WE, Nuttall CE, Luke RG. The effects of amphotericin B therapy on the intrarenal vasculature and renal tubules in man. A study of renal biopsies by light, electron, and immunofluorescence microscopy. Clin Nephrol 1978;9:103–110.
156. Branch RA. Prevention of amphotericin B-induced renal impairment. A review on the use of sodium supplementation. Arch Intern Med 1988;48:2389–2394.
157. Llanos A, Cieza J, Bernardo J, et al. Effect of salt supplementation on amphotericin B nephrotoxicity. Kidney Int 1991;40:302–308.
158. Drutz DJ. Rapid infusion of amphotericin B: Is it safe, effective, and wise? Am J Med 1992;93:119–121.
159. Ralph ED, Barber KR, Grant CWM. Clinical experience with multilamellar liposomal amphotericin B in patients with proven and suspected fungal infections. Scand J Infect Dis 1993;25:487–496.
160. Ng TTC, Denning DW. Liposomal amphotericin B (AmBisome) therapy in invasive fungal infections. Arch Intern Med 1995;155:1093–1098.
161. Moreau P, Milpied N, Fayette N, et al. Reduced renal toxicity and improved clinical tolerance of amphotericin B mixed with Intralipid compared with convention amphotericin B in neutropenic patients. J Antimicro Chemother 1992;30:535–541.
162. Brouhard BH, Baetz-Greenwalt B. Calcium-channel blocking agents as therapy for amphotericin B nephrotoxicity. Cleve Clin J Med 1992;59:263–264.
163. Sattler FR, Cowan R, Nielsen DM, Ruskin J. Trimethoprim-sulfamethoxazole compared with pentamidine for treatment of *Pneumocystis carinii* pneumonia in the acquired immunodeficiency syndrome. A prospective, noncrossover study. Ann Intern Med 1988;109:280–287.
164. Lachaal M, Venuto RC. Nephrotoxicity and hyperkalemia in patients with acquired immunodeficiency syndrome treated with pentamidine. Am J Med 1989;87:260–263.
165. Cantor ES, Kimmel PL, Bosch JP. Effect of race on expression of acquired immunodeficiency syndrome associated nephropathy. Arch Intern Med 1991;151:125–128.
166. Shah GM, Alvarado P, Kirschenbaum MA. Symptomatic hypocalcemia and hypomagnesemia with renal magnesium

wasting associated with pentamidine therapy in a patient with AIDS. Am J Med 1990;89:380–382.
167. Antoniskis, Larsen RA. Acute, rapidly progressive renal failure with simultaneous use of amphotericin B and pentamidine. Antimicrob Agents Chemother 1990;34:470–472.
168. Deray G, Martinez F, Katlama C, et al. Foscarnet nephrotoxicity: Mechanism, incidence and prevention. Am J Nephrol 1989;9:316–321.
169. Smith GH. Treatment of infections in the patient with acquired immunodeficiency syndrome. Arch Intern Med 1994;154:949–973.
170. Toto RD. Review: Acute tubulointerstitial nephritis. Am J Med Sci 1990;299:392–410.
171. Linton AL, Clark WF, Driedger AA, et al. Acute interstitial nephritis due to drugs. Review of the literature with a report of nine cases. Ann Intern Med 1980;93:735–741.
172. Ditlove J, Weidmann P, Bernstein M, Massry SG. Methicillin nephritis. Medicine 1977;56:483–491.
173. Kleinknecht D, Vanhille P, Morel-Maroger L, et al. Acute interstitial nephritis due to drug hypersensitivity. An up-to-date review with a report of 19 cases. Adv Nephrol 1983;12:277–308.
174. Ten RM, Torres VE, Milliner DS, et al. Acute interstitial nephritis: Immunologic and clinical aspects. Mayo Clin Proc 1988;63:921–930.
175. Nolan CR, Anger MS, Kelleher SP. Eosinophiluria—a new method of detection and definition of the clinical spectrum. N Engl J Med 1986;315:1516–1519.
176. Averbuch SD, Austin HA III, Sherwin SA, et al. Acute interstitial nephritis with the nephrotic syndrome following recombinant leukocyte A interferon therapy for mycosis fungoides. N Engl J Med 1984;310:32–35.
177. Feinfeld DA, D'Agati V, Dutcher JP, et al. Interstitial nephritis in a patient receiving adoptive immunotherapy with recombinant interleukin-2 and lymphokine-activated killer cells. Am J Nephrol 1991;11:489–492.
178. Hansen PB, Johnsen HE, Hippe E. Hypereosinophilic syndrome treated with alpha-interferon and granulocyte colony-stimulating factor but complicated by nephrotoxicity. Am J Hematol 1993;43:66–68.
179. Cryst C, Hammar SP. Acute granulomatous interstitial nephritis due to co-trimoxazole. Am J Nephrol 1988;8:483–488.
180. Shear NH, Spielberg SP, Grant DM, et al. Differences in metabolism of sulfonamides predisposing to idiosyncratic toxicity. Ann Intern Med 1986;105:179–184.
181. Walker RG. Lithium nephrotoxicity. Kidney Int 1993;44(suppl 42):S93–S98.
182. Simard M, Gumbiner B, Lee A, Lewis H, Norman D. Lithium carbonate intoxication. A case report and review of the literature. Arch Intern Med 1989;149:36–46.
183. Fenves AZ, Emmett M, White MG. Lithium intoxication associated with acute renal failure. South Med J 1984;77:1472–1474.
184. Batlle DC, von Riotte AB, Gaviria M, Grupp M. Amelioration of polyuria by amiloride in patients receiving long-term lithium therapy. N Engl J Med 1985;312:408–414.
185. Bendz H. Kidney function in lithium-treated patients. A literature survey. Acta Psychiatr Scand 1983;68:303–324.
186. Hestbech J, Hensen HE, Amdisen A, Olsen S. Chronic renal lesions following long-term treatment with lithium. Kidney Int 1977;12:205–213.
187. Kincaid-Smith P, Burrows GD, Davies BM, et al. Renal biopsy findings in lithium and prelithium patients. Lancet 1979;2:700–701.
188. Lokkegaard H, Andersen NF, Henriksen E, et al. Renal function in 153 manic-depressive patients treated with lithium for more than five years. Acta Psychiatr Scand 1985;71:347–355.
189. Jorkasky DK, Amsterdam JD, Oler J, et al. Lithium-induced renal disease: A prospective study. Clin Nephrol 1988;30:293–302.
190. Waller DG, Edwards JG, Papasthatis-Papayanni S. A longitudinal assessment of renal function during treatment with lithium. Q J Med 1988;255:553–558.
191. Simon G. Combination angiotensin converting enzyme inhibitor/lithium therapy contraindicated in renal disease. Am J Med 1988;85:893–894.
192. Dubach UC, Rosner B, Sturmer T. An epidemiologic study of abuse of analgesic drugs. Effects of phenacetin and salicylate on mortality and cardiovascular morbidity (1968 to 1987). N Engl J Med 1991;324:155–160.
193. Nanra RS. Analgesic nephropathy in the 1990s—an Australian perspective. Kidney Int 1993;44(suppl 42):S86–S92.
194. Hoffbrand BI. Dapsone and renal papillary necrosis. Br Med J 1978;1:78.
195. Buckalew VM, Schey HM. Analgesic nephropathy: A significant cause of morbidity in the United States. Am J Kidney Dis 1986;7:164–168.
196. Piper JM, Tonascia J, Matanoski GM. Heavy phenacetin use and bladder cancer in women aged 20 to 49 years. N Engl J Med 1985;313:292–295.
197. Bennett WM, DeBroe ME. Analgesic nephropathy—a preventable renal disease. N Engl J Med 1989;320:1269–1271.
198. Pommer W, Bronder E, Greiser E, et al. Regular analgesic intake and the risk of end-stage renal failure. Am J Nephrol 1989;9:409–412.
199. Sandler DP, Smith JC, Weinberg CR, et al. Analgesic use and chronic renal disease. N Engl J Med 1989;320:1238–1243.
200. Segasothy M, Samad SA, Zulfigar A, Bennett WM. Chronic renal diseases and papillary necrosis associated with the long-term use of nonsteroidal anti-inflammatory drugs as the sole or predominant analgesic. Am J Kidney Dis 1994;24:17–24.
201. Bach PH, Hardy TL. Relevance of animal models to analgesic-associated renal papillary necrosis in humans. Kidney Int 1985;28:605–613.
202. Eknoyan G. Analgesic nephrotoxicity and renal papillary necrosis. Semin Nephrol 1984;4:65–76.
203. Zenser TV, Mattammal MB, Rapp NS, Davis BB. Effect of aspirin on metabolism of acetaminophen and benzidine by renal inner medulla prostaglandin hydroperoxidase. J Lab Clin Med 1983;101:58–65.
204. McCredie M, Stewart JH, Mathew TH, et al. The effect of withdrawal of phenacetin-containing analgesics on the incidence of kidney and urothelial cancer and renal failure. Clin Nephrol 1989;31:35–39.

205. Hauser AC, Derfler K, Balcke P. Progression of renal insufficiency in analgesic nephropathy: Impact of continuous drug abuse. J Clin Epidemiol 1991;44:53–56.
206. Fer MF, McKinney TD, Richardson RL, et al. Cancer and the kidney: Renal complications of neoplasms. Am J Med 1981;71:704–718.
207. Strom BL, West SL, Sim E, Carson JL. The epidemiology of the acute flank pain syndrome from suprofen. Clin Pharmacol Ther 1989;46:693–699.
208. Cadnapaphornchai P, Taher S, McDonald FD. Acute drug-associated rhabdomyolysis: An examination of its diverse renal manifestations and complications. Am J Med Sci 1980;280:66–72.
209. Patel R, Connor G. A review of 30 cases of rhabdomyolysis-associated acute renal failure among phencyclidine users. Clin Toxicol 1985–86;23:547–556.
210. Rumpf KW, Henning HV. Rhabdomyolysis and β-adrenoceptor agonists. Nephron 1990;55:346–347.
211. Roth D, Alarcón FJ, Fernandez JA, et al. Acute rhabdomyolysis associated with cocaine intoxication. N Engl J Med 1988;319:673–677.
212. Affarah HB, Mars RL, Someren A, et al. Myoglobinuria and acute renal failure associated with intravenous vasopressin infusion. South Med J 1984;77:918–921.
213. Alejandro DSJ, Peterson J. Myoglobinuric acute renal failure in a cardiac transplant patient taking lovastatin and cyclosporine. J Am Soc Nephrol 1994;5:153–160.
214. Rossert J, Rondeau E, Jondeau G, et al. Tamm-Horsfall protein accumulation in glomeruli during acetazolamide-induced acute renal failure. Am J Nephrol 1989;9:56–57.
215. Hein R, Brunkhorst R, Thon WF, et al. Symptomatic sulfadiazine crystalluria in AIDS patients: a report of two cases. Clin Nephrol 1993;39:254–256.
216. Krieble BF, Rudy DW, Glick MR, Clayman MD. Case report: Acyclovir neurotoxicity and nephrotoxicity—the role for hemodialysis. Am J Med Sci 1993;305:36–39.
217. Eck P, Silver SM, Clark EC. Acute renal failure and coma after a high dose of oral acyclovir. N Engl J Med 1991;325:1178.
218. Lawton JM, Conway LT, Crosson JT, et al. Acute oxalate nephropathy after massive ascorbic acid administration. Arch Intern Med 1985;145:950–951.
219. Coggins CH, Fang LS-T. Acute renal failure associated with antibiotics, anesthetic agents, and radiographic contrast agents, In Brenner BM, Lazarus JM (eds): Acute Renal Failure. Philadelphia, WB Saunders, 1983, pp 283–320.
220. Feest TG. Low molecular weight dextran: A continuing cause of acute renal failure. Br Med J 1976;2:1300.
221. Roy LF, Villeneuve J-P, Dumont A, et al. Irreversible renal failure associated with triamterene. Am J Nephrol 1991;11:486–488.
222. Biberstein M, Parker BA. Enema-induced hyperphosphatemia. Am J Med 1985;79:645–646.
223. Wilson C, Azmy AF, Beattie TJ, Murphy AV. Hypermagnesemia and progression of renal failure associated with renacidin therapy. Clin Nephrol 1986;25:266–267.
224. Critchley JAJH, Smith MF, Prescott LF. Distalgesic abuse and retroperitoneal fibrosis. Br J Urol 1985;57:486–487.
225. Danziger LH, Horn JR. Disopyramide-induced urinary retention: Report of nine cases and review of the literature. Arch Intern Med 1983;143:1683–1686.
226. Hricik DE, Goldsmith GH. Uric acid nephrolithiasis and acute renal failure secondary to streptozotocin nephrotoxicity. Am J Med 1988;84:153–156.
227. Kranen S, Keough D, Gordon RB, Emerson BT. Xanthine-containing calculi during allopurinol therapy. J Urol 1985;133:658–659.
228. Millette CH, Snodgrass GL. Acute renal failure associated with chronic antacid ingestion. Am J Hosp Pharm 1981;38:1352–1355.
229. Dick WH, Lingeman JE, Preminger GM, et al. Laxative abuse as a cause for ammonium urate renal calculi. J Urol 1990;143:244–247.
230. Birnbaum J, Kahan FM, Kropp H, MacDonald JS. Carbapenems, a new class of β-lactam antibiotics. Discovery and development of imipenem/cilastatin. Am J Med 1985;78(suppl 6A):3–21.

Chapter 48

Nephrolithiasis

Charles L. Smith, MD, and David R. P. Guay, PharmD, FCP

Renal stone disease is a common disorder estimated to occur in approximately 12% of the population with an annual incidence in the United States of 1.6/1000.[1] The recurrence rate is 70–81% in males and 47–60% in females.[2] For these reasons, an understanding of the pathophysiology and treatment of stone disease is warranted.

Stone Formation

There are three requirements for clinical stone disease to occur. First, a nidus must form. Second, this nidus must be retained within the urinary tract. Third, the nidus must grow to sufficient size to become radiologically apparent or to obstruct the ureter. Three theories have been proposed to explain nidus formation. The first is the matrix theory.[3] All stones, regardless of their crystalline composition, consist of 2–3% organic material. The matrix theory proposes that this organic material is the initiating mechanism of calculus formation. A mucoprotein unique to stone formers condenses in the urine to serve as the core for mineral precipitation. Conflicting studies have appeared regarding the uniqueness of this protein to stone formers. Furthermore it now appears that the mucoprotein found in stones is not essential to the initiation of stone formation but is simply adsorbed to the surface of crystals.[4] Currently most people working in this area do not accept a role for matrix as an initiating event. It may, however, play a role in protecting crystals from dissolution.

The second theory is the inhibitor deficiency theory.[5] Urine is a complex fluid that contains a number of inhibitors of crystallization.[6] Some of these are citrate, sulphate, pyrophosphate, magnesium, glycosaminoglycans, ribonucleotides, and nephrocalcin. These inhibitors have been shown to inhibit nucleation, crystal growth, and crystal aggregation, all of which are processes considered important to stone formation. The inhibitor deficiency theory proposes there is a decrease in inhibitor activity in the urine of stone formers that allows precipitation to occur.

Two potential inhibitors, citrate and nephrocalcin, have been extensively studied. Urinary citrate excretion has been reported to be low in from 12%[7] to 55%[8] of stone formers. There is considerable overlap between stone formers and non-stone formers in urinary citrate excretion and sequential studies suggest that hypocitraturia is not present consistently.[9] Thus, the true prevalence of hypocitraturia and its significance to stone formation awaits further study. Nephrocalcin is an acid glycoprotein that inhibits calcium oxalate crystal growth.[10] This macromolecule may provide 90% of the inhibitory potential of human urine for calcium oxalate crystal growth.[10] The glycoprotein from non-stone formers contains γ-carboxyglutamic acid residues, whereas none can be found in stone formers.[11] The potential role of this abnormal macromolecule in stone formation is still being studied.

The third theory is the precipitation–crystallization theory. This theory relies on the recognized regions of saturation that exist in an aqueous solution containing minerals.[12] These regions are defined by the solubility product and the formation product. The solubility product is that level of saturation where the liquid phase is in equilibrium with solid phase. The formation product is the level of saturation where spontaneous nucleation occurs. Below the solubility product, the solution is undersaturated. Between the solubility product and the formation product, the solution is supersaturated, a region called metastable. Above the formation product, the solution is oversaturated and spontaneous nucleation (or crystal nidus formation) occurs. The precipitation–crystallization theory proposes that periods of oversaturation occur that result in precipitation of a crystalline nidus that initiates stone disease. When levels of saturation between stone formers and non-stone formers have been compared, the levels in stone formers are higher. However, extensive overlap between the two groups is present, suggesting that the level of saturation is not a sufficient explanation for stone formation. The level of saturation is nevertheless important. Crystallization cannot occur, whether matrix is present or absent and whether inhibitors are present or absent, if a state of supersaturation does not exist.

The renal papilla is considered to be the site where stone formation occurs.[13] Crystals form within the nephron and abnormalities in the mucin layer of the urinary tract could result in adherence of crystals to the epithelial lining[14] and, thus, stone formation.[15] The particles become fixed and grow by continuous exposure to supersaturated urine. Randall plaques are areas of papillary subepithelial calcification that may also serve as a site for stone formation.[16]

Crystal growth, crystal aggregation, and epitaxy are processes that can increase the crystalline mass. Since crystal growth rate is related to the degree of supersaturation of the urine, the higher the level of supersaturation the more rapidly crystals grow. Inhibitors have also been described that prevent or retard crystal growth and could play a role in stone formation by altering the rate of crystal growth. When the formation product is exceeded, many nuclei are formed and these can aggregate to increase the crystalline mass. Inhibitors of crystal aggregation have been described but their role, if any, in stone formation is not known. Aggregates of crystals tend to be found more in stone formers than non-stone formers, and this has been interpreted as evidence for an abnormality in crystal aggregation.[17] Epitaxy involves the growth of crystals of one material on the surface of a different material. This process is also poorly understood, although many possible combinations based on the fit of crystal surfaces are possible.[18] Most kidney stones grow by a combination of all three of these processes.

Calcium-Containing Stones

Four primary types of stones are recovered from patients (Table 48.1). Approximately 90% of all stones analyzed contain calcium.[19] Although pure calcium oxalate or calcium phosphate stones occur, most calcium stones (50–65%) are a mixture of both types of stone material.[19,20] This section deals with the risk factors for and management of calcium oxalate/calcium phosphate stone disease[21] (Table 48.2).

PATHOGENESIS

The precipitation of calcium oxalate and calcium phosphate is dependent on the concentrations of calcium and oxalate or phosphorous in the urine and the presence or absence of inhibitors of precipitation. In addition, calcium phosphate precipitation is pH sensitive; that is, solubility decreases as the urine pH increases. Thus, hypercalciuria predisposes to both calcium oxalate and calcium phosphate precipitation, while hyperoxaluria predisposes to calcium oxalate precipitation and increased urine pH to calcium phosphate precipitation. Hypercalciuria is the most common risk factor identified in calcium stone formers: It is present in 40–75% of patients.[22,23] Disorders associated with hypercalciuria are listed in Table 48.3.

TABLE 48.1. STONE COMPOSITION

Component(s)	%[a]
Calcium (both oxalate and phosphates)	77
Uric acid	9
Struvite	8
Cystine	2
Others	4

[a]Based on Refs. 19 and 20.

TABLE 48.2. RISK FACTORS FOR CALCIUM STONE DISEASE

Hypercalciuria
Hyperoxaluria
Hyperuricosuria
Alkaline urine
Decreased inhibitors
Low urine volume

Hypercalciuria

Idiopathic hypercalciuria occurs in 40–60% of all stone formers,[24,25] is characterized by urinary calcium excretion in excess of that expected for the level of calcium intake, a normal level of total serum calcium, and the absence of systemic disorders that could lead to excessive calcium excretion.[26] There is controversy surrounding the pathophysiology of this condition. Most agree that there is increased intestinal absorption of calcium.[26,27] Whether this is a primary abnormality of intestinal transport or secondary to an abnormality in vitamin D metabolism or renal handling of calcium or phosphorus remains controversial.

Intestinal transport of calcium occurs by both active and passive processes. Active transport occurs in the duodenum, whereas passive transport occurs in the jejunum, ileum, and colon. The active transport system in the duodenum is stimulated by vitamin D.[28] The role of vitamin D in the more distal segments is unclear, but studies in humans suggest that this can be stimulated by 1,25-dihydroxyvitamin D_3.[29] Intestinal hyperabsorption of calcium in idiopathic hypercalciuria is not dependent on vitamin D; this suggests a primary abnormality in permeability of the brush

TABLE 48.3. DISORDERS ASSOCIATED WITH HYPERCALCIURIA

Idiopathic hypercalciuria	Renal tubular acidosis
Dietary calcium excess	Sarcoidosis
Dietary sodium excess	Thyrotoxicosis
Dietary protein excess	Hypervitaminosis D
Immobilization	Glucocorticoid excess
Primary hyperparathyroidism	Paget's disease of bone

border membrane.[30,31] Balance studies, however, have demonstrated that for the same net intestinal absorption of calcium, the calcium excretion is higher in patients with idiopathic hypercalciuria than in normal individuals.[32] This finding is not compatible with a simple abnormality in brush border membrane permeability. To account for this balance data, a more widespread abnormality in calcium metabolism would have to exist and derangements in vitamin D metabolism have been suggested.

The three major circulating metabolites of vitamin D are 25-hydroxyvitamin D, 1,25-dihydroxyvitamin D, and 24,25-dihydroxyvitamin D.[33] The serum level of 25-hydroxyvitamin D is considered the best measurement of nutritional vitamin D status. 1,25-dihydroxyvitamin D is considered the most active metabolite in stimulating intestinal calcium absorption, while 24,25-dihydroxyvitamin D is probably biologically inactive.[33] The level of 25-hydroxyvitamin D has been found by most investigators to be normal in idiopathic hypercalciuria[34] but a few studies have shown elevated levels.[35,36] The mild elevations found in these latter studies would not be expected to stimulate intestinal calcium transport directly, and, in this range, there is no relation between serum concentrations of 25-hydroxyvitamin D and 1,25 dihydroxyvitamin D.[34] A lack of correlation between the serum concentration of 25-hydroxyvitamin D and urinary calcium excretion[35] suggests that these mild elevations are not of pathogenic significance.

Intestinal calcium absorption is stimulated primarily by 1,25-dihydroxyvitamin D. Studies have revealed elevated levels of this metabolite in calcium stone formers.[34,37,38] Although there is disagreement as to the cause of the elevated levels of 1,25-dihydroxyvitamin D, increased parathyroid hormone and decreased phosphorus levels alter 1,25-dihydroxyvitamin D levels[33] and both have been implicated in the pathogenesis of idiopathic hypercalciuria. Early in the description of idiopathic hypercalciuria, it was proposed that the cause was abnormal calcium handling by the kidney.[26] Approximately 99% of calcium filtered at the glomerulus is reabsorbed by the renal tubule. A primary defect in tubular reabsorption of calcium would result in an increased excretion of calcium. This defect would lower the serum ionized calcium and stimulate parathyroid hormone secretion, which in turn would increase the production of 1,25-dihydroxyvitamin D resulting in increased intestinal calcium absorption. This is the proposed mechanism of the renal leak form of idiopathic hypercalciuria.[39] Others have questioned the existence of the renal leak form of idiopathic hypercalciuria.[40] Hypophosphatemia results in increased 1,25-dihydroxyvitamin D levels, increased intestinal calcium absorption, and hypercalciuria.[33] Although renal tubular phosphate wasting also has been proposed as the mechanism for hyperabsorption of dietary calcium,[38] others have not been able to confirm this.[37,41]

A primary abnormality in vitamin D metabolism with increased production of 1,25-dihydroxyvitamin D has also been considered.[32,37] When 1,25-dihydroxyvitamin is administered to healthy non-stone formers, there is an increase in intestinal calcium absorption, a suppression of parathyroid hormone secretion, a decrease in renal tubular reabsorption of calcium, an increase in the fasting calcium excretion, and hypercalciuria.[42] When combined with a low calcium diet, large doses of 1,25-dihydroxyvitamin D may result in a negative calcium balance and bone resorption.[42,43] This model in many aspects resembles idiopathic hypercalciuria. The serum phosphorus, however, tends to be high, while in idiopathic hypercalciuria it tends to be low.[43]

Pak et al.[39] have proposed the following subclassification of idiopathic hypercalciuria. Absorptive hypercalciuria is divided into three types. Type I absorptive hypercalciuria is due to intestinal hyperabsorption, and these individuals remain hypercalciuric on a low-calcium diet. Type II absorptive hypercalciuric individuals have normal calcium excretion when eating a calcium-restricted diet. Type III absorptive hypercalciuria is intestinal hyperabsorption associated with hypophosphatemia. Renal leak hypercalciuria is evidenced by an elevated fasting calcium–creatinine ratio along with evidence of increased parathyroid hormone activity—while resorptive hypercalciuria is due to primary hyperparathyroidism.

Dietary Factors Associated with Stone Formation

A number of dietary factors have been implicated in calcium stone formation.[44] Excessive dietary calcium is seldom a cause of hypercalciuria. Although net absorption increases as dietary calcium goes up, this is moderated by a decrease in fractional absorption. Intakes must be in excess of 2000 mg/d to result in hypercalciuria.[45] Dietary sodium intake also influences urinary calcium excretion. In normal individuals, for each 100 mEq/d increase in urinary sodium, there is approximately a 25 mg/d increase in urinary calcium.[46] However, some patients show a remarkable sensitivity to sodium with hypercalciuria that is virtually unrelated to calcium intake but dependent on a high sodium intake.[47] High dietary animal protein intake has been related to an increase in urinary calcium and oxalate concentration and an increased risk of stone disease.[48] Similarly, glucose loading has been suggested to increase urinary calcium and oxalate excretion.[49]

Patient Activity

Immobilization (e.g., prolonged bed rest) results in an increase in urinary calcium excretion secondary to bone resorption.[50] This results in a suppression of parathyroid hormone and a fall in the circulating levels of 1,25-dihydroxyvitamin D.[51] The suppression of parathyroid hormone results in a fall in renal tubular calcium reabsorption and a rise in the fasting calcium excretion. There is also a fall in intestinal calcium absorption secondary to decreased levels of 1,25-dihydroxyvitamin D,[52] which makes dietary therapy of limited usefulness.

Primary Hyperparathyroidism

Around 5% of stone formers seen at referral centers have primary hyperparathyroidism.[25] Excessive parathyroid hormone secretion from either a single adenomatous gland or four hyperplastic glands results in increased bone resorption. The high parathyroid hormone also stimulates the production of 1,25-dihydroxyvitamin D and, therefore, intestinal absorption of calcium. Hypercalciuria thus has an absorptive component as well as a bone resorptive component. Supersaturation of the urine for both calcium oxalate and calcium phosphate occurs with subsequent stone formation.[53]

Although most patients with primary hyperparathyroidism have hypercalciuria, only 50% develop stones.[54] Those who form stones have been found by some to have a higher urinary calcium excretion.[52,55] This may be due to the presence of higher levels of 1,25-dihydroxyvitamin D in the stone formers, which leads to an augmented intestinal absorption of calcium.[55] Other investigators have been unable to demonstrate differences between stone formers and non-stone formers in levels of urinary calcium excretion, circulating levels of 1,25-dihydroxyvitamin D, or fractional intestinal calcium absorption.[56] The possibility of changes in inhibitor activity between the stone forming and non-stone forming patients with primary hyperparathyroidism has been suggested.[56] However, citrate excretion has been found to be the same or lower in stone formers, and magnesium excretion has been similar in both groups.[57,58] Excretion of pyrophosphate is controversial.[59,60] An interesting observation is that although the excretion of total acid mucopolysaccharide is not different between stone formers and non-stone formers with primary hyperparathyroidism, the potency of these substances to prevent calcium oxalate precipitation is less in the stone formers.[61]

In summary, most patients with primary hyperparathyroidism have hypercalciuria, which is secondary to resorptive and absorptive changes. This hypercalciuria results in supersaturation of the urine for calcium oxalate and calcium phosphate. Only 50% of patients with primary hyperparathyroidism form stones; this may be due to higher circulating levels of 1,25-dihydroxyvitamin D and thus a larger absorptive component to the hypercalciuria in those forming stones. The degree of hypercalciuria thus becomes diet dependent, introducing variability in the expression of renal stone disease.

Renal Tubular Acidosis

Renal tubular acidosis (RTA) can be defined as a reduction in the kidney's ability to excrete sufficient hydrogen ions to maintain a normal acid–base balance that is out of proportion to any reduction in renal mass. The three basic types of RTA are distal (classic, type I, or gradient limited), proximal (bicarbonate wasting or type II), and hyperkalemic renal tubular acidosis (type IV).[62] Renal stone disease has not been associated with type IV RTA. This is surprising since these individuals tend to have persistently acid urine with low urinary ammonia levels reminiscent of idiopathic uric acid stone formers (see section on Urates and Stones).[62]

Likewise, type II RTA, which occurs most often in children and usually with other abnormalities in proximal tubular transport, such as phosphaturia, glycosuria, uricosuria, and aminoaciduria (known as the Fanconi syndrome), is generally not considered to result in stone formation.[63] The underlying defect in type II RTA is a decrease in the threshold for proximal tubular reabsorption of bicarbonate. This resetting of the threshold for bicarbonate reabsorption results in a wasting of bicarbonate in the urine until the threshold is reached. When the threshold is reached, no more bicarbonate is lost in the urine, but hypobicarbonatemia and hyperchloremia are present. Acid–base balance is restored,[64] accounting for the lack of hypercalciuria in this form of RTA. This and the presence of normal to high urinary citrate levels[65] as well as the potential of calcium complexation by amino acids[66] may explain the rarity of nephrolithiasis in type II RTA.

Acetazolamide and dichlorphenamide are carbonic anhydrase inhibitors that produce a tubular abnormality in bicarbonate reabsorption similar to proximal RTA and both have been associated with calcium stone formation.[67] Unlike isolated proximal RTA or that associated with Fanconi's syndrome, drug-induced proximal tubular bicarbonate wasting is associated with low citrate excretion.[68] Despite this decrease in urinary citrate in virtually all patients, only 4–8% develop nephrolithiasis.[69,70] Hypercalciuria existing prior to the administration of a carbonic anhydrase inhibitor may thus be required before stone formation will occur.[70]

Distal renal tubular acidosis (type I) is associated with nephrocalcinosis, nephrolithiasis, and metabolic bone disease.[62] This type of RTA is characterized by an inability to generate and/or maintain a steep hydrogen-ion gradient across the collecting duct epithelium. Thus, there is an inability to lower the urine pH maximally, even when a systemic acidosis is present and plasma bicarbonate is markedly reduced.[62] Distal RTA can present in the complete form with a depression of plasma bicarbonate and elevation of plasma chloride or, more commonly, it can present with normal serum electrolytes (incomplete form).[62,71]

The risk factors for stone disease associated with distal RTA are hypercalciuria, persistently alkaline urine, and hypocitraturia.[71] The calcium excretion in patients with distal RTA has varied from normal to markedly elevated.[72] It would appear that those with marked hypercalciuria have an associated idiopathic hypercalciuria.[72] Indeed, it has been proposed that the hypercalciuria results in tubular damage leading to renal tubular acidosis.[73] Many patients with distal RTA, however, either do not have hypercalciuria or it is mild.[72]

Several mechanisms have been proposed to explain the mild hypercalciuria associated with distal RTA. Balance studies in normal individuals with induced metabolic acidosis suggest that there is an ongoing positive net balance of acid.[74] It was proposed that the acid not excreted by the kidneys and not buffered by the bicarbonate buffer system was disposed of by buffers fixed in tissues, namely, bone. This would result in the mobilization of calcium from bone and account for both the hypercalciuria and the osteopenia that has been described. This proposal is supported by the finding that the administration of alkali leads to a reversal of the positive acid balance[75] and to a decrease in urinary calcium excretion.[76] Against this mechanism of hypercalciuria is the finding that parathyroid hormone levels are elevated in distal RTA.[77] Suppressed levels would be expected if acidosis was mobilizing calcium from bone.

Metabolic acidosis may decrease renal tubular reabsorption of calcium resulting in an increase in urinary calcium excretion.[78] This mechanism could explain the development of secondary hyperparathyroidism and the reversal of excess parathyroid hormone secretion and hypercalciuria with alkali therapy. However, it should lead to the development of osteitis fibrosa cystica or hyperparathyroid bone disease while, in fact, rickets in children and osteomalacia in adults are the lesions usually present.[79] These defects in the mineralization of bone suggest an abnormality in vitamin D metabolism. Indeed, the generation of 1,25-dihydroxyvitamin D in the kidney has been found to be impaired in the presence of metabolic acidosis.[80] Thus metabolic acidosis could lead to low circulating levels of 1,25-dihydroxyvitamin D and result in impaired intestinal calcium absorption and bone mineralization.

Hypocitraturia is a common if not universal finding in both complete and incomplete distal RTA.[81] Citrate is an inhibitor of calcium phosphate precipitation, and citrate deficiency represents a major risk factor for calcium stone disease. Urinary citrate excretion is altered by changes in systemic pH with acidosis leading to a decrease and alkalosis to an increase in excretion.[82] Calcium phosphate is the most common component of stones formed in distal RTA.[83] Alkaline urine as found in distal RTA markedly decreases the solubility of calcium phosphate, thus contributing to the stone formation.

Hyperoxaluria and Other Risk Factors

Hyperoxaluria results in an increase in urinary supersaturation for calcium oxalate. Hyperoxaluria can be either primary or secondary (Table 48.4). Primary hyperoxaluria is a rare disorder of glyoxylate metabolism; it occurs primarily in children and leads to renal failure secondary to oxalate deposition, usually before the second decade of life.[84] Two types of this disorder exist and two distinct biochemical abnormalities have been identified. Both lead to marked hyperoxaluria and follow an autosomal recessive mode of inheritance.

TABLE 48.4. CAUSES OF HYPEROXALURIA

Primary
Type I: glycolic aciduria
Type II: L-glyceric aciduria
Secondary
Increased dietary intake
Decreased dietary calcium intake
Excessive vitamin C intake (?)
Enteric
Pyridoxine deficiency
Ethylene glycol
Methoxyflurane
Xylitol

Hyperoxaluria more commonly develops as the result of a high dietary intake of oxalate. Foods such as rhubarb, spinach, chocolate, tea, nuts, and peanut butter have been found to have high levels of oxalate. Unfortunately, few studies have been done to assess bioavailability of the oxalate from these foods. Another dietary factor that can increase oxalate excretion is a low dietary calcium intake.[85] Any decrease in available dietary calcium will result in more oxalate being available for absorption. There seems to be greater augmentation of urinary oxalate excretion on a low calcium diet in those patients with underlying idiopathic hypercalciuria.[86]

Although vitamin C ingestion in excess of 4 g/d has been reported to increase urinary oxalate levels,[87] a subsequent assessment in normal individuals failed to show an effect of vitamin C (8 g/d) on urinary oxalate excretion.[88] The possibility exists that there is a difference between stone formers and non-stone formers in how they handle ascorbic acid. Evidence has been presented suggesting a greater rise in urinary oxalate in stone formers than in non-stone formers following oral ascorbate loading.[89] Although pyridoxine deficiency in experimental animals results in hyperoxaluria,[90] hyperoxaluria in humans based on this etiology is rare.

Intestinal disease associated with fat malabsorption may also result in hyperoxaluria. This "enteric" hyperoxaluria occurs when malabsorbed fat binds dietary calcium, thus freeing oxalate for absorption. Although this has been a major complication of jejunoileal bypass operations for obesity or blood lipid control, it may also develop secondary to fat malabsorption from any bowel disease.

Inhibitor deficiency has been proposed[5] as an etiology for calcium stone disease; the occurrence of this condition in the presence of hypocitraturia associated with distal RTA,[81] acetazolamide therapy,[68] and enteric hyperoxaluria[91] support the hypothesis. Idiopathic hypocitraturia has been described[92] but as yet not confirmed. A role for hyperuricosuria to decrease inhibitor activity of glycosaminoglycans is discussed in the section on uric acid stone disease. Deficiencies of magnesium, pyrophosphate, or glycosaminoglycans have not been convincingly demonstrated. Low urine volume is also a risk factor for calcium stone disease[21] in that it increases the level of supersaturation for both calcium phosphate and calcium oxalate.[93] Because urine volumes are an obvious continuum in any population, it is difficult to define "low urine volume." In our experience, urine volumes of less than 1000 mL/d represent a significant independent risk factor.

CLINICAL CHARACTERISTICS

Calcium stone disease constitutes approximately 80% of all stone disease and can occur in newborns and the very elderly. The highest incidence, however, is in adults between 20–40 years of age. Idiopathic hypercalciuria is the most common etiology in all age groups. However, in children, inherited disorders such as primary hyperoxaluria or distal RTA should be considered[94] as should primary hyperparathyroidism and drug-induced (i.e., acetazolamide) stone disease in the elderly.

Clinical presentation can be totally asymptomatic or be accompanied by the severe pain of renal colic. Whether or not a stone passes is related to the size of the stone.[95] Stones less than 4 mm pass spontaneously 93% of the time, stones 4–6 mm pass in 53% of cases, and stones greater than 6 mm rarely pass spontaneously. Calcium stone disease seldom leads to renal damage even in those patients with frequent stone passage. The exceptions to this are patients with primary hyperoxaluria, enteric hyperoxaluria, distal RTA, or superimposed infection. These patients need aggressive management to prevent loss of renal function. Recurrence of calcium stone disease is the rule. There is a recurrence rate of 70–80% within 20 years[2] and the rate does not appear to decrease with age.[96]

MANAGEMENT

Maintenance treatment of calcium stone disease is usually focused on reversing the metabolic defect(s) responsible for stone formation. The five elements of the "selective approach" to therapy are that it (1) corrects the physicochemical abnormality in urine, (2) overcomes physiological derangements in patients with stones, (3) inhibits stone formation, (4) does not cause significant side effects, and (5) prevents extrarenal manifestations of the disease process. Utilization of the selective treatment approach to calcium stone disease has been documented to reduce significantly new stone formation and the need for operative intervention.[97,98]

In general, therapeutic intervention revolves around reducing the urinary concentration of stone forming materials and/or increasing the urinary concentration of inhibitors (Table 48.5). Fluid intake is important in reducing the urinary concentration of stone forming substances. A fluid intake sufficient to ensure a urine output of at least 2 L/d is recommended and has been shown to reduce the level of urinary saturation.[93] However, a recent study has questioned the ability of a large diuresis to prevent stone formation in recurrent stone formers.[99] Tea and cola drinks should be avoided due to their oxalate content. Diuresis due to xanthine-containing beverages may also be problematic due to the dehydration risk. Salt intake should be reduced to modest levels through the avoidance of high-salt foods and use of salt after food preparation.[100] The use of a low-calcium diet as discussed below is controversial.[101] Even bringing calcium intake to the RDA (800 mg/d) should be accompanied by a restriction in dietary oxalate. Dietary calcium restriction below 800 mg/d should be avoided since a low-calcium diet will worsen the already decreased bone mineral content in such patients.[102]

Hyperabsorption of calcium due to absorptive hypercalciuria type I can be treated by means of a 800 mg/d calcium diet plus pharmacotherapy with a thiazide diuretic or an agent that will bind calcium in the gut to prevent its absorption, such as sodium phytate[103] or sodium cellulose phosphate.[104] Thiazide diuretics and an 800 mg/d calcium diet is the recommended approach for absorptive hypercalciuria type I in individuals at risk of bone disease (example, pediatric patients or postmenopausal females). Sodium cellulose phosphate may be a useful temporary substitute for thiazide diuretics if thiazide tachyphylaxis occurs (Table 48.5). After a period of 6 months, thiazide diuretic therapy can then be resumed. Results with sodium phytate have been disappointing, with little alteration in the natural history of calcium stone disease and a high incidence of diarrhea leading to noncompliance with therapy. Sodium cellulose phosphate, an ion-exchange resin in doses of 2.5–5 g with each meal, has been documented to reduce calcium absorption from the gut. This leads to a decrease in urinary calcium, thus reducing urine brushite saturation and decreasing the propensity for spontaneous nucleation.[105] Not all investigators have reported successful therapy with cellulose phosphate in absorptive hypercalciuria.[106] This treatment does not stimulate parathyroid function or induce bone disease when used in usual therapeutic doses[104] but may cause hyperoxaluria and reduced magnesium excretion.[104,106] Because magnesium is one of the purported inhibitors of stone formation and hyperoxaluria is a major risk factor, it is recommended that oral magnesium supplementation be given separately from cellulose phosphate and that dietary oxalate be restricted.[107] This agent should not be used in patients with renal hypercalciuria or those with low or normal calcium absorption because secondary hyperparathyroidism may ensue. Absorptive hypercalciuria

TABLE 48.5. DRUGS USED IN THE MANAGEMENT OF CALCIUM STONE DISEASE

Agent	Dose	Proposed Action
Thiazide (hydrochlorothiazide)	12.5–100 mg/d	Reduces urinary calcium excretion
Sodium phytate	12.0 mg/kg–21.0 mg/kg/d	Reduces intestinal calcium absorption
Sodium cellulose phosphate	2.5–5.0 g with meals	Reduces intestinal calcium absorption
Magnesium oxide	600 mg/d	Increases inhibitor capacity
Orthophosphate	1250–2250 mg/d[a]	Reduces urinary calcium excretion Increases inhibitor capacity
Potassium citrate	60–80 mEq/d	Increases inhibitor capacity Increases urinary pH
Cholestyramine	4 g with meals	Decreases urinary oxalate excretion
Pyridoxine	200–400 mg/d	Decreases urinary oxalate excretion

[a]Of elemental phosphorus.

type II usually responds to a reduction of dietary calcium to 800 mg/d.

Orthophosphate is indicated for patients with hypophosphatemic or type III absorptive hypercalciuria. In this disorder, phosphate supplementation is logical because it will suppress 1,25-dihydroxyvitamin D synthesis, thereby reducing calcium absorption and hence excretion.[108] It has, however, been used in all patients with idiopathic hypercalciuria and in patients with calcium stone disease of undefined etiology. The urinary saturation of calcium oxalate decreases because of the fall in urinary calcium excretion. The major benefit may be an increase in pyrophosphate excretion, an inhibitor of both calcium phosphate and calcium oxalate stone formation.[109] Orthophosphates are available as acid, neutral, or alkaline salts of sodium or potassium phosphates. All have proven effective in the treatment of recurrent calcium calculi, although the acid preparation may be somewhat inferior to the other preparations. The acid load may result in an increase in urinary calcium and a decrease in urinary citrate.[110] Dosages utilized have ranged from 1250–2250 mg of elemental phosphorus per day administered in divided doses. Several studies have documented the efficacy of orthophosphates in preventing calcium-containing calculi.[111–113] Patients with gastrointestinal disorders do not tolerate phosphate therapy, the sodium load may be deleterious in patients with heart failure or hypertension, and diarrhea may limit attainable drug dosage. Dystrophic calcification has been noted by one group of investigators[114] but not verified by others. Phosphate therapy should not be utilized in patients with renal insufficiency and is contraindicated in patients with infection-induced stone disease. The related diphosphonate compounds are exceptionally potent inhibitors of the formation and aggregation of calcium oxalate and calcium phosphate crystals.[115] However, the large doses required to modify crystalluria cause bone disease in humans and thus, for the present, oral diphosphonates hold little promise of usefulness in stone disease.

Patients with enteric hyperoxaluria have been treated with cholestyramine[116] or diethylaminoethanol-cellulose (DEAE-cellulose),[117] both of which act as oxalate binders. Cholestyramine, although safely used for many years as a hypolipidemic agent, has physical characteristics that contribute to a high degree of noncompliance. In addition, it may bind various vitamins, other nutrients, and drugs. DEAE-cellulose, although safe and effective in reducing elevated urinary oxalate excretion, has not received approval for this indication in United States. Hyperoxaluria can be reduced by limiting the intake of oxalate-rich foods such as spinach, rhubarb, strawberries, peppers, parsley, tea, nuts, chocolate, beet greens, currants, endive, figs, grapes, green beans, okra, plums, poppy seeds, raspberries, sorrel, sweet potatoes, and swiss chard. It is important to counsel patients to avoid coffee, tea, or chocolate beverages as part of their fluid therapy. In addition, the ingestion of large doses of ascorbic acid should be avoided because of the potential relationship to hyperoxaluria. Additional therapeutic modalities include dietary fat restriction, oral calcium and/or magnesium supplements (to precipitate oxalate in the gut and increase the inhibitor capacity of the urine), and oral citrate salts.[118] It is preferable to use a combination of these modalities rather than a single modality at its maximum level.

Another agent that could potentially reduce the *in vivo* generation of oxalate is pyridoxine. Pyridoxine is thought to act by decreasing endogenous oxalate production and hence excretion by stimulating the conversion of glyoxylic acid to glycine rather than to oxalic acid.[119] Pyridoxine therapy has been reported to be successful in cases of primary hyperoxaluria.[120,121] Oral orthophosphate combined with pyridoxine has been documented to be effective.[122] If the glomerular filtration rate is between 30 and 50 mL/min, phosphate must be used cautiously with careful monitoring of serum creatinine, phosphorus, and calcium. It should not be used if the glomerular filtration rate is less than 30 mL/min. Magnesium oxide or hydroxide salts have also been used with good results.[123] Although calcium carbimide can theoretically reduce glyoxylate (and hence oxalate) formation by inhibiting the oxidation of glycolaldehyde via aldehyde dehydrogenase in primary hyperoxaluria,[124] this agent has not been found to decrease urinary oxalate excretion in clinical practice.[125] In addition, succinate is thought to decrease the formation of oxalate by bringing more C_2 metabolites into the Krebs cycle. Although succinate has been documented to reduce hyperoxaluria in 74% of patients in one series,[126] poor results were noted in the treatment of hyperoxaluria in another.[127] Thus succinate therapy should be regarded as experimental at this time.

Thiazides represent the "ideal" treatment program for renal leak hypercalciuria because they increase renal tubular reabsorption of calcium[128] and restore normal parathyroid function, serum 1,25-dihydroxyvitamin D, and calcium absorption.[129] However, many clinicians use these agents for hypercalciuria of any etiology, because the fall in urinary calcium leads to a decrease in the level of saturation of brushite and calcium oxalate.[130] The mechanism by which renal calcium excretion is reduced by thiazides is unknown. Although it seems that volume contraction and parathyroid hormone are required,[131] increased tubular reabsorption of calcium would appear to be the major mechanism. In addition, thiazides have been reported to reduce the urinary excretion of oxalate and increase excretion of zinc and magnesium, two potential stone formation inhibitors.[132,133] However, thiazide-induced potassium depletion may occur, leading to hypocitraturia. This may be deleterious in lieu of the inhibitor effects of citrate but can be prevented by potassium supplementation with the chloride or citrate salts.[134] Serum calcium may rise but this effect is generally mild.

Although open nonrandomized, noncontrolled, or poorly controlled studies have documented the efficacy of thiazides in hypercalciuric stone formers,[135,136] two randomized, well-controlled studies questioned the value of thiazides in this disorder.[137,138] One controlled double-blind study has documented the superiority of chlorthalidone compared to placebo and magnesium hydroxide in the prevention of recurrent calcium oxalate nephrolithiasis.[139] The thiazides used most commonly in renal stone disorders include hydrochlorothiazide, trichlormethiazide, bendroflumethiazide, chlorthalidone, and chlorothiazide.

Potassium citrate has recently been evaluated in the treatment of all forms of calcium nephrolithiasis, although it is primarily indicated for the treatment of hypocitraturic calcium stone disease. Favorable results have been noted due to its effects on both urinary pH and calcium salt crystallization.[140,141] Renal citrate excretion is enhanced in the presence of increased urinary pH. Potassium citrate would seem advantageous over sodium alkali since it is free of the potential complications of sodium-induced hypercalciuria and sodium urate-induced crystallization of calcium oxalate. Ingestion of orange juice (400 mL thrice daily) has been demonstrated in preliminary studies to be potentially beneficial by increasing urinary pH and citrate excretion. Unlike potassium citrate, calcium excretion is unchanged and oxalate excretion is increased in patients ingesting orange juice.[142]

Citrate salts may also be beneficial following extracorporeal shock-wave lithotripsy (ESWL) to enhance calcium stone fragment clearance and prevent fragment growth and reaggregation in patients unable to clear stone fragments.[143] As with all potassium-containing preparations, patients should be followed for hyperkalemia and gastrointestinal upset and bleeding.

The administration of oral magnesium has been evaluated since magnesium inhibits calcium stone crystallization.[144] Although a few studies of magnesium oxide or hydroxide therapy have documented some benefit in calcium stone formers,[144–146] data are too limited to recommend this as a first-line treatment. Investigators have found no significant beneficial effect on urinary formation product or on the rate of crystal growth of calcium oxalate or brushite.[147] However, its use in conjunction with cellulose phosphate therapy may improve the therapeutic response to this calcium-binding agent. Caution should be exercised in its use in patients with renal impairment, and dosage may be limited by the appearance of diarrhea.

URATES AND STONES

Between 5 and 10% of renal stones in the United States are composed of uric acid. A similar percentage applies to most of Europe, but higher figures are reported from Germany, Spain, and Israel[148–150] and lower figures from Sweden.[151] Urates have also been proposed to play a role in calcium stone disease so both uric acid stone disease and urate involvement in calcium stone disease are discussed.

PATHOGENESIS

Uric Acid Stone Disease

Uric acid is the end product of purine metabolism. Purines are derived from endogenous sources or the diet and are converted to hypoxanthine and xanthine. Hypoxanthine is then oxidized to xanthine, and this compound in turn is oxidized to uric acid by xanthine oxidase. In many animals, uric acid is then oxidized by uricase to allantoin, a water-soluble end product. Humans, reptiles, and birds are deficient in uricase activity and cannot convert uric acid to allantoin. Uric acid thus becomes the end product of purine metabolism and must be excreted. However, uric acid is not as soluble as allantoin in an aqueous medium and, thus, tends to precipitate. Uric acid is excreted by renal and extrarenal mechanisms. Two-thirds of the uric acid excreted per day is cleared through the kidneys and one-third by the intestine. The uric acid lost in the intestine is degraded by uricase containing bacteria.[152]

Uric acid is cleared by the kidney by four mechanisms. As protein binding is less than 5%, it is freely filtered at the glomerulus. It is thought that virtually all filtered uric acid is reabsorbed. Tubular secretion adds approximately 50% of the original filtered load to the tubule lumen before subsequent tubular reabsorption. This postsecretory reabsorption accounts for 40–45% of the original filtered load. Thus, total excretion of urate is 5–10% of the original filtered load, but most if not all of the urate appearing in the urine is derived from that urate secreted by the nephron that escaped postsecretory reabsorption.[153] The site in the nephron of excretion and reabsorption is controversial but is probably in the proximal tubule.[154]

The risk factors for uric acid stone formation are (1) hyperuricosuria, (2) low urine volume, and (3) persistently acid urine. Although inhibitors of uric acid precipitation have been proposed,[155] as well as promoters of precipitation,[156] studies on uric acid solubility have shown similar levels required for precipitation in non-stone formers and stone formers.[157] This suggests that the most important factors governing uric acid precipitation are uric acid concentration and pH. Uric acid solubility in the urine is determined by the concentration of undissociated uric acid. Undissociated uric acid concentration can be calculated using the following equation:

$$[A] = [T] \div (1 + 10^{pH-pK})$$

where [A] is the concentration of undissociated uric acid in mg/L, [T] is the concentration of total uric acid in mg/L, pH is the pH of the urine, and the value of p*K* is 5.345.[158] Examination of this formula reveals a marked effect of urine pH on the solubility of uric acid.

Hyperuricosuria is not the most common of the three risk factors, being present in only 31% of uric acid stone formers in one large series.[150] It is always a manifestation of the overproduction of uric acid and occurs in the conditions listed in Table 48.6. Hyperuricosuria is observed most commonly in patients with high dietary protein intake and gout. Low urine volume secondary to high environmental temperatures may be a contributing factor to the high incidence of uric acid stones seen in the Middle East.[150] It is also seen as an important risk factor in ileostomy patients and any patient with large gastrointestinal losses of fluids.[159]

The most common risk factor for uric acid stone disease is a persistently acid urine,[160] that is, urine pH that remains below 6 throughout the day.[161] Although there is controversy as to the mechanism, early studies proposed that there was an impairment in ammonium excretion by the kidney.[162] Others attributed the finding of decreased ammonium excretion to differences in the age of the patients and controls (the patients were older than the controls and ammonium excretion decreased with age) and/or renal impairment in the patients that is known to decrease ammonium excretion.[163,164] Subsequent studies suggested decreased ammonium excretion but with an elevated titratable acid excretion that was sensitive to changes in dietary protein intake.[165,166] Current data suggest that patients with uric acid stones have a persistently acid urine, which is related to an abnormal partitioning of hydrogen ion between ammonium and titratable acid. This abnormality is more prominent as the level of protein in the diet increases.

TABLE 48.6. CLASSIFICATION OF URIC ACID STONE DISEASE

Associated with Hyperuricosuria:

1. Gout secondary to overproduction of uric acid
   a. Lesch-Nyhan syndrome (hypoxanthine–guanine phosphoribosyl-transferase deficiency)
   b. Type I glycogen storage disease (glucose-6-phosphatase deficiency)
   c. Phosphoribosyl pyrophosphate synthetase overactivity
   d. Glutathione reductase overactivity

Associated with Persistently Acid Urine:

1. Idiopathic uric acid stone disease
2. Gout
3. Gastrointestinal losses of bicarbonate
   a. Chronic diarrhea
   b. Ileostomy
   c. Fistulas

Associated with Low Urine Volume:

1. Excessive sweating
2. Low fluid intake
3. Gastrointestinal losses

Urate and Calcium Stone Disease

Calcium-containing stones occur more commonly among individuals with gout than in the general population.[167] In addition, calcium stone formers with hyperuricosuria or hyperuricemia but with no abnormalities in calcium metabolism have been described.[168] An increased prevalence of hyperuricosuria in calcium stone formers compared to non-stone formers has also been reported.[169] Hyperuricosuria has been identified as a risk factor in 9–15% of calcium stone formers.[25,96] Patients with calcium stone disease associated with hyperuricosuria have a more aggressive disease with higher stone formation rates, shorter intervals between stone events, and a higher frequency of stones requiring operative management.[96,169] The etiology of the hyperuricosuria has been attributed to a high dietary purine intake, a higher uric acid production for any given purine intake, and alterations in renal handling of uric acid,[166,170,171] although the latter proposed mechanism has not been found by all investigators.[172]

Urates exist in the urine in several forms; in an acid urine, urates exist predominantly as undissociated uric acid. However, when the urine pH is greater than 6.0, urates associate with monovalent cations, the most abundant being sodium, to form monosodium urate.[173] Potentially, either uric acid or monosodium urate could play a role in calcium stone formation. Epitaxy is a process by which one crystal form serves as a nidus for a second type of crystal. It has been proposed that either uric acid or monosodium urate could serve as a substrate for calcium oxalate precipitation.[18] *In vitro* studies showed that monosodium urate readily initiated nucleation of calcium oxalate whereas uric acid failed to do so.[174] This process was slowed by pyrophosphate, a known inhibitor of calcium oxalate precipitation.[175]

A second proposed mechanism is that urates interfere with the inhibitory action of glycosaminoglycans on calcium oxalate precipitation. Glycosaminoglycans have been shown to be potent inhibitors of the nucleation of calcium oxalate[176] as well as crystal growth and aggregation.[177] Monosodium urate decreases this inhibitory action of glycosaminoglycans.[176] Furthermore, hyperuricosuria leads to supersaturation of the urine for monosodium urate and results in a decrease in the level of supersaturation required for spontaneous precipitation of calcium oxalate.[178]

CLINICAL CHARACTERISTICS

In addition to renal colic, uric acid gravel is common. This gravel is characteristically reddish in appearance due to adsorption of urochromes. Passage of gravel is frequently asymptomatic but can be associated with dysuria and hematuria. Occasionally massive deposition can occur with bilateral ureteral obstruction and acute renal failure. The age of onset and sex distribution of uric acid stone disease depends on whether or not it is associated with gout. Uric acid stone disease unassociated with gout is termed idiopathic and can occur at any age, having a male to female ratio of 3 to 1. When associated with gout, this stone disease occurs almost exclusively after the age of 40 with a male to female ratio of 12 to 1.[150]

Uric acid stones are radiolucent. Renal colic with no stone seen on a routine flat plate of the abdomen should suggest uric acid stones. They can be seen with an intravenous pyelogram where they appear as negative filling defects. They are dense in appearance with computerized tomography and appear echogenic with an acoustic shadow on ultrasound.

MANAGEMENT

Treatment of uric acid stone disease is dictated by the risk factors present in the individual patient. Treatment is designed to reduce the level of undissociated uric acid to less than 90 mg/L.[158] A daily urine output of 2.5–3 L/d should be maintained with an emphasis on evening intake to guarantee a high urine flow during the night. The emphasis should be on the volume of urine excreted, not on the volume of fluid consumed. Excessive amounts of animal protein should be avoided by limiting daily fish, meat, and poultry portions to less than 8 ounces. In addition, foods rich in purines should be avoided.[100]

Allopurinol therapy should be used if hyperuricosuria (>800 mg/d) is present but should be utilized in conjunction with fluid and alkali therapy[179,180] (Table 48.7). This drug inhibits xanthine oxidase, thus decreasing the conversion of xanthine and hypoxanthine to uric acid. Although the usual starting dose is 200–300 mg once daily, dosage should be adjusted in patients with significant renal dysfunction.[181] Patients should be monitored for the appearance of potentially serious side effects such as precipitation of acute gouty attacks, skin rash (may progress to toxic epidermal necrolysis), vasculitis, blood dyscrasias, and hepatitis. As well, xanthine and oxypurinol stones may develop in patients receiving allopurinol, especially those patients with extremely high purine loads (neoplasia, Lesch–Nyhan syndrome).[182,183]

Alkali therapy is required in patients with persistently acid urine. Urine pH should be maintained between 6.0 and 7.0 and not be allowed to drop below 5.5. Also, urine pH should not be allowed to exceed 7.0 to reduce the risk of calcium phosphate precipitation. Unless obstruction is complete, systemic alkalinization with intravenous sodium bicarbonate or sodium lactate titrated to produce a urine pH of 6.0 to 7.0 may be sufficient to result in stone dissolution.[184,185] Lactate may be the preferred intravenous agent due to a lesser propensity to induce metabolic alkalosis as

TABLE 48.7. DRUGS USED IN THE MANAGEMENT OF URATE STONE DISEASE

Agent	Dose	Proposed Action
Allopurinol	200–300 mg/d	Reduces uric acid excretion
Alkalinizing agents	Titrate to urine pH 6.0–7.0	Increases uric acid solubility
Sodium bicarbonate		
Sodium lactate		
Potassium citrate		

well as the theoretical advantage of lactate providing the antiketogenic effect of glycogen that may potentiate the acid neutralizing effect of the sodium ion. Controlled comparative trials, however, have not been done. Intravenous alkalinization may produce dissolution within 1 to 2 days. During intravenous alkalinization, patients should be monitored for the development of fluid overload, hypernatremia, pulmonary edema, metabolic alkalosis and hypertension. Oral alkalinization may also be adequate for the treatment of incompletely obstructing uric acid stones. Therapy should be monitored with pH strips to assure that the desired pH is maintained. Alkalinization may be achieved with sodium bicarbonate, sodium or potassium citrate, or acetazolamide. Acetazolamide is only recommended if troublesome sodium or fluid retention occurs with sodium salts or if nocturnal pH cannot be raised above 6.0 with conventional therapy.[186] Citrate salts may be preferable to bicarbonate due to better gastrointestinal tolerance. Potassium citrate may be preferable to sodium citrate because of a reduced potential for the development of calcium stones that may arise from sodium citrate or sodium bicarbonate therapy.[187] Also, monopotassium urate is more soluble than monosodium urate.

Treatment of acute urinary obstruction secondary to uric acid stones requires either open lithotomy or irrigation with or without extraction via percutaneous nephrostomy or stint placement followed by ESWL.[188] Irrigation therapy may be used as primary therapy after decompression of the urinary tract. It may also be used as an adjunct to ESWL, lithotomy, or nephrostomy extraction to ensure dissolution of residual stone fragments or stones inaccessible to removal. Irrigation solutions have included 0.1 *M* sodium bicarbonate (pH 8.4)[185,189] and tromethamine.[190,191] Bicarbonate is recommended because of greater clinical experience and a much lower cost. One to 3 weeks of therapy has generally been required to effect total stone dissolution.

Infection-Induced Stones

Stones due to infection are composed of magnesium-ammonium-phosphate (struvite) usually combined with carbonate-apatite. Between 9% and 19% of stones analyzed will contain struvite.[19,20] Although urinary tract infection has been reported in 10–12% of stone patients,[192,193] the fraction of stone disease attributed to infection is only 2–3%.[25,192] One can conclude from these figures that stones due to infection are probably analyzed more frequently than other stones, that urinary tract infections in stone formers are more common than stone formation due to infections, and that infection is not a common cause of renal stone disease. However, it is important to recognize this type of stone disease since it can result in the loss of renal function, be associated with urosepsis, and has a high rate of recurrence.

PATHOGENESIS

Infection stones are associated with an alkaline urine containing a high concentration of ammonia. Struvite solubility is pH sensitive; it precipitates in an alkaline environment (pH ≥7.0) and is soluble in an acid solution.[194] Carbonate-apatite, a form of calcium phosphate plus carbonate, is also pH sensitive, precipitating in an alkaline solution. Ammonia excretion generally falls in an alkaline urine and would therefore not be expected to reach sufficient concentration to precipitate as struvite. Therefore, any explanation of the pathogenesis of these stones must account for the high urine pH as well as an increase in the urine concentration of ammonia.

This type of stone disease only occurs in the presence of infection with urease producing bacteria. Sterile urine from stone formers and non-stone formers has been shown to be undersaturated for struvite.[195] The addition of urease to sterile urine, which is undersaturated for struvite, results in alkalinization of the urine and supersaturation for struvite.[196] The enzyme urease hydrolyzes urea to form ammonia and carbon dioxide, which on further hydrolysis yields ammonium and bicarbonate plus carbonate. In addition to the generation of the ionic species required for stone formation, the hydrolysis of urea also results in the alkalinization of the urine. Thus the requirements for precipitation of struvite and carbonate-apatite (alkaline pH with high ammonia and carbonate concentrations) are met.

Many gram-positive and gram-negative organisms as well as yeasts and T-strain mycoplasma are urease producers.[197] Virtually all *Proteus* sp. are urease producers whereas *Escherichia coli* seldom, if ever, produces urease. The T-strain mycoplasma, *Ureaplasma urealyticum,* has been shown to produce urease[198] and has been cultured from struvite stones.[199]

Matrix has also been suggested to play a role in the infection of stones. Ultrastructural studies have demonstrated the production of a bacterial glycocalyx, which is proposed to facilitate bacterial adhesion to either uroepithelium or preexisting stone material and to trap mucoproteins (matrix material), struvite, and carbonate-apatite crystals to form the infection stone.[200] Bacteria have been demonstrated to reside within the substance of the stone and not just be adherent to the surface.[201] This makes therapy difficult since antibiotics do not penetrate the stone to reach the bacteria and any fragment left after surgery constitutes infected material and may result in recurrence.

Infection-induced stone disease is unlike other stone disease in that it is more common in women than men.[202] Also renal colic, the most frequent presentation of other types of stone disease, is uncommon in infection stones, which usually present with resistant urinary tract infections or urosepsis. Any patient predisposed to urinary tract infection is at risk for this type of stone disease. This would include those with a history of recurrent urinary tract infections with intact anatomy (most commonly women), individuals with bladder dysfunction or obstruction, and those with urinary tract diversions or indwelling bladder catheters. Patients with underlying metabolic stone disease also appear to be at risk. Stones in the urinary tract can serve as foreign bodies but probably more important is that patients with metabolic stone disease are frequently subjected to urologic instrumentation, which can introduce bacteria into an otherwise sterile system.[202]

CLINICAL CHARACTERISTICS

Infection-induced stones can be either radiolucent or radiopaque depending on the proportion of matrix material. Stones that are predominantly matrix with little or no crystalline material will be radiolucent whereas stones with a great deal of carbonate-apatite will be radiodense. These stones are the most common to present as staghorn calculi. Staghorn stones have one or more branches extending from the pelvis into the calyces of the kidney.

The natural history of untreated unilateral infection stones indicates that 71% ultimately required a nephrectomy with a mortality rate, primarily from renal failure, of 22%. Bilateral disease appears to fare even less well; nephrectomy was required in 44% with a mortality rate of 80%.[203] A second study found that in bilateral infection-induced stone disease there was a 25% mortality within 5 years and a 40% mortality within 10 years.[204] The severe nature of this stone disease is demonstrated by the fact that 77% of patients requiring nephrectomy for treatment of renal stone disease had infection-induced stones.[205]

MANAGEMENT

Treatment of infection (struvite) stones is directed toward (1) surgical removal of all stone material and correction of anatomic abnormalities, (2) eradication and/or long-term suppression of urinary infection, (3) the maintenance of an acid urine, and (4) specific treatment of any underlying metabolic disorder.

Surgical removal of stone material is the major therapeutic modality in struvite stone disease. A review of the surgical techniques involved in the removal of struvite calculi is beyond the scope of this chapter, but calculi are commonly removed using standard or extended pyelolithotomy, anatrophic nephrolithotomy, pyelonephrolithotomy, and partial nephrectomy.[206,207] The surgical goal is removal of all stone fragments. Numerous adjunctive surgical techniques have been developed to improve surgical success rates. These include regional renal hypothermia, operative radiography, operative nephroscopy, and postoperative irrigations with stone solvents. Surgical removal results in "cure" of infection in only approximately 60% of cases.

Recent reports have stressed the value of postoperative stone solvent irrigations to remove inaccessible macroscopic and microscopic fragments left behind after surgery.[206,208] Suby's G solution[209] and hemiacidrin (Renacidin)[208,210–213] have been used successfully, although currently hemiacidrin is the solvent of choice due to better patient tolerance (Table 48.8). Both agents contain citric acid and magnesium with a pH of 4. Whether pH is the only important effect or complexes between calcium and citrate and magnesium are additive has not been resolved. Complications in the early years of hemiacidrin use, including death due to sepsis and hypermagnesemia,[214] prompted the Food and Drug Administration (FDA) to withdraw approval for use within the kidney. However, these complications were thought to be due to irrigation of an infected urinary tract at high intrarenal pressure. Investigations since 1962 have documented the relative safety of hemiacidrin irrigation provided the urinary tract is kept sterile using systemic antibiotics throughout irrigation therapy, blood magnesium levels are monitored, and intrarenal pressures are kept below 25 cm H_2O to prevent pyelovenous reflux. Hemiacidrin irrigation therapy can result in urothelial irritation and mucosal changes but these are of unknown clinical significance.[215] Informed consent should be obtained prior to this patient therapy. Oral citrate salts may play a role following ESWL in enhancing struvite stone fragment clearance and preventing fragment growth and reaggregation in patients unable to clear stone fragments.[143] The theoretical risk of increased struvite precipitation due to increased pH may

TABLE 48.8. DRUGS USED IN THE MANAGEMENT OF INFECTION-INDUCED STONE DISEASE

Agent	Dose	Proposed Action
Culture-specific antibiotics	—	—
Suby's G solution	Irrigation of renal pelvis	Increases solubility of stone material
Hemiacidrin (10%)	Irrigation of renal pelvis	Increases solubility of stone material
Ammonium chloride	Titrate urine pH to <6.0	Acidifies urine
Acetohydroxamic acid	250–1500 mg/d	Inhibits bacterial urease
Hydroxyurea	500–1000 mg/d	Inhibits bacterial urease

be mitigated by reduced renal ammoniagenesis (by the citrate-induced alkaline tide) and by reduced ammonia production due to urease (by antibiotic sterilization).

Irrigation therapy may also be useful as primary therapy of struvite stones, especially in those patients who are high risk or are nonsurgical candidates.[188] Primary dissolution therapy is generally very slow, may not be cost effective, and risks sepsis and renal damage in patients with large stones unless scrupulous technique is used.

Traditional medical therapy plays an adjunctive role to surgery in the management of infection-induced stones. Antibiotics chosen on the basis of culture and sensitivity results are given preoperatively, intraoperatively, and postoperatively in an attempt to eradicate the attendant infection. Long-term culture-specific antibiotics are indicated if cessation of therapy results in recurrence of urinary tract infection. Periodic and routine bacteriologic and radiographic follow-up is necessary.

Acidification of the urine results in an undersaturated urine with respect to struvite and significantly reduces the level of calcium phosphate saturation. Ammonium chloride appears to be the only effective means of acidifying the urine. Results of urine acidification with ascorbic acid have been quite variable, with some authors citing that 1–6 g/d will significantly lower the urine pH,[216] while others have reported no significant reduction.[217] Also, there is the risk of precipitating calcium oxalate stone disease by increasing urinary oxalate excretion as a by-product of ascorbic acid metabolism. However, even with ammonium chloride, it may not be possible to acidify the urine in the presence of urease-producing bacteria.

Hydroxyurea and acetohydroxamic acid, which are structurally similar to urea, act by inhibiting the bacterial enzyme urease.[218] Acetohydroxamic acid forms a stronger, noncompetitive, more slowly reversible bond than hydroxyurea. The reduction in urinary ammonia and pH produced by these agents is said to enhance the effectiveness of concurrent antibiotic therapy, reduce the virulence of bacteria, and permit nonpathologic colonization of the urinary tract (in experimental animal models).[219,220] However, *in vivo* confirmation of these findings in humans is lacking. Although hydroxyurea (in doses of 500–1000 mg/d) and acetohydroxamic acid (in doses of 250–1500 mg/d) have been documented to reduce ammonia and urinary alkalinity, convincing evidence of total or even partial stone dissolution in a substantial proportion of patients is lacking.[221,222] In most patients, stone growth will cease while on inhibitor therapy. Increases in magnesium and phosphate excretion may counteract the effects of the large falls in pH and urinary ammonium excretion on the saturation of struvite and brushite.[223] Of the two agents, acetohydroxamic acid appears to be superior based on its more potent urease-inhibitor activity.[218]

Acetohydroxamic acid therapy may be accompanied by side effects in a significant proportion of patients. These include mild headaches, gastrointestinal upset, Coombs' negative hemolytic anemia (dose-related, seen more frequently in patients with renal impairment), thrombophlebitis, and psychiatric disturbances (including depression, anxiety, tremulousness). This drug is also teratogenic and should not be used in women of childbearing age without adequate birth control measures. Hydroxyurea therapy has been associated with bone marrow suppression (primarily leukopenia), gastrointestinal upset, skin rashes, and rare CNS disturbances such as headache, drowsiness, dizziness, and hallucinations. It is recommended not to use these agents in patients with significant renal impairment (creatinine clearance <20 mL/min) due to reduced efficacy and increased risk of toxicity. Studies with the investigational urease inhibitors propionohydroxamic acid (PHA)[224] and flurofamide[225] have documented findings similar to those with hydroxyurea and acetohydroxamic acid. Alopecia with PHA has been reported in a number of treated subjects. PHA does not appear to be a significant advance over available urease inhibitors and flurofamide requires further study.

The role of urease inhibitors is thus undefined at this time. These agents should always be used in conjunction with antibiotic therapy. These agents should be reserved for those patients unable to undergo more definitive operative or irrigation procedures, those patients who have recurrent stones despite optimal management with traditional medical therapy, those patients who have not responded to ammonium chloride acidification therapy, and those patients who fail to sterilize their urine despite adequate courses of culture-specific antibiotics.

CYSTINE STONES

Cystine stone disease accounts for approximately 1% of stones.[19] It is the result of excess cystine excretion in the urine due to an inherited abnormality in cystine transport in the kidney. Cystinuria is transmitted as an autosomal recessive gene with an incidence in the population of 1/4000 to 1/15,000.

PATHOGENESIS

Amino acids are freely filtered at the glomerulus and virtually 100% reabsorbed in the proximal tubule. In cystinuria, there is a transport defect in the proximal tubule of the kidney for the amino acids cystine, lysine, arginine, and ornithine, which results in excess excretion of these amino acids. There is also a transport abnormality in the intestine for these same amino acids leading to a decrease in their intestinal absorption. These combined abnormalities would result in no clinical problems if it were not for the limited solubility of cystine, which is the primary reason for the development of renal stone disease.[226]

The normal excretion of cystine is less than 60 mg per 24 hours. Homozygotes will excrete over 400 mg per 24 hours while heterozygotes excrete intermediate values. Of the amino acids excessively excreted in this disease, cystine is the least soluble. Urine pH has an influence on the solubility of cystine. However, this effect is minimal between pH values of 5.0–7.0 with solubility in this range being 300–400 mg/L. The solubility rises rapidly above a pH of 7.0, but these pH values can only be accomplished with alkali therapy. There is a good correlation between the level of saturation of the urine for cystine and crystalluria, and thus inhibitors appear to play no role in the pathophysiology of cystine stone formation.[226]

CLINICAL CHARACTERISTICS

The disease presents most frequently in the second to third decade of life. However, it has been reported to be present as late as the sixth decade.[227] Since there is impairment of intestinal absorption and renal conservation, there has been concern that deficiency of the involved amino acids could lead to other clinical problems. Cystinuria has been reported to occur more frequently in individuals with mental illness or retardation. However, when cystinurics were compared to their normal sibs, no difference in intelligence could be demonstrated, and there was no difference from intelligence test norms. Similarly some investigators have found shorter stature among cystinurics where others have not been able to demonstrate a difference. It would appear that the only significant clinical problem associated with cystinuria is renal stone disease and its consequences, particularly loss of renal function. The risk factors for cystine stone formation include excess cystine excretion, acid urine, and low urine volume. Cystine solubility, as noted above, is pH sensitive and an acid pH decreases its solubility. Excess excretion and low urine volume lead to increased levels of saturation at any urine pH.

The finding of cystine on stone analysis is diagnostic of cystinuria. Likewise, finding cystine crystals, which have a characteristic hexagonal "benzene-ring" appearance, on urinalysis is diagnostic of cystinuria. When no stone is available nor crystals present on urinalysis, a qualitative test for cystine is the least expensive way to make a presumptive diagnosis. The cyanide-nitroprusside test is simple to perform and is only positive with excess cystine excretion. When the qualitative test is positive, it should be followed by a quantitative determination. Excess excretion of cystine can also occur in Fanconi's syndrome but in this condition cystine excretion is usually less than 200 mg/d and accompanied by diffuse aminoaciduria, glycosuria, and phosphaturia. Cystine stones are radiopaque on x-ray due to their sulfur content. They have a homogenous, smooth appearance and are less dense than calcium-containing stones.

MANAGEMENT

Therapy is aimed at prevention of new stone formation and, when necessary, dissolution of stones. A very low protein diet (0.5 g/kg/d or less) that will reduce the intake of methionine, a precursor of cystine, has been demonstrated to reduce urinary cystine output.[228] However, such protein restriction is impractical for most patients. Furthermore, the diet is difficult to prepare and frequently unacceptable. Attempts to reduce the breakdown of methionine to cystine using added dietary choline has also been unsuccessful.[229] Intravenous and oral glutamine has also been reported to reduce urinary cystine[230,231] but this observation has not been confirmed in other studies.[232]

In patients with no stones present in the kidney, treating the risk factors of acid urine and low urine volumes may be sufficient. Hydration to ensure a urine output of 3 to 4 L/d and alkalinization with sodium bicarbonate, sodium citrate, or potassium citrate to achieve a urine pH of 7.0–7.5 will usually prevent new stone formation.[227] Urine flow must be maintained at night as well as in the daytime. This will usually entail sufficient hydration to cause the patient to arise once nightly to void and drink fluid.

If cystine stones are present in the kidney, the hydration/alkalinization protocol is usually inadequate for medical dissolution and oral Penicillamine is usually required[227] (Table 48.9). Penicillamine acts by forming a disulfide complex with cystine that is 50 times more soluble than cystine alone. Penicillamine therapy is not tolerated by a

TABLE 48.9. DRUGS USED IN THE MANAGEMENT OF CYSTINE STONE DISEASE

Agent	Dose	Proposed Action
Penicillamine	1–4 g/d	Reduces urinary cystine excretion
α-Mercaptopropionyl-glycine	300–1200 mg/d	Reduces urinary cystine excretion
Alkalinizing agents	Titrate urine pH to 7.0–8.0	Increases cystine solubility
Sodium bicarbonate		
Sodium citrate		
Potassium citrate		

substantial proportion of patients due to the development of serious side effects such as systemic lupus erythematosus, proteinuria, nephrotic syndrome, blood dyscrasias, myasthenia gravis, skin rashes, mucositis, and dysgeusia.[233]

Oral α-mercaptopropionyl-glycine will also form a disulfide complex with cystine and increase its solubility. It has been effective in stone dissolution and reported to have a lower incidence of side effects.[234,235] Therapy with the investigational agent, mercaptoethane sulfonate (MESNA), has shown promise in significantly reducing cystinuria.[236] Similar findings have been noted with the use of captopril.[237] However, the ability of this class of agents to reduce the frequency of stone recurrence and promote stone dissolution has not been studied. Oral *N*-acetylcystine may reduce the frequency of stone recurrence and possibly promote stone dissolution,[238] but further studies to confirm and extend these observations are necessary before this mode of therapy can be recommended.

While some stones dissolve with treatment, the natural course of cystinuria often involves multiple surgical procedures to alleviate obstruction and colic. Irrigation therapy may be used as primary therapy after nephrostomy tube insertion to decompress the urinary tract. It may also be used as an adjunct to lithotomy or nephrostomy extraction to ensure dissolution of residual stone fragments or stones inaccessible to removal. Irrigation solutions have included penicillamine (pH 8.0),[239] α-mercaptopropionyl-glycine,[240] and tromethamine-E.[241] Tromethamine-E appears superior to the other irrigants with regard to decreasing the duration of therapy but controlled comparative trials are lacking. Primary dissolution therapy has usually required 2–13 weeks of treatment time, a definite disadvantage compared to surgical procedures.

REFERENCES

1. Sierakowski R, Finlayson B, Landes RR, et al. The frequency of urolithiasis in hospital discharge diagnoses in the United States. Invest Urol 1978;15:438–441.
2. Smith CL. When should the stone patient be evaluated? Early evaluation of single stone formers. Med Clin North Am 1984;68:455–459.
3. Boyce WH. Organic matrix of human urinary concretions. Am J Med 1968;45:673–683.
4. Vermeulen CW, Lyon ES, Gill WB. Artificial urinary concretions. Invest Urol 1964;1:370–386.
5. Thomas WC, Howard IE. Studies on the mineralizing propensity of urine from patients with and without renal calculi. Trans Assoc Am Physicians 1959;72:181–187.
6. Fleisch H. Inhibitors and promoters of stone formation. Kidney Int 1978;13:361–371.
7. Goldberg H, Grass L, Vogl R, et al. Urine citrate and renal stone disease. Can Med Assoc J 1989;141:217–221.
8. Nicar MJ, Skurla C, Sakahee K, et al. Low urinary citrate excretion in nephrolithiasis. Urol 1983;21:8–14.
9. Hosking DH, Wilson JWL, Liedtke RR, et al. Urinary citrate excretion in normal persons and patients with idiopathic calcium urolithiasis. J Lab Clin Med 1985;106:682–689.
10. Nakagawa Y, Abram V, Kezdy FJ, et al. Purification and characterization of the principal inhibitor of calcium oxalate monohydrate crystal growth in human urine. J Biol Chem 1983;258:12594–12600.
11. Nakagawa Y, Abram V, Parks JH, et al. Urine glycoprotein crystal growth inhibitors: Evidence for a molecular abnormality in calcium oxalate nephrolithiasis. J Clin Invest 1985;76:1455–1462.
12. Pak CYC. Physical chemistry of stone formation, in Calcium Urolithiasis: Pathogenesis, Diagnoses, and Management. New York, Plenum, 1978, p 5.
13. Vermeulen CW, Lyon ES, Ellis JE, et al. The renal papilla and calculogenesis. J Urol 1967;97:573–582.
14. Hering F, Lueoend G, Briellman T, et al. Calcification sites in human kidneys: A REM study, in Scharille PO, Smith LH, Robertson WG, et al (eds): Urolithiasis and Related Clinical Research. New York, Plenum, 1985, p 205.
15. Smith C. ^{14}C-calcium oxalate (CAOX) adherence in the rat bladder, in Scharille PO, Smith LH, Robertson WG, et al (eds): Urolithiasis and Related Clinical Research. New York, Plenum 1985, p 949.
16. Randall A. The initiating lesions of renal calculus. Surg Gynecol Obstet 1937;64:201–208.
17. Robertson WG, Peacock M, Nordin BEC. Calcium crystalluria in recurrent renal-stone formers. Lancet 1969;2:21–24.
18. Lonsdale K. Epitaxy as a growth factor in urinary calculi and gallstones. Nature 1968;217:50–58.
19. Herring, LC. Observations on the analysis of ten thousand urinary calculi. J Urol 1962;88:545–562.
20. Prien EL, Prien EL. Composition and structure of urinary stone. Am J Med 1968;45:654–672.
21. Robertson WG, Peacock M, Heyburn PJ, et al. Risk factors in calcium stone disease in urinary calculus, in Brockus JG, Finlayson B (eds): International Urinary Stone Conference. Littleton, MA, PSG Publishing, 1981, pp 265–273.
22. Pak CYC. Medical management of nephrolithiasis. J Urol 1982;128:1157–1164.
23. Smith LH, Van Den Berg CJ, Wilson DM. Nutrition and urolithiasis. N Engl J Med 1978;298:87–89.
24. Ljunghall S. Renal stone disease: Studies of epidemiology and calcium metabolism. Scand J Urol Nephrol 1977;S41:4–96.
25. Pak CYC, Britton F, Peterson R, et al. Ambulatory evaluation of nephrolithiasis: Classification, clinical presentation and diagnostic criteria. Am J Med 1980;69:19–30.
26. Henneman PH, Benedict PH, Forbes AP, et al. Idiopathic hypercalciuria. N Engl J Med 1958;259:802.
27. Jackson WPU, Dancaster CA. Consideration of the hypercalciuria in sarcoidoses, idiopathic hypercalciuria, and that produced by vitamin D. A new suggestion regarding calcium metabolism. J Clin Endocrinol 1959;19:658–680.
28. Avioli LV. Intestinal absorption of calcium. Arch Intern Med 1972;129:345–355.
29. Krejs GJ, Nicar MJ, Zerwekh JE, et al. Effect of 1,25-dihydroxyvitamin D_3 on calcium and magnesium absorption in the healthy human jejunum and ileum. Am J Med 1983;75:973–976.

30. Brannan PG, Marauski G, Pak CYC, et al. Selective jejunal hyperabsorption of calcium in absorptive hypercalciuria. Am J Med 1979;66:425–428.
31. Zerwekh JE, Pak CYC, Kaplan RA, et al. Pathogenic role of 1 alpha,25-dihydroxyvitamin D in sarcoidosis and absorptive hypercalciuria: Different response to prednisolone therapy. J Clin Endocrinol Metab 1980;51:381–386.
32. Coe FL, Bushinksy DA. Pathophysiology of hypercalciuria. Am J Physiol 1984;247:F1–F13.
33. DeLuca HF. The transformation of a vitamin into a hormone: The vitamin D story. Harvey Lect 1979–80;75:333–379.
34. Caldas AE, Gray RW, Lemann J. The simultaneous measurement of vitamin D metabolites in plasma: Studies in healthy adults and in patients with calcium nephrolithiasis. J Lab Clin Med 1978;91:840–849.
35. Berlin T, Bjorkhem I, Collste L, et al. Relation between hypercalciuria and vitamin D_3—status in renal stone formers, in Schwille PO, Smith LH, Robertson WG, et al (eds): Urolithiasis and Related Clinical Research. New York, Plenum, 1985, p 253.
36. Elomaa I, Karonen S-L, Kairento A-L, Pelkonen R. Seasonal variation of urinary calcium and oxalate excretion, serum $25(OH)D_3$ and albumin level in relation to renal stone formation. Scand J Urol Nephrol 1982;16:155–161.
37. Broadus AE, Insogna KL, Lang R, et al. A consideration of the hormonal basis and phosphate leak hypothesis of absorptive hypercalciuria. J Clin Endocrinol Metab 1984;58:161–169.
38. Shen FH, Baylink DJ, Nielsen RL, et al. Increased serum 1,25-dihydroxyvitamin D in idiopathic hypercalciuria. J Lab Clin Med 1977;90:955–962.
39. Pak CYC, Ohata M, Lawrence EC, et al. The hypercalciurias: Causes, parathyroid functions and diagnostic criteria. J Clin Invest 1974;54:387–400.
40. Burckhardt P, Jaeger P. Secondary hyperparathyroidism in idiopathic renal hypercalciuria: Fact or theory? J Clin Endocrinol Metab 1981;53:550–555.
41. Barilla DE, Zerwekh JE, Pak CYC. A critical evaluation of the role of phosphate in the pathogenesis of absorptive hypercalciuria. Miner Electrolyte Metab 1979;2:302–309.
42. Broadus AE, Erickson SB, Gertner JM, et al. An experimental human model of 1,25-dihydroxyvitamin D-mediated hypercalciuria. J Clin Endocrinol Metab 1984;59:202–206.
43. Maierhofer WH, Gray RW, Cheung HS, et al. Bone resorption stimulated by elevated serum $1,25\text{-}(OH)_2$-vitamin D_3 concentrations in healthy men. Kidney Int 1983;24:555–560.
44. Smith CL, Davis M, Berkseth RO. Dietary factors in calcium nephrolithiasis. J Renal Nutrition 1992;2:146–153.
45. Nordin BEC. Hypercalciuria. Clin Sci Mol Med 1977;52:1–8.
46. Lemann J, Adams ND, Gray RW. Urinary calcium excretion in human beings. N Engl J Med 1979;301:535–541.
47. Silver J, Friedlaender MM, Rubinger D, et al. Sodium-dependent idiopathic hypercalciuria in renal-stone formers. Lancet 1983;2:484–486.
48. Robertson WG, Heyburn PJ, Peacock M, et al. The effect of high animal protein intake on the risk of calcium stone formation in the urinary tract. Clin Sci 1979;57:285–288.
49. Nguyen NV, Dumoulin G, Wolf JP, et al. Urinary oxalate and calcium excretion in response to oral glucose load in man. Horm Metab Res 1986;18:869–870.
50. Donaldson CL, Hulley SB, Vogel JM, et al. Effect of prolonged bed rest on bone mineral. Metabolism 1970;19:1071–1084.
51. Stewart AF, Ader M, Byers CM, et al. Calcium homeostasis in immobilization: An example of resorptive hypercalciuria. N Engl J Med 1982;306:1136–1140.
52. Heaney RP. Radiocalcium metabolism in disuse osteoporosis in man. Am J Med 1962;33:188–200.
53. Peacock M, Marshall RW, Robertson WG, et al. Renal stone formation in primary hyperparathyroidism and idiopathic stone disease: Diagnosis, etiology and treatment, in Finlayson B, Thomas WC (eds): Colloquium on Renal Lithiasis. Gainesville, University Press of Florida, 1976, p 339.
54. Parnell DC, Smith LC, Scholz DA, et al. Primary hyperparathyroidism: A prospective clinical study. Am J Med 1971;50:670–678.
55. Broadus AE, Horst RL, Lang R, et al. The importance of circulating 1,25-dihydroxyvitamin D in the pathogenesis of hypercalciuria and renal stone formation in primary hyperparathyroidism. N Engl J Med 1980;302:421–426.
56. Pak CYC, Nicar MI, Peterson R, et al. A lack of unique pathophysiologic background for nephrolithiasis of primary hyperparathyroidism. J Clin Endocrinol Metab 1981;53:536–542.
57. Pak CYC, Holt K. Nucleation and growth of brushite and calcium oxalate in urine of stone formers. Metabolism 1976;25:665–673.
58. Smith LH, Van Den Berg CJ, Wilson DM, et al. Urolithiasis in primary hyperparathyroidism. Proc Am Soc Nephrol 1977;9 [abstract].
59. Avioli LV, McDonald JE, Signer RA. Excretion of pyrophosphate in disorders of bone metabolism. J Clin Endocrinol Metab 1965;25:912–915.
60. Russell RGG, Hodgkinson A. The urinary excretion of inorganic pyrophosphate in hyperparathyroidism, hyperthyroidism, Paget's disease and other disorders of bone metabolism. Clin Sci 1969;36:435–443.
61. Robertson WG, Knowles F, Peacock M. Urinary acid mucopolysaccharide inhibitors of calcium oxalate crystallization, in Fleisch H, Robertson WG, Smith LH, et al (eds): Urolithiasis Research. New York, Plenum, 1976, p 331.
62. Battle DC, Arruda JAL. Renal tubular acidosis syndromes. Miner Electrolyte Metab 1981;5:83–99.
63. Brenner RJ, Spring DB, Sebatian A, et al. Incidence of radiographically evident bone disease, nephrocalcinosis and nephrolithiasis in various types of renal tubular acidosis. N Engl J Med 1982;307:217–221.
64. Leman J, Wilz DR, Brenes LG. Acid, calcium and phosphorus balances in proximal renal tubular acidosis. Kidney Int 1976;10:561.
65. de Toni E, Nordio S. The relationship between calcium-phosphorus in metabolism, the "Krebs cycle" and steroid metabolism. Arch Dis Child 1959;34:371–382.
66. Milne MD, Stanbury SW, Thomson AE. Observations on the Fanconi syndrome and renal hyperchloremic acidosis in the adult. Q J Med 1952;21:61–82.

67. Mackenzie AR. Acetazolamide-induced renal stone. J Urol 1960;84:453–455.
68. Harrison HE, Harrison HC. Inhibition of urine citrate excretion and the production of renal calcinosis in the rat by acetazolamide (Diamox) administration. J Clin Invest 1955;34:1662–1670.
69. Becker B, Middleton WH. Long-term acetazolamide (Diamox) administration in therapy of glaucoma. AMA Arch Ophthalmol 1955;54:187–192.
70. Sutton RAL, Dewar J, Walker VR, et al. Renal calculi and acetazolamide (ACZ) therapy. Pro Am Soc Nephrol 1982;44 [abstract].
71. Buckalew VM, McCurdy DK, Ludwig GD, et al. Incomplete renal tubular acidosis: Physiologic studies in three patients with a defect in lowering urine pH. Am J Med 1968;45:32–442.
72. Buckalew VM, Purvis ML, Shulman MG, et al. Hereditary renal tubular acidosis: Report of a 64 member kindred with variable clinical expression including idiopathic hypercalciuria. Medicine 1974;53:229–254.
73. Hamed IA, Czerwinski AW, Coats B, et al. Familial absorptive hypercalciuria and renal tubular acidosis. Am J Med 1979;67:385–391.
74. Lemann J, Lennon EJ, Goodman AD, et al. The net balance of acid in subjects given large loads of acid or alkali. J Clin Invest 1965;44:507–517.
75. Goodman AD, Lemann J, Lennon EJ, et al. Production, excretion and net balance of fixed acid in patients with renal acidosis. J Clin Invest 1965;44:495–506.
76. Coe FL, Parks JH. Stone disease in hereditary distal renal tubular acidosis. Ann Intern Med 1980;93:60–61.
77. Coe FL, Firpo JJ. Evidence for mild reversible hyperparathyroidism in distal renal tubular acidosis. Arch Intern Med 1975;135:1485–1489.
78. Sutton RAL, Wong NLM, Dirks JH. Effects of metabolic acidosis and alkalosis on sodium and calcium transport in the dog kidney. Kidney Int 1979;15:520–533.
79. Dent CE, Stamp TCB. Vitamin D, rickets and osteomalacia, in Avioli LV, Krane SM (eds): Metabolic Bone Disease. New York, Academic Press, 1977, p 237.
80. Lee SW, Russell J, Avioli LV. 25-hydroxycholecalciferol to 1,25-dihydroxychlecalciferol: Conversion impaired by systemic metabolic acidosis. Science 1977;195:994–996.
81. Dedmon RE, Wrong O. The excretion of organic anion in renal tubular acidosis with particular reference to citrate. Clin Sci 1962;22:19–32.
82. Simpson DP. Citrate excretion: A window on renal metabolism. Am J Physiol 1983;244:F223–F234.
83. Coe FL. Renal tubular acidosis, in Nephrolithiasis: Pathogenesis and Treatment. Chicago, Year Book Medical Publishers, 1978, p 116.
84. Williams HE. Oxalic acid and the hyperoxaluric syndromes. Kidney Int 1976;13:410–419.
85. Zarembski PM, Hodgkinson A. Some factors influencing the urinary excretion of oxalic acid in man. Clin Chim Acta 1969;25:1–10.
86. Jaegger P, Portman L, Jacquet A-F, et al. Influence of the calcium content of the diet on the incidence of mild hyperoxaluria in idiopathic renal stone formers. Am J Nephrol 1985;5:40–44.
87. Lamden MP, Chrystowski GA. Urinary oxalate excretion in man following ascorbic acid ingestion. Proc Soc Exp Biol Med 1954;85:190–192.
88. Fituri N, Allavi N, Bently M. Urinary and plasma oxalate during ingestion of pure ascorbic acid: A re-evaluation. Eur Urol 1983;9:312–315.
89. Chalmers AH, Cowley DM, Brown JM. A possible etiological role for ascorbate in calculi formulation. Clin Chem 1986;32:333–336.
90. Gershoff SN, Faragalla FF, Nelson DA, et al. Vitamin B_6 deficiency and oxalate nephrocalcinosis in the cat. Am J Med 1959;27:72–80.
91. Smith CL. Renal complication following jejunoileal bypass surgery, in Linner J (ed): Surgery for Obesity. New York, Springer-Verlag, 1984, pp 42–48.
92. Pak CYC, Fuller C. Idiopathic hypocitraturic calcium-oxalate nephrolithiasis successfully treated with potassium citrate. Ann Intern Med 1986;104:33–37.
93. Pak CYC, Sakhaee K, Crowther C, et al. Evidence justifying a high fluid intake in treatment of nephrolithiasis. Ann Intern Med 1980;93:36–39.
94. Malek RS, Kelalis PP. Pediatric nephrolithiasis. J Urol 1975;113:545–551.
95. Sandegaard E. Prognosis of stone in the ureter. Acta Chir Scand 1956; (suppl 219):1–67.
96. Coe FL, Keck J, Norton ER. The natural history of calcium urolithiasis. JAMA 1977;239:1519–1523.
97. Pak CYC, Peters P, Hunt G, et al. Is selective therapy of recurrent nephrolithiasis possible? Am J Med 1981;71:615–622.
98. Elomaa I, Ala-Opas M, Porkka L. Five years of experience with selective therapy in recurrent calcium nephrolithiasis. J Urol 1984;132:656–661.
99. Ljunghall S, Fellstrom B, Johansson G. Prevention of renal stones by a high fluid intake? Eur Urol 1988;14:381–385.
100. Hughes J, Norman RW. Diet and calcium stones. Can Med Assoc J 1992;146:137–143.
101. Curhan GC, Willett WC, Rimm EB, Stampfer MJ. A prospective study of dietary calcium and other nutrients and the risk of symptomatic kidney stones. N Engl J Med 1993;328:833–838.
102. Fuss M, Pepersack T, VanGeel J, et al. Involvement of low-calcium diet in the reduced bone mineral content of idiopathic renal stone formers. Calcif Tissue Int 1990;46:9–13.
103. Boyce WH, Garvey FK, Goven CE. Abnormalities of calcium metabolism in patients with "idiopathic" urinary calculi. Effect of oral administration of sodium phytate. JAMA 1958;166:1577–1583.
104. Pak CYC. Clinical pharmacology of sodium cellulose phosphate. J Clin Pharmacol 1979;451–457.
105. Pak CYC. Effects of cellulose phosphate and sodium phosphate on formation product and activity product of brushite in urine. Metabolism 1972;21:447–455.
106. Backman U, Danielson BG, Johansson G, et al. Treatment of recurrent calcium stone formation with cellulose phosphate. J Urol 1980;123:9–13.
107. Pak CYC. A cautious use of sodium cellulose phosphate in the management of calcium nephrolithiasis. Invest Urol 1981;19:187–190.

108. Van den Berg CJ, Kumar R, Wilson DM, et al. Orthophosphate therapy decreases urinary calcium excretion and serum 1,25-dihydroxyvitamin D concentrations in idiopathic hypercalciuria. J Clin Endocrinol Metab 1980;51:998–1001.
109. Fleisch H, Bisaz S, Core AD. Effect of orthophosphate on urinary pyrophosphate excretion and the prevention of urolithiasis. Lancet 1964;1:1065–1067.
110. Lau K, Wolf C, Nussbaum C, et al. Differing effects of acid versus neutral phosphate therapy of hypercalciuria. Kidney Int 1979;16:736–742.
111. Thomas Jr WC. Effectiveness and mode of action of orthophosphates in patients with calcareous renal calculi. Trans Am Clin Climatol Assoc 1971;83:113–124.
112. Edwards NA, Russell RGG, Hodgkinson A. The effect of oral phosphate in patients with recurrent renal calculus. Br J Urol 1965;37:390–398.
113. Oliver I, Weinberger A, Boi-Meir S, et al. Orthophosphate treatment of calcium lithiasis associated with idiopathic hypercalciuria. Urol Int 1974;29:414–420.
114. Dudley FJ, Blackburn CRB. Extraskeletal calcification complicating oral neutral phosphate therapy. Lancet 1970;2:628–630.
115. Fleisch H, Russell RGG, Bisoy S, et al. The inhibitory effect of phosphanates on the formation of calcium phosphate crystals in vitro and on aortic and kidney calcification in vivo. Eur J Clin Invest 1970;1:12–18.
116. Hofmann AF, Poley JR. Role of bile acid malabsorption in pathogenesis of diarrhea and steatorrhea in patients with ileal resection. I. Response to cholestyramine or replacement of dietary long chain triglyceride by medium chain triglyceride. Gastroenterology 1972;62:918–934.
117. Pinto B, Bernshtam J. Diethylaminoethanol-cellulose in the treatment of absorptive hyperoxaluria. J Urol 1978;119:630–632.
118. Ito H, Suzuki F, Yamaguchi K, et al. Reduction of urinary oxalate by combined calcium and citrate administration without increase in urinary calcium oxalate stone formers. Clin Nephrol 1992;37:14–18.
119. Gershoff SN, Mayer AL, Kulczycki LL. Effect of pyridoxine administration on the urinary excretion of oxalic acid, pyridoxine, and related compounds in mongoloids and nonmongoloids. Am J Clin Nutr 1959;7:76–79.
120. Will EJ, Bijvoet OLM. Primary oxalosis: Clinical and biochemical response to high-dose pyridoxine therapy. Metabolism 1979;28:542–548.
121. Gibbs DA, Watts RWE. The action of pyridoxine in primary hyperoxaluria. Clin Sci 1970;38:277–286.
122. Smith Jr LH, Williams HE. Treatment of primary hyperoxaluria. Mod Treat 1967;4:522–530.
123. Dent CE, Stamp TCB. Treatment of primary hyperoxaluria. Arch Dis Child 1970;45:735–745.
124. Solomons CC, Goodman SI, Riley CM. Calcium carbimide in the treatment of primary hyperoxaluria. N Engl J Med 1967;276:207–210.
125. Zarembski PM, Hodgkinson A, Chochran M. Treatment of primary hyperoxaluria with calcium carbimide. N Engl J Med 1967;277:1000–1002.
126. Hautmann R, Hering FJ, Lutzeyer W. Calcium oxalate stone disease: Effects and side effects of cellulose phosphate and succinate in long-term treatment of absorptive hypercalciuria or hyperoxaluria. J Urol 1978;120:712–715.
127. Pinto B, Ruiz-Marcellan FJ, Bernshtam J. Effect of a 5-year treatment program in patients with hyperoxaluric stones. J Urol 1983;130:943–945.
128. Yendt ER, Gagne RJA, Cohanim M. The effects of thiazides in idiopathic hypercalciuria. Am J Med Sci 1966;251:449–460.
129. Zerwekh JE, Pak CYC. Selective effects of thiazide therapy on serum 1α,25-dihydroxyvitamin D and intestinal calcium absorption in renal and absorptive hypercalciurias. Metabolism 1980;29:13–17.
130. Pylypchuk G, Ehrig U, Wilson DR. Effect of hydrochlorothiazide on urine saturation with brushite, in vitro collagen calcification by urine, and urinary inhibitors of collagen calcification. Can Med Assoc J 1978;118:792–797.
131. Jorgensen FS. Effect of thiazide diuretics upon calcium metabolism. Dan Med Bull 1976;23:223–230.
132. Yendt ER, Cohanim M. Prevention of calcium stones with thiazides. Kidney Int 1978;13:397–409.
133. Pak CYC, Ruskin B, Diller E. Enhancement of renal excretion of zinc by hydrochlorothiazide. Clin Chim Acta 1972;39:511–517.
134. Nicar MJ, Peterson R, Pak CYC. Use of potassium citrate as potassium supplement during thiazide therapy of calcium nephrolithiasis. J Urol 1984;131:430–433.
135. Yendt ER, Guay GF, Garcia DA. The use of thiazides in the prevention of renal calculi. Can Med Assoc J 1970;102:614–624.
136. Scott R, Levi H. Therapeutic management of upper urinary tract stone disease in 172 subjects. Urology 1989;33:277–281.
137. Brocks P, Dahl C, Wolf H, Trousbol I. Do thiazides prevent idiopathic renal calcium stones? Lancet 1981;2:124–125.
138. Scholz D, Schurlle PO, Siegel A. Double-blind study with thiazide in recurrent calcium lithiasis. J Urol 1982;128:903–907.
139. Ettinger B, Citron JT, Livermore B, et al. Chlorthalidone reduces calcium oxalate calculous recurrence but magnesium hydroxide does not. J Urol 1988;139:679–684.
140. Pak CYC, Sakhaee K, Fuller CJ. Physiological and physicochemical correction and prevention of calcium stone formation by potassium citrate therapy. Trans Assoc Am Physicians 1983;96:294–305.
141. Barcelo P, Wuhl O, Servitoge E, et al. Randomized double-blind study of potassium citrate in idiopathic hypocitraturic calcium nephrolithiasis. J Urol 1993;150:1761–1764.
142. Wabner C, Pak CYC. Effect of orange juice consumption on urinary stone risk factors. J Urol 1993;149:1405–1408.
143. Cicerello E, Merol F, Gambaro G, et al. Effect of alkaline citrate therapy on clearance of residual renal stone fragments after extracorporeal shock wave lithotripsy in sterile calcium and infection nephrolithiasis patients. J Urol 1994;151:5–9.
144. Prien Sr EL, Gershoff SF. Magnesium oxide-pyridoxine therapy for recurrent calcium oxalate calculi. J Urol 1974;112:509–512.
145. Johansson G, Backman U, Danielson BG, et al. Biochemical and clinical effects of the prophylactic treatment of

renal calcium stones with magnesium hydroxide. J Urol 1980;124:770–774.
146. Melnick I, Landes RR, Hoffman AA, et al. Magnesium therapy for recurring calcium oxalate urinary calculi. J Urol 1971;105:119–122.
147. Fetner CD, Barilla DE, Townsend J, et al. Effects of magnesium oxide on the crystallization of calcium salts in urine in patients with recurrent nephrolithiasis. J Urol 1978;120:399–401.
148. Scholz D, Schwiller PO, Engelhardt W, et al. Idiopathic uric acid lithiasis—some less known epidemiologic and metabolic findings, in Sperling O, Vahlensieck W (eds): Advances in Urology and Nephrology, vol 16. Darmstadt, Steinkopff, 1981, pp 66–69.
149. Cifuentes-Delatte L, Rapado A, Abehsera A, et al. Uric acid lithiasis and gout, in Cifuentes-Delatte L, Rapado A, Hodgkinson A (eds): Urinary Calculi International Symposium Renal Stone Research. Basel, Karger, 1973, pp 115–118.
150. Frank M, Lazebrik J, DeVries A. Uric acid lithiasis: A study of six hundred and twenty-two patients. Urol Int 1970;25:32–46.
151. Backman U, Danielson BG, Fellstrom B, et al. Kidney stone disease. Experiences from Uppsala, Sweden. Scand J Urol Nephrol 1980;53(suppl):207–211.
152. Sorenson LB. Role of the intestinal tract in the elimination of uric acid. Arthritis Rheum 1965;8:694–703.
153. Steele TH. Renal excretion of uric acid. Arthritis Rheum 1975;18(suppl):793–804.
154. Weinman EJ, Knight TF. Renal tubular transport of urate. Miner Electrolyte Metab 1978;1:121–128.
155. Sperling O, deVries A, Kedem O. Studies on the etiology of uric acid lithiasis. IV. Urinary non-dialyzable substances in idiopathic uric acid lithiasis. J Urol 1965;94:286–292.
156. Pinto B. Isolation and identification of uricine and its effect on uric acid precipitation, in Finlayson B, Thomas WC (eds): Colloquium on Renal Lithiasis. Gainesville, University Press of Florida, 1976, pp 131–135.
157. Sperling O, deVries A. Studies on the etiology of uric acid lithiasis. II. Solubility of uric acid in urine specimens from normal subjects and patients with idiopathic uric acid lithiasis. J Urol 1964;92:331–334.
158. Coe FL, Strauss AL, Tembe V, Dun SL. Uric acid saturation in calcium nephrolithiasis. Kidney Int 1980;17:662–668.
159. Bennett RC, Jepson RP. Uric acid stone formation following ileostomy. Aust NZ J Surg 1966;36:153–158.
160. Henneman PH, Wallach S, Demsey EF. The metabolic defect responsible for uric acid stone formation. J Clin Invest 1962;41:537–542.
161. Pak CYC, Poy RK. Urinary pH in gout. Aust Ann Medicine 1965;4:35–39.
162. Barzel US, Sperling O, Frank M, deVries A. Renal ammonium excretion and urinary pH in idiopathic uric acid lithiasis. J Urol 1964;92:1–5.
163. Metcalfe-Gibson A, McCallum FM, Morrison RBI, Wrong O. Urinary excretion of hydrogen ion in patients with uric acid calculi. Clin Sci 1965;28:325–342.
164. Rapoport A, Crassweller PO, Hudson H, et al. The renal excretion of hydrogen ion in uric acid stone formers. Metabolism 1967;16:176–188.
165. Plank GE, Durivage J, Lemieux G. Renal excretion of hydrogen in primary gout. Metabolism 1968;17:377–385.
166. Falls WF. Comparison of urinary acidification and ammonium excretion in normal and gouty subjects. Metabolism 1972;21:433–445.
167. Yu T-F, Gutman AB. Uric acid nephrolithiasis in gout: Predisposing factors. Ann Intern Med 1967;67:1133–1148.
168. Coe FL, Raisen L. Allopurinol treatment of uric-acid disorders in calcium-stone formers. Lancet 1973;1:129–131.
169. Fellstrom B, Bachman U, Danielson BG, et al. Urinary excretion of urate in renal calcium stone disease and in renal tubular acidification disturbances. J Urol 1982;127:589–592.
170. Coe FL, Kavalach AG. Hypercalciuria and hyperuricosuria in patients with calcium nephrolithiasis. N Engl J Med 1974;291:1344–1350.
171. Anton FM, Puig JG, Gaspar G, et al. Renal handling of uric acid in patients with recurrent calcium nephrolithiasis and hyperuricosuria. Nephron 1984;37:123–127.
172. Fellstrom B, Backman U, Danielson BG, et al. Renal handling of urate in patients with calcium stone disease. Nephron 1982;31:31–36.
173. Pak CYC, Waters O, Arnold L, et al. Mechanism for calcium urolithiasis among patients with hyperuricosuria: Supersaturation of urine with respect to monosodium urate. J Clin Invest 1977;59:426–431.
174. Pak CYC, Arnold LH. Heterogenous nucleation of calcium oxalate by seeds of monosodium urate (38929). Proc Soc Exp Biol Med 1975;149:930–932.
175. Coe FL, Lawton RL, Goldstein RB, Tembe V. Sodium urate accelerates precipitation of calcium oxalate in vitro (38928). Proc Soc Exp Biol Med 1975;149:926–929.
176. Pak CYC, Holt K, Zerwekh JE. Attenuation by monosodium urate of the inhibitory effect of glycosaminoglycans on calcium oxalate nucleation. Invest Urol 1979;17:138–140.
177. Bowyer RC, Brockis JG, McCulloch RK. Glycosaminoglycans as inhibitors of calcium oxalate crystal growth and aggregation. Clin Chim Acta 1979;25:23–28.
178. Pak CYC, Barilla DE, Holt K, et al. Effect of oral purine load and allopurinol on the crystallization of calcium salts in urine of patients with hyperuricosuric calcium urolithiasis. Am J Med 1978;65:593–599.
179. Smith MJV. Placebo versus allopurinol for renal calculi. J Urol 1977;117:690–692.
180. deVries A, Frank M. Prophylaxis of idiopathic and gouty uric acid lithiasis by allopurinol. Urol Int 1967;22:506–516.
181. Hande KR, Noone RM, Stone WJ. Severe allopurinol toxicity. Description and guidelines for prevention in patients with renal insufficiency. Am J Med 1984;76:47–56.
182. Landgrebe AR, Nyhan WL, Coleman M. Urinary-tract stones resulting from the excretion of oxypurinol. N Engl J Med 1975;292:626–627.
183. Kranen S, Keough D, Gordon RB, et al. Xanthine-containing calculi during allopurinol therapy. J Urol 1985;133:658–659.
184. Lewis RW, Roth Jr JK, Polanco EJ, et al. Molar lactate in the management of uric acid renal obstruction. J Urol 1981;125:87–90.
185. Sharma SK, Indudhara R. Chemodissolution of urinary uric acid stones by alkali therapy. Urol Int 1991;48:81–86.

186. Freed SZ. Alternating use of an alkalinizing salt and acetazolamide in the management of cystine and uric acid stones. J Urol 1975;113:96–99.
187. Sakhaee K, Nicar M, Hill K, et al. Contrasting effects of potassium citrate and sodium citrate therapies on urinary chemistries and crystallization of stone forming salts. Kidney Int 1983;24:348–352.
188. Smith AD, Lee WJ. Percutaneous stone removal procedures including irrigation. Urol Clin North Am 1983;10:719–727.
189. Spataro RF, Linke CA, Basbaric ZL. Use of percutaneous nephrostomy and urinary alkalinization in the dissolution of obstructing uric acid stone. Diagn Radiol 1978;129:629–632.
190. Ebisuno S, Fukatani T, Yoshida M, et al. Percutaneous dissolution of uric acid calculi with THAM irrigation. Urol Radiol 1987;9:146–148.
191. Mills GD, Morrison ND, Walker RJ. Local dissolution of uric acid calculi using THAM-E. Renal Fail 1993;15:539–543.
192. Bailey RR, Dann E, Greenslade NF, et al. Renal stones: A prospective study of 350 patients. NZ Med J 1974;79:961–965.
193. Modlin M. Renal stone: A study of 520 patients with special reference to the pattern of recurrence. S Afr Med J 1957;312:824–828.
194. Griffith DP, Musker DM. Prevention of infected urinary stones by urease inhibition. Invest Urol 1973;11:228–233.
195. Robertson WG, Peacock M, Nordin BEC. Activity products in stone forming and non-stone forming urine. Clin Sci 1968;34:579–594.
196. Griffith DP, Musker DM, Itin C. Urease: The primary cause of infection-induced urinary stones. Invest Urol 1976;13:346–350.
197. Griffith DP, Bruce RR, Fishbein WN. Infection (urease)-induced stones, in Coe FL, Brenner M, Stein JH (eds): Contemporary Issues in Nephrology, vol 5, Nephrolithiasis. New York, Churchill Livingstone, 1980, p 230.
198. Masover GK, Sawyer JE, Hayflick L. Urea-hydrolyzing activity of a T-strain mycoplasma: *Ureaplasma urealyticum.* J Bacteriol 1976;125:581–587.
199. Petterson S, Bronson JE, Grenbaro L, et al. *Ureaplasma urealyticum* in infectious urinary tract stones. Lancet 1983;1:526–527.
200. McLean RJC, Nickel JC, Noakes VC, et al. An in vitro ultrastructural study of infectious kidney stone genesis. Infect Immun 1985;49:805–811.
201. Nemoy NJ, Stamey TA. Surgical, bacteriological and biochemical management of "infection stones." JAMA 1971;215:1470–1476.
202. Cox CE. Urinary tract infection and renal lithiasis. Urol Clin North Am 1974;1:279–297.
203. Singh M, Chapman R, Tresidder GC, et al. The fate of unoperated staghorn calculus. Br J Urol 1973;45:581–585.
204. Wojewski A, Zajaczkowski T. The treatment of bilateral staghorn calculi of the kidneys. Int Urol Nephrol 1974;5:249–260.
205. Androulakis P, Frangoulis E, Lefkidis C, et al. Kidney damage in recurrent lithiasis: A survey of 175 cases with clinicopathological observations. Eur Urol 1982;8:261–264.
206. Silverman DE, Stamey TA. Management of infection stones: The Stanford experience. Medicine 1983;62:44–51.
207. Bueschen AJ, Zahm MJ, Lloyd LK. Adjuvant surgical techniques in the removal of staghorn calculi. J Urol 1980;123:342–344.
208. Wall I, Tiselius H-G, Larsson L. Hemiacidrin: A useful component in the treatment of infectious renal stones. Eur Urol 1988;15:26–30.
209. Suby HI, Albright F. Dissolution of phosphatic urinary calculi by the retrograde introduction of a citrate solution containing magnesium. N Engl J Med 1943;228:81–91.
210. Streem SB, Geisinger MA. Combination therapy for staghorn calculi in solitary kidneys: Functional results with long-term follow-up. J Urol 1993;149:449–452.
211. Saad F, Faucher R, Mauffette F, et al. Staghorn calculi treated by percutaneous nephrolithotomy: Risk factors for recurrence. Urology 1993;41:141–143.
212. Streem SB, Lammert G. Long-term efficacy of combination therapy for struvite staghorn calculi. J Urol 1992;147:563–566.
213. Angermeier K, Streem SB, Yost A. Simplified infusion method for 10% hemiacidrin irrigation of renal pelvis. Urology 1993;41:243–246.
214. Fostvedt GA, Barnes RW. Complications during lavage therapy for renal calculi. J Urol 1963;89:329–331.
215. Kohler FP. Renocidrin and tissue reaction. J Urol 1962;87:102–105.
216. Murphy FJ, Zelman S, Man W. Ascorbic acid as a urinary acidifying agent: Its adjunctive role in chronic urinary infection. J Urol 1965;94:300–305.
217. Nahata MC, Shimp L, Lampman T. Effect of ascorbic acid on urine pH in man. Am J Hosp Pharm 1977;34:1234–1237.
218. Fishbein WN, Carbone PP. Urease catalysis. II. Inhibition of the enzyme by hydroxyurea, hydroxylamine and acetohydroxamic acid. J Biol Chem 1965;240:2407–2414.
219. Musker DM, Saenz C, Griffith DP. Interaction between acetohydroxamic acid and 12 antibiotics against 14 gram-negative pathogenic bacteria. Antimicrob Agents Chemother 1974;5:106–110.
220. Maclaren DM. Influence of acetohydroxamic acid on experimental proteus pyelonephritis. Invest Urol 1974;12:146–149.
221. Smith MJV. Management of infected stone disease with hydroxyurea: A five year follow-up. Proc Eur Dial Transplant Assoc 1983;20:466–468.
222. Williams JJ, Rodman JS, Peterson CM. A randomized, double-blind study of acetohydroxamic acid in struvite nephrolithiasis. N Engl J Med 1984;311:760–764.
223. Burr RG, Naseibeh I. Effect of oral acetohydroxamic acid on urinary saturation in stone forming spinal cord patients. Br J Urol 1983;55:162–165.
224. Martelli A, Buli P, Cortecchia V, et al. Urease inhibition in the treatment of infected renal stones: Propionohydroxamic acid. Contr Nephrol 1987;58:196–200.
225. Milliner OE, Anderson JA, Appler ME, et al. Fluropamide: A potent inhibitor of bacterial urease with potential clinical utility in the treatment of infection induced urinary stones. J Urol 1982;127:340–350.
226. Labeeuw C, Gerbaulet C, Pozet C, et al. Cystine crystalluria and urinary saturation in cystine and non-cystine stone formers. Urol Res 1981;9:163–168.

227. Dahlberg PJ, Van Den Berg CJ, Kurtz SB, et al. Clinical features and management of cystinuria. Mayo Clin Proc 1977;52:533–542.
228. Kolb FO, Earll JM, Harper HA. "Disappearance" of cystinuria in a patient treated with prolonged low methionine diet. Metabolism 1967;16:378–381.
229. Zinnser HA. Effect of oral choline in reducing cystine excretion in cystinuria. J Urol 1950;63:929–935.
230. Miyagi K, Nakada F, Oshiro S. Effect of glutamine on cystine excretion in a patient with cystinuria. N Engl J Med 1977;30:196–198.
231. Miyagi K, Nakoda F. Amino acid reabsorption in cystinuria: The effects of monoaminodicarboxylic acids and amidogroup amino acids with special reference to glutamine. J Jpn Soc Intern Med 1978;67:694–702.
232. Skouby R, Rosenberg LE, Thier SO. No effect of L-glutamine on cystinuria. N Engl J Med 1980;302:236–237.
233. Kean WF, Dwosh IL, Anastassiades TP, et al. Toxicity pattern of D-penicillamine therapy. Arthritis Rheum 1980;23:158–164.
234. Koide T, Yoshioka T, Yamaguchi S, et al. A strategy of cystine stone management. J Urol 1992;147:112–114.
235. Hautmann R, Terhorst B, Stuhlsatz HW, et al. Mercaptopropionylglycine: A progress in cystine stone therapy. J Urol 1977;117:628–630.
236. DiSilverio F, Gallucci M, Ricciutti GP, et al. Mercaptoethane sulphonate in cystinic calculosis therapy. Contr Nephrol 1987;58:193–195.
237. Al-Hariri SO, Elzouki AY. Captopril: A new treatment for cystinuria in children. Pediatr Nephrol 1989;3:196 [abstract].
238. Mulvaney WP, Quilter T, Montera A. Experiences with acetylcysteine in cystinuric patients. J Urol 1975;114:107–108.
239. Stark H, Savir A. Dissolution of cystine calculi by pelviocaliceal irrigation with D-penicillamine. J Urol 1980;124:895–898.
240. Smith AD, Lange PH, Miller RP, et al. Dissolution of cystine calculi by irrigation with acetylcystine through percutaneous nephrostomy. Urology 1979;13:422–423.
241. Tseng CA, Talwalkon YB, Tank EJ, et al. Dissolution of cystine calculi by pelviocaliceal irrigation with tromethamine-E. J Urol 1982;128:1281–1284.

Chapter 49

Glomerulonephritis

Alan H. Lau, PharmD, FCCP,
and Ignatius Y. S. Tang, PharmD, BCPS

Clinical and pathologic findings associated with primary glomerular injury were first reported in the nineteenth century. The natural history of many glomerular diseases was not described until the 1950s when percutaneous diagnostic kidney biopsy became available. The development of immunofluorescence microscopy and advances in immunopathology in the 1960s and 1970s further expanded our understanding of the antibody-related immune mechanisms that are responsible for the different types of glomerular injury.[1] Recent advances in cell and molecular biology afford us a plethora of new information concerning the disease processes.[2] However, the precise pathogenetic mechanisms for many glomerular diseases remain unknown and the available therapeutic regimens are still far from optimal.

Glomerulonephritis is now the third most common cause of end-stage renal disease (ESRD) and accounts for 12.6% of all new cases, or about 5000 patients each year.[3] The median age of glomerulonephritis patients with ESRD (54 years old) is considerably less than their diabetic (61 years) and hypertensive (68 years) counterparts.

This chapter provides an overview of the pathogenetic mechanisms of glomerular injury and the clinical presentations of glomerulonephritis. The specific characteristics of and the treatment approach for each of the more common forms of glomerulonephritis are also discussed. Although diabetes mellitus and amyloidosis are important secondary causes of glomerular diseases, we have limited the scope of this chapter to the primary causes of glomerulonephritis.

Pathophysiology/Mechanisms of Glomerular Injury

NORMAL ANATOMY AND FUNCTION

The glomerulus is a unique capillary bed that allows small nonprotein plasma constituents up to the size of inulin, which has a molecular weight of 5200, to pass freely while excluding macromolecules equal to or larger than albumin, which has a molecular weight of 69,000 (Fig. 49.1). Both the size and charge of the molecules affect the ease of passage through the glomerular membrane.[4] For molecules with similar effective molecular radii, those that are anionic tend to experience more difficulties in passing through the membrane than molecules that are cationic (Fig. 49.2).[4]

The glomerulus, which is enclosed within the Bowman's capsule, consists of two important components: the filtration barrier and the mesangium (Fig. 49.3). Blood flow in the glomerular capillary bed is supplied by the afferent arteriole while the efferent arterioles channel the flow leaving the glomerular tuft. The capillary wall, which serves as a filtration barrier, consists of three well-defined layers: fenestrated endothelium, glomerular basement membrane (GBM), and epithelial cells. The epithelial cells, also known as podocytes, have specialized foot processes embedded in the outer layer of the GBM. It is across this barrier that fluid flows and ultimately forms ultrafiltrate. Under normal conditions, the GBM appears to function as a compact hydrated gel of matrix proteins with a porelike structure. The mesangium provides support for the glomerular capillaries and also modulates blood flow through the capillaries. It consists of mesangial cells embedded in an extracellular matrix.

Fixed, negatively charged sites have been demonstrated within the glomeruli. These charged sites are detectable in all three layers of the capillary wall: the endothelium, the epithelium, and the GBM. Biochemical and cytochemical studies have shown that the epithelial cell coat is composed of a negatively charged glycoprotein (podocalyxin), made up largely of sialic acid. In addition, the GBM contains an abundance of negatively charged sulfated glycosaminoglycans. These charged entities can affect the passage of ionic molecules through the capillary wall. The movement of negatively charged molecules is restricted more than that of neutral or positively charged molecules (Fig. 49.2).[4] The different glomerular diseases affect this size- and charge-selective barrier to different extents and the glomerulopathies therefore present with varied clinical features and solute excretion patterns.

Aside from being a barrier for solute excretion, some of the glomerular cells, such as the epithelial cells, have phagocytic function that can remove macromolecules trapped within the filtration barrier. They are also capable

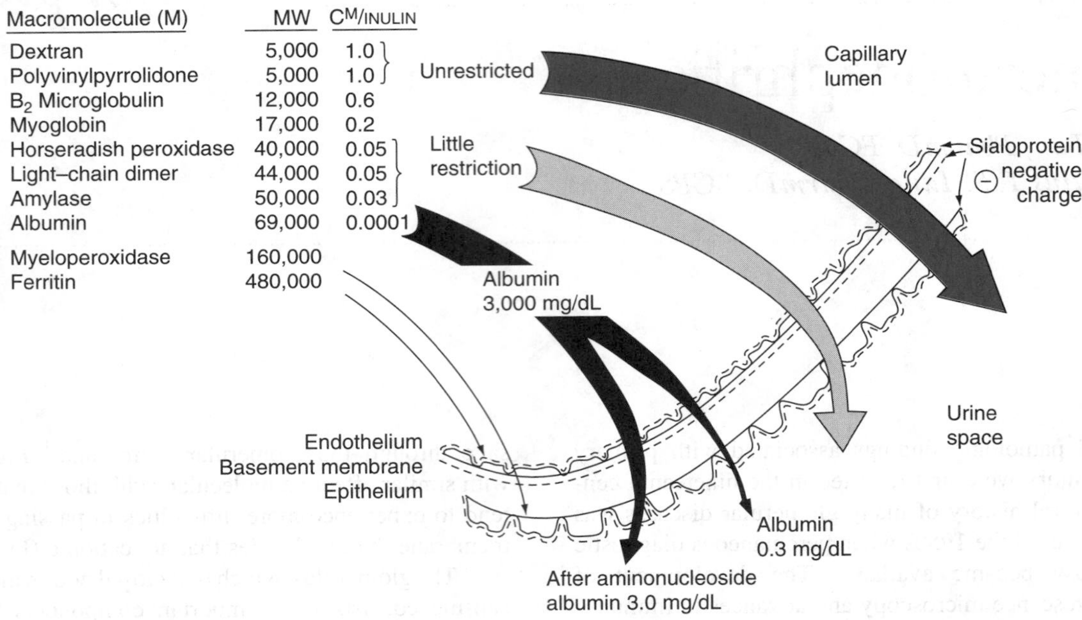

Figure 49.1. Movement of various macromolecules across the glomerular capillary. The thicker the arrow, the less restriction on movement. The fractional clearance of each macromolecule as compared to inulin (C^M/INULIN) decreases as molecular weight (MW) increases. The disproportionately greater restriction of albumin movement indicates importance of factors other than size, such as the negative charge of albumin. *(Reprinted from Hutt MP, Kelleher SP. Proteinuria and the nephrotic syndrome, in Schrier RW (ed): Renal and Electrolyte Disorders, 3rd ed. Boston, Little, Brown and Co, 1986.)*

of synthesizing the GBM. In contrast, the mesangial cells regulate glomerular hemodynamics, by responding to angiotensin II and producing prostaglandins. They also synthesize and respond to various cytokines and thus play a key role in immune-mediated glomerular diseases. There are also resident phagocytes in the mesangium. They remove macromolecules trapped in the basement membrane and move them into the urinary space. These phagocytes are involved in the development of both immune and nonimmune glomerular injury.[5]

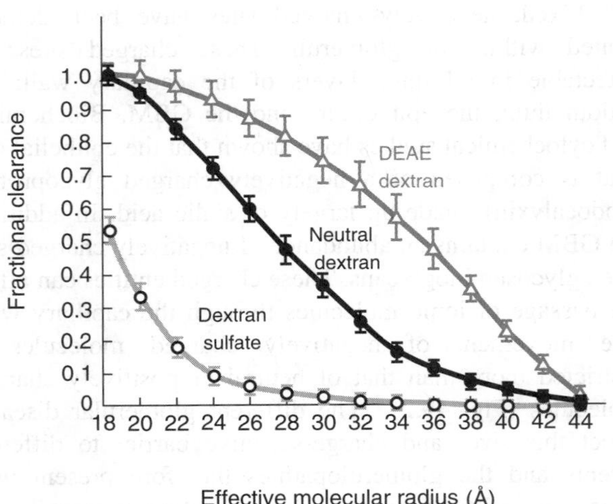

Figure 49.2. Fractional clearances of DEAE dextran (cationic), neutral dextran, and dextran sulfate (anionic), plotted as a function of effective molecular radius in normal rats. Values are expressed as means±SEM. *(Reprinted from Ref. 4.)*

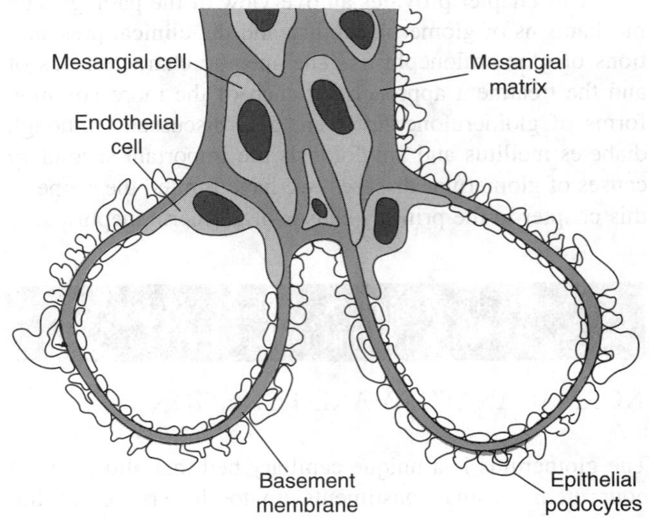

Figure 49.3. Schematic representation of glomerulus.

PATHOGENESIS OF GLOMERULAR INJURY AND PATHOLOGIC MANIFESTATIONS

The etiology of most human glomerulonephritides is unknown. However, humoral and cellular immunologic mechanisms are implicated in the pathogenesis. Abnormalities in coagulation and metabolism, as well as hereditary and vascular diseases, have also contributed to glomerular damage. The histopathologic manifestations vary substantially among the different types of glomerulonephritis. Although this section provides an overview of the primary pathogenetic mechanisms, those specific for each of the primary types of glomerulonephritis are presented in subsequent sections.

The glomerular lesion may be diffuse (involving all glomeruli), focal (involving some but not all glomeruli), or segmental, also known as local (involving part of the individual glomeruli).[6] Glomerular pathologic manifestations may also be described as proliferative (overgrowth of epithelium, endothelium, or mesangium), membranous (thickening of GBM), and/or sclerotic.[6]

The glomerular capillary wall is particularly susceptible to immune-mediated injury. Antigen and antibody tend to localize in the glomerulus probably because of its high blood flow and capillary hydrostatic pressure. Parenchymal damage can be induced as a result of humoral- and cell-mediated immune reactions (Table 49.1). Antibodies and sensitized T lymphocytes are the primary mediators of glomerular injury.[7,8]

Production of antibodies to endogenous or exogenous antigens that are recognized as foreign by the host is the first step in humoral immunologic damage to the glomerulus. Endogenous antigens may be intrinsic glomerular antigens, such as Heymann antigen on the epithelial cell or Goodpasture antigen on the GBM; or previously sequestered antigens, such as DNA or thyroglobulin. Exogenous antigens are most often viral, bacterial, parasitic, or fungal in origin (Table 49.2). Recently, antineutrophil cytoplasmic autoantibodies (ANCAs) have been found in patients with idiopathic crescentic glomerulonephritis and also in those with different forms of accompanying vasculitis.[9] ANCAs are autoantibodies that react to the cytoplasmic components of neutrophils and monocytes.

Classically, it has been considered that antigen– antibody complexes are formed in the circulation and then passively entrapped in the glomerular capillary or mesangium.

TABLE 49.1. IMMUNOLOGIC MECHANISMS OF GLOMERULAR INJURY

Circulating immune complexes
In situ antigen-antibody interaction
Intrinsic glomerular antigen, e.g., GBM antigens
Exogenous planted antigens
Cell-mediated mechanism

TABLE 49.2. ANTIGENS POSSIBLY INVOLVED IN IMMUNE-MEDIATED GLOMERULAR INJURY

Source of Antigen	Clinical Example
Endogenous Antigens	
Released sequestered cellular antigens	DNA, thyroglobulin
Endogenous antigens modified by exogenous source	IgG modified by streptococcal neuraminidase
Tumor antigens	CEA[a] in bronchial and other solid tumors
Intrinsic glomerular antigens	Goodpasture's syndrome
Neutrophil granule constituents	ANCA[b]-associated glomerulonephritis
Exogenous	
Viral	Hepatitis B
Bacterial	Streptococcal organisms
Parasitic	Malaria
Fungal	*Candida*

[a]CEA, carcinoembryonic antigen.
[b]ANCA, antineutrophil cytoplasmic antibody.

Recent experimental data, however, have shown that antibodies may combine with endogenous glomerular antigens or exogenous antigens entrapped in the glomerulus to form complexes locally, or *in situ.*[7] Regardless of the mechanism of formation, these antigen–antibody complexes are often localized along the capillary loop or the mesangium (Fig. 49.3) and detected by immunofluorescence microscopy. The type and extent of glomerular damage is dependent on the location of the immune complex formation and the rate at which it is removed. Hence, subendothelial and mesangial deposits have direct access to inflammatory cells in the circulation, and result in their activation. On the other hand, subepithelial deposits are separated from circulating cells by the GBM, and a noninflammatory lesion is produced. Impaired removal of the immune complex facilitates the growth of the complex and thus increases the likelihood of glomerular damage.

Subsequent to antigen–antibody formation, a series of biologic events is triggered that ultimately leads to glomerular injury. Both inflammatory and noninflammatory lesions can be induced by antibody deposition. Noninflammatory lesions can be a result of noncomplement fixing antibody to the glomerular epithelial cell (type 1), or activation of the complement system to form the C5b-9 membrane attack complex (type 2).[7,8] Both these mechanisms damage the glomerular epithelial cell and result in capillary wall injury and proteinuria (Fig. 49.4). Inflammatory lesions are induced by glomerular infiltration of circulating inflammatory cells such as neutrophils, monocytes/macrophages, and platelets (type 3), or proliferation of resident glomerular mesangial cells (type 4), resulting in GBM damage[7] (Fig. 49.4). The migration of neutrophils and

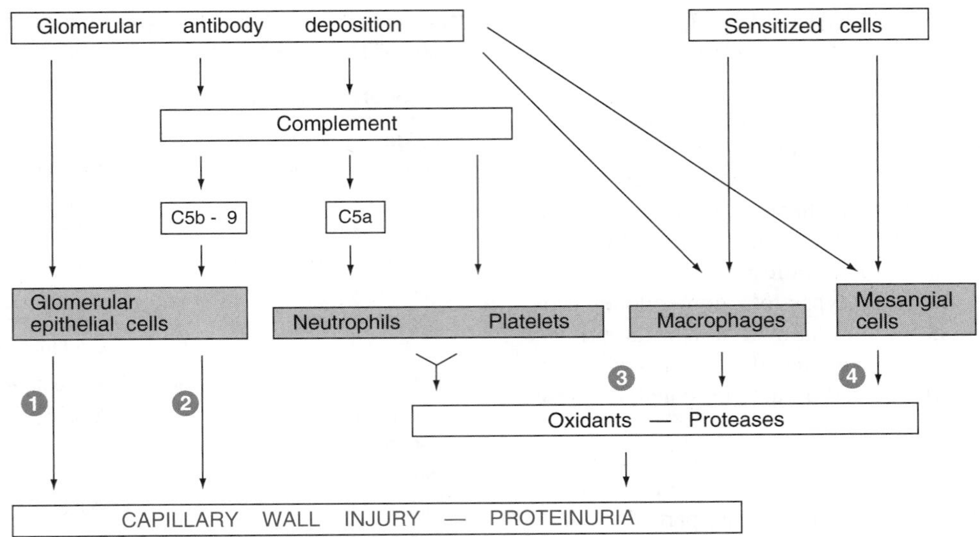

Figure 49.4. The major pathways of immune-mediated glomerular injury. Mechanisms 1 and 2 primarily act on the glomerular epithelial cell and result in noninflammatory lesions. Mechanisms 3 and 4 involve participation of effector cells and result in glomerular inflammation and structural damage. *(Reprinted from Ref. 7.)*

monocytes to the glomerular tufts is promoted by chemoattractants such as complement fragments (C3a, C5a), platelet activating factor, interleukin-8, and monocyte chemotactic protein-1.[10]

T cells sensitized to glomerular antigen, macrophages, and resident mesangial cells are important participants in cell-mediated injury. Sensitized T cells can cause glomerular hypercellularity in the absence of antibody deposition.[7,8,10,11] Cytotoxic T cells may bind with the target cells and destroy them. Alternatively, a delayed-type hypersensitivity reaction may be initiated by activated T cells, through the release of lymphokines, to attract, activate, and transform monocytes into macrophages.[7,11] These humoral and cellular mediators, in conjunction with a host of toxic molecular entities, including reactive oxygen species, proteinases, eicosanoids, and procoagulants, which are secreted by neutrophils, macrophages, platelets, and resident glomerular cells, can alter the permeability, blood flow, and function of the glomeruli. Vascular constriction and occlusion follow to result in the eventual destruction of the glomeruli.

Acute forms of glomerular injury may frequently lead to chronic and persistent renal dysfunction even though the original immune factors that induce glomerular injury have resolved. Progression to end-stage renal failure may become inevitable. Recent experimental and clinical investigations have suggested that a variety of factors may participate in the progression of renal injury.[12] These include systemic and glomerular hypertension,[13] high dietary protein intake, proteinuria,[14–16] glomerular hypertrophy, hyperlipidemia,[17] activation of the coagulation system,[13] abnormalities of calcium and phosphorous balance,[13] and tubulointerstitial injury.[15] The latter is considered an important factor in the progression of glomerular disease (Fig. 49.5). How these nonimmunologic factors contribute to renal injury is not well defined. Much interest has been focused on the role of proteinuria in causing glomerular and tubulointerstitial damage. The degree of proteinuria not only is an index of the severity of glomerular diseases, but also provides a measure of the rate of progression of renal injury. Heavy proteinuria is an indicator of poor prognosis in various glomerular diseases.[16] Although there is no direct evidence to substantiate that proteinuria per se results in progression of renal impairment,[14,15] there are many possible mechanisms through which proteinuria directly or indirectly causes renal damage. Proximal tubular uptake and metabolism of albumin may lead to unregulated intracellular release of potentially toxic fatty acids, which may provoke secretion of a lipid macrophage chemotactic factor, resulting in interstitial inflammation.[16] Tubular hypermetabolism may lead to increased reactive oxygen species production and renal ammoniagenesis, resulting in complement activation and consequent tubular injury.[15] Proteinuria is also accompanied by an increased flux of macromolecules across the mesangium. The mesangial overload may then lead to structural damage. The passage of serum components, such as complement, across the GBM may have a pathophysiologic effect on the glomerular epithelial cells and alter the integrity of the glomerular filtration barrier.[14] The damaging effects of macromolecules other than albumin, such as immunoglobulins, lipoproteins, transferrin, and complement, remain to be characterized.[15]

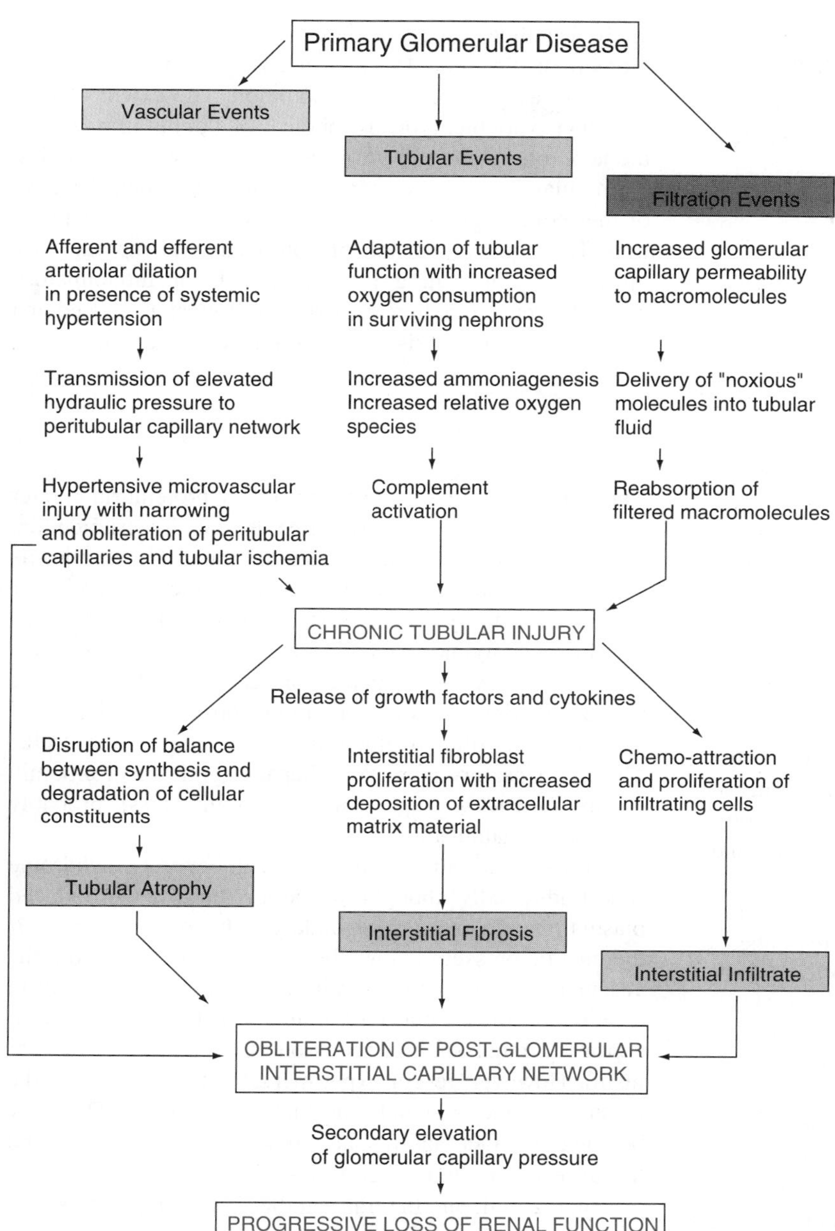

Figure 49.5. Proposed sequence of events leading from primary glomerular disease to progressive loss of renal function through tubulointerstitial injury. *(Reprinted from Ref. 15.)*

Clinical Presentation

Patients with glomerular disease may present with a nephritic or a nephrotic syndrome (Table 49.3). Nephritic syndrome reflects glomerular inflammation and frequently results in hematuria. White cells and cellular and granular casts are also commonly found in the urine. In contrast, nephrotic syndrome reflects noninflammatory injury to the glomerular structures, and thus results in few cells or cellular casts in the urine. Initially, there may be limited or no reduction in renal excretory function.

Hematuria occurs when red blood cells leak through the openings of the GBM. The presence of red cell casts is highly indicative of glomerulonephritis or vasculitis. The presence of dysmorphic red blood cells in the urine is also suggestive of glomerular disease. The red blood cells are damaged as they pass through the openings in the GBM or the cells may sustain osmotic injury as they travel through the different osmotic environments within the lumen of the kidney tubules.

The presence of proteinuria indicates a defect of the size- and/or charge-selective barriers within the GBM. Nor-

TABLE 49.3. TENDENCIES OF GLOMERULAR DISEASES TO MANIFEST NEPHROTIC AND NEPHRITIC FEATURES

	Nephrotic Features	Nephritic Features
Minimal change nephropathy	++++	–
Membranous nephropathy	++++	+
Diabetic glomerulosclerosis	++++	+
Amyloidosis	++++	+
Focal segmental glomerulosclerosis	+++	++
Mesangioproliferative glomerulonephritis	++	++
Membranoproliferative glomerulonephritis	++	+++
Proliferative glomerulonephritis	++	+++
Acute post-streptococcal glomerulonephritis	+	++++
Crescentic glomerulonephritis[a]	+	++++

[a]Can be immune complex-mediated, antiglomerular basement membrane antibody-mediated, or associated with antineutrophil cytoplasmic autoantibodies.

mal urinary protein excretion is usually between 40–80 mg/d, with a maximum of 150 mg. Fewer than 20 mg of the excreted proteins are albumin. Most of the albumin that enters the glomerular filtrate is either reabsorbed or catabolized by the tubular epithelium. The dipsticks that are commonly used to identify proteinuria detect only albumin and they only become positive when the protein excretion is more than 300–500 mg/d. The test is therefore not useful to detect early stages of renal injury secondary to diabetes mellitus or hypertension. These conditions are often associated with microalbuminuria with urinary albumin excretion ranging between 30–300 mg/d. Recently, a simple immunoassay on a dipstick has been introduced (Micral, Boehringer Mannheim Diagnostics, Indianapolis, IN). This device permits the specific and semiquantitative determination of urinary albumin concentrations at five levels: 0, 10, 20, 50, and 100 mg/L. It showed no cross-reactivity with other human proteins that may possibly be present in urine, and storage of the urine specimen for up to 7 days at 4°C and bacterial contamination did not alter the results.

Hypertension is a common feature in patients with glomerular diseases. Expansion of plasma volume is a frequent cause of hypertension, especially during acute disease. In contrast, the increased activity of vasoconstrictors, such as angiotensin II, is often responsible for elevated blood pressure in patients with chronic glomerular diseases.[18] Scarring of the glomerulus resulting in regional ischemia is thought to be responsible.

NEPHRITIC SYNDROME

Glomerular bleeding resulting in hematuria is a typical finding in nephritic syndrome. Dysmorphic red cells, especially acanthocytes, are a sensitive and specific marker of glomerular bleeding. The presence of pus and cellular and granular casts in the urine is common. The extent of proteinuria is variable, typically about 1–3 g/d, but it may be in the nephrotic range (>3 g/d). Patients with severe nephritic glomerular injury have renal function impairment because of the reduced glomerular surface area available for filtration. The latter is a result of constriction of the capillary lumen by proliferating mesangial cells or inflammatory cells. As renal function declines hypertension and edema may develop or preexisting conditions may worsen.

NEPHROTIC SYNDROME

Nephrotic syndrome is characterized by proteinuria greater than 3.0–3.5 g/d, hypoproteinemia, edema, hyperlipidemia, and, sometimes, a hypercoagulable state. The syndrome may be the result of primary diseases of the glomerulus or associated with systemic diseases such as diabetes mellitus, lupus, amyloidosis and preeclampsia. The hypoproteinemia, especially hypoalbuminemia, results from the increased urinary loss of albumin and increased rate of catabolism of filtered albumin by proximal tubular cells. The compensatory increase in hepatic synthesis of albumin is insufficient to replenish the protein loss, probably because of malnutrition.[19]

Edema formation in patients with nephrotic syndrome was traditionally thought to be driven by the reduced plasma oncotic pressure secondary to hypoalbuminemia. If the oncotic pressure is low, the movement of fluid from the vascular space to the interstitial compartment will result in a reduction of the plasma volume, which can cause compensatory renal sodium retention (the "underfill" mechanism). However, recent experimental data suggest that the plasma volume is actually normal or elevated.[20] This may be due to the fact that hypoalbuminemia has not been found to cause edema until the serum albumin concentration is less than 2 g/dL and the transcapillary oncotic pressure gradient is not as high as previously thought since increased lymphatic flow reduces the interstitial oncotic pressure by removing protein and fluid from the interstitium.[21] Thus, fluid retention is likely mediated by a primary increase in sodium reabsorption at the distal nephron, which is probably caused by tubular resistance to the action of atrial natriuretic peptide (the "overflow" mechanism).[22] It is still possible, however, that an interaction between the underfill and overfill mechanisms ultimately produces edema in the nephrotic patient.[22]

Although albuminuria below the nephrotic range appears to have a minor influence on serum cholesterol in patients with primary glomerular disease, daily urinary albumin excretion of greater than 3 grams is associated with a significant increase in serum cholesterol concentrations.[23] Hyperlipidemia in nephrotic syndrome is characterized by elevated serum total cholesterol and triglyceride concentrations, with increased very-low-density lipoprotein (VLDL) and low-density lipoprotein (LDL) cholesterol concentrations. Although high-density lipoprotein (HDL) cholesterol concentrations are normally distributed, there is a maldistribution of HDL subtypes, with a reduction in HDL_2 and an increase in HDL_3.[24,25] Furthermore, lipoprotein(a) levels may also be increased. Oval fat bodies and fatty casts are also found in the urine. The mechanisms for nephrotic hyperlipidemia are not well defined. A reduction in plasma oncotic pressure as a result of hypoalbuminemia may stimulate hepatic synthesis of lipids and lipoproteins. The increased VLDL production and increased liver cholesterol synthesis along with a decrease in LDL receptor activity can then lead to an increase in LDL cholesterol concentrations. In addition, reduced serum albumin or the loss of a liporegulatory substance may result in reduced VLDL clearance[24,25] (see Fig. 44.18). Nephrotic patients with hyperlipidemia, especially those with concomitant hypertension, are presumed to have an increased risk for atherosclerotic vascular disease. Hyperlipidemia has also been shown to promote the progression of glomerular injury, as evidenced by glomerosclerosis, mesangial expansion, and hyalinosis.[17,24,25]

Many patients with nephrotic syndrome have a hypercoagulable state due to defects of several control proteins in the coagulation cascade. Antithrombin III concentration is reduced because of increased loss in the urine.[26] A reduced amount of the coagulation inhibitors protein C and S, abnormal concentrations of clotting factors, increased fibrinogen concentrations, and abnormal platelet function may also contribute to the hypercoagulable state.[26] The net result of these alterations in coagulation is an increased risk for arterial and venous thrombosis, especially in the deep veins and renal veins.

Diagnostic Considerations

Patients with suspected glomerular disease should first be evaluated for a potential systemic cause. A thorough medical history should be obtained to identify symptoms of diabetes mellitus, amyloidosis, systemic lupus erythematosus, and other familial conditions associated with renal disease. Reduced appetite, fatigue, weight gain, and edema are all suggestive of nephrotic syndrome. Thorough medication, environmental, and occupation histories should be obtained to identify possible exposure to drugs, toxins, or chemicals that are known to be nephrotoxic. A carefully conducted physical examination may reveal signs and symptoms associated with systemic diseases, such as hypertension, rash, arthritis, retinopathy, neuropathy, lymphadenopathy, and hepatomegaly, as well as evidence of malignancy.

Examination of urine for active sediments, such as red blood cells, white blood cells, and casts, can differentiate the nephrotic and nephritic nature of the disease. The patient may present with normal urinalysis, isolated hematuria, or proteinuria, or significant abnormalities, such as nephrotic range proteinuria, hematuria, pyuria, lipiduria, and the presence of different casts.[27] Nephrotic sediment is characterized by heavy proteinuria (usually more than 3 g/d) and lipiduria. The patient's total urinary protein excretion can be quantified by a 24-hour urine collection or estimated by measuring the total protein:creatinine ratio in a random daytime urine specimen. This ratio correlates closely with the total urinary protein excretion. A ratio of 250 mg/dL:100 mg/dL represents 2.5 grams of protein excreted a day per 1.73 m^2 of body surface area.[28] In contrast, nephritic sediment includes hematuria, pyuria, cellular and granular casts, and variable degrees of proteinuria. When glomerular diseases progress to advanced renal insufficiency and result in a significant reduction in the glomerular filtration rate (GFR), the urinalysis may show less proteinuria and hematuria. The presence of broad waxy casts in the urinary sediment suggests chronicity of the glomerular disease.

GFR in patients with glomerular disease may be variable. In the early stages of the disease, the GFR may remain within the normal range. Initial injury to the glomerulus primarily lowers the permeability coefficient (K_f) of the GBM, by reducing the surface area available for filtration and/or the unit permeability of the membrane.[29] The reduced permeability is compensated by an elevation in the glomerular capillary hydrostatic pressure through afferent arteriolar dilation and efferent arteriolar constriction.[30] Extensive glomerular damage may therefore be present before a substantial reduction of total GFR is evident.

Patients who present with glomerulonephritis may be categorized according to the presence or absence of evidence for systemic disease (Fig. 49.6). Determination of the serum complement concentration is frequently helpful in defining the specific type of glomerular disease (Table 49.4). Measurement of antinuclear and anti-DNA antibodies, antistreptolysin antibodies, circulating anti-GBM antibodies, and cryoglobulins is useful in identifying the etiology (Fig. 49.7).

The patient's age is often helpful in pinpointing the specific type of glomerular disease. Many of the conditions are more prevalent in certain age groups, though they may occur at any age. Benign hematuria, for example, is primarily a disease of children. Lupus and idiopathic membranoproliferative glomerulonephritis are seen primarily in 15- to 40-year-old patients, and primary amyloidosis affects adults over the age of 40.

Although the cause of proteinuria and glomerular disease may be established from clinical and laboratory evaluation, more often uncertainty persists. In addition, specific treatment of the glomerular disease depends on the underlying pathology. Percutaneous renal biopsy is, therefore, often needed to provide a definitive diagnosis. One notable excep-

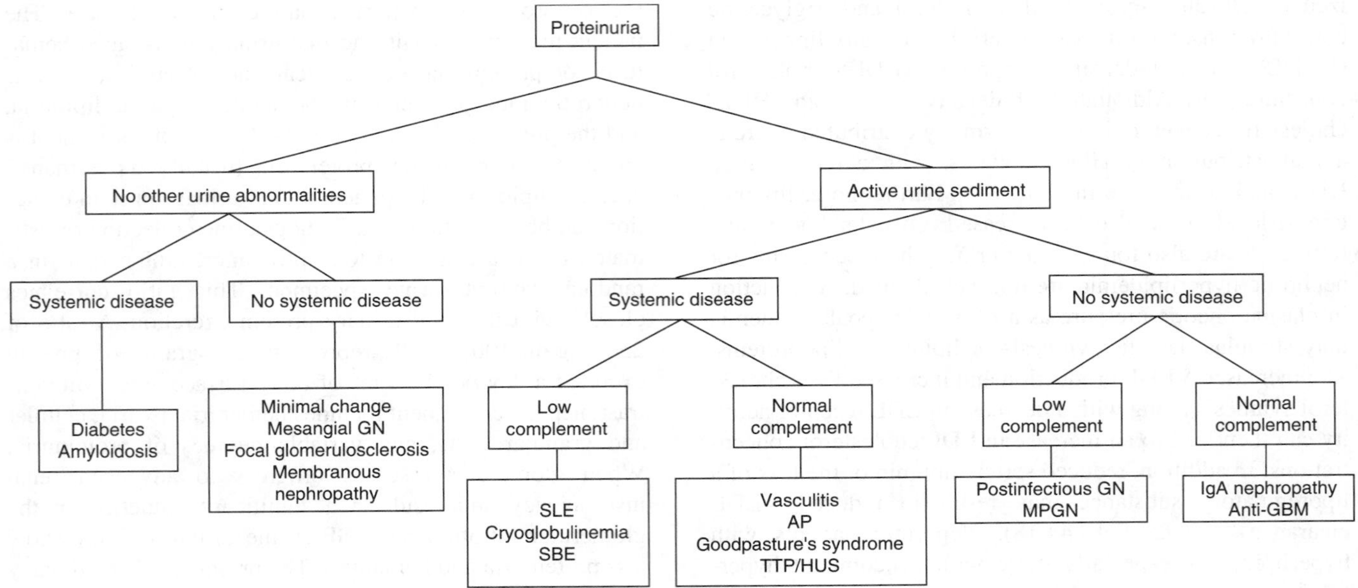

Figure 49.6. Clinical presentations of glomerulonephritis. GN, glomerulonephritis; MPGN, membranoproliferative glomerulonephritis; SLE, systemic lupus erythematosus; SBE, subacute bacterial endocarditis; GBM, glomerular basement membrane; TTP, thrombotic thrombocytopenic purpura; HUS, hemolytic–uremic syndrome; AP, anaphylactoid purpura.

tion is minimal-change disease (lipoid nephrosis), which is the most common etiology for nephrotic syndrome in children between 1 and 6 years of age. An empiric trial of corticosteroids is indicated for these patients without the need for histologic diagnosis. Biopsy is only indicated for those who fail to respond to a therapeutic trial of corticosteroids.

The decision to perform a biopsy should be based on an evaluation of the potential risks of the procedure against the anticipated benefits of knowing the underlying pathology as the basis for rational therapy. The most common complication of biopsy is bleeding, which may present as hematuria or perinephric hematoma. About 10% of the patients will have gross hematuria, which usually resolves in several days. However, blood transfusion may be needed in up to 1.0% of patients and nephrectomy or therapeutic embolic infarction may be necessary in 0.1% of the patients because of severe bleeding. Mortality from renal biopsy is probably less than 0.1%.[31] Biopsy is contraindicated in patients with a solitary kidney, polycystic kidney disease, uncontrolled hypertension, coagulation defects, or poor cooperation. Morphologic diagnosis can usually be made if tissue is examined with light, immunofluorescence, and electron microscopic techniques.

TABLE 49.4. DIAGNOSTIC CONSIDERATIONS OF RENAL DISEASES BASED ON SERUM COMPLEMENT LEVELS

Low Serum Complement Level	Normal Serum Complement Level
Systemic Diseases	**Systemic Diseases**
Systemic lupus erythematosus	Vasculitis group
Infection-related glomerulonephritis	Polyarteritis nodosa
Subacute bacterial endocarditis	Hypersensitivity vasculitis
"Shunt" nephritis	Wegener's granulomatosis
Cryoglobulinemia	Henoch–Schönlein purpura
Primary Renal Diseases	Goodpasture's syndrome
Acute poststreptococcal glomerulonephritis	**Primary Renal Diseases**
Membranoproliferative glomerulonephritis	IgA nephropathy
	Idiopathic rapidly progressive glomerulonephritis
	Idiopathic nephrotic syndrome

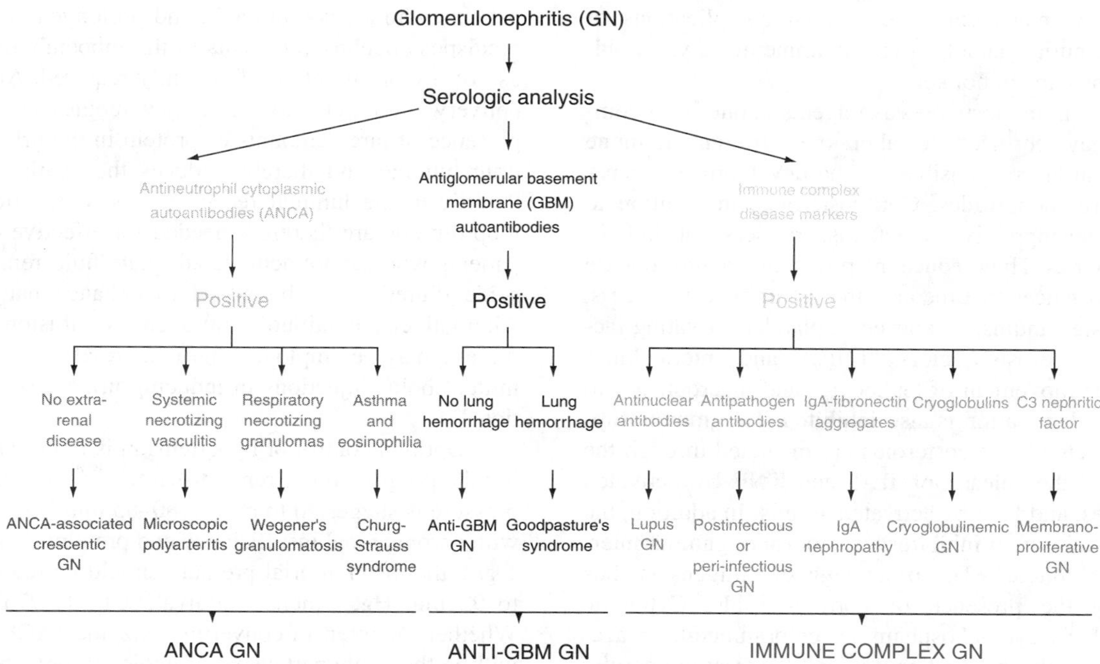

Figure 49.7. Schematic diagram depicting the serologic analysis of patients with glomerulonephritis. GN, glomerulonephritis; GBM, glomerular basement membrane; ANCA, antineutrophil cytoplasmic antibody. *(Reprinted from Jennette JC, Falk R. Glomerular clinicopathologic syndromes, in Greenburg A (ed): Primer on Kidney Diseases. Academic Press, San Diego, 1994.)*

Course and Prognosis

The course and prognosis of the different glomerular diseases are extremely variable and depend on the underlying etiology. In glomerular diseases with a secondary cause, once the initiating factor is removed, the prognosis of the renal disease is often good. In contrast, the rates of renal function deterioration among the primary glomerulonephritides vary according to the form of glomerulonephritis. Most patients with minimal-change disease, IgA nephropathy, and membranous nephropathy have a fairly good prognosis. However, those with focal segmental glomerulosclerosis who are resistant to therapy as well as those with rapidly progressive glomerulonephritis who are untreated are likely to experience a rapid loss of renal function. The latter group of patients may lose half of their renal function within 3 months.

The variable courses exhibited by the different glomerulonephritides require that specific treatment approaches be developed for each disease. The natural history of each type of glomerulonephritis has to be well delineated before a promising regimen can be evaluated. Otherwise, patients will be exposed to unnecessary drug toxicities if they have a type of glomerulonephritis that is likely to undergo spontaneous remission. It is therefore imperative to identify patients who are most likely to benefit from treatment, especially those who have other risk factors that may contribute to the deterioration of their renal function. In those instances where satisfactory regimens are not available to treat the primary disease, supportive measures should be identified to retard the rate of renal function loss. Optimization of systemic and glomerular pressure, reducing proteinuria, and possibly controlling hyperlipidemia may all improve the long-term outcome of these patients.

Prospective, randomized, controlled comparative trials need to be conducted in a sizable patient population before the efficacy of a new regimen can be established. This type of large-scale study is quite feasible for the more common forms of glomerulonephritis such as minimal-change disease, IgA nephropathy, and membranous nephropathy. In contrast, prospective, controlled trials are difficult to conduct for the relatively uncommon glomerulonephritides such as membranous proliferative glomerulonephritis.

Overview of Treatment

The management of patients with glomerulonephritis involves specific pharmacologic therapy for the glomerular disease, and supportive measures to prevent and/or treat the pathophysiologic sequelae, namely, hypertension, edema, and progression of renal disease. In addition, in patients with nephrotic syndrome, supportive therapy should also address the management of extrarenal complications of heavy proteinuria, namely, hypoalbuminemia, hyperlipidemia, and thromboembolism.

Multiple immunosuppressive agents, alone or in combination, may be used to alter the different immune processes that are responsible for the development of specific glomerulonephritides. Corticosteroids, in addition to their immunosuppressive effect, also possess anti-inflammatory activities. They reduce the production and/or release of many substances that mediate the inflammatory process, such as prostaglandins, leukotrienes, platelet activating factors, tumor necrosis factors (TNFs), and interleukin-1 (IL-1).[32] The movement of leukocytes and macrophages to the site of inflammation is also inhibited. The immunosuppressive effects of corticosteroids are mediated through the inhibition of the release of IL-1 and TNF by activated macrophages, and IL-2 by activated T cells. In addition, the actions of migration-inhibitory factor and gamma-interferon are inhibited.[32] The processing of antigens is thus affected by the presence of corticosteroids. Cytotoxic agents, such as cyclophosphamide, chlorambucil, or azathioprine, may also be used occasionally to treat glomerular diseases. Cyclosporine has been used recently to treat glomerulonephritis. The drug can reduce lymphokine production by activated T lymphocytes. It may also decrease proteinuria by improving the permselectivity of the GBM.

Since many immune factors are implicated in the pathogenesis of glomerulonephritis, plasmapheresis has been used to remove these mediators. Platelets have been shown to be activated in glomerular disease and platelet factors can cause arteriolar smooth muscle cell proliferation and alter vascular permeability. Antiplatelet agents are therefore used in some of these patients. Nonsteroidal anti-inflammatory agents (NSAIDs) are used because of their antiplatelet effect and their ability to alter capillary wall permeability, that often results in an improvement of proteinuria. They may also affect the arachidonic acid metabolism; however, the specific mechanisms of the beneficial effect remain to be established.

Supportive Therapy

In patients with nephrotic syndrome, dietary measures involve restriction of sodium intake to 50–100 mEq/d,[21,33] protein intake of 0.8–1.0 g/d,[33–35] and a low lipid diet of less than 200 mg cholesterol. Total fat should account for less than 30% of daily total calories.[33,34] Sodium restriction is important not only in the control of edema, but also hypertension and proteinuria. Similarly, protein restriction not only helps to reduce proteinuria, but also has a potential role in retarding the progression of renal disease.[34,36]

Management of nephrotic edema involves salt restriction, bedrest, and use of support stockings and diuretics.[22] However, severe salt restriction is difficult to achieve in patients who are sodium-avid and prolonged bedrest could predispose nephrotic patients to thromboembolism. Hence, use of a loop diuretic is frequently required. Although the delivery of diuretic to the kidney tubules is normal, the presence of large amounts of protein in the urine promotes drug binding and thereby reduces the availability of the diuretic to the luminal receptor sites. Large doses of the loop diuretic are therefore needed for effective diuresis. In patients who cannot achieve adequate fluid removal, a thiazide diuretic may be added to enhance natriuresis.[33,37] Alternatively, continuous intravenous infusion of a loop diuretic may be employed and is more effective than intermittent bolus injections in inducing urinary sodium excretion.[38]

Optimal control of hypertension is important in reducing the progression of renal disease.[35,39,40] The target blood pressure is suggested to be 130/80–85 mm Hg.[39] In patients with chronic renal insufficiency and proteinuria greater than 1 g/d, the mean arterial pressure should be reduced further to 92 mm Hg, which is equivalent to 125/75 mm Hg.[40] Whether angiotensin-converting enzyme (ACE) inhibitors will be the antihypertensive of choice to prevent and delay progression of renal disease as shown in type I diabetes mellitus[41] awaits further studies. However, it may be useful in patients with more than 3 grams of daily urinary protein excretion.[40]

Dietary protein restriction reduces proteinuria and may retard renal function deterioration. However, data from the Modification of Diet in Renal Disease (MDRD) study in patients with a moderate loss of renal function, i.e., a GFR of 25–55 mL/min/1.73 m^2, are inconclusive regarding the efficacy of a low-protein diet in slowing renal disease progression. Subgroup analyses of the MDRD data are under way. The current recommendation is to prescribe a standard protein diet, i.e., greater than 0.8 g/kg/d for these patients. In those who have GFRs of 13–25 mL/min/1.73 m^2, dietary protein intake should be reduced to 0.6 g/kg/d since it can retard the rate of renal function loss and also the time to reach end-stage renal disease.[35]

Since heavy proteinuria is the underlying cause for hypoalbuminemia and other complications of nephrotic syndrome, various strategies including protein restriction to 0.6–0.8 g/kg/d, plus an additional gram of protein for each gram of protein lost in the urine,[34,35] ACE inhibitors,[42–45] and NSAIDs,[46,47] have been shown to be effective in reducing proteinuria. An additive antiproteinuric effect has been shown with the combination of a low-protein diet and ACE inhibition,[45] as well as combined therapy with ACE inhibitors and NSAIDs.[48] Serum albumin concentrations were also improved during treatment.[44,45] ACE inhibition may also allow the use of a high-protein diet without risks of decreased albumin synthesis.[19,49] A reduction in proteinuria is usually apparent within the first few weeks of therapy while the maximal effect is attained after 8–12 weeks.[50] The initial antiproteinuric effect of ACE inhibitors is associated with a fall in filtration fraction, suggesting a reduction in intraglomerular pressure. However, an improvement of GBM permselectivity may be responsible for the long-term effect of ACE inhibitors.[50]

NSAIDs probably reduce proteinuria through an alteration of intrarenal hemodynamics, a decrease in GFR, and also the restoration of the barrier size-selectivity of the GBM.[33,50] Indomethacin and meclofenamate are the two NSAIDs that have been evaluated the most. Their antiproteinuric effect occurs within 1–2 weeks of the initiation of therapy.[33,51] NSAID therapy is indicated for patients with severe steroid-resistant nephrotic syndrome who have greater than 50% residual renal function.[51] The agents should be avoided in those with poor renal function because of their potential detrimental effect on kidney function and also the increased susceptibility of these patients to nephrotoxicity.[33,51] Long-term treatment is indicated for those who have greater than 40% reduction in urinary protein excretion and/or those whose serum albumin concentrations are doubled during therapy.[51] In conjunction with dietary sodium restriction, the antiproteinuric efficacy of protein restriction, ACE inhibition, and NSAIDs is enhanced.[50]

The abnormal lipoprotein profile seen in nephrotic patients may increase the risk of atherosclerosis. Even though the clinical sequelae of the dyslipidemia of nephrotic syndrome are unknown, it is prudent to treat patients with persistent nephrotic syndrome and sustained dyslipidemia, i.e., those with high VLDL and LDL cholesterol levels in the presence of a normal or low HDL cholesterol level. Therapy is especially needed for those with concurrent atherosclerotic cardiovascular disease, or with additional risk factors for atherosclerosis, such as smoking and hypertension.[24] Whether correction of lipoprotein abnormalities will slow the progression of renal disease as demonstrated in animal studies requires clinical confirmation.[24,25]

A low-fat diet is usually not sufficient to correct hyperlipoproteinemia.[17,33,52] Lipid-lowering agents are usually required. Probucol, bile acid resins, fibric acid derivatives, and hydroxymethylglutaryl coenzyme A (HMG CoA) reductase inhibitors have all been evaluated in patients with nephrotic syndrome.[24] HMG CoA reductase inhibitors, such as lovastatin, pravastatin, and simvastatin, are considered the drug of choice.[17,24,33] These agents inhibit the rate-limiting step in cholesterol biosynthesis, namely, the conversion of HMG CoA to mevalonate.[25] In short-term studies, they reduce total plasma cholesterol concentration by 22–36%, LDL cholesterol by 27–45%, and total plasma triglyceride concentration by 19–40%.[24] The increase in HDL cholesterol and/or decrease in atherogenic lipoprotein(a) is variable.[50,53,54] A recent meta-analysis showed that use of HMG CoA reductase inhibitors resulted in the greatest and most consistent decrease in LDL cholesterol levels.[52] Interestingly, the reduction in proteinuria with ACE inhibitors is accompanied by a reduction in total plasma cholesterol and the lipoprotein(a) level.[43,55] Combined use of an ACE inhibitor with an HMG CoA reductase inhibitor may therefore be more effective in controlling nephrotic hyperlipidemia.

Intravascular thrombosis is a serious and common complication of nephrotic syndrome, particularly in membranous nephropathy. While it is generally agreed that patients who have documented thromboembolic episodes should be anticoagulated with warfarin until remission of nephrotic syndrome, the use of prophylactic anticoagulation is controversial.[33] Recently, a decision analysis study suggested that prophylactic anticoagulation is beneficial in patients with membranous nephropathy.[56] However, prospective controlled studies should be conducted to confirm these findings. Anticoagulation should also be considered in patients with increased risks for thrombosis, such as prolonged bedrest, surgery, episodes of dehydration, or use of high-dose intravenous steroids.[33] The role of low molecular weight heparin in preventing thromboembolism is uncertain but preliminary results are encouraging.[57]

Pathophysiology and Pharmacotherapy of Individual Glomerulopathies

MINIMAL-CHANGE NEPHROPATHY

Minimal-change nephropathy (also termed minimal-change disease) is commonly found in children between 3 months and 6 years of age. It is in fact one of the most common chronic diseases in childhood. In children between 1 and 4 years of age, minimal-change disease accounts for more than 90% of all cases of nephrotic syndrome. The percentage drops gradually to less than 50% after 10 years old and only accounts for 10–15% of all cases of idiopathic nephrotic syndrome in adults.

Pathology and Pathogenesis

Minimal-change disease is also known as "nil" disease primarily because of the absence of definitive pathologic changes observed under light microscopy. The characteristic lesion in patients with minimal-change disease is the spreading and fusion of the foot processes of epithelial cells over an unchanged GBM. Lipoid nephrosis is another term that has been used to describe this type of glomerular disease because lipids, as well as renal tubular cells, are found in the urine. The pathogenesis of minimal-change disease is still unknown. Altered cell-mediated immunologic response, specifically T-cell dysfunction, is suspected to be responsible. The activated lymphocytes are thought to secrete lymphokines that reduce the production of anions in the GBM. The permeability of the GBM to plasma albumin is therefore increased through a reduction of electrostatic repulsion. The loss of anionic charges also results in fusion of the foot processes of the epithelial cells. Other conditions that involve T-cell abnormalities, such as Hodgkin's disease, T-cell lymphoma, and nephritis induced by NSAIDs, are also associated with minimal-change disease.

Clinical Manifestations

Most patients present initially with edema, frequently acute in onset, following a nonspecific upper respiratory tract infection which might have activated the T lymphocytes.[58] Nephrotic syndrome with massive proteinuria (substantially more than 40 $mg/m^2/h$ for children and 3 g/d for adults), edema, hypoalbuminemia, and hyperlipidemia is common. The patient's weight may be increased dramatically because of sodium and fluid retention. Gross hematuria is uncommon although microscopic hematuria may be seen in up to 20–25% of patients. Hypertension and decreased renal function are uncommon. However, volume depletion may result in mild to moderate azotemia in some patients.

Pharmacotherapy and Prognosis

Among all the causes of nephrotic syndrome, minimal-change disease is the most responsive to corticosteroid treatment. In children, steroid therapy is expected to reduce proteinuria in about 90% of the patients. The 10-year renal survival is greater than 95%.[59] Because of the excellent response to initial therapy with steroids and the prevalence of this glomerular disease in children, reduction of proteinuria secondary to steroid treatment is considered diagnostic for minimal-change disease without the need for biopsy. In the International Study of Kidney Disease in Children (ISKDC), remission was induced, as evidenced by diuresis, loss of edema, and resolution in proteinuria, within 8 weeks of therapy in over 93% of the 363 children.[60] Prednisone was administered at a dose of 60 $mg/m^2/d$, with a maximum 80 mg daily, in divided doses during the first 4 weeks. The dose was then reduced to 40 $mg/m^2/d$, or a maximum of 60 mg daily, in divided doses for three consecutive days every 7 days for another 4 weeks. An alternate-day dosage regimen can be used instead in the second 4 weeks, after which the prednisone dosage is tapered over several months.[59] Single daily doses of prednisone, instead of multiple daily doses, may result in faster and more sustained response with less frequent and less severe side effects.[59]

For adults, the dose of prednisone is 1 mg/kg/d during the initial 4 weeks with a reduction to 0.75 mg/kg/d every other day for the next 4 weeks. Proteinuria will disappear in 50–60% of patients after 8 weeks of treatment, and complete remission will be attained in 80% of patients after 28 weeks of therapy.[58] In some patients, 16 weeks of therapy may be needed before remission is induced.[58,60]

As many as 75–85% of the patients who respond to initial steroid therapy (steroid sensitive) will experience a relapse of proteinuria, mostly within 6–12 months after disease onset. However, some patients may not have the first relapse until 24–30 months later.[61] The risk of relapse is affected by the duration of initial steroid therapy.[33] Children who were asymptomatic with proteinuria diagnosed on a urinary screening program tend to have less frequent relapses and a more favorable clinical course.[62] In those who relapse, 50–65% may have steroid-responsive relapse episodes over the subsequent 3- to 5-year period.[61] The dose and duration of steroid treatment for the relapse do not influence the subsequent rate of relapse.[33] The remaining patients become steroid-dependent, requiring continuous low-dose alternate-day prednisone to maintain an extended relapse-free period.[58] A small number of patients will eventually develop resistance to steroids and a biopsy done at that time often reveals another pathology such as focal segmental glomerular sclerosis. It is controversial whether minimal-change disease progresses into focal segmental glomerular sclerosis or whether the glomerulosclerosis that was present at the time of initial diagnosis was inadvertently diagnosed as minimal-change nephropathy because of a tissue sampling error during the renal biopsy.

For patients who are steroid resistant as well as those who require large doses of steroids to sustain remission (steroid dependent), alternative therapy should be considered. Furthermore, in pediatric patients, the growth inhibition associated with long-term steroid use often necessitates the use of alternative agents. Cyclophosphamide at 2.0–2.5 mg/kg/d for 8–12 weeks given alone or with prednisone (50–75 mg/m^2) is very effective in inducing remission and restoring steroid responsiveness in patients who were previously steroid dependent and became steroid resistant recently. Alternately, chlorambucil at 0.1–0.2 mg/kg/d may be used. This agent, however, has been associated with more adverse effects than cyclophosphamide.[63] Azathioprine has also been used; however, favorable response is often not seen until therapy is continued for more than 6–12 months.[64] Thus the use of these cytotoxic agents should be reserved for patients who are clearly steroid resistant, or steroid dependent (relapse within 14 days after termination of steroid treatment or dosage reduction) with significant adverse effects, or those who have two or more relapses within 6 months after the first episode or three or more relapses within 12 months.[33] The immunosuppressive effect of these agents, with or without the concurrent use of steroids, can result in serious infections, which are the primary cause of death in patients with minimal-change nephropathy.[65] Other toxicities associated with cyclophosphamide include gonadal fibrosis, which results in sterility, hemorrhagic cystitis, alopecia, and a potential to develop malignancy in those on long-term treatment.

Cyclosporine has been used recently in adult and pediatric patients. The drug decreases lymphokine production by activated T lymphocytes[66] and thus reduces proteinuria by reversing the lymphokine-induced alterations in the anionic charge and permeability of the GBM to albumin. Cyclosporine can also reduce proteinuria by improving the permselectivity of the GBM. In patients with steroid-sensitive or steroid-dependent minimal-change disease, cyclosporine induces remission in 80–85% of the patients. However, the disease-free period is frequently not sustained, and relapse, which is usually not as responsive to cyclosporine retreatment, may occur as soon as the drug is tapered or discontinued.[67] Patients with high IL-2 concentrations tend to have more sustained remission.[68] The rate of relapse is also reduced when the dose tapering is gradual or when the cyclosporine treatment period is prolonged. Although only 10–20% of patients who have steroid-resistant disease respond to cyclosporine, combination treatment with low-dose steroid increases the effectiveness in some patients.[67,69] A 2-month trial treatment with cyclosporine may therefore be warranted in steroid-resistant patients. The steroid-sparing effect of cyclosporine is also useful in steroid-dependent patients, especially those who have experienced significant adverse effects. The usual starting dose of cyclosporine for remission induction is 5 mg/kg for adults and 6 mg/kg for children. The need to monitor cyclosporine blood concentrations is controversial. No correlation has been found between the severity of the cyclosporine-induced tubulointerstitial lesions with either the mean dose or trough drug concentration.[67] However, the incidence of these lesions increases with the duration of treatment and cyclosporine should therefore not be given for more than 4 months in the absence of any beneficial effect.[67] Other nonrenal adverse effects associated with cyclosporine treatment include hypertrichosis, gum hyperplasia, gastrointestinal symptoms, and hypertension.[70]

Levamisole, an immunostimulant, has also been evaluated for the treatment of patients with steroid-dependent nephrotic syndrome. The agent can promote the maturation of young T cells and restore the function of T cells and phagocytes when the immune system is depressed.[71] It may also inhibit the production of an immunosuppressive lymphokine that is associated with minimal-change nephrotic syndrome. However, its precise mechanisms of action in immunocompetent patients with glomerulonephritis remain to be identified. Levamisole was found in a placebo-controlled study to have a steroid-sparing effect in children who had steroid-responsive and steroid-dependent nephrotic syndrome.[72] About half of the 31 children in the levamisole group remained in remission 16 weeks into therapy while prednisolone was tapered in the initial 8 weeks. The most serious adverse effect of levamisole is neutropenia, which is generally reversible. Rarely, agranulocytosis has been reported in patients with connective tissue or neoplastic diseases. Levamisole has also been shown to have a favorable effect when used in conjunction with BCG and dipyridamole in adult patients with different types of primary glomerulonephritis.[73] At present, further controlled studies are needed to define precisely the benefit of this agent in the treatment of glomerulonephritis.

The long-term prognosis of most patients with minimal-change disease is good. The majority of pediatric patients will not experience any relapse of the disease 10 years after the initial onset, and most will be free of the proteinuria after puberty.[61] In adults, an 85–90% survival rate is seen 10 years after the disease onset.[61] Spontaneous remission may be present in up to 70% of untreated adults.[74] Development of renal failure is uncommon in both adult and pediatric patients. Only in those patients who are steroid resistant or steroid dependent is significant deterioration of renal function observed. Because of the overall favorable outcome of the disease and the relatively uncommon progression into chronic renal failure, aggressive use of cytotoxic agents is not indicated even in most patients with frequent relapses. Toxicities associated with aggressive therapy do not justify the need to induce remission in these patients who fail to respond to steroids and the nonaggressive use of cytotoxic agents. Symptomatic therapy with diuretics to control edema, in conjunction with a low-salt diet and albumin infusion as needed for acute development of anasarca, is often a more rewarding therapeutic approach. NSAIDs and ACE inhibitors may also be used to reduce the proteinuria.

FOCAL SEGMENTAL GLOMERULOSCLEROSIS

Focal segmental glomerulosclerosis (FSGS) is a histologic lesion that can be idiopathic (primary) or secondary to a variety of causes. Conditions such as sickle cell disease, cyanotic congenital heart disease and morbid obesity can induce hemodynamic stress on an initially normal nephron population and result in FSGS.[75] Severe glomerular injury can also be seen in patients with nephropathy associated with heroin abuse and human immunodeficiency (AIDS) virus infection.[75,76] The primary and secondary sclerotic lesions may be morphologically similar, but they represent diseases with different courses and response to therapy.

Pathology and Pathogenesis

Sclerotic lesions are characteristically found in some of the glomeruli (focal) and usually involve only a portion of the glomeruli (segmental).[77] Similar to the minimal-change disease, fusion of foot processes is commonly seen in those glomeruli that are not sclerotic. It is thought that both minimal-change disease and FSGS share similar pathogenetic mechanisms, with FSGS resulting in severe injury to the glomerular epithelial cells. During the early stage of FSGS, only a small number of glomeruli may have the segmental sclerotic lesion and the disease may be confined to the juxtamedullary region. If an inadequate number of glomeruli is sampled during renal biopsy, the diagnosis of FSGS may be missed or the patient may be thought to have minimal-change disease. Resistance to steroid therapy may thus be one of the first clues that the patient indeed has FSGS rather than minimal-change disease. Alternately, a patient may have the steroid-sensitive minimal-change disease initially, which subsequently progresses to steroid-resistant FSGS.

Clinical Manifestations

FSGS accounts for less than 15% of the cases of idiopathic nephrotic syndrome in children and about 15–20% in adults. Almost all the patients present with proteinuria, and many of them have all the features of nephrotic syndrome.[78] The proteinuria is nonselective, containing albumin and other higher molecular weight proteins, and is usually less severe when compared with patients who have minimal-change disease. Hypertension, microscopic hematuria, and renal dysfunction may be seen in up to half of the patients. The reduced renal function becomes more prevalent as the disease progresses. FSGS is more common in black patients who tend to present with proteinuria more frequently in the nephrotic range. They are also more likely to have rapid decline in renal function.

Pharmacotherapy and Prognosis

Since the pathophysiology of primary FSGS is unknown, it is not possible to direct pharmacologic treatment against any specific pathologic processes. Furthermore, the treatment of FSGS remains controversial due to the lack of data from randomized, prospective, controlled trials. A course of prednisone (1–2 mg/kg/d) may be considered initially. Urinary protein excretion and serum albumin concentration should be monitored to assess efficacy. The average time to induce complete remission is 3–4 months and up to 6 months may be needed in some patients.[78] A longer duration of treatment (6 months or more) has resulted in complete remission in more than 40% of patients while older studies reported a response rate of less than 20% using regimens of a shorter duration.[78,79]

Cytotoxic agents such as cyclophosphamide, chlorambucil, and azathioprine have not been found effective in the treatment of FSGS. However, combining prednisone therapy with cyclophosphamide and/or azathioprine over an extended period of time has been reported to result in complete or partial remission in 60% of 59 adult patients in one study.[80] Using an aggressive regimen incorporating pulse methylprednisolone infusions with long-term immunosuppression using oral prednisone and cytotoxic agents, a remission rate of over 50% was reported in children with steroid-resistant FSGS in a retrospective, uncontrolled trial.[81] Despite the encouraging results of these recent studies, additional randomized, controlled trials will be needed to confirm the efficacy and assess the risks for adverse effects before these approaches become generally accepted.

Short-term cyclosporine may reduce proteinuria in some patients who have FSGS resistant to corticosteroid and cytotoxic agents.[78] However, relapse of proteinuria is frequent, especially if treatment is withdrawn abruptly.[82] The relapse may occur within 2 months of tapering or drug discontinuation.[78] A recent study was conducted to evaluate long-term cyclosporine therapy in 21 black and hispanic children who had steroid-resistant FSGS.[83] These patients tend to have more rapid renal function deterioration than white children. The cyclosporine dosage was titrated to the serum cholesterol concentration. Higher doses were given to patients with severe hypercholesterolemia.[83,84] This aggressive regimen (4–20 mg/kg/d for 3–97 months) produced a reduction in proteinuria from 6.2 to 2.0 g/day, and the percentage of patients who developed ESRD (78% in the historical controls to 24% in these treated patients).[83] Although histologic evidence of cyclosporine nephrotoxicity was not seen in the study patients, the drug should only be used cautiously, especially in patients with tubulointerstitial and/or vascular lesions.

Due to the lack of a consistently effective regimen for primary FSGS, many patients with mild disease are treated conservatively for symptomatic control. ACE inhibitors have been found to be effective in reducing proteinuria and stabilizing renal function in patients with primary or secondary FSGS.[75,85] The constriction of afferent arterioles by these agents reduces intraglomerular pressure, which may diminish the potential effect of glomerular hypertension in promoting the development of FSGS.[85] The driving force for proteinuria may also be reduced without necessarily correcting the primary defect in glomerular wall permselectivity.[75] The NSAID meclofenamate has been found to be effective in reducing proteinuria in patients with steroid-resistant FSGS.[51] These favorable results have, however, not been confirmed in studies using a larger number of patients. Thus, their role in the overall scheme of therapy remains to be defined. For patients with more severe disease, corticosteroids with or without immunosuppressive agents should be considered. Treatment should not be continued for more than 3–4 months unless the patient experiences a remission. In this case, therapy may be continued for 12–24 months to maintain the therapeutic response.[80]

Patients with primary FSGS are at risk for developing ESRD. For the 30–50% of adults and children who had attained complete remission, ESRD develops in about 10% at 10 years.[78] For those patients who are resistant to therapy, the rate of renal function deterioration to ESRD may be rapid, within 1 year, or slow, over as long as 10–20 years. About 50% of them develop ESRD in 10 years. Those patients with severe proteinuria (>10–15 g/d), high serum creatinine concentration at diagnosis, initial steroid resistance, or interstitial fibrosis on renal biopsy are likely to have a more rapid decline in renal function. Kidney transplantation is often indicated for those patients who develop ESRD; however, FSGS has reoccurred in 20–50% of the renal allografts soon after transplantation. Children and those with severe disease or rapid progression to ESRD prior to transplantation are more likely to experience a recurrence. The proteinuria may reappear within hours after transplantation and graft failure may occur in one-third to half of the patients. The median time to recurrence was reported to be 14 days in one study.[86] Although cyclosporine is not effective in preventing the recurrence of nephrotic syndrome after transplantation, a high dose of the agent (up to 35 mg/kg/d) has been shown to induce a remission of the recurrent disease.[87] ACE inhibitors and plasmapheresis have also been used to prolong graft survival. The effectiveness of these therapies and the rapid recurrence of the disease in the transplanted kidney substantiate the possibility that a circulating humoral mediator is responsible for the nephropathy.[88]

MEMBRANOUS NEPHROPATHY

Membranous nephropathy is the most common disorder responsible for idiopathic nephrotic syndrome in adults, accounting for about 25% of cases.[89–91] The hallmark histologic features of membranous nephropathy are glomerular capillary wall thickening with subepithelial deposits under light and electron microscopy.[91,92] Most cases are idiopathic, but up to 30% of patients have secondary causes.[91,93] The most common etiologies are autoimmune diseases (e.g., lupus), infection (e.g., hepatitis B),[94,95] syphilis, neoplasm[96] (e.g., carcinoma of the lung, breast, gastrointestinal tract, or kidney), and medications (e.g., organic gold,[97] penicillamine,[98] mercury, and captopril.[91] *De novo* membranous nephropathy can also occur in the allografts of renal transplant patients.[99] It is important to identify any potential underlying causes because the treatment and prognosis of patients with idiopathic or secondary membranous nephropathy are different. Although this glomerular disease can occur at any age, over 80% of patients are more than 30 years old at the time of diagnosis.[100] The peak incidence is in those over 50 years of age.[91]

Pathology and Pathogenesis

Examination of kidney tissue under light microscopy reveals normal mesangium and normocellularity.[92] The glomerular capillary wall may be thickened in well-developed lesions. Trichome stain shows subepithelial deposits, and silver stain reveals spike-like projections between deposits.[91,92] These projections gradually fuse to engulf the deposits such that, in the advanced stage, the capillary wall is markedly thickened and intramembranous deposits are found. Progressive changes in capillary lumen patency parallel those in the GBM, resulting in glomerulosclerosis with capillary collapse, and tubular atrophy in end-stage membranous nephropathy.[91,92] Immunofluorescence microscopy shows strong capillary wall staining of IgG and C3 on the epithelial side of the basement membrane.[92] Secondary membranous nephropathy exhibits similar lesions except for the additional presence of mesangial expansion and hypercellularity with fewer deposits.[100] In patients with membranous nephropathy induced by lupus, subendothelial and extraglomerular deposition can also be seen.

Antibody-mediated immune injury appears to be the main pathogenetic mechanism. Animal models of membranous nephropathy, particularly Heymenn nephritis in rats, provide evidence that it is an autoimmune disease with immune complex deposition in the subepithelium of the GBM.[101] The immune complex can be formed in-situ or deposited from circulating immune complexes. In Heymenn nephritis,[101] the intrinsic antigen is a glycoprotein gp330 produced by the visceral epithelial cells. The anti-gp330 antibodies traverse across the glomerular basement membrane to form immune complexes in the coated pits of the glomerular epithelial cells. These anti-gp330 immune complexes then become anchored to the glomerular basement membrane and detached from the podocyte cell membrane. These processes repeat themselves, resulting in accumulation of more immune complexes in the GBM until they become morphologically apparent.[101] Although the antigen responsible for primary human membranous nephropathy is not known, the mechanism for disease progression is thought to be similar.

Clinical Manifestations

The majority of patients with membranous nephropathy present with heavy proteinuria exceeding 3.5 g/d.[100] However, fewer than 30% of them suffer from nephrotic syndrome[102] and its extrarenal complications, namely, edema, hypoalbuminemia, hyperlipidemia, and hypercoagulability.[103] The signs and symptoms are usually insidious in onset, and consist of anorexia, malaise, edema, occasionally anasarca, ascites, and pericardial and pleural effusions.[100] Pulmonary embolism is the most serious complication, but resultant death is rare.[103] Renal vein thrombosis may also be found; the reported incidence varies from 5–62%.[26,93,100,103] Renal vein thrombosis should be suspected when there is a sudden onset of hematuria, loin pain, pulmonary embolus, fluctuating or worsening proteinuria or glomerular filtration rate, renal tubular acidosis, or an increase in leg edema.[91] Hypertension is usually not seen until the disease is advanced.

In addition to heavy proteinuria, urinalysis often reveals lipiduria and oval fat bodies. Microhematuria is seen in fewer than 25% of patients while gross hematuria and red cell casts are rare.[91,100] In idiopathic membranous nephropathy, the serum complement concentrations are normal. Low levels of complement should alert one to search for secondary causes or an alternative diagnosis. Similarly, antinuclear antibodies, anti-DNA antibodies, rheumatoid factor, hepatitis B serologies, and serum cryoglobulins are generally negative in idiopathic membranous nephropathy.[100] Occult malignancy has been found in up to 10% of elderly patients with membranous nephropathy.[91,96]

Pharmacotherapy and Prognosis

The natural course of idiopathic membranous nephropathy is variable. About 25% of patients experience spontaneous remission of the disease over a mean of 5.5 years.[91–93] Twenty-five percent will progress to end-stage renal failure over 10 years. The other 50% have various degrees of renal insufficiency and proteinuria. Heavy proteinuria (>10 g/d), male gender, elevated serum creatinine concentration at the time of presentation, poorly controlled hypertension, old age at onset of disease, non-Oriental race, certain HLA antigens, and tubulointerstitial fibrosis on initial renal biopsy are associated with progressive renal disease.[91,93,100] Overall, patients with idiopathic membranous nephropathy have a relatively benign course. The mean 10-year survival is about 70%.[102] Those who present with persistent non-nephrotic proteinuria seldom develop renal insufficiency and have a normal life expectancy. Fewer than 10% of patients develop a remitting and relapsing course.[93]

The prognosis for secondary membranous nephropathy depends on the underlying cause. Remission occurs when the infection resolves[94,95] or when the causative medication is withdrawn.[100]

The treatment of idiopathic membranous nephropathy has been controversial and has ranged from supportive therapy to immunosuppression with steroids alone, or in combination with alkylating agents.[93] Conservative management of membranous nephropathy includes control of edema with salt restriction and diuretics,[104] and reduction of proteinuria with protein restriction and ACE inhibitors.[19,100,105] Management of hypertension and hyperlipidemia[106] will be required for most, while long-term anticoagulation is usually only necessary for patients with renal vein thrombosis or a documented pulmonary embolus.[93,106]

Since remission of proteinuria, whether spontaneously or treatment related, may confer a good prognosis,[93,107] most studies have focused on treatment in patients with nephrosis and normal or stable renal function. Numerous uncontrolled and controlled studies have yielded conflicting results regarding the efficacy of corticosteroids.[93] The U.S. prospective randomized collaborative trial demonstrated a beneficial effect of high-dose oral prednisone 120 mg given every other day for 8 weeks in 72 patients with idiopathic membranous nephropathy.[108] Advanced renal failure occurred in only 1 of the treated patients but 10 of 38 control patients progressed to ESRD. However, the unusually poor prognosis of the placebo group has cast doubts on the favorable results of the study. Indeed, the British Medical Research Council, using the same steroid protocol as the American study, did not demonstrate a difference in the incidence of ESRD between treatment and placebo groups.[109] The benefits of steroids were also not shown in a Canadian study, which used moderate doses of prednisone, 40 mg/m^2 daily for 6 months.[110] These later studies suggest that daily or alternate-day oral steroids, in the doses and duration used, have a limited role in the treatment of idiopathic membranous nephropathy. In contrast, high doses of intravenous steroids may improve renal function, particularly in patients with a superimposed crescentic glomerulonephritis.[93,111]

Conflicting results have also been reported with the use of alkylating agents alone, or in combination with steroids.[112–117] In a retrospective study of 36 patients with idiopathic membranous nephropathy, oral prednisolone 60 mg daily for 8–10 weeks and subsequent taper was compared with combination therapy of the same regimen of steroid and oral cyclophosphamide (1.5–2.0 mg/kg/d) for a mean period of 3.6 months. No differences were noted with respect to the induction of complete or partial remission, or the percentage of patients who developed ESRD.[112] Similarly, a randomized, controlled trial of oral cyclophosphamide 1.5–2.5 mg/kg/d for 1 year did not show benefits over supportive therapy.[113] Nonetheless, a 2-year randomized controlled trial with daily oral cyclophosphamide for 6 months with dipyridamole and warfarin for 2 years showed significant improvement in proteinuria with no significant change in renal function in either group.[114] The most impressive results to date were reported by Ponticelli et al. who administered intravenous methylprednisolone 1 g/d for 3 days, followed by 0.4 mg/kg/d orally for 27 days, and then alternated every other month with chlorambucil 0.2 mg/kg/d for a total of 6 months.[115,116] This immunosuppressive regimen resulted in remissions in 67% of the treated patients, compared to only 23% of those receiving supportive care alone.[116] Only 10% of the treated patients had elevated serum creatinine concentrations, compared to 49% of those in the supportive care group. Interestingly, when the combination regimen of alternating chlorambucil and methylprednisolone was compared with methylprednisolone alone, more remission occurred in the combination treatment group than the steroid-only group in the first 3 years of follow-up.[117] However, no difference in outcome was demonstrated at the fourth year of follow-up.[117]

When the data from the prospective trials with steroids and those with cytotoxic agents were evaluated by meta-analysis, treatment with cytotoxic agents but not steroids was associated with an increased likelihood of complete or partial remission.[118,119] The recent analysis of 10 prospective trials and 22 case series involving treatment of new-onset biopsy-proven idiopathic membranous nephropathy also support the findings of the meta-analyses.[119] Even though cytotoxic agents appear to induce remission more frequently in patients with idiopathic membranous nephropathy, they are associated with complications, such as leukopenia, infection, malignancy, and sterility. Treatment-associated adverse events were reported in 3% of the steroid-treated and in 12% of alkylating agent-treated patients.[119]

Since only about 25% of patients with new-onset idiopathic membranous nephropathy ultimately develop ESRD over a 20- to 30-year period, it is prudent not to treat all patients with new-onset membranous nephropathy.[120–122] Patients who have low risk factors for renal disease progression can be managed with observation and symptomatic therapy. These include children 2–16 years of age, adult males with proteinuria less than 2 g/d, or adult females with proteinuria less than 5 g/d and normal renal function.[120,122] Patients who have high risks of developing renal failure, including those with proteinuria greater than 10 g/d with or without impaired renal function, and patients with symptomatic nephrotic syndrome with a plasma albumin of less than 2 g/dL, should be aggressively treated to induce remission.[93,100,120,122] Alkylating agents, chlorambucil or cyclophosphamide, combined with steroids[122,123] or the high-dose steroid regimen in the Italian study[117] can be used to induce remission after considering the benefits and risks of treatment.[33,123]

In patients with deteriorating renal function, several trials using either cyclophosphamide[124,125] or chlorambucil[126–128] in conjunction with steroids have shown variable effects. While some patients' disease remitted, that is, proteinuria decreased and renal function stabilized,[124–127] others did not.[128,129] In addition, the rate of complications appeared higher.[126,128] Therefore, cytotoxic therapy should be avoided in patients whose serum creatinine concentration at diagnosis is greater than 3 mg/dL.[102,120,122] Doses of cytotoxic agents should also be adjusted downward in patients with mild renal impairment to reduce side effects.[33]

Patients with severe nephrotic syndrome who did not respond to this therapy are candidates for treatment with cyclosporine. Cyclosporine may benefit some patients with idiopathic membranous nephropathy[130]; however, the potential of developing cyclosporine nephrotoxicity, especially during long-term therapy is of concern.[131] Recently, a 12-month course of cyclosporine (mean dose of 3.8 mg/kg/d) was shown to reduce proteinuria as well as the rate of renal deterioration.[132] However, for many patients, hypertension was exacerbated and/or a transient rise in serum creatinine concentration was noted.

The treatment of secondary membranous nephropathy is directed at removing the underlying cause. For instance, membranous nephropathy secondary to syphilis can be treated with penicillin.[100] Alpha-interferon has been shown to be beneficial in the management of hepatitis B-induced membranous nephropathy.[133] Corticosteroids are of no benefit in this setting and have been shown to induce transient viral replication with increased serum concentrations of hepatitis B virus antigen and hepatitis B virus DNA.[134]

Both *de novo*[99] and recurrent membranous nephropathy may occur in the renal allograft.[135] The incidence of membranous nephropathy in the allograft appears to be three times greater in patients for whom membranous nephropathy was the original primary cause of renal failure. The frequency of recurrence ranges from 2–7%.[136] Recurrence is typically associated with nephrotic syndrome and a high risk of allograft failure from disease and/or rejection.[135]

MEMBRANOPROLIFERATIVE GLOMERULONEPHRITIS

Membranoproliferative glomerulonephritis (MPGN) is a morphologic entity that occurs in older children and adults. Although Caucasians are more frequently affected, there is no gender difference in incidence. Many diseases and disorders, such as infections and neoplasms, may result in secondary MPGN. The several types of MPGN are classified according to the pathologic features. Type I MPGN, also known as mesangiocapillary glomerulonephritis, is characterized by diffuse thickening of glomerular capillary walls and mesangial hypercellularity. Subendothelial dense deposits that frequently contain immunoglobulins and C3 of the complement system are responsible for the capillary wall thickening. Immune complexes are therefore presumed to have a major role in the pathogenesis of type I MPGN, which is the most common type of primary, idiopathic MPGN. Type I MPGN may also be secondary to systemic immune complex-mediated disease (lupus), chronic infection (infected ventriculoatrial shunt, endocarditis, malaria), chronic liver disease (hepatitis B, C; cirrhosis), and malignancy (leukemia, lymphoma).[137]

Type II MPGN is also known as dense deposit disease because of the presence of dense deposits of C3 within the glomerular basement membrane, which gives rise to a ribbon-like appearance. The deposit contains C3, but without immunoglobulins. Other variants of the disease include type III MPGN, which is seen rarely and consists of subendothelial and subepithelial deposits with lamination and disruption of the lamina densa of the GBM.[138]

Type I MPGN is a slowly progressive disease that accounts for 80% of all cases of MPGN, but only 5–15% of all cases of nephrotic syndrome seen in pediatric and adult patients. It occurs most frequently in patients between 5–30 years of age, and since remissions are rare patients develop ESRD in 9–12 years. Type II MPGN is a more aggressive disease that constitutes about 15% of all patients with MPGN. Only 20% of patients remain stable for more than a few years and the median time before the development of ESRD is 7 years. There is an impression that the incidence of idiopathic MPGN has declined recently worldwide. Nephrotic syndrome is the most common presenting condition and some patients may also have a nephritic component (hematuria), hypertension, and renal insufficiency. Hypocomplementemia is commonly seen. Renal survival 10 years after biopsy is about 60–65% for type I MPGN while the prognosis for type II disease is generally less favorable.[139]

Pharmacotherapy and Prognosis

The efficacy of corticosteroids, cyclophosphamide, antiplatelet drugs, and anticoagulants has been evaluated in patients with MPGN. Five prospective, randomized clinical trials, using prednisone and different combinations of cyclophosphamide, dipyridamole, warfarin, and aspirin did not reveal any long-term improvement in renal function or reduction in proteinuria.[140] Two additional multicenter trials involving more than 200 patients each, likewise did not demonstrate any consistent beneficial effects of steroids, cyclophosphamide, and azathioprine.[141,142] Cyclosporine has only been evaluated in a limited number of patients with MPGN. Some beneficial effect was suggested; however, the trials were not controlled nor randomized.[143] In addition, the risks for developing adverse effects were high.

It is difficult to conduct large-scale controlled trials for MPGN due to the low incidence of the disease. Based on the available studies, none of the drugs evaluated has been shown to have any consistent, beneficial effect on renal function and proteinuria. Renal transplantation is another alternative for patients with MPGN. Recurrence of the disease has been seen in patients with both types of MPGN; however, less than 10% of the transplanted patients have graft failure due to recurrent disease.

IgA NEPHROPATHY

IgA nephropathy, also known as Berger's disease, was first described by Berger in France in 1968. It is now recognized to be the most common glomerulonephritis in the world and accounts for 10% of patients with ESRD in many countries. The prevalence varies around the world from as high as 50% in Japan to 10–30% in Europe. In the United States, the overall prevalence is about 5% but is as high as 35% among Native Americans.[144] The disease has a male predominance (two to three times that of females) and is more frequently seen in younger adults. It is uncommon in blacks both in the United States and Africa.[144] IgA nephropathy was once thought to be a benign disease presenting with asymptomatic hematuria. It is now recognized that IgA nephropathy can present with any clinical syndrome associated with glomerular disease.

Pathology and Pathogenesis

Henoch–Schönlein purpura (HSP) is a systemic disease that is believed to be closely linked to IgA nephropathy because they share similar immunohistologic features. HSP may therefore be the systemic form of the disease process causing IgA nephropathy in which only the joint, skin, and gastrointestinal tract are involved rather than the kidneys. Mesangial deposition of IgA immune complex is also seen in patients with celiac disease and dermatitis herpetiformis, possibly due to an increased exposure to antigens. Patients with chronic liver disease may have IgA nephropathy because of reduced clearance of IgA immune complexes. Secondary IgA nephropathy may also be present in patients with different connective tissue diseases, carcinomas, and HIV infection.[145]

The diagnosis of IgA nephropathy can be established by immunofluorescence examination of the kidney biopsy. The hallmark feature is the dominance or codominance of IgA deposition in the mesangium. IgG and/or IgM as well as C3 may also be present. The IgA immune complex is presumed to be deposited from the systemic circulation or formed *in situ*. However, the precise pathogenetic mechanisms for IgA nephropathy remain unknown. Conditions that stimulate the release of IgA are believed to cause IgA deposition in the mesangium. In fact, infections of the upper respiratory tract or intestinal mucosa are known to correlate with the onset or exacerbation of IgA nephropathy. IgA production is likely to be increased through antigenic stimulation of IgA-producing mucosal lymphoid tissue by microorganisms as well as ingested or inhaled substances.

Clinical Manifestations

IgA nephropathy frequently presents as gross hematuria concurrent with an infection, most commonly pharyngitis or tonsillitis and less often pneumonia, gastroenteritis, or urinary tract infection.[144] In contrast to the 10- to 14-day delay after the pharyngitis in poststreptococcal glomerulonephritis, the hematuria of IgA nephropathy occurs 1–2 days after the onset of infection symptoms. The hematuria lasts from 24 hours to a few days and it may recur with a febrile illness months or years later. Frequently, there is persistent microscopic hematuria in between episodes of gross hematuria. Proteinuria is common and sometimes it can be in the nephrotic range. In contrast, hypertension and edema that are frequent in poststreptococcal glomerulonephritis are infrequent in IgA nephropathy. Renal dysfunction is uncommon at the initial presentation. However, about 10–20% of the patients will develop ESRD within 10 years after diagnosis.[146] Hypertension, severe proteinuria, renal function impairment, old age and the severity of histologic lesions are all predictive factors for poor long-term outcome.[146,147] The alternative but less common clinical presentations are asymptomatic, microscopic hematuria with variable degrees of proteinuria or nephrotic syndrome.

Pharmacotherapy and Prognosis

No therapy is known to be consistently effective for the treatment of IgA nephropathy. Due to the slow progression of the disease to ESRD, it is very difficult to conduct trials to evaluate the long-term effectiveness of specific treatments. The lack of understanding of the pathogenetic mechanisms and the unavailability of appropriate animal models have severely limited the development of rational treatment regimens.[148] Several different therapeutic approaches have been taken. The first is to prevent the formation of IgA immune complex or to increase its elimination. Restriction of dietary gluten is effective in patients with celiac disease but not in other patients with no identifiable nephritogenic antigens. Phenytoin was evaluated because of its ability to reduce the amount of polymeric IgA in the circulation.[149] Although phenytoin resulted in a reduction in serum IgA concentrations and in the frequency of macroscopic hematuria, the glomerular lesions deteriorated in some of the patients despite treatment. Removal of the tonsils, which produce IgA1 and may contribute to IgA nephropathy, should be considered for patients with recurrent infections.[150]

The second approach is to reduce IgA production. Corticosteroids with or without immunosuppressive agents have been used in several studies. Prednisone does not appear to preserve renal functions although a modest amelioration of proteinuria has been reported.[144] A meta-analysis of randomized trials reveals that heavy proteinuria (greater than 3 g/d) may be reduced by steroids and/or cytotoxic drugs in 66.7% of the patients.[151] In contrast, such an effect was not seen in patients with moderate proteinuria.

The third approach is to reduce glomerular inflammation induced by IgA deposits. Anti-inflammatory agents, antiplatelet drugs, and anticoagulants have been tried without success to decrease the production or action of mediators responsible for IgA immune complex-induced glomerular damage. However, the n-3 fatty acids in fish oil, which limit the production or action of cytokines and eicosanoids, have been shown recently in a randomized, placebo-controlled trial of 106 patients to delay the progression of renal failure and to reduce proteinuria slightly.[152] These patients had marked proteinuria and serum creatinine concentrations were less than 3 mg/dL prior to study enrollment. Since the majority of patients with IgA nephropathy do not have severe proteinuria, the efficacy of fish oil in these patients remains to be determined.[153]

ACE inhibitors can reduce proteinuria in patients with IgA nephropathy through its effect on the filtration barrier in the glomerular membrane.[154] In addition, they have been shown to be superior to other antihypertensive agents, including β-adrenergic antagonists, in reducing the progression of renal failure as well as proteinuria in both normotensive and hypertensive patients with IgA nephropathy.[154–156] Patients with IgA nephropathy were found to have abnormal production of IgA and several different immunoglobulins. High-dose immunoglobulins, initially administered intravenously, followed by the intramuscular route, for over 9 months arrested the decline of renal function and reduced hematuria and proteinuria in all of the 11 patients evaluated.[157] The efficacy of this regimen must be confirmed in a larger number of patients before it is used as primary therapy.

Urokinase, danazol, dapsone, sodium cromoglycate, and plasma exchange have also been evaluated but none is consistently effective.[144,158] Cyclosporine treatment for 12 weeks was evaluated in nine patients. Proteinuria was reduced and plasma albumin concentrations increased. However, the creatinine clearance decreased during treatment and did not return to baseline after termination of cyclosporine therapy.[159] Cyclosporine is therefore not indicated for patients with IgA nephropathy.

Based on the available studies, there is no regimen that is consistently effective for IgA nephropathy. Since corticosteroids have been found to reduce proteinuria, a course of alternate-day prednisone is therefore indicated for patients with proteinuria greater than 1 g/d.[144] If the patient experiences rapid GFR decline of more than 2 mL/min/month, immunoglobulin therapy should be considered despite the fact that only limited data are available.[144] If the patient is hypertensive, ACE inhibitors, instead of other antihypertensive agents, ought to be used to control the blood pressure as well as the proteinuria.

For those patients who develop end-stage renal failure secondary to IgA nephropathy, transplantation is an effective alternative with excellent allograft survival. Recently, it has been reported that patients with IgA nephropathy who had IgA antibodies to HLA antigens actually had better graft survival when compared with those without the antibodies.[160] It is hypothesized that the improved graft survival might be related to the blockade of IgG antibodies or inhibition of cellular immune response by the autoantibodies to the HLA class I molecules.

LUPUS NEPHRITIS

Glomerulonephritis is one of the most serious complications of systemic lupus erythromatosus (SLE) and accounts for much of the morbidity and mortality of patients afflicted with the disease.[161] The renal manifestations of lupus nephritis are variable and encompass a wide spectrum of histopathologic lesions.[161–163] The underlying histopathology has been associated with different prognosis and response to therapy, which cannot be predicted solely based on clinical manifestations. A renal biopsy is therefore required to assess the severity of the disease and to predict the short-term and long-term outcomes associated with therapy.

Pathology and Pathogenesis

Lupus nephritis is the prototype of all immune complex-mediated glomerulonephritis. It is characterized by the pleomorphic histologic presentations.[162] Immune complex deposits can be found in the mesangial, subendothelial, and subepithelial regions of the glomerulus, as well as the peritubular interstitium and vasculature outside the glomerulus.[163] Based on light, immunofluorescence, and electron microscopy findings, lupus nephritis can be categorized into five classes: I–normal; II–mesangial; III–focal proliferative; IV–diffuse proliferative; and V–membranous.[91,163,164] Semiquantitative assessment of active lesions and sclerotic changes is incorporated into an activity index and chronicity index, respectively, in an attempt to enhance the predictive values of the histologic findings.[163,164] However, the usefulness of these indices is still controversial.[165,166]

The hallmark feature in the pathogenesis of SLE is the dysregulated production of antibodies against multiple antigens in the body.[161,162] Circulating immune complexes can be deposited in the glomerulus or formed *in situ*. The size and location of the immune complexes in the glomerulus correlate with the nature and severity of renal injury.[163] Deposition of small numbers of stable immune complexes of intermediate size in the mesangium tends to produce less severe inflammation in the glomerulus. The sequestration of the immune complexes in the mesangium prevents them from activating inflammatory mediators. Hence, the lesion is noninflammatory in nature. In contrast, large numbers of intermediate-sized or large immune complexes can overload the mesangial clearing system. The eventual accumulation of these complexes in the subendothelial region allows them access to plasma inflammatory mediators, resulting in infiltration of inflammatory cells and release of necrotizing enzymes. Since subepithelial deposits are denied access to circulating inflammatory mediators, there is disproportionally more disturbance of glomerular capillary permeability than inflammatory response. Heavy proteinuria is therefore the primary clinical picture in lupus-induced membranous nephropathy.[163]

Clinical Manifestations

The onset of nephritis is usually seen within the first 4 years of diagnosis of SLE but may also be the first manifestation of the disease.[164] The clinical presentation ranges from minimal hematuria and proteinuria to severe, rapidly progressive diffuse glomerulonephritis. Proteinuria is common and most patients with the membranous lesion also present with the nephrotic syndrome.[91] An active urinary sediment (red cell casts, dysmorphic red cells, hematuria) is suggestive of the diffuse proliferative lesion. However, the urinary sediments are not a reliable indicator of the underlying glomerular lesion.[161] Hypertension is present in 25–45% of patients[164] and is associated with a worse prognosis.[167] Most patients have hypocomplementemia and increased anti-double-stranded DNA antibody titers, particularly those with focal or diffuse proliferative lesions.[91] Serum creatinine concentration at the time of diagnosis is most predictive of short-term outcome.[163,168]

Pharmacotherapy and Prognosis

The treatment of lupus nephritis has evolved over the past several decades.[169] The choice of therapy depends on the underlying lesion, and the activity as well as the chronicity indices. Corticosteroids have been the cornerstone of therapy. However, for severe lupus nephritis, primarily the diffuse proliferative type, alkylating agents may be needed to reduce or prevent the progression to ESRD.[170,171]

Patients with normal renal function and less than 2 grams of proteinuria usually do not require therapy, except for the management of extrarenal lupus manifestations. Renal biopsy can be delayed in these patients.[164] However, close follow-up of renal function and urinalysis is required. Those with more than 2 grams of proteinuria, deteriorating renal function, and/or an active urinary sediment require a renal biopsy to define the underlying lesion and determine the activity and chronicity of disease. Most patients with classes I, II, III, and V lesions can be treated with oral steroids 1 mg/kg/d for 8 weeks with subsequent tapering to maintain remission.[164] Patients with class IV lesion, and those with class III lesion associated with subendothelial deposits and signs of severe disease activity, should be treated with a cytotoxic agent, either azathioprine and cyclophosphamide, and steroids.

In a long-term randomized NIH study of 107 patients with active lupus nephritis, the likelihood of renal failure in patients taking oral prednisone alone was found to increase substantially after 5 years of observation.[170] Renal function was more frequently preserved in patients who received cytotoxic drugs, but a statistically significant difference was only found for the group receiving both intravenous cyclophosphamide (0.5–1.0 g/m^2) quarterly and low-dose oral prednisone. The benefit of therapy was particularly evident in the subgroup with chronic histologic changes on renal biopsy. Furthermore, hemorrhagic cystitis or malignancy was not reported among patients receiving intravenous cyclophosphamide. However, the small number of at-risk patients in each treatment group at the 5-year follow-up period raises doubts as to the superiority of intravenous cyclophosphamide over other cytotoxic agents.[169]

Favorable effects also have been reported when the intravenous cyclophosphamide regimen was modified from quarterly administration to monthly administration for 6 months.[172–174] Two regimens of pulse cyclophosphamide (monthly for 6 months versus monthly for 6 months followed by quarterly pulses for 2 additional years) were compared to pulse methylprednisolone in 65 patients with severe lupus nephritis.[175] Patients treated with the short-course cyclophosphamide had a higher probability of exacerbations than those treated with the prolonged regimen. Both regimens, however, were associated with a lower risk of doubling of serum creatinine concentration than those treated with pulse methylprednisolone alone.[175] It should be noted that combination therapy with steroids and cytotoxic agents is associated with increased morbidity, including major infections, malignancies (azathioprine- and cyclophosphamide-treated groups), herpes zoster, hemorrhagic cystitis (oral cyclophosphamide group), and secondary amenorrhea (particularly patients treated with cyclophosphamide).[169,170,174,175] Indeed, the longer course of cyclophosphamide treatment has been associated with a higher incidence of secondary amenorrhea, particularly in females over 25 years old.[176]

In patients who do not respond to cyclophosphamide and steroid therapy, cyclosporine has produced favorable results in some.[177,178] However, the number of patients studied was small and the follow-up period was short. Treatment with plasmapheresis in addition to a standard regimen consisting of a short course of oral cyclophosphamide and oral prednisone did not improve the clinical outcome of patients with severe lupus nephritis when compared to standard regimen alone.[179]

Lupus nephropathy with membranous lesion (type V) generally carries a good prognosis and a trial of steroids may be used to obtain remission of nephrotic syndrome. If treatment is unsuccessful after 6 months, it should be stopped to avoid infectious complications.[91] If progressive renal dysfunction occurs, or steroid therapy is not tolerated, oral cyclophosphamide 2 to 3 mg/kg/d can be used.[164] In 10 patients with lupus membranous nephropathy, cyclosporine, 4–6 mg/kg/d, given alone, or in combination with low-dose steroids, for a period of 6–43 months, has been shown to decrease proteinuria and induce remission of nephrotic syndrome.[180]

The survival of patients with lupus nephritis has improved during the last 2–3 decades, and now ranges from 74–80% at 10 years.[162,167] This improvement cannot be explained solely by the use of cytotoxic agents. The lower steroid dosage and better management of complications such as hypertension, infections, hyperlipidemia, and other metabolic complications of the disease also likely have contributed to the more favorable long-term outcome of this disease.[169] Lupus patients with ESRD on dialysis fare as well as those with non-lupus-related renal disease.[181] In those patients who received a renal transplant, the allograft outcome of patients with lupus nephritis is favorable.[182] Recurrence of lupus in the renal allograft can occur but is usually of minor clinical importance.[135]

RAPIDLY PROGRESSIVE GLOMERULONEPHRITIS

Rapidly progressive glomerulonephritis (RPGN) describes a clinicopathologic syndrome of rapid loss of renal function, usually over 50% decrement of the glomerular filtration rate within 3 months. The predominant histologic finding of RPGN is extensive crescent formation, usually in more than 50% of the glomeruli.[183–187] Hence, it is also known as crescentic glomerulonephritis. RPGN accounts for 2–7% of all renal biopsy findings and is responsible for up to 5% of patients with ESRD.[188] Though a rare disease, RPGN usually leads to renal demise within weeks or months if left untreated.

RPGN is not a single disease entity. A variety of glomerulonephritides with or without systemic diseases may present as RPGN, including anti-GBM glomerulonephritis, Goodpasture's syndrome, lupus nephritis, post-streptococcal glomerulonephritis, membranoproliferative glomerulonephritis, IgA nephropathy, polyarteritis nodosa, Wegener's granulomatosis, and idiopathic crescentic glomerulonephritis.[183–185] RPGN may also be found superimposed on an underlying primary glomerulopathy such as membranous nephropathy.

Besides the hallmark feature of extensive crescents, severe endocapillary proliferation and segmental necrosis can also be seen on light microscopy.[184] Based on immunofluorescence microscopic findings, three types of primary RPGN can be identified.[183,184] Type I RPGN is characterized by the linear localization of immunoglobulins, mainly IgG, along the GBM, signifying anti-GBM antibody-induced injury. Type II is defined by the coarse granular deposition of immunoglobulins and complement within the capillary walls and mesangium, denoting immune complex-mediated injury. Type III is characterized by scanty or lack of immune complex deposits; therefore, it is also known as pauci-immune RPGN. Circulating ANCA is often detected in type III RPGN. This immunohistologic classification of RPGN also reflects the immunopathogenesis of the different types of crescentic glomerulonephritis.

Pathology and Pathogenesis

Though the causal relationships are not firmly established, several etiologic factors have been implicated in RPGN, including toxins, drugs,[189] viral and bacterial infections, neoplasm, autoimmune mechanisms, and various immunogenetic factors.[183]

Irrespective of the etiology and type of RPGN, the disruption in the glomerular capillary wall seems to be the common lesion in crescentic glomerulonephritis.[183] Various mechanisms have been proposed to account for the severe damage to the capillary wall. Both humoral and cellular pathways of inflammation are involved. Activation of the terminal C5b-9 (membrane attacking complex) of the complement system produces severe capillary wall injury.[183] Both neutrophils and macrophages release proteinases and reactive oxygen species and may thereby produce severe glomerular injury.[183] Platelets and the coagulation system are activated and result in capillary thrombosis.[184] Fibrinogen and procoagulants that are released from ruptured capillaries may come into contact with thrombogenic tissue debris and lead to fibrinoid changes.[184] In anti-GBM glomerulonephritis, the direct attack of the anti-GBM antibody on the noncollagenous region of the type IV collagen molecule of the GBM is responsible for the capillary wall injury.[183,187] ANCAs may also play an important role in mediating the vascular injury in patients with ANCA-associated disease.[9] The interaction of ANCAs with neutrophils and monocytes, which have been primed by concurrent infections or inflammatory processes, can lead to activation of these leukocytes and release of toxic oxygen species and lytic enzymes, resulting in vascular injury.[9,190]

The disruption of the capillary wall allows movement of macrophages and other plasma constituents into Bowman's space, and stimulates the formation of crescents, which are composed mainly of parietal epithelial cells, as well as macrophages and fibroblasts.[183] Crescent formation indicates the severity of the glomerular capillary disease but not its pathogenesis. The age of crescents can serve as a marker for disease duration and the likelihood of successful therapeutic intervention.[183]

Clinical Manifestations

Among the crescentic glomerulonephritides, the pauci-immune RPGN is the most frequent, accounting for over 50% of cases, whereas the anti-GBM antibody-mediated RPGN is the least frequent, occurring in roughly 10% of patients.[183,184,187] Sixty to 70% of patients with type I RPGN may have concurrent pulmonary hemorrhage and Goodpasture's syndrome.[184,187] Most patients with immune complex-mediated RPGN have collagen vascular disease, systemic infections, or a severe form of primary glomerular disease.[187] Approximately 70% of patients with type III RPGN also present with evidence of systemic vasculitis, such as Wegener's granulomatosis and polyarteritis nodosa, but some have only renal manifestations, and the terms idiopathic crescentic glomerulonephritis or renal vasculitis have been used.[183–186]

The clinical presentation is dominated by progressive renal insufficiency with complaints of tea-colored urine, malaise, anorexia, low-grade fever, and migratory polyarthropathy.[187] Mild hypertension is usually present. Uremic signs and symptoms may develop as renal function worsens. Type I RPGN is more commonly found in the third and sixth decade of life.[187] Patients with ANCA-mediated disease tend to be older, with peak incidence occurring between 50–60 years of age.[191–193] The age-related incidence varies among the immune complex-mediated RPGN; for example, poststreptococcal glomerulonephritis and Henoch–Schönlein purpura nephritis are more common in young children, whereas membranoproliferative glomerulonephritis is more common in older children.[184] Urinalysis shows a nephritic sediment with hematuria, erythrocyte casts, and proteinuria. Overt nephrotic syndrome is rare, however.

Serologic analysis is very useful in distinguishing the different types of RPGN. The detection of serum anti-GBM antibodies with the appropriate clinical presentation confirms the diagnosis of anti-GBM glomerulonephritis.[184] Over 80% of patients with pauci-immune or idiopathic crescentic glomerulonephritis have circulating ANCAs.[9,184,187] ANCAs are autoantibodies specific for the cytoplasmic constituents of neutrophil granules and monocyte lysosomes.[9] Patients with ANCA-associated disease limited to renal involvement often have P-ANCA (perinuclear staining), while patients with Wegener's granulomatoses tend to have C-ANCA (cytoplasmic staining).[9,184,192,193] Both the anti-GBM antibody and the ANCAs are absent in patients with type II RPGN.[187] Measurements of circulating immune complexes are not useful for making a specific diagnosis, but detection of specific serum antibodies known to mediate immune complex-associated nephritis is helpful; e.g., anti-DNA antibody as a marker for lupus nephritis, and elevated anti-streptolysin-O titers for poststreptococcal glomerulonephritis.[184,187] The serum complement levels are normal in RPGN, although they can be low in the immune complex-mediated category.[187]

Pharmacotherapy and Prognosis

Early aggressive therapy has improved the renal prognosis of patients with crescentic glomerulonephritis.[194] Though no controlled prospective studies have been performed, type II and III RPGN appear to respond well to high-dose steroid therapy. Immunosuppressive therapy alone appears to be ineffective in type I RPGN.[183,195,196] Irrespective of the type of RPGN, poor response to therapy and an ominous renal survival are expected if the patient presents with oliguria, has a serum creatinine concentration greater than 6 or 7 mg/dL, is dialysis dependent, or the renal biopsy shows advanced chronic parenchymal disease.[184]

Anti-GBM Glomerulonephritis

The data on the treatment of anti-GBM glomerulonephritis are limited. Pulse intravenous administration of corticosteroids has been used successfully to alleviate pulmonary hemorrhage,[187] but the results are not as convincing for the treatment of glomerulonephritis.[183,195,196] Plasmapheresis, in combination with steroids and cytotoxic agents, may be more beneficial than immunosuppression alone.[183] Plasmapheresis may confer its benefits by removing the circulating pathogenetic anti-GBM antibody.[183,188] Compared to historical controls, an improved outcome is observed with addition of plasmapheresis to immunosuppressive therapy.[187] Plasma exchange is usually continued for at least 2 weeks[183] or until the circulating anti-GBM antibody concentrations decrease to undetectable levels.[187] The immunosuppression should be maintained for 8 weeks to prevent antibody rebound.[183] Plasmapheresis has been useful in treating pulmonary hemorrhage. However, the long-term benefits on renal function are not known.[183] Treatment should be started early. When the serum creatinine concentration is already 6 mg/dL or above, or the patient is oliguric, or requires dialysis, the response to therapy is usually poor.[183,187]

Immune Complex-Mediated Glomerulonephritis

The treatment of this category of RPGN varies with the underlying glomerulonephritis. Patients with postinfectious RPGN generally have a favorable prognosis even without treatment.[183,184] Complete spontaneous recovery occurs in 50% of cases, while chronic renal failure develops in 32%.[183] Pulse doses of methylprednisolone have been shown to be beneficial in type II RPGN,[183,195,196] with an overall response rate of 50–60%.[183] Plasmapheresis does not appear to provide any additional benefit.[183,195]

Antineutrophil Cytoplasmic Autoantibody (ANCA)-Associated Glomerulonephritis

Type III RPGN has been treated successfully with pulse doses of steroid.[183,185,187,192,195,196] The effectiveness of cyclophosphamide in systemic vasculitis, the detection of ANCAs, and the recognition that pauci-immune necrotizing crescentic glomerulonephritis is part of the spectrum of necrotizing vasculitides have led to the use of cyclophosphamide combined with steroids in ANCA-mediated RPGN.[9,191,192,197] Both oral (2–3 mg/kg/d) and intravenous (500–1000 mg/m^2) cyclophosphamide have been used. In a prospective study of 70 patients with ANCA-associated disease, no difference in renal or patient survival was detected between the oral and intravenous cyclophosphamide regimens. Similarly, there was no difference in response between the steroid-treated and the cyclophosphamide-treated groups.[191] The serum ANCA levels can be monitored to determine the efficacy of therapy.[187] To date, plasmapheresis has not been demonstrated in prospective trials to be of additional benefit in type III RPGN.[188,198]

Anti-GBM nephritis has been reported to recur in up to 55% of patients who received a renal transplant.[135] However, only 25% of these patients showed clinical disease activity, with rare allograft failure. Since the frequency of recurrence and its severity are related to the presence of circulating anti-GBM antibody, it is recommended that transplantation should not be performed until the anti-GBM antibody is undetectable for at least 6–12 months.[135,136] The recurrence rate in idiopathic crescentic glomerulonephritis, including ANCA-associated nephritis, is unknown and is thought to be low.[135,187] Thus, the outcome of the renal allograft appears favorable.[135]

Patient Outcomes

A better understanding of the pathogenetic mechanisms leading to glomerular injury has improved the management of glomerulonephritis. However, the glomerulonephritides are a heterogeneous group of immune disorders with different clinical courses, prognoses, and responses to current immunologic and nonimmunologic therapies. The clinician should understand the natural history and prognosis of each subgroup of glomerulonephritis, the efficacy of different immunomodulating regimens in inducing disease remission and preserving renal function, and the characteristics of at-risk patients who warrant aggressive therapy. Judicious use of immunosuppressive agents with careful monitoring of their adverse effects cannot be overemphasized. In addition, treatment of the disease complications and control of factors that lead to progression of renal disease are important in reducing the morbidity and mortality of patients with glomerulonephritis.

References

1. Couser WG. Research opportunities and future directions in glomerular disease. Semin Nephrol 1993;13:457–471.
2. Miller DE, Noble NA, Yu X, Border WA. Molecular and cellular biological techniques in the study of glomerular diseases. Semin Nephrol 1992;12:506–515.
3. US Renal Data System 1995 Annual Data Report. National Institutes of Health and National Institute of Diabetes and Digestive and Kidney Diseases.
4. Bohrer MP, Baylis C, Humes HD, et al. Permselectivity of the glomerular capillary wall: Facilitated filtration of circulating polycations. J Clin Invest 1978;72–78.
5. Schreiner GF. The mesangial phagocyte and its regulation of contractile cell biology. J Am Soc Nephrol 1992;2:S74–S82.
6. Llach F. Papper's Clinical Nephrology. Boston, Little, Brown and Company, 1993, pp 135–183.
7. Couser WG. Mediation of immune glomerular injury. J Am Soc Nephrol 1990;1:13–29.
8. Makker SP. Mediators of immune glomerular injury. Am J Nephrol 1993;13:324–336.
9. Jennette JC, Falk RJ. Antineutrophil cytoplasmic autoantibodies and associated diseases: A review. Am J Kidney Dis 1990;15:517–529.
10. Remuzzi G, Zoji C, Perico N. Proinflammatory mediators of glomerular injury and mechanisms of activation of autoreactive T cells. Kidney Int 1994;45(suppl 44):S8–S16.
11. Foster MH, Neilson EG. Immunopathogenesis of renal disease, in Greenburg A (ed): Primer on Kidney Diseases. San Diego, Academic Press, 1994, pp 59–67.
12. Klahr S, Schreiner G, Ichikawa I. The progression of renal disease. N Engl J Med 1988;318:1657–1666.
13. Ritz E, Orth S, Wennich T, et al. Systemic hypertension versus intraglomerular hypertension in progression. Kidney Int 1994;45:438–442.
14. Williams JD, Coles GA. Proteinuria: A direct cause of renal injury morbidity? Kidney Int 1994;45:443–450.
15. Ong ACM, Fine LG. Loss of glomerular function and tubulointerstitial fibrosis: Cause or effect? Kidney Int 1994;45:345–351.
16. Thomas ME, Schreiner F. Contribution of proteinuria to progressive renal injury: Consequences of tubular

uptake of fatty acid bearing albumin. Am J Nephrol 1993;13:385–398.
17. Keane WF. Lipids and the kidney. Kidney Int 1994;46:910–920.
18. Rodríguez-Iturbe B, Colic D, Parra G, Gutkowska J. Atrial natriuetic factor in the acute nephritic and nephrotic syndromes. Kidney Int 1990;38:512–517.
19. Kaysen GA. Albumin metabolism in the nephrotic syndrome: The effect of dietary protein intake. Am J Kidney Dis 1988;12:461–480.
20. Geers AB, Koomans HA, Roos JC, Dorhout Mees EJ. Preservation of blood volume during edema removal in nephrotic subjects. Kidney Int 1985;28:652–657.
21. Humphreys MH. Mechanisms and management of nephrotic edema. Kidney Int 1994;45:266–281.
22. Koomans HA, Kortlandt W, Geers AB, Dorhout Mees EJ. Lowered protein content of tissue fluid in patients with the nephrotic syndrome: Observations during disease and recovery. Nephron 1985;40:391–395.
23. Warwick GL, Fox JG, Boulton-Jones JM. The relationship between urinary albumin excretion rate and serum cholesterol in primary glomerular disease. Clin Nephrol 1994;41:135–137.
24. Wheeler DC, Bernard DB. Lipid abnormalities in the nephrotic syndrome: Causes, consequences, and treatment. Am J Kidney Dis 1994;23:331–346.
25. Keane WF, St Peter JV, Kasiske BL. Is the aggressive management of hyperlipidemia in nephrotic syndrome mandatory? Kidney Int 1992;42(suppl 38):S134–S141.
26. Llach F. Hypercoagulability, renal vein thrombosis, and other thrombotic complications of the nephrotic syndrome. Kidney Int 1985;28:429–439.
27. Lee HS, Mujais SK, Kasinath BS, et al. Course of renal pathology in patients with systemic lupus erythematosus. Am J Med 1984;77:612–620.
28. Ginsberg JM, Chang BS, Matarese RA, et al. Use of single voided urine samples to estimate quantitative proteinuria. N Engl J Med 1983;309:1543–1546.
29. Chang RLS, Deen WM, Robertson CR, et al. Permselectivity of the glomerular capillary wall: Studies of experimental glomerulonephritis in the rat using neutral dextran. J Clin Invest 1976;57:1272–1286.
30. Sakai T, Harris FH, Marsh DJ, et al. Extracellular fluid expansion and autoregulation in nephrotoxic serum nephritis in rats. Kidney Int 1984;25:619–628.
31. Gault MH, Meuhrcke RC. Renal biopsy: Current views and controversies. Nephron 1983;34:1–34.
32. Haynes RC. Adrenocorticotropic hormone; adrenalcortical steroids and their synthetic analogs: Inhibitors of the synthesis and actions adrenocortical hormones, in Gilman AG, Rall TW, Nies AS, Taylor P (eds): Goodman and Gilman's The Pharmacological Basis of Therapeutics, 8th ed. Pergamon Press, New York, pp 1431–1462.
33. Ponticelli C, Passerini P. Treatment of the nephrotic syndrome associated with primary glomerulonephritis. Kidney Int 1994;46:595–604.
34. Ahmed K, Kopple JD. Nutritional management of renal disease, in Greenburg A (ed): Primer on Kidney Diseases. San Diego, Academic Press, 1994, pp 287–293.
35. Klahr S, Levey A, Beck G, et al. The effects of dietary protein restriction and blood pressure control on the progression of chronic renal disease. N Engl J Med 1994;330:877–884.
36. Ihle BU, Becker GJ, Whitworth JA, et al. The effect of protein restriction on the progression of renal insufficiency. N Engl J Med 1989;321:1173–1177.
37. Fliser D, Schroter M, Neubeck M. Coadministration of thiazides increases the efficacy of loop diuretics even in patients with advanced renal failure. Kidney Int 1994;46:482–488.
38. Rudy DW, Voelker JR, Greene PK, et al. Loop diuretics for chronic renal insufficiency: A continuous infusion is more efficacious than bolus therapy. Ann Intern Med 1991;115:360–366.
39. National High Blood Pressure Education Program. National high blood pressure education program working group report on hypertension and chronic renal failure. Arch Intern Med 1991;151:1280–1287.
40. Jacobson HR, Striker GE. Report on a workshop to develop management recommendations for the prevention of progression in chronic renal disease. Am J Kidney Dis 1995;25:103–106.
41. Lewis EJ, Hunsicker LG, Bain RP, et al. The effect of angiotensin-converting-enzyme inhibition on diabetic nephropathy. N Engl J Med 1993;329:977–986.
42. Jeeg JE, De Jong PE, Van der Hem GK, et al. Reduction of proteinuria by angiotensin converting enzyme inhibition. Kidney Int 1987;32:78–83.
43. Remuzzi A, Perticucci E, Ruggenenti P, et al. Angiotensin converting enzyme inhibition improves glomerular size-selectivity in IgA nephropathy. Kidney Int 1991;39:1267–1273.
44. Praga M, Hernandez E, Montoyo C, et al. Long-term beneficial effects of angiotensin-converting enzyme inhibition in patients with nephrotic proteinuria. Am J Kidney Dis 1992;20:240–248.
45. Gansevoort RT, deZeeuw D, de Jong PE. Additive antiproteinuric effect of ACE inhibition and a low-protein diet in human renal disease. Nephrol Dial Transplant 1995;10:497–504.
46. Vriesendorp R, Donker AJM, de Zeeuw D, et al. Effects of nonsteroidal anti-inflammatory drugs on proteinuria. Am J Med 1986;81(suppl 2B):84–94.
47. Golbetz H, Black V, Shemesh O, et al. Mechanism of the antiproteinuric effect of indomethacin in nephrotic humans. Am J Physiol 1989;256:F44–F51.
48. Heeg JA, de Jong PE, de Zeeuw D. Additive antiproteinuric effect of angiotensin converting enzyme inhibition and nonsteroidal anti-inflammatory drug therapy: A clue to the mechanism of action. Clin Sci 1991;81:367–372.
49. Don BR, Kaysen GA, Hutchinson FN, et al. The effect of angiotensin-converting enzyme inhibition and dietary protein restriction in the treatment of proteinuria. Am J Kidney Dis 1991;27:1017.
50. ter Wee PM, Donker AJM. Pharmacologic manipulation of glomerular function. Kidney Int 1994;45:417–424.
51. Velosa JA, Torres VE. Benefits and risks of nonsteroidal antiinflammatory drugs in steroid-resistant nephrotic syndrome. Am J Kidney Dis 1986;8:345–350.
52. Massy ZA, Ma JZ, Louis TA, Kasiske BL. Lipid-lowering

therapy in patients with renal disease. Kidney Int 1995;48:188–198.

53. Elisaf M, Dardamanis M, Pappas M, et al. Treatment of nephrotic hyperlipidemia with lovastatin. Clin Nephrol 1991;36:50–52.
54. Thomas ME, Harris KPG, Ramaswamy C, et al. Simvastatin therapy for hypercholesterolemic patients with nephrotic syndrome or significant proteinuria. Kidney Int 1993;44:1124–1129.
55. Keilani T, Schlueter WA, Levin ML, et al. Improvement of lipid abnormalities associated with proteinuria using fosinopril, an angiotensin-converting enzyme inhibitor. Ann Intern Med 1993;118:246–254.
56. Sarasin FP, Schifferli JA. Prophylactic oral anticoagulation in nephrotic patients with idiopathic membranous nephropathy. Kidney Int 1994;45:578–585.
57. Rostoker G, Durand-Zaleski I, Petit-Phar M, et al. Prevention of thrombotic complications of the nephrotic syndrome by the low-molecular-weight heparin enoxaparin. Nephron 1995;69:20–28.
58. Nolasco F, Cameron JS, Heywood EF, et al. Adult-onset minimal change nephrotic syndrome: A long-term follow-up. Kidney Int 1986;29:1215–1223.
59. Jennette JC, Mandal AK. The nephrotic syndrome, in Mandal AK, Jennette JC (eds): Diagnosis and Management of Renal Disease and Hypertension, 2nd ed. Durham, NC, Carolina Academic Press, 1994, pp 235–272.
60. A report of the international study of kidney disease in children: The primary nephrotic syndrome in children. Identification of patients with minimal change nephrotic syndrome for initial response to prednisone. J Ped 1981;98:561–564.
61. Siegel NJ. Minimal change nephropathy, in Greenberg A (ed): Primer on Kidney Diseases. San Diego, Academic Press, 1994, pp 67–70.
62. Hiraoka M, Takeda N, Tsukahara H, et al. Favorable course of steroid-responsive nephrotic children with mild initial attack. Kidney Int 1995;47:1392–1393.
63. Kleinknecht C, Guesry P, Lenoir G, Broyer M. High-cost benefit of chlorambucil in frequently relapsing nephrosis. N Engl J Med 1977;296:48.
64. Cade R, Mars D, Privette M, et al. Effect of long-term azathioprine administration in adults with minimal-change glomerulonephritis and nephrotic syndrome resistant to corticosteroids. Arch Intern Med 1986;146:737.
65. A report of the international study of kidney disease in children: Minimal change nephrotic syndrome in children: Deaths during the first 5 to 15 years' observation. Pediatrics 1984;73:497–501.
66. Shevach EM. The effects of cyclosporin A on the immune system. Ann Rev Immunol 1985;3:397–423.
67. Niaudel P, Habib R. Cyclosporine in the treatment of idiopathic nephrosis. J Am Soc Nephrol 1994;5:1049–1056.
68. Tejani A, Suthanthiran M, Pomrantz A. A randomized controlled trial of low-dose prednisone and ciclosporin versus high-dose prednisone in nephrotic syndrome of children. Nephron 1991;59:96–99.
69. Meyrier A, Condamin M-C, Broneer D, and the Collaborative Group of the French Society of Nephrology. Treatment of adult idiopathic nephrotic syndrome with cyclosporin A: Minimal-change disease and focal-segmental glomerulosclerosis. Clin Nephrol 1991;35(suppl 1):S37–S42.
70. Collaborative Study Group of Sandimmun in Nephrotic Syndrome. Safety and tolerability of cyclosporin A (Sandimmun) in idiopathic nephrotic syndrome. Clin Nephrol 35(suppl 1):48–60, 1991.
71. Amery WK, Gough DA. Levamisole and immunotherapy: Some theoretic and practical considerations and their relevance to human disease. Oncology 1981;38:168–181.
72. British Association for Paediatric Nephrology. Levamisole for corticosteroid-dependent nephrotic syndrome in childhood. Lancet 1991;337:1555–1557.
73. Xu J, Qian T, Jiang J, et al. Clinical studies in the use of BCG and levamisole in the treatment of glomerulonephritis. Nephrol Dial Transpl 1991;6:548–553.
74. Black DAK, Rose G, Brewer DB. Controlled trial of prednisone in adult patients with the nephrotic syndrome. Br Med J 1970;3:421–426.
75. D'Agati V. The many masks of focal segmental glomerulosclerosis. Kidney Int 1994;46:1223–1241.
76. Rennke HG, Klein PS. Pathogenesis and significance of nonprimary focal and segmental glomerulosclerosis. Am J Kidney Dis 1989;13:443–456.
77. Schwartz MM, Korbet SM. Primary focal segmental glomerulosclerosis: Pathology, histological variants and pathogenesis. Am J Kidney Dis 1993;22:874–883.
78. Korbet SM, Schwartz MM, Lewis EJ. Primary focal segmental glomerulosclerosis: Clinical course and response to therapy. Am J Kidney Dis 1994;23:773–783.
79. Pei Y, Cattran D, Delmore T, et al. Evidence suggesting under-treatment in adults with idiopathic focal segmental glomerulosclerosis. Am J Med 1987;82:938–944.
80. Banfi G, Moriggi M, Sabadini E, et al. The impact of prolonged immunosuppression on the outcome of idiopathic focal-segmental glomerulosclerosis with nephrotic syndrome in adults. A collaborative retrospective study. Clin Nephrol 1991;36:53–59.
81. Mendoza SA, Reznik VM, Griswold WR, et al. Treatment of steroid-resistant focal segmental glomerulosclerosis with methylprednisolone and alkylating agents. Pediatr Nephrol 1990;4:303–307.
82. Ponticelli C, Rizzoni G, Edefonti A, et al. A randomized trial of cyclosporine in steroid-resistant idiopathic nephrotic syndrome. Kidney Int 1993;43:1377–1384.
83. Ingulli E, Singh A, Baqi N, et al. Aggressive, long-term cyclosporine therapy for steroid-resistant focal segmental glomerulosclerosis. J Am Soc Nephrol 1995;5:1820–1825.
84. Ingulli E, Tejani A. Severe hypercholesterolemia inhibits cyclosporin A efficacy in a dose-dependent manner in children with nephrotic syndrome. J Am Soc Nephrol 1992;3:254–259.
85. Keane WF, Anderson S, Aurell M, et al. Angiotensin converting enzyme inhibitors and progressive renal insufficiency. Ann Intern Med 1989;11:503–516.
86. Tejani A, Stablein DH. Recurrence of focal segmental glomerulosclerosis posttransplantation: A special report of the North American Pediatric Renal Transplant Cooperative Study. J Am Soc Nephrol 1992;2:S258–S263.
87. Mowry J, Marik J, Cohen A, et al. Treatment of recurrent focal segmental glomerulosclerosis with high dose

ciclosporine and plasmapheresis. Transplant Proc 1993;25:1345–1346.

88. Artero M, Biava C, Amend W, et al. Recurrent focal glomerulosclerosis: Natural history and response to therapy. Am J Med 1992;92:375–383.
89. Schieppati A, Mosconi L, Perna A, et al. Prognosis of untreated patients with idiopathic membranous nephropathy. N Engl J Med 1993;329:85–89.
90. Donadio JV Jr, Torres VE, Velosa JA, et al. Idiopathic membranous nephropathy: The natural history of untreated patients. Kidney Int 1988;33:708–715.
91. Mann R, Neilson EG. Pathogenesis and treatment of immune-mediated renal disease. Med Clin N Am 1985;69:715–749.
92. Austin HA. Membranous nephropathy. Ann Intern Med 1992;116:672–682.
93. Glassock RJ. The therapy of idiopathic membranous glomerulonephritis. Semin Nephrol 1991;11:138–147.
94. Gilbert RD, Wiggelinkhuizen J. The clinical course of hepatitis B virus-associated nephropathy. Pediatr Nephrol 1994;8:11–14.
95. Wong SN, Yu ECL, Chan KW. Hepatitis B virus associated membranous glomerulonephritis in children—experience in Hong Kong. Clin Nephrol 1993;40:142–147.
96. Burstein DM, Korbert SM, Schwartz MM. Membranous glomerulonephritis and malignancy. Am J Kidney Dis 1993;22:5–10.
97. Katz WA, Blodgett RC Jr., Putrusko RG. Proteinuria in gold-treated rheumatoid arthritis. Ann Intern Med 1984;101:176–179.
98. Hall CL, Jawad S, Harrison PR, et al. Natural course of penicillamine nephropathy: A long term study of 33 patients. Br Med J 1988;296:1083–1086.
99. Heidet L, Gagnadoux ME, Beziau A, et al. Recurrence of de novo membranous glomerulonephritis on renal grafts. Clin Nephrol 1994;41:314–318.
100. Adler SG, Nast CC. Membranous nephropathy, in Greenburg A (ed): Primer on Kidney Diseases. San Diego, Academic Press, 1994, pp 78–83.
101. Kerjaschi D. Molecular pathogenesis of membranous nephropathy. Kidney Int 1992;41:1090–1105.
102. Winerals CG, Sanderson F. Treatment of aggressive idiopathic membranous glomerulonephritis. Q J Med 1994;87:109–201.
103. Bernard DB. Extrarenal complications of the nephrotic syndrome. Kidney Int 1988;33:1184–1202.
104. Humphreys MH. Mechanisms and management of nephrotic edema. Kidney Int 1994;45:266–281.
105. Rostoker G, Maadi AB, Remy P, et al. Low-dose angiotensin-converting-enzyme inhibitor captopril to reduce proteinuria in adult idiopathic membranous nephropathy: A prospective study of long-term treatment. Nephrol Dial Transplant 1995;10:25–29.
106. Wheeler DC, Bernard DB. Lipid abnormalities in the nephrotic syndrome: Causes, consequences, and treatment. Am J Kidney Dis 1994;23:331–346.
107. Ponticelli C, Passerini P. The natural history and therapy of idiopathic membranous nephropathy. Nephrol Dial Transplant 1990(suppl 1):37–41.
108. Collaborative study of the adult idiopathic nephrotic syndrome. A controlled study of short-term prednisone treatment in adults with membranous nephropathy. N Engl J Med 1979;301:1301–1306.
109. Cameron JS, Healy MJR, Adu D. The Medical Research Council trial of short-term high-dose alternate day prednisolone in idiopathic membranous nephropathy with nephrotic syndrome in adults. Q J Med 1990;74:133–156.
110. Cattran DC, Delmore T, Roscoe J, et al. A randomized controlled trial of prednisone in patients with idiopathic membranous nephropathy. N Engl J Med 1989;320:210–215.
111. Ponticelli C, Fogazzi GB. Methylprednisolone pulse therapy for primary glomerulonephritis. Am J Nephrol 1989;9(suppl 1):41–46.
112. Alexopoulos E, Sakellariou G, Memmos D, et al. Cyclophosphamide provides no additional benefit to steroid therapy in the treatment of idiopathic membranous nephropathy. Am J Kidney Dis 1993;21:497–503.
113. Donadio JV Jr, Holley KE, Anderson CF, et al. Controlled trial of cyclophosphamide in idiopathic membranous nephropathy. Kidney Int 1974;6:431–439.
114. Murphy BF, McDonald I, Fairley KF, et al. Randomized controlled trial of cyclophosphamide, warfarin and dipyridamole in idiopathic membranous glomerulonephritis. Clin Nephrol 1992;37:229–234.
115. Ponticelli C, Zucchelli P, Imbasciati E, et al. Controlled trial of methylprednisolone and chlorambucil in idiopathic membranous nephropathy. N Engl J Med 1984;310:946–950.
116. Ponticelli C, Zucchelli P, Passerini P, et al. A randomized trial of methylprednisolone and chlorambucil in idiopathic membranous nephropathy. N Engl J Med 1989;320:8–13.
117. Ponticelli C, Zucchelli P, Passerini P, et al. Methylprednisolone plus chlorambucil as compared with methylprednisolone alone for the treatment of idiopathic membranous nephropathy. N Engl J Med 1992;327:599–603.
118. Imperiale TF, Goldfarb S, Berns JS. Are cytotoxic agents beneficial in idiopathic membranous nephropathy? A meta-analysis of the controlled trials. J Am Soc Nephrol 1995;5:1553–1558.
119. Hogan SL, Muller KE, Jennette C, et al. A review of therapeutic studies of idiopathic membranous glomerulopathy. Am J Kidney Dis 1995;25:862–875.
120. Glassock RJ. Therapy of idiopathic nephrotic syndrome in adults. A conservative or aggressive approach? Am J Nephrol 1993;13:422–428.
121. Cameron JS. Membranous nephropathy is still a treatment dilemma. N Engl J Med 1992;327:639–640.
122. Hebert LA. Therapy of membranous nephropathy: What to do after (meta) analyses. J Am Soc Nephrol 1995;5:1543–1545.
123. Piccoli A, Pillon L, Passerini P, et al. Therapy for idiopathic membranous nephropathy: Tailoring the choice by decision analysis. Kidney Int 1994;45:1193–1202.
124. Bruns FJ, Adler S, Fraley DS, et al. Sustained remission of membranous glomerulonephritis after cyclophosphamide and prednisone. Ann Intern Med 1991;114:725–730.
125. Mathieson PW, Turner AN, Maidment CGH, et al. Prednisolone and chlorambucil treatment in idiopathic membranous nephropathy with deteriorating renal function. Lancet 1988;2:869–872.

126. Jindal K, West M, Bear R, et al. Long-term benefits of therapy with cyclophosphamide and prednisone in patients with membranous glomerulonephritis and impaired renal function. Am J Kidney Dis 1992;19:61–67.
127. Reichert LJM, Huysmans FTM, Assmann K, et al. Preserving renal function in patients with membranous nephropathy: Daily oral chlorambucil compared with intermittent monthly pulses of cyclophosphamide. Ann Intern Med 1994;121:328–333.
128. Warwick GL, Geddes CG, Boulton-Jones JM. Prednisolone and chlorambucil therapy for idiopathic membranous nephropathy with progressive renal failure. Q J Med 1994;87:223–229.
129. Falk RJ, Hogan SL, Muller KE, et al. Treatment of progressive membranous glomerulopathy. A randomized trial comparing cyclophosphamide and corticosteroids with corticosteroids alone. The Glomerular Disease Collaborative Network. Ann Intern Med 1992;116:438–448.
130. Guasch A, Suranyl M, Newton L, et al. Short-term responsiveness of membranous glomerulopathy to cyclosporine. Am J Kidney Dis 1992;20:472–481.
131. Habib R, Niaudet P. Comparison between pre- and post-treatment renal biopsies in children receiving ciclosporine for idiopathic nephrosis. Clin Nephrol 1994;42:141–146.
132. Cattran DC, Greenwood C, Ritchie S, et al. A controlled trial of cyclosporine in patients with progressive membranous nephropathy. Kidney Int 1995;47:1130–1135.
133. Lin CY. Treatment of hepatitis B virus-associated membranous nephropathy with recombinant alpha-interferon. Kidney Int 1995;47:225–230.
134. Lai KN, Tam JS, Lin HJ, et al. The therapeutic dilemma of the usage of corticosteroid in patients with membranous nephropathy and persistent hepatitis B virus surface antigenaemia. Nephron 1990;54:12–17.
135. Mathew TH. Recurrence of disease following renal transplantation. Am J Kidney Dis 1988;12:85–96.
136. Ramos EL, Tisher CC. Recurrent diseases in the kidney transplant. Am J Kidney Dis 1994;24:142–154.
137. Rennke HG. Secondary membranoproliferative glomerulonephritis. Kidney Int 1995;643–656.
138. D'Amico G, Ferrario F. Mesangiocapillary glomerulonephritis. J Am Soc Nephrol 1992;2:S159–S166.
139. Cameron JS, Turner DR, Heaton J, et al. Idiopathic mesangiocapillary glomerulonephritis. Comparison of types I and II in children and adults and long-term prognosis. Am J Med 1983;74:175–192.
140. Donadio JV, Offord KP. Reassessment of treatment results in membranoproliferative glomerulonephritis. Am J Kidney Dis 1989;14:445–451.
141. Schmitt H, Bole A, Reineke T, et al. Long-term prognosis of membranoproliferative glomerulonephritis type I. Nephrol 1990;55:242–250.
142. Confalonieri P, Schena P, Fellin F, et al. Evoluzione, indici prognostici e terapia in 294 casi di glomerulonefrite idiopatica. Giorn It Nefrologia 1990;7:89–95.
143. Cattran DC. Current status of cyclosporin A in the treatment of membranous, IgA and membranoproliferative glomerulonephritis. Clin Nephrol 1991;35(suppl 1):S43–S47.
144. Galla JH. IgA nephropathy. Kidney Int 1995;47:377–387.
145. Mustonen J, Pasternack A. Associated diseases in IgA nephropathy, In Clarkson AR (ed): IgA Nephropathy. Boston, Martin Nijhoff Publishing, 1987, pp 47–65.
146. D'Amico G. Influence of clinical and histological features on actuarial renal survival in adult patients with idiopathic IgA nephropathy, membranous nephropathy, and membranoproliferative glomerulonephritis: Survey of the recent literature. Am J Kidney Dis 1992;20:315–323.
147. Donadio JV, Bergstralh EJ, Offord KP, et al. Clinical and histopathologic associations with impaired renal function in IgA nephropathy. Clin Nephrol 1994;41:65–71.
148. Glassock RJ. Treatment of immunologically mediated glomerular disease. Kidney Int 1992;42(suppl 38):S121–S126.
149. Egido J, Rivera F, Sancho J, Barat A, Hernando L. Phenytoin in IgA nephropathy: A long-term controlled trial. Nephron 1984;38:30–39.
150. Béné MC, Hurault de Ligny B, Kessler M, et al. Tonsils in IgA nephropathy. Contrib Nephrol 1993;104:153–161.
151. Schena FR, Montenegro M, Scivittaro V. Meta-analysis of randomized controlled trials in patients with IgA nephropathy (Berger's disease). Nephrol Dial Transpl 1990;5(suppl 1):47–52.
152. Donadio JV, Bergstralh EJ, Offord KP, et al. A controlled trial of fish oil in IgA nephropathy. N Engl J Med 1994;331:1194–1199.
153. Strihou CY. Fish oil for IgA nephropathy. N Engl J Med 1994;331:1227–1229.
154. Maschio G, Cagnoli L, Claroni F, et al. ACE inhibition reduces proteinuria in normotensive patients with IgA nephropathy: A multicentre, randomized, placebo-controlled study. Nephrol Dial Transplant 1994;9:265–269.
155. Cattran DC, Greenwood C, Ritchie S. Long-term benefits of angiotensin-converting enzyme inhibitor therapy in patients with severe immunoglobulin A nephropathy: A comparison to patients receiving treatment with other antihypertensive agents and to patients receiving no therapy. Am J Kidney Dis 1994;23:247–254.
156. Rekola S, Bergstrand L, Bucht H. Deterioration rate in hypertensive IgA nephropathy: Comparison of a converting enzyme inhibitor and β-blocking agents. Nephron 1991;59:57–60.
157. Rostoker G, Desvaux-Belghiti D, Pilatte Y, et al. High-dose immunoglobulin therapy for severe IgA nephropathy and Henoch-Schoenlein purpura. Ann Int Med 1994;120:476–484.
158. Clarkson AR, Woodroffe AJ, Bannister KM, Odum J. Therapy in IgA nephropathy. Contrib Nephrol 1993;104:189–197.
159. Lai KN, Lai FM, Li PKT, Vallance-Owen J. Cyclosporin treatment of IgA nephropathy. Brit Med J 1987;195:1165–1168.
160. Lim EC, Chai D, Gjertson DW, et al. In vitro studies to explain high renal allograft survival in IgA nephropathy patients. Transplantation 1993;55:996–999.
161. Mills JA. Systemic lupus erythromatosus. N Engl J Med 1994;330:1871–1879.
162. Balow JE. Lupus nephritis. Ann Intern Med 1987;106:79–94.
163. Kashgarian M. Lupus nephritis: Lessons from the path lab. Kidney Int 1994;45:928–938.

164. Couser W, Striker GE. Systemic lupus erythematosus, in Jacobson HR, Striker GE, Klahr S (eds.): The Principles and Practice of Nephrology. St. Louis, Mosby–Year Book, 1991, pp 302–306.
165. Schwartz MM, Bernstein J, Hill GS, et al. Predictive value of renal pathology in diffuse proliferative lupus glomerulonephritis. Kidney Int 1989;36:891–896.
166. Schwartz MM, Lan SP, Bernstein J, et al. Role of pathology indices in the management of severe lupus glomerulonephritis. Kidney Int 1992;42:743–748.
167. Gruppo Italiano per lo Studio della Neffrite Lupica (GISNEL) Lupus nephritis: Prognostic factors and probability of maintaining life-supporting renal function 10 years after the diagnosis. Am J Kidney Dis 1992;19:473–479.
168. Progression and remission of renal disease in the lupus nephritis collaborative study. Results of treatment with prednisone and short-term oral cyclophosphamide. Ann Intern Med 1992;116:1114–1123.
169. Donadio JV, Glassock RJ. Immunosuppressive drug therapy in lupus nephritis. Am J Kidney Dis 1993;21:239–250.
170. Austin HA, Klippel JH, Balow JE, et al. Therapy of lupus nephritis: Controlled trial of prednisone and cytotoxic drugs. N Engl J Med 1984;314:614–619.
171. Steinberg AD, Steinberg SC. Long-term preservation of renal function in patients with lupus nephritis receiving treatment that includes cyclophosphamide versus those treated with prednisone only. Arthritis Rheum 1991;34:945–950.
172. Balow JE. Treatment and monitoring of patients with lupus nephritis. Nephrol Dial Transplant 1990(suppl 1):58–59.
173. Eiser AR, Grishman E, Dreznin S. Intravenous pulse cyclophosphamide in the treatment of type IV lupus nephritis. Clin Nephrol 1993;40:155–159.
174. Valleri A, Radhakrishnan J, Estes D, et al. Intravenous pulse cyclophosphamide treatment of severe lupus nephritis: A prospective five-year study. Clin Nephrol 1994;42:71–78.
175. Boumpas D, Austin HA, Vaughn EM, et al. Controlled trial of pulse methylprednisolone versus two regimens of pulse cyclophosphamide in severe lupus nephritis. Lancet 1992;340:741–745.
176. Boumpas DT, Austin HA, Vaughan EM, et al. Risk for sustained amenorrhea in patients with systemic lupus erythromatosus receiving intermittent pulse cyclophosphamide therapy. Ann Intern Med 1993;119:366–369.
177. Favre H, Miescher PA, Huang YP, et al. Ciclosporin in the treatment of lupus nephritis. Am J Nephrol 1989;9(suppl 1):57–60.
178. Hussein MM, Mooij JMV, Roujouleh H. Cyclosporine in the treatment of lupus nephritis including two patients treated during pregnancy. Clin Nephrol 1993;40:160–163.
179. Lewis EJ, Hunsicker LG, Lan SP, et al. A controlled trial of plasmapheresis therapy in severe lupus nephritis. N Engl J Med 1992;326:1373–1379.
180. Radhakrishnan J, Kunis CL, D'Agati V, et al. Cyclosporine treatment of lupus membranous nephropathy. Clin Nephrol 1994;42:147–154.
181. Coplon NS, Diskin CJ, Peterson J, et al. The long-term clinical course of systemic lupus erythromatosus in end-stage renal disease. N Engl J Med 1983;308:186–190.
182. Roth D, Milgrom M, Esquenazi V, et al. Renal transplantation in systemic lupus erythromatosus: One center's experience. Am J Nephrol 1987;7:367–374.
183. Couser WG. Rapidly progressive glomerulonephritis: Classification, pathogenetic mechanisms, and therapy. Am J Kidney Dis 1988;11:449–464.
184. Jennette JC, Falk RJ. Diagnosis and management of glomerulonephritis and vasculitis presenting as acute renal failure. Med Clin North Am 1990;74:893–908.
185. Levy JB, Winearls CC. Rapidly progressive glomerulonephritis: What should be first-line therapy. Nephron 1994;657:402–407.
186. Ferrario F, Tadros MT, Napodano P, et al. Critical reevaluation of 41 cases of "idiopathic" crescentic glomerulonephritis. Clin Nephrol 1994;41:1–9.
187. Johnson JP. Rapidly progressive glomerulonephritis, in Greenburg A (ed): Primer on Kidney Diseases. San Diego, Academic Press, 1994, pp 94–99.
188. Cole E, Cattran D, Magil A, et al. A prospective trial of plasma exchange as additive therapy in idiopathic crescentic glomerulonephritis. Am J Kidney Dis 1992;20:261–269.
189. Kohler IJ, Gohara AF, Hamilton RW, et al. Crescentic fibrillary glomerulonephritis associated with intermittent rifampin therapy for pulmonary tuberculosis. Clin Nephrol 1994;42:263–265.
190. Kallenberg CGM, Brouwer E, Weening JJ, et al. Antineutrophil cytoplasmic antibodies: Current diagnostic and pathophysiological potential. Kidney Int 1994;46:1–15.
191. Falk RJ, Hogan S, Carey TS, et al. Clinical course of antineutrophil cytoplasmic autoantibody-associated glomerulonephritis and systemic vasculitis. Ann Intern Med 1990;113:656–663.
192. Bindi P, Mougenot B, Mentre P, et al. Necrotizing crescentic glomerulonephritis without significant immune deposits: A clinical and serological study. Q J Med 1993;86:55–68.
193. Gans ROB, Kuizinga MC, Goldschmeding R, et al. Clinical features and outcome in patients with glomerulonephritis and antineutrophil cytoplasmic autoantibodies. Nephron 1993;64:182–188.
194. Bruns FJ, Adler S, Fraley DS, et al. Long-term follow-up of aggressively treated idiopathic rapidly progressive glomerulonephritis. Am J Med 1989;86:400–406.
195. Ponticelli C, Fogazzi GB. Methylprednisolone pulse therapy for primary glomerulonephritis. Am J Nephrol 1989;9(suppl 1):41–46.
196. Bolton W, Couser WG. Intravenous pulse methylprednisolone therapy of acute crescentic rapidly progressive glomerulonephritis. Am J Med 1979;66:495–502.
197. Kunis CL, Kiss B, Williams G, et al. Intravenous "pulse" cyclophosphamide therapy of crescentic glomerulonephritis. Clin Nephrol 1992;37:1–7.
198. Pusey CD, Rees AJ, Evans DJ, et al. Plasma exchanges in focal necrotizing glomerulonephritis without anti-GBM antibodies. Kidney Int 1991;40:757–763.

Chapter 50

Drug Therapy Individualization for Patients with Renal Insufficiency

Gary R. Matzke, PharmD, FCP, FCCP, and Reginald F. Frye, PharmD, PhD

Renal insufficiency is accompanied by progressive alterations in several other organ systems and results in the development of anemia, hyperparathyroidism, bleeding abnormalities, hyperlipidemia, hypertension, and gastrointestinal (GI) tract integrity (Chapter 44, Chronic Renal Failure and End-Stage Renal Disease). It should not be surprising then that there are now many reports that document changes in the disposition of some drugs in patients with renal insufficiency as the result of changes in bioavailability,[1] protein binding,[2,3] distribution volume,[4] and metabolic activity.[5,6]

Drug therapy individualization for patients with renal insufficiency may only require a simple dose adjustment based on the fractional reduction in creatinine clearance.[7,8] However, the use of medications that are extensively metabolized or for which dramatic changes in protein binding and/or distribution volume have been noted may require a more complex adjustment.[4,9] Furthermore, because of the physiologic and biochemical changes associated with progressive renal insufficiency, patients may respond to a given dose or serum concentration of a drug differently than patients with normal renal function.[9,10]

Knowledge of basic pharmacokinetic principles combined with the drug disposition properties of a particular compound and the degree and type of pathophysiologic alterations associated with renal insufficiency will make it possible for the pharmacotherapist to design an individualized therapeutic regimen. The objectives of this chapter are to describe the influence of renal insufficiency on drug absorption, distribution, metabolism, and elimination and to provide a practical approach for drug dosage individualization for patients with reduced renal function as well as those receiving continuous renal replacement therapy, continuous ambulatory peritoneal dialysis, and hemodialysis.

Effect of Renal Insufficiency on Drug Absorption

There is little quantitative information regarding the influence of impaired renal function on drug absorption and bioavailability. Several factors, such as alterations in GI emptying time, gastric pH, and antacid administration, could affect drug bioavailability in this patient population. Edema of the GI tract, as well as vomiting and diarrhea, which are frequent complications of severe renal insufficiency, may also alter drug bioavailability. The assessment of bioavailability in this patient population is further complicated, because most patients with severe renal insufficiency receive multiple medications, many of which cannot be discontinued during the course of a bioavailability study.

Some of the drug absorption "bioavailability" studies in patients with renal failure have not provided an assessment of absolute bioavailability (i.e., they have not included intravenous administration of the drug). Rather, they have documented alterations in the peak concentration (C_{max}) and the time at which peak concentration was attained (t_{max}) or in the fractional amount of drug recovered in the urine in a finite time period. Unfortunately, this limited information has been extrapolated to suggest that drug absorption is slowed and/or that the extent of absorption is reduced.[1,11,12]

The absolute bioavailability of only a few drug compounds is affected and for several the increase in bioavailability is due to a decrease in metabolism during the first pass through the GI tract and liver. Balant et al.[13] reported an increased bioavailability of three β blockers, tolamolol, bufuralol, and oxprenolol, in patients with renal failure. These data confirm the observations of increased systemic bioavailability of propranolol,[14] dextropropoxyphene,[15] and dihydrocodeine[16] in patients with renal insufficiency.

Although the bioavailability of all these compounds was increased, clinical consequences (development of excessive or unexpected adverse effects) have been demonstrated only with dextropropoxyphene[15] and dihydrocodeine.[17,18] The lack of association between the pharmacokinetic profile and clinical consequences of the β blockers may be a result of an alteration in the responsiveness of patients with renal disease to these agents, as has been reported with propranolol in the elderly.[19]

Effect of Renal Insufficiency on Drug Distribution

Although most clinicians assume that the volume of distribution of a drug is unaltered in patients with renal disease, recent evidence has indicated that the volume of distribution of many drugs may be significantly increased or decreased (Table 50.1).[4,20,21] Alterations in distribution volume may result from increased or decreased protein binding; altered tissue binding; pathophysiologic alterations in body composition, for example, the fractional contribution of total body water to total body weight; or be an artifact of the volume term used in the comparison.

Generally, the plasma protein binding of acidic drugs (warfarin, phenytoin) is decreased in uremia[2,3,22,23] (Table 50.2), whereas the binding of basic drugs (quinidine, lidocaine) is usually normal or slightly decreased or increased[2,3,24,25] (Table 50.3). The decrease in binding of acidic drugs in uremic plasma has been attributed to qualitative changes in the binding sites, accumulation of endogenous inhibitors of binding, and decreased concentrations of albumin. The first two of these mechanisms appear to account for most of the observed changes in binding.[26,27] In addition, the high concentrations of metabolites of some compounds that accumulate in patients with renal insufficiency may interfere with the protein binding of the parent compound.

Currently, clinical laboratories measure total rather than "free" or unbound concentrations of most drugs. Consequently, if one could predict the degree of protein binding in individuals, the ability to interpret total concentrations would improve. Liponi et al.[26] have suggested a method by

TABLE 50.1. EFFECT OF ESRD ON THE VOLUME OF DISTRIBUTION OF SELECTED DRUGS[a]

	Normal	ESRD
Increased		
Amikacin	0.20	0.29
Azlocillin	0.21	0.28
Bretylium	3.58	4.48
Cefazolin	0.13	0.16
Cefonicid	0.11	0.14
Cefoxitin	0.16	0.26
Cefuroxime	0.20	0.26
Clofibrate	0.14	0.24
Cloxacillin	0.14	0.26
Dicloxacillin	0.08	0.18
Erythromycin	0.57	1.09
Furosemide	0.11	0.18
Gentamicin	0.20	0.32
Isoniazid	0.6	0.8
Minoxidil	2.6	4.9
Nalmefene	7.9	14.7
Phenytoin	0.64	1.4
Sisomicin	0.19	0.25
Sulfamethopyrazine	0.21	0.38
Trimethoprim	1.36	1.83
Vancomycin	0.64	0.85
Decreased		
Chloramphenicol	0.87	0.60
Digoxin	513 L	280 L
Ethambutol	3.7	1.6
Methicillin	0.45	0.30
Pindolol	150 L	80 L
Pipemidic acid	2.0	0.84

[a]All data are in liters per kilogram unless otherwise stated.

TABLE 50.2. PROTEIN BINDING OF ACIDIC DRUGS IN PATIENTS WITH NORMAL RENAL FUNCTION AND ESRD

	Normal	ESRD
Abecarnil	94–98	85
Azlocillin	35–40	25
Cefazolin	84	71
Cefoxitin	73	41
Ceftriaxone	90	80
Clofibrate	97	91
Cloxacillin	95	80
Diazoxide	94	84
Dicloxacillin	97	91
Diflunisal	88	56
Doxycycline	88	72
Furosemide	96	94
Methotrexate	42.8	36.2
Metolazone	95	90
Moxalactam	52	36
Naproxen	99.8	99.2
Pentobarbital	66	59
Phenylbutazone	93–96	82–86
Phenytoin	90	74–85
Piretanide	94	88
Salicylate	92	80
Sulfamethoxazole	66	42
Valproic acid	92	77
Warfarin	99	98
Zomepirac	98.7	96.2

TABLE 50.3. PROTEIN BINDING OF BASIC DRUGS IN PATIENTS WITH NORMAL RENAL FUNCTION AND ESRD

	Normal	ESRD
Amphotericin B	96.5	95.9
Bepridil	99.7	99.9
Chloramphenicol	55	36
Clonazepam	86.1	84.0
Clonidine	44.4	52.4
Clorazepate	98	95
Diazepam	98	92
Disopyramide	68	72
Fluoxetine	94.5	93.5
Ketoconazole	99	98.5
Morphine	35	29
Prazosin	94	89.9
Propafenone	96.6	97.6
Triamterene	81	57

which the total phenytoin concentration (C_m^{total}) in patients with creatinine clearance values of 10 to 24 mL/min and less than 10 mL/min can be equated to the concentration that would be observed if plasma protein concentrations and phenytoin-binding characteristics were normal. A patient's "equated" total phenytoin concentration (C_e^{total}) would thus equal:

$$C_e^{\text{total}} = \left(\frac{1}{[1] + [(nK_a)(p)]}\right)(C_m^{\text{total}})(10)$$

where nK_a is the binding parameter based on the patient's renal function (10–24 mL/min = 1.5, and <10 mL/min = 1.0), and p is the measured serum albumin concentration. This methodology allows one to approximate the equivalent "total" phenytoin concentration in a patient with reduced renal function and can be used to predict dosage requirements via a standard nonlinear approach (see Chapter 3).

The principal binding protein for several basic drug compounds is α_1-acid glycoprotein (AAG), an acute-phase reactant whose plasma concentration is increased in a wide variety of patients, including renal transplant patients and hemodialysis patients.[27,28] The fraction of those drugs principally bound to AAG, for example, bepridil[25] and propafenone,[24] may be significantly increased in uremic patients. Thus, patients with renal insufficiency may experience increased or decreased protein binding depending on the principal binding protein for the drug in question.

Altered tissue binding may also affect the apparent volume of distribution of a drug. The distribution volume of digoxin has been reported to be reduced by 30–50% from normal values in patients with renal disease.[29,30] It has been postulated that this reduction in the distribution volume is secondary to a decrease in tissue binding as a result of competitive inhibition by endogenous or exogenous substances. This factor must therefore be taken into consideration in the design of individualized dosage regimens. Multiple methods have been proposed to estimate the degree of reduction in digoxin's distribution volume.[29] Jusko et al.[30] have reported that the volume of distribution of digoxin is related to creatinine clearance in the following way:

$$Vd_{\text{(liters)}} = [226] + \left[\frac{(298)(\text{CL}_{\text{cr}})}{29.1 + \text{CL}_{\text{cr}}}\right]$$

For a patient weighing 60 kg with a creatinine clearance of approximately 15 mL/min, the volume of distribution for digoxin would be:

$$Vd = [226] + \left[\frac{(298)(15)}{29.1 + 15}\right]$$

$$= 327 \text{ L or } 5.5 \text{ L/kg TBW}$$

This represents a 30% reduction from the volume of distribution that would have been anticipated in a patient with normal renal function. Acidosis or the presence of digoxin-like immunoreactive substances that bind to and inhibit membrane ATPase may also contribute to this phenomenon.[31,32] In this situation, the absolute amount of digoxin bound to the receptor would be reduced and the resultant serum digoxin concentration from any dose would be greater.

Knowledge of protein and tissue binding changes in patients with renal insufficiency is critically important in the interpretation of serum drug concentrations. Numerous investigations have shown that the unbound concentration of several drugs in plasma correlates more closely with the concentration of drug at the receptor site and, therefore, with the pharmacologic effect, than does the total concentration of drug in plasma.[33] Since an alteration in plasma protein or tissue binding of a drug will likely alter the total drug concentration, the usual expected relationship between total drug concentration and pharmacologic response will be perturbed but the relationship to unbound drug should be unaffected.

Thus, in patients with renal insufficiency, particularly those with end-stage renal disease (ESRD), a "normal" total drug concentration may be associated with either serious adverse reactions secondary to elevated unbound drug concentrations or subtherapeutic responses because of an altered plasma/tissue drug concentration ratio. The monitoring of unbound drug concentrations in this patient population is therefore suggested for those drugs that have a narrow therapeutic range, are highly protein bound (free fraction of <20%), and for which marked variability in the free fraction has been reported, for example, phenytoin and disopyramide.

Finally, the method utilized to calculate the volume of distribution may be influenced by renal disease. The three most commonly used volume of distribution terms are volume of the central compartment (V_c), volume of the terminal phase (V_β, V_{area}), and volume of distribution at steady state (V_{SS}). The central compartment volume is calculated as the intravenous bolus dose divided by the initial plasma concentration. V_c for many drugs approximates extracellular fluid volume and thus may be increased or decreased by shifts in this physiologic volume. Renal insufficiency, especially oliguric acute renal failure, is often accompanied by fluid overload and a resultant increased V_c due to reduced renal elimination of water and sodium. V_{area} (V_β) is calculated as the total body clearance divided by the terminal elimination rate constant (k or β). This volume term represents the proportionality constant between plasma concentrations in the terminal elimination phase and the amount of drug remaining in the body. V_β is affected by both distribution characteristics, as well as the elimination rate constant. The third volume term, the steady-state volume of distribution (V_{SS}), is determined by (AUMC • Dose)/AUC^2, where AUMC is the area under the first moment of the concentration time curve and AUC is the area under the concentration time curve. V_β and V_{SS} will often be similar in magnitude with V_β being slightly larger. In situations in which V_β is much larger than V_{SS}, V_β may reflect the elimination rate more than the distribution volume. Since V_{SS} has the advantage of being independent of drug elimination, it may be the most appropriate volume term to use when one desires to compare drug distribution volumes between patients with renal insufficiency and those with normal renal function.[34,35]

Effect of Renal Insufficiency on Metabolism

Although the role of the kidneys as an excretory organ for drugs and chemicals and their polar metabolites is well described, the fact that the kidney is very metabolically active in the biotransformation of a variety of drugs is not well appreciated.[36–38] The renal cytochrome P-450 system catalyzes the metabolism of a variety of chemicals and drugs with an activity that may equal that of the liver on an activity per gram of tissue basis. Whole kidney homogenate cytochrome P-450 activity has varied from 14–18% of that observed in the liver. Glucuronide, glutathione, and sulfate conjugation activity has also been documented in kidney homogenates. Finally, glucuronyl transferase activity of the kidney in various animal species has been reported to range from 8–120% of the liver activity.[36] Prescott et al.[39] and van Olden et al.[40] recently demonstrated that *p*-aminohippurate (PAH), a compound frequently used to estimate effective renal plasma flow, is converted to *n*-acetyl-PAH by the human kidney and liver. This metabolism accounts for up to 25% of the total elimination of PAH. These studies clearly suggest that the kidney possesses considerable drug-metabolizing capability; however, the contribution to the total metabolic activity is generally low, because total kidney weight is far less than liver weight.

Investigations of the effect of chronic renal failure on hepatic enzyme activity in animals have also demonstrated alterations in certain pathways of hepatic drug metabolism.[41,42] Chronic renal failure was associated with a 26–71% decrease in hepatic enzyme activity. In each case, the alteration in enzyme activity declined as the extent of renal failure increased.[41] These data suggest that chronic renal impairment may have a detrimental effect not only on drug metabolism in the kidney but also on drug metabolism within the liver.

Drug metabolism may be increased, decreased, or unaffected by renal failure depending on the drug and the species (animals versus man) investigated[5,6,37–40,43] (Table 50.4). These studies should be interpreted cautiously since concurrent drug intake, age, smoking habit, and alcohol intake often were not controlled. Furthermore, the possibility of pharmacogenetic variation must be considered.

TABLE 50.4. EFFECT OF ESRD ON NONRENAL (HEPATIC) CLEARANCE

	Decreased		
Acyclovir	Aztreonam	Bufuralol	Captopril
Cefmenoxime	Cefmetazole	Cefonicid	Cefotaxime
Cefotiam	Cefsulodin	Ceftizoxime	Cilastatin
Cimetidine	Cortisol	Encainide	Erythromycin
Erythromycin	Imipenem	Isoniazid	Methylprednisolone
Metoclopramide	Moxalactam	Nicardipine	Nimodipine
Nitrendipine	Procainamide	Quinapril	Verapamil
Zidovudine			
	Unchanged		
Acetaminophen	Chloramphenicol	Clonidine	Codeine
Diflunisal	Indomethacin	Insulin[a]	Isradipine
Lidocaine	Morphine	Metoprolol	Nisoldipine
Nortriptyline	Pentobarbital	Propafenone	Quinidine
Theophylline	Tocainide	Tolbutamide	
	Increased		
Antipyrine	Bumetanide	Cefpiramide	Fosinopril
Nifedipine	Phenytoin	Sulfadimidine	

[a]May be unchanged or decreased.

TABLE 50.5. PHARMACOLOGIC ACTIVITY OF SELECTED DRUG METABOLITES

Parent Drug	Metabolite	Pharmacologic Activity of Metabolites
Acetaminophen	*N*-acetyl-*p*-benzo-quinoneimine	Responsible for hepatotoxicity
Allopurinol	Oxipurinol	Metabolite primarily responsible for suppression of xanthine oxidase
Azathioprine	Mercaptopurine	All of the immunosuppressive activity resides in the metabolite
Cefotaxime	Desacetyl cefotaxime	Similiar antimicrobial spectrum, but one-fourth to one-tenth as potent
Chlorpropamide	2-Hydroxychlorpropamide	Similar *in vitro* insulin-releasing activity
Clofibrate	Chlorophenoxyisobutyric acid	Primarily responsible for hypolipidemic effect and direct muscle toxicity
Codeine	Morphine-6-glucuronide	Possibly more active than parent compound; may contribute to prolonged narcotic effect in renal failure patients
Imipramine	Desmethylimipramine	Similar antidepressant activity
Meperidine	Normeperidine	Less analgesic activity than parent, but more CNS-stimulatory effects
Morphine	Morphine-6-glucuronide	Possibly more active than parent compound; may contribute to prolonged narcotic effect in renal failure patients
Procainamide	*N*-acetyl procainamide	Distinct antiarrhythmic activity, the mechanism of which is different from that of the parent compound
Sulfonamides	Acetylated metabolites	Devoid of antibacterial activity, but elevated concentrations are associated with increased toxicity
Theophylline	1,3-Dimethyl uric acid	Cardiotoxicity has been demonstrated
Zidovudine	Zidovudine triphosphate	Primarily responsible for antiretroviral activity

Prediction of the effect of renal impairment on the metabolism of a particular drug is thus difficult; for example, nifedipine, nitrendipine, and nisoldipine are all apparently metabolized *in vivo* by cytochrome P-450 3A4, yet the metabolism of nifedipine is increased,[44] nitrendipine decreased,[45] and nisoldipine is unaffected by renal failure.[46] If the metabolism of a drug is known to be increased or decreased in patients with renal failure, then the dose will need to be adjusted appropriately in order to achieve the desired effect. If the effect of renal failure on metabolism is unknown, then the agent should be utilized with extreme caution.

Patients with severe renal insufficiency receiving chronic treatment with some agents may experience accumulation of metabolite(s) as well as parent compound. Although metabolites of several drugs have been reported to have significant pharmacologic and/or toxicologic activity in general, the pharmacokinetics and pharmacology of metabolites are not often fully elucidated in humans. In a sense, the patient with severe renal impairment is being exposed to a "new pharmacologic entity" if the serum concentrations of the metabolite exceed those reported in patients with normal renal function.

The metabolite may have pharmacologic activity similar to that of the parent drug and thus contribute significantly to clinical response, for example, oxipurinol and desacetyl cefotaxime.[47] Alternatively, the metabolite may have qualitatively dissimilar pharmacologic action, for example, normeperidine has a CNS-stimulatory activity that has been reported to produce seizures, while meperidine has CNS-depressant actions.[48,49] Because of the multiplicity of potential interactions of compounds that are primarily metabolized, the practical consequences of metabolite accumulation are difficult to predict and are most often identified in those patients at risk by trial and error (Table 50.5).

Effect of Renal Insufficiency on Renal Excretion

Measurement of endogenous creatinine clearance is the usual clinical means of determining a patient's renal function (see Chapter 42, Quantification of Renal Function). This measurement, however, provides only an index of glomerular function. Tubular secretion and tubular reabsorption are also key mechanisms involved in the renal excretion of many drug compounds.[50] Alterations in one or more of these three mechanisms secondary to reduction in functional nephron mass may have a dramatic effect on the pharmacokinetics of a drug.

Kamiya et al.[51] and Hori et al.[52] demonstrated that the type of renal disease may explain in part the differences in pharmacokinetic parameters observed among patients with similar reductions in glomerular filtration rate. The disposition of antibiotic agents extensively secreted by the proximal renal tubules (e.g., ampicillin, cephalexin) was altered to a greater degree in patients with tubulointerstitial disease compared to those with primary glomerular disease. These data suggest that dosage-adjustment methodologies may need to be developed to take into consideration the impact of altered tubular as well as glomerular function.[53] Quantitative investigations of renal handling of new drugs will be required to elucidate the relative contribution of tubular and glomerular function to renal drug clearance. The availability of these data should provide a more rational approach to dosage regimen design for those agents that undergo extensive tubular secretion or reabsorption.

In the absence of data delineating the contribution of tubular function to renal elimination, the clinical measurement or estimation of creatinine clearance remains the guiding factor for drug dosage regimen design.[4,7–9] The importance of an alteration in renal function on drug elimination thus depends on two factors: the fraction of drug normally eliminated by the kidney unchanged and the degree of renal insufficiency.

Quantitation of the patient's renal function can be accomplished by measurement of creatinine clearance or estimation based on the stable serum creatinine (see Chapter 42, Quantitation of Renal Function). Because of the time delay involved and problems in obtaining complete urine collections, measured creatinine clearance values are infrequently used for initial drug dosage regimen design. Therefore, the calculation of initial drug dosage regimens relies on the estimation of creatinine clearance (CL_{cr}) in adults and children from such routinely available clinical data as age, sex, height, weight, and serum creatinine.[54–58] We should emphasize that these relationships are most accurate for individuals of average muscle mass for their age, weight, and height. The creatinine clearance of emaciated and obese adult patients is difficult to predict and incorrect estimates have been obtained with most methods.

Several methods are also available for estimating creatinine clearance in adults with acute renal insufficiency utilizing age, height, weight, serum creatinine, and time data.[59,60] These methods have not been as rigorously validated as the equations for patients with stable renal function. However, they are one of the few methods we have to approximate renal function in this complex patient situation.

Drug Dosage Regimen Design for Patients with Renal Insufficiency

Most dosage adjustment guidelines have proposed the use of a fixed dose or interval for patients with broad ranges of renal function.[21,61–65] For example, moderate renal insufficiency may encompass a creatinine clearance range of 10–50 mL/min, while severe renal insufficiency is often defined as a creatinine clearance of less than 10 mL/min. These categories encompass up to a tenfold range in renal function and, thus, the drug regimen may not be optimal for all patients whose renal function lies within the range.

The design of the optimal dosage regimen for patients with renal insufficiency requires an individualized assessment and is dependent on the availability of an accurate characterization of the relationship between the pharmacokinetic parameters of the drug and renal function and an accurate assessment of the patient's renal function (i.e., creatinine clearance). Secondary references such as the *Physicians' Desk Reference* (PDR),[61] *AHFS Drug Information,*[62] and textbooks[66] are excellent sources of information about a drug's pharmacokinetic characteristics in subjects with normal renal function. They, however, often do not provide the explicit relationships of the kinetic parameters of interest (total body clearance, elimination rate constant, and distribution volume) with a continuous index of renal function, such as creatinine clearance. To find this information, you may need to identify the original research study that assessed the drug's disposition or a comprehensive review article on the class of drugs of interest. Ideally one should be able to identify a relationship between total body clearance (CL), elimination rate constant (k), or distribution volume (V_d) with CL_{cr} (see Table 50.6). This information along with the patient's CL_{cr} will allow prediction of the patient's kinetic parameters and then formulation of a therapeutic regimen to attain the desired therapeutic outcome.

If specific literature recommendations and/or the relationship of kinetic parameters to CL_{cr} are not available, then one can estimate the kinetic parameters of the patient with the method of Welling et al.[8] or Tozer,[7,9] provided you know the fraction of the drug that is eliminated renally unchanged (f_e) in subjects with normal renal function. These approaches assume that the decrease in CL and k are proportional to CL_{cr}, that renal disease does not alter the drug's metabolism, that the metabolites if formed are inactive and nontoxic, that the drug obeys first-order (linear) kinetic principles, and that it is adequately described by a one-compartment model. If these assumptions are true then

TABLE 50.6. RELATIONSHIP BETWEEN RENAL FUNCTION AND PHARMACOKINETIC PARAMETERS OF SOME DRUGS

Drug	Total Body Clearance	Elimination Rate Constant
Acyclovir	$CL = 3.37 (CL_{cr}) + 0.41$	
Amikacin	$CL = 0.6 (CL_{cr}) + 9.6$	$k_{el} = 0.0026 (CL_{cr}) + 0.02$
Cefazolin		$k_{el} = 0.003 (CL_{cr}) + 0.02$
Cefmetazole	$CL = 1.18 (CL_{cr}) - 0.29$	
Ceftazidime	$CL = 1.15 (CL_{cr}) + 10.6$	$k_{el} = 0.004 (CL_{cr}) + 0.004$
Ciprofloxacin	$CL = 2.83 (CL_{cr}) + 363$	
Digoxin	$CL = 0.88 (CL_{cr}) + 23$	
Gentamicin	$CL = 0.983 (CL_{cr})$	$k_{el} = 0.00315 (CL_{cr})$
Netilmicin	$CL = 0.65 (CL_{cr}) + 3.72$	$k_{el} = 0.003 (CL_{cr}) + 0.013$
Ofloxacin	$CL = 1.04 (CL_{cr}) + 38.7$	
Piperacillin	$CL = 1.36 (CL_{cr}) + 1.50$	
Procainamide	$CL = 3 (CL_{cr}) + 0.23 (ABW)$	
Teicoplanin	$CL = 7.09 (CL_{cr}) - 16.2$	
Tobramycin	$CL = 0.801 (CL_{cr})$	$k_{el} = 0.00382 (CL_{cr})$
Vancomycin	$CL = 0.69 (CL_{cr}) + 3.7$	$k_{el} = 0.00083 (CL_{cr}) + 0.0044$

(Compiled from Refs. 20 and 64–66.)

the kinetic parameter/dosage adjustment factor (Q) can be calculated as:

$$Q = 1 - [f_e(1 - KF)]$$

where KF is the ratio of the patient's CL_{cr} to the assumed normal value of 120 mL/min. Thus, for a drug that is 85% eliminated renally unchanged in a patient who has a CL_{cr} of 10 mL/min, the Q factor would be:

$$\begin{aligned} Q &= 1 - \{0.85(1 - [10/120])\} \\ &= 1 - [0.85(0.92)] \\ &= 1 - 0.78 \\ &= 0.22 \end{aligned}$$

The estimated total body clearance for this patient would then be calculated as $CL_{PT} = CL_{norm} \cdot Q$, where CL_{norm} is the mean value in patients with normal renal function as reported in the literature.

Once the kinetic parameters for the patient have been estimated, the best method for dosage regimen adjustment should be selected. Specifically, one must determine if the desired goal is the maintenance of a similar peak, trough, or average steady-state drug concentration. If there is a significant relationship between peak or trough concentration and clinical response[67–70] (e.g., aminoglycosides and vancomycin) or toxicity[71–73] (e.g., quinidine and phenytoin), then attainment of the specific target values is critical. If, however, no specific target values for peak or trough concentrations have been reported (e.g., antihypertensive agents, benzodiazepines), then a regimen goal of attaining the same average steady-state concentration may be appropriate.

Although several methods have been proposed to attain the desired average steady-state concentration profile, the principal choices are to decrease the dose or prolong the dosing interval. If the size of the dose is reduced while the dosing interval remains unchanged, the desired average steady-state concentration will be similar; however, the peak will be lower and the trough higher (Fig. 50.1). Alternatively, if the dosing interval is increased and the dose size remains unchanged, the peak and trough concentrations in the patient with reduced renal function will be similar to those in the patient with normal renal function. This dosage adjustment method is generally preferred because it is likely to yield significant cost savings as a result of a reduction in nursing and pharmacy time as well as in the supplies associated with frequent drug administration. Finally, the dose and dosing interval may both need to be changed to attain a desired peak or trough serum concentration time profile.

Regardless of the approach chosen to adjust the dosage regimen, the first step in the process, as previously mentioned, is to estimate the drug disposition parameters in the patient with renal insufficiency. The ratio (Q) of the estimated elimination rate constant or total body clearance of the patient relative to subjects with normal renal function (CL_{cr} = 120 mL/min) may then be calculated. This parameter may be used to determine the dose or dosing interval alterations necessary for the patient.

For example, the following relationship between total clearance (CL) and creatinine clearance has been reported for ganciclovir[74]:

$$CL\ (mL/min/1.8\ m^2) = 1.25(CL_{cr}) + 8.57$$

Thus, CL for a subject with normal renal function (CL_{norm}) would be calculated as:

$$\begin{aligned} CL_{norm} &= [1.25(120)] + 8.57 \\ &= 158.6\ mL/min/1.8\ m^2 \end{aligned}$$

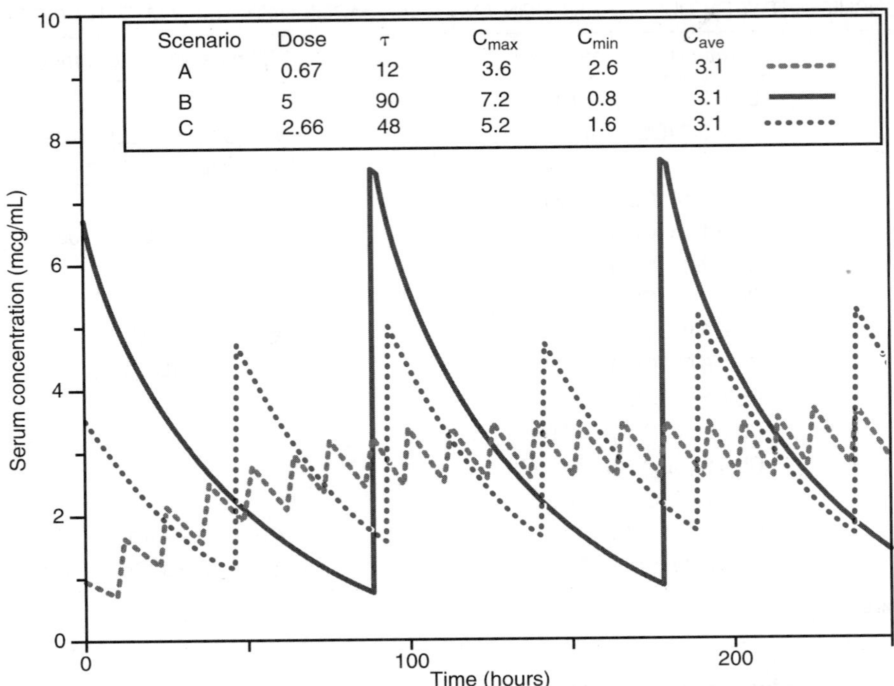

Figure 50.1. Although the average steady-state concentrations (C_{ave}) are identical, the concentration-time profile will be markedly different if one changes the dose and maintains the dosing interval (τ) constant (scenario A), versus changing τ and maintaining the dose constant (scenario B), or changing both (scenario C).

Clearance (CL_{fail}) for a patient with a creatinine clearance of 10 mL/min would be:

$$CL_{fail} = [1.25\ (10)] + 8.57$$
$$= 21.1\ \text{mL/min/1.8 m}^2$$

Neutropenia has been associated with ganciclovir trough concentrations exceeding 10 μmol/L.[75] If this patient received the typical ganciclovir dose for a patient with normal renal function, the predicted trough concentrations would approach 20 μmol/L. Therefore, a dosage modification in this patient is necessary to avoid potential toxicity. The dosing regimen can be modified using the ratio of the predicted clearance values. Therefore, the quotient or Q, for this patient is calculated as:

$$Q = CL_{fail}/CL_{norm}$$
$$= 21.1/158.6$$
$$= 0.133$$

where CL_{norm} is the clearance in a patient with normal renal function and CL_{fail} is the clearance of the patient with impaired renal function.

The maintenance dose (D_f) for the patient or the adjusted dosing interval (τ_f) may then be calculated from the following relationships, where D_n is the normal dose and τ_n is the normal dosing interval:

$$D_f = D_n \times Q$$
$$\tau_f = \tau_n/Q$$

For this patient situation, the normal dose of ganciclovir would be 5 mg/kg (D_n) and the $\tau_n = 12$ hours. If we wanted to maintain the dosing interval at 12 hours, then D_f would be calculated as:

$$D_f = (5\ \text{mg/kg}) \times 0.133 = 0.67\ \text{mg/kg}$$

This regimen would result in decreased peak and increased trough concentrations compared to patients with normal renal function (Fig. 50.1, scenario A).

If we want to maintain D_n and extend the dosing interval, τ_f would be calculated as:

$$\tau_f = \tau_n/Q = 12/0.133 = 90.2\ \text{hours}$$

This regimen would yield similar peak and trough concentrations in the renally impaired patient as the normal renal function patient but there is a risk of missed doses with such an unorthodox interval (Fig. 50.1, scenario B). In addition, the prolonged period below the C_{ss} average concentration may be less than optimal.

Finally, a practical dosing interval may be selected and then a dose based on that interval can be calculated (Fig. 50.1, scenario C). If a dosage interval τ_f of 48 hours was selected, since in many institutions there is an increased risk of missed doses with longer dosing intervals, then the D_f would be calculated as follows:

$$D_f = [D_n \times Q \times \tau_f]/\tau_n$$
$$= [(5\ \text{mg/kg}) \times (0.133) \times (48)]/12$$
$$= 2.66\ \text{mg/kg}$$

This method would likely be most appropriate in this case; prolonged subtherapeutic concentrations are avoided and troughs are reduced from the first method. The selection of which dosage adjustment method to use to calculate an optimal regimen depends on the drug characteristics and the patient care situation. This dosage adjustment method assumes that the protein binding and volume of distribution of the drug are not significantly altered by renal insufficiency. Thus, this approach cannot be used with accuracy for those drugs with demonstrated differences in these pharmacokinetic parameters.

If the volume of distribution (V_d) of a drug is significantly altered in patients with renal insufficiency or one desires to attain a specific maximum or minimum concentration, the estimation of a dosage regimen becomes more complex. If the relationship between V_d and creatinine clearance has been characterized, then V_d may be estimated. If one assumes the drug can be described by a one-compartment linear model, the predicted V_d may then be used with the predicted elimination rate constant (k) of the drug to yield an adjusted dosing interval and intravenous or oral dose.

For example, the following relationships between CL_{cr} and elimination rate constant and V_d have been reported for the aminoglycoside netilmicin[76]:

$$k_f\,(h^{-1}) = 0.003(CL_{cr}) - 0.013$$

$$V_f\,(L/kg) = -\,0.0017(CL_{cr}) + 0.354$$

where k_f is the elimination rate constant and V_f is the volume of distribution of the patient with renal insufficiency.

Therefore, if a 65-kg patient with a CL_{cr} of 24 mL/min is to receive netilmicin infused over 0.5 hour, the adjusted interval necessary to yield a C_{peak} of 8 mg/L at 0.5 hour after a 0.5-hour infusion and C_{trough} of 1 mg/L could be calculated as:

$$k_f = 0.003(24) - 0.013 = 0.059\ h^{-1}$$

$$\begin{aligned}\tau_f &= -1/k_f\,[\ln C_{trough}/C_{peak}] + t' \\ &= [-1/(0.059)][\ln 1/8] + 0.5 \\ &= 35.7 \text{ hours (or a more practical 36 hours)}\end{aligned}$$

where τ_f is the dosing interval and t' is the infusion duration. The volume of distribution would be:

$$V_f = [(-0.0017)\,(24)] + 0.354 = 0.313\ L/kg = 20.3\ L$$

The dose to be administered every 36 hours could then be calculated as:

$$\begin{aligned}Dose_{IV} &= (k_f)(V_f)(C_{peak})t'\,[(1 - e^{-k_f\tau_f}/(1 - e^{-k_f t'}))]e^{-k_f t_z} \\ &= (0.059)(20.3)(8)(0.5) \\ &\quad [(1 - e^{-(0.059)(36)})/(1 - e^{-(0.059)(0.5)})]/e^{-(0.059)(0.5)} \\ &= 149.4 \text{ mg (or a more practical 150 mg)}\end{aligned}$$

where t_z is the time after the end of the intravenous infusion. If the change in distribution volume reported by Luft et al.[76] were not taken into consideration and a volume of distribution of 0.184 L/kg (12 L) were utilized, a volume appropriate for an individual with a CL_{cr} of 100 mL/min, the calculated dose would be about 80–90 mg.

For orally administered drugs, the τ_f can be calculated as $\tau_f = [(-1/k_f)(\ln[C_{min}/C_{max}])] + t_{peak}$, and the dose can be approximated as:

$$Dose_{PO} = [SFC_p^t V_d\,(k_a - k)]/ \\ [k_a((e^{-kt}/1 - e^{-k\tau}) - (e^{-k_a t}/1 - e^{-k_a\tau}))]$$

where C_p^t equals the desired plasma concentration at time t and k_a is the absorption rate constant. This approach allows for the individualization of a dosage regimen for attainment of specific peak and trough serum concentrations. If the drug is absorbed extremely rapidly, one can approximate the τ_f as $\tau_f = (-1/k_f)(\ln\,[C_{min}/C_{max}])$ and the dose as Dose = $V_d \cdot (C_{max} - C_{min})$.

Digoxin is a frequently utilized oral medication for which the V_d is decreased in patients with renal insufficiency and for which one usually desires to closely control the plasma concentration time profile. The V_d and CL_T of digoxin can be estimated for a 70-kg patient with a CL_{cr} of 12 mL/min as follows[29,30]:

$$\begin{aligned}V_d &= 226 + \{(298[CL_{cr}]/[29.1 + CL_{cr}])\} \\ &= 226 + \{(298[12]/[29.1 + 12]\} \\ &= 226 + 87.0 = 313\ L\end{aligned}$$

$$\begin{aligned}CL_f &= (0.88CL_{cr}) + 23\ mL/min \\ &= 10.6 + 23 = 33.6\ mL/min\end{aligned}$$

$$\begin{aligned}k_f &= CL_f/V_d \\ &= (33.6\ mL/min \cdot 1440\ min/d)/313\ L \\ &= (48.3\ L/d)/313\ L = 0.154\ d^{-1}\end{aligned}$$

The t_{peak} is generally at 2 hours and the k_a from the literature is about 0.76 h^{-1} or 18 d^{-1}.[77] Thus one now has all the information needed to calculate the τ_f and dose for this patient:

$$\begin{aligned}\tau_f &= \{(-1/k_f)(\ln[C_{min}/C_{max}])\} + t_{peak} \\ &= [(-1/0.154)(\ln 0.8/1.4)] + 2 \text{ hours} \\ &= [(-6.49)(-0.56)] \\ &= 3.6 \text{ days} + 2 \text{ hours} \\ &\quad \sim 4 \text{ days}\end{aligned}$$

$$Dose_{PO} = [(1.4)(313)(18 - 0.154)]/[18((e^{-0.154(0.083)}/ \\ 1 - e^{-0.154(4)}) - (e^{-18(0.083)}/1 - e^{-18(4)}))]$$

Dose = 0.226 mg or 0.25-mg oral capsules every 4 days

Alternately, the predicted volume of distribution and elimination rate constant or the total body clearance may be used to calculate a dose regimen that will maintain the desired average steady-state concentration of the drug (C_{ss}).

$$Dose\,(mg/h) = C_{ss}\,[(k_f\,V) \text{ or } (CL_f)]$$

Depending on how much variance about the average steady state one desires, the dosing interval may range from hourly to as infrequent as every 48 hours or longer. For example, if the calculated dose were 10 mg/h, the desired average steady-state concentration would be maintained with a dosing interval of 60 mg every 6 hours or 480 mg every 48 hours.

Drug Dosage Regimen Design for Patients Receiving Continuos Renal Replacement Therapy

Continuous renal replacement therapy (CRRT) is utilized for the management of fluid overload and the removal of uremic toxins in patients with acute renal failure and other conditions.[78] The several forms of CRRT are extensively described in Chapter 43, Acute Renal Failure. Which of these therapies will be optimal for a given patient is dependent on several factors including bleeding risk, degree of hypercatabolism, acid–base balance, and experience of the health care provider.

Drug therapy individualization for the patient receiving CRRT is complicated by the fact that patients with acute renal failure may have a higher residual nonrenal clearance of some drugs than patients with chronic renal insufficiency who have a similar CL_{cr}.[79,80] For example, the nonrenal clearance of imipenem in patients with acute renal failure (95 mL/min) is between the values observed in chronic renal failure patients (50 mL/min) and normal values (130 mL/min).[80] This may occur due to less exposure to or accumulation of uremic by-products that may alter hepatic function. A nonrenal clearance value in a patient with acute renal failure that is higher than anticipated based on chronic renal failure data would result in lower than expected, possibly subtherapeutic, serum concentrations.

In addition to patient-specific differences, there are marked differences between intermittent hemodialysis and the three primary types of CRRT (i.e., continuous arteriovenous ultrafiltration (CAVU) or slow continuous ultrafiltration (SCUF), continuous arteriovenous or venovenous hemofiltration (CAVH or CVVH), and continuous arteriovenous or venovenous hemodiafiltration (CAVHD/CVVHD) with regard to drug removal).

During CAVU/SCUF and CAVH/CVVH drug removal primarily occurs via convection/ultrafiltration (i.e., the passive transport of drug molecules at the concentration at which they exist in plasma water into the plasma ultrafiltrate). The clearance of a drug by either of these methods is thus a function of the membrane permeability for the drug, which is called the sieving coefficient (SC) and the rate of ultrafiltrate formation (UFR). The SC can be calculated as:

$$SC = (2C_{UF})/[(C_a/1 - \theta) + (C_v/1 - \theta)]$$

where C_a and C_v are the concentration in the plasma going into and returning from the filter, respectively, and θ is 0.0107 times the total protein concentration in plasma. The SC is often approximated by the fraction unbound (f_{ub}) since this information may be more readily available. Thus the clearance by these two modes of CRRT can be calculated as:

$$CL_{CAVU} = UFR \cdot SC \quad \text{or} \quad UFR \cdot f_{ub}$$

Clearance of a drug by CAVHD/CVVHD (CL_{CAVHD}/CL_{CVVHD}) is generally greater than by CAVU/SCUF or CAVH/CVVH since in addition to the convection/ultrafiltration process drug is removed by diffusion from the plasma water into the dialysate. The CL_{CVVHD} can be mathematically approximated as:

$$CL_{CVVHD} = (UFR \cdot f_{ub}) + CL_{diffusion}$$

In the clinical setting it is often not possible to separate these two components of CL_{CVVHD}. In essence the CL_{CVVHD} is calculated as the product of the combined ultrafiltrate and dialysate volume (V_{df}) and the concentration of the drug in this fluid (C_{df}) divided by the plasma concentration (C_p^{mid}) at the midpoint of the V_{df} collection period:

$$CL_{CVVHD} = (V_{df} \cdot C_{df})/C_p^{mid}$$

There are not only differences in the rate of drug removal between the three primary modes of CRRT but also within each mode. This is due to differences in the filter membrane composition as the result of variable degrees of drug binding to the membrane[81,83] and the permeability characteristics of the membrane.[82,84]

Reliable recommendations on drug dosage during CRRT require the measurement of drug concentrations in ultrafiltrate and/or dialysate plus plasma. Estimates of SC based solely on f_{ub} are unreliable because of the large interindividual variability of protein binding in patients who are critically ill especially those with renal insufficiency.[85] Furthermore, since f_{ub} data are rarely available from patients with chronic renal insufficiency, data from patients without renal disease may need to be utilized. The predictability of CL_{CVVHD} is even more complicated because the diffusive properties of most drugs with these new filter membranes are unknown.

Individualization of therapy for a patient receiving CRRT therapy is dependent on the patient's residual renal function and the clearance of the drug by the mode of CRRT they are receiving. The patient's residual drug clearance can be predicted as described in the previous section of this chapter. The CRRT clearance can also be ascertained from published literature reports.[86,87] The SCs of frequently used drugs are summarized in Table 50.7, while the clearance by CVVHD at various dialysate flow rates is listed in Table 50.8. These data can be utilized to design initial dosage regimens for patients receiving CRRT.

For example, WT is a 48-year-old, 60-kg male in acute renal failure with a serum creatinine of 7.2 mg/dL, which has increased from 2.3 mg/dL over 3 days. The residual creatinine clearance value in this patient, calculated using the Jelliffe and Jelliffe equation[59] for changing serum cre-

TABLE 50.7. PREDICTED AND MEASURED SIEVING COEFFICIENTS OF SELECTED DRUGS

Drug	Predicted	Measured
Amikacin	0.95	0.88
Amphotericin	0.01	0.32–0.4
Ampicillin	0.8	0.6–0.69
Cefoperazone	0.10	0.27–0.69
Cefotaxime	0.62	0.55–1.1
Cefoxitin	0.30	0.32
Ceftazidine	0.90	0.38–0.78
Ceftriaxone	0.10	0.71–0.82
Clindamycin	0.25	0.49–0.98
Digoxin	0.75	0.96
Erythromycin	0.25	0.37
5-Flurocytosine	0.96	0.98
Gentamicin	0.95	0.81–0.75
Imipenem	0.80	0.78
Metronidazole	0.80	0.80
Mezlocillin	0.68	0.68
Nafcillin	0.20	0.47
N-acetyl procainamide	0.80	0.92
Netilmicin	—	0.85
Oxacillin	0.05	0.02
Phenobarbital	0.60	0.86
Phenytoin	0.10	0.45
Procainamide	0.80	0.86
Theophylline	0.47	0.85
Tobramycin	0.95	0.78–0.86
Vancomycin	0.90	0.5–0.8

(Adapted from Refs. 81–87.)

atinines (see Chapter 42, Quantification of Renal Function), is 4.8 mL/min. The consulting nephrologist recommends that CVVHD be initiated using a Fresenius F-40 filter at a blood and dialysis flow rate of 100 and 33.3 mL/min, respectively. The patient is to receive ceftazidime while on CVVHD. The patient's residual ceftazidime clearance can be estimated using the regression equation in Table 50.6 relating CL_{cr} and clearance.

$$\begin{aligned} CL\ (mL/min) &= 1.15\ (CL_{cr}) + 10.6 \\ &= 1.15\ (4.8) + 10.6 = 16.1\ mL/min \end{aligned}$$

The total clearance while on CVVHD would be the sum of the patient's residual clearance and the ceftazidime clearance associated with CVVHD (CL_{CVVHD}; Table 50.8) as follows:

$$\begin{aligned} CL_{PT} &= CL + CL_{CVVHD} \\ &= 16.1\ mL/min + 15.2\ mL/min = 31.3\ mL/min \end{aligned}$$

This patient clearance value can be used to adjust the ceftazidime dose as described earlier. The ceftazidime clearance in a patient with normal renal function would be calculated as:

TABLE 50.8. CLEARANCE OF SELECTED DRUGS BY CAVHD/CVVHD

	Dialysate Flow Rate (mL/min)				
	5	**10**	**16.7**	**33.3**	**50–60**
Ceftazidime	—	—	13–17	15.2	24
Cefuroxime	—	—	14–19	16.2	35
Ciprofloxacin	—	—	16.3	19.9	—
Digoxin	2.6	4.2	6.4–10.0	11	—
Gentamicin	—	—	20.5	26.0	—
Phenytoin	1.4	3.0	6.5	—	—
Theophylline	4.0	7.8	14.8	—	—
Tobramycin	—	—	11.1–29	14.9	16–37
Urea	—	—	13–28	18–36	27–40
Vancomycin	3.3	6.7	8.1–11.7	23–28	—

(Adapted from Refs. 81–87.)

$$\begin{aligned} CL_{norm}\ (mL/min) &= 1.15(CL_{cr}) + 10.6 \\ &= 1.15(120) + 10.6 = 148.6\ mL/min \end{aligned}$$

The dosage adjustment factor would then be:

$$\begin{aligned} Q &= CL_{PT}/CL_{norm} \\ &= 31.3/148.6 = 0.21 \end{aligned}$$

For this patient situation, the normal regimen of ceftazidime would be 1000 mg (D_n) every 8 hours (τ_n). If we wanted to maintain D_n and extend the dosing interval, then τ_f would be calculated as:

$$\begin{aligned} \tau_f &= \tau_n/Q \\ &= 8\ \text{hours}/0.21 \\ &= 38\ \text{hours or a more practical 36 hours} \end{aligned}$$

Therefore, this patient should receive 1000 mg every 36 hours. If the additional clearance associated with CVVHD (15.2 mL/min) was not considered, the dosing interval would have been considerably longer at approximately 72 hours.

Drug Dosage Regimen Design for Patients Receiving Chronic Ambulatory Peritoneal Dialysis

Although the majority of patients with ESRD receive treatment with hemodialysis, approximately 15% of dialysis patients are maintained with chronic ambulatory peritoneal dialysis (CAPD). A more detailed discussion of CAPD therapeutic principles is provided in Chapter 46, Principles and Practice of Chronic Renal Replacement Therapy. Peritoneal dialysis, like other dialysis modalities, has the potential to affect drug disposition; however, drug therapy individualization is often less complicated in these patients due to the continuous nature of the CAPD procedure.

Many of the factors that are important in determining drug dialyzability for other treatment modalities pertain to peritoneal dialysis as well.[88–90] Peritoneal dialysis involves the instillation of 1 to 3 L of dialysis solution into the peritoneal cavity. Waste products and other substances, potentially including drugs, move from the blood and surrounding tissues into the dialysis solution by means of diffusion and ultrafiltration. Factors that influence drug dialyzability in peritoneal dialysis include drug-specific characteristics such as molecular weight, solubility, degree of ionization, protein binding, and volume of distribution. The intrinsic properties of the peritoneal membrane that affect drug removal include blood flow, pore size, and peritoneal membrane surface area, which is approximately equal to the body surface area. There is an inverse relationship between peritoneal drug clearance and molecular weight, protein binding, and volume of distribution. Also, drug compounds that are ionized at physiologic pH will diffuse across the membrane more slowly than unionized compounds. In general, hemodialysis is more effective in removing drug substances than peritoneal dialysis such that if a drug is not removed by hemodialysis, it is not likely to be removed by peritoneal dialysis.

Peritonitis is a major complication associated with CAPD therapy and has an incidence of approximately 1.3 episodes per patient per year.[91] Treatment algorithms have been developed for peritonitis that provide guidelines for selection of appropriate antibiotic therapy.[92] The half-life of several antibiotics in CAPD patients, as well as those with normal renal function and ESRD are presented in Table 50.9. Detailed reviews of the disposition of other drugs in CAPD patients are reported elsewhere.[88,89] Table 50.9 also provides the proposed treatment regimens for CAPD-associated peritonitis recommended by the *ad hoc* advisory committee.[92]

Drug Dosage Regimen Design for Chronic Hemodialysis Patients

The number of patients with ESRD who receive chronic hemodialysis has steadily increased since the early 1970s and currently almost 200,000 patients receive this life-sustaining therapy.[93] Although considerable advances in hemodialysis filter technology have been made in the last 20 years and the efficiency of the hemodialysis procedure has been increased,[94] the effect of hemodialysis on drug disposition once reported has rarely been reevaluated. Thus most of the literature probably represents an underestimation of the impact of hemodialysis on drug disposition.

The impact of hemodialysis on a patient's drug therapy is dependent on several factors, including the characteristics of each drug, the dialysis conditions, and the clinical situation for which dialysis is performed. Drug-related factors that affect dialyzability include the molecular weight, protein binding, and distribution volume of each drug.[4] The impact of distribution volume (V_d) on drug removal by dialysis is evident in the following example where drug A has a 10-L V_d, while drug B has a V_d of 80 L. Both drugs are not bound to plasma proteins, are exclusively eliminated unchanged by the kidney, have a molecular weight of 300, and a dialyzer clearance of 40 mL/min (2.4 L/h). The half-life in an anuric patient during dialysis ($t_{1/2} = [V_d \times 0.693]/\text{CL}$) will be markedly different for these two drugs (2.9 hours versus 23 hours) and thus approximately 50% of drug A but only 10% of drug B would be removed during 3 hours of dialysis as a direct result of the larger distribution volume. Prior to the mid-1980s these were the primary factors that needed to be known to assess the degree of dialyzability of a given drug since the vast majority of dialysis filters were composed of cellulose, cellulose acetate, or regenerated cellulose (cuprophane). These "conventional" filter materials were generally impermeable to drugs with a molecular weight over 1000 and the clearance by hemodialysis tended to decline dramatically (by up to 60%) as molecular weight increased from 100 to 500.[95] Drugs that are small but highly protein bound are also not well dialyzed since both of the principal binding proteins, AAG and albumin, have a very high molecular weight (Fig. 50.2).[96] Finally, those drugs that are widely distributed throughout the body are poorly removed by hemodialysis.

The dialysis prescription for the patient can also dramatically affect the degree of drug removal. The primary factors that can vary between patients are the type of hemodialysis they are prescribed, which is reflected in the composition of the dialysis membrane, the filter surface area, blood and dialysate flow rates, and whether or not the dialysis unit reuses the dialysis filter. During the mid to late 1980s, two additional modes of hemodialysis were introduced: rapid high-efficiency hemodialysis (RHED) and high-flux dialysis (HFD), the characteristics of which are described in Chapter 46, Principles and Practice of Chronic Renal Replacement Therapy. HFD filters more closely mimic the filtration characteristics of the human kidney than the filters used to deliver conventional or RHED. They allow the free passage of most solutes including drugs, which have a molecular weight of 20,000 or less.[95] Thus high molecular weight drugs such as vancomycin are likely to be removed by this mode of dialysis while they are not by conventional dialysis. An increase in removal has also been reported with several other drugs that have lower molecular weights (Table 50.10).[97–106]

Two of the primary factors that are increased in RHED compared to conventional dialysis are the blood and dialysate flow rates. These changes have been reported to increase significantly the dialyzer clearance of many endogenous solutes and drugs, especially those with molecular weights of 500 or less. Changes in blood flow rate appear to have the most dramatic impact. Increases in gentamicin clearance of 50–100% have been associated with

TABLE 50.9. PHARMACOKINETICS OF ANTIBIOTICS IN CAPD PATIENTS AND PROPOSED REGIMENS FOR THE TREATMENT OF CAPD PERITONITIS

	Half-Life (h)				Maintenance Dose (per 70-kg adult)	
	Normal	ESRD	CAPD	Initial Dose (mg/2-L bag)	Intermittent (mg/2-L bag per dosing interval)	Continuous (mg/2-L bag)
Aminoglycosides						
Amikacin	1.6	39	40	500	120–150/d	12–15
Gentamicin	2.2	53	32	70–140	50/d	8–16
Netilmicin	2.1	42	18	70–140	60/d	8–16
Tobramycin	2.5	58	36	70–140	50/d	8–16
Cephalosporins						
First Generation						
Cefazolin	2.2	28	30	500–1000	1000/d	250–500
Cefonicid	4.0	68	50	250	ND	50
Cephalothin	0.2	3.7	ND	1000	ND	200
Cephradine	0.9	12	ND	500	ND	250
Cephalexin	0.8	19	9	1000 PO	500/QID PO	NA
Second Generation						
Cefamandole	1.0	10	8.0	1000	1000/d	500
Cefmenoxime	1.3	11.3	6.0	2000	1000/d	100
Cefoxitin	0.8	20	15	1000	ND	200
Cefuroxime	1.3	18	15	1000	ND	150–400
Third Generation						
Cefixime	3.2	11.5	15	400 PO	400/d PO	NA
Cefoperazone	1.8	2.3	2.2	2000	ND	400–1000
Cefotaxime	0.9	2.5	2.4	2000	2000/d	500
Cefsulodin	1.8	11	11	1000	500/d	50
Ceftazidime	1.8	26	13	1000	1000/d	100–250
Ceftizoxime	1.6	28	11	1000	10000/d	250
Ceftriaxone	8.0	15	12	1000	1000/d	250–500
Moxalactam	2.2	20	16	1000	1000/d	350
Penicillins						
Azlocillin	0.9	5.1	ND	500	ND	500
Mezlocillin	1.0	4.3	ND	3000 IV	3000/BID IV	500
Piperacillin	1.2	3.9	2.4	4000 IV	4000/BID IV	500
Ticarcillin	1.2	15	ND	1000–2000	2000/BID	250
Quinolones						
Ciprofloxacin	4.0	8.0	11	750 PO	750/BID PO	50
Fleroxacin	13.0	27	27	800 PO	400/d PO	NA
Ofloxacin	7.0	30	25	400 PO	200/d PO	ND
Vancomycin and Others						
Vancomycin	6.9	161	92	1000–2000	1000–2000/7d	30–50
Teicoplanin	50	260	260	400	ND	40[b]
Aztreonam	2.0	7.0	9.3	1000	ND	500
Clindamycin	2.8	2.8	ND	300	ND	300
Erythromycin	2.1	4.0	ND	ND	500/QID PO	150
Metronidazole	7.9	7.7	11	500 PO/IV	500/TID PO/IV	ND
Rifampin	4.0	8.0	ND	600 PO	600/d PO	NA
Antifungal Agents						
Amphotericin	360	360	ND	NA	20–30/d IV	100
Flucytosine	4.2	115	ND	2000–3000 PO	1000/d PO	100
Fluconazole	22	125	72	NA	150/2d	ND
Ketoconazole	2.0	1.8	2.4	400 PO	200–800/d PO	NA
Miconazole	24	25	ND	200	ND	100–200
Combinations						
Ampicillin	1.3	15	9.5	1000–2000	1000/BID	100
Sulbactam	1.0	19	9.7	1000–2000	500/BID	100
Imipenem	0.9	3.0	6.4	500–1000	500/BID	100–200
Cilistatin	0.8	15	19	500–1000	500/BID	100–200
Sulfamethoxazole	10	13	14	1600 PO	1600/1–2 d PO	200–400
Trimethoprim	14	33	34	320 PO	320/1–2 d PO	40–80

Key: ESRD, creatinine clearance <10 mL/min, patient not on dialysis; NA, not applicable; ND, no data; IV, intravenous; PO, oral; d, once a day; 2d, every other day; 7d, once a week; BID, twice a day; TID, three times a day; QID, four times a day.

[a]The route of administration is intraperitoneal unless otherwise specified. There is no evidence that mixing different antibiotics in dialysis fluid (except for aminoglycosides and pencillins) is deleterious for the drugs or patients. Do not use the same syringe to mix antibiotics.

[b]This is in each bag for 7 days, then in 2 bags/day for 7 days, and then in 1 bag/day for 7 days. (Data from Ref. 92.)

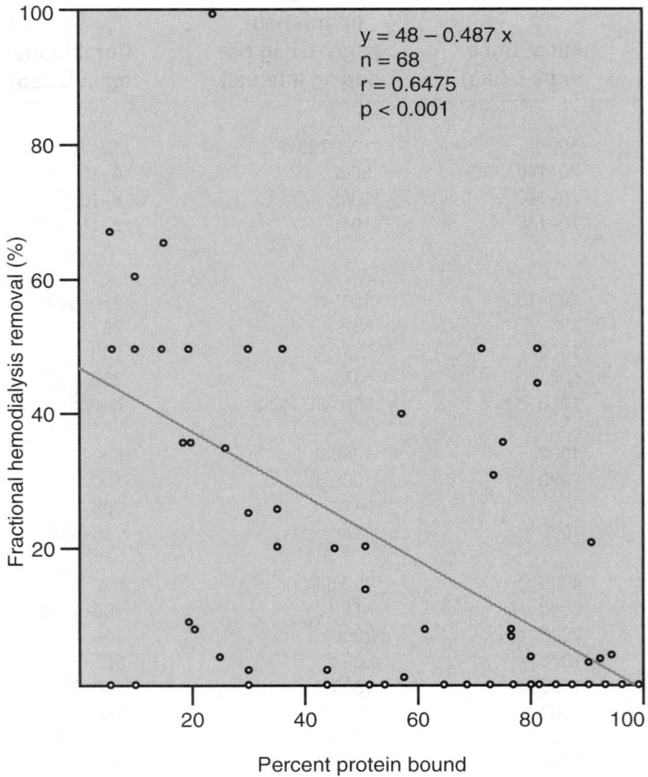

Figure 50.2. Linear regression between the dialyzability (HD%) and the percentage of plasma protein binding (PB%) of 89 drugs.[96] (From Ref. 96.)

an increase in blood flow rate from 100 to 300 mL/min.[98] Dialysate flow rates are fairly standardized now at 500 mL/min unless patients are receiving RHED where the dialysate flow rate may be as high as 1000 mL/min. Although no direct comparisons of drug clearances have been reported at these two different dialysate flow rates, urea clearance is only increased by about 11–12%.[95] Thus, it is unlikely that changes in this component of the dialysis prescription will significantly alter pharmacokinetic projections.

The final component of the dialysis prescription that may affect drug clearance by dialysis is whether or not the patient has authorized the unit to reuse his/her dialysis filter. Currently more than 75% of all dialysis units in the United States utilize this procedure to reduce the cost of chronic hemodialysis.[93] Only one center has prospectively evaluated the clearance of a drug (ceftazidime) in patients following the first and twelfth use of both cuprophane and polysulfone filters.[100] Their results indicate that ceftazidime clearance decreased by up to 30% with the polysulfone filter. In contrast, no significant change in clearance was observed with the cuprophane filter.

The impact of hemodialysis on drug therapy should thus not be viewed as a generic procedure such that a certain percentage of drug in the body is removed with each dialysis session; neither should simple "yes–no" answers on the dialyzability of drug compounds be considered sufficient information for therapeutic decisions. Reference materials that indicate "yes–no" status regarding the dialyzability of drug compounds provide no quantification of the impact of hemodialysis and are thus of little value to the clinician who is attempting to design a rational dosing regimen. Compounds considered nondialyzable may in fact be significantly removed by high-flux hemodialysis filters. Characteristics of the dialysis prescription such as membrane composition and surface area, and blood and dialysis flow rates, are critical data for the design of drug dosing regimens for chronic hemodialysis patients.

The effect of hemodialysis on drug disposition can be estimated in several ways. The determination of drug concentrations at the start and end of dialysis, with the subse-

TABLE 50.10. DRUG DISPOSITION DURING DIALYSIS DEPENDS ON FILTER CHARACTERISTICS

	Hemodialysis Clearance (mL/min)		Half-Life During Dialysis (h)	
Drug	**Conventional**	**High-Flux**	**Conventional**	**High-Flux**
Ceftazidime	55–60	155[a]	3.30	1.2[a]
Cefuroxime	NR	103[b]	3.75	1.6[b]
Gentamicin	58.2	41.7[b]	3.0	4.3[b]
Netilmicin	46	87–109	5.0–5.2	2.9–3.4
Vancomycin	9–21	31–60[c]	35–38	12.0[c]
		40–150[b]		4.5–11.8[b]
		72–116[d]		NR[d]

Key: NR, not reported.
[a]Polyamide filter.
[b]Polysulfone filter.
[c]Polyacrylonitrile filter.
[d]Polymethylmethacrylate.

TABLE 50.11. REBOUND IN DRUG CONCENTRATIONS AFTER THE END OF HEMODIALYSIS

	t_{max}	% Rebound
Cefmetazole	0.9	17.9
Ceftibuten	0.58	45.9
Gentamicin	1.3	23.3
Netilmicin	1.9	38.3
Tobramycin	1.7	18.3
Vancomycin	6.4	52.4

quent calculation of the half-life during dialysis ($t_{1/2,\text{onHD}}$), has frequently been utilized as an index of drug removal by dialysis. Unfortunately, the $t_{1/2,\text{onHD}}$ may not be interpretable because declining plasma drug concentrations during dialysis represent elimination by the body as well as by dialysis. Furthermore, recent reports of a significant rebound in drug concentrations after dialysis suggest that in some cases the removal of drug by the dialysis procedure may be artificially high depending on when, after dialysis, the concentration is determined (Table 50.11).[99,107–111]

An alternative and more accurate means of assessing the effect of hemodialysis is to calculate the dialyzer clearance of the drug. The dialyzer clearance (CL_D) can be calculated by several approaches. The C_D^b from blood can be calculated as $C_D^b = Q_b[(A_b - V_b)/A_b]$, where Q_b is blood flow through the dialyzer, A_b is the concentration of drug in blood going into the dialyzer filter, and V_b is the blood concentration of drug leaving the filter. This equation is only valid if the drug concentrations are measured in whole blood or if the drug rapidly and completely distributes into red blood cells. Since drug concentrations are generally determined in plasma, the previous equation is usually modified to $C_D^p = Q_p[(A_P - V_p)/A_p]$, where p represents plasma and Q_p is plasma flow, which equals Q_b (1 − hematocrit). This clearance calculation accurately reflects dialysis drug clearance only if the drug does not penetrate red blood cells or bind to formed blood elements.

Because of potential problems in accurately determining Q_b or Q_p, the dialysate recovery method is widely used. In addition, venous plasma concentrations may be concentrated, since plasma water is generally removed from the blood at a faster rate than drug when ultrafiltration is performed simultaneously with diffusion during dialysis. Thus, the recovery clearance approach described as follows has become the benchmark for the determination of dialyzer clearance.[4]

Dialyzer clearance can thus be calculated as:

$$\text{CL}_D^r = R/\text{AUC}_{0-t}$$

where R is the total amount of drug recovered unchanged in the dialysate and AUC_{0-t} is the area under the prefilter plasma concentration–time curve during hemodialysis. To determine the AUC_{0-t} at least two and preferably three to four plasma concentrations should be obtained during dialysis.

The hemodialysis clearance values reported in the literature may vary significantly depending on which of the previous methods was utilized to calculate CL_D. The principal reason for this is that for most medications we do not know the degree and rapidity with which the drug crosses the red blood cell membrane. Since the CL_D^r method incorporates no assumption of the degree of RBC permeability it can be reliably utilized as the benchmark value. Comparisons of CL_D^p and CL_D^b values to the CL_D^r benchmark thus provide valuable insight to a given drug's dialyzability.[112] Since the CL_D^b and CL_D^r of the cephalosporins listed in Table 50.12 agree, it can be concluded that these three cephalosporins readily distributed into and out of RBCs. In contrast, since the CL_D^p and CL_D^r of netilmicin are approximately the same, one can conclude that netilmicin does not readily penetrate the RBCs. Thus to evaluate the CL_D of a new dialysis filter in the clinical setting, the CL_D^b method would be preferred for these cephalosporins and tobramycin but the CL_D^p method may be best for netilmicin.

The following principles may be applied to drug dosage regimen design by using a value of CL_D that is reported in the literature.[4,20,21,64,65] Because clearance terms are additive, the total clearance during dialysis can be calculated as the sum of total body clearance during the interdialytic period (CL) and dialyzer clearance (CL_D):

$$\text{CL}_T = \text{CL} + \text{CL}_D$$

The half-life during the period between dialysis treatments and during dialysis can then be calculated from the following relationships using an estimate of the drug's distribution volume (V), which can be obtained from review articles[4,20,21,64,65]:

$$t_{1/2,\,\text{offHD}} = 0.693\ [V/\text{CL}]$$

$$t_{1/2,\,\text{onHD}} = 0.693\ [V/(\text{CL} + \text{CL}_D)]$$

Once the key pharmacokinetic parameters (CL, CL_D, and V) have been estimated/calculated, they may be used to simulate the plasma concentration–time profile of the drug for the individual patient and ascertain how much drug to administer and when.

TABLE 50.12. VARIATION IN CL_D DETERMINATIONS ARE DEPENDENT ON THE METHOD OF CALCULATION[a]

	CL_D^b	CL_D^p	CL_D^r
Cefepime	166	116	158
Cefmetazole	83	55	86
Ceftibuten	62	43	77
Netilmicin	78	63	62
Tobramycin	55	44	55

[a]All values are mL/min.

This approach to drug therapy individualization can be accomplished in a stepwise fashion assuming first-order elimination of the drug and a one-compartment model. For example, a 34-year-old male with ESRD was admitted to your institution from the outpatient hemodialysis unit where he experienced shaking, chills, and had a temperature of 40°C. He weighed 70 kg and was 69 inches tall, had a residual creatinine clearance of 3 mL/min, and received conventional dialysis for 4 hours TIW on a CA170 cellulose acetate filter. He received 140 mg of tobramycin at the end of his hemodialysis treatment.

The first step is to estimate this patient's pharmacokinetic parameters of tobramycin on the basis of published population data. The volume of distribution in this patient would be 23.1 L (0.33 L/kg × 70 kg) based on the recent report of Fish et al.[113] The patient's residual total body clearance (CL) can be estimated from the relationship between CL and creatinine clearance, such as the one reported by Matzke et al.[114]:

$$\begin{aligned} CL &= CL_{cr} \times 0.801 \\ &= 3\ \text{mL/min} \times 60\ \text{min/h} \times (1\ \text{L}/1000\ \text{mL}) \times 0.801 \\ &= 0.144\ \text{L/h} \end{aligned}$$

The hemodialysis clearance of tobramycin is dialysis filter dependent (Table 50.12) and a value of 69 mL/min can be extrapolated from the report of Fish et al.[113] for the CA170 filter.

Once the patient's kinetic parameters have been approximated, one can predict what the plasma concentrations of tobramycin will be over the next 24–48 hours. The concentration at the end of the 30-minute infusion (C_{max}) would be:

$$\begin{aligned} C_{max} &= \frac{(\text{Dose}/t')\ 1 - e^{-kt'}}{CL} \\ &= \frac{(140\ \text{mg}/0.5\ \text{h})\ 1 - e^{-(CL/V)t'}}{0.144\ \text{L/h}} \\ &= \frac{(280\ \text{mg/h})\ 1 - e^{-(0.0062)0.5}}{0.144\ \text{L/h}} \\ &= (1944\ \text{mg/L})\ (0.003) = 5.8\ \text{mg/L} \end{aligned}$$

The plasma concentration prior to the next dialysis session (C_{bD}), which is 44 hours away, and the concentration after dialysis (C_{aD}) can be calculated as:

$$\begin{aligned} C_{bD} &= C_{max} \cdot e^{-(CL/V) \cdot t} \\ &= 5.8 \cdot e^{-0.0062 \cdot 44} = 4.4\ \text{mg/L} \end{aligned}$$

$$\begin{aligned} C_{aD} &= C_{bD} \cdot e^{-(CL + CL_D)/Vt} \\ &= 4.4 \cdot e^{-([0.144 + 4.14]/23.1) \cdot 4} \\ &= 4.4 \cdot e^{-0.185 \cdot 4} = 2.1\ \text{mg/L} \end{aligned}$$

On the basis of these data, one could feel confident that no further therapy would likely be required until after the next dialysis treatment. During this interdialytic interval, however, several blood samples should be collected to characterize this patient's residual tobramycin clearance, distribution volume, and lastly the clearance of tobramycin during dialysis. Blood samples were therefore collected at the following times after the first dose:

Day 1	7 PM (2 hours after dose)	6.5 mg/L
Day 2	8 AM (39 hours after dose)	4.1 mg/L
Day 3	12 noon (after HD)	2.0 mg/L

The C_{max} can be calculated by back extrapolation to the end of the infusion. The elimination rate during the interdialytic period (k_{ID}) and during dialysis (k_{DD}), and the V_d can be calculated as:

$$\begin{aligned} k_{ID} &= (\ln C_1/C_2)/\Delta t \\ &= (\ln 6.5/4.1)/37 = 0.0125\ \text{h}^{-1} \end{aligned}$$

$$\begin{aligned} k_{DD} &= (\ln C_2/C_3)/\Delta t \\ &= (\ln 4.1/2.0)/4 = 0.179\ \text{h}^{-1} \end{aligned}$$

$$\begin{aligned} V_d &= \frac{\text{Dose}/t'}{k_{ID}} \ \frac{1 - e^{-k_{ID}t'}}{(C_{max} - C_{min}\ e^{-k_{ID}t'})} \\ &= \frac{140/0.5}{0.0125} \ \frac{1 - e^{-(0.0125)0.5}}{(6.7 - 0.0\ e^{-(0.0125)0.5})} \\ &= \frac{134.4}{6.7} = 20\ \text{L} \end{aligned}$$

The patient's clearance (CL) and the dialyzer clearance (CL_D) of tobramycin can then be calculated as:

$$\begin{aligned} CL &= V_d \times k_{ID} \\ &= 20.0\ \text{L} \times 0.0125 = 0.25\ \text{L/h or } 4.2\ \text{mL/min} \end{aligned}$$

$$\begin{aligned} CL_D &= CL_T - CL \\ &= (k_{DD} \times V_d) - 4.2\ \text{mL/min} \\ &= (0.179\ \text{h}^{-1} \times 20.0\ \text{L}) - 4.2\ \text{mL/min} \\ &= (3.6\ \text{L/h or } 59.6\ \text{mL/min}) - 4.2\ \text{mL/min} = 55.4\ \text{mL/min} \end{aligned}$$

This case illustrates the need for individualizing drug therapy for hemodialysis patients since this patient's V_d was 13% smaller, CL was 75% greater, and CL_D was 19.7% less than the estimates based on population parameters. The ultimate reason for measuring the plasma concentrations of aminoglycosides and several other agents is to design the patient's dosage regimen. Thus there remains one important step in our evaluation (i.e., the calculation of the dose this patient should receive next). The two factors that enter into this decision are the desired peak and trough concentrations and the degree of rebound in drug concentrations, after the end of dialysis. Since tobramycin concentrations have been noted to increase by about 20% within 1.5–2 hours after the end of hemodialysis (Table 50.11) the trough concentration of this patient can be considered to be 2.4 mg/L (2.0 mg/L × 1.2). Although this value is higher than one might like to maintain in an individual with normal renal function, a prolonged period of almost 24 hours would be required just to have the concentration drop below 2.0

mg/L. It is frequently necessary in critically ill individuals to redose the patient even though the postdialysis trough values are between 2 and 3 mg/L. Assuming the desired peak concentration was 7.0 mg/L, the postdialysis dose this patient would need can then be calculated as follows since the elimination half-life is extremely prolonged relative to the infusion time and thus minimal drug is eliminated during the infusion period:

$$\text{Dose} = V_d \times (C_{\max} - C_{\min})$$
$$= 20.0\text{ L} \times (7.0 - 2.4) = 92\text{ mg}$$

Combination antibiotic therapy with aminoglycosides and extended-spectrum penicillins are frequently prescribed for ESRD patients to provide wider antibacterial coverage against gram-negative bacilli through a synergistic effect. It is known, however, that the combined use may result in *in vitro* chemical inactivation of the aminoglycoside, leading to a loss in antibiotic activity. The rate of inactivation is related to the incubation period, temperature, presence of solutes, and β-lactam concentration.[115–117]

The extent of aminoglycoside inactivation *in vivo* may not be clinically significant in human subjects with normal or slightly impaired renal function due to the short contact time.[118,119] However, in patients with significant renal insufficiency, subtherapeutic aminoglycoside concentrations and a decreased aminoglycoside elimination half-life during combination therapy with broad-spectrum β-lactam penicillins have been reported and will require appropriate dosage modification to maintain the desired serum concentrations.[120,121] The inactivation of aminoglycosides in patients receiving chronic dialysis therapy has been reported for gentamicin in combination with carbenicillin,[120] ticarcillin,[122] and piperacillin.[123] Inactivation of tobramycin given in combination with ticarcillin and piperacillin has also been described,[121,124] while netilmicin disposition is not affected by piperacillin administration.[124]

Tobramycin serum concentrations declined at a faster rate when tobramycin was given with piperacillin, 4 g q 12 hours (half-life alone = 60 ± 25 hours, half-life combined = 25 ± 5 hours) while no significant change was noted in the half-life of netilmicin (41.8 versus 40.0 hours). A similar study recently evaluated the degree of inactivation of isepamicin and gentamicin when they are administered concomitantly with piperacillin.[125] The half-life of gentamicin was reduced significantly from 48 ± 21 hours to 36 ± 11 hours, while no significant difference was noted in the half-life of isepamicin (48 versus 45 hours). No significant changes in V_d were noted for any of the aminoglycosides and thus the inactivation clearances of netilmicin and isepamicin were significantly less than those of tobramycin and gentamicin. From these data tobramycin appears to be affected to the greatest degree followed by gentamicin, netilmicin, and isepamicin in descending order.

Thus the elimination of aminoglycosides in renal failure patients also receiving antipseudomonal penicillins will be increased; therefore, frequent serum concentration monitoring should be performed. To eliminate any *in vitro* inactivation of aminoglycosides that would complicate assessment of the *in vivo* effects, serum samples should be assayed as soon as possible after collection. If this is not possible, serum samples should be frozen (preferably at −70°C) until they can be assayed.

Conclusion

Subtherapeutic or supratherapeutic responses to drugs in uremic patients are often misinterpreted and not recognized as such. The adverse outcomes associated with inappropriate drug use and dosing has not been quantified but does warrant future investigations. Sound pharmacokinetic principles as illustrated in this chapter used in concert with reliable population pharmacokinetic estimates should ultimately yield the optimal approach to drug dosage regimen design for patients with impaired renal function. Individualization of therapy should be undertaken whenever clinical therapeutic monitoring tools are available.

References

1. Ritschel WA, Denson DD. Influence of disease on bioavailability, in Pharmacokinetics: Regulatory, Industrial, Academic Perspectives. New York, Marcel Dekker, 1995.
2. Zini R, Riant P, Barre J, et al. Disease-induced variations in plasma protein levels: Implications for drug dosage regimens (Part I). Clin Pharmacokinet 1990;19(2):147–159.
3. Zini R, Riant P, Barre J, et al. Disease-induced variations in plasma protein levels: Implications for drug dosage regimens (Part II). Clin Pharmacokinet 1990;19(3):218–229.
4. Matzke GR, Millikin SP. Influence of renal disease and dialysis on pharmacokinetics, in Evans WE, Schentag JJ, Jusko WJ (eds): Applied Pharmacokinetics: Principles of Therapeutic Drug Monitoring, 3rd ed. Spokane, WA, Applied Therapeutics, 1992.
5. Tochette MA, Slaughter RL. The effect of renal failure on hepatic drug clearance. DICP Ann Pharmacother 1991;25:1214–1224.
6. Elston AC, Bayliss MK, Park GR. Effect of renal failure on drug metabolism by the liver. Br J Anaesth 1993;71:282–290.
7. Tozer TN. Nomogram for modification of dosage regimens in patients with chronic renal impairment. J Pharmacokinet Biopharm 1974;2:13–28.
8. Welling PG, Craig WA, Kunin CM. Prediction of drug dosage in patients with renal failure using data derived from normal subjects. Clin Pharmacol Ther 1975;18:45–52.
9. Rowland M, Tozer TN. Clinical Pharmacokinetics: Concepts and Applications, 3rd ed. Philadelphia, Lea & Febiger, 1995, pp 248–266.

10. Piergies AA, Worwag EM, Atkinson AJ. A concurrent audit of high digoxin plasma levels. Clin Pharmacol Ther 1994;55:353–358.
11. Tilstone WJ, Dargie H, Dargie EN, et al. Pharmacokinetics of metolazone in normal subjects and in patients with cardiac or renal failure. Clin Pharmacol Ther 1974;16:322–329.
12. Tilstone WJ, Fine A. Furosemide kinetics in renal failure. Clin Pharmacol Ther 1978;23:644–650.
13. Balant LP, Dayer P, Fabre J. Consequences of renal insufficiency on the hepatic clearance of some drugs. Int J Clin Pharmacol Res 1983;3:459–474.
14. Bianchetti G, Graziani G, Brancaccio D, et al. Pharmacokinetics and effects of propranolol in terminal uremic patients and in patients undergoing regular dialysis treatment. Clin Pharmacokinet 1976;1:373–384.
15. Gibson TP, Giancomini KM, Briggs WA, et al. Propoxyphene and norpropoxyphene plasma concentrations in the anephric patient. Clin Pharmacol Ther 1980;27:665–670.
16. Barnes JN, Williams AJ, Tomson MJF, et al. Dihydrocodeine in renal failure: Further evidence for an important role of the kidney in the handling of opioid drugs. Br Med J 1985;290:740–742.
17. Barnes JN, Goodwin FJ. Dihydrocodeine narcosis in renal failure. Br Med J 1983;286:438.
18. Redfern N. Dihydrocodeine overdose treated with naloxone infusion. Br Med J 1983;287:751–752.
19. Vestal RE, Wood AJ, Shand DG. Reduced β-receptor sensitivity in the elderly. Clin Pharmacol Ther 1979;26:181–186.
20. St. Peter WL, Redic-Kill KA, Halstenson CE. Clinical pharmacokinetics of antibiotics in patients with impaired renal function. Clin Pharmacokin 1992;22:169–210.
21. St. Peter WL, Halstenson CE. Pharmacologic approach in patients with renal failure, in Chernow B (ed): The Pharmacologic Approach to the Critically Ill Patient. Baltimore, William & Wilkins, 1994, pp 41–79.
22. Vanholder R, Van Landsehoot N, De Smet R, et al. Drug protein binding in chronic renal failure: Evaluation of nine drugs. Kidney Int 1988;33:996–1004.
23. Karara AH, Frye RF, Hayes PE, et al. Pharmacokinetics of abecarnil in patients with renal insufficiency. Clin Pharmacol Ther (in press).
24. Chan GLC, Axelson JE, Price JDE, et al. *In vitro* protein binding of propafenone in normal and uraemic human sera. Eur J Clin Pharmacol 1989;36:495–499.
25. Pritchard JF, Matzke GR, Opsahl JA, et al. Effects of hemodialysis on plasma protein binding of bepridil. J Clin Pharmacol 1995;35(2):137–141.
26. Liponi DF, Winter ME, Tozer TN. Renal function and therapeutic concentrations of phenytoin. Neurology 1984;34:395–397.
27. Haughey DB, Kraft CJ, Matzke GR, et al. Protein binding of disopyramide and elevated alpha-1-acid glycoprotein concentrations in serum obtained from dialysis patients and renal transplant recipients. Am J Nephrol 1985;5:35–39.
28. Docci D, Bilancioni R, Pistocchi E, et al. Serum alpha-1-acid glycoprotein in chronic renal failure. Nephron 1985;39:160–163.
29. Job ML. Digoxin, in Murphy J (ed): Clinical Pharmacokinetics Pocket Reference. Bethesda, MD, ASHP, 1993, pp 71–80.
30. Jusko WJ, Szefler SJ, Goldfarb AL. Pharmacokinetic design of digoxin dosage regimens in relation to renal function. J Clin Pharmacol 1974;14:525–535.
31. Malini PL, Strocchi E, Feliciangeli G, et al. Digitalis receptors and digoxin sensitivity in renal failure. Clin Pharm Physiol 1985;12:115.
32. Rambausek M, Ritz E. Digitalis in chronic renal insufficiency. Blood Purif 1985;3:4–9.
33. Levy RH, Moreland TA. Rationale for monitoring free drug levels. Clin Pharmacokinet 1984;9(suppl 1):1–9.
34. Jusko WJ, Gibaldi M. Effects of change in elimination on various parameters of the two-compartment open model. J Pharm Sci 1972;61(8):1270–1273.
35. Koup J. Disease states and drug pharmacokinetics. J Clin Pharmacol 1989;29:674–679.
36. Anders MW. Metabolism of drugs by the kidney. Kidney Int 1980;18:636–647.
37. Gibson TP. Renal disease and drug metabolism: An overview. Am J Kidney Dis 1986;8:7–17.
38. Milad MA, Ludwig EA, Lew KH, et al. The pharmacokinetics and pharmacodynamics of methylprednisolone in chronic renal failure. Am J Ther 1994;1:49–57.
39. Prescott LF, Freestone S, McAuslane JAN. The concentration-dependent disposition of intravenous p-aminohippurate in subjects with normal and impaired renal function. Br J Clin Pharmacol 1993;35:20–29.
40. van Olden RW, van Acker BAC, Koomen GCM, et al. Urinary recovery of p-aminohippuric acid (PAH) and acetyl-PAH (PACAH) in haemodialysis patients [abstract]. Nephrol Dial Transplant 1994;9:574.
41. Patterson SE, Cohn VH. Hepatic drug metabolism in rats with experimental long-term renal failure. Biochem Pharmacol 1984;35:711–716.
42. Terner UK, Wiebe LI, Noujaim AA, et al. The effects of acute and chronic uremia in rats on their hepatic microsomal enzyme activity. Clin Biochem 1978;4:156–158.
43. Kim Y-G, Shin J-G, Shin S-G, et al. Decreased acetylation of isoniazid in chronic renal failure. Clin Pharmacol Ther 1993;54:612–620.
44. van Bortel L, Bohm R, Mooij J, et al. Total and free steady-state plasma levels and pharmacokinetics of nifedipine in patients with terminal renal failure. Eur J Clin Pharmacol 1989;37:185–189.
45. Aronoff GR. Pharmacokinetics of nitrendipine in patients with renal failure: Comparison to normal subjects. J Cardio Pharmacol 1984;6(suppl):S974–S976.
46. van Harten J, Burggraaf J, van Brummelen P, et al. Influence of renal function on the pharmacokinetics and cardiovascular effects of nisoldipine after single and multiple dosing. Clin Pharmacokin 1989;16:55–64.
47. Jones RN, Barry AL. Antimicrobial activity of ceftriaxone, cefotaxime, desacetylcefotaxime, cefotaxime-des acetylcefotaxime in the presence of human serum. Antimicrob Agents Chemother 1987;31:818–820.
48. Wolfert AI, Sica DA. Narcotic usage in renal failure. Int J Artif Organs 1988;11(6):411–415.

49. Kaiko RF, Foley KM, Grabinski PY, et al. Central nervous system excitatory effects of meperidine in cancer patients. Ann Neurol 1982;13:180–185.
50. Rowland M, Tozer TN. Clinical Pharmacokinetics: Concepts and Applications, 3rd ed. Philadelphia, Lea & Febiger, 1995, pp 156–183.
51. Kamiya A, Okumura K, Hori R. Quantitative investigation of renal handling of drugs in dogs with renal insufficiency. J Pharm Sci 1984;74:892–896.
52. Hori R, Okumura K, Kamiya A, et al. Ampicillin and cephalexin in renal insufficiency. Clin Pharmacol Ther 1983;34:792–798.
53. Hori R, Okumura K, Nihria H, et al. A new dosing regimen in renal insufficiency: Application to cephalexin. Clin Pharmacol Ther 1985;38:290–295.
54. Cockroft DW, Gault MH. Prediction of creatinine clearance from serum creatinine. Nephron 1976;16:31–41.
55. Hull JH, Hak LJ, Koch GG, et al. Influence of range of renal function and liver disease on predictability of creatinine clearance. Clin Pharmacol Ther 1981;29:516–521.
56. Dechaux M, Gonzalez G, Broyer M. Creatinine plasmatique, clearance et excretion urinaire de la creatinine chez l'enfant. Arch Fr Ped 1978;35:53–62.
57. Luke DR, Halstenson CE, Opsahl JA, et al. Validity of creatinine clearance estimates in the assessment of renal function. Clin Pharmacol Ther 1990;48:503–508.
58. Paap CM, Nahata MC. Prospective evaluation of ten methods for estimating creatinine clearance in pediatric patients with varying degrees of renal dysfunction [abstract]. Pharmacotherapy 1991;11:271.
59. Jelliffe RW, Jelliffe SM. A computer program for estimation of creatinine clearance from unstable serum creatinine concentration. Math Biosci 1972;14:17–24.
60. Chiou WL, Hsu FH. A new simple and rapid method to monitor renal function based on pharmacokinetic considerations of endogenous creatinine. Res Com Chem Path Pharmacol 1975;10:315.
61. Physicians' Desk Reference. Oradell, NJ, Medical Economics Data, 1995.
62. McEvoy GK, Litvak K, Welsh OH, et al. American Hospital Formulary Service, Drug Information. Bethesda, MD, American Society of Hospital Pharmacists, 1994.
63. Bennett WM, Aronoff GR, Golper TA, et al. Drug Prescribing in Renal Failure: Dosing Guidelines for Adults, 2nd ed. Philadelphia, American College of Physicians, 1991.
64. Brater DC. Pocket Manual of Drug Use in Clinical Medicine, 3rd ed. Philadelphia, BC Becker, 1987.
65. Murphy JE, ed. Clinical Pharmacokinetics Pocket Reference. Bethesda, MD, ASHP, 1993.
66. Benet LZ, Williams RL. Design and optimization of dosage regimens: pharmacokinetic data, in Goodman GA, Rall TW, Nies AS, Taylor P (eds): The Pharmacological Basis of Therapeutics, 8th ed. Elmsford, NY, Pergamon Press, 1990, pp 1650–1735.
67. Moore RD, Lietman PS, Smith CR. Clinical response to aminoglycoside therapy: Importance of the ratio of peak concentration to minimal inhibitory concentration. J Infect Dis 1987;155:93–99.
68. McLean AJ, Ioannides-Demos LL, Li SC, et al. Bactericidal effect of gentamicin peak concentration provides a rationale for administration of bolus doses. J Antimicrob Chemo 1993;32:301–305.
69. McLean AJ, Bastone EB, Ioannides-Demos LL, et al. Bactericidal effect of gentamicin trough concentration provides a rationale for administration of bolus doses and maintenance of trough levels. J Antimicrob Chemo 1994;33:999–1004.
70. Zimmermann AE, Katona BG, Plaisance KI. Association of vancomycin serum concentrations with outcomes in patients with gram-positive bacteremia. Pharmacotherapy 1995;15(1):85–91.
71. Zaske DE. Aminoglycosides, in Evans WE, Schentag JJ, Jusko WJ (eds): Applied Pharmacokinetics: Principles of Therapeutic Drug Monitoring, 3rd ed. Vancouver, WA, Applied Therapeutics, 1992.
72. Gram L, Lensen PK. Carbamazepine—toxicity, in Levy R, Mattson R, Meldrum B, et al. (eds): Antiepileptic Drugs, 3rd ed. New York, Raven Press, 1989, pp 555–565.
73. Kim SY, Benowitz NL. Poisoning due to class IA antiarrhythmic drugs. Quinidine, procainamide and disopyramide. Drug Saf 1990;5:393–420.
74. Sommadossi JP, Bevan R, Ling T, et al. Clinical pharmacokinetics of ganciclovir in patients with normal and impaired renal function. Rev Infect Dis 1988;10(suppl 3):S507–S514.
75. Balfour HH. Management of cytomegalovirus disease with antiviral drugs. Rev Infect Dis 1990;12(suppl 7):S849–S860.
76. Luft FC, Brannon DR, Stropes LL. Pharmacokinetics of netilmicin in patients with renal impairment and patients on dialysis. Antimicrob Agents Chemother 1978;14(3):403–407.
77. Ohnhaus EE, Vozeh S, Nüesch E. Absolute bioavailability of digoxin in chronic renal failure. Clin Nephrol 1979;11(6):302–306.
78. Paganini EP. General application of continuous therapeutic techniques, in Henrich WL, (ed): Principles and Practice of Dialysis. Baltimore, William & Wilkins, 1994, pp 98–110.
79. Macias WL, Mueller BA, Scarim SK. Vancomycin pharmacokinetics in acute renal failure: Preservation of non-renal clearance. Clin Pharmacol Ther 1991;50:688–694.
80. Mueller BA, Scarim SK, Macias WL. Comparison of imipenem pharmacokinetics in patients with acute or chronic renal failure treated with continuous hemofiltration. Am J Kidney Dis 1993;21:172–179.
81. Kirschner T, Bohler J, Krumme B, et al. Drug kinetics in hemodialysis (HD)–Netilmicin elimination by absorption to the polyacrylonitrile (PAN) membrane. Kidney Int 1995;47(3):982.
82. Joy MS, Matzke GR, Palevsky PM, et al. Dialysate and blood flow dependence of vancomycin clearance during CVVHD [abstract]. Pharmacotherapy 1995;15(3):380.
83. Kronfol NO, Lau AH, Barakat MM. Aminoglycoside binding to polyacrylonitrile hemofilter membranes during continuous hemofiltration. ASAIO Transactions 1987;33(3):300–303.
84. Lau AH, Kronfol NO. Determinants of drug removal by continuous hemofiltration. Int J Artif Organs 1994;17(7):373–378.
85. Golper TA. Drug removal during continuous hemofiltration or hemodialysis. Contrib Nephrol 1991;93:110–116.

86. Reetze-Bonorden P, Böhler J, Keller E. Drug dosage in patients during continuous renal replacement therapy. Clin Pharmacokinet 1993;24:362–379.
87. Bressolle F, Kinowski JM, de la Coussaye JE, et al. Clinical pharmacokinetics during continuous hemofiltration. Clin Pharmacokinet 1994;26:457–471.
88. Paton TW, Cornish WR, Manuel MA, Hardy BG. Drug therapy in patients undergoing peritoneal dialysis: Clinical pharmacokinetic considerations. Clin Pharmacokinet 1985;10:404–425.
89. Keller E. Peritoneal kinetics of different drugs. Clin Nephrol 1988;30(suppl 1):S24–S28.
90. Golper TA, Bennett WM. Drug usage in dialysis patients, in Nissenson AR, Fine RN, Gentile DE (eds): Clinical Dialysis, 2nd ed. Norwalk, CT, Appleton & Lange, 1990, pp 608–630.
91. Millikin SP, Matzke GR, Keane WF. Antimicrobial treatment of peritonitis associated with continuous ambulatory peritoneal dialysis. Perit Dial Int 1991;11:252–260.
92. Keane WF, Everett ED, Golper TA, et al. Peritoneal dialysis-related peritonitis treatment recommendations: 1993 update. Perit Dial Int 1993;13:14–28.
93. US Renal Data Systems, USRDS 1995 annual data report. Bethesda, MD, The National Institutes of Health, Institute of Diabetes and Digestive and Kidney Diseases, March 1995.
94. Matzke GR. Pharmacotherapeutic consequences of recent advances in hemodialysis therapy. Ann Pharmacother 1994;28:512–514.
95. Konstantin P. Newer membranes: cuprophane versus polysulfone versus polyacrylonitrile, in Bosch JP (ed): Contemporary Issues in Nephrology. Hemodialysis: High Efficiency Treatments, vol. 27. New York, Churchill Livingstone, 1993, pp 63–78.
96. Keller F. Effect of plasma protein binding, volume of distribution and molecular weight on the fraction of drugs eliminated by hemodialysis. Clin Nephrol 1983;19:201–205.
97. Golper TA, Vincent HH, Gleason JR, Vos MC. Drug removal during high efficiency and high-flux hemodialysis, in Bosch JP (ed): Contemporary Issues in Nephrology. Hemodialysis: High Efficiency Treatments, vol 27. New York, Churchill Livingstone, 1993, pp 175–209.
98. Agarwal R, Cronin RE. Heterogeneity in gentamicin clearance between high-efficiency hemodialyzers. Am J Kid Dis 1994;23(1):47–51.
99. Pollard TA, Lampasona V, Mullins RE, et al. Vancomycin redistribution: Dosing recommendations following high flux hemodialysis. Kidney Int 1994;45:232–237.
100. Toffelmire EB, Reymond JPH, Broudar R, et al. Dialysis clearance in high flux hemodialysis with reuse using ceftazidime as the model drug [abstract]. Clin Pharmacol Ther 1989;45:160.
101. Herrero A, Alarco FR, Garcia-Diez JM, et al. Pharmacokinetics of netilmicin during hemodialysis: Comparison of four artificial kidneys. Int J Clin Pharmacol Ther Toxicol 1988;26:605–609.
102. Weiss LG, Cars O, Danielson BG, et al. Pharmacokinetics of intravenous cefuroxime during intermittent and continuous arteriovenous hemofiltration. Clin Nephrol 1988;30(5):282–286.
103. Bastani B, Spyker DA, Minocha A, et al. *In vivo* comparison of three different hemodialysis membranes for vancomycin clearance: Cuprophan, cellulose acetate, and polyacrylonitrile. Dial Transplant 1988;17:527–543.
104. Lanese DM, Alfrey PS, Molitoris BA, Gal J. Markedly increased clearance of vancomycin during hemodialysis using polysulfone dialyzers. Kidney Int 1989;35:1409–1413.
105. Minakata T, Fukazawa A, Ikeda Y. Comparison of vancomycin clearance during hemodialysis between high flux and conventional membranes [abstract]. J Am Soc Nephrol 1991;2:339.
106. Torras J, Cao C, Rivas MC, et al. Pharmacokinetics of patients undergoing hemodialysis and polyacrylonitrile. Clin Nephrol 1991;36:35–41.
107. Barbhaiya RH, Knupp CA, Forgue ST, et al. Pharmacokinetics of cefepime in subjects with renal insufficiency. Clin Pharmacol Ther 1990;48:268–276.
108. Halstenson CE, Guay DRP, Opsahl JA, et al. Disposition of cefmetazole in healthy volunteers and patients with impaired renal function. Antimicrob Agents Chemother 1990;34:519–523.
109. Matzke GR, O'Connell ME, Collins AJ, Keshaviah PR. Disposition of vancomycin during hemofiltration. Clin Pharmacol Ther 1986;40:425–430.
110. Kelloway JS, Awni WM, Lin CC, et al. Pharmacokinetics of ceftibuten-cis and its trans metabolite in healthy volunteers and in patients with chronic renal insufficiency. Antimicrob Agents Chemother 1991;35:2267–2274.
111. Halstenson CE, Berkseth RO, Mann HJ, Matzke GR. Aminoglycoside redistribution phenomenon after hemodialysis: Netilmicin and tobramycin. Int J Clin Pharmacol Ther Tox 1987;25:50–55.
112. Matzke GR, Halstenson CE, Frye RF. Hemodialysis clearance of aminoglycosides and cephalosporins [abstract]. Pharmacother 1992;11:41.
113. Fish JT, St. Peter WL. Population pharmacokinetics of vancomycin, netilmicin, amikacin, tobramycin and gentamicin in patients receiving hemodialysis [abstract]. Pharmacotherapy 1993;13:681.
114. Matzke GR, Millikin SP Kovarik JM. Variability in pharmacokinetic values for gentamicin, tobramycin, and netilmicin in patients with renal insufficiency. Clin Pharm 1989;8:800–806.
115. Flournoy DJ. Factors influencing the inactivation of aminoglycosides by β-lactams. Methods Find Exp Clin Pharmacol 1979;1:233–238.
116. Henderson JL, Polk RE, Kline BJ. In vitro inactivation of gentamicin, tobramycin, and netilmicin by carbenicillin, azlocillin, or mezlocillin. Am J Hosp Pharm 1981;38:1167–1170.
117. Waitz JA, Drube CG, Moss EL, et al. Biological aspects of the interaction between gentamicin and carbenicillin. J Antibiot 1972;25:291–295.
118. Lau A, Lee M, Flascha S, et al. Effect of piperacillin on tobramycin pharmacokinetics in patients with normal renal function. Antimicrob Agent Chemother 1983;24:533–537.
119. Riff LJ, Jackson GG. Laboratory and clinical conditions for gentamicin inactivation by carbenicillin. Arch Intern Med 1972;130:887–891.

120. Blair DC, Duggan DO, Schroeder ET. Inactivation of amikacin and gentamicin by cabenicillin in patients with end-stage renal failure. Antimicrob Agent Chemother 1982;22:376–379.
121. Matzke GR, Luckham DR, Collins AJ, Halstenson CE. Effect of ticarcillin on gentamicin and tobramycin pharmacokinetics in a patient with end-stage renal disease. Pharmacotherapy 1984;4:158–160.
122. Russo ME, Atkin-Thor E. Gentamicin and ticarcillin in subjects with end-stage renal disease. Clin Nephrol 1981;15:175–180.
123. Thompson MIB, Russo ME, Saxon BJ, et al. Gentamicin inactivation by piperacillin or carbenicillin in patients with end-stage renal disease. Antimicrob Agent Chemother 1982;21:268–273.
124. Halstenson CE, Hirata CAI, Heim-Duthoy KL, et al. Effect of concomitant administration of piperacillin on the dispositions of netilmicin and tobramycin in patients with end-stage renal disease. Antimicrob Agent Chemother 1990;34:128–133.
125. Halstenson CE, Wong MO, Herman CS, et al. Effect of concomitant administration of piperacillin on the dispositions of isepamicin and gentamicin in patients with end-stage renal disease. Antimicrob Agent Chemother 1992;36:1832–1836.

Chapter 51

Body Electrolyte Homeostasis

Nathan J. Schultz, PharmD, BCPS,
and Kerri K. Chitwood-Dagner, PharmD, BCPS

Electrolyte disorders are associated with many disease states and are thus frequently encountered in the acute care setting. A basic understanding of the pathophysiology of these disorders is necessary to determine etiology, properly classify, and adequately treat these syndromes. In this chapter, we review the etiology, classification, symptomatology, and therapy of disorders of sodium, potassium, calcium, magnesium, and phosphorus homeostasis.

Disorders of Sodium Homeostasis

Sodium metabolism and water metabolism are intimately coupled. Sodium is actively excluded from the intracellular milieu, creating an osmotic gradient that maintains water distribution between the intracellular fluid (ICF) and extracellular fluid (ECF). Sodium, accompanied by chloride and bicarbonate, accounts for more than 90% of the osmolality of the extracellular compartment, while potassium is the major osmotic force within the cell.[1]

The kidney has the remarkable ability to maintain body homeostasis over a wide range of dietary sodium intake. A change in effective circulating volume promotes an afferent response from pressure receptors in the renal juxtaglomerular apparatus. This causes an efferent response in which glomerular filtration rate (GFR), aldosterone, oncotic pressure, adrenergic activity, renal hormones, and atrial natriuretic factor contribute to volume expansion through both water and sodium retention.[1] These processes result in the maintenance of adequate ECF volume.

The proper assessment of serum sodium requires recognition that the serum sodium concentration may bear no relationship to total body sodium content. The serum sodium concentration is equal to the amount of total body sodium divided by the amount of ECF water, with normal concentrations ranging from 135–145 mEq/L.[2] Hypernatremia and hyponatremia may be associated with conditions of high, low, or normal ECF water and high, low, or normal total body sodium. Because sodium is the major determinant of ECF osmolality, disorders of sodium homeostasis result in disorders of plasma tonicity.

HYPONATREMIA

Hyponatremia (serum sodium <135 mEq/L) is the most common electrolyte abnormality in hospitalized patients, with a reported incidence of about 1%. Brain damage is the cause of the majority of morbidity associated with hyponatremia. Patient age and sex appear to be major determinants of brain damage.[3]

Etiology

The first step in the proper assessment of hyponatremia is to measure serum osmolality. Hyponatremia associated with normal serum osmolality (isotonic hyponatremia) may be observed in patients with hyperlipidemia or hyperproteinemia. Sodium-free lipid or protein displaces sodium-rich serum water. While the concentration of sodium in serum water remains normal, the laboratory assessment assumes normal plasma solid content, resulting in a falsely decreased serum sodium concentration, termed pseudohyponatremia.[4]

Isotonic hyponatremia may also occur during intravenous infusion of isotonic, sodium-free solutions. Initially, these solutions (e.g., glucose, mannitol, glycerol) are restricted to the intravascular space, where they dilute serum sodium and result in isotonic hyponatremia.[4] Hyponatremia caused by isotonic fluids is usually mild and readily reversible with the addition of sodium-containing fluids.

Hyponatremia in the presence of elevated serum osmolality suggests the presence of excess measured or unmeasured osmoles in the serum. This is most frequently encountered in the settings of hyperglycemia or the administration of hyperosmolar glycerin or mannitol solutions. Serum sodium falls by 1.6 mEq/L for each 100 mg/dL increase in blood glucose.[4] These effective osmoles create an osmotic gradient between the isotonic ICF and the hyperosmolar ECF, drawing sodium-free water into the extracellular fluid, diluting the serum sodium, and resulting in hyponatremia.[4] The presence of a milliosmolar gap (measured mosm/L – calculated mosm/L >10) suggests the presence of hyperosmolar compounds not normally measured and provides a clue as to the cause of hyponatremia.

The second step in determining the cause of hyponatremia is the clinical assessment of extracellular fluid volume. Hypotonic hyponatremia may be classified as hypovolemic hyponatremia, hypervolemic hyponatremia, or isovolemic hyponatremia (Fig. 51.1).

Hypovolemic hyponatremia is associated with a deficit of ECF volume and sodium with a proportionally greater deficit of sodium than water. Replacement of sodium-rich fluid losses with sodium-free fluids results in hyponatremia. Hypovolemia is clinically detected by the presence of poor skin turgor, tachycardia, orthostatic hypotension, oliguria, and azotemia. The ECF volume contraction stimulates the activation of the renin-angiotensin, aldosterone, and antidiuretic hormone (ADH) systems and also changes certain aspects of renal hemodynamics.[5] In patients with extrarenal sodium losses, these changes result in a low urinary sodium concentration (<20 mEq/L). Sodium losses through the kidney are associated with an impairment of water excretion as a result of the body's attempt to maintain volume even at the expense of tonicity.[5]

Diuretic-induced hypovolemic hyponatremia is one of the most common causes of drug-induced hyponatremia. Diuretic action causes a decrease in free water excretion by blocking sodium reabsorption in the thick ascending loop of Henle, thereby decreasing the kidney's ability to dilute urine; causing extracellular fluid volume depletion, which decreases sodium delivery to the proximal tubule and stimulates ADH secretion; causing magnesium and potassium losses in the urine, which decreases renal sensitivity to ADH; and causing urinary sodium excretion.[6] Diuretic-induced hyponatremia may have a quick onset, particularly in elderly females, and may occur as soon as 3–15 days after the start of therapy. Diuretic-induced hyponatremia is commonly associated with hypokalemia.

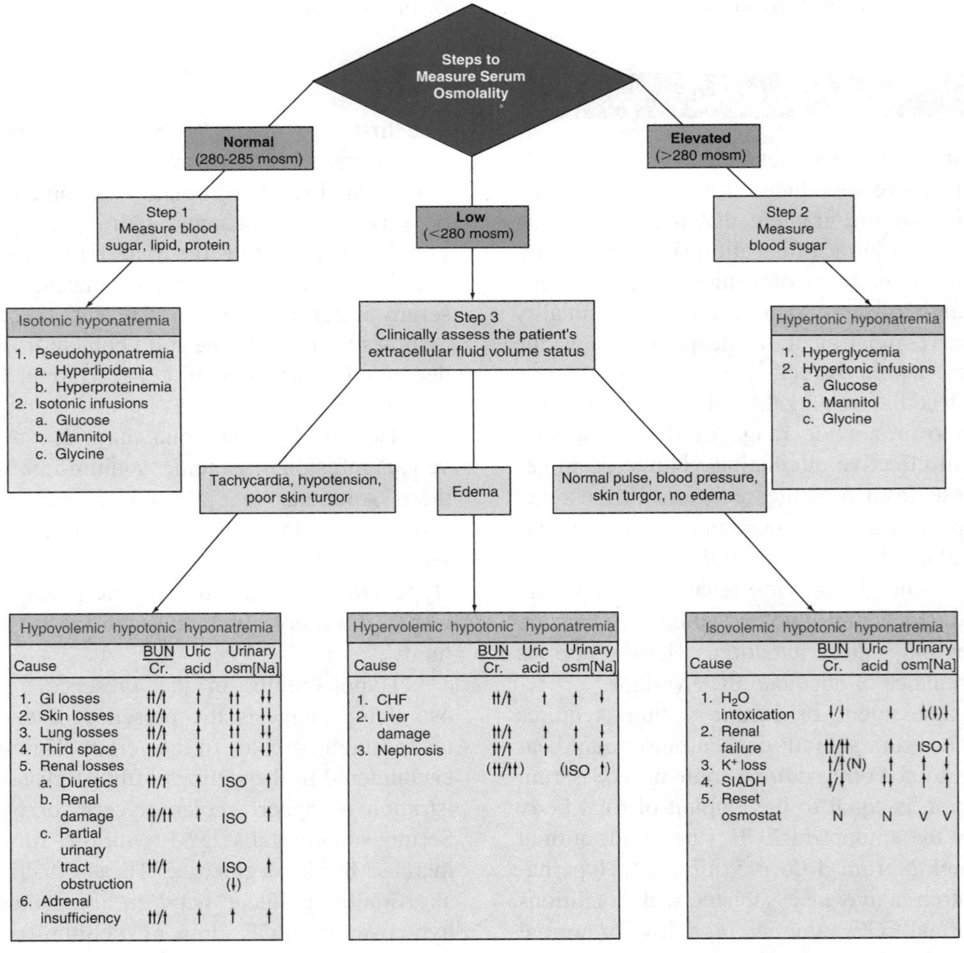

Figure 51.1. Diagnostic approach to hyponatremia. Arrows indicate direction of change. Single and double arrows define the magnitude of change. Iso, isotonic; N, normal; V, variable. *(From Narins RG, Jones RE, Stom MC, et al. Diagnostic strategies and disorders of fluid, electrolyte and acid base homeostasis. Am J Med 1982;72(3):498. Reprinted with permission from American Journal of Medicine.)*

Isovolemic hyponatremia is associated with a normal total body sodium content and small increases in ECF volume. Therefore, the retention of free water present in the setting of isovolemic hyponatremia is always the result of an imbalance of water intake and excretion.[4] Isovolemic hyponatremia is thus due to a combination of altered thirst, ADH secretion, and defective renal diluting mechanisms causing water retention and hyponatremia in patients who appear clinically euvolemic. Conditions associated with isovolemic hyponatremia are listed in Table 51.1.

The most common cause of isovolemic hyponatremia is the syndrome of inappropriate antidiuretic hormone secretion (SIADH). SIADH is defined as a sustained or intermittently elevated level of ADH that is inappropriate in the face of osmotic and volume stimuli that normally inhibit ADH secretion.[5] SIADH has been found to be the most common cause of hyponatremia in hospitalized patients.[4] SIADH may occur in a wide variety of clinical diseases (Table 51.1). Drugs are an important cause of SIADH and act by either sensitizing the kidney to ADH or stimulating the release of ADH (Table 51.2).[4] Drugs that inhibit prostaglandin synthesis, such as nonsteroidal anti-inflammatory drugs, have demonstrated potentiation of antidiuretic hormone in both animals and humans and thus are likely to contribute to hyponatremia, particularly in the elderly or neonates.[7]

Hypervolemic hyponatremia is associated with an elevated total body sodium content and an expanded ECF volume, clinically apparent as edema and weight gain. Diseases such as congestive heart failure and the hypoalbuminemic syndromes (cirrhosis, nephrotic syndrome, malnutrition, etc.) are associated with a decreased effective circulating plasma volume, resulting in secretion of renin, angiotensin, aldosterone, and ADH, causing sodium and water retention.[4] Even though total body sodium is elevated, the disproportionate accumulation of water results in hyponatremia. Hypervolemic hyponatremia is thus often termed dilutional hyponatremia.

TABLE 51.1. DISORDERS ASSOCIATED WITH THE SYNDROME OF INAPPROPRIATE ANTIDIURETIC HORMONE SECRETION

Carcinomas
Lung
Duodenum
Pancreas
Pulmonary disorders
Viral pneumonia
Bacterial pneumonia
Pulmonary abscess
Tuberculosis
Aspergillosis
Central nervous system disorders
Encephalitis, viral or bacterial
Meningitis, viral, bacterial, or tuberculosis
Acute psychosis
Stroke (cerebral thrombosis or hemorrhage)
Acute intermittent porphyria
Brain tumors
Brain abscess
Subdural or subarachnoid hematoma or hemorrhage
Guillain–Barré syndrome
Head trauma

Clinical Presentation

In hypovolemic hyponatremia, most of the clinical manifestations are due to hypovolemia and not hypotonicity. In contrast, the hypotonicity associated with isovolemic and hypervolemic hyponatremia may result in symptoms. Symptoms of hypotonicity can be related to the development of cellular swelling, with CNS symptoms of cerebral edema with increased intracranial pressure being the most severe. The severity of symptoms appears to be related to both the degree and the rapidity of development of hyponatremia.[8]

A decrease in serum sodium concentration from 140 to 130 mEq/L over a period of minutes to hours may be accompanied by moderate symptoms, such as bloating, headache, anorexia, muscle cramps, nausea, and vomiting.[5] A decrease of greater than 10 mEq/L over a similar time period however may be associated with more severe syndromes such as headache, lethargy, and disorientation, which may progress to seizures and coma.[5] There is considerable overlap between serum sodium values and symptomatology; this may be partially related to the ECF volume status of the patient and its role in the development of cerebral edema. Patients with serum sodium concentrations of 115–120 mEq/L may be free of symptoms, particularly in chronic cases in which hyponatremia developed slowly. While there is a wide overlap in the serum sodium concentration at which symptoms appear, the occurrence of seizures and coma carries grave prognostic significance.[5]

Treatment

The appropriate treatment of hyponatremia is dependent on the correct classification of hyponatremia, severity of symptoms, concurrent disease states, ECF volume, rate of decline of serum sodium concentration, and degree of hyponatremia. Treatment begins with attention to possible reversible causes of hyponatremia and identification of underlying disorders. Specific therapies are then determined by the type of hyponatremia present in the patient.

Because hypovolemic hyponatremia is rarely associated with hypotonic symptoms, therapy is directed at replacing the sodium and volume losses with normal saline over a period of 6–12 hours.[5] It is rarely necessary to infuse hypertonic saline (3 or 5% NaCl), because isotonic saline corrects the pathophysiologic factors that lead to impaired free water excretion.[5] Ongoing sodium losses must be accounted for by appropriate maintenance fluid adjustments.

TABLE 51.2. DRUGS CAUSING HYPONATREMIA

	Mechanism of Action			
Drugs	**Sensitize Kidney to ADH**[a]	**Stimulate Release of ADH**	**Other**	**Comments**
Hypoglycemic agents				
Chlorpropamide	+	+(?)		Hyponatremia found in 3–4% of patients taking chlorpropamide
Tolbutamide	+			Tolbutamide rarely causes hyponatremia
Antineoplastic drugs				
Cyclophosphamide		+	? Direct ADH effect of cyclophosphamide metabolite	Cystitis and uric acid lithiasis demand H_2O intake
Vincristine				Associated with vincristine neurotoxicity
Sedatives				
Barbiturates		+		
Morphine		+		
Psychotropic agents				
Thioridazine			Thirst	SIADH[b] associated with psychosis without drugs; role of drugs is
tenuous				
Thiothixine			Thirst	
Amitriptyline				
Fluphenazine			Thirst	
Diuretics		+		All diuretics may cause hyponatremia; volume contraction stimulates ADH release; furosemide, ethacrynic acid, and thiazides block diluting mechanisms
Miscellaneous				
Indomethacin	+			Hyponatremia not yet described with indomethacin and acetaminophen
Acetaminophen	+			
Clofibrate		+		Clofibrate is useful in partial central diabetes insipidus
Nicotine		+		
Oxytocin			Direct ADH effect	Leads to hyponatremia when pregnant woman receives oxytocin with excess water

[a]ADH, antidiuretic hormone.
[b]SIADH, syndrome of inappropriate antidiuretic hormone. (From Narins RG, Jones RE, Stom MC, et al. Diagnostic strategies and disorders of fluid, electrolyte and acid base homeostasis. Am J Med 1982;72(3):500. Reprinted with permission from American Journal of Medicine.)

Isovolemic hyponatremia associated with a nonacute reduction of serum sodium concentrations to values not less than 115 mEq/L and an absence of symptoms may be treated conservatively by water restriction. Fluids are provided to allow for mandatory urinary solute excretion, allowing insensible water loss to correct the hyponatremia. Because the kidney can concentrate urine up to an osmolality of 1200 mOsm/L, and the average solute load excreted per day is 600 mOsm, a minimum of 500 mL/d is necessary to meet obligatory urine excretion. Fluid restrictions of 500 mL/d or less may be necessary to correct hyponatremia over a 3- to 5-day period.[5] Isovolemic hyponatremia resulting from chronic SIADH may require pharmacologic intervention in addition to water restriction. Demeclocycline, a tetracycline antibiotic, interferes with the action of ADH at the renal collecting duct, resulting in a nephrogenic diabetes insipidus-like picture. Demeclocycline is effective chronic therapy for isovolemic hyponatremia when SIADH is not self-limiting and when the underlying cause cannot be corrected. Demeclocycline therapy is indicated when hyponatremia is due to an inability to excrete free water, the serum sodium is <125 mEq/L, and the patient is symptomatic and unresponsive to rigorous fluid restriction and/or fluid restriction is not possible because of other management requirements.[9] Demeclocycline doses of 600–1200 mg/d have been effective, with the onset of action ranging from 5–8 days.[10] Because of the delay in onset of action, demeclocycline has no role in the acute treatment of severe hyponatremia. Adverse effects of demeclocycline include photosensitivity, an antianabolic effect, and nephrotoxicity. The antianabolic effect worsened azotemia in patients with underlying renal disease.[11] Direct nephrotoxicity has occurred, and patients with cirrhosis or congestive heart failure (CHF) are at the greatest risk.[10] Nephrotoxicity may occur as a result of accumulation of excessively high serum concentrations in liver disease patients.[10]

Treatment of hypervolemic hyponatremia is centered on the correction of the underlying disease and the restriction of both water and salt.[5] Loop diuretics may be necessary to elicit a loss of free water. Improvement of hemodynamics and renal plasma flow and glomerular filtration rate may also promote a water and sodium diuresis. Therapy for hypervolemic hyponatremia is often difficult secondary to the severity of the associated illness (i.e., CHF, cirrhosis, nephrotic syndrome).

The rapidity of sodium concentration correction has been the subject of some controversy. The term *osmotic demyelinization syndrome* has been used to describe a delayed neurologic deterioration (quadriparesis, mutism, pseudobulbar palsy) that sometimes follows the treatment of symptomatic hyponatremia.[12] Clinical and experimental evidence suggest that this syndrome is most likely to follow a rapid increase in serum sodium concentration in patients with severe hyponatremia of more than 2 days' duration.[12] Patients with acute, rapid development of hyponatremia (acute water intoxication or hypotonic fluid intake in the setting of impaired water excretion) usually tolerate rapid correction (absolute change in serum sodium concentration of 15 mEq/L in 12 hours, 26 mEq/L in 48 hours).[13] However, osmotic demyelination syndrome has occasionally occurred in patients with acute hyponatremia as well.[12] Slow correction of serum sodium concentration (an increase of less than 12 mEq/L/d) is recommended for most cases of nonemergent symptomatic hyponatremia; this treatment approach has been associated with complications even in severe cases of hyponatremia.[12] Rapid correction of hyponatremia should be reserved for true emergencies (seizures or coma in any hyponatremic patient) or in cases of known rapid onset of severe hyponatremia (water intoxication).[12] Treatment of symptomatic hyponatremia may require administration of parenteral hypertonic saline (3% NaCl, which contains 513 mEq/L) in addition to water restriction.

HYPERNATREMIA

Hypernatremia (serum sodium >150 mEq/L) is always associated with hypertonicity and results from a state of relative water deficit.[14] Because the thirst mechanism is so effective in correcting the hypertonic state, hypernatremia results only when hypotonic fluid loss occurs in combination with a disturbance of water intake.[6] Therefore, patients who cannot express their thirst (infants, unconscious patients) or who are unable to ambulate (elderly and disabled patients) to obtain fluids are at the highest risk for developing hypernatremia. Hypernatremia occurs less frequently than does hyponatremia. Mortality from acute hypernatremia in children ranges from 10–70%, while chronic hypernatremia in children has a mortality rate of 10%.[6] In adults an acute increase in serum sodium to more than 160 mEq/L is associated with a 75% mortality rate, with chronic cases resulting in a 60% mortality rate.[6] Hypernatremia in adults is often associated with serious underlying illness, which may contribute to the high mortality rates.

Etiology

Hypernatremia may be classified according to the status of the ECF volume (Fig. 51.2). Unlike hyponatremia, which may be associated with low, normal, or even high osmolality, hypernatremia is always associated with hyperosmolality.[4]

Hypernatremia that occurs in the setting of ECF volume depletion is termed hypovolemic hypernatremia. It is caused by losses of both sodium and water, with water deficit being of a greater magnitude. Loss of sodium and water from renal and extrarenal sources, when replaced with fluids containing more sodium than present in the fluid lost, will result in the development of hypernatremia (Fig. 51.2). Common extra renal causes of hypernatremia include profound diarrhea and excessive sweating.[15] Important drug-induced causes include osmotic diuresis with mannitol, diuretics, and laxative-induced diarrhea.

Isovolemic hypernatremia is associated with an isolated pure water loss and is the most common presentation of hypernatremia.[15] Because pure water loss is shared equally across total body water, the ratio of ICF to ECF is not changed; thus, signs of ECF volume depletion are rare unless water losses are massive (serum sodium 160–170 mEq/L).[4] Total body sodium content is normal in patients with isovolemic hypernatremia.[14] Mechanisms of pure water loss are listed in Fig. 51.2. Iatrogenic causes include failure to replace insensible water loss or the replacement of insensible water losses with relatively hypertonic solutions. Excessive insensible water loss may occur with fever or high ambient temperatures. Insufficient fluid intake may result from lack of access to water (e.g., elderly patients with decreased levels of consciousness). Isovolemic hypernatremia associated with the production of large amounts of hypotonic urine characterizes diabetes insipidus (DI). Severe, life-threatening hypernatremia may develop if free water intake is not maintained. DI may be categorized as central DI (characterized by low levels of circulating ADH and an inability to produce a maximally concentrated urine)

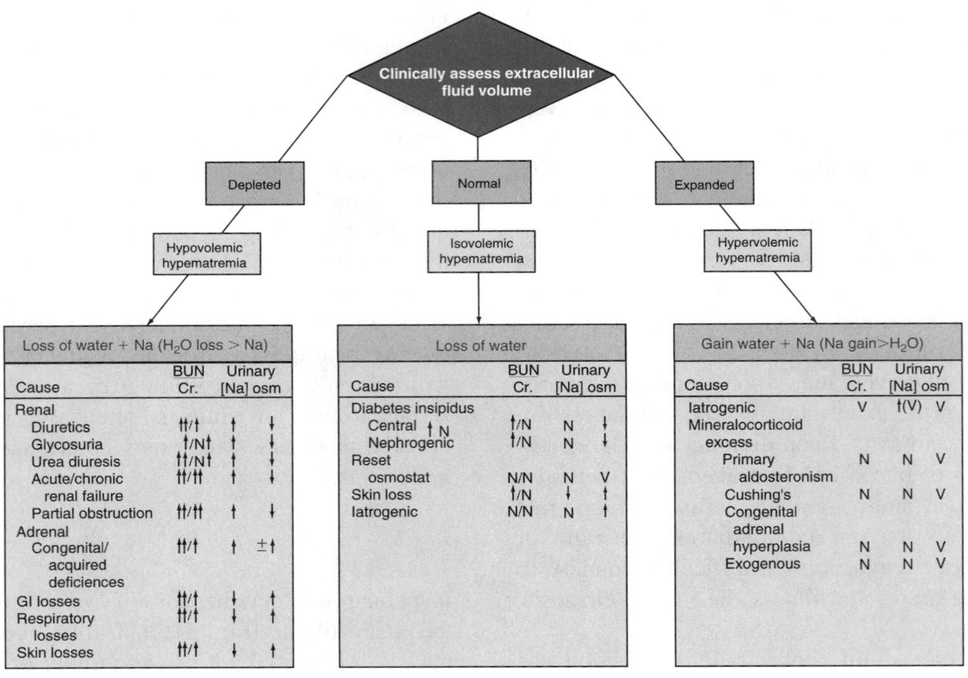

Figure 51.2. Diagnostic approach to hypernatremia. Arrows indicate direction of change. Single and double arrows define the magnitude of change. Iso, isotonic; N, normal; V, variable. *(From Narins RG, Jones RE, Stom MC, et al. Diagnostic strategies and disorders of fluid, electrolyte and acid base homeostasis. Am J Med 1982;72(3):501. Reprinted with permission from American Journal of Medicine.)*

and nephrogenic DI (characterized by an ADH-resistant defect in the renal concentrating mechanism).[14] The causes of both central and nephrogenic DI are listed in Table 51.3. Central DI and nephrogenic DI can be distinguished by characteristic responses to water deprivation and exogenous ADH administration.

Central DI is associated with an initial diuretic phase, an antidiuretic phase in which urine output normalizes because of the release of ADH from injured axons, and resumption of the polyuric phase.[6] The degree of polyuria may range from 3–15 L/24 h; serum sodium is increased only if water intake is inhibited.[6]

Nephrogenic DI is usually associated with less severe polyuria (3–4 L/24 h) than is central DI, especially in the acquired causes of nephrogenic DI (underlying renal disease and drugs).[6] Drugs causing nephrogenic DI include demeclocycline, lithium, methoxyflurane, colchicine, phenytoin, vinblastine, and amphotericin B.[6] While maximal urine concentrating ability is impaired in nephrogenic DI, a hypertonic urine may still be produced; thus the risk of hypernatremia is considerably less than in central DI.

Hypervolemic hypernatremia results from an increase in total body sodium and water, with the gain of sodium exceeding that of water. The increment in sodium results in an expansion of the ECF and the intravascular space, concurrent with a decrease in ICF volume.[14] In patients with renal failure, the inability to diurese the expanded ECF may result in vascular overload and pulmonary edema. Hypervolemic hypernatremia is commonly iatrogenic, because of excessive sodium administration.[14] Some examples include sodium bicarbonate therapy, inadvertent intravenous administration of intra-amniotic hypertonic saline for therapeutic abortion, and inadvertent use of salt instead of sugar in preparation of infant formulas. Patients with conditions associated with primary mineralocorticoid excess may also develop hypervolemic hypernatremia, usually of less severity than that caused iatrogenically.

Clinical Presentation

Most of the signs and symptoms of hypernatremia represent central nervous system (CNS) dysfunction and can be attributed to the effect of hypertonicity on brain cells. Cellular dehydration may lead to symptoms of thirst, restlessness, irritability, tremulousness, spasticity, hyperreflexia, ataxia, seizures, coma, and death.[15] In addition, the shrinking effect of hypernatremia may result in the tearing of cerebral blood vessels, leading to intracranial bleeding.[6] The severity of symptoms is related to both the degree and the rate of rise of serum osmolality; thus, acute hypernatremia is more dangerous than chronic hypernatremia.[14] In an attempt to preserve intracellular volume, brain cells form new intracellular solutes, called idiogenic osmoles. Idiogenic osmoles are effective in restoring intracellular brain

TABLE 51.3. CAUSES OF DIABETES INSIPIDUS

Cause	Character of Urine: Volume (L/24 h)	Character of Urine: Tonicity	Comments
Central Diabetes Insipidus (CDI)			"Complete" defects: highest volume and lowest osmolarity; "partial" defects; relatively normal volume with mildly hypertonic urine
Primary			
Familial	Variable (<3 to >10)	Variable, usually hypotonic	Less than 1% of cases
Idiopathic	Variable	Variable, usually hypotonic	50% of all cases
Secondary			
Trauma	Variable	Variable	Neoplasm and trauma account for vast majority of secondary causes; other secondary causes are quite rare
Neoplasms: lung, breast most common	Variable	Variable	
Granulomatous diseases: lues, tuberculosis, sarcoid	Variable	Variable	Sarcoid may also cause NDI
Eosinophilic granuloma, Hand–Schuller–Christian disease	Variable	Variable	
Cardiovascular: aneurysm, thrombosis, Sheehan syndrome	Variable	Variable	Sheehan syndrome more commonly affects anterior pituitary function
Nephrogenic Diabetes Insipidus (NDI)			
Primary			
Congenital	>3–5	Hypotonic	NDI usually associated with mild polyuria but for congenital NDI; seen in Novia Scotia Scottish
Secondary			
Electrolyte disorders Hypercalcemia Hypokalemia	2–4	Isotonic	K^+ depletion of > 200 mEq required
Renal: ATN,[a] postobstruction, partial obstruction, posttransplantation	Variable, usually <2–4	Isotonic	Excretion of retained fluid and urea diuresis play important roles in diuretic phase of ATN and postobstruction diuresis
Hematologic: sickle cell trait and disease	Variable, usually 2–3	Isotonic	
Drugs: lithium, demeclocycline, methoxyflurane	Variable, usually 2–3	Isotonic to hypotonic	Lithium also causes distal RTA[b]; methoxyflurane causes calcium oxalate crystalluria
Miscellaneous: amyloid, myeloma, Sjögren syndrome, malnutrition	Variable, usually 2–4	Variable, usually isotonic	

[a]ATN, acute tubular necrosis.
[b]RTA, renal tubular acidosis. (From Narins RG, Jones RE, Stom MC, et al. Diagnostic strategies and disorders of fluid, electrolyte and acid base homeostasis. Am J Med 1982;72:(3):502. Reprinted with permission from American Journal of Medicine.)

water to normal during a 7-day period in the presence of chronic hypernatremia.[14] The presence of idiogenic osmoles has important implications with regard to the rate of correction of serum hypertonicity.

Treatment

The goal of hypernatremia therapy is the normalization of serum tonicity. The approach to therapy consists of correction of reversible causes of hypernatremia, attention to underlying disorders, and normalization of ECF volume status.

In patients with hypovolemic hypernatremia, restoration of intravascular volume with isotonic 0.9% NaCl solution over 30–45 minutes should be accomplished to reverse the hemodynamic alteration.[16] Note that 0.9% NaCl solution will be hypotonic relative to the hypernatremic plasma and thus will aid in correcting hypertonicity as well as intravascular volume. Once intravascular volume is replaced, the water deficit can be replaced. Free water deficit can be estimated by the following formula[14]: water deficit = normal TBW − current TBW, where TBW = total body water (normal TBW = 0.60 × normal body weight in kilograms, and current TBW = normal TBW × 140/current measured Na concentration). The free water deficit can be replaced with 5% dextrose or 0.45% NaCl solution. Serum sodium concentration must be decreased slowly to avoid the development of cerebral edema, seizures, permanent neurologic damage, or even death.[8] The presence of idiogenic osmoles inside brain cells causes an osmotic gradient to develop between the brain and plasma, and rapid lowering of plasma osmolality may result in the movement of water from plasma into the intracellular space, leading to cerebral edema and increased intracranial pressure. An acceptable rate of decrease in osmolality is 2 mOsm/h (1 mEq/L Na per hour) over a period of 48–72 hours.[8,16] Hypernatremia greater than 175 mEq/L should not be corrected by more than 15 mEq/L during the first 24 hours.[8]

Treatment of isovolemic hypernatremia is targeted at replacing water deficit, as outlined earlier, with 5% dextrose or 0.45% NaCl solutions. Initial therapy with 0.9% NaCl is not necessary, because ECF volume is usually not decreased. In addition, potentially reversible or treatable underlying conditions must be addressed. Patients with central DI will respond to administration of natural and synthetic ADH (vasopressin) preparations (Table 51.4). Parenteral products are usually used for acute management; intranasally administered agents are usually reserved for

TABLE 51.4. COMPARISON OF ANTIDIURETIC AGENTS

	Desmopressin (DDVAP)	Vasopressin (ADH,[a] AVP)	Lypressin (DIAPID)
Pharmacology			
Vasoconstriction/ADH ratio	+	+++	±
ACTH release	−	++++	−
Oxytocicity	+	++++	+
ADH activity	+++ (IV 10 × nasal)	+	+++
Factor VIII	+++	−	?
Pharmacokinetics	(Nasal)	(Parenteral)	(Nasal)
Onset	1 h		Minutes
Peak	1–5 h		0.5–2 h
Duration	8–20 h	Aqueous SC 2–8 h: oil IM 48–72 h	3–8 h
Route of administration			
Parenteral	IV/SC	Oil IM/SC Aqueous IM/IV/SC	−
Intranasal	+	—	+
Dose	Nasal: 0.05–0.4 mL (0.01% solution); 5–40 μg in 1–3 doses Parenteral: 2–4 μg/d in 2 doses	Aqueous: 5–10 U SC/IM 2–4 × day prn Oil: 1.5–5 U IM every 2–3 d	1–2 sprays qid

[a]ADH, antidiuretic hormone.

long-term management. Drugs with antidiuretic properties such as chlorpropamide, carbamazepine, and clofibrate have also been successfully used to manage patients with partial central DI.[17]

Hypervolemic hypernatremia should be treated by replacement of water deficit in conjunction with diuretics to eliminate sodium excess. Patients with hypervolemic hypernatremia and renal failure may be treated by hemodialysis against a relatively hypotonic dialysate.[6] The rate of correction of hypernatremia should not exceed those previously proposed for hypovolemic and isovolemic hypernatremias.

Disorders of Potassium Homeostasis

Potassium has two major physiologic functions: cell metabolism, participating in such processes as protein and glycogen synthesis and determination of the resting potential across cell membranes based on the intracellular to extracellular concentration ratio.[18] Potassium disorders can thus be expected to influence adversely cellular metabolism and neural and muscular function.

Potassium is the primary intracellular cation at a concentration of approximately 150–160 mEq/L, while the ECF contains 3.5–5 mEq/L. There is approximately 50–75 mEq of potassium in ECF (serum), in contrast to 3400 mEq in ICF.[19] Muscle tissue represents the major site of intracellular potassium and varies with age (decreased in elderly), sex (males > females), and muscle mass.[19] Even though the serum potassium represents only a small percentage of total body potassium, it is the ratio of intracellular potassium to serum potassium that is important in maintaining the resting membrane potential, responsible for normal action potential generation in cardiac and noncardiac tissue.[18]

Potassium homeostasis and the maintenance of normal serum potassium concentration (3.5–5.0 mEq/L) depend on complex extrarenal and renal factors. Because only 2% of total body potassium resides in the serum (ECF), and the serum potassium level is influenced by shifts between the ICF and ECF as well as potassium balance, estimation of the magnitude of an excess or deficit of total body potassium balance extrapolated from the serum potassium concentration is imprecise.[20] Figure 51.3 depicts the approximate relationship between serum potassium concentration and total body potassium. For each 1 mEq/L decrease in serum, the potassium deficit is approximately 150–200 mEq. In addition, it can be seen that relatively small incremental increases in total body potassium may result in fatal increases in serum potassium concentration. Thus, the evaluation of serum potassium concentration requires the consideration of factors influencing redistribution of potassium across cell membranes, as well as factors influencing total body potassium balance. Factors influencing the intracellular–extracellular movement of potassium are listed in Table 51.5. The Na^+/K^+-ATPase pump is responsible for main-

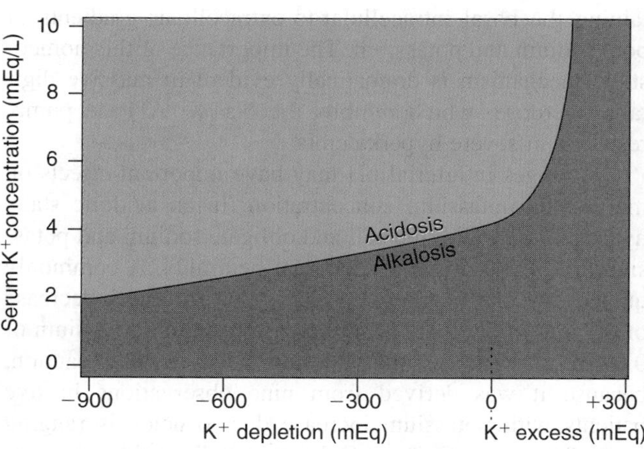

Figure 51.3. Approximate relationship between changes in total body potassium and serum potassium concentration in an adult. The graph depicts a rough gauge of the degree of negative or positive potassium balance with hypokalemia or hyperkalemia and the effect of acidosis to raise, and alkalosis to lower, the serum potassium concentration. *(From Brown RS. Potassium homeostasis and clinical implications. Am J Med Suppl 1984;77(5A):4. Reprinted with permission from American Journal of Medicine Supplement.)*

TABLE 51.5. FACTORS INFLUENCING REDISTRIBUTION OF POTASSIUM

	Serum K^+ Concentration
Serum pH	
Metabolic acidosis (mineral acids)	↑
Metabolic alkalosis	↓
Respiratory acidosis	↔
Respiratory alkalosis	↔
Adrenergic system	
β_2 agonists (epinephrine terbutaline)	↓
β_2 blockade (propranolol)	↑
α_1 agonists (phenylephrine)	↑
α_1 blockade (phentolamine)	↓
Insulin	
Excess	↓
Deficit	↑
Hyperosmolarity	↑
Cellular disruption	↑
Trauma/injury	
Nutrition	
Anabolism	↓
Catabolism	↑
Exercise	↑
Na^+/K^+-ATPase pump	
Stimulate (catecholamines)	↓
Inhibit (digitalis toxicity)	↑

taining the basal intracellular-to-extracellular gradients of both sodium and potassium. The importance of this homeostatic mechanism is dramatically evident in massive digitalis overdose, which inhibits the Na^+/K^+-ATPase pump, resulting in severe hyperkalemia.

Changes in arterial pH may have important effects on the plasma potassium concentration. In an acidotic state, hydrogen ions enter the cell and obligate sodium and potassium to exit to preserve electrical neutrality. A commonly quoted estimate of the pH effect is that for every decrease of 0.1 unit of pH there is an increase in serum potassium of 0.6 mEq/L. This estimate should be used with caution, because it was derived from nine observations in five patients with potassium increase due to acidosis ranging from 0.4–1.3 mEq/L.[21] Only metabolic acids such as hydrochloric acid cause this increase in serum potassium. Organic acids, such as lactic acid, do not produce a change in potassium concentration because with H^+ entry, lactate follows, thereby preserving electroneutrality.[21] Respiratory acidosis does not produce large changes in serum potassium concentration.[18]

Metabolic alkalosis causes a shift of potassium into cells; however, this effect is considerably less prominent than the opposite effect produced by metabolic acidosis.[18] The potassium shift associated with alkalosis may not be entirely pH dependent. Experimental work in animals has documented that increases in serum bicarbonate with no change in pH also move potassium intracellularly.[21] Respiratory alkalosis does not appreciably influence serum potassium.[21]

β-Adrenergic agonists stimulate the activity of the Na^+/K^+-ATPase pump via stimulation of cyclic AMP.[22] α-Adrenergic stimulation has the opposite effect and inhibits potassium movement into the cell. The mechanism of α-medicated inhibition of intracellular potassium movement is not known.[23]

Insulin increases potassium uptake by both skeletal muscle and hepatic cells by stimulating the Na^+/K^+-ATPase pump.[18,24] Insulin release is stimulated by hyperkalemia and serves as a primary defense against pathologic potassium elevations. Hyperkalemia also causes a concurrent release in glucagon as protection from insulin-associated hypoglycemia. Hypokalemia inhibits insulin release and accounts for the hyperglycemia associated with diuretic use.[24]

Osmolality increases of 10 mOsm/kg can raise serum potassium 0.3–0.6 mEq/L.[21] Potassium leaves the cell to lower the intracellular osmolality caused by water loss. This hypertonic movement of potassium and possible hyperkalemia are more likely in diabetics who lack insulin and who develop an inadequate aldosterone response.[21]

In addition to the intracellular–extracellular redistribution of potassium, the regulation of serum potassium by renally controlled potassium excretion is paramount in the pathogenesis of potassium disorders. Almost all of the potassium that is filtered in the glomerulus is reabsorbed in the proximal tubule and ascending loop of Henle.[18] Potassium excretion into the urine by secretion from the distal tubule and collecting duct is regulated primarily by aldosterone and plasma potassium concentration.[18] These regulators act to increase tubular intracellular potassium concentration, resulting in increased secretion. Distal tubule urine flow may also influence potassium secretion. Increased distal flow results in a reduced concentration gradient, thus increasing potassium secretion; conversely, decreased tubular flow results in decreasing potassium secretion.[18] The transepithelial potential difference across tubular cell membranes is influenced by sodium reabsorption. Sodium reabsorption makes the tubular lumen relatively electronegative. The enhanced electronegativity favors the movement of positively charged potassium from the cell into the lumen.[18]

HYPOKALEMIA

Hypokalemia is a common disorder and occurs with greater frequency than does hyperkalemia. Hypokalemia may be classified as moderate (serum potassium 2.5–3.5 mEq/L) or severe (serum potassium less than 2.5 mEq/L). An approach to evaluation of the hypokalemic patient is depicted in Fig. 51.4.

Etiology

The multifactorial causes of hypokalemia can be classified on the basis of body stores; normal body stores (laboratory error, redistribution) or decreased total body stores (gastrointestinal loss, renal loss, other) (Table 51.6). The most frequent causes of hypokalemia are gastrointestinal and diuretic-induced renal losses.[18] Gastrointestinal (GI) losses may be due to direct loss of potassium from GI fluids (vomiting, diarrhea, draining fistulas, etc.); metabolic alkalosis from hydrogen ion loss (vomiting, nasogastric suction), resulting in intracellular potassium shift; and plasma volume contraction, leading to secondary increase in aldosterone. Diuretics cause hypokalemia by increasing distal tubular flow, resulting in potassium loss down its concentration gradient.[18]

Clinical Presentation

Hypokalemia may cause a wide variety of physiologic abnormalities, resulting in a symptomatology involving several organ systems (Table 51.7). The severity of symptoms is related to the degree and acuteness of hypokalemia, although substantial interindividual variability does exist.[18] Marked symptoms are unusual unless serum potassium concentration is less than 3.0 mEq/L.[18]

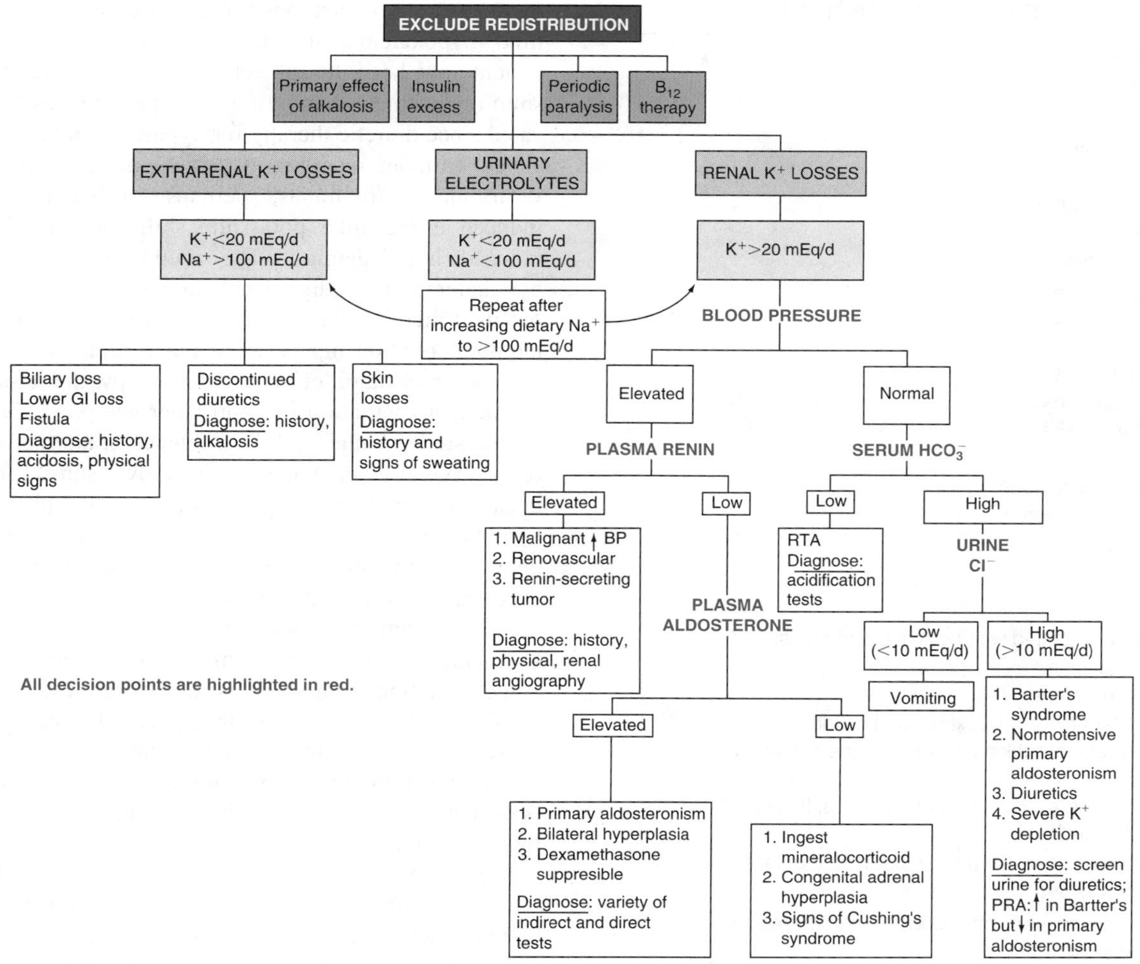

Figure 51.4. Diagnostic approach to hypokalemia. PRA, plasma renin activity; RTA, renal tubular acidosis. *(From Narins RG, Jones RE, Stom MC, et al. Diagnostic strategies and disorders of fluid, electrolyte, and acid base homeostasis. Am J Med 1982;72(3)506. Reprinted with permission from American Journal of Medicine.)*

The association between serum potassium and arrhythmias can be explained by the effect of potassium on resting membrane potential (RMP) in cardiac tissue. The RMP is proportional to the log of the ratio of extracellular to intracellular potassium; therefore, small changes in serum potassium can have a significant effect on this ratio. Hypokalemia results in an increase in RMP while hypokalemia decreases RMP.[25]

The electrocardiographic effects of hypokalemia (Fig. 51.5) are characterized by ST segment lowering or flattening, inversion of the T wave, and elevation of the U wave. A widening of the PR interval, an increase in P-wave amplitude, and widening of the QRS complex may also occur, most frequently when serum potassium concentration is less than 2.7 mEq/L.[26] Hypokalemia-associated arrhythmias include bradyarrhythmias, heart block, atrial flutter, paroxysmal atrial tachycardia with block, atrioventricular dissociation, premature ventricular contractions, and ventricular fibrillation. It is well accepted that hypokalemia lowers the threshold for digitalis cardiotoxic arrhythmias.

The neuromuscular effects of hypokalemia can be attributed to decreased muscular excitability, as a result of increased RMP. Because the ratio of extracellular to intracellular potassium determines membrane potential, acute reductions of serum potassium have been associated with more severe neuromuscular changes.[19] Both smooth muscle and skeletal muscle may be affected, resulting in the symptoms listed in Table 51.7. The pattern of muscle weakness is relatively characteristic, first involving the lower extremities and subsequently ascending to the trunk, upper extremities, and muscles of respiration.[18,19] The smooth muscle of the GI tract is often involved, resulting in paralytic ileus.[18,19]

Treatment

Serum potassium levels of less than 3.5 mEq/L in the digitalized patient or when associated with symptoms require

TABLE 51.6. SYNDROMES OF HYPOKALEMIA

Normal Body K^+
Laboratory error
Redistribution
Metabolic alkalosis
Insulin
β_2-Adrenergic agonists
B_{12} therapy
Barium poisoning
Periodic paralysis
Athletes (exercise)
Low Body K^+
Gastrointestinal losses
Nasogastric drainage
Poor dietary intake
Protracted vomiting
Diarrhea (laxative abuse)
Ureterosigmoidostomy
Biliary drainage
Skin losses
Sweat
Renal losses associated with normal blood pressure
Hypomagnesemia
Bartter's syndrome
Renal tubular acidosis (proximal and distal)
Vomiting (metabolic alkalosis and volume depletion)
Drugs
Diuretics (acetazolamide, loop diuretics, thiazides)
Amphotericin B
Carbenicillin, ticarcillin (nonreabsorbable anion)
Aminoglycosides
Renal losses associated with increased blood pressure
Hyperreninemic
Renovascular hypertension
Renin tumor
Malignant essential hypertension
Hyporeninemic steroid dependent
Exogenous mineralocorticoid
Licorice
Desoxycorticosterone
Fludrocortisone
Chewing tobacco
Carbenoxolone
Endogenous mineralocorticoid
Adrenal adenoma
Adrenal glomerulosa hyperplasia
Enzyme deficiency (17-hydroxylase, 11-hydroxylase)
Liddle's syndrome
Exogenous glucocorticoid
Endogenous glucocorticoid
Excessive ACTH[a]
Cushing's syndrome

[a]ACTH, adrenocorticotropic hormone. (Adapted from Narins RG, Jones RC, Stom MC, et al. Diagnostic strategies and disorders of fluid, electrolyte and acid base homeostasis. Am J Med 1982;72(3):505. Reprinted with permission from American Journal of Medicine.)

treatment. The indications for the treatment of moderate to mild hypokalemia in the asymptomatic, nondigitalized patient have been the subject of much controversy.[27] Potassium replacement therapy for these patients has been advocated since diuretic therapy for hypertension has been associated with an increase in sudden death, attributable to ventricular arrhythmias, perhaps mediated by stress-induced intracellular potassium shifts on top of diuretic-induced hypokalemia.[28] The routine treatment of mild hypokalemia in nondigitalized patients however is not without its critics.[27] These criticisms include the lack of a firm temporal relationship between the serum potassium level and the observation of ventricular ectopy, the possibility of spontaneous variation of ventricular ectopic activity influencing study results, and the influence of alternative causes of ventricular ectopic activity on study results.[27] It has also been suggested that the possibility of life-threatening hyperkalemia in certain at-risk groups may outweigh the benefits of therapy.[29] Further controlled clinical trials are necessary to resolve this controversy.

Potassium replacement therapy is indicated under the following conditions: symptomatic hypokalemia, starvation and debilitation, potassium loss associated with vomiting or diarrhea, acidosis leading to increased renal potassium excretion, digitalis intoxication leading to cardiac arrhythmias, myocardial infarction with low serum potassium, diabetic ketoacidosis treated with insulin, and adrenocortical hyperactivity.[30] Potassium replacement therapy is commonly required for patients on diuretic therapy. Suggested guidelines for potassium administration in nonedematous patients include monitoring serum potassium concentration prior to and at 1- to 2-month intervals during diuretic therapy until a pattern is identified. No treatment is required while serum potassium remains >3.0 mEq/L unless symptoms develop. If serum potassium falls below 3.0 mEq/L, use 50–60 mEq/d KCl oral solution or wax matrix. If potassium-sparing diuretics are used, monitor carefully. Caution should be used in patients with renal impairment. For the edematous patient (i.e., congestive heart failure, cirrhosis with ascities, severe aldosteronism), potassium replacement should be considered when the risks of treatment with replacement therapy are outweighed by the value of restoring potassium balance. Oral therapy at a dose of 40–80 mEq/d should be used to correct mild deficits. With more severe deficits, use up to 100–120 mEq/d with careful monitoring. If oral potassium replacement therapy does not increase serum potassium, a potassium-sparing diuretic may be used.[30]

A variety of potassium salts are available for replacement and prophylactic therapy: chloride, bicarbonate (acetate and citrate are rapidly metabolized to bicarbonate), phosphate, and gluconate. The most frequently utilized potassium salt is potassium chloride. Metabolic alkalosis is often associated with hypokalemia, and because the causes of metabolic alkalosis (vomiting and diuretics) also cause chloride depletion, the administration of chloride is essen-

TABLE 51.7. CLINICAL PROBLEMS ASSOCIATED WITH POTASSIUM DEFICIENCY

Cardiovascular	Muscular	Metabolic	Renal
Arrhythmias Reentry phenomena Delayed conductance Ventricular escape rhythms Increased risk of digitalis toxicity Increased risk of complications after myocardial infarction Ventricular tachycardia or fibrillation Increased ischemia Orthostatic hypotension Impaired pressor responsiveness to catecholamine or angiotensin infusions Decreased cardioacceleration in response to postural change	Myalgia Weakness Cramps Akathisia Paralysis Rhabdomyolysis with myoglobinuria Hypodynamic ileus Decreased ureteral peristalsis Elevated serum enzymes Creatine kinase (MM isoenzyme) AST Aldolase	Abnormal carbohydrate metabolism Reduced muscle glycogen content and synthesis Precipitation of overt diabetes mellitus Increased glucose intolerance in diabetes mellitus Reduced normal insulin release during hyperglycemia Increased risk of complications from electrolyte abnormalities Hypercalcemia Hypomagnesemia Achlorhydria Hyperlipidemia Impotence	Increased production of ammonia by the kidneys Decreased protein synthesis Negative nitrogen balance Growth retardation Hepatic encephalopathy or coma in susceptible patients with end-stage liver disease Nephrogenic diabetes insipidus Increased risk of pyelonephritis

(From Knochel JP. Diuretic-induced hypokalemia. Am J Med Suppl. 1984;77(5A):20. Reprinted with permission from American Journal of Medicine Supplement.)

tial for correction of both the alkalosis and the potassium deficit.[18] Nonchloride salts of potassium are indicated only in treating hypokalemia associated with metabolic acidosis (e.g., renal tubular acidosis).

The route of administration depends on feasibility, severity of hypokalemia, and presence of symptoms. Intravenous potassium is indicated when the oral route is not feasible and/or in the presence of life-threatening hypokalemia (paralysis, arrhythmias). Because of the many factors influencing the internal distribution of potassium, rapid administration of potassium directly into the plasma can potentially result in hyperkalemia. In general, potassium can be intravenously administered safely at a rate of 10–20 mEq/h.[18] Potassium administration at rates greater than 10 mEq/h should be accompanied by electrocardiographic monitoring for the signs of hyperkalemia. In rare instances, severe hypokalemia associated with paralysis or life-threatening arrhythmias has been treated by the administration of parenteral potassium at a rate of 40–100 mEq/h. This necessitates careful electrocardiographic monitoring and the frequent determination of serum potassium concentration.[25] The generally accepted maximally tolerated potassium concentration for peripheral-vein intravenous administration is 40–60 mEq/L.[18,31] Potassium concentrations greater than 50–60 mEq/L are often not tolerated by patients because of burning pain and peripheral venous sclerosis. Thus, more centrally located, larger veins are more appropriate sites of administration if large potassium doses are needed. The use of central venous lines for administration of potassium has been discouraged by some authors, because of the potential for adverse cardiac effects as the result of locally high potassium concentrations.[18,31] Data supporting these warnings are scarce, however, and many institutions safely use central line access for the controlled administration of 10–20 mEq potassium mixed in 100 mL of dextrose or saline solution given over 1 hour in electrocardiographically monitored ICU patients.[31] Because the rate of intracellular movement and the total body deficit of potassium are unpredictable, caution is advised when parenteral potassium therapy is initiated.

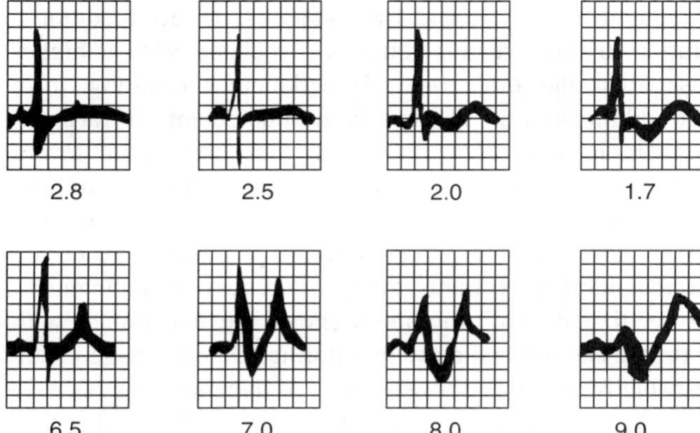

Figure 51.5. ECG patterns in hypokalemia (top) and in hyperkalemia (bottom). Serum potassium in mEq/L. *(From* The Merck Manual of Diagnosis and Therapy, *Edition 16, p. 1000, edited by Robert Berkow. Copyright 1992 by Merck & Co., Inc., Rahway, NJ. Used with permission.)*

Oral administration, when feasible, is the preferred route for potassium replacement in hypokalemia not associated with life-threatening symptoms and for prophylaxis of diuretic-induced hypokalemia. Factors influencing the choice of an oral potassium chloride dosage form include product effectiveness, adverse effects, cost, and the patient's ability to comply with the prescribed regimen since no comprehensive study has shown that any one dosage form is more effective than another.[30,32,33] Liquid potassium preparations are inexpensive, but are often poorly tolerated by patients because of unpleasant taste, aftertaste, nausea, heartburn, and diarrhea.[18,30] Enteric-coated tablets should be avoided, because a high incidence of small-bowel ulceration and scarring is associated with their use.[34,35] Nonetheless, because of poor patient acceptance of liquid potassium preparations and the small-bowel toxicity of enteric-coated potassium products, sustained-release potassium products have enjoyed immense popularity. Potassium crystals embedded in a wax matrix or microencapsulated in polymers result in dosage forms that release potassium in the gut in a sustained, gradual manner, thereby minimizing gastric irritation and ulceration. However, recent studies have shown that even these products may cause endoscopic GI ulceration.[36] Because of their palatability and low side-effect profile, the sustained-release potassium chloride products are excellent dosage forms for oral potassium therapy.

Alternatives to pharmaceutical dosage forms of potassium chloride include salt substitutes and potassium-rich food sources (i.e., bananas, orange juice). Salt substitutes are an effective, inexpensive potassium supplement, which is usually better tolerated than liquid potassium chloride products.[18] Food sources of potassium are generally not recommended for chronic potassium supplementation because they often contain less chloride than other potassium sources and may add unwanted calories to the diets of patients who may benefit from caloric restriction.[18]

Potassium-sparing diuretics are an alternative to exogenous potassium supplementation during diuretic therapy. These agents are widely used in combination with thiazide diuretics. Spironolactone, which antagonizes aldosterone and thereby reduces potassium exchange in the distal tubule, is especially effective as a potassium-sparing agent in conditions associated with primary and secondary hyperaldosteronism. Triamterene and amiloride act by an aldosterone-independent but unknown method to reduce potassium excretion.[37]

Combined use of potassium chloride supplements and potassium-sparing diuretics is generally contraindicated, except during the initial phase of therapy for disorders requiring replenishment of total body potassium stores along with prevention of ongoing potassium losses. The risk of hyperkalemia with combined use is significant, especially in patients with renal dysfunction or diabetes mellitus or the elderly.[32]

HYPERKALEMIA

Hyperkalemia is defined as serum potassium greater than 5.5 mEq/L. Hyperkalemia may be classified as mild (serum potassium 5.5–6.5 mEq/L without electrocardiographic changes), moderate (6.5–8.0 mEq/L), and severe (>8.0 mEq/L).[38] The incidence of hyperkalemia in hospitalized patients is 3–8%, with greater prevalence in elderly patients, most likely because of the frequency in this population of diseases and conditions associated with hyperkalemia.[39]

Etiology

Hyperkalemia may be associated with normal or elevated total body stores of potassium. Hyperkalemia associated with normal total body stores includes redistribution of potassium and "pseudohyperkalemia." Pseudohyperkalemia is an *in vitro* phenomenon in which the measured serum potassium level is falsely elevated compared with the actual *in vivo* level, usually as a result of release from red blood cells (RBCs), white blood cells (WBCs), or platelets, which may occur in myeloproliferative or hemolytic disorders.[38] Redistribution of potassium from the intracellular to the extracellular space may occur *in vivo*. Acidosis and insulin deficiency may result in ECF movement of potassium as previously discussed. Release of potassium from ischemic, injured, or lysed cells may occur secondary to crush injury, rhabdomyolysis, burns, and chemotherapy (tumor lysis syndrome).[18] Drugs may cause redistribution of potassium by disruption of the Na^+/K^+-ATPase pump (digitalis intoxication),[40] release of potassium from muscle cells following depolarizing muscle relaxant administration (succinylcholine),[41] β_2 blockade (propranolol),[42] positively charged molecules entering cells to displace potassium (lysine and arginine),[43] inhibition of potassium secretion in a dose-dependent manner (trimethoprim-sulfamethoxazole),[44] and hyporeninemic hypoaldosteronism (NSAIDs and cyclosporine).[45]

Hyperkalemia associated with elevated total body potassium stores is due to excessive potassium ingestion, potassium excretion, or both. Although all potassium supplements may cause hyperkalemia, reduced administration by intravenous route is associated with a higher risk than the oral route. Hyperkalemia resulting from the administration of potassium supplements is rare unless rapid intravenous administration occurs, or severe kidney dysfunction, inhibition of renal tubular secretion, or the renin-angiotensin-aldosterone axis coexists.[4] Exogenous administration of potassium to patients receiving concomitant potassium-sparing diuretics or angiotensin-converting enzyme inhibitors should be undertaken with extreme caution and close monitoring. Diabetic patients are especially at risk for development of hyperkalemia because they lack insulin and its vital role in potassium redistribution. Diabetics also have a tendency toward hyporeninemic hypoaldosteronism, which decreases the kidney's ability to excrete potassium. The combination of insulin deficiency and attenuated aldosterone response places the diabetic at greater risk for the development of hyperkalemia.[40]

Clinical Presentation

The clinical presentation of hyperkalemia is limited primarily to muscle weakness and abnormalities of cardiac conduction, in addition to the symptoms associated with underlying disease. As the resting potential approaches the threshold potential, the cell is unable to sustain an action potential, and weakness or paralysis results.[18] Symptoms often begin in the lower extremities, ascending to the trunk and upper extremities.[18] At serum concentrations of 6.5 mEq/L and above muscle twitching, weakness, nausea, and cramping can occur.[46]

The cardiac rhythm disturbances associated with hyperkalemia pose the greatest danger to the patient, because they may lead to ventricular fibrillation or cardiac standstill (asystole). The earliest electrocardiogram (ECG) changes are peaked T waves and shortening of the QT interval, reflecting an increased rate of repolarization with occasional ST depression.[46] These changes are seen typically when serum potassium concentrations are 5.5–6 mEq/L. With serum concentrations between 6 and 7 the PR interval and QRS duration are prolonged (Fig. 51.5). When the serum concentration exceeds 7–8 mEq/L, electrocardiographic manifestations of delayed depolarization occur, resulting in slowed cardiac conduction, and appear as widening of the QRS complex and decreased amplitude, widening, and eventual loss of the P wave.[18] When serum concentrations exceed 9–10 mEq/L, the QRS complex merges with the T wave, resulting in a sine-wave pattern, which may deteriorate to ventricular fibrillation or asystole at concentrations from 10–12 mEq/L.[46] Depolarization slowing is the result of a reduction in sodium permeability into the cell, caused by a hyperkalemia-induced reduction of resting membrane potential.[18] Note that the serum concentrations at which the characteristic electrocardiographic changes occur are variable since hypocalcemia, acidosis, hyponatremia, and the rapidity of elevation of serum potassium all may enhance the cardiotoxicity of hyperkalemia.[18] Acute hyperkalemia is generally more dangerous than chronic hyperkalemia, because the protective mechanisms for rapid intracellular movement of potassium may be overwhelmed. When hyperkalemia develops gradually, electrocardiographic changes are usually not observed until serum potassium levels exceed 7–7.5 mEq/L.[42] Ventricular fibrillation usually results from rapidly progressive hyperkalemia, while asystole is most often observed in patients with slow progression to severe hyperkalemia.[43]

Treatment

Severe hyperkalemia (>8 mEq/L) or moderate hyperkalemia (6.5–8 mEq/L), when associated with clinical symptoms or electrocardiographic changes, requires immediate treatment. Treatment of hyperkalemia is achieved by antagonism of the membrane actions of hyperkalemia (calcium), decrease in extracellular potassium concentration by promotion of intercellular movement of the cation (glucose, insulin, beta-2 agonists, bicarbonate), and removal of potassium from the body (hemodialysis, cation-exchange resins)[19] (Table 51.8). Exogenous potassium must be withheld, and potentially reversible causes of hyperkalemia must be reversed as well.

Calcium administration is an effective rapidly acting but short-lived therapy that dramatically reverses the electrocardiographic manifestations and arrhythmias of hyperkalemia.[19] Calcium changes the relationship between mem-

TABLE 51.8. TREATMENT OF HYPERKALEMIA

Medication	Dose	Route of Administration	Mechanism of Action	Expected Result	Onset/Duration
Albuterol	10–20 mg	Nebulized over 10 min	Stimulates Na^+/K^+-ATPase pump	Redistribution of K^+ into the cell	30 min/1–2 h
Calcium chloride	1 g (13.5 mEq)	IV over 5–10 min	Raises threshold potential and reestablishes cardiac excitability	Reverses ECG effects	1–2 min/10–30 min
Dextrose 50%	50 mL (25 g)	IV over 5 min	Increases insulin release	Redistribution of K^+ into the cell	30 min/2–6 h
Dextrose 10%	1000 mL (100 g)	IV over 1–2 h	Increases insulin release	Redistribution of K^+ into the cell	30 min/2–6 h
Sodium bicarbonate	50–100 mEq	IV over 2–5 min	Increases serum pH	Redistribution of K^+ into the cell	30 min/2–6 h
Insulin (regular)	1 unit per 3–5 g dextrose	IV with 10% dextrose SC	Potassium intracellular uptake	Redistribution of K^+ into the cell	30 min/2–6 h
Sodium polystyrene sulfonate	15–60 g	Orally or rectally	Exchanges resin Na^+ for K^+	Increase in K^+ elimination	1 h/variable
Hemodialysis	2–4 h	—	Removal from plasma	Increase in K^+ elimination	Immediate/variable

brane potential and threshold potential, restoring normal conduction in the heart.[18] Calcium administration does not in any way lower serum potassium concentration and, because it is so short acting, must be repeated if symptoms recur, until serum potassium can be lowered. The frequency of repeat administration is dependent on the rate of symptom recurrence.

Promoting intracellular movement of potassium is an effective mechanism for lowering extracellular potassium serum levels. Intravenous glucose enhances endogenous insulin release in nondiabetics, thus promoting intracellular uptake of potassium. Insulin is often administered with glucose to facilitate the effect of endogenous insulin. Glucose administration may be omitted and insulin alone administered to the hyperglycemic patient. Albuterol alone or in combination with insulin may substantially decrease plasma potassium.[22] Sodium bicarbonate also promotes the intracellular movement of potassium, by increasing extracellular pH and also by a direct action of the bicarbonate anion itself.[18]

Sodium polystyrene sulfonate, a cation-exchange resin, is effective when given orally or rectally. Each gram of resin may bind as much as 1 mEq of potassium and release 1–2 mEq of sodium.[18] The resin remains in the GI tract and must be removed to be effective. Sodium polystyrene sulfonate should be administered with sorbitol to prevent constipation and retention of the resin. Prepackaged suspensions in sorbitol are commercially available. Sodium polystyrene sulfonate doses of 40 g given orally in four divided doses may decrease serum potassium concentrations by 1.0 mEq/L in 24 hours in patients with renal failure.[19]

If hyperkalemia persists, especially if the patient is in renal failure (acute or chronic), hemodialysis is indicated.[46] Peritoneal dialysis is less effective due to the lower efficiency of potassium elimination compared to hemodialysis (see Chapter 43, Acute Renal Failure).[45]

DISORDERS OF CALCIUM HOMEOSTASIS

The control and maintenance of calcium concentration in the intracellular and extracellular spaces is vital for the preservation and function of cell membranes, propagation of neuromuscular activity, regulation of endocrine and exocrine secretory functions, blood coagulation cascade, platelet adhesion process, bone metabolism, muscle cell excitation/contraction coupling, and mediation of the electrophysiologic slow channel response in cardiac and smooth muscle tissue. Because of the biologic importance of calcium, the concentration of this cation is closely regulated by a complex system involving parathyroid hormone, vitamin D, calcitonin, and their target. Disruption of these homeostatic mechanisms results in the clinical manifestations of hypercalcemia or hypocalcemia.

The disorders of calcium homeostasis are related to the calcium content of the extracellular fluid, which contains less than 0.5% of the total body stores of calcium. Skeletal bone contains more than 99.5% of total body stores of calcium. ECF calcium is bound to plasma proteins to an extent of about 46%, with albumin being the primary binding protein. Unbound or ionized calcium is the only physiologically active form and is the fraction that is homeostatically regulated. Extracellular calcium is most commonly measured as the total serum calcium level, which includes both bound and unbound calcium.[47] The normal total calcium serum concentration range is 8.5–10.5 mg/dL.[2]

Any factor that alters the concentration of albumin or its binding of calcium may be expected to change the fraction of total serum calcium in the ionized form. The most significant cause of alteration in extent of calcium binding to albumin occurs in the setting of changing extracellular fluid pH. Metabolic alkalosis and respiratory alkalosis favor an increased binding of calcium to albumin, thus lowering the ionized free calcium fraction while leaving total serum calcium unchanged. This may result in clinically evident, symptomatic hypocalcemia.[47] Conversely, metabolic or respiratory acidosis decreases calcium-protein binding and results in increased ionized calcium. Hypoalbuminemic states are probably the most common cause of low laboratory values of serum calcium. Because of the decreased protein content, however, ionized calcium concentration may be normal. Thus, total serum calcium concentration must be evaluated in light of the serum albumin concentration. A general rule of thumb is that for each 1 g/dL that the serum albumin concentration is below 4 g/dL, total serum calcium concentration decreases by 0.8 mg/dL.[47,48]

HYPERCALCEMIA

Hypercalcemia (total serum calcium >10.5 mg/dL) may be due to a multitude of causes (Table 51.9). The most common causes of hypercalcemia are cancer and primary hyperparathyroidism. The incidence of hypercalcemia of cancer is 150 new cases per million persons per year, compared with an incidence of approximately 250 new cases of primary hyperparathyroidism per million persons per year.[49] Cancer-associated hypercalcemia is most commonly encountered in hospitalized patients, while primary hyperparathyroidism is often asymptomatic and first diagnosed in the ambulatory/outpatient environment.[49,50]

Etiology

Hypercalcemia of malignancy is most commonly observed in squamous cell carcinomas of the lung, head, and neck, hematologic malignancies such as myeloma and T-cell lymphomas, and carcinomas of ovary, kidney, bladder, and

TABLE 51.9. CAUSES OF HYPERCALCEMIA

Neoplasms	Drug induced
Bone metastasis	Thiazides
Breast	Lithium
Multiple myeloma	Vitamin A toxicity
Lymphoma	Vitamin D toxicity
Leukemia	Milk–alkali syndrome
Humoral induced	Calcium supplements
Ovary	Granulomatous disease
Kidney	Sarcoidosis
Lung	Tuberculosis
Head and neck	Berylliosis
Esophagus	Histoplasmosis
Cervix	Coccidiodomycosis
Lymphoproliferative disease	Endocrine disorders
Multiple endocrine neoplasia	Hyperthyroidism
Pheochromocytoma	Adrenal insufficiency
Hyperparathyroidism	Miscellaneous
Primary	Immobilization
Tertiary	Paget's disease
After renal transplant	Familial hypocalciuric hypercalcemia

breast.[51] Ten to 20% of cancer patients develop hypercalcemia during the course of the disease.[52] The most frequent types of malignancy-associated with hypercalcemia are carcinomas of the lung and breast.[49] The most common example of a hematologic cancer associated with hypercalcemia is multiple myeloma, with 20–30% of patients developing hypercalcemia.[49] In most patients with malignancy-associated hypercalcemia, there is evidence for an increase in resorption of calcium from bone.[51] Both metastatic involvement of the skeleton and humoral factors produced by tumors thus contribute to the increase in calcium.[51]

Hyperparathyroidism is the most common cause of hypercalcemia in the general population. Increased levels of circulating parathyroid hormone are associated with increased gastrointestinal calcium absorption, renal tubular calcium reabsorption, and calcium resorption from bone. Primary hyperparathyroidism is the result of parathyroid carcinoma in only 5% of cases. Benign parathyroid adenomas account for 70–85% of cases of hyperparathyroidism, with parathyroid hyperplasia accounting for the remaining 15%.[47,53]

Clinical Presentation

Mild to moderate hypercalcemia with serum calcium concentrations of less than 13 mg/dL may often be asymptomatic, as is usually the case in drug-induced hypercalcemia and the vast majority of patients with hyperparathyroidism.[47] The signs and symptoms of hypercalcemia may differ depending on the acuteness of onset of elevated serum calcium levels.[54] Symptoms of hypercalcemia associated with malignancy usually have an acute presentation, because the onset of hypercalcemia is often very rapid. The patients may infrequently present in hypercalcemic crisis, manifested by the acute onset of severe hypercalcemia, acute renal failure, and obtundation.[47] If untreated, hypercalcemic crisis may progress to oliguric renal failure, coma, and malignant ventricular arrhythmias, which may result in death.[47] Hypercalcemia more frequently presents with a symptom complex characterized by anorexia, nausea and vomiting, constipation, polyuria, polydipsia, and nocturia.[47] Polyuria and polydipsia secondary to a urinary concentrating defect constitute one of the most frequent renal effects of hypercalcemia.[47] Disorders associated with long-standing hypercalcemia (i.e., hyperparathyroidism) are more likely to present with metastatic calcification, nephrolithiasis, and chronic renal insufficiency caused by deposition of calcium phosphate in soft tissue.[47]

The electrocardiographic changes associated with hypercalcemia include shortening of the QT interval, and coving of the ST-T wave.[47] Very high serum calcium concentrations may cause T-wave widening, indicating a repolarization defect that may be associated with spontaneous ventricular tachyarrhythmias.[47] Sensitivity to the pharmacologic and toxic actions of digitalis may be enhanced in the setting of hypercalcemia.[55]

Treatment

The indications for treatment of hypercalcemia are dependent on the degree of hypercalcemia, acuteness of development of hypercalcemia, and presence or absence of symptoms. Patients with hypercalcemic crisis or symptomatic hypercalcemia should be treated immediately. Asymptomatic patients with mild hypercalcemia may be carefully observed, especially if treatment for the underlying condition (i.e., malignancy) is initiated.

A rational treatment approach to therapy for hypercalcemia is outlined in Fig. 51.6. Effective treatment begins with attention to the underlying disorder. Patients with primary hyperparathyroidism often require surgery, patients with malignancy often require reduction of tumor load, while patients with drug-associated hypercalcemia generally respond to discontinuation of the offending agent. The pharmacologic therapy of hypercalcemia should be individualized according to the patient's presentation, symptoms, and underlying disease.

Few comparative studies of the different agents available for treatment of hypercalcemia exist; thus, treatment modalities vary from center to center. In patients with functioning kidneys, the cornerstone of treatment is rehydration with normal saline. Patients with symptomatic hypercalcemia are often dehydrated secondary to vomiting and polyuria; thus rehydration with saline-containing fluids

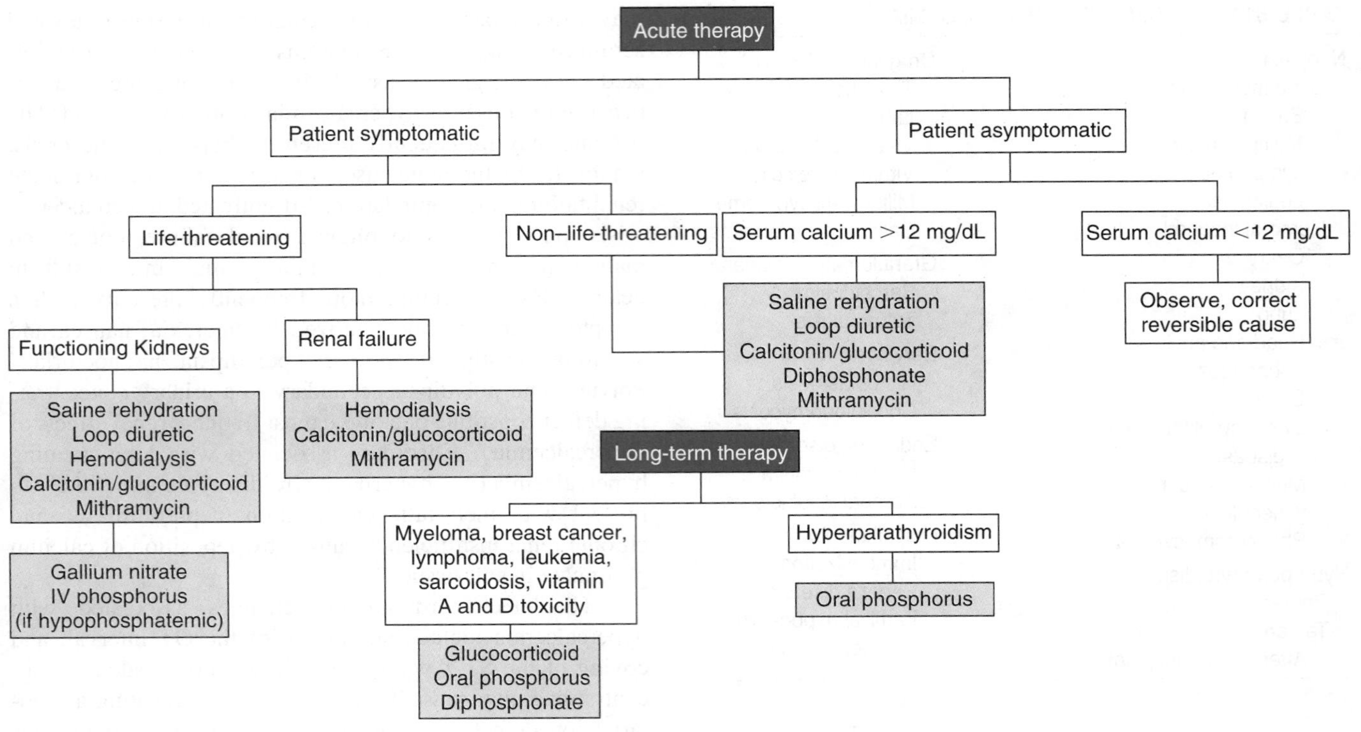

Figure 51.6. Approach to the hypercalcemic patient.

is necessary to interrupt the stimulus for sodium and calcium reabsorption in the kidney tubule. Rehydration can be accomplished by the infusion of normal saline at rates of 200–300 mL/h, checking for continued dehydration or fluid overload by monitoring fluid intake and output or by central venous pressure monitoring. Once rehydration has been accomplished, loop diuretics such as furosemide (40–80 mg intravenously every 1–4 hours) may be instituted to increase urine output to a goal of 200–250 mL/h.[54] Loop diuretics, such as furosemide, block calcium reabsorption in the thick ascending loop of Henle and augment the calciuric effect of saline alone.[52] Loop diuretics should be employed only after the patient has been fully rehydrated, because the use of a diuretic may lead to further reduction in glomerular filtration rate and a consequential reduction in clearance of calcium.[50,54] Potassium chloride should be added to the saline solution after rehydration is accomplished to maintain normokalemia. Serum magnesium levels should also be monitored, and magnesium replacement instituted if diuretic-induced hypomagnesemia occurs. Rehydration with saline and administration of furosemide often leads to decreases of 2–3 mg/dL in total serum calcium within 24–48 hours.[50]

Patients with acute life-threatening hypercalcemia crisis will require rapid reduction of serum calcium concentration. The chelating agent ethylenediaminetetraacetate (EDTA) reduces ionized calcium immediately; however, use of this agent is not recommended because of the possibility of renal tubular damage.[54] Intravenous phosphate may rapidly reduce ionized calcium concentrations through the formation of insoluble calcium phosphate salts. Intravenous phosphate is extremely hazardous, because extraskeletal precipitation of calcium phosphate may result in metastatic calcification, hypotension, acute renal failure, or death.[47,52] Intravenous phosphates should be reserved for the extraordinary patient with severe hypercalcemia and hypophosphatemia unresponsive to other measures. If employed, doses of intravenous phosphorus should be initiated at 400–800 mg of elemental phosphorus infused over 12–24 hours. Therapy must be monitored carefully with measurement of calcium, phosphorus, and creatinine on a daily basis; therapy should be withheld when serum phosphorus values reach a midnormal range.[50] If rapid reduction of ionized calcium levels is indicated, hemodialysis with calcium-free dialysate solutions may rapidly reduce serum calcium concentrations.[50]

Fortunately, life-threatening hypercalcemic crisis is rare; thus, agents that decrease bone resorption or decrease intestinal calcium absorption are preferred over the more toxic EDTA and intravenous phosphorus therapies. Therapy can be subdivided into agents employed in the acute situation versus those utilized chronically. Acute, short-term therapy with calcitonin is effective in rapidly reducing serum calcium levels. Calcitonin may be administered subcutaneously or intramuscularly in doses of four Medical Research Council (MRC) units/kg every 12 hours, or intravenously by a constant infusion at rates of 10–12 MRC units per hour. Calcitonin administration is rarely accompanied by nausea and/or allergic reaction.[50] Calcitonin has a rapid onset of action (within 1–2 hours); however, the degree and extent of serum calcium level reduction are often unpredictable.[56] Calcitonin therapy is frequently associated with tachyphylaxis, however, combination of corticosteroid therapy with calcitonin may prolong calcitonin's actions.[56]

Mithramycin (plicamycin), a potent cytotoxic antibiotic, inhibits osteoclast-mediated bone resorption by inhibition of DNA-directed RNA synthesis of proteins.[54] Mithramycin may be administered at a dose of 25 mcg/kg via intravenous infusion over 1–3 hours in saline or 5% dextrose solution.[50,52,54] Serum calcium levels begin to fall within 12 hours of a mithramycin dose with the peak effect generally occurring within 48–96 hours.[50,51] The most common adverse effects associated with mithramycin are thrombocytopenia, inhibition of platelet function, renal toxicity, and hepatotoxicity.[56] Toxicity has not been reported with single antihypercalcemic doses in patients with normal bone marrow, renal, and hepatic function.[50] Mithramycin should probably be limited to short-term therapy in patients who have not responded to hydration and diuretics.[52] Safe long-term therapy with mithramycin has been reported; however, therapy should probably be limited to a period of 2–3 weeks to minimize toxicity.[50,57] Repeated doses may be given every 3–4 days as needed, along with frequent determinations of complete blood count, liver function, and renal function. Mithramycin should be avoided in patients with thrombocytopenia, liver disease, or renal disease.

Biphosphonates (etidronate and pamidronate) and the bisphosphonate (alendronate) block bone resorption very efficiently, render the hydroxyapatite crystal of bone mineral resistant to hydrolysis by phosphatases, and also inhibit osteoclasts and their precursors via an intracellular mechanism.[50] Etidronate when administered in doses of 7.5 mg/kg/d by slow intravenous infusion over 3 hours has been shown to be effective in the therapy of hypercalcemia of malignancy.[58] Treatment may be necessary for 4–5 days to decrease serum calcium levels to normal, thus calcitonin therapy may be necessary if rapid serum level reduction is required.[58] Pamidronate is very effective in controlling hypercalcemia associated with malignancy and slightly more effective than etidronate.[51] The usual dose of pamidronate is 60–90 mg as an IV infusion given over 24 hours. Pamidronate also has the advantage of single-dose therapy and is currently the biphosphonate of choice.[51] Data on the use of these agents for maintenance therapy are limited; however, pamidronate has demonstrated more promise than etidronate.[51]

Gallium nitrate is indicated for the treatment of symptomatic hypercalcemia of malignancy not responsive to hydration therapy. Gallium nitrate inhibits bone resorption, and may be superior to calcitonin in inducing normocalcemia.[51] Gallium nitrate may provide a longer duration of normocalcemia compared to etidronate; however, further studies are needed to clarify the duration of these agents.[51] Gallium nitrate is usually administered as a continuous IV infusion at a dose of 200 mg/m^2/d for 5 consecutive days. Gallium nitrate is potentially nephrotoxic, especially if administered with other nephrotoxic drugs.

Glucocorticoids are usually effective in the treatment of hypercalcemia resulting from multiple myeloma, leukemia, lymphoma, sarcoidosis, and hypervitaminoses A and D.[50,57] The mechanisms of glucocorticoid actions include direct tumor lysing, interference in production of osteoclast-activating factor, and interference in metabolism of vitamin D_2 to calcitriol.[47,50,52] Daily doses of 40–60 mg of prednisone or the equivalent have been effective. The disadvantages of glucocorticoid therapy are a lag time of 5–10 days before onset of hypocalcemic effect, potential immunosuppressive and catabolic effects, and skeletal demineralization and osteolysis.[50] Treatment of hypercalcemia with inhibitors of prostaglandin synthesis, such as indomethacin, is rarely effective and thus not recommended.[52] The administration of oral phosphorus is minimally effective in the chronic treatment of hypercalcemia associated with hyperparathyroidism and malignancy.[56] Long-term administration of oral phosphorus should be used cautiously because the calcium-phosphate crystals may precipitate in the kidneys or other major organs; thus serum calcium, phosphorus, and creatinine should be monitored closely.

HYPOCALCEMIA

Hypocalcemia (total serum calcium less than 8.5 mg/dL) occurs when the normal homeostatic mechanisms are disrupted. The incidence of total serum hypocalcemia in ICU patients ranges from 70–90%; however, the occurrence rate of ionized hypocalcemia is more variable and ranges from 15–50% in different reports.[59]

Etiology

Hypocalcemia results from alteration of the effect of parathyroid hormone and vitamin D on the target end organs (bone, gut, and kidney) (Table 51.10). The majority of cases of hypocalcemia are due to vitamin D deficiency states and hypoparathyroidism.

Vitamin D and its metabolites play an important role in the maintenance of extracellular calcium concentrations and in normal skeletal structure and mineralization. On a worldwide basis, the most common cause of hypocalcemia is nutritional vitamin D deficiency. In malnourished populations, this is manifested by rickets and osteomalacia. Nutritional vitamin D deficiency is uncommon in Western societies because of the supplementation of milk with ergo-

TABLE 51.10. CAUSES OF HYPOCALCEMIA

Hypoalbuminemia
Hypoparathyroidism
- Surgical
- Infiltrative
- Idiopathic
- Pseudohypoparathyroidism
- Pseudoidiopathic

Hypomagnesemia
Hyperphosphatemia
Pancreatitis
Intestinal malabsorption
Drugs
- Oral phosphorus
- Furosemide
- Calcitonin
- Mithramycin
- Drugs causing hypomagnesemia
- Phenytoin
- Barbiturates

Hungry bone syndrome
- Recovery from parathyroid surgery

Vitamin D deficiency
- Nutritional
- Malabsorption
- Liver disease
  - Decreased production of 25-OH-vitamin D_3
- Increased metabolism of 25-OH-vitamin D_3
  - Phenytoin, barbiturates
  - Accelerated loss of 25-OH-vitamin D_3
  - Nephrotic syndrome
- Decreased production of 1,25-$(OH)_2$-vitamin D_3
  - Renal disease
  - Hereditary vitamin D–dependent rickets
- Decreased end-organ response of 1,25-$(OH)_2$-vitamin D_3
  - Hereditary

calciferol.[60] The most common cause of vitamin D deficiency is GI disease resulting in vitamin D and calcium malabsorption.[61] Gastric surgery, chronic pancreatitis, small-bowel disease, and intestinal resection and bypass surgery have all been associated with decreased levels of vitamin D and metabolites.[47] Decreased production of 1,25-dihydroxyvitamin D_3 may occur as a result of a hereditary defect resulting in vitamin D-dependent rickets. It also can occur secondary to chronic renal insufficiency where insufficient 1 α-hydroxylase enzyme is available for the production of the most active metabolite.[62,63] Treatment of hypocalcemia associated with chronic renal failure is reviewed in Chapter 44.

Symptomatic hypocalcemia most commonly occurs because of parathyroid gland dysfunction secondary to surgical procedures involving the thyroid, parathyroid, and neck.[60] Hypocalcemia in these postsurgical patients is generally transient in nature.[60] Serum calcium concentration should be monitored carefully during the first 24 hours following such surgeries.

Proper assessment of total serum calcium levels includes measurement of serum albumin concentrations. Hypoalbuminemia, which may be associated with many disease states, is probably the most common cause of laboratory hypocalcemia. Patients remain asymptomatic because the ionized fraction of serum calcium remains normal. Serum albumin concentration is a vital consideration in the assessment of the cause of hypocalcemia.

Hypomagnesemia of any cause may be associated with severe symptomatic hypocalcemia that is unresponsive to calcium replacement therapy (see section on Disorders of Magnesium Homeostasis). The magnesium cation plays an important role in the secretion of and skeletal response to parathyroid hormone. Serum magnesium levels are important in determining the cause of hypocalcemia.

Clinical Presentation

The clinical manifestations of hypocalcemia are characterized by a large degree of individual variability. The acuteness of the development of hypocalcemia plays a large role in whether or not symptoms will occur.[60] The more acute the drop in ionized calcium concentration, the more likely the patient will develop symptoms. Thus, acid–base balance plays a significant role in the likelihood of development of hypocalcemic symptoms, with alkalosis predisposing and acidosis inhibiting symptom development.

Hypocalcemia may manifest as neuromuscular, CNS, dermatologic, and cardiac sequelae.[47] Acute hypocalcemia is more likely to manifest as neuromuscular and cardiovascular symptoms, while chronic hypocalcemia may often present as CNS and dermatologic symptoms associated with an underlying chronic disease (i.e., hypoparathyroidism) (Table 51.11). The hallmark sign of acute hypocalcemia is tetany, due to enhanced peripheral neuromuscular irritability.[47] Tetany manifests as paresthesias around the mouth and in the extremities, muscle spasms and cramps, carpopedal spasms, and rarely as laryngospasm and bronchospasm.[47,60]

The cardiovascular manifestations of hypocalcemia result in electrocardiographic changes characterized by a prolonged QT interval and symptoms of decreased myocardial contractility often associated with congestive heart failure.[64] Both acute and chronic hypocalcemia may result in a reversible syndrome characterized by acute myocardial failure. Refractory congestive heart failure may also be precipitated by hypocalcemia.

Treatment

Treatment of hypocalcemia is dependent on identification of the pathogenesis of the disorder, acuteness of onset, and presence and severity of symptoms. Hypocalcemia associated with hypoalbuminemia requires no treatment, because

TABLE 51.11. SIGNS AND SYMPTOMS OF HYPOCALCEMIA

Central nervous system
- Fatigue
- Irritability
- Memory loss
- Depression
- Confusion
- Delusion
- Hallucinations
- Areflexia
- Seizures

Neuromuscular tetany
- Perioral paresthesias
- Carpopedal spasm
- Muscle spasms
- Cramps

Latent tetany
- Positive Chvostek's sign
- Positive Trousseau's sign
- Weakness

Ocular
- Cataracts

Cardiovascular
- Prolonged QT interval
- Acute myocardial failure
- Hypotension

Skin
- Hair loss
- Brittle, grooved nails
- Eczema
- Psoriasis
- Hyperpigmentation with dermatitis

ionized plasma calcium concentrations are normal. Acute, symptomatic hypocalcemia requires parenteral administration of soluble calcium salts. The initial goal of therapy is to administer doses of 200–300 mg of elemental calcium intravenously and repeat until symptoms (i.e., tetany) are fully controlled.[47] This may be provided by the administration of 1 g of calcium chloride or 2–3 g of calcium gluconate. Calcium gluconate is generally preferred over calcium chloride for peripheral venous administration because extravasation of calcium chloride may result in tissue necrosis.[47] Disadvantages to the use of calcium gluconate are the small amounts of elemental calcium per volume and a less predictable, slightly smaller increase in plasma ionic calcium compared with calcium chloride. Intravenous calcium should be administered no faster than 30–60 mg of elemental calcium per minute, since rapid administration may be associated with hypotension, bradycardia, or cardiac asystole. Calcium should not be added to bicarbonate-containing solutions because of the possibility of precipitation. If symptoms recur after initial IV calcium replacement, a slow IV infusion of 15 mg/kg of elemental calcium over 4–6 hours may be administered.[47] Intravenous calcium administration should be used with caution in patients receiving digitalis glycosides, because of the possibility of cardiac arrhythmias.

Once acute hypocalcemia is corrected by parenteral administration, further treatment modalities should be individualized according to the cause of hypocalcemia. If hypomagnesemia is present, magnesium supplementation is indicated (see Disorders of Magnesium Homeostasis). Chronic hypocalcemia associated with hypoparathyroidism and vitamin D-deficient states may be managed by oral calcium and vitamin D supplementation. Therapy is begun with 2–4 g/d of elemental calcium.[47] Elemental calcium content differs among the available oral calcium salts (Table 51.12). Flavored calcium carbonate antacids such as Tums are often preferred as calcium supplements. These products contain a higher elemental calcium content compared with other salts and the flavoring may increase palatability.[65] If serum calcium does not normalize, a vitamin D preparation should be added. A comparison of vitamin D preparations is found in Chapter 44.

Treatment of hypocalcemia associated with vitamin D-deficient states should be individualized. In patients with malabsorption, vitamin D requirements vary markedly, and large doses may be required. In contrast, vitamin D deficiency associated with anticonvulsant medication may be corrected with smaller doses of vitamin D (e.g., 5000–10,000 units of ergocalciferal per day).[47] The treatment of vitamin D deficiency associated with chronic renal failure is discussed in Chapter 44. Situations in which 25-hydroxylase activity is reduced (e.g., hepatic disease) may require treatment with calcitriol (1,25-dihydroxyvitamin D_3). In selected cases, calcium supplementation may be required if vitamin D replacement alone is ineffective in returning calcium concentrations to normal.

Adverse effects of oral calcium and vitamin D supplementation include hypercalcemia and hypercalciuria, especially in the hypoparathyroid patient, where the renal calcium-sparing effect of parathyroid hormone is absent. Hypercalciuria may increase the risk of calcium stone formation and nephrolithiasis in susceptible patients (see Chapter 48). Addition of thiazide diuretics in patients at risk for stone formation may result in reduction of both urinary calcium excretion and vitamin D requirement.[66]

TABLE 51.12. CALCIUM PREPARATIONS

Calcium salt	*Elemental Calcium per Gram of Salt* (mg)	(mEq)	Route
Calcium carbonate	400	20.0	PO
Calcium chloride	270	13.5	IV
Calcium citrate	211	10.6	PO
Calcium glubionate	64	3.2	PO
Calcium gluceptate	82	4.1	IV
Calcium gluconate	90	4.5	IV/PO
Calcium glycerophosphate	191	9.6	IV
Calcium lactate	130	6.5	PO
Calcium phosphate (dibasic anhydrous)	290	14.5	PO
Calcium phosphate (dibasic dihydrate)	230	11.5	PO
Calcium phosphate (tribasic)	400	20.0	PO

DISORDERS OF MAGNESIUM HOMEOSTASIS

Magnesium is ionically bound to the center of chlorophyll molecules; thus, the entire food chain and transfer of energy in biologic systems are dependent on its presence. Magnesium is an important cofactor for hundreds of enzyme systems, including all phosphate transfer reactions involving ATP.[67] Magnesium appears to modulate the neuromuscular activity of the calcium ion; indeed, magnesium has been called "nature's physiologic calcium blocker."[68] Magnesium is the fourth most plentiful cation and the second most abundant intracellular cation behind potassium. As the clinical significance of magnesium disorders becomes more clearly defined, the need for an understanding of the appropriate therapy for these disorders becomes vital.

Because only about 1% of total body magnesium resides in the ECF space, serum magnesium concentration provides only a rough index of total body magnesium stores. Magnesium is 30% bound to albumin; thus, in contrast to calcium, changes in albumin concentration have much less effect on serum magnesium concentration. Normal serum magnesium concentration is 1.5–2.0 mEq/L (1.8–2.4 mg/dL).[2]

The kidney is the primary regulator of magnesium balance in the body. Magnesium homeostasis is maintained by a balance of glomerular filtration and tubular reabsorption. Renal handling of magnesium seems to follow a tubular maximum mechanism similar to the renal handling of glucose. This tubular maximum is set very close to the filtered load of magnesium that is present at normal serum concentrations. Thus, small increases in serum magnesium concentration are associated with a rise in magnesium excretion.[69] Conversely, decreases in serum magnesium concentration result in the near disappearance of magnesium from the urine.

HYPERMAGNESEMIA

Hypermagnesemia results when magnesium intake exceeds the elimination capacity of the kidneys. Because of the tubular maximum threshold mechanism, hypermagnesemia occurs only in the setting of renal dysfunction or excessive exogenous administration of magnesium. The prevalence of hypermagnesemia (serum magnesium >2 mEq/L) in hospital patients has been reported to range from 5.7–9.3%.[70,71] Fortunately, symptomatic hypermagnesemia is an uncommon clinical problem.[72]

Etiology

Hypermagnesemia most commonly occurs in the setting of renal insufficiency, when glomerular filtration rates are less than 30 mL/min.[47] Use of magnesium-containing laxatives or antacids can lead to hypermagnesemia in renal failure patients.[68] Patients in the intensive care unit with multiple-system organ failure receiving magnesium-containing antacids for stress ulcer prophylaxis or magnesium-containing parenteral fluids (i.e., total parenteral nutrition) constitute a population of patients particularly at risk for developing hypermagnesemia. Parenteral treatment of eclampsia with magnesium sulfate or its use in the therapy of preterm labor can potentially cause hypermagnesemia.[68] Other causes of hypermagnesemia are listed in Table 51.13.

Clinical Presentation

Hypermagnesemia manifests as neuromuscular, cardiovascular, and endocrine effects (Table 51.14). Signs and symptoms of hypermagnesemia occur when plasma magnesium concentration exceeds 4 mEq/L. The neuromuscular manifestations of hypermagnesemia can be ascribed to neuromuscular blockade. Hypermagnesemia may cause hypotonic, diminished, or absent deep tendon reflexes, varying degrees of muscle weakness, and complete flaccid paralysis with resultant respiratory depression, depending on the serum concentration of magnesium attained.[47,67,72] Because deep tendon reflexes disappear before the appearance of paralysis of voluntary muscle, monitoring of the deep tendon reflex is a useful tool to evaluate magnesium toxicity. CNS depression may result in varying degrees of lethargy and sedation, which may progress to stupor and coma, especially at high (≥6 mEq/L) serum magnesium concentrations.[73]

Excessively high magnesium concentrations may affect heart rate, cardiac conduction, and blood pressure. Hypotension and cutaneous vasodilation may occur above serum levels of 3 mEq/L.[47,74] A variety of mechanisms have been implicated, including vascular smooth muscle relaxation and sympathetic blockade.[67] Sinus bradycardia, first-degree heart block, nodal rhythms, or bundle branch block may occur at serum magnesium concentrations of 5–10 mEq/L or greater.[72] Complete heart block progressing to asystole and cardiac arrest may occur at serum concentrations greater than 14–15 mEq/L.[72,74]

TABLE 51.13. CAUSES OF HYPERMAGNESEMIA

Decreased renal excretion	Other
Acute renal failure	Lithium therapy
Chronic renal failure with exogenous intake	Hypothyroidism
	Milk–alkali syndrome
Excessive intake	Addison's disease
Treatment of toxemia of pregnancy	Viral hepatitis
Ureteral irrigants (hemiacidrin)	Acute diabetic ketoacidosis
Cathartics	

TABLE 51.14. CLINICAL FINDINGS ASSOCIATED WITH HYPERMAGNESEMIA

Serum Magnesium Level (mEq/L)	Cardiovascular	Neuromuscular	Other
>3	Hypotension		Nausea
	Cutaneous vasodilation		Vomiting
>4	QT interval prolongation		Skin warmth
>4.5	Bradycardia		
	First-degree heart block		
	Nodal rhythms		
	Bundle branch block		
>5	QRS interval prolongation	Sedation	
	PR interval prolongation	Hypotonia	
		Hyporeflexia	
>7		Somnolence	
>10		Coma	
		Muscle paralysis	
		Respiratory depression	
>14	Complete heart block		
>15	Asystole		

Treatment

Guidelines for the treatment of hypermagnesemia are based on clinical signs and symptoms and the degree of elevation of serum magnesium. Treatment is indicated in symptomatic patients with serum magnesium levels of 5–8 mEq/L, and in all patients whose serum level is greater than 8 mEq/L regardless of symptoms.[74] Because calcium directly antagonizes the neuromuscular and cardiovascular effects of magnesium, intravenous administration of calcium in doses of 100–200 mg of elemental calcium is indicated.[74] Reversal of symptomatic hypermagnesemia after calcium administration is rapid but transient in nature; thus, repeated doses of calcium may be necessary in life-threatening situations. Hemodialysis is the treatment of choice in all patients with renal dysfunction.[72] Supportive care with mechanical ventilation, pressors, and cardiac pacemakers may be necessary until serum magnesium concentrations are lowered. In patients with adequate renal function and non–life-threatening hypermagnesemia, promotion of renal magnesium excretion may be accomplished by administering IV saline and furosemide.

HYPOMAGNESEMIA

Hypomagnesemia occurs when magnesium intake is less than renal excretion, or when the renal magnesium-conserving mechanisms fail. Hypomagnesemia (serum magnesium <1 mEq/L) is a common clinical disorder but is frequently overlooked because of the typically complex clinical setting in which it occurs.[47] Because less than 1% of total body magnesium is extracellular, serum magnesium concentration may not always reflect the true amount of magnesium in the body.[75] The prevalence of hypomagnesemia among patients admitted to a hospital is approximately 10% with up to a 65% prevalence in intensive care units.[75]

Etiology

Magnesium depletion is almost always secondary to disturbances of either the intestinal tract or the kidney. Table 51.15 illustrates many of the potential causes of hypomagnesemia. Magnesium conservation in normal subjects is extremely effective; therefore, dietary magnesium deprivation rarely leads to significant magnesium depletion unless it is prolonged.[47] Generalized malabsorption syndromes associated with hypomagnesemia occur in various intestinal mucosal diseases (e.g., coeliac sprue, Whipple's disease, radiation enteritis), massive intestinal resection, and pancreatic insufficiency.[47,72,76] Magnesium losses exceeding intake may produce hypomagnesemia. GI disorders may result in hypomagnesemia, secondary to the loss of intestinal fluids (magnesium 14 mEq/L) or biliary, gastric, and pancreatic fluids (0.4–1.1 mEq/L).[47]

Renal magnesium wasting may be due to intrinsic tubular disorders and drug-induced, hormone-induced, and ion- or nutrient-induced renal tubular magnesium losses. Particularly severe hypomagnesemia may occur during the diuresis associated with the recovery phase of oliguric acute tubular necrosis, the postobstructive period, and the postrenal transplantation period.[77]

The most frequent cause of renal magnesium wasting is long-term diuretic therapy.[47] Fifty percent of patients

TABLE 51.15. CAUSES OF HYPOMAGNESEMIA

Gastrointestinal	Drug-induced renal losses
Reduced intake	Aminoglycosides
Protein-calorie malnutrition	Amphotericin B
Total parenteral nutrition without magnesium	Cyclosporine
Prolonged parenteral fluid administration without magnesium	Diuretics
Alcoholism	Digitalis
Reduced absorption	Cisplatin
Primary hypomagnesemia	Alcohol
Malabsorption syndromes (e.g., tropical sprue, celiac disease, radiation enteritis, intestinal lymphectasia)	Hormone-induced renal losses
Short-bowel syndrome (e.g., small-bowel resection, ileal bypass)	Hyperparathyroidism
Pancreatic insufficiency	Hyperthyroidism
Increased loss	Aldosteronism
Excessive vomiting	Hypoparathyroidism
Prolonged nasogastric suction	"Hungry bone syndrome" after parathyroidectomy
Excessive laxative use	**Internal redistribution**
Intestinal and biliary fistulas	Diabetic ketoacidosis
Prolonged diarrhea (ulcerative colitis, Crohn's disease, cancer of the colon)	Glucose, amino acid, insulin administration
Renal	Massive blood transfusion (citrate)
Primary tubular disorders	Pancreatitis with lipidemia (magnesium soap)
Primary renal magnesium wasting	**Other**
Bartter's syndrome	Excessive sweating and lactation
Renal tubular acidosis	Hypercalcemia and hypercalciuria
Diuretic phase of acute tubular necrosis	Phosphate depletion
Postobstructive diuresis	Chronic alcoholism
Post–renal transplant diuresis	ECF volume expansion
Glomerulonephritis	
Pyelonephritis	
Nephrotic syndrome	

receiving long-term diuretic therapy develop hypomagnesemia.[78] Patients at highest risk for development of hypomagnesemia from chronic diuretic therapy include elderly patients, alcohol abusers, and patients consuming diets low in magnesium.[78] Other therapeutic agents associated with magnesium wasting include aminoglycosides, amphotericin B, foscarnet, pentamidine, *cis*-platinum, and cyclosporine.[79,80]

The most common clinical setting for hypomagnesemia is acute and chronic alcoholism.[47,81] The causes of hypomagnesemia in the alcoholic are multifactorial and include malnutrition, dietary magnesium deficiency, vomiting and diarrhea, increased urinary magnesium excretion, hypophosphatemia, hyperaldosteronism, and pancreatic insufficiency.[81] In addition, upon entry of alcoholic patients into the hospital, acute ethanol withdrawal and IV glucose therapy may lead to further reductions in ECF magnesium levels.[47] It appears likely that magnesium deficiency along with other metabolic disorders associated with alcoholism and alcohol withdrawal contribute to the delirium tremens associated with alcohol withdrawal.[47,81] Monitoring of serum magnesium concentration is indicated in alcoholic patients, and supplementation is recommended in all patients undergoing acute alcohol withdrawal.[81]

Clinical Presentation

Clinical manifestations of hypomagnesemia are generally not seen until serum magnesium concentrations approach 1 mEq/L (Table 51.16).[8] Patients with magnesium depletion may develop symptoms suddenly and without warning, even if hypomagnesemia has been chronic.[82] Magnesium deficiency can result in various nonspecific neuromuscular signs and symptoms. Concomitant hypocalcemia and hypokalemia may contribute as well. Neuromuscular signs and symptoms of hypomagnesemia are the converse of those of hypermagnesemia. Neuromuscular hyperactivity is often the predominant complaint of patients with magnesium deficiency.[75]

Several studies have suggested an association between dietary magnesium deficiency from drinking water with decreased magnesium content ("soft water") and sudden death from coronary artery disease.[83] Atrial or ventricular arrhythmias may occur in magnesium deficiency.[75] Magnesium may play an important etiologic role in atypical

TABLE 51.16. CLINICAL MANIFESTATIONS OF HYPOMAGNESEMIA

Neuromuscular	Cardiac
Muscle twitching and tremor	Premature ventricular beats
Muscle weakness	Ventricular fibrillation
Hyperreflexia	Ventricular tachycardia
Paresthesias	Torsades de pointes
Positive Chvostek's and Trousseau's signs	Predisposition to digitalis-mediated arrhythmias
Tetany	Supraventricular tachycardia
Seizures	Electrocardiographic changes (PR, QT prolongation, widened QRS)
Coma	Coronary artery spasm
Nystagmus, ataxia, vertigo	Calcium and potassium
Choreoathetoid movements	Refractory hypocalcemia
Psychiatric	Refractory hypokalemia
Apathy	
Depression	
Delirium	
Agitation	
Confusion	
Hallucinations	

ventricular tachycardia (i.e., torsades de pointes), and successful therapy of this potentially lethal arrhythmia with magnesium has been reported.[84] Hypomagnesemia may also exacerbate digitalis toxicity-induced arrhythmias. The finding of a 19% frequency of hypomagnesemia in hospitalized patients receiving digitalis combined with the potential life-threatening manifestations of digitalis toxicity has prompted recommendations for routine monitoring and supplementation of both potassium and magnesium in patients receiving digitalis.[85]

The electrocardiograph changes associated with hypomagnesemia are nonspecific and include wide QRS complexes and tall, peaked T waves in moderate magnesium deficiency, and prolonged PR, QRS, and QT intervals, ST-segment depression, and flat, broad T waves with prominent U waves in severe magnesium deficiency.[76] These electrocardiographic changes probably reflect alterations in intracellular potassium and calcium in the myocardium.

Magnesium is important in regulating intracellular potassium content.[75] Movement of these intracellular cations appears to be closely linked; attempts to replace potassium deficits in the presence of magnesium deficiency are difficult. Magnesium deficiency impairs the Na^+/K^+-ATPase pump and allows potassium to escape from the cell.[81] It is estimated that the incidence of hypomagnesemia in hypokalemic patients ranges from 38–42%.[85]

Hypocalcemia is a prominent manifestation of magnesium deficiency perhaps due to an altered equilibrium between calcium in extracellular fluid and bone, impaired release of parathyroid hormone, impaired formation of parathyroid hormone, and end-organ resistance to parathyroid hormone.[81] Serum calcium concentration should be assessed if hypomagnesemia is discovered.

Treatment

Magnesium supplementation may be administered via the intravenous, intramuscular, or oral route (depending on severity of hypomagnesemia, presence of symptoms, and patient tolerance) (Table 51.17). Patients with nonsymptomatic hypomagnesemia, levels greater than 1 mEq/L (1.2 mg/dL) may be treated with oral magnesium supplements. However, diarrhea may be a limiting factor with oral magnesium therapy. Patients with serum magnesium levels less than 1 mEq/L (1.2 mg/dL) or who are symptomatic should receive parenteral magnesium therapy.

Regardless of route of administration, assessment of renal function is indicated. Patients with renal insufficiency should be treated with lower doses and must be monitored by measuring serum or plasma levels frequently.[75] Even if severe magnesium deficiency is present, approximately 50% of an administered dose is excreted in the urine.[47] Magnesium replacement must thus be continued over 3–5 days, and subsequent maintenance magnesium administration should continue in patients who are unable to eat or who have continuing magnesium losses. Rapid IV injection of magnesium may be associated with flushing, sweating, and a sensation of warmth; thus, rapid bolus injection of magnesium should be avoided. Direct IV administration of 50% magnesium sulfate may produce pain and venosclerosis; therefore, it should be diluted to 20% before administration. Because intramuscular injections are painful, involve multiple punctures, and have no therapeutic advantage over the IV route, intramuscular therapy should be

TABLE 51.17. GUIDELINES FOR TREATMENT OF MAGNESIUM DEFICIENCY IN ADULTS

1. Serum magnesium <1 mEq/L (1.2 mg/dL) with life-threatening symptoms (seizure, arrhythmia)

   Day 1

   a. 2 g $MgSO_4$[a] mixed with 6 mL 0.9% NaCl in 10-mL syringe and administer IV push over 1 min
   b. Follow with 0.5 mEq Mg^{2+}/kg lean body weight IV infusion over 5–6 h, then 0.5 mEq Mg^{2+}/kg lean body weight IV infusion over 17–18 h

   Days 2–5

   0.5 mEq Mg^{2+}/kg lean body weight per day divided in maintenance IV fluids
2. Serum magnesium <1 mEq/L (1.2 mg/dL) without life-threatening symptoms

   Day 1

   Total of 1 mEq Mg^{2+}/kg lean body weight per day as continuous IV infusion, or divided and given IM every 4 h for five doses

   Days 2–5

   Total of 0.5 mEq Mg^{2+}/kg lean body weight IV infusion per day as continuous IV infusion or divided and given IM every 6–8 h
3. Serum magnesium >1 mEq/L (1.2 mg/dL) and <1.5 mEq/L (1.8 mg/dL) without symptoms

   As in No. 2, or

   a. Milk of Magnesia 5 mL four times daily as tolerated
   b. Magnesium-containing antacid 15 mL three times daily as tolerated
   c. Magnesium oxide tablets 300 mg four times daily, increase to two tablets four times daily as tolerated

[a] 1 g $MgSO_4$ = 8.1 mEq Mg^{2+}.

reserved for situations in which peripheral venous access is not readily available.

Disorders of Phosphorus Homeostasis

Phosphorus is an essential element in phospholipid cell membranes, nucleic acids, and phosphoproteins required for mitochondrial function.[86] Phosphorus regulates the intermediary metabolism of carbohydrates, fats, and proteins. Phosphorus also regulates enzymatic reactions including glycolysis, ammoniogenesis, and the 1-hydroxylation of 25-hydroxyvitamin D.[86] In addition, phosphorus regulates the amount of 2,3-diphosphoglycerate (2,3-DPG) in red blood cells. 2,3-DPG promotes the release of oxygen by hemoglobin thus delivering oxygen to tissues.[87] Phosphorus is the source of the high-energy bonds of ATP, thus fueling a wide variety of physiologic processes, including muscle contractibility, electrolyte transport, neurologic function, and other important biochemical reactions.[86] Considering its diverse biologic importance, it is not difficult to appreciate the clinical implications of disorders of phosphorus homeostasis.

Phosphorus is present in living organisms mainly as inorganic phosphate and organic phosphate esters. Because potassium is the major intracellular cation, phosphorus is the major intracellular anion. The majority of intracellular phosphorus exists as organic esters, mainly 2,3-DPG, adenosine and guanosine triphosphate, and fructose 1,6-diphosphate.[88] Only a small fraction of intracellular phosphorus exists as inorganic phosphate; however, this fraction is critical because it is the source from which ATP is resynthesized.[88] The majority of inorganic phosphate is located in the extracellular space. Normal serum phosphorus concentration in the adult is 3.0–4.5 mg/100 mL.[2] Extracellular inorganic phosphate is the prime determinant of intracellular phosphate; thus, small increments in the organic phosphate pool can profoundly alter both the extracellular and intracellular phosphate pools. Metabolic disturbances, hydrogen ion shifts, and hormones all can cause important syndromes. Because of these phenomena, the serum phosphorus level does not accurately reflect total body stores.[89]

Phosphorus excretion by the kidney is the single most important regulator of steady-state serum phosphorus levels. Renal excretion of phosphorus is regulated by glomerular filtration and active tubular reabsorption. Under normal conditions, 85–90% of filtered phosphate is reabsorbed, the majority in the early proximal tubule. Renal tubular reabsorption of phosphorus is inhibited by parathyroid hormone and 1,25-dihydroxyvitamin D_3.[86] Conversely, phosphorus reabsorption is increased by growth hormone and thyroxine.[90,91] Internal phosphorus balance (transcellular phosphate distribution) is also of importance in the maintenance of normal serum phosphorus, which may vary by as much as 2 mg/dL throughout the day, as the result of acute changes in transcellular distribution of phosphate influenced primarily by carbohydrate intake and insulin secretion.[86]

HYPERPHOSPHATEMIA

Hyperphosphatemia (serum phosphorus concentration greater than 4.5 mg/dL) occurs much less frequently than hypophosphatemia. Serum phosphorus concentration is so closely regulated by the kidneys that it is unusual for hyperphosphatemia to develop in patients with normal renal function. The most frequent causes of hyperphosphatemia are increases in phosphate entrance into the extracellular fluid via either exogenous administration or endogenous intracellular phosphate release, and decreased renal excretion of phosphate.

Etiology

The most common cause of hyperphosphatemia is a decrease in urinary phosphorus excretion secondary to decreased glomerular filtration rate.[92] Patients with excessive exogenous phosphorus administration or endogenous intracellular phosphorus release in the setting of acute renal failure may develop profound hyperphosphatemia. In patients with chronic progressive renal insufficiency, severe hyperphosphatemia is usually encountered in patients with advanced disease, when the glomerular filtration rate is less than 25 mL/min.[92] Patients with renal dysfunction thus have the greatest risk for developing hyperphosphatemia of any patient group.

Hypoparathyroidism results in increased renal tubular reabsorption of phosphorus and may result in hyperphosphatemia. Hyperphosphatemia associated with hypoparathyroidism is usually less severe than that associated with severe renal failure or excessive exogenous or endogenous introduction of phosphorus into the ECF space. Hypoparathyroidism is the most important cause of increased tubular phosphorus reabsorption.

Iatrogenic causes of hyperphosphatemia have been widely reported, and awareness of the phosphorus content of intravenous, oral, and rectally administered phosphorus-containing drugs can aid in the prevention of this cause of hyperphosphatemia. Sodium phosphate enemas may cause severe symptomatic hyperphosphatemia when administered to children.[93] In adults, hyperphosphatemia has been observed in patients ingesting laxatives containing phosphate salts.[94] Administration and retention of phosphate-containing enemas in patients with moderate and severe renal insufficiency has also been reported to cause hyperphosphatemia with severe symptoms.[95] Large doses of phosphorus administered intravenously to treat patients with hypercalcemia have also been reported to cause severe life-threatening hyperphosphatemia.[96]

Any disorder that causes disruption of skeletal muscle cells can release large amounts of phosphorus into the systemic circulation and cause hyperphosphatemia. Rhabdomyolysis (destruction of skeletal muscle) of any cause may result in the release of large amounts of phosphorus from intracellular stores. This condition is frequently associated with acute renal failure as well; thus, hyperphosphatemia of a severe degree may result.

Hyperphosphatemia is not uncommonly observed in patients undergoing treatment for acute leukemia and lymphomas.[92] Chemotherapeutic treatment of acute lymphoblastic leukemia may result in the release of large amounts of phosphorus into the systemic circulation secondary to lysis of lymphoblasts. Initiation of chemotherapy for Burkitt's lymphoma may also result in a rapid lysis of malignant cells, resulting in hyperphosphatemia, hyperuricemia, hyperkalemia, and hypocalcemia (tumor lysis syndrome).[92]

Diabetic ketoacidosis is an unappreciated but common cause of hyperphosphatemia. In one study, hyperphosphatemia was present in 94.7% of patients with diabetic ketoacidosis prior to the initiation of treatment.[97] However, with the institution of treatment, serum phosphorus levels decrease and patients may ultimately develop hypophosphatemia.

Clinical Presentation

Signs and symptoms of hyperphosphatemia can be related to the solubility of phosphorus and calcium. It has been estimated that the *in vivo* solubility product of calcium phosphate in mg/dL is about 70.[98] *In vivo* calcium phosphate solubility products greater than 58 pose a significant risk of calcium phosphate precipitation. Because of this relationship, the major effect of hyperphosphatemia is related to the development of hypocalcemia with its related consequences, as well as damage resulting from the deposition of calcium phosphate crystals. The calcium phosphate solubility relationship may be influenced by the acid–base status of the patient. An alkaline environment would be predicted to decrease the solubility product; conversely, an acidic environment would increase the solubility product of calcium phosphate.

Hypocalcemia associated with hyperphosphatemia is thought to be caused by deposition of calcium phosphate in the bone, in soft tissues, or possibly both.[48] Metastatic calcification leading to band keratopathy, "red eye," pruritus, vascular calcification, and periarticular calcification is most common in renal failure patients (see Chapter 44). In addition, soft tissue calcifications in the conjunctiva, skin, heart, cornea, lung, gastric mucosa, and kidney have been observed primarily in chronic renal failure patients.[92] Hyperphosphatemia associated with chronic renal disease may result in azotemic osteodystrophy (osteitis fibrosis cystica and osteomalacia) and is discussed in Chapter 44.

Treatment

The treatment of hyperphosphatemia should initially be directed at the correction of reversible factors and the treatment of the disease states associated with its development. Severe symptomatic hyperphosphatemia manifesting as hypocalcemia and tetany should be treated by the IV administration of calcium salts. In general, the most effective way to treat hyperphosphatemia itself is to decrease phosphate absorption in the lumen of the GI tract by the use of phosphate binders.[92] Antacids containing divalent cations are the agents most frequently used in the prevention and treatment of hyperphosphatemia. Magnesium salts should be avoided in patients with renal failure, and aluminum hydroxide and aluminum carbonate gels should be frequently utilized with caution because they are associated with anemia and CNS and bone disease (see Chapter 44). Short-term therapy with these agents is effective, the most frequent adverse effect being constipation. However, long-term treatment with aluminum-containing antacids in patients with chronic renal failure has led to concern over the toxic effects of aluminum accumulation. Thus, calcium salts are now the preferred phosphate binders in this population (see Chapter 44).

HYPOPHOSPHATEMIA

Hypophosphatemia can be differentiated on the basis of severity: Moderate hypophosphatemia is defined as serum phosphorus concentrations from 1–2.5 mg/dL, whereas severe hypophosphatemia is serum phosphorus concentrations of less than 1 mg/dL. Hypophosphatemia is an extremely common finding. Hypophosphatemia is found in approximately 2–3% of hospital admissions.[99] Hypophosphatemia has been reported to be present in 50% of hospitalized alcoholics.[99] Moderate hypophosphatemia is much more common than severe hypophosphatemia, and seldom causes recognizable effects.[100]

Etiology

The causes of hypophosphatemia are many, but can be divided into those associated with phosphate depletion, such as decreased intake or excess renal excretion; those associated with transcellular shifts, resulting in a redistribution of phosphate; or a combination of both[86] (Table 51.18). Patients with moderate hypophosphatemia generally lack significant symptomatology. While the causes of severe hypophosphatemia are relatively few, these conditions are frequently encountered in patients in the acute care setting and can be associated with life-threatening symptoms.

Phosphate-binding substances such as sucralfate, calcium carbonate, and aluminum/magnesium-containing antacids have the potential to bind large amounts of phosphorus in the gut. If phosphate-binding agents are ingested on a chronic basis in conjunction with a dietary phosphorus deficiency, severe hypophosphatemia may result.[100] Patients who are receiving long-term phosphate-binding agents, those with peptic ulcer disease or chronic renal failure, and those who may already possess moderate hypophosphatemia (alcoholics) are at highest risk for the development of severe hypophosphatemia.

TABLE 51.18. CONDITIONS CAUSING HYPOPHOSPHATEMIA

Inadequate phosphate intake
- Starvation
- Diet deficiency
- Malabsorption
- Vitamin D deficiency
- Vomiting
- Gastrectomy
- Phosphate-binding drugs[a]
  - Sucralfate
  - Antacids
  - Calcium salts

Intracellular phosphate shift
- Respiratory alkalosis[a]
  - Gram-negative bacteremia
  - Salicylate poisoning
  - Hepatic coma
  - Heat stroke
  - Thyrotoxicosis
  - Primary hyperventilation
  - Correction of respiratory acidosis
- Hyperalimentation[a]
- Nutritional recovery syndrome[a]
- Rapid tumor growth[a]
- Exogenous administration of
  - Insulin
  - Glucose
  - Fructose
  - Glycerol
  - Epinephrine
  - Gastrin
  - Lactate
  - Corticosteroids

Increased phosphate excretion
- Recovery from severe burns[a]
- Glucagen
- Diuretics
- Volume expansion
- Hypomagnesemia
- Hyperparathyroidism
- Hypothermia[a]
- Diabetic ketoacidosis[a]
- Acute gout
- Renal tubular defects
  - Heavy metal toxicity
  - Fanconi syndrome
  - Nephrotic syndrome
  - Multiple myeloma
  - Amyloidosis
- Aldosteronism
- Alcohol withdrawal[a]

[a]May be associated with severe hypophosphatemia.

The healing process associated with recovery from extensive third-degree burns is associated with a marked diuretic phase. This marked diuresis may be associated with an impressive loss of phosphate through the urine.[88,89,100] This recovery may also be associated with the development of an anabolic state as stress levels decrease and nutritional therapies take effect. Phosphorus is rapidly taken up by the new cells and severe hypophosphatemia may result.

Rapid refeeding of malnourished patients with high-carbohydrate, high-calorie nutritional diets with inadequate amounts of supplemental phosphorus may result in severe symptomatic hypophosphatemia. This phenomenon is especially significant in patients with other underlying risk factors for the development of hypophosphatemia such as alcoholism.[101] The etiology of severe hypophosphatemia associated with hyperalimentation and nutritional recovery may be separated into several phases: acute, rapid hypophosphatemia secondary to intracellular shifts of phosphorus resulting from glucose-induced insulin secretion and transcellular shift, and the gradual decrease in serum phosphorus concentration over 5–10 days secondary to tissue repair in the presence of phosphorus deprivation.[88] The development of severe hypophosphatemia secondary to hyperalimentation can be prevented by the administration of 12–15 mmol of phosphorus per liter of hyperalimentation solution or 15 mmol per 1000 Cal of dextrose administered.[101]

Severe and prolonged respiratory alkalosis may cause profound hypophosphatemia.[101] The mechanism of hypophosphatemia associated with respiratory alkalosis is thought to be secondary to intracellular shifts of phosphorus. Respiratory alkalosis is thought to contribute significantly to the hypophosphatemia observed during alcohol withdrawal.

Patients with diabetic ketoacidosis may present with hyperphosphatemia. With the institution of therapy, however, serum phosphorus levels may rapidly drop as phosphorus shifts back into the intracellular compartment. As the acidosis associated with the diabetic ketoacidotic state causes decomposition of organic compounds inside the cell, inorganic phosphorus is released into the plasma and subsequently excreted into the urine.[88] The combination of intracellular phosphorus loss and intracellular shift of phosphorus on initiation of treatment may cause severe hypophosphatemia.

Chronic ethanol abusers are prone to a variety of serum electrolyte disorders including hypocalcemia, hypomagnesemia, hypokalemia, and hypophosphatemia. The etiology of hypophosphatemia in the alcoholic patient is multifactorial. Malnutrition, poor dietary intake, diarrhea, vomiting, and the use of phosphate-binding antacids may contribute to the hypophosphatemia of alcoholism.[88,89,100] In addition, serum phosphorus levels may decrease after 2 or 3 days of hospitalization in the alcoholic patient with the institution of dextrose-containing IV fluids, as a result of an intracellular shift of phosphorus.[89] Hyperventilation associated with the alcohol withdrawal syndrome may also contribute to the development of hypophosphatemia in the alcoholic patient.[102] Alcoholic patients are particularly susceptible to the complications of hypophosphatemia such as rhabdomyolysis, which occur with great frequency in these patients.[102] Because this complication can be prevented by the administration of phosphorus, particular awareness of serum phosphorus concentration is indicated when dealing with the alcoholic patient.

Clinical Presentation

The clinical manifestations of severe hypophosphatemia are diverse and may affect many major organ systems (Table 51.19). It is likely that two primary biochemical abnormalities are responsible for most of the clinical manifestations of severe hypophosphatemia.[86] First, intracellular energy stores may be decreased secondary to depletion of intracellular ATP, which in itself is dependent on inorganic intracellular phosphate. Second, reduced RBC 2,3-diphosphoglycerate levels are associated with a shift to the left of the oxyhemoglobin saturation curve. This shift to the left is associated with a decrease in the release of oxygen to peripheral tissues and may result in tissue hypoxia.[100] These metabolic disorders can be seen in a wide variety of organ systems.

CNS manifestations of severe hypophosphatemia are compatible with a syndrome of metabolic encephalopathy.[88] A progressive syndrome of irritability, apprehension, weakness, numbness, paresthesias, dysarthria, confusion, obtundation, seizures, and coma has been described in patients with severe hypophosphatemia secondary to parenteral nutrition lacking phosphorus.[103]

Severe hypophosphatemia may result in significant dysfunction of skeletal muscle ranging from myalgia and weakness, with chronic hypophosphatemia, to potentially fatal rhabdomyolysis, with severe, acute hypophosphatemia.[99] Hypophosphatemia has resulted in acute respiratory failure secondary to respiratory muscle weakness and diaphragmatic contractile dysfunction has been demonstrated in patients with acute respiratory failure associated with concomitant hypophosphatemia.[104,105] Correction of hypophosphatemia has resulted in an increase in diaphragmatic function and reversal of acute respiratory failure.[104] Close assessment of serum phosphorus concentration is thus indicated in patients at risk for respiratory failure. Treatment of hypophosphatemia in respiratory failure patients may aid in successful weaning from the ventilator.

Cardiac muscle function has also been reported to be impaired in the setting of hypophosphatemia and has resulted in congestive cardiomyopathy.[99] Hypophosphatemia is a potentially reversible cause of heart failure and thus should be considered in patients with acute deterioration in ventricular function.

The hematologic abnormalities of hypophosphatemia constitute a major manifestation of the syndrome.[86] RBC manifestations of hypophosphatemia include decreased levels of 2,3-diphosphoglycerate, decreased RBC ATP, and alteration of RBC structure.[86,89,100] When RBC ATP

TABLE 51.19. MANIFESTATIONS OF SEVERE HYPOPHOSPHATEMIA

Central nervous system
Irritability
Apprehension
Weakness
Numbness
Paresthesias
Dysarthria
Confusion
Obtundation
Seizures
Coma
Pulmonary
Acute respiratory failure
Slow weaning from ventilator
Respiratory muscle fatigue
Cardiac
Congestive cardiomyopathy
Decreased contractility
Hepatic
Exacerbation of underlying hepatic insufficiency
Hepatocellular dysfunction
Gastrointestinal
Anorexia
Nausea
Emesis
Skeletal/muscle
Weakness
Myalgia
Rhabdomyolysis
Osteomalacia
Hematologic
Decreased RBC 2,3-diphosphoglycerate
Hemolysis
WBC dysfunction
Platelet dysfunction
Renal
Acute tubular necrosis if myoglobinemia and rhabdomyolysis are present
Bicarbonate and glucose wasting

decreases to below 15% of normal, cells become spherocytic and rigid and are trapped and destroyed in the spleen.[88,106] Therefore, hemolysis may be a manifestation of severe hypophosphatemia.

Reduction in ATP content of WBC may cause dysfunction of white blood cell mobility, chemotaxis, phagocytosis, and bacteria-killing ability.[86,88,89,100] WBC dysfunction may contribute to an increased risk of infection in hypophosphatemia patients.[99] Animal studies have demonstrated thrombocytopenia, shortened platelet survival time, alteration of clot retraction, and hemorrhage as manifestations of platelet dysfunction in the setting of hypophosphatemia.[89] The implications of hypophosphatemia on human platelet function however have not been determined.

Treatment

Treatment is guided by the presence or absence of symptoms and the severity of hypophosphatemia. Awareness of the clinical situations in which hypophosphatemia may be anticipated (alcoholism, diabetic ketoacidosis, glucose infusion) is of vital importance in preventing iatrogenic hypophosphatemia. Frequent serum phosphorus determinations should be made in patients at risk. The routine addition of phosphorus in concentrations of 12–15 mmol/L of IV hyperalimentation solution is of utmost importance for the prevention of severe hypophosphatemia, which may be associated with phosphorus-free hyperalimentation solutions.

Mild to moderate asymptomatic hypophosphatemia can be treated orally by the administration of oral phosphorus salts (Table 51.20). The dose-limiting adverse effect associated with oral phosphorus replacement is the development of an osmotic diarrhea. Patients with moderate hypophosphatemia and concomitant renal dysfunction should receive reduced daily oral doses (i.e., 1 g or approximately 30 mmol of phosphorus) with careful monitoring of serum phosphorus concentration.

Severe symptomatic hypophosphatemia should be treated with parenteral phosphorus replacement. Similar to potassium, estimation of total body phosphorus deficit is extremely difficult because phosphorus is an intracellular element. Recommendations for parenteral phosphorus replacement have evolved from a theoretical base as well as clinical experience.[107–110] Response to IV serum phosphorus supplementation is highly variable. The infusion of 9–15 mmol of phosphorus (0.15–0.25 mmol/kg) over 4–12 hours has been shown to be safe and effective treatment for severe hypophosphatemia.[108,109]

Parenteral phosphorus supplementation is associated with the risks of hyperphosphatemia, metastatic soft tissue deposition of calcium phosphate, hypocalcemia, and hyperkalemia or hypernatremia, depending on the salt employed. Inappropriate administration of large doses of parenteral phosphorus administered over relatively short time periods has resulted in symptomatic hypocalcemia and soft tissue calcification.[92] The rate of infusion and choice of initial dosage should therefore be based on severity of hypophosphatemia and presence of symptoms. Patients should be closely monitored with frequent serum phosphorus determinations. Monitoring should also include assessment of serum calcium concentrations, and therapy with parenteral phosphorus should be undertaken with great caution and at reduced dosage for patients with baseline hypercalcemia, renal dysfunction, or evidence of tissue injury.[88]

TABLE 51.20. PHOSPHORUS REPLACEMENT THERAPY

Moderate hypophosphatemia (serum phosphorus 1.0–2.5 mg/dL)
Oral therapy
1.5–2 g (50–60 mmol) phosphorus per day, divided into three or four doses
Parenteral therapy
0.15 mmol/kg lean body weight infused in 250–1,000 mL D_5W over 12 h; repeat until serum phosphorus > 2 mg/dL
Severe hypophosphatemia (serum phosphorus <1 mg/dL)
Parenteral therapy
0.25 mmol/kg lean body weight infused in 250–500 mL D_5W by infusion pump over 4–6 h; repeat until serum phosphorus >2 mg/dL

Patient Outcome

The pharmacist can play an integral part in the management of electrolyte abnormalities and thus improve the patient's outcome. Most important, the pharmacist is responsible for reviewing the patient's medication history and determining if any of the patient's current drug therapy may have contributed to the existing electrolyte abnormalities. The patient's drug therapy should not be assessed in a vacuum. The acute clinical conditions or chronic diseases the patient has can have a great impact on both existing and future drug therapy. The pharmacist should also assume responsibility for new drug therapy recommendations to reduce the risk of developing new electrolyte problems and to optimize the outcome of the current management plan.

Pharmacists in ambulatory settings may identify existing or potential drug-related electrolyte abnormalities and then suggest dosage adjustments or new drug therapies when appropriate. It is hoped that this proactive interventional approach will facilitate the management of mild disorders in the community and reduce the need for hospitalization. It is critical that the pharmacist be aware of the signs and symptoms of electrolyte problems that patients may have. Pharmacists should attempt to ascertain the presence of mild symptoms due to electrolyte problems in those patients at high risk (e.g., the elderly or the renally impaired).

References

1. Bichet DG, Anderson RJ, Schrier RW. Renal sodium excretion, edematous disorders and diuretic use, in Schier RW (ed): Renal and Electrolyte Disorders, 4th ed. Boston, Little, Brown and Co, 1992, pp 89–159.
2. Scully RE, McNeely BV, Mark EJ. Normal reference laboratory values. N Engl J Med 1986;314:39–49.
3. Arieff AI. Management of hyponatraemia. Br Med J 1993;307:305–308.
4. Narins RG, Chung HM, Kluge R, et al. Hyponatremia: A prospective analysis of its epidemiology and the pathogenic role of vasopressin. Ann Intern Med 1985;102:164–168.
5. Goldberg M. Hyponatremia. Med Clin North Am 1981;65:251–269.
6. Berl T, Schier RW. Disorders of water metabolism, in Schier RW (ed): Renal and Electrolyte Disorders, 4th ed. Boston, Little, Brown and Co, 1992, pp 1–87.
7. Rault RM. Case report: Hyponatremia associated with nonsteroidal antiinflammatory drugs. Am J Med Sci 1993;305:318–320.
8. Rose BD. Clinical Physiology of Acid Base and Electrolyte Disorders, 4th ed. New York, McGraw-Hill, 1994, pp. 651–694.
9. Trump DL. Serious hyponatremia in patients with cancer: Management with demeclocycline. Cancer 1981;47:2908–2912.
10. Forrest JN, Cox M, Hong C, et al. Superiority of demeclocycline over lithium in the treatment of chronic syndrome of inappropriate secretion of antidiuretic hormone. N Engl J Med 1978;298:173–177.
11. De Troyer A. Demeclocycline: Treatment of syndrome of inappropriate antidiuretic hormone secretion. JAMA 1977;237:2723–2726.
12. Sterns RH. The treatment of hyponatremia: First, do no harm. Am J Med 1990;88:557–560.
13. Cheng JC, Zikos D, Skopicki HA, et al. Long-term neurologic outcome in psychogenic water drinks with severe symptomatic hyponatremia: The effect of rapid correction. Am J Med 1990;88:561–566.
14. Feig PU. Hypernatremia and hypertonic syndromes. Med Clin North Am 1981;65:271–290.
15. Devita MV, Michelis MF. Perturbations in sodium balance. Hyponatremia and hypernatremia. Clin Lab Med 1993;13:135–148.
16. Gabow PA. Fluids and Electrolytes: Clinical Problems and Their Solutions. Boston, Little, Brown & Co, 1983, pp 69–75.
17. Weitzman RE, Kleeman CR. The clinical physiology of water metabolism. II. Renal mechanisms for urinary concentration: Diabetes insipidus. West J Med 1979;131:486–515.
18. Rose BD. Clinical Physiology of Acid-Base and Electrolyte Disorders. 4th ed. New York, McGraw-Hill, 1994, pp 346–378.
19. Gabow AP, Peterson LN. Disorders of potassium metabolism, in Schrier RW (ed): Renal and Electrolyte Disorders, 4th ed. Boston, Little, Brown and Co, 1992, pp 231–287.
20. Brown RS. Potassium homeostasis and clinical implications. Am J Med 1984;77(5A):3–10.
21. Stearns RH, Cox M, Feig PU. Internal potassium balance and the control of the plasma potassium concentration. Medicine 1981;60:339–354.

22. Allon M, Copkney C. Albuterol and insulin for treatment of hyperkalemia in hemodialysis patients. Kidney Int 1990;38:869–872.
23. Williams ME, Rosa RM, Silva P, et al. Impairment of extra-renal potassium disposal by α-adrenergic stimulation. N Engl J Med 1984;311:145–149.
24. Knochel JP. Role of glucoregulatory hormones in potassium homeostasis. Kidney Int 1977;11:443–452.
25. Freedman BI, Burkart JM. Hypokalemia. Crit Care Clin 1991;7:143–153.
26. Surawicz B. Relationship between electrocardiogram and electrolytes. Am Heart J 1967;73:814–834.
27. Harrington JT, Isner JM, Kasirer JP. Our national obsession with potassium. Am J Med 1982;73:155–159.
28. Isaac G, Holland OB. Drug-induced hypokalemia. Drugs Aging 1992;2:35–41.
29. Lawson DH. Adverse reactions to potassium chloride. Q J Med 1974;63:433–440.
30. Stanaszek WF, Romankiewica JA. Current approaches to management of potassium deficiency. Drug Intell Clin Pharm 1985;19:176–183.
31. Kruse JA, Carlson RW. Rapid correction of hypokalemia. Using concentrated intravenous potassium chloride infusions. Arch Intern Med 1990;150:613–617.
32. Bia MJ, Defronzo RA. Potassium chloride therapy. JAMA 1981;246:2501.
33. Sherlock P. Cardiovascular and Renal Drugs and Gastrointestinal Drugs Advisory Committee Meeting. Bethesda, MA, Food and Drug Administration, 1983, pp 1–273.
34. Boley SJ, Allen AC, Schultz L, et al. Potassium induced lesions of the small bowel: I. Clinical aspects. JAMA 1965;193:997–1000.
35. Allen AC, Boley SJ, Schultz L, et al. Potassium-induced lesions of the small bowel: II. Pathology and pathogenesis. JAMA 1965;193:1001–1006.
36. Latta K, Hisano S, Chan JCM. Perturbations in potassium balance. Clin Lab Med 1993;13:149–156.
37. Weiner IM, Hays RM. Drugs affecting renal function and electrolyte metabolism, in Gilman AG, et al (eds): The Pharmacologic Basis of Therapeutics. New York, Pergamon, 1991, pp 708–748.
38. Martin ML, Hamilton R, West MF. Potassium. Emerg Med Clin North Am 1986;4:131–144.
39. Walmsley RN, White GH, Cain M, et al. Hyperkalemia in the elderly. Clin Chem 1984;30:1409–1412.
40. DeFronzo RA, Ria M, Smith D. Clinical disorders of hyperkalemia. Ann Rev Med 1982;33:521–554.
41. Kunis CL, Lowenstein J. The emergency treatment of hyperkalemia. Med Clin North Am 1981;65:165–176.
42. Smith JD, Bia MJ, DeFronza RA. Clinical disorders of potassium metabolism, in Arieff AI, DeFronzo RA (eds): Fluid, Electrolyte, and Acid-Base Disorders, vol 1. New York, Churchill Livingstone, 1985, pp 413–510.
43. Janson CL. Fluid and electrolyte balance, in Rosen P (ed): Emergency Medicine: Concepts and Clinical Practice, vol 2. St. Louis, CV Mosby, 1983, pp 1419–1465.
44. Greenberg S, Reiser IW, Chou S, Porush JG. Trimethoprim-sulfamethoxazole induces reversible hyperkalemia. Ann Intern Med 1993;119:291–295.
45. Williams ME. Hyperkalemia. Crit Care Clin 1991;7:155–174.
46. Innerarity SA. Hyperkalemic emergencies. Crit Care Nurs Q 1992;14:32–39.
47. Agus ZS, Wasserstein A, Goldfarb S. Disorders of calcium and magnesium homeostasis. Am J Med 1982;72:473–488.
48. Popovtzer MM, Knochel JP, Kumar R. Disorders of calcium, phosphorus, vitamin D, and parathyroid hormone activity, in Schreir RW (ed): Renal and Electrolyte Disorders, 4th ed. Boston, Little, Brown and Co, 1992, pp 287–370.
49. Mundy GR, Ibbotson KJ, D'Souze SM, et al. The hypercalcemia of cancer, clinical implications and pathogenic mechanisms. N Engl J Med 1984;310:1718–1727.
50. Stewart AF. Therapy of malignancy-associated hypercalcemia: 1983. Am J Med 1983;74:475–480.
51. Hall TG, Burns Schaiff RA. Update on the medical treatment of hypercalcemia of malignancy. Clin Pharm 1993;12:117–125.
52. Ritch PS. Treatment of cancer-related hypercalcemia. Semin Oncol 1990;17(suppl 5):26–33.
53. Mallette LE, Bilezikian JP, Heath DA, et al. Primary hyperparathyroidism: Clinical and biochemical features. Medicine 1974;53:127–146.
54. Purnell DC, VanHoerden JA. Management of symptomatic hypercalcemia and hypocalcemia. World J Surg 1982;6:702–709.
55. Bajorunas DR. Clinical manifestations of cancer-related hypercalcemia. Semin Oncol 1990;17(suppl 5):16–25.
56. Nussbaum SR. Pathophysiology and management of severe hypercalcemia. Endocrinol Metab Clin North Am 1993;22:343–362.
57. Lebbin D, Ryan WG, Schwartz TB. Outpatient treatment of Paget's disease of bone with mithramycin. Ann Intern Med 1984;81:635–637.
58. Budyr AA, Nissenson RA, Kelin RF, et al. Increased serum levels of a parathyroid hormone-like protein in malignancy-associated hypercalcemia. Ann Intern Med 1989;111:807–812.
59. Zaloga GP. Hypocalcemia in critically ill patients. Crit Care Med 1992;20:251–262.
60. Juan D. Hypocalcemia: Differential diagnosis and mechanisms. Arch Intern Med 1979;139:1166–1171.
61. Sitrin M, Meredith S, Rosenberg IH. Vitamin D deficiency and bone disease in gastrointestinal disorders. Arch Intern Med 1978;138:886–888.
62. Fraser D, Kooh SW, Kind HP, et al. Pathogenesis of hereditary vitamin D-dependent rickets: An inborn error of vitamin D metabolism involving defective conversion of 25-hydroxy vitamin D to I-alpha,25-dihydroxy vitamin D. N Engl J Med 1973;289:817–822.
63. Coburn JW, Hartenbower DL, Brickman AS. Advances in vitamin D metabolism as they pertain to chronic renal disease. Am J Clin Nutr 1976;29:1292–1299.
64. Lebowitz MR, Moses AM. Hypocalcemia. Semin Nephrol 1992;12:146–158.
65. Keyler D, Peterson CD. Oral calcium supplements. How much of what, for whom, and why? Postgrad Med 1985;78:123–125.

66. Porter RH, Cox BA, Heaney D. Treatment of hypoparathyroid patients with chlorthalidone. N Engl J Med 1978;298:577–581.
67. Graber TW, Yee AS, Baker FJ. Magnesium: Physiology, clinical disorders, and therapy. Ann Emerg Med 1981;10:49–57.
68. Van Hook JW. Endocrine crises. Hypermagnesemia. Crit Care Clin 1991;7:215–223.
69. Alfrey AC. Normal and abnormal magnesium metabolism, in Schreir RW (ed): Renal and Electrolyte Disorders, 4th ed. Boston, Little, Brown and Co, 1992, pp 371–405.
70. Whang R, Ryder KW. Frequency of hypomagnesemia and hypermagnesemia. JAMA 1990;263:3063–3064.
71. Wong ET, Rude RK, Singer FR, et al. A high prevalence of hypomagnesemia and hypermagnesemia in hospitalized patients. Am J Clin Pathol 1983;79:348–352.
72. Rude RK, Singer FR. Magnesium deficiency and excess. Ann Rev Med 1981;32:245–259.
73. Clark BA, Brown RS. Unsuspected morbid hypermagnesemia in elderly patients. Am J Nephrol 1992;12:336–343.
74. Mordes JP, Waker WC. Excess magnesium. Pharmacol Rev 1978;29:273–300.
75. Abbott LG, Rude RK. Clinical manifestations of magnesium deficiency. Miner Electrolyte Metab 1993;19:314–322.
76. Berkelhammer C, Benir RA. A clinical approach to common electrolyte problems. 4. Hypomagnesemia. Can Med Assoc J 1985;1321:360–368.
77. Davis BB, Preuss HG, Murdaugh JV Jr. Hypomagnesemia following the diuresis of post-renal obstruction and renal transplant. Nephron 1975;14:275–280.
78. Sheehan J, White A. Diuretic-associated hypomagnesemia. Br Med J 1982;285:1157–1159.
79. Gearhart MO, Sorg TB. Foscarnet-induced severe hypomagnesemia and other electrolyte disorders. Ann Pharmacother 1993;27:285–289.
80. Shah GM, Kirschenbaum MA. Renal magnesium wasting associated with therapeutic agents. Miner Electrolyte Metab 1991;17:58–64.
81. Cronin RE, Knochel JP. Magnesium deficiency. Adv Intern Med 1983;28:509–533.
82. Flink EB. Magnesium deficiency. Etiology and clinical spectrum. Acta Med Scand 1980;647(suppl):125–137.
83. Anderson TW, Neri LC, Schreiber GB, et al. Ischemic heart disease, water hardness and myocardial magnesium. Can Med Assoc J 1975;113:199–203.
84. Topac EJ, Lerman EB. Hypomagnesemic torsades de pointes. Am J Cardiol 1983;52:1367–1368.
85. Whang R, Oei TO, Watanabe A. Frequency of hypomagnesemia in hospitalized patients receiving digitalis. Arch Intern Med 1985;145:655–656.
86. Stoff JS. Phosphate homeostasis and hypophosphatemia. Am J Med 1982;72:489–495.
87. Levine BS, Kleeman CR. Hypophosphatemia and hyperphosphatemia: Clinical and pathophysiologic aspects, in Narins RG (ed): Clinical Disorders of Fluid and Electrolyte Metabolism, 5th ed. New York, McGraw-Hill, 1994, pp 1045–1097.
88. Knochel JP. The pathophysiology and clinical characteristics of severe hypophosphatemia. Arch Intern Med 1977;137:203–220.
89. Janson C, Birnbaum G, Baker FJ. Hypophosphatemia. Ann Emerg Med 1983;12:107–116.
90. Corvilain J, Abramow M. Effect of growth hormone on tubular transport of phosphate in normal and parathyroidectomized dogs. J Clin Invest 1964;34:1608–1612.
91. Bommer J, Bonjour JP, Ritz E, et al. Parathyroid independent changes in renal handling of phosphate in hyperthyroid rats. Kidney Int 1979;15:325.
92. Bourke E, Yanagawa N. Assessment of hyperphosphatemia and hypophosphatemia. Clin Lab Med 1993;13:183–207.
93. Davis RF, Eichner JM, Bleyer WA, et al. Hypocalcemia, hyperphosphatemia and dehydration following a single hypertonic phosphate enema. J Pediatr 1977;90:484–485.
94. McConnell TH. Fatal hypocalcemia from phosphate absorption from laxative preparation. JAMA 1971;216:147–148.
95. Biberstein M, Parker BA. Enema-induced hyperphosphatemia. Am J Med 1985;79:645–646.
96. Breuer RI, LeBauer J. Caution in the use of phosphates in the treatment of severe hypercalcemia. J Clin Endocrinol 1967;27:695–698.
97. Kebler R, McDonald FD, Cadnapaphornchai P. Dynamic changes in serum phosphorus levels in diabetic ketoacidosis. Am J Med 1985;79:571–576.
98. Herbert LA, Lemann Jr J, Petersen JR, et al. Studies of the mechanism by which phosphate infusion lowers serum calcium concentration. J Clin Invest 1966;45:1886–1894.
99. Rubin MR, Narins RG. Hypophosphatemia: Pathophysiological and practical aspects of its therapy. Semin Nephrol 1990;10:536–545.
100. Knochel JP. Hypophosphatemia. Clin Nephrol 1977;4:131–137.
101. Silvis SE, DiBartolomeo AG, Aaker HM. Hypophosphatemia and neurological changes secondary to oral caloric intake. Am J Gastroenterol 1980;73:215–222.
102. Knochel JP. Hypophosphatemia in the alcoholic. Arch Intern Med 1980;140:613–615.
103. Silvis SE, Paragas PD. Paresthesias, weakness, seizures and hypophosphatemia in patients receiving hyperalimentation. Gastroenterology 1972;62:513–520.
104. Newman JH, Neff TA, Ziporin P. Acute respiratory failure associated with hypophosphatemia. N Engl J Med 1977;296:1101–1103.
105. Aubier M, Murciano D, Lecocguic Y, et al. Effect of hypophosphatemia on diaphragmatic contractility in patients with acute respiratory failure. N Engl J Med 1985;313:420–424.
106. Jacob HS, Amsden T. Acute hemolytic anemia with rigid red cells in hypophosphatemia. N Engl J Med 1971;285:1446–1450.
107. Vannatta JB, Whang R, Papper S. Efficacy of intravenous phosphorous therapy in severely hypophosphatemic patients. Arch Intern Med 1981;141:885–887.
108. Kingston M, Badawi Al-Sibai M. Treatment of severe hypophosphatemia. Crit Care Med 1985;13:16–18.
109. Andress DL, Vannatta JB, Whang R. Treatment of refractory hypophosphatemia. South Med J 1982;75:767–770.
110. Wilson HK, Keuer SP, Lea AS, et al. Phosphate therapy in diabetic ketoacidosis. Arch Intern Med 1982;142:517–520.

Chapter 52

Acid–Base Disorders

Robert A. Kilroy, PharmD, BCPS

Acid–base disorders constitute a common, widespread, and often serious problem affecting patients that may result in significant morbidity and mortality. This chapter reviews the principles and pathophysiology of acid–base disorders, provides guidelines for assessment, and outlines specific treatments.

The pharmacist can play an important role in the management of patients with acid–base disorders. Since acid–base homoestasis is affected by many drugs and disease states and since many acid–base abnormalities are potentially preventable, there is an opportunity for the pharmacist to have a considerable positive impact on patient outcome. The pharmacist's responsibility to the patient to anticipate drug-related problems, avoid or minimize clinical consequences, and design appropriate treatment regimens requires an understanding of the basic physiology of respiratory and metabolic acid–base regulation. In addition, this chapter reviews the etiology, pathophysiology, assessment, treatment, and prevention of acid–base abnormalities.

Acid–Base Chemistry and Physiology

An acid is a substance that can donate hydrogen ions, H^+. A base is a substance that can accept hydrogen ions, for example,

$$\underset{\text{(acid)}}{HCl \rightarrow H^+ + Cl^-}$$

$$\underset{\text{(base)}}{NH3 + H^+ \rightarrow NH_4^+}$$

The acid–base pairs commonly encountered in the body are listed in Table 52.1. A substance capable of accepting and donating hydrogen ions is a buffer. Buffering refers to the ability of a solution containing a weak acid and its anion (a base) to resist a change in pH upon addition of a strong acid or base. The principal buffer system utilized by the body is the carbonic acid/bicarbonate (H_2CO_3/HCO_3^-) system. Other buffers include phosphate, hemoglobin, and protein.

The degree of acidity of body fluids is expressed in terms of the hydrogen ion concentration. The normal concentration of hydrogen ions in blood is 0.00004 mEq/L or 0.40×10^{-7} Eq/L.[1] By convention, the degree of acidity is often expressed as pH, or the negative logarithm (base 10) of the hydrogen ion concentration. pH and hydrogen ion concentration are inversely related. Figure 52.1 shows the nonlinear relationship between pH and hydrogen ion concentration. Normally, the pH of blood is maintained at 7.40, with a range of 7.35–7.45. A pH of less than 6.8 or greater than 7.8 is considered incompatible with life.[1]

The hydrogen ion concentration in blood may not be indicative of that in other areas of the body. For example, the pH within cells, within cerebrospinal fluid, and on the surface of bone may all be altered without causing an alteration in blood pH.[2] The blood pH is critically important in determining acid–base status within the body and in diagnosing acid–base disorders. The relationship between pH, pK (the negative logarithm of the dissociation constant for the acid–base buffer pair), and the concentration of the acid [acid] and the base [base], is described by the Henderson–Hasselbach equation:

$$pH = pK + \log \frac{[\text{base}]}{[\text{acid}]}$$

BUFFERS

Because the carbonic acid/bicarbonate buffer system is the body's most abundant and measurable buffer, bicarbonate and carbonic acid are most commonly used to assess acid–base status. The equation describing the dissociation of carbonic acid is thus:

$$\text{Dissolved } CO_2\ (P_{CO_2}) + H_2O \xleftrightarrow[\text{anhydras}]{\text{carbonic}} H_2CO_3 \rightarrow H^+ + HCO_3^- \quad (1)$$

$$K = \frac{[H^+]\,[HCO_3^-]}{[H_2CO_3^-]} \quad (2)$$

where K is the dissociation constant for the buffer system.

TABLE 52.1. ACID–BASE PAIRS

Carbonic acid/bicarbonate	H_2CO_3/HCO_3^-
Monobasic/dibasic phosphate	H_2PO_4/HPO_4^-
Ammonium/ammonia	NH_4^+/NH_3
Lactic acid/lactate	$H_6C_3O_2/H_5C_3O_2^-$

Rearrangement of Eq. (2) gives:

$$[H^+] = K\frac{[H_2CO_3]}{[HCO_3^-]} \tag{3}$$

By taking the negative logarithm of each term, Eq. (3) appears in the form of the Henderson–Hasselbach equation:

$$pH = pK + \log (HCO_3^-/H_2CO_3) \tag{4}$$

The concentration of carbonic acid is directly proportional to the amount of CO_2 dissolved in blood, which is directly proportional to the partial pressure of CO_2 gas, P_{CO_2}. The dissolved CO_2, ($P_{CO_2} \cdot 0.03$), can be substituted into Eq. (4) because it is more readily measurable than carbonic acid, and along with substitution of the appropriate value for pK (6.1), the resultant equation is:

$$pH = 6.1 + \log(HCO_3^-/0.03\ P_{CO_2}) \tag{5}$$

Hydrogen ion concentration and pH are determined not by the absolute amounts of bicarbonate and P_{CO_2}, but by their ratio.[2] Examples of calculations using the Henderson–Hasselbach equation are shown as follows:

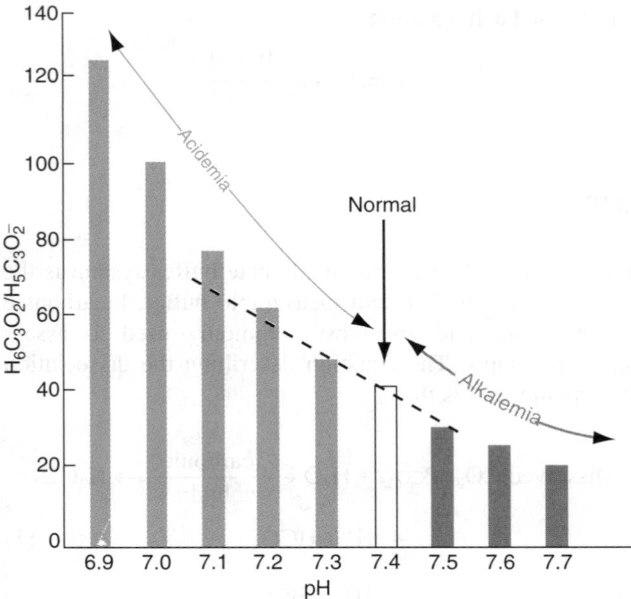

Figure 52.1. Relationship of pH to hydrogen ion concentration. *(From Narins RG, Emmett M. Simple and mixed acid–base disorders: A practical approach. Medicine 1980;59:161–187, with permission.)*

1. Normal
   P_{CO_2} = 40 mm Hg HCO_3 = 24 mEq/L
   $pH = 6.1 + \log [24/(0.03 \cdot 40)]$
   $= 6.1 + 1.3 = 7.4$
2. Uncompensated respiratory acidosis
   P_{CO_2} = 60 mm Hg HCO_3 = 24 mEq/L
   $pH = 6.1 + \log [24/(0.03 \cdot 60)]$
   $= 6.1 + 1.12 = 7.22$

Cellular metabolism of neutral dietary and tissue components results in the production of hydrogen ions and fixed acid anions, both of which need to be excreted to maintain acid–base balance. Small amounts of acid and alkali are presented as such to the body through the diet. On the average, 0.8 mEq/kg/d or 50–100 mEq of acid is consumed as part of our normal American diet.[3] Digestion of dietary substances and tissue metabolism also result in the production of nonvolatile acids. These acids are derived primarily from the sulfur-containing amino acids, cysteine and methionine, as well as from ingested sulfur. In addition, phosphate is produced from metabolism of proteins and phospholipids. Neutral substances such as glucose are metabolized to intermediates, lactic and pyruvic acids, with the production of hydrogen ion. These intermediates are then metabolized to H_2O and CO_2. Other organic anions, such as citrate and acetoacetate, are also metabolized to CO_2. When respiratory function is normal, the blood CO_2 concentration remains constant, and the amount of CO_2 produced metabolically is equal to the amount lost by respiration. The average adult produces 15,000–20,000 mmol of CO_2 each day.[3]

Three mechanisms collectively maintain acid–base balance: extracellular buffering, renal regulation of hydrogen ion and bicarbonate, and ventilatory regulation of carbon dioxide elimination. Extracellular buffering is the body's first defense against an increase in hydrogen ion concentration. The body's buffering system can be broken down into three components: bicarbonate/carbonic acid, proteins, and phosphates. The bicarbonate buffer is the most important of the body's buffers, because, (1) there is more bicarbonate present in the extracellular fluid (ECF) than any other buffer component, (2) the supply of carbon dioxide is unlimited, and (3) the acidity of ECF can be regulated by controlling either the bicarbonate concentration or the P_{CO_2}.

Carbonic acid represents the respiratory component of the buffer pair because its concentration is directly proportional to the partial pressure of CO_2 (P_{CO_2}), which is determined by ventilation. Bicarbonate represents the metabolic component because the kidney may alter its concentration by reabsorption, generating new bicarbonate, or elimination. The bicarbonate buffer system easily adapts to changes in acid–base status by alterations in ventilatory elimination of acid (P_{CO_2}) and renal elimination of base (HCO_3^-).[3]

The phosphate buffer system consists of serum inorganic phosphate (3.5–5.0 mg/dL), intracellular organic phosphate, and calcium phosphate in bone. Extracellular phosphate is present only in low concentrations so that its usefulness as a buffer is limited; however, as an intracellular buffer, phosphate is more useful. Calcium phosphate in bone is relatively inaccessible as a buffer, but prolonged metabolic acidosis will result in the release of phosphate from bone.

Intracellular and extracellular proteins also act as buffering systems. The charged side chains of amino acids provide the buffering action. Because the concentration of protein is much greater intracellularly than extracellularly, protein is much more important as an intracellular buffer.

Renal regulation of H^+ and HCO_3^- is a second mechanism by which the body maintains acid–base balance. The kidney is responsible for reabsorption of filtered HCO_3^- and elimination of H^+ to regulate the daily acid load. Essentially all of the approximately 4000 mEq of HCO_3^- filtered daily is reabsorbed, primarily in the proximal tubule. The filtered bicarbonate is reabsorbed in combination with secreted H^+. The HCO_3^- and H^+ combine to form H_2CO_3, which later dissociates to HCO_3^- and H^+. The hydrogen ion is secreted back into the tubule.[2]

The final mechanism of acid–base balance is ventilation. Both the rate and depth of ventilation can be varied to allow for excretion of CO_2 generated by diet and tissue metabolism. Medullary chemoreceptors sense changes in P_{CO_2} or in pH controlling ventilation. This system rapidly adjusts, within minutes, to changes in acid–base balance so that ventilation can be altered.

LABORATORY ASSESSMENT OF ACID–BASE STATUS

Several pieces of information must be considered in order to determine the type of acid–base disorder, ascertain the underlying cause, and plan desired treatment. Arterial blood gases, along with serum electrolytes, medical history, medication history, and the clinical condition of the patient, are the primary tools to determine the cause of the acid–base disorder and to design a course of therapy.

BLOOD GASES

Arterial blood gases are measured to determine the patient's oxygenation and acid–base status. Arterial blood rather than venous blood should be utilized because venous blood obtained from an extremity provides information only about that extremity. Extrapolating the information from that extremity to the entire body can be misleading if the metabolism in the extremity is altered by hypoperfusion, exercise, infection, or some other cause. In addition, arterial blood provides the added information of how well the lungs are oxygenating the blood (i.e., an accurate measurement of P_{O_2}).

Under normal circumstances, there is no clinically significant difference in pH between arterial and mixed venous blood (Table 52.2). However, in shock and during cardiopulmonary resuscitation with poor blood flow, the differences between arterial and venous blood can be dramatic. Weil and associates[4] reported average mixed venous pH of 7.15 and P_{CO_2} of 74 mm Hg during cardiopulmonary resuscitation, even though the arterial pH was 7.41 and arterial P_{CO_2} was 32 mm Hg. This indicates a severe tissue acidosis from CO_2 accumulation despite adequate arterial blood gases. Therefore, the use of mixed venous blood gases and end-tidal CO_2 monitoring during prolonged cardiopulmonary resuscitation may be a more useful guide to correcting tissue acidosis, rather than arterial blood gases.

The most accessible sites for direct arterial puncture are the brachial, radial, and femoral arteries. The brachial artery is preferred, although the radial is also used. The femoral should be avoided if possible; however, it is sometimes used in hypotensive patients.

All methods of arterial blood gas analysis currently used in hospital laboratories are similar and measure pH, P_{CO_2}, and P_{O_2} of the sample directly. The bicarbonate values and O_2 saturation are calculated. The apparatus for measuring blood gases consists of a pH electrode for measuring the hydrogen ion concentration of the sample, an electrode designed for measuring the partial pressure or tension of carbon dioxide (P_{CO_2}) and an electrode that measures the partial pressure of oxygen (P_{O_2}) in the arterial sample.[5] The temperature of the blood has an effect on pH. For this reason, the analyzer warms the samples to 37°C. Most systems also allow for corrections in temperature when the patient's body temperature differs from 37°C (e.g., during hypothermia for coronary artery bypass).

Clotted samples, samples with air bubbles, and small samples cannot be used to obtain blood gas measurements and should be discarded. Clotted samples may provide misleading information and damage the machinery. Samples that contain air bubbles will also provide distorted blood gas information. Inadequate samples, less than 1 mL, may also provide distorted information because of the concentration of heparin, an acid that is added to anticoagulate the sample.[5] Arterial samples are designated with the letter "a" (Pa_{O_2} and Pa_{CO_2}), while venous samples are labeled with

TABLE 52.2. NORMAL BLOOD GAS VALUES

	Arterial Blood	Mixed Venous Blood
pH	7.40 (7.35–7.45)	7.38 (7.33–7.43)
P_{O_2}	80–100 mm Hg	35–40 mm Hg
Sa_{O_2}	≥95%	70%–75%
P_{CO_2}	35–45 mm Hg	45–51 mm Hg
HCO_3	22–26 mEq/L	24–28 mEq/L

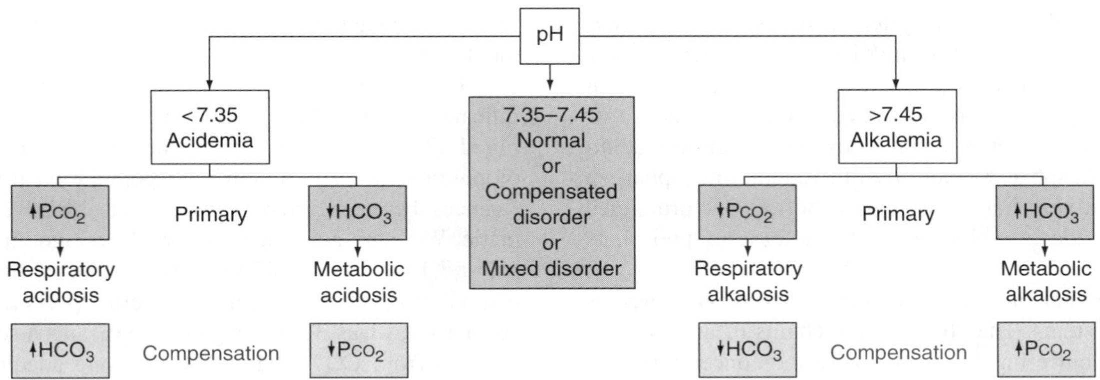

Figure 52.2. Analysis of arterial blood gases.

the letter "v" (Pv_{O_2} and Pv_{CO_2}). The normal values for arterial and venous blood gases are shown in Table 52.2.

ANALYSIS OF ARTERIAL BLOOD GASES

Arterial blood gases provide an assessment of the patient's acid–base status. Low pH values (less than 7.35) indicate an acidemia, while high pH values (higher than 7.45) indicate an alkalemia (see Fig. 52.2). The Pa_{CO_2} value helps one to determine if there is a primary respiratory abnormality, while the HCO_3^- concentration enables the assessment of a metabolic component.

Two conditions are associated with an abnormal Pa_{CO_2}: respiratory acidosis and respiratory alkalosis. *Acute respiratory acidosis* is characterized by an elevated Pa_{CO_2}, a moderately elevated HCO_3^- concentration (25–30 mEq/L), and a decreased pH. The renal compensatory response to acute respiratory acidosis is an increase in reabsorption and generation of bicarbonate, leading to a further increase in serum bicarbonate (HCO_3^-) over time. While buffering occurs almost immediately, the renal response to conserve bicarbonate does not exert a noticeable influence for 12–24 hours and requires several days for maximal renal compensation to occur. *Acute respiratory alkalosis* is characterized by a decreased Pa_{CO_2}, a decreased HCO_3^- concentration, and an increased pH. The renal compensatory response is increased renal bicarbonate excretion, ultimately leading to an additional decrease in serum bicarbonate (HCO_3^-).

An examination of the bicarbonate concentration helps to determine if there is a primary metabolic abnormality. The two conditions that occur with altered bicarbonate concentration are metabolic acidosis and metabolic alkalosis. *Metabolic acidosis* is characterized by a decrease in serum bicarbonate concentration. The body's compensatory response is to increase ventilation, leading to a decrease in Pa_{CO_2}. *Metabolic alkalosis* is characterized by an increase in serum bicarbonate concentration; compensatory hypoventilation results in a subsequent increase in Pa_{CO_2}.

Occasionally acid–base reports may be significantly different from those expected on the basis of the patient's clinical condition and previous laboratory determination. For this reason, it is a good idea when drawing blood for blood-gas studies to draw additional blood for electrolyte determinations. Then, the bicarbonate associated with the patient's Pa_{CO_2} and pH can be compared with the bicarbonate value estimated from the total CO_2 content (the amount of CO_2 gas extractable from plasma, consisting of HCO_3^-, H_2CO_3, and Pa_{CO_2}). Ordinarily, the bicarbonate estimated from the pH and Pa_{CO_2} will be approximately 1.0–2.0 mEq/L less than total CO_2 content.[6] If these values are not similar, the results should be interpreted with caution since it may reflect an error in the blood collection or storage of the sample, or in the calibration of the blood-gas analyzer.

ACID–BASE DISTURBANCES

Primary alterations in pH may be metabolic or respiratory in origin. Metabolic acid–base disturbances result from processes that alter pH primarily by changing the plasma bicarbonate concentration (HCO_3^-), the metabolic component of the Henderson–Hasselbach equation. Respiratory acid–base disturbances result from primary changes in the arterial carbon dioxide tension (Pa_{CO_2}), the respiratory component of the Henderson–Hasselbach equation. The changes in pH resulting from these metabolic and respiratory disturbances are dictated by the HCO_3^-/Pa_{CO_2} ratio.[2] The remainder of this chapter focuses on the pathophysiology and treatment of these acid–base disturbances.

A nomogram such as the one shown in Fig. 52.3 can be used to differentiate between the various acid–base disorders. In this nomogram, each pathologic acid–base disorder, together with the appropriate range of *in vivo* physio-

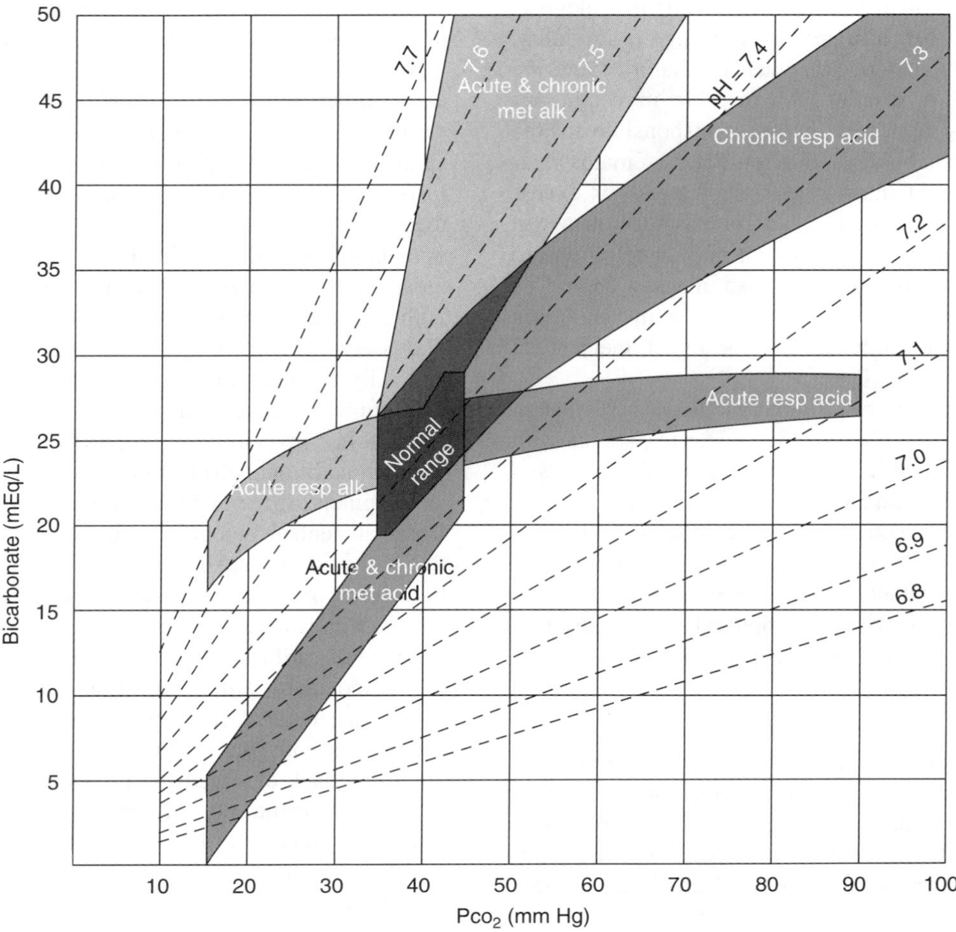

Figure 52.3. Acid–base nomogram. Chr resp acid, chronic respiratory acidosis; Ac & chr met alk, acute and chronic metabolic alkalosis; Ac resp acid, acute respiratory acidosis; Ac resp alk, acute respiratory alkalosis; Ac & chr met acid, acute and chronic metabolic acidosis. *(Reprinted from, by permission of the publisher, CMAJ 1973;109:291–293.)*

logic compensation, is represented as a shaded band. Acid–base values falling within a band usually represent a single disturbance; however, such values may represent a combination of acid–base disorders, a mixed disturbance. Acid–base values falling outside any band almost certainly represent a mixed acid–base disturbance.[7]

Respiratory Acid–Base Disorders

There are two types of simple respiratory acid–base disturbances: acidosis and alkalosis. These disorders are generated by a primary alteration in carbon dioxide excretion, which changes the concentration of carbon dioxide and, therefore, the carbonic acid concentration in body fluids. A primary reduction in $Paco_2$ causes a rise in pH (respiratory alkalosis) and a primary increase in $Paco_2$ causes a decrease in pH (respiratory acidosis).

RESPIRATORY ALKALOSIS

Pathophysiology

Respiratory alkalosis is characterized by a primary decrease in $Paco_2$, hypocapnia, that raises pH and results in a secondary decrease in plasma bicarbonate concentration. This disorder is one of the most commonly found acid–base disturbances among hospitalized patients. Mazarra et al.[8] reviewed 8607 blood gas samples from critically ill patients. Respiratory alkalosis, defined as pH greater than or equal to 7.45 and a $Paco_2$ less than 35 mm Hg without metabolic alkalosis, was observed in 46% of patients. The incidence of shock and sepsis was significantly higher in patients with spontaneous extreme hypocapnia ($Paco_2$ of $\leq$15 mm Hg). Mortality from sepsis and shock correlated inversely with the $Paco_2$ concentration and a $Paco_2$ concentration of 15 mm Hg or less was a morbid prognostic sign. While respiratory alkalosis occurs in a significant number of critically ill patients, treatment of the alkalosis itself has not been shown to produce a change in mortality.

A decrease in $Pa{CO_2}$ occurs when ventilatory excretion exceeds metabolic production. An increase in ventilatory excretion of $Pa{CO_2}$, hyperventilation, is responsible for the decrease, as the metabolic production $Pa{CO_2}$ remains relatively constant except during periods of stress or excess carbohydrate administration (i.e., parenteral nutrition) when it may be increased. Hyperventilation may develop due to an increase in neurochemical stimulation via a central or peripheral mechanism or a physical increase in ventilation either voluntarily or artificially by means of mechanical ventilation.

Specific causes for respiratory alkalosis are listed in Table 52.3. A decrease in $Pa{CO_2}$ may occur in patients with cardiogenic, hypovolemic, or septic shock since oxygen delivery to the carotid and aortic chemoreceptors is reduced. This relative deficit in PaO_2 compared to demand stimulates an increase in ventilation. Hyperventilation-induced respiratory alkalosis with an elevation in cardiac index and hypotension without peripheral vasoconstriction may therefore be an early sign of sepsis.

Clinical Presentation

Respiratory alkalosis may cause adverse neuromuscular, cardiovascular, and gastrointestinal effects. During periods of decreased $Pa{CO_2}$, there is a decrease in cerebral blood flow, which may be responsible for symptoms of lightheadedness, confusion, decreased intellectual functioning, syncope, and seizures. Nausea and vomiting may occur, probably as a result of cerebral hypoxia. In severe respiratory alkalosis, cardiac arrhythmias may occur.[9] Lawson et al.[10] studied nine post-traumatic patients who developed cardiac arrhythmias during periods of inadvertent severe alkalosis. Four of the patients had a simple respiratory alkalosis and the remaining five had a mixed respiratory and metabolic alkalosis. The authors concluded that the development of arrhythmias in the presence of alkalosis was independent of preexisting heart disease, although patients with heart disease and those taking digitalis were at an increased risk. Arrhythmias occurring during alkalosis were generally resistent to antiarrhythmic therapy and required correction of the alkalosis. Correction of the alkalosis itself resulted in conversion of these arrhythmias to sinus rhythm without additional drug therapy. The mechanism for the development of the arrhythmia is unknown, but may result from an enhancement of automaticity by hypoxia or hypokalemia. Alkalosis may also sensitize the myocardium to the arrhythmogenic effects of circulating catecholamines.

TABLE 52.3. CAUSES OF RESPIRATORY ALKALOSIS

Central stimulation of respiration
Anxiety
Pain
Fever
Brain tumors, vascular accidents
Head trauma
Pregnancy
Progesterone
Catecholamines, theophylline, nicotine
Salicylates
Peripheral stimulation of respiration
Pulmonary emboli
Congestive heart failure
Altitude
Asthma
Pulmonary shunts
Hypotension
Pneumonia
"Stiff lungs" without hypoxemia
Multiple mechanisms
Hepatic cirrhosis
Gram-negative sepsis
Mechanical or voluntary hyperventilation

Acute respiratory alkalosis has no effect on blood pressure or cardiac output in awake individuals. There is an associated tachycardia indicating a decreased stroke volume. Anesthetized humans, however, may experience a decrease in both cardiac output and blood pressure possibly due to the lack of a tachycardic response.[11]

The concentration of serum electrolytes may also be altered secondary to the development of respiratory alkalosis. The serum chloride concentration is usually slightly increased and serum potassium concentration may be slightly decreased. Clinically significant hypokalemia has been reported as a consequence of extreme respiratory alkalosis, although most studies of both acute and chronic respiratory alkalosis report very small or negligible effects on plasma potassium concentration.[12] Serum phosphorus concentration may decrease by as much as 1.5–2.0 mg/dL because of the movement of inorganic phosphate into cells.[13] The amount of ionized calcium is reduced in respiratory alkalosis, which may be partially responsible for symptoms such as muscle cramps and tetany. Approximately 50% of calcium is bound to albumin and an increase in pH results in an increase in binding secondary to conformational changes in the albumin molecule.[11]

Compensation

The initial response, during the first 6 hours, of the body to acute respiratory alkalosis is to chemically buffer the excess bicarbonate. Hydrogen ions from intracellular proteins, phosphates, and hemoglobin move extracellularly to titrate bicarbonate. Acutely, the bicarbonate concentration is decreased by a maximum of no more than 3.5 mEq/L for each 10 mm Hg decrease in $Pa{CO_2}$.[1]

The second, or compensatory, phase of the body's response to the increase in pH occurs when respiratory alkalosis is prolonged for longer than 6 hours. During this stage, the kidneys attempt to compensate for the decrease in the respiratory acid component, $Paco_2$, by increasing bicarbonate elimination. This compensation consists of a decrease in reabsorption of filtered bicarbonate and net acid excretion. The bicarbonate concentration can be reduced by up to 5 mEq/L for each 10 mm Hg drop in $Paco_2$.[1] For example, a sustained decrease in $Paco_2$ of 20 mm Hg will lower serum bicarbonate from 24 to 14 mEq/L with a resultant pH of 7.46. Bicarbonate concentrations differing from those anticipated using the preceding guideline would suggest a mixed acid–base disorder (refer to Fig. 52.3).

Treatment

The first consideration in the treatment of respiratory alkalosis is the identification and correction of the underlying cause. Relief of pain, correction of hypovolemia with volume, treatment of fever or infection, treatment of salicylate overdose, and other direct measures may prove effective. A rebreathing device, such as a paper bag, may be useful in controlling hyperventilation in some patients. Oxygen therapy should be initiated in patients with severe hypoxemia. Patients with life-threatening alkalosis (pH > 7.55) and complications such as arrhythmia or seizures, may require mechanical ventilation. They may also require sedation and paralysis to control hyperventilation.[9] Simple respiratory alkalosis rarely requires such aggressive therapy, but it may be helpful in mixed respiratory and metabolic alkalosis.

Respiratory alkalosis in patients receiving mechanical ventilation is usually iatrogenic. It may often be corrected by decreasing the minute ventilation (i.e., the number of mechanical breaths per minute), although other measures can also be employed. The use of a capnograph and spirometer in the breathing circuit enables a more precise adjustment of the ventilator settings. Another method of treating a respiratory alkalosis is to increase the amount of dead space in the ventilator circuit. This involves placing a known length of tubing between the artificial airway and the "Y" piece of the ventilator. This results in "rebreathing" of expired gas and, therefore, an increase in the inspired carbon dioxide concentration. This should increase the carbon dioxide tension of the patient and thereby correct the respiratory alkalosis.

RESPIRATORY ACIDOSIS

Pathophysiology

This disorder is caused by a primary retention of carbon dioxide that lowers the pH and produces a compensatory increase in plasma bicarbonate concentration. Respiratory acidosis was found to occur in 13.4% of critically ill hospitalized patients in one large review.[8]

Respiratory acidosis results from a failure of carbon dioxide excretion secondary to a disorder that restricts ventilation or an increase in CO_2 production (Table 52.4). Acute respiratory acidosis with hypoxemia, hypercarbia, and acidosis is life threatening. Those disorders that produce an increase in $Paco_2$ and hypoxemia to a degree compatible with life, (e.g., chronic obstructive pulmonary disease) with or without oxygen therapy, may result in chronic respiratory acidosis (Table 52.5). These patients can function normally without noticeable neurologic defects with $Paco_2$ concentrations in the range of 90–100 mm Hg (normal 40 mm Hg), provided adequate oxygenation is maintained.[11]

Clinical Presentation

Neuromuscular symptoms include altered mental status, abnormal behavior, seizures, stupor, and coma. Hypercapnia may mimic stroke or central nervous system (CNS) tumor by producing headache, papilledema, focal paresis, and abnormal reflexes. Carbon dioxide acts as a vasodilator in the brain, thus causing an increase in cerebral blood flow. This increase in cerebral blood flow is thought to be partially responsible for the CNS symptoms of respiratory acidosis. The CNS response to hypercapnia is extremely variable between patients and is also influenced by the acuity of presentation. Chronic hypercapnia alters the usual respiratory stimulus of increasing $Paco_2$ and the drive for respiration in these patients is hypoxemia rather than hypercapnia.[11]

The degree to which cardiac contractility and heart rate are altered depends on the severity of acidosis, whether metabolic or respiratory, and the rapidity with which acidosis develops. Acute hypercapnia stimulates a stress-like response, with elevated catecholamines and corticosteroid hormone levels. The physiologic response is modified by a blunting of receptor sensitivity to catecholamines.[11]

TABLE 52.4. CAUSES OF ACUTE RESPIRATORY ACIDOSIS

Perfusion abnormalities
- Massive pulmonary embolism
- Cardiac arrest

Airway and pulmonary abnormalities
- Severe pulmonary edema
- Severe pneumonia
- Smoke inhalation
- Bronchospasm
- Adult respiratory distress syndrome
- Airway obstruction: foreign body, laryngeal edema
- Aspiration of vomitus

Neuromuscular abnormalities
- Trauma, stroke
- Brainstem or cervical cord injury
- Guillain-Barré syndrome
- Myasthenia gravis
- Narcotic or sedative overdose

Mechanical ventilator
- Ventilator malfunction
- Inadequate frequency or tidal volume settings
- Large dead space

TABLE 52.5. CAUSES OF CHRONIC RESPIRATORY ACIDOSIS

Neuromuscular abnormalities
Brainstem infarct
Obesity-hypoventilation (Pickwickian) syndrome
Tumors
Poliomyelitis
Multiple sclerosis
Diaphragmatic paralysis
Pulmonary abnormalities
Chronic obstructive pulmonary disease
Kyphoscoliosis
Interstitial pulmonary disease
Overzealous parenteral feeding

In respiratory acidosis, serum concentrations of sodium and chloride remain normal or increase slightly. The serum potassium concentration increases secondary to intracellular movement. The increases are less than inorganic metabolic acidosis but have low predictive value in individual patients.[11]

Compensation

The body responds to acute respiratory acidosis with chemical buffering. Nonbicarbonate buffers, (i.e., proteins, phosphate, hemoglobin) take up the hydrogen ions from the carbonic acid formed as a result of the increase in $Paco_2$. This allows the bicarbonate concentration to increase. Buffering begins almost immediately after an acute increase in $Paco_2$. In general, the bicarbonate concentration will increase by 1 mEq/L above 24 for each 10 mm Hg increase in $Paco_2$ above 40 in acute respiratory acidosis.[1]

When respiratory acidosis is prolonged beyond 12–24 hours or becomes chronic, renal excretion of hydrogen ion also increases to compensate for acidosis. The kidneys excrete hydrogen ion, which generates new bicarbonate and raises the pH toward normal. Renal compensation for chronic hypercapnia generally results in the plasma bicarbonate concentration increasing by 4 mEq/L above 24 for each 10 mm Hg increase in $Paco_2$ above 40 in compensated respiratory acidosis.[1] A new steady state in acid–base values generally occurs within 5 days of the onset of hypercapnia in dogs, but the time interval necessary for establishing chronic (i.e., compensated) respiratory acidosis in humans has not been established.

Treatment

The treatment of respiratory acidosis is dependent on the chronicity of the condition of the patient. Acute respiratory acidosis, and acute respiratory acidosis superimposed on chronic respiratory acidosis, are discussed in detail here. The treatment of chronic respiratory acidosis is discussed in Chapter 26.

Acute Respiratory Acidosis

When carbon dioxide excretion is severely impaired and life-threatening hypoxia is present ($Po_2 < 40$ mm Hg), the immediate therapeutic goal is to provide adequate ventilation. This involves maintaining a patent airway, which may necessitate emergency tracheotomy, bronchoscopy, or intubation. In addition, excessive secretions must be cleared from the airway. Oxygen should be administered to restore adequate oxygenation. Mechanical ventilation may be required in cases of life-threatening hypoxia.

The underlying cause of the acidosis should be treated aggressively (i.e., bronchodilators for treatment of severe bronchospasm, discontinuing or reversing respiratory depressant drugs such as narcotics and benzodiazepines). Bicarbonate administration is rarely necessary in the treatment of respiratory acidosis. Furthermore, rapid correction of acidosis with bicarbonate may eliminate the patient's respiratory drive or precipitate a metabolic alkalosis. Arterial blood gases should be monitored closely to ensure that the respiratory acidosis is resolving without creating a metabolic alkalosis as the result of the compensatory elevation in HCO_3^- and decrease in $Paco_2$. Arterial blood gases should be obtained every 2–4 hours during the acute phase and less frequently (every 12–24 hours) as the acidosis improves.

Acute Respiratory Acidosis in a Compensated Chronic Respiratory Acidotic Patient

Patients with a history of chronic respiratory acidosis (e.g., those with chronic obstructive pulmonary disease) may experience an acute worsening of their respiratory acidosis. This may result in severe life-threatening hypoxemia. As with acute respiratory acidosis, the goals of therapy are maintenance of a patent airway and adequate oxygenation. Individuals with chronic respiratory acidosis are routinely able to tolerate a low Pao_2 and an elevated $PaCO_2$ because of compensation (increased red blood cells, hemoglobin, and 2,3-diphosphoglycerate). The drive to breathe in these patients is dependent on hypoxemia rather than hypercarbia. Administration of oxygen to a patient with chronic respiratory acidosis can eliminate this drive to breathe and result in the syndrome of carbon dioxide narcosis. In this case, if the Pao_2 is greater than or equal to 50 mm Hg, no oxygen treatment is necessary. If the Pao_2 is less than 50 mm Hg, oxygen therapy should be initiated carefully.[9]

Arterial blood gases should be checked periodically to ensure adequate oxygenation. If the $Paco_2$ increases during oxygen therapy, it may be a sign of impending carbon dioxide narcosis and oxygen therapy may need to be discontinued. If the pH remains less than 7.2 and the $Paco_2$ remains elevated and/or the patient develops symptoms of acidosis, bicarbonate may be given. The amount of bicarbonate given should increase the pH to no more than 7.25. Arterial blood gases should be monitored to avoid precipitation of metabolic alkalosis.

Measures should be taken to treat the underlying cause of the acute exacerbation. Pulmonary infections should be treated with the appropriate antibiotics and bronchodilators as necessary. Excess secretions should be cleared from the airway to allow proper gas exchange. This may involve increasing oral fluid intake to decrease secretion viscosity, deep breathing and postural drainage, suction, or bronchoscopy.

METABOLIC ACID–BASE DISORDERS

The two metabolic acid–base disorders, acidosis and alkalosis, are generated by a primary change in bicarbonate concentration. In metabolic acidosis, bicarbonate is lost or a nonvolatile acid is gained, whereas metabolic alkalosis is characterized by a gain in bicarbonate or a loss of nonvolatile acid.

METABOLIC ACIDOSIS

Pathophysiology

Metabolic acidosis is characterized by a decrease in pH and a low serum bicarbonate concentration. This can result from an addition of organic acid to the ECF (e.g., lactic acid, ketoacids), loss of bicarbonate stores (e.g., in diarrhea), or progressive accumulation of endogenous acids secondary to impaired renal function (e.g., phosphates, sulfates).[3] Patients with metabolic acidosis may have an elevated anion gap or a normal anion gap (i.e., hyperchloremic metabolic acidosis).

In the serum, the total concentration of cations must equal the total concentration of anions. The cation concentration is equal to the sodium concentration plus the unmeasured cations (UC)—magnesium, calcium, and potassium—which is normally 11 mEq/L. The anion concentration is equal to the concentration of chloride and bicarbonate and the unmeasured anions (UA)—proteins, sulfates, phosphate, and organic acid—which normally total 23 mEq/L. Therefore,

$$Na^+ + UC = (Cl^- + HCO_3^-) + UA$$

$$\text{Anion gap} = Na^+ - (Cl^- + HCO_3^-) = UA - UC$$

The normal value for the anion gap is approximately 12 mEq/L with a range of 8–16 mEq/L. The potassium concentration may be included with the sodium concentration in the calculation of the anion gap, in which case the normal range is 12–16 mEq/L. As the potassium concentration varies over a narrow range, it rarely increases the accuracy of the equation and, therefore, may be excluded from the calculation. In most clinical situations, an increase in the anion gap can be equated with accumulation of unmeasured anions in ECF. Normal anion gap metabolic acidosis occurs when bicarbonate losses from the ECF are replaced by chloride. This decrease in bicarbonate results from losses from the gastrointestinal tract, dilution of bicarbonate in the ECF space by the addition of sodium chloride solution, or addition of chloride-containing acids to the ECF, which titrates the bicarbonate and replaces it with chloride. Common causes of metabolic acidosis with an increased anion gap or a normal anion gap are listed in Table 52.6. The increase in unmeasured anions may result from accumulation of endogenous organic acids, such as lactic acid, acetoacetic acid, or β-hydroxybutyric acid, or from ingestion of such toxins as methanol or ethylene glycol.

Normal Anion Gap Metabolic Acidosis

Gastrointestinal disorders such as diarrhea and pancreatic fistula can result in hyperchloremic metabolic acidosis. Diarrhea is by far the most common cause. Severe diarrhea can lead to a daily loss of 5–10 L of fluid. Each liter of stool contains 100–140 mEq of sodium, 20–40 mEq of potassium, 80–100 mEq of chloride, and 30–50 mEq of bicarbonate.[14] Those patients with diseases of the lower urinary tract who require removal of the bladder and urinary diversion into the sigmoid colon may also develop a hyperchloremic metabolic acidosis. While urine is retained in the colon, water reabsorption, passive chloride reabsorption, and active bicarbonate secretion occur, resulting in a net loss of bicarbonate.

Renal tubular acidosis (RTA) causes a metabolic acidosis with a normal anion gap because the kidneys fail to excrete sufficient hydrogen ion to generate new bicarbonate that must replace bicarbonate lost in titrating the daily acid load. There are three major types of RTA: type I, classic, distal, or gradient limited; type II, proximal or quantity limited; and hyperkalemic type IV (see Chapter 48, Nephrolithiasis). In type I, a defect in the distal nephron prevents the kidney from acidifying the urine to a pH of less than 5.4. A mild to moderate metabolic acidosis results from failure to excrete the endogenous acid load and from the bicarbonate leak. In the presence of metabolic acidosis, up to 3–5% of the filtered load of bicarbonate may be

TABLE 52.6. COMMON CAUSES OF METABOLIC ACIDOSIS

Increased Anion Gap	Normal Anion Gap
Alcoholic ketoacidosis	Acid ingestion
Diabetic ketoacidosis	Carbonic anhydrase inhibitors
Lactic acidosis	Diarrhea
Chronic renal failure	Dilutional acidosis
Methanol ingestion	Gastrointestinal disorders
Ethylene glycol ingestion	Pancreatic fistula
Salicylate overdose	Renal acidification defects
Starvation	Ureterosigmoidostomy, ileostomy

excreted in the urine when the plasma bicarbonate is normal. Hypokalemia may occur because of an increase in potassium excretion.[3,14–16]

In type II RTA (proximal RTA), there is a defect in the ability of the proximal tubule to reclaim bicarbonate. Normally, 85% of the filtered load of bicarbonate is reabsorbed in the proximal tubule. Due to the defect in proximal tubule reabsorption, bicarbonate is shunted to the distal nephron, which has a limited capacity for bicarbonate reabsorption. Thus, up to 15% of the filtered bicarbonate load may be lost in the urine when plasma bicarbonate concentration is normal, resulting in a metabolic acidosis. The bicarbonaturia also leads to hypovolemia and hypokalemia secondary to sodium and potassium losses.[3,14–16]

Elevated Anion Gap Metabolic Acidosis

Metabolic acidosis with an increased anion gap is most often present when bicarbonate losses are replaced by an anion other than chloride. This type of acidosis commonly results from increased endogenous acid production, such as lactic acidosis or ketoacidosis induced by diabetes mellitus, starvation, or alcohol (see Table 52.6). In uremia, accumulation of organic anions (amino acids, proteins, sulfate, and phosphate) is responsible for the increased anion gap, which is usually less than 24 mEq/L.[17] The severe metabolic acidosis seen in myoglobinuric acute renal failure due to rhabdomyolysis may be caused by the metabolism of large amounts of sulfur-containing amino acids released from myoglobin.[18]

The presence of an elevated anion gap cannot be automatically attributed to an increase in organic acids.[19] Twenty-nine percent of patients with anion gaps of 20–29 mEq/L may have no increase in identifiable organic acids.[19] Further, lactic acidosis was not the culprit in 60% of patients with a high anion gap without azotemia or ketonemia. Identifiable organic anions contributed an average of only 62% to the increment in anion gap. In contrast, the diagnosis of an organic acidosis has been shown to be highly likely when the anion gap exceeds 30 mEq/L.

Another helpful diagnostic parameter, particularly for mixed acid–base disorders, is the ratio of the change in anion gap (AG) to change in bicarbonate ($\Delta AG/\Delta HCO3$). The ratio is usually 1.0 for the common organic acidoses (diabetic ketoacidosis or lactic acidosis). However, when the ratio is greater than 1.2 or less than 0.8, a mixed acid–base disorder is probably present.[17]

Lactic acidosis is one of the most common causes of metabolic acidosis. Lactic acid is the end product of anaerobic metabolism of glucose (glycolysis). In normal individuals, lactic acid, derived from pyruvate, enters the circulation in small amounts and is promptly removed by the liver. In the liver, lactic acid is reoxidized to pyruvic acid, which is then metabolized to CO_2 and H_2O. Plasma lactate concentration in normal, healthy subjects is approximately 1 mEq/L.[20]

Normally, the concentration of lactate in blood is 10 times the concentration of pyruvate (L/P ratio). If pyruvate is elevated (e.g., by increased glucose intake), lactate increases, but the L/P ratio remains unchanged. If anaerobic glycolysis increases (e.g., because of tissue hypoxia) and sufficient oxidized nicotinamide adenine dinucleotide (NAD) is not available to reconvert lactate to pyruvate, lactate will increase more than pyruvate and an increase in L/P ratio will result. This increase in L/P ratio is associated with metabolic acidosis. The basic cause of lactic acid overproduction is inadequate oxygen delivery to cells or the inability of the cells to utilize oxygen.[16]

The definitive diagnosis of lactic acidosis is made by measuring serum lactate concentrations. The serum lactate threshold necessary for a diagnosis of lactic acidosis has not been defined, although lactate concentrations of 4.0–5.0 mEq/L or greater with a simultaneous decrease in bicarbonate and arterial pH are highly suggestive of lactic acidosis. Each 1 mEq/L increase in plasma lactate will cause an equivalent decrease in serum bicarbonate.[20]

The causes of lactic acidosis can be divided into two types: those associated with tissue hypoxia, type A; and those associated primarily with systemic disorders, type B (Table 52.7). The most frequent form of lactic acidosis is type A. Cardiovascular collapse with resultant tissue hypoperfusion is the most common cause of type A lactic acidosis. Poor tissue perfusion and hypoxia influence enzymatic pyruvate and lactate metabolism to stimulate anaerobic glycolysis and decrease lactate utilization. This leads to hyperlactatemia and lactic acidosis. The mortality rate of type A lactic acidosis may be as great as 80% and appears to be related to blood lactate concentrations. Lactate concentrations of 4.4–8.9 mEq/L were associated with a mortality of 75% while the mortality rate was only 18% when lactate concentrations ranged between 1.3 and 4.4 mEq/L.[20]

Type B lactic acidosis may result from a variety of causes, including drugs, toxins, and congenital enzyme deficiency. The exact role of diabetes mellitus in the induction of lactic acidosis is not clear. It may involve a decrease in pyruvate dehydrogenase activity, the enzyme responsible for pyruvate metabolism. Lactic acidosis in neoplastic disease is uncommon and reported mostly in patients with myeloproliferative disorders. Leukocytes and neoplastic cells in general have high rates of glycolysis. In the case of a large tumor or tightly packed bone marrow, oxygenation can be decreased, favoring the accumulation of lactate. Lactic acidosis has been reported in patients with massive liver tumors, and it has been postulated that the liver uptake of lactate is decreased in these patients. Type B lactic acidosis associated with seizures is usually transient and occurs because of excessive muscle activity.[14]

TABLE 52.7. CAUSES OF LACTIC ACIDOSIS

Type A (associated with tissue hypoxia)
Shock
Cardiogenic
Endotoxic
Hypovolemic
Severe anemia
Congestive heart failure
Asphyxia
Carbon monoxide poisoning
Type B (associated with systemic disorders)
Diabetes mellitus
Neoplastic disease
Liver failure
Renal Failure
Convulsions
Abnormal gut flora
Type B1
Biguanides (phenformin, buformin, metformin)
Fructose, sorbitol, xylitol
Ethanol
Methanol, ethylene glycol
Salicylates
Type B3 (associated with inborn errors of metabolism)
Glucose-6-phosphatase deficiency (type 1 glycogen storage disease)
Fructose-6-diphosphatase deficiency
Pyruvate dehydrogenase and carboxylase deficiency
Defective oxidative phosphorylation

(From Frommer JP. Lactic acidosis. Med Clin North Am 1983;67:815–829, with permission.)

Clinical Presentation

Metabolic acidosis can result in alterations in the cardiovascular, gastrointestinal, and central nervous systems. Hyperventilation is often the first sign of metabolic acidosis. At a pH of 7.2, pulmonary ventilation increases about fourfold and an increase of eightfold has been noted at a pH of 7.0.[1] In extremely severe acidosis (pH <6.8), the function of the CNS is disrupted to such a degree that the respiratory center is depressed. Respiratory compensation may occur as Kussmaul's respirations—the deep, rapid respirations seen commonly in patients with diabetic ketoacidosis.

CNS depression has been found to correlate more closely with spinal fluid pH than with blood pH. For this reason, neurologic symptoms tend to occur more frequently and to a greater degree in patients with respiratory acidosis, because the CO_2 accumulated in the respiratory form readily crosses the blood–brain barrier to cause acidosis in the CNS.[2] Because of the slow penetration of administered bicarbonate into the CNS, the CNS pH fails to normalize as rapidly as blood pH. Therefore, patients continue to hyperventilate because of sustained CNS acidity and severe respiratory alkalosis may occur. Sustained lowering of Pa_{CO_2} within 12–36 hours is to be anticipated during the correction of any metabolic acidosis.[2]

Systemic acidosis can cause peripheral vasodilation, characterized by flushing, a rapid heart rate, and wide pulse pressure. Initially, cardiac output may be increased, but as acidosis becomes more severe, it falls as hypotension becomes more pronounced. Experimental work in animals has demonstrated that cardiac contractility decreased as pH declined to values of 7.0 or less by infusion of lactic acid.[21] In contrast, the effects of vagal stimulation were enhanced at pH levels lower than 7.1, probably as a consequence of inhibition of acetylcholinesterase. This increases the danger of vagally mediated bradycardia or arrest during acidosis.

Gastrointestinal symptoms of metabolic acidosis include loss of appetite, nausea, and vomiting. These symptoms occur commonly in patients with renal insufficiency who experience a mild acidosis.[1] Severe acidosis (pH <7.1) interferes with carbohydrate metabolism and insulin utilization and results in hyperglycemia.

The effect of metabolic acidosis on serum potassium depends on the type of acidosis: The effects of mineral acids (e.g., hydrochloric acid) differ from those of organic acids (e.g., lactic acidosis). In dogs, during a steady-state metabolic acidosis produced by the infusion of hydrochloric acid, the change in plasma potassium concentration per 0.1 unit change in pH was a rather consistent increase, averaging 0.6 mEq/L. In contrast, the experimental infusion of organic acid (acetic, lactic, or betahydroxybutyric acid) into animals produced much smaller increments in the plasma potassium concentrations.[12]

Compensation

The patient's primary means to compensate for metabolic acidosis is to increase carbon dioxide excretion and thereby decrease Pa_{CO_2} by increasing their respiratory rate. This ventilatory compensation is initiated as the result of stimulation of the respiratory center due to the changes in cerebral bicarbonate concentration and pH.[2] Arterial blood compensation begins rapidly, but does not reach a steady state for 12–24 hours after the onset of metabolic acidosis. For every 1 mEq/L decrease in bicarbonate concentration below the average of 24, the Pa_{CO_2} decreases by 1.0–1.5 mm Hg from the normal value of 40.[1]

Treatment

Treatment for metabolic acidosis can be approached from two different perspectives depending on the patient's anion gap (Fig. 52.4). Unfortunately, the effectiveness of exogenous alkalizing agents in changing patient outcomes is in doubt. A recent clinical trial in critically ill patients comparing sodium chloride and sodium bicarbonate therapy reported similar changes in cardiac output, arterial pressure, and pulmonary capillary wedge with both agents, despite

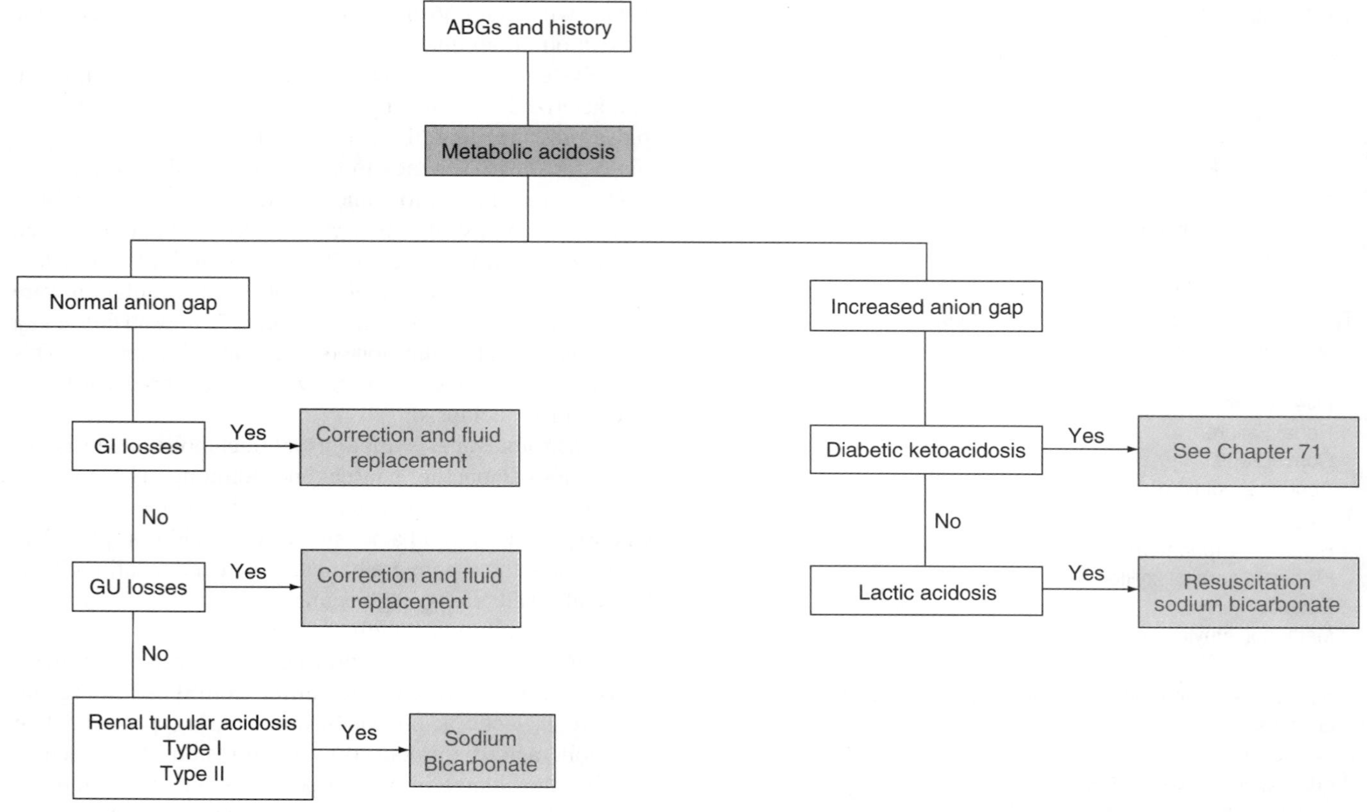

Figure 52.4. Treatment of metabolic acidosis.

significant increases in arterial pH and bicarbonate associated with sodium bicarbonate administration.[22]

Sodium Bicarbonate

Although it has been recommended that sodium bicarbonate be administered to raise the arterial pH to about 7.15–7.20, there are no controlled clinical trials demonstrating that sodium bicarbonate administration is significantly better than general supportive care in reducing morbidity and mortality in these patients.[23,24] In theory, sodium bicarbonate administration provides fluid and electrolyte replacement and increases arterial pH, thereby improving cardiac function, perfusion and oxygenation of peripheral tissues, intracellular pH, and therefore lactate metabolism. However, sodium bicarbonate administration can actually have an adverse effect on intracellular pH. When bicarbonate is given by IV infusion, the carbon dioxide generated diffuses more readily than bicarbonate across cell membranes and into cerebrospinal fluid. Therefore, the intracellular pH can actually be decreased by administration of bicarbonate.[23]

Excessive sodium bicarbonate administration during rescusitation may result in (1) metabolic alkalosis and subsequent impairment of oxygen release from hemoglobin to tissues, (2) sodium and water overload with subsequent hypernatremia and hyperosmolality, and (3) decreased ionized calcium with resultant decreased myocardial contractibility. If there is an endogenous source of bicarbonate, such as can occur in the case of ketoacidosis or lactic acidosis, a bicarbonate "overshoot" may develop since the ketoacids (acetoacetic acid and betahydroxybutyric) or lactic acid are converted in the liver to bicarbonate once the underlying cause of acidosis is corrected. Serum bicarbonate is then increased as regenerated bicarbonate adds to exogenous bicarbonate and an alkalosis may result. Bicarbonate should be administered cautiously in these patients with frequent monitoring of blood gases and serum electrolytes.[23]

In an acute situation (e.g., treatment of metabolic acidosis in cardiac arrest), sodium bicarbonate administration may be necessary. The standards and guidelines from the National Conference on Cardiopulmonary and Emergency Cardiac Care state that sodium bicarbonate is useful in cardiac life support when combined with ventilation in an attempt to maintain near-normal arterial pH during an arrest.[25] It has become apparent that less sodium bicarbonate is needed to provide adequate acid–base control during an arrest than had previously been assumed.

A major component of depressed pH (respiratory acidosis) can be managed without sodium bicarbonate if one maintains adequate ventilation. Keep in mind that administration of sodium bicarbonate is followed by release of carbon dioxide, which requires adequate alveolar activity to ensure continued excretion of this source of potential acid. Thus, the importance of adequate ventilation in the control of pH must be emphasized, as well as the need for repeated arterial measurements of blood pH and $PaCO_2$.

During a cardiac arrest, sodium bicarbonate (initial dose 1 mEq/kg) may be administered by rapid, direct intravenous injection. It should be used only after more proven interventions such as defibrillation, cardiac compression, support of ventilation including intubation, and drug therapies such as epinephrine and antiarrhythmic agents have been employed. Subsequent doses of sodium bicarbonate should be based on measurements of arterial blood pH and $PaCO_2$. Bicarbonate therapy is generally thought not to be necessary in the routine patient with cardiac arrest, even if the initial arrest was unmonitored. Sodium bicarbonate therapy is clearly indicated, however, in hyperkalemia-induced cardiac arrest.[26]

Other alkalinizing agents include lactate, acetate, and citrate ions. These agents are converted in the liver to bicarbonate and may have an advantage over bicarbonate because of their compatibility and stability in parenteral solutions. In patients already receiving total parenteral nutrition, sodium or potassium acetate may be substituted for the usual chloride salts to provide a source of bicarbonate. Ringer's lactate solution has been found to be useful in the resuscitation period of patients in shock. In theory, it would appear that Ringer's lactate solution would be contraindicated for two reasons: (1) The level of excess lactate may increase and compound the lactic acidosis already present, and (2) blood pH may be decreased because the pH of Ringer's lactate is 6–6.5. Canizaro et al.[27] studied 69 patients with hemorrhagic, septic, cardiogenic, or neurogenic shock and 15 injured patients not in shock, all of whom received Ringer's lactate solution during the resuscitation. Initial lactate concentrations correlated well with the clinical impression of the depth of shock. These concentrations rapidly returned to normal after successful resuscitation. This was attributed to reestablishment of tissue perfusion resulting in cessation of excess production of lactate. The remaining lactate would then be rapidly metabolized by the liver after restoration of adequate hepatic blood flow.

Tromethamine

Tromethamine (THAM, TRIS) has also been used to correct metabolic acidosis. It is a highly alkaline, sodium-free organic amine that acts as a proton acceptor to prevent or correct acidosis. Tromethamine combines with hydrogen ions from carbonic acid to form bicarbonate and a cationic buffer. THAM also acts as an osmotic diuretic to increase urine flow, urine pH, and the excretion of fixed acids, CO_2, and electrolytes. At pH 7.4, 30% of THAM is not ionized and therefore is capable of reaching equilibrium with total body water.[28] This portion may penetrate into cells and may neutralize acidic anions of the intracellular fluid. Intracellular pH increases have been noted within 1 hour after the infusion of THAM. There is no clinical or physiologic evidence that this action is beneficial and there are theoretical reasons for believing that it may be undesirable.

When THAM is used, it must be administered slowly and with careful monitoring to avoid alkalosis. Large doses may cause respiratory depression because of a decrease in ventilation secondary to an increase in blood pH and decrease in $PaCO_2$ concentration. Tromethamine solution is highly alkaline and may cause severe inflammation, vascular spasm, or tissue damage (necrosis, sloughing, pain, chemical phlebitis, thrombosis) if infiltration occurs. The usual dosage range for tromethamine is 1–5 mmol/kg administered intravenously during 1 hour, but doses up to 1.25 mmol/kg may be given over 5–15 minutes in acute situations. The dose of tromethamine can be calculated using the following equation[28]:

$$\text{Milliliters of } 0.3\ M \text{ tromethamine} = 1.1\ (\text{body weight in kg})(\text{normal } HCO_3^- - \text{pt's } HCO_3^-)$$

The need for additional tromethamine is determined by serial measurements of the serum bicarbonate concentration and calculation of the base deficit.

Carbicarb

The investigational agent Carbicarb, an equimolar mixture of sodium carbonate (Na_2CO_3) and sodium bicarbonate ($NaHCO_3$), acts to buffer hydrogen ion without the generation of excess CO_2. This theoretically reduces the adverse reaction potential associated with the conversion of CO_2 to carbonic acid.[29–35] In a prospective, double-blind, randomized, multicenter trial, Leung et al.[36] compared Carbicarb versus sodium bicarbonate in surgical patients with mild intraoperative metabolic acidosis. Carbicarb proved as effective as sodium bicarbonate in correcting mild metabolic acidosis. There was also a tendency to increase cardiac output when compared to sodium bicarbonate, a potential therapeutic advantage. However, additional studies are needed to validate these findings, especially in patients with more severe acidosis. Until these studies are completed, the role of Carbicarb remains to be determined.

Dichloroacetate

Another investigational agent, dichloroacetate (DCA), has been shown to significantly lower serum lactate levels and increase blood pH in patients with lactic acidosis.[37,38] DCA facilitates aerobic lactate metabolism by stimulating the activity of lactate dehydrogenase, reverses hyperlactatemia, and decreases morbidity in acquired and congenital forms of lactic acidosis. In a randomized, multicenter, placebo-controlled trial, Stacpoole et al.[37] studied the effects of 50–100 mg/kg of DCA in 252 patients with lactic acidosis. Serum lactate was significantly lowered and blood pH increased, but there was no effect on patient mortality. The drug also improves cardiac output and left ventricular mechanical efficiency under conditions of myocardial ischemia or failure, probably by facilitating myocardial glucose utilization and inhibiting gluconeogenesis, and also inhibits lipogenesis and cholesterolgenesis. Vary and associates[39] reported that DCA administration reversed the abnormal glucose metabolism, branch chain amino acid utilization, and muscle catabolism in septic patients. DCA can cause a reversible peripheral neuropathy that may be ameliorated or prevented with thiamine supplementation. Mild drowsiness has been reported in approximately half of the adult recipients, but no other drug-related adverse effects have been reported.[37] Due to the lack of improvement in patient mortality, the routine use of DCA cannot be recommended at this time.

Treatment of Renal Tubular Acidosis

Both type I and type II RTA are treated with the administration of alkali; in type I RTA, 1–3 mEq/kg/d may be needed to correct the metabolic acidosis. Potassium supplementation may also be necessary (e.g., potassium citrate, which would provide both potassium and alkali). In type II RTA, 10–25 mEq of alkali per kilogram per day may be needed to maintain the bicarbonate concentration in the normal range. Potassium supplementation is also necessary because of urinary potassium losses that increase with the increasing bicarbonaturia following alkali treatment.[14,15]

METABOLIC ALKALOSIS

The second type of simple nonrespiratory, or metabolic, acid–base disorder is metabolic alkalosis. This disorder, which is characterized by a primary increase in bicarbonate concentration, is a common acid–base disturbance among hospitalized patients. Wilson et al.[40] reported that 33% of the more than 1000 critically ill patients with acid–base disturbances experienced metabolic alkalosis. Forty-one percent of the patients who had pH values between 7.54 and 7.56 died and more than 80% of those with pH values greater than 7.56 died. The mortality was highest among those patients experiencing severe sepsis with metabolic alkalosis and respiratory alkalosis. Although a significant correlation between degree of alkalosis and incidence of mortality was reported, this does not indicate that reversal of the alkalosis would have altered the mortality rate.

Pathophysiology

A primary elevation of bicarbonate concentration can be generated by three mechanisms: (1) a net loss of hydrogen ion from the ECF space; (2) a net addition of bicarbonate or its precursors (i.e., carbonate, citrate, acetate) to the ECF space; or (3) loss of chloride-rich bicarbonate-poor fluid. Disturbances that initiate metabolic alkalosis can be divided into two categories on the basis of their response to treatment with saline volume expansion. Those categories are sodium chloride-responsive disorders and sodium chloride-resistant disorders (see Table 52.8).

The most common initiating event for metabolic alkalosis is the loss of chloride-rich, bicarbonate-poor fluid from the body as seen with diuretic use, nasogastric suctioning, or vomiting. Gastric secretory volume is usually less than 50 mL/h in the basal state but may increase fivefold with stimulation. One or more liters of gastric fluid may be lost daily with persistent vomiting. The 24-hour gastric juice output in a 70-kg adult includes 1–2 L of fluid, 40–160 mEq of sodium, 10 mq of potassium, 200 mq of chloride, and 25–100 mEq of hydrogen ion. Hydrogen ion and bicarbonate are formed from CO_2 and water by gastric parietal cells.[41] The hydrogen ion is secreted into gastric fluid and the bicarbonate is retained in the ECF. Normally, an amount of bicarbonate equal to the bicarbonate generated in the stomach is eliminated in the alkaline pancreatic and small bowel secretions, maintaining hydrogen ion balance. With vomiting and nasogastric suctioning, hydrogen ion is lost externally. Bicarbonate is not eliminated and metabolic alkalosis results.

Diuretic therapy, with agents acting on the cortical and medullary ascending limb of the loop of Henle (e.g., furosemide, bumetamide, torsemide, and thiazides) is a common cause of metabolic alkalosis. These agents pro-

TABLE 52.8. CAUSES OF METABOLIC ALKALOSIS

Sodium chloride responsive (urinary chloride concentration <10 mEq/L)
Gastrointestinal disorders
Vomiting
Gastric drainage
Villous adenoma of the colon
Chloride diarrhea
Diuretic therapy
Correction of chronic hypercapnia
Cystic fibrosis
Sodium chloride resistant (urinary chloride concentration >20 mEq/L)
Excess mineralocorticoid activity
Hyperaldosteronism
Cushing's syndrome
Bartter's syndrome
Excessive licorice intake
Profound potassium depletion
Unclassified
Alkali administration
Milk–alkali syndrome
Massive blood or plasmanate transfusion
Nonparathyroid hypercalcemia
Glucose ingestion after starvation
Large doses of penicillin

mote the excretion of sodium and potassium almost exclusively in association with chloride without a proportionate increase in bicarbonate excretion. Net acid excretion is also frequently increased during the diuresis because of both the disproportionate loss of chloride and the loss of hydrogen ion in the urine by increasing tubular flow and sodium delivery to the distal tubule for sodium–hydrogen exchange. Patients at risk from metabolic alkalosis are those with a combined volume depletion, in which the distal tubule exchange sites are stimulated to reabsorb sodium; those on a low-salt diet, which limits the sodium chloride available for reabsorption, and those on diuretics, which continue to deliver sodium to the distal exchange site. Alkalosis caused by diuretic use is usually mild, but the accompanying hypokalemia may be serious.[41]

Other causes of metabolic alkalosis are those that are resistant to sodium chloride administration. Many of these are associated with excess mineralocorticoid activity. Increased mineralocorticoid activity may result from (1) primary adrenal overproduction, as in primary hyperaldosteronism, or oversupply of endogenous mineralocorticoids as in licorice ingestion; and (2) oversecretion of mineralocorticoid secondary to increased renin activity. In the sodium chloride-resistant group, renin secretion is driven by stimuli other than ECF depletion such as renal artery stenosis, magnesium deficiency, or Bartter's syndrome, a renal tubular reabsorptive defect. Mineralocorticoids act on the distal segment of the renal tubule where they increase sodium reabsorption and enhance secretion of potassium and hydrogen ion into the tubular lumen. For example, in hyperaldosteronism, an increase in aldosterone leads to stimulation of the distal renal tubular exchange of sodium for hydrogen. The increased hydrogen ion secreted into the renal tubular causes the generation of new bicarbonate or the reclamation of filtered bicarbonate.[1]

Miscellaneous causes of metabolic alkalosis include large doses of penicillins (e.g., ticarcillin) since they act as a nonreabsorbable anion. High concentrations of the poorly reabsorbable anion in the distal renal tubule result in an increased flow rate and electrical negativity within the tubular lumen. These changes enhance the secretion of potassium and hydrogen ion, producing increased plasma bicarbonate concentration and hypokalemia.

No matter which condition initiated the metabolic alkalosis, the kidney is responsible for its maintenance. Normally, the kidneys are capable of excreting all bicarbonate presented to them, even during periods of increased bicarbonate loads. The kidney senses changes in the blood bicarbonate concentration and excess bicarbonate is excreted in the urine to return the blood bicarbonate concentration to normal. If the kidneys are working properly, excess bicarbonate will be excreted and metabolic alkalosis will not occur.[41]

Several mechanisms tend to increase bicarbonate reabsorption by the kidney, thereby maintaining a metabolic alkalosis. The combination of decreased ECF volume, hypochloremia, and hypokalemia associated with diuretic use or nasogastric suction can maintain a metabolic alkalosis.[3] During periods of decreased ECF volume, sodium reabsorption is enhanced in the proximal and distal tubules. Sodium reabsorption from the renal tubule must be associated with an ion with a negative charge, such as chloride, or it must be exchanged for an ion in the tubular cell that has a positive charge, such as potassium or hydrogen. Normally, 80% of sodium is reabsorbed along with chloride and 20% is exchanged for hydrogen or potassium. In hypochloremia, there is less chloride available for reabsorption and therefore more sodium must be exchanged for potassium or hydrogen. Only a small amount of potassium is available for exchange with sodium and when the patient becomes hypokalemic, hydrogen is exchanged instead. This loss of hydrogen ions results in hypochloremic metabolic alkalosis.

Metabolic alkalosis may also be maintained by persistent hypokalemia, independent of hypovolemia. Hypokalemic metabolic alkalosis is frequently associated with excess mineralocorticoid activity since mineralocorticoids promote sodium reabsorption and enhance potassium and hydrogen ion excretion in the urine.[41]

Clinical Presentation

There are no unique signs or symptoms associated with metabolic alkalosis, but patients may complain of symptoms related to the underlying cause of the disorder (e.g., muscle weakness with hypokalemia or postural dizziness with volume depletion). They may have a history of vomiting, gastric drainage, or diuretic use, all of which contribute to the development of metabolic alkalosis. Neuromuscular irritability may be present with signs of tetany or hyperactive reflexes possibly caused by the decreased ionized calcium concentration that occurs secondary to the increase in pH. This decrease in ionized calcium may be caused by a conformational change in the albumin molecules, to which the calcium is bound, resulting in increased binding, or by decreased competition from hydrogen ions for binding sites on the albumin molecule.[41] Mental confusion, muscle cramping, and paresthesia may also occur. Severe alkalemia (blood pH >7.55) has been associated with cardiac arrhythmias in patients with normal hearts, but particularly in those with heart disease (see Respiratory Alkalosis).[42]

Compensation

After the plasma bicarbonate has been elevated by one of the three basic mechanisms that generate metabolic alkalosis, the body attempts to restore the pH to normal. The immediate response to elevated bicarbonate is chemical buffering. This buffering involves the movement of hydrogen ions from within the cells to the ECF in exchange for potassium and sodium. This system is immediate in onset but limited in its capacity to protect the body from sudden life-threatening changes in extracellular pH.

The second phase of the body's response to metabolic alkalosis is respiratory compensation (i.e., hypoventilation to raise the $Pa{CO_2}$). Using the Henderson–Hasselbach equation one can see that an increase in the $Pa{CO_2}$ will return the $Pa{CO_2}$/bicarbonate ratio, and therefore the pH, toward normal. Respiratory compensation is initiated when the central and peripheral chemoreceptors sense an increase in pH and occurs over 1 to several hours. The $Pa{CO_2}$ increases 6–7 mm Hg for each 10 mEq/L increase in bicarbonate, up to a $Pa{CO_2}$ of about 50–60 mm Hg,[1] before hypoxia sensors react to prevent further hypoventilation. If the $Pa{CO_2}$ is normal or less than normal, one should consider the presence of a superimposed respiratory alkalosis, which may be secondary to fever, gram-negative sepsis, or pain.

Treatment

Treatment should be aimed at correcting the underlying cause. However, unlike respiratory acidosis, the treatment of the cause may not correct the acid–base disorder. Metabolic alkalosis may persist until the renal mechanism responsible for maintaining the disorder is eliminated, despite the fact that the original cause of the elevated plasma bicarbonate may have susbsided. For example, hypovolemia must be treated with sodium chloride in certain cases (i.e., diuretic abuse, nasogastric suction) to allow excretion of bicarbonate by the kidney. Therapy for metabolic alkalosis is divided into two treatment categories: sodium chloride-responsive disorders and sodium chloride-resistant disorders (Fig. 52.5).

Sodium Chloride-Responsive Disorders

Sodium chloride-responsive disorders are those resulting from volume depletion and chloride loss as occurs with severe vomiting or nasogastric suction. Initially, therapy is directed at expanding intravascular volume and replenishing chloride stores. Sodium chloride and potassium solutions should be administered to patients who can tolerate the administration of fluid and sodium.[43] Patients with a metabolic alkalosis who are volume expanded or intolerant to sodium volume loads, as in congestive heart failure, may benefit from the carbonic anhydrase inhibitor, acetazolamide. This agent inhibits the action of carbonic anhydrase in the kidney tubule cell and promotes renal bicarbonate and potassium excretion, resulting in a decreased concentration of bicarbonate in the ECF. Administration of one or two doses of acetazolamide, 250 or 500 mg, may promote a sufficient bicarbonate diuresis to return the pH toward normal.

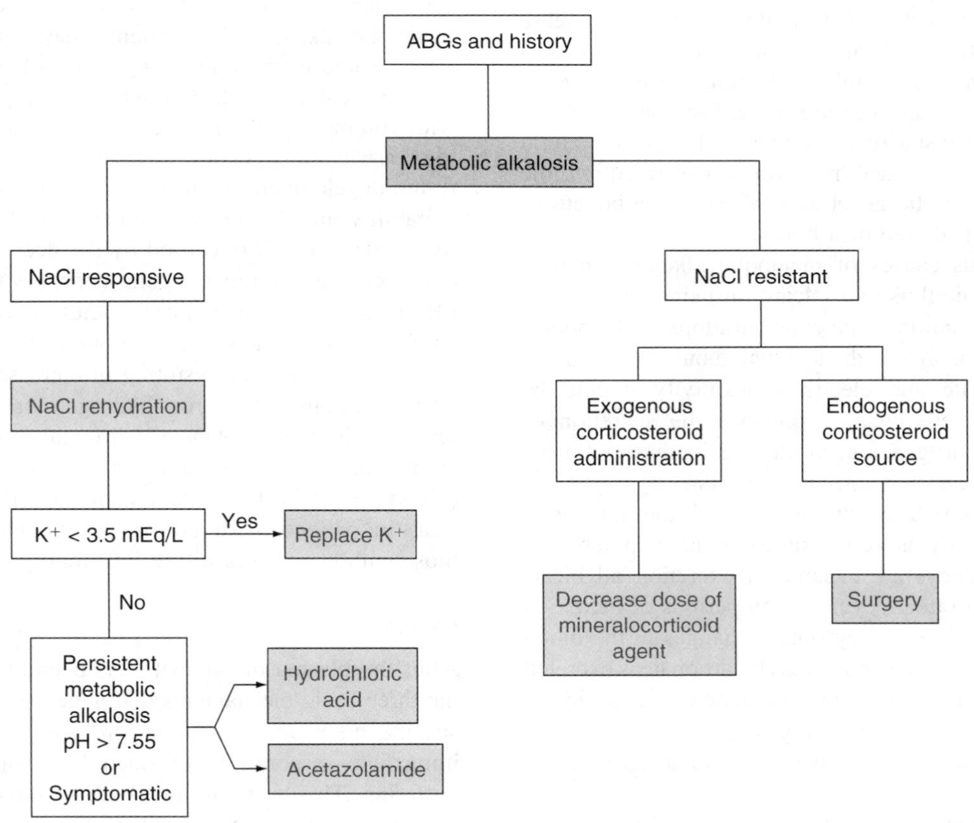

Figure 52.5. Treatment algorithm for patients with primary metabolic alkalosis.

Other agents sometimes used to treat sodium chloride-responsive metabolic alkalosis include hydrochloric acid, ammonium chloride, and arginine monohydrochloride. Indications for the use of hydrochloric acid include severe metabolic alkalosis (pH >7.55), symptoms of alkali toxicity unresponsive to fluid and electrolyte administration, and the patient's inability to tolerate a large sodium and fluid load (i.e., decompensated CHF or renal failure with oliguria).[43] The dose of hydrochloric acid may be based on an estimate of the chloride deficit:

$$\text{Dose HCl (mEq)} = [0.2 \text{ L/kg} \times \text{Body weight (kg)}] \times [103 - \text{Observed serum chloride}]$$

where the estimated chloride space is 0.2 times the body weight and the average serum chloride is 103 mEq/L. The duration of infusion of hydrochloric acid has ranged from 4–24 hours, although the total dose is usually administered over 12–24 hours. Improvement is usually seen within 24 hours of initiating therapy. Arterial blood gases and serum electrolytes should be drawn every 4–12 hours to evaluate and adjust therapy. If the $Paco_2$ is markedly elevated because of respiratory compensation, the estimated dose of hydrochloric acid should be infused over at least 24 hours.[44] Otherwise, a severe transient respiratory acidosis may occur because of the slower reduction of the elevated bicarbonate concentration in the cerebrospinal fluid than in the extracellular fluid.[45]

Hydrochloric acid is usually infused intravenously via a large central vein as a 0.1–0.25 *N* HCl solution in either 5% dextrose or normal saline, although sterile water has also been used. Extemporaneously prepared solutions can be made by adding 100–250 mEq of HCl through a 0.22-μm filter into a glass container of saline or dextrose. Mirtallo et al.[46] demonstrated that hydrochloric acid may also be added to parenteral nutrient solutions and administered via a central line without serious degradation of proteins. The rate of infusion should be 100–125 mL/h (10–25 mEq/h) with frequent monitoring of arterial blood gases. The infusion should be stopped when the arterial pH falls to 7.45, in order to prevent overcorrection.[43]

Ammonium chloride has a limited role in the treatment of metabolic alkalosis. Ammonium chloride is converted by the liver to urea and free hydrochloric acid[28]:

$$2NH_4^+ + 2Cl^- + 2HCO_3^- \rightarrow CO\,(NH_2)_2 + CO_2 + 3H_2O + 2Cl^-$$

The dose of ammonium chloride can also be calculated on the basis of the chloride deficit (using the same method as dosing HCl), but only half of the calculated dose of ammonium chloride should be administered to avoid ammonia toxicity.[27] Ammonium chloride is available as a 26.75% solution containing 100 mEq in 20 mL, which should be further diluted prior to administration. A dilute solution may be prepared by adding 100 mEq of ammonium chloride to 500 mL of normal saline and infusing it at a rate not exceeding 1 mEq/min. Improvement in metabolic status is usually seen within 24 hours of ammonium chloride administration. CNS toxicity, marked by confusion, irritability, seizures, and coma, has been associated with faster rates of administration. It must be administered cautiously to patients with renal or hepatic impairment, because serum ammonia and urea levels may increase. This may lead to encephalopathy in patients with hepatic dysfunction because of impaired conversion of ammonia to urea, and for patients with renal impairment, it may worsen their uremia.[28]

Arginine monohydrochloride is available as a 10% solution, which contains 0.475 mEq/mL of both hydrogen and chloride. A dose of 10 g/h given intravenously has been used to treat metabolic alkalosis, although it is not FDA-approved for this purpose.[27,42] Like ammonium chloride, arginine must undergo metabolism by the liver to produce hydrogen ions. Unlike ammonium chloride, arginine combines with ammonia in the body to synthesize urea; thus, it may be used in patients with relative hepatic insufficiency. Patients with renal insufficiency should not receive arginine monohydrochloride because it may significantly elevate blood urea nitrogen and has been associated with severe hyperkalemia.[15,27] The increase in potassium is caused by arginine-induced shifts of potassium from the intracellular to the extracellular space.

In patients with metabolic alkalosis caused by nasogastric suction, histamine H_2-receptor antagonists and omeprazole have been used to decrease the volume and hydrogen ion content in gastric fluids. Standard doses of H_2 antagonists produce a marked reduction in volume of gastric aspirate and acid production and demonstrate a significantly decreased H^+ loss during nasogastric suctioning.[16,47,48]

Sodium Chloride-Resistant Disorders

Sodium chloride-resistant disorders are commonly associated with hypermineralocorticoidism and are characterized by plasma volume expansion, hypertension, and a high urinary chloride concentration. Treatment of these disorders involves the removal of the source of excess mineralocorticoid activity. Patients who are taking corticosteroids may have to have their dose decreased or may need to be switched to a corticosteroid with less mineralocorticoid activity. Patients with an endogenous source of excess mineralocorticoid activity may require surgery. Restriction of dietary sodium also helps prevent metabolic alkalosis.

MIXED ACID–BASE DISORDERS

When two or more primary acid–base disturbances occur simultaneously, a mixed acid–base disorder results. A mixed disturbance can be suspected from the clinical setting and medical history and can be diagnosed with this information together with arterial blood gas and electrolyte data.

TABLE 52.9. MIXED RESPIRATORY AND METABOLIC ACIDOSIS

	Normal	Uncomplicated Metabolic Acidosis	Mixed: Severe	Mixed: Mild
HCO_3^- (mEq/L)	24	15	17	16
Pco_2 (mm Hg)	40	30	50	37
pH	7.40	7.32	7.15	7.26
Anion gap (mEq/L)	10	20	20	21

Clinical example: Patient with cardiopulmonary arrest or COPD plus shock.

Diagnosis

The diagnosis of a mixed disorder depends on an understanding of the appropriate quantitative response of the defense mechanisms in the primary, uncomplicated acid–base disorders. To diagnose mixed disorders, one must know how each of the four simple disorders alters pH, $Paco_2$, and HCO_3. If a given set of blood gases does not fall within the range of expected responses for a simple acid–base disorder according to the nomogram (Fig. 52.3), a mixed disorder should be suspected. In addition to laboratory information, a clinical evaluation of the patient is important. A thorough history and physical examination will often lead to the diagnosis, even before the laboratory data are available. Examples of common mixed disorders follow.

Respiratory Acidosis and Metabolic Acidosis

In mixed respiratory and metabolic acidosis there is a failure of compensation. The respiratory disorder prevents the compensatory decrease in $Paco_2$ expected in the defense against metabolic acidosis. The metabolic disorder prevents the buffering and renal mechanisms from raising the bicarbonate concentration as expected in the defense against respiratory acidosis. In the absence of compensatory mechanisms, the pH decreases markedly (Table 52.9).

A mixed respiratory and metabolic acidosis may develop in patients with cardiorespiratory arrest, in chronic lung disease patients who are in shock, and in metabolic acidosis patients who develop respiratory failure. This mixed disorder should be treated by responding to both the respiratory and metabolic acidosis. Improved oxygen delivery must be initiated to improve hypercarbia and hypoxia. Mechanical ventilation may be needed to reduce $Paco_2$. During the initial stage of therapy, appropriate amounts of $NaHCO_3$ should be given to reverse the metabolic acidosis (see section on Treatment, under Metabolic Acidosis).

Respiratory Alkalosis and Metabolic Alkalosis

The combination of respiratory and metabolic alkalosis is the most common mixed acid–base disorder. This mixed disorder occurs frequently in critically ill surgical patients with respiratory alkalosis caused by mechanical ventilation, hypoxia, sepsis, hypotension, neurologic damage, pain, or drugs, and with metabolic alkalosis caused by vomiting or nasogastric suctioning and massive blood transfusions. It may also occur in patients with hepatic cirrhosis, hyperventilation, diuretic use, or vomiting, and in patients with chronic respiratory acidosis and an elevated plasma bicarbonate concentration who are placed on mechanical ventilation and undergo a rapid fall in $Paco_2$ to hypocapnic levels.

The decrease in bicarbonate concentration that usually compensates for respiratory alkalosis is prevented by the complicating metabolic alkalosis. Likewise, the increase in $Paco_2$ expected to compensate for metabolic alkalosis is prevented by primary respiratory alkalosis. Sample laboratory values found in mixed respiratory and metabolic alkalosis are listed in Table 52.10. The failure of compensation that occurs with mixed respiratory and metabolic alkalosis may result in a severe alkalosis.

Correction of the metabolic component by administration of sodium chloride and potassium chloride solutions should be undertaken, and readjustment of the ventilator or treatment of an underlying disorder causing hyperventila-

TABLE 52.10. MIXED RESPIRATORY AND METABOLIC ALKALOSIS

	Normal	Uncomplicated: Metabolic Alkalosis	Uncomplicated: Respiratory Alkalosis	Mixed: Severe	Mixed: Mild
HCO_3^- (mEq/L)	24	35	17	32	32
Pco_2 (mm Hg)	40	47	25	30	39
pH	7.40	7.49	7.45	7.65	7.53

Clinical example: Patient with hepatic cirrhosis plus hyperventilation, use of diuretics, or emesis.

TABLE 52.11. MIXED RESPIRATORY ALKALOSIS AND METABOLIC ACIDOSIS

	Normal	Uncomplicated Metabolic Acidosis	Mixed	
			Severe	Mild
HCO_3^- (mEq/L)	24	15	13	14
P_{CO_2} (mm Hg)	40	30	15	24
pH	7.40	7.32	7.56	7.39

Clinical examples: (1) Salicylate intoxication, (2) hepatic failure leading to renal failure and hyperventilation.

tion may correct or ameliorate the respiratory component of this mixed disorder.

Metabolic Acidosis and Respiratory Alkalosis

This mixed disorder may be seen in patients with advanced liver disease, salicylate intoxication, and patients with pulmonary-renal syndromes. The combination of respiratory alkalosis and metabolic acidosis is a disorder of excessive compensation. The respiratory alkalosis decreases the Pa_{CO_2} beyond the appropriate range of the respiratory compensation for metabolic acidosis. The plasma bicarbonate concentration also falls below the level expected in primary respiratory alkalosis. In a sense, the defense of pH for either disorder alone is enhanced; thus, the pH may be normal or close to normal, with a low Pa_{CO_2} and a low HCO_3^- (Table 52.11). Treatment of this disorder should be directed at the underlying cause. Because of the enhanced compensation, the pH is usually closer to normal than in either of the two simple disorders.

Metabolic Alkalosis and Respiratory Acidosis

This mixed disorder may occur in patients with chronic obstructive pulmonary disease (COPD) and respiratory acidosis who are treated with salt restrictions, diuretics, and possibly glucocorticoids. COPD patients with CO_2 retention and respiratory acidosis often develop congestive heart failure requiring diuretics. When diuretics are initiated, the plasma bicarbonate may increase due to renal bicarbonate production and reabsorption, providing mechanisms for both generating and maintaining metabolic alkalosis. The elevated pH diminishes respiratory drive and may therefore worsen the pulmonary disease (Table 52.12).

Although the pH may not deviate significantly from normal, treatment may need to be initiated in order to maintain Pa_{O_2} and Pa_{CO_2} at acceptable levels. Since it is often difficult to correctly identify this mixed disorder, it is helpful to observe the patient's response to discontinuation of diuretics and administration of sodium and potassium chloride. This treatment will correct the metabolic alkalosis component if it is a simple metabolic alkalosis, but will only minimally affect the Pa_{CO_2} if it is a mixed disorder. Treatment should be aimed at decreasing plasma bicarbonate with sodium and potassium chloride therapy, allowing the renal excretion of retained bicarbonate from the diuretic-induced metabolic alkalosis. This therapy should be used cautiously to avoid exacerbating the congestive heart failure.

PATIENT OUTCOME

Since acid–base disorders are such a common and widespread problem, pharmacists may play a key role in identifying, preventing, and properly treating acid–base abnormalities in patients. Some pharmacists mistakenly believe that acid–base disorders only occur in the ICU setting, but patients in ambulatory and extended care settings have many chronic conditions and drug therapies that commonly affect acid–base balance. Thus, pharmacists in all practice settings should utilize their knowledge to identify patients at high risk for developing drug-related problems and to undertake appropriate prevention and treatment measures to improve their patients' quality of life.

TABLE 52.12. MIXED METABOLIC ALKALOSIS AND RESPIRATORY ACIDOSIS

	Normal	Uncomplicated		Mixed Disorder
		Metabolic Alkalosis	Respiratory Acidosis	
HCO_3^- (mEq/L)	24	36	36	40
P_{CO_2} (mm Hg)	40	48	70	67
pH	7.40	7.49	7.33	7.40

Clinical example: A COPD/CHF patient receiving diuretic therapy.

References

1. Narins RG, Emmett M. Simple and mixed acid–base disorders: A practical approach. Medicine 1980;59:161–187.
2. Narins RG. Acid–base disorders: Definitions and introductory concepts, in Narins RG (ed): Maxwell & Kleeman's Clinical Disorders of Fluid and Electrolyte Metabolism, 5th ed. New York, McGraw-Hill, 1994, pp 765–768.
3. Laske ME. Normal regulation of acid–base balance. Med Clin North Am 1983;67:771–780.
4. Weil MH, Rackow EC, Trenio R, et al. Difference in acid–base state between venous and arterial blood during cardiopulmonary resuscitation. N Engl J Med 1986;315:153–155.
5. Fell WL. Sampling and measurement of blood gases, in Lane EE, Walker JF (eds): Clinical Arterial Blood Gas Analysis. St. Louis, CV Mosby, 1987, p 202.
6. Broughton JO. Understanding Blood Gases. Madison, WI, Ohmeda, 1980.
7. Arbus GS. An in-vivo acid–base nomogram for clinical use. Can Med Assoc J 1973;109:291–293.
8. Mazzara JR, Ayers SM, Grace WJ. Extreme hypocapnia in the critically ill patient. Am J Med 1974;56:450–456.
9. Kaehny WD. Pathogenesis and management of respiratory and mixed acid–base disorders, in Schrier RW (ed): Renal and Electrolyte Disorders, 4th ed. Boston: Little, Brown, and Co, 1992, pp 211–230.
10. Lawson NW, Butler GH, Ray CT. Alkalosis and cardiac arrhythmias. Anesth Analgesia 1973;52:951–964.
11. Gennari FJ. Respiratory acidosis and alkalosis, in Narins RG (ed): Maxwell & Kleeman's Clinical Disorders of Fluid and Electrolyte Metabolism, 5th ed. New York, McGraw-Hill, 1994, pp 957–990.
12. Stearns RH, Cox M, Feig PU, Singer I. Internal potassium balance and the control of the plasma potassium concentration. Medicine 1981;60:339–354.
13. Okel BB, Hurst JW. Prolonged hyperventilation in man: Associated electrolyte changes and subjective symptoms. Arch Intern Med 1961;108:757–762.
14. Narins RG, Krishna GG, Yee J, et al. The metabolic acidoses, in Narins RG (ed): Maxwell & Kleeman's Clinical Disorders of Fluid and Electrolyte Metabolism, 5th ed. New York, McGraw-Hill, 1994, pp 769–826.
15. Halperin ML, Carlisle EJ, Donnelly S, et al. Renal tubular acidosis, in Narins RG (ed): Maxwell & Kleeman's Clinical Disorders of Fluid and Electrolyte Metabolism, 5th ed. New York, McGraw-Hill, 1994, pp 875–910.
16. Shapiro JI, Kaehny WD. Pathogenesis and management of metabolic acidosis and alkalosis, in Schrier RW (ed): Renal and Electrolyte Disorders, 4th ed. Boston, Little, Brown, and Co, 1992, pp 175–181.
17. Oster JR, Perez GO, Materson BJ. Use of the anion gap in clinical medicine. South Med J 1988;81:229–237.
18. McCarron DA, Elliot WC, Rose JS, et al. Severe mixed metabolic acidosis secondary to rhabdomyolysis. Am J Med 1979;67:905–908.
19. Gabow PA, Kaehny WD, Fennessey PV, et al. Diagnostic importance of an increased serum anion gap. N Engl J Med 1980;303:854–858.
20. Frommer JP. Lactic acidosis. Med Clin North Am 1983;67:815–829.
21. Teplinsky K, O'Toole M, Olman M, et al. Effect of lactic acidosis on canine hemodynamics and left ventricular function. Am J Physiol 1990;258:H1193–H1199.
22. Cooper DJ, Walley KR, Wiggs BR, Russell JA. Bicarbonate does not improve hemodynamics in critically ill patients who have lactic acidosis: A prospective controlled clinical study. Ann Intern Med 1990;112:492–498.
23. Stacpoole PW. Lactic acidosis: The case against bicarbonate therapy. Ann Intern Med 1986;105:276–278.
24. Narins RG, Cohen JJ. Bicarbonate therapy for organic acidosis: The case for its continued use. Ann Intern Med 1987;106:615–618.
25. Emergency Cardiac Care Committee and Subcomittees, American Heart Association. Guidelines for cardiopulmonary resuscitation and emergency cardiac care. JAMA 1992;268:2171–2302.
26. Raehl CL. Advances in drug therapy of cardiopulmonary arrest. Clin Pharm 1987;6:118–139.
27. Canizaro PC, Prager MD, Shires GT. The infusion of Ringer's lactate solution during shock. Surg Forum 1971;122:494–501.
28. Drug Information. American Hospital Formulary Service. 1994;1575–6,1638–9,1645–6.
29. Gazmuri RJ, von Planta M, Weil MH, Rackow EC. Cardiac effects of carbon dioxide-consuming and carbon dioxide-generation buffers during cardiopulmonary resuscitation. J Am Coll Cardiol 1990;15(2):482–490.
30. Bersin RM, Arieff AI. Improved hemodynamic function during hypoxia with Carbicarb, a new agent for the management of acidosis. Circulation 1988;77:227–233.
31. Kucera RR, Shapiro JI, Whalen MA, et al. Brain pH effects of $NaHCO_3$ and Carbicarb in lactic acidosis. Crit Care Med 1989;17:1320–1323.
32. Shapiro JI. Functional and metabolic responses of the isolated heart during acidosis: Effects of sodium bicarbonate and Carbicarb. Am J Physiol 1990;258:H1835–H1839.
33. Shapiro JI, Mathew A, Whalen M, et al. Different effects of sodium bicarbonate and an alternate buffer [Carbicarb] in normal volunteers. J Crit Care 1990;5:1.
34. Shapiro JI, Whalen M, Kucera R, et al. Brain pH responses to sodium bicarbonate and Carbicarb during systemic acidosis. Am J Physiol 1989;256:H1316–H1321.
35. Rhee KH, Toro LO, McDonald GG, et al. Carbicarb, sodium bicarbonate, and sodium chloride in hypoxic lactic acidosis. Chest 1993;104:913–918.
36. Leung JM, Landow L, Franks M, et al. Safety and efficacy of intravenous Carbicarb in patients undergoing surgery: Comparison with sodium bicarbonate in the treatment of mild metabolic acidosis. Crit Care Med 1994;22:1540–1549.
37. Stacpoole PW, Wright EC, Baumgartner TG, et al. A controlled clinical trial of dichloroacetate for treatment of lactic acidosis. N Engl J Med 1992;327:1564–1569.
38. Stacpoole PW. The pharmacology of dichloroacetate. Metabolism 1989;38:1124–1144.
39. Vary TC, Siegel JH, Zechnich A, et al. Pharmacologic reversal of abnormal glucose regulation, BCAA utilization, and muscle catabolism in sepsis by dichloroacetate. J Trauma 1988;28:1301–1311.

40. Wilson RF, Gibson D, Percinel AK, et al. Severe alkalosis in critically ill patients. Arch Surg 1972;105:197–203.
41. Sabatini S, Kurtzman NA. Metabolic alkalosis, in Narins RG (ed): Maxwell & Kleeman's Clinical Disorders of Fluid and Electrolyte Metabolism, 5th ed. New York, McGraw-Hill, 1994, pp 933–956.
42. Lawson NW, Butler GH, Ray CT. Alkalosis and cardiac arrythmias. Anesth Analg 1973;52:951–964.
43. Martin WJ, Matzke GR. Treating severe metabolic alkalosis. Clin Pharm 1982;1:42–48.
44. Harken AH, Gabel RA, Fencl A, et al. Hydrochloric acid in the correction of metabolic alkalosis. Arch Surg 1975;110:819–821.
45. Brimioulle S, Berre J, Dufaye P, et al. Hydrochloric acid infusion for treatment of metabolic alkalosis associated with respiratory acidosis. Crit Care Med 1989;17:232–236.
46. Mirtallo JM, Rogers KR, Johnson JA, et al. Stability of amino acids and the availability of acid in total parenteral nutrition solutions containing hydrochloric acid. Am J Hosp Pharm 1981;38:1729–1731.
47. Rowlands BJ, Tindall SF, Elliot DJ. The use of dilute hydrochloric acid and cimetidine to reverse severe metabolic alkalosis. Postgrad Med J 1978;54:118–123.
48. Barton CH, Vaziri ND, Ness RL, et al. Cimetidine in the management of metabolic alkalosis induced by nasogastric drainage. Arch Surg 1979;1:70–74.

Section 5
NEUROLOGIC DISORDERS

Chapter 53

Introduction to Neurology

Christina Dalmady-Israel, PharmD, BCPS

The complexity of the nervous system, with its vast number of neurotransmitters and intricate neuronal pathways and a unique approach to diagnosis, make the study of neurology challenging. In most subspecialties, a patient's signs and symptoms point to a diagnosis (e.g., the triad of polydipsia, polyphagia, and polyuria directs one toward a diagnosis of diabetes mellitus). In contrast, various neurologic diseases may affect the same part of the brain and cause identical symptoms (e.g., weakness may be seen with ischemic cerebrovascular disease, multiple sclerosis, myasthenia gravis, tumor, etc.). Thus, in neurologic patients, symptomatology is used to determine the anatomic structure or system of neurons affected ("location of the lesion") rather than a particular diagnosis. Additional information, such as patient and family history, mode of onset, evolution of symptoms, and laboratory findings, is used in concert with symptomatology to ascertain an etiologic diagnosis.

Further challenges are encountered in approaching the treatment of these diseases. In some cases (e.g., Parkinson's disease, multiple sclerosis), treatment is primarily symptomatic and may not alter the progression of the disease or affect the underlying disease process. Clinical trials performed in patients with some of the less common neurologic syndromes often do not include large numbers of patients and are not well designed. This is partly because the exact pathophysiology of many neurologic syndromes remains unclear. In addition, the prevalence is low when compared, for example, with cardiovascular disease and diabetes. Despite these problems, the field of neurology is exciting and dynamic. The advent of more sophisticated imaging techniques such as magnetic resonance imaging, positron emission tomography, and single photon emission computed tomography has led to advances in diagnosis and a better understanding of the pathophysiology of many neurologic disorders. The decade of the 1990s has been declared the "decade of the brain," and new funding initiatives have been implemented to advance basic scientific and clinical knowledge in several neurobiologic areas.[1] This decade has already witnessed the approval of new drugs to treat Parkinson's disease, headaches, seizure disorders, and multiple sclerosis. Many other drugs are currently under evaluation for these and other disorders.

THE NEUROLOGIC EXAMINATION

To fully understand the various neurologic syndromes, it is important for the clinician to have a basic understanding of the neurologic examination. In addition to the patient history, which is an essential part of any medical examination, the neurologic examination can be classified into eight basic components, as listed in Table 53.1. It is beyond the scope of this introduction to give a detailed review of each of these components; however, each is briefly discussed in the following sections. For more detailed information, the reader can refer to a variety of textbooks of neurology.[2]

HISTORY

Obtaining an accurate and complete history is of utmost importance in the evaluation of neurologic diseases. In

TABLE 53.1. BASIC COMPONENTS OF THE NEUROLOGIC EXAMINATION

1. History
2. Cerebral function (mental status)
3. Cranial nerve function
4. Cerebellar function
5. Motor function
6. Sensory function
7. Reflex function
8. Gait and stance

many instances the diagnosis is made on the basis of the history and the rest of the examination serves to confirm this diagnosis and aid in localizing the problem. In addition to information important for any medical history, the mode of onset, evolution, and course of illness often help to differentiate between different neurologic syndromes.

TESTS FOR CEREBRAL FUNCTION (MENTAL STATUS EXAMINATION)

Cerebral function is usually tested while obtaining the medical history, whereas the rest of the neurologic examination is performed as the last part of the physical examination. During the course of the examination, the clinician assesses the patient's behavior, emotional state, intellect, perceptions, personality, thought content, and any physiological changes. In addition to watching for clues regarding the patient's general mental and emotional status, speech should be carefully evaluated. Clinicians should assess the patient's ability to communicate in light of his or her desire to do so. Many neurologic syndromes may include problems with memory, so the clinician should evaluate the possibility of confabulations, as well as loss of memory.

General cerebral functions can be evaluated by observing the patient's appearance and behavior throughout the examination. The level of consciousness (i.e., alert, lethargic, etc.) and orientation to person, place, and time should be noted. Attention span and cognitive function are also assessed. It is important to differentiate between alertness and the ability to focus attention. The clinician should also note any evidence of perseveration (the incorrect or inappropriate repetition of a response), which indicates diffuse brain disease except in the very young or very old where this response is normal.

In evaluating intellectual or cognitive function, the patient's educational level and socioeconomic background should always be considered. Functions usually tested include short- and long-term memory, abstract reasoning, thought content, and emotional status. Specific cerebral functions can be evaluated by assessing the interpretation of sensory stimuli, motor integration, and language. An example of the first is having the patient identify common objects by sight or touch (e.g., identify a pen by sight or identify the value of a coin by touch). Motor integration is assessed by asking the patient to follow simple commands. This requires that the patient understand the command, remember it, and carry it out. Last, the clinician tries to evaluate the patient's ability to understand and communicate spoken or written language or gestures.

The Modified Mini-Mental State Test (3MS) is an efficient and frequently used tool to assess many aspects of cerebral function including orientation, short- and long-term memory, attention, naming, repetition, writing, visual-language comprehension, abstraction ability, and visuospatial ability. The 3MS cannot test nonlanguage memory or judgment. The 3MS provides an outline for the clinician to use, and a score is given based on the patient's responses. The maximum score is 100 and scores lower than 80 suggest a deficiency.[2]

CRANIAL NERVE TESTS

The cranial nerves and the functions tested to evaluate them are listed in Table 53.2.

CEREBELLAR FUNCTION TESTS

Several tests are used to evaluate balance and coordination, which are controlled in part by the cerebellum. During the finger–nose test, the patient must touch, in rapid succession, his or her nose and the examiner's finger, which is held at arm's length in front of him or her. He or she does this first with his or her eyes open and then closed. Past-pointing or irregular movements may indicate cerebellar disease. Similarly, in the heel–shin test, the patient is asked to lift one heel to the patella and slowly run it down the shin to the ankle. Shaky movements may be seen if there is a cerebellar abnormality.

While not diagnostic, the drifting of an arm after a patient has been asked to hold his arms outstretched in front of him with his eyes closed may also indicate cerebellar problems. Additional tests used to assess cerebellar function include asking the patient to repeat rapidly alternating movements with their hands or fingers, and tandem (heel-to-toe) walking. Inability to perform these tests suggests an abnormality in the cerebellar pathways. However, the clinician should consider the possible influence of weakness, pain, involuntary movements, proprioception problems, and joint disorders on movements before attributing symptoms to a cerebellar disorder.

TABLE 53.2. THE CRANIAL NERVE EXAMINATION

Cranial Nerve	Function and Examples of Testing
I. Olfactory nerve	Smell: Identify odors (coffee, cinnamon, lemon; test each nostril separately)
II. Optic nerve	Visual acuity: Eye card Visual fields: Peripheral vision and blind spot Funduscopic exam Color vision (rarely done)
III. Oculomotor IV Trochlear V. Abducens (*similar functions and are tested as a unit*)	(Cranial nerves III, IV, and V have similar functions and are tested as a unit) Eye movements: Patient is asked to watch and follow a light as it moved up, down, and on both sides, while eye movements are observed
VI. Trigeminal nerve	Motor: Tests power of jaw opening and sideways deviation against the resistance of a hand placed against the jaw Sensory: Test corneal reflex by touching cornea with a wisp of cotton
VII. Facial nerve	Observe asymmetry of face at rest or on speaking, baring teeth, raising eyebrows, or wrinkling forehead Reflex eye closure to a threatening movement Glabellar tap: Repetitive tapping over bridge of nose—initial blinking should cease after the first few taps
VIII. Auditory nerve	Vestibular division: Observe for nystagmus, positional testing Auditory division: Test acuity with light sound; watch, whisper, rubbing of fingers close to ear
IX. Glossopharyngeal X. Vagus nerve	Test for gag reflex by touching back of throat with tongue depressor; test swallowing and coughing and note any drooling or pooling of saliva
XI. Spinal accessory nerve	Trapezius and sternomastoid muscles: Test power of shrugging shoulders and turning the head to one side against resistance
XII. Hypoglossal nerve	Motor function of tongue

MOTOR FUNCTION TESTS

Abnormalities of the motor system are assessed by evaluating the patient's muscle size, tone, and strength, as well as involuntary muscle movements. The temples, limbs, and pelvic and shoulder girdles are examined for wasting, fasciculations, or hypertrophy. Tone, the muscular resistance to passive stretch, is assessed by quickly moving the patient's limb after the patient is relaxed. Spasticity is noted if there is increasing resistance to the stretching force that then gives way, whereas rigidity is increased tone that remains constant while passively moving the limb. Muscle strength is usually graded on a scale from 0 to 5 as listed in Table 53.3.

TABLE 53.3. GRADING SCALE FOR MUSCLE STRENGTH

0	No evidence of movement
1	Trace movement—no joint motion
2	Complete movement, but not against gravity
3	Movement against gravity, but not against added resistance
4	Complete motion against gravity and some resistance
5	Complete movement against gravity and full resistance

SENSORY SYSTEM TESTS

Sensation is tested by evaluating the patient's ability to perceive a light touch, superficial pain (pin prick), differences in temperature, vibration, positional sense, and motion. More complex forms of sensation that require cortical interpretation also are tested. These may be tested by asking a patient to close his or her eyes and locate the spot where he or she was touched (point localization), differentiate between different textures, identify familiar objects by touch, and identify a number that is traced in the palm of his or her hand (graphesthesia). If any deficit is found, it is important to demarcate the area of deficit clearly and find a point where the abnormal sensation becomes normal again. This point is referred to as a level.

REFLEX STATUS TESTS

Deep tendon reflexes are usually tested by tapping on a tendon with fingers or a reflex hammer, which causes a stretching of certain muscles and results in contraction. Reflexes are most commonly rated on a scale from 0 to 4 as seen in Table 53.4. The rapidity and strength of the reflexes should

TABLE 53.4. RATING SCALE FOR DEEP TENDON REFLEXES

0	Not present
1+	Present but diminished
2+	Normal
3+	Hyperactive, may have clonus but not sustained
4+	Hyperactive with sustained clonus

be symmetrical when comparing one side with the other. The reflexes most often tested are the biceps, brachioradialis (wrist), triceps, patellar (knee), and Achilles (ankle). Certain superficial reflexes (abdominal, cremasteric, plantar) are also commonly tested by stroking the skin with a moderately sharp object and watching for a response.

The Babinski reflex is a pathologic reflex that indicates a disturbance of the pyramidal system. It is elicited by stroking the lateral aspect of the sole of the foot and observing dorsiflexion (upward movement) of the big toe along with fanning of the other toes. Pyramidal lesions are usually associated with increased deep tendon reflexes, decreased superficial reflexes and a positive Babinski reflex.

GAIT AND STANCE

The act of walking is a complex activity that requires the integration of various elements in the peripheral and central nervous systems. The rate, rhythm, and character of the movements used are observed and may aid in the identification of a particular neurologic syndrome. For example, a shuffling gait is characteristically seen in Parkinson's disease, whereas ataxia is commonly associated with cerebellar disorders.

Stance is usually tested by asking the patient to stand with his or her feet together, head erect, eyes open, and arms outstretched. When stable in this position, the patient is asked to close his or her eyes and any tendency to sway or fall is noted. An increase in unsteadiness when closing the eyes is known as a positive Romberg test.

Performing a neurologic examination in children or the elderly poses additional challenges. Children younger than 5 years of age may not be able to cooperate with the exam as outlined. With infants, much of the exam may be performed without actually touching the child. Spontaneous movement and activity should be noted. Some of the major differences include the presence of developmental reflexes such as the Moro reflex, flexor withdrawal reflex, and tonic neck reflex.

Normal aging may also result in changes on the neurologic examination. The senses of smell, taste, vision, and hearing may be less acute, and extraocular movements may be impaired. Muscle mass and strength decrease with age, and muscle reflexes become less brisk. Superficial abdominal reflexes may be absent and peripheral sensations may be decreased in the elderly. For modifications in the neurologic examination in these specific populations, the reader is referred to a neurologic text.[2]

OTHER TESTS USED IN NEUROLOGIC INVESTIGATIONS

In addition to the neurologic examination, certain imaging techniques and procedures may be essential in the diagnosis of neurologic syndromes. Some of the more commonly used procedures are described next.

Lumbar puncture (LP) and cerebrospinal fluid (CSF) evaluation are used in the diagnostic evaluation of a variety of neurologic disorders including meningitis, subarachnoid hemorrhage, multiple sclerosis, and dementia.[2,3] The CSF pressure is usually less than 200 mm CSF, if measured appropriately. Low readings may result from excessive removal of CSF prior to measurement, a CSF leak around the needle, or herniation. An LP should be avoided if there is any evidence of increased intracranial pressure. Normal CSF is clear and should not contain any red blood cells or polymorphonuclear cells. The presence of up to 10 mononuclear cells is considered normal.[2] If the white blood cell (WBC) count is high, one must consider whether blood was introduced during the procedure (traumatic tap), which would lead to a falsely elevated WBC count.

CSF glucose should always be compared to a simultaneous blood glucose measurement. The normal CSF glucose concentration is approximately 20 mg/dL below the blood glucose and is considered abnormal if less than 50% of the blood glucose reading. Protein in the CSF is usually 0.4–0.6 g/L with IgG making up less than 13% of total protein. Protein may increase with infection, cerebral tumors, stroke, and diabetes. An increase in IgG is observed in multiple sclerosis and neurosyphilis. Bacteriologic, cytologic, and serologic evaluations are also often performed on the CSF.

Electroencephalography (EEG) is used to record the electrical activity of the brain and is used primarily in the assessment of seizure disorders. Some centers have epilepsy monitoring units, where patients can be monitored around the clock by EEG and video in an attempt to characterize a particular seizure disorder. The EEG recording is evaluated for basic waveform patterns, symmetry of the cerebral activity, transient discharges, and the changes when stimulatory techniques are used. EEG is also used in localizing cerebral tumors and in assessing organic brain syndromes and coma. Functional imaging techniques are now being used in some centers and in the future may provide more useful information than EEG.

Three types of evoked potentials (EP)[2,3] are used clinically: visual, auditory (brainstem), and somatosensory.

EEG responses to repetitive stimuli (visual patterns, auditory clicks, or electrical skin stimulation) are averaged to produce the evoked potentials. Abnormalities in the latency and amplitude may indicate a lesion in a particular sensory pathway, but give no information regarding the nature of the lesion. EP may be useful in the diagnosis of multiple sclerosis, acoustic neuromas, and spinal cord lesions.

Cerebral arteriography is used to visualize the intracranial vasculature by injecting a radio-opaque material into the bloodstream, similar to what is done with coronary arteriography. This technique is particularly useful to identify the location of aneurysms, vascular occlusions, and arteriovenous malformations.[2]

The advent of computed tomography (CT) technology revolutionized the practice of neurology and allowed clinicians a three-dimensional noninvasive view of the brain.[2–6] X-ray information processed by a computer allows the evaluation of 3- to 12-mm-thick "slices" of brain. CT scans are used, among other things, in differentiating cerebral infarction from cerebral hemorrhage and on identification of cerebral tumors and cerebral edema. A second CT using intravenous contrast medium (a contrast-enhanced scan) is often done to enhance the image of blood vessels and areas of blood–brain barrier damage such as tumors or cerebral edema.

Magnetic resonance imaging (MRI) uses the magnetic properties of the hydrogen atom nucleus and proton to produce computer-processed scans that provide greater anatomic accuracy than CT scans. MRI offers the advantages of differentiating between white and gray matter, delineating lesions close to bone, and offering no radiation risk; however, it is not as readily available as CT and is more expensive. MRI has a proven advantage over CT in detecting plaques in multiple sclerosis and is also useful in the diagnosis of tumors and vascular infarction changes.[2,3,7]

Newer investigational imaging techniques include positron emission tomography (PET) and single photon emission computed tomography (SPECT), which are considered tests of brain function. These tests are being studied extensively in epilepsy as well as in cerebrovascular disorders, cerebral tumors, movement disorders, and dementia.

PET scans use a positron-emitting isotope to display chemical activity and the rates of biologic processes within the brain. This method can assess metabolic changes within different areas of the brain and, thus, is considered to evaluate brain function rather than structure.[2,6,8] The expense and complexity (cyclotron is needed) of this technique may limit its clinical utility.

SPECT scans measure radiotracer uptake by tissues and provide cross-sectional images of the brain. This technique has been used extensively to assess cerebral blood flow. While the resolution with SPECT is not as good as with PET scanners, the lesser complexity may lead it to have wider clinical use.[2,6,9] SPECT is being studied in cerebrovascular disease, Alzheimer's disease, epilepsy, and migraine.

References

1. Anonymous. Implementation plan for the decade of the brain: Executive summary. Neurology 1990;40:1483–1486.
2. Pryse-Phillips WEM, Murray TJ. Essential Neurology. New York, Medical Examination Publishing Company, 1991, pp 1–70.
3. Warlow C. Handbook of Neurology. Boston, Blackwell Scientific Publications, 1991, pp 39–44.
4. Pryse-Phillips WEM, Murray TJ. Essential Neurology. New York, Medical Examination Publishing Company, 1991, pp 88–122.
5. Gibby WA, Zimmerman RA. X-ray computed tomography, in Mazziota JC, Gilman S (eds): Clinical Brain Imaging: Principles and Applications. Philadelphia, FA Davis Company, 1992, pp 3–38.
6. Theodore WH. Introduction, in Theodore WH (ed): Clinical Neuroimaging. New York, Alan R Liss, 1988, pp 1–9.
7. Lufkin RB. Magnetic resonance imaging, in Mazziota JC, Gilman S (eds): Clinical Brain Imaging: Principles and Applications. Philadelphia, FA Davis Company, 1992, pp 39–70.
8. Phelps ME. Positron emission tomography (PET), in Mazziota JC, Gilman S (eds): Clinical Brain Imaging: Principles and Applications. Philadelphia, FA Davis Company, 1992, pp 71–107.
9. Lassen NA, Holm S. Single photon emission computerized tomography (SPECT), in Mazziota JC, Gilman S (eds): Clinical Brain Imaging: Principles and Applications. Philadelphia, FA Davis Company, 1992, pp 108–134.

Chapter 54

Multiple Sclerosis

Christina Dalmady-Israel, PharmD, BCPS

Multiple sclerosis (MS) is an inflammatory disease of the central nervous system (CNS) that affects between 250,000 and 350,000 persons in the United States.[1] It is one of the major causes of neurologic disability in young and middle-age adults. The term *multiple sclerosis* refers to two characteristics of the disease: the numerous affected areas of the brain producing multiple neurologic symptoms that accrue over time, and the characteristic plaques or sclerosed areas that are the hallmark of the disease. The variable clinical presentation and the lack of specific diagnostic tests create difficulties in the diagnosis of MS and in the evaluation of disease activity and treatment efficacy.

Although MS was first described almost 130 years ago, the cause remains a mystery, and a cure is still unavailable. Nevertheless, many advances have been made in treating and managing the complications of the disease and improving the quality of life of those individuals affected by MS.

Epidemiology

MS is usually diagnosed in patients between the ages of 20 and 45 years, with the peak incidence occurring in the fourth decade.[2] Onset can occur as early as age 10 and into the eighth decade.[3] Women are afflicted more than men by a ratio of approximately 2:1.[3] Men usually develop the first signs of MS at a later age than women, and are also more likely to develop the chronic progressive form of the disease.[3,4] The most important factors in the determination of individuals at risk for developing the disease are geography, age, environmental influences, and genetics.[2,5,6]

Based on rates of prevalence of MS, the globe can be divided into three geographic zones[7] (Table 54.1). In general, the greater the distance from the equator, the higher the prevalence of the disease.[2,7,8] Within the United States, the prevalence of MS is higher in those states above the 37th parallel. Ethnic differences in prevalence are also observed within the described geographic areas, with MS occurring more frequently in Caucasians of Scandinavian or "North Sea" ancestry than in other ethnic groups.[8,9] Asian-Americans, African-Americans, American Hispanics living in California, Australian aborigines, Polynesian Maoris, Lapps, and Hungarian gypsies are among the ethnic groups that have a very low reported incidence of MS, sometimes despite being located in what are considered high-risk areas.[8,9]

The geographic distribution of MS suggests the influence of an environmental factor in the development of the disease. The nature of this factor remains unknown; however, most hypotheses point to a viral agent. The MS epidemics that were reported in the Faroe Islands, Orkney Islands, and Iceland seem to support this hypothesis.[10]

MS is thought to be contracted by susceptible individuals between the ages of 10 and 15 years[4,11] that have usually lived in a high-risk area for at least 2 years.[4] Interestingly, an individual that migrates from a low-risk area to a high-risk area prior to the age of 15 years has the same chance of developing MS as those who have lived in a high-risk area all of their lives.[4] If the move is made in the opposite direction, from a high- to a low-risk area, the individual retains the high risk if the move is made after the age of 15 years, but acquires the lower risk if the move is made prior to this age.[11,12]

The familial recurrence rate of MS is approximately 15%, with siblings being the most commonly reported relationship.[9] Concordance data show a higher prevalence of MS between monozygotic than between dizygotic twins. While these data support a genetic influence in the development of MS, the numbers of monozygotic twins that are discordant for the disease, and the variability in the severity and expression of the disease between members of concordant pairs, also point to the fact that genetics alone may not be sufficient for the development of disease.[9,10,13]

Genetic studies also have determined an association between MS and the major histocompatibility complex (MHC) and, in particular, with the human leukocyte antigen (HLA) region on the sixth chromosome that is associated with the genetic control of immune mechanisms.[9,14] Currently, the strongest association appears to be with the MHC class II alleles DR15 and DQ6.[9] Although the significance of the association between MS and the MHC remains unclear, the fact that certain HLA antigens are neither necessary nor sufficient to lead to the development of MS suggests that inheritance is most likely polygenic.[8,9]

TABLE 54.1. GEOGRAPHIC PREVALENCE OF MULTIPLE SCLEROSIS

High Frequency (>30 per 100,000)	Medium Frequency (5–30 per 100,000)	Low Frequency (<5 per 100,000)
Northern Europe	Southern Europe	Asia
Northern U.S.	Southern U.S.	Parts of South America
Canada	Northern Australia	
Southern Australia		
New Zealand		

(From Ref. 3.)

PATHOLOGY

The basic pathologic derangement in MS is the stripping of the myelin sheath surrounding neurons in the CNS. Demyelination, coupled with an inflammatory response, leads to the formation of the characteristic MS lesions or plaques that are found primarily in the brain, spinal cord, and optic nerves. Neuronal axons, although stripped bare of their myelin sheath, are usually well preserved.[15]

Demyelination causes disruption in the transmission of nerve impulses, which leads to neurologic symptoms reflecting the area of the brain affected. A single plaque may extend across several nerve pathways producing symptoms involving several nervous system functions.[4] Smaller plaques may cause isolated disturbances; however, typically, several plaques develop at the same time, causing multiple but unrelated problems such as disturbed vision and decreased sensation.

The pathology of MS lesions is different in early stages of the disease, during chronic MS, and during acute exacerbations.[16] Active and inactive lesions can be found side by side in the brain. Both types of lesions display some degree of perivascular inflammation, but it is much more pronounced and usually associated with blood–brain barrier (BBB) damage in active lesions.[16]

Decreased numbers of oligodendrocytes (myelin-producing cells) are observed within the MS plaques, causing speculation as to whether myelin or the oligodendrocyte is the target of an immunologic attack.[10,13,15] Oligodendrocyte destruction appears to occur in a nonspecific manner in early or acute MS, whereas selective destruction of myelin and oligodendrocytes occurs in chronic stages of MS.[16] The observed differences in pathology between lesions formed in the early or late stages of MS suggests that the immune response may change with chronicity of disease.[16,17] Plaques range in size from 1 mm to 4 cm and are located preferentially in perivenular areas. Plasma cells, immunoglobulins, lymphocytes, and macrophages are characteristically found within the active plaques and in proximate perivenular areas. These elements, as well as hypertrophied astrocytes (gliosis), also are observed at the outer margins of the lesions where progression may occur.[15] To date it is unclear whether the inflammatory response is a result or the cause of the demyelinating process.

ETIOLOGY

Even though the exact cause and pathophysiology of MS remain a mystery, the disease is postulated to be autoimmune in nature and/or related to a viral process.[18]

AUTOIMMUNE ETIOLOGY

In this theory (Fig. 54.1), MS results from an autoimmune attack against self-myelin or self-oligodendrocyte antigens. The actual mediator of myelin destruction has not been established, but this activity has been attributed to the action of macrophages, killer T cells, lymphokines, antibodies, or a combination of these elements.[10,13,18] Impaired T suppressor cell function also may play a role in the immunologic process.[19]

A reduction in T suppressor cells has been reported during active MS and in patients with progressive disease[10,13,19]; however, a relative increase in the T helper/suppressor ratio is not consistently found and does not always correlate with disease activity.[13,20]

VIRAL ETIOLOGY

Although the exact mechanism has not been found, there are several ways in which a virus could play a role in the pathogenesis of MS. In the simplest scenario, the virus directly attacks myelin and/or the oligodendrocyte. Second, the virus could cause a change in the nervous system that would elicit an autoimmune response leading to demyelination. Third, the virus could have an effect on the immune system, causing an autoimmune attack on the nervous system. Last, in a more complex theory, the virus alters the immune process in a susceptible individual with a subsequent attack on the nervous system by another virus.[4,15]

Evidence to support a viral etiology includes increased IgG synthesis in the CNS, increased antibody titers to certain viruses (in particular the measles virus), and epidemiologic studies indicating a childhood exposure factor and suggesting that "viral" infections may precipitate exacerbations. In addition, viruses have been shown to cause diseases with prolonged incubation periods, myelin destruction, and a relapsing/remitting course in humans and in experimental animal models.[2,21]

The most compelling evidence against a viral etiology is the fact that no single infectious agent has been identi-

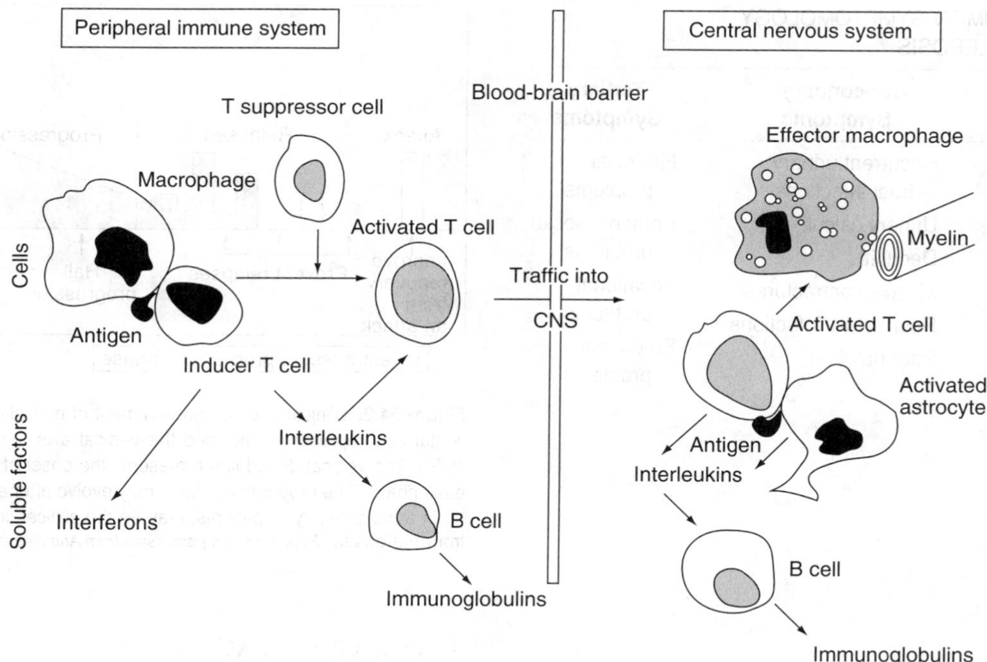

Figure 54.1. Autoimmune theory of the pathogenesis of MS. The immune response is initiated in the peripheral immune compartment when antigen is processed and presented to an inducer cell by a macrophage or antigen-presenting cell. The inducer cell becomes activated and releases a number of soluble factors including interleukins and interferons, which act on both B cells and T cells to augment the immune response. T suppressor cells act to dampen the immune response. Activated T cells traffic into the central nervous system (CNS), where they again release factors, presumably after having antigen presented to them. In this regard, astrocytes are capable of presenting antigens to T cells. Other cellular elements also enter the CNS (macrophages, B cells), where the potential for a local immune response occurs. B cells are known to produce immunoglobulin locally within the CNS, and macrophages function within the CNS to phagocytose myelin, in addition to their antigen-presenting properties. *(Reprinted with permission from Ann Neurol, vol 23, p 214, 1988.)*

fied as the causative agent of MS. Many agents, including mycoplasma, spirochetes, rabies virus, herpes simplex, canine distemper virus, coronavirus, human T-cell leukemia virus (HTLV)-1, and measles have been implicated; however, studies have been unable to establish a causal relationship.[10,15,21]

Clinical Presentation

The clinical presentation of MS is extremely variable among patients and may vary over time in a given patient. The transient nature of initial symptoms and the characteristic exacerbations and remissions make diagnosis difficult.

The signs and symptoms of MS are usually divided into three categories as shown in Table 54.2. Primary symptoms are a direct consequence of conduction disturbances produced by demyelination and reflect the area of the brain or spinal cord that is damaged. Secondary symptoms are complications resulting from primary symptoms. For example, urinary retention, a primary symptom, may lead to frequent urinary tract infections, considered a secondary symptom. Tertiary symptoms relate to the effect of the disease on the patient's everyday life.[22] The most widely used clinical rating scale in MS is the Expanded Disability Status Scale (EDSS) in which a numerical value ranging from 0 (no disability) to 10 (death from MS) is assigned based on the evaluation of several neurologic functions.[23] The limitations to this scale are the relative insensitivity to clinical changes that do not impair gait at the higher ends of the scale and interevaluator inconsistency. Increasingly, magnetic resonance imaging (MRI) is being used as a measure of disease activity and as a predictor of future disability.[24,25]

PRECIPITATING FACTORS

The unpredictable nature of MS makes it impossible to anticipate when an exacerbation will occur. However, certain factors have been reported to aggravate symptoms or

TABLE 54.2. COMMON SYMPTOMOLOGY OF MULTIPLE SCLEROSIS

Primary Symptoms	Secondary Symptoms	Tertiary Symptoms
Visual complaints	Recurrent urinary tract infections	Financial problems
Gait problems	Urinary calculi	Personal/social problems
Paresthesias	Decubiti	Vocational problems
Pain	Muscle contractures	Emotional problems
Spasticity	Respiratory infections	
Weakness	Poor nutrition	
Ataxia		
Speech difficulty		
Psychologic changes		
Cognitive changes		
Fatigue		
Bowel/bladder dysfunction		
Sexual dysfunction		
Tremor		

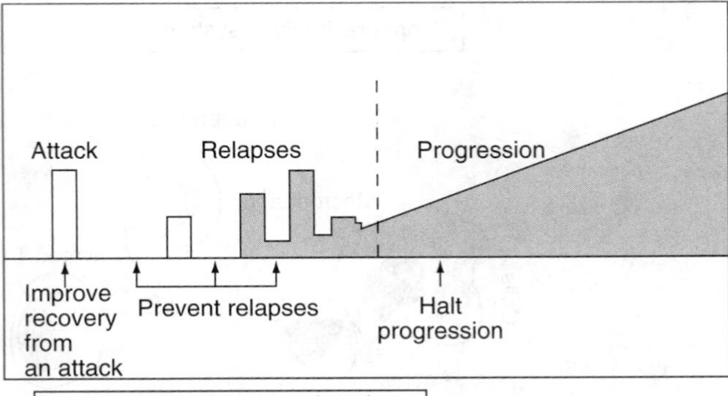

Figure 54.2. Clinical course and treatment of multiple sclerosis. The horizontal axis represents time, and the vertical axis represents level of disability. The vertical dotted line represents the onset of the progressive disease phase. The progressive phase may evolve after a number of relapses or, in a subcategory of patients, may be the clinical course of the disease from the onset. *(Reprinted with permission from Ann Neurol, vol 23, p 212, 1988.)*

even lead to an acute attack (new episode of demyelination). These implicated factors include infections, hyperventilation, heat, sleep deprivation, malnutrition, anemia, concurrent organ dysfunction, exertion, heavy metals, and childbirth.[2–4,26] It is currently thought that physical trauma does not play a major role in the onset or exacerbation of MS.[27]

CLINICAL COURSE

The clinical course of MS is variable, but seems to follow a general pattern of exacerbations and remissions (Fig. 54.2). Based on the course of the disease, MS may be classified into four clinical categories.[4,18,28] A benign course, characterized by an abrupt onset, few exacerbations, and no permanent disability, is seen in approximately 20% of patients. Another 20–30% of patients develop relapsing/remitting MS, which also begins abruptly, but is subsequently characterized by partial or total remissions, which may last months or years. A large portion of patients (40%) will eventually develop the secondary progressive (or relapsing/progressive) form of the disease in which a period of initial remissions is followed by progressive disability. The primary progressive (chronic progressive) form of MS, characterized by the slow onset of symptoms, relatively few attacks, and disability that continually worsens over time, is seen in 10–20% of patients. In all patients, attack frequency tends to decrease over time, independently of the development of worsening disabilities.[28]

PROGNOSTIC FACTORS

MS does not directly diminish life expectancy; however, the development of complications may lead to a shorter than expected life span. Suicide rates as high as seven times greater than expected in the general population have been reported.[28] Clinical and demographic factors that have been used to predict prognosis of MS are listed in Table 54.3.[28,29]

DIAGNOSIS

MS is often referred to as "the great masquerader" because its symptoms can be attributed to other neurologic diseases, just as many syndromes can mimic MS. The unpredictable nature of MS and the lack of laboratory tests and imaging techniques specific for the disease add to the difficulties in making this diagnosis, especially in the early stages of the disease. Ultimate diagnosis is made only at autopsy, and even then plaques are found in a significant number of patients with no clinical evidence of the disease.[15]

Although MRI techniques have aided in the detection of MS lesions, the diagnosis remains primarily a clinical one that requires the demonstration of "lesions separated in space and time." This statement refers to the occurrence of at least two episodes of neurologic disturbance reflecting distinct sites of damage in the CNS that cannot be explained by another mechanism.[30] MS is currently classified into four major categories based on clinical evidence as well as laboratory studies[29,31] (Table 54.4). Prior to these criteria, which were developed primarily for research purposes, diagnosis was based exclusively on clinical evi-

TABLE 54.3. PROGNOSTIC INDICATORS IN MULTIPLE SCLEROSIS

Indicator	Favorable Prognosis	Unfavorable Prognosis
Age at onset	<40 years	>40 years
Gender	Female	Male
Initial symptoms	Optic neuritis or sensory symptoms	Motor or cerebellar symptoms
Attack frequency in early disease	Low	High
Course of disease	Relapsing/remitting	Progressive

(Table based on information in Ref. 28.)

dence. For purposes of diagnostic classification, an attack is defined as an episode of neurologic dysfunction lasting at least 24 hours. The terms "relapse," "exacerbation," and "bout" also are used synonymously with "attack." The two attacks specified in the criteria must affect different parts of the CNS and must be separated in time by at least 1 month. Clinical evidence refers to objective signs found on neurologic examination, whereas paraclinical evidence relates to information provided by neuroimaging procedures and other tests besides physical examination.[29–31] It is not uncommon to detect lesions that have not produced clinical signs or symptoms, and these are referred to as subclinical or silent lesions.[30]

LABORATORY STUDIES

To date there are no tests specific for MS. Tests that are frequently used include cerebrospinal fluid (CSF) evaluation, MRI, computed tomography (CT) scans, and evoked potentials. Evidence provided by these studies, used in conjunction with the clinical history, may aid in establishing the diagnosis of MS.

TABLE 54.4. CLASSIFICATION OF MULTIPLE SCLEROSIS

A. Clinically definite MS
   1. Two attacks and clinical evidence of two separate lesions
   2. Two attacks with clinical evidence of one lesion and paraclinical evidence of another (separate) lesion

B. Laboratory-supported definite MS
   1. Two attacks with either clinical or paraclinical evidence of one lesion and demonstration, in cerebrospinal fluid (CSF), of IgG oligoclonal bands (OB) or increased CNS synthesis of IgG
   2. One attack, clinical evidence of two separate lesions and demonstration of CSF OB/IgG
   3. One attack, clinical evidence of one lesion, paraclinical evidence of another (separate) lesion, and demonstration of CSF OB/IgG

C. Clinically probable MS
   1. Two attacks and clinical evidence of one lesion
   2. One attack and clinical evidence of two separate lesions
   3. One attack, clinical evidence of one lesion, and paraclinical evidence of another (separate) lesion

D. Laboratory-supported probable MS
   1. Two attacks and presence of CSF OB/IgG

(From Swanson JW. Multiple sclerosis: Update in diagnosis and review of prognostic factors. Mayo Clin Proc 1989;64:579, with permission.)

Cerebrospinal Fluid Evaluation

CNS synthesis of IgG is increased, while serum IgG levels are normal. Electrophoretic studies of the CSF show that the IgG separates into a small number of discrete bands called "oligoclonal bands."[29] While oligoclonal banding of IgG is present in 90–95% of patients with clinically definite MS, it is significant only if banding is not found in the serum.[29,32] The increase in CSF IgG synthesis is usually reported as a CSF IgG–albumin index, which can be calculated after determining CSF and serum concentrations of IgG and albumin:

CSF IgG–albumin index
= (CSF IgG/CSF albumin) (serum IgG/serum albumin)

A CSF IgG–albumin index of greater than 0.77 is considered abnormal and is observed in 70–90% of patients with MS. A CSF IgG synthesis rate of greater than 3 g/d is also reported in more than 90% of MS patients. This synthesis rate is considered to be more sensitive than the IgG–albumin index; however, in practice it is not used as often. It is important to remember that CSF IgG elevations are not specific for MS and may be seen in a variety of other diseases. Myelin basic protein is detected in the CSF of 90% of patients shortly after an acute attack. Additional CSF abnormalities may include increased CSF protein concentrations in approximately 25% of patients and a mild CSF leukocytosis.[29] The presence of greater than 50×10^6 mononuclear cells in the CSF usually indicates a diagnosis other than MS.[32]

Imaging Studies

MRI, especially with gadolinium enhancement, is much more sensitive than CT scans in the detection of MS lesions and is currently considered the preferred imaging method.[29,33] Lesions are observed on MRI in 70–95% of patients with clinically definite MS. More important, they are observed in 65–85% of patients with suspected MS.[29]

Although CT scans are not as sensitive as MRI, they are usually performed at some point in the course of the patient's diagnosis, and may be useful in the diagnosis of other disease processes included in the differential diagnosis.

Evoked Potentials

These electrophysiologic studies measure an electric response to the stimulation of a nerve pathway. Visual evoked potentials (VEP), which record responses following visual stimulation such as flashing lights or a checkerboard pattern, are useful in confirming the presence of a lesion when the symptoms are equivocal.[29]

THERAPEUTIC MANAGEMENT

The therapeutic management of MS is by no means straightforward. To date, no therapy has been shown to cure MS and, until recently, no therapy had shown the ability to halt the progression of the disease, nor was specifically indicated for the treatment of MS. Symptomatic management of the disease is of utmost importance to maintain the patient's quality of life. The very nature of MS makes evaluation of therapeutic agents difficult. A variety of different treatment modalities have been studied; however, many trials are plagued with flaws in design or interpretation.[34] The lack of specific indicators for disease activity and the unpredictable course of the disease make assessment of various therapies difficult. There are no universally accepted treatment protocols, and treatments will vary among clinicians and treatment centers. Great strides have been made in attempting to establish better methods for assessment of disease activity and treatment effects.[24,33]

GOALS OF THERAPY

Therapy of MS may be attempted at different stages during the course of the disease as shown in Fig. 54.2. The basic goals of therapy are to decrease the severity and intensity of exacerbations, enhance recovery from exacerbations, prevent relapses and the onset of progressive disease, halt or even reverse progressive disease, and provide symptomatic relief from the complications of MS.[18] Various treatment modalities are presented in Table 54.5.

DISEASE-MODIFYING MODALITIES

Treatment of Acute Exacerbations

Treatment of an acute exacerbation varies depending on the severity of the attack. Mild exacerbations that do not produce functional decline, may not require any treatment.[35,36]

TABLE 54.5. OVERVIEW OF DISEASE-MODIFYING MODALITIES IN THE TREATMENT OF MS

Acute Exacerbations	Prevention of Progression
Mild	Interferon β-1b[a]
No therapy	Cyclophosphamide
Oral steroids	Azathioprine
Moderate–Severe	Other experimental modalities
IV Methylprednisolone	
ACTH	
Rehabilitation (e.g., physical therapy)	

[a]Patient selection according to advisory panel guidelines.[48]

When functional ability is affected, treatment is usually started with corticosteroids. In milder cases, oral prednisone is used in a variety of dosing regimens.[35] Adrenocorticoid hormone (ACTH) or intravenous methylprednisolone are the most commonly used agents in the treatment of severe, acute exacerbations.[35,36] Because effects of steroids may be transient and tend to diminish with repeated use, some clinicians stress that steroid therapy should not be used for symptom fluctuations without any functional consequence.[36]

The mechanism of action for corticosteroids in MS is unknown; however, it is speculated that steroids improve recovery by decreasing edema in the area of demyelination.[18,36] In addition, steroids have been shown to reduce blood–brain barrier abnormalities observed by CT, reduce CSF IgG synthesis, and decrease concentrations of myelin basic protein during acute exacerbations. Unfortunately, the relationship between these parameters and disease activity has not been established.[35–37]

High-dose methylprednisolone and ACTH have been shown to shorten the duration of acute exacerbations,[38–40] although neither has been shown to affect the progression of disease.[18,35,41] Investigators disagree on which agent is superior, and there is no consensus on optimal dose or duration of therapy for acute exacerbations.[34,36] One study, performed in 25 patients, showed more rapid clinical improvement with high-dose methylprednisolone when compared with ACTH[36,42]; however, others have not demonstrated a difference between the two agents.[41,43]

No formal dosing guidelines exist for the use of corticosteroids in the treatment of MS. ACTH is given in doses ranging from 20–100 IU twice daily, either intramuscularly or intravenously. Although the manufacturer recommends that large intravenous doses of ACTH be infused over 8 hours, it is this author's experience that doses of 100 units in 100 mL of a suitable solution given over 1 hour are well tolerated.

Methylprednisolone doses may range from 250–500 mg intravenously every 6 hours. The duration of therapy with either agent is also extremely variable and may range from 3 days to 3 weeks depending on clinical response. If improvement occurs it is usually seen in the first 3–5 days, so it is common to see ACTH or methylprednisolone given for 5 days and then followed by an oral steroid taper.[37] Repeat treatments with corticosteroids may not produce the same improvement as initial therapy, and long-term therapy, which has not been shown to have a beneficial effect, is not recommended.[18,36]

Oral steroid regimens usually begin with 60 mg or more of prednisone for 3–7 days, and then the dosage is tapered over 7 days or longer depending on the patient's symptoms.[36]

Prevention of Relapses and Progression

Interferon β-1b

Evidence of significant reductions in the frequency of MS-related exacerbations and in the number of new lesions detected by serial MRI scans following treatment with interferon β-1b (Betaseron), led to the July 1993 FDA approval of the use of this agent in ambulatory patients with relapsing-remitting MS.[44,45] This is the first agent that has shown ability to halt and even reverse the progression of the disease. Interferon β-1b is a synthetic analogue of recombinant interferon beta produced in *Escherichia coli.* Although the exact mechanism of action is unknown, its effect in MS may be due to its immunomodulating properties, including the ability to augment suppressor cell function, increase cytotoxicity of natural killer cells, increase phagocytic activity of macrophages, reduce interferon γ secretion by activated lymphocytes, and reduce the expression of interferon γ induced class II MHC antigens on antigen-presenting glial cells.[46,47] Interferon γ has been shown to exacerbate MS.

Interferon β-1b is administered every other day subcutaneously at a dose of 8 million IU. An advisory panel has published guidelines for selection of patients for treatment with interferon β-1b (Table 54.6).[48] These recommendations are much broader than the initial treatment guidelines, which suggest using interferon β-1b only in ambulatory patients with frequent attacks of relapsing-remitting MS. The patient's motivational level and perceived ability to comply with this therapy are also considered during patient selection.

TABLE 54.6. PATIENT SELECTION CRITERIA FOR TREATMENT WITH INTERFERON β-1b

A. Class I experimental evidence and expert consensus suggest interferon β-1b may be helpful:
   1. Relapsing-remitting course in patients with clinically definite or laboratory supported MS
   2. Age 18–50 years
   3. Ambulatory with EDSS ≤ 5.5
   4. At least two exacerbations in last 2 years

B. Expert consensus suggests interferon may be helpful:
   1. Relapsing-remitting disease and age >50 years
   2. Relapsing-remitting disease and EDSS ≥ 6.0
   3. Relapsing-progressive (secondary progressive) disease with clinically definite or laboratory supported MS and at least two exacerbations in last 2 years

C. Neither Class I[a] evidence nor expert consensus supports therapy with interferon β:
   1. Primary chronic progressive disease

D. Avoid interferon in patients
   1. At risk for poor compliance
   2. With concurrent illness that will substantially reduce life expectancy

E. Reasons to consider discontinuation of interferon beta:
   1. Steady progression of disability for 6 months
   2. Three courses of ACTH or corticosteroids during a 1-year period despite treatment with interferon
   3. Severe depression or suicidal ideation
   4. Consistent noncompliance
   5. Severe adverse reactions
   6. Planned pregnancy or becoming pregnant

[a]Class I: Evidence provided by one or more well-designed clinical trials. (Table compiled from Ref. 48.)

Baseline hemoglobin, complete blood counts, platelets, and liver function tests should be documented before starting therapy with interferon β-1b, which costs approximately $10,000/year. The most common adverse effects include injection site redness and swelling and flu-like symptoms (fever, chills, myalgias). These symptoms can be mild or severe and are seen in the majority of patients. Injection site reactions may be lessened by using appropriate injection technique, including site rotation and hydrocortisone cream. Ice applied before and/or after the injection may also decrease the pain and the redness. Some clinicians begin therapy at half the recommended dose for 1–2 weeks, to decrease the incidence of flu-like symptoms. Nonsteroidal agents taken before and at regular intervals for 24 hours after administration may also alleviate the flu-like symptoms. Less commonly reported side effects include shortness of breath, tachycardia, and depression. Patients who become depressed should be closely monitored because there may be a risk for suicide. The other side effects are usually transient.

Most patients will not feel better when taking this drug, and most will experience side effects, thus compliance may become a major issue. Patients should be reminded that some of the side effects are transient, and they should be counseled to minimize problems associated with local reactions.

Interferon β-1b was granted expedited approval under the condition that additional clinical data supporting the drug's efficacy be documented "within a reasonable amount of time."[46] The trial used a surrogate endpoint of MRI activity (number of active scans that showed new, recurrent, or enlarging lesions) that to date has not been proven to have a direct relationship with disability.[49] Trials are ongoing to establish a firm relationship between administration of this drug and decrease in disease progression. Interferon β-1a is also undergoing investigation for possible use in the treatment of MS.

Other Therapies

Apart from interferon β-1b, few studies have evaluated the efficacy of therapy in the prevention of relapses, and there is more evidence regarding what does not work, as opposed to what does work. Frequency of exacerbations, which is often used as an endpoint in these studies, may not be a valid outcome measure, because it does not correlate with prognosis and tends to decrease over time.

Short-term, intensive pulse doses of corticosteroids, similar to those used in acute exacerbations, may initially decrease disability; however, prolonged steroid therapy has minimal effects on the progression of disease.[36,41] If progression continues, an immunosuppressive agent may be tried. Cyclophosphamide has been studied alone and in combination with other treatment modalities in attempts to halt progression of MS.[37] Short, intensive courses of cyclophosphamide (500 mg/d for 2–3 weeks or until the leukocyte count drops to less than 4000 cells/mm^3) followed by ACTH therapy for 21 days have shown stabilization and/or improvement of symptoms in a majority of patients after 12–24 months; however, progression invariably recurred.[37,50] Maintenance therapy with intermittent pulse doses of cyclophosphamide may slow the progression of disease in younger patients with secondary progressive disease.[47] Prolonged therapy with cyclophosphamide is usually intolerable; however, it appears that some form of maintenance is necessary.[33,51] Although cyclophosphamide appears beneficial, toxicities may limit its long-term use.

Conflicting results have been shown when azathioprine is used alone or in combination with other therapies. It is usually given in doses of 2–3 mg/kg until the white blood cell count drops to less than 4000/mm^3 and is then followed with corticosteroid therapy.[35] Although not without serious side effects, azathioprine may be less toxic than cyclophosphamide and may be tolerated for a longer period of time.

Cyclosporine appears to produce only a modest delay in the progression of disability in chronic progressive MS. A significant number of patients may develop severe side effects, in particular nephrotoxicity and hypertension,[52] which may limit the usefulness of this agent.

Following initial encouraging results, further studies are being performed with copolymer-1 (Cop-1), an investigational agent structurally related to myelin basic protein.[35,53] Other experimental modalities include total lymphoid irradiation (TLI), α-interferon, monoclonal antibodies, mitoxantrone, and oral myelin.[35] Plasmapheresis does not appear to be of benefit, but is still under study, and hyperbaric oxygen is probably of no value.

SYMPTOMATIC MANAGEMENT

Many of the symptoms of MS do not require pharmacologic management or do not respond to it. The following section covers those primary symptoms in which pharmacologic management may be of benefit (Table 54.7).

Gait Difficulties—Spasticity

Problems with gait may be due to spasticity, weakness, ataxia, defective proprioception, or a combination of these factors. Spasticity is amenable to pharmacologic intervention, whereas physical therapy may be required in treating gait disturbances due to any of the other factors. The increased muscle tone of a spastic limb often lends strength to patients with underlying weakness. Therefore, when using muscle relaxants, one must be careful not to decrease the tone to an extent where ambulation is actually hindered.[22,26,54] Baclofen (Lioresal), a γ-aminobutyric acid (GABA) inhibitor, is the preferred agent and is usually started in dosages of 5 mg tid and titrated upward to achieve the desired response. Most patients will achieve a satisfactory response with dosages between 40 and 80 mg/d; however, dosages higher than the recommended daily maximum of 80 mg are required by some patients.[22,36,54] Baclofen should not be abruptly discontinued to avoid the possibility of seizures.[54] Small doses of diazepam (e.g., 0.5–1 mg) are often added to baclofen in patients in whom optimal response has not been achieved. In patients who are unable to tolerate baclofen, diazepam may be used alone, starting at 1–2 mg tid and slowly increasing to dosages of up to 30 mg/d.[54] However, the somnolence caused by diazepam is not acceptable for many of these patients who often experience

TABLE 54.7. TREATMENT OF SELECTED SECONDARY MS SYMPTOMS

Spasticity	Bladder Symptoms	Sensory Symptoms	Fatigue
Baclofen	Propantheline	Carbamazepine	Amantadine
Dantrolene	Oxybutinin	Phenytoin	Pemoline
Diazepam	Dicyclomine	Amitriptyline or other TCAs	Antidepressants
	DDAVP		
	Self-catheterization		

MS-related fatigue.[22] Dantrolene sodium (Dantrium) may be an alternative for patients experiencing CNS side effects from baclofen, especially at higher doses. However, it is usually used when baclofen and diazepam are ineffective, or in nonambulatory patients. Its peripheral mechanism of action produces more muscle weakness than baclofen and may cause more problems with walking in ambulatory patients.[36,54] In addition, dantrolene is not recommended for long-term use due to the potential hepatotoxic effects, especially in the young female population. Severe spasticity, refractory to medical therapy, may require the use of chemical neurectomy (nerve blocks). Intrathecal baclofen is currently under investigation for use in patients with refractory spasticity or who have had severe complications from oral therapy.[36,54]

Bowel/Bladder Symptoms

Patients commonly complain of incontinence, urgency, frequency, and nocturia, which are indications of a hyperreflexic bladder (i.e., inability to store urine). A number of anticholinergic agents including propantheline bromide (Probanthine 45–90 mg/d), oxybutinin chloride (Ditropan 10–30 mg/d), and dicyclomine hydrochloride (Bentyl 30–80 mg/d) are used to treat this problem, if postvoid residual urine volumes are not too large.[55] In addition, tricyclic antidepressants such as imipramine (Tofranil) and amitriptyline (Elavil) also have been used for their anticholinergic properties, and a rather expensive alternative, desmopressin (DDAVP), also has been reported effective in the treatment of urgency and incontinence.[55] Intermittent self-catheterization with or without a concomitant anticholinergic agent is recommended in patients with large postvoid urine residual volumes or when the urinary problem is hyporeflexic in nature (i.e., failure to empty).[36,54] This technique requires adequate manual dexterity and may not be possible in patients with severe symptoms. Patients with large postvoid residual volumes are at risk for developing urinary tract infections and are often prescribed urinary acidifiers or antiseptics in an attempt to prevent their occurrence.

Constipation due to either inactivity or medication side effects is the most common bowel complaint. Increases in dietary fiber and hydration may alleviate this problem; however, in some instances laxatives or enemas may be necessary.[22]

Sensory Symptoms

Numbness and paresthesias are frequent sensory complaints, but usually do not require treatment. Some MS patients may develop acute or chronic pain syndromes,[56] such as trigeminal neuralgia and painful dysasthesias for which treatment is necessary. Carbamazepine is the preferred agent for the treatment of trigeminal neuralgia; however, phenytoin may also be effective. Both agents are used in the same doses that are used for the treatment of seizure disorders. Painful dysasthesias are burning sensations that commonly occur in the extremities. These sensory complaints are difficult to treat, but may sometimes respond to treatment with tricyclic antidepressants.[22,36,56] Excruciating pain may also be the result of severe spasticity, which should be treated with muscle relaxants.

Fatigue

Fatigue, one of the most common complaints in MS patients, can be severely disabling. It usually worsens before and during a flare, and with increases in ambient temperature. Spasticity, weakness, and depression may also contribute to MS-related fatigue. Amantadine hydrocholoride 100 mg bid is sometimes used and may offer modest relief.[54] Studies evaluating this agent are subjective and do not show conclusive evidence as to the efficacy of this agent. Pemoline (Cylert) has also been used in doses starting at 18.75–37.5 mg/d.[36,54] Antidepressants may also be helpful, especially if the patient has some symptoms of depression.

The aminopyridines, 4-aminopyridine and 3,4-diaminopyridine,[22,54,57] are potassium channel blockers that are currently under investigation in the symptomatic treatment of MS. These agents appear to improve conduction in demyelinated axons and may improve strength and decrease heat sensitivity.[35]

Evaluation of Therapeutic Outcomes

Because of the relapsing-remitting nature of MS, it is often difficult to assess whether improvement is due to treatment or due to the course of the disease. The paucity of conclusive evidence for many of the described treatments and the lack of specific guidelines make treatment choices difficult. Each symptom should be assessed individually, and therapy with available agents tried and modified when needed. In addition to counseling patients regarding the adverse effects associated with medications, pharmacists should also actively encourage patients to comply with their prescribed regimens. Support is extremely important for MS patients and their families. Patients should be referred to the National Multiple Sclerosis Society (1-800-FIGHTMS) or a local chapter for information about local support services. Presently, the disease is assessed by the EDSS; however, in the future serial MRI scans may be used to assess disease activity and treatment efficacy.

Conclusion

MS is an inflammatory disease of the CNS that appears to strike young, genetically susceptible individuals living in high-risk geographic areas. Although the exact etiology of MS is unknown, it is likely that MS is an autoimmune disease triggered by a viral infection. There is no cure for MS;

however, quality of life can be improved through symptomatic management. Currently only one agent, interferon β-1b, is indicated in the primary treatment of MS, and further trials are needed to show if it can reduce MS-related disability. Other therapies to modify the disease process are aimed at altering immune function; however, the use of these therapies remains primarily empirical.

References

1. Anderson DW, Ellenberg JH, Leventhal CM, et al. Revised estimate of the prevalence of multiple sclerosis in the United States. Ann Neurol 1992;31:333–336.
2. Wynn DR, Rodriguez M, O'Fallon WM, et al. Update on the epidemiology of multiple sclerosis. Mayo Clin Proc 1989;64:808–817.
3. Sadovnick AD, Ebers GC. Epidemiology of multiple sclerosis: A critical overview. Can J Neurol Sci 1993;20:17–29.
4. Lechtenberg R. Multiple Sclerosis Fact Book. Philadelphia, FA Davis, 1988.
5. Ebers GC, Bulman D. The geography of MS reflects genetic susceptibility. Neurology 1986;36(suppl 1):108.
6. Compston A. Risk factors for multiple sclerosis: Race or place? (editorial). J Neurol Neurosurg Psychiatry 1990;53:821–823.
7. Kurtzke JF. Epidemiologic contributions to multiple sclerosis: An overview. Neurology (NY) 1980;30(suppl 2):61–79.
8. Ebers GC. Genetics and multiple sclerosis: An overview. Ann Neurol 1994;36:S12–S14.
9. Compston A. The epidemiology of multiple sclerosis: Principles, achievements, and recommendations. Ann Neurol 1994:36;S211–S217.
10. Rodriguez M. Multiple sclerosis. Basic concepts and hypothesis. Mayo Clin Proc 1989;64:570–576.
11. Wolfson C, Wolfson EB, Zielinski JM. On the estimation of the distribution of the latent period of multiple sclerosis. Neuroepidemiology 1989;8:239–248.
12. Detels R, Visscher BR, Haile RW, et al. Multiple sclerosis and age at migration. Am J Epidemiol 1978;108:386–393.
13. McDonald WI. The mystery of the origin of multiple sclerosis. J Neurol Neurosurg Psychiatry 1989;49:113–323.
14. Hillert J. Human leukocyte antigen studies in multiple sclerosis. Ann Neurol 1994;36:S15–S17.
15. Silberberg DH. Pathogenesis of demyelination, in McDonald WI, Silberberg DH (eds): Multiple Sclerosis. Boston, Butterworth, 1986, p 99.
16. Lassman H, Suchanek G, Ozawa K. Histopathology and the blood–cerebrospinal fluid barrier in multiple sclerosis. Ann Neurol 1994;36:S42–S46.
17. Raine CS. The Dale E. McFarlin memorial lecture: The immunology of the multiple sclerosis lesion. 1994;36:S61–S72.
18. Weiner HL, Hafler DA. Immunotherapy of multiple sclerosis. Ann Neurol 1988;23:211–222.
19. De Keyser J. Autoimmunity in multiple sclerosis. Neurology 1988;38:371–374.
20. Poser CM. Pathogenesis of multiple sclerosis. A critical reappraisal. Acta Neuropathol 1986;71:1–10.
21. Johnson RT. The virology of demyelinating diseases. Ann Neurol 1994;36:S54–S60.
22. Schapiro RT. Symptom management in multiple sclerosis. Ann Neurol 1994;36:S123–S129.
23. Kurtzke JF. Rating neurologic impairment in multiple sclerosis: An expanded disability status scale (EDSS). Neurology 1983;33:1444–1452.
24. Noseworthy JH. Clinical scoring methods for multiple sclerosis. Ann Neurol 1994;36:S80–S85.
25. Miller DH. Magnetic resonance imaging in monitoring the treatment of multiple sclerosis. Ann Neurol 1994;36:S91– S94.
26. Abramsky O. Pregnancy and multiple sclerosis. Ann Neurol 1994;36:S38–S41.
27. Kurland LT. Trauma and multiple sclerosis. Ann Neurol 1994;36:S33–S37.
28. Weinshenker BG. Natural history of multiple sclerosis. Ann Neurol 1994;36:S6–S11.
29. Swanson JW. Multiple sclerosis: Update in diagnosis and review of prognostic factors. Mayo Clin Proc 1989;64:577– 586.
30. McDonald WI, Silberberg DH. The diagnosis of multiple sclerosis, in McDonald WI, Silberberg DH (eds): Multiple sclerosis. Boston, Butterworth, 1986, p 1.
31. Poser CM, Paty DW, Scheinberg L, et al. New diagnostic criteria for multiple sclerosis: Guidelines for research protocols. Ann Neurol 1983;13:227–231.
32. Olsson T. Cerebrospinal fluid. Ann Neurol 1994;36:S100– S102.
33. Weiner HL, Paty DW. Diagnostic and therapeutic trials in multiple sclerosis: A new look. Summary of Jekyll Island workshop. Neurology 1989;39:972–979.
34. Myers LW, Ellison GW. The peculiar difficulties of therapeutic trials for multiple sclerosis. Neurol Clin 1990;8:119–141.
35. Bansil S, Troiano R, Dowling PC, et al. Advances in the pharmacological and neurological treatment of patients with multiple sclerosis. Neuro Rehabil 1993;3(4):1–8.
36. Rudnick RA, Goodkin DE, Ransohoff RM. Pharmacotherapy of multiple sclerosis: Current status. Cleve Clin J Med 1992; 59:267.
37. Carter JL, Rodriguez M. Immunosuppressive treatment of multiple sclerosis. Mayo Clin Proc 1989;64:664–669.
38. Rose AS, Kuzma JW, Kurtzke JF, et al. Co-operative study in the evaluation of therapy in multiple sclerosis: ACTH versus placebo, final report. Neurology 1970;20(suppl):1–19.
39. Durelli L, Cocito A, Riccio C, et al. High-dose intravenous methylprednisolone in the treatment of multiple sclerosis: Clinical immunologic correlations. Neurology 1986;36:238–243.
40. Milligan NM, Newcombe R, Compston DAS. A double-blind controlled trial of high-dose methylprednisolone in patients with multiple sclerosis. 1. Clinical effects. J Neurol Neurosurg Psychiatry 1987;50:511–516.
41. Goodin DS. The use of immunosuppressive agents in the treatment of multiple sclerosis: A critical review. Neurology 1991;41:980–985.
42. Barnes MP, Bateman DE, Cleland PG, et al. Intravenous methylprednisolone for multiple sclerosis in relapse. J Neurol Neurosurg Psychiatry 1985;48:157–159.

43. Thompson AJ, Kennard C, Swash M, et al. Relative efficacy of intravenous methylprednisolone and ACTH in the treatment of acute relapse in MS. Neurol 1989;39:969–971.
44. The IFNB Multiple Sclerosis Study Group. Interferon beta-1b is effective in relapsing-remitting multiple sclerosis. I. Clinical results of a multi-center, randomized, double-blind, placebo-controlled trial. Neurology 1993;43:655–661.
45. The IFNB Multiple Sclerosis Study Group. Interferon beta-1b is effective in relapsing-remitting multiple sclerosis. II. MRI analysis results of a multicenter, randomized, double-blind, placebo-controlled trial. Neurology 1993;43:662–667.
46. Goodkin DE. Interferon β-1b. Lancet 1994;344:1057–1060.
47. Weiner HL, Mackin GA, Orav EJ, et al. Intermittent cyclophosphamide pulse therapy in progressive multiple sclerosis: Final report of the Northeast Co-operative Multiple Sclerosis Treatment Group. Neurology 1993;43:910–918.
48. Quality Standards Subcommittee of the American Academy of Neurology. Practice advisory on selection of patients with multiple sclerosis for treatment with betaseron. Neurology 1994;44:1537–1540.
49. McDonald WI, Miller DH, Thompson AJ. Are magnetic resonance findings predictive of clinical outcome in therapeutic trials of multiple sclerosis? The dilemma of interferon-β. Ann Neurol 1994;36:14–18.
50. Carter JL, Hafler DA, Dawson DM, et al. Immunosuppression with high-dose IV cyclophosphamide and ACTH in progressive multiple sclerosis: Cumulative 6-year experience in 164 patients. Neurology 1988;38(suppl 2):9–14.
51. Goodkin DE, Plencner S, Palmer-Saxerud J, et al. Cyclophosphamide in chronic progressive multiple sclerosis. Maintenance versus nonmaintenance therapy. Arch Neurol 1987;44:823–827.
52. The Multiple Sclerosis Study Group. Efficacy and toxicity of cyclosporine in chronic progressive multiple sclerosis: A randomized, double-blinded, placebo-controlled clinical trial. Ann Neurol 1990;27:591–605.
53. Johnson KP. Experimental therapy of relapsing-remitting multiple sclerosis with copolymer-1. Ann Neurol 1994;36:S115–S117.
54. Mitchell G. Update on multiple sclerosis therapy. Med Clin North Am 1993;77(1):231–249.
55. Kinn AC, Larsson PO. Desmopressin: A new principle for symptomatic treatment of urgency and incontinence in patients with multiple sclerosis. Scand J Urol Nephrol 1990;24:109–112.
56. Moulin DE. Pain in multiple sclerosis. Neurol Clin 1989;7:321–331.
57. Beaver CT Jr. The current status of studies of aminopyridine in patients with multiple sclerosis. Ann Neurol 1994;36: S118–S121.

Chapter 55

Epilepsy

William R. Garnett, PharmD

Epilepsy has been recognized for at least 2400 years. It is derived from the Greek *epilepsia* meaning "to come upon, to be grabbed hold of or thrown down, to attack, to seize hold of."

Today epilepsy is viewed as a symptom of disturbed electrical activity in the brain caused by a wide variety of disorders. Epilepsy is a general name given to the wide range of symptoms that reflect the manifold functions of the brain in a pathologically disturbed manner. It is a collection of many different types of seizures that vary widely in severity, appearance, cause, consequence, and management. Epilepsy implies a periodic recurrence of seizures with or without convulsions.[1]

A seizure results from an excessive discharge of neurons and is characterized by changes in electrical activity as measured by the electroencephalogram (EEG). In addition, there may be disturbances in consciousness, sensory systems, motor systems, subjective well-being, and objective behavior. A seizure is episodic, is brief, has a beginning and an end, may produce postseizure impairment, and is involuntary. A convulsion implies a violent, involuntary contraction or series of contractions of the voluntary muscles.

Epilepsy is a chronic disorder. In selected patients, surgery may offer a cure. Although drug therapy can often control the manifestations of the disease, antiepileptic drugs (AEDs) do not cure epilepsy. The proper treatment of epilepsy begins with a careful classification of the seizure type and selection of the most effective AED. The major determinant of AED selection may be toleration of the drug by the patient. Therefore, avoidance of side effects rather than superior efficacy may be the main criterion for drug selection.[2] Quality of life is an important determinant in directing the therapy of patients with epilepsy.[3] Quality of life is an assessment of the health status, social, community and civic activities, economics variables, family life, and personal development of a patient. In epilepsy quality of life takes into account the factors that patients are concerned about other than the disease and the AEDs.[3] Monotherapy is preferred and about 70% of all patients with epilepsy can be maintained on one drug.[1] However, not all of these patients are seizure free. The percentage of patients who are seizure free on one drug varies by seizure type. For example, the second VA Collaborative Trial demonstrated that fewer than 40% of patients with partial seizures were seizure free after 1 year.[4] Drugs may be combined in rational combinations in an attempt to help the patient become seizure free. Although epilepsy is a chronic disorder, some patients may be successfully discontinued from AEDs after an extended seizure-free period. The success of AED therapy depends on careful dosage titration based on pharmacokinetic principles to a desired patient response, the patient's ability to tolerate side effects, and long-term patient monitoring to ensure compliance, prevent drug interactions, and minimize toxicity.[5]

After a 15-year hiatus with no major new drugs approved for epilepsy therapy, three new drugs were approved in 1993–1994. Three others are pending approval with the FDA.[6] The availability of new drugs for the therapy of epilepsy offers new opportunities to improve treatment and makes it essential that clinicians review all of their patients to ensure that they are achieving the best outcomes possible.[7]

EPIDEMIOLOGY

Each year 120 per 100,000 people in the United States will come to medical attention because of a newly recognized seizure. At least 8% of the general population will have at least one seizure in a lifetime. However, it is possible to have a seizure and not have epilepsy.[8] Recurrence of a first unprovoked seizure at 5 years ranges between 23 and 80%. Children with an idiopathic first seizure and a normal EEG have a particularly favorable prognosis.[9] Some seizures may occur as single events resulting from withdrawal of central nervous system (CNS) depressants (e.g., alcohol, barbiturates, and other drugs) or during acute illnesses (e.g., meningoencephalitis) or toxic conditions (e.g., uremia or eclampsia). Some patients will only have seizures associated with fever. These seizures do not constitute epilepsy. Epilepsy is a chronic disorder indicating recurrent seizures.[1] The age-adjusted incidence of epilepsy was 44 per 100,000 person-years. This represents about 125,000 new cases per year; of these, 30% will be under the age of

18 at the time of diagnosis. The frequency of epilepsy in the elderly has increased. There is a bimodal distribution to the occurrence of the first seizure with one peak occurring in newborn and young children and the second peak occurring in patients older than age 65.[10] At least 10% of patients in long-term care facilities are taking AEDs.[11] The seizure type and the cause of the seizure change with age.[10]

PATHOPHYSIOLOGY

MECHANISM OF A SEIZURE

Seizure activity is characterized by paroxysmal discharges occurring synchronously in a large population of cortical neurons. This is characterized on the EEG as a sharp wave or "spike." The basic physiology of a seizure episode is traceable to an unstable cell membrane or its surrounding, supportive cells. The seizure originates from the gray matter of any cortical or perhaps subcortical area. Initially, a small number of neurons fire abnormally. Normal membrane conductances and inhibitory synaptic currents break down and excess excitability spreads, either locally to produce a focal seizure or more widely to produce a generalized seizure.[12] This onset propagates by physiologic pathways to involve adjacent or remote areas. The clinical manifestations depend on the site of the focus, on the degree of irritability of the surrounding area of the brain, and on the intensity of the impulse.[13]

The normal firing of neurons is controlled by excitatory and inhibitory neurotransmitters. The development of an action potential in a neuron is similar to that in a cardiac cell. Sodium concentration is high in the extracellular space and low in the intracellular space. The concentrations of potassium are reversed. The major ion species involved in burst activity appears to be calcium. An abnormality of potassium conductance, a defect in the voltage-sensitive calcium channels, or a deficiency in the membrane ATPases linked to ion transport may result in neuronal membrane instability and a seizure.[13] Neurotransmitters (e.g., glutamate, aspartate, acetylcholine, norepinephrine, histamine, corticotropin-releasing factor, purines, peptides, cytokines, and steroid hormones) enhance the excitability and propagation of neuronal activity, whereas gamma-aminobutyric acid (GABA) and dopamine inhibit neuronal activity and propagation. Normal neuronal activity also depends on an adequate supply of glucose, oxygen, sodium, potassium, calcium, and amino acids. Systemic pH is also a factor in precipitating seizures. There may be primary defects in the GABA-ergic inhibitory system or in the sensitivity or arrangement of the receptors involved in excitatory neurotransmission that result in a seizure.[12,13]

Most of what is known about abnormal neuronal activity is derived from *in vitro* models such as the hippocampal slice model or from animal studies. The generation of epileptogenic discharges appears to depend on the interplay of three major factors. Some neurons must have an inherent ability to elaborate responses leading to paroxysmal bursts. Abnormal neurons recruit normal neurons to propagate the discharge of a seizure. This is augmented by the failure of normal inhibitory activities or by an enhancement of normal excitatory synaptic activities. Thus, a deficiency of inhibitory neurotransmitters such as GABA or an increase in excitatory neurotransmitters would promote abnormal neuronal activity. Interference with normal metabolic processes also promotes seizure activity; however, neither a failure of inhibition nor an enhancement of excitation completely explains the promotion of abnormal propagation. The most recent *in vitro* experiments suggest that modulation of neuronal activity in favor of the pathologic discharge is also important. This modulation appears to be under cholinergic control. In hippocampal neurons, acetylcholine causes an initial hyperpolarization, followed by a long-lasting depolarization with decreased conductance that leads to prolonged bursting. Differences between acute and chronic foci probably depend more on the degree and intensity of these factors than on fundamentally different mechanisms.[12] The different kinds of epilepsies probably arise from different physiologic abnormalities.[13]

Control of abnormal neuronal activity with AEDs is accomplished by elevating the convulsive threshold of neurons to electrical or chemical stimuli or by limiting the propagation of the seizure discharge from its origin. Raising the threshold most likely involves stabilization of neuronal membranes, whereas limiting the propagation involves depression of synaptic transmission and reduction of nerve conduction.[12] The newer AEDs approved in the 1990s appear to have a different mechanism of action than the older AEDs. The newer AEDs focus more on inhibiting the neuroexcitatory mechanisms.[6]

CONSEQUENCES OF A SEIZURE

The maintenance of the neuronal membrane action potential requires energy from adenosine triphosphate (ATP). Cellular respiration generates ATP and synthesizes neurotransmitters. During a seizure there is a large increase in the demand for brain blood flow to carry off CO_2 and to bring substrates for neuronal metabolic activity. The brain has a limited capacity to increase blood flow and during a seizure the brain may use more energy than it can manufacture. The more prolonged the seizure, the more likely the brain is to suffer ischemia that may result in neuronal destruction and brain damage. The developing brain is especially vulnerable and susceptible to damage. Seizure disorders per se do not cause a significant decrease in intelligence.[14]

Seizures beget seizures. There appears to be a positive correlation between the initiation of appropriate AED therapy and the ability to control seizure activity. The failure to control seizures seems to lead to an increase in seizure activity and also to the occurrence of other seizure types. Therefore, appropriate therapy should be initiated early after the diagnosis of epilepsy. However, a single unprovoked seizure is not epilepsy. Longitudinal studies indicated that about 70% of patients who receive a diagnosis of epilepsy will become seizure free and that the majority can have their AEDs withdrawn.[1,2]

ETIOLOGY AND PRECIPITATION OF SEIZURES

Seizures occur because small numbers of neurons discharge abnormally. Anything that disrupts the normal homeostasis of the neuronal cell and disturbs its stability may trigger abnormal activity and seizures. As shown in Table 55.1, these disruptions include mechanical disturbances, metabolic disturbances, sudden withdrawal of CNS drugs, and toxins. A hereditary predisposition to seizures has been suggested. Patients with mental retardation and cerebral palsy are at increased risk for seizures. The more profound the degree of mental retardation as measured by IQ, the greater the incidence of epilepsy.[14] In the elderly, seizures are primarily (67%) partial from onset. The causes of seizures in the elderly are cerebrovascular disease, tumor, head trauma, metabolic disorders, CNS infections, and multifactorial etiology.[10] In some cases if an etiology can be found, it can be corrected, and the patient will not require chronic AEDs; however, most patients who present with seizures do not have an identifiable cause and have idiopathic epilepsy.[10] The incidence of idiopathic epilepsy is higher in children.[1,2]

Many factors have been shown to precipitate seizures in susceptible individuals.[15] Hyperventilation may precipitate absence seizures. Sleep, sleep deprivation, sensory stimuli, and emotional stress may initiate seizures. Hormonal changes occurring around the time of menses, puberty, or pregnancy have been associated with the onset of, or an increase in, seizure activity. The risk of catamenial epilepsy (i.e., the situation whereby at least 75% of seizures each month occur during menstruation) is estimated at 12.5%.[16] Birth control pills should be administered with caution to patients with epilepsy. Other precipitating factors include fever, trauma, lack of food, and drugs. A careful history for theophylline, alcohol, phenothiazines, antidepressants (especially maprotiline), and street drug use should be obtained from patients presenting with seizures. Also, AEDs in excessive concentrations may cause seizures. Perinatal factors and subsequent events have been identified as risk factors for the later development of epilepsy. Children who are "small for gestational age" or with neonatal seizures are at increased risk for developing epilepsy. Children with febrile seizures are at increased risk for developing epilepsy later in life. The most clearly established risk factors for epilepsy are severe head trauma, CNS infections, and stroke. Brain surgery increases the risk of developing epilepsy although the extent of the risk is unknown. Immunizations have not been associated with an increased risk of epilepsy.[10] However, pertussis immunization has been associated with an increase in febrile seizures.

TABLE 55.1. COMMON CAUSES OF SEIZURES

Mechanical	Sudden Withdrawal of Drugs
Trauma	Alcohol
Birth injury	Street drugs
Neoplasms	Antipsychotics
Vascular abnormalities	Antidepressants
Metabolic	Antiepileptic drugs
Electrolytes	Toxins
Water	Fever
Glucose	Infection
Amino acids	Hereditary
Lipids	Idiopathic
pH	

CLINICAL PRESENTATION

DIAGNOSIS OF SEIZURES

The diagnosis of seizures begins with a careful and accurate patient history.[17] The best evaluation of a seizure occurs if the patient has an episode in the presence of a trained observer; however, the frequency may be such that this is impossible. Therefore, the patient and the patient's family should be interviewed carefully to obtain a description of the seizure.

Information that should be obtained includes (1) frequency and duration of episodes, (2) precipitating factors, (3) times at which episodes occur, (4) presence of an aura, (5) ictal activity, and (6) postictal state. Patients may use terms to describe seizures that have no real meaning in seizure classifications. For example, patients may refer to "the little ones" or to "petit mal seizures" that are partial seizures and not absence. The patient's own terms need to be translated into the appropriate seizure classification. Also, the patient may be having more than one seizure type. Patients may not recognize some events as seizures, especially if there are no convulsions or no loss of consciousness. Seizure patients may experience anxiety for various reasons.[17] True panic attacks should be identified and treated separately.

The physical, neurologic, and laboratory evaluations may help identify an underlying etiology. The physical and neurologic examinations may reveal head trauma or signs of other diseases that manifest as seizures. Laboratory tests (e.g., SMA-20, complete blood cell count [CBC] , urinalysis, and special blood chemistries) may identify a metabolic etiology for the seizures (e.g., hypoglycemia, electrolyte abnormalities, or amino acid disturbances). The suspicion of systemic diseases (e.g., lead ingestion, sickle-cell anemia, and infections) may be confirmed by laboratory evaluation. A lumbar puncture may be required if the patient has seizures and a fever. In many patients with idiopathic epilepsy, the physical, neurologic, and laboratory evaluations will be normal.[17]

An EEG should be done as soon after the seizure as possible. The EEG is essential in properly classifying seizure types.[1] For example, differentiation between generalized absence seizures and complex partial seizures with loss of consciousness may be best accomplished by the EEG. The best time to obtain an EEG is while the patient is having a seizure. The EEG may be done under normal conditions, in a sleep-induced state, or in a sleep-deprived state. Clinicians should remember that a patient may have a normal EEG between seizures, while other patients have an abnormal EEG without having epilepsy. EEG results should be combined with the clinical description to classify the seizure type. To facilitate seizure classification, it may be necessary to hospitalize some patients and place them on simultaneous EEG and video monitoring. The use of epilepsy monitoring units (EMUs) is increasing for difficult-to-control patients or for patients who may be surgical candidates.[17]

Additional tests used in seizure evaluation include computed tomography (CT), positron emission tomography (PET), single photon emission CT (SPECT), and magnetic resonance imaging (MRI). These neurologic imaging studies may identify structural brain disorders that may be causally related to seizures. An MRI has been recommended for all patients with refractory seizures that may prompt consideration for surgery. A brain imaging study has also been recommended for all patients older than 18 years of age and in all children with partial seizures, abnormal findings on neurologic examination, or focal slow-wave function on EEG. Functional imaging (e.g., PET, SPECT) may identify interictal abnormalities but they are not routine or generally available procedures.[1]

A psychologic evaluation may be required if the patient is thought to have pseudoseizures or hysterical epilepsy. This disorder mimics epilepsy but is emotionally based and does not result from paroxysmal abnormal dysfunction. It may coexist with epilepsy and may occur in perhaps 20% of patients referred to epilepsy centers. EMUs may be useful in diagnosing this type of disorder.[18]

CLASSIFICATION OF SEIZURES

The International League Against Epilepsy has developed a classification system that combines clinical description with EEG findings (Table 55.2). More than 90% of seizure patients may be classified using this system.[19,20] This classification has helped demonstrate that all seizures should not be treated with the same AEDs.[21] The therapeutic range of the AEDs may differ depending on the seizure classification.[22] Elaboration of the classification of seizures into those localized to the six-layered isocortex and those whose elaboration involves regions of the brain involved with consciousness and memory has provided the focus for the increasing use of epilepsy surgery. Therefore, proper seizure classification is essential to therapeutic drug monitoring. Further refinements in seizure classification may result in better drug and dosing selection.

Using the international classification scheme, seizures may be divided into partial, generalized, or unclassified. Recent attempts have been made to subdivide the partial seizure classification in terms of where the seizure foci are localized. This is predominantly for clinical description. For pharmacologic treatment decisions, the classification of generalized versus partial and simple versus complex provides the most essential information regarding the drugs to select.[23]

Partial seizures begin in one hemisphere of the brain and, unless they become secondarily generalized, result in an asymmetric seizure. Partial seizures may be described as focal or unilateral seizures and may be subdivided into simple and complex. Partial seizures manifest as alterations in motor functions, sensory or somatosensory symptoms, or autonomic symptoms (automatisms). If there is no loss of

TABLE 55.2. INTERNATIONAL CLASSIFICATION OF SEIZURES

- I. Partial seizures (seizures begin locally)
  - A. Simple (without impairment of consciousness)
    - 1. With motor symptoms
    - 2. With special sensory or somatosensory symptoms
    - 3. With psychic symptoms
  - B. Complex (with impairment of consciousness)
    - 1. Simple partial onset followed by impairment of consciousness—with or without automatisms
    - 2. Impaired consciousness at onset—with or without automatisms
  - C. Secondarily generalized (partial onset evolving to generalized tonic–clonic seizures)
- II. Generalized seizures (bilaterally symmetrical and without local onset)
  - A. Absence
  - B. Myoclonic
  - C. Clonic
  - D. Tonic
  - E. Tonic–clonic
  - F. Atonic
  - G. Infantile spasms
- III. Unclassified seizures
- IV. Status epilepticus (prolonged partial or generalized seizures without recovery between attacks)

(Compiled from Ref. 19)

consciousness, the seizures are classified as simple partial. If there is loss of consciousness, the seizures are described as complex partial. With complex partial seizures, the patient may have automatisms, periods of memory loss, or aberrations of behavior.[24] Some patients with complex partial epilepsy have been mistakenly diagnosed as having psychotic episodes.[25] Complex partial seizures may progress to a generalized seizure.[24] Partial epilepsy in young children and infants is reported to be rare, but this may reflect misdiagnosis. It is now recognized that partial epilepsy may begin in infancy.[26] Complex partial epilepsy may be difficult to recognize in an elderly population.

Generalized seizures have clinical manifestations that indicate involvement of both hemispheres. Motor manifestations are bilateral, and there is a loss of consciousness. Generalized seizures may be further subdivided by EEG and clinical manifestations.[17] A partial seizure that becomes generalized is referred to as a secondarily generalized seizure.

Absence seizures are manifested by a sudden onset, interruption of ongoing activities, a blank stare, and possibly a brief upward rotation of the eyes. The EEG during the seizure has a characteristic 2–4 cycle/s spike and slow-wave complex.[27] It is important to differentiate absence seizures from complex partial seizures.[28]

Tonic–clonic seizures, formerly known as grand mal, are what many people think of as epilepsy. Although they may be preceded by premonitory symptoms known as an aura, the majority of patients lose consciousness without warning. A tonic–clonic seizure that is preceded by an aura is likely a partial seizure that secondarily generalized. The seizure results in a sudden sharp tonic contraction of muscles followed by a period of rigidity. During this period the patient may fall and be injured. During the seizure the patient may cry or moan, lose sphincter control, bite his or her tongue, or develop cyanosis. After the seizure the patient may be unconscious for a variable period of time, and frequently goes into a deep sleep. Tonic and clonic seizures may occur separately.[17]

Brief shocklike muscular contractions of the face, trunk, and extremities are known as myoclonic jerks. They may be isolated events or rapidly repetitive.[29]

A sudden loss of muscle tone is known as an atonic seizure. This may be described as a head drop, the dropping of a limb, or a slumping to the ground.[17] These patients often wear protective headware to prevent trauma.

Unclassified seizures include all seizures that cannot be classified because of inadequate or incomplete data.

Seizures are classified on the basis of clinical and EEG characteristics. The epilepsies and epilepsy syndromes are classified by clusters of signs and symptoms that customarily occur together (see Table 55.3).[23] The classification of the epileptic syndromes considers the predominant seizure type, age of onset, natural history, EEG, response to AEDs, etiology (idiopathic or primary versus symptomatic or secondary), family history, and prognosis.[28] Some of the more common syndromes are West syndrome, which is characterized by infantile spasms, arrested psychomotor development, and hypsarrhythmia; Lennox–Gastaut syndrome, which includes tonic, atonic, atypical absence, myoclonic, generalized tonic–clonic, partial seizures with a characteristic EEG, febrile convulsions, and neonatal seizures; and juvenile myoclonic epilepsy, which is characterized by myoclonic jerks, generalized tonic–clonic, and absence seizures. Rolandic epilepsy is a well-defined epileptic syndrome that begins between the ages of 3 and 13. It is characterized by a high-voltage centrotemporal spike focus, which may shift from side to side. The patient has simple partial seizures with sensory and motor symptoms, and there is often secondary generalization. Rolandic epilepsy tends to be benign and may not require AED therapy.[30] It is difficult to classify patients into specific syndromes early in the process of diagnosis but it is important to help predict prognosis.[28]

TREATMENT

GOALS

The first treatment goal is to control or reduce the frequency of seizures, allowing the patient to live an essentially normal life. Ideally, seizure frequency should be reduced to zero; however, all AEDs have some side effects, and the complete suppression of seizures must be balanced against side effects.[31,32]

Thus, the second treatment goal would be the absence of side effects and drug–drug interactions. Because therapy is extended for many years, often a lifetime, chronic side effects must be considered.[33–35] If the patient is overly sedated or develops other significant side effects, some seizure control may have to be sacrificed to improve functioning.[36] The patient should be involved in deciding the balance between frequency of seizures and the occurrence of side effects. Some patients (e.g., patients who have seizures only while they are sleeping) may prefer a greater number of seizures and fewer drug side effects. The newer AEDs offer alternatives for balancing seizure frequency and drug side effects.[37,38]

The third treatment goal is to provide the best quality of life possible for the patient. This concept goes beyond balancing the number of seizures and the occurrence of side effects. It involves assessing all of the concerns that a patient with epilepsy has. For example, epilepsy patients are concerned about their future, forming relationships, housing, social isolation, social stigma, and so on.[39] Despite public awareness programs, there are still many misconceptions about epilepsy. These misconceptions often liken epilepsy to mental retardation, to possession by demons, or to punishment by God. Knowledge of epilepsy has been

TABLE 55.3. INTERNATIONAL CLASSIFICATION OF EPILEPSIES, EPILEPTIC SYNDROMES, AND RELATED SEIZURE DISORDERS (ICES)

1. Localization-related (focal, local, partial)		
Idiopathic (primary)	1.1	Benign childhood epilepsy with centrotemporal spike Childhood epilepsy with occipital paroxysms Primary reading epilepsy
Cryptogenic	1.2	Defined by: Seizure type (see ICES) Clinical features Etiology Anatomic localization
Symptomatic (secondary)	1.3	Temporal lobe epilepsies Frontal lobe epilepsies Parietal lobe epilepsies Occipital lobe epilepsies Chronic progressive epilepsia partialis continua of childhood Syndromes characterized by seizures with specific modes of precipitation
2. Generalized	2.1	Benign neonatal familial convulsions Benign neonatal convulsions Benign myoclonic epilepsy in infancy Childhood absence epilepsy (pyknolepsy) Juvenile absence epilepsy Juvenile myoclonic epilepsy (impulsive petit mal) Epilepsies with grand mal seizures (GTCS) on awakening Other generalized idiopathic epilepsies Epilepsies with seizures precipitated by specific modes of activation
Cryptogenic or symptomatic	2.2	West syndrome (infantile spasms, Blitz Nick–Salaam Krämpfe) Lennox–Gastaut syndrome Epilepsy with myoclonic–astatic seizures Epilepsy with myoclonic absences
	2.3.1	Nonspecific etiology: Early myoclonic encephalopathy Early infantile epileptic encephalopathy with suppression bursts Other symptomatic generalized epilepsies
	2.3.2	Specific syndromes Epileptic seizures may complicate many disease states
3. Undetermined epilepsies	3.1	With both generalized and focal seizures: Neonatal seizures Severe myoclonic epilepsy in infancy Epilepsy with continuous spike-waves during slow wave sleep Acquired epileptic aphasia (Landau–Kleffner syndrome) Other undetermined epilepsies
	3.2	Without unequivocal generalized or focal features
4. Special syndromes	4.1	Situation-related seizures (gelegenheitsanfälle) Febrile convulsions Isolated seizures or isolated status epilepticus Seizures occurring only when there is an acute or toxic event due to factors such as alcohol, drugs, eclampsia, nonketotic hyperglycemia

(From Dreifuss FE. The epilepsies: Clinical implications of the international classification. Epilepsia 1990;31(suppl 3):S3–S10, with permission.)

shown to correlate with quality of life.[40] Patients may be encouraged to join the Epilepsy Foundation of America or other support groups that encourage patients with epilepsy to lead normal lives. Because some AEDs may cause behavioral and cognitive abnormalities, these side effects should be considered in selecting a drug of choice.[33–35]

PRINCIPLES

Establish Diagnosis and Exclude Remedial Causes

Some seizures result from correctable etiologies, for example, metabolic disturbances. Therefore, while AEDs may be used acutely, they would not be indicated for chronic use if the etiology could be identified and corrected (see Table 55.4). There are no data to support the prophylactic use of AEDs in patients who have had neurologic injuries but have not developed epilepsy.[41]

Select Primary Drug Most Appropriate for Seizure Type

Classification of seizure types and epilepsy syndromes has improved the ability of clinicians to select drugs of choice for specific seizures (Table 55.5). Absence seizures are pharmacologically different from other seizure types. Phenytoin, phenobarbital, and carbamazepine, although effective in generalized and partial seizures, are ineffective in treating absence seizures and in some cases may precipitate an increase in seizure activity. Absence seizures are best treated with ethosuximide or valproic acid. Ethosuximide is effective only in absence seizures and is ineffective against other generalized and partial seizures. If the patient has a combination of absence and other generalized or partial seizures, valproic acid is the preferred first choice because it is the only AED effective against absence and other seizure types. If valproic acid is ineffective in treating a mixed seizure disorder that includes absence, ethosuximide should be used in combination with another AED.[31,32]

The traditional treatment of tonic–clonic seizures is phenytoin or phenobarbital; however, the use of carbamazepine and valproic acid is increasing because these AEDs have a lower incidence of side effects and equal efficacy. Valproic acid is the drug of first choice for atonic seizures and for juvenile myoclonic epilepsy.[31,32]

TABLE 55.4. PRINCIPLES OF THERAPY

Establish diagnosis and exclude remedial causes
Select primary drug most appropriate for seizure type
Titrate dose to achieve desired response
Monotherapy is preferred
Consider rational polytherapy
Provide patient education
Consider discontinuing AEDs

Carbamazepine is recognized as the AED of first choice for partial seizures. Alternatives to carbamazepine are phenytoin, gabapentin, and lamotrigine.[31,32] The newer antiepileptic drugs, (e.g., gabapentin and lamotrigine) are approved as adjunctive therapy for patients with refractory partial seizures. Monotherapy trials with these drugs are under way.[37,38] Phenobarbital and valproic acid have also been used in partial seizures. Felbamate, which has monotherapy approval for partial seizures, is very effective but has been associated with some significant side effects.[7]

Recent data suggest that the therapeutic range for AEDs may be different for different seizure types. Blood concentrations may need to be higher to control complex partial seizures than to control tonic–clonic seizures.[22] If initial therapy fails to control seizures, alternative AEDs or a combination of AEDs should be tried to accomplish seizure control.

Titrate AED Dose to Achieve Adequate Patient Response

All AEDs are associated with depressed CNS function (e.g., drowsiness, lethargy, tiredness) early in the course of treatment, but some tolerance usually develops in 7–10 days. Therefore, except in life-threatening situations (e.g., status epilepticus), AEDs should be started in low doses and gradually increased until seizure control is achieved or intolerable side effects occur. A general rule is to initiate therapy with one-fourth to one-third of the anticipated maintenance dose and increase the dose to maintenance over 3–4 weeks.[42]

Although doses of AEDs are frequently cited in milligrams per kilogram, the individual patient's response is a more definitive therapeutic endpoint. There is a large interpatient variability in pharmacokinetic parameters, which results in a large variation in the milligram-per-kilogram dose required to achieve adequate blood concentrations.[42] Therefore, the concentration of the drug in the serum or plasma may be a guideline in assessing drug dosing. In compliant patients with low plasma concentrations who are receiving a normal milligram-per-kilogram dose, the dosage may need to be increased.

A therapeutic range has been described for the older AEDs. The blood concentration is a target that should be correlated with clinical outcome. However, the blood concentration is not the endpoint. The desired response is the cessation of seizures without side effects. Seizure control may occur before the "minimum" of the range is achieved, and side effects may appear before the "maximum" of the range is achieved. Some patients may need and tolerate concentrations beyond the "maximum." Therefore, while the blood concentration is a guideline, it is not dogma. Clinicians should treat patients and not numbers.[42]

Many AEDs are highly bound to plasma proteins. The unbound or "free" concentration is the active drug capable

TABLE 55.5. DRUGS OF CHOICE FOR SPECIFIC SEIZURE DISORDERS

New International	Commonly Used Major Drugs	Commonly Used Alternative Drugs
Simple partial	Carbamazepine Phenytoin	Lamotrigine Gabapentin
Complex partial	Carbamazepine Phenytoin	Lamotrigine Gabapentin
Tonic–clonic	Phenytoin Valproic acid Carbamazepine	Phenobarbital
Absence	Ethosuximide Valproic acid	Clonazepam Acetazolamide
Mixed seizures	Phenytoin Phenobarbital + ethosuximide or valproic acid	Primidone Carbamazepine + clonazepam Acetazolamide
Bilateral massive epileptic myoclonus, atonic, infantile spasms[a]	Clonazepam ACTH	Phenytoin Phenobarbital Benzodiazepines Acetazolamide

[a]Difficult group to treat; combinations are the rule.

of penetrating the blood–brain barrier and interacting at the receptor site. Equilibrium dialysis used to be the only method available to determine free drug concentration. This technique is still the standard used in research, but is too time consuming to be clinically useful.[42]

Several companies have marketed ultrafiltration systems that are capable of more rapid separation of free from protein-bound drug. The availability of these systems makes determination of free drug concentrations potentially clinically useful. Despite the ease of using ultrafiltration devices, however, free level monitoring is not indicated for routine use in all patients. In patients who are not responding or having side effects at "therapeutic" concentrations of total drug, a free concentration may explain the unusual response. For populations known to have altered plasma protein binding (Table 55.6), free rather than total drug concentrations should be measured for highly protein-bound drugs.[43] Free concentration monitoring is especially useful for phenytoin.

TABLE 55.6. CONDITIONS ALTERING ANTIEPILEPTIC DRUG[a]—PROTEIN BINDING

Chronic renal failure
Liver disease
Hypoalbuminemia
Burns
Pregnancy
Malnutrition
Displacing drugs
Age—neonates and elderly

[a]Phenytoin and valproic acid are highly protein bound; carbamazepine has variable binding; phenobarbital and primidone are minimally bound; and ethosuximide is not bound to plasma proteins.

Monotherapy and Rational Polytherapy

It was once common to start patients with seizures on combination AEDs (e.g., phenytoin and phenobarbital). Numerous studies have demonstrated that many patients can be effectively managed on one AED alone. The reduction in polypharmacy is correlated with a subsequent decrease in side effects. Therefore, the initial treatment of seizures should begin with the most potentially effective single drug.[31,32]

The initial agent should be titrated until maximum benefit is achieved (i.e., until seizure control is achieved or intolerable side effects occur). Patient compliance must be assessed to evaluate the usefulness of the initial agent. Efficacy may be assessed by seizure frequency.

A second medication may be added if the patient is having continued seizure activity despite good plasma concentrations. The second AED may replace or be added to the initial therapy. If the initial AED is replaced, it should be gradually tapered after the second drug has been titrated to the desired dose.

The concept of "rational polytherapy" suggests that a second drug can be better selected by combining drugs with different mechanisms of actions, different side effects, and a lack of drug interactions. The AEDs introduced in the 1990s potentially have different mechanisms of action than the older AEDs and have been approved as adjunctive therapy.[6]

Provide Patient Education

To promote compliance, assess safety and efficacy, and prevent behavioral aberrations, the patient must understand the disease and prescribed medications. This requires patient education. Knowledge of epilepsy has been correlated with an improved quality of life.[40]

Noncompliance may be the single most common reason for treatment failure.[2] It is estimated that up to 60% of patients with epilepsy are noncompliant.[44] Physicians overestimate compliance by 50%.[2] The rate of noncompliance is increased by the complexity of the drug regimen and by three and four times a day dosing.[2] Noncompliance is not influenced by age, sex, psychomotor development, seizure type, or seizure frequency.[42] Compliant patients achieve better seizure control.[45] Patient education should be continuous and compliance stressed at each clinic visit.

Consider Discontinuing AEDs

AEDs may not need to be given for a lifetime. Polypharmacy may be reduced and some patients can discontinue AEDs altogether. In reducing polypharmacy, the drug considered less appropriate for the seizure type should be discontinued first and the possibility of drug interactions considered. Reduction of polypharmacy has resulted in a decrease in side effects and an increase in cognitive abilities.[46] Other researchers have reported that the improvement in cognition is small, especially if the patient is on one drug and that the effect is primarily on psychomotor speed with less effect on higher order cognitive functioning.[47]

Factors promoting complete withdrawal of AEDs include a seizure-free period of 2–4 years, complete seizure control within 1 year of onset, an onset of seizures after age 2 but before age 35, a normal EEG, and use of AEDs for inappropriate reasons. Factors associated with a poor prognosis in discontinuing AEDs despite a seizure-free interval include a history of a high frequency of seizures, repeated episodes of status, combination of seizure types, and development of abnormal mental functioning. A 2-year seizure-free period is suggested for absence and rolandic epilepsy, while a 4-year seizure-free period is suggested for simple partial, complex partial, and absence associated with tonic–clonic convulsions. Withdrawal is generally not suggested for patients with juvenile myoclonic epilepsy, absence with clonic–tonic–clonic seizures, or clonic–tonic–clonic seizures.[48]

The withdrawal of AEDs should be gradual. Some patients will have a recurrence of seizures as the AEDs are withdrawn. The risk of seizure relapse has been estimated at 10–70%. A recent meta-analysis determined that the relapse rate was 25% after 1 year and 29% after 2 years.[49] Seizure relapses occur most often within the first several months of drug removal. Seizure relapse has been reported to be more common if the AEDs are withdrawn over 1–3 months than over 6 months. However, another study found no difference in the rate of seizure recurrence in a 6-week taper versus a 9-month taper.[50] In addition to seizure relapse, the withdrawal of AEDs was associated with the emergence of anxiety and depression.[51] Sudden withdrawal is to be avoided because this is associated with the precipitation of status epilepticus.

The patient should agree to any plan to reduce or withdraw AED therapy. Some patients may be reluctant to stop medications because of fear of a seizure. There may be a significant psychosocial benefit to the patient from AED withdrawal.[52] Withdrawal may need to be scheduled at the convenience of the patient (e.g., during a summer vacation). A follow-up of 5 years is suggested for any patient successfully withdrawn from AED therapy.

Therapeutic Outcomes

Much of the financing of health care is centering on outcome assessment. The treatment goals and principles can be used to develop desirable treatment outcomes for patients with epilepsy. Some desirable therapeutic outcomes for the treatment of epilepsy are (1) the patient is seizure free; (2) the patient has no side effects or drug interactions; (3) the patient, the caregivers, and society are educated about epilepsy; (4) the patient achieves the best quality of life possible; (5) the patient receives the best care at the least cost; and (6) the patient is satisfied with the care provided.

SPECIFIC ANTIEPILEPTIC DRUGS

The control of most seizure disorders can usually be accomplished by the careful selection and monitoring of the major AEDs. Reasons for treatment failure are outlined in Table 55.7. (See also Tables 55.8–55.10.) In compliant refractory patients therapy with the "newer" AEDs may be tried as rational polypharmacy.[6]

Phenytoin

Therapeutics

Phenytoin may be used for any generalized seizure type except absence, where it may worsen the condition. Partial seizures may also be treated with phenytoin.

Phenytoin blocks post-tetanic potentiation by influencing synaptic transmission. Proposed mechanisms include altering ion fluxes associated with depolarization, repolarization, and membrane stability, altering calcium uptake in presynaptic terminals, influencing calcium-dependent synaptic protein phosphorylation and transmitter release, altering the sodium-potassium ATP-dependent ionic membrane pump, and preventing cyclic nucleotide buildup and cerebellar stimulation.[53]

TABLE 55.7. REASONS FOR TREATMENT FAILURE

Inappropriate drug selection
- Ubiquitous use of phenytoin and phenobarbital for all seizure types
- Failure to recognize antiepileptic drug of choice

Inappropriate dose
- Failure to evaluate serum drug concentration
- Failure to maximize serum drug concentration

Poor compliance

Refractory patients
- Some patients do not respond despite maximal therapy

Pharmacokinetics

(See Table 55.8.) Phenytoin is absorbed primarily from the duodenum; little absorption occurs in the stomach or ileum. Absorption is almost complete, with dissolution being the rate-limiting step. Absorption may be prolonged and secondary peaks may be seen. The absorption of phenytoin may be saturable. Enterohepatic cycling of phenytoin occurs, but there is no first-pass metabolism.[54]

The absorption of orally administered phenytoin is affected by the particle size of the administered formulation. Therefore, some brands may be absorbed faster than others. Preparations intended for single daily dosing are identified as "extended-release" preparations. The brand of phenytoin that a patient receives should not be switched without careful monitoring.[42] The intramuscular administration of phenytoin is problematic and best avoided.

Phenytoin enters the brain quickly, where it is redistributed to other body tissues including saliva and breast milk. It crosses the placenta to reach an equilibrium between mother and fetus. Phenytoin distributes to serum and tissue proteins. Obesity may increase the volume of distribution.[42]

In the blood, phenytoin is highly (90%) protein bound, primarily to albumin. For most patients, this binding is predictable and is proportional throughout the therapeutic range; however, special populations have altered protein binding (Table 55.6). The equations that have been used to normalize the phenytoin concentration in patients with hypoalbuminemia or renal failure have been found to be unreliable. The equation underpredicted the phenytoin concentration in patients with hypoalbuminemia and over- and underprediction occurred in patients with renal failure.[55] A

TABLE 55.8. ANTIEPILEPTIC DRUG PHARMACOKINETIC DATA

AED	$t_{1/2}$ (h)	Time to Steady State (d)	% Unchanged	V_D (L/kg)	% Bioavailability	Clinically Important Metabolite	% Removed by Dialysis	% Protein Binding
Phenytoin	A[a] 10–34 C 5–14	7–28	<5	0.6–8.0	90–95	No	4% (H)[b]	90
Phenobarbital	A 46–136 C 37–73	14–21	20–40	0.6	90–100	No	30% (H)[b]	50
Primidone	A 3.3–19 C 4.5–11	1–4	40	0.43–1.1	90–100	PB[c] PEMA[c]	30% (H)[b]	80
Carbamazepine	12 h if monotherapy; 5–14 h if combination; chronic dosing undergoes autoinduction	21–28 for completion of auto-induction	<1	1–2	>75	10,11-epoxide	<20	40–90
Valproic acid	A 8–20 C 7–14	1–3	<5	0.1–0.5	100	May contribute to toxicity	—	90–95 binding saturates
Ethosuximide	A 60 C 30	6–12	10–20	0.67	Assumed 100	No	~50	0
Felbamate	22	5	50%	0.73–0.82	790	No	?	~25%
Gabapentin	5.3	1	0	58 L	[d]	No	Y	0
Lamotrigine	22	0	1.28	798	No	?	40–50	

[a]A, adult; C, child.
[b]H, hemodialysis.
[c]PB, phenobarbital; PEMA, phenylethylmalonamide.
[d]The bioavailability of gabapentin is dose dependent.

good correlation has been shown between the free phenytoin concentration and the ratio of total phenytoin to albumin in patients with normal albumin or hyperalbuminemia. The ratio was not predictive for patients with hypoalbuminemia.[56]

Phenytoin is metabolized in the liver primarily by parahydroxylation to 5-(*p*-hydroxyphenyl)-5-phenylhydantoin (HPPH). HPPH is conjugated and excreted in the urine as a glucuronide. About 80% of an oral dose of phenytoin appears in the urine as HPPH. Abnormally low percentages of HPPH in the urine would indicate a problem with absorption. Phenytoin is a low-extraction drug and its metabolism is not greatly influenced by changes in liver blood flow; however, because the major route of metabolism is hydroxylation, the clearance may be influenced by drugs that stimulate or inhibit liver microsomal enzymes.[54]

Phenytoin displays Michaelis–Menten elimination (i.e., the metabolism changes from first order to zero order) because the enzyme system is saturable. Therefore, increasing the serum concentration above a certain point does not increase the amount of drug that can be metabolized. Thus, any change in dosage produces significantly disproportional changes in serum concentrations. The process may be described by the equation

$$D = \frac{V_{max} \times C_p}{K_m + C_p}$$

where D is the dose (in mg/d), V_{max} is the maximum rate of metabolism, K_m is the serum concentration at which the rate of metabolism is half-maximal, and C_p is the serum concentration.

Because V_{max} and K_m are both highly and independently variable, the metabolism of phenytoin may saturate at any concentration and may occur within the therapeutic range. V_{max} has been shown to decline with age and the K_m may be affected by concurrent drug therapy. It is very difficult to predict the resulting outcome of a dosage increase of phenytoin. Also, serum concentrations do not decline by a constant percentage upon discontinuation. Therefore, any dosage change should be followed with careful patient monitoring and serum concentration determinations.[54]

Because of the saturable metabolism, the clinically useful concept of half-life may be inappropriate for phenytoin. Half-life assumes concentration-independent elimination. A better term for phenytoin is the time required to eliminate 50% ($t_{50\%}$). The average $t_{50\%}$ for phenytoin is 22 hours, but may range from 7–42 hours. Because of saturation, the $t_{50\%}$ increases with increasing serum concentrations and the time to reach steady state may be prolonged.[54]

Less than 5% of a dose of phenytoin is excreted unchanged. Renal impairment does not affect the excretion of HPPH. While an inhibitory effect of HPPH on phenytoin metabolism has been suggested, it has not been documented in humans. Neither hemodialysis nor peritoneal dialysis affects the clearance of phenytoin. Clinically insignificant amounts of phenytoin are removed by plasmapheresis.[42]

Therapeutic Range/Dosing

The accepted therapeutic range of phenytoin is 10–20 mcg/mL in otherwise healthy patients receiving no other medications. This range has evolved from observations that patient response is enhanced as concentrations increase, with 50% of patients showing a decrease in seizures at concentrations greater than 10 mcg/mL and 86% at concentrations greater than 15 mcg/mL. The incidence of side effects begins to increase as the phenytoin concentration exceeds 20 mcg/mL. At this range the free fraction is 10% of total drug concentration in most patients. Therefore, the therapeutic range of free drug is 1–2 mcg/mL. Serum concentrations should be interpreted in concert with clinical response.[42]

Because of the intersubject variability in the nonlinear elimination of phenytoin, serum concentration is a much better endpoint than total daily dose. The common practice of placing everyone on phenytoin 300 mg/d results in plasma concentrations above and below the desired therapeutic range.[54] The dose of phenytoin must be individually titrated. Loading doses are needed only in status epilepticus. In nonacute situations, phenytoin may be initiated in doses of 3–6 mg/kg/d and titrated upward.

Because of the saturable metabolism, dose prediction of phenytoin is difficult. Several attempts have been made to estimate phenytoin dosing. Bayesian regression-analysis computer programs are the most useful in predicting non–steady-state and steady-state dosing; however, this method requires sophisticated computer support. Other forecasting methods require one or two doses with resulting steady-state concentrations. The one-point methods fix either V_{max} or K_m and estimate the other. Population clearance and nomogram methods are clinically useful if used judiciously. Because they fix one independent variable, all one-point methods have the potential for estimating the wrong dose. The reliability of dosage prediction can be enhanced if two different doses and the resulting steady-state values are known.[54] The two values allow for calculation of both V_{max} and K_m. Empirically, doses of phenytoin may be increased by 100 mg/d if concentrations are less than 7 mcg/mL, and by 50 mg/d if concentrations are >7 but <12 mcg/mL, and by 30 mg/d if the concentration is >12 mcg/mL.[57] Any dosage forecasting should be accompanied by careful clinical monitoring.

Based on an average "half-life" of 22 hours, once-a-day dosing has been postulated for phenytoin. A single daily dose should be easier to schedule and could be taken at night if CNS depression accompanies the dose. Most adult patients can be maintained on a single daily dose of phenytoin; however, children may have more rapid elimination requiring more frequent administration. Adults also have variable elimination rates so everyone cannot be adequately controlled on once-a-day dosing. The larger the dose, the more likely split dosing will be required.[42]

Dosage Forms

Three dosage forms are used for oral administration of phenytoin. The tablet and suspension contain phenytoin acid, while the capsule contains phenytoin sodium. Phenytoin sodium is 92% phenytoin. The parenteral solution is phenytoin sodium. The salt content should be considered in dosage form changes.

If given in equal amounts of phenytoin acid, the tablets, capsules, and suspension have the same bioavailability. Phenytoin capsules are designated as immediate-release or extended-release. Only the extended-release should be used in once-a-day dosing. A single-dose study indicated that phenytoin suspension has the potential for once-a-day dosing.[58] Particle size rather than formulation may determine the rate of absorption.

Phenytoin suspension will settle, producing unequal concentration distribution. A recent study indicated that resuspension could be accomplished without overzealous agitation.[59] Clinicians should remember that there are two different strengths of phenytoin suspension.

If oral administration is not feasible, intravenous administration of phenytoin is preferred over intramuscular administration. Fosphenytoin is a prodrug for phenytoin and is under investigation as a parenteral dosage form. It is very water soluble and is rapidly converted to phenytoin systemically. This allows the development of a dosage form that can be given rapidly intravenously and that may be given intramuscularly with reliable absorption and minimal pain.[38]

Adverse Effects

The side effects of phenytoin may be described as acute, concentration dependent, and chronic. When phenytoin is initiated, the CNS-depressant effects may result in lethargy, fatigue, incoordination, visual blurring, higher cortical dysfunction, and drowsiness. These effects are usually transient and may be minimized by slow dosage titration (Tables 55.9 and 55.10).

When serum concentrations exceed 20 mcg/mL, a significant number of patients exhibit nystagmus at a 45° lateral gaze. Ataxia frequently occurs at concentrations greater than 30 mcg/mL. Phenytoin levels greater than 30 mcg/mL may induce seizures. At concentrations greater than 40 mcg/mL, mental status changes including coma occur. At very high concentrations, phenytoin can exacerbate seizures or precipitate generalized status epilepticus.[33–35]

It is difficult to determine whether the chronic side effects of phenytoin are concentration or duration dependent. One of the more common chronic side effects is gingival hyperplasia, which occurs in up to 50% of the patients. Suppression of cognitive abilities is also a concern. Other chronic effects include vitamin D deficiency, osteomalacia, folic acid deficiency, carbohydrate intolerance, immunologic disturbances, hypothyroidism, and peripheral neuropathy. Phenytoin is associated with rare hypersensitivity or idiosyncratic reactions resulting in rashes, Stevens–Johnson syndrome, pseudolymphoma, bone marrow suppression, lupus-like reactions, and hepatitis.[33–35]

Drug Interactions

Phenytoin is prone to many drug interactions (Table 55.10) and these have been extensively reviewed. The effects of phenytoin may be enhanced or reduced by drugs that affect its pharmacokinetic parameters. Phenytoin is highly protein bound and may be displaced by other highly protein-bound drugs. A decrease in binding results in an increase in free phenytoin. The initial increase in free phenytoin is followed by an increase in clearance, a fall in total phenytoin concentrations, and the reestablishment of normal free phenytoin concentrations. Usually no dosage adjustment is necessary. Problems arise when clinicians react to the lower total phenytoin concentration without considering the free concentration. If protein-binding interactions are suspected, free rather than total phenytoin concentrations are a better therapeutic guideline.[60] Drug interactions affecting absorption, metabolism, or excretion are potentially more significant because total and free concentrations are affected. The metabolism of phenytoin can be inhibited (e.g., cimetidine) as well as increased (e.g., phenobarbital).

Phenytoin may alter the pharmacokinetics of other drugs. The AEDs frequently interact with each other via complex mechanisms. Caution should be used when they are added to or withdrawn from a patient's drug regimen.

Nutritional factors may also interfere with phenytoin. The rate of absorption of phenytoin may be decreased if it is given simultaneously with food. The bioavailability of phenytoin suspension was recently reported to be decreased in patients receiving continuous enteral nutrient tube feedings. A single-dose study of simultaneous administration of enteral feeding found no difference in phenytoin bioavailability, indicating that the mechanism was something other than physical contact.[42] A complex interaction of phenytoin with folic acid has also been described, making vitamin ingestion an important part of the drug history. Phenytoin reportedly decreases folic acid absorption, but folic acid enhances the clearance of phenytoin.[67] Replacement of folic acid can reduce phenytoin concentrations and result in loss of efficacy.

Therapeutic Monitoring

The dose of phenytoin should be individualized using serum concentrations of total or free drug in relationship to the patient's clinical response.[42] The unbound drug should be measured in any patient in whom altered protein binding is suspected. A trough level is preferred for evaluation, but because of the usually long $t_{50\%}$, minimal peak-to-trough fluctuation is expected. For a patient experiencing side

TABLE 55.9. SUMMARY OF ANTIEPILEPTIC DRUG PHARMACOLOGIC DATA

AED	Initial Dose (mg/kg/d)	Therapeutic Range (μg/mL Total)	Side Effects Dose Related	Side Effects Not Dose Related	Manufacturer
Phenytoin	Loading dose; 20 in status	10–20	Nystagmus, ataxia, cognitive impairment, lethargy	Gingival hyperplasia, increase in body hair, coarsening of facial features, acne, folate deficiency, skin rash	Parke-Davis, others
Phenobarbital	Loading dose; 20 in status	15–40	Sedation, mental dullness, cognitive impairment, hyperactivity, ataxia	Hyperactivity, change in sleep problems, skin rashes	Multiple
Primidone	50–125 mg initial dose; no loading dose required	5–20			Ayerst
Carbamazepine	2–8 mg; no loading dose required	4–12	Double vision, blurred vision, lethargy	Fluid retention, leukopenia, bone marrow suppression, skin rash, GI distress	Ciba-Geigy, others
Valproic acid	7.5–15; no loading dose required	50–150(?)	GI upset, lethargy	Weight gain, nausea, alopecia, hepatitis	Abbott, others
Ethosuximide	5–7; no loading dose required	40–100	GI distress, nausea, drowsiness, hiccups	Headache	Parke-Davis
Felbamate		—	—	Anorexia, insomnia, aplastic anemia, acute liver failure	Carter Wallace
Gabapentin		—	—	CNS	Parke-Davis
Lamotrigine		—	—	CNS, rash	Glaxo Wellcome

effects, a peak may be indicated. The initial peak of phenytoin is usually seen in 3–12 hours. A secondary peak may also be observed.[54]

Because of the long $t_{50\%}$, the time to reach steady state with phenytoin is prolonged and variable. There usually is no need to obtain serum concentrations on hospitalized patients any more often than every 3–4 days, except in critical situations where loading and supplemental doses are given. Outpatients can be monitored every 2–4 weeks after a judicious dosage increase. If patients experience signs of toxicity (e.g., nystagmus, ataxia) serum concentrations should be evaluated.[42,54]

Phenobarbital/Primidone

Therapeutics

These AEDs may be considered together because primidone is metabolized to phenobarbital. Primidone is an active

TABLE 55.10. CNS EFFECTS OF ANTIEPILEPTIC DRUGS

	Behavioral/Motor	Cognitive
Phenytoin	Tiredness, ataxia, involuntary movements, alteration of emotional state	Impaired cognitive functioning, decreased attention, decreased problem solving and visuomotor tasks
Phenobarbital	Hyperactivity, lethargy, irritability, fussiness, disobedience, altered sleep	Impaired cognitive functioning, impaired short-term memory, decreased memory concentration
Carbamazepine	Irritability, difficulty sleeping, agitation, emotional liability	Minimal
Valproic acid	Drowsiness	Minimal

AED and has a second metabolite that may be active—phenylethylmalonamide (PEMA). In general, because of costs and dosing frequency, phenobarbital should be tried first and primidone reserved for refractory patients. In some patients, primidone will be effective where phenobarbital has failed because of additional AED activity.

Phenobarbital is the drug of choice for neonatal seizures. It is also useful in generalized seizures (except absence) and may be useful in patients with partial seizures. Primidone shares the same indications but is less useful in partial seizures.[62] The widespread use of phenobarbital in the prophylaxis of febrile seizures has recently been questioned.[63]

These agents are CNS depressants. They elevate seizure threshold by decreasing postsynaptic excitation, possibly by stimulating postsynaptic GABA-ergic inhibitor responses.[53]

Pharmacokinetics

Phenobarbital is rapidly and completely absorbed regardless of whether it is given orally, intramuscularly, or rectally. The rate of absorption appears to be independent of dose, with peak concentrations being reached 0.5–4.0 hours after a dose. The bioavailability of primidone is approximately 90–100% (Table 55.8).[42]

Phenobarbital has a biphasic distribution. Initially, phenobarbital penetrates highly perfused organs including the brain. Phenobarbital penetrates the brain at a rate comparable to that of phenytoin, and peak concentrations are achieved 3–20 minutes after an intravenous dose. Phenobarbital then distributes evenly to all body tissues including fat. Decreasing the systemic pH drives phenobarbital into body tissues. Phenobarbital is only about 50% bound to plasma proteins but the free fraction was reported to be 93% in a burn patient with uremia.[42]

Drugs affecting liver enzymes may alter phenobarbital metabolism, but phenobarbital clearance is not affected by liver blood flow. Despite the fact that phenobarbital is a potent enzyme inducer, there is no evidence in humans that it is an autoinducer. The elimination of phenobarbital is linear. Neonates have a longer half-life than adults and children have a shorter half-life. About 20–40% of a dose of phenobarbital is excreted in the urine unchanged. Because tubular reabsorption of phenobarbital is pH dependent, the amount excreted renally can be increased by giving diuretics and urinary alkalinizers.[42]

Primidone is metabolized to phenobarbital (3–5%) and PEMA (30–45%). The primidone–phenobarbital ratio is highly variable. A significant portion of primidone is excreted unchanged. The half-life of primidone may become shorter after chronic therapy because the phenobarbital metabolite may induce the metabolism of primidone.[42]

Therapeutic Range/Dosing

The therapeutic range of phenobarbital for the treatment of seizures is between 15 and 40 mcg/mL. Occasionally, patients respond at lower or higher plasma concentrations. Because of the low plasma protein binding, determination of free concentrations are seldom necessary (Table 55.9).[42]

The accepted therapeutic range of primidone is 5–20 mcg/mL. At this concentration, most patients have a phenobarbital concentration that is in the therapeutic range. It is rare that a patient on primidone needs supplemental doses of phenobarbital. PEMA concentrations are not routinely monitored.[42]

In emergency situations phenobarbital may be given by intravenous loading doses (as discussed in Chapter 56). In nonacute situations, phenobarbital should be started in low doses and titrated upward. The dose–concentration effect is linear and maintenance doses can be estimated from the first dose and resulting steady-state concentration. Phenobarbital meets the criteria for predicting maintenance dose with a single serum concentration obtained after the first dose. Because the half-life of phenobarbital is so long, the dose can be given as a single daily dose.[64] Giving the drug at bedtime sometimes minimizes the consequences of CNS depression. Because of its long half-life phenobarbital takes 3–4 weeks to reach steady state. Therefore, rapid dosage adjustments should be avoided in a nonacute situation.

Primidone is not administered as a loading dose. An initial dose of 50–125 mg may be increased every 2 to 4 days until the desired concentration is reached. Because of the short half-lives of primidone and PEMA, the drug should be given in divided doses.

Adverse Effects

CNS side effects are the primary factors limiting use of phenobarbital. Tolerance usually develops to initial complaints of fatigue, drowsiness, sedation, and depression.[65] In children, paradoxically, the primary side effect is hyperactivity. Phenobarbital impairs higher cortical function and depresses cognitive performance.[63] In susceptible patients phenobarbital may precipitate porphyria. Other rare side effects include rashes, osteomalacia, and hypotension (Tables 55.9 and 55.10).

The side effects of primidone and phenobarbital are similar and may be difficult to separate. The initial side effects of sedation, nystagmus, and ataxia may be minimized by starting at a low dose and gradually titrating the dose.[65]

Drug Interactions

Phenobarbital is a potent enzyme inducer and will increase the elimination of any drug metabolized by phase I oxidative processes. Other drugs may alter the concentrations of phenobarbital by altering its metabolism. Valproic acid, phenytoin, cimetidine, and chloramphenicol inhibit phenobarbital metabolism, necessitating a decrease in dose. Ethanol increases the metabolism of phenobarbital. The interactions of primidone are similar.[42]

Therapeutic Monitoring

Because of its long half-life, there are minimal peak-to-trough fluctuations with phenobarbital. Trough levels are preferred unless patients complain of side effects. Except after loading doses, there is no need to obtain a phenobarbital concentration until steady state has been reached, 3–4 weeks after initiating therapy, or until side effects occur. The guidelines for primidone are similar.

Carbamazepine

Therapeutics

This drug was originally approved for the treatment of trigeminal neuralgia; however, clinical trials have shown it to be a safe and effective AED. Carbamazepine's relative lack of side effects compared to phenytoin and phenobarbital has resulted in an increased use in a variety of seizure disorders. It may also be useful in selected psychiatric disorders, as discussed in Chapter 68, Bipolar Disorders. Carbamazepine is considered the AED of first choice for partial seizures, especially complex partial seizures. It is also useful for generalized seizures other than absence.[66]

Animal studies indicate that carbamazepine depresses transmission in the nucleus ventralis anterior of the thalamus. This area has been associated with the generalization and spread of seizure discharge. There is some depression of post-tetanic potentiation (PTP) by carbamazepine, but it is of a lesser magnitude than occurs with phenytoin. The exact mechanism by which carbamazepine suppresses seizure spread is obscure. It affects ionic conductance only at concentrations far above those normally produced in man. It may inhibit an increase in cyclic AMP. Other biochemical effects are unknown.[53]

Pharmacokinetics

Based on bioavailability studies using a reference solution, the absorption of carbamazepine tablets is greater than 75%. The absorption of carbamazepine from immediate-release tablets is slow and erratic because of its low water solubility. Absorption is dissolution rate dependent. Therefore, dose-dependent absorption may occur, resulting in less bioavailability at higher doses. The variable absorption results in times to peak of 2–24 hours (average 6 hours). There is also a large variability in the peak-to-trough concentrations of up to 40%. There is no first-pass metabolism. Food may enhance the bioavailability of carbamazepine. The suspension dosage form is absorbed faster than the tablets.[42]

Carbamazepine is a neutral and highly lipophilic drug that results in high body tissue binding. Carbamazepine binds to α_1-acid glycoprotein with high affinity and to albumin to a lesser extent. The percentage bound may decrease at higher concentrations within the therapeutic range. The usefulness of free carbamazepine concentrations remains to be defined.[42]

Most (98–99%) of an administered dose of carbamazepine is metabolized by the liver. Although 33 metabolites have been identified for carbamazepine, the major metabolite is 10,11-epoxide carbamazepine.[42] This metabolite has significant anticonvulsant activity in animals and has demonstrated activity in humans. In a recent pilot study patients were switched from carbamazepine to 10,11-epoxide carbamazepine with no loss of seizure control.[67] The formation of 10,11-epoxide carbamazepine is influenced by the presence of other enzyme-inducing or enzyme-inhibiting drugs. The 10,11-epoxide carbamazepine concentration may change with no change in parent carbamazepine concentration.[68]

Carbamazepine has the unique ability to induce its own metabolism. The half-life after a single dose is much longer than the half-life after chronic therapy. The presence of enzyme-inducing drugs reduces the half-life even more. The enzyme induction effect begins within 3–5 days after the initiation of therapy and takes 21–28 days to complete. Therefore, it is possible to achieve initial concentrations that are within the therapeutic range but have concentrations fall despite continued therapy with good compliance. Some patients who respond well to initial therapy may be labeled refractory or noncompliant if the autoinduction phenomenon is not considered. The autoinduction rapidly reverses if therapy with carbamazepine is temporarily discontinued.[69] This would be very important in epilepsy monitoring units where all drugs are stopped in an attempt to precipitate seizures in patients being evaluated for seizure surgery.

Therapeutic Range/Dosing

Clinical trials indicate that the therapeutic range of carbamazepine is between 4 and 12 mcg/mL.[66] Concentrations higher than 12 mcg/mL are associated with an increase in the incidence of CNS-related side effects. The variable contributions of the 10,11-epoxide metabolite and free carbamazepine concentrations have restricted a precise definition of the therapeutic range.

Loading doses of carbamazepine are indicated only for critically ill patients. Carbamazepine suspension has been used to administer a loading dose of 7.4–10.4 mg/kg in critically ill patients.[70] Oral loading has also been accomplished with a controlled-release formulation of carbamazepine.[71] There are significant CNS-depressant effects and gastrointestinal (GI) complaints (e.g., nausea and vomiting) associated with large initial doses, but these may be minimized by slow, gradual dosage adjustment. During dosage titration, it should be remembered that carbamazepine clearance increases with time. Doses may be started at one-fourth to one-third of the anticipated maintenance dose and increased every 2–3 weeks. The ranges for maintenance doses are 7–15 mg/kg/d for adults and 11–40 mg/kg/d for children less than 15 years of age (Table 55.9).[42]

Because of the autoinduction and heteroinduction of carbamazepine metabolism, it is necessary to administer the drug two to four times per day. While some patients, especially those on monotherapy, can be maintained on twice-a-day therapy, others may require more frequent dosage administration. Children are likely to need more frequent administration. The occurrence of annoying CNS and GI side effects may be minimized by giving larger doses at bedtime.[42]

Dosage Forms

Generic dosage forms of carbamazepine were approved by the FDA in the summer of 1986. Anecdotal reports suggest that some patients may have breakthrough seizures or side effects when brands are switched. Patients should be stabilized on one brand and continued on that therapy. If brands are switched, the patient should be carefully monitored. It may be necessary to administer the suspension dosage form more frequently than the tablet to prevent excessive peak-to-trough fluctuations. The chewable tablet may be preferable for some children. The controlled-release dosage form will significantly reduce the peak-to-trough variability and may improve seizure control and patient tolerance.[42] A controlled-released dosage form (Tegretol XR) is being reviewed by the FDA. The controlled-release dosage form given twice a day had comparable pharmacokinetics to immediate-release carbamazepine given four times a day.[72] Carbamazepine tablets should not be stored in places where they would be exposed to high heat and high humidity.[73]

Adverse Effects

Side effects (Tables 55.9 and 55.10) of carbamazepine may fluctuate daily, paralleling the rise and decline of serum concentrations. The side effect profile may also follow a circadian rhythm.[74]

Neurosensory side effects (e.g., diplopia, blurred vision, nystagmus, ataxia, unsteadiness, dizziness, and headache) are the most common, occurring in 35–50% of the patients. They are more common during initiation of therapy and may dissipate with continued treatment. Patients have variable threshold concentrations for the occurrence of CNS side effects. If the carbamazepine concentration is kept below the individual threshold, the CNS side effects can be minimized. The patient may become tolerant to these effects, or they may abate with a reduction in dose. They may also be minimized by giving larger bedtime doses. Dosage manipulation should be tried before the patient is considered to be intolerant of carbamazepine.

Carbamazepine may induce a hyponatremic hyposmolar condition that is similar to the syndrome of inappropriate antidiuretic hormone secretion.[75] The incidence may increase with age. Periodic determinations of serum sodium are recommended. GI discomfort is also frequently reported with carbamazepine.

Until recently, the concern over carbamazepine-induced bone marrow suppression was reinforced by a "black-box" warning in the package insert requiring frequent CBC monitoring. Only a few cases of aplastic anemia, the most serious complication, have been reported since 1964. In many cases there were confounding factors that precluded a definite cause-and-effect relationship. Thrombocytopenia and anemia have an incidence of less than 5% and usually respond to a cessation of drug therapy. Leukopenia is the most common hematologic side effect of carbamazepine. An incidence as high as 10% has been reported. Leukopenia is usually transient even when the drug is continued. In about 2% of patients, the leukopenia is persistent, but even patients with white blood cell (WBC) counts of 3000/mL or less do not seem to have an increased incidence of infection. A clinical guide is to continue carbamazepine therapy unless the WBC count drops to less than $2500/mm^3$ and the absolute neutrophil count drops to less than $1000/mm^3$.[5]

Rashes are the most frequent hypersensitivity response. An incidence of 9.9% has been reported.[76] These are usually mildly eczematous but may progress to a Stevens–Johnson syndrome. Other rare side effects reported with carbamazepine include hepatitis, osteomalacia, cardiac conduction defects, and lupus-like reactions. Carbamazepine appears to have no or minimal effects on cognitive functioning.[77]

Drug Interactions

Because of concentration-dependent efficacy and side effects, drug interactions with carbamazepine are often clinically very significant. Drugs may interact with carbamazepine by enzyme induction (e.g., phenytoin, phenobarbital, and primidone) or enzyme inhibition (e.g., valproic acid, erythromycin, cimetidine, propoxyphene, and isoniazid). Valproic acid appears to reduce the formation of the 10,11-epoxide metabolite without affecting the concentration of carbamazepine. Because of the empiric use of erythromycin, the interaction of erythromycin with carbamazepine is particularly significant. Carbamazepine may interact with other drugs by inducing their metabolism; for example, carbamazepine increases the metabolism of valproic acid, theophylline, warfarin, and ethosuximide (Tables 55.11 and 55.12).[42] The absorption of carbamazepine suspension is slower and diminished when it is given during nasogastric feeding. This may result from adherence to the nasogastric tube. It is recommended that carbamazepine suspension be mixed with an equal volume of diluent before being administered through nasogastric feeding tubes.[78]

TABLE 55.11. INTERACTIONS BETWEEN ANTIEPILEPTIC DRUGS

AED	Added Drug	Effect
Phenytoin	Carbamazepine	↓ Concentration
	Methsuximide	↑ Concentration
	Valproic acid	↓ Total
Phenobarbital	Phenytoin	↑ Concentration
	Valproic acid	↑ Concentration
Primidone	Carbamazepine	↑ Phenobarbital
	Phenytoin	↑ Phenobarbital
Carbamazepine	Phenobarbital	↓ Concentration
	Phenytoin	↓ Concentration
	Primidone	↓ Concentration
Valproic acid	Carbamazepine	↓ Concentration
	Phenobarbital	↓ Concentration
	Primidone	↓ Concentration
	Phenytoin	↓ Concentration
Lamotrigine	Phenytoin	↓ Concentration
	Carbamazepine	
	Valproic acid	↑ Concentration
Phenytoin	Felbamate	↑ Concentration
Carbamazepine	Felbamate	↑ Concentration of active metabolite
Phenobarbital	Felbamate	↑ Concentration

Therapeutic Monitoring

Therapeutic monitoring of carbamazepine should reflect the autoinduction and time to reach steady state. Trough levels are preferred. Samples may be collected at the time of reported side effects. The relationship between time of last dose and sample collection should be noted.

Valproic Acid

Therapeutics

Valproic acid is a branched-chain carboxylic acid first synthesized in 1881. Until 1963, it was used primarily as an organic solvent, but has since shown efficacy against a variety of seizure disorders. Its relative lack of toxicity compared to phenytoin and phenobarbital has contributed to its expanded use.[79]

Valproic acid is the drug of first choice for most generalized seizures[79] and is also useful in the treatment of partial seizures.[80] It is the only AED that is effective against absence and other types of generalized seizures. It may also be useful in neonatal seizures.[79]

Initially it was believed that valproic acid increased GABA by inhibiting its degradation or by activating its synthesis. Although this may explain some of valproic acid effects, the time course for the increase in GABA compared with anticonvulsant effects of valproic acid indicates that inhibition of GABA synthesis does not fully explain how valproic acid prevents seizures. In 1994, it was proposed that valproic acid may potentiate postsynaptic GABA responses, may have a direct membrane-stabilizing effect, and may affect the potassium channel.[79]

Pharmacokinetics

Valproic acid appears to be completely absorbed from available oral dosage forms when administered on an empty stomach.[79] Peak concentrations occur in 0.5–1 hour with the syrup, 1–3 hours with the capsule, and 2–6 hours with the enteric-coated tablet.[79] There is a diurnal decrease in absorption of the enteric-coated preparation following an evening dose. Food delays, but does not decrease, the amount of valproic acid absorbed.[42]

TABLE 55.12. INTERACTIONS OF ANTIEPILEPTIC DRUGS WITH OTHER DRUGS

AED	Altered by	Result	Alters	Result
Phenytoin	Antacids	↓ Absorption	Oral contraceptives	↓ Efficacy
	Disulfiram	↑ Concentration	Bishydroxycoumarin	↓ Anticoagulation
	Isoniazid	↑ Concentration	Quinidine	↓ Concentration
	Chloramphenicol	↑ Concentration	Vitamin D	↓ Concentration
	Propoxyphene	↑ Concentration	Folic acid	↓ Concentration
	Cimetidine	↑ Concentration		
	Ethanol	↓ Concentration		
Phenobarbital			Oral contraceptives	↓ Efficacy
Primidone			Quinidine	↑ Metabolism
			Tricyclics	↑ Metabolism
			Corticosteroids	↑ Metabolism
			Chlorpromazine	↑ Metabolism
			Furosemide	↓ Renal sensitivity
Carbamazepine	Propoxyphene	↑ Concentration	Warfarin	↓ Concentration
	Cimetidine	↑ Concentration	Theophylline	↓ Concentration
	Isoniazid	↑ Concentration	Doxycycline	↓ Concentration
	Erythromycin	↑ Concentration		
Valproic acid	Salicylates	↑ Free concentration		

Valproic acid distributes widely throughout the body. It is 90–95% protein bound, primarily to albumin. The binding sites for valproic acid are saturable and the free fraction may increase as the total concentration increases. The saturable binding may indicate that the free concentration is a better monitoring parameter than the total valproic acid concentration, especially at higher concentrations.[42] The protein binding of valproic acid is decreased in patients with head trauma.[81]

Valproic acid is metabolized primarily by the liver. There is no first-pass metabolism, and the clearance is independent of hepatic blood flow. As with other highly protein-bound drugs, an increase in free drug results in an increase in clearance. Thus, the clearance of valproic acid changes at higher concentrations.[42]

The primary route of valproic acid metabolism is β-oxidation, although up to 40% of a dose may be excreted as the glucuronide. At least 10 metabolites of valproic acid have been identified. Some of these may have weak anticonvulsant activity, and at least 1 metabolite may be responsible for the hepatotoxicity reported with valproic acid. One of the lesser oxidative metabolites, 4-*en*-valproic acid, causes significant hepatotoxicity in rats. The formation of this metabolite is increased when valproic acid is given with enzyme-inducing drugs like phenobarbital.[79]

Therapeutic Range/Dosing

The minimal effective concentration of valproic acid is 50 mcg/mL; however, there is disagreement on the upper end of the therapeutic range.[79] Although 100 mcg/mL is widely quoted as the upper end of the therapeutic range, experience indicates that a significant number of patients have improved seizure control when the concentration is increased. Although some reports have linked drowsiness, stupor, and decreases in fibrinogen to concentrations greater than 80–100 mcg/mL, there are very few clearly defined concentration-dependent side effects of valproic acid. In refractory or partially responding patients, the concentration of valproic acid may cautiously be titrated upward, provided the patient is closely monitored. As the concentration is pushed upward, the saturable protein binding of valproic acid may become significant, and free concentration monitoring may be helpful.[42]

In normal circumstances, loading doses of valproic acid are not indicated. Doses of 15–20 mg/kg daily usually produce concentrations of 75–100 mcg/mL. The more common dosing procedure is to start patients on 7.5–15 mg/kg/d in divided doses and increase the dose in 2–3 days. Some patients may experience GI distress or CNS depression if the initial dose is too high or increased too quickly.[42]

Although some patients may have a half-life sufficiently long to permit once-a-day dosing with valproic acid, more frequent dosing is the norm. Based on half-life data, twice-a-day dosing is feasible with any valproic acid dosage form; however, children and other patients taking enzyme inducers may require dosing three to four times per day.[42]

The serum concentration–dose relationship is curvilinear (i.e., the concentration–dose ratio decreases with increasing dose), probably because of increasing free concentrations and a resulting increase in clearance.[42]

Dosage Forms

Valproic acid is available as a soft gelatin capsule, an enteric-coated tablet, a syrup, and a "sprinkle." The sprinkle is designed to be opened and mixed with food. The soft gelatin capsule is available in several generic forms. The syrup is absorbed more rapidly than either solid. The enteric-coated tablet is not a sustained-release dosage form. The tablet consists of sodium divalproex, which must be metabolized in the gut to valproic acid, and is enteric coated to reduce the incidence of GI distress. The enteric coating does cause delayed absorption, although once the enteric coating dissolves, sodium divalproex has absorption, metabolism, and elimination rates similar to those for other dosage forms of valproic acid. There is decreased absorption from the enteric-coated preparation following an evening dose. The sprinkle formulation has a slower rate of absorption, which results in fewer fluctuations in the peak-to-trough ratio. Its absorption is unaffected by food. An intravenous formulation is under development.[42]

Adverse Effects

The most common side effects may cause mild patient discomfort, but are not life threatening.[79] The most frequently reported side effects are GI complaints (up to 20%) including nausea, vomiting, anorexia, and weight gain. Pancreatitis is very rare. The GI complaints may be minimized but not totally alleviated with the enteric-coated formulation or by giving the drug with food. Other frequently reported side effects are drowsiness (10%), ataxia (15%), and tremor (10%). These may respond to a modification of dose (Tables 55.9 and 55.10). Alopecia and hair changes occur but are temporary. Peripheral edema may also occur. Weight gain can be a significant side effect to many patients. Valproic acid causes minimal cognitive impairment.[79]

The most serious side effect reported with valproic acid is hepatotoxicity. Hyperammonemia is common (50%) but does not necessarily imply liver damage; however, at least 67 fatalities have been attributed to valproic acid hepatotoxicity. Patients dying with valproic acid-associated hepatotoxicity share certain features. Most deaths have occurred in patients who were less than 2 years of age, mentally retarded, and receiving multiple therapy. The hepatotoxicity occurred early in the course of therapy.[82] The multiple therapy may have altered the normal metabolism, leading to increased formation of the potentially liver-toxic 4-*en*-valproic acid. Valproic acid has been shown to alter carnitine metabolism,[83] and it has been postulated that a deficiency of carnitine alters fatty acid oxidation that could lead to liver toxicity. However, valproic acid hepatotoxicity has occurred in a patient taking supplemental carnitine, and a prospective study demonstrated no effect on well-being when carnitine was added. Carnitine is expensive, and there are no data to support routine supplemental carnitine therapy in patients taking valproic acid.[83]

Thrombocytopenia occurs in 6–40% of the patients receiving valproic acid, but is responsive to a decrease in dose. Other hematologic toxicities including leukopenia with transient neutropenia, transient erythroblastopenia, and bone marrow changes have been reported. More recently, a series of severe hematologic side effects that included thrombocytopenia, macrocytic red cells with or without anemia, and the Pelger–Huet anomaly in segmented neutrophils, along with elevated vitamin B_{12} levels, normal serum folic acid levels, and elevated fetal hemoglobin values with abnormal bone marrow findings were reported in patients with severe cerebral palsy, mental retardation, and seizures.[84] High-dose valproic acid therapy was reported to suppress the growth of hematopoietic progenitors, resulting in bone marrow failure.[85]

Drug Interactions

Drugs that affect liver enzymes may alter valproic acid kinetics by increasing or decreasing clearance; for example, phenytoin, phenobarbital, primidone, and carbamazepine all increase valproic acid clearance. Because it is highly protein bound, other highly protein-bound drugs may displace valproic acid. Free fatty acids, aspirin, and phenytoin may alter valproic acid binding.

Valproic acid is an enzyme inhibitor. The most significant reported interaction is with phenobarbital. The addition of valproic acid to patients taking phenobarbital results in a 30–50% decrease in the clearance of phenobarbital and toxicity if the dose of phenobarbital is not reduced.[42] Valproic acid may increase concentrations of 10,11-diepoxide carbamazepine without affecting concentrations of the parent drug.

Therapeutic Monitoring

Valproic acid displays diurnal variations in serum concentrations. Therefore, the serum samples should be collected at the same time of day; trough levels are preferred. Because the enteric coating on the sodium divalproex tablets delays absorption, the trough with this formulation may not occur for 2–4 hours after a dose. At higher concentrations, the curvilinear serum concentration–dose relationship and saturable protein binding should be considered.[42]

Ethosuximide

Therapeutics

This is the most effective, least toxic representative of the succimide class of AEDs. It was developed from a systematic search for a more effective treatment of absence seizures.

The only indication for the use of ethosuximide is the treatment of absence seizures, for which it is the treatment of choice. It may be used in combination with valproic acid for difficult-to-control absence patients.[86]

The exact mechanism of action of ethosuximide remains elusive. It may inhibit the sodium-potassium ATPase system. Ethosuximide also inhibits NADPH-linked aldehyde reductase necessary for the formation of γ-hydroxybutyrate, which has been associated with the induction of absence seizures. Ethosuximide is not believed to have a direct membrane effect or to affect brain metabolism.[53]

Pharmacokinetics

The absorption of ethosuximide is essentially complete. The syrup and the capsule forms are equally bioavailable, but the rate of absorption of the syrup is faster. The time to peak ranges between 3 and 7 hours, and there is little first-pass metabolism. Ethosuximide is not bound to plasma proteins or tissues. Only 10–20% of a dose of ethosuximide is excreted unchanged in the urine. Metabolism occurs in the liver by hydroxylation, and the metabolites are believed to be inactive. There is some evidence of a nonlinear metabolic process.[42] Ethosuximide has a chiral center, and there may be some stereochemical aspects to its metabolism.[87]

Therapeutic Range/Dosing

The therapeutic range of ethosuximide was defined in a relatively small number of patients. Many unresponsive patients became responders when their drug concentrations were raised to equal those of the responsive patients. The accepted therapeutic range is 40–100 mcg/mL, although higher concentrations are occasionally needed.[86]

A loading dose of ethosuximide is not required. The most common dosing procedure is to start patients on 5–7 mg/kg/d in divided doses and increase the dose in 1–2 weeks. Doses of 20 mg/kg/d usually result in concentrations of approximately 50 mcg/mL. Doses can then be titrated to individual response. Data suggest that patients can be successfully managed on once-a-day therapy; however, GI distress appears to be dose related and the total daily dose is usually divided into two equal doses.[86]

Adverse Effects

Ethosuximide is a relatively benign anticonvulsant. The most frequently reported side effects are nausea and vomiting (up to 40%), and these symptoms may be minimized by administration of smaller doses. Other common side effects include drowsiness, fatigue, lethargy, dizziness, hiccups, and headaches. Rarely, idiosyncratic reactions such as rashes, lupus, and blood dyscrasias are reported.[8]

Drug Interactions

Because ethosuximide is not protein bound, displacement interactions cannot occur. The metabolism of ethosuximide may be induced by carbamazepine. A complex interaction between valproic acid and ethosuximide has been reported. Valproic acid may inhibit the metabolism of ethosuximide, but only if the metabolism of ethosuximide is near saturation.[42]

Therapeutic Monitoring

Because efficacy is associated with concentrations greater than 50 mcg/mL, trough levels are preferred. Because of the long half-life, minimal peak-to-trough fluctuations are expected.[42]

"NEW" ANTIEPILEPTIC DRUGS

No major antiepileptic drug was approved by the FDA between 1978 and 1993. Recently three AEDs have been approved. These drugs have used novel study design primarily as adjunctive therapy.[88] These trials have been done primarily in patients with refractory partial seizures who have failed therapy with one or more AEDs. There are limited data in children and in the elderly and monotherapy trials are now being conducted. There have been no comparative studies on the new AEDs. These new drugs appear to have a mechanism of action that is different from those of the older drugs,[89] and they have unique pharmacokinetics.[90]

Felbamate

Therapeutics

Felbamate is a structural analogue of meprobamate but does not display any of the tolerance or dependency associated with meprobamate. Felbamate appears to act as an antagonist of the glycine receptor site on the *N*-methyl-D-aspartate (NMDA) receptor. This action inhibits the initiation and propagation of seizures.[89] Felbamate has been approved for use in adults 14 years and older as monotherapy and adjunctive therapy in partial seizures with and without secondary generalization and for children 2 years and older as adjunctive therapy for the Lennox–Gastaut syndrome.[91] Because of the association of aplastic anemia and acute liver failure with felbamate postmarketing, felbamate is now recommended for patients refractory to other AEDs.[7]

Pharmacokinetics

Felbamate is rapidly and well absorbed orally with a T_{max} of 1–4 hours and an apparent oral bioavailability exceeding 90%. The absorption is unaffected by food or antacids. About 40–50% of a dose of felbamate is metabolized by hydroxylation and conjugation pathways in the liver with the rest being excreted unchanged in the urine. The half-life of felbamate is between 20 and 23 hours in drug naive subjects. In patients taking enzyme-inducing drugs the half-life is shorter. Felbamate displays linear pharmacokinetics and the concentrations are dose proportional. Felbamate is not bound to plasma proteins and has a volume of distribution of 0.7 L/kg.[6,90]

Therapeutic Range/Dosing

A therapeutic range for felbamate has not been established. The drug is dosed to clinical response. If felbamate is used as monotherapy, the dose is initiated at 1200 mg/day (15 mg/kg in children) and then is increased by 600 mg every 2 weeks up to a maximum dose of 3600 mg (45 mg/kg in children). When felbamate is used in combination with other AEDs, the dose of the concurrent AED should be reduced by 30–50% at the initiation of felbamate, and further reductions should occur as the dose is increased.[91]

Adverse Effects

The most frequently reported side effects reported with felbamate prior to marketing were anorexia, weight loss, insomnia, nausea, and headache. Less common side effects included diarrhea, rash, diplopia, ataxia, rhinitis, and taste disturbances. The side effects of felbamate are more common with polytherapy than monotherapy.[91] After about 1 year of general use and 100,000 patient care exposures, the use of felbamate was found to be associated with aplastic anemia and acute liver failure. As of December 1994, there were 27 (19 females, 8 males) reported cases of aplastic anemia with 8 deaths and 14 (11 females, 3 males) cases of acute liver failure with 8 deaths. The onset was between 68 and 354 days of therapy. There was no relationship with dose and no predictors of who is more likely to develop these life-threatening reactions. This clearly demonstrates the need to continue to monitor the side effects of drugs postmarketing.[7]

Drug Interactions

Significant drug interactions have been reported with felbamate. Felbamate inhibits the clearance of phenytoin, carbamazepine, and valproic acid,[92] and the concentrations of phenytoin and valproic acid increase in patients in whom felbamate is added. The concentration of carbamazepine decreases in patients on concurrent therapy with felbamate. However, the concentration of the 10,11-epoxide metabolite increases.[93] It is recommended that the dose of phenytoin, carbamazepine, and valproic acid be decreased by about 30% when felbamate is added.[91] These interactions are dose proportional and there is a further change in clearance with each dosage increase of felbamate. Phenytoin and carbamazepine are enzyme inducers and have been shown to increase the clearance of felbamate. Interactions with phenobarbital and warfarin have also been reported.[94,95]

Therapeutic Monitoring

It is not necessary to monitor the blood levels of felbamate. However, because of the association of aplastic anemia and acute liver failure with felbamate, it is necessary to obtain laboratory tests to monitor for these side effects. It is suggested that liver function tests be obtained weekly and that a CBC be obtained at least every other week in patients taking felbamate. In monitoring the CBC, it appears that felbamate causes a decrease in WBCs and platelets before it causes a decrease in red blood cells. Other side effects such as weight loss and insomnia should be assessed as well as seizure frequency and severity.[7]

Gabapentin

Therapeutics

Gabapentin was designed to be a GABA agonist. However, it has been demonstrated that gabapentin does not react at either GABA receptor, does not alter GABA uptake, and does not interfere with GABA transaminase. Gabapentin appears to bind to an amino acid carrier protein and appears to act at a unique receptor.[96,97] Although several mechanisms have been proposed, gabapentin appears to alter amino acid metabolism, possibly l-leucine. Gabapentin is approved for the adjunctive therapy for partial seizures with or without secondary generalization in adults with epilepsy.[98]

Pharmacokinetics

Gabapentin binds to an amino acid carrier protein in the gut, as well as in the CNS. This amino acid carrier protein transports the drug across the gut membrane by an active process. The binding of gabapentin to this system saturates and the bioavailability decreases with an increase in dose.[97] The bioavailability of a 400-mg dose is about 25% less than a 100-mg dose. The bioavailability of doses (300 to 600 mg) that are likely to be used clinically is about 60%. At doses greater than 1200 mg three times per day, there appears to be a plateauing of the achieved concentration.[99] Gabapentin is rapidly absorbed with a T_{max} between 2 and 4 hours. The absorption of gabapentin is unaffected by food.[97,99]

The half-life of gabapentin is about 5.3 hours. About 77% of a given dose is excreted unchanged in the urine with the rest being excreted in the feces.[99] Therefore, gabapentin is eliminated exclusively by renal elimination, and dosage adjustments will be necessary in patients with significantly impaired renal function.[100] For patients with a creatinine clearance greater than 60 mL/min the dose is 1200 mg/d; for patients with a creatinine clearance between 30 and 60 mL/min the dose is 600 mg/d; for patients with a creatinine clearance of 15 to 30 mL/min the dose is 300 mg/d; and for patients with a creatinine clearance less than 15 mL/min the dose is 150 mg/d (300 mg every other day).[97] The Cockroft and Gault equation may be used to estimate creatinine clearance in the elderly and in patients with chronic renal failure.

Therapeutic Range/Dosing

The dosing of gabapentin is initiated at 300 mg at bedtime on the first day. The dose is increased to 300 mg twice a day on the second day and 300 mg three times a day on the third day. The dose is then titrated as needed up to 1800 mg/d.[91] The package insert recommends doses up to 2400 or 3600 mg/d but higher doses (e.g., 5000–10,000 mg/d) have been used safely. It is unclear if higher doses of gabapentin should be given more frequently than three times per day because of saturable absorption.

Adverse Effects

Fatigue, somnolence, dizziness, and ataxia are the most frequently reported side effects. Other side effects reported more frequently than placebo include nystagmus, tremor, and diplopia. The CNS effects of gabapentin are less than or equal to the CNS side effects of traditional AEDs.[98]

Drug Interactions

Gabapentin is not metabolized by the liver and is not bound to plasma proteins. It does not induce or inhibit liver enzymes. Therefore, drug interactions are not likely to occur with gabapentin.[97] There is a 10% reduction in the clearance of gabapentin in patients taking cimetidine and a 20% reduction in the bioavailability if aluminum antacids are taken simultaneously with gabapentin.

Therapeutic Monitoring

The clinical response of patients taking gabapentin should be assessed. The frequency and severity of seizures should be monitored. A serum creatinine should be obtained for estimating creatinine clearance.

Lamotrigine

Therapeutics

Lamotrigine appears to act as an AED by regulating the release of glutamate and aspartate, which are excitatory neurotransmitters.[101] Lamotrigine is approved as adjunctive therapy in adult patients with partial epilepsy refractory to other agents.[102] In open and small controlled trials, lamotrigine also appears to be effective against many generalized seizure types.[103]

Pharmacokinetics

Lamotrigine is rapidly absorbed with a T_{max} of 1–3 hours. The oral bioavailability is 98%. It is about 55% bound to plasma proteins and has a V_d of 1.1 L/kg. About 70% of a dose of lamotrigine is metabolized in the liver by glucuronide conjugation. The glucuronide conjugate accounts for about 90% of the total drug recovery. Less than 1% of the drug is excreted renally. The half-life of lamotrigine is about 20–24 hours in drug naive subjects. There is no first-pass metabolism, and there is no evidence of saturable pharmacokinetics.[104] One report suggests that there may be some autoinduction in healthy male volunteers, but this has not been seen in patients.[102] The pharmacokinetics in the elderly are not different from those of younger subjects.[105] There is significant intersubject variability in the pharmacokinetic profile of lamotrigine.[106]

Therapeutic Range/Dosing

A therapeutic range for lamotrigine has not been established. The drug should be dosed to individual patient response. In patients who are taking enzyme-inducing drugs lamotrigine should be started at a dose of 50 mg/d for 2 weeks and then increased to 100 mg/d for 2 weeks. Then the dose can be titrated by 100 mg/d at weekly intervals up to a total dose of 500 mg/d. In patients taking valproic acid and other enzyme inhibitors, the dose should be started at 25 mg/d for 2 weeks and then increased to 50 mg/d for 2 weeks. Then the dose can be titrated to a maximum of 150 mg/d.[102]

Adverse Effects

The most frequently reported side effects of lamotrigine include diplopia, drowsiness, ataxia, and headache.[107] It may cause several types of rash, which usually appears in the first 3–4 weeks of therapy. The rash is typically generalized, erythematous, and morbilliform and is generally mild to moderate in severity. However, the Stevens–Johnson reaction has also been reported. Some of these rashes may necessitate the withdrawal of lamotrigine. The incidence of rash appears to be increased in patients who are also receiving valproic acid and who have a rapid dosage titration. The incidence may be higher in children than in adults.[107]

Drug Interactions

Lamotrigine does not inhibit or induce liver enzymes. However, the metabolism of lamotrigine may be altered by concurrent therapy with other drugs. Phenytoin and carbamazepine enhance and valproic acid inhibits the clearance of lamotrigine.[104] A pharmacodynamic interaction may occur with carbamazepine leading to an increase in CNS side effects.

Therapeutic Monitoring

Patients taking lamotrigine should be monitored clinically. Blood levels of lamotrigine are not indicated at this time. The seizure frequency and severity should be assessed, and the patient should be monitored for side effects especially for rash.[102]

MISCELLANEOUS ANTIEPILEPTIC DRUGS

Benzodiazepines

Some benzodiazepines (e.g., diazepam and lorazepam) are used in the acute treatment of status epilepticus (discussed in Chapter 56). On a chronic basis, other benzodiazepines such as clonazepam, nitrazepam (not available in the United States), and clobazam (not available in the United States) are more useful, especially in the treatment of seizure types that occur primarily in children.

Clonazepam is an effective adjunctive agent in the treatment of myoclonic seizures, atonic seizures, atypical absence seizures, and infantile spasms. Although clonazepam is effective in the treatment of absence seizures, its use is limited because it has a higher incidence of side effects than conventional AEDs. Clonazepam may also be effective in the treatment of partial seizures. It is also useful in treating neonatal seizures.[108] Despite initial response, tolerance to the anticonvulsant effects of clonazepam may occur. CNS side effects have limited the use of clonazepam. Drowsiness, ataxia, and changes in behavior are common, although some tolerance may develop. The correlation between therapeutic effect and serum clonazepam concentration is undefined. Dosing begins with 0.01–0.03 mg/kg/d given in two to three doses and is increased until the desired response or side effects occur.

Acetazolamide

The exact role of carbonic anhydrase inhibitors in decreasing brain excitability is not completely defined. The effect may be secondary to the induction of a systemic metabolic acidosis similar to the ketogenic diet. Although acetazolamide has been shown to be effective in a variety of seizure disorders, including generalized tonic–clonic, absence, and complex partial, its use has been limited by the rapid emergence of tolerance. Intermittent use has been more effective, and it may be particularly useful in treating the increase in seizures present during menses (catamenial epilepsy).[109]

Adrenocorticotropic Hormone (ACTH)

ACTH is the standard treatment for infantile spasms. Dosages used range between 5–180 U, administered in variable dosing regimens, but most clinicians recommend 20–40 units of corticotropin per day. Clinical and EEG improvement are usually evident within 3 weeks in 70–90% of the patients but relapses are common. The duration of therapy has ranged from 2 weeks to 18 months.[110] ACTH has not been shown to be superior to oral steroids. ACTH can induce Cushing's syndrome.

INVESTIGATIONAL ANTIEPILEPTIC DRUGS

The Antiepileptic Drug Development program developed by The Epilepsy Branch of the National Institute of Neurologic Disorders and Stroke has resulted in three new drugs approved for epilepsy. There are still a number of drugs in various stages of clinical trials. The most promising of these are vigabatrin,[111] oxcarbazepine,[112] tiagabine,[113] zonisamide,[114] topirimate,[115] and stiripentol.[115]

CHRONIC SIDE EFFECTS OF ANTIEPILEPTIC DRUGS

The selection of an anticonvulsant depends on the side effects as well as efficacy. The effectiveness of monitoring serum drug concentrations is controversial. Although many clinicians routinely measure drug concentrations, there are differences of opinion as to what is the therapeutic range for some AEDs.[116] Chronic side effects can occur despite serum concentrations within the therapeutic range.[42] The incidence of chronic side effects is greatest with phenytoin (33%), phenobarbital (23%), carbamazepine (15%), and valproic acid (12%). Side effects are lowest in patients on monotherapy and increase with the addition of each additional drug.[117] The risk of side effects must always be balanced with the benefit of preventing seizure activity.[1,2]

Cognitive Impairment

The occurrence of nonfebrile seizures has not been associated with a significant change in full-scale IQ. However, seizures have an immediate effect on cognitive function, and the effect is more distinct if the seizures occur in series.[118] Problems of learning and behavior are overrepresented in children with epilepsy. The AEDs all affect mental functioning in normal volunteers. Therefore, concern over impairment of cognitive or intellectual abilities by chronic use of AEDs, especially in children, must be considered (Table 55.10).[119] Impairment of cognition has lead to a rethinking of the value of prophylactic AED therapy in patients with head trauma and febrile seizures.

The comparative effects on cognition have been difficult to evaluate because of differences in study design, seizure types, control of drug concentrations, and neuropsychologic tests used.[120] Some drugs, such as phenytoin, may have a greater effect on motor function while others, such as carbamazepine, may have a greater effect on speed. On balance, carbamazepine and valproate cause less impairment of cognition. Improvement in cognition has been reported in patients switched from phenytoin or phenobarbital to these agents.[121] However, these effects are subtle and may not be pronounced if patients are in the same relative area of the therapeutic range.[122,123] Patients reduced from polytherapy to monotherapy also demonstrate improvement in cognition.[124] The newer agents are believed to cause less neurobehavioral effects.[125]

Behavioral Effects

The most significant, non–concentration-dependent behavioral abnormality is phenobarbital-induced hyperactivity.[126] Tolerance, dosage titration, and serum concentration monitoring reduce the sleepiness, lethargy, and tiredness reported with AEDs. Reports of beneficial effects of carbamazepine on mood and behavior in seizure patients need additional confirmation. Epilepsy per se may cause everyday memory failure, and the effects of antiepileptic drugs on memory are not well studied.[127] While the majority of patients with epilepsy lead normal lives, neurobehavioral problems are found in a substantial subset. These neurobehavioral problems include psychiatric disorders, anxiety, depression, dissociative disorders, disorders of impulse control, and personality disorders.[128]

Teratogenicity/Lactation

Exposure to AED treatment *in utero* occurs in 1 of every 250 newborns. The absolute risk of major malformations in these infants is about 7–10%, which is 3–5% higher than in the general population.[129] More than 90% of pregnancies in epileptic mothers have satisfactory outcomes. Barbiturates and phenytoin are associated with congenital heart malformations, facial clefts, and other malformation. Valproic acid and carbamazepine are associated with spina bifida and hypospadias. Other adverse pregnancy outcomes associated with, but not necessarily caused by AEDs, are growth, psychomotor, and mental retardation. There may be a genetic link to the occurrence of teratogenic effects. Guidelines have been developed for counseling and managing the pregnant woman with epilepsy.[130,131] While AEDs pass into the breast milk, the concentrations are very low and the infant will receive a subtherapeutic dose. Treatment with AEDs is not necessarily a reason to discourage breast-feeding.[132]

Drug-Induced Seizures

An often overlooked toxic effect of AEDs is the potential for AED-induced seizures (Table 55.13).[133] EEG telemetry combined with an enhanced knowledge of pharmacokinetics has increased understanding of this adverse effect. Other drugs that the patient may be taking may also cause seizures. The most commonly reported drugs to cause

TABLE 55.13. EXACERBATION OF SEIZURES BY ANTICONVULSANTS

Acute or chronic toxicity
High concentrations of phenytoin or carbamazepine
Use of AED in a seizure type for which it is not indicated
Phenytoin exacerbates absence
Phenobarbital exacerbates atonic, myoclonic, and absence
Carbamazepine may precipitate generalized convulsive, atonic, and myoclonic seizures when used in children with atypical absence seizures
Unmasking one seizure type when another is controlled
Attributed to ethosuximide
Drug-induced somnolence
Phenobarbital and benzodiazepines
Sudden withdrawal
All anticonvulsants
Indirect effects
Carbamazepine-induced water intoxication and hyponatremia secondary to inappropriate ADH secretion

seizures are meperidine, phenothiazines, clozapine, contrast agents, flumazenil, and vaccines (febrile seizures). Other drugs also reported to cause seizures are general anesthetics, β-lactam antibiotics, isoniazid, theophylline, alkylating agents, and butyrophenones.[134]

SPECIAL PROBLEMS IN EPILEPSY

QUALITY OF LIFE IN EPILEPSY

Providing the best quality of life possible is a treatment goal for patients with epilepsy. This concept is more than a balance between side effects and the number of seizures. The concept of quality of life takes into account all of the concerns of the patient with epilepsy as well as their social and economic concerns. This can best be assessed by the patient. Quality of life in epilepsy has been described as "not how many seizures you have but how you feel about the number of seizures that you have."[135]

There are now three disease-specific rating scales that have been validated for patients with epilepsy to measure quality of life in epilepsy (QUOLIE). A 10-question short version (QUOLIE-10) can be used in the clinic for patient assessment. The 31-question (QUOLIE-31) and an 89-question (QUOLIE-89) versions are more suitable for research. Assessment of quality of life is a therapeutic outcome. It may ultimately be more meaningful than measuring the blood levels of the AEDs.

COSTS

The direct costs of epilepsy include the cost of the drug, treatment for adverse events, emergency room visits, drug levels and other laboratory tests, physician visits, rehabilitation, and transportation. Indirect costs include the costs associated with time lost from work, the inability to get a job, decreased productivity, and mortality.

It has been difficult to assess the entire cost of epilepsy to society. Pashko et al.[136] used a cohort of Pennsylvania Medicaid patients to estimate that the total direct cost of epilepsy is in excess of $10 billion annually. Another study suggested that the direct costs of epilepsy made up about 37% of the total costs with indirect costs accounting for about 63% of the total costs.[137] This study also indicated that the costs were much less for a patient who is well controlled than for a patient who is poorly controlled. Drug costs in the Pashko study accounted for about 10% of the total costs of epilepsy. It is clear that the cheapest drug in epilepsy (e.g., phenobarbital) is not the best drug because of the number of side effects. Further, drug therapy that would control seizures, decrease side effects, improve the quality of life, and reduce the utilization of other health care resources would be cost effective.

DRUG INTERACTIONS

AEDs have narrow therapeutic ranges, are given chronically, and are frequently given in combination with other drugs. Drug interactions may occur by a variety of mechanisms that include displacement from protein binding, induction or inhibition of metabolism, self-induction or self-inhibition of metabolism, and altered elimination or altered absorption. Drug interactions are frequent and significant. Some of the interactions between AEDs are summarized in Table 55.11; the interactions between AEDs and other drugs are summarized in Table 55.12. (For more detail the reader should consult Chapter 7.) The clinician should remember that drug interactions may occur by pharmacokinetic and pharmacodynamic mechanisms. The pharmacodynamic interactions are not well studied.

FEBRILE CONVULSIONS

Febrile seizures are the most common seizures of childhood and are defined as seizures precipitated by fever in young children. Only 2–4% of all children have a febrile seizure. Febrile seizures do not increase the risk of death, injury, mental retardation, or cerebral palsy. In patients who have experienced a febrile seizure, there is a chance of having further febrile seizures and a 2% chance of having epilepsy by age 7.[138] Febrile seizures occurring before age 6 months and after age 5 years are not considered benign febrile seizures. It should be determined that the patient has febrile seizures and not seizures with a fever. Febrile status epilepticus may also occur.[139] The risk factors for a first febrile seizure include first- or second-degree relative with a history of febrile seizures, neonatal discharge at 28 days or later, parental report of "slow" development, and day-care attendance. The risk of febrile seizures increases with the number of risk factors. The risk factors for the recurrence of febrile seizures are previous febrile seizures, a first-degree family member with a history of febrile or unprovoked seizures, and a relatively low temperature at the time of the first seizure. A young age of onset (<12 months), a family history of unprovoked seizures, and a partial initial febrile seizure were associated with an increased risk of complex seizures.[138]

Although it was once routine to give prophylactic phenobarbital to patients with febrile seizures, this is no longer recommended.[138] Phenobarbital does not prevent the recurrence of febrile seizures, and it may impair the mental development of children with a history of febrile seizures.[63] Oral diazepam, given only when fever is present, is safe and reduces the risk of recurrent febrile seizures.[140] The rectal administration of diazepam may also be effective. Benign febrile seizures are best treated by talking to the parents and providing reassurance that intensive AED therapy is not needed.[138]

Patients with a history of febrile convulsions should have ready access to an antipyretic when their temperature is greater than 101°F.

NEONATAL SEIZURES

Neonatal seizures are seizures that occur during the newborn period. The incidence of neonatal seizures is 1.5–15 per 1000 live births, but in the neonatal intensive care unit, this increases to 25%.[141]

The diagnosis of neonatal seizures is complex. Abnormal body movement may be difficult to recognize, especially if the brain has been severely damaged; therefore, an EEG may greatly aid in the diagnosis. Neonatal seizures may be caused by a variety of disorders that include trauma and anoxia, congenital abnormalities, metabolic disorders, infections, drug withdrawal, pyridoxine dependency, amino acid disturbances, kernicterus, toxins, and familial seizures. The presence of seizures should be determined by EEG before treatment is begun. Risk factors making initial therapy necessary are asphyxia, bacterial meningitis, herpes encephalitis, and brain trauma.[141]

Treatment of neonatal seizures requires identifying and correcting the precipitating cause if possible. Phenobarbital is the most commonly used AED. Other AEDs include phenytoin, diazepam, paraldehyde, and primidone.

There is significant controversy over the duration of therapy for neonatal seizures. Chronic AED therapy, primarily phenobarbital, is often continued for at least 1 year in the hope of preventing afebrile seizures; however, this is empiric therapy and is not supported by data from controlled clinical trials. Long-term treatment is often unnecessary for neonatal seizures caused by hypoglycemia, hypocalcemia, local anesthetic injections, drug withdrawal, pyridoxine deficiency, and electrolyte imbalance but is often necessary if the seizures are caused by cortical dysgenesis.[141] In the absence of high-risk factors, phenobarbital may be discontinued after initial seizure control because of its effects on cognitive functioning.

ALCOHOL AND EPILEPSY VERSUS ALCOHOL WITHDRAWAL SEIZURES

On the basis of limited data, the prevalence of epilepsy in alcoholics is three times that of the general population, and alcoholism appears to be more prevalent in epileptics than in the general population. There is general agreement that alcohol abuse increases seizure frequency; however, the exact incidence of alcohol-provoked seizures is unknown. The mechanism of alcohol-provoked seizures is also undetermined. Small amounts of alcohol do not appear to induce seizures and may have transient anticonvulsant effects. Alcohol may stimulate liver enzymes and alter AED clearance. In alcoholics with liver disease, protein synthesis may be decreased, altering the binding of AEDs.[142]

The sudden withdrawal of any CNS depressant drug may induce seizures. The clinician must differentiate alcohol withdrawal seizures from epilepsy. Alcohol withdrawal seizures usually occur within the first 24 hours of cessation of drinking. The seizures are generally tonic–clonic and are frequently accompanied by signs of tremulousness, anorexia, GI disturbances, insomnia, weakness, and hallucinations. Epileptics usually do not have these symptoms.[142]

Epileptics suffering from alcoholism require AEDs; however, alcohol withdrawal seizures are not epilepsy. Most alcohol withdrawal seizures occur before admission. In a recent study, 90 nonepileptic patients were randomized to receive either phenytoin or placebo within 6 hours after the onset of alcohol withdrawal seizures. The phenytoin was found to show no benefit over placebo in preventing subsequent seizures. It was concluded that the risk of the phenytoin therapy outweighed the benefit in the short-term treatment of alcohol withdrawal.[142] The liberal use of benzodiazepines in alcoholics to prevent delirium tremens may decrease the incidence of alcohol withdrawal seizures. On a chronic basis there are no data to suggest that AEDs prevent alcohol withdrawal seizures. Chronic dosing of AED therapy to prevent alcohol withdrawal seizures in nonepileptics has recently been shown to possibly enhance seizures because of erratic compliance and sudden cessation of the AEDs.[142]

PREGNANCY/SEX HORMONES/ CONTRACEPTION

Pregnancy and treatment with sex hormones complicate the treatment of epilepsy. About 50% of epileptic women have no change in seizure activity during pregnancy, 40% have an increase, and about 10% have fewer seizures. Seizure activity fluctuates during the menstrual cycle.[143] Seizures decrease during the luteal phase and increase when progesterone levels decline.

Increased seizure activity during pregnancy may result from either a direct effect on seizure threshold or a reduction in AED concentration. An increase in clearance has been reported for phenytoin, carbamazepine, phenobarbital, ethosuximide, and clorazepate. The postulated mechanisms for the increased clearance include enhanced metabolic clearance and altered protein binding. The altered disposition of AEDs may begin as early as the first 10 weeks of pregnancy and may take up to 4 weeks postpartum to return to normal. The return to the nonpregnant situation takes longer for carbamazepine and phenobarbital than it does for phenytoin.[144] Full seizure control before pregnancy is associated with a more favorable outcome during pregnancy. Oral contraceptives may also increase the clearance of AEDs.

AEDs affect the pharmacokinetics of sex hormones. The enzyme-inducing AEDs shorten hormone half-life, increase levels of sex hormone-binding globulin, and lower free hormone concentrations. Although decreased libido, potency, and fertility and altered menstrual cycles have been attributed to AEDs, a direct cause-and-effect relationship has not been shown.

The enzyme-inducing AEDs may cause treatment failures in females taking oral contraceptives. Valproic acid and benzodiazepines are not enzyme inducers and have not been associated with this effect. The degree of increased metabolism of estrogen and progesterone is highly variable and unpredictable. Women taking AEDs may require higher doses of oral contraceptives for adequate contraceptive effect. A supplemental form of birth control in addition to oral contraceptives is advised.[145]

HEAD TRAUMA

Head trauma may be associated with seizures that develop immediately or have a latent period. Seizures occurring immediately (e.g., within the first week) differ in character and carry a different prognosis. Late seizures occur up to 4 years following the trauma presumably from scar tissue. The incidence in civilians is around 5–7% but is higher in combat-associated trauma. The risk factors for early seizures include intracranial hematoma (subdural), age <5 years, post-traumatic amnesia >24 hours, depressed skull fracture, focal neurologic deficit, and a linear skull fracture. The risk factors for late seizures are early seizures, intracranial hematoma, depressed skull fracture, CT consistent with intracerebral bleed, post-traumatic amnesia, and the duration of coma. The incidence of post-traumatic epilepsy increases with the severity of the head injury.[146]

The practice of treating everyone who has head trauma with chronic AEDs has been questioned because of the low rate of incidence of true epilepsy. Two recent studies suggest that the benefit of chronic AED therapy does not exceed the risk. Temkin et al.[147] randomized 404 patients with head trauma to phenytoin or placebo upon admission and followed them for at least 2 years. Their data showed that phenytoin reduced seizures in the first 7 days but had no effect on the occurrence of late seizures despite serum concentrations that were considered in the therapeutic range. Dikmen et al.[148] assessed the neurobehavioral effects in 244 patients randomized to phenytoin or placebo following trauma. The severely injured patients receiving phenytoin had impaired performance at 1 month. There was no difference in the moderately injured patients. Patients who stopped receiving phenytoin between 1 and 2 years improved on the neurobehavioral assessment more than the placebo group. The efficacy of other drugs in post-traumatic seizures has not been evaluated.

CEREBROVASCULAR DISEASE, CRANIOTOMY, AND STROKE

The increasing incidence of seizures in patients older than 60 years of age has been attributed to cerebrovascular disease and stroke.[10] Seizures in acute strokes generally occur within the first 48 hours, and tend to be single, partial, and easily controlled. These seizures are not associated with an increase in mortality or morbidity. The incidence of seizures after stroke is reported to be about 10%, and patients with hemorrhagic stroke, cortical lesions, and lesions involving more than one lobe are at higher risk. About 27% of the patients have a recurrence of the seizure or epilepsy.[149] Therefore, the chronic use of AED therapy in stroke patients has been questioned. It has recently been suggested that AED therapy be reviewed at 2–4 weeks after the seizure due to stroke and that AEDs be tapered in the absence of an underlying cortical hemorrhage, epileptiform activity on the EEG, or recurrent seizures.[150] If AEDs are given to stroke patients, the impairment of cognitive functioning should be considered.

The incidence of seizures after craniotomy may depend on the site of surgery. No data are available to suggest that chronic AED therapy is indicated in these patients.[151]

SPECIAL POPULATIONS

While all patients on AEDs require monitoring, some populations require special monitoring because of particular variability in pharmacokinetic properties and hence their response to AEDs. Neonates may metabolize drugs more slowly but eliminate unchanged drug more rapidly. Infants and children may metabolize drug rapidly.[152] The volume of distribution changes as children grow.

The ability to metabolize drugs decreases with age, and lower doses of AEDs are required as patients age.[152] Gabapentin is dependent on renal function for elimination. Because renal function declines as a function of age, the dose of gabapentin may need to be reduced in the elderly.[100] While pharmacokinetic differences can be anticipated, pharmacodynamic changes with the AEDs have not been studied in the elderly. However, some CNS drugs (e.g., opiates and benzodiazepines) have an increased receptor sensitivity in the elderly. A change in the pharmacodynamics would mean that the therapeutic range for younger patients would be invalid in the elderly. Because of pharmacokinetic and potential pharmacodynamic changes in the elderly, the patient response rather than blood levels is the most important clinical outcome.[153] There may be an overestimation of generalized seizures in the elderly, and the diagnosis of partial seizures with secondary generalization may be missed.

Disease states may alter the pharmacokinetics of AEDs. Liver disease may decrease drug metabolism. In addition, if synthesis of albumin decreases, the protein binding of highly bound AEDs will decrease. Patients with chronic renal failure may have decreased elimination of unchanged drug as well as altered protein binding.[11]

SURGERY FOR EPILEPSY

The use of surgery for intractable epilepsy that interferes with patients' lives and functioning is increasing. The success rate of this surgery is reported to be between 80 and 90% in properly selected patients. The procedure involves identifying and removing the site of seizure foci. The recent National Institutes of Health Consensus Conference identified three absolute requirements for surgery. They are an absolute diagnosis of epilepsy, failure on an adequate trial of drug therapy, and definition of the electroclinical syndrome.[154] A foci in the temporal lobe has the best chance for a positive outcome; however, extratemporal foci may be successfully excised in more than 75% of the patients. The procedure is not without risk. Learning and memory are most susceptible to impairment postoperatively, and general intellectual abilities are also affected in a small number of patients. It is estimated that 20% of patients with epilepsy may benefit from seizure surgery. It may be particularly useful in children with intractable epilepsy.[155]

KETOGENIC DIET

The ketogenic diet was devised in the 1920s. It is high in fat and low in carbohydrate and protein. The protein and calorie intake is set at levels that will meet requirements for growth. Most of the calories are provided in the form of heavy cream and butter. No sugar is allowed. Vitamins and minerals are supplemented.[156] Medium-chain triglycerides may be substituted for the dietary fats. Fluids are also controlled. The diet induces ketosis. It requires strict control and parent compliance.[157] Although some centers find this useful for refractory patients, others have found that it is poorly tolerated by patients.

SUDDEN DEATH IN EPILEPSY

Patients with epilepsy have a reduced life span. About one-third of recorded deaths are sudden. The estimated incidence of sudden death in epilepsy is 1:500–1000. The incidence may be higher in the population between the ages of 20–40 years. The underlying mechanisms are unknown but may involve autonomically mediated cardiac arrhythmias alone or in combination with neurogenic pulmonary edema and heart failure. The cause of death in epilepsy should be carefully evaluated.[158]

ASSESSMENT OF THERAPEUTIC OUTCOMES

Patients should be monitored to assure that the treatment principles are followed. The treatment of epilepsy begins with a careful identification of the seizure type and selection of the most appropriate ADE. Therapy should be initiated slowly, except in life-threatening situations, to avoid acute toxicity. The pharmacokinetics and therapeutic plasma concentration range of the AED should be integrated into the clinical monitoring of seizure control to identify the appropriate dose. The patient's response is more important than the drug concentration. Patients should be chronically monitored for seizure control, social adjustment, drug interactions, compliance, dosage adjustments, and toxicity.

Outcomes can be assessed by prospective clinical monitoring, drug utilization review, and by quality of life assessments. Clinical monitoring involves identifying the number and type of seizures. Patients should be given a seizure diary and the severity as well as the frequency of seizures should be monitored. There should be a decrease in the number or in the severity of the seizures. Other clinical monitoring parameters include side effects unique to each drug, drug dosing, compliance, and drug interactions. Drug utilization reviews can be done for a given drug or a disease utilization review could be done for all patients with epilepsy. In a utilization review, criteria for acceptable practice are developed and a given population is measured to determine if these standards are met. Finally, there is a disease-specific quality of life rating scale for epilepsy and the quality of life of epilepsy patients can be screened or assessed in depth.

CONCLUSION

Uncontrolled seizures can be a socially devastating disease resulting in impaired progress in school or loss of work. If the seizures are repetitive and prolonged, there is the possibility of brain injury or death.

While most patients can be successfully managed on monotherapy, some patients' seizures remain uncontrolled despite use of multiple AEDs. There is a need for new antiepileptic drugs and continued research in this area.

REFERENCES

1. Chadwick D. Epilepsy. J Neurol Neurosurg Psychiatry 1994;57:264–277.
2. French J. The long-term therapeutic management of epilepsy. Ann Int Med 1994;120:411–422.
3. Herman BP. Quality of life in epilepsy. J Epilepsy 1992;5:153–165.

4. Mattson RH. Current challenges in the treatment of epilepsy. Neurology 1994;44(suppl 5):S4–S9.
5. Pugh CB, Garnett WR. Current issues in the treatment of epilepsy. Clin Pharm 1991;10:335–358.
6. Ramsey RE. Advances in the pharmacotherapy of epilepsy. Epilepsia 1993;34(suppl 5):S9–S16.
7. Garnett WR. New opportunities for the treatment of epilepsy. Am J Health-Syst Pharm 1995;52:88–91.
8. Hauser WA. The prevalence and incidence of convulsive disorders in children. Epilepsia 1994;35(suppl 2):S1–S6.
9. Shinnar S, Berg AT, Moshe SL, et al. Risk of seizure recurrence following a first unprovoked seizure in childhood: A prospective. Pediatrics 1990;85:1076–1085.
10. Hauser WA. Seizure disorders: The changes with age. Epilepsia 1992;33(suppl 4):S6–S14.
11. Cloyd JC, Lackner TE, Leppik IE. Antiepileptics in the elderly. Arch Fam Med 1994;3:589–598.
12. Dichter MA. Emerging insights into mechanisms of epilepsy: Implications for new antiepileptic drug development. Epilepsia 1994;35(suppl 4):S51–S57.
13. Meldrum BS. Anatomy, physiology, and pathology of epilepsy. Lancet 1990;336:231–234.
14. Ellenberg JH, Hirtz PG, Nelson. Do seizures in children cause intellectual deterioration? N Engl J Med 1986;314:1085–1088.
15. Janz D. Epilepsy: Seizures and syndromes, in Freg HH, Janz D (eds): Antiepileptic Drugs. New York, Springer-Verlag, 1985, pp 3–34.
16. Duncan S, Read CL, Brodie MJ. How common is catamenial epilepsy? Epilepsia 1993;34:827–831.
17. Murphy JV, Dehkharghani F. Diagnosis of childhood seizure disorders. Epilepsia 1994;35(suppl 2):S7–S17.
18. Ozkara C, Dreifuss FE. Differential diagnosis in pseudoepileptic seizures. Epilepsia 1993;34:294–298.
19. Commission on Classification and Terminology of the International League Against Epilepsy. Proposal for revised clinical and electroencephalographic classification of epileptic seizures. Epilepsia 1981;22:489–501.
20. Commission on Classification and Terminology of the International League Against Epilepsy. Proposal for classification of epilepsies and epileptic syndromes. Epilepsia 1985;26:268–278.
21. Mattson RH, Cramer JA, Collins JF, et al. Comparison of carbamazepine, phenobarbital, phenytoin and primidone in partial and secondary generalized tonic–clonic seizures. N Engl J Med 1985;313:145–151.
22. Schmidt D, Einicke I, Haenel F. The influence of seizure type on the efficacy of plasma concentrations of phenytoin, phenobarbital and carbamazepine. Arch Neurol 1986;43:263–265.
23. Luders HO, Burgess R, Noachtar S. Expanding the international classification of seizures to provide localization information. Neurology 1993;43:1650–1655.
24. Sveinbjornsdottir S, Duncan JS. Parietal and occipital lobe epilepsy: A review. Epilepsia 1993;34:493–521.
25. Schachter SC. Brainstorms: Epilepsy in Our Words. New York, Raven Press, 1993.
26. Bye AME, Foo S. Complex partial seizures in young children. Epilepsia 1994;35:482–488.
27. Porter RJ. The absence epilepsies. Epilepsia 1993;34(suppl 3):S42–S48.
28. Pellock JM. The classification of childhood seizures and epilepsy syndromes. Neurol Clin 1990;8:619–632.
29. Grunewald RA, Panayiotopoulos CP. Juvenile myoclonic epilepsy: A review. Arch Neurol 1993;50:594–598.
30. Holmes GL. Benign focal epilepsies of childhood. Epilepsia 1993;34(suppl 3):S49–S61.
31. Pellock JM. Standard approach to antiepileptic drug treatment in the United States. Epilepsia 1994;35(suppl 4):S11–S18.
32. Chadwick D. Standard approach to antiepileptic drug treatment in the United Kingdom. Epilepsia 1994;35(suppl 4):S3–S10.
33. Bruni J. Antiepileptic drug selection and adverse effects: An overview. Can J Neurol Sci 1994;21(suppl 3):S3–S6.
34. Camfield P, Camfield C. Acute and chronic toxicity of antiepileptic medications: A selective review. Can J Neurol Sci 1994;21(suppl 3):S7–S11.
35. Bourgeois BFD. Pharmacologic intervention and treatment of childhood seizure disorders: Relative efficacy and safety of antiepileptic drugs. Epilepsia 1994;35(suppl 2):S18–S23.
36. Meador KJ. Cognitive side effects of antiepileptic drugs. Can J Neurol Sci 1994;21(suppl 3):S12–S16.
37. Kalviainen R, Keranen T, Riekkinen PJ. Place of newer antiepileptic drugs in the treatment of epilepsy. Drugs 1993;46:1009–1024.
38. Harden CL. New antiepileptic drugs. Neurology 1994;44:787–795.
39. Chaplin JE, Yepez R, Shorvon SP, Floyd M. National general practice study of epilepsy: The social and psychological effects of recent diagnosis of epilepsy. Br Med J 1992;304:1416–1418.
40. Cimmino A, Garnett WR, Carroll NV, et al. Relationship between knowledge of epilepsy (KE) and quality of life (QOL) in patients with epilepsy. Epilepsia 1994;35(suppl 8):58.
41. Treiman DM. Current treatment strategies in selected situations in epilepsy. Epilepsia 1993;34(suppl 5):S17–S23.
42. Garnett WR. Antiepileptics, in Schumacher GE (ed): Therapeutic Drug Monitoring. Norwalk, CT, Appleton & Lange, 1995, pp 345–395.
43. Commission on Antiepileptic Drugs, International League Against Epilepsy. Guidelines for therapeutic monitoring on antiepileptic drugs. Epilepsia 1993;34:585–587.
44. Cramer JA. Optimizing long-term patient compliance. Neurology 1995;45(2 suppl 1):S25–S28.
45. Peterson GM, McLean S, Millinger KS. A randomized trial of strategies to improve patient compliance with anticonvulsant therapy. Epilepsia 1984;25:412–417.
46. Duncan JS, Shorvon SD, Trimble MR. Effects of removal of phenytoin, carbamazepine, and valproate on cognitive function. Epilepsia 1990;31:584–591.
47. Aldenkamp AP, Alpherts WCJ, Blennow G, et al. Withdrawal of antiepileptic medication in children—Effects on cognitive function: The multicenter Holmfrid study. Neurology 1993;43:41–50.
48. Holmes GL. Stopping antiepileptic drugs in children: When and why. Ann Neurology 1994;35:509–510.

49. Berg AT, Shinnar S. Relapse following discontinuation of antiepileptic drugs: A meta-analysis. Neurology 1994;44:601–608.
50. Tennison M, Greenwood R, Lewis, Thorn M. Discontinuing antiepileptic drugs in children with epilepsy: A comparison of a six-week and a nine-month taper period. N Engl J Med 1994;330:1407–1410.
51. Ketter TA, Malow BA, Flamini R, et al. Anticonvulsant withdrawal—Emergent psychopathology. Neurology 1994;44:55–61.
52. Jacoby A, Johnson A, Chadwick D. Psychosocial outcomes of antiepileptic drug discontinuation. Epilepsia 1992;33:1123–1131.
53. Macdonald RL, Kelly KM. Antiepileptic drug mechanisms of action. Epilepsia 1993;34(suppl 5):S1–S8.
54. Tozer TN, Winter ME. Phenytoin, in Evans WE, Schentag JJ, Jusko WJ (eds): Applied Pharmacokinetics, 3rd ed. Spokane, WA, Applied Therapeutics, 1992, pp 25-1–25-44.
55. Mauro LS, Mauro VF, Bachmann KA, et al. Accuracy of two equations in determining normalized phenytoin concentrations. DICP 1989;23:64–68.
56. Dasgupta A, Dennen DA, Dean R, et al. Prediction of free phenytoin levels based on (total phenytoin)/(albumin) ratios: Potential errors with hypoalbuminemia. Am J Clin Pathol 1991;95:253–256.
57. Privitera MD. Clinical rules for phenytoin dosing. Ann Pharmacotherapy 1993;27:1169–1173.
58. Fitzsimmons WE, Garnett WR, Comstock TJ, et al. Single dose comparison of the relative bioavailability of phenytoin suspension and extended capsules. Epilepsia 1986;27:464–468.
59. Sarkar MA, Garnett WR, Karnes HT. The effects of storage and shaking on the settling properties of phenytoin suspension. Neurology 1989;39:207–209.
60. Phelps SJ, Baldree LA, Boucher BA, Hogue SL. Neuropsychiatric toxicity of phenytoin: Importance of monitoring phenytoin levels. Clin Pediatrics 1993;107–110.
61. Berg MJ, Fincham RW, Ebert BE, et al. Decrease of serum folates in healthy male volunteers taking phenytoin. Epilepsia 1988;29:67–73.
62. Painter MJ. Benzodiazepines and the barbiturates in the treatment of childhood epilepsy, in Dodson WE, Pellock JM (eds): Pediatric Epilepsy: Diagnosis and Treatment. New York, Demos Publications, 1993, pp 281–289.
63. Farwell JR, Lee YJ, Hirtz DG, et al. Phenobarbital for febrile seizures—effects on intelligence and on seizure recurrence. N Engl J Med 1990;322:364–369.
64. Wroblewski BA, Garvin WH. Once-daily administration of phenobarbital in adults. Arch Neurol 1985;42:699–700.
65. Mattson RH, Cramer JA. Phenobarbital: Toxicity, in Levy RH, Mattson RH, Meldrum BS, Penry JK (eds): Antiepileptic Drugs, 3rd ed. New York, Raven Press, 1989, pp 341–355.
66. Dodson WE. Carbamazepine and oxycarbazepine, in Dodson WE, Pellock JM (eds): Pediatric Epilepsy: Diagnosis and Treatment. New York, Demos Publications, 1993, pp 303–314.
67. Tomson T, Almkvist O, Nilsson BY. Carbamazepine-10,11-epoxide in epilepsy: A pilot study. Arch Neurol 1990;47:888–892.
68. Robbins DK, Wedlund PJ, Buhn R, et al. Inhibition of epoxide hydrolase by valproic acid in epileptic patients receiving carbamazepine. Br J Clin Pharmacol 1990;29:759–762.
69. Schaffler L, Bourgeois BRD, Luders HO. Rapid reversibility of autoinduction of carbamazepine metabolism after temporary discontinuation. Epilepsia 1994;35:195–198.
70. Miles MV, Lawless ST, Tennison MB, et al. Rapid loading of critically ill patients with carbamazepine suspension. Pediatrics 1990;86:263–266.
71. Van Der Meyden CH, Kruger AJ, Muller FO, et al. Acute oral loading of carbamazepine-CR and phenytoin in a double-blind randomized study of patients at risk of seizures. Epilepsia 1994;35:189–194.
72. Thakker KM, Mangat S, Garnett WR, et al. Comparative bioavailability and steady state fluctuations of Tegretol commercial and carbamazepine OROS tablets in adult and pediatric epileptic patients. Biopharm Drug Dispos 1992;24:839–841.
73. Wang JT, Shiu GK, Ong-Chen T, et al. Effects of humidity and temperature on in vivo dissolution of carbamazepine tablets. J Pharm Sci 1993;83:1002–1005.
74. Haefeli WE, Meyer PG, Luscher TF. Circadian carbamazepine toxicity. Epilepsia 1994;35:400–402.
75. Van Amelsvoort TH, Bakshi R, Devaus CB, Schwabe S. Hyponatremia associated with carbamazepine and oxcarbazepine therapy: A review. Epilepsia 1994;35:181–188.
76. Konishi T, Naganuma Y, Hongo K, et al. Carbamazepine-induced skin rash in children with epilepsy. Eur J Pediatr 1993;152;605–608.
77. Andrews DG, Bullen JG, Tomlinson L, et al. A comparative study of the cognitive effects of phenytoin and carbamazepine in new referrals with epilepsy. Epilepsia 1986;27:128–134.
78. Clark-Schmidt AL, Garnett WR, Lowe DR, et al. Loss of carbamazepine suspension through nasogastric feeding tubes. Am J Hosp Pharm 1990;47:2034–2037.
79. Davis R, Peters DH, McTavish D. Valproic acid: A reappraisal of its pharmacological properties and clinical efficacy in epilepsy. Drugs 1994;47:332–372.
80. Seino M. A comment on the efficacy of valproate in the treatment of partial seizures. Epilepsia 1994;35(suppl 5):S101–S104.
81. Anderson GD, Gidal BE, Hendryx RJ, et al. Decreased plasma protein binding of valproate in patients with acute head trauma. Br J Clin Pharmacol 1994;37:559–562.
82. Dreifuss FE, Santilli N. Valproic acid hepatic fatalities: A retrospective review. Neurology 1987;37:379–385.
83. Kelley RI. The role of carnitine supplementation in valproic acid therapy. Pediatrics 1994;93:891–892.
84. Ganick DJ, Sunder T, Finley JL. Severe hematologic toxicity of valproic acid. Am J Pediatr Hematol Oncol 1990;12:80–85.
85. Kishi T, Fujita N, Kawaguchi H, et al. Bone marrow suppression induced by high dose valproic acid. Arch Dis Child 1994;71:153–155.
86. Garnett WR. Ethosuximide, in Taylor WJ, Caviness MHD (eds): A Textbook for the Clinical Application of Therapeutic Drug Monitoring. Irving, TX, Abbott Laboratories, 1986, pp 225–236.

87. Millership JS, Mifsud J, Collier PS. The metabolism of ethosuximide. Eur J Drug Metab Pharmacokinet 1993;18:349–353.
88. Pledger GW, Schmidt D. Evaluation of antiepileptic drug efficacy: A review of clinical trial design. Drugs 1994;48:498–509.
89. Macdonald RL, Kelly KM. Mechanisms of action of currently prescribed and newly developed antiepileptic drugs. Epilepsia 1994;35(suppl 4):S41–S50.
90. Bialer M. Comparative pharmacokinetics of the newer antiepileptic drugs. Clin Pharmacokinet 1993;24:441–452.
91. Graves NM. Felbamate. Ann Pharmacotherapy 1993;27:1073–1081.
92. Graves NM, Holmes GB, Fuerst RH, et al. Effect of felbamate on phenytoin and carbamazepine serum concentrations. Epilepsia 1989;30:225–229.
93. Wagner ML, Remmel RP, Graves NM et al. Effect of felbamate on carbamazepine and its major metabolites. Clin Pharmacol Ther 1993;53:536–543.
94. Gidal BE, Upanc ML Potential pharmacokinetic interaction between felbamate and phenobarbital. Ann Pharmacother 1994;28:455–458.
95. Tisdel KA, Israel DS, Kolb KW. Warfarin–felbamate interaction: First report. Ann Pharmacother 1994;28:805.
96. Taylor CP. Emerging perspectives on the mechanism of action of gabapentin. Neurology 1994;44(suppl 5):S10–S16.
97. Goa KL, Sorkin EM. Gabapentin: A review of its pharmacological properties and clinical potential in epilepsy. Drugs 1993;46:409–427.
98. Ramsay RE. Clinical efficacy and safety of gabapentin. Neurology 1994;44(suppl 5):S23–S30.
99. McLean MJ. Clinical pharmacokinetics of gabapentin. Neurology 1994;44(suppl 5):S17–S22.
100. Blum RA, Comstock TJ. Sica DA, et al. Pharmacokinetics of gabapentin in subjects with various degrees of renal function. Clin Pharmacol Ther 1994;56:154–159.
101. Peck AW. Clinical pharmacology of lamotrigine. Epilepsia 1991;(suppl 2):S9–S12.
102. Garnett WR, Pellock JM. Critical drug appraisal: Lamotrigine—Effective oral add-on therapy. P & T 1995;20:156–170.
103. Yuen AWC. Lamotrigine: A review of antiepileptic efficacy. Epilepsia 1994;35(suppl 5):S33–S36.
104. Rambeck B, Wolf P. Lamotrigine clinical pharmacokinetics. Clin Pharmacokinet 1993;25:433–443.
105. Posner J, Holdich CP. Comparison of lamotrigine pharmacokinetics in young and elderly healthy volunteers. J Pharm Med 1991;1:121–128.
106. Ramsay RE, Pellock JM, Garnett WR, et al. Pharmacokinetics and safety of lamotrigine (Lamictal) in patients with epilepsy. Epilepsy Rev 1991;10:191–200.
107. Richens A. Safety of lamotrigine. Epilepsia 1994;35(suppl 5):S37–S40.
108. Andre M, Boutroy MJ, Bianchetti G, et al. Clonazepam in neonatal seizures: Dose regimens and therapeutic efficacy. Eur J Clin Pharmacol 1991;40:193–195.
109. Woodbury DM. Sulfonamides and derivatives: Acetazolamide, in Levy RH, Mattson RH, Meldrum BS, Penry JK (eds): Antiepileptic Drugs, 3rd ed. New York, Raven Press, 1989, pp 855–875.
110. Shields WD, Shewmon DA, Chugani HT, Peacock WJ. Treatment of infantile spasms: Medical or surgical? Epilepsia 1992;33(suppl 4):S26–S31.
111. Mumford JP, Cannon DJ. Vigabatrin. Epilepsia 1994;35(suppl 5):S25–S28.
112. Lloyd P, Flesch G, Dieterle W. Clinical pharmacology and pharmacokinetics of oxcarbazepine. Epilepsia 1994;35(suppl 3):S10–S13.
113. Gram L. Tiagabine: A novel drug with a GABAergic: Mechanism of action. Epilepsia 1994;35(suppl 5):S85–S87.
114. Peters DH, Sorkin EM. Zonisamide: A review of its pharmacodynamic and pharmacokinetic properties, and therapeutic potential in epilepsy. Drugs 1993;45:760–787.
115. Leppik IE. Antiepileptic drugs in development: Prospects for the near future. Epilepsia 1994;35(suppl 4):S29–S40.
116. Dooley JM, Camfield PR, Camfield CS, et al. The use of antiepileptic drug levels in children: A survey of Canadian pediatric neurologists. Can J Neurol Sci 1993;20:217–221.
117. Collaborative Group for Epidemiology of Epilepsy. Adverse reactions to antiepileptic drugs: A follow-up study of 355 patients with chronic antiepileptic drug treatment. Epilepsia 1988;29:787–793.
118. Dam M. Children with epilepsy: The effect of seizures, syndromes, and etiological factors on cognitive functioning. Epilepsia 1990;31(suppl 4):S26–S29.
119. Committee on Drugs. Behavioral and cognitive effects of anticonvulsant therapy. Pediatrics 1985;76:644–647.
120. Dodrill CB. Problems in the assessment of cognitive effects of antiepileptic drugs. Epilepsia 1992;33(suppl 6):S9–S32.
121. Albright P, Bruni J. Reduction of polypharmacy in epileptic patients. Arch Neurol 1985;42:797–799.
122. Meador KJ, Loring DW, Huh K, et al. Comparative cognitive effects of anticonvulsants. Neurology 1990;40:391–394.
123. Dodrill CB, Troupin AS. Neuropsychological effects of carbamazepine and phenytoin: A reanalysis. Neurology 1991;41:141–143.
124. Ludgate J, Keating J, O'Dwyer R, et al. An improvement in cognitive function following polypharmacy reduction in a group of epileptic patients. Acta Neurol Scand 1985;71:448–452.
125. Dreifuss FE. Cognitive function—Victim of disease or hostage to treatment? Epilepsia 1992;33(suppl 1):S7–S12.
126. Reynolds EH, Trimble MR. Adverse neuropsychiatric effects of anticonvulsant drugs. Drugs 1985;29:570–581.
127. Thompson PJ. Antiepileptic drugs and memory. Epilepsia 1992;33(suppl 6):S37–S40.
128. Perrine K, Congett S. Neurobehavioral problems in epilepsy. Neurol Clin 1994;12:129–152.
129. Lindhout D, Omtzigt JGC. Teratogenic effects of antiepileptic drugs: Implications for the management of epilepsy in women of childbearing age. Epilepsia 1994;35(suppl 4):S19–S28.
130. Delgado-Escueta AV, Janz D. Consensus guidelines: Preconception counseling, management, and care of the pregnant woman with epilepsy. Neurology 1992;42(suppl 5):149–160.
131. Commission on Genetics, Pregnancy and the Child, International League Against Epilepsy. Guideline for the care of women of childbearing age with epilepsy. Epilepsia 1993;34:588–589.

132. Brodie MJ. Management of epilepsy during pregnancy and lactation. Lancet 1990;336:426–427.
133. Lerman P. Seizures induced or aggravated by anticonvulsants. Epilepsia 1986;27:706–710.
134. Garcia PA, Alldredge BK. Drug-induced seizures. Neurol Clin 1994;12:85–99.
135. Cramer JA. Quality of life for people with epilepsy. Neurol Clin 1994;12:1–13.
136. Pashko S, McCord A, Sena MM. The cost of epilepsy and seizures in a cohort of Pennsylvania Medicaid patients. Medical Interface 1993;November:79–84.
137. Begley CE, Annegers JF, Lairson DR, et al. Cost of epilepsy in the United States: A model based on incidence and prognosis. Epilepsia 1994;35:1230–1243.
138. Freeman JM. The best medicine for febrile seizures. N Engl J Med 1992;327:1161–1163.
139. Smith MC. Febrile seizures: Recognition and management. Drugs 1994;47:933–944.
140. Rosman NP, Colton T, Labazzo, et al. A controlled trial of diazepam administered during febrile illnesses to prevent recurrence of febrile seizures. N Engl J Med 1993;329:79–84.
141. Young RSK. Controversies in treatment of neonatal seizures. Pediatr Neurol 1993;9:331–332.
142. McMicken DB, Freedland ES. Alcohol-related seizures: Pathophysiology, differential diagnosis, evaluation, and treatment. Emerg Med Clin North Am 1994;12:1057–1079.
143. Dalessio DJ. Seizure disorders and pregnancy. N Engl J Med 1985;312:359–363.
144. Lander CM, Eadie MJ. Plasma antiepileptic drug concentrations during pregnancy. Epilepsia 1991;32:257–266.
145. Mattson RH, Cramer JA, Darney PD, et al. Use of oral contraceptives by women with epilepsy. JAMA 1986;256:238–240.
146. Dalmady-Israel C, Zasler ND. Post-traumatic seizures: A critical review. Brain Inj 1993;7:263–273.
147. Temkin NR, Dikmen SS, Wilensky AJ, et al. A randomized double-blind study of phenytoin for the prevention of posttraumatic seizures. N Engl J Med 1990;323:497–502.
148. Dikmen SS, Temkin NR, Miller B, et al. Neurobehavioral effects of phenytoin prophylaxis of posttraumatic seizures. JAMA 1991;265:1271–1277.
149. Lancman ME, Golimstok A, Norscini J, Granillo R. Risk factors for developing seizures after a stroke. Epilepsia 1993;34:141–143.
150. Armon C, Radtke RA, Massey EW. Therapy of seizures associated with stroke. Clin Neuropharmacol 1991;14:17–27.
151. Shaw MDM, Foy PM. Epilepsy after craniotomy and the place of prophylactic anticonvulsant drugs: Discussion paper. J Royal Soc Med 1991:221–223.
152. Leppik IE. Metabolism of antiepileptic medication: Newborn to elderly. Epilepsia 1992;33(suppl 4):S32–S40.
153. Burns JMA, McAlpine CH. Audit of the use of anticonvulsant level monitoring in the elderly. J Clin Exp Gerontol 1992;14:197–206.
154. National Institutes of Health Consensus Development Conference Statement. Surgery for epilepsy. Epilepsia 1990;31:806–812.
155. Morrison G, Duchowny M, Resnick T, et al. Epilepsy surgery in childhood. Pediatr Neurosurg 1992;18:291–297.
156. Kinsman SL, Vining EPG, Quaskey SA, et al. Efficacy of the ketogenic diet for intractable seizure disorders: Review of 58 cases. Epilepsia 1992;33:1132–1136.
157. Anonymous. The Johns Hopkins ketogenic diet factsheet. Epilepsy USA, Oct–Nov 1994, p 10.
158. Lip GYH, Brodie MJ. Sudden death in epilepsy: An avoidable outcome? J Royal Soc Med 1992;85:609–611.

Chapter 56

Status Epilepticus

William R. Garnett, PharmD

Status epilepticus (SE) is one of the most common neurologic emergencies. The earliest reference to SE is found in a Babylonian medical diagnostic series that was written in the middle of the first millennium B.C. This describes what is now known as convulsive SE.[1] The syndrome most commonly associated with the name SE is tonic–clonic or "convulsive" status; however, SE may also be nonconvulsive. Today, generalized convulsive SE is a neurologic emergency that carries a significant risk of permanent brain damage and death when not promptly and appropriately treated. The longer the generalized convulsive SE continues, the higher the morbidity and mortality. The sequelae of nonconvulsive SE remain to be defined.[2] Because of rapid treatment, the mortality of convulsive SE has declined.[3] The mortality in children is lower than in adults.[4] SE accounts for about one-half of the deaths caused by epilepsy.[5]

Definition/Classification

SE is defined as more than 30 minutes of (1) continuous seizure activity, or (2) two or more sequential seizures without full recovery of consciousness between seizures.[6] SE may be convulsive or nonconvulsive, generalized or partial.[1,7–12] Nonconvulsive SE may be composed of complex partial, absence, myoclonic, or atonic seizures.[8] The hallmark of nonconvulsive SE is altered mental status, which has an extensive and complex differential diagnosis. Some patients in nonconvulsive SE will be correctly diagnosed only if an electroencephalogram (EEG) is obtained at the time of the epileptic event.[13]

The international classification of SE is provided in Table 56.1, and the terms are compared with traditional terms previously used to describe SE. Controversy exists about the urgency with which nonconvulsive SE needs to be treated. However, it has been suggested that nonconvulsive SE may result in permanent neuronal damage.[13]

Incidence

A recent estimate using prospective epidemiological data suggested that more than 250,000 cases of SE may occur annually.[14] Assuming that the incidence is similar in other parts of the world, the annual incidence of convulsive SE worldwide is between 1.2 and 5 million cases per year.[15] Convulsive SE accounts for about 3–5% of admissions to a neurologic intensive care unit (ICU).[16] The frequency of SE in patients diagnosed with epilepsy is between 0.5 and 6.6%.[5] About one-third of the cases represent the initial presenting symptoms of epilepsy, one-third occur in patients with previously diagnosed epilepsy, and one-third occur at the time of an acute insult with no history of epilepsy.[5] The greatest number of cases occur in children, although the risk is equally high in the over 60 population.[6] In young children, 21% of the cases were reported in the first year of life and 64% were reported in the first 5 years of life.[9] SE is more likely to occur in patients with partial seizures and in those with remote symptomatic epilepsy. The presence of an underlying neurologic abnormality increases the risks of developing SE and the mortality of SE.[2] The large discrepancy among reported incidence data may be related to the different populations being studied, the inclusion of diverse seizure types and etiologies, and variability in the duration of seizure activity accepted as SE.

Nonconvulsive SE accounts for approximately one-quarter of all cases of SE. However, the actual proportion may be higher because patients with nonconvulsive SE may go unidentified.[8] Absence SE is considered more frequent but complex partial SE is more common than generally recognized.[8,12] Focal SE and epilepsia partialis continua are most frequently seen with chronic focal progressive encephalitis. They may also be associated with multiple sclerosis, primary or metastatic brain tumor, benign epilepsy of childhood, and acquired aphasia.[11]

Etiology

SE can arise from diverse etiologies in either a normal brain or in a previously epileptic brain.[17] A recent study indicated that the primary etiologies for SE have not changed during the last two decades.[18] The most frequent precipitating factors for SE are withdrawal of antiepileptic drugs (AEDs), alcohol-withdrawal SE, drug toxicity, cerebrovascular disease, CNS infection, and metabolic disor-

TABLE 56.1. INTERNATIONAL CLASSIFICATION OF STATUS EPILEPTICUS

International	Traditional
Generalized SE	
Convulsive	
Tonic–clonic	Grand mal, epilepticus convulsivus
Tonic	
Clonic	
Myoclonic	
Nonconvulsive	
Absence	Spike-and-wave stupor, spike and slow-wave or 3/s spike-and-wave SE, petit mal, epileptic fugue, epilepsia minora continua, epileptic twilight state, minor SE
Partial SE	Focal motor status, focal sensory, epilepsia partialis continuans, adversive SE
Elementary	
Somatomotor	
Dysphasic	
Other types	
Complex partial	Epileptic fugue state, prolonged epileptic stupor, prolonged epileptic confusional state, temporal lobe SE, psychomotor SE, continuous epileptic twilight state
Unilateral SE	Hemicolonic SE, hemiconvulsion—hemiplegia—epilepsy, hemigrand mal SE, grand mal dimidie
Erratic SE (unclassified)	Neonatal status epilepticus

(Compiled from Ref. 7.)

ders.[18,19] A recent report found that low AED levels or withdrawal can explain some causes of SE but cautioned that other causes of SE must not be overlooked.[20] There is a significant interaction between organic brain disease and a history of epilepsy and SE.[21] Age correlates with etiology.[22] In the newborn and up to the first year of life, the majority of seizures are the result of acute encephalopathy or metabolic disease.[22] In young children the cause is frequently idiopathic but may be associated with fever or a viral illness.[22] A 10-year review of patients 0–16 years who were admitted to a pediatric ICU for SE revealed that most cases of SE were caused by epilepsy, atypical febrile seizures, encephalitis, meningitis, or metabolic disease.[23] In adults the cause is more likely to be related to AED, alcohol withdrawal, head trauma, or due to an underlying neurologic disorder.[24] In elderly patients who had their first seizures after age 60, cerebrovascular disease was the leading cause of SE. This was followed by head trauma, multifactorial etiology, metabolic disorders, brain tumors, and central nervous system (CNS) infection.[25] Table 56.2 lists the most frequent causes of SE. Other precipitating factors include emotional stress, sleep deprivation, and drug toxicity.[23] Recreational drug use is reported to cause prolonged SE.[26]

TABLE 56.2. CAUSES OF STATUS EPILEPTICUS

Etiology	Percent
Withdrawal of AEDs	21
Cerebrovascular disease	21
Alcohol withdrawal	19
Metabolic disorders	13
Hemorrhage	7
Infectious disorders	4
Hypotension	4
Tumors	3
Anorexia	2
Other	7

The initiating events of nonconvulsive SE have not been well characterized.[8] Absence SE has been associated with carbamazepine therapy[27] and benzodiazepine withdrawal.[28]

Mechanism of Status Epilepticus

SE may result from dysfunction in the extracellular space, in neurons, or in the glia. Both alterations in inhibitory and excitatory neurotransmitters have been studied. In animal models a diminution of gaba-aminobutyric acid (GABA)-ergic inhibition in the hippocampus after a single, short-lived seizure can be demonstrated. This may explain in part the evolutionary nature of SE. Excitatory neurotransmitters, free radical formation, and toxic calcium flux may also be involved in SE. Glutamate activates postsynaptic neurons. Quisqualate and kainic acid activate non-*N*-methyl-D-aspartate (NMDA) receptors that give rise to fast excitatory postsynaptic potentials. Also, NMDA receptors that are linked to an ionic channel may be important in SE.[17] More research has been done on the consequences of SE than on the basic underlying cause. A single seizure occurs when a few neurons reach an electronegative potential that allows them to discharge abnormally. The reasons that the seizure may be of short duration or may progress to SE are unknown. SE may progress over time beginning with a premonitory stage of minutes or hours and progressing to continuous convulsions.[16]

Diagnosis

The definition of SE is applied to clinical or electrical seizures, or both.[29] Therefore, the diagnosis must include a clinical and an EEG evaluation because electrical SE may not always be clinically apparent (e.g., when a patient is comatose). It was recently pointed out that paralysis makes it difficult to diagnoses SE.[30] The EEG is also useful in making an accurate identification of the subvariety of SE, which will determine the type and promptness of therapy. Patients with primary generalized tonic–clonic SE resulting from a preexisting epileptic condition respond much better to standard therapy than those with secondary generalized tonic–clonic SE caused by acute CNS impairment.[31]

The diagnosis of convulsive SE should not be made until a trained clinician has witnessed at least one generalized tonic–clonic seizure occurring in a patient with a depressed state of consciousness who has a history of repeated seizures without regaining consciousness between episodes.[29] For nonconvulsive or focal motor SE, the diagnosis should not be made until 30 minutes of continuous seizure activity has been observed.[29] If these guidelines for proper diagnosis are followed, the premature administration of large doses of potentially toxic medications may be avoided. Occasionally, a person with intermittent decorticate or decerebrate posturing is mistakenly identified and treated as having SE.[32] Often, by the time the patient is evaluated, he or she has been treated in the ambulance or by an emergency room staff. Because of the significant morbidity and mortality associated with SE, patients need to be carefully monitored for a period of time after seizures have stopped. A careful history of the nature and duration of the seizure should be obtained from the ambulance crew, the emergency room personnel, the family, and other observers.[19] Also, many physiologic consequences of SE (e.g., leukocytosis, pleocytosis, and hyperthermia) produce symptoms that may be confused with other conditions such as infections.[17]

Diagnostic tests are done in a biphasic fashion.[24] The first phase includes blood sugar and serum chemistries. Hypoglycemia, hyponatremia, hypernatremia, hypomagnesemia, hypocalcemia, and renal failure can all cause seizure activity as can thyrotoxicosis. A toxicology screen should be obtained to determine if drugs of abuse are involved. A complete blood cell count (CBC) should be obtained and all women of child-bearing potential should have a pregnancy test done.[24]

A second phase of diagnostic tests is conducted after the seizures have stopped and the patient has stabilized. These tests are employed to identify a possible cause of the SE and include a screening test for drugs of abuse, a lumbar puncture, especially in young children with fever, and brain imaging. The computed tomography (CT) scan is generally adequate and can be done in emergency situations but some patients will require magnetic resonance imaging (MRI).[6]

PHYSIOLOGIC CONSEQUENCES

Generalized convulsive SE is accompanied by a marked increase in plasma catecholamines. This produces a number of changes in the general systemic physiology, which may include hypertension, tachycardia, cardiac arrhythmias, hyperglycemia, acidosis, and hyperpyrexia.[33] The physiologic consequences of SE that result from the increased motor activity due to the abnormal neuronal activity may be divided into two phases.[16,22] Table 56.3 summarizes these sequelae. The first phase is manifested by tachycardia (as high as 200 beats/min) and an increase in blood pressure, which results in a parasympathetic response to maintain cerebral perfusion and provide the muscles with adequate energy supplies. Other responses to parasympathetic stimulation are increased salivation, vomiting, and incontinence. The airway may be obstructed and the patient may become cyanotic or hypoxic at any time, with a low PaO_2. Respira-

TABLE 56.3. PHYSIOLOGIC CONSEQUENCES OF STATUS EPILEPTICUS

Phase I	Phase II
Tachycardia	Decrease in CO
Hypertension	Hypotension
Increased cardiac output	Raise in cerebral venous pressure
Pallor	Hypoglycemia
Hyperglycemia	Metabolic acidosis
Increase in central venous pressure	Hyperkalemia
Cerebral venous oxygen, raised or normal	Cerebral congestion
Lactic acidosis	Cerebral edema
Hyperkalemia or normokalemia	Increase in intracranial pressure
Hypersalivation	Increase in liver enzymes
Incontinence	Increase in plasma muscle enzymes
Vomiting	Water intoxication
	Hyperpyrexia
	Consumptive coagulopathy

(From Brown JK, Hussain IHMI. Status epilepticus. 1: Pathogenesis. Dev Med Child Neurol 1991;33:3–17, with permission.)

tory acidosis with or without metabolic acidosis is common in patients with convulsive SE and is reported to occur in 84% of patients. Lactic acid accumulation develops as well as an increase in body heat and hyperpyrexia. There may be alterations in blood glucose, potassium, and phosphate. Rhabdomyolysis may occur. During phase I, the body adequately compensates for the increased metabolic demands placed on it.[16,22]

If SE continues for longer than 30 minutes, the body loses the ability to compensate. In phase II there is an excessive consumption of oxygen and glucose, and the blood flow is inadequate to remove the accumulated lactic acid and carbon dioxide. There is a fall in cardiac output and a drop in systemic blood pressure, producing hypoxia and ischemia.

Thus SE involves a gradual worsening of the patient's condition.[15] The patient will have systemic symptoms that include hyperthermia, leukocytosis, pleocytosis, hemodynamic alterations, and respiratory defects.[33,34] While pleocytosis may occur after convulsive SE, it should not be attributed to SE alone until other causes have been ruled out.[35] The cardiovascular system will be especially stressed. Rhabdomyolysis may lead to myoglobinuria, which may cause renal failure. There may be metabolic and biochemical complications including respiratory and metabolic acidosis, hyperkalemia, hypoglycemia, hyponatremia, anoxemia, and hyperazotemia.[33] There is increased sweating and salivation. Marked elevations in plasma prolactin, glucagon, growth hormone, and adrenocorticotropic hormone have recently been identified.[36]

Thus SE represents a medical emergency because significant morbidity and mortality may result from the physiologic sequelae. Also, there is evidence that SE itself, independent of its metabolic and physiologic sequelae, may lead to lasting brain dysfunction.[17]

Cerebral Consequences

SE has an adverse effect on brain development and on the functioning of the mature brain.[37] The CNS sequelae of SE include excessive oxygen and energy demands and accumulation of excitatory amino acids and toxic metabolites, with resultant edema and cellular death.[24] Neuronal damage after an episode of SE is probably related to excessive metabolic activity of vulnerable neurons in the presence of inadequate energy supplies. Neuronal damage may also occur because of transient local hypoxia, which occurs during seizures and is caused by a metabolic transition of oxygen sufficiency to insufficiency in the cerebral cortex.[29] Excitotoxic mechanisms mediated by both NMDA and non-NMDA glutamate receptors open ionic channels permeable to calcium and play a major role in neuronal injury from SE.[38] The most vulnerable areas of the brain are the neocortex, hippocampus, and cerebellum.[24] Neuronal damage probably occurs during the late phase of SE, which suggests that hyperpyrexia, arterial hypotension, hypoxia, and hypoglycemia may be associated with its development.[38] Some patients may escape SE with no discernable effects by physical, neurologic, and mental status examination; however, others definitely have neurologic impairment, which results in decreased performance on intelligence quotient (IQ) tests and subtle neuropsychometric tests.[37] SE exerts an epileptogenic effect that persists.[39] Nonconvulsive SE is also believed to result in brain damage in some cases.[13,38]

Morbidity and Mortality

The morbidity and mortality associated with convulsive SE depend on the underlying causes and precipitating factors as well as the response to treatment.[5] Patients may die of seizures, but more frequently they die as a result of the acute illness that precipitated the attack.[16] The morbidity and mortality of SE are related to CNS damage caused by the acute insult precipitating the SE, systemic stress from repeated convulsions, and injury from repetitive electrical discharges within the CNS.[38]

Recent estimates of mortality suggest a 3–10% rate in children and a 20–30% rate in adults.[1,7] In the elderly, the mortality rate is reported to be 35%.[25] Predictors of mortality include seizure duration, specific etiologies, and age.[14] SE lasting less than 60 minutes had a lower mortality than seizures lasting longer than 60 minutes. Low mortality rates were seen in SE cases involving alcohol and AED discontinuation whereas there was a higher mortality rate reported in cases involving anoxia and increasing age. Race and sex did not affect mortality.[40] Blood cortisol levels have been noted to be significantly higher in patients with SE with a poor outcome compared to a control group and a group of patients with SE and a good outcome.[41] The mortality rate for SE appears to be decreasing, which probably reflects a greater understanding of the need to initiate immediate therapy to decrease seizure duration. There does not appear to be a difference in the mortality rates for SE between community hospitals and major medical centers.[14]

The morbidity for patients surviving SE may be significant. While some patients may have no sequelae, others may have impaired mental abilities or neurologic deficits. Patients who have experienced SE are more likely to have continued seizures and are less likely to have a remission of their epilepsy.[2] Morbidity may be highest in children under 2 years of age in whom SE is primarily a manifestation of symptomatic epilepsy. In a study of 239 children with SE, defined as 60 minutes or more of predominantly generalized tonic–clonic or unilateral clonic convulsions, there was an 11% mortality during the first or subsequent episode of SE. Of the survivors, 67% had sequelae of epilepsy, mental retardation, or neurologic deficits. The younger the child at the time of onset, the greater the chance of significant sequelae.[42]

Patients having febrile SE may not have significant sequelae unless they have an underlying neurologic abnormality.[43] In a study of 44 children with febrile convulsions lasting more than 30 minutes, the occurrence of febrile SE in an otherwise normal child did not significantly increase the risk of subsequent febrile or afebrile seizures within the first few years following the episode. There was a risk of recurrent seizures in the group that had a prior neurologic abnormality.[44]

Of the various subtypes of SE, generalized convulsive SE clearly causes the most morbidity and mortality. However, other types of SE can also cause residual damage.[8] Complex partial SE may continue for a prolonged period of time before the seizures are controlled.[45] It is imperative that focal SE and nonconvulsive SE be regarded as urgent situations requiring prompt treatment.[13,46]

Treatment

CONVULSIVE STATUS EPILEPTICUS

The most common form of SE in adults is tonic–clonic with bilateral motor activity. Many of the same principles and therapeutic modalities are utilized to treat other, less common forms of convulsive SE (e.g., tonic SE, clonic SE).

The treatment goals for convulsive SE are (1) assure adequate brain oxygenation and cardiorespiratory function, (2) terminate clinical and electrical seizure activity as rapidly as possible, (3) prevent seizure recurrence, (4) identify precipitating factors, (5) correct metabolic imbalance, (6) prevent systemic complications, and (7) further evaluate and treat the etiology of SE.[5]

Table 56.4 outlines the currently recommended management of convulsive SE. Rapid treatment is necessary to reduce morbidity and mortality.[5,6,15,16,24,47] Particular attention must be paid to supportive measures, including adequate oxygenation and correction of metabolic anomalies to prevent chronic sequelae. The treatment guidelines were developed by the Professional Advisory Board of The Epilepsy Foundation of America. Approximately 100 experts in the treatment of convulsive SE were involved in the development of these guidelines.[6]

Supportive Care

While AEDs will be necessary to stop the convulsions, the initial concerns for the patient with SE are vital signs in the priority of (1) maintenance of a patent airway with adequate ventilation, (2) maintenance of an intact cardiovascu-

TABLE 56.4. MANAGEMENT OF TONIC–CLONIC STATUS EPILEPTICUS

Time[a] (min)	Action[b]
0–5	Diagnose status epilepticus by observing continued seizure activity or one additional seizure.
	Give oxygen by nasal cannula or mask; position patient's head for optimal airway patency; consider intubation if respiratory assistance is needed.
	Obtain and record vital signs at onset and periodically thereafter; control any abnormalities as necessary; initiate ECG monitoring.
	Establish an IV; draw venous blood samples for glucose level, serum chemistries, hematology studies, toxicology screens, and determinations of antiepileptic drug levels.
	Assess oxygenation with oximetry or periodic arterial blood gas determinations.
6–9	If hypoglycemia is established or a blood glucose determination is unavailable, administer glucose; in adults, give 100 mg of thiamine first, followed by 50 mL of 50% glucose by direct push into the IV; in children, the dose of glucose is 2 mL/kg of 25% glucose.
10–20	Administer either 0.1 mg/kg of lorazepam at 2 mg/min or 0.2 mg/kg of diazepam at 5 mg/min by IV; if diazepam is given, it can be repeated if seizures do not stop after 5 min; if diazepam is used to stop the status, phenytoin should be administered next to prevent recurrent status.
21–60	If status persists, administer 15–20 mg/kg of phenytoin no faster than 50 mg/min in adults and 1 mg/kg/min in children by IV; monitor ECG and blood pressure during the infusion; phenytoin is incompatible with glucose-containing solutions; the IV should be purged with normal saline before the phenytoin infusion.
>60	If status does not stop after 20 mg/kg of phenytoin, give additional doses of 5 mg/kg to a maximal dose of 30 mg/kg.
	If status persists, give 20 mg/kg of phenobarbital by IV at 100 mg/min; when phenobarbital is given after benzodiazepine, the risk of apnea or hypopnea is great and assisted ventilation is usually required.
	If status persists, give anesthetic doses of drugs such as phenobarbital or pentobarbital; ventilatory assistance and vasopressors are virtually always necessary.

[a]Time starts at seizure onset. Note that a neurologic consultation is indicated if the patient does not wake up, convulsions continue after the administration of a benzodiazepine and phenytoin, or confusion exists at any time during evaluation and treatment.
[b]ECG, electrocardiogram; IV, intravenous line. (From Treatment of convulsive status epilepticus. JAMA 1993;270(7):857 with permission.)

lar system as demonstrated by pulse rate and blood pressure, (3) regulation of blood sugar, and (4) prevention of an elevated temperature that would indicate toxic or metabolic processes.[6,24] Specific supportive measures should be instituted simultaneously with AED therapy. Airway management to provide adequate ventilation, oxygenation, and protection from aspiration is essential. The patient should be positioned so that aspiration, suffocation, and physical injury are avoided. A plastic oral airway may be placed if possible. Excessive oral secretions should be suctioned to prevent impairment of airway functioning. The patient should be intubated if airway exchange status is questionable. Unfortunately, these manipulations are often quite difficult to perform on a patient who is actively seizing. Managing the airway is easier after the seizure has stopped.

Blood pressure, pulse rate, and temperature should be carefully monitored. Excessive fluid loss and the subsequent decrease in blood pressure may necessitate increased administration of intravenous fluids. However, it is suspected that all patients with convulsive SE have some degree of cerebral edema and overhydration should be avoided.[6] Placing a bladder catheter may also be helpful to monitor the patient's fluid output. If possible, electrocardiographic (ECG) and EEG monitoring should be used. An indwelling intravenous catheter should be immediately placed and a sample of venous blood obtained for estimates of serum glucose, electrolytes, blood urea nitrogen (BUN), calcium, serum AED concentrations (if appropriate), and a toxicology screen (if adequate suspicion exists).

Hypoglycemia is a rare cause of convulsive SE and hyperglycemia may be present in the early phases of SE. However, SE can cause a secondary hypoglycemia.[6] Initially, administration of 50 mL of 50% glucose in adults (1–2 mL/kg in children) is recommended. In addition, blood glucose testing using finger stick methods (e.g., Dextrostix, Visidex, Chemstrip bG) is needed to determine if additional glucose should be administered. IV thiamine should be administered prior to glucose in adults.[6]

An arterial blood sample for measurement of pH, Pao_2, $PaCo_2$, and HCO_3 should be obtained to assure adequate oxygenation and to determine if the patient is becoming acidotic. An acidotic condition (pH <7.35) is corrected by administration of 50 mEq of sodium bicarbonate ($NaHCO_3$). Repeat blood gas measurements and additional doses of $NaHCO_3$ may be required in patients with compromised respiratory status.

Significant hyperpyrexia may develop in convulsive SE. This may occur as a result of increased motor activity and may contribute to brain damage. It is imperative that significant hyperpyrexia be prevented in convulsive SE. Rectal temperatures should be monitored, and specific treatment may be required.[6,16]

For the patient experiencing a convulsive SE attack outside the hospital environment, every effort should be made to get medical assistance as quickly as possible. In the interim, the patient should be eased to the floor and constrictive clothing should be loosened. Any objects that might harm the patient should be removed. Nothing hard should be forced between the patient's teeth as this may cause injury. The patient's head should be turned to the side to prevent aspiration if vomiting occurs. An accurate summary of the details surrounding the onset of the attack and the duration of seizure activity should be recorded and provided to medical personnel as soon as possible.

Drug Therapy

The characteristics of an "ideal drug" to treat SE have been proposed by Treiman[29] (Table 56.5). Although an ideal drug presently does not exist, these properties are useful in determining a rational therapeutic plan for treating SE.

The drug should be available for intravenous administration because of the necessity for rapidly achieving therapeutic plasma concentrations at the effector site (i.e., brain). Intramuscular, nasogastric, and rectal routes are less desirable, as they depend on adequate tissue perfusion for drug absorption and subsequent distribution. The ideal drug should be administered rapidly without concern for adverse effects (e.g., hypotension, cardiac arrhythmias, respiratory depression). The agent chosen should rapidly enter the brain and remain for a sufficient duration to prevent further seizure activity.

Table 56.6 describes some pharmacologic and pharmacokinetic parameters of AEDs routinely used in the treatment of convulsive SE. The therapeutic plasma concentrations are those specific for generalized convulsive SE and are not based on controlled, prospective dose-ranging studies. Dose–response curves have not been adequately characterized, and many of these recommendations are based only on experience or are extrapolated from studies evaluating drug treatment of chronic epilepsy. The $t_{1/2}\alpha$ and $t_{1/2}\beta$ terms represent distribution and elimination half-lives, respectively. The "effective" half-life is an estimation of the length of time a particular agent will exert a therapeutic

TABLE 56.5. PROPERTIES OF AN IDEAL DRUG FOR TREATMENT OF STATUS EPILEPTICUS

Rapidly effective against all types of status
Available for intravenous administration
Potent, so that small volumes can be given rapidly
Safe: no cardiorespiratory depression, no depression of consciousness, no systemic side effects
Rapidly enters the brain
Long distribution half-life
Short elimination half-life
Useful in oral form as a chronic antiepileptic drug

(Modified from Treiman DM. General principles of treatment: Responsive and intractable status epilepticus in adults, in Delgado-Escueta AV, Wasterlain CG, Treiman DM, et al (eds): Status Epilepticus. New York, Raven Press, 1983, p 381.)

TABLE 56.6. PHARMACOKINETIC AND DOSING GUIDELINES FOR AEDS COMMONLY USED IN STATUS EPILEPTICUS

Drug	Usual Initial IV Dose	Administration Rate	Time to Stop SE, $t_{1/2}\alpha^a$ (min)	Mean $t_{1/2}\beta^b$ (h)	Estimated Effective Half-Life	Initial Plasma Concentration[c] (μg/mL)
Diazepam	5–10 mg (0.25–0.4 mg/kg)[d]	1–2 mg/min (same)	3–5	30–40	1.5 min	0.5–0.8
Phenytoin	18–20 mg/kg (same)	≤50 mg/min (0.5–1.5 mg/kg/min)	30	22[e]	22 h	20–25
Phenobarbital	300–800 mg (20 mg/kg)	25–50 mg/min (same)	20	86	50–120 h	20–45
Lorazepam	4–8 mg (—)	<2 mg/min (—)	3	15	2 h	0.3–1.0
Paraldehyde[f]	0.2–0.4 mL/kg[g] (0.1–0.15 mL/kg)	Repeat initial IV dose every 2–4 h prn	—[h]	7.5	6 h	150–300
Lidocaine	50–100 mg (0.5–1 mg/kg)	1–2 mg/min (20–50 μg/kg/min)	1	1.5–2.5	—	—

[a] $t_{1/2}\alpha$, distribution half-life.
[b] $t_{1/2}\beta$, elimination half-life.
[c] Plasma concentrations have generally not been well established for treatment of SE.
[d] Information in parentheses for children.
[e] Phenytoin displays nonlinear elimination; this value will change depending on the concentration.
[f] Injectable form is no longer commercially available.
[g] Can also be given intramuscularly at a dose of 5–10 mL for adults.
[h] Dashes are used for data that could not be extracted from the literature.

response after a single dose. This last parameter takes into account relative lipid solubilities, pK_α, and distribution characteristics, and can be used when making decisions regarding dosing intervals or the need for continuous infusions.[29,48]

The use of rectal or intramuscular AEDs may allow for the initiation of drug therapy before the arrival of the patient at the emergency room.[16] In the emergency room, AED therapy is initiated usually with a benzodiazepine (BZ), which can be given rapidly intravenously and which has an immediate onset of activity. This is followed by another AED, usually phenytoin, which is given intravenously but which has a much longer duration of effect. Some patients are nonresponsive to this approach; they will require greater CNS suppression, which may be provided by phenobarbital, paraldehyde, or even general anesthetics.[6,16,24,47]

Benzodiazepines (BZs)

The BZs have been shown to be one of the most potent classes of drugs on a mg/kg basis in the acute treatment of SE.[47] They enhance GABA-ergic inhibition and reduce repetitive firing. They distribute quickly into the brain and have a rapid onset of anticonvulsant activity. Some BZs are available in a dosage form that does not require reconstitution so it can be injected intravenously by rapid bolus injection. Therefore, BZs are frequently the AED of first choice in SE. The rapid distribution into the brain is followed by redistribution to other compartments and a diminution of anticonvulsant activity.[49] Tolerance commonly develops with chronic administration.[47] Thus, while BZs may be used to stop SE, another AED with longer lasting effects will also be needed.[49]

The BZs most often used in convulsive SE in the United States are diazepam and lorazepam. There is no unequivocal evidence of superior efficacy for either drug. The choice is based on pharmacokinetic parameters and the longer effective duration of lorazepam.[50] Recently, midazolam, a water-soluble benzodiazepine used as a preanesthetic medication, has been used in convulsive SE[51] and has been reported to be effective in refractory generalized SE.[15,52]

Diazepam

Diazepam stops convulsions within 3 minutes in 33% of patients, and within 5 minutes in 80%.[47] Unfortunately, despite rapid cessation of seizure activity, seizures frequently recur after 15–20 minutes.[5] The rapid initial response followed by loss of seizure control is due to the pharmacokinetic characteristics of the drug. Diazepam is extremely lipophilic and rapidly penetrates the brain after intravenous administration. This initial distribution phase is followed by a rapid and extensive redistribution of diazepam into body fat stores, thus decreasing the concentration of drug at the receptor sites.[53] There is a greater than 70% fall in serum concentration of diazepam in the first 2 hours after intravenous administration despite a half-life that is approximately 60 hours.[48] This phenomenon necessitates repeated administration of diazepam or the use of a second drug (e.g., phenytoin) to prevent seizure recurrence.

Intravenous diazepam should be administered at a rate of 2–5 mg/min (Table 56.4).[16] Complications associated with the intravenous administration of diazepam include respiratory depression, hypotension, and arrhythmias. Because of the poor solubility of diazepam in water, the commercially available diazepam injection is formulated with 40% propylene glycol and 10% ethyl alcohol. Therefore, rapid infusion may potentiate propylene glycol-induced hypotension and possibly arrhythmias. At an infusion rate of 2 mg/min, no episodes of hypotension occurred in a series of 50 patients with SE.[54] The maximum rate of infusion is 5 mg/min.[6]

The recommended initial dose of diazepam is 10–20 mg IV.[47] The expected time for seizures to stop after diazepam administration is 1–3 minutes.[8] If seizures have not stopped after 5 minutes, another dose should be given.[47] The maximum recommended total dose is 40 mg.[16] Diazepam is a safe drug and can be administered in larger doses with minimal concern for toxicity (provided the rate of administration is appropriate). The significant acute adverse effects include CNS and respiratory depression. CNS depression may hamper clinical assessment of the patient's response, especially when absence SE is being treated. Both CNS and respiratory depression may be potentiated by the coadministration of other agents, particularly barbiturates; however, because the primary objective in SE is seizure control and because artificial ventilation should be available, diazepam should be administered in doses large enough to induce seizure cessation.

Other possible adverse effects caused by the administration of intravenous diazepam include laryngospasm and local complications, such as thrombophlebitis. If proper administration techniques are used and adequate venous access is secured, local complications are negligible.[55] Finally, paradoxical effects have been reported after intravenous diazepam administration. In patients with Lennox-Gastaut syndrome, BZs and other AEDs have induced brief episodes of tonic SE.[55]

Continuous diazepam infusion is indicated for patients whose seizures are not adequately controlled after appropriate intravenous doses of diazepam and phenytoin (Table 56.4). Despite the paucity of large, controlled clinical trials, intravenous infusion of diazepam appears to be a safe and effective therapy in these treatment-resistant patients.[56] Other therapies may be more effective for refractory convulsive SE.

Stability and compatibility problems with intravenous diazepam infusions have created some confusion and hesitancy in the use of this form of therapy. Contrary to the manufacturer's recommendations, diazepam can be safely diluted and administered as an infusion. The drug is soluble in NaCl 0.9%, Ringer's, lactated Ringer's, and dextrose solutions. Diazepam does not adhere to glass containers but may adhere to polyvinyl chloride (PVC) administration sets.[57] Adsorption of diazepam to the tubing of some infusion sets can be minimized by using glass containers and volume control sets containing cellulose propionate. Plastic containers and infusion sets made of PVC appear to produce the greatest amount of drug adsorption.[56] Solutions of diazepam at a concentration of 0.125 mg/mL are stable for 6–8 hours in glass containers.[58]

Suggested doses and administration rates for diazepam infusions are provided in Table 56.4. The duration of the diazepam infusion should be determined by the clinical situation, but infusion is usually continued at least 3 hours after seizure cessation. Tolerance may develop with prolonged use. Patients should be continuously monitored clinically and by EEG for seizure activity. If breakthrough seizures occur, an additional bolus dose should be administered and the infusion rate increased.[56] Patients must also be monitored for signs of toxicity, including respiratory depression, hypotension, and arrhythmias.

Rectal diazepam has shown efficacy in stopping SE.[59] It should be considered as an alternative to intravenous diazepam for patients who cannot be given the drug intravenously.[60] It may be particularly useful when given by a caregiver when SE first starts.[60,61] The dose rectally is 0.5 mg/kg. Rectal therapy is effective in the treatment of febrile convulsions and absence SE.[62,63] Intramuscular diazepam is erratically absorbed (especially in adults and those with poor hemoperfusion) and should not be used in the treatment of SE.

Diazepam is cleared from plasma primarily by hepatic (phase I) metabolism. After its redistribution into adipose tissue, diazepam demonstrates a slow elimination half-life of 1–2 days. This elimination is age dependent, longer in premature newborns than newborns, and shorter in infants and children than adults. Elderly patients show a longer elimination half-life, caused in part by a change in volume of distribution.[64] The dose of diazepam need not be altered in renal failure, though patients with impaired hepatic metabolism and/or hypoperfusion require close clinical monitoring and possible reduction in infusion rate over time.[64] For a more complete discussion of BZ pharmacokinetics, the reader is referred to Chapter 3.

Diazepam plasma concentrations between 0.2 and 0.8 mg/L are probably effective in the treatment of SE (Table 56.4), but this therapeutic range has not been rigorously studied.[54] Diazepam assays are not readily available and are impractical to use in the acute clinical setting. Objective measures of response and toxicity should be used in titrating the appropriate diazepam dose in patients with SE.

Lorazepam

Lorazepam has been shown to be effective in both generalized and partial SE, can be rapidly administered by intravenous push and is relatively safe.[65]

Lorazepam is less lipid soluble than diazepam and is much less extensively tissue bound. This property allows clinically effective CNS concentrations to remain at the receptor site for a longer time after a single dose than is the case with diazepam. Phase II metabolic processes are responsible for the elimination of lorazepam. The elimination half-life of lorazepam is shorter than that of diazepam, and accumulation of lorazepam after repeated administration does not occur.[66] In an animal model it was demonstrated that lorazepam remains in the brain longer than in the serum, leading to an increasing brain:serum ratio over time once the peak concentration has been reached. These data indicated that a target concentration of 200 ng/mL would provide seizure protection for 24 hours after a single dose in most cases.[67] Lorazepam is now frequently the initial AED administered because of its rapid onset and long duration of effect.

The efficacy data for lorazepam in SE are largely limited to case reports that suggest the drug is very effective.[65,68] One large, well-controlled, double-blind comparative trial between lorazepam and diazepam found the drugs to be virtually identical in efficacy and adverse effects.[69] Despite the differences in lipophilicity, no statistical differences existed between median times of onset for lorazepam (3 minutes) and diazepam (3–5 minutes). Adverse effects consisted of respiratory depression and respiratory arrest, and occurred in less than 15% in each group. Subjects experiencing adverse effects in the lorazepam group had more underlying medical problems, which possibly predisposed them to adverse drug effects.[69] One shortcoming of this trial was the need to coadminister phenytoin to patients in both groups for ethical reasons. This prevented the assessment of duration of activity for lorazepam when given alone.[69] In a series of 77 patients, lorazepam stopped the SE in 79% of the patients. Effectiveness was not altered by acute or chronic use of other AEDs. The duration of effect was independent of dose. Patients requiring more than one dose had a diminished response suggesting tachyphylaxis with repeated doses.[70] In a retrospective study of 45 episodes of SE occurring in patients 2 weeks to 18 years of age, 27 episodes were treated with lorazepam and 18 were treated with diazepam. Lorazepam was effective in stopping the SE in 82% of the patients and there was no difference between lorazepam and diazepam in either efficacy or side effects.[71]

The most common adverse effect reported for lorazepam when used to treat SE is sedation.[65] Other effects include confusion, tremor, hallucinations, and respiratory depression.[65,69]

Before intravenous administration, lorazepam must be diluted with an equal volume of compatible diluent, such as sterile water for injection, 0.9% sodium chloride injection, or 5% dextrose injection. Lorazepam injection is available in prefilled syringes that can accommodate diluent directly in the syringe. Once diluted, the solution should be mixed gently, but not shaken vigorously.

Lorazepam may be administered by rapid intravenous push over 2 minutes. Doses for the treatment of SE have ranged from 2–10 mg.[65] The recommended initial dose of lorazepam is 4–8 mg administered over 2 minutes. If the seizures do not stop within 5 minutes, the dose should be repeated.[47] Tachyphylaxis develops, making repeated doses less useful. Lorazepam is less useful in patients exposed to chronic BZ therapy.[5] Refractory SE has been successfully treated with a continuous infusion of 0.3–9 mg/h of lorazepam. There were no reports of hypotension.[72]

Phenytoin

Phenytoin is an effective agent in the treatment of both partial and generalized convulsive SE, but it is not indicated in the treatment of absence SE.[5] Between 56 and 90% of patients with convulsive SE can be controlled with phenytoin.[47] With respect to effectiveness in terminating a convulsive SE episode, intravenous phenytoin is similar to diazepam, although diazepam has a quicker onset of action.[73,74] BZs are usually given before phenytoin because they can be given more quickly. Phenytoin is not available in a solution that can be given by rapid intravenous injection; it must be given slowly to avoid side effects. A loading dose of 18 mg/kg for a 70-kg man will take close to 30 minutes to administer at the maximally recommended rate of 50 mg/min. Phenytoin is frequently given after a BZ because it provides a longer duration of effect. Brain phenytoin concentrations peak in 15–20 minutes, with maintenance of effective brain concentrations and subsequent seizure control for 24 hours or longer after an intravenous loading dose of 18–20 mg/kg (Table 56.6).[73–75] Loading doses of 10–14 mg/kg will result in plasma concentrations within the therapeutic range, but additional doses will be needed in the first 24 hours.[44,48]

Adverse effects are associated with the intravenous administration of phenytoin, because the injectable formulation of phenytoin also contains 40% propylene glycol and 10% ethanol. The potential complications of hypotension and cardiac arrhythmias can be minimized by not exceeding an administration rate of 50 mg/min.[76]

Elderly patients and those with unstable cardiopulmonary function require an even slower infusion rate.[16,75] In a study of patients over the age of 50, those patients with a history of atherosclerotic cardiovascular disease (ASCVD) had more cardiovascular side effects (hypotension and bradycardia) when phenytoin was infused at a rate of 50 mg/min. For patients with ASCVD, the infusion rate should not exceed 25 mg/min.[77] ECG monitoring and frequent blood pressure determinations should be performed during and for 1 hour after the infusion.

Intramuscular administration of phenytoin is painful and results in erratic and slow absorption because phenytoin precipitates at the injection site. Fosphenytoin is a prodrug of phenytoin. It is rapidly converted systemically to phenytoin. It is less irritating than phenytoin when administered intramuscularly or intravenously. It may be administered rapidly intravenously and may replace parenteral phenytoin if it becomes available (see discussion later in this section).

Intravenous infusion of phenytoin as a large-volume parenteral also creates difficulties because of its poor solubility with other fluids and the potential formation of a phenytoin acid precipitate.[76] Phenytoin is soluble in 0.45% and 0.9% sodium chloride and lactated Ringer's solution. Admixtures with other drugs or base fluids containing dextrose should be avoided. Sodium chloride 0.9% is an acceptable diluent if the final phenytoin sodium admixture concentration is no less than 100 mg/100 mL and, preferably, 100 mg per 25–50 mL.[78] In addition to the mixing and administration procedure outlined in Table 56.4, the use of an in-line filter (0.22 or 0.45 m) is advocated to prevent minor drug crystals from entering the vein.[75] The solution should be prepared immediately prior to use and infused within 1 hour.[78] The stability of Dilantin was compared to three generic phenytoin formulations. Dilantin had the lowest interlot variability and significantly higher mean apparent pH. Microscopic evidence of crystallization was seen in the generic formulations with the lower apparent pH values.[79]

Local reactions to intravenous phenytoin include painful sensations (burning, aching) and, less frequently, extravasation.[80,81] These effects are thought to be dependent on concentration and rate of administration, and may be minimized by not exceeding a phenytoin concentration of 6.7 mg/mL (in the intravenous admixture fluid) and not administering the drug at a rate greater than 40–50 mg/min.[80] To avoid extravasation, phenytoin should be infused only through a free-flowing, well-positioned intravenous site. Smaller veins (hand, wrist, foot) are best avoided.[80,81]

Patients who have not previously received phenytoin, or those noncompliant patients whose drug concentrations are virtually nonexistent, should be given an intravenous loading dose of 18–20 mg/kg. This dose should produce initial serum concentrations in the range of 20–25 mcg/mL and 24-hour concentrations greater than 10 mcg/mL.[82] Phenytoin exhibits an increased volume of distribution in obese subjects.[83] For very obese patients, phenytoin loading doses should be calculated on the basis of ideal body weight (IBW) plus the product of 1.33 times the excess weight over IBW.[83]

For patients with subtherapeutic phenytoin concentrations, the following equation may be used to rapidly estimate an appropriate dose to provide therapeutic serum concentrations:

$$\text{Dose (mg)} = (Cp_d - Cp_m)(0.7)(W_{kg})$$

Here Cp_d is the desired serum concentration (generally considered to be between 20 and 25 mcg/mL for SE); Cp_m is the measured subtherapeutic serum concentration; the constant 0.7 represents an approximation of the average volume of distribution; and W_{kg} is the patient's weight in kilograms. Thus, for a 70-kg patient with a known phenytoin concentration of 4 mg/L who is experiencing an SE attack, a calculated dose of 780 mg should raise the serum concentration to approximately 20 mcg/mL.

A cautionary note should be emphasized when interpreting serum phenytoin concentrations. Phenytoin is a weak acid and is highly protein bound (approximately 90%) to albumin. In a patient with a normal serum albumin who is not taking other drugs known to displace phenytoin from protein binding sites, a "total" concentration in the range of 10–20 mcg/mL corresponds to a "free" (unbound) concentration of 1–2 mcg/mL. Although the free phenytoin concentration is responsible for the therapeutic effect, total phenytoin concentrations are generally obtained, because they are simpler and less expensive to quantify.[76]

A low total serum phenytoin concentration in the face of a therapeutic free concentration may be caused by decreased serum protein binding or displacement of phenytoin from protein binding sites. Thus, in interpreting phenytoin concentrations, factors altering protein binding (discussed in Chapter 55) should be considered. Measurement of a serum free phenytoin concentration may be indicated in patients with decreased serum albumin or those taking other highly protein-bound drugs. Toxic phenytoin concentrations (i.e., free concentrations greater than 4.0 mcg/mL or total concentrations greater than 40 mcg/mL) may cause seizure activity and should be avoided.

The decision to initiate chronic phenytoin therapy depends on the clinical situation and the patient's history. For patients with readily correctable causes of their seizures, chronic AED therapy is not warranted. Avoidance of precipitating factors may be all the therapy that is required. The noncompliant patient should be placed back on phenytoin (or other AEDs) and counseled intensively on the importance of compliance. Potential drug interactions should be investigated and doses of phenytoin adjusted accordingly. Any patient presenting with tonic–clonic SE and no identifiable causes should probably be placed on a chronic regimen of phenytoin, at least until a full diagnostic workup is performed. After the initial intravenous loading dose and seizure cessation, a serum phenytoin concentration should be obtained within 12–24 hours. A recent study gave a loading dose of phenytoin and measured the phenytoin blood concentration at 4, 8, 16, 24, 28, 32, and 36 hours after the initial administration. The levels were used for dosage adjustment.[84] Chronic oral administration of phenytoin should be instituted at a dose between 6 and 7 mg/kg/d, 24 hours after the loading dose. The complexities and maintenance dose requirements of phenytoin are reviewed in Chapter 55.

Fosphenytoin. Fosphenytoin is the disodium phosphate ester of phenytoin. It is water soluble and can be given by IM and IV injection. It does not cause pain following IM injection and is rapidly absorbed reaching effective concentrations within 20–30 minutes. It can also be given at a faster rate of injection than phenytoin because it does not require propylene glycol for solubilization. Fosphenytoin 150 mg is equivalent to phenytoin 100 mg. This drug is pending FDA review.[47,85,86]

Phenobarbital

Phenobarbital was among the first effective pharmacologic therapies used in the treatment of SE; it replaced ether and chloroform.[87] Despite the availability of newer agents (e.g., diazepam, lorazepam, and phenytoin), phenobarbital is still an important drug in SE, and remains the drug of choice in some institutions.[24,87]

Barbiturates raise the threshold of many neuronal pathways to direct and indirect stimulation, and cause general CNS depression. The ability of phenobarbital to suppress cortical seizure activity at doses that do not cause excessive sedation is an advantage when compared with other barbiturates.[87] Highest brain concentrations occur 5–15 minutes after intravenous infusion.[88] Although reported to have the slowest onset of action because of low lipid solubility, a recent study reported a median onset time of 5.5 minutes. This study compared the combination of diazepam and phenytoin to phenobarbital with optional phenytoin. Eleven of 18 patients in the phenobarbital group responded to phenobarbital as monotherapy. Phenobarbital was found to be at least as effective and comparable in safety to the combination.[89]

An intravenous loading dose of 20 mg/kg (and possibly up to 25 mg/kg) administered at a rate not exceeding 100 mg/min is recommended.[6,16,24,47,90] A slower rate of infusion (i.e., 30 mg/min) has been recommended for children.[48] One author suggested a dose of 250–300 mg be given intravenously and, if the patient has not stopped seizing within 20–30 minutes, a second dose may be administered. Only occasionally, a third dose is given after an additional 20 minutes.[87] This protocol has produced adequate seizure control with serum concentrations well below the therapeutic range of 25–40 mcg/mL, without problems of respiratory failure (Table 56.6).[87]

Phenobarbital can be administered rapidly by intravenous push over several minutes. Absorption by the intramuscular route is too slow to be effective in convulsive SE.[47] It is soluble in common intravenous fluids and can be mixed without concern of precipitation. A major problem with phenobarbital use is respiratory depression, and ventilatory assistance must be readily available. The coadministration of phenobarbital and diazepam may cause additive respiratory depression. Special precautions should be observed when the two drugs are given concurrently. Also, decreased blood pressure and altered sensorium may occur with phenobarbital administration.

Advantages of using phenobarbital over diazepam are that the depressant effects on respiration, blood pressure, and sensorium are more gradual than those of diazepam and the therapeutic effects of phenobarbital are longer lasting.[16] Also, phenobarbital displays linear kinetics.[48] The main disadvantage is that phenobarbital has a slower onset of action than diazepam, although this has recently been questioned.[89] Patients who have been taking phenobarbital may have developed tolerance. Phenobarbital is a potential alternative to phenytoin; however, use of phenytoin results in less respiratory and sensorium depression.[16] For the treatment of neonatal SE, phenobarbital is the drug of choice.

Phenobarbital may be used to induce coma for refractory generalized convulsive SE.[91,92] Caution should be used to avoid hypotension.[92]

Paraldehyde

Paraldehyde has been used in the treatment of SE for over 100 years. It is an extremely potent anticonvulsant in the acute treatment of seizures but the intravenous form is no longer manufactured in the United States and its future as an AED is uncertain.[47] Poor understanding of its physicochemical properties has led to compatibility problems and adverse effects.[93] The water solubility of paraldehyde decreases with increasing temperature, and the change from room to body temperature may cause precipitation of paraldehyde in the bloodstream, resulting in pulmonary embolization.[93] The drug can be safely administered as a 4% solution in saline.

Paraldehyde is very sensitive to light and air; improper storage leads to decomposition.[93] The revised USP specifications state that paraldehyde must be maintained in well-filled, tight, light-resistant containers not exceeding 30 mL. Any unused portions must be discarded 24 hours after opening.[93]

The pharmacokinetics of paraldehyde make it a desirable agent for SE. After intravenous administration, the drug rapidly distributes to the brain. The drug is 70–80% metabolized by the liver and has an elimination half-life between 6 and 7.5 hours.[93]

Paraldehyde can be administered intramuscularly, orally, or rectally. The intravenous formulation is no longer available. Peak plasma levels occur within 30 minutes to 1 hour following intramuscular injection.[88] When paraldehyde is administered intramuscularly, caution should be exercised to avoid severe sciatic nerve damage. Also, skin sloughing and sterile abscesses may occur. The drug should be given by deep intramuscular injection into the buttocks. A glass syringe must be used when injecting paraldehyde because the drug decomposes plastic syringes and tubing.[93]

For rectal administration, paraldehyde can be diluted 2:1 in oil (olive or cottonseed) or mixed in 200 mL 0.9% NaCl. The slow rectal absorption limits the rectal utility of paraldehyde in SE. However, in some situations it may be the only route available. Because paraldehyde is irritative to oral mucosa, it should be given in a diluted form when administered orally.[47]

Adverse effects reported with paraldehyde include pulmonary hemorrhage, pulmonary edema, metabolic acidosis, hepatitis, and erythematous rash.[47] Oral paraldehyde can cause irritation and ulceration of the mouth and stomach and often produces foul breath (from exhaled paraldehyde).[93]

Despite the many shortcomings of paraldehyde, it is useful for patients with refractory SE not responding to standard therapy. Situations in which paraldehyde offers particular benefit include the need for initial intramuscular drug administration, SE caused by alcohol withdrawal, and when allergies to safer agents preclude their use.[16]

Lidocaine

Lidocaine is recommended as an alternative drug in the treatment of refractory SE (Table 56.4) and may control seizures when diazepam, phenytoin, phenobarbital, and/or paraldehyde have failed.[94] Lidocaine is easy to administer intravenously and has a rapid onset of action, often noted within 20–30 seconds. The effectiveness of lidocaine in the treatment of convulsive SE has been studied in small groups of patients,[95–97] but it is generally perceived to be effective.[96]

The recommended initial dose is 2–3 mg/kg, but most clinicians administer 50–100 mg. Because initial seizure control is lost after 20 minutes, lidocaine infusion at a rate of 1–2 mg/min is recommended, although higher infusion rates (3–10 mg/kg/h) may be necessary.[93] The usually quoted therapeutic range for lidocaine is 2–6 mcg/mL.[98] This range has been established for the antiarrhythmic effects of the drug; the therapeutic range for SE has not been established. CNS toxicity (e.g., fasiculations, visual disturbances, tinnitus) may occur at concentrations between 6 and 8 mcg/mL; seizures and obtundation may develop when concentrations exceed 8 mcg/mL.[98] Serum lidocaine concentrations should be monitored to avoid drug accumulation and toxicity.

Valproic Acid

Although not generally recommended, rectal administration of valproic acid represents an alternative second-line agent in SE. Less experience exists with this form of therapy as compared with paraldehyde or lidocaine. No comparative trials are available assessing valproic acid versus other AEDs in the treatment of SE. A suppository formulation of valproic acid evaluated in a small number of patients was found to be effective when administered with intravenous phenytoin.[99] The slow absorption of valproic acid from the rectal route limits its clinical usefulness in the immediate control of seizure activity.[24] An intravenous dosage form of valproic acid is not currently available but is being investigated.

Until more experience is gained, rectal administration of valproic acid in the acute setting of an SE episode is not generally recommended.[24]

Chloral Hydrate

A recent report used rectal chloral hydrate in five adult patients who were refractory to intravenous diazepam and phenytoin. Excellent clinical and EEG results were achieved.[100]

Refractory SE

If convulsive SE does not respond to recommended initial doses of a BZ, phenytoin, and phenobarbital, the condition is considered refractory and consideration should be given to anesthetizing the patient to suppress the cerebral ictal discharge.[6,15] One estimate is that about 9% of patients with generalized convulsive SE will fail therapy with these agents and about 30% with subtle manifestations of SE remain in status after administration of these three drugs.[15] Convulsive SE becomes harder to treat the longer it lasts.[101]

Midazolam has recently been suggested as the third-line agent to use if the patient does not respond to lorazepam or phenytoin. If the patient is not adequately responding after 24–48 hours and the dosage requirements are increasing, consideration should be given to pentobarbital coma.[15] Therapy with pentobarbital is initiated with a loading dose of 5–8 mg/kg over 40–60 minutes followed by an infusion of 3 mg/kg/h. The dose should be titrated until there is evidence of burst suppression on EEG. The patient should be continuously monitored; intubation and respiratory support are essential. The duration of barbiturate coma in most studies has been 2–3 days. Underlying CNS pathology may decrease the response to pentobarbital.[102] Neurologic side effects and tolerance have been reported.[103]

SE resistant to barbiturate coma has been treated with halothane and neuromuscular blockade.[47] Recently, isoflurane and propofol have been used. Isoflurane has no reported organ toxicity and produces EEG suppression at clinically useful concentrations. The dose should be titrated to prevent burst suppression. In addition to respiratory depression, hypotension may occur.[104,105] Propofol is extremely soluble in lipids and has a high volume of distribution. Its onset is very quick, and there is a quick recovery after the infusion is discontinued.[106,107] In addition to respiratory and cerebral depression, seizures have also been reported to occur with the administration of propofol.[108]

NONCONVULSIVE STATUS EPILEPTICUS

Absence Status Epilepticus

Absence SE represents the most frequently observed form of nonconvulsive SE. Rarely is absence SE the initial manifestation of a generalized seizure disorder. About 3% of all patients with absence have SE.[8] The longest reported episode of absence SE is 60 days.[13] The clinical manifestations of this disorder include an altered state of consciousness and/or behavior (lethargy, decreased mental function) and manifestation of the classic 3 per second spike-and-wave pattern on EEG.[109] Attacks are frequently caused by precipitating factors (similar to tonic–clonic SE) and avoidance of these factors may be the only therapy required. Correction of identifiable causes, such as structural or metabolic aberrations, is paramount.[13]

Absence SE should be treated as a medical emergency.[8] The acute absence SE attack can be treated by the administration of intravenous diazepam. Rectal valproic acid may also be useful. Acetazolamide IV in doses of 250–500 mg has also been used to stop absence SE.[8] Seizure cessation may be more difficult in patients with secondary generalized epilepsy than those with primary generalized epilepsy.[110] Chronic therapy to prevent recurrent attacks should be instituted with ethosuximide or valproic acid, as discussed in Chapter 55.

Atypical Absence and Myoclonic Status Epilepticus

Minor motor seizures are difficult to treat. Valproic acid is probably the drug of choice for atypical absence. Combined therapy with ethosuximide or clonazepam may be useful for refractory patients.[111] Generalized myoclonic SE is rare but may occur during absence or atypical SE. Valproic acid is probably the drug of first choice.[8]

Complex Partial Status Epilepticus

Complex partial SE occurs when clinical and electroencephalic seizure activity is focal in onset and consciousness is impaired during the attack.[112] Complex partial SE is now believed to be more common than originally thought.[12] Clinically, the difference between absence SE and complex partial SE is that absence SE manifests as a prolonged state of one attack, whereas complex partial SE is a continuous series of repeated attacks. Also, patients with complex partial SE experience phases of total unresponsiveness with stereotypical automatisms, whereas patients with absence SE do not.[112] There are distinct differences on the EEG, and the EEG is an essential part of the diagnosis.[8]

Complex partial SE should be treated aggressively because there are clinical and experimental data to suggest that memory and behavioral alterations may occur as sequelae.[8] Treatment recommendations for complex partial SE are similar to those described for convulsive SE, and include identifying the underlying cause and removing precipitating factors. The combination of intravenous diazepam and phenytoin appears to be effective. But in complex partial SE, phenytoin alone may be more beneficial, because it does not produce sedation.[110] This may represent an important advantage when evaluating a disease state with subtle symptoms.

Lorazepam may be a reasonable alternative to the diazepam-phenytoin combination in the treatment of nonconvulsive SE,[113] although sedation limits its usefulness in many instances. Therefore, although intravenous lorazepam is possibly effective, its sedative properties make intravenous phenytoin (as a single agent) a superior choice.

SPECIAL POPULATIONS

Neonates

Neonates, infants, and children represent unique patient populations with different etiologies for SE episodes. Neonatal SE is an ominous prognostic indicator. Because of the immature cortical organization of the CNS, seizure activity in the neonate is often subtle and abstruse.[114] Clinical manifestations may be limited to abnormal eye movement, repetitive eye blinking, and repetitive oral buccolingual movements such as sucking or swallowing. The classic tonic and/or clonic movements of the extremities may not be present.[114] Seizure activity must be distinguished from clonus or jitteriness that is not convulsive. The major distinguishing traits of clonus are that it is rhythmic, the alternating movements are of equal amplitudes, it is positional and thus responds to changes in position, it may be ablated by restraining the moving part, and the abnormal eye movements and sucking or swallowing common with seizures do not occur with clonus.[114]

The causes of seizures in neonates are similar to those in adults, but also include amino acid disturbances and drug withdrawal (resulting from addicted mothers).[114] A pyridoxine deficiency may exist, and an intravenous dose of 100 mg of pyridoxine may be given with EEG monitoring. If there is a pyridoxine deficiency, the EEG should become normal within several hours. Once correctable causes of seizure activity have been rectified, anticonvulsant therapy should be instituted. AEDs commonly used in the neonate include phenobarbital, phenytoin, diazepam, and paraldehyde.

Phenobarbital, the AED most commonly used in the neonatal period, is given as an intravenous loading dose of 20 mg/kg followed by a maintenance dose of 3.5–5 mg/kg/d.[89,114] Though a maintenance dose of 5 mg/kg/d might be expected to produce toxic serum phenobarbital concentrations based on the neonate's ability to metabolize the drug, the half-life drops significantly between the first and fourth week of life. Serum concentration monitoring and dosage adjustment should be instituted with chronic phenobarbital administration to maintain concentrations between 20 and 40 mcg/mL.

If phenobarbital alone is ineffective in stopping seizure activity, despite a serum concentration of 40 mcg/mL, phenytoin should be added. The intravenous route is the most desirable mode of administration for phenytoin, because of unreliable absorption from the oral route and irritation and unpredictable absorption from intramuscular administration.[114] A phenytoin loading dose of 20 mg/kg should be given.

Seizures in the neonatal period are associated with higher mortality and neurologic sequelae (e.g., mental retardation, cerebral palsy, epilepsy).[115] The best predictors of morbidity and mortality include a 5-minute Apgar score of less than seven, the need for resuscitation during the first 5 minutes after birth, early onset of seizures, seizures lasting longer than 30 minutes, and the number of days on which seizures occurred.[115]

The decision to institute chronic AED therapy in a neonate poses a therapeutic dilemma. The high frequency of neurologic toxicity from long-term AED therapy may outweigh the low risk of subsequent seizure activity.[115] Some clinicians recommend phenobarbital prophylaxis for neonates with risk factors such as severe asphyxia, intraventricular hemorrhage, and structural brain abnormalities.[116] Until controlled clinical trials are performed, the decision to institute phenobarbital (or other AED) prophylaxis will be based on clinical judgment.

Infants and Children

The pediatric doses and rates of administration for the AEDs commonly used in the treatment of SE are provided in Table 56.6. The principles of drug administration and monitoring outlined in the previous sections for adults apply to this patient population. Unlike neonates, children tend to have better capacities for metabolic and renal clearance of drugs than adults. Pediatric patients generally tolerate more rapid IV drug administration than older patients, but IV access can be a problem.[6] Close monitoring of serum concentrations and clinical response with subsequent dose titration is warranted.

Administration of intravenous phenytoin (9–21 mg/kg) eradicated seizure activity within 3 minutes in 12 out of 13 pediatric patients in SE.[117] This rapid response was produced without concomitant diazepam or phenobarbital administration. The anticipated benefit of lack of sedation was evident, and neurologic status was unaltered in all cases. Until these data are replicated in larger clinical trials, the coadministration of intravenous diazepam and phenytoin will remain the treatment of choice in pediatric patients with convulsive SE.[5]

When intravenous access is not readily available, rectal paraldehyde[6,118] and rectal valproic acid[8,119] may offer reasonable alternatives as first-line agents in the treatment of SE. Rectal paraldehyde may be given at a dose of 0.3 mL/kg. A second dose should be given within 20 minutes if seizures persist.[6,118] Valproic acid should be administered rectally at a dose of 20 mg/kg to produce serum concentrations of approximately 50 mcg/mL.[6,119] When the rectal route of administration is used to treat SE, careful monitoring of serum AED concentrations and clinical response is paramount because of the potential for hypoperfusion and poor absorption.

Pregnant Women

Seizures in pregnancy pose a risk to the mother and the fetus. While AEDs have a teratogenic risk, this is less than the risk of uncontrolled seizures. Good seizure control is associated with better fetal outcome. The treatment of the pregnant woman with SE is the same as that for a nonpregnant woman. The use of magnesium is controversial.[120]

Elderly

Changes in the pharmacokinetics of AEDs associated with aging should be considered when elderly patients are treated. Decreases in renal clearance and hepatic metabolism of AEDs may occur, resulting in toxic serum AED concentrations in this population. Pharmacodynamic or receptor site changes may also occur. Therefore, close monitoring of serum concentrations and clinical response is warranted.

Many elderly patients have decreased serum albumin concentrations, and an increase in the free/total ratio of highly bound AEDs (i.e., phenytoin) should be considered. Monitoring of both free and total serum AED concentrations may be helpful in making therapeutic decisions in this patient population. The free serum concentration should be emphasized over the total serum concentration, because the free (unbound) drug is available for diffusion to the pharmacologic receptors in the brain. Therefore, it is common for the elderly to have "subtherapeutic" total concentrations, yet "therapeutic" free concentrations. Clinical response should be monitored carefully.

Evaluation of Therapeutic Outcomes

Convulsive SE is a life-threatening condition. Therefore, therapy of SE must be aggressive. There is a tendency to underdose many of the AEDs used in the treatment of SE and priority should be given to stopping the seizures. There is less concern about drug-induced side effects in SE and more concern about preventing brain damage or death. The priority for treatment and drug administration is provided in Table 56.4. Therefore, the primary outcome for SE is to stop the seizure activity. The patient must also receive supportive care. After the seizure activity has terminated, plans for chronic AED therapy should be developed using the principles discussed in Chapter 55.

Conclusion

Although SE has been identified for more than 150 years, it remains a serious and emergent clinical entity with a high morbidity and mortality. Efforts to more precisely define and classify the various forms of SE have led to greater universal understanding and recognition of the manifestations of the disease. Convulsive SE is the most common and ominous of the various forms of SE and requires immediate treatment. Nonconvulsive SE is now recognized as producing residual morbidity if not appropriately treated. Identification and removal of the causes or precipitating factors of SE are important aspects of therapy. Equal attention must be paid to the systemic physiologic aberrations as well as the seizure activity when treating SE. The long-term follow-up of the patient with SE is very important. However, a lack of continuity of care from the emergency room to the clinic has been reported.[121]

AEDs are the mainstay of therapy. Therapy should be initiated with a drug that can be given quickly and has a rapid onset of effect. Lorazepam is becoming the agent used initially to stop seizure activity. It must be followed with an AED with a more prolonged anticonvulsant effect such as phenytoin or phenobarbital. Refractory SE may be treated with paraldehyde, lidocaine, valproic acid, and chloral hydrate. For extreme cases of refractory response, barbiturate coma or general anesthesia may be required. New agents, such as fosphenytoin, a prodrug for phenytoin, and parenteral valproic acid will offer additional therapeutic options.

The therapy for SE has evolved over time, and is not always supported by data from large, controlled clinical trials. Drugs chosen on a theoretical basis appear to be effective. Formal study is required to determine if other currently available agents, or investigational agents, offer advantages over traditional treatment choices.

References

1. Treiman DM. Generalized convulsive status epilepticus in the adult. Epilepsia 1993;34(suppl 1):S2–S11.
2. Hauser WA. Status epilepticus: Epidemiologic considerations. Neurology 1990;40(suppl 2):9–13.
3. Phillips SA, Shanahan RJ. Etiology and mortality of status epilepticus in children: A recent update. Arch Neurol 1989;46:74–76.
4. Maytal J, Shinnar S, Moshe SL, et al. Low morbidity and mortality of status epilepticus in children. Pediatrics 1989;83:323–331.
5. Pellock JM. Status epilepticus, in Dodson WE, Pellock JM (eds): Pediatric Epilepsy: Diagnosis and Therapy. New York, Demos Publications, 1993, pp 197–206.
6. Working Group on Status Epilepticus. Treatment of convulsive status epilepticus: Recommendations of the Epilepsy Foundation of America's Working Group on Status Epilepticus. JAMA 1993;270:854–859.
7. Gross-Tsur V, Shinnar S. Convulsive status epilepticus in children. Epilepsia 1993;34(suppl 1):S12–S20.
8. Cascino GD. Nonconvulsive status epilepticus in adults and children. Epilepsia 1993;34(suppl 1):S21–S28.
9. Granner MA, Lee SI. Nonconvulsive status epilepticus: EEG analysis in a large series. Epilepsia 1994;34:42–47.
10. Tomson T, Lindbom U, Nilsson BY. Nonconvulsive status epilepticus in adults: Thirty-two consecutive patients from a general hospital population. Epilepsia 1992;33:829–835.
11. Schomer DL. Focal status epilepticus and epilepsia partialis continua in adults and children. Epilepsia 1993;34(suppl 1):S29–S36.
12. Cockerell OC, Walker MC, Sander JWAS, Shorvon SD. Complex partial status epilepticus: A recurrent problem. J Neurol Neurosurg Psychiatry 1994;57:835–837.
13. Jagoda A. Nonconvulsive seizures. Emerg Med Clin North Am 1994;12:963–971.
14. DeLorenzo RJ, Towne AR, Pellock JM, Ko D. Status epilepticus in children, adults, and the elderly. Epilepsia 1992;33(suppl 4):S15–S25.
15. Bleck TP. Advances in the management of refractory status epilepticus. Crit Care Med 1993;21:955–957.
16. Shorvon S. Tonic clonic status epilepticus. J Neurol Neurosurg Psychiatry 1993;56:125–134.
17. Lothman E. The biochemical basis and pathophysiology of status epilepticus. Neurology 1990;40(suppl 2):13–23.
18. Lowenstein DH, Alldredge BK. Status epilepticus at an urban public hospital in the 1980s. Neurology 1993;43:483–488.
19. DeLorenzo RJ. Status epilepticus: Concepts in diagnosis and treatment. Semin Neurol 1990;10:396–405.
20. Barry E, Hauser WA. Status epilepticus and antiepileptic medication levels. Neurology 1994;44:47–50.
21. Barry E, Hauser WA. Status epilepticus: The interaction of epilepsy and acute brain disease. Neurology 1993;43:1473–1478.
22. Brown JK, Hussain IHMI. Status epilepticus. I: Pathogenesis. Dev Med Child Neurol 1991;33:3–17.
23. Lacroix J, Deal C, Gauthier M, et al. Admissions to a pediatric intensive care unit for status epilepticus: A 10 year experience. Crit Care Med 22:827–832.
24. Shepherd SM. Management of status epilepticus. Emerg Med Clin North Am 1994;12:941–961.
25. Sung CY, Chu NS. Status epilepticus in the elderly: Etiology, seizure type and outcome. Acta Neurol Scand 1989;80:51–56.
26. Alldredge BK, Lowenstein DH, Simon RP. Seizures associated with recreational drug abuse. Neurology 1990;39:1037–1039.
27. Callahan DJ, Noetzel MJ. Prolonged absence status epilepticus associated with carbamazepine therapy, increased intracranial pressure, and transient MRI abnormalities. Neurology 1992;42:2198–2201.
28. Thomas P, Lebrun C, Chatel M. De novo absence status epilepticus as a benzodiazepine withdrawal syndrome. Epilepsia 1993;34:355–358.
29. Treiman DM. General principles of treatment: Responsive and intractable status epilepticus in adults, in Delgado-Escueta AV, Wasterlain CG, Treiman DM, Porter RJ (eds): Status Epilepticus. New York, Raven Press, 1983, pp 377–384.
30. Munn RI, Farrell K. Failure to recognize status epilepticus in a paralysed patient. Can J Neurol Sci 1993; 20:234–236.
31. Cranford RE, Leppik IE, Patrick B, et al. Intravenous phenytoin in acute treatment of seizures. Neurology 1979;29:1474–1479.
32. Leppik IE. Status Epilepticus (State of the Science in EEG and Epilepsy—1986). Seattle, WA, American Electro-

encephalographic Society and American Epilepsy Society, 1986.
33. Walton NY. Systemic effects of generalized convulsive status epilepticus. Epilepsia 1993;34(suppl 1):S54–S58.
34. Wijdicks EFM, Hubmayr RD. Acute acid–base disorders associated with status epilepticus. Mayo Clin Proc 1994;69:1044–1046.
35. Barry E., Hauser WA. Pleocytosis after status epilepticus. Arch Neurol 1994;51:190–193.
36. Leppik IE. Status epilepticus: The next decade. Neurology 1990;40(suppl 2):4–9.
37. Dodrill CB, Wilensky AJ. Intellectual impairment as an outcome of status epilepticus. Neurology 1990;40(suppl 2):23–27.
38. Wasterlain CG, Fujikawa DG, Penix L, Sankar R. Pathophysiological mechanisms of brain damage from status epilepticus. Epilepsia 1993;34(suppl 1):S37–S53.
39. Lothman EW, Bertram EH. Epileptogenic effects of status epilepticus. Epilepsia 1993;34(suppl 1):S59–S70.
40. Towne AR, Pellock JM, Ko D, DeLorenzo RJ. Determinants of mortality in status epilepticus. Epilepsia 1994;35:27–34.
41. Calabrese VP, Gruemer HD, Tripathi HL, et al. Serum cortisol and cerebrospinal fluid beta-endorphins in status epilepticus. Arch Neurol 1993;50:689–693.
42. Aicardie J, Chevrie JJ. Convulsive status epilepticus in infants and children. A study of 239 cases. Epilepsia 1970;11:187–197.
43. Verity CM, Ross EM, Golding J. Outcome of childhood status epilepticus and lengthy febrile convulsions: Findings of national cohort study. Br Med J 1993;307:225–228.
44. Maytal J, Shinnar S. Febrile status epilepticus. Pediatrics 1990;86:611–616.
45. Hou JW, Wang PJ, Lin MY, et al. Complex partial status epilepticus: Report of one case. Acta Paediatr Scand 1989;30:254–260.
46. Desbiens R, Berkovic SF, Dubeau F, et al. Life-threatening focal status epilepticus due to occult cortical dysplasia. Arch Neurol 1993;50:695–700.
47. Ramsay RE. Treatment of status epilepticus. Epilepsia 1993;34(suppl 1):S71–S81.
48. Browne TR. The pharmacokinetics of agents used to treat status epilepticus. Neurology 1990;40(suppl 2):28–32.
49. Treiman DM. Pharmacokinetics and clinical use of benzodiazepines in the management of status epilepticus. Epilepsia 1989;30(suppl 2):S4–S10.
50. Treiman DM. The role of benzodiazepines in the management of status epilepticus. Neurology 1990;40(suppl 2):32–42.
51. Rivera R, Segnini M, Baltodano A, Perez V. Midazolam in the treatment of status epilepticus in children. Crit Care Med 1993;21:991–994.
52. Parent JM, Lowenstein DH. Treatment of refractory generalized status epilepticus with continuous infusion of midazolam. Neurology 1994;44:1837–1840.
53. Shader RI, Greenblatt DJ. The use of benzodiazepines in clinical practice. Br J Clin Pharmacol 1981;11:55–95.
54. Delgado-Escueta AV, Enrile-Bascal F. Combination therapy for status epilepticus: Intravenous diazepam and phenytoin, in Delgado-Escueta AV, Wasterlain CG, Treiman DM, Porter RJ (eds): Status Epilepticus. New York, Raven Press, 1983, pp 477–485.
55. Tassinari CA, Michelucci DR, Bureau M, et al. Benzodiazepines: Efficacy in status epilepticus, in Delgado-Escueta AV, Wasterlain CG, Treiman DM, Porter RJ (eds): Status Epilepticus. New York, Raven Press, 1983, pp 465–475.
56. Bell HE, Bertino JS. Constant diazepam infusion in the treatment of continuous seizure activity. Drug Intell Clin Pharm 1984;18:965–970.
57. Arruda WO, Brito FD, Rosa SL, et al. Factors affecting diazepam availability from intravenous admixture solutions. Arq Neuropsiquiatr 1989;47:291–294.
58. Mason NA, Cline S, Hyneck ML, et al. Factors affecting diazepam infusion: Solubility, administration-set composition, and flow rate. Am J Hosp Pharm 1981;38:1449–1554.
59. Devilat M, Demarta JC, Masafierro MP, et al. Treatment of status epilepticus with rectally administered diazepam. Rev Chil Pediatr 1990;61:127–130.
60. Albano A, Reisdorff EJ, Wiegenstein JG. Rectal diazepam in pediatric status epilepticus. Am J Emerg Med 1989;7:168–172.
61. Camfield CS, Camfield PR, Smithe E, et al. Home use of rectal diazepam to prevent status epilepticus in children with convulsive disorders. J Child Neurol 1989;4:125–126.
62. Milligan N, Dhillon S, Richens A, et al. Rectal diazepam in the treatment of absence status: A pharmacodynamic study. J Neurol Neurosurg Psychiatry 1981;41:914–917.
63. Knudsen FU. Rectal administration of diazepam in solution in the acute treatment of convulsions in infants and children. Arch Dis Childhood 1979;54:855–857.
64. Schmidt D. Benzodiazepines: Diazepam, in Levy RH, Dreifuss FE, et al. (eds): Antiepileptic Drugs, 3rd ed. New York, Raven Press, 1989, 735–764.
65. Levy RJ, Krall RL. Treatment of status epilepticus with lorazepam. Arch Neurol 1984;41:605–611.
66. Greenblatt DJ, Divoll M. Diazepam versus lorazepam: Relationship of drug distribution to duration of clinical action, in Delgado-Escueta AV, Wasterlain CG, Treiman DM, Porter RJ (eds): Status Epilepticus. New York, Raven Press, 1983, pp 487–491.
67. Walton NY, Treiman DM. Lorazepam treatment of experimental status epilepticus in the rat: Relevance to clinical practice. Neurology 1990;40:990–994.
68. Homan RW, Walker JE. Clinical studies of lorazepam in status epilepticus, in Delgado-Escueta AV, Wasterlain CG, Treiman DM, Porter RJ (eds): Status Epilepticus. New York, Raven Press, 1983, pp 493–498.
69. Leppik IE, Derivan AT, Homan RW, et al. Double-blind study of lorazepam and diazepam in status epilepticus. JAMA 1983;249(11):1452–1454.
70. Crawford TO, Mitchell WG, Snodgrass SR. Lorazepam in childhood status epilepticus and serial seizures: Effectiveness and tachyphylaxis. Neurology 1987;37:190–195.
71. Giang DW, McBride MC. Lorazepam versus diazepam for the treatment of status epilepticus. Pediatr Neurol 1988;4:358–361.
72. Labar DR, Ali A, Root J. High-dose intravenous lorazepam for the treatment of refractory status epilepticus. Neurology 1994;44:1400–1403.

73. Wilder BJ. Efficacy of phenytoin in treatment of status epilepticus, in Delgado-Escueta AV, Wasterlain CG, Treiman DM, Porter RJ (eds): Status Epilepticus. New York, Raven Press, 1983, pp 441–446.
74. Leppik IE, Patrick BK, Cranford RE. Treatment of acute seizures and status epilepticus with intravenous phenytoin, in Delgado-Escueta AV, Wasterlain CG, Treiman DM, Porter RJ (eds): Status Epilepticus. New York, Raven Press, 1983, pp 447–451.
75. Cloyd JC, Gumnit RJ, McLain LW. Status epilepticus: The role of intravenous phenytoin. JAMA 1980;244(13):1479–1481.
76. Tozer TN, Winter M. Phenytoin, in Evans WE, Schentag JJ, Jusko WJ (eds): Applied Pharmacokinetics, 3rd ed. Spokane, WA, Applied Therapeutics, 1992, pp 25-1–25-44.
77. Donovan PJ, Cline D. Phenytoin administration by constant intravenous infusion: Selective rates of administration. Ann Emerg Med 1991;20:139–142.
78. Carmichael RR, Mahoney DC, Jeffrey LP. Solubility and stability of phenytoin sodium when mixed with intravenous solutions. Am J Hosp Pharm 1980;37:95–98.
79. Markowsky SJ, Kohls PR, Ehresman D, et al. Compatibility and pH variability of four injectable phenytoin sodium products. Am J Hosp Pharm 1991;48:510–514.
80. Earnest MP, Marx JA, Drury LR. Complications of intravenous phenytoin for acute treatment of seizures: Recommendations for usage. JAMA 1983;249(6):762–765.
81. Comer JB. Extravasation from intravenous phenytoin. Am J IV Ther Clin Nutr 1984;11(1):23–29.
82. Cranford RE, Leppik IE, Patrick B, et al. Intravenous phenytoin: Clinical and pharmacokinetic aspects. Neurology 1978;28:874–880.
83. Abernathy DR, Greenblatt DJ. Phenytoin disposition in obesity: Determination of loading dose. Arch Neurol 1985;42:468–471.
84. Richard MO, Chiron C, d'Athis P, et al. Phenytoin monitoring in status epilepticus in infants and children. Epilepsia 1993;34:144–150.
85. Garnett WR, Kugler AR, O'Hara KA, et al. A five-day randomized, double-blind, placebo-controlled, parallel-group clinical study of tolerance, safety, and pharmacokinetics of multiple doses of intramuscularly administered fosphenytoin sodium substituted for oral Dilantin in epilepsy patients. Neurology 1995;45(suppl 4):-A248.
86. Wilder BJ, Campbell K, Ramsay RE, et al. Safety and tolerance of multiple doses of intramuscularly administered fosphenytoin (Cerebyx) substituted for oral phenytoin (Dilantin) in epilespy or neurosurgery patients. Neurology. In press.
87. Goldberg MA, McIntyre HB. Barbiturates in the treatment of status epilepticus, in Delgado-Escueta AV, Wasterlain CG, Treiman DG, Porter RJ (eds): Status Epilepticus. New York, Raven Press, 1983, pp 499–503.
88. Ramsay RE. Pharmacokinetics and clinical use of parenteral phenytoin, phenobarbital, and paraldehyde. Epilepsia 1989;30(suppl 2):S1–S3.
89. Shaner DM, McCurdy SA, Herring MO, et al. Treatment of status epilepticus: A prospective comparison of diazepam and phenytoin versus phenobarbital and optional phenytoin. Neurology 1988;38:202–207.
90. Holmes GL. Phenobarbital bolus dose for status epilepticus [letter]. Am J Hosp Pharm 1994;51:1578.
91. Mirski MA, William MA, Hanley DF. Prolonged pentobarbital and phenobarbital coma for refractory generalized status epilepticus. Crit Care Med 1995;23:400–404.
92. Yaffe K, Lowenstein DH. Prognostic factors of pentobarbital therapy for refractory generalized status epilepticus. Neurology 1993;43:895–900.
93. Browne TR. Paraldehyde, chlormethiazole, and lidocaine for treatment of status epilepticus, in Delgado-Escueta AV, Wasterlain CG, Treiman DM, Porter RJ (eds): Status Epilepticus. New York, Raven Press, 1983, pp 509–517.
94. Aggarwal P, Wali JP. Lidocaine in refractory status epilepticus: A forgotten drug in the emergency department. Am J Emerg Med 1993:11:243–244.
95. DeGiorgio CM, Altman K, Hamilton-Byrd E, Rabinowicz AL. Lidocaine in refractory status epilepticus: Confirmation of efficacy with continuous EEG monitoring. Epilepsia 1992:33:913–916.
96. Pascual J, Sedano MJ, Polo JM, Berciano J. Intravenous lidocaine for status epilepticus. Epilepsia 1988;29:584–589.
97. Pascual J, Ciudan J, Berciano J. Role of lidocaine (lignocaine) in managing status epilepticus. J Neurol Neurosurg Psychiatry 1992;55:49–51.
98. Pieper JA, Johnson KE. Lidocaine, in Evans WE, Schentag JJ, Jusko WJ (eds). Applied Pharmacokinetics, 3rd ed. Spokane, WA, Applied Therapeutics, 1992, pp 21-1–21-37.
99. Vajda FJ. Valproic acid in the treatment of status epilepticus, in Delgado-Escueta AV, Wasterlain CG, Treiman DM, Porter RJ (eds): Status Epilepticus. New York, Raven Press, 1983, pp 519–529.
100. Lampl Y, Eshel Y, Gilad R, et al. Chloral hydrate in intractable status epilepticus. Ann Emerg Med 1990;19:674–676.
101. Walton NY, Treiman DM. Motor and electroencephalographic response of refractory experimental status epilepticus to treatment with MK-801, diazepam, or MK-801 plus diazepam. Brain Res 1991;553:97–104.
102. Van Ness PC. Pentobarbital and EEG burst suppression in treatment of status epilepticus refractory to benzodiazepines and phenytoin. Epilepsia 1990;31:61–67.
103. Osorio I, Reed RC. Treatment of refractory generalized tonic–clonic status epilepticus with pentobarbital anesthesia after high-dose phenytoin. Epilepsia 1989; 30:464–467.
104. Kofke WA, Young RS, Davis P, et al. Isoflurane for refractory status epilepticus: A clinical series. Anesthesiology 1989;71:653–659.
105. Meeke RI, Soifer BE, Gelb AW. Isoflurane for the management of status epilepticus. DICP 1989;23:579–581.
106. Borgeat A, Wilder-Smith OHG, Jallon P, Suter PM. Propofol in the management of refractory status epilepticus: A case report. Intensive Care Med 1994;20:148–149.
107. Pitt-Miller PL, Elcock BJ, Maharaj M. The management of status epilepticus with a continuous propofol infusion. Anesth Analg 1994;78:1193–1194.
108. Makela JP, Iivanainen M, Pieninkeroinen IP, et al. Seizures associated with propofol anesthesia. Epilepsia 1993;34:832–835.

109. Porter RJ, Penry JK. Petit mal status, in Delgado-Escueta AV, Wasterlain CG, Treiman DM, Porter RJ (eds): Status Epilepticus. New York, Raven Press, 1983, pp 61–67.
110. Thomson T, Svanborg E, Wedlund JE. Nonconvulsive status epilepticus: High incidence of complex partial status. Epilepsia 1986;27(3):276–285.
111. Yasuhara A, Yoshide H, Hatanaka T, et al. Epilepsy with continuous spike-waves during slow sleep and its treatment. Epilepsia 1991;32:59–62.
112. Treiman DM, Delgado-Escueta AV. Complex partial status epilepticus, in Delgado-Escueta AV, Wasterlain CG, Treiman DM, Porter RJ (eds): Status Epilepticus. New York, Raven Press, 1983, pp 69–81.
113. Walker JE, Homan RW, Crawford IL. Lorazepam: A controlled trial in patients with intractable partial complex seizures. Epilepsia 1984;25(4):464–466.
114. Painter MJ. General principles of treatment: Status epilepticus in neonates, in Delgado-Escueta AV, Wasterlain CG, Treiman DM, Porter RJ (eds): Status Epilepticus. New York, Raven Press, 1983, pp 385–393.
115. Gal P. Anticonvulsant therapy after neonatal seizures: How long should it be continued? I. A case for early discontinuation of anticonvulsants. Pharmacotherapy 1985;5(5):268–273.
116. Hodson A. Anticonvulsant therapy after neonatal seizures: How long should it be continued? II. A case for long-term treatment with anticonvulsants. Pharmacotherapy 1985;5(5):274–277.
117. Koren G, Brand N, Halkin H, et al. Kinetics of intravenous phenytoin in children. Pediatr Pharmacol 1984;4:31–38.
118. Curless RG, Holzman BH, Ramsay RE. Paraldehyde therapy in childhood status epilepticus. Arch Neurol 1983;40:477–480.
119. Snead OC, Miles MV. Treatment of status epilepticus in children with rectal sodium valproate. J Pediatr 1985;106(2):323–325.
120. Jagoda A, Riggio S. Emergency department approach to managing seizures in pregnancy. Ann Emerg Med 1991;20:80–85.
121. Krumhola A, Grufferman S, Orr ST, et al. Seizures and seizure care in an emergency department. Epilepsia 1989;30:175–181.

Chapter 57

Acute Management of the Head Injury Patient

Bradley A. Boucher, PharmD, and Stephanie J. Phelps, PharmD, FCCP

The incidence of head injury in the United States is approximately 200 per 100,000, resulting in more than 420,000 new cases in 1980.[1] Motor vehicle accidents account for approximately 50% of all adult cases while falls, assaults, gunshot wounds, occupational accidents, and other miscellaneous causes account for the remaining cases.[1] In small children, falls are the most common cause of head injury followed by motor vehicle accidents. The majority of head trauma occurs in early adult life in persons who are free of medical problems; peak age for acute neurotrauma is 15–24 years.[1] Productivity losses secondary to trauma, in general, exceed that of heart disease, stroke, and cancer combined.[2] In addition to extensive morbidity and mortality, the economic cost of acute neurotrauma is also staggering. It is estimated that the lifetime costs of trauma cases in the United States in 1985 exceeded $64 billion.[2] The mean first-year treatment costs of managing a patient with an acute severe head or spinal cord injury are $105,000.[3] Considering the excessive physical, emotional, and economic costs associated with severe neurotrauma, even small improvements in the management of these patients should bring great dividends to individuals and society.

PATHOPHYSIOLOGY

PRIMARY HEAD INJURY

The neurologic sequelae of head trauma can occur instantaneously as a consequence of the primary injury or can result from secondary injuries that follow within minutes to days. Primary injury involves the external transfer of kinetic energy to various structural components of the head (e.g., nerve cells, nerve synapses, supporting cells of the brain [glial cells], and cerebral blood vessels).[4] The biomechanical forces responsible for primary head injury can be broadly classified as concussive/compressive (e.g., blunt object blow, penetrating missile injuries) and acceleration–deceleration (e.g., motor vehicle accidents). Primary injuries are further categorized as focal or diffuse.[4] The latter are usually associated with shearing forces, which affect axons within the brain.

SECONDARY BRAIN INJURY

A complex sequence of secondary pathophysiologic events precipitated by primary head injury may seriously disrupt the normal central nervous system (CNS) balance between oxygen supply and demand.[5] Specific causes of secondary head injury include cerebral edema, expanding mass lesions (e.g., epidural, subdural, and intracerebral hematomas), and cerebral vasospasm. Seizures, agitation, and temperature elevation may further disrupt this balance. The key pathophysiologic process triggering secondary brain injury is cerebral ischemia.[5] The brain is particularly susceptible to ischemia because it has little capacity to store oxygen, glucose, and high-energy phosphate compounds [e.g., adenosine triphosphate (ATP)]. Careful study of ischemia following head injury has documented that it is typically an early event that occurs less than 6 hours after the insult.[6] Patients studied after this 6-hour window frequently have hyperemia (i.e., "luxury perfusion"). This latter phenomenon is the result of an uncoupling of oxygen delivery (CDo_2) and consumption ($CMRo_2$) in the brain, a process that is closely autoregulated by the brain under normal conditions.[5]

One of the major effects of cerebral ischemia is hypoxia and alterations in cellular homeostasis. Hypoxia can also develop from systemic causes such as acute respiratory failure and hypotension. Loss of cellular integrity can lead to major intracellular and extracellular ionic shifts, resulting in cytotoxic edema and disruption of neuronal electrical conduction.[5] Vasogenic cerebral edema can also occur as a consequence of cerebral capillary endothelial damage.[5] Cytotoxic and vasogenic edema result in expansion of the intracellular and interstitial fluid spaces, respectively. Elevated intracranial pressure (ICP) is the most detrimental consequence of cerebral edema formation and occurs as the brain tissue volume increases within the nondistensible skull. Expanding CNS hematomas and cerebral contusions may also elevate ICP. A significant increase in ICP may further compromise cerebral blood flow (CBF) and extend cytotoxic edema. Hence, an increase in ICP may be self-perpetuating unless this cycle is reversed. Extreme elevations in ICP may also cause brain herniation, which is associated with substantial morbidity and mortality. Another pathophysiologic consequence of ischemia is intracerebral acidosis, which may further contribute to neurologic dysfunction.[7,8]

The failure of cerebral cellular ionic pumps is thought to be an important event in perpetuating secondary brain injury. Specifically, there is a cellular influx of sodium, chloride, and water with a corresponding efflux of potassium when the Na^+/K^+-ATPase pump begins to fail.[5] Another important ionic alteration that occurs following severe head injury is cellular efflux of magnesium. Depletion of magnesium has the potential to affect a number of metabolic processes (e.g., glucolysis, oxidative phosphorylation, protein synthesis), and enzymatic reactions. Magnesium depletion also affects regulation of calcium transport that results in accumulation.[7] Calcium transport is also modulated by other mediators including the excitatory amines, glutamate and aspartate, and acetylcholine, which increase dramatically following acute head injury.[7,9] The rise in glutamate, aspartate, and acetylcholine may be stimulated by the increase in extracellular potassium following pump failure.[9] Opiate receptor activation may also modulate the release of these "excitotoxins."[10] Specifically, activation of the μ and Δ opiate receptors may attenuate the excitotoxic effects following head injury. In contrast, K-receptor activation by endogenous opiates may have a detrimental effect on cerebral microcirculatory blood flow following head injury. The influx of calcium across the cell membrane induced by glutamate and aspartate occurs through their agonist activity at the *N*-methyl-D-aspartate (NMDA) receptor.[11] It is at the NMDA receptor that normal extracellular concentrations of magnesium act to block or gate the influx of calcium.

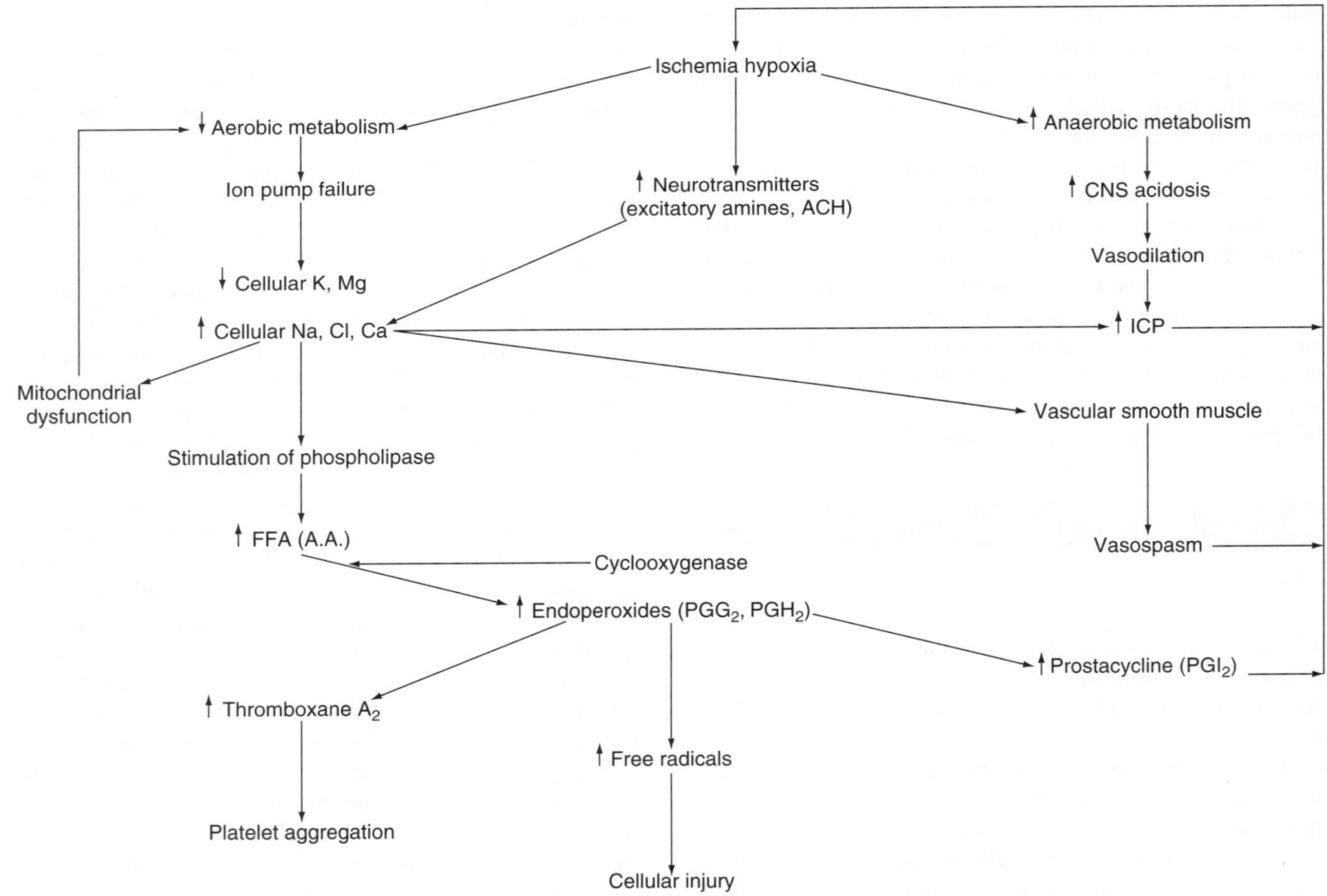

Figure 57.1. Schematic illustration of the cascade of biochemical events proposed to occur following severe neurotrauma. *(From Kirsch JR, Dean JM, Rogers MC. Current concepts in brain resuscitation. Arch Intern Med 1986;146:1415. Copyright 1986, American Medical Association.)*

The effect of calcium influx and accumulation is thought to initiate a number of pathologic events. One of these events is cerebral vasospasm, which could lead to further ischemia.[5] High intracellular concentrations of calcium can also result in mitochondrial dysfunction, which inhibits cellular respiration, a process already affected by ischemic and/or hypoxic insults.[7,9] A third major deleterious effect of calcium is to stimulate activation of proteases and lipases including calpains, phospholipase A2, lipooxygenase, and cyclooxygenase.[7] Calpain I is thought to interact with several substrates in the CNS to degrade major structural proteins. The effect of lipase stimulation includes formation of several arachidonic acid metabolites derived from membrane lipids: thromboxane A_2, prostaglandin G_2, prostaglandin H_2, prostacyclin, and leukotrienes. The subsequent effects of these metabolites include platelet aggregation, vasoconstriction, and lipid peroxidation. A by-product of lipid peroxidation is the formation of oxygen free radical species.[12] Iron released from damaged red blood cells may be a key component of this process. Lipid peroxidation is an especially damaging event since the formation of oxygen free radicals can be a self-perpetuating event resulting in further cellular membrane destruction unless quenched by endogenous antioxidants (e.g., vitamin E, superoxide dismutase). This process can also be fueled by introduction of oxygen into a previously ischemic region (i.e., "reperfusion injury").[13] Figure 57.1 summarizes the processes that constitute secondary brain injury and their various interrelationships.

In addition to CNS effects, head injury also results in a graded, complex, systemic metabolic response believed to be mediated by the neuroendocrine system and the sympathetic nervous system.[14] Trauma causes an increase in serum and urinary catecholamine concentrations. Also, increases in pituitary and adrenocorticoid activity cause an elevation in serum glucocorticoid concentration. The overall result of this response is a hypermetabolic state characterized by an elevation of energy expenditures and urinary nitrogen excretion.[14] Additional features of this condition include increased liver synthesis of acute-phase proteins, increased gluconeogenesis, decreased synthesis of constitutive protein, and leukocytosis. Thyroid function may also be altered; however, the influence of thyroid hormones on the observed metabolic rate and oxygen consumption after injury is not clearly defined.

Initial Assessment

An initial neurologic examination is important for assessing the extent of brain injury in trauma patients and establishing a baseline for future comparison. The level of consciousness of head injury patients on admission ranges from awake and alert to completely unresponsive. The Glasgow Coma Scale (GCS) is the most widely used system to grade the arousal and functional capacity of the cerebral cortex.[15] The GCS defines the level of consciousness according to eye opening, motor response, and verbal response (Table 57.1). A GCS of 15 is equivalent to a normal neurologic examination. A GCS of 3–8, 9–12, and 13–14 is consistent with severe, moderate, and minor head injury, respectively. In addition to the GCS, an assessment of pupillary response to light and any eye movement abnormalities provides a measure of brainstem function.[16] A dilated pupil and contralateral hemiparesis are strong indicators of increased ICP. The possibility of ethanol, or drug intoxication, or hypotension altering the neurologic examination should always be considered. Because narcotic and muscle relaxants affect the neurologic examination, they should not be administered until the initial examination is complete. Patients with mild head injuries may present with dizziness, drowsiness, headache, nausea, or vomiting, and a history of transient loss of consciousness. Significant post-traumatic amnesia (e.g., >1 hour), increasing dizziness, a moderate to severe headache, limb weakness or paresthesia, CSF otorrhea or rhinorrhea, and seizures indicate more severe injury.[16] A rapid deterioration in mental status strongly suggests the presence of an expanding lesion within the skull.

In addition to a profoundly abnormal neurologic examination, patients with severe head injury also may have significant alterations or instability in their vital signs including abnormal breathing patterns (e.g., apnea, Cheyne–Stokes respiration, tachypnea), hypertension, or bradycardia. Hypotension is rarely caused by the primary head injury but usually occurs as a result of blood loss, spinal cord injury (e.g., neurogenic shock), or impaired cardiac function.[16] After stabilization of vital signs, a thorough physical examination and patient history should be performed. A history of the traumatic event as reported by the patient or eyewitnesses can also provide valuable information. The physical examination should identify injuries that may result in secondary brain injury. For example, airway obstruction and aspiration may compromise pulmonary gas exchanged, chest trauma may affect both pulmonary and cardiac function (e.g., rib fractures, tension pneumothorax, cardiac tamponade), and substantial blood loss from intra-abdominal or vascular injuries may decrease the blood's oxygen-carrying capacity. Examination of the head and skull may reveal penetrating brain injuries (e.g., missile entrance wound, depressed skull fracture) or the presence of periorbital ecchymosis ("raccoon eyes"), hemotympanum, and retroauricular ecchymosis (Battle's sign), common signs of a basilar skull fracture.

Computed tomography (CT) of the head and spine is an important diagnostic tool for detecting the presence of mass lesions. Radiographs are also used to detect spinal injuries, skull fractures, and injuries to other sites. Initial and follow-up laboratory tests should include serum electrolytes, blood glucose, complete blood count, and arterial

TABLE 57.1. GLASGOW COMA SCALE

	Response	Score
Eyes	Open spontaneously	4
	To verbal command	3
	To pain	2
	No response	1
Best Motor Response		
To verbal command	Obeys	6
To painful stimulus (pressure to nailbeds)	Localizes pain	5
	Flexion-withdrawal	4
	Flexion-abnormal (decorticate rigidity)	3
	Extension (decerebrate rigidity)	2
	No response	1
Best Verbal Response		
(Arouse patient with painful stimulus if necessary)	Oriented and converses	5
	Disoriented and converses	4
	Inappropriate words	3
	Incomprehensible sounds	2
	No response	1
	Total	3–15

(From Ref. 15.)

blood gases (in patients with evidence of respiratory compromise), blood ethanol level, and a urine drug screen.

A continuous ICP monitor (e.g., intraventricular catheter, intracranial subarachnoid bolt, subdural bolt, or epidural monitor) should be employed in patients at risk for elevated ICP based on physical examination, or in patients with a GCS ≤8. Continuous ICP monitoring decreases the morbidity and mortality following head injury by enabling the diagnosis of important increases in ICP in the absence of clinical findings. It also provides an objective measurement of the therapeutic success of strategies used to decrease ICP. Normal ICP ranges from 0–10 mm Hg; ICP is generally considered elevated when values exceed 20 mm Hg. An increase in ICP occurs in 54% of patients with severe head injury.[17] The ICP may be within the normal range initially and rise over a period of hours to days, or be markedly elevated upon presentation (e.g., intracranial hemorrhage). Only 37% of patients with ICP exceeding 40 mm Hg for more than 15 minutes have favorable outcomes.[18]

Clinical Course/Prognosis

The clinical course of head injury depends on the severity of the insult, concurrent injuries, and development of complications. Most patients with mild head injury recover without significant neurologic complications. In contrast, among the 400,000 patients who are hospitalized secondary to severe head injury, approximately 25,000 will die during their hospitalization and another 150,000 will have significant permanent neurologic disabilities.[4] Poor prognostic signs of survival include GCS <5, uncontrolled ICP elevation, and the presence of flaccidity, decerebrate posturing, or fixed dilated pupils.[19] Associated complications are another major source of morbidity and mortality and include development of nosocomial pneumonia, acute respiratory distress syndrome (ARDS), deep venous thrombosis, pulmonary emboli, bacterial meningitis, urinary tract infections, severe sepsis, diabetes insipidus, syndrome of inappropriate antidiuretic hormone secretion (SIADH), and acute gastritis.[20] The rapid attenuation of the processes of secondary brain injury and aggressive management of associated complications offer the most promise for improving the short- and long-term prognosis for patients following moderate to severe head injury.

Therapeutic Management

EVALUATION OF THERAPEUTIC OUTCOMES

The overall therapeutic goals in patients with acute head trauma are (1) establishment of an adequate airway, maintenance of breathing and circulation during the initial period of evaluation; (2) maintenance of balance between $C\dot{D}O_2$ and $CMRO_2$; (3) prevention or attenuation of secondary injury pathophysiologic processes; and (4) prevention and/or treatment of associated medical complications. Collectively, the first three of these goals constitute the process of *cerebral resuscitation.* Achievement of these goals by successfully managing the patient and returning them ideally to their preinjury neurologic status is the benchmark on which all therapies to be discussed are measured. For patients surviving their acute event, the relative long-term success or failure for each of the available treatment modalities must then be measured against the patient's return to their baseline neurologic state. One of the most commonly used assessment tools for this purpose in head injury patients is known as the Glasgow Outcome Scale. This straightforward scale categorizes patient outcome as (1) death, (2) persistent vegetative state, (3) severe disability (conscious but disabled), (4) moderate disability (disabled but independent), and (5) good recovery. Other quality of life outcome measurements used in head injury patients include cognitive tests (e.g., language, verbal learning, memory), level of productive activity (e.g., return to work or school), residential status, and hours/day of attendant care or supervision. These objective outcome criteria, typically measured at least 6 months postinjury, are particularly useful to clinicians and payers in evaluating the relative merits of costly available rehabilitation programs for these patients.

INITIAL RESUSCITATION

The first priority in the unconscious head injury patient is to establish an airway, which is of paramount importance to ensure adequate oxygenation and prevent aspiration. The cervical spine should also be immobilized in any patient with a suspected spinal cord injury to prevent extension of the injury. Patients with severe head injury should be hyperventilated during the first 24 hours to acutely reduce elevated ICP. Another empiric maneuver to reduce increased ICP is to elevate the head of the bed to 30° thereby promoting cerebral venous drainage.

Maintenance of adequate systemic blood pressure in a normotensive range is another immediate priority during the initial resuscitative and intensive care periods.[5] Prolonged hypotension will compromise CBF further, exacerbating cerebral ischemia; whereas excessively high blood pressure may result in elevation of ICP, especially if autoregulatory mechanisms have been compromised. Although hypotension is not a common consequence of an isolated head injury, it is frequently present secondary to other concurrent injuries causing hypovolemia. In those head injury patients with hypotension, controversy exists as to the optimal resuscitative fluid. Based on available data, it is recommended that the more economical alternative, isotonic saline, be routinely used over colloids (e.g., albumin).[21] Regardless of the fluid used, the goal of therapy in these patients should be euvolemia or mild dehydration. Vasopressors and inotropic agents may be needed to maintain adequate mean arterial pressure (MAP) if hypotension persists after adequate restoration of intravascular volume.[22]

In contrast to hypotension, hypertension is a relatively common clinical finding in head injury patients.[23] The major problem with excessively high blood pressure (systolic blood pressure >200 mm Hg) is the potential for further ICP elevation. This detrimental effect relates to an increase in cerebral perfusion pressure (CPP), which occurs from an increase in MAP in patients who have lost autoregulation (i.e., CPP = MAP − ICP). Choice of antihypertensive treatment following brain injury is controversial. Nonetheless, the following general principles are offered. Use of the venodilators, nitroprusside and nitroglycerine, and selected calcium channel blockers (e.g., nicardipine, diltiazem) should be avoided since they may have the undesirable effect of increasing cerebral venous capacitance and, hence, cerebral blood volume.[22] Alternatively, α and β blockers may be the preferred agents since they do not affect ICP.[5] Angiotensin-converting enzyme inhibitors (ACEIs) may also be useful in shifting the lower autoregulatory limit downward, preserving CBF at a lower MAP.[5] Use of sedatives (e.g., benzodiazepines, barbiturates) and opiate analgesics may also be effective in lowering transiently increased blood pressure; however, the ability to assess the patient's neurologic status accurately may be affected.[5] Individualization of therapy and setting of appropriate blood pressure targets should take into account the degree of ICP control by other methods, erring on the side of mild to moderate hypertension versus iatrogenic hypotension.

Once the patient is hemodynamically stable, total daily fluid intake is limited to 60–80% of calculated maintenance requirements (or by administering normal amounts of maintenance fluid accompanied by the judicious use of diuretics) to prevent the exacerbation of cerebral edema or hyponatremia (e.g., SIADH). In either management scheme, the daily fluid intake and output must be monitored very closely in order to maintain a slightly negative fluid balance. Medications should be maximally concentrated and administered in 0.9% sodium chloride whenever possible. Aggressive nutritional support of the head injury patient is another important therapeutic consideration.[14,24] Figure 57.2 is an algorithm for the initial management of acute head injury that outlines treatment priorities in these patients. Similarly, Fig. 57.3 summarizes the stepwise management of increased ICP using the strategies outlined in the following section.

ELEVATED INTRACRANIAL PRESSURE

Surgical Intervention

Approximately 40% of all patients with severe head injury have an intracranial mass lesion that often results in an elevation in ICP. Early surgical repair of correctable lesions (e.g., evacuation of hematomas, elevation of depressed skull fractures, debridement of penetrating wound tracts) is important in preventing and managing increased ICP.

Posture

A 30° elevation of the patient's head promotes venous drainage and decreases ICP. The decrease in ICP is most significant when the head is elevated and maintained in the midline position, thus avoiding obstruction of the internal

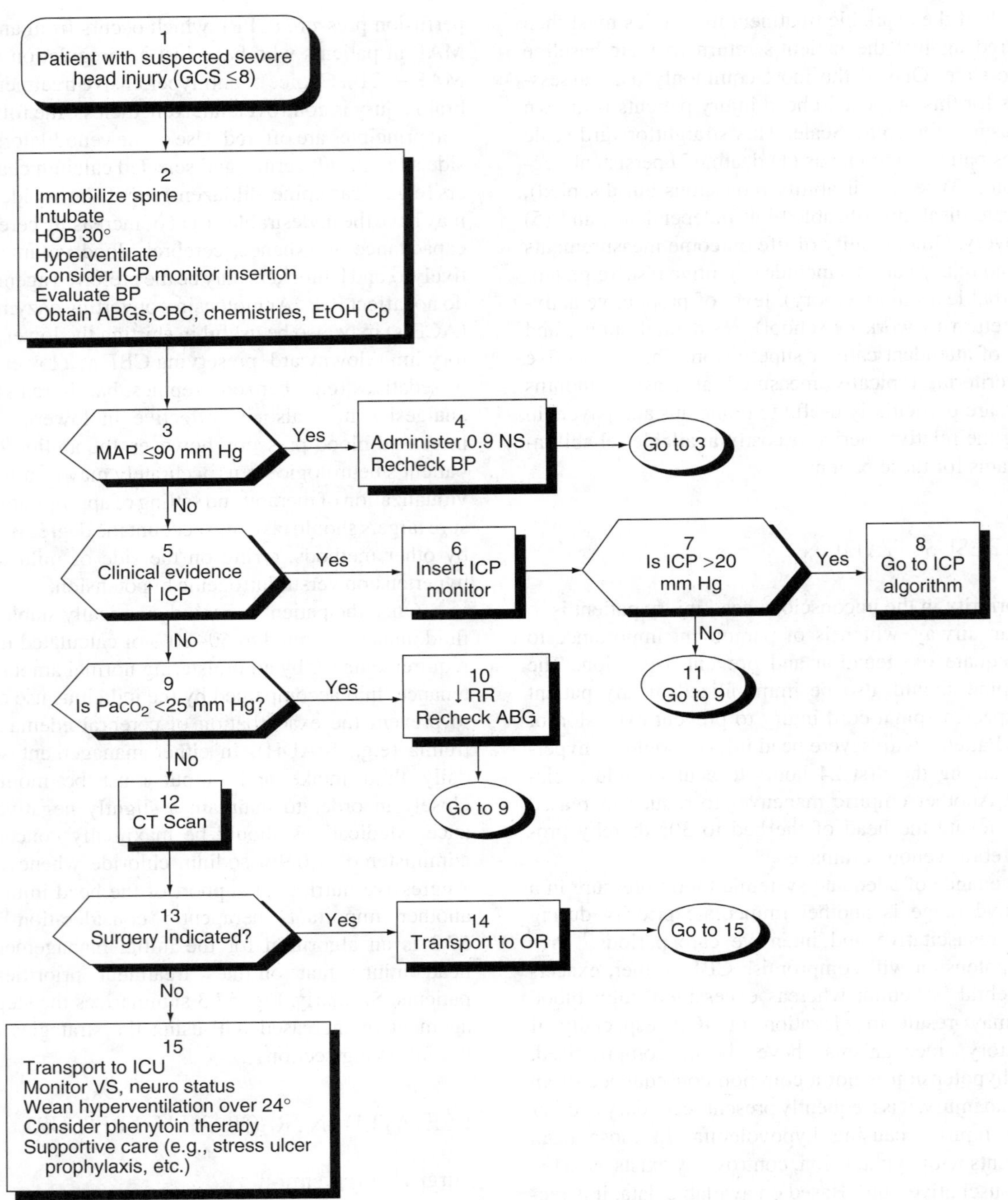

Figure 57.2. Algorithm for the acute management of the head injury patient. *(Adapted from Boucher BA. Neurotrauma. Pharmacotherapy Self Assessment Program, 3rd ed. Module 2 (Critical Care); pp 215–238, 1995. By permission of the American College of Clinical Pharmacy).*

jugular veins. If possible, jugular catheters should be avoided because these may restrict CBF.

Hyperventilation

Controlled hyperventilation is the most effective means of preventing and controlling ICP elevations. Hyperventilation requires the patient to be intubated and may necessitate the administration of sedatives or muscle relaxants. Hyperventilating the patient will cause a decrease in systemic and cerebral P_{CO_2}, resulting in cerebral vasoconstriction and a decrease in CBF. By reducing CBF, cerebral blood volume will also be reduced, thereby decreasing ICP. In these patients, the P_{CO_2} should be maintained between 25 and

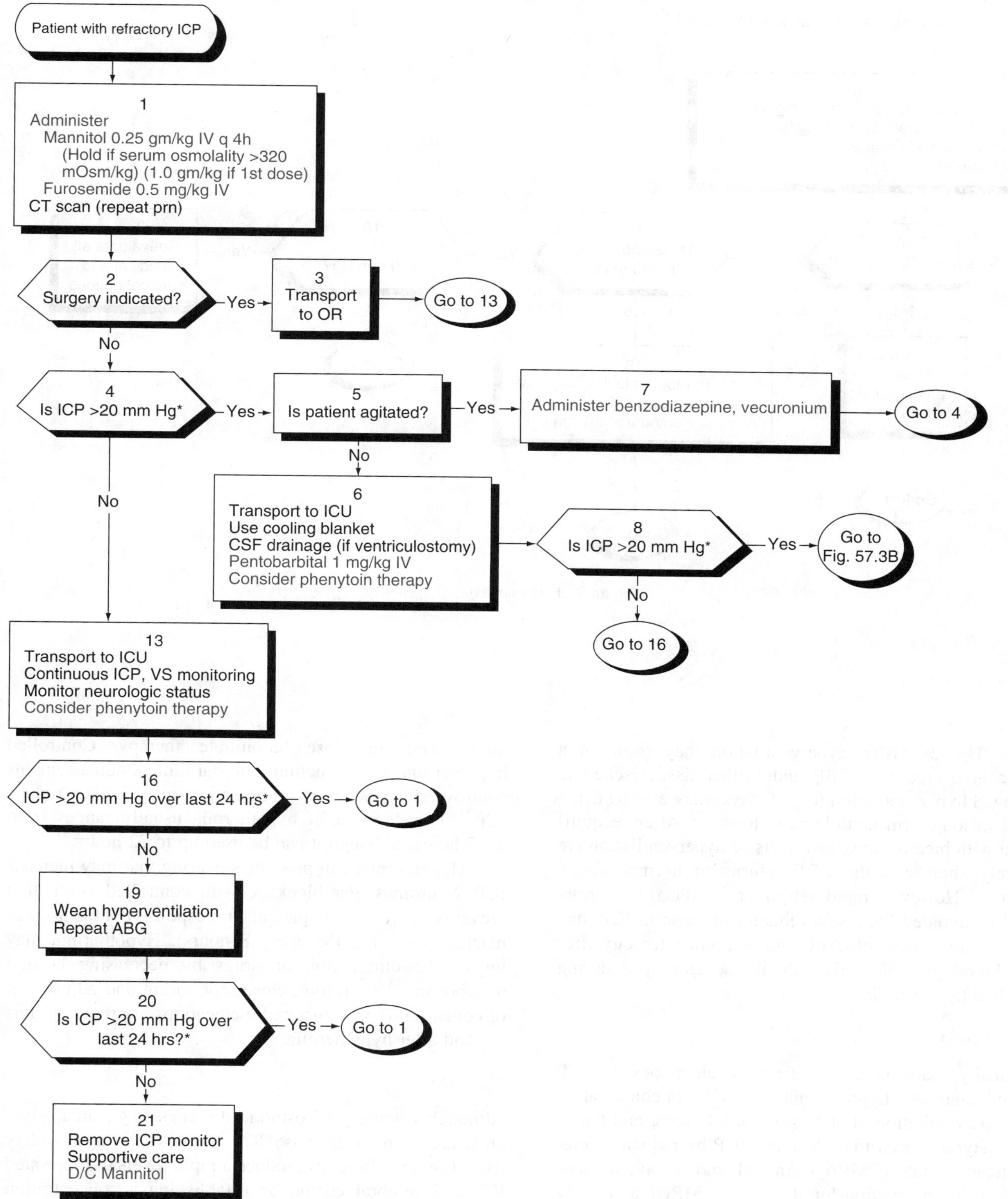

Figure 57.3. Algorithm for the management of ICP. *(Adapted from Boucher BA. Neurotrauma. Pharmacotherapy Self Assessment Program, 3rd ed. Module 2 (Critical Care); pp. 215–238, 1995. By permission of the American College of Clinical Pharmacy.)* **Treatment Thresholds: ICP 20–29 mm Hg for > 15 minutes; ICP 30–39 mm Hg for > 2 minutes; ICP ≥ 40 mm Hg for > 1 minute. Note: Transient increases may occur following respiratory procedures (e.g., suctioning, chest physiotherapy, bronchoscopy, intubation).*

†Partial Penobarbital loading dose (mg) = (20 mg/L − measured Cp)(1L/kg × wt [kg]).

(continued)

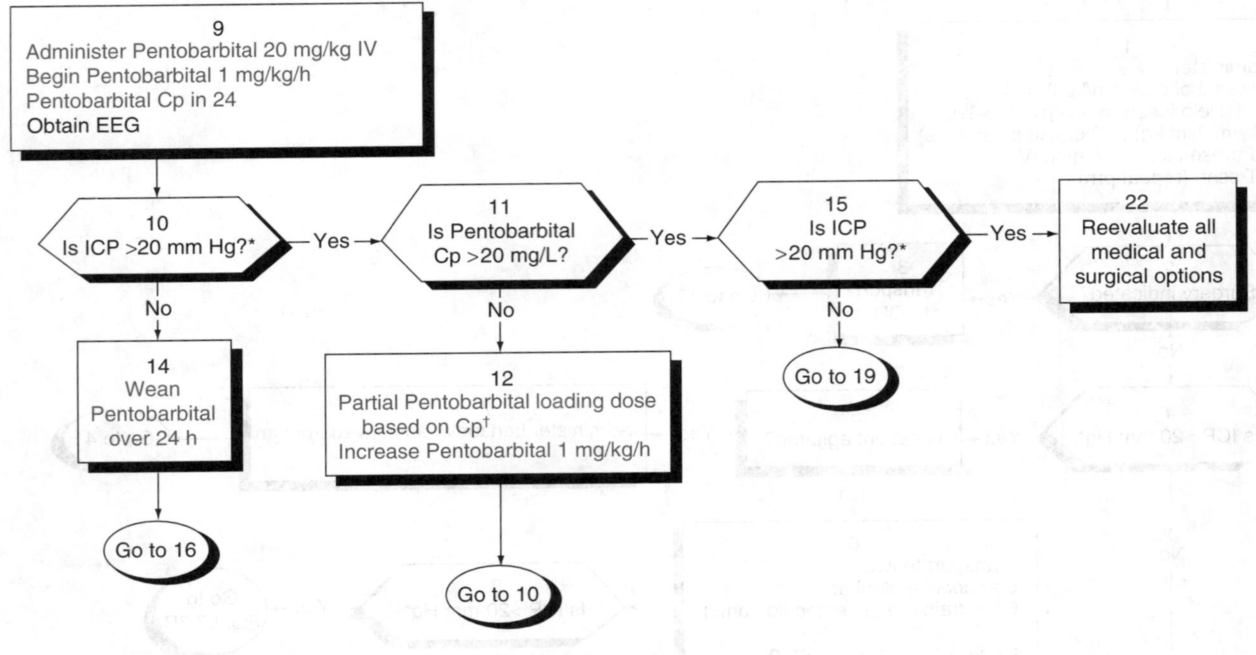

Figure 57.3. *(continued)*

35 mm Hg; excessive hyperventilation may result in a significant decrease in CBF and further tissue ischemia. Prolonged hyperventilation (e.g., 5 days) may also be detrimental to long-term neurologic outcome.[25] After reequilibration with bicarbonate, the effects of hyperventilation are relatively short and the CBF returns to normal within 6 hours.[26] However, rapid return of the P_{CO_2} to normal should be avoided because a rebound increase in ICP may occur. To maximize efficacy and minimize toxicity, frequent blood gas monitoring should be employed during controlled hyperventilation.

Hypothermia

Historically, patients with refractory elevations in ICP received controlled hypothermia (30–32°C) in combination with hyperventilation, diuretics, corticosteroids, and barbiturates. Hypothermia may decrease ICP by reducing cerebral metabolic rate (CMR_{O_2}). Animal studies have demonstrated a linear relationship between CMR_{O_2} and body temperature such that a 5°C decrease in body temperature produces a 10% decrease in the CMR_{O_2}. However, the use of controlled hypothermia alone has not been successfully used to decrease ICP.[27,28] Nonetheless, two studies have recently reported that mild hypothermia improves mortality and morbidity rates in patients with uncontrolled ICP.[29,30] In these studies, ICP, CBF, and CMR_{O_2} were significantly reduced in patients who failed fluid restriction, hyperventilation, and high-dose barbiturate therapy. Controlled hypothermia in conjunction with barbiturate coma remains controversial since this combination may further reduce ICP.[31] The duration of hypothermia usually ranges from 3–12 hours, although it can be used up to 72 hours.[31]

Hypothermia can produce shivering that may increase ICP. Neuromuscular blockade with controlled ventilation prevents shivering in patients unresponsive to chlorpromazine (5–25 mg IM every 8 hours). Hypothermia may impair the elimination of drugs by decreasing hepatic metabolism.[32] Therefore, close monitoring and adjustment of concurrently administered medications are required during and after hypothermia.

Mannitol

Although a variety of osmotic diuretics (e.g., urea, glycerol) are used to decrease ICP, mannitol is most widely used. Osmotic diuretics produce a rapid reversal of elevated ICP and cerebral edema by establishing a concentration gradient across an intact blood–brain barrier. As water diffuses from the brain into the intravascular compartment, ICP decreases. If the blood–brain barrier is disrupted as a result of injury, rebound elevations of ICP may occur as the osmotic agent accumulates in the brain tissue, resulting in an increase in intracellular brain volume.

Although some practitioners use an initial dose of 1 g/kg IV, decreases in ICP can be achieved with starting doses of 0.25 g/kg IV every 4 hours.[33] Monitoring serum osmolality is vital since the continued use of mannitol is not associated with a decrease in ICP when osmolality values exceed 325 mOsm/kg.[33] An elevated ICP is reduced within minutes of the mannitol infusion and the duration of action ranges from 2–4 hours depending on the administered dose.[33] When an immediate reduction in ICP is needed, mannitol can be safely infused over 3–5 minutes; however, in nonemergent situations mannitol should be administered over 20–30 minutes to avoid transient increases in CBF.

Several adverse effects are associated with mannitol. A reversible acute renal dysfunction may occur in adults with previously normal renal function after long-term, high-dose administration.[34] Exacerbation of underlying congestive heart failure and pulmonary edema may also occur as the result of intravascular volume expansion. Mannitol may increase the CBF and worsen intracranial hypertension in children who develop a generalized cerebral hyperemia during the first 24–48 hours postinjury.[35] Furosemide is recommended as an alternative agent for lowering ICP in these latter two patient groups.

Glycerol

Glycerol is effective in lowering ICP by osmotic brain dehydration, decreasing CSF production, and increasing CBF to ischemic brain tissue. Although glycerol promotes diuresis, its mechanism of action is not dependent on the degree of diuresis. Generally, glycerol is not administered orally in these patients since they may have decreased bowel perfusion that could limit bioavailability. Intravenous glycerol can be given intermittently (0.5–1 g/kg every 4–6 hours) or continuously (0.2–1 g/kg/h); however, the lack of a sterile glycerol preparation is a limitation to its use.[36] Glycerol's onset of effect occurs within 0.5–1 hour while its duration of action is not well established. Rebound cerebral edema may occur when glycerol is given more frequently than every 4 hours.[37] The rebound in ICP is attributed to an increase in intracranial glycerol concentration and osmolality. Possible mechanisms for intracranial accumulation of glycerol include an increase in glycerol diffusion into the brain as a result of a defective blood–brain barrier or aggressive dosing of glycerol.[37] Some investigators have also speculated that these patients may produce "idiogenic" organic molecules when amino acids are released from neuronal cells, abolishing the osmotic gradient established by glycerol.

Furosemide/Other Diuretics

Compared with osmotic diuretics, furosemide does not produce significant changes in serum osmolality or increase intravascular or cerebral volume. The proposed mechanisms for furosemide lowering ICP include (1) the suppression of cerebral sodium uptake, (2) carbonic anhydrase inhibition resulting in decreased CSF production, and (3) inhibition of the cellular membrane cation-chloride pump, thereby affecting transport of water into astroglial cells.

Following intravenous furosemide (0.5–1 mg/kg), a drop in ICP occurs within minutes, and maximal decreases occur within 25 minutes.[38] Adverse effects include hyponatremia, hypocalcemia, hypokalemia, and decreased intravascular volume. Ethacrynic acid and acetazolamide can decrease ICP; however, these agents are either more toxic (e.g., ethacrynic acid) or have a delayed onset (e.g., acetazolamide), making them less useful than furosemide or the osmotic diuretics.

Corticosteroids

Although steroids are effective in preventing or reducing cerebral edema in patients with structural brain damage (e.g., tumors), studies assessing their efficacy in head trauma have documented beneficial effects, no effect, or possibly detrimental effects.[39–43] Criticisms of these studies include a lack of controls or blinding, inadequate sample size, incomplete patient descriptors (e.g., outcome), incomplete experimental data (e.g., ICP, CBF), or dosing inconsistencies. Despite these conflicting reports, there persists an impression among some clinicians that steroids may be beneficial. Possible therapeutic benefits of steroids include vascular membrane stabilization against free radical peroxidation, decreased vascular permeability, decreased CSF production, lysosomal membrane stabilization, improved neuronal metabolism, and improved brain compliance.

Advocates of steroids recommend dexamethasone because it enhances anti-inflammatory action and has minimal mineralocorticoid activity. The initial recommended IV doses vary widely ranging between 4 mg every 6 hours to 100 mg every 6 hours.[40] Discontinuation after 72 hours is recommended in nonresponders.[41] The beneficial effects of steroids are not seen for 12–18 hours and maximal effect may not be evident until 24 hours. Because of the delay in onset, steroids should not be used in patients experiencing acute intermittent ICP elevations. Complications of steroid therapy include gastrointestinal (GI) irritation and hemorrhage, glucose intolerance, electrolyte abnormalities, and infection.[44]

Barbiturates

Numerous studies have demonstrated the effectiveness of barbiturates in reducing ICP refractory to hyperventilation, diuretics, steroids, and hypothermia.[45–48] Comparison of these studies is difficult because of differences in inclusion criteria, therapy used before and during barbiturate therapy, barbiturate dosing, monitoring parameters, and definition of therapeutic outcome between studies. The mechanism for barbiturate reduction of ICP is unknown. Barbiturates increase cerebral ATP concentrations, which may aid in maintaining the sodium-potassium pump, thus preserving the transmembrane ion potential and cell membrane integrity. Barbiturates also may cause vasoconstriction and reduce cerebral metabolism, resulting in decreased CBF or shunting of blood toward ischemic areas. Finally, barbiturates may interrupt the formation of free radicals, or act as oxygen free radical scavengers.

Normal doses of barbiturates may be used intermittently to decrease an acute elevation in ICP (e.g., thiopental 3 mg/kg IV), whereas higher doses of barbiturates are used to induce coma. Before inducing barbiturate coma, the patient must be mechanically ventilated with continuous monitoring of arterial blood pressure, ECG, and ICP. The goal of barbiturate coma is to maintain ICP <15 mm Hg, achieve pentobarbital serum concentrations of 20 to 40 mcg/mL, maintain MAP between 60 and 90 mm Hg, and mean CPP >50 mm Hg.[45,47] Because pentobarbital concentrations ≥20 mcg/mL are associated with an isoelectric EEG, this value is considered the lower limit for barbiturate coma. Concentrations ≥40 mcg/mL may cause cardiac depression and should be avoided.[49]

Pentobarbital and thiopental are the most commonly used agents for induction of coma. Thiopental is more lipid soluble and achieves rapid therapeutic brain concentrations; however, because of rapid redistribution, it has a shorter duration of coma. Although thiopental has several theoretical advantages, there does not appear to be any significant clinical advantage of thiopental versus pentobarbital. Although initial pentobarbital loading doses range from 3–35 mg/kg IV administered over 10 minutes to 3 hours, an initial loading dose of 20–30 mg/kg IV is recommended as pentobarbital's estimated volume of distribution is 1 L/kg. This should be followed by maintenance doses ranging from 0.5–3.5 mg/kg/h.[45–47] Although thiopental coma has not been well studied, a loading dose of 20 mg/kg IV administered over 1 hour with maintenance doses of 2 to 12 mg/kg/h is recommended.[46]

Side effects associated with high-dose barbiturate therapy involve primarily the cardiovascular system. Hypotension, caused by peripheral vasodilation, may occur and necessitate decreasing the barbiturate dose, or the administration of fluids and vasopressors to maintain blood pressure. GI effects include decreased GI muscular tone and decreased amplitude of contraction. On emergence from coma, there may be a period of GI hypermotility. In addition, barbiturates induce hepatic microsomal enzyme activity affecting drug metabolism. Care should be taken to avoid extravasation of pentobarbital and thiopental solutions because severe tissue damage may occur. Because of many known drug incompatibilities, the barbiturates should be administered by continuous infusion through a central line designated for this purpose.

Criteria for discontinuing high-dose barbiturate therapy include normalization of the intracranial volume-pressure response, ICP ≤15 mm Hg for 72 hours, and systolic arterial blood pressure ≤160 mm Hg without vasodilator therapy.[45,47] In addition, coma should be discontinued if a reduction in ICP from baseline does not occur, if signs of progressive neurologic impairment are evident, or arbitrarily after 5 days of therapy. Barbiturates are tapered over 24–72 hours to prevent ICP spikes; however, because of the prolonged elimination half-life of pentobarbital and thiopental, systemic elimination of the drug occurs over several days. The persistence of detectable barbiturate concentrations can delay a determination of brain death. Mild symptoms of barbiturate withdrawal include tremors, agitation, delirium, and visual hallucinations. These symptoms may persist for 2–7 days and usually resolve without pharmacologic intervention.

Other Agents

Intravenous lidocaine is often effective in preventing ICP spikes caused by surgical stimulation, endotracheal intubation, or endotracheal suctioning.[50,51] A lidocaine bolus of 1.5 mg/kg IV produces a gradual and prolonged reduction in ICP without affecting MAP.[50] Dimethyl sulfoxide (DMSO) may be used as an osmotic diuretic to lower ICP; however, reports are limited to patients with refractory elevations in ICP.[52] The long-term effects of intravenous administration and its effects on other organ systems are unknown, and DMSO is not approved for intracranial hypertension. Etomidate, a nonhistamine-releasing anesthetic agent, is used to control moderately elevated ICP. It may be given continuously (5–25 mcg/kg/min IV) or intermittently (0.2 mg/kg IV). Hypotension limits its use particularly in hypovolemic patients.[53]

POST-TRAUMATIC SEIZURES

Seizures greatly increase $CMRo_2$. Therefore, it is generally agreed that patients who have experienced ≥1 seizure following a moderate to severe head injury should receive anticonvulsant therapy to avoid further increases in $CMRo_2$ for at least 1 week postinjury. Initial therapy in these persons should consist of incremental intravenous doses of diazepam (5–40 mg) or lorazepam (2–8 mg) to terminate any active seizure activity followed by intravenous phenytoin to prevent seizure recurrence.[5] The merits of preventive anticonvulsant therapy in patients who have not had a seizure postinjury is more controversial. Risk factors for early seizures (<7 days postinjury) include intracranial hematoma, focal neurologic deficit, amnesia lasting >24 hours, linear or depressed skull fracture, and age <5 years.[54] In 1990, a landmark randomized, placebo-controlled study was published providing the strongest evidence to date relative to the benefits of phenytoin in preventing early seizures following head trauma.[55] The incidence of early post-traumatic seizures in patients receiving placebo was 14.2% compared to 3.6% in patients receiving phenytoin ($p<0.05$). The data from this study do not support the use of prophylactic phenytoin beyond 7 days, however, since there was no significant difference in seizure incidence between the placebo and phenytoin groups during this period.

Aggressive phenytoin therapy is recommended during the treatment period to maintain total concentrations in the range of 10–20 mg/L. This can generally be achieved using an IV loading dose of 18–20 mg/kg followed by an initial adult daily maintenance dose of 2.5–3.0 mg/kg/day q12h and a pediatric dose of 7–10 mg/kg/day (administered q6–8h). Nonetheless, the potential for phenytoin's metabolism to increase as a function of time should also be considered in these patients.[56,57] Monitoring of phenytoin trough concentrations should occur every other day to assure that concentrations are being maintained in the target range. The possibility of the total phenytoin concentration falling as a consequence of decreased protein binding secondary to hypoalbuminemia and/or renal insufficiency should also be considered. The use of unbound (i.e., free) phenytoin concentrations is strongly encouraged if available. If chronic therapy is indicated, patients may be switched to oral phenytoin or to another anticonvulsant (e.g., carbamazepine, valproic acid), based on the relative side-effect profile for these agents. However, no clinical evaluations have been conducted to date to support the use of these alternative anticonvulsants in this setting.

INVESTIGATIONAL THERAPY

The steady decrease in morbidity and mortality following severe neurotrauma over the last three decades can be largely attributed to expeditious and aggressive management of those processes resulting in secondary injury (i.e., ischemia, hypoxia, increased ICP). Clinical and experimental approaches are now being investigated to prevent or attenuate the effects of secondary injury mediators (treatment goal 3) in patients with head injury that will ideally further decrease morbidity and mortality.

Antioxidants

The potential role of oxygen free radicals in the pathophysiology of head injury has stimulated interest in the use of antioxidants to interrupt the self-perpetuating cycle of membrane destruction in these patients. Tirilazad, a 21-aminosteroid, is one such antioxidant that was in phase III testing in head injury patients until December 1994.[57,58] At that time, the trial was halted by the FDA due to unexpected and unexplained differences in mortality rates between tirilazad and the placebo groups. This steroid analog, although a potent inhibitor of lipid peroxidation, is essentially devoid of glucocorticoid activity. Another antioxidant in clinical trials is superoxide dismutase (SOD). Interest in SOD in the treatment of neurotrauma has been renewed following enhancement of its intracellular availability as a complexed product with the carrier compound, polyethylene glycol (PEG).

Modulation of Calcium Influx

In light of the integral role calcium has in the pathophysiology of acute neurotrauma, it is logical that a significant amount of attention be given to pharmacologically modulating calcium influx in acute head injury. Magnesium, an endogenous calcium channel antagonist, is thought to exert its effects via a gating effect on the NMDA receptor. Experimental evidence in head injury models suggests that (1) magnesium deficiency exacerbates traumatic brain injury and (2) administration of magnesium limits the extent of neurologic dysfunction.[59,60] In addition to these positive results, the fact that magnesium is readily available for clinical use makes this strategy very appealing. Randomized, controlled clinical studies are currently under way to substantiate the findings of experimental head injury. Specific competitive and noncompetitive NMDA receptor antagonists include phencyclidine, ketamine, dextrophan and dizocilpine, CGS 19755, and D-CPP-ene.[61,62] A significant amount of experimental evidence has been accumulated confirming the efficacy of NMDA receptor antagonists in attenuating the development of cerebral edema, motor dysfunction, and cellular electrolyte and metabolic disturbances following model head injury. Although many of these drugs have side effects that limit their utility in humans, preclinical development of other NMDA receptor antagonists is currently under way. In addition to the excitotoxic amines, glutamate, and aspartate, increased concentrations of acetylcholine (ACh) has also been demonstrated following head injury. Thus, use of muscarinic cholinergic receptor antagonists has been studied as a potentially beneficial adjunct in the treatment of model head injury.[63] The calcium channel blockers are obvious candidates for attenuating the deleterious effects of calcium influx in acute neurotrauma patients. Unfortunately, experimental studies using conventional calcium channel blockers in head injury models have been disappointing overall. Nonetheless, a recent study of (S)-emopamil, a calcium channel blocker with potent serotonin-2 receptor antagonist properties, was also found effective in attenuating cerebral edema and postinjury cognitive dysfunction and in improving functional motor recovery in experimental head injury compared to placebo.[64]

Opiate Antagonists

A substantial amount of experimental evidence has implicated endogenous opioid peptides in the pathophysiology of severe neurotrauma, probably via activation of the K receptor. These results are complicated by the finding that endogenous opiate activity at the μ and Δ receptors following neurotrauma has neuroprotective effects. Thus, dosing of a nonspecific opiate antagonist such as naloxone may be very critical since at high dosages (10 mg/kg), it appears to exhibit its antagonistic effects at the μ, Δ, and K receptors, whereas at lower dosages (0.1 mg/kg), its effects are primarily through inhibition at the μ receptor.[62] Use of alternative agents such as nalmefene, an opiate antagonist with greater specificity for the K receptor, may alleviate some of the problems surrounding naloxone dosing in neurotrauma.[65]

Modulators of Arachidonic Acid Metabolism

Formation of inflammatory mediators including the metabolites of arachidonic acid have been implicated in the latter stages of tertiary injury following neurotrauma. Since nonsteroidal anti-inflammatory drugs (NSAIDs) act by blocking the formation of these metabolites (e.g., prostaglandins, leukotrienes, thromboxane), an adjunctive role for these agents has been postulated for patients with head injury. Limited studies with indomethacin in animals following model injury[66] and patients[67] have been promising relative to reducing mortality and managing refractory cases of increased ICP, respectively.

Conclusion

The management of patients with severe head injury involves the control and prevention of secondary brain injuries, and the accompanying medical complications. Traditional pharmacologic management includes normalization of blood pressure, treatment of increased ICP, and anticonvulsant therapy to prevent post-traumatic seizures. Preliminary studies with several investigational agents directed at attenuating the complex pathophysiology of brain injury are encouraging. Future management of head injury will likely entail administering a combination of drugs in an attempt to diminish the devastating morbidity and mortality seen in this patient population. Close attention to dose, timing and sequencing of administration, and duration of therapy relative to the traumatic event will be essential in optimizing the beneficial effects of pharmacologic interventions.

References

1. Kalsbeek WD, McLaurin RL, Harris BSH III, et al. The national head and spinal cord injury survey: Major findings. J Neurosurg 1980;53:S19–S31.
2. Centers for Disease Control and Prevention (CDC). Cost of injury—U.S.: A report to Congress, 1989. MMWR 1989;743–746.
3. MacKenzie EJ, Shapiro S, Siegel JH. The economic impact of traumatic injuries. One-year treatment-related expenditures. JAMA 1988;260:3290–3296.
4. Gennarelli TA. Mechanisms of brain injury. J Emerg Med 1993;11:5–11.
5. Hayek DA, Veremakis C. Physiologic concerns during brain resuscitation, in Civetta JM, Taylor RW, Kirby RR (eds): Critical Care, 2nd ed. Philadelphia, JB Lippincott, 1992, pp 1449–1466.
6. Bouma GJ, Muizelaar JP, Choi SC, et al. Cerebral circulation and metabolism after severe traumatic brain injury: The elusive role of ischemia. J Neurosurg 1991;75:685–693.
7. Pitts LH, McIntosh TK. Dynamic changes after brain trauma, in Vinken PJ, Bruyn GW, Klawans HL (eds): Handbook of Clinical Neurology, Vol 57, Head Injury. New York, Elsevier Science Publishing, 1990, pp 65–100.
8. Marmarou A. Intracellular acidosis in human and experimental brain injury. J Neurotrauma 1992;9(suppl 2):S551–S562.
9. Kelly BJ, Luce JM. Current concepts in cerebral protection. Chest 1993;103(12):1246–1254.
10. Lyeth BG, Hayes RL. Cholinergic and opioid mediation of traumatic brain injury. J Neurotrauma 1992;9(suppl 2):S463–S474.
11. Faden AI, Demediuk P, Panter SS, Vink R. The role of excitatory amino acids and NMDA receptors in traumatic brain injury. Science 1989;244:798–800.
12. Hall ED. The role of oxygen radicals in traumatic injury: Clinical implications. J Emerg Med 1993;11:31–36.
13. Hallenbeck JM, Dutka AJ. Background review and current concepts of reperfusion injury. Arch Neurol 1990;47:1245–1254.
14. Young B, Ott L, Yingling B, McClain C. Nutrition and brain injury. J Neurotrauma 1992;9(suppl 1):S375–S383.
15. Teasdale G, Jennett B. Aspects of coma after severe head injury. Lancet 1977;1:878–881.
16. Narayan RK. Emergency room management of the head-injured patient, in Becker DP, Gudeman SK (eds): Textbook of Head Injury. Philadelphia, WB Saunders, 1989, pp 23–66.
17. Miller JD, Becker DP, Ward JD, et al. Significance of intracranial hypertension in severe head injury. J Neurosurg 1977;47:503–516.
18. Marshall LF, Smith RW, Shapiro HM. The outcome with aggressive treatment in severe head injuries. Part I: The significance of intracranial pressure monitoring. Neurosurg 1979;50:20–25.
19. Jennett B, Bond M. Assessment of outcome after severe brain damage. Lancet 1975;1:480–484.
20. Pacult A, Gudeman SK. Medical management of head injuries, in Becker DP, Gudeman SK (eds): Textbook of Head Injury. Philadelphia, WB Saunders, 1989, pp 192–220.
21. Schmoker JD, Shackford SR, Wald SL, Pietropaoli JA. An analysis of the relationship between fluid and sodium administration and intracranial pressure after head injury. J Trauma 1992;33:476–481.
22. Borel C, Hanley D, Diringer MN, Rogers MC. Intensive management of severe head injury. Chest 1990;98:180–189.
23. Ruben BH, Greenberg J. Neurologic injury: Prevention and initial care, in Civetta JM, Taylor RW, Kirby RR (eds): Critical Care, 2nd ed. Philadelphia, JB Lippincott, 1992, 725–745.
24. Cochran EB, Kamper CA, Phelps SJ, et al. Parenteral nutrition in the critically ill patient. Clin Pharm 1989;8:783–797.

25. Muzelaar JP, Marmarou A, Ward JD, et al. Adverse effects of prolonged hyperventilation in patients with severe head injury: A randomized clinical trial. J Neurosurg 1991;75:731–739.
26. Raichle ME, Posner JB, Plum F. Cerebral blood flow during and after hyperventilation. Arch Neurol 1970;23:394–403.
27. Steen PA, Soul EM, Michenfelder JD. Detrimental effect of prolonged hypothermia in cats and monkeys with and without cerebral regional cerebral ischemia. Stroke 1979; 10:522–529.
28. Lakowski EJ, Klatzo I, Baldwin M. Experimental study of the effects of hypothermia on local brain injury. 1960;10:499–505.
29. Shiozaki T, Sugimoto H, Taneda M, et al. Effect of mild hypothermia on uncontrolled intracranial hypertension after severe head injury. J Neurosurg 1993;79:363–368.
30. Marion DW, Obrist WD, Carlier PM, et al. The use of moderate therapeutic hypothermia for patients with severe head injuries: A preliminary report. J Neurosurg 1993;79:354–362.
31. Shapiro HM, Wyte SR, Loeser J. Barbiturate-augmented hypothermia for reduction of persistent intracranial hypertension. J Neurosurg 1974;40:90–100.
32. McAllister JR, Tan TG. Effect of hypothermia on drug metabolism. In vitro studies with propranolol and verapamil. Pharmacology 1980;20:95–100.
33. Marshall LF, Smith RW, Rauscher LA, et al. Mannitol dose requirements in brain-injured patients. J Neurosurg 1978;48:169–172.
34. Goldwasser P, Fotino S. Acute renal failure following massive mannitol infusion: Appropriate response of tubuloglomerular feedback? Arch Intern Med 1984;144:2214–2216.
35. Bruce DA, Langfitt TW, Miller JD. Regional cerebral flow, intracranial pressure and brain metabolism in comatose patients. J Neurosurg 1973;38:131–144.
36. Tourtellotte WW, Reinglass JL, Newkirk TA. Cerebral dehydration action of glycerol. 1. Historical aspects with emphasis on the toxicity and intravenous administration. Clin Pharm Ther 1972;13:159–171.
37. Rottenberg DA, Hurwitz BJ, Posner JB. The effect of oral glycerol on intraventricular pressure in man. Neurology 1977;27:600–608.
38. Cottrell JE, Robustelli A, Post K, et al. Furosemide- and mannitol-induced changes in intracranial pressure and serum osmolality and electrolytes. Anesthesiology 1977;47:28–30.
39. Sapolsky RM, Pulsinelli WA. Glucocorticoids' potential ischemic injury of neurons: Therapeutic implications. Science 1985;229:1397–1400.
40. Hoffman JR, Orban DJ, Podolsky S. Pharmacologic therapeutic modalities: Corticosteroids. Crit Care Qtr 1983;1:52–62.
41. Braakman R, Schouten HJA, Dishoeck MB, Minerhoud JM. Megadose steroids in severe head injury. Results of a prospective double-blind clinical trial. J Neurosurg 1983;58:326–330.
42. Saul TG, Ducker TB, Salcman M, Carro E. Steroids in severe head injury. A prospective randomized clinical trial. J Neurosurg 1981;54:596–600.
43. Dearden NM, Gibson JS, McDowell DG, et al. Effect of high dose dexamethasone on outcome from severe head injury. J Neurosurg 1986;64:81–88.
44. DeMaria EJ, Reichman W, Kenney PR, et al. Septic complications of corticosteroid administration after central nervous system trauma. Ann Surg 1985;202:248–252.
45. Rockoff MA, Marshall LF, Shapiro HM. High-dose barbiturate therapy in humans: A clinical review of 60 patients. Ann Neurol 1979;6:194–199.
46. Quandt CM, de los Reyes RA, Diaz FG. Barbiturate-induced coma for the treatment of cerebral ischemia: Review of outcome. Clin Pharm 1982;1:549–551.
47. Marshall LF, Smith RW, Shapiro HM. The outcome with aggressive treatment in severe head injuries. Part II: Acute and chronic barbiturate administration in the management of head injury. J Neurosurg 1979;50:26–30.
48. Eisenberg HM, Frankowski RF, Contant CF, et al. High-dose barbiturate control of elevated intracranial pressure in patients with severe head injury. J Neurosurg 1988;69:15–23.
49. Heinemeyer G, Roots I, Dennhardt R. Monitoring of pentobarbital plasma levels in critical care patients suffering from increased intracranial pressure. Ther Drug Monit 1986;8:145–150.
50. Bedford RF, Persing JA, Pobereskin L, et al. Lidocaine or thiopental for rapid control of intracranial hypertension. Anesth Analg 1980;59:435–437.
51. Donegan MF, Bedford RF, Dacey R. Lidocaine for prevention of intracranial hypertension. Anesthesiology 1979;51:S201.
52. Waller FT, Tanabe CT, Paxton HD. Treatment of elevated intracranial pressure with dimethyl sulfoxide. Ann NY Acad Sci 1983;411:286–292.
53. Prior JGL, Hinds CJ, Williams J, et al. The use of etomidate in the management of severe head injury. Intensive Care Med 1983;9:313–320.
54. Kuhl DA, Boucher BA, Muhlbauer MS. Prophylaxis of posttraumatic seizures. DICP Ann Pharmacother 1990;24:277–285.
55. Temkin NR, Dikmen SS, Wilensky AJ, et al. A randomized, double-blind study of phenytoin for the prevention of posttraumatic seizures. N Engl J Med 1990;323:497–502.
56. Boucher BA, Rodman JH, Jaresko GS, et al. Phenytoin pharmacokinetics in critically ill trauma patients. Clin Pharmacol Ther 1988;675–683.
57. Braughler JM, Hall ED, Jacobsen J, et al. The 21-aminosteroids: Potent inhibitors of lipid peroxidation for the treatment of central nervous system trauma and ischemia. Drugs Future 1989;14:143–152.
58. Hall ED. Lipid antioxidants in acute central nervous system injury. Ann Emerg Med 1993;22:1022–1027.
59. Vink R, McIntosh TK. Pharmacological and physiological effects of magnesium on experimental traumatic brain injury. Magnesium Res 1990;3:163–169.
60. McIntosh TK, Vink R, Yamakami I, Faden AI. Magnesium protects against neurological deficit after brain injury. Brain Res 1989;482:257–260.
61. Gentile NT, McIntosh TK. Antagonists of excitatory amino acids and endogenous opioid peptides in the treatment of experimental central nervous system injury. Ann Emerg Med 1993;22:1028–1034.
62. Faden AI, Salzman S. Pharmacological strategies in CNS trauma. Trends Pharmacol Sci 1992;13:29–35.
63. Jenkins LW, Lyeth BG, Lewelt W, et al. Combined pretrauma scopolamine and phencyclidine attenuate posttraumatic

increased sensitivity to delayed secondary ischemia. J Neurotrauma 1988;5:275–287.

64. Okiyama K, Smith DH, Thomas MJ, McIntosh TK. Evaluation of a novel calcium channel blocker, (S)-emopamil, on regional cerebral edema and neurobehavioral function after experimental brain injury. J Neurosurg 1992;77:607–615.
65. Vink R, McIntosh TK, Rhomhanyi R, Faden AI. Opiate antagonist nalmefene improves intracellular free Mg^{2+}, bioenergetic state, and neurologic outcome following traumatic brain injury in rats. J Neurosci 1990;10:3524–3530.
66. Kim HY, Levasseur JE, Patterson JL Jr, et al. Effect of indomethacin pretreatment on acute mortality in experimental brain injury. J Neurosurg 1989;71:565–572.
67. Jensen K, Ohrstrom J, Cold GE, Astrup J. The effects of indomethacin on intracranial pressure, cerebral blood flow, and cerebral metabolism in patients with severe head injury and intracranial hypertension. Acta Neurochir 1991;108:116–121.

Chapter 58

Parkinson's Disease

Merlin V. Nelson, PharmD, MD, Richard C. Berchou, PharmD, and Peter A. LeWitt, MD

While its clinical manifestations had previously escaped attention in the medical literature, *paralysis agitans* (the "shaking palsy") became an unmistakable presence after the 1817 publication of a monograph by an obscure British physician. James Parkinson's account of six patients with this disorder[1] is difficult to improve on in the acuity of observation, although only some of the major characteristics of *paralysis agitans* (now termed Parkinson's disease) are described in "An Essay on the Shaking Palsy." Parkinson provided vivid descriptions of features such as an "involuntary tremulous motion" and the tendency to "pass from a walking to a running pace." Later observers recognized a greater variety of signs and symptoms, and added rigidity and instability of balance to the list of cardinal manifestations. Idiopathic Parkinson's disease (IPD), which is sometimes referred to as *Lewy body parkinsonism* on the basis of its highly characteristic neuropathological findings, is just one of several types of neurologic disorders known to present this clinical picture.

Diagnosis

Although the disorder is unmistakable in its advanced form, the subtle features of a mild case of IPD can present a challenge in distinguishing it from changes seen with normal aging. Diagnostic criteria for IPD have been developed,[2] which emphasize that bradykinesia should be present with at least two of the following features: limb muscle rigidity, resting tremor (at 4–6 Hz and abolished by movement), or postural instability (not caused by primary visual, vestibular, cerebellar, or proprioceptive dysfunction). For the accurate diagnosis of IPD, other conditions causing secondary parkinsonism must be considered (Table 58.1). The most common of these is the effect of dopamine receptor blocking drugs. Drug-induced parkinsonism can fully resemble the idiopathic disorder, so it is important to establish if antipsychotics, antiemetics, or metoclopramide have been used. Focal infarcts of the brain rarely cause the abrupt onset of parkinsonism. Earlier in the twentieth century, there was a pandemic of *encephalitis lethargica,* which was commonly associated with the development of parkinsonism and other movement disorders. Although once an extremely widespread disorder, *encephalitis lethargica* has not occurred in more than 50 years. Other neurodegenerative conditions may resemble the clinical picture of IPD. These include progressive supranuclear palsy, striatonigral degeneration, olivopontocerebellar degeneration, and, rarely, Huntington's and Wilson's diseases. To distinguish IPD from secondary causes, other diagnostic criteria include slow progression, lack of additional types of neurologic impairment, and responsiveness to levodopa (L-dopa).

IPD has a characteristic pathological picture that permits its differentiation from similar clinical syndromes. In the pars compacta of the substantia nigra, the Lewy body (a neuronal inclusion body composed of amyloid neurofilaments) is always found.[2] Lewy bodies and some adjacent gliosis appear to be produced by the degeneration of neurons. The loss of pars compacta neurons is the basis for loss of dopamine found at the sites of their projects to the caudate nucleus and putamen. Lewy bodies can be found in other neurologic disorders and in normal aging (in from 3.8–12.8% of patients from age 60–100 years).[2] Conceivably, the occurrence of Lewy bodies in patients without parkinsonism might be an indication that the disease can exist as a pathologic entity with far less involvement than is necessary to bring out clinical signs and symptoms (incidental Parkinson's disease). Recent studies have shown that even cases whose clinical features strongly suggest IPD may lack its characteristic pathology. In a series of 100 autopsied cases of patients diagnosed as IPD during life, 24 had pathological findings of disorders other than IPD.[3] The condition most commonly mistaken for IPD was progressive supranuclear palsy.[3]

Clinical Features

IPD develops insidiously and progresses slowly in most patients. It is often difficult for a patient to discern exactly when the motor disorder began. Initial complaints may include one or more sensory symptoms. These can include

TABLE 58.1. DIFFERENTIAL DIAGNOSIS OF PARKINSONISM

Idiopathic Parkinsonism (Parkinson's Disease, Lewy Body Parkinsonism)
Secondary Parkinsonism
- Drug-Induced
  - Antipsychotics (phenothiazines, butyrophenones, others)
  - Antiemetics (metoclopramide, prochlorperazine)
  - Other drugs (reserpine, alpha-methyldopa)
- Toxic
  - Carbon monoxide poisoning
  - Manganese
  - MPTP
  - Petrochemicals
- Neoplasms or strokes in the regions of the nigrostriatal pathways
- Traumatic lesions interrupting substantia nigra projections
- Normal pressure hydrocephalus

Parkinsonism with Other Neuronal System Degenerations
- Wilson's disease (copper deposition in the brain)
- Progressive supranuclear palsy
- Pallidonigral degeneration
- Corticobasalganglionic degeneration
- Alzheimer's disease
- Multiple system atrophy
  - Striatonigral degeneration
  - Shy–Drager syndrome
  - Olivopontocerebellar atrophy

aching pains, paresthesias, numbness, and coldness. As the disease progresses the patient will exhibit one or more of the classic clinical features: resting tremor, rigidity, bradykinesia, or change in posture. Characteristic problems even in mildly affected patients include small handwriting (micrographia), decreased facial animation and blink rate, diminished arm swing while walking, shuffling of gait, soft or indistinct speech, and decreased dexterity in everyday activities.

Other clinical characteristics of IPD are listed in Table 58.2. Bradykinesia, a term referring to the slowness of movement, is only one of the facets of motor impairment in IPD. Movement in IPD is often slow throughout an intended action, but the start of the movement may display a hesitation out of proportion to slowness affecting the rest of the movement. In addition to hesitancy of starting gait, a progressive slowing and decline in dexterity with repetition may impair tasks, as exemplified by repeated performance of finger tapping. Intermittent immobility ("freezing") is another common characteristic in some Parkinsonians. "Freezing" is especially likely to occur in situations such as when walking in a crowd or when walking through a narrow doorway. Patients may also experience difficulty at halting their steps while walking, a condition that has been termed *festination.* Bradykinesia manifested in the facial muscles results in hypomimia or a masked quality to facial expression. In such situations, there can be a staring quality to the gaze (associated, in part, with a decrease in blink rate).

The pathophysiology of bradykinesia appears to be an impairment in the execution of learned or semireflex sequential motor plans. This has been attributed to a disconnection between basal ganglia structures and the supplementary motor cortex. Many inputs influence the functioning of this system and bradykinesia can on occasion be reversed by sudden changes in emotional state. This type of response, termed *kinesia paradoxica,* suggests that the intrinsic program for these movements is intact in IPD.

Tremor occurring at rest is highly typical of IPD and rarely is due to other disorders. Often, tremor is the sole presenting feature of IPD, however, only two-thirds of Parkinsonian patients have tremor on diagnosis, and some will never develop this sign.[4] Tremor is often seen with IPD onset at a younger age and is associated with less functional decline and decreased risk of dementia.[5] Tremor in IPD is present most commonly in the hands, sometimes with a characteristic "pill-rolling" quality. It can also involve the jaw or legs. Sometimes, the sensory equivalent is perceived as an "internal" sensation of vibration without outward

TABLE 58.2. CLINICAL FEATURES

Primary
- Bradykinesia
- Postural instability
  - Propulsion
  - Retropulsion
- Resting tremor (may have postural and action components)
- Rigidity

Motor Symptoms
- Dysarthria
- Dysphagia
- Festinating gait
- Flexed posture
- "Freezing" at initiation of movement
- Hypomimia
- Hypophonia
- Micrographia
- Slow turning

Autonomic Symptoms
- Bladder and anal sphincter disturbances
- Constipation
- Diaphoresis
- Orthostatic blood pressure changes
- Paroxysmal flushing
- Sexual disturbances

Mental Status Changes
- Confusional state
- Dementia
- Psychosis (paranoia, hallucinosis)
- Sleep disturbance

Other
- Fatigue
- Oily skin
- Pedal edema
- Seborrhea
- Weight loss

manifestations. Electromyographic recordings usually show resting tremor to occur in the range of 4–7 Hz. Similar to other symptoms of IPD, resting tremor often begins unilaterally and may persist in this distribution. Occasionally, maintaining a position of the limbs or volitional movement will bring out tremor. Stressful situations or use of limbs in other activities may increase tremor amplitude in a limb at rest. Usually, resting tremor is abolished by volitional movement, and it is absent during sleep.

Rigidity (increased muscular resistance to passive range of motion) is another characteristic sign of parkinsonism, although not pathognomonic for this disorder. Together with increased tone there can be "cog wheel-like" resistance to movement. Another condition that produces increased tone in IPD is the occurrence of dystonic postures (especially in the feet).

Because it can lead to falls, postural instability is one of the most disabling problems of parkinsonism. A disturbance of appropriate responses to the perturbation of balance is common in advanced IPD. Testing for impaired postural responses by means of the "pull test" (in which a patient is unable to recover balance after sudden backward displacement at the shoulders) can help to identify the risk for falling. Many patients with impaired postural responses also have tendencies for propulsive gait (festination) and a forward flexed posture of their axial structures along with partial flexion of the extremities. This pattern has been described as a simian posture.

Other characteristics of IPD are closely related to the bradykinesia and decreased precision of movement. These features include *micrographia* (handwriting that slows and decreases in size as the task proceeds), and *hypophonia* (a gradual decrease in volume and clarity of speech). A decreased rate of involuntary swallowing and a forward tilt of the head can result in drooling. Some Parkinsonian patients experience various autonomic impairments that coincide with the onset of motor impairments, including excessive sweating, constipation, and postural hypotension. Some of these problems can also be induced by medications used to treat parkinsonism.

In most instances, IPD is predominantly a disorder of motor capabilities. Certain neuropsychological abnormalities can be detected in IPD patients, even with early and mild forms of the disorder in the absence of any cognitive impairments. Although intellectual deterioration is not inevitable in IPD, some patients deteriorate in a manner indistinguishable from Alzheimer's disease and other dementing conditions. It has been hard to estimate the number of patients at risk, since medications and other concomitant illnesses can confound determination of the degree of cognitive decline due specifically to IPD.[6] Another problem for which IPD patients may have increased risk is depression. Although the disabilities of IPD may provoke some instances of depression, the biochemical changes in the brain due to IPD may also predispose for endogenous depression.

EPIDEMIOLOGY

In a series of 100 pathologically proven cases of IPD, the mean age of disease onset was 62.5 years (range: 31–83 years).[3] The annual incidence of IPD is about 20 per 100,000 in North America.[7] Extensive research into the epidemiology of the disorder has not identified occupations, regional clusters, or incidence trends implicating specific environmental factors in the etiology of IPD although rural living may be one of the few characteristics enhancing the risk for IPD.[8]

While IPD appears to be a sporadic disorder in most instances, there may be some role(s) for genetic factors in its etiology. In rare patients with otherwise typical IPD, studies of their families have provided evidence for an inherited disorder. An autosomal dominant pattern with decreased penetrance and variable age of onset has been described.[9] The onset of IPD in later life implies that cumulative exposures to putative toxins, factors associated with central nervous system aging, or other as yet uncharacterized cell death mechanisms are responsible for the onset and progression of the disease.

PATHOPHYSIOLOGY

Dopaminergic neurons project from the pars compacta of the substantia nigra to the striatum via the nigrostriatal pathway. Dopamine is synthesized in the cell bodies of neurons in the substantia nigra and transported for storage in synaptic vesicles until release into the synaptic cleft. Virtually all the motor deficits of IPD occur from the marked loss in dopaminergic nerve terminals projecting primarily to the putamen. The basal ganglia have specific patterns of activation in the initiation, sequencing, and modulating of motor activity. The synaptic organization of the basal ganglia involves a variety of neurotransmitters, including acetylcholine, dopamine, GABA, glutamate, substance P, and serotonin. These are all possible targets for interventions in IPD. Drugs enhancing dopaminergic neurotransmission and inhibiting acetylcholine effects have been successful in IPD therapeutics; the role for drug modulation of other neurotransmitters active in the basal ganglia has not been well explored.

The greatest attention for the treatment of IPD has been focused on the loss of dopaminergic neurons projecting to caudate and putamen. The model of dopaminergic depletion (with reserpine) or blockade in producing Parkinsonian features provided much of the impetus for development of therapies to augment stimulation of striatal dopamine receptors. Five classes of human dopamine receptors (D_1, D_2, D_3, D_4, and D_5) have been cloned.[10] Stimulation of D_1 dopamine receptors (which are the most abundant class in the striatum) is linked to activation of adenylate cyclase. D_2 dopamine receptors are coupled to a guanosine triphosphate (GTP)-binding protein, which opens potassium channels to hyperpolarize neurons, thereby reducing the excitability of striatal cells.[11] In IPD, activation of the D_2 receptor appears to be of primary importance for mediating both clinical improvements and adverse effects (such as dyskinesias or hallucinations).

Pathologic findings reveal a markedly decreased number of nigrostriatal dopamine neurons and a positive correlation between the degree of nigrostriatal dopamine loss and the severity of clinical features.[6] The threshold for onset of parkinsonism appears to be the loss of 80% or more of these neurons (Fig. 58.1).[12] ^{18}F-fluorodopa positron emission studies clearly demonstrate decreased uptake and utilization of fluorodopa in IPD.[13] There has been suggestion of a compensatory increase in striatal dopamine receptors in response to the decreased capabilities for dopamine release, although positron emission studies with dopamine antagonists have shown no difference in dopamine receptor density between sides in hemiparkinsonian subjects.[14] Some *in vivo* imaging studies suggest that chronic dopaminergic stimulation may cause downregulation of postsynaptic dopamine receptors, leading possibly to a lack of response or else fluctuating responses to dopaminergic drugs.[15] Other evidence suggests that fluctuations in stimulation of receptors may predispose to agonist tolerance.[16] Progressive supranuclear palsy and other "Parkinson-plus" disorders are not responsive to dopamine replacement or dopamine agonist therapies, presumably on the basis of decreased dopamine receptors or, more likely, damage to postsynaptic elements of striatal function and other neuropathologic changes beyond those found in IPD.

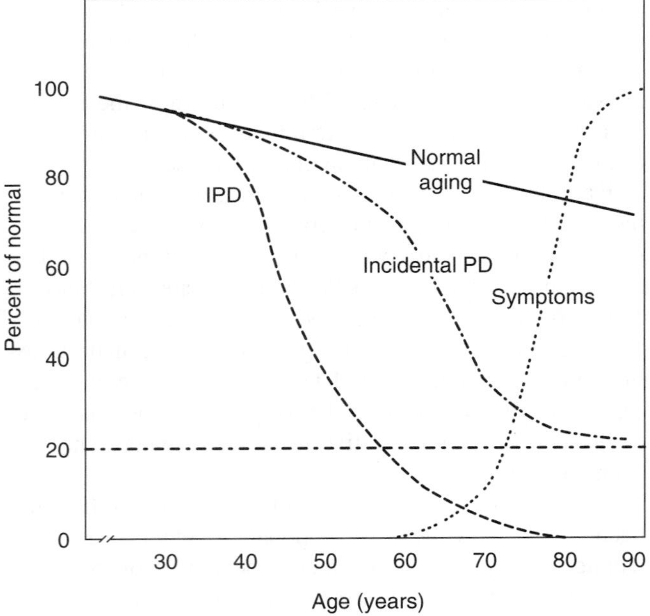

Figure 58.1. There is a loss of dopaminergic neurons with normal aging (———). Either an endogenous or exogenous insult results in premature dropout of neurons (— — —). Symptoms develop when about 20% of neurons remain (• • •). Patients with incidental Parkinson's disease have premature loss of neurons and Lewy bodies but symptoms never develop (—•—).

Dopamine metabolism is shown in Fig. 58.2, and the range of therapeutic interventions for IPD are summarized in Table 58.3. Tyrosine, the metabolic precursor of dopamine, is converted by tyrosine hydroxylase (TH) to L-dihydroxyphenylalanine (L-dopa) in a highly regulated synthetic process. Tetrahydrobiopterin is the cofactor required for this process. Attempts to augment synthesis for dopamine by supplementation with this cofactor have not been effective.[17] L-dopa is decarboxylated to dopamine by the enzyme L-amino acid decarboxylase (L-AAD). L-AAD is present outside of the central nervous system (CNS) and in some nonaminergic neurons, while tyrosine hydroxylase is found exclusively in aminergic neurons. Peripheral L-AAD can be blocked by administering antagonists such as carbidopa or benserazide, which do not pass the blood–brain barrier. Use of these drugs with L-dopa therefore can increase the CNS penetration of exogenously administered L-dopa, thereby decreasing adverse effects from peripheral L-dopa metabolism to dopamine. Dopamine is stored in synaptic vesicles until stimulated to be released into the synapse by calcium-dependent mechanisms. Dopamine activity is terminated primarily by reuptake into the presynaptic neuron by means of a specific dopamine transporter. In the presynaptic neurons, sequestration into the storage granules or the actions of catabolic pathways involving monoamine oxidase (MAO) or catechol-O-methyl transferase (COMT) lead to inactivation of dopamine.

Since dopamine tonically inhibits acetylcholine neurons in the striatum, the degeneration of nigrostriatal dopamine neurons results in a relative increase of striatal cholinergic interneuron activity. This increased cholinergic activity contributes especially to the tremor of IPD, as evidenced by symptomatic improvement with the use of anticholinergics and worsening with cholinergic agents.

The pathogenesis of IPD is not known, but neurotoxins highly selective to dopaminergic neurons have been instructive. Animal models of parkinsonism can be created with 6-hydroxydopamine and 1-methyl-4-phenyl-1,2,3,6-tetrahydropyridine (MPTP). The latter compound is converted by MAO type B to the toxic 1-methyl-4-phenylpyridinium (MPP^+) ion, and inhibition of the oxidase by a drug such as selegiline eliminates the toxicity of MPTP. MPP^+ is toxic to neurons because of its interference with mitochondrial metabolism. Another mechanism of toxicity also under consideration for the pathogenesis of IPD is cellular damage from oxyradicals. Dopamine metabolism generates free radicals from both auto-oxidation and as a by-product of MAO (Fig. 58.3). Several antioxidative mechanisms are

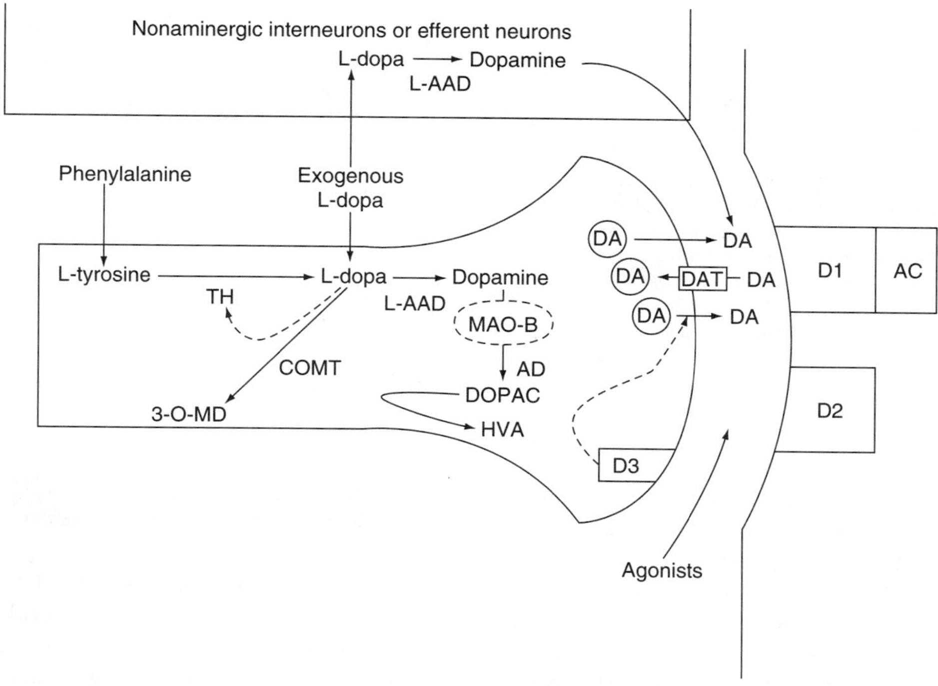

Figure 58.2. Dopamine metabolism in presynaptic dopamine neuron. 3-O-MD, 3-O-methyldopa; AC, adenylate cyclase; AD, aldehyde dehydrogenase; COMT, catechol-O-methyl transferase; D1–D3, dopamine receptors; DA, dopamine; DAT, dopamine transporter; DOPAC, 3,4-dihydroxyphenylacetic acid; HVA, homovanillic acid; L-AAD, L-aromatic amine decarboxylase; MAO-B, monamine oxidase B; and TH, tyrosine hydroxylase.

TABLE 58.3. MECHANISMS FOR POTENTIAL IPD TREATMENTS

Increase Endogenous Dopamine
- Increase tyrosine hydroxylase
  - Tetrahydrobiopterin
- L-dopa
  - Inhibit peripheral metabolism by dopa decarboxylase
    - Carbidopa
    - Benserazide
  - Sustained release products
  - Infusions
    - Intravenous
    - Duodenal
  - Inhibit peripheral and central metabolism by catechol-O-methyl transferase
    - Entacapone (peripheral only)
    - Tolcapone
  - Inhibit central and peripheral metabolism by monoamine oxidase B
    - Selegiline (deprenyl)

Dopamine Agonists
- D_2 specific
  - Bromocriptine
  - Lisuride
- D_1 and D_2 nonspecific
  - Pergolide
  - Apomorphine
    - Intravenous
    - Subcutaneous infusions
    - Intranasal
    - Sublingual
- Partial agonists
  - Terguride

Anticholinergic
- Benztropine
- Trihexyphenidyl

Preventative
- Selegiline (deprenyl)

Surgical Options
- Autologous adrenal tissue transplantation
- Fetal tissue transplantation
- Thalamotomy
- Pallidotomy
- Thalamic electrical stimulation

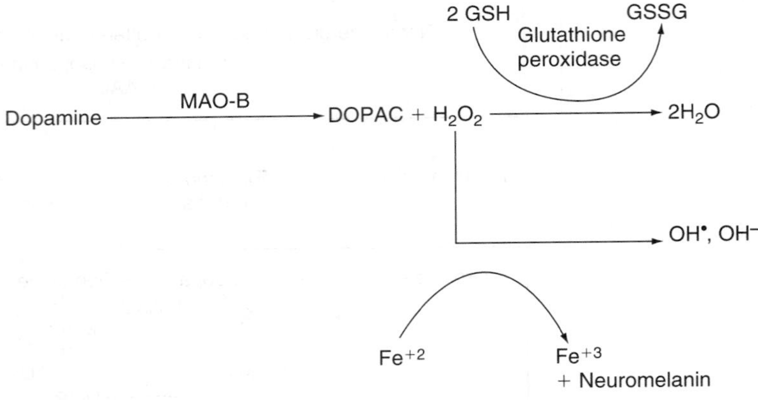

Figure 58.3. Dopamine metabolism results in hydrogen peroxide (H_2O_2) formation. If the glutathione system is deficient or excess hydrogen peroxide is present, hydrogen peroxide accepts an electron from ferrous iron (Fe^{+2}) forming ferric iron (Fe^{+3}) and the hydroxyl free radical ($OH^{\bullet}$). The hydroxyl free radical can cause lipid peroxidation thereby damaging cell membranes. MAO-B, monoamine oxidase B; DOPAC, 3,4-dihydroxyphenylacetic acid; H_2O, water; GSH, glutathione; GSSG, glutathione disulfide; and OH^-, the hydroxide ion.

present within and outside of neurons to limit any damage that might be produced by free radical attack, but it is possible that such protection might be overwhelmed or impaired in IPD. Another unique feature of the substantia nigra neuron is the presence of neuromelanin and accumulation of iron. Each of these substances catalyzes the conversion of hydrogen peroxide (derived from MAO catabolism of dopamine) to the superoxide and hydroxyl radicals.[18] Free radicals or other types of cellular damage may also be the consequence of a defect in mitochondrial complex 1 functions in the substantia nigra.[19]

Therapeutics

A general algorithm for treatment of IPD is shown in Fig. 58.4, however, more complete algorithms covering virtually every aspect of IPD management have recently been published.[20] The optimal management of IPD is best determined by individualized considerations of a patient's disability profile. The classification system developed by Hoehn and Yahr[21] is used most frequently to stage disease severity (Table 58.4). The only established pharmacologic

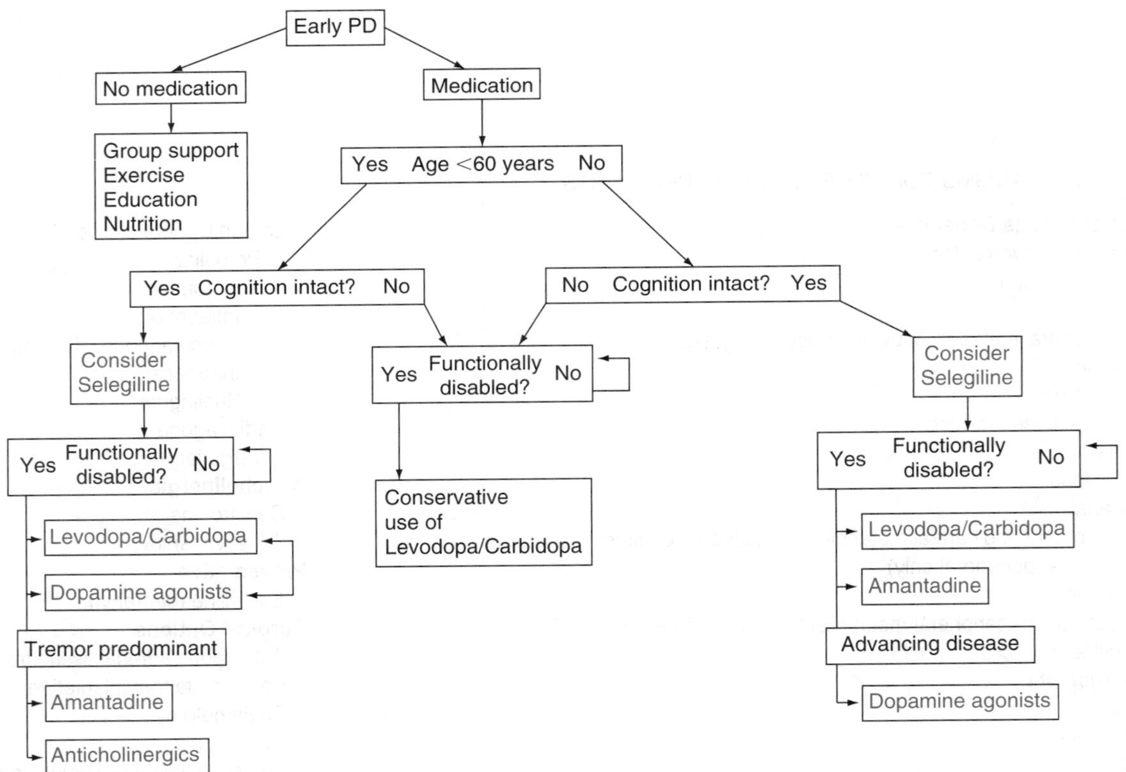

Figure 58.4. General algorithm for treating IPD.

TABLE 58.4. HOEHN AND YAHR STAGING OF SEVERITY OF PARKINSON'S DISEASE

Stage 0:	No clinical signs evident
Stage I:	Unilateral involvement
Stage II:	Bilateral involvement but no postural abnormalities
Stage III:	Bilateral involvement with mild postural imbalance on examination or history of poor balance or falls; patient leads independent life
Stage IV:	Bilateral involvement with postural instability; patient requires substantial help
Stage V:	Severe, fully developed disease; patient restricted to bed or wheelchair

(Compiled from Ref. 20.)

therapy for IPD is medication that can transiently reverse signs and symptoms. Although these symptomatic treatments can be highly effective, the major loss of nigrostriatal neurons by the time that the first symptoms arise means that definitive treatment of the underlying disease would need to have been instituted much earlier. In addition to drugs, regular exercise can have a major impact on quality of life with IPD. Referrals for speech, occupational, and physical therapies are sometimes quite helpful. In patients with mild features of IPD, use of medications is often not needed if disabilities have not evolved. Many patients will never have more than mild slowness and resting tremor, circumstances that often can be managed effectively with anticholinergics or amantadine (see the following paragraph).

The most effective drug therapy for IPD involves enhancement of dopaminergic activity. This can be accomplished in several ways (Table 58.3). The most efficacious treatment is replacement of the natural neurotransmitter, dopamine, by the use of its immediate precursor, L-dopa. Although L-dopa is more effective than other medications currently available, there has been considerable concern with respect to the possible risks from long-term use. Hence, minimal use of L-dopa is widely advocated at present. As indicated in the treatment algorithm, anticholinergic drugs or amantadine can be used as an alternative to L-dopa for treating resting tremor. While these drugs are not highly effective against bradykinesia, gait disturbance, or other features of advanced parkinsonism, they can be useful for relieving mild disabilities experienced by patients in the first few years after the onset of parkinsonism. The decision to incorporate L-dopa therapy comes from advancing disability and ineffectiveness of these alternative medications to provide adequate symptomatic control. Depending on profession and lifestyle, the same basic Parkinsonian features may result in different degrees of disability, and drug therapy goals may need to be adjusted accordingly. A summary of available anti-Parkinsonian medications is listed in Table 58.5.

TABLE 58.5. DRUGS USED IN PARKINSON'S DISEASE

Generic Name	Trade Name	Manufacturer	Dosage Range (mg/d)	Dosage Forms (mg)	Cost Index[a]
Amantadine	Symmetrel	DuPont	200–300	100,50/5mL	8,8
		Various generic brands			3,7
Carbidopa/L-dopa	Sinemet	DuPont	[b]	10/100,25/100,25/250	6,7,8
	Atamet	Athena			
Controlled-release carbidopa/L-dopa	Sinemet CR	DuPont	[b]	25/100,50/200	7,14
L-dopa	Larodopa	Roche	[b]	100,250,500	2,3,6
	Dopar	Roberts Pharm			
Selegiline	Eldepryl	Somerset	10	5	21
Agonists					
Bromocriptine	Parlodel	Sandoz	[b]	2.5, 5	14,22
Pergolide	Permax	Athena	[b]	0.05,0.25,1	2,25,82
Anticholinergic Drugs					
Benztropine	Cogentin	Merck and Co.	0.5–6	0.5,1,2	2,2,2
		Various generic brands			1,1,1
Biperiden	Akineton	Knoll	2–16	2	2
Diphenhydramine	Benadryl	Parke-Davis	25–100	25,50	2,3
		Various generic brands			1,1
Procyclidine	Kemadrin	Burroughs-Wellcome	2.5–20	5	4
Trihexyphenidyl	Artane	Lederle	1–15	2,5,2/5mL,5 LA	1,3,3,4
		Various generic brands			1,3

[a]Cost index calculated from June 1994 Average Wholesale Price per 100. Approximate cost per 100 (or per pint for solutions) equivalent to index × $10.00.
[b]Dosage must be individualized.

SELEGILINE

Selegiline (Eldepryl, Somerset), an MAO-B inhibitor also known as deprenyl, is marketed for producing extension of L-dopa effects. By blocking the breakdown of dopamine, it can extend the duration of action from each dose of L-dopa, and often permits reduction in the dose of L-dopa needed for optimal effect. Patients undergoing L-dopa "wearing-off" actions may experience an hour or more of increased action from each L-dopa dose (just as they might by use of sustained-release L-dopa).[22] Selegiline also increases the peak concentrations of L-dopa, and so can enhance adverse reactions such as worsening of preexisting dyskinesias or psychiatric symptoms such as delusions and hallucinations. Often, selegiline permits reduction of L-dopa intake to as little as one-half of its previous dose without loss of efficacy.

Selegiline has been widely used at a dose of 10 mg/d, although its irreversible inhibition of MAO-B may occur at lower doses.[23] In addition, renewal of the enzyme proceeds at a slow rate, so that the effect of the drug lingers for weeks. Selegiline is lipophilic and penetrates the blood–brain barrier rapidly. The metabolic pathway of selegiline leads to end-products of L-methamphetamine and L-amphetamine.[24] Adverse effects of selegiline are minimal and include insomnia and jitteriness. The hypertensive "cheese effect," which occurs from ingesting tyramine with the use of MAO-A inhibitors, does not occur with selegiline.[25] However, there have been a few case reports of an adverse reaction characterized by hypertension, diaphoresis, and shivering associated with concomitant use of the selective serotonin reuptake blocker fluoxetine.[26] A similar reaction has been reported with meperidine.[27]

In addition to its symptomatic effects at enhancing L-dopa action, selegiline may have neuroprotective properties. As mentioned previously, the oxidative deamination of dopamine by MAO-B generates hydrogen peroxide, which is converted to free radicals capable of damaging nigrostriatal neurons. Because MAO-B inhibition diverts dopamine catabolism away from the generation of peroxide, selegiline therapy has been proposed as one means for sparing these neurons from oxidative stress. Several studies have investigated the role of selegiline as a means to slow the progression of IPD by its blockade of MAO-B. Although initial findings were quite promising, the application of selegiline gives only partial protection against the advance of Parkinsonian disability, and the effect has not been demonstrated to last for more than a year.[28–31]

ANTICHOLINERGIC MEDICATIONS

The anticholinergic drugs can be effective against tremor but rarely show much benefit for bradykinesia or other disabilities of IPD. Even with respect to tremor not all patients respond. Dystonic features associated with IPD can also be improved with anticholinergic drugs. Adverse effects of these drugs include dry mouth, blurred vision, constipation, and urinary retention. More serious reactions include forgetfulness, sedation, depression, and anxiety. An encephalopathic state can also gradually evolve in some patients. Patients with preexisting cognitive deficits and advanced age are at greater risk for central anticholinergic effects.[32] A number of anticholinergic drugs are available (Table 58.5). These differ little in their adverse effects and have essentially the same therapeutic potential. Anticholinergic drugs can be useful for monotherapy when tremor is the major clinical symptom, and these drugs can be used in conjunction with L-dopa and the other anti-Parkinsonian agents.

AMANTADINE

Amantadine (Symmetrel, Du Pont; various generic brands) is often effective for relief of most mild signs and symptoms of IPD.[33] Similar to anticholinergics, it can be especially effective against tremor. The drug is used at 200–300 mg/d. Adverse effects associated with initiation of amantadine (sedation and vivid dreams) may disappear with time. Dry mouth is a common adverse effect reminiscent of anticholinergic drugs, although amantadine does not block cholinergic receptors. Other adverse central effects seen uncommonly include depression, hallucinations, anxiety, dizziness, psychosis, and confusion.

A frequent (and reversible) adverse effect of amantadine is livedo reticularis, a diffuse mottling of the skin. Amantadine is eliminated renally and a decreased dose should be administered when renal dysfunction is present (100 mg/d with creatinine clearances from 30–50 mL/min, 100 mg every other day for creatinine clearances from 15–29 mL/min, and 200 mg every 7 days for creatinine clearances less than 15 mL/min and patients on hemodialysis). Unlike other drugs for IPD, the precise mechanism of action of amantadine is unknown. An increase in presynaptic dopamine synthesis, an increase in dopamine release, and inhibition of dopamine reuptake were initially suggested as possible mechanisms; however, recently nondopaminergic mechanisms have been proposed.[34]

L-DOPA AND CARBIDOPA/L-DOPA

L-dopa (Larodopa, Roche; Dopar, Norwich-Eaton; various generic brands) was first studied for parkinsonism in the early 1960s, and recognition of its unequivocal benefit was reported in 1967.[35] It is still the most effective drug available for the management of IPD. L-dopa, the immediate precursor of dopamine, crosses the blood–brain barrier, whereas dopamine does not. In the striatum and elsewhere, the conversion of L-dopa is via L-AAD. The peripheral conversion of L-dopa to dopamine is responsible for adverse effects such as nausea, vomiting, cardiac arrhythmias, and postural hypotension. By combining L-dopa with the peripherally acting L-AAD inhibitors, carbidopa (Sinemet, Merck Sharp & Dohme; various generic brands) or benserazide (Madopar, not available in the United States), peripheral conversion of L-dopa to dopamine is blocked. As a result, increased amounts of L-dopa are transported into the brain.[36]

As of the mid-1990s, L-dopa is used almost exclusively in combination with carbidopa. Starting L-dopa doses of 200–300 mg/d in combination with carbidopa often achieves adequate relief of disability. Some patients require larger amounts on a daily basis, possibly as a result of less complete absorption. The usual maximal dose of L-dopa needed by patients even with severe parkinsonism is 800 mg/d. Slow buildup of dose (e.g., increments of 100 mg of L-dopa per week) can help to determine the lowest effective dose and minimizes the risk of adverse effects, such as postural hypotension, nausea, vomiting, sedation, and vivid dreams.

Several formulations of carbidopa/L-dopa are available. Carbidopa has a maximum effective daily dose of 100–125 mg beyond which there is little increase in dopa decarboxylase inhibitory effect. Carbidopa/L-dopa is most widely used in a 25 mg/100 mg tablet form, although 25 mg/250 mg and 10 mg/100 mg dosage forms are also available. Controlled-release preparations of carbidopa/L-dopa are available in 50 mg/200 mg and 25 mg/100 mg strengths.[37] If peripheral adverse effects are prominent, 25-mg carbidopa (Lodosyn, Merck and Co.) tablets are available from the manufacturer by physician request and can be used to supplement the fixed combination products.

After 3 or more years of treatment, one-third or more of L-dopa-treated patients develop involuntary movements or short-duration responses to the drug. Movement complications associated with long-term treatment with carbidopa/L-dopa treatment and their suggested treatments are listed in Table 58.6. Debate exists whether these complications are related to treatment or are intrinsic to the disease process itself.

End-of-dose deterioration (the "wearing-off" effect) has been related to increasing loss of neuronal storage capability for dopamine. Initially, exogenous L-dopa is taken up by the remaining presynaptic neurons, converted to dopamine, and stored in synaptic vesicles. With progressive loss of presynaptic neurons, storage capacity declines, and patients become more dependent on the rate of L-dopa delivery to the brain for the generation of dopamine. Hence, the peripheral pharmacokinetics of L-dopa increasingly become the determinants of dopamine synthesis.

With advance of IPD and chronicity of L-dopa therapy, motor response fluctuations tend to become more prominent. A single carbidopa/L-dopa dose may produce benefits for as little as 1.5–2 hours. In this instance, carbidopa/L-dopa needs to be given more frequently in order to prevent the "wearing-off" of its benefits. Rather than give carbidopa/L-dopa more frequently, the sustained-release prod-

TABLE 58.6. MOTOR FLUCTUATIONS AND POSSIBLE INTERVENTIONS IN IPD

Effect	Possible Treatments
End of dose deterioration ("wearing off")	Increase frequency of doses, controlled-release carbidopa/L-dopa, consider agonists, selegiline, or amantadine, duodenal or intravenous L-dopa infusions, carbidopa/L-dopa oral solution, subcutaneous apomorphine infusions, transdermal dopamine agonists
Delayed onset of response	Give on empty stomach before meals, crush or chew and take with a full glass of water, reduce dietary protein intake, antacids, morning standard-release carbidopa/L-dopa if on sustained-release carbidopa/L-dopa, infusions of L-dopa or dopamine agonists
Drug resistant "off" periods	Increase carbidopa/L-dopa dose and/or frequency, give on empty stomach before meals, crush or chew and take with a full glass of water, infusions of L-dopa or dopamine agonists, apomorphine intranasal spray
"Random" oscillations ("on-off")	Dopamine agonists, selegiline, infusions of L-dopa or dopamine agonists, consider drug holiday
Start hesitation ("freezing")	Increase carbidopa/L-dopa dose, dopamine agonists, gait modifications (tapping, rhythmic commands, stepping over objects, rocking)
Peak dose dyskinesia ("I-D-I" response[a])	Smaller more frequent doses of carbidopa/L-dopa, controlled-release carbidopa/L-dopa
Diphasic dyskinesias ("D-I-D" response[b])	Reduce anticholinergic medication
Dystonia	Baclofen, nighttime carbidopa/L-dopa, morning standard-release carbidopa/L-dopa if on sustained-release carbidopa/L-dopa, dopamine agonists, anticholinergics
Myoclonus	Decrease nighttime L-dopa doses, clonazepam
Akathisia	Benzodiazepines, propranolol

[a]I-D-I is the "improvement-dyskinesia/dystonia-improvement" pattern of response.
[b]D-I-D is the "dyskinesia-improvement-dyskinesia" pattern of response.

uct can extend the duration of the L-dopa effect. A more gradual "wearing-off" of the L-dopa effect and a need for fewer daily doses are associated with the use of this product.[38] Some patients will require an increase of L-dopa intake when switched to the sustained-release form because of its decreased bioavailability. Patients maintained on the sustained-release product may also require a conventional carbidopa/L-dopa dose in the morning for its more rapid absorption and response.[39]

Dopamine agonists also can be added to a carbidopa/L-dopa regimen in an attempt to treat "wearing off." In addition, either intravenous or duodenal L-dopa infusions will produce constant serum L-dopa concentrations (and presumably striatal dopamine concentrations) and thus reduce response fluctuations.[40,41] Although some patients have been maintained on duodenal and intravenous infusions for long periods of time, these invasive methods of administration require careful planning and are generally not used outside the research setting. Sipping small amounts of carbidopa/L-dopa solution is an easier way to noninvasively titrate drug intake to optimal effect.[42] Finally, MAO-B inhibitors (e.g., selegiline) and COMT inhibitors currently under development extend the action of L-dopa.[43]

Drug-resistant "off" periods or delayed response to carbidopa/L-dopa can be due to delayed stomach emptying or decreased absorption in the upper GI tract. Chewing a tablet or crushing it and then drinking a full glass of water may decrease disintegration time and facilitate gastric emptying. Antacids also facilitate gastric emptying. Meals delay gastric emptying, and high protein content in ingested food sometimes leads to decreased L-dopa absorption. The latter effect is the result of competition between L-dopa and large neutral amino acids (LNAAs), which can compete for absorption of the drug in the proximal duodenum. Circulating LNAA can also compete with facilitated uptake of L-dopa into the brain through a saturable transport system.

Rapid fluctuations from "on" to "off" states can occur in patients receiving L-dopa chronically. Rapid transitions from normal or dyskinetic "on" motor activity to bradykinetic or "off" states can occur. Concentration versus effect data after sustained-release carbidopa/L-dopa use reveal nonlinear (sigmoid E_{max} model) relationships such that small changes in serum L-dopa concentrations may lead to large effect responses.[44] Indeed, sudden "off" states have been associated with a decline in L-dopa plasma concentrations.[45] With progression of the disease, motor skill performance decreases so that there will be larger differences between baseline capabilities and maximum therapeutic effect; hence, there will be a steep slope at the EC50 (concentration at half-maximal effect). These circumstances contribute to rapid fluctuations in motor responses. Infusions of L-dopa or regimens of drugs with long-acting dopaminergic effects tend to alleviate these fluctuations.

Dopaminergic agonists can also be added to L-dopa as a means for treating "on–off" fluctuations. Other strategies include MAO-B inhibitors and inhibitors of COMT, which can decrease the clearance of L-dopa. A drug-free period (drug holiday) has been investigated in an attempt to modify postsynaptic dopamine receptors and thus decrease "on–off" fluctuations.[46,47] The discontinuation regimens studied involved tapering L-dopa and discontinuing the drug for 7–14 days. During the holiday period, there can be a dramatic worsening of functional status, sometimes necessitating hospitalization. Neuroleptic malignant syndrome can occur after abrupt anti-Parkinsonian drug withdrawal.[48,49] After the holiday, therapy can be reinstituted at doses much less than those needed previously. Because of the discomforts and risks as well as the limited gains achieved for most patients, drug holiday is not currently used as a therapeutic intervention.

Another complication of L-dopa therapy is dyskinesias (choreiform abnormal involuntary movements usually involving the neck, trunk, and upper extremities) and dystonias (sustained muscle spasm and posturing). These involuntary movements are usually associated with peak anti-Parkinsonian benefit (peak-effect dyskinesia), although they can also develop during the rise and fall of L-dopa effects (the "improvement-dyskinesia/dystonia-improvement" [I-D-I] pattern of response). In the case of peak-effect dyskinesias or dystonias, smaller, more frequent doses of L-dopa or use of the sustained-release preparations can be beneficial. Treatment for the "dyskinesia-improvement-dyskinesia" (D-I-D) pattern is unknown and can actually worsen with strategies useful for the other pattern. Simplistically, dyskinesias can be thought of as "too much movement" secondary to an extension of the pharmacologic effect or "too much" striatal dopamine receptor stimulation. However, the phenomenology is actually far more complex, as demonstrated by the occasional patient simultaneously demonstrating Parkinsonian features and dyskinesias. An interaction between different classes of dopamine receptors may be involved. In some studies, the rate of decrease in dyskinetic movements after an intravenous infusion of L-dopa has been stopped differs from the rate of increase in Parkinsonian features.[50,51] The amelioration of dyskinesias is usually achieved by decreasing the size of each dose as well as the total daily dose and increasing the dosage frequency. A partial dopamine agonist, terguride, has been found to have specific activity at suppressing dyskinesias without worsening Parkinsonian symptoms, suggesting that some pharmacologic approaches may differentiate the effects of dopaminergic stimulation on different aspects of motor system activation.[52]

Dystonias are especially common in the distal lower extremities. Clenching of the toes or turning of the foot can precede the development of IPD. L-dopa therapy can be associated with the occurrence of these spasms in the early morning hours and improve after the first L-dopa dose. Remedies for this problem include bed-time administration of sustained-release L-dopa, dopaminergic agonists, or baclofen. Another problem that can occur during sleep is exaggerated myoclonus. Lowering nighttime L-dopa doses or use of clonazepam can be beneficial. Benzodiazepines or propranolol can be used for treating akathisia, another adverse effect of L-dopa. Akathisia is the sensation of inner restlessness resulting in the need to make movements.

L-dopa and dopaminergic agonists do not only act in the nigrostriatal system, but also facilitate other dopamine pathways (including those in the mesolimbic dopaminergic projections). Activation of the latter system may result in occurrence of psychiatric manifestations including delirium, agitation, paranoia, delusions, and hallucinations. These effects occur even more frequently (up to 85%) in older patients and in those with underlying confusion or dementia.[53] Clozapine (Clozaril, Sandoz), an atypical antipsychotic, improves most of these psychotic symptoms without worsening Parkinsonian symptoms.[54] There is even some suggestion that clozapine may improve Parkinsonian motor symptoms.[55]

The decision whether to start L-dopa early (as soon as the diagnosis of IPD is made) or late (only when symptoms compromise social, occupational, or psychological well-being) has generated controversy.[56,57] Proponents for delaying treatment point to evidence suggesting that long-term L-dopa therapy is associated with increased risk of response fluctuations, increased risk of dementia, and loss of L-dopa efficacy.[58] L-dopa therapy may also increase oxidative stress in dopaminergic neurons and thus increase dopaminergic neuronal loss.

The counterargument is that response fluctuations are secondary to disease progression, not L-dopa therapy. Studies comparing early and late treatment with L-dopa have shown similar Hoehn and Yahr staging scores at the time of L-dopa intervention, suggesting that the reason L-dopa was started sooner in the early L-dopa treatment group was because of more rapid disease progression from the time of diagnosis.[59] Thus, it is not unexpected that this group would continue to have disease progression at a more rapid rate. In addition, a multicenter study found that withholding L-dopa therapy for more than 3 years after diagnosis resulted in a doubling of the excess mortality rate compared to early treatment.[60]

Despite these conflicting views, there is general consensus that the proper time to initiate L-dopa therapy is when the disease interferes with the patient's occupation or activities of daily living or when the patient makes a rational decision to begin therapy after considering all risks and benefits. Arbitrary dosage limits should not be set and L-dopa dosage must be individualized.

L-dopa pharmacokinetic properties help explain some of the clinical effects seen. There is marked intra- and intersubject variability in the time to peak plasma concentrations after oral L-dopa. Often there may be more than one peak plasma concentration after a single dose, which is attributed to erratic gastric emptying. Meals delay gastric emptying, while antacids that decrease gastric acidity promote gastric emptying.[61] Recently, cisapride has been shown to increase peak plasma concentrations and the area under the L-dopa plasma concentration versus time curve (AUC) presumably by increasing gastric emptying.[62] L-dopa is primarily absorbed in the proximal duodenum by a saturable LNAA transport system. Competition for this site by dietary or supplemental LNAAs can reduce L-dopa plasma concentrations. The gut wall also contains a saturable decarboxylase, which limits the bioavailability of L-dopa unless a peripheral decarboxylase inhibitor such as carbidopa is combined with the L-dopa dose.

L-dopa is not bound to plasma proteins. It crosses the blood–brain barrier by stereospecific saturable facilitated diffusion. Thus, L-dopa also competes with LNAA for transport into the brain. Infusions of phenylalanine and leucine decrease clinical response to L-dopa without altering L-dopa plasma concentrations.[63] This has led to special diets being recommended for these patients.[64] A metabolite of L-dopa, 3-O-methyldopa (3OMD), also competes for transport, but it is not clear how this affects L-dopa clinical response. Drug holidays may allow the body to clear this longer half-life metabolite thus restoring better L-dopa responsiveness.

L-dopa elimination is primarily by decarboxylation to dopamine. Additional pathways are by 3-O-methylation and transamination. When a decarboxylase inhibitor is used, increased amounts of L-dopa are metabolized by the other pathways. The elimination half-life of L-dopa is about 1 hour and this is extended to about 1.5 hours with the addition of carbidopa. 3OMD has a half-life of about 15 hours and will accumulate with chronic dosing. Dose versus AUC suggests a nonlinear relationship for L-dopa that is suggestive of a saturable elimination process.[65] There do not appear to be any peripheral pharmacokinetic differences between patients with stable responses, response fluctuations, and "on–off" fluctuations.[66]

Poor correlations between L-dopa plasma concentrations and clinical response were noted initially because of a lag time in clinical response resulting in timewise hysteresis.[67] Subsequent studies using an effect compartment model have revealed nonlinear relationships between effect compartment concentrations and clinical responses.[68,69]

L-dopa should be administered cautiously with nonselective MAO inhibitors (possible hypertensive crisis), antihypertensive agents (possible additive hypotensive effect), phenytoin (possible reversal of anti-Parkinsonian effect), and antipsychotic agents (possible antagonism of L-dopa effect).

DOPAMINE AGONISTS

The use of the dopamine agonists pergolide (Permax, Athena) and bromocriptine (Parlodel, Sandoz) as adjuncts to L-dopa therapy is beneficial in prolonging the effective treatment period in patients with deteriorating response to L-dopa,[70–72] in patients who are experiencing fluctuations in response to L-dopa,[73,74] and in patients with limited clinical response to L-dopa secondary to inability to tolerate higher doses.[69] The dopamine agonists also decrease the frequency of "off" periods and provide an L-dopa sparing effect. Bromocriptine and pergolide are considered equally efficacious in producing these beneficial effects.[75] Limited data suggest that pergolide may improve functional status in patients with deteriorating response to bromocriptine,[76] whereas bromocriptine does not appear to improve function in patients with a deteriorating response to pergolide.[77] The dopamine agonists also are effective as monotherapy in previously untreated Parkinson's disease patients[78–81]; however, there is a high incidence of adverse effects and treatment failure necessitating either a lower dose or the addition of L-dopa. These results have led some investigators to examine the combination of low-dose L-dopa with low-dose dopamine agonists in hopes of decreasing the development of response fluctuations. These investigations have had mixed results.[82–84]

A recommended initial dose of bromocriptine is 1.25 mg once or twice daily. The dose of bromocriptine should be escalated slowly by 1.25 to 2.5 mg/d every week and maintained at the minimum amount necessary to accomplish the desired therapeutic effect. Average daily dosages less than 30 mg may be effective for several years in many patients, however, some patients may require dosages of up to 120 mg per day. Comparison of rapid and slow titration regimens have shown that rapid escalation in dosage produces more adverse effects but has less of a delay in reaching an effective dosage in *de novo* patients.[85]

A recommended initial dose for pergolide (which is about 13 times more potent than bromocriptine) is 0.05 mg/d for 2 days, gradually increasing the dose by approximately 0.1–0.15 mg/d every 3 days over a 12-day period. Should more drug be needed, the dose may then be increased by 0.25 mg every 3 days until symptoms are eliminated or adverse effects occur. The mean therapeutic dose in most clinical trials was approximately 3 mg/d.

The limiting factor of dopamine agonist therapy is adverse effects. These occur in 30–50% of patients and are more frequent at higher doses and with rapid escalation of dose. Nausea is the most frequently reported GI effect, occurring in greater than 50% of patients taking the drug; vomiting rarely occurs. Cardiovascular effects occur infrequently, with the exception of postural hypotension, which is common. CNS effects are the most common dose-limiting side effects and occur in as many as one-third of patients taking dopamine agonists. These include confusion, hallucinations, and sedation. The addition of a dopamine agonist to L-dopa therapy will increase the frequency and severity of dyskinesias during periods of good functional status. Pergolide, in addition to its arrhythmogenic effect, has a reported bradycardic effect.[86] The clinical significance of these cardiovascular effects in Parkinson's disease patients without underlying cardiac disease is considered insignificant.

Bromocriptine is fairly rapidly absorbed, exhibits high first-pass metabolism, is highly protein bound, and has multiple metabolites primarily excreted through the bile.[87] The elimination half-life is about 3 hours. A slow-release bromocriptine product has been investigated but is not clinically available.[88] A significant increase in bromocriptine plasma concentrations has been documented with the addition of erythromycin but not with caffeine.[89] A precise assay has not been developed for pergolide at this time because of its high potency and low serum concentrations.

Apomorphine and lisuride are dopamine agonists being investigated but not available in the United States. Apomorphine and lisuride have both been administered as subcutaneous infusions,[90] and a variety of formulations including sublingual and intranasal apomorphine are being investigated.[91,92] Specific D_1 receptor agonists do not at this time appear to have much anti-Parkinsonian effect.[93] Domperidone is a peripheral dopamine receptor blocker (not available in the United States) that can be used to block some of the peripheral adverse effects of the dopamine agonists.[94]

Evaluation of Therapeutic Outcomes

A summary of assessment parameters in determining anti-Parkinsonian drug response is given in Table 58.7. It is important to educate patients, spouses, or significant others regarding what to expect with treatment. They can also participate in treatment by recording medication administration times as well as duration of "on" and "off" times, which can be reviewed at each office visit. If a bothersome symptom or dystonia only occurs infrequently, it can be videotaped by the family and reviewed in the office.

The history should always include a detailed medication history since patients may often improvise and adjust their own medication schedule. It is important to determine the times of the day that may be most difficult for them to function. Assessment of general level of functioning including activities of daily living will help determine when L-dopa or dopamine agonists should be added. A history of falls should be investigated further as to the circumstances surrounding the falls to determine whether falls are secondary to IPD or some other etiology. The most common adverse effects of the anti-Parkinsonian medications should be surveyed for. These include nausea, hypotension, and psychiatric difficulties.

A focused neurologic examination as listed in Table 58.7 should be undertaken keeping in mind the timing of the examination in relation to the last dose of medication. Findings should always be considered in view of the patient's perception of severity of symptoms.

TABLE 58.7. ASSESSMENT OF A PARKINSONIAN PATIENT

History
- Precise medications and frequency
- General level of functioning
- History of falls, circumstances of any falls
- Problems with activities of daily living: eating/swallowing, dressing, hygiene
- Hallucinations
- Sleep, vivid dreams
- Depression
- Freezing

Physical Assessment
- Appearance: face, salivation, seborrhea
- Speech
- Tremor
- Rigidity/dyskinesia
- Finger tapping
- Rapid alternating movements
- Foot tapping
- Arise from chair with outstretched hands
- Standing posture
- Stability
- Gait
- Handwriting
- Intellectual assessment

Surgical Options

The transplantation of autologous adrenal medulla tissue or the implantation of dopamine-rich dissociated mesencephalic fetal tissue into the caudate nucleus of patients with Parkinson's disease has been investigated. Autologous tissue transplantation results have been disappointing in view of the risks associated with surgery. Fetal tissue transplantation is fraught with ethical issues and still highly investigational. Functional neurosurgical techniques include ventrolateral thalamotomy for tremor reduction and ventroposterior pallidotomy for reducing akinesia and rigidity.[95,96]

Conclusion

Although the cause of Parkinson's disease remains unknown, the identification of a neurotoxin, and a mechanism to protect against the neurotoxin, have advanced the knowledge of the disease. Pharmacologic therapy through manipulation of the dopaminergic system can significantly improve a patient's functional status and prolong meaningful life. Despite the multiple problems associated with L-dopa therapy, it remains the standard of therapy for patients with Parkinson's disease. The goal of management remains maintaining acceptable functional control with the minimum amount of anti-Parkinsonian drug necessary.

References

1. Tyler KL. A history of Parkinson's disease, in Koller WC (ed): Handbook of Parkinson's Disease, 2nd ed. New York, Marcel Dekker, 1992, pp 1–34.
2. Gibb WRG, Lees AJ. The relevance of the Lewy body to the pathogenesis of idiopathic Parkinson's disease. J Neurol Neurosurg Psychiatry 1988;51:745–752.
3. Hughes AJ, Daniel SE, Kilford L, Lees AJ. The accuracy of the clinical diagnosis of Parkinson's disease: A clinicopathological study of 100 cases. J Neurol Neurosurg Psychiatry 1992;55:181–184.
4. Martin WE, Loewenson RB, Resch JA, Baker AB. Parkinson's disease. Clinical analysis of 100 patients. Neurology 1973;23:783–790.
5. Zetusky WJ, Jankovic J, Pirozzolo FJ. The heterogeneity of Parkinson's disease: Clinical and prognostic implications. Neurology 1985;35:522–526.
6. Hughes AJ, Daniel SE, Blankson S, Lees AJ. A clinicopathologic study of 100 cases of Parkinson's disease. Arch Neurol 1993;50:140–148.
7. Rajput AH, Offord KP, Beard CM, Kurland LT. Epidemiology of parkinsonism: Incidence, classification and mortality. Ann Neurol 1984;16:278–282.
8. Rajput AH. Environmental causation of Parkinson's disease. Arch Neurol 1993;50:651–652.
9. Lazzarini AM, Myers RH, Zimmerman TR, et al. A clinical genetic study of Parkinson's disease: Evidence for dominant transmission. Neurology 1994;44:499–506.
10. Jarvie KR, Caron MG. Heterogeneity of dopamine receptors. Adv Neurology 1993;60:325–333.
11. Mercuri NB, Calabresi P, Bernardi G. Physiology and pharmacology of dopamine D_2 receptors: Their implications in dopamine-substitute therapy for Parkinson's disease. Neurology 1989;39:1106–1108.
12. Bernheimer H, Birkmayer W, Hornykiewicz O, et al. Brain dopamine and the syndrome of Parkinson's and Huntington: Clinical, morphological, and neurochemical correlations. J Neurol Sci 1973;20:415–455.
13. Calne DB, Snow BJ. PET imaging in parkinsonism. Adv Neurology 1993;60:484–487.
14. Rutgers AWF, Lakke JPWF, Paans AMJ, et al. Tracing of dopamine receptors in hemiparkinsonism with positron emission tomography. J Neurol Sci 1987;80:237–248.
15. Pizzolato G, Chierichetti F, Rossato A, et al. Dopamine receptor SPECT imaging in Parkinson's disease: A [^{123}I]-IBZM and [^{99m}Tc]-HM-PAO study. Eur Neurol 1993;33:143–148.
16. Post RM. Intermittent versus continuous stimulation: Effect of time on the development of sensitization or tolerance. Life Sci 1980;26:1275–1282.
17. Curtius HC, Niederwieser A, Levine R, Muldner H. Therapeutic efficacy of tetrahydrobiopterin in Parkinson's disease. Adv Neurol 1984;40:463–466.
18. Olanow CW. Oxidative reactions in Parkinson's disease. Neurology 1990;40(suppl 3):32–37.
19. Schapira AHV. Mitochondrial complex I deficiency in Parkinson's disease. Adv Neurology 1993;60:288–291.

20. Koller WC, Silver DE, Lieberman A. An algorithm for the management of Parkinson's disease. Neurology 1994;44 (suppl 10):1–52.
21. Hoehn MH, Yahr MD. Parkinsonism: Onset, progression and mortality. Neurology 1967;17:427–442.
22. Golbe LI, Lieberman AN, Muenter MD, et al. Deprenyl in the treatment of symptom fluctuations in advanced Parkinson's disease. Clin Neuropharmacol 1988;11:45–55.
23. Hubble JP, Koller WC, Waters C. Effects of selegiline dosing on motor fluctuations in Parkinson's disease. Clin Neuropharmacol 1993;16:83–87.
24. Heinonen EH, Myllyla V, Sotaniemi K, et al. Pharmacokinetics and metabolism of selegiline. Acta Neurol Scand 1989;80(suppl 126):93–99.
25. Elsworth JD, Glover V, Reynolds GP, et al. Deprenyl administration in man: A selective MAO-B inhibitor without "cheese-effect." Psychopharmacology 1987;57:33–38.
26. Montastruc JL, Chamotin B, Senard JM, et al. Pseudophaeochromocytoma in parkinsonian patient treated with fluoxetine plus selegiline [letter]. Lancet 1993;341:555.
27. Zornberg GL, Bodkin JA, Cohen BM. Severe adverse interaction between pethidine and selegiline. Lancet 1991;337:246.
28. The Parkinson Study Group. Effect of deprenyl on the progression of disability in early Parkinson's disease. N Engl J Med 1989;321:1364–1371.
29. The Parkinson Study Group. Effects of tocopherol and deprenyl on the progression of disability in Parkinson's disease. N Engl J Med 1993;328:176–183.
30. Landau WM. Clinical neuromythology IX. Pyramid sale in the bucket shop: DATATOP bottoms out. Neurology 1990;40:1337–1339.
31. Schulzer M, Mak E, Calne DB. The antiparkinsonian efficacy of deprenyl derives from transient improvement that is likely to be symptomatic. Ann Neurol 1992;32:795–798.
32. van Spaendonick KPM, Berger HJC, Hortink MWI, et al. Impaired cognitive shifting in Parkinsonian patients on anticholinergic therapy. Neuropsychologia 1993;31:407–411.
33. Fahn S, Isgreen W. Long-term evaluation of amantadine and levodopa combination in parkinsonism by double-blind crossover analysis. Neurology 1975;25:695–700.
34. Jackisch R, Link T, Neufang B, Koch R. Studies on the mechanism of the antiparkinsonian drugs memantine and amantadine: No evidence for direct dopaminomimetic or antimuscarinic properties. Arch Int Pharmacodyn Ther 1992;320:21–42.
35. Cotzias CG, Van Woert MH, Schiffer LM. Aromatic amino acids and modification of parkinsonism. N Engl J Med 1967;276:374–379.
36. Papavasilou PS, Cotzias GC, Duby SE, et al. Levodopa in parkinsonism: Potentiation of central effects with a peripheral inhibitor. N Engl J Med 1972;285:8–14.
37. Ward CD, Trombley LK, Calne DB, et al. L-dopa decarboxylation in chronically treated patients. Neurology 1984;34:198–201.
38. LeWitt PA, Nelson MV, Berchou RC, et al. Controlled-release carbidopa/levodopa (Sinemet 50/200 CR4): Clinical and pharmacokinetic studies. Neurology 1989;39 (suppl 2):45–53.
39. Stocchi F, Quinn NP, Barbato L, et al. Comparison between a fast and a slow release preparation of levodopa and a combination of the two: A clinical and pharmacokinetic study. Clin Neuropharmacol 1994;17:38–44.
40. Quinn N, Parkes JD, Marsden CD. Control of on/off phenomenon by continuous intravenous infusion of levodopa. Neurology 1984;34:1131–1136.
41. Kurth MC, Tetrud JW, Tanner CM, et al. Double-blind, placebo-controlled crossover study of duodenal infusion of levodopa/carbidopa in Parkinson's disease patients with 'on–off' fluctuations. Neurology 1993;43:1698–1703.
42. Kurth MC, Tetrud JW, Irwin I, et al. Oral levodopa/carbidopa solution versus tablets in Parkinson's patients with severe fluctuations: A pilot study. Neurology 1993;43:1036–1039.
43. LeWitt PA. Treatment strategies for extension of levodopa effect. Neurol Clin 1992;10:511–526.
44. Nelson MV, Berchou RC, LeWitt PA, et al. Pharmacodynamic modeling of concentration-effect relationships after controlled release carbidopa/levodopa (Sinemet CR4) in Parkinson's disease. Neurology 1990;40:70–74.
45. Fahn S. 'On–off' phenomenon with levodopa therapy in parkinsonism: Clinical and pharmacological correlations and the effect of intramuscular pyridoxine. Neurology 1974;24:431–441.
46. Feldman RG, Kaye JA, Lannon MC. Parkinson's disease: Follow-up after drug holiday. J Clin Pharmacol 1986;26:663–667.
47. Mayeux R, Stern Y, Mulvey K, et al. Reappraisal of temporary levodopa withdrawal ("drug holiday") in Parkinson's disease. N Engl J Med 1985;313:724–728.
48. Friedman JH, Feinberg SS, Feldman RG. A neuroleptic malignantlike syndrome due to levodopa therapy withdrawal. JAMA 1985;254:2792–2795.
49. Hirschorn KA, Greenberg HS. Successful treatment of levodopa-induced myoclonus and levodopa withdrawal-induced neuroleptic malignant syndrome: A case report. Clin Neuropharmacol 1988;2:278–281.
50. Mouradian MM, Heuser IJE, Baronti F, et al. Pathogenesis of dyskinesias in Parkinson's disease. Ann Neurol 1989;25:523–526.
51. Nutt JG. Levodopa-induced dyskinesia: Review, observations, and speculations. Neurology 1990;40:340–345.
52. Baronti F, Mouradian MM, Conant KE, et al. Partial dopamine agonist therapy of levodopa-induced dyskinesias. Neurology 1992;42:1241–1244.
53. Girotti F, Soliveri P, Carella F, et al. Dementia and cognitive impairment in Parkinson's disease. J Neurol Neurosurg Psychiatry 1988;51:1498–1502.
54. Pinter MM, Helscher RJ. Therapeutic effect of clozapine in psychotic decompensation in idiopathic Parkinson's disease. J Neural Transm [Park Dis Dement Sect] 1993;5:135–146.
55. Arevalo GJG, Gershanik OS. Modulatory effect of clozapine on levodopa response in Parkinson's disease: A preliminary study. Mov Disord 1993;8:349–354.
56. Fahn S, Bressman SB. Should levodopa therapy for parkinsonism be started early or late? Evidence against early treatment. Can J Neurol Sci 1984;11:200–206.
57. Muenter MD. Should levodopa therapy be started early or late? Can J Neurol Sci 1984;11:195–199.

58. Rajput AH, Stern W, Laverty WH. Chronic low-dose levodopa therapy in Parkinson's disease: An argument for delaying levodopa therapy. Neurology 1984;34:991–996.
59. Cedarbaum JM, Gandy SE, McDowell FH. "Early" initiation of levodopa treatment does not promote the development of motor response fluctuations, dyskinesias, or dementia in Parkinson's disease. Neurology 1991;41:622–629.
60. Diamond SG, Markham CH, Hoehn MM, et al. Multicenter study of Parkinson mortality with early versus later dopa treatment. Ann Neurol 1987;22:8–12.
61. Rivera-Calimlim L, Dujovne CA, Morgan JP, et al. L-dopa treatment failure: Explanation and correction. BMJ 1970;4:93–94.
62. Neira WSD, Sanchez V, Mena MA, et al. Effect of cisapride on levodopa pharmacokinetics and clinical response in patients with Parkinson's disease. Neurology 1994;44(suppl 2):A245.
63. Nutt JG, Woodward WR, Hammerstad JP, et al. The 'on–off' phenomenon in Parkinson's disease: Relation to levodopa absorption and transport. N Engl J Med 1984;310:483–488.
64. Berry EM, Growdon JH, Wurtman JJ, et al. A balanced carbohydrate:protein diet in the management of Parkinson's disease. Neurology 1991;41:1295–1297.
65. Sasahara K, Nitanai T, Habara T, et al. Dosage form design for improvement of bioavailability of levodopa III: Influence of dose on pharmacokinetic behavior of levodopa in dogs and Parkinsonian patients. J Pharm Sci 1980;69:1374–1378.
66. Fabbrini G, Juncos JL, Mouradian MM, et al. Levodopa pharmacokinetic mechanisms and motor fluctuations in Parkinson's disease. Ann Neurol 1987;21:370–376.
67. Nutt JG. On–off phenomenon: Relation to levodopa pharmacokinetics and pharmacodynamics. Ann Neurol 1987;22:535–540.
68. Nelson MV, Berchou RC, LeWitt PA, et al. Pharmacokinetic and pharmacodynamic modeling of L-dopa plasma concentrations and clinical effects in Parkinson's disease after Sinemet. Clin Neuropharmacol 1989;12:91–97.
69. Contin M, Riva R, Martinelli P, et al. Pharmacokinetic modeling of oral levodopa: Clinical application in Parkinson's disease. Neurology 1993;43:367–371.
70. Jansen ENH. Bromocriptine in levodopa response-losing parkinsonism double-blind study. Eur Neurol 1978;17:92–99.
71. Lieberman A, Kupersmith M, Estey E. Treatment of Parkinson's disease with bromocriptine. N Engl J Med 1976;295:1400–1404.
72. Lang AE, Quinn N, Brincat S, et al. Pergolide in late-stage Parkinson disease. Ann Neurol 1982;12:243–247.
73. Grimes JD, King DB, Kofman OS, et al. Bromocriptine in the management of end of dose deterioration in Parkinson's disease. Can J Neurol Sci 1984;11:452–456.
74. Jankovic J. Long-term study of pergolide in Parkinson's disease. Neurology 1985;35:296–299.
75. LeWitt PA, Ward CD, Larsen TA, et al. Comparison of pergolide and bromocriptine therapy in parkinsonism. Neurology 1983;33:1009–1014.
76. Lieberman A, Neophytides A, Liebowitz M, et al. Comparative efficacy of pergolide and bromocriptine in patients with advanced Parkinson's disease. Adv Neurol 1983;37:95–108.
77. Olanow CW. Pergolide, Parlodel crossover study. Neurology 1988;38:314–316.
78. Lees AJ, Stern GM. Sustained bromocriptine therapy in previously untreated patients with Parkinson's disease. J Neurol Neurosurg Psychiatry 1981;44:1020–1023.
79. Teychenne PF, Bergsrud D, Elton RL, et al. Bromocriptine: Long-term low-dose therapy in Parkinson's disease. Clin Neuropharmacol 1986;9:138–145.
80. Bergamasco B, Benna P, Scarzella L. Long-term bromocriptine treatment of *de novo* patients with Parkinson's disease. A 7-year follow-up. Acta Neurol Scand 1990;81:383–387.
81. Montastruc JL, Rascol O, Rascol A. A randomized controlled study of bromocriptine versus levodopa in previously untreated parkinsonism patients: A 3-year follow-up. J Neurol Neurosurg Psychiatry 1989;52(6):773–775.
82. Rinne UK. Combined bromocriptine-levodopa therapy early in Parkinson's disease. Neurology 1985;35:1196–1198.
83. Weiner WJ, Factor SA, Sanchez-Ramos JR, et al. Early combination therapy (bromocriptine and levodopa) does not prevent motor fluctuations in Parkinson's disease. Neurology 1993;43:21–27.
84. Horstink MWIM, van't Hof MA, Berger HJC. Combination therapy for PD [letter]. Neurology 1993;43:2725.
85. UK Bromocriptine Research Group. Bromocriptine in Parkinson's disease: A double blind study comparing "low-slow" and "high-fast" introductory dosage regimens in *de novo* patients. J Neurol Neurosurg Psychiatry 1989;52:77–82.
86. Kurlan R, Miller C, Knapp R, et al. Double-blind assessment of potential pergolide-induced cardiotoxicity. Neurology 1986;36:993–995.
87. Cedarbaum JM. Clinical pharmacokinetics of anti-Parkinsonian drugs. Clin Pharmacokinet 1987;13:141–178.
88. Mannen T, Mizuno Y, Iwata M, et al. A multi-center, double-blind study on slow release bromocriptine in the treatment of Parkinson's disease. Neurology 1991;41:1598–1602.
89. Nelson MV, Berchou RC, Kareti D, LeWitt PA. Pharmacokinetic evaluation of erythromycin and caffeine administered with bromocriptine. Clin Pharmacol Ther 1990;47:694–697.
90. Stocchi F, Bramante L, Monge A, et al. Apomorphine and lisuride infusion: A comparative chronic study. Adv Neurol 1993;60:653–655.
91. Montastruc JL, Rascol O, Senard JM, et al. Sublingual apomorphine in Parkinson's disease: A clinical and pharmacokinetic study. Clin Neuropharmacol 1991;14:432–437.
92. van Laar T, Jansen ENH, Essink AWG, Neef C. Intranasal apomorphine in Parkinsonian on-off fluctuations. Arch Neurol 1992;49:482–484.
93. Tsui JKC, Wolters EC, Peppard RF, Calne DB. A double-blind, placebo controlled, dose ranging study to investigate the safety and efficacy of CY 208-243 in patients with Parkinson's disease. Neurology 1989;39:856–858.
94. Quinn N, Illas A, Lhermitte F, Agid Y. Bromocriptine and domperidone in the treatment of Parkinson's disease. Neurology 1981;31:662–667.
95. Goetz CG, DeLong MR, Penn RD, Bakay RAE. Neurosurgical horizons in Parkinson's disease. Neurology 1993;43:1–7.
96. Widner H, Rehncrona S. Transplantation and surgical treatment of Parkinsonian syndromes. Curr Opin Neurol 1993;6:344–349.

Chapter 59

Pain Management

Terry J. Baumann, PharmD

Although the world is full of suffering, it is also full of the overcoming of it.

—Helen Keller[1]

Humans have always known and sought relief from pain. In fact, the act of relieving pain is probably as old as the medical profession itself. Today, pain's impact on society is still great and, indeed, pain complaints are the number one reason patients seek medical advice. Most Americans experience three or four different types of pain every year. More than 50 million people are partially or totally disabled because of pain. The annual cost of pain to American society is an estimated $79–$90 billion.[2,3]

Unfortunately, pain is often undertreated and pain management greatly misunderstood.[4–8] Marks and Sacher[4] studied hospitalized medical patients receiving narcotic analgesia and found 73% in severe or moderate distress despite their analgesic regimen. Caregivers' misconceptions regarding narcotic doses, duration of analgesic effect, and fear of addiction were reportedly responsible for this undertreatment.[4] Cohen[5] demonstrated that despite narcotic analgesics, 75% of postsurgical patients were in moderate or marked distress and 45% "cried out" in pain. Fear of addiction and inadequate knowledge of pharmacologic agents were again considered major factors contributing to pain mismanagement.[5] Similar problems are reported in ambulatory patients.[8]

Regrettably, many health care providers do not receive adequate training in this area, and new information is not widely disseminated and/or understood. Clearly, pain management is enhanced when a multidisciplinary approach is applied. Thus, understanding the pathophysiology and concepts of pain therapy and maintaining a working knowledge of individual pain regimens are important to pharmacists and are key factors in reversing the problem of inadequate pain control.

Definition

An acceptable definition of pain remains an enigma. Once thought to be a punishment from the gods, the word is derived from the Latin *peone* and the Greek *poine,* meaning "penalty" or "punishment."[8] This punishment theory was advanced by Aristotle, who considered pain a feeling and classified it as a passion of the soul. Two thousand years later Descartes, Galen, and Vaselius postulated that pain was a sensation in which the brain played an important role. In the nineteenth century, Mueller, Van Frey, and Goldscheider hypothesized the concepts of neuroreceptors, nociceptors, and sensory input.[8] These theories developed into this century's definition of pain: "an unpleasant sensory and emotional experience associated with actual or potential tissue damage or described in terms of such damage."[9] Pain is often so subjective, however, that many clinicians define pain as whatever the patient says it is.

Pathophysiology

The pathophysiology of pain involves a complex series of afferent and efferent neuronal connections that have not been fully elucidated; however, research during the last 20 years has greatly advanced our understanding of pain transmission.

AFFERENT PAIN TRANSMISSION

Peripheral Stimulation

The first step leading to the sensation of pain is the stimulation of receptors known as nociceptors. These free nerve endings are found in skin, blood vessels, subcutaneous tissues, muscle fascia, periosteum, viscera, joints, and other structures. They may be specific (responding only to mechanical, thermal, chemical, or ischemic processes alone) or polymodal (responding to one or more of these processes). The exact mechanism that underlies the stimulation of nociceptors is poorly understood; however, bradykinins, H^+, K^+, prostaglandins, leukotrienes, histamine, and serotonin sensitize these receptors. Receptor activation leads to action potentials that are transmitted along afferent nerve fibers to the spinal cord.[10–16]

Somatostatin, cholecystokinin, and substance P have been identified as possible neurotransmitters in afferent nociceptive neurons.[17,18] In addition, substance P may play a role in enhancing the effectiveness of nociceptive neurotransmitters that promote pain.[16] In fact, when substance P is blocked by the neurotoxin capsaicin, pain transmission is significantly reduced, making substance P antagonists a separate class of analgesics.[19,20] Topical creams containing capsaicin (0.025%, 0.075%, and 0.25%) are available for the treatment of painful neuralgias.[21]

Afferent fibers are classified as A, B, or C. Large, fast, myelinated A fibers are further divided into alpha, beta, gamma, and delta subfibers. In comparison, C fibers are small, slow, and myelinated and are not subgrouped. Nociceptive transmission takes place in the A–delta or C fibers.[15] Stimulation of A–delta fibers evokes bright, well-localized pain, whereas stimulation of C fibers produces dull, poorly localized, and persistent pain.[15]

Gate Control Theory

These afferent, nociceptive pain fibers synapse in the dorsal horn of the spinal cord along with many other non–pain-transmitting or non-nociceptive neurons (Fig. 59.1). Synapses are made directly onto pain transmission neurons (PTNs) or onto interconnecting neurons (ICNs) that excite PTNs. In addition, large non-nociceptive fibers originating either in the periphery or in neurons descending from the spinal cord may inhibit both PTNs and ICNs in the dorsal horn. When large myelinated fibers are stimulated they have an inhibitory effect on pain transmission. Therefore, perception of pain is a complex summation of non-nociceptive and nociceptive neuronal stimulation (Fig. 59.2).[10,22]

Functionally, the importance of the interplay between these different fibers is evident in the analgesic response produced by treatments that stimulate large non-nociceptive neurons, for example, topical irritants, acupuncture, or transcutaneous electrical nerve stimulation. Although modified, this theory was first explained by Melzack and Wall[23] and is referred to as the *gate control theory* of pain transmission.

Spinal Cord Transmission

These pain-initiated processes reach the brain through a complex array of ascending spinal cord pathways. In addition, information other than pain impulses is carried along these pathways. Thus, pain is influenced by many factors supplemental to nociception and precludes simple schematic representation; however, one major ascending pathway, the spinothalamic tract, is known to have a major influence on pain transmission and is classically divided into lateral and ventral pathways. The lateral pathway is associated with sharp localized pain and is responsible for the spatial and temporal discriminative aspects of nociception.[8] The ventral pathway makes possible the perception of aching, dull, nonlocalized pain and the reflexes responsible for aversion motivation.[8] Both pathways eventually merge in the thalamus and connect with the cortex.

PAIN MODULATION

The brain modulates pain through a system that we are just beginning to understand. First evidence of this system was the analgesia produced by selected electrical stimulation of animal brains,[24,25] with subsequent similar results in patients with intractable clinical pain.[26] Almost simultaneously, other investigators discovered opiate receptors within the central nervous system (CNS).[27–29] Dense clusters of opiate receptors are found in the ascending and descending pain pathways and in portions of the brain believed to be essential to the pain-modulating system.[8] In 1975, researchers[30,31] identified two pentapeptides (Metenkephalin and Leu-enkephalin) whose actions were similar to morphine. These enkephalins interact with opiate receptors to form, in part, what is known as the endogenous opiate system.[8] Three classes of opioid peptides are known: the enkephalins, dynorphins, and β-endorphins. Although all three are important in the endogenous opiate system, each class originates from a different precursor and has a distinct anatomical distribution.[16] All are generically referred to as endorphins. As the knowledge of endorphins has expanded, so has the understanding of opiate receptors. Five such receptors, mu (sometimes split into two subpopulations mu-1 and mu-2), delta, sigma, kappa, and epsilon (whose identity and existence is still being debated)[32] have been recognized. These receptors display similar chemical properties but have varying affinities and functions (Table 59.1).[8]

The development of narcotic antagonists (substances that block endogenous opiate receptors) led to the discovery of a highly integrated network associating pain, opiate receptors, and endorphins. Although the endogenous opioid relationship is still not completely defined, it may moderate pain through a positive and negative feedback system. Thus, a given nociceptive stimulus activates both peripheral pain transmission pathways (causing pain and termed *positive feedback*) and the brain's modulatory network (inhibiting pain and termed *negative feedback*), making the sensation of pain a partial summation of these two processes.[10] Other neurotransmitter substances known to play a role in pain regulation include acetylcholine,[33] dopamine,[34] norepinephrine,[35] and serotonin.[36]

EFFERENT PAIN TRANSMISSION

The CNS also contains a highly organized descending system for control of pain transmission. This system influences synaptic transmission of sensory fibers at the dorsal horn level of the spinal cord and is dependent on the biogenic amine neurotransmitters and other networks previously mentioned.[8]

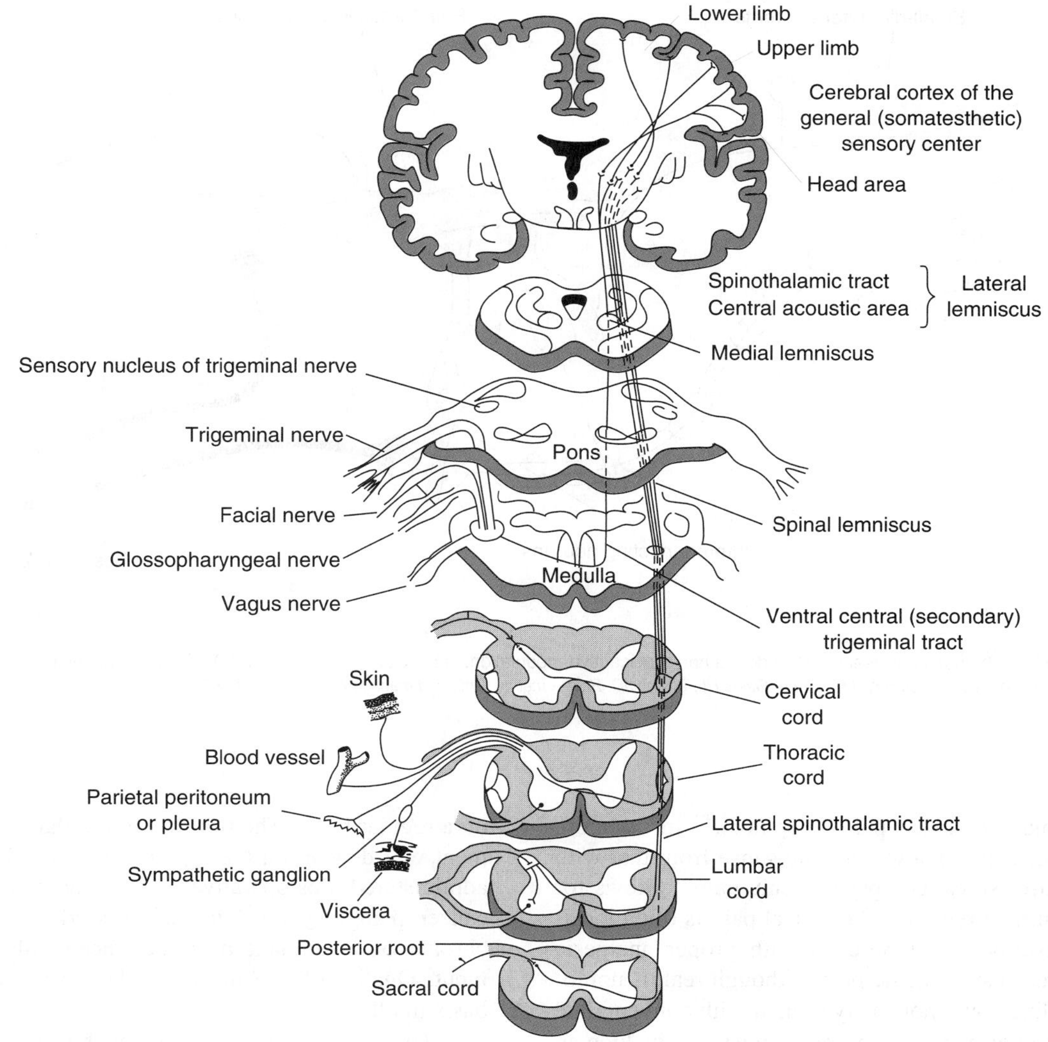

Figure 59.1. Afferent pain conduction pathway. *(Reproduced with permission. Special Reports in the Management of Acute Pain Considerations. New York, HP Publishing, January 1977, p 5. Illustration by Ms. Carol Donner.)*

In summary, although progress has occurred in unraveling the pain transmission mystery, understanding of this complex pathway is still limited. Pain without nociception (algodynia), neuropathic pain, sympathetically maintained pain, and phantom limb pain (pain in a limb that has been amputated) are very real phenomena, but defy explanation using our present knowledge of neurophysiology.[8] Additional research is needed to clarify the roles of neuromodulaters and neurotransmitters. Although the current pain model is not incorrect, it is certainly incomplete.[3]

Pain Assessment

Pain is a complex concept,[37] and a proper pain assessment and an accurate diagnosis of the underlying cause are often major obstacles in effective treatment. A patient-oriented approach is essential, and evaluation methods should not differ from those used in other medical conditions.[8] Therefore, a comprehensive history and physical examination are imperative to thoroughly evaluate underlying diseases and possible contributing factors.[8] A baseline description of pain can be obtained by assessing PQRST characteristics (Table 59.2).[38] Attention must also be given to mental factors that alter the pain threshold. Anxiety, depression, fatigue, anger, and fear are particularly noted to lower this threshold, whereas rest, mood elevation, sympathy, diversion, and understanding raise the pain threshold.[38]

Clinicians must evaluate all components of the pain experience, for example, behavioral (much of our reaction to pain is learned),[39] cognitive (thinking processes alter pain experiences),[15] social (pain expression differs in accordance with social environments),[40] and cultural (cultural

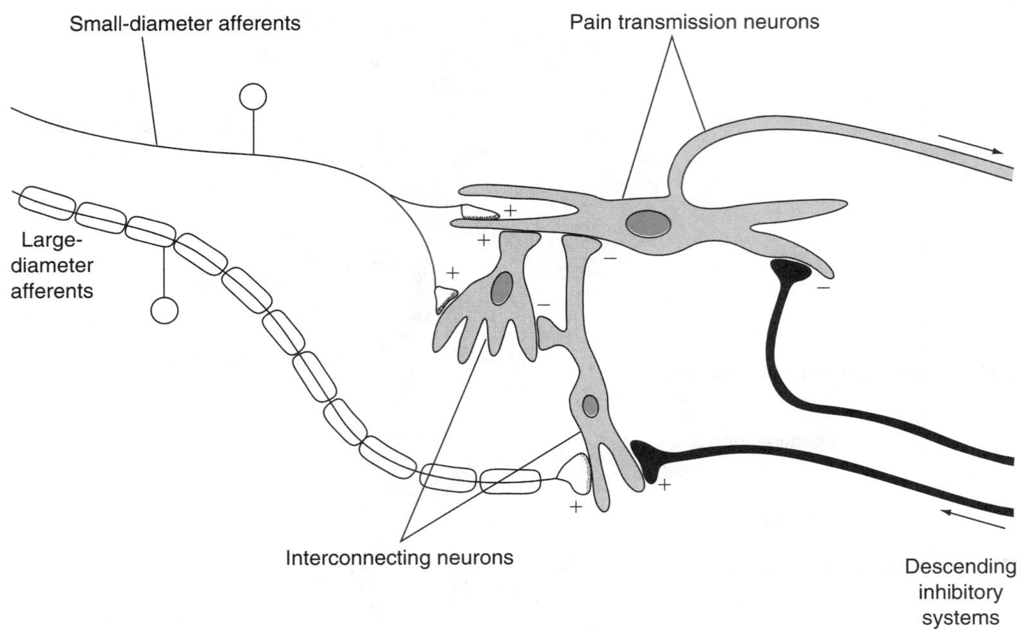

Figure 59.2. Schematic representation of dorsal horn nociceptive modulation. (+) excitatory connection, (–) inhibitory connection. *(Reprinted by permission of the Western Journal of Medicine. Fields HL, Levine JD. Pain— mechanisms and management. 1984;141:349.)*

background may influence pain tolerance).[40] In addition, separating pain with a known organic cause from that with no known cause (so-called "psychogenic pain") allows for improved treatment regimens.[8] Physical pain is often localized, well described, and relieved with proper analgesic therapy, whereas psychogenic pain, although real, is nonlocalized, ill defined, and not easily treated with conventional analgesics.[8] Proper patient assessment must also include an evaluation of pain management. Pain intensity, pain relief, and medication side effects must be assessed and reassessed on a regular basis. The timing and regularity of this assessment will depend on the type of pain and the medications administered. Postoperative pain and acute exacerbation of cancer pain may need to be assessed every hour, while chronic nonmalignant pain may need only daily assessment. Quality of life must also be assessed on a regular basis in all patients.

TABLE 59.1. OPIATE RECEPTORS AND FUNCTION

Opiate Receptor	Function
Mu-1	Analgesia
Mu-2	Respiratory depression Euphoria Physical dependence Constipation
Delta	Analgesia
Sigma	Autonomic stimulation Dysphoria Hallucinations
Kappa	Analgesia Sedation Miosis
Epsilon	Analgesia

(Modified from Ref. 8.)

The clinician must remember, however, that "pain is always subjective. Objective observations of grimacing, limping, and tachycardia may be useful in assessing the patient, but these signs are often absent in patients with chronic pain known to be caused by structural lesions. There is no neurophysiological or chemical test that can measure pain. The clinician does well in the absence of strong contrary evidence to accept the patient's report of pain."[41]

TABLE 59.2. PQRST CHARACTERISTICS OF PAIN

P	Palliative factors Provocative factors	What makes the pain better? What makes the pain worse?
Q	Quality	Describe the pain.
R	Radiation	Where is the pain?
S	Severity	How does this pain compare with other pain you have experienced?
T	Temporal factors	Does the intensity of the pain change with time?

(Modified from Ref. 38, p. 499.)

ACUTE AND CHRONIC PAIN

Acute pain may be a useful physiologic process warning individuals of disease states and potentially harmful situations. Unfortunately, severe, unremitting, undertreated acute pain, when it outlives its biologic usefulness, can produce many deleterious effects (e.g., psychological problems). When pain is not effectively treated, the stress and concurrent reflex reactions often cause hypoxia, hypercapnia, hypertension, excessive cardiac activity, and permanent emotional difficulties. The problems associated with these reactions range from a prolonged recovery time to death.[3]

Under normal conditions, acute pain quickly subsides as the healing process decreases the pain-producing stimuli; however, in some instances, pain may persist for months to years, leading to a chronic pain state with features quite different from those of acute pain (Table 59.3). Typically, chronic pain is divided into four subtypes: pain that persists beyond the normal healing time for an acute injury, pain related to a chronic disease, pain without identifiable organic cause, and pain that involves both the chronic and acute pain associated with cancer.[42] Patients in chronic pain often develop severe psychologic problems caused by fear and memory of past pain. In addition, chronic pain patients may develop dependence and tolerance to analgesics, have trouble sleeping, and more readily react to environmental changes that can intensify the pain response. Distinguishing between chronic and acute pain states is very important because of differing management techniques.[41]

TABLE 59.3. CHARACTERISTICS OF ACUTE AND CHRONIC PAIN

Characteristic	Acute Pain	Chronic Pain
Relief of pain	Highly desirable	Highly desirable
Dependence and tolerance to medication	Unusual	Common
Psychologic component	Usually not present	Often a major problem
Organic cause	Common	Often not present
Environmental contributions and family involvement	Small	Significant
Insomnia	Unusual	Common component
Treatment goal	Cure	Rehabilitation not a cure

(Modified from Ref. 8, p. 256.)

ACUTE PAIN MANAGEMENT

The obvious way to relieve pain is to eliminate the underlying cause. This is often not possible, however, and symptomatic relief is usually indicated. Therapeutic interventions include pharmacologic treatment, stimulation therapies, and psychologic therapies.

PHARMACOLOGIC TREATMENT

Although pharmacologic agents that effectively treat acute pain are available, they are not always appropriately used. Inadequate dose titration, fear of analgesic side effects, varying analgesic requirements, inadequate application of current available therapies, and failure to appreciate the complications of untreated pain contribute to ineffective and inappropriate pain management. Adherence to the basic principles of the pharmacologic treatment of pain (Table 59.4) will promote rational pain control decisions. Analgesic agents should be given an adequate trial and often require individual dosage titration. Even in acute pain, administering analgesics as needed (PRN) may promote anxiety and contribute to future drug dependence. In most cases, these drugs should be administered on a regular dosing schedule and not on an as-needed schedule. This is especially true in the initial stage of great pain. As the painful state subsides, pain schedules can be used. Side effects should be well understood and excessive sedation avoided. Finally, placebo therapy should never be used to diagnose psychogenic pain and the route of administration should always be geared to the analgesic needs of the patient.

Non-Narcotic Agents

Analgesia should be initiated with the weakest effective analgesic agent having the fewest side effects. Acetaminophen, acetylsalicylic acid (aspirin), and nonsteroidal anti-inflammatory drugs (NSAIDs) are often preferred over narcotic agents in the treatment of acute, mild to moderate pain (Tables 59.5 and 59.6). These drugs (with the excep-

TABLE 59.4. PHARMACOLOGIC TREATMENT OF PAIN

Identify the source of pain.
Use the least potent analgesic with the fewest side effects.
Properly titrate the dose and administer for an adequate duration.
Initially, do not use analgesics on an as-needed basis.
Recognize side effects of analgesics.
Avoid excessive sedation.
Adjust the route of administration to the needs of the patient.
Use equianalgesic doses.
Do not use placebo therapy to diagnose psychogenic pain.

(Modified from Ref. 8, p. 245.

TABLE 59.5. PHARMACOKINETIC AND PHARMACODYNAMIC PROFILES OF FDA-APPROVED NON-NARCOTIC ANALGESICS

Agent	Time to Peak Concentration (h)	Elimination Half-Life (h)	Analgesic Onset (h)	Analgesic Duration (h)
Aspirin	0.25–2	0.25–0.33	0.5	3–6
Choline salicylate	1.5–2	—[a]	—[a]	4
Magnesium salicylate	1.5–2	—[a]	—[a]	4
Sodium salicylate	0.67	—[a]	—[a]	4
Diflunisal	2–3	8–12	1	8–12
Acetaminophen	0.5–2	1–4	0.5–1	3–6
Meclofenamate	0.5–2	2.3–3.3	—[a]	4–6
Mefenamic acid	2–4	2–4	—[a]	6
Etodoloc	1	7	0.5–1.0	6–8
Diclofenac potassium	0.5–1	2	0.5	6–8
Ibuprofen	1–2	1–2.5	0.5	4–6
Fenoprofen	1–2	2–3	0.25–0.5	4–6
Ketoprofen	0.5–2	2–4	1	3–4
Naproxen	2–4	12–15	1	Up to 7
Naproxen sodium	1–2	12–13	1	Up to 7
Ketorolac (parenteral)	0.5–1	4–6	0.17	6
Ketorolac (oral)	0.5–1	4–6	0.5–1	4–6

[a]Data not available. (Compiled from Refs. 43, 45, 46, 97, 98, 101, and 102.)

tion of acetaminophen) affect the prostaglandins produced by the arachidonic acid cascade in response to noxious stimuli,[43] thereby decreasing the number of pain impulses received by the CNS. Patient response to mild analgesics varies, with the best results evident in low-grade, somatic-type pain (e.g., headache, myalgia, neuralgia, and dysmenorrhea).[44] Results are poor for intense or sharp visceral pain present after surgery or with headaches of vascular origin.[44] Therapeutic outcomes are also less than desired in those who do not expect "mild" analgesics to relieve pain. Studies comparing the efficacy of these agents have been inconsistent because of problems in presentation, perception, and reproducibility of pain.[44] Therefore, the choice of a particular agent often depends on availability, cost, and pharmacokinetic and pharmacologic characteristics (Tables 59.5 and 59.6), and the side-effect profile (Table 59.7). It should be noted that all NSAIDs have some analgesic effects, but only the ones that are FDA approved for mild to moderate pain are compared in the tables.

Aspirin or aspirin-like compounds are the most widely used peripherally acting analgesics in the world.[43] This may be because they impart antipyretic and anti-inflammatory action, as well as analgesic effects; however, problems with platelet aggregation defects and direct gastrointestinal (GI) irritation leading to nausea, dyspepsia, and epigastric burning have limited their use.[43] Other problems connected with the use of aspirin include a strong association with gastric ulcers (dose related), GI bleeding (even with normal doses), tinnitus (dose related), and hypersensitivity reactions in patients with asthma.[44] Caution is advised when these agents are used concurrently with other peripherally acting NSAIDs because they may increase the potential for side effects.[43]

In addition, these compounds (especially aspirin) should not be given to children or teenagers who have influenza or chicken pox. This combination has been associated with Reye's syndrome.[45] The salicylate salts differ from aspirin in that they have fewer GI effects and do not inhibit platelet aggregation.[46]

NSAIDs have effective analgesic and anti-inflammatory properties, but generally cause fewer GI problems than aspirin. Particular attention must be given to the effects that NSAIDs have on renal function. Prostaglandins play an important role in counteracting the deleterious effects that release of renin-angiotensin, catecholamines, and vasopressin has on the kidney. When prostaglandin synthesis is inhibited by NSAIDs or by aspirin-like compounds in patients with poor renal function, this control mechanism is lost, and severe renal damage may result.[47] Patients suspected of minimal renal function (creatinine clearances below 50 mL/min) who receive NSAIDs or aspirin-like compounds must be carefully monitored for further kidney damage. NSAIDs can also cause rash, tinnitus, nausea, vomiting, a burning sensation in the esophagus and stomach, diarrhea, edema, hypertension, constipation, and vertigo.[43,46] In addition, all NSAIDs inhibit platelet aggregation. In contrast to aspirin, however, the

TABLE 59.6. FDA-APPROVED NON-NARCOTIC ANALGESICS

Class and Generic Name	Trade Name and Manufacturer	Usual Dosage Range (mg)	Maximal mg/d
Salicylates			
Acetylsalicylic acid[a] (aspirin)	Various	325–650 every 4 h	5400
Choline[a]	Arthropan (Purdue Fedrick)	870 every 3–4 h	5220
Magnesium[a]	Original Doan's (Ciba Consumer)	500 every 4 h	4800
	Generic (various)		
Sodium[a]	Generic (various)	325–650 every 4 h	5400
Diflunisal	Dolobid (MSD)	250–500 every 8–12 h	1500
***para*-Aminophenol**			
Acetaminophen[a]	Tylenol (McNeil-CPC)	325–650 every 4–6 h	4000
	Generic (various)		
Fenamates			
Meclofenamate	Meclomen (Park-Davis)	50 every 4–6 h	400
	Generic (various)		
Mefenamic acid	Ponstel (Park-Davis)	250 every 6 h	1000
Acetic Acid			
Etodoloc	Lodine (Wyeth-Ayerst)	200–400 every 6–8 h	1200
Diclofenac potassium	Cataflam (Geigy)	50 three times a day	150[c]
Propionic Acids			
Ibuprofen[a]	Motrin (Upjohn)	200–400 every 4–6 h	3200
	Generic (Various)		
Fenoprofen	Nalfon (Dista)	200 every 4–6 h	3200
	Generic (various)		
Ketoprofen[a]	Orudis (Wyeth-Ayerst)	25–50 every 6–8 h	300
	Orudis KT (Wyeth-Ayerst)		
	Generic (various)		
Naproxen	Naprasyn (Syntex/Roche)	250 every 6–12 h	1250
	Generic (various)		
Naproxen sodium[a]	Anaprox (Syntex/Roche	220 every 8–12 h	660[d]
	Aleve (Procter & Gamble)		
	Generic (various)		
Ketorolac (parenteral)	Toradol (Syntex/Roche)	15–30 every 6 h	120[e]
Ketorolac (oral)	Toradol (Syntex/Roche)	10 every 4–6 h	40[e]

[a]Available both as an over-the-counter preparation and as a prescription drug.
[b]Up to 1250 mg on the first day.
[c]Up to 200 mg on the first day.
[d]Over-the-counter dose.
[e]Maximum of 5 days. (Compiled from Refs. 43, 45, and 46.)

aggregation lasts only as long as drug concentrations are sustained.[41] There appears to be a great deal of variability from one patient to another in the therapeutic response seen with the NSAIDs. After an adequate drug trial of any of these agents, it is considered rational therapy to switch to another member of this drug group for an additional trial period.

The *para*-aminophenols (acetaminophen and phenacetin) inhibit prostaglandin synthesis in the CNS and manifest both analgesic and antipyretic activity with little anti-inflammatory action.[43] Acetaminophen exhibits a linear dose–response curve, with doses larger than 1000 mg showing greater efficacy than doses of 650 mg.[43] Phenacetin therapy was linked to renal papillary necrosis and has been removed from the worldwide market.[43] Acetaminophen is relatively free from side effects, although in overdose situations it is highly liver toxic. It can also be used in cases of aspirin allergy.

Narcotic Agents

Most clinicians consider the use of narcotic analgesics to be the next logical step in the management of acute pain. The classification of these agents, their equianalgesic doses, and dosing guidelines are outlined in Tables 59.8 and 59.9.

The pharmacologic activity of narcotics depends on their affinity for opiate receptors.[48] Therapeutic activities and side effects range from those exhibited by the pure opiate agonists or stimulators (e.g., morphine), to those seen with the pure opiate antagonists or blockers (e.g., naloxone) (Table 59.1). Partial agonists and antagonists (e.g., pentazocine) compete with agonists for opiate receptor sites and,

TABLE 59.7. RELATIVE SIDE EFFECTS OF FDA-APPROVED NON-NARCOTIC ANALGESICS

Agent	GI Irritation	CNS Effects	Hepatic Toxicity	Renal Toxicity
Aspirin	++++++	+	++	++
Choline salicylate	+++	—[a]	—[a]	—[a]
Magnesium salicylate	+++	—[a]	—[a]	—[a]
Sodium salicylate	+++	—[a]	—[a]	—[a]
Diflunisal	++	++	+	+
Acetaminophen	+	+	++	+
Meclofenamate	+++	++	+	++
Mefenamic acid	++	+	+	++
Etodolac	++	++	+	++
Diclofenac potassium	++	++	+	++
Ibuprofen	++	++	+	++
Fenoprofen	++	+++	+	+++
Ketoprofen	+	+	+	++
Ketorolac[b]	++	++	+	+
Naproxen	++	++	+	++

[a]Data not available.
[b]Five-day use only. (Compiled from Refs. 43, 45, 46, and 102.)

depending on the inherent ability to either stimulate or block these sites, exhibit mixed agonist–antagonist activity. Mixed agonist–antagonist agents with analgesic activity appear to exhibit selectivity for analgesic receptor sites (Table 59.1).[8] This may result in analgesia with fewer undesirable side effects.

In usual doses, narcotic analgesics do not eliminate pain; instead, they decrease its unpleasantness. Patients report that although their pain is still present, it no longer bothers them. The effects of the analgesics are also relatively selective and, at normal therapeutic concentrations, these agents do not decrease sensitivity to touch, sight, or hearing, or impair intellectual functioning[8]; however, as the dosage increases, so do the undesirable side effects (Table 59.10).

Narcotic analgesics share related pharmacologic attributes and exert their most profound effects on the CNS and GI tract.[49] Mood changes, sedation, respiratory depression, nausea, vomiting, decreased GI motility, dependence, and tolerance are evident in varying degrees with all agents. Consideration of efficacy and side-effect profile assists in the selection of the most appropriate agent.

The route of administration depends on individual patient needs. Oral codeine, oxycodone, hydrocodone, propoxyphene, and pentazocine are used in moderate pain. Peak analgesic effect usually occurs 1.5 to 2 hours after oral administration and must be considered when immediate relief is needed.[41] The narcotics differ greatly in equianalgesic dose (Table 59.8). Table 59.8 should be used only as a guide because the nature of pain makes it necessary to individualize pain regimens. True narcotic allergies are rare, but Table 59.8 can also be used when treating a patient hypersensitive to narcotics. Although caution is always advised, cross sensitivity between the morphine-like agonists, meperidine-like agonists, and methadone-like agonists is unlikely. When considering cross sensitivity, the mixed agonist-antagonist class acts much like the morphine-like agonists.[50]

In the initial stages of acute pain, analgesics should be given around the clock. This should commence after administering a typical starting dose and titrating up or down depending on the patient's degree of pain and demonstrated side effects (e.g., sedation).[41] As-needed schedules often produce wide swings in analgesic plasma concentrations that create wide swings in pain and sedation. This may initiate a vicious cycle where increasing amounts of pain medications are needed for relief.[51] As the painful state subsides and the need for medication decreases, however, as-needed schedules can be used. Continuous intravenous and subcutaneous methods of narcotic infusion are effective in some postoperative pain,[41,52] but the probability of unwanted side effects is high. An alternative method that has gained prominence is patient-controlled analgesia. With this technique, patients can self-administer preset amounts of intravenous narcotics via a syringe pump electronically interfaced with a timing device. Using this procedure, patients balance pain control with sedation.

Administration of narcotics directly into the CNS (epidural and intrathecal) has shown considerable promise in the control of acute pain (Table 59.11)[53] and is becoming prominent in both large and small institutions throughout the United States. Because of reports of marked sedation, pruritis, nausea, vomiting, urinary retention, and hypotension,[54] these methods of analgesia require careful monitoring and are best employed by experienced practitioners. Respiratory depression is of concern and can occur within the first 2 hours of opioid administration or manifest as late as 24 hours (especially shown with morphine) after single doses of spinal analgesia.[54] Naloxone is used to antagonize this effect, but repeated doses may be required.[54] Analgesia as well as side effects are evident at lower doses when the opioids are administered intrathecally instead of epidurally. Intrathecally, single morphine doses of 0.25–1 mg are common, whereas epidurally 5- to 10-mg doses are the norm. All opioids administered directly into the CNS should be preservative free.

Morphine and Congeners

Despite the availability of several newer agents, morphine remains the prototype narcotic analgesic. As new narcotic and non-narcotic compounds are developed, their efficacy and side-effect profiles are compared, with morphine as the standard. Many clinicians consider morphine the first-line agent when treating moderate to severe pain. Morphine can be given parenterally, orally, or rectally.

TABLE 59.8. NARCOTIC ANALGESICS

Class and Generic Name	Trade Name	Manufacturer	Route	Equianalgesic Dose (mg)
Morphine-Like Agonists				
Morphine	Generic	Various	IM, SQ	10
			PO	30–60
Hydromorphone	Dilaudid (generic)	Knoll (various)	IM, SQ	1.3
			PO	7.5
Oxymorphone	Numorphan	Du Pont	IM, SQ	1.0
			R	5
Levorphanol	Levo-Dromoran	Roche	IM, SQ	2.0
			PO	4.0
Codeine	Generic	Various	IM	130[a]
			PO	200[a]
Hydrocodone	Generic	Various	PO	30[a]
Oxycodone	Roxicodone (generic)	Roxane (various)	PO	30[a]
Meperidine-Like Agonists				
Meperidine	Demerol (generic)	Winthrop (various)	IM, SQ	75
			PO	300[c]
Fentanyl	Sublimaze (generic)	Janssen (various)	IM	0.1–0.2
	Duragesic	Janssen	Transdermal	25 mcg/h[c]
Methadone-Like Agonists				
Methadone	Dolophine (generic)	Lilly (various)	IM	10
			PO	20
Propoxyphene	Darvon (generic)	Lilly (various)	PO	130[a]
Mixed Agonist–Antagonists				
Pentazocine	Talwin	Sanofi	IM, SQ	30–60
		Winthrop	PO	180[a]
Butorphanol	Stadol	Mead Johnson	IM	2.0
	Stadol NS	Mead Johnson	Intranasal	1.0[b] (one spray)
Nalbuphine	Nubain (generic)	Du Pont (various)	IM	10
Buprenorphine	Buprenex	Norwich-Eaton	IM	0.3–0.4
Dezocine	Dalgan	Astra	IM	10
Antagonists				
Naloxone	Narcan (generic)	Du Pont (various)	IV	0.4–1.2[d]
Central Analgesic (not considered a narcotic)				
Tramadol	Ultram	Ortho-McNeil	PO	50–100[b]

[a]Starting doses lower (codeine, 30 mg; oxycodone and hydrocodone, 5 mg; meperidine, 50 mg; propoxyphene, 65–130 mg; pentazocine, 50 mg).
[b]Starting dose only (equianalgesia not shown).
[c]Equivalent IM morphine dose = 8–22 mg day.
[d]Starting doses to be used in cases of opioid overdose. (Compiled from Refs. 41, 45, 49, 73, 89, 94–96, 100, and 103.)

Morphine's CNS effects are numerous. Through direct stimulation of the chemoreceptor trigger zone, morphine causes nausea and vomiting. This is observed more often in ambulatory patients, often subsides after the initial dose, and may be counteracted by drugs that block postsynaptic dopamine action (e.g., phenothiazine derivatives).[55] Although euphoria and dysphoria have been reported, morphine's unpleasant effects are more frequent when administered to those not experiencing pain.[49] As doses of morphine are increased, the respiratory center becomes less responsive to carbon dioxide, resulting in progressive respiratory depression. This effect is less pronounced in those being treated for severe pain. Respiratory depression is most often manifested as a decrease in respiratory rate and is further compounded because the cough reflex is also depressed. Morphine-induced respiratory depression can be reversed by pure narcotic antagonists.[55] In patients with emphysema, kyphoscoliosis, and cor pulmonale, extreme caution must be employed when using morphine or any related opioid. Although these patients may be functioning normally, they are already using compensatory breathing mechanisms and are at risk for further respiratory compromise.[55] Precaution is also urged when using narcotic analgesics with alcohol or other CNS depressants. This combination amplifies CNS depression and is potentially quite harmful and possibly lethal.

Therapeutic doses of morphine have minimal effects on blood pressure, cardiac rate, or cardiac rhythm when

TABLE 59.9. DOSING GUIDELINES

Agent(s)	Doses (titrate up or down based on patient response)	Notes
NSAIDs/acetaminophen/aspirin	Dose to maximum before switching to another agent (see Table 59.6)	• Regular alcohol use and high doses of acetaminophen may result in liver dysfunction • Used in mild to moderate pain • May use in conjunction with narcotic agents to decrease doses of each • Care must be exercised to avoid overdose when combination products containing these agents are used
Morphine	PO 10–30 mg q 3–4 h[a] IM 5–10 mg q 3–4 h[a] IV 1–2.5 mg q 5 min PRN[a] SR 15–30 mg q 12 h (may need to be q 8 in some patients) Rectal 10–20 mg q 3–4 h[a]	• Drug of choice in severe pain • Use immediate-release product with SR product to control "breakthrough" pain
Hydromorphone	PO 2–4 mg q 3–4 h[a] IM 0.5–1 mg q 3–4 h[a] IV 0.1–0.5 mg q 5 min PRN[a] Rectal 2–4 mg q 3–4 h[a]	• Use in severe pain • More potent than morphine, otherwise no advantages
Oxymorphone	IM 1–1.5 mg q 3–4 h[a] IV 0.5 mg initially[a] Rectal 5 mg q 3–4 h[a]	• Use in severe pain • No advantages over morphine
Levorphanol	PO 2–4 mg q 6–8 h IM 2 mg q 6–8 h IV 2 mg q 6–8 h	• Use in severe pain • Extended half-life useful in cancer patients
Codeine	PO 15–60 mg q 3–4 h[a] IM 15–60 mg q 3–4 h[a] IV 15–60 mg q 3–4 h[a]	• Use in moderate pain • Weak analgesic, use with NSAIDs or aspirin or acetaminophen
Hydrocodone	PO 5–10 mg q 3–4 h[a]	• Use in moderate/severe pain • Most effective when used with NSAIDs or aspirin or acetaminophen
Oxycodone	PO 5–10 mg q 3–4 h[a]	• Use in moderate/severe pain • Most effective when used with NSAIDs or aspirin or acetaminophen
Meperidine	PO 50–150 mg q 3–4 h[a] IM 75–100 mg q 3–4 h[a] IV 5–10 mg q 5 min PRN[a]	• Use in severe pain • Oral not recommended • Do not use in renal failure • May precipitate tremors, myoclonus, and seizures • Monoamine oxidase inhibitors can induce hyperpyrexia and/or seizures
Fentanyl	IM 0.05–0.1 mg q 1–2 h[a] Transdermal 25 mcg/h	• Used preoperative, intraoperative, postoperative • Used in severe pain • Do not use transdermal in patient with acute pain
Methadone	PO 10–20 mg q 6–8 h IM 5–10 mg q 6–8 h	• Effective in severe chronic pain • Sedation can be major problem • Some patients with chronic pain can be dosed q 12 h
Propoxyphene	PO 65–100 mg q 3–4 h[a]	• Use in moderate pain • Weak analgesic, most effective when used with NSAIDs or aspirin or acetaminophen • Will cause carbamazepine levels to increase
Pentazocine	PO 50–100 mg q 3–4 h[b] IM 30 mg q 3–4 h[b]	• Third-line agent for moderate to severe pain • May precipitate withdrawal in opiate-dependent patients
Butorphanol	IM 1–4 mg q 3–4 h[b] IV 0.5–2 mg q 3–4 h[b] Intranasal 1 mg (1 spray) q 3–4 h[b]	• Second-line agent for moderate to severe pain • May precipitate withdrawal in opiate-dependent patients

(continued)

TABLE 59.9. DOSING GUIDELINES (*continued*)

Agent(s)	Doses (titrate up or down based on patient response)	Notes
Nalbuphine	IM 10 mg q 3–6 h[b] IV 10 mg q 3–6 h[b]	• Second-line agent for moderate to severe pain • May precipitate withdrawal in opiate-dependent patients
Buprenorphine	IM 0.3 mg q 6 h[b] IV 0.3 mg q 6 h[b]	• Second-line agent for moderate to severe pain • May precipitate withdrawal in opiate-dependent patients
Dezocine	IM 5–20 mg q 3–6 h[b] IV 2.5–10 mg q 2–4 h[b]	• Second-line agent for moderate to severe pain • May precipitate withdrawal in opiate-dependent patients
Naloxone	IV 0.4–1.2 mg	• When reversing opiate side effects in patients needing analgesia, dilute and titrate (0.1–0.2 mg q 2–3 minutes) so as not to reverse analgesia
Tramadol	PO 50–100 mg q 4–6 h[a]	• Maximum dose is 400 mg/24 h • Decrease dose in renal impairment and in the elderly

[a]May start with an around-the-clock regimen and switch to PRN if/when the painful signal subsides.
[b]May reach a ceiling analgesic effect. (Compiled from Refs. 45, 46, 73, 89, 104, and 105.)

patients are supine; however, morphine does produce venous and arteriolar vessel dilation, and orthostatic hypotension may result. Hypovolemic patients, those whose blood pressure is being maintained by sympathetic outflow, and patients with acute myocardial infarction are more susceptible to morphine-induced cardiovascular changes (e.g., decreases in blood pressure).[55] Because morphine prompts a decrease in myocardial oxygen demand in ischemic cardiac patients, it is often considered the narcotic of choice when using opioids to treat pain associated with myocardial infarction.

TABLE 59.10. MAJOR ADVERSE EFFECTS OF THE NARCOTIC ANALGESICS

Effect	Manifestation
Mood changes	Dysphoria, euphoria
Somnolence	Lethargy, drowsiness, apathy, inability to concentrate
Stimulation of chemoreceptor trigger zone	Nausea, vomiting
Respiratory depression	Decreased respiratory rate
Interference with hypothalamic function (mostly morphine)	Increase in ADH; decrease in CRF, GnRF, TSH, GH, LRF, and FSH; disordered temperature regulation
Decreased gastrointestinal motility	Constipation
Increase in sphincter tone (mostly morphine)	Biliary spasm, urinary retention
Histamine release (mostly morphine and meperidine)	Urticaria, pruritus, rarely exacerbation of asthma
Tolerance	Larger doses for same effect
Dependence	Withdrawal symptoms upon abrupt discontinuation

(Compiled from Refs. 8 and 55.)

Morphine decreases the motility of the entire GI tract, in turn reducing biliary and pancreatic secretions. The end result, especially when administered over extended time periods, is constipation. Morphine-induced spasms of the sphincter of Oddi have been observed. Atropine can partially reduce these spasms,[55] but the clinical significance of such an occurrence should be assessed on an individual basis. Although morphine's effect on the urinary bladder varies, urinary retention can become a problem; this is especially true in patients with prostate disease.[8] Morphine-induced histamine release often manifests as pruritus and, although not seen often, may exacerbate bronchospasm in patients with a history of asthma.[8] Special attention must be given to patients with increased intracranial pressure and those with head injury secondary to trauma. In these patients morphine can markedly exaggerate this pressure and more readily produce respiratory depression[55] while clouding the neurologic examination results.

Hydromorphone is more potent, has better oral absorption characteristics, and is more soluble than morphine; however, its overall pharmacologic profile parallels that of morphine. Oxymorphone can be administered rectally and by injection. Although it is more potent than morphine, it offers no real pharmacologic advantages. Although levorphanol has an extended half-life, its overall therapeutic effects are similar to those of morphine.

Codeine is an analgesic that is effective in mild to moderate pain. It is often combined with other analgesic

TABLE 59.11. EPIDURAL OPIOIDS

Agent	Dose (mg)	Onset of Pain Relief (min)	Duration of Pain Relief (h)
Morphine	5–10	24	20
Hydromorphone	1	13	12
Fentanyl	0.1	4–10	2.5–6

(Modified from Cousins MJ, Mather LE. Intrathecal and epidural administration of opioids. Anesthesiology 1984;61:299.)

products and enjoys a popularity that makes it the standard for other oral narcotics. Unfortunately, codeine has the same propensity to produce tolerance, dependence, and constipation as morphine. Hydrocodone, a derivative of codeine, is also most often seen in combination products and has pharmacologic properties similar to those of morphine. Oxycodone is equal in potency to morphine and is an excellent oral analgesic for moderate to severe pain. This is especially true when the product is used in combination with a non-narcotic agent; however, its predilection for causing tolerance and dependence, along with its basic opioid characteristics, likens it to morphine.

Meperidine and Congeners (Phenylpiperidines)

The prototype phenylpiperidine, meperidine, has a pharmacologic profile comparable to that of morphine; however, it is not as potent and has a shorter half-life. This necessitates larger doses that must be administered more frequently; however, several studies have shown that this is often not done.[4,5] Although meperidine is effective orally, larger doses must be administered to achieve the same effect that is obtained with the parenteral form (Table 59.8). With high doses or in patients with renal failure, the metabolite normeperidine accumulates, causing CNS excitability manifested as tremor, muscle twitching, and possibly seizures.[46] Meperidine's effects on the cardiovascular system, GI tract, and smooth muscle are less severe than those of morphine, causing considerably less biliary spasm and urinary retention. The combination of monoamine oxidase inhibitors and meperidine should not be used because this mixture can produce an excitation syndrome, hyperpyrexia, and convulsions. In most clinical settings, meperidine offers no real advantage over morphine.[49]

Fentanyl is a synthetic opioid structurally related to meperidine and is most often used in anesthesiology for induction of anesthesia.[56] These agents are more potent and shorter acting than meperidine (Tables 59.8 and 59.12) and at high doses can produce marked muscle rigidity.[45,56] A fentanyl lozenge on a plastic handle is currently available as a premedication in children before anesthesia. A fentanyl transdermal system is also available for the treatment of chronic pain in patients requiring opioid analgesics. One patch can provide analgesic support for 72 hours but it takes 12–24 hours to obtain steady-state levels after a patch is initially applied. In addition, it may take 6 days after increasing a dose before new steady-state levels accumulate. Thus, the patch should not be used in patients with acute pain.[45]

Methadone and Congeners

Methadone has gained considerable popularity because of its oral efficacy, extended duration of action, low cost, and ability to suppress withdrawal symptoms in heroin addicts. With repeated doses the analgesic duration of action is prolonged, but because of metabolite accumulation, excessive sedation may also result. Although methadone is quite effective in acute pain,[46] it is usually used to treat chronic pain. The pharmacologic profile resembles that of morphine.

Propoxyphene is one-half as potent as codeine, and is more effective than placebo when 65–100 mg is ingested.[57] It is usually used in combination with aspirin or acetaminophen in the treatment of moderate pain. The toxicity profile of propoxyphene is similar to that of codeine.

Mixed Narcotic Agonist–Antagonists

Analgesic agents that stimulate the analgesic portion (mu-1, delta, kappa, epsilon) of opioid receptors while blocking the toxicity portion (mu-2, sigma) would be considered ideal (Table 59.1). The mixed agonist–antagonist agents were developed with this ideal in mind. This analgesic class is effective in the treatment of moderate to severe pain and has a ceiling effect on respiratory depression (e.g., after a dose of 30 mg in adults, progressively higher doses of nalbuphine do not affect respiratory rate).[58] They have a low abuse potential, cause decreased constipation, and show less biliary spasmotic effects than morphine; however, psychotomimetic responses (e.g., hallucinations and vivid dreams, seen more often with pentazocine and butorphanol), a ceiling analgesic effect, and a propensity to cause pain and initiate withdrawal in narcotic-dependent populations have diminished their widespread clinical use.

Pentazocine, the first agonist–antagonist clinically available, is a good oral and parenteral analgesic in moderate to severe pain but causes the most psychotomimetic effects. The oral form has been melted down and used illicitly in combination with tripelennamine; however, the addition of small amounts of naloxone has countered this illegitimate use by blocking the euphoric but not the analgesic effects.

Although decreased in intensity, butorphanol shares pentazocine's tendency to produce hallucinations and increase cardiac workload. Both must be used with caution in patients with myocardial ischemia. Butorphanol, however, is the only analgesic available in an intranasal dosage form. Nalbuphine acts similarly to pentazocine and butorphanol but causes a reduced myocardial oxygen demand in patients after myocardial infarction, compared with pentazocine and butorphanol. Because nalbuphine blocks the mu receptor and produces analgesia by stimulating the kappa receptor, nalbuphine has been used postoperatively to treat opioid-induced respiratory depression and pain simultaneously.[59]

Buprenorphine acts as a partial opioid receptor agonist and may offer a longer duration of analgesic effect with less respiratory depression than previously mentioned agents.[58] It binds quite strongly to opioid receptors and very large doses of narcotic receptor antagonists (e.g., naloxone) may be needed to reverse the agonist activities.[58] Dezocine is the newest mixed agonist–antagonist. Its advantage over existing agents, however, remains to be demonstrated. Unlike the previously mentioned narcotics, butorphanol, nalbuphine, and dezocine are not controlled substances.[59] Considering the high cost of storing, recording, and dispensing

TABLE 59.12. NARCOTIC ANALGESIC PHARMACOKINETICS[a]

Agent	Time to Peak (h)	Half-Life (h)	Analgesic Onset (min)	Analgesic Duration (h)
Morphine	0.5–1	2–4	15–30, 60[b]	4–5
Hydromorphone	0.5–1	2–3	15–30	4–5
Oxymorphone	0.5–1	2–3	5–15	3–6
Levorphanol	0.5–1	12–16	30–90	6–8
Hydrocodone	1.3	4	—[c]	4–5
Codeine	0.5–1	2–4	15–30	4–6
Oxycodone (PO)	0.5–1	3–4	15–30	4–5
Meperidine	0.5–1	3–4	10–45	3–5
Fentanyl	—[c]	1.5–6	7–8	1–2
Methadone	0.5–1	15–40	30–60	4–5 (acute) >8 (chronic)
Propoxyphene (PO)	2.0–2.5	6–12	30–60	4–6
Pentazocine	0.25–1	4–5	15–20	3–6
Butorphanol	0.5–1	2.5–3.5	<10	4–6
Nalbuphine	1	2–3	<15	3–6
Buprenorphine	1	5	15	6
Dezocine	0.17–1.5	0.6–5	15–30	2–4
Naloxone[d]	0.5–2	0.5–1.5	2–5	0.5–1
Tramadol (PO)	2–3	6–7	<60	6

[a]Based on intramuscular data unless otherwise indicated.
[b]Data based intrathecal or epidural administration.
[c]Data not available.
[d]Narcotic antagonist. (Compiled from Refs. 45, 46, 49, 56, 94–96, 99, 100, 103, and 106.)

scheduled drugs, these agents may offer hidden potential economic benefits.

Narcotic Antagonists

The pure opioid antagonist naloxone binds competitively to opioid receptors but does not produce an analgesic response. Therefore, it is most often used to reverse the toxic effects of agonist and mixed agonist–antagonist narcotics.

Central Analgesic

Tramadol is the first centrally acting binary analgesic available in the United States. It is not derived from natural sources and is not related chemically to the opiates or NSAIDs. Its efficacy has compared favorably with acetaminophen and codeine and it is indicated for the relief of moderate to moderately severe pain.

Tramadol has two basic modes of action: weak opiate receptor binding (predominantly on the μ-receptor) and inhibition of norepinephrine and serotonin reuptake.

Although associated with minimal dependency and tolerance, tramadol has a side effect profile similar to that of opiates: dizziness, somnolence, nausea, constipation, sweating, pruritus, and increased sedation and/or respiratory depression when used with CNS depressants such as alcohol, other opiates, phenothiazines, tranquilizers, or sedative hypnotics. Tramadol also may enhance the risk of seizure in patients taking MAOIs, neuroleptics or other drugs that can reduce the seizure threshold, and in patients with seizure disorders.

Tramadol may have a place in treating patients with chronic pain when avoidance of the dependence and tolerance of opiates is desired. However, this agent has little advantage over opiates when treating patients for acute pain and is more expensive.

Combination Therapy

The combination of narcotic and non-narcotic oral analgesics often results in analgesia superior to that produced by either agent alone.[60] Attacking pain on two fronts, prostaglandins and opiate receptors enhance pain relief and facilitate the use of lower doses of each agent. This frequently produces a more favorable side-effect profile and is the reason there are so many aspirin and/or acetaminophen–narcotic analgesic combination products marketed. The addition of an injectable NSAID (ketorolac) also makes this combination possible in patients who cannot take oral medications. The clinician should not be limited by the availability of commercially established fixed-ratio combinations. For example, the administration of around-the-clock acetaminophen, aspirin, or other NSAIDs in combination

TABLE 59.13. LOCAL ANESTHETICS

Agent	Trade Name	Manufacturer	Onset (min)	Duration (h)
Esters				
Procaine	Novocain	SanofiWinthrop	2–5	0.25–1
	Generic	Various		
Chloroprocaine	Nesacaine	Astra	6–12	0.50
Tetracaine	Pontocaine	SanofiWinthrop	15	2–3
Amides				
Mepivacaine	Carbocaine	SanofiWinthrop	3–5	0.75–1.5
	Generic	Various		
Bupivacaine	Marcaine	SanofiWinthrop	5	2–4
	Generic	Various		
Lidocaine	Generic	Various	<2	0.5–1
Prilocaine	Citanest	Astra	<2	≥1
Etidocaine	Duranest	Astra	3–5	5–10

(Compiled from Ref. 45.)

with scheduled narcotic regimens is often very effective in the treatment of pain resulting from bone metastases in advanced cancer.

Not all analgesic combinations are clearly effective. Caffeine in combination with aspirin may offer a slight analgesic advantage over aspirin alone in treating moderate pain[61,62]; however, caffeine's additive analgesic effects are controversial and the benefits of caffeine in combination with aspirin or acetaminophen remain unclear.[63]

Agents shown to potentiate the analgesic efficacy of parenteral narcotics include hydroxyzine and dextroamphetamine.[64,65] Phenothiazines, with the exception of methotrimeprazine, once thought to possess this potentiating property, apparently offer no inherent analgesic or potentiating characteristics when combined with narcotics, although unwanted sedation may be greatly increased.[8,66] Methotrimeprazine (Levoprome 10–20 mg, available in parenteral form only) does not seem to cause constipation or respiratory depression and may be useful in narcotic-tolerant cancer patients. Its use has been limited, however, due to sedation and orthostatic hypotension.[41]

Regional Analgesia

Regional analgesia with properly administered local anesthetics can provide complete relief of pain and block acute pain reflex responses often deleterious in acute pain (Table 59.13).[67] These agents have also been applied directly onto surgical wounds and have substantially decreased postoperative narcotic requirements.[68] They are also used epidurally in both acute and chronic pain. Regional analgesics relieve pain by blocking nociceptive transmission, interrupting sympathetic reflexes, and preventing increased skeletal muscle activity.[46] Their lipid solubility, protein-binding characteristics, pK_a, and vasodilator behavior determine the mechanism of action.[69] Although safe, they readily cross the blood–brain barrier, causing signs of CNS excitation and depression, including dizziness, tinnitus, drowsiness, disorientation, muscle twitching, seizures, and respiratory arrest.[69] Cardiovascular effects include myocardial depression, hypotension, hypertension, decreased cardiac output, heart block, bradycardia, ventricular arrythmia, and cardiac arrest.[45] Disadvantages of such methods incorporate the need for skillful technical application, the need for frequent administration, and highly specialized follow-up procedures.

STIMULATION THERAPY

Transcutaneous electrical nerve stimulation (TENS) and electroacupuncture have shown moderate success in managing postoperative pain.[70] Although narcotic-like side effects are certainly prevented, a lack of well-controlled studies has prevented this technique from gaining wide acceptance.

PSYCHOLOGIC INTERVENTION

Even though the cognitive, behavioral, and social aspects of pain are well established, psychologic techniques for the treatment of acute pain are not widely employed. Simple interventions (e.g., introductory information about sensations to expect after certain procedures) reduce patient distress and greatly reduce postprocedure suffering.[71] Other successful psychologic techniques include relaxation training, controlled mental imagery, controlled attention or distraction, reinforcement of appropriate actions, hypnosis, and biofeedback.

CHRONIC PAIN MANAGEMENT

CANCER PAIN

Managing the pain of malignant diseases encompasses both acute and chronic management techniques. Thus, the phar-

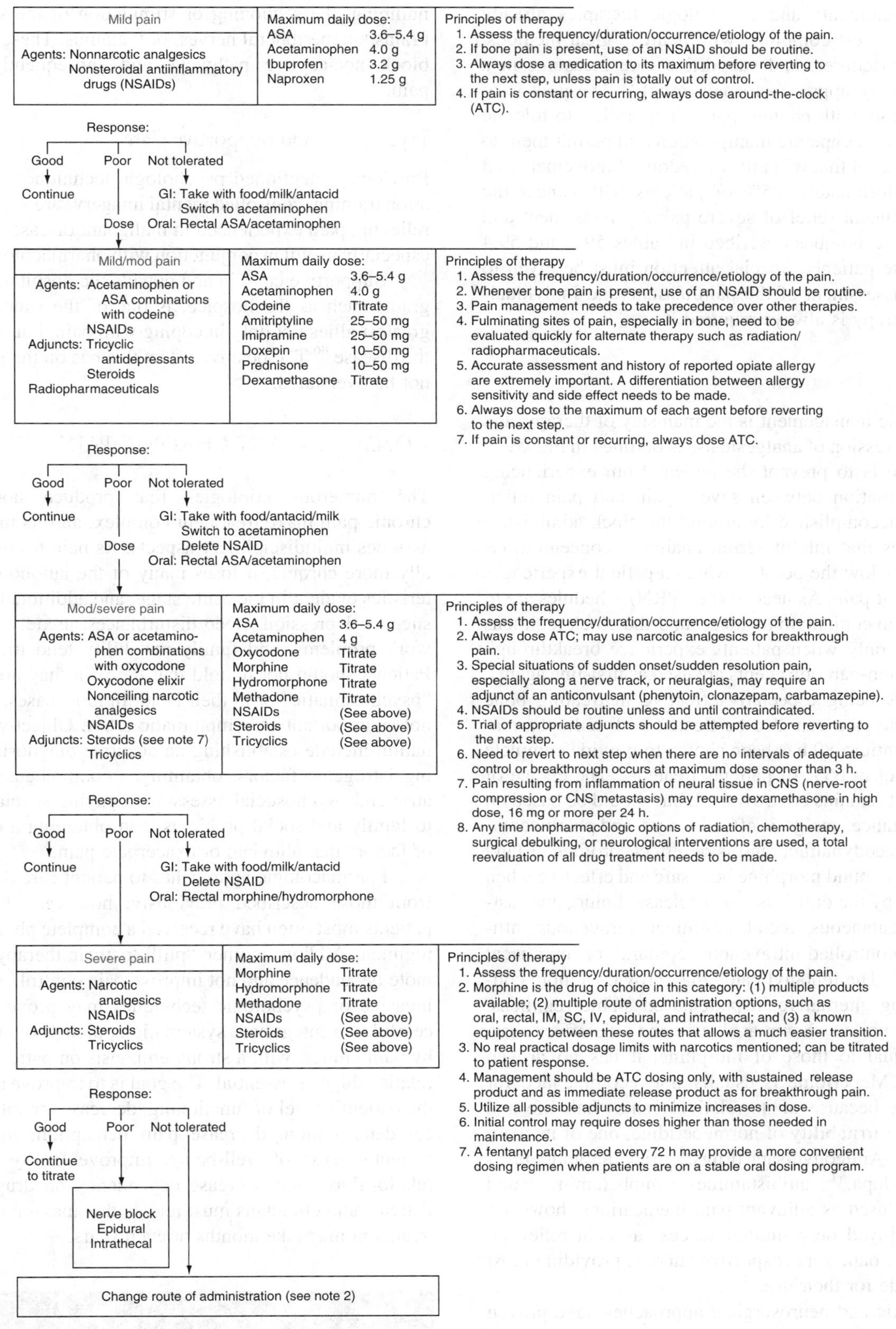

Figure 59.3 Algorithm for pain management in oncology patients. *(Adapted from the Kaiser Permanente Algorithm for Pain Management in Patients with Advanced Malignant Disease.)*

macologic treatments and psychologic therapies already mentioned are best combined with neurosurgical methods, anesthetic procedures, and supportive care measures in a multidisciplinary approach to pain relief.[72] The goal is to provide patients with enough pain amelioration to tolerate diagnostic and therapeutic manipulation and permit them to function at a level that will allow freedom of movement and choice.[72] Unfortunately, 25% of patients with cancer die without significant relief of severe pain.[72] Assessment and management techniques described in Tables 59.2 and 59.4 apply to these patients. Special attention must be given to continual reassessment of the painful state and individualization of therapy is always required.[72]

Pharmacologic Treatment

Pharmacologic management is the mainstay of therapy, and a typical progression of analgesic use is outlined in Fig. 59.3. The objective is to prevent the patient from experiencing constant fluctuation between severe pain and pain relief. This is best accomplished by around-the-clock administration schedules that inhibit serum analgesic concentrations from falling below the point at which a patient experiences the suffering of pain. As needed (i.e., PRN) schedules are to be employed in conjunction with around-the-clock regimens and are used only when patients experience breakthrough pain. Again, non-narcotic agents are used as first-line agents, with NSAIDs being especially effective in treating bone pain.[73,74] Bone pain can also be treated with radiopharmaceuticals. Stontium-89 has been shown to provide complete to partial relief in 65% of patients treated.[73] The choice of narcotic agent remains controversial, but should be based on patient acceptance, analgesic effectiveness, and pharmacokinetic, pharmacodynamic, and side-effect profiles. Many clinicians have found morphine both safe and effective when administered by the oral (sustained-release, liquid, and fast-release), subcutaneous, rectal, continual intravenous infusion, patient-controlled intravenous, epidural, or intrathecal route.[54,73,75–80] The fentanyl patch may provide a more convenient dosing alternative in patients on stable regimens. Although heroin has shown analgesic and side-effect characteristics equal to those of morphine, it has no proven superiority.[81] Meperidine is usually not recommended for long-term use because of its relatively short half-life and the CNS hyperirritability of normeperidine, one of its main metabolites.[82] Anticonvulsant drugs,[72] tricyclic antidepressants,[83] levodopa,[84] antihistamines, amphetamines, and steroids[85] are used as adjuvant pain medications; however, they have enjoyed only limited success as pain relievers, with anecdotal data or retrospective surveys providing most of the rationale for their use.[72]

Anesthetic and neurosurgical approaches have proven successful in alleviating pain but require special expertise and are usually reserved for patients who are refractory to conventional analgesics. They most commonly involve, numbing, the sectioning or stimulation of the spinal cord, brainstem, peripheral nerves, or thalamus. These techniques block nociceptive pathways and subsequently alleviate pain.[72]

Psychologic and Supportive Care

Previously mentioned psychologic techniques (e.g., relaxation training, controlled mental imagery) are very helpful in relieving pain experienced in malignant disease[72] and prove especially useful in conjunction with pharmacologic therapy.

Supportive care, in and outside the hospital, using programs such as the hospice, is one of the cancer patient's greatest allies not only in coping with pain, but in accepting the disease.[86] The positive effect this has on the patient cannot be overstated.

NONMALIGNANT CHRONIC PAIN

The numerous etiologies that produce nonmalignant chronic pain make treatment complex, and its management assumes multidisciplinary aspects. As pain becomes gradually more chronic, it loses many of the autonomic characteristics evident in the acute stage, and additional symptoms such as depression, sleep disturbances, anxiety, irritability, work problems, and family instability tend to dominate.[8] Patients should not be told that the pain they are feeling is "psychosomatic" or in their head. In most cases, etiology is not as important as symptomatic relief. Objectives in evaluation include establishing an accurate diagnosis, identifying iatrogenic factors, obtaining a comprehensive psychiatric and psychosocial assessment, paying special attention to family and social problems, and obtaining a description of factors that alleviate or exacerbate pain.[8]

Pharmacologic approaches to patient care do not differ from those described previously; however, chronic pain patients most often have received a complete pharmacologic regimen. Adding another "pill" to their therapy will promote dependence and not improve pain control.[8] Other noninvasive or psychologic techniques may prove more successful. An integrated, systematic approach often provided by pain clinics, with a strong emphasis on patient–clinician relationships, is essential. The goal is to improve or maintain the patient's level of functioning, decrease the rate of physical deterioration, decrease pain perception, improve the patient's sense of well-being, improve family and social relationships, and decrease dependency on drug therapy.[8] Patients and clinicians must realize that maximum effective treatment may take months or even years.

EVALUATION OF THERAPEUTIC OUTCOMES

The key to treating pain effectively is to adhere to the basic principles of the pharmacologic treatment of pain (Table

59.4), consistently monitor effectiveness (i.e., pain relief) versus side effects (i.e., sedation), and titrate treatment accordingly (see Tables 59.6 and 59.9). As stated previously, in acute pain this often needs to be done several times a day (in the early stages, hourly), while in chronic pain this may take place daily or even weekly. The frequency of evaluation depends also on the drug, the administration route, and other therapies being utilized. When patients cannot evaluate their own pain, monitoring agitation and heart rate is appropriate. Given the subjective nature of pain, the most successful therapies will involve not only frequent patient assessment, but a large degree of patient control (i.e., patient-controlled analgesia).

All narcotic analgesics can cause constipation. The best management of constipation is prevention. Patients should be counseled on the proper intake of fluids and fiber. A laxative may be added if needed. As noted earlier, CNS depressants (i.e., alcohol, benzodiazepines) amplify CNS depression when used with narcotic analgesics and should be closely monitored and discouraged when possible.

It must be remembered that pain is whatever the patient says it is. In acute pain and cancer pain, when patients tell you they are hurting, aggressive drug therapy should be considered. In chronic pain, aggressive assessment and understanding may be more appropriate. If acute pain does not subside within the anticipated duration of the insult (often 1–2 weeks), further investigation of the cause is warranted. Cancer pain and chronic pain may need treatment for years.

Drug Misuse, Abuse, Tolerance, and Dependence

The tendency of narcotic analgesics to be abused and the problems of tolerance, dependence, and withdrawal have left clinicians with an understandable but often unfounded fear regarding the appropriate use of these agents. Porter and Jick[87] studied 12,000 patients who had received narcotic analgesics for acute pain and found only four cases of medically induced dependence. Cohen[5] investigated 109 pain patients in five different hospitals and reported that house officers consistently underdosed narcotics and nursing staffs interpreted PRN orders to mean "as little as possible." Their overwhelming concern was the fear of addiction.

The problem associated with dependence and withdrawal is real but often overstated, especially with short-term use. An improper fear of addiction, therefore, promotes inappropriate pain management. The term "addiction" is often misused in the patient care setting in that it refers to individuals who are abusing drugs. Even those patients who develop dependence and tolerance to narcotic analgesics seldom become "drug abusers." The word "addiction" should never be used in place of the terms dependence or tolerance if abuse is not taking place. This confuses patients and causes them needless anxiety. With a better understanding of rational analgesic therapy, these problems will certainly be minimized.

Special Pain Populations

ELDERLY

Aging causes degeneration of neurons in the dorsal column accompanied by diminished sensory awareness, which may change pain perception[88]; however, study results are inconclusive, and no age differences have been noted in pain thresholds.[89] In general, the elderly are more sensitive to the effects of analgesics, and individualization of treatment to ensure efficacy and monitoring for adverse effects becomes even more important than in younger individuals.[8]

CHILDREN

For years it was assumed that younger children are less likely to experience pain because their CNS is less advanced.[90] Recent work disputes this theory.[91] Children react to painful stimuli based on their cognitive, social, and emotional development.[90] In acute pain, older children may display discomfort more readily than younger ones, because they have experienced previous pain, and the present suffering reminds them of former discomforts and their unpleasant consequences.[92] Children of all ages respond to chronic pain by withdrawal and regression to an earlier stage of development.[90] Pain in children should be treated vigorously with the pharmacologic and nonpharmacologic methods and procedures previously mentioned. Special attention should be given to the anxiety suffered because of separation from parents and to the developmental level of the child reacting to painful stimuli.

NARCOTIC-DEPENDENT PATIENTS

Patients dependent on street narcotics, those taking methadone to prevent narcotic withdrawal, and medically dependent patients should be treated for acute or chronic pain with the same pharmacologic concepts used for other populations. Traditionally, these patients are among those least favored by clinicians[8] and are often the cause of patient–caregiver conflict and hostility. Rather than using punishment techniques and withholding narcotics, caregivers should treat this group with aggressive pharmacologic methods because of probable tolerance and withdrawal problems not seen in other populations. Care must be taken to adequately meet the individual's immediate need for pain relief. The chronic narcotic problems can be dealt with later, realizing that often, even with good patient–caregiver relations, long-term therapy may not be successful.

Conclusion

The importance of proper pain management has been examined by several reviewers and has received national prominence by a consensus panel assembled to study the problem by the National Institutes of Health (NIH)[93] and by the publication of clinical practice guidelines in both acute and cancer pain by the Agency for Health Care Policy and Research.[73,89] Many of the deficiencies noted were attributed to poor training of health care practitioners in pain assessment and management, improper patient education, and inadequate communication among health care professionals.[93] The NIH panel suggested an integrated approach, utilizing the expertise of many disciplines, as well as individualized pharmacologic and nonpharmacologic strategies as a way of better addressing the problem. Pain relief assessment as part of a quality assurance program was also suggested as a means of ensuring proper therapy.[93] Indeed, it is the responsibility of the pharmacist and all health care professionals who deal with pain to communicate therapies and assure proper management in an effort to relieve treatable suffering and pain.

References

1. Hazelden Foundation. Touchstones. New York, Harper & Row, 1986, page listed as June 19.
2. Bonica JJ, Procacci P. General considerations of acute pain. General considerations of chronic pain, in Bonica JJ, Loeser JD, Chapman CR, Fordyce WE (eds): The Management of Pain. Philadelphia, Lea & Febiger, 1990, pp 159–196.
3. Chapman CR, Bonica JJ. Acute pain, in Current Concepts. Kalamazoo, MI, Scope Publications, 1983.
4. Marks RM, Sacher EJ. Undertreatment of medical inpatient pain with narcotic analgesics. Ann Intern Med 1973;78:173–181.
5. Cohen FL. Postsurgical pain relief: Patients' status and nurses' medication choices. Pain 1980;9:265–274.
6. Perry SW. The undertreatment of pain. Psychiatr Ann 1984;14:808–811.
7. Weis OF, Sriwatanakul K, Alloza JL, et al. Attitudes of patients, housestaff, and nurses toward postoperative analgesic care. Anesth Analg 1983;62:70–74.
8. Stimmel B. Pain, Analgesia and Addiction: The Pharmacology of Pain. New York, Raven Press, 1983.
9. Bonica JJ. Definitions and taxonomy of pain, in Bonica JJ, Loeser JD, Chapman CR, et al (eds): The Management of Pain. Philadelphia, Lea & Febiger, 1990, pp 18–27.
10. Fields HL, Levine JD. Pain—Mechanisms and management. West J Med 1984;141:347–357.
11. Gilfoil TM, Klavins I. 5-Hydroxytryptamine, bradykinin and histamine as mediators of inflammatory hyperesthesia. Am J Physiol 1965;204:867–876.
12. Ignelzi RJ, Atkinson JH. Pain and its modulation. Part 1. Afferent mechanisms. Neurosurgery 1980;6:577–583.
13. Bessou P, Burgess PR, Perl ER, Taylor CB. Dynamic properties of mechanoreceptors with unmyelinated (C) fibers. J Neurophysiol 1971;34:116–131.
14. Bessou P, Perl ER. Response of cutaneous sensory units with unmyelinated fibers to noxious stimuli. J Neurophysiol 1969;32:1025–1043.
15. Chapman CR. New directions in the understanding and management of pain. Soc Sci Med 1984;19:1261–1277.
16. Bonica JJ. Biochemistry and modulation of nociception and pain, in Bonica JJ, Loeser JD, Chapman CR, et al (eds): The Management of Pain. Philadelphia, Lea & Febiger, 1990, pp 95–121.
17. Hokfelt T, Johansson O, Ljungdahl A, Schultzberg M. Peptidergic neurones. Nature 1980;284:515–521.
18. Hunt SP, Kelly JS, Emson PC, et al. An immunohistochemical study of neuronal populations containing neuropeptides or aminobutyrate within the superficial layers of the rat dorsal horn. Neurosciences 1981;6:1883–1898.
19. Yaksh TL, Farb DH, Leeman SE, Jessell TM. Intrathecal capsaicin depletes substance P in the rat spinal cord and produces prolonged thermal analgesia. Science 1979; 206:481–488.
20. Rosell S, Olgart L, Gazelius B, et al. Inhibition of antidromic and substance P induced vasodilation by a substance P antagonist. Acta Physiol Scand 1981;111:381–382.
21. Schweyen DH. The use of fluoxetine and capsaicin for diabetic peripheral neuropathy. Hosp Pharm 1990;25:402–408.
22. Cervero F, Iffo A. The substantia gelatinosa of the spinal cord—A critical review. Brain 1980;103:717–772.
23. Melzack R, Wall PD. Pain mechanisms: A new theory. Science 1965;150:971–979.
24. Mayer DJ, Leibeskind JC. Pain reduction by focal electrical stimulation of the brain: An anatomical and behavioral analysis. Brain Res 1974;68:73–93.
25. Mayer DJ, Wolfe TL, Akil H, et al. Analgesia from electrical stimulation in the brain stem of the rat. Science 1971; 174:1351–1354.
26. Basbaum AL, Fields HL. Endogenous pain control mechanisms: Review and hypothesis. Ann Neurol 1978;4:451–462.
27. Goldstein A, Lowney LL, Pal BK. Stereospecific and nonspecific interactions of morphine narcotic congener levorphanol in subcellular fractions of mouse brain. Proc Natl Acad Sci USA 1971;68:1742–1747.
28. Pert CB, Pasternak G, Snyder SH. Opiate agonists and antagonists discriminated by receptor binding in brain. Science 1973;182:1359–1361.
29. Simon EJ, Hiller JM, Edelman I. Stereospecific binding of the potent narcotic analgesic (3-H) etorphine to rat-brain homogenate. Proc Natl Acad Sci USA 1973;38:377–384.
30. Hughes F, Smith TW, Kosterlitz HW, et al. Identification of two related pentapeptides from the brain with potent opiate agonist activity. Nature 1975;258:577–580.
31. Li CH, Chung D. Isolation and structure of an untriakontapeptide with opiate activity from camel pituitary glands. Proc Natl Acad Sci USA 1976;73:1145–1148.
32. Benedetti C, Butler SH. Systemic analgesics, in Bonica JJ, Loeser JD, Chapman CR, et al (eds): The Management of Pain. Philadelphia, Lea & Febiger, 1990, pp 1640–1675.

33. Armstrong D, Dry RML, Keele CA. Observations on chemical excitants of cutaneous pain in man. J Physiol 1953;120:326–351.
34. Starke K, Taube HD, Borowski E. Presynaptic receptor systems in catecholaminergic transmission. Biochem Pharmacol 1977;26:259–268.
35. Pepeu G. Involvement of central transmitters in narcotic analgesia, in Bonica JJ, Albe-Fessard D (eds): Advances in Pain Research and Therapy vol 1. New York, Raven Press, 1976, pp 595–600.
36. Tenen SS. Antagonism of the analgesic effect of morphine and other drugs by *p*-chlorophenylalanine, a serotonin depleter. Psychopharmacology (Berlin) 1968;12:31–50.
37. Turk DC, Kerns RD. Conceptual issues in the assessment of clinical pain. Int J Psychiatry Med 1983;84;13:57–68.
38. Twycross RG. Pain and analgesics. Curr Med Res Opin 1978;5:497–505.
39. Fordyce WE. Learning processes in pain, in Sternbach RA (ed): The Psychology of Pain. New York, Raven Press, 1978, pp 49–72.
40. Craig KD. Social modeling influences on pain, in Sternbach RA (ed): The Psychology of Pain. New York, Raven Press, 1978, pp 73–109.
41. American Pain Society. Principles of analgesic use in the treatment of acute pain and chronic cancer pain. Clin Pharm 1990;9:601.
42. Chapman CR, Bonica JJ. Chronic Pain. Current Concepts. Kalamazoo, MI, Scope Publications, 1985.
43. Amadio P. Peripherally acting analgesics. Am J Med 1984;77:17–26.
44. Pittman AW, Rudd GD. Analgesic Therapy. Carrboro, NC, Health Sciences Consortium, 1984.
45. Facts and Comparisons. Philadelphia, JB Lippincott, 1986, 1991, 1994, 1995.
46. American Hospital Formulary Service. McVoy GK (ed). Drug Information. Bethesda, MD, American Society of Hospital Pharmacists, 1987, 1991, 1994, 1995.
47. Zarro V. Nonsteroidal anti-inflammatory drugs: A review. Clin Pharmacol 1984;30:243–246.
48. Pert CB, Snyder SH. Opiate receptor binding of agonists and antagonists affected differentially by sodium. Mol Pharmacol 1974;10:868–879.
49. Hare BD. The opioid analgesics: Rational selection of agents for acute and chronic pain. Hosp Form 1987;22:64–86.
50. Ginsberg GS. Managing a patient with a morphine allergy. Drug Therapy 1985;June:18–23.
51. Graves DA, Foster TS, Batenhorst RL, Baumann TJ. The evolution of patient-controlled analgesia: A review. Ann Intern Med 1983;99:360–366.
52. Stapleton JV, Austin KL, Mather LE. A pharmacokinetic approach to postoperative pain: Continuous infusion. Anaesth Intern Care 1979;7:25–32.
53. Shafer AL, Donnelly AJ. Management of postoperative pain by continuous epidural infusion of analgesics. Clin Pharm 1991;10:745–764.
54. Cousins MJ, Mather LE. Intrathecal and epidural administration of opioids. Anesthesiology 1984;61:276–310.
55. Jaffe JH, Martin WR. Opioid analgesics and antagonists, in Gilman AG, Goodman LS, Rall TW, et al (eds): The Pharmacological Basis of Therapeutics. New York, Macmillan, 1985, pp. 491–531.
56. Larijani GE, Goldberg ME. Alfentanil hydrochloride: A new short-acting narcotic analgesic for surgical procedures. Clin Pharm 1987;6:275–282.
57. Beaver WT. Mild analgesics: A review of their clinical pharmacology (part II). Am J Med Sci 1966;251:576–599.
58. Zola EM, McLeod DC. Comparative effects and analgesic efficacy of the agonist–antagonist opioids. Drug Intell Clin Pharm 1983;17:411–417.
59. Magruder MR, Delaney RD, Difazio CA. Reversal of narcotic-induced respiratory depression with nalbuphine hydrochloride. Anesth Rev 1982;9:34–37.
60. Beaver WT. Combination analgesics. Am J Med 1984; 77(3a):38–53.
61. DeKornfeld TJ, Lasagna L, Frazier TM. A comparative study of five proprietary analgesic compounds. JAMA 1962;182:1315–1318.
62. Laska EM, Sunshine A, Mueller F, et al. Caffeine as an analgesic adjuvant. JAMA 1984;251:1711–1718.
63. Beaver WT. Caffeine revisited. JAMA 1984;251:1732–1733.
64. Beaver WT, Feise G. Comparison of the analgesic effects of morphine, hydroxyzine and their combinations in patients with postoperative pain, in Bonica JJ, Albe-Fessard D (eds): Advances in Pain Research and Therapy. New York, Raven Press, 1976, pp 553–565.
65. Forrest WH, Brown BW, Brown CR, et al. Dextroamphetamine with morphine for the treatment of postoperative pain. N Engl J Med 1977;296:712–715.
66. Moore J, Dundee JW. Alterations in response to somatic pain associated with anaesthesia. VII: The effects of nine phenothiazine derivatives. Br J Anaesth 1961;33: 422–431.
67. Moore DC. Intercostal nerve block for postoperative somatic pain following surgery of thorax and upper abdomen. Br J Anaesth 1975;47:284–286.
68. Patel JM, Lanzafave RJ, Williams JS, et al. The effect of incisional infiltration of bupivacaine hydrochloride upon pulmonary functions, atelectasis and narcotic need following elective cholecystectomy. Surg Gynecol Obstet 1983;157:338–340.
69. Covino BG. Pharmacology of local anesthetics. Resident Staff Phys 1982;28:60–70.
70. Tyler E, Caldwell C, Ghia JN. Transcutaneous electrical nerve stimulation: An alternative approach to the management of postoperative pain. Anesth Analg 1982; 61:449–456.
71. Johnson JE, Rice VH, Fuller SS, Endress MP. Sensory information, instructions in a coping strategy and recovery from surgery. Res Nurs Health 1978;1:4–17.
72. Foley KM. The treatment of cancer pain. N Engl J Med 1985;313:84–95.
73. Clinical Practice Guideline No. 9. Management of cancer pain. U.S. Department of Health, Public Health Service, Agency for Health Care Policy and Research, 1994.
74. Kantor TG. Nonsteroidal anti-inflammatory analgesic agents in management of cancer pain, in Symposium on the Management of Cancer Pain. Hosp Prac 1984;Summer: 30–34.

75. Citron ML, Johnston-Early A, Fossieck BE, et al. Safety and efficacy of continuous intravenous morphine for severe cancer pain. Am J Med 1984;77:199–204.
76. Sawe J, Dahlstrom B, Rane A. Steady state kinetics and analgesic effect of oral morphine in cancer patients. Eur J Clin Pharmacol 1983;24:537–542.
77. Meed SD, Kleinman PM, Kantor TG, et al. Management of cancer pain with oral controlled-release morphine sulfate. J Clin Pharmacol 1987;27:155–161.
78. Baumann TJ, Batenhorst RL, Graves DA, et al. Patient-controlled analgesia in the terminally ill cancer patient. Drug Intell Clin Pharm 1986;20:297–301.
79. Nahata MC, Miser AW, Miser JS, Reuning RH. Analgesic plasma concentrations of morphine in children with terminal malignancy receiving a continuous subcutaneous infusion of morphine to control severe pain. Pain 1984;18:109–114.
80. Ellison NM, Lewis GO. Plasma concentrations following single oral doses of morphine sulfate in oral solution and rectal suppository. Clin Pharm 1984;3:614–617.
81. Health and Public Policy Committee, American College of Physicians. Drug therapy for severe chronic pain in terminal illness. Ann Intern Med 1983;99:870–873.
82. Kaiko RF, Foley KM, Grabinski PY, et al. Central nervous system excitatory effects of meperidine in cancer patients. Ann Neurol 1983;13:180–185.
83. Walsh TD. Antidepressants in chronic pain. Clin Neuropharmacol 1983;6:271–295.
84. Minton JP. The response of breast cancer patients with bone pain to L-dopa. Cancer 1974;33:358–363.
85. Schell HW. The risk of adrenal corticosteroid therapy with far advanced cancer. Am J Med Sci 1966;252:641–649.
86. Kane RL, Bernstein L, Wales J, et al. Hospice effectiveness in controlling pain. JAMA 1985;253:2683–2686.
87. Porter J, Jick H. Addiction is rare in patients treated with narcotics[letter] . N Engl J Med 1980;302:123.
88. Procacci P, Bozza G, Buzelli G, Corte MD. The cutaneous pricking pain threshold in old age. Gerontol Clin 1970; 12:213–218.
89. Clinical Practice Guideline. Acute pain management: Operative or medical procedures and trauma. U.S. Department of Health and Human Services, Public Health Service, Agency for Health Care Policy and Research, 1992.
90. Schechter NL. Symposium on recurrent pains in children: An overview and an approach. Pediatr Clin North Am 1984;31:949–968.
91. Bhatt-Mehta V, Rosen DA. Management of acute pain in children. Clin Pharm 1991;10:667–685.
92. Beales JG, Kean JH, Lennox-Holt PJ. The child's perception of the disease and the experience of pain in juvenile chronic arthritis. J Rheumatol 1983;10:61–65.
93. News: Panel cites need for improved pain management. Clin Pharm 1986;5:777–778.
94. Inturrisi CE. Role of opioid analgesics. Am J Med 1984; 77(3a):27–37.
95. Gourlay GK, Cousins MJ. Strong analgesics in severe pain. Drugs 1984;28:79–91.
96. Clotz MA, Nahata MC. Clinical use of fentanyl, sufentanil, and alfentanil. Clin Pharm 1991;10:581–593.
97. Hopkinson JH, Smith MT, Bare WW, et al. Acetaminophen (500 mg) versus acetaminophen (325 mg) for relief of pain in episiotomy patients. Curr Ther Res 1974;16:194–200.
98. Levy G. Comparative pharmacokinetics of aspirin and acetaminophen. Arch Intern Med 1981;141:279–281.
99. Schoenle JR, Mullins PM. Dezocine. PT 1990;November: 1357–1371.
100. Jaffe JH, Martin WR. Opioid analgesics and antagonists, in Gilman AG, Roll TW, et al (eds): The Pharmacological Basis of Therapeutics. New York, Pergamon Press, 1990, pp 485–521.
101. Gaston GW, Mallow RD, Frank JE. Comparison of etodolac, aspirin, and placebo for pain after oral surgery. Pharmacotherapy 1986;6:199–205.
102. Package Insert. Diclofenac potassium. Geigy Pharmaceuticals, c93–c94.
103. Package insert. Tramadol. Ortho-McNeil. 1995.
104. Drugs for pain. The Medical Letter 1993;35:4.
105. Maurer PM, Bartkowski RR. Drug interactions of clinical significance with opioid analgesics. Drug Safety 1993; 8:30–48.
106. Sunshine A. New clinical experience with tramadol. Drugs 1994;47(Suppl 1): 8–18.

Chapter 60

Headache Disorders

Brian E. Beckett, PharmD

Headache is one of the most common complaints presenting to health care practitioners. An estimated 24 million U.S. citizens have experienced a migraine headache and this population accounts for 18 million physician visits per year.[1,2] Headaches have been extensively classified by the International Headache Society according to etiology (Table 60.1).[3] This classification is different from previous ones and has resulted in name changes for some of the headache types (e.g., classic migraine is now migraine with aura; common migraine is migraine without aura). Establishing the headache profile, pattern, and history is essential to establish an accurate diagnosis. Unfortunately, many people with headache disorders are not diagnosed, and, therefore, they either do not receive medical treatment or they attempt to treat themselves with over-the-counter (OTC) medications.[1–4]

The most common of the headache disorders is migraine headaches. Tension-type headaches, formerly known as muscle contraction headaches, and cluster headaches also occur frequently. This chapter focuses on the epidemiology, pathophysiology, symptomology, management, and prevention of migraine and cluster headaches.

Migraine Headache

EPIDEMIOLOGY

Migraine headache accounts for 10–20% of all headaches in adults. It is three times more prevalent in women (18%) than men (6%). The usual age of onset is 15–35 years of age, but prevalence is highest in the 35–45 age group. Incidence tends to decrease in those >45 years of age. An estimated 8.7 million females and 2.6 million males experience moderate to severe migraine-associated disability. Approximately 40% of these patients suffer more than one attack per month. Migraine headaches are more common in lower socioeconomic groups; this may be related to diet, stress, increased use of OTC medications, and/or reduced access to the health care system. Lower income households are also more likely to use emergency care services to treat migraines than are other economic groups. Gender differences in migraine occurrence have been linked to menstruation, but even postmenopausal women have a higher incidence of migraines than males. The exact cost of migraine is difficult to ascertain but has been estimated to be between $5.6 and $17.8 billion per year in direct costs and lost productivity.[5]

Migraine headaches have been defined as "a familial disorder characterized by recurrent attacks of headache widely variable in intensity, frequency, and duration. Attacks are commonly unilateral and are usually associated with anorexia, nausea, and vomiting. In some cases, they are preceded by, or associated with neurological and mood disturbances."[6] Migraines are a type of vascular headache. Migraine with aura can be distinguished from migraine without aura by the presence of neurologic symptoms (aura or prodrome) prior to the onset of the headache. Migraines without aura occur more frequently than migraines with aura (85% versus 15%) and usually have a longer duration. A discussion of ophthalmologic and retinal migraines and the complications of migraine headache is beyond the scope of this chapter.

PATHOPHYSIOLOGY

The precise pathophysiologic mechanism that results in migraine headache is poorly understood. Migraine results from the interplay between brain tissue and the cranial circulation. Two theories of the pathophysiologic origin of migraines reflect the thinking that migraines are either of vascular or neuronal origin. The vascular theory postulates that headaches are a result of stimulation of sensory nerves in the large cerebral arteries and meningeal circulation.[7] The neuronal theory focuses on the interplay between the trigeminal (fifth cranial) nerve and a variety of inflammatory neurotransmitters, resulting in plasma protein extravasation, which stimulates nerve endings resulting in pain.[8] The precise pathophysiology underlying induction of migraines is unknown but probably involves interplay of both vascular and neuronal mechanisms.[9,10]

Induction of migraines appears to be triggered by interactions between precipitating events and specific brain

TABLE 60.1. INTERNATIONAL HEADACHE SOCIETY CLASSIFICATION OF HEADACHE

1. Migraine
   a. Migraine with aura
   b. Migraine without aura
   c. Ophthalmologic migraine
   d. Retinal migraine
   e. Childhood periodic syndromes
   f. Complications of migraine
   g. Migrainous disorder not meeting these criteria
2. Tension-type headache
   a. Episodic tension-type headache
   b. Chronic tension-type headache
3. Cluster headache
4. Miscellaneous headaches not associated with structural lesion
5. Headache associated with head trauma
6. Headache associated with vascular disorders
   a. Acute ischemic cerebrovascular disorder
   b. Intracranial hemorrhage
   c. Subarachnoid hemorrhage
   d. Others
7. Headache associated with nonvascular intracranial disorder
   a. Intracranial infection
   b. Intracranial sarcoidosis and other noninfectious inflammatory disorders
   c. Intracranial neoplasms
8. Headache associated with substances or their withdrawal
9. Headache associated with noncephalic infection
10. Headache associated with metabolic disorder
   a. Hypoxia
   b. Hypercapnia
   c. Hypoglycemia
   d. Dialysis
   e. Others
11. Headache or facial pain associated with disorder of cranium, neck, eyes, ears, nose, sinuses, teeth, mouth, or other facial or cranial structures
12. Cranial neuralgias, nerve trunk pain, and deafferentation pain
13. Headache not classifiable

(Adapted from Ref. 3.)

areas. The cerebral cortex, thalamus, hypothalamus, and the internal and external carotid arteries respond to emotions, stress, excessive afferent stimulation (glaring lights, noise, or smells), changes in the internal clock, and vasodilator therapy to induce brainstem mechanisms responsible for migraine. These factors appear to induce a period of arterial vasoconstriction with a corresponding drop in cranial blood flow to 16–23 mL/100 g of brain tissue/min (normal is 50–100 mL/100 g of brain tissue/min).[7] This reduction in cerebral blood flow may induce periods of ischemia sufficient enough to result in neurologic dysfunction. The aura associated with migraine may be the result of this ischemic event. Cerebral vasodilation and neurogenic inflammation usually follow any ischemic event producing the painful event.

An initial vasospasm has been postulated to occur because of the increased release and/or production of prostaglandins, epinephrine, norepinephrine, tyramine, and, most important, serotonin.[11] Reduced destruction of these vasoactive amines by platelet monoamine oxidase accounts for some increase in their activity. Norepinephrine released from the adrenal medulla, in response to stimulation of the locus ceruleus, may cause the release of serotonin-releasing factor, thus causing platelets to release serotonin and produce further platelet aggregation. Serotonin metabolism and platelet aggregation are altered in patients with migraine.[12–14] Platelet serotonin concentrations decrease dramatically at the onset of a migraine while free serotonin concentrations in the plasma may increase by as much as 100% during a migraine attack. Serotonin appears to be critical in vascular changes resulting in migraine; altering serotonin activity is an important approach in the pharmacotherapy of migraine.[10,11]

Four types of serotonin receptors have been identified, 5-HT_1, 5-HT_2, 5-HT_3, and 5-HT_4, that are widely distributed throughout the body.[10] Each of these receptor types has numerous subtypes (Table 60.2).[15] The primary serotonin receptors in the cerebral circulation are the 5-HT_1 subtypes: 5-HT_{1A}, 5-HT_{1C}, 5-HT_{1D}, and 5-$HT_{1\text{-Like}}$. There appears to be a high density of the 5-HT_{1D} receptors in the central nervous system (CNS), especially in the substantia nigra and the basal ganglia. The 5-$HT_{1\text{-Like}}$ receptor subtype is found in high quantities in the intracranial vasculature and may be involved in the mediation of vasoconstriction.

Neurogenic inflammation resulting from the ischemia is mediated by the release of vasoactive neuropeptides.[8] Substance P, neurokinin A, and calcitonin gene-related peptide (CGRP) enhance the permeability of plasma proteins in the dura mater after trigeminal nerve stimulation. Trigeminal nerve stimulation can occur in paroxysms, lasting only a few seconds and producing "ice pick pain" or for seconds to minutes resulting in "ice cream headaches."[7] The release of chemical mediators from platelets and injured tissues alters sensory transmission. Chemical mediators including potassium, serotonin, leukotrienes, bradykinin, histamine, and prostaglandins alter blood flow and the cellular response to the inflammatory event.[16]

Numerous factors have been investigated as possible etiologic agents in migraine (Table 60.3).[17–27] Common to all of these is probably a disturbance in secretion and/or response to the vasoactive amines previously described. Dietary and psychological disorders may elevate norepinephrine and epinephrine, leading to altered concentrations of serotonin and ultimately migraine symptoms. Tyramine

TABLE 60.2. CLASSIFICATION OF SEROTONIN RECEPTORS AND SUMMARY OF FUNCTIONAL RESPONSES

Receptor Subtype	Location	Functional Response
5-HT_{1A}	Neuronal (CNS)	Hypotension; neuronal hyperpolarization
5-HT_{1B}	Found in humans and rats	Undetermined
5-HT_{1C}	CNS (choroid plexus)	Increased turnover of PI
5-HT_{1D}	CNS/sensory fibers	Inhibition of neuropeptide and transmitter release
5-HT_{1E}	CNS	Unknown
5-$HT_{1\text{-Like}}$	Intracranial vasculature	Contraction of cephalic arteries
	Vascular and GI smooth muscle	Vasodilation
5-HT_2	Vascular smooth muscle	Vasoconstriction
	Platelets	Platelet aggregation
	Lung/GI/CNS	Bronchoconstriction
5-HT_3	Peripheral/central neurons	Membrane depolarization and activation of sensory afferents
5-HT_4	Heart/CNS/GI	Increase in cAMP
		Activation of neurotransmitter release

Key: PI, phosphoinositol; cAMP, cyclic AMP. (Adapted from Ref. 15.)

containing foods such as chocolate, caffeinated beverages, red wines, and aged cheeses have been reported to cause migraine. Monosodium glutamate (MSG) added as a flavor enhancer to many Chinese foods has also been linked with migraines. Genetic disturbances in tyramine metabolism might also be a cause. Medication-induced causes of migraine are important to identify. Proposed mechanisms for drug-induced causes include the inhibition of granular reuptake and storage of serotonin (reserpine), blocking neuronal reuptake of serotonin (fluoxetine), altering platelet aggregation (ethinyl estradiol and mestranol), and vasodilation (nitroglycerin and nifedipine).

CLINICAL PRESENTATION

Migraine without aura (previously known as common migraine and hemicrania simplex) occurs in about 85% of

TABLE 60.3. PROPOSED ETIOLOGIC FACTORS ASSOCIATED WITH MIGRAINE

Psychological Factors
- Stress
- Depression
- Personality

Environmental Factors
- Tobacco smoke
- Sensory stimulation (e.g., light glare, odors, etc.)
- Weather changes

Dietary Factors
- Alcohol
- Tyramine-containing foods (e.g., red wine, aged cheese)
- Citrus fruit
- Aspartame
- Food additives
- Chocolate
- Caffeine

Physiologic Factors
- Autonomic nervous system dysfunction
- Atherosclerosis
- Epilepsy
- Autosomal tract defect
- Immunologic response
  - Hypersensitivity reaction
  - Allergy

Medications
- Cimetidine
- Cocaine
- Ethinyl estradiol
- Fenfluramine
- Fluoxetine
- Histamine
- Hormone replacement therapy
- Indomethacin
- Mestranol
- Nicotine
- Nifedipine
- Nitroglycerin
- Oral contraceptives
- Reserpine

Others
- Hormonal changes
  - Menses
  - Pregnancy
- Hypoglycemia
- Excessive or inadequate sleep
- Strenuous exercise
- Alterations in intracellular magnesium and calcium concentrations

patients with migraines. Migraine with aura (also known as classic or classical migraine) occurs in approximately 10% of migraineurs. The remaining 5% are caused by other migraine types (Table 60.1). Females are more commonly afflicted than males (18 versus 6%, respectively).[1] Risk factors have been previously discussed. A higher incidence of migraines is seen in patients with multiple risk factors and a strong family history of migraines. A higher incidence of migraines is seen during menstruation while pregnancy may lower the incidence in 60–80% of female migraineurs. Migraines can begin during childhood and adolescence, peak during the 35- to 45-year age range, and decline with advancing age.[1,2,4] Headaches beginning later in life have been associated with organic etiologies such as cerebrovascular disease, cancer, and temporal arteritis.

As its name states, migraine with aura begins with an aura or prodrome occurring 15–60 minutes prior to the onset of the headache. The aura is a result of neurologic ischemia in the brain producing such symptoms as aphasia, visual field defects, scotomas, and hemisensory disturbances (tingling or numbness in the extremities). Alterations in mood and motor functions may also occur. The aura is usually conspicuous to the migraineur; however, some patients are not able to identify their prodrome. In some patients, the prodrome may not be easily identified. Migraine without aura does not begin with prodromal features.

Migraines usually occur in the early morning hours. Peak intensity of the migraine occurs typically within 1 hour of onset. Pain is usually unilateral and can occur anywhere on the face or head, but is most often in the temple. Pain is predominately right or left sided, but may be bilateral and is usually localized. Typical headache pain is described as pounding, pulsating, or throbbing. Headaches may be of moderate to severe intensity and may inhibit many activities of daily living. Physical activity may worsen the headache pain. Patients often complain of being incapacitated during the migraine and will seek a dark quiet place for rest or sleep. Patients may complain of a variety of other symptoms such as increased sensitivity to light or sound, anorexia, nausea, vomiting, and constipation or diarrhea. Headache duration can range from 4–72 hours. Headache-free periods occur between attacks.[4]

Migraine pain may cause changes in mood or personality and should be closely monitored by the patient or a family member. Migraineurs may be withdrawn, irritable, depressed, and suffer from insomnia, fatigue, and changes in libido.[4,9] These alterations in lifestyle may be more severe than the pain itself. Migraine patients typically want to be left alone. The postheadache syndrome is characterized by exhaustion, scalp tenderness, and recurrence of headache with sudden head movements.

TABLE 60.4. THE HEADACHE PROFILE

Time of day when attacks occur
Aura present or absent
Description of the aura
Intensity of attack
Description of the pain
Location of the pain
Precipitating factors
Factors that provide relief or improvement
Associated symptoms
Significance to the patient
Duration of attack

TREATMENT

Management of migraine is directed at altering the attack once it is under way (symptomatic or abortive therapy) or by preventing the attack altogether (prophylactic therapy).[28,29] Before therapy is chosen as accurate a diagnosis as possible must be made.

The initial step in establishing appropriate treatment for patients with migraine should be a thorough evaluation of the headache profile (Table 60.4). The physical exam, common laboratory tests, including an erythrocyte sedimentation rate, and diagnostic procedures (computed tomography [CT scan], magnetic resonance imaging [MRI]) performed should all be within normal limits to accurately diagnose migraine and rule out any organic causes of headache pain (Table 60.5).

Patient education is essential to the adequate treatment of migraine pain. Abortive therapies must begin at the onset of the attack to achieve their full potential. Altering the neurovascular changes that occur early in the headache phase with abortive therapies may act to eliminate or reduce the pain. Once the migraine's vasodilatory phase has begun, abortive therapies are less likely to be effective. Only 50–80% of patients taking abortive therapies will receive significant relief.

TABLE 60.5. EVALUATION OF PATIENTS WITH HEADACHE

Obtain the headache profile (see Table 60.4).
Perform a neurologic examination.
Obtain a computed tomography (CT) of the head if tumor, abscess, or hemorrhage is suspected.
Perform a lumbar puncture if an infection is suspected.
Identify metabolic or electrolyte abnormalities and drug effects or drug withdrawal.
Identify any emotional disturbances.
In elderly patients with new onset of headaches, obtain an erythrocyte sedimentation rate and consider a temporal artery biopsy to rule out temporal arteritis.

For patients with infrequent migraine attacks (one or two attacks per month) abortive therapy and/or treatment of associated symptoms can be sufficient. Table 60.6 describes medications used for abortive therapy of migraine headaches.

Abortive Therapy

Simple Analgesics

Initial therapy for patients with infrequent migraines should be with simple analgesics such as aspirin or acetaminophen; mild migraines often respond well to these agents.[28–30] Aspirin should be considered the drug of choice, but acetaminophen can be used when aspirin is contraindicated or is not well tolerated. Both aspirin and acetaminophen have been combined with a barbiturate, butalbitol, to induce sleep, with narcotics for additional pain relief, and with caffeine to help improve gastrointestinal absorption. Caffeine, however, may interfere with sleep. Butalbitol and narcotics have been associated with rebound headaches caused by a pattern of increasing use that induces migraine.[17,31–33] Increasing use of combination preparations may fail to provide pain relief and worsen headache symptoms when the narcotic wears off, leading to additional medication consumption.

Nonsteroidal Anti-Inflammatory Drugs (NSAIDs)

Many of the NSAIDs are as effective as aspirin and acetaminophen. NSAIDs may alleviate migraine pain by inhibiting prostaglandin synthesis, blocking platelet aggregation,

TABLE 60.6. ABORTIVE MIGRAINE THERAPIES

Medication	Dosage
Simple Analgesics	
Acetaminophen	650 mg at onset; repeat q4h as needed
Aspirin	650 mg at onset; repeat q4h as needed
Aspirin/acetaminophen with butalbital	1–2 tablets every 4–6 h, but not more than 4 tablets/day or usage more than twice per week
Aspirin/acetaminophen with narcotics	Sparingly and infrequently
NSAIDs[a]	
Diclofenac	50–100 mg at onset
Ibuprofen	400–600 mg at onset; repeat in 1–2 h
Flurbiprofen	50–100 mg at onset; repeat in 1–2 h
Ketorolac	15–60 mg IM at onset
Mefanamic acid	500 mg at onset
Meclofenamate sodium	100 mg at onset; repeat in 1 h up to 500 mg/d
Naproxen	750 mg at onset; 250 mg PRN up to 1375 mg/d
Naproxen sodium	550–750 mg at onset; repeat in 1–2 h
Ergotamine Preparations	
Ergotamine 1 mg with 100 mg caffeine	2 tablets at onset; then 1 tablet every 30 min PRN to a maximum of 6 tablets/day or 10 tablets/week
Ergotamine 2 mg SL tablets	1 tablet every 30 min as needed to a maximum of 6 tablets/day or 10 tablets/week; do not swallow, chew, or crush tablets
Ergotamine 2 mg with 100 mg caffeine suppositories	Insert 1 at onset; repeat in 1 h as needed to a maximum of 2/day or 5/week
Ergotamine MDI (0.36 mg/puff)	1 puff every 5 min as needed to a maximum of 6 puffs/day or 12–15/week
Dihydroergotamine 1 mg/mL injection	0.5–1 mg IV or IM every hour as needed to a maximum of 2 mg/day, 6 mg/week IV or 3 mg/week IM
Sumatriptan	
Sumatriptan 6 mg SQ autoinjector	6 mg SQ at onset; repeat in 1 h as needed but not more than 12 mg/24 h
Sumatriptan 25-mg tablets	1 tablet at onset; repeat in 2 h as needed to a maximum of 300 mg/d
Miscellaneous Agents	
Butorphanol nasal spray	1 spray in 1 nostril only; repeat 1 time in 60–90 min if needed
Chlorpromazine	0.1–1 mg/kg IV at onset
Isometheptene/dichloralphenazone/acetaminophen (Midrin)	2 capsules at onset; repeat one capsule every hour to a maximum of 5/day or 12/week
Metoclopramide	10 mg IV or PO at onset
Prochlorperazine	10 mg IV at onset

[a]Usage should be limited to three times weekly. (Adapted from Refs. 28 and 29.)

and reducing serotonin release.[34,35] NSAIDs have not been associated with rebound headaches; however, NSAIDs are more expensive than simple analgesics and may cause more side effects. Naproxen sodium has been compared with both placebo and ergotamine in clinical trials in patients with migraine.[34–36] Naproxen was superior to placebo and more efficacious than ergotamine in controlling acute migraine attacks. Rapidly acting NSAIDs (e.g., naproxen, naproxen sodium, ibuprofen) may prove to be superior to agents with a longer onset of action or those used primarily for inflammation. Indomethacin should not be used because of its propensity to cause headaches in a significant number of patients. Migraines that occur before, during, or after menstruation may respond well to NSAIDs. Injectable ketorolac has been used in patients with drug-seeking behavior and in patients with severe nausea and vomiting that prohibit oral therapy.[37]

Ergotamine

Ergotamine was first used for migraines in 1926. Ergotamine is a direct vasoconstrictor of smooth muscle in cranial blood vessels, an α-adrenergic blocker and a nonselective 5-HT agonist. Activity of ergotamine depends on the CNS vascular tone at the time of administration. Ergotamine and its derivatives are more effective when given early in the migraine attack.[28,29,38] Ergotamine tartrate is available as an oral and sublingual tablet, and as suppositories. Dihydroergotamine (DHE-45) is available in an injectable form.[39,40] Inhaled ergotamine can be useful in patients properly instructed on inhalation technique. Caffeine is added to oral preparations to increase absorption, but may interfere with sleep. Other drugs used in combination with ergotamine include antispasmodics, antiemetics, sedatives, analgesics, and CNS stimulants.

Oral ergotamine has poor oral bioavailability, due primarily to extensive first-pass metabolism; sublingual administration may not provide appreciable blood levels.[41,42] Rectal administration has been used for patients suffering from nausea and vomiting, but increased absorption may lead to a worsening of the symptoms due to stimulation of the vomiting center. Intravenous administration is the fastest way to achieve therapeutic drug concentrations and may be preferred by some patients or in more severe attacks.

Ergotamine dosage requirements should be strictly titrated to determine the necessary dose for future attacks. Repeated dosing or exceeding the maximum dosage guidelines should be avoided to prevent rebound headaches resulting from persistent vasodilation. Rebound headaches may last several days and may require hospitalization to adequately wean the patient from ergotamine and treat the headache pain. Naproxen may be effective for ergotamine withdrawal.[43] Daily use of ergotamine should be discouraged. Ergotamine addiction and dependency have been reported.[44]

Side effects to the ergot products include vasoconstriction leading to elevation in blood pressure and severe peripheral ischemia. The syndrome of ergotism is manifested by nausea, diarrhea, thirst, pruritus, vertigo, muscle cramps, paresthesia, cold skin, and decreased pulses in the extremities. Gastrointestinal vascular ischemia requiring intensive vasodilator therapy has been described.[45] Severe peripheral ischemia has occurred when beta blockers and ergot alkaloids are used together, therefore, extreme caution is warranted if these agents must be used concomitantly.[46] Contraindications to use include coronary artery disease, peripheral vascular disease, hypertension, liver or kidney disease, and pregnancy. They are also contraindicated in patients with prolonged auras (>60 minutes).

Sumatriptan

Sumatriptan is a selective 5-HT_1 receptor agonist. It is highly specific for 5-HT_{1D} and to a lesser extent 5-HT_{1A} receptors.[10,15,47] Stimulation of the 5-HT_{1D} receptors produces a direct vasoconstrictive effect. Sumatriptan also appears to inhibit the release of tachykinins and subsequently blocks neurogenic plasma protein extravasation and inflammation. Sumatriptan has been evaluated in a number of controlled clinical trials.[48–57] Efficacy of sumatriptan is consistently superior to placebo in alleviating migraine attacks. Comparisons to ergotamine/caffeine combinations[50] and to aspirin plus metoclopramide[57] have shown sumatriptan to be statistically better at producing migraine pain relief. Patients usually need fewer rescue medications and report fewer problems with nausea, vomiting, and sensitivity to light and noise. Sumatriptan is generally well tolerated. Adverse effects associated with oral use include bad taste, nausea, vomiting, malaise, fatigue, dizziness, and vertigo but are usually of short duration. Subcutaneous administration has been associated with minor injection site reactions; chest tightness and pressure have occurred in 3–5% of patients.

Sumatriptan is contraindicated in patients with a history of ischemic heart disease, angina pectoris, Prinzmetal's angina, previous myocardial infarction, and uncontrolled hypertension. Clinicians should evaluate patients for contraindications and recommend that the initial dose of sumatriptan be given in the presence of a health care practitioner. Administration of sumatriptan within 2 weeks of therapy with monamine oxidase inhibitors is not recommended. Therapy with sumatriptan should not be used if ergotamine derivatives have been used within the previous 24 hours. Presently, the tablet formulation of sumatriptan is awaiting FDA approval, and a nasal spray formulation is under investigation.

Miscellaneous Agents

Midrin. Midrin is a combination of isometheptene mucate 65 mg, a sympathomimetic amine acting as a vasoconstrictor, dichloralphenazone 100 mg, a mild sedative, and acetaminophen 325 mg.[58] Midrin can be used in patients who cannot take or do not respond to ergotamine or sumatriptan. Midrin is less effective than ergotamine, but also has fewer side effects. The most frequent side effects are dizziness, insomnia, nausea, vomiting, and transient numbness.

Metoclopramide. Metoclopramide may be useful in preventing or treating the nausea and vomiting associated with migraines when given with abortive therapies, and metoclopramide may be beneficial as a single agent for pain relief.[59] Metoclopramide may also help to increase absorption of medications by decreasing gastric stasis.[60] Metoclopramide should be given 15–30 minutes before the antimigraine therapy and can be repeated in 4–6 hours. Extrapyramidal reactions may occur, but acute dystonic reactions are rare with intermittent use. Anticholinergic agents and narcotics may antagonize the increased gastric emptying seen with metoclopramide.

Others. Chlorpromazine is effective when used parenterally (IM or IV) for severe migraine unresponsive to ergotamine.[61] An exact mechanism of action for this agent in migraine therapy is unknown. Side effects include sedation, extrapyramidal effects, and orthostatic hypotension. Tardive dyskinesia can occur after long-term use, but is unusual with lower doses and in younger patients afflicted with migraines.

Intravenous prochlorperazine has been shown to be effective for the treatment of severe headaches.[62] Corticosteroids may help control prolonged migraines and reduce narcotic requirements.[29] Therapy should be short term with rapid dosage reductions to minimize long-term side effects associated with their use. Reduced inflammation is their probable mechanism of action, and onset of action is within 8–12 hours. Sodium cromoglycate[63] and aerobic exercise[64,65] have also been shown to be beneficial for abortive therapy. Parenteral narcotics can be used for pain relief and may allow the patient to sleep through the attack. Use of narcotics should be minimized, however, to prevent abuse. Transnasal butorphanol is an alternative to injectable narcotics.[29] It has a rapid onset of action and induces sleep in many patients. Use of butorphanol should be monitored closely in patients prone to drug abuse.

Summary

Patients may respond to rest or sleep in a darkened room. Overall, management should be individualized based on the patient and his or her presentation. Simple analgesics and NSAIDs should be considered the drugs of choice for abortive therapy. Sumatriptan or ergotamine preparations can be used as secondary agents if initial therapies have not been effective. Failure of abortive agents to provide adequate relief should be an indication for prophylactic therapy.

Prophylactic Therapy

Prophylactic or preventive therapy is appropriate when a headache of moderate to severe intensity occurs more than twice a month, when they are less frequent but prolonged or refractory to acute therapy, or if they are predictable in occurrence.[28,29] Patients unable to take abortive therapy are also candidates for prophylactic therapy. Daily, or in some cases scheduled (i.e., pre- and postmenstruation), medication use can reduce both the incidence and severity of migraine attacks. In all cases, a trial of 2–3 months is necessary before an agent can be considered ineffective. Table 60.7 describes medications used for prophylactic therapy.

Beta Blockers

Propranolol, atenolol, metoprolol, nadolol, and, to a lesser extent, timolol and acebutolol are effective for migraine prophylaxis.[66–69] The precise mechanism of action is unknown, but blocking vasodilator receptors, membrane

TABLE 60.7. PROPHYLACTIC MIGRAINE THERAPIES

Medications	Dosage
NSAIDs/Aspirin	
Aspirin	650 mg BID
Ibuprofen	300–600 mg TID
Meclofenamate	50 mg TID
Ketoprofen	50–75 mg BID or TID
Naproxen	250–750 mg daily, or 250 mg TID
Naproxen sodium	250–750 mg daily, or 250 mg TID
Beta Blockers	
Atenolol	50–150 mg/d in divided doses
Metoprolol	50–300 mg/d in divided doses[a]
Nadolol	20–240 mg/d in divided doses
Propranolol	40–320 mg/d in divided doses[a]
Timolol	20–60 mg/d in divided doses
Calcium Channel Blockers	
Diltiazem	90–180 mg/d in divided doses[a]
Nifedipine	30–120 mg/d in divided doses[a]
Nimodipine	40 mg TID
Verapamil	120–360 mg/d in divided doses[a]
Antidepressants	
Amitriptyline	10–200 mg at bedtime
Doxepin	10–200 mg at bedtime
Fluoxetine	10–20 mg daily
Imipramine	10–200 mg at bedtime
Nortriptyline	10–150 mg at bedtime
Phenelzine	15 mg BID to QID
Miscellaneous Agents	
Clonidine	0.1 mg BID or TID
Cyproheptadine	4–8 mg daily
Ergonovine	0.2 mg BID to TID
Methysergide	4–8 mg daily
Valproic acid	250–1500 mg/d[a]

[a]Extended release preparations may be given in single daily doses. (Adapted from Refs. 28 and 29.)

stabilization, decreased platelet adhesiveness, decreased platelet aggregation, and enhanced release of oxygen to tissues have been proposed. Beta blockers with intrinsic sympathomimetic activity are ineffective for migraine prophylaxis. Side effects of beta blockers include fatigue, dizziness, sleep disturbances, hypotension, and GI alterations. Nonselective beta blockers are relatively contraindicated in patients with asthma, congestive heart failure, and diabetes.

Antidepressants

Tricyclic antidepressants are effective agents for migraine prophylaxis, even in patients who are not clinically depressed.[28,29,67,70] Tertiary amines (amitriptyline and imipramine) with potent inhibition of the reuptake of serotonin are more effective than secondary amines (nortriptyline and desipramine) with less serotonergic activity. Initiation with low doses and gradual dosage titration is usually effective. The anticholinergic side effects of these agents are the major problem with therapy. Drowsiness is better tolerated if the patient takes the medication at night.

Fluoxetine, a serotonin specific reuptake inhibitor, has been shown to be safe and effective for migraine prophylaxis; however, fluoxetine has also been implicated as a potential trigger for migraine induction.[71,72]

Phenelzine, a monoamine oxidase inhibitor, can be used in migraines not responding to other preventive therapies. Phenelzine blocks serotonin metabolism, which increases serotonin availability. Patients must be carefully counseled regarding dietary restrictions (avoidance of tyramine-containing foods) and sympathomimetic and other drug usage to avoid hypertensive crisis and central serotonergic syndrome. For a complete review of phenelzine side effects and dietary restrictions, refer to the chapter on depressive illness.

Calcium Channel Blockers

Calcium channel blocking agents, through their ability to alter calcium concentrations, are capable of inhibiting the initial vasoconstrictive phase of the migraine. Additional therapeutic effects include vasodilation and inhibition of platelet aggregation and serotonin release.[73] However, intravenous verapamil appears to be ineffective for abortive therapy.[74] Nifedipine, verapamil, nimodipine, diltiazem, and the investigational agent flunarizine have been shown to be effective for prophylactic therapy of migraine.[75–79] Calcium channel blockers are usually well tolerated with constipation, flushing, increased or decreased heart rate, fluid retention, and rash being common side effects.

NSAIDs

Aspirin and naproxen sodium, through their effects on prostaglandin synthesis, inhibition of platelet aggregation, and reduced serotonin release can decrease the frequency of migraines.[28,29,34,35,80,81] Patients may benefit from daily administration or from intermittent use with predictable headaches. Administration 1 week prior to menses and continued throughout menstruation may effectively eliminate migraines. Although generally well tolerated, long-term continuous usage should be discouraged because of GI and renal toxicity associated with chronic prostaglandin inhibition. Monitoring of renal function and occult blood loss should be provided.

Clonidine

Clonidine is a central sympatholytic agent that may stabilize CNS vasculature after α- and β-adrenergic receptor stimulation. However, clonidine does not appear to be any more effective than placebo.[29] A potential role is for the management of migraine associated with dietary triggers or for patients who are hypertensive. Common side effects are drowsiness, dry mouth, and orthostatic hypotension with initiation of therapy. A rebound headache may occur with abrupt withdrawal of clonidine.

Cyproheptadine

Cyproheptadine, an antihistamine with 5-HT_2 receptor antagonist activity and antiplatelet effects, has been effective in hormone-related migraine.[29] Administration of a large dose at bedtime with a smaller morning dose may minimize sedation. Weight gain is also possible. Overall, clinical response to this agent is unpredictable.

Anticonvulsants

Phenytoin, carbamazepine, and valproic acid may be efficacious in certain migraine types, especially if there is an association with epilepsy. Valproic acid has been effective for migraine prophylaxis.[28] Rebound headache may occur with these agents; therefore, use should be closely monitored and prescribed according to clearly defined guidelines.

Calcitonin

Calcitonin is a polypeptide hormone used primarily in calcium homeostasis. Calcitonin has been shown to influence serotonin concentrations, to act directly on CNS circulation to influence vascular tone, and to alter pain thresholds. Calcitonin may also be a neurotransmitter or neuromodulator. Chronic treatment with either salmon calcitonin or a synthetic eel-calcitonin analogue has been efficacious for migraine prophylaxis.[82,83] Side effects (flushing and GI disturbances) are mild and transient.

Methysergide

Methysergide is a potent 5-HT_2 receptor antagonist with a complex pharmacologic profile. Additional effects include inhibition of histamine release from mast cells, potentiation of norepinephrine-induced vasoconstriction, reduced platelet serotonin release, and central serotonin agonist activity. Methysergide has been one of the most efficacious agents for migraine prophylaxis, but because of potential side effects it is no longer a first-line agent.[28,29] Continuous use of methysergide for more than 7 months can cause proliferation of fibrous tissue in the retroperitoneal, pleural, pericardial, and subendocardial spaces. Because of this unwanted effect, a drug holiday of 2 weeks every 3 months or 1 month every 6 months is recommended. Patient monitoring for flank pain, dysuria, and chest discomfort is recommended to help minimize fibrotic changes. Early recognition and discontinuation of therapy will reverse fibrotic changes. Methysergide should be tapered slowly to prevent rebound headaches. Because of the potential problems associated with its use, methysergide should be reserved for patients refractory to other therapeutic modalities.

Summary

Prophylactic therapy is indicated for patients with two or more migraines per month, migraines refractory to abortive therapy, or migraines occurring in a predictable manner. Therapy should be individualized based on the patient and the migraine presentation. Reassessment of therapeutic efficacy should be done periodically. Prolonged headache-free intervals could allow for dosage reduction or discontinuation of therapy.

CLUSTER HEADACHES

EPIDEMIOLOGY

Cluster headaches produce one of the most severe forms of headache pain.[84] Cluster headaches are described as short, severe, episodic, clustering pain over the eyes and the forehead. Clustering of the headaches is the predominant feature. Episodes seem to be more common in the spring and fall.[4] Cluster periods last between 2–3 months in most patients. Periods of remission may last from 2 months to 20 years but are usually of approximately 2 years duration. Unlike migraine, more men are afflicted than women. Onset of cluster headaches can occur at any age, but they are more common in the late twenties. Whereas migraines occur most commonly in the early morning hours, cluster headaches are more common at night. A family history of migraine or cluster headache is usually not present. Cluster headaches are labeled chronic when remissions last less than 14 days or if the cluster period lasts longer than 1 year without remission.

PATHOPHYSIOLOGY

The pathophysiology of cluster headaches has not been adequately defined.[84] An initial vasoconstrictive phase of the internal carotid artery has been identified by angiography and radionuclide imaging of the brain. Decreased blood flow in supraorbital and frontal arteries occurs before the headache, but vasodilation occurs during the headache phase. Extracranial vasodilation has also been observed and may distend against pain-sensitive structures surrounding the brain. Sustained dilation may render vessels less responsive to therapy. Stimulation of the trigeminal nerve results in release of substance P, CGRP, and other vasoactive polypeptides, resulting in vasodilation, pain, and neurogenic inflammation. Extravasation of plasma proteins may also occur. Periodic discharges of the trigeminal vascular system caused by cluster triggers result in cluster headache pain. Since cluster headaches occur with regularity, alterations in the hypothalamic control of circadian rhythms may be involved in the pathogenesis. Changes in cortisol, prolactin, beta endorphins, and melatonin have been noticed between cluster attacks and remission. Neurohormonal changes in the hypothalamus are mediated by the serotonin system, so as in migraine, serotonin may play a significant role in cluster pathophysiology. Triggers for cluster headaches include vasodilators and hypoxemia. High-altitude hypoxia may also induce cluster headaches.

CLINICAL PRESENTATION

The location of pain is almost always unilateral and described behind or around the eye or in the temples.[4,84] Pain is described as excruciating, penetrating, but does not throb. Tenderness over the carotid arteries has been described. Whereas migraine patients retreat to a quiet dark room, cluster headache patients will often pace, beat their head against objects, and attempt suicide in rare instances. Patients with cluster headaches tend to work through the attack. During a cluster attack, patients may exhibit signs of sympathetic system paresis and parasympathetic overreaction. Features are ipsilateral and include lacrimation, nasal stuffiness, rhinorrhea, ptosis, miosis, and conjunctival injection. Scalp and facial tenderness or flushing occurs on the same side as the headache. Associated clinical features include tobacco and alcohol abuse. Peptic ulcer disease and cluster headache are inversely related.[84] Auras are not present with cluster headaches.

TREATMENT

As in migraine, therapy for cluster headaches involves both abortive and prophylactic therapy. Daily administration of medication may be needed for headaches of moderate to severe intensity that occur several times a month.

Abortive Therapy

Ergotamine

The ergot preparations are effective for aborting cluster headache attacks. Ergotamine dosing guidelines for cluster headaches are the same as for migraine headache therapy. Aerosol ergot preparations may be effective when used properly. Dihydroergotamine given IM or IV can terminate cluster attack, but effectiveness may be limited by side effects and/or excessive use.[85] Self-injection of IM DHE-45 is effective in some patients. Oral ergot alkaloids are often inadequate in acute attacks, but are often effective if taken an hour before the anticipated time of the attack. If the patient is awakened at night with headache, ergotamine either orally or by suppository at bedtime remains an alternative. Because of the self-limiting nature of cluster attacks in most patients, long-term continuous therapy is not recommended and often unnecessary.

Oxygen

Oxygen, a potent cerebral vasoconstrictor, has also been effective in the symptomatic treatment of cluster headache. Inhalation of 100% oxygen through a facial mask at a rate of 6–8 L/min for no longer than 15 minutes is a safe and effective alternative to ergotamine therapy.[86,87]

Topical Anesthetics

A less commonly used abortive therapy for cluster headache consists of topical anesthetic agents.[88] Application of cocaine in a 5–10% solution or 4% lidocaine to the nasal mucosa and sphenopalatine ganglion is sometimes beneficial. The use of topical anesthetic agents has been studied in only a few patients. Lidocaine is a safe, nonaddicting agent; however, cocaine poses a risk of addiction and should be avoided.

Sumatriptan

Sumatriptan has been reported to be safe and effective for abortive therapy of cluster headaches.[89] A reduction in the severity of headache attacks can occur within 15 minutes, and sumatriptan is generally well tolerated. Oral sumatriptan has not been well studied for cluster headaches.

Miscellaneous Agents

Capsaicin[90] (a 0.025% cream swabbed intranasally twice daily), prednisone[91] 30 mg daily, and leuprolide[92] 3.75 mg IM (depot formulation) have all been used successfully for abortive therapy of cluster headaches.

Prophylactic Therapy

Lithium

Lithium carbonate is effective in treating episodic and chronic cluster headache attacks.[84,93] Lithium was initially suggested as a therapeutic option because the cyclical nature of cluster headaches is similar to the cyclical episodes in bipolar disorder. Currently, the mechanism of action of lithium in cluster headache is unknown, but effects on platelets as well as on the CNS are postulated. Lithium is initiated in a dose of 300–600 mg/d and increased to 600–1200 mg/d as necessary in two to four divided doses. Prophylaxis is usually started when the attacks begin, and a favorable clinical response often occurs during the first week of therapy. Plasma lithium concentrations should be monitored, because symptoms of toxicity correlate with plasma levels. A lithium level between 0.6 and 1.2 mEq/L measured at steady state, 12 hours after the last dose, is usually sought but optimal plasma levels of lithium for prevention of cluster headache have not been established.

Initial side effects are mild and include tremor, lethargy, nausea, diarrhea, and abdominal discomfort. Treatment with lithium may result in headache symptoms, but these headaches are easily distinguishable from the cluster headache. Lithium-induced headaches are episodes of moderately severe, throbbing occipital pain lasting 6–12 hours. They disappear when lithium is withdrawn. Lithium should be administered with caution to patients with significant renal or cardiovascular disease, dehydration, pregnancy, or concomitant diuretic use. For a complete review of lithium use, please refer to the chapter on bipolar disorders.

Ergotamine

Ergotamine can be an efficacious agent for abortive as well as prophylactic therapy of cluster headaches.[84] Dosing ergotamine at bedtime may prove beneficial for nocturnal attacks. Ergotamine 1–2 mg in one to two daily doses has been beneficial and ergotism is unlikely. Ergotamine can be safely used with lithium therapy.

Methysergide

In patients unresponsive to lithium, methysergide, 2 mg three or four times a day, is usually effective in shortening the course of cluster headaches.[84] Response to treatment usually occurs within 1 week of initiation of the drug. Doses may be tapered after 2–3 weeks of freedom from headaches. Precautions regarding methysergide use were described earlier in this chapter.

Corticosteroids

Corticosteroids are effective for cluster headaches not responsive to either lithium or methysergide.[84] High doses of injectable or oral steroids begin to ease pain within 8–12 hours, with maximum effectiveness in 2–3 days. Prednisone is often given in an initial dosage of 40–60 mg orally, administered in divided doses, and rapidly tapered over a 2-week to 1-month period. Steroids seem to suppress and not eliminate the factors producing the headaches; therefore, their usefulness is limited to short-lasting cluster attacks. Long-term use is not recommended to avoid steroid-induced complications.

Miscellaneous Agents

Other prophylactic measures advocated in the management of cluster headache include β blockers, tricyclic antidepressants, histamine blockers, nonprescription analgesics, cyproheptadine, calcium channel blockers (primarily verapamil), and chlorpromazine, but well-designed, controlled studies are lacking. Narcotics should not be used in the management of migraine headaches.

Evaluation of Therapeutic Outcomes

Due to the prevalence of migraine and cluster headaches, pharmacists need to be actively involved in patient care issues. All headache patients should be monitored for frequency, intensity, and duration of headaches, but also for any change in the headache pattern. Careful monitoring of therapy is essential to initiate the most appropriate agent or agents for the patient, evaluate therapeutic failures, document successful therapy, identify medication contraindications, and prevent and/or minimize adverse events. Patients taking abortive therapy should be monitored for frequency of medication use of both prescription and OTC medications. Strict adherence to dosing guidelines should be stressed to minimize potential toxicity. Success of the abortive interventions should also be documented. Changes in abortive medication use can be documented to establish the need for prophylactic therapy. Prophylactic therapies should also be monitored closely for adverse reactions, abortive therapy needs (and any change from baseline), and dosing guidelines. Regardless of the type of therapy, medications and doses should be monitored by the pharmacist to ensure appropriateness. Patient counseling is necessary to allow for proper medication use (e.g., self-injection with sumatriptan), to encourage early use of medications in the headache cycle, and to enhance patient compliance. Consultation with other health care practitioners should be encouraged when changes in headache patterns or medication use appear.

Conclusion

Migraine and cluster headaches occur due to complex interactions between the cranial blood flow and neurologic influences. Alterations in platelet function and serotonin activity play major roles. A careful patient workup, including patient history, physical examination, and appropriate laboratory tests, identifies most headache patients with major disease. A variety of strategies can be helpful for managing both migraines and cluster headaches (Table 60.8). Management of vascular headaches is directed at suppressing an acute attack and preventing recurrences.

The wide range of available symptomatic and prophylactic treatment options in managing vascular headaches indicates that none is wholly effective. Prophylactic medication is warranted when headache of moderate or greater severity recurs with a frequency of two or more attacks per month. Treatment failures may result when patients receive an insufficient dosage of the drug or an inadequate drug trial. Therapy should be continued for 6–8 weeks before an agent is considered to be ineffective. Continuing research into the problem of headache disorders will better define pathophysiologic mechanisms and aid the search for less toxic and more efficacious pharmacologic agents.

TABLE 60.8. SUMMARY OF MIGRAINE AND CLUSTER HEADACHE MANAGEMENT

1. Migraine
   a. Abortive therapy
      1. Acetaminophen
      2. Aspirin
      3. Ergotamine preparations
      4. NSAIDs
      5. Midrin
      6. Sumatriptan
      7. Others (chlorpromazine, prochlorperazine, metoclopramide)
   b. Prophylactic therapy
      1. Antidepressants
      2. Aspirin
      3. Beta blockers
      4. Calcium channel blockers
      5. Ergotamine preparations
      6. Methysergide
      7. NSAIDs
      8. Others (cyproheptadine, clonidine, anticonvulsants, steroids, calcitonin)
2. Cluster headaches
   a. Abortive therapy
      1. Ergotamine preparations
      2. Local anesthetic agents
      3. Oxygen
      4. Sumatriptan
   b. Prophylactic therapy
      1. Calcium channel blockers
      2. Corticosteroids
      3. Ergotamine preparations
      4. Lithium
      5. Methysergide
      6. Others (capsaicin, leuprolide)

References

1. Stewart WF, Lipton RB, Celentano DD, Reed ML. Prevalance of migraine headache in the United States: Relation to age, income, race, and other sociodemographic factors. JAMA 1992;267:64–69.
2. Linet MS, Stewart WF, Celentano DD, et al. An epidemiologic study of headache among adolescents and young adults. JAMA 1989;261:2211–2216.
3. Dalessio DJ. Diagnosing the severe headache. Neurology 1994;44(s3):6–12.

4. Lipton RB, Stewart WF. Migraine in the United States: A review of epidemiology and health care use. Neurology 1993;43(s3):6–12.
5. de Lissovoy G, Lazarus SS. The economic cost of migraine: Present state of knowledge. Neurology 1994;44:(s4):56–62.
6. Silberstein SD. Treatment of headache in primary care practice. Am J Med 1984;77(3A):65–72.
7. Lance JW. Current concepts of migraine pathogenesis. Neurology 1993;43(s3):11–15.
8. Moskowitz MA. Neurogenic inflammation in the pathophysiology and treatment of migraine. Neurology 1993;43(s3):16–19.
9. Martin JB. Headache, in Wilson JD, Braunwald E, Isselbacher KJ, et al (eds): Harrison's Principles of Internal Medicine, 12th ed. New York, McGraw-Hill, 1991, p 108.
10. Plosker GL, McTavish D. Sumatriptan: A reappraisal of its pharmacology and therapeutic efficacy in the acute treatment of migraine and cluster headache. Drugs 1994;47(4):622–651.
11. Peroutka SJ. 5-Hydroxytryptamine receptor subtypes and the pharmacology of migraine. Neurology 1993;43(s3):34–38.
12. Hanington E, Jones RJ, Amess JAL, Wachowicz B. Migraine: A platelet disorder. Lancet 1981;2:720–723.
13. Hanington E. The platelet and migraine. Headache 1986;26:411–415.
14. Coppen A, Swade C, Wood K, Carroll JD. Platelet 5-hydroxytryptamine accumulation and migraine. Lancet 1979;2:914.
15. Dechant KL, Clissold SP. Sumatriptan: A review of its pharmacodynamic and pharmacokinetic properties, and therapeutic efficacy in the acute treatment of migraine and cluster headache. Drugs 1992;43(5):776–798.
16. Delessio DJ. Headache, in Wall PD, Melzack R (eds): Textbook of Pain. New York, Churchill Livingstone, 1984, pp 277–292.
17. Edmeads J. Four steps in managing migraine. Postgrad Med 1989;85(6):121–134.
18. Edmeads J. Aspartame and headache. Headache 1988;28:64–65.
19. Glover V, Littlewood J, Sandler M, et al. Biochemical predisposition to dietary migraine: The role of phenosulphotransferase. Headache 1983;23:53–58.
20. Mauskop A, Altura BT, Cracco RQ, Altura BM. Deficiency in serum ionized magnesium but not total magnesium in patients with migraines. Possible role of ICa^{2+}/IMg^{2+} ratio. Headache 1993;33:135–138.
21. Krabbe AA, Olesen J. Headache provocation by continuous intravenous infusion of histamine. Clinical results and receptor mechanisms. Pain 1980;8:253–259.
22. Dhuna A, Pascual-Leone A, Belgrade M. Cocaine-related vascular headaches. J Neurology, Neurosurgery, and Psych 1991;54:803–806.
23. Ziegler DK, Hassanein RS, Ward DF. Migraine, tyramine and blood serotonin. Headache 1976;5:53–57.
24. Littlewood JT, Glover V, Davies PTG, et al. Red wine as a cause of migraine. Lancet 1988;1:558–559.
25. Mansfield, LE. Food allergy and headache: Whom to evaluate and how to treat. Postgrad Med 1988;83(7):46–55.
26. Monro J, Carini C, Brostoff J, et al. Food allergy in migraine: Study of dietary exclusion and RAST. Lancet 1980;2:1–4.
27. Kohlenberg RJ. Tyramine sensitivity in dietary migraine: A critical review. Headache 1982;22:30–34.
28. Welch KMA. Drug therapy of migraine. N Engl J Med 1993;329(20):1476–1483.
29. Baumel B. Migraine: A pharmacologic review with newer options and delivery modalities. Neurology 1994;44(s3):13–17.
30. Peters BH, Fraim CJ, Masel BE. Comparison of 650mg aspirin and 1000mg acetaminophen with each other, and with placebo in moderately severe headache. Am J Med 1983;75:36–42.
31. Rapoport AM. Analgesic rebound headache. Headache 1988;28:662–665.
32. Mendelson G, Little TF. Narcotic analgesics in headache. Med J Aust 1981;2(10):518.
33. Hering R, Steiner TJ. Abrupt outpatient withdrawal of medication in analgesic-abusing migraineurs. Lancet 1991;337:1442–1443.
34. Diamond S, Freitag FG. Do non-steroidal anti-inflammatory agents have a role in the treatment of migraine headaches? Drugs 1989;37:755–760.
35. Pradalier A, Clapin A, Dry J. Treatment review: Non-steroidal anti-inflammatory drugs in the treatment and long-term prevention of migraine attacks. Headache 1988;28:550–557.
36. Treves TA, Streiffler M, Korczyn AD. Naproxen sodium versus ergotamine tartrate in the treatment of acute migraine attacks. Headache 1992;32:280–282.
37. Klapper JA, Stanton JS. Ketorolac versus DHE and metoclopramide in the treatment of migraine headaches. Headache 1991;31:523–524.
38. Goldstein J. Ergot pharmacology and alternative delivery systems for ergotamine derivatives. Neurology 1992;42(s2):45–46.
39. Raskin NH. Repetitive intravenous dihydroergotamine as therapy for intractable migraine. Neurology 1986;36:995–997.
40. Callaham M, Raskin NH. A controlled study of dihydroergotamine in the treatment of acute migraine headaches. Headache 1986;26:168–171.
41. Ibraheem JJ, Paalzow L, Tfelt-Hansen P. Low bioavailability of ergotamine tartrate after oral and rectal administration in migraine sufferers. Br J Clin Pharmacol 1983;16:695–699.
42. Tfelt-Hansen P, Paalzow L, Ibraheem JJ. Bioavailability of sublingual ergotamine [Letter]. Br J Clin Pharmacol 1982;13:239–240.
43. Mathew NT. Amelioration of ergotamine withdrawal symptoms with naproxen. Headache 1987;27:130–133.
44. Saper JR. Ergotamine dependency—A review. Headache 1987;27:435–438.
45. Rogers DA, Mansberger JA. Gastrointestinal vascular ischemia caused by ergotamine. South Med J 1989;82(8):1058–1059.
46. Venter CP, Joubert PH, Buys AC. Severe peripheral ischaemia during concomitant use of beta blockers and ergot alkaloids. Br Med J 1984;289:288–289.
47. Hsu VD. Sumatriptan: A new drug for vascular headache. Clin Pharm 1992;11:919–929.
48. Doenicke A, Brand J, Perrin VL. Possible benefit of GR 43175, a novel $5\text{-}HT_1$-like receptor agonist, for the acute treatment of severe migraine. Lancet 1988;1:1309–1311.
49. Visser WH, Ferrar MD, Bayliss EM, Ludlow S, Pilgrim AJ for the Subcutaneous Sumatriptan International Study Group. Treatment of migraine attacks with subcutaneous sumatriptan: First placebo controlled study. Cephalagia 1992;12:308–313.

50. The Multinational Oral Sumatriptan and Cafergot Comparative Study Group. A randomized, double-blind comparison of sumatriptan and Cafergot in the acute treatment of migraine. Eur Neurol 1991;31:314–322.
51. Bousser MG, D'Allens J, Richard A, and the Early-Morning Migraine Sumatriptan Study Group. Efficacy of subcutaneous sumatriptan in the acute treatment of early-morning migraine: A placebo-controlled trial. J Int Med 1993;234:211–216.
52. The Sumatriptan Auto-Injector Study Group. Self-treatment of acute migraine with subcutaneous sumatriptan using an auto-injector device. Eur Neurol 1991;31:323–331.
53. Goadsby PJ, Zagami AS, Donnan GA, et al. Oral sumatriptan in acute migraine. Lancet 1991;338:782–783.
54. Patten JP. Clinical experience with oral sumatriptan: A placebo-controlled, dose-ranging study. J Neurol 1991;238:S62–S65.
55. Nappi G, Sicuteri F, Byrne M, et al. Oral sumatriptan compared with placebo in the acute treatment of migraine. J Neurol 1994;241:138–144.
56. Ferrari MD, James MH, Bates D, et al. Oral sumatriptan: Effect of a second dose, and incidence and treatment of headache recurrences. Cephalalgia 1994;14:330–338.
57. The Oral Sumatriptan and Aspirin Plus Metoclopramide Comparative Study Group. A study to compare oral sumatriptan with oral aspirin plus oral metoclopramide in the acute treatment of migraine. Eur Neurol 1992;32:177–184.
58. Diamond S. Treatment of migraine with isometheptene, acetaminophen, and dichloralphenazone combination: A double–blind, crossover trial. Headache 1976;15:282–287.
59. Tek DS, McClellan DS, Olshaker JS, et al. A prospective, double-blind study of metoclopramide hydrochloride for the control of migraine in the emergency department. Ann Emerg Med 1990;19:1083–1087.
60. Voans GN. The effect of metoclopramide on the absorption of effervescent aspirin in migraine. Br J Clin Pharmacol 1975;2:57–63.
61. Iserson KV. Parenteral chlorpromazine treatment of migraine. Ann Emerg Med 1983;12:756–758.
62. Jones J, Sklar D, Dougherty J, White W. Randomized double-blind trial of intravenous prochlorperazine for the treatment of acute headache. JAMA 1989;261:1174–1176.
63. Monro J, Carini C, Brostoff J. Migraine is a food-allergic disease. Lancet 1984;2:719–720.
64. Lockett DM, Campbell JF. The effects of aerobic exercise on migraine. Headache 1992;32:50–54.
65. Darling M. The use of exercise as a method of aborting migraine. Headache 1991;31:616–618.
66. Corelli R, Hart LL. Beta-blocking agents for migraine. DICP, Ann Pharmacother 1989;23:248–249.
67. Ziegler DK, Hurwitz A, Preskorn S, Hassanein R. Propranolol and amitriptyline in prophylaxis of migraine: Pharmacokinetic and therapeutic effects. Arch Neurol 1993;50:825–830.
68. Stellar S, Ahrens SP, Meibohm AR, Reines SA. Migraine prevention with timolol: A double-blind crossover study. JAMA 1984;252(18):2576–2580.
69. Dalessio DJ. Beta-blockers and migraine [Editorial]. JAMA 1984;252(18):2614.
70. Couch JR, Hassanein RS. Amitriptyline in migraine prophylaxis. Arch Neurol 1979;36:695–699.
71. Adly C, Straumanis J, Chesson A. Fluoxetine prophylaxis of migraine. Headache 1992;32:101–104.
72. Larson EW. Migraine with typical aura associated with fluoxetine therapy: A case report. J Clin Psychiatry 1993;54(6):235–236.
73. Schuler ME, Goldman MP, Munger MA. The role of calcium channel blocking agents in the prevention of migraine. DICP 1988;21:187–191.
74. Molaie M, Olson CM, Koch J. The effect of intravenous verapamil on acute migraine headache. Headache 1987;27:51–53.
75. Jonsdottir M, Meyer JS, Rogers RL. Efficacy, side effects, and tolerance compared during headache treatment with three different calcium blockers. Headache 1987;27:364–369.
76. Smith R, Schwartz A. Diltiazem prophylaxis in refractory migraine. N Engl J Med 1984;310(20):1327–1328.
77. McArthur JC, Marek K, Pestronk A, et al. Nifedipine in the prophylaxis of classic migraine: A crossover, double-masked, placebo-controlled study of headache frequency and side effects. Neurology 1989;39:284–286.
78. Stewart DJ, Gelston A, Hakim A. Effect of prophylactic administration of nimodipine in patients with migraine. Headache 1988;28:260–262.
79. Bassi P, Brunati L, Rapuzzi E, et al. Low dose flunarizine in the prophylaxis of migraine. Headache 1992;32:390–392.
80. O'Neil BP, Mann JD. Aspirin prophylaxis in migraine. Lancet 1978;2:1179–1181.
81. Welch KMA, Ellis DJ, Keenan PA. Successful migraine prophylaxis with naproxen sodium. Neurology 1985;35:1304–1310.
82. Patti F, Scapagnini U, Nicoletti F, et al. Calcitonin and migraine. Headache 1986;26:172–174.
83. Patti F, Scapagnini U, Nicoletti F, et al. A short-term trial of an analogue of eel-calcitonin in headache. Headache 1987;27:334–339.
84. Mathew N. Cluster headache. Neurology 1992;42 (suppl 2):22–31.
85. Mather PJ, Silberstein SD, Schulman EA, Hopkins MM. The treatment of cluster headache with repetitive intravenous dihydroergotamine. Headache 1991;31:525–532.
86. Sabato FD, Fusco BM, Pelaia P, Giacovazzo M. Hyperbaric oxygen therapy in cluster headache. Pain 1993;52:243–245.
87. Fogan L. Treatment of cluster headache: A double-blind comparison of oxygen v. air inhalation. Arch Neurol 1985;42:362–363.
88. Kittrelle JP, Grouse DS, Seybold ME. Cluster headache: Local anesthetic abortive agents. Arch Neurol 1985;42:496–497.
89. The Sumatriptan Cluster Headache Study Group. Treatment of acute cluster headache with sumatriptan. N Engl J Med 1991;325:322–326.
90. Marks DR, Rapoport A, Padla D, et al. A double-blind placebo-controlled trial of intranasal capsaicin for cluster headache. Cephalalgia 1993;13:114–116.
91. Jammes J. The treatment of cluster headaches with prednisone. Dis Nerv Syst 1975;36:375–376.
92. Nicolodi M, Sicuteri F, Poggioni M. Hypothalamic modulation of nociception and reproduction in cluster headache. I. Therapeutic trials of leuprolide. Cephalalgia 1993;13:253–257.
93. Mathew NT. Clinical subtypes of cluster headache and response to lithium therapy. Headache 1978;18:26–30.

Section 6
Psychiatric Disorders

Chapter 61

Assessment of Psychiatric Illness

Patricia A. Marken, BS Pharm, PharmD,
and Mark E. Schneiderhan, BS Pharm, PharmD

Certain patient assessment skills are common across specialties, however, psychiatry uses additional procedures that are less objective than traditional laboratory tests and physical examination techniques. Mental health clinicians need training in psychiatric assessment in order to participate meaningfully on the treatment team and to provide patient care for the mentally ill. This chapter provides an overview of the assessment of the psychiatric patient in order to facilitate pharmaceutical care planning.

Overview of the Diagnostic and Statistical Manual of Mental Disorders

The *Diagnostic and Statistical Manual of Mental Disorders*, fourth edition (DSM-IV), provides a common language for mental health practitioners to describe psychiatric disorders.[1] Common language is essential because there is considerable overlap of symptoms between many diagnoses. DSM-I was introduced in 1952 and was the first manual on mental disorders to contain a description of diagnostic categories. The most recent edition, DSM-IV, was released in 1994.

The DSM-IV is widely accepted as the most important diagnostic reference for mental illness. It contains many components that provide a comprehensive understanding of the illness and assist clinicians in making an accurate diagnosis. For example, the multiaxial patient evaluation ensures that most factors that could contribute to, or modify, the condition are considered during a patient assessment. Axis I lists the principal psychiatric disorder or disorders, or provisional diagnoses. Axis II lists developmental and personality disorders. Axis III describes existing physical disorders or conditions. Axis IV describes the severity of psychosocial stressors that may have contributed to a new or recurrent mental disorder, or exacerbation of an existing condition. Stressors are rated on a scale of 1 (none) to 6 (catastrophic) and can be acute (lasting less than 6 months) or enduring (lasting longer than 6 months). They include difficulties with interpersonal relationships, parenting, occupation, living circumstances, finances, the legal system, and health. Axis V describes the global assessment of functioning (GAF). GAF is rated on a scale from 1 (persistent danger to self or others) to 90 (minimal or absent symptoms). A GAF rating should be made for the current level of functioning and the highest level of functioning in the past months to a year prior to the current evaluation. The GAF assists the clinician in documenting the baseline level of functioning, which helps in establishing ultimate therapeutic goals.

DSM-IV provides information on all mental disorders recognized by the American Psychiatric Association, including age of onset, clinical course, complications, predisposing factors, prevalence, and differential diagnoses. The specific diagnostic criteria for each mental illness and the number of symptoms required to establish a diagnosis are also listed. The DSM-IV also includes decision trees for differential diagnosis and a glossary of technical terms. *The Clinical Interview Using the DSM-IV* is a companion book that provides extensive information on interviewing techniques to allow the clinician to establish the presence of a DSM-IV diagnosis.[2] Additional information besides the DSM-IV diagnosis is required before a comprehensive treatment plan is developed.[1]

Mental Status Examination

The mental status examination in psychiatry can be conceptualized as the counterpart to the physical examination in medicine. However, conducting a mental status exam does not obviate the need for a physical exam in a psychiatric patient. The mental status examination creates a description of current patient behavior, thoughts, perceptions, and functioning and provides an objective evaluation used for diagnosis, assessment of course of the illness, and response to treatment. The interview should be completed in a quiet, private, and comfortable area where the patient and the interviewer feel at ease. The interviewer should introduce him- or herself and explain the procedure in order to facilitate establishment of a trusting relationship. Generally, open-ended questions should come first followed by questions focused on more specific or personal data. Open-ended questions ask the patient to provide descriptions and other information in his or her own words. Even though more specific questions may then be necessary to fill in the gaps, beginning in this manner minimizes the risk of "leading" the patient. Patients may respond to specific questions and "yes" or "no" questions with answers they think the interviewer wants to hear. The interviewer must be nonjudgmental in order to develop trust and rapport with the patient and to ensure completeness and accuracy of the information. A mental status examination has several components.[2,3]

APPEARANCE

The appearance of the patient throughout the interview should be noted, including age, dress, grooming and hygiene, use of cosmetics, and facial expressions. A description of appearance should also include unusual physical characteristics and the general state of physical health.

ACTIVITY

Changes in motor activity include overactivity, underactivity, and catatonia. Overactivity includes an increase in purposeful movements or agitation, where the movements appear purposeless to the observer. Examples of overactivity include pacing, hand wringing, picking at clothing, skin or hair, inability to sit still during the interview, and excessive hand gestures. Underactive patients move less than expected. Patients described with rigid posture, an absence of movement, and failure to communicate with surroundings may be catatonic.

ATTITUDE TOWARD EXAMINER

The interviewer should note whether the patient is cooperative, mute, hostile, paranoid, or withdrawn.

SPEECH AND LANGUAGE

The quantity, content, and speed of speech and whether the patient makes eye contact should be noted. Speech should be assessed as to whether it proceeds logically toward a goal-directed ideal or whether the content is vague and poorly organized. Abnormal speech characteristics include blocking, whereby the person suddenly stops speaking without any obvious reason. Thought blocking usually occurs when a hallucination or delusion has intruded into the person's thinking, or upsetting issues are discussed. Circumstantial speech lacks a clear direction because of excess unnecessary information, but the circumstantial patient will eventually make his or her point. In tangential speech, however, the ultimate point is never made. Perseveration is repetition of speech despite the patient trying to produce a new answer. Flight of ideas is overproductive, rapid speech during which patients jump rapidly from one idea to the next. Mutisum is when the patient does not respond even though she or he is aware of the discussion.

MOOD AND AFFECT

Affect describes the prevailing emotional tone, while mood describes more sustained feelings. To properly evaluate a patient's mood and affect, their appearance and the content of speech must be considered. Change in facial expression and the presence of tears, flushing, sweating, or tremors should be noted. Affect can further be described by its range, appropriateness, intensity, and stability. For example, in schizophrenia or depression, the affect may be flat whereby no change in expression occurs throughout the interview. In contrast, during a manic episode the affect is very intense and often labile. The range of emotional expression is reduced but not absent with blunted affect. An example of inappropriate affect is when a patient laughs when they are depressed, or cries when stating they are happy. A rapidly shifting affect from one extreme to the other is described as labile.

THOUGHT AND PERCEPTUAL DISTURBANCES

A variety of thought disturbances can occur in mental illness. Delusions are fixed, false beliefs that are not based in reality, religion, or culture. They can be paranoid, somatic, or grandiose in nature, and patients may be deluded that they are controlled by an outside force. Delusions are often unshakable, and one should not attempt to talk a patient out of a delusion. Obsessions are unwanted thoughts, ideas, or impulses that intrude into a person's thinking, whereas compulsions are actions often performed in response to the obsessions or to control anxiety associated with the obsession. Thought broadcasting is the belief that one's thoughts are audible to others. Hallucinations are false sensory impressions or perceptions that occur in the absence of an external stimulus. Hallucinations may be auditory, visual, olfactory, or gustatory and may be continuous or intermittent. In contrast, illusions are visual perceptions that are misinterpreted, but have a real sensory stimulus. For example, a patient who perceives a chair sitting in a dark corner to be a threatening figure is experiencing an illusion.

NEUROPSYCHIATRIC EVALUATION

A neuropsychiatric evaluation assesses senorium, attention, concentration, memory, and higher cognitive functions such as orientation, abstraction, and calculation. Prior to initiation of the neuropsychiatric evaluation, it should be documented whether the patient has been prescribed medications with sedative properties, because the outcome of the examination could be altered if central nervous system depressants have been taken.

Sensorium, or level of consciousness, refers to the alertness of the patient and, if they are not fully alert, the amount of stimulation needed to awaken them. Attention and concentration can be assessed using serial "7's" or "3's," whereby the patient subtracts backwards from 100 in increments of 7 or 3, respectively. Another concentration test is to have a patient spell a five-letter word backwards. Language skills are initially assessed by having a patient read something aloud and silently. General intelligence can be loosely assessed by asking factual information about current news items, recent presidents, or popular television shows or sporting events. Memory is the ability to recall past experiences and is classified as immediate, recent (past events leading to the patient's current situation), and remote (historical facts). Orientation to time, place, person and situation assesses immediate and recent memory. Asking a patient to recall three objects 5 minutes after they are learned is another test for recent memory. Remote memory is assessed by asking the patient to recall old facts of their life, such as where they were born or where they went to school. Remote memory usually stays intact the longest in patients with intellectual decline. Abstraction is the ability to interpret information such as a proverb (e.g., "people in glass houses shouldn't throw stones") or identify similarities or differences between words (*apple* and *orange*). Abstraction ability is influenced by education and linguistic fluency, thus inability to abstract is not always a sign of a thought disorder.

INSIGHT AND JUDGMENT

Insight refers to patients' awareness that they have a mental illness and the consequences of that illness on their life. Patients typically have a lack of insight when they are psychotic. Patients with poor insight are often noncompliant with prescribed medications. Judgment is the ability to make decisions appropriate to the situation and may be impaired in a variety of mental illnesses.

A mental status exam is usually completed upon admission to a hospital or intake into a psychiatric facility. The mental status exam should be used to identify initial target symptoms that are monitored during the course of drug therapy. Table 61.1 provides examples of questions that can be used to gather some information in the mental status exam. Note that these are additional questions that can be asked for probing and clarification after as much information as possible has been gathered using open-ended (nonleading) questions.

PSYCHIATRIC HISTORY

Both the patient's and the family's history of mental illness provides important information when formulating a diagnosis. Information should be descriptive and include the current and previous psychiatric diagnoses, presentation of each illness, time frame between episodes, level of functioning between episodes, length of each episode, total duration of illness, and treatment given during each episode. Baseline functioning or the highest level of functioning achieved in the past few years is important information because it provides a target or goal for treatment. Information on the history of the current episode and reasons for coming to the clinician should also be gathered. A family history should include a medication history of the immediate relatives, because a family member's response to a given medication may predict an individual patient's response to that same medication.

A social history should include educational and occupational background, religion, martial status, substance use patterns, including smoking, and current living situation. By understanding a patient's living environment and social situation, strategies to prevent noncompliance and to reduce stress and increase social support can be developed.

MEDICATION HISTORY

A thorough medication history is one of the most important contributions a pharmacist can make to treatment planning.

TABLE 61.1. EXAMPLES OF INTERVIEW QUESTIONS FOR ASSESSING MENTAL ILLNESSES

Mania
1. Do your thoughts go faster than you can say them?
2. Have you noticed a change in the amount of sleep that you require?
3. Have you spent a lot of money lately and what did you spend it on?
4. Do you have a lot of extra energy?

(To assess hallucinations and delusions see Schizophrenia section below.)

Depression
1. Do you cry without any reason?
2. Do you still enjoy the same hobbies/activities that you once did?
3. Has your weight changed recently?
4. Have you had changes in your energy level recently?
5. Do you have any guilty feelings?
6. Do you find it difficult to remember phone numbers, names of friends, appointments, etc.?

(To assess sleep and suicidal potential, see Sleep and Suicide sections below.)

Schizophrenia

Delusions:
1. Do you feel that people plot against you?
2. Do you feel that you are ever watched or spied on?
3. Do you have any special abilities?
4. Does anyone ever try to mess with you or bother you?
5. Do others read your thoughts?

Hallucinations:
1. Does the TV/radio ever tell you things?
2. Do you hear voices that other people don't hear?
3. What do they say? How many voices?
4. How often do they bother you?
5. Do the voices ever tell you to hurt yourself or someone else?
6. Have you ever heard your name called when there is no one there?
7. Have you ever seen anything strange that you can't explain?
8. Do you ever see things that bother you and no one else?
9. Do you want to act on what the voices say?

Thought Broadcasting/Insertion:
1. If I stood by you could I hear your thoughts?
2. Does your head ever act like a radio?
3. Do you feel that others can put thoughts in your head?

Insight
1. What reasons did your family give you for coming here?
2. What brought you here?
3. Do you consider yourself in need of help?
4. What does your medication do for you?

Sleep
1. Tell me about your sleep?
2. How many hours do you sleep each night at present?
3. How many hours do you usually sleep at night?
4. Do you sleep all through the night?
5. Is there a reason for your waking up?
6. Do you have trouble falling asleep?
7. How do you feel when you wake up?

Suicide Potential
1. Do you feel your life is worth living?
2. Do you ever think of hurting yourself?
3. Do you see things improving in the future?
4. Do you think you will try to hurt yourself now?
5. How would you do it?
6. Do you have the means to hurt yourself?

The history should include medication for both psychiatric and medical conditions. The medication history should note not only which medications have been taken, but how they were tolerated and how well the patient responded to them. Because most psychiatric medications have a delay in the onset of effect and many mental illnesses are chronic, it is important to determine whether an adequate trial (adequate duration and adequate dose) was provided before the patient is considered nonresponsive. If a patient has a history of noncompliance, specific causes such as cost, complicated dosing schedules, lack of insight, and adverse effects should be investigated.

MEDICAL ASSESSMENT IN PSYCHIATRY

A careful medical assessment of patients who present with psychiatric symptoms is important for many reasons.[4] Both medical illnesses and medications can cause psychiatric symptoms, making accurate diagnosis very difficult. Patients with psychiatric illnesses, especially depressive and anxiety disorders may describe only physical complaints. In addition, many patients with chronic psychiatric illnesses receive poor medical care and need medical referral.

Medical illnesses may be misdiagnosed as psychiatric illnesses for reasons identified in Table 61.2.[5] An important clue that a physical illness may be causing or contributing to psychiatric symptoms is rapidity of onset of psychiatric symptoms. Most chronic mental illnesses have a prodromal period, whereas medically based psychiatric symptoms often have a more rapid onset of symptoms. Patients over age 40 at first presentation are more likely to have a medical cause for their psychiatric symptoms, because major psychiatric illnesses such as schizophrenia and bipolar affective disorder usually first present at an earlier age. A family history of physical illnesses with a psychiatric component, such as Huntington's chorea and systemic lupus erythematosus, provides an additional clue. Patients with fluctuating levels of consciousness, disorientation, memory impairment, or visual, tactile, or olfactory hallucinations are more likely to have a medical basis for their illness.

Routine laboratory screening in psychiatry is useful for ruling out medical causes of psychiatric illnesses, but extensive testing is usually unnecessary and not cost effective. Laboratory tests should be individualized to the age and physical health of the patient. A complete physical examination along with a detailed medical history and routine blood chemistry (34 panel) are most likely to identify possible

TABLE 61.2. REASONS FOR MISDIAGNOSIS OF MEDICAL ILLNESSES IN THE MENTALLY ILL

Disease-Related
- Psychiatric symptoms may precede physical signs and symptoms of illness
- Impaired memory or perception prevents patients from providing accurate history

Patient-Related
- Appearance (dirty, strange dress)
- Behavior (hostile, threatening, uncooperative)

Physician-Related
- Incomplete assessments: incomplete medical history, cursory physical examination, failure to interview other informants (old records, friends, family), lack of current physical exam or laboratory tests
- Incorrect assumptions: absence of delirium, memory impairment, or disorientation rules out physical disease, psychiatric symptoms imply psychiatric diagnosis, psychosocial stressors explain current symptoms

(Adapted with permission from Sternberg DE. Testing for physical illness in psychiatric patients. *The Journal of Clinical Psychiatry* 1986;47(1, suppl):3–9. Copyright 1986, Physicians Postgraduate Press.)

medical-related causes.[5] Urine drug screens and blood alcohol tests play an important role in identifying the contribution of substances of abuse to the presenting symptoms. In some cases, if available, recent laboratory tests can be used, provided that no change in physical status has occurred. A blood chemistry panel and a complete blood count are usually needed to assess contraindications and complications to drug therapy. Serum concentration monitoring of selected medications is also helpful in increasing probability of response and minimizing the likelihood of adverse effects.

PSYCHOLOGICAL TESTING

Although pharmacists are not directly involved in psychological testing, they can use the results to evaluate the role of medication in relationship to the diagnosis. Psychological testing alone cannot establish a firm diagnosis, but can be a useful diagnostic tool when coupled with clinical judgment. Types of psychological testing include personality tests, intelligence tests, and neuropsychological tests.[6] Table 61.3 describes common psychological tests.

PSYCHIATRIC RATING SCALES

Psychiatric rating scales have multiple uses including, research, patient care, and education.[7] The purpose of a rating scale is to provide objective data to answer a clinical or research question. A single psychiatric rating scale score provides only a limited picture or snapshot of a complex clinical situation. However, repeated ratings can objectively describe longitudinal change over a defined treatment period. For example, the Hamilton Anxiety Rating Scale (HAM-A) can be used to assess baseline symptoms of anxiety and the change produced by an intervention or time.[8]

Global rating scales, such as the Clinical Global Impression (CGI) scale, assess the overall severity of illness based on a rater's clinical experience.[9] The HAM-A can detect features of somatic and psychic anxiety (e.g., anxious mood, tension, fears, insomnia, somatic, cardiovascular symptoms). The rating scale will not determine the reason for the symptoms; for example, a patient's anxiety may be secondary to paranoia or a primary anxiety disorder. Second, a patient may have a 15% drop in a rating scale score from one week to the next, but remain severely ill. Sensitivity, specificity, reliability, and validity are important considerations when selecting a rating scale. The sensitivity of a test refers to its ability to detect a symptom or illness, given that the symptom or illness is present. Specificity refers to a test's ability to determine that a symptom or illness is absent given that the person does not have the illness.

Reliability is the extent to which the score on the scale reflects the hypothetical "true" score and how much interference occurs from outside influences.[10] Reliability is reported by the correlation coefficient, which represents a chance correlation (zero) or perfect correlation (one). Rating scales with correlation coefficients of less than 0.7 are usually considered unreliable for clinical studies. Interrater reliability, agreement in rating scores among clinicians, is important to achieve when multiple people rate the same patient or population. Interrater reliability is established by having all raters independently rate individual patients at the same time to determine the correlation of their scores. Other types of reliability include test–retest reliability (assesses the stability of the scale in producing the same

TABLE 61.3. COMMON PSYCHOLOGICAL TESTS

Wechsler Intelligence Scales (WAIS-R for adults; WISC-R for children)
- Measures abstract thinking, learning from experience, problem solving, adjustment to new situations
- Score less than 70 denotes mental retardation

Bender Visual Motor Gestalt Test
- Screening test for brain damage, learning problems, emotional difficulties, nonverbal intelligence
- Person is asked to reproduce nine geometric designs

Interpretation of Projective Drawings
- Patient draws a person, house-tree-person, family, or spontaneously to assess unconscious feeling, conflicts, and strengths

Rorschach
- Patient interprets 10 inkblots and explains what they mean
- Assesses personality structure

Minnesota Multiphasic Personality Inventory (MMPI)
- Measures personality traits from 566 true/false questions
- Can be affected by intelligence, education, socioeconomic status

results with repeated use) and internal consistency (degree to which items in the scale measure different aspects of the same condition without overlap).

Validity, in contrast, is the ability of a scale to measure what it was designed to measure. Content validity measures the extent to which the scale assesses appropriate aspects of the problem's characteristics. Concurrent validity is a measure of the correlation of the rating scale to an external measure such as diagnosis or clinical change. Construct validity is the extent to which the test appears to measure symptom traits in contrast to measuring a more limited, specific symptom.

Psychiatric rating scales should not be confused with psychological tests such as neuropsychological and intellectual assessments and are best used as only one part of a comprehensive diagnostic plan. Tables 61.4, 61.5, and 61.6 describe commonly used patient-rated and clinician-rated scales for a variety of disease states.[11–16] In clinical research, a combination of clinician- and self-rated rating scales and diagnostic tests provides the most accurate measurement of drug efficacy and treatment outcome.

Patient assessment is the backbone from which a pharmaceutical care plan evolves. Problem identification and therapeutic monitoring cannot occur unless a thorough assessment is first completed. The initial assessment is also the basis of evaluating response to therapy throughout the course of treatment. Psychiatric assessment requires sensitivity and good listening skills on the part of the clinician because it is primarily based on a subjective interview and not objective tests. With careful data collection, pharmacists can make substantial contributions to care that improve patient outcomes.

TABLE 61.4. SCHIZOPHRENIA RATING SCALES

Rating Scale	Type	Scoring	Comments
Brief Psychiatric Rating Scales (BPRS)	Clinician-rated	18 items with a 7-point severity scale: BPRS ≥ 38 indicates moderate severity.	The anchored BPRS provides descriptions of each severity rating to increase the interrater reliability. The BPRS has four clusters of symptoms: thinking disturbance, anxious depression, withdrawal–retardation, hostility–suspiciousness.
Scale for Assessment of Negative Symptoms (SANS)	Clinician-rated	30 items, 6-point severity scale: 0 = normal 5 = severe	Measures degree of affect, alogia, avolition, anhedonia, and attention.
Schedule for Affective Disorders and Schizophrenia–Change version (SADS–C)	Clinician-rated	29 items, 6-point scale and Global Assessment Scale. Subsets of items can be combined to score specific affective symptoms	Structured interview to measure change in symptoms and assess anxiety, depression, manic features, and delusions or disorganization.
Positive and Negative Syndrome Scale (PANSS)	Clinician-rated	30 items, 7-point severity scale	Based on the 18-item BPRS.
Nurses Observations Scale for Inpatient Evaluation (NOSIE)	Observational	30 items, 4-point severity scale: 0 = never 1 = sometimes 2 = often 3 = usually 4 = always	Patient's behavior is rated daily.
Clinical Global Impression Scale (CGI)	Observational	Severity of illness, 7-point rating scale Global improvement, 7-point rating scale Efficacy index: 1–4 = marked improvement 5–8 = moderate 9–12 = minimal 13–16 = unchanged/worse	Observational rating scale to compare severity of illness compared to other similar patients and measures improvement from baseline. The efficacy index measures therapeutic effect and side effects to determine the score.

TABLE 61.5. DEPRESSION RATING SCALES

Rating Scale	Type	Scoring	Comments
Hamilton Psychiatric Rating Scale for Depression (HAM-D)	Clinician-rated	17-item scale: < 6 = normal mood 17–25 = mild depression > 25 = severe depression	Used to screen patients for drug studies and to determine severity of symptoms, treatment outcome, and the standard to compare other depression rating scales.
Montgomery–Asberg Depression Rating Scale (MADRS)	Clinician-rated	10 items, 7-point scale. For each item: 0 = no symptoms 6 = severe symptoms	Differentiates between all the intermediate grades of depression. Decreases bias in patients with other medical illness and increased somatization.
Beck Depressive Inventory (BDI)	Patient-rated	21-item scale: 0–9 = normal 10–15 = mild depression 16–19 = mild-moderate 20–29 = moderate-severe 30–63 = severe depression	The standard for self-rating scales and an objective measure of change in symptoms as a result of treatment.
Zung Self-Rating Depression Scale (SDS)	Patient-rated	20-item scale, 4-point severity: < 50 = normal 50–59 = minimal–mild 60–69 = moderate-marked ≥ 70 = severe depression	Severity rated by frequency of occurrence of symptoms. May not be as sensitive in measuring changes in severity of symptoms.
Raskin's Mood Scales and Modified Mood Scales for Depression (RMS)	Patient-rated	53-item scale	Measures the presence or absence of symptoms. Sensitive in measuring changes resulting from treatment.

TABLE 61.6. ANXIETY RATING SCALES

Rating Scale	Type	Scoring	Comments
Hamilton Anxiety Scale (HAM A or HAMAS or HAMRS)	Clinician-rated	14 items, 5-point scales: scores of ≥18–20 for moderate anxiety	Consists of subscales to measure somatic and psychic anxiety.
Self-Rating Anxiety Scale (SAS) (Zung)	Patient-rated	20 items, 4-point intensity ratings	Correlates to the clinician-rated Anxiety Status Inventory (ASI), however, there is little information on the validity of either test.
State-trait Anxiety Inventory (STAI)	Patient-rated	20 items state anxiety (A-state) and 20 items trait anxiety (A-trait), 4-point intensity ratings: total scores range from 20 to 80	A-trait scale reflects the patient's general or baseline anxiety. A-state scale reflects the patient's most current anxiety and measures changes in anxiety. The A-state score is sensitive to stress-induced testing.
Sheehan Panic and Anticipatory Anxiety Scale (SPAAS)	Patient- and clinician-rated	Three-part scale	Measures panic attacks, anticipatory anxiety, and limited symptom attacks.
Yale-Brown Obsessive Compulsive Scale (YBOCS)	Clinician-rated	Semistructured interview	Consists of several clusters of obsessions and compulsions. Used to assess change in treatment studies.

REFERENCES

1. American Psychiatric Association. Diagnostic and Statistical Manual of Mental Disorders 4th ed. (DSM-IV). Washington, DC, Author, 1994.
2. Othemer E, Othmer SC. The Clinical Interview Using DSM-IV. Volume 1: Fundamentals. Washington, DC, American Psychiatric Press, 1994.
3. Leon RL, Bowden CL, Faber RA. The psychiatric interview, history and mental status examination, in Kaplan HI, Sadock BJ (eds): Comprehensive Textbook of Psychiatry/V, 5th ed. Vol 1. Baltimore, Williams & Wilkins, 1989, p 475.
4. Kirch DG. Medical assessment and laboratory testing and psychiatry, in Kaplan HI, Sadock BJ (eds): Comprehensive Textbook of Psychiatry/V, 5th ed. Vol 1. Baltimore, Williams & Wilkins, 1989, p 525.
5. Sternberg DE. Testing for physical illness in psychiatric patients. J Clin Psychiatry 1986;47(suppl 1):3–9.
6. Bulter RW, Satz P. Psychological assessment of personality of adults and children, in Kaplan HI, Sadock BJ (eds): Comprehensive Textbook of Psychiatry/V, 5th ed. Vol 1. Baltimore, Williams & Wilkins, 1989, p 449.
7. Grebb JA. Psychiatric rating scales, in Kaplan HI, Sadock BJ (eds): Comprehensive Textbook of Psychiatry/V, 5th ed. Vol 1. Baltimore, Williams & Wilkins, 1989, p 534.
8. Hamilton M. The assessment of anxiety states by rating. Br J Med Psychol 1959;32:50–55.
9. Guy W. ECDEU assessment manual for psychopharmacology, rev ed, DHWE Publication (ADM) 76-338. Washington, DC, US Government Printing Office, 1976, pp 158–169.
10. Thompson C. Introduction, in Thompson C (ed): The Instruments of Psychiatric Research. New York, John Wiley & Sons, 1989, pp 1–16.
11. Fankhauser MP, German ML. Understanding the use of behavioral rating scales in studies evaluating the efficacy of antianxiety and antidepressant drugs. Am J Hosp Pharm 1987;44:2087–2100.
12. Andreasen NC. The scale for assessment of negative symptoms (SANS): Conceptual and theoretical foundations. Br J Psychiat 1989;155(suppl 7):49–58.
13. Kay SR, Opler LA, Lindenmayer JP. The positive and negative syndrome scale (PANSS): Rationale and standardization. Br J Psychiat 1989;155(suppl 7):59–65.
14. Montgomery SA, Asberg M. A new depression scale designed to be sensitive to change. Br J Psychiat 1979;134:382–389.
15. Sheehan DV. The Anxiety Disease. New York, Bantam Books, 1983, pp 114–115.
16. Goodman WK, Price LH, Rasmussen SA, et al. The Yale-Brown Obsessive Compulsive Scale (Y-BOCS): Part II. Validity. Arch Gen Psychiatry 1989;46:1006–1011.

Chapter 62

Disorders of Childhood

Karen A. Theesen, PharmD, and Julie A. Dopheide, PharmD

The *Diagnostic and Statistical Manual of Mental Disorders,* 4th ed.[1] (DSM-IV), confirms that all of the major psychiatric disorders, including schizophrenia, major depression, and anxiety disorders, can occur in children; however, the onset of these disorders is usually in late adolescence or adulthood. A substantial scientific base has been established for psychopharmacology of these major disorders in adults. Much less research, however, has been done in children.

Using psychotropic drugs to treat children and adolescents often requires a very different approach than when the same drugs are used for psychiatric disorders among adults. A child's neurologic, physiologic, and psychosocial status is different from that of an adult, and these are undergoing constant changes throughout the developmental period. Age-related pharmacodynamic and pharmacokinetic differences can alter drug disposition and response. Well-defined diagnostic criteria guide drug selection; however, frequent comorbid disorders present treatment challenges. In addition, children may not be able to verbalize their symptom response or adverse effects of a medication. All factors considered, children are given psychotropic drugs to control a group of symptoms or behavior in order to facilitate the child's learning and development.

The psychiatric assessment of a child requires obtaining information from the child, the parents or caregivers, and teachers. The overall diagnostic impression is formed from psychiatric, social, neuropsychologic, and educational evaluations. Before the initiation of psychotropic drugs, the child, family, and caregivers need to be familiar with the risks and benefits of drug therapy and with alternate non-drug therapies. In addition, an explanation of the drug monitoring techniques and the possible adverse effects including drug withdrawal should be presented. The risks associated with untreated illness and the possibly related issues of low self-esteem and impaired academic and social functioning should also be discussed.

Pharmacotherapy for children and adolescents is usually administered in conjunction with other therapies (e.g., psychotherapy, family therapy, or behavioral therapy). Medication should not be used in place of other therapies or only because other therapies have failed. Careful documentation of baseline symptoms is necessary before initiating drug therapy to identify the responsive symptoms and establish a realistic expectation for treatment outcome.

Attention-Deficit Hyperactivity Disorder (ADHD)

CLINICAL PRESENTATION

The three essential features of ADHD are signs of developmentally inappropriate inattention, impulsivity, and hyperactivity. Inattention typically involves the child failing to finish tasks, not seeming to listen, being easily distracted, having difficulty concentrating on schoolwork, and having difficulty sticking to a play activity. Impulsivity is often manifested as acting before thinking, shifting excessively from one activity to another, difficulty in organizing work, needing much supervision, frequently calling out in class, and difficulty awaiting a turn in games or group situations. Hyperactivity typically includes excessive running about or climbing on things, difficulty sitting still or staying seated, and excessive movement during sleep. Symptom presence and severity vary with the situation. It is unusual for a child to display signs of the disorder in all settings or even in the same setting at all times.[1] The onset of ADHD is typically by the age of 3 and must be by age 7, although the disorder may not require professional attention until the child enters school. Approximately 10% of boys and 2% of girls have ADHD, with the general prevalence in school-age children estimated at 6%.[2] It is necessary to differentiate the etiologies of the observed clinical behaviors. Inattention and distractibility can be symptoms of an anxiety and/or depressive disorder.[3] In addition, children with ADHD frequently present with comorbid anxiety, depression, learning deficiencies, and/or conduct/oppositional disorder.[4,5]

ETIOLOGY/PATHOPHYSIOLOGY

ADHD involves multiple etiologies. Family studies indicate a genetic component.[2] In addition, children with central nervous system (CNS) disorders including fetal alcohol syndrome, lead poisoning, and meningitis have a higher incidence of ADHD. Dietary causes are unlikely.[6] Early investigators proposed etiologies of under- or overarousal. More recently it has been proposed that ADHD is neither a high or low arousal state but a dysequilibratory disorder of the frontal-neostriatial dopamine systems with widely varying states of arousal. Children with ADHD tend to have phasic outbursts of activity and inactivity, resulting in insufficient alertness during dull and repetitive tasks, and overarousal at other times, resulting in ineffective performance. Stimulant drugs may serve as a homeostat to stabilize arousal and thereby temper the spontaneous fluctuations that are characteristic of ADHD.[7,8] The positive effect of the stimulants is not paradoxical and is not specific for ADHD because normal children also experience increased attention, decreased motor activity, and improvement on learning tasks when given stimulants.[9] Long-term studies indicate that a significant proportion of children with ADHD (30–70%) continue to have impulsivity and inattentiveness in adolescence and as adults.[8,10,11] Hyperactivity, however, does not usually present beyond middle childhood.

TREATMENT

The primary factor in the decision to initiate drug treatment is severity of symptoms. Drug treatment is reserved for moderate to severe symptom intensity; milder cases can often be successfully treated with environmental manipulation alone. Although drug treatment can often successfully ameliorate symptoms of ADHD and certain comorbid disorders, educational, social, and family consequences of this disorder need to be addressed by nondrug treatment approaches.

Stimulants are the most effective drug treatment options. Dextroamphetamine and methylphenidate are equally effective when a trial of either drug is given using wide dosage ranges.[12] Pemoline is either slightly less effective than or equal in efficacy to dextroamphetamine and methylphenidate. Caffeine has been found to be inferior in efficacy to dextroamphetamine, methylphenidate, and pemoline.[13,14]

Despite knowledge of the effects of stimulants on neurotransmitter activity, how these drugs affect the primary symptoms of ADHD is unclear. The CNS stimulants, in varying degrees, inhibit the reuptake of dopamine and norepinephrine; release dopamine, norepinephrine, and serotonin from the presynaptic neuron; or inhibit the enzyme monoamine oxidase (MAO). Because stimulants work through slightly different mechanisms, nonresponse to one stimulant does not preclude response to another.

Although initiation and dosage titration procedures vary, the following scheme is based on published recommendations of experienced clinicians.[15] The initial dose is 2.5 mg of dextroamphetamine or 5.0 mg methylphenidate. Drug response is maximal during the absorption phase, is evident in 15–30 minutes, and lasts 2–6 hours. Future dosing increments should be 2.5 and 5 mg, respectively. The dosing schedule can be determined by observing when the loss of positive drug effect occurs during the 2–6 hours after an oral dose. Most patients require a two- or three-times-daily dosing schedule due to the short half-lives: 2–4 hours for methylphenidate and approximately 6 hours for dextroamphetamine. Sustained-release products are reported to be either equally or less effective than short-acting products. The convenience of once-daily dosing must be weighed against the increased likelihood of difficulty falling asleep with sustained-release products.[16,17] The dose should be titrated for maximum individual efficacy and minimum side effects. Doses range from 0.3–1.0 mg/kg/d for methylphenidate. Maximum daily doses are 40 mg of dextroamphetamine and 60 mg of methylphenidate.

For pemoline, 18.75 mg is the usual starting dose and the amount of subsequent dosing increments, with optimal benefit usually achieved with 56.25 to 75 mg/d. The maximum dose of pemoline is 112.5 mg/d. The onset of action of pemoline is controversial. Recent observations suggest that when pemoline is initiated at higher doses 2–3 mg/kg/d or 56.25–75 mg/d, a clinical effect can be seen within 1–3 hours after dosing.[16,18] A potential advantage of pemoline is a longer duration of action, allowing once-daily dosing. Pemoline displays a wide interindividual variability in metabolism. The plasma half-life varies from 2–12 hours acutely and extends to 14–34 hours on chronic dosing. Pemoline may accumulate after weeks to months of chronic dosing.[19]

Imipramine and desipramine are the most systematically studied tricyclic antidepressants (TCAs) in the treatment of ADHD, although nortriptyline is also effective.[20] The onset of TCA effect occurs within the first 2 weeks, with full effect achieved by week three, but drug tolerance develops in many patients after several months of therapy. The initial dose of a TCA is 10 mg twice daily or 25 mg in the morning. Therapeutic doses of a TCA are 1–5 mg/kg/d administered in divided doses.[21] The variability in dosage requirements may be due to the tenfold interpatient variability in resultant drug plasma concentrations, which are achieved at a given dose.

TCAs are second-line alternatives to the stimulants for treatment of ADHD. The potential benefits of TCAs in comparison with stimulants include a longer duration of action, less sleep disturbance, reduced risk of abuse, lack of growth suppression, and reduced likelihood of exacerbating tics,[22] whereas their negative aspects include decreased efficacy, emergence of tolerance in some patients, more adverse effects, and the risk of death in overdose.[23]

Because stimulants inhibit the enzyme MAO, monoamine oxidase inhibitors (MAOIs) have been evaluated for their potential efficacy in ADHD. Tranylcypromine, a nonselective MAOI and clorgyline, an investigational drug specific for the MAO type A isoenzyme, have been compared with dextroamphetamine in the treatment of ADHD.[24] The MAOI's onset of activity and clinical efficacy were indistinguishable from that of dextroamphetamine. A preliminary study suggests that selegiline, a MAOI selective for isoenzyme B, is also effective in reducing the symptoms of ADHD in children with both ADHD and Tourette's disorder.[25]

Bupropion, a monocyclic antidepressant, is a weak dopamine uptake inhibitor with no significant direct effect on serotonin, norepinephrine, or MAO. Bupropion was compared to placebo in a 6-week controlled trial in 30 children with ADHD.[26] Bupropion was initiated at 3 mg/kg and titrated to 6 mg/kg over 15 days of therapy. The response to bupropion was better than placebo on the overall assessment and the hyperactivity rating scales, but the conduct rating scales did not improve. Bupropion is associated with exacerbation of tics and therefore should be used with caution in children with tics or a family history of tics.[27] In an open trial, fluoxetine, a selective serotonin reuptake inhibitor antidepressant, was associated with overall improvement in 11 of 19 children with ADHD who were considered refractory to stimulants and TCAs.[28] These studies point to the need for further investigations using more rigorous methodological design.

Clonidine, a central α_2-adrenergic agonist, inhibits noradrenergic activity by decreasing the release of norepinephrine from the presynaptic neuron. Clonidine reduces the firing rate of the locus coeruleus and decreases excessive arousal. A preliminary controlled study suggests that clonidine is more effective than placebo in reducing hyperactivity and impulsivity in children with ADHD.[29] Clonidine was initiated at 0.05 mg/d and increased by 0.05 mg every other day until a divided daily dose of 0.004–0.005 mg/kg was administered. Clonidine is an alternative to stimulants, particularly in children with comorbid tic disorder, extreme overactivity, or oppositional/conduct disorder.

Antipsychotic drugs decrease hyperactivity in ADHD but do not improve attention and concentration.[30] Although the pathophysiology of ADHD is controversial, a lack of dopamine activity in the CNS is the primary proposed etiology and, therefore, the use of dopamine-blocking drugs would appear to be disadvantageous. Major concerns with the use of antipsychotic drugs are the deleterious effects on learning and cognitive functioning and the potential for extrapyramidal effects such as dystonia and tardive dyskinesia. For most children, the disadvantages far outweigh any possible advantage.

In 1973, Feingold reported a significant reduction of hyperactivity with use of a diet free of salicylates and food additives.[31] Controlled studies indicate these diets are only occasionally efficacious; however, this directly contrasts with parental reports of dramatic improvements.[32] In 1982, a National Institutes of Health (NIH) Consensus Development Conference on Defined Diets and Childhood Hyperactivity concluded that defined diets should be described to parents as an option, although scientific evidence supports efficacy in only a small proportion of children.[33,34]

EVALUATION OF THERAPEUTIC OUTCOMES

Careful documentation of baseline symptoms and complaints over a 1-month predrug period is essential to the evaluation of therapeutic and adverse outcomes. Baseline symptoms can be measured using videotapes, clinician rating scales, or both. In addition, height, weight, and eating and sleeping patterns should be recorded. After the initiation and titration of any drug treatment, it is necessary that parents, teachers, and clinicians assess the overall functioning of the child to determine if significant therapeutic benefit justifies continuing the medication.

Therapeutic effects of the stimulants include decreased motor activity and impulsivity and increased attention span. In addition to behavioral effects, stimulants may improve cognitive performance (e.g., reading and arithmetic performance). Improved cognitive performance may result from an overall increase in attention and concentration, and may not be a specific effect on cognition.[8] This suggests that the stimulants are indicated for the target behaviors and not for primary learning disorders.

The benefits of drug therapy must outweigh the risks involved, namely, the adverse effects. Adverse effects, such as anorexia, insomnia, stomachaches, and headaches, are frequent but usually mild with stimulant use in children.[35] Anorexia and insomnia can be minimized with proper scheduling of doses. Although many children will have no appetite for breakfast, lunch and dinner can usually be minimally affected if the morning dose is given after breakfast and the last dose given near midday. Insomnia is specifically a delay in onset of sleep and can be minimized by adjusting the dosing schedule and/or the child's bedtime. Occasionally, insomnia persists so that dosage reduction is necessary. Headache and abdominal pain occur particularly in the first few weeks of drug treatment and can be treated with dosage reduction. Rare effects include hallucinations (visual or tactile) or delusions. A past history of motor tics or a family history of Tourette's syndrome is a relative contraindication to the use of stimulants, because they may unmask or exacerbate tics. Heart rate and blood pressure are increased with stimulants, but the magnitude is rarely of clinical importance.[12,36] Long-term use of pemoline may cause hepatotoxicity, elevated transaminases, and bilirubin or even cause hepatic failure.[37] Routine liver function tests are recommended every 3–6 months or as clinical symptoms warrant (fatigue, nausea, vomiting) during pemoline therapy.[36]

Growth suppression from stimulants represents the side effect of most concern. Proposed mechanisms of stimulant-induced growth suppression include alterations in growth hormone secretion and suppression of appetite leading to reduced calorie intake.[36] Some tolerance may develop after the first year, with growth catching up if treatment is interrupted. Heights and weights should be assessed every 3 months for all patients receiving stimulants.

A more controversial aspect of stimulant use concerns drug holidays and duration of treatment. Drug holidays are important because they provide time to reassess treatment and allow for growth catchup, if necessary. All children should be given a drug-free trial every year. One convenient method is to discontinue the drug during summer vacation and the first 2 weeks of school. If the drug must be restarted, then it can often be restarted and adjusted at a lower dose than was used at the end of the last school year. Drug dosage often varies from year to year, largely due to age-related pharmacokinetic changes. As a child develops, hepatic metabolism slows and volume of distribution increases.

TCAs are effective for control of behavior (impulsivity, hyperactivity) but they are not as effective as stimulants in increasing attention.[38] Stimulant nonresponders may improve on TCAs, but whether children who respond to the TCAs represent a subpopulation of ADHD is controversial and needs further investigation.[39,40] Children with ADHD and concurrent symptoms of conduct disorder, depression, or anxiety may respond better to a TCA than to stimulants, although it is controversial whether these additional symptoms respond or not.[40]

Therapeutic drug plasma concentrations for imipramine or desipramine have not been established in treating ADHD. Plasma level monitoring may be useful to detect noncompliance in addition to subtherapeutic or toxic levels. A plasma level less than 75 ng/mL may warrant a dose increase while plasma levels higher than 250 ng/mL may be associated with increased risk of toxicity. Parents should provide doses of TCAs throughout the week and not just during school days, because TCA withdrawal effects including nausea, vomiting, and diarrhea are common in children.

Common adverse effects of TCAs include sedation, anticholinergic, and cardiovascular effects. Anticholinergic effects include constipation, stomachache, dry mouth, and decreased appetite. Common cardiovascular effects include orthostatic hypotension and tachycardia,[41] whereas toxic effects include the potential for various arrhythmias and first-degree heart block. The effects of TCAs on the electrocardiogram (ECG) should be carefully monitored. Of more recent concern are reports of sudden death in three children taking desipramine for ADHD.[42] Desipramine plasma concentrations for these children were in the usually accepted therapeutic or subtherapeutic range documented for depression. Children and adolescents given TCAs should have pretreatment and follow-up ECGs to assess the effects of TCA therapy on cardiac rate and rhythm. Possible CNS effects include dizziness, aggressiveness, excitement, nightmares, insomnia, forgetfulness, and irritability. Signs of CNS toxicity are confusion, disorientation, impaired concentration, hallucinations, and delusions.

Despite comparable onset and efficacy to stimulants in treating ADHD, MAOIs are not routinely used. If MAOIs are given, caregivers and children need to be instructed regarding a low-tyramine diet and the need to avoid the use of sympathomimetic drugs. The ability of children to follow a low-tyramine diet in unsupervised situations is a concern.

Clonidine is a reasonable alternative treatment for children with ADHD, particularly if tics are present. The main side effect of clonidine is dose-dependent sedation that usually subsides after 2–3 weeks of therapy. Careful blood pressure monitoring is necessary. In one study of 10 children, the mean blood pressure dropped 10% and was associated with light-headedness upon standing or strenuous exertion.[29] One child with symptoms of mild depression became more tearful and unhappy on clonidine. Clonidine withdrawal was associated with marked deterioration in overall behavior.

SUMMARY

At this time, the best drug therapy for ADHD is either methylphenidate or dextroamphetamine. The TCAs are good options for those unresponsive to or unable to tolerate stimulants. Clonidine is a reasonable alternative, particularly if a tic disorder is present. Other agents, MAOIs, and fluoxetine require further investigation before their status in the treatment of ADHD can be fully determined.

ENURESIS

CLINICAL PRESENTATION/ ETIOLOGY/PATHOPHYSIOLOGY

The essential feature of enuresis is repeated involuntary or intentional voiding of urine by day or night not caused by any physical disorder. Rare physical causes of enuresis (e.g., diabetes mellitus, diabetes insipidus, seizure disorders, or urinary tract infections) should be ruled out. Diagnostic criteria for enuresis include the repeated voiding of urine that is characterized by either a frequency of at least twice per week for at least 3 months or the presence of clinically significant distress, or impairment in social, academic, or other important areas of functioning. The child must be at least 5 years of age.[1] There are two types of enuresis, primary and secondary. The most common type, primary enuresis, is diagnosed if the child has never established urinary continence. Secondary enuresis follows an established period (3–6 months) of urinary continence. At age 5, prevalence is 7% for boys and 3% for girls, and at age 10, it is 3% for boys and 2% for girls. The spontaneous remission rate is between 5 and 15% per year.[43] At age 18 only 1% of boys and virtually no girls still have the condition.[1]

Factors that predispose a child to either type of enuresis include a positive family history, delayed or lax toilet training, and psychosocial stress. The psychiatric disorders most commonly associated with enuresis are depression and developmental delays.[44] In addition, children with nocturnal enuresis lack the normal diurnal nighttime increase in antidiuretic hormone (ADH).[45] Nocturnal enuresis is not associated with a particular sleep stage; it typically occurs in the deeper stages of nonrapid eye movement (non-REM) sleep, but also can occur during the REM stage of sleep.[46]

TREATMENT

The first step in treating the child with enuresis is to educate the family about the high frequency of the problem, dispel any misconceptions, provide emotional support, and strongly discourage punishment.[47] For younger children who have not been properly toilet trained, the conditioning technique of dry bed training should be tried first. This technique encourages extra fluids during the day and restricts fluids close to bedtime. Children are encouraged to use the toilet before bedtime. If this method is unsuccessful, then a bedwetting alarm can be utilized. Teaching continence skills and various behavioral and conditioning methods remain the primary treatment for enuresis, and drug treatment remains a secondary approach.[48]

The exact mechanism of action of TCAs in treating enuresis is unknown; proposals include an anticholinergic effect, an α-adrenergic agonist effect, and an increase in ADH.[47] Imipramine is the most studied TCA, although desipramine, amitriptyline, and nortriptyline are also effective. For children 6 years and older, the initial dose of imipramine should be 25 mg at bedtime, with weekly increases of 25 mg, if necessary. A nightly dose greater than 75 mg is rarely necessary, although doses up to 150 mg have been required in teenagers.

Desmopressin acetate, a synthetic analogue of the natural human ADH, arginine vasopressin, is currently available in a nasal spray for the treatment of nocturnal enuresis. Desmopressin raises overnight urinary osmotic concentration by increasing water reabsorption and reducing the volume of urine entering the bladder. For children 6 years of age and older, the initial recommended nasal dose is 20 mcg at bedtime, increasing to 40 mcg per night after 3 days if there is no response. Some patients may respond to as little as 10 mcg. One-half of each dose is administered in each nostril. About 10% of the dose of desmopressin is absorbed from the nasal mucosa; plasma concentrations reach a maximum about 45 minutes after administration. Biologic half-life is 4–6 hours, and the duration of action varies from 6–24 hours.[49]

EVALUATION OF THERAPEUTIC OUTCOMES

Before treatment begins, an accurate baseline of bedwetting frequency must be obtained. It usually takes 3–4 months of using a bedwetting alarm to stop bedwetting, but more than 70% of the children are cured using this method. Drug treatment is necessary when nondrug methods fail. Drug therapy is preferred when intermittent treatment is desired, for example, while camping or on overnight trips away from home. Unfortunately, therapeutic efficacy does not extend beyond drug administration.[50] If drug treatment is required for more than several weeks, attempts to discontinue the drug every 3–6 months are advisable to assess for spontaneous remission.

TCA efficacy is often immediate and is usually evident within 7 days. Drug plasma concentrations of imipramine plus desipramine do correlate with clinical response, and although individual variation exists, a higher percentage of patients responds to higher plasma levels.[51] In addition, true nonresponders exist at therapeutic doses.[52] Imipramine efficacy is about 85%; one-half of patients experience total elimination of bedwetting, and the other half, a significant decrease in the number of episodes. An initially effective dose often becomes ineffective in 2–6 weeks, but increasing the dose usually re-establishes control. One week is needed to evaluate the efficacy of a new dose. Refer to ADHD and the TCAs for monitoring parameters and adverse effects.

Desmopressin is effective in reducing the number of wet nights in 70% of children. In short-term, 2-week studies, 24.5% of children became completely dry.[53] The best response rate to desmopressin appears to occur in children older than 9 years.[54] Patients with colds or allergies that affect the nasal mucosa may have a less-than-optimal response to desmopressin.[55] Infrequent adverse effects include nasal irritation, epistaxis, rhinitis, nasal congestion, transient headache, chills, dizziness, nausea, and abdominal pain. Rare effects of water intoxication, hyponatremia, and subsequent tonic–clonic seizures have been reported in children with concurrent physical disorders, intentional overdoses, or excessive fluid intake.[56]

SUMMARY

Overall, both TCAs and desmopressin are effective in the treatment of nocturnal enuresis as long as the drug is maintained. Drug selection is based on adverse effect profiles, ease of administration, and cost. Imipramine has a higher incidence of adverse effects than desmopressin, and the risk of accidental TCA overdose is of concern, especially in very disorganized families. In contrast, desmopressin nasal spray requires a specific administration technique and is markedly more expensive than imipramine.

Tourette's Disorder

CLINICAL PRESENTATION

Once considered rare, this CNS disorder is present in as many as 1 out of every 100 male children and 1 out of every 800 female children.[57] The essential features of Tourette's disorder are multiple motor tics and one or more vocalizations. A tic is a sudden, rapid, recurrent, nonrhythmic, stereotyped motor movement or vocalization. A motor tic includes eye blinking, facial twitching, lip licking, shoulder shrugging, moving hair out of eyes, and coughing. A vocal tic includes throat clearings, hissing, barking, snorting, echolalia, and coprolalia.[1] Any or all of these motor and vocal tics may be voluntarily suppressed from minutes to hours. The clinical presentation may vary from just noticeable to debilitating, and the type of tic expressed may change over time.[58]

Presence of both motor and vocal tics are necessary for more than 1 year before the diagnosis of Tourette's disorder is made. The median age of onset of motor tics is 7 years, with most patients having the onset of symptoms before age 14. Transient tic disorder is diagnosed if motor or vocal tics occur for less than 1 year. If either motor or vocal tics are present for longer than 1 year, chronic motor or vocal tic disorder is diagnosed.[1]

ETIOLOGY/PATHOPHYSIOLOGY

Tourette's disorder is genetically transmitted in an autosomal dominant pattern, however, the symptoms and severity of the disorder vary from one generation to another.[1] Several behavioral disorders commonly occur in association with Tourette's disorder including ADHD (50% of cases) and obsessive–compulsive disorder (40% of cases). Family studies of Tourette's disorder show that obsessive–compulsive disorder is genetically related, while ADHD may or may not be.[57,58] Tourette's disorder itself does not cause diminished intellectual functioning, however, the severity of tics and associated attentional and behavioral disorders can result in impaired neuropsychological performance.[59] The neurochemical pathophysiology involves an imbalance in the interaction of dopaminergic, serotonergic, and noradrenergic systems in multiple brain regions. The imbalance may cause a lack of regulation of the brain's inhibitory mechanisms, resulting in tics and associated behavior disorders. This multisystem etiology best explains the success of a variety of effective treatment options.[57,60]

TREATMENT

Whenever symptoms are severe enough to impair the child's ability to function or whenever symptoms are particularly troublesome to the child, drug therapy should be initiated. The drug of choice for Tourette's disorder is controversial. Many clinicians choose haloperidol or pimozide first because they are FDA approved and highly effective with a relatively rapid onset. Other clinicians suggest giving a trial of clonidine first in order to avoid possible extrapyramidal side effects, particularly the risk of tardive dyskinesia. Psychotherapy and behavior management are useful adjuncts.

Although other high potency neuroleptics can be effective in relieving tics, haloperidol is the most appropriate choice for Tourette's disorder because it is low in sedation, cardiovascular, and anticholinergic effects.[57,60] Haloperidol's efficacy in Tourette's disorder may be due to central dopamine-2 receptor blocking effects in the basal ganglia or the indirect effect such blockade has on facilitation of serotonergic function.[57] Despite its long history of use, there is only one adequately controlled study supporting the efficacy and superiority of haloperidol over placebo.[61] Haloperidol is effective in decreasing the frequency of tics but has limited or no effect on comorbid disorders such as ADHD.

Therapy with haloperidol should be initiated at very low doses of 0.25–0.5 mg/d given at bedtime and then increased gradually. The therapeutic effects of haloperidol are typically sustained enough to permit once-daily dosing, however, on occasion, divided doses are required for a more continuous control of tics. Gradual titration over 2–3 weeks helps minimize extrapyramidal and sedative effects while permitting careful assessment of response. Symptoms may regress within 48–72 hours after dosage initiation. Doses less than 5 mg/d are effective in controlling tics for most patients, but occasionally doses approaching 10 mg/d are required.[57,61]

Approved for marketing in the United States in 1984 as an orphan drug, pimozide represents an alternative to haloperidol for Tourette's disorder. Like haloperidol, pimozide causes central dopamine-2 receptor blockade, which can modulate serotonergic functioning. Unlike haloperidol, it causes calcium channel antagonism, which may contribute to its greater association with ECG abnormalities. Pimozide is one-half as potent as haloperidol. The starting dose is higher, 0.5 to 1 mg/d with gradual increase to 10 mg if needed. The maximum daily dose is

0.3 mg/kg/d or 20 mg/d. Its elimination half-life in children with Tourette's disorder ranges from 24–142 hours, allowing once-daily dosing. Most efficacy studies show pimozide to be equal or slightly less effective than haloperidol.[57,61]

Clonidine response rates vary from 20–70% in clinical studies, and it is generally effective for approximately half of Tourette's disorder patients.[57,62,63] In some patients the response is limited to attentional and behavioral problems with no changes in the frequency of tics. Clonidine's mechanism of action in treating Tourette's disorder is unknown, but as an α-adrenergic agonist, it modulates serotonergic, dopaminergic, noradrenergic, and opioid systems. Clonidine is generally well tolerated in healthy children as long as treatment is initiated with a single test dose, usually 0.05 mg given in the morning with gradual titration every 4–7 days to the usual therapeutic dose of 0.15–0.25 mg/d. Doses usually need to be divided during maintenance therapy for more continuous symptom control and to minimize adverse effects. The onset of therapeutic effects is slow, ranging from 2 weeks to a few months. Though not well studied, Comings[57,64] recommends the clonidine patch over oral dosage forms. The starting dose is one-fourth of a 0.1-mg transdermal patch applied every 4–7 days, then gradually increased over weeks to months as needed. Comings suggests that the patch can be effective when oral doses are not.

EVALUATION OF THERAPEUTIC OUTCOMES

Once a drug is selected, Comings'[57] general principles for pharmacological management of patients with Tourette's disorder are useful: (1) Tourette's disorder patients are very sensitive to medication. Medication should be started at a very low dose with gradual (weekly) dosage increases as tolerated. (2) A plateau effect is normal. A patient may be quite sensitive to the effects of a medicine, and tics may remit at a very low dose. However, as the body adjusts to this state, tics may slowly return, requiring upward adjustments after 2–4 weeks. (3) The treatment goal is not necessarily total elimination of all tics. (4) If tics disappear for a number of weeks, the dose can be decreased. Tics can spontaneously disappear for weeks to months at a time. If the tics reappear, the medication can be increased gradually. (5) Medication should not be abruptly stopped. Withdrawal effects can be intolerable in children.

Medication does not impair neuropsychological performance according to one controlled study; however, the assessment of the individual risk versus benefit is necessary.[65] The use of regular videotaped assessments in conjunction with a standardized rating scale (Yale Global Tic Severity Scale) is helpful in objectively evaluating symptoms and side effects.[66] Adult patients with Tourette's disorder may still be responsive to drug treatments that were effective during childhood, although the dose and schedule may require adjustment.[57,60]

Common side effects of the antipsychotics include drowsiness, weight gain, and extrapyramidal effects including dyskinesias, dystonias, akathisia, akinesia, and pseudoparkinsonism. These side effects have been reported to occur in almost all patients once haloperidol doses of 2 mg/d or greater are used. Because extrapyramidal side effects can mimic symptoms of Tourette's disorder and impair the child's ability to function, frequent attempts to lower the dose are warranted. If the dose cannot be lowered, then an anti-Parkinsonian agent such as benztropine (at a starting dose of 0.5 mg orally twice daily) will generally reverse side effects. Discontinuation of the anti-Parkinsonian agent should be attempted after 4 weeks of effective treatment of extrapyramidal symptoms. Whether a patient with Tourette's disorder is developing a new symptom or is developing tardive dyskinesia can be very difficult to determine. Dosage titration of the medication and careful monitoring will assist in this clinical decision-making process. Additional side effects of haloperidol include dysphoria, crying spells, irritability, social withdrawal, fearfulness, preoccupation with morbid subject matter, whiny or clinging behavior, and phobic symptoms.

Pimozide was originally proposed to offer an alternative to haloperidol with fewer adverse effects (e.g., extrapyramidal effects and cognitive impairment), but this has not been demonstrated. Pimozide also commonly causes anticholinergic effects. ECG changes, including T- and U-wave abnormalities and prolongation of the QT (corrected) interval, are rarely found in recommended therapeutic doses for Tourette's disorder, however, patients given pimozide should receive baseline and follow-up ECGs. Some clinicians continue to recommend pimozide for patients who become too sedated on haloperidol because, subjectively, some patients prefer it.[57,60] Patients with Tourette's disorder may be more susceptible to all side effects of antipsychotic drugs than children or adults treated for psychotic disorders.[57,60,67] Abrupt discontinuation of haloperidol or pimozide can result in worsening of Tourette's symptoms and withdrawal dyskinesia for as long as 2–3 months.

For clonidine, the most common adverse effect is sedation. Fortunately, tolerance usually develops to this effect over days to weeks. The most potentially serious side effect is orthostatic hypotension, which requires careful blood pressure monitoring and dosage adjustments. Other side effects include dry mouth, headache, mood changes, and even a temporary worsening of tics in 10% of patients. The clonidine patch has the additional adverse effect of skin irritation, which can be minimized by changing the position of the patch every few days or pretreating the skin with beclomethazone dipropionate aerosolized spray.[68] Clonidine should never be abruptly discontinued due to the risk of rebound hypertension and abrupt re-emergence of tics.[62] Gradual tapering at 5- to 7-day intervals prevents withdrawal symptoms.

COMORBIDITY/ALTERNATIVES

When Tourette's disorder coexists with other behavioral disorders, the pharmacotherapy can be more challenging, possibly requiring medication combinations. Often the behavioral problems precede and are more disturbing than the involuntary movements. The use of stimulant drugs that increase dopaminergic activity often aggravates or precipitates tics. Interestingly, the clinical use of methylphenidate in patients with Tourette's disorder has no predictable result; tics may be exacerbated, reduced, or remain unchanged. Patients and caregivers should be aware of the risks of using stimulants in children with Tourette's, and careful monitoring is essential.[69]

Clonidine is an effective alternative to stimulants in the treatment of children with Tourette's disorder and ADHD. A review of 54 children with ADHD treated over a 4-year period showed that children with a comorbid tic disorder more frequently had a positive response to clonidine.[70] In another investigation, clonazepam demonstrated efficacy in decreasing tics to an acceptable level in seven patients in whom ADHD was under control with clonidine. Clonazepam was well tolerated at doses of 0.5–1.0 mg/d with only mild sedation and no behavioral disinhibition.[71] Guanfacine, a central α-adrenergic agonist with a longer half-life than clonidine, is under study. Clearly, further investigations are needed to determine the most effective and safest method of treating Tourette's disorder with ADHD.

Fluoxetine treatment of comorbid Tourette's disorder and obsessive–compulsive disorder is under investigation. In an open trial, 10 patients took 20–40 mg/d of fluoxetine for at least 6 weeks and one-half were considered responders.[72] Another small but better controlled study evaluated fluoxetine doses of 20–40 mg/d in 11 children older than 4 months. Some improvement was noted in tic severity, attentional abilities, and social functioning; however, obsessive–compulsive symptoms remained largely unchanged.[73] Both studies revealed high incidences (20–40%) of mild to moderate behavioral agitation or activation; otherwise, fluoxetine was well tolerated.

Several case reports have demonstrated the positive effects of the calcium channel antagonists in Tourette's disorder; however, well-controlled studies are needed before these agents can be recommended.[74] Nicotine administration by gum or patch may potentiate the effects of haloperidol in relieving tics according to small open trials and case reports. The adverse effects of nicotine on overall health may limit usefulness and, clearly, further investigations are needed.[75]

SUMMARY

At this time the best approach for the treatment of Tourette's disorder is either haloperidol or clonidine. Haloperidol has the advantage of greater efficacy and rapid onset, while the advantage of clonidine is its lack of extrapyramidal side effects. Drug treatment must be highly individualized, considering comorbid disorders and side-effect sensitivity.

REFERENCES

1. American Psychiatric Association. Diagnostic and Statistical Manual of Mental Disorders, 4th ed (DSM-IV). Washington, DC, Author, 1994, pp 37–121.
2. Popper CW. Disorders usually first evident in infancy, childhood, or adolescence, in Talbott JA, Hales RE, Yudofsky SC, (eds): Textbook of Psychiatry. Washington, DC, American Psychiatric Press, 1988, pp 649–735.
3. Halperin JM, Matier K, Bedi G, et al. Specificity of inattention, impulsivity and hyperactivity to the diagnosis of attention-deficit hyperactivity disorder. J Am Acad Child Adolesc Psychiatry 1992;31:190–196.
4. Jensen PS, Shervette RE, Xenakis SN, Richters J. Anxiety and depressive disorders in attention deficit disorder with hyperactivity: New findings. Am J Psychiatry 1993;150:1203–1209.
5. Biederman J, Newcorn J, Sprich S. Comorbidity of attention deficit hyperactivity disorder with conduct, depressive, anxiety and other disorders. Am J Psychiatry 1991;148:564–577.
6. Wolraich ML, Lindgren SD, Stumbo PJ, et al. Effects of diets high in sucrose or aspartame on the behavior and cognitive performance of children. N Engl J Med 1994;330:301–307.
7. Evans RW, Gualtieri CT, Hicks RE. A neuropathic substrate for stimulant drug effects in hyperactive children. Clin Neuropharmacol 1986;9:264–281.
8. Jacobvitz D, Sroufe LA, Stewart M, Leffert N. Treatment of attentional and hyperactivity problems in children with sympathomimetic drugs: A comprehensive review. J Am Acad Child Adolesc Psychiatry 1990;29:677–688.
9. Rapoport JL, Buchsbaum MS, Weingartner H, et al. Dextroamphetamine: Its cognitive and behavioral effects in normal and hyperactive boys and normal men. Arch Gen Psychiatry 1980;37:933–943.
10. Bellak L, Black RB. Attention-deficit hyperactivity disorder in adults. Clinical Therap 1992;14:138–147.
11. Mannuzza S, Klein RG, Bessler A, et al. Adult outcome of hyperactive boys: Educational achievement, occupational rank and psychiatric status. Arch Gen Psychiatry 1993;50:565–576.
12. Calis KA, Grothe DR, Elia J. Attention-deficit hyperactivity disorder. Clin Pharm 1990;9:632–642.
13. Arnold LE, Christopher J, Huestis R, Smeltzer DJ. Methylphenidate vs dextroamphetamine vs caffeine in minimal brain dysfunction. Arch Gen Psychiatry 1978;35:463–473.

14. Firestone P, Davey J, Goodman JT, Peters S. The effects of caffeine and methylphenidate on hyperactive children. J Am Acad Child Psychiatry 1978;17:445–456.
15. Barkley RA, DuPaul GJ, Costello A. Stimulants, in Werry JS, Aman MG (eds): Practitioners Guide to Psychoactive Drugs for Children and Adolescents. New York, Plenum Publishing, 1993, pp 224–227.
16. Pelham WE, Greenslade KE, Vodde-Hamilton M, et al. Relative efficacy of long-acting stimulants on children with ADHD: A comparison of standard methylphenidate, sustained-release methylphenidate, sustained-release dextroamphetamine, and pemoline. Pediatrics 1990;86:226–237.
17. Fitzpatrick PA, Klorman R, Brumaghim JT, Borgstedt AD. Effects of sustained-release and standard preparations of methylphenidate on attention deficit disorder. J Am Acad Child Adolesc Psychiatry 1992;31:226–234.
18. Sallee FR, Stiller RL, Perel JM. Pharmacodynamics of pemoline in attention deficit disorder with hyperactivity. J Am Acad Child Adolesc Psychiatry 1992;31:244–251.
19. Sallee F, Stiller R, Perel J, Bates T. Oral pemoline kinetics in hyperactive children. Clin Pharmacol Ther 1985;37:606–609.
20. Wilens TE, Biederman J, Geist DE, et al. Nortriptyline in the treatment of ADHD: A chart review of 58 cases. J Am Acad Child Adolesc Psychiatry 1993;32:343–349.
21. Biederman J, Baldessarini RJ, Wright V, et al. A double-blind placebo controlled study of desipramine in the treatment of ADD: I. Efficacy. J Am Acad Child Adolesc Psychiatry 1989;28:777–784.
22. Riddle MA, Hardin MT, Cho SC, et al. Desipramine treatment of boys with attention-deficit hyperactivity disorder and tics: Preliminary clinical experience. J Am Acad Child Adolesc Psychiatry 1988;27:811–814.
23. Spencer T, Biederman J, Wilens T, et al. Nortriptyline treatment of children with attention-deficit hyperactivity disorder and tic disorder or Tourette's syndrome. J Am Acad Child Adolesc Psychiatry 1993;32:205–210.
24. Zametkin A, Rapoport JL, Murphy DL, et al. Treatment of hyperactive children with monoamine oxidase inhibitors: I. Clinical efficacy. Arch Gen Psychiatry 1985;42:962–966.
25. Jankovic J. Deprenyl in attention deficit associated with Tourette's syndrome. Arch Neurol 1993;50:286–288.
26. Casat CD, Pleasants DZ, Van Wyck Fleet J. A double-blind trial of bupropion in children with attention deficit disorder. Psychopharmacol Bull 1987;23:120–122.
27. Spencer T, Biederman J, Steingard R, Wilens T. Bupropion exacerbates tics in children with attention-deficit hyperactivity disorder and Tourette's syndrome. J Am Acad Child Adolesc Psychiatry 1993;32:211–214.
28. Barrickman L, Noyes R, Kuperman S, et al. Treatment of ADHD with fluoxetine: A preliminary trial. J Am Acad Child Adolesc Psychiatry 1991;30:762–767.
29. Hunt RD, Minderaa RB, Cohen DJ. The therapeutic effect of clonidine in attention deficit disorder with hyperactivity: A comparison with placebo and methylphenidate. Psychopharmacol Bull 1986;22:229–236.
30. Rapoport J, Abramson A, Alexander D, Lott, I. Playroom observations of hyperactive children on medication. J Am Acad Child Psychiatry 1971;10:524–534.
31. Feingold BF. Why Your Child Is Hyperactive. New York, Random House, 1975.
32. Mattes JA, Gittelman R. Effects of artificial food colorings in children with hyperactive symptoms. A critical review and results of a controlled study. Arch Gen Psychiatry 1981;38:714–718.
33. National Institutes of Health Consensus Development Conference, Vol. 4, No. 3. Defined Diets and Childhood Hyperactivity. Bethesda, MD, National Institutes of Health, 1982.
34. Carter CM, Urbanowicz M, Hemsley R, et al. Effects of a few foods in attention deficit disorder. Arch Dis Child 1993;69:564–568.
35. Barkley RA, McMurray MB, Edelbrock CS, Robbins K. Side effects of methylphenidate in children with attention deficit hyperactivity disorder: A systemic, placebo-controlled evaluation. Pediatrics 1990;86:184–192.
36. Greenhill LL. Pharmacologic treatment of attention deficit hyperactivity disorder. Psychiatr Clin North Am 1992;15:1–27.
37. Pratt DS, Dubois RS. Hepatotoxicity due to pemoline: A report of two cases. J Pediatr Gastroenterol Nutr 1990;10:239–241.
38. Rapport MD, Carlson GA, Kelly KL, Pataki C. Methylphenidate and desipramine in hospitalized children: I. Separate and combined effects on cognitive function. J Am Acad Child Adolesc Psychiatry 1993;32:333–342.
39. Biederman J, Baldessarini RJ, Wright V, et al. A double-blind placebo controlled study of desipramine in the treatment of ADD: III. Lack of impact of comorbidity and family history factors on clinical response. J Am Acad Child Adolesc Psychiatry 1993;32:199–204.
40. Pliszka SR. Tricyclic antidepressants in the treatment of children with attention deficit disorder. J Amer Acad Child Adolesc Psychiatry 1987;26:127–132.
41. Biederman J, Baldessarini RJ, Wright V, et al. A double-blind placebo controlled study of desipramine in the treatment of ADD: II. Serum drug levels and cardiovascular findings. J Am Acad Child Adolesc Psychiatry 1989;28:903–911.
42. Riddle MA, Nelson JC, Kleinman CS, et al. Sudden death in children receiving norpramin: A review of three reported cases and commentary. J Am Acad Child Adolesc Psychiatry 1991;30:104–108.
43. Forsythe WI, Redmond A. Enuresis and spontaneous cure rate: Study of 1129 enuretics. Arch Dis Child 1974;49:259–263.
44. Garfinkel BD. The elimination disorders, in Garfinkel BD, Carlson GA, Weller EB, (eds): Psychiatric Disorders in Children and Adolescents. Philadelphia, WB Saunders, 1990, pp 325–336.
45. Norgaard JP, Rittig S, Djurhuus JC. Nocturnal enuresis: An approach to treatment based on pathogenesis. J Pediatr 1989;114:705–710.
46. Mikkelsen EJ, Rapoport JL, Nee L, et al. Childhood enuresis. I. Sleep patterns and psychopathology. Arch Gen Psychiatry 1980;37:1139–1144.
47. Miller K, Atkin B, Moody ML. Drug therapy for nocturnal enuresis. Drugs 1992;44:47–56.
48. Kaplan SL, Breit M, Gauthier B, Busner J. A comparison of three noctural enuresis treatment methods. J Am Acad Child Adolesc Psychiatry 1989;28:282–286.

49. Richardson DW, Robinson AG. Desmopressin. Ann Intern Med 1985;103:228–239.
50. Wille S. Comparison of desmopressin and enuresis alarm for nocturnal enuresis. Arch Dis Child 1986;61:30–33.
51. Fritz GK, Rockney RM, Yeung AS. Plasma levels and efficacy of imipramine treatment for enuresis. J Am Acad Child Adolesc Psychiatry 1994;33:60–64.
52. Rapoport JL, Mikkelsen EJ, Zavadil A, et al. Childhood enuresis II. Psychopathology, tricyclic concentration in plasma, and antienuretic effect. Arch Gen Psychiatry 1980;37:1146–1152.
53. Moffatt ME, Harlos S, Kirshen AJ, Burd L. Desmopressin acetate and nocturnal enuresis: How much do we know? Pediatrics 1993;92:420–425.
54. Dimson SB. DDAVP and urine osmolality in refractory enuresis. Arch Dis Child 1986;61:1104–1107.
55. Miller K, Goldberg S, Atkin B. Nocturnal enuresis: Experience with long-term use of intranasally administered desmopressin. J Pediatr 1989;114:723–726.
56. Bamford MF, Cruickshank G. Dangers of intranasal desmopressin for nocturnal enuresis. J Royal College Gen Pract 1989;39:345–346.
57. Comings DE. Tourette Syndrome and Human Behavior. Duarte, CA, Hope Press, 1990, pp 1–792.
58. Cohen DJ, Leckman JF. Developmental psychopathology and neurobiology of Tourette's syndrome. J Am Acad Child Adolesc Psychiatry 1994;33:2–15.
59. Randolph C, Hyde TM, Gold JM, et al. Tourette's syndrome in monozygotic twins. Arch Neurol 1993;50:725–728.
60. Cohen DJ, Riddle MA, Leckman JF. Pharmacotherapy of Tourette's syndrome and associated disorders. Psychiatr Clin North Am 1992;15:109–129.
61. Shapiro E, Shapiro AK, Fulop G, et al. Controlled study of haloperidol, pimozide, and placebo for the treatment of Gilles de la Tourette's syndrome. Arch Gen Psychiatry 1989;46:722–730.
62. Cohen DJ, Detlor J, Young JG, Shaywitz BA. Clonidine ameliorates Gilles de la Tourette's syndrome. Arch Gen Psychiatry 1980;37:1350–1357.
63. Goetz CG, Tanner CM, Wilson RS, et al. Clonidine and Gilles de la Tourette's syndrome: Double blind study using objective rating methods. Ann Neurol 1987;21:307–310.
64. Comings DE, Comings BG, Tacket T, Li SZ. The clonidine patch and behavior problems [letter]. J Am Acad Child Adolesc Psychiatry 1990;29:667–668.
65. Bornstein RA, Yang V. Neuropsychological performance in medicated and unmedicated patients with Tourette's disorder. Am J Psychiatry 1991;148:468–471.
66. Leckman JF, Riddle MA, Hardin MT, et al. The Yale global tic severity scale: I Initial testing of a clinician-rated scale of tic severity. J Am Acad Child Adolesc Psychiatry 1989;28:566–573.
67. Bruun RD. Subtle and underrecognized side effects of neuroleptic treatment in children with Tourette's disorder. Am J Psychiatry 1988;145:621–624.
68. McChesney JA. Preventing the contact dermatitis caused by a transdermal clonidine patch. Western J Med 1991;154:736.
69. Sverd J, Gadow KD, Paolicelli LM, et al. Methylphenidate treatment of attention-deficit hyperactivity disorder in boys with Tourette's syndrome. J Am Acad Child Adolesc Psychiatry 1989;28:574–579.
70. Steingard R, Biederman J, Spencer T, et al. Comparison of clonidine response in the treatment of attention-deficit hyperactivity disorder with and without comorbid tic disorders. J Am Acad Child Adolesc Psychiatry 1993;32:350–353.
71. Steingard RJ, Goldberg M, Lee D, DeMaso DR. Adjunctive clonazepam treatment of tic symptoms in children with comorbid tic disorders and ADHD. J Am Acad Child Adolesc Psychiatry 1994;33:394–399.
72. Riddle MA, Hardin MT, King R, et al. Fluoxetine treatment of children and adolescents with Tourette's and obsessive compulsive disorders: Preliminary clinical experience. J Am Acad Child Adolesc Psychiatry 1990;29:45–48.
73. Kurlan R, Como PG, Deeley C, et al. A pilot controlled study of fluoxetine for obsessive compulsive symptoms in children with Tourette's syndrome. Clin Neuropharmacol 1993;16:167–172.
74. Walsh TL, Lavenstein B, Licamele WL, et al. Calcium antagonists in the treatment of Tourette's disorder. Am J Psychiatry 1986;143:1467–1468.
75. McConville BJ, Fogelson MH, Norman AB, et al. Nicotine potentiation of haloperidol in reducing tic frequency in Tourette's disorder. Am J Psychiatry 1991;148:793–794.

Chapter 63

Eating Disorders

Patricia A. Marken, BSPharm, PharmD, and Roger W. Sommi, PharmD

The initial descriptions of anorexia nervosa (AN) were published over a century ago[1,2]; however, bulimia nervosa (BN) was only recently described as a distinct disorder.[3] Recently, extensive research has significantly improved our understanding of these severely disabling and potentially fatal disorders. Once thought to be primary disorders of the pituitary gland or variants of another psychiatric disorder (e.g., depression or obsessive–compulsive disorder), eating disorders may encompass several biologic, psychologic, and developmental etiologies. Unfortunately, pharmacologic management of these disorders remains disappointing.

EPIDEMIOLOGY

ANOREXIA NERVOSA

AN occurs predominantly in females (95%), and usually presents in late adolescence.[4] Most patients develop the disorder before the age of 25.[5]

The reported prevalence of AN in the United States ranges from 1 in 100 to 1 in 800 for females between the ages of 12–18 years.[4] The prevalence of AN may have increased over time, as noted by one epidemiologic study that reported a sixfold increase in the number of documented cases of AN for the period of 1970–1976 compared with the period of 1960–1969.[6] A study of 300 suburban female shoppers showed that 0.7% suffered from AN at some point in time.[7]

BULIMIA NERVOSA

BN also occurs predominantly in females (90%), and usually presents in adolescence or early adult life.[4] This disorder has been studied primarily in college students and, therefore, knowledge of its prevalence may be limited by the lack of data from other populations. Overall, studies report that between 8 and 20% of young females and 0.5 and 2% of young males meet diagnostic criteria for BN.[8] The wide discrepancies in these prevalence figures is most likely due to changes in the diagnostic criteria for BN that have occurred since the mid-1980s.

EATING DISORDER NOT OTHERWISE SPECIFIED/BINGE EATING DISORDER

Recognizing that the current taxonomy of eating disorders does not encompass all potential presentations, the American Psychiatric Association's *Diagnostic and Statistical Manual of Mental Disorders,* 4th ed. (DSM-IV) includes the diagnosis of eating disorder not otherwise specified (NOS).[4] Individuals with eating disorder NOS manifest symptoms characteristic of eating disorders (e.g., persistent concern over body image), but they do not meet the diagnostic criteria for a specific eating disorder. In addition, research diagnostic criteria have been established for further consideration and elaboration of a binge-eating disorder (BED). The diagnostic criteria for BED describe binge eating without the purging behavior requisite for the bulimia diagnosis. The epidemiology of these disorders is unknown, but is likely to be reflective of eating disorders in general—affecting primarily adolescent to young adult females and upper-middle- and middle-class students.[9] The increased recognition of variants and subtypes will likely result in an overall increase in the reported prevalence of eating disorders.

CLINICAL PRESENTATION

Figure 63.1 lists the common clinical signs and symptoms for AN and BN. Definitive diagnosis is often difficult in patients presenting with symptoms of both disorders because of the number of overlapping signs and symptoms. Many patients initially present with either AN or BN and alternate from one eating disorder to the other along a continuum of symptoms between the disorders. The clinician should pay particular attention to these fluctuations and alter therapy accordingly, because patients with AN and BN respond differently to treatment interventions.

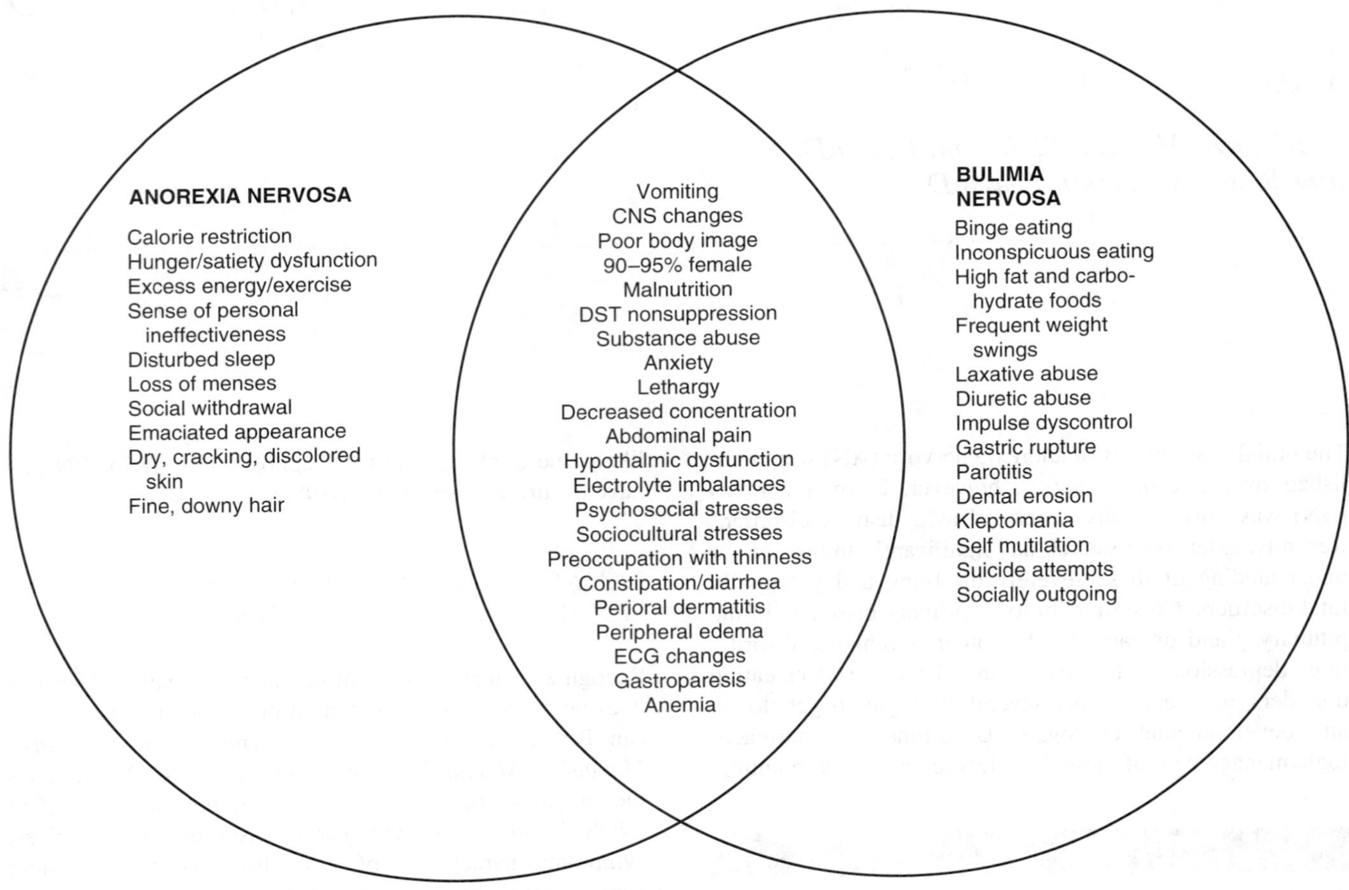

Figure 63.1. Signs and symptoms of anorexia nervosa and bulimia nervosa.

The medical consequences of an eating disorder are vast and are related primarily to self-induced starvation and chronic vomiting. Patients commonly present with vague complaints of lethargy and pain. Metabolic and electrolyte disturbances and dehydration are common and occur because of poor dietary intake, self-induced vomiting, or chronic laxative or diuretic abuse. Severe electrolyte disturbances may result in cardiac disturbances and even sudden death. Abnormalities of the hypothalamic-pituitary axes are also common and are likely the result of starvation. These abnormalities include effects on estradiol, the gonadotropins [luteinizing hormone (LH), follicle stimulating hormone (FSH), and gonadotropin releasing hormone (GnRH)], thyroid function, adrenal function, and growth hormone.[10] Vomiting can result in oral and dental problems, leading to decalcification, erosion of the enamel and dentin layers, and staining of the surfaces of the teeth.[11]

Eating abnormalities are present in other psychiatric disorders such as depression, schizophrenia, obsessive–compulsive disorders, and conversion disorders. These disorders should be included in the differential diagnosis of AN and BN, and the clinician should be alert to symptoms of irritability, moodiness, and social withdrawal that may precede or coincide with the changes in weight or eating behavior.[12] The salient difference between these psychiatric disorders and eating disorders is the overriding drive for thinness, a disturbed body image, increased energy level directed toward losing weight, and binge-eating episodes that are relatively specific for the eating disorders. Many patients will experience relief of the psychiatric symptoms upon refeeding, while others may find relief of depressive symptoms with antidepressant medication.[9]

Psychiatric comorbidity occurs in patients with eating disorders and includes depression, substance abuse (especially alcohol and stimulant abuse), and kleptomania (impulsive stealing not necessarily due to need or value of object stolen), particularly in patients with BN. Eating disorder patients commonly have a history of physical and sexual abuse. Attention should be given to these psychiatric complications when diagnostic and treatment decisions are considered.

ANOREXIA NERVOSA

The DSM-IV diagnostic criteria for AN are listed in Table 63.1.[4] The essential features include refusal to maintain a minimal normal body weight, intense fear and obsession

TABLE 63.1. DSM-IV DIAGNOSTIC CRITERIA FOR ANOREXIA NERVOSA AND BULIMIA NERVOSA

Anorexia Nervosa:

1. Refusal to maintain body weight over a minimal normal weight for age and height; or failure to make expected weight gain during period of growth, leading to a body weight 15% lower than expected normal weight for age and height.
2. Intense fear of gaining weight or becoming fat, even though underweight.
3. Disturbance in the way one's body weight, size, or shape is experienced, undue influence of body weight or shape on self-evaluation, or denial of the seriousness of the current low body weight.
4. In postmenarcheal females, amenorrhea (i.e., absence of at least three consecutive menstrual cycles when otherwise expected to occur [primary or secondary amenorrhea]).

Subtypes are based on findings during the current episode with regard to binge-eating or purging behavior (i.e., self-induced vomiting or the misuse of laxatives, diuretics, or enemas):

Restricting Type: The person has not regularly engaged in binge-eating or purging behavior.

Binge-Eating/Purging Type: The person has regularly engaged in binge-eating or purging behavior.

Bulimia Nervosa:

1. Recurrent episodes of binge eating characterized by both of the following:
   A. Eating, in a discrete period of time, an amount of food that is definitely larger than most people would consume during a similar period of time and under similar circumstances.
   B. A feeling of lack of control over eating behavior during the episode.
2. Recurrent compensatory behavior to prevent weight gain such as self-induced vomiting, misuse of laxatives, diuretics, enemas, or other medications, strict dieting or fasting, or vigorous exercise.
3. Binge-eating episodes and compensatory behaviors occur on average at least twice weekly for 3 months.
4. Self-evaluation is unduly influenced by body shape and weight.
5. Symptoms do not occur exclusively during episodes of AN.

Subtypes are based on findings during the current episode with regard to binge-eating or purging behavior (i.e., self-induced vomiting or the misuse of laxatives, diuretics, or enemas):

Purging Type: The person has regularly engaged in self-induced vomiting or the misuse of laxative, diuretics, or enemas.

Nonpurging Type: The person has used other inappropriate compensatory behaviors, such as fasting or excessive exercise, but has not engaged in self-induced vomiting or the misuse of laxatives, diuretics, or enemas.

(Modified and reprinted with permission from the Diagnostic and Statistical Manual of Mental Disorders, Fourth Edition. Copyright 1994 American Psychiatric Association.)

about weight gain or being "fat," a distorted body image, and amenorrhea (in females). Patients typically lack an appreciation for the degree of weight loss experienced or are preoccupied with the idea that a part of their body is too large, the key feature of a distorted body image. The DSM-IV allows the clinician to further differentiate an episode of AN into restricting type or binge-eating/purging type, depending on the patient's recent behavior. Specific criteria for these subtypes can be found in Table 63.1.[4] The AN patient also has difficulty in sensing when he or she is full (satiety) and commonly complains of feeling bloated or early fullness. AN patients feel as though they are not in control of various aspects of their life and, in particular, caloric intake.[13]

The course of AN most commonly consists of a single episode with subsequent return to normal weight. Some may experience an unremitting course leading to death, or episodic periods of anorexic behavior.[4] About 40% of patients who, upon follow-up, were asymptomatic continued to be symptom free after 6 years; 30% had significant clinical improvement; and 5% died.[14,15] In addition, up to 40% of treated patients have a primary mood disorder.[16] Approximately 50% of patients with AN (those who achieve and maintain low weight through food restriction, the so-called "restrictors") also suffer from BN (those who alternate between restriction and overeating).[17]

Although predictors of outcome have not been well studied, some trends have emerged. A poorer prognosis is associated with a longer duration of illness, hospitalization, poor response to previous treatment, being married, having a lower initial weight, having a premorbid history of poor family relationships, and the presence of BN or additional symptoms such as vomiting and laxative abuse.[9,18] Long-term follow-up shows that over a period of 20 years, 20% of AN patients died, primarily from cardiac arrest or suicide.[19] Patients with a high need to conform but who are self-accepting and have a sense of well-being tend to have a better treatment outcome than patients with low ego strength (a decreased ability to react and cope with the environment around them), impulsivity, addictive behaviors, poor interpersonal abilities, poor family dynamics, and a history of obesity and binge eating.[20]

BULIMIA NERVOSA

The DSM-IV diagnostic criteria for BN are listed in Table 63.1.[4] The essential feature is binge eating—an excessive intake of calorie-laden food over a short period of time. As with AN, persons with BN are overly concerned with body image. Most have normal weight; however, others may be slightly underweight or overweight for body size and age. DSM-IV allows the clinician to further differentiate an episode of BN into purging type or nonpurging type, depending on the patient's recent use of purging methods to offset the effects of binge eating. Specific criteria for these subtypes can be found in Table 63.1.[4]

Patients typically binge one or more times daily and vomit at least once daily. Patients may consume 5000 to 20,000 calories in a single bingeing episode. Not all persons with BN, however, consume such large quantities of food. Patients tend to consume foods that are easy to ingest, do not require much chewing or preparation, and are high in carbohydrates or fat (e.g., ice cream, bread, candy, or doughnuts). Binge eating is typically secretive, and episodes are often precipitated by a stressful event. Patients experience a loss of control over their eating behavior and are often remorseful after a binge. Although binges typically last less than 2 hours, they are reported to last as long as 8 or more hours.[8] To compensate for the excessive caloric intake, many patients fast for prolonged periods, resulting in frequent weight fluctuations. Persons with BN, similar to individuals with AN, are very sensitive about their weight and have a distorted body image.

Psychiatric comorbidity includes depression (up to 80%), impulse control problems, and substance abuse. Substance abuse and the abuse of food observed in patients with BN have many common characteristics. Approximately 25–30% of bulimic patients report a personal or family history of substance abuse. Kleptomania (another impulse control disorder) is more commonly reported in patients with BN than in the general public.[8]

The prognosis of BN has not been well studied. On average, a 70% reduction in binge eating and purging episodes has been reported following any treatment intervention. Patients with milder presenting symptoms who can be treated on an outpatient basis tend to do better. Hospitalized patients followed for 3 years showed a good outcome in 27% of patients (binge/purge less than once per month), intermediate outcome in 40%, and poor outcome in 33% (daily binge/purge episodes or ongoing cathartic/laxative abuse).[9]

EATING DISORDERS IN CHILDREN

Special considerations should be noted when dealing with eating disorders in children. Children, because of their relatively lower body weights, lower percentage of body fat, and increased tendency to restrict water, have a higher propensity to experience the morbidity associated with AN than adults. The clinician should, therefore, react more promptly to smaller decrements in weight loss in children. Secondary effects of malnutrition in children include delayed puberty, delayed growth, and delayed breast development. Early onset AN (under 13 years of age) tends to have a poorer prognosis. Anorexia in children is associated with higher amounts of depression relative to the adult population. Triggers for AN include stressors (moving, divorce, births, illnesses, deaths), identity issues, changing sex roles, seeking the ideal body image, and anxiety about maturation. In general, prepubertal AN is associated with a higher degree of family and environmental issues, whereas pubertal onset may be more associated with the role changes associated with puberty as well as the biologic aspects of sexual development.[21]

PATHOPHYSIOLOGY

The potential etiologic or exacerbating factors for eating disorders represent an array of physiological, biochemical, developmental, psychological, and psychiatric phenomenon. It is unlikely that one single event is responsible for the development of AN or BN. The wide spectrum of the clinical presentation reflects dysfunction in biologic, psychological, and developmental systems. It is difficult to delineate the biologic basis for eating disorders, because it is unclear whether the observed biologic changes are causing the aberrant eating behavior, or are a result of the eventual starvation. In addition, AN and BN, although distinct diagnostically, occur together in a subpopulation of patients. Therefore, the eating disorders may not be distinct diagnostic entities, but may occur along a continuum between AN and BN.[22,23]

Early descriptions of the pathology of AN suggested a primary dysfunction of the pituitary gland.[24] Since that time, abnormalities of the hypothalamic-pituitary-gonadal (HPG), hypothalamic-pituitary-adrenal (HPA), and hypothalamic-pituitary-thyroid (HPT) axes have been described. (An extensive review of the psychoendocrinology of AN is provided in Ref. 9).

The finding of amenorrhea in the majority of females with AN suggests an important role for the HPG axis, and in particular the function of the gonadotropins (LH, FSH, and GnRH). Amenorrhea is common in anorexia; however, up to 25% of females had amenorrhea before the onset of anorexia, and the return of menses lags behind weight normalization. These findings suggest the possibility of a functional hypothalamic defect in persons who develop anorexia. Although many endocrine abnormalities occur in other forms of starvation, a primary difference with AN is that the dysfunction may not correct despite weight normalization. In addition, the potential for abnormal functioning of dopaminergic, nonadrenergic, and opioid systems, which normally function as inhibitory or stimulatory control mechanisms for the endocrine system, needs further exploration to define the interplay of these systems with the HPG axis findings.

The role of the neurotransmitter serotonin in eating disorders has been extensively reviewed because it plays an important role in feeding. The primary location of serotonin-mediated eating activity is the medial hypothalamus. Serotonin activity in the paraventricular and ventromedial nuclei controls energy balance, while activity in the suprachiasmatic nucleus controls the circadian pattern of feeding. Stimulation of serotonin receptors in these areas decreases carbohydrate intake, enhances satiety, and terminates feeding. In contrast, stimulation of presynaptic serotonin autoreceptors initiates feeding, presumably by inhibiting the release of serotonin. In anorexia, plasma tryptophan (a serotonin precursor), urinary concentration of the major serotonin metabolite (5-HIAA), platelet serotonin binding, and basal cerebrospinal fluid (CSF) 5-HIAA concentrations are reportedly decreased. These abnormalities all correct with weight normalization.[25]

The role of other neurotransmitters should also be considered. In the presence of decreased food intake, norepinephrine is released in the paraventricular nucleus, which inhibits satiety, while at the same time release of norepinephrine is inhibited at the lateral hypothalamus, which increases the sensation of hunger. Dopamine is associated with self-administration and self-stimulatory behaviors in other disorders, and similarly may be etiologically related to the eating binges observed in BN. Taste and food cues are also regulated by neurotransmitters within the hypothalamus. Hypothalamic dysfunction may account for the food preferences present in BN and the food dislikes exhibited by persons with AN.

A great deal of emphasis is placed on psychological and developmental issues in the pathogenesis of eating disorders, especially regarding the role of the family. These issues are important when considering nondrug treatments. A comprehensive review of the issues surrounding the role of the family is beyond the scope of this chapter. Issues surrounding family separations, losses, and dysfunction may trigger abnormal eating behavior. These issues include divorce, death, household moves, prolonged illness, infidelity, pregnancy or birth of a sibling, and leaving home for school. The individual may have a sense of personal failure associated with an event that precedes the illness.[26] Whether family-related issues are truly etiologic for eating disorders remains controversial. It is interesting, however, to note that the prognosis is better in persons with a relatively healthy family environment.[27] In summary, the eating disorders are very complex and will probably not be explained by any simple physiological, biochemical, developmental, psychological, or psychiatric model. Instead, a multifaceted view of potential etiologies will best serve the clinician in making decisions about treatment alternatives for eating disorders.

TREATMENT

Various treatment modalities are used to improve the quality of life for patients with AN and BN. Although the approach to individual patients may differ, the basic goals of therapy are to reduce distorted body image, restore and maintain healthy body weight, reestablish normal eating patterns, improve associated psychological and physical problems, resolve contributory family problems, and prevent relapse.

The first treatment decision, whether to hospitalize, is usually based on the results of a comprehensive assessment including nutritional status, current signs and symptoms of the eating disorder, comorbid psychiatric conditions, current physical health, and a family assessment.[9] Criteria for hospitalization are shown in Table 63.2. An individual treatment plan is based on the specific core and associated features of the eating disorder. Such multifaceted plans require a team approach to care. Medications are never indicated as a sole treatment for eating disorders.

ANOREXIA NERVOSA (TABLE 63.3)

Antipsychotics

Antipsychotics were the first medications used to treat AN, based on reports of weight gain and reduced eating-related anxiety, agitation, and obsessions.[28] Clinical experience has found little specific improvement from antipsychotic treatment in AN patients. The limited benefit, along with the sensitivity of AN patients to antipsychotic-induced adverse effects, limits their usefulness.

Cyproheptadine

Cyproheptadine (Periactin), a histamine and serotonin antagonist, is used with variable success to stimulate

TABLE 63.2. CRITERIA FOR HOSPITALIZATION OF PATIENTS WITH EATING DISORDER(S)

1. Significant weight loss (30% less than normal weight or greater), particularly if weight loss has been recent and rapid, and severe starvation symptoms are present
2. Medical complications and metabolic abnormalities, especially hypokalemic alkalosis from bulimic complications
3. Overriding psychiatric problems including clinical depression and/or thought or intents of suicide
4. Nonresponsiveness to outpatient treatment (after 3–4 months)
5. Demoralized, nonfunctioning family
6. Lack of outpatient facilities

(Compiled from Refs. 9 and 55.)

TABLE 63.3. MEDICATION MANAGEMENT OF ANOREXIA NERVOSA

Drug	Benefits	Limitations
Antipsychotics	Short-term weight gain; decreased eating-related anxiety, agitation, and obsessions	Rarely used today; no long-term benefit; anticholinergic, orthostatic cardiac adverse effects; risk of tardive dyskinesia
Cyproheptadine	Weight gain; decreased depression; fewer adverse effects than antidepressants; efficacious in controlled trial	Long-term benefit unknown; sedation
Antidepressants (TCAs, FLX)	Limited benefit from TCAs in some controlled trials; FLX increased and maintained weight gain; reserved for depression that persists postrestoration of normal weight	Anticholinergic, orthostatic cardiac effects with TCAs; FLX reported to be abused
Lithium	Marginal results and limited data	Adverse effects especially in metabolically unstable patients; weight gain, fluid retention
Metoclopramide	Adjunct to relief of gastrointestinal distress	Long-term benefit unknown

appetite and decrease depression in AN patients. Early studies using relatively low doses (12 mg/d) found no difference compared with placebo.[29] A double-blind study by Halmi compared cyproheptadine in doses up to 32 mg/d to amitriptyline (AMI), up to 160 mg/d and placebo in 72 subjects. Cyproheptadine-treated patients, especially the severe cases, experienced weight gain and improvement in depression.[30] However, cyproheptadine decreased the rate of weight gain in a bulimic subgroup of anorexics.[30] Cyproheptadine is not effective in all AN patients, but its low incidence of adverse effects and efficacy in severe cases and in patients without bulimia, makes it a useful adjunct to promote weight gain and decrease depression when used at higher doses.

Antidepressants

Antidepressants are targeted at improving depression and promoting weight gain. The Halmi trial found mild improvement in the AMI group when compared to placebo and cyproheptadine. A double-blind comparison of clomipramine (CLO) 100 mg at bedtime and placebo in 16 subjects found that the CLO-treated subjects had significantly more hunger and energy than the placebo subjects. Rate of weight gain was slower in CLO-treated subjects, perhaps due to increased activity.[31] The CLO-treated subjects maintained a more stable weight than the placebo patients after discontinuation from the study. Open trials giving fluoxetine (FLX) 20–60 mg/d showed reduction in obsessions and depression, maintenance of the target body weight, and restoration of normal eating behavior[32,33]; however, controlled and long-term trials are needed before FLX can be routinely recommended.

The overall role of antidepressants in managing AN remains limited because many patients do not respond to any type of medication.[9] Antidepressants should be initiated only if depression persists after a target weight has been achieved, because many symptoms of mood disturbance will remit with improved nutrition.[9,34] Patients with AN are sensitive to anticholinergic and cardiovascular effects, necessitating low starting doses and slow titration toward an antidepressant dose. The risk of cardiotoxicity in an often malnourished population must not be underestimated, especially in chronic purgers who may have hypokalemia. A baseline electrocardiogram (ECG) must be obtained before beginning an antidepressant. Antidepressants with a low anticholinergic profile, such as desipramine (DSI), at doses of 150 mg/d, are better tolerated and should be tried first.

Miscellaneous

Several additional agents have been used for treating AN. The effectiveness of lithium has been unimpressive, and the risk of serious adverse effects in patients with AN-induced metabolic and cardiac abnormalities limits its use.[35] Metoclopramide (Reglan), 10 mg four times a day 30 minutes before meals, is used as an adjunct to increase the rate of gastric emptying and reduce the bloating and abdominal pain often seen in AN.[36] Short-acting benzodiazepines, given before meals, may be useful when severe anxiety limits eating.[5] Clomiphene citrate (Clomid) 50–100 mg daily for 1 week can be used in AN patients who remain amenorrheic after achieving their optimum weight.[37] However, return of the menstrual cycle has little effect on the eventual outcome of AN. Estrogen replacement (conjugated estrogens 0.3–1.25 mg/d) to reduce calcium loss in adult patients with chronic amenorrhea has also been used.[38] Finally, total parenteral nutrition (TPN) is needed during the initial management of severely malnourished patients; however, the decision to administer TPN must be made carefully because of the potentially devastating psychological effect on patients who do not wish to gain weight.

Nondrug Treatment

Nondrug treatment is critical to the successful outcome of AN therapy. Cognitive- and behavioral-based psychotherapy is used to maintain healthy eating behavior, while interpersonal therapy is used to improve coping skills and relationships. Family participation in psychotherapy for younger patients and marital therapy for married patients is usually necessary to improve outcome. Support groups conducted by professionals trained in treatment of eating disorders can serve as useful adjunct therapy. However, 12-step programs that focus only on abstinence and not on the nutritional and behavioral changes associated with AN are discouraged.[9]

Evaluation of Therapeutic Outcomes

The overall treatment goals in AN are to restore healthy weight and eating habits, resolve other physical complications from AN, correct behavioral problems, dysfunctional thoughts and psychological problems, improve family relationships, and prevent relapse.[9] Medications are likely to assist only in appetite stimulation (cyproheptadine) and in alleviation of depression and maintenance of target weight (cyproheptadine and antidepressants). Cyproheptadine may actually supress weight gain in AN patients with bulimic behavior. Improvement in mood should occur within approximately 8 weeks. Return to and maintenance of target weight is evaluated by regular weight checks, return of menses, and the absence of compulsive exercising and purging. Patients receiving tricyclic antidepressants (TCAs) should be evaluated for anticholinergic effects, especially dry mouth and constipation, hypotension, and sedation. Patients receiving FLX should be monitored for agitation, nausea, and insomnia. Follow-up laboratory tests and ECGs are not part of routine monitoring, unless signs and symptoms persist necessitating their collection, or the patient continues to lose weight despite treatment. The decision to use long-term medication must be based on specific and sustained improvement in aforementioned target symptoms balanced with tolerance of adverse effects.

BULIMIA NERVOSA (TABLE 63.4)

Anticonvulsants

The pharmacotherapy of BN is based on two pathophysiologic models: a relationship to seizure disorders and a relationship to affective disorders. Anticonvulsants were the first medications specifically targeted to treat BN. Green and Rau[39] noted that 38 of 59 patients with binge eating had abnormal electroencephalograms. They subsequently administered phenytoin (Dilantin) to 47 BN patients and achieved a 57% improvement in bulimic symptoms. Wermuth et al.,[40] in contrast, found no significant difference between placebo and the phenytoin-treated groups. Kaplan and colleagues,[41] in a placebo-controlled, double-blind trial of six BN patients treated with carbamazepine (Tegretol), found a dramatic response in one patient in both bulimic and affective symptoms. Valproic acid (Depakene) produced a dramatic response in a patient with concurrent bulimia and bipolar affective disorder in a single case report. Subsequent bulimic episodes occurred only after the serum concentration decreased to subtherapeutic values.[42] Anticonvulsants are reserved for the subgroup of BN patients with a comorbid bipolar affective disorder. Doses used and serum concentrations sought are similar to those used for patients with seizure disorders.

Antidepressants (Table 63.5)

Antidepressants have been extensively evaluated for BN, although benefit varies between studies, and methodologic shortcomings are present in several trials. Antidepressants are reported to reduce binge eating, vomiting, and depression, and improve eating habits, although their impact on body dissatisfaction remains unclear.[43–45] The prevalence of major depression is 15% or less in most studies, suggesting an antibulimic effect independent of an antidepressant effect.

Imipramine (IMI), DSI, and phenelzine demonstrated clear superiority over placebo in double-blind trials for treating specific symptoms of BN. Doses for BN are the same as those used to treat depression, although slow titration is needed to allow time to develop tolerance to adverse effects. Serum concentration monitoring targeting the range used for depression is recommended when using TCAs. Phenelzine should be used only if the patient will reliably follow a tyramine-free diet and observe the required dietary restrictions.

FLX has received attention because of its specific effects on serotonin and its efficacy in comorbid conditions such as depression, obsessive–compulsive disorder, and kleptomania.[46] The Fluoxetine Bulimia Nervosa Collaborative Study Group conducted the largest trial to evaluate FLX in BN. They found FLX 60 mg/d to be superior to

TABLE 63.4. MEDICATION MANAGEMENT OF BULIMIA NERVOSA

Drug	Benefits	Limitations
Anticonvulsants (carbamazepine, valproic acid)	Possible benefit in subpopulations of bipolar bulimics	Limited data
TCAs (IMI, DSI)	Decrease in bingeing, vomiting, depression; efficacious in controlled clinical trials; extensive clinical experience; plasma concentration monitoring may reduce toxicity and improve efficacy	Anticholinergic effects, orthostatic hypotension cardiac effects; low therapeutic index in overdose; long-term efficacy unknown
Phenelzine	Decrease in binge eating	Dietary restrictions; potential for hypertensive crisis; orthostatic hypotension; long-term efficacy unknown
Trazodone	Fewer anticholinergic effects than TCAs	Limited controlled data; dizziness and drowsiness
FLX	Reduction in bingeing, purging, depression, and carbohydrate craving in large controlled trial; fewer adverse effects than tertiary amine TCAs and MAOIs	Cost at 60 mg a day can be prohibitive
Fenfluramine	Fewer adverse effects than antidepressants; decrease in depression, binge eating, and vomiting; possible decreased urge to vomit	Limited data
Lithium	Decrease binge eating and vomiting episodes; reserve for comorbid bipolar affective disorder	Weight gain and fluid retention; adverse effects, especially in metabolically unstable patients; limited data

both placebo and FLX 20 mg/d for reducing vomiting, bingeing, depression, carbohydrate craving, and pathologic eating habits. The drug was well tolerated, and weight changes were minimal, even at 60 mg/d.[47]

Adverse effects reduce the usefulness of antidepressants because patients with BN have a heightened sensitivity to side effects. Selection of an agent with minimal anticholinergic effects, sedation, weight gain, or orthostatic hypotension may improve compliance and outcome. DSI and FLX have a lower incidence of adverse effects than tertiary amine TCAs and monoamine oxidase inhibitors (MAOIs), making them good first-line agents. A careful baseline physical examination with laboratory workup is essential because underlying ECG changes (U waves, increased Q–T interval, flat T waves) secondary to hypokalemia or bradycardia and arterioventricular block from starvation may be present. All antidepressants can cause seizures, thus a careful risk–benefit assessment is warranted if the patient has predisposing factors such as a personal or family history of seizures, cerebral vascular disease, and alcohol or sedative-hypnotic withdrawal.[48,49] Table 63.6 describes medication management guidelines for BN.

Miscellaneous Agents

Lithium has shown limited benefit and should be used cautiously in the BN population because of toxicity risks from associated behaviors such as purging and laxative abuse. Serum concentrations should be maintained between 0.6–0.8 mEq/L to minimize adverse effects. Fenfluramine (Pondimin), an indirect serotonin agonist and anorectic agent, given at 60 mg/d appears to be a promising alternative, although the data are limited. Nutritional support plays a role in metabolically disturbed patients, although the decision to use such an intervention must be weighed against the psychologic risks. Low-dose benzodiazepines, such as alprazolam 0.25 mg three times a day, administered before meals may also help reduce anxiety associated with refeeding, although long-term use is not warranted for most patients because of the risk of abuse.

Nondrug and Combination Therapy

Psychosocial intervention is critical to improving outcome; however, appropriate studies are sorely lacking. Psychosocial interventions include family therapy and interpersonal, cognitive and psychoanalytic based psychotherapy. As

TABLE 63.5. SUMMARY OF DRUG TRIALS IN BULIMIA NERVOSA

Author/Year	Drug/Dose	Size of Sample	Design	Outcome	Comments
Pope, 1983 Pope, 1985 (follow-up)	Imipramine (IMI) 200 mg/d	22 normal weight females	Double-blind, placebo-controlled, 6-week study	IMI group averaged 70% decrease in bingeing, 35% binge-free, 50% decrease in depression; no change in placebo group	8-month follow-up (Pope 1985) in 20 patients; majority changed to MAOIs or trazodone, 50% still in remission, and 45% partially improved
Hughes, 1986	DSI 200 mg/d	22 females with BN, but not major depression; 10 received DSI, 12 received placebo	Double-blind, placebo-controlled, 6-week study with open-label phase	19 of 22 had 80% or greater decrease in weekly binge frequency; 15 of 22 complete abstinence at 10 weeks	6 of 22 had therapeutic serum concentration; 3 dropped out due to adverse effects
Barlow, 1988	DSI 150 mg/d	47 normal weight bulimics	15-week, double-blind crossover with placebo	Significant decrease in bingeing and vomiting in the DSI group, but overall effect was modest; no effect on fatigue, depression, and eating attitudes	Onset was apparent at 1 week with maximum effect at 6 weeks; benefits lost when DSI was discontinued
McCann, 1990	DSI 100–300 mg/d (average 188 mg)	23 females with nonpurging BN	Double-blind, placebo-controlled, 12-week study	63% decrease in binge eating in DSI group and 16% increase in binge eating in placebo group; 60% of DSI group had not binged at 12 weeks	No difference in bulimic thoughts, body weight, image, or depression between the two groups; 5 DSI patients dropped out due to adverse effects
Freeman, 1987	FLX 60–80 mg/d	10 females with BN	Open 4-week trial	7 stopped bingeing and vomiting completely and 2 improved; no significant change in body dissatisfaction	At 1 yr, 4 remained binge-free, 2 binged only occasionally, and 2 switched to fenfluramine
Pope, 1989	Trazodone to maximum of 400 mg/d	42 females with DSM-III-R criteria for BN	Double-blind, placebo-controlled, 6-week trial after 2 weeks of washout placebo phase	41% of trazodone group had a 50% decrease in frequency of bingeing and vomiting after 4 weeks; placebo group worsened	Trazodone group had significantly more dizziness and drowsiness; follow-up in 36 patients at 9–19 months found 26 continued on medication, although many switched to other antidepressants; 18 remained in remission and 26 had at least moderate improvement
Mitchell, 1984	AMI 150 mg/d	32 females, nonpurging BN	Double-blind, placebo-controlled, 8-week study	Same degree of improvement in both groups; therapeutic concentration of AMI correlated to improvement in depression only	Lack of response possibly due to subtherapeutic concentrations (0–220 ng/mL, average 103 ng/mL)
Solyom, 1990	FLX 80 mg	10 females, low weight BN	3-month open trial	2 patients had complete remission of bingeing and vomiting, 2 had 75% improvement, 2 had 50% improvement, and 4 less than 50% improvement	Adverse drug reactions were minimal and did not result in discontinuation; 5 had concurrent depression, 4 had obsessive-compulsive disorder; no long-term data available

(continued)

TABLE 63.5. SUMMARY OF DRUG TRIALS IN BULIMIA NERVOSA *(Continued)*

Author/Year	Drug/Dose	Size of Sample	Design	Outcome	Comments
Walsh, 1988	Phenelzine up to 90 mg/d	50 females with BN; 23 received phenelzine, 27 received placebo	Double-blind, placebo-controlled, 8-week trial with open-label phase	Phenelzine superior to placebo for reducing binge frequency and inducing remission; 42 subjects received phenelzine; 36 were 75% improved at 6 months, but 24 stopped medications due to adverse drug reactions	9 of 31 phenelzine were unable to complete due to orthostatic hypotension and sedation; average subject was only mildly depressed
Hsu, 1987	Lithium to serum concentration between 0.6–1.0 mEq/L	13 females with BN	Double-blind, placebo-controlled, 8-week trial	70% decrease in binge/purge episodes in both groups	Both groups had weekly 30-min sessions with a psychiatrist and dieting instruction
Blouin, 1988	DSI 150 mg/d; fenfluramine 60 mg/d	10 fenfluramine/12 DSI	Double-blind, placebo-controlled, crossover trial with DSI for 6 weeks then placebo for 6 weeks or fenfluramine for 6 weeks and placebo for 6 weeks	Both groups had a significant decrease in bingeing and vomiting, although more were improved in fenfluramine group; both groups had a reduction in the urge to vomit and in feelings of depression	Fenfluramine had fewer adverse effects than DSI
Fluoxetine Bulimia Nervosa Collaborative Study Group, 1992	FLX 60 mg/d; fluoxetine 20 mg/d	387 females with BN by DSM-III-R, not depressed by Hamilton Depression Rating Scale	Double-blind, placebo-controlled 8-week study; 1-week placebo run-in phase to exclude placebo responders	FLX 60 mg/d superior to placebo in reducing frequency of weekly binge/vomiting episodes. FLX 20 mg/d had effect between that of 60 mg/d and placebo	Most dropouts were in placebo group with most common reason being lack of efficacy; adverse drug reactions were greater in FLX groups than in placebo group, but no statistical difference in adverse drug reactions-related rate of dropouts between groups

TABLE 63.6. GUIDELINES FOR MEDICATION USE IN BULIMIA NERVOSA

1. Assess baseline frequency of binge and vomiting episodes, laxative abuse, and self-image.
2. Assess baseline mood disturbance and anxiety.
3. Assess baseline physical status (especially nutritional status, ECG, fluid and electrolytes).
4. Consider a mood stabilizer if comorbid bipolar affective disorder is present. Consider an antidepressant as part of a comprehensive treatment plan.
5. Start antidepressant at a low dose and titrate upward slowly as tolerated to dose used for depression (except for fluoxetine).
6. Monitor carefully for response, adverse effects, and compliance. Response usually seen after 6–12 weeks. Serum concentration assessment for TCAs.
7. If response occurs, continue treatment for at least 12 months then reassess.
8. If poor response, evaluate compliance and whether patient is vomiting medication.
9. Multiple trials of antidepressants or a trial of fenfluramine may be needed before optimal response is obtained.

with AN, support groups should be limited to those run by trained professionals. Cox and Merkel[50] evaluated 32 studies of individual and group therapy techniques used to manage BN. Most studies had methodological shortcomings (e.g., failure to use a control group, overreliance on self-reporting as an outcome, and small sample sizes). Approximately 40% of patients were totally abstinent from binge eating and purging at follow-up. None of these interventions was shown to be clearly superior. A comparison of IMI and psychotherapy found that the three groups receiving active treatment (IMI, IMI plus psychotherapy, or placebo plus psychotherapy) showed a better response than did those taking placebo alone and that combination treatment was superior to IMI alone. IMI reduced depression and anxiety, but did not improve eating behavior.[51] Angras et al.[52] compared the effectiveness of DSI, cognitive–behavioral therapy, and their combination for 16 or 24 weeks in outpatients with BN. He found DSI and cognitive–behavioral therapy in combination for 24 weeks to be superior to any other treatment or duration for reducing bingeing, purging, dietary preoccupation, and hunger. The combination of medication and psychotherapy appears to produce the best outcome for a patient with BN.

Evaluation of Therapeutic Outcomes

Any individual treatment plan using medication should carefully describe frequency and severity of medication responsive target symptoms and routinely assess changes from baseline in mood, anxiety, eating behaviors, and laxative abuse.[9] The time to onset of effect is unclear; however, a 1-month trial after a therapeutic dose is achieved should be tried to fully evaluate response. Optimal duration of treatment after response is also poorly defined. There is some suggestion that 2 years of continuous treatment is needed in responders to ensure a sustained remission.[44] The impact of antidepressants on the long-term prognosis of BN is also ill defined. Twenty to 40% of subjects are estimated to have a poor or inadequate response to antidepressants.[53] Careful evaluation for binge–purge behavior is necessary to ensure that treatment failure is not secondary to vomiting. Evaluation of previously described adverse effects should also be part of the treatment plan. Supportive counseling that encourages compliance may be needed early in treatment while the patient becomes tolerant to adverse effects. If early adverse effects remain intolerable after approximately 1 month of treatment, a change in medication or discontinuation may be needed.

The eating disorder patient presents a challenge to the community pharmacist. Impulsivity associated with BN may increase the risk for suicide. Small supplies of medication should be dispensed. In addition, the pharmacist should be alert to identify persons who make large or frequent purchases of laxatives and/or ipecac syrup. If such activity is noted, possible laxative abuse and bulimic behaviors should be considered. Finally, a single case of FLX abuse was reported in a patient with AN, indicating the need for attention to the frequency of refills.[54]

CONCLUSION

Our understanding of the pathophysiology and symptomatology of eating disorders has improved significantly over the past several years. Although various models are used to explain the etiology of eating disorders, it is unlikely that any single model will sufficiently explain these complex disorders. Medication serves an adjunctive role to a variety of psychosocial therapies in AN, while it plays a more central role in BN. By gaining a greater understanding of the underlying physiologic changes and the psychosocial complications associated with eating disorders, treatment plans can be specifically designed for an individual patient with the goal of improving the quality of life.

REFERENCES

1. Gull WW. Anorexia nervosa. Trans Clin Soc (Lond) 1874;7:22–28. In Kaufman RM, Heifman M (eds): Evolution of Psychosomatic Concepts. Anorexia Nervosa: A Paradigm. New York, International Universities Press, 1964.
2. Lesegue C. De l'anorexic hysterique. Arch Gen Med 1873: 385. In Kaufman RM, Heifman M (eds): Evolution of Psychosomatic Concepts. Anorexia Nervosa: A Paradigm. New York, International Universities Press, 1964.

3. Russel G. Bulimia nervosa: An ominous variant of anorexia nervosa. Psychol Med 1979;9:429–448.
4. American Psychiatric Association. Diagnostic and Statistical Manual of Mental Disorders, 4th ed. (DSM-IV). Washington, DC, Author, 1994, pp 539–550.
5. Kennedy S, Garfinkel PE. Anorexia nervosa, in Hales RE, Frances AJ (eds): Psychiatry Updates: Annual Review, Vol 4. Washington, DC, American Psychiatric Press, 1985, pp 438–463.
6. Jones DJ, Fox MM, Babigian HM, Hutton HE. Epidemiology of anorexia nervosa in Monroe County, New York, 1960–1976. Psychosom Med 1980;42:551–558.
7. Pope HG, Hudson JI, Yurgelun-Todd D. Anorexia nervosa and bulimia among 300 suburban women shoppers. Am J Psychiatry 1984;141:292–294.
8. Mitchell JE, Pyle RL, Eckert ED. Bulimia, in Hales RE, Frances AJ (eds): Psychiatry Updates: Annual Review, Vol 4. Washington, DC, American Psychiatric Press, 1985, p 464.
9. Work Group on Eating Disorders. American Psychiatric Association practice guidelines. Practice guidelines for eating disorders. Am J Psychiatry 1993;150:208–228.
10. Weiner H. Psychoendocrinology of anorexia nervosa. Psychiatr Clin North Am 1989;12:187–206.
11. Stege P, Visco-Dangler L, Rye L. Anorexia nervosa: Review including oral and dental manifestations. J Am Dent Assoc 1982;104:648–652.
12. Garfinkel PE, Kaplan AS. Anorexia nervosa—diagnostic conceptualizations, in Brownell KD, Foreyt JP (eds): Handbook of Eating Disorders: Physiology, Psychology, and Treatment of Obesity, Anorexia, and Bulimia. New York, Basic Books, 1986, pp 262–282.
13. Bruch H. Perceptual and conceptual disturbances in anorexia nervosa. Psychosom Med 1962;24:187–194.
14. Morgan HG, Russel GFM. Value of family background and clinical features as predictors of long-term outcome in anorexia nervosa: A four-year follow up of 41 patients. Psychol Med 1975;5:355–371.
15. Hsu LKG. Outcome of anorexia nervosa: A review of the literature (1954–1978). Arch Gen Psychiatry 1980;37:1041–1046.
16. Cantwell DP, Sturzenberger S, Burroughs J, et al. Anorexia nervosa: An affective disorder? Arch Gen Psychiatry 1977;34:1087–1093.
17. Garfinkel PE, Moldofsky H, Garner DM. The heterogeneity of anorexia nervosa: Bulimia as a distinct subgroup. Arch Gen Psychiatry 1980;37:1036–1040.
18. Eckert ED. Characteristics of anorexia nervosa, in Mitchel JE (ed): Anorexia Nervosa and Bulimia: Diagnosis and Treatment. Minneapolis, University of Minnesota Press, 1985.
19. Theander S. Outcome and prognosis in anorexia nervosa and bulimia: Some results of previous investigations, compared with those of a Swedish long-term study. J Psychiatric Res 1985;19:493–508.
20. Strober M. An empirically derived typology of anorexia nervosa, in Darby PL, Garfinkel PE, Garner DM (eds): Anorexia Nervosa: Recent Developments in Research. New York, Alan R Liss, 1983, pp 185–196.
21. DiNicola VF, Roberts N, Oke L. Eating and mood disorders in young children. Psychiatr Clin North Am 1989;12:873–893.
22. Garner DM, Olmsted MP, Garfinkel PE. Does anorexia nervosa occur on a continuum? Subgroup of weight-preoccupied women and their relationship to anorexia nervosa. Int J Eating Dis 1983;2:11–20.
23. Garner DM, Garfinkel PE, O'Shaughnessy M. Validity of the distinction between bulimia with and without anorexia nervosa. Am J Psychiatry 1985;142:581–587.
24. Simmonds M. Ueber embolische prozesse in des hypophysis. Arch F Pathol Anat 1914;217:226–239.
25. Liebowitz SF. The role of serotonin in eating disorders. Drugs 1990;39(suppl 3):33–48.
26. Foreyt JP, McGavin JK. Anorexia nervosa and bulimia, in Mash EJ, Terdel LG (eds): Behavioral Assessment of Childhood Disorders, 2nd ed. New York, Guilford Press, 1988, pp 776–805.
27. Rosenvinge JH, Mouland SO. Outcome and prognosis of anorexia nervosa. Br J Psychiatry 1990;156:92–97.
28. Dally PJ, Sargant W. A new treatment for anorexia nervosa. Br Med J 1960;1:1770–1773.
29. Vigersky RA, Loriaux DL. The effect of cyproheptadine in anorexia nervosa: A double-blind trial, in Vigersky RA (ed): Anorexia Nervosa. New York, Raven Press, 1977, pp 346–356.
30. Halmi KA, Eckert E, LaDu TJ, Cohen J. Anorexia nervosa. Treatment efficacy of cyproheptadine and amitriptyline. Arch Gen Psychiatry 1986;43:177–181.
31. Lacey JH, Crisp AH. Hunger, food intake and weight: The impact of clomipramine on refeeding an anorexia nervosa population. Postgrad Med J 1980;56:79–85.
32. Gwirtsman HE, Guze BH, Yager J, Gainsley B. Fluoxetine treatment of anorexia nervosa: An open clinical trial. J Clin Psychiatry 1990;51:378–382.
33. Kay WH, Weltzin TE, Hsu G, Bulik CM. An open trial of fluoxetine in patients with anorexia nervosa. J Clin Psychiatry 1991;52:464–471.
34. Anderson AE, Morese C, Santymer K. Inpatient treatment for anorexia nervosa, in Garner DM, Garfinkel PE (eds): Handbook of Psychotherapy for Anorexia Nervosa and Bulimia. New York, Guilford Press, 1985, pp 311–343.
35. Gross HA, Ebert M, Faden VB, et al. A double-blind controlled trial of lithium carbonate in primary anorexia nervosa. J Clin Psychopharmacol 1981;1:376–381.
36. Saleh JW, Lebwohl SF. Metoclopramide-induced gastric emptying in patients with anorexia nervosa. Am J Gastroenterol 1980;74:127–132.
37. Russell GF, Checkley SA, Robinson PH. The limited use of drugs in the treatment of anorexia and bulimia nervosa, in Carruba MD, Blundell JE (eds): Pharmacology of Eating Disorders: Theoretical and Clinical Developments. New York, Raven Press, 1986.
38. Bachrach LK, Katzman DK, Guido D, Marcus R. Recovery from osteopenia in adolescent girls with anorexia nervosa. J Clin Endocrinol Metab 1991;72:602–606.
39. Green RS, Rau JH. Treatment of compulsive eating disorders with anticonvulsant medication. Am J Psychiatry 1974;131:428–432.
40. Wermuth BM, Davis KL, Hollister LE, Stunkard AJ. Phenytoin treatment of binge eating syndrome. Am J Psychiatry 1977;136:1249–1253.

41. Kaplan AS, Garfinkel PE, Darby PL, Garner DM. Carbamazepine in the treatment of bulimia. Am J Psychiatry 1983;140:1225–1226.
42. Herridge PL, Pope HG. Treatment of bulimia and rapid cycling bipolar disorder with sodium valproate: A case report. J Clin Psychopharmacol 1985;5:229–230.
43. Pope HG, Hudson JI, Jonas JM, Yurgelun-Todd D. Bulimia treated with imipramine: A placebo-controlled, double-blind study. Am J Psychiatry 1983;140:554–558.
44. Pope HG, Hudson JI, Jonas JM, Yurgelun-Todd D. Antidepressant treatment of bulimia: A two-year follow-up study. J Clin Psychopharmacol 1985;5:320–327.
45. Mitchell JE, Pyle RL, Eckert ED, et al. Response to alternative antidepressants in imipramine nonresponders. J Clin Psychopharmacol 1989;9:291–293.
46. McElroy SL, Keck PE, Pope HG, Hudson JI. Pharmacological treatment of kleptomania and bulimia nervosa. J Clin Psychopharmacol 1989;9:358–360.
47. Fluoxetine Bulimia Nervosa Collaborative Study Group. Fluoxetine in the treatment of bulimia nervosa. A multicenter, placebo-controlled, double-blind trial. Arch Gen Psychiatry 1992;49:139–147.
48. Davidson J. Seizures and buproprion. J Clin Psychiatry 1989;50:256–261.
49. Betts TA, Kabra PL, Cooper R, Jeavons DM. Epileptic fits as a probable side effect of amitriptyline. Lancet 1968;1:390–392.
50. Cox GL, Merkel WT. A qualitative review of psychosocial treatments for bulimia. J Nerv Ment Dis 1989;177:77–83.
51. Mitchell JE, Pyle RL, Eckert ED, et al. A comparison study of antidepressants, structured interview and group psychotherapy in the treatment of bulimia nervosa. Arch Gen Psychiatry 1990;47:149–157.
52. Angras WS, Rossiter EM, Arnow B, et al. Pharmacological and cognitive-behavioral treatment for bulimia nervosa: A controlled comparison. Am J Psychiatry 1992;149:82–87.
53. Solyom L, Solyom C, Ledwidge B. The fluoxetine treatment of low-weight chronic bulimia nervosa. J Clin Psychopharmacol 1990;10:421–425.
54. Wilcox JA. Abuse of fluoxetine by a patient with anorexia nervosa. Am J Psychiatry 1987;144:1100.
55. Anderson AE. Inpatient and outpatient treatment of anorexia nervosa, in Brownell KD, Foreyt JP (eds): Handbook of Eating Disorders: Physiology, Psychology, and Treatment of Obesity, Anorexia and Bulimia. New York, Basic Books, 1986, pp 333–352.

Chapter 64

Alzheimer's Disease

Andrea Eggert, PharmD, M. Lynn Crismon, PharmD, FCCP, and Larry Ereshefsky, PharmD, FCCP

I now begin the journey that will lead me into the sunset of my life.

—Ronald Reagan

Alzheimer's disease (AD), first characterized by Alois Alzheimer in 1907, is a type of progressive dementia for which no cause is known and no cure exists.[1] Currently, all treatments for AD are palliative. Although newer drugs such as tacrine may retard the progression of Alzheimer's symptoms for a time, they do not affect the underlying illness, and the disease remains eventually fatal. If the reader of this chapter has never personally known anyone with AD, it will be difficult to fathom the devastation this illness produces on the patient and affected family. The Alzheimer's *family* is stressed because this disease has a tremendous negative effect on the family as well as the patient. Persons with AD eventually lose their very identity, not just memories, but all associated cognitive, analytical, and physical functioning.[1]

Persons with AD experience something akin to traveling through a time warp; they are dropped into a foreign universe in which they no longer know how to function. They gradually lose sense of time, date, or year, and become unable to operate simple appliances such as ovens, microwaves, or telephones. Simple day-to-day things like paying bills, mailing letters, or picking out items in a grocery store become beyond their comprehension. Calculation of simple figures becomes impossible, such as how much change to expect when paying for a $4 item with a $5 bill. Men and women with AD slowly become strangers in their own environments, increasingly unable to recognize their homes, neighborhoods, friends, or family members. Language and speech become difficult. Personality, memory, and functional ability progressively fade away until the person becomes essentially like a small child, robbed of the ability to dress him- or herself, feed him- or herself, bathe, or even use the bathroom. The need for supervision and assistance increases until the late stages of the disease, when Alzheimer's sufferers become totally dependent on a family member, spouse, or other caregiver for all their basic needs. These are all experiences of the more than 4 million people in the United States who have AD.[1]

In the *Diagnostic and Statistical Manual of Mental Disorders, 3rd ed., Revised* (DSM-III-R),[2] AD was classified under the heading of Organic Mental Syndromes and Disorders. Since all types of mental disorders have some basis in biology (i.e., all mental disorders are to some degree "organic"), this classification was discarded for the new edition, DSM-IV, in favor of the more specific heading Delirium, Dementia and Amnestic and Other Disorders.[3] Dementias are neuropsychiatric disorders defined by widespread symptoms of memory loss and deficits in cognition or reasoning.[3] *Dementia* is a nonspecific term used to describe cognitive deficits of a wide variety of causes, much like the word *senility* is a popular layperson's term used to describe cognitive deficits of old age. Because the severity, course, and treatment of dementia depends almost entirely on the underlying cause, an accurate diagnosis is essential.

AD is the most common cause of dementia (senility), accounting for 60% of all cases of late life cognitive dysfunction.[1] Other DSM-IV subclasses of dementia are based on etiology and listed in Table 64.1. This chapter focuses exclusively on dementia of the Alzheimer's type. The reader is encouraged to use the nonspecific treatment portions of this chapter to assist in management of noncognitive behavioral problems associated with other forms of dementia.

EPIDEMIOLOGY

Approximately 100,000 individuals die every year from AD, the fourth leading cause of death in the United States.[4] Generally, it is thought of as a disease of old age since most cases present after age 65, but in about 5% of cases of AD onset can be as early as age 40, resulting in the arbitrary age classifications of early (age 40–64) and late onset (≥ age 65) disease.[5] The incidence of AD increases exponentially with age, affecting 3% of individuals ages 65–74, and rising dramatically to almost 50% of persons ages 85 and older[6] (Fig. 64.1). The overall prevalence was 10.3% in

TABLE 64.1. DSM-IV SUBCLASSIFICATIONS OF DEMENTIA

- Dementia of the Alzheimer's type
- Vascular dementia (formerly multi-infarct dementia)
- Dementia due to other medical conditions
    - Dementia due to HIV disease
    - Dementia due to head trauma
    - Dementia due to Parkinson's disease
    - Dementia due to Huntington's disease
    - Dementia due to Pick's disease
    - Dementia due to Creutzfeldt–Jakob disease
    - Dementia due to general medical conditions (indicate condition, e.g., B_{12} deficiency, hypothyroidism, etc.)
- Substance-induced persisting dementia (persistent dementia resulting from exposure to toxins, drugs of abuse or medications)
- Dementia due to multiple etiologies
- Dementia not otherwise specified (reserved for dementia that cannot be attributed to any other subtype)

(Adapted from Ref. 3.)

a large community sample of persons older than age 65.[6] The disease affects two times as many women as men, and while genetic inheritance is the primary mode of transmission, several environmental factors may contribute. Factors determining age of onset and rate of progression remain largely undefined.

The economic and social costs of AD are staggering. It is the third most expensive illness in the United States after heart disease and cancer. Currently most insurance plans do not cover AD, and much of the cost of caring for these patients is left to their families. In 1991 the average cost of caring for an Alzheimer's patient was about $33,600 per year.[7] This estimate includes direct costs as well as unpaid caregiver cost. Add to this the cost associated with loss of earnings due to disability and premature death, and the total annual cost of AD in the United States was $67.3 billion.[7] To put these numbers in perspective, in 1991, the estimated medical cost of acquired immune deficiency syndrome (AIDs) was $4.2 billion. Medicaid costs alone of AD totaled $5.7 billion.[7]

The average life expectancy in 1900 was 47 years. Few people lived long enough to experience the onset of AD. Life expectancy is now 75 years; 4 million people are afflicted with AD, and 250,000 more cases are diagnosed annually.[4] By the year 2050, one out of four people will be older than age 65, and the number of Alzheimer's patients is projected at 14 million. AD has become a major public health concern, yet in comparison to other major illnesses such as AIDS, heart disease, and cancer, it has received relatively little attention. The potential financial burden of this disease on the health care system could reach crisis proportions unless more effective avenues are developed to provide care for these individuals, prevent the disease from occurring, or slow its progress.

PATHOPHYSIOLOGY

STRUCTURAL CHANGES IN ALZHEIMER'S DISEASE

Alzheimer's disease destroys neurons in the cortex and limbic structures of the central nervous system (CNS), particularly the basal forebrain, amygdala, hippocampus, and cerebral cortex. These areas of the brain are associated with

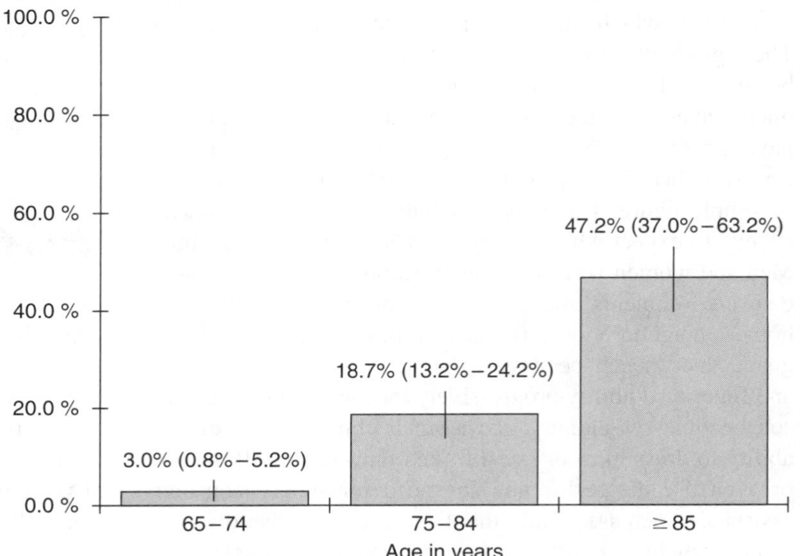

Figure 64.1. Increasing prevalence of Alzheimer's disease with age. Illustrates the disproportional increase in Alzheimer's disease prevalence with age. Percentages on top of bars indicate prevalence estimates (95% confidence limits). *(Adapted with permission from JAMA 1989;262(18):2551–2556. Copyright 1989, American Medical Association.)*

functions of higher learning, memory, reasoning, behavior, and emotional control. Four major alterations in these brain structures define AD: cortical atrophy, degeneration of cholinergic and other neurons, presence of neurofibrillary tangles (NFTs), and the accumulation of neuritic plaques.[8–10] Neurofibrillary tangles (NFTs) and neuritic plaques are considered the signature lesions of AD. Central to recent Alzheimer's pathophysiology research is an attempt to discover how neuritic plaques and NFTs form, and how two proteins, beta amyloid protein and apolipoprotein E, contribute to their genesis.[1,11]

NEUROFIBRILLARY TANGLES AND NEURITIC PLAQUES

NFTs and neuritic plaques are both present in normal brains, their numbers increasing with age. In AD, however, the quantity of these lesions is drastically increased, particularly in areas associated with memory and cognition, namely, the hippocampus, amygdala, and cerebral cortex.[1,12,13]

NFTs are located intracellularly, within the cytoplasm of neurons. NFTs are comprised of paired neurofilaments adopting a helical shape, unlike normal neurofilaments. The paired helical filaments aggregate in dense bundles, which appear microscopically like tiny flames filling the neuronal cell body. Comprising these paired helical filaments is an abnormally phosphorylated form of tau protein, a naturally occurring cell protein commonly associated with microtubules.[1,10,12,13] Microtubules are important in cellular transport. Abnormalities of tau protein and the presence of NFTs disrupt the cell structure, resulting in improper cell function and eventual cell death. NFTs and associated abnormal tau protein products are found in other disease states where symptoms of dementia are present and may represent a common method by which various inciting factors culminate in cell death.[9]

Neuritic plaques (also termed amyloid or senile plaques) differ from NFTs in both location and composition. Neuritic plaques are extracellular lesions found in the brain and cerebral vasculature. Plaques are comprised of a core of beta amyloid protein, surrounded by a snarled mass of broken neurites (axon and dendrite projections of neurons).[1,10,12] Many of these broken neurites contain neuropil filaments made up of the abnormally phosphorylated tau protein found in NFTs.[9,10] Also surrounding and entwined in the plaques are two types of glial cells, astrocytes and microglia.[12,13] Among other functions, glial cells secrete inflammatory mediators and serve as scavenger cells, which may be important in considering inflammatory mechanisms of AD. The number of neuritic plaques parallels disease severity, making the study of these lesions a popular topic of Alzheimer's research.

Neuritic plaques and NFTs significantly interfere with neuronal transmission. To use an analogy, think of a network of optic fibers carrying millions of telephone calls. Just as telephone calls are interrupted, slowed, or rerouted when sections of optic fiber are damaged, relay of brain messages crucial for information recall and integration cannot travel properly through snarled neurites gummed with plaques and cells clogged with tangles.[1]

Neuritic plaques and NFTs appear in brain areas where cholinergic and other brain neuronal pathways have been destroyed. Plaque accumulation, tangle formation, and cholinergic pathway destruction are all steps in a process eventually leading to the vast memory loss characterizing AD.[1,10]

BETA AMYLOID PROTEIN

Forming the center of the neuritic plaque is a roughly 4-kDa, 39–43 amino acid protein segment called beta amyloid protein (βAP).[9,14–16] The amyloidoses are a set of diseases marked by amyloid protein deposition in various target organs. The βAP accumulating in the brain and cerebral blood vessels in AD is different from other disease-producing amyloid proteins.[13]

The process by which βAP cleaves from its parent protein, deposits extracellularly, and aggregates to form a plaque is an important key to unraveling the mystery of Alzheimer's pathogenesis. Occasionally referred to by the generic term *amyloid,* βAPs are named for their beta-pleated sheet structure, referring to the tertiary folding of the protein. Following release into the extracellular space, βAP protein fragments can adhere to one another, forming insoluble aggregates that are relatively resistant to destruction by proteases. As extracellular deposits of βAP develop into mature neuritic plaques, they create physical barriers between nerve cells.[8] Plaque formation seems to precede the accumulation of NFTs and neuropil threads eventually causing nerve cell breakdown.[9]

Other evidence supports the theory that βAP deposits initiate the widespread structural damage associated with dementia. For example, more than 20 years prior to the development of clinical symptoms of AD, βAP deposits can be seen in Down syndrome patients.[9,17,18] (Most Down syndrome patients develop AD early in life.) In animal experiments, mice genetically engineered to produce βAP secondarily developed amyloid plaques, dystrophic neurites, loss of synaptic connections, and activated glial cells.[9,19] Injection of beta amyloid into rats' brains causes neuronal breakdown in the exposed areas.[9,19] *In vitro,* hippocampal cells exposed to βAP aggregates develop abnormally phosphorylated tau protein and begin to degenerate.[9,20] Taken as a whole, these data suggest that βAP deposition occurs early in the disease process and, rather than being simply an end product of neuronal death, could initiate the process of plaque formation and eventual nerve cell destruction.

How is βAP formed? βAP is cleaved from a larger protein, the amyloid precursor protein (APP) containing either 695, 751, or 770 amino acids[9,10,15] (Fig. 64.2). APP is a transmembrane protein. The βAP portion of APP is partially anchored within the cell membrane, with one portion extending extracellularly.[9,12,13,15] Proteases cleave APP in several different ways. APP may be cleaved within the βAP region so that intact βAP protein is not released into the extracellular fluid.[10,21] However, an alternative pathway is also followed in which APP is cleaved on either side of the beta region, leaving unbroken βAP to be released. Intact βAP can aggregate into fibrils, forming the precursors to neuritic plaques[9,10,12,13,15] (Fig. 64.3). The composition of proteases responsible for the alternative cleavage of APP, and the process causing βAP to aggregate are unknown.[9] There is some speculation that the site of APP cleavage is influenced by the presence of certain protease inhibitors. For example, these could include increased proportions of APP carrying the Kunitz protease inhibitor, a protease inhibitor built into some forms of APP, or possibly acute phase proteins such as α_1-antichymotrypsin and α_2-macroglobulin, whose increased presence in AD is thought to be due to activation of an immune response.[9,22] Other factors, including the degree lipophilicity of the βAP carboxyl-terminal and the length of the cleaved βAP fragment, are important in controlling the rate of βAP fibril formation *in vitro*.[9] Therapies designed to modify the βAP protein C-terminal or alter its site of cleavage from APP should reduce plaque precursor formation and ultimately disease progression.

APP is found in many cells in the body, yet its function is not well understood. It is not known why βAP selectively deposits in the brain in AD as opposed to other anatomic sites. APP is encoded on chromosome 21. Patients with Down syndrome or trisomy 21 almost uniformly develop AD during the fifth decade of life.[10] Some cases of familial AD have also been associated with mutations in the APP, but these appear to account for only a small number of early-onset Alzheimer's cases. Genetic abnormalities of the APP gene on chromosome 21 can lead to overproduction of βAP.[9,10,23] Other early-onset cases may be attributed to an Alzheimer's gene located on chromosome 14, which may play a role in the production and cleavage of APP.[9,24] Late-onset AD was previously thought to occur spontaneously; however, recently, inheritance of certain apolipoprotein E isoforms has been shown to influence susceptibility to late-onset cases, the most common form of AD.

APOLIPOPROTEIN E

The discovery of an apolipoprotein E (apo E) subtype as a genetic marker for late-onset AD is considered one of the most important advances in recent Alzheimer's research.[1,11,25,26] Apo E is well known for its role as a shuttle of cholesterol in the blood. However, apo E is also produced in the brain by glial cells, and its production is increased following injury of neuronal tissue. The gene responsible for the production of apo E is located on chromosome 19 in a region previously noted to be associated with late-onset AD. There are three major subtypes or isoforms of apo E termed apo E2, apo E3, and apo E4. Apo E3 is the most common type (90% of individuals have at least one copy), with E2 and E4 occurring less frequently.[11] Each individual has two copies of the gene responsible for the manufacture of apo E as a result of inheriting one allele from each parent. Investigators have found an unexpectedly high relationship between the number of copies of apo E4 and one's risk for late-onset AD. Ninety percent of persons inheriting two copies of apo E4 will develop AD by age 80 years. Moreover, onset of symptoms will occur at a relatively younger age compared with patients having no or only one copy of apo E4 in their genotype[11,27] (Fig. 64.4). Conversely, apo E2 appears to be protective, conferring a relative resistance to AD.[28,29] Apo E binds tightly to the βAP deposits located in neuritic plaques and cerebral vessels in Alzheimer patients' brains and is also associated with NFTs. At present the exact role of apo E in the genesis of AD is unclear. Apo E binds to βAP *in vitro*. One theory is that apo E4 stabilizes βAP, facil-

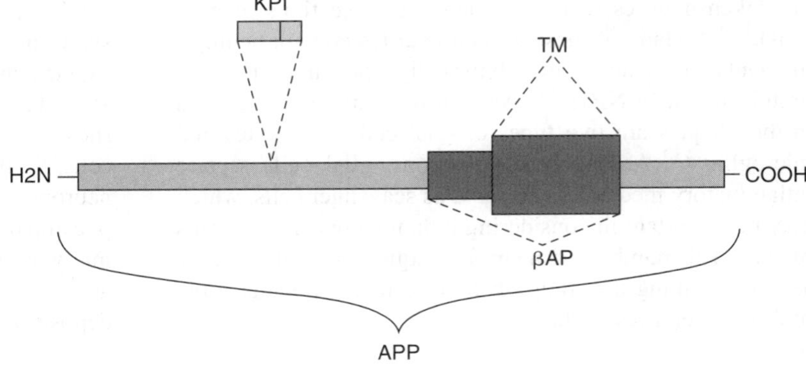

Figure 64.2. Representation of the amyloid precursor protein (APP), containing the beta amyloid protein (βAP) subunit. The transmembrane spanning unit (TM) of the protein is located within the βAP subunit. The presence of the Kunitz protease inhibitor (KPI) increases the size of APP from 695 to either 751 or 770 amino acids. *(Adapted from Ref. 9.)*

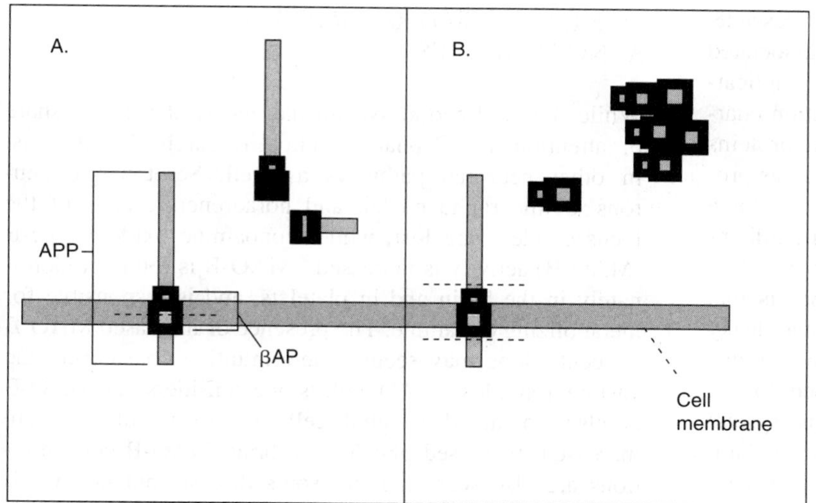

Figure 64.3. Representation of two physiologic cleavage sites of APP. APP is pictured as a transmembrane protein, with the βAP subunit anchored within the membrane. In section A, proteases cut APP through the βAP region. In section B, proteases cut βAP on either side of the βAP subunit. βAP is then released intact into the extracellular fluid, where it can aggregate, forming insoluble preamyloid plaques. *(Adapted from Ref. 12.)*

itating its incorporation into neuritic plaques. Another theory involves tau protein. Tau protein is said to lend structural support to microtubules within neurons and may be aided in this task by apo E3. It is hypothesized that apo E4 may not be as efficient at binding tau protein to microtubules, thus facilitating destruction of the microtubule network and subsequent cell death.[11] It is important to remember that while inheritance of the apo E4 subtype might facilitate the development of AD, it is not essential for disease presence. AD does occur in persons with no copies of apo E4.

INFLAMMATORY MEDIATORS

Inflammatory mediators and other immune system constituents are present near areas of plaque formation, suggesting that the immune system plays an active role in the pathogenesis of AD. While perhaps not the initial disease-producing event, an immune response generated against some unknown factor or insult could foster disease progression. Evidence supporting significant involvement of the immune system includes the increased presence of acute phase proteins, such as α_1-antichymotrypsin and α_2-macroglobulin, both in the serum and within amyloid plaques of patients with AD.[22] Glial cells (microglial cells and astrocytes), the cytokines interleukin-1 and interleukin-6, and components of the classic complement cascade are also markedly increased in plaque-infested areas.[22] Microglial cells located around and within amyloid plaques are thought to release inflammatory mediators, which locally destroy nerve tissue. Glial cells also function as phagocytes, similar to macrophages and monocytes in the

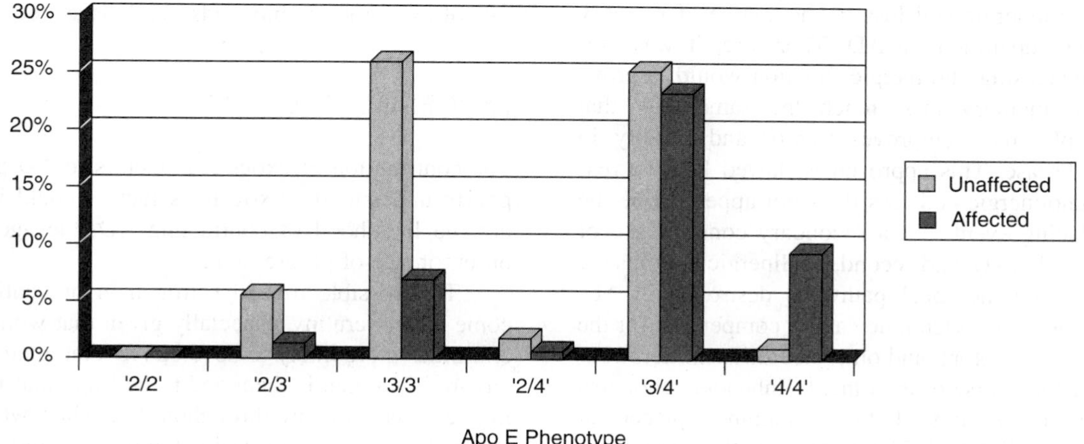

Figure 64.4. Percent of family members categorized by apo E phenotype and disease presence in 42 families (total N=234) with late-onset Alzheimer's disease. Prevalence of Alzheimer's disease increases with number of inherited copies of apo E4. Phenotype legends indicate apo E subtypes (e.g., '2/3' signifies one copy of the apo E2 allele, and one copy of apo E3). *(Adapted from Ref. 27.)*

periphery. Another component of the complement cascade, the membrane attack complex (MAC), is found associated with broken neurites and areas containing NFTs, implicating MAC as promoting the vast neuronal destruction characterizing AD.[22] As stated earlier, the acute phase proteins α_1-antichymotrypsin and α_2-macroglobulin also act as protease inhibitors, and could influence proteolytic breakdown of APP into βAP.[13] As is the case in many chronic inflammatory illnesses, specific factors responsible for initiating the immune response are not known. One theory is that breaks in the blood–brain barrier due to trauma, leaky endothelial cells, or other conditions trigger an immune response to brain proteins previously unexposed to the periphery.[22] Another possibility is that the immune system is activated by plaque precursors or by-products of damaged cells, resulting in further destruction of adjacent neurons.[30]

THE CHOLINERGIC SYSTEM

Multiple neuronal pathways are destroyed in AD. Determining which cells are destroyed and which are preserved is governed mostly by location. Basically, damage occurs in any nerve cell population located in or traveling through plaque-laden areas.[9,13] Widespread cell destruction results in a variety of neurotransmitter deficits. Most profoundly damaged are the cholinergic pathways, particularly a large system of neurons located at the base of the forebrain in the nucleus basalis of Mynert, a brain area believed to be involved in thought integration.[13] Axons of these cholinergic neurons project to the frontal cortex and hippocampus, areas strongly associated with memory and cognition.

The discovery of vast cholinergic cell loss led to the development of a cholinergic hypothesis and to a major thrust of drug development in AD being directed toward augmenting cholinergic function. The cholinergic hypothesis targeted cholinergic cell loss as the source of memory and cognitive impairment in AD. Therefore, it was presumed that increasing cholinergic function would improve symptoms of memory loss, much the same way that dopamine replacement improves tremor and rigidity in Parkinson's disease. This approach is flawed for two reasons. First, cholinergic cell loss does not appear to be the disease-producing event, but a secondary consequence of Alzheimer's pathology, and second, cholinergic neurons are only one of many neuronal pathways destroyed in AD. Simple addition of acetylcholine cannot compensate for the loss of neurons, receptors, and other neurotransmitters consumed during the course of the illness. Enhancing cholinergic activity no more cures AD than dopamine replacement cures Parkinson's disease.[31] The principle is the same, however: to minimize or improve dementia symptoms through augmentation of cholinergic transmission at remaining synapses.

OTHER NEUROTRANSMITTER ABNORMALITIES

While the cholinergic system has received a lion's share of attention in AD pharmaceutical research, deficits exist in other neuronal pathways as well. Serotonergic neurons of the raphe nuclei, and noradrenergic cells of the locus ceruleus are lost, while monoamine oxidase type-B (MAO-B) activity is increased.[8] MAO-B is found predominately in the brain and in platelets, and is responsible for metabolizing dopamine. The presence of increased MAO-B concentrations may seem counterintuitive considering the vast neuronal loss in AD, unless one considers that MAO-B is also contained in glial cells whose populations are increased. Increased platelet and brain MAO-B concentrations are also seen in Parkinson's disease, but not multi-infarct dementia.[32]

Other abnormalities appear in glutamate pathways of the cortex and limbic structures, where a loss of neurons leads to a focus on excitotoxicity models as possible contributing factors to AD pathology.[8] Glutamate is a major excitatory neurotransmitter in the cortex and hippocampus. Many neuronal pathways essential to learning and memory use glutamate as a neurotransmitter, including the pyramidal neurons (a layer of neurons with long axons carrying information out of the cortex), hippocampus, and entorhinal cortex. Glutamate and other excitatory amino acid neurotransmitters have been implicated as potential neurotoxins in AD.[33,34] If glutamate is allowed to remain in the synapse for extended periods of time, it can act as a toxin, destroying nerve cells. Toxic effects are thought to be mediated through increased intracellular calcium and accumulation of free radicals.[35] The presence of βAP renders cells more susceptible to glutamate-mediated excitotoxicity *in vitro*.[9] Dysregulated glutamate activity is thought to be one of the primary mediators of neuronal injury after stroke or acute brain injury. Although intimately involved in cell injury, the role of excitatory amino acids in AD is as yet unclear.

EXOGENOUS FACTORS

The contribution of exogenous factors to AD pathology is poorly understood.[5] Exogenous factors could influence, if not the likelihood of contracting AD, the age of disease onset, or rate of progression.

The possible role of estrogen in preventing AD has come under scrutiny, especially given that women are several times more likely to develop AD than their male counterparts. Estrogen is theorized to be important in maintaining neuronal structure throughout life. Thus, when estrogen levels drop postmenopausally, the brain would become less able to stimulate neuritic growth and form new synapses, rendering it less able to compensate for structural damage. Because circulating testosterone is converted to estrogen in the brain, and men do not undergo drastic changes in testosterone levels with age, they would be relatively protected compared with females.

Several case-control epidemiological studies have examined the role of post-menopausal estrogen supplementation in preventing AD. Although epidemiological studies cannot prove causality, they can indicate relationships between exposure to an agent and disease presence. Study results are contradictory, with two studies showing a positive relationship between estrogen consumption and reduced prevalence of AD (up to a 40% decrease),[36,37] and one showing no relationship.[38] It is difficult to draw definitive conclusions from these studies since data regarding estrogen use were either gathered indirectly, or through reliance on patient recall. Also, disease prevalence was generally compared with recent estrogen use, without a reliable means of examining the effects of long-term estrogen therapy, making it difficult to examine potential relationships among estrogen dose, duration of therapy, and presence or severity of AD. Only one study has followed women prospectively over time using ongoing monitoring of estrogen use, and standard measures to assess cognitive function. Barrett-Conner and Kritz-Silverstein[39] measured multiple areas of cognitive function using standard scales after 15–20 years of follow-up in 800 women older than 65 (80% of the surviving cohort). They could find no relationship between estrogen use and cognitive function despite multiple comparisons, testing different definitions of estrogen use, across six cognitive tests. While the study does not show a relationship between estrogen use and cognitive function, the cohort was well educated and few patients showed signs of dementia at follow-up, suggesting this sample may not be representative of a population with AD. Based on the available studies, it is currently premature to suggest a role for estrogen in the routine treatment or prevention of AD.

History of repeated or severe head trauma (dementia pugilistica) is also said to predispose to AD.[5] Increased risk in this population is interesting from the standpoint that glial cells and apo E are more prevalent in injured brain areas. If inflammatory pathways promote neuronal damage in AD, the increased presence of inflammatory mediators following head injury could explain increased prevalence of dementia in this population. Excitotoxicity has been also implicated as a source of neuronal damage in patients with head trauma, similar to AD.

Aluminum exposure was once thought to promote AD, causing a media-driven public scare that resulted in many people throwing away aluminum cookware. Although aluminum has been found in association with NFTs, even persons with high exposure, such as aluminum factory workers, do not have a higher prevalence of AD, and it is no longer thought to play a role in disease pathogenesis. Patients with AD do not need to avoid aluminum-containing antacids or deodorants. Likewise, there is no evidence to suggest EDTA chelation therapy is an effective treatment of AD.[40]

Another heavy metal ion, zinc, has recently become of interest as a potential facilitator of plaque formation. Following a small study in which Alzheimer's patients treated with zinc showed a rapid deterioration in cognition, Bush and colleagues[41] performed *in vitro* experiments to more closely examine the role of zinc in promoting neuritic plaques. They found zinc accelerated plaque formation from soluble βAP and hypothesized that abnormalities of zinc homeostasis in the brain could lead to plaque formation. This research is preliminary, and experiments conducted *in vitro* may not represent *in vivo* occurrences. Although the use of zinc supplements should be discouraged in patients with AD, at this time zinc should not be considered a cause of the disease.

One conclusion emanating from the multitude of research into AD pathogenesis is that there does not seem to be a single common mechanism for producing disease in all cases. Regardless of the source, however, the features remain the same: degeneration of neurons in higher brain areas; accumulation of NFTs and neuritic plaques; profound destruction of cholinergic pathways; and an insidious dementia, slowly progressive until death. Until a method is found to arrest the neuronal degeneration causing dementia symptoms, AD will not be cured.

Clinical Presentation

Unlike dementia due to stroke, the onset of AD is almost imperceptible, without abrupt changes in cognition or function. Deficits occur progressively over time and are global, affecting multiple areas of cognition.[1,42,43] The majority of cases occur after age 65, but onset can be as early as age 40.

Loss of memory is typically the presenting patient complaint. Memory, however, is a nonspecific term representing many diverse areas of cognitive function (e.g., recall, recognition, calculation, and orientation). Crucial to understanding the plight of persons with AD is to understand that "loss of memory" means substantially more than the simple inability to reminisce; it means the inability to extract and use all previously learned information, activity, and experience. Patients' initial complaints of "memory loss" typically refer to disorientation for time, or an inability to recall recent events. In early AD the ability to lay down new memory (learn) and recall recent events is severely impaired, whereas recall for remote events (childhood/adolescent years) is spared until later in the disease process. Common early problems include forgetting appointments, misplacing items such as keys, purse/wallet, or eyeglasses, getting lost traveling to familiar locations, and difficulties handling money or balancing a checkbook. Patients may notice an increasing need for lists, problems recalling the date or day of the week, and difficulty performing routine tasks at home or work. Anomia is a problem, with difficulty recalling names of familiar objects or people. Speech becomes difficult as details and content words are lost, and patients resort to confabulation or circumlocution (nonspecific, evasive speech) to compensate for their deficits. For example, when asked how he or she spends a typical day, the patient may respond, "Oh, there's always plenty to do," but he may be unable to provide further detail. Problems with speech, recall of events, and comprehension result in decreased socialization and withdrawal from casual conversation. Persons with AD often conceal their memory problem well at first. Problems may not be noticed by those unfamiliar with the patient until the disease has progressed well into its moderate stage. At this point, the patient may deny or "forget" he or she has a memory problem. Common symptoms include the inability to use objects properly even though the patient may be able to name the object or even describe how it should be used (apraxia), loss of the ability to draw complex figures or conceptualize their orientation in space (constructional apraxia) (Fig. 64.5), inability to work or do routine household chores, forgetting to eat or change clothes, disorientation to place, and difficulty initiating activities. For example, the patient may voice a desire to mow the lawn, but may be unable to undertake the steps to initiate this activity without assistance. Patients also become unable to determine the appropriate time of day for accomplishing activities and are generally unable to plan or independently follow a daily schedule. This may result in the patient following the caregiver around the house or rifling through drawers looking for environmental clues as to what he or she should be doing. As dementia progresses, patients become lost in their own homes, unable to recognize family or spouses, and unable to speak (aphasia). Judgment and reasoning are extremely impaired and, without supervision, patients may burn themselves on appliances, leave water running, wander outside and become lost, or engage in

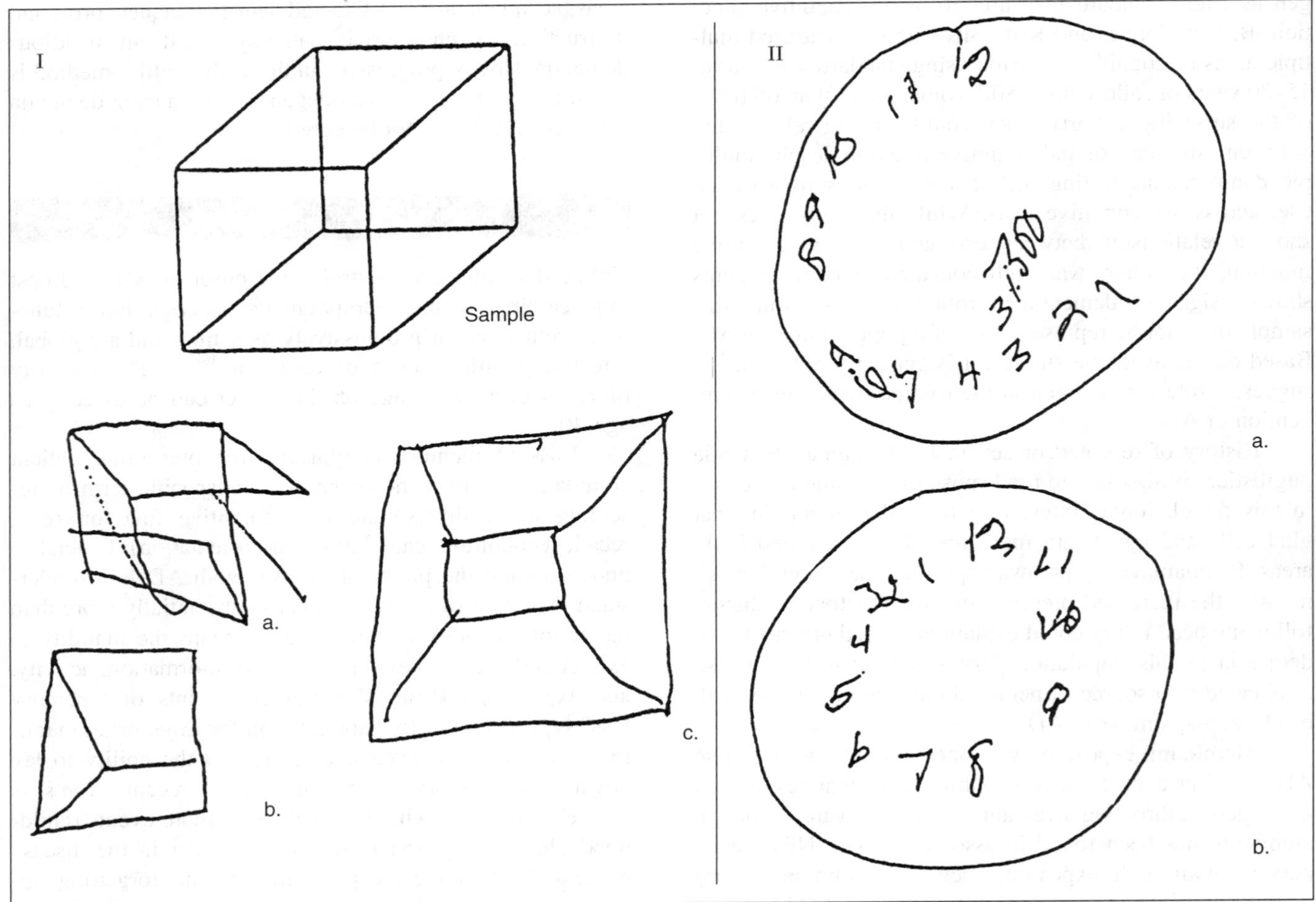

Figure 64.5. Constructional apraxia in patients with mild to moderate AD. Diagram I (a, b, c) Patients were instructed to copy the sample box. Diagram II (a, b) Patients were instructed to draw the face of a clock. The patient in (a) was then asked to draw hands on the clock representing 3:30.

TABLE 64.2. FUNDAMENTAL SYMPTOM CATEGORIES IN ALZHEIMER'S DISEASE

Cognitive Deficits[a]	Noncognitive Psychiatric Symptoms and Disruptive Behaviors[b]
• Memory loss: *poor recall; agnosia; losing items* • Dysphasia: *anomia; circumlocution; aphasia* • Dyspraxia • Disorientation: *impaired perception of time; poor sense of direction; cannot recognize acquaintances, family, or self* • Impaired calculation • Impaired judgment and problem-solving skills	• Depression • Psychotic symptoms: *hallucinations; delusions; suspiciousness* • Nonpsychotic disruptive behaviors: *physical and verbal aggression; motoric hyperactivity; uncooperativeness; wandering; repetitive mannerisms/activities; combativeness*

[a]Cognitive deficits: symptoms occurring in all patients as disease progresses.
[b]Noncognitive symptoms: symptoms that are variably present, consisting mainly of psychiatric and behavioral problems. (Compiled from Ref. 44.)

other dangerous activities. Wandering, combativeness, and incontinence are common reasons for placement in a long-term care facility. In the final stages of the disease, patients lose the ability to eat, walk, or communicate. Choking, aspiration, or infection generally results in death within 3 to 20 years after disease onset.

For treatment and assessment purposes it is helpful to divide Alzheimer's symptoms into two basic categories: cognitive symptoms and noncognitive (behavioral) symptoms[43] (Table 64.2). Cognitive symptoms are present in all patients reaching the final stages of the illness; whereas behavioral symptoms are less predictable.[43]

Noncognitive symptoms such as mood disturbances, disruptive behavior, and psychosis are present at one time or another in most patients and can pose significant management problems for caregivers. Early in the course of the illness, the patient may become depressed, frustrated, or irritable. Anxiety, hostility, misinterpretations, and delusions are common in moderate stages of AD. Personality changes and changes in emotional expression are also frequently reported. Disruptive behaviors and psychosis are most often seen in the moderate to severe stages of AD, with severity fluctuating over time. Common disruptive behaviors include wandering, agitation, aggression, uncooperativeness, and purposeless activity. Examples of the latter include rummaging through clothing or drawers, repetitive asking of questions, perpetual humming or grunting, fingernail clicking, and picking at clothes. Patients frequently experience "sundowning," or worsening of symptoms at night because of decreased sensory input and fewer orienting stimuli. Suspiciousness, nonsystematized paranoid delusions, and misinterpretation of actual phenomena (illusions) are the most common psychotic symptoms. It is important to recognize that the psychotic symptoms characterizing AD are substantially different from those seen in nondemented patients, such as those with schizophrenia. Delusions in AD more often appear to be an attempt to explain things that have been forgotten. For example, the patient may misplace an item, and upon being unable to find it, reason it has been stolen. Based on this belief, he or she may accuse family members of stealing lost items, or become agitated, believing that intruders are entering the home. Other delusions may stem from an inability to recognize friends and family members, combined with preferential loss of recent memories. Common delusions include the belief that the house one is living in is not one's real home, deceased persons (such as parents) are still living, the caregiver has been replaced by an impostor, or that a spouse is being unfaithful (delusional jealousy). Common hallucinations and illusions include seeing or hearing imaginary people in the house, mistaking one's own reflection in a mirror for an intruder, or misinterpreting shadows as people or objects. As a consequence of these phenomena, the patient may become agitated, physically or verbally aggressive, or attempt to leave the residence in search of missing persons or to "go home."[44]

Because patients are frequently unaware of their deficits, it can be difficult to appreciate the full morbidity of AD without talking to the primary caregiver. Persons with AD become extraordinarily dependent on those around them. Family and direct caregivers may experience considerable psychological distress through role changes, time commitments, cost, and the hassles of day-to-day care. Patients become progressively childlike, relying on caregivers for provision of all their basic needs. It is extremely difficult for caregivers to cope with the transformation of someone from an able-bodied companion or parent to a dependent stranger. Any attempts at therapeutic management must take into account the effect of treatment on the caregiver, both with respect to cost and ease of use versus expected therapeutic gain.

DIAGNOSIS

Minor memory loss, sometimes called *age-associated memory impairment,* is a common complaint associated with normal aging and is not a cause for concern. However, if memory loss affects social or occupational functioning, or is noticed by friends and co-workers, patients should be encouraged to visit a neurologist for a formal evaluation. At present, the only way to definitively diagnose AD is through direct examination of brain tissue at autopsy or biopsy. Because no definitive diagnostic laboratory, clinical, or imaging tests are available, AD remains a diagnosis of exclusion. In early research, as many as 20% of cases thought to be AD would later be found to be caused by other diseases. To design criteria that would minimize inaccurate diagnosis, a workgroup was established in 1984 by the National Institute of Neurological and Communicative Disorders and Stroke (NINCDS) and the Alzheimer's Disease and Related Disorders Association (ADRDA). Utilization of the workgroup's explicit criteria has reduced the percentage of erroneously diagnosed AD cases to under 10%, and the NINCDS–ADRDA criteria (Table 64.3) are now standardly employed for selecting patients in pharmaceutical research trials.[45] Patient's fulfilling these criteria are given a diagnosis of probable AD. The first step in this diagnostic process is a thorough history and physical exam. The history should be obtained from the patient and reliable caregivers and confirm a slowly progressive and not precipitous deterioration of functioning. Questions should include review of prescription drug use, history of alcohol or other substance use, family medical history, and history of trauma, depression, or head injury. It is important to rule out medication use as contributing to dementia symptoms, especially medications with anticholinergic or other CNS side effects. An established dementia screening scale, such as the Folstein Mini-Mental Status Exam (MMSE),[46] can aid in confirming a history of deficits in two or more areas of cognition.[45,46] Other causes of dementia must be excluded, including cerebral vascular disease, subcortical stroke, alcoholism, or vitamin B_{12} deficiency, to name a few (Table 64.1). Routine laboratory tests and physical and neurologic exams should rule out other disorders. Brain imaging tools help rule out multi-infarct dementia, and although atrophy or other nonspecific abnormalities are often seen on computed tomography (CT) scans or magnetic resonance imaging (MRI), these are not sufficient to confer an AD diagnosis. Following diagnosis, AD is staged using a scale such as the Global Deterioration Scale (GDS)[47] (Table 64.4). This seven-point system is widely used, has been validated as correlating to psychometric measures and changes in CT or positron emission tomography (PET) scans, and is useful to monitor the global changes in the patient with AD. This NINCDS–ADRDA diagnostic workup, while fairly accurate, is tedious and costly. It is easy to understand why simpler methods for early diagnosis would be highly desirable.

TABLE 64.3. NINCDS–ADRDA CRITERIA AND DIAGNOSTIC WORKUP FOR PROBABLE ALZHEIMER'S DISEASE

1. History of progressive cognitive decline of insidious onset
   - In-depth interview of patient and caregivers
2. Deficits in at least two or more areas of functioning
   - Confirmation with use of dementia rating scale (i.e., Mini-Mental Status Exam [MMSE[a]] or Blessed Dementia Scale)
3. No disturbance of consciousness
4. Age between 40 and 90 (usually >65)
5. No other explainable cause of symptoms
   - Normal laboratory tests including hematology, full chemistries, B_{12} and folate, thyroid function tests, VDRL (to rule out venereal disease or syphilis)
   - Normal electrocardiogram and electroencephalogram
   - Normal physical exam, including thorough neurologic exam
   - Neuroimaging: CT or MRI scanning; no focal lesions signifying other possible causes of dementia are allowed. Abnormalities that are common, but not diagnostic for Alzheimer's disease include general cerebral wasting, widening of sulci, widening of the ventricles, and lesions of white matter surrounding the ventricle deep in the brain.

[a]The Folstein Mini-Mental Status Exam (MMSE)[46] is a commonly used scale that measures orientation, recall, short-term memory, concentration, constructional praxis, and language. The MMSE is scored from 0 to 30, with a score of 10 to ~28 typical of moderate to very early Alzheimer's disease. (Adapted from Ref. 45.)

Early diagnosis of AD is important from a treatment standpoint, in that cognition enhancing drugs are more likely to be effective early in the course of the illness, before neurons are extensively destroyed. Two potential methods of early diagnosis deserve mention, and are currently undergoing further research. The first uses the anticholinergic eyedrop tropicamide. Since the cholinergic system is known to be damaged in AD, it would naturally follow that these patients would be more sensitive to anticholinergic medications. In a double-blind, drug versus placebo study, using subjects as their own controls, Scinto et al.[48] demonstrated that patients with AD could be distinguished from normal controls and persons with non–Alzheimer's dementia by measuring changes in pupil size following application of a dilute 0.01% tropicamide solution (standard concentrations are 0.5–1.0%). Although the sample size was small (58 subjects), the test showed a sensitivity of 95%, selecting patients in even mild stages of cognitive decline. This test appeared useful in distinguishing Alzheimer's patients from other types of dementia; however, research with a larger patient sample will be required to determine specificity. The low cost of the method is also encouraging, and further research is under way to validate this potential diagnostic tool.

Another strategy for early diagnosis combines two less specific tests, genetic testing for the apo E4 gene and PET scan measures for decreased parietal glucose metabolism and left–right asymmetry.[49] The predictive ability of this method is unclear at present. Currently apo E typing is not available on a routine clinical basis. Concern exists regarding potential discrimination by insurance companies and employers toward individuals who possess one or more copies of apo E4. Until either a cure for AD is found or measures are in place to prevent discrimination against these patients, there is resistance to testing becoming widely available.

THERAPEUTIC MANAGEMENT

Pharmacotherapy in AD addresses two areas, cognitive symptoms and noncognitive symptoms. Cognition-enhanc-

TABLE 64.4. STAGES OF COGNITIVE DECLINE: THE GLOBAL DETERIORATION SCALE (GDS)

Stage 1	Normal	No subjective or objective change in intellectual functioning.
Stage 2	Forgetfulness	Complaints of losing things or forgetting names of acquaintances. Does not interfere with job or social functioning. Generally a component of normal aging.
Stage 3	Early confusion	Cognitive decline causes interference with work and social functioning. Anomia, difficulty remembering right word in conversation, and recall difficulties are present and noticed by family members. Memory loss may cause anxiety for patient.
Stage 4	Late confusion (early Alzheimer's)	Patient can no longer manage finances or homemaking activities. Difficulty remembering recent events. Begins to withdraw from difficult tasks and give up hobbies. May deny memory problems.
Stage 5	Early dementia (moderate Alzheimer's)	Patient can no longer survive without assistance. Frequently disoriented with regard to time (date, year, season). Difficulty selecting clothing. Recall for recent events is severely impaired; may forget some details of past life (i.e., school attended or occupation). Functioning may fluctuate from day to day. Patient generally denies problems. May become suspicious or tearful. Loses ability to drive safely.
Stage 6	Middle dementia (moderately severe Alzheimer's)	Patients need assistance with activities of daily living (i.e., bathing, dressing, and toileting). Patients experience difficulty interpreting their surroundings; may forget names of family and caregivers; forgets most details of past life; difficulty counting backward from 10. Agitation, paranoia, and delusions are common.
Stage 7	Late dementia	Patient loses ability to speak (may only grunt or scream), walk, and feed self. Incontinent of urine and feces. Consciousness reduced to stupor or coma.

(Adapted from Ref. 47.)

ing medications are intended to treat core dementia symptoms and are designed to reverse or retard the rate of cognitive decline. Psychotropic medications are used to treat noncognitive psychiatric target symptoms and disruptive behaviors accompanying AD. Psychotropic medications generally have no effect on cognition and may negatively impact cognition in some cases.

PHARMACOTHERAPY OF COGNITIVE SYMPTOMS

Research Methodology in Alzheimer's Disease

Early studies with potential cognition-enhancing agents in AD are difficult to interpret. Significant variation existed from study to study with respect to methodology and patient assessments, and in many cases consistency in diagnosis could be questioned. Criticisms of study methodology, including the questionable ability to determine clinically significant effects of a drug in AD, led the Food and Drug Administration (FDA) to reject the initial New Drug Application (NDA) for tacrine. Subsequent to this decision and considerable discussions and publicity among both professionals and the lay public, the FDA recommended uniform criteria for conducting efficacy studies in patients with AD.

At a minimum, studies in support of a NDA for treatment of AD must be double blind, placebo controlled, randomized, and of parallel group design. Efficacy must be indicated by statistically significant differences between groups on both the Alzheimer's Disease Assessment Scale—Cognitive Portion (ADAS–Cog) and the Clinical Interview-Based Impression of Change (CIBIC).[50] The ADAS–Cog is a structured psychometric assessment measuring patient performance on multiple, discrete areas of cognitive function. The CIBIC is a clinician's assessment based solely on an interview with the patient, and without access to any other patient information. Efficacy based on the CIBIC is deemed important because it is thought to represent a clinically distinguishable change in cognition and more closely mimic the manner in which a clinician might evaluate a patient in the office setting.[51] More recently, the CIBIC–Plus, a clinical assessment based on interviews with both the patient and the caregiver, is being used in lieu of the CIBIC by many investigators.[52]

Tacrine

The development of the cholinergic hypothesis in the early 1980s led to significant interest in developing drug therapies for AD. Just as levodopa was developed as replacement therapy for dopaminergic deficiency in Parkinson's disease, researchers began to examine means in which to enhance cholinergic activity in patients with AD. Tacrine was the first such drug to be examined in a systematic fashion.

Tacrine is a competitive, reversible inhibitor of both acetylcholinesterase and butylcholinesterase. Inhibition of acetylcholinesterase increases the amount of acetylcholine available for binding to muscarinic receptors, thereby enhancing muscarinic effects, and theoretically improving memory and cognition. Tacrine's muscarinic activity produces secondary effects on other neurotransmitter systems. The synthesis, turnover, and release of serotonin, norepinephrine, and dopamine have all been shown to be increased by tacrine in animal studies. The contribution of these effects to the drug's clinical activity in humans is unknown.[52]

The efficacy of tacrine has been proven in two large multicenter clinical trials.[53,54] The second of these is a 30-week trial comparing the effects of tacrine 80 mg, 120 mg, and 160 mg daily with placebo. Currently, this clinical trial represents the best long-term treatment information of a cognitive agent in patients with AD.[54] Although the study demonstrates the efficacy of tacrine in AD, a number of other important points can be gleaned from the study. Primarily because of elevated hepatic enzymes, but also due to peripheral cholinergic side effects, many patients cannot tolerate tacrine. Therefore, the dropout rate with treatment is high. After 6 months of treatment, only 11–12% of the patients started on tacrine were still taking it and demonstrating clinical improvement. An additional 10–11% tolerated the drug and showed no cognitive decline.[52,54] A positive dose–response relationship exists for efficacy as well as side effects.

Significant placebo response is observed in AD, and cognition declines slowly in many untreated patients.[51,54] After 30 weeks of treatment, more than 50% of placebo-treated patients either showed minimal improvement or no change on the CIBIC. Although there was a significant drug placebo difference, this causes one to question how long one must evaluate a drug in treatment of AD in order to assess adequately the effects of the agent on progression of the disease. This also provides minimal guidance to the clinician with respect to treatment decisions, particularly regarding how long to use tacrine in a patient demonstrating no change in cognition or functional status.

Adverse effects with tacrine are significant, with the potential for hepatotoxicity being of most concern. Elevated transaminases, as defined by an alanine aminotransferase (ALT) or aspartate aminotransferase (AST) concentration greater than three times the upper limits of normal, occurred in 636 of 2706 (23.5%) patients receiving tacrine in all trials.[1,52] Liver function test (LFT) elevations tend to occur during the first 8 weeks of tacrine therapy and are more common in females. The rise in ALT is more often abrupt than gradual and does not appear to be dose related. During the course of clinical trials, there were no reports of permanent hepatotoxicity; in fact, most patients were asymptomatic.[55] However, in this setting, LFTs were closely monitored, and the drug discontinued if the ALT exceeded predetermined limits. The frequency and extent of serious liver damage if tacrine were to be continued despite elevated LFTs is unknown. This reinforces the importance of closely monitoring patients' LFTs during tacrine treatment. Liver enzymes generally return to normal within 4–6 weeks following dosage decrease or discontinuation. Of patients developing LFT elevations during clinical trials, five developed jaundice.[1,52] Among these five, all had ALTs of more than 3 times the upper limit of normal. All recovered with drug discontinuation. Biopsy data in six other patients with elevated transaminases showed histology consistent with hepatocellular necrosis.[52]

In patients experiencing LFT elevations, rechallenge with tacrine has been attempted after the ALT has returned to normal. Of 145 patients rechallenged, tacrine had to be discontinued again in 18 (12%) because of persistently elevated LFTs.[55] In those patients who developed recurrence, elevated ALTs occurred more rapidly than originally (mean time = 22 days). If rechallenge is considered, the recommended initial dose is 10 mg four times daily, with weekly LFT monitoring.

Table 64.5 lists the frequency of adverse effects occurring in greater than 2% of 2706 patients receiving tacrine in all phases of controlled and open clinical trials.[1] Adverse events occurred in 81–87% of patients receiving tacrine as compared with 75% of patients receiving placebo. Although the overall reported incidence of adverse effects with tacrine is high, it is important to point out the high frequency of physical complaints that naturally occur in this patient population. With the exception of elevated transaminases, the common adverse experiences reported with tacrine are those expected from a drug with cholinergic properties, namely, nausea and vomiting, diarrhea, abdominal pain, and dyspepsia.

Significant interindividual variation exists with respect to tacrine's dose–response relationship. Much of this is associated with the drug's pharmacokinetics, and tacrine serum concentrations have been shown to more closely correlate with both efficacy and cholinergic-related adverse effects than does dose.[52,56] Tacrine pharmacokinetics are illustrated in Table 64.6. Of special note is the fact that tacrine has a low bioavailability with significant interindividual variation. Bioavailability is also nonlinear, with disproportionately greater AUCs occurring with increasing doses. The rate and extent of tacrine absorption is decreased when it is taken within 2 hours after a meal. Absorption does not appear to be affected by aluminum/magnesium-containing antacids. Tacrine is metabolized in the liver, primarily through cytochrome P-450 isoenzyme IA2. The metabolite, 1-hydroxytacrine, contributes significantly to the drug's activity. The half-life is short, thus requiring multiple doses daily. A sustained-release form of tacrine is currently under investigation. Pharmacokinetics are unaffected by renal insufficiency.[52]

Drug interactions with tacrine have been poorly studied. Centrally acting anticholinergics would be expected to antagonize its efficacy, and other cholinergic agents would

TABLE 64.5. INCIDENCE OF ADVERSE DRUG REACTIONS WITH TACRINE USE IN CLINICAL TRIALS

Adverse Event	Incidence	
Hepatotoxicity (during weekly monitoring in 2446 patients):		
Maximum ALT		
Within normal limits	1243 (50.8%)	
Above normal	1203 (49.2%)	
>3× upper normal limit	621 (25.4%)	
>10× upper normal limit	172 (7%)	
>20× upper normal limit	40 (1.6%)	
Other Adverse Events Occurring in ≥2% of Patients in New Drug Application		
Adverse Event[a]	**Placebo ($N = 342$) (%)**	**Tacrine ($N = 2706$) (%)**
Nausea/vomiting	1.5	28.2
Diarrhea	5.3	13.9
Headache	15.2	12.5
Agitation	8.8	9.9
Anorexia	3.2	8.9
Abdominal pain	7.0	8.9
Dyspepsia	6.4	8.7
Rhinitis	6.4	8.2
Myalgia	5.3	7.5
Insomnia	5.3	7.4
Ataxia	3.5	7.4
Rash	5.3	7.2
Confusion	7.0	7.1
Depression	4.1	5.7
Urinary tract infection	5.8	5.1
Constipation	2.3	4.7
Coughing	5.3	4.0
Anxiety	2.0	4.0
Hallucinations	3.5	3.8
Fatigue	2.6	3.5
Flatulence	1.5	3.5
Back pain	4.1	3.5
Upper respiratory infection	3.2	3.3
Urinary frequency	3.5	3.2
Somnolence	3.2	3.1
Purpura	2.3	2.8
Urinary incontinence	2.6	2.7
Hostility	1.5	2.7
Weight decrease	1.2	2.7
Tremor	0.6	2.7
Abnormal thinking	4.1	2.5
Chest pain	5.3	2.3
Asthenia	2.0	2.1
Any event	74.9	80.9

[a]Table indicates all adverse events reported, without assessment of severity or causal relationship to drug administration. *(Adapted from Ref. 52, with permission.)*

TABLE 64.6. TACRINE PHARMACOKINETICS

Bioavailability (F)	17%
Range (increases with increasing dose)	(2.4–36%)
Area under the curve (AUC)	
10 mg q 6 h	19.7 ng/ml/h
20 mg q 6 h	82.9 ng/ml/h
30 mg q 6 h	139 ng/ml/h
Volume of distribution (V_d)	349 ± 193 L (5.02 L/kg)
Clearance (Cl)	2.42 ± 0.77 L/min
Half-life ($t_{1/2}$)	
Single dose	
25 mg	1.59 ± 0.15 h
50 mg	2.14 ± 0.24 h
Multiple dose	
10 mg q 6 h	3.4 h
20 mg q 6 h	3.6 h
30 mg q 6 h	3.2 h

(Adapted from Ref. 52, with permission.)

be expected to have additive side effects. Tacrine decreases theophylline clearance by approximately 50% but has no effects on digoxin, diazepam, or warfarin. Cimetidine decreases tacrine clearance by approximately 30%. Until more is known about drug interactions involving tacrine, careful patient monitoring should occur when it is used in combination with other drugs metabolized through hepatic microsomal pathways.[52]

Clinical Use

Tacrine should be used only in patients with mild to moderate dementia. The efficacy of tacrine has not been studied in patients with severe dementia (i.e., MMSE scores <10). Based on its mechanism of action and the pathophysiology of AD, the likelihood of clinically significant improvement in the severely demented patient is poor. Patients can be easily screened using an objective assessment tool such as MMSE,[46] with patients scoring ≥10 being placed on the drug. Because of its cholinergic activity, tacrine should be used cautiously in patients with other disease states where cholinergic stimulation may be problematic. The initial dosage should be 10 mg PO four times daily with the dose titrated, if tolerated, in 40 mg/d increments every 4–6 weeks up to a maximum of 40 mg four times daily. As per the approved product labeling, LFTs, particularly the ALT, should be monitored weekly for the first 18 weeks, and weekly for 6 weeks after any increase in dose. The manufacturer recommends decreasing the dose if the ALT exceeds three times the upper limit of normal and discontinuing the drug if the ALT exceeds five times the upper limit of normal.[1,52]

If tolerated, patients should be treated for a minimum of 3 months in order to assess therapeutic response. The question of how long to treat with tacrine is an important one. As mentioned earlier, no change in symptoms may be a positive response. In the 30-week study, mean peak improvement occurred after 24 weeks and began to decline after that, but still remained superior to the placebo group.[54] How long to expect a positive response from tacrine is unknown. Based on these facts, tacrine should be continued as long as the patient is tolerating the drug and showing no rapid decline. If tacrine is discontinued, tapering is recommended because there are case reports of patients rapidly deteriorating upon discontinuation. This is not thought to be a rebound deterioration, but rather a decline to the point the patient would have been at if he or she had never been treated with the drug.

Caregivers should be carefully counseled about having realistic expectations with respect to response from tacrine. Economic factors must be considered, as well. Depending on the patient's age, physical health, severity of dementia, and financial status, a decision to use tacrine may not always be in the patient's or the caregiver's best interests. But given a motivated family and no contraindications to the use of tacrine, a therapeutic trial is a reasonable decision.

Investigational Agents

A large number of agents are being investigated as potential therapeutic agents in the treatment of AD. Physostigmine, a short-acting cholinesterase inhibitor, is being developed in a sustained-release form. However, it has a high incidence of gastrointestinal (GI) side effects, particularly nausea and diarrhea. Other cholinesterase inhibitors, particularly ones such as Eisai 20-20[57] and CP-118,954,[58] which may have no hepatotoxicity, are being developed. Hepatotoxicity appears to be associated with the aminoacridine moiety, and cholinesterase inhibitors without this structure appear not to cause LFT elevations. It has been suggested that cholinesterase inhibitors that are specific for acetylcholinesterase may augment central muscarinic activity with a lower incidence of peripheral cholinergic side effects.

Since AD involves dysfunction in multiple neurotransmitter systems, agents are being developed that affect neurotransmitters such as serotonin, norepinephrine, or dopamine in addition to augmenting cholinergic activity. Acetyl-L-carnitine and besipridine are such agents.[59] Acetyl-L-carnitine is structurally similar to acetylcholine, and it promotes acetylcholine synthesis and acts as a cholinergic facilitator in experimental studies. Besipridine enhances cholinergic activity by acting postsynaptically at a site separate from the muscarinic receptor. It also inhibits the reuptake of norepinephrine and dopamine. The first multicenter trial with besipridine showed significant improvement on the ADAS–Cog but not on the CIBIC–Plus. Studies in larger populations and of longer duration are currently in progress. These two drugs are also alleged to have "neuroprotective" effects, meaning they facilitate natural neuronal protective mechanisms that guard the cell from oxidative damage and/or promote membrane stabilization and repair of neuronal processes.

Nerve growth factor (NGF) or neurotrophins have sparked significant interest because animal studies indicate that they can halt chemical injury to neurons and promote restitution.[60] NGF can be thought of as part of the brain's maintenance department, helping to restore damaged neurons. Animal studies also suggest NGF causes hypertrophy of remaining cholinergic neurons in the nucleus basalis. One case report in a patient with AD indicates reason for promise,[60] but problems in delivering these agents to the CNS provide a challenge for clinical investigators.

Drugs approved by the FDA for other indications have also been tried in AD. Based on the presence of inflammatory mediators in Alzheimer's plaques, and reduced prevalence of AD in arthritic patients receiving long-term anti-inflammatory drugs, indomethacin was studied in a small, double-blind pilot trial with positive results.[61] While patients treated with indomethacin 100–150 mg/d did not appear to show cognitive decline during the 6-month trial, about one-third dropped out due to GI side effects. In a retrospective chart review, patients with AD treated with various nonsteroidal anti-inflammatory drugs (NSAIDs), including ibuprofen, aspirin, and naproxen, for other indications showed better performance on cognitive tests and a slower rate of decline than controls.[62] However, NSAID-treated patients had a shorter duration of illness than non–NSAID-treated controls at baseline. While these preliminary trials are encouraging, large prospective trials using conventional rating assessments are needed to determine the utility of NSAIDs in AD. Nimodipine, a calcium blocker, has been tried in patients with AD. Its use is justified based on the theory that prolonged calcium influx may be associated with cell injury in AD. In one small study, nimodipine 90 mg daily, but not 180 mg daily, showed statistically significant improvement on selected memory tests.[63] Although these studies have shown promising results, they need to be replicated in larger scale, better controlled studies.

Another strategy to treat AD involves antioxidants. Theoretically, it is hoped that antioxidants might be effective in binding free radicals associated with cell injury. Glial cell proliferation occurs in AD, resulting in increased concentrations of MAO. Data from a multicenter trial with L-deprenyl and vitamin E, modeled after the Datatop study in Parkinson's disease, will soon be available.[64] L-Deprenyl is a relatively selective inhibitor of MAO-B. In a 15-month double-blind study in mildly demented patients, the only demonstrated effect with L-Deprenyl 10 mg daily was a mild decrease in Brief Psychiatric Rating Scale scores. The clinical significance of this effect was questioned by the investigators.[65] Other studies with L-Deprenyl alone have shown mixed results. Some studies have shown improvement in cognition while others have shown improvement in behavior or mood.[65,66] It appears that patients who are more severely demented and those with behavioral symptoms are more likely to receive benefit than patients with milder disease presentation.

PHARMACOTHERAPY OF NONCOGNITIVE SYMPTOMS

The majority of patients with AD will manifest noncognitive symptoms at some point in the illness. These symptoms are detailed in the section on clinical presentation[43,44] in this chapter and can be roughly divided into three categories: psychotic symptoms, disruptive behavior, and depression. Effective management of these problems is important because behavioral symptoms are distressing to both the patient and the caregiver, necessitate increased caregiver supervision and patience to manage, and are a leading reason for nursing home placement. Despite the widespread nature of these symptoms in AD, there has been surprisingly little formal research on psychotropic drug efficacy in these patients. Most treatment recommendations come from small trials, case reports, and clinical experience. Although information can be extrapolated from studies using psychotropic drugs for similar symptoms in nondemented patients, the widespread neuronal loss seen in AD and different underlying pathology suggests that this approach may not be valid. General guidelines governing therapy can be summarized as follows: reduced doses, close monitoring, and careful documentation. Periodic attempts to reduce medication are also recommended, as symptoms change with disease progression. Many psychotropic medications have anticholinergic effects, which may actually worsen cognition. These anticholinergic effects, as well as sedative effects, medication-induced postural instability, and extrapyramidal side effects also decrease the clinical utility of many traditional psychotropic agents in this population. An outline of suggested doses of medications is provided in Table 64.7.[66]

Prior to implementing pharmacotherapy for behavioral problems, persons caring for the patient should have the necessary information on how best to communicate and work with the patient. For example, overly technical or detailed directions may confuse and upset patients. Simple instructions or a demonstration of the desired activity is easier for the patient to understand. Caregivers with good intentions may also try to push patients to continue doing familiar tasks in hopes this will preserve existing memory as long as possible. As the patient becomes increasingly unable to accomplish a task due to disease progression, he or she may easily become frustrated and upset. A simple change to a less demanding lifestyle may decrease agitated behaviors substantially. Family members may not realize at first the degree of impairment in the Alzheimer's patient's memory and ability to reason. The patient, for example, may accuse a family member of stealing an item that has been misplaced. The family member becomes upset at this accusation and attempts to rationalize or argue with the patient. This frequently causes agitated behavior to escalate. Although difficult, the caregiver may find that by ignoring accusations or changing the subject, the patient will calm down. Helpful resources for caregivers are provided in Table 64.8.

TABLE 64.7. MEDICATIONS USED IN TREATING NONCOGNITIVE SYMPTOMS OF DEMENTIA

Drugs	Suggested Dosage in Dementia (mg/d)	Indications
Antipsychotics		Psychosis: hallucinations, delusions, suspiciousness
Haloperidol	0.5–5 mg	Disruptive behaviors: agitation, aggression
Thioridazine	30–150 mg	
Antidepressants[b]		Depression: poor appetite, insomnia, hopelessness, anhedonia, withdrawal, suicidal thoughts, agitation
Desipramine	50–100[a] mg	
Nortriptyline	25–100[a] mg	
Fluoxetine	5–20 mg	
Sertraline	50–200 mg	
Paroxetine	10–40 mg	
Trazodone	150–400[a] mg	
Anticonvulsants		
Carbamazepine	100–1000[a] mg	
Valproic acid	1000–2500[a] mg	
Others		
L-Deprenyl	10 mg	Disruptive behaviors, agitation, anxiety, depression
Buspirone	10–45 mg[a]	Disruptive behaviors
Oxazepam	10–60 mg[a]	Disruptive behaviors

[a]Administer in divided doses.

[b]Newer antidepressants such as venlafaxine and nefazodone theoretically could be used but have not been reported. Concurrent use of fluroxamine with tacrine should be avoided due to fluroxamine's capacity to inhibit cytochrome P=450–IA2. (Adapted from Refs. 65, 66, and 67.)

TABLE 64.8. RESOURCES FOR CAREGIVERS OF PERSONS WITH ALZHEIMER'S DISEASE

The following organizations provide educational literature, information on diagnosis, treatment, and ongoing research in Alzheimer's disease:

- Alzheimer's Disease Education and Referral Center (ADEAR)
  PO Box 8250
  Silver Spring, MD 20907
  1-800-438-4380
- Alzheimer's Disease and Related Disorders Association (ADRDA or The Alzheimer's Association)
  919 N. Michigan
  Chicago, IL 60601
  1-800-272-3900
- Alzheimer's Disease Society of Canada
  491 Lawrence Ave. West, #501
  Toronto, Ontario, Canada M5M1C7

Further Reading:

- *Failure-Free Activities for the Alzheimer's Patient.* San Francisco, CA: Cottage Books, 1987.
- *Reminiscence: Uncovering a Lifetime of Memories.* San Francisco, CA: Elder Press, 1991.
- *Living in the Labyrinth. A Personal Journey Through the Maze of Alzheimer's.* San Francisco, CA: Elder Press, 1993.
- *The 36 Hour Day.* Baltimore, MD: Johns Hopkins University Press, 1981.

Depression

Prevalence rates of depression in AD have been estimated to range from <10–80%. The inconsistency in these figures may be ascribed to the overlap of symptoms in these two disorders and the fact that patients with AD are often poor historians. Symptoms common to both disorders include apathy, decreased initiative and socialization, decreased concentration, psychomotor retardation, agitation, and changes in appetite and sleep patterns.[67] An interview with the patient's caregiver can be helpful in obtaining a more accurate record of symptoms. Depression may be more common in the early stages of AD as the patient adjusts to limitations such as having to retire from employment and relinquishing other intellectually demanding activities.

The bulk of literature examining antidepressant use in AD is made up of case reports and uncontrolled studies. Most of these report a favorable response to antidepressants.[67] The only available placebo-controlled study, an 8-week trial of imipramine versus placebo, showed significant response in both treatment groups, but no advantage of imipramine over placebo.[68] The available literature also suggests that antidepressant response, as measured by reductions in Hamilton Depression Rating (HAM-D) scores, is not as dramatic as in depressed nondemented patients. Since depressive target symptoms are difficult to distinguish from dementia, it is unclear whether this modest decrease in HAM-D scores is due to poor drug response or difficulty in assessing symptoms in this population.[67,68] Based on the available literature, it would be desirable to document symptoms of depression for several weeks prior to initiating antidepressant therapy in a patient with AD. There appears to be a significant placebo response in this population, and it is possible that simply visiting with a clinician or increasing the patient's activity level may be sufficient to improve symptoms. If this approach fails, a limited trial of an antidepressant could be initiated. Pharmacotherapy should be initiated with an antidepressant possessing a favorable side-effect profile. Acceptable antidepressants in this patient population include secondary amine tricyclic antidepressants such as nortriptyline or desipramine, which have a lower incidence of anticholinergic and cardiovascular side effects than the tertiary amines, or serotonin specific reuptake inhibitors (SSRI) such as fluoxetine, paroxetine, or sertraline.[69] Trazodone, which lacks anticholinergic effects, tends to cause sedation and orthostasis, which may pose disadvantages over other available agents. Because of their low propensity to cause anticholinergic effects, orthostatic hypotension, and sedation, the SSRIs are often considered to be preferred antidepressants in this population. SSRIs can often be dosed once daily. These medications are not without risk however. GI adverse effects, confusion, agitation, dizziness, and insomnia have been reported in patients with AD taking fluoxetine, especially at higher doses (>20 mg daily).[70] For a more complete discussion, refer to Chapter 67.

Antipsychotics

Antipsychotic medications have traditionally been used to treat disruptive behaviors and psychosis in AD patients. Rationale for use of these medications is partly derived from their beneficial effects in treating psychosis in schizophrenia, even though the quality of these symptoms is quite different in AD.[44,67] Despite widespread use, available placebo-controlled studies suggest that antipsychotics are only moderately effective at best.[71–73] Symptoms responding include assaultiveness, extreme agitation and hyperexcitability, hallucinations, delusions, suspiciousness, hostility, and uncooperativeness.[71–73] Symptoms not responding include withdrawal, apathy, cognitive deficits, and incontinence.[67] Patients with AD are more sensitive to antipsychotic side effects than other patient groups. Particularly problematic side effects are extrapyramidal side effects, postural instability due to alpha-adrenergic blockade, and anticholinergic effects, including increased confusion, urinary retention, constipation, and dry mouth.[8,67,69] These side effects and worsening cognition seriously limit the usefulness of these medications, especially when behavioral problems are minor. Effective doses of antipsychotic medications are much lower than those typically used to treat schizophrenia. For example, the suggested starting dose of haloperidol is 0.5 mg/d.[1,8]

Increased sensitivity to antipsychotic agents appears to be the result of altered pharmacodynamics rather than altered pharmacokinetics.[67,74] The suggested therapeutic range for haloperidol serum concentrations, 5–12 ng/mL, should not be used as a guide for dosing in AD because efficacy and adverse effects occur well below this range in many patients.[74] Pharmacotherapy with antipsychotics should be guided by several key concepts. First, if the delusions or behaviors are not particularly disturbing to the patient or caregiver, they may not require treatment. Second, many caregivers have erroneous expectations regarding the effects of these medications, and it should be assured that the anticipated benefits and risks of therapy are understood. Third, disruptive behaviors and delusions wax and wane with disease progression. Attempts to taper and discontinue antipsychotic medication should be undertaken frequently (at least every 3 months), since many patients who initially respond to these medications show no change in symptoms and occasionally improve on medication withdrawal.[1,67] The most widely used antipsychotic in Alzheimer's is haloperidol, likely due to its relatively low incidence of anticholinergic effects, sedation, and orthostatic hypotension as compared with other typical neuroleptics. However, if extrapyramidal effects are bothersome, thioridazine in low doses is an acceptable substitute.

Miscellaneous Therapies

Because antipsychotic therapy has shown only modest efficacy and poses a substantial risk of undesirable side effects, medications traditionally used to treat disruptive behaviors and aggression in other psychiatric and neurologic disorders have been suggested as potential alternatives. These include benzodiazepines, buspirone, lithium, carbamazepine, L-deprenyl, valproate, and fluoxetine. Unfortunately, few of these agents have been studied in a controlled fashion in patients with AD. Doses of selected medications are listed in Table 64.7. Benzodiazepines, particularly oxazepam, have been used to treat anxiety, agitation, and aggression, but generally show inferior efficacy when compared to antipsychotics. Because benzodiazepines impair cognition and increase the risk of falls in AD patients, their routine use is not advised.[67] Conversely, the 5-HT_{1A} partial agonist, buspirone, has shown benefit in treating agitation and aggression in a limited number of patients with minimal adverse effects.[75,76] L-Deprenyl has been shown to decrease anxiety, depression, and agitation in open-label and controlled studies.[65,77,78] Although a longer term double-blind study using L-Deprenyl in mildly demented patients showed no benefit, the more typical patient with AD (i.e., greater disease severity) may be more likely to respond.[66] Should antipsychotics fail to manage noncognitive behaviors, a trial of buspirone or L-Deprenyl might be reasonable alternatives. There is less documentation to support use of carbamazepine or valproate, and lithium thus far has shown no benefit.[67] Clearly, more rigorous placebo-controlled studies would assist in determining the place in therapy, and relative efficacy of these alternative medications.

Evaluation of Therapeutic Outcomes

An evaluation of therapeutic outcomes in the patient with AD begins with a thorough assessment at baseline and a clear definition of therapeutic goals. Cognitive status, physical status, functional performance, mood, thought processes, and behavior all need to be evaluated before initiation of drug therapy. The clinician should interview both the caregiver and the patient to assess the patient's response to the drug. Because caregivers often have difficulty giving honest and frank information about their loved one's condition in his or her presence, it is best to interview caregivers and their loved ones separately when possible. In evaluating response to tacrine or other cognitive agents, the clinician should ask questions about the patient's ability to perform daily functional tasks and about mood and behavior as well as questions about memory and orientation. The MMSE[46] or a variation of it can be used to more objectively assess multiple spheres of cognition.

Since target symptoms of psychiatric disorders may respond differently in demented patients, a detailed list of symptoms to be treated should be documented in the pharmaceutical care plan to aid in monitoring. These could include, for example, "striking at spouse because patient believes spouse is an impostor," "verbal threats and refusal to allow clothes to be changed," and so on, as opposed to documenting vague symptoms such as "aggression" or "delusions." To make an accurate assessment of depression, multiple symptoms, including sleep, appetite, activity and interest levels, need to be assessed in addition to the patient's stated mood.

In addition to laboratory monitoring (e.g., LFTs with tacrine), the patient should be observed carefully for potential side effects of drug therapy. Depending on the therapeutic agent being employed, patients should be assessed for potential side effects such as diarrhea, GI distress, dizziness, sedation, extrapyramidal side effects, or worsening of behavior. The specific side effects to be monitored and the method and frequency of monitoring should be documented. Periodic assessments for drug efficacy, compliance, need for dosage adjustment, or change in treatment should occur at least monthly. However, patients need to be treated for an adequate duration to see a therapeutic effect from a given intervention. Since the effects of cognition-enhancing medications are not great, a treatment period of 6 months to 1 year may be necessary before it can be determined whether therapy is beneficial. Often effects of the drug are noticed only as deterioration following drug discontinuation. If there is doubt, the patient can be monitored off the drug for 4 to 6 weeks to determine the need for continued therapy. Efficacy monitoring for behavioral interventions can be performed more frequently, every 1–2 weeks.

Conclusion

Significant advances have been made in our knowledge of the pathophysiology of AD. However, much additional study will be required to allow for development of therapies that will "cure" or arrest progression of the disease. Tacrine represents the first of hopefully many therapeutic agents that will have the potential to improve the cognition and hopefully the quality of life of these patients. As tacrine is not likely to be effective in patients with severe disease and because it has significant side effects, the clinician must carefully screen the patient for appropriateness of treatment, and the family should be active participants in treatment decisions. The clinician should closely monitor tacrine therapy, being mindful of changes in the patient's clinical status, liver enzyme changes, cholinergic side effects, and the potential for drug interactions. Lastly, and most important, families must be educated about the appropriate use of tacrine, its side effects, and the realistic expectations they should have regarding response.

Behavioral and psychiatric manifestations of AD can add significantly to the morbidity of the disease. Carefully chosen psychotropic drugs in combination with consistent behavioral and environmental interventions can often be effective in ameliorating these symptoms.

As new findings become available to unravel the Alzheimer's puzzle, more and more treatments will become available to treat symptoms, and hopefully to slow or halt progression of the disease. In future editions, perhaps we will even have the opportunity to discuss genetic treatments that prevent onset of this devastating illness.

References

1. Eggert A, Crismon ML. Current concepts in understanding Alzheimer's disease. Clin Pharm Newswatch 1994;1:1–8.
2. American Psychiatric Association, Diagnostic and Statistical Manual for Mental Disorders, 3rd ed., Revised (DSM-III-R). Washington, DC, Author, 1987, pp 97–163.
3. American Psychiatric Association, Diagnostic and Statistical Manual for Mental Disorders, 4th ed. (DSM-IV). Washington, DC, Author, 1994, pp 123–174.
4. Evans D. Estimated prevalence of Alzheimer's disease in the United States. Milbank Q 1990;68:267–289.
5. Rocca WA, Amaducci LA, Schoenberg BS. Epidemiology of clinically diagnosed Alzheimer's disease. Ann Neurol 1986;19:415–424.
6. Evans DA, Funkenstein HH, Albert MS, et al. Prevalence of Alzheimer's disease in a community population of older persons: Higher than previously reported. JAMA 1989;262:2551–2552.
7. Ernst RL, Hay JW. The US economic and social costs of Alzheimer's disease revisited. Am J Pub Health 1994;84:1261–1264.
8. Ereshefsky L, Anderson CB. Organic brain syndromes, in Dipiro JT, Talbert RL, Hayes PE, et al. (eds): Pharmacotherapy: A Pathophysiologic Approach, 2nd ed. Norwalk, CT, Appleton and Lange, 1992; pp 973–1000.
9. Cordell B. β-amyloid formation as a potential therapeutic target for Alzheimer's disease. Annu Rev Pharmacol Toxicol 1994;34:69–89.
10. Yankner BA, Mesulam MM. β-amyloid and the pathogenesis of Alzheimer's disease. N Engl J Med 1991;325:1849–1857.
11. Travis J. New piece in Alzheimer's puzzle. Science 1993;261:828–829.
12. Selkoe D. Amyloid protein and Alzheimer's disease. Sci Am 1991;265:68–71, 74–76, 78.
13. Goldman J, Cote L. Aging of the brain: Dementia of the Alzheimer's type, in Kandel ER, Scwartz JH, Jessell TM (eds): Principles of Neural Science, 3rd ed. New York, Elsevier Science Publishing Co, 1991, pp 974–983.
14. Masters CL, Simms G, Multhaup G, et al. Amyloid plaque core protein in Alzheimer's disease and Down's syndrome. Proc Natl Acad Sci USA 1985;82:4245–4249.
15. Shoji M, Golde TE, Ghiso J, et al. Production of the Alzheimer amyloid β protein by normal proteolytic processing. Science 1992;258:126–129.
16. Gleener GG, Wong CW. Alzheimer's disease: Initial report of the purification and characterization of a novel cerebrovascular amyloid protein. Biochem Biophys Res Commun 1984;120:885–890.
17. Giaccone G, Tagliavini F, Linoli G, et al. Down syndrome patients: Extracellular preamyloid deposits precede neuritic degeneration and senile plaques. Neurosci Lett 1989;97:232–238.
18. Mann DMA, Esiri MM. The pattern of acquisition of plaques and tangles in brains of patients under 50 years of age with Down's syndrome. J Neurol Sci 1989;89:169–179.
19. Quon D, Wang Y, Catalino R, et al. Formation of β-amyloid deposits in brains of transgenic mice. Nature 1991;357:239–241.
20. Pike CJ, Walencewicz AJ, Glabe CG, Cotman CW. Aggregation-related toxicity of synthetic β-amyloid protein in hippocampal cultures. Eur J Pharmacol 1991;207:367–368.
21. Esch FS, Keim PS, Beattie EC, et al. Cleavage of amyloid β-peptide during constitutive processing of its precursor. Science 1990;248:1122–1124.
22. Aisen PS, Davis KL. Inflammatory mechanisms in Alzheimer's disease: Implications for therapy. Am J Psychiatry 1994;151:1105–1113.
23. Rosenberg RN. A causal role for amyloid in Alzheimer's disease: The end of the beginning. Neurology 1993;43:851–856.
24. Harrison P. Alzheimer's disease and chromosome 14. Different gene, same process? Br J Psychiatry 1993;163:2–5.
25. Saunders AM, Strittmatter WJ, Schmechal D, et al. Association of apolipoprotein E allele E4 with late-onset familial and sporadic Alzheimer's disease. Neurology 1993;43:1467–1472.

26. Strittmatter WJ, Saunders AM, Schmechel D, et al. Apolipoprotein E: High-avidity binding to β-amyloid and increased frequency of type 4 allele in late-onset familial Alzheimer's disease. Med Sci 1993;90:1977–1981.
27. Corder EH, Saunders AM, Strittmatter WJ, et al. Gene dose of apolipoprotein type 4 allele and the risk of Alzheimer's disease in late onset families. Science 1993;261:921–923.
28. Talbot C, Lendon C, Craddock N, et al. Protection against Alzheimer's disease with Apo E E2. Lancet 1994;343:1432–1433.
29. Corder EH, Saunders AM, Risch NJ, et al. Protective effect of apolipoprotein E type 2 allele for late-onset Alzheimer's disease. Nat Genet 1994;7:180–184.
30. Blass JP. Pathophysiology of the Alzheimer's syndrome. Neurology 1993;43(suppl 4):S25–S38.
31. Schneider LS. Clinical pharmacology of aminoacridines in Alzheimer's disease. Neurology 1993;43(suppl 4):S64–S79.
32. Piccini GL, Finali G, Piccirilli M. Neuropsychological effects of L-deprenyl in Alzheimer's type dementia. Clin Neuropharmacol 1990;13:147–163.
33. Francis PT, Sims NR, Procter AW, Bowen DM. Cortical pyramidal neurone loss may cause glutamatergic hypoactivity and cognitive impairment in Alzheimer's disease: Investigative and therapeutic perspectives. J Neurochem 1993;60:1589–1604.
34. Pomara N, Singh R, Deptula D, et al. Glutamate and other CSF amino acids in Alzheimer's disease. Am J Psychiatry 1992;149:251–254.
35. Choi WD. Glutamate neurotoxicity and diseases of the nervous system. Neuron 1988;1:623–634.
36. Henderson VW, Paganini-Hill A, Emanuel CK, et al. Estrogen replacement therapy in older women: Comparisons between Alzheimer's disease cases and nondemented control subjects. Arch Neurol 1994;51:896–900.
37. Paganini-Hill A, Henderson VW. Estrogen deficiency and risk of Alzheimer's disease in women. Am J Epidemiol 1994;140:256–261.
38. Brenner DE, Kukull WA, Stergachis A, et al. Postmenopausal estrogen replacement therapy and the risk of Alzheimer's disease: A population based case-control study. Am J Epidemiol 1994;140:262–267.
39. Barrett-Connor E, Kritz-Silverstein D. Estrogen replacement therapy and cognitive function in older women. JAMA 1993;269:2637–2641.
40. Hamdy RC. Aluminum toxicity and Alzheimer's disease. Is there a connection? Postgrad Med 1990;88:239–240.
41. Bush AI, Pettingell WH, Multhaup G, et al. Rapid induction of Alzheimer Aβ amyloid formation by zinc. Science 1994;265:1464–1467.
42. McKhann G, Drachman D, Folstein M, et al. Clinical diagnosis of Alzheimer's disease. Neurology 1984;34:939–944.
43. Mohs RC. Neuropsychological assessment of patients with Alzheimer's disease, in Bloom FE, Kupfer DJ (eds): Psychopharmacology: The Fourth Generation of Progress. New York, Raven Press, 1995, pp 1377–1388.
44. Raskind MA. Geriatric psychopharmacology: Management of late-life depression and the noncognitive behavioral disturbances of Alzheimer's disease. Psychiatr Clin North Am 1993;16:815–827.
45. McKhann G, Drachman D, Folstein M, et al. Clinical diagnosis of Alzheimer's disease: Report of the NINCDS–ADRDA work-group under the auspices of the department of health and human services task force on Alzheimer's disease. Neurology 1984;34:939–944.
46. Folstein MF, Folstein SE, McHugh PR. Mini mental state: A practical method for grading the cognitive state of patients for the clinician. J Psychiatr Res 1975;12:189–198.
47. Reisberg B, Ferris SH, DeLeon MJ, Crook T. The global deterioration scale for assessment of primary degenerative dementia. Am J Psychiatry 1982;139:1136–1139.
48. Scinto LFM, Daffner KR, Dressler D, et al. A potential noninvasive neurobiological test for Alzheimer's disease. Science 1994;266:1051–1054.
49. Small GW, Mazziotta JC, Collins MT, et al. Apolipoprotein E type 4 allele and cerebral glucose metabolism in relatives at risk for familial Alzheimer's disease. JAMA 1995;273:942–947.
50. Cognex expanded access proposed by FDA as part of "program of further study": Warner-Lambert will support NDA studies with other data by April 1. F-D-C Reports, March 25, 1991, 4–9.
51. Knopman DS, Knapp MJ, Gracon SI, Davis CS. The clinical interview-based impression (CIBI): A clinician's global change rating scale in Alzheimer's disease. Neurology 1994;44:2315–2321.
52. Crismon ML. Tacrine: First drug approved for Alzheimer's disease. Ann Pharmacother 1994;28:744–751.
53. Farlow M, Gracon SI, Hershey LA, et al. A controlled trial of tacrine in Alzheimer's disease. JAMA 1992;268:3523–3529.
54. Knapp MJ, Knopman DS, Solomon PR, et al. A 30-week randomized controlled trial of high-dose tacrine in patients with Alzheimer's disease. JAMA 1994;271:985–991.
55. Watkins PB, Zimmerman HJ, Knapp MJ, et al. Hepatotoxic effects of tacrine administration in patients with Alzheimer's disease. JAMA 1994;271:992–998.
56. Ford JM, Truman CA, Wilcock GK, Roberts CJC. Serum concentrations of tacrine hydrochloride predict its adverse effects in Alzheimer's disease. Clin Pharmacol Ther 1993;53:691–695.
57. Mihara M, Ohnishi A, Tomono Y, et al. Pharmacokinetics of E2020, a new compound for Alzheimer's disease, in healthy male volunteers. Int J Clin Pharmacol Ther Toxicol 1993;31:223–229.
58. Pfizer Pharmaceuticals, personal communication, July 26, 1994.
59. Spagnoli A, Lucca U, Menasce G, et al. Long-term acetyl-L-carnitine treatment in Alzheimer's disease. Neurology 1991;41:1726–1732.
60. Olson L. NGF and the treatment of Alzheimer's disease. Exp Neurol 1993;124:5–15.
61. Rogers J, Kirby LC, Hempelman SR, et al. Clinical trial of indomethacin in Alzheimer's disease. Neurology 1993;43:1609–1611.
62. Rich JB, Rasmusson DX, Folstein MF, et al. Nonsteroidal anti-inflammatory drugs in Alzheimer's disease. Neurology 1995;45:51–55.
63. Tollefson GD. Short-term effects of the calcium channel blocker nimodipine (Bay-e-9736) in the management of pri-

mary degenerative dementia. Biol Psychiatry 1990;27:1133–1142.
64. Marin DB, Davis KL. Experimental therapeutics, in Bloom FE, Kupfer DJ (eds): Psychopharmacology: The Fourth Generation of Progress. New York, Raven Press, 1995, pp 1417–1426.
65. Burke WJ, Roccaforte WH, Wengel SP, et al. L-Deprenyl in the treatment of mild dementia of the Alzheimer type: Results of a 15-month trial. JAGS 1993;41:1219–1225.
66. Schneifer LS, Tariot PN. Emerging drugs for Alzheimer's disease: Mechanisms of action and prospects for cognitive enhancing medications. Med Clin North Am 1994;78:911–934.
67. Raskind MA. Alzheimer's disease: Treatment of noncognitive behavioral abnormalities, in Bloom FE, Kupfer DJ (eds): Psychopharmacology: The Fourth Generation of Progress. New York, Raven Press, 1995, pp 1427–1435.
68. Reifler BV, Raskind MA, Veith R, et al. Double-blind trial of imipramine in Alzheimer's disease patients with and without depression. Am J Psychiatry 1989;146:45–49.
69. Crismon ML. Psychotropic drugs in the elderly: Principles of use. Am Pharm 1990;NS30(12):57–63.
70. Geldmacher DS, Waldman AJ, Doty L, Heilman KM. Fluoxetine in dementia of the Alzheimer's type: Prominent adverse effects and failure to improve cognition. J Clin Psychiatry 1994;55:161.
71. Devanand DP, Sackeim HA, Brown RP, Mayeux R. A pilot study of haloperidol treatment of psychosis and behavioral disturbance in Alzheimer's disease. Arch Neurol 1989;46:854–857.
72. Petrie WM, Ban TA, Berney S, et al. Loxapine in psychogeriatrics: A placebo and standard-controlled clinical investigation. J Clin Psychopharmacol 1982;2:122–126.
73. Barnes R, Veith R, Okimoto J, et al. Efficacy of antipsychotic medications in behaviorally disturbed dementia patients. Am J Psychiatry 1982;139:1170–1174.
74. Dysken MW, Johnson SB, Holden L, et al. Haloperidol concentrations in patients with Alzheimer's disease. Am J Geriatr Psychiatry 1994;2:124–133.
75. Sakuye KM, Camp CJ, Ford PA. Effects of buspirone on agitation associated with dementia. Am J Geriatr Psychiatry 1993;1:82–84.
76. Hermann N, Eryavec G. Buspirone in the management of agitation and aggression associated with dementia. Am J Geriatr Psychiatry 1993;1:249–253.
77. Tariot PN, Cohen RM, Sunderland T, et al. L-Deprenyl in Alzheimer's disease. Arch Gen Psychiatry 1987;44:427–433.
78. Schneider LS, Pollock VE, Zemansky MF, et al. A pilot study of low-dose L-deprenyl in Alzheimer's disease. J Geriatr Psychiatry Neurol 1991;4:143–148.

Chapter 65

Substance-Related Disorders

Brian L. Crabtree, PharmD, and Alexis Polles, MD

Drug abuse and drug dependence are among the most common of medical problems. Nearly 50% of all highway fatalities involve alcohol. Up to 30% of all patients with short stay admissions to general hospitals have alcohol problems, regardless of diagnosis.[1,2] Approximately 41% of youths (age 12–17 years) have tried alcohol, and about 12% have tried marijuana. Overall, about 37% of the U.S. population have tried marijuana, cocaine, or another illicit drug at least once.[3] Approximately 7% of the adult population of the United States is considered alcohol dependent, with males being more than twice as likely as females to meet criteria for diagnosis.[4] Recent trends in the use of alcohol and other drugs show a reversal of the decline in drug use that peaked in 1979. Prevalence of drug use has increased slightly over the last 2 years, particularly among youth.[5] In addition, perceived risk of drug use has decreased and perceived availability of drugs has increased.[6] Purity and potency of drugs have increased in recent years. Although problems associated with drug use are virtually ubiquitous, there is perhaps no other area of medicine that is more variably practiced, understood, and misunderstood.

Historical Perspective

A complete discussion of the history of drug abuse is beyond the scope of this chapter. Although attempts to control drug use have been in practice only since the end of the nineteenth century, the use of drugs for mood-altering purposes is almost as old as human beings themselves. The Bible makes mention of wine and intoxication. Peyote cactus containing mescaline and mushrooms containing psilocybin have been used for centuries. Cocaine has been used for more than 2000 years by the Indians of South America in the form of the coca leaf. Cocaine itself was first isolated from the coca leaf in 1860 with its original use medically as an anesthetic. Sigmund Freud, the father of modern psychoanalysis, felt cocaine could be used therapeutically. Cocaine was part of the soft drink *Coca-Cola* until replaced by caffeine in 1903.[7] Gasoline sniffing has been a common drug use pattern for many years. Recent trends of drug use have included the use of crack, a form of cocaine, and "look-alike" or designer synthetic drugs.

Terminology

An important step in understanding substance-related disorders and their treatment is the establishment of a standardized working vocabulary. A consensus agreement among scientists and the treatment community with regard to definitions of terms has been difficult. Until recently, there have been no standardized credentials for individuals wishing to offer treatment. As a result, progress in treatment and understanding has been slow, and interpretation of scientific literature difficult. A list of important terms relative to substance-related disorders is given below. Although there are no universally accepted definitions, these are widely used and accepted by clinicians.

Drug abuse: Use of a drug in a manner inconsistent with social norms with the intent of altering mood or feeling state.

Drug misuse: Inappropriate use of a drug intended for therapeutic purposes (e.g., inappropriate prescribing, use of a prescription drug not under the supervision of a physician, self-medication with a nonprescription drug inconsistent with label information).

Addiction or drug dependence: Behavioral patterns of compulsive drug use in which obtaining and using a drug constitute the principal focus of the user's life. There is continued use of a drug to alter feelings or prevent withdrawal effects despite medical, social, or occupational contraindications. Although drug dependence is a type of drug abuse (i.e., use of a drug with the intent of altering mood or feeling state), it is possible to be a drug abuser without being drug dependent.

Physical dependence: State of physiologic adaptation to chronic use of a drug such that abrupt dosage reduction or discontinuation results in a characteristic abstinence syndrome.

Tolerance: State of physiologic adaptation to a drug such that higher-than-usual dosages are required to achieve the usual effect.

Withdrawal or abstinence syndrome: Characteristic physical and emotional signs and symptoms precipitated by the abrupt reduction or discontinuation of a drug on which an individual is physically dependent.

Cross-tolerance and cross-dependence: Ability of one drug to suppress the manifestations of physical withdrawal produced by another drug and to maintain the physically dependent state.

Chemically Impaired Health Care Professionals

Health care professionals, including pharmacists, are among the highest risk occupational categories for the development of drug dependency. Data from studies of the epidemiology of controlled substance use among pharmacists and physicians indicate that 46% of pharmacists and 62% of pharmacy students have used a controlled substance with a prescription, with the pharmacy students using controlled substances more often for recreational purposes than for self-treatment.[8] Data from the mid-1980s indicate that of practicing pharmacists, 19% are occasional or regular users of controlled substances without a prescription and 41% of pharmacy students are occasional or regular users (i.e., at least once per month). Physicians and medical students show similar patterns of drug use, with 59% of physicians and 77% of medical students having tried a controlled substance for recreational or self-treatment purposes.[9]

In a more recent national survey, medical students and resident physicians reported lower rates of cocaine and marijuana use than age- and gender-matched cohorts in the general population. Residents were more likely to use benzodiazepines and opiates than students, which they indicated was for self-treatment rather than recreation. This pattern of self-treatment is disturbing because this may contribute to future impairment.[10] Residents also had higher rates of alcohol use than their peers of the same age and gender. The overall prevalence of resident substance use in this study was lower than in all previous studies.[11] Although 3% of U.S. physicians are anesthesiologists, 13% of drug-dependent physicians who had been treated listed this as their specialty.[12] Surveys show that about 33% of pharmacy students have one or more family members who are drug dependent.[13,14]

Pharmacists and physicians are not well sensitized to their increased risk for the development of drug dependence. As shown above for anesthesiologists, the prevalence of drug dependence among health care professionals, including pharmacists, is between 10–15%.[15,16] Theories about why this occurs include stressful professional responsibilities, ready accessibility to alcohol and other drugs, and a false feeling of invincibility associated with an increased knowledge of drug effects. Although health care professionals are often quite knowledgeable about therapeutics, they often know little about drug dependence.

Substance-Related Disorders in the Elderly

Only in the last 20 years has substance abuse in the elderly been recognized as a problem. Clinicians are becoming increasingly aware of this problem in the geriatric population, and substance abuse, misuse, and chemical dependency should be considered by physicians in the differential diagnosis of the elderly. Illegal drug use is still much lower among the elderly than among the general population, but this may change as the population ages.

Alcohol dependence is more common among the elderly than previously thought. Compared with a prevalence of 8–10% among the general population, alcoholism has a prevalence of between 3–15% among elderly in the community and as high as 44% in the general medical and psychiatric elderly population.[17] Approximately one-third of elderly individuals who are alcohol dependent began drinking after the age of 60.[18] A complicating factor is that a large percentage of the elderly are on medications that may adversely interact with alcohol.

Prescription drugs are also commonly misused and abused. In addition to the usual problems with abuse, the elderly are more likely to experience adverse drug reactions from all drugs. Approximately 25% of the elderly use psychoactive drugs, with central nervous system (CNS) depressants being most common.[19] It is clear that drug abuse and misuse among the elderly are more common than previously thought, and that the prevalence will increase with the aging of the population. The elderly are at greater risk for complications related to drug abuse because of concomitant physical disease and use of multiple drugs.

Patterns of Use, Clinical Presentation, Pharmacology, and Diagnostic Classification

There are many diagnostic classifications of disorders of drug abuse and drug dependence. The system presented here is that of the American Psychiatric Association's *Diagnostic and Statistical Manual of Mental Disorders,* 4th ed. (DSM-IV).[4] Substance-related disorders are divided into two broad categories: substance use disorders and substance-induced disorders.

The substance use disorders include dependence and abuse. The substance-induced disorders to be discussed here mainly include intoxication and withdrawal. Other substance-induced disorders, including dementia, psychosis, mood disorders, and anxiety, are discussed elsewhere.

The essential feature of substance dependence is the continued use of the substance despite adverse substance-related problems. Repeated use of the drug is often associated with the development of tolerance, withdrawal, and compulsive use, but it is possible to meet criteria for dependence in the absence of physical dependence. The criteria for substance dependence are the same for each of the drugs or drug classes, varying only to fit the unique pharmacologic properties of each drug. To meet criteria for the diagnosis of substance dependence, at least three of the following must be present at any time in a 12-month period: (1) tolerance; (2) withdrawal, indicated by the appearance of the characteristic withdrawal syndrome or the use of the same or related drug to relieve or avoid withdrawal symptoms; (3) the substance is taken in larger amounts or over a longer period of time than was intended; (4) persistent desire or unsuccessful efforts to cut down or control substance use; (5) time spent in activities necessary to obtain the substance, use the substance, or recover from its effects; (6) social, occupational, or recreational activities are given up or reduced because of substance use; and (7) substance use is continued despite knowledge of having a persistent or recurrent physical or psychological problem that has been caused or exacerbated by the substance.

The essential feature of substance abuse is a maladaptive pattern of substance use indicated by repeated adverse consequences related to the repeated use of substances. Examples include failure to fulfill important obligations at work, school, or home; repeated use in situations in which it is physically dangerous such as driving under the influence; legal problems; and social or interpersonal problems such as arguments and fights.

Intoxication refers to the development of a substance-specific syndrome after recent ingestion and presence in the body of a substance and is associated with maladaptive behavior during the waking state caused by the effect of the substance on the CNS. Examples include belligerence, mood lability, impaired judgment, and impaired social or occupational functioning. Evidence for recent intake of the substance can be obtained from the history, physical examination, or laboratory examination. The most common changes involve disturbances in perception, wakefulness, attention, thinking, judgment, motor behavior, and interpersonal behavior.

Withdrawal, as defined previously, is the development of a substance-specific syndrome after cessation of or reduction in intake of a substance that was regularly used by the individual to induce a state of intoxication. Withdrawal causes significant distress to the individual and is associated with impairment in social, occupational, or other areas of functioning. Withdrawal is usually associated with substance dependence. Withdrawal is generally also associated with a craving to readminister the drug to relieve the symptoms.

As with most illnesses, the course and prognosis of the disorders of substance use and dependence are variable. Acute intoxication associated with many drugs, especially opiates and cocaine, is potentially fatal. Untreated physical withdrawal from the CNS depressants is potentially life threatening; however, withdrawal can almost always be successfully managed with proper medical care. Getting patients who are drug dependent to stop using drugs is very difficult, and many patients return to drug use even after treatment. As many as 75% of treated substance-dependent patients relapse at least once. Many patients are, however, able to obtain recovery with treatment and continued care in programs such as Alcoholics Anonymous (AA). Substance dependence or addiction can be viewed as a chronic illness that can be successfully controlled with treatment, but cannot be cured and is associated with a high relapse rate. Without treatment, the course can progress to life-threatening severity, resulting from the effects of the drug, drug contaminants, or medical complications of use.

CENTRAL NERVOUS SYSTEM DEPRESSANTS

ALCOHOL

In Western culture, alcohol is the only drug with which obvious self-induced intoxication is socially acceptable under certain circumstances. In the United States, about 88% of the adult population has voluntarily consumed alcohol. Approximately 59% of young adults (age 18–25) and 49% of older adults (35 or older) are at least monthly users of alcohol.[3] Approximately 7% of the adult population has met criteria for alcohol dependence within the last year while 14% meet the criteria sometime in their lives.[4] Medical complications of alcoholism are common and varied, with virtually all organ systems affected. Common examples of medical complications are liver disease (e.g., cirrhosis, fatty liver), cardiomyopathy, pancreatitis, gastrointestinal (GI) disease (e.g., ulcer, varices), anemia, CNS disturbances, and fetal alcohol syndrome.[20]

Signs and symptoms of alcohol intoxication and alcohol withdrawal are summarized in Table 65.1.[4] Alcohol is a CNS depressant drug that historically has been thought to exert its actions by disrupting neuronal membrane function and, secondarily, membrane-mounted proteins including receptors, ion channels, and enzymes.[21] More recent research has shown that alcohol also has actions on the major inhibitory and excitatory brain neurotransmitter systems and that these effects may better explain the effects of lower doses such as decreased anxiety, incoordination, and impaired cognition. Alcohol potentiates gamma-aminobutyric acid type A ($GABA_A$) receptor function, the major inhibitory system, and inhibits the function of the *N*-methyl-D-aspartate (NMDA) subtype of glutamate receptors, a major excitatory system.[22] Decreases in the synthesis of $GABA_A$ and increases in NMDA syn-

TABLE 65.1. SIGNS AND SYMPTOMS OF ALCOHOL INTOXICATION AND WITHDRAWAL

Intoxication	Withdrawal
Slurred speech	Tremor
Ataxia	Tachycardia
Nystagmus	Diaphoresis
Sedation	Labile blood pressure
Flushed face	Anxiety
Mood change	Nausea and vomiting
Irritability	Hallucinations
Euphoria	Seizures
Loquacity	Hyperthermia
Impaired attention	Delirium

thesis during chronic exposure to alcohol may help to explain tolerance and the hyperexcitability of the CNS during alcohol withdrawal. Inhibitory functions of the brain (e.g., impulse control) are more depressed at lower alcohol concentrations than are excitatory functions (e.g., consciousness and respiration). Although individuals with mild alcohol intoxication may appear stimulated, an effect known as a *disinhibition effect,* this behavior is a CNS depressant effect.

Alcohol withdrawal is a cumulative phasic process, that is, symptoms of the initial phases do not diminish as withdrawal progresses to advanced phases. The extent of phasic progression is determined by the amount of alcohol consumed, the abruptness of discontinuation, and overall physical health. Although alcoholics do not uniformly fit the stereotype of the "skid row" individual, patients who are nutritionally deficient, dehydrated, or have compromised organ system status or other debilitating factors are at risk for more severe withdrawal.

Phase I acute alcohol withdrawal begins within hours of cessation of drinking, lasts for 3–5 days, and consists of tremor, autonomic hyperactivity including tachycardia, diaphoresis, labile blood pressure, anxiety, nausea, and vomiting. Phase II withdrawal includes perceptual disturbances that are most commonly auditory or visual, but may be of any type. Phase III includes seizures, usually the generalized clonic–tonic type, lasting 30 seconds to 4 minutes and progressing to status epilepticus in approximately 3% of cases. Between 10–15% of untreated alcohol withdrawal patients experience withdrawal seizures. Phase IV is called *delirium tremens,* a syndrome of acute autonomic hyperactivity and delirium, including severe hyperthermia. This occurs in less than 1% of patients. The mortality rate for patients who progress to phase IV is approximately 20%. Deaths are frequently related to stroke or cardiovascular collapse. Most alcohol withdrawal patients do not progress beyond phase I, even when they are untreated.[23,24]

BENZODIAZEPINES AND OTHER SEDATIVE–HYPNOTICS

In clinical practice, the benzodiazepines and zolpidem (Ambien) have largely replaced the short-acting barbiturates and other nonbarbiturate sedative–hypnotics. Barbiturates such as pentobarbital and amobarbital remain drugs of abuse, however. The incidence and prevalence of use of sedative–hypnotic drugs remains low. Of interest is the fact that the source of most sedative–hypnotic abuse is prescriptions. Approximately 3% of adults have tried a sedative drug for nonmedical use, with 0.2–0.3% having used a sedative in the past month.[4] These figures are contrasted with 1982 prevalence data reporting that 19% of adults had tried sedatives, with 2.6% having used them within the past month. Shorter acting barbiturates (e.g., pentobarbital, secobarbital) are generally preferred over longer acting drugs (e.g., phenobarbital). A combination of secobarbital and amobarbital, an intermediate-acting barbiturate, is popular among barbiturate users. Shorter acting nonbarbiturate sedative–hypnotics including meprobamate, methyprylon, ethchlorvynol, and glutethimide are also abused. Among the benzodiazepines, faster onset drugs, especially diazepam, which has the highest lipophilicity among the benzodiazepines, are often preferred. Alprazolam has acquired a reputation among some clinicians for being particularly associated with dependency, but confounding variables relating to the types of patients often treated with alprazolam compared to other benzodiazepines make a conclusive judgment difficult. Because all benzodiazepines have abuse and dependence liability, however, patients cannot be switched from one benzodiazepine drug to another in hopes of decreasing a pattern of drug abuse or dependence behavior. A nonbenzodiazepine, nonbarbiturate sedative, zolpidem, has been suggested to have little liability for physical dependence, but tolerance and withdrawal have been reported in association with its use as well.[25]

An important difference between the barbiturate-like drugs and benzodiazepines is the potential for toxicity at very high doses. Benzodiazepines do not generally cause significant respiratory depression as do the barbiturate-like drugs.[26] Signs and symptoms of withdrawal are similar in many respects to those of alcohol withdrawal, but the time courses may be quite different. While withdrawal from shorter acting agents (e.g., lorazepam and alprazolam) has an onset within 12–24 hours of the last dose, others (e.g., diazepam, chlordiazepoxide, clorazepate, phenobarbital, amobarbital) have elimination half-lives or active metabolites with elimination half-lives of 24 to greater than 100 hours. As a result, the onset of withdrawal symptoms may be delayed for several days after discontinuation of the drug.[27] Dependence on sedative–hypnotics and benzodiazepines is summarized in Table 65.2.

TABLE 65.2. DEPENDENCE ON SEDATIVE–HYPNOTICS[a]

Generic Name	Common Trade Names (Manufacturer)	Oral Sedating Dose (mg)	Physical Dependence Dose and Time Needed to Produce Dependence	Time Before Onset of Withdrawal (h)	Peak Withdrawal Symptoms (d)
Benzodiazepines					
Diazepam	Valium (Roche)	5–10	40–120 mg × 42–120 d	12–24	5–8
Chlordiazepoxide	Librium, Libritabs (Roche)	10–25	75–600 mg × 42–120 d	12–24	5–8
Clorazepate	Tranxene (Abbott)	7.5–15	45–180 mg × 42–120 d (est.)	12–24	5–8
Alprazolam	Xanax (Upjohn)	0.25–8	8–16 mg × 42 d (est.)	8–24	2–3
Barbiturates					
Secobarbital	Seconal, Seco-8 (Lilly)	100	800–2200 mg × 35–37 d	6–12	2–3
Pentobarbital	Nembutal (Abbott)	100	Same	6–12	2–3
Equal parts of seco- and amobarbital	Tuinal (Lilly)	100	Same	6–12	2–3
Amobarbital	Amytal (Lilly)	65–100	Same	8–12	2–5
Nonbarbiturate Sedative–Hypnotics					
Ethchlorvynol	Placidyl (Abbott)	200	1–1.5 g × 30 d	6–12	2–3
Chloral hydrate	Noctec (various)	250	Exact dose unknown: 12 g/d chronically has led to delirium upon sudden withdrawal	6–12	2–3
Meprobamate	Equanil, Miltown, Meprotabs (various)	400	1.6–3.2 g × 270 d	8–12	3–8

[a]Withdrawal symptoms are tremor, tachycardia, diaphoresis, nausea, vomiting, blood pressure lability, delirium, seizures, and hallucinations.

Long-term use of even therapeutic doses of benzodiazepines may cause physical dependence and withdrawal symptoms after abrupt discontinuation.[27] The likelihood and severity of withdrawal is a function of both dose and duration of exposure. Individuals who have taken approved dosages would be expected to experience less severe withdrawal than those who have taken much higher than prescribed amounts. Gradual tapering of dosage is also associated with less withdrawal and rebound anxiety than upon abrupt discontinuation. Patients who have taken benzodiazepines for the treatment of anxiety often experience a rebound increase in anxiety after discontinuation of the antianxiety drug. The heightened autonomic activity of severe anxiety can be easily mistaken for drug withdrawal. A combination of withdrawal and increased anxiety may also occur, and each may intensify the other. Occurrence of hallucinations or seizures would indicate severe physical withdrawal. (For additional information on benzodiazepine withdrawal refer to Chapter 69.)

OPIATES

Intravenous injection of an opiate causes a warm flushing of the skin and a lower abdominal sensation often described as similar to sexual orgasm. Tolerance may develop rapidly, possibly after the first dose, because many users say they are never able to achieve the same experience again, although a heightened sense of anticipation may also explain the perceived decrease in effect. Following the initial "rush," there is a period of apathetic detachment for a few hours before the effect of the drug wears off.[28]

Incidence and prevalence of opiate use are widely variable depending on the drug. Heroin, which gained widespread notoriety during the 1960s and 1970s and which remains the single most commonly used illicit opiate, has been tried by about 1% of the adult population with less than 0.1% having used it in the last month.[3] The number of heroin-dependent individuals nationally is estimated at around one-half million, a number that pales somewhat in comparison with the approximately 13 million alcohol-dependent individuals.

Collectively, use of opiates other than heroin is far more common. Approximately 6% of adults have tried an opiate or opiate-like analgesic for nonmedical use with around 1% having used an analgesic within 1 month.[3] Hydromorphone has become widely used among the opiate-using population, with single 4-mg tablets selling for as much as $70. Hydromorphone has a pharmaceutical profile very similar to heroin, with the advantage of purity. Drug combinations involving opiates are quite popular. Pentazocine combined with tripelennamine, an antihistamine (so-called "Ts and blues"), is an example, although use of the combination has declined significantly with the addition of naloxone, an opiate receptor antagonist, to pentazocine tablets. Naloxone is not absorbed when given orally, thus it antagonizes pentazocine's narcotic effect only when injected. Opiates are commonly combined with stimulant drugs, especially cocaine, a combination known as a "speedball," although any sedative combined with any stimulant is often referred to as a speedball. Opiate users frequently also drink alcohol, especially when their use of opiate drugs declines because of lack of availability or sometimes following treatment.

Many of the complications of opiate use, especially intravenous use, are related not only to the drug itself, but also to varying purity, contaminants, and techniques of administration such as dirty equipment and use of shared needles. Overdoses, anaphylactic reactions to impurities, nephrotic syndrome, septicemia, endocarditis, and acquired immune deficiency syndrome (AIDS) are examples.[29]

Not all opiate use is street drug use. Some opiate-dependent individuals first obtained their drug during medical treatment and progressed to compulsive drug use and an inability to tolerate the drug-free state, although the number of these individuals appears to be extremely small. The prevalence of opiate-dependent health care professionals is quite high relative to other groups of comparable educational and socioeconomic status. Most impaired health care professionals initially use the drug to relieve depression or fatigue and not generally to achieve an intense euphoria. There are many opiate-dependent individuals who initially used street drugs, but do not obtain methadone as part of their treatment. A more recent development is the availability of levo-alpha-acetylmethadol (LAAM), a prodrug that is closely related to methadone and is converted to a metabolite that is very slowly inactivated and excreted.[28] LAAM is available for use instead of methadone in treatment programs, but the extent to which programs have switched from methadone to LAAM is not known at present.

Signs and symptoms of opioid intoxication and withdrawal are summarized in Table 65.3.[4] Onset of the acute phase of withdrawal varies with the drug consumed, but ranges from a few hours after stopping the drug with heroin to 3–5 days with methadone. The time course of withdrawal ranges from 3–14 days. Opioid withdrawal is significantly different from withdrawal from alcohol or other sedative–hypnotics. Of greatest importance is that opioid withdrawal is not fatal unless there is a concurrent medical problem of major concern. This has significant treatment implications, especially where drug therapy is concerned. Although patients in opioid withdrawal may be in great discomfort and incapacitated, they are not delirious. The presence of delirium should raise the question of concurrent withdrawal from another drug, such as alcohol, or another cause of delirium possibly secondary to drug use.

TABLE 65.3. SIGNS AND SYMPTOMS OF OPIOID INTOXICATION AND WITHDRAWAL

Intoxication	Withdrawal
Euphoria	Lacrimination
Dysphoria	Rhinorrhea
Apathy	Mydriasis
Motor retardation	Piloerection
Sedation	Diaphoresis
Slurred speech	Diarrhea
Attention impairment	Yawning
Miosis	Fever
	Insomnia
	Muscle aching

CENTRAL NERVOUS SYSTEM STIMULANTS

COCAINE

Cocaine is perhaps the most behaviorally reinforcing of all drugs of abuse. That is not to say that dependence on other drugs (e.g., alcohol) is any less "powerful" than that on cocaine, but the pharmacology, pharmacokinetics, and the route of administration of cocaine causes intense drug-seeking behavior. The most characteristic systemic effect of cocaine is stimulation of the CNS.[29] In the CNS, cocaine appears to mediate its effects primarily by blocking reuptake of catecholamine neurotransmitters such as norepinephrine and dopamine. The most common clinical manifestations of cocaine stimulation of the CNS are intense euphoria, decreased fatigue, and increased alertness. Common slang terms for cocaine are "coke," "snow," "girl," and "nose candy."

Recent research has helped clarify certain patterns of cocaine use such as combining cocaine and alcohol. Such drug use would seem counteractive since cocaine is a CNS stimulant and alcohol a CNS depressant. In the presence of alcohol, cocaine is metabolized to cocaethylene, a longer acting but equally potent psychoactive compound as compared to the parent drug.[30] Cocaethylene is more potent than cocaine in terms of lethality.[31] The cocaine–alcohol combination is one of the most commonly identified among individuals who come to hospital emergency departments with acute substance abuse problems.

Cocaine is rapidly absorbed from virtually all sites of application. For many years, cocaine has been administered as the hydrochloride salt form, usually by inhalation, but also by injection. In the last 15 years as the purity of cocaine hydrochloride obtained on the street declined, many users converted the cocaine hydrochloride to cocaine base, also known as "crack" or "rock." Conversion to cocaine base is accomplished by creating an alkaline environment, such as with the addition of sodium bicarbonate and heat. The cocaine base clumps together into rocklike formations, which are then melted to form vapors and inhaled.[32] Crack cocaine receives its name from the crackling sound that occurs when the rocks are melted into vapors.

This form of administration of the drug leads to almost instant absorption and intense euphoria. Peak plasma concentrations of greater than 900 ng/mL have been achieved following inhalation of cocaine base vapors. Peak concentrations of 150–200 ng/mL have been achieved after inhalation of 96 mg of pure cocaine hydrochloride powder.[33]

Cocaine is rapidly metabolized and eliminated. The elimination half-life of cocaine is approximately 1 hour, and the duration of effect is very short.[32] Coupled with the compensatory CNS depression commonly experienced when the effect of the drug is diminished, the short duration of effect provides a powerful incentive for repeated use of the drug. Many users experience intense drug use cycling, sometimes lasting days, characterized by rapidly repeating doses of cocaine until their supply is exhausted. Laboratory monkeys, given a choice between food and cocaine around the clock for 8 days, consistently choose cocaine.[34]

Complications of cocaine use frequently involve cardiovascular system events.[35] Even in small doses, cocaine slows the heart through a vagal stimulation. At higher doses, it increases heart rate because of an overall systemic increase in sympathetic tone. At toxic doses, cocaine causes cardiac failure due to a direct effect on myocardial contractility. Cocaine is also pyrogenic, and hyperthermia is frequently observed in cocaine poisoning. Death is usually related to arrhythmias, shock, or convulsions.

Cocaine is a psychotomimetic drug, sometimes even at systemically nontoxic doses. A kindling phenomenon has been described with cocaine in which neuronal function becomes altered with each dose of the drug. This causes a type of reverse tolerance with increased receptor sensitivity to cocaine, and psychosis may be caused by doses that formerly did not cause psychosis. A toxic psychosis caused by cocaine is characterized by auditory, visual, and frequently tactile hallucinations, paranoid thinking, and looseness of associations. The psychosis is qualitatively very similar to a paranoid schizophrenic psychosis.[36]

Incidence and prevalence of cocaine use increased significantly in the early 1980s. In the mid-1980s, the advent of "crack" at low prices, sometimes $5 to $10 for a single dose, increased use among lower socioeconomic groups. Eleven percent of adults have tried cocaine, with approximately 1% having used it in the past month.[3] Even more ominous, the percentage of cocaine users who use the drug daily, almost daily, or weekly has remained steady or increased slightly while overall use fell during the last several years.

Signs and symptoms of cocaine intoxication are summarized in Table 65.4. Although there is some controversy as to whether cocaine is associated with physical withdrawal upon abrupt discontinuation, most clinicians feel that there is a characteristic syndrome of withdrawal effects although they are not life threatening.[4] Cocaine withdrawal consists primarily of fatigue, sleep disturbance, nightmares, and depression; it begins within hours of discontinuing the drug and lasts up to several days.

TABLE 65.4. SIGNS AND SYMPTOMS OF COCAINE INTOXICATION AND WITHDRAWAL

Intoxication	Withdrawal
Motor agitation	Fatigue
Elation/euphoria	Sleep disturbance
Grandiosity	Nightmares
Loquacity	Depression
Hypervigilance	Increased appetite
Tachycardia	
Mydriasis	
Elevated or lowered blood pressure	
Sweating or chills	
Nausea and vomiting	

AMPHETAMINES AND OTHER STIMULANTS

The physiologic and psychologic effects of amphetamines and other stimulants are qualitatively the same as those of cocaine (i.e., they diminish fatigue, increase alertness, suppress appetite). Amphetamines are psychotomimetic and amphetamine-induced psychosis is a principal experimental model for schizophrenia. Pharmacologically, amphetamines increase the activity of catecholamine neurotransmitters (e.g., norepinephrine, dopamine) by blocking reuptake, increasing release of neurotransmitters, and inhibiting the degradative enzyme monoamine oxidase.[37] The primary differences between cocaine and amphetamines are pharmacokinetic. The onset and duration of effect of amphetamines are not as abrupt as those of cocaine.

The incidence and prevalence of stimulant use (other than cocaine) continues to decrease slightly. Approximately 6% of adults have tried stimulants other than cocaine at least once, with less than 1% having used them in the past month.[3] In addition to use of stimulants for their euphoric effects, amphetamines and similar drugs are sometimes used by long-distance drivers and students to maintain alertness. The intravenous use of methamphetamine and amphetamine is known as "speed." A potent form of methamphetamine base called "ice" has also been reported.[38] Like cocaine base, methamphetamine base can be smoked, and the duration of effect of methamphetamine is much longer than that of cocaine. An increased awareness by state and federal regulatory authorities of diversion of stimulants via so-called weight control clinics has led to efforts to control distribution of these drugs. Many states now prohibit prescribing stimulants for obesity.

Stimulants include many of the so-called "designer" and "look-alike" drugs. A common example is 3,4-

methylenedioxymethamphetamine (MDMA), usually called "ecstasy."[39] Nonprescription stimulant drugs, such as caffeine and phenylpropanolamine, are frequently packaged in dosage forms designed to resemble more potent amphetamine stimulant drugs. Designer drugs are the result of efforts by amateur organic chemists to manipulate the chemical structure of controlled substances to create drugs with similar effects. Designer drugs are not subject to legal prescription controls, although the Food and Drug Administration (FDA) is able to rapidly classify these substances as class I drugs (i.e., no approved medical use and subject to regulatory authority).

PHENCYCLIDINE

Phencyclidine was first used as a veterinary anesthetic and briefly as an anesthetic in humans. Phencyclidine is a member of the arylcyclohexylamines. Another member compound, ketamine, is still used clinically as an anesthetic and has many of the same effects as phencyclidine.[29] Phencyclidine, commonly referred to as PCP, "angel dust," and "crystal," was popular in the 1970s, but as its adverse effects became better known, use declined. Phencyclidine is most often a substitute for or contaminant of other drugs, and its most common pattern of use may now be unintentional. The actual extent of its use is unclear. It is often misrepresented as lysergic acid diethylamide (LSD) or Δ^9-tetrahydrocannabinol (THC). THC is virtually unavailable on the street because it is highly unstable when isolated from the marijuana plant. When used intentionally, PCP is commonly smoked with marijuana and referred to as a "crystal joint," but may also be taken orally or intravenously.

Phencyclidine has widely varied actions including CNS stimulation, depression, and hallucinogenic properties. Pharmacologically, it is known to block reuptake of serotonin, dopamine, and norepinephrine, but neurotransmitter antagonists do not effectively block its effects. Phencyclidine blocks the activity of the NMDA subtype of the glutamate receptor and binds at an opiate receptor associated with psychotomimetic properties, the σ-opiate receptor. In low doses, phencyclidine causes sedation, ataxia, nystagmus, slurred speech, and paresthesias. At higher doses, users experience an increase in heart rate, blood pressure, temperature, diaphoresis, and muscle rigidity. At acutely toxic doses, coma and seizures may occur.[40]

Behavioral effects of phencyclidine range from sleep to catatonic detachment to paranoid psychosis to violent hostility. Users are sometimes amnestic for events that occur under the influence of the drug. Psychoses sometimes last for weeks. Users with a previous history of schizophrenia are especially susceptible to the psychotomimetic effects of the drug. The only truly characteristic behavioral effect of phencyclidine use is its high unpredictability. The signs and symptoms of phencyclidine intoxication are summarized in Table 65.5.

TABLE 65.5. SIGNS AND SYMPTOMS OF PHENCYCLIDINE INTOXICATION

Nystagmus	Euphoria
Increased blood pressure	Motor agitation
Tachycardia	Anxiety and emotional lability
Paresthesias	Hostility
Ataxia	Delusions
Slurred speech	Hallucinations
Muscle rigidity	

HALLUCINOGENS

The drugs commonly thought of as being within this category are LSD, psilocybin, dimethyltryptamine (DMT), mescaline, and other related compounds. The incidence and prevalence of hallucinogen use has remained steady over the past few years. Approximately 9% of adults have tried the drugs, with less than 0.5% having used them within a month.[3] Hallucinogenic activity is certainly not unique to these drugs, as discussed for cocaine, amphetamine, phencyclidine, and marijuana. If there is a characteristic effect of hallucinogens, it is the so-called psychedelic effect, a heightened awareness of sensation with a diminished ability to differentiate boundaries of objects or the self from the environment. Pharmacologically, LSD and related drugs stimulate both presynaptic (5-HT_{1A}, 5-HT_{1B}) and postsynaptic (5-HT_2) serotonin recognition sites in the brain, which may functionally cause either agonist or antagonist effects on serotonin activity.[41] Precisely how the hallucinogens exert their effects remains unclear. LSD, often referred to as "acid," is an extraordinarily potent compound, producing observable CNS effects at doses as low as 25 μg.[29]

Signs and symptoms of hallucinogen intoxication are summarized in Table 65.6. Psychological symptoms of intoxication include a subjective intensification of perceptions, depersonalization, illusions, hallucinations, and synthesias, the overflow of one sensory modality to another (i.e., colors are heard and sounds are seen). Among the hallucinogenic drugs, LSD is the most potent and long acting; it is hundreds of times more potent than both psilocybin and mescaline. DMT is inactive when ingested orally, but can be smoked, inhaled, or injected. There is cross-tolerance among LSD, psilocybin, and mescaline. There is not an observable physical withdrawal syndrome after abrupt discontinuation of hallucinogenic drugs.[42]

TABLE 65.6. SIGNS AND SYMPTOMS OF HALLUCINOGEN INTOXICATION

Psychologic	Physical
Perceptual intensification	Mydriasis
Depersonalization	Tachycardia
Derealization	Diaphoresis
Illusions	Palpitations
Hallucinations	Blurred vision
Synesthesias	Tremor
	Incoordination
	Dizziness
	Weakness
	Drowsiness
	Paresthesias

Complications from hallucinogen use are primarily psychologic. Users sometimes experience prolonged episodes of panic, the so-called "bad trip." Hallucinogen drug flashbacks are common, occurring in approximately 15% of users and occurring episodically up to several years after the last exposures to the drug. Flashbacks may occur spontaneously, but are also triggered by other drugs, including marijuana, and by anxiety-provoking stimuli. Physical effects of hallucinogen use are relatively nontoxic. Deaths are generally accidents related to intoxication but not to direct effects of the drug. There is no evidence that hallucinogen use causes chromosome damage or genetic defects.[29]

Marijuana

Marijuana, referred to as reefer, pot, grass, or weed, remains the most commonly used illicit drug. Approximately 34% of adults have tried the drug, with 4% having used it within the last month.[3] Among youth aged 12–17, 12% have tried marijuana, with 5% having used it within a month. *Cannabis sativa,* the marijuana plant, has been produced with increasingly sophisticated growing techniques to produce a plant of greater potency. The principal psychoactive component of marijuana is THC. Hashish, the dried resin of the top of the plant, is much more potent than the plant itself. The pharmacologic mechanism of THC is unknown.[29]

Marijuana has been widely used and is believed by many to be a relatively harmless, nonaddictive intoxicant. Chronic exposure to marijuana is not associated with significant physical withdrawal upon abrupt discontinuation, but many chronic users exhibit compulsive drug-seeking and drug use behavior characteristic of addiction or dependence. As experience with the drug is gained, it is clear that marijuana is far from harmless. Acutely, marijuana has many of the effects of alcohol—sedation, a decrease in reactivity and ability to perform complex tasks, and disinhibition. Marijuana also causes hallucinations. Chronic use is associated with all of the risks of tobacco smoking, although marijuana smokers are commonly also tobacco smokers and thus differentiation of effects is often difficult. Endocrine effects including amenorrhea, decreased testosterone production, and inhibition of spermatogenesis have been demonstrated. Although controversial, marijuana is associated with an amotivational syndrome, characterized by a behavioral pattern of apathy, dullness, impaired judgment, decreased concentration and memory, loss of interest in personal hygiene, and a general reduction of goal-directed behavior.[43]

TABLE 65.7. SIGNS AND SYMPTOMS OF MARIJUANA INTOXICATION

Tachycardia	Euphoria
Conjunctival congestion	Sensory intensification
Increased appetite	Apathy
Dry mouth	Hallucinations

The signs and symptoms of marijuana intoxication are summarized on Table 65.7. Cardiovascular effects and reddened conjunctivae are the most prominent physical effects with acute use (e.g., tachycardia, increased blood pressure with large orthostatic changes). Although the duration of effect of marijuana may be only several hours, THC is detectable upon toxicologic screening for up to 4–5 weeks, especially in chronic users.[29]

Inhalants

Inhalation of organic solvents including gasoline, glue, aerosols, amyl nitrite, and nitrous oxide has remained fairly constant over the past few years. Approximately 10% of young adults (age 18–25) and 6% of youth (age 12–17) have tried inhalant drugs. The 1-month use prevalence is about 1% for young adults and 1.4% for youth.[3]

Toluene is a common solvent component. A trend in inhalants is the use of typewriter correction fluid, referred to as "whiting out," which contains trichloroethane and trichloroethylene. Several sudden-death reactions related to inhalation of fumes of typewriter correction fluid have been reported.[44]

Inhalants are CNS depressants, and symptoms of intoxication are similar to those of alcohol. Intoxication is often accompanied by headache and nausea, and users may experience hallucinations and delusions. The most serious physical risk of acute use is sudden death, usually from cardiac arrhythmias. Some users die from suffocation by plastic bags that contain the solvent. With chronic use, the drugs are toxic to virtually all organ systems. Psychologic impairment, impaired pulmonary, renal, and hepatic function, neuropathies, encephalopathy, and brain damage have all been observed.[44]

Tobacco

Tobacco is the second most commonly used recreational drug in the United States behind alcohol. Approximately 71% of the adult population has smoked tobacco, with 24% smoking regularly. Twenty percent of young adults and 9% of teenagers have tried smokeless tobacco.[3] The health consequences of tobacco use are enormous and well known. A characteristic withdrawal syndrome associated with nicotine, the principal psychoactive component of tobacco, has been observed. Nicotine withdrawal consists of headache, increased appetite, sleep disturbance, anxiety, irritability, difficulty concentrating, and restlessness. Withdrawal begins within 24 hours of last exposure to nicotine, with some symptoms, such as increased appetite, lasting for weeks.[4]

Caffeine

Caffeine is widely consumed in coffee, tea, soft drinks, chocolate, and many analgesic preparations. Health consequences remain controversial. Caffeinism secondary to excessive intake of caffeine has been well documented but is treated clinically only by discontinuation of the drug. Caffeinism may be observed following the ingestion of as little as 300 mg (equivalent to about 2 to 3 cups of coffee) in sensitive individuals, but is more often associated with doses near 1 g. Caffeine intoxication is characterized by restlessness, anxiety, insomnia, flushed face, diuresis, GI complaints, muscle twitching, palpitations, and motor agitation.[4]

Physical dependence may occur when daily intake exceeds approximately 500 mg of the drug, about 5 cups of coffee. It is estimated that approximately 25% of the adult population consumes this much caffeine per day. Physical withdrawal from caffeine, beginning around 24 hours after last exposure and lasting several days, consists primarily of headache, anxiety, and restlessness.[45]

Anticholinergic Drugs

Scopolamine, trihexyphenidyl, benztropine, and other anticholinergic drugs have potentially intoxicating effects. Symptoms of an anticholinergic drug-induced toxic psychosis include euphoria, disorientation, hallucinations, and paranoid ideation. Physical symptoms include mydriasis, warm dry skin, tachycardia, dry mouth, ataxia, and constipation with absence of bowel sounds. Users of anticholinergic drugs describe a "buzz" associated with the drugs, and there are reports of individuals presenting to emergency rooms asking for the drugs by name or feigning extrapyramidal symptoms in order to obtain them.[46]

Anabolic Steroids

Synthetic derivatives of the male sex hormone testosterone have become increasingly abused for their athletic performance-enhancing properties, also known as ergogenic potential. Estimates of use prevalence are not precise and range from 2–20%. Adverse effects occur frequently and most commonly involve the hepatic and endocrine systems. These include infertility, gynecomastia, and masculinization in women. Other adverse effects include irritability, aggression, psychosis, mania, and psychologic dependence.[47]

Pathophysiology

MECHANISMS OF TOLERANCE, DEPENDENCE, AND WITHDRAWAL

Many factors influence the development of drug dependence. As with any disease, a susceptible host must be combined with favorable conditions. Western society is unquestionably drug oriented. Advertising encourages the reward of good behavior and productivity by the use of alcohol, tobacco, and caffeine. Use of drugs, especially alcohol, is often depicted in the context of boisterous camaraderie and good times following a hard day's work or play.

Drug dependence depends on the reinforcing properties of the drug being used (i.e., the drug satisfies a need that demands repetition). Drug dependence most likely evolves in a phasic manner. The euphoriant or other pleasant properties of a drug act initially as reinforcers of drug-seeking behavior; but as tolerance develops, the pleasant effects of the drug are reduced, and higher doses are required to produce the same desirable feelings. Also, the user becomes aware of the need to avoid the pain and discomfort associated with the abstinence syndrome, or drug withdrawal. Many drug-dependent individuals state that their principal motivation for drug use turns relatively quickly from seeking of pleasurable effects to avoidance of unpleasant effects.[48]

Mechanisms of physical dependence involve homeostasis. Drugs disturb biochemical and physiologic systems, and systems, therefore, adapt to reduce those effects. Such compensatory adaptation leads to the development of tolerance. Therefore, when the drug is withdrawn, the compensatory changes dominate, and the user experiences withdrawal symptoms. The clinical manifestations of withdrawal syndromes are generally opposite to those effects produced by the drugs. In many cases, the disturbance in homeostatic mechanisms may be long lasting. Withdrawal may consist of an acute, relatively short phase lasting several days, followed by a more subacute, protracted withdrawal syndrome. Protracted withdrawal has been most consistently reported for alcohol and opiates. Opiate dependence, for example, is associated with a "conditioned abstinence syndrome" lasting up to several months or longer after cessation of intake and may be precipitated by environmental stimuli previously associated with drug use.[48] Opiate-dependent individuals have reported the onset of physical withdrawal symptoms after merely coming into contact with their previous environment (e.g., the user's neighborhood, the sight of heroin, or the observation of other individuals who are using drugs). Conditioned abstinence may be described as a heightened sensitivity to stimuli, abnormal autonomic responses, dysphoria, and intense craving for the effects of the drug.

There are two types of physiologic tolerance to drugs.[29] The first, dispositional tolerance, also called *metabolic* or *pharmacokinetic tolerance,* results from changes in the pharmacokinetics of drugs. Usually, the tolerance is related to increased metabolism. Examples of drugs associated with dispositional tolerance are barbiturates and alcohol. The second type of tolerance is pharmacodynamic tolerance, also known as a *cellular* or *functional tolerance.* Pharmacodynamic tolerance results from adaptive changes at the site of action of drugs, such as changes in receptor system binding sensitivity. Examples of drugs that exhibit pharmacodynamic tolerance are alcohol and opiates.

CNS DEPRESSANTS

Alcohol tolerance develops through both dispositional and pharmacodynamic mechanisms.[49] Alcohol is an inducer of liver enzymes and enhances its own metabolism, but the principal mechanism of tolerance appears to be pharmacodynamic. Acute effects of alcohol are mediated by the lipid membrane permeability of cell membranes as well as membrane-mounted proteins that regulate neurotransmitter activity and ion transport. With chronic exposure to alcohol, the structural integrity of the cell membrane appears to change in such a way as to resist the actions of alcohol. In addition, changes in cell function mediated by neurotransmitter substances, such as gamma-aminobutyric acid (GABA) and ion transport may also account for alcohol tolerance. Alcohol has a depressing, disordering effect on cell function, and cells compensate by increasing sympathetic activity. In the abrupt absence of alcohol, sympathetic nervous system overactivity appears to cause withdrawal.

The principal mechanism of barbiturate tolerance appears to be dispositional.[29] All barbiturates are potent inducers of liver enzymes and induce their own metabolism. Tolerance to benzodiazepines appears to be primarily pharmacodynamic.[29] The precise cellular mechanism of tolerance to benzodiazepines is not clear, but may be a decrease in the number or sensitivity of benzodiazepine receptors.

Tolerance to opiates appears to be pharmacodynamic.[29] The primary center in the brain for both opiate and noradrenergic-mediated neurons appears to be the locus coeruleus in the midbrain. Neurons from the locus coeruleus project throughout the cerebral cortex. Although there are multiple subtypes of opiate receptors, the opiate receptor appears to be primarily a presynaptic receptor and has an inhibitory effect on the noradrenergic nerve terminal (i.e., stimulation of the presynaptic opiate receptor inhibits neuronal release or norepinephrine). The endogenous ligand for the opiate receptor is enkephalin. Another presynaptic receptor that serves as an inhibitory receptor for noradrenergic activity is the α_2-adrenergic receptor.[50] The presynaptic α_2 receptor is a norepinephrine autoreceptor.

Chronic use of exogenous opiates, such as heroin, hydromorphone, and methadone, causes a decrease in production of the endogenous substance enkephalin, just as administration of exogenous corticosteroids causes a decrease in endogenous production of cortisol. Greater than normal activity at the receptor is associated with a compensatory decrease in the binding sensitivity of the opiate receptor system, also known as down-regulation. Because the opiate receptor is inhibitory to noradrenergic activity, a down-regulation effect would diminish the effect of opiates; thus larger doses would be required to achieve the same degree of inhibition of noradrenergic activity. Abrupt discontinuation of exogenous opiates produces a down-regulated inhibitory opiate receptor system and diminished levels of endogenous ligand, enkephalin. Therefore, opiate withdrawal can be conceptualized as a syndrome of noradrenergic hyperactivity.[51]

CNS STIMULANTS

Tolerance to the stimulants, including cocaine, is pharmacodynamic in nature,[29] but the precise cellular mechanism is unclear; however, tolerance to different pharmacologic effects of stimulants develops at different rates. Tolerance to appetite suppression, for example, develops within days to weeks, whereas tolerance to the euphoric effects and increased alertness develops more slowly. A type of reverse pharmacodynamic tolerance, kindling, was described earlier and has been observed with both cocaine and amphetamines. The neuropharmacology of cocaine and amphetamine withdrawal is not well understood; however, such withdrawal effects as depression, fatigue, and increased sleep and appetite are the opposite of the usual effects of the drug, as is the case with most drugs. Chronic cocaine use may cause a catecholamine depletion in the brain.

Tolerance develops to phencyclidine and the LSD-type hallucinogens, although the mechanisms are not clearly understood. Phencyclidine may be associated with a dispositional tolerance. Tolerance to marijuana appears to be more pharmacodynamic than dispositional, although marijuana is known to induce microsomal liver enzymes.[52] The mechanism of tolerance to inhalants is not understood.

THE DISEASE MODEL OF ADDICTION

Individuals who are drug dependent are frequently regarded as constitutionally weak people who have brought their problems upon themselves and deserve the consequences of their behavior. Even when the lay public and health care professionals acknowledge addiction as a disease process, it is often felt to be self-induced. The disease concept of addiction, using alcoholism as a model, states that addiction is a disease and that individuals who suffer from the disease do not choose to contract the disease any more than someone who suffers from heart disease or diabetes mellitus chooses to contract that illness. A *disease* is defined as "any deviation from or interruption of the normal structure or function of any part, organ, or system (or combination thereof) of the body that is manifested by a characteristic set of symptoms and signs and whose etiology, pathology, and prognosis may be known or unknown."[53] Alcoholism, which is discussed as a prototype, meets all of the definition criteria. Diagnostic criteria for alcoholism do not specify frequency of drinking or amount of alcohol consumed. For example, episodic binge drinkers may still be severely alcohol dependent. The key determinant is whether drinking is compulsive, out of control, and consequential *when one drinks*.

Numerous biologic differences between alcoholics and normals have been demonstrated, but discussions of the disease of alcoholism usually focus on three points. The first point involves interindividual differences in response to alcohol, based on the animal model. When a community of rats is offered two sources of water, one of a solution of glucose, the other of alcohol, approximately 90% of the animals selectively choose glucose–water after testing both supplies. The remainder prefer alcohol. If the alcohol-preferring rats are separated from the remainder of the population, their offspring are significantly more likely to be alcohol preferring.[54] Data suggest that there is significant interindividual variation in how animals prefer and respond to alcohol, and that these differences can be selectively inbred.

The experience of the animal studies led researchers to examine family trends in alcoholism and the possibility that alcoholism can be genetically transmitted. Data in human subjects suggest an association between a dopamine D_2-receptor gene and alcoholism,[55] although not all similar studies have replicated these results. More recent data suggest a similar genetic predisposition to polysubstance abuse.[56] A preliminary study in male veterans also showed an association of the D_2-receptor gene with cocaine dependence.[57] Although many researchers think it unlikely that there is a specific gene for addiction, it is possible that interactions among several genes combine in such a way as to be conducive to making a drug an effective reinforcer.[58]

The prevalence of alcoholism among the first-degree relatives of alcoholics (i.e., parents, siblings, children) is approximately 25%, versus 8% in the adult population. Concordance for alcoholism among fraternal twins is approximately 31%, but among identical twins concordance is approximately 54%,[59] although there are conflicting data on this point. When children of alcoholic parents are separated at birth and placed in nonalcoholic homes, they remain three to five times more likely to become alcoholic than adoptees whose biologic parents are not alcoholic.[60–63] The opposite is also true (i.e., offspring of nonalcoholics adopted by alcoholics do not have elevated rates of alcohol problems).[64]

The difference in concordance between fraternal and identical twins and the greater likelihood of developing alcoholism among adoptees whose biological parents are alcoholic argue for what some clinicians have called a genetic *predisposition.* A genetically predisposed individual will not necessarily manifest alcoholic drinking behavior. As stated previously, a susceptible host and favorable conditions must combine in order for a disease process to occur. Sons of men with early-onset alcoholism appear especially predisposed to developing alcoholism.[65] Research into genetic influences on other forms of drug dependence is limited owing to their being less prevalent, a greater difficulty in recruiting subjects, lack of restriction of use to one class of drugs, and the changes in availability of illicit substances.

A third point regarding the disease of alcoholism regards possible biochemical abnormalities. Research findings are necessarily limited to animal trials and remain controversial. Animal models are used to determine gene sequences controlling alcohol sensitivity, conditions under which learning to overcome aversion to alcohol's taste occurs, the role of learning in the development of tolerance, and improved ways to manage withdrawal and maintain abstinence. Behavioral genetics studies in drug self-administration in rats across different drugs and genotypes suggest that the drug-seeking behaviors maintained by alcohol, cocaine, and opiates may have some common biological determinants.[58] Advances in techniques for analysis of brain electrophysiology suggest that alcoholics and their alcohol-naive offspring have similar electroencephalography (EEG) profiles.[66] If these findings are borne out with additional studies, it would support the concept of biological differences between alcoholics and normals that are innate rather than a consequence of exposure to alcohol. In addition, a family history of alcoholism has been shown to be associated with decreased subjective feelings of acute intoxication, less alcohol-induced anxiety, and fewer alcohol-induced decrements in psychomotor and cognitive test performance. EEGs done on this population of nonalcohol-dependent sons of alcoholics also showed less intense EEG alpha activity in response to ethanol challenge than did matched controls.[67] Other suggested biologic markers for alcoholism include differences in the activity of liver transaminase enzymes and platelet monoamine oxidase activity.

The belief that addiction is a self-induced disease or a constitutional weakness has been dismissed by clinicians in the addiction treatment field. Willpower and self-discipline cannot control genetics and possible biochemical abnormalities. Given that almost all the population will try alcohol and that over half drink alcohol regularly, the determination of who becomes alcoholic is based on more factors than environmental precipitants. It is highly likely the many "susceptible hosts" will at some time find themselves in favorable circumstances for the clinical expression of alcohol or other drug dependence.

TREATMENT

INTOXICATION

Treatment of drug intoxication, summarized in Table 65.8, is primarily supportive, and vital functions are maintained while waiting for the drug to be eliminated. When absolutely necessary, physical restraint may be required temporarily while a diagnostic evaluation is initiated to rule out other causes for the behavior (e.g., metabolic or fluid and electrolyte disturbances). Whenever possible, drug therapy should be avoided, because psychotropic drug therapy has the potential for worsening a toxic reaction to another psychoactive agent; however, when patients are agitated, combative, assaultive, hallucinatory, or delusional, drug therapy may be required. Drug therapy may also be indicated in the treatment of an acute, potentially fatal drug overdose. Toxicology screens are useful in the evaluation and treatment process, but many drugs, including cocaine and heroin, are eliminated so rapidly that drug screens may become negative in a matter of hours, although the benzoylecognine metabolite of cocaine is present for a longer period of time. When toxicology screens are desired, blood or urine should be collected immediately upon the patient's arrival.

For alcohol and barbiturate intoxication, supportive treatment is the rule. For benzodiazepine intoxication, the benzodiazepine antagonist flumazenil (Mazicon, Roche) can be used to reverse toxic effects. It is not universally indicated in all cases of suspected drug overdosage, however, and is specifically contraindicated in cases in which cyclic antidepressant involvement is known or suspected because of the risk of seizures. In addition, it should be used with caution in patients when benzodiazepine physical dependence is suspected because of the risks of induction of benzodiazepine withdrawal.[68] In the case of opiate intoxication, if the patient is unconscious and respiration is depressed, the opiate antagonist naloxone (Narcan, Du Pont) can be used to revive the patient. The usual dosage for naloxone in acute opiate toxicity is 0.4–2.0 mg intravenously, given approximately every 3 minutes as necessary.[69] Although naloxone is effective in reversing opiate overdose, it may also precipitate physical withdrawal in physically dependent patients. Patients who fail to respond to a total dosage of 10 mg of naloxone probably have a cause of acute intoxication other than an opiate.

Intoxication with stimulants, including cocaine, is treated pharmacologically only if the patient is overtly psychotic and agitated. Injectable benzodiazepine antianxiety drugs, usually lorazepam (Ativan, Wyeth) 2–4 mg IM every 30 minutes to 6 hours as necessary, can be used for agitation. As a backup to lorazepam, antipsychotic drugs can be used on a short-term basis, primarily in patients with psychotic symptoms, and usually at relatively low doses (e.g., haloperidol [Haldol, McNeil] 2–5 mg IM every 30 minutes to 6 hours as necessary, followed by 5–15 mg orally per day in single or divided doses if the patient is still psychotic

TABLE 65.8. TREATMENT OF SUBSTANCE INTOXICATION

Drug Class	Pharmacologic Therapy	Nonpharmacologic Therapy
Benzodiazepines	Flumazenil 0.1–0.2 mg/min IV up to 1 mg	Support vital functions
Alcohol, barbiturates, and sedative–hypnotics (nonbenzodiazepines)	None	Support vital functions
Opiates	Naloxone 0.4–2.0 mg IV every 3 min	Support vital functions
Cocaine and other CNS stimulants	Lorazepam 2–4 mg IM every 30 min to 6 h prn agitation	Monitor cardiac function
	Haloperidol 2–5 mg (or other antipsychotic agent) every 30 min to 6 h prn psychotic behavior	
Hallucinogens, marijuana, and inhalants	Lorazepam and/or haloperidol as above	Reassurance; "talk-down therapy"; support vital functions
Phencyclidine	Lorazepam and/or haloperidol as above	Minimize sensory input

after initial treatment.)[6] Cardiovascular complications are treated symptomatically with antiarrhythmic agents or other intervention as necessary. Seizures are generally treated supportively. Intravenous lorazepam or diazepam can be used if seizures progress to status epilepticus.

Hallucinogen intoxication is treated in a manner similar to stimulant intoxication. Drug therapy can often be avoided, because patients may respond to careful reassurance, or so-called talk-down therapy. When necessary, short-term antianxiety and/or antipsychotic drug therapy can be used as described previously. The same approach applies to marijuana and inhalant intoxication.

Phencyclidine intoxication is more unpredictable and more difficult to treat than other psychosis-producing drugs. Most clinicians suggest that sensory input be minimized to the extent possible; thus, "talk-down" therapy is not recommended and may in fact make the patient worse. If phencyclidine intoxication is suspected, patients should be left alone in a quiet, dimly lit room. If behavior is uncontrollable, antianxiety and/or antipsychotic drug therapy may be necessary.

WITHDRAWAL

Treatment of drug withdrawal is the primary indication for drug therapy in substance-related disorders. Goals of drug therapy include prevention of progression of withdrawal to life-threatening severity, enabling the patient to be sufficiently comfortable and functional in order to participate in a behavioral treatment program, and supportive drug therapy. The clinician should remember that withdrawal is usually part of a substance dependence disorder. Patients with drug dependence generally cope with almost any stress through the use of a drug. In drug therapy for withdrawal, it is important to avoid reinforcing the patient's drug-seeking and drug use behavior to the extent possible. Drug withdrawal in the best of circumstances is uncomfortable. Patients must be educated to deal with the stress of withdrawal without seeking drugs. The use of drugs as needed for anxiety or insomnia should be avoided. Treatment of drug withdrawal is summarized in Table 65.9.

CNS DEPRESSANT WITHDRAWAL

Alcohol

Supportive drug therapy for alcohol withdrawal consists of treatment such as replacement of B vitamins, especially thiamine, to treat or prevent Wernicke's encephalopathy, and fluid and electrolyte replacement to correct dehydration and electrolyte disturbances. Thiamine 100 mg IM is frequently administered, followed by thiamine 100 mg orally once daily. A multivitamin supplement is also often given. Electrolyte replacement often includes an injection of magnesium sulfate 1 g IM (2 mL of a 50% solution) daily for 1–3 days.[70]

TABLE 65.9. TREATMENT OF WITHDRAWAL FROM COMMON DRUGS OF ABUSE

Drug or Drug Class	Pharmacologic Therapy
Alcohol	
Detoxification	Chlordiazepoxide 50 mg tid-qid or lorazepam 2 mg tid-qid; taper over 5–7 d
Withdrawal hallucinations	Lorazepam 2 mg IM, may be repeated; higher detoxification dosage and slower taper may be needed
Withdrawal seizures	Supportive treatment only during seizure unless condition progresses to status epilepticus; lorazepam 2 mg IM after seizure ends; use higher detoxification dosage and slower taper
Supportive drug therapy	Thiamine 100 mg IM, then 100 mg PO daily; multivitamin, one daily; magnesium sulfate 1 g IM × 1–3 d
Benzodiazepines	
Short- to intermediate-acting	Chlordiazepoxide 50 mg tid-qid or lorazepam 2 mg tid-qid; taper over 5–7 d
Long-acting	Chlordiazepoxide 50 mg tid-qid or lorazepam 2 mg tid-qid; taper over additional 5–7 d
Barbiturates and other sedative–hypnotics	Pentobarbital tolerance test (Table 65.11); initial detoxification at upper limit of tolerance test; decrease dosage by 100 mg every 2–3 d
Opiates	Methadone 20–80 mg PO daily; taper by 5–10 mg daily or clonidine 2 μg/kg tid × 7 d; taper over additional 3 d
Mixed-substance withdrawal	
Drugs are cross-tolerant	Detoxify according to treatment for longer acting drug used
Drugs are not cross-tolerant	Detoxify from one drug while maintaining second drug (cross-tolerant drugs), then detoxify from second drug
CNS stimulants	Supportive treatment only; pharmacotherapy often not used; bromocriptine 2.5 mg tid or higher may be used for severe craving associated with cocaine withdrawal

Detoxification, the treatment of acute withdrawal from alcohol, can be accomplished with any drug that is cross-tolerant to alcohol. All sedative–hypnotic drugs are cross-tolerant to alcohol, and most have been used to treat alcohol withdrawal. Most clinicians now agree that the benzodiazepines are the drugs of choice in the treatment of alcohol withdrawal.[71] Compared with the barbiturates and other sedative–hypnotics, benzodiazepines are safer at high doses and have fewer adverse effects on the liver and other organ systems. The choice of benzodiazepine drug is much less clear, because all are effective. Many clinicians use long-acting drugs (e.g., chlordiazepoxide, diazepam) that effectively control withdrawal with few rebound effects after discontinuation. Short- to intermediate-acting drugs (e.g., oxazepam, lorazepam) can also be used and have the advantages of having no active metabolites, being less affected by liver impairment, and have few residual sedative effects after discontinuation. Once a drug is selected, the patient is begun on a dose adequate to control the major symptoms of withdrawal, then the drug is gradually tapered over 5–7 days. Representative detoxification regimens using benzodiazepines for treatment of alcohol withdrawal are described in Table 65.10. Patients with more severe withdrawal symptoms may require higher doses and longer tapering periods. Monitoring parameters should include the patient's vital signs, presence of tremor, sweating, and other signs and symptoms of withdrawal.

Unless the patient has a concurrent psychotic disorder, antipsychotic drug therapy is not generally indicated for alcohol withdrawal, even if withdrawal hallucinations occur. Antipsychotic drugs create the additional risk of further lowering the seizure threshold in patients in severe withdrawal. More aggressive treatment with a benzodiazepine, often by injection (e.g., lorazepam 2–4 mg IM or IV, or diazepam 10 mg IV), may be required to bring alcohol withdrawal under better control. When the intramuscular form of a benzodiazepine is needed, lorazepam should be used.[70] Intramuscular injections of diazepam and chlordiazepoxide are both erratically and poorly absorbed.[72] The benzodiazepine treatment regimen may require a higher initial dosage and a slower tapering schedule to maintain adequate control of withdrawal symptoms.

TABLE 65.10. ALCOHOL DETOXIFICATION

Chlordiazepoxide
50 mg tid × 1 d
50 mg bid × 1 d
25 mg tid × 1 d
25 mg bid × 1 d
25 mg daily × 1 d, then discontinue
Lorazepam
2 mg tid × 2 d
2 mg bid × 2 d
2 mg daily × 1 d, then discontinue

(Compiled from Ref. 70.)

Alcohol withdrawal seizures do not require treatment with an anticonvulsant drug unless the patient progresses to status epilepticus, because seizures usually end before diazepam or another drug can be administered.[70] Phenytoin, which is not cross-tolerant to alcohol, does not prevent or treat withdrawal seizures, and without an intravenous loading dose, therapeutic blood levels of phenytoin are not reached until acute withdrawal is complete. Patients experiencing seizures should be treated supportively. An increase in the dosage and tapering schedule of the benzodiazepine used in detoxification or a single injection of a benzodiazepine may be necessary to prevent further seizure activity. Patients with a history of withdrawal seizures can be predicted to experience an especially severe withdrawal syndrome. In such patients, a higher initial dosage of a benzodiazepine drug and a slower tapering period of 7–10 days are advisable.

Alternative medications tried for alcohol withdrawal include clonidine (Catapres, Boehringer-Ingleheim), carbamazepine (CBZ) (Tegretol, Ciba-Geigy) and propranolol (Inderal, Wyeth-Ayerst).[71] Clonidine is an agonist of the presynaptic α_2-adrenergic receptor, an autoreceptor with a negative feedback inhibitory effect on noradrenergic discharge. Alcohol withdrawal, indeed withdrawal from most drugs associated with physical dependence, is associated with marked autonomic nervous system hyperactivity. By activating a negative feedback mechanism to decrease adrenergic activity, withdrawal symptoms may be relieved. Studies of clonidine for alcohol withdrawal remain inconclusive, and clonidine has not been demonstrated to prevent or treat severe withdrawal symptoms, such as seizures. At the present time, clonidine must not be regarded as first-line treatment for alcohol withdrawal. Carbamazepine, an antiepileptic drug, has been used commonly in Europe for treatment of alcohol withdrawal. It has been studied in the United States on a limited basis, but is not considered first-line treatment. CBZ is not considered a drug that is cross-tolerant to alcohol. CBZ's mechanism of action is not known, but may involve a cell membrane stabilizing effect known as *antikindling*. Kindling is an increase in excitability with multiple stimuli of constant magnitude. Propranolol and other β-adrenergic receptor blockers reduce the symptoms of withdrawal associated with autonomic hyperactivity, but like clonidine, do not prevent or treat the most severe withdrawal features. In addition, they may exacerbate hypoglycemia associated with malnutrition, a common problem in alcoholism.

Benzodiazepines

Treatment of benzodiazepine withdrawal is very similar to the treatment of alcohol withdrawal, and the same drugs and dosages may be used.[27] The major difference in management is the length of treatment. The onset of withdrawal symptoms in patients physically dependent on the long-acting benzodiazepines may be delayed up to 7 days after discontinuation of the drug. A common approach in detoxification of such patients is to initiate treatment at usual dosages (e.g., chlordiazepoxide 50 mg three times a day, lorazepam 2 mg three times a day) and to maintain the initial dosage for 5 days, with gradual tapering over an additional 5 days. Detoxification in patients physically dependent on shorter acting benzodiazepines is similar to treatment of alcohol withdrawal. Among the benzodiazepines, alprazolam has been suggested to be more difficult to taper and discontinue than the other benzodiazepines.[73] Whether the difficulty is related to a different patient population commonly treated with alprazolam (e.g., panic disorder) or to intrinsic differences between alprazolam and other benzodiazepines is not clear. A longer, more gradual taper of the benzodiazepine used for detoxification may be needed. With all benzodiazepines, protracted minor abstinence symptoms, such as anxiety, insomnia, irritability, sensitivity to light and sound, and muscle spasms, may remain for several weeks in patients with a history of long exposure, even after the acute phase of benzodiazepine withdrawal is complete. As with alcohol, clonidine and CBZ have been used in the treatment of benzodiazepine withdrawal, but are not considered first-line treatments.

Barbiturates and Other Sedative–Hypnotic Drugs

Because of the unpredictability and frequently greater severity of withdrawal from barbiturates and other sedative–hypnotic drugs, it is useful to attempt to determine the patient's level of tolerance before initiating detoxification. Tolerance testing is most often done with pentobarbital (Nembutal, Abbott).[29] The patient is given 200 mg of pentobarbital orally and observed for 2–3 hours for signs of a mild intoxication, including sedation, slurred speech, ataxia, and nystagmus. The procedure is repeated until one or more signs of intoxication are observed. The total dosage of pentobarbital required to reach the lower levels of the patient's limit of tolerance can be used as an approximate initial daily starting dosage for detoxification. The daily dosage can be reduced in decrements of 100 mg every third day at first, then every other day if the patient tolerates initial dosage reductions without difficulty. The reliability of the test is influenced by the dosage and interval since ingestion of the sedative drug, prior to administering the tolerance test. The pentobarbital tolerance test is summarized in Table 65.11. Monitoring parameters for barbiturate detoxification are the same as for alcohol and benzodiazepine detoxification.

Opiates

As mentioned previously, opiate withdrawal is unlike alcohol and sedative–hypnotic drug withdrawal with respect to potential lethality. Opiate withdrawal is not life threatening unless there is a concurrent life-threatening medical condition. In addition, some patients who are addicted to opiates (i.e., compulsive drug seekers and drug users) are not physically dependent. The purity of street drugs, especially heroin, is often very low. The average volume of usage of street drugs may be insufficient to maintain physical dependence in many patients. Although most patients complain of symptoms of withdrawal, such as cramping or insomnia, these symptoms are tolerable, and initiation of drug therapy may be avoided. Because opiate withdrawal is not life threatening, observable signs of withdrawal, such as mydriasis, pilomotor erection, diaphoresis, or diarrhea, should be noted before initiation of drug therapy. Unnecessary detoxification with drugs, especially methadone, should be avoided if possible.

TABLE 65.11. PENTOBARBITAL TOLERANCE TEST

1. Administer pentobarbital 200 mg PO every 2–3 h until tolerance is observed (sedation, slurred speech, nystagmus, ataxia).
2. Begin detoxification at cumulative dosage required to observe intolerance.
3. Taper daily dosage by 100 mg every 2–3 d.

The conventional drug therapy for opiate withdrawal has been methadone, a synthetic opiate. Usual starting dosages have been 20–80 mg/d orally; but treatment of withdrawal from heroin usually requires no more than 20 mg of methadone, owing to the low purity of street heroin. The dosage of methadone can be tapered in decrements of 5–10 mg/d until discontinued. Most patients in withdrawal continue to complain of mild symptoms after detoxification is completed. Some patients who are unable to discontinue methadone completely or habitually return to drug use whenever methadone is discontinued are placed in methadone-maintenance treatment programs and receive methadone chronically.[29] LAAM (Orlaam, Biometric Research Institute) has been approved by the FDA as a potential alternative to methadone maintenance. LAAM forms two long-acting metabolites, which allow three times a week dosing.[74]

An increasingly accepted method of opiate detoxification is the use of clonidine. Use of clonidine can attenuate the noradrenergic hyperactivity of opiate withdrawal without interfering significantly with activity at the opiate receptors. Production of enkephalin and the return of receptors to normal levels of sensitivity can occur as rapidly as possible. Advantages of detoxification with clonidine include a somewhat more rapid detoxification and an absence of the euphoria sometimes observed with methadone.[29,51,75]

Clonidine is often given in an initial dosage of 6 μg/kg/d, in three divided doses. Dosage can be increased if necessary to as high as 17 μg/kg/d. The patient is maintained on the same dosage for 7 days, which is then tapered and discontinued over the next 3 days. A common clonidine side effect is orthostatic hypotension, and the patient's blood pressure should be monitored in the supine and standing positions at least daily. If blood pressure drops to an unacceptably low level (e.g., lying systolic blood pressure less than 90 mm Hg), the dose should be held. If blood pressure has risen in time for the next dose, clonidine can be resumed. Clonidine for treatment of opiate withdrawal has also been administered transdermally, but this method has not been well studied.

Less well established opiate detoxification strategies include the combination of clonidine and naltrexone. Naltrexone, an opiate antagonist, is used to rapidly induce withdrawal that is then attenuated with clonidine. The potential advantage of this method is the shortening of detoxification to as little as 2 days. A similar detoxification regimen using buprenorphine, a partial opiate agonist, and naltrexone has been tried.[75] Buprenorphine has been used as an alternative to methadone maintenance, as well.[76]

WITHDRAWAL FROM OTHER SUBSTANCES

Withdrawal from other drugs, including cocaine and other stimulants, is primarily supportive. Pharmacotherapy has, however, recently assumed a greater role in treating cocaine withdrawal and dependence. Bromocriptine (Parlodel, Sandoz), a dopamine antagonist at low dosages and agonist at high dosages, usually used in the treatment of parkinsonism and hyperprolactinemia, has been used to treat cocaine withdrawal symptoms and to reduce the craving for cocaine.[7] Use of bromocriptine is based on the hypothesis that chronic use of cocaine causes dopamine depletion; therefore, higher dosages should be utilized (i.e., 2.5 mg three times daily or higher). Use is generally short term.

Nicotine withdrawal has been treated with nicotine transdermal patches and a chewing gum containing a nicotine resin (Nicorette, Marion-Merrell-Dow).[77] Patients should be instructed to briefly hold the saliva produced by chewing the gum under the tongue before swallowing, to maximize absorption. Clonidine, using both oral and transdermal routes of administration, has been used in treating nicotine withdrawal.[77] Several studies have demonstrated relief of nicotine withdrawal symptoms and nicotine craving. Not all trials have confirmed this finding, however, and some of the studies with positive effects had significant methodologic problems such as small sample sizes and preexisting differences between study groups. Because of these issues, efficacy has not been conclusively established, and use of clonidine for nicotine withdrawal and smoking cessation is not considered a primary therapy.

MIXED SUBSTANCE WITHDRAWAL

Many drug users practice polypharmacy, and it is common for a patient to experience withdrawal from more than one drug. Treatment of withdrawal depends on the individual drug combination. If the drugs are cross-tolerant (e.g., alcohol and diazepam), treatment for withdrawal from diazepam, the longer acting of the two drugs, will also concurrently treat alcohol withdrawal. If the drugs are not cross-tolerant (e.g., alcohol and opiates), withdrawal from each drug must be treated separately. Withdrawal from both drugs can be treated concurrently in a young, otherwise healthy patient, but a more conservative approach is needed to treat withdrawal from each drug consecutively. While detoxification for one drug is under way, treatment with the second drug (or a drug that is cross-tolerant to the second drug) must be maintained. When detoxification from the first drug is complete, the second drug can be tapered and discontinued according to usual procedures.

SUBSTANCE DEPENDENCE

The treatment of drug dependence, or addiction, is primarily behavioral. The patient is generally taught that complete abstinence is the only realistic alternative to a life of uncontrollable drug use and despair that will ultimately end in death. There is no intermediate, controllable level of drinking or use of another drug. Complete and permanent abstinence as the sole route to recovery is controversial. There may be an extremely few individuals who can return to controllable levels of drinking alcohol, but it is impossible to predict who these individuals are; thus, most treatment programs continue to advocate complete abstinence. The prospect of life without alcohol or other drugs is incomprehensible to many patients. Entry into treatment is often facilitated by some type of leverage that the drug-dependent person associates with negative consequences, such as potential loss of job, divorce, legal problems, or deteriorating physical health. Early treatment is directed at penetrating the denial of a problem that is always present. The patient must be educated as to the disease of addiction, the effects of drugs, and the permanence of the condition. Although treatment may help patients to reorganize their lives in the absence of the drug, they are generally unable to return to controlled drug use.

In recent years, there has been a trend toward outpatient treatment for drug dependence, due, in part, to cost-containment efforts. Inpatient treatment programs can cost as much as $20,000 for a 4-week stay. When withdrawal symptoms are mild to moderate and there are no other medical indications for hospitalization, outpatient treatment may be an attractive alternative to inpatient treatment. One critical criterion for outpatient treatment is the patient's compliance with complete abstinence from the drug on which he is dependent during the treatment experience.

Families must be involved in treatment, not only for the good of the drug-using family member, but for themselves. The course of the patient's illness often has a devastating effect on other family members. Severely depleted self-esteem, denial of the family member's addiction, feelings of responsibility for the family member's drug use, and other behaviors that parallel the addiction process itself are often present. Treatment must be a lifelong process. Aftercare, or what is now being called continued care, should include regular and frequent treatment in some form. Most drug-dependence treatment programs embrace a treatment approach based on Alcoholics Anonymous (AA). AA is one of the most successful of all self-help groups. Associated groups include Alanon (a group for family members of alcoholics), Narcotics Anonymous (self-help groups based on the AA concept for users of other drugs), Overeaters Anonymous (a group for individuals with eating disorders), Gamblers Anonymous, and several other similar programs. Among chemically dependent health care professionals, treatment that incorporates both AA and peer-led self-help groups may be most effective.[78]

Drug Therapy

As previously stated, drug therapy for drug-dependent patients should be minimized to the extent possible. There are, however, several pharmacologic approaches in drug dependency.

Disulfiram (Antabuse, Ayerst) is an inhibitor of the enzyme aldehyde dehydrogenase.[29] In the absence of alcohol, disulfiram has minimal effects. In the presence of alcohol, however, the metabolism of acetaldehyde produced by dehydrogenation of alcohol is inhibited, thus causing an acute increase in acetaldehyde levels. Acetaldehyde causes a characteristic reaction consisting of flushing, nausea, vomiting, headache, palpitations, sweating, fever, and hypotension. Severe reactions may include respiratory depression, arrhythmias, myocardial infarction, cardiovascular collapse, and death. The reaction lasts from 30 minutes to several hours. Supportive measures is the only treatment. The patient is made aware of the likelihood of the disulfiram reaction when treatment with disulfiram is initiated, thus providing a disincentive to drink alcohol. If the alcoholic drinks, the experience of the reaction is intended to serve as aversive conditioning to discourage further alcohol consumption. Binding of disulfiram to aldehyde dehydrogenase is irreversible, thus inhibition of the enzyme continues for as long as 2 weeks after discontinuing disulfiram while new enzyme is synthesized.

Patients taking disulfiram should be educated regarding risks of unsuspected alcohol consumption. Many nonprescription products, including cough syrups and elixirs, contain alcohol. Disulfiram reactions have also been associated with the use of alcohol-containing mouthwashes and even the topical application of alcohol-containing aftershaves. The usual dosage of disulfiram is 250–500 mg/d. The likelihood of a disulfiram reaction is a function of the dose of both disulfiram and alcohol. The most common side effects of disulfiram include rash, headache, lethargy, a metallic taste, and impotence, although impotence caused by alcohol is far more common than impotence caused by disulfiram.[29]

Disulfiram is not a cure for alcoholism. It is not intended to be the sole or primary treatment modality for alcoholism, but is intended to serve as an adjunct to behavioral treatment. The efficacy of disulfiram for maintaining abstinence from alcohol among alcoholics is controversial. Studies show conflicting results and generally indicate that factors such as compliance to treatment may correlate better with abstinence than use of disulfiram.[71]

Naltrexone has been approved as an adjunctive treatment for alcoholism. Two controlled trials show that subjects given naltrexone report less alcohol craving and fewer drinking days.[79,80] The mechanism of naltrexone's effect in alcoholism is not clear, but animal studies show an interaction between alcohol and opiates. Naltrexone blocks stress-induced alcohol preference in rats.[81] There is also an association between alcohol preference and high endogenous opioid activity in rats bred for alcohol preference.[82] The dosage of naltrexone is generally 50 mg daily. The most common side effect of naltrexone is GI disturbance. Laboratory values should be monitored for hepatic toxicity.

Naltrexone is an opiate receptor antagonist that blocks the euphoric effects of opiates.[29] Although it causes no aversive reaction, blockade of the effects of opiates can interrupt the reinforcement process that leads to further drug use. This can be especially useful during the conditioned abstinence syndrome associated with the first several months after initial withdrawal from opiates, when return to drug use is most likely. Naltrexone is orally active and long acting. The usual dosage is 50 mg daily or 350 mg per week in three divided doses. Patients should be started on naltrexone after detoxification to avoid unintentional precipitation of withdrawal, which would provide a powerful incentive for opiate use. As with disulfiram, naltrexone is not a cure for opiate dependence and should be used as an adjunct to behavioral treatment. Compliance is critical to a positive outcome.

Tricyclic antidepressants, primarily desipramine (Norpramin, Marion-Merrill-Dow), have been used in the last several years to decrease cocaine craving.[7] In addition to treating the depression associated with cocaine withdrawal, desipramine may block cocaine-induced euphoria, although data on this question are conflicting. Both desipramine and cocaine block reuptake of brain catecholamines. Competition for common receptor binding sites may decrease the euphoric effect of cocaine. With chronic use, desipramine and cocaine have opposite effects on brain neurotransmitter levels and receptor binding sensitivity, thus possibly relieving the craving for cocaine. Several other drugs have been tried in cocaine dependency, but a paucity of controlled studies limits conclusions regarding efficacy. Examples are dopamine agonists (e.g., bromocriptine, amantadine), carbamazepine, and buprenorphine, a partial opiate antagonist that has been given to prevent cocaine use in methadone-maintained opiate addicts.[83]

COEXISTENT DRUG DEPENDENCE AND PSYCHIATRIC DISORDERS: THE DUAL DIAGNOSIS PATIENT

Although the majority of chemical dependence is primary (i.e., no evidence of a preexisting major psychiatric problem prior to the first life problem related to addiction), a significant percentage, up to 50%, coexists with another psychiatric disorder.[24] One way to conceptualize this is that there are two broad categories of persons who receive diagnoses of two or more conditions that occur together. In one type, chemical dependence might be secondary to a complication of a psychiatric disorder. In these individuals, the onset of the psychiatric disorder significantly predated the regular abuse of substances.

A second type of patient has two concurrent primary diagnoses, chemical dependence and a psychiatric disorder. Recognition of this type of patient has been increasing in recent years. A study of 55 male schizophrenic patients showed that 55% abused some type of drug with alcohol, cocaine, and marijuana comprising 88% of the total drug use.[84] In a study of 401 involuntarily hospitalized patients, however, only 8% of the patients with schizophrenia had a positive urine screen.[85] This points out the frequently profound variation among studies that attempt to examine the prevalence of comorbid psychiatric disorders in substance abusers due to the variations in diagnostic methodology, examiner bias, study design, study length, and patient population.[86,87]

When dual problems of a psychiatric disorder and substance use disorder coexist, they are interactive and may be interdependent. This may be particularly true when personality disorder and substance abuse or dependence coexist.[88] Of the personality disorders, antisocial personality disorder (APD) has been subject to the most extensive validity and reliability testing in patients with substance abuse.[86] Even so, there continues to be controversy about the reliability and stability in the APD diagnosis, particularly when substance abuse is involved. The overall prevalence of substance dependence in clinical psychiatric settings is about 50%, but the prevalence of psychiatric disorders in addiction treatment populations is much lower, approximating levels found in the general population.[87]

Treatment of the patient with coexisting substance use and psychiatric disorders involves initial treatment of the substance use disorder, especially when the patient is in physical withdrawal. If symptoms of psychiatric disorder continue after the patient has been drug free for a minimum of 2 weeks, then treatment of the psychiatric disorder must be considered. Psychotropic drug therapy appropriate to the diagnosis may be indicated. Improved relations between psychiatrists and chemical-dependence treatment professionals have led to cooperative efforts to treat all aspects of the patient's illness.

CONCLUSION

Substance use disorders remain one of the great public health issues of contemporary society. Dependence on drugs is a powerful emotional and political issue. Because we live in a chemically oriented society, everyone is affected in some way by drug abuse and drug dependence. Health care professionals must be particularly vigilant for problems associated with drug use, not only for our patients, but also for themselves.

REFERENCES

1. Accident facts. Chicago, National Safety Council, 1993, 59.
2. Dufour MC, Fe Caces M. Epidemiology of the medical consequences of alcohol. Alcohol Health and Research World 1993;17:265–271.
3. National household survey on drug abuse. Rockville, MD, US Department of Health and Human Services, Substance Abuse and Mental Health Services Administration, 1994.
4. American Psychiatric Association. Diagnostic and Statistical Manual of Mental Disorders, 4th ed (DSM-IV). Washington, DC, Author, 1994.
5. Monitoring the future study: National high school senior drug abuse survey. Rockville, MD, National Institute on Drug Abuse, 1994.
6. Perceived availability and risk of harm of drugs: Estimates from the national household survey on drug abuse. Rockville, MD, US Department of Health and Human Services, Substance Abuse and Mental Health Services Administration, 1994.
7. Gold MS. Cocaine (and crack): Clinical aspects, in Lowinson JH, Ruiz P, Millman RB, Langrod JG (eds): Substance Abuse: A Comprehensive Textbook, 2nd ed. Baltimore, Williams & Wilkins, 1992, p 205.
8. McAuliffe WE, Santangelo SL, Gingras J, et al. Use and abuse of controlled substances by pharmacists and pharmacy students. Am J Hosp Pharm 1987;44:311–317.
9. McAuliffe WE, Rohman M, Santangelo S, et al. Psychoactive drug use among practicing physicians and medical students. N Engl J Med 1986;315:805–810.
10. Hughes PH, Storr C, Baldwin DC, et al. Patterns of substance use in the medical profession. Maryland Med J 1992;41:311–314.
11. Hughes PH, Scott EC, Baldwin DC, et al. Resident physician substance use in the United States. JAMA 1991;265:2069–2073.
12. Lutsky I, Hopwood M, Abram SE, et al. Psychoactive substance use among American anesthesiologists: A 30-year retrospective study. Can J Anesthes 1993;40:915–921.
13. Miller CJ, Banahan BF, Borne RF. A comparison of alcohol and illicit drug use between pharmacy students and the

general college population. Am J Pharm Educ 1990;54:27–30.
14. Tucker DR, Gurnee MC, Sylvestri MF, et al. Psychoactive drug use and impairment markers in pharmacy students. Am J Pharm Educ 1988;52:42–47.
15. Bissell L, Haberman PW. Alcoholism in the Professions. New York, Oxford University Press, 1984, p 21.
16. Crosby LR, Bissell L. To care enough. Intervention with chemically dependent colleagues: A guide for healthcare and other professionals. Minneapolis, Johnson Institute, 1989, p 9.
17. Gambert SR. Substance abuse in the elderly, in Lowinson JH, Ruiz P, Millman RB, Langrod JG (eds): Substance Abuse: A Comprehensive Textbook, 2nd ed. Baltimore, Williams & Wilkins, 1992, p 843.
18. Guterman A, Eisdorfer C. Geriatric psychiatry: Other psychiatric conditions of the elderly, in Kaplan HI, Sadock BJ (eds): Comprehensive Textbook of Psychiatry, 5th ed. Baltimore, Williams & Wilkins, 1989, p 2031.
19. Abrams RC, Alexopoulos GS. Substance abuse in the elderly: Alcohol and prescription drugs. Hosp Community Psychiatry 1987;38:1285–1287.
20. Goodwin DW. Alcohol: Clinical aspects, in Lowinson JH, Ruiz P, Millman RB, Langrod JG (eds): Substance Abuse: A Comprehensive Textbook, 2nd ed. Baltimore, Williams & Wilkins, 1992, p 144.
21. Harris RA, Schroeder F. Ethanol and the physical properties of brain membranes: Fluorescence studies. Mol Pharmacol 1981;20:128–137.
22. Tabakoff B, Hoffman PL. The neurochemistry of alcohol. Curr Opin Psychiatry 1993;6:388–394.
23. Charness ME, Simon RP, Greenberg DA. Ethanol and the nervous system. N Engl J Med 1989;321:442–454.
24. Schuckit MA. Drug and Alcohol Abuse: A Clinical Guide to Diagnosis and Treatment, 3rd ed. New York, Plenum, 1989, p 84.
25. Cavallaro R, Regazzetti MG, Covelli G, Smeraldi E. Tolerance and withdrawal with zolpidem. Lancet 1993;342:868–869.
26. Rall TW. Hypnotics and sedatives; ethanol, in Gilman AG, Rall TW, Nies AS, Taylor P (eds): The Pharmacological Basis of Therapeutics, 8th ed. New York, Pergamon, 1990, p 345.
27. Smith DE, Wesson DR. Benzodiazepines and other sedative-hypnotics, in Galanter M, Kleber HD (eds): Textbook of Substance Abuse Treatment. Washington, DC, American Psychiatric Press, 1994, p 179.
28. Jaffe JH. Opiates: Clinical aspects, in Lowinson JH, Ruiz P, Millman RB, Langrod JG (eds): Substance Abuse: A Comprehensive Textbook, 2nd ed. Baltimore, Williams & Wilkins, 1992, p 186.
29. Jaffe JH. Drug addiction and drug abuse, in Gilman AG, Rall TW, Nies AS, Taylor P (eds): The Pharmacological Basis of Therapeutics, 8th ed. New York, Pergamon, 1990, p 522.
30. Hearn WL, Flynn DD, Hime GW, et al. Cocaethylene: A unique cocaine metabolite displays high affinity for the dopamine transporter. J Neurochem 1991;56:698–701.
31. Hearn WL, Rose W, Wagner J, et al. Cocaethylene is more potent than cocaine in mediating lethality. Pharmacol Biochem Behav 1991;3:531–533.
32. Gold MS, Miller NS, Jonas JM. Cocaine (and crack): Neurobiology, in Lowinson JH, Ruiz P, Millman RB, Langrod JG (eds): Substance Abuse: A Comprehensive Textbook, 2nd ed. Baltimore, Williams & Wilkins, 1992, p 222.
33. Fischman MW. The behavioral pharmacology of cocaine in humans. Natl Inst Drug Abuse Res Monogr Ser 1984;50:72–91.
34. Aigner TG, Balster RL. Choice behavior in rhesus monkeys: Cocaine versus food. Science 1978;201:534–535.
35. Van Dette JM, Cornish LA. Medical complications of illicit cocaine use. Clin Pharm 1989;8:401–411.
36. Brady DT, Lydiard RB, Malcolm R, Ballenger JC. Cocaine-induced psychosis. J Clin Psychiatry 1991;52:509–512.
37. King GR, Ellinwood EH. Amphetamines and other stimulants, in Lowinson JH, Ruiz P, Millman RB, Langrod JG (eds): Substance Abuse: A Comprehensive Textbook, 2nd ed. Baltimore, Williams & Wilkins, 1992, p 247.
38. Jackson JG. Hazards of smokable methamphetamine. N Engl J Med 1989;321:907.
39. Morgan JP. Controlled substance analogues: Current clinical and social issues, in Lowinson JH, Ruiz P, Millman RB, Langrod JG (eds): Substance Abuse: A Comprehensive Textbook, 2nd ed. Baltimore, Williams & Wilkins, 1992, p 328.
40. Zukin SR, Zukin RS. Phencyclidine, in Lowinson JH, Ruiz P, Millman RB, Langrod JG (eds): Substance Abuse: A Comprehensive Textbook, 2nd ed. Baltimore, Williams & Wilkins, 1992, p 290.
41. Glennon RA. Do classical hallucinogens act as 5-HT_2 agonists or antagonists? Neuropsychopharmacology 1990;3:509–517.
42. Ungerleider JT, Pechnick RN. Hallucinogens, in Lowinson JH, Ruiz P, Millman RB, Langrod JG (eds): Substance Abuse: A Comprehensive Textbook, 2nd ed. Baltimore, Williams & Wilkins, 1992, p 280.
43. Grinspoon L, Bakalar JB. Marihuana, in Lowinson JH, Ruiz P, Millman RB, Langrod JG (eds): Substance Abuse: A Comprehensive Textbook, 2nd ed. Baltimore, Williams & Wilkins, 1992, p 236.
44. Sharp CW, Rosenberg NL. Volatile substances, in Lowinson JH, Ruiz P, Millman RB, Langrod JG (eds): Substance Abuse: A Comprehensive Textbook, 2nd ed. Baltimore, Williams & Wilkins, 1992, p 303.
45. Greden JF, Walters A. Caffeine, in Lowinson JH, Ruiz P, Millman RB, Langrod JG (eds): Substance Abuse: A Comprehensive Textbook, 2nd ed. Baltimore, Williams & Wilkins, 1992, p 357.
46. Smith JM. Abuse of the antiparkinson drugs: A review of the literature. J Clin Psychiatry 1980;41:351–354.
47. Brower KJ. Addictive potential of anabolic steroids. Psychiatr Ann 1992;22:30–34.
48. Wikler A. Conditioning factors in opiate addiction and release, in Wilner DI, Kossebaum GG (eds): Narcotics. New York, McGraw-Hill, 1965, p 85.
49. Tabakoff B, Hoffman PL. Alcohol: Neurobiology, in Lowinson JH, Ruiz P, Millman RB, Langrod JG (eds): Substance Abuse: A Comprehensive Textbook, 2nd ed. Baltimore, Williams & Wilkins, 1992, p 152.
50. Lefkowitz RJ, Hoffman BB, Taylor P. Neurohumoral transmission: The autonomic and somatic motor nervous systems, in Gilman AG, Rall TW, Nies AS, Taylor P (eds): The Pharmacological Basis of Therapeutics, 8th ed. New York, Pergamon, 1990, p 84.

51. Gold MS, Redmond DE, Kleber HD. Noradrenergic hyperactivity in opiate withdrawal supported by clonidine reversal of opiate withdrawal. Am J Psychiatry 1979;136:100–102.
52. Dewey WL. Cannabinoid pharmacology. Pharmacol Rev 1986;38:151–178.
53. Dorland's Illustrated Medical Dictionary, 28th ed. Philadelphia, WB Saunders, 1994, p 478.
54. Li TK, Lumeng L, McBride WJ, Murphy JM. Rodent lines selected for factors affecting alcohol consumption. Alcohol Alcohol 1987;(suppl 1):91–96.
55. Blum K, Noble EP, Sheridan PJ, et al. Allelic association of human dopamine D_2 receptor gene in alcoholism. JAMA 1990;263:2055–2060.
56. Smith SS, O'Hara BF, Persico AM, et al. Genetic vulnerability to drug abuse: The D_2 dopamine receptor taq I B1 restriction fragment length polymorphism appears more frequently in polysubstance abusers. Arch Gen Psychiatry 1992;49:723–727.
57. Noble EP, Blum K, Khalsa ME, et al. Allelic association of the D_2 dopamine receptor gene with cocaine dependence. Drug Alcohol Depend 1993;33:271–285.
58. George FR. Genetic models in the study of alcoholism and substance abuse mechanisms. Prog Neuropsychopharmacol Biol Psychiatry 1993;17:345–361.
59. Goodwin DW. Alcoholism and heredity. Arch Gen Psychiatry 1979;36:57–61.
60. Devor EJ, Cloninger CR. Genetics of alcoholism. Ann Rev Genet 1989;23:19–36.
61. Cadoret RJ, Cain CA, Grove WM. Development of alcoholism in adoptees raised apart from alcoholic biologic relatives. Arch Gen Psychiatry 1980;37:561–563.
62. Cloninger CR, Bohman M, Sigvardsson S. Inheritance of alcohol abuse: Cross-fostering analysis of adopted men. Arch Gen Psychiatry 1981;38:861–868.
63. Bohman M, Sigvardsson S, Cloninger CR. Maternal inheritance of alcohol abuse: Cross-fostering analysis of adopted women. Arch Gen Psychiatry 1981;38:965–969.
64. Goodwin DW. Alcoholism and genetics. Arch Gen Psychiatry 1985;42:171–174.
65. Cloninger CR. Neurogenetic adaptive mechanisms in alcoholism. Science 1987;236:410–416.
66. Begleiter H, Porjesz B, Bihari B, Kissin B. Event-related brain potentials in boys at risk for alcoholism. Science 1984;225:1493–1496.
67. Ehlers CL, Schuckit MA. EEG response to ethanol in sons of alcoholics. Psychopharmacol Bull 1988;24:434–437.
68. Hoffman EJ, Warren EW. Flumazenil: A benzodiazepine antagonist. Clin Pharm 1993;12:641–656.
69. Jaffe JH, Martin WR. Opioid analgesics and antagonists, in Gilman AG, Rall TW, Nies AS, Taylor P, (eds): The Pharmacological Basis of Therapeutics, 8th ed. New York, Pergamon, 1990, p 485.
70. Guthrie KS. The treatment of alcohol withdrawal. Pharmacotherapy 1989;9:131–143.
71. Gallant D. Alcohol, in Galanter M, Kleber HD, ed. Textbook of Substance Abuse Treatment. Washington, DC, American Psychiatric Press, 1994, p 67.
72. Hillestad L, Hansen T, Melsom H, Drivenes A. Diazepam metabolism in normal man. I. Serum concentrations and clinical effects after intravenous, intramuscular, and oral administration. Clin Pharmacol Ther 1974;16:479–484.
73. Browne JL, Hauge KJ. A review of alprazolam withdrawal. Drug Intell Clin Pharm 1986;20:837–841.
74. Greenstein RA, Fudala PJ, O'Brien CP. Alternative pharmacotherapies for opiate addiction, in Lowinson JH, Ruiz P, Millman RB, Langrod JG (eds): Substance Abuse: A Comprehensive Textbook, 2nd ed. Baltimore, Williams & Wilkins, 1992, p 562.
75. Kleber HD. Opioids: detoxification, in Galanter M, Kleber HD (eds): Textbook of Substance Abuse Treatment. Washington, DC, American Psychiatric Press, 1994, p 191.
76. Strain EC, Stitzer ML, Liebson IA, Bigelow GE. Comparison of buprenorphine and methadone in the treatment of opioid dependence. Am J Psychiatry 1994;151:1025–1030.
77. Jarvik ME, Schneider NG. Nicotine, in Lowinson JH, Ruiz P, Millman RB, Langrod JG (eds): Substance Abuse: A Comprehensive Textbook, 2nd ed. Baltimore, Williams & Wilkins, 1992, p 334.
78. Galanter M, Talbott D, Gallegos K, Rubenstone E. Combined Alcoholics Anonymous and professional care for addicted physicians. Am J Psychiatry 1990;147:64–68.
79. O'Malley SS, Jaffe AJ, Chang G, et al. Naltrexone and coping skills therapy for alcohol dependence. Arch Gen Psychiatry 1992;49:881–887.
80. Volpicelli JR, Alterman AI, Hayashida M, O'Brien CP. Naltrexone in the treatment of alcohol dependence. Arch Gen Psychiatry 1992;49:876–880.
81. Volpicelli JR, Davis MA, Olgin JE. Naltrexone blocks the post-shock increase of ethanol consumption. Life Sci 1986;38:841–847.
82. Myers RD, Melchior CL. Alcohol drinking: Abnormal intake caused by tetrahydropapaveroline in brain. Science 1977;196:554–556.
83. Kosten TR, Kleber HD, Morgan C. Treatment of cocaine abuse with buprenorphine. Biol Psychiatry 1989;26:637–639.
84. Miller FT, Tenebaun JH. Drug abuse in schizophrenia. Hosp Community Psychiatry 1989;40:847–849.
85. Sanguineti VR, Samuel SE. Comorbid substance abuse and recovery from acute psychiatric relapse. Hosp Community Psychiatry 1993;44:1073–1076.
86. Weiss RD, Mirin SM, Griffin ML. Methodological considerations in the diagnosis of coexisting psychiatric disorders in substance abusers. Br J Addiction 1992;87:179–187.
87. Raskin VD, Miller NS. The epidemiology of the comorbidity of psychiatric and addictive disorders: A critical review. J Addict Dis 1993;12:45–57.
88. Walker R. Substance abuse and B-cluster disorders. I: Understanding the dual diagnosis patient. J Psychoactive Drugs 1992;24:223–232.

Chapter 66

Schizophrenia

M. Lynn Crismon, PharmD, FCCP, and Peter G. Dorson, PharmD

Schizophrenia is one of the most complex and challenging of psychiatric disorders. It represents a heterogeneous syndrome of disorganized and bizarre thoughts, delusions, hallucinations, inappropriate affect, and impaired psychosocial functioning. From the time that Kraepelin first described dementia praecox in 1896 until the *Diagnostic and Statistical Manual of Mental Disorders, 4th ed.* (DSM-IV) in 1994,[1] the description of this illness has continued to evolve. With technological advances increasing our abilities to understand central nervous system (CNS) physiology and pathophysiology, this will likely continue in the future.

Epidemiology

Depending on the criteria used in studies, the worldwide prevalence of schizophrenia is between 0.2–2% of the population, with the actual lifetime prevalence probably being close to 1%. With only a few possible exceptions, the prevalence of schizophrenia appears remarkably similar among all cultures. Schizophrenia most commonly has its onset in late adolescence or early adulthood and rarely occurs before adolescence or after the age of 40. Although the prevalence of schizophrenia is equal in males and females, the onset of illness tends to be earlier in males. Males typically have the first hospitalization between 15 and 24 years of age, whereas females usually experience their first admission between 25 and 34 years.[1,2]

Pathophysiology

During the past 30 years, the most common pathophysiologic theories associated with the etiology of schizophrenia have involved the dopaminergic (DAergic) system. Since the discovery of dopamine's (DA) role as a neurotransmitter in 1958 and the observations that antipsychotic (AP) drugs are postsynaptic DA receptor antagonists, there has been interest in a DAergic hypothesis for the pathophysiology of schizophrenia. However, these theories are more appropriately oriented toward the etiology of psychosis than the disease schizophrenia itself.

There are four DAergic tracts of primary interest (Table 66.1). The extrapyramidal tract originates with cell bodies from the A9 area in the substantia nigra, and their axons terminate with synapses in the caudate nucleus and putamen of the basal ganglia. The second tract, the mesolimbic pathway, projects from A10 in the midbrain ventral tegmentum to the cingulate gyrus and to limbic regions such as the amygdala, olfactory tubercle, and septal nuclei. The mesocortical tract extends from A10 to the prefrontal and frontal cortex. The tuberoinfundibular tract projects from the hypothalamus to the pituitary. Each is thought to have a functional correlate that relates to its anatomic projections (Table 66.1). A basic knowledge of these anatomic/functional relationships is important to understanding the therapeutic and adverse effects of both typical and atypical AP drugs.[3]

Data on DA metabolism in schizophrenic patients have yielded inconsistent results. Homovanillic acid (HVA) is a metabolite of dopamine. HVA concentrations in the cerebrospinal fluid (CSF) are thought to reflect DAergic turnover in the synapse (and, therefore, HVA formation). A hyperactive DA system should result in increased DA release from the presynaptic terminal and increased metabolite formation. However, HVA concentrations are not increased in most chronic schizophrenics, and a subgroup of schizophrenics appears to have decreased CSF HVA. This subgroup of patients may have a more chronic, degenerative disease process that is refractory to AP drug therapy. In these same schizophrenic patients, an increase in CSF HVA, reflecting increased DA turnover, is observed during acute psychotic episodes.[4]

Increasing evidence supports a hypothesis that a DA receptor defect may exist in schizophrenia. Numerous positron emission tomography (PET) studies, measuring glucose metabolism, have shown regional brain abnormalities, especially increased glucose metabolism in the caudate

TABLE 66.1. DOPAMINERGIC TRACTS AND EFFECTS OF ANTIPSYCHOTICS

Dopamine Tract	Origin	Innervation	Function	Antipsychotic Drug Effect
Nigrostriatal	Substantia nigra (A9 area)	Caudate nucleus Putamen	Extrapyramidal system—movement	Movement disorders
Mesolimbic	Midbrain ventral tegmentum (A10 area)	Limbic areas (e.g., amygdala, olfactory tubercle, septal nuclei), Cingulate gyrus	Arousal, memory, stimulus processing, motivational behavior, etc.	Relief of psychosis
Mesocortical	Midbrain ventral tegmentum (A10 area)	Frontal and prefrontal lobe cortex	Cognition, communication, social function, response to stress, etc.	Relief of psychosis Akathisia?
Tuberoinfundibular	Hypothalamus	Pituitary gland	Regulates prolactin release	Increased prolactin concentrations

nucleus. However, other data suggest that blood flow and glucose metabolism in the frontal lobe and left temporal lobe are decreased.[2,4] This may indicate DAergic hyperactivity in the head of the caudate nucleus and DAergic hypofunction in the frontotemporal regions. PET studies utilizing D_2-specific ligands, such as raclopride, provide information regarding receptor density studies in schizophrenia. These data suggest increased densities of D_2 receptors in the head of the caudate nucleus with decreased densities in the prefrontal cortex.[3] One study has also shown an increased density of D_4 receptors in the dorsal striatum.[5] PET studies assessing D_1 function suggest that subpopulations of schizophrenics may have decreased densities of D_1 receptors in the caudate nucleus and the prefrontal cortex. Additional evidence for prefrontal lobe hypoactivity is provided by computerized electroencephalogram (EEG) (brain mapping) studies that show an increase in prefrontal lobe slow wave activity in schizophrenic brains. Hypofrontality may be associated with lack of volition, one of the core symptoms seen in schizophrenia.[2,6] It is important to emphasize that it is unknown whether these changes represent a primary event or whether they are merely compensatory changes secondary to other pathophysiologic abnormalities in schizophrenia. Because of the heterogeneity in the clinical presentation of schizophrenia, it has also been suggested that the DA hypothesis may be more applicable in "neuroleptic-responsive psychosis," with other abnormalities being primarily responsible in treatment-resistant patients.[4]

Attempts have been made to develop relationships between these abnormal findings and behavioral symptoms present in schizophrenic patients. The positive symptoms are possibly more closely associated with receptor hyperactivity in the mesocaudate, whereas negative symptoms are most closely related to DA receptor hypofunction in the prefrontal cortex.

The potential for phospholipid abnormalities has been investigated in schizophrenia. Of particular interest, phosphoinositide (PI) serves as a second messenger system for the D_2 receptor, and D_2 stimulation decreases PI turnover. It has been suggested that this may be the mechanism through which chronic neuroleptic treatment may produce modification of D_2 receptor mediated transduction.[4]

A dysregulation hypothesis has been invoked to explain the divergent findings in biochemical and receptor studies.[3,7] The dysregulation hypothesis maintains that aberrant homeostatic control mechanisms cause erratic neurotransmission; that is, the homeostatic mechanisms that control the relationships among neurotransmitter synthesis, release, reuptake, metabolism, activity at receptors, and second messenger systems are defective. This lack of homeostasis can be pictured as having dysfunction in several different processes, including basal neurotransmission, biological rhythm, and return to the basal rate after perturbations on the system. One hypothesis is that a primary problem exists with presynaptic release of DA from the neuron and ineffective feedback mechanisms. This may lead to postsynaptic DA receptor hypersensitivity. This is reflected by the decreased DA turnover and increased D_2 density seen in several studies. During acute psychotic exacerbations, DA turnover may increase, perhaps even returning to normal.[7]

Other neurotransmitter systems have been implicated in schizophrenia. Serotonergic receptors are present on DAergic axons, and it is known that stimulation of these receptors will decrease DA release, at least in the striatum.[3] Although somewhat more diffuse, the distribution of serotonergic neurons is similar to that of dopaminergic neurons, thus allowing interaction between these two neurotransmitter systems. Increased peripheral serotonin concentrations have been found in schizophrenics in some studies, and atypical antipsychotics such as clozapine and risperidone are potent serotonin-2 (5-HT_2) receptor antagonists. These types of drugs have also been shown to reverse worsening of symptomatology induced by serotonin agonists in schizophrenic patients.[4] Increased concentrations of norepinephrine have been observed in limbic structures of patients with chronic paranoid schizophrenia, but not in patients with other subtypes.[4] The relationship of these neurotransmitters to the function of the limbic filtering system is unclear. However, it is possible that they have important functions in modulating the corticostriatal loop, thus modulating limbic input.

A role for glutamatergic neuron involvement in the pathophysiology of schizophrenia has been advocated. Dopaminergic innervations from the ventral striatum decrease the limbic system's inhibitory activity, thus DAergic stimulation increases arousal. The corticostriatal glutamate pathways have the opposite effect, inhibiting DAergic function from the ventral striatum, therefore, allowing the limbic system to have increased inhibitory activity. It is not known whether glutamate pathways impinge directly on dopaminergic neurons or act through GABA interneurons. Glutamatergic deficiency produces symptoms similar to those with DAergic hyperactivity and possibly those seen in schizophrenia. Clinical support for this hypothesis comes from the fact that phencyclidine, a potent psychotomimetic, is a noncompetitive antagonist at the NMDA receptor, a major glutamate receptor. It is proposed that schizophrenia may involve an imbalance in activity between DAergic and glutamatergic neurons, with a relative deficiency of glutamatergic activity being at least partially responsible for psychotic symptomatology.[8]

Schizophrenia is a complex syndrome, and multiple etiologies may exist, producing similar clinical phenotypes. Based on current knowledge, it is naive to think that any one etiology can adequately explain the genesis of this complex disease. In particular, it should not be assumed that because dopaminolytic drugs are effective in decreasing psychotic symptoms or even because abnormalities in DAergic function exist in schizophrenia that this is proof that a DAergic abnormality is the sole or even the primary dysfunction in the illness.

Computerized axial tomography (CAT) scans and magnetic resonance imaging (MRI) show increased ventricular size, particularly in the third and lateral ventricles, in subtypes of schizophrenics. Recent studies also show a small but definite decrease in brain size as compared with matched controls. These changes appear to be consistent with brain asymmetry, the ventricular enlargement being most pronounced in the left temporal horn, and the decreased cortical thickness being most obvious in the left temporal lobe.[9] Although results are inconsistent, some studies report that patients with enlarged ventricles are more likely to demonstrate abnormal findings on neuropsychologic testing. Patients with enlarged ventricles may respond more poorly to AP medications. Consistent with PET studies showing decreased metabolism, there is also evidence indicating decreased left temporal lobe size in schizophrenia.[9]

Although a specific abnormality has not been discovered, increasing evidence suggests a genetic basis for schizophrenia. Although the risk of developing schizophrenia is 0.5–1.5% in the general population, this increases to approximately 10% if a first-degree relative has the illness and 3% for second-degree relatives.[1,2,10] If both parents have schizophrenia, the risk of producing a schizophrenic offspring increases to approximately 40%. Twin studies in dizygotic twins report that the risk of the second twin developing schizophrenia if one twin has the illness is between 12–14%. However, in monozygotic twins the risk increases to 48%.[10] Numerous adoption studies indicate that the risk for schizophrenia lies with the biological parents, and change in the environment during the child's developmental stages does not alter this. If schizophrenia occurs in siblings, the onset of illness tends to occur at the same age in each, thus lessening the possibility of an environmental precipitant. The lack of a difference in incidence of schizophrenia among different cultures also weighs against a strong environmental influence.

A neurodevelopmental model has recently been evoked as a possible explanation for the etiology of schizophrenia. This model proposes that a genetic predisposition exists for schizophrenia and that an unknown *in utero* disturbance occurs, probably in the second trimester of pregnancy. Evidence for this is provided by the abnormal neuronal migration demonstrated in some studies of schizophrenic brains. This cortical maldevelopment is thought to lead to the development of abnormal brain circuits. The resulting secondary "synaptic disorganization" is thought not to produce clinical manifestations until adolescence or early adulthood because this is the corresponding time period of neuronal maturation. Additional support for a developmental model is provided by the fact that while studies have shown decreased brain mass and increased ventricular size in many schizophrenics, this occurs in the absence of gliosis. Gliosis, or the proliferation of glial cells, is thought to always occur as a compensatory change in degenerative diseases of the brain. Although this model for the etiology of schizophrenia is far from conclusive, it does provide a useful framework for additional research into the etiology of the disease.[11,12]

Antipsychotic Drug Mechanism of Action

AP medications are putative DAergic antagonists. Among the typical dopaminolytic compounds, although there are some differences in their affinities for D_1 and D_2 receptors, these differences do not appear to be clinically significant. During chronic treatment with these agents, between 70–89% of D_2 receptors in the striatum are usually occupied.[6] Shortly after beginning treatment with AP drugs, several compensatory processes begin to occur in the brain, particularly in the basal ganglia. These include an increase in metabolite formation, increased rate of DA synthesis, and increased rate of cell firing.[13] However, within 21 days of continuous treatment, depolarization block occurs, which is the term for the decreased release of DA or inactivation of DAergic neurons occurring with continuous treatment. With typical APs, depolarization block occurs in both A9 and A10 areas, with the exception of neurons projecting to the prefrontal or cingulate cortex. With at least some atypical APs, depolarization block appears to occur only in the A10 region.[3,14]

Multiple DA receptor subtypes exist, with D_1 and D_2 being the best studied. Even with these two subtypes, their functioning has not been adequately elucidated. D_1 receptors are at least partially responsible for AP activity, and may serve as a permissive or modulating receptor for extrapyramidal side effects (EPS). The D_2 receptor is also associated with AP efficacy; in fact, most studies with typical APs show a high correlation between D_2 blockade and AP efficacy. D_2 receptors also appear to be the primary receptor involved in the pathogenesis of EPS. However, some D_1 blockade appears to be necessary to produce EPS. D_3, D_4, and D_5 receptors have been isolated as well. D_4 and D_5 receptors appear to have significantly higher levels in frontal cortex and limbic areas than in the basal ganglia, whereas the distribution of D_3 appears more similar to D_2.[15–17]

DA receptors are subtyped by their effects on adenylate cyclase. D_1 and D_5 receptors are linked to adenylate cyclase and cause an activation of the adenylate cyclase, cAMP system. D_2 receptors, however, are either not linked to adenylate cyclase or agonists cause an inhibition of adenylate cyclase activity.[3] Available data suggest that the D_3 receptor may not be linked to adenylate cyclase.[16]

Autoreceptors are important in regulating DAergic function. Autoreceptors are thought to be D_2 receptors and are located on all parts of the DA neuron: at the axonal terminal, on the cell body, and the dendrites. Depending on location, DA autoreceptors have differing functions. Those on the presynaptic nerve terminal may be primarily involved with DA synthesis and/or release, whereas the somatodendritic autoreceptors are thought to regulate cell firing. Whereas autoreceptors regulating DA release are present on all DA neurons, autoreceptors regulating DA synthesis and cell firing are absent in those cells projecting to cortical structures. Their densities are also probably lower in limbic neurons than in striatal ones. These differences in autoreceptor distribution serve as one explanation for the development of tolerance to the acute-occurring EPS, but rarely to the AP therapeutic effects of typical APs. The D_3 receptor appears to be present in the limbic system as an autoreceptor as well as a postsynaptic receptor. The clinical implications of the D_3 autoreceptor are, as yet, poorly understood.[16]

Based on the binding affinities and clinical profiles of various APs, it may be necessary to have D_2 blockade and at least some D_1 antagonism to produce EPS, at least on a predictable basis.[3] For example, haloperidol (HPD) has high D_2 affinity, but some D_1 binding, and produces a high incidence of extrapyramidal reactions. Sulpiride and raclopride, both investigational highly specific D_2 antagonists, have a low incidence of EPS, and clozapine (CLZ), a relatively D_1 and D_4 specific drug, with high non-DA affinity, causes almost no EPS.[17]

Typical APs have effects on all four DAergic tracts (Table 66.1). However, because of differences in receptor subtypes, autoreceptors, and feedback loops in the various brain areas, there are distinct differences in the clinical effects of these drugs. This is important because the primary therapeutic effects of APs are thought to occur in the limbic system, including the ventral striatum, whereas the EPS are thought to be related to DA blockade in the dorsal striatum. Tolerance usually develops to the acutely occurring extrapyramidal effects within a few weeks, but tolerance to the AP effects would appear to be uncommon, if not rare. It is also noteworthy that tolerance develops to an AP drug-induced increase in DA turnover in the striatum and limbic system, but not in the prefrontal lobe cortex.[3] This latter finding is consistent with autoreceptor distribution and with depolarization block not being produced by APs in the prefrontal lobe. It may explain a relative lack of tolerance to the AP effects. In the tuberoinfundibular system, APs block prolactin inhibitory factor, which is DA, at D_2 sites. Tolerance does not appear to develop to this effect, even with long-term treatment.[13]

APs affect other neurotransmitter receptor systems. APs have effects on cholinergic, α_1-adrenergic, and histaminic receptors. As a rule, the lower potency APs (e.g., chlorpromazine [CPZ] and thioridazine [TRD]) are less specific for DA receptors and block other receptors as well.[18] These differences in affinity for nondopaminergic receptors are at least partially responsible for the varying side effect profiles among AP agents. This offers a rational explanation for the side effects, such as dry mouth, constipation, sinus tachycardia, and orthostatic hypotension, seen more commonly with the "low-potency" APs.

Atypical is the term applied to AP neuroleptics that produce little or no EPS, and potentially have clinical response patterns different than traditional APs. The atypical APs' exact mechanism of action is unknown, and it likely differs among drugs. It may be related to one or more of the following pharmacodynamic effects: relative D_1, D_4, or D_5 specificity; relative selectivity for limbic DAergic receptors; 5-HT_2, 5-HT_6, and 5-HT_7 antagonism; or α_1-adrenergic antagonism.[3,5,15,18] For example, CLZ has relative D_1 and D_4 selectivity and is an antagonist for 5-HT_2, 5-HT_6, and 5-HT_7 receptors. CLZ is also the only AP, at present, that has been shown to affect long-term responsivity and adaptation of prefrontal cortex neurons.[19] Risperidone has approximately equal affinity as an antagonist for D_2 and D_4 receptors and is a potent antagonist at 5-HT_2 receptors.[5,18] This has led some investigators to believe that the ratio between 5-HT_2 blockade and D_2 blockade is important in producing an atypical profile.

Risperidone causes EPS less often than typical APs, particularly at low to moderate doses. Risperidone, similar to clozapine, also appears to be more effective in improving negative symptoms than traditional APs. However, clozapine and risperidone do differ clinically. Clozapine produces a significantly lower incidence of EPS than risperidone, and clozapine does not elevate serum prolactin concentrations (through blocking D_2-mediated prolactin inhibitory factor) while risperidone does.[20]

Ironically, at one time a lack of specificity for DA receptors (particularly D_2) was considered a disadvantage for AP drugs because of the systemic side effects associated with blocking nondopaminergic receptors. However, the discovery that some atypical APs have an extremely low prevalence of EPS and perhaps more efficacy on negative symptoms has caused this position to be reexamined.

Pharmacokinetics

Absorption of AP drugs can be variable, depending on the specific agent and the dosage formulation. In particular, low-potency APs are prone to a large first-pass effect, secondary to both gut wall and hepatic metabolism, and the systemic bioavailability is significantly higher with the concentrate than with tablet formulations.[21] Peak plasma concentrations (Cps) after intramuscular CPZ administration may be four to ten times higher, and the area under the curve two to four times greater than after administration of an equivalent oral dose.[13] Among the APs, mean relative bioavailability between oral and intramuscular administration ranges from a low of 25% with CPZ to a high of 65% with HPD.[21]

The APs are highly lipophilic and highly bound to membranes and plasma proteins. They distribute readily into most tissues with a high blood supply and may accumulate in tissues; therefore, they have large volumes of distribution. APs are largely metabolized, primarily through microsomal enzyme processes in the liver. Primary pathways are oxidative, and depending on the drug, metabolites may be active or inactive. The specific hepatic isoenzymes responsible for metabolism has not been identified for most antipsychotics. APs have fairly long elimination half-lives, most in the range of 20–40 hours. Thus after dosage stabilization, most APs can be dosed once daily. APs exhibit multiple compartment pharmacokinetic models.[13,21] Because of tissue accumulation and a high degree of membrane binding, some drugs or metabolites may be slowly eliminated from the body over a prolonged period. AP metabolites in the urine may be detected for several months after drug discontinuation.

Efforts to develop relationships between AP Cps and clinical response have been hampered by several factors, including the variable lag time between beginning AP treatment and symptom change, the subjective and relatively imprecise methods of measuring symptom change in schizophrenia, the extremely low concentrations of drug present in plasma requiring sensitive analytical methodologies, and the presence of multiple metabolites. The most successful research assessing the relationship between AP Cps and response has been performed with HPD, fluphenazine (FPZ), and CLZ.

With HPD, the most well-controlled, fixed-dose studies suggest that the approximate therapeutic Cp range is between 5 and 12 ng/mL. A daily dosage of HPD HCl 10 mg usually results in a HPD Cp in this range in about 50% of patients. HPD may possess a curvilinear Cp response relationship, with less efficacy at Cps higher than the therapeutic range. It is uncertain whether this truly exists or whether patients' clinical presentation is worse at higher Cps because of increased side effects. Regardless, research indicates that the above proposed range maximizes the therapeutic relationship of efficacy and adverse effects.[22] An HPD metabolite, reduced HPD, may function as a partial antagonist and has been suggested to interfere with HPD's efficacy, particularly at higher reduced HPD concentrations. However, these data have been disputed. Most patients with high reduced HPD concentrations also have high HPD concentrations, and this may not be a significant factor in patients if HPD Cps are kept within the suggested therapeutic range.

Although the research with FPZ is not nearly as extensive, preliminary results suggest that the lower end of the FPZ therapeutic range is approximately 0.5 ng/mL.[23] As the Cp increases, efficacy may improve, but adverse effects worsen. The upper end of the suggested therapeutic range is approximately 3 ng/mL.

Two different studies have examined the relationship between clozapine plasma concentrations and clinical response in typical AP treatment refractory patients.[24,25] In both studies, a clozapine plasma concentration greater than approximately 350 ng/mL was associated with a significantly greater probability of efficacy. In one study, a daily dose of approximately 400 mg achieved a Cp ≥350 ng/mL in only 11 of 29 patients, indicating significant interindividual variation in clozapine pharmacokinetics.[24] This combined with the higher risk of seizures at clozapine doses greater than 600 mg daily suggests a possible role for the monitoring of clozapine plasma concentrations.

Recommendations for obtaining Cps with APs remain controversial. It is probably not cost effective to monitor AP Cps routinely in all patients. Cp monitoring should be considered in patients who do not respond to reasonable doses within a 6-week period, patients who develop unusual or severe adverse experiences, patients who are taking concomitant medications that may cause drug interactions, patients who have age or pathophysiologic changes suggesting a change in pharmacokinetics, and assessment of patient compliance. However, considering the interindividual variation in pharmacokinetics, lag time in therapeu-

TABLE 66.2. PHARMACOKINETIC PARAMETERS OF DEPOT ANTIPSYCHOTICS

Drug	t_{max} (days)	$t_{1/2}$ Single Dose (days)	$t_{1/2}$ Multiple Dose (days)	$t_{90\%}$ (weeks)
Fluphenazine enanthate	2–3	3.5–4	N/A[a]	3
Fluphenazine decanoate	0.3–2	6–10	14.3 ± 2.2	4–8
Haloperidol decanoate	4–11	N/A	3	12

[a]Indicates data not available.

tic response, severity of side effects, and cost of hospitalization, if laboratory results for HPD, FPZ, and CLZ plasma determinations can be obtained promptly and economically, a rational argument can be made for routine monitoring of these drugs. Data with other APs are sparse, and Cp monitoring is of little value on a routine basis.

The depot APs, FPZ decanoate (also available in an enanthate salt), and HPD decanoate are esterified APs formulated in sesame seed oil for deep intramuscular injection. Their absorption from the muscle and metabolism to the free base is sufficiently slow to cause absorption to be the rate-limiting step in determining their respective, apparent half-lives. Thus, their pharmacokinetics follow a flip-flop model. Table 66.2 lists comparative pharmacokinetic information for these drugs.[26]

The pharmacokinetics of the depot APs lend themselves to significant usefulness in the outpatient treatment of schizophrenia, where noncompliance with medications is a significant problem causing relapse. Patients may be dosed with FPZ decanoate on a 1- to 3-week interval, and with HPD decanoate usually once a month. Patients may come to the clinic for their injections or receive them at home from a visiting nurse. A study with FPZ decanoate reports a lower incidence of psychotic exacerbation at 6 and 12 months of treatment if patients' predose FPZ Cps are kept greater than 1 ng/mL. A dose of 25 mg IM every 2 weeks achieved a mean steady-state Cp of approximately 1.4 ng/mL. These results indicate that Cps may be useful in the long-term maintenance treatment of schizophrenia.[27]

Clinical Presentation, Diagnosis, and Prognosis

Schizophrenia is the most common functional psychosis, and its clinical presentation can be extremely varied. Despite numerous attempts to portray a stereotype in movies and on television, the stereotypic schizophrenic essentially does not exist. Moreover, schizophrenia does not mean "split personality." Schizophrenia is a chronic disorder of thought and affect with the individual having a significant disturbance in interpersonal relationships and the ability to function in society on a daily basis.

The first psychotic episode may be sudden in onset with few premorbid symptoms, or commonly may be preceded by withdrawn, suspicious, peculiar behavior (schizoid). During the acute psychotic episodes, the patient loses touch with reality, and, in a sense, the brain creates a false reality to replace it. The patient experiences a variety of acute psychotic symptoms, including hallucinations (especially hearing voices), delusions (fixed false beliefs), ideas of influence (actions controlled by external influences), and so on. These are sometimes called Schneiderian symptoms and are outlined in Table 66.3. Thought processes are disconnected (loose associations), the patient may not be able to carry on logical conversation, and may have simultaneous, contradictory thoughts (ambivalence). The patient's affect may be flat (no emotional expression), or it may be inappropriate and labile. The patient is often withdrawn and inwardly directed (autism). Uncooperativeness, hostility, and verbal or physical aggression may be seen because of the patient's misperception of reality. Self-care skills are impaired, and the patient is frequently dirty, unkempt, and, in general, has poor hygiene. Sleep and appetite are often disturbed.

When the acute psychotic episode remits, the patient typically has residual features. This is an important point in differentiating schizophrenia from other psychotic disorders. Although residual symptoms and their severity vary, patients may have difficulty with anxiety management, suspiciousness, and lack of volition, motivation, insight, and judgment. Therefore, they often have difficulty living independently in the community. Because of poor anxiety management and suspiciousness, they are frequently withdrawn socially, and have difficulty forming close relationships with others. Most do not marry. In addition, impaired voli-

TABLE 66.3. SCHNEIDER'S FIRST-RANK SYMPTOMS OF SCHIZOPHRENIA

- Complete hallucinations
  - Audible voices
  - Voices arguing
  - Voices commenting on one's behavior
- Somatic passivity
- Thought withdrawal
- Thought insertion
- Thought broadcasting
- Ego boundary disruptions
  - Experiences feelings not his or her own
  - Experiences powerful influence not his or her own, but actual performance of the act is his or hers
- Experiences actions under control of external influence
- Delusional perception

TABLE 66.4. DSM-IV DIAGNOSTIC CRITERIA FOR SCHIZOPHRENIA

A. Characteristic symptoms: Two or more of the following, each persisting for a significant portion of at least a 1-month period
   (1) delusions
   (2) hallucinations
   (3) disorganized speech
   (4) grossly disorganized or catatonic behavior
   (5) negative symptoms
   Note: Only one criterion A symptom required if delusions are bizarre or if hallucinations consist of a voice keeping a running commentary on the person's behavior or two or more voices conversing with each other.

B. Social/occupational dysfunction: For a significant portion of the time since onset of the disorder, one or more major areas of functioning such as work, interpersonal relations, or self-care are significantly below the level prior to onset.

C. Duration: Continuous signs of the disorder for at least 6 months. This must include at least 1 month of symptoms fulfilling criterion A (unless successfully treated). This 6 months may include prodromal or residual symptoms.

D. Schizoaffective or mood disorder has been excluded.

E. Disorder is not due to a medical disorder or substance use.

F. If a history of a pervasive developmental disorder is present, there must be symptoms of hallucinations or delusions present for at least 1 month.

tion and motivation contribute to poor self-care skills and make it difficult for the schizophrenic patient to maintain employment. Schizophrenics frequently experience a lack of historicity, or difficulty in learning from their experiences. They may repeatedly make the same mistakes in social conduct and situations requiring judgment. They have difficulty understanding the importance of treatment, including medications, in maintaining their ability to function in society. Therefore, they tend to discontinue medications and other treatments, and this increases the risk of relapse and rehospitalization.

Although the course of the illness is variable, the long-term prognosis for many schizophrenic patients is poor. The disease is marked by intermittent acute psychotic episodes and impaired psychosocial functioning between acute episodes. By the time they reach late life, some schizophrenics become "burned out," that is they cease to have acute psychotic episodes but residual symptoms, as previously described, usually persist. However, functional skills may actually improve as compared with earlier in the patient's life. Although AP drugs effectively treat the acute psychotic symptoms and aid in preventing relapse, they do not affect the impairment in psychosocial functioning seen with the disease. In a subpopulation of patients, probably 5–15%, psychotic symptoms are nearly continuous, and response to typical antipsychotics poor.[2]

DSM-IV places a greater emphasis on the chronicity of schizophrenia and negative symptoms than do previous editions. Schizophrenia is a chronic disorder, and the patient's history must be carefully assessed for dysfunction that has persisted for greater than 6 months. After their first episode, schizophrenics rarely have a level of adaptive functioning as high as before the onset of the disorder. The DSM-IV criteria are summarized in Table 66.4, and this reference should be consulted for a more detailed discussion of the differential diagnosis.[1]

DSM-IV classifies the symptoms of schizophrenia into two categories—positive and negative (Table 66.5). Utilizing positive and negative symptoms, numerous authors have attempted to construct subtypes of schizophrenia, and it has been suggested that symptom complexes may correlate with prognosis, cognitive functioning, structural abnormalities in the brain, and response to typical AP drugs (Table 66.6).[3] Negative symptoms may be more closely associated with prefrontal lobe dysfunction and positive symptoms with temporolimbic abnormalities. Many patients demonstrate both positive and negative symptoms. Andreasen and associates[28] found that patients with negative symptoms may have more antecedent cognitive dysfunction, poor premorbid adjustment, low level of educational achievement, and a poorer overall prognosis. However, they were unable to confirm results that patients with negative symptoms have increased ventricle : brain ratios.[28] Many patients present with different types of symptoms at different points in the course of their illness, and this is a potential conflicting variable in these types of studies.

General Treatment Guidelines

ASSESSMENT PRIOR TO TREATMENT

The importance of initial assessment for accurate diagnosis cannot be underestimated in a patient presenting with acute psychosis. A thorough mental status examination, physical and neurologic examination, a complete family and social history, and laboratory workup must be performed to exclude medical or substance-induced causes of psychosis, such as acute or chronic drug ingestion. Laboratory tests, biological markers, and commonly available brain imaging techniques do not assist in diagnosis or selection of med-

TABLE 66.5. POSITIVE AND NEGATIVE SYMPTOMS OF SCHIZOPHRENIA

Positive Symptoms	Negative Symptoms
Delusions	Alogia (poverty of speech)
Disorganized speech (association disturbance)	Avolition
Hallucinations	Affective flattening
Behavior disturbance (disorganized or catatonic)	Anhedonia
Illusions	Social isolation

(Compiled from Refs. 1 and 3.)

ication. A pretreatment patient workup should include the following areas of baseline studies: vital signs, complete blood count, electrolytes, hepatic function, renal function, cardiac function, thyroid function, and toxicology.

RELATIVE EFFICACY AND SAFETY

All typical APs are equal in efficacy when used in equipotent doses. Interindividual variation does occur between individual APs, such that a relatively responsive patient may not respond to each AP. Intraindividual variation has been described but the contributing factors, other than progression of disease state, have not been delineated. Selection of medication should be based on the need to avoid certain side effects in concurrent medical or psychiatric disorders. There are no differences in efficacy between low- and high-potency APs. High-potency drugs (e.g., HPD) are as effective in treating acute agitation as low-potency, highly sedating APs (e.g., CPZ) providing evidence of this category of medications' calming effect in the psychotic patient. Despite practice trends, no proof exists that agitation responds best to sedating drugs or that withdrawn patients respond best to nonsedating drugs.

Recent controlled trials suggest that atypical antipsychotics such as risperidone, have superior efficacy for the treatment of negative symptoms; the clinical relevance of these findings in the "average" antipsychotic-responsive patient remains to be determined. To date, no maintenance treatment studies have been performed with atypical agents to know if improved clinical outcomes, relapse rates, or cost-effectiveness will result from their widespread use.

Previous patient or family history of response to an AP is helpful in the selection of an agent. Traditional dosage equivalents (expressed in "CPZ equivalent dosages"—the equipotent dosage of any AP compared with 100 mg of CPZ) may assist in determining the range of effective dosage when the need arises to treat a patient with another AP drug. However, dosage equivalents were obtained in early studies based on the blinded prescribing of investigators using empiric dosing. Despite the possibility of numerical imprecision, they provide a fairly accurate yardstick by

TABLE 66.6. FEATURES OF SCHIZOPHRENIC SUBTYPES BASED ON THE POSITIVE AND NEGATIVE MODELS

Characteristic	Syndrome Type I (Good Prognosis)	Syndrome Type II (Poor Prognosis)
Premorbid adjustment	Good	Poor
Precipitating factors	Present	Not obvious
Onset	Abrupt (<6 months)	Insidious
Family history of schizophrenia	Less frequent	More frequent
Family history of affective disorder	More frequent	Less frequent
Sensorium	Dream-like or "spacy"	Clear
Symptoms	Predominance of positive symptoms	Predominance of negative symptoms
Outcome of treatment	Potentially reversible	More chronic course
Intellectual impairment dysfunction	Absent	Neurocognitive
Postulated pathophysiology	D_2 overactivity	D_2 hypoactivity (?), cell loss in prefrontal cortex and temporal lobes
Ventricle: brain ratio	Normal	Increased
Response to antipsychotics	Marked to moderate	Variable response
Response to clozapine	Marked to moderate	Marked to moderate
Response to dopamine agonists and stimulants	Exacerbation common	Little effect or symptoms are improved
Importance of dopamine dysfunction	Highly important	Possibly implicated

which to measure the adequacy of different treatments and dosages of AP drugs.

APs, as listed in Table 66.7, are a relatively safe class of medications when used in normal therapeutic doses. Physicians are usually familiar with one drug from every major subgroup. However, monitoring patients who are being treated by a variety of practitioners, each with different treatment philosophies, requires that the pharmacist be familiar with all commonly used APs.

EVALUATION OF THERAPEUTIC OUTCOMES

A pharmacotherapeutic treatment plan should be developed that delineates drug-related aspects of therapy. Explicit endpoints should be defined, including realistic goals of the target symptoms most likely to respond and the relative time course for response. Other goals include avoiding unwanted side effects, using the minimum effective dose, an emphasis on time as the primary determinant of response (outweighing dosage), and the limitation of adjunctive medications to severely ill or nonresponsive patients. Assessment of response has traditionally been done subjectively or empirically (a relative sense of how the assessor feels the patient is doing). A formal mental status examination (MSE) is used to structure the patient interview and focus on items related to appearance, mood, sensorium, intellectual functioning, and thought processes. However, the MSE is not specific for the measurement of drug response. Realistically, clinicians should be trained to use standardized psychiatric rating scales to assist in objectively rating patients' drug responses.[29] The Brief Psychiatric Rating Scale (BPRS), although not specific for schizophrenia or any other illness, is accepted by the Food and Drug Administration (FDA) as the primary instrument to determine AP drug efficacy in phase II and III clinical trials. Other scales (such as the Comprehensive Psychiatric Rating Scale, Positive and Negative Syndrome Scale) are also available but less commonly used or not validated in this population. Objectively, the use of a numeric indicator (e.g., 20% reduction in BPRS score) can be used to quantify overall symptom reduction. However, individual symptoms considered socially disabling, such as fixed delusions or unusual posturing, which do not improve,

TABLE 66.7. AVAILABLE ANTIPSYCHOTICS: DOSES AND DOSAGE FORMS

Generic Name	Trade Name	Manufacturer	Traditional Equivalent Dose (mg)	Dosage Range (mg/d)	Geriatric Maximum Dose (mg/d)	Dosage Forms[a]
Aliphatic Phenothiazines						
Chlorpromazine	Thorazine, others	SmithKline Beecham	100	60–2000	800	T,L,LC,I,C-ER,S
Piperazine Phenothiazines						
Fluphenazine	Prolixin, Permitil	Princeton, Schering	2	2–40	20	T,L,LC,I
Perphenazine	Trilafon	Schering	10	8–64	32	T,LC,I
Trifluoperazine	Stelazine, others	SmithKline Beecham	5	2–80	40	T,LC,I
Piperidine Phenothiazines						
Mesoridazine	Serentil	Boehringer Ingelheim	50	50–500	250	T,LC,I
Thioridazine	Mellaril	Sandoz	100	50–800	400	T,LC
Thioxanthenes						
Chlorprothixene	Taractan	Roche	100	100–1600	800	T,LC,I
Thiothixene	Navane	Roerig	4	5–60	30	C,LC,I
Butyrophenone						
Haloperidol	Haldol, others	McNeil	2	1–100	50	T,LC,I
Dibenzoxapine						
Clozapine	Clozaril	Sandoz	50	75–900	NL[b]	T
Loxapine	Loxitane	Lederle, others	10	20–250	125	C,LC,I
Dihydroindolone						
Molindone	Moban	Du Pont	10	15–225	112	T,LC
Benzisoxazole						
Risperidone	Risperdal	Janssen	ND[c]	2–16	8	T

[a]T, tablet; C, capsule; ER or SR, extended or sustained release; I, injection; L, liquid solution, elixir, or suspension; LC, liquid concentrate; R, rectal suppositories; S, syrup.
[b]NL, not listed.
[c]ND, no data available.

may become the focus of treatment despite an overall rating scale improvement.

Similarly, the pharmacotherapeutic plan should include specific monitoring parameters for potential side effects. The plan should include the side effects to be monitored (e.g., EPS), how the potential side effect will be monitored (e.g., observation, Simpson Angus scale) and the frequency of assessment (e.g., daily, weekly).

PREDICTORS OF RESPONSE

The patient's medication history is critical in determining his or her treatment. Previous AP treatment should help guide the selection of future drug therapy, in that either a good response will favor the use of the same agent, or a negative response should influence the selection of a dissimilar drug. Nonprescription and illicit drug use may influence psychiatric presentation and, thus, diagnosis or AP response. Amphetamine and other CNS stimulants, cocaine, corticosteroids, digitalis glycosides, indomethacin, marijuana, pentazocine, phencyclidine, and other drugs can induce psychosis in susceptible individuals or exacerbate psychosis in patients with preexisting psychiatric illness.[30] Schizophrenic patients who continue to abuse alcohol or drugs usually have poor response to medications. Alcohol, caffeine, and nicotine use potentially result in drug interactions.

Individual differences in patient response have been either proposed or identified, which may be clinically useful predictors of response.[31] Lower socioeconomic status is associated with poor response, but may be a reflection of access to care or compliance. Acute onset and short duration of illness, presence of acute stressors or precipitating factors, later age of onset, family history of affective illness, and good premorbid adjustment as reflected in stable interpersonal relationships or employment are predictors of good response in a schizophrenic's social history.[31]

Negative schizophrenic symptoms are less responsive to AP therapy. Although controversial, affective symptoms may correlate with good response. However, other than these caveats, there are little data to support a relationship between drug response and schizophrenic subtypes. Neuropsychologic deficits related to cognition and neurologic soft signs may correlate with poor AP response.[31]

A patient's subjective response within the first 48 hours after being administered an AP may be associated with drug responsiveness.[32] A dysphoric response, demonstrated by stating a dislike of the medication, feeling worse or zombie-like, combined with anxiety or akathisia-like symptoms results in poor drug response, and if continued on the same medication, the patient will likely be noncompliant.

The importance of developing a therapeutic alliance between the patient and the clinician cannot be underestimated. Patients who form good alliances are more likely to be compliant with all aspects of therapy, experience a better outcome at 2 years, and generally require smaller doses of AP medications.[33]

A certain minority of patients fail to benefit from AP therapy, and their psychosocial functioning may actually worsen. Unfortunately, there is no accepted method to identify these people before treatment.[31]

INITIAL TREATMENT

Initial dosing should follow goals described in the pharmacotherapeutic treatment plan. The goals during the first 7 days should be decreased agitation, hostility, combativeness, anxiety, tension, aggression, and normalization of sleep and eating patterns. The usual recommendation is to initiate therapy with 400 to 600 CPZ equivalents unless the patient's physiologic status or history indicates that this dose may result in unacceptable adverse effects.

Low-dose strategies, including so-called threshold doses, have been recently reviewed.[22] The dosage of AP was titrated until mild, subclinical rigidity was physically detected, the dosage slightly lowered, and that dosage maintained for the remainder of the study, at which time a majority of patients responded to a mean haloperidol dose of 2.1 mg daily for drug naive patients and 4.3 mg daily for previously treated patients.

Although some practitioners believe that larger daily doses are necessary in more severely symptomatic patients, fixed-dose studies of low versus high daily doses do not reveal any major differences in time to response or length of hospitalization.[22,34] Randomized comparisons of HPD 5, 10, or 20 mg/d, FPZ 10, 20, or 30 mg/d, and HPD 10, 30, or 80 mg/d demonstrate little difference in efficacy based on dose. Some symptoms, such as agitation, tension, aggression, and increased motor activity, may respond more quickly. However, side effects, especially EPS, may be more common with higher doses, as well.

High doses or megadoses are used in theory to produce a faster response or as an intervention in poorly responding patients. A popular assumption has been that nonresponsive patients have low Cps of APs due to poor systemic availability or rapid metabolism. However, these theories have not been scientifically validated, and most of the literature with megadoses is anecdotal. Studies with doses upward of CPZ 5 g or FPZ 1200 mg daily show no greater and sometimes lesser efficacy when compared with standard doses, whereas other large dose studies report symptom worsening.[22] Currently, the use of megadoses cannot be advocated unless low plasma concentrations indicate the need for higher doses.

Rapid neuroleptization is the administration of repeated doses of a high-potency AP (e.g., HPD 5 mg IM) every 30–60 minutes over a period of less than 24 hours. The goal is to obtain a rapid calming effect (not sedation) in severely agitated patients. Agitation can be manifested by loud, physically or verbally threatening behavior, motor hyperactivity, or physical aggression. Although this technique may assist in calming an acutely agitated, psychotic patient, it does not improve the extent of or time to remission or the length of hospitalization.

Adjunctive benzodiazepines absorbed rapidly after intramuscular administration (e.g., lorazepam) are equivalent to intramuscular APs in the management of acute agitation or aggression. If the patient is receiving a reasonable daily dose of an AP (as previously described), the use of lorazepam 2 mg IM as needed in combination with the maintenance antipsychotic may actually be more effective in controlling agitation than using additional doses of the antipsychotic. In addition, it may assist in decreasing the overall incidence of side effects in the patient, especially acute EPS.

After the first week of therapy, a modest increase in dosage may be considered if the goals of treatment for that time period have not been met (i.e., decreased agitation and uncooperativeness). If "cheeking" of medication is suspected, liquid formulations of most APs are available (see Table 66.7).

STABILIZATION OF THERAPY

Improvement is usually a slow but steady and gradual process over 6–8 weeks or longer. During the first 2 weeks, goals should include increased socialization and improvement in self-care habits and mood. Improvement in formal thought (i.e., Schneiderian symptoms) should follow and may take an additional 6–8 weeks to respond. However, therapeutic onset and time course of AP effects are based mostly on clinicians' impressions and experience, not on placebo-controlled trials.

Most clinicians feel that the dose necessary to bring about response in the acute phase of illness is approximately two times the dose needed for maintenance treatment. The older literature recommends that the average patient will require a dosage of 500–800 mg of CPZ equivalents daily for the acute stabilization phase. An optimum dose of the chosen drug should be predetermined in the initial treatment plan. If the patient begins to show adequate response before or at this dosage, then typically the patient should remain at this dosage as long as symptoms continue to improve. If necessary, dose titration may continue every week or two as long as the patient has no side effects. Titration should not continue until the patient can no longer tolerate side effects. During this stage in treatment, most patients can also be switched to once-daily dosing, which can positively affect compliance, cost, and incidence of certain side effects.

An adequate trial to evaluate clinical response is at least 6 weeks of treatment with an AP dose of 800 mg CPZ equivalents. However, a fixed-dose study indicated that 50% of patients nonresponsive at 6 weeks of treatment responded by 12 weeks when continued on the same dose of FPZ.[35] If response is not considered satisfactory after 6 to 12 weeks, other considerations are necessary before a change in AP is made. When faced with a poorly responsive patient, the clinician should ask the following questions: Would an AP Cp be helpful? Were the initial target symptoms indicative of psychosis or did they represent manifestations of a long-standing behavioral problem? Are the symptoms unresponsive to AP drugs (e.g., impaired insight or judgment, or fixed delusions)? How does the patient's current status compare with response during previous hospitalizations? Would this patient potentially benefit from a change to an AP of a different chemical class? Does this patient qualify as a refractory schizophrenic patient? However, treatment goals must be realistic. Medications are effective at decreasing some of the symptoms of schizophrenia (and are thus referred to as *palliative*), but they are not curative, and all symptoms may not abate.

MAINTENANCE THERAPY

Maintenance drug therapy prevents relapse, as shown in numerous double-blind studies. The average relapse rate after 1 year is 20% with active drug (including some noncompliant patients) versus 60–80% for placebo.[36]

Targeted medication administration has been recommended as an alternative to continuous AP treatment in stabilized patients.[37] The rationale for this technique is to (1) decrease lifetime exposure to APs and subsequently long-term side effects, (2) address the concept that APs treat the illness only during an exacerbation of acute symptoms, otherwise acting prophylactically, and (3) minimize the potential for worsening negative schizophrenic symptoms and psychosocial function. AP medication is reintroduced based on the appearance of prodromal symptoms (greater degrees of tension, difficulty in sleep or concentration, anxiety) that can be seen immediately before relapse. These symptoms can often be recognized by both the patient, family, and clinician. However, studies have shown continuous medication to be more effective than targeted medication in preventing decompensation and decreasing need for hospitalization, and improving the extent and quality of employment. The effectiveness of targeted medication treatment is enhanced in a patient who has insight and in the context of a supportive environment.

Based on the available literature, after the treatment of the first psychotic episode in a schizophrenic patient, medication should be continued for not less than 12 months after remission.[38] Maintenance treatment in patients with multiple acute episodes is more difficult to define. However, it would appear that good medication responders should be treated for at least 5 years, then low-dose strategies or complete drug withdrawal should be attempted to determine the need for continued treatment.

Antipsychotics should be tapered slowly before discontinuation. Abrupt discontinuation of APs, especially low-potency agents, can occasionally result in withdrawal symptoms, felt to be a manifestation of rebound cholinergic outflow. Insomnia, nightmares, headaches, gastrointestinal (GI) symptoms (such as abdominal cramps, stomach pain, nausea, vomiting, and diarrhea), restlessness, increased salivation, and sweating are reported.

METHODS TO ENHANCE PATIENT COMPLIANCE

The chronic mentally ill may be noncompliant with medications based on denial of illness, lack of insight, grandiosity or paranoia, no perceived need for medication, perceived lack of input into choice of medication or dosage, side effects, misperceived "allergies," or the number of medications prescribed or doses received daily.[39] Education geared toward patients becoming more informed about the effectiveness and risks of treatment may help increase compliance. Self-medication administration in the hospital helps reinforce the patient's perception of their active role in their own treatment. Psychosocial programming and the involvement of family members encourages patients to monitor their responses to medication and become more active in reporting their success in attaining treatment goals.

Depot APs are recommended for patients who are unreliable in taking oral medication on a daily basis. However, the patient's motivation is still a major factor influencing outcome. Conversion from oral therapy to depot therapy is most successful in patients who have been stabilized first on oral therapy. Most clinicians recommend the first dose of depot medication be administered immediately before hospital discharge. The ideal patient for depot therapy is the patient who does not like the daily reminder of oral medication or is unreliable in taking medications. Depot medications should not be used as "forced compliance" in uncooperative patients who refuse to consent to treatment.

Guidelines for the conversion from oral antipsychotics to their respective depot formulation are outlined. Although it has not been well studied, deviation from these protocols may result in poor outcome, adverse effects, or increased hospitalization. The primary principles are stabilization on an oral dosage form of the same agent, or at least a short trial (3–7 days) to determine if the patient tolerates the medication without significant side effects; use of an appropriate conversion factor, taking into account whether the patient is still acutely ill or relatively stable; and overlap with the oral agent until adequate Cps can be achieved with the depot agent alone. For fluphenazine, the simplest conversion is the Stimmel method, which uses 1.2 times the oral daily dose for stabilized patients, rounding up to the nearest 12.5-mg interval, administered in weekly doses for the first 4–6 weeks; or 1.6 times the oral daily dose for more acutely ill patients.[26] Subsequently, fluphenazine decanoate may be administered once every 2–3 weeks. Oral fluphenazine may be overlapped for 1 week. For haloperidol, a factor of 10–15 times the oral daily dose is commonly recommended, rounding up to the nearest 50-mg interval, administered in a once-monthly dose with oral haloperidol overlap for the first month. However, this may be inadequate in more acutely ill patients. Ereshefsky et al.[40] performed an inpatient conversion study using the standard conversion from European trials (20 times the oral daily dose), but dividing the injection into consecutive doses of 100–200 mg every 3–7 days until the entire amount was given. With this method, oral medication overlap was not necessary. The depot dose was decreased by 25% at the second and third months. The method was as safe as other methods, and had a lower relapse rate than the most commonly recommended guidelines.

Injection site reactions have been reported with HPD decanoate, consisting of painful pruritic swelling at the injection site when the 100 mg/mL preparation is used.[41] Acute EPS can be seen following injections with FPZ decanoate. Despite the fear of severe or persistent side effects occurring during depot therapy, research indicates that similar depot and oral doses result in a similar incidence of side effects. These issues are also less relevant if patients are stabilized on oral medication before conversion to an appropriate depot dose.

Depot APs should be administered by a deep, "Z-tract" intramuscular method, although there is some evidence that FPZ decanoate can be administered subcutaneously with similar results. Using anticholinergics (AChs) routinely upon administration of a depot AP should be reserved for patients who consistently experience EPS around the time of their injections.

MANAGEMENT OF THE REFRACTORY PATIENT

As mentioned earlier, somewhere between 10–30% of schizophrenic patients receive minimal therapeutic response with APs.[20,22] An additional group of patients either receives less than optimal response or has unacceptable side effects associated with AP use. This has lead to attempts to develop new approaches for the treatment of the disease.

ATYPICAL ANTIPSYCHOTICS

There is no universally accepted definition for atypical AP. Common to all definitions, however, is the ability of the drug to produce antipsychotic response with little or no acutely occurring EPS. Other attributes that have been ascribed to atypical APs include enhanced efficacy, particularly on negative symptoms; absence of TD; and lack of effect on serum PRL. To date the only approved atypical AP that fulfills all of these criteria is clozapine, the prototypical drug.[20]

In the classic study evaluating drug efficacy in refractory schizophrenia,[42] CLZ was effective in approximately 32% of refractory schizophrenic patients as compared with only 2% treated with a combination of CPZ and benztropine. Rating-scale scores suggest that CLZ may be more effective against negative symptoms than typical APs. However, it is unclear whether this clinical improvement represents a true superior efficacy against negative symptoms or the absence of extrapyramidal effects that often blunt the patient's appearance and affective responses.[43]

This study is considered a "classic" because not only did it prove the efficacy of CLZ in this population, but it also provided a definition for refractory schizophrenia. This definition includes treatment failures on three different APs from at least two different chemical classes and a history of poor social functioning for the past 5 years.[42] It is significant that when using these criteria for treatment-resistant patients, almost no patients improved with a trial of HPD or CPZ. These criteria have been subsequently modified to require only two treatment failures. Other treatment candidates for CLZ include those patients who are neuroleptic intolerant and cannot tolerate even conservative doses of typical APs.[20]

To minimize orthostasis and sedation, a clozapine test dose of 12.5–25 mg should be given, followed by slow titration until a daily dose of 300–450 mg is reached. If inadequate response is obtained after 6 weeks of treatment, then further titration may occur. However, many of CLZ's side effects are dose related, and patients receiving greater than 600 mg daily must be carefully monitored.

Response with CLZ in the refractory patient may occur more slowly in many patients. As many as 60% of treatment refractory patients may improve if CLZ is used for longer time periods; Meltzer recommends individual patient trials of at least 6 months.[20] Cost-effectiveness studies have shown that clozapine use is associated with a decrease in total patient care costs of nearly $10,000 per patient annually.[20] Although the response in CLZ-treated patients is significant, these treatment refractory patients usually experience a moderate response at best, not a complete remission of the disorder. This in combination with clozapine's adverse effects profile provides sufficient information to conclude that CLZ is not a panacea for schizophrenia. However, as the only FDA-approved AP showing efficacy in the treatment-resistant population, a therapeutic trial of clozapine is justified in all patients who meet clinical criteria for use.

Risperidone fulfills the atypical criterion of having a low incidence of EPS at low to moderate doses. In studies of randomly selected groups of schizophrenic patients in acute exacerbation, risperidone has proven efficacy, and may be superior to haloperidol in treatment of negative symptoms. The mean optimal dose in parallel, fixed-dose studies was 4–6 mg daily. At doses greater than 10 mg daily, risperidone's profile is more similar to a typical AP.[44,45] Since risperidone appears to lose its atypical profile at higher doses, the lowest possible dose should be used in treatment. This may include dose titration downward if patients do not respond initially, rather than upward titration as has been the traditional approach to dosing APs.[20]

Risperidone has not been systematically evaluated in treatment refractory patients, but there are reports of patients' symptoms worsening after being changed from clozapine.[46] However, because of drug acquisition cost differences and the agranulocytosis associated with clozapine, clinicians will often use risperidone before proceeding on to clozapine.

A wide variety of investigational atypical AP compounds are currently in clinical trials.[20] Some of these include HP 873 (Hoechst), olanzapine (Lilly), sertindole (Abbott), seroquel (Zeneca), zaprisidone (Pfizer), and zotepine (Knoll). It is hoped that one or more of these will provide positive enhancements to clinicians' AP armamentarium.

AUGMENTATION THERAPY

Augmentation therapy involves the addition of a "non-AP" drug to an AP in a poorly responsive patient. Theoretically, the approach is based on the assumption that the mechanism of action of the augmentation agent will interact synergistically with the dopaminolytic to produce efficacy. Although inadequately controlled research data are available concerning most augmentation regimens, there is suggestive information indicating potential efficacy with some interventions.[47] Several guidelines should be followed regarding augmentation: (1) augmentation should only be used in poorly responding patients; (2) augmentation agents are rarely effective in most treated patients; (3) augmentation agents rarely are effective when used alone in treating schizophrenia; (4) augmentation responders usually improve rapidly; and (5) if augmentation does not improve symptomatology, the augmenting agent should be discontinued.

Lithium augmentation is one of the better evaluated augmentation interventions.[22] In patients with significant aggression, lithium may assist in calming behavior. However, lithium has no AP activity, and there are little data to support its use in treating schizophrenic patients without aggressive behavior. It should be emphasized that this is not a diagnosis-specific effect, and patients need not have a bipolar or schizoaffective disorder to benefit from lithium's antiaggression effects. Dosing of lithium in schizophrenics should be approached in the same manner as for bipolar disorder patients.

Alprazolam has been evaluated as an augmentation agent in double-blind studies using the patient as his or her own control.[47,48] When added to FPZ at an average optimal alprazolam dose of 2.88 mg daily, clinically significant decreases in global psychosis, thought disorder, and paranoia scores occurred in 5 of 12 patients. However, a few patients worsened with this intervention; therefore, patients must be carefully monitored for a change in symptoms when alprazolam is added to an AP.

Published experiences with other benzodiazepines have been mixed.[22] Overall, the reports are not encouraging, and the development of violent behaviors was reported in 4 of 13 patients treated with clonazepam in a placebo-controlled study.

Reportedly, propranolol has an antiaggression effect when used in a variety of psychiatric disorders, but particularly when used in the organic aggressive syndrome. As with other augmentation agents, propranolol does not have an AP effect when given alone. Although its efficacy is probably associated with its pharmacodynamic effects, concomitant use may increase AP plasma concentrations as well.[22] Patients should receive a test dose of 20 mg to evaluate tolerance, and, if it is acceptable, initial propranolol dosing should be 20 mg three times daily. Dose increases should be in 60 mg/d increments, every 3 days. Patients should be monitored carefully for side effects related to β-adrenergic blockade. Once the patient is β-blocked, the dose may be increased more rapidly as tolerated. Patients may need to be treated with adequate doses for 6–8 weeks in order to evaluate an antiaggression response. If appropriate response is not received with a daily dose of 1000 mg, additional response is not usually achieved at higher doses.[49]

Some researchers suggest that the improvement observed in schizophrenia with propranolol is primarily due to a lessening of akathisia symptoms. The basis for this hypothesis is that most studies demonstrating efficacy for propranolol in schizophrenia have been in combination with a neuroleptic, whereas studies with propranolol alone have not demonstrated efficacy.[50] Whether propranolol has efficacy in schizophrenic patients without symptoms of aggression or akathisia remains unclear.

Because of its efficacy in bipolar mood disorder, carbamazepine has been used as an augmenting agent in schizophrenia, especially in patients with aggressive behavior. Although research in this area is inconclusive, it appears that carbamazepine may be a helpful adjunctive agent in decreasing aggressive behavior in schizophrenic patients. However, there are no data to support that it is efficacious in improving core schizophrenic symptoms.[51] Furthermore, its enzyme-induction properties may cause a decrease in plasma concentration and potentially a worsening of symptoms in some patients.[22]

Antipsychotic Adverse Effects

Table 66.8 presents the relative incidence of common categories of AP side effects. The precise incidence of many of these side effects has not been systematically evaluated. Side effects will be discussed with respect to organ system affected. Also, most of the side effects can be categorized by the neurotransmitter system affected, as listed in Table 66.9. A general approach to monitoring and assessing side effects requires prospective monitoring by clinicians, preferably using a thorough review of systems approach. Patient-oriented self-rating side-effect scales may also be helpful, because many schizophrenics do not readily complain of side effects, due to lack of volition, lack of perception of having input into their treatment, poor understanding, or because of the actual interference of side effects themselves (e.g., sedation).[29]

TABLE 66.8. RELATIVE SIDE EFFECTS INCIDENCE OF COMMONLY USED ANTIPSYCHOTICS

	Sedation	EPS	Anticholinergic	Cardiovascular
Chlorpromazine	++++	+++	+++	++++
Clozapine	+++++	+	+++++	++++
Fluphenazine	++	+++++	++	++
Haloperidol	+	+++++	+	+
Loxapine	+++	++++	++	+++
Molindone	+	+++	++	++
Perphenazine	++	++++	++	++
Risperidone	+	++	+	++
Thioridazine	++++	++	++++	++++
Trifluoperazine	++	++++	++	++
Thiothixene	++	++++	++	++

Key: +, very low; ++, low; +++, moderate; ++++, high; +++++, very high.

TABLE 66.9. ADVERSE EFFECTS BY RECEPTOR BLOCKADE

Receptor Type	Adverse Effects
Histamine H_1	Sedation Weight gain Potentiation of CNS depressant drugs
Muscarinic	Urinary retention Cognition and memory effects Sinus tachycardia Dry mouth Blurred vision Constipation
α_1 adrenergic	Orthostatic hypotension Reflex tachycardia Potentiation of antihypertensives
Dopamine D_2 receptor	Extrapyramidal side effects Prolactin elevation

AUTONOMIC NERVOUS SYSTEM

Patients receiving APs (or APs in combination with AChs) have frequent difficulties with ACh side effects (dry mouth, constipation, tachycardia, blurred vision, inhibition or impairment of ejaculation, urinary retention). Lower potency agents are typical offenders, and the elderly are especially sensitive to these effects.[41,52] System-specific effects are discussed under the appropriate heading.

Dry mouth can be managed with increased intake of fluids, oral lubricants (Xerolube), ice chips, or use of sugarless chewing gum or hard candy. Constipation, caused by slowed peristaltic movement and decreased intestinal fluid content, should be closely monitored and treated, especially in the elderly. Paralytic ileus may also occur. Constipation can be treated with increases in fluid and dietary fiber intake, and exercise.

CENTRAL NERVOUS SYSTEM

Extrapyramidal System

Dystonia

Dystonia is defined as a state of abnormal tonicity, sometimes described simplistically as a severe "muscle spasm."[53] Dystonias may be dramatic, frightening, and painful. More accurately, they are prolonged tonic contractions, with a rapid onset, usually within 24–96 hours of dosage administration or dosage increase. They may be life threatening, as in the case of pharyngeal-laryngeal dystonias, and can contribute to noncompliance. Types of dystonic reactions include trismus, glossospasm, tongue protrusion, pharyngeal-laryngeal dystonia, blepharospasm, oculogyric crisis, torticollis, and retrocollis.

Two pathophysiologic theories for dystonia are proposed[54]: (1) DA release from presynaptic receptors transiently increases (increased synthesis and release) in compensatory response to DA blockade, and (2) heightened sensitivity of postsynaptic DA receptors (as brain AP concentration decreases), such that DA release has an enhanced effect. The actual mechanism may be a combination of these two theories.

Risk factors include younger patients (especially males), the use of high-potency agents, and high dosage. An overall incidence from the 1960s through the mid-1970s ranged from 2.3%–10%, but as higher potency agents became more widely used, the rate has increased to as high as 64%.

Pharmacotherapeutic treatment options are effective and straightforward, with the choice of intramuscular or intravenous AChs (Table 66.10) or benzodiazepines. Benztropine mesylate 2 mg or diphenhydramine 50 mg may be given intramuscularly or intravenously, with the options of diazepam 5–10 mg slow intravenous push or lorazepam 1–2 mg intramuscularly. Relief is typically seen within 15–20 minutes of an intramuscular injection and within 5

TABLE 66.10. ANTI-PARKINSONIAN AGENTS

Generic Name	Trade Name	Manufacturer	Equivalent Dose (mg)	Dosage Range (mg)	Dosage Forms[a]
Antimuscarinics					
Benztropine	Cogentin	MSD	1	1–8[b]	T,I
Biperiden	Akineton	Knoll	2	2–8	T,I
Orphenadrine	Various	Various	50	50–250	T
Procyclidine	Kemadrine	Burroughs Wellcome	2	7.5–20	T
Trihexyphenidyl	Artane	Lederle, others	2	2–15	T,C-ER,L
Antihistaminic					
Diphenhydramine	Benadryl	Parke-Davis	50	50–400	C,T,L,I
Dopamine agonist					
Amantadine	Symmetrel	Du Pont	N/A	100–400	C,L

[a]Abbreviations as per Table 66.7.
[b]Dosage may be titrated to 12 mg with care; nonlinear pharmacokinetics have been demonstrated.

minutes of intravenous administration. This dose should be repeated if no response is seen within 15 minutes of intravenous injection or within 30 minutes of intramuscular injection. AP medication may be continued, with concomitant short-term use of oral ACh agents. A promising, but as yet unproven treatment may be botulinum toxin type A, a potent agent that irreversibly inhibits release of ACh; it has been successfully used in blepharospasm.

A controversial and complex issue arises regarding the question of prophylaxis of dystonia with ACh medications. Many clinicians prescribe AChs routinely when initiating AP therapy, whereas others do so only in patients who may be at greater risk for dystonic reactions or in those patients with a history of dystonic reactions. Studies available to help resolve this issue are contradictory and vary considerably in design. In a prospective study of 202 patients given a variety of APs, no significant difference was found between the prophylactic ACh group versus those treated without prophylaxis.[55] However, of the 95 patients given HPD, the incidence of dystonia was 11.5% for those receiving prophylactic AChs, whereas the group without prophylactic treatment had a 38.2% incidence. A recent analysis of pooled data from nine studies concluded there was a fivefold to eightfold reduction in dystonia when ACh prophylaxis was used, especially in young males on high-potency APs, a 1.9-fold reduction when taking all APs into account, and, no benefit in patients older than 45 years or in patients treated with low-potency agents (e.g., CPZ, TRD).[56] A recent World Health Organization (WHO) consensus statement does not recommend routine prophylaxis with AChs.[57]

A case-by-case approach in decisions involving the use of ACh prophylaxis seems most prudent, with selection based on risk factors. Dystonias may also be minimized by the use of lower initial doses of APs. The AChs are good choices for prophylaxis, whereas amantadine has not been proven effective for this purpose. A trial of risperidone or clozapine may be indicated in patients who have dystonic reactions to low doses of both high- and low-potency APs.

Akathisia

Akathisia is defined as the inability to sit still and as being functionally motor restless. The most accurate diagnosis is made by combining subjective complaints with objective symptoms (pacing, shifting, shuffling, or tapping feet). Subjectively, patients may describe a feeling of inner restlessness or disquiet, a compulsion to move or remain in constant motion. Akathisia occurs in 25–36% of patients treated with high-potency agents.[58] Some clinicians believe that the majority of patients experience akathisia, but the reported incidence only reflects patients who can verbalize their feelings, or recognize akathisia as being different from psychosis. Akathisia is frequently accompanied by dysphoria. Detection of akathisia requires a high degree of interviewer sensitivity.

The pathophysiology of akathisia is uncertain, but there are two current theories.[54] Theory 1 states that when the presynaptic DA receptor antagonism is greater than the postsynaptic receptor blockade, the net effect is increased synthesis and release of DA. Akathisia could then be explained by the behavioral effects of increased DA. However, this theory appears unlikely considering the frequency of concurrent pseudoparkinsonism, which occurs by an opposite mechanism. Theory 2 appears more likely, based on differential effects of DA in the brain. From studies involving the destruction of distinct portions of rat brain, it has been proposed that mesocortical postsynaptic DA blockade leads to increased locomotor activity, unlike the cataleptic effect in the striatum.

Many treatments for akathisia, although accepted to be effective, are based on anecdotal data. Akathisia research is particularly difficult as the nature of the illness is subjective. Treatment with ACh agents, usually considered the standard treatment for all acute EPS, is disappointing for akathisia.[58] Reduction in AP dosage is perhaps the best intervention; however, this may not be a realistic goal in an acutely psychotic patient. Another alternative is to switch to a lower potency agent or an AP previously used in the patient without adverse effect. Chronic akathisia that does not respond to multiple interventions including changes in antipsychotic agent may warrant a trial of clozapine therapy.[59]

Benzodiazepines are commonly used for akathisia, probably due to their sedative and anxiolytic properties. Efficacy using diazepam 5 mg three times per day was reported in patients who failed to respond to AChs, whereas other researchers failed to demonstrate efficacy in a series of 25 patients.[58] Diazepam 5 mg administered by slow intravenous push is reportedly as efficacious as diphenhydramine (Benadryl) 50 mg IV as an acute treatment.

β-Blockers are being used with increasing frequency. Most studies are flawed in allowing concurrent benztropine despite "failure" on ACh agents. Propranolol in doses up to 160 mg daily, nadolol in doses up to 80 mg daily, and metoprolol in β_2-selective doses of 100 mg daily or less were reported as effective doses.[60] The use of β-blockers may indicate a role for norepinephrine in the pathophysiology of this syndrome. The effectiveness of clonidine lends further support to this reasoning. A mean dose of 0.43 mg/d produced response in six patients, with maximum response within 24–48 hours of the previous dosage increase. Hypotension and sedation were the only observed side effects. No specific preventive measures exist for akathisia; however, the use of the lowest possible AP doses should minimize the incidence and severity of this side effect.

Pseudoparkinsonism

Pseudoparkinsonism, an AP-induced extrapyramidal side effect, resembles idiopathic Parkinson's disease. A patient with pseudoparkinsonism may present with any of four cardinal symptoms[53]: (1) akinesia, bradykinesia, or decreased motor activity including difficulty initiating movement as well as extreme slowness, mask-like facial expression, micrographia, slowed speech, and decreased arm swing; (2) tremor, known as pill-rolling type, predominant at rest, decreases with movement, usually involves the fingers and hands, although it may be seen in the arms, legs, neck, head, and chin (it may often be activated by having the patient perform mechanical movements with one extremity); (3) cogwheel rigidity, seen as the patient's limbs yield in jerky, rachet-like fashion when passively moved by the examiner (a mild form may present as stiffness); and (4) postural abnormalities and instability manifested as stooped posture, difficulty in maintaining stability when changing body position, and a gait that ranges from slow and shuffling to festinating (a result of dysfunction in autonomic stability combined with a shift in the center of gravity due to the stooped posture). Accessory symptoms include the autonomic manifestations seborrhea, sialorrhea, and hyperhidrosis. Fatigue and weakness may be noted, as well as speech abnormalities including dysphagia and dysarthria, and abnormal palmomental and glabellar reflexes. A variant of pseudoparkinsonism is rabbit syndrome, a perioral tremor.

The overall incidence ranges from 15.4–36%, but differs depending on the AP used. Akinesia alone can be seen in 59% of patients on high-potency agents. Other risk factors include increasing age and possibly female gender. The onset of symptoms is usually 1–2 weeks after initiation of AP therapy or dose increase.

The pathophysiology involves a deficiency of DA. Normal motor function is dependent on a balance between cholinergic and DAergic systems. AP blockade of postsynaptic DA receptors leads to a relative functional DA deficiency and cholinergic excess in the striatum resulting in motor abnormalities approximating those seen in Parkinson's disease.[54]

The efficacy of ACh medications in alleviating or attenuating pseudo-Parkinsonian symptoms is well established.[61] Benztropine is advantageous in that its longer half-life allows twice-daily dosing, and in many patients it may be given once daily.[53] Typical dosing is 1–2 mg twice a day up to a usual maximum dosage of 8 mg daily, although some patients will continue to respond to doses up to 12 mg. Dosage increases above 6 mg must be slow, as benztropine displays nonlinear pharmacokinetics. Trihexyphenidyl (2–5 mg tid), diphenhydramine (25–50 mg tid), and biperiden (2 mg tid) usually require three-times daily administration. Diphenhydramine produces more sedation than the other agents. Although it has been suggested that trihexyphenidyl is more likely to be abused, all of the anticholinergics have been abused for their euphorant effects.[62] With all of these agents, symptoms will typically begin to resolve in 3–4 days after initiation of treatment, but a minimum of at least 2 weeks of treatment is normally required for full response.

Amantadine is generally as efficacious for pseudoparkinsonism as AChs, with significantly less effect on memory function. Amantadine has less potential than other DA agonists (bromocriptine and levodopa) for significant adverse effects. Its mechanism involves enhancement of DAergic tone in the striatum. Excessive doses may produce anxiety, agitation, and restlessness, as well as exacerbation of psychosis. Dosage adjustment is necessary with renal insufficiency.

The need for prophylactic use of these agents against pseudoparkinsonism is less convincing than with dystonias. Trials examining this issue are typically retrospective reviews calculating the incidence of development of pseudoparkinsonism in patients treated with prophylactic agents versus those who were not, or trials examining withdrawal of anti-Parkinsonian medications in patients on maintenance AP therapy.

The long-term treatment of pseudoparkinsonism with anti-Parkinsonian medication is controversial. Most investigators believe that it is seldom necessary with maintenance AP therapy, whereas others demonstrate a population of patients who have recurrence or worsening of pseudo-Parkinsonian symptoms upon discontinuation of ACh medication, even if the medication is withdrawn gradually. An attempt should be made to taper and discontinue these agents 6 weeks to 3 months after symptoms resolve. If symptoms reappear, then a longer treatment period may be necessary.

Risperidone, when used in doses of 10 mg/d or less, demonstrates significantly less pseudoparkinsonism than haloperidol.[44] Clozapine is also a reasonable alternative for those patients with moderate to severe extrapyramidal symptoms for which a multitude of interventions have failed.[59]

Tardive Dyskinesia

Tardive dyskinesia (TD) is a syndrome characterized by abnormal involuntary movements occurring late in onset in relation to initiation of AP therapy. TD is sometimes irreversible and continues to be a controversial issue, legally and ethically, and one of the major challenges facing psychiatry.

The classical description of TD is the bucco-lingual-masticatory (BLM) syndrome, or orofacial movements.[53] The onset of BLM movements is usually insidious. Typically, they are the first detectable signs of TD, and begin with mild forward, backward, or lateral movements of the tongue. As the disorder progresses, more obvious or frank BLM movements appear, including tongue thrusting, rolling, or fly-catching movements, and chewing or lateral jaw movements. TD symptoms may interfere with the patient's ability to chew, speak, or swallow. Further complications include oral ulcerations, inability to wear dentures, and inflammation and loosening of mandibular joints. Eating difficulties and malnutrition may be primary physical complications of TD. Weight loss may be seen in patients with esophageal or respiratory manifestations but not in those with truncal movements.

Facial movements include frequent blinking, brow arching, grimacing, upward deviation of the eyes, and lip smacking. Involvement of the extremities occurs in later stages with the appearance of restless choreiform (irregular spasmodic) and distal athetosis (slow, writhing movement) of limbs including twisting, spreading, flexion (bending) and extension of fingers, toe tapping, and toe dorsiflexion (upward turning). The final area of involvement is the truncal movements. Unusual posture, hyperextension, pelvic thrusting, axial hyperkinesia (excessive muscular activity of head and trunk), ballismus (jerking or shaking), exaggerated lordosis (bending backward), rocking, and swaying are observed. Among the more common differential diagnoses are withdrawal dyskinesias occurring after short-term use of APs, spontaneous orofacial dyskinesias in the elderly, orofacial dyskinesias in the edentulous, stereotypic movements in schizophrenics, Huntington's disease, and congenital torsion dystonia.

Orofacial movements are reported more commonly in older patients, whereas the truncal axial movements are classically reported in young adults. Movements may worsen with stress, decrease with sedation, and disappear during sleep. Concentration on motor tasks or attempts to suppress the movements voluntarily may actually increase them.

Early signs of TD may be reversible, but if allowed to persist or if not detected in the early stages, they may be irreversible, even with discontinuation of drug. When the AP dose is decreased or tapered and discontinued, there is usually a worsening of abnormal movements and then possibly a slow improvement after months or years if the patient remains on lower doses or discontinues treatment.

There are no standardized criteria for the diagnosis of TD. Abnormal involuntary movements can be detected early through physical assessment and the use of rating scales. Instrumentation and frequency counts are infrequently used. The failure of clinicians to recognize TD until it is clinically obvious is a strong case for using comprehensive rating scales, because choreiform movements of the extremities are frequently missed in unstructured clinical assessments. The most commonly used and recognized scale is the Abnormal Involuntary Movement Scale (AIMS).[63] The AIMS may be used for general screening, but contrary to popular belief, is not diagnostic by itself. The Dyskinesia Identification System: Condensed User Scale (DISCUS) represents the first involuntary movement scale to be psychometrically valid.[64]

The pathophysiology of TD is complex and remains to be satisfactorily explained. The traditional theory is that postsynaptic DA receptor blockade in the nigrostriatum leads to disuse hypersensitivity or denervation. This is usually considered in conjunction with a cholinergic hypofunction relative to DAergic activity or the classic DA/acetylcholine imbalance. With DA receptor blockade, there is either an increase in the number of binding sites or an alteration in the sensitivity of the receptor to DA through adenylate cyclase activity. These DA receptors are generally considered to have an inhibitory effect on acetylcholine function in the corpus striatum. DA function may be modulated by a negative feedback system involving two sets of GABA-mediated neurons. GABA output to the thalamus and motor cortex is reduced as a result, and this causes the movement disorder. Deficiencies of this theory include the following: (1) It explains withdrawal dyskinesias or a transient movement disorder, but not persistent symptoms; (2) it does not explain concurrent TD and parkinsonism in the same patient; (3) it does not account for the presence of presynaptic DA autoreceptors; (4) postsynaptic receptor hypersensitivity usually develops soon after beginning APs, whereas TD develops after prolonged use; and (5) postmortem studies have found no increase in DA receptors in brains of TD patients.[65] Lack of site specificity and differential effects of APs on D_1 versus D_2 receptors may explain why traditional APs cause TD while some atypical APs do not (see section on Mechanism of Action). DA receptor antagonists' effects on decreasing GABA turnover and resulting GABA receptor hypersensitivity have also been theorized as a potential mechanism for TD.[65] Although neuronal degeneration and gliosis in the brain is a frequent finding on postmortem examination of patients with TD, it is uncertain whether neurocellular change is related to cause or effect of TD.

Risk factors include increasing age, female gender, and diagnoses of organic mental disorder or mood disorders.[66] It is uncertain if the history of significant unresolved acute EPS or lengthy treatment with ACh agents is the real risk factor, although the role of AChs has been disputed.[67] Duration of AP therapy, daily dosage, and possibly total cumulative dosage are probably the most significant risk factors. However, persistent dyskinesias occur with as little as 6 months of therapy. Altered drug metabolism may also play a part in the development of TD, as higher Cps on fixed dosages of thiothixene were seen in patients with TD than in dyskinesia-free schizophrenics.[68] Overall morbidity and mortality is greater in TD patients, and patients with TD show a greater incidence of respiratory tract infections and cardiovascular illness, leading some to propose that patients who develop TD may, in general, constitute a more biologically disadvantaged group.

The incidence of TD ranges from 0.5–62% with the mean being approximately 20%.[65] Factors causing variation in epidemiologic studies are patient population characteristics, drug dosage, duration of therapy, varieties of methods used in the assessment of TD, inadequacies in differentiating TD from other movement disorders, and bias. In a longitudinal study, Kane and colleagues showed an incidence of 4% per year of drug treatment for the first 4 years.[69] These cases usually were in younger patients (mean age = 29 years) and were mild; follow up after 2–3 years indicates dyskinesia scores did not increase.

Dosage reduction alone may have a significant effect on outcome, with a complete disappearance of symptoms in some.[70] If patients with TD are kept on AP therapy, many are concerned about the possibility of TD symptoms worsening. In a recent series of patients, however, the syndrome remained stable over the years, and while a few patients worsened or only modest changes were seen, many improved on lower doses.[71] However, an increase in the incidence of pseudoparkinsonism was seen in all patients. In another recent longitudinal study, remissions were seen in 25% of patients with TD after 5 years of continued treatment. The authors also reported an increased incidence of pseudoparkinsonism, believed to be a risk factor toward the development of TD.[72]

Possibly only a small subgroup of patients with TD will develop a clinically severe form.[73] Although it is difficult to predict who will develop severe TD, one sample of patients was characterized by a greater number of affective/schizoaffective patients; frequent eye blinking was a prodromal sign in 37%.

Prevention is the single most important aspect of TD, because treatment of movements once they have become manifest is difficult. APs should be used only when they are drugs of choice (i.e., when used for AP target symptoms), and they should be used at the minimum effective dose. When a patient is treated with APs for more than 3 months for an initial episode of illness, the need for continued treatment should be assessed. When treatment is continued, regular neurologic examination (AIMS or other scales) should be performed to assess for early signs of TD, at least quarterly. When possible, APs should be discontinued at the earliest symptoms of TD. Schizophrenic patients should occasionally have a trial of drug tapering and possible discontinuation if the patient's clinical status allows. Theoretically, this might prevent receptor hypersensitization. It also allows the clinician to assess for further need of the drug and may detect mild TD symptoms masked by the drug, although this procedure may not be possible in patients who have a history of rapid relapse with drug discontinuation. In nonpsychotic patients, APs should only be used acutely to abort an aggressive behavior crisis, and then always in combination with a behavioral treatment program.

There are no FDA-approved agents for treatment of TD. Numerous drugs have been used representing various biochemical alterations in the CNS. Strategies are aimed at altering the DA, GABA, and cholinergic systems.[65] Any particular patient may respond to all, some, or none of the categories, and the most efficacious interventions are only partially successful. A summary of potential treatments appears in Table 66.11.[74] Long-term treatment with most of these agents has not been examined.

TABLE 66.11. MISCELLANEOUS PHARMACOTHERAPIES FOR TARDIVE DYSKINESIA

Agents That Alter Dopaminergic Activity
- Dopamine blocking agents
  - Clozapine
- Dopamine depletors
  - Reserpine
- Dopamine synthesis antagonists
  - Alpha-methyldopa
- Dopamine receptor agonists
  - Amantadine
  - Bromocriptine
  - Levodopa

Cholinergic Agents
- Physostigmine
- Choline
- Lecithin (phosphatidylcholine)

GABA Facilitators
- Baclofen
- Valproic acid
- Benzodiazepines

Miscellaneous Agents
- Lithium
- Adrenergic blocking agents
  - Beta blockers
  - Clonidine
- Papaverine
- Cyproheptadine
- Alpha-tocopherol
- Calcium channel blockers

Agents that alter DAergic activity have been utilized, including the DA depletor reserpine, which produces presynaptic depletion of DA by interfering with intraneuronal vesicular uptake and storage, therefore allowing greater DA degradation by monoamine oxidase (MAO). In doses of 0.75–5 mg daily, its effects are usually temporary, and dosage increases are necessary to maintain effect. DA receptor agonists have been used and are postulated to work by modulating intraneuronal DA release via presynaptic autoreceptors. Amantadine has theoretical protective effects when used concurrently with APs, causing D_2 receptors to conform in a high-affinity binding state. It, along with bromocriptine and levodopa, requires further study.

The use of cholinergic agents is based on the traditional restoration of a DAergic cholinergic balance. Physostigmine has been used as a predictor of response to oral cholinergics in a test dose of 1 g IV. Oral agents include choline, a precursor to acetylcholine, which increases levels of acetylcholine but which imparts to many patients a distinctive fishy odor caused by the breakdown of choline to trimethylamine by GI bacteria; and lecithin (phosphatidylcholine), which is the primary dietary source of choline and is not degraded by gut bacteria. Doses up to 24 g daily are usually necessary. Although lecithin demonstrated a statistically significant treatment effect in a double-blind crossover trial, the clinical significance is questionable.[75]

The use of agents that facilitate GABA should result in decreased DA release and decreased motor transmission to the thalamus, based on the role that GABA plays in negative feedback inhibition to modulate DA release. Baclofen in doses of 60–75 mg/d has been partially effective, but limited by severe and common side effects of muscular hypotonia and sedation. Valproic acid, an anticonvulsant with psychotropic properties, has been used in doses of 600–900 mg. Although there are successful reports of benzodiazepines improving symptoms of TD, recent analyses have not shown any greater effect than placebo; their success probably represents only the effects of sedation.

α-Tocopherol (vitamin E) in doses of 1200–1600 IU has been used based on its antioxidant properties. Results from short-term treatment studies have variously shown significant reduction in movements,[76] no significant difference from placebo with minor benefit in select patients,[77] and no effect.[78] Based on its safety and low cost, vitamin E is a reasonable treatment option for TD.

CLZ does not appear to cause TD. Although only recently introduced in the United States, it has been used in some European countries since the early 1970s. To date, there are no reports of TD with CLZ monotherapy. CLZ reduced abnormal involuntary movements by 50% or greater in 43% of patients with TD, but controlled trials have yet to be performed.[59]

Sedation

Sedation must be recognized as an AP side effect and not as an indication of therapeutic effect. It occurs more frequently with low-potency APs through their antihistaminic properties. CPZ, TRD, mesoridazine, and CLZ are most frequently implicated. Administration of most or all of the daily dosage at bedtime can decrease daytime sedation and in some patients eliminate the need for hypnotic agents. Sedation occurs early in treatment and may decrease over time. Oversedation plays a large role in cognitive, perceptual, and motor dysfunction.[79] With acute dosing, tasks requiring vigilance, attention, or motor behavior may be affected. However, the positive effects of medication are seen with chronic administration, evidenced by improvements in tasks involving visual-motor skills and attention. Neuropsychologic testing is not affected by chronic drug administration. However, many of these improvements appear to be inversely proportional to dose.

Seizures

APs lower the seizure threshold through GABA depletion, changes in CNS permeability leading to enhanced conduction of a discharge, disruption of DA–acetylcholine balance, or the activation of a latent seizure focus. There is an increased risk of drug-induced seizures in all patients treated with APs. However, this risk is greater if the following predisposing factors are present: preexisting seizure disorder, history of drug-induced seizure, abnormal EEG, and preexisting CNS pathology or head trauma. Seizures are more closely associated with the use of higher doses, rapid dosage increases, and upon initiation of treatment. When an isolated seizure occurs, a dosage decrease is first recommended; anticonvulsant therapy is not recommended. The highest potential seizure risk by an AP drug is with the use of CPZ or CLZ, followed by trifluoperazine and perphenazine. Addition of lithium to a stable CLZ regimen has resulted in seizures in two reported cases.[80] If a change in AP therapy is required in the management of AP-induced seizures, molindone, TRD, HPD, and FPZ are associated with the lowest potential.[81]

Thermoregulation

Poikilothermia, the body temperature adjusting to the ambient temperature, can be a serious side effect of AP therapy in temperature extremes. Hyperpyrexia can be a danger in hot weather or during exercise. Inhibition of sweating, a result of ACh properties impairing the peripheral mechanisms of heat dissipation, can also contribute to this problem, which in its severest form can lead to heat stroke. Hypothermia is also a risk, particularly in the elderly. All patients receiving APs should be educated about these potential problems. Thermoregulatory problems are reportedly more common with the use of low-potency APs.[82]

Neuroleptic Malignant Syndrome

Neuroleptic malignant syndrome (NMS) occurs in 0.5–1% of patients receiving APs. NMS may occur more frequently in patients receiving high-potency, injectable, or depot APs, and in patients who are dehydrated, with physical exhaustion, or organic mental disorders.[83] The onset of symptoms varies from early in treatment to months later. It develops rapidly, over the course of 24–72 hours. NMS may occur after AP discontinuation, especially when depot agents are used. Possible mechanisms of NMS include disruption of the central thermoregulatory process or excess production of heat secondary to skeletal muscle contractions. The differential diagnosis includes heat stroke, lethal catatonia, anesthetic-associated malignant hyperthermia, ACh toxicity, and MAO inhibitor drug interactions.

Cardinal signs and symptoms of NMS are body temperature exceeding 38°C, altered level of consciousness, autonomic dysfunction (tachycardia, labile blood pressure, diaphoresis, tachypnea, urinary or fecal incontinence), and rigidity. Laboratory evaluation, although considered nonspecific, frequently shows leukocytosis with or without left shift, increases in creatine kinase (CK), aspartate aminotransferase (AST), alanine aminotransferase (ALT), lactate dehydrogenase (LDH), and myoglobinuria.

Treatment should always begin with AP discontinuation and supportive care. The DA agonist bromocriptine, used in theory to reverse DA blockade, reduces rigidity, fever, or CK in up to 94% of patients, whereas the use of another DA agonist, amantadine, has been successfully used in up to 63% of patients.[84] Dantrolene has been used as a skeletal muscle relaxant, with effects on temperature, heart, respiratory rate, and CK in up to 81% of patients. AChs and benzodiazepines have been tried but appear to have little effect in most patients, and ACh use can complicate the clinical presentation with possible delirium. Wide recognition and rapid AP discontinuation has drastically reduced mortality from 20% one decade ago to 4% in the mid-1990s.

Many schizophrenics, despite having had NMS, will require future AP pharmacotherapy. Patient selection for rechallenge is important, as only those patients in greatest need of reinstitution of APs (e.g., those who pose risk of harm to society or self) should receive future trials. A review of AP rechallenges suggests that the risk of rechallenge is acceptable in most patients, provided there is careful monitoring, patient selection is appropriate, and the patient is observed for an extended period of time (2 weeks or more is suggested) without APs.[85] Neither patient-specific demographic variables nor AP agent used (neither same or dissimilar, low or high potency) assist in predicting recurrence. Using the lowest effective AP dose is also suggested.

The absence of NMS was also thought to be a potential advantage of atypical agents. However, cases of NMS associated with clozapine and risperidone therapy have been reported.[20,86]

Psychiatric Side Effects

AP-induced akathisia, akinesia, and dysphoria may have unfortunate sequelae, resulting in what has been termed "behavioral toxicity."[32] Akathisia has resulted in impulsivity and, in extreme cases, violence and suicide. Akinesia, characterized by "diminished spontaneity," results in symptoms of apathy and withdrawal, often mistaken for the negative symptoms of schizophrenia; these patients may actually appear depressed on formal evaluation. Dysphoric subjective responses by patients after the initiation of AP therapy affect ratings of patient response, making the patient appear to be doing less well, although many will eventually experience a fair level of improvement.

Catatonia (characterized by symptoms of mutism, immobility, staring, rigidity, withdrawal, posturing, grimacing, negativism, waxy flexibility, echolalia, echopraxia, stereotypes, or verbigeration) has been described as a AP-induced reaction or variant of severe pseudoparkinsonism.[87]

Delirium and psychosis are reported with larger doses of APs or combinations of AChs with APs. Chronic confusion and disorientation can occur in the elderly as a result of AP treatment.[52] Unfortunately, the link is not always made between initiation of AP therapy, and the patient may be misdiagnosed with an organic mental disorder. This clinical presentation, called a "pseudodementia," is easily reversible on discontinuation of the AP.

ENDOCRINE SYSTEM

DA blockade in the tuberoinfundibular tract results in increased prolactin levels, because DA is the major prolactin-inhibiting factor. Galactorrhea may occur in up to 57% of women, and menstrual irregularities or amenorrhea in up to 97%. These effects may be dose related and appear more commonly with the use of high-potency APs. Gynecomastia and galactorrhea are reported in men as well. Tolerance does not appear to develop to these effects.[88] Switching AP agents, bromocriptine in doses up to 15 mg daily or amantadine in doses up to 300 mg daily, are possible management strategies.

Weight gain is frequently reported in patients receiving APs.[88] APs can induce weight gain, but dietary factors and activity levels may play a significant role in this population, as does renourishment after a period of poor self-care.

APs may affect glucose levels and response, a consideration in diabetic patients, although studies in diabetics show little effect in the successful management of their illness.

CARDIOVASCULAR SYSTEM

Orthostatic Hypotension

Postural or orthostatic hypotension, defined as a greater than 20 mm Hg drop in systolic pressure, is caused by α-adrenergic blockade, which inhibits reflex vasoconstriction when rising to a sitting or standing position; this appears to be a combination of local vasodilatory effects and central inhibition of the vasomotor center, as well as sympatholysis leading to unopposed β-adrenergic effect.[82] Patients may experience lightheadedness or syncope. Associated with lower potency APs (especially on intramuscular or intravenous administration), orthostatic hypotension can occur in any patient, but diabetics, patients with preexisting cardiovascular disease, and the elderly seem particularly predisposed. For the mild case, patient education should address slow changes in posture to allow for adaptation or the use of support hose. For most patients, tolerance to this effect occurs within 2–3 months. If this does not occur, lower doses or a change to a higher potency AP can be attempted. Low-potency agents and clozapine should be used with caution in patients with underlying cardiovascular disease.

Severe hypotensive episodes require more vigorous treatment. The patient should be placed in a Trendelenburg position. Volume expansion through intravenous fluids should be attempted before the use of pressor agents. Pure α-adrenergic pressor agents, such as phenylephrine (Neo-Synephrine) or metaraminol (Aramine), can be used, as well as norepinephrine (Levophed), which has β_1-adrenergic properties. Epinephrine (Adrenalin), with α- and β-adrenergic effects, should never be used because unopposed β-adrenergic stimulating effects will further lower a patient's blood pressure, potentially leading to cardiovascular collapse. Isoproterenol (Isuprel), which also has β-adrenergic stimulating effects, should be avoided.

Electrocardiogram (ECG) Changes

APs have both antiarrhythmic and arrhythmogenic effects. They produce direct myocardial depression and quinidine-like effects on cardiac conduction, and they also antagonize sympathetic nervous system activity in the hypothalamus and stabilize cardiac tissue through local anesthetic properties. Low-potency agents, especially piperidine phenothiazines (such as TRD) and clozapine, are more likely to cause these effects. ECG changes include increased heart rate (through sinus tachycardia, from ACh effects, or reflex tachycardia, from α-adrenergic blockade), flattened T waves, ST segment depression, and prolongation of QT and PR intervals. Torsades de pointes has been reported with TRD, perhaps through its sulfoxide metabolite, which may be a cause of cardiac sudden death. However, most ECG changes are not usually clinically significant at normal therapeutic doses in physically healthy patients.[89] Greater caution is necessary in the elderly and patients with preexisting cardiac disease.[52] In patients older than 40 years, a pretreatment ECG is recommended.

OPHTHALMIC SIDE EFFECTS

Impairment in visual accommodation results from paresis of ciliary muscles, an ACh effect. Although bothersome, the effect is temporary in most cases. Photophobia may also result. Pilocarpine ophthalmic solution may be necessary in severe cases.

Exacerbation of narrow-angle (angle closure) glaucoma can result from increases in intraocular pressure, another ACh effect. High-potency APs should be used with great caution in susceptible individuals.

Opaque deposits in the cornea and lens occur with chronic phenothiazine treatment, most frequently with CPZ. Although visual acuity is not usually affected, periodic slit-lamp ophthalmologic examinations are frequently recommended in patients receiving long-term treatment with phenothiazines.

Retinitis pigmentosis can result from use of TRD doses greater than 800 mg daily (the manufacturer's recommended maximum dose). It is caused by melanin deposits, and can result in permanent visual impairment or blindness. There is no evidence that it is a function of dosage accumulation.[90]

HEPATIC SYSTEM

Liver function test (LFT) abnormalities (elevated aminotransferases and alkaline phosphatase) are reported in up to 50% of patients on APs, and may occur without clinical symptoms.[91] This occurs most commonly in patients less than 50 years of age and does not appear to be dose related. Mild LFT elevations are typically not significant, although they should be followed closely. If aminotransferases are greater than three times the upper limit of normal, AP therapy should be changed to a chemically unrelated AP.

Cholestatic hepatocanalicular jaundice can occur in up to 2% of patients receiving phenothiazines. It may be a hypersensitivity reaction, or due to either the effects on bile composition or the direct toxic effect of a metabolite on biliary ductile hepatocytes impairing bile flow.[91] The onset is usually within the first 2 weeks of therapy, with prodromal symptoms of malaise, fatigue, fever, chills, arthralgias, myalgias, GI symptoms, and severe pruritis. Symptoms resolve without residual liver damage within 2–8 weeks upon discontinuation of the offending AP. Palliative treatment of pruritis with topical or oral antihistamines is frequently necessary. Resumption of AP therapy should be delayed as long as reasonably possible, and it should be done with a nonphenothiazine AP.

GENITOURINARY SYSTEM

Urinary hesitancy and retention is commonly reported with low-potency APs. ACh effects cause smooth muscle slowing and paralyze the detrusor muscle of the bladder, requiring greater urine volume to evoke muscle contraction. Men with benign prostatic hypertrophy are especially prone to this effect.[52]

Urinary incontinence is felt by some to be unrelated to urinary retention, as many patients do not complain of problems before it occurs. Instead, it may be mechanistically similar to a dystonic reaction. It is reported more frequently in older patients, especially women.[92]

The AP effects on sexual dysfunction can be frightening or devastating to most schizophrenics and can significantly affect compliance. Erectile dysfunction and impotence, considered an ACh effect, occurs in 25–60% of patients, most frequently with TRD. Although this can occur in a large number of untreated psychotic patients, it is most certainly compounded by AP drugs. Anorgasmia and decreased libido in women have also been proposed to be ACh in nature. α-Adrenergic blockade is proposed to be the mechanism behind priapism, and retarded and retrograde ejaculation. Again, TRD is the most frequently reported AP for these effects and is a potent α-blocker. Decreased libido may also be caused by sedation. In men, another possible, although not fully explored, mechanism of sexual dysfunction is decreased testosterone production secondary to hyperprolactinemia. Using lower AP doses, changing to high-potency APs, or discontinuation of ACh medications are potential interventions.[93]

HEMATOLOGIC SYSTEM

Transient leukopenia may occur during initial treatment with APs; however, it typically does not progress to clinically significant parameters.[94] If the white blood cell (WBC) count is less than 3000/mm^3 or the absolute neutrophil count (ANC) is <1000/mm^3, the AP should be discontinued, and the WBC monitored closely until it returns to normal. Agranulocytosis reportedly occurs in 0.01% of patients receiving APs, and of the typical APs may occur most frequently with CPZ and piperazine phenothiazines. The onset is usually within the first 8 weeks of therapy. Agranulocytosis may initially manifest clinically as a local infection, with sore throat, leukoplakia, and erythema and ulcerations of the pharynx. These symptoms in any patient receiving APs should signal the immediate need for a WBC. If either the WBC or ANC falls below these parameters, the drug should be discontinued immediately and the patient monitored closely for the development of secondary infections. There are also isolated, rare case reports of thrombocytopenia and eosinophilia.

Agranulocytosis is the CLZ-related adverse effect receiving the most publicity, from both the medical and political perspectives. Data on the incidence since the release of clozapine in February 1990, following stringent monitoring guidelines, reveal that the 1-year treatment risk of developing agranulocytosis with CLZ appears to be approximately 0.8%, with the 18-month risk at 0.91%.[95] Increasing age and female gender are associated with greater risk. Based on available data, the time period for greatest risk appears to be between months 1 and 6 of treatment.[96] WBC monitoring, as currently mandated in the labeling, is once weekly. If the total WBC count drops to less than 2000/mm^3, or the ANC is less than 1000/mm^3, CLZ should be discontinued and the patient monitored closely. Some clinicians have used the granulocyte colony stimulating factor, filgrastim, with hopes of improving the outcome by hastening resolution or decreasing morbidity. One case series, using filgrastim (starting dose of 300 mcg/d sc increased by 300 mcg/d until 900 mcg/d is reached, which is then continued until the agranulocytosis is resolved), demonstrated a decrease in time to resolution and decreased intensive care bed costs when compared with historical controls.[97] In cases of mild to moderate neutropenia (granulocytes between 2000–3000/mm^3, or ANC between 1000–1500/mm^3), which occurs in up to 2% of patients, CLZ should be discontinued with daily monitoring of complete blood counts until values return to normal.

DERMATOLOGIC SYSTEM

Allergic reactions are rare and usually occur within 8 weeks of therapy, manifesting as maculopapular, erythematous, pruritic rashes that are evident on the face, neck, trunk, or extremities. Drug discontinuation and topical steroids are recommended.

Contact dermatitis, including the oral mucosa, may occur in patients or medical personnel. For patients, mixing the concentrate in a sufficient quantity of a nonacidic liquid and swallowing it quickly decreases problems in susceptible patients. Care should be taken in the handling and preparation of liquid APs.

Phenothiazine structures can absorb ultraviolet light and energy, resulting in the formation of free radicals, which can have damaging effects on the skin. Erythema and severe sunburns can occur. Exposure to sunlight should be limited, and patients should be educated about the use of a maximally blocking sunscreen, hats, protective clothing, and sunglasses.[82]

Blue-gray or purplish skin coloration in areas exposed to sunlight occurs in patients receiving higher doses of low-potency phenothiazines during long-term administration, especially with CPZ. It commonly occurs with concurrent corneal or lens pigmentation.

SUDDEN DEATH SYNDROMES

Although fewer sudden deaths occurred before AP use, it has been reported in schizophrenics before and after the advent of APs. Most theories emphasize a pharmacologic etiology. The most common theory is that ventricular arrhythmias progress to ventricular fibrillation and death. Another common hypothesis is that an impaired gag reflex from a laryngeal-pharyngeal dystonia leads to aspiration, hypoxia, and death, a syndrome known as "obstructive asphyxia" or "café coronary." Other potentially drug-related theories include hyperpyrexia, NMS, seizures, and toxic megacolon, whereas nondrug-related theories include acute exhaustive mania or Bell's mania, lethal catatonia, coronary artery disease, and the sequelae of alcohol and substance abuse.[98]

TOXICITY ON OVERDOSE

Acute overdose with APs rarely results in serious symptomatology. Mild intoxication manifests as sedation, hypotension, and miosis, whereas with severe intoxication, agitation, and delirium may typically progress to motor retardation, seizures, cardiac arrhythmias, respiratory arrest, and coma. Dystonias and pseudo-Parkinsonian symptoms also occur. Supportive measures, gastric lavage, and activated charcoal are recommended. Induction of emesis may be difficult due to effects on the chemoreceptor trigger zone, and dialysis is ineffective due to the degree of drug-protein binding. Phenytoin or sodium bicarbonate are useful in the treatment of quinidine-like cardiac conduction effects on the QRS or QTc intervals. Physostigmine is not generally recommended to reverse anticholinergic toxicity because of deleterious effects on arrhythmias and seizure threshold.[90]

MISCELLANEOUS ADVERSE EFFECTS

A particularly curious and sometimes troubling side effect with CLZ is sialorrhea; this drooling, possibly adrenergic in etiology, occurs in the absence of Parkinson's symptoms.[96] Some cases respond to the addition of the α-adrenergic blocker clonidine, in doses of 0.1–0.2 mg/d.[99] It may also abate with benztropine therapy.

USE IN PREGNANCY AND LACTATION

Currently available data assessing the risk of teratogenesis with AP agents are insufficient. HPD was studied in the treatment of hyperemesis gravidarum without negative effect; it and other high-potency agents appear to be preferred, but unfortunately this is primarily due to a lack of published reports over decades of use. Case reports implicating limb malformations are rare, but should be considered in deciding on the need for first-trimester AP use. The risks of AP use must be weighed against the benefits of pharmacotherapy in patients who may be experiencing disorganized thoughts, delusions about change in body image or pregnancy, or who are unable to provide adequate prenatal care.[100] Other potential but largely unknown risks of APs throughout pregnancy are the incidence of behavioral teratogenicity on the neonate, receptor changes, perinatal effects (e.g., tonicity, strength, sucking), EPS, jaundice, respiratory depression, and intestinal obstruction.

APs appear in breast milk with milk to plasma ratios of 0.5 to 1. Little is known about the effects of these drugs on the neonate. Although not contraindicated, the lowest dosage should be used in the mother, and the infant should be carefully monitored.

DRUG INTERACTIONS

Most AP drug interactions are relatively minor in severity and often involve additive CNS side effects. The most common drug interactions seen in schizophrenia involve anticholinergics and drugs causing sedation. The concurrent use of lithium with APs is generally safe; however, a handful of case reports of irreversible encephalopathy (including delirium, ataxia, rigidity, tremors, fever, weakness, lethargy, etc.) have been reported.[101,102] Although anecdotal data report this more commonly with HPD, this is poorly substantiated. Although this interaction can appear similar to NMS, patients recovering from an AP/lithium interaction may more commonly suffer sequelae.

AP pharmacokinetics can be significantly affected by concomitant enzyme inducers or inhibitors. Anticonvulsants, particularly carbamazepine, are the most commonly used enzyme inducers in schizophrenics. However, smoking is a potent inducer of hepatic enzymes and may increase AP clearance by as much as 50%.[21] Commonly used enzyme inhibitors in this population include cimetidine, tricyclic antidepressants, some anticonvulsants, and perhaps fluoxetine. See Table 66.12 for a listing of additional drug interactions.[78]

USE IN PEDIATRIC AND GERIATRIC POPULATIONS

The dosing of APs in children and geriatric patients is empirically based. Many who treat children feel as if more frequent dosing (or shorter dosing intervals) is necessary due to rapid metabolism. Very low doses are also advocated, with most children requiring less than one-fourth of the adult dose. In the elderly, an arbitrary guideline for dosing is one-half the adult acute or maintenance dose. This guideline has long been promulgated by regulatory standards, and Medicare Long Term Care Standards recently reaffirmed these doses.[52] Not having a physiologic definition of either of these populations presents difficulties in defining pharmacokinetic differences, and thus the standard "under 12" and "over 65" definitions are used by pharmacists to monitor patients. Cp monitoring may be helpful in determining the need for doses outside of these guidelines.

CONCLUSION

Schizophrenia is a complex disease with multiple ramifications for patients and their families. Treatment issues remain clouded by the fact that the etiology of the illness is unknown. It is clear, however, that no single treatment modality is adequate to properly manage a patient with schizophrenia. APs are not a panacea and have multiple adverse effects in addition to the limitations of their efficacy. However, when used within the context of multidisciplinary treatment, they usually assist in keeping psychotic symptoms under control so that patients can appropriately participate in other therapies. Although the philosophy of

TABLE 66.12. DRUG INTERACTIONS INVOLVING ANTIPSYCHOTICS[a]

Interacting Medication	Mechanism of Interaction	Clinical Effect or Result Reported
Part A: Drug interactions that are established, probable, or suspected, regardless of severity, along with possible interactions whose severity is felt to be major:		
Anticholinergics	Decreased AP concentrations	Decreased antipsychotic effect
	Additive anticholinergic effect	See discussion under autonomic effects
Barbiturates	APs increase neuromuscular excitation with barbiturate anesthesia	Involved only those phenothiazines used as preanesthetic agents
	Phenobarbital induces AP metabolism	Decreased AP concentrations
Beta blockers	Synergistic pharmacologic effect or increases in AP concentrations	Case report of severe hypotension
	APs inhibit metabolism of propranolol, increase plasma concentrations	Increased pharmacologic effects, clinical effect not documented
	Unknown	Potentiated antipsychotic effect
Carbamazepine	Carbamazepine induces AP metabolism	Up to 50% reduction in AP concentrations
Charcoal	Reduces GI absorption of AP and adsorbs drug during enterohepatic circulation	May reduce antipsychotic effect; toxicity when used during overdose or for GI disturbances
Epinephrine, norepinephrine	APs antagonize pressor effect	Hypotension (see discussion of orthostatic hypotension in text)
Ethanol	Additive CNS depression	Impaired psychomotor skills
Guanethidine	APs antagonize guanethidine reuptake	Impaired antihypertensive effect
Lithium	Unknown	Rare reports of neurotoxicity
Meperidine	Additive CNS depression	Hypotension and sedation
Metrizamide	Lowered seizure threshold	Two case reports of seizures
Part B: Possible interactions assessed to have minor to moderate severity:		
Angiotensin-converting enzyme inhibitors	Additive hypotensive effects	One case of marked hypotension, postural intolerance
Aluminum-containing antacids	Forms insoluble complexes in GI tract	Possible reduced antipsychotic effect
Amphetamines, anorexiants	Decreased pharmacologic effect of amphetamine	Diminished weight loss effect
	Drug-disease state interaction	Amphetamines may exacerbate psychosis
		Amphetamines have been reported to improve psychotic symptoms in treatment-refractory schizophrenics
Antidepressants	Decreased metabolism of antidepressants through competitive inhibition	Increased antidepressant concentration, possible increased effect or adverse effect
Benzodiazepines	Increased pharmacologic effect of the benzodiazepine	Case reports of respiratory depression, stupor, hypotension; these effects, along with ataxia and sialorrhea, may be pronounced with clozapine
Bromocriptine	APs antagonize dopamine receptor stimulating effect; increases prolactin	Should not be coadministered during treatment of prolactin-secreting tumors
Caffeinated beverages	Form precipitates with oral antipsychotic solutions; should not be mixed despite product labeling	Possible diminished antipsychotic effect
Cimetidine	Reduced AP absorption; increased AP Cps	Decreased AP effect; impairs AP metabolism
Clonidine	APs potentiate alpha-adrenergic hypotensive effect	Hypotension
Disulfiram	Impairs AP metabolism	Increased AP concentrations
Fluoxetine	Impairs AP metabolism	Sudden onset of EPS; also, 20% increase in haloperidol Cps
Methyldopa	Unknown	Blood pressure elevations
Phenytoin	Induction of AP metabolism	Decreased AP concentrations
	Increased phenytoin metabolism	Decreased phenytoin levels
Valproic acid	APs inhibit valproic acid metabolism	Increases valproic acid half-life and levels

[a]Drug interactions that have been reported but assessed as unlikely are not included in this table.

deinstitutionalization has provided the initiative to allow schizophrenic patients to live in the community rather than in hospitals, implementation of this philosophy would have been impossible without the introduction of AP medications. Hopefully, the introduction of new technologies will allow clinicians to have a better understanding of brain function and the pathophysiology of schizophrenia. This, in turn, will aid greatly in the design of safer and more effective medications. In the interim, however, it is mandatory that clinicians have a thorough understanding of APs, their indications, knowledge of adverse effects, and appropriate use in psychotic patients.

REFERENCES

1. Schizophrenia and other psychotic disorders, in Diagnostic and Statistical Manual of Mental Disorders, Fourth Edition (DSM-IV), Washington, DC, American Psychiatric Association, 1994, pp 273–290.
2. Carpenter WT, Buchanan RW. Schizophrenia. N Engl J Med 1994;330:681–690.
3. Ereshefsky L, Tran-Johnson TK, Watanabe MD. Pathophysiologic basis for schizophrenia and the efficacy of antipsychotics. Clin Pharm 1990;9:682–707.
4. Lieberman JA, Koreen AR. Neurochemistry and neuroendocrinology of schizophrenia: A selective review, in Shore D (ed): Schizophrenia 1993. Rockville, MD, National Institute of Mental Health, 1993, pp 197–255.
5. Pickar D. Serotonin and dopamine abnormalities in schizophrenia. J Clin Psychiatry Monograph Series 1994;12(2):10–15.
6. Gur RF. Functional brain-imaging studies in schizophrenia, in Bloom FE, Kupfer DJ (eds): Psychopharmacology: The Fourth Generation of Progress. New York, Raven Press, 1995, pp 1185–1192.
7. Heritch AJ. Evidence for reduced and dysregulated turnover of dopamine in schizophrenia. Schizophr Bulletin 1990;16:605–615.
8. Bunney BG, Bunney WE, Carlsson A. Schizophrenia and glutamate, in Bloom FE, Kupfer DJ (eds): Psychopharmacology: The Fourth Generation of Progress. New York, Raven Press, 1995, pp 1205–1214.
9. Gur RE, Pearlson GD. Neuroimaging in schizophrenia research, in Shore D (ed): Schizophrenia 1993. Rockville, MD, National Institute of Mental Health, 1993, pp 163–179.
10. Kendler KS, Diehl SR. The genetics of schizophrenia: A current, genetic, epidemiologic perspective, in Shore D (ed): Schizophrenia 1993. Rockville, MD, National Institute of Mental Health, 1993, pp 87–111.
11. Bogerts B. Recent advances in the neuropathology of schizophrenia, in Shore D (ed): Schizophrenia 1993. Rockville, MD, National Institute of Mental Health, 1993, pp 257–271.
12. Weinberger DR. Neurodevelopmental perspectives on schizophrenia, in Bloom FE, Kupfer DJ (eds): Psychopharmacology: The Fourth Generation of Progress. New York, Raven Press, 1995, pp 1171–1183.
13. Baldessarini RJ. Drugs and the treatment of psychiatric disorders, in Gilman AG, Rall TW, Nies AS, et al (eds): Goodman and Gilman's The Pharmacological Basis of Therapeutics, 8th ed. New York, Pergamon, 1990, pp 383–435.
14. The ad hoc committee on schizophrenia. Report on schizophrenia of the American College of Neuropsychopharmacology. Neuropsychopharmacology 1987;1:89–99.
15. Kahn RS, Davis KL. New developments in dopamine and schizophrenia, in Bloom FE, Kupfer DJ (eds): Psychopharmacology: The Fourth Generation of Progress. New York, Raven Press, 1995, pp 1193–1203.
16. Sokoloff P, Giros B, Martres MP, et al. Molecular cloning and characterization of a novel dopamine receptor (D3) as a target for neuroleptics. Nature 1990;347:146–151.
17. Waddington JL. Sight and insight: Brain dopamine receptor occupancy by neuroleptics visualised in living schizophrenic patients by positron emission tomography. Br J Psychiatry 1989;154:433–436.
18. Richelson E. Preclinical pharmacology of antipsychotic drugs: Relationship to efficacy and side effects. J Clin Psychiatry Monograph Series 1994;12(2):17–23.
19. Weinberger DR. Biological basis of schizophrenia: Structural/functional considerations relevant to potential for antipsychotic drug response. J Clin Psychiatry Monograph Series 1994;12(2):4–9.
20. Meltzer HY. Atypical antipsychotic drugs, in Bloom FE, Kupfer DJ (eds): Psychopharmacology: The Fourth Generation of Progress. New York, Raven Press, 1995, pp 1277–1286.
21. Ereshefsky L, Jann MW, Saklad SR, Davis CM. Bioavailability of psychotropic drugs: Historical perspective and pharmacokinetic overview. J Clin Psychiatry 1986;47(suppl 9):6–15.
22. Wirshing WC, Marder SR, Van Putten T, Ames D. Acute treatment of schizophrenia, in Bloom FE, Kupfer DJ (eds): Psychopharmacology: The Fourth Generation of Progress. New York, Raven Press, 1995, pp 1259–1266.
23. Van Putten T, Marder SR, Wirshing C, et al. Fluphenazine, its metabolites and clinical response. Presented at the National Institute of Mental Health 30th annual NCDEU meeting, Key Biscayne, FL, June 1, 1990.
24. Perry PJ, Miller DD, Arndt SV, Cadoret RJ. Clozapine and norclozapine plasma concentrations and clinical response of treatment-refractory schizophrenic patients. Am J Psychiatry 1991;148:231–235.
25. Hasegawa M, Gutierrez-Esteinou R, Way L, Meltzer H. Relationship between clinical efficacy and clozapine concentrations in plasma in schizophrenia: Effect of smoking. J Clin Psychopharmacol 1993;13:383–390.
26. Ereshefsky L, Saklad SR, Jann MW, et al. Future of depot neuroleptic therapy: Pharmacokinetics and pharmacodynamic approaches. J Clin Psychiatry 1984;45(5) (sec 2):50.
27. Marder SR, Van Putten T, Aravagiri M, et al. Fluphenazine plasma levels and clinical response. Psychopharmacol Bull 1990;26:256–259.
28. Andreasen NC, Flaum M, Swayze VW, et al. Positive and negative symptoms in schizophrenia. Arch Gen Psychiatry 1990;47:615–621.

29. Wetzler S. Measuring mental illness: Psychometric assessment for clinicians. Washington DC, American Psychiatric Association Press, 1988.
30. Anonymous. Drugs that cause psychiatric symptoms. Med Lett Drugs Ther 1993;35:65–70.
31. Awad AG. Drug therapy in schizophrenia: Variability of outcome and prediction of response. Can J Psychiatry 1989;34:711–720.
32. Van Putten T, Marder SR. Behavioral toxicity of antipsychotic drugs. J Clin Psychiatry 1987;48(suppl 9):13–19.
33. Frank AF, Gunderson JG. The role of the therapeutic alliance in the treatment of schizophrenia: Relationship to course and outcome. Arch Gen Psychiatry 1990;47:228–236.
34. Levinson DF, Simpson GM, Singh H, et al. Fluphenazine dose, clinical response, and extrapyramidal symptoms during acute treatment. Arch Gen Psychiatry 1990;47:761–768.
35. Schooler N. Presented at the New Clinical Drug Evaluation Unit (NCDEU) 30th annual meeting. Key Biscayne, FL, May 1990.
36. Csernansky JG, Newcomer JG. Maintenance drug treatment for schizophrenia, in Bloom FE, Kupfer DJ (eds): Psychopharmacology: The Fourth Generation of Progress. New York, Raven Press, 1995, pp 1267–1275.
37. Herz MI, Glazer WM, Mostert MA, et al. Intermittent vs maintenance medication in schizophrenia: Two year results. Arch Gen Psychiatry 1991;48:333–339.
38. Johnson DAW. Pharmacological treatment of patients with schizophrenia: Past and present problems and potential future therapy. Drugs 1990;39:481–488.
39. Chen A. Noncompliance in community psychiatry: A review of clinical interventions. Hosp Community Psychiatry 1991;42:282–287.
40. Ereshefsky L, Toney G, Saklad SR, Seidel DR. A loading-dose strategy for converting from oral to depot haloperidol. Hosp Comm Psychiatry 1993;44:1155–1161.
41. Hamann GL, Egan TM, Wells BG, et al. Injection site reactions after intramuscular administration of haloperidol decanoate 100 mg/mL. J Clin Psychiatry 1990;51:502–504.
42. Kane J, Honigfeld G, Singer J, et al. Clozapine for the treatment-resistant schizophrenic: A double blind comparison with chlorpromazine. Arch Gen Psychiatry 1988;45:789–796.
43. Baldessarini RJ, Frankenburg FR. Clozapine: A novel antipsychotic agent. N Engl J Med 1991;324:746–754.
44. Marder SR, Meibach RC, and the Risperidone Study Group. Risperidone in the treatment of schizophrenia. Am J Psychiatry 1994;151:825–835.
45. Risperdal, risperidone. Approved product labeling. Titusville, NJ, Janssen Pharmaceutica, August 1994.
46. Still DJ, Dorson PG, Crismon ML. The effects of risperidone in clozapine-treated schizophrenic patients. Abstracts of the 35th annual New Clinical Drug Evaluation Unit (NCDEU) program. 1995;35:P-68.
47. Pickar D, Litman RE, Konicki PE, et al. Neurochemical and neural mechanisms of positive and negative symptoms in schizophrenia, in Andreason NC (ed): Schizophrenia: Positive and Negative Symptoms and Syndromes. Modern Problems in Pharmacopsychiatry. Basel, Karger, 1990, 24, pp 124–151.
48. Wolkowitz OM, Breier A, Doran A, et al. Alprazolam augmentation of the antipsychotic effects of fluphenazine in schizophrenic patients. Arch Gen Psychiatry 1988;45:664–671.
49. Yudolfsky SC, Silver JM, Hales RE. Pharmacologic management of aggression in the elderly. J Clin Psychiatry 1990;5(suppl 10):22–28.
50. Lipinski JF, Keck PE, McElroy SL. β-Adrenergic antagonists in psychosis: Is improvement due to treatment of neuroleptic-induced akathisia? J Clin Psychopharmacol 1988;409–416.
51. Elphick M. Clinical issues in the use of carbamazepine in psychiatry: A review. Psychol Medicine 1989;19:591–604.
52. Crismon ML. Psychotropic drugs in the elderly: Principles of use. Am Pharm 1990;NS30(12):57–63.
53. Crismon ML. Drug induced extrapyramidal syndromes. US Pharmacist 1982;7(1):33–42.
54. Marsden CD, Jenner P. The pathophysiology of extrapyramidal side-effects of neuroleptic drugs. Psychol Med 1980;10:55–72.
55. Sramek JJ, Simpson GM, Morrison RL, Heiser JF. ACh agents for prophylaxis of neuroleptic-induced dystonic reactions: A prospective study. J Clin Psychiatry 1986;47:305–309.
56. Arana GW, Goff DC, Baldessarini RJ, Keepers GA. Efficacy of ACh prophylaxis for neuroleptic-induced acute dystonia. Am J Psychiatry 1988;145:993–996.
57. World Health Organization (WHO). Prophylactic use of anticholinergics in patients on long-term neuroleptic treatment: A consensus statement. Br J Psychiatry 1990;156:412.
58. Braude WM, Barnes TRE, Gore SM. Clinical characteristics of akathisia: A systematic investigation of acute psychiatric inpatient admissions. Br J Psychiatry 1983;143:139–150.
59. Lieberman JA, Saltz BL, Johns CA, et al. The effects of clozapine on tardive dyskinesia. Br J Psychiatry 1991;158:503–510.
60. Fleischhacker WW, Roth SD, Kane JM. The pharmacologic treatment of neuroleptic-induced akathisia. J Clin Psychopharmacol 1990;10:12–21.
61. McEvoy JP. The clinical use of ACh drugs as treatment for extrapyramidal side effects of neuroleptic drugs. J Clin Psychopharmacol 1983;3:288–302.
62. Wells BG, Marken PA, Rickman LA, et al. Characterizing anticholinergic abuse in community mental health. J Clin Psychopharmacol 1989;9:431–435.
63. Anonymous. Tardive dyskinesia scales in current use, in Fann W, Smith RC, Davis JM, et al. (eds): Tardive Dyskinesia Research and Treatment. Jamaica, NY, Spectrum Publications, 1980, pp 243–267.
64. Sprague RL, Kalachnik JE. Reliability, validity, and a total score cutoff for the Dyskinesia Identification System Condensed User Scale (DISCUS) with mentally ill and mentally retarded populations. Psychopharmacol Bull 1991;27:51–58.
65. Gerlach J, Casey DE. Tardive dyskinesia. Acta Psychiatr Scand 1988;77:369–378.
66. Kane JM, Smith J. Tardive dyskinesia: Prevalence and risk factors 1959–1979. Arch Gen Psychiatry 1982;39:473–481.

67. Gardos G, Cole JO. Tardive dyskinesia and anticholinergic drugs. Am J Psychiatry 1983;140:200–202.
68. Yesavage JA, Tanke ED, Sheikh JI. Tardive dyskinesia and steady-state serum levels of thiothixene. Arch Gen Psychiatry 1987;44:913–915.
69. Kane JM, Woerner M, Borenstein M, et al. Integrating incidence and prevalence of tardive dyskinesia. Psychopharmacol Bull 1986;22:254–258.
70. Yagi G, Itoh H. Follow-up study of 11 patients with potentially reversible tardive dyskinesia. Am J Psychiatry 1987;144:1496–1498.
71. Casey DE, Povisen UJ, Meidahl B, et al. Neuroleptic-induced tardive dyskinesia and parkinsonism: Changes during several years of continuing treatment. Psychopharmacol Bull 1986;22:250–253.
72. Chouinard G, Annable L, Mercier P, Ross-Chouinard A. A five year follow-up study of tardive dyskinesia. Psychopharmacol Bull 1986;22:259–263.
73. Gardos G, Cole JO, Salomon M, Schniebolk S. Clinical forms of severe tardive dyskinesia. Am J Psychiatry 1987;144:895–902.
74. Jeste DV, Wyatt RJ. Therapeutic strategies against tardive dyskinesia: Two decades of experience. Arch Gen Psychiatry 1982;39:803–816.
75. Gelenberg AJ, Dorer DJ, Wojcik JD, et al. A crossover study of lecithin treatment of tardive dyskinesia. J Clin Psychiatry 1990;51:149–153.
76. Dabiri LM, Pasta D, Darby J, Mosbacher D. Effectiveness of vitamin E for treatment of long-term tardive dyskinesia. Am J Psychiatry 1994;151:925–926.
77. Egan MF, Hyde TM, Albers GW, et al. Treatment of tardive dyskinesia with vitamin E. Am J Psychiatry 1992;149:773–777.
78. Shriqui CL, Bradwejn J, Annable L, Jones BD. Vitamin E in the treatment of tardive dyskinesia: A double-blind, placebo-controlled study. Am J Psychiatry 1992;149:391–393.
79. Cassens G, Inglis AK, Appelbaum PS, Gutheil TG. Neuroleptics: Effects on neuropsychological function in chronic schizophrenic patients. Schizophr Bull 1990;16:477–499.
80. Garcia G, Crismon ML, Dorson PG. Seizures in two patients after the addition of lithium to a clozapine regimen. J Clin Psychopharmacol 1994;14:426–428.
81. Cold JA, Wells BG, Froemming JH. Seizure activity associated with AP therapy. DICP Ann Pharmacother 1990;24:601–606.
82. Simpson GM, Pi EH, Sramek JJ. Adverse effects of AP agents. Drugs 1981;21:138–151.
83. Guze BH, Baxter Jr LR. Neuroleptic malignant syndrome. N Engl J Med 1985;313:163–166.
84. Sakkas P, Davis JM, Hua J, et al. Pharmacotherapy of neuroleptic malignant syndrome. Psychiatr Ann 1991;21:157–164.
85. Wells AJ, Sommi RW, Crismon ML. Neuroleptic rechallenge after neuroleptic malignant syndrome: Case report and literature review. Drug Intell Clin Pharm 1988;22:475–480.
86. Webster P, Wijeratne C. Risperidone-induced neuroleptic malignant syndrome. Lancet 1994;344:1228–1229.
87. Gelenberg AJ, Mandel MR. Catatonic reactions to high-potency neuroleptic drugs. Arch Gen Psychiatry 1977;34:947–950.
88. Zito JM, Sofair JB, Jaeger J. Self-reported neuroendocrine effects of APs in women: A pilot study. DICP Ann Pharmacother 1990;24:176–180.
89. Risch SC, Groom GP, Janowsky DS. The effects of psychotropic drugs on the cardiovascular system. J Clin Psychiatry 1982;43:5(sec 2)16–31.
90. Perry PJ, Alexander B, Liskow B. Psychotropic Drug Handbook, 6th ed. Cincinnati, OH, Harvey Whitney Books, 1991, pp 3–34, 247–248.
91. Regal RE, Billi JE, Glazer HM. Phenothiazine-induced cholestatic jaundice. Clin Pharm 1987;6:787–794.
92. Nurnberg HG, Ambrosini PJ. Urinary incontinence in patients receiving neuroleptics. J Clin Psychiatry 1979;40:271–274.
93. Sullivan G, Lukoff D. Sexual side effects of AP medication: Evaluation and interventions. Hosp Community Psychiatry 1990;41:1238–1241.
94. Balon R, Berchou R. Hematologic side effects of psychotropic drugs. Psychosomatics 1986;27:119–120, 125–127.
95. Alvir JMJ, Lieberman JA, Safferman AZ, et al. Clozapine-induced agranulocytosis: Incidence and risk factors in the United States. N Engl J Med 1993;329:162–167.
96. Ereshefsky L, Watanabe MD, Tran-Johnson TK. Clozapine: An atypical antipsychotic agent. Clin Pharm 1989;8:691–709.
97. Gullion G, Yeh HS. Treatment of clozapine-induced agranulocytosis with recombinant granulocyte colony-stimulating factor. J Clin Psychiatry 1994;55:401–405.
98. Dorson PG, Crismon ML. CPZ accumulation and sudden death in a patient with renal insufficiency. Drug Intell Clin Pharm 1988;22:776–778.
99. Grabowski J. Clonidine treatment of clozapine-induced hypersalivation. J Clin Psychopharmacol 1992;12:69–70.
100. Mortola JF. The use of psychotropic drugs in pregnancy and lactation. Psychiatr Clin North Am 1989;12:69–87.
101. Karkji SD, Holden JM. Combined use of HPD and lithium. Psychiatric Ann 1990;20:154–161.
102. Callahan AM, Fava M, Rosenbaum JF. Drug interactions in psychopharmacology. Psychiatric Clin N Am 1993;16:647–671.

Chapter 67

Depressive Disorders

Barbara G. Wells, PharmD, FASHP, FCCP, Laura A. Mandos, PharmD, and Peggy E. Hayes, PharmD

Mood disorders (affective disorders) are among the most common mental disorders encountered in clinical practice and are divided into bipolar disorders and depressive disorders. The essential feature of these disorders is a major disturbance in mood. Mood is defined as a pervasive and sustained emotion that, in the extreme, markedly affects the person's perception of the world. A mood disorder occurs when a mood disturbance is combined with certain associated symptoms that impair the person's ability to function for a minimal duration of time. Bipolar disorders (discussed in Chapter 68) refer to patients who have episodes of mania and/or hypomania usually alternating with episodes of depression.[1]

Patients with depressive disorders do not have a history of mania or hypomania. Various names (or classifications) used to describe depressive disorders have included reactive, unipolar, psychotic and neurotic, exogenous and endogenous, agitated and retarded, primary and secondary, and involutional melancholia.[2] Clinicians are currently using the diagnostic criteria for depressive disorders listed in the *Diagnostic and Statistical Manual of Mental Disorders, Fourth Edition* (DSM-IV), published by the American Psychiatric Association in 1994.[1] The use of these standardized criteria has greatly improved clinicians' ability to diagnose correctly and appropriately treat depressive disorders. Major depressive disorder and dysthymic disorder are types of depressive disorders listed in the DSM-IV. Dysthymic disorder is a chronic disturbance of mood involving depressed mood and at least two other symptoms such as appetite or sleep disturbance, low energy, low self-esteem, hopelessness, poor concentration, and indeciveness. There is a history of a depressed mood more days than not, for at least 2 years.[2] However, these symptoms are not of sufficient severity or duration to meet the criteria for major depression. This chapter focuses on the diagnosis and treatment of major depressive disorder.

Major depressive disorder is one of the most common health problems of patients seen in primary care settings. It is associated with a high level of functional disability and increased use of medical services.[3] Recently, the functioning and well-being of depressed patients was compared with that of patients with chronic medical conditions (e.g., hypertension, diabetes, and arthritis). Depressed patients had significantly worse social, role, and physical functioning, spent more days in bed, and had more bodily pain (except arthritic patients) than medical patients.[4] A 2-year follow-up study concluded that depressed patients have substantial and long-lasting impairments of functioning and well-being that equal or exceed those of patients with chronic medical conditions.[5] A large part of the costs of depression comes from work days lost each year.[2]

The most frequent complication of depression is suicide. Approximately 15% of patients with unrecognized or inadequately treated depression commit suicide; this is approximately 30 times the rate of occurrence in nondepressed patients.[2,6] Although adequate treatment reduces the risk of suicide and improves functioning and well-being, studies conducted in primary care settings reported that even when depression is accurately diagnosed, few patients receive an adequate dose and duration of antidepressant treatment. The gap between research findings and clinical practice is especially wide in the management of depression.[3]

Fortunately, depression is no longer viewed as a disease that can be cured by "pulling oneself up by the bootstraps." The introduction of effective antidepressant drugs with distinctly different side-effect profiles and relatively greater safety in an overdose situation has enabled more patients to be successfully managed in the community.

EPIDEMIOLOGY

The true prevalence of depressive disorders in the United States is unknown. The National Institute of Mental Health Epidemiologic Catchment Area (ECA) study, an extensive community survey, reported that the 6-month prevalence rates for mood disorders were 6% (the lifetime rate was 8.3%), while only 31% of depressed adults sought treatment.[7] A recent survey, the National Comorbidity Survey (NCS), reported that 17% of the population had a history of major depressive disorder in their lifetime, and more than 10% had an episode in the past 12 months.[8] Evidence supports increasing rates and a decreasing age of onset of depression in persons born after World War II.[9]

Depression is two to three times as frequent in females as males.[1,8,9] Although depression can occur at any age, the highest rates of major depression occurred in adults 25–44 years old.[8,9] Depressive symptoms occur in about 15% of those 65 and older living in the community[7,8] and the prevalence of major depression is approximately 10–20% among elderly persons in institutions.[6] Depressive disorders are quite common during adolescence. Rates of alcoholism, substance abuse, and suicide attempts and deaths have increased in these young patients.[9] Patients with depressive disorder have a high risk of developing another psychiatric illness (comorbidity), especially anxiety disorders and alcoholism.[2,8]

Depressive disorders and suicide tend to cluster in families, and first-degree relatives of patients with depression are one and a half to three times more likely to develop depression than controls.[1,9,10] Approximately 8–18% of patients with major depression have at least one first-degree relative (father, mother, brother, or sister) with a history of depression compared with 5.6% of the first-degree relatives of a normal control group.[10,11] Twin studies of major depression estimate the concordance rate for monozygotic (identical) twins to be 54–65% and the rate for dizygotic (fraternal) twins to be 14–24%.[11]

PATHOPHYSIOLOGY

The etiology of depressive disorders is too complex to be totally explained by a single social, developmental, or biologic theory. A variety of factors appear to work together to cause or precipitate depressive disorders. Patients with major depression have symptoms that reflect changes in brain monoamine neurotransmitters, specifically norepinephrine (NE), serotonin (5-HT), and dopamine (DA).[12]

Although life is filled with unexpected events that cause pain (death of a loved one, loss of a job, major illness, loss of functioning through advancing age), not everyone becomes depressed. Most individuals adjust to life's challenges and suffer only mild, transient dysphoric feelings. However, some individuals exposed to these psychosocial stressors or unfortunate life events experience a major depressive episode. The initial episodes of depression are more likely to be associated with stressful life events than are later episodes.[12] Certain factors (e.g., stressful events, medical illness, monoamine-depleting drugs) may place predisposed individuals, especially those with a family or personal history of depression, at high risk for developing a major depressive episode.[12]

BIOGENIC AMINE HYPOTHESIS

A generation ago, it was known that most effective antidepressants increased the availability of monoamines at the synapse.[13] Also, early studies reported that reserpine, an antihypertensive drug that depleted neuronal storage granules of NE, 5-HT, and DA, produced clinically significant depression in 15% or more of patients.[14] These observations lead to the early hypothesis that depression was caused by inadequate monoamine neurotransmission, most notably NE.[15] However, this early hypothesis failed to explain the actual cause of depression. While reuptake blockade or monoamine oxidase inhibition occurs immediately upon administration of an antidepressant medication, antidepressant clinical effects are generally not observed until after 4 weeks of dosing.[16]

PERMISSIVE HYPOTHESIS

In the early 1970s, Prange and colleagues put forth the "permissive hypothesis of affective illness" to accommodate observations in the literature on both NE and 5-HT and to explain the results of their carefully controlled trial that showed an antimanic effect of L-tryptophan, a precursor of 5-HT.[17]

As the theory states, low 5-HT permits the expression of the affective state, but the type is governed by the level of NE. Low NE levels cause depression; high NE levels cause mania. According to this hypothesis, correcting the low 5-HT activity corrects the affective disease.

THEORIES OF POSTSYNAPTIC CHANGES IN RECEPTOR SENSITIVITY

One of the more perplexing aspects of the observed effects of antidepressants is the discrepancy in the time course between monoamine reuptake blockade and measurable improvement in depressive symptomatology. Accordingly, theories that focus on adaptive changes in amine receptor systems have emerged.

In the mid-1970s, Vetulani and coworkers presented data to help explain this observation.[18] Chronic, but not acute, administration of antidepressants in animals caused desensitization of NE-stimulated cyclic AMP synthesis. In fact, for most antidepressants, down-regulation of β-adrenergic receptors accompanies this desensitization.

Studies of many antidepressants have demonstrated that either desensitization or down-regulation of NE receptors corresponds to a clinically relevant time course for antidepressant effects.[19] Other studies have revealed down-regulation of 5-HT_2 receptors following chronic administration of antidepressants.[19,20] Thus, a theory based on postsynaptic changes in receptor sensitivity provides a cogent explanation of the delayed onset of activity of antidepressant drugs.[19]

DYSREGULATION HYPOTHESIS

The dysregulation hypothesis incorporates the diversity of antidepressant activity with the adaptive changes occurring in receptor sensitization over several weeks.[21] In this theory, emphasis is placed on a failure of homeostatic regulation of neurotransmitter systems, rather than on absolute increases or decreases in their activities.[21,22] According to this hypothesis, effective antidepressant agents restore efficient regulation to the dysregulated neurotransmitter system.[21,22]

5-HT/NE LINK HYPOTHESIS

As clinical evidence accumulates, it is apparent that no single neurotransmitter theory of depression is adequate. The 5-HT/NE link hypothesis was proposed by Sulser[23]; it maintains that both the serotonergic and noradrenergic systems need to be intact for an antidepressant effect to be exerted. The 5-HT/NE link hypothesis is also consistent with the rationale of the postsynaptic alteration theory of depression, which emphasizes the importance of β-adrenergic receptor down-regulation for achieving an antidepressant effect.[19] Again, it has been proposed that both NE and 5-HT are necessary for homologous desensitization of central β-adrenergic receptors by antidepressants.[23,24]

ROLE OF DOPAMINE IN DEPRESSION

Traditional explanations of the biological basis of depressive disorders have focused largely on NE and 5-HT; however, most of the evidence that coalesced into the biogenic amine hypothesis of depression does not clearly distinguish between NE and DA.[25]

Several reviews suggest that elevation of DA neurotransmission in the nucleus accumbens may represent a final common pathway for at least part of the mechanism of action of antidepressant medications.[26,27] The mechanisms by which antidepressant drugs sensitize dopamine transmission remain unclear, but may be indirectly mediated by primary actions at NE or 5-HT terminals.

The evidence supporting a dopaminergic mechanism of antidepressant action is entirely preclinical: Clinical studies evaluating the role of DA mechanisms in the action of classical antidepressants have not been articulated.[25]

The complexity of the interaction between 5-HT, NE, and possibly DA is gaining greater appreciation, but a more in-depth understanding of the precise mechanism is needed.

BIOLOGIC MARKERS

Investigators continue to search for biologic markers to assist in the diagnosis and treatment of depressed patients. Although no biologic marker has been discovered, several interesting biologic abnormalities are present in many depressed patients. Approximately 45–60% of patients with major depression have a neuroendocrine abnormality, including hypersecretion of cortisol, lack of cortisol suppression after dexamethasone administration (i.e., a positive dexamethasome suppression test [DST]), or an abnormal or diminished thyroid-stimulating hormone (TSH) response to the administration of thyrotropin-releasing hormone (TRH).[12] The DST is the most specific measure of hypothalamic–pituitary–adrenal (HPA) axis overactivity. Dexamethasone administration suppresses adrenal corticosteroid production in normal subjects for 24 hours. Failure of dexamethasone to suppress plasma cortisol concentrations indicates overactivity or dysregulation of the HPA axis, and in depressed patients this also reflects an increased vulnerability to suicide.[12] The DST is reserved for patients whose diagnosis is in doubt, and then only to confirm clinical impressions. Unfortunately, the high rate of false positives and false negatives limits the usefulness in testing for these markers.

The results of sleep studies in patients with major depression have reported several abnormalities that become more pronounced with advancing age. The onset of rapid eye movement (REM) sleep occurs sooner in depressed patients (decreased REM latency) than in the normal population. There may also be a decrease in slow-wave sleep, a shift of REM sleep activity to the first half of the night, increased disruption of sleep, and early morning awakening.[28] Sleep abnormalities occur in other psychiatric disorders and are not diagnostic for major depression.

CLINICAL PRESENTATION

DIAGNOSIS

When a patient presents with depressive symptoms, it is necessary to investigate the possibility of a medical, psychiatric, and/or drug-induced cause (Table 67.1).[29] Up to 25% of patients with chronic medical conditions (e.g., diabetes, myocardial infarction, carcinomas, stroke) will develop a major depressive episode during the course of their medical condition, and the diagnosis is often missed, especially in the elderly.[1,6]

Clinicians should also be alert for major depression in some patients with alcoholism. Patients often self-medicate with alcohol or other drugs to mask or partially mask their symptoms of depression. Concomitant depressive symptoms may be present in patients with Alzheimer's disease,

TABLE 67.1. COMMON MEDICAL DISORDERS, PSYCHIATRIC DISORDERS, AND DRUG THERAPY ASSOCIATED WITH DEPRESSION

Medical Disorders		Psychiatric Disorders
Endocrine diseases	Systemic lupus erythematosus	Alcoholism
Hyperthyroidism	Metabolic disorders	Anxiety disorders
Hypothyroidism	Electrolyte imbalance	Eating disorders
Addison's disease	Hypokalemia	Schizophrenia
Cushing's disease	Hyponatremia	**Drug Therapy**
Deficiency states	Hepatic encephalopathy	Alcohol
Pernicious anemia	Cardiovascular disease	Antihypertensives
Wernicke's encephalopathy	Cerebral arteriosclerosis	Reserpine
Severe anemia	Congestive heart failure	Methyldopa
Infections	Myocardial infarction	Propranolol hydrochloride
Encephalitis	Neurologic disorders	Guanethidine sulfate
Influenza	Alzheimer's disease	Hydralazine hydrochloride
Mononucleosis	Huntington's disease	Clonidine hydrochloride
Tuberculosis	Multiple sclerosis	Diuretics
AIDS	Parkinson's disease	Oral contraceptives
Collagen disorders	Poststroke	Steroids/ACTH
	Malignant disease	

(Compiled from Ref. 29.)

and untreated major depression is frequently the cause of intellectual or cognitive difficulties in the elderly.[2,6]

The differential diagnosis of a major depressive episode and normal grief caused by the death of a loved one (bereavement) is often difficult, because of overlapping symptoms. Grief is characterized as a self-limited reaction to loss that requires no intensive medical intervention. Bereavement should be considered a major depressive episode only if the symptoms are still present 2 months after the loss or if there are suicidal thoughts, psychomotor retardation, marked functional impairment, feelings of worthlessness, and psychotic symptoms.[1]

All depressed patients, especially the elderly, should have a complete physical examination, mental status examination, and basic laboratory workup, including a complete blood count with differential, thyroid function tests, and electrolyte determinations to identify any potential medical problems. A complete medication review should be performed, since many drugs (e.g., propranolol)[30] can precipitate or worsen a depressive episode (Table 67.1).

Major depressive disorder is characterized by one or more episodes of major depression. A major depressive episode is characterized by five or more of the symptoms described in Table 67.2. At least one of the symptoms is depressed mood (often an irritable mood in children or adolescents) or loss of interest or pleasure in nearly all activities.[1] The five symptoms must have been present nearly every day for at least 2 weeks and must represent a change from previous functioning. The clinician must consider presenting symptoms, their duration, and the patient's current level of social, occupational, or other important areas of functioning. Significant stressors or life events may trigger depression in some, but not others, and there may be an important precipitant at the beginning of the disorder.[1,2]

EMOTIONAL SYMPTOMS

Major depressive episode is characterized by a persistent, diminished ability to experience pleasure. A loss of interest and pleasure in usual activities, hobbies, or work is common. Patients appear sad or depressed, and they are often

TABLE 67.2. DSM-IV CRITERIA FOR MAJOR DEPRESSIVE EPISODE

A. Five (or more) of the following symptoms have been present during the same 2-week period and represent a change from previous functioning; at least one of the symptoms is either (1) depressed mood or (2) loss of interest or pleasure.
   1. Depressed mood most of the day, nearly every day
   2. Markedly diminished interest or pleasure in all, or almost all, activities
   3. Significant weight loss (not dieting) or weight gain, or decrease or increase in appetite nearly every day
   4. Insomnia or hypersomnia nearly every day
   5. Psychomotor agitation or retardation nearly every day (observable)
   6. Fatigue or loss of energy nearly every day
   7. Feelings of worthlessness or excessive or inappropriate guilt (may be delusional) nearly every day
   8. Diminished ability to think or concentrate, or indecisiveness
   9. Recurrent thoughts of death, recurrent suicidal ideation without a specific plan, or a suicide attempt or a specific suicide plan

B. The symptoms cause clinically significant distress or impairment in social, occupational, or other important areas of functioning.

C. The symptoms are not due to the direct physiologic effects of a substance or a general medical condition (e.g., hypothyroidism).

(Modified from American Psychiatric Association. *Diagnostic and Statistical Manual of Mental Disorders, Fourth Edition.* Washington, DC, American Psychiatric Association, 1994, p 327.)

pessimistic and believe that nothing will help them feel better. Patients often weep or report crying spells. The presence of intense hopelessness and complete or near total loss of interest and pleasure in usual activities may identify patients at risk for suicide.[31] Anxiety symptoms are present in almost 90% of depressed outpatients.

Patients often feel they have let others down. These guilt feelings are unrealistic and may reach delusional proportions. Patients may feel they are responsible for the sins of the world and that they deserve punishment; they may view their present illness as a punishment. A depressed patient may hear voices (auditory hallucinations) saying that he or she is a bad person and that he or she should commit suicide. Depression with psychotic features usually requires hospitalization, especially if the patient becomes a danger to self or others.

PHYSICAL SYMPTOMS

These symptoms often motivate the patient, especially the elderly, to seek medical attention. Chronic fatigue is a common complaint, and patients complain of loss of energy and feeling tired with a decreased ability to perform normal, daily tasks. Fatigue often seems worse in the morning and does not improve with rest. Complaints of pain, especially headache, often accompany fatigue.

Sleep disturbances generally present as frequent early morning awakening (terminal insomnia), with difficulty returning to sleep. This may coexist with difficulty falling asleep (initial insomnia) and frequent nighttime awakening. Less frequently, depressed patients complain of increased sleep or hypersomnia, although they experience daytime exhaustion or fatigue.

Appetite disturbances, including complaints of decreased appetite, often result in substantial weight loss, especially in the elderly.[6] Some patients lose two or more pounds per week without dieting. Other patients, especially in the ambulatory setting, may overeat and gain weight, although they may not actually enjoy eating. They may crave specific foods.

Some patients exhibit gastrointestinal complaints, others cardiovascular complaints, especially heart palpitations. Patients frequently present with a loss of sexual interest or libido.

INTELLECTUAL OR COGNITIVE SYMPTOMS

These symptoms include a decreased ability to concentrate, slowed thinking, and a poor memory for recent events. Patients may appear confused and indecisive. Depression should be considered when cognitive symptoms are present in the elderly.[6]

PSYCHOMOTOR DISTURBANCES

Patients may appear noticeably slowed or retarded in physical movements, thought processes, and speech (psychomotor retardation). Conversely, depression may be accompanied by psychomotor agitation manifesting as purposeless, restless motion (e.g., pacing, wringing of hands, outbursts of shouting).

SUICIDE RISK EVALUATION AND MANAGEMENT

Depressed patients should be assessed for suicidal thoughts. Widely held myths regarding suicide include the belief that people are more likely to commit suicide if they are asked about it; that people who attempt or talk about suicide are just looking for attention and are not serious; that suicidal people are crazy; and that most suicides are caused by a sudden traumatic event.

Factors that increase the risk for suicide include increasing age, being widowed, being unmarried, being unemployed, living alone, a history of a previous psychiatric admission, substance abuse, depression, and feelings of hopelessness.[31] The presence of a very detailed plan with the intention and ability to carry it out indicates strong intent and a high risk of suicide. Although women attempt suicide two to three times more often than men, men succeed about three times more frequently. Completed suicide rates in 80- to 84-year-olds are more than twice the ratio in the general population (i.e., 26.5 versus 12.4/100,000).[32] Additional factors that increase suicide risk are prior attempts, family history of suicide, anniversary of a loss, presence of a serious medical problem, lack of a social support system, and refusal to seek help.

In assessing the severity of suicidal thoughts, the clinician must be sensitive to hints of suicidal ideation including a change in personality, a sudden decision to make a will or give away possessions, and recent purchase of a gun or obtaining (or hoarding) a large supply of medications or other potentially toxic substances. It must be recognized that it is not possible to predict accurately whether or when a depressed person will attempt suicide.

When suicidal intent is suspected, it is important to ask, "Are you thinking about harming or killing yourself?" If the risk is determined to be significant, the patient must be referred to the appropriate health care professional, and a family member must be contacted.

CLASSIFICATION/PROGNOSIS

A major depressive episode is subclassified in the DSM-IV according to severity (mild, moderate, or severe). A severe episode of depression may present with or without psychotic symptoms. Psychotic symptoms include delusions (a false fixed belief) and hallucinations (a sensory perception in the absence of an actual stimulus) that are entirely consistent with the depressed mood (mood-congruent).[1]

A major depressive episode may be further described as chronic (the current episode has lasted for 2 years), with melancholic features, or with a seasonal pattern. Major depression with melancholic features is usually severe and particularly responsive to drug therapy or electroconvulsive therapy (ECT). Melancholic features include a nearly complete absence of the capacity for pleasure, diurnal mood swings (symptoms are worse in the morning), early morning awakening, marked psychomotor retardation or agitation, excessive or inappropriate guilt, and significant weight loss.[1] In depression with a seasonal pattern, there is a regular temporal relationship between the onset of the depression and a particular time of the year (onset in the winter, remission in spring or summer).[1]

Depressive episodes may be further described as having catatonic features. These features could include (1) motoric immobility, (2) excessive motor activity, (3) extreme negativism or mutism, (4) peculiarities of voluntary movement, and (5) ecolalia or echopraxia. In major depression with atypical features, the mood is responsive to actual or potential positive events. In addition, the patient exhibits two or more of the following: (1) weight gain or increase in appetite, (2) hypersomnia, (3) heavy feelings in arms or legs, and/or (4) interpersonal rejection sensitivity. Postpartum onset major depression is an episode with onset within 4 weeks postpartum.[1]

The natural course of a major depressive episode is variable, but is generally characterized by remissions and relapses. Although 30% of patients have only a single episode, relapse occurs in about 70%. Most treated episodes last approximately 3 months, while untreated episodes last about 6–12 months.[1,2] Although most individuals usually function well between episodes, in about 20–35% of the patients even with treatment, the disease is chronic with considerable residual symptoms and social impairment. Older persons are less likely to recover fully from an episode of depression.[6]

TREATMENT

The goals of treatment of the acute depressive episode are to reduce the symptoms of depression and facilitate the patient's return to a premorbid level (before the onset of the illness) of functioning. Whether or not to hospitalize the patient is the first decision in the treatment plan. This decision is made in consideration of the patient's risk of suicide, physical state of health, social support system, and the presence of a psychotic and/or catatonic depression.

Studies comparing the efficacy of antidepressants have found that antidepressants are equivalent when administered in comparable doses. Because one cannot predict which antidepressant will be the most effective, the initial choice is made empirically. Factors that often influence the choice of an antidepressant include the patient's past history of response, pharmacogenetics (the history of familial antidepressant response), the subtype of depression, the patient's concurrent medical history, the potential for drug–drug interactions, the adverse events profile of the various antidepressants, and drug cost.

Because of the various treatment options, depression in a sense has become to psychiatry what hypertension is to internal medicine.[33] Although the pathophysiology of major depression remains elusive, the clinician can now select from multiple drug therapies with different mechanisms of action. Failure to respond to one antidepressant class does not predict a failed response to another drug class.

Approximately 65–70% of patients with varying types of depression improve with drug therapy compared with 30–40% who improve with placebo. Melancholic depression appears to respond well to tricyclic antidepressants (TCAs) and selective serotonin reuptake inhibitors (SSRIs).[33] A preferential response to monoamine oxidase inhibitors (MAOIs) has been reported in patients with atypical depression.[34] Psychotically depressed individuals generally require either ECT or combination therapy with an antidepressant plus an antipsychotic agent.[35]

CLASSIFICATION OF ANTIDEPRESSANTS

Antidepressants can be classified in several ways. One approach is by chemical structure, and another is by the presumed mechanism of antidepressant activity (Table 67.3). Although the link between the presumed mechanism of drug action and antidepressant response is tenuous, this classification has the advantage of being based on established pharmacology and clearly explains some of the actions (i.e., adverse effects) of the antidepressants. The knowledgeable clinician can use these facts to tailor treatment to individual patient needs and thereby optimize treatment outcome. Currently available antidepressants, their manufacturers, and initial dosages are shown in Table 67.4.

TABLE 67.3. CLASSIFICATION OF ANTIDEPRESSANT PHARMACOTHERAPY BY PRESUMED MECHANISM OF ACTION

Mixed 5-HT/NE reuptake inhibitors	TCAs, venlafaxine
SSRIs	Fluoxetine, paroxetine, sertraline, fluvoxamine
Mixed serotonin effects	Trazodone, nefazodone
Mixed NE/DA reuptake inhibitors	Bupropion
MAOIs	Phenelzine, tranylcypromine

TABLE 67.4. ADULT DOSAGES FOR CURRENTLY AVAILABLE ANTIDEPRESSANT MEDICATIONS

Generic Name	Trade Name	Manufacturer	Suggested Therapeutic Plasma Concentration Range (ng/mL)	Initial Dose[a] (mg/d)	Usual Dosage Range[a] (mg/d)
Tricyclic antidepressants					
Tertiary amines					
Amitriptyline	Elavil	Stuart	120–250[b]	50–75	100–300
	Endep	Roche			
	Generic	Various			
Clomipramine	Anafranil	Basel		25	100–250
Doxepin	Adapin	Lotus Biochemical	110–250[b]	50–75	100–300
	Sinequan	Roerig			
	Generic	Various			
Imipramine	Tofranil	Geigy	200–300[b]	50–75	100–300
	Generic	Various			
Trimipramine	Surmontil	Wyeth-Ayerst		50–75	100–300
Secondary amines					
Desipramine	Norpramin	Marion Merrell Dow	125–300	50–75	100–300
	Generic	Various			
Nortriptyline	Pamelor	Sandoz	50–150	25–50	50–150
	Generic	Various			
Protriptyline	Vivactil	Merck	70–240	10–20	15–60
Dibenzoxazepine					
Amoxapine	Asendin	Lederle	200–400[c]	50–150	100–400
	Generic	Various			
Tetracyclic					
Maprotiline	Ludiomil	Ciba	200–300[b]	50–75	100–225
	Generic	Various			
Triazolopyridines					
Nefazodone	Serzone	Bristol-Myers Squibb		200	300–600
Trazodone	Desyrel	Apothecon		50–150	150–400
	Generic	Various			
Aminoketone					
Bupropion	Wellbutrin	Burroughs Wellcome	50–100	200	300–450
Monoamine oxidase inhibitors					
Phenelzine	Nardil	Parke-Davis		15	15–90
Tranlycypromine	Parnate	SmithKline Beecham		20	20–60
Selective serotonin reuptake inhibitors					
Fluoxetine	Prozac	Dista		10–20	10–80
Fluvoxamine	Luvox	Solvay		50	50–300
Paroxetine	Paxil	SmithKline Beecham		20	20–50
Sertraline	Zoloft	Roerig		50	100–200
Serotonin/norepinephrine reuptake inhibitor					
Venlafaxine	Effexor	Wyeth-Ayerst		75	75–375

[a]Doses listed are total daily doses; elderly patients are usually treated with approximately one-half of the dose listed.
[b]Parent drug plus demethylated metabolite.
[c]Parent drug plus hydroxymetabolite. (Modified from Refs. 16, 21, 40, 47, 49, and 73.)

Mixed Serotonin and Norepinephrine Reuptake Inhibitors

Among the TCAs, amitriptyline and imipramine are the most extensively studied, either directly against placebo or as an active control for another antidepressant. Studies comparing the secondary amine TCAs (desipramine and nortriptyline) to the tertiary amine TCAs (amitriptyline and imipramine) found no clinically important difference in efficacy; however, the secondary amines were more potent on a milligram to milligram basis.[36]

The TCAs are effective in treating all depressive subtypes, especially the severe melancholic subtype of major depressive disorder. All TCAs potentiate the activity of NE and 5-HT by blocking their reuptake. However, the potency and selectivity of TCAs for the inhibition of NE and 5-HT vary greatly among these agents (Table 67.5). Because TCAs affect other receptor systems, anticholinergic, neurologic, and cardiovascular adverse events are frequently reported during TCA therapy.[21]

Venlafaxine, a structurally novel antidepressant, is a potent inhibitor of 5-HT and NE reuptake and a weak inhibitor of dopamine reuptake. Unlike the TCAs, it has virtually no affinity for muscarinic, histaminergic, and α_1-adrenergic receptors.[37]

Maprotiline and amoxapine are both inhibitors of NE reuptake, with less effect on 5-HT reuptake. Maprotiline is associated with a higher incidence of seizures than is imipramine or amitriptyline.[21] Amoxapine, while less sedating than some antidepressants, blocks cholinergic receptors, causing clinically significant anticholinergic effects.

Selective Serotonin Reuptake Inhibitors

The impetus for the development of the SSRIs was the perceived need for antidepressants with an improved efficacy and adverse effect profile compared with the traditional TCAs. There is a substantial body of knowledge to indicate that the efficacy of SSRIs is superior to placebo and equal

TABLE 67.5. RELATIVE POTENCIES OF NOREPINEPHRINE AND SEROTONIN REUPTAKE BLOCKADE AND SIDE-EFFECTS PROFILE OF ANTIDEPRESSANT DRUGS

	Reuptake Antagonism		Anticholinergic		Orthostatic		Conduction
	Norepinephrine	Serotonin	Effects	Sedation	Hypotension	Seizures	Abnormalities
Tertiary amines							
Amitriptyline	++	++++	++++	++++	+++	+++	+++
Clomipramine	++	+++	++++	++++	++	++++	+++
Doxepin	++	++	+++	++++	++	+++	++
Imipramine	+++	+++	+++	+++	++++	+++	+++
Trimipramine	++	++	++++	++++	+++	+++	+++
Secondary amines							
Desipramine	++++	+	++	++	++	++	++
Nortriptyline	+++	++	++	++	+	++	++
Protriptyline	+++	++	++	+	++	++	+++
Dibenzoxazepine							
Amoxapine[a]	+++	++	+++	++	++	+++	++
Tetracyclic							
Maprotiline	+++	+	+++	+++	++	++++	++
Triazolopyridines							
Nefazodone	0	++	0	+++	+++	++	+
Trazodone	0	++	0	++++	+++	++	+
Aminoketone							
Bupropion	+	+	+	0	0	++++	+
Monoamine oxidase inhibitors							
Phenelzine			++	++	++	++	+
Tranylcypromine			++	+	++	++	+
Selective serotonin reuptake inhibitors							
Fluoxetine	0	+++	0	0	0	++	0
Fluvoxamine	0	++++	0	0	0	++	0
Paroxetine	0	++++	+	+	0	++	0
Sertraline	0	++++	0	0	0	++	0
Serotonin/norepinephrine reuptake inhibitor							
Venlafaxine	++++	++++	+	+	0	++	+

Key: ++++, high; +++, moderate; ++, low; +, very low; 0, none.
[a]Also blocks dopamine receptors. (Modified from Refs. 16, 21, 40, 47, 48, 52, and 64.)

to the TCAs in treating patients with major depression.[33] Patients who fail to respond to a TCA may well respond to an SSRI and vice versa.

Triazolopyridines

Trazodone and nefazodone are the marketed antidepressants from the triazolopyridine class. Both have dual actions on serotonergic neurons, acting as both a 5-HT_2 antagonist and 5-HT reuptake inhibitor,[38] and appear to enhance 5-HT_{1A}-mediated neurotransmission. These drugs have negligible affinity for cholinergic and histaminergic receptors. Nefazodone also has low affinity for α_1-adrenergic receptors. Similar to TCAs and SSRIs, the triazolopyridines are effective agents in treating major depression with no substantial evidence to support a unique spectrum of therapeutic activity.

Aminoketone

Bupropion, the only marketed aminoketone antidepressant, appears to have a unique mechanism of drug action.[39] It has no appreciable effect on the reuptake of 5-HT, and its most potent neurochemical action is blockade of DA reuptake.

Monoamine Oxidase Inhibitors

The MAOIs increase the concentrations of NE, 5-HT, and DA within the neuronal synapse, through inhibition of the monoamine oxidase enzyme. Studies of several MAOIs have demonstrated that, similar to the TCAs, chronic therapy causes changes in receptor sensitivity (i.e., down-regulation of β-adrenergic, α-adrenergic, and serotonergic receptors).[40,41]

The spectrum of activity for MAOIs differs from the TCAs. Clinical features that predict preferential response to MAOIs include mood reactivity, irritability, hypersomnia, hyperphagia, psychomotor agitation, and hypersensitivity to rejection.[34] These features are collectively referred to as the defining features of atypical depression.

The MAOIs currently marketed in the United States are nonselective inhibitors of monoamine oxidase A and monoamine oxidase B. Phenelzine and tranylcypromine inhibit both of these forms (isozymes) of monoamine oxidase. Moclobemide, an antidepressant marketed in Europe, is a selective and reversible inhibitor of monoamine oxidase A. Clinical trials of moclobemide conducted in Europe have reported efficacy equal to TCAs and superior to placebo.[42]

ADVERSE EFFECTS

Tricyclic Antidepressants and Other Heterocyclics

The most commonly reported adverse effects of antidepressant therapy are summarized in Table 67.5. The TCAs affect several neurotransmitters and produce a wide range of pharmacologic actions, sometimes causing many unwanted adverse effects. The side effects most frequently associated with the TCAs (e.g., dry mouth, constipation, blurred vision, urinary retention, dizziness, tachycardia, memory impairment, and, at higher doses, delirium) may result from blockade of cholinergic receptors.[43] These adverse effects often impact patient tolerance and compliance, particularly in the elderly and those receiving long-term maintenance therapy. In general, anticholinergic effects and sedation are more severe during therapy with tertiary amine TCAs than with secondary amine TCAs.[43]

A common and potentially serious side effect of the TCAs is orthostatic hypotension, which has been attributed to the affinity of the TCAs for α_1-adrenergic receptors.[43] Orthostatic hypotension may be symptomatic resulting in syncope, a particular concern when treating elderly patients due to the increased risk of falls and subsequent fractures.[44] Patient education is important in reducing the risk associated with orthostatic hypotension. Patients should be advised to rise slowly from a supine position, and prolonged bed rest should be avoided because of the deconditioning and volume-contracting effect. Tilting the head of the bed upward can be helpful for some patients. Adequate fluid intake should be maintained, and blood pressure should be monitored both supine and upright. Antigravity support garments can also be helpful. The risk of symptomatic orthostatic hypotension can be minimized by adequate ambulation and hydration along with proper drug selection, gradual dose increases, and patient education.[45]

TCAs also cause cardiac conduction delays and may even induce heart block in patients with preexisting conduction disease. TCA overdose can produce severe arrhythmias.[43] Due to these potential cardiovascular effects, caution should be exercised when prescribing these agents to patients with clinically significant cardiac disease. Other adverse effects that lead to noncompliance include weight gain, excessive perspiration, and sexual dysfunction.[43]

Abrupt withdrawal of TCAs is associated with symptoms suggestive of cholinergic rebound (e.g., dizziness, nausea, diarrhea, insomnia, and restlessness), especially if the daily dose exceeds 300 mg.[46]

Clomipramine is a tertiary amine TCA with 5-HT reuptake inhibiting properties. Although it is a commonly used antidepressant in Europe, in the United States it is approved only for the treatment of obsessive–compulsive disorder (OCD). For an indepth discussion of clomipramine, the reader is referred to Chapter 70.

Amoxapine, the demethylated metabolite of loxapine, has intermediate sedative and anticholinergic potency.[47] Because of its postsynaptic receptor DA-blocking effects, its use is associated with extrapyramidal side effects including pseudoparkinsonism, dystonia, akathisia, and tardive dyskinesia.[21] Amoxapine offers no advantage over standard TCAs or other antidepressants.

Maprotiline, a tetracyclic drug, blocks reuptake of NE with little effect on 5-HT. It has intermediate sedative and anticholinergic effects and may cause less orthostatic hypotension than imipramine; however, an exanthemous rash occurs in approximately 4% of patients.[21] Maprotiline is also associated with a higher incidence of seizures than standard TCAs and is contraindicated in patients with a history of seizure disorder.

Venlafaxine

The most commonly reported adverse effects with venlafaxine include nausea, constipation, somnolence, dry mouth, dizziness, nervousness, sweating, asthenia, abnormal ejaculation/orgasm, and anorexia.[37] These side effects are believed to be dose related. Venlafaxine may cause a dose-related increase in diastolic blood pressure, and baseline blood pressure is not a useful predictor of the occurrence of this phenomenon. Blood pressure should be monitored regularly during venlafaxine therapy, and dosage reduction or discontinuation may be necessary if sustained hypertension occurs.[48]

Selective Serotonin Reuptake Inhibitors

Four SSRIs have been introduced in the United States—fluoxetine, sertraline, paroxetine, and fluvoxamine. Fluvoxamine has been approved by the FDA for the treatment of OCD, and a more in-depth discussion can be found in Chapter 70. In general, the SSRIs have a low affinity for histamine, α_1-adrenergic, and muscarinic receptors. They produce fewer anticholinergic and cardiovascular adverse effects than the TCAs, and they are not associated with weight gain.[49] The main adverse effects, which are generally mild and short lived, are gastrointestinal symptoms (nausea, vomiting, diarrhea) and sexual dysfunction in both males and females.

Although the SSRIs as a group are known to improve the anxiety symptoms associated with depression, a few patients experience an increase in anxiety symptoms or agitation early in treatment. This occurrence may be reported most frequently with fluoxetine.[50] Headache, insomnia, and fatigue also are reported commonly with these agents.[49]

Triazolopyradines

The adverse effect profile for trazodone and nefazodone is different from the other antidepressants. Trazodone and nefazodone have minimal anticholinergic effects or 5-HT agonist side effects, but can cause orthostatic hypotension. Sedation and cognitive slowing are the most frequent dose-limiting side effects associated with trazodone.[36]

A rare but potentially serious adverse effect of trazodone is priapism, which is reported to occur in approximately 1 in 6000 male patients. Some cases have required surgical intervention (1 in 23,000), and permanent impotence may result.[51] There have been no reports of priapism associated with nefazodone use.

Common adverse effects associated with nefazodone use include lightheadedness, dizziness, orthostatic hypotension, somnolence, dry mouth, nausea, and asthenia.[38] These side effects tend to lessen with continued treatment.

Aminoketone

Adverse effects associated with bupropion include nausea, dizziness, tremor, insomnia, vomiting, constipation, dry mouth, and skin reactions. The occurrence of seizures in patients taking bupropion appears to be strongly associated with dose and may be increased by predisposing factors such as history of head trauma and CNS tumor. At daily doses of 450 mg or less, the incidence of seizures is 0.4%. At 600 mg/d the incidence is 2.3%, and at doses between 600 and 900 mg/d, the incidence is 2.8% of patients.[52]

Monoamine Oxidase Inhibitors

The most common adverse effect of MAOIs is postural hypotension; this is more significant with phenelzine than tranylcypromine.[40] Hypotensive reactions may be minimized through divided dosage scheduling. Anticholinergic side effects, especially dry mouth and constipation, are common, but are mild compared with those associated with the TCAs.

Phenelzine, the most frequently prescribed MAOI, has mild to moderate sedating effects. Tranylcypromine may exert a stimulating effect and insomnia may occur, so the last dose of the day should be administered in the early afternoon.

Dose-related impotence and anorgasmia in males and orgasmic inhibition in females have been reported.[53,54] In addition, fever, myoclonic jerking, and brisk deep tendon reflexes may occur.[40,55,56]

Phenelzine has been associated with hepatocellular damage and weight gain. Tranylcypromine is a nonhydrazine MAOI and should be selected for patients with a history of liver disease if an MAOI is to be used.[40]

Hypertensive crisis, a potentially fatal but rare adverse reaction, occurs when MAOIs are taken concurrently with certain foods, especially those high in tyramine (Table 67.6) or drugs (Table 67.7). Ten milligrams of tyramine can cause a marked pressor effect, and 25 mg can result in serious hypertensive crisis.[57] These incidents may culminate in cerebrovascular accident and death.[40] Symptoms of hypertensive crisis include occipital headache, stiff neck, nausea, vomiting, sweating, and sharply elevated blood pressure. The hypertensive crisis can be treated with 10–20 mg of nifedipine sublingually or swallowed or 5 mg of phentolamine IV.[58]

Education of patients taking MAOIs regarding dietary and medication restrictions is extremely important. Printed and verbal patient instructions should be provided. Patients

TABLE 67.6. DIETARY RESTRICTIONS FOR PATIENTS TAKING MONOAMINE OXIDASE INHIBITORS

Aged cheeses[a]	Liver (chicken or beef, more than 2 days old)
Sour cream[b]	Fermented foods
Yogurt[b]	Canned figs
Cottage cheese[b]	Raisins
American cheese[b]	Pods of broad beans[a] (fava beans)
Mild Swiss cheese[b]	Yeast extract[a] and other yeast products
Wine[c] (especially Chianti and sherry)	Meat extract (Marmite)
Beer	Soy sauce
Herring[a] (pickled, salted, dry)	Chocolate[b]
Sardines	Coffee[d]
Snails	Ripe avocado
Anchovies	Sauerkraut
Canned, aged, or processed meats	Licorice
Monosodium glutamate	

[a]Clearly warrants absolute prohibition (e.g., English Stilton, blue, Camembert, cheddar).
[b]Up to 2 oz. daily is acceptable.
[c]3 oz. white wine or a single cocktail is acceptable.
[d]Up to 2 oz. daily is acceptable; larger amounts of decaffeinated coffee are acceptable.

TABLE 67.7. MEDICATION RESTRICTIONS FOR PATIENTS TAKING MONOAMINE OXIDASE INHIBITORS

Amphetamines	Guanethidine
Appetite suppressants	Levodopa
Asthma inhalants	Local anesthetics containing sympathomimetic vasoconstrictors
Buspirone	Meperidine
Carbamazepine	Methyldopa
Cocaine	Methylphenidate
Cyclobenzaprine	Other antidepressants
Decongestants (topical and systemic)	Other MAOIs
Dextromethorphan	Reserpine
Dopamine	Stimulants
Ephedrine	Sympathomimetics
Epinephrine	Tryptophan

unable to read and those with difficulty understanding or remembering medication instructions should not be given MAOIs unless they have competent caregivers. Patients should be instructed regarding the necessity of consulting a health professional before taking over-the-counter medications. Patients should also be informed of the symptoms of hypertensive crisis and be advised about what to do should those symptoms occur.

PHARMACOKINETICS

The pharmacokinetics of the antidepressants are summarized in Table 67.8. In general, the TCAs are rapidly absorbed after oral administration. Bioavailability is low (30–70% for most TCAs) as a result of the first-pass effect, which shows great interindividual variation.[59]

The TCAs have a large volume of distribution and concentrate in brain and cardiac tissue in laboratory animals. Substantial amounts of TCAs pass into breast milk, and breast feeding is, therefore, inadvisable. The TCAs are bound extensively and strongly to plasma albumin, erythrocytes, α_1-acid glycoprotein, and lipoprotein.[59]

The major metabolic pathways are demethylation, aromatic and aliphatic hydroxylation, and glucuronide conjugation. Enterohepatic cycling has been described.[59] Metabolism of TCAs appears to be linear within the usual dosage range. The elimination half-lives of the TCAs vary greatly among individual patients, and this may be genetically determined.[59]

The diversity of the SSRIs is evident not only in their chemical structures but also in their pharmacokinetic profiles. Fluoxetine has an elimination half-life of 2–3 days (4–5 days with multiple dosing). The single dose half-life of norfluoxetine, the active metabolite, is 7–9 days. Paroxetine and sertraline have half-lives of approximately 1 day. Unlike paroxetine, sertraline has an active metabolite, but the metabolite contributes minimally to the pharmacologic effects. The SSRIs, with the exception of fluvoxamine are extensively bound to plasma proteins (94–99%). The SSRIs are extensively distributed to the tissues, and all may have a nonlinear pattern of drug accumulation with long-term administration.[60]

Nefazodone and trazodone have elimination half-lives considerably shorter than the standard antidepressants, 2–4 hours and 6–11 hours, respectively. The time to reach peak plasma concentration is short (1–2 hours). Venlafaxine also has a short elimination half-life (5 hours), and is unique in that it is only 27–30% bound to plasma proteins.

Altered Pharmacokinetics

Factors reported to influence TCA plasma concentrations include disease states, genetics, age, cigarette smoking, and concurrent drug administration. Hepatic disease may reduce metabolic clearance of TCAs.[59] Renal failure does not alter nortriptyline metabolism, but the 10-hydroxy metabolite may accumulate, and protein binding may be diminished, with resultant enhanced sensitivity to the drug.[59] Clinicians should be alert to the possibility of higher-than-expected plasma concentrations of some TCAs in the elderly. Because dose-related kinetics cannot be ruled out in the elderly, dosage adjustments based on plasma concentration monitoring may be difficult.

TABLE 67.8. PHARMACOKINETIC PROPERTIES OF ANTIDEPRESSANTS

Generic Name	Elimination Half-Life (h)[a]	Time of Peak Plasma Concentration (h)	Plasma Protein Binding (%)	% Bioavailable	Clinically Important Metabolites
Tricyclic antidepressants					
Tertiary amines					
Amitriptyline	9–46	1–5	90–97	30–60	Nortriptyline
Clomipramine	20–24	2–6	97	36–62	10-Hydroxynortriptyline
Doxepin	8–36	1–4	68–82	13–45	Desmethyldoxepin
Imipramine	6–34	1.5–3	63–96	22–77	2-Hydroxyimipramine; desipramine; 2-hydroxydesipramine
Trimipramine	7–40	3	94–96	18–63	None
Secondary amines					
Desipramine	11–46	3–6	73–92	33–51	2-Hydroxydesipramine
Nortriptyline	16–88	3–12	87–95	46–70	10-Hydroxynortriptyline
Protriptyline	54–198	6–12	90–94	75–90	None
Dibenzoxazepine					
Amoxapine	8–30[b]	1–2	90	—[c]	8-Hydroxyamoxapine
Tetracyclic					
Maprotiline	28–105	4–24	88	79–87	Desmethylmaprotiline
Triazolopyridines					
Nefazodone	2–4	1	99	20	*meta*-Chlorophenylpiperazine; hydroxynefazodone; triazole-dione
Trazodone	6–11	1–2	92	—[c]	*meta*-Chlorophenylpiperazine
Aminoketone					
Bupropion	10–21	3	82–88	—[c]	Bupropion threo-amino alcohol; bupropion morpholinol
Monoamine oxidase inhibitors					
Phenelzine	1.5–4	—[c]	—[c]	—[c]	
Tranylcypromine	1.5–3	—[c]	—[c]	—[c]	
Selective serotonin reuptake inhibitors					
Fluoxetine	24–120	4–8	94	95	Norfluoxetine
Fluvoxamine	15–26	2–8	77	53	None
Paroxetine	24–31	5–7	95		None
Sertraline	27	6–8	99	36[d]	*N*-Desmethylsertraline
Serotonin/norepinephrine reuptake inhibitor					
Venlafaxine	5	2	27–30		*O*-Desmethylvenlafaxine

[a]Biologic half-life in slowest phase of elimination.
[b]Amoxapine, 8 hours; 8-hydroxyamoxapine, 30 hours.
[c]No data available.
[d]Increases 30–40% when taken with food.

In cirrhotics, the half-lives of fluoxetine and norfluoxetine increased to 7.6 and 12 days, respectively.[61] Patients with hepatic impairment had a twofold increase in plasma concentrations of paroxetine.[62] Similarly, in patients with mild stable cirrhosis, the half-life of sertraline was two and one-half times greater than in patients without liver disease.[63] Patients with renal impairment had a two- to fourfold increase in paroxetine plasma concentrations compared to normal volunteers.[62] Plasma concentrations of SSRIs in the elderly are reported to be greater than in younger patients.[62,63]

The AUC of nefazodone and hydroxynefazodone is 25% greater in cirrhotics than in normal volunteers.[64] Patients with cirrhosis accumulate metabolites of bupropion to concentrations two to three times those in normals.[52]

Plasma Concentration and Clinical Response

Studies in acutely depressed patients have demonstrated a correlation between antidepressant effect and plasma concentrations for some TCAs. The patient's clinical response, not plasma concentration, dictates dosage adjustments. Some patients with plasma concentrations outside the suggested therapeutic plasma concentration range respond, whereas others are nonresponsive regardless of their plasma concentration. See Table 67.4 for a listing of suggested therapeutic plasma concentration ranges.

For four TCAs (nortriptyline, desipramine, imipramine, and amitriptyline) there is more consistent evidence of a minimal plasma concentration for clinical response. The best established therapeutic range is for nortriptyline.[65]

Studies suggest a curvilinear plasma concentration/antidepressant response relationship for nortriptyline with a suggested therapeutic range of 50–150 ng/mL. Using logistic regression analysis of data from multiple published studies, it was found that within this range, 70% of patients with major depression responded versus only 29% of patients with plasma concentrations outside this range. Interestingly, the response rate was generally higher at the lower end of this range than at the upper limit.[66]

In the same analysis, the therapeutic window for desipramine was 110–160 ng/mL. The remission rate was 50% within this range versus only 20% outside the range.[66] Many clinicians, however, feel that the data better support a minimal threshold plasma concentration for clinical response, and a more commonly accepted range is 125–300 ng/mL.

The data for the tertiary amine TCAs are less convincing, and most investigators conclude that the desired plasma concentration range is defined by a threshold level below which patients are less likely to respond and an upper limit that is associated with increased risk for CNS and cardiac toxicity.[32]

Studies suggest that optimal response in patients taking bupropion is most likely at plasma concentrations of 50–100 ng/mL.[32] For the newer antidepressants, a correlation has not been established between plasma concentration and clinical response.

Plasma Concentration Monitoring

Because of interindividual variations in plasma concentrations achieved by a given dose, approximately 40% of patients given standard doses of TCAs may not obtain plasma concentrations within the desired therapeutic range.[67] Although plasma level monitoring is not routinely performed, some indications include inadequate response, relapse, serious or persistent adverse effects, use of higher than standard doses, suspected toxicity, elderly patients, pregnant patients, patients of African or Asian descent (because of slower metabolism), cardiac disease, suspected noncompliance, suspected pharmacokinetic drug interactions, and changing brands. Plasma concentration monitoring of TCAs when used appropriately can improve efficacy and minimize drug-related problems associated with antidepressant therapy. Plasma concentrations should be obtained at steady state, usually after a minimum of 1 week at constant dosage. Sampling should be done during the elimination phase, usually in the morning, 12 hours after the last dose. Samples collected in this manner are comparable for patients on once-daily, twice-daily, or three-times-daily regimens.[59]

DRUG INTERACTIONS

Tricyclic Antidepressants

Since the TCAs are metabolized in the liver through the cytochrome P-450 system, they may interact with other drugs that modify hepatic enzyme activity or hepatic blood flow.[21] TCAs are also extensively protein bound, which can cause drug interactions through displacement from protein binding sites. Many commonly used medications can interact when given concurrently with TCAs. Pharmacokinetic and pharmacodynamic drug interactions involving TCAs are shown in Tables 67.9 and 67.10, respectively.

Barbiturates induce the cytochrome P-450 system to increase metabolism of TCAs, resulting in lower TCA plasma concentrations.[68] Drugs that inhibit microsomal enzymes (e.g., oral contraceptives, cimetidine, methylphenidate, and the SSRIs) may increase TCA plasma concentrations.[68]

TABLE 67.9. PHARMACOKINETIC DRUG INTERACTIONS INVOLVING TRICYCLIC ANTIDEPRESSANTS

Elevates plasma concentrations of TCAs
Cimetidine
Diltiazem
Ethanol, acute ingestion
SSRIs
Haloperidol
Labetalol
Methylphenidate
Phenothiazines
Propoxyphene
Quinidine
Verapamil
Lowers plasma concentrations of TCAs
Barbiturates
Carbamazepine
Ethanol, chronic ingestion
Phenytoin
Elevates plasma concentrations of interacting drug
Hydantoins
Oral anticoagulants
Phenytoin
Lowers plasma concentrations of interacting drug
Levodopa

(Compiled from Ref. 68.)

TABLE 67.10. PHARMACODYNAMIC DRUG INTERACTIONS INVOLVING TRICYCLIC ANTIDEPRESSANTS

Interacting Drug	Effect
Alcohol	Increased CNS depressant effects
Amphetamines	Increased effect of amphetamines
Androgens	Delusions, hostility
Anticholinergic agents	Excessive anticholinergic effects
Bethanidine	Decreased antihypertensive efficacy
Clonidine	Decreased antihypertensive efficacy
Disulfiram	Acute organic brain syndrome
Estrogens	Increased or decreased antidepressant response; increased toxicity
Guanadrel	Decreased antihypertensive efficacy
Guanethidine	Decreased antihypertensive efficacy
Insulin	Increased hypoglycemic effects
Lithium	Possible additive lowering of seizure threshold
Methyldopa	Decreased antihypertensive efficacy; tachycardia; CNS stimulation
Monoamine oxidase inhibitors	Increased therapeutic and possibly toxic effects of both drugs; hypertensive crisis; delirium; seizures; hyperpyrexia; serotonin syndrome
Oral hypoglycemics	Increased hypoglycemic effects
Phenytoin	Possible lowering of seizure threshold and reduced antidepressant response
Sedatives	Increased CNS depressant effects
Sympathomimetics	Increased pharmacologic effects of direct-acting sympathomimetics; decreased effects of indirect acting sympathomimetics
Thyroid hormones	Increased therapeutic and possibly toxic effects of both drugs; CNS stimulation; tachycardia

(Compiled from Ref. 68.)

TCAs may reverse the hypotensive effects of certain sympatholytic antihypertensives (e.g., guanethidine, methyldopa, clonidine) because of inhibition of presynaptic uptake of the antihypertensive or desensitization of the α_2-adrenergic receptor.[68] Similarly, because of inhibition of presynaptic uptake, TCAs may increase the vasopressor response to direct-acting sympathomimetics such as phenelephrine, epinephrine, and NE. The vasopressor response to indirect-acting sympathomimetics, such as ephedrine, is decreased.[68] Adverse effects of any TCA would be additive with those of other drugs with similar pharmacologic effects (e.g., anticholinergic, sedative, or hypotensive drugs).[68]

Although MAOIs and TCAs may be safely coadministered in refractory patients with apparent increased efficacy compared with monotherapy, severe reactions and fatalities have occurred. These reactions include hypertensive crises, hyperpyrexia, excitation, and convulsions, and they usually occur when TCAs are added to established MAOI therapy.[69]

Selective Serotonin Reuptake Inhibitors

Table 67.11, on pages 1410–1411, summarizes the drug interactions of non-TCA antidepressants. Drug–drug interactions may occur when an SSRI is coadministered with another drug metabolized through the cytochrome P-450 system.[68] The long half-lives of fluoxetine (2–5 days in young healthy subjects) and of its active metabolite, norfluoxetine (7–9 days), ensure that, following discontinuation of the drug, these active compounds will persist in the body for weeks. The very slow elimination of fluoxetine makes it critical to ensure a 5-week washout after fluoxetine discontinuation before starting an MAOI.[70] Serious and potentially fatal reactions may occur when any SSRI is coadministered with an MAOI.[68]

Patients given concurrent fluoxetine and warfarin should be monitored for a possible increased risk of bleeding. Patients prescribed concomitant phenytoin or carbamazepine with fluoxetine may have increased anticonvulsant plasma concentrations and symptoms of toxicity.[68] Markedly increased plasma concentrations of TCAs with resultant symptoms of toxicity have been reported in patients taking fluoxetine.

Phenytoin, which induces hepatic enzymes, has been reported to decrease paroxetine levels, but no significant changes occurred when paroxetine was given with diazepam, phenobarbital, or digoxin.[49] Although no significant pharmacokinetic changes were seen with coadministration of warfarin, an increased bleeding time was noted.[71] Careful monitoring of prothrombin time is recommended when warfarin and paroxetine are administered concomitantly. No clinically significant drug interactions occurred during coadministration of paroxetine with haloperidol, amobarbital, oxazepam, or alcohol, indicating that paroxetine does not potentiate the central nervous system depressant effects of such agents.[49] Plasma lithium levels were also unaffected by concurrent administration of paroxetine.[72] Cimetidine was shown to increase paroxetine concentrations by 50% in healthy volunteers, but the importance of this effect is unclear.[71] Paroxetine was found to increase the half-life and plasma concentrations of desipramine.[68]

Sertraline administration had no clinically significant effects on the pharmacokinetics and protein binding of diazepam or digoxin.[49] Bleeding time was increased with the concurrent administration of sertraline and warfarin, so the prothrombin time should be closely monitored.[49] Sertraline has been reported to increase significantly the plasma concentrations of secondary amine TCAs (e.g., desipramine, nortroptyline) and carbamazepine.

Newer Agents

Venlafaxine and its active metabolite, O-desmethylvenlafaxine, are only 30% protein bound, so coadministration with other highly protein bound drugs should not cause a significant drug interaction.[48] Venlafaxine did not cause any significant changes in the pharmacokinetics of ethanol, diazepam, or lithium when administered concomitantly.[48] Cimetidine inhibited the first-pass metabolism of venlafaxine, but the significance of this interaction is not known. *In vitro* studies have demonstrated that venlafaxine is metabolized to its active metabolite by the cytochrome P-450IID6 isoenzyme, which is the source of the genetic polymorphism seen in the metabolism of many antidepressants. Therefore, the potential exists for interaction between venlafaxine and drugs that inhibit the P-450IID6 system.[48]

Nefazodone is highly protein bound to human plasma proteins *in vitro*. While nefazodone does not alter the *in vitro* protein binding of chlorpromazine, desipramine, diazepam, phenytoin, lidocaine, prazosin, propranolol, verapamil, or warfarin, it is unknown whether or not displacement of either nefazodone or other drugs occurs *in vivo*.[64] Triazolobenzodiazepines, such as triazolam and alprazolam, interacted significantly with nefazodone. If triazolam is to be coadministered with nefazodone, a 75% dose reduction of the triazolam is recommended. If alprazolam is coadministered with nefazodone, a 50% reduction in the initial dose of alprazolam is recommended.[64] Terfenadine and astemizole are both metabolized by the cytochrome P-450IIIA4 isoenzyme, and it has been demonstrated that ketoconazole, erythromycin, and other inhibitors of IIIA4 can block the metabolism of terfenadine and astemizole, resulting in increased plasma concentrations of parent drug. Increased plasma concentrations of terfenadine and astemizole are associated with QT prolongation and with rare cases of serious cardiovascular adverse events, including death. Nefazodone has been shown to be an *in vitro* inhibitor of IIIA4. Consequently, it is recommended that nefazodone not be used concomitantly with either terfenadine or astemizole.[64] Concurrent administration of MAOIs and nefazodone is also contraindicated.[64]

SPECIAL POPULATIONS

Elderly Patients

Depression in the aging and the aged is a major public health problem. Many elderly depressed patients are undiagnosed or inadequately treated. Diagnosis is often missed or mistaken for another disorder, such as dementia. Depressed mood, the typical signature symptom of depression, may be less prominent than the other depressive symptoms such as loss of appetite, cognitive impairment, sleeplessness, anergia, and loss of interest in and enjoyment of the normal pursuits of life.[73] Somatic complaints are frequent in elderly depressed patients.

It is important to screen for medical conditions, psychiatric conditions, and drug therapies that may underlie depression (Table 67.1). Before initiating antidepressant treatment, the elderly patient should undergo a complete physical examination including cardiovascular, cerebrovascular, ophthalmologic, gastrointestinal, and urinary systems.

Elderly depressed patients are often over- or undertreated. Overtreatment often occurs when age-related pharmacokinetic and pharmacodynamic factors are overlooked. Undertreatment often results from an overly conservative approach as a result of the patient's advanced age or medical problems. Plasma concentration monitoring can be a useful tool in managing drug therapy in this patient population. A TCA would not be an appropriate first choice for a depressed patient with cardiac conduction delay. However, in the healthy elderly, cautious use of a secondary amine TCA (desipramine or nortriptyline) may be appropriate because of their defined therapeutic plasma concentration ranges, well-established efficacy, and well-known adverse effect profiles.[32]

The SSRIs are often selected as first-choice antidepressants, and they may enable the clinician to avoid some of the more serious adverse effects commonly associated with the TCAs (e.g., sedative, anticholinergic, and cardiovascular side effects). Trazodone, nefazodone, and bupropion are also often chosen because of their milder anticholinergic and less frequent cardiovascular side effects.[32]

Although phenelzine has been used safely and effectively in well-selected patients, the MAOIs are usually not recommended for elderly patients because of hypotensive side effects and uncertainty of patients' likelihood of adherence to dietary and medication restrictions.[32]

Pediatric Patients

Several common myths exist concerning depression and children. One myth is that depression among children is an unusual phenomenon; accumulating evidence indicates that childhood depression occurs quite commonly. Another myth is that children do not commit suicide; again, there is increasing evidence that suicide among children is a significant public health problem. A final myth is that the symptoms of childhood depression are different than the symptoms of depression in adults; a growing body of evidence suggests that the symptoms are similar to those experienced by adults.[74]

Data collected under controlled conditions supporting the efficacy of antidepressants in children and adolescents are sparse. In the double-blind study by Preskorn et al.,[75]

TABLE 67.11. DRUG INTERACTIONS OF NON-TCA ANTIDEPRESSANTS

Non-TCA	Interacting Drug/Drug Class	Effect
Dibenzoxazepine		
Amoxapine	Many of the drugs that interact with the TCAs	Similar response to that seen with TCA interaction
Tetracyclic		
Maprotiline	Many of the drugs that interact with the TCAs	Similar response to that seen with TCA interaction
Triazolopyridine		
Nefazodone	Alprazolam	Increased plasma concentrations of alprazolam
	Astemizole	Theoretically increased plasma concentrations of astemizole with potentially serious cardiovascular adverse effects
	Digoxin	Increased C_{max}, C_{min}, and AUC of digoxin by 29, 27, and 15%, respectively
	Haloperidol	Decreased clearance of haloperidol by 35%
	MAOIs	Hypertensive crisis; serotonin syndrome; delirium; coma; seizures; hyperpyrexia
	Propranolol	Decreased C_{max} and AUC of propranolol; increased C_{max}, C_{min}, and AUC of *m*-CPP metabolite of nefazodone
	Terfenadine	Theoretically increased plasma concentrations of terfenadine with potentially serious cardiovascular adverse effects
	Triazolam	Increased plasma concentrations of triazolam; increased psychomotor impairment
Trazodone	CNS depressants	Increased CNS depression
	Digoxin	Increased serum concentrations of digoxin
	Ethanol	Additive impairment in motor skills
	Fluoxetine	Increased plasma concentrations of trazodone
	MAOIs	Theoretically central serotonin syndrome could occur
	Neuroleptics	Increased hypotension
	Phenytoin	Increased serum concentrations of phenytoin
	Tryptophan	Agitation, restlessness, poor concentration, nausea
	Warfarin	Decreased hypoprothrombinemic response
Aminoketone		
Bupropion	MAOIs	Increased toxicity of bupropion
	Medications that lower seizure threshold	Increased incidence of seizures
	Levodopa	Increased incidence of adverse experiences
Selective serotonin reuptake inhibitors		
Fluoxetine	Alprazolam	Increased plasma concentrations and half-life of alprazolam; increased psychomotor impairment
	Anticoagulants	Possible increased risk of bleeding
	β-Adrenergic blockers	Increased metoprolol serum concentrations and bradycardia; possible heart block
	Buspirone	Decreased therapeutic response to buspirone
	Carbamazepine	Increased plasma concentrations of carbamazepine with symptoms of carbamazepine toxicity
	Dextromethorphan	Visual hallucinations (one patient only)
	Haloperidol	Increased haloperidol concentrations and increased extrapyramidal side effects
	Lithium	Neurotoxicity—confusion, ataxia, dizziness, tremor, absence seizures
	MAOIs	Severe or fatal reactions—confusion, nausea, double vision, hypomania, hypertension, tremor, serotonin syndrome
	Phenytoin	Increased plasma concentrations of phenytoin and symptoms of phenytoin toxicity
	TCAs	Markedly increased TCA plasma concentration with symptoms of TCA toxicity
	Terfenadine	Arrhythmias, shortness of breath and orthostasis

TABLE 67.11. DRUG INTERACTIONS OF NON-TCA ANTIDEPRESSANTS *(Continued)*

Non-TCA	Interacting Drug/Drug Class	Effect
	Trazodone	Headaches, dizziness, sedation
	Tryptophan	Agitation, restlessness, poor concentration, nausea
	Valproate	Increased valproate serum concentrations
Fluvoxamine	Alprazolam	Increased AUC of alprazolam by 96%, increased alprazolam half-life by 71%, and increased psychomotor impairment
	Astemizole	Theoretically increased plasma concentrations of astemizole with potentially serious cardiovascular effects
	β-Adrenergic blockers	Fivefold increase in propranolol serum concentrations; bradycardia and hypotension with combined fluvoxamine and metoprolol
	Carbamazepine	Possible carbamazepine toxicity, although a controlled study did not support this
	Clozapine	Increased clozapine serum concentrations and increased risk for seizures and orthostatic hypotension
	Diazepam	Decreased clearance of diazepam and its active metabolite
	Diltiazem	Bradycardia
	Haloperidol	Increased haloperidol plasma concentrations
	Lithium	Increased serotonergic effects; seizures, nausea, tremor
	MAOIs	Potential for hypertensive crisis, serotonin syndrome, seizures, delirium
	Methodone	Increased methodone plasma concentrations with symptoms of methodone toxicity
	TCAs	Increased TCA plasma concentration
	Terfenadine	Theoretically increased plasma concentrations of terfenadine with potentially serious cardiovascular effects
	Theophylline	Increased serum concentrations of theophylline with symptoms of theophylline toxicity
	Tryptophan	Increased serotonergic effects and severe vomiting
	Warfarin	Increased hypoprothrombinemic response to warfarin
Paroxetine	Cimetidine	Increased paroxetine serum concentrations
	Desipramine	Increased plasma concentrations and half-life of desipramine
	MAOIs	Potential for hypertensive crisis, serotonin syndrome, seizures, delirium
	Warfarin	Possible increased risk for bleeding
Sertraline	Carbamazepine	Increased plasma concentrations of carbamazepine
	Diazepam	Small decrease in clearance of diazepam
	MAOIs	Serotonin syndrome, myoclonus, violent shaking
	TCAs	Increased plasma concentrations of secondary amine TCAs (desipramine, nortriptyline)
	Tolbutamide	Decreased clearance of tolbutamide (16%)
	Warfarin	Increased protime
Serotonin/norepinephrine reuptake inhibitor		
Venlafaxine	Cimetidine	Reduced clearance of venlafaxine by 43%; AUC and peak serum concentration of venlafaxine increased by 60%
	MAOIs	Potential for hypertensive crisis, serotonin syndrome, seizures, delirium

(Compiled from Ref. 68.)

sample size was small (N = 15 in each cell), but plasma concentration monitoring was used to adjust doses. Nonetheless, imipramine was superior in efficacy to placebo only through the first 3 weeks of treatment.[75] Demonstration of efficacy in this population is confounded by the high placebo response rate. Similar studies with other antidepressants, including SSRIs, have been negative. The SSRIs, however, are better tolerated than the TCAs and relatively safer on overdose. Toxicity on overdose is important in the adolescent population, where suicide is the second leading cause of death.[32]

TCAs and other antidepressant compounds are used to treat depressed children and adolescents, because no other definitive therapies are available. Plasma concentration monitoring of TCAs is important to ensure safety. As in the adult population, plasma concentrations above 450 ng/mL are associated with increased risk of serious adverse effects including delirium, seizures, delayed cardiac conduction, and sudden death.[32]

Several cases of sudden death have been reported in children and adolescents taking desipramine. A baseline ECG is recommended before initiating a TCA in children and adolescents, and many clinicians recommend an additional ECG when steady-state plasma concentrations are achieved.[32]

The only FDA-approved antidepressant for children over 6 years of age is imipramine, but it is approved only for the treatment of enuresis. Antidepressants should be initiated in this patient population at a dosage somewhat lower than that in adults; however adolescents usually require adult doses, and 6–8 weeks may be required before an antidepressant response is seen. A typical dosing regimen is a starting dose of 1.5 mg/kg/d that is increased by 1.0 to 1.5 mg/kg every third day. The daily dose should not exceed 5 mg/kg.[76]

Pregnant/Lactating Patients

Approximately 10% of pregnant women develop serious depression. No major teratogenic effects have been identified for the TCAs. Although the MAOIs have demonstrated teratogenicity in animals, there are insufficient data in humans to permit firm conclusions. Similarly, there are inadequate data on the use of the newer antidepressants during pregnancy. As a general rule, nondrug approaches to the treatment of depression in the pregnant patient are preferred. The TCAs are usually given preference, and nortriptyline or desipramine may be the treatment of choice because of the experience that has been gained with these agents in pregnant patients and because therapeutic plasma concentrations have been established. If a TCA is withdrawn during pregnancy, it should be gradually tapered to avoid maternal or fetal withdrawal symptoms. If possible, drug tapering is usually begun 5–10 days before the estimated day of confinement.[32]

CLINICAL APPLICATION

Dosing

Recommended initial doses and dosage ranges are shown in Table 67.4. The usual initial adult dose of most TCAs is 50 mg at bedtime, and the dose may be increased by 25–50 mg every third day. The recommended initial dose for fluoxetine is 10–20 mg in the morning, the recommended starting dose for paroxetine is 20 mg in the morning, and the recommended initial dose for sertraline is 50 mg in the morning.

Bupropion is usually initiated at 100 mg twice daily, and this dose may be increased to 100 mg three times daily after 3 days. Most patients will respond at 300 mg/d; however, an increase to 450 mg/d, given as 150 mg three times daily, may be considered in patients with no clinical response after several weeks of treatment at 300 mg/d.

Typically, phenelzine is initiated at 15 mg in the morning and then increased by 15 mg every third day up to 60 mg daily. The dose should be given three times daily to minimize postural hypotension, with the last dose given in the early afternoon to lessen the likelihood of insomnia. Maintenance doses may be as low as 15 mg/d.

The usual starting dose of venlafaxine is 75 mg/d given in two or three divided doses, taken with food. Depending on tolerability, the dose is then increased to 150 mg/d. If needed, the dose can then be further increased to 225 mg/d. Certain patients, including severely depressed patients, may need a dose up to 375 mg/d.

The starting dose of nefazodone is 100 mg given twice daily. Dose increases should occur in increments of 100 mg/d, on a twice daily schedule, at intervals of no less than 1 week, with the usual effective dose range being between 300–600 mg/d.

Caution is urged when switching from one antidepressant to another. It is important to remember that 3–4 weeks is usually required before a mood elevating response is seen. A 6-week trial at a maximum dosage is considered an adequate trial.[77] It is crucial to explain to the patient about the expected lag time before the onset of clinical response. Patients uneducated in this regard often fail to comply with their prescribed regimens.

In elderly patients, as a general rule, dosing is initiated at half the initial dose given to younger adults, and the dose is increased at a slower rate. Thus, desipramine or nortriptyline may be initiated at 10–25 mg/d or fluoxetine at 10–20 mg/d or alternatively 20 mg every second or third day. Six to 12 weeks of treatment may be required to achieve the desired antidepressant response.[32]

A remission is achieved when symptoms of depression are no longer present. A relapse is a return of symptoms within 6 months after remission. To prevent relapse, antidepressants should be continued at full therapeutic doses for 4–9 months after remission.[78] This period of treatment is termed *continuation therapy.* A recurrence is a separate episode of depression, which may occur after years of normal functioning. Five years after the first episode of depression, only 25% of patients had recovered and remained well.[79] The risk of recurrence increases as the number of past episodes and age at onset of the first episode increases.[80] The duration of antidepressant therapy depends on the risk of recurrence. Some investigators recommend life-long maintenance therapy for persons at greatest risk for recurrence (e.g., persons >50 years of age at onset of the first episode, persons >40 years of age and with 2 or more prior episodes, and persons of any age with 3 or more prior episodes).[65]

Refractory Patients

The majority of "treatment-resistant" depressed patients are likely the result of inadequate therapy (i.e., relative resistance).[32] Issues to be addressed in assessing the patient who has not responded to treatment include the following: (1) Is the diagnosis correct? (2) Does the patient have a psychotic depression? (3) Has the patient received an adequate dose and adequate duration of treatment? (4) Do adverse effects preclude adequate dosing? (5) Has the patient been compliant with the prescribed regimen? (6) Was a stepwise approach to treatment used? (7) Was treatment outcome adequately measured? (8) Is there a coexisting or preexisting medical or psychiatric disorder? (9) Are there other factors that interfere with treatment?[32]

When a patient has failed to respond to one antidepressant, an alternate antidepressant with a different profile can often bring about an antidepressant response. In addition, other modalities including environmental manipulation, family counseling, cognitive therapy, or interpersonal psychotherapy are often beneficial.[32]

Three primary approaches are used when dealing with treatment nonresponse. The current antidepressant may be stopped and a trial with an unrelated agent initiated. For example, the patient may be switched from a TCA to an SSRI or an MAOI. Second, the current antidepressant can be augmented (potentiated) by the addition of lithium, liothyronine, or an anticonvulsant such as carbamazepine or valproic acid. A third approach to the treatment-resistant patient is to use concurrently two different classes of antidepressants (e.g., a TCA plus an MAOI).[32] As previously discussed, the combination of an SSRI and an MAOI should never be used.

There are accumulating data to support that 50–60% of previously treatment-resistant depressed patients respond to adequate doses of SSRIs.[32] When separate adequate trials of a heterocyclic antidepressant and an SSRI have failed, many clinicians would switch to an MAOI, especially for the patient with atypical features.[32]

Augmenting strategies, such as the addition of lithium to a TCA regimen has been found to benefit many previously unresponsive patients, including those with psychotic depression. Lithium augmentation of fluoxetine benefitted five refractory patients. Several trials support that addition of liothyronine to a TCA regimen may induce antidepressant response.[32]

Concurrent use of a TCA and MAOI should be undertaken only by a prescriber experienced in the use of such combinations. When this is undertaken, the MAOI is slowly added to the TCA. Desipramine is not recommended to be used in combination with an MAOI. When the combination is discontinued, the MAOI should be stopped first.[32] Patients with psychotic depression usually require the combination of an antidepressant and an antipsychotic.[32]

The Agency for Health Care Policy and Research offers guidelines in managing patients who fail to respond. They advise that when patients fail to respond to medication by week six, the adequacy of the diagnosis and treatment should be reassessed. Comorbid medical or psychiatric conditions should be identified and treated, because they may complicate treatment. Before changing a patient's treatment, the clinician is advised to evaluate the adequacy of the medication dosage and compliance with the prescribed regimen. A combination of two drugs should not be used when one drug will suffice. Therefore, switching medications is often preferred over augmentation as an initial strategy.[65] An algorithm for treatment of depression, including refractory patients, is shown in Fig. 67.1.

Evaluation of Therapeutic Outcomes

Several monitoring parameters, in addition to plasma concentrations, are useful in managing patients. Patients must be monitored for adverse effects (e.g., sedation, anticholinergic effects, sexual dysfunction) and remission of previously documented target symptoms. The presence of side effects does not indicate adequate dosage. In addition, changes in social and occupational functioning should be assessed. When TCAs are given concurrently with adrenergic neuronal blocking antihypertensives (e.g., guanethidine, methyldopa, clonidine), blood pressure should be regularly monitored. Patients receiving venlafaxine should have their blood pressure monitored at regular intervals. Patients older than 40 should receive a pretreatment ECG before starting TCA therapy, and follow-up ECGs should be performed periodically. Patients should be monitored for the emergence of suicidal ideation after initiation of any antidepressant.

In addition to the clinical interview, psychometric rating instruments (e.g., patient-rated and clinician-rated scales) allow for rapid and reliable measurement of the nature and severity of depressive and associated symptoms (see Chapter 61). Interviewing a family member or friend (with the patient's permission) regarding symptoms and daily functioning can also assist in assessment of progress. It is recommended that patients be monitored closely for relapse or recurrence if the brand of antidepressant is changed. Patients should be monitored at more frequent intervals early

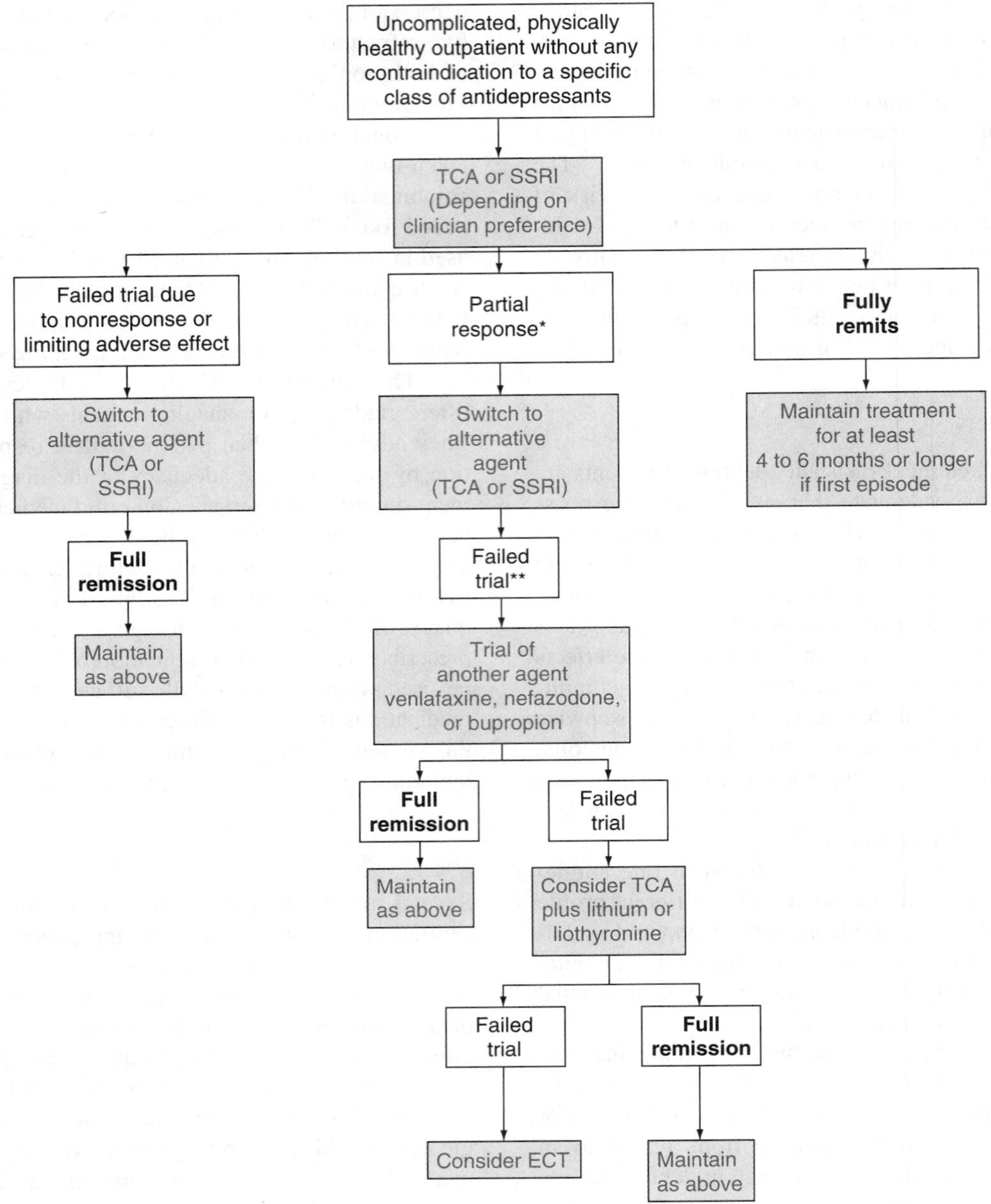

Figure 67.1. Algorithm for treatment of uncomplicated major depression. *Be certain patient is receiving an adequate dose and treatment duration has been at least 3 to 4 weeks; **some clinicians attempt augmentation (with lithium or liothyronine) at this point. *(Modified from Ref. 33.)*

in treatment. Monitoring is then continued at regular intervals throughout the continuation and maintenance phases of treatment. Regular monitoring should also be assured for several months after antidepressant therapy is discontinued.

Electroconvulsive Therapy

Electroconvulsive therapy (ECT) is a safe and very effective treatment for certain severe mental illnesses. Patients receive ECT when a rapid response is needed, risks of other treatments outweigh potential benefits, there has been a poor response to drugs and a good response to ECT, and the patient expresses a preference for ECT.[81] It is effective for all subtypes of major depressive disorder as well as other selected psychiatric illnesses.

A course of ECT generally consists of 6–12 treatments administered either unilaterally or bilaterally two to three times weekly. A rapid therapeutic response (10–14 days) has been reported.

Although there are no absolute contraindications to the use of ECT, several conditions are associated with increased risk. These include increased intracranial pressure, cerebral lesions, recent myocardial infarction, recent intracerebral hemorrhage, bleeding, or otherwise unstable vascular condition. The use of an anesthetic as well as a nondepolarizing neuromuscular blocking agent decreases the morbidity associated with ECT.[82]

Adverse effects of ECT include cognitive dysfunction, cardiovascular dysfunction, prolonged apnea, treatment emergent mania, headache, nausea, and muscle aches. Cognitive changes associated with ECT include confusion immediately after the seizure and retrograde and anterograde memory disturbance. Most of these cognitive disturbances are transient, but some patients may have permanent loss of memory of some events occurring over the months before, after, or during treatment.[81]

Relapse rates during the year following ECT are high unless maintenance antidepressant medications are prescribed. The guidelines for the use of ECT developed by the American Psychiatric Association include indications and contraindications for the use of ECT, procedures for obtaining informed consent, and issues in administering ECT.[81]

Psychotherapy

The comparative value of psychotherapy and pharmacotherapy in the treatment of depression has not been adequately studied. The efficacy of psychotherapy and antidepressant medications is considered to be additive.

Psychotherapy alone is not recommended for the acute treatment of patients with severe and/or psychotic major depressive disorders, but it may be first-line therapy if the episode is mild to moderate in severity.[65] Combined treatment may be advantageous for patients with partial responses to either treatment alone and for those with a chronic course of illness. However, for uncomplicated, nonchronic major depressive disorder, combined treatment may provide no unique advantage.[65] Although not well studied, cognitive therapy, behavioral therapy, and interpersonal psychotherapy appear to be equal in efficacy.[65] Maintenance psychotherapy as the sole treatment to prevent recurrence is generally not recommended unless the patient needs to avoid medication. If there was a full response to combined medication and psychotherapy in the acute or continuation phases of treatment, medication may be all that is necessary in the maintenance phase of treatment to prevent a recurrence.[65]

Conclusion

Major depressive disorder remains one of the most commonly occurring mental illnesses in adults, and it is often undiagnosed and untreated. Pharmacologic intervention remains the cornerstone of antidepressant treatment. Antidepressant medications have a broad spectrum of neurochemical effects and influence a variety of receptors peripherally and centrally. Safe and effective use of antidepressants requires a thorough understanding of the pharmacology of these drugs and of the principles for monitoring efficacy and adverse effects. In addition, clinicians must have a thorough understanding of antidepressant drug interactions and other factors that may influence the pharmacokinetics of antidepressant drugs. Plasma concentration monitoring is unnecessary for most patients, but can improve the outcome in some situations. The search for more effective antidepressants with more favorable adverse effect profiles must continue.

References

1. American Psychiatric Association. Diagnostic and Statistical Manual of Mental Disorders, 4th ed. (DSM-IV). Washington, DC, American Psychiatric Association, 1994, pp 317–391.
2. Keller MB, Hanks DL. The natural history and heterogeneity of depressive disorder disorders: Implications for rational antidepressant therapy. J Clin Psychiatry 1994;55: (9, suppl A):25–31.
3. Katon W, Von Korff M, Lin E, et al. Collaborative management to achieve treatment guidelines: Impact on depression in primary care. JAMA 1995;273(13):1026–1031.
4. Wells KB, Stewart A, Hays RD, et al. The functioning and well-being of depressed patients. Results from the medical outcomes study. JAMA 1989;262:914–919.
5. Hays RD, Wells KB, Sherbourne CD, et al. Functioning and well-being outcomes in patients with depression compared with chronic general medical illnesses. Arch Gen Psychiatry 1995;52:11–19.
6. Blazer D. Depression in the elderly. N Engl J Med 1989;320:164–166.
7. Regier DA, Burke JD, Burke KC. Comorbidity of affective and anxiety disorders in NIMH epidemiologic catchment area program, in Maser JD, Cloninger CR, (eds): Comorbidity of Mood and Anxiety Disorders. Washington, DC, American Psychiatric Press, 1990, pp 113–122.
8. Kessler RC, McGonagle KA, Zhao S, et al. Lifetime and 12-month prevalence of DSM-III-R psychiatric disorders in the United States. Results from the National Comorbidity Survey. Arch Gen Psychiatry 1994;51:8–19.
9. Klerman GL, Weissman MM. Increasing rates of depression. JAMA 1989;261:2229–2235.
10. Weissman MM, Gershon ES, Kidd KK, et al. Psychiatric disorders in the relatives of probands with affective disorder. Arch Gen Psychiatry 1984;41:13–21.
11. McGuffin P, Katz R. The genetics of depression and manic-depressive disorder. Brit J Psychiatry 1989;155:294–304.
12. Gold PW, Goodwin FK, Chrousus GP. Clinical and biochemical manifestations of depression in relation to the neurobiology of stress: Part I. N Engl J Med 1988;319: 348–353.

13. Alpers HS, Himwich HE. An *in vitro* study of effects of tricyclic antidepressant drugs on the accumulation of C-14 serotonin by rabbit brain. Biol Psychiatry 1969;1:81–85.
14. Goodwin FK, Bunney WE. Depressions following reserpine: A reevaluation. Sem Psychiatry 1971;3:435–448.
15. Maas JW. Biogenic amines and depression. Arch Gen Psychiatry 1975;32:1357–1361.
16. Baldessarini RJ. Drugs and the treatment of psychiatric disorders II: Drugs used in the treatment of disorders of mood, in Gilman AG, Rall TW, et al (eds): Goodman and Gilman's The Pharmacologic Basis of Therapeutics, 8th ed. New York, Pergamon Press, 1990, pp 404–435.
17. Prange AJ, Wilson IC, Lynn CW, et al. L-tryptophan in mania. Arch Gen Psychiatry 1974;30:56–62.
18. Vetulani J, Stawarz RJ, Dingell JV, Sulser F. A possible common mechanism of action of antidepressant treatments; reduction in the sensitivity of the noradrenergic cyclic AMP generating system in the rat limbic forebrain. Naunyn-Schmiedeberg's Arch Pharmacol 1976;293:109–114.
19. Richelson E. Biological basis of depression and therapeutic relevance. J Clin Psychiatry 1991;52(6 suppl):4–10.
20. Synder SH, Peroutka SJ. A possible role of serotonin receptors in antidepressant drug action. Pharmacopsychiatry 1982;15:131–134.
21. Bryant SG, Brown CS. Current concepts in clinical therapeutics: Major affective disorders, part 1. Clin Pharm 1986;5:304–318.
22. Siever LJ, Davis KL. Overview: Toward a dysregulation hypothesis of depression. Am J Psychiatry 1985;142: 1017–1031.
23. Sulser F. Mode of action of antidepressant drugs. J Clin Psychiatry 1983;44:14–20.
24. Kalus O, Asnis GM, Van Praag HM. The role of serotonin in depression. Psychiatric Ann 1989;19:348–353.
25. Willner P. Dopaminergic mechanisms in depression and mania, in Bloom FE, Kupfer DJ (eds): Psychopharmacology: The Fourth Generation of Progress. New York, Raven Press, 1995, pp 921–931.
26. Reddy PL, Khanna S, Subhash MN, et al. CSF amine metabolites in depression. Biol Psychiatry 1992;31:112–118.
27. Willner P. Dopamine and depression: A review of recent evidence. Brain Res Rev 1983;6:211–246.
28. Meltzer HY. Role of serotonin in depression, In Witaker-Azsmitia PM, Peroutka SJ (eds): The Neuropharmacology of Serotonin. New York, Annals of the New York Academy of Sciences, 1990, pp 486–499.
29. Katon W, Sullivan MD. Depression and chronic medical illness. J Clin Psychiatry 1990;51(suppl):3–11.
30. Thiessen BQ, Wallace SM, Blackburn JL, et al. Increased prescribing of antidepressants subsequent to beta-blocker therapy. Arch Intern Med 1990;150:2286–2290.
31. Vaillant GE, Blumenthal SJ. Suicide over the life cycle: Risk factors and life span development, in Blumenthal SJ, Kupfer DJ (eds): Suicide Over the Life Cycle. Washington, DC, American Psychiatric Press, 1990, pp 1–16.
32. Janicak PG, Davis JM, Preskorn SH, Ayd FJ. Principles and practice of psychopharmacotherapy. Baltimore, Williams & Wilkins, 1993, pp 209–292, 488–489, 506–507.
33. Preskorn SH, Burke MJ. Somatic therapy for major depressive disorder: selection of an antidepressant. J Clin Psychiatry 1992;53(9, suppl):5–18.
34. Liebowitz M, Quitkin F, Stewart J, et al. Antidepressant specificity in atypical depression. J Clin Psychiatry 1984;45:19–21.
35. Parker G, Roy K, Hadzi-Pavlovic D, Pedic F. Psychotic (delusional) depression: A meta-analysis of physical treatments. J Affect Disord 1992;24:17–24.
36. Burke MJ, Preskorn SH. Short term treatment of mood disorders with standard antidepressants, in Bloom FE, Kupfer DJ (eds): Psychopharmacology: The Fourth Generation of Progress. New York, Raven Press, 1995, pp 1053–1065.
37. Montgomery SA. Venlafaxine: A new dimension in antidepressant pharmacotherapy. J Clin Psychiatry 1993;54:119–126.
38. Fontaine R. Novel serotonergic mechanisms and clinical experience with nefazodone. Clin Neuropharmacol 1993; 16(suppl 3):45–50.
39. Zung W. Review of placebo controlled trials with bupropion. J Clin Psychiatry 1983;44(5, suppl):104–114.
40. Bryant SG, Brown CS. Current concepts in clinical therapeutics: Major affective disorders, part 2. Clin Pharm 1986;5:385–395.
41. Peroutka SJ, Snyder SH. Long term antidepressant treatment decreases spiroperidol-labeled serotonin receptor binding. Science 1980;210:88–90.
42. Berwish N, Amsterdam J. An overview of investigational antidepressants. Psychosomatics 1989;30:1–17.
43. Cole JO, Bodkin JA. Antidepressant side effects. J Clin Psychiatry 1990;51(suppl):21–26.
44. Ray WA, Griffin MR, Schaffner W, et al. Psychotropic drug use and the risk of hip fracture. N Engl J Med 1987;316:363–369.
45. Jefferson JW. Cardiovascular effects and toxicity of anxiolytics and antidepressants. J Clin Psychiatry 1989;50:368–378.
46. Dilsaver SC, Feinberg M, Greden JF. Antidepressant withdrawal symptoms treated with anticholinergic agents. Am J Psychiatry 1983;140:249–251.
47. Bernstein JG. Handbook of Drug Therapy in Psychiatry. Boston, John Wright PSG, 1983, pp 74–76.
48. Venlafaxine prescribing information. Philadelphia PA, Wyeth-Ayerst Laboratories, 1995.
49. Grimsley SR, Jann MW. Paroxetine, sertraline, and fluvoxamine: New selective serotonin reuptake inhibitors. Clin Pharm 1992;11:930–957.
50. Levinson ML, Lipsy RJ, Fuller DK. Adverse effects and drug interactions associated with fluoxetine therapy. DICP Ann Pharmacother 1991;25:657–661.
51. Aranoff GM. Trazodone associated with priapism. Lancet 1984;1:856.
52. Bupropion prescribing information. Research Triangle Park, NC, Burroughs Wellcome Co, 1995.
53. Nierenberg AA, Cole JO. Antidepressant adverse drug reactions. J Clin Psychiatry 1991;52(suppl):40–47.
54. Rapp MS. Two cases of ejaculatory impairment related to phenelzine. Am J Psychiatry 1979;136:1200–1201.
55. Barton JL. Orgasmic inhibition by phenelzine. Am J Psychiatry 1979;136:1616–1617.
56. Rabkin JG, Quitkin FM, McGrath P, et al. Adverse reactions to monoamine oxidase inhibitors, II: treatment correlates and clinical management. J Clin Psychopharmacol 1985;5:2–9.
57. Neil JF, Licata SM, May SJ, Himmelhoch JM. Dietary noncompliance during treatment with tranylcypromine. J Clin Psychiatry 1979;40:33–37.

58. Clary C, Schweizer E. Treatment of MAOI hypertensive crisis with sublingual nifedipine. J Clin Psychiatry 1987;48:249–250.
59. Wells BG. Tricyclic antidepressants, in Taylor WJ, Caviness MHD (eds): A Textbook for the Clinical Application of Therapeutic Drug Monitoring. Irving, TX, Abbott Laboratories, 1986, pp 449–465.
60. DeVane CL. Pharmacokinetics of the selective serotonin reuptake inhibitors. J Clin Psychiatry 1992;53(suppl 2):13–20.
61. Fluoxetine prescribing information. Indianapolis, IN, Dista Products Co, 1995.
62. Paroxetine prescribing information. Philadelphia, PA, SmithKline Beecham Pharmaceuticals, 1995.
63. Sertraline prescribing information. New York, Roerig Division, 1994.
64. Nefazodone prescribing information. Wallingford, CT, Bristol-Myers Squibb, 1995.
65. Depression Guideline Panel. Depression in Primary Care: Vol 2. Treatment of Major Depression. Rockville, MD, Agency for Health Care Policy and Research, 1993, pp 40–41, 71, 84, 92, 118, 124.
66. Perry PJ, Pfohl BM, Holstad SC. The relationship between antidepressant response and tricyclic antidepressant plasma concentrations. Clin Pharmacokinet 1987;13:381–392.
67. Anonymous. Tricyclic antidepressants—blood level measurements and clinical outcomes: An APA task force report. Am J Psychiatry 1985;142:155–162.
68. Hansten PD, Horn JR. Drug interactions and updates. Vancouver, WA, Applied Therapeutics, 1995, pp 127–842.
69. Hansten PD. Drug Interactions, 6th ed. Philadelphia, PA, Lea and Febiger, 1989.
70. DeVane CL. Pharmacokinetics of the selective serotonin reuptake inhibitors. J Clin Psychiatry 1992;53(suppl):13–20.
71. Bannister SJ, Houser VP, Hulse JD, et al. Evaluation of the potential interactions of paroxetine with diazepam, cimetidine, warfarin, and digoxin. Acta Psychiatr Scand 1989;90(suppl):102–106.
72. Stellamans G. A study to investigate the efficacy, adverse events, safety, and pharmacokinetic effects of coadministration of paroxetine and lithium [abstract]. Biol Psychiatry 1991;29:628S.
73. NIH Consensus Development Panel on Depression in Late Life. Diagnosis and treatment of depression in late life. JAMA 1992;268:1018–1024.
74. Kelly GL. Childhood depression and suicide. Nursing Clin North Am 1991;26:545–558.
75. Preskorn S, Weller E, Hughes C, et al. Depression in prepubertal children: DST nonsuppression predicts differential response to imipramine versus placebo. Psychopharmacol Bull 1987;23:128–133.
76. Weller EB, Weller RA. Depressive disorders in children and adolescents, in Garfinkel BD, Carlson GA, Weller EB (eds): Psychiatric Disorders in Children and Adolescents. Philadelphia, PA, WB Saunders, 1990, pp 17–19.
77. Hollister LE. Treatment of depression with drugs. Ann Intern Med 1978;89:78.
78. Montgomery SA, Dunbar G. Paroxetine is better than placebo in relapse prevention and the prophylaxis of recurrent depression. Int Clin Psychopharmacol 1993; 8:189–195.
79. Keller MB, Lavori PW, Mueller TI. Time to recovery, chronicity, and levels of psychopathology in major depression: A five year prospective followup of 431 subjects. Arch Gen Psychiatry 1992;49:809–816.
80. Greden JF. Antidepressant maintenance medications: When to discontinue and how to stop. J Clin Psychiatry 1993; 54(8, suppl):39–45.
81. Anonymous. APA announces development of guidelines for effective use of electroconvulsive therapy. Hosp Community Psychiatry 1991;41:208–209.
82. Krueger RB, Sackheim HA, Ganzu ER. Pharmacological treatment of the cognitive side effects of ECT: A review. Psychopharmacol Bull 1992;28:409–424.

Chapter 68

Bipolar Disorders

Martha P. Fankhauser, MS,
and William H. Benefield, Jr., PharmD, FASCP

Bipolar disorder (previously known as manic–depressive illness) is a cyclical disorder with recurrent fluctuations in mood, energy, and behavior encompassing the extremes of human experiences. This disorder differs from recurrent major depression (or unipolar depression) in the presence of a manic, hypomanic, or mixed episode during the course of the illness. Bipolar disorder is an intriguing psychiatric disorder because it is genetically based, environmentally influenced, and the clinical presentation differs widely from individual to individual.[1]

EPIDEMIOLOGY

Epidemiologic studies report the lifetime prevalence rate of a manic episode is 1.6% ± 0.3 for men and 1.7% ± 0.3 for women in the United States.[2] The onset of the illness is rare before puberty, but its prevalence increases during adolescence and into adulthood (usually between the ages of 18 and 44). Onset of mania after age 65 is rare and may be related to comorbid neurologic causes instead of a genetic risk for the disorder.[3]

PATHOPHYSIOLOGY

GENETICS

Bipolar disorder has a higher genetic risk than do major depressive disorders.[4] Approximately 80–90% of bipolar patients have a relative, parent, sibling, or child with a mood disorder (e.g., major depressive, cyclothymic, dysthymic). Twin studies show a 78–80% concordance in monozygotic twins compared with 20% in dizygotic twins.[4] Adoption studies found that 38% of adopted children (if one biological parent has bipolar disorder) have a mood disorder, whereas only 7% of control, adopted children develop a mood disorder. The exact mechanism of genetic transmission is not known and may involve multifactorial inheritance.[4] Early reports of a genetic marker on chromosome 11 were not substantiated; research is now focusing on genetic abnormalities on chromosome 18. Currently, there is no widely accepted genetic linkage finding for mood disorders.

NEUROTRANSMITTER THEORIES

Several biologic theories have been proposed to account for the underlying pathophysiology of bipolar disorder, but so far none has been confirmed.[5] The most prominent and oldest hypotheses regarding mood disorders are those proposing an alteration in monoamine neurotransmitter concentrations in the central nervous system (CNS). These hypotheses suggest a functional deficit of neurotransmitters [primarily norepinephrine (NE) and/or serotonin (5-HT)] in depression and an excess of catecholamines (primarily NE) in mania. NE and 5-HT are highly interdependent and interact or modulate other neurotransmitter and hormone systems. The "permissive serotonin hypothesis" proposes that there is low central 5-HT in both mania and depression and that 5-HT plays a critical role in modulating CNS activity.

Mood disorders may be caused by a dysregulation between neurotransmitter systems that produces a cyclical rhythm disturbance.[6] NE dysregulation may play an important role in the development of mania. One hypothesis of the switch phenomenon from depression to mania involves the balance of dopamine (DA) to NE activity.[5] When NE activity is decreased (as in depression), the DA activity predominates and this may account for the switch to hypomania or mania. Hyperdopaminergic activity may play a role in causing hyperactivity and psychosis associated with the severe stages of mania.

γ-Aminobutyric acid (GABA), the main inhibitory neurotransmitter in the CNS, is involved in the inhibition of NE and DA activity.[5] A GABA deficiency hypothesis has been proposed for mood disorders, and GABA activity may be related to the sensitization–kindling model for mood disorders.[5] Several antimania drugs [e.g., lithium, carbamazepine (CBZ), valproic acid (VPA), clonazepam, and lorazepam] enhance GABA-ergic activity.

SENSITIZATION AND KINDLING THEORIES

A supersensitivity and kindling model has been proposed as causing cyclical mood disorders.[5] Recurrences of the illness may result in behavioral sensitivity and electrophysiologic kindling (similar to amygdala kindling models in animals for seizures). Initially, psychosocial or physical stressors trigger episodes, but later, the episodes occur spontaneously due to the increased sensitivity and kindling of the CNS. Support for the sensitization–kindling theory arises from the actions of antimanic drugs.[7] In animals, lithium prevents behavioral sensitization caused by cocaine (e.g., decreased dopaminergic and β-adrenergic supersensitivity), but does not prevent amygdala kindling. CBZ does not block behavioral sensitization to cocaine, but can inhibit amygdala kindling.[7] Lithium is most effective in the early course of bipolar illness, but may not be as effective later in the illness or for rapid cycling/mixed states. In contrast, anticonvulsants such as CBZ and VPA are effective in rapid cyclers/mixed states and may be additive if combined with each other or with lithium. Electroconvulsive therapy (ECT) can also inhibit kindling and is used for rapid cyclers/mixed states and in nonresponders to lithium or CBZ. Early recognition and successful treatment of initial episodes of bipolar disorder may decrease the likelihood that patients will develop rapid or continuous cycling.

ELECTROLYTE THEORIES

Changes in electrolyte balance may be related to mood fluctuations observed in bipolar disorder.[5] High serum and cerebrospinal fluid (CSF) calcium concentrations were found in patients with depression, whereas low CSF levels were reported in manic patients. Calcitonin, a CSF peptide that affects calcium metabolism, was lower during mania than in the bipolar-depressed phase or in euthymia. Changes in extracellular and intracellular calcium concentrations can affect the excitability of neuronal firing and may be related to emotional variations and "switches" from depression to mania.[5] Recent studies of calcium secondary messenger systems may help clarify the neurobiologic abnormalities associated with bipolar disorder.[8]

Several antimanic drugs have calcium antagonist effects (e.g., calcium channel blockers, phenothiazine antipsychotics).[5] CBZ may decrease serum sodium and calcium concentrations. Lithium decreases calcium transport into cells and may interfere with the calcium–sodium active transport system. Lithium also increases renal tubular reabsorption of calcium, which may result in hypercalcemia and hyperparathyroidism.

MEMBRANE/SECONDARY MESSENGER SYSTEM THEORIES

Abnormalities in the membrane transport and secondary messenger system indicate a genetic vulnerability in bipolar patients.[5] A reduction in erythrocyte sodium-potassium-activated adenosine triphosphatase (Na^+/K^+-ATPase) activity has been suggested as a marker for bipolar disorder. ATPase maintains ionic gradients across the cell membranes and responds to neurotransmitter activation. If ATPase activity is reduced, another secondary messenger system involving phosphatidylinositol may become more active, resulting in excessive release of monoaminergic neurotransmitters. Initial studies report that bipolar manic patients have elevated platelet membrane phosphatidy linositol-4, 5, biphosphate. Lithium blocks the enzyme inositol-1-phosphatase (an enzyme that converts inositol-1-phosphatase to inositol), that decreases the neurons' ability to restore normal phosphatidylinositol biphosphate (PIP2) concentrations. By affecting this secondary messenger system, lithium reduces the responsiveness of neurons to muscarinic, cholinergic, α-adrenergic, and other stimuli. Lithium interferes with the adenyl cyclase-catalyzed conversion of ATP to cyclic AMP that results in a decrease in cellular responses to neurotransmitters.

ENVIRONMENTAL, SEASONAL, OR CIRCADIAN RHYTHM THEORIES

Circadian rhythm desynchronization or seasonal rhythms may cause diurnal variations in mood, sleep disturbances, and seasonal recurrences of episodes.[9] Changes in the sleep–wake or light–dark cycle have precipitated episodes of mania or depression.[10] Seasonal peaks of depression are highest in the spring (March to May) and next in the fall (September to November), which parallels the same peaks for suicide.[2] There is less seasonal data for manic episodes, but there appears to be an increased incidence of mania during the summer months when there is more exposure to light and heat.[11] Bright light therapy has been used for the treatment of depression and may precipitate hypomanic, manic, or mixed episodes. Switches from depression to mania can happen when patients miss a night's sleep. Sleep deprivation is sometimes used to cause a remission in depressed patients temporarily, but the clinical response is usually brief.

Environmental, psychosocial, or physical stressors may precipitate mood changes, particularly in vulnerable patients with a genetic predisposition.[3] Approximately two-thirds of bipolar patients report a significant stressful life event (especially difficulty at work or interpersonal conflicts) preceding their first manic episode.

Classification/Clinical Presentation

The American Psychiatric Association's *Diagnostic and Statistical Manual of Mental Disorders, Fourth Edition* (DSM-IV), represents our present understanding of mood (or affective) disorders.[12] DSM-IV divides bipolar disorder into four subtypes: bipolar I, bipolar II, cyclothymic disorder, and bipolar disorder not otherwise specified (NOS). The mood states are further separated into four subcategories to differentiate the current or most recent mood episode: major depressive, manic, mixed, or hypomanic. *Bipolar I* is characterized by one or more manic or mixed episodes and is usually accompanied by major depressive episodes. Bipolar I patients have episodes that are severe enough to require treatment or hospitalization. *Bipolar II* is characterized by one or more major depressive episodes and at least one hypomanic episode (Table 68.1). *Cyclothymic disorder* is characterized by at least 2 years (1 year for children and adolescents) of numerous episodes or periods of both hypomanic and depressive symptoms, but they do not meet the criteria for a manic or major depressive episode. Patients with cyclothymic disorder have a 15–50% risk of later developing a bipolar I or II disorder. *Bipolar disorder NOS* is a category for patients with bipolar features whose symptoms do not meet the criteria for any specific bipolar disorder (e.g., recurrent hypomanic episodes without recurrent depressive symptoms or a manic episode superimposed on residual schizophrenia).

The essential feature of bipolar disorder is a history of mania or hypomania that is not caused by any other medical condition, substance (medications or drugs of abuse), or mental disorder.[12] Bipolar disorder is characterized by mood swings (mania and depression) that are outside the range of normal mood changes. Patients usually experience periods of mood elevation (mania or hypomania) that alternate with normal mood states (euthymia). The diagnosis of bipolar disorder does not require a history of depression, but approximately 95% of bipolar patients experience episodes of depression during their lifetime. Unipolar mania (with no depressive episodes) accounts for less than 5–9% of bipolar patients.

Bipolar disorder has diverse clinical manifestations that can differ in symptoms, course, severity, and response to treatment among individuals.[13] Descriptions of the four subcategories of mood episodes (major depressive, manic, mixed, and hypomanic) are given as follows.

TABLE 68.1. COMPARISON OF BIPOLAR I AND BIPOLAR II DISORDERS

	Bipolar I	Bipolar II
Episodes	Manic Hypomanic Mixed Major depression	Hypomanic Major depression
Lifetime prevalence	0.4–1.6%	0.5%
Sex differences	Female = male First episode in males more likely manic episode First episode in females more likely depressive episode	Female > male
Clinical course	60–70% of manic episodes occur just before/after a depressive episode; interval between episodes decreases with age	60–70% of hypomanic episodes occur just before/after a depressive episode
Lifetime episodes	More episodes than major depressive disorder	More episodes than major depressive disorder
Rapid cycling	5–15% of patients	5–15% of patients
% of patients that do not recover between episodes	20–30%	15%
Precipitants of episodes	Changes in sleep-wake cycle Sleep deprivation	Postpartum period
Familial pattern	First-degree biological relatives with mood disorder: Bipolar I (4–24%) Bipolar II (1–5%) Major depression (4–24%)	Higher rates of mood disorder than general population

(Adapted from Refs. 12 and 70.)

MAJOR DEPRESSIVE EPISODE

The clinical presentation and diagnostic criteria for bipolar depression are the same as those for major depressive episode, as discussed in Chapter 67. During a major depressive episode, there is a depressed mood and a marked decrease in pleasure or interest in almost all activities.[12] Bipolar depressed patients tend to have an increased need for sleep, low energy, psychomotor retardation, decreased sexual activity, slowed speech, carbohydrate craving, and weight gain (also called atypical depressive features).[14] Approximately 10–15% of patients first diagnosed as having major depressive illness will later experience an episode of mania or hypomania.

MANIC EPISODE

The DSM-IV diagnostic criteria for a manic episode are listed in Table 68.2.[12] A manic episode is defined by a distinct period when the mood is abnormally and persistently elevated, expansive, or irritable. Acute mania usually begins abruptly and symptoms escalate over several days.[3] Seasonal changes, stressors, antidepressants, bright light, or electroconvulsive therapy (ECT) can precipitate a manic episode.[13] Mania is characterized by heightened mood (euphoria), quicker thoughts (flight of ideas), more and faster speech (pressured speech), increased energy, increased physical and mental activities (psychomotor excitement), decreased need for sleep, anger or irritability, heightened perceptual acuity, increased sexual activity, and impulsivity.

Manic patients frequently become involved in foolish business ventures, illegal activities, or buying sprees.[13,14] Their impulsive and irrational spending behavior often causes significant financial consequences. A change in the sleep cycle (with a decreased need for sleep) is often the first clue to the beginning of an episode. Attention span is usually very short resulting in impairment of concentration and "flight of ideas" (thoughts that change rapidly from one topic to another).

The severe stages of a manic episode may resemble paranoid schizophrenia with symptoms of bizarre behavior, hallucinations, and delusions. Approximately two-thirds of bipolar patients have psychotic symptoms at some point, primarily paranoid or grandiose delusions. Up to 20% of bipolar patients have a formal thought disorder and 5% are later diagnosed with schizophrenia.[3] Bipolar patients with psychotic features are frequently misdiagnosed as having schizophrenia.[2]

TABLE 68.2. DSM-IV DIAGNOSTIC CRITERIA FOR MANIC EPISODE

A. At least a 1-week period of abnormal and persistent elevated mood (expansive or irritable).

B. During the mood disturbance, at least three (or more) of the following symptoms persisted (four if the mood was only irritable) and were present to a significant degree:
   (1) Inflated self-esteem (grandiosity)
   (2) Decreased need for sleep
   (3) Increased talking (pressure of speech)
   (4) Racing thoughts (flight of ideas)
   (5) Distractable (poor attention)
   (6) Increased activity (either socially, at work, or sexually) or increased motor activity or agitation
   (7) Excessive involvement in activities that are pleasurable but have a high risk for serious consequences (e.g., buying sprees, sexual indiscretions, poor judgment in business ventures)

C. The above symptoms must not meet the criteria for a mixed episode.

D. Marked impairment in functioning (social, occupational) or need for hospitalization due to potential for self-harm, harm of others, or psychotic symptoms.

E. The above symptoms are not due to a medical condition or substance-induced disorder.

(Adapted from Ref. 12.)

MIXED EPISODE

Bipolar "mixed episode" (previously known as mixed state, dysphoric mania, or depressive mania) occurs when symptoms of a manic episode and a major depressive episode occur nearly every day for at least a 1-week period.[12] There must be variability and lability in mood that is severe enough to cause impairment in social or occupational functioning or to require hospitalization. Mixed episodes may be more common in younger and older patients and occur more frequently in males.[12] The disturbance should not be due to the effects of medications (e.g., antidepressants, cocaine, corticosteroids) or any medical condition such as hyperthyroidism.

Bipolar disorder is a dynamic and constantly changing illness so that manifestations of either phase may occur simultaneously or patients may cycle or "switch" from one mood state to another. *Rapid cyclers* are defined as having four or more episodes per year (major depressive, manic, mixed, or hypomanic).[3,13] Mixed episodes and rapid cycling are often difficult to diagnose and treat because of the fluctuating clinical presentation. Rapid-cycling and mixed states are associated with a poorer prognosis and nonresponse to antimanic agents.[15] A rare form of bipolar disorder is characterized by "ultrarapid" cycles (e.g., every 48 hours) or "continuous" cycles with no free interval between episodes.[13] Tricyclic antidepressants (TCAs) and monoamine oxidase inhibitors (MAOIs) or subclinical hypothyroidism may exacerbate rapid cycling or convert rapid cyclers to a continuous form of the illness.[1]

HYPOMANIC EPISODE

Hypomania describes a less severe form of mania in which the patient's mood is elevated, expansive, or irritable and there are associated symptoms such as increased psychomotor activity, decreased need for sleep, pressure of speech, flight of ideas, and distractibility. The hypomanic episode does not fit the DSM-IV criteria for a manic episode because there is no marked impairment in social or occupational functioning to necessitate a hospitalization and no delusions or hallucinations are present.[12] Symptoms found in hypomanic episodes are similar to cocaine- or antidepressant-induced mood disorders, thus the differential diagnosis should rule out any substance-induced or medical conditions that present with elevated mood.

During a hypomanic episode, patients may function better and be more productive and creative.[16] Patients find the hypomanic state very desirable because they have a sense of well-being, happiness, exhilaration, feel more powerful and productive, and have increased energy. Hypomanic states are usually associated with euphoria, but some patients have emotional fluctuations with irritability, outburst, rage, and intolerance. Hypomanic states should be closely monitored because 5–15% of patients may rapidly "switch" to a manic episode.[12]

Course of Illness

The average age of onset of a first manic episode is the early twenties, although some episodes may start in adolescence or after age 50. Most bipolar patients have more than one episode during their lifetime (i.e., greater than 80% of patients have more than four episodes).[3,12] For bipolar I disorder, 90% of individuals with a manic episode later have multiple recurrent episodes of either major depression, mania, hypomania, or mixed episodes alternating with a normal mood state. Usually there is a period of normal functioning between episodes, but approximately 25–60% of patients have no period of euthymia due to switching to the opposite polarity.[3,12]

The length and severity of an episode and the interval between episodes vary from patient to patient. The recurrences may become more frequent as the disease progresses, particularly if there was an early age of onset. Manic episodes are usually briefer and end more abruptly than major depressive episodes.[12] The average length of untreated manic episodes ranges from 4 to 13 months.[3] Episodes may occur regularly (at the same time or season of the year) and often cluster at 12-month intervals. If a manic episode occurs postpartum, the woman may have an increased risk for recurrences during subsequent postpartum periods.[12]

In children, the clinical presentation is usually one of lability of mood before the onset of bipolar disorder.[3] Attention-deficit/hyperactivity disorder (ADHD) and a manic episode have similar characteristics (hyperactivity, impulsivity, poor judgment) so ADHD should be ruled out if there is an early onset (i.e., before age 7 years).[12] Early onset bipolar disorder has an increased risk of psychotic features, mixed states, and rapid cycling.[17] Often adolescents use alcohol or drugs, which can mask the symptoms and make diagnosis difficult, to self-treat the mood swings. Individuals with early onset bipolar disorder, rapid cycling, and mood-incongruent psychotic features have a more chronic course and a less favorable response treatment.

Morbidity and Mortality

Bipolar disorder can have devastating long-term effects because recurring episodes may cause deterioration in functioning.[1] Bipolar patients have a high lifetime prevalence rate for alcohol abuse/dependence (46%) and for drug abuse/dependence (41%).[18] Alcohol or drug abuse can precipitate or modify bipolar episodes (e.g., cocaine can lengthen or intensify euphoria, whereas alcohol can cause depression). Bipolar patients tend to self-medicate during episodes resulting in impaired judgment, poor impulse control, and a worsening of the clinical course.

Bipolar disorder is considered a life-threatening illness, particularly if it is not diagnosed and treated.[1] Untreated, depressed bipolar patients have a high risk of suicide (i.e., one in four to five patients commits suicide and approximately 25–50% of patients attempt suicide at least once).[3,19] Inadequately treated bipolar disorder places a significant strain on interpersonal relationships, career, and financial status. Because bipolar disorder is usually evident by the mid-twenties, education may be interrupted and some patients have difficulty keeping a job.[2]

Acutely manic patients may need protection (or hospitalization) because they lack appropriate judgment and insight. Bipolar manic patients may not think that anything is wrong with their thinking or behavior, therefore, they may resist treatment. Often, collaboration with the patient's family is needed for them to receive help.

Fortunately, the majority of bipolar patients are adequately controlled on medication and function well. Those who relapse may do so because of medication noncompliance. Some patients have difficulties accepting that they have a serious, chronic illness and do not receive appropriate treatment until late in the illness or after several hospitalizations. It is estimated that only 33% of bipolar patients receive treatment (due to either failure to recognize the disorder or reluctance to acknowledge the disorder).

DIFFERENTIAL DIAGNOSIS

LABORATORY TESTS/ DIAGNOSTIC PROCEDURES

There are no specific, sensitive diagnostic tests available to assist in the diagnosis of bipolar disorder; however, several potential biologic markers are being investigated. Hypercortisolemia (or elevated urinary cortisol metabolites) is more frequently found in depression than in euthymia, hypomania, or mania.[5] The majority of bipolar patients with depression or mixed episodes are nonsuppressors to the dexamethasone suppression test (DST), but there is disagreement regarding the manic phase. Several studies have reported that hypercortisolemia and the DST return to normal when bipolar patients are recovered from either mania or depression.[5]

A blunted thyroid-stimulating hormone (TSH) response to the thyrotropin-releasing hormone (TRH) stimulation test has been reported in mania.[5] The TRH stimulation test may be useful in differentiating mania from other psychotic states. Provocative challenge tests have been used to determine dysfunctioning in the HPA or HPT axis, but are rarely used as diagnostic tests for bipolar disorder. The DST and TRH tests may predict recovery from episodes because patients have an increased risk of relapse if both tests do not return to normal.[5]

MEDICAL CONDITIONS AND MEDICATIONS ASSOCIATED WITH BIPOLAR DISORDERS

The differential diagnosis for bipolar disorder often includes ruling out other psychiatric disorders including schizophrenia.[20] An accurate diagnosis requires longitudinal psychiatric data, family history, and documentation of signs and symptoms (e.g., premorbid functioning, course of the illness, presence of affective symptoms, mood-congruent delusions or hallucinations, and duration of symptoms). Several medical conditions, medications, and drug withdrawal syndromes can induce or present as mania (Table 68.3). The diagnostic workup should include a thorough medical, drug, and alcohol history, a complete physical examination, and appropriate laboratory tests.

TABLE 68.3. NONPSYCHIATRIC CAUSES OF MANIC AND HYPOMANIC SYMPTOMS

Medical Conditions
AIDS (HIV)
Addison's disease
Carcinoid tumors
Cushing's disease
Epilepsy (temporal lobe)
Hemodialysis
Huntington's disease
Hyperthyroidism
Multiple sclerosis
Neoplasm
Neurosyphilis
Postconcussion
Postinfection (viral, encephalitis, influenza)
Postcerebrovascular accident
Subarachnoid hemorrhage
Surgical trauma

Medications
Alcohol
Amantadine
Amphetamines
Anabolic steroids
Anticholinergics
Anticonvulsants
Antidepressants (TCAs, MAOIs, SSRIs)
Baclofen
Benzodiazepines
Bronchodilators
Caffeine
Calcium replacement
Captopril
Cimetidine
Cocaine
Corticosteroids (ACTH)
Disulfiram
Ephedrine
Hallucinogens
Indomethacin
Isoniazid
Levodopa
Methylphenidate
Phenylpropanolamine
Procainamide
Procarbazine
Quinacrine
Sympathomimetics (decongestants)
Theophylline
Thyroid supplements
Tolmetin
Yohimbine

Drug Withdrawal Syndromes
Antidepressants (TCAs, MAOIs)
Baclofen
Benzodiazepines
Clonidine
Corticosteroids
Guanabenz
Guanfacine
Methyldopa

Somatic Treatments
Electroconvulsant therapy
Bright light therapy

TREATMENT

NONPHARMACOLOGIC THERAPY

Because of the chronicity and recurrence of bipolar illness, patients (and family members) need education and supportive therapy. Bipolar disorder is most effectively treated with a combination of medications and adjunctive "supportive" or "insight-oriented" psychotherapy (individual, group, or family).[21] After a manic episode, bipolar patients often feel ashamed of their behavior during the episode (e.g., inappropriate behavior, aggression, spending of money, sexual indiscretions). They may lack self-confidence, question their judgment, and have difficulties with interpersonal relationships. Bipolar patients often worry about recurrent episodes and fear they will transmit the illness to their offspring.

Patients should be educated about psychosocial or physical stressors that may precipitate episodes (e.g., changing jobs, moving, childbirth, sleep deprivation, jet lag, bereavement) and counseled about how to cope with stressful life events.[3] Patients should be educated about recognizing the signs and symptoms of mania and depression and the importance of complying with treatment. Patients should be encouraged to chart target symptoms to help them recognize mood changes and to seek treatment as soon as possible.

PHARMACOLOGIC THERAPY

The pharmacologic treatment of bipolar disorder must be individualized because the clinical presentation, severity, and frequency of episodes vary widely among patients.[22–26] Hypomanic episodes may not require treatment unless the patient has a previous history of manic episodes. Manic episodes are usually first treated with lithium (plus short-term adjunctive agents, such as benzodiazepines for sleep). Recurrent manic episodes can be treated with either lithium, CBZ, or VPA along with adjunctive benzodiazepines for anxiety/insomnia. The more severe manic episodes, with psychosis or agitation, often require longer term adjunctive benzodiazepines and/or antipsychotics along with lithium, CBZ, or VPA until the mania subsides. If the patient has not responded within 2–3 weeks, a second mood stabilizer can be added to the regimen for augmentation. If patients are nonresponsive to these pharmacologic approaches, ECT may be used to reduce acute manic symptoms rapidly.[22]

Once the patient is stabilized, most patients are placed on long-term (or prophylactic) therapy to prevent or attenuate future episodes.[24] Maintenance therapy is recommended for any patient with at least two major episodes. Although CBZ and VPA are usually reserved as alternative agents for patients who do not tolerate lithium or are nonresponders, these agents are gaining popularity and are widely prescribed.

Despite adequate maintenance treatment, some patients may have "breakthrough" episodes of hypomania or depression that require short-term adjunctive medication (e.g., benzodiazepines or antipsychotics for mania and antidepressants for depression).[24] Depressed patients on lithium should always be evaluated for lithium-induced hypothyroidism, because thyroid supplementation may reverse the depression without the risk of inducing mania.[23] Rapid cyclers may have subclinical hypothyroidism and require thyroid supplements (depending on thyroid indices) before resorting to alternative treatment approaches.

Monotherapy is preferred for long-term maintenance, however, combinations of drugs may be necessary for patients with mixed episodes or rapid cyclers (e.g., lithium plus CBZ, lithium plus VPA, CBZ plus VPA).[25,26] The concomitant use of multiple drugs is often needed to stabilize refractory patients or continuous cyclers (e.g., lithium plus CBZ, clonazepam, or VPA plus an antipsychotic and/or benzodiazepine). Discontinuation of effective prophylaxis with lithium therapy has been associated with an increased risk of relapse (and possibly a more severe and nonresponsive type of disorder). The risk of relapse after discontinuation of maintenance therapy with CBZ or VPA is not known.

LITHIUM

Lithium is considered the first truly antimanic drug.[27] In the late 1800s and early 1900s, it was advocated as a mild tonic, a sedative, an anticonvulsant, and a diuretic. In the early 1940s, lithium-chloride was introduced in the United States as a salt substitute for cardiac patients. After numerous reports of severe toxicity and several deaths, it was withdrawn from the U.S. market. In 1949 John Cade, an Australian physician, reintroduced lithium for the treatment of mania after noting that guinea pigs became lethargic and unresponsive to stimuli after intraperitoneal injection of lithium-urate. In 1954, Mogens Shou, a physician from Denmark, reported the first controlled study of lithium's antimanic effects. In 1970, lithium-carbonate was reintroduced in the United States for the treatment of acute mania, and in 1974 lithium was approved for maintenance therapy of bipolar disorder.[1]

Efficacy in Bipolar Disorder

Extensive clinical experience and well-controlled studies show that lithium is effective in preventing both manic and depressive episodes.[1,25–27] Lithium is generally 70–80% effective in aborting an acute manic or hypomanic episode within 7–14 days after starting therapy.[22,27] Prophylactic lithium therapy is approximately 70–80% effective in preventing or attenuating recurrences of mania, hypomania, and depression in unipolar and bipolar patients.[24] Long-term lithium therapy may be more effective in patients with fewer prior episodes, with a history of euthymia or good functioning between episodes, and with a family history of bipolar illness with a positive response to lithium.[1] Patients maintained on "standard" plasma concentrations of lithium (between 0.8–1.0 mEq/L) may have fewer relapses than patients maintained on lower plasma concentrations (0.4–0.6 mEq/L).[28] Lithium has antidepressant effects and is sometimes used to augment other antidepressants in refractory patients.[24] Lithium may be less effective for severe mania with psychotic features, mixed episodes, rapid/continuous cycling, and in organic-induced mood states.[25,27]

Other Therapeutic Uses

Lithium carbonate has been used in the treatment of schizophrenia, schizoaffective disorder, impulse control disorders, aggression, self-injurious behavior, pervasive developmental disorders, mental retardation, alcoholism, substance abuse, bulimia nervosa, premenstrual syndrome, and for steroid-induced mania. Nonpsychiatric uses of lithium include the treatment of neutropenia, granulocytopenia, syndrome of inappropriate secretion of antidiuretic hormone (SIADH), hyperthyroidism, migraine, and cluster headaches.

Proposed Mechanism of Action

Despite numerous investigations into the biologic and clinical properties of lithium, there is no unified theory for its mechanism of action.[7,27] Lithium is a monovalent cation and belongs to the group of alkali metals. Lithium competes with other monovalent and divalent cations, such as calcium, magnesium, potassium, and sodium, in body tissues and at binding sites. Lithium affects the synthesis, storage, release, and reuptake of central monoamine neurotransmitters including NE, 5-HT, DA, ACh, and GABA.[27] Neuropharmacologic effects of lithium include blockade of dopamine-receptor supersensitivity, decreases of β-adrenoceptor stimulation of adenylate cyclase, and increases of 5-HT, ACh, and GABA function.

Lithium stabilizes postsynaptic receptor sensitivity and has properties similar to calcium channel antagonists. Lithium may decrease neurotransmitter activity by acting at the postsynaptic secondary-messenger system (e.g., decreases neurotransmitter-coupled adenylate cyclase activity and cyclic AMP formation; decreases receptor-G protein coupling; and decreases phosphoinositide metabolism).[27] Lithium inhibits the enzyme inositol-1-phosphatase within neurons that are linked to phosphatidylinositol and blocks 3′, 5′, cyclic adenosine monophosphate (cAMP) stimulation by adrenergic agonists (as reviewed in the Pathophysiology section).[5]

Pharmacokinetics

Absorption

The rate and extent of absorption of lithium from the gastrointestinal tract varies depending on the dosage formulation and whether the dose is taken on an empty or full stomach.[29] Regular-release tablets or capsules are 95–100% absorbed. Peak plasma concentrations occur within 1–3 hours after an oral dose, and absorption is usually complete within 6–8 hours.[27] Slow- or controlled-release tablets are 80–97% absorbed and have a slower absorption with lower and delayed peak plasma concentrations (within 2–6 hours) and complete absorption in 6–10 hours.[29] Oral solutions of lithium-citrate are rapidly and completely absorbed with peak concentrations occurring within 15–60 minutes. Patients who ingest lithium on an empty stomach absorb it more rapidly and may have higher peak plasma concentrations than patients who take it after meals. Administering lithium with meals or using an extended-release product significantly delays absorption, but has no effect on the total amount absorbed. Concurrent administration of antacids does not affect lithium plasma concentrations.

Distribution

Lithium is widely distributed into most body tissues and fluids. The distribution phase follows a biphasic or two-compartment model. The initial distribution phase has a central compartment of 25–40% of body weight, and the final distribution space is approximately 50–100% of body weight.[29] The volume of distribution ranges from 0.5–1.2 L/kg. Elderly patients have a smaller volume of distribution of about 90% body weight compared with 120% for younger patients. Distribution is usually complete 6–10 hours after oral administration of regular-release tablets or capsules. It may take up to 25–30 hours for complete distribution of extended-release preparations.[29]

Lithium is unevenly distributed into tissues and fluids throughout the body and is not bound to plasma proteins. The plasma concentration equals that found in muscle, heart, lung, and kidney. Concentrations more than twice the plasma concentration are found in the thyroid gland, bone, and some areas of the brain, whereas liver, spinal fluid, and erythrocyte concentrations are 50% or less of the plasma concentration.

Elimination

Lithium is primarily renally excreted and is not metabolized.[29] Less than 5% of a lithium dose is excreted through the feces, sweat, and saliva. In patients with normal renal function, about 30–70% of a single dose is excreted in urine within 6–12 hours and 50–80% within 24 hours. Lithium has biphasic elimination with an α half-life of 0.8–1.2 hours and a β half-life of 20–27 hours. The average half-life is approximately 24 hours in adults and 36 hours in geriatric patients. Patients with impaired renal function may have plasma half-lives of 40–50 hours.

Lithium clearance is directly proportional to glomerular filtration rate and renal blood flow.[29] Approximately 80% of the lithium filtered through the glomeruli is reabsorbed in the proximal renal tubules. Renal clearance is about 20% of the glomerular filtration rate (GFR) or about 25 mL/min (range: 10–40 mL/min). Because GFR decreases with age, renal clearance of lithium is reduced in the elderly.

Initiation of Therapy

Baseline Assessment

Before beginning lithium therapy, the patient's medical and medication history should be assessed, looking particularly for evidence of renal, thyroid, cardiovascular or neurologic disease, electrolyte imbalance, potentially significant drug interactions, and for pregnancy. The recommended guidelines for baseline laboratory testing are listed in Table 68.4.[27]

Dosing

Dosing of lithium should be individualized and depends on age, weight, salt intake, renal clearance, and the clinical state.[22] Therapy is usually initiated with moderate doses (900–1200 mg/d) for prophylaxis and higher doses (1200–1800 mg/d) for acute mania, using a two to four times a day dosing regimen. Divided dosing regimens help to minimize the early, dose-related side effects of nausea and tremor. The dose should be adjusted based on the plasma steady-state concentration drawn 12 hours ± 30 minutes after the last dose. Approximately 300 mg of lithium-carbonate will raise the plasma concentration by 0.3 ± 0.1 mEq/L. A therapeutic trial (lithium plasma concentrations of 0.8–1.2 mEq/L) should last a minimum of 4 to 6 weeks. If lithium therapy must be stopped, a gradual tapering over several days is recommended instead of abrupt discontinuation since this may reduce the risk of relapse.[30]

Choosing a Product Formulation

Lithium is available in several salt forms, but only the citrate and carbonate salts are marketed in the United States (Table 68.5). Lithium-citrate is available as a syrup (5 mL contains 8 mEq of lithium). Lithium-carbonate is available in regular-release tablets (300 mg) and capsules (150, 300, and 600 mg), and as extended-release tablets (300 and 450 mg). Selection of a product is based on patient preference, tolerance of side effects, and cost. Patients may prefer capsules if they cannot tolerate the taste of the tablets or have difficulty swallowing them. The syrup is used primarily for patients who refuse to take medication or who have difficulty swallowing tablets or capsules. Lithium oral solution should not be mixed with an antipsychotic (particularly chlorpromazine concentrate) or antidepressant liquid since it may form an insoluble citrate salt. Extended-release products are more expensive and are usually reserved for patients who are experiencing side effects such as nausea or hand tremor with the regular-release products.

TABLE 68.4. RECOMMENDATIONS FOR BASELINE AND ROUTINE LABORATORY TESTING FOR LITHIUM THERAPY

	Baseline	12 Months
Cardiac		
ECG[a]	*	
Pulse and blood pressure	*	
Hematologic		
CBC with differential	*	*
Metabolic/endocrine		
Weight	*	*
Serum electrolytes (sodium, potassium, calcium, phosphate)	*	*
T_3, T_4, free thyroxine index, TSH[b]	*	*
Renal function		
Serum creatinine[c]	*	*
24-hour creatinine clearance[d]	*	*
Urinalysis/osmolality/specific gravity	*	*
Pregnancy test		
In women of childbearing age	*	
Plasma lithium concentrations[e]		

[a]Patients older than 50 or those with preexisting cardiovascular disease; measure at baseline and every 6–12 months as indicated.
[b]TSH is a better indicator of hypothyroidism and should be obtained every 3–6 months during maintenance therapy if thyroid function tests change, if TSH >4 mIU/mL, or if symptoms of hypothyroidism occur.
[c]Measure every 3 months in patients with impaired renal functioning.
[d]Indicated at baseline for patients with a history of renal disease or abnormally high serum creatinine or significant increases in serum creatinine.
[e]Measure every 1–3 months during maintenance therapy; every 5–7 days after any dosage change or possible drug interactions; less frequent monitoring in stable patients (every 6–12 months). (Adapted from Ref. 27.)

TABLE 68.5. LITHIUM PREPARATIONS AVAILABLE IN THE UNITED STATES

Product	Manufacturer
Regular-Release Capsules	
150 mg lithium carbonate (4.06 mEq)	
Lithium carbonate	Roxane
300 mg lithium carbonate (8.12 mEq)	
Eskalith	SmithKline Beecham
Lithonate	Solvay
Lithium carbonate	Roxane
600 mg lithium carbonate (16.24 mEq)	
Lithium carbonate	Roxane
Regular-Release Tablets	
300 mg lithium carbonate (8.12 mEq)	
Eskalith (scored)	SmithKline Beecham
Lithonate (scored; with tartrazine)	Miles
Lithium carbonate (scored)	Roxane, generic brands, various
Lithotabs (scored; film-coated)	Solvay
Extended-Release Tablets	
300 mg lithium carbonate (8.12 mEq)	
Lithobid (film-coated)	Solvay
450 mg lithium carbonate (12.18 mEq)	
Eskalith CR (scored)	SmithKline Beecham
Oral Solution	
8 mEq/5 mL as lithium citrate	
Cibalith-S (sugar-free)	Ciba
Lithium citrate (sugar-free)	Roxane, generic brands, various

Special Considerations for Dosing

Lower initial doses should be prescribed in the elderly or in clinical situations of impaired lithium excretion (e.g., concomitant diuretic therapy, low-salt diet, renal disease, dehydration, or decreased cardiac output). Because of poorer compliance with multiple-dose regimens, the frequency of dosing should be minimized during maintenance therapy. Single-daily dosing at bedtime with extended-release products may be used in patients with polyuria, because lower urine volume may occur with the once-per-day schedule than with multiple doses per day.[24,31]

Lithium is not approved by the Food and Drug Administration (FDA) for children under 12 years of age, but it has been used to treat children with bipolar disorder or aggressive behavior. When therapy is initiated in children, the dose should be low (e.g., 300–900 mg/d or 30 mg/kg/d in divided doses) with gradual increases after laboratory monitoring. Children normally have a higher renal clearance and a shorter elimination half-life of lithium, thus, they may require doses relatively higher than those used in adults to achieve therapeutic plasma concentrations.[22] When lithium is used in children, height and weight measurements should be obtained at baseline and repeated every 3 months.

Dose Prediction Methods

Several dose prediction methods have been developed to obtain therapeutic lithium concentrations more rapidly and with fewer blood level determinations.[22,24] Cooper et al. in 1973 were the first to develop a single-point prediction method (based on a single lithium concentration drawn 24 hours after administering a 600-mg test dose).[32] Other pharmacokinetic methods include a modified Cooper method using a 900-mg test dose, a single- and multiple-point method by Perry, a 4-hour urine and a blood sample method by Norman et al., and the Zetin and Pepin method that does not utilize lithium concentrations.[22,32]

Blood Level Monitoring

Therapeutic Plasma Concentrations

Lithium has a narrow therapeutic index in comparison with other psychotropic medications that necessitates close monitoring of plasma concentrations.[22,27] The usual therapeutic range of lithium is 0.6–1.2 mEq/L, measured 12 hours after the last dose.[24] Acutely manic patients should have a plasma concentration of at least 0.8 mEq/L, and some patients may require plasma concentrations of 1.2–1.5 mEq/L to achieve a therapeutic response. In general, treatment of acute mania requires higher plasma concentrations than maintenance therapy.[22] Onset of the acute antimanic effect of lithium usually occurs within 5–7 days; the full antimanic effect may require 10–21 days and up to 28 days for full antidepressant effect. When mania begins to resolve, the dose should be adjusted downward to decrease the risk of toxicity. Patients should be monitored more closely when they are changing from mania to euthymia or depression because changes in lithium distribution and clearance have been reported in different mood states.[24,27]

Currently, there is no therapeutic reference range for single-daily dosing with lithium. The 12-hour postdose value may be 12–33% higher with extended-release preparations and lower with regular-release tablets compared with divided dosage schedules.

Initial Monitoring of Lithium Plasma Concentrations

When lithium is first started, a nonsteady-state plasma concentration is recommended every 2–3 days in patients prone to toxicity. The standardized "therapeutic" lithium concentration requires the patient to receive the same daily dosage for at least 4–5 days preceding the blood test (until steady state is reached). When the desired plasma concentration has been achieved (after dosage adjustments), blood level monitoring should be done weekly for 3–4 weeks or until lithium concentrations are stabilized.[24]

Blood sampling should be done at the same time and interval so that plasma concentrations are comparable (i.e., 12 hours plus or minus 30 minutes after the last evening dose).[24,29] Blood samples drawn before or after the 12-hour postdose time can be significantly higher or lower than the reference range. Numerous variables influence the accuracy of plasma lithium concentrations and should be assessed if abnormal results occur (Table 68.6).[24]

Red Blood Cell and Saliva Lithium Concentrations

RBC and saliva concentrations have been used as alternative methods for monitoring lithium.[24] Patients with RBC concentrations greater than 0.6 mEq/L or an RBC:plasma ratio greater than 0.5 may have an increased risk of neurotoxicity. Saliva concentrations have been used in children to avoid multiple venipunctures once the exact saliva:plasma ratio is determined (approximately 2 : 1 to 3 : 1 ratio).

Maintenance Therapy

Plasma Concentrations for Maintenance Therapy

Recommended lithium plasma concentrations for maintenance therapy are controversial. Standard therapeutic plasma concentrations (approximately 0.8–1.0 mEq/L) may decrease the risk of relapses,[28] but lower concentrations of 0.4–0.6 mEq/L are better tolerated and may be effective for some patients.[24] The NIMH/NIH Consensus Development Conference on Mood Disorders recommended a maintenance range of 0.6–0.8 mEq/L for most patients.[33] Elderly patients should be maintained on lower plasma concentrations to avoid neurotoxicity (0.6 mEq/L or less).[24] Because more adverse effects (and noncompliance) are associated with higher lithium concentrations, the maintenance concentrations should be individualized and the patient maintained on the lowest possible dose to prevent relapses.[27] Breakthrough episodes during maintenance therapy should be treated by increasing the dose of lithium to achieve higher plasma concentrations (1.0–1.2 mEq/L).[24]

During maintenance therapy, lithium plasma concentrations should be obtained every 1–3 months depending on the individual and the frequency of episodes.[24] If a patient has been stable for a year, lithium concentrations may be checked less frequently (every 6–12 months).[27] Individuals who are prone to toxicity or who have intercurrent illnesses should be carefully supervised by monitoring lithium concentrations more frequently. In addition, lithium concentrations should be obtained 5–7 days after any change in the dose, whenever there is suspected toxicity, a possible drug interaction, a major change in diet or significant weight fluctuations.

TABLE 68.6. FACTORS THAT CAN AFFECT THE ACCURACY AND RELIABILITY OF PLASMA LITHIUM CONCENTRATIONS OR ALTER DOSE/BLOOD RELATIONSHIP

Compliance before the blood test
Timing of blood sampling after last dose
Inadequate time to reach steady state
Product formulation and bioequivalency differences
Accuracy and reliability of the laboratory
Changes in sodium intake or excretion
Caffeine and alcohol intake
Concomitant drugs that alter lithium clearance
Medical illnesses (renal disease, dehydration, diarrhea, vomiting, anorexia, etc.)
Alterations in diet or physical activity
Pregnancy and delivery

Routine Laboratory Monitoring

During maintenance therapy with lithium, it is important to monitor several laboratory indices to minimize potential long-term side effects. The recommended guidelines for laboratory tests and monitoring are listed in Table 68.4.[27]

Duration of Treatment

Bipolar patients who have had only one manic episode and have responded to treatment should be continued on a mood stabilizer for 9–12 months and gradually tapered off over several months with close monitoring for recurrences of symptoms.[24] Lifetime prophylactic antimanic therapy should be given to any patient with two or three previous episodes, with frequent episodes (greater than one per year), or with rapid onset of manic episodes.[24]

Adverse Effects

Side effects of lithium are divided into those that occur early in therapy but are generally innocuous and transient, those that occur with long-term therapy and are usually not dose related, and toxic effects that occur with high plasma concentrations (Table 68.7).[27,34,35]

Early Side Effects

Gastrointestinal disturbances, such as nausea, diarrhea, anorexia, abdominal pain, and bloating, occur in 10–30% of patients but are usually mild and transient.[34,35] Nausea is associated with the rate of increase in plasma lithium concentrations or with high peak concentrations after the dose. If nausea is significant, patients should take lithium after a meal or snack. Other approaches to alleviate nausea include giving a smaller dose more frequently (e.g., 300 mg four times a day rather than 600 mg twice a day) or switching to an extended-release product.

Muscle weakness and lethargy are reported in about 30% of patients, but these symptoms are usually transient, and no intervention is generally needed. Polydipsia with polyuria and nocturia occur in up to 70% of patients initially; these side effects are usually innocuous and diminish with time. Many patients respond to polydipsia with weight gain, probably because of increased consumption of high-calorie fluids or fluid retention. As many as 40% of patients may complain of headache, memory impairment, mental confusion, a decreased ability to concentrate, and impaired fine motor performance.

TABLE 68.7. ADVERSE EFFECTS ASSOCIATED WITH LITHIUM THERAPY

Early Onset	Long Term	Toxicity
GI upset	Weight gain	Severe drowsiness
Nausea	Altered taste	Coarse hand tremor
Polydipsia	Decreased libido	Muscle twitching
Polyuria	Hypothyroidism	Myoclonus
Nocturia	Rash	Choreoathetosis
Dry mouth	Acne	Cogwheel rigidity
Fine hand tremor	Psoriasis	Vomiting
Leukocytosis	Alopecia	Loss of appetite
Muscle weakness	Nonspecific T-wave changes	Confusion
Difficulty concentrating	Premature ventricular beats (rare)	Ataxia
Impaired memory	Nephrogenic diabetes insipidus	Hyperreflexia
	Nephrotoxicity (rare)	Nystagmus
	Fine hand tremor	Seizures
		Coma

A fine hand tremor may be observed in up to 50% of patients during the first week of lithium therapy, and this usually decreases in intensity with time.[34,35] The tremor is seen at rest and increases with voluntary movement. Patients often complain that they are unable to write or to perform fine motor skills. The tremor is worsened by stress, concomitant use of antidepressants or antipsychotics, caffeine, sympathomimetics, and impending toxicity.[24] Tremors may persist in up to 4% of patients and be more severe in patients with a preexisting essential tremor. Strategies to reduce the tremor include lowering the dose, dividing the dose to decrease peak plasma concentrations, switching to an extended-release product, or adding a β blocker. Propranolol in divided doses of 20–80 mg daily is commonly used to treat lithium-induced tremor. Propranolol's effect is usually evident within 30 minutes, and the antitremor action may last up to 6 hours.[24] Other β blockers (e.g., atenolol 50 mg/d, metoprolol 20–80 mg/d) have also been used. Lithium-induced tremor should be differentiated from the constant, coarse, resting tremor (pseudoparkinsonian) caused by antipsychotics since it is not responsive to anticholinergic or antiparkinson drugs.

Long-Term Side Effects

Renal Effects. Lithium reduces the kidney's ability to concentrate urine and in some patients produces a nephrogenic diabetes insipidus (NDI) manifested as polyuria (urine output greater than 3 L/d).[34,35] Polyuria may persist for more than 1 year in up to 10–25% of patients taking lithium. Lithium blocks the action of antidiuretic hormone (ADH) by interfering with cAMP production in the distal renal tubule cells, thus, it decreases reabsorption of water in the distal tubules and collecting ducts. Lithium-induced NDI is associated with normal or elevated plasma concentrations of ADH and does not respond to exogenous vasopressin. NDI is characterized by low urine specific gravity and low osmolality polyuria (e.g., urine volumes of 5–6 L/d). NDI may cause hypernatremia, hypovolemia, and mental changes that can be life-threatening.

Reduction of the lithium dose, changing to single-daily dosing with an extended-release product, adding a potassium supplement (10–20 mEq/d), or discontinuation of therapy may alleviate polyuria or NDI.[24,36] Occasionally, the syndrome persists even after lithium is discontinued. Lithium-induced NDI has been treated with loop diuretics, thiazide diuretics, or triamterene that paradoxically decreases water excretion (see section on Drug Interactions: Diuretics).[24] Thiazide diuretics increase water reabsorption in the proximal tubule, thereby decreasing the amount of water delivered to the distal tubules. Amiloride, a potassium-sparing diuretic, has been used to treat lithium-induced polyuria in doses of 10–20 mg/d (or in combination with hydrochlorothiazide). Amiloride has weaker natriuretic effects than thiazides and appears to be relatively safe with minimal effect on lithium clearance.[37] Frequent monitoring of serum electrolytes and lithium concentrations are required for patients who develop NDI. Fluid restriction is not recommended since dehydration increases the risk of lithium toxicity.

In 1977, there was a report that renal damage may occur from chronic lithium therapy (e.g., glomerulosclerosis, tubular atrophy, interstitial nephritis, presence of urinary casts).[38] During long-term lithium therapy, there may be a slight decrease in GFR that is related to normal aging processes.[23] Numerous studies have examined the issue of lithium-induced renal effects. In general, lithium causes minimal nephrotoxicity if patients are maintained on the lowest effective dose, if adequate hydration is maintained, and if toxicity is avoided.[35] A small percent of patients receiving chronic lithium therapy develop rising levels of serum creatinine, therefore, creatinine levels should be monitored every 6–12 months.[39]

Thyroid Effects. Lithium is concentrated by the thyroid gland and interferes with thyroid hormone synthesis.[34,35] Lithium blocks the release of thyroxine (T_4) and triiodothyronine (T_3) mediated by thyrotropin, inhibits the organification of iodine, decreases the sensitivity of cell surface receptors to TSH, inhibits the peripheral conversion of T_4 to T_3, and stimulates the formation of antithyroid antibodies in some patients.[34,35] Up to 30% of patients on maintenance lithium therapy develop transiently elevated TSH concentrations and 5–15% of patients develop a goiter and/or hypothyroidism.[24] Lithium-induced hypothyroidism is not dose related, is observed 10 times more frequently in women, and usually occurs after at least 18 months of therapy.[34] Lithium may exacerbate a preexisting autoimmune thyroid disease (i.e., Hashimoto's thyroiditis).[40] This condition is diagnosed by the presence of serum thyroid autoantibodies (antithyroglobulin and antimicrosomal Abs).[35]

Symptoms of hypothyroidism (e.g., weight gain, fatigue, low energy, slowed mental functioning) may go unrecognized and are confused with lithium side effects or symptoms of a major depressive episode. Subclinical hypothyroidism (normal total and free T_4 with TSH >6 mIU/mL) is indicative of insufficient thyroid functioning.[35] Hypothyroidism does not require discontinuation of lithium, because exogenous thyroid hormone can be added to the regimen.[24] If the TSH is >5.0 mIU/mL, levothyroxine (LT_4) 0.05 mg/d can be added (followed by a TSH level in 1 month) and increased up to 0.2 mg/d or higher (to achieve TSH >0.1 and <5.0). When lithium is discontinued, patients should be reassessed for the need of exogenous thyroid hormone since hypothyroidism is almost always reversible and since hyperthyroidism has been reported upon discontinuation of lithium therapy.

Cardiac Effects. Lithium may cause a variety of benign and reversible cardiac effects, particularly T-wave flattening or inversion in up to 30% of patients.[24,34,35] The cardiac effects of lithium may be secondary to displacement of potassium from intracellular myocardial sites. Lithium rarely causes myocarditis, sinus node dysfunction, or sinoatrial block, but may aggravate ventricular arrhythmias and atrial premature contractions.[24,35] During lithium intoxication, the ST segment may be depressed, and/or the QT interval prolonged. If a patient has significant preexisting cardiac disease, consultation with a cardiologist is recommended before initiation of lithium therapy.[34]

Miscellaneous Effects. Other long-term lithium side effects include benign reversible leukocytosis, weight gain (20% of patients gain more than 10 kg), and a variety of dermatologic effects (e.g., acne and acneiform eruptions, alopecia, psoriasis, pruritic dermatitis, maculopapuloeruptions, folliculitis).[24,34,35] Decreased libido, sexual dysfunction, dry mouth, alterations in taste, changes in glucose tolerance, hypercalcemia, and hyperparathyroidism have been reported. Severe neuromuscular disturbances such as myasthenia gravis, extrapyramidal symptoms, pseudotumor cerebri, and papilledema are occasionally observed. Cogwheel rigidity that is unresponsive to anti-Parkinson medications has been reported with lithium administration but these patients have usually been treated with antipsychotics.[35,41] Muscular hyperirritability (including fasciculations, twitching, clonic movements of limbs), and hyperactive deep-tendon reflexes may occur in some patients. Permanent neurologic sequelae, including cerebellar ataxia, choreoathetoid movements, and disturbances in gait and speech are rare and usually associated with chronic lithium toxicity.[41]

Toxicity

Lithium is an extremely toxic drug if accidentally or intentionally taken in overdose. Table 68.7 lists the most common signs and symptoms of toxicity. There are several situations that predispose patients to the risk of elevated lithium concentrations and potential toxicity (Table 68.8). Physically ill patients often become dehydrated or have electrolyte imbalances secondary to poor fluid intake, vomiting, and diarrhea. Concomitant medications that interfere with lithium clearance may lead to toxicity. High-risk patients (e.g., the elderly and those with renal impairment) should be monitored closely for signs of toxicity.

Initial signs of mild toxicity (1.2–1.5 mEq/L) include difficulty with memory and concentration, fine hand tremor, gastrointestinal upset, muscle weakness, and fatigue.[42] An organic brain syndrome (or neurotoxicity) manifested by confusion, memory impairment, agitation, electroencephalogram (EEG) changes, and extrapyramidal symptoms (cogwheel rigidity) may be present at therapeutic concentrations, especially in the elderly.[41] Moderate to severe toxic side effects are usually observed at concentrations greater than 1.5 mEq/L. These include agitation, confusion, lethargy, ataxia, dysarthria, aphasia, speech impediments, nystagmus, headache, emesis, increased deep-tendon reflexes, coarse tremors, involuntary choreoathetosis, and muscle fasciculations. Above 3.0 mEq/L, the syndrome progresses with clonic–tonic twitching, seizures, irreversible brain damage, respiratory complications, coma, and death.[42]

TABLE 68.8. SITUATIONS THAT MAY INCREASE PLASMA LITHIUM CONCENTRATIONS

Decreased sodium intake or increased sodium excretion
Low-sodium diet
Diuretics
Excessive exercise/sweating
Protracted diarrhea/vomiting
Salt deficiency
Decreased water intake or increased water excretion
Dehydration
Diuretics (thiazide and potassium sparing)
Fever
Physical illness (flu, surgery, diarrhea, vomiting)
Postpartum fluid changes
Slimming diets
Renal disease or decreased renal blood flow
Renal dysfunction
Nonsteroidal anti-inflammatory agents

If severe lithium intoxication occurs (concentrations higher than 2.5 mEq/L taken 12 hours after the last dose), lithium therapy should be discontinued.[24] Treatment of lithium toxicity depends on the severity of the poisoning, but should include supportive care with monitoring of vital signs, cardiac, pulmonary and neurologic status, electrolytes, and plasma lithium concentrations.[42] The primary goal of treatment should be to correct any fluid or electrolyte imbalance and to lower lithium concentrations. Alkalinization of the urine along with diuretics (e.g., acetazolamide, mannitol, and aminophylline) is not recommended except in cases of severe overdose when dialysis is not available. Sodium loading without evidence of sodium depletion may cause hyperosmolality and is not recommended as a method to enhance lithium elimination.

When lithium concentrations are above 3.5–4.0 mEq/L, the plasma concentration should be measured every 3 hours until it is below 1.0 mEq/L. If the concentration does not drop greater than 10% every 3 hours or the lithium half-life is greater than 36 hours, intermittent hemodialysis (12 hours on and 12 hours off) should be started and continued until the lithium plasma concentration is below 1.0 mEq/L taken 12 hours after the last dialysis. Peritoneal dialysis may be used if hemodialysis facilities are not available. Hemodialysis can increase lithium clearance by 50 mL/min and peritoneal dialysis by 15 mL/min.[42] Because of slow equilibrium between intracellular and extracellular compartments, rebound increases in plasma lithium concentrations may occur 5–8 hours after dialysis. Generally, signs of toxicity disappear slowly within 6–7 days of lithium poisoning. Several reports of irreversible neurologic deficits with dementia, ataxia, deficits in memory and concentrating ability, and kidney damage with reduced GFR have been reported with lithium intoxication.[42]

Special Considerations for Adverse Effects

Pregnancy and Lactation. For many years, lithium was considered to have serious teratogenic effects, and women of childbearing age were encouraged to use contraception and to gradually taper off and discontinue lithium prior to pregnancy. However, lithium may have a lower incidence of causing cardiovascular defects (particularly Epstein's anomaly) if taken during the first trimester than was previously thought.[43] Several studies have reported a more modest teratogenic risk associated with first-trimester exposure to lithium, thus, physicians may have more choices in weighing the risk versus benefits of using lithium in pregnant women. Alternatives to lithium during pregnancy include antipsychotics, CBZ, VPA, and benzodiazepines, although problems have also been associated with the use of these agents during pregnancy.[22] In general, ECT (and possibly a calcium channel blocker such as verapamil) may be safer than lithium, CBZ, and VPA in pregnant women who are manic, depressed, or psychotically depressed.

If lithium is prescribed during pregnancy or is restarted during the latter part of pregnancy, several precautions are necessary. During pregnancy, GFR increases 30–50%, and plasma volume increases 50%, thus lithium dosages should be adjusted based on regular monitoring of plasma concentrations.[24] At parturition, there is a rapid decrease in GFR, and plasma volume returns to normal, thus lithium dosages should be reduced by one-half either a week before the delivery or discontinued 2–3 days before the expected delivery date.[44] Lithium therapy can be restarted a few days after delivery at the normal dosage to decrease the risk of postpartum mania and/or depression.[24]

Lithium freely crosses the placenta and is found in equal concentrations in maternal and fetal blood.[35,44] The clinical features of neonatal lithium toxicity include hypotonia, bradycardia, cyanosis, and low Apgar scores. Lithium may impair thyroid function in the fetus, and goiters have been reported. Lithium passes easily from blood into breast milk. Concentrations in the milk range from 30–100% of the mother's plasma concentration, and plasma concentrations in the nursing infant are 10–50% of the mother's.[44] For these reasons, breast-feeding is discouraged.

Drug Combinations and Drug Interactions

Patients receiving lithium frequently require the addition of other medications during the course of therapy. Several drug–drug interactions have been reported and are summarized in Table 68.9.[27,35]

Antidepressants

Patients with bipolar depression may require antidepressants (TCAs, heterocyclics, or MAOIs) along with lithium to treat episodes of major depression.[23] Increased cycling or induction of mania or hypomania has occurred when some bipolar patients are treated with antidepressants alone or in combination with mood stabilizers, but this has not been substantiated by all studies.[23] To decrease the risk of inducing mania or rapid cycling, it is recommended that higher plasma concentrations of the mood stabilizer be tried first to determine clinical response before adding an antidepressant.[1] Patients with a history of developing mania after a depressive episode or who have frequent cycling should be treated cautiously with antidepressants.[23] Once the depressive episode has resolved, antidepressants should be gradually withdrawn and the patient can be maintained on a mood stabilizing agent. There appears to be no long-term prophylactic value in combining lithium and antidepressants for maintenance therapy over lithium alone.[24]

Little information is available comparing the various antidepressants to determine if specific agents are better for bipolar depression and have a lower potential for precipitating mania (reports that bupropion has a lower risk of inducing mania need to be substantiated in larger studies).[45] Because psychomotor retardation is more common in bipolar depression, a less sedating antidepressant may be better tolerated (e.g., desipramine, nortriptyline, bupropion, phenelzine, tranylcypromine, serotonin reuptake

TABLE 68.9. DRUG INTERACTIONS WITH LITHIUM

Class/Generic Name	Effect on Plasma Lithium Concentration	Significance
Antibiotics		
Erythromycin Metronidazole Spectinomycin Tetracycline	Unclear	Case report of possible increase in lithium concentrations (from nephrotoxic effect of antibiotics); tetracycline may be safe, as drug interaction not substantiated
Antidepressants		
Fluoxetine	Increase	Case reports of increased lithium concentrations and neurotoxicity
Tricyclic Monoamine oxidase inhibitors	Unknown	May cause switch to mania; increase in tremors
Anti-inflammatory drugs		
Diclofenac Ibuprofen Indomethacin Mefenamic acid Naproxen Phenylbutazone Piroxicam	Increase	All nonsteroidals (except sulindac) interfere with clearance and increase lithium concentrations
Sulindac	No effect	May be used with lithium
Antipsychotics		
Chlorpromazine Fluphenazine Haloperidol Perphenazine Thioridazine	Unclear	All antipsychotics may increase lithium's neurotoxicity; may increase RBC lithium concentrations; haloperidol may increase plasma lithium concentrations
Cardiovascular drugs		
ACE inhibitors		
Lisinopril Captopril Enalapril	Increase	Case reports of increased lithium concentrations due to decreased renal elimination
Calcium channel blockers		
Verapamil Diltiazem	Unclear	Case reports of neurotoxicity and bradycardia; case reports of decreased lithium concentrations
Digoxin	Unknown	Case report of CNS confusion and bradycardia
Methyldopa	Unclear	Case reports of neurotoxicity at low lithium concentrations
Diuretics		
Carbonic anhydrase inhibitors Acetazolamide	Decrease	Increase lithium excretion
Loop diuretics		
Ethacrynic acid Furosemide	Possible increase	May increase lithium concentrations; less likely than distal tubule diuretics
Distal tubule diuretics		
Chlorthalidone Metolazone Thiazides	Increase	Well-documented interaction with increase in lithium concentrations
Osmotic diuretics		
Mannitol Urea	Decrease	Increase lithium excretion
Potassium-sparing diuretics		
Amiloride	No effect	May be used to treat lithium-induced polyuria
Spironolactone Triamterene	Increase	May increase lithium concentrations
Xanthines		
Caffeine Theophylline	Decrease	Increase lithium excretion
Neuromuscular blocking drugs		
Pancuronium bromide Succinylcholine	Unknown	May prolong neuromuscular blockade

(continued)

TABLE 68.9. DRUG INTERACTIONS WITH LITHIUM (*Continued*)

Class/Generic Name	Effect on Plasma Lithium Concentration	Significance
Miscellaneous		
Alcohol	Unknown	Increased lithium toxicity in animals; acute alcohol ingestion may increase peak lithium concentration
Carbamazepine	Unknown	May have synergistic effect in treating mania and depression; case reports of neurotoxicity
Clonazepam	Unknown	May potentiate lithium toxicity and neurotoxicity
Insulin and oral hypoglycemics	Unclear	Careful monitoring of glucose is needed as lithium can alter glucose tolerance
Metoclopramide	Unknown	Case report of extrapyramidal symptoms
Metronidazole	Unknown	May increase lithium concentrations
Phenytoin	Unknown	Case reports of lithium toxicity even at therapeutic concentrations and changes in phenytoin concentrations
Sodium bicarbonate	Decrease	Alkalinization of urine increases lithium excretion
Sodium chloride	Decrease	Increase lithium excretion

(Adapted from Refs. 27, 35, and 50–52.)

inhibitors).[23,24,45] The use of selective serotonin reuptake inhibitors (fluoxetine, sertraline, paroxetine, and fluvoxamine) and the serotonin/norepinephrine reuptake inhibitor, venlafaxine, in treating major depressive episodes is very popular, but little information is available about their safety and efficacy in bipolar depression. Nonpharmacologic treatments for bipolar depression include partial sleep deprivation or phase-advance sleep schedule, high-intensity light therapy, or ECT.[23,24] ECT is considered to be more effective than TCAs and MAOIs for severe bipolar depression.[45]

Antipsychotics

An acute manic episode may be treated with antipsychotics or a combination of an antipsychotic and mood stabilizer for additive or synergistic effects.[46] Low-potency agents (e.g., chlorpromazine, thioridazine) are more sedating and cause more orthostatic hypotension, but have the advantage of causing fewer extrapyramidal side effects (EPS). The high-potency agents (e.g., haloperidol, fluphenazine, thiothixene) cause less sedation and fewer blood pressure changes but have increased risk of causing EPS. Atypical antipsychotics (e.g., clozapine, risperidine) cause less EPS and have been used in combination with mood stabilizers.

Antipsychotics are often prescribed for acute mania, however, other alternatives such as CBZ, VPA, clonazepam, or lorazepam are gaining popularity. Antipsychotics (and possibly CBZ and VPA) may have a more rapid onset of action than lithium (during the first week or two) to control the psychotic symptoms and increased psychomotor activity of acute mania.[25,46] Lower doses of antipsychotics are usually effective but higher doses (e.g., haloperidol 5–10 mg intramuscularly or 10–25 mg orally every 4–6 hours as needed) may be required for psychotic or agitated patients.[25] Once acute mania is controlled (usually within 7–14 days), the antipsychotic should be gradually tapered and discontinued, and the patient maintained on the mood stabilizer alone to avoid neurotoxicity, post-mania depression, EPS, supersensitivity psychosis, and tardive dyskinesia.[22] Intermittent use of antipsychotics has been associated with an increased risk of tardive dyskinesia in bipolar patients, therefore, exposure to antipsychotics should be minimized and only used in patients with psychotic symptoms.[46]

Cases of neurotoxicity (e.g., confusion, hyperthermia, severe rigidity, mutism, incontinence of urine, tremor, and irreversible tardive dyskinesia) have been reported with the combined use of lithium and antipsychotics.[22] Neurotoxicity is more common with higher lithium and antipsychotic doses if there is preexisting encephalopathy, or in elderly patients. Symptoms usually disappear if both drugs are discontinued and if lithium is reinstituted at lower doses. Lithium and antipsychotics may be safely administered together if lower doses are used and if lithium plasma concentrations are maintained below 1.0 mEq/L.[22] The exact mechanism for increased neurotoxicity is not known but may be related to increased intracellular lithium concentrations or a neuroleptic malignant syndrome. Patients receiving both lithium and phenothiazines may have a higher RBC/plasma lithium ratio, and haloperidol has been reported to increase plasma lithium concentrations.

Benzodiazepines

An alternative to antipsychotic therapy in acutely manic patients is the use of benzodiazepines that facilitate GABA-ergic transmission. Clonazepam and lorazepam have been used in conjunction with lithium, CBZ, and VPA during acute mania.[22,47,48] Benzodiazepines cause minimal adverse effects and at higher doses rapidly sedate agitated patients.[25] Benzodiazepines have efficacy in the treatment of acute mania or breakthrough mania, but they may not be as effective for prophylactic therapy.[24]

The dosing of lorazepam is approximately 1–4 mg three times daily with gradual increases of doses to achieve maximum effects (approximately 0.5–1.0 mg clonazepam equals 2.0 mg lorazepam). Lower doses (up to 4 mg/d) may be used with benzodiazepine–antipsychotic combinations.[25] Lorazepam is available by parenteral injection (2 and 4 mg/mL), and lower doses are required if administered IM or IV. Once the patient is stabilized, the dose can be gradually reduced to avoid daytime oversedation or administered at bedtime to promote sleep. Benzodiazepines should be gradually tapered over several weeks and discontinued to avoid withdrawal symptoms. A potential drug interaction may occur between lithium and clonazepam resulting in lithium toxicity (either a pharmacokinetic interaction resulting in increased lithium concentrations or a synergistic neurotoxic effect).[49]

Diuretics

Because approximately 80% of lithium is reabsorbed at the proximal tubule, any drug that affects proximal sodium resorption can significantly alter lithium clearance. Thiazide diuretics decrease tubular reabsorption of sodium and indirectly increase lithium reabsorption at the proximal tubule.[22] Thiazide diuretics decrease lithium renal clearance by 24% and increase plasma lithium concentrations by one-third. Diuretics and lithium may be given concomitantly as long as lithium doses are lowered and plasma concentrations and electrolytes are monitored closely. Before a patient is started on a thiazide diuretic, the plasma lithium concentration should be within the therapeutic range (0.6–1.2 mEq/L), and the lithium dose should be reduced by about 50%.[50] Plasma lithium concentrations should be ordered biweekly until the concentration restabilizes.

Loop diuretics have less effect on lithium clearance and may not significantly alter lithium concentrations.[22] The effect of potassium-sparing diuretics on lithium clearance has not been sufficiently studied so patients should be closely monitored. Amiloride, a potassium-sparing diuretic, has been used concomitantly with lithium to reduce lithium-induced polyuria without increasing lithium concentrations.[37] Osmotic and xanthine diuretics have been shown to increase lithium clearance.

Nonsteroidal Anti-Inflammatory Drugs

Pharmacokinetic studies found a significant decrease in lithium clearance and a clinically important increase in steady-state plasma concentrations when lithium was combined with nonsteroidal anti-inflammatory drugs (NSAIDs) (e.g., indomethacin, 30–60% increase; phenylbutazone, 20% increase; naproxen, up to 40% increase; and ibuprofen, 12–66% increase).[51] The NSAIDs reduce renal prostaglandin synthesis and thus decrease the urinary excretion of prostaglandins and sodium. Plasma lithium concentrations should be monitored every 4–5 days when a NSAID is added or discontinued to determine the significance of the interaction. Sulindac, an NSAID with no effect on the renal prostaglandin system in therapeutic doses, may not increase lithium concentrations.[52] Aspirin and acetaminophen have minimal effect on lithium plasma concentrations and may be used in patients who require an anti-inflammatory or analgesic agent.

Sodium Intake

Low-sodium diets or restriction of sodium intake significantly increases plasma lithium concentrations. Heavy exercise, sauna baths, hot weather, and fever may promote sodium loss. Patients should be cautioned to maintain adequate sodium and fluid intake. Increases in sodium consumption via high-sodium diets may increase lithium clearance. When drugs with a high sodium content are used concomitantly with lithium, plasma lithium concentrations should be monitored.

Patient Education

Bipolar patients taking lithium (or other mood stabilizers), require patient counseling and medication education. Because most bipolar patients take mood stabilizers for many years, the clinician must address the psychologic implications of long-term therapy.[24] Patients should be informed about the need to take medication regularly and the importance of monitoring plasma concentrations. It is essential that patients and family members know the symptoms of toxicity as well as the early and long-term side effects. The most frequently cited reason for noncompliance is adverse side effects (e.g., weight gain, polyuria, tremor, and cognitive changes).[24] Patients should be instructed on how to minimize side effects and what to do if they experience symptoms of toxicity.

For patients taking lithium, the need for ample fluid and sodium intake should be discussed, because dehydration and low-sodium diets may precipitate toxicity. Patients should drink at least 2.5–3 quarts of fluid each day and avoid excessive use of coffee, tea, cola, and other caffeine-containing beverages. Patients should be warned that alcohol intake may increase the potential for toxicity. Women of childbearing age should be educated about the possible teratogenic effects of mood stabilizers and advised of appropriate birth control methods. Because of lithium's numerous drug interactions, patients should be instructed to inform their physician that they are taking lithium and should avoid taking diuretics and NSAIDs unless under close medical supervision.

Alternative Treatments for Bipolar Disorder

Although lithium has been considered the drug of choice for bipolar disorder, anticonvulsants such as CBZ and VPA are now being used as first-line mood stabilizers. Approximately 20–40% of patients cannot tolerate the adverse effects or do not respond to lithium despite therapeutic plasma concentrations.[25] Rapid cycling, mixed episodes, or severe manic stages are often resistant to monotherapy with lithium.[24,27] Several alternative medications (or adjunctive therapies) are being investigated and are now commonly prescribed in bipolar illness.

CARBAMAZEPINE

CBZ is the first medication that was extensively studied as an alternative treatment for bipolar disorder.[1] CBZ is marketed as an anticonvulsant and for paroxysmal pain syndromes, such as trigeminal neuralgia. Studies show that CBZ has acute antimanic, antidepressant, and prophylactic effects comparable with lithium in bipolar disorder.[25] Preliminary evidence suggests that CBZ may be more effective than lithium in severe mania, rapid/continuous cycling, and in mixed episodes.[1,22] Approximately 60% of patients with acute mania respond to CBZ, 50–60% of patients show good to moderate antidepressant response, and effective prophylaxis is provided in approximately 60–75% of patients. There are some reports that CBZ may lose effectiveness over time, thus, further studies are needed to determine its long-term efficacy compared to lithium.[53]

In most studies, approximately 60% of manic subjects who were first unresponsive to lithium responded to CBZ within the first several days (faster than the antimanic response with lithium).[22] The addition of CBZ to lithium should be tried in rapid cycling patients or in those who have failed on lithium therapy alone.[25] Once patients have responded, the lithium should be slowly withdrawn over several months (to minimize the risk of relapse), and the patient continued on CBZ therapy alone. CBZ is also beneficial in managing aggressive behavior and has been used for alcohol and benzodiazepine withdrawal syndrome. CBZ is recommended over lithium for patients with dementia and organic causes of mania (e.g., hypomania induced by levodopa, head trauma, CNS pathology, multiple sclerosis, myasthenia gravis).[22] Positive predictors for response with CBZ include severe manic episodes, anxiety, dysphoria, schizoaffective/psychotic features, brain damage (abnormal EEG), patients with early onset manic episodes, and a negative family history for mood disorders.[54]

Proposed Mechanism of Action

CBZ, a dibenzazepine derivative, is structurally related to TCAs. The precise mechanism of action of CBZ in affective disorders remains to be elucidated.[7] CBZ blocks the reuptake of NE, decreases the release of NE, increases acetylcholine in the striatum, decreases DA and GABA turnover, and decreases the activity of adenylate cyclase.[7] In animal models, CBZ is effective in inhibiting amygdala kindling in the temporal lobe (as discussed in the Pathophysiology section).[7,22,25]

Baseline Assessment

Baseline laboratory testing should include a complete blood count (CBC) with differential and platelet count (possibly a reticulocyte count and serum iron), liver enzymes, thyroid function (T_3, T_4, and TSH), serum electrolytes, blood urea nitrogen, urine specific gravity, serum creatinine, neurologic assessment, and ECG if the patient is older than 40 years old or has preexisting cardiac disease.[24]

Dosing

CBZ should be administered with meals to minimize gastrointestinal side effects. Severe drowsiness and dizziness may occur when the dose is increased rapidly, therefore, the dose should be gradually increased according to response and tolerance of adverse effects.[25] During an acute manic episode, CBZ should be started at 200–400 mg/d and increased by 200 mg every 3 or 5 days up to 600–1200 mg/d in divided doses (two to four times daily).[22] If there is no response after 2 weeks, then the dose can be gradually increased to obtain plasma concentrations between 6 and 12 mcg/mL.[22] Some treatment-resistant patients may require higher plasma concentrations (up to 12–14 mcg/mL) to achieve a response. When patients are symptom free, CBZ can be initiated with lower initial doses (e.g., 100 to 200 mg/d, and increased by 100 to 200 mg/d every 3 or 5 days until 600–1200 mg/d).

In general, children ages 13–15 should not receive >1 g/d of CBZ and those older than 15 years of age should not receive >1.2 g/d. Most patients respond to low to moderate doses of CBZ, but some patients (especially rapid cyclers or mixed states) require higher doses (1.6–3.0 g/d) to achieve therapeutic plasma concentrations. When CBZ is combined with lithium, VPA, or antipsychotics, lower doses and blood levels of CBZ should be used to minimize neurotoxicity. CBZ should be withdrawn slowly to avoid precipitating recurrence of bipolar symptoms or seizures in epileptic patients.

Plasma Concentrations

There appears to be no direct relationship between doses of CBZ and plasma concentration, or is there any significant correlation between plasma concentration and degree of antimanic or antidepressant response.[25] Despite the poor correlation between plasma concentration and clinical response, most clinicians attempt to maintain plasma concentrations of CBZ between 6 and 12 mcg/mL. During the first month of therapy, plasma concentrations of CBZ may decrease (due to autoinduction of hepatic oxidative enzymes that increases CBZ metabolism) and the dose may need to be increased to maintain therapeutic plasma concentrations. Autoinduction of CBZ may begin by day 3 and can continue up to 30 days after the last dosage change. Steady-state concentrations should initially be obtained twice a month during the first 2 months of treatment. Once steady-state concentrations are stabilized, plasma CBZ concentrations can be monitored every 2–3 months. For patients stabilized for over a year, less frequent monitoring may be indicated (e.g., 2–3 times per year).

Routine Laboratory Monitoring

Because bone marrow suppression is rare, the guidelines for monitoring hematologic changes with CBZ are now less extensive than previous recommendations.[55] Patients with low-normal or below-normal pretreatment white blood cell (WBC) and neutrophil counts should be monitored more closely due to increased risks of developing leukopenia (e.g., every 2 weeks for the first 1–3 months of treatment).[24,55] A transient decrease in WBC and platelets can occur during the first few months of treatment (approximately 12% of children and 7% of adults) and does not require discontinuation of the drug.[55] CBZ-induced leukopenia has been reversed in some patients by adding lithium, which causes a leukocytosis.[56] If symptoms of bone marrow suppression occur (sores, infections, fever, fatigue, petechiae, or easy bruising), a CBC with differential, platelet count, and liver enzymes should be done to rule out aplastic anemia, agranulocytosis, or thrombocytopenia.[22] If leukopenia occurs (WBC <3000/mm^3 or neutrophil counts <1000/mm^3), then the dose of CBZ should be decreased or discontinued.[55] CBZ may be restarted at lower doses when WBC and neutrophils return to normal ranges. The highest period of risk for hematologic reactions is during the first year of treatment so patients should be monitored more closely during this time.

Adverse Effects

Neurologic

CNS toxicity can occur in up to 60% of patients receiving CBZ.[57] Neurologic side effects include drowsiness, dizziness, fatigue, clumsiness, ataxia, vertigo, blurred vision, diplopia, nystagmus, dysarthria, confusion, and headache. These side effects usually occur during the first few weeks of therapy (when plasma concentrations are >4 mcg/mL) and may be minimized by initiating therapy with low doses and gradually increasing the dose to achieve the desired therapeutic response. Side effects may also be alleviated rapidly by dose reduction or giving a larger bedtime dose.

Gastrointestinal

Gastrointestinal (GI) side effects occur early in therapy in up to 15% of patients and include nausea, vomiting, abdominal pain, diarrhea, constipation, and anorexia.[57] The GI side effects may be minimized by administering the drug with food or reducing the daily dose.

Dermatologic

Approximately 8–15% of patients develop hypersensitivity reactions including various types of dermatologic reactions (e.g., pruritic and erythematous rashes, urticaria, photosensitivity reactions, a lupus erythematosus-like syndrome).[57] Mild to moderate skin rashes may be treated with 20–30 mg of prednisone and/or antihistamines (diphenhydramine or hydroxyzine) for a few weeks, then gradually decreased and discontinued.[22] More serious and life-threatening skin reactions reported with CBZ include erythema multiforme, Stevens–Johnson syndrome, lichenoid or eczematous rashes, bullous eruptions, exfoliative dermatitis, and toxic epidermal necrolysis.

Hematologic

While transient decreases in leukocyte counts are common, the more serious CBZ-induced hematologic toxicities appear to be rare. Idiosyncratic hematologic effects reported with CBZ include aplastic anemia, agranulocytosis, thrombocytopenia, leukopenia, eosinophilia, and hemolytic anemia.[57] Agranulocytosis and aplastic anemia occur in approximately 1 in 125,000 patients, and fatal toxicity is uncommon. Patients should be informed of early signs of hematologic problems (e.g., sore throat, fever, mouth ulcers, easy bruising) and instructed to contact their physician if any symptoms occur during treatment. If there is any evidence of significant bone marrow suppression, CBZ should be discontinued and the patient monitored closely. Patients with a history of bone marrow suppression and concomitant use of medications that have an increased incidence of causing agranulocytosis (such as clozapine) should not receive CBZ.

Hyponatremia

CBZ may cause SIADH or water intoxication secondary to its antidiuretic activity.[57] Patients who have low baseline serum sodium concentrations or who complain of fatigue, irritability, or decreased concentration should be evaluated for hyponatremia/hyposmolarity.

Hepatic

A mild transient elevation of liver enzymes is commonly seen during initial CBZ treatment but does not necessitate drug discontinuation.[22] A fairly rare and potentially fatal hepatic reaction (granulomatous hepatitis) has been reported with CBZ, so yearly monitoring of liver function tests is recommended.

Pregnancy and Lactation

The safe use of CBZ during pregnancy and lactation has not been established. CBZ may cause craniofacial defects, fingernail hypoplasia, and developmental delays (but usually no major birth defects) among children whose mothers took CBZ during pregnancy.[58] Maternal plasma concentrations and umbilical cord concentrations of CBZ are identical.

Concentrations of CBZ in breast milk are about 60% of the mother's plasma concentration. CBZ has been considered an alternative drug of choice instead of lithium during pregnancy, but caution should be used in prescribing it during the first trimester of pregnancy and during breast-feeding.

Drug Combinations

CBZ is known to interact with numerous drugs because of its effect on enhancing the hepatic microsomal enzyme system.[59,60] For a more complete description of drug interactions with CBZ, see Chapter 55.

Lithium and CBZ may be synergistic in the treatment of refractory bipolar patients (e.g., CBZ can be added to lithium therapy for nonresponsiveness and lithium may potentiate the antidepressant response for CBZ nonresponders). Neurotoxicity has been observed when lithium and CBZ are combined despite therapeutic plasma concentrations of both drugs.[35] Clinical symptoms included confusion, drowsiness, generalized weakness, lethargy, coarse tremor, hyperreflexia, and cerebellar signs. The neurotoxic syndrome usually resolves quickly when one or both agents are discontinued. Lithium and CBZ may have additive effects in suppressing thyroid function, so regular monitoring of thyroid indices is advisable during combination therapy.[56]

In the majority of clinical trials, CBZ has been combined with antipsychotics or antidepressants with no adverse effects. Neurotoxicity has been reported with the combination of CBZ and haloperidol (e.g., lethargy, confusion, slurred speech, disorientation), but these symptoms usually clear quickly with discontinuation of the drugs. Concomitant drug therapies that may result in CBZ toxicity include cimetidine, erythromycin, isoniazid, verapamil, diltiazem, propoxyphene, and fluoxetine.[24,35,57–60] CBZ may increase the oxidative metabolism of other drugs (e.g., antipsychotics, antidepressants, phenytoin, VPA, benzodiazepines, doxycycline, warfarin, theophylline, oral contraceptives), thus patients should be closely monitored for loss of efficacy of concomitant medications.

Divalproex Sodium, Sodium Valproate, or Valproic Acid

VPA, a branched-chain fatty acid, originally was marketed as an anticonvulsant (as discussed in Chapter 55). VPA is manufactured as sodium valproate, valproic acid, and divalproex sodium. Valproate sodium is rapidly converted to VPA in the stomach, whereas divalproex sodium delayed-release tablets must pass into the small intestine to be converted to VPA.

In 1995, divalproex sodium was approved by the FDA as a mood stabilizer for the treatment of mania associated with bipolar disorder. In several controlled studies, divalproex sodium has been shown to be as effective as lithium in patients with pure mania and may be more effective than lithium in certain subtypes of bipolar disorder (e.g., rapid cycling, mixed mania, secondary bipolar disorder, comorbid substance abuse.)[61–67] Predictors of positive response with VPA include rapid cycling, a high level of dysphoria or depression during the manic episode (mixed episode), concomitant panic attacks, mania associated with organic features (abnormal EEG) or organic mental disorders, history of head trauma, and mental retardation.[54, 62, 66–67] Antimanic effects may be augmented when VPA is given with lithium, CBZ, antipsychotics, or benzodiazepines.[61] Low-dose VPA (125–500 mg/d) has been reported to be effective in reducing mood cycling in bipolar II disorder and cyclothymia.[68] VPA may also have anxiolytic, antimigraine, and analgesic effects.[61]

Proposed Mechanism of Action

The exact mechanism of action of VPA is not known, but may be related to the inhibition of GABA metabolism, stimulation of GABA synthesis and release, and augmentation of the postsynaptic inhibitory effect of GABA.[7,61]

Dosing

The initial starting dose of VPA is 250–750 mg/d (5–10 mg/kg/d) in divided doses, and the dose is adjusted up by 250 mg every 2–3 days to 750–3000 mg/d (maximum of 60 mg/kg/d).[22] Higher initial doses (20 mg/kg/d or 1200–1500 mg/d in divided doses) have been used as a loading dose in acutely agitated manic patients. The half-life of VPA is about 8 hours, thus doses should be administered three times daily to maintain stable plasma concentrations.

Therapeutic plasma concentrations have not been established for VPA in bipolar disorder, therefore, most clinicians use the anticonvulsant therapeutic range of 50–150 mcg/mL taken 12 hours after the last dose. VPA concentrations up to 200 mcg/mL have been tried in some resistant bipolar cases but may increase the risk of adverse effects.[25]

Adverse Effects

Compared with other anticonvulsants, VPA has a lower incidence of adverse effects and is generally well tolerated.[61] The most frequent adverse effects reported with VPA are GI complaints (nausea, vomiting, epigastric cramping, dyspepsia, indigestion, and anorexia) and sedation. The GI complaints are usually transient and minimized by (1) giving the drug with food, (2) using lower initial doses with gradual increases in doses, or (3) switching to the delayed-release product (divalproex sodium).

Other adverse effects of VPA include drowsiness, ataxia, lethargy, fine hand tremor, alopecia, changes in the texture or color of hair, pruritus, prolonged bleeding due to inhibition of platelet aggregation, transient increases in liver enzymes (transaminase and lactic dehydrogenase), and weight gain.[61,62] Thrombocytopenia may occur at higher doses, and patients should be monitored for bleeding and bruising. Since thrombocytopenia may be dose related, this could be managed by reducing the dose and closely monitoring platelet counts. Rare cases of hepatitis have been reported (1 in 20,000 patients), and most cases were in children with severe seizure disorders that were receiving multiple-drug combinations. Liver function tests should be obtained at baseline and at 6- to 12-month intervals; younger patients in particular should be monitored for clinical signs of hepatic dysfunction. VPA should not be administered to patients with hepatic disease or significant hepatic dysfunction. VPA is not recommended during the first trimester of pregnancy (1–2% risk of neural tube birth defects, primarily spina bifida). VPA is excreted into human breast milk in low concentrations (up to 15% of the mother's serum concentrations); so far, no adverse effects in the nursing infant from VPA exposure have been reported.

Drug Interactions

There are several complex drug–drug interactions between VPA and other drugs. The concomitant administration of VPA with other CNS depressants or anticonvulsants may cause additive CNS depressant effects. VPA may displace CBZ from plasma protein binding sites, and thereby cause CBZ toxicity. CBZ may decrease VPA plasma concentrations due to induction of hepatic metabolism. If CBZ and VPA are administered together, blood levels of both agents should be monitored closely due to changes in liver enzyme metabolism and competition for protein binding.[22,24,61,69] The hematologic effects of VPA may potentiate the anticoagulant effects of warfarin and aspirin. VPA also interferes with laboratory tests (e.g., falsely elevates urine ketones and causes abnormal thyroid function tests).

ELECTROCONVULSIVE THERAPY

ECT is an effective alternative treatment for severe mania, psychotic depression, and mixed states with high suicidal risk. It may also be used in pregnant women who cannot take lithium, CBZ, or VPA.[22,23] ECT has approximately an 80% response rate. Preliminary data suggest that bilateral ECT may be more effective than unilateral treatment in mania.[25] Acute neurotoxicity and delirium have been reported in patients receiving ECT with lithium (even at reduced doses). Lithium should be withdrawn and discontinued at least 2 days before ECT and should not be resumed until 2–3 days after the last ECT.[25] Since CBZ, VPA, and benzodiazepines have anticonvulsant properties, these drugs should also be tapered down and discontinued prior to ECT.

OTHER INVESTIGATIONAL THERAPIES

Drugs that reduce the availability of NE have been suggested for use in bipolar disorder. Both clonidine and propranolol have been utilized in a few patients with some success.[22,24] GABA-mimetic agents such as clonazepam may be effective in high doses for controlling acute mania, but this may be secondary to sedation instead of a specific antimanic effect. Little is known about the efficacy of atypical antipsychotics such as clozapine and risperidone (both have dopamine and serotonin antagonist effects). These agents may be effective for bipolar mania, mixed episodes, schizoaffective disorder, and psychosis associated with bipolar disorder without causing significant extrapyramidal reactions or tardive dyskinesia.

If the calcium hypothesis of bipolar disorder is correct, then calcium channel blockers, such as verapamil (that act by lowering calcium influx intracellularly), should be effective.[22,70] Preliminary data suggest that verapamil has acute antimanic effects, although an open trial of verapamil in lithium-resistant mania did not show positive results.[25] Verapamil and diltiazem may increase plasma concentrations of CBZ, lower plasma lithium concentrations, and the lithium–verapamil combination may increase cardiotoxicity due to additive calcium antagonist effects. Little information is available about the efficacy of other calcium antagonists (diltiazem, nifedipine, and nimodipine) but a few case reports suggest they also have antimanic effects.[23] Verapamil may be considered a fourth-line agent if patients cannot be treated with lithium, CBZ, or VPA.

GUIDELINES FOR TREATMENT OF BIPOLAR DISORDER

Pharmacologic treatment must be individualized based on the target symptoms, response to treatment, and development of adverse effects. Bipolar disorder is a dynamic illness and constantly changes, thus different treatment approaches and strategies must be tried to optimize patient outcomes and functioning. Several algorithms have been proposed for selecting different mood stabilizers and combination therapies, but no decision-making tree can accurately reflect the diversity and complexity of bipolar disorder. In 1994, The American Psychiatric Association (APA) published practice guidelines for the treatment of patients with bipolar I disorder.[71] These guidelines provide basic information about the diagnosis, clinical course, epidemiology, and treatment strategies for bipolar I disorder. However, the APA guidelines are not considered to be the standard of care due to the variability of bipolar disorder and the need to individualize therapy.

EVALUATION OF THERAPEUTIC OUTCOMES

The evaluation of therapeutic outcomes for bipolar disorder requires frequent patient and laboratory monitoring and regular office visits (every 1–3 months depending on stability).[71] Patients should be actively involved with their treatment and help to monitor target symptoms and adverse effects. Because some patients have a rapid onset or "switching" in episodes, they should be encouraged to call their physician (or mental health professional involved with their care) in order to receive prompt treatment. Treatment goals should be to minimize toxicity and the adverse effects of medications while optimizing the patient's social and occupational functioning.

CONCLUSION

Despite the advances in the treatment of bipolar disorder over the past 30 years, there are still many questions to be answered about the pathophysiology, differences in subtypes of the disorder, and comparison of various treatment approaches.[1] More research is needed to compare monotherapy versus combination therapy in patients with mixed episodes or rapid/continuous cycling because these are often the most difficult patients to treat.[71] Bipolar disorder remains a challenge for clinicians because it is a constantly changing illness that requires close monitoring and different treatment approaches depending on the clinical state of the patient.

REFERENCES

1. Prien RF, Potter WZ. NIMH workshop report on treatment of bipolar disorder. Psychopharmacol Bull 1990;26:409–427.
2. Kessler RC, McGonagle KA, Zhao S, et al. Lifetime and 12-month prevalence of DSM-III-R psychiatric disorders in the United States: Results from the national comorbidity survey. Arch Gen Psych 1994;51:8–19.
3. Goodwin FK, Jamison KR (eds). Course and outcome, in Manic-Depressive Illness. New York, Oxford University Press, 1990, pp 127–156.
4. Goodwin FK, Jamison KR (eds). Genetics, in Manic-Depressive Illness. New York, Oxford University Press, 1990, pp 373–401.
5. Goodwin FK, Jamison KR (eds). Biochemical and pharmacological studies, in Manic-Depressive Illness. New York, Oxford University Press, 1990, pp 416–502.
6. Siever LJ, Davis KL. Overview: Toward a dysregulation hypothesis of depression. Am J Psychiatry 1985;149:1017–1031.
7. Post RM, Weiss SRB, Chuang D. Mechanisms of action of anticonvulsants in affective disorders: Comparisons with lithium. J Clin Psychopharmacol 1992;12:23S–35S.
8. Dubovsky SL, Murphy J, Christiano J, et al. The calcium second messenger system in bipolar disorders: Data supporting new research directions. J Neuropsychiatr Clin Neurosci 1992;4:3–14.
9. Goodwin FK, Jamison KR (eds). Sleep and biological rhythms, in Manic-Depressive Illness. New York, Oxford University Press, 1990, pp 541–574.
10. Wehr TA, Sack DA, Rosenthal NE, et al. Sleep and biological rhythms in bipolar illness, in Hales RE, Frances AJ (eds): American Psychiatric Association Annual Review. Washington DC, American Psychiatric Press, 1987, pp 61–80.
11. Blehar MC, Lewy AJ. Seasonal mood disorders: Consensus and controversy. Psychopharmacol Bull 1990;26:465–494.
12. Mood disorders, in Diagnostic and Statistical Manual of Mental Disorders, 4th ed. (DSM-IV). Washington DC, American Psychiatric Press, 1994, pp 317–390.
13. Goodwin FK, Jamison KR (eds). The manic-depressive spectrum, in Manic-Depressive Illness. New York, Oxford University Press, 1990, pp 74–84.
14. Goodwin FK, Jamison KR (eds). Clinical description, in Manic-Depressive Illness. New York, Oxford University Press, 1990, pp 15–55.
15. Dilsaver SC, Swann AC, Shoaib AM, et al. Depressive mania associated with nonresponse to antimanic agents. Am J Psychiatry 1993;150:1548–1551.
16. Goodwin FK, Jamison KR (eds). Manic-depressive illness, creativity, and leadership, in Manic-Depressive Illness. New York, Oxford University Press, 1990, pp 332–367.
17. Goodwin FK, Jamison KR (eds). Childhood and adolescence, in Manic-Depressive Illness. New York, Oxford University Press, 1990, pp 186–209.
18. Goodwin FK, Jamison KR (eds). Alcohol and drug abuse in manic-depressive illness, in Manic-Depressive Illness. New York, Oxford University Press, 1990, pp 210–226.
19. Goodwin FK, Jamison KR (eds). Suicide, in Manic-Depressive Illness. New York, Oxford University Press, 1990, pp 227–246.
20. Goodwin FK, Jamison KR (eds). Diagnosis, in Manic-Depressive Illness. New York, Oxford University Press, 1990, pp 85–126.
21. Goodwin FK, Jamison KR (eds). Psychotherapy, in Manic-Depressive Illness. New York, Oxford University Press, 1990, pp 725–745.
22. Goodwin FK, Jamison KR (eds). Medical treatment of manic episodes, in Manic-Depressive Illness. New York, Oxford University Press, 1990, pp 603–629.
23. Goodwin FK, Jamison KR (eds). Medical treatment of acute bipolar depression, in Manic-Depressive Illness. New York, Oxford University Press, 1990, pp 630–664.
24. Goodwin FK, Jamison KR (eds). Maintenance medical treatment, in Manic-Depressive Illness. New York, Oxford University Press, 1990, pp 665–724.
25. Chou JC. Recent advances in treatment of acute mania. J Clin Psychopharmacol 1991;11:3–21.
26. Gerner RH, Stanton A. Algorithm for patient management of acute manic states: Lithium, valproate, or carbamazepine? J Clin Psychopharmacol 1992;12:57S–63S.
27. Price LH, Henninger GR. Lithium in the treatment of mood disorders. N Engl J Med 1994;331:591–598.
28. Gelenberg AJ, Kane JM, Lavori P, et al. Comparison of standard and low serum levels of lithium for maintenance treatment of bipolar disorder. N Engl J Med 1989;321:1489–1493.
29. Carson S. Lithium, in Evans WE, Schentag JJ, Jusko WJ (eds): Applied Pharmacokinetics: Principles of Therapeutic Drug Monitoring, 3rd ed. Spokane, WA, Applied Therapeutics, 1992, pp 34:1–26.
30. Faedda GL, Tondo L, Baldessarini RJ, et al. Outcome after rapid discontinuation of lithium treatment in bipolar mood disorders. Arch Gen Psych 1993;50:448–455.

31. Bowen RC, Grof P, Grof E. Less frequent lithium administration and lower urine volume. Am J Psychiatry 1991;148:189–192.
32. Carson SW. Lithium, in Murphy JE (ed): Clinical Pharmacokinetics. Bethesda, MD, American Society of Hospital Pharmacists, 1993, pp 145–156.
33. Consensus Development Panel. NIMH/NIH consensus development conference statement, mood disorders: Pharmacologic prevention of recurrences. Am J Psychiatry 1985;142:469–476.
34. Jefferson JW, Griest JH, Ackerman DL, et al. (eds). Lithium Encyclopedia for Clinical Practice, 2nd ed. Washington, DC, American Psychiatric Press, 1987.
35. Kane JM, Lieberman JA (eds). Adverse Effects of Psychotropic Drugs. New York, The Guilford Press, 1992.
36. Jefferson JW. Potassium supplementation in lithium patients: A timely intervention or premature speculation. J Clin Psychiatry 1992;53:370–372.
37. Martin A. Clinical management of lithium-induced polyuria. Hosp Community Psychiatry 1993;44:427–428.
38. Hestbech J, Hansen HE, Amidsen A, et al. Chronic renal lesions following long-term treatment with lithium. Kidney Int 1977;12:205–213.
39. Gitlin MJ. Lithium-induced renal insufficiency. J Clin Psychopharmacol 1993;13:276–279.
40. Calabrese JR, Gulledge Ad, Hahn, et al. Autoimmune thyroiditis in manic-depressive patients treated with lithium. Am J Psychiatry 1985;142:1318–1321.
41. Ghadirian AM, Lehman HE. Neurological side effects of lithium: Organic brain syndrome, seizures, extrapyramidal side effects and EEG changes. Compr Psychiatry 1980;21:327–335.
42. Simard M, Gumbier B, Lee A, et al. Lithium carbonate intoxication: A case report and review of the literature. Arch Intern Med 1989;149:36–46.
43. Cohen LS, Friedman JM, Jefferson JW, et al. A reevaluation of risk of in utero exposure to lithium. JAMA 1994;271:146–150.
44. Schou M. Lithium treatment during pregnancy, delivery, and lactation: An update. J Clin Psychiatry 1990;51:410–413.
45. Zornberg GL, Pope HG. Treatment of depression in bipolar disorder: New directions for research. J Clin Psychopharmacol 1993;13:397–408.
46. Kane JM. The role of neuroleptics in manic-depressive illness. J Clin Psychiatry 1988;49(suppl 11):12–14.
47. Chouinard G. The use of benzodiazepines in the treatment of manic-depressive illness. J Clin Psychiatry 1988;49 (suppl 10):15–19.
48. Bradwejn J, Shriqui C, Koszycki D, et al. Double-blind comparison of the effects of clonazepam and lorazepam in acute mania. J Clin Psychopharmacol 1990;10:403–408.
49. Koczerginski D, Kennedy SH, Swinson RP. Clonazepam and lithium: A toxic combination in the treatment of mania? Int Clin Psychopharmacol 1989;4:195–199.
50. Ayd FA. Drug–drug interactions that matter: Lithium/diuretics. Int Drug Ther News 1984;19:32.
51. Ragheb M. The clinical significance of lithium-nonsteroidal anti-inflammatory drug interactions. J Clin Psychopharmacol 1990;10:350–354.
52. Ragheb MA, Powell AL. Lithium interaction with sulindac and naproxen. J Clin Psychopharmacol 1986;6:150–154.
53. Frankenburg FR, Tohen M, Cohen BM, et al. Long-term response to carbamazepine: A retrospective study. J Clin Psychopharmacol 1988;8:130–132.
54. Dilsaver SC. The manic syndrome: Factors which may predict a patient's response to lithium, carbamazepine, and valproate. J Psychiatry Neuroscience 1993;18:61–66.
55. Sobotka JL, Alexander B, Cook BL. A review of carbamazepine's hematologic reactions and monitoring recommendations. DICP Ann Pharmacother 1990;24:1214–1219.
56. Kramlinger KG, Post RM. Addition of lithium carbonate to carbamazepine: Hematologic and thyroid effects. Am J Psychiatry 1990;147:615–620.
57. McEvoy GK, Litvak K, Welsh OH, et al (eds). Carbamazepine, in AHFS Drug Information 95. Bethesda, MD, American Society of Hospital Pharmacists, 1995, pp 1449–1453.
58. Jones KL, Lacro RV, Johnson KA, et al. Pattern of malformations in the children of women treated with carbamazepine during pregnancy. N Engl J Med 1989;320:1661–1666.
59. Ketter TA, Post RM, Worthington K. Principles of clinically important drug interactions with carbamazepine. Part I. J Clin Psychopharmacol 1991;11:198–203.
60. Ketter TA, Post RM, Worthington K. Principles of clinical important drug interactions with carbamazepine. Part II. J Clin Psychopharmacol 1991;11:306–313.
61. Balfour JA, Bryson HM. Valproic acid. A review of its pharmacology and therapeutic potential in indications other than epilepsy. CNS Drugs 1994;2:144–173.
62. McElroy SL, Keck Jr PE. Treatment guidelines for valproate in bipolar and schizoaffective disorder. Can J Psychiatry 1993;38:S62–S66.
63. Schaff MR, Fawcett J, Zajecka JM. Divalproex sodium in the treatment of refractory affective disorders. J Clin Psychiatry 1993;54:380–384.
64. Calabrese JR. Rapid cycling bipolar disorder and its treatment with valproate. Can J Psychiatry 1993;38:S57–S61.
65. Bowden CL, Brugger AM, Swann AC, et al. Efficacy of divalproex vs lithium and placebo in the treatment of mania. The Depakote Mania Study Group. JAMA 1994;271:918–924.
66. Calabrese JR, Woyshville MJ. A medication algorithm for treatment of bipolar cycling? J Clin Psychiatry 1995;56(suppl 3):11–18.
67. Bowden CL. Predictors of response to divalproex and lithium. J Clin Psychiatry 1995;56(suppl 3):25–30.
68. Jacobsen FM. Low-dose valproate: A new treatment for cyclothymia, mild rapid cycling disorders, and premenstrual syndrome. J Clin Psychiatry 1993;54:229–234.
69. Tohen M, Castillo J, Pope HG, Herbstein J. Concomitant use of valproate and carbamazepine in bipolar and schizoaffective disorder. J Clin Psychopharmacol 1994;14:67–70.
70. Dubovsky SL. Calcium antagonists in manic-depressive illness. Neuropsychobiology 1993;27:184–192.
71. Practice Guideline for the Treatment of Patients with Bipolar Disorder. American Psychiatric Association Practice Guidelines. Am J Psychiatry 1994;151(suppl):1–36.

Chapter 69

Anxiety Disorders

Cynthia K. Kirkwood, PharmD, and Peggy E. Hayes, PharmD

Anxiety is a universal feeling state that is part of the fabric of everyday life. Feelings of anxiety and fear are often unpleasant emotions commonly caused by the perception of actual or potential (anticipatory) danger that threatens the security of the individual.

Everyone experiences a certain amount of nervousness and apprehension when faced with a stressful situation. Usually the response is reasonable and adaptive, enabling individuals to "rise to the occasion," and contains a built-in control mechanism to return to a normal physiologic state. Some persons, however, experience anxiety-like symptoms and possess fears that are frequently abnormal, irrational, and severely impair normal daily functioning. These persons often suffer from an anxiety disorder.[1]

Anxiety disorders are among the most frequent mental disorders encountered in clinical practice. The lifetime prevalence for anxiety disorders was recently estimated at 24.9% (or one-fourth of the population).[2] Unfortunately, the majority of patients with anxiety disorder received no professional treatment.[2,3]

The health consequences of persons with untreated or inadequately treated anxiety disorders are not well researched. Untreated anxious patients tend to be high utilizers of health care facilities for nonpsychiatric reasons.[4] In community, primary care, and outpatient settings, patients with major depression, panic disorder, and generalized anxiety disorder showed higher levels of disability.[5] Furthermore, patients with anxiety disorders are at high risk for developing another anxiety disorder, depression, substance abuse, or suicide attempts.[2,6,7]

Differential Diagnosis

The differential diagnosis of anxiety disorders includes medical and psychiatric illnesses and certain drugs. Evaluation of the anxious patient requires a complete physical and mental status examination, appropriate laboratory tests, and a thorough knowledge of the patient's medical, psychiatric, and drug history.[8–10]

To treat anxiety appropriately, the clinician must make a reliable diagnosis. It is essential that the distinction between short-term symptoms of anxiety and anxiety disorders be understood. Common or situational anxiety, probably more accurately termed "worry" or "apprehension," is a normal response to a stressful situation (e.g., problems at work, interpersonal conflict, or financial difficulties). Although the symptoms are severe, they are temporary and usually last no more than 2 or 3 weeks. Situational anxiety is not classified as an anxiety disorder. Although short-term, "as-needed" treatment with an anxiolytic agent such as a benzodiazepine (BZ) is very common and may provide some symptomatic relief, prolonged drug therapy is unnecessary and discouraged.[9,10]

MEDICAL DISEASES ASSOCIATED WITH ANXIETY

Anxiety symptoms are an inherent part of the initial clinical presentation in several medical disorders, thus complicating the distinction between anxiety disorders and medical disorders.[9–11] If the anxiety symptoms are secondary to a medical illness, they will usually subside as the illness improves.[11] However, the knowledge that one has a physical illness may trigger anxious feelings, especially in the elderly, and further complicate therapy.

Symptoms of anxiety frequently present in medical disorders include palpitations, tachycardia, chest pain or tightness, shortness of breath, and hyperventilation.[9] Medical disorders most closely associated with anxiety involve the endocrine, cardiovascular, digestive, and respiratory systems (Table 69.1).[11,12] "Functional" gastrointestinal (GI) disorders (e.g., irritable bowel syndrome) account for 50–60% of the GI complaints seen by physicians. Often these patients have a complicating illness such as an anxiety disorder.[12]

Clinically significant anxiety is present as a reaction to postmyocardial infarction (MI), postcardiac surgery, irritable bowel syndrome, and asthma, which may influence treatment outcomes. After hospital discharge of MI

TABLE 69.1. COMMON MEDICAL DISORDERS ASSOCIATED WITH ANXIETY SYMPTOMS

Cardiovascular/Respiratory System

Arrhythmias, chronic obstructive lung disease, hyperdynamic beta-adrenergic state, hypertension, hyperventilation, mitral valve prolapse, myocardial infarction, angina, pulmonary embolus

Endocrine System

Cushing's disease, hyperthyroidism, hypothyroidism, hypoglycemia, pheochromocytoma

Gastrointestinal System

Colitis, irritable bowel syndrome, peptic ulcer, ulcerative colitis

Miscellaneous

Epilepsy, migraine, pain, pernicious anemia, porphyria

(Compiled from Refs. 8 and 10.)

patients, anxiety and depression may interfere with patients' recovery and subsequent return to work. These patients often require medication for anxiety symptoms.[9,12]

PSYCHIATRIC DISEASES ASSOCIATED WITH ANXIETY

Anxiety may be a concomitant symptom of several major psychiatric illnesses. Anxiety symptoms are extremely common in patients with mood disorders, schizophrenia, organic mental syndromes, and substance use disorders.[12] The majority of psychiatric patients will have two or more concurrent psychiatric disorders (comorbidity) within their lifetime. Therefore, a patient with one anxiety disorder is highly predisposed to develop another anxiety disorder, a depression, or a substance use disorder. To appropriately treat patients with anxiety disorders, it is important to adequately assess and diagnose all comorbid psychiatric and medical conditions.[2,5]

DRUG-INDUCED ANXIETY

The two major drug classes that cause anxiety symptoms are the central nervous system (CNS) stimulants and depressants (Table 69.2). CNS stimulants include nicotine, caffeine, cocaine, sympathomimetic amines, amphetamines, and other anorexic agents including nonprescription products containing phenylpropanolamine.[11] Anxiety occurs during the use of these drugs in a dose-dependent manner, but ingestion of minimal amounts may result in marked anxiety, including panic attacks, in some individuals.[7,8] Caffeine and nonprescription drugs are especially important as possible inducers of anxiety in the elderly. Patients with panic disorder may be hypersensitive to even small doses of caffeine and other CNS stimulants.[10,11]

Anxiety occasionally occurs during the use of CNS depressants (e.g., ethanol, barbiturates, meprobamate, and BZs), especially in children and the elderly; however, anxiety complaints including panic attacks are more common as complications of drug withdrawal after the abrupt discontinuation of these agents.[10]

TABLE 69.2. DRUGS ASSOCIATED WITH ANXIETY SYMPTOMS

CNS Depressants

Anxiolytics/sedatives, ethanol, narcotic agonists (withdrawal)

CNS Stimulants

Prescription products

Albuterol (Proventil, Ventolin), amphetamine sulfate, cocaine, diethylpropion (Tenuate), fenfluramine (Pondimin), isoproterenol (Isuprel, Medihaler-Iso), methylphenidate (Ritalin)

Nonprescription products

Caffeine (NoDoz, Vivarin), ephedrine (Efedron Nasal), naphazoline (Privine, Allerest Eye Drops), oxymetazoline (Afrin, Dristan), phenylephrine (Neo-Synephrine, Sinex), phenylpropanolamine (Dexatrim, Acutrim), pseudoephedrine (Sudafed, Novafed)

Miscellaneous

Anticholivergic toxicity, baclofen (Lioresal), digitalis toxicity, dapsone (Avlosulfon), cycloserine (Seromycin)

EPIDEMIOLOGY

The National Comorbidity Survey (NCS), a congressionally mandated survey, provides the most up-to-date, comprehensive data regarding the prevalence of psychiatric disorders. In this extensive community survey of noninstitutionalized persons aged 15–54 years, the 12-month prevalence rate for anxiety disorders averaged 17.2% and the lifetime rate was 24.9%. Social phobia was the most common anxiety disorder reported with a 12-month prevalence rate of 7.9% and a lifetime rate of 13.3%.[2]

In general, anxiety disorders are a group of heterogeneous illnesses that develop before age 30, and are more common in women and those with a family history of anxiety and depression. Patients often develop another anxiety disorder, major depression, or substance abuse.[1,2] Anxiety disorders are generally chronic in nature, and although symptoms wax and wane over time, patients are rarely completely symptom free.[1,4] Most patients with anxiety disorders can be treated effectively. However, long-term treatment may be required and relapse after drug discontinuation is common.[4]

CLASSIFICATION AND CLINICAL PRESENTATION

The *Diagnostic and Statistical Manual of Mental Disorders,* 4th ed. (DSM-IV), published by the American Psychiatric Association (APA) in 1994, classifies anxiety disorders into several categories (Table 69.3).[1] The characteristic features of these illnesses are anxiety and avoidance behavior. Obsessive–compulsive disorder is discussed in Chapter 70.

GENERALIZED ANXIETY DISORDER

The DSM-IV diagnostic criteria (Table 69.4) for generalized anxiety disorder (GAD) require that symptoms occur more days than not for a period of at least 6 months.[1] The essential feature of GAD is unrealistic or excessive anxiety and worry about a number of events or activities (e.g., finances, illness, misfortune) without panic or phobic symptoms. In children and adolescents this may be worry about academic, athletic, and social performance. Symptoms of GAD are both psychological (tension, fear, difficulty concentrating, and apprehension) and somatic or physical (tachycardia, palpitations, tremor, sweating, and GI upset).[1] The lifetime prevalence of GAD is 5.1%, with the illness more common in women than men (6.6% versus 3.6%).[2,13]

GAD has a gradual onset, usually in the early twenties, but may be precipitated in later life by severe psychologic stressors. Stressful life events may also play a role in the persistence of symptoms. The course of the illness is chronic with multiple spontaneous exacerbations and remissions.[1,2,13] Patients report substantial interference with their lives and have a high probability of seeking treatment.[13] The majority of GAD patients will eventually develop another mental disorder (e.g., affective disorder, panic disorder).[2,13]

SOCIAL PHOBIA

The essential feature of a social phobia is a marked and persistent fear of social or performance situations in which embarrassment may occur. Fear is a disturbing feeling that danger is close at hand. Unlike most anxiety disorders, the object of this fearful feeling is clearly recognized. Although adolescents and adults recognize that their fear is excessive or unreasonable, this may not be the case in children. Most often, the social or performance situation is avoided, but it is sometimes endured with dread. The fear and avoidance of the situation must interfere significantly with the person's daily routine, occupational functioning, or social life.[1]

The lifetime prevalence rate for social phobia is 13.3%, with the illness being more common in women than men (15.5% versus 11.1%).[2] Specific social activities such as public speaking, eating in a restaurant, or using a public restroom are avoided or endured with intense discomfort.[1]

TABLE 69.3. DSM-IV CLASSIFICATION OF ANXIETY DISORDERS

A. Generalized anxiety disorder
B. Panic disorder
   With agoraphobia
   Without agoraphobia
C. Agoraphobia without a history of panic disorder
D. Phobic disorders
   Social phobia
   Specific phobia
E. Obsessive–compulsive disorder
F. Post-traumatic stress disorder
G. Acute stress disorder

(Compiled from Ref. 1.)

TABLE 69.4. DSM-IV DIAGNOSTIC CRITERIA FOR GENERALIZED ANXIETY DISORDER

A. Excessive anxiety and worry (apprehensive expectation), occurring more days than not for at least 6 months, about a number of events or activities (such as work or school performance).
B. The person finds it difficult to control the worry.
C. The anxiety and worry are associated with three (or more) of the following six symptoms (with at least some symptoms present for more days than not for the past 6 months):
   1. Restlessness or feeling keyed up or on edge
   2. Being easily fatigued
   3. Difficulty concentrating or mind going blank
   4. Irritability
   5. Muscle tension
   6. Sleep disturbance
D. The anxiety and worry is not confined to features of another psychiatric illness (e.g., having a panic attack, being embarrassed in public).
E. The constant worry causes significant distress, and significant impairment in social, occupational, or other important areas of functioning.
F. The excessive anxiety and worry are not caused by a drug substance (e.g., drugs of abuse or medications), or a general medical disorder, and do not occur exclusively as part of another psychiatric disorder (e.g., an affective disorder).

(Adapted from the *Diagnostic and Statistical Manual of Mental Disorders*, Fourth Edition. Washington, DC: American Psychiatric Association, 1994; 435–436.)

SPECIFIC PHOBIA

Specific phobia is marked and persistent fear of a specific object or situation such as thunderstorms, snakes, insects, or heights. Apart from contact with the feared object or situation, the patient is usually free of symptoms. Most persons simply avoid the feared object and adjust to certain restrictions on their activities.[1] Although specific phobia has a lifetime prevalence rate of 11.3%, patients are not seriously impaired in terms of daily functioning and few persons seek treatment.[1,2]

PANIC DISORDER

Panic disorder begins as a series of unexpected (spontaneous) panic attacks, involving an intense, terrifying fear, similar to that caused by life-threatening danger. The unexpected panic attacks are followed by at least 1 month of persistent concern about having another panic attack, worry about the possible consequences of the panic attack, or a significant behavioral change related to the attacks. Patients often describe an overwhelming sense of doom, a fear of dying or losing control, and numerous physical symptoms (Table 69.5).[1] Although the panic attacks may seem interminable to the patient, they usually last no more than 20–30 minutes, with the peak intensity of symptoms within the first 10 minutes. Often patients seek help at a nearby physician's office or emergency room, only to have their symptoms resolve prior to or upon arrival. Because panic symptoms mimic those present in several medical conditions (e.g., hyperthyroidism, pheochromocytoma, atypical chest pain), patients are often misdiagnosed and multiple referrals are common.[1,6]

Secondary to the panic attacks, many patients eventually develop agoraphobia (diagnosed as panic disorder with agoraphobia). Agoraphobia is anxiety about being in places or situations where escape might be difficult (or embarrassing) or where help might not be available in the event of having a panic attack or panic-like symptoms.[1] As a result, patients often avoid specific situations (e.g., crowded places, stores, bridges, and traveling away from home) where they fear a panic attack might occur.[1]

Panic disorder has an adverse impact on the patient's quality of life, including a significant degree of social and work impairment. Complications include suicide attempts, depression (50–65% have major depressive disorder), alcohol abuse, and increased use of medications, health services, and emergency room use.[7,14] Patients with panic disorder have a high lifetime risk for suicide attempts (18%), compared with 1% for the general population.[7] The usual course is chronic but waxing and waning.

The lifetime prevalence of panic disorder is 3.5%, with the illness more common in women than men (5% versus 2%).[2] The illness usually begins between late adolescence and the mid thirties. First-degree relatives of patients with panic disorder have a four to seven times greater chance of developing panic disorder. Twin studies indicate that genetic factors contribute to the underlying cause.[15]

TABLE 69.5. DSM-IV DIAGNOSTIC CRITERIA FOR PANIC ATTACK

A discrete period of intense fear or discomfort, in which at least four (or more) of the following symptoms developed abruptly and reached a peak within 10 minutes:

1. Palpitations or accelerated heart rate
2. Sweating
3. Trembling or shaking
4. Sensations of shortness of breath or smothering
5. Feeling of choking
6. Chest pain or discomfort
7. Nausea or abdominal distress
8. Feeling dizzy, unsteady, lightheaded, or faint
9. Derealization or depersonalization
10. Fear of losing control or going crazy
11. Fear of dying
12. Numbness or tingling sensations (paresthesias)
13. Chills or hot flushes

(Adpated from the *Diagnostic and Statistical Manual of Mental Disorders*, Fourth Edition. Washington, DC: American Psychiatric Association, 1994; 395.)

PATHOPHYSIOLOGY

Although the pathophysiology of anxiety disorders is unknown, scientists have explored several interesting neurochemical theories. Current evidence strongly suggests that anxiety disorders are primarily biologic illnesses associated with an underlying genetic vulnerability. Anxiety may not reflect an imbalance in a single neurotransmitter system, but may be the result of multiple interactions among various neurotransmitters including norepinephrine (NE), γ-aminobutyric acid (GABA), and serotonin (5-HT).

NORADRENERGIC MODEL

The basic premise of the noradrenergic theory is that the autonomic nervous system of anxious patients (especially those with panic disorder) is hypersensitive and overreacts to various stimuli. Many anxious patients clearly display symptoms of peripheral autonomic hyperactivity (e.g., hyperventilation, palpitations, and tremulousness).[10] The locus coeruleus (LC), a small midbrain nucleus, may play a major role in regulating anxiety. The LC contains neurons that supply 50–70% of the brain's NE with widespread projections to many brain areas (e.g., limbic system, cerebral, and cerebellar cortices). In response to anxiety or fearful situations, the LC serves as an alarm center activating NE release and stimulating the sympathetic nervous system. The presynaptic α_2-adrenergic autoreceptor plays a significant role in controlling the release of NE from the synapse.[16] Chronic, central noradrenergic overactivity down-regulates α_2 adrenoreceptors in GAD patients. This receptor may also be abnormal in some patients with panic disorder.[17,18]

By administering drugs that have a relatively specific effect on the LC, researchers have further explored the NE theory of anxiety and panic disorder. Drugs with anxiogenic effects (e.g., yohimbine, isoproterenol, and caffeine) stimulate LC firing and increase noradrenergic activity. These agents often produce subjective feelings of anxiety and can precipitate a panic attack in those with panic disorder, but not in normal volunteers or those with other psychiatric illnesses.[18] Drugs with anxiolytic or antipanic effects (e.g., BZs, antidepressants, and clonidine) inhibit LC firing, decrease noradrenergic activity, and block the effects of anxiogenic drugs.[17,18]

BENZODIAZEPINE RECEPTOR MODEL

Studies to determine the mechanism of action of BZs led to the discovery of specific BZ receptor sites in rat and human brain tissue.[19,20] The BZ receptor is functionally (and perhaps structurally) linked to the GABA type A ($GABA_A$) receptor and a chloride ion channel; this is referred to as the supramolecular receptor complex.[19,20] The therapeutic effects of BZs (e.g., anxiolytic, anticonvulsant, sedative, and muscle relaxant actions) are mediated through the $GABA_A$ receptor.

GABA, the major inhibitory neurotransmitter in the CNS, is involved in nerve transmission in nearly one-third of brain impulses. In addition, the GABA system has a strong regulatory or inhibitory effect on the 5-HT and NE systems. When GABA binds to its receptor, the adjacent chloride ion channel opens and permits the influx of negatively charged chloride ions; this results in hyperpolarization of the cell membrane and causes a decrease in nerve cell excitability. When BZs bind to their receptor, GABA's inhibitory effects are potentiated via an increase in the frequency of chloride ion channel openings. BZs in the absence of GABA have little effect on nerve cell excitability. Other anxiolytics (e.g., barbiturate and alcohol) also enhance GABA effects.[19,20]

SEROTONIN MODEL

Although there is increasing evidence that the 5-HT system is altered (disturbed) in patients with anxiety disorders, as well as other psychiatric illnesses, definitive evidence that shows a clear abnormality in 5-HT function remains to be demonstrated. 5-HT is primarily an inhibitory neurotransmitter that is used by neurons having their origin in the raphe nuclei of the brainstem and projecting diffusely throughout the brain (e.g., cortex and limbic system).[21,22] The diverse actions of 5-HT are regulated by approximately eight different receptor subtypes. The azapirone, buspirone, is a selective 5-HT_{1A} partial agonist that is effective for GAD, but not for panic disorder.[23] Although the therapeutic properties of other 5-HT_{1A} partial agonists (e.g., gepirone, ipsapirone, and tandospirone) have been extensively researched, only buspirone has been approved for marketing in the United States. Because the 5-HT_{1A} partial agonists reduce serotonergic activity, GAD symptoms may reflect excessive 5-HT transmission or overactivity of the stimulatory 5-HT pathways.[23] The role of 5-HT in panic disorder is unclear. Although buspirone is not an effective antipanic agent, the 5-HT reuptake inhibitors (SSRIs) are effective antipanic compounds.[21,22]

TREATMENT

GENERALIZED ANXIETY DISORDER

Once GAD is diagnosed, a patient-oriented treatment plan, which usually consists of both psychotherapy and drug therapy, is developed. The treatment plan depends on the patient's degree of emotional distress and incapacitation, age, medication history, medical status, personality, and the potential outcomes of pharmacologic treatment. Clinical drug trials in outpatients with GAD indicate a high placebo response rate (50–60%), which suggests that some patients have a mild syndrome that may respond to psychotherapy alone.[8] Psychotherapy is the least invasive and safest treatment modality. For those patients experiencing anxiety symptoms severe enough to produce functional disability or discomfort, antianxiety medication is indicated.[8,24]

The BZs are the most effective and widely prescribed medications for the amelioration of anxiety symptoms. Buspirone, autonomic blocking agents, and antidepressants are additional anxiolytic options (Table 69.6). Because of the high risk of adverse effects and toxicity, barbiturates, antipsychotics, antipsychotic/antidepressant combinations, and antihistamines are generally not indicated in the treatment of GAD.[24] An algorithm for the management of GAD is shown in Fig. 69.1.

Nonpharmacologic Therapy

Nonpharmacologic treatment modalities in GAD include short-term counseling, stress management, psychotherapy, meditation, or exercise. Anxious patients should be instructed to avoid caffeine, nonprescription stimulants, and diet pills. Most GAD patients require psychologic therapy, alone or in combination with antianxiety medication, to overcome fears and learn to improve coping abilities.[8] Consideration of the patient's clinical symptoms, personality, and life problems aids in the choice of psychologic therapy. Cognitive therapy is the most effective psychological therapy in GAD patients. Supportive psychotherapy provides explanations and encouragement, and allows formulation of strategies to effectively manage anxiety-provoking situations. Behavioral therapy is indicated in patients with avoidance behavior. Patients with anxiety secondary to impaired interpersonal relations may benefit from group therapy. Although relaxation therapy (biofeedback, relaxation exercises, meditation) may aid in the relief of ten-

TABLE 69.6. NONBENZODIAZEPINE ANTIANXIETY AGENTS

Class/Generic Name	Brand Name	Manufacturer	Approved for Anxiety	Usual Dosage Range (mg/d)[a]
Diphenylmethanes				
Diphenhydramine	Benadryl	Parke-Davis	No	25–200
	Generics	Various		
Hydroxyzine	Vistaril	Pfizer	Yes	50–400
	Atarax	Roerig		
	Generics	Various		
β-Blockers				
Propranolol	Inderal	Wyeth-Ayerst	No	80–160
	Generics	Various		
Azapirones				
Buspirone	BuSpar	Mead Johnson	Yes	15–60[b]

[a]Elderly patients are usually treated with approximately one-half of the dose listed.
[b]The dosage range in elderly patients appears to be the same, but is not established.

sion,[8] it is usually inadequate treatment when used alone in patients with severe anxiety.

Benzodiazepine Therapy

The BZs are the drugs of choice for treating GAD. Discovered in the 1930s, these agents were not marketed in the United States until 1960. Chlordiazepoxide and diazepam dominated the BZ market until the 1980s when the prescribing pattern shifted to lorazepam and alprazolam (the most commonly prescribed BZ since 1987).[25] More recently, prescriptions for clonazepam have risen.[24] Most prescriptions for BZs are written by general practitioners and internists.[26]

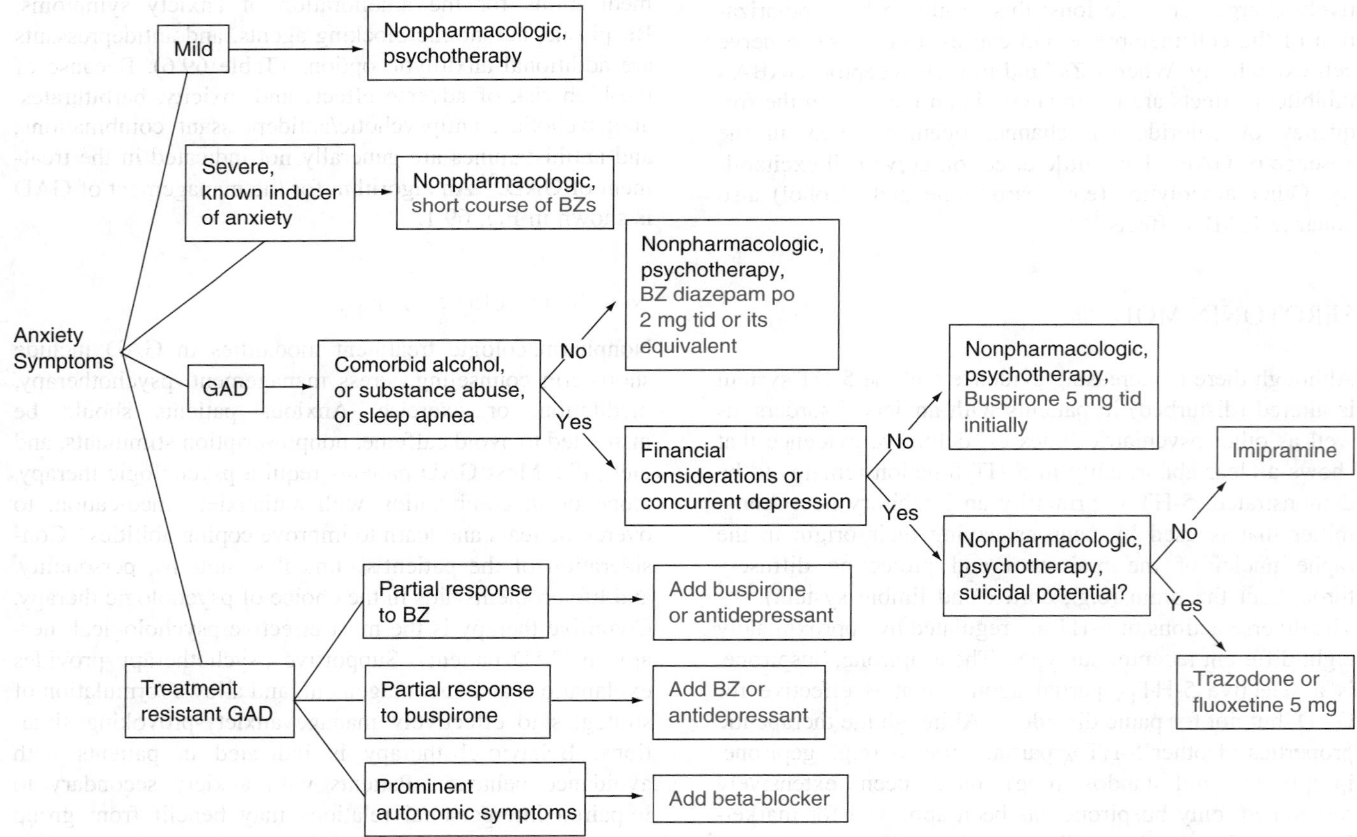

Figure 69.1. Algorithm for the management of generalized anxiety disorder. *(Developed from Refs. 8, 62, and 63.)*

TABLE 69.7. BENZODIAZEPINE ANTIANXIETY AGENTS

Generic Name	Brand Name	Manufacturer	Approved Indications	Approved Dosage Range (mg/d)[a]	Approximate Equivalent Dose (mg)
Alprazolam	Xanax	Upjohn	Anxiety Anxiety-depression Panic disorder	0.75–4 1.5–10	0.5
Chlordiazepoxide	Librium Generics	Roche Various	Anxiety Alcohol withdrawal Pre-op sedation	25–200	10
Clorazepate	Tranxene Generics	Abbott Various	Anxiety Seizure disorders	7.5–90	7.5
Diazepam	Valium Generics	Roche Various	Anxiety Alcohol withdrawal Muscle spasm Pre-op sedation Status epilepticus	2–40	5
Halazepam	Paxipam	Schering	Anxiety	20–160	20
Lorazepam	Ativan Generics	Wyeth-Ayerst Various	Anxiety Pre-op sedation	0.5–10	1
Oxazepam	Serax Generics	Wyeth-Ayerst Various	Anxiety Anxiety-depression Alcohol withdrawal	30–120	15
Prazepam	Centrax	Parke-Davis	Anxiety	20–60	10

[a]Elderly patients are usually treated with approximately one-half of the dose listed.

Indications

Although all BZs possess anxiolytic properties, only 8 of the 16 currently marketed agents have Food and Drug Administration (FDA)-approved labeling for the treatment of GAD (Table 69.7). Estazolam, flurazepam, temazepam, quazepam, and triazolam are marketed as sedative–hypnotic agents. Clonazepam is marketed as an anticonvulsant and midazolam is labeled for preoperative sedation. In addition to GAD, alprazolam is indicated for the treatment of panic disorder with or without agoraphobia.[27] Differences in marketed clinical indications often represent the manufacturers' marketing strategy rather than any major inherent differences in pharmacologic properties.[28]

Mechanism of Action

The BZ receptor model of anxiety (described under section on Pathophysiology) theorizes that BZs ameliorate anxiety through potentiation of the inhibitory activity of GABA.[19] BZ binding sites are present in high density in the cortical and limbic-forebrain areas of the CNS.[19] The BZ receptor is structurally and functionally coupled to the $GABA_A$ receptor and the associated Cl ion channel in the postsynaptic nerve cell membrane. The receptor complex is composed of three protein subunits that form an intrinsic Cl ion channel and BZs bind to the γ_2 subunit.[29] When the BZ receptor is activated in the presence of GABA, the frequency of the Cl ion channels opening and influx of Cl ions into the neuronal cell is increased. The resultant negatively charged, hyperpolarized membrane prevents further depolarization by excitatory neurotransmitters. Other neurotransmitters (e.g., 5-HT, NE, dopamine) may be involved in BZ activity. Animal studies support serotonergic involvement in the anxiolytic effect of BZs downstream from the BZ–$GABA_A$–Cl complex.[19]

Pharmacokinetics

A wide difference in milligram potency exists between the BZ compounds; however, when dosage adjustments are made, all agents share similar anxiolytic and sedative–hypnotic activity.[19] Variations in lipid solubility between compounds may influence BZ pharmacokinetic properties. Differences in BZ pharmacokinetic and pharmacodynamic properties may assist the clinician in choosing an appropriate anxiolytic (Table 69.8). After a single dose, the onset, intensity, and duration of pharmacologic effects are important factors to consider when using BZs for the short-term, intermittent, or as-needed treatment of anxiety.

The primary determinant of a drug's onset of effect after a single oral dose is the rate of drug absorption. Because of high lipophilicity, diazepam and clorazepate are rapidly absorbed and quickly distributed into the CNS. Therefore, the onset of anxiolytic effect occurs within 30–60 minutes and produces a rapid and intense relief of anxiety. High lipophilicity increases the extent of drug redistribution into the periphery, particularly adipose tissue, resulting in a shorter duration of effect after a single dose

TABLE 69.8. PHARMACOKINETICS OF BENZODIAZEPINE ANTIANXIETY AGENTS

Generic Name	Peak Plasma Level (h)	Elimination Half-Life, Parent (h)	Metabolic Pathway	Clinically Significant Metabolites	Protein Binding (%)
Alprazolam	1–2	12–15	Oxidation	None	80
Chlordiazepoxide	1–4	5–30	*N*-Dealkylation Oxidation	Desmethylchlordiazepoxide Demoxepam *N*-DMDZ[a]	96
Clorazepate	1–2	Prodrug	Oxidation	*N*-DMDZ	97
Diazepam	0.5–2	20–80	Oxidation	*N*-DMDZ	98
Halazepam	1–3	14	Oxidation	*N*-DMDZ	97
Lorazepam	2–4	10–20	Conjugation	None	85
Oxazepam	2–4	5–20	Conjugation	None	97
Prazepam	6	Prodrug	Oxidation	*N*-DMDZ	97

[a]*N*-desmethyldiazepam half-life 36–200 h. (Compiled from Refs. 28 and 30.)

than indicated by single-dose elimination half-life studies.[19,30] Clinically, patients perceive a rapid onset of action, but some may experience an unpleasant feeling of drowsiness, relaxation, or loss of control.[30] This "rush" may be euphoric and may contribute to an individual BZ's abuse potential. Chlordiazepoxide's onset of action is much slower because of decreased lipophilicity, slower absorption, and delayed passage into the CNS.

Compared with diazepam, lorazepam, oxazepam, and prazepam are relatively less lipophilic and have a slower onset of effect. These BZs have smaller volumes of distribution and a resultant longer duration of action.[19] Oxazepam absorption is slow and peak levels are not obtained until 2–4 hours after a single dose; however, like lorazepam, oxazepam's anxiolytic effects are long lasting because extensive distribution does not occur. Prazepam, a prodrug, is very slowly absorbed and requires hepatic dealkylation to *N*-desmethyldiazepam (*N*-DMDZ), with peak levels delayed until 6 hours after a single dose. BZs with slow absorption rates are not recommended for the immediate (acute) relief of anxiety symptoms.

Parenteral administration through the intramuscular route should be avoided with diazepam and chlordiazepoxide secondary to variability in the rate and extent of drug absorption. Intramuscular lorazepam provides rapid, reliable, and complete absorption; however, the preparation requires refrigeration.[30]

After multiple dosing, the rate and extent of drug accumulation are functions of the drug's elimination half-life in relation to dosing intervals, clearance, and formation of active metabolites. Differences in clinical effects that occur during and after repeated dosage with the BZs are related in part to variability in metabolism and metabolite accumulation. With dosing intervals less than 24 hours, long-elimination half-life BZs accumulate extensively.[24]

The BZs undergo two primary metabolic processes, hepatic microsomal oxidation (*N*-dealkylation or aliphatic hydroxylation) and glucuronide conjugation. With the exception of lorazepam and oxazepam (which are conjugated only), all BZs are oxidized first, then conjugated, and excreted renally. Oxidation may be impaired in such clinical situations as liver disease, in the elderly, and with the simultaneous use of drugs that inhibit oxidation. Impaired oxidation results in higher levels of the parent drug and/or an active metabolite.[30] BZ conjugation is not affected by these factors.

Many BZs (e.g., diazepam, halazepam, and chlordiazepoxide) are converted (through *N*-demethylation) to *N*-DMDZ, an active metabolite with a long-elimination half-life of 36–200 hours (Table 69.8).[28] *N*-DMDZ is further oxidized to oxazepam, then conjugated, and excreted. After multiple dosing, accumulation of *N*-DMDZ is slow and extensive, providing a long-lasting antianxiety effect. If oxidation of *N*-DMDZ is impaired, the half-life is prolonged, and complications of drug accumulation (e.g., drowsiness, sedation) may result over time with repeated dosing.[30]

Clorazepate and prazepam are prodrugs and possess no anxiolytic effects until they are metabolized into *N*-DMDZ. This metabolite is primarily responsible for the anxiolytic effects. Before absorption, clorazepate is rapidly metabolized in the stomach through a pH-dependent process under acidic conditions.[30] Alterations of stomach pH (e.g., administration of antacids) may decrease the rate of *N*-DMDZ formation. Prazepam requires first-pass liver transformation before *N*-DMDZ is formed.

BZs with short half-lives (e.g., alprazolam, lorazepam, oxazepam) reach steady-state plasma concentrations rapidly, and drug accumulation after repeated dosing is minimal. Alprazolam is oxidized to α-hydroxyalprazolam, which probably contributes little to the clinical effects. Neither oxazepam nor lorazepam is converted into active metabolites.[30]

BZ protein binding is extensive, especially those with long-elimination half-lives. Patients with hypoalbuminemia often have increased sensitivity to clinical effects and BZs with lower protein binding (e.g., lorazepam, alprazolam) should be used.

Clinical Use

A knowledge of the pharmacokinetic and pharmacodynamic properties of the BZs may assist the clinician in selecting an agent for a particular clinical situation. After a single dose of a long-elimination half-life BZ, the expected duration of clinical activity may not parallel the drug's pharmacokinetic half-life because of drug redistribution.[19] After multiple dosing, drugs with long-elimination half-lives and active metabolites may require 1–2 weeks to reach steady state. In the elderly, secondary to a decreased capacity for oxidation and alterations in the volume of distribution, drug accumulation may result. Patients with hepatic disease also are at risk for drug accumulation and subsequent complications. Therefore, intermediate- or short-acting BZs are preferred for chronic use in the elderly and those with liver disorders because of minimal accumulation and achievement of steady state within 1–3 days.

BZs with long-elimination half-lives may be dosed once a day at bedtime and may provide both hypnotic and daytime anxiolytic activity. Agents with shorter elimination half-lives should be administered in divided daily doses.

Drug Interactions

Drug interactions with the BZs generally fall into two categories—pharmacodynamic and pharmacokinetic (Table 69.9).[31–40] Simultaneous use of alcohol and a BZ results in additive CNS depressant effects (sedation and psychomotor impairment) and lowers the therapeutic index of the BZ. In addition, concurrent use of a BZ and drugs with CNS depressant properties (e.g., antipsychotics, antihistamines, narcotics, barbiturates, anticonvulsants, antidepressants) may potentiate the adverse sedative effects. When ingested alone in an overdose attempt, BZs are rarely life-threatening; however, the combination of BZs with alcohol or other CNS depressant agents is potentially fatal. The concomitant use of intravenous lorazepam during clozapine therapy was associated with respiratory suppression and death.[32]

Cimetidine, an H_2-receptor antagonist, competitively inhibits the metabolism of drugs that require oxidation through the hepatic microsomal P-450 enzyme system. A prolonged elimination half-life and decreased plasma clearance for single doses of diazepam, chlordiazepoxide, and alprazolam occurred after treatment with cimetidine; however, cimetidine failed to inhibit metabolism of oxazepam and lorazepam because these agents are conjugated.[33] Greenblatt and associates[34] did not demonstrate adverse psychomotor effects when cimetidine was added to diazepam therapy, despite a mean increase in diazepam and *N*-DMDZ plasma concentrations of 62% and 54%, respectively. Thus, the clinical importance of this interaction is minimal in healthy patients on chronic BZ therapy; however, when chronic therapy is indicated in the elderly or debilitated patient receiving cimetidine, oxazepam or lorazepam is the BZ of choice. Ranitidine (Zantac)[35] and famotidine (Pepcid) are H_2-receptor antagonists that do not inhibit oxidative metabolism and are alternatives to cimetidine for patients on BZs that undergo oxidative metabolism.

TABLE 69.9. DRUG INTERACTIONS WITH THE BENZODIAZEPINES

Drug	Effect
Alcohol	Decreased clearance of chlordiazepoxide and diazepam; additive psychomotor impairment
Antacids	Decreased rate and extent of clorazepate absorption; decreased rate of diazepam and chlordiazepoxide absorption
Cimetidine	Decreased clearance of alprazolam, diazepam, chlordiazepoxide, and clorazepate and increased elimination half-life
Clozapine	Respiratory suppression, possibly death
Disulfiram	Decreased clearance of chlordiazepoxide and diazepam by 40–50%, and probably alprazolam, clorazepate, halazepam, prazepam
Fluoxetine	Decreased clearance of diazepam
Fluvoxamine	Decreased clearance of alprazolam and prolonged half-life
Isoniazid	Decreased metabolism of diazepam
Nefazodone	Decreased clearance of alprazolam, AUC doubled and half-life prolonged
Omeprazole	Decreased clearance of diazepam
Oral contraceptives	Increased free concentration of chlordiazepoxide and slightly decreased clearance; decreased clearance and increased half-life of diazepam and alprazolam
Rifampin	Increased metabolism of diazepam
Theophylline	Decreased alprazolam concentrations

(Compiled from Refs. 28, 30–40.)

Antacids may decrease the rate of clorazepate absorption. The rate, but not extent, of diazepam and chlordiazepoxide absorption is decreased by concurrent antacid ingestion.[28] Other agents that may impair BZ metabolism include theophylline, disulfiram, fluoxetine, isoniazid, omeprazole, rifampin, and low-dose estrogens.[28,36–38] Nefazodone and fluvoxamine increased alprazolam concentrations by 100%.[39,40] Therefore, the alprazolam dose should be reduced by 50% when these agents are added.[39,40]

Adverse Drug Reactions

The most common adverse events associated with BZ therapy involve CNS depression. This is clinically manifested as drowsiness, sedation, psychomotor impairment, and ataxia.[24] A transient mild drowsiness is commonly experienced by patients during the first few days of treatment; however, tolerance often develops. Disorientation, confusion, irritability, aggression, and excitement have been reported.[24]

Impairment of memory and recall may also occur during BZ treatment. The memory loss induced by the BZs and barbiturates is typically limited to events occurring after drug ingestion (or anterograde amnesia).[41] The anterograde amnesia is secondary to disordered consolidation processes that store information and is not an impairment in the perception or retrieval of information.[24,41] BZs with high affinity for binding to the BZ receptor appear to possess a higher potential for amnesia (e.g., lorazepam). The extent of BZ-induced memory impairment is unknown and may go unrecognized by both the clinician and the patient. Complaints of forgetfulness in patients receiving BZs, especially the elderly, should be explored for drug-induced amnesia.

Abuse, Dependence, Withdrawal, and Tolerance

The widespread use of BZs has generated public concern regarding the potential for abuse. The long-term use of BZs has caused increased interest regarding the development of physical dependence. Most BZ users consume these agents for brief periods, but 15% report daily use that exceeds 1 year. The use of BZs peaked from 1973–1975, and the annual prescription volume (1985–1987) has remained at 61 million (the equivalent of 1970 data). These data fail to provide evidence for increases in prescription volume and prevalence of usage.[25]

Drug abuse is defined by the World Health Organization (WHO) as the persistence of sporadic, excessive drug use inconsistent with or unrelated to acceptable medical practice. BZ abuse is rare in the general population of users; however, individuals with a history of multiple drug abuse (e.g., alcohol, sedatives) are at the greatest risk for becoming BZ abusers.[24,25]

BZ dependence is a physiologic phenomenon demonstrated by the appearance of a predictable abstinence syndrome (withdrawal symptoms) upon abrupt discontinuation of therapy. Although initially reported in patients taking excessive doses, it is now recognized that a mild withdrawal syndrome may occur in up to 44% of patients ingesting therapeutic doses of BZs for only 4–6 weeks.[42] Withdrawal symptoms may result because of the abrupt dissociation of a BZ from its receptor site. After abrupt BZ discontinuation, an acute decrease in GABA neurotransmission results, producing a less inhibited CNS.[25]

Benzodiazepine Discontinuation

After BZ therapy is abruptly discontinued, several events can occur (i.e., post-BZ phenomenon). Rebound symptoms represent an immediate, but transient return of original symptoms having an increased intensity compared with baseline. Recurrence or relapse is the return of original symptoms having the same intensity as before treatment. In patients treated with BZs for over 1 year, a recurrence of GAD is reported in 50–65%. Withdrawal symptoms are the emergence of new symptoms as well as a worsening of preexisting symptoms after BZ discontinuation (e.g., photophobia, seizures, auditory hypersensitivity, tinnitus). Withdrawal symptoms may occur with rebound and recurrence, persist for days to weeks, and may be so severe that they interfere with normal functioning.

Common symptoms of BZ withdrawal include anxiety, insomnia, restlessness, agitation, muscle tension, and irritability. Less frequently occurring symptoms are nausea, malaise, coryza, blurred vision, diaphoresis, nightmares, depression, hyperreflexia, and ataxia. Tinnitus, confusion, paranoid delusions, hallucinations, seizures, and psychosis rarely occur.[25] Seizures occur with both therapeutic and high doses of short-elimination half-life BZs, usually within 3 days of drug discontinuation or approximately 1 week for long-elimination half-life agents. High BZ doses, a long duration of therapy, and concurrent ingestion of drugs that lower the seizure threshold are risk factors for withdrawal seizures.[25]

BZ pharmacokinetics influence the time course of the development of symptoms.[25] The onset of withdrawal symptoms in patients ingesting BZs with short-elimination half-lives occurs much earlier (within 24–48 hours) than in those taking BZs with long-elimination half-lives, where symptoms begin 3–8 days later.[43] Other factors associated with an increased incidence or severity of BZ withdrawal include high doses and long-term BZ therapy. Abrupt discontinuation after using short-elimination half-life BZs (e.g., lorazepam, oxazepam, and alprazolam) may produce a more severe withdrawal[44] than long-elimination half-life agents. The difference in half-life is less distinct when BZs are gradually tapered.[45]

Factors that increase the likelihood of BZ dependence include high doses for up to 4–6 weeks or therapeutic doses for extended periods of time. Rebound symptoms are more intense after the ingestion of short-elimination relative to long-elimination half-life BZs. In patients who ingest BZs for more than 4 months, withdrawal symptoms are more likely and more severe; patients who experience withdrawal at this time usually do not wish to stop therapy. Therefore, continuous daily usage of BZs for 4–8 months may increase the development of dependency. The risk of developing dependence and a withdrawal syndrome in patients ingesting BZs for over 1 year is considerably higher.[25]

Several strategies to minimize the severity of BZ withdrawal include a 25% per week reduction in dosage until 50% of the dose is reached, then dosage reduction by one-eighth every 4–7 days. The patient should be observed drug free for 3 weeks to monitor for the presence of withdrawal symptoms versus recurrence of original symptoms. Tapering will not entirely eliminate the emergence of withdrawal symptoms, but will prevent severe withdrawal (e.g., convulsion, psychosis). Slow drug taper is extremely important for the short-elimination half-life drugs because some individuals have greater difficulty with discontinuation.[25,44] Results of studies performed to evaluate the use of adjunctive carbamazepine, clonidine, propranolol, and antidepressants to attenuate BZ withdrawal have been inconclusive.[46] If patients experience difficulties, especially with the short-elimination half-life agents, then substitution of a long-elimination half-life BZ should be considered. Diazepam can be initiated as a loading dose (40% of daily consumption), followed by daily tapering of 10%. Clonazepam is an alternative agent. Phenobarbital could be used especially if the patient has mixed BZ and alcohol dependence. Dosage conversion charts are available and the loading dose should be maintained for 2 days, then the phenobarbital dose decreased by 30 mg/d.[25]

If BZ therapy exceeds 6 weeks, a slow dosage taper over several weeks is recommended.[28] A long-elimination half-life BZ (e.g., diazepam) may be substituted for agents with short-elimination half-lives (e.g., lorazepam, oxazepam, alprazolam), and patients should receive these drugs for several weeks before gradual drug discontinuation begins. In patients receiving alprazolam, carbamazepine may be a useful alternative to diazepam.[45]

Although tolerance develops to the sedative, muscle relaxant, and anticonvulsant activities, the BZs do not appear to lose anxiolytic or antipanic efficacy.[25] The anxiolytic efficacy of BZs in long-term clinical trials (i.e., greater than 4–6 months of chronic use) has not been reported; however, some patients obtain beneficial anxiolytic effects from chronic BZ ingestion.

General Prescribing Guidelines

The goals of BZ therapy in GAD are to reduce the severity, duration, and frequency of the anxiety symptoms and to improve the patient's overall functioning. All BZs are equally effective anxiolytics, and consideration of pharmacokinetic properties and the patient's clinical situation will assist in the selection of the most appropriate agent. Pharmacokinetic differences vary, and the clinician must monitor the patient's response to the initial treatment regimen.

Diazepam, clorazepate, and alprazolam are preferable in situations where a rapid onset of drug effect is necessary. Agents with short-elimination half-lives are recommended for the elderly, for patients with hepatic disorders, and for those receiving drugs that impair oxidative metabolism. Drug and metabolite accumulation and toxicity may result if long-elimination half-life BZs are used in these situations, however, this can be minimized by lowering the dosage or decreasing the frequency of drug administration.

BZ dosage requirements vary widely among patients and must be individualized and carefully titrated to avoid adverse effects. Therapy should be initiated using low doses (e.g., diazepam 2 mg three times per day or its equivalent), and titrated upward to relieve anxiety symptoms and avoid the appearance of adverse events (diazepam, maximum 40 mg/d). After an initial treatment response is achieved, agents with long-elimination half-lives may be dosed at bedtime and dosage adjustments should be made on a weekly basis. Side effects such as drowsiness and sedation can be managed by a decrease in dosage or an increase in dosage frequency.[28]

The duration of BZ therapy should be monitored and should not exceed 4 months. However, some patients require longer treatment.[8] Intermittent therapy is indicated in patients with intermittent symptoms or anxiety induced by a known cause. Individuals with persistent symptoms may require continuous treatment. Use of an intermittent schedule with interruptions of BZ therapy every 6–8 weeks to reevaluate the diagnosis and need for treatment has been proposed.[47] Problems with drug withdrawal rarely occur in patients receiving the usual therapeutic doses of BZs for less than 4 months, especially when the BZ is tapered. The overall incidence of abuse is rare among anxious patients, but may occur in patients with alcohol or sedative–hypnotic dependence.

The elderly anxious patient requires additional monitoring when a BZ is prescribed. These patients have an enhanced sensitivity to BZ response, both to therapeutic and CNS depressant effects, that may possibly be related to pharmacokinetic alterations (e.g., decreased clearance).[48] The elderly may be susceptible to sedation, impaired daytime functioning, and memory problems, which also may be enhanced by other drugs with CNS depressant effects. Thus dosages should be low and short-elimination half-life agents (e.g., oxazepam, lorazepam) prescribed.[48]

Patient education should include the anticipated length of drug therapy, potential side effects, and consequences of the ingestion of alcohol and other CNS depressants. Patients should understand that medications provide symptomatic relief, but do not solve underlying psychological problems. Patients should be told not to decrease or discontinue BZ usage without contacting their physician.

Buspirone Therapy

Buspirone, an azapirone anxiolytic, is structurally and pharmacologically unlike the BZs—it lacks anticonvulsant, muscle relaxant, hypnotic, motor impairment, and dependence properties. For the treatment of GAD, clinical trials found buspirone superior to placebo and as efficacious as BZs after 4 weeks.[49]

Mechanism of Action

Buspirone's anxiolytic mechanism of action is unknown; however, it does not interact with the BZ–$GABA_A$–Cl receptor complex nor decrease noradrenergic neuron firing in the LC (it slightly increases firing). Buspirone possesses activity as a 5-HT_{1A} partial agonist binding presynaptically to the receptors in the dorsal raphe and postsynaptically to receptors in the hippocampus and cortical brain areas.[50] Buspirone also possesses both dopamine agonist and indirect dopamine antagonist properties.[50]

Pharmacokinetics

After an oral dose, buspirone is rapidly and completely absorbed, and undergoes extensive first-pass metabolism. The mean systemic bioavailability is approximately 4%. Buspirone is 95% protein bound to both albumin and α_1-acid glycoprotein.[51] The mean elimination half-life of buspirone is 2.1–2.7 hours.[52]

Buspirone is eliminated primarily by oxidative metabolism and is converted into both active and inactive metabolites. One pharmacologically active metabolite, 1-pyrimidinylpiperazine, possesses approximately one-fifth the anxiolytic activity of buspirone.[51] Buspirone's metabolites lack postsynaptic dopamine receptor-binding properties, thus metabolism may play a major role in minimizing both clinical (i.e., antipsychotic) and adverse effects associated with postsynaptic dopaminergic blockade.[53] Although unaffected by age, buspirone's clearance is markedly decreased in patients with cirrhosis and to a lesser extent in patients with renal impairment.[51]

Adverse Drug Reactions

A major advantage of buspirone is its lack of sedative properties. The incidence of sedation is much less than with BZs at equipotent doses. Other adverse effects include dizziness, nausea, headaches, nervousness, and dysphoria (especially with large single doses of 20–40 mg).[54] Potential problems secondary to postsynaptic dopaminergic blockade (e.g., gynecomastia, galactorrhea, extrapyramidal symptoms) are rare.

Drug Interactions

Buspirone reportedly increases the area under the concentration-versus-time curve of haloperidol and the manufacturer recommends avoidance of this combination.[55] In comparative trials with BZs, buspirone (but not the BZs) lacked a pharmacokinetic interaction with alcohol and failed to potentiate performance impairment.[28] Six occurrences of elevated blood pressure were reported in patients taking a monoamine oxidase inhibitor (MAOI) and buspirone concurrently, thus this combination is not recommended.[56] Fluoxetine is reported to antagonize buspirone's anxiolytic activity.[57]

Abuse, Physical Dependence, and Withdrawal

Buspirone has a low potential for abuse.[58] Physical dependence and withdrawal symptoms have not been reported.[49]

General Prescribing Guidelines

The recommended initial dose of buspirone is 5 mg three times a day with dosage increments of 5 mg/d every 2–3 days as needed.[55] The usual therapeutic dose of buspirone is 20–30 mg/d, with a maximum dose of 60 mg/d.[55] The onset of anxiolysis is not immediate, requiring a week or more before clinical effects occur; maximum therapeutic benefit may not be evident for 4–6 weeks.[49]

Buspirone possesses specific characteristics that distinguish it from other anxiolytic agents. Thus different guidelines must be used for successful therapy. Buspirone has minimal sedating properties and is not useful in clinical situations requiring immediate anxiolytic effects or for situations requiring as-needed anxiolytic therapy. Therefore, buspirone is an alternative for GAD patients who are unable to tolerate the sedative effects and psychomotor impairment of BZs, especially the elderly.

Buspirone is not cross-tolerant with BZs and thus will not prevent or treat symptoms of BZ withdrawal.[59] When a patient is switched from a BZ to buspirone, the BZ should be tapered slowly before buspirone is initiated.

Previous BZ therapy may lead to certain expectations of anxiolytic drug effects (immediate response and sedation) that buspirone does not demonstrate.[43] Therefore, patients who have received BZs should be advised of these differences, particularly at the outset of therapy. Buspirone is an appropriate choice for patients with a history of alcohol or drug abuse because of its low potential for abuse. Other azapirones (e.g., gepirone and ipsapirone) are currently under investigation as anxiolytics.[60]

Adrenergic Blocking Agents

Propranolol and other β-blocking agents may be useful in patients with prominent cardiovascular symptoms of anxiety (e.g., palpitations, tremors). β-Blocking drugs are less effective anxiolytics than BZs[61] and their usefulness may be entirely restricted to those anxiety patients whose physical symptoms, especially cardiovascular complaints, have not adequately responded to BZ therapy. Propranolol therapy is usually well tolerated with few adverse effects, provided a complete medical examination is performed and medical contraindications are observed (e.g., heart block, asthma, Raynaud's disease).

Doses of propranolol ranging from 40–360 mg/d are used in managing GAD.[28] Although propranolol has a short-elimination half-life (2–6 hours), β-blockade usually lasts for 8–12 hours after a single dose. Propranolol should be dosed at least twice a day.[61] Propranolol 10 mg twice a day should be used initially and gradually titrated to anxiolytic response. Doses can be titrated to a reduction in heart rate (e.g., 5–10 beats per minute).[8] The usual duration of therapy is not well defined, but response should be observed within 1 week of therapy.[8] The emergence of adverse effects (e.g., depression, fatigue, decreased concentration) may limit the clinical usefulness of these agents. Upon discontinuation of therapy, the propranolol dosage should be tapered to avoid rebound anxiety and cardiovascular effects.[61]

Antidepressants

Because of their adverse events profile, antidepressants are not considered first-line agents in the management of GAD. Recent studies indicated that imipramine, a tricyclic antidepressant (TCA), and trazodone are effective in GAD after 3–8 weeks of therapy.[62] The mean daily dosages of imipramine at the end of 1 and 8 weeks were 92 and 143 mg, respectively. The mean daily dosages of trazodone at the end of weeks 1 and 8 were 175 and 235 mg, respectively.[62] Low doses of SSRIs (e.g., fluoxetine 5 mg) have been successful in some GAD patients.[8,63] Antidepressants are alternatives for individuals with contraindications to BZ use. They are also useful adjuncts in the treatment of patients with a partial response to BZs or buspirone.[8,63]

Evaluation of Therapeutic Outcomes

Initially, anxious patients should be monitored twice weekly for a reduction in the frequency, duration, and severity of anxiety symptoms and improvement in occupational, social, and interpersonal functioning. The goals of treatment and duration of therapy should be discussed with the patient at the beginning of therapy. The pharmacist should assess the patient for response to treatment by asking about the target symptoms of anxiety and emergence of adverse drug events. After achieving an optimal drug dosage, the patient can be evaluated monthly until drug discontinuation. Use of an objective measurement of anxiety symptoms (e.g., a Visual Analogue Scale to rate the severity, frequency, and duration of symptoms on scales of 1 to 10 or a standard rating instrument such as the State-Trait Anxiety Inventory or Zung Self-Rating Anxiety Scale[26]) may assist in the evaluation of drug response.

PANIC DISORDER

Panic disorder is effectively treated with several drugs including the TCA imipramine, the BZ alprazolam, the MAOI phenelzine, and SSRIs (Table 69.10).[8,63] Alprazolam is currently the only drug approved for this indication. Therapeutic options include a single pharmacologic agent, concurrent psychotherapy, or psychotherapy followed by pharmacotherapy. Most patients without agoraphobia will improve with pharmacotherapy alone; however, if agoraphobia is present, cognitive–behavioral therapy is typically initiated concurrently. With all effective drug therapies, resolution of phobic avoidance tends to occur slowly, and many patients require concurrent cognitive–behavioral therapy. When imipramine or alprazolam were combined with behavioral therapy, approximately 66–75% of patients reported a marked global improvement after short-term treatment, but at follow-up long-term outcome was poor in alprazolam-treated patients.[64] Goals of therapy include a complete resolution of panic attacks, marked reduction in anticipatory anxiety and phobic fears, and maintenance of a clinical response that allows the patient to resume normal activities.[65]

Nonpharmacologic Therapy

Patients should be educated to avoid substances that may precipitate panic attacks including caffeine, drugs of abuse, and nonprescription stimulants. Patients often require behavioral therapy (specifically exposure) to alleviate their phobic-avoidance behavior.[66] Patients usually acknowledge that, although their panic attacks resolve with proper drug therapy, fears and avoidance of situations (crowded places, stores, bridges, and travel) remain firm. Patients need to learn they can reenter feared situations safely without having a panic attack by actually confronting the situation. Exposure requires patients to confront phobic situations gradually, starting with the least feared situation and progressing to the most feared situation.[66]

For patients who cannot or will not take medication, behavioral treatment alone is certainly indicated with approximately two-thirds of patients reporting clinically significant improvement.[64,66] Unfortunately, behavioral therapy does not alleviate the panic attacks that may be experienced during exposure, which may further reinforce phobic-avoidance behavior. Cognitive therapy is effective in reducing panic attacks in approximately 83% of patients.[66] Combined cognitive–behavioral therapy is associated with short-term improvement in 66% of patients and 6-month improvement in 75% of patients.[67]

Pharmacotherapy

Antidepressants

TCAs. Double-blind, placebo-controlled studies have demonstrated the efficacy of imipramine in blocking panic attacks.[68,69] It is effective in 75% of patients with panic disorder.[8,68,69] Imipramine effectively blocks panic attacks within 3–5 weeks; however, maximal improvement (including antiphobic response) does not occur until 6–10 weeks. The sequence of patient response is an initial decrease in the number of panic attacks, then diminution of anticipatory anxiety, followed by a reduction in phobic avoidance. Approximately 20–30% of patients experience stimulatory (amphetamine-like) side effects including insomnia, jitteriness, irritability, and unusual energy.[65] These side effects often significantly affect patient compliance, prevent medication dosage increases, and interfere with the overall treatment outcome. Reducing the dose may eliminate these unpleasant effects.[69,70]

Although imipramine is the most studied antidepressant for panic disorder, other TCAs, especially desipramine and clomipramine,[71] may possibly be effective. Trazodone and maprotiline were effective in some patients, but bupropion was ineffective.[8,63,70]

TABLE 69.10. DRUGS USED IN THE TREATMENT OF PANIC DISORDER

Class/Generic Name	Brand Name	Manufacturer	Antipanic Dosage[a] Range (mg)	Comments
Benzodiazepines				
Alprazolam	Xanax Generics	Upjohn Various	4–10[b]	Effective in high doses, rapid response *Problems:* side effects, withdrawal
Diazepam	Valium Generics	Roche Various	30–40	Possibly effective, needs more study
Clonazepam	Klonopin	Roche	3–6	Possibly effective, needs more study
Lorazepam	Ativan Generics	Wyeth-Ayerst Various	3–4	Possibly effective, needs more study
Tricyclic antidepressants				
Imipramine	Tofranil Generics	Ciba-Geigy Various	150–300	Effective *Problems:* lag time, side effects
Monoamine oxidase inhibitors				
Phenelzine	Nardil	Parke-Davis	45–90	Effective *Problems:* patient acceptance, dietary restrictions, side effects
Serotonin reuptake inhibitors				
Fluoxetine	Prozac	Dista	2.5–20	Effective *Problems:* lag time, expensive
Fluvoxamine	Luvox	Solvay	150–300	Effective *Problems:* lag time, expensive
Paroxetine	Paxil	SmithKline Beecham	10–60	Possibly effective, needs more study *Problems:* lag time, expensive
Sertraline	Zoloft	Roerig	25–100	Possibly effective, needs more study *Problems:* lag time, expensive
Miscellaneous agents				
Clonidine	Catapres Generics	Boehringer Ingelheim Various	0.2–0.5	Reserved as last-line agent; tolerance develops to antipanic effects
Valproic acid	Depakene Generics	Abbott Various	500–2000	Reserved as last-line agent

[a]Dosage used in clinical trials but not FDA approved.
[b]Dosage is FDA approved.

SSRIs. The SSRIs are commonly used in the management of panic disorder. In a limited number of controlled[72] and uncontrolled[73] trials, fluvoxamine and fluoxetine, respectively, have shown efficacy. Approximately 40–50% of patients respond to fluoxetine.[73] Other SSRIs may also be effective. The antipanic effect of SSRIs is delayed for 3–5 weeks.

MAOIs. The majority of studies assessing the efficacy of MAOIs in treating panic disorder were poorly designed, lacked sufficient dosage and duration of treatment, sufficient sample size, and valid ratings of panic attacks. Sheehan et al.[74] conducted the most definitive trial comparing phenelzine (45 mg/d) and imipramine (150 mg/d) with placebo. Both drugs were found effective and superior to placebo; however, phenelzine was slightly superior on several rating scales. As with imipramine, the antipanic effect of phenelzine is delayed for 3–5 weeks, and the antiphobic effect does not occur for 6–10 weeks.[74] Side effects and dietary restrictions adversely affect patient acceptance.[70,74] MAOIs are usually reserved for the most refractory or difficult patient.[8,70]

Benzodiazepines

During the past decade, several placebo-controlled studies have documented the efficacy of high-dose alprazolam in treating panic disorder.[69,75] This finding is of clinical importance because originally it was believed that BZs (e.g., diazepam and chlordiazepoxide) were ineffective in blocking panic attacks. This assumption was based on the historical observation that patients who received BZs continued to have panic attacks that subsequently cleared after treatment with imipramine or phenelzine. In these cases, BZs may have failed because they were prescribed in insufficient doses and because patients were instructed to take as little medication as possible. In addition to alprazolam, the BZs diazepam, lorazepam, and clonazepam are possibly effective in treating panic disorder when taken in sufficiently high doses (Table 69.10).[8,69,75,76] Therapeutic response to BZs occurs in 1–2 weeks, with further improvement occurring at weeks 4 to 6.[8] It is estimated that 80% of panic disorder patients respond to BZs. Alprazolam is an ideal agent for patients who need immediate relief. Patient acceptance of alprazolam is not usually a problem and, except for sedation, side effects are rarely reported.[77]

Clinical Guidelines

Choice of Agent

The emergence of depressive symptoms during BZ treatment has been reported.[78] Since most panic disorder patients experience at least one episode of depression, the association with BZ therapy may be coincidental.[76] However, because some antidepressants are superior to BZs in treating depression, they should be selected first for patients with panic disorder who are clinically depressed or have a history of depression. In patients whose illness is complicated by a history of alcohol or drug abuse, BZs should be cautiously used and a TCA, SSRI, or MAOI would be more appropriate.[8,79]

Problems with using imipramine in panic disorder are well documented and include stimulatory side effects, anticholinergic effects, orthostatic hypotension, delayed onset of antipanic effects (3–5 weeks), and toxicity in an overdose. For patients who cannot tolerate the anticholinergic side effects of imipramine, a switch to an SSRI may be helpful.[8] Some clinicians view SSRIs as first-line agents because of their improved tolerability;[8] however, these agents are significantly more expensive than the generically available TCAs and BZs.

The medication and dietary restrictions and the side effects associated with phenelzine adversely affect patient acceptance. This clear disadvantage places phenelzine as a last-line medication.[8,63] Only the most compliant and reliable patients should receive phenelzine.

Before antipanic drug therapy begins, it is important to obtain a thorough and complete medication history. Alcohol abuse and psychoactive drug use may present a problem in treating certain patients.

Acute Phase. The main goal of therapy in the acute phase is reduction of symptoms (e.g., resolution of panic attacks, reduction in anxiety and phobic fears, and resumption of the patient's usual activities).[65] The duration of this phase is generally 1–3 months depending on the choice of medication. The guiding principle for using medication in panic disorder is to start low, use an adequate dose, and treat for an appropriate period of time.[65] Side effects with the antidepressants, often from too high an initial dose, may prevent achievement of an optimal dosage, compromise treatment response, and contribute to patient noncompliance.[8,75]

The duration of the acute phase with antidepressants requires a minimum of 8–12 weeks. When using imipramine, treatment should be initiated with 10 mg/d at bedtime and slowly increased by 10 mg every 2–4 days as tolerated to 100–200 mg/d over a 2- to 4-week period.[8,65,70] Although an occasional patient will respond to 50 mg/d or less, most require at least 150 mg/d of imipramine (or a combined imipramine/desipramine plasma concentration of 100–150 ng/mL).[65] If this dose is not effective, a higher dose (up to 300 mg/d) should be used.[70] Many patients with panic disorder are extremely sensitive to imipramine (experienced as an immediate stimulatory feeling or motor restlessness) and the starting dose, therefore, is very conservative. Stimulatory side effects are transient and generally dissipate after several weeks of therapy.[65] Approximately 25–35% of patients reportedly discontinue treatment because of side effects or nonresponse.[8,65] Weight gain is a problematic side effect associated with long-term therapy and is the most frequent reason given for discontinuing treatment.[80]

Low initial doses of SSRIs are recommended to avoid stimulatory side effects (e.g., insomnia, nervousness). Starting doses of fluoxetine are 2.5–5 mg/d with dosage increases every 2 or 3 days to a dosage range of 10–20 mg/d by the end of 2 weeks.[8,73] A starting dose of fluvoxamine 50 mg/d increased to 150 mg/d, in divided doses, over 2 weeks was used in clinical trials (range of 100–300 mg/d).[72] Despite the lack of published controlled trials, anecdotal evidence suggests that sertraline initiated at 25 mg/d and titrated to 100 mg/d and paroxetine daily doses of 10–60 mg are also effective in panic disorder.[8,81]

The starting dose of phenelzine is 15 mg/d after the evening meal, increased by 15 mg/d every 3–4 days until 60 mg/d is reached. A dose of less than 45 mg/d is rarely effective. Dosages may be increased (up to 90 mg/d) if improvement is not achieved after 8–12 weeks.[74] If a patient has previously been receiving an antidepressant, 2 weeks should lapse before phenelzine is started to prevent a potential drug interaction. Fluoxetine must be stopped 5 weeks before phenelzine (or another MAOI) can be started. Phenelzine doses taken after meals lessens the risk of orthostatic hypotension. Anticholinergic side effects are less severe with phenelzine than with TCAs, but orthostatic hypotension and insomnia are often more of a problem. After 3 weeks, most unpleasant side effects subside.

Hypertensive crisis following the ingestion of tyramine-containing foods or sympathomimetic drugs is the most serious, potentially life-threatening event encountered with phenelzine.[82,83] Symptoms include a severe headache, usually accompanied by throbbing, flushing, and a heavy "thumping" of the heart. Patients should be instructed that if symptoms occur, they must go immediately to the nearest emergency room. They must never lie down, because this serves only to increase intracranial pressure. (Refer to the chapter on Depressive Disorders for a complete list of the food and drug restrictions and a more complete discussion of side effects.) Patients should observe the food, drink, and drug restrictions for at least 24 hours before starting the first dose of phenelzine, and for 2 weeks after stopping therapy.[82,83]

The duration of the acute phase with BZs is approximately 1 month because response is rapid and occurs within 1–3 weeks. The starting dose of alprazolam is 0.25 or 0.5 mg/d in three divided doses, slowly increased over several weeks. During the initial weeks of therapy, patients may pass through two or three dosage plateaus followed by some tolerance to side effects and some loss of benefit before reaching an ideal dose. The duration of action may be as little as 4–6 hours, causing some patients to experience "breakthrough" symptoms. Although a few patients may respond to doses as low as 2–3 mg/d, many patients require 3–6 mg/d, and some need doses of 6–10 mg/d to obtain a full therapeutic (antipanic and antiphobic) response.[8,65,69,75,84] Patients appear to tolerate the initial side effects of alprazolam (e.g., sedation) much better than those of imipramine or phenelzine.[69,77] Because of its long half-life, clonazepam is an alternative if patients experience breakthrough panic symptoms at the end of a dosing interval.

Continuation Phase. The goals of therapy during the continuation phase are to complete and extend the treatment response obtained in the acute phase, especially with regards to phobic avoidance.[65] During this time the drug dosage necessary to optimally maximize response and minimize adverse drug effects is obtained. Depending on response, this phase lasts for 2–4 months.

Maintenance Phase and Discontinuation. The duration of the maintenance phase is 3–12 months. In some patients, especially those experiencing adverse events, the drug dosage may be reduced without loss of improvement.[65] The goals of treatment are to maintain response and allow the patient to resume normal functioning.[65] The optimal length of therapy is unknown, however, the total optimal duration of therapy appears to be 8–12 months before drug discontinuation is attempted.[65] The rate of relapse, measured 6 months after a 3-month imipramine discontinuation, was 83% in panic disorder patients with agoraphobia treated for 6 months and 25% in those treated for 18 months with imipramine.[85] Thus, longer periods of treatment are associated with more sustained response. When medications are discontinued too early, a high rate of relapse (or reemergence of panic attacks) occurs.[79] Reinstitution of medication usually results in renewed clinical response.[65] After 3 months, medication taper may be attempted again. Many patients may be successfully tapered off medication during the second year of therapy.[65] Approximately 20–40% of patients will require chronic therapy.[79]

Patients have taken alprazolam or imipramine for up to 8 months with no reported loss of antipanic efficacy and no increase in the dose prescribed.[68] This indicates that tolerance does not develop to the antipanic effects of alprazolam or imipramine.[68]

Some patients receiving high-dose alprazolam (>4 mg/d) may have an extremely difficult time with drug taper, and the withdrawal schedule for all patients should be individualized. In patients receiving alprazolam doses greater than 3 mg/d, dosage reduction should proceed by 0.5 mg every 2 weeks until 3 mg/d is obtained, then 0.25 mg every 2 weeks until 1 mg is obtained, then 0.125 mg every 2 weeks.[86] The taper phase is most successful when it is accomplished over a 3- to 6-month period.[65] Approximately 30% of the patients receiving high doses, even with slow taper, may experience transient, mild to moderate withdrawal symptoms (as discussed under section on Benzodiazepines) and relapse of panic attacks.[79,84] Also, if a TCA is discontinued abruptly, a substantial number of patients will develop severe cholinergic rebound with upset stomach, nausea, vomiting, and abdominal cramping, thus TCAs should be reduced by 25 mg every 2–4 weeks.[79] The dose of phenelzine should be reduced by 15 mg every 2–4 weeks.

Treatment Resistance. Common reasons for treatment failures are comorbid psychiatric disorders, rapid dosage increases with resultant intolerable side effects, and underdosage. All standard treatments should be tried before using augmentation strategies. The most common strategy used in patients with a partial response to one agent is to augment with low doses of another agent. Limited data support the use of valproate.[87] Clonidine has shown improvement in a few treatment-resistant patients, however tolerance developed to its therapeutic effect.[88]

Patient Education. Many patients are reluctant to take medications for fear that drugs will worsen their illness or that they will become addicted. Adverse events are often perceived as a worsening of the illness and may contribute to noncompliance and prevent necessary medication increases. Patients should be informed regarding the lag time before a therapeutic response will occur and any problematic side effects. Patients taking phenelzine should be instructed about possible food and drug interactions. Patients receiving alprazolam or another BZ should be told not to decrease or discontinue therapy unless authorized by their physician.

Evaluation of Therapeutic Outcomes

During the first 2 weeks of the acute phase of therapy, patients with panic disorder should be seen twice weekly to adjust medication doses based on improvement in panic symptoms and to monitor for adverse events. Once stabilized, the patient can be seen on a weekly basis until antipanic response is achieved. After this, monthly visits should suffice. The patient should be counseled to maintain a diary to record the date, time, frequency, and duration of panic episodes and the severity of panic symptoms, anticipatory anxiety, and phobic avoidance. At scheduled visits the pharmacist should inquire about the level of disability experienced by the patient. Ratings of functional disability can be achieved by using the Sheehan Disability Scale.[89] During drug discontinuation, the frequency of appointments should be increased to evaluate for emergence of withdrawal symptoms and monitor for relapse.

OTHER ANXIETY DISORDERS

Specific Phobias

Specific phobia is considered unresponsive to drug therapy, although highly responsive to behavioral therapy. The use of antidepressant medications may be detrimental in patients with specific phobia.

Social Phobia

Although there is no approved treatment for social phobia, patients with generalized social phobia may respond to MAOIs, BZs, or SSRIs. Three double-blind, placebo-controlled trials have documented the efficacy of phenelzine in the acute management of social phobia.[90] Approximately 65% of patients treated with phenelzine (doses similar to those used in panic disorder) responded to treatment after 8–12 weeks.[90] The BZs, clonazepam 1.5–2 mg/d or alprazolam 3 mg/d, have shown effectiveness after 2 weeks.[8,91] β-Blocking agents are not effective in the management of generalized social phobia, however evidence supports their use in the management of performance anxiety (discrete phobia). Propranolol 40 mg, one hour before the performance may be quite helpful, as physical symptoms of anxiety frequently add to the patient's distress. Results of 12-week, open clinical trials indicate that fluoxetine (range of 10–80 mg/d) and sertraline (range of 50–200 mg/d) reduce avoidance and social anxiety, and improve social functioning.[8,90] Fluvoxamine 150 mg/d, evaluated under controlled conditions, significantly improved social and general anxiety compared with placebo.[92] Further controlled evaluations of the SSRIs are necessary to define their role in the management of social phobia. Behavioral therapy has also been found useful in controlled studies.[8] Most patients require 6–12 months of therapy. Slow medication taper, especially with the BZs, is required to prevent relapse (estimated to be 90% with fast tapers).

CONCLUSION

Theories about anxiety disorders have undergone major revisions over the past several years. Anxiety disorders are quite common, occurring in approximately 25% of the population during their lifetime. The proper management of anxiety disorders begins with the correct diagnosis; not all patients should receive antianxiety agents. Nonpharmacologic interventions are often effective alone or when combined with drug therapy.

The current classification for anxiety disorders includes several subtypes. The diagnosis determines the type of drug and nonpharmacologic intervention selected. While BZs remain the drugs of choice for GAD and situational anxiety, other agents may be preferable for other types of anxiety. The anxiolytic agent buspirone may be useful for patients who need chronic therapy for GAD or who cannot tolerate BZs. Antidepressants, including the SSRIs, and the BZ, alprazolam, are extensively used in patients with panic disorder. The pharmacologic treatment of phobic disorders and post-traumatic stress disorder is not as well studied, and further research is needed to better define appropriate pharmacologic treatment.[93]

REFERENCES

1. American Psychiatric Association. Diagnostic and statistical manual of mental disorders, 4th ed (DSM-IV). Washington, DC, Author, 1994, pp 393–444.
2. Kessler RC, McGonagle KA, Zhao S, et al. Lifetime and 12-month prevalence of DSM-III-R psychiatric disorders in the United States. Results from the National Comorbidity Survey. Arch Gen Psychiatry 1994;51:8–19.
3. Regier DA, Burke JD, Burke KC. Comorbidity of affective and anxiety disorders in the NIMH epidemiologic catchment area program, in Maser JD, Cloninger CR (eds): Comorbidity of Anxiety and Mood Disorders. Washington, DC, American Psychiatric Press, 1990, p 113.
4. Rickels K, Schwiezer E. The clinical course and long-term management of generalized anxiety disorder. J Clin Psychopharmacol 1990;10:101S–110S.
5. Ormel J, VonKorff M, Ustun TB, et al. Common mental disorders and disability across cultures: Results from the WHO collaborative study on psychological problems in general health care. JAMA 1994;272:1741–1748.
6. Pounds R. A review of the medical and social consequences of generalized anxiety disorder and panic disorder. J La State Med Soc 1992;144:479–483.
7. Markowitz JS, Weissman MM, Oullette R, et al. Quality of life in panic disorder. Arch Gen Psychiatry 1989;46:984–992.

8. Roy-Burne P, Wingerson D, Cowley D, Dager S. Psychopharmacologic treatment of panic, generalized anxiety disorder, and social phobia. Psychiatric Clin N Am 1993;16:719–735.
9. Wise MG, Rieck SO. Diagnostic considerations and treatment approaches to underlying anxiety in the medically ill. J Clin Psychiatry 1993;54(suppl 5):22–26.
10. Hayes PE, Dommisse CS. Current concepts in clinical therapeutics: Anxiety disorders, part I. Clin Pharm 1987;6:140–147.
11. Wise MG, Taylor SE. Anxiety and mood disorders in medically ill patients. J Clin Psychiatry 1990;51(suppl 1):27–32.
12. Weiner H. The psychobiology and pathophysiology of anxiety and fear, in Tuma AH, Maser JD (eds): Anxiety and the Anxiety Disorders. Hillsdale, NJ, Lawrence Erlbaum Associates, 1985, pp 333–354.
13. Wittchen H, Zhao S, Kessler RC, Eaton WW. DSM-III-R generalized anxiety disorder in the National Comorbidity Survey. Arch Gen Psychiatry 1994;51:355–364.
14. Johnson J, Weissman MM, Klerman GL. Panic disorder, comorbidity, and suicide attempts. Arch Gen Psychiatry 1990;47:805–808.
15. Kendler KS, Walters EE, Neale MC, et al. The structure of the genetic and environmental risk factors for six major psychiatric disorders in women. Arch Gen Psychiatry 1995;52:374–383.
16. Redmond DE, Huang YH. New evidence for a locus coeruleus-norepinephrine connection with anxiety. Life Sci 1979;25:2149–2162.
17. Gorman JM, Liebowitz MR, Fyer AJ, et al. A neuroanatomical hypothesis for panic disorder. Am J Psychiatry 1989;146:148–161.
18. Heninger GR, Charney DS. Monoamine receptor systems and anxiety disorders. Psychiatric Clin North Am 1988;11:309–326.
19. Teboul E, Chouinard G. A guide to benzodiazepine selection. Part I: Pharmacologic aspects. Can J Psychiatry 1990;35:700–710.
20. Paul SM. The GABA and glycine, in Bloom FE, Kupfer DJ (eds): Psychopharmacology: The Fourth Generation of Progress. New York, Raven Press, 1995, pp 87–94.
21. Dubovsky SL. Beyond the serotonin reuptake inhibitors: Rationale for the development of new serotonergic agents. J Clin Psychiatry 1994;55(suppl 2):34–44.
22. Dubovsky SL, Thomas M. Serotonergic mechanisms and current and future psychiatric practice. J Clin Psychiatry 1995;56(suppl 2):38–48.
23. Coplan JD, Wolk SI, Klein DF. Anxiety and the serotonin receptor, in Bloom FE, Kupfer DJ (eds): Psychopharmacology: The Fourth Generation of Progress. New York, Raven Press, 1995, p 1301.
24. Shader RI, Greenblatt DJ. Use of benzodiazepines in anxiety disorders. N Engl J Med 1993;328:1398–1405.
25. American Psychiatric Association. Benzodiazepine dependence, toxicity, and abuse: A task force report of the American Psychiatric Association. Washington, DC, American Psychiatric Press, 1990, p 1.
26. Hollister LE, Müller-Oerlinghausen B, Rickels K, Shader RI. Clinical uses of benzodiazepines. J Clin Psychopharmacol 1993;13(suppl 1):1S–169S.
27. Upjohn Company. Xanax package insert. Kalamazoo, MI, June 1993.
28. Dommisse CS, Hayes PE. Current concepts in clinical therapeutics: Anxiety disorders, part II. Clin Pharm 1987;6:196–215.
29. Sigel E, Baur R, Trube G, et al. The effect of subunit composition of rat brain $GABA_A$ receptors on channel function. Neuron 1990;5:703–711.
30. Greenblatt DJ, Shader RI, Abernethy DR. Current status of benzodiazepines, part I. N Engl J Med 1983;309:354–358.
31. Stoehr GP, Kroboth PD, Juhl RP, et al. Effect of oral contraceptives on triazolam, temazepam, alprazolam, and lorazepam kinetics. Clin Pharmacol Ther 1984;36:683–690.
32. Klimke A, Klieser E. Sudden death after intravenous application of lorazepam in a patient treated with clozapine. Am J Psychiatry 1994;151:780.
33. Greenblatt DJ, Abernethy DR, Koepke HH, et al. Interaction of cimetidine with oxazepam, lorazepam, and flurazepam. J Clin Pharmacol 1984;24:187–193.
34. Greenblatt DJ, Abernethy DR, Morse DS, et al. Clinical importance of the interaction of diazepam and cimetidine. N Engl J Med 1984;310:1639–1643.
35. Abernethy DR, Greenblatt DJ, Eshelman FN, et al. Ranitidine does not impair oxidative or conjugative metabolism: Noninteraction with antipyrine, diazepam, and lorazepam. Clin Pharmacol Ther 1984;35:188–192.
36. Tuncok Y, Akpinar O, Guven H, Akkaclu A. The effects of theophylline on serum alprazolam levels. Int J Clin Pharmacol Ther 1994;32:642–645.
37. Massoomi F, Savage J, Destache CJ. Omeprazole: A comprehensive review. Pharmacotherapy 1993;13:46–59.
38. Borcherding SM, Baciewicz AM, Self TH. Update on rifampin drug interactions. Arch Intern Med 1992;152:711–716.
39. Fleishaker JC, Hulst LK. A pharmacokinetic and pharmacodynamic evaluation of the combined administration of alprazolam and fluvoxamine. Eur J Clin Pharmacol 1994; 46:35–39.
40. Serzone (nefazodone hydrochloride), Bristol-Myers Squibb Company, January 1995.
41. Barbee JG. Memory, benzodiazepines, and anxiety: Integrations of theoretical and clinical perspectives. J Clin Psychiatry 1993;54(suppl 10):86–97.
42. Power KG, Jerrom DWA, Simpson RJ, et al. Controlled study of withdrawal symptoms and rebound anxiety after 6-week course of diazepam for generalized anxiety. Br Med J 1985;290:1246–1248.
43. Busto U, Sellers EM, Naranjo CA, et al. Withdrawal reaction after long-term therapeutic use of benzodiazepines. N Engl J Med 1986;315:854–859.
44. Rickels K, Schweizer E, Case G, et al. Long-term therapeutic use of benzodiazepines: Effects of abrupt discontinuation. Arch Gen Psychiatry 1990;47:899–907.
45. Rickels K, Case W, Schweizer E, et al. Benzodiazepine dependence: Management of discontinuation. Psychopharmacol Bull 1990;26:63–68.
46. Roy-Burne PP, Sullivan MD, Cowley DS, Ries R. Adjunctive treatment of benzodiazepine discontinuation syndromes: A review. J Psychiatric Res 1993;27(suppl 1):143–153.
47. Rickels K. Antianxiety therapy: Potential value of long-term treatment. J Clin Psychiatry 1987;48(suppl 12):7–11.

48. Markovitz PJ. Treatment of anxiety in the elderly. J Clin Psychiatry 1993;54(suppl 5):64–68.
49. Sussman N. The uses of buspirone in psychiatry. J Clin Psychiatry Monograph 1994;12:3–19.
50. Yocca FD. Neurochemistry and neurophysiology of buspirone and gepirone: Interactions at presynaptic and postsynaptic 5-HT_{1A} receptors. J Clin Psychopharmacol 1990;10(suppl 10):6–12.
51. Gammans RE, Mayol RF, Labudde JA. Metabolism and disposition of buspirone. Am J Med 1986;80:41S–51S.
52. Gammans RE, Mayol RF, Mackenthun AV, et al. The relationship between buspirone bioavailability and dose in healthy subjects. Biopharm Drug Dispos 1985;6:139–145.
53. Temple DL, Yevich JP, New JS. Buspirone: Chemical profile of a new class of anxioselective agents. J Clin Psychiatry 1982;43:4S–9S.
54. Newton RE, Marunycz JD, Alderdice MT, et al. Review of the side effect profile of buspirone. Am J Med 1986;80:17S–21S.
55. Mead Johnson Pharmaceutical Division/Bristol Myers. BuSpar package insert. Evansville, IN, January 1995.
56. Ciraulo DA, Shader RI. Question the expert: Buspirone and MAOI interaction. J Clin Psychopharmacol 1990;10:306.
57. Bodkin JA, Teicher MH. Fluoxetine may antagonize the anxiolytic action of buspirone. J Clin Psychopharmacol 1989;9:150.
58. Baughman OL. The safety record of buspirone in generalized anxiety disorder. J Clin Psychiatry Monograph 1994;12:37–43.
59. Lader M, Olajide D. A comparison of buspirone and placebo in relieving benzodiazepine withdrawal symptoms. J Clin Psychopharmacol 1987;7:11–15.
60. Glitz DA, Pohl R. 5-HT_{1A} partial agonists: What is their future? Drugs 1991;1:11–18.
61. Lader M. β-Adrenoreceptor antagonists in neuropsychiatry: An update. J Clin Psychiatry 1988;49:213–223.
62. Rickels K, Downing R, Scheizer E, Hassman H. Antidepressants for the treatment of generalized anxiety disorder. Arch Gen Psychiatry 1993;50:884–895.
63. Hollander E, Cohen LJ. The assessment and treatment of refractory anxiety. J Clin Psychiatry 1994;55(suppl 2):27–31.
64. Telch MJ, Lucas RA. Combined pharmacological and psychological treatment of panic disorder: Current status and future directions, in Wolfe BE, Maser JD (eds): Treatment of Panic Disorder: A Consensus Development Conference. Washington, DC, American Psychiatric Press, 1994, p 177.
65. Ballenger JC. Long-term pharmacologic treatment of panic disorder. J Clin Psychiatry 1991;52(suppl 2):18–23.
66. Chambless DL, Gillis MM. A review of psychosocial treatments for panic disorder, in Wolfe BE, Maser JD (eds): Treatment of Panic Disorder: A Consensus Development Conference. Washington, DC, American Psychiatric Press, 1994, p 149.
67. Shear MK, Pilkonis PA, Cloitre M, Leon AC. Cognitive behavioral treatment compared with nonprescriptive treatment of panic disorder. Arch Gen Psychiatry 1994;51:395–401.
68. Schweizer E, Rickels K, Weiss S, Zavodnick S. Maintenance drug treatment of panic disorder. Arch Gen Psychiatry 1993;50:51–60.
69. Cross-National Collaborative Panic Study, Second Phase Investigators. Drug treatment of panic disorder: Comparative efficacy of alprazolam, imipramine, and placebo. Br J Psychiatry 1992;160:191–202.
70. Liebowitz MR. Antidepressants in panic disorder. Br J Psychiatry 1989;155(suppl 6):46–52.
71. Modigh K, Westberg P, Eriksson E. Superiority of clomipramine over imipramine in the treatment of panic disorder: A placebo-controlled trial. J Clin Psychopharmacol 1992;12:251–261.
72. Hoehn-Saric R, McLeod DR, Hipsley PA. Effect of fluvoxamine on panic disorder. J Clin Psychopharmacol 1993;13:321–326.
73. Schneier FR, Liebowitz MR, Davies SO, et al. Fluoxetine in panic disorder. J Clin Psychopharmacology 1990;10:119–121.
74. Sheehan DV, Ballenger JC, Jacobsen G. Treatment of endogenous anxiety with phobic, hysterical, and hypochondriacal symptoms. Arch Gen Psychiatry 1980;37:51–59.
75. Tesar GE. High-potency benzodiazepines for short-term management of panic disorder: The U.S. experience. J Clin Psychiatry 1990;51(suppl 5):4–10.
76. Tesar G, Rosenbaum JF, Pollack MH, et al. Double-blind, placebo-controlled comparison of clonazepam and alprazolam for panic disorder. J Clin Psychiatry 1991;52:69–76.
77. Noyes R, DuPont RL, Pecknold JC, et al. Alprazolam in panic disorder and agoraphobia: Results from a multicenter trial II. Patient acceptance, side effects, and safety. Arch Gen Psychiatry 1988;45:423–428.
78. Lydiard RD, Laraia MT, Ballenger JC, et al. Emergence of depressive symptoms in patients receiving alprazolam for panic disorder. Am J Psychiatry 1987;144:664–665.
79. Schatzberg AF, Ballenger JC. Decisions for the clinician in the treatment of panic disorder: When to treat, which treatment to use, and how long to treat. J Clin Psychiatry 1991;52(suppl 2):26–31.
80. Noyes R, Garvey MJ, Cook BL, et al. Problems with tricyclic antidepressant use in patients with panic disorder or agoraphobia: Results of a naturalistic follow-up study. J Clin Psychiatry 1989;50:163–169.
81. Judge R, Ohrstrom J, Manniche P, et al. Paroxetine in the treatment of panic disorder. Eur Neuropsychopharmacol 1993;3:374–375.
82. Brown CS, Bryant SG. Monoamine oxidase inhibitors: Safety and efficacy issues. Drug Intell Clin Pharmacy 1988;22:232–235.
83. Blackwell B. Monoamine oxidase inhibitor interactions with other drugs. J Clin Psychopharmacol 1991;11:55–59.
84. Pecknold JC, Swinson RP, Kuch K, et al. Alprazolam in panic disorder and agoraphobia: Results from a multicenter trial III. discontinuation effects. Arch Gen Psychiatry 1988;45:429–436.
85. Mavissakalian M, Perel J. Protective effects of imipramine maintenance in panic disorder with agoraphobia. Am J Psychiatry 1992;149:1053–1057.
86. Noyes R, Garvey MN, Cook B, Suelzer M. Controlled discontinuation of benzodiazepine treatment for patients with panic disorder. Am J Psychiatry 1991;148:517–523.

87. Keck PE, McElroy SL, Tugrul KC, et al. Antiepileptic drugs for the treatment of panic disorder. Neuropsychobiology 1993;27:150–153.
88. Puzantian T, Hart LL. Clonidine in panic disorder. Ann Pharmacotherapy 1993;27:1351–1352.
89. Perugi G, Akiskal HS, Musetti L, et al. Social adjustment in panic-agoraphobic patients reconsidered. Br J Psychiatry 1994;164:88–93.
90. Marshall RD, Schneier FR, Fallon BA, et al. Medication therapy for social phobia. J Clin Psychiatry 1994;55 (suppl 6):33–37.
91. Davidson JR, Tupler LA, Potts NLS. Treatment of social phobia with benzodiazepines. J Clin Psychiatry 1994;55(suppl 6):28–32.
92. Van Vliet IM, den Boer JA, Westenberg HGM. Psychopharmacological treatment of social phobia: A double blind placebo controlled study with fluvoxamine. Psychopharmacol 1994;115:128–134.
93. Silver JM, Sandberg DP, Hales RE. New approaches in the pharmacotherapy of posttraumatic stress disorder. J Clin Psychiatry 1990;51(suppl 10):33–38.

Chapter 70

Obsessive–Compulsive Disorder

Barbara G. Wells, PharmD, FASHP, FCCP, and Peggy E. Hayes, PharmD

Although symptoms of obsessive–compulsive disorder (OCD) have been recognized for centuries, OCD has been only recently the focus of extensive research. These investigations have advanced greatly our understanding of the epidemiology, etiology, and pharmacologic treatment of OCD. Since the mid-1980s, the Food and Drug Administration (FDA) has approved three drugs (clomipramine [Anafranil], fluoxetine [Prozac], and fluvoxamine [Luvox]), as effective for the treatment of OCD. Although OCD is officially classified as an anxiety disorder, it is presented as a separate illness because of its unique clinical presentation and treatment approach. OCD is the most disabling of the anxiety disorders and rarely remits without specific pharmacologic treatment. Unfortunately despite treatment, many patients suffer disabling symptoms and a lifelong disability.[1]

Epidemiology

The National Institute of Mental Health Epidemiologic Catchment Area (ECA) study provides the most up-to-date, comprehensive data regarding the prevalence of mental illness including OCD. The ECA study was an extensive community survey conducted from 1980 to 1984 in five metropolitan areas across the United States, involving more than 18,500 interviews. This study estimated the prevalence of psychiatric illness among community populations and included persons not seeking psychiatric treatment.[2]

A most surprising finding was that OCD is approximately 50 times more common than previously reported by surveys conducted using clinical populations (or persons seeking treatment). OCD was once considered extremely rare and treatment resistant. However, the ECA study found a lifetime prevalence of 2.5% in adults and 1% in children and a 1-year prevalence rate of 1.5–2.1%.[1,2] OCD is the fourth most common psychiatric disorder following phobias, substance abuse, and major depression. Unfortunately, many patients do not seek treatment.[2,3]

OCD usually begins in late adolescence or early adulthood, but it may begin in childhood. Childhood-, adolescent- and adult-onset OCD have a similar clinical presentation. The incidence of OCD is higher in females than males; however, males tend to have a slightly earlier modal age of onset (between ages 6 and 15 years for males versus between ages 20 and 29 years for females). The onset is usually gradual with a chronic waxing and waning course.[1,3] OCD may have a familial component to its etiology.[4,5] Approximately 10% of first-degree relatives (mother, father, sibling) of patients with OCD have OCD, and another 8% have a subclinical form of the disorder. In a comparison group of first-degree relatives of normal subjects, there was a prevalence of only 2% for OCD and another 2% for the subclinical form.[4] When one twin has OCD, the concordance rate is higher for monozygotic twins than for dizygotic twins.[5]

The familial and clinical overlap between tic disorders (e.g., Tourette's syndrome) and OCD is well documented. Tourette's syndrome, a neurologic disorder that begins in childhood, is characterized by repetitive, involuntary multiple motor and vocal tics.[6] In a recent study of adolescents with Tourette's, approximately 40% of these individuals were diagnosed with OCD.[7] In addition, almost 20% of the relatives of patients with Tourette's have OCD.[3] Approximately 38% of OCD patients met the criteria for a tic disorder.[8]

Clinical Presentation

The *Diagnostic and Statistical Manual of Mental Disorders,* Fourth Edition (DSM-IV), requires the presence of either obsessions and/or compulsions (although most patients have both) that are severe enough to cause marked distress, to be time consuming (occupy more than 1 hour a day), and to cause significant impairment in social or occupational functioning (Table 70.1).[1] These individuals often recognize that their obsessions or compulsions are excessive or unreasonable. An obsession is a recurrent, persistent idea, thought, impulse, or image that is experienced as intrusive and inappropriate, and produces marked anxiety. Common obsessions involve thoughts about contamination (such as a concern about germs, dirt, or toxic chemicals),

TABLE 70.1. DSM-IV DIAGNOSTIC CRITERIA FOR OBSESSIVE–COMPULSIVE DISORDER

A. Either obsessions or compulsions:
Obsessions as defined by (1), (2), (3), and (4):
(1) Recurrent and persistent thoughts, impulses, or images that are experienced, at some time during the disturbance, as intrusive and inappropriate and that cause marked anxiety or distress
(2) The thoughts, impulses, or images are not simply excessive worries about real-life problems
(3) Attempts are made to ignore or suppress the thoughts, impulses, or images or to eliminate them
(4) It is recognized that the obsessional thoughts, impulses, or images are a product of the person's own mind (not imposed from without)
Compulsions as defined by (1) and (2):
(1) Repetitive behaviors (e.g., hand washing, ordering, checking) or mental acts (e.g., praying, counting, repeating words silently) that the person is driven to perform in response to an obsession, or according to certain rules
(2) The behaviors or mental acts are aimed at preventing or reducing distress or preventing some dreaded event or situation; however, these behaviors or mental acts either are not connected in a realistic way with what they are designed to eliminate or they are clearly excessive

B. The person has recognized that the obsessions or compulsions are excessive or unreasonable.

C. The obsessions or compulsions cause marked distress, are time consuming (take more than 1 hour per day), or significantly interfere with the person's normal routine, occupational (or academic) functioning, or usual social activities or relationships.

(Modified from American Psychiatric Association: *Diagnostic and Statistical Manual of Mental Disorders, Fourth Edition.* Washington, DC. American Psychiatric Association, 1994, pp 422–423, with permission.)

repeated doubts (e.g., whether a door was left unlocked), and needing to have things in a particular order.[1,3] Individuals recognize obsessions as products of their own mind and attempt to ignore or suppress them. "No matter how hard I try, I cannot get this crazy thought out of my mind." An obsession produces an intense feeling of anxiety and is not simply excessive worry about a real-life situation.[1,3]

A compulsion is a repetitive, purposeful, intentional behavior or mental act usually performed in response to an obsession. The most common compulsions involve washing and cleaning, counting, checking, and requesting or demanding assurances. Compulsive behavior is not pleasurable and is designed to prevent discomfort or the occurrence of a dreaded event that is often unknown. For example, many patients are obsessed with feelings of doubt (e.g., whether a door was left unlocked), causing them marked distress, and leading to repetitive checking (or compulsive behaviors). These behaviors are usually performed according to certain rules or in a stereotyped fashion.[1,3]

Compulsions are also recognized by the individual as senseless. Because patients recognize their behavior as silly, they become extremely adept at denying symptoms, disguising their rituals, and concealing their illness from friends and family members.[1,3] In addition to primary symptoms, about 20–40% of patients have involuntary motor movements (e.g., facial tics and grimaces).[5,8]

Many patients experience disabling symptoms for several years before seeking treatment.[2,3] Typically, almost 7.5 years elapse between the onset of clinical symptoms and the first psychiatric visit.[2,3] Although the consequences of untreated OCD have not been systematically studied, OCD produces significant work and social disability. Depression and anxiety symptoms are also present in many patients with OCD, and depression often prompts patients to seek treatment.[1,3] The ECA study reported that approximately 50% of patients with OCD had another major psychiatric disorder (e.g., major depression, alcohol abuse or dependence, panic disorder, schizophrenia). In most patients, OCD occurred first.[2,3] This means that certain illnesses (e.g., major depression, alcohol abuse, panic disorder) might be consequences of untreated OCD or part of the natural course of OCD. Therefore, OCD patients seeking treatment commonly require treatment for a comorbid psychiatric disorder. OCD is a chronic disorder that for most patients continues throughout adult life.[1,3]

Differential Diagnosis

Patients with OCD are aware of the irrationality of their symptoms, are often ashamed to admit their symptoms, and are skilled at hiding them.[1–3] Therefore, most cases of OCD are not recognized by the primary care physician. Certain disorders have symptoms resembling OCD, including trichotillomania (an urge to pull out one's hair), Tourette's syndrome, bowel and urinary obsessions, eating disorders (15% of adult women with OCD had anorexia in adolescence), compulsive gambling, compulsive sexual behaviors, and monosymptomatic hypochondriasis.[1,3] Patients with OCD often initially seek treatment from primary care physicians or dermatologists because of severe dermatitis from excessive washing.[3]

A distinction should be made between OCD and obsessive–compulsive personality disorder. Obsessions and compulsions are not present in obsessive–compulsive personality disorder. These individuals are preoccupied with orderliness, perfectionism, and control beginning early in childhood. Unlike individuals with OCD, those with obsessive–compulsive personality disorder do not view their behavior as irrational and do not wish to change, because they consider these personality features to be beneficial.[1,3]

Pathophysiology

Although OCD can occasionally begin following a brain injury (e.g., encephalitis or trauma), there is usually no neurologic precipitant. The most compelling evidence suggesting a biologic basis for OCD is the consistent successful treatment using potent serotonin (5-HT) reuptake blocking drugs. Therefore, 5-HT effects are important for the antiobsessional effects of medications.[9,10] Studies of 5-HT function have dominated research into the pathophysiology of OCD since the mid-1980s. Unfortunately, a clear model of serotonergic dysfunction to explain the pathophysiology of OCD is lacking. (For example, is there a decrease or increase in serotonergic function and what specific subtypes of 5-HT receptors are involved?)

SEROTONERGIC PROBES

Important evidence for an abnormality in 5-HT functioning comes from pharmacologic challenge studies that assess serotonergic responsiveness in OCD patients.[11–13] *m*-Chlorophenylpiperazine (*m*-CPP) has been the most frequently used probe in studies of OCD. *m*-CPP, a nonspecific postsynaptic 5-HT agonist and metabolite of the antidepressant trazodone, produced very limited behavioral effects in normal volunteers. In untreated OCD patients, *m*-CPP produced a marked, but transient, increase in obsessions, depression, and anxiety symptoms.[11,12] These findings indicate an increased sensitivity to *m*-CPP in untreated OCD patients. Treatment with clomipramine[11] and fluoxetine[12] abolished the pretreatment *m*-CPP-induced exacerbation of obsessive–compulsive symptoms. Several other 5-HT probes have been studied in OCD patients (e.g., MK212, ipsapirone, L-tryptophan, fenfluramine). The serotonergic probes have been disappointing in their failure to identify a consistent 5-HT defect in OCD.[13]

BRAIN-IMAGING STUDIES

Structural brain-imaging studies (computed tomography [CT] and magnetic resonance imaging [MRI]) have not identified the presence of a clear lesion (structural pathology) in patients with OCD.[14,15] However, brain-imaging studies to assess the biochemical and physiologic function of the brain (single photon emission computed tomography [SPECT] and positron emission tomography [PET]) have produced consistent findings that identify three areas of increased/abnormal metabolic activity (e.g., orbitofrontal cortex, cingulate cortex, and head of the caudate nucleus).[14–17] These areas may be involved in the pathophysiology of OCD symptoms and may form a circuit that is "hyperactive" in OCD. (However, these areas of increased metabolic activity may be merely compensating for areas of decreased brain activity.) It is of interest that successful pharmacologic treatment of OCD patients with increased metabolic activity in the caudate nucleus (with fluoxetine or behavioral therapy)[16] as well as the orbitofrontal cortex (with clomipramine or fluoxetine)[17] was associated with a return to normal metabolic functioning.

DOPAMINE MODEL

Because neurologic symptoms (tics) are part of the clinical presentation in some OCD patients and because some patients have a family history of Tourette's syndrome (a disorder of dopamine [DA] dysfunction), DA dysregulation may contribute to some forms of OCD. The neurotransmitter DA is found in high concentrations in the caudate nucleus, an area believed to be "hyperactive" in OCD. These patients often benefit from the addition of an antipsychotic to their treatment regimen.[18]

TREATMENT

Although a few OCD patients respond to tricyclic antidepressants (TCAs), such as imipramine or amitriptyline, or the monoamine oxidase inhibitor (MAOI) tranylcypromine, the only medications demonstrating efficacy in controlled clinical trials are 5-HT reuptake inhibitors. Double-blind trials support the thinking that clomipramine is more effective than placebo and other antidepressants.[9,19,20] These studies confirm the gradual improvement of obsessive and compulsive symptoms with clomipramine over a 4- to 10-week treatment period. Similarly, fluvoxamine has consistently shown efficacy superior to placebo[21–24] and to desipramine.[25] Fluoxetine was effective in reducing obsessive–compulsive symptoms in several open trials,[26–28] and in a multicenter double-blind trial.[29] Sertraline has also demonstrated efficacy in double-blind placebo-controlled trials.[30,31] In a controlled comparative trial, fluoxetine and clomipramine demonstrated similar therapeutic efficacy.[32] Jenike et al.[24] retrospectively compared clomipramine, fluoxetine, fluvoxamine, and sertraline using a meta-analysis of open and controlled trials of these drugs. Clomipramine seemed to produce a greater therapeutic effect than the other three drugs, but no statistical analysis was possible.[24] In a small unblinded nonrandomized trial in 23 patients, clomipramine and fluvoxamine were shown to be equally effective after 12 weeks of treatment.[33]

Jenike and colleagues[34] reported six cases in which an MAOI produced improvement and four cases in which there was no response. Patients who responded had associated panic attacks or severe anxiety.[34] Based on limited data, the MAOIs may be beneficial for some OCD patients with concurrent phobic anxiety or panic attacks, but their efficacy in OCD appears limited.[34] Benzodiazepines are rarely useful despite occasional case reports of response.[35] Although there are no placebo-controlled trials, limited evidence suggests that buspirone, a 5-HT_{1A} partial agonist, may be occasionally beneficial in the treatment of OCD.[36,37]

PHARMACOLOGIC APPROACHES

MECHANISMS OF ACTION

Current evidence strongly indicates that 5-HT is important for the antiobsessional effects of medications. Clomipramine, fluoxetine, fluvoxamine, and sertraline inhibit 5-HT reuptake into the presynaptic neuron. Reuptake is the first and most important step in reducing 5-HT neurotransmission. Inhibiting reuptake of 5-HT makes more 5-HT available to postsynaptic receptors and reduces formation of the 5-HT metabolite, 5-hydroxyindoleacetic acid (5-HIAA). Although other antidepressants, such as imipramine and amitriptyline, inhibit 5-HT reuptake, they are less potent and selective than clomipramine, fluoxetine, fluvoxamine, or sertraline. Prolonged exposure to increased amounts of 5-HT following chronic antidepressant treatment (2–3 weeks) leads to altered responsiveness of postsynaptic 5-HT receptors or presynaptic autoregulatory receptors that may govern 5-HT release in specific brain regions.[38]

The most impressive and consistent evidence to support a role for 5-HT in treating OCD is that only potent 5-HT reuptake inhibitors appear to be consistently effective. Further, an improvement in obsessional symptoms may correlate with plasma concentrations of clomipramine but not desmethylclomipramine, the metabolite of clomipramine having less selectivity for 5-HT reuptake inhibition. With clomipramine treatment, the decrease in obsessional symptoms correlates with a decrease in the concentration of 5-HIAA in cerebrospinal fluid, and a decrease in platelet 5-HT content.[38] The effectiveness of serotonergic agents in treating OCD lends support to the role of 5-HT in the etiology of OCD. However, since many patients fail to respond to these agents, the role of other neurotransmitter systems in the pathophysiology of OCD must continue to be explored.

ADVERSE EFFECTS

Clomipramine

The most frequently reported adverse effects with clomipramine are similar to those reported with other TCAs (refer to Chapter 67, Depressive Disorders). In the U.S. premarketing trials, the Clomipramine Collaborative Study Group treated 520 patients with OCD and reported the following clomipramine-related adverse effects: dry mouth (80%), dizziness (53%), tremor (53%), fatigue (38%), somnolence (49%), constipation (44%), and nausea (27%). Other adverse effects included weight gain and sexual dysfunction such as ejaculation failure (41%), libido change (18%), and impotence (7%).[9,39] Another study reported that approximately 70% of OCD patients were anorgasmic at therapeutic doses, with men and women equally affected.[40] In a retrospective study, Jenike et al.[41] reported that clomipramine had a higher incidence of sedation, dry mouth, dizziness, nausea, constipation, headache, sweating, and blurred vision than fluoxetine.

The risk of seizures with clomipramine appears dose-related, although duration of treatment exposure may also be a factor. In U.S. premarketing trials, OCD patients receiving clomipramine in doses up to 300 mg/d had an incidence of seizures of 0.64% at 90 days, 1.12% at 180 days, and 1.45% at 365 days. Data from more than 4000 patients (those receiving clomipramine for OCD, as well as other indications) who were enrolled in U.S. clinical trials reported a higher seizure rate with clomipramine dosages that exceeded 250 mg/d (2.2%) versus lower dosages (0.5%). Therefore, the maximum daily dosage should not exceed 250 mg/d, and caution should be exercised in prescribing clomipramine to patients with a history of seizures, alcoholism, or brain damage.[9,39] Caution should also be used when prescribing clomipramine concomitantly with other drugs known to lower the seizure threshold.[39]

In foreign postmarketing evaluations, rare reports of severe liver injury, some fatal, were recorded. Therefore, caution is advised when prescribing clomipramine for patients with a history of liver disease.[9,39]

Fluoxetine

In depressed patients, fluoxetine-related side events have been well documented (see Chapter 67, Depressive Disorders); however, fluoxetine is less well studied in patients with OCD. Fluoxetine was the second drug approved by the FDA for the treatment of OCD. Although published reports have described depressed patients who developed suicidal preoccupation after receiving fluoxetine, there is no evidence to suggest this is more common with fluoxetine than with TCAs. Although this has not been reported in patients with OCD, clinicians should remain vigilant for the emergence of suicidal thoughts following initiation of any antidepressant in this population.

The most commonly reported fluoxetine-related adverse effects in OCD patients include nausea, headache, anxiety, sedation, insomnia, diarrhea, sexual dysfunction, and tremor.[28] Jenike et al.[41] combined data from several protocols and found that 43% of OCD patients taking fluoxetine reported no side effects, whereas only 3% of OCD patients taking clomipramine reported none. However, the dropout rate for patients taking clomipramine (16%) was not significantly different from the fluoxetine dropout rate (15%).[41]

Fluvoxamine

In controlled OCD trials at a dose range of 50–300 mg/d, the most commonly observed fluvoxamine-related adverse effects were insomnia (31.3%), nausea (29.4%), somnolence (28.1%), fatigue (28.1%), abnormal ejaculation (17.9%), nervousness (15.6%), dry mouth (11.9%), tremor (8.1%), anorexia (8.1%), anorgasmia (7.7%), sweating (7.5%), and decreased libido (5.6%).[42]

PHARMACOKINETICS

Oral clomipramine is rapidly absorbed, and absorption is not affected by food. The major route of clomipramine's metabolism is demethylation followed by hydroxylation and conjugation. Protein binding is approximately 97% and is unaffected by plasma clomipramine concentration. The elimination half-life of clomipramine ranges from 31 to 37 hours. However, given reports of non-first-order clomipramine elimination kinetics, these estimates should be viewed with caution.[43]

Studies have reported that plasma clomipramine concentrations positively correlated with improvement in compulsions[44] and obsessions,[45] whereas plasma desmethylclomipramine levels were related to improvement in depression.[44] Mavissakalian and others[46] reported that plasma concentrations of clomipramine, but not desmethylclomipramine, correlated significantly with clinical response. Responders had significantly higher clomipramine levels and a trend toward lower ratios of desmethylclomipramine/clomipramine in the plasma. In children and adolescents, plasma concentrations of neither clomipramine nor desmethylclomipramine predicted response to clomipramine treatment.[47] Additional studies using a fixed-dose study design are required to confirm the existence of a relationship between plasma concentrations of clomipramine and antiobsessive compulsive response.

Fluoxetine is well absorbed from the gastrointestinal tract after oral administration and peak plasma concentrations are achieved in 6–8 hours. Absorption is delayed when it is administered with food. It is approximately 95% bound to plasma proteins. After a single oral dose, the elimination half-life for fluoxetine averages 1.9 days and that of norfluoxetine averages 7 days. With multiple daily dosing the half-life of fluoxetine increases to 5.7 days, and that of norfluoxetine has been reported to be 7–15 days. The drug is extensively metabolized, and limited data from animal studies suggest that fluoxetine undergoes first-pass metabolism.[48] No relationship has been established between plasma concentrations of fluoxetine or norfluoxetine and clinical response in treatment of depression or OCD.

Fluvoxamine is absorbed well when administered orally, and peak plasma concentrations are achieved within 2–8 hours. The half-life of elimination of the parent compound is 15 hours, and there are no known active metabolites. After multiple dosing, the half-life of fluvoxamine is increased by 30–50%. Fluvoxamine is 77% plasma protein bound, and the primary route of elimination is metabolism in the liver. The pharmacokinetics of fluvoxamine are not affected by concomitant food intake.[49]

DRUG INTERACTIONS

Clomipramine's drug–drug interactions are similar to those of the other TCAs. Caution should be exercised when administering clomipramine with other drugs having sedative or anticholinergic properties because additive effects would be expected. Clomipramine should not be administered concomitantly with MAOIs. Like other TCAs, clomipramine may block the antihypertensive effects of clonidine, guanethidine, reserpine, and similar sympatholytic agents. The concurrent administration of haloperidol reportedly increases plasma concentrations of clomipramine. The administration of methylphenidate, cimetidine, or fluoxetine increases plasma concentrations of other TCAs, and a similar interaction may occur with clomipramine. Clomipramine increased plasma concentrations of concurrently administered phenobarbital. Clomipramine may displace other highly protein bound drugs (warfarin, digoxin) from binding sites, resulting in adverse effects. Similarly, clomipramine may be displaced from its binding site by other highly bound drugs.[39,43,50]

Several fatal reactions have occurred with coadministration of MAOIs and fluoxetine. Therefore, MAOIs should not be administered until at least 5 weeks after discontinuation of fluoxetine. Carbamazepine toxicity, parkinsonism, and a "serotonin syndrome" (shivering, agitation, incoordination, hyperreflexia, and myoclonus) have been reported with the concurrent use of carbamazepine and fluoxetine. Twenty-six patients receiving phenytoin experienced increased plasma concentrations of phenytoin with symptoms of phenytoin toxicity after beginning fluoxetine therapy.[51] Complaints of irregular heart beats, shortness of breath, and orthostasis were attributed to the addition of fluoxetine therapy in a patient taking terfenadine.[51] Case reports suggested increased metoprolol serum concentrations and bradycardia as a result of adding fluoxetine.[51] Plasma concentrations of TCAs or trazodone may be markedly increased by the addition of fluoxetine to the regimen. Adverse effects reported with these combinations include lethargy, fatigue, increased sedation, anticholinergic symptoms, dizziness, seizures, and delirium.[51] The metabolism of both methylated and demethylated TCAs is impaired by fluoxetine. Therefore, the TCA dosage should be reduced by 75% when fluoxetine is added, and 3 months should be allowed for a new steady-state TCA plasma concentration to be attained.[48] The mechanism underlying this interaction is fluoxetine's inhibition of hepatic cytochrome P-450IID6, an enzyme involved in the metabolism of many cyclic antidepressants. Although some patients tolerate lithium plus fluoxetine without difficulty, others have developed neurotoxicity manifested as confusion, ataxia, stiffness of arms and legs, dysarthria, tremor, and absence seizures.[51] Although fluoxetine does not appear to affect the pharmacokinetics of clonazepam or triazolam, it may increase plasma concentrations of alprazolam and diazepam. This interaction may result in an increase in benzodiazepine-induced psychomotor impairment in some patients.[51] Agitation, restlessness, poor concentration, nausea, and diarrhea have been reported following addition of tryptophan to fluoxetine therapy. Symptoms resolved when tryptophan was discontinued.[51] Several cases of reduced therapeutic response to buspirone have been reported when used in combination with fluoxetine.[51] There is theoretical evidence to limit the use of dextromethorphan, which is metabolized by cytochrome P-450IID6, in patients taking fluoxetine. A patient receiving fluoxetine developed visual hallucinations after dextromethorphan was added to treat her cough.[51] Caution is advised in using fluoxetine in patients undergoing vigorous diuresis and others at risk of hyponatremia. Two patients receiving fluoxetine and furosemide died unexpectedly, and it was speculated that the combination may have contributed to their death. Fluoxetine occasionally is associated with hyponatremia and may have additive hyponatremic effects when given with loop diuretics such as furosemide.[51] Limited evidence suggests that fluoxetine does not increase the hypoprothrombinemic response to warfarin, but fluoxetine could increase the risk of bleeding through another mechanism. Bleeding has been reported with fluoxetine in the absence of warfarin.[51] Patients receiving fluoxetine concomitantly with haloperidol should be monitored for worsening of extrapyramidal side effects.[51]

The addition of fluvoxamine for 2 weeks resulted in a 98% increase in warfarin plasma concentrations and an increase in the hypoprothrombinemic response.[42] As previously noted, some selective serotonin reuptake inhibitors may impair hemostasis by other mechanisms as well. Accordingly, caution is warranted when using these two drugs concurrently. Several cases of theophylline toxicity due to fluvoxamine have been reported. Due to the serious nature of theophylline toxicity, patients receiving theophylline should be monitored closely, including plasma concentration monitoring as appropriate, when fluvoxamine is initiated, discontinued, or changed in dosage.[51] As is the case with other 5-HT reuptake inhibitors, fluvoxamine should not be given within 2 weeks of the administration of a MAOI. Three patients taking carbamazepine experienced increased carbamazepine plasma concentrations and symptoms of toxicity when fluvoxamine was added.[51] Isolated cases of neurologic effects have been reported in patients taking lithium and fluvoxamine concurrently.[51]

Fluvoxamine reduced the clearance of both diazepam and its active metabolite desmethyldiazepam, significantly increasing the likelihood of accumulation of both these drugs. Similarly, clearance of alprazolam was reduced by 50% when fluvoxamine 100 mg/d was added. Decreased psychomotor performance and impaired memory resulted.[51]

Fluvoxamine is likely a potent inhibitor of cytochrome P-450IIIA4. Ketoconazole, another inhibitor of P-450IIIA4, increases plasma concentrations of terfenadine and astemizole, which can cause potentially fatal ventricular arrhythmias. It is, therefore, recommended that fluvoxamine not be administered in combination with terfenadine or astemizole.[42]

Coadministration of fluvoxamine and propranolol resulted in a five-fold increase in propranolol plasma concentrations, but only a slight potentiation of propranolol-induced reductions in heart rate and in exercise diastolic blood pressure.[51] In three patients, plasma concentrations of amitriptyline and clomipramine were sharply increased by the addition of fluvoxamine. However, these patients manifested no symptoms of toxicity.[48] Fluvoxamine has been reported to increase the serum concentrations of haloperidol markedly in three schizophrenic patients. Fluvoxamine may increase the risk of extrapyramidal symptoms and other haloperidol side effects as a result.[51]

Crewe et al.[52] reported that the ability to interact with cytochrome P-450IID6 is a common feature of the selective serotonin reuptake inhibitors *in vitro,* and that these compounds are likely to interact with human P-450IID6 *in vivo,* thus having the potential to cause drug interactions. Their *in vitro* study using human liver microsomes demonstrated that fluvoxamine is a less potent inhibitor of P-450IID6 than paroxetine, fluoxetine, or sertraline, but the clinical importance of this finding remains to be shown.[52]

SPECIAL POPULATIONS

Hepatic and Renal Disease

Clomipramine, fluoxetine, and fluvoxamine are extensively metabolized in the liver, and patients with significant liver disease should be prescribed these drugs cautiously and in lower doses than those used in healthy subjects. The pharmacokinetics of fluoxetine and fluvoxamine were similar in patients with renal failure and in healthy subjects. However, the manufacturer recommends starting with a lower dose in patients with renal impairment.

Elderly Patients

There is little available information on treating OCD in the elderly. Approximately 150 elderly patients received clomipramine in U.S. clinical trials. Although no unusual age-related adverse effects were identified, age-related differences in efficacy or safety cannot be ruled out. This is especially true for elderly patients with coexisting diseases and those receiving concurrent drugs. Elderly patients receiving clomipramine may experience more sedation and anticholinergic adverse effects than younger adults.[9,39]

Plasma concentrations of fluoxetine are 127% higher in the elderly than in younger individuals receiving the same dose.[53] The safety of fluoxetine has not been adequately studied in unselected elderly patients or in patients with cardiovascular disease.[48] The overall cardiovascular profile of fluoxetine appears quite favorable. However, Buff and associates[54] reported that atrial fibrillation and bradycardia developed in an 87-year-old woman shortly after fluoxetine was initiated. On fluoxetine rechallenge, these dysrhythmias recurred.

The multiple dose elimination half-life of fluvoxamine was 17.4 and 25.9 hours in the elderly compared to 13.6 and 15.6 hours in young subjects at steady state for 50- and 100-mg doses, respectively.[42] The safety of fluvoxamine has not been adequately studied in the elderly and patients with cardiovascular disease. Dosage should be titrated slowly during initiation of fluvoxamine therapy in elderly patients.

Children and Adolescents

Flament and others[55] treated 19 children and adolescents (ages 6–18 years) with clomipramine in a double-blind, placebo-controlled, crossover trial of 10 weeks' duration (two 5-week treatment periods). Clomipramine was significantly better than placebo in ameliorating OCD symptoms at week 5, with 75% of patients having a moderate to marked improvement, whereas 16% were unchanged. Male subjects responded significantly better than females. In an additional double-blind, crossover study comparing clomipramine with desipramine, 48 children and adolescents (ages 7–19 years) completed the 10-week trial (two 5-week treatment periods). Clomipramine was superior to desipramine in ameliorating OCD symptoms, and desipramine was no more effective than placebo.[47] Clomipramine was well tolerated at doses of 3 mg/kg/d.[47,55] The safety and efficacy of fluoxetine and fluvoxamine for the treatment of OCD in pediatric patients have not been established.

Pregnant/Lactating Patients

There are no adequate studies using clomipramine, fluoxetine, or fluvoxamine in pregnancy, and these drugs should, therefore, be used only when clearly indicated. Two cases of neonatal convulsions due to maternal withdrawal of clomipramine were reported. In both cases, parenteral phenobarbital failed to control seizures adequately. Clomipramine, fluoxetine, and fluvoxamine are excreted into breast milk and, therefore, a decision must be made whether to discontinue nursing or discontinue drug therapy, weighing the potential benefits against risks. The milk to plasma concentration ratio for fluvoxamine is 0.29, and that of fluoxetine is 0.29. In contrast the milk to plasma ratio for paroxetine is approximately 1. Paroxetine would, therefore, appear to be a particularly poor choice for the breast-feeding mother.[48]

TOXICITY

The lethality of clomipramine in overdose is considered to be similar to that of other closely related TCAs. Although patients ingesting 5000 mg of clomipramine have survived, the lowest dose associated with fatality was 750 mg.[39] Although death has occurred with overdose of fluoxetine alone, it is generally considered to be less toxic than clomipramine. Prominent symptoms of fluoxetine overdose include nausea, vomiting, agitation, restlessness, and hypomania.[56] Of the 354 cases of overdose with fluvoxamine, there were 19 deaths, 2 of whom ingested fluvoxamine alone. The highest reported overdose of fluvoxamine involved in a nonlethal ingestion was 10,000 mg. Signs and symptoms associated with fluvoxamine overdose include somnolence, coma, tachycardia, bradycardia, hypotension, ECG abnormalities, and convulsions.[42] Consult the toxicology literature for details regarding the treatment of overdose with these drugs.

CLINICAL APPLICATION

Patient Response

Clomipramine, fluoxetine, and fluvoxamine are superior to placebo, but their comparative efficacies are more difficult to assess. Jenike and colleagues[41] compared clomipramine and fluoxetine across studies, and concluded that clomipramine is slightly more effective, but causes more side effects. However, a randomized double-blind crossover study[57] and a clomipramine-to-fluoxetine substitution study[58] showed equal efficacy for the two drugs. It is unlikely that clinical trials will be able to demonstrate significant differences in efficacy between the 5-HT reuptake inhibitors, because 600–700 patients would likely be required to show a statistically significant difference.[20] A meta-analysis suggested that the efficacy of clomipramine was slightly superior to that of fluvoxamine, which was slightly superior to that of sertraline.[59] These data must be viewed with caution, because of varying methodologies between studies and differences in numbers of treatment-resistant patients and placebo responders between studies.

Patients responding to clomipramine, fluoxetine, or fluvoxamine generally have a symptom reduction far short of total symptom relief.[9] Responders often experience only 50% reduction in symptom severity. A patient showing partial response after 4–5 weeks of treatment may improve considerably if treatment is continued for several more weeks. Based on a clinical global rating of much or very much improved, about 60% of patients responded to clomipramine.[9] Approximately 65–70% of treatment-naive patients will demonstrate at least a moderate response to the 5-HT reuptake inhibitors.[20] Therefore, most OCD patients continue to have symptoms severe enough to limit their functioning. Although this degree of improvement seems modest, patients usually find this improvement clearly preferable to their pretreatment condition and are often willing to tolerate substantial adverse effects to maintain partial remission of their symptomatology. The goal of treatment is to achieve as great a level of symptom reduction as possible while recognizing that a cure is unlikely.[9,38]

Approximately 89% of 18 OCD patients chronically treated with clomipramine had a substantial recurrence of symptoms after a 7-week placebo period.[60] In a study of 35 OCD patients who discontinued fluoxetine after a good response, only 23% relapsed without medication during the first year.[61] Behavior therapy that accompanies pharmacotherapy may not only increase the extent of symptom reduction, but may also enhance the persistence of improvement after drug therapy is discontinued. No predictors of response to pharmacotherapy have been identified. Most investigators agree that factors failing to predict response include severity of illness, presence of depression, duration of illness, type of symptoms (obsessions versus compulsions), dexamethasone resistance, reduced rapid-eye movement (REM) sleep latency, and platelet 5-HT measures.[38] Alarcon et al.,[62] however, found that higher initial scores on the Yale–Brown Obsessive–Compulsive Scale (Y–BOCS) were associated with poorer response to clomipramine. Further, this group reported that the presence of cleaning rituals, such as washing or cleaning sinks, bathtubs, walls, ovens, and so on, was a predictor of poor or modest response to clomipramine.[62] An additional report found that the presence of panic or phobia with OCD is a positive predictor of response to clomipramine.[63]

Patients beginning drug therapy for OCD should be told that antiobsessive compulsive response may not occur for several weeks, and the importance of compliance should be emphasized. Patients should not discontinue their medication, because nausea and headache may occur with abrupt discontinuation. Patients should be advised to exercise caution in driving or operating machinery. Patients should be made familiar with the common adverse effects of their medication and advised not to take other medications concurrently without first checking with their physician or pharmacist.

Treatment Guidelines

First-line pharmacotherapy should be a trial of a 5-HT reuptake inhibitor. If the patient is treatment resistant, then a second 5-HT reuptake inhibitor should be substituted, and if necessary a third such agent should be substituted. Treatment resistance can be defined as failure to achieve at least a 25% reduction in baseline score on the Y–BOCS. According to Jenike, at least one of these three drugs should be clomipramine.[64] An adequate trial entails titration to optimal or maximal tolerated doses with a minimal total trial duration of 10–12 weeks. There are no adequate guidelines on when to discontinue drug therapy in the patient who has responded to treatment, and there is no way to determine which patients will maintain their improvement after drug discontinuation.

Many clinicians treat drug responders for a year, but often at a reduced dosage. When patients are discontinued, the dose should be gradually tapered perhaps as slowly as 50 mg of clomipramine or 20 mg of fluoxetine every 2 months. These recommendations are based on anecdotal evidence, and definitive answers regarding treatment discontinuation await further systematic study.

Dosing Guidelines

Clomipramine should be initiated at a dose of 25 mg/d (usually at bedtime) and gradually increased during the first 2 weeks to approximately 100 mg/d. Initially, clomipramine should be administered in divided doses with meals to reduce gastrointestinal adverse effects. Over the next several weeks, the dose may be increased gradually to a maximum of 250 mg/d. After titration, the total daily dose may be given once daily at bedtime to minimize sedation.[9,39,65] After acute therapy, many patients may have their dose reduced by 25–50% for maintenance therapy. In children and adolescents, the starting dose is 25 mg/d with a gradual dosage increase during the first 2 weeks up to a daily maximum of 3 mg/kg or 100 mg/d, whichever is smaller. These initial doses should be divided and taken with meals. Thereafter, the dose may be increased over the next several weeks to a maximum of 3 mg/kg/d or 200 mg/d, whichever is smaller. After titration, the dose may be given once daily at bedtime.[65]

The effective dose for fluoxetine in treating OCD is 20–80 mg/d. The manufacturer recommends an initial dose of fluoxetine of 20 mg/d given in the morning. If improvement is insufficient, a dose increase may be considered after several weeks. Doses greater than 20 mg/d may be administered once daily in the mornings or on a twice-daily schedule (i.e., morning and noon).[56] Fixed-dose studies revealed no significant difference in efficacy between the 20-, 40-, and 60-mg doses of fluoxetine or between the 50, 100, and 200 mg/d doses of sertraline. However, individual patients may have a better response at higher doses.

The recommended initial dose of fluvoxamine is 50 mg at bedtime. This should be increased in 50-mg increments every 4–7 days, as tolerated, until maximal response is achieved, not to exceed 300 mg daily. The recommended dosage range is 100–300 mg/d. The manufacturer recommends that total daily doses of more than 100 mg be given in two divided doses. In many cases, a larger dose is given at bedtime.[42]

Maximum response to pharmacotherapy typically requires at least 6–8 weeks. Before nonresponding patients are switched to another drug, they should have taken the maximum tolerated dose for at least 10 weeks. The maximum dosage for clomipramine is 250 mg/d; for fluoxetine, 80 mg/d; and for fluvoxamine, 300 mg/d. If one 5-HT reuptake inhibitor is ineffective, then another should be tried. Although the appropriate maintenance dose of the 5-HT reuptake inhibitors is unknown, it is notable that one investigator was successful in reducing the dose of clomipramine from a mean of 270 mg/d to 165 mg/d in the maintenance phase.

Evaluation of Therapeutic Outcomes

OCD patients receiving pharmacotherapy should be monitored for target symptom response, adverse effects (including the emergence of suicidal ideas), and drug interactions. Symptom severity can be effectively monitored through periodic assessment using the Y–BOCS.

Although controversial, patients failing to respond to clomipramine may benefit from having the dose adjusted to bring the plasma concentration of clomipramine between 100 and 250 ng/mL. Patients taking clomipramine who develop fever and sore throat should have leukocyte and differential white blood counts assessed to evaluate for agranulocytosis. In patients with a history of liver disease, baseline and periodic liver function tests are recommended if clomipramine treatment is undertaken. When clomipramine is given concurrently with sympatholytic antihypertensives, blood pressure should be regularly monitored.

Refractory Patients

Approximately 20% of patients fail to respond to first-line therapies, behavioral therapy, and pharmacologic therapy.[64] Unfortunately, there are few controlled data to guide the clinician in managing these refractory patients. As an initial step, the diagnosis should be reviewed for accuracy. OCD symptoms often do not respond to treatment if a concurrent psychiatric condition (schizophrenia, mood disorders, other anxiety disorders, or personality disorders) remains untreated. It is essential to assess the adequacy of previous drug trials. As a rule, first-line pharmacotherapy should include at least three separate trials with different 5-HT reuptake inhibitors, and at least one of these trials should be clomipramine. An adequate trial involves titration to optimal or maximal tolerated doses with a total trial duration of at least 10 weeks.[64] Figure 70.1 summarizes pharmacologic management of the treatment-resistant patient.

Adding an augmenting agent to ongoing 5-HT reuptake inhibitor therapy will sometimes improve response. Unfortunately, data supporting use of this strategy come

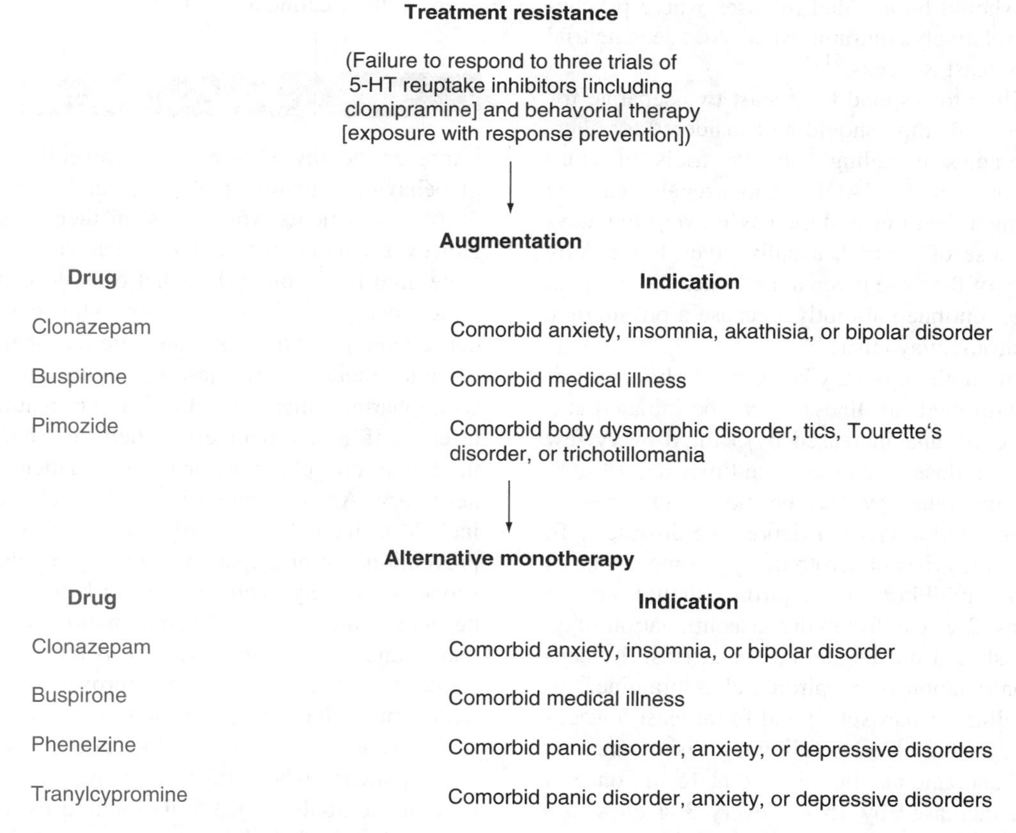

Figure 70.1. Pharmacologic management of treatment-resistant obsessive–compulsive disorder. *(Compiled from Refs. 64 and 74.)*

from case studies and open trials. The augmentation agents used most frequently are clonazepam, buspirone, or neuroleptics.[64] Clonazepam can be added to any 5-HT reuptake inhibitor at a dose of 0.5 mg once or twice daily. The dose can be increased every few days if necessary to a maximal dose of 5 mg/d. It may be less well tolerated by patients who are anergic or depressed. An adequate trial of clonazepam augmentation should last a minimum of 4 weeks.[64]

Buspirone may be used to augment fluoxetine therapy, beginning with a buspirone dose of 5 mg three times daily and increased as tolerated to a usual therapeutic dose of 30–60 mg/d. An adequate trial of buspirone augmentation should last at least 8 weeks.[64]

Augmentation with antipsychotics has been useful in patients whose OCD is accompanied by tics, Tourette's disorder, body dysmorphic disorder, or trichotillomania. Similarly, in patients with comorbid psychosis (OCD with delusions) a trial of antipsychotic augmentation is reasonable. Pimozide can be added to 5-HT reuptake inhibitor therapy at a dose of 1 mg/d, or haloperidol at 0.5 mg/d, and increased every 2 weeks to a maximum of 3 mg/d. Prior to initiating antipsychotic therapy, tardive dyskinesia and other risks should be discussed with the patient. An adequate trial of neuroleptic augmentation should last at least 4 weeks.[64]

Fenfluramine may be added to a 5-HT reuptake inhibitor starting at a dose of 5 mg/d and increasing to 20–60 mg/d. It should be avoided in cases where psychostimulant use is relatively contraindicated. An adequate trial should last for at least 8 weeks.[64]

Patients failing to respond to at least two separate trials of augmentation therapy should be considered for alternative monotherapies including separate trials of clonazepam, buspirone, and MAOIs. Clonazepam can be initiated at 0.5 mg at bedtime and increased every few days to a maximum dose of 5 mg/d, usually given twice daily with the majority of the dose given at bedtime. Clonazepam should not be discontinued abruptly, because a physiologic withdrawal syndrome may ensue.[64]

Buspirone monotherapy may be particularly appropriate in patients with medical illness. It can be initiated at 5 mg three times daily and increased by 5 mg/d every few days to a maximum dose of 20 mg three times daily.[64]

Phenelzine monotherapy may be most appropriate in patients with comorbid anxiety or depressive disorders. To prevent hypertensive crisis or serotonin syndrome, a trial of a 5-HT reuptake inhibitor or buspirone should not be started for at least 2 weeks following discontinuation of an MAOI. MAOIs should not be started for at least 2 weeks following discontinuation of buspirone, clomipramine, fluvoxamine, sertraline, or paroxetine and for at least 5 weeks (probably longer in the elderly) following discontinuation of fluoxetine. Phenelzine can be initiated at 15 mg once or twice daily and increased by 15 mg every 3–4 days to a dose of 60–90 mg/d.

Tranylcypromine can be started at 10 mg once or twice daily and increased to a maximum of 60 mg/d.[64]

OTHER AGENTS

Preliminary evidence suggests that sertraline may also be effective in treating OCD. In a double-blind study of 10 weeks' duration, sertraline was dosed 50–200 mg/d in 77 OCD patients and was found to be significantly more effective than placebo, with 56% of sertraline-treated patients improved after 8 weeks of treatment.[66] More recently, 12 weeks of once-daily treatment with sertraline 50, 100, or 200 mg/d was significantly more effective than placebo in 325 nondepressed OCD patients, and there were no significant differences in efficacy between sertraline dosage groups.[67]

An open trial in only 10 patients concluded that buspirone was ineffective,[37] but a small double-blind placebo-controlled trial found that buspirone (mean dose = 58 mg/d) had efficacy equal to that of clomipramine (mean dose = 225 mg/d) in the acute treatment of OCD.[36] Although a type II error may have occurred in this small study, a later meta-analysis suggested that buspirone in that study had a greater effect size than fluoxetine and sertraline in a previous meta-analysis.[68] These findings must be considered preliminary, and further controlled studies with larger sample sizes are needed to assess whether buspirone is an effective agent in the treatment of OCD.

NONDRUG APPROACHES

Exposure therapy with response prevention is the mainstay of behavioral treatment of OCD, and two-thirds to three-fourths of patients who persist in therapy may respond.[69] However, patients who agree to behavior therapy must tolerate high levels of anxiety that often lead them to discontinue therapy.[20] OCD patients who have concomitant depression, psychosis, or mania are not likely to respond to behavior therapy until these symptoms are well controlled with pharmacotherapy.[70] Behavioral treatments are most effective if family members participate. Behavior therapy in the home, on field trips, or in the inpatient setting may be necessary. An adequate trial of behavior therapy should include at least 20 hours of actual exposure and response prevention.[64] Some patients with compulsive rituals respond completely to either drugs or behavior therapy alone, but most patients require a combination of the two for optimal clinical response.[70] Eighty percent of patients will experience at least moderate improvement with combined treatment. Behavior therapy has little to offer the patient with severe obsessions who does not have compulsions. In OCD patients who suffer from obsessive thoughts only (without compulsions), a trial of antiobsessional medication is a reasonable first choice.[70]

For patients who have suffered for years with disabling OCD and have responded poorly to most conventional therapies, psychosurgery offers a reasonable chance for favorable outcome.[71,72] Response rates of 25–90% have been claimed, but the efficacy of psychosurgery remains unproven.[64] These findings should be interpreted with caution, because negative results are rarely reported.[72] Reviews of these neurosurgical procedures are published elsewhere.[73]

Conclusion

OCD is a chronic and often profoundly disabling anxiety disorder with a lifetime prevalence rate ranging from 1.9–3.3%. Traditional psychotherapies have failed to offer significant benefit to OCD patients. The effectiveness of behavior therapy and the 5-HT reuptake inhibitors is well established. These complementary treatments effect a substantial reduction in symptomatology in most patients. Although currently available medications are far superior to placebo, many patients are left with significant symptomatology even after successful pharmacologic intervention. Further, the 5-HT reuptake-inhibiting drugs are associated with an adverse effect profile that is problematic for a significant percentage of patients. If response is inadequate, an alternate 5-HT reuptake inhibitor should be tried or augmentation strategies should be employed. A high rate of relapse is reported after medication discontinuation, indicating that OCD may be a chronic condition requiring continued treatment. Only after all treatments have failed and if the disorder is very severe should psychosurgery be considered.

References

1. American Psychiatric Association. Diagnostic and Statistical Manual of Mental Disorders, 4th ed (DSM-IV). Washington, DC: American Psychiatric Press, 1994, pp 417–423.
2. Karno M, Golding J, Sorenson S, Burnam A. The epidemiology of obsessive–compulsive disorder in five U.S. communities. Arch Gen Psychiatry 1988;45:1094–1099.
3. Rasmussen SA, Eisen JL. Epidemiology and differential diagnosis of obsessive–compulsive disorder. J Clin Psychiatry 1992;53(4 suppl):4–10.
4. Pauls DL, Alsobrook JP, Goodman W, et al. A family history of obsessive–compulsive disorder. Am J Psychiatry 1995;152:76–84.
5. Pauls DL, Towbin KE, Leckman JF, et al. Tourette's syndrome and obsessive–compulsive disorder. Arch Gen Psychiatry 1986;43:1180–1182.
6. Hyde TM, Weinberger DR. Tourette's syndrome. A model neuropsychiatric disorder. JAMA 1995;273(6):498–501.
7. Apter A, Pauls DL, Bleich A, et al. An epidemiologic study of Gilles de la tourette's syndrome in Israel. Arch Gen Psychiatry 1993;50:734–738.
8. Pitman RK, Green RC, Jenike MA, Mesulam MM. Clinical comparison of Tourette's disorder and obsessive–compulsive disorder. Am J Psychiatry 1987;144:1166–1171.
9. The Clomipramine Collaborative Study Group. Clomipramine in the treatment of patients with obsessive–compulsive disorder. Arch Gen Psychiatry 1991;48:730–738.
10. Greist JH, Jefferson JW, Kobak KA, et al. Efficacy and tolerability of serotonin transport inhibitors in obsessive–compulsive disorder. Arch Gen Psychiatry 1995;52:53–60.
11. Zohar J, Insel TR, Zohar-Kadouch RC, et al. Serotonergic responsivity in obsessive–compulsive disorder: Effects of chronic clomipramine treatment. Arch Gen Psychiatry 1988;45:167–172.
12. Hollander E, DeCaria CM, Nitescu, A, et al. Serotonic function in obsessive–compulsive disorder: Behavioral and neuroendocrine responses to oral *m*-chlorophenylpiperazine and fenfluramine in patients and healthy volunteers. Arch Gen Psychiatry 1992;49:21–28.
13. Barr LC, Goodman WK, Price LH, et al. The serotonin hypothesis of obsessive compulsive disorder: Implications of pharmacologic challenge studies. J Clin Psychiatry 1992;53(suppl 4):17–28.
14. Insel TR. Toward a neuroanatomy of obsessive–compulsive disorder. Arch Gen Psychiatry 1992;49:739–744.
15. Baxter LR. Neuroimaging studies of human anxiety disorders: Cutting paths of knowledge through the field of neurotic phenomena, in Bloom FE, Kupfer DJ, (eds): Psychopharmacology: Fourth Generation of Progress. New York, Raven Press, 1995, pp 1287–1300.
16. Baxter LR Jr, Schwartz JM, Bergman KS, et al. Caudate glucose metabolic rate changes with both drug and behavior therapy for obsessive–compulsive disorder. Arch Gen Psychiatry 1992:49;681–689.
17. Swedo SE, Pietrini P, Leonard HL, et al. Cerebral glucose metabolism in childhood-onset obsessive–compulsive disorder: Revisualization during pharmacotherapy. Arch Gen Psychiatry 1992:49;690–694.
18. McDougle CJ, Goodman WK, Price LH. Dopamine antagonists in tic-related and psychotic spectrum obsessive compulsive disorder. J Clin Psychiatry 1994;55(3 suppl):24–31.
19. Rapoport JL. The neurobiology of obsessive compulsive disorder. JAMA 1988;260:2888–2890.
20. Rasmussen SA, Eisen JL, Pato MT. Current issues in the pharmacologic management of obsessive compulsive disorder. J Clin Psychiatry 1993;54(6, suppl):4–9.
21. Perse T, Greist JH, Jefferson JW, et al. Fluvoxamine treatment for obsessive compulsive disorders. Am J Psychiatry 1987;144:1543–1548.
22. Goodman WK, Price LH, Rasmussen SA, et al. Efficacy of fluvoxamine in obsessive compulsive disorder: A double-blind comparison with placebo. Arch Gen Psychiatry 1989;46:36–44.
23. Rasmussen SA. A multicenter controlled trial of fluvoxamine in the treatment of OCD. Presented at the 145th annual meeting of the American Psychiatric Association, May 5, 1992, Washington, DC.
24. Jenike MA, Hyman S, Baer L, et al. A controlled trial of fluvoxamine in obsessive compulsive disorder: Implications for a serotonergic theory. Am J Psychiatry 1990;147:1209–1215.

25. Goodman WK, Price LH, Delgado PL, et al. Specificity of serotonin reuptake inhibitors in the treatment of obsessive–compulsive disorder: Comparison of fluvoxamine and desipramine. Arch Gen Psychiatry 1990;47:577–585.
26. Turner SM, Jacob RG, Beidel DC, Himmelhoch J. Fluoxetine treatment of obsessive compulsive disorder. J Clin Psychopharmacol 1985;5:201–212.
27. Fontaine R, Chouinard G. Fluoxetine in the treatment of obsessive compulsive disorder. Prog Neuropsychopharmacol Biol Psychiatry 1985;9:605–608.
28. Jenike MA, Buttolph L, Baer L, et al. Open trial of fluoxetine in obsessive compulsive disorder. Am J Psychiatry 1989;146:909–911.
29. Dominguez RA. Serotonergic antidepressants and their efficacy in obsessive compulsive disorder. J Clin Psychiatry 1992;53(10, suppl):56–59.
30. Jenike MA, Baer L, Summergrad P, et al. Sertraline in obsessive compulsive disorder: A double-blind comparison with placebo. Am J Psychiatry 1990;147:923–928.
31. Chouinard G, Goodman W, Greist J, et al. Results of a double-blind placebo controlled trial of a new serotonin uptake inhibitor, sertraline, in the treatment of obsessive compulsive disorder. Psychopharmacol Bull 1990;26:279–284.
32. Pigott TA, Pato MT, Bernstein SE, et al. Controlled comparisons of clomipramine and fluoxetine in the treatment of obsessive–compulsive disorder: Behavioral and biological results. Arch Gen Psychiatry 1990;47:926–932.
33. Tamimi RR, Mavissakalian MR, Jones B, Olson S. Clomipramine versus fluvoxamine in obsessive-compulsive disorder. Ann Clin Psychiatry 1991;3:275–279.
34. Jenike MA, Surman OS, Cassem NH, et al. Monoamine oxidase inhibitors in obsessive–compulsive disorder. J Clin Psychiatry 1983;44:131–132.
35. Hewlett WA, Vinogradov S, Agras WS. Clonazepam treatment of obsessions and compulsions. J Clin Psychiatry 1990;51:158–161.
36. Pato MT, Pigott TA, Hill JL, et al. Controlled comparison of buspirone and clompramine in obsessive compulsive disorder. Am J Psychiatry 1991;148:127–129.
37. Jenike MA, Baer L. An open trial of buspirone in obsessive compulsive disorder. Am J Psychiatry 1988;145:1285–1286.
38. Insel TR. New pharmacologic approaches to obsessive compulsive disorder. J Clin Psychiatry 1990;51(suppl 10):47–51.
39. Ciba-Geigy Corporation. Anafranil package insert. Summit, NJ, 1992.
40. Monteiro WO, Noshirvani HF, Marks IM, Lelliott PT. Anorgasmia from clomipramine in obsessive compulsive disorder. A controlled trial. Br J Psychiatry 1987;151:107–112.
41. Jenike MA, Baer L, Greist JH. Clomipramine versus fluoxetine in obsessive compulsive disorder: A retrospective comparison of side effects and efficacy. J Clin Psychopharmacol 1990;10:122–124.
42. Solvay Pharmaceuticals, Incorporated. Luvox package insert. Marietta, GA, 1994.
43. Jermain DM, Crismon LC. Pharmacotherapy of obsessive compulsive disorder. Pharmacotherapy 1990;10:175–198.
44. Stern RS, Marks IM, Mawson D, Luscombe DK. Clomipramine and exposure for compulsive rituals: II. Plasma levels, side effects, and outcome. Br J Psychiatry 1980;136:161–166.
45. Insel TR, Murphy DL, Cohen RM, et al. Obsessive compulsive disorder. Arch Gen Psychiatry 1983;40:605–612.
46. Mavissakalian MR, Jones B, Olson S, Perel JM. Clomipramine in obsessive compulsive disorder: Clinical response and plasma levels. J Clin Psychopharmacol 1990;10:261–268.
47. Leonard HL, Swedo S, Rapoport JL, et al. Treatment of obsessive compulsive disorder with clomipramine and desipramine in children and adolescents. Arch Gen Psychiatry 1989;46:1088–1092.
48. van Harten J. Clinical pharmacokinetics of selective serotonin reuptake inhibitors. Clin Pharmacokinet 1993;24:203–220.
49. Finley PR. Selective serotonin reuptake inhibitors: Pharmacologic profiles and potential therapeutic distinctions. Ann Pharmacotherapy 1994;28:1359–1369.
50. Hansten PD. Drug Interactions, 6th ed. Philadelphia, Lea and Febiger, 1989.
51. Hansten PD, Horn JR. Drug Interactions and Updates. Vancouver, WA, Applied Therapeutics, 1993, pp 476–480, 490–492, 597, 721–726, 744.
52. Crewe HK, Lennard MS, Tucker GT, et al. The effect of selective serotonin re-uptake inhibitors on cytochrome $P_{450}2D_6$ (CYP2D6) activity in human liver microsomes. Br J Clin Pharmacol 1992;34:262–265.
53. Preskorn SH. Recent pharmacologic advances in antidepressant therapy for the elderly. Am J Med 1993;94(suppl SA):2S–12S.
54. Buff DD, Brenner R, Kirtane SS, Gilboa R. Dysrhythmia associated with fluoxetine treatment in an elderly patient with cardiac disease. J Clin Psychiatry 1991;52:174–176.
55. Flament MF, Rapoport JL, Berg CJ, et al. Clomipramine treatment of childhood compulsive disorder. Arch Gen Psychiatry 1985;42:977–983.
56. Dista Products Company. Prozac package insert. Indianapolis, IN, 1994.
57. Murphy DL, Pato MT, Pigott TA. Obsessive–compulsive disorder: Treatment with serotonin-selective uptake inhibitors, azapirones, and other agents. J Clin Psychopharmacol 1990;10(suppl):91–100.
58. Pigott TA, Pato MT, Berstein SE. Controlled comparisons of clomipramine and fluoxetine in the treatment of obsessive-compulsive disorder: Behavioral and biological results. Arch Gen Psychiatry 1990;47:926–932.
59. Jenike MA, Hyman S, Baer L, et al. A controlled trial of fluvoxamine in obsessive compulsive disorder: Implications for a serotonergic theory. Am J Psychiatry 1990;147:1209–1215.
60. Pato MT, Zohar-Kadouch R, Zohar J, Murphy DL. Return of symptoms after discontinuation of clomipramine in patients with obsessive compulsive disorder. Am J Psychiatry 1988;145:1521–1525.
61. Fontaine R, Chouinard G. Fluoxetine in the long-term maintenance treatment of obsessive compulsive disorder. Psychiatr Annals 1989;19:88–91.
62. Alarcon RD, Libb JW, Spitler D. A predictive study of obsessive compulsive disorder response to clomipramine. J Clin Psychopharmacol 1993;13:210–213.
63. Austin LS, Lydiard B, Fossey MD. Panic and phobic disorders in patients with obsessive compulsive disorder. J Clin Psychiatry 1990;51:456–458.

64. Jenike MA, Rauch SL. Managing the patient with treatment-resistant obsessive compulsive disorder: Current strategies. J Clin Psychiatry 1994;55(3, suppl):11–17.
65. Micromedex, Inc. Denver, CO, Vol 68, May 31, 1991.
66. Chouinard G, Goodwin W, Greist J, et al. Results of a double-blind placebo-controlled trial of a new serotonin uptake inhibitor, sertraline, in the treatment of obsessive compulsive disorder. Psychopharmacol Bull 1990;26:279–284.
67. Greist J, Chouinard G, DuBoff E, et al. Double-blind comparison of three doses of sertraline and placebo in the treatment of outpatients with obsessive–compulsive disorder. Poster presented at the 18th Collegium Internationale Neuro-Psychopharmacologicum Congress, Nice, France, June 28–July 2, 1992.
68. Pato MT, Gluhoski V. Serotonin and effect sizes of antiobsessive agents [letter]. Am J Psychiatry 1992;149:420–421.
69. Baer L. Behavior therapy for obsessive compulsive disorder in the office-based practice. J Clin Psychiatry 1993;54(6, suppl):10–15.
70. Jenike MA. Approaches to the patient with treatment-refractory obsessive compulsive disorder. J Clin Psychiatry 1990;51(suppl 2):15–21.
71. Tippin J, Henn FA. Modified leukotomy in the treatment of intractable obsessional neurosis. Am J Psychiatry 1982;139:1601–1603.
72. Jenike MA, Baer L, Ballantine HT, et al. Cingulotomy for refractory obsessive compulsive disorder: A long-term follow-up of 33 patients. Arch Gen Psychiatry 1991;48:548–555.
73. Mindus P, Jenike MA. Neurosurgical treatment of malignant obsessive–compulsive disorder, in Jenike MA, ed. Psychiatric Clinics of North America: Obsessional Disorders. vol 15, no 4. Philadelphia, WB Saunders, 1992, pp 921–938.
74. Goodman WK, McDougle CJ, Barr LC, et al. Biological approaches to treatment-resistant obsessive compulsive disorder. J Clin Psychiatry 1993;54(6, suppl):16–26.

Chapter 71

Sleep Disorders

Cynthia K. Kirkwood, PharmD, and Rakesh K. Sood, MD

Approximately one-third of our lives is spent sleeping. There is a wide interindividual variability in the amount of sleep required per night (i.e., 3–10 hours).[1] Although largely an enigma, sleep is an important component of human behavior and provides an emotional and physical restoration for the body. Abnormalities in the normal physiology of sleep often cause patients to complain of three types of sleep problems: insomnia, excessive daytime sleepiness, and abnormal sleep behaviors.[2] The prevalence of sleep difficulties in the general population is estimated to be 30–35%.[3] Approximately 4–5% of the population report excessive sedation.[3] Untreated sleep disturbances are associated with high rates of serious accidents, impaired occupational functioning, and morbidity and mortality.[2,4]

Normal Human Sleep

A circadian rhythm of sleep and waking is established shortly after birth and changes over the life cycle. Two oscillators with different period lengths control the circadian rhythm of sleep. One oscillator is located in the suprachiasmic nucleus (i.e., biological clock) and the other occurs through neurobiologic mechanisms. Two peptides, δ-sleep-inducing peptide and factor S also appear to be involved in the biochemical regulation. Synchronization of the sleep–wake cycle, which naturally lasts 25 hours, with the 24-hour cycle imposed by the earth's rotation requires routinely occurring zeitgebers or cues (e.g., clock, light, shower, breakfast time) to set the internal clock.[1]

Neurochemistry

Sleep is a complex psychophysiologic phenomenon that ensues as wakefulness abates. Neuronal complexes involved in regulating the cyclic alteration of sleep and wakefulness are located in the brainstem, basal forebrain, and hypothalamus with projections into the cortex and thalamus. The reticular activating system (RAS) is responsible for maintaining wakefulness. Neurochemically, norepinephrine (NE) and acetylcholine in the cortex and histamine and neuropeptides (e.g., substance P, corticotropin-releasing factor) in the hypothalamus modulate neuronal activity during wakefulness.[5] Neuron systems in the brainstem raphe nuclei, solitary tract, ventricular thalamus, anterior hypothalamus, and basal forebrain are involved in sleep promotion. As the RAS decelerates, information transfer to the cortex ceases and serotonin (5-HT) neurotransmission in the raphe nuclei reduces sensory input to inhibit motor activity.[5] NE is involved in dreaming, while 5-HT is active during nondreaming sleep.

Sleep Physiology

During sleep the brain is extremely active and produces a characteristic pattern of stages that cycle during the night.[2] Polysomnography (PSG) is a procedure that measures multiple electrophysiologic parameters simultaneously during sleep such as an electroencephalogram (EEG), electrooculogram (EOG), and electromyogram (EMG).[2] Two EOGs, one EEG, and one EMG are the minimal recordings utilized in scoring sleep stages.[6] Commonly measured objective parameters of sleep include the latency to sleep onset (amount of time to fall asleep), number of awakenings, number of stage shifts during the night, and latency to the first rapid eye movement (REM) period. Other polysomnographic measures (e.g., oral and nasal airflow, respiratory effort, oxygen [O_2] desaturation, periodic leg movements [PLM], gross motor activity, and nocturnal penile tumescence) may be used to diagnose sleep disorders.[2,7]

Wakefulness is characterized by an EEG of low voltage, fast activity, random eye movements and blinks, and a high muscle tone. The two types of sleep are non-REM (NREM, stages 1–4) and REM. During NREM sleep skeletal muscle tone and eye movements are low in comparison with wakefulness, and respiratory activity occurs at a slow, regular pace. Stage 1 sleep represents a transition between wakefulness and sleep that lasts between 0.5 and 7 minutes; the EEG reveals low-voltage (3- to 7-Hz), desynchronized activity. Stage 2 sleep is characterized by a low-voltage EEG, and frequent "sleep spindles" (10- to 16-Hz spindle-shaped waves) and "K-complexes" (high-voltage spikes).

Stages 3 and 4 are called delta sleep and consist of high-amplitude, slow waves.[7]

REM sleep is marked by the onset of a low-voltage, mixed frequency EEG and bursts of bilaterally conjugate REMs.[7] During REM sleep muscle tone is low, but autonomic fluctuations (e.g., heart rate, perspiration, penile erection) are active.[8] Dream reports occur in 80–90% of subjects if awakened during or at the end of a REM period.

SLEEP CYCLE

The architecture of sleep in a healthy young adult is cyclic. From wakefulness, the passage through stages 1 to 4 occurs in 45 minutes. Within 90 minutes of falling asleep, the first REM period commences and lasts only 5–7 minutes. The cycle lasts approximately 70–120 minutes and is repeated 4–6 times during the night.[7] Most delta sleep occurs during the first half of the night. REM periods progressively lengthen throughout the night.[9] A typical young adult spends approximately 75% of the night in NREM sleep and the remainder in REM sleep.[7] A sleep histogram for a normal young adult is depicted in Figure 71.1.

In elderly individuals the sleep pattern is altered with a considerable decrease in delta sleep, REM sleep, and total sleep time.[7] Correspondingly, there is an increase in the number of awakenings and total time spent awake at night.[10] The contribution of daytime napping and specific sleep pathology (e.g., sleep apnea, PLM) to this apparent decrease in sleep is unclear; however, in randomly selected, noncomplaining, elderly individuals, the incidence of sleep pathology may be as high as 40%.[11]

CLASSIFICATION

Progression in sleep disorders medicine and research has resulted in several classification systems. The Association of Sleep Disorders Center's *International Classification of Sleep Disorders* (ICSD) organizes more than 80 sleep disorders based on pathophysiology under the major headings of dyssomnias, parasomnias, medical/psychiatric sleep disorders, and proposed sleep disorders.[12] Similar to the ICSD, the *Diagnostic and Statistical Manual of Mental Disorders,* Fourth Edition (DSM-IV), classifies sleep disorders based on presumed etiology into three major categories (Table 71.1) and requires a period of duration of 1 month before a sleep disorder is diagnosed.[13] Primary sleep disorders result from endogenous abnormalities in the sleep–wake timing or generating processes and are further classified as dyssomnias (abnormalities in the amount, timing, or quality of sleep) or parasomnias (abnormal behaviors associated with sleep). Sleep disorders secondary to another mental disorder, medical condition, or substance (concurrent use or dis-

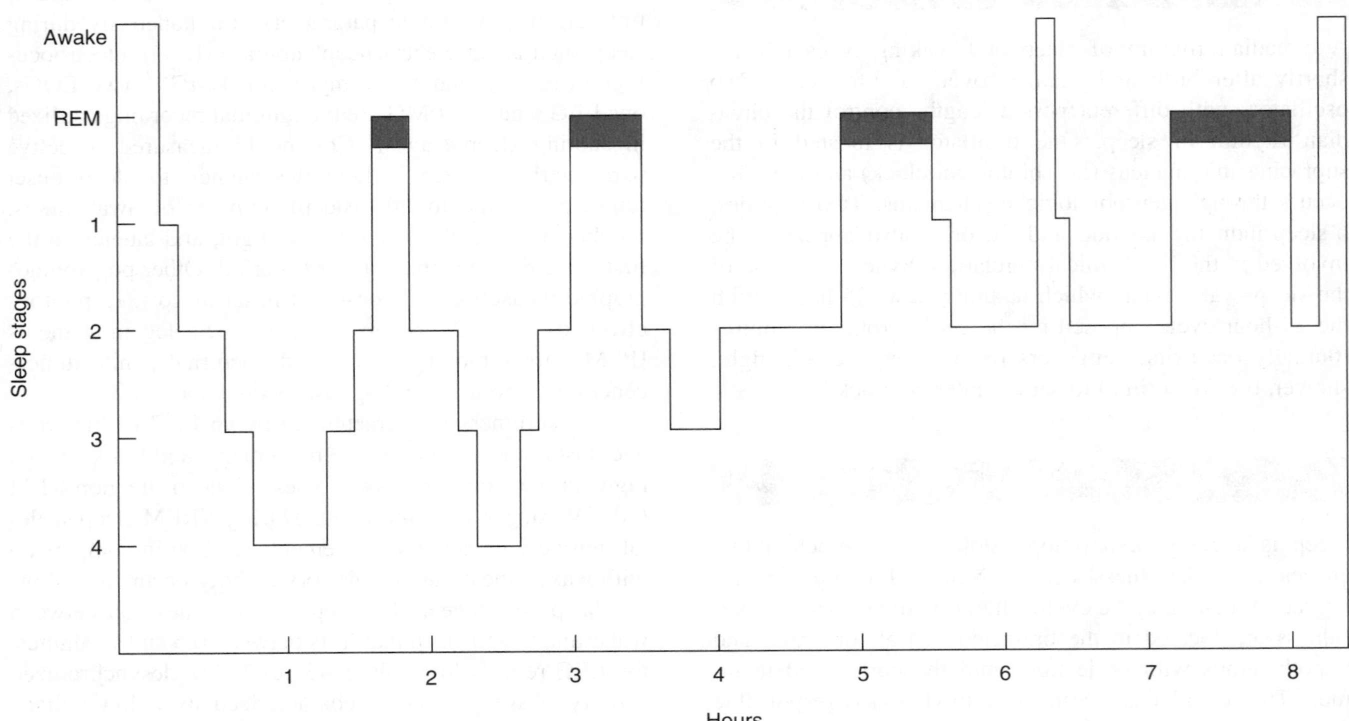

Figure 71.1. Sleep histogram showing a typical night's sleep of a young adult. (Red areas indicate REM sleep.) *(Reprinted with permission from Ref. 9.)*

TABLE 71.1. DSM-IV CLASSIFICATION OF SLEEP DISORDERS

Primary Sleep Disorders
- Dyssomnias
  - Primary insomnia
  - Primary hypersomnia
  - Narcolepsy
  - Breathing-related sleep disorder
  - Circadian rhythm sleep disorder
    - Delayed sleep phase type
    - Jet lag type
    - Unspecified type
  - Dyssomnias not otherwise specified
- Parasomnias
  - Nightmare disorder
  - Sleep terror disorder
  - Sleepwalking disorder
  - Parasomnias not otherwise specified

Sleep Disorders Related to Another Mental Disorder
- Insomnia related to another mental disorder
- Hypersomnia related to another mental disorder

Other Sleep Disorders
- Sleep disorder due to a general medical condition
- Substance-induced sleep disorder

(Compiled with permission from Ref. 13.)

continuation of a substance or a drug) are classified separately.

INSOMNIA

Insomnia is a subjective complaint of difficulty falling asleep, maintaining sleep, or of not feeling rested despite a sufficient opportunity to sleep.[13,14] A concurrent disturbance of daytime functioning (e.g., decreased concentration, fatigue, myalgia) usually accompanies the sleep complaint.[15] Younger individuals usually complain of delays in sleep onset, while older patients complain of nocturnal awakening and shorter time periods of sleep.[13] The most important aspect in evaluating a sleep complaint is its duration. Transient (2–3 nights) and short-term (less than 3 weeks) insomnia are typical of individuals without a history of sleep problems; however, long-term or chronic insomnia has a duration exceeding 3 weeks and may be related to medical or psychiatric disorders, or may be psychophysiologic in nature.[14] Psychophysiologic insomnia is caused by arousal or anxiety at bedtime, usually surrounding a negative expectation about sleep. Patients possess tension and maladaptive, conditioned behavior typified by a marked overconcern about their inability to fall asleep.[2,10,14]

It is estimated that the total cost of insomnia is $92.5 to $107.5 billion annually.[4] Direct and indirect costs include medications and treatment, absenteeism, decreased productivity, accidents, hospitalizations, and increased morbidity (both psychiatric and nonpsychiatric) and mortality. Improved recognition and treatment of insomnia may ease the economic burden and prevent progression to other psychiatric disorders, especially depression.[4,16]

EPIDEMIOLOGY

Insomnia is the most prevalent sleep complaint in the general population and one of the most commonly expressed to the physician.[2] More than 50% of the population report insomnia during their lifetimes.[15] A 1-year prevalence study of insomnia in the United States reported that one-third of individuals surveyed complained of insomnia and 17% reported the symptoms to be serious.[17] The most common types of insomnia are sleep maintenance and difficulty falling asleep.[18] Data from the National Institute of Mental Health Epidemiologic Catchment Area (ECA) study indicates that the 6-month prevalence of insomnia, defined as symptoms for 2 weeks, was 10.2%. Females; individuals who are unemployed, elderly, separated, or widowed; and those in the lower socioeconomic sector reported significantly higher rates of insomnia. Forty percent of those with insomnia had a concurrent psychiatric disorder (e.g., anxiety, depression, alcohol or substance abuse).[16]

Despite the widespread prevalence of insomnia, only 5% of individuals seek medical assistance for management.[15] Approximately 10–20% of insomniacs use nonprescription drugs or alcohol to alleviate symptoms. Of the 3% of the population who ingest hypnotics for insomnia, 11% report a duration of use exceeding 1 year.[17,19]

DIFFERENTIAL DIAGNOSIS

The causes of insomnia may be multidimensional and related to underlying situational stressors, medical or psychiatric illnesses, or medication use. Common identifiable causes of insomnia are listed in Table 71.2. Evaluation of the patient with a complaint of transient insomnia should focus on possible acute stress, environmental disruptions (e.g., change in job, recent surgery, examinations), and drug-related causes. In patients with a complaint of chronic sleep disturbances, a complete diagnostic evaluation should include physical and mental status examinations and routine laboratory tests, as well as medication and substance abuse histories to rule out medical and psychiatric etiologies.

TREATMENT

The assessment of insomnia should include a history of the specific symptomatology, time course of onset of insomnia, duration, frequency, daytime symptoms, sleep hygiene habits, and history of previous treatments. The therapeutic

TABLE 71.2. COMMON ETIOLOGIES OF INSOMNIA

Situational
- Work or financial stress
- Interpersonal conflicts
- Major life events
- Jet lag, shift work

Medical
- Cardiovascular (angina, arrhythmias, heart failure)
- Respiratory (asthma, sleep apnea)
- Chronic pain
- Endocrine disorders (diabetes, hyperthyroidism)
- Gastrointestinal (gastroesophageal reflux, ulcers)
- Neurologic (delirium, epilepsy, Parkinson's disease)
- Pregnancy

Psychiatric
- Mood disorders (depression, mania)
- Anxiety disorders (generalized anxiety disorder, obsessive–compulsive disorder, panic disorder)
- Substance abuse (alcohol or sedative/hypnotic withdrawal)

Pharmacologically Induced
- Anticonvulsants
- Central adrenergic blockers
- Diuretics
- Selective serotonin reuptake inhibitors
- Steroids
- Stimulants

(Adapted from Refs. 2, 5, and 18.)

management of insomnia is determined by the duration of insomnia and may consist of a combination of general measures to improve sleep, psychotherapy, and pharmacotherapy. A treatment plan should be individualized based on the type of insomnia, severity of daytime impairment in functioning, patient age, and concurrent medical conditions.

General therapeutic measures should be used for all patients with insomnia. Such measures include treatment of all identified causes of insomnia and patient education on sleep hygiene and stress management techniques. All unnecessary or high dosages of medications should be discontinued.[14,15] Psychotherapy and behavioral techniques are effective in many individuals, especially those with chronic insomnia. The adjunctive use of hypnotics for intermittent or short-term use is effective in relieving insomnia.[7,15] The expected duration of therapy and desired pharmacologic profile must be considered when choosing a hypnotic.[18]

Nonpharmacologic Therapy

General measures to improve insomnia are useful adjuncts to the specific treatment of identifiable etiologies. Cognitive, behavioral, and educational interventions include cognitive therapy, relaxation therapy (e.g., progressive muscle relaxation), stimulus control therapy, light therapy, sleep deprivation, and sleep hygiene education.[20,21] Results of a meta-analysis of nonpharmacologic treatments for chronic insomnia indicate that stimulus control and sleep restriction were the most effective treatment modalities compared with placebo or no treatment, and improvements were sustained for 6 months.[20] Changes in sleep hygiene habits can improve the patient's sleep–wake routine and augment recovery from transient or short-term insomnia (Table 71.3).[14]

TABLE 71.3. NONPHARMACOLOGIC RECOMMENDATIONS FOR INSOMNIA

Stimulus Control Procedures
1. Establish a regular time to wake up and to go to sleep (including weekends).
2. Sleep only as much as necessary to feel rested.
3. Avoid long periods of wakefulness in bed. Use the bed only for sleep or intimacy; do not read or watch television in bed.
4. Avoid trying to force sleep. If you do not fall asleep within 20–30 minutes, leave the bed and perform a relaxing activity (e.g., read, listen to music, watch television) until drowsy. Repeat this as often as necessary.
5. Avoid daytime naps.

Sleep Hygiene Recommendations
1. Exercise routinely (e.g., three to four times weekly), but not close to bedtime because this may cause arousal.
2. Create a comfortable sleep environment by avoiding temperature extremes, loud noises, and illuminated clocks.
3. Discontinue or reduce the use of alcohol, caffeine, and nicotine.
4. Avoid excessive fullness or hunger at bedtime.
5. Avoid drinking large quantities of liquids in the evening to prevent nighttime trips to the restroom.

(Adapted from Ref. 18, with permission.)

Alcohol, stimulants, and nicotine use should be avoided by patients with insomnia. Although alcohol enhances sleep onset, the subsequent sleep is disturbed and fragmented. Alcoholics frequently have insomnia for months to years after recovery.[5] Individuals with insomnia are sensitive to the arousal effects of mild stimulants and should avoid all caffeine-containing products and chocolate for at least 8 hours before bedtime. Nicotine withdrawal often arouses smokers from quiescence.[22]

Hypnotic Agents

Table 71.4 lists the commonly prescribed hypnotic agents. The benzodiazepines (BZs) are the drugs of choice for the symptomatic relief of insomnia because of their favorable therapeutic index. The BZs have largely replaced barbiturates (e.g., butalbital, pentobarbital, secobarbital) because of the latter's propensity for the rapid development of tolerance, fatalities by overdose, development of physical and psychological dependence, withdrawal syndromes, and significant drug interactions.[7] Because of safety considerations the barbiturates have few indications for use as hypnotics.[5,14]

Excluding zolpidem, the nonbarbiturate, non-BZ hypnotics have associated risks identical to those of the barbi-

TABLE 71.4. CLASSIFICATION AND DOSAGES OF HYPNOTICS

Generic Name	Trade Name (Manufacturer)	Daily Dosage Range (mg)
Benzodiazepines		
Estazolam	ProSom (Abbott)	1–2
Flurazepam	Dalmane (Roche)	15–30
Generics (various)		
Quazepam	Doral (Baker Cummins)	7.5–15
Temazepam	Restoril (Sandoz)	15–30
	Generics (various)	
Triazolam	Halcion (Upjohn)	0.125–0.25
Nonbarbiturate, Nonbenzodiazepines	Generics (various)	
Chloral hydrate	Noctec (Squibb Mark)	500–2000
	Generics (various)	
Zolpidem	Ambien (Searle)	5–10
Antidepressants[a]		
Trazodone	Desyrel (Mead Johnson)	50–100
	Generics (various)	
Antihistamines		
Diphenhydramine	Benadryl (Parke–Davis)	25–100
	Generics (various)	
Doxylamine	Unisom (Leeming)	25–100

[a]Non-FDA-approved for insomnia.

turates and thus offer no clinical advantages. Chloral hydrate therapy may be complicated by gastrointestinal irritation, drug interactions, and fatalities in overdosage. Chloral hydrate interacts with other sedatives, and the combination of chloral hydrate and alcohol has been termed a "Mickey Finn" or "knockout drops."[14] Because of glutethimide's disproportionately high rate of abuse and fatalities by overdosage it is not recommended as a hypnotic for outpatients.

The antidepressants (e.g., amitriptyline, doxepin, trazodone) are alternatives in patients who complain of nonrestorative sleep and should not receive BZs.[23,24] Prescriptions for antidepressants as hypnotics doubled from 11.6% in 1987 to 26.4% of all hypnotic prescriptions in 1991.[19] Trazodone is an effective hypnotic in patients with fluoxetine- or bupropion-induced insomnia.[24]

Antihistamines are less effective than the BZs and their use may be complicated by anticholinergic side effects.[14] Nonprescription sleep aids commonly contain antihistamines and analgesics. The amino acid L-tryptophan is no longer recommended for use as a hypnotic because of reports of eosinophilia-myalgia syndrome.[25]

Zolpidem, an imidazolpyridine chemically unrelated to BZs or barbiturates, was approved for the short-term treatment of insomnia in December 1992. Zolpidem acts selectively at the BZ_1 receptor and has minimal anxiolytic and no muscle relaxant or anticonvulsant effects. It is comparable in effectiveness to BZ hypnotics, reducing latency to sleep, and increasing total sleep time and efficiency.[26] Oral doses of 10 mg to greater than 20 mg have been associated with increased stages 2, 3, and 4 sleep and decreased REM.[26] Zolpidem is metabolized by methyloxidation and hydroxylation to inactive metabolites. Its half-life is approximately 2.5 hours, and duration of effect is 6–8 hours. Lower dosages should be used in elderly patients and those with hepatic impairment.[27]

The most common adverse effects of zolpidem are drowsiness, amnesia, dizziness, headache, and gastrointestinal complaints.[26] Compared with BZs, zolpidem use is not associated with the development of tolerance or rebound insomnia after 35 days of continuous use[28]; however, it is more expensive. The recommended daily dosage is 10 mg, and 5 mg in elderly patients. The dosage can be increased up to 20 mg nightly; yet, the incidence of adverse events is dose related.[27]

Benzodiazepine Therapy

In the United States five BZs are marketed with a therapeutic indication for insomnia (Table 71.4); however, other BZs also are effective. Between 1987 and 1991 the number of prescriptions for BZ hypnotics fell from 6.1 million to 4.3 million.[19] Despite a decline in prescribing frequency, triazolam remained the most widely prescribed BZ hypnotic.[19]

The BZs relieve insomnia by reducing the latency to sleep onset and number of awakenings, and increasing the total sleep time. BZs decrease the duration of stages 1 and 4 sleep, and increase stage 2 sleep. Unlike the barbiturates, BZs do not decrease REM sleep to cause a severe REM withdrawal syndrome.[29]

Pharmacokinetics

BZ onset and duration of activity are dependent on pharmacokinetics and are the most important characteristics to be considered when choosing an agent.[8,30] If a BZ hypnotic is to be administered as a single dose, its extent of distribution and elimination half-life are important in predicting its duration of action. However, after multiple dosing the BZ elimination half-life and formation of active metabolites will determine the extent of drug accumulation and resultant clinical effects.[30]

BZ pharmacokinetic properties are summarized in Table 71.5. The rapidity of onset of action is dependent on the drug's rate of absorption. Flurazepam and triazolam are rapidly absorbed. Because of high lipophilicity, sedation after triazolam is intense in its severity and maximal at approximately 1 hour. Temazepam is less lipophilic and has a slower onset of effect. Sedation after flurazepam occurs within 1–2 hours after ingestion and is not as intense as that with the previous two agents.[31] Estazolam and quazepam are similar to flurazepam in their onset of effect.[32,33]

TABLE 71.5. PHARMACOKINETICS OF BENZODIAZEPINE HYPNOTIC AGENTS

Generic Name	Time to Peak Plasma Concentration (h)	Elimination Half-Life Parent (h)	Metabolic Pathway	Clinically Significant Metabolites
Estazolam	2	12–15	Oxidation	—
Flurazepam	1	8	Oxidation	Hydroxyethylflurazepam Flurazepam aldehyde
			N-Dealkylation	*N*-DAF[a]
Quazepam	2	39	Oxidation	2-Oxo-quazepam
			N-Dealkylation	*N*-DAF[a]
Temazepam	1.5	10–15	Conjugation	—
Triazolam	1	2	Oxidation	—

[a]*N*-desalkylflurazepam, mean half-life 47–100 hours.

Triazolam is redistributed quickly because of its high lipophilicity and thus has a short duration of effect.[30] Estazolam and temazepam are intermediate in their duration of action. The therapeutic effects of flurazepam and quazepam are long in comparison with the other BZs because of the formation of active metabolites with long-elimination half-lives.

With the exception of temazepam, which is eliminated via conjugation, all BZ hypnotics are metabolized by hepatic microsomal oxidation and then undergo glucuronide conjugation. Oxidation may be inhibited in patients with impaired liver function, advanced age, or concurrent use of drugs that inhibit oxidation. Drugs that inhibit the cytochrome P-450IIIA4 enzyme (e.g., erythromycin, nefazodone, ketaconazole) reduce the clearance of triazolam and increase its plasma concentrations.[34,35]

Triazolam (short-elimination half-life BZ), estazolam, and temazepam (intermediate-elimination half-life BZs) lack clinically significant metabolites. Flurazepam and quazepam are long-elimination half-life BZs. Flurazepam is rapidly metabolized to two short-acting metabolites, hydroxyethylflurazepam and flurazepam aldehyde. These metabolites contribute to sleep induction on the first night of therapy but are eliminated within 12 hours. *N*-Desalkylflurazepam (*N*-DAF) is an active metabolite that peaks 10 hours after a single dose and accumulates extensively during multiple dosing.[36] *N*-DAF accounts for most of flurazepam's pharmacologic effects. Quazepam and one of its metabolites, 2-oxo-quazepam, have elimination half-lives of 39 hours. Quazepam's oxo-quazepam metabolite is metabolized to *N*-DAF.[37] If oxidation of *N*-DAF is impaired, its half-life becomes prolonged, and compli-cations of drug accumulation may result with repeated dosing; however, tolerance may develop to these effects.[30] *N*-DAF is beneficial when daytime anxiety or early morn-ing awakening are patient complaints, but daytime sedation and impaired psychomotor performance may complicate therapy.[14]

Adverse Effects

The appearance of residual daytime central nervous system (CNS) effects is dependent on the dose and pharmacokinetic characteristics of the BZ hypnotic. High dosages of BZs with long- or intermediate-elimination half-lives have a greater potential for producing daytime sedation and performance decrements. Residual or carryover daytime effects include excessive drowsiness, psychomotor incoordination, decreased concentration, and cognitive deficits.[38] Tolerance to the CNS carryover effects may develop with time in some individuals. Rapidly eliminated BZs have less potential for producing daytime sedation.

Tolerance to BZ hypnotic effect develops sooner with triazolam (after 2 weeks of continuous use) than with other BZ hypnotics.[8] Laboratory studies indicate that the hypnotic efficacy of flurazepam, quazepam, and temazepam is maintained for 1 month of continuous nightly use.[39] Estazolam reportedly maintains the duration and quality of sleep at the maximum dosage (i.e., 2 mg nightly) for up to 12 weeks.[40] The efficacy of long-term continuous use of BZ hypnotics has not been established. Long-term use (greater than 6 months) of low doses of BZs was associated with loss of efficacy and worsened sleep (suppression of delta and REM sleep) in chronic insomniacs.[41]

Anterograde amnesia is an impairment of memory and recall after drug ingestion reported to occur during BZ therapy. Anterograde amnesia occurs more frequently with triazolam than with temazepam[42]; however, flurazepam demonstrated more anterograde effects than triazolam in one study.[43] Use of the lowest possible dosage is recommended to avoid adverse effects on memory. When compared with temazepam, triazolam usage was associated with a higher reported rate of confusion, bizarre behavior, agitation, and hallucinations. These CNS effects occurred with higher doses (68% of patients ingested 0.5–1.5 mg) and in older patients (mean of 63 years).[42] Because of the high incidence of CNS adverse effects, the United Kingdom temporarily suspended sales of triazolam in October 1991, until the manufacturer addressed cautions regarding the CNS adverse effects through product relabeling and repackaging into a 10-day blister package.[44]

Daytime anxiety and rebound insomnia are associated with use of the short-elimination half-life agent triazolam.[14]

Rebound insomnia is characterized by increased wakefulness beyond baseline amounts that usually lasts for one to two nights after abrupt discontinuation of BZ hypnotics with short- or intermediate-elimination half-lives. Rebound insomnia occurs more frequently after high doses of triazolam, even when intermittently ingested.[45] The occurrence of rebound insomnia can be minimized by utilizing the lowest effective dose and tapering the dose upon discontinuation.[46]

The incidence of CNS side effects increases with age because of increased sensitivity to pharmacologic effects and prolonged BZ half-lives in the elderly with resultant increased potential for drug accumulation. The result is often impaired judgment, excessive daytime sedation, and confusional states.[47] Short- and intermediate-elimination half-life drugs are associated with fewer performance deficits; however, they may increase the chance of daytime anxiety in elderly patients. There is an association between falls and hip fractures and the use of long-elimination half-life BZs, thus prescription of flurazepam and quazepam should be avoided in elderly patients.[48]

Guidelines

Hypnotic therapy is indicated in individuals with transient or short-term insomnia.[2] Patients should receive counseling to the effect that sleep will return to normal when the precipitating stressor is eliminated and also be educated on strategies for stimulus control and good sleep hygiene (Table 71.3). If the stressor is expected to last more than 1 week, intermittent hypnotic use (three or four nights per week) should be prescribed for no more than 3 weeks. For patients with chronic insomnia, medical, psychiatric, and pharmacologic causes should be identified and managed.[14] If treatment of an underlying disorder fails to result in improvement, intermittent pharmacotherapy should be initiated. If the insomnia is psychophysiologic, several months of supervised hypnotic therapy may help alleviate anxiety and re-establish a regular sleep pattern upon drug discontinuation; however, patients require nonpharmacologic therapy as well.[20]

Tolerance and dependence can be avoided by using hypnotics at the lowest possible dose, intermittently, for the shortest duration possible. Patients should receive instruction on frequency of drug use and the expected duration of therapy to prevent development of dependence. Withdrawal symptoms can be diminished by gradually tapering the dosage. Patients should be counseled on rebound insomnia when BZ therapy is terminated.

Patients with difficulty initiating sleep and those who require daytime alertness should receive the short-acting BZ hypnotics. Those with difficulty maintaining sleep or early morning awakening may benefit from intermediate-elimination half-life agents if daytime performance is required. Long-elimination half-life BZs should be considered if management of daytime anxiety is required. There is no rationale for the concurrent use of two BZs to treat anxiety and insomnia.

BZ hypnotics should not be prescribed for individuals with sleep apnea, a history of substance abuse, or during pregnancy. Patients should be instructed to avoid alcohol; even alcohol on the day after ingestion of a long-elimination half-life BZ can result in additive CNS impairment. Prescriptions for BZ hypnotics should be accompanied by printed information and counseling on precautions.

Sleep Apnea

Sleep-related respiratory abnormalities are commonly diagnosed in sleep labs using PSG. Apnea is defined as the cessation of air flow at the nose and mouth lasting at least 10 seconds and is classified into two major categories, obstructive and central. Patients with sleep apnea have a high risk of morbidity and mortality.[49]

OBSTRUCTIVE SLEEP APNEA

Obstructive sleep apnea (OSA) is a potentially life-threatening condition characterized by repeated episodes of nocturnal breathing cessation with loud snoring and gasping, often reported by the bed partner.[50] OSA is estimated to occur in 1–9% of the population, predominantly in males.[2] OSA is caused by an occlusion of the upper airway (e.g., obesity, polyps, enlarged tonsils, adenoids, or tongue) that occurs only during sleep.[50]

In OSA patients, electrophysiologic recording of airflow through the nose and mouth and thoracic respiratory efforts demonstrate that airflow ceases while respiratory effort continues. The apneic episode is terminated by a reflex action to the fall in O_2 saturation that causes a brief "mini-arousal" during which breathing resumes. Patients may be unaware of the "mini-arousals"; however, the EEG clearly indicates an activation that may cause fragmented sleep. Thus, patients with OSA usually present with complaints of excessive daytime sleepiness. In severe cases, excessive somnolence may cause sleep attacks that can result in decrements in performance (e.g., motor vehicle accidents). Additional daytime symptoms include morning headache, poor memory, and irritability.[50] Most individuals with OSA are overweight. Complications of OSA include arrhythmias, hypertension, cor pulmonale, and sudden death during somnolence.[50]

Treatment of OSA must be individualized and depends on the severity of the disordered breathing and the amount of sleep disruption.[51] Patients with severe apnea (greater than 20 apneas/h on PSG and excessive daytime somnolence) and those with moderate apneas (5–20 apneas/h on PSG and excessive daytime sleepiness or other daytime symptoms) have shown significant improvement and reduction in mortality with treatment.[50] Nonpharmacologic measures are the treatments of choice in patients with OSA. Weight loss may eliminate the apnea and reduce daytime hypersomnia[51]; however, improvement is only limited. Treatment of underlying causes of obstruction (e.g., tonsillectomy, nasal septal repair, nonsedating antihistamines for allergic rhinitis) may eliminate apneas during sleep. In patients with mild apnea and snoring with no daytime symptomatology, management may include avoidance of a supine sleep position.[51]

Nasal continuous positive airway pressure (CPAP) during sleep is the standard treatment for most patients with OSA.[49] CPAP elevates the pressure in the oropharyngeal space to maintain positive airway pressure during the respiratory cycle. Patient tolerance and compliance are the major limitations of CPAP. Although tracheostomy is an effective surgical procedure, it is reserved for use in treatment-resistant patients. Uvulopalatopharyngoplasty is a surgical procedure to enlarge the pharyngeal airspace that successfully reduces apnea in 50% of patients and snoring in 90%.[49,51] Upper airway resection can also be performed with new laser surgical techniques.[49]

The single most important pharmacologic intervention in the treatment of sleep apnea is the avoidance of all CNS depressants (e.g., alcohol, anxiolytics, hypnotics, narcotics).[49] CNS depressant use is potentially lethal because it interferes with the brain's ability to produce the resumption of breathing. Pharmacologic intervention should be reserved for patients with mild forms of OSA and in those who have failed other treatments. The TCA protriptyline, in doses of 10–30 mg daily, reduces the frequency of apneas and increases O_2 saturation.[49] The antidepressant mechanism of action may be related to a decrease in REM sleep or an increase in the tonus of the musculature of the oropharynx; however, anticholinergic side effects often complicate therapy.[51] Fluoxetine 20 mg/d was effective in reducing apneas in some patients.[52] Respiratory stimulants, such as theophylline[53] and clonidine (in males),[54] also have been tried; however, efficacy is limited and research has not documented long-term effectiveness.

CENTRAL SLEEP APNEA

Central sleep apnea (CSA) is characterized by repeated episodes of apnea caused by temporary loss of respiratory effort during somnolence. It accounts for less than 10% of all apneas. Hypercapnic patients usually present with morning headache and daytime somnolence, while nonhypercapnic patients complain of insomnia and nocturnal awakenings with shortness of breath or gasping. Although the majority of CSA cases are idiopathic, identifiable causes are nasal obstruction, autonomic system lesions (e.g., cervical cordotomy), neurologic diseases (e.g., poliomyelitis, encephalitis, myasthenia gravis), and congestive heart failure.[55] The primary treatment approach for the hypercapnic CSA patient is ventilatory support with O_2 and CPAP; acetazolamide, theophylline, and medroxyprogesterone have shown mixed results.[55] In refractory cases diaphragmatic pacing, tracheostomy, or positive pressure ventilation are helpful. In nonhypercapnic CSA patients, treatment may consist of BZs (triazolam or temazepam) to reduce arousals, and acetazolamide, CPAP, and O_2 to stabilize breathing patterns.[55]

NARCOLEPSY

Narcolepsy is a chronic disease that typically begins before the age of 25 years. About 0.5% of the adult population has narcolepsy, with men and women being equally affected. There appears to be a genetic predetermination for narcolepsy; 3% of patients have a first-degree relative with the disorder.[56] An association between narcolepsy and the human leukocyte antigens (HLA) HLA-DR2 and HLA-DQ1 (HLA-DR15 and HLA-DQ6 under new nomenclature) has been identified.[57]

The essential feature of narcolepsy is excessive daytime sleepiness with sleep attacks that may last up to 30 minutes. Individuals often complain of hypersomnia, fatigue, impaired performance, and disturbed nighttime sleep. Excessive daytime sleepiness occurs before the second decade of life and the auxiliary symptoms (cataplexy, hypnagogic hallucinations, sleep paralysis) appear several years later.[56]

Cataplexy occurs in 70–80% of narcoleptics and is characterized by brief episodes (seconds to several minutes) of muscle weakness and/or paralysis that may cause the individual to collapse while remaining conscious. Cataplectic episodes are often precipitated by emotionally charged stimuli (e.g., laughter, anger, excitement). Sleep paralysis and hypnagogic and hypnopompic hallucinations manifest during the onset of sleep or upon awakening. Sleep paralysis is a loss of muscle tone while the patient is still awake. Hypnagogic (at the threshold of sleep) and hypnopompic (upon awakening) hallucinations are brief dreamlike experiences with more fragmentation and bizarre features than a typical dream.[56]

Sleep laboratory evaluation of the narcoleptic confirms the existence of excessive daytime sleepiness, disturbed nighttime sleep, and sleep-onset REM periods. The occurrence of sleep paralysis, cataplexy, and sleep-onset REM indicates that narcolepsy represents an abnormality in the regulatory mechanisms of REM sleep (possibly in the cholinergic system).[56]

TREATMENT

Management of narcolepsy is symptomatic and consists of both nonpharmacologic and pharmacologic interventions.

TABLE 71.6. STIMULANT DRUGS USED TO TREAT NARCOLEPSY

Generic Name	Trade Name (Manufacturer)	Daily Dosage Range (mg)
Dextroamphetamine	Dexedrine (SmithKline Beecham) Generics (various)	5–60
Dextroamphetamine/amphetamine salts[a]	Adderall (Richwood)	5–60
Methamphetamine[b]	Desoxyn (Abbott)	5–15
Methylphenidate	Ritalin (Ciba) Generics (various)	30–80
Pemoline	Cylert (Abbott)	37.5–112.5

[a]Dextroamphetamine sulfate, dextroamphetamine saccharate, amphetamine aspartate, amphetamine sulfate.
[b]Not available in some states. (Compiled from Refs. 57 and 59.)

Counseling the patient and significant others is essential, because family members often think that narcolepsy is voluntary and the patient is lazy and nonproductive. Good sleep habits should be encouraged. If the patient's daily schedule allows, at least two daytime naps can be beneficial. Following a 15-minute nap, the patient may be refreshed for several hours. Long-term support groups exist locally and nationally for narcoleptics.[58]

Pharmacologic treatment consists of the use of psychostimulants (Table 71.6) for excessive daytime sleepiness and antidepressants for cataplexy.[56] Stimulants exert their effects by enhancing norepinephrine release from presynaptic neurons.[56] Only methylphenidate and dextroamphetamine are labeled for use in narcolepsy. Amphetamines and methylphenidate have a fast onset of effect and durations of 3–4 hours and 6–10 hours, respectively. Divided daily doses are recommended; however, more expensive sustained-release formulations are available. Pemoline has a delayed onset of effect, but its duration is 8–10 hours; maximal effect may take several weeks. Liver function tests must be monitored (at 1 month and yearly) during pemoline therapy. Amphetamine use is associated with more likelihood of abuse and tolerance, especially when prescribed in high doses.[59]

The TCAs, through blockade of NE and 5-HT reuptake, are effective in reducing cataplexy and sleep paralysis. Imipramine (50–250 mg/d), protriptyline (5–30 mg/d), and nortriptyline (50–200 mg/d) are effective in approximately 80% of patients.[59] Selegiline (Eldepryl) in daily doses of 20–40 mg improves hypersomnolence and cataplexy, presumably through REM suppression.[60] γ-Hydroxybutyrate, 60 mg/kg/night, is a therapeutic option without anticholinergic side effects.[61]

GUIDELINES

General principles of drug therapy for narcolepsy include using the lowest effective dose possible, employing gradual titration, and carefully monitoring for therapeutic and adverse events. The goal of therapy is to maximize alertness during normal waking hours or at selected times of the day. Scheduled naps can help to maintain wakefulness.[57] In addition, cataplexy may be treated on an as-needed basis in some patients. If the patient can predict the occurrence of cataplexy (associated with an anticipated specific stimulus), then a TCA can be ingested for only the day or two before and during the expected occurrence.

CIRCADIAN RHYTHM DISORDERS

Most behavioral and psychological processes (e.g., endocrine secretions, body temperature regulation) are characterized by a temporal structure that matches the 24-hour day/night cycle or the "circadian." This daily cyclicity establishes a pattern of sleep and wakefulness. Humans studied in isolation demonstrate a "free running" sleep–wake cycle that lasts approximately 25 hours. Zeitgebers synchronize the biological clock to a 24-hour cycle.[62] The etiology of circadian rhythm disorders is a mismatch between an individual's biologic clock and the external time cues of the environment. Two commonly occurring circadian rhythm sleep disorders are jet lag and shift work sleep problems.

JET LAG

Jet lag follows rapid travel over multiple time zones and results in varying degrees and durations of sleep onset or maintenance insomnia complaints and daytime sleepiness. Insomnia usually occurs every other night. Sleep disturbances last for 2–3 days, but may prevail for 7–10 days if time zone changes are 8–12 hours. Compared with westward travel, eastward travel is associated with a longer duration of jet lag. Affected individuals also may suffer from decreased performance and alertness and gastrointestinal disturbances.[62]

Treatment of jet lag may consist of preventive measures and pharmacologic management. Jet lag can be avoided during coast-to-coast travel in the United States for durations of stay less than 7 days in a new time zone by adhering to the normal sleep–wake schedule from home. For longer lengths of stay, adjustment to a westbound time zone can be made by staying up and arising 1–2 hours later several days before the trip. Eastbound travelers also can adjust their schedule by retiring and arising earlier for several days before the trip.[62]

Pharmacologic treatment of jet lag includes the use of short-acting BZs. The lowest dose of triazolam (i.e., 0.125 mg) should be taken on alternate nights. Patients should be instructed to avoid ingestion of alcohol and counseled on rebound insomnia once triazolam is stopped. High doses of triazolam (i.e., 0.5 mg) were associated with next-day anterograde amnesia[63] and morning drowsiness in jet-lagged individuals. The pineal hormone, melatonin, has been used investigationally to rapidly entrain the circadian rhythm.[5,62]

SHIFT WORK SLEEP PROBLEMS

Shift workers comprise approximately 20% of the workforce.[62] Working at night causes a misalignment in the sleep–wake cycle and circadian rhythms associated with a decrease in alertness, performance, and quality of daytime sleep. On nonworking nights many night-shift workers experience insomnia.[62] Treatment may consist of recommending a daytime job, extending daytime sleep by sleeping in the afternoon, or scheduling a 2- to 3-hour afternoon nap on days off from work. Hypnotics should be used cautiously, if at all. Daytime doses of triazolam were associated with cognitive performance deficits in shift workers.[64] Scheduled exposure to bright lights at night and darkness during the daytime improves psychologic and behavioral adaptation to night work and daytime sleep.[65]

PARASOMNIAS

Parasomnias refer to a group of acute, episodic, physical phenomena that occur either exclusively during sleep or are exaggerated by sleep. Sleep walking (somnambulism) and sleep terrors are seen in children and may be considered normal to some degree at a certain age. Although a number of miscellaneous parasomnias have been identified, only three are discussed.

SOMNAMBULISM

Somnambulism is generally a delta sleep phenomenon that occurs during the first third of the night. About 10–30% of children experience at least one sleepwalking episode, but the prevalence of repeated episodes is estimated to be 1–5%. In adults, the prevalence of sleepwalking episodes is 1–7%.[13] The etiology of somnambulism is unknown, but may involve genetic (family history is positive in 80% of patients), developmental, organic, or psychologic factors (especially in adults). The initial episode of somnambulism usually occurs between the ages of 4 and 8 years with peak prevalence at about 12 years of age. It abates spontaneously in early adolescence, usually around the age of 15 years.[13] Although the patient appears to be navigating well during an episode, there is a significant impairment of motor skills and reactivity. Individuals have reduced alertness and responsiveness and stare blankly during an episode; afterward, there may be a period of confusion or difficulty with orientation.[13] If awakened, there is limited recall of the event.

Treatment of somnambulism consists primarily of protecting the individual from injury (e.g., safety latches on doors and windows, removal of hazardous objects from the bedroom, covering glass doors with heavy curtains). Theoretically, sleepwalking may be prevented by suppressing delta sleep. Although BZs suppress delta sleep, the risks of long-term, continuous exposure of a developing child to delta sleep suppressants is unknown. BZs or TCAs may be beneficial in adults.[66]

SLEEP TERRORS

Sleep terrors are characterized by extreme vocalizations, motility, and autonomic changes (e.g., tachycardia, sweating) coupled with severe panic and fear. Usually sleep terrors start in the first half of the night and last for 1–10 minutes. Individuals are inconsolable and difficult to awaken; however, if awakened, they typically do not recall dream content. Sleep terror episodes are prevalent in 1–6% of children. The onset of sleep terror episodes occurs between ages 4 and 12 years and usually resolves during adolescence. Adult-onset sleep terrors occur between 20–30 years of age and may follow a chronic course with episodic waxing and waning.[13] Treatment consists of counseling the parents to wait until the disorder is outgrown. As with somnambulism, sleep terrors occur during delta sleep; BZs may be useful in adults secondary to delta sleep suppression.[66]

NIGHTMARES

The lifetime prevalence of nightmares in the general population is 10%. Nightmares are a REM phenomenon and are associated with frequent and elaborate recall of frightening dream content (e.g., dreams of physical attacks and death). Less motility and variability in autonomic parameters are present in nightmares than with sleep terrors. Once REM-suppressant drug withdrawal has been ruled out as a causative factor, the usual treatment consists of psychologic intervention. This may be as simple as a parent providing comfort and reassurance to a child with an occasional nightmare or as complex as intensive psychotherapy for an adult with frequent, highly disturbing nightmares.[66]

Evaluation of Therapeutic Outcomes

Patients with short-term or chronic insomnia should be evaluated after 1 week of therapy to assess for drug effectiveness and adverse events and for adherence to nonpharmacologic recommendations. Patients should be instructed to maintain a daily sleep diary. The diary provides a measure of baseline severity and allows the pharmacist to monitor hypnotic therapy over the course of treatment. It requires daily recording of bedtime, arising time, sleep onset latency, number and durations of awakenings, medication ingestion, naps, and an index of sleep quality.[67]

Individuals with sleep apnea treated with weight reduction and CPAP or drug therapy should be evaluated after 2–4 weeks of treatment for improvement in alertness and daytime symptoms (e.g., reduction in headache frequency and severity, improvement in memory, decreased irritability), and weight reduction. The bed partner can be consulted regarding reduced snoring and gasping episodes. A repeat PSG is indicated if the patient has not shown clinical improvement. Overall, the goals of therapy are to reduce the number of apneic episodes and improve O_2 saturation.

Monitoring parameters for the pharmacotherapy of narcolepsy include reduction in daytime sleepiness, cataplexy, hypnogogic and hypnopompic hallucinations, and sleep paralysis. Patients should be evaluated monthly until an optimal dose is achieved, then every 6–12 months to assess for the development of adverse drug events (e.g., mood changes, sleep disturbances, cardiovascular abnormalities). If symptoms increase during therapy, PSG should be performed.

Conclusion

Disturbances of sleep affect approximately one-third of the population. Effective management of sleep disturbances is dependent on a proper diagnosis. Treatment of sleep disorders includes both pharmacologic and nonpharmacologic modalities.

Identifiable causes of insomnia should be managed before pharmacologic therapy is considered. BZs are the preferable agents for the short-term treatment of insomnia; however, their use is contraindicated in sleep apnea. Antidepressants are an alternative for insomnia and effectively manage sleep apnea and symptoms of narcolepsy. The psychostimulants and TCAs are effective treatments for patients with narcolepsy. Parasomnias and circadian rhythm disorders are usually managed nonpharmacologically.

References

1. Hauri PJ, Orr WC. Current Concepts: The Sleep Disorders. Kalamazoo, MI, The Upjohn Company, 1982, p 6.
2. Farney RJ, Walker JM. Office management of common sleep–wake disorders. Med Clin North Am 1995;79:391–414.
3. Bixler EO, Kales A, Soldatos CR, et al. Prevalence of sleep disorders in the Los Angeles metropolitan area. Am J Psychiatry 1979;136:1257–1262.
4. Stoller MK. Economic effects of insomnia. Clin Ther 1994;16:873–897.
5. Culebras A. Update on disorders of sleep and the sleep–wake cycle. Psychiatric Clin North Am 1992;15:467–489.
6. Rechtschaffen A, Kales A. A manual of standardized terminology, techniques and scoring system for sleep stages of human subjects. Publication 204, Public Health Service Publications. Washington, DC, US Government Printing Office, 1968, p 1.
7. Neylan TC, Reynolds CF, Kupfer DJ. Sleep disorders, in Hales RE, Yudofsky SC, Talbott JT (eds): American Psychiatric Press Textbook of Psychiatry, 2nd ed. Washington, DC, American Psychiatric Press, 1994, p 833.
8. Lader MH. Management of insomnia. Br J Clin Prac 1990;44:125–130.
9. Morin CM. Insomnia: Psychological Assessment and Management. New York, Guilford Press, 1993, p 16.
10. Prinz PN, Vitiello MV, Raskind MA, et al. Geriatrics: Sleep disorders and aging. N Engl J Med 1990;323:520–526.
11. Ancoli-Israel S, Kripke DF, Mason WJ, et al. Sleep apnea and nocturnal myoclonus in a randomly selected elderly population: Final prevalence results. Sleep Res 1986;15:101.
12. American Sleep Disorders Association Diagnostic Classification Steering Committee. International Classification of Sleep Disorders: Diagnostic and Coding Manual. Rochester, NY, American Sleep Disorders Association, 1990, p 1.
13. American Psychiatric Association. Sleep Disorders. Diagnostic and Statistical Manual of Mental Disorders, 4th ed. Washington, DC, American Psychiatric Press, 1994, p 551.
14. Gillin JC, Byerley WF. The diagnosis and management of insomnia. N Engl J Med 1990;322:239–248.
15. Dement WC. The proper use of sleeping pills in the primary care setting. J Clin Psychiatry 1992;53(12 suppl):50–56.
16. Ford DE, Kamerow DB. Epidemiologic study of sleep disturbances and psychiatric disorders. JAMA 1989;262:1479–1484.
17. Mellinger GD, Balter MB, Uhlenhuth EH. Insomnia and its treatment: Prevalence and correlates. Arch Gen Psychiatry 1985;42:225–232.
18. Hartmann PM. Drug treatment of insomnia: Indications and newer agents. Am Fam Physician 1995;51:191–194.
19. Walsh JK, Engelhardt CL. Trends in the pharmacologic treatment of insomnia. J Clin Psychiatry 1992;53(12 suppl):10–17.
20. Morin CM, Culbert JP, Schwartz SM. Nonpharmacological interventions for insomnia: A meta-analysis of treatment efficacy. Am J Psychiatry 1994;151:1172–1180.
21. Bootzin RR, Perlis ML. Nonpharmacologic treatments of insomnia. J Clin Psychiatry 1992;53(6 suppl):37–41.

22. Soldatos CR, Kales JD, Scharf MB, et al. Cigarette smoking associated with sleep difficulty. Science 1980;207:551–553.
23. Ware JC. Tricyclic antidepressants in the treatment of insomnia. J Clin Psychiatry 1983;44:25–28.
24. Nierenberg AA, Alder LA, Peselow E, et al. Trazodone for antidepressant-associated insomnia. Am J Psychiatry 1994;151:1069–1072.
25. Hertzman PA, Blevins WL, Mayer J. Association of eosinophilia-myalgia syndrome with the ingestion of tryptophan. N Engl J Med 1990;322:869–873.
26. Hoehns JD, Perry PJ. Zolpidem: A nonbenzodiazepine hypnotic for treatment of insomnia. Clin Pharm 1993;12:814–828.
27. Zolpidem package insert. Chicago, IL, GD Searle & Co, May 1993.
28. Scharf MB, Roth T, Vogel GW, Walsh JK. A multi-center, placebo-controlled study evaluating zolpidem in the treatment of chronic insomnia. J Clin Psychiatry 1994;55:192–199.
29. Ashton H. Guidelines for the rational use of benzodiazepines: When and what to use. Drugs 1994;48:25–40.
30. Greenblatt DJ. Benzodiazepine hypnotics: Sorting the pharmacokinetic facts. J Clin Psychiatry 1991;52(9 suppl):4–10.
31. Greenblatt DJ, Harmatz JS, Engelhart N, et al. Pharmacokinetic determinants of dynamic differences among three benzodiazepine hypnotics. Arch Gen Psychiatry 1989;46:326–332.
32. Dominguez RA, Goldstein BJ, Jacobson AF, et al. Comparative efficacy of estazolam, flurazepam, and placebo in outpatients with insomnia. J Clin Psychiatry 1986;47:362–365.
33. Kales A, Bixler EO, Soldatos CR, et al. Quazepam and flurazepam: Long-term use and extended withdrawal. Clin Pharm Ther 1982;32:781–788.
34. Serzone package insert. Princeton, NJ, Bristol-Myers Squibb Co, January 1995.
35. Greenblatt DJ, von Moltke LL, Harmatz JS, et al. Interaction of triazolam and ketaconazole. Lancet 1995;345:191.
36. Greenblatt DJ, Divoll M, Harmatz JS, et al. Kinetics and clinical effects of flurazepam in young and elderly noninsomniacs. Clin Pharmacol Ther 1981;30:475–486.
37. Ankier SI, Goa KL. Quazepam. A preliminary review of its pharmacodynamic and pharmacokinetic properties, and therapeutic efficacy in insomnia. Drugs 1988;35:42–62.
38. Roth T, Roehrs TA. Issues in the use of benzodiazepine therapy. J Clin Psychiatry 1992;53(6 suppl):14–18.
39. Mendelson WB. Hypnotics in the treatment of chronic insomnia, in Thorpy MJ (ed): Handbook of Sleep Disorders. New York, Marcel Dekker, 1990, p 737.
40. ProSom package insert. Chicago, IL, Abbott Labs, October 1991.
41. Schneider-Helmert D. Why low-dose benzodiazepine dependent insomniacs can't escape their sleeping pills. Acta Psychiatr Scand 1988;78:706–711.
42. Wysowski DK, Barash D. Adverse behavioral reactions attributed to triazolam in the Food and Drug Administration's spontaneous reporting system. Arch Intern Med 1991;151:2003–2008.
43. Juhl RP, Daugherty VM, Kroboth PD. Incidence of next-day anterograde amnesia caused by flurazepam hydrochloride and triazolam. Clin Pharm 1984;3:622–625.
44. Ghaeli P, Dufresne RL, Stoukides CA. Triazolam treatment controversy. Ann Pharmacotherapy 1994;28:1038–1040.
45. Kales A, Manfredi RL, Vgontzas AN, et al. Rebound insomnia after only brief and intermittent use of rapidly eliminated benzodiazepines. Clin Pharmacol Ther 1991;49:468–476.
46. Roehrs T, Vogel G, Roth T. Rebound insomnia: Its determinants and significance. Am J Med 1990;88(suppl 3A):39–42.
47. Monane M. Insomnia in the elderly. J Clin Psychiatry 1992;53(6 suppl):23–28.
48. Ray WA, Griffin MR, Schaffner W. Psychotropic drug use and the risk of hip fracture. N Engl J Med 1987;316:363–369.
49. Rapoport DM. Treatment of sleep apnea syndromes. Mt Sinai J Med 1994;61:123–130.
50. Brown LK. Sleep apnea syndromes: Overview and diagnostic approaches. Mt Sinai J Med 1994;61:99–112.
51. Kaplan J, Staats BA. Obstructive sleep apnea syndrome. Mayo Clin Proc 1990;65:1087–1094.
52. Hanzeol DA, Proia NG, Hudgel DW. Response of obstructive sleep apnea to fluoxetine and protriptyline. Chest 1991;100:416–421.
53. Mulloy E, McNicholas WT. Theophylline in obstructive sleep apnea: A double-blind evaluation. Chest 1992;101:753–757.
54. Issa FG. Effect of clonidine in obstructive sleep apnea. Am Rev Respir Dis 1992;145:435–439.
55. Hanly PJ. Mechanisms and management of central sleep apnea. Lung 1992;170:1–17.
56. Aldrich MS. Narcolepsy. Neurol 1992;42(suppl 6):34–43.
57. Mitler MM, Aldrich MS, Koob GF, Zarcone VP. ASDA standards of practice: Narcolepsy and its treatment with stimulants. Sleep 1994;17:352–371.
58. Garma L, Murchand F. Non-pharmacological approaches to the treatment of narcolepsy. Sleep 1994;17:S97–S102.
59. Standard of Practice Committee of the American Sleep Disorders Association. Practice parameters for the use of stimulants in the treatment of narcolepsy. Sleep 1994;17:348–351.
60. Hublin C, Partinen M, Heinonen EF, et al. Selegiline in the treatment of narcolepsy. Neurol 1994;44:2095–2101.
61. Lammers GJ, Arends J, Declerck AC, et al. Gammahydroxybutyrate and narcolepsy: A double-blind placebo-controlled study. Sleep 1993;16:216–220.
62. Wagner DR. Circadian rhythm sleep disorders, in Thorpy MJ (ed): Handbook of Sleep Disorders. New York, Marcel Dekker, 1990, p 493.
63. Seidel WF, Cohen SA, Bliwise NG, et al. Treatment of jet lag with triazolam. Sleep Res 1987;16:140.
64. Walsh JK, Muehlbach MJ, Schweitzer PK. Acute administration of triazolam for the daytime sleep of shift workers. Sleep 1984;7:223–229.
65. Czeisler CA, Johnson MP, Duffy JF, et al. Exposure to bright light and darkness to treat physiologic maladaptation to night work. N Engl J Med 1990;322:1253–1259.
66. Kales A, Soldatos CR, Kales JD. Sleep disorders: Insomnia, night terrors, nightmares, and enuresis. Arch Intern Med 1987;106:582–592.
67. Morin CM. Insomnia: Psychological Assessment and Management. New York, Guilford Press, 1993, p 61.

Section 7
Endocrinologic Disorders

Chapter 72

Diabetes Mellitus

Condit F. Steil, PharmD, CDE

The term *diabetes mellitus* describes a series of complex and chronic metabolic disorders characterized by symptomatic glucose intolerance. Because diabetes appears to be a heterogeneous group of disorders, there is no commonality with regard to the age of onset, genetic predisposition, or development of complications. It is known, however, that all diabetics eventually show abnormalities of insulin secretion and complications of the disease, such as vascular and neurologic abnormalities and most manifest some degree of cellular resistance to insulin in non–insulin-dependent diabetes mellitus.

Recent data from the American Diabetes Association shows some dramatic trends in the incidence of diabetes. Approximately 14 million people in America have diabetes, but more than 6 million of these individuals have not been diagnosed. It is especially troublesome in minority populations, including Hispanics, African Americans, American Indians, and Asian Americans, where there is a two to five times higher rate of diabetes and a subsequently greater burden from its complications. As detection and screening methods become more common, the identification of patients will increase.

The annual costs of diabetes care during 1992 were estimated at $91.8 billion for both direct and indirect costs, with $46.7 billion of this total representing direct costs of care. Diabetes is the leading cause of blindness in adults ages 20–74, the leading cause by category of end-stage renal disease, and accounts for approximately 55,000 lower extremity amputations annually.[1] This is true even though new technology provides opportunity for early intervention, treatment, and limitation of the complications.

Pathogenesis/Classification

Historically, diabetes was classified primarily by age of onset and ease of control. Such terms as *juvenile onset, adult onset, brittle, chemical, overt,* and *latent* often made the understanding of diabetes difficult. In 1979, the National Diabetes Data Group reclassified diabetes into two main types: insulin-dependent diabetes mellitus (IDDM or type I) and non–insulin-dependent diabetes mellitus (NIDDM or type II).[2] The American Diabetes Association has adopted this classification, but is presently reviewing it for possible revision. Specifically, a method of differentiating insulin-sensitive and insulin-resistant type II disease is being planned. Smaller groups of persons' diabetes etiologies include diabetes secondary to various drugs and diseases, impaired glucose tolerance (IGT), and gestational diabetes mellitus. (See Table 72.1 for a more complete classification.)

TYPE I

Type I diabetes usually develops in childhood or early adulthood and accounts for up to 10% of all diabetics. These patients are often thin, have an absolute lack of insulin, and are prone to develop diabetic ketoacidosis (DKA) if insulin is withheld. This is probably a heterogeneous disorder; heredity, viruses, and autoimmune syndromes have been linked to its development.

TABLE 72.1. CLASSIFICATION OF DIABETES MELLITUS AND IMPAIRED GLUCOSE TOLERANCE

Diabetes mellitus
- Type I: insulin-dependent diabetes mellitus (IDDM)
- Type II: non–insulin-dependent diabetes mellitus (NIDDM)

Secondary causes of diabetes mellitus
- Pancreatic disease and endocrinopathies
  - Chronic pancreatitis, cystic fibrosis, pancreatectomy, hemochromatosis
  - Acromegaly, Cushing's disease, glucagonoma, pheochromocytoma, primary aldosteronism
- Drugs: catecholamines, glucocorticoids, oral contraceptives, thiazide and loop diuretics
- Genetic syndromes: Huntington's chorea, hyperlipidemia, muscular dystrophy

Causes of impaired glucose tolerance
- Pre–diabetes mellitus
- Secondary to pancreatic disease, drugs, and genetic syndromes (see secondary causes of diabetes mellitus above)
- Gestational glucose intolerance

TYPE II

Type II diabetes usually manifests in adulthood around age 40 or later. About 90% of patients with diabetes develop type II diabetes. Type II diabetes also appears to be a heterogeneous group, although it is more genetically linked than is type I diabetes with some HLA linking (DR3 and DR4) identified.[3] About 90% of patients with NIDDM are obese and may not display the classic symptoms of diabetes. They may initially be hyposecretors, normal secretors, or hypersecretors of insulin; however, the insulin does not appear to be effective in the transport of glucose into cells. Inactive receptors, desensitized receptors, or inadequate insulin action may produce this condition. NIDDM patients do not usually progress to ketoacidosis except during periods of stress; therefore, insulin replacement is not an absolute necessity for initial therapy, but may ultimately be needed as their insulin production declines. Many clinicians are beginning to group NIDDM patients as *insulin sensitive* and *insulin resistant* to more accurately describe their disease. This classification is under current study. (See Table 72.2 for a more thorough differentiation between type I and II diabetes.)

OTHER TYPES

Some people develop diabetes as a result of preexisting pancreatic disease or a hormone excess (e.g., ACTH, cortisol) resulting from endocrine disease or hormone treatment. Diabetes may also result from the use of certain medications (e.g., thiazide diuretics) or from insulin receptor abnormalities.

Gestational diabetes mellitus (GDM) refers to the onset of glucose intolerance during pregnancy, usually in the second or third trimester. Those patients who require drug therapy must use insulin, but usually return to normal glucose tolerance postdelivery. Most clinicians recommend general screening by weeks 24–28 of the pregnancy, and subsequent follow-up due to the risk that up to 40% of persons with GDM will develop diabetes within the next 10 years.[4]

IMPAIRED GLUCOSE TOLERANCE

Impaired glucose tolerance (IGT) is the term given to patients who have higher than normal plasma glucose lev-

TABLE 72.2. GENERAL CHARACTERISTICS OF TYPE I AND TYPE II DIABETICS

Characteristic	Type I Diabetes	Type II Diabetes
Age of onset	Usually during childhood or adolescence	Usually age 40 or older
Rapidness of onset	Usually abrupt	Usually gradual
Family history	Usually little family history of diabetes	Positive history for diabetes is common
Etiology	Unknown; postulated causes include heredity, autoimmune diseases, and viral infections	Unknown, but heredity is highly associated with occurrence
Body weight	Usually thin and undernourished	Obesity is common
Insulin	Secretion is markedly diminished early in the disease and may be totally absent later in the disease; insulin therapy is mandatory	Levels may be low (indicating deficiency), normal, or high (indicating insulin resistance); insulin therapy may not be required, decreasing as the disease progresses, indicating the pancreas loses its insulin production capacity
Ketosis	Common, especially with proper insulin control	Uncommon; if present, usually associated with severe stress or infection
Symptoms	Polyuria, polydipsia, polyphagia, weight loss	May be asymptomatic, polyuria and/or polydipsia may be present

els but are not diagnostic for diabetes. Although about 25% of these patients will develop diabetes mellitus, it is important not to label these patients as diabetic until a definite diagnosis has been made because social, insurance, and job limitations often result for persons with diabetes. Medications may be identified as the cause of IGT (Table 72.3).

METABOLISM AND UTILIZATION OF CARBOHYDRATES, PROTEINS, AND FATS

INSULIN: DIABETES-RELATED CHANGES

Before understanding the etiology, manifestations, or complications of diabetes, one must first be familiar with normal carbohydrate, protein, and fat metabolism. Carbohydrates are metabolized in the body to glucose, the body's main source of glucose. The glucose is absorbed from the gastrointestinal (GI) tract into the bloodstream, where it is oxidized in skeletal muscle to produce energy. Glucose is also stored in the liver in the form of glycogen and is converted in adipose tissue to fats and triglycerides. Insulin, which is produced in, stored in, and released from the β cells of the pancreas, facilitates these processes. It increases uptake of glucose by the tissues, increases liver glycogen levels, decreases glycogen breakdown (glycogenolysis) by the liver, increases synthesis of fatty acids, decreases breakdown of fatty acids into ketone bodies, and promotes incorporation of amino acids into proteins.[5]

Insulin is released from a functioning pancreas at a rate of 0.5–1 U/h. Additional insulin is also released when the blood sugar is in excess of 100 mg/dL. The normal adult pancreas secretes 25–50 U of insulin per day. Insulin is cleared metabolically by the liver, peripheral tissues, and kidneys. Hence, it is not unusual for patients with renal disease to require less insulin simply because insulin is not being cleared totally by metabolism.

Glucose can diffuse into the brain without the aid of insulin, but muscle and fat require the presence of insulin to receive glucose for energy. Glucose is the primary energy source for the body's cells. If glucose is not available to muscle and adipose tissue, these tissues will convert amino acids and fatty acids to carbohydrates (called gluconeogenesis). If this tissue deprivation continues, the tissue will eventually metabolize stored fats, resulting in the production of free fatty acids that are eventually oxidized to ketone bodies.[5]

The body normally maintains plasma glucose concentrations between 40 and 160 mg/dL. A plasma glucose concentration of at least 40 mg/dL is necessary for brain function. Symptoms of hypoglycemia will usually be present at these concentrations. A high plasma concentration implies that glucose is not being transported into cells for energy production. Plasma concentrations in excess of 180 mg/dL usually exceed the renal tubular maximal reabsorption rate or "threshold" for reabsorption; consequently, glucose, which is not normally present in the urine, spills into the urine. Higher concentrations may actually cause an osmotic diuresis. Of course, because these plasma values are only averages, there may be significant interpatient variation, especially when considering the trend for the threshold to increase with aging.

COUNTERREGULATORY HORMONES

In addition to insulin, other substances in the body play a role in the regulation of blood glucose levels.[5]

TABLE 72.3. DRUGS CAUSING SIGNIFICANT ELEVATIONS IN PLASMA GLUCOSE CONCENTRATION

Drug	Mechanism of Action	Clinical Significance
Alcohol	Chronic ingestion increases tolbutamide metabolism	+
Asparaginase	Related to inhibition of insulin synthesis	++
β-adrenergic antagonists	Inhibit insulin secretion	++
Calcium channel blockers	Inhibit insulin secretion	+/–
Combination oral contraceptives	Unknown	++
Diazoxide	Inhibits insulin secretion	+++
Diuretics	May be related to hypokalemia	++
Glucocorticoids	Increase gluconeogenesis, depress insulin action	+++
Glycerol	Unknown	++
Lithium salts	May decrease insulin secretion	+
Niacin	Unknown	++
Pentamidine isethionate	Promotes pancreatic toxicity	+++
Phenytoin sodium	Inhibits insulin secretion	++
Rifampin	Enhances metabolism of tolbutamide	+
Sympathomimetics	Increase glycogenolysis and gluconeogenesis	++

+ = relative significance, not quantitative. (From White J, Hartman J, Campbell RK. Drug interactions in diabetic patients. Postgrad Med 1993;93:137.)

Glucagon

The α cells of the endocrine pancreas produce glucagon, which opposes the effects of insulin. Glucagon secretion is stimulated during fasting to prevent blood glucose values from dropping too low. Glucagon increases blood glucose by increasing glycogenolysis and gluconeogenesis in the liver.

Growth Hormone

Secreted from the anterior pituitary, growth hormone also opposes the action of insulin by interfering with the body's ability to utilize glucose. One stimulus for growth hormone secretion is hypoglycemia.

Somatostatin

Somatostatin is produced in the γ cells of the pancreas. It inhibits both insulin and glucagon secretion and suppresses growth hormone. This results in a fall in blood glucose levels because of the suppression of glucagon. In addition, somatostatin inhibits absorption of glucose from the GI tract.

Epinephrine

Epinephrine, secreted by the adrenal medulla, acts to increase blood glucose levels by stimulating the conversion of glycogen to glucose in the liver. Similarly, drugs, such as ephedrine and phenylpropanolamine, which stimulate the release of epinephrine and other catecholamines, can also produce an elevation in plasma glucose levels via the same mechanism.

Glucocorticoids

Compounds with glucocorticoid activity elevate plasma glucose by stimulating gluconeogenesis, thereby causing a marked increase in liver glycogen. They do not, however, increase glycogen in any other body cells. In fact, glucocorticoids decrease glycogen stores in all other cells because they decrease glucose uptake and utilization by these cells.

Thyroid Hormone

Thyroid hormone elevates blood glucose by increasing the rate of absorption of glucose from the GI tract. Moreover, thyroid hormone increases liver gluconeogenesis and glycogenolysis. Some similarity between the autoimmune reactions of Hashimoto's thyroiditis and diabetes has been identified.

CLINICAL PRESENTATION

The classic symptoms of diabetes include polyuria (excessive urination), polydipsia (increased thirst), and polyphagia (increased appetite with increased calorie intake). As plasma glucose levels increase to about 180 mg/dL, the reabsorptive capacity of the kidneys for glucose is exceeded, resulting in spillage of glucose into the urine. Higher urine glucose levels then result in an osmotic diuresis. This diuresis produces the symptom of polyuria, which can lead to dehydration with accompanying polydipsia. Because glucose cannot be adequately transported into cells, the "hunger sensation" is triggered, resulting in polyphagia. These symptoms are common in type I patients along with weight loss, weakness, and dry skin. The onset of these symptoms is rapid, and secondary ketoacidosis is common.[6]

Type II diabetes, however, presents gradually and may be present without symptoms. Because the type II patient is usually obese (except for the elderly who are usually of normal weight), weight loss and/or polyphagia may be absent or go unnoticed. Polyuria may be a presenting complaint, but most type II diabetics are discovered because of an abnormal blood or urine glucose on routine physical examination or screening.

SCREENING TESTS

It has been estimated that about 2.5% of the U.S. population may have diabetes that will go undetected unless screening tests are performed. Persons who should be screened for diabetes include those with a strong family history of diabetes mellitus; persons who are markedly obese; women with an obstetrical history resulting in morbidity or a history of babies of over 9 pounds at birth, and all women between 24 and 28 weeks of pregnancy; anyone with recurrent skin, genital, or urinary tract infections, older than 65 years of age, of certain races (American Indian, Hispanic, African American), or who have had previous impaired glucose tolerance.[1,2,7] Table 72.4 lists a questionnaire for screening utilized by the American Diabetes Association for identifying persons at risk who may need a blood test.

TABLE 72.4. DIABETES SCREENING QUESTIONNAIRE

Could You Have Diabetes and NOT Know It?	Point Values
1. My weight is equal to or above that listed in the chart (chart lists 20% heavier than recommended weights).	Yes 5 ______
2. I am under 65 years of age and I get little or no exercise during a usual day.	Yes 5 ______
3. I am between 45 and 64 years of age.	Yes 5 ______
4. I am 65 years old or older.	Yes 9 ______
5. I am a woman who has had a baby weighing more than 9 pounds at birth.	Yes 1 ______
6. I have a sister or brother with diabetes.	Yes 1 ______
7. I have a parent with diabetes.	Yes 1 ______

TABLE 72.5. DIAGNOSTIC CRITERIA FOR DIABETES MELLITUS

Nonpregnant adults—must display ONE

a. Random plasma glucose ≥200 mg/dL **plus** classic signs and symptoms (polyuria, polydipsia, polyphagia, weight loss)
b. Fasting plasma glucose level ≥140 mg/dL on at least two occasions
c. Fasting plasma glucose <140 mg/dL **plus** at least two sustained glucose levels during the OGTT (one 0- to 2-h glucose level and the 2-h level should be ≥200 mg/dL)

Children—must display ONE

a. Random plasma glucose ≥200 mg/dL **plus** classic signs and symptoms (polyuria, polydipsia, ketonuria, weight loss)
b. Fasting plasma glucose ≥140 mg/dL on at least two occasions **plus** at least two sustained glucose levels during the OGTT (one 0- to 2-h glucose level and the 2-h level should be ≥200 mg/dL)

Pregnant women—diagnosis of gestational diabetes is made if two plasma glucose values equal or exceed the following:

Fasting	105 mg/dL
1 h	190 mg/dL
2 h	165 mg/dL
3 h	145 mg/dL

TABLE 72.6. CRITERIA FOR IMPAIRED GLUCOSE TOLERANCE

Children—must display BOTH

a. Fasting plasma glucose <140 mg/dL
b. 2-h OGTT plasma level >140 mg/dL

Nonpregnant adults—must display ALL

a. Fasting plasma glucose <140 mg/dL
b. 2-h OGTT level between 140 and 200 mg/dL
c. 0- to 2-h OGTT level ≥200 mg/dL

The recommended screening test for nonpregnant adults and children is a fasting plasma glucose level. The patient should fast 10–14 hours prior to the test and should have discontinued any medications that may lower or raise plasma glucose 3 days before testing if possible. Other screening tests have included urine glucose determinations, 2-hour postprandial plasma glucose determinations, or random plasma glucose levels. In pregnant women, a 50-g oral glucose load is recommended for screening.[8]

DIAGNOSTIC TESTS

Most patients can be diagnosed with diabetes on the basis of classic signs and symptoms plus a positive screening test (see the following criteria); however, those patients who have only one of the following should undergo diagnostic testing with an oral glucose tolerance test (OGTT):

1. Positive screening test
2. Presence of obvious signs and symptoms of diabetes such as polydipsia, polyuria, polyphagia, or weight loss
3. Inconclusive findings of a random plasma glucose level

For a meaningful glucose tolerance test, the patient should have fasted for the past 10–14 hours and should have discontinued glucose-altering medications 3 days before the test day if possible. The patient must not be carbohydrate depleted and should have an adequate carbohydrate intake 3 days prior to testing. He or she should be instructed not to smoke or drink coffee just before and during the test, because misleading elevations in plasma glucose may occur. A fasting plasma glucose is then drawn. The patient is administered a standard glucose-containing solution (75 g for adults, and 1.75 g/kg ideal body weight up to 75 g for children). In nonpregnant adults and children, blood samples are drawn every 30 minutes for 2 hours. In pregnant women, blood samples are drawn every hour for 3 hours. Plasma glucose values should peak in about 1 hour, remain under 200 mg/dL throughout the test, and return to fasting values by the 2-hour interval.[2,6] (See Table 72.5 for specific diagnostic criteria.) Those patients who have abnormal test results and cannot be diagnosed as diabetic are classified as having IGT. The criteria for the diagnosis of IGT are listed in Table 72.6.

Once the diagnosis of diabetes has been made, it is important to classify the patient as having either type I or type II diabetes. Usually the classification can be made on the basis of age, suddenness of onset, and physical characteristics of the patient. C-peptides have also been used to distinguish between type I and II diabetics. Proinsulin is cleaved in the pancreas to form insulin and C-peptide molecules. Therefore, patients with no insulin production have little, if any, production of C-peptides.[9] Regardless of the criteria used to classify the diabetic, it is important to remember that the type I diabetic has an absolute lack of insulin and must be given exogenous insulin to sustain life and prevent ketoacidosis. Therapy for type II diabetes, however, can often be started without oral medication or insulin.

TREATMENT

GOALS AND THE DCCT

The basic goals of diabetes therapy had remained largely unchanged for several years. Many clinicians assumed that tighter management of glucose was beneficial to the patient's welfare, although little clinical data supported this belief. The results of a large, multicenter, long-term study, which studied the basic premise of tight management making a difference, were reported in 1993. The study was the

TABLE 72.7. TREATMENT PLAN—DIABETES CONTROL AND COMPLICATIONS TRIAL

Treatment Parameter	Treatment Groups: Conventional	Treatment Groups: Intensive
Insulin	1 or 2 daily injections	3 or > injections or insulin pump
Testing	Daily monitoring, urine or blood	Blood monitoring several times per day
Diet and exercise instruction	Quarterly	Monthly
Follow-up exam	Quarterly	Monthly
Care contact	PRN, by patient	Weekly by nurse

Diabetes Control and Complications Trial (DCCT) and involved 1441 patients treated for more than 7000 patient-years. The two hypotheses for the study were as follows: "Does tight management prevent the initiation of complications?" (primary prevention) and "Does tight management prevent or limit the progression of diabetes complications?" (secondary intervention). Retinopathy was the complication used for assigning patients to the prevention or intervention cohort. The patients had type I diabetes and were divided into intensive and conventional treatment groups with their therapy plan noted in Table 72.7. The study results are listed in Table 72.8. Note the significant improvement in microvascular and neurologic complication progression. The primary adverse event in the intensive treatment group was a two- to threefold increase in severe hypoglycemia.[10]

The dramatic findings of the study have changed the therapy goals—certainly for IDDM patients—and triggered planning to apply the same principles to NIDDM therapy since the cellular changes causing complication development are similar. However, application to NIDDM patients directly is difficult due to their insulin resistance and other disorders that may be present. Some limitations to applying the same intensive principles to all patients exist. Persons who already have significant hypoglycemia unawareness or significant cardiovascular disease may be poor candidates due to the potential for hypoglycemia. Young patients, while clinicians desire good control, may be challenges due to the rapid changes that occur. Add to this equation the very intense intervention that occurred, and one can see the motivation for the statement by the DCCT staff that innovative approaches in providing intensive care must be studied. However, the best information provided by the DCCT is that by separating the cohorts by individuals who achieved similar levels of glycemic improvement, any improvement in glucose control helped![10]

TABLE 72.8. RESULTS—DIABETES CONTROL AND COMPLICATIONS TRIAL: RISK REDUCTIONS FROM CONVENTIONAL TO INTENSIVE COHORTS (BOTH PRIMARY AND SECONDARY INTERVENTIONS)

Complication	Reduction (%)
>3 step sustained retinopathy	63
Macular edema	26
Severe nonproliferative or proliferative retinopathy	47
Laser treatment	51
Urinary albumin excretion (mg/24 h)	
>40	39
>300	54
Clinical neuropathy at 5 years	60

The treatment of diabetes varies considerably between type I and type II diabetes. Type I diabetics have an absolute lack of insulin, so that diet, exercise, self-monitoring of blood glucose, and insulin are necessary for proper management. The therapy for type II diabetes also consists of diet and exercise; however, oral medications or insulin may or may not be required. The goals of diet for the two types of diabetics are often quite different. The overall goal of therapy, however, is consistent—to maintain the plasma glucose in an acceptable range throughout the day so that the patient remains asymptomatic. Desirable plasma glucose concentrations are listed in Table 72.9.

PATIENT EDUCATION

Successful treatment of diabetes involves lifestyle changes for the patient (e.g., diet, exercise, self-monitoring of blood and possibly urine, and/or taking medication). The patient, therefore, must be involved in the decision-making process. He or she must learn as much as possible about diabetes, including why the symptoms of diabetes are occurring and how a controlled blood glucose concentration will alleviate the symptoms. The long-term complications of diabetes

TABLE 72.9. GOALS OF THERAPY

Parameter	Normal	Acceptable	Fair	Poor
Fasting plasma glucose (mg/dL)	115	140	200	>200
Postprandial plasma glucose (mg/dL)	140	175	235	>235
Glycosylated hemoglobin[a] (%)	6	<8	8–9.5	>10

[a]Increase limits 10% for elderly patients.

must be explained to the patient, stressing that newer evidence indicates that many of these complications can be curtailed or prevented with a well-controlled blood glucose concentration. The DCCT was carried out at each center by a team that included nurse and dietitian educators. Long-term control was achieved with an intensive treatment regimen *and* a team approach to follow up and positive support. Recognition of this need for proper patient involvement in care has spawned a new specialty practice of diabetes education, including a certification process whose requirements are noted in Table 72.10. Most educators follow a two-phase education structure, with survival skills taught initially and then self-care management, which mandates behavior change and patient motivation.[11]

DIET

Recent changes in the American Diabetes Association's nutrition guidelines have created some alteration in the approach of dietary management of diabetes. Effective self-management requires an individualized approach for building a diet plan, usually involving the input of a dietitian. The goal of the diet plan for type I patients is to build a healthy daily nutrition intake into a regimen that allows flexibility in insulin therapy and home monitoring. The emphasis on dietary therapy for type II patients should be placed on achieving blood glucose, lipid, and blood pressure goals. Weight loss usually improves short-term glucose levels. Few patients achieve long-term weight loss. Therefore, the emphasis shifts to glucose and lipid goals. Healthy food choices may be the first step used for the type II patient, who needs to obtain the calories with less saturated fat and protein.

Data are limited with regard to establishing firm protein nutritional recommendations for diabetes patients. The recommendation is the same as for the general population, about 10–20% of total calories. This is reduced for patients with renal failure. Less than 10% of the total daily intake should come from saturated fats, and up to 10% from polyunsaturated fats, leaving 60–70% of the total calories between carbohydrates and monounsaturated fats. The distribution of calories between these two remaining categories varies from patient to patient depending on the assessment and treatment goals. For individuals with near-normal body weight and lipid levels, the recommendations of 30% or less of the calories from total fat could be implemented, leaving 50–60% of the calories as carbohydrates. If obesity and weight loss are major issues, a reduction in dietary fat can be effective in achieving positive change. One may also want to consider the Step II diet guidelines of the National Cholesterol Education Program, which calls for <7% of the total calories from saturated fat, with <200 mg cholesterol.

TABLE 72.10. CERTIFIED DIABETES EDUCATOR REQUIREMENTS

1. Professional education: currently hold a U.S. license as an RN, RD, RPh, MD, licensed PA, podiatrist, registered PT, registered OT *or* hold at least a master's level education in the chosen health profession.
2. Experience: at least 2000 hours of direct diabetes patient education in the United States in an organized education program in at least 2 years and within the past 10 years.
3. Successfully pass the certification examination.
4. Recertification by examination every 5 years.

The percentage of calories from carbohydrates will vary and should be individualized with the patient's eating habits and therapy goals. For many years, patients with diabetes were taught to avoid simple sugars. There is little evidence that the assumed rapid absorption and increase in glucose actually occurs when the sugar is part of the basic meal plan. Rather than a concern for the type of carbohydrate source (starch, bread, etc.), one should be concerned with the total amount consumed.

The patient should understand the need for attention to the amount of other nutritive sweeteners (fructose, sorbitol, etc.) consumed and their being "hidden" in several foods. The polyols of course carry the potential for a laxative effect. Sodium intake should receive attention with the risk link for hypertension. Similar precautions for alcohol consumption apply to persons with diabetes as with the public at large. The risk for hypoglycemia acutely can be enhanced when alcohol is consumed on an empty stomach. Although it has no nutritional value, its calories must be accounted for, and moderation is the key, avoiding binges. One should consider the potential for combinations of concurrent pancreatitis, neuropathy, and alcohol consumption as well as individual occurrences.[12,13]

It is becoming increasingly evident that all diabetics (type I and type II) should begin monitoring blood glucose concentrations at home to see which foods adversely affect the control of their blood glucose (see section on Monitoring Therapy). Unless the patient has some way of monitoring progress, diet usually fails as a means of controlling diabetes.

EXERCISE

Unless contraindicated, appropriate physical activity should be recommended to improve insulin sensitivity and possibly improve glucose tolerance. Exercise can also help promote weight loss and maintain ideal body weight when combined with restricted caloric intake.[14] Exercise, however, is not recommended if the patient has poorly controlled, labile blood glucose levels or is at increased risk from diabetic complications (discussed later). Strenuous exercise is usually not wise in the patient prone to developing hypoglycemia unless the patient is well educated about the symptoms and consequences of hypoglycemia and has taken proper measures to anticipate and treat this condition. Diabetics having progressive complications involving the eyes or feet should avoid strenuous activity that may cause further damage.[15]

ORAL HYPOGLYCEMICS

For the type II diabetic who has successfully lost weight and has maintained proper diet and caloric distribution but has still failed to control blood glucose adequately, the clinician is faced with initiating drug therapy. The dilemma of whether to prescribe an oral hypoglycemic agent or insulin now arises. In the late 1960s, the University Group Diabetes Program (UGDP) study examined diet alone versus diet plus oral hypoglycemia (tolbutamide) versus diet plus insulin in controlling short- and long-term diabetes.[16] The doses of each of the medications were fixed, and of course no home blood glucose monitoring was available. One of the conclusions of the study was that prolonged use of an oral hypoglycemic agent greatly increased cardiovascular mortality. Physicians were advised against using oral hypoglycemics in most patients, especially in younger type II diabetics. Since that time, however, numerous flaws in the design and conclusions of the study were uncovered, and patients on sulfonylureas are not believed to have a greater risk. Although controversy regarding the overall safety and long-term efficacy of oral hypoglycemic agents still exists, this form of therapy is preferred by most clinicians and type II patients. Insulin resistance, hyperlipidemia, hypertension, and hyperinsulinemia may induce these reactions with a condition termed Syndrome X, causing a higher risk of cardiovascular problems.[17]

The sulfonylureas have been the only class of oral hypoglycemics marketed in the United States until recently. In late 1994, a biguanide known as metformin was approved for use by the FDA and released in April 1995. While structurally in the same class as a product called phenformin, its ability to induce the life-threatening lactic acidosis is much lower. A possible protocol or plan for implementing therapy of NIDDM is shown in Figure 72.1. The sulfonylureas are classified into two groups or generations based on their potency, duration of action, and drug interaction/side-effect profiles. All oral agents exert their initial effect by increasing β-cell insulin secretion. After several months, insulin levels return to pretreatment values but glucose levels remain improved. This suggests that sulfonylureas exert extrapancreatic as well as pancreatic effects on glucose metabolism. The extrapancreatic mechanisms of action may include reducing the rate of hepatic glucose production, increasing the insulin receptor sensitivity, and increasing the number of insulin receptors—although little convincing evidence for these mechanisms is presented and enhancing insulin release remains their action.[18]

Approximately 60–70% of all patients with type II diabetes have an initial response to sulfonylurea therapy. Primary failure with an oral hypoglycemic medication occurs when a patient does not respond initially to the drug;

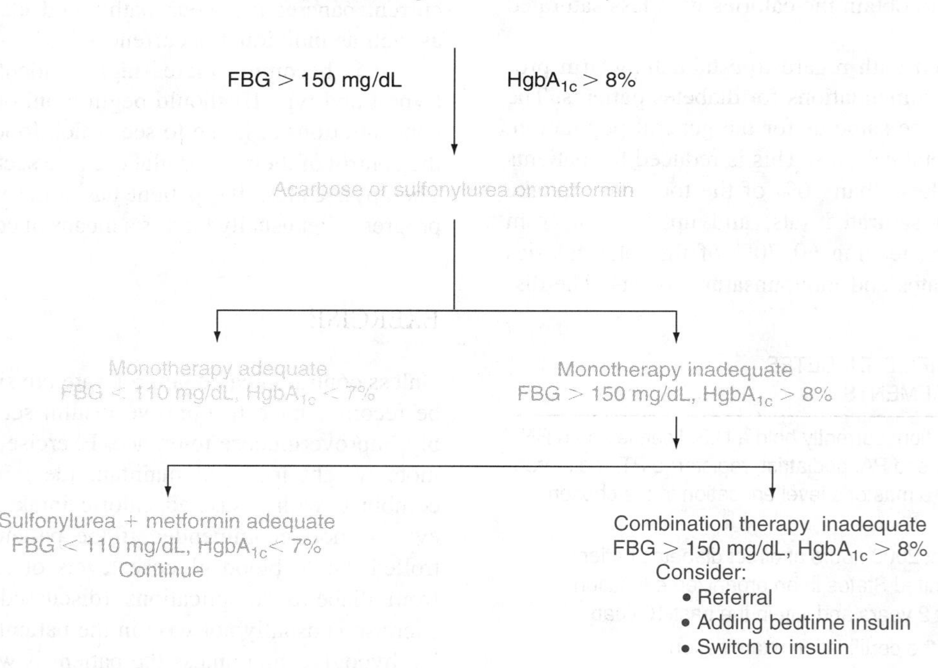

Figure 72.1. Proposed treatment algorithm for type II diabetes.

however, when initial glycemic control has been achieved with an oral agent and then lost, the patient is considered to be a secondary drug failure. About 5–20% of patients experience secondary failure because of the patient's failure to follow a dietary plan, because of the insulin-sensitive group previously mentioned, or because of the occurrence of an underlying stressful condition or disease. If a patient fails to respond to sulfonylureas because of progression of the disease, then the clinician may increase the dose of the present drug, switch to metformin, switch the patient to insulin, or prescribe combined insulin–oral hypoglycemic therapy. Note that only about 10% of patients will respond when changed from one sulfonylurea to another.[7] If the patient fails to respond to sulfonylurea therapy because of underlying stress or disease, he or she should receive insulin at least until termination of the stressful period, at which time oral therapy can usually be successfully reinitiated.

All sulfonylureas have similar mechanisms of action, pharmacologic effects, and side-effect profiles. Generally, there are few therapeutic differences among the agents. Any of these drugs should be administered 30 minutes before breakfast for maximum absorption, with glipizide more affected than the others. Since these drugs have structural similarities to sulfonamides, dermatologic side effects are relatively common, occurring in approximately 3% of patients. Hypoglycemia is the major side effect of these drugs. The duration of action of the parent compound plus the formation of active metabolites determine the degree of hypoglycemia expected with each agent.[18]

First-Generation Agents

The first-generation oral hypoglycemics include tolbutamide, acetohexamide, tolazamide, and chlorpropamide (Table 72.11). Tolbutamide is the shortest acting sulfonylurea (6–12 hours) and is metabolized in the liver to inactive metabolites, which are excreted in the urine. On a weight basis, tolbutamide is the least potent of the first-generation hypoglycemics, but the net hypoglycemic effect from the maximum dose is usually equivalent. Although some

TABLE 72.11. ORAL AGENTS FOR DIABETES

Generic (trade)	Onset (h)	Half-Life (h)	Duration (h)	Recommended Starting Dose: Nonelderly	Recommended Starting Dose: Elderly	Maximum Dose per Day	Metabolism/ Elimination
Sulfonylureas							
First-generation agents							
Tolbutamide (orinase)	1	5.6	6–12	1–2 g/d	500 mg/d to 500 mg twice daily	2–3 g	Metabolized in liver to inactive metabolites that are excreted renally
Acetohexamide (Dymelor)	1	5	10–14	250 mg–1.5 g/d	125–250 mg/d	1.5 g	Metabolized in liver; metabolite's potency is equal to or greater than that of parent compound; renally eliminated
Tolazamide (Tolinase)	4–6	7	10–14	100–250 mg/d	100 mg/d	750 mg–1 g	Metabolized in liver; metabolite less active than parent compound; renally eliminated
Chlorpropamide (Diabinese)	1	35	72	250 mg/d	100 mg/d	500 mg	Metabolized in liver; also excreted unchanged in the urine
Second-generation agents							
Glyburide (Diaβeta, Micronase)	1.5	2–4	18–24	2.5 mg/d	1.25–2.5 mg/d	20 mg	Metabolized in liver; 50% of metabolites eliminated in urine, 50% in feces
Glyburide, micronized (Glynase)	1.5	2–4	18–24	1.5 mg	1.5–3 mg	12 mg	Metabolized in liver; 50% metabolites eliminated in urine, 50% in feces
Glipizide (Glucotrol)	1	3–7	10–24	5 mg/d	2.5–5 mg/d	40 mg	Metabolized in liver to inactive metabolites; renally eliminated
Biguanides							
Metformin (Glucophage)	1.5	1.5–4.9	16–20	500 mg	500–1000 mg	2550 mg	Urinary excretion

patients, particularly the elderly, respond to once-daily dosing, tolbutamide is usually administered two to three times a day to control plasma glucose. Many clinicians consider this drug safer than other agents, in patients with renal impairment or in the elderly.[17,18]

Tolazamide (Tolinase) and acetohexamide (Dymelor) are intermediate-acting sulfonylureas that are metabolized by the liver. Exhibiting a duration of action of 12–24 hours, tolazamide is usually administered once or twice a day.[17,18] Because its three active metabolites are eliminated renally, hypoglycemia may result in the patient with renal failure. Acetohexamide's primary metabolite is 2 to 2.5 times more potent than the parent compound. Both acetohexamide and its metabolite exhibit diuretic and potent uricosuric activity. Like tolazamide, acetohexamide is usually administered once or twice daily and can accumulate in patients with renal failure.

Chlorpropamide has the longest duration of action of any of the oral hypoglycemic agents (60–72 hours) and is usually prescribed once per day. The drug is more than 80% metabolized in the liver to active compounds; the other 20% is excreted unchanged in the urine. In elderly or renally impaired patients, chlorpropamide has been associated with more side effects than any other first- or second-generation sulfonylurea. In addition to problems of hypoglycemia due to its long duration of action, it can cause significant water retention and hyponatremia, primarily by promoting the release of antidiuretic hormone (syndrome of inappropriate antidiuretic hormone [SIADH] secretion); this has also been demonstrated less often with tolbutamide. In addition, a disulfiram-like reaction is experienced in 30% of patients who ingest alcohol while using this medication. Because of chlorpropamide's long half-life, accumulation of metabolites in the elderly and in patients with renal failure, and its side-effect profile, there is no pharmacologic advantage in using this drug as a first-line agent in the treatment of type II diabetes; however, the drug is generically available.

Second-Generation Agents

Currently, the two second-generation agents marketed in the United States include glyburide (Diaβeta, Micronase), its micronized form (Glynase), and glipizide (Glucotrol) and a longer acting form (Glucotrol XL). These agents are at least 100 times more potent on a weight basis than first-generation drugs and have a duration of action of up to 24 hours. Moreover, except for hypoglycemia, the second-generation oral hypoglycemics appear to produce fewer side effects than do the older drugs.

Glyburide has an onset of action of approximately 1.5 hours and is more effective when administered at least 30 minutes before breakfast.[19] The pharmacokinetic half-life has been reported as 2–10 hours (more specific assays show the half-life to be closer to 2–4 hours), whereas the biologic half-life is much longer. The micronized preparation provides a higher plasma level and perhaps more predictable absorption, thus the recommended dose is 60% of the regular glyburide. The duration of activity is approximately 24 hours, and many patients require only one dose per day.

Glyburide is metabolized completely by the liver with 50% of the metabolites excreted renally and the other 50% eliminated via the biliary/gastrointestinal tract. Elderly patients are usually started on 1.25 mg/d, and younger patients are usually started on a daily dose of 2.5 mg. Because of the long duration of activity of glyburide, several case reports of glyburide-induced hypoglycemia (some of which have been fatal) have been reported.[20] Other side effects of glyburide include a mild diuresis with an increase in free-water clearance.

Glipizide has a half-life similar to that of glyburide but a duration of action of only 10–24 hours. The absorption of glipizide is impaired by meals, so it should be administered 30 minutes before meals. The drug is hydroxylated in the liver to inactive compounds that are renally excreted. Once-daily dosing can be achieved with doses of 15 mg or less; larger doses should be divided and administered twice a day.

It is generally accepted that glyburide is twice as potent as glipizide on a weight basis[21]; therefore, the maximum daily dose of glyburide is reported to be 20 mg and that of glipizide 40 mg. More recent studies have shown that adequate glycemic control can be produced by equal doses.[22] Further controversy surrounds long-term control with these agents. Glipizide has been associated with better postprandial control, whereas glyburide has demonstrated better 24-hour glycemic control.[22]

Side Effects

Hypoglycemia is the major complication of all sulfonylurea drugs. It is particularly troublesome with chlorpropamide because of the drug's long duration of action. Elderly patients are more susceptible to the hypoglycemia, especially when they skip meals or when there is some degree of renal or liver impairment. Other side effects of sulfonylureas include hematologic reactions such as leukopenia, thrombocytopenia, and hemolytic anemia; skin reactions, particularly rashes, purpura, and pruritus; antithyroid activity; and diffuse pulmonary reactions.[23] Renal side effects of these drugs include mild diuresis, seen especially with tolazamide and acetohexamide, as well as significant fluid retention and hyponatremia occurring with chlorpropamide.[7,18] Gastrointestinal side effects include nausea, vomiting, and cholestasis (with or without jaundice). Cholestatic jaundice has been identified more often with chlorpropamide than with any other oral agent. If jaundice results from any of these drugs, it is recommended that the patient be switched to insulin therapy rather than to another oral agent.[7]

Those patients who are at least 40 years of age at the onset of NIDDM, have been diabetic for less than 5 years prior to the initiation of sulfonylurea therapy, and have a fasting plasma glucose concentration of less than 300 mg/dL appear to be the best candidates for sulfonylurea therapy.[7,24] The dosage of these agents should be increased every 1–2 weeks until satisfactory control has been achieved or until the maximum dose has been reached.

Biguanide

As noted earlier, metformin became available for clinical use in 1995. This drug is a biguanide and has a twofold mechanism to enhance peripheral muscle glucose uptake and inhibit glucose release from the liver. A drug with a similar structure, phenformin, was removed from the U.S. market in the 1970s secondary to the production of lactic acidosis. However, metformin does not interfere with glucose oxidation and undergoes little mitochondrial binding unlike phenformin. Metformin is also observed to induce some increased insulin sensitivity more consistently in obese versus lean NIDDM patients. This may explain the modest weight loss in some patients. The most frequent side effects of metformin are gastrointestinal, with diarrhea incidence as high as 30% and up to 4% of patients stopping the therapy due to this action. A severe but uncommon action of metformin is the production of lactic acidosis. Worldwide incidence over the past four decades indicates the incidence of lactic acidosis is about 3 cases per 100,000 patient-years of use. The product will carry some prescribing restrictions in patients with renal disease (SCr >1.5 for males, >1.4 for females), liver disease, history of alcohol abuse, acute/chronic metabolic acidosis, and patients with conditions that predispose them to renal insufficiency or hypoxia. This new alternative is best classified as an "antihyperglycemic" agent because it does not induce hypoglycemia when used alone.[25,26]

Acarbose

Absorption of starch and disaccharides such as sucrose requires the action of α-glucosidase enzymes on the brush border of the intestine. Inhibition of these enzymes will decrease the absorption rate of carbohydrate, slowing or lowering the peak postprandial blood glucose concentration. The first product that can be considered an α-glucosidase inhibitor approved for use in the United States is acarbose, which competitively inhibits both glucoamylase and sucrose.[27] Studies have demonstrated a decrease in postprandial blood glucose with some improvement of glycosylated hemoglobin. The usually recommended dose is 50–100 mg with each large meal, and is most effective when given with a starchy high-fiber meal. The most common side effects are increased flatulence and abdominal bloating. When used in combination with a hypoglycemic agent (sulfonylurea or insulin), patients must be taught the importance of treating hypoglycemia with glucose-based product since acarbose will block absorption of more complex disaccharide sugars.[28]

Oral Hypoglycemic Combinations

With the addition of metformin, combined sulfonylurea–metformin regimens are possible. This combination has demonstrated the capability of lowering blood glucose by a greater amount than one of the agents alone. Several investigators have studied insulin versus the combination of insulin plus an oral agent to control plasma glucose. Most of these studies have found a statistically significant improvement in fasting glucose concentrations utilizing combination therapy.[29–31] The proposed mechanism is the oral agent's ability to increase endogenous insulin secretion rather than to improve the insulin sensitivity of tissues. Nighttime insulin is administered to suppress hepatic glucose production. Whether this slight improvement in control is clinically important long term or economically worthwhile remains to be shown.

INSULIN

Characteristics

Insulins are categorized according to their strength, onset of duration of action, species source, and purity. Each of these factors plays a role in determining the insulin type and dose best suited to an individual patient.

Strengths

Most patients in the United States utilize U-100 insulin, although U-500 is also available. (The numeral following the "U" indicates the number of units of insulin per milliliter.) In an attempt to purify and standardize the various insulin products, production of U-80 was discontinued in the early 1980s with U-40 insulin dropped in 1994. Although subject to debate, it had been reported that U-40 had a more rapid onset of action.[32] U-500 is available for patients who require greater than 100 units of insulin as a single injection. For those patients who require other strengths of insulin (e.g., U-10), special diluents and empty sterile vials are available from the manufacturer to prepare appropriate dilutions.

Species Source

All insulins currently on the market are of three types: pork, beef–pork mixture, or "biosynthetic" human. Beef insulin differs from human insulin by three amino acids, whereas pork insulin differs from human insulin by one amino acid. Consequently, it has been cited that beef insulin is more antigenic than pork insulin, although rarely has this proven to be clinically significant.[33] Biosynthetic insulins are also known as "human" insulins because their amino acid structure is identical in composition to human insulin and they are less antigenic than either beef or pork insulins. The biosynthetic insulins are produced by recombinant DNA technology using yeast or bacteria. There may be slight differences in pharmacokinetics between pork and human insulins or between human insulins from different manufacturers. If these differences are significant, they would be more noticeable in the type I patient.[34] The ability to use recombinant DNA technology to produce human insulin has stimulated research for other products, so-called insulin analogs. Altering the insulin molecule to improve the monomeric state while retaining the physiologic action on blood glucose provides an insulin analog that can be administered immediately before a meal. This analog is currently in phase three study, with others under investigation.[35] A more detailed listing of the current insulins is given in Table 72.12.

Purity

Purity refers to the amount of proinsulin and other impurities present in a given insulin product. Prior to 1980, most insulins contained enough impurities (300–10,000 ppm) to cause local reactions upon injection as well as systemic adverse effects from antibody induction. This led to production of a "purified" insulin, containing fewer than 10 parts per million (ppm) of proinsulin. Because of the expense of this purification technique, these insulins were initially more expensive than "standard" insulin. Modern technology, however, has made the purification process less expensive; consequently, all "purified" insulins produced in the United States contain 10 or less ppm of proinsulin, and none is considered to be antigenic.[36] Only purified insulins are now marketed in the United States. The term *standard insulin* referred to any product containing 10–25 ppm of proinsulin.

Pharmacokinetics

Table 72.13 compares the onset, peak, and duration of various insulin preparations. Regular insulin is a clear, colorless solution. Until the advent of the insulin infusion pump, regular insulin was rarely used by itself for maintenance therapy because of its short duration of action. Regular insulin with added buffers (Velosulin) is recommended for the pump to avoid crystal formation in the microbore tubing and possible plugging. It was found that the addition of acetate buffers, protamine, and/or zinc to regular insulin could greatly prolong its effect. Consequently, the addition of protamine and zinc led to Protamine Zinc & Iletin (PZI) insulin, with a predetermined amount of protamine and zinc in a neutral fluid-producing NPH. The addition of acetate buffers and zinc led to the Lente series to avoid allergic reactions to protamine. Because regular insulin is a solution, it can be administered by the intravenous, intramuscular, or subcutaneous route. All other types of insulin, however, are suspensions and can be administered subcutaneously only.[37] Note that both PZI and SemiLente insulins were discontinued in 1994.

NPH and Lente insulins are considered "intermediate-acting" insulins. Because their duration of action usually lies between 18 and 24 hours, a single injection of either NPH or Lente was usually the first step in chronic maintenance of the insulin-dependent diabetic. NPH is produced by combining zinc, protamine, and regular insulins. Protamine is a foreign protein and can produce high-antibody titers and symptoms of allergy in a small number of patients. Lente insulin is produced by adding acetate buffers and zinc to regular insulin. The resultant product may produce local allergic manifestations in patients with metal allergies.[38]

Although NPH and Lente are essentially identical in their onset, peak, duration of action, and cost, they differ in their ability to be mixed with other types of insulin. NPH and regular insulins can be combined in the same syringe and refrigerated for up to 21 days without changes in potency.[39] If larger quantities of NPH and regular insulins are mixed in a vial, the preparation is stable for 1 month if unrefrigerated or for 3 months under refrigeration.[40]

There is a well-documented and clinically significant interaction between regular and Lente insulins.[41] Lente insulin is formed by adding zinc to regular insulin, with an excess of zinc in the mixture. The addition of regular insulin in the same syringe produces an interaction within 15 minutes. This interaction lasts for 24 hours. The zinc binds with the regular insulin and delays the absorption. Moreover, this interaction produces more Lente insulin, possibly causing hypoglycemia when the absorption of Lente reaches its peak. To avoid the effects of this interaction, patients should be instructed either to inject the mixture immediately or to wait 24 hours before administration consistently. Patients who use syringes that have been prefilled and stored in the refrigerator should be instructed to use only those that have been prepared at least 24 hours in advance.[42] These patients should also be instructed to store prefilled syringes with the needle tips facing upward to prevent insulin suspensions from settling and plugging the needle.

In addition, phosphate-buffered insulins (e.g., NPH and PZI) should not be combined with insulins in the Lente series. Zinc is precipitated by the phosphate buffer, thus forming a product that acts similar to regular insulin. Predictable interactions also occur with the human insulins. It appears that human NPH and human regular preparations can be mixed with no consequences.

Dosing

Insulin doses can range anywhere from 0.1 U/kg to more than 2.5 U/kg of actual body weight (Table 72.14). Because the type II patient is usually not prone to ketoacidosis, there is less urgency to initiate aggressive therapy. He or she can

TABLE 72.12. INSULINS[a]

Brand Name	Manufacturer	Origin
Short-acting insulins		
Animal		
Single peak		
Iletin I, regular	Lilly	Beef–pork
Insulin, regular	Novo-Nordisk	Pork
Semilente Iletin I	Lilly	Beef, pork
Semilente insulin	Novo-Nordisk	Beef
Purified		
Iletin II, regular pork[b]	Lilly	Pork
Iletin II, regular beef	Lilly	Beef
Regular purified pork	Novo-Nordisk	Pork
Velosulin	Novo-Nordisk	Pork
Semilente purified pork	Novo-Nordisk	Pork
Human (purified)		
Humulin R	Lilly	Recombinant DNA
Velosulin Human R	Novo-Nordisk	Semisynthetic
Novolin R	Novo-Nordisk	Recombinant DNA
Novolin R Penfill	Novo-Nordisk	Recombinant DNA
Intermediate-acting insulins		
Animal		
Isophane (NPH)		
Single Peak		
Iletin I, NPH	Lilly	Beef, pork
NPH	Novo-Nordisk	Beef
Purified		
Iletin II, NPH	Lilly	Beef, pork
Insulatard NPH	Novo-Nordisk	Pork
NPH purified pork	Novo-Nordisk	Pork
Mixtard	Novo-Nordisk	Pork
Zinc (Lente)		
Single peak		
Iletin I, Lente	Lilly	Beef–pork
Lente	Novo-Nordisk	Beef
Purified		
Iletin II, Lente	Lilly	Beef–pork
Lente	Novo-Nordisk	Pork
Human		
Isophane (NPH)		
Humulin N	Lilly	Recombinant DNA
Novolin N	Novo-Nordisk	Recombinant DNA
Novolin N Penfill	Novo-Nordisk	Recombinant DNA
Insulatard Human N	Novo-Nordisk	Semisynthetic
Zinc (Lente)		
Humulin L	Lilly	Recombinant DNA
Novolin L	Novo-Nordisk	Recombinant DNA
Isophane (NPH)-regular combinations		
Animal		
Mixtard	Novo-Nordisk	Pork
Human		
Humulin 70/30	Lilly	Recombinant DNA
Novolin 70/30	Novo-Nordisk	Recombinant DNA
Humulin 50/50	Lilly	Recombinant DNA
Novolin 70/30 Penfill	Novo-Nordisk	Recombinant DNA
Mixtard Human 70/30	Novo-Nordisk	Semisynthetic
Long-acting insulins		
Animal		
Single peak		
Iletin I, Ultralente	Lilly	Beef–pork
Ultralente	Novo-Nordisk	Beef
Purified		
Ultralente purified beef	Novo-Nordisk	Beef
Human		
Humulin U Ultralente	Lilly	Recombinant DNA

[a]All insulins are available in U-100 concentration (100 units per ml).
[b]Available as U-100 and U-500 concentrations.

TABLE 72.13. ONSET, PEAK, AND DURATION OF VARIOUS INSULIN PREPARATIONS

Type of Insulin	Onset (h)	Peak (h)	Duration (h)
Short acting			
Regular	0.5–1	2–4	5–7
Intermediate acting			
NPH	1–2	6–14	18–24
Lente	1–2	6–14	18–24
Long acting			
Ultralente	4–6	18–26	36+

be started on a single injection of 15–20 U/d of an intermediate-acting insulin, and dosage adjustments can be made according to plasma glucose levels. Studies have shown that almost 90% of type II diabetics can be initially controlled on less than 20 U/d.[7,43] Either NPH or Lente insulin can be selected as the intermediate-acting insulin; however, many patients will eventually require regular insulin added to the regimen. To avoid the problems associated with the regular–Lente interaction, NPH may be a better initial choice, with premixed NPH and regular being available. Patients receiving insulin for the first time should be started on human insulin, whereas those who were started on a pork or a beef–pork combination can remain on that product unless resistance or other complications arise.

Although daily insulin doses can be up to 2.5 U/kg, most type I and type II diabetics generally require 0.5–1.2 U/kg of insulin per day. Many diabetologists discourage single daily injections of intermediate-acting insulin, citing evidence that the majority of their patients do not exhibit 24-hour control on this regimen. The first injection, consisting of an intermediate-to-regular ratio of 2 : 1, is given 30 minutes before breakfast. The second injection is given 30 minutes before the evening meal; the ratio of intermediate-acting to regular insulin is 1 : 1. These regimens are known as "intensive dose" regimens.[24,44] The basic reason for the dosing regimen development for intensive therapy is to mimic the activity of a functioning pancreas. Figure 72.2 illustrates the effects of a nondiabetic glucose/insulin

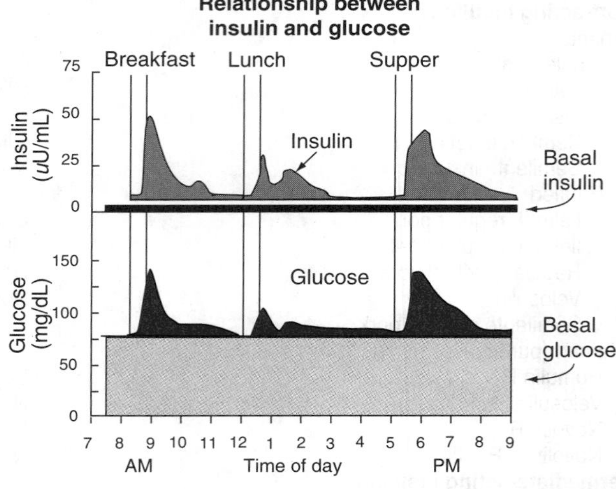

Intensive insulin therapy regimens

	7A	11A	4–5P	HS
1. 2 Doses, intermediate	X		X	
2. 2 Doses, regular or intermed.	Reg. & intermed.		Reg. & intermed.	
3. 3 Doses, regular or regular and intermed.	Reg. & intermed.	Reg.	Reg. & intermed.	
4. 4 Doses, regular and long acting	Reg.	Reg.	Reg.	Long acting

Figure 72.2. Insulin actions. *(From Schade DS, Santiago JV, Skyler JS, Rizza RA. Intensive Insulin Therapy. Amsterdam, Excerpta Medica, 1983, p 24.)*

release pattern around meals and throughout the day. The goal of the therapy is to fit the schedule to the patient's needs. The regimen for a scholarship swimmer with variable practice schedules will differ from a schoolteacher with a very predictable schedule.

A second intensive dose regimen utilizes regular insulin only. The patient's total daily insulin requirement is divided into four equal doses, each given 30 minutes before meals and at bedtime. This regimen attempts to mimic insulin release that occurs in nondiabetics with ingestion of meals. The bedtime dose is given with a snack and is used to suppress glycogen and fat metabolism, which occur at night during the fasting state.

A different method utilizes regular insulin via an insulin pump, termed a continuous subcutaneous insulin infusion (CSII). Insulin is administered continuously and as bolus doses before meals. A high incidence of complications, including hypoglycemia, ketoacidosis, dermatologic problems, and mechanical pump problems occur with this regimen. As a result, the American Diabetes Association recommends restricting insulin pump use to those patients who are knowledgeable, stable, and well motivated and who are receiving care from a physician properly trained in

TABLE 72.14. AVERAGE DAILY INSULIN REQUIREMENTS

Diabetes Type	Dosage in U/kg Actual Body Weight
Type I	
Initial dose	0.5–0.6
Honeymoon phase	0.1–0.4
Split-dose therapy	0.5–1.2
With ketosis or during acute illness	0.5–1.0
Type II	
Initial dose	0.2–0.6
Split-dose therapy	0.5–1.2
With insulin resistance	0.7–2.5

the use of these pumps. Figure 72.2 lists several options to dosing regimens.[45]

Of course, there are other approaches to begin insulin dosing. For the hospitalized patient, some clinicians prefer a "sliding scale" approach. Blood glucose concentrations are ordered several times a day (e.g., every 4 hours, every 6 hours, or at specified times: 7 AM, 11 AM, 4 PM, and midnight) such that fasting values and values before meals are obtained. Subcutaneously administered regular insulin is then ordered in an amount that increases with the increase in blood glucose. When the patient's insulin requirement has stabilized over 2–3 days, the number of units required during the last 24 hours is totaled. The patient can then be started on an insulin regimen, perhaps a split dose of regular insulin and NPH starting with about three-fourths of the 24-hour sliding scale insulin needs. The dose would then be "fine-tuned" over the next several days. While sliding scale regimens have long been used, many clinicians now initiate therapy on the patient's previous dose or their estimated requirements, and adjust the therapy from that starting point.

New technology is leading to the development of novel insulin delivery systems, including sustained-release injections and nasal insulin administration. Amylin is a substance produced by the pancreas that apparently aids in facilitating insulin's action. Perhaps amylin should be replaced along with insulin; current studies are assessing the usefulness of this concept.

Dosing Insulin During the "Honeymoon" Phase

It is important to note that type I diabetics often go through a "honeymoon phase" after the initial diagnosis of diabetes. During this period, insulin requirements diminish so that the patient is taking a very low dose of insulin. Regardless of how low the dose may become, patients should be encouraged to remain on insulin during this period to decrease the likelihood of producing antibodies to the insulin and becoming insulin resistant.[46]

Storage, Preparation, and Administration

Patients should be taught proper storage, dosage preparation, and administration techniques for their insulin. These guidelines are presented in Table 72.15.

MONITORING THERAPY

Regardless of whether the patient's therapy consists of diet and exercise, diet and exercise plus an oral agent(s), or diet and exercise plus insulin, the success of the therapy must be closely monitored. Monitoring instruments such as home-based urine testing and blood or plasma glucose testing can be used. Glycosylated hemoglobins, C-peptides, and blood glucose levels are more suited for clinic-based assessments. The choice of method depends on the severity of the diabetes, the progression of the disease, economic factors, and the patient's willingness and ability to monitor therapy.

In the home setting, urine glucose concentrations had been the mainstay of assessing diabetic control until recent years. Most patients now use whole-blood glucose determinations as a means of monitoring diabetic control. Urine testing is the least expensive monitoring device, but the results are not always easily interpretable. The tests, listed in Table 72.16, utilize either the glucose oxidase or the copper reduction method to detect glucose in the urine. The glucose oxidase method is a qualitative test, which is specific for glucose and yields few false-positive results. The copper reduction method is a better quantitative test, but will react with any reducing substance, thereby producing false-positive results (Table 72.17). With either test, the presence of glucose results in a color change that can then be correlated with a relative urine glucose concentration.

Urine glucose tests, although inexpensive and relatively easy to perform, have several limitations. First, a randomly collected urine specimen may correspond to a blood glucose concentration several hours previously. One tries to overcome this obstacle by using a "double-voided" specimen, whereby the patient urinates, drinks a full glass of water, and in approximately 30 minutes recollects and tests a second urine specimen. Urine testing may lack correlation between urine and blood glucose values. The tests are technique dependent, and the patient must read the results at the appropriate time.

Although it is commonly stated that the average person begins to spill glucose into the urine when the serum glucose approaches 180 mg/dL, this figure actually fluctuates greatly among patients. In addition, there can even be intrapatient variation depending on the progression of the disease and day-to-day stress factors. A negative urine glucose cannot discern among the adequately controlled patient, the person who is hypoglycemic, and the patient who is hyperglycemic but whose blood glucose value has not exceeded the renal threshold for spilling into the urine. While urine glucose is used less frequently for patient monitoring, urine ketone determination is commonly recommended to patients with IDDM or who are ketosis prone (Ketostix, etc). These home-based tests can indicate during episodes of increased glucose if the patient's metabolism has shifted.[47]

Blood glucose determination has become the standard for diabetes monitoring. In the laboratory, serum or plasma is utilized for glucose determinations. These concentrations may be slightly higher than those obtained on whole blood, although in almost all cases, the differences have no clinical significance. More recent advances in blood glucose monitoring have allowed patients and health professionals to monitor glucose levels using chemically impregnated strips or hand-held electronic glucose monitoring machines that utilize many of these strips. These

TABLE 72.15. PATIENT INFORMATION ON THE STORAGE AND ADMINISTRATION OF INSULIN

1. Unopened vials of insulin should be stored in the refrigerator but should not be frozen, storage on the refrigerator door is preferred usually. Freezing may alter the desired effect of the insulin. An opened vial of insulin that is being used daily should be stored at room temperature (59–85°F), away from windows, lamps, or any other places in which temperature could be altered. Insulin injected at room temperature causes less pain and fewer local reactions than does refrigerated insulin. Insulin that is refrigerated is usable until the expiration date stamped on the vial. Insulin stored at room temperature loses 1.5% of its activity each month; many clinicians recommend use within a month.
2. All supplies for administering an insulin dosage should be close at hand. These include insulin syringes, cotton balls, and 70% isopropyl alcohol or alcohol swabs, and the insulin. The alcohol should be clear in appearance and should not contain any soaps or perfumes that might cause a local irritation resembling an insulin allergy. U-100 syringes are available as standard or Lo-Dose. The Lo-Dose (25 U, 30 U, 50 U) syringes can accurately measure single units of insulin, and the numbers on the barrel of the syringe are easy to read; these syringes are useful for patients who are administered lower doses of insulin per injection. Syringes can be capped after use, stored in the refrigerator, and reused until the needle starts to dull.
3. All insulins except "Regular" are cloudy—like skim milk—in appearance and need to be gently agitated before a dosage is drawn. If the insulin appears to be different (color change, particles sticking to the vial, clumps in the vial, or the suspension settles after agitation momentarily), the insulin should be replaced. The vial should not be shaken vigorously but should be gently agitated or rolled between the palms of the hands.
4. The plunger on the syringe should be pulled back to the appropriate number of units desired.
5. The insulin vial should be inverted and the needle should be inserted into the rubber stopper in the vial. The plunger should be pressed all the way into the barrel of the syringe; the plunger should then be pulled back, allowing the correct number of units of insulin to enter the barrel of the syringe.
6. Air bubbles should be tapped toward the needle and gently expelled from the syringes. Injecting an air bubble subcutaneously is not harmful; however, air in the syringe indicates that the full dose of insulin has not been properly drawn up. Therefore, every attempt should be made to ensure that air bubbles have been expelled from the syringe, leaving the correct number of units of insulin in the syringe for injection.
7. A subcutaneous injection is made into fat (not merely "under the skin" as many people think). The most popular places for injecting insulin are the backs of the arms (triceps area), the abdomen, and the inner thigh areas. Patients who administer their own injections usually prefer the abdomen or thighs. Absorption is usually fastest from the abdomen, slowest from the thigh inducing some changes in injection site use recommendations. Many centers advocate use of one site with rotation before switching (example: several injections in the left leg, then to the right leg), although some centers now have patients rotate around the abdomen only. Not alternating sites with each injection may lead to a "calloused" area, affecting the actual subcutaneous tissue and altering insulin's absorption from that area.
8. After the site for injection is chosen, the area should be cleaned with alcohol. This should be done in a circular fashion, beginning in the center of the circle working outward about 2 in. Allow a few seconds for the alcohol to evaporate.
9. If you are right-handed, pinch up the fat at the site of injection with your left hand, being careful not to touch the area where the needle will enter the skin. Hold the syringe in your right hand as you would a pencil. The needle should be aimed perpendicular (90°) to the skin unless the patient is very thin and has too little subcutaneous tissue (in which case the needle should be inserted at a 45° angle). Using a slight wrist action, quickly insert the needle through the skin into the subcutaneous tissue. The entire length of the needle should be below the skin surface.
10. While the needle is still in the subcutaneous tissue, gently pull back on the plunger about 2 units—this is called aspirating. (If you are right-handed, this can be done by using the thumb of your right hand or by letting go of the pinched up area with your left hand and using your left hand to aspirate.) If any blood comes back into the syringe, you may have inserted the needle into a vein—DO NOT INJECT! If no blood appears in the syringe after aspirating, you can assume it is okay to inject. Note: Many health professionals are no longer teaching the technique of aspiration, because they claim it is rare for the needle to be inserted into a large vein. Check with providers in your practice setting.
11. Slowly push the plunger in all the way until it stops. Gently pull out the needle. You may use a cotton ball to GENTLY wipe the injected area after pulling out the needle, but do NOT massage the area of injection because this will alter the rate of insulin absorption.

strips or machines are designed to be able to monitor whole-blood glucose from several drops of blood obtained by a fingerstick.[48]

There are several differences in the various commercially available strips. The strip itself cannot monitor a true blood glucose concentration but measures a range within which the patient's value lies, similar to the ranges of glucose spilling into the urine ranges. Many of these strips, however, can be inserted into a machine that can then measure and display an accurate blood glucose value. When used without the machine, the patient's blood interacts with the chemicals on the strip to produce a color change that corresponds to a range of blood glucose values. Some strips maintain this color for several hours or days, whereas other strips begin to fade after a few minutes. A drawback to the use of either strips or the glucose monitoring machine is the relative expense, especially if the patient has to monitor blood values several times a day.[47]

TABLE 72.16. TESTS FOR URINE GLUCOSE DETERMINATION

Product	Detection Method	Range Detected (%)
Chemstrip μG	Glucose oxidase	0, ¼, ½, 1, 2, 3, 5
Clinitest (5-drop)	Copper reduction	0, ¼, ½, ¾, 1, ≥2
Clinitest (2-drop)	Copper reduction	0, ≤½, ½, 1, 2, 3, 5
Diastix	Glucose oxidase	0, ⅒, ¼, ½, 1, ≥2
TesTape	Glucose oxidase	0, ⅒, ¼, ½, ≥2

The monitors have become increasingly user friendly, in large part as a result of two conferences reviewing their use. These monitors have allowed patients to become involved in the day-to-day management of their disease.[49] Also, keep in mind the need for maintaining a good quality assurance program for the use of the monitors as noted in a user error study.[50] In addition, the strips or machines are not useful in detecting ketones, although strips are available to detect urine ketones.

The glycosylated hemoglobin (hemoglobin A1c) may be useful for monitoring long-term control of diabetes. Glucose can react in a concentration-dependent manner with groups of amino acids to produce glycosylated products.[51] For example, chronic elevation of blood glucose results in an increase in the presence of glycosylated hemoglobins, of which hemoglobin A1c is a major component. Hemoglobin A1c usually constitutes 4–8% of the total hemoglobin, but may constitute up to 15% of the total with chronic hyperglycemia. Since the life span of an average red blood cell is 120 days, bringing the blood glucose under control for 4–6 weeks will result in a fall in the percentage of hemoglobin A1c. However, a patient must have experienced hyperglycemia for 1–4 weeks before the hemoglobin A1c concentration rises substantially.[51,52] Methods for measuring glycosylated hemoglobins have become more standardized. Some tests that measure other glycosylated derivatives may be affected by short periods of hyperglycemia. Other conditions, such as sickle cell anemia, bleeding, or hemolysis, that affect the average life span of the red blood cell can also yield misleading results.

TABLE 72.17. DRUGS THAT CAUSE FALSE-POSITIVE RESULTS WITH COPPER REDUCTION TESTS FOR GLUCOSURIA

para-Aminosalicyclic acid	Methyldopa
Ascorbic acid	Nalidixic acid
Cephalosporins	Penicillins (large doses)
Chloral hydrate	Probenecid
Isoniazid	Salicylates
Levodopa	Streptomycin
Metaxalone	

Most patients show an interest in monitoring their urine or blood glucose initially but seem to lose interest after a short time. Factors contributing to this loss of interest include expense and lack of knowledge as to what to do with the results of these tests. Therefore, patients must be educated as to the short- and long-term benefits of day-to-day monitoring of glucose. Daily monitoring of glucose allows the patient to fine-tune dietary constraints. Follow-up visits to review the patient's monitoring technique are recommended.[50] For example, some patients can eat peanuts but find that peanut butter substantially raises their blood glucose concentration. Other patients find that they can eat certain types of bread but must avoid others. Still other patients find that small amounts of sucrose do not significantly affect their blood or urine glucose concentrations. Thus, patients become more involved in their own therapy.

Exercise also affects daily blood glucose concentrations. Monitoring daily urine or blood glucose values allows the patient to define how much and what kind of exercise is appropriate. For the insulin-dependent diabetic, the amount and type of exercise may dictate which parts of the body are best for insulin injections. Running may increase the absorption of insulin that has been injected into the thighs, resulting in hypoglycemia or shorter duration of action of the insulin.[34]

Certain prescription and nonprescription drugs can alter blood glucose concentrations (listed in Table 72.3). Daily monitoring of glucose allows the patient to determine if taking one or more of these drugs causes individual loss of diabetic control. In addition, other short-term factors affect daily insulin requirements. Factors that increase insulin requirements include infection, trauma, stress, and the second and third trimesters of pregnancy.[17] Conversely, exercise and early pregnancy decrease insulin requirements in most individuals. Consequently, daily monitoring of blood glucose not only can detect the aforementioned factors but can also help to define to what extent they affect an individual patient.

Self-monitoring of blood glucose, therefore, is essential in helping the patient and physician detect acute and chronic factors that affect the patient's overall control of diabetes. Moreover, daily monitoring involves the patient in his or her own therapy, which is essential to the overall success of any therapeutic regimen. Most important, home glucose monitoring allows the patient to adjust his or her insulin on a daily basis to achieve "tight" glucose control. Without monitoring the patient really is not an active participant in his or her care.

ADJUSTING THERAPY

Recognizing, Treating, and Preventing Hypoglycemia

Hypoglycemia is the most common side effect from sulfonylurea or insulin therapy. During the waking hours, the usual symptoms of hypoglycemia include sweating, tachycardia, palpitations, and tremor. When the blood glucose level falls below 40 mg/dL, central nervous system signs such as headache, confusion, visual disturbances, irritability or other personality changes, seizures, or unconsciousness may occur. Hypoglycemia may occur during the night or early morning hours while the patient is asleep, producing such symptoms as nightmares, night sweats, and headache. All of these symptoms result from a release of epinephrine, which is triggered by low-plasma glucose concentrations. Patients who have had diabetes for 5 years or more often lose this counterregulatory response and are asymptomatic with a fall in plasma glucose concentrations.

In some diabetics (especially the elderly diabetic) and nondiabetic individuals, a mildly depressed blood glucose level (50–70 mg/dL) can produce epinephrine release with resulting symptoms. It is often hard in these cases to document the hypoglycemia; consequently, the patient may experience these episodes for months or years before a definitive diagnosis is made. Unexplained hypoglycemia in previously well-controlled diabetics may also result from microinfarcts of the pituitary gland with loss of growth hormone secretion.

Although there are several causes of hypoglycemia, by far the most frequent cause in the insulin-dependent diabetic is not eating at the proper times. Other possible causes of hypoglycemia could include a high level of exercise or too much insulin or sulfonylurea. Many patients let their lifestyle dictate their eating habits just like other people in society. It is not uncommon for someone to skip breakfast because he or she is late for work. Working through lunch or making a late dinner engagement are other common causes. Intensive insulin management and self-monitoring of blood glucose allow patients to achieve some flexibility in their life's activities.

Other causes of hypoglycemia, especially in the insulin-dependent diabetic, include a defect in glucagon secretion and renal insufficiency leading to prolonged insulin action.[53] Other counterregulatory mechanisms may also be adversely affected, such as the impairment of epinephrine's action resulting from the administration of a β-adrenergic blocking drug or from hypopituitarism.

Hypoglycemia occurring in the early morning hours can produce a rebound hyperglycemia because of the release of counterregulatory hormones (glucagon, cortisol, or growth hormone). This rebound hyperglycemia, often accompanied by glucosuria and possibly ketonuria, is known as the Somogyi phenomenon.[54,55] Although often hard to diagnose, this phenomenon must be distinguished from the "dawn phenomenon," a relative resistance to the effect of insulin during the early morning hours. The dawn phenomenon also results in hyperglycemia and is thought to result from excessive action of growth hormone and cortisol.[56]

The immediate treatment of hypoglycemia in a conscious patient involves the administration of food, preferably sugar. Eight Lifesavers, 4–6 ounces of a sugar-containing soft drink, a piece of fruit (equivalent to ¼ to ⅓ cup raisins), ½ cup fruit juice, 2–3 glucose tablets (5 g each), a tube of glucose gel, or 1 cup skim milk usually reverses the symptoms in 10–20 minutes. In the unconscious patient, 1 mg of glucagon injected subcutaneously should provide relief within 10–15 minutes. Patients who weigh less than 20 kg should receive 0.5 mg. Common side effects are nausea and vomiting. Once the patient regains consciousness, oral liquids containing sugar should then be administered. In the hospitalized hypoglycemic patient, 50 mL of $D_{50}W$ provides rapid reversal of symptoms.

The long-term prevention of hypoglycemia involves altering the patient's dietary habits, exercise patterns, or medication dosage. If insulin has been implicated as the cause of hypoglycemia, the dosage regimen may have to be altered to deliver the proper effect when needed. Hypoglycemia (ultimately leading to hyperglycemia) resulting from the Somogyi phenomenon can be corrected by decreasing the insulin dose by 10% in the insulin-dependent patient and by 30–40% in the non–insulin-dependent diabetic.[24]

Correcting Hyperglycemia with Oral Hypoglycemics

Many patients taking sulfonylureas mistakenly assume that the drug by itself will adequately control their diabetes. Therefore, any patient taking an oral agent who has been controlled but who is now hyperglycemic should be asked the following questions:

1. Tell me how you have been taking your medication.
2. Have you run out of your medication during the past several days?
3. Tell me about your diet and exercise plan and how you have followed it since you were last here.
4. Have you experienced any recent "stresses" (infection, trauma, altered lifestyle, increased pressures)?
5. Are you self-monitoring your blood sugar? If so, show me how you do this. Is this hyperglycemia a new phenomenon or has it evolved over the past few weeks?
6. Have you experienced any symptoms of low blood sugar (i.e., increased heart rate, irritability, night sweats, nightmares) recently?
7. Have you experienced any symptoms of high blood sugar (i.e., increased urination, increased thirst) recently?
8. Have you taken any new medicine—prescription or nonprescription—during the past month?

Correctable factors should first be determined. If the patient has deviated from the prescribed diet and exercise plans, every attempt should be made to reinstitute these programs or determine if the original goals of these control steps are too rigid. If increased work or family pressures have triggered the hyperglycemia, whether these pressures are acute or will continue to exist for an indefinite period of time must be ascertained. If there is evidence of infection or other "stress," then many times the patient will not respond to an oral agent. In such cases, the patient must be started on short-term insulin therapy (preferably "human" insulin to minimize production of antibodies)[36] until the problem subsides, at which time the patient can be restarted on an oral agent. At this point, blood glucose determinations performed three or four times per day will be beneficial in deciding if the dose needs to be increased and/or administered more than once a day, if the patient needs a trial with a different oral agent, or if the patient must be converted to insulin therapy.

Usually if the patient's blood glucose is not adequately controlled with maximum doses of one oral agent then use of the other category is indicated (sulfonylurea–biguanide). Note that the protocol also provides a timing recommendation for use of insulin.

Correcting Hyperglycemia with Insulin

It is not uncommon for patients who have begun insulin therapy, whether they have type I or type II diabetes, to reject the course of treatment—insulin injections, finger glucose sticks, diet adherence, exercise plans, and so on. This nonadherence results from a set of reactions to the diagnosis including fear, anger, denial, and guilt. Sometimes a patient becomes overwhelmed with the demands of working to control their diabetes. Therefore, in the patient who is no longer controlled on his or her current insulin regimen, an attempt should be made to find answers to the following questions:

1. Are you administering the correct number of units of the correct insulin(s) at the correct time(s) per day and visually inspecting the insulin vial(s) to assure its quality?
2. How do you store your insulin?
3. If the patient is using an insulin suspension, have him or her show you how it is swirled for resuspending.
4. Have the patient show you how he or she draws up a dose.
5. What site do you use? How do you alternate the sites?
6. Is the patient injecting the insulin correctly? Check the technique.
7. Have you experienced any itching or redness at the site of injection, or any other evidence of insulin allergy?
8. Have there been any recent dietary modifications (time of meals, type of food consumed, amount of food consumed)?
9. Have you continued to follow the same exercise plan during the past month?
10. Have you gained or lost any weight during the past month?
11. Have you experienced any daytime or nocturnal symptoms of hypoglycemia recently?
12. Have you experienced any recent "stresses" (infection, trauma, altered lifestyle, increased pressures, etc.)?
13. Have you tested your urine or blood consistently during the past month? Is the hyperglycemia a new phenomenon or has it evolved over several weeks?
14. Have you experienced any recent symptoms of hyperglycemia?
15. Have you taken any new medications—prescription or nonprescription—during the past month?

Weight

A weight gain may indicate that the patient's insulin dosage is too large. Excess insulin promotes fat storage and hypoglycemia, which results in rebound hyperglycemia, thus seeming to require extra insulin to reduce the high blood glucose.[24,57] This can be a caveat to intensive therapy, ultimately resulting in the patient remaining hyperglycemic while simultaneously gaining weight. Symptoms of hypoglycemia and hyperglycemia can verify this suspicion. In this case, the insulin dosage must actually be adjusted downward.

Somogyi Effect

Hyperglycemia occurring during the early morning hours may be caused by a shorter-than-anticipated duration of action of the insulin with a pronounced dawn effect to raise glucose or by nocturnal hypoglycemia resulting from rebound hyperglycemia (Somogyi effect). Blood glucose levels measured during the early morning hours (3 AM) will determine the cause of the morning hyperglycemia. Often more than one 3 AM measurement is needed. Questioning the patient about symptoms of nocturnal hypoglycemia (nightmares, night sweats) may also help to differentiate between the two causes of the problem. If a Somogyi reaction is confirmed, the insulin dose should be changed.

Times of Hyperglycemia

This is by far the most important factor in determining how to adjust insulin therapy. Blood glucose levels collected at various times throughout the day can pinpoint the times at which the patient consistently loses control. The simplest way of starting to determine insulin dose issues is to examine blood glucose patterns, and "fall back" from the abnormal glucose. That is, fall back to the most recent insulin peak action. If a patient experiences hyperglycemia during

TABLE 72.18. ADJUSTING INSULIN DOSAGES BASED ON CLINICAL RESPONSE

Problem	Time Problem Experienced	Possible Solutions
Hyperglycemia	Fasting	If the patient is receiving a single dose of an intermediate-acting insulin, split into 2 doses—⅔ of total dose before breakfast, ⅓ of dose before supper If the patient is receiving split-dose intermediate insulin, increase presupper dose or move present dose to a later time in the evening
	Midmorning	Add Regular to morning dose
	Midafternoon	Increase morning NPH or Lente dose *or* add Regular at lunch time
	Bedtime	Add Regular with presupper dose if not currently receiving *or* increase Regular at presupper dose
	Early morning (2:00–3:00 AM)	If using Regular/intermediate dose before the evening meal, split the dose and give the Regular dose before the meal and the intermediate dose at bedtime (consider the dawn effect)
Hypoglycemia	Fasting	Decrease evening insulin dose, but first check timing of AM test and dose
	Midmorning	Decrease or omit prebreakfast dose of Regular insulin
	Midafternoon	Decrease morning NPH or Lente dose Be sure patient is withdrawing correct dosage into syringe in the correct order if he/she is receiving more than one type of insulin
	Bedtime	Instruct patient to eat a bedtime snack and/or check dose of PM NPH/Lente (again, "fall back") Decrease presupper dose of Regular insulin Decrease presupper dose of intermediate-acting insulin if it is being administered earlier in the afternoon
	Early morning (2:00–3:00 AM)	Consider Somogyi effect—decrease the evening dose of intermediate-acting insulin

Note: If more than one monitoring time throughout the day is abnormal, try to adjust only one insulin dose at a time. Adequately titrating more than one dose adjustment and gauging the effects is quite difficult and often creates more adjustment problems.

the night and/or has a high fasting value using one dose daily, splitting the dose of intermediate-acting insulin such that the patient received two-thirds of the total dose before breakfast and one-third before supper will help achieve tighter control. A patient who exhibits hyperglycemia during the evening hours may benefit from a dose of regular insulin just before supper. Examples of the "fall back" principle for multiple daily injections are included in Table 72.18.

COMPLICATIONS

Much of the concern for optimal treatment of diabetes is focused around the long-term complications of the disease. Diabetes, especially when untreated, can induce complications involving numerous organ systems through changes in neurologic and macro- and microvascular function. Most diabetes-related deaths appear to result from the long-term complications of the disease with only 10% or less resulting from direct causes such as ketoacidosis and hypoglycemia.[1,58] The results of the DCCT confirm that good diabetes management is perhaps the best current method for preventing the progression of the complications.[10] Further study is needed to determine the reasons and potential therapy differences for patient susceptibility variance. This may allow clinicians to predict the relative individual patient risk for complications. The knowledge that some large macromolecules are altered in diabetes patients and undergo glycation during high blood glucose episodes may play a large role in setting treatment options for the future. These macromolecule–glucose complexes undergo further change to form advanced glycation end products (AGE products), which appear to deposit in tissue and induce much of the complication problems.[59] Some medications, notably aminoguanidine, have been noted to prevent the formation of AGE products, and are currently in clinical research.[60]

MACROVASCULAR

Diabetic complications are generally categorized as either neurologic, macrovascular, or microvascular. Macrovascular complications involve large blood vessels such as coronary, cerebral, or peripheral vessels. With diabetes, these vessels are more prone to occlusion leading to coronary heart disease, stroke, or peripheral vascular disease. Although uncontrolled chronic hyperglycemia may be causal, most clinicians believe macrovascular complications are secondary to alterations in lipid metabolism and hypertension.[58,61]

Hyperlipidemia

A relationship between obesity, hyperlipidemia, hypertension, and diabetes seems to exist and accelerates the long-term complications of the disease. Specifically, people with diabetes develop a unique dyslipidemia including a high VLDL, small dense LDL, and low HDL. Hypertension is also about two times more common in diabetes. Data suggest that these metabolic changes may be related to increased abdominal fat. The glycation of proteins and lipoproteins is now recognized during this state of abnormal metabolism. Free fatty acids also seem to inhibit liver metabolism of insulin, which may, in turn, predispose patients to hypertension and contribute to peripheral insulin resistance causing glucose derangements.[59,61]

The obese diabetic is most often associated with type II diabetes. In fact, 60% of deaths in type II diabetes result from macrovascular complications, whereas there is only a 30% mortality rate in type I diabetes.[62,63] Evidence now shows that increases in glucose correlate with coronary heart disease, and the glycosylated hemoglobin may be a predictor of myocardial infarction.[64] There is also a recognized association between blood glucose control and cholesterol levels. Controllable risk factors (smoking, hypertension) should be controlled along with attention to weight reduction. Reduced intake of saturated fats and cholesterol will decrease atherogenic proteins, especially LDL. The National Cholesterol Education Program has set the goal for LDL-cholesterol reduction in patients with multiple risk factors, including diabetes, at 130 mg/dL. If a diabetic patient also has coronary heart disease, the goal is lower (100 mg/dL).[58,61] The use of lipid-lowering agents in the diabetic patient may prove beneficial in decreasing the risk of coronary heart disease; however, available data have not substantiated this claim. Currently five product choices are available, including nicotinic acid, bile acid sequestrants, HMG CoA reductase inhibitors, fibric acids, and probucol. Nicotinic acid use is limited in persons with diabetes due to its ability to increase blood glucose. The CoA reductase inhibitors are often used as initial agents when the LDL cholesterol is elevated with the additional changes described in HDL and triglycerides. In addition, estrogen replacement therapy can be considered for postmenopausal women. The clinician should realize the potential for these agents to aggravate other complications common to the diabetic (Table 72.19).[63]

Hypertension

Diabetics with hypertension represent a challenge to the clinician when choosing appropriate antihypertensive therapy. Many of the available agents can induce adverse effects that can potentiate the risk of long-term complications. Beta blockers and diuretics can increase serum glucose and lipid levels and increase the incidence of sexual dysfunction. In addition, β blockers exacerbate claudication and block the normal physiologic response to hypoglycemia, making them potentially dangerous additions to the diabetic drug regimen. Orthostasis is worsened by many of the antiadrenergic agents. Other antihypertensive medications that can aggravate diabetic-induced complications include guanethidine, guanadrel, methyldopa, and reserpine. Many of the newer agents, such as angiotensin-converting enzyme (ACE) inhibitors, calcium channel blockers, and α_1 blockers (e.g., prazosin, terazosin), do not potentiate the adverse complications of diabetes and thus are drugs of choice for diabetic patients. Recent data have demonstrated that ACE inhibitors are also beneficial in slowing the progression of nephropathy.[65,66]

Additional possible influences leading to the development of atheromatous macrovascular complications include genetic predisposition, racial characteristics, stressful personality types, obesity, and smoking.[67] Therefore, important aspects that should be addressed to help prevent macrovas-

TABLE 72.19. POSSIBLE COMPLICATIONS ASSOCIATED WITH ANTILIPIDEMICS

Drug	Possible Complication	Notes
Bile acid-binding resins	Hypertriglyceridemia	Increased triglycerides is a major risk factor for diabetic vascular disease
	Constipation, abdominal pain	Diabetics are predisposed to GI disease
Nicotonic acid	Hyperuricemia	Diabetics are predisposed to hyperuricemia and gout
	Glucose intolerance	May increase blood glucose, can be significant
	Constipation, abdominal pain	Diabetics are predisposed to GI disease
Gemfibrozil	Gallstone formation	Diabetics are predisposed to cholelithiasis
Clofibrate	Gallstone formation	Diabetics are predisposed to cholelithiasis
Probucol	Lowers HDL cholesterol	Diabetics are predisposed to having lower HDL than nondiabetics
	Loose stools, diarrhea	Diabetics are predisposed to GI disease

cular complications include cholesterol control, treatment of hypertension, diet and weight control, stress management, and smoking cessation.

MICROVASCULAR

Aberrations of arterioles and capillaries result in microvascular complications. Data from the DCCT demonstrate that microvascular complications arise from the degree and duration of hyperglycemia and limitation is possible. Although microvascular complications occur in both types of diabetes, their prevalence increases with the progression and duration of the disease and eventually can lead to diabetic nephropathy, retinopathy, and neuropathy. Although the mechanism for the development of these complications is unclear, data suggest that hyperglycemia induces metabolic aberrations that lead to structural tissue damage and long-term complications. Recent studies have implicated alterations in the polyol (sorbitol) pathway and the aforementioned protein glycosylation (AGE products) as major mechanisms for inducing metabolic complications. This results in damaged, leaky capillary wall vessels, causing capillary membrane thickening and functional impairment. The capillary abnormality primarily affects the eyes and kidneys as well as autonomic nerves, leading to painful neuropathies.[68,69]

Neuropathy

Up to 50% of diabetics will experience painful neuropathies after several years postdiagnosis with diabetes. The neuropathies can be categorized as motor/sensory or autonomic neuropathies. Symptoms may begin as tingling, or burning sensations, particularly in the distal tissues with a definite loss in vibratory sensation.[70] As these neuropathic problems progress, the patient may lose all sensation in a particular area, thus not being able to detect hot, cold, or pain. Circulation is usually impaired to these areas because of diabetes-related vascular changes. Diabetes is the leading cause of nontraumatic amputations in America.[1] Again, the DCCT demonstrated the real value to intensive diabetes care in preventing and limiting neuropathy.[10,71]

Treatment for painful neuropathy remains symptomatic and unsatisfactory. Many drugs have been tried for the treatment of diabetic peripheral neuropathy, but none has proven very effective. The wide variety of analgesic and anti-inflammatory agents can provide some relief for this painful complication. These include narcotics, nonsteroidal anti-inflammatory agents, anticonvulsants, and psychotropic agents. Of the anticonvulsants used, phenytoin and carbamazepine have been effective at doses ranging from 100–200 mg three or four times daily. Because of the incidence of side effects, such as dizziness, drowsiness, GI disturbances, and ataxia, and because of inconsistent therapeutic benefits, these agents should not be used routinely for the treatment of diabetic peripheral neuropathy.[70,71] A short trial may be warranted only in severe cases that have been resistant to other treatments.[58,72,73] Psychotropic drugs, such as tricyclic antidepressants, trazodone, fluoxetine, and phenothiazines, have mixed favorable responses but seem to provide greater pain relief than do anticonvulsant agents. Doses for the treatment of painful neuropathies should be initially low and titrated to effect.[74–76] In addition, antiarrhythmics such as mexiletine have been beneficial in resistant cases of neuropathy. Capsaicin (Axasin-Galen Pharma, Inc.) is an over-the-counter preparation indicated for painful neuropathies. Capsaicin, obtained from red chili peppers, is an approved FDA, category 1 counterirritant, for external use. Few data support benefit from this product; however, subjective response from patients appears promising.[77]

Because impairment of nerve conduction is thought to be due, in part, to abnormalities in the polyol pathway, newer therapy has focused on the pathway's rate-limiting enzyme, aldose reductase.[68] One should keep in mind that this enzymatic path is only one that plays a role in development of neuropathy, thus not inhibiting neuropathic change totally. Alteration to the polyol pathway results in sorbitol accumulation in peripheral nerves with fluid accumulation, capillary membrane thickening, and functional impairment leading to axonal degeneration, myelin damage, and decreased nerve conduction with painful neuropathies. Aldose reductase inhibitors, such as tolrestat and sorbinil, prevent the conversion of glucose to sorbitol, thus minimizing these effects.[69] The initial studies with these investigational agents indicated promising improvements in motor and sensory nerve conduction and reduction in pain and weakness. However, a more recent study suggests that these agents may be less effective with more chronic neuropathic syndromes, perhaps due to the incomplete block.[78] Generally, the incidence of side effects is low with these agents. Hypersensitivity reactions, such as skin rash and fever, are the most common and can occur in up to 10% of patients. More severe reactions have included Stevens–Johnson syndrome and adult respiratory distress syndrome (ARDS). Other reported adverse effects include liver enzyme elevation, dizziness, and postural hypotension.[68]

Autonomic neuropathies are the other form of nerve changes in diabetes.[79,80] These complications may induce changes in the function of organ systems controlled by the autonomic nervous system. Neurogenic bladder, with loss of autonomic mediated urinary continence, requiring bethanechol and/or anticholinergics will be experienced. Most data indicate that as many as 50% of men with diabetes duration for 25 years may become impotent. The symptoms of hypoglycemia may not be sensed by many patients, especially the elderly. This so called "hypoglycemia unawareness" is a significant danger in attempting an aggressive intensive control program in such a patient. Vision changes affecting eye focus are reported. Orthostasis can be a significant problem in patients who develop significant autonomic neuropathy. In its final stages, drops in pressure of more than 30 mm Hg are not uncommon upon standing.

Gastroparesis is a complication that affects approximately 20–30% of patients with diabetes, but is often overlooked. It is most common in the type I patient, and is believed to be autonomically induced. Symptoms include nausea, vomiting, and abdominal distension from delayed gastric emptying. This gastric emptying variance can lead to fluctuation of blood glucose levels, with glycemic control believed to be linked to limiting the gastroparesis. The goals of therapy are generally to provide good glycemic control and relief of symptoms. While antiemetics have been used with some success, most clinical attention has centered on use of agents to stimulate gastric emptying. Two agents currently in use in the United States are metoclopramide (Reglan), an antidopaminergic agent, and cisapride (Propulsid), a cholinergic stimulant with apparently more potency.[81] Many clinicians will switch patients from one agent to the other because their systems seem to develop some resistance to the action. Cisapride may induce fewer side effects, such as extrapyramidal action.[79] Other agents such as clonidine and erythromycin have shown limited success.[80]

Diabetic diarrhea occurs in about 20% of patients and may also be a neuropathic disorder.[84] It is characterized as episodic, with voluminous watery brown stools alternating with normal bowel function. This is most common in middle-age people with long-standing diabetes. Treatment has included anticholinergic agents, dietary change, antibiotics, bulk and bile salt resins, kaolin/pectin, and diphenoxylate/atropine. Somatostatin analogues have shown some promise in this disorder.[85]

Retinopathy

Diabetic retinopathy is the leading cause of new blindness in the United States.[86] The DCCT demonstrated that good glycemic control slowed by 54% the progression of retinopathy. Diabetes-related retinopathy may be either nonproliferative or proliferative. Nonproliferative reintopathy develops with little vision impairment, whereas proliferative retinopathy can greatly diminish vision or cause sudden blindness.[62] It is estimated that after 15 years duration of type I diabetes, 75% of patients will develop some degree of retinopathy. All persons with diabetes should be encouraged to have annual eye examinations. The majority will have little significant visual impairment, however, because the retinopathy is minimal. Only 5% or less of insulin-dependent diabetics in the United States are totally blind from diabetic-induced retinopathy.[2,58] The prevalence for developing significant retinopathy in patients with type II diabetes is much less than it is in type I diabetics. Nonproliferative retinopathy presents with microaneurysms progressing to hard yellow exudates, retinal edema, and hemorrhage. Nonproliferative retinopathy can be treated with laser photocoagulation therapy that may help to arrest progression and decrease the loss of vision associated with macular edema. Because hypertension and smoking lead to more rapid progression of ocular damage, it is very important to halt or to eliminate these risk factors.[87]

Aldose reductase inhibitors may prove beneficial in progressive retinopathy by preventing sorbitol-induced osmotic swelling and halting lenticular cataract development.[68] Because platelet aggregation may play a role in occluding retinal capillaries, there is some evidence that aspirin therapy may help to prevent the development of diabetic retinopathy. Debate in the diabetes clinical community also speculates the positive value of low-dose aspirin for the vascular changes.[88] Once retinopathy has developed, aspirin is contraindicated due to the increased risk of retinal hemorrhage. The patient should be cautioned to avoid strenuous physical activity, such as heavy lifting, that might increase venous pressure causing hemorrhage from the weakened ocular vessels.[58]

Nephropathy

Diabetic nephropathy syndrome, defined as persistent proteinuria, decreased glomerular filtration, and increased arterial blood pressure, is the primary cause of increased morbidity and mortality in the IDDM patient. The DCCT demonstrated the positive benefits of glycemic control in limiting progression of nephropathy.[10] Again, one must weigh the relative risks of increased incidence of hypoglycemia and the patient's skill and motivation against their limitations for participating in their control. Roughly, 35% of all diabetic patients will develop this syndrome, and the accumulated death rate is 50–75% 10 years after the diagnosis of diabetic nephropathy is made. Data indicate that this means that about 13,000 patients develop end-stage diabetic renal disease annually. Factors such as hypertension, hyperlipidemia, poor diet control, and smoking can all contribute to the development of progressive renal insufficiency.[1,58,66]

Treatment of diabetic nephropathy with aldose reductase inhibitors has shown some promise, though far less than originally anticipated. Sorbinil, an aldose reductase inhibitor, has been demonstrated in rats to reduce proteinuria and diminish thickening of the glomerular basement membrane. Further data will help to determine the usefulness of these agents in inhibiting the progression of diabetic-induced kidney disease. Other agents that may play a role in preventing and reversing kidney disease include aspirin, dipyridamole, somatostatin analogues, and certain antihypertensive medications. In addition, data from rats show these agents prevented thickening in the glomerular basement membrane.[89] The somatostatin analogue octreotide has demonstrated some effect in reducing glomerular filtration rate and kidney hypertrophy. However, long-term studies are needed to determine its clinical usefulness.

The renin–angiotensin system's function in the kidney involves the regulation of glomerular and tubular function and the regulation of systemic blood pressure. As diabetes-related changes evolve in the kidney, hyperfiltration will be the initial alteration in glomerular filtration. With progression of the diabetes the filtration rate shifts to normal and then to loss of renal function. Hypertension results in greater glomerular capillary pressure, which, in turn, leads to progressive glomerular damage, proteinuria, and azotemia, a common risk link with diabetes. ACE inhibitors seem to normalize systemic and glomerular capillary pressures, resulting in reduced proteinuria and glomerulosclerosis, as demonstrated in some recent studies. When the ACE inhibitors are started the patient may have a transient rise in serum creatinine, which usually returns to baseline within a few days. Caution must be advised, however, when using these agents in severe renal disease, since ACE inhibitors can worsen or cause renal impairment. ACE inhibitors, therefore, seem to be most useful during the early stages of diabetic nephropathy.[65,66]

The American Diabetes Association estimates that more than 10 million persons with diabetes have experienced long-term complications. Once these conditions develop, they are irreversible. Strong support to achieve optimal glycemic control and identifying therapies to prevent the progression of the complications must be a priority. Foot care and lower extremity complications are a particular worry. At least half of all amputations from diabetes-related disease can be prevented with good self-care and monitoring. This combined neurologic/vascular complication requires very close monitoring.

Special Problems Associated with Therapy

DIABETIC KETOACIDOSIS/HYPERGLYCEMIC HYPEROSMOLAR NONKETOTIC SYNDROME

Hyperglycemia from uncontrolled diabetes can lead to two types of metabolic crises that may result in a medical emergency. Diabetic ketoacidosis is more common in type I diabetics, resulting from complications from inadequate glycemic control, concurrent stress (e.g., infection, myocardial infarction, stroke), failure to take insulin, or as an acute reaction of previously undiagnosed diabetes mellitus. Another abnormality is termed hyperglycemic hyperosmolar nonketotic syndrome (HHNS). This is a life-threatening emergency usually seen in the elderly or undiagnosed person. HHNS is characterized by four principal features: severe hyperglycemia (>800 mg/dL), absence of ketoacidosis, profound dehydration, and neurologic signs or depressed sensorium to coma. Plasma insulin concentrations are usually higher in HHNS than in DKA. Because the mortality associated with these conditions averages 5–10%,[90] they should be regarded as a medical emergency that requires immediate diagnosis and prompt treatment.

Pathophysiology of DKA

For DKA to develop, a relative insulin deficit must be present plus increased levels of stress hormones (glucagon, cortisol, catecholamines, or growth hormone) along with a precipitating factor.[91] Insulin deficiency produces hyperglycemia post-meal, impaired protein synthesis, and increased protein degradation. Consequently, there is usually some internal or external stress causing increases in counterregulatory factors, thus creating either direct hyperglycemia or insulin resistance. Examples of precipitating events are listed in Table 72.20.

The counterregulatory hormones cause increased glucose production by the liver, and glycerol is an important gluconeogenic precursor. Figure 72.3 presents the pathways of DKA and HHNS. These two events in tandem produce moderate to severe hyperglycemia. Insulin deficiency also causes glycogen to be catabolized to glucose in the liver, and glycogen is depleted within several hours. There is a subsequent mobilization of fatty acids from peripheral tissues that undergo hepatic lipolysis. Insulin deficiency also reduces peripheral clearance of glucose, causing increased hyperglycemia. Moreover, protein from muscles is metabolized in the liver to amino acids. Increased levels of glucagon can also increase glucose and ketone production by altering hepatic metabolism.[92] This series of events results in ketosis and metabolic acidosis. Hyperglycemia, ketosis and ketonemia, and acidosis comprise the triad producing diabetic ketoacidosis.[91]

TABLE 72.20. FACTORS PRECIPITATING DIABETIC KETOACIDOSIS

Relative insulin deficiency—50% of cases
Insulin withdrawal or noncompliance
Insulin resistance/inappropriate dose
β-cell dysfunction, undiagnosed patient
Triggers diabetes diagnosis—25% of cases
Production of excess counterregulatory hormones
Dehydration
Infection, illness—25% of cases
Surgery
Psychologic stress
Sustained strenuous exertion
Pregnancy
Trauma
Pancreatitis
Hyperthyroidism
Hyperthermia
Acute myocardial infarction

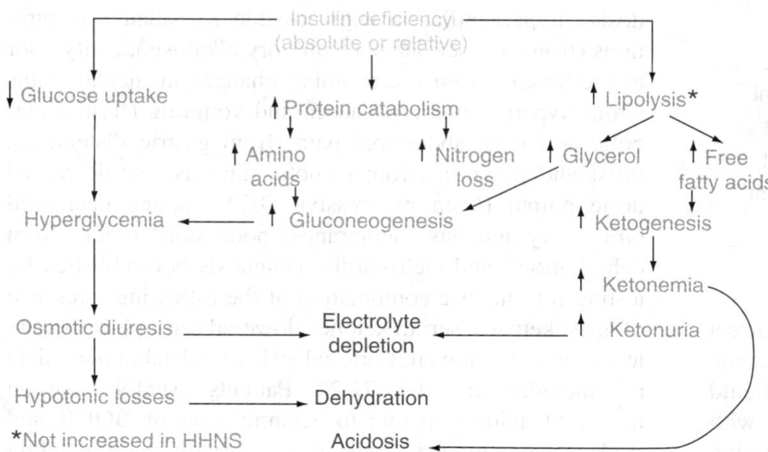

Figure 72.3. DKA–HHNS pathways. *(Adapted from Davidson MB. Diabetic ketoacidosis and hyperosmolar non-ketotic coma, in Davidson MB (ed.) Diabetes Mellitus: Diagnosis and Treatment, 3rd ed. New York, Churchill Livingstone, 1991,175–212.)*

Diabetic ketoacidosis profoundly affects the body's fluid and electrolyte status, renal function, and central nervous system. Renal tubular glucose levels surpass the threshold to "spill" into the urine producing an osmotic diuresis and dehydration. Because the plasma glucose cannot be transported into cells, an osmotic gradient between intracellular and extracellular compartments is established. Thus a movement of fluid from the intracellular to extracellular space ensues, diminishing hemodynamic signs of dehydration.[91] Many patients with DKA experience vomiting, which worsens the dehydration and prevents patients from ingesting enough fluids to improve their fluid status. Osmotic diuresis and dehydration lead to a decrease in glomerular filtration rate (GFR). This further impairs glucose, free fatty acid, and ketone elimination and leads to serum hyperosmolality. Kussmaul respiration pattern may occur, which is a deep, rapid respiratory pattern in response to metabolic acidosis. Kussmaul respiration results in hyperventilation to reduce $P\text{CO}_2$ and a secondary respiratory alkalosis.

Hypovolemia causes decreased tissue perfusion, leading to lactic acidosis. Some estimate that 25% of the acidemia seen in DKA may be due to lactic acid accumulation.[93] Decreased GFR impairs the excretion of organic acids and ketones. β-Hydroxybutyric acid (BOHB) and acetoacetate (AcAc) are precursors of acetone as depicted by Figure 72.4.

BOHB is converted to AcAc by oxidation; AcAc is further decarboxylated to acetone. Normally the ratio of BOHB to AcAc in the serum is 3 : 1, but the ratio in DKA increases from 6 : 1 to 12 : 1; acetone concentration is much lower. Because the common method of measuring serum or urinary ketones (nitroprusside method) detects only AcAc, the quantification of ketones will most likely be low prior to therapy and not reflect the true contribution of BOHB to the acidosis. Ketone concentration may appear to increase during therapy as oxidative metabolism improves and converts BOHB to AcAc.[91,94] The osmotic diuresis causes losses of electrolytes, primarily sodium, potassium, phosphate, and bicarbonate. Typical losses of fluid and electrolytes are quantitated in Table 72.21. Serum sodium may appear normal or low in patients in DKA, even though dehydration may be severe. This is due partially to fluid shifts from the intravascular to extravascular compartments caused by the increased osmotic pressure exerted by hyperglycemia. Each 100 mg/dL elevation of plasma glucose lowers the serum sodium by 1.6 mEq/L.[95] Consequently, the following equation is often utilized for "correcting" the serum sodium concentration:

$$\text{Na}^+ = \text{Na}^+(\text{measured}) + 1.6 \times (\text{Glucose} - 100)100$$

Potassium is shifted to the extracellular compartment during acidosis and is lost through osmotic diuresis; stimulation of aldosterone secretion by dehydration may also lead to hypokalemia. The patient's serum potassium concentration may appear to be normal or elevated during the early stages of DKA due to the shift of potassium to the extracellular compartment and the decreased GFR. Rehy-

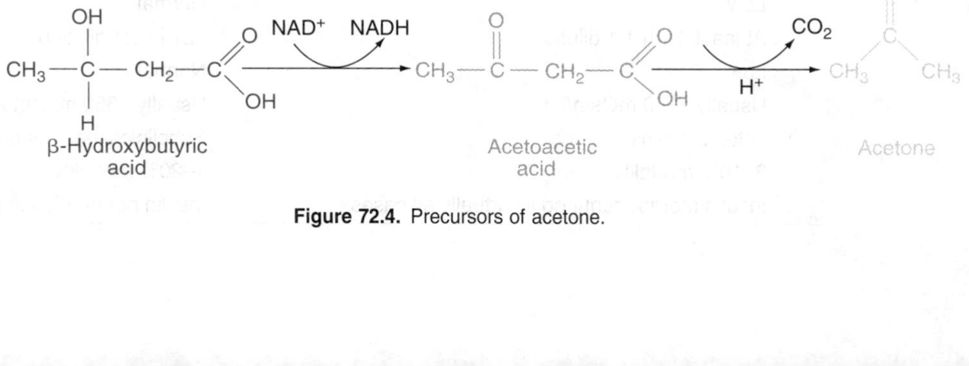

$$CH_3-CH(OH)-CH_2-COOH \xrightarrow{NAD^+ \rightarrow NADH} CH_3-CO-CH_2-COOH \xrightarrow[H^+]{CO_2} CH_3-CO-CH_3$$

β-Hydroxybutyric acid — Acetoacetic acid — Acetone

Figure 72.4. Precursors of acetone.

TABLE 72.21. FLUID AND ELECTROLYTE LOSSES IN DIABETIC KETOACIDOSIS

Free water	50–150 mL/kg body weight
Sodium	4–11 mEq/kg body weight
Potassium	3–10 mEq/kg body weight
Phosphate	0.1–2 mmol/kg body weight
Bicarbonate	3–6 mEq/kg body weight

dration and insulin therapy improve the GFR and correct the acidosis, thereby producing evidence of hypokalemia. If serum potassium prior to therapy is low, one should expect a precipitous drop in potassium during therapy with fluids and insulin. In such instances, potassium-containing intravenous fluids should be administered prior to insulin. The patient should have a heart monitor at all times secondary to the effects of potassium swings to induce arrhythmias.

Phosphate is depleted due to acidosis and diuresis, although serum phosphate concentrations in patients with DKA are usually normal or somewhat decreased. The clinical significance of phosphate depletion in patients with DKA is unclear.

Serum bicarbonate concentrations in patients with DKA are low because the bicarbonate buffer system is one of the body's defenses against metabolic acidosis. Although the serum bicarbonate concentration appears low, ketoacids and lactic acid are eventually metabolized via the Corey cycle to regenerate bicarbonate so that serum bicarbonate is restored to a near-normal level and the anion gap is reduced.[91]

Clinical Manifestations

Patients in diabetic ketoacidosis often present with lethargy (from hyperglycemia, hyperosmolality, ketonemia, and acidosis), hyperventilation with possible Kussmaul's respirations (from compensatory respiratory alkalosis), fruity odor to the breath (from acetonemia), changes in mental status (from hyperosmolality), nausea and vomiting (from metabolic acidosis), abdominal pain (from gastric distention), thirst and polyuria (from osmotic diuresis), or decreased urine output (from progressive DKA causing decreased GFR), dry mucous membranes, poor skin turgor (from dehydration), and tachycardia. Diagnosis is established by testing for one or a combination of the following: presence of urine ketones, serum ketones, lowered serum bicarbonate level, and/or a lowered arterial pH. Initial laboratory data are included in Table 72.22. Patients usually have an increased anion gap due to accumulation of BOHB and AcAc. Thereafter, acid–base status is usually determined by calculating the anion gap as a marker for acidemia. In addition, over three-fourths of patients in DKA will exhibit an increased serum amylase, although the cause and significance of this is unclear.[96]

Treatment

If DKA is diagnosed, it is imperative for the physician to initiate immediate treatment and to search for and correct the precipitating event. Treatment of DKA should be targeted toward correcting dehydration, reducing the plasma glucose concentration to normal, reversing the acidosis and ketosis, replenishing electrolyte and volume losses, and identifying the underlying cause.

Patients in ketoacidosis have fluid deficits of 4–10 L (with an average deficit of 5 L).[96] Administration of the proper type and amount of intravenous fluids will correct the dehydration and hyperglycemia associated with DKA. Plasma glucose concentrations greater than 600 mg/dL denote dehydration greater than 10%. Plasma glucose concentrations of this magnitude can be reduced to 300 mg/dL by administering fluids alone without insulin.[97] Volume

TABLE 72.22. DIABETIC KETOACIDOSIS AND HYPERGLYCEMIC HYPEROSMOLAR NONKETOTIC SYNDROME—COMPARISON CONDITIONS

Feature	DKA	HHNS
Age of patients	Usually <40 years	Usually >60 years
Duration of symptoms	Usually <2 days	Usually >5 days
Glucose level	Usually <600 mg/dL	Usually >800 mg/dL
Sodium concentration	More likely to be normal or low	More likely to be normal or high
Potassium concentration	High, normal, or low	High, normal, or low
Bicarbonate concentration	Low	Normal
Ketone bodies	At least 4+ in 1:1 dilution	<2+ in 1:1 dilution
pH	Low	Normal
Serum osmolality	Usually <350 mOsm/kg	Usually >350 mOsm/kg
Cerebral edema	Often subclinical	Subclinical has not been evaluated
Prognosis	3–10% mortality	1–20% mortality
Subsequent course	Insulin therapy required in virtually all cases	Insulin not needed in many cases

replacement lowers the plasma glucose concentration by increasing urine flow and glucose excretion, through a dilutional effect, and by decreasing circulating levels of counterregulatory hormones. There is some consensus regarding fluid replacement in these patients, with such factors as the patient's hemodynamic status, age, concurrent medical problems, and suspected precipitating event influencing the decision. Most clinicians believe, however, that 0.9% sodium chloride should be administered initially. Normal saline should be administered at a rate of 1 L/h for 2–3 hours.[91,96] After the patient's vascular status has been stabilized, with heart rate rhythm and blood pressure normalized, intravenous fluids can be changed to 0.45% sodium chloride. When the patient's plasma glucose concentration has dropped to approximately 250 mg/dL, the intravenous fluid should be changed to 5% dextrose in 0.45% sodium chloride. This change is to prevent hypoglycemia and to avoid hyperchloremic acidosis.

Insulin lowers plasma glucose and ketone levels. Large doses of insulin were utilized in DKA to overcome a perceived insulin resistance. Inhibition of lipolysis and ketogenesis is much more sensitive than glucose lowering effects. Now, investigators have discovered that a relatively low dose of insulin is just as effective without producing postrecovery hypoglycemia.[91,97] Counterregulatory hormone activity diminishes at similar rates with high-dose versus low-dose regimens. Consequently, most clinicians now use low-dose intravenous regular insulin to treat DKA.

Because the half-life of insulin is approximately 20 minutes,[96] giving a loading dose is probably not needed. Nevertheless, to avoid time delays encountered in preparing intravenous fluids containing insulin, some practitioners prefer administering a bolus of 0.1 U/kg before starting a continuous infusion. The maintenance infusion may be prepared by adding 100 units of regular to 100 mL of 0.9% sodium chloride piggybacked and infusing the drug at an initial rate of 0.1 U/kg/h.[91] Plasma glucose determinations should be made hourly. If there has been less than a 10% drop in 2 hours, then the insulin drip rate should be doubled.[98] The need for increased levels of insulin in some patients is believed to indicate insulin resistance, which will improve with continued therapy and reversal of the acidosis.

When the patient's plasma glucose concentration approaches 250 mg/dL, the primary intravenous fluid should be changed from 0.45% sodium chloride to 5% dextrose in 0.45% sodium chloride, and the infusion rate of the insulin drip should be cut in half.[91] It is important to emphasize that the endpoint of insulin therapy is not euglycemia but correction of acidosis and ketonemia. The insulin infusion should be continued until the acidosis has been corrected (arterial pH, >7.30; plasma glucose concentration, <250 mg/dL; anion gap, 13–17; serum bicarbonate, >15 mEq/L; no ketonemia).[91]

Electrolytes depleted from osmotic diuresis and acidosis should be replaced as quickly as possible to prevent development of cardiovascular problems. Sodium and potassium are the primary electrolytes that need to be replaced, although some clinicians also replace phosphate, magnesium, and bicarbonate. Sodium is generally replaced by administering 2–4 L of normal saline during the initial management of DKA. Sodium balance is maintained by changing the patient's intravenous fluids to 0.45% sodium chloride and later to 5% dextrose in 0.45% sodium chloride.

Osmotic diuresis produces a total body deficit of potassium ranging from 300–600 mEq. Generally, the serum potassium concentration falls to its lowest point approximately 1–4 hours after treatment of ketoacidosis is initiated. Potassium levels should be monitored closely every hour initially, then every 2–4 hours because hypokalemia can induce cardiac arrhythmias. Potassium can be replaced by adding 40–60 mEq to each liter of intravenous fluid and administering it at a rate of 10–20 mEq/h.[96] Electrocardiogram (ECG) monitoring is necessary to monitor the patient's status. Oral potassium replacement is possible provided the patient is not experiencing nausea or vomiting and is not comatose.[98]

There is no agreement on the routine administration of phosphate, bicarbonate, or magnesium in DKA. Phosphate is necessary to maintain adequate levels of 2,3-dephosphoglycerate in red blood cells to improve tissue oxygenation by shifting the oxygen–hemoglobin dissociation curve to the right. Phosphate is also necessary to produce ATP and enhance proper function of cardiac and respiratory tissues. Serum phosphate concentrations may drop during treatment of ketoacidosis. Therefore, phosphate replacement should be instituted when the serum level approaches the lower end of the normal range.[98] If phosphate is replaced as the potassium salt, keep in mind that each milliliter of potassium phosphate contains 3 mM phosphate and 4.4 mEq potassium. Doses of 1.5 mmol/L/kg in 24 hours can induce hypocalcemia.

Significant amounts of bicarbonate are lost in ketoacidosis. However, most clinicians agree that replacement of this electrolyte has the potential to cause hypokalemia, acidification of cerebrospinal fluid, systemic alkalosis, impaired oxygen delivery to tissues, increased carbon dioxide production, and ketoacid overproduction.[93] During therapy, ketoacids and lactic acid are metabolized by the liver to bicarbonate. Generally, bicarbonate is administered only to patients whose arterial pH is below 7.0. When indicated, bicarbonate should be administered via infusion of 50 mEq (or 1 mEq/Kg) over 1 hour. The goal of therapy is to raise the arterial pH to 7.10–7.15.[98]

Monitoring

Plasma or whole-blood glucose concentrations should be monitored hourly until they have stabilized below 250 mg/dL. At least one study has shown that fingerstick glucose testing does not accurately represent venous glucose concentrations in severely hypotensive patients.[91] Electrolytes, especially potassium, should be monitored every hour until stabilized within the normal range, then every 2–4 hours until the acidosis has been corrected. Heart rhythm should be monitored, especially in comatose patients. Patients with HHNS are managed in a manner similar to that used for patients who have DKA, with fluid and electrolyte replacement the cornerstone of treatment. Usually lower doses of insulin are needed for treating HHNS due to higher circulating insulin levels. The troubling component of HHNS is that many times the diagnosis is missed due to the patient's history. Refer to Table 72.22 for some differentiating features.

INSULIN REQUIREMENTS OF THE SURGICAL PATIENT

Diabetics scheduled for surgery usually do not receive breakfast on the day of surgery, and administration of insulin might lead to profound hypoglycemia; however, the "stress" of surgery has a tremendous hyperglycemic effect such that withholding insulin can lead to dehydration, an impaired inflammatory response, and possible ketoacidosis (in the type I diabetic). Therefore, plasma glucose values should ideally be less than 250 mg/dL, usually with IV glucose infusion preoperatively with the morning insulin. This can be followed with glucose monitoring and insulin infusion during surgery and postoperatively.

The diet-controlled diabetic usually needs no exogenous insulin but should at least be covered by a sliding scale order should the need for insulin arise. "Human" insulin should be utilized to minimize the formation of insulin antibodies. The patient controlled with oral hypoglycemics should have the medication held on the day of surgery and needs a sliding scale order. The insulin-dependent diabetic should receive one-half of his or her usual dose of an intermediate-acting insulin and should likewise have an order for sliding scale insulin after surgery.[99]

"SICK-DAY" GUIDELINES FOR INSULIN-DEPENDENT DIABETICS

When a patient with IDDM is too ill to eat, the question often arises as to how much (if any) insulin is needed. Insulin needs may vary, but the stress of the infection or causative event will increase blood glucose. Extra clear fluids (up to 12 glasses) should be consumed, especially if the patient has a fever. Patients should be instructed to record the amount of fluid they consume as well as the number of times they urinate, vomit, or have loose stools. Blood glucose concentrations should be measured several times during the day up to hourly, and urine should be tested for ketones with each urination. Most patients are instructed to contact their health provider when a "sick day" starts for specific guidelines, and consider their mentation in the monitoring. If the blood glucose concentration is greater than 300 mg/dL and urine ketones are present, the patient needs to be formally evaluated. Similarly, any patient having difficulty breathing or breathing over 24 times/min (symptoms of respiratory compensation for metabolic acidosis) should seek medical attention. Although it is normal to feel tired or sleepy when sick, any patient who is very sleepy or cannot pay attention should seek medical help immediately.[100]

REFERENCES

1. American Diabetes Association. Diabetes 1993 Vital Statistics. Alexandria, VA, Author, 1993.
2. National Diabetes Group. Classification and diagnosis of diabetes mellitus and other categories of glucose tolerance. Diabetes 1979;28:1039–1057.
3. Rifkin H, Porte D, Jr., eds. Ellenberg and Rifkin's Diabetes Mellitus: Theory and Practice, 4th ed. New York, Elsvier Science Publishing, 1990.
4. Metzger BE, Organizing Committee. Summary and recommendations of the Third International Workshop–Conference on Gestational Diabetes Mellitus. Diabetes 1991;40(suppl 2):197–201.
5. Cahill GF. Disorders of carbohydrate metabolism: Diabetes mellitus, in Wyngaarden JB, Smith LH (eds): Cecil Textbook of Medicine. Philadelphia, WB Saunders, 1982, pp 1054–1056.
6. Gerich JE. Insulin-dependent diabetes mellitus: Pathophysiology. Mayo Clin Proc 1986;61:787–791.
7. American Diabetes Association. The Physician's Guide to Type II Diabetes (NIDDM): Diagnosis and Treatment. New York, Author, 1984, pp 1–112.
8. Standards of medical care, Diabetes Care 1994;17:616.
9. Hoekstra JBL, van Rijn HJM, Erkelens DW, et al. Review: C-peptide. Diabetes Care 1982;5:438–446.
10. The Diabetes Control and Complications Trial Research Group. The effect of intensive treatment of diabetes on the progression of long-term complications in insulin-dependent diabetes mellitus. N Engl J Med 1993;319:977–986.
11. Funnell MM, Anderson RM, Arnold MS, et al. Empowerment: An idea whose time has come in diabetes education. Diabetes Educ 1991;17:37–41.
12. Franz MJ, Horton ES, Bantle JP, et al. Technical review: Nutrition principles for the management of diabetes and related complications. Diabetes Care 1994;17:490–518.
13. Crapo PA. Nutrition update. Clin Diabetes 1983;1:12–14.
14. Bogardus C, Ravussin E, Robbins DC, et al. Effects of physical training and diet therapy on carbohydrate metabolism in patients with glucose intolerance and non–insulin-dependent diabetes mellitus. Diabetes 1984;33:311–318.
15. Zimman B. Exercise in diabetes treatment. Clin Diabetes 1983;1:18–22.

16. The University Group Diabetes Program. A study of the effects of hypoglycemic agents on vascular complications in patients with adult onset diabetes. Diabetes 1970;19(suppl 2):1–26.
17. Lebovitz HE, Feiglos MN. The oral hypoglycemic agents, in Ellenberg M, Rifkin H (eds): Diabetes Mellitus: Theory and Practice. New Hyde Park, NY, Medical Examination Publishing, 1983, pp 591–610.
18. Lebovitz HE. Sulfonylurea drugs, in Lebovitz HE (ed): Therapy for Diabetes Mellitus and Related Disorders. Alexandria, VA, American Diabetes Association, 1991, pp 114–122.
19. Antidiabetic agents, in American Hospital Formulary Service Drug Information 95. Bethesda, MD, American Society of Hospital Pharmacists, 1995, pp 1742–1789.
20. Gavin JR. Dual actions of sulfonylureas and glyburide: Receptor and post-receptor effects. Am J Med 1985;79(suppl 3B):34–43.
21. Melander A, Bitzen P-O, Faber O, et al. Sulphonylurea antidiabetic drugs: An update of their clinical pharmacology and rational therapeutic use. Drugs 1989;37:58–72.
22. Kilo C. Multicenter comparison of glyburide and glipizide in the treatment of non–insulin-dependent diabetes mellitus. Clin Ther 1988;10:294–302.
23. Zavaroni I, Bonora E, Pagliara M, et al. Risk factors for coronary artery disease in healthy persons with hyperinsulinemia and normal glucose tolerance. N Engl J Med 1989;320:702–706.
24. Gregerman RI. Diabetes mellitus, in Barker LR, Burton JR, Zieve PD (eds): Principles of Ambulatory Medicine. Baltimore, Williams & Wilkins, 1986, pp 951–986.
25. Bailey CJ. Biguanides and NIDDM. Diabetes Care 1992;15:755–772.
26. Klip A, Leiter LA. Cellular mechanism of action of metformin. Diabetes Care 1990;13:696–704.
27. Johnson DG, Bressler R. Short-term efficacy of acarbose in obese patients with non–insulin-dependent diabetes mellitus, in Creutzfeldt W (ed): Acarbose. Effects on Carbohydrate and Fat Metabolism. Amsterdam, Excerpta Medica, 1982, pp 355–390.
28. Bressler R, Johnson D. New pharmacological approaches to therapy of NIDDM. Diabetes Care 1992;15:792–805.
29. Goodman A. The Metformin Investigators Group. Efficacy and safety of metformin in NIDDM: Results of a multicenter trial. Diabetes 1993;42(suppl 1):1–57A. (53rd annual meeting of the American Diabetes Association, Las Vegas, Nevada.)
30. Reaven GM, Johnston P, Hollenbeck CB, et al. Combined metformin–sulfonylurea treatment of patients with non–insulin-dependent diabetes in fair to poor glycemic control. J Clin Endocrinol Metab 1992;74:1020–1026.
31. Lewitt MS, Yu VKF, Rennie GC, et al. Effects of combined insulin–sulfonylurea in type II patients. Diabetes Care 1989;12:379–383.
32. Galloway JA, Spradlin CT, Nelson RL, et al. Factors influencing the absorption, serum insulin concentration, and blood glucose responses after injections of regular insulin and various mixtures. Diabetes Care 1981;4:366–376.
33. Deckert T. The immunogenicity of new insulins. Diabetes 1985;34(suppl 2):94–96.
34. Krosnick A. Newer insulin, insulin allergies, and the clinical use of insulins, in Bergman M (ed): Principles of Diabetes Management. New Hyde Park, NY, Medical Examination Publishing, 1987, pp 123–135.
35. Brange J, Owens DR, Kang S, Valund A. Monomeric insulins and their experimental and clinical implications. Diabetes Care 1990;13:923–954.
36. Galloway JA. Insulin treatment for the early 80's: Facts and questions about old and new insulins and their usage. Diabetes Care 1980;3:615–622.
37. Skyler JS. Insulin dependent diabetes mellitus. Postgrad Med 1987;81(6):163–174.
38. Heine RJ, Bilo HJG, Fonk T, et al. Absorption kinetics and action profiles of mixtures of short- and intermediate-acting insulins. Diabetologia 1984;27:558–562.
39. Peters AL, Davidson MB. Effect of storage on action of NPH and regular insulin mixtures. Diabetes Care 1986;14:180–183.
40. Jawadi MH, Ho LS. Stability and reproducibility of the biologic activity of premixed short-acting and intermediate-acting insulins. Am J Med 1986;81:467–471.
41. White J, Campbell RK. Guide to mixing insulins. Hosp Pharm 1991;26:1046–1048.
42. Colaguiri S, Villalbos S. Assessing effect of mixing insulins by glucose-clamp technique in subjects with diabetes mellitus. Diabetes Care 1986;9:579–586.
43. Olsson PO, Arnqvist H, Von Schenck H. Miscibility of human semisynthetic regular and Lente insulin and human biosynthetic regular and NPH insulin. Diabetes Care 1987;10:473–477.
44. Genuth S. Insulin use in NIDDM. Diabetes Care 1990;13(12):1240–1264.
45. Schade D, Santiago J, Skyler J, Rizza R. Intensive Insulin Therapy. Geneva, Excerpta Medica, 1983.
46. Cahill GF, McDevitt HO. Insulin-dependent diabetes mellitus: The initial lesion. N Engl J Med 1981;304:1454–1465.
47. Guthrie D, Guthrie R, Hinnen D. Urine tests: Still useful after all these years. Diabetes Forecast 1985;38(2):43–45.
48. Peterson CM, ed. Diabetes Management in the 1980's: The Role of Home Blood Glucose Monitoring and New Insulin Delivery Systems. New York, Praeger Publishers, 1982, pp 184–197.
49. American Diabetes Association. Consensus statement. Self-monitoring of blood glucose. Diabetes Care 1994;17:76–87.
50. National Steering Committee for Quality Assurance in Capillary Blood Glucose Monitoring. Proposed strategies for reducing user error in capillary blood glucose monitoring. Diabetes Care 1993;16(2):493–498.
51. Goldstein DE, Parker KM, England JD, et al. Clinical application of glycosylated hemoglobin measurements. Diabetes 1982;31(suppl 3):70–78.
52. Bunn HF. Evaluation of glycosylated hemoglobin in diabetic patients. Diabetes 1981;30:613–617.
53. Gossain VV, Rovner DR. Pancreatic glucagon: Possible implications of the hyperglycemic hormone in diabetes control. Postgrad Med 1982;72:87–96.
54. Galloway JA. The complications of insulin therapy, in Bressler R., Johnson DG (eds): Management of Diabetes Mellitus. Boston, John Wright—PSG, 1982, pp 91–114.

55. Stephenson JM, Schernthaner G. Dawn phenomenon and Somogyi effect in IDDM. Diabetes Care 1989;12:245–251.
56. Bolli GB, Gerich JE. The dawn phenomenon—a common occurrence in both non–insulin-dependent and insulin-dependent diabetes mellitus. N Engl J Med 1984;310:746–750.
57. Reaven GM. Clinician's Guide to Non–Insulin-Dependent Diabetes Mellitus: Pathogenesis and Treatment. New York and Basel, Marcel Dekker, 1989.
58. Nathan DM. Long-term complications of diabetes mellitus. N Engl J Med 1993;328:1676–1685.
59. Brownlee M. Glycation of macromolecules, in Alberti KGM, DeFronzo RA, Keen H, Zimmet P (eds): International Textbook of Diabetes Mellitus. West Sussex, England, John Wiley and Sons, 1993, pp 669–684.
60. Brownlee M. Glycation products and the pathogenesis of diabetic complications. Diabetes Care 1992;15:1835–1843.
61. Kaplan NM. The deadly quartet: Upper-body obesity, glucose intolerance, hypertriglyceridemia, and hypertension. Arch Intern Med 1989;149:1514–1519.
62. Feingold KR. Preventing the Vascular Complications of Diabetes. New York, HIP Publishing, 1987, pp 2–16.
63. Lyons T. Lipoprotein glycation and its metabolic consequences. Diabetes 1992;41(suppl 2):67–76.
64. Stanlee J. Glycosylated hemoglobin and predictive data (MRFIT study analysis). Diabetes Care 1993;16:434–445.
65. Lewis EJ, Hunsicker LG, Bain RP, et al. The effect of angiotensin-converting-enzyme inhibition on diabetic nephropathy. N Engl J Med 1993;328:1456–1462.
66. Houston MC. New insights and new approaches for the treatment of essential hypertension. Am Heart J 1989;117:911–951.
67. Mitchell BD, Hawthorne VM, Vinik AI. Cigarette smoking and neuropathy in diabetic patients. Diabetes Care 1990;13:434–437.
68. Zenon GJ, Abobo CV, Carter BL, et al. Potential use of aldose reductase inhibitors to prevent diabetic complications. Clin Pharm 1990;9:446–457.
69. Masson EA, Boulton AJM. Aldose reductase inhibitors in the treatment of diabetic neuropathy. Drugs 1990;39(2):190–202.
70. Daniels JS. Abnormal nerve conduction in impotent patients with diabetes mellitus. Diabetes Care 1989;12:449–454.
71. Zimmerman BR. Influence of the degree of control of diabetes on the prevention, postponement and amelioration of late complications. Drugs 1989;38(6):941–956.
72. Greene DA, Sima AAF, Albers JW, Pfeifer MA. Diabetic neuropathy, in Rifkin H, Porte D (eds): Diabetes Mellitus, 4th ed. New York, Elsevier Science Publishing, 1990, pp 710–755.
73. Vinik AI, Holland MT, LeBeau JM, et al. Diabetic neuropathies. Diabetes Care 1992;15:1926–1975.
74. Theesan KA, Marsh WR. Relief of diabetic neuropathy with fluoxetine. DICP: Annals Pharmacother 1989;23:572–574.
75. Mendel CM, Klein RF, Chappell DA, et al. A trial of amitriptyline and fluphenazine in the treatment of painful diabetic neuropathy. JAMA 1986;255:637–639.
76. Krinesdal B, Molin J, Froland A, et al. Imipramine treatment of painful diabetic neuropathy. JAMA 1984;251:1727–1730.
77. Capsaicin Study Group. Effect of treatment with Capsaicin on daily activities of patients with painful diabetic neuropathy. Diabetes Care 1992;15:159–165.
78. Jennings PE, Nightingale S, Guen CL, et al. Prolonged aldose reductase inhibition in chronic peripheral diabetic neuropathy: Effects on microangiopathy. Diabetic Med 1990;7:63–68.
79. Cahill GF, Arky RA, Perlman AJ. Diabetes mellitus, in Rubenstein E, Federman DD (eds): Scientific American Medicine. New York, Scientific American, 1987, pp 1–19.
80. Cyrus J, Broadstone VL, Pfeifer MA, Greene DA. Diabetic peripheral neuropathy. Part II. Autonomic neuropathies. Diabetes Educ 1987;13:111–114.
81. Brown CK, Khanderia U. Use of metoclopramide, domperidone, and cisapride in the management of diabetic gastroparesis. Clin Pharm 1990;9:357–363.
82. Horowitz M, Roberts AP. Long-term efficacy of cisapride in diabetic gastroparesis. Am J Med 1990;88:195–196.
83. Jassens J, Peeters TL, Vantrappen J, et al. Improvement of gastric emptying in diabetic gastroparesis by erythromycin. N Engl J Med 1990;322(15):1028–1031.
84. Ogbonnaya KI, Arem R. Diabetic diarrhea pathophysiology, diagnosis, and management. Arch Intern Med 1990;150:262–267.
85. Rosenberg JM. Octreotide: A synthetic analog of somatostatin. DICP 1988;22:748–754.
86. Merimee TJ. Diabetic retinopathy: A synthesis of perspectives. N Engl J Med 1990;322:978–983.
87. The Prevention and Treatment of Complications of Diabetes: A Guide for Primary Care Practitioners. Atlanta, GA, Department of Health and Human Services, Centers for Disease Control and Prevention, 1991.
88. Colwell JA. Vascular thrombosis in type II diabetes mellitus. Diabetes Care 1993;42:8–11.
89. Reddi AS, Camerini-Davalos RA. Diabetic nephropathy. Arch Intern Med 1990;150:31–34.
90. Krane EJ. Diabetic ketoacidosis: Biochemistry, physiology, treatment, and prevention. Pediatr Clin North Am 1987;34:935–960.
91. Davidson MB. Diabetic ketoacidosis and hyperosmolar nonketotic coma, in Davidson MB (ed): Diabetes Mellitus: Diagnosis and Treatment, 3rd ed. New York, Churchill Livingstone, 1991, pp 175–212.
92. Walker M, Marshall SM, Alberti KGMM. Clinical aspects of diabetic ketoacidosis. Diabetes/Metab Rev 1989;5:651–663.
93. Morris LR, Murphy MB, Kitabchi AG. Bicarbonate therapy in severe diabetic ketoacidosis. Ann Intern Med 1986;105:836–840.
94. Kandel G, Aberman A. Selected developments in the understanding of diabetic ketoacidosis. Can Med Assoc J 1983;128:392–397.
95. Sabo CE, Michael SR. Diabetic ketoacidosis: Pathophysiology, nursing diagnosis and interventions. Focus Crit Care 1989;16:21–28.
96. Israel RS. Diabetic ketoacidosis. Emerg Med Clin North Am 1989;7:859–871.

97. Peragallo-Dittko V, Godley K, Meyer J (eds). A Core Curriculum for Diabetes Education, 2nd ed. Chicago, American Association of Diabetes Educators, 1993.
98. Pecoraro RE, Reiber GE, Burgess EM. Pathways to diabetic limb amputation: Basis for prevention. Diabetes Care 1990;13:513–531.
99. Gill GV, Alberti KGMM. The care of the diabetic patient during surgery, in Alberti KGMM, DeFronzo RA, Keen H, Zimmet P (eds): International Textbook of Diabetes Mellitus. West Sussex, England, John Wiley & Sons, 1993.
100. Ley B, Goldman D. Sick-day management: Preparing for the unexpected. Diabetes Spectrum 1991;4:173–176.

Chapter 73

Thyroid Disorders

Charles A. Reasner II, MD, FACE,
and Robert L. Talbert, PharmD, FCCP

Thyroid hormones affect the function of virtually every organ system. In the child, thyroid hormone is critical for normal growth and development. In the adult, the major role of thyroid hormone is to maintain metabolic stability. Substantial reservoirs of thyroid hormone in the thyroid gland and blood provide constant thyroid hormone availability. In addition, the hypothalamic–pituitary–thyroid axis is exquisitely sensitive to small changes in circulating thyroid hormone concentrations, and alterations in thyroid hormone secretion maintain peripheral free thyroid hormone levels within a narrow range. Patients seek medical attention for evaluation of symptoms due to abnormal thyroid hormone levels or because of diffuse or nodular thyroid enlargement.

Thyroid Hormone Physiology

THYROID HORMONE SYNTHESIS

The thyroid hormones thyroxine (T_4) and triiodothyronine (T_3) are formed on thyroglobulin, a large glycoprotein synthesized within the thyroid cell (Fig. 73.1). Because of the unique tertiary structure of this glycoprotein, iodinated tyrosine residues present in thyroglobulin are able to bind together to form active thyroid hormones.[1]

IODIDE TRANSPORT AND ORGANIFICATION

Iodide is actively transported from the extracellular space into the thyroid follicular cell against both electrical and biochemical gradients. Structurally related anions such as SCN^- (thiocyanate), ClO_4^- (perchlorate), and TcO_4^- (pertechnetate) are competitive inhibitors of iodine transport. In addition, bromine, fluorine, and lithium block iodide transport into the thyroid (Table 73.1). Inorganic iodide, which enters the thyroid follicular cell, is oxidized by thyroid peroxidase and is covalently bound (organified) to tyrosine residues of thyroglobulin (Fig. 73.2). It is interesting that while salivary glands and the gastric mucosa are able to actively transport iodide, they are unable to effectively incorporate iodide into proteins. Similarly, when tyrosine molecules are iodinated on proteins other than thyroglobulin, they lack the proper tertiary structure needed to allow the formation of active thyroid hormones.

IODOTYROSINE COUPLING

The iodinated tyrosine residues monoiodotyrosine (MIT) and diiodotyrosine (DIT) combine to form iodothyronines (Fig. 73.3). Thus, DIT and DIT combine to form T_4, while MIT and DIT constitute T_3. In addition to its role in iodine organification, the hemoprotein thyroid peroxidase also catalyses the formation of iodothyronines (coupling).

Iodine deficiency causes an increase in the ratio of MIT to DIT in thyroglobulin and leads to a relative increase in the production of T_3. Because T_3 is more potent than T_4, the increase in T_3 production in iodine-depleted areas may be beneficial. The thionamide drugs used to treat hyperthyroidism inhibit thyroid peroxidase and thus block thyroid hormone synthesis.

THYROID HORMONE SECRETION

Thyroglobulin is stored in the follicular lumen and must reenter the cell where the process of proteolysis liberates thyroid hormone into the bloodstream. Thyroid follicles active in hormone synthesis are identified histologically by columnar epithelial cells lining follicular lumens, which are depleted of colloid. Inactive follicles are lined by cuboidal epithelial cells and are replete with colloid. Both iodide and lithium block the release of preformed thyroid hormone through poorly understood mechanisms.

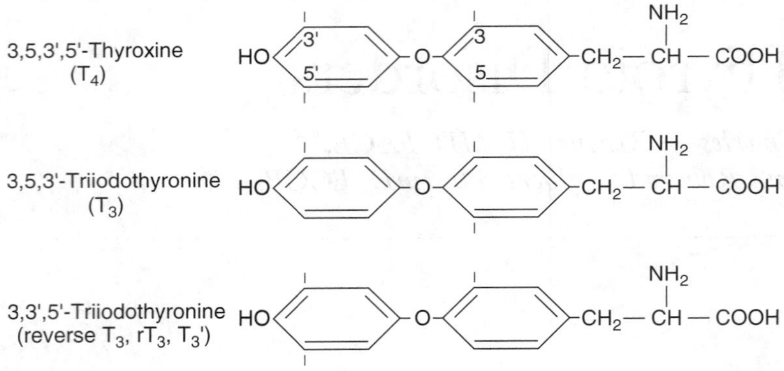

3,5,3',5'-Thyroxine (T_4)

3,5,3'-Triiodothyronine (T_3)

3,3',5'-Triiodothyronine (reverse T_3, rT_3, T_3')

Figure 73.1. Structure of thyroid hormones. *(From Hershman JM. Endocrine Pathophysiology. Philadelphia, Lea and Febiger, 1980, with permission.)*

CHARACTERISTICS OF CIRCULATING THYROID HORMONES

T_4 and T_3 are transported in the bloodstream by three proteins: thyroid-binding globulin (TBG), thyroid-binding prealbumin (TBPA), and albumin. It is estimated that 99.96% of T_4 and 99.5% of T_3 are bound to these proteins. Only the unbound (free) thyroid hormone is able to diffuse into the cell, elicit a biologic effect, and regulate thyroid-stimulating hormone (TSH) secretion from the pituitary.

Whereas T_4 is secreted solely from the thyroid gland, less than 20% of T_3 is produced in the thyroid. The majority of T_3 is formed from the breakdown of T_4 catalyzed by the enzyme 5′-monodeiodinase found in peripheral tissues. Because T_3 may be five times more active than T_4, the deiodinase enzymes play a pivotal role in determining overall metabolic activity. Two different 5′-monodeiodinase enzymes are present in the body. Type I enzymes are present in peripheral tissues; whereas, type II enzymes are found in the central nervous system. The principal characteristics of these enzymes are listed in Table 73.2. T_4 may also be acted on by the enzyme 5-monodeiodinase to form reverse T_3. Reverse T_3 has no known significant biologic activity. T_3 is removed from the body by deiodinative degradation and through the action of sulfotransferase enzymes systems to T_3 sulfate and 3,3-diiodothyronine sulfate.[2]

TABLE 73.1. THYROID HORMONE SYNTHESIS AND SECRETION INHIBITORS

Mechanism of Action	Substance
Blocks iodide transport into thyroid	Bromine Fluorine Lithium
Impairs organification and coupling of thyroid hormones	Thionamides Sulfonylureas Sulfonamide (?) Salicylamide (?) Antipyrine (?)
Inhibits thyroid hormone secretion	Iodide (large doses) Lithium

THYROID HORMONE RECEPTORS[3]

Thyroid hormone receptors regulate the transcription of target genes in the presence of physiologic concentrations of T_3. Thyroid receptors translocate from the cytoplasm to the nucleus and interact in the nucleus with T_3, target genes, and other proteins required for basal and T_3-dependent gene transcription. Thyroid receptors exist in multiple isoforms such as TRb2, TRb1, TRa1, and others in man and animals.

REGULATION OF THYROID HORMONE PRODUCTION

The production of thyroid hormone is regulated in two main ways. First, thyroid hormone is regulated by TSH

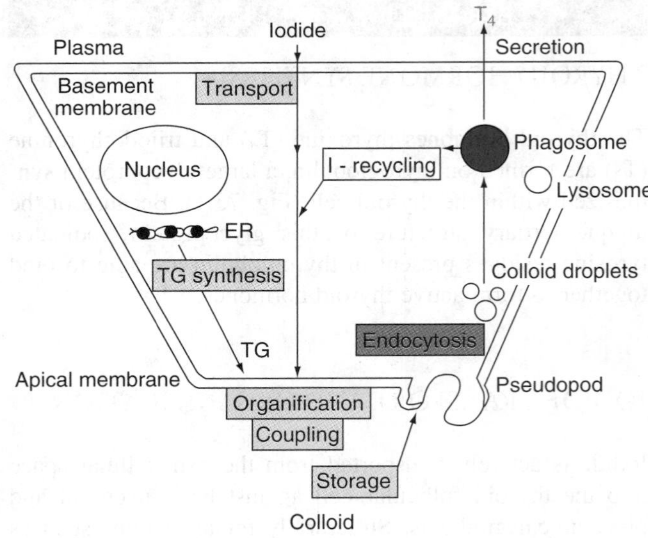

Figure 73.2. Thyroid hormone synthesis. Iodide is transported from the plasma, through the cell, to the apical membrane, where it is organified and coupled to thyroglobulin (TG) synthesized within the thyroid cell. Hormone stored as colloid reenters the cell through endocytosis and moves back toward the basal membrane where T_4 is secreted. Nonhormonal iodide is recycled. *(From Becker KL [ed]. Principles and Practice of Endocrinology and Metabolism. Philadelphia, JB Lippincott, 1990, with permission.)*

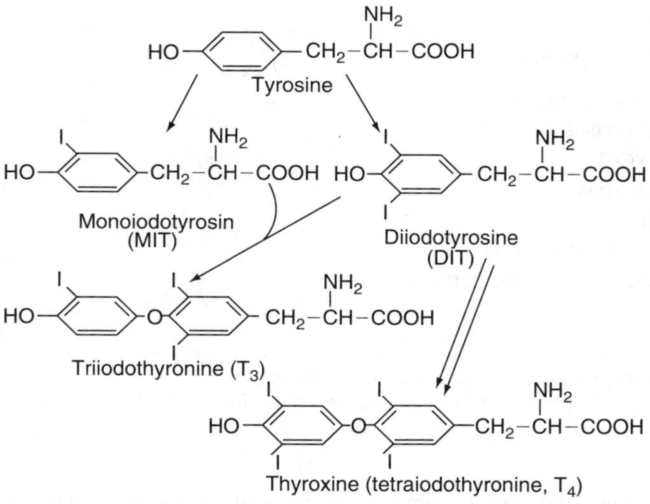

Figure 73.3. Scheme of coupling reactions. After tyrosine is iodinated to form MIT or DIT (organification of the iodine), MIT and DIT combine to form T_3, or two molecules of DIT form T_4. *(From Cryer PE. Diagnostic Endocrinology. New York, Oxford University Press, 1979, with permission.)*

secreted by the anterior pituitary. The secretion of TSH is itself under negative feedback control by the circulating level of free thyroid hormone and the positive influence of hypothalamic thyrotropin-releasing hormone (TRH). Second, extrathyroidal deiodination of T_4 to T_3 is regulated by a variety of factors including nutrition, nonthyroidal hormones, drugs, and illness.

THYROTOXICOSIS

Thyrotoxicosis results when tissues are exposed to excessive levels of T_4, T_3, or both. Like many endocrine disorders, thyrotoxicosis occurs more frequently in women, with an estimated annual incidence of 3 per 1000.

CLINICAL PICTURE

The clinical manifestations of thyrotoxicosis include nervousness, emotional lability, easy fatigability, and heat intolerance. A cardinal sign is loss of weight concurrent with an increased appetite. In the elderly patient and in the patient with very severe disease, anorexia may be present as well. The frequency of bowel movements may increase but frank diarrhea is unusual. Palpitations are a prominent and distressing symptom, particularly in the patient with preexisting heart disease. Proximal muscle weakness is common and is noted on climbing stairs or in getting up from a sitting position. Women may note their menses are becoming scanty and irregular.

A variety of physical signs may be elicited including warm, smooth, moist skin and unusually fine hair. Separation of the end of the fingernails from the nail beds (onycholysis) may be noted. Ocular signs that result from thyrotoxicosis include retraction of the eyelids and lagging of the upper lid behind the globe when the patient looks downward (lid lag). Physical signs of a hyperdynamic circulatory state are common and include tachycardia at rest, a widened pulse pressure, and a systolic ejection murmur. Gynecomastia is sometimes noted in men. Neuromuscular examination often reveals a fine tremor of the protruded tongue and outstretched hands. Deep tendon reflexes are generally hyperactive.

DIFFERENTIAL DIAGNOSIS OF THYROTOXICOSIS (TABLE 73.3)

Measurement of the radioactive iodine uptake (RAIU) is critical in the evaluation of the clinically thyrotoxic patient. The normal 24-hour RAIU ranges from 10–30% with some regional variation due to differences in iodine intake. An elevated RAIU indicates *true hyperthyroidism,* i.e., the patient's thyroid gland is actively overproducing T_4, T_3, or both. Conversely, a low RAIU indicates the excess thyroid hormone is not a consequence of thyroid gland hyperfunction. The importance of differentiating true hyperthyroidism from other causes of thyrotoxicosis lies in the widely different prognosis and treatment of the diseases in these two categories. Therapy of thyrotoxicosis associated with thyroid hyperfunction is mainly directed at decreasing the rate of thyroid hormone synthesis, secretion, or both. Such measures are ineffective in treating thyrotoxicosis that is not the result of true hyperthyroidism, because hormone synthesis and regulated hormone secretion are already at a minimum.

TABLE 73.2. CHARACTERIZATION OF 5′-IODOTHYRONINE DEIODINASE

	Type I	Type II
Effect of propylthiouracil	Inhibition	None
K_m for T_4	"High"	"Low"
Tissue localization	Liver, kidney	Pituitary, CNS
Response to hypothyroidism	Decrease	Increase
Possible physiologic role	Provides T_3 to serum	Provides T_3 to serum

(From Burrow GN, Oppenheimer SH, Volpé R (eds). Thyroid Function and Disease. Philadelphia, WB Saunders, 1989, with permission.)

TABLE 73.3. DIFFERENTIAL DIAGNOSIS OF THYROTOXICOSIS

Increased RAIU	Decreased RAIU
TSH-induced hyperthyroidism	Inflammatory thyroid disease
TSH-secreting tumors	Subacute thyroiditis
Selective pituitary resistance to T_4	Painless thyroid
Thyroid simulators other than TSH[a]	Ectopic thyroid tissue
TSAb (Graves' disease)	Struma ovarii
HCG (trophoblastic diseases)	Metastatic follicular carcinoma
Thyroid autonomy	Exogenous sources of thyroid hormone
Toxic adenoma	Medication
Multinodular goiter	Food

Key: RAIU, radioactive iodine uptake; TSH, thyroid-stimulating hormone; TSAb, thyroid-stimulating antibodies; HCG, human chorionic gonadotropin.
[a]The RAIU may be decreased if the patient has been recently exposed to excess iodine. (Adapted from Ingbar SH, Braverman LE, Werners SC. The Thyroid, 5th ed. Philadelphia, JB Lippincott, 1986, with permission.)

CAUSES OF THYROTOXICOSIS ASSOCIATED WITH AN ELEVATED RAIU

TSH-Induced Hyperthyroidism

To better understand these syndromes we must first review TSH biosynthesis and secretion. TSH is synthesized in the anterior pituitary as separate α- and β-subunit precursors. The α subunits from luteinizing hormone (LH), follicle-stimulating hormone (FSH), human chorionic gonadotropin (HCG), and TSH are similar whereas the β subunits are unique and confer immunologic and biologic specificity. Free β subunits are devoid of receptor binding and biologic activity and require combination with an α subunit to express their activity. Criteria for the diagnosis of TSH-induced hyperthyroidism include (1) evidence of peripheral hypermetabolism, (2) diffuse thyroid gland enlargement, (3) elevated free thyroid hormone levels, and (4) elevated serum immunoreactive TSH concentrations.[4] Because the pituitary gland is extremely sensitive to even minimal elevations of free T_4, a detectable TSH level in any thyrotoxic patient indicates the inappropriate production of TSH.

TSH-Secreting Pituitary Adenomas[5]

TSH-secreting pituitary tumors occur sporadically and release biologically active hormone that is unresponsive to normal feedback control. The mean age at diagnosis is around 40 years with women being diagnosed more commonly than men (8:7). These tumors may cosecrete prolactin or growth hormone; therefore, the patients may present with amenorrhea/galactorrhea or signs of acromegaly. Most patients present with classic symptoms and signs of thyrotoxicosis. Visual field defects may be present due to impingement of the optic chiasm by the tumor. Tumor growth and worsening visual field defects have been reported following treatment of thyrotoxicosis.

Diagnosis of a TSH-secreting adenoma should be made by demonstrating lack of response to TRH stimulation, elevated α-subunit levels, and radiologic imaging. Note that some small tumors are not identified by MRI. Moreover, 10% of "normal" individuals may have pituitary tumors noted on pituitary imaging.[6]

Transphenoidal pituitary surgery is the treatment of choice for TSH-secreting adenomas. Pituitary gland irradiation is often given following surgery to prevent tumor

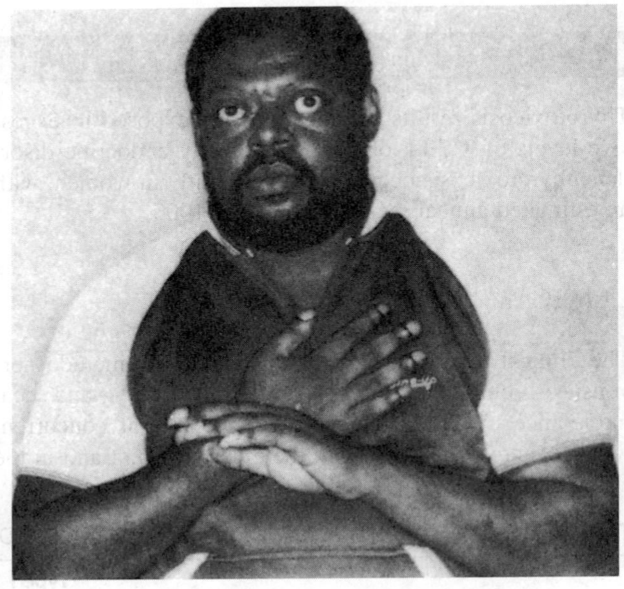

Figure 73.4. A 33-year-old man with Graves' disease manifested by bilateral exophthalmos, achropacy (clubbing), extensive pretibial myxedema, and insulin-dependent diabetes mellitus. When this photograph was taken, he already had been treated with radioactive ^{131}I, had become hypothyroid, and was receiving replacement therapy with exogenous L-thyroxine. *(From Becker KL [ed]. Principles and Practice of Endocrinology and Metabolism. Philadelphia, JB Lippincott, 1990, with permission.)*

recurrence. Treatment with bromocryptine has been useful in tumors that cosecrete prolactin.

Pituitary Resistance to Thyroid Hormone (PRTH)[5]

PRTH refers to selective resistance of the pituitary thyrotrophs to thyroid hormone. About twice as many women as men have been reported with this rare, probably familial syndrome. Multiple abnormalities have been reported in the initial 50 reported cases including schizophrenia (3 patients), mental retardation (2 patients), short fourth metacarpals (1 patient), and Marfanoid habitus (1 patient). About 90% of the patients studied have an appropriate increase in TSH in response to TRH; conversely, the TSH will be suppressed by T_3 administration.

Patients with PRTH require treatment to reduce their elevated thyroid hormone levels. Determining the appropriate serum T_4 level is difficult since TSH cannot be used to evaluate adequacy of therapy. Any reduction in thyroid hormone carries the risk of inducing thyrotroph hyperplasia. Ideally, agents that suppress TSH secretion could be used to treat these individuals. Glucocorticoid, dopaminergic drugs, somatostatin and its analog, and thyroid hormone analogs with reduced metabolic activity have all been tried. None is ideal.

THYROID STIMULATORS OTHER THAN TSH

Graves' Disease

Graves' disease is a syndrome that may include hyperthyroidism, diffuse thyroid enlargement, exophthalmus, pretibial myxedema, and thyroid acropachy (Figs. 73.4 and 73.5). The prevalence of Graves' disease is estimated to be 3 per 1000 population in the United States. Hyperthyroidism results from the action of thyroid-stimulating antibodies (TSAb), which are directed against the thyrotropin receptor on the surface of the thyroid cell. When these immunoglobulin G (IgG) antibodies bind to the receptor they activate the enzyme adenylate cyclase in the same manner as TSH. The reason for production of IgG antibodies in Graves' disease is unknown. Likewise, the causes of the extrathyroidal manifestations of this syndrome are not known. Clinically, the extrathyroidal disorders may not appear at the same time that hyperthyroidism develops. Autoantibodies that react with orbital muscle and fibroblast tissue in the skin are responsible for the extrathyroidal manifestations of Graves' disease and these autoantibodies are encoded by the same germline genes that encode for other autoantibodies for striated muscle and thyroid peroxidase.[7] The defect leading to abnormal antibody production may be a genomic point mutation in the extracellular domain of the thyrotropin receptor.[8]

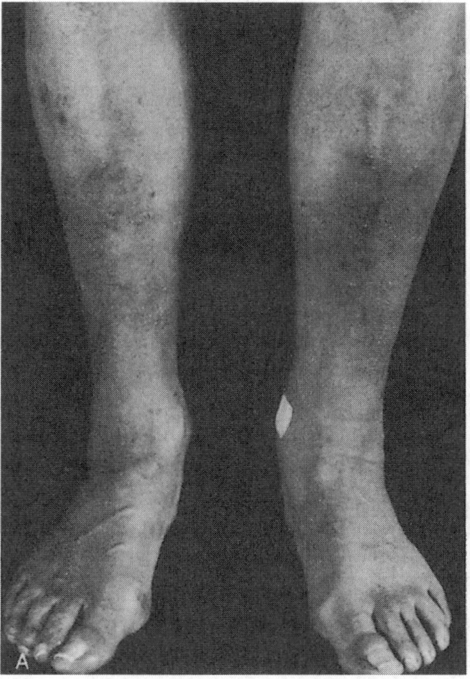

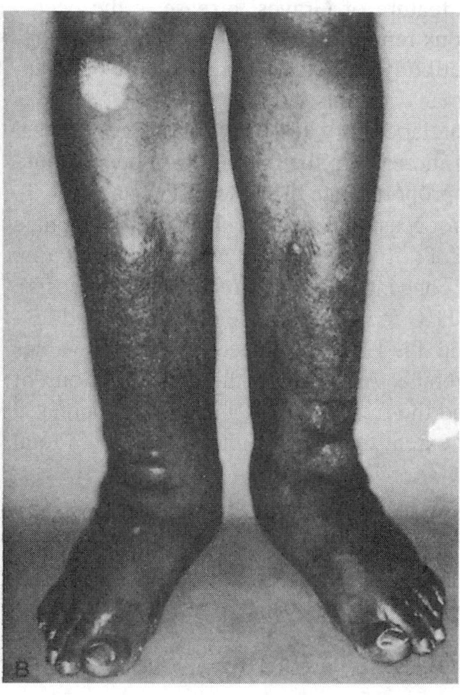

Figure 73.5. (A–B): Different degrees of involvement of tissues with pretibial myxedema. *(From Becker KL [ed]. Principles and Practice of Endocrinology and Metabolism. Philadelphia, JB Lippincott, 1990, with permission.)*

There is now compelling evidence that heredity and gender both play a role in the development of clinically overt thyroid disease. Several lines of evidence support a role for heredity. First, there is a well-recognized clustering of Graves' disease within some families. Twin studies in patients with Graves' disease have revealed that a monozygotic twin has a 50% likelihood of ultimately developing the disease compared to a 9% likelihood for a dizygotic twin. Second, the occurrence of other autoimmune diseases, including Hashimoto's thyroiditis, is also increased in families of patients with Graves' disease. Third, several studies have demonstrated an increased frequency of certain human leukocyte antigens (HLAs) in patients with Graves' disease. In Caucasians, HLA-D3 is present in at least one-half of patients, and the presence in an individual of both HLA-B8 and -D3 confers a fourfold greater risk for developing Graves' disease. A role for gender in the emergence of Graves' disease is suggested by the fact that hyperthyroidism is approximately eight times more common in women than men.

The thyroid gland is diffusely enlarged in the majority of patients and is commonly 40–60 g (two to three times the normal size). The surface of the gland is smooth and the consistency varies from soft to firm. In patients with severe disease, a thrill may be felt and a systolic bruit may be heard over the gland. The presence of any of the extrathyroidal manifestations of this syndrome including exophthalmus, thyroid acropachy, or pretibial myxedema in a thyrotoxic patient is pathognomonic of Graves' disease (Fig. 73.4). An important clinical feature of Graves' disease is the occurrence of spontaneous remissions. The abnormalities in thyroid-stimulating antibody production may decrease or disappear over time in many patients.

The results of laboratory tests in thyrotoxic Graves' disease include an increase in the overall hormone production rate with a disproportionate increase in T_3 relative to T_4 (Table 73.4). In an occasional patient, the disproportionate overproduction of T_3 is exaggerated with the result that only the serum T_3 concentration is increased (T_3 toxicosis). The saturation of TBG is increased due to the elevated levels of serum T_4 and T_3. This is reflected in elevated values for the T_3 resin uptake. As a result, the concentrations of free T_4, free T_3, and the free T_4 and T_3 indices are increased to an even greater extent than are the measured serum total T_4 and T_3 concentrations. The TSH level will be undetectable due to negative feedback by elevated levels of thyroid hormone at the pituitary.

In the patient with manifest disease, measurement of the serum T_4 concentration, T_3 resin uptake (or free T_4), and the TSH value will confirm the diagnosis of thyrotoxicosis. If the patient is not pregnant, a 24-hour RAIU should be obtained. An increased RAIU documents that the thyroid gland is inappropriately utilizing the iodine to produce more thyroid hormone at a time when the patient is thyrotoxic.

Hypokalemic periodic paralysis is a rare complication of hyperthyroidism commonly observed in Asian and Hispanic populations. It presents as recurrent proximal muscle flaccidity ranging from mild weakness to total paralysis. The paralysis may be asymmetrical and usually involves muscle groups that are strenuously exercised before the attack. Cognition and sensory perception are spared while deep tendon reflexes are commonly markedly diminished. Hypokalemia results from a shift of potassium from extracellular to intracellular sites. High carbohydrate loads and exercise provoke the attacks. Treatment includes correcting the hyperthyroid state, potassium administration, spironolactone to conserve potassium and propranolol to minimize intracellular shifts.[9]

Trophoblastic Diseases

In the past decade several lines of evidence have shown that HCG is a thyroid stimulator and may cause hyperthyroidism.[10] The basis for the thyrotropic effect of HCG is the molecular similarity of HCG to TSH (similar α subunits and unique β subunits). In hyperthyroid patients with very high HCG levels, serum TSH may be inappropriately detectable due to the weak cross-reactivity of HCG in the radioimmunoassay for TSH. In patients with hyperthyroidism due to trophoblastic tumors, serum HCG levels usually exceed 300 U/mL and always exceed 100 U/mL. The mean peak HCG level in normal pregnancy is 50 U/mL. On a molar basis, HCG has only 1/10,000th the activity of pituitary TSH in mouse bioassays. Nevertheless, this thyrotropic activity may be very substantial in patients with trophoblastic tumors whose serum HCG concentrations may reach 2000 U/mL.

TABLE 73.4. THYROID FUNCTION TEST RESULTS IN DIFFERENT THYROID CONDITIONS

	Total T_4	Free T_4	Total T_3	T_3 Resin Uptake	Free Thyroxine Index	TSH
Normal	4.5–12.5 μg/dL	0.8–2.8 ng/dL	80–220 ng/dL	22–34%	1.0–4.3 U	0.25–6.7 μU/mL
Hyperthyroid	↑↑	↑↑	↑↑↑	↑	↑↑↑	↓↓
Hypothyroid	↓↓	↓↓	↓	↓↓	↓↓↓	↑↑
Increased TBG	↑	Normal	↑	↓	Normal	Normal

Key: TSH, thyroid-stimulating hormone; TBG, thyroid-binding globulin.

THYROID AUTONOMY

Toxic Adenoma

An autonomous thyroid nodule is a discrete thyroid mass whose function is independent of pituitary control. These nodules may be referred to as a toxic adenoma or a "hot" nodule because of their appearance on a radioiodine thyroid scan (Fig. 73.6). The amount of thyroid hormone produced by an autonomous nodule is mass related. Therefore, hyperthyroidism usually occurs with larger nodules, i.e., those more than 4 cm in diameter. Older patients are more likely to be thyrotoxic from autonomous nodules than are younger patients. Among 239 patients with autonomous nodules reported by Hamburger,[11] 56% of those more than 60 years old were hyperthyroid while only 12% of those less than 60 years of age were hyperthyroid. There are many reports of isolated elevation of serum T_3 in patients with autonomously functioning nodules. Therefore, if the T_4 level is normal, a T_3 level must be measured to rule out T_3 toxicosis. Once a radioiodine scan has demonstrated that the toxic thyroid adenoma would collect more radioiodine than the surrounding tissue, independent function may be documented by a failure of the autonomous nodule to decrease its iodine uptake during exogenous T_3 administration. RAI ablation or subtotal thyroidectomy are both effective in treating this condition. Because thyroid carcinoma is not a practical consideration in an autonomously functioning thyroid nodule, observation is usually recommended for patients with autonomously functioning nodules who are euthyroid. Burman et al.[12] followed 54 patients with solitary autonomous thyroid nodules for an average of 2 years. The course of the disease was completely benign and none of the patients developed hyperthyroidism during the follow-up period.

Multinodular Goiters

In multinodular goiters (MNGs), follicles with a very high degree of autonomous function coexist with normal or even nonfunctioning follicles. Thyrotoxicosis in a multinodular goiter occurs when the follicles with a high degree of autonomy generate enough thyroid hormone to exceed the needs of the patient. It is not surprising that this type of hyperthyroidism develops insidiously over a period of several years and predominantly affects older individuals with long-standing goiters. Often, elderly women present with subtle signs of hyperthyroidism which are superimposed on underlying heart disease. The patient's complaints of weight loss, depression, anxiety, and insomnia may be attributed to old age. Any unexplained chronic illness in an elderly patient presenting with a multinodular goiter calls for the exclusion of hidden thyrotoxicosis.

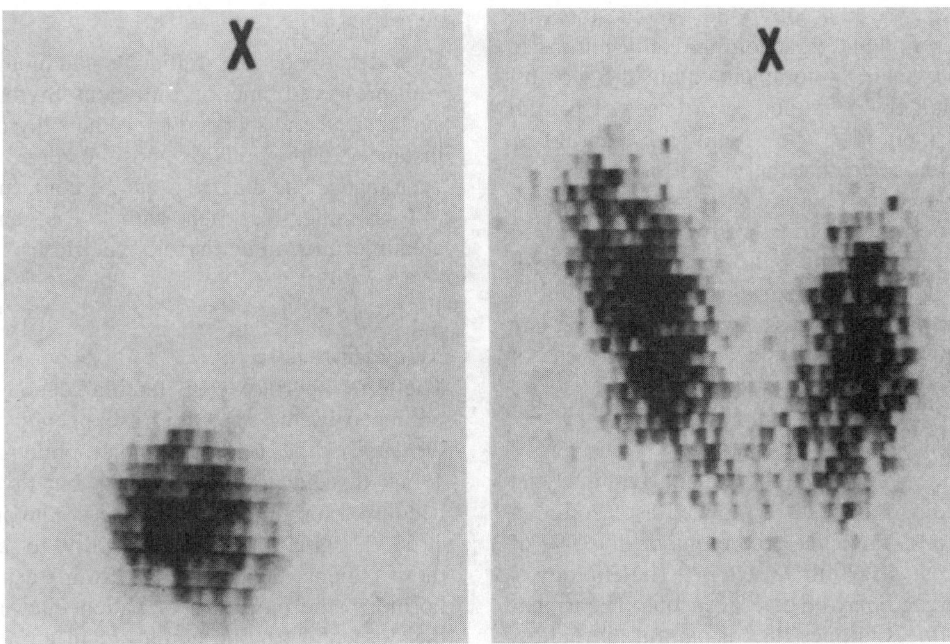

Figure 73.6. Left, autonomously functioning nodule is suppressing the remainder of thyroid gland. Right, previously suppressed lobes of thyroid gland are visualized 3 months after radioiodine treatment of hyperfunctioning nodule. The "X" is a marker for thyroid cartilage. *(From Becker KL [ed]. Principles and Practice of Endocrinology and Metabolism. Philadelphia, JB Lippincott, 1990, with permission.)*

A thyroid scan will show patchy areas of autonomously functioning thyroid tissue. The preferred treatment for toxic MNG is RAI or surgery. Surgery is usually selected for younger patients and patients in whom large goiters impinge on vital organs.

CAUSES OF THYROTOXICOSIS ASSOCIATED WITH A SUPPRESSED RAIU

Inflammatory Thyroid Disease

Subacute Thyroiditis

Painful subacute (viral, or DeQuervain's) thyroiditis is felt to be caused by viral invasion of thyroid parenchyma. Typically, patients complain of severe pain in the thyroid region, which often extends to the ear on the affected side. With time, the pain may migrate from one side of the gland to the other. Low-grade fever is common. Systemic symptoms due to thyrotoxicosis are present. On physical examination, the thyroid gland is firm and exquisitely tender. Signs of thyrotoxicosis are present.

Thyroid function tests typically run a triphasic course. Initially, serum thyroxine levels are elevated due to release of preformed thyroid hormone from disrupted follicles. The 24-hour RAIU during this time is less than 2% due to thyroid inflammation and TSH suppression by the elevated thyroxine level. As the disease progresses, intrathyroidal hormone stores are depleted and the patient may become mildly hypothyroid with an appropriately elevated TSH level. During the recovery phase thyroid hormone stores are replenished and serum TSH elevation gradually returns to normal. Recovery is generally complete within 2–6 months. Most patients remain euthyroid and recurrences of painful thyroiditis are extremely rare. The patient with painful thyroiditis should be reassured that the disease is self-limited and is unlikely to recur. Thyrotoxic symptoms may be relieved with β blockers. Aspirin (650 mg orally every 6 hours) will usually relieve the pain. Occasionally, prednisone (20 mg orally three times a day) must be used to suppress the inflammatory process. Antithyroid drugs are not indicated because they do not decrease the release of preformed thyroid hormone.

Painless Thyroiditis

Since its description in 1975, painless (silent, lymphocytic, postpartum) thyroiditis has been recognized as a common cause of thyrotoxicosis and may represent up to 15% of cases of thyrotoxicosis in North America.[13] The etiology is not fully understood and may be heterogeneous. The triphasic course of this illness mimics that of painful thyroiditis. Most patients present with mild thyrotoxic symptoms. Lid retraction and lid lag are present while exophthalmos is absent. The thyroid gland may be diffusely enlarged but thyroid tenderness is absent.

The 24-hour RAIU will be suppressed to less than 2% during the thyrotoxic phase of painless thyroiditis. Antithyroglobulin and antimicrosomal antibody levels are elevated in more than 50% of patients. Painless thyroiditis frequently occurs during the immediate postpartum period and individual patients may experience recurrence of the disease with subsequent pregnancies. Patients with mild hyperthyroidism and painless thyroiditis should be reassured that they have a self-limited disease. Adrenergic symptoms may be ameliorated with propranolol. Antithyroid drugs are not indicated because they do not decrease the release of preformed thyroid hormone.

Ectopic Thyroid Tissue

Struma Ovarii

Struma ovarii is a teratoid tumor of the ovary which is capable of making thyroid hormone. This extremely rare cause of thyrotoxicosis is suggested by the absence of thyroid enlargement in a thyrotoxic patient with a suppressed RAIU. The diagnosis is established by localizing functioning thyroid tissue in the ovary with whole body radioactive iodine (^{131}I) scanning. Interestingly, struma ovarii without associated hyperthyroidism is much more common than struma ovarii associated with hyperthyroidism. Only 9 of 233 patients mentioned in an extensive review of struma ovarii had signs of thyrotoxicosis, which were relieved by tumor resection.[14] Because the tissue is neoplastic and potentially malignant, surgical resection is the recommended treatment.

Follicular Cancer

In widely metastatic follicular carcinomas with relatively well-preserved function, sufficient thyroid hormone can be synthesized and secreted to produce thyrotoxicosis. In most instances, a previous diagnosis of thyroid malignancy has been made. The diagnosis can be confirmed by whole body ^{131}I scanning. Treatment with ^{131}I is generally effective at ablating functioning thyroid metastases.

Exogenous Sources of Thyroid Hormone

Medication

The term "thyrotoxicosis factitia" denotes hyperthyroidism produced by the ingestion of exogenous thyroid hormone. Obesity is the most common nonthyroidal disorder for which thyroid hormone is used, but thyroid hormone has been used for almost every conceivable problem from menstrual irregularities and infertility to baldness. Because these patients do not benefit from treatment with thyroid hormone, the physician or patient may gradually increase the dose of hormone employed in an attempt to gain the desired effect. Obviously, thyrotoxicosis factitia can also occur when too large a dose of thyroid hormone is employed for conditions in which it is likely to be beneficial, such as hypothyroidism or nontoxic goiter. Rarely, thyrotoxicosis factitia is caused by the purposeful and secretive ingestion of thyroid hormone by disturbed patients (usually with a medical background) who wish to obtain attention or lose weight.

Thyrotoxicosis factitia should be suspected in a thyrotoxic patient without infiltrative ophthalmopathy or thyroid enlargement. The RAIU uptake is at low levels because the patient's thyroid gland function is suppressed by the exogenous thyroid hormone. Measurement of plasma thyroglobulin (TG) is a valuable laboratory aid in the diagnosis of thyrotoxicosis factitia.[15] TG is normally secreted in small amounts by the thyroid gland; however, when thyroid hormone is taken orally, very low amounts of thyroglobulin are detectable in the plasma. In other entities characterized by a low RAIU, such as silent thyroiditis, leakage of preformed thyroid hormone results in elevated thyroglobulin levels. If a history of thyroid hormone ingestion is elicited or deduced, exogenous thyroid hormone should be withheld between 4–6 weeks and thyroid function tests repeated to document that the euthyroid state has been restored.

Amiodarone may induce thyrotoxicosis (2–3% of patients) or hypothyroidism. Amiodarone contains 37.2% iodine by weight and approximately 6 mg/d of iodine is released for each 200 mg of amiodarone. The recommended daily amount of iodine is 200 μg/d. Thyroid cytotoxicity produced by amiodarone is mainly due to a direct effect of the drug on thyroid cells, but excess iodide released from the drug may contribute to its toxic action. Iodine-induced thyroid dysfunction occurs primarily in patients with preexisting thyroid disease (Graves' disease, nodular goiter, Hashimoto's thyroiditis). An inflammatory process induced by amiodarone or iodine, which also leads to follicular cell damage and subacute thyroiditis with leakage of thyroid hormones into the circulation, is associated with elevated interleukin-6 levels. The manifestations may be untypical symptoms such as ventricular tachycardia and exacerbation of underlying chronic obstructive pulmonary disease. Prednisone has been reported to normalize IL-6 and thyroid hormone values.[16–19]

Iodinated glycerol has recently been found useful in the symptomatic treatment of chronic obstructive pulmonary disease. This compound contains 15 mg of organic iodine per tablet or 25 mg/mL of solution. Thyroid dysfunction has been reported with this preparation and patients with underlying thyroid disease need to be monitored carefully if iodinated glycerol is used.[20]

Food

An outbreak of thyrotoxicosis occurred between April 1984 and August 1985 among residents of southwestern Minnesota and adjacent areas of South Dakota and Iowa. One hundred twenty-one cases were identified through surveillance at medical clinics, laboratories, hospitals, and physicians' offices. Investigation of the outbreak demonstrated an association between the occurrence of thyrotoxicosis and the consumption of ground beef prepared from neck trimmings processed by a single slaughtering plant. The cause was confirmed by finding bovine thyroid tissue and high concentrations of thyroid hormone in samples of ground beef.[21] Bovine thyroid tissue had been introduced into the neck trimmings inadvertently during the process of "gullet trimming," a procedure that harvests muscles from bovine larynx. The outbreak resolved after this procedure was discontinued. The clinical features of the illness suggested a diagnosis of silent thyroiditis and it is possible that sporadic cases or even outbreaks of a similar nature have occurred in the past but were not recognized. Permanent prohibition of the use of livestock glands in the preparation of edible meat products has been proposed by the U.S. Department of Agriculture.

TREATMENT OF HYPERTHYROIDISM (TABLE 73.5)

Three common treatment modalities are used in the management of hyperthyroidism: antithyroid medications, radioactive iodine (RAI), and surgery. The overall therapeutic objectives are to eliminate the excess thyroid hormone and minimize the symptoms and long-term consequences of hyperthyroidism. Therapy must be individualized based on the type and severity of hyperthyroidism, patient age and gender, existence of nonthyroidal conditions, and response to previous therapy.[22]

Antithyroid Medications

Thiourea Drugs

Two drugs within this category, propylthiouracil (PTU) and methimazole, are approved for the treatment of hyperthyroidism in the United States. They are classified as thioureylenes (thioamides), which incorporate a N–C–S=N group into their ring structures.

Mechanism of Action. PTU and methimazole share several mechanisms to inhibit the biosynthesis of thyroid hormone.[23] These drugs inhibit the peroxidase enzyme system of the thyroid gland, thus preventing oxidation of trapped iodide and subsequent incorporation into iodotyrosines and ultimately iodothyronine ("organification"). Second, they inhibit coupling of monoiodotyrosine and diiodotyrosine to form T_4 and T_3. The coupling reaction may be more sensitive to these drugs than the iodination reaction. Experimentally, these drugs exhibit immunosuppressive effects although the clinical relevance of this finding is unclear. In patients with Graves' disease, antithyroid drug treatment has been associated with lower thyroid-stimulating antibody titers and restoration of normal suppressor T-cell function. However, perchlorate, which has a different mechanism action, also decreases thyroid-stimulating anti-

TABLE 73.5. MANAGEMENT OF HYPERTHYROIDISM

Modality	Maintenance Dose (mg/d)	Maximal Dose (mg/d)	Actions	Indications
Thiourea drugs			Inhibit thyroid hormone synthesis (PTU also inhibits peripheral conversion of T_4 to T_3); may exert immunosuppressive actions	First-line therapy for Graves' hyperthyroidism, short-term therapy before ^{131}I or surgery
Propylthiouracil (PTU) 50 mg tablets	200–600	1200		
Methimazole (Tapazole) 5 and 10 mg tablets	10–60	120		
β-Adrenergic antagonists[a]			Ameliorate action of thyroid hormone in tissues	Adjunctive therapy; often therapy required for thyroiditis
Propranolol	80–160	480		
Nadolol	80–160	320		
Iodine-containing compounds			Inhibit T_4 and T_3 release	Preparation for surgery; thyrotoxic crisis
Lugol's solution	750	750		
Potassium iodide (SSKI)	10–300	400		
Miscellaneous				
Potassium perchlorate	NA	NA	Inhibits iodine transport	No routine indications
Lithium carbonate	NA	NA	Inhibits thyroid hormone synthesis and release	No routine indications
Glucocorticoids			Ameliorates actions of thyroid hormones in tissues; exerts immunosuppressive action (Graves' disease)	Severe subacute thyroiditis; thyrotoxic crisis
Radioactive iodine (RAI, ^{131}I)	NA	2–10 mCi	Ablation of thyroid gland	First-line therapy for Graves' hyperthyroidism, treatment of choice for recurrent thyrotoxicosis; young adults to elderly; contraindicated in pregnancy, children, and active ophthalmopathy
Surgery	NA	NA	Removal of thyroid gland	Patients should be euthyroid prior to surgery; caution in elderly; cold iodine given prior to surgery

Key: SSKI, Saturated solution of potassium iodide; NA, not applicable.
[a]Not approved in the United States by the FDA for the treatment of thyrotoxicosis.

bodies suggesting that normalization of the thyroid hormone level may itself improve the abnormal immune function. PTU inhibits the peripheral conversion of T_4 to T_3.[24] This effect is acutely dose related and occurs within hours of PTU administration. Methimazole does not have this effect. Over time, depletion of stored hormone and lack of continuing synthesis of thyroid hormone results in the clinical effects of these drugs.

Pharmacokinetics. Both antithyroid drugs are well absorbed (80–95%) from the gastrointestinal tract, with peak serum concentrations about 1 hour after ingestion. The plasma half-life ranges of PTU and methimazole are 1–2.5 hours and 6–9 hours, respectively, and are not appreciably affected by thyroid status. Urinary excretion is about 35% for PTU and less than 10% for methimazole. These drugs are actively concentrated in the thyroid gland, which may account for the disparity between their relatively short plasma half-lives and the effectiveness of once-daily dosing regimens even with PTU. Approximately 60–80% of PTU is bound to plasma albumin while methimazole is not protein bound. Methimazole readily crosses the placenta and appears in breast milk. Older studies suggested that PTU crosses the placental membranes only one-tenth as well as methimazole; however, these studies were done in the course of therapeutic abortion early in pregnancy.[25] More recently, Gardner et al.[26] have shown that PTU mean maternal and cord concentrations at term were 0.19 and 0.36 g/mL, respectively, for a fetal : 3 maternal ratio of 1.89. Higher fetal concentrations may be consistent with either reduced clearance in the fetus or an ion trapping or pH partitioning effect. TSH was 0.8 mIU/mL in maternal blood while the concentration in cord blood was 10.2 mIU/mL, which is consistent with subclinical hypothyroidism in the infant, as the T_3 and T_4 concentrations were in the normal range. Additionally, they found that PTU concentrations were lower in the third trimester compared with postpartum values suggesting altered pharmacokinetics of PTU during pregnancy.

Dosing/Monitoring. PTU is available as 50-mg tablets and methimazole as 5- and 10-mg tablets. Methimazole is approximately 10 times more potent than PTU. Initial therapy with PTU ranges from 300–600 mg daily, usually in four divided doses. Methimazole is given in three divided doses totaling 30–60 mg/d. Although the traditional recommendation is for divided doses, evidence exists that both drugs can be given as single daily doses.[27] Patients with severe hyperthyroidism may require larger initial doses and some may respond better at these larger doses if the dose is divided. The maximal blocking doses of PTU and methimazole are 1200 and 120 mg daily, respectively. Once the intrathyroidial pool of thyroid hormone is reduced and new hormone synthesis is sufficiently blocked, clinical improvement should ensue. Usually within 4–8 weeks of initiating therapy, symptoms are diminished and circulating thyroid hormone levels are returning to normal. At this time the tapering regimen can be started. Changes in dose for each drug should be made on a monthly basis, as the endogenously produced T_4 will reach a new "steady-state" concentration in this interval. Typical ranges of daily maintenance doses for PTU and methimazole are 50–300 mg and 5–30 mg, respectively. If clinical improvement is not observed, the following factors should be considered: (1) noncompliance, (2) insufficient dosage to block hormone synthesis, and (3) inadequate dosing interval if a single daily dose has been used.

If the objective of therapy is to induce a long-term remission, the patient should remain on continuous antithyroid drug therapy for 12–24 months. Antithyroid drug therapy induces permanent remission rates of 31–77% with an overall average of about 46%. This is much higher than the remission rate seen with propranolol alone which is reported to range from 22–36%. Possible explanations for induction of a permanent remission include alteration of TSAb to a nonstimulating form of immunoglobulin, the development of immune complexes that block the antibody or its actions, or alteration in the underlying immunologic defect that allowed TSAb to be produced initially. The latter may occur in the setting of a partial defect in immunoregulation that is aggravated by stress of some type. Restoration of the euthyroid state may cause reversal of this partial defect and allow the functional capacity of the immune system to return to normal. The presence of TSAb predicts relapse, in that about 75% of patients who are antibody positive will relapse while only 25% who are negative will relapse.[28] Those patients who relapse after the initial course are less likely to have a remission with subsequent courses of therapy. Patient characteristics for a favorable outcome include a small goiter (less than 50 g), short duration of disease (less than 6 months), no previous history of relapse with antithyroid drugs, and low maintenance dosage requirements of antithyroid drug therapy.[29] Based on the T_3 suppression tests, relapse occurs in 72% of patients with nonsuppressed TSH levels within 1 year. In those patients who suppressed following T_3 administration, 30% of recurrences occurred in the first year, 60% between 1 and 5 years and 10 years.[30] Relapse at 5 years was less common in patients experiencing suppression (34 versus 74%). It is important that patients be followed every 6–12 months after remission occurs. If a relapse occurs, alternate therapy with RAI is preferred to a second course of antithyroid drugs.

One of the clinical controversies surrounding the use of the thionamide drug in Graves' disease is whether the dosage or duration of therapy affects the remission rate. Romaldini et al.[31] compared remission rates in a prospective study of patients receiving high doses of PTU (mean dose of 693 mg/d) or methimazole (60 mg/d) for 1–2 years. Findings revealed that the high-dose group had a nearly twofold higher remission rate (75.4 versus 41.6%) after a mean follow-up period of 42 months; however, this high-dose group had a higher incidence of side effects, especially hepatotoxicity. Thus, the high-dose regimen has not received widespread clinical use. Others have found no relationship between dose and response.[30,32]

Greer et al.[33] found that remission rates of 30–40% with therapy continuing for only 2–6 months versus the conventional 1–2 years. Hedley et al.[30] found the rate of a remission and relapse favored antithyroid drug use for 1 year rather than 6 months. Today, most clinicians administer antithyroid medications for at least 12 months.

Past recommendations for the use of T_4 along with antithyroid drugs were that concurrent therapy was not needed. Hashizume et al.[34] have reported a dramatic decrease in relapse rates in a group of Japanese patients with Graves' disease treated with methimazole and thyroxine for 1 year, followed by thyroxine alone for 3 years. The relapse rate for those given thyroxine was only 1.7%, compared 34.7% in those given methimazole and placebo. It is theorized that the low relapse rate reflects thyroxine-induced suppression of thyroid antigens.

Adverse Effects. Minor adverse reactions to PTU and methimazole have an overall incidence of 5–16% depending on the dose and the drug, while major adverse effects occur in 1.5–4.6% of patients receiving these drugs.[35] Pruritic maculopapular rashes (sometimes associated with vasculitis based on skin biopsy), arthralgias, and fevers occur in up to 5% of patients and may occur at greater frequency with higher doses and in children. Rashes often disappear spontaneously, but if persistent, may be managed with antihistamines.

Perhaps one of the most common side effects is a benign transient leukopenia characterized by a white blood cell (WBC) count of less than 4000/mm.[36] This condition occurs in up to 12% of adults and 25% of children and sometimes can be confused with mild leukopenia seen in Graves' disease. This mild leukopenia is not a harbinger of the more serious adverse effect of agranulocytosis, so therapy can usually be continued. If a *minor* adverse reaction occurs with one antithyroid drug, the alternate thiourea may be tried, but cross-sensitivity occurs in about 50% of patients.[37]

Agranulocytosis is the most serious adverse effect of thiourea drug therapy and is characterized by fever, malaise, gingivitis, oropharyngeal infection, and a granulocyte count of less than 250/mm.[36] These drugs are concentrated in granulocytes and this reaction may represent a direct toxic effect rather than hypersensitivity. This toxic reaction has occurred with both thioureas, and the incidence varies from 0.5–6%. It is higher in patients over age 40 receiving a methimazole dose greater than 40 mg/d or the equivalent dose of PTU. Agranulocytosis almost always develops in the first 3 months of therapy. Since the onset is sudden, routine monitoring is not recommended. Peripheral lymphocytes obtained from patients with PTU-induced agranulocytosis undergo transformation in the presence of other thioamides suggesting that these severe reactions are immunologically mediated and patients should not receive other thionamides.[38] Aplastic anemia has been reported with methimazole, and in one report this was associated with an inhibitor to colony-forming units.[39] Once antithyroid drugs are discontinued, clinical improvement is seen over several days to weeks. Patients should be counseled to discontinue therapy and contact their physician when flu-like symptoms such as fever, malaise, or sore throat develop.

Arthralgias and a lupus-like syndrome (sometimes in the absence of antinuclear antibodies) has been reported in 4–5% of patients. This generally occurs after 6 months of therapy. Uncommonly, polymyositis, presenting as proximal muscle weakness and elevated creatine phosphokinase, has been reported with PTU administration.[40] Gastrointestinal intolerance is also reported to occur in 4–5% of patients. Hepatotoxicity, which usually occurs within the first 3 months of therapy, may be seen with both methimazole and PTU with a prevalence of about 1.3%.[35] In a cohort study of 54 patients placed on PTU 100–150 mg/d, Liaw et al.[41] found that elevation in alanine aminotransferase and alkaline phosphatase occurred in 28% of patients and that with continued therapy, the enzyme levels normalized in most patients. High doses of PTU are more likely to produce severe hepatitis and even death. Discontinuation of therapy usually results in complete resolution of hepatitis. Although older reports suggested that congenital skin defects (aplasia cutis) may be caused by methimazole and carbimazole, a recent registry review from the Netherlands could not find an association between maternal use of these drugs and skin defects.[42] Hypoprothrombinemia is a rare complication of thionamide therapy. Patients who have experienced a *major* adverse reaction to one thiourea drug should not be converted to the alternate drug because of cross-sensitivity.

Iodides

Iodide was the first form of drug therapy for Graves' disease. Its mechanism of action is to acutely block thyroid hormone release, inhibit thyroid hormone biosynthesis by interfering with intrathyroidal iodide utilization (the Wolff–Chaikoff effect), and decrease the size and vascularity of the gland. This early inhibitory effect provides symptom improvement within 2–7 days of initiating therapy, and serum T_4 and T_3 concentrations may be reduced for a few weeks. Despite the reduced release of T_4 and T_3, thyroid hormone synthesis continues at an accelerated rate, resulting in a gland rich in stored hormones. The normal and hyperfunctioning thyroid soon escapes from this inhibitory effect by decreasing the active transfer of iodide into the gland. However, large doses of iodine may exacerbate hyperthyroidism or indeed precipitate hyperthyroidism in some previously euthyroid individuals (Jod–Basedow disease). This Jod–Basedow phenomenon is most common in iodine-deficient areas, particularly in patients with preexisting nontoxic goiter. Iodides are often used as adjunctive therapy to prepare a patient with Graves' disease for surgery, to acutely inhibit thyroid hormone release and quickly attain the euthyroid state in severely thyrotoxic patients with cardiac decompensation,[37] or to inhibit thyroid hormone release following radioactive iodine therapy.

Potassium iodide is available either as a saturated solution (SSKI), which contains 40 mg of iodide per drop, or as Lugol's solution, which contains 8 mg of iodide per drop. The typical starting dose of SSKI is 3–10 drops daily (120–400 mg) in water or juice. There is no documented advantage to using doses in excess of 6–8 mg/d. When used to prepare a patient for surgery, it should be administered 7–14 days preoperatively. As an adjunct to RAI, SSKI should not be used before, but rather 3–7 days after RAI treatment so that the radioactive iodide can concentrate in the thyroid. The most frequent toxic effect with iodide therapy is hypersensitivity reactions (skin rashes, drug fever, rhinitis, conjunctivitis); salivary gland swelling; "iodism" (metallic taste, burning mouth and throat, sore teeth and gums, symptoms of a head cold, and sometimes stomach upset and diarrhea); and gynecomastia.

Other compounds containing organic iodide have also been used therapeutically for hyperthyroidism. These include various radiologic contrast media that share a triiodo- and monoaminobenzene ring with a propionic acid chain (e.g., iopanoic acid and sodium ipodate). The effect of these compounds is due to the iodine content inhibiting thyroid hormone release as well as competitive inhibition of 5′-monodeiodinase conversion related to their structures, which resemble thyroid analogues.[43] Bal and Nair[44] have advocated the use of iopanoic acid, 1 g daily for 21 days, in the preoperative control of thyrotoxicosis and following RAI ablative therapy.

Adrenergic Blockers

Because many of the manifestations of hyperthyroidism are mediated by β-adrenergic receptors, β blockers (especially propranolol) have been used widely to ameliorate thyrotoxic symptoms such as palpitations, anxiety, tremor, and heat intolerance. Although β blockers are quite effective for symptom control, they have no effect on the urinary excretion of calcium, phosphorus, hydroxyproline, creatinine, or various amino acids, suggesting a lack of effect on peripheral thyrotoxicosis and protein metabolism.[45,46] Furthermore, β blockers do not reduce TSAb nor prevent thyroid storm. Propranolol and nadolol partially block the conversion of T_4 to T_3 but this contribution to the overall therapeutic effect is small in magnitude. Inhibition of conversion of T_4 to T_3 is mediated by D-propranolol, which is devoid of β-blocking activity, and L-propranolol, which is responsible for the antiadrenergic effects, has little effect on the conversion.[47]

Beta blockers are usually used as adjunctive therapy with antithyroid drugs, RAI, or iodides when treating Graves' disease or toxic nodules; in preparation for surgery; or in thyroid storm. The only conditions for which β blockers are primary therapy for thyrotoxicosis are thyroiditis and iodine-induced hyperthyroidism. The dose of propranolol required to relieve adrenergic symptoms is variable but an initial dose of 20–40 mg four times daily is effective (heart rate less than 90 beats/min) for most patients. A comparable dose for nadolol would be 80 mg daily.[48] Younger or more severely toxic patients may require as much as 240–480 mg/d because there seems to be an increased clearance rate in these patients. Beta blockers are contraindicated in patients with congestive heart failure unless it is due solely to tachycardia (high output) and in patients who have developed cardiomyopathy and heart failure. Nonselective agents and those lacking intrinsic sympathomimetic activity (ISA) should be used with caution in patients with asthma, chronic obstructive lung disease, and diabetes mellitus (particularly insulin-dependent diabetes). Cardioselective and ISA β blockers may have a slight margin of safety in these situations. Other patients in whom contraindications exist are those with sinus bradycardia, those receiving monoamine oxidase inhibitors or tricyclic antidepressants, and those with spontaneous hypoglycemia. Beta blockers may also prolong gestation and labor during pregnancy. Other side effects include nausea, vomiting, anxiety, insomnia, lightheadedness, bradycardia, and hematologic disturbances.

Historically important antiadrenergic agents such as reserpine and guanethidine have been usurped by β blockers but other antiadrenergic agents such as centrally acting sympatholytics and calcium channel antagonists may have some role in the symptomatic treatment of hyperthyroidism. These drugs might be useful when contraindications to β blockade exist. When compared to nadolol 40 mg twice daily, clonidine 150 g twice daily reduced plasma catecholamines, whereas nadolol increased both epinephrine and norepinephrine after 1 week of treatment.[49] Diltiazem 120 mg given every 8 hours reduced heart rate by 17%; fewer ventricular extrasystoles were noted after 10 days of therapy and diltiazem has been shown to be comparable to propranolol in lowering heart rate and blood pressure.[50,51] The findings for diltiazem may not apply to verapamil and nifedipine due to their disparate effects on blood pressure and contractility when compared to diltiazem.

Radioactive Iodine

Although other radioisotopes have been used to ablate thyroid tissue, sodium iodide 131 (^{131}I) is considered to be the agent of choice. RAI is administered as a colorless and tasteless liquid that is well absorbed and concentrates in the thyroid. Sodium iodide 131 is a β emitter with a tissue penetration of 2 mm and a half-life of 8 days. Other organs take up ^{131}I but the thyroid gland is the only organ in which organification of the absorbed iodine takes place. Initially, RAI disrupts hormone synthesis by incorporating into thyroid hormones and thyroglobulin. Over a period of weeks, follicles that have taken up RAI and surrounding follicles develop evidence of cellular necrosis, breakdown of follicles, development of bizarre cell forms, nuclear pyknosis, and destruction of small vessels within the gland leading to edema and fibrosis of the interstitial tissue. Pregnancy is an absolute contraindication to the use of RAI.

Beta blockers may be given anytime without compromising RAI therapy, accounting for their role as a mainstay of adjunctive therapy to RAI treatment. If iodides are administered, they should be given 3–7 days *after* RAI to prevent interference with the uptake of RAI in the thyroid gland. Thioamides should not routinely be administered after RAI, because their use is associated with a lower rate of hypothyroidism and a higher incidence of early post-treatment recurrence or persistence of hyperthyroidism.[52] The slow onset of effect with RAI warrants symptomatic control with adjunctive thionamides to attain a euthyroid state up until 1 week prior to RAI in the patient whose symptoms are not controlled with β blockers alone. Because thyroid hormone levels will transiently increase following RAI treatment due to release of performed thyroid hormone, patients with cardiac disease and elderly patients are often treated with thionamides prior to RAI ablation. Occasionally, in patients with underlying cardiac disease, it may be necessary to reinstitute antithyroid drug therapy following radioactive iodine abalation. The standard practice is to withdraw the thionamide 4 days prior to RAI treatment and to reinstitute it 4 days following therapy. Administering antithyroid drug therapy following RAI treatment may result in a higher rate of post-treatment recurrence or persistent hyperthyroidism.[52]

Corticosteroid administration will blunt and delay the rise in antibodies to the TSH receptor, thyroglobulin, and thyroid peroxidase while reducing T_3 and T_4 concentrations following RAI.[53] Some have suggested that corticosteroids be used in conjunction with RAI treatment of patients with Graves' disease. Theoretically, if shared thyroidal and orbital antigen is involved in the pathogenesis of Graves' ophthalmopathy, antigen released with RAI treatment could aggravate preexisting eye disease. Note also that thyroid ablation may decrease eye disease in the long term by removing the source of antigen.[54]

Destruction of the gland attenuates the hyperthyroid state and hypothyroidism commonly occurs months to years following RAI. The goal of therapy is to destroy overactive thyroid cells and a single dose of 4000–8000 rads results in a euthyroid state in 60% of patients at 6 months or less. The remaining 40% become euthyroid within 1 year, requiring two or more doses. It is advisable that a second dose of RAI be given 6 months after the first RAI treatment if the patient remains hyperthyroid. Variables that influence the outcome of RAI include gender (men are less likely to develop hypothyroidism), race (blacks are more resistant to ^{131}I), the size of the thyroid, severity of disease, and perhaps the level of TSAb. The acute, short-term side effects of ^{131}I therapy are minimal and include mild thyroidal tenderness and dysphagia. Concern over the development of thyroid carcinoma and leukemia and increased risk of mutations and congenital defects now appears to be unfounded as long-term follow-up studies have not revealed increased risk for these complications.[55,56]

A common approach to Graves' hyperthyroidism is to administer a single dose of 5–10 mCi. Larger doses are likely to induce hypothyroidism and are seldom given outside the United States due to the imposition of stringent safety restrictions. For example, in the United Kingdom, a nursery school teacher is advised to stay out of school for 3 weeks following a 15-mCi dose of ^{131}I.[57]

Surgery

Surgical removal of the thyroid gland became feasible in 1923 when Plummer discovered that iodine reduced the gland's vascularity, making this definitive procedure possible. Traditional preparation of the patient for thyroidectomy includes PTU or methimazole until the patient is biochemically euthyroid (usually 6–8 weeks), followed by the addition of iodides (500 mg/d) for 10–14 days before surgery to decrease the vascularity of the gland. Levothyroxine may be added to maintain the euthyroid state while the thionamides are continued. **Levothyroxine has also been suggested to prevent postoperative recurrence of goiter; however, recent studies show a nonsignificant trend for levothyroxine.**[58] Propranolol for several weeks preoperatively and 7–10 days after surgery has also been used to maintain a pulse rate less than 90 beats/min. Combined pretreatment with propranolol and 10–14 days of potassium iodide also has been advocated.[59]

The overall morbidity rate with surgery is 2.7%. Hyperthyroidism persists or recurs in 0.6–17.9% of patients after thyroidectomy for Graves' disease and is more common in children. The most common complications of surgery include hypothyroidism (up to about 49%), hypoparathyroidism (up to 3.9%), and vocal cord abnormalities (up to 5.4%). The frequent occurrence of hypothyroidism following surgery requires periodic follow-up for identification and treatment of these patients.[60,61]

EVALUATION OF THERAPEUTIC OUTCOMES—HYPERTHYROIDISM

There is no single best treatment for all patients with Graves' disease. Treatment is individualized on the basis of the patient's age and health condition. Often the treatment decision is empiric. The thionamides are the preferred treatment for children and pregnant women. The increased risk of hypothyroidism following RAI or surgery make thionamides a reasonable treatment alternative in young adults. Patients with a large gland, diffuse goiter, and long duration of disease are unlikely to have a long-term remission with thionamide therapy. Noncompliant patients and those with swallowing difficulty may require surgery or RAI therapy. RAI is the preferred treatment of debilitated, cardiac, and elderly patients and patients who have had a failure or toxic reaction on drug therapy. RAI is also used in patients who relapse after surgery. Thyroidectomy is considered the treatment of choice for coexisting cold nodules, extremely large goiters (over 80 g), and patients with contraindications to thionamides (i.e., allergy or adverse effects) and RAI (i.e., pregnancy).

After therapy (thionamides, RAI, or surgery) for hyperthyroidism has been initiated, patients should be evaluated on a monthly basis until they reach a euthyroid condition. Clinical signs of continuing thyrotoxicosis (tachycardia, weight loss, heat intolerance, etc.) or the development of hypothyroidism (bradycardia, weight gain, lethargy, etc.) should be noted. Beta blockers may be used to control symptoms of thyrotoxicosis until the definitive treatment has returned the patient to a euthyroid state. Titration of the thionamide dose should be done as outlined in the Dosing/Monitoring section of this chapter. The goal is to maintain the patient's free thyroxine level and TSH concentration in the "normal range" until a remission is induced. If the patient was treated with RAI or surgically, the patient must be observed for the development of hypothyroidism. Clinical evaluation and the results of thyroid function testing will allow you to determine when thyroxine replacement is indicated. We typically begin thyroxine replacement when the free T_4 level is "below normal" and the TSH concentration is above 10. Once thyroxine replacement is initiated, the goal is to maintain both the free thyroxine level and the TSH concentration in the "normal range." Once a stable dose of thyroxine is identified, the patient may be followed every 6–12 months.

Finally, a common, potentially confusing clinical situation should be mentioned. Why are the TSH concentrations suppressed in some patients who are clinically hypothyroid and who have a low free T_4 level? In patients with long-standing hyperthyroidism, the pituitary thyrotrophs responsible for making TSH become atrophic. The average amount of time required for these cells to resume normal functioning is 6–8 weeks. (Uy H, Reasner C, Samuels M. Pattern of recovery of the hypothalamic–pituitary–thyroid axis following radioactive iodine therapy in patients with Graves' disease, submitted.) Therefore, if a thyrotoxic patient has his/her free T_4 concentration lowered rapidly, before the thyrotrophs resume normal function, a period of "transient central hypothyroidism" will be observed.

SPECIAL CONDITIONS

Graves' Disease and Pregnancy

Hyperthyroidism during pregnancy is almost solely due to Graves' disease, with approximately 0.2% of pregnancies affected. The increased metabolic rate is usually well tolerated in pregnant women and there is no increase in maternal mortality or morbidity in treated patients; however, postpartum thyroid storm has been reported in untreated individuals. Fetal loss is also more common due to spontaneous abortion and premature delivery in untreated pregnant women. Transplacental passage of thyroid-stimulating antibodies may occur, causing fetal as well as neonatal hyperthyroidism.[62]

Because RAI is contraindicated in pregnancy and surgery is usually not recommended (especially during the first trimester), antithyroid drug therapy is usually the treatment of choice. Methimazole readily crosses the placenta and appears in breast milk. Older studies suggested that PTU should be the drug of choice in pregnancy; however, based on the study performed by Gardner et al.,[26] this is no longer the case.

PTU is considered to be the drug of choice in pregnancy with the lowest possible doses used to maintain the maternal T_4 level in the high-normal range for pregnancy, which is usually 12–17 g/dL (somewhat higher than the usual 4–12 g/dL because of high TBG concentrations). To prevent goiter and suppression of fetal thyroid function, PTU is usually prescribed in daily doses of 300 mg or less and tapered to 50–150 mg daily after 4–6 weeks. PTU doses of less than 200 mg daily are unlikely to produce fetal goiter. During the last trimester, TSAbs fall spontaneously and some patients will go into remission so that antithyroid drug doses may be reduced. A rebound in maternal hyperthyroidism may require more intensive treatment postpartum than in the last trimester of pregnancy.

Long-term administration of iodides (even vaginal povidone-iodine) may lead to iodine crossing the placenta and fetal goiter. Momotani et al.[63] have recently shown that iodine given during pregnancy to women with mild to moderate Graves' disease resulted in reduction in maternal and fetal cord free T_4 concentrations and that most of the fetal T_4 concentrations were in the normal range at delivery. Concomitant thyroid hormone given to the mother does prevent fetal goiter since thyroxine does not cross the placenta well due to its extensive protein binding. Thyroxine has been shown to reduce the level of antibodies to the TSH receptor and to prevent the recurrence of hyperthyroidism following delivery.[64] Long-term use of propranolol should be avoided because of its association with fetal respiratory depression, small placenta, intrauterine growth retardation, postnatal bradycardia, and hypoglycemia. If acute symptoms occur or preoperative preparation is required, propranolol or iodides may be used cautiously for less than 7 days. Surgery should be delayed until after the first trimester to avoid spontaneous abortion.[65]

Neonatal and Pediatric Hyperthyroidism

Following delivery, some babies will be hyperthyroid due to placental transfer of TSAb, which stimulates thyroid hormone production *in utero* and postpartum. This is likely if the maternal TSAb titers were quite high. The disease is usually expressed 7–10 days postpartum and treatment with antithyroid drugs may be needed for as long as 8–12 weeks until the antibody is cleared (IgG half-life is about 2 weeks). Iodide and sodium ipodate may be used for the first few days to acutely inhibit hormone release.[66]

Childhood hyperthyroidism is usually managed with either PTU or methimazole. Long-term follow-up studies suggest that this form of therapy is quite acceptable with 25% of a cohort experiencing remission every 2 years.[67,68]

Thyroid Storm

Thyroid storm is a life-threatening medical emergency characterized by severe thyrotoxicosis, high fever (often greater than 103°F), tachycardia, tachpnea, dehydration, delirium, coma, nausea, vomiting, and diarrhea. Precipitating factors for thyroid storm include infection, trauma, surgery, RAI treatment, and withdrawal from antithyroid drugs. It may occur at any age and has an average duration of 72 hours, although symptoms may persist up to 8 days if treatment is not aggressive. With aggressive treatment, the mortality rate has been lowered to 20%. The following therapeutic measures should be instituted promptly: (1) suppression of thyroid hormone formation and secretion, (2) antiadrenergic therapy, (3) administration of cortico-

TABLE 73.6. DRUG DOSAGES USED IN THE MANAGEMENT OF THYROID STORM

Drug	Regimen
Propythiouracil	900–1200 mg/d PO in four or six divided doses
Methimazole	90–120 mg/d PO in four or six divided doses
Sodium iodide	Up to 2 g/d IV in single or divided doses
Lugol's solution	5–10 drops TID in water or juice
Saturated solution of potassium iodide	1–2 drops TID in water or juice
Propranolol	40–80 mg every 6 h
Reserpine	0.25 mg PO every 8 h 2.5–50 mg IV or IM every 8 h
Guanethidine	10–50 mg PO every 8 h
Lithium	600–1500 mg/d PO in three or four divided doses
Dexamethasone	5–20 mg/d PO or IV in divided doses
Prednisone	25–100 mg/d PO in divided doses
Methylprednisolone	20–80 mg/d IV in divided doses
Hydrocortisone	100–400 mg/d IV in divided doses

steroids, and (4) treatment of associated complications or coexisting factors that may have precipitated the storm. Specific agents used in thyroid storm are outlined in Table 73.6. PTU in large doses is the preferred thionamide because it interferes with the production of thyroid hormones and blocks the peripheral conversion of T_4 to T_3. If patients are unable to take medications orally, the tablets can be crushed into suspension and instilled by gastric tube. Iodides, which rapidly block the release of preformed thyroid hormone, should be administrated *after* PTU is initiated to inhibit iodide utilization by the overactive gland. If iodide is administered first, it may provide the substrate permitting the synthesis and storage of a large amount of thyroid hormone in the thyroid gland, which would prolong the duration of hyperthyroidism thereafter.

Antiadrenergic therapy with the short-acting agent esmolol may be used in the patient with pulmonary disease or at risk for cardiac failure because its effects may be rapidly reversed.[69] Reserpine and guanethidine are no longer recommended for the acute treatment of thyroid storm because their onset of action is long relative to β blockers. Corticosteroids are generally recommended although Rosenberg[70] has pointed out that there is no convincing evidence of adrenocortical insufficiency in thyroid storm, and the benefits derived from steroids may be due to their antipyretic action and their effect of stabilizing blood pressure. Lithium has effects that are qualitatively and quantitatively similar to iodine but with significant toxicity; therefore, its use is not recommended routinely. General supportive measures, including acetaminophen as an antipyretic (do not use aspirin or other nonsteroidal anti-inflammatory agents since they may displace bound thyroid hormone), fluid and electrolyte replacement, sedatives, digitalis, antiarrhythmics, insulin, and antibiotics should be given as indicated. Plasmapheresis and peritoneal dialysis have been used to remove excess hormone when the patient has not responded to more conservative measures.[71,72]

HYPOTHYROIDISM

Hypothyroidism is defined as the clinical and biochemical syndrome resulting from decreased thyroid hormone production. Overt hypothyroidism occurs in 1.5–2% of women and 0.2% of men and its incidence increases with age.[73] The vast majority of hypothyroid patients have thyroid gland failure (primary hypothyroidism). Pituitary failure is an uncommon cause of hypothyroidism but should be suspected in a patient with decreased levels of thyroxine and inappropriately normal or low TSH levels. Most patients with secondary hypothyroidism will have clinical signs of more generalized pituitary insufficiency such as abnormal menses and decreased libido, or evidence of a pituitary adenoma such as visual field defects, galactorrhea, or acromegaloid features. Generalized (peripheral and central) resistance to thyroid hormone is extremely rare.

Thyroid hormone is essential for normal growth and development during embryonic life. Thyroid hormone deficiency during fetal and neonatal development results in mental retardation. In the child thyroid hormone deficiency may manifest as growth retardation. In the adult manifestations of hypothyroidism are varied and nonspecific. There is slowing of physical and mental activity as well as cardiovascular, gastrointestinal, and neuromuscular function. Common symptoms of hypothyroidism include dry skin, cold intolerance, weight gain, constipation, and weakness. Complaints of lethargy and fatigue or loss of ambition and energy are also common but are less specific. Depression may result from untreated hypothyroidism. Speech is often slow as well as hoarse.

The most common signs of decreased levels of thyroid hormone include coarse skin and hair, cold skin, periorbital puffiness, and bradycardia. Reversible neurologic syndromes such as carpal tunnel syndrome, polyneuropathy, and cerebellar dysfunction may also occur. Muscle cramps, myalgia, and stiffness are frequent complaints of the hypothyroid patients. Objective weakness is common with proximal muscles being affected more than distal muscles. Slow relaxation of deep tendon reflexes is common.

A rise in the TSH level is the first evidence of primary hypothyroidism. Many patients will have a T_4 level within the normal range (compensated hypothyroidism) and few, if any, symptoms of hypothyroidism. As the disease progresses the T_4 concentration will drop below the normal level. Interestingly, the T_3 concentration will often be maintained in the normal range in spite of a low T_4. The RAIU is not a useful test in the evaluation of a hypothyroid patient.

CAUSES OF HYPOTHYROIDISM (TABLE 73.7)

Chronic Autoimmune Thyroiditis (Hashimoto's Disease)

Autoimmune thyroiditis is the most common cause of spontaneous hypothyroidism in the adult. Patients may present with either goitrous thyroid gland enlargement and mild hypothyroidism or thyroid gland atrophy and more severe thyroid hormone deficiency. Both forms of autoimmune thyroiditis probably result from cell- and antibody-mediated thyroid injury. The bulk of evidence suggests that the presence of specific defects in suppressor T-lymphocyte function leads to the survival of a randomly mutating clone of helper T lymphocytes, which are directed against normally occurring antigens on the thyroid membrane. Once these T lymphocytes interact with thyroid membrane antigen, B lymphocytes are stimulated to produce thyroid antibodies.[74]

Antimicrosomal antibodies are present in virtually all patients with Hashimoto's thyroiditis and appear to be directed against the enzyme thyroid peroxidase and other thyroid cell membrane antigens. These antibodies are capable of fixing complement and inducing cytotoxic changes in thyroid cells. Antibodies that are capable of stimulating thyroid growth are also present in the goitrous variety of Hashimoto's disease; conversely, antibodies that inhibit the trophic effects of TSH are present in the atrophic type.

TABLE 73.7. CAUSES OF HYPOTHYROIDISM

Primary Hypothyroidism
Hashimoto's disease
Iatrogenic hypothyroidism
Others
Iodine deficiency
Enzyme defects
Thyroid hypoplasia
Goitrogens
Secondary Hypothyroidism
Pituitary disease
Hypothalamic disease

Iatrogenic Hypothyroidism

Iatrogenic hypothyroidism follows exposure to radiation (radioiodine or external radiation) or surgery. Hypothyroidism occurs within a year after ^{131}I therapy in most patients treated for Graves' disease. Thereafter, it occurs at a rate of approximately 2.5% each year. External radiation therapy to the region of the thyroid using doses of greater than 2500 rads for therapy of neck carcinoma also causes hypothyroidism. This effect is dose dependent with more than 50% of patients developing hypothyroidism who have received more than 4000 rads to the thyroid bed. Total thyroidectomy causes hypothyroidism within 1 month.

Other Causes of Primary Hypothyroidism

Iodine deficiency, enzymatic defects within the thyroid gland, thyroid hypoplasia, and maternal ingestion of goitrogens during fetal development may cause cretinism. Early recognition and treatment of the resultant thyroid hormone deficiency is essential for optimal mental development. Large-scale screening programs in North America, Europe, Japan, and Australia are now in place. The frequency of congenital hypothyroidism in North America and Europe is between 1 per 3500 to 4000 live births. In the United States, there are racial differences in the incidence of congenital hypothyroidism with whites being affected seven times as frequently as blacks.[75]

In the adult, hypothyroidism may rarely be caused by iodine deficiency and goitrogens. Rarely, iodine ingestion in the form of expectorants can lead to hypothyroidism. In sensitive persons, the iodide blocks the synthesis of thyroid hormone leading to an increased secretion of TSH which causes thyroid enlargement.[76] Thus, both iodine excess and iodine deficiency can cause decreased secretion of thyroid hormone.

Causes of Secondary Hypothyroidism

Pituitary Disease

TSH is required for normal thyroid secretion. Thyroid atrophy and decreased thyroid secretion follow pituitary failure. Pituitary insufficiency may be caused by destruction of thyrotrophs by either functioning or nonfunctioning pituitary tumors, surgical therapy, external pituitary radiation, postpartum pituitary necrosis (Sheehan's syndrome), infiltrative processes of the pituitary such as metastatic tumors, tuberculosis, histiocytosis, and autoimmune mechanisms. In all these situations, TSH deficiency most often occurs in association with other pituitary hormone deficiencies.

In most hypothyroid patients with pituitary disease, serum TSH concentrations are low or normal. A serum TSH concentration in the normal range is clearly inappropriate if the patient's T_4 is low.

Note that pituitary enlargement in hypothyroidism does not invariably indicate the presence of a primary pituitary tumor. Pituitary enlargement is seen in patients with severe primary hypothyroidism due to compensatory hyperplasia and hypertrophy of the thyrotrophs. These patients are easily separated from patients with primary pituitary failure by measuring a TSH. Serum TSH concentrations and pituitary enlargement decline during thyroid hormone replacement therapy, indicating that the TSH secretion is not autonomous.

Hypothalamic Hypothyroidism

TRH deficiency also causes hypothyroidism. Hypothalamic hypothyroidism occurs predominantly in children unaccompanied by any anatomic abnormality. In both adults and children it may occur as a result of cranial irradiation, trauma, infiltrative diseases, neoplastic diseases, or occasionally pituitary lesions that interrupt the hypothalamic pituitary circulation. Fortunately, hypothalamic hypothyroidism is rare.

TREATMENT

The goals of therapy are to restore thyroid hormone concentration in tissue, provide symptomatic relief, prevent neurologic deficits in newborns and children, and reverse the biochemical abnormalities of hypothyroidism. Any of the commercially available thyroid preparations accomplish this goal (Table 73.8); however, levothyroxine (L-thyroxine) is considered the drug of choice. The thyroid preparations are either natural (i.e., desiccated thyroid, thyroglobulin) or synthetic (levothyroxine, liothyronine, liotrix) in origin. The availability of sensitive and specific assays for total and free hormone levels as well as TSH now allow more definitive dose titration to allow adequate replacement without inadvertent overdose. The response of TSH to TRH had been advocated by some for "fine-tuning" thyroid replacement but this is not necessary if the sensitive immunoradiometric assays (IRMA) for TSH are used.

Natural Thyroid Hormones

Desiccated thyroid is derived from hog, beef, or sheep thyroid gland. The *United States Pharmacopeia,* 11th edition, requires Thyroid USP to contain 38 μg (±15%) of levothyroxine and 9 μg (±10%) of liothyronine for each 65 mg (1 grain) of the labeled content of thyroglobulin. Thyroglobu-

TABLE 73.8. THYROID PREPARATIONS USED IN THE TREATMENT OF HYPOTHYROIDISM

Drug/Dosage Form	Content	Relative	Comments/Equivalency
Thyroid, USP Aromour Thyroid, USV ¼-, ½-, 1-, 1½-, 2-, 3-, 4-, and 5-grain tablets	Desiccated hog, beef, or sheep thyroid gland	1 grain (equivalent to 60 μg of T_4)	Unpredictable hormonal stability, inexpensive generic brands may not be bioequivalent
Thyroglobulin 32 mg (½ grain), 65 mg (1 grain), 100 mg (1½ grain), 130 mg (2 grain), and 200 mg (3 grain)	Partially purified hog thyroglobulin	1 grain	Standardized biologically to give T_4T_3 ratio of 2.5 : 1 ; more expensive than thyroid extract; no clinical advantage
L-Thyroxine Synthroid, Flint; Levothyroid, USV 25, 50, 75, 100, 125, 150, 175, 200, and 300 g tablets; 100 g/mL, 5 mL	Synthetic T_4	100 μg	Stable; predictable potency; generics may be bioequivalent; when switching from natural thyroid to L-thyroxine, lower dose by ½ grain; variable absorption between products; $t_{1/2}$ = 7 days, so daily dosing
Liothyroine Cytomel, Smith Kline and French 5-, 25-, and 50-μg tablets	Synthetic T_3	25 μg	Uniform absorption; rapid onset; $t_{1/2}$ = 1.5 days, multiple daily dosing; monitor response with TSH assays
Liotrix Euthyroid, Parke-Davis; Thyrolar, USV ¼, ½, 1, 2, and 3 strength tablets	Synthetic T_4T_3 in 4 : 1 ratio		Stable, predictable, expensive; lacks therapeutic rationale because T_4 is converted to T_3 peripherally

lin USP should contain 36 μg (±15%) of levothyroxine and 12 μg (±10%) of liothyronine for each 65 mg (1 grain) of the labeled content of thyroglobulin. Not all generic brands may be bioequivalent and switching among brands in patients stabilized on one product should be discouraged. Thyroid USP, as an animal protein-derived product, may be antigenic in allergic or sensitive patients. Even though desiccated thyroid is inexpensive, its limitations preclude it from being considered as a drug of choice for hypothyroid patients. Thyroglobulin is a purified hog gland extract but it has no clinical advantages and is not widely used.

Synthetic Thyroid Hormones[77]

Levothyroxine (T_4, L-thyroxine) is the drug of choice for thyroid replacement and suppressive therapy because it is chemically stable, relatively inexpensive, free of antigenicity, and has uniform potency. Whereas T_3 and not T_4 is the biologically active form of thyroid hormone, levothyroxine administration results in a pool of thyroid hormone that is readily and consistently converted to T_3; in this regard levothyroxine may be thought of as a prohormone. The half-life of levothyroxine is approximately 7 days. This long half-life is responsible for a stable pool of prohormone and the need for only once-daily dosing with levothyroxine. Older studies with levothyroxine suggested that bioavailability was low and erratic; however, this product has been reformulated and the average bioavailability is now approximately 80%.[78] The time to maximal absorption is 2 hours and this should be considered when T_4 and TSH concentrations are determined.[79] The average increase in serum T_4 concentrations with levothyroxine is 10–15% and T_4 levels remain above the basal concentration for about 6 hours. Ileojejunal bypass and short bowel syndrome significantly reduce the amount of levothyroxine absorbed and the use of high doses or concurrent medium-chain triglycerides may be used to overcome lack of absorption.[80,81] Mucosal diseases such as sprue and diabetic diarrhea may also reduce absorption. Cholestyramine, sucralfate, aluminum hydroxide,[82] ferrous sulfate, soybean formula, and possibly lovastatin may also impair the absorption of levothyroxine from the gastrointestinal tract. Drugs that increase nondeiodinative T_4 clearance include rifampin, carbamazepine, and possibly phenytoin. Selenium deficiency and amiodarone may block the conversion of T_4 to T_3.

Generic preparations may not be bioequivalent with brand name products and have resulted in inadequate thyroid replacement. One study has shown that Synthroid and Levothroid are bioequivalent.[83] Substitution of other multisource thyroid preparations should be undertaken with caution as the product content of levothyroxine as well as its bioavailability may not be equivalent.[78,84] When doses of levothyroxine exceeding 2 μg/kg/d are used, the clearance of levothyroxine is increased.[78]

Liothyronine (T_3) is chemically pure with known potency and has a shorter half-life of 1.5 days. Although it is widely used diagnostically in the T_3 suppression test, T_3 has some clinical disadvantages including a higher incidence of cardiac adverse effects, higher cost, and difficulty in monitoring with conventional laboratory tests. Liotrix is a combination of synthetic T_4 and T_3 in a 4:1 ratio that attempts to mimic the natural hormonal secretion. It is chemically stable, pure, and has a predictable potency. The major limitations to this product are high cost and lack of therapeutic rationale, because about 35% of T_4 is peripherally converted T_3.

Dosing/Monitoring

During the mid-1980s the average dose of levothyroxine was about 160 μg/d. With the advent of more sensitive assay methods for TSH and the reformulation of levothyroxine, it is now apparent that many patients have been treated with excessive amounts of levothyroxine. More recent studies suggest that the average maintenance dose for most adults should be closer to about 110–120 μg/d.[85–87] Indeed, as many as one-third of patients receiving levothyroxine 150 μg daily will be overreplaced.[88] There is, however, a wide range of replacement doses, necessitating individualized therapy and appropriate monitoring to determine an adequate but not excessive dose.

The initial dose of levothyroxine is dependent on the patient's age, the presence of associated disorders, and the severity and duration of hypothyroidism. In young patients with long-standing disease and patients over age 45 without known cardiac disease, therapy should be initiated with 50 μg daily of levothyroxine and increased to 100 μg daily after 1 month. The recommended initial daily dose for older patients or those with known cardiac disease is 25 μg/d titrated upward in increments of 25 μg at monthly intervals to prevent stress on the cardiovascular system. Some patients may experience an exacerbation of angina with higher doses of thyroid hormone.

Patients with subclinical hypothyroidism (seen more commonly in the elderly and particularly in women) have no or few signs or symptoms, normal serum T_3 and T_4 concentrations, and an elevated basal TSH concentration. The prevalence of this disorder is thought to be about 8% but the reported range is quite wide.[25,89] Although the treatment of subclinical hypothyroidism is controversial, patients presenting with marked elevations in TSH (>10 mU/L) and high titers of TSAb or prior treatment with ^{131}I may be most likely to benefit from treatment.[89] Other patients who may improve with replacement include those with mild symptoms of hypothyroidism and depression. It should be noted that some studies find that only one of four treated patients experienced improvement.[90] Conservative treatment goals in this situation would be to maintain serum T_4 and T_3 levels in the normal range and reduce TSH to a midrange value. This is usually accomplished with a subreplacement dose of levothyroxine of 50–75 μg per day.

Once euthyroidism is attained, the daily maintenance dose of levothyroxine does not fluctuate greatly. As patients age, the dosing requirement may need to be reduced.[91] The ability to measure serum TSH concentrations has improved the accuracy with which thyroid hormone replacement can be monitored. Many clinicians now consider serum TSH concentration to be the most sensitive and specific monitoring parameter for adjustment of levothyroxine dose.[91–93] Plasma TSH concentrations begin to fall within hours and are usually normalized within 2 weeks but may take up to 6 weeks in some patients, depending on the baseline value.[92] Children receiving levothyroxine may also be monitored with TSH concentrations.[94] TSH and T_4 concentrations are both used to monitor therapy and they should be checked monthly until a euthyroid state is achieved. Serum T_4 concentrations can be useful in detecting noncompliance, malabsorption, or changes in levothyroxine product bioequivalence. TSH may also be used to check for noncompliance.[95] The expected range of serum T_4 concentrations in patients receiving replacement therapy is higher than that of a normal person. This may occur because the biologic effect of T_3 is absent and must be supplemented by a higher thyroxine dose. The usual serum range in thyroxine-treated patients is 6–17 μg/dL (mean: 11 μg/dL) compared with the normal range of 5–12 μ/dL (mean: 8.5 μg/dL).[78,96] An elevated TSH concentration indicates insufficient replacement. The appropriate dose maintains the TSH concentration in the normal range.

In patients with hypothyroidism caused by hypothalamic or pituitary failure, alleviation of the clinical syndrome and restoration of serum T_4 to the normal range are the only criteria available for estimating the appropriate replacement dose of levothyroxine. Concurrent use of dopamine, dopaminergic agents (bromocriptine), somatostatin or somatostatin analogues (octreotide), and corticosteroids suppresses TSH concentrations and may confound the interpretation of this monitoring parameter.[97]

Thyroid-stimulating hormone suppressive levothyroxine therapy may also be given to patients with nodular thyroid disease and diffuse goiter, to patients with a history of thyroid irradiation, and to patients with thyroid cancer. The rationale for suppressive therapy is to reduce TSH secretion, which promotes growth and function in abnormal tissue. In patients with soliditary nodules who have not received radiation, TSH should be suppressed to 0.05–0.1 mU/L in premenopausal women and in men <60 years old. A dose of levothyroxine of 100–150 μg/d is usually sufficient. In men over 60 years of age and postmenopausal women, TSH should be reduce to 0.1–0.3 mU/L due to the risk of more serious adverse effects in this population and reduced clearance of levothyroxine with advanced age. Levothyroxine may be given in nontoxic multinodular goiter to suppress the TSH to low normal levels of 0.5–1.0 mU/L if the baseline TSH is >1.0 mU/L. Goiter size and thyroid volume may be reduced with suppression therapy. Diffuse goiter associated with autoimmune thyroiditis may also be treated with levothyroxine to reduce goiter size and thyroid volume. In patients with follicular or papillary thyroid cancer, current recommendations are to suppress the TSH to <0.1 mU/L for the initial postoperative period (up to 5 years) and then to reduce the levothyroxine dose, allowing the TSH to rise into the range of 0.1–0.3 mU/L to minimize the risk of long-term adverse effects such as osteoporosis. Doses of levothyroxine of up to 2.2–2.5 μg/kg may be needed to provide TSH levels of <0.1 mU/L in this population.[98]

Patients have been given thyroid hormone for long periods without sufficient justification, often in an ill-advised effort to aid weight loss. A single TSH determination 8 weeks after thyroid hormone therapy is withdrawn may be used to separate euthyroid individuals from patients with primary thyroid failure.[99]

Adverse Effects

Serious untoward effects are unusual if dosing is appropriate and the patient is carefully monitored during initial treatment. Patients with an underlying or past history of bipolar affective disorders may exhibit manic behavior on thyroid supplementation. Levothyroxine replacement in athyreotic hypothyroid patients restores systolic and diastolic left ventricular performance within 2 weeks and the use of levothyroxine may increase the frequency of atrial premature beats but not necessarily ventricular premature beats.[100,101] Excessive doses of thyroid hormone may lead to congestive heart failure, angina pectoris, and myocardial infarction; rarely, the latter may be caused by coronary artery spasm.[102,103] Allergic or idiosyncratic reactions can occur with the natural animal-derived products such as desiccated thyroid and thyroglobulin, but these are extremely rare with the synthetic products used today. The 0.05-mg Synthroid tablet is the least allergenic (due to lack of dye and few excipients) and should be tried in the patient suspected to be allergic to thyroid hormone.

Hyperremodeling of cortical and trabecular bone due to hyperthyroidism leads to reduced bone density and may increase the risk of fracture. Excess exogenous thyroid hormone results in similar histomorphometric changes to those observed in hyperthyroidism.[104–106] The risk for this complication of therapy seems to be related to the dose of levothyroxine, patient age, and gender. Markers for bone turnover include pyridinoline cross-link urinary excretion, osteocalcin, and bone-specific alkaline phosphatase. When doses of levothyroxine are used to suppress TSH concentrations to below normal values (less than 0.3 mTU/L) in postmenopausal women, this adverse effect is more likely to be seen. In contrast, it appears to be much less likely in men and in premenopausal women.[107] Maintaining the TSH between 0.7–1.5 mU/L with approximately 150 μg/d of levothyroxine does not alter bone mineral density in premenopausal women.[108]

EVALUATION OF THERAPEUTIC OUTCOMES—HYPOTHYROIDISM

A patient with uncomplicated hypothyroidism receiving a typical dose of levothyroxine of 100–125 μg daily will have an increase in metabolic activity and be out of the myxedematous zone within 1 week of initiating therapy. Plasma TSH concentrations begin to drop within hours and may be in the normal range within 2–6 weeks. An impressive diuresis usually occurs within 2–3 days, with an improvement in the puffy facial appearance and weight loss. Speech, skin temperature, mental alertness, and physical activity show improvement within 72 hours. Long-term replacement therapy with levothyroxine does not adversely affect morbidity or mortality and the quality of life for these patients is similar to a euthyroid control group.[109]

In children with hypothyroidism developing beyond 2–3 years of age, normal CNS and physiologic development are expected with thyroid replacement therapy; however, in congenital or neonatal hypothyroidism, CNS development is dependent on the severity of disease and the time at which therapy is begun. Three months of age seems to be a critical time after which treatment may not normalize intellectual development.[110]

SPECIAL CONDITIONS

Myxedema Coma

Myxedema coma is the end stage of long-standing uncorrected hypothyroidism. Clinical features include hypothermia, advanced stages of hypothyroid symptoms, and altered sensorium ranging for delirium to coma. Mortality rates of 60–70% necessitate immediate and aggressive therapy with intravenous bolus thyroxine 300–500 μg. Glucocorticoid therapy with intravenous hydrocortisone 100 mg every 8 hours should be given until coexisting adrenal suppression is ruled out. Consciousness, lowered TSH concentrations, and normal vital signs are expected within 24 hours. Maintenance doses are typically 75–100 μg given intravenously until the patient stabilizes and oral therapy is begun. Supportive therapy must be instituted to maintain adequate ventilation, euglycemia, blood pressure, and body temperature. Any underlying disorder, such as sepsis, myocardial infarction, etc., must obviously be diagnosed and treated.[111]

Congenital Hypothyroidism

In congenital hypothyroidism, full maintenance therapy should be instituted early to improve the prognosis for mental and physical development. The average maintenance dose in infants and children depends on the age and weight of the child. Several studies demonstrate that aggressive therapy with levothyroxine is important for normal development and current recommendations are for initiation of therapy within 45 days of birth at a dose of 10–15 μg/kg/d.[112] This dose is used to keep T_4 concentrations at about 10 μg/dL within 30 days of starting therapy and is associated with improved IQs in treated infants. The dose is progressively decreased as the child ages to a typical adult dose, which occurs in the age range of 11–20 years. *In utero* treatment of fetal goiter and hypothyroidism has been accomplished with the injection of thyroxine into the amniotic fluid.[113]

Hypothyroidism in the Pregnant Patient

Hypothyroidism is not commonly diagnosed in the pregnant patient.[114] Hypothyroidism during pregnancy leads to an increased rate of stillbirths and possibly lower psychologic scores in infants born of women who received inadequate replacement during pregnancy.[115] Thyroid hormone is necessary for fetal growth and must come from the maternal side during the first 2 months of gestation. Although liothyronine may cross placental membrane slightly better than levothyroxine, the latter is considered to be the drug of choice. The objective of treatment is to decrease TSH to less than 6 U/mL and maintain T_4 concentrations in the range of about 2–4 μg/dL. Based on elevated TSH levels during pregnancy, Mandel et al.[116] found that the mean dose of levothyroxine had to be increased from 102 to 148 μg/d in 9 to 12 pregnant patients to suppress TSH into the normal range. Increased need for thyroid hormone during pregnancy may be due to pharmacokinetic alterations, although this has not been studied. Increase in thyroxine metabolism by the fetal–placental unit also contributes to increased thyroid hormone demand, as the need for increased doses decreases after delivery. Consequently, after delivery the dose of levothyroxine may need to be reduced based on T_4 concentrations and measurement of TSH.

Effects of Hypothyroidism on Selected Medications

Hypothyroidism may affect the metabolism and clinical efficacy of several medications. Digitalis preparations have a decreased volume of distribution in the hypothyroid state, resulting in increased sensitivity to the digitalis effect. Therefore, many hypothyroid patients achieve a therapeutic effect at lower digitalis doses. Insulin degradation may be delayed in hypothyroidism, thereby requiring a lower insulin dose.[117] Hypothyroidism delays the catabolism of clotting factors and if a patient stabilized on warfarin is made euthyroid with levothyroxine the patient may become excessively anticoagulated. Respiratory depressants such as barbiturates, phenothiazines, and opioid analgesics should be avoided, because increased sensitivity may increase carbon dioxide retention and precipitate myxedema coma.

Nonthyroidal Illness

A wide variety of abnormalities of pituitary–thyroid function, serum thyroid hormone binding, and extrathyroidal thyroid hormone metabolism occur in patients with nonthyroidal illness. These abnormalities frequently result in decreased serum T_3 concentrations and less often lead to a decreased serum T_4 concentration. Serum TSH concentrations are usually within the normal range. Nonthyroidal illness does not cause significant reductions in serum TSH concentration. Therefore, the presence of coexisting primary hypothyroidism can be recognized in patients who have other illnesses by an elevation in the TSH concentration.

The degree and extent of the abnormality in thyroid function generally correlates with the severity of the nonthyroidal illness. These conditions are frequently referred to as the "euthyroid sick syndrome." It is likely that these changes represent adaptive forms of hypothyroidism that serve to reduce the availability of thyroid hormones in order to lessen the impact of the nonthyroidal illness.

Decreased serum T_3 concentrations occur in patients with both acute and chronic illnesses. The fundamental cause of decreased serum T_3 concentrations in these situations is decreased extrathyroidal conversion of T_4 to T_3. This reaction is normally mediated by T_4-5′-deiodinase. A circulating inhibitor of this enzyme is present in patients with nonthyroidal illness. Serum total and free T_4 concentrations are usually normal. The serum reverse T_3 concentration is characteristically high because the same enzyme, 5′-deiodinase, which is necessary to convert T_4 to T_3 is necessary to convert reverse T_3 to its breakdown products. In children with acute respiratory infection interleukin-6 is acutely elevated and inversely correlated with temporal changes in T_3 concentration.[118]

Low serum T_4 is seen in most critically ill patients. The free T_4 concentration is generally normal. This change is due to diminished serum T_4 binding resulting either from decreased serum concentrations of TBG, TBPA, albumin, or from inhibitors of T_4 binding. This more severe degree of hypothyroidism, which occurs in severely ill patients, produces a greater reduction in thyroid hormone availability. The low serum T_4 concentrations in patients with nonthyroidal illness indicate a grave prognosis. In two studies, more than 60% of patients with a low serum free-T_4 index died before leaving the hospital. T_4 or T_3 supplementation has been of no benefit in this situation and in fact has increased morbidity.[119]

To confuse matters, some patients with nonthyroidal illness have elevation of their serum T_4 concentration. Most commonly, this is seen in patients with psychiatric disorders during acute psychotic breaks. Thyroid hormone levels return to normal within 2 weeks after successful treatment of the underlying psychiatric disease. The occurrence of these abnormalities requires that care be taken in diagnosing hypothyroidism or hyperthyroidism in patients who have nonthyroidal illnesses.

Goitrous Thyroid Disease

Endemic goiter is the major thyroid disease throughout the world, affecting more than 200 million people. Many goitrous glands contain one or more nodules. The introduction of iodide supplementation has eliminated goiter as a major medical problem in developed countries, though it continues to be a problem in developing countries whose geographic position makes them more susceptible to iodide deficiency. In 1924, Marine[120] postulated that periods of iodide deficiency resulted in cyclic hyperplasia and involution of thyroid follicular cells with eventual development of nodular hyperplasia. This hypothesis is still used to explain goiter formation today. Whatever the specific cause, the final common pathway appears to result from an inadequate thyroid hormone secretion with compensatory TSH secretion and eventual thyroid gland enlargement. The essential factor for the conversion of a hyperplastic iodine deficiency goiter into a colloid goiter appears to be an acute reduction of TSH stimulation; therefore, any situation that would result in a cyclical increase and decrease in TSH secretion might eventually result in the production of a nodular goiter.

There has been an interest in the possibility that growth factors other than TSH play a role in the development of a goiter. Immunoglobulin fractions capable of stimulating thyroid growth have been found in patients with nontoxic goiter and Graves' disease. The thyroid growth promoting immunoglobulin titers correlates with goiter size rather than with the thyroid hormone concentration.

Sporadic goiter is defined as a goiter occurring in a nonendemic goiter region. Although a number of known goitrogens and errors in thyroid hormone biosynthesis may cause goiter, the majority of cases of sporadic goiter have no known etiology.

Treatment of all goiters is a trial of thyroid hormone suppression in an effort to eliminate TSH as a possible stimulus for continued thyroid growth. Large, long-standing goiters seldom undergo significant reduction in size. If the patient is symptomatic (dysphagia or dyspnea) or there is a question of malignant thyroid involvement, surgery is recommended.

Conclusion

Although the exact etiology of thyroid disorders is unknown, recent research indicates that the two most common disorders, Graves' disease and Hashimoto's thyroiditis, are associated with antibody production directed toward specific antigens within the thyroid gland. Regardless of etiology, the treatment objectives are to normalize the production of thyroid hormone and minimize the associated systemic symptoms of hypothyroidism and hyperthyroidism. While many patients present with "textbook" clinical manifestations, thyroid disorders are often nonspecific or subclinical in the neonate and elderly. The diagnosis must be based on biochemical findings in addition to clinical presentation. Effective treatment must be individualized and take into consideration the patient's age, gender, overall health status, and severity of thyroid disease.

References

1. DeGroot LJ, Niepomniszcze H. Biosynthesis of thyroid hormone. Basic and clinical aspects. Metabolism 1977;26:665.
2. LoPresti J, Nicoloff JT: 3,5,3′triiodothyronine (T3) sulfate: A major metabolite in T3 metabolism in man. J Clin Endocrinol Metab 1994;78:688–692.
3. Lazar MA. Thyroid hormone receptors: Multiple forms, multiple possibilities. Endocrinol Rev 1993;14:184–193.
4. Weintraub BD, Gershengorn MC, Kourides IA. Inappropriate secretion of thyroid stimulating hormone. Ann Intern Med 1981;95:339–351.
5. Refetoff S, Weiss RE, Usala SJ. The syndromes of resistance to thyroid hormone. Endocrin Rev 1993;14:348–399.
6. Hall WA, Luciano MG, Doppman JL, et al. Pituitary magnetic resonance imaging in normal human volunteers. Occult adenomas in the general populations. Ann Intern Med 1994;120:817–820.
7. Jaume JC, Portolano S, Prummel MF, et al. Molecular cloning and characterization of genes for antibodies generated by orbiral tissue-infiltrating B-cells in Graves' ophthalmorpathy. J Clin Endocrinol Metab 1994;78:348–352.
8. Rahn RS, Dutton CM, Heufelder AR, Sakar G. A genomic point mutation in the extracellular domain of the thyrotropin receptor in patients with Graves' ophthalmorpathy. J Clin Endocrinol Metab 1994;78:256–260.
9. Ober KP. Thyrotoxic periodic paralysis in the United States. Report of 7 cases and review of the literature. Medicine 1992;71:109–120.
10. Higgins HP, Hershman JM. The hyperthyroidism due to trophoblastic hormone. Clin Endocrinol Metab 1978;7:167–175.
11. Hamburger JI. Evolution of toxicity in solitary nontoxic autonomously functioning thyroid nodules. J Clin Endocrinol Metab 1980;50:1089–1093.
12. Burman KD, Earll JM, Johnson MC. Clinical observations on the solitary autonomous thyroid nodule. Arch Intern Med 1974;134:915–919.
13. Nikolai TF, Brosseau JU, Kethrick MA. Lymphocytic thyroiditis with spontaneously resolving hyperthyroidism (silent thyroiditis). Arch Intern Med 1980;140:478–482.
14. Brocq P, Rouvillois C, Gaughzz J. A propos des varietes, del'avenir, du diagnostic des temeurs thyroidiennes de l'ovaire. Presse Med 1959;67:165.
15. Mariotti S, Martino E, Cupinin C. Low serum thyroglobulin as a clue to the diagnosis of thyrotoxicosis factitia. N Engl J Med 1982;307:410–412.
16. Bartalena L, Grasso L, Brogioni S, et al. Serum interleukin-6 in amiodarone-induced thyrotoxicosis. J Clin Endocrinol Metab 1994;78:423–427.
17. Mulligan DC, McHenry CR, Kinney W, Esselstyn CBJ. Amiodarone-induced thyrotoxicosis: Clinical presentation and expanded indications for thyroidectomy. Surgery 1993; 114:1114–1119.
18. Chiovato L, Martino E, Tonacchera M, et al. Studies on the *in vivo* cytotoxic effect of amiodarone. Endocrinology 1994;134:2277–2282.
19. Roti E, Minelli R, Gardini E, et al. Thyrotoxicosis followed by hypothyroidism in patients treated with amiodarone. Arch Intern Med 1993;153:886–892.
20. Becker CB, Gordon JM. Iodinated glycerol and thyroid dysfunction. Four cases and a review of the literature. Chest 1993;103:188–192.
21. Hedberg CW, Fishbein DB, Janssen RS. An outbreak of thyrotoxicosis caused by the consumption of bovine thyroid gland in ground beef. N Engl J Med 1980;316:993–998.
22. Stockight JR, Topliss DJ. Hyperthyroidism current drug therapy. Drugs 1989;37:375–381.
23. Farwell AP, Baverman LE. Thyroid and antithyroid drugs, in Hardman JG, Limbird LE, Molinoff PB, Ruddon RW, Gilman AG (eds): Goodman and Gilman's The Pharmacological Basis of Therapeutics. New York, McGraw-Hill, 1996.
24. Chopra IJ. A study of extrathyroidal conversion of thyroxine (T_4) to 3′, 3′, 5-triiodothyronine (T_3) in vitro. Endocrinology 1977;101:453–463.
25. Cooper DS, Bode HH, Nath B. Methimazole pharmacology in man: Studies using a newly developed radioimmunoassay for methimazole. J Clin Endocrinol Metabol 1984;58:473–479.
26. Gardner DF, Cruikshank DP, Hays PM. Pharmacology of propylthiouracil (PTU) in pregnant hyperthyroid women: Correlation of maternal PTU concentrations with cord serum thyroid function test. J Clin Endocrinol Metab 1986;62:217–220.
27. Roti E, Gardini E, Minelli R. Methimazole and serum thyroid hormone concentrations in hyperthyroid patients: Effects of single and multiple daily doses. Ann Intern Med 1989;111:181–182.
28. Feldt-Rasmussen U, Schleusener H, Carayon P. Meta-analysis evaluation of the impact of thyrotropin receptor antibodies on long term remission after medical therapy of Graves' diseases. J Clin Endocrinol Meta 1994;78:98–102.
29. Wartofsky L. Guidelines for the treatment of hyperthyroidism. Am Fam Phys 1984;30:199–210.
30. Hedley AJ, Young RE, Jones SJ. Antithyroid drugs in the treatment of hyperthyroidism of Graves' disease: Long-term follow up of 434 patients. Clin Endocrinol 1989;31:209–218.

31. Romaldini JH, Bromberg N, Werner RS. Comparison of effect of high and low dosage regimens of antithyroid drugs in the management of Graves' hyperthyroidism. J Clin Endocrinol Metab 1983;57:563–570.
32. Reinwein D, Benker G, Lazarus JH, Alexander WE, European Multicenter Study Group on Antithyroid Drug Treatment: A prospective randomized trial of antithyroid drug dose in Graves' disease therapy. J Clin Endocrinol Metab 1993;76:1516–1521.
33. Greer MA, Kammer H, Bouma DJ. Short-term antithyroid drug therapy for the thyrotoxicosis of Graves' disease. N Engl J Med 1977;297:173–176.
34. McIver B, Rae P, Beckett G, et al. Lack of effect of Thyroxin in patients with Graves' hyperthroidism who are treated with an antithyroid drug. N. Engl J Med 1996;334:220–234.
35. Werner MC, Romaldini JH, Bromberg N. Adverse effects related to thionamide drugs and their dose regimen. Am J Med Sci 1989;297:216–219.
36. Refetoff S. Syndromes of thyroid hormone resistance. Am J Physiol 1982;243:88.
37. Cooper DS, Ridgway EC. Clinical management of patients with hyperthyroidism. Med Clin North Am 1985;69:953–971.
38. Wall JR, Fang SL, Kuroki T. In vitro immunoreactivity to propylthiouracil, methimazole, and carbimazole in patients with Graves' disease: A possible cause of antithyroid drug-induced agranulocytosis. J Clin Endocrinol Metab 1984;58:868–872.
39. Moreb J, Shemesh O, Shilo S. Transient methimazole-induced bone marrow aplasia: In vitro evidence for a humoral mechanism of bone marrow suppression. Acta Haematol (Basel) 1983;69:127–131.
40. Shergy WM, Caldwell DS. Polymyositis after propylthiouracil treatment for hyperthyroidism. Ann Rheum Dis 1988;47:340–343.
41. Liaw YF, Huang MJ, Fan KD, et al. Hepatic injury during propylthiouracil therapy in patients with hyperthyroidism. Ann Intern Med 1993;118:424–428.
42. Van Dijke CP, Heydendael RJ, De Kleine MJ. Methimazole, carbimazole, and congenital skin defects. Ann Intern Med 1987;106:60–61.
43. Wenzel KW. Pharmacological interference with in vitro tests of thyroid function. Metabolism 1981;30:717–732.
44. Bal C, Nair N. The therapeutic efficacy oral cholecystographic agent (iopanoic acid) in the management of hyperthyroidism. J Nucl Med 1990;31:1180–1182.
45. Adlerberth A, Angeras U, Jagenburg R. Urinary excretion of 3-methylhistidine and creatinine and plasma concentrations of amino acids in hyperthyroid patients following preoperative treatment with antithyroid drug of β-blocking agent: Results from a prospective, randomized study. Metabolism 1987;36:637–642.
46. Georges LP, Santangelo RP, Mackin JF. Metabolic effects of propranolol in thyrotoxicosis. I, nitrogen, calcium and hydroxypoline. Metabolism 1975;24:11–21.
47. Eber O, Buchinger W, Lindner W. The effect of D- versus L-propranolol in the treatment of hyperthyroidism. Clin Endocrinol 1990;32:363–372.
48. Lazarus JH, Kingswood JC, John R: The effect of nadolol on heart rate in hyperthyroidism. Acta Endocrinol 1987;114:102–106.
49. Herman VS, Joffe BI, Kalk WJ. Clinical and biochemical responses to nadolol and clonidine in hyperthyroidism. J Clin Pharmacol 1989;29:1117–1120.
50. Roti E, Montermini M, Roti S. The effect of diltiaze, a calcium channel-blocking drug, on cardiac rate and rhythm in hyperthyroid patients. Arch Intern Med 1988;148:1919–1921.
51. Milner MR, Phillips RA, Gelman KM. Are calcium antagonists as effective as beta blockers for the treatment of thyrotoxicosis? J Am Coll Cardiol 1987;1:1127–1129.
52. Velkeniers B, Cytryn R, Vanhaelst L. Treatment of hyperthyroidism with radioiodine: Adjunctive therapy with antithyroid drugs reconsidered. Lancet 1988;1:1127–1129.
53. Gamstedt A, Karlsson A. Pretreatment with betamethasone of patients with Graves' disease given radioiodine therapy: Thyroid autoantibody responses and outcome of therapy. J Clin Endocrinol Metab 1991;73:125–131.
54. Bahn RS, Heufelder AE. Pathogenesis of Graves' ophthalmopathy. N Eng J Med 1993;329:1468–1475.
55. Dobyns BM, Sheline GE, Work JB. Malignant and benign neoplasms of the thyroid in patients treated for hyperthyroidism in a report of the cooperative thyrotoxicosis therapy follow-up study. J Clin Endocrinol Metab 1974;38:976–1002.
56. Robertson JS, Gorman CA. Gonadal radiation dose and its genetic significance in radioiodine therapy of hyperthyroidism. J Nucl Med 1976;17:826–835.
57. Franklyn JA: The management of hyperthyroidism. N Engl J Med 1994;330:1731–1738.
58. Bistrup C, Nielsen JD, Gregersen G, Franch P. Preventive effect of levothyroxine in patients operated for non-toxic goitre: A randomized trial of one hundred patients with nine years follow-up. Clin Endocrinol 1994;40:323–337.
59. Feek CM, Sawers JS. Combination of potassium iodide and propranolol in preparation of patients with Graves' disease for thyroid surgery. N Engl J Med 1980;302:883–885.
60. Menegaux F, Ruprecht T, Chigot JP. The surgical treatment of Graves' disease. Surgery 1992;176:277–282.
61. Kuma K, Matsuzuka F, Kobayashi A, et al. Natural course of Graves' disease after subtotal thyroidectomy and management of patients with postoperative thyroid dysfunction. Am J Med Sci 1991;302:8–12.
62. Burrow GN. Thyroid function and hyperfunction during gestation. Endocrinol Rev 1993;14:194–202.
63. Momotani N, Hisaoka T, Noh J, et al. Effects of iodine on thyroid status of fetus versus mother in treatment of Graves' disease complicated by pregnancy. J Endocrinol Metab 1992;75:738–744.
64. Kashizume K, Ichikawa K, Nishil Y, et al. Effect of administration of thyroxine on the risk of postpartum recurrence of hyperthyroid Graves' disease. J Clin Endocrinol Metab 1992;75:6–10.
65. Burrow GM. The management of thyrotoxicosis in pregnancy. N Engl J Med 1985;313:562–565.

66. Karpman BA, Rapoport B, Feletti S. Treatment of neonatal hyperthyroidism due to Graves' disease with sodium ipodate. J Clin Endocrinol Metab 1987;64:119–123.
67. Lippe BM, Landaw EM, Kaplan SA. Hyperthyroidism in children treated with long-term medical therapy: Twenty-five percent remission every two years. J Clin Endocrinol Metab 1987;64:1241–1245.
68. Gorton C, Sadeghi-Nejad A, Senior B. Remission in children with hyperthyroidism treated with propylthiouracil. Am J Dis Child 1987;141:1084–1086.
69. Reasner C, Isley W: Thyrotoxicosis in the critically ill. Crit Care Clin 1991;7:57–94.
70. Rosenberg IN. Thyroid storm, in Hershman JM, Bray GA (eds): The Thyroid. Physiology and Treatment of Disease. International Encyclopedia of Pharmacology and Therapeutics. New York, Pergamon Press, 1979.
71. Ashkar FS, Katims RB, Smoak WM. Thyroid storm treatment with blood exchange and plasmapheresis. JAMA 1970;214:1275–1279.
72. Herman J, Kruskemper JL, Grosser KD. Peritonealdialyse in der Behandlung der thyrotoxischen Krise. Duetsch Med Woch 1971;95:742–747.
73. Mandel SJ, Brent GA, Larsen PR. Levothyroxine therapy in patients with thyroid disease. Ann Intern Med 1993; 119:492–502.
74. Volpé R. Autoimmune thyroiditis in thyroid function and disease, in Burrow GN, Oppenheimer JA, Volpé R (eds): Thyroid Function and Disease. Philadelphia, WB Saunders, 1989.
75. Dussault JH. Hypothyroidism in infants and children—neonatal screening, in Ingbar SH, Braverman LE, (eds): The Thyroid. Philadelphia, JB Lippincott, 1986.
76. Wolff J. Iodide goiter and the pharmacologic effects of excess iodide. Am J Med 1969;47:101.
77. Roti E, Minelli R, Gardini E, Braverman LE. The use and misuse of thyroid hormone. Endocrin Rev 1993;14: 401–423.
78. Fish LH, Schwartz HL, Cavanaugh J. Replacement dose, metabolism, and bioavailability of levothyroxine in the treatment of hypothyroidism. Role of triiodothyronine in pituitary feedback in humans. N Engl J Med 1987;316: 764–770.
79. Wennlund A. Variation in serum levels of T_3, T_4, FT_4 and TSH during thyroxine replacement therapy. Acta Endocrinol 1986;113:47–49.
80. Bevan JS, Munro JF. Thyroxine malabsorption following intestinal bypass surgery. Int J Obesity 1986;10: 245–246.
81. Smallridge RC, Burman KD. Malabsorption of thyroxine, calcium, and vitamin D in thyroparathyriodectomized women: Efficacy of therapy with medium-chain triglyceride oil. Mil Med 1990;155:156–158.
82. Sperber AD, Liel Y. Evidence of interference with the intestinal absorption of levothyroxine sodium by aluminum hydroxide. Arch Intern Med 1992;152:183–184.
83. Blouin RA, Clifton GD, Adams MA. Biopharmaceutical comparison of two levothyroxine sodium products. Clin Pharm 1989;8:588–592.
84. Ingbar JC, Braverman LE, Ingbar SH. Equivalence of thyroid preparations. JAMA 1980;244:1095.
85. Frey H, Johannesen O, Kapelrud H. Appropriate replacement dose of thyroxine in primary hypothyroidism. Acta Med Scand 1987;222:163–167.
86. Grund FM, Niewoehner CB. Hyperthyroxinemia in patients receiving thyroid replacement therapy. Arch Intern Med 1989;149:921–924.
87. Carr D, McLeod DT, Parry G. Fine adjustment of thyroxine replacement dosage: Comparison of the thyrotrophin releasing hormone test using a sensitive thyrotrophin assay with measurement of free thyroid hormones and clinical assessment. Clin Endocrinol 1988;28:325–333.
88. Symons RG, Murphy LJ, Cai W-Y. Effect of thyroid hormone dosage on thyroid function test in T_4-replaced hypothyroid patients. Clin Med J 1987;100:211–215.
89. Drinka PJ, Nolten W. Review: Subclinical hypothyroidism in the elderly: To treat or not to treat? Am J Med Sci 1988;101:18–24.
90. Nystrom E, Caidahl K, Fager G. A double-blind cross-over 12 month study of L-thyroxine treatment of women with 'subclinical' hypothyroidism. Clin Endocrinol 1988;29:63–76.
91. Kabadi VM. Optimal daily levothyroxine dose in primary hypothyroidism. Its relation to pretreatment thyroid hormone levels. Arch Intern Med 1989;149:2209–2212.
92. England ML, Hershman JM. Serum TSH concentration as an aid to monitoring compliance with thyroid hormone therapy in hypothyroidism. Am J Med Sci 1986;292:264–266.
93. Garces J, Barsano CP. Immunoradiometric assay for basal thyroid-stimulating hormone levels: Strategy for the management of thyroxine replacement. South Med J 1988;81:1127–1131.
94. Radetti G, Pasquino B, Franzellin F. Thyrotropin (TSH) secretion in L-thyroxine treated children: Assessment by an ultrasensitive TSH immunoradiometric assay. Helv Paediatr Acta 1987;42:413–418.
95. McClelland P, Stott A, Howel-Evans W. Hyperthyrotrophinaemia during thyroxine replacement therapy. Postgrad Med J 1989;65:205–207.
96. Stock JM, Surks MI, Oppenheimer JH. Replacement dosage of L-thyroxine in hypothyroidism. N Engl J Med 1974;290:529–533.
97. Surks MI, Chopra IJ, Mariash CN. American Thyroid Association guidelines for use of laboratory tests in thyroid disorders. JAMA 1990;263:1529–1532.
98. Burmesiter LA, Goumaz MO, Mariash CN, Oppenheimer JH. Levothyroxine dose requirements for thyrotropin suppression in the treatment of differentiated thyroid cancer. J Clin Endocrinol Metab 1992;75:344–350.
99. Rubinoff H, Fireman BH. Testing for recovery of thyroid function after withdrawal of long-term suppression therapy. J Clin Epidemiol 1989;42:417–420.
100. Punzengruber CH, Weissel M. Influence of L-thyroxine on cardiac function in athyreotic thyroid cancer patients—an echophonocardiographic study. Klinische Wochenschrift 1988;66:729–735.

101. Polikar R, Feld GK, Dittrich HC. Effect of thyroid replacement therapy in the frequency of benign atrial and ventricular arrhythmias. J Am Coll Cardiol 1989;14:999–1002.
102. Klein AH, Meltzner S, Kenny FM. Improved prognosis in congenital hypothyroidism treated before age three months. Am J Med 1981;71:887–890.
103. Hiasa Y, Ishida T, Aihara T. Acute myocardial infarction due to coronary spasm associated with L-thyroxine therapy. Clin Cardiol 1989;12:161–163.
104. Coindre JM, David JP, Riviere L. Bone loss in hypothyroid patients overtreated with L-thyroxine. Arch Intern Med 1986;146:48–53.
105. Ribot C, Tremollieres F, Pouilles JM. Bone mineral density and thyroid hormone therapy. Clin Endocrinol 1990;33:143–153.
106. Stall GM, Harris S, Sokoll LJ. Accelerated bone loss in hypothyroid patients overtreated with L-thyroxine. Ann Intern Med 1990;113:265–269.
107. Toh SH, Brown PH. Bone mineral content in hypothyroid male patients with hormone replacement: A 3-year study. J Bone Min Res 1990;5:2077–2081.
108. Marcocci C, Golia F, Bruno-Bossio G, et al. Carefully monitored levothyroxine suppressive therapy is not associated with bone loss in premenopausal women. J Clin Endocrinol Metab 1994;78:818–823.
109. Petersen K, Bengtsson C, Lapidus L. Morbidity, mortality, and quality of life for patients treated with levothyroxine. Arch Intern Med 1984;101:18–21.
110. Bhasin S, Wallace W, Lawrence JB. Sudden death associated with thyroid hormone abuse. J Pediatr 1972;81:912–915.
111. Siafakas NM, Salesiotou V, Filaditaki V, et al. Respiratory muscle strength in hypothyroidism. Chest 1992;102:189–194.
112. Fisher DA, Foley BL. Early treatment of cogenital hypothroidism. Pediatrics 1989;83:785–789.
113. Davidson KM, Richards DS, Schatz DA. Successful in utero treatment of fetal goiter and hypothyroidism. N Engl J Med 1991;324:543–546.
114. Burrow GN. Thyroid diseases in pregnancy, in Burrow GN, Oppenheimer JH, Volpe R (eds): Thyroid Function and Disease. Philadelphia, WB Saunders, 1989.
115. Man EB, Jones WS, Holden RH. Thyroid function in human pregnancy. VIII. Retardation of progeny aged 7 years: Relationships to maternal age and maternal thyroid function. Am J Obstet Gynecol 1971; 111:905–916.
116. Mandel SJ, Larsen R, Seely EW. Increased need for thyroxine during pregnancy in women with primary hypothyroidism. N Engl J Med 1990;323:91–96.
117. Reasner CA. Autoimmune thyroid disease and type I diabetes. Diabetes Rev 1993;1:343–351.
118. Hasimoto H, Igarashi N, Yachie A, et al. The relationship between serum levels of interleukin-6 and thyroid hormone in children with acute respiratory infection. J Clin Endocrinol Metab 1994;78:288–291.
119. Brent GA, Hershman JM. Thyroxine therapy in patients with severe nonthyroidal illnesses and low serum thyronine concentration. J Clin Endocrinol Metab 1986; 63:1.
120. Marine D. Etiology and prevention of simple goiter. Medicine 1924;3:453–479.

Chapter 74

Disorders of the Adrenal Gland

John G. Gums, PharmD, and Vickie M. Wilt, PharmD

The adrenal glands were first characterized by Eustachius in 1563 (Table 74.1). After Addison identified a case of adrenal insufficiency in man, adrenal anatomy and physiology flourished. Most of the work done in the early and mid-1900s centered on the glucocorticoid cortisol. With the discovery of aldosterone by Simpson and Tait in 1952, adrenal pharmacology turned toward the mineralocorticoid. Conn[1] followed with his classical description of primary aldosteronism in 1955, and numerous clinicians and investigators have continued the discovery of the variety of disease processes promoted through the adrenal gland.

Physiology, Anatomy, and Biochemistry

There are two adrenal glands located extraperitoneally to the upper poles of each kidney (Fig. 74.1). On average, each adrenal gland weighs 4 g and is 2–3 cm in width and 4–6 cm in length. The gland is fed by small arteries from the abdominal aorta and renal and phrenic arteries. Drainage of the adrenal gland occurs via the renal vein on the left and the inferior vena cava on the right.

The adrenal cortex occupies 90% of the total gland. The adrenal medulla accounts for the remaining 10% and is responsible for the secretion of catecholamines. The adrenal cortex comprises three separate zones.[2] The zona glomerulosa, 15% of the total adrenal cortex, is responsible for aldosterone production. The zona reticularis, the innermost zone, makes up 60% of the cortex and is responsible for basal and stimulated cortisol production. The zona fasiculata occupies 25% of the adrenal cortex, is highly cholesterol bound, and is responsible for all androgen production.

The adrenal cortex is responsible for the secretion of three types of hormones (Fig. 74.2). The first of these is the glucocorticoids. Cortisol, the end metabolite, is responsible for the regulation of fat, carbohydrate, and protein metabolism. The second group is the mineralocorticoids, of which aldosterone is the principal end product. Aldosterone maintains electrolyte and volume homeostasis by altering potassium and magnesium secretion and renal tubular sodium reabsorption. The androgens, testosterone and estradiol, are the major end products of the third type. Androgens have influence within the reproductive system and affect primary and secondary sex characteristics.

HORMONE PRODUCTION AND METABOLISM

Cortisol production is accomplished via two successive hydroxylations: the first at the 21-position by 21-hydroxylase (yielding 11-deoxycortisol) and the second at the 11-position by 11-hydroxylase, yielding cortisol or hydrocortisone.

Aldosterone is a by-product of the 21-hydroxylation of pregnenolone to form deoxycorticosterone. The oxidation of 18-hydroxycorticosterone to aldosterone is a unique feature of the zona glomerulosa, explaining why aldosterone is not affected during disease processes limited to the fasiculata and/or reticularis.

Androgens have a 19-carbon nucleus and serve as precursors to more potent analogues produced in the periphery. The adrenal gland can synthesize estradiol and estrone from testosterone and androstenedione, respectively; however, the quantities are extremely small. The relative rates of production for the various steroids produced by the adrenal gland are listed in Table 74.2.

Metabolism of glucocorticoids is responsible for converting inactive steroids to active metabolites as well as deactivating the active steroids to less active or inactive metabolites. Most steroid products administered are active; however, in the case of prednisone and cortisone, metabolism is necessary for the conversion to the active prednisolone and cortisol, respectively. Following metabolic conversion, renal elimination of the glucocorticoids is responsible for the excretion of the less active or inactive metabolites.

After metabolic conversion, glomerular filtration is primarily responsible for the elimination of endogenously produced glucocorticoids. The half-life of cortisol is 70–120 minutes; with aldosterone, the half-life is only 15 minutes because of an extremely high first-pass effect.

Metabolism and conversion of the various steroids can be altered by a variety of disease states and medicinal com-

TABLE 74.1. LANDMARKS IN ADRENAL CORTICAL HISTORY

Date	Discovery	Investigator
1563	Adrenal described	Eustachius
1855	Adrenal insufficiency in man	Addison
1856	Adrenalectomy fatal in dog	Brown
1895–1904	Discovery of epinephrine	Oliver
1910	Hypoglycemia of Addison's disease	Porges
1927	First active adrenal cortical extract	Hartman
1932	Life of patient with Addison's disease prolonged with salt	Loeb
1936	The "alarm reaction"	Selye
1938	Synthesis of deoxycorticosterone	Reichstein
1948	Partial synthesis of cortisone	Sarrett
1949	First anti-inflammatory use of cortisone	Hench/Kendall
1952	Discovery of aldosterone	Simpson/Tait
1955	Discovery of primary aldosteronism	Conn

pounds. Drugs and diseases known to result in enhanced clearance of steroids include phenytoin, phenobarbital, rifampin, mitotane, aminoglutethimide, hyperthyroidism, and renal disease (dexamethasone only). Drugs and diseases known to result in reduced clearance of steroids include estrogens and estrogen-containing oral contraceptives, liver disease, age, pregnancy, hypothyroidism, anorexia nervosa, protein-calorie malnutrition, and renal disease (prednisolone only).

Plasma glucocorticoids are bound to one of three plasma proteins in varying degrees. Corticosteroid-binding globulin (CBG), albumin, and α_1 glycoprotein are capable of binding glucocorticoids, with CBG being the principal binding protein. While CBG is the principal binding site for endogenous cortisol, albumin maintains the largest capacity for binding cortisol. At physiologic temperature, approximately 15% of the cortisol is bound to plasma albumin. However, more than 20,000 mcg % cortisol-binding capacity is available on the albumin receptor sites. This correlates to only 25 mcg % cortisol-binding capacity with CBG. In patients with hypoalbuminemia, the proportion of non–CBG-bound cortisol that is free will increase.

The function of steroid binding is to serve as a reservoir of steroids in their inactive state. This binding may change the availability of glucocorticoids to receptor-activating sites. Therefore, a final but important variable in altered plasma concentration of free (active) steroids is concentration of plasma proteins.

REGULATION OF HORMONE SECRETION

The regulation of glucocorticoid secretion is accomplished by the pituitary hormone, adrenocorticotropic hormone (ACTH). Under normal conditions, ACTH is released from the anterior pituitary in response to corticotropin-releasing factor (CRF), which is secreted by the median eminence of the hypothalamus (Fig. 74.3).

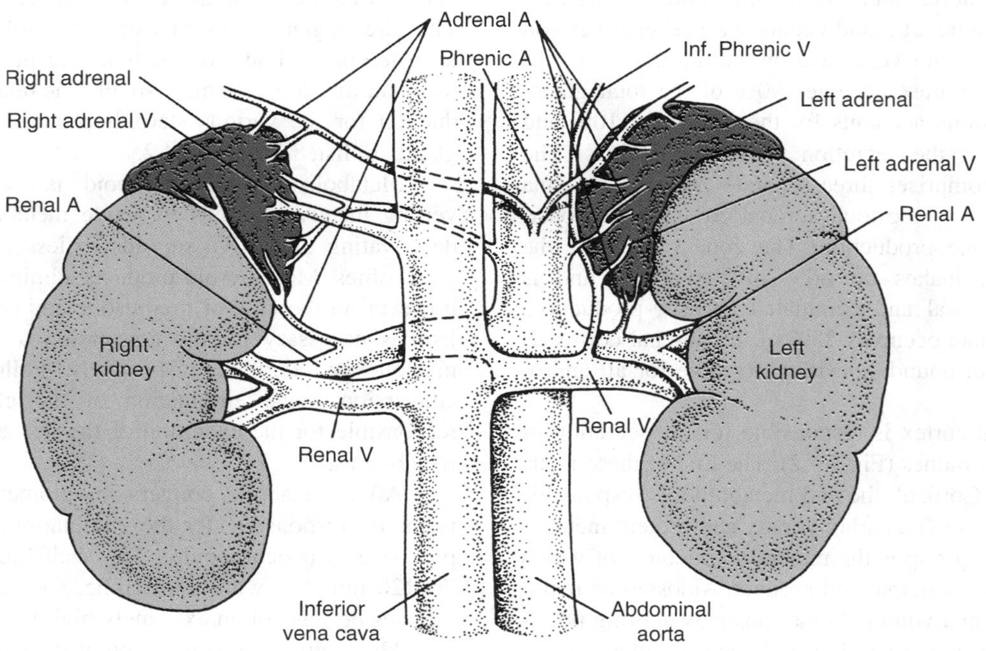

Figure 74.1. Anatomy of the adrenal gland. A, artery; V, vein.

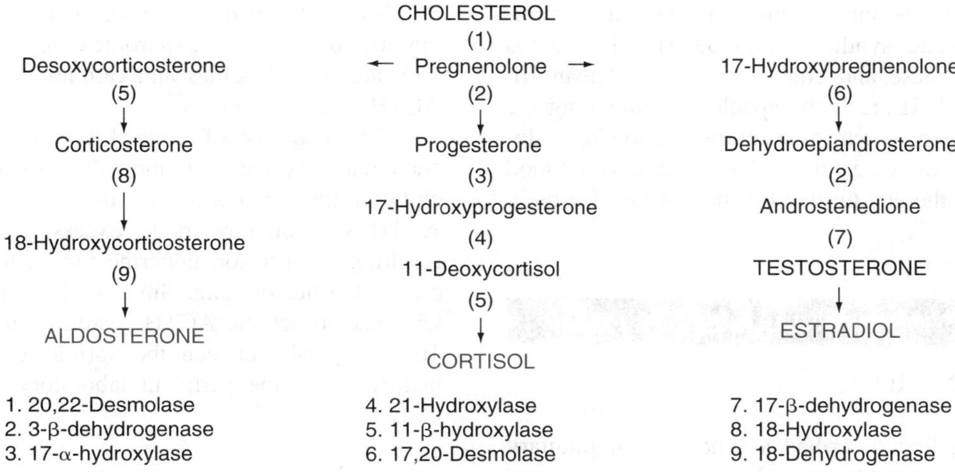

Figure 74.2. The cholesterol pathway with the major enzymes and endpoints. *(From Conn JW. Primary aldosteronism, a new clinical syndrome. J Lab Clin Med 1955;45:6–17, with permission.)*

Additionally, histochemical studies have demonstrated that certain neurotransmitters have unique ability to stimulate production of CRF or ACTH directly. 5-Hydroxytryptamine (5-HT) and norepinephrine (NE) have both been shown to increase levels of ACTH. 5-HT causes a release of CRF through excitation of a cholinergic intervention. NE can cause direct stimulation of ACTH release, although this effect is still controversial. After release, ACTH stimulates the adrenal gland to release cortisol and to a lesser extent aldosterone and androgens. The rising cortisol concentration inhibits the secretion of CRF and ACTH through a negative-feedback mechanism.

TABLE 74.2. RATES OF PRODUCTION OF PLASMA CONCENTRATIONS OF VARIOUS STEROIDS

Steroid	24-Hour Secretion (mg)	Plasma Concentration (ng/mL)
Aldosterone	0.15	0.15–0.17
Androstenedione	2.50 (female) 2.20 (male)	1.80 ± 0.21 (female) 1.14 ± 0.21 (male)
Corticosterone	1–4	2.4 ± 1.5 (female) 4.2 ± 2.2 (male)
Cortisol	8.00–25.00	85.00 (female) 116.00 (male)
11-Deoxycorticosterone	0.60	0.15–0.17
11-Deoxycortisol	0.40	0.95–2.50
Progesterone	0.0	0.20 ± 0.09 (female)[a] 11.80±7.00 (female)[b] 0.18 ± 0.10 (male)
Testosterone	0.23	0.48 ± 0.14 (female) 5.59 ± 1.51 (male)

[a]Follicular phase of menstrual cycle.
[b]Luteal phase of menstrual cycle.

Regulation of adrenal androgens is accomplished in a manner similar to cortisol regulation. Therefore, when plasma androgen reaches sufficient concentrations, production is terminated via a negative-feedback loop. Androgen release is increased during puberty and in women with hirsutism. Adrenal androgen release is decreased in fasting, anorexia nervosa, and aging.

Regulation of aldosterone secretion is considerably more complex. The renin–angiotensin system has the ability to respond to electrolyte and volume changes to increase or decrease aldosterone secretion. Renin production and subsequent aldosterone secretion is stimulated by blood pressure lowering, erect posture, salt depletion, β-adrenergic stimulation, and central nervous system excitation. It is inhibited by salt loading, angiotensin II, vasopressin, potassium, calcium, blood pressure increases, and a variety of drugs. The conversion of renin substrate to angiotensin

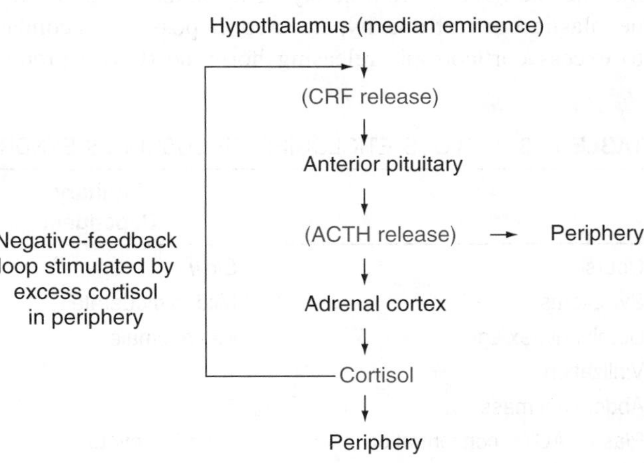

Figure 74.3. Regulation of cortisol secretion under normal conditions. CRF, corticotropin-releasing factor; ACTH, adrenocorticotropic hormone.

I and subsequently to angiotensin II is the initial stimulus for aldosterone synthesis. Angiotensin II is acted on by aminopeptidase and converted to angiotensin III. Angiotensin II and III are both capable of stimulating the zona glomerulosa to secrete aldosterone. Following aldosterone secretion, increases in sodium, water, and blood pressure are seen, thereby turning off the stimulus for renin release.

Hyperfunction of the Adrenal Gland

CUSHING'S SYNDROME

In 1932, Cushing first described a syndrome of pituitary basophilism that attracted national attention. It was not until this time that patients with unexplained central obesity, cutaneous striae, osteoporosis, weakness, hypertension, and diabetes mellitus had a definite diagnosis. Cushing emphasized that the disease was of pituitary origin. Ten years later, Albright[3] focused his attention on the sugar hormone, which he believed originated from the adrenal cortex.

After the development of the method for measuring urinary steroids, Daughaday discovered elevated steroids in the urine of Cushing's disease patients. Finally, the end product was identified and Cushing's disease was correctly explained as an excess of cortisol in the plasma (hypercortisolism).

Etiology

Cushing's syndrome results from the effects of supraphysiologic levels of glucocorticoids originating either from overproduction by the adrenal glands (endogenous) or from exogenous administration. Overproduction of ACTH by the pituitary gland causing adrenal hyperplasia (Cushing's disease) accounts for 70% of Cushing's cases. Pituitary adenomas account for approximately 85% of these cases. Nonneoplastic corticotrope hypersecretion possibly secondary to excess corticotropin-releasing hormone (CRH) production is felt to be responsible for the remainder. The remaining 30% of Cushing's syndrome cases are divided between 15% adrenal adenomas and carcinomas, and 15% ectopic ACTH-secreting tumors.[4]

The majority of adrenal cortex tumors are benign adenomas. Adrenal carcinoma is found more often in children than adults with Cushing's syndrome. Ectopic ACTH syndrome refers to excessive ACTH production resulting from a nonendocrine tumor, usually of the pancreas, thyroid, or lung. Small cell carcinoma of the lung will lead to ectopic ACTH secretion in 0.5–2% of cases. To distinguish between the various etiologies, a careful history and some pertinent laboratory work are required (Table 74.3).

Clinical Presentation

The clinical symptoms most commonly seen with Cushing's syndrome are listed in Table 74.4.[5] The most common of these findings include central obesity and facial rounding. Patients often are described as having moon facies with a buffalo hump. Fat accumulation often is noted at the supraclavicular and dorsocervical areas as well.

About 50% of patients will exhibit some peripheral obesity and fat accumulation. Facial plethora is caused by an underlying atrophy of the skin and connective tissue. Striae take on a red to purple color and are usually present along the lower abdomen. Excess androgen secretion is responsible for the 80% of female patients who present with hirsutism.

Hypertension is seen in 75–85% of patients with Cushing's syndrome. Ross et al.[6] noted that more than 50% of patients with Cushing's syndrome had diastolic blood pressures greater than 100 mm Hg. Hypertensive complications have traditionally been major contributors to the mortality and morbidity of Cushing's syndrome.

Gonadal dysfunction is common in patients with hypercortisolism. The abnormalities are principally due to elevated levels of androgens in the females and cortisol in the males. Most common in females is amenorrhea, which is seen in up to 75% of females with the diagnosis.

TABLE 74.3. VARIOUS ETIOLOGIES OF CUSHING'S SYNDROME AND THEIR RESPECTIVE DIFFERENCES

	Pituitary Dependent	Adrenal Adenoma	Adrenal Carcinoma	Ectopic ACTH Syndrome
Course	Slow	Slow	Rapid	Rapid
Symptoms	Mild to moderate	Mild to moderate	Severe	Atypical
Dominant sex/age	Female/male	None noted	Children	Male
Virilization	+	+	+++	+
Abdominal mass	0	0	++	0
Plasma ACTH concentration	Slightly elevated	0	0	0
Dexamethasone suppression test	50% suppression or greater	No suppression	No suppression	No suppression
Iodocholesterol scan	Bilateral uptake	Unilateral uptake	No uptake	Bilateral uptake

TABLE 74.4. CLINICAL FEATURES IN PATIENTS WITH HYPERCORTISOLISM

Feature	% Patients
Obesity	90
Hypertension	85
Facial plethora	84
Glucose intolerance	80
Menstrual dysfunction	76
Hirsutism	72
Striae	67
Myopathy	65
Muscular weakness	58
Osteoporosis	55
Psychiatric changes	55

Approximately 50–60% of patients will develop Cushing's-induced osteoporosis. Forty percent of these patients will present with back pain and about 20% of these will progress to compression fractures of the spine.

Diagnosis

Diagnosis of Cushing's syndrome is relatively easy, but the differentiation between etiologies can be difficult.[4,7] The diagnostic evaluation involves two steps. First, the presence of hypercortisolism must be established via one or both of the following tests: 24-hour urine free cortisol and the low-dose dexamethasone-suppression test (using 1 mg for the overnight test or 0.5 mg/6 h for the "classic" 2-day study). Second, since these tests cannot determine the etiology of Cushing's syndrome, other tests and procedures will be employed and may include any of the following: high-dose dexamethasone-suppression test (DST); plasma ACTH via radioimmunoassay (RIA); adrenal vein catheterization; iodocholesterol nuclear scan; metyrapone testing; adrenal, chest, or abdominal computerized tomography (CT); CRH stimulation test; inferior petrosal sinus sampling; and pituitary magnetic resonance imaging (MRI).[4,8–11]

Elevated urinary free cortisol (UFC) concentrations are highly suggestive of Cushing's syndrome. Normal reference values for urinary free cortisol are 20–90 μg per 24-hour period. It is not unusual to detect a twofold or threefold increase in urine cortisol in the patient with hyperfunction of the adrenal gland. Starvation, topical steroid application, hydration from water loading, and acute stress all are capable of falsely elevating the urine cortisol concentrations. Because other pathologic conditions can increase the amount of free cortisol, additional tests should be performed to confirm the diagnosis, or the diagnostic evaluation should be repeated when the acute stress has resolved. Of all urinary measures, UFC is the most useful for assessment of any patient with suspected Cushing's syndrome.[8]

In the overnight dexamethasone suppression test, 1 mg of dexamethasone is administered at 11:00 PM. The following morning at 8:00 AM plasma cortisol is obtained for analysis. The Cushing's patient will not exhibit a suppressed cortisol concentration via the negative-feedback loop, and the morning cortisol concentration will be elevated (greater than 5 μg/100 mL).[7] The overnight dexamethasone test is useful only as a screening tool for Cushing's syndrome because of a high sensitivity, but a rather low specificity. Phenytoin, rifampin, phenobarbital, and other drugs that induce liver enzymes may cause an increase in the clearance rate of the dexamethasone, causing decreased levels and leading to a falsely positive suppression test.[8]

Urinary examination of steroids can be used in the diagnosis of Cushing's syndrome. The normal circadian rhythm of cortisol will demonstrate a 60–80% decline between 8:00 AM and 11:00 PM. This rhythm is lost in the Cushing's syndrome patient. Critics of the use of urinary steroids in the diagnosis of Cushing's syndrome point out that urinary 17-OHCS levels may be decreased in the presence of starvation, renal failure, liver disease, pregnancy, and hypothyroidism. Additionally, drugs that induce hepatic microenzymes such as phenytoin, phenobarbital, carbamazepine, and mitotane may indirectly reduce levels of urinary 17-OHCS. Drugs that have direct assay interference with urinary 17-OHCS include spironolactone, hydroxyzine, chlordiazepoxide, phenothiazines, and troleandomycin.[12] The false-negative and false-positive rates from clinical studies of 11% and 27%, respectively, exclude urinary 17-OHCS from being a screening test.[8]

Additionally, plasma ACTH concentrations can be measured via RIA.[11] In the pituitary and ectopic Cushing's syndromes, ACTH may be normal or elevated. Very high levels of ACTH do favor the ectopic production. ACTH values are low in adrenal Cushing's syndrome. ACTH levels may appear artificially low in some ectopic ACTH-producing tumors because ACTH can be secreted as an active prohormone that is not detected by the assay.

The high-dose dexamethasone suppression test operates under the same principle as the low-dose test.[13] The main difference is in total dose (16 mg) and the time to test the patient (48 hours). The high-dose test has its main application in differentiating the adrenal hyperplasia patient from the patient with another form of hypercortisolism. The adrenal hyperplasia patient will generally demonstrate a 50% reduction in urinary steroids over baseline, whereas the others will generally not suppress. The high-dose test is based on the principle that patients with Cushing's syndrome not due to adrenal tumors or ectopic ACTH production will suppress their hypothalamic–pituitary axis in the presence of glucocorticoids, but it takes higher than normal doses. Recently, an overnight high-dose DST has been developed. The patient has a serum cortisol drawn at 8:00 AM and dexamethasone 8 mg is taken at 11:00 PM. The next morning, another serum cortisol is drawn.[11] The high-dose test is most useful when the low-dose test and other diagnostic studies have confirmed the diagnosis of Cushing's syndrome. The high-dose DST has recently been studied in combination with ACTH and metyrapone testing and results in better specificity than either test alone.

Two other diagnostic tests include the metyrapone and the new CRH stimulation tests. The CRH stimulation test can successfully distinguish between pituitary and adrenal causes of Cushing's syndrome. Also, distinguishing pituitary from ectopic causes can be reliably accomplished. The metyrapone test can be used to help in the differential diagnosis of ACTH-dependent Cushing's syndrome. Two days before the test, patients must be free of all medication. It has been suggested that the metyrapone test is as effective as the high-dose DST for differentiating pituitary Cushing's syndrome from ectopic ACTH syndrome. In the future, through combination of the metyrapone and dexamethasone tests (and the CRH test when it becomes more widely available), it may be possible to diagnose Cushing's syndrome nonivasively with high accuracy without positive pituitary imaging. Also, the need for inferior petrosal sinus sampling may be reduced.[8–11]

Two techniques for substantiating the diagnosis and differentiating an etiology in Cushing's syndrome are the adrenal catheterization and the nuclear scan. Selective adrenal vein catheterization can distinguish adrenal adenoma from adrenal hyperplasia. The procedure is invasive and requires skill and quality equipment. Intra-adrenal hemorrhage follows this procedure in as many as 10% of patients. Nuclear scanning uses a cholesterol compound, iodocholesterol, which is taken up by the adrenal gland. Once in the gland the iodinated cholesterol can be scanned and read for uptake percentage. Following the nuclear scan, a differential diagnosis can be made between hyperplasia and tumor-producing Cushing's syndrome.

Abnormal adrenal anatomy is effectively identified using high-resolution CT scanning and perhaps MRI. Nodules as small as 1 cm on the adrenal cortex are easily identified by CT. With the use of thin-section scanning, nodules as small as 3–5 mm can be visualized.[14]

Differential Diagnosis of Cushing's Syndrome

Although the diagnosis of Cushing's disease is not a difficult one, at times the clinician will need to differentiate it from syndromes that mimic Cushing's signs and symptoms. Pseudo-Cushing's syndrome refers to a group of diseases that can mimic Cushing's disease. Patients with obesity, chronic alcoholism, depression, and acute illness of any type can cloud the diagnosis of Cushing's disease. Depressed patients, while mimicking the urinary steroid abnormalities of Cushing's disease, will not resemble a Cushinoid patient in appearance. The chronic alcoholic will have his laboratory panel returned to baseline after he or she stops drinking. The obese patient often will have normal cortisol concentrations of both serum and urinary screening. Iatrogenic Cushing's syndrome, induced by glucocorticoid administration, often can be indistinguishable from Cushing's disease. A careful history and serum determination in a basal state can aid the clinician in making the diagnosis. If the patient is factitiously taking glucocorticoids and the basal plasma or urine cortisol level is low, screening the urine for synthetic glucocorticoids is useful. If the patient is using cortisol, basal urine and plasma levels may not be low. Administering ACTH may then be helpful. If exogenous glucocorticoids are being taken, plasma cortisol levels may increase while corticosterone levels remain low.[15]

Several additional tests and procedures are being evaluated for use in the diagnosis of Cushing's syndrome. These include insulin-induced hypoglycemia,[8] loperamide test,[8] somatostatin receptor scintigraphy,[16] and the desmopression stimulation test.[17] Table 74.5 summarizes the tests used to diagnose Cushing's syndrome.

TABLE 74.5. SUMMARY OF TESTS USED IN CUSHING'S SYNDROME

Test	Normal	Hyperplasia	Adenoma	Carcinoma
Plasma				
Cortisol (μg/100 mL, AM/PM)	17/8	30/25	35/35	50/50
ACTH (pg/mL)	150	50–500	50	10
Urine				
17-Hydroxycorticosteroid (mg/d)				
Basal	2–10	15	30	50
After ACTH	2–5x ↑	3–5x ↑	↕	↕
Dexamethasone 2 mg/d	3	4	30	50
Dexamethasone 8 mg/d	3	3	30	50
Nuclear				
Iodocholesterol uptake pattern	B	B	U	N

Key: ↑, increase; ↕, no change; B, bilateral; U, unilateral; N, no uptake.

TABLE 74.6. POSSIBLE TREATMENT PLANS IN CUSHING'S DISEASE BASED ON ETIOLOGY

Etiology	Treatment
Adrenal adenoma	Surgery plus postoperative replacement therapy
Adrenal carcinoma	Surgery Mitotane (*o, p'*DD)
Ectopic ACTH syndrome	Surgery Chemotherapy Irradiation Adrenal inhibitors (metyrapone, aminoglutethimide, trilostane)
Pituitary dependent	Surgery Irradiation Cyproheptadine, metyrapone, trilostane, or mitotane

TABLE 74.7. ALTERNATIVE STEROID REPLACEMENT REGIMENS IN THE ADRENAL ADENOMA PATIENT

	Hydrocortisone Dose (mg)		
Time	IV	IM	PO
Operation day	300	50 mg before surgery/ 50 mg after surgery	
Postoperative day			
1	200	50 q 12 h	
2	150	50 q 12 h	
3	100	50 q 12 h	
4		50 q 12 h	25 q 6 h
5		25 q 12 h	25 q 6 h[a]
7			25 q 6 h
8–10			25 q 8 h
11–20			25 q 12 h
21+			20 at 8 AM 10 at 4 PM

[a]Add fludrocortisone 0.05–0.2 mg PO daily starting on day 5 and adjust dose based on blood pressure, body weight, and serum electrolytes.

Treatment

The treatment of Cushing's syndrome is dependent on the etiology of the hypercortisolism.[4,7] If left untreated, Cushing's syndrome is associated with a high percentage of morbidity and mortality. If left untreated, associated disorders such as diabetes mellitus, cardiovascular disease, and electrolyte disorders limit the survival of the Cushing's syndrome patient to 4–5 years following initial diagnosis. Many treatment plans are available depending on the etiology of the disease (Table 74.6).

Adrenal Adenoma

The treatment of choice for benign adrenal adenoma is surgical resection. Surgical resection is associated with relatively few side effects and a high cure rate (95%). The contralateral gland in the patient with adrenal adenoma is usually atrophic. Therefore, steroid replacement is needed both perioperatively and postoperatively. Table 74.7 outlines an approach to steroid replacement for three separate routes of hydrocortisone. Therapy should be continued for 6–12 months following surgery. Before replacement therapy is discontinued, recovery of the adrenal axis may be assessed by administering ACTH (Cortrosyn) and measuring cortisol response at 30 and 60 minutes. Cortisol levels should exceed 18 μg/dL before discontinuance of the steroids.[4]

Adrenal Carcinoma

The treatment of adrenal carcinoma is surgical resection.[7] However, unlike the benign adenoma patient, patients with adrenal carcinoma have an unpredictable and unfavorable outcome. Often, the complete tumor cannot be excised, leaving the patients with some degree of symptomatology and extra-adrenal involvement. Irradiation can be used if metastases are discovered. In the patient with adrenal carcinoma who is not a surgical candidate, the focus of treatment is on palliative pharmacologic intervention (e.g., mitotane).

The adrenolytic agent mitotane (*ortho, para,* dichlorodiphenyldichloroethane, Lysodren, Bristol-Myers), is a cytotoxic drug that structurally resembles the insecticide chlorophenothane (DDT).[18] Mitotane appears to selectively inhibit adrenocortical function without causing cellular destruction. Degeneration of cells within the zona fasiculata and reticularis occurs with resultant atrophy of the adrenal cortex. The zona glomerulosa is minimally affected during acute therapy but can become damaged following long-term treatment. Mitotane decreases the cortisol secretion rate, plasma cortisol concentrations, urinary free cortisol, and plasma concentrations of the 17-substituted steroids. Mitotane inhibits the 11-β-hydroxylation of 11-desoxycortisol and 11-desoxycorticosterone in the cortex. The net result is a reduced synthesis of cortisol and corticosterone.

Mitotane appears to be the drug of choice in inoperable functional and nonfunctional adrenal carcinoma. Tumor regression is seen in approximately 35–50% of the patients, with most regression occurring between the second and fourth month of therapy. Seventy-five percent of patients will exhibit a 30% fall in urinary steroids, with 50% of patients showing an improved clinical response after 5 months of treatment. Patient survival appears prolonged, although no adequate clinical trials are available to support this assumption. Approximately 80% of mitotane-treated patients develop lethargy and somnolence, and other central nervous system adverse drug reactions occur in approximately 40% of patients.

Because mitotane can severely reduce urinary excretion of 17-OHCS, before initiating therapy the patient should be hospitalized. The recommended dose of mitotane is 9–10 g/d, divided into three or four doses. If a higher dose is tolerated dosage increases should be attempted every 3–7 days. The maximum daily dose is approximately 16 g. Pediatric dosing of mitotane is accomplished by using 0.5–1.0 g/d. Mitotane should be continued as long as clinical benefits occur. Cortisol secretion rate, plasma cortisol concentration, urinary free cortisol, and urinary steroid production should be monitored to assess mitotane response. If necessary, steroid replacement therapy can be given.

Metyrapone, aminoglutethimide, and ketoconazole may be given to attempt control of steroid hypersecretion. 5-Fluorouracil has also been used in combination therapy.[19]

Ectopic ACTH Syndrome

Surgical removal of the responsible tumor is the treatment of choice in the ectopic ACTH syndrome. Multiple sources of tumors exist, and location of the ectopic site is essential but often difficult. Approximately 10% of patients are cured following surgery; the remaining 90% receive postoperative medication.

Pharmacologic management with metyrapone (Metopirone, Ciba) was shown to be effective and remains the agent of choice.[19,20] In the ectopic ACTH syndrome patient, metyrapone inhibits 11-β–hydroxylase activity, resulting in cortisol-synthesis inhibition. Initially, patients may demonstrate an increase in plasma ACTH concentrations because of a sudden drop in cortisol. Metyrapone is biologically active following oral administration. Nausea, lethargy, ataxia, dizziness, edema, and skin rash have been reported following administration.[21]

Adults are given 750 mg orally every 4 hours for six doses. Urine samples are obtained for 17-hydroxyketosteroids, and plasma ACTH concentrations are measured. In the patient with adrenal hypercortisolism, the steroid production in the urine will be depressed following metyrapone administration. Patients with ectopic-producing ACTH syndrome will maintain elevated concentrations of cortisol in the urine even after inhibition within the adrenal gland.

A second agent used in the treatment of ectopic ACTH syndrome is aminoglutethimide.[4,22] Initially, aminoglutethimide (Cytadren, Ciba) was used to treat refractory forms of epilepsy, but it was later discovered to be a potent inhibitor of cortisol synthesis. Aminoglutethimide inhibits the conversion of cholesterol to pregnenolone early in the cortisol pathway.[22,23] Plasma cortisol concentrations are reduced by up to 50% following aminoglutethimide therapy. Side effects include severe sedation, nausea, ataxia, fever, and skin rashes. Most of the reactions are dose dependent, and they limit its use in most patients. Aminoglutethimide may decrease the anticoagulant effect of warfarin. Alone, aminoglutethimide is indicated for short-term use in inoperable Cushing's disease with ectopic-ACTH syndrome as the suspected underlying etiology. Aminoglutethimide is available as 250-mg tablets.

Aminoglutethimide may be used in combination with metyrapone. Smaller doses of both drugs can be used, therefore minimizing the toxicity associated with either agent. The combination therapy appears effective for various etiologies of Cushing's syndrome and is useful in the inoperable patient.

A third alternative agent in the treatment of Cushing's syndrome caused by a disturbance in the hypothalamic–pituitary axis is trilostane.[22] Trilostane (Modrastane, Breon) is a synthetic steroid that blocks the adrenal cortical enzymes responsible for cortisol synthesis. The most common adverse reactions include diarrhea, stomach upset, bloating, belching, mucosal burning, and headache.[18] Initial therapy should be started at 30 mg four times a day with dosage titration every 3–4 days with urinary steroid and electrolyte measurements. Dosages above 480 mg/d are not recommended. Trilostane (Modrastane) is available as 30- and 60-mg capsules.

Mitotane has been tried in patients with ectopic ACTH syndrome; however, its side-effect profile generally limits its use.

Spironolactone has been used for its competitive antagonism of aldosterone in the treatment of Cushing's syndrome. Spironolactone can provide symptomatic relief of the hypertension and hypokalemia often seen in Cushing's syndrome.

Recently, RU-486 (mitepristone), ketoconazole, and the somatostatin analogue (octreotide) have been reported to reduce the clinical signs of ectopic ACTH syndrome.[19] Further evaluation of these agents is needed. Steroid secretion should be monitored with all of these drugs and steroid replacement given as needed.

PITUITARY-DEPENDENT CUSHING'S SYNDROME (CUSHING'S DISEASE)

The etiology of Cushing's disease of pituitary origin is unknown. A solitary corticotroph adenoma is almost always the cause.[4] The tumor is usually a microadenoma (<1 cm in diameter) with macroadenomas being rare and corticotroph hyperplasia and carcinomas extremely rare.[7] A minority of cases may be due to excessive ACTH secretion by non-neoplastic corticotrope cells.[22] Currently the optimal form of therapy for Cushing's disease utilizes the hypothalamic, pituitary, and adrenal glands as avenues for intervention.

Therapeutic Management

Surgery

During the last decade, the treatment of choice for Cushing's disease has been transsphenoidal resection of the pituitary microadenoma.[4,7,19] The advantages to this procedure include preservation of pituitary function, low complication rate, and high clinical improvement rate. The overall cure rate of histologically proven tumors approaches 90%.

Bilateral adrenalectomy surgery had been the mainstay of therapy for years. It is only used now in patients for whom transsphenoidal surgery and pituitary irradiation have failed or cannot be used.[7,22] Bilateral adrenalectomy rapidly reverses hypercortisolism. However, patients may develop Nelson's syndrome, which involves sella turcica enlargement and hyperpigmentation, caused by postoperative hypothalamic stimulation. Therefore, if bilateral adrenalectomy is used, it should be accompanied by some form of hypothalamic inhibition.

Irradiation

Irradiation (4000–5000 rads) of the pituitary has provided favorable results in approximately 50% of patients.[22] Improvement is usually not seen until 6–12 months after therapy and can create pituitary-dependent hormone deficiencies. Most clinicians will reserve pituitary irradiation for the patient with a mild case of Cushing's disease or as an adjunct to another therapy.

Pharmacotherapy

Pharmacotherapy of Cushing's disease can be divided into three categories based on the anatomic site of action of the agent including (1) steroidogenic inhibitors; (2) neuromodulators of ACTH release, and (3) glucocorticoid receptor blocking agents.[21]

Steroidogenic inhibition may be accomplished with the following agents: mitotane, metyrapone, aminoglutethimide, trilostane, and ketoconazole. Pharmacologic therapy may be attempted with either metyrapone or aminoglutethamide. Either agent used alone has limited efficacy with relapse occurring after discontinuation of therapy. Neither agent should be used after successful surgery. Their use should be restricted to the refractory patient who is not a surgical candidate. Combination therapy with these agents appears more effective than single-agent therapy and may cause fewer side effects.

The imidazole derivative antifungal, ketoconazole[19,21,22] (Nizoral, Janssen), is highly effective in lowering cortisol in Cushing's disease resulting in normal corticosteroid values in 84% of the patients with an additional 11% of patients reporting improvement. In addition to lowering serum cortisol levels, ketoconazole has been noted to cause gynecomastia and lower plasma testosterone values. All of these effects are attributed to its inhibition of a variety of cytochrome P-450 enzymes including 11 β-hydroxylase and 17 α-hydroxylase.

Dosage regimens of ketoconazole range from 200–1200 mg/d with most studies reporting response at 600–800 mg/d administered twice daily. Treatment failures have mainly been reported at doses of 600 mg/d or less. The most common adverse effects are reversible elevation of hepatic transaminases, gynecomastia, and gastrointestinal upset. Treatment-related hypoadrenalism has been reported at dosages as low as 200–400 mg/d.

Neuromodulatory agents include cyproheptadine, bromocriptine, valproic acid, and octreotide. None of the neuromodulatory agents has demonstrated consistent clinical efficacy in the treatment of Cushing's disease. The existence of a bromocriptine-responsive subset of patients remains controversial.[21]

Cyproheptadine (Periactin, Merck, Sharp and Dohme) can decrease ACTH secretion in the Cushing's disease patient. The initial dose should be 4 mg, given twice daily. However, doses of 24–32 mg/d are generally required to control symptoms. Morning plasma cortisol concentrations and 24-hour urinary cortisol (free) concentrations should be monitored. Side effects are minor and include sedation and hyperphagia. Cyproheptadine should be reserved for nonsurgical candidates who fail more conventional therapy. Because the response rate is no more than 30%, patients should be followed closely for relapses.

Glucocorticoid receptor antagonism may be accomplished via RU-486 (mifepristone). RU-486[19,21,22] is a progesterone and glucocorticoid receptor antagonist that inhibits dexamethasone suppression and raises endogenous cortisol and ACTH values in normal subjects. Limited clinical experience in Cushing's suggests that RU-486 is highly effective in reversing the manifestation of hypercortisolism. Because of its novel site of action as a receptor antagonist leading to higher cortisol and ACTH levels, the diagnosis of treatment-induced glucocorticoid insufficiency must rest on clinical signs only. The efficacy and long-term effects of RU-486 remain to be determined.

Whatever the choice, pharmacologic therapy in pituitary-dependent disease is mainly centered around patient stabilization prior to surgery or in patients waiting for potential response to other therapies.

The focal point in the management of Cushing's disease is proper diagnosis of the underlying etiology. Figure 74.4 provides an algorithm for the proper diagnosis of the disease and accurate identification of the correct etiology.

HYPERALDOSTERONISM

Excess aldosterone is categorized as either primary or secondary forms of hyperaldosterone (Table 74.8).[24–26]

Primary Aldosteronism

Etiology

Primary aldosteronism implies that the physiologic abnormality is within the adrenal cortex. Etiologies include a solitary adrenal adenoma, multiple adenomas, hyperplastic tissue, or adrenal cortex carcinoma.[24] Of the possible etiologies responsible for primary aldosteronism, 65% are accounted for by adrenal adenomas, 30% by bilateral

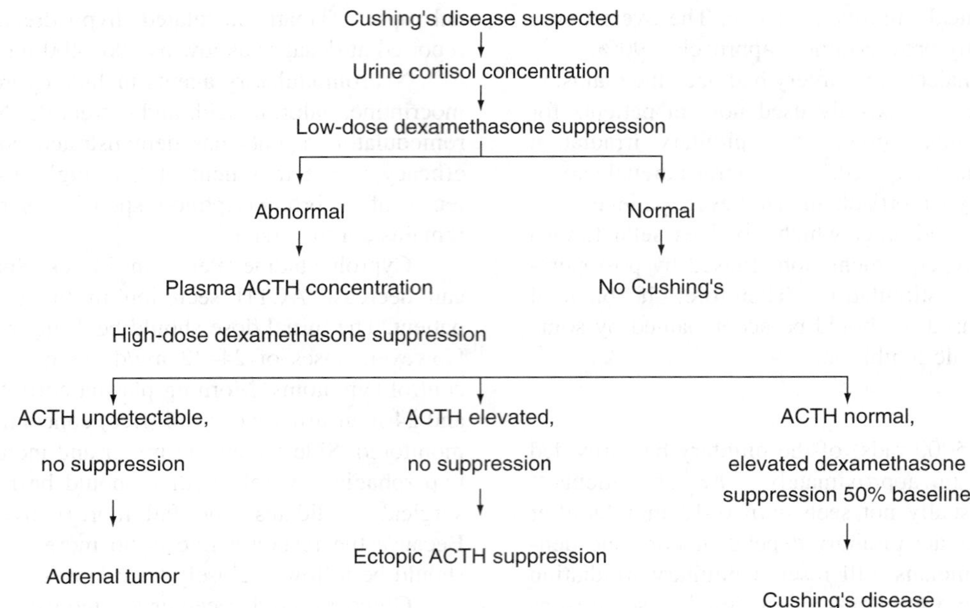

Figure 74.4. Algorithm for diagnosing Cushing's disease. ACTH, adrenocorticotropic hormone.

hyperplasia, and the remaining 5% by unilateral (primary) hyperplasia.[27]

Clinical Presentation

The incidence of primary aldosteronism is relatively uncommon, occurring in approximately 0.05–2% of all hypertensive patients. The disease is more common in women aged 30–50 years. Signs and symptoms include arterial hypertension, muscle weakness, fatigue, nocturnal polyuria, polydipsia, reduced glucose tolerance (25%), metabolic alkalosis, and headache.[24] Hypokalemia (80–90%), suppressed renin activity, elevated plasma aldosterone concentrations, hypernatremia (>142 mEq/L), hypomagnesemia, and an elevated bicarbonate concentration (>31 mEq/L) are characteristics of laboratory findings in primary aldosteronism.[25]

TABLE 74.8. SYNDROMES OF MINERALOCORTICOID EXCESS

Primary Aldosteronism
- Aldosterone-producing adenoma (APA)
- Bilateral adrenal hyperplasia (BAH), idiopathic
- Adrenal carcinoma
- Glucocorticoid-remediable hyperaldosteronism

Secondary Aldosteronism
- Nonhypertensive
  - Sodium depletion
  - Hemorrhage
  - Pregnancy
  - Edema
  - Bartter's syndrome
  - Diuretic therapy
- Hypertensive
  - Accelerated and renal vascular hypertension
  - Renin-secreting tumors
  - Necrotizing vasculitis
  - Estrogen therapy

Diagnosis

The absolute diagnosis is relatively easy based on clinical findings and pertinent laboratory findings.[28–34] However, as in Cushing's disease, the discovery of the underlying etiology is mandatory to ensure proper treatment. Table 74.9 lists the various abnormalities that must be ruled out when suspicion of hyperaldosteronism is high.

A serum potassium concentration of less than 3.5 mEq/L with a concurrent urinary potassium content greater than 30 mEq per 24 hours is suggestive of primary aldosteronism.[35] Normokalemia does not exclude the diagnosis of primary aldosteronism. Between 7–38% of patients with primary aldosteronism will have serum potassium concentrations greater than 3.6 mEq/L.[35]

Differentiating between an aldosterone-producing adenoma (APA) and bilateral adrenal hyperplasia (BAH) is imperative to formulate a proper treatment plan. A majority of the adenomas are singular and small, less than 1 cm. The left adrenal gland is affected at a higher rate than the right. Patients with APA generally have more severe hypertension, more profound hypokalemia, and higher plasma and urinary aldosterone levels compared to patients with BAH.[35]

The underlying abnormality in BAH remains a mystery, but some investigators feel a hormone factor stimulates the zona glomerulosa, resulting in increased sensitivity to angiotensin II.[36] In contrast to APA patients,

TABLE 74.9. DIFFERENTIAL DIAGNOSIS OF PRIMARY ALDOSTERONISM

Disease	Plasma Renin Concentration	Plasma Aldosterone Concentration	Blood Pressure
Primary aldosteronism	Low	High	High
Edematous disorders	High	High	Normal
Malignant hypertension	High	High	High
Congenital adrenal hyperplasia	Low	Low	High
Cushing's syndrome	Low to normal	Low to normal	High
Liddle's syndrome	Low	Low	High
Bartter's syndrome	High	High	Low to normal
Licorice ingestion	Low	Low	High
Low-renin essential hypertension	Low	Low to normal	High

patients with BAH are able to maintain control of the renin–angiotensin system with little effect following doses of ACTH. The use of 50 mg of captopril given orally with subsequent determination of plasma renin and plasma aldosterone has been suggested as a useful method of screening for primary aldosternism.[37] The false-negative rate was 6.3% and the false-positive rate was 0.6%.

To distinguish APA from BAH, numerous methods have been tried, but the most accurate method appears to be adrenal localization. The two methods used to localize the adenoma are adrenal vein catheterization and adrenal imaging.[24] Because adrenal vein catheterization is invasive and has a significant morbidity, clinicians are using this procedure less often. Adrenal imaging involves pretreatment with dexamethasone and the cholesterol derivatives, ^{131}I-19-iodocholesterol and I-19-10 iodomethylnorcholesterol.[24,26,35] Iodocholesterol is taken up by the adrenal gland similar to cholesterol. Following uptake, the adrenals can be visualized for "hot" areas of increased or sustained uptake. Patients with APA will normally have unilateral visualization compared with a bilateral visualization seen with patients who have BAH.[36]

To use iodocholesterol scanning, the patient must be imaged over 2–5 days. Diagnostic accuracy is approximately 72% and the cost exceeds that of CT of the adrenal glands. Why is the differentiation between APA and BAH so important if both are producing excess aldosterone? The answer is treatment.[38] Surgical resection of the adenoma is generally the treatment of choice. In patients with BAH, pharmacologic innervention is useful in controlling or limiting the symptoms.

Therapeutic Management: BAH-Dependent Hyperaldosteronism

Spironolactone, a competitive inhibitor of aldosterone, is the drug of choice in BAH-dependent hyperaldosteronism.[38] Spironolactone (Aldactone, Searle) has the capability of inhibiting aldosterone biosynthesis within the adrenal gland, making it extremely useful in overstimulated BAH patients.[24] Spironolactone is orally available, with most patients responding to doses in the 200–400 mg/d range. The clinician should wait 4–8 weeks before reassessing the patient for urinary electrolytes and blood pressure control since spironolactone has an active metabolite that has a long half-life and can accumulate. Adverse effects of spironolactone include gastrointestional discomfort, impotence, gynecomastia, and menstrual irregularities. In addition, because salicylates increase the renal secretion of canrenone, the active metabolite, patients should be advised to avoid concomitant therapy with salicylates. Because spironolactone also blocks testosterone biosynthesis, it often is not used in men. The drug of choice in men and patients intolerant of spironolactone is amiloride (Midamor, MSD).[39] The usual dose is 5 mg twice a day up to 30 mg/d if necessary.

Second-line therapy is often required to control the patient's blood pressure with BAH. Agents useful as second-line choices include the calcium channel blockers, nifedipine and verapamil; the ACE inhibitors, captopril, enalapril, or lisinopril; and low-dose diuretics, HCTZ.

Therapeutic Management: APA-Dependent Hyperaldosteronism

The treatment of choice for APA-dependent aldosteronism remains surgical resection of the adenoma. If no primary lesion is found, resection of one and a half of the adrenal glands can be attempted with supplemental spironolactone therapy.

Summary

The diagnosis of primary aldosteronism is made through the observation of elevated blood pressure, low serum potassium, high urinary potassium, and elevated serum and urinary aldosterone (Fig. 74.5).

Differentiating between the various etiologies is mandatory. Patients with adrenal adenomas can be distinguished from patients with hyperplasia by CT scan. Treatment depends on the etiology with surgical resection, well accepted as the treatment of choice in adenomas and

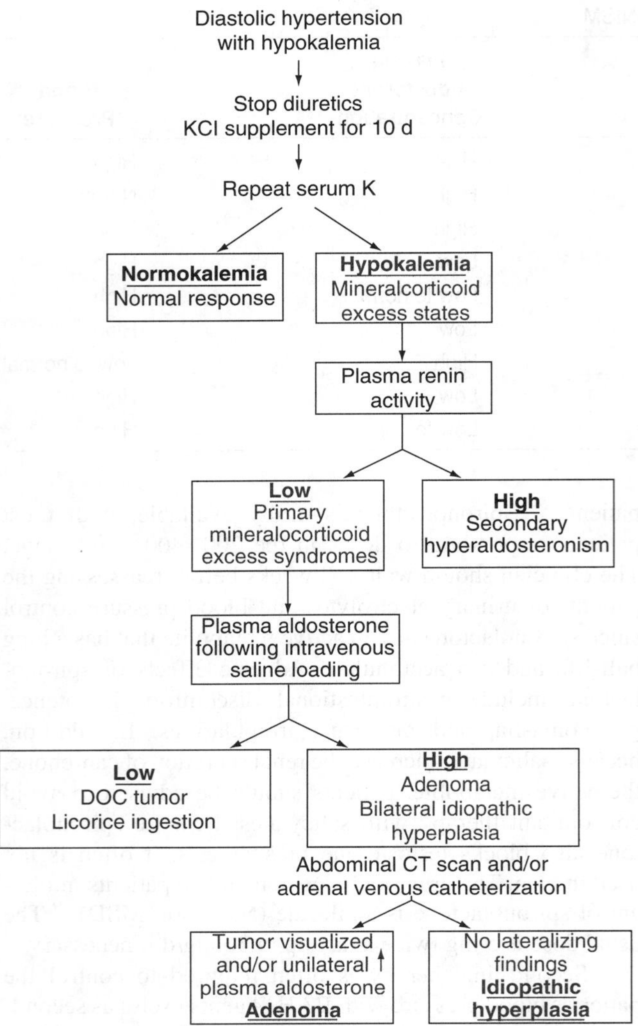

Figure 74.5. Flowchart in the diagnosis of primary aldosteronism.

spironolactone or amiloride plus second-line agents in patients with hyperplasia.

Secondary Aldosteronism

Secondary hyperaldosteronism results from stimulation of the zona glomerulosa by an extra-adrenal factor, usually the renin–angiotensin system. Excessive potassium intake can create a physiologic increase in aldosterone, as can oral contraceptive use, pregnancy (10 times normal by third trimester), and menses. Congestive heart failure, cirrhosis, renal artery stenosis, and Bartter's syndrome also can lead to elevated aldosterone concentrations.

Treatment of secondary aldosteronism is dictated by etiology. Removal of the extra-adrenal source of the excess aldosterone should resolve the disorder. Medical therapy with spironolactone is the mainstay of treatment until an exact etiology can be located.

Hypofunction of the Adrenal Gland

Primary adrenal insufficiency, or Addison's disease, involves the destruction of all regions of the adrenal cortex.[40] Deficiencies arise in cortisol, aldosterone, and the various androgens. Approximately 40–53% of patients with idiopathic primary adrenal insufficiency present with one or more clinical disorders involving multiple organs. This polyglandular failure syndrome is only associated with the idiopathic etiology and has not been seen with adrenal insufficiency associated with tuberculosis or other invasive diseases. The organs involved can include ovary, thyroid, pancreas, and parathyroid gland.

Secondary insufficiency most commonly results from exogenous steroid use, leading to suppression of the hypothalamic–pituitary axis, resulting in a deficiency of ACTH, producing low concentrations of androgen and cortisol. Secondary disease classically presents with normal concentrations of mineralocorticoids.

Approximately 90% of the adrenal cortex must be destroyed before adrenal insufficiency symptoms will occur.[40] Specific etiologies for both primary and secondary insufficiency are listed in Table 74.10.

Symptoms common in patients with adrenal insufficiency include weakness (100%), weight loss (100%), increased pigmentation (95%), hypotension (90%), and vitiligo (20%).

Adrenal hemorrhage can result from multiple etiologies, but septicemia is the most common.[41] Symptoms include shaking, chills, headache, vertigo, vomiting, rash, and death in 6–48 hours if not treated. The most common organisms found on autopsy are *Pneumococcus, Staphylococcus,* and *Haemophilus influenzae.*

TABLE 74.10. ETIOLOGIES OF PRIMARY AND SECONDARY ADRENAL INSUFFICIENCY

Primary Insufficiency	Secondary Insufficiency
Autoimmune adrenalitis[a]	Tumors of the third ventricle
Tuberculosis[b]	Craniopharyngioma
Fungal infection	Hypopituitarism
Amyloidosis	Corticosteroid administration
Sarcoidosis	Cure of Cushing's syndrome
Hemochromatosis	
Congenital adrenal hypoplasia	
Adrenal vein thrombosis	
Adrenal hemorrhage	
Bilateral adrenalectomy	
Acquired immune deficiency syndrome	
Metastatic neoplasia	

[a]Accounts for approximately 70% of total cases.
[b]Accounts for approximately 20% of total cases.

ADDISON'S DISEASE

Distinguishing Addison's disease from secondary insufficiency is difficult; however, the following guidelines may be helpful:

1. Hyperpigmentation usually is not seen in secondary adrenal insufficiency because of low amounts of melanocyte-stimulating hormone (MSH). Low amounts of MSH are present due to a deficient pituitary secretion of ACTH and β-lipotropin.
2. Aldosterone secretion usually is preserved in secondary insufficiency.
3. Weight loss, dehydration, hyponatremia, hyperkalemia, and elevated blood urea nitrogen are common in primary insufficiency.
4. Primary adrenal insufficiency will have an abnormal response to the rapid ACTH-stimulation test. Plasma ACTH levels are usually 400–2000 pg/mL in primary insufficiency versus 0–50 pg/mL in secondary insufficiency. Patients who are maintained on cortisone, hydrocortisone, prednisone, or methylprednisolone will have assay interference and possible obscuring of the results. A normal ACTH-stimulation test does not rule out secondary adrenal insufficiency. The short cosyntropin stimulation test can be used to assess patients suspected of hypocortisolism. Patients are given 250 μg of synthetic ACTH IV or IM, with serum cortisol levels drawn at baseline and 60 minutes after the injection. An increase of 7 μg/dL in serum cortisol and an absolute cortisol level above 20 μg/dL rules out adrenal insufficiency.[42]

Treatment of Addison's disease must include adequate patient education, so that the patient is aware of treatment complications, expected outcome, missed doses, and drug side effects. The agents of choice are prednisone, hydrocortisone, and cortisone, with the treatment objective being the establishment of the lowest effective dose while mimicking the normal diurnal adrenal rhythm[40] (Table 74.11). Usually, a twice-daily dosing schedule is adequate, with the dose used dependent on the steroid chosen. A morning dose of cortisone (25 mg), hydrocortisone (20 mg), or prednisone (5 mg) followed by an evening dose of the same agent at 50% of the morning dose is usually sufficient to duplicate the normal circadian rhythm of cortisol production. To replace the mineralocorticoid loss, 9-α-fluohydrocortisone can be used. A dose of 0.05–0.2 mg by mouth once a day is adequate. If parenteral therapy is needed, 2–5 mg of deoxycorticosterone trimethylacetate in oil intramuscularly every 3–4 weeks can be used. The main reason for adding the mineralocorticoid is to minimize the development of hyperkalemia.

Adverse effects must be monitored closely. Symptoms include gastric upset, edema, hypertension, hypokalemia, insomnia, excitability, and diabetes mellitus. In addition, patient weight, blood pressure, and electrocardiogram should be monitored regularly.

The endpoint of therapy is difficult to assess in most patients, but a reduction in excess pigmentation is a good clinical marker. Treatment of secondary adrenal insufficiency is identical to primary disease treatment with the exception that mineralocorticoid replacement usually is not necessary. Patient education still should be stressed with emphasis placed on establishing an alternate-day regimen.

Acute Adrenal Insufficiency

Adrenal crisis, or Addisonian crisis, is characterized by an acute adrenocortical insufficiency. Adrenal crisis represents a true endocrine emergency. Anything that increases adrenal requirements dramatically can precipitate an adrenal crisis. Stressful situations, surgery, infection, and trauma are potential triggering events, especially in the patient with some underlying adrenal or pituitary insufficiency. The most common cause of adrenal crisis is adrenal insufficiency brought on by chronic use of glucocorticoids.

Early symptoms of acute adrenal insufficiency include myalgias, malaise, anorexia, weakness, and weight loss. As the situation continues, vomiting, fever, hypotension, and

TABLE 74.11. RELATIVE POTENCIES OF GLUCOCORTICOIDS

Glucocorticoid	Anti-Inflammatory Potency	Equivalent Potency (mg)	Approximate Half-Life (min)	Sodium-Retaining Potency
Hydrocortisone	1.0	20.0	90	2.0
Prednisolone	4.0	5.0	200	1.0
Prednisone	3.5	5.0	60	1.0
Cortisone	0.8	25.0	30	2.0
Triamcinolone	5.0	4.0	300	0.0
Methylprednisolone	5.0	4.0	180	0.0
Betamethasone	25.0	0.60	100–300	0.0
Dexamethasone	30.0	0.75	100–300	0.0

shock will develop. Hyponatremia, hypoglycemia, and hypercalcemia also may be present.

Treatment of adrenal crisis in patients with documented Addison's disease involves the administration of parenteral glucocorticoids. Hydrocortisone (Solu-cortef, Upjohn) is the agent of choice due to its mineralocorticoid activity plus glucocorticoid effects. Hydrocortisone is started at 100 mg intravenously through rapid infusion and followed by a continuous infusion of 100 mg over an 8-hour interval. Intravenous administration is continued for 24–48 hours, at which time, if the patient is stable, oral hydrocortisone may be started at a dose of 50 mg every 8 hours for another 48 hours. Following oral maintenance therapy, a hydrocortisone taper is initiated until the dosage is 30–50 mg/d in divided doses. Fluid replacement often is required and may be accomplished with 5% dextrose and isotonic saline (D_5NS) at a rate to support blood pressure. If hyperkalemia is present after the hydrocortisone maintenance phase, additional mineralocorticoid usually is required. Fludrocortisone acetate (Florinef, Squibb) in a dose of 0.1 mg by mouth daily is the agent of choice.

HYPOALDOSTERONISM

Hypoaldosteronism is rare and usually is associated with low renin status, diabetes, complete heart block, or severe postural hypotension, or it may occur postoperatively following tumor removal.[2]

Hypoaldosteronism may be part of a larger adrenal insufficiency or be the only defect the patient has. In nonselective hypoaldosteronism, the etiology of the low aldosterone is most likely generalized adrenalcortical insufficiency (see section on Addison's Disease). In selective hypoaldosteronism, the etiology is usually a specific defect in the stimulation of adrenal aldosterone secretion (21-hydroxylase deficiency—most common) or a defect in peripheral aldosterone action (decreased aldosterone receptors).

Laboratory analysis reveals low serum sodium and high serum potassium concentrations. Patients often will present with hyperchloremic metabolic acidosis. Because the deficiency is in the mineralocorticoid, replacement with 9-α-fluohydrocortisone in a dose of 0.1–0.3 mg is usually effective. Patients should be followed for blood pressure response as well as electrolyte status.

Congenital Adrenal Hyperplasia

ADRENAL VIRILISM

Virilism, excessive secretion of androgens from the adrenal gland, is more commonly seen in females, with hirsutism being the dominant feature.[43] Women who present with hirsutism also may have voice deepening, increased muscle mass, menstrual abnormalities, or clitoral enlargement.[44] While virilism may be easy to diagnose based on clinical symptoms, making the diagnosis on a biochemical basis is difficult. The most common etiology of virilism involves one of many possible congenital enzyme defects. Depending on the enzyme deficiency, accumulation of a variety of androgens, notably testosterone, can develop.

Treatment of virilism centers around suppression of the pituitary–adrenal axis with exogenous glucocorticoids. Choice of steroids is variable with the focus of treatment being the establishment of an alternate-day therapy. In adults, the usual steroid used is dexamethasone (0.23 mg/m^2 per 24 hours) or hydrocortisone (18 mg/m^2 per 24 hours).

HIRSUTISM

Hirsutism (hypertrichosis) is defined as more hair than is cosmetically acceptable. The majority of cases occur in women with no underlying endocrine abnormality. Some cases of hypertrichosis are related to a wide variation in hairiness as well as hereditary factors. In general, people who are dark-haired, pigmented Caucasians of either sex from the Mediterranean and southern European stock are more prone to genetic hypertrichosis. If virilism and/or defeminization are concurrently present, the chances of the hirsutism arising from an endocrine abnormality increase.[45]

Endocrinopathies without masculinization can predispose to hirsutism in patients with documented pituitary tumors, Cushing's disease, or excessive use of steroids/androgens.[45] Certain drug-related hirsutisms have been documented, namely phenytoin, oral contraceptives, minoxidil, and diazoxide. In the patient with hirsutism, congenital adrenal hyperplasia, adrenal tumors, and ovarian tumors should be ruled out.[45]

In patients whose etiology suggests ovarian or adrenal tumor, a laboratory examination should consist of urinary 17-ketosteroids. To exclude ovarian tumor, blood testosterone and androstenedione concentrations should be measured. To exclude Cushing's disease, a routine Cushing's disease workup should be performed.

Only when cosmetic surgery is ineffective should suppressive therapy be used. Glucocorticoids, such as dexamethasone, can be used, but may induce Cushingnoid symptoms even in doses of 0.5 mg/d. Oral contraceptives can be used in patients who require contraception concurrently. If oral contraceptives are used, a progestin with low androgen activity (norethynodrel or ethynodiol diacetate) should be employed.

Because many enzyme systems are needed to complete the complex cholesterol to cortisol pathway, enzyme deficiencies may lead to disruptions of the normal cascade of events (Fig. 74.2). This group of enzyme disorders is known as congenital adrenal hyperplasia, mainly because of the resultant chronic adrenal gland stimulation that occurs following enzyme deficiency.[46] Any enzyme deficiency is capable of affecting any one or all three of the steroid pathways.[47] Therefore, treatment should be focused on replacement of the deficient hormone as well as cessation of chronic stimulation causing the hyperplasia. Below, six of the most common enzyme deficiencies are briefly discussed.

20-HYDROXYLASE DEFICIENCY ("NONVIRILIZING CONGENITAL ADRENAL HYPERPLASIA")

A deficiency of 20-hydroxylase will lead to an enlarged adrenal gland that is almost always full of cholesterol. Infants with this disorder generally present with enlarged female genitalia and have a poor prognosis. Blood and urine concentrations of all steroids are low, with elevated ACTH concentrations.

3-β-HYDROXYSTEROID DEHYDROGENASE DEFICIENCY ("MIXED CONGENITAL ADRENAL HYPERPLASIA")

Patients with this disorder present with both cortisol and aldosterone deficiencies. Increased concentrations of pregnenolone and cholesterol commonly are seen. The defect involves the adrenals and the gonads and results in decreased secretion of cortisol, aldosterone, androgens, and estrogens.

17-α-HYDROXYLASE DEFICIENCY ("NONVIRILIZING CONGENITAL ADRENAL HYPERPLASIA")

Following progesterone synthesis, one major pathway for the production of cortisol and estradiol is dependent on 17-α-hydroxylase. Since the aldosterone pathway is not affected, replacement of the mineralocorticoid is not necessary. Hypertension is usually present. Patients with this disorder are generally hypertensive, with low concentrations of cortisol and estrogens.

21-HYDROXYLASE DEFICIENCY ("VIRILIZING CONGENITAL ADRENAL HYPERPLASIA")

This is the most common form of congenital adrenal hyperplasia, causing approximately 90% of all congenital adrenal hyperplasias. The incidence of classic 21-hydroxylase deficiency is approximately 1 in 10,000.[48] This disorder results in excessive concentrations of progesterone, 17-α-hydroxyprogesterone, and ACTH and low concentrations of cortisol and aldosterone. Patients who exhibit this disorder may not be diagnosed until later in life, when the pubertal irregularities become clinically evident. In milder forms of this disorder, children may go undiagnosed for 2–10 years when acne, early appearance of pubic hair, voice lowering, or increased muscularity become bothersome. Patients with classic 21-hydroxylase deficiency usually have high levels of adrenal androgens, low aldosterone levels, high plasma renin activity, and hyponatremia. Once replacement therapy begins, most children mature normally. Patients are followed by measuring serial plasma renin activity and plasma 17-α-hydroxyprogesterone levels, and by monitoring growth velocity and bone age.

11-β-HYDROXYLASE DEFICIENCY ("VIRILIZING CONGENITAL ADRENAL HYPERPLASIA")

This enzyme marks the final step in the biosynthesis of cortisol and corticosterone. The enzyme is found only in the adrenal cortex. This disorder is the second most common cause of congenital adrenal hyperplasia (CAH). It is responsible for 9% of the cases of CAH and is seen in approximately 1 in 100,000 births.[48] Patients with this disorder will exhibit low plasma cortisol and aldosterone concentrations. In addition, high ACTH and MSH concentrations will be present. Patients will classically present with hypertension, secondary aldosterone excess, and virilism from androgen excess. Often this disorder is mistaken for Cushing's disease, but no glucose intolerance, often seen with Cushing's disease, occurs.

18-HYDROXYSTEROID DEHYDROGENASE DEFICIENCY (CORTICOSTERONE METHYLOXIDASE DEFICIENCY)

This enzyme disorder is restricted to the zona glomerulosa and results in a sole aldosterone-synthesis defect. The deficiency results in sodium depletion, potassium retention, hypotension, and increased plasma renin activity. Therapy should be identical to that of Addison's disease with mineralocorticoid replacement but no glucocorticoid replacement.

PRINCIPLES OF GLUCOCORTICOID ADMINISTRATION

Originally, the term glucocorticoid was given to these agents to describe their glucose-regulating properties. However, carbohydrate metabolism is only one of a multitude of effects that steroids can exhibit.

Glucocorticoids are natural products of the adrenal gland. In physiologic doses they affect many of the cells and tissues in the body. The pharmacologic doses of these agents, however, can produce a wide and complex range of activities. The activity produced is a function of the receptor activated (glucocorticoid versus mineralocorticoid) as well as the agent and dose prescribed.

The mechanism of steroids is complex and not fully known. The steroid probably enters the cell through passive diffusion and binds to the steroid receptor. There are between 5000 to 100,000 receptors per cell. Steroids exhibit various binding affinities to the receptor and therefore elicit various biologic effects.

After binding to the receptor, a structural change occurs in the receptor; this process is called activation. After activation, the receptor–steroid complex binds to DNA sites in the cell called glucocorticoid regulatory elements (GREs). This binding to the GREs affects transcription of nearby genes. Transcription can either be stimulated or inhibited by this binding.

This sequence of activation followed by binding to GREs is most likely responsible for the physiologic action of systemic steroids. The wide variability in effects is most likely a function of the vast number of receptors in almost every body tissue.

The pharmacokinetics of the glucocorticoids varies with the agent given and the route of administration. In general, most steroids given by the oral route are well absorbed. Water-soluble agents are more rapidly absorbed following intramuscular injection than are lipid-soluble agents. Intravenous administration is recommended when a quick onset of action is needed. A summary of the steroids is provided in Table 74.11.

Complications of systemic steroids can affect a variety of organ systems. Long-term complications tend to be insidious and less likely to respond to steroid withdrawal.

In addition to causing iatrogenic Cushing's syndrome, systemic steroids can also lead to increased susceptibility to infection, osteoporosis,[49] sodium retention with resultant edema, hypokalemia, hypomagnesemia, cataracts, peptic ulcer disease, seizures, and generalized suppression of the hypothalamic–pituitary–adrenal (HPA) axis.

Suppression of the HPA axis is a major concern whenever systemic steroids are tapered or withdrawn. Single doses of glucocorticoids can prevent the axis from responding to major stressors for several hours. In general, the longer the steroid is administered and the higher the dose used, the more suppression of the axis that occurs.

The possibility of HPA axis suppression occurs anytime the patient is exposed to supraphysiologic doses of a steroid. Symptoms of steroid withdrawal resemble those seen in a patient with adrenalcortical deficiency.

A variety of recommendations for steroid tapering are available. In general, patients who have been on long-term steroid therapy will need to be gradually withdrawn toward physiologic doses over months. On average, the normal adult produces approximately 20–30 mg of cortisol per day with the peak concentration occurring around 8:00 AM. As the steroid or steroid-equivalent dose approaches the 20- to 30-mg level, the taper should be slowed and the patient checked for axis function. The primary mode to test HPA integrity is the rapid ACTH test. A normal ACTH test would indicate that daily steroid maintenance therapy is not needed. More recently, the use of exogenous human CRH was found to be nearly as useful in the assessment of pituitary–adrenal function.[50] Pituitary–adrenal function was studied in 279 patients who were receiving between 5–30 mg of prednisone per day and in 50 normal subjects. Stimulation tests using 100 μg of CRH were performed and referenced to the standard of an insulin hypoglycemia test. The investigators concluded that pituitary–adrenal function cannot be reliably estimated from the dose of glucocorticoid, the duration of therapy, or the plasma cortisol concentration. Stimulation testing with CRH is nearly as useful as an insulin hypoglycemia test to assess pituitary–adrenal function. Caution should be used to prevent disease exacerbation during the steroid taper so as not to end up rebolusing the patient with another course of high-dose steroids.

The dilemma of prolonged steroid administration is sometimes lessened by the use of an alternate-day therapy (ADT) regimen.[41] ADT minimizes the hypothalamic–pituitary suppression as well as some of the adverse effects seen with once-daily therapy. This can be especially important in the treatment of the child and young adult, in whom growth suppression is a major concern. ADT is not recommended for initial management, but rather in the management of the stabilized patient who needs long-term therapy.[51] The transfer of a patient from a once-daily steroid to once every other day is a gradual process. The patient will be exposed to "on" and "off" days, with the "on" day dose gradually increased with concurrent reduction in the "off" day dose over a period of 14 days. By the 14th day, the patient will be consuming medication only on the "on" day.

THERAPEUTIC OUTCOMES

Successful glucocorticoid therapy involves counseling the patient, monitoring the patient, and recognizing complications of therapy (see Table 74.12). The risk–benefit of glucocorticoid administration should always be considered especially with concurrent disease states such as hypertension, diabetes mellitus, peptic ulcer disease, and uncontrolled systemic infections.

TABLE 74.12. FACTORS IN SUCCESSFUL GLUCOCORTICOID THERAPY

Monitoring
- Blood pressure
- Glucose concentrations (blood and urine)
- Ophthalmologic exams
- Serum electrolytes
- Urine electrolytes
- Stool tests for occult blood loss
- Growth and development (children and adolescents)

Counseling
- Take with food to minimize gastrointestinal upset
- Never discontinue medication on your own; check with physician—gradual dosage reduction is usually necessary
- Carry or wear medical identification indicating that you are on long-term glucocorticoid therapy
- Dosage increases may be necessary at times of increased stress (surgery or emergency treatments). A prepared syringe of 4 mg dexamethasone for intramuscular use should be available for home administration. A family member needs to be trained on the use and administration of dexamethasone.
- Be aware of potential side effects (i.e., visual disturbances, bruising, delayed wound healing, etc.)
- What to do if you miss a dose:
  - If dosing schedule is every other day: Take as soon as possible if remembered that morning; if not remembered until later, skip that day; take the next morning, then skip a day.
  - If dosing schedule is every day: Take as soon as possible but skip if almost time for the next dose; never double dose.

Recognizing complications
- Early in therapy and essentially unavoidable: insomnia, enhanced appetite and/or weight gain
- Common in patients with underlying risk factors: hypertension, diabetes mellitus, peptic ulcer disease
- Long-term intense treatment: Cushingoid habitus, hypothalamic–pituitary adrenal suppression, impaired wound healing
- Delayed and insidious: osteoporosis, cataracts, atherosclerosis
- Rare and unpredictable: psychosis, glaucoma, pancreatitis

(From Refs. 52 and 53.)

REFERENCES

1. Conn JW. Primary aldosteronism, a new clinical syndrome. J Lab Clin Med 1955;45:6–17.
2. Liddle GW. The adrenals, in Williams RH (ed): Textbook of Endocrinology. Philadelphia, WB Saunders, 1981, pp 249–290.
3. Albright F. Cushing syndrome. Harvey Lect 1942–1943;38:123–186.
4. Neiman L, Cutler GB. Cushing's syndrome, in Degroot LJ (ed): Endocrinology, 3rd ed. Philadelphia, WB Saunders, 1995, pp 1741–1769.
5. Vagnucci AH, Evans E. Cushing's disease with intermittent hypertension. Am J Med 1986;80:83–88.
6. Ross EJ, Marshall-Jones P, Friedman M. Cushing's syndrome: Diagnostic criteria. Q J Med 1966;35:149.
7. Orth DN. Cushing's syndrome. N Engl J Med 1995;332:791–803.
8. Trainer PT, Grossman A. The diagnosis and differential diagnosis of Cushing's syndrome. Clin Endocrin 1991;34:317–330.
9. Snow K, Nai-Siang J, Kao P, Scheithauer BW. Biochemical evaluation of adrenal dysfunction: The laboratory perspective. Mayo Clin Proc 1992;67:1055–1065.
10. Avgerinos PC, Yanovski JA, Oldfield EW, et al. The metyrapone and dexamethasone suppression tests for the differential diagnosis of the adrenocorticotropin-dependent Cushing's syndrome: A comparison. Ann Intern Med 1994;121:318–327.
11. Kaye TB, Crapo L. The Cushing's syndrome: An update on diagnostic tests. Ann Intern Med 1990;112:434–444.
12. Boruskek S, Gold JJ. Commonly used medications that interfere with routine endocrine laboratory procedures. Clin Chem 1964;10:41.
13. Tyrrell JB, Findling JW, Arno DC, et al. An overnight high-dose dexamethasone suppression test for rapid differential diagnosis of Cushing's syndrome. Ann Intern Med 1986;104:180–186.
14. Dunnick NR, Doppman JL, Gill JR, et al. Localization of functional adrenal tumors by computed tomography and venous sampling. Radiology 1982;142:429–433.
15. Cook DM, Meikle AW. Factitious Cushing's syndrome. J Clin Endocrin Metab 1985;61:385–387.
16. DeHerder WW, Krenning EP, Malchoff CD, et al. Somatostatin receptor scintigraphy: Its value in tumor localization in patients with Cushing's syndrome caused by ectopic corticotropin or corticotropin-releasing hormone secretion. Am J Med 1994;96:305–312.
17. Malerbi DA, Liberman B, Corradini MC, et al. The desmopressin stimulation test in the differential diagnosis of Cushing's syndrome. Clin Endocrin 1993;38:463–472.
18. McEvoy GK (ed). American Hospital Formulary Service (AHFS) Drug Information. American Society of Hospital Pharmacists, Inc 1994:670–673, 2489–2494.
19. Atkinson AB. The treatment of Cushing's syndrome. Clin Endocrin 1991;34:507–513.
20. Dickstein G, Lahar M, Shen-Orr, et al. Primary therapy for Cushing's disease with metyrapone. JAMA 1986;255:1167–1169.
21. Miller JW, Crapo L. The medical treatment of Cushing's syndrome. Endocrine Rev 1993;14(4):443–458.
22. Schteingart DE. Cushing's syndrome. Endocrine Metab Clin North Am 1989;18(2):311–338.
23. Cocconi G. First generation aromatase inhibitors—aminoglutethimide and testololactone. Breast Cancer Res Treatment 1994;30:57–80.
24. Weinberger MM, Grim CE, Mollified JW, et al. Primary aldosteronism: Diagnosis, localization, and treatment. Ann Intern Med 1979;90:386–395.
25. Ferriss H, Beevers G, Brown J. Clinical, biochemical and pathological features of low-renin ("primary") hyperaldosteronism. Am Heart J 1978;95:375–388.
26. Ganguly A, Donohue JP. Primary aldosteronism: Pathophysiology, diagnosis, and treatment. J Urol 1983;129:241–247.
27. White PC. Disorders of aldosterone biosynthesis and action. N Engl J Med 1994;331:250–258.

28. Lyons DF, Kern DC, Brown RD, et al. Single-dose captopril as a diagnostic test for primary aldosteronism. J Clin Endocrinol Metab 1983;57:892–896.
29. Stokes GS, Monaghan JC, Menme BA. Use of an intravenous sodium load in screening for primary hyperaldosteronism. Aust NZ J Med 1984;14:201–207.
30. Noth RH, Biglieri EG. Primary hyperaldosteronism. Med Clin North Am 1988;72:1117–1131.
31. Ganguly A. Glucocorticoid—suppressible hyperaldosteronism: An update. Am J Med 1990;88:321–324.
32. Lotgering FK, Derkx FMH, Wallenburg HCS. Primary hyperaldosteronism in pregnancy. Am J Obstet Gynecol 1986;155:986–988.
33. Arteaga E, Klein R, Biglieri EG. Use of the saline infusion test to diagnose the cause of primary aldosteronism. Am J Med 1985;79:722–728.
34. Gordon RD. The diagnosis of primary hyperaldosteronism. Aust NZ J Med 1984;14:195–196.
35. Young WF, Hogan MJ, Klee GG, et al. Primary aldosteronism: Diagnosis and treatment. Mayo Clinic Proc 1990;65:96–110.
36. Banks WA, Kastin AJ, Biglier EG, et al. Primary adrenal hyperplasia: A new subset of primary hyperaldosteronism. J Clin Endocrinol Metab 1984;58:783–785.
37. Iwaoka T, Umeda T, Naomi S, et al. The usefulness of the captopril test as a simultaneous screening for primary aldosteronism and renovascular hypertension. Am J Hypertens 1993;6:899–906.
38. Siragy H, Carey RM. Management of primary aldosteronism. Drug Ther 1986;16:89–103.
39. Blumenfeld JD, Sealey JE, Schlussel Y, et al. Diagnosis and treatment of primary hyperaldosteronism. Ann Intern Med 1994;121:877–885.
40. Nerup J. Addison's disease—clinical studies. A report of 108 cases. Acta Endocrinol 1974;76:127–141.
41. Claman HN. Glucocorticoids II: The clinical responses. Hosp Pract 1983;18:143–151.
42. Reasner CA. Adrenal disorders. Crit Care Nurs Q 1990;13(3):67–73.
43. Kenney FM, Hashida Y, Askari AH, et al. Virilizing tumors of the adrenal cortex. Am J Dis Child 1968;115:445–458.
44. Thorn GW. The adrenal cortex. Johns Hopkins Med J 1968;123:49–77.
45. Kuttenn F, Couillin P, Girard F, et al. Late-onset adrenal hyperplasia in hirsutism. N Engl J Med 1985;313:224–231.
46. Bongiovanni AM, Root AW. The adrenogenital syndrome. N Engl J Med 1963;268:1283–1289, 1342–1351, 1391–1399.
47. Finkelstein M, Shaefer JM. Inborn errors of steroid biosynthesis. Physiol Rev 1979;59:353–406.
48. Stewart PM, Edwards CRW. The medical treatment of adrenal disease. Br J Hosp Med 1989;42:25–29.
49. Zelissen PM, Croughs RJ, van Rijk PP, et al. Effects of glucocorticoid replacement therapy on bone mineral density in patients with Addison's disease. Ann Intern Med 1994;120:207–210.
50. Schlaghecke R, Kornely E, Santen RT, et al. The effect of long-term glucocorticoid therapy on pituitary–adrenal responses to exogenous corticotropin-releasing hormone. N Engl J Med 1992;326:226–230.
51. Federman DD. The adrenal, in Ribensten E, Federman DD (eds): Medicine. New York, Scientific American, 1986, pp 3(IV)1–3(IV)14.
52. Balow JE. Complications of therapy, pp 1205–1206, in Boumpas DT, moderator. Glucocorticoid therapy for immune mediated diseases: Basic and clinical correlates. Ann Intern Med 1993;119:1198–1208.
53. U.S. Pharmacopeial Convention, Inc. USP DI: Drug Information for the Health Care Professional, Vol I, 15th ed. Taunton, MA, Rand McNally, 1995, pp 878–908.

Section 8

Gynecologic and Obstetric Disorders

Chapter 75

Therapeutic Considerations in Pregnancy and Lactation

Janet McCombs, PharmD

Pregnancy is a normal, natural life event through which most women progress with minimal problems. Although modern medicine and updated technology have improved obstetric risks and decreased complications, new problems such as the teratogenicity of medications have emerged. Since the thalidomide tragedy in 1956 and, more recently, the diethylstilbestrol problems, medical practitioners are more cautious about recommending medication for their pregnant patients.

Most medications have an unknown risk of teratogenicity, and fewer than 10 are specifically indicated for use during pregnancy.[1] Although very little information is available about drug effects on the fetus, many women ingest both prescription and nonprescription medications during pregnancy. The patient may have an acute or chronic medical problem that requires medication, and though it would be best to avoid all medications, the well-being of the mother must also be considered. A mother who is uncomfortable and ill for the duration of her pregnancy is less likely to approach delivery and the newborn with a positive attitude. Also, a patient may take medication before realizing that she is pregnant or before consulting a physician. Other patients may assume that because of easy availability, nonprescription medications are safe during pregnancy.

Diagnosis

Amenorrhea is usually the first symptom of pregnancy in most patients; however, in early pregnancy, women may also experience morning nausea and vomiting, frequent urination, and tender breasts with enlargement and increased pigmentation of the nipple and areola. Early pregnancy may be confirmed by the presence of human chroionic gonadotropin (HCG), and some assays for HCG are sensitive enough to detect its presence 7–9 days after fertilization. HCG is produced by the placenta very early in pregnancy and the concentration doubles approximately every 2 days in a normal pregnancy. HCG is comprised of α and β subunits. The α subunit is identical to the α subunit of luteinizing hormone (LH), thyroid-stimulating hormone (TSH), and follicle-stimulating hormone (FSH). In some of the earlier tests, cross-reactivity with these hormones occasionally produced a false-positive result. The β subunit is unique to HCG, and the newer pregnancy tests specifically detect the β subunit. Serum tests such as radioimmunoassay (RIA) and enzyme linked immunosorbent assay (ELISA) can detect concentrations of HCG as low as 5 mIU/mL (present about 6–10 days after implantation).[2] Urine tests using monoclonal antibodies can usually detect concentrations of HCG in the 20–40 mIU/mL range (1–2 weeks after conception). Ectopic pregnancies may not produce enough HCG to be detected by the urine tests, and a negative urine test should not be used as the sole diagnostic test for pregnancy. Quantitative serum assays for HCG should be used in the diagnosis of ectopic pregnancies or suspected pregnancy loss. The current home pregnancy tests using monoclonal antibodies are very sensitive and specific and are useful for detecting normal pregnancies when used correctly. Again, these home tests fail to detect 50% of ectopic pregnancies, and women who observe a negative result should be counseled about this possibility and encouraged to repeat the test again in 7 days if menses have not begun. A second negative test should prompt the patient to make an appointment with her physician for evaluation.

Normal Course of Pregnancy

The normal duration of human gestation is 267 days from conception or 280 days from the first day of the last menstrual period. Thus, pregnancy usually spans 40 weeks. There are charts and "wheels" developed to aid the practitioner in determining the expected date of confinement (EDC), but Nagele's rule also provides a reasonable estimate of the delivery date. To apply Nagele's rule, take the date of the first day of the last menstrual period, subtract 3 months, then add 7 days[3] (for example, June 20 − 3 months = March 20 + 7 days = March 27). This method is usually correct to within 2 weeks of delivery and works best with patients who have regular 28-day cycles.

Gestational age is the number of completed weeks of pregnancy beginning with the first day of the last menstrual period. The product of conception is referred to as an embryo for the first 8 weeks and thereafter is termed *fetus.* The gravidity of a female patient is the total number of pregnancies including ectopic, premature, and aborted pregnancies. A gravid patient is pregnant; a primigravida is pregnant for the first time and a nulligravida has never been pregnant. The parity of a patient refers to the number of deliveries after the twentieth week of gestation.

Parity may be further defined for an individual patient by a series of four numbers. In order, these numbers indicate the number of term deliveries, number of premature deliveries, number of aborted and/or ectopic pregnancies, and number of living children. Deliveries involving multiple births add only one parous experience to the mother's obstetric history.

The average weight gain during pregnancy is 24 pounds. Patients gaining 24 pounds or less usually have more success returning to their prepregnancy weight after delivery. Patients who gain more than 24 pounds have often consumed a diet too high in calories. The gain during the first trimester is about 3 pounds, but during the last 16 weeks, a gain of 1 pound per week may be expected. Adequate protein intake is especially important during pregnancy because it is essential for normal fetal development. Normally, a pregnant patient requires an increase of 300 cal/d, including an additional 30 grams of protein. The lactating patient requires an additional 500 calories daily including 20 grams of protein.

During pregnancy, it is common to give a multivitamin supplement though this may not be necessary in a patient consuming a well-balanced diet. Many pregnant patients also require supplemental iron, and this 200 mg of elemental iron is included in most prenatal vitamins. Pregnant patients should also make sure to ingest at least 1.2 grams of elemental calcium daily either in their diet or with calcium supplementation. Adequate calcium intake is necessary for normal growth of fetal bones and teeth.

The Committee on Genetics of the American Academy of Pediatrics currently recommends that all women of childbearing age who are capable of becoming pregnant take at least 0.4 mg of folic acid daily to reduce the incidence of neural tube defects.[4] Studies indicate that maximal benefit is received when women receive supplemental folic acid at least 1 month prior to conception and through the first trimester. Most prescription prenatal vitamins contain 1 mg of folic acid, which meets this recommendation. Women who have had a previous neural tube defect-affected pregnancy are at higher risk and should receive prenatal counseling and testing in addition to treatment with 4 mg of folic acid daily.[5] Patients should never take more than 0.8 mg of folic acid daily without physician supervision.

Physiologic Changes in Pregnancy

Many physiologic changes occur in the pregnant patient, altering the use of medications in this population. Total blood volume in pregnancy increases 30–40% (1500–1800 mL). The cellular components increase about 20% and the fluid portion, about 40–50%. This disparity may be erroneously interpreted as an anemia in the third trimester when the hemoglobin and hematocrit fall. Also, during the second and third trimesters the extravascular volume increases; this could cause decreased plasma concentrations of some drugs.

Serum proteins are often 1–1.5 grams lower in pregnancy, and the albumin-to-globulin ratio falls by about 50%. Renal function is improved during gestation as the renal blood flow increases about 30% and the glomerular filtration rate is increased about 50%. Drugs excreted primarily by glomerular filtration would be expected to have an increased rate of excretion. Because of improved renal filtration, serum urea, creatinine, and uric acid are decreased in pregnancy.

The cardiovascular system also undergoes several significant changes during pregnancy. Cardiac output increases about 32% due to an increased heart rate of 10–15 beats per minute and an increased stroke volume; however, the blood pressure remains relatively constant during most pregnancies.

In the gastrointestinal (GI) tract, motility and acidity are decreased. The tone of the bowel is also decreased; thus, symptoms of a hiatal hernia are common but resolve after delivery. The decreased peristalsis of the GI tract often leads to constipation in the pregnant patient. Nausea and vomiting in the early weeks of pregnancy may contribute to the decreased absorption of medications, and the decreased motility of the lower GI tract may delay the fecal excretion of some drugs.

Although the metabolism of drugs may be increased or decreased at various stages of gestation, it is unlikely that this would have a profound effect on the plasma clearance of drugs during pregnancy.[6]

During pregnancy, a hypercoagulable state develops, with higher levels of fibrinogen and factors VII, VIII, IX, and X. The risk of disseminated intravascular coagulation (DIC) is increased during pregnancy, but the incidence of deep vein thrombosis is not increased.

PREGNANCY-INDUCED DISEASES

Physiologic and functional changes during pregnancy may lead to exacerbation or development of medical problems commonly diagnosed in the general population. Pregnancy and concern for the fetus may dictate management of these disorders in a manner different than in the nonpregnant patient. On the other hand, there are several pregnancy-induced disorders that also demand treatment during pregnancy with consideration for the fetus.

NAUSEA AND VOMITING

The nausea and vomiting associated with pregnancy are usually mild and are often referred to as "morning sickness." About half of all pregnant patients experience some degree of nausea and vomiting during the first trimester of pregnancy. The symptoms usually begin within a few weeks after conception and continue through the 12th to 14th weeks of gestation. Nausea is often apparent upon arising but abates as the day progresses. Some women, however, experience nausea throughout the day and in some patients it persists throughout the pregnancy. Severe nausea and vomiting that cannot be controlled and result in dehydration and malnutrition are termed hyperemesis gravidarum. Hyperemesis gravidarum can be a life-threatening problem and requires immediate therapy. Complications include nutritional deficiencies, weight loss, and starvation. Left untreated, maternal neurologic, renal, retinal, and hepatic damage may occur and are similar to changes observed in starvation. These patients are generally hospitalized and treated with intravenous fluids, electrolytes, antiemetics, and sedation. In very severe cases, peripheral or central parenteral nutrition may be useful.[7,8] Treatment with total parenteral nutrition has been shown to be effective in providing the mother and fetus with adequate nutrition as evidenced by birth weight and lack of adverse effects.[7,8]

The cause of nausea and vomiting in pregnancy is unknown. Proposed mechanisms include increased levels of hormones during pregnancy and emotional or psychological factors. Because the etiology is yet undetermined, treatment is directed at the symptoms. A patient who experiences only early morning nausea may be instructed to eat two or three soda crackers upon awakening, then wait 15–20 minutes before arising. Often keeping the stomach from becoming completely empty is helpful and dietary management would include small, dry meals high in carbohydrates and avoidance of spicy foods and those with noxious odors.

Medication must be considered for patients whose nausea persists despite dietary alterations. Although teratogenic risk cannot be ruled out for any drug, the risk involved with the antiemetic agents currently used for nausea and vomiting in pregnancy seems to be minimal.[9–12] Medications used most often include the phenothiazines, meclizine, cyclizine, dimenhydrinate, doxylamine, and pyridoxine. Bendectin (Merrell-Dow; doxylamine 10 mg, pyridoxine 10 mg) was the most widely used agent for morning sickness until its withdrawal from the market by the manufacturer in 1983. Despite lack of evidence associating Bendectin with birth defects, damaging publicity and decreasing patient confidence prompted the decision to stop manufacture of the medication. This tablet had a special coating that delayed activity, making a bedtime dose effective during the morning hours.

Antihistamines and phenothiazines have been used often to treat nausea and vomiting during pregnancy without any evidence of association with teratogenic effects.[11,12] When considering the use of medications for nausea and vomiting during pregnancy, the possible effects of malnutrition and dehydration and the electrolyte status of the mother and her general health must be considered in the risk-to-benefit ratio.

HEARTBURN

Many patients experience heartburn during the latter half of pregnancy. This usually results from relaxation of the cardiac sphincter and increased pressure in the stomach caused by the enlarging uterus, allowing regurgitation of the stomach contents into the lower esophagus. Relaxation of the lower esophageal sphincter is probably caused by a combination of mechanical and intrinsic factors.[13] Dietary management of heartburn should be attempted before drug therapy. Smaller, more frequent meals often help to alleviate the symptoms. Some women find that avoiding food and liquids other than water for at least 3 hours before bedtime and elevating the head of the bed with blocks help relieve discomfort that is exacerbated when they lie down.

Antacids may be used judiciously in patients who do not respond to dietary alterations. Magnesium and/or aluminum hydroxides are usually effective for relieving the pain and their duration of activity is several hours. Sodium bicarbonate is not recommended due to its short duration of effect, possible rebound symptoms, and metabolic alkalosis with chronic use. Sucralfate is poorly absorbed by the GI tract and has been suggested as a reasonable treatment for heartburn in pregnancy. Although sucralfate is an aluminum salt and aluminum has been associated with neurobehavioral and skeletal toxicity in animals, there is no evidence that aluminum is absorbed from the GI tract, and there have been no reports of associated congenital defects.[9,13]

CONSTIPATION

Constipation is a common problem in pregnancy and is most likely a result of decreased peristalsis. Patients experiencing constipation should be encouraged to add bulky, high-fiber foods to their diet and increase their fluid intake. Moderate exercise, such as walking, is also helpful for most patients.

Surfactants and bulk laxatives are the agents of choice for the pregnant patient. Bulk laxatives are not absorbed and thus would pose the least threat to the fetus. Adequate intake of fluids should be stressed to the patient to prevent possible intestinal obstruction with the fiber laxatives. Mineral oil should be avoided because there is a possibility of impairment of vitamin K absorption, which could decrease availability to the fetus and result in hypoprothrombinemia.

HEMORRHOIDS

Hemorrhoids often develop or worsen during pregnancy. The causes are usually a combination of increased venous pressure below the uterus and constipation.

Correction of constipation, use of stool softeners and sitz baths are usually helpful in reducing discomfort from hemorrhoids. External medications are preferred over those inserted into the rectum because many drugs are readily absorbed from the rectal mucosa. Products containing topical anesthetics and steroids should be avoided except under supervision of a physician due to possible systemic absorption with consequent effect on the fetus.

COAGULATION DISORDERS

Thromboembolic phenomena are uncommon during pregnancy, the incidence being about 0.2–0.4%. The mortality associated with thromboembolism may reach 13%, but with adequate anticoagulation this can be reduced to 1% or less.[14] Patients who have a cardiac valve prosthesis will also require anticoagulation during pregnancy.

Standard protocols are unacceptable for use in the pregnant patient because oral anticoagulants pose a significant risk to the fetus. About 30% of pregnancies exposed to oral anticoagulants result in fetal malformations, developmental deficiencies, stillbirths, or hemorrhage.[9] The teratogenic risk appears to be greatest during the first trimester; although ophthalmic abnormalities and mental retardation are associated with the use of coumarin anticoagulants in the second and third trimesters.[14–16] Another concern is the risk of fetal hemorrhage if delivery occurs while the mother is taking oral anticoagulants.

The anticoagulant of choice during pregnancy is subcutaneous (SQ) heparin,[17] although it too has risks. The large molecular weight of heparin prevents it from crossing the placenta,[14,16] thus the fetal risks associated with heparin are indirect, such as maternal hemorrhage, or from the underlying disease requiring anticoagulation. There are no reports of congenital defects associated with heparin.[9] Another reason heparin is preferred in pregnancy is because the effect of the medication can be antagonized by administering protamine sulfate. This is advantageous because the onset of labor and the necessity of an operative delivery are not always predictable.

Although heparin appears to be the safest anticoagulant for the mother and fetus, the risk of osteoporosis in the mother must be considered. Demineralization of bone occurs with long-term heparin therapy; unfortunately, the reversibility of this effect has not been established.[18]

Reproductive-age females requiring long-term anticoagulation with oral agents should be counseled about the risks of pregnancy and provided with effective contraception. Conversion from oral anticoagulants to SQ heparin should be considered for those patients desiring pregnancy despite the possible risks. Ambulatory patients should be capable of self-administering SQ heparin and compliant with appointments for follow-up monitoring.

PREGNANCY-INDUCED HYPERTENSION

Pregnancy-induced hypertension can be a serious and life-threatening obstetric complication. Recently, definitions of hypertensive disorders in pregnancy have been revised.[10] Gestational hypertension is diagnosed when the blood pressure exceeds 140/90 mm Hg in the absence of proteinuria or pathologic edema. Preeclampsia is further divided into mild and severe forms. Mild preeclampsia is hypertension accompanied by proteinuria (≥300 mg/24 h or 100 mg/dL in two random samples 6 hours apart) and/or pathologic edema. Preeclampsia is determined to be severe when proteinuria exceeds 4 g/24 h or persistent dipstick values of 2+ are present, blood pressure is 160/110 mm Hg, and/or severe headache, visual disturbances, or epigastric pain is noted. Eclampsia is the development of generalized tonic–clonic seizures in a patient with pregnancy-induced hypertension. Pregnancy-aggravated hypertension is diagnosed in a patient with preexisting essential hypertension who experiences a 15 mm Hg increase in diastolic or 30 mm Hg increase in systolic blood pressure after the 24th week of gestation. If pathologic edema or proteinuria develop, the patient has superimposed preeclampsia.

The incidence of preeclampsia in the United States is 5–8%.[10,19] Hypertensive disorders induced by pregnancy are diagnosed after the 20th week of gestation but can also occur within 48 hours of delivery and in the presence of trophoblastic disease. Eighty-five percent of patients diagnosed with the disorder are primiparas, particularly those who are very young or at the upper end of the reproductive age group.[20] Other risk factors include essential hypertension, diabetes, familial history, multiple fetuses, and molar pregnancies.

Although the specific cause(s) of preeclampsia are as yet unknown, three mechanisms are likely to be involved in the development of this disorder. Increased vasospasm, an immunologic reaction, and an imbalance of vasoactive prostaglandins probably contribute to this problem. The hypertension in preeclamptic and eclamptic patients is caused by vasospasm and increased vascular resistance. The etiology of the vasospasm is unknown, but preeclamptic patients are more sensitive to angiotensin II than normal pregnant patients. The immunologic factor is suggested by the fact that most cases of preeclampsia are noted in the first pregnancy that continues past the first trimester, suggesting that exposure to fetal antigens provides subsequent protection. An abnormal balance in prostaglandins has also been documented in preeclamptic patients.[21] Prostacyclin, which causes vasodilation, inhibits platelet aggregation, and decreases uterine contractility, increases about fivefold in normal pregnancies but is less in preeclamptic women. This lower concentration appears to increase sensitivity to angiotensin II as early as the 18th week of pregnancy.[22] Thromboxane A_2, another prostaglandin, is also increased in normal pregnancies and has activity that opposes prostacyclin. Thromboxane A_2 causes vasoconstriction, platelet aggregation, and uterine contractility. It has been suggested that in the preeclamptic patient there is an imbalance of these two prostaglandins in favor of thromboxane A_2.[21] This imbalance would likely cause increased vasoconstriction, platelet aggregation, and decreased uteroplacental blood flow, all of which have been reported in the preeclamptic patient. Until the mechanism(s) for the development of the disorder is identified, the problem cannot be prevented or treated specifically. The only cure for preeclampsia/eclampsia is termination of the pregnancy.

Prevention of preeclampsia with low-dose aspirin has been suggested for patients at high risk for development of the disorder. If an imbalance of prostaglandins is a causative factor in this state, then perhaps prophylactic aspirin would be useful in some women. Low-dose aspirin has been shown to decrease thromboxane A_2 synthesis to a greater degree than the decrease in prostacyclin synthesis,[23,24] which would theoretically normalize the ratio of prostacyclin and thromboxane A_2. The dose of aspirin used in the most recent and ongoing studies is 60 mg/d and is usually given from the 24th to 28th week of gestation and continued until the onset of labor.[25,26] The usefulness of low-dose aspirin in preventing preeclampsia has now been verified in a number of studies,[25–27] but further investigation is needed to determine which patients are at the highest risk for preeclampsia and might benefit from prophylaxis. While there have been no adverse effects noted in infants or mothers exposed to low-dose aspirin during pregnancy,[27] pregnancies at low risk for development of preeclampsia should not be exposed to any medication unnecessarily. Low-dose aspirin has not been shown to be useful in the treatment of existing preeclampsia/eclampsia.

Patients exhibiting mild preeclampsia should be placed on strict bedrest. Diuresis usually begins within 36–48 hours with regression of symptoms in 4–5 days. Compliant patients may be allowed to remain at home and instructed to do daily measurements for proteinuria and to check their blood pressure twice daily. Patients should bring these records to twice-weekly office visits. Patients who are unable or unwilling to comply with necessary restrictions and monitoring must be hospitalized. Antihypertensive medications have not been shown to be useful in prolonging gestation in pregnancies complicated by pregnancy-induced hypertensive states.[10]

Severely preeclamptic women must be hospitalized and begun on a regimen of parenteral magnesium sulfate to prevent seizures, and plans for delivery should be discussed. Several different methods for the administration of magnesium sulfate in preeclamptic patients have been described.[10,20] Both IM and IV routes of administration are effective in achieving adequate serum concentrations, and both have advantages and disadvantages in the treatment of the preeclamptic/eclamptic patient. IV administration may be preferred because magnesium does carry some risk of toxicity, and an IV infusion may be discontinued immediately should the serum level become excessive. If IV administration is chosen, a loading dose of 4 g is followed by an infusion of 1–3 g/h and must be delivered via a reliable controlled infusion pump. Another regimen begins with a 4-gram IV loading dose with simultaneous IM injection of 10 grams (5 grams in each buttock) followed by 5 grams IM every 4 hours. The disadvantages of IM administration are the large volume of solution required to administer the dose and the pain associated with the injection. Lidocaine may be used to minimize the discomfort of the injection. Convulsions not controlled by adequate serum concentrations of magnesium may respond to IV diazepam or phenytoin.

It is extremely important that the patient receiving magnesium sulfate be closely monitored for signs of toxicity. The optimum serum concentration for prevention of convulsions is 4–7 mEq/L.[10] At 9–10 mEq/L the patellar reflexes become hypoactive and may disappear; reflexes should be checked every 30 minutes. Urine output should be greater than 25 mL/h because magnesium is only excreted renally and impaired excretion can result in toxicity. Respirations should be greater than 10/min and respiratory depression and cardiac conduction abnormalities may occur if the magnesium serum concentration reaches 13–15 mEq/L. The IV administration of 1 gram of calcium gluconate (10 mL of 10% solution) usually reverses mild magnesium toxicity. An ampule of calcium gluconate should be kept at the bedside of any patient receiving magnesium therapy for preeclampsia/eclampsia. Reversal of respiratory depression occurs rapidly in the mother, but calcium gluconate administration to the mother may not be effective for hypermagnesemia in the infant. Magnesium does cross the placenta and magnesium levels should be determined in "floppy" neonates exposed to magnesium prior to delivery.

Magnesium sulfate is not an antihypertensive, and blood pressure should continue to be monitored frequently. A systolic reading of 160–180 mm Hg or greater or a diastolic reading of 110 mm Hg or greater should be treated with an intravenous antihypertensive medication to prevent cerebral hemorrhage. Intravenous hydralazine in a dose of 5–10 mg should be given initially, followed by 10 mg every 20 minutes as needed to decrease diastolic blood pressure below 100 mm Hg. An IV infusion may also be used if necessary. To avoid shock, it is important not to decrease blood pressure too quickly. Parenteral hydralazine often produces tachycardia, palpitations, flushing, and headache, and propranolol may be useful in opposing the cardiac side effects of hydralazine but should not be used alone for the treatment of hypertension. Labetalol, an α- and β-adrenergic blocking agent may be an alternative choice to hydralazine in the acute treatment of hypertension in preeclampsia/eclampsia.[10,28] The drug is given intravenously at a dose of 10–20 mg, doubling the dose every 10 minutes until blood pressure is controlled or a cumulative dose of 300 mg is reached. Labetalol can also be given by IV infusion at a rate of 1–2 mg/min until blood pressure is controlled, then decreasing to 0.5 mg/min to maintain control. It seems to have a faster onset of effectiveness than IV hydralazine with less reflex tachycardia but IV hydralazine tends to be somewhat more effective. In the absence of IV hydralazine, labetalol appears to be a good alternative choice.[10,28]

Diazoxide is not recommended for control of blood pressure in the preeclamptic/eclamptic patient due to multiple, serious adverse effects. It causes sodium and water retention, serious hyperglycemia in the mother and neonate, and may produce irreversible hypotension when given with other antihypertensive agents. The drug has a relaxant effect on the uterus and is likely to inhibit labor; thus, the use of diazoxide to control blood pressure in the obstetric patient is best reserved for postpartum hypertension. Diuretics are not recommended for use in preeclampsia/eclampsia because of the possibility of decreasing placental perfusion following intravascular fluid depletion. Calcium channel blockers may be useful for acute hypertensive episodes in pregnancy but further investigation is required. Nitroprusside is not used in this population due to lack of experience with the drug in pregnancy and concern about fetal thiocyanate toxicity.[29] It is used only when all other medications fail or when left ventricular failure is present.

The goal of therapy in preeclampsia/eclampsia is to decrease blood pressure, prevent or control convulsions, and deliver a viable infant. In most cases, the response to any treatment is temporary. Labor often begins spontaneously in these patients but, if not, plans for induction of labor or cesarean surgery should be made. The only cure for preeclampsia/eclampsia is delivery.

ANEMIAS

The most common anemia detected during pregnancy results from iron deficiency. Common causes include frequently recurring pregnancies, abnormal blood loss, and nutritional inadequacies. Hemoglobin values should be expected to drop during pregnancy because of the increase in blood volume with a smaller proportional increase in red blood cell mass. Iron deficiency anemia should be ruled out in pregnancy when the hemoglobin falls below 10 g/dL or the hematocrit is below 30%. Decreased blood levels of serum iron and total iron binding capacity are diagnostic. To prevent the development of iron deficiency anemia in pregnancy, all pregnant patients should receive approximately 30–60 mg of elemental iron daily. This may be achieved by the administration of prenatal vitamins.

CHRONIC MEDICAL DISORDERS IN PREGNANCY

DIABETES

Because of the significant metabolic changes during pregnancy, the management of the pregnant diabetic patient differs from that in the nonpregnant state. The White classification system of diabetes in pregnancy[30] is used for determining the prognosis and management of the pregnant diabetic (Table 75.1). This classification is based on the duration and severity of the disease and remains in use for describing the pathologic complications of the disease.

When possible, pregnancy in the diabetic patient should be planned, because prevention of complications provides the best management. The patient should be assessed for other risk factors, undergo ophthalmic evaluation and electrocardiography, and have a 24-hour urine collected for creatinine and protein values. The incidence of congenital abnormalities in diabetics is 3–22% depending on the degree of glycemic control,[31] compared with 2% in the normal population. It is especially important that the

TABLE 75.1. WHITE CLASSIFICATION OF DIABETES IN PREGNANCY

Class A: Chemical diabetes
Class B: Maturity onset (age older than 20 years), duration under 10 years, no vascular lesions
Class C^1: Age 10–19 years at onset
Class C^2: 10–19 years duration
Class D^1: Under 10 years at onset
Class D^2: Over 20 years duration
Class D^3: Benign retinopathy
Class D^4: Calcified vessels of legs
Class D^5: Hypertension
Class E: No longer sought
Class F: Nephropathy
Class G: Many failures
Class H: Cardiomyopathy
Class R: Proliferating retinopathy
Class T: Renal transplant added by Tagatz and colleagues of the University of Minnesota

(From White P. Classification of obstetric diabetes. Am J Obstet Gynecol 1978; 130(2):229, with permission.)

patient be normoglycemic before conception and during the first trimester, because the congenital malformations associated with diabetes seem to be related to poor control during the first 8 weeks of gestation.[32] Determination of glycosylated hemoglobin (A_1C) before conception helps to determine the degree of glucose control.

Patients with the highest risk of complications include those with vasculopathy, poor glucose control, a previous stillbirth, and noncompliance. The complications of diabetic pregnancies include fetal macrosomia, polyhydramnios, malformations, and respiratory distress syndrome. Patients with vascular disease are more likely to have a fetus with intrauterine growth retardation. With good prenatal management, diabetic patients now have a 96% chance of delivering a healthy child.[33]

During pregnancy, diabetic patients have an increased risk of hypoglycemia and ketoacidosis. Thus, the goal of therapy is the avoidance of fasting and postprandial hyperglycemia and hypoglycemia. The quality of maternal glucose control is the best indicator of perinatal risk, and use of the newer home glucose reflectance meters has significantly improved control. Tests using whole-blood determinations of glucose are preferred over urine tests during pregnancy because the renal threshold for glucose is decreased in pregnancy, giving an inaccurate estimate of blood sugar. Glucose should be monitored fasting, before meals, and at bedtime daily. Some physicians also ask their patients to monitor glucose 1 hour after meals 1 day per week. Evaluation of glycosylated hemoglobin once each trimester helps assess control.

Pregnant patients usually require a diabetic diet of 35 kcal/kg ideal body weight daily, or about 2200–2400 calories; only intermediate-acting and fast-acting insulins should be used. Long-acting insulins should not be used because of the variable rates of onset and prolonged duration of activity. NPH or Lente insulin combined with regular insulin should be given SQ in two divided doses daily. Optimal management is usually achieved by administering two-thirds the total dose of each insulin before breakfast and the remaining one-third before the evening meal. Split dosing includes using a 2:1 ratio of NPH to regular insulin in the morning injection and a 1:1 mixture in the evening injection. The dose should be adjusted to maintain rigid control, and with multiple dosing of insulin and careful monitoring of glucose, most women should be able to maintain glucose levels between 60–120 mg/dL.[34] About 70% of pregnant patients have increased insulin requirements after the 24th week, and requirements will usually double by the end of pregnancy. Insulin has a large molecular weight, thus it crosses the placenta minimally; the effects on the fetus are indirect.

Oral hypoglycemic agents are contraindicated during pregnancy because they cross the placenta and stimulate the fetal pancreas and can produce fetal and neonatal hypoglycemia. They may also cause some teratogenic effects[9] and do not appear to have any advantage in the control of blood sugar in the pregnant patient over insulin except avoidance of the injection. These agents should be discontinued before conception if at all possible. Should pregnancy occur in a patient taking one of these medications, the drug should be stopped when pregnancy is confirmed, and insulin therapy initiated.

Prenatal visits should be scheduled with the patient's internist and obstetrician every 2 weeks during the first half of pregnancy and weekly thereafter. This aids in compliance and early recognition of possible problems.

Glucose intolerance of pregnancy (gestational diabetes) develops during the second half of pregnancy in about 2–3% of patients.[31] Initially, the patient is placed on a diabetic diet and home glucose monitoring; if this does not control glucose, insulin therapy should be started and the patient managed as a pregnant diabetic.

Tight control should be maintained during labor and delivery to reduce the risk of neonatal hypoglycemia. This may be accomplished by an IV infusion of 1 L of 5% dextrose injection with 10 units of regular insulin given at a rate of 100 mL/h. Additional glucose or insulin is given to maintain glucose at approximately 100 mg/dL. Another regimen includes IV administration of 50 g of glucose every 6 hours, with regular insulin given SQ as needed. In either case, blood glucose should be checked every 1–2 hours with a portable glucose monitor.

Immediately after delivery of the placenta, insulin requirements drop and remain lower for 24–72 hours. During this period, hypoglycemic shock is common, and the patient must be monitored very closely. Breastfeeding is encouraged in the diabetic patient; lower insulin requirements during lactation are expected.[32]

THYROID DISEASE

The incidence of hyperthyroidism in pregnancy is 0.1–0.2%.[35] It is important that these patients be treated to minimize maternal and fetal morbidity and mortality. Preeclampsia, maternal heart failure, and stillbirths are more common in hyperthyroid pregnancies than normal pregnancies or those adequately treated.

Thioamides, methimazole and propylthiouracil (PTU), have both been used with equal efficacy in pregnancy.[35] Both medications cross the placenta and have the potential for causing fetal hypothyroidism and goiter. However, PTU is generally the preferred drug due to a dual mechanism of action not produced by methimazole and some belief that it crosses the placenta to a lesser degree. There are also reports of aplasia cutis in infants exposed to methimazole.[9] The dose is empirical and may need to be adjusted in pregnancy. The dose should be adequate to maintain the total serum T_4 level in the upper range of normal and the patient clinically minimally thyrotoxic.

Hypothyroidism in pregnancy should be treated with thyroxine replacement sufficient to maintain the patient in the euthyroid state. Patients with uncorrected hypothyroidism have a greater incidence of preeclampsia, placental abruption, low-birth-weight and stillborn infants, and heart failure. Infants born to hypothyroid mothers are usually healthy. All infants in the United States are screened for congenital hypothyroidism at birth.[10]

CHRONIC HYPERTENSION

Chronic hypertension in pregnancy is described as hypertension present at conception or developing before the 20th week of gestation. Obstetric patients with chronic hypertension are considered high risk and require close observation during pregnancy with prenatal visits scheduled every 1–2 weeks. Hypertensive patients have a greater incidence of decreased fetal weight and fetal growth retardation because of decreased placental function. At delivery, the placenta is small and multiple infarcts may be present. About one-third of hypertensive patients have superimposed preeclampsia,[10] which occurs earlier and progresses more rapidly than in otherwise normal pregnancies. These patients have higher maternal and fetal mortality rates and are less responsive to treatment. Abruptio placentae (premature separation of the placenta) occurs more often in patients with vascular disease than in patients with uncomplicated pregnancies. Cerebral hemorrhage is a more common cause of maternal mortality than preeclampsia in these patients. To minimize complications, blood pressure should be controlled during pregnancy. It is common for blood pressure to decrease in the second trimester, and it may be possible to discontinue therapy at this time and reinstate it if necessary.

Given the relatively young age of many pregnant patients, most chronic hypertension is usually mild and with minimal sequelae. Mild hypertension should first be treated with bedrest and home blood pressure monitoring. The patient should have complete bedrest for at least 1 hour at lunchtime and 1 hour in the afternoon in addition to 10 hours of bedrest each night.

Blood pressure not responding satisfactorily to bedrest may be treated with methyldopa. Methyldopa is the most commonly used antihypertensive medication in pregnancy. It is effective with no significant fetal or neonatal problems reported.[9] Using methyldopa reportedly increases fetal survival rates and decreases midtrimester fetal loss.[36]

Either propranolol or hydralazine is the second-line drug of choice. There are reports of intrauterine growth retardation, bradycardia, neonatal respiratory distress syndrome, and hypoglycemia with the use of propranolol. The true incidence of these effects is not known and may be more likely when used immediately prior to delivery. If using propranolol during pregnancy becomes necessary, when possible, the drug should be discontinued 1–2 weeks before delivery and the neonate observed closely for adverse effects. Trials using β blockers including atenolol, labetalol, and metoprolol are ongoing and may give more definitive information about the efficacy and safety of these drugs in pregnancy. Oral hydralazine may be less effective than propranolol, but it may be useful in controlling blood pressure if the patient is near delivery.

Cardiac output and intravascular volume are often reduced in hypertensive pregnancies; therefore, diuretics are to be avoided during pregnancy because these drugs cause a 5–10% decrease in plasma volume that may be detrimental to the fetus if uteroplacental blood flow is altered. Diuretics also cause fluid depletion and electrolyte imbalance and decrease carbohydrate tolerance in the mother. Decreased cardiac output may also decrease blood flow to the fetus. Reserpine is also avoided during pregnancy because of the possibility of fetal and neonatal bradycardia, congenital abnormalities, and alteration of thermal equilibrium at birth.

Calcium channel blockers are being used extensively in the treatment of chronic hypertension in the nonpregnant population but there are no published, large, controlled studies using these drugs in pregnancy. Until more data are available, calcium channel blockers should be avoided during pregnancy. Angiotensin-converting enzyme (ACE) inhibitors are contraindicated during pregnancy due to reports of fetal and neonatal renal impairment, oligohydramnios, congenital malformations, and neonatal death.[28,37,38]

Although fetal loss is about 16% in mild hypertension and may reach 40% in severe hypertension,[20] the primary goal of blood pressure management is to prevent maternal complications.

EPILEPSY

The incidence of pregnancies complicated by epilepsy is about 1%.[39,40] The primary goal in managing these patients is prevention of seizures with the fewest possible effects on the fetus. Pregnancy has unpredictable effects on the frequency and severity of seizures. About 40–50% of patients experience an exacerbation of the disease, 40–50% do not change, and the remaining 5–10% improve.[41] Patients with epilepsy, both those taking medication and those not taking medication, have a higher incidence of delivering an infant with congenital abnormalities and mental retardation.[39,41] Though it is difficult to separate the effects of medication from the effects of the disease, most evidence supports the role of anticonvulsants in causing congenital problems.[40] The most common abnormalities include orofacial clefts, skeletal anomalies, central nervous system (CNS) malformations, and cardiac abnormalities,[9,39,41] as well as mental retardation. Although teratogenicity does occur with anticonvulsants, the risk of a seizure is considered more harmful to the fetus.

The American Academy of Pediatrics Select Committee on Anticonvulsants in Pregnancy recommends that a patient seizure free for several years undergo a trial of medication withdrawal before becoming pregnant. A patient with recurrent epilepsy on medication should be advised that she has a 90% chance of having a normal child, but that the risk of congenital abnormalities and mental retardation is twice that of the normal population.[42]

Treatment with one medication is preferred when possible to decrease fetal exposure, thus minimizing teratogenic risk. When monotherapy fails, an assessment of compliance and evaluation of serum concentrations, with adjustment of dose if necessary, should be performed. If the first drug does not successfully control seizures, a second drug should be initiated and the first drug gradually withdrawn over 7 days. A trial using a third drug may be tried. If monotherapy with the third drug does not succeed, this indicates a trial with two medications simultaneously.

Serum concentrations of most anticonvulsants are lower during pregnancy despite maintenance of prepregnancy dosage.[39,41] Although serum concentrations may be decreased, seizure frequency may not increase because free concentrations of the drug do not decline proportionally with total concentration.[39] Reasons for decreased serum concentrations include noncompliance because of fears of teratogenic potential of the medication, inadequate dosage, incomplete absorption secondary to nausea and vomiting, increased hepatic clearance, abnormally rapid excretion, and an increased volume of distribution resulting from passage into fetal tissues. The increased extracellular fluid volume occurring in pregnancy may cause dilutional lowering of serum concentrations. Anticonvulsant serum concentrations should be evaluated at least bimonthly during pregnancy and dose adjusted according to the concentration and frequency of seizures and adverse effects.[39]

Phenytoin dosages may need to be increased during pregnancy, and serum concentrations should be monitored because of individual variation.[40] Although teratogenicity, coagulopathy, and vitamin deficiencies occur, phenytoin is not associated with neonatal depression and withdrawal reported with other anticonvulsants (e.g., barbiturates).[43]

Phenytoin does cause the fetal hydantoin syndrome. The fetal hydantoin syndrome includes craniofacial abnormalities, growth retardation, limb defects, cardiac lesions, hernias, and distal digital and nail hypoplasias. Many congenital malformations are surgically correctable. About 10% of infants exposed to phenytoin will manifest the full syndrome and about 30% have some features. The teratogenic potential of phenytoin may be more closely related to the metabolites than to the parent drug. Genetic variations would help explain why some infants are affected and others are not after exposure to phenytoin. Phenytoin is probably more teratogenic than phenobarbital, suggesting that phenobarbital should be used in reproductive-age women when possible.

In a large percentage of neonates exposed to anticonvulsants, a severe coagulopathy occurs during the first 24 hours after delivery.[44] This is because of a deficiency of the vitamin K-dependent clotting factors, and all exposed infants should be treated with 2 mg vitamin K_1 at birth.[41] Cord blood should be sent for clotting studies and, if necessary, additional vitamin K administered. Some physicians give pregnant patients receiving anticonvulsants prophylactic oral vitamin K during the last 3 weeks before expected delivery.[39] Prophylaxis is required because treatment may not be successful once there is clinical evidence of bleeding. Folate deficiency also occurs in patients on anticonvulsants and prophylaxis is suggested to prevent megaloblastic anemia.

Phenobarbital is the anticonvulsant of choice in women of childbearing age because it appears to have less teratogenic potential than phenytoin.[42] During pregnancy, higher dosages are usually required to maintain serum levels.[45] The coagulopathy and folate deficiency seen in patients taking phenytoin can also develop with phenobarbital. Neonates exposed to phenobarbital may experience depression at delivery and may experience withdrawal symptoms. Because of the long half-life in neonates, withdrawal symptoms do not usually begin for 4–7 days after delivery; thus, it is likely that symptoms will begin after hospital discharge. Parents should be advised to report neuromuscular excitability, hyperactivity or sleep disturbances, excessive crying, tremulousness, or persistent vomiting or diarrhea, because these symptoms may indicate withdrawal. The withdrawal may last 2–6 months[46] and may be treated by avoiding excessive stimulation of the infant and sedation with phenobarbital if necessary.

Phenobarbital is an active metabolite of primidone, and thus primidone would be expected to be associated with the same problems.

Carbamazepine was thought to be less teratogenic than other anticonvulsants and was often considered the drug of choice for pregnant epileptics. Recent reports, however, indicate that carbamazepine is teratogenic.[47,48] Defects reported include spina bifida, craniofacial defects, nail hypoplasia, and developmental delays.

Valproic acid is associated with cleft palate, renal defects, and neural tube defects, which are often not surgically correctable.[41] Its use should be avoided in women of childbearing age.

Trimethadione is the most potent teratogen in the anticonvulsant class. There is an approximate 83%[39] incidence of major malformations including developmental delays, low set ears, palatal abnormalities, V-shaped eyebrows, and speech impediments.[41] It should never be used in pregnancy. Felbamate and gabapentin, the mostly recently approved anticonvulsants for partial seizures, have not been studied in pregnancy and have been assigned a pregnancy risk category of C.

ASTHMA

Approximately 1% of pregnant patients have asthma.[10] The effect of pregnancy on asthma is not predictable; one-third of patients experience improvement of their disease, one-third worsen, and one-third do not change. The effect of asthma on pregnancy is generally not a problem in mild cases. Severe asthmatics who have impairment of respiratory function or medical complications may experience an adverse effect on pregnancy outcome.

Of the drugs used to treat asthma in the nonpregnant population, only the iodides are absolutely contraindicated in pregnancy. Iodides cross the placenta and may cause congenital thyroid problems.[9] Cromolyn sodium is not recommended by the manufacturer for use in pregnancy because of a lack of evidence confirming safety.

In the patient with mild and/or infrequent attacks, aerosol albuterol, metaproterenol, or isoetharine should be chosen. These drugs have fewer cardiac side effects than isoproterenol and epinephrine. Reportedly, congenital abnormalities do not occur with these agents.[9]

Patients with more severe or more frequent asthma attacks may receive oral theophylline. Fetal serum concentrations approximate maternal levels, but no adverse effects are reported.[9] Oral terbutaline may be added to theophylline if symptoms persist. Metaproterenol is used, but there is more experience using terbutaline in pregnancy, because it is often used to inhibit preterm labor. Aerosolized steroids are added if necessary to control the frequency and severity of attacks. When oral steroids are required, prednisone and prednisolone are suggested because the fetal serum concentration appears to be only 10% of the maternal level; other steroids appear in the fetal circulation at greater concentrations.[49]

Severe attacks and status asthmaticus are managed as in the nonpregnant population.

TREATMENT OF PRETERM LABOR

Uterine contractions with cervical changes beginning before the 37th week of gestation are considered premature labor.[50] There is some controversy as to the earliest gestational age at which premature labor should be treated. Labor occurring before the 20th week of amenorrhea usually results in expulsion of an imperfect fetus; inhibition of labor should not be attempted before the 20th week.

Many patients in premature labor respond to bedrest, hydration, and sedation; however, pharmacologic treatment should not be delayed because of the possibility of unsuccessful treatment or treatment of false labor. Pharmacologic intervention is most successful when the cervix is dilated less than 4 cm and the membranes are intact. Certain maternal and fetal conditions preclude the use of tocolytic agents (medications that inhibit uterine contractions). Although premature rupture of membranes is usually considered a contraindication to inhibition of labor, it may be advantageous to administer pharmacologic agents to delay delivery 24–48 hours to give glucocorticoids to enhance fetal lung maturity.

Recently, several investigators have questioned the efficacy of tocolytic agents, β agonists specifically, to prolong gestation, decrease perinatal mortality and increase birth weight.[51] Most clinicians, however, choose to treat preterm labor in order to give the fetus the greatest chance of survival. Tocolytic agents that delay labor for at least 48 hours allow the mother to receive glucocorticoids and may provide time for transfer to a facility with a neonatal intensive care department.

BETA AGONISTS

The most widely used tocolytic agents are the β agonists. Ritodrine is the only β-adrenergic drug approved in the United States for the treatment of premature labor, but terbutaline is used as well. No data are available to suggest that one agent is more efficacious or has fewer side effects than the other. Isoxsuprine is not widely used because it is associated with significant tachycardia and hypotension.

Before ritodrine was released in 1980, terbutaline was the drug used most often for the inhibition of premature labor. Terbutaline is effective[52] and much less expensive than ritodrine.

Terbutaline and ritodrine have similar side effects including hypotension and tachycardia. In many patients, hypokalemia occurs secondary to an intracellular shift of potassium, but resolves after discontinuation of the drug. This intracellular shift occurs only with parenteral therapy and unless hypokalemia is detrimental to the patient for other medical reasons, no treatment is required. Other side effects include palpitations, tremor, nervousness, angina, and headache.

Hyperglycemia is a common side effect of the β-agonist drugs, but it is usually not clinically important unless the patient is diabetic. Diabetic patients should be closely followed and use of an insulin pump should be considered. Some women receiving terbutaline maintenance dosing develop hyperglycemia or unmasking of gestational diabetes, and evaluating glucose tolerance after a week of therapy is suggested.

Pulmonary edema has occurred with the β-agonist agents.[53] The incidence is greater when the infusion solution is isotonic saline.[54] Therefore, the fluid of choice is 5% dextrose in water injection. Limiting the fluid intake to 2500 mL per 24 hours may also decrease the likelihood of pulmonary edema. Preparing a concentrated solution of ritodrine (300 mg in 500 mL D_5W) will help minimize fluid intake.

The intravenous infusion of ritodrine or terbutaline is usually continued for 12 hours after contractions cease. Oral medication is initiated 30 minutes before the infusion is stopped to allow for absorption. Some investigators have used terbutaline via subcutaneous pump for maintenance.[55,56] It has been suggested that some failures of β agonists are due to β-receptor down-regulation and that using very small doses of terbutaline continuously with a subcutaneous pump may prevent this occurrence.[10] Oral ritodrine does not seem to have the effectiveness of oral terbutaline,[57] and inadequate dosing of ritodrine may be the difference. The effectiveness of using these drugs prophylactically has not been investigated for use in single or twin gestations.

MAGNESIUM SULFATE

Though most often used as an anticonvulsant in severe eclampsia, magnesium sulfate is also effective in inhibiting premature labor. Magnesium sulfate probably antagonizes calcium to prevent the actin–myosin interaction, thus reducing uterine activity. Serum magnesium levels of 6–8 mEq/L are effective in suppressing uterine contractions.[50]

The patient should be closely observed for signs of hypermagnesemia. In addition to monitoring the patellar reflex, urine output, and respirations, some protocols require serial magnesium levels every 6 hours as an added precaution (see section on Preeclampsia/Eclampsia). Magnesium sulfate does not alter carbohydrate metabolism and may be the agent of choice in the diabetic patient.[50]

Magnesium sulfate crosses the placenta and can produce serum levels comparable to the maternal level.[9] Serious neonatal effects are uncommon unless the treatment fails and the delivery occurs during the infusion. Respiratory depression in the mother can be reversed by administration of 10 mL of 10% calcium gluconate.

PROSTAGLANDIN SYNTHETASE INHIBITORS

Prostaglandins are present in amniotic fluid during labor and delivery but are absent during pregnancy. The production and release of prostaglandins is postulated as a key factor in the initiation of labor. Therefore, the prostaglandin synthetase inhibitors may be useful in stopping labor. Oral and rectal indomethacin are effective in the treatment of preterm labor[58]; however, its usefulness is limited by serious potential side effects in the fetus. The possibility of premature closure of the ductus arteriosus and poor cardiopulmonary adaptation after delivery are of great concern.[58] Other reported problems in premature neonates exposed to indomethacin include necrotizing enterocolitis, intracranial hemorrhage, and renal dysfunction.[59] Oligohydramnios has also been reported in pregnancies exposed to these drugs.[60] Maternal side effects are the same as those in the nonpregnant patient.

CALCIUM CHANNEL BLOCKERS

Because calcium is necessary for muscle contraction, calcium channel blocking agents should be useful in the treatment of preterm labor. Two agents, verapamil and nifedipine, relax the myometrium *in vitro*[58]; however, the large doses of verapamil required to stop contractions are not tolerated by the mother. Nifedipine is effective in decreasing uterine contractions in severe dysmenorrhea[61] and during prostaglandin-induced abortions.[62] These results support further investigative studies into the usefulness of nifedipine as a tocolytic agent. No significant side effects were noted, but studies in animals indicate that metabolic alterations in the fetus may occur.

OXYTOCIN ANTAGONISTS

Oxytocin antagonists, a new class of drugs, are being studied for tocolysis. Atosiban is currently undergoing trials to demonstrate its effectiveness in inhibiting premature labor in humans.[63] Atosiban appears to lack cardiovascular, pulmonary and CNS effects; side effects such as nausea and vomiting are minimal.

Induction of Labor

Labor is not usually induced in normal pregnancies because the uterus is the preferred environment for the fetus. Induction is most successful when the cervix is soft, effaced, partially dilated, and in the center of the vagina. Induction should not be attempted unless an operative delivery would be appropriate should induction fail. Appropriate indications include severe maternal infection, uterine bleeding (usually caused by partial placenta previa or abruptio placentae), preeclampsia/eclampsia or chronic hypertension, diabetes mellitus, maternal renal insufficiency, premature rupture of membranes after the 36th week, polyhydramnios, evidence of placental insufficiency, isoimmunization, and postdate pregnancy.

Three classes of drugs are effective for stimulating uterine contractions: oxytocin, ergot alkaloids, and prostaglandins. The ergot alkaloids are only used to terminate pregnancy. They are not used to induce labor because of the possibility of violent, sustained uterine contractions that could compromise the fetus or rupture the uterus. The ergot alkaloids are orally absorbed and are most often used to decrease postpartum or postabortion bleeding.

The prostaglandin suppositories and solution that are currently available are used only for the termination of pregnancy, because their fetal effects are unknown. Prostaglandin E_2 is now approved in a gel that is applied to the cervix to promote cervical ripening prior to induction of labor. The gel is applied to the cervix in the afternoon or evening before planned induction. It is supplied in prefilled applicators for application by the obstetrician in the labor and delivery area because there is some chance of uterine hyperstimulation. Fetal and uterine monitors are utilized to evaluate the efficacy of the medication and monitor the fetal response. Hyperstimulation can be reversed with the use of β-adrenergic tocolytic therapy.

Oxytocin is the drug used most often to induce labor and to augment inadequate labor, as well as to decrease postpartum bleeding. The risks and benefits of oxytocin therapy must be considered before administration. The initial dose is 2 milliunits (mU) per minute by intravenous infusion. The infusion is usually mixed by adding 10 units of oxytocin to 1 liter of fluid. A controlled pump must be used for accurate dosing when administered by this route. IV infusion is recommended because the drug's absorption, distribution, and response are more predictable. IM administration is not recommended because the absorption is not consistent, and the medication cannot be discontinued if complications or side effects arise.

The dose may be increased by 2 mU/min every 15–20 minutes if needed to achieve adequate contractions; however, the dose should not exceed 20 mU/min. The goal of treatment is contractions lasting 45–60 seconds at intervals of 2–3 minutes.

The patient should be attended, and monitoring of uterine contractions (frequency, duration, and intensity) and fetal heart rate is essential for the early recognition and treatment of side effects. It is very important to monitor the intensity of resting uterine contractions because a resting pressure greater than 15–20 mm H_2O increases the incidence of complications such as uterine rupture, uteroplacental hypoperfusion, and fetal distress from hypoxia.[64] If the resting pressure exceeds this level, the medication should be discontinued. Maternal blood pressure and pulse rate should also be checked frequently.

Side effects of oxytocin are limited if appropriate monitoring is performed. Oxytocin does not cross the placenta[64]; any effects on the fetus are indirect secondary to the drug effects on the uterus. The most notable, but infrequent, side effect is uterine rupture. Oxytocin can reduce uteroplacental blood flow, resulting in decelerations of fetal heart rate and possible fetal hypoxia. Other side effects are maternal hypotension, hypoglycemia, and fluid retention. Oxytocin is structurally very similar to antidiuretic hormone, and some fluid retention is unavoidable.

Contraindications include abnormal fetal positions or presentations, cephalopelvic disproportion, repeat cesarean section or other previous uterine surgery, or a firm, closed, uneffaced, posterior cervix. Patients with functional class III or IV heart disease are not good candidates for oxytocin use. Grand multiparas (greater than seven previous deliveries) have a significantly increased risk of uterine rupture when oxytocin is used.

Lactation Suppression

Lactation is a complex, neuroendocrine-mediated process. Prolactin produced in the hypophysis stimulates the production of milk in breast tissue, whereas oxytocin causes ejection of milk from the nipple.

Recently, there has been renewed interest and greater participation in breast-feeding; however, there remain patients who choose not to nurse because of personal preference, working conditions, or because their babies are unable to nurse (e.g., babies who require intensive care or who have palate abnormalities). These mothers can pump their breasts to establish lactation in the event the baby can later breast-feed. Maternal drug therapy deleterious to the nursing infant would preclude nursing, as would other problems such as inverted nipples not successfully corrected.

Breast engorgement is usually self-limiting, begins about the third to fourth day postpartum, and resolves within 48–72 hours. During this time, the breasts are swollen, firm, and tender. Some patients relate severe pain, while others have only mild discomfort. Nondrug treatment includes application of ice packs and binding of the breasts. The patient should be reminded not to express the milk as this will only result in further production.

Until recently, two classes of medications were used for lactation suppression. Hormonal therapy, both androgenic and estrogenic substances, and bromocriptine mesylate were indicated for lactation suppression. Use of either type of medication was controversial because of reports of serious side effects when using these medications for treatment of a self-limiting problem.

Although many estrogenic and androgenic substances were once used, chlorotrianisene, a synthetic proestrogen, and a testosterone enanthate/estradiol valerate combination injection were the most frequently used. Both products have a local effect on breast tissue.

Concern regarding the use of estrogenic substances for postpartum lactation suppression stems from the hypercoagulable state that exists in the later stages of pregnancy and during parturition. Use of estrogenic agents could possibly potentiate the development of thromboemboli in this population. The British literature reported that deep vein thromboembolic events were not increased in women less than 25 years of age who had normal vaginal deliveries and received estrogenic medication. The incidence was increased in women over 25 years of age and in women undergoing cesarean delivery.[65]

Bromocriptine mesylate acts centrally to inhibit prolactin secretion and will thus prevent postpartum breast engorgement. While bromocriptine mesylate in a dose of 2.5 mg twice daily is effective, there appears to be several "pertinent negatives" associated with its use in postpartum lactation suppression. First, the drug must be taken for 14 days to treat a problem, which if left untreated, would not persist for more than a few days. The incidence of rebound lactation after discontinuation of the bromocriptine is as high as 40%.[66] The most significant concern recently reported with this medication is the risk of stroke, seizure, and myocardial infarction after its use postpartum.[66,67] However, a causal relationship with bromocriptine and these serious side effects has neither been confirmed nor ruled out, although several cases of litigation have resulted in awards to affected patients. Less serious side effects reported include headache, nausea, dizziness, and nasal congestion. Most obstetric centers have discontinued the pharmacologic suppression of lactation; however, if bromocriptine is used for this indication, the patient should be stabilized and at least 4 hours should elapse after delivery before beginning the medication. The incidence of hypotension is greater if the drug is administered too soon after delivery.

In summary, postpartum breast engorgement is a self-limiting problem that resolves in a few days. Current evidence suggests that nonpharmacologic treatment and analgesics are the best choice until more information is available.

Drug Effects on the Fetus

Any medication administered to a pregnant patient may affect the fetus directly or indirectly. Drugs and environmental agents that have the potential to cause abnormal fetal growth and development are called teratogens. Teratogenicity is the capability to produce congenital abnormalities that include not only major and minor malformations but also functional abnormalities. The incidence of major structural abnormalities (defects incompatible with life or requiring major surgery or correction) in the United States is 2–4%. If minor malformations, such as ear tags or extra digits are included, this could increase to as much as 10%.[68] Approximately 10% of children have either abnormal physical or mental development. About 25% of abnormalities are probably due to genetic predisposition, 2–3% are drug induced, and in the remainder the causes are unknown.[68]

Although the number of infants with defects due to drug exposure seems to be relatively small, any defect that can be avoided should be. The use of any drug, prescription or nonprescription, should be avoided during pregnancy unless absolutely necessary. Studies cannot be performed in pregnant women to ascertain outcome and, unfortunately, animal studies do not always correlate with human fetal risk. A prime example is thalidomide, a sedative marketed in Europe that was very close to being approved in the United States when its teratogenic potential was recognized. This drug is extremely teratogenic in humans; up to one-third of all infants exposed *in utero* to thalidomide developed abnormalities, but standard animal studies failed to demonstrate this risk. Thus, there is no good method of predicting or determining the safety of a particular drug given during pregnancy. Most reports of teratogenicity are case reports following the birth of a child exposed to a particular medication.

Drugs may be placed in categories that describe their potential risk in pregnancy based on available animal and human studies. The FDA published definitions for pregnancy risk categories in 1980[69] (Table 75.2). Unfortunately, the regulation applies only to drugs marketed after December 1983; thus, most drugs currently available are not required to have risk categories assigned. Practitioners who need to assess teratogenic risk for particular medications are referred to the primary literature and selected references.[9,12,14,20,70]

While there is a great deal of concern about the risks associated with medication use during pregnancy, drugs are a welcome addition to managing the obstetric patient with chronic medical disorders. An example is the use of insulin in diabetic patients. In the past, many diabetic patients had virtually no chance of a successful pregnancy without complications; today with close monitoring of glucose and control with insulin, these patients have a much improved pregnancy outcome.

TABLE 75.2. FDA CATEGORIES FOR DRUG USE IN PREGNANCY

Category A: Controlled studies in women fail to demonstrate a risk to the fetus in the first trimester, and the possibility of fetal harm appears remote.

Category B: Either animal studies do not indicate a risk to the fetus and there are no controlled studies in pregnant women or animal studies have indicated fetal risk, but controlled studies in pregnant women failed to demonstrate a risk.

Category C: Either animal studies indicate a fetal risk and there are no controlled studies in women or there are no available studies in women or animals.

Category D: There is positive evidence of fetal risk but there may be certain situations where the benefit might outweigh the risk (life-threatening or serious diseases where other drugs are ineffective or carry a greater risk).

Category X: There is definite fetal risk based on studies in animals or humans or based on human experience and the risk clearly outweighs any benefit in pregnant women.

(From Federal Register 1980;44:37434–37467.)

Timing of exposure to medication is of the utmost importance when considering the teratogenic risk. Exposure around the time of conception and implantation may kill the fetus, and the patient may never realize that she was pregnant. If the exposure occurs in the first 12–15 days after conception when the cells are still totipotential, meaning if one cell is damaged or killed, another can assume its function, the fetus may not be damaged.[71,72] The first 3 months are the most critical in terms of malformations.[9] More recently, functional and behavioral defects have been associated with exposure to drugs or other environmental factors later in gestation while the brain was still growing and developing.[9] These effects are both more difficult to recognize and to establish cause and effect.

Before any drug is prescribed during pregnancy, several factors should be considered. First, the risk-to-benefit ratio must be weighed. The practitioner must be confident that the selected drug is indicated and is the most effective with the least risk of teratogenicity. To make this determination, appropriate references should be consulted to ascertain whether or not there are any reports of abnormalities and the nature of possible problems. The gestational age and the long-term effects may not be recognized for many years (i.e., the carcinogenic potential of diethylstilbestrol [DES] in exposed daughters did not become evident until after puberty). Once the decision has been made to use medication, the lowest effective dose should be prescribed for the shortest possible duration.

Often a patient has already taken a medication before she seeks professional advice about the teratogenic risk. In this situation, it is important to accurately determine the drug, dose, route of administration, exact gestational age at exposure, and any other drugs taken concurrently. The patient's general health, previous obstetric history, and family history may also be helpful. In this case, the physician can be helpful in giving the patient all the information he or she has available and even give an opinion about the actual risk; but, ultimately, the decision to continue the pregnancy should be made by the patient.

The extent to which drugs cross the placenta varies, and many drugs reach concentrations in the fetus at 50–100% of maternal blood levels. The total concentration of blood protein is less in the fetus and often results in more free drug, especially for drugs that are highly protein bound in maternal blood. Excretion of medications by the fetus occurs primarily via the fetal liver and the placenta and clearance may be slower than in adults.

Factors that influence the teratogenicity of a drug include the genotypes of the mother and fetus, the embryonic stage at exposure, dose, the specificity of the agent and simultaneous administration or exposure to other drugs, or environmental agents that may increase or decrease potential abnormalities.[72] Teratogens may cause spontaneous abortion, congenital abnormalities, intrauterine growth retardation, mental retardation, carcinogenesis, and mutagenesis.

Late in pregnancy, effects of medication on labor and delivery should be considered. For example, salicylate use late in gestation can cause increased bleeding at delivery or even delay the onset of labor by decreasing prostaglandins. Very near delivery, the effect of a medication on the neonate must be considered because medication present in the infant at delivery is metabolized and excreted by the neonate resulting in prolonged exposure and possible toxicity.

Pregnancy is a time for nurturing the developing fetus, but it also brings a time of great physical change for the mother. These changes cause symptoms in the pregnant patient that often cause her to actually increase her medication use. All patients who are considering pregnancy or have a confirmed pregnancy should be informed about the risk involved with using any medication during pregnancy.

Every parent both expects and desires a normal, healthy baby. This includes not only a child free of malformations but one who also has normal physical and mental development. The birth of a child with an abnormality is a personal tragedy for both the parents and for the medical professionals caring for the family. In searching for a reason, the mother often tries to recall any medication taken during pregnancy. As discussed previously, medications are probably implicated only in a very small number of abnormalities but for legal reasons, all medications prescribed or recommended for a pregnant patient should be carefully documented in the patient's medical record.

PLACENTAL TRANSPORT

The amount of drug reaching the fetus depends on many factors, factors that vary from patient to patient, and on the stage of gestation.

Drugs with molecular weights of less than 400 cross the placenta more readily as do highly unionized and lipophilic drugs. Since most drugs have molecular weights between 250 and 400, they have the potential to cross the placenta and enter the fetal circulation. Other factors that influence the placental transfer of drugs include the degree of protein binding, maternal and fetal blood flow, the area available for exchange, and amount of placental metabolism. Most drugs cross the placenta by simple diffusion. Because simple diffusion depends on the concentration gradient, fetal serum concentrations usually equal maternal levels. However, in some cases, the fetal serum concentrations are as low as 50% of maternal levels, but in other cases, the fetal concentration may actually exceed maternal levels.

In the past, the placenta was referred to as a barrier; however, the placenta does not protect the fetus from effects of drugs.

SPECIFIC AGENTS

Several classes of drugs and their effects on the fetus are discussed in this chapter. The following section discusses other potentially teratogenic medications. Because this is not an all-inclusive list, the reader is referred to the primary literature and specific references about drug use in pregnancy.

Benzodiazepines

These drugs cross the placenta and are associated with congenital malformations. The incidence of malformations is greater when exposure occurs within the first trimester. The association most often reported is with diazepam and facial clefts. Large studies both refute and confirm the teratogenicity of benzodiazepines.[9]

The floppy infant syndrome, neonatal depression, and withdrawal may occur following chronic benzodiazepine use during the last trimester and when large doses are administered shortly before delivery.[73]

Lithium

Infants exposed to lithium during the first trimester of pregnancy have an increased risk of developing abnormalities; 75% are cardiovascular. Epstein's anomaly, a rare heart defect, accounts for most cardiovascular problems.[72] When lithium is administered late in pregnancy, manifestations of neonatal toxicity include cyanosis, hypotonia, bradycardia, and electrocardiographic abnormalities. These toxic effects usually reverse as the lithium is excreted by the infant.[9]

Sex Hormones

Estogrens, progestogens, and androgens are associated with congenital abnormalities. Progestins and androgens, including danazol, are associated with masculinization of the female fetus. Abnormalities found in female infants exposed *in utero* to progestogenic or androgenic agents include ambiguous genitalia, clitoral hypertrophy, and labial fusion.[9,74]

Progestogens, primarily those present in oral contraceptives, may produce the VACTERL syndrome. This syndrome was associated with vertebral, anal, cardiovascular, esophageal, renal, and limb defects. Recent studies indicate that if a fetus is exposed to these agents, the risk for this syndrome is very small (0.07%).[9] The more likely problem is abnormal sexual organ development.

DES causes a number of reproductive tract abnormalities in both female and male infants exposed *in utero.*[9] Vaginal clear cell adenocarcinoma is the most common problem seen in offspring of mothers taking DES. Estrogens and progestogens are contraindicated in pregnancy due to reports of congenital abnormalities.

Isotretinoin

Isotretinoin (Accutane), a vitamin A isomer, is a potent human teratogen. Indicated only for the treatment of severe cystic acne, the drug should never be used in pregnancy. Recognized as a teratogen before marketing, the manufacturer issued warnings about its use in pregnant women or in women who might become pregnant while taking isotretinoin. Women of childbearing age should have a negative pregnancy test before initiating treatment and must use at least two reliable methods of contraception during the course of therapy and for 1 month after the last dose. Major malformations reported with isotretinoin include craniofacial, CNS, and cardiac defects.

Antineoplastic Agents

All the drugs in this class, except cyclosporin A, have teratogenic potential in animals. Fortunately, the occurrence of anomalies in exposed infants is not as great as in animals. The highest rate of malformations occurs with first trimester exposure. Since most treatment regimens for neoplasms include several drugs, it is difficult to ascertain cause and effect for individual agents. Limited use of these medications during pregnancy is due to a high rate of elective and spontaneous abortions during treatment.

Because these drugs are designed to kill rapidly proliferating malignant cells, it is logical to assume that the rapidly growing fetus might be subject to the same effect.

TABLE 75.3. MEDICATIONS KNOWN TO BE TERATOGENS

ACE inhibitors
Alcohol
Androgens
Anticonvulsants
Antineoplastics
Cocaine
Diethylstilbestrol
Iodides
Isotretinoin
Lithium
Live vaccines
Tetracycline
Warfarin

TABLE 75.4. MEDICATIONS SUSPECTED TO BE TERATOGENS

Benzodiazepines
Estrogens
Methimazole
Quinolones
Oral hypoglycemic agents
Progestogens
Tricyclic antidepressants

TABLE 75.5. MEDICATIONS WITH NO KNOWN ADVERSE EFFECTS IN PREGNANCY[a]

Acetaminophen
Cephalosporins
Corticosteroids
Docusate sodium
Erythromycin
Multiple vitamins
Narcotic analgesics
Penicillin
Phenothiazines
Thyroid hormones

[a]No drug is absolutely without risk during pregnancy. These drugs appear to have a minimal risk when used judiciously in usual doses under the supervision of a medical professional.

Handling of chemotherapeutic agents by those health care professionals in the reproductive age group should be done with caution to minimize direct contact with these drugs.

Summary

The use of medications during pregnancy and their effect on the fetus is at best an inexact science. No drug is absolutely safe with no risk to the fetus and no drug produces abnormalities in all exposed infants. Drugs with known, suspected, and no known teratogenic effect are listed in Tables 75.3 through 75.6. Every patient must be treated individually. Possible risks and benefits should be carefully weighed before the patient and physician make a decision to use medication during pregnancy.

TABLE 75.6. MEDICATIONS WITH NONTERATOGENIC ADVERSE EFFECTS IN PREGNANCY

Antithyroid drugs
Aminoglycosides
Aspirin
Barbiturates (chronic use)
Beta blockers
Benzodiazepines (chronic use)
Caffeine
Chloramphenicol
Cocaine
Diuretics
Isoniazid
Narcotic analgesics (chronic use)
Nicotine
Nonsteroidal anti-inflammatory agents
Oral hypoglycemic agents
Propylthiouracil
Sulfonamides

MEDICATION USE DURING LACTATION

The renewed interest in breast-feeding in recent years is favorable, but it has also presented clinicians with a new challenge (i.e., what medications are transferred into breast milk, to what extent, and with what effect on the infant?). When using medications in lactating women, the effect on both quality and quantity of milk produced must be considered.

Drugs that decrease milk production include sympathomimetics, nicotine, levodopa, bromocriptine, ergot alkaloids, pyridoxine, monoamine oxidase inhibitors, and androgens. Drugs that decrease prolactin inhibitory factor may increase milk production and often have galactorrhea as a side effect. Examples are the antipsychotics, cimetidine, metoclopramide, reserpine, amoxapine, and methyldopa.

A patient with a chronic medical problem requiring medication should consult her physician before delivery to determine if she may consider nursing. Women who require short-term medication for acute problems while nursing may pump their breasts and discard the milk if the drug is contraindicated. Once the course of therapy is completed, nursing may resume.

To minimize the effects of drugs during breast-feeding, sustained-release products or drugs with long half-lives should be avoided. Scheduling a dose immediately after a feeding or before a long sleep would help decrease the dose reaching the infant depending on the drug's half-life. If several drugs are appropriate, the drug that is excreted in breast milk in the lowest concentration, with the least effect on the infant, should be selected. As a general guide, the practitioner could consider whether or not the medication is typically given to neonates. The infant should be observed closely for problems after a nursing mother has taken any medication.

Drugs contraindicated by the American Academy of Pediatrics include amphetamines, bromocriptine, cocaine, ergotamine, lithium, nicotine, and most antineoplastic drugs and drugs of abuse.[70]

SELECTED AGENTS

Alcohol

There is no evidence that occasional, moderate intake of alcohol during lactation is harmful to the infant. However, ingestion of large quantities or chronic use may cause sedation, CNS depression, weakness, and abnormal growth.

Caffeine

Caffeine is excreted in breast milk at low levels. Mothers who are breast-feeding should be cautioned about ingestion of large amounts of beverages containing caffeine. Moderate use (1–2 cups/d) of caffeine-containing beverages is considered acceptable if tolerated by the infant. Caffeine can cause irritability and sleeplessness in breast-fed infants.

Nicotine

Nicotine causes a decrease in milk production and is excreted in breast milk. Nausea, vomiting, diarrhea, tachycardia, and restlessness may occur in nursing infants exposed to nicotine. Both smoking and nicotine gum should be avoided in lactating women.

Analgesics

Most analgesics, both narcotic and non-narcotic, are excreted in breast milk in low concentrations and, as such, should not be harmful to the baby. However, large doses or chronic use should be considered with more caution. For example, a mother taking antiarthritic doses of aspirin may excrete enough drug to alter a baby's prothrombin time. Chronic use of narcotic analgesics may cause sedation, CNS depression, and dependence.

Antibiotics

Antibiotics are perhaps the drugs most often required by nursing mothers. All cross into breast milk but at less than pharmacologic doses; however, there remains the potential to cause candidiasis, diarrhea, and thrush in the infant. Penicillins, cephalosporins, and erythromycins are usually considered to be permissible for nursing mothers. Sulfonamides are permitted in healthy, full-term infants. Chloramphenicol, tetracycline, and isoniazid should be avoided. If metronidazole is required, a single 2-gram dose should be used and the breasts pumped for 24–48 hours to allow for excretion of the drug before nursing is resumed.

Anticonvulsants

Anticonvulsants are generally considered permissible during breast-feeding, although the drugs appear in breast milk at low concentrations. Infants should be observed for sedation and poor feeding.

Laxatives

All laxatives, with the exception of bulk-forming products, potentially cross into breast milk. Infants should be observed for diarrhea; however, occasional use is not likely to be harmful.

Hypoglycemic Agents/Insulin

There is little information available about oral hypoglycemic agents and breast-feeding. Diabetic mothers using insulin may breast-feed because the large molecular weight of insulin prevents its excretion into breast milk. The diabetic mother may have an increased incidence of nipple candidiasis with accompanying thrush in the baby. This is usually treated with topical nystatin applied to the nipple and concurrent suspension given to the nursing infant. Keeping the nipples clean and dry will decrease the potential for fungal infections.

Summary

As with using medications during pregnancy, the possible risks and benefits of drug therapy should be assessed. There are few controlled studies documenting drug levels in breast milk and its subsequent effects on the infant. Most available information is from case reports or small studies.

CONCLUSION

Medication use in pregnancy and lactation is a complex issue, and physicians and pharmacists must work together to provide the patient with the most effective and least potentially harmful medication when treatment is indicated. All medication use in pregnancy, during labor and delivery, and during breast-feeding should include patient education and patient consent.

References

1. Berlin CM. Pregnancy and childbirth. Presented at the National Conference on Women's Health, Bethesda, MD, June 17, 1986.
2. Jacobs DS, Kasten Jr BL, Demott WR, Wolfson WL. Laboratory Test Handbook, 2nd ed. Baltimore, Williams & Wilkins, 1990, pp 224–225, 305–307.
3. Taylor CM, Pernoll ML. Normal pregnancy & prenatal care, in Pernoll ML (ed): Current Obstetric and Gynecologic Diagnosis and Treatment, 7th ed. Norwalk, CT, Appleton & Lange, 1991, pp 179–197.
4. Committee on Genetics of the American Academy of Pediatrics. Folic acid for the prevention of neural tube defects. Pediatrics 1993;92:493–494.
5. Centers for Disease Control. Recommendations for use of folic acid to reduce number of spina bifida cases and other neural tube defects. JAMA 1993;269:1233–1238.
6. Juchau MR, Faustman-Watts E. Pharmacokinetic considerations in the maternal–placental–fetal unit. Clin Obstet Gynecol 1983;26:379–390.
7. Watson LA, Bommarito AA, Marshall JF. Total peripheral parenteral nutrition in pregnancy. J Parenter Enteral Nutr 1990;14:485–489.
8. Levine MG, Esser D. Total parenteral nutrition for the treatment of severe hyperemesis gravidarum: Maternal nutritional effects and fetal outcome. Obstet Gynecol 1988;72:102–107.
9. Briggs GG, Freeman RK, Yaffe SJ. Drugs in pregnancy and lactation, 4th ed. Baltimore, Williams & Wilkins, 1994.
10. Cunningham FG, MacDonald PC, Gant NF, et al. Williams Obstetrics, 19th ed. Norwalk, CT, Appleton & Lange, 1993.
11. Milkovich L, Van Den Berg BJ. An evaluation of the teratogenicity of certain antinauseant drugs. Am J Obstet Gynecol 1976;125:244–248.
12. Lewis JH, Weingold AB, Committee on FDA-Related Matters, American College of Gastroenterology. The use of gastrointestinal drugs during pregnancy and lactation. Am J Gastroenterol 1985;80:912–923.
13. Baron TH, Richter JE. Gastroesophageal reflux disease in pregnancy. Gastroenterol Clin North Am 1992;21:777–791.
14. Goldberg E. Anticoagulants in pregnancy, in Niebyl J (ed): Drug Use in Pregnancy, 2nd ed. Philadelphia, Lea & Febiger, 1988, pp 83–88.
15. Hirsh J, Fuster V. Guide to anticoagulant therapy. Part 2: Oral anticoagulants. Circulation. 1994;89:1469–1480.
16. Greaves M. Anticoagulants in pregnancy. Pharmacol Ther 1993;59:311–327.
17. Hirsh J, Fuster V. Guide to anticoagulant therapy. Part 1: Heparin. Circulation 1994;89:1449–1468.
18. Barbour LA, Kick SD, Steiner JF, et al. A prospective study of heparin-induced osteoporosis in pregnancy using bone densitometry. Am J Obstet Gynecol 1994;170:862–869.
19. Mabie SC, Sabai BM. Hypertensive states of pregnancy, in Pernoll ML (ed): Current Obstetric and Gynecologic Diagnosis and Treatment, 7th ed. Norwalk, CT, Appleton & Lange, 1991, pp 373–387.
20. Zuspan FP, Zuspan KJ. Antihypertensive therapy during pregnancy, in Rayburn WF, Zuspan FP (eds): Drug Therapy in Obstetrics and Gynecology, 3rd ed. St. Louis, MO, Mosby–Year Book, 1992, pp 105–126.
21. Friedman SA. Preeclampsia: A review of the role of prostaglandins. Obstet Gynecol 1988;71:122–137.
22. Walsh SW. Preeclampsia: An imbalance in placental prostacyclin and thromboxane production. Am J Obstet Gynecol 1985;152:335–340.
23. Lubbe WF. Low-dose aspirin in prevention of toxaemia of pregnancy. Does it have a place? Drugs 1987;34:515–518.
24. Sibai BM, Mirro R, Chesney CM, Leffler C. Low-dose aspirin in pregnancy. Obstet Gynecol 1989;74:551–557.
25. Sibai BM, Caritis SN, Thom E, et al. Prevention of preeclampsia with low-dose aspirin in healthy, nulliparous pregnant women. N Engl J Med 1993;329:1213–1218.
26. Hauth JC, Goldenberg RL, Parker CR, et al. Low-dose aspirin therapy to prevent preeclampsia. Am J Obstet Gynecol 1993;168:1083–1093.
27. Imperiale TF, Petrulis AS. A meta-analysis of low-dose aspirin for the prevention of pregnancy-induced hypertensive disease. JAMA 1991;266:261–265.
28. Kyle PM, Redman CWG. Comparative risk-benefit assessment of drugs used in the management of hypertension in pregnancy. Drug Saf 1992;7:223–234.
29. Shoemaker CT, Meyers M. Sodium nitroprusside for control of severe hypertensive disease of pregnancy: A case report and discussion of potential toxicity. Am J Obstet Gynecol 1984;149:171–173.
30. White P. Classification of obstetric diabetes. Am J Obstet Gynecol 1978;130:228–230.
31. Barss VA. Diabetes and pregnancy. Med Clin North Am 1989;73:685–700.
32. Gabbe SG. Management of diabetes mellitus in pregnancy. Am J Obstet Gynecol 1985;153:824–828.
33. Schneider JM. Pregnancy complicated by diabetes mellitus, in Pernoll ML (ed): Current Obstetric and Gynecologic Diagnosis and Treatment, 7th ed. Norwalk, CT, Appleton & Lange, 1991, pp 364–372.
34. Landon MB, Gabbe SG. Diabetes mellitus and pregnancy. Obstet Gynecol Clin North Am 1992;19:633–654.
35. Wing DA, Millar LK, Koonings PP, et al. A comparison of propylthiouracil methimazole versus in the treatment of hyperthyroidism in pregnancy. Am J Obstet Gynecol 1994;170:90–95.
36. Redman CWG, Beilin LJ, Bonnar J, Ounsted MK. Fetal outcome in trial of antihypertensive treatment in pregnancy. Lancet 1976;2:753–756.
37. Sabai BM. Diagnosis and management of chronic hypertension in pregnancy. Obstet Gynecol 1991;78:451–461.
38. Shotan A, Widerhorn J, Hurst A, Elkayan U. Risks of angiotensin-converting enzyme inhibition during pregnancy: Experimental and clinical evidence, potential mechanisms, and recommendations for use. Am J Med 1994;96:451–456.
39. Yerby MS, Devinsky O. Epilepsy and pregnancy. Adv Neurol 1994;64:45–63.
40. Buehler BA, Stempel LE. Anticonvulsant therapy during pregnancy, in Rayburn WF, Zuspan FP (eds): Drug Therapy in Obstetrics and Gynecology, 3rd ed. St. Louis, MO, Mosby–Year Book, 1992, pp 147–163.

41. Dalessio DJ. Seizure disorders and pregnancy. N Engl J Med 1985;312:559–563.
42. Committee on Drugs of the American Academy of Pediatrics. Anticonvulsants and pregnancy. Pediatrics 1979;63:331–333.
43. Mirkin BL. Diphenylhydantoin: Placental transport, fetal localization, neonatal metabolism and possible teratogenic effect. J Pediatr 1971;78:329–337.
44. Mountain KR, Hirsh J, Gallus AS. Neonatal coagulation defect due to anticonvulsant drug treatment in pregnancy. Lancet 1970;1:265–268.
45. Lander CM, Edwards VE, Eadie MJ, Tyrer JH. Plasma anticonvulsant concentrations during pregnancy. Neurology 1977;27:128–131.
46. Desmond MM, Schwanecke RP, Wilson GS, et al. Maternal barbiturate utilization and neonatal withdrawal symptomatology. J Pediatr 1972;80:190–197.
47. Rosa FW. Spina bifida in infants of women treated with carbamazepine during pregnancy. N Engl J Med 1991;324:674–677.
48. Jones KL, Lacro RV, Johnson KA, Adams J. Pattern of malformations in the children of women treated with carbamazepine during pregnancy. N Engl J Med 1989;320:1661–1666.
49. Romero R, Berkowitz R. The use of anti-asthmatic drugs in pregnancy, in Niebyl J (ed): Drug Use in Pregnancy, 2nd ed. Philadelphia, Lea & Febiger, 1988, pp 67–82.
50. Gonik B, Creasy RK. Preterm labor: Its diagnosis and management. Am J Obstet Gynecol 1986;154:3–8.
51. The Canadian Preterm Labor Investigators Group. Treatment of preterm labor with the beta-adrenergic agonist ritodrine. N Engl J Med 1992;327:308–312.
52. Beall MH, Edgar BW, Paul RH, Smith-Wallace T. A comparison of ritodrine, terbutaline, and magnesium sulfate for the suppression of preterm labor. Am J Obstet Gynecol 1985;153:854–859.
53. Guernsey BG, Villareal Y, Snyder MD, et al. Pulmonary edema associated with the use of betamimetic agents in preterm labor. Am J Hosp Pharm 1981;38:1942–1948.
54. Philipsen T, Eriksen PS, Lynggard F. Pulmonary edema following ritodrine-saline infusion in premature labor. Obstet Gynecol 1981;58:304–308.
55. Lam F, Gill P, Smith M, et al. Use of the subcutaneous terbutaline pump for long-term tocolysis. Obstet Gynecol 1988;72:810–813.
56. Fischer JR, Kaatz BL. Continuous subcutaneous infusion of terbutaline for suppression of preterm labor. Clin Pharm 1991;10:292–296.
57. Caritis SN, Toig G, Heddinger LA, Ashmead G. A double-blind study comparing ritodrine and terbutaline in the treatment of preterm labor. Am J Obstet Gynecol 1984;150:7–14.
58. Souney PF, Kaul AF, Osathanondoh R. Pharmacotherapy of preterm labor. Clin Pharm 1983;2:29–44.
59. Norton ME, Merrill J, Cooper BAB, et al. Neonatal complications after the administration of indomethacin for preterm labor. N Engl J Med 1993;329:1602–1607.
60. Schoenfeld A, Bar Y, Merlob P, Ovadia Y. NSAIDs: Maternal and fetal considerations. Am J Reprod Immunol 1992;28:141–147.
61. Andersson KE, Ulmsten U. Effects of nifedipine on myometrial activity and lower abdominal pain in women with primary dysmenorrhea. Br J Obstet Gynecol 1978;85:142–148.
62. Andersson KE, Ingemarrson I, Ulmsten U, Wingerup L. Inhibition of prostaglandin-induced uterine activity by nifedipine. Br J Obstet Gynecol 1979;86:175–179.
63. Goodwin TM, Paul R, Silver H, et al. The effect of the oxytocin antagonist atosiban on preterm uterine activity in the human. Am J Obstet Gynecol 1994;170:474–478.
64. Thurnau GR, Rayburn WF. Cervical ripening agents and uterine stimulants, in Rayburn WF, Zuspan FP: Drug Therapy in Obstetrics and Gynecology, 3rd ed. St. Louis, Mosby Year Book, 1992, pp 229–246.
65. Jeffcoate TNA, Miller J, Roos RF, Tindall VR. Puerperal thromboembolism in relation to the inhibition of lactation by oestrogen therapy. Br Med J 1968;4:19–25.
66. Katz M, Kroll D, Pak I, et al. Puerperal hypertension, stroke, and seizure after suppression of lactation with bromocriptine. Obstet Gynecol 1985;66:822–824.
67. Iffy L, Ten Hove W, Frisoli G. Acute myocardial infarction in the puerperium in patients receiving bromocriptine. Am J Obstet Gynecol 1986;155:371–372.
68. Oakley GP. Frequency of human congenital malformations. Clin Perinatol 1986;13:545–554.
69. Federal Register. 1980;44:37434–37467.
70. Committee on Drugs of the American Academy of Pediatrics. Transfer of drugs and other chemicals into human milk. Pediatrics 1994;93:137–150.
71. Blake DA, Niebyl JR. Requirements and limitations in reproductive and teratogenic risk assessment, in Niebyl JR: Drug Use in Pregnancy, 2nd ed. Philadelphia, Lea & Febiger, 1988, pp 1–9.
72. Dicke JM. Teratology: Principles and practice. Med Clin North Am 1989;73:567–582.
73. Scialli AR. Anticonvulsants in pregnancy, in Niebyl JR: Drug Use in Pregnancy, 2nd ed. Philadelphia, Lea & Febiger, 1988, pp 45–54.
74. Willson RJ, Carrington ER. Obstetrics and Gynecology, 8th ed. St. Louis, CV Mosby, 1987, p. 457.

Chapter 76

Infertility

Deborah Stier Carson, PharmD, BCPS, and Kathryn K. Bucci, PharmD, BCPS

Comprehension of mechanisms involved in the hormonal regulation of the normal menstrual cycle are essential to understanding contraception and infertility in women. Undeveloped follicles in the ovaries are present during early fetal development. Each follicle consists of an oocyte (undeveloped ovum) surrounded by a single layer of cells. The oocytes remain in a resting phase until puberty, when the stimulus for further development occurs. At puberty, hypothalamic and pituitary activation cause cyclic changes in the ovary that in turn affect the endometrium and cervix. Manipulation of the hormonal relationships during the menstrual cycle is the basis for hormonal contraception. Infertility can result from quantitative or chronological alterations in the normal hormonal cycle.

Until their numbers (about 2 million) are exhausted, follicles grow under a variety of physiologic circumstances, including ovulatory and anovulatory cycles. The stimulus for follicular development and the normal menstrual cycle depends on pulsatile secretion of gonadotropin-releasing hormone (GnRH) from the hypothalamus in a changing but critical range frequency and concentration. GnRH is responsible for stimulating the synthesis, storage, and secretion of the specific hormones (gonadotropins) from the anterior pituitary. These gonadotropins, follicle-stimulating hormone (FSH) and luteinizing hormone (LH), direct events in the ovarian follicles that result in the production of a fertile ovum. Prolactin is also secreted from the anterior pituitary. Whereas a low concentration of prolactin is expected in the normal menstrual cycle, elevated prolactin concentrations can alter the menstrual cycle leading to ovulation failure. Although follicles begin to grow independent of control of the gonadotropins, FSH and LH are necessary for a follicle to more fully develop and produce estrogen (specifically estradiol) and progesterone. Each month of a normal female menstrual cycle, gonadotropins and ovarian hormones cyclically increase and decrease as depicted in Fig. 76.1. The ovarian hormones cause sequential changes in the endometrium which sustain a suitable environment for growth of a fertilized ovum within the uterus if conception occurs. With relation to events in the ovary, the cycle can be divided into three phases: the follicular phase, ovulation, and the luteal phase. Events in the uterus can be divided into the menstrual, proliferative, and secretory phases with the first two corresponding temporally to the follicular phase and the latter coinciding with the luteal phase.

Follicular (Menstrual and Proliferative) Phase

Follicular development begins during the menstrual flow when FSH concentrations are high. The follicular or proliferative phase ends with ovulation of usually only one follicle called the dominant follicle. As the concentration of FSH rises at the end of the previous cycle, a series of hormonal events over 10–14 days matures the dominant follicle and causes the degeneration or atresia of the remaining follicles recruited during the cycle.

Once a follicle has received FSH stimulation, it must continue to be stimulated by FSH or die. Once gonadotropin-dependent growth is initiated in the follicle, the follicle enlarges and develops other layers of cells capable of further developing receptors for FSH and LH, as well as synthesizing estradiol, progesterone, and androgen. Estradiol increases its own follicular receptors, stimulates cell growth (independent of FSH), and amplifies the effect of FSH action in the follicle. The developing follicles cause a rise in the estradiol level that serves to stop the menstrual flow from the previous cycle, thicken the endometrial lining of the uterus, increase the uterine gland size, and thin the cervical mucus. Follicles receiving the most FSH stimulation will have the greatest rate of cell proliferation and produce the highest estradiol concentrations. FSH also regulates an aromatase enzyme system that converts androgens to estrogens in the follicles. Follicles that become androgenic do not survive. Therefore, follicles with the most FSH stimulation have the lowest androgen/estrogen ratios.

Although estrogen positively influences FSH action within the maturing follicle, a rising serum estradiol concentration has a negative feedback for FSH release at the hypothalamic–pituitary level, leading to diminished FSH

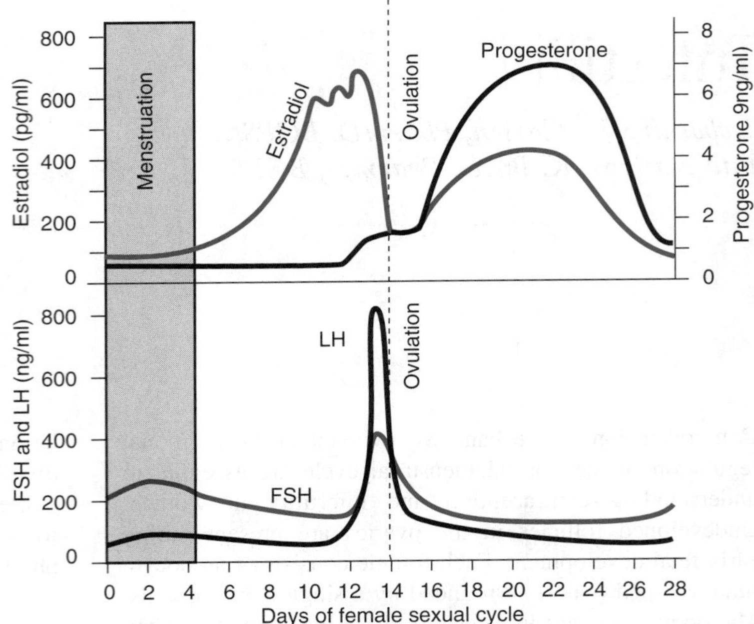

Figure 76.1. Approximate plasma concentrations of the gonadotropins and ovarian hormones during the normal female menstrual cycle. *(From Guyton AC (ed). Textbook of Medical Physiology, 8th ed. Philadelphia, WB Saunders, 1991, p 900 with permission.)*

support for the other less developed follicles (Fig. 76.2). Follicular atresia of the nondominant follicles parallels the rise in plasma estrogen concentration. The dominant follicle can be observed as early as cycle days 5–7, corresponding with the gradual fall of FSH levels observed at midfollicular phase. However, exposure to exogenous estrogen in concentrations found in oral contraceptives (OCPs) can induce atresia of the dominate follicle by reducing FSH concentrations below the critical sustaining level.[1]

FSH, with estrogen as a coordinator, is also responsible for the production of LH receptors on the dominant follicle. The dominant follicle produces increasing amounts of estradiol, reaching a peak approximately 24–36 hours before ovulation. As the estrogen concentration slowly increases, gonadotropin secretion diminishes, but accumulation continues within the pituitary. At a critical estradiol concentration (greater than 200 pg for at least 50 hours), GnRH is triggered, leading to a midcycle LH and FSH

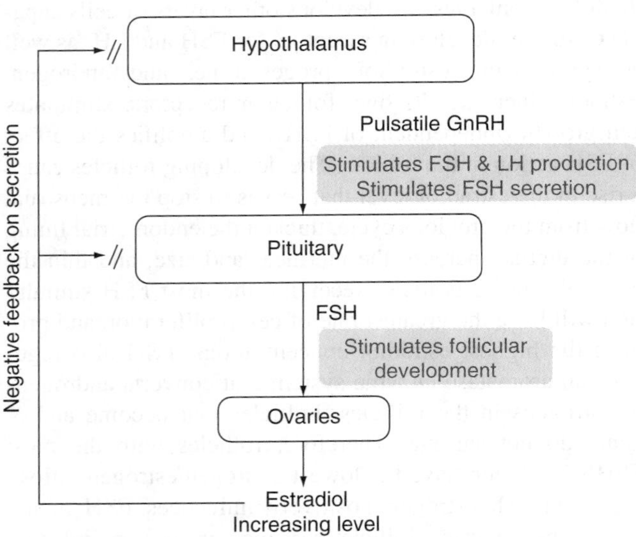

Figure 76.2. Hypothalamic–pituitary–ovarian (HPO) feedback loop during the follicular phase of the normal menstrual cycle.

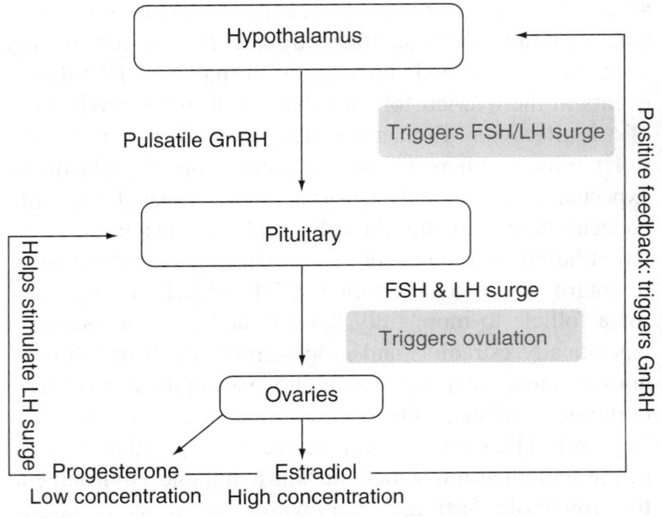

Figure 76.3. HPO feedback loop just prior to ovulation in a normal menstrual cycle.

surge (Fig. 76.3). If LH is prematurely presented to a maturing follicle, cell proliferation decreases, degenerative changes ensue, and intrafollicular androgen levels rise. While providing the ovulatory stimulus to the dominant follicle, the LH surge ensures atresia of the remaining follicles with their lower estrogen and FSH content. LH also promotes production of progesterone from the dominant follicle. An increase in circulating levels of progesterone, specifically 17-OH progesterone, occurs 12–24 hours before ovulation. This small amount of preovulatory progesterone enhances the LH surge at the level of the pituitary. However, if large amounts of progesterone, such as that in OCPs, are administered before sufficient estrogen priming or in high doses, the midcycle LH surge can be blocked at the level of the hypothalamus.

Ovulation

Ovulation is dependent on both adequate gonadotropin levels and a follicle being sufficiently mature to respond to an appropriate stimulus. Though considerable variation exists from cycle to cycle, ovulation is estimated to occur approximately 10–12 hours after the LH peak and 24–36 hours after peak estradiol concentrations. The LH surge, occurring 28–32 hours before follicle rupture, is the most clinically useful indicator of approaching ovulation.

Progesterone may increase the distensibility of the follicle wall, which is necessary to accommodate the accumulating fluid. Proteolytic enzymes and prostaglandins appear necessary for induction of follicular rupture from the ovary.

As soon as the follicle ruptures, releasing the ovum, the plasma estradiol concentration dramatically decreases because the fluid surrounding the follicle, or the antrum, is the primary source of estrogen. This drop in estrogen may be related to LH-induced down-regulation of its own receptors on the follicle or to an inhibitory action of midcycle progesterone on further cell proliferation. The actual mechanism for LH withdrawal is not known.

Luteal or Secretory Phase

After rupture of the follicle and release of the ovum, the remaining luteinized follicular cells become the corpus luteum, which is able to synthesize androgen, estrogen, and progesterone. Concentrations of progesterone and estradiol from the corpus luteum peak by day 8 or 9 after ovulation. Progesterone, the most abundant ovarian hormone during the luteal phase, antagonizes estrogen action through depletion of estrogen receptors as well as inhibiting gonadotropin release at the hypothalamic level. Negative feedback actions of both estrogen and progesterone on gonadotropins inhibit new follicular growth during the luteal phase. Progesterone also stimulates glands in the endometrium to release a glycogen-rich secretion, which prepares the uterus to receive a fertilized ovum and causes cervical mucus to become more viscous.

The life span and hormone-producing capacity of the corpus luteum are dependent on the continuous presence of small amounts of LH. Although the length of the follicular phase varies greatly from cycle to cycle, the time period from the LH midcycle surge to menses (13–15 days) is the least variable portion of the cycle. The corpus luteum function rapidly declines 9–11 days after ovulation by an unknown mechanism thought to involve estrogen. Luteal phase estrogen may also be necessary to prepare the endometrium for progesterone stimulation after ovulation. Estrogen is necessary for synthesis of progesterone receptors. Without adequate estrogen priming, progesterone receptor content may be inadequate and cause infertility or early abortion.

Unless fertilization occurs, the corpus luteum usually degenerates. As progesterone concentration decreases, the endometrial lining cannot be maintained and partially sloughs, thus beginning another menstrual cycle. With pregnancy, the corpus luteum is maintained by the emergence of human chorionic gonadotropin (HCG), which first appears 9–13 days after ovulation, thus preventing luteal regression. HCG maintains the vital hormonal production from the corpus luteum until placental progesterone production is well established by week 6 to week 8 of gestation.

Infertility

Infertility is defined as 1 year of unprotected coitus without conception. Conception rates of 20–25% per month are expected in normal couples trying to achieve pregnancy. Therefore, within 13 months approximately 95% of normal couples should conceive.[2] If couples had been using OCPs previously, this period may be extended to 15 months.[3] A series of complex and interrelated events must occur for successful conception, implantation and maintenance of a pregnancy (Table 76.1). Dysfunction in one or more of these events can result in infertility.

Impaired ability to have children occurs in an estimated 8.4% of women 15–44 years of age in the United States, with about 25% of women having an episode of infertility at some point in their reproductive lives.[4] The prevalence of infertility has increased in the past 15 years. Contributing factors are a delay in childbearing, contraceptive practices, sexual practices, and an increased use of therapeutic abortions. Male factors are wholly or partially responsible for 40–50% of infertility problems. These factors include individuals who have normal semen that fails to penetrate the ovum, sperm antibodies, and infection with *Ureaplasma urealyticum.* Although assessment and treatment of these factors are beyond the scope of this chapter, they should be investigated before an extensive workup and hormonal

TABLE 76.1. COMPLEX AND INTERRELATED EVENTS THAT MUST OCCUR FOR NORMAL FERTILIZATION, IMPLANTATION, AND MAINTENANCE OF PREGNANCY

1. The male must produce an adequate number of viable spermatozoa and must be able to deposit them in the upper vagina at the time when a mature oocyte has been released from the ovary.
2. The female's ovulatory cycle must be normal, including sufficient estrogen in the proliferative phase to stimulate the endometrial lining and produce the quantity and quality of cervical mucus necessary to allow passage of spermatozoa and enough progesterone in the secretory phase to support implantation and maintenance of pregnancy.
3. The oviducts must be patent and sufficiently mobile to allow fertilization as well as transport of the ovum from the ovary to the uterus.
4. The uterus must be capable of supporting implantation and fetal growth throughout pregnancy.

(Adapted from Ref. 3, p 1.)

manipulation begins in the woman. Uterine and tubal disease (including endometriosis) are present in 20–50% of female infertility patients. Cervical and immunologic factors and various infectious diseases cause infertility in approximately 5–10% of infertility cases and failure to ovulate occurs in 30–40%. While new assisted reproduction techniques, including *in vitro* fertilization (IVF), gamete intrafallopian transfer (GIFT), zygote intrafallopian transfer (ZIFT), and surgical correction of abnormalities contribute greatly to successful pregnancies in previously infertile couples, drug therapy directed toward induction of ovulation still plays an important role in treating infertility.

PATHOGENESIS OF FEMALE INFERTILITY

Numerous causes of infertility exist and the more common ones are listed in Table 76.2. More than one cause can be found in 10–30% of infertile couples.[4] Failure to ovulate or anovulation secondary to chronic hypothalamic dysfunction is probably the most frequent cause of menstrual disorders in women with normal prolactin and androgen levels. Stress, trauma, alterations in body weight, or excessive athletic activity often contribute. Patients with hypothalamic dysfunction exhibit a variety of patterns ranging from luteal phase defects to amenorrhea.

Another common cause of chronic anovulation is polycystic ovary disease (PCOD). Patients with PCOD have chronically increased LH secretion, which continuously stimulates follicles to produce excess androgen. Elevated androgen levels may lead to prolonged periods of anovulation by enhancing follicular atresia and estrogen overproduction from peripheral conversion of the androgens to estrogens. Ovarian cysts, amenorrhea, or oligomenorrhea, acne, obesity, and hirsutism in association with normal or elevated testosterone concentrations and an inappropriately high LH : FSH ratio (often greater than 3 : 1) are classically associated with this disease.

Age-related changes in the reproductive system eventually result in loss of ovulatory function. During the peri-

TABLE 76.2. COMMON CAUSES OF INFERTILITY, ESTIMATED PREGNANCY RATES, AND CONVENTIONAL TREATMENTS

Cause of Infertility	Pregnancy Rate in a Couple with a Single Infertility Factor: Actual[a](%)	Pregnancy Rate in a Couple with a Single Infertility Factor: Life-Table Expected with Indefinite Follow-Up[a] (%)	Conventional Treatment
Endometriosis	31	52	Ablation of ectopic endometrial tissue, danazol; sex steroids; GnRH analogs; assisted reproduction
Male factor	38	74	Assisted reproduction or donor insemination
Anovulation	44	79	Clomiphene, gonadotropins, GnRH
Tubal factor	26	48	Tubal surgery
Luteal phase abnormalities	46	58	Correction of cause, progesterone, clomiphene citrate, gonadotropins
Cervical factor	26	45	Estrogen; guiafenesin, intrauterine insemination
Uterine factor (congenital anomalies, adhesions, polyps, hyperplasia)	33	38	Surgical correction of congenital abnormalities; cerclage; dilation and curettage; appropriate antibiotic therapy

[a]Pregnancy rate is a function of time. Actual rates are based on conventional measures (i.e., number of patients achieving pregnancy compared to number of patients treated in a defined period of time) while life-table rates are calculated based on the assumption that patients are followed indefinitely. (Adapted from Refs. 3 and 4.)

menopausal period, a woman may still have follicular growth, but she does not consistently ovulate because of potential refractoriness to FSH and LH. Although changes in fertility rates related to age are difficult to quantify, fertility rates decline after age 30; however, the rate does not fall dramatically until a woman enters her forties. Approximately one-third of the women who defer pregnancy to their mid to late thirties have infertility problems.

Luteal phase deficiency or inadequacy is linked to inappropriate or inadequate LH support. The inability of the corpus luteum to maintain the luteal phase causes recurrent miscarriages and contributes to infertility. A deficient luteal phase is (1) the production of adequate progesterone concentrations, but not for an appropriate length of time (less than 11 days) or, more commonly, (2) progesterone produced in suboptimum quantities for the full luteal phase. Whether luteal deficiency causes infertility is controversial since sporadic luteal deficiency occurs in fertile women and treatment is not always beneficial.[4] Premature luteinization, another defect related to the luteal phase, is an untimely LH surge in response to rising estrogen when the follicle is still immature and unable to ovulate. This defect may represent an exaggerated sensitivity of the pituitary to rising levels of estrogen, resulting in a premature LH surge.

Infectious processes that result in scarring of the reproductive system are increasingly identified as a cause of infertility and ectopic pregnancy in young women. Each episode of pelvic inflammatory disease (PID) is associated with an increasing risk of infertility. *Neisseria gonorrhea* and *Chlamydia trachcomatis* are the most common causes of PID. Tubal damage contributing to later infertility problems may occur in women who have had a septic abortion or a ruptured appendix, used an intrauterine device, or had tubal surgery. In addition, *U. urealyticum* and *Mycoplasma hominis* are more commonly found in couples with unexplained infertility than in fertile couples.[5,6]

Endometriosis is a disease indicating the presence of ectopic endometrial tissue. Although endometriosis at any stage of the disease is associated with infertility, the mechanism is not fully understood. Postulated mechanisms include disease-related mechanical interference with ovulation, ovum pick-up by the fallopian tube, ovum transport, or implantation of a fertilized egg. Recent data suggest that the peritoneal fluid contains factors that inhibit gamete function.[7,8] Patients may avoid coitus or have inadequate penile penetration because of discomfort. Additional factors include intratubal polyps or other conditions capable of decreasing the chances of fertility (e.g., increased age at the time of desired pregnancy, luteal phase problems, and secretion of substances from the endometrium).

The most common drugs patients associate with infertility are the OCPs. This concept is most likely related to post-pill amenorrhea, which may not be related to OCP use. Non-OCP factors frequently contributing to post-pill amenorrhea, include previous menstrual irregularities, conditions of stress, psychiatric disorders, and marked weight loss. The incidence of post-pill amenorrhea is low (1–3%) with the use of low-dose OCPs. However, women who stop taking OCPs to become pregnant may have to wait longer to conceive than women who have been using non-OCP methods.

Prostaglandins are involved in the mechanism for causing the rupture of the mature follicle. Because inhibition of prostaglandin synthesis may block follicle rupture, the use of drugs that inhibit prostaglandin synthesis should be avoided near the time of expected ovulation if failure to ovulate is causing infertility. Other drugs commonly implicated in causing menstrual disturbances or female infertility are listed in Table 76.3.

Endocrine abnormalities such as thyroid disease, prolactinoma, diabetes, excessive adrenal androgen production, and hepatic disease can alter the metabolism or feed-

TABLE 76.3. DRUGS ASSOCIATED WITH FEMALE INFERTILITY OR MENSTRUAL IRREGULARITIES

Agent	Type of Problem
Nonsteroidal anti-inflammatory agents	Block release of mature follicle through inhibition of prostaglandin
Opiates	Hyperprolactinemia, suppresses LH secretion
Corticosteroids	Amenorrhea with high doses; inhibition of ovulation if given early in cycle
Coumarin derivatives	Follicular (corpus luteum) bleeding, ovarian hemorrhage
Cyproterone acetate	Inhibition of ovulation
Reserpine	Hyperprolactinemia
Oral contraceptives	Inhibition of ovulation
Progestogens	Alter FSH/LH ratio
Spironolactone	Menorrhagia, metrorrhagia, amenorrhea
Cannabis	Increase in HCG when used in testicular cancer; concerns are mostly related to male fertility
Cytostatics/cytotoxic agents	Amenorrhea, early menopause, dyspareunia, decreased libido
Antipsychotic	Hyperprolactinemia, galactorrhea, hirsutism, amenorrhea
Licorice (glycyrrihiza glabra)	Amenorrhea and hyperprolactinemia
Diethylstilbestrol (history of exposure *in utero*)	Cervical, uterine, and vaginal changes resulting in infertility, spontaneous abortion, and premature labor

(Adapted from Dukes MNG (ed). Meyler's Side Effects of Drugs. Amsterdam, Elsevier, 1988.)

back of hormones on the hypothalamus or pituitary, thus preventing follicular development, ovulation, or the survival of the corpus luteum. Diseases that cause increased prolactin concentrations can cause luteal phase inadequacy, progressing to anovulation and amenorrhea with complete GnRH suppression. Prolactin may work both centrally and in the ovaries to prevent ovulation. The presence of galactorrhea, with or without elevated serum prolactin levels, tends to indicate the presence of excessive prolactin stimulation. Prolactin levels are normally elevated during lactation but can also be increased in response to prolactin-producing tumors, stress, and drugs (e.g., antipsychotics, opiates, and reserpine derivatives).

Although sperm are very antigenic, only a small percentage of infertility cases can be explained by an immunologic reaction to sperm. The treatment options are controversial, and include sperm washing, high-dose corticosteroids, vitamin C, and assisted reproductive technologies such as GIFT and IVF.

DIAGNOSIS OF INFERTILITY

An estimated 43% of infertile couples seek help for infertility problems.[9] The history and physical examination are important, and close attention should be paid to details that provide clues to ovulation, previous infections or surgery, androgenicity, or other factors that could contribute to infertility.[10] In addition to history and physical exam of both partners, the current workup of the infertile couple consists of (1) semen analysis after 2–3 days of abstinence; (2) evaluation of pelvic anatomy and tubal patency via laparoscopy, fluoroscopically controlled hysterosalpingography (HSG), and/or hysteroscopy; (3) postcoital testing (PCT); and (4) evaluation of ovulatory function. Other tests such as sperm penetration assay, immune screen, karyotype, and human leukocyte antigen (HLA) screening may be employed in certain cases.

If an approximate time of ovulation can be determined, coitus can be scheduled (or avoided if contraception is desired) 3–4 days prior to and 2–3 days after expected ovulation. The human egg is fertilizable for 12–24 hours after ovulation and sperm may retain ability to fertilize for 24–48 hours. Although serial ultrasound examination by an experienced operator is an accurate noninvasive method of determining follicular growth and ovulation, ovulatory function can be evaluated with home test kits for detection of increase in urinary LH, measurement of serum progesterone concentration, endometrial biopsy or measurement of basal body temperature (BBT) (Fig. 76.4). BBT, the body temperature after a night's rest, is often lower than 98.6°F and varies throughout the menstrual cycle. Although not completely reliable, charting BBT allows indirect confirmation that ovulation has taken place. BBT can be taken orally or rectally with a regular thermometer or with special thermometers that show a range of only a few degrees making it easier to read small differences. It is very important that women take the reading upon arising and before any activity. In women who have an ovulatory menstrual cycle, BBT will reach a nadir at about the time of the LH surge and rise about 0.5°F at the time of ovulation when progesterone is secreted from the corpus luteum.

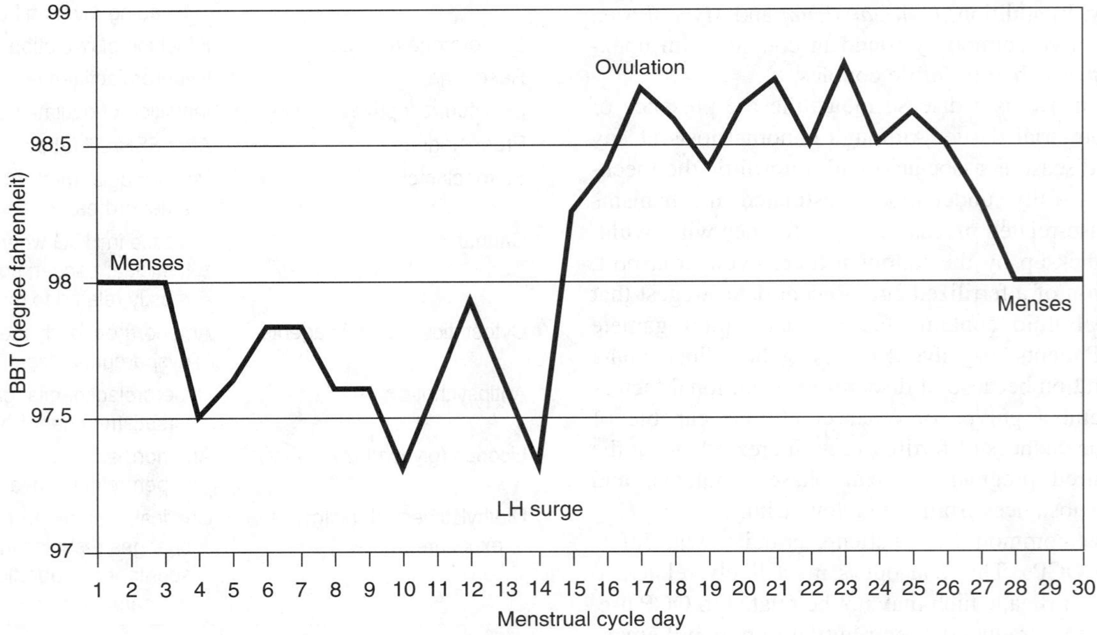

Figure 76.4. Basal body temperature over a normal ovulatory cycle.

PRINCIPLES OF OVULATION INDUCTION

When infertility is related to anovulation or luteal phase defects, hormonal manipulation is often successful. Some therapeutic agents augment the patient's natural endocrine process, while other agents will take control of, and in some cases replace, the natural cycle (Table 76.4). To induce ovulation, FSH is necessary in the early phase of the cycle to recruit and select follicles. For follicular growth and maturation, both FSH and LH are necessary. Adequate estrogen is necessary in the follicular phase to stimulate the endometrial lining and alter the cervical mucus, making it favorable

TABLE 76.4. DRUGS USED TO INDUCE OVULATION

Category	Trade Name (Manufacturer)	Content	How Supplied	Indications/Adjunct Therapy
Estrogen agonist/ antagonist	Clomid (Marion Merrell Dow), Milophene (Milex), Serophene (Serono)	Clomiphene citrate	50-mg tablet	Anovulation or oligo-ovulation with intact pituitary/ovarian response and endogenous estrogen
Human chorionic gonadotropin (HCG)	Various	HCG from human placenta and urine of pregnant women (activity is essentially identical to activity of LH)	Reconstituted products available in following strengths: 200, 500, 1000, and 2000 IU/mL	Used after pretreatment with clomiphene, human menotropins, and other agents in women with secondary ovarian failure
Menotropin (HMG)	Pergonal (Serono)	FSH and LH (human urine)	• 75 IU FSH, 75 IU LH activity/2 mL ampule • 150 IU FSH, 150 IU LH activity/2 mL ampule	Hypothalamus–pituitary failure; ovaries must be responsive (secondary ovarian failure)/stimulates follicular growth and maturation; HCG needed for ovulation
Urofollitropin	Metrodin (Serono)	FSH	0.83 mg (75 IU FSH activity)/2 mL ampule	Women with PCOD where LH: FSH is elevated; used sequentially with HCG
Synthetic GnRH	Lutrepulse (Ortho)	Gonadorelin acetate	0.8 and 3.2 mg powder (lyophilized) for injection, available in complete kits including pump	Anovulation due to primary hypothalamic failure or dysfunction; must be given in a pulsatile fashion
	Factrel (Ayerst)	Gonadorelin HCl	100 µg (as HCl)/vial 500 µg (as HCl)/vial	Same as above, but does not have FDA approval for this indication
Synthetic GnRH agonist/analog	Synarel (Syntex)	Nafarelin acetate	2 mg/mL nasal spray	Endometriosis; adjunct to HMG/HCG for ovulation induction (not an FDA approved use)
	Lupron (TAP Pharmaceuticals)	Leuprolide acetate	5 mg/mL for SC injection (Depot formulation should NOT be used for ovulation induction.)	Endometriosis; adjunct to HMG/HCG for ovulation induction (neither are FDA approved uses)
	Superfact (Hoechst AG,FRG)	Buserilin	Nasal spray, subcutaneous injection	Adjunct to HMG/HCG for ovulation induction (not available in U.S.)
	Tryptorelin pamoate (Organon)	Decapeptyl	Injection	Orphan drug; palliative treatment for ovarian carcinoma of epithelial origin; may be more prone to ovarian hyperstimulation than other GnRH-a
	Zoladex (ICI Pharma)	Goserelin acetate	3.6-mg implant	Not used for ovulation induction because of duration of effect

for sperm penetration. The aim is to develop one or two mature follicles; therefore, gonadotropin stimulation should be delayed until the dominant follicle has been selected. Once ovulation has occurred, progesterone is required in the luteal phase to maintain and transform the endometrial lining into one suitable for implantation by a fertilized ovum. In cases of IVF where the aim is to obtain many oocytes, increased gonadotropin stimulation is commenced before or during the early follicular recruitment phase. Pregnancy rates achieved in patients with single infertility factors are listed in Table 76.2.

SPECIFIC AGENTS

Clomiphene

Clomiphene, a triphenylchloroethylene derivative, is available as a racemic mixture (zuclomiphene and enclomiphene) in the United States. As a nonsteroidal estrogen agonist–antagonist, clomiphene is capable of interacting with hypothalamic estrogen receptors. The hypothalamus releases GnRH as if estrogen concentrations were low. The FSH and LH pulse frequency (but not amplitude) rise, increasing the peripheral serum concentrations of FSH and LH (Fig. 76.5). Enhancement of the natural HPO axis is recognized as the primary mechanism of action, although pituitary and ovarian effects may occur. The primary indication for clomiphene is for anovulatory or oligo-ovulatory infertility, including PCOD. Suitable patients are likely to have a chronic anovulatory disorder often dating back to puberty. Appropriate candidates for clomiphene therapy have endogenous estrogen activity and an intact HPO axis. Although generally less successful in inducing ovulation in women with reduced estrogen levels, a trial of clomiphene therapy may be warranted unless galactorrhea or hyperprolactinemia suggest other therapy (see section on Bromocriptine). Patients with FSH at or above 40 mIU/mL have absent or resistant follicles and are not likely to respond to ovulation induction.

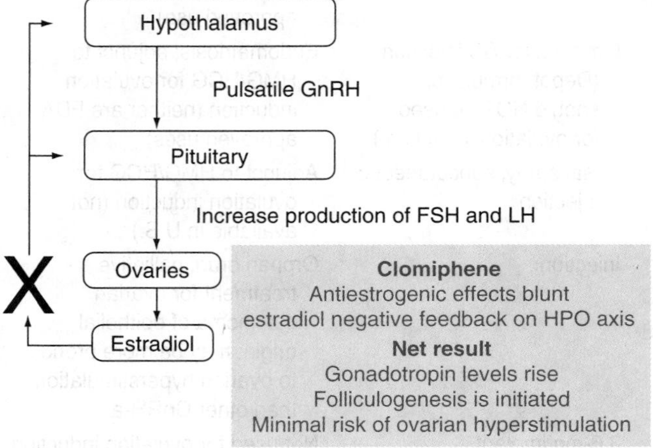

Figure 76.5. Effects of clomiphene on HPO axis.

Because there is a possible association between clomiphene dosage and multiple birth, a low dose of clomiphene should be used initially and then increased, if necessary, with each cycle. The recommended starting dosage is 50 mg/d for 5 days. Because women with PCOD may be ultrasensitive, the starting dose may be lowered to 25 mg. Treatment is most commonly started on or about the 5th day of the cycle after the start of progestin-induced bleeding or spontaneous uterine bleeding. An earlier starting date (day 3 or 4) is sometimes used, but waiting until day 9 may be too late to induce ovulation. Ovulation is expected 5–10 days after the last dose and is determined by BBT charts, urinary LH monitoring, plasma progesterone assay, or endometrial histology.

If the initial clomiphene dosage is ineffective, the dosage is usually increased by 50 mg/d for the next cycle. Once an ovulatory dosage is identified, the treatment cycle may be repeated for 4–6 months or longer unless pregnancy occurs. To ensure optimal timing for conception, intercourse can be timed according to results of ultrasound or urinary LH monitoring kits or should occur every other day for 1 week beginning 4–5 days after the last day of clomiphene administration. The vast majority of pregnancies occur at dosages of 150 mg/d or less and within 6 months after ovulation begins. A lack of response to 200 or 250 mg daily for 5 days suggests that other treatment measures are needed. However, an increased duration of clomiphene therapy may improve chances of ovulation in women who are unresponsive to standard therapy.[11-13] If pregnancy fails to occur when ovulation appears to be present and prolactin and androgen levels are normal, clomiphene-associated antiestrogen effects may cause thick, tenacious cervical mucus that can hinder sperm migration. Treatment with estrogen may reduce this unwanted effect (see section below on Corticosteroids, Estrogens, Tamoxifen, and Others).

Clomiphene should not be given if pregnancy is suspected or to those patients with a history of significant liver disease. Because clomiphene is capable of stimulating follicular and endometrial growth, further enlargement of preexisting ovarian and endometrial cysts may prove potentially harmful. Abnormal uterine bleeding should be evaluated to rule out neoplastic lesions and other disorders before clomiphene therapy is begun. Multiple-births rates have ranged from 5–12.3%, with the vast majority being twins.

The adverse effects of clomiphene do not usually interfere with treatment and are generally reversible. Most occur at the initial starting dose of 50 mg/d. When higher doses are required to induce ovulation, the woman is thought to be less sensitive to the drug, including adverse reactions. The antiestrogenic properties of clomiphene cause reversible hot flushes in 11% of patients. Visual disturbances occur at an estimated rate of less than 2%. "Blurring," or spots or flashes (scintillating scotomata), are dose related and are an indication to discontinue therapy. Although midcycle pain (mittelschmerz) may be accentuated, abnormal ovarian enlargement is infrequently associated with normal doses of clomiphene. However, clomiphene is capable of causing ovarian enlargement and cyst formation with high or prolonged doses. Abdominal symptoms (discomfort, distention, bloating, and abnormal uterine bleeding) occur in 5–6% of patients. Miscellaneous symptoms including nausea, vomiting, breast tenderness, headache, and dizziness occur in 1–2.5% of patients.

The use of clomiphene generally does not require intense monitoring. BBT charting as an adjunctive measure is recommended. Some experts employ pelvic ultrasound with dosage increases or serum progesterone concentrations in an attempt to ascertain an adequate luteal phase.[10] Approximately 70–80% of well-selected patients treated with clomiphene are expected to ovulate with a conception rate of approximately 40%.[10] When no other causes of infertility are identified, conception rates approaching 90% are reported.[14,15]

Human Chorionic Gonadotropin

In some cases, clomiphene and other agents cause follicular maturation with an adequate rise in the follicular phase estradiol concentration, but ovulation fails to occur. If a lack of a midcycle gonadotropin surge is causing ovulation failure, that can be bypassed by exogenous administration of HCG (5000–10,000 IU intramuscularly) 3 or 4 days after the last dose of clomiphene or when follicular diameter is 20 mm or greater by ultrasound.[10] The activity of HCG is essentially identical to that of LH, but with a longer half-life (>24 hours versus 60 minutes). Hormonal monitoring and follicle ultrasound measurements help determine the appropriate timing of HCG administration.

Gonadotropin Therapy (HMG, FSH, and LH)

Clomiphene, with or without the addition of HCG, has been both a safe and effective drug for the induction of ovulation for more than 20 years. However, if clomiphene is to induce ovulation, the HPO axis must be responsive. For women without an intact HPO axis, replacement or supplementation of the pituitary gonadotropins and HCG is an effective alternative for ovulation induction.

Gonadotropins are relatively safe when administered as ovulation-inducing drugs to properly selected patients, in correct dosages, and with appropriate monitoring. Gonadotropins are expensive, must be administered parenterally on a daily basis, and require more extensive monitoring than other methods. They are indicated only after a thorough infertility workup and careful counseling of the couple. *These agents should only be prescribed and monitored by individuals who are expert in their use.* Once exogenously administered gonadotropins are employed, the menstrual cycle, including the follicle selection process (ovarian stimulation) and ovulation, is controlled by external manipulation. Without proper monitoring, women may be at risk for severe consequences. Gonadotropin replacement therapy is indicated in amenorrheic women with anovulation due to hypothalamic–pituitary insufficiency or failure. The ovaries must be able to respond normally to FSH and LH stimulation.

Human menopausal gonadotropin (HMG), obtained from the urine of postmenopausal women, contains both FSH and LH. Each vial of HMG for intramuscular administration should contain equal amounts of FSH and LH activity; however, radioimmunoassay suggests a dominance of FSH. HMG is used to induce ovulation in women with primary hypothalamic–pituitary insufficiency, but it also has been used for follicular recruitment for IVF. Purified FSH is available and may be of particular benefit for women with PCOD with increased LH : FSH ratio who have failed clomiphene therapy.

Administration of HMG or purified FSH may override the normal mechanism of ovarian follicular selection and produce more than one mature follicle (Fig. 76.6). Apparently, the earlier exogenous FSH stimulation occurs during the cycle (before the follicle selection process), the more recruited follicles. HMG or purified FSH is administered daily until at least one follicle is ready to ovulate; then HCG is delivered to induce ovulation. The effective gonadotropin dose, the length of time required for follicular maturation, and the appropriate time to trigger ovulation with HCG are determined by monitoring ovulation induction. Because a variation in gonadotropin concentration may occur as a result of human origin, ampules produced in the same lot are recommended for each cycle.

The usual effective dose (based on FSH) is 150 IU/d IM beginning the third or fourth day of the cycle, but lower doses (75 IU/d) may induce ovulation in a few women who are hypersensitive to gonadotropin therapy. Once the serum

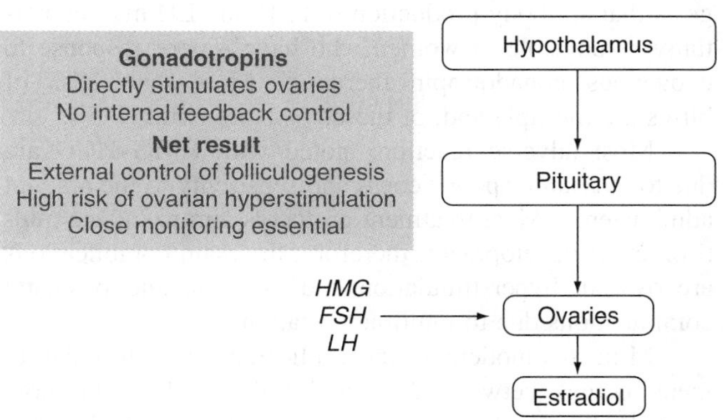

Figure 76.6. Effects of exogenous gonadotropins on HPO axis.

estrogen concentration has risen steadily and is not excessive (<1500 pg/mL), the same dosage is continued until the serum concentration is between 500 and 1500 pg/mL and one or two follicles have reached a diameter of 18–25 mm via ultrasound monitoring. The injections should be given at a consistent time each day and can be administered by the patient or her partner, if properly trained. Generally, gonadotropin administration should not exceed 12 days, although a longer time may be required. Ovulation is triggered by the intramuscular administration of HCG 5000–10,000 IU 1 day after the last dose of gonadotropin. Intercourse is advised the day after HCG administration and for the next 2 days. Because of the sustained half-life of HCG compared to LH, multiple corpus lutea can develop and supraphysiologic concentrations of estradiol and progesterone can occur throughout the luteal phase.

Monitoring is not only necessary for adjusting therapy, but helps prevent or recognize ovarian hyperstimulation. Monitoring includes ultrasonography, serum estrogen concentrations, and cervical mucus changes. In addition, the patient is usually examined clinically at least every other day during the administration of HMG and for at least 2 weeks post-treatment for signs of ovarian hyperstimulation.

When many large follicles (18–25 mm) are present or when serum estradiol concentrations are excessive (>1500 pg/mL), HCG administration is generally withheld and the treatment cycle terminated in order to prevent multiple gestations and/or ovarian hyperstimulation. In centers that perform assisted reproductive procedures, such as IVF, multiple follicles pose less risk of ovarian hyperstimulation syndrome because excess follicles are punctured during the surgical procedure thus reducing the estrogen stimulation.

The pregnancy rate with HMG–HCG therapy in amenorrheic patients with hypothalamic–pituitary insufficiency or failure may be as high as 80%, but the success rate is lower in patients with PCOD.[10] The cumulative pregnancy rate is significantly affected by age with 95% of patients younger than 35 years of age conceiving after six treatment cycles while only 60% of patients older than 35 conceive. Overall, women older than 35 years of age have a relatively poor chance of becoming pregnant. Recent evidence suggests that antibody production to FSH and LH may be partially responsible in women who have a poor response to exogenous gonadotropin therapy.[16] More than 25% of births are multiple and, of these, 74% are twins.

Most adverse reactions noted with HMG–HCG are due to ovarian responsiveness and sensitivity to the amount administered. Most treatment protocols aim to induce multifollicular development; therefore, the main complications are ovarian hyperstimulation and obstetric and postnatal complications due to multiple gestation.

Mild to moderate uncomplicated ovarian enlargement ranges between 20% and 60% in different large series.[17] Severe hyperstimulation develops rapidly over 3–4 days and generally within 2 weeks after HCG administration. If ovarian hyperstimulation results in rupture of ovarian cysts, serious complications may arise from the subsequent hemoperitoneum, ascites, hypovolemia, and electrolyte imbalance. If moderate or severe hyperstimulation is detected, treatment must be discontinued, supportive fluid and electrolyte therapy begun, and hospitalization may be required.[18] The ovaries slowly return to normal within 2–3 weeks in nonpregnant women, but will take longer in pregnant women because of endogenous HCG stimulation. A baseline ultrasound in patients who have experienced hyperstimulation in previous cycles should be performed before a new cycle of HMG stimulation is started. The incidence of severe hyperstimulation has declined and with proper monitoring is rare.

Clinical evidence does not indicate that HMG–HCG ovulation induction places fetuses at any greater risk of malformation than the normal population. However, fetal loss due to abortion or premature delivery of multiple gestations is of concern. Hypersensitivity and febrile reactions are also reported with HMG–HCG.

Gonadotropin-Releasing Hormone for Ovulation Induction

GnRH, also commonly known as luteinizing hormone-releasing hormone (LH–RH) or luteinizing hormone-releasing factor (LRF), is normally released in a pulsatile fashion. Continuous stimulation with GnRH results in down-regulation of the normal FSH/LH response. Early efforts to induce ovulation with GnRH were not encouraging because of the lack of understanding of these pulsatile requirements. The availability of portable pulsatile infusion pumps for GnRH provides the necessary technology to more closely mimic natural physiology. GnRH therapy is most successful in women who are infertile because of hypothalamic dysfunction; however, therapy is effective in women with hyperprolactinemia who are resistant to traditional therapy and to a lesser degree in women with PCOD.

If GnRH is given as a constant infusion, gonadotropins will peak at 30 minutes (release of secretory pool), plateau, then rise a second time in approximately 230 minutes.[19] Subsequently, gonadotropin concentrations fall due to down-regulation of the pituitary gonadotropes. In terms of ovulation induction, a theoretical but unproven advantage of this self-regulation is the reduced likelihood of ovarian hyperstimulation.

GnRH for ovulation induction is administered via a programmable pump in a pulsatile fashion either intravenously (usually 3 to 5 μg/bolus) or subcutaneously (10–20 μg/bolus) for 10–20 days. The pulse interval may range from 60- to 120-minute intervals, with a 90-minute interval recommended most often. However, the 90-minute interval is associated with a higher rate of multiple pregnancies than the 120-minute interval. The dose (intravenous or subcutaneous) may be increased by 3- to 5-μg increments if the patient fails to ovulate. Multiple pregnancies generally occur with intravenous dosages of 5 μg and greater. Hyperphysiologic responses occur at intravenous dosages of 4–5 μg (75 ng/kg).[20] The clinical usefulness of this method of delivery is limited by the need for constant care of the pump system and expense.

Although the subcutaneous route is better tolerated and is effective in most women with hypothalamic dysfunction,[21] higher doses are necessary and this route does not appear to be as successful in inducing ovulation in patients with PCOD[22] or obesity.[23] Heparin (1000 IU/mL diluent) should be added if GnRH is to be administered via the intravenous route. After reconstitution, GnRH can remain biologically potent for more than 1 month.[24] Regardless of the route of administration, GnRH given at a fixed interval can produce normal gonadotropin stimulation resulting in follicular development, adequate LH surge, ovulation, and development of a healthy corpus luteum (Fig. 76.7). Also, GnRH is currently being considered as a potential treatment for infertility due to luteal phase deficiency in women who are refractory to the more established treatments.[25,26]

The administration of a combined OCP or medroxyprogesterone acetate (5–10 mg) for 7–10 days to induce withdrawal bleeding serves as a useful reference point to begin treatment. GnRH is begun 7 days after the first day of flow. Ovulation should occur within 14–21 days of treatment. HCG in low doses (1500–2500 IU IM), beginning the day after ovulation and administered every third day thereafter for three doses, is often used following pulsatile GnRH to support the luteal phase. However, continuous treatment with pulsatile GnRH alone is effective for maintaining the corpus luteum.[1] Progesterone is also given intramuscularly or by suppository during the luteal phase.[27] Ultrasound monitoring is recommended to decrease the risk of unrecognized ovarian hyperstimulation and multiple pregnancy (5%) even though the risk is small with this therapy. Ultrasound monitoring may be used to adjust the GnRH dosage in hyporesponders.

Ovulation rates of more than 90% are observed in hypothalamic insufficiency, and most patients become pregnant within 6 months of subcutaneous GnRH therapy. In women with PCOD, the ovulation rates are about 50% per treatment cycle. The addition of clomiphene citrate, glucocorticoids, or low-dose HMG may increase GnRH responsiveness in otherwise resistant patients.

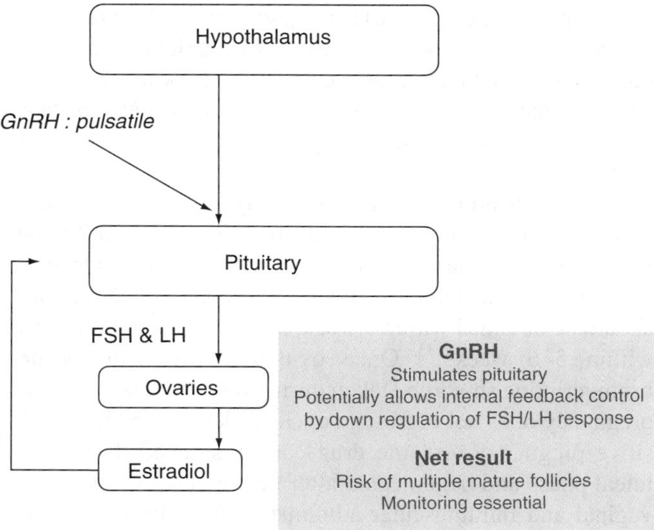

Figure 76.7. Effects of pulsatile GnRH administration on HPO axis.

GnRH Analogues

Analogues of GnRH are more potent with a longer half-life than GnRH. Clinical experience is far greater with GnRH agonists than the more recently developed antagonists. GnRH agonists initially cause gonadotropin stimulation during the first week followed by suppression that results from hypothalamic desensitization. Antagonists appear to more rapidly produce gonadotropin suppression through direct receptor blockade and may have potential in reproductive medicine. Research on antagonists has been delayed because of allergic reactions in the first-generation agents. Basic differences between GnRH analogues are presented in Table 76.5.[28] Because of the longer duration of effect, intermittent administration of GnRH analogues results in a profound suppression in gonadotropin secretion of the magnitude produced by constant GnRH infusion with subsequent suppression of pituitary–gonadal function (Fig. 76.8). The effect of GnRH analogues on pituitary and ovarian function is temporary and persists only as long as continued administration of the analogue. HPO function returns to baseline within 1–2 months after discontinuation of the GnRH analogue.

Although not FDA approved for ovulation induction, GnRH agonists are frequently used in combination with gonadotropins in women who have failed clomiphene or who are undergoing assisted reproduction.[29] GnRH agonists are administered via nasal spray or by subcutaneous injection for up to 3 weeks starting in the luteal phase of the previous cycle or early in the follicular phase. Administration beginning in the luteal phase effectively blocks endogenous gonadotropin secretion, especially the LH surge, which could prove detrimental if premature. When a hypogonadotropic hypogonadal state is achieved, ovulation can be induced with gonadotropins. Complete suppression of endogenous gonadotropin secretion allows better follicular synchronization with exogenous HMG and improves the predictability of ovarian response, especially in clomiphene-resistant patients with PCOD and in superovulation regimens used with IVF. Beginning GnRH agonist therapy in the follicular phase takes advantage of the initial gonadotropin stimulating effects and reduces the

TABLE 76.5. COMPARISON OF GnRH ANALOGUES

GnRH Analogues	Agonists	Antagonists
Mechanism of gonadotropin suppression	Desensitization with repeated use	Competitive receptor blockade
Acute response	Stimulation of LH and FSH	Inhibition of LH; partial inhibition of FSH
Chronic response	Inhibition of LH and FSH	Inhibition of LH and FSH
Clinical experience	Extensive	Limited
Safety	Long history of safety	Initial histamine release problem
Cost	Relatively low	High
Agents	Buserilin, Leuprolide, Nafarelin	Nal-glu, Nal-lys

amount of exogenous gonadotropin that is necessary to induce ovulation.[29] Monitoring with ultrasound and measuring estradiol response to screening tests with a GnRH agonist may help individualize ovarian stimulation and possibly reduce the risk of ovarian hyperstimulation or multiple pregnancy.[30,31] Typical regimens are summarized in Table 76.6. GnRH analogues are also useful in the treatment of sex steroid-hormone-dependent disorders (e.g., precocious puberty, endometriosis, uterine fibroids, prostate disease, hyperandrogenic states).

Adverse Effects

Adverse effects of GnRH and its analogues can be classified into the effects caused by the drugs themselves (allergic reactions with production of antibodies), by changes in the gonadotropins, particularly with GnRH analogues (symptoms of decreased estrogen production, including hot flushes, vaginal dryness, and decreased libido), and by the route of administration (local irritation at the site of injection, or nasal irritation and bad taste in the mouth after nasal sprays). Most adverse risks involve pump function or local reactions to the needle placement and to the concurrent use of HMG. Women with myocardial valvular disease that is prone to microbial seeding of the valve should be evaluated prior to pump use. Multiple pregnancy occurs in 5% of patients. Ovarian hyperstimulation, although rare, may occur with GnRH doses greater than 10 μg/pulse intravenously or 20 μg/pulse subcutaneously. Allergic reactions may occur in patients receiving long-term treatment. The development of anti-GnRH antibodies may reduce treatment effectiveness and contribute to the slightly higher than expected miscarriage rate (about 20%) that occurs in GnRH-induced pregnancies.

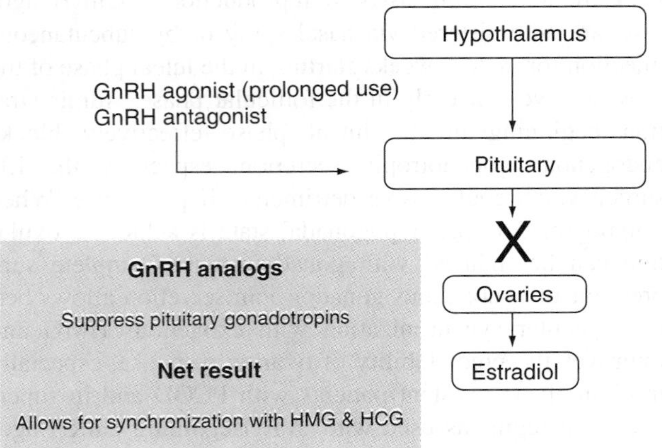

Figure 76.8. Effects of GnRH analogues on HPO axis.

Bromocriptine

Bromocriptine is clearly indicated for women whose infertility is related to hyperprolactinemia with or without galactorrhea (80% fertility rate after therapy). Bromocriptine, a semisynthetic ergotamine derivative, acts as a dopamine agonist to directly inhibit pituitary prolactin secretion. Normalizing prolactin concentration restores central gonadotropin function. The use of bromocriptine over many years may reduce the size of prolactin-producing pituitary tumors and return serum prolactin concentrations to normal. Hyperprolactinemia also occurs in up to 20–40% of patients with PCOD. Bromocriptine may help correct the inappropriate release of LH in these patients by normalizing prolactin. It is sometimes used with variable success in combination with clomiphene in patients who appear to have normal prolactin levels with or without galactorrhea. These anovulatory women may have nocturnal elevations of prolactin.[32]

Bromocriptine treatment is usually initiated with a bedtime dose of 1.25 mg for 1 week then titrated up to 2.5 mg three times daily based on prolactin concentrations. Once an effective dose is achieved, normal prolactin concentrations should be obtained within 1 week, and menses should follow within 5–6 weeks.[33] Once ovulation begins to occur, bromocriptine should be taken during the follicular phase. If pregnancy does not occur in a cycle as determined by a sensitive pregnancy test, the drug can be stopped during the luteal phase and begun again after next menses starts. Intravaginal and intramuscular administration of bromocriptine may also prove to be beneficial and reduce the incidence of side effects.[34] In patients with galactorrhea or hyperpro-

TABLE 76.6. TYPICAL REGIMENS OF GnRH ANALOGUE ADMINISTRATION

Diagnosis	GnRH-a	HMG/FSH	HCG
PCOD or assisted reproduction	Leuprolide 0.5–1 mg SQ QD until HCG	*Luteal phase protocol:* 2–4 amps QD after 1–2 weeks of GnRH-a; adjust dose as indicated by ultrasound and E_2 level *Follicular phase protocol:* 2 amps QD after 3 days of GnRH-a; adjust dose as indicated by ultrasound and E_2 level	5000–10000 IU IM when leading follicle measures >15–18 mm; intercourse advised for the day after HCG and for the next 2 days or assisted reproductive technology employed such as IVF; may need luteal phase support (i.e., low-dose HCG [1000–2500 IU] every third day for 3 doses)
Disorders of either hypothalamic or pituitary origin	Leuprolide 0.5–1 mg SQ QD, followed by pulsatile GnRH, 2.5–5 μg IV QH		
Premature ovarian failure	Leuprolide 0.2–0.5 mg SQ QD until HCG	HMG 1–6 amps IM QD after 2–3 weeks of GnRH-a; adjust dose as indicated by ultrasound and E_2 level	5000–10,000 IU IM when leading follicle measures >15–18 mm; intercourse advised for the day after HCG and for the next 2 days; may need luteal phase support such as low-dose HCG [1000–2500 IU] every third day for 3 doses)

Key: PCOD, polycystic ovary disease; GnRH-a, gonadotropin-releasing hormone agonists; E_2, estradiol; HMG/FSH, human menopausal gonadotropin/follicle-stimulating hormone; HCG, human chorionic gonadotropin.

lactinemia, ovulatory menses and pregnancy occurs in 80%. The average time to initiation of menses is 5–6 weeks. If there is no objective indication that ovulation is occurring within 3 months despite normal prolactin, then clomiphene and/or gonadotropins may be added.

Nausea, headache, and faintness are common side effects. Psychiatric symptoms may occur in less than 1% of patients. Other complaints reported by bromocriptine-treated patients include dizziness, orthostatic hypotension, nasal congestion, vomiting, constipation, and abdominal cramps. Side effects from oral administration can be minimized by slow dosage titration and by taking the dose at bedtime and with food. There is no evidence of increased teratogenicity with use of bromocriptine.

Corticosteroids, Estrogen, Tamoxifen, and Others

Corticosteroid supplementation may act synergistically with clomiphene to promote ovulation by lowering the circulating levels of adrenal androgens that might otherwise inhibit folliculogenesis or aromatase activity. Dexamethasone (0.5–1 mg/d) or prednisone (5–10 mg/d) should be taken at bedtime until pregnancy occurs. The dose of clomiphene usually remains unchanged from the previous cycle. Low-dose dexamethasone may be a beneficial adjuvant to HMG–HCG regimens in women with PCOD (usually excess androgen from ovaries), but is more likely to be useful in women who have excessive adrenal androgen production.[35]

Clomiphene has associated antiestrogen effects causing thick, tenacious cervical mucus that can hinder sperm migration. Although the increased amount of estrogen being produced by multiple maturing follicles usually overrides this effect, exogenous estrogen (ethinyl estradiol, 10–20 μg/d, or conjugated equine estrogens 0.3–2.5 mg/d on cycle days 10–16) in combination with clomiphene may improve the quality of the cervical mucus. The lower doses (conjugated equine estrogens 0.3 mg) may be begun as early as cycle day 4. Other therapeutic attempts to improve the cervical mucus quality include guaifenesin and potassium iodide. If sperm penetration through the cervical mucus remains a problem, artificial intrauterine insemination with the partner's sperm may be attempted. On rare occasions, estrogen replacement is associated with the return of fertility in women who were sterile because of elevated gonadotropin concentrations (premature ovarian failure).[36,37]

Tamoxifen, a nonsteroidal antiestrogen primarily indicated for adjuvant treatment of breast cancer, has successfully treated infertility in anovulatory women who have failed clomiphene. The usual dose is 20–40 mg/d for 4–5 days commencing after menstruation, or at any time in amenorrheal women.[38] A proposed mechanism is lowering prolactin levels by reducing estrogen stimulation.[22]

Although data are limited and await further clarification, tamoxifen may reduce infertility in men with oligospermia (5–40 mg daily).[38]

Evaluation of Therapeutic Outcomes

Few pharmacists are directly involved with therapeutic management of infertility because most of the treatment and close monitoring occurs within the setting of the infertility center. With the exception of clomiphene and bromocriptine, which are relatively safe, the drugs that do need to be monitored require high technology and expert supervision. Similarly, the treatment regimens, including drug and dose, are often based on a complex combination of the underlying disorder and the individual patient's response to follicular development and ovulation as indicated by ultrasound or laboratory parameters. However, pharmacists need to understand and respect the psychological component of the patient and/or couple receiving treatment for infertility. The process of diagnosing and treating infertility has a widespread impact on the lives of the couple. The emotional pain and impact of infertility, combined with the time-consuming and expensive therapeutic manipulations and monitoring procedures can take a toll on relationships, self-esteem, health, and security. Couples seeking treatment often experience severe anxiety, grief, and depression as a result of the process. In addition to being understanding and supportive, pharmacists may help relieve some of the fears and frustration by explaining the purpose of drugs being used, side effects to expect, and the importance of adhering to the prescribed monitoring regimen. If properly trained, pharmacists could assist in the administration of or education regarding intramuscular gonadotropin therapy. Pharmacists can also educate patients on proper method for obtaining and interpreting basal body temperature and using home kits for detecting LH surge. Pharmacists should also be alert to serious psychological disturbances that may manifest in the infertile couple, encourage them to discuss these issues with each other and their infertility therapist, or refer patients for appropriate psychological consultation.

References

1. Speroff L, Glass RH, Kase NG. Clinical Gynecologic Endocrinology and Infertility, 4th ed. Baltimore, William & Wilkins, 1989.
2. Cramer DW, Walker AM, Schiff I. Statistical methods in evaluating the outcome of infertility therapy. Fertil Steril 1979;32:80–86.
3. Talbert LM. Overview of the diagnostic evaluation, in Hammond MG, Talbert LM (eds): Infertility: A Practical Guide for Physicians, 3rd ed. Boston, Blackwell Scientific Publications, 1993, pp 1–10.
4. Jones HW, Toner JP. The infertile couple. N Engl J Med 1993;329:1710–1712.
5. Wessels PH, Viljoen GJ, Marais NF, et al. The prevalence, risks and management of Chlamydia trachomatis infection in fertile and infertile patients from the high socioeconomic bracket of the South African population. Fertil Steril 1991;56:485–488.
6. Risi GF, Sanders CV. The genital mycoplasmas. Obstet Gynecol Clin North Am 1989;16:611–626.
7. Halme J. Role of peritoneal inflammation in endometriosis-associated infertility. Ann NY Acad Sci 1991;622:266–274.
8. Coddington CC, Oehninger S, Cunningham DS, et al. Peritoneal fluid from patients with endometriosis decreases sperm binding to the zona pellucida in the hemizona assay: A preliminary report. Fertil Steril 1992;57:783–786.
9. Wilcox L, Mosher W. The use of infertility services in the United States [abstract], in Proceedings and Abstracts of the 48th Annual Meeting of the American Fertility Society, New Orleans, Louisiana, October 31–November 5, 1992. Birmingham, AL: American Fertility Society, 1993:S138.
10. American College of Obstetrics and Gynecologists. (ACOG) Infertility. ACOG Technical Bulletin 125. Washington, DC, Author, 1989.
11. Lobo RA, Granger LR, Davajan V, Mishell DR Jr. An extended regimen of clomiphene citrate in women unresponsive to standard therapy. Fertil Steril 1982;37:762–766.
12. O'Herlihy C, Pepperell RJ, Brown JB, et al. Incremental clomiphene therapy: A new method for treating persistent anovulation. Obstet Gynecol 1981;58:535–542.
13. Kelly AC, Jewelewicz R. Alternate regimens for ovulation induction in polycystic ovarian disease. Fertil Steril 1990;54:195–202.
14. Rust LA, Israel R, Mishell DR Jr. An individualized graduated therapeutic regimen for clomiphene citrate. Am J Obstet Gynecol 1974;120:785.
15. Drake TS, Tredway DR, Buchanan GC. Continued clinical experience with an increasing dosage regimen of clomiphene citrate administration. Fertil Steril 1978;30:274–277.
16. Meyer WR, Lavy G, DeCherney AH, et al. Evidence of gonadal and gonadotropin antibodies in women with a suboptimal ovarian response to exogenous gonadotropin. Obstet Gynecol 1990;75:795–799.
17. Lunenfeld B, Blankenstein J, Ron E, et al. Short- and long-term survey of patients treated with HMG/HCG and follow-up of offspring, in Genazziani AR, Volpe AF (eds): Proceedings of the First International Congress on Gynecological Endocrinology. Lancanshire, Parthenon, 1987, p 459.
18. Borenstein R, Elhalah U, Lunenfeld B, Schwartz ZS. Severe ovarian hyperstimulation syndrome: A reevaluated therapeutic approach. Fertil Steril 1989;51:791–795.
19. Claman P, Seibel MM. Ovulation induction: GnRH, in Seibel MM (ed): Infertility: A Comprehensive Text. Norwalk, CT, Appleton & Lange, 1990, pp 333–350.
20. Santoro N, Wierman ME, Filicori M, et al. Intravenous administration of pulsatile gonadotropin-releasing hormone in hypothalamic amenorrhea: Effects of dosage. J Clin Endocrinol Metab 1986;62:109–116.
21. Mason P, Adams J, Morris DV, et al. Induction of ovulation with pulsatile luteinizing hormone releasing hormone. Br Med J 1984;288(6412):181–185.

22. Sakamoto H, Den K, Kondo Y, et al. Evidence that estrogen may be a key factor in hyperprolactinemic anovulation: A case report. Am J Obstet Gynecol 1987;157:318–319.
23. Lyles R, Elkind-Hirsch K, Goldzieher, Besch PK. Plasma gonadotropin releasing hormone profiles after intravenous and subcutaneous bolus injection in thin and obese women. Obstet Gynecol 1988;71:44–48.
24. Hahn PM, Van Vugt DA, Reid RL. The stability of synthetic gonadotropin-releasing hormone in solution. Fertil Steril 1987;48:155–158.
25. Loucopoulos A, Ferin M. The treatment of luteal phase defects with pulsatile infusion of gonadotropin-releasing hormone. Fertil Steril 1987;48:933–936.
26. Jansen RP, Handelsman DJ, Boylan LM, et al. Pulsatile intravenous GnRH for ovulation induction in infertile women. Fertil Steril 1987;48:33–38.
27. Hammond MG. Management of ovulatory dysfunction, in Hammond MG, Talbert LM (eds): Infertility: A Practical Guide for Physicians, 3rd ed. Boston, Blackwell Scientific Publications, 1993, pp 151–181.
28. Hall JE. Gonadotropin-releasing hormone antagonists: Effects on the ovarian follicle and corpus luteum. Clin Obstet Gynecol 1993;36:744–752.
29. Grosskinsky CM, Hammond MG. Ovulation induction in the anovulatory woman with GnRH agonists. Sem Reproductive Endocrinol 1993;11:136–141.
30. Itskovitz-Eldor J, Levron J, Kol S. Use of gonadotropin-releasing hormone agonist to cause ovulation and prevent ovarian hyperstimulation syndrome. Clin Obstet Gynecol 1993;36:701–710.
31. Garcia JE. Gonadotropin-releasing hormone and its analogs: Applications in gynecology. Clin Obstet Gynecol 1993;36:719–723.
32. Suginami H, Hamada K, Yano K, et al. Ovulation induction with bromocriptine in normoprolactinemic anovulatory women. J Clin Endocrinol Metab 1986;62:899–903.
33. American College of Obstetrics and Gynecologists (ACOG). Medical induction of ovulation. ACOG Technical Bulletin 120. Washington, DC, Author, 1988.
34. Katz E, Adashi EY. Treatment of infertility using bromocriptine mesylate, in Seibel MM (ed): Infertility: A Comprehensive Text. Norwalk, CT, Appleton & Lange, 1990, pp 351–362.
35. Evron S, Navot D, Laufer N, Diamant YZ. Induction of ovulation with combined human gonadotropins and dexamethasone in women with polycystic ovarian disease. Fertil Steril 1983;40:183–186.
36. Aiman J, Smentek C. Premature ovarian failure. Obstet Gynecol 1985;66:9–14.
37. Rebar RW, Erickson GF, Yen SSC. Idiopathic premature ovarian failure: Clinical and endocrine characteristics. Fertil Steril 1982;37:35–41.
38. Buckley MM-T, Goa KL. Tamoxifen, a reappraisal of its pharmacodynamic and pharmacokinetic properties and therapeutic use. Drugs 1989;37:451–490.

Chapter 77

Contraception

Kathryn K. Bucci, PharmD, BCPS, and Deborah Stier Carson, PharmD, BCPS

Comprehension of mechanisms involved in the hormonal regulation of the normal menstrual cycle are essential to understanding contraception and infertility in women. Please refer to the chapter on Infertility (Chapter 76) for a review of the menstrual cycle.

Comparative Effectiveness of Various Methods of Contraception

The most commonly used methods of reversible contraception include oral contraceptives, long-acting injectable or implantable progestins, condoms, spermicides, withdrawal, the diaphragm, periodic abstinence, and the intrauterine device.[1,2] These methods differ in their relative effectiveness, safety, and patient acceptability.[3]

The actual effectiveness of any contraceptive method is difficult to determine because many factors affect contraceptive failure. An important determinant of contraceptive failure is the user's motivation to prevent pregnancy.[2] Other factors include the inherent biologic capacity of the couple to conceive, the frequency of intercourse, and how well the user follows instructions. Failure inherent in the proper use of the contraceptive alone is considered a "method failure" or "perfect use failure." "User failure" or "typical use failure" takes into account inaccuracies in the user's abilities to follow directions, such as skipping an oral contraceptive pill (Table 77.1).[4]

Hormonal Methods of Contraception

Oral contraceptives (OCs) are used by approximately 13.2 million women, thus making them the most popular method of reversible contraception in the United States.[2] These agents are also highly effective for birth control (Table 77.1).

COMPOSITION AND FORMULATIONS

The currently available OCs contain either a combination of a synthetic estrogen and synthetic progestin, or a progestin alone.[5] Estrogen and/or progestin inhibit ovulation and alter cervical mucus and the endometrium by suppressing the production of follicle-stimulating hormone (FSH) and the lutenizing hormone (LH) surge.[1,5,6]

The first OC, Enovid 10, introduced in 1960, contained both estrogen and progestin given in constant doses throughout the cycle.[7] The use of this combination monophasic increased until 1963, when numerous cases of thromboembolism were reported.[7] Adverse effects were originally attributed to the estrogen component and, as a result, the dose was progressively decreased.[8]

In the 1960s, the "sequential" form of OCs (e.g., Oracon, C-Quens) was released containing only estrogen in the first portion of the cycle with progestin added during the second phase. This type of OC was associated with an increased risk of pregnancy and endometrial carcinoma, and as a result in 1976 the manufacturer voluntarily removed these products from the market.[8–10]

The progestin-only "minipill" was also introduced in 1960 and is still available, but its use is generally for women who have contraindications or intolerance to estrogens, smokers older than 35 years of age, and women who are breast feeding.[1] This pill is less effective than the combination pill and is associated with irregular bleeding and an increased frequency of functional ovarian cysts.[3,8,11–13] Progestin-only pills are believed to thicken and decrease the amount of cervical mucus (making it more difficult for sperm to penetrate), create a thin, atrophic endometrium, and possibly inhibit ovulation.[1,3] In that the dose of progestin may not block ovulation, there is an increased risk of ectopic pregnancy associated with using the progestin-only pills when compared to combination pills.[4,8] The progestin-only pill must be administered daily (with no days off) to maintain contraceptive efficacy.[8] Irregular and unpredictable menstrual cycles indicate that ovulation has been inhibited; however, this is one of the most frequent reasons for discontinuation of this method.[1,3]

The currently available "combination" OCs on the market are modifications of the original products, containing approximately one-fifth the estrogen and one-tenth the progestin dose found in earlier pills.[10] More recently, the

TABLE 77.1. COMPARISON OF REVERSIBLE METHODS OF CONTRACEPTIVES

Method	Contraindications	Advantages	Disadvantages	Failure Rates (%)[a]	
				Perfect Use	Typical Use
Episodic Contraceptive Methods					
Spermicides alone	Allergy to spermicide Abnormal vaginal anatomy	Inexpensive No office visit required Some protection against STDs	May enhance HIV transmission High user failure rate Must be reapplied before each act of intercourse May cause local irritation in either partner	6	21
Condoms, male	Allergy to latex	Inexpensive Readily available STD protection, including HIV (latex only) No office visit required	Poor acceptance Possibility of breakage Efficacy decreased by oil-based lubricants Latex can cause allergic reactions in either partner	3	12
Condoms, female (Reality)	Allergy to polyurethane Hx of toxic shock syndrome (?)	Stronger than latex STD protection, including HIV Protects outside the vagina and base of penis Not affected by oil-based lubricants No office visit required Can be inserted up to 8 hours before intercourse	Dislike ring hanging outside vagina Cumbersome	5	21
Sponge	Allergy to spermicide Hx of toxic shock syndrome	Moderate cost No office visit required Can be inserted just before intercourse or ahead of time; provides protection for 24 hours	Decreased efficacy with parity Difficulty in removal Causes vaginal dryness Increased incidence of vaginal yeast and UTI infections Increased incidence of toxic shock syndrome USA manufacturer stopped production in early 1995	20 (parous) 9 (nulliparous)	36 (parous) 18 (nulliparous)
Diaphragm with spermicide	Allergy to rubber or spermicide Recurrent UTIs Hx of toxic shock syndrome Abnormal gynecologic anatomy	Low cost Decreased incidence of cervical neoplasia STD protection, including HIV Can be inserted up to 6 hours before intercourse	Office visit required Decreased efficacy with increased frequency of intercourse Increased incidence of vaginal yeast and UTI infections. Increased incidence of toxic shock syndrome	6	18

			Efficacy affected by oil-based lubricants Cervical irritation		
Cervical cap (Prentif)	Allergy to rubber or spermicide Hx of toxic shock syndrome Abnormal gynecologic anatomy Abnormal Pap smear	Low cost STD protection, including HIV Can be inserted just before intercourse or ahead of time; provides protection for 48 hours	Office visit required May be difficult for patient to use correctly Decreased efficacy with parity Not possible to fit all patients	26 (parous) 9 (nulliparous)	36 (parous) 18 (nulliparous)
Hormonal Methods					
OCPs	Hepatic adenomas Thromboembolic disorders or history thereof Cerebrovascular or coronary artery disease Known or suspected breast cancer Undiagnosed abnormal gynecologic bleeding Cardiovascular risk factors (relative contraindication) Jaundice with pregnancy or previous pill use	Decreased menstrual flow Decreased menstrual cramping Decreased rate of ectopic pregnancy Decreased rate of PID (except chlamydia) Protection against ovarian and endometrial cancer Protection against iron deficiency anemia, fibrocystic breast disease, and ovarian cysts	Increased risk of benign hepatocellular adenomas Mild increased risk of thromboembolism and stroke Increased elevation of blood pressure No protection against most STDs Estrogenic side effects (nausea, breast tenderness, fluid retention) Progestogen side effects (acne, increased appetite, depression) Increased risk of myocardial infarction in older smokers, nausea, headache, depression	0.1	3
Progestin-only OCPs	Undiagnosed abnormal gynecologic bleeding	May be used by lactating women and women with cardiovascular risk Allows avoidance of estrogen-related side effects Protection against PID, iron deficiency anemia, and dysmenorrhea	Frequent spotting/ amenorrhea Increased risk of ectopic pregnancy Must take every day at the same time	0.5	3
Norplant (Levonorgestrel)	Undiagnosed abnormal gynecologic bleeding Acute liver disease Hx of MI, cerebrovascular accident or breast cancer Active thrombophlebitis or pulmonary emboli Relative contraindications: diabetes mellitus, migraine, epilepsy, depression, gallbladder or kidney disease, predisposition to SBE	Passive contraception Effective for 5 years Effects are quickly reversible Less menstrual cramping/mittelschmerz pain No suppression of lactation No metabolic disturbances	Requires outpatient surgical procedure Irregular menstrual bleeding, headaches, weight gain, acne Progestin side effects Local infection or bruising on insertion; removal may be difficult Expensive initially High discontinuation rate Unacceptable in patients using some anticonvulsants	0.09	0.09
Depo-Provera	Breast cancer Liver disease Thrombophlebitis	No suppression of lactation No increased risk of thromboembolism	Irregular menstrual bleeding, headache, weight gain, acne	0.3	0.3

(*continued*)

TABLE 77.1. COMPARISON OF REVERSIBLE METHODS OF CONTRACEPTIVES *(Continued)*

Method	Contraindications	Advantages	Disadvantages	Failure Rates (%)[a]	
				Perfect Use	Typical Use
Hormonal Methods (cont.)					
	Undiagnosed abnormal gynecologic bleeding	Passive contraception No drug interactions May decrease seizures Effective for 3 months	Possible increased risk of breast cancer in younger users Decreased HDL Progestin side effects Decreased bone density in long term users Office visit required		
Intrauterine Devices (Hormonal and Nonhormonal)					
Copper-T 380 (Paragard)	Multiple sexual partners/ partner with multiple partners (high risk for STDs) Hx of PID or ectopic pregnancy, acute pelvic infection Abnormal uterine cavity/pelvic surgery/undiagnosed vaginal bleeding Uterine or cervical cancer Postpartum endometritis or infected abortion in previous 3 months	Passive contraception Long-term contraception (can remain in place up to 10 years) Less expensive per year and easier for some patients	Increased fertility rate after removal Increased heavy bleeding Spotting between periods Increased cramping and dysmenorrhea Increased risk of ectopic pregnancy Office visit required Rarely uterine perforation		
Progesterone T (Progestasert)	Acute cervicitis or vaginitis, (including BV) until infection controlled	Remains in place for 1 year Decreased cramping and dysmenorrhea Decrease in menstrual blood loss	Office visit required Must be changed each year Increased risks of ectopic pregnancy Rarely uterine perforation	< 2	< 2

Levonorgestrel IUD	Conditions associated with increased susceptibility to infections, including leukemia, AIDS, IV drug abuse, and corticosteroid use Valvular heart disease (+/–) Nulliparity (+/–) Genital actinomyces Wilson's disease Allergy to copper	Constant rate of hormone release for 5 years Possibly, the single most effective reversible contraceptive method over 5-year period Decreased cramping and dysmenorrhea Reduced incidence of PID and menorrhagia Combines benefits of Norplant and Copper-T	Office visit required Irregular menstrual bleeding (?) Rarely uterine perforation

[a]% failure during first year of use.

[b]Contraindicated with Copper-T IUD. (Adapted from Hatcher RA, Trussell J, Stewart F, et al. Contraceptive Technology, 16th ed. New York, Irvington, 1994, p 129; Heath CB. Helping patients choose appropriate contraception. Am Fam Physician 1993;48:(6)1116; and Anonymous. Choice of contraceptives. Med Lett Drug Ther 1995;37:9, with permission.)

recognition that many side effects are progestin related has resulted in attempts to further lower the progestin dose. This is the rationale behind the development of combination multiphasic (biphasic and triphasic) formulations, which vary the dose of estrogen and progestin over two or three portions of the cycle; however, this has not been demonstrated as a clinical advantage.[1,8]

COMPONENTS OF ORAL CONTRACEPTIVES

Two estrogenic compounds are commonly used in OCs in the United States: ethinyl estradiol (EE) and mestranol. Both of these compounds are synthetic estrogens that differ only by the presence of a methyl group attached to mestranol at the C-3 site. Mestranol, which must be converted by the liver to EE before it is pharmacologically active, is estimated to be 50% less potent than EE.[3,14]

Progestins currently used in OCs include ethynodiol diacetate, desogestrel, norgestimate, norethindrone, norethynodrel, norethindrone, acetate, norgestrel, and its active isomer levonorgestrel.[8] Progestins vary in their progestational activity. Progestins differ in their inherent estrogenicity and antiestrogenic and androgenic effects.[3] Estrogenic and antiestrogenic properties are secondary to the extent of progestin's metabolism to estrogenic substances, whereas androgenic activity is determined by structural similarity of the progestin to testosterone (Table 77.2).[15] Norgestimate and desogestrel are new progestins with no estrogenic effect and less androgenicity when compared to levonorgestrel. When compared to norethindrone, norgestimate and desogestrel have higher androgenic activity.[14,16] Unfortunately, properly controlled clinical trials comparing norethindrone, norgestimate, and desogestrel are scarce, so determining actual relevance of these purported improvements in progestational selectivity and lower androgenic activity (such as acne, hirsutism, and weight gain) remains unknown.[1] Table 77.3 (pages 1608–1609) lists available OC products by brand name and specifies hormonal composition and pill activity.

CONSIDERATIONS WITH ORAL CONTRACEPTIVE USE

Oral contraceptives are highly effective and, when used properly, extremely safe.[8] However, a complete medical history and physical examination should be obtained before a patient is started on an OC, and the risks and contraindications to OC use must be carefully considered (Tables 77.4, 77.5, and 77.6).[3,8,15,17]

Generally, OCs are an acceptable form of birth control for women younger than 50 years of age who do not smoke.[2,3,17] Patients who may benefit from OC use include those at risk for pelvic inflammatory disease and those with ovarian cysts, benign breast disease, ectopic pregnancy, or severe dysmenorrhea.[17] Conversely, there are patient-specific characteristics that increase the patient's risk for adverse drug effects.[17] For example, hypertension, even when well controlled by antihypertensives, is a relative contraindication to OC use.[3,17,18] The incidence of hypertension (diastolic blood pressure greater than 90 mm Hg) while taking an OCP increases with the patient's age and duration of OC use.[14] Blood pressure monitoring is recommended in all users of OCs.[2] In OC users hypertension may be associated with the progestin component, such that mild increases in blood pressure may be initially managed by switching to an OC with less progestin activity.[14] However, there are women receiving progestins without estrogen who do not experience increases in blood pressure over time.[2,19] Therefore, the estrogen component is the major determinant in the development of hypertension in certain OC users.[2] If hypertension develops, discontinuing the OC usually results in a return to pretreatment blood pressure values within 3 months.[14,17]

TABLE 77.2. PHARMACOLOGIC EFFECTS OF PROGESTOGENS USED IN HORMONAL CONTRACEPTIVES

	Progestational	Estrogenic	Antiestrogenic	Androgenic
Norgestrel/levonorgestrel	+++	0	++	++++
Ethynodiol diacetate	++	+[a]	+[a]	+
Norethindrone acetate	+	+	+++	+
Norethindrone	+	+[a]	+[a]	+
Norethynodrel	+	+++	0	0
Gestodene	++++	0	++	++
Norgestimate	+	0	N/A	++
Desogestrel	+++	0[b]	+	+++

Key: ++++, highest effect; +++, pronounced effect; ++, moderate effect; +, minimal effect; 0, no effect; N/A, data not available.

[a]Estrogenic effects at low doses; may have antiestrogenic effect at higher doses.

[b]The 3-β OH metabolite has affinity at the estrogen receptor, but probably does not contribute significantly to activity. (Adapted from Facts and Comparisons, July 1994; and Dickey RP. Managing Contraceptive Pill Patients, 7th ed. Durant, OK, Essential Medical Information Systems, 1993, pp 128–129, with permission.)

OCs may affect carbohydrate and lipid metabolism.[19] These effects are possibly related to the dose and potency of the progestin component in the OC.[2] Specifically, when high doses of progestins are administered, 4–16% of women (depending on their age) respond abnormally to a glucose-tolerance test.[1,20,21] Although conflicting evidence exists, formulations containing a low dose of progestin do not alter insulin, glucose, or glucagon release after a glucose load in healthy women[22] or in those with a history of gestational diabetes.[2,23] The new progestins (i.e., desogestrel and norgestimate) are believed to have little if any effect on carbohydrate metabolism.[6] When an OC is prescribed for a patient with a history of glucose intolerance, a product containing one of the new progestins (i.e., desogestrel and norgestimate) or a low dose of a norethindrone-type progestin is recommended, and glucose tolerance should be periodically monitored to reduce the risk of hastening the onset of permanent diabetes in these women.[2]

Generally, synthetic progestins decrease high-density lipoprotein (HDL) and increase low-density lipoprotein (LDL).[2] Estrogens have an opposite effect (beneficial) on lipid metabolism, and recent studies of low-dose estrogen-progestin formulations, including levonorgestrel, found no adverse alterations in the levels of HDL, LDL, or total cholesterol.[2,8,24,25] However, the triphasic products with norgestrel (not norethindrone) may significantly lower HDL cholesterol.[2,26,27] Although the lipid effects of OCPs must be considered, the cause of the increased incidence of both venous and arterial cardiovascular disease, including myocardial infarction, is believed to be the result of thrombosis, not atherosclerosis.[2]

Early studies reported the incidence of venous thromboembolic disease to be 3 to 11 times greater in OC users than in nonusers.[8,18] However, more recent studies indicate the relative risk of venous thrombosis is 2.8 times the nonuser rate, with a very low absolute risk.[8] For this reason, OCs are contraindicated in patients with a history of deep venous thrombosis (Table 77.4).[3,18] Venous thrombosis and pulmonary embolism appear to be directly related to the dose of estrogen.[2,8] Proposed mechanisms include an increase in blood viscosity, adhesiveness of platelets, and levels of clotting factors and fibrinogen, as well as a decrease in antithrombin III activity.[17,28]

Both thrombotic and hemorrhagic stroke are associated with OC use, with 5–10% of OC-associated deaths attributed to stroke.[8] The relative risk is estimated to be 3.1 times the nonuser rate. Cerebrovascular accidents (CVAs) are often preceded by persistent headaches (for weeks or months) and/or by temporary hemiparesis.[14] Patients should be carefully screened and counseled to recognize warning signs of CVAs in order to decrease its risk of occurrence.[8]

Myocardial infarction (MI) primarily occurs in OC users who have additional risk factors for cardiovascular disease.[17,28] Cigarette smoking, advancing age, and OC use is more than cumulative in the risk of MI.[18] Specifically, the relative risk increases in smokers at age 35.[8,29] Myocardial infarction is a rare complication in OC users under 25 years of age even if they smoke.[2,8] Furthermore, OC use is a much less significant risk factor for MI than smoking.[18]

Until recently, OCs were generally not recommended for use in women over the age of 35 because of the potential for cardiovascular disease.[2,19] However, new data indicate that use of OCs containing less than 50 μg of estrogen by healthy, nonsmoking women up to the age of 50 is not associated with an increased risk of serious cardiovascular disease.[2,8] The American College of Obstetricians and Gynecologists states that healthy nonsmoking women 35–44 years of age may continue using OCs. However, OCs should not be used by women with preexisting systemic disease that may affect the cardiovascular system (e.g., hypertension, insulin-dependent diabetes mellitus, hyperlipidemia) or by women over 35 years who smoke.[2,19]

OCs appear to have a protective effect against the development of ovarian and endometrial cancer.[2,18] Not only is the risk for these cancers decreased by 50%, but the beneficial effect is believed to persist for at least 15 years after OC use ceases.[2,5,18]

Based on an exhaustive review of the literature[2] examining the association between OC use and the incidence of breast cancer, the data did not provide sufficient evidence that the long-term use of OCs increases the risk of breast cancer overall or in any specific subgroup of women.[2,30] It is unclear, however, whether OC use increases the risk of cervical cancer. Thus, OC users should receive at least annual cytology screening.[2,30]

Epidemiologic studies have recently documented beneficial health effects from OC use (Table 77.7).[18] Combination OCs provide significant protection against pelvic inflammatory disease (PID) (not including PID caused by *Chlamydia trachomatis*),[3] benign breast disease,[3,31] ovarian cysts (triphasic and low-dose OCs may provide less protection),[3] and ectopic pregnancies.[32] The severity of dysmenorrhea is also decreased among OC users.[5]

CHOICE OF AN ORAL CONTRACEPTIVE

Before prescribing an OC, several issues must be addressed. Are there any contraindications to the use of OCs (Tables 77.4, 77.5, and 77.6)? Does this form of contraception fit the patient's lifestyle, and will the patient be compliant? Are there any other forms of contraception that would be better suited, better tolerated, or more acceptable (Table 77.1)? The advantages and disadvantages of all available forms of contraception should be discussed with the patient to ensure that an informed choice can be made.[8] If OCs are the preferred medication, a specific formulation must be prescribed.[18]

TABLE 77.3. COMPOSITION AND ACTIVITY OF COMMONLY PRESCRIBED ORAL CONTRACEPTIVES[a]

	Composition				Relative Activities			
Product	Estrogen	μg	Progestin	mg	Estrogenic	Progestational	Androgenic	Spotting & BTB[b] (%)
50 μg Estrogen								
Ovral	E. estradiol	50	Norgestrel	0.5	++++	++++	+++	4.5
Norlestrin 2.5/50	E. estradiol	50	Nor. acetate	2.5	+	+++++	++++	5.1
Genora/Norethin/Norinyl/ Ortho-Novum 1/50	Mestranol	50	Norethindrone	1.0	+++	+++	++	10.6
Ovcon 50	E. estradiol	50	Norethindrone	1.0	++++	+++	++	11.9
Demulen 50	E. estradiol	50	Ethy. diacetate	1.0	++	++++	++	13.9
Norlestrin 1/50	E. estradiol	50	Nor. acetate	1.0	+++	+++	+++	13.6
Sub 50 μg Estrogen Monophasic								
Lo-Ovral	E. estradiol	30	Norgestrel	0.3	++	++	++	9.6
Desogen/Ortho-Cept	E. estradiol	30	Desogestrel	0.15	++	++++	+	9.9
Ovcon 35	E. estradiol	35	Norethindrone	0.4	++++	+	+	11.0
Levlen/Nordette/Min-Ovral[c]	E. estradiol	30	Levonorgestrel	0.15	++	++	++	14.0
Ortho-Cyclen	E. estradiol	35	Norgestimate	0.25	+++	+	+	14.3
Brevicon/Modicon/Nelova 0.5/35 Brevicon/Ortho 0.5/35[c]	E. estradiol	35	Norethindrone	0.5	++++	+	+	14.6
Genora/Nelova/Norethin/Norinyl/ Ortho-Novum 1/35 Ortho 1/35[c]	E. estradiol	35	Norethindrone	1.0	+++	+++	++	14.7
Loestrin 1.5/30	E. estradiol	30	Nor. acetate	1.5	+	+++++	+++	25.2
Loestrin/Minestrin[c] 1/20	E. estradiol	20	Nor. acetate	1.0	+	+++	+++	29.7
Demulen 1/35	E. estradiol	35	Ethy. diacetate	1.0	+	++++	++	37.4

Sub 50 μg Estrogen Multiphasic[d]								
Ortho Novum 7/7/7	E. estradiol	35(7)	Norethindrone	0.5(7)	++++	++	++	12.2
	E. estradiol	35(7)	Norethindrone	0.75(7)				
	E. estradiol	35(7)	Norethindrone	1.0(7)				
Jenest	E. estradiol	35(7)	Norethindrone	0.5(7)	+++	++	++	14.1
	E. estradiol	35(14)	Norethindrone	1.0(14)				
Tri-Levlen/TriPhasil	E. estradiol	30(6)	Levonorgestrel	.05(6)	++	+	++	15.1
Triquilar[c]	E. estradiol	40(5)	Levonorgestrel	.075(5)				
	E. estradiol	30(10)	Levonorgestrel	.125(10)				
Tri-Norinyl	E. estradiol	35(7)	Norethindrone	.5(7)	++++	++	++	14.7
Synphasic[c]	E. estradiol	35(7)	Norethindrone	1.0(9)				
	E. estradiol	35(7)	Norethindrone	.5(5)				
Tri-Cyclen	E. estradiol	35(7)	Norgestimate	0.180(7)	+++	+	++	17.5
	E. estradiol	35(7)	Norgestimate	0.215(7)				
	E. estradiol	35(7)	Norgestimate	0.250(7)				
Ortho Novum 10-11	E. estradiol	35(10)	Norethindrone	0.5(10)	++++	++	++	19.6
	E. estradiol	35(11)	Norethindrone	1.0(11)				
Progestin Only								
Ovrette	none		Norgestrel	0.075	—	+	+	34.9
Micronor/Nor Q.D.	none		Norethindrone	0.35	—	+	+	42.3

Key: E. estradiol, ethinyl estradiol; Ethy. diacetate, ethynodiol diacetate; Nor. acetate, norethindrone acetate; BTB, breakthrough bleeding; +, very low; ++, low; +++, moderate; ++++, high; +++++, very high.

[a]Oral contraceptives containing greater than 50 μg of estrogen are not included in this chart. These products are generally not necessary to prevent conception and are associated with an increase in serious complications. Women who may need to use the higher strength estrogen include women who have had a contraceptive failure while *properly* taking a product containing 50 μg of estrogen, women who are concomitantly taking a medication which decreases the efficacy of the estrogen, or in women who have severe acne. The higher dose estrogen products are also used to treat other conditions such as ovarian cysts, endometriosis, and dysfunctional uterine bleeding.

[b]Reported prevalence of breakthrough bleeding (BTB) and spotting in the third cycle of use. Information should not be precisely compared.

[c]Canadian trade name.

[d]Number in parentheses indicates number of tablets (days) in each phase. (Adapted from Dickey RP. Managing Contraceptive Pill Patients, 7th ed. Durant, OK, Essential Medical Information Systems, pp 128–135, 146–147, with permission.

TABLE 77.4. ABSOLUTE CONTRAINDICATIONS TO THE USE OF ORAL CONTRACEPTION

1. Thrombophlebitis, thromboembolic disorders, cerebral vascular disease, coronary occlusion, or a past history of these conditions, or conditions predisposing to these problems.
2. Markedly impaired liver function. Steroid hormones are contraindicated in patients with hepatitis until liver function tests return to normal.
3. Known or suspected breast cancer.
4. Undiagnosed abnormal vaginal bleeding.
5. Known or suspected pregnancy.
6. Smokers over the age of 35.

(From Speroff L, Darney P. A Clinical Guide for Contraception. Baltimore, Williams & Wilkins, 1992, pp 70–71, with permission.)

Most clinicians routinely prescribe a combination OC that possesses hormonal activity equivalent to 50 μg or less of ethinyl estradiol (Table 77.3). This strategy is based on evidence that the most serious side effects of combination OCs (e.g., thromboembolic stroke, MI) result from the OC's estrogen content.[5,8,18,33] The specific biologic activities (i.e., progestational, estrogenic, androgenic) of the currently available products are determined by biologic assay (Table 77.3).[14,18] Endometrial activity, a combination of biologic activities, is related to the ratio of estrogen to progestin and is expressed as a percentage of patients taking the drug who experience spotting or bleeding during the third cycle of OC use.[14,18] High endometrial activity coincides with a low frequency of bleeding (i.e., the lower the number, the higher the activity).[14,18]

Patients may be "sensitive" to the estrogen, progestin, or androgenic effects of OCs. For example, an estrogen-sensitive woman frequently has a history of migraine, heavy menstrual cramps, severe nausea and vomiting during pregnancy, and, occasionally, pregnancy-induced hypertension. These patients may benefit from an OC containing a very low dose of estrogen. However, these patients should be cautioned that spotting may occur, menses may be light or skipped, and missed pills could result in breakthrough ovulation.[18]

A progestin-sensitive woman may have a history of excessive weight gain, tiredness, varicose veins, or toxemia during pregnancy. This patient may benefit from a pill with low progestational activity.[14,18]

Androgenic-sensitive patients may present with a history of irregular, heavy menses. On physical exam, these patients demonstrate oily skin, hirsutism, and acne. Such patients tend to respond better to a pill with high progestational activity and low androgenic activity. A patient with severe acne may benefit from an OC with high estrogenic activity and almost no androgenic activity (e.g., Enovid-E).[18]

There are specific situations where "high"-dose estrogen OCs may be indicated. Women who experience contraceptive failure or who have symptoms of low estrogen content while receiving a 50-μg pill may benefit from a pill with greater estrogenic activity. Patients taking anticonvulsants on a chronic basis have an increased metabolism of estrogen. Although these patients may benefit from an OC containing greater estrogenic activity, other forms of contraception are strongly recommended.[18]

TABLE 77.5. RELATIVE CONTRAINDICATIONS TO THE USE OF OCs REQUIRING CLINICAL JUDGMENT AND INFORMED CONSENT

1. Migraine headaches. In retrospective studies of high-dose pills, migraine headaches have been associated with an increased risk of stroke, however some women report an improvement in their headaches.
2. Hypertension. A woman under 35 who is otherwise healthy and whose blood pressure is controlled by medication can elect to use oral contraception.
3. Uterine leiomyoma. This is no longer a contraindication with the low-dose formulations. There is evidence that the risk of leiomyomas is decreased by 31% in women who used higher dose oral contraception for 10 years.
4. Gestational diabetes. Low-dose formulations do not produce a diabetic glucose tolerance response in women with previous gestational diabetes, and there is no evidence that oral contraception increases the incidence of overt diabetes mellitus. We believe that women with previous gestational diabetes can use oral contraception with annual assessment of the fasting glucose level.
5. Elective surgery. The recommendation that oral contraception should be discontinued 4 weeks before elective surgery to avoid an increased risk of postoperative thrombosis is based on data derived from high-dose pills. If possible, it is safer to follow this recommendation, but it is probably less critical with low-dose oral contraceptives. It is more prudent to maintain contraception right up to the performance of a sterilization procedure, and this short, outpatient operation probably carries very minimal risk.
6. Epilepsy. Oral contraceptives do not exacerbate epilepsy, and in some women, improvement in seizure control has occurred. Antiepileptic drugs, however, may decrease the effectiveness of oral contraception.
7. Obstructive jaundice in pregnancy. Not all patients with this history will develop jaundice on oral contraception, especially with the low-dose formulations.
8. Sickle cell disease or sickle C disease. Patients with sickle cell trait can use oral contraception. The risk of thrombosis in women with sickle cell disease or sickle C diseases is theoretical (and medical-legal). We believe effective protection against pregnancy in these patients warrants the use of low-dose oral contraception.
9. Diabetes mellitus. Effective prevention of pregnancy outweighs the small risk in diabetic women who are under age 35 and otherwise healthy.
10. Gallbladder disease.

(From Speroff L, Darney P. A Clinical Guide for Contraception. Baltimore, Williams & Wilkins, 1992, pp 70–71, with permission.)

TABLE 77.6. OC USE AND MEDICAL PROBLEMS

Gestational Diabetes. There is no contraindication to oral contraceptive use following gestational diabetes.

Diabetes Mellitus. Oral contraception can be used by diabetic women less than 35 years old, who do not smoke and are otherwise healthy (especially an absence of diabetic vascular complications).

Hypertension. Low-dose oral contraception can be used in women less than 35 years old with hypertension controlled by medication, and who are otherwise healthy and do not smoke.

Pregnancy-Induced Hypertension. Women with pregnancy-induced hypertension can use oral contraception as soon as the blood pressure is normal in the postpartum period.

Gallbladder Disease. Oral contraception use may precipitate a symptomatic attack in women known to have stones or a positive history for gallbladder disease, and therefore, should either be used very cautiously or not at all.

Obesity. An obese woman who is otherwise healthy can use low-dose oral contraception.

Hepatic Disease. Oral contraception can be utilized when liver function tests return to normal. Follow-up liver function tests should be obtained after 2–3 months of use.

Seizure Disorders. There is no impact of oral contraceptives on pattern or frequency of seizures; anticonvulsant doses can decrease. The concern is that anticonvulsant-induced hepatic enzyme activity can increase the risk of contraceptive failure. Some clinicians advocate the use of higher dose (50 µg estrogen) products.

Mitral Valve Prolapse. Oral contraception use is limited to patients who have only the echocardiographic diagnosis and are free of the clinical findings of mitral regurgitation.

Systemic Lupus Erythematosus. Oral contraceptive use can exacerbate systemic lupus erythematosus, and the vascular disease associated with lupus represents a contraindication to estrogen-containing oral contraceptives. The progestin-only methods can be considered.

Migraine Headaches. Low-dose oral contraception can be tried with careful surveillance. Daily administration can prevent menstrual migraine headaches.

Sickle Cell Disease. Patients with sickle cell trait can use oral contraception. The risk of thrombosis in women with sickle cell disease or sickle C diseases is theoretical (and medical-legal). We believe effective protection against pregnancy in these patients warrants the use of low-dose oral contraception.

Benign Breast Disease. Benign breast disease is not a contraindication for oral contraception; with 2 years of use, the condition can improve.

Congenital Heart Disease or Valvular Heart Disease. Oral contraception is contraindicated only if there is marginal cardiac reserve or a condition that predisposes to thrombosis.

Hyperlipidemia. Because low-dose oral contraceptives have negligible impact on the lipoprotein profile, hyperlipidemia is not a contraindication, with the exception of very high levels of triglycerides (which can be made worse by oral contraception). Of course, if vascular disease is already present, oral contraception should be avoided.

Depression. Low-dose oral contraceptives have minimal, if any, impact on mood.

Smoking. Oral contraception is absolutely contraindicated in smokers over the age of 35. In patients 35 years old and less, heavy smoking (15 or more cigarettes per day) is a relative contraindication. The data indicate no increased risk of dying of a cardiovascular event in smokers under the age of 30. An ex-smoker should be regarded as a nonsmoker. Risk is only linked to active smoking.

Pituitary Prolactin-Secreting Adenomas. Low-dose oral contraception can be used in the presence of microadenomas.

Infectious Mononucleosis. Oral contraception can be used as long as liver function tests are normal.

Ulcerative Colitis. There is no association between oral contraception and ulcerative colitis; women with this problem can use oral contraceptives. Oral contraceptives are absorbed mainly in the small bowel.

(From Speroff L, Darney P. A Clinical Guide for Contraception. Baltimore, Williams & Wilkins, 1992, pp 80–82, with permission.)

Many symptoms occurring in the first cycle of OC use (e.g., breakthrough bleeding and side effects related to estrogen excess) improve spontaneously by the second or third cycle of use as the body adjusts to the altered hormonal level (Table 77.8).[14] Therefore, initial OC use should be reevaluated during the first 3–6 months of therapy to determine if the patient is experiencing any adverse effects and if the patient wishes to continue medication.[4,14]

If the patient complains of symptoms related to OC use, the first step is to determine if the symptom indicates the presence or potential development of a serious illness (Table 77.9).[14] Any serious symptom requires that the OC be discontinued immediately. Symptoms considered potentially serious may not necessitate the immediate discontinuation of OCs while the patient undergoes evaluation.[14]

Symptoms relating to the estrogen or progestin content of OCs may benefit from adjustments in the pill activity, because nearly all OC-induced side effects parallel the symptoms and physiologic changes of pregnancy (hormone excess) or premenopausal and postmenopausal period (hormone deficiency).[14] OC activity reflects the unique combination of the estrogen and progestin used since progestins can contribute to estrogenic and antiestrogenic activity. For example, if a woman complains of nausea and vomiting while taking an OC (e.g., Ortho Novum 1/35) for longer than 3 months and pregnancy has been ruled out, switching the patient to an OC of lower estrogenic activity (e.g., TriLevlin/Triphasil) may minimize this complaint (Tables 77.3 and 77.8). Also, recommending the patient take the OC with food or at bedtime can minimize nausea and vom-

TABLE 77.7. NONCONTRACEPTIVE BENEFITS OF ORAL CONTRACEPTIVES

Decreased incidence of disease
Pelvic inflammatory disease
Ovarian cancer
Endometrial cancer
Ovarian cysts
Ectopic pregnancy
Fibrocystic breast disease
Premenstrual tension syndrome
Toxic shock syndrome
Anemia
Rheumatoid arthritis
Duodenal ulcer
Significant improvement in menstrual symptoms
Fewer cramps
Less flow for fewer days
More predictable menses
Elimination of mittelschmerz

(Reprinted from the October 1990;42(4) issue of *American Family Physician*, published by the American Academy of Family Physicians, with permission.)

iting.[18] Several handbooks and articles are useful to the practitioner in managing side effects associated with OCs.[3,10,14] These resources provide helpful nonpharmacologic measures, in addition to recommendations on how to alter the hormonal content of the OCs. Furthermore, effective patient education enables the OC user to recognize the difference between the two major types of side effects so that they may receive appropriate medical attention.

DRUG INTERACTIONS

The effectiveness of OCs is sometimes limited by several drug interactions, which may result from a variety of mechanisms, such as interference with gastrointestinal absorption; increased intestinal motility by alteration of gut bacteriologic flora; and alterations in the metabolism, excretion, or binding of the OC.[5,14,34] Several articles reviewing OC drug interactions, with information for the patient, have been published.[10,34,35] Table 77.10 provides a summary of clinically significant drug interactions, including examples of drugs, proposed mechanisms of action, and management.

PATIENT INSTRUCTIONS

The majority of women who take OCs are poorly informed about the proper use of this medication.[18] This represents a unique opportunity for the pharmacist, who is in an ideal position to provide useful information. The patient should first be given the patient package insert (PPI), the product information required for all estrogen products, and be instructed to read it carefully.[3] The written information in the PPI should be supplemented by additional information: (1) This medication works primarily by inhibiting ovulation (stopping the release of the egg from the ovary) and provides no physical barrier to the transmission of sexually transmitted diseases (including acquired immunodeficiency syndrome).[3] (2) The medication is contained in a "compact." "Active" medication is taken for 21 days and the last seven pills are inactive/placebo. Usually, the patient is instructed to take the first table on the first day of the next menses or on the Sunday following the onset of menses (to avoid weekend periods).[5,18] The patient should be instructed to swallow one pill a day until she finishes the pack.[3] Taking the pill at the same time each day promotes consistent plasma concentrations and often increases compliance as administration becomes a routine.[18] The patient should expect her period during the 7 inactive pill days (usually starting within 2 days after taking the last active pill). The patient should expect to start the second pack of pills immediately after finishing a 28-day pack (no days between) and whether or not her period is completed. If a 21-day pack is used, the patient should be instructed to start the new pack 1 week after finishing the previous pack.[3] (3) The patient should be instructed on management strategy for missed pills. If the patient forgets to take one pill, instruct her to take it as soon as she remembers. If she does not remember to take the pill until the next scheduled pill, she may take two pills at once. If the patient misses two pills in a row, she may take two pills for the next 2 days. If the patient misses more than two pills, she should be instructed to call her physician. If the patient misses one or more pills in any given cycle, an additional (barrier) method of contraception should be used for the rest of that cycle. An additional method should be recommended during the first pack of pills and during any time that the patient experiences severe diarrhea or vomiting for several days.[17] (4) Instruct the patient on the recognition of side effects and their management. Although there are often several transient self-limiting side effects, such as breast tenderness, bloating, breakthrough bleeding (BTB) or spotting, nausea, and vomiting, there are pill danger signals that should not be ignored (Table 77.9).[3] If the patient experiences any of these effects (i.e., ACHES, see Table 77.11), she should contact her physician immediately.[3] (5) Instruct the patient about drug interactions. Nonprescription medications are usually no problem; however, some prescription drugs, including certain antibiotics, may decrease OC effectiveness. Instruct the patient to inform her physician or dentist that she is taking an OC. Explain to the patient that if she receives antibiotics, she may need to use an additional method of contraception for the course of antibiotics and the rest of that cycle.

TABLE 77.8. RELATION OF SIDE EFFECTS TO HORMONE CONTENT

Estrogen Excess		Progestin Excess: Progestational	Progestin Excess: Androgenic	Estrogen Deficiency	Progestin Deficiency
General symptoms Cholasma Chronic nasal pharyngitis Gastric influenza and varicella Hay fever and allergic rhinitis Urinary tract infection	**Reproductive system** Breast cystic changes Cervical extrophy Dysmenorrhea Hypermenorrhea, menorrhagia, and clotting Increase in breast size Mucorrhea Uterine enlargement Uterine fibroid growth	**General symptoms** Appetite increase Depression Fatigue, tiredness Hypoglycemia symptoms Libido decrease Neurodermatitis Weight gain (noncyclic) Breast regression	**Androgenic symptoms** Acne Cholestatic jaundice Hirsutism Libido increase Oily skin and scalp Rash and pruritus Edema	Absence of withdrawal bleeding Early or midcycle bleeding and spotting (pill days 1 to 9) Continuous bleeding and spotting Flow decrease, hypomenorrhea Nervousness Pelvic relaxation symptoms Vaginitis atrophic Vasomotor symptoms	Late breakthrough bleeding and spotting (pill days 10 to 21) Delayed withdrawal bleeding Dysmenorrhea (also estrogen excess) Heavy flow and clots (also estrogen excess), hypermenorrhea, menorrhagia
Premenstrual syndrome Bloating Dizziness, syncope Edema Headache (cyclic) Irritability Leg cramps Nausea, vomiting Visual changes (cyclic) Weight gain (cyclic)	**Cardiovascular system** Capillary fragility Cerebrovascular accident Deep vein thrombosis hemiparesis (unilateral weakness and numbness) Telangiectasias Thromboembolic disease Vascular headaches (migraine)	**Cardiovascular symptoms** Hypertension Leg vein dilation			
		Reproductive system Cervicitis Flow length decrease Moniliasis			

(Adapted from Dickey RP. Managing Contraceptive Pill Patients, 7th ed. Durant, OK, Essential Medical Information Systems, 1993, pp 146–147; and Facts and Comparisons. Monthly updates. Nov 1989.)

TABLE 77.9. SYMPTOMS OF A SERIOUS OR POTENTIALLY SERIOUS NATURE

Symptom	Possible Cause
Serious: OCPs Should Be Stopped Immediately	
Loss of vision, proptosis, diplopia, papilledema	Retinal artery thrombosis
Unilateral numbness, weakness, or tingling	Hemorrhagic or thrombotic stroke
Severe pains in chest, left arm, or neck	Myocardial infarction
Hemoptysis	Pulmonary embolism
Severe pains, tenderness or swelling, warmth, or palpable cord in legs	Thrombophlebitis
Slurring of speech	Hemorrhagic or thrombotic stroke
Hepatic mass or tenderness	Liver neoplasm
Potentially Serious: OCPs May Be Continued with Caution While Patient Is Being Evaluated	
Absence of menses	Pregnancy
Spotting or breakthrough bleeding	Cervical, endometrial, or vaginal cancer
Breast mass, pain, or swelling	Breast cancer
Right upper-quadrant pain	Cholecystitis, cholelithiasis, or liver neoplasm
Midepigastric pain	Thrombosis of abdominal artery or vein, myocardial infarction, or pulmonary embolism
Migraine (vascular or throbbing) headache	Vascular spasm which may precede thrombosis
Severe nonvascular headache	Hypertension, vascular spasm
Galactorrhea	Pituitary adenoma
Jaundice, pruritus	Cholestatic jaundice
Depression	Vitamin B_6 deficiency
Uterine size increase	Leiomyomata, adenomyosis, pregnancy

(From Dickey RP. Managing Contraceptive Pill Patients, 7th ed. Durant, OK, Essential Medical Information Systems, 1993, pp 148–149, with permission.)

STOPPING THE OC AND RETURN OF FERTILITY/OCS IN NURSING MOTHERS

The rate of return of fertility is lower for previous users of OCs than for women who have used barrier contraception methods.[3] Eventually, the percentage of women who conceive after stopping OCs becomes the same as for barrier-method users.[36]

Traditionally, women are counseled to allow for two to three normal menstrual periods before becoming pregnant, to permit the reestablishment of menses and ovulation.[3] However, in several cohort and case-controlled studies of large numbers of babies born to women who stopped using the OC, for the infants conceived in the first month after the OC was discontinued, there was no greater chance of the infant being born with a birth defect than for those infants born in the general population.[2,37–39]

Lactation is generally regarded as a relative contraindication to using combination OCs because the hormones in OCs are excreted into breast milk.[8] This contraindication, which was based on earlier formulations containing higher doses of estrogen and progestin, may not apply to current formulations. Estrogens also inhibit the action of prolactin in breast tissue receptors resulting in decreased milk production and protein content.[2] Furthermore, the risk of thromboembolic disease is increased in women prescribed an OC less than 3 weeks after delivery.[16,40] For these reasons, many practitioners recommend formulations containing only a progestin, because this product does not diminish the amount of breast milk and is an effective contraceptive in the mother who is breast feeding.[2]

PROGESTIN-ONLY "MINIPILLS"

Progestin-only agents, although less effective and likely to produce more side effects than combination OCs, may be considered appropriate for nursing mothers and patients with sickle cell hemoglobinopathies.[3,5] Minipills may also be a good choice in patients at risk for estrogen-related side effects (e.g., those with a history of headache, hypertension, or varicose veins)[3]; women who report premenstrual weight gain, nausea, or acne may also benefit.[3,5] Drug administration is always begun on the first day of menses and continued every day.[5] Many women experience a change in their menstrual cycle (e.g., an increase in the number of days of light bleeding).[3]

POSTCOITAL "MORNING-AFTER" PILLS

High doses of various estrogen products are used to prevent pregnancy after unprotected intercourse.[41] It is believed that high-dose estrogens cause almost immediate shedding of the endometrium and prevent implantation of the fertilized

TABLE 77.10. PILL INTERACTIONS WITH OTHER DRUGS

Interacting Drugs	Adverse Effects (Probable Mechanism)	Comments and Recommendations
Acetaminophen (Tylenol and others)	Possible decreased pain-relieving effect (increased metabolism)	Monitor pain-relieving response
Alcohol	Possible increased effect of alcohol	Use with caution
Anticoagulants (oral)	Decreased anticoagulant effect	Use alternative contraceptive
Antidepressants (Elavil, Norpramin, Tofranil, and others)	Possible increased antidepressant effect	Monitor antidepressant concentration
Barbiturates (phenobarbital and others)	Decreased contraceptive effect	Avoid simultaneous use; use alternative contraceptive for epileptics
Benzodiazepine tranquilizers (Ativan, Librium, Serax, Tranxene, Valium, Xanax, and others)	Possible increased or decreased tranquilizer effects including psychomotor impairment	Use with caution Greatest impairment during menstrual pause in oral contraceptive dosage
Beta blockers (Corgard, Inderal, Lopressor, Tenormin)	Possible increased blocker effect	Monitor cardiovascular status
Carbamazepine (Tegretol)	Possible decreased contraceptive effect	Use alternative contraceptive
Corticosteroids (cortisone)	Possible increased corticosteroid toxicity	Clinical significance not established
Griseofulvin (Fulvicin, Grifulvin V, and others)	Decreased contraceptive effect	Use alternative contraceptive
Guanethidine (Esimil, Ismelin)	Decreased guanethidine effect (mechanism not established)	Avoid simultaneous use
Hypoglycemics (Tolbutamide, Diabinese, Orinase, Tolinase)	Possible decreased hypoglycemic effect	Monitor blood glucose
Methyldopa (Aldoclor, Aldomet, and others)	Decreased antihypertensive effect	Avoid simultaneous use
Penicillin	Decreased contraceptive effect with ampicillin	Low but unpredictable incidence; use alternative contraceptive
Phenytoin (Dilantin)	Decreased contraceptive effect Possible increased phenytoin effect	Use alternative contraceptive Monitor phenytoin concentration
Primidone (Mysoline)	Decreased contraceptive effect	Use alternative contraceptive
Rifampin	Decreased contraceptive effect	Use alternative contraceptive
Tetracycline	Decreased contraceptive effect	Use alternative contraceptive
Theophylline (Bronkotabs, Marax, Primatene, Quibron Tedral, Theor-Dur, and others)	Increased theophylline effect	Monitor theophylline concentration
Troleandomycin (TAO)	Jaundice (additive)	Avoid simultaneous use
Vitamin C	Increased serum concentration and possible increased adverse effects of estrogens with 1 g or more per day of vitamin C	Decrease vitamin C to 100 mg/d

(From Hatcher RA, Trussell J, Stewart F, et al. Contraceptive Technology, 16th ed. New York, Irvington, 1994, with permission.)

ovum.[1] Although no drug is currently approved by the Food and Drug Administration (FDA) for this use, Ovral (containing 50 μg of EE and 0.5 mg of norgestrel) is recommended by some practitioners as a "morning-after" pill.[3,41] Ovral has a low failure rate as a morning-after pill when two tablets are taken within 72 hours (preferably within 12–24 hours) after unprotected intercourse and two more tablets are taken 12 hours later or two pills daily for 2 days.[1,3] Begun more than 72 hours after intercourse, the efficacy of this regimen declines, and treatment is totally ineffective by 7 days, when implantation usually occurs.[41] Patients may experience nausea, vomiting, and breast ten-

TABLE 77.11. WHICH ACHES AND PAINS MAY BE WARNINGS OF SERIOUS TROUBLE?

Five Signals	Possible Problem
Abdominal pain (severe)	Gallbladder disease, hepatic adenoma, blood clot, pancreatitis
Chest pain (severe), shortness of breath, or coughing up blood	Blood clot in lungs or myocardial infarction (heart attack)
Headaches (severe)	Stroke or hypertension or migraine headache
Eye problems: blurred vision, flashing lights, or blindness	Stroke or hypertension or temporary vascular problem of many possible sites
Severe leg pain (calf or thigh)	Blood clot in legs

See your clinician if you have any of these problems, or if you develop depression, yellow jaundice, or a breast lump. (From Hatcher RA, Trussell J, Stewart F, et al. Contraceptive Technology, 16th ed. New York, Irvington, 1994, with permission.)

derness with this regimen. Although some clinicians will prescribe antiemetics prophylactically, others will recommend simply repeating the dose if the patient vomits within an hour of taking the pills.[41]

LONG-ACTING INJECTABLE OR IMPLANTABLE PROGESTINS

Steroids are useful for long-term contraception when injected or implanted into the skin. The most commonly used steroids for contraception are progestogens. Sustained progestogen exposure blocks the LH surge, thus preventing ovulation. Should ovulation occur, progestogens reduce ovum motility in the fallopian tubes and, even if fertilization occurs, progestogens thin the endometrium, reducing the chance of implantation. Progestogens also thicken the cervical mucus, producing a barrier for sperm penetration. However, FSH is not intensely suppressed by progestogen-only contraception, therefore, follicular growth and estrogen concentrations, although lower than normal at times, are maintained. Pregnancy failure rates with long-acting progestogen contraception are comparable to female sterilization.[1] These methods of contraception do not offer protection from sexually transmitted diseases, but the thickened cervical mucus may help prevent PID.

MEDROXYPROGESTERONE ACETATE

Medroxyprogesterone is a C21-17 acetoxy-progestogen that is similar in structure to naturally occurring progesterone. Depomedroxyprogesterone acetate (DMPA), 150 mg administered by deep intramuscular (IM) injection in the gluteal or deltoid muscle within 5 days after the onset of menstrual bleeding, inhibits ovulation for over 3 months. The half-life of DMPA is approximately 50 days after IM injection.[42] Peak plasma concentrations (1–7 ng/mL) are reached within 3 weeks, followed by exponentially decreasing concentrations that are undetectable (<100 pg/mL) 120–200 days after injection. Although DMPA 150 mg IM may inhibit ovulation for up to 14 weeks, the dose should be repeated every 3 months to ensure continuous contraception.[43] No apparent weight restrictions apply in women using DMPA.[42] Although two strengths of DMPA are available (Depo-Provera 100 and 400 mg/mL suspensions), the 400 mg/mL concentrated form has inconsistent bioavailability, may be less effective, is more painful, and is not approved for contraception.[3,43]

DMPA can be used in lactating women and may even increase the length of time a woman can breast-feed.[3] Although DMPA is safe postpartum and no adverse effects have occurred in infants exposed to DMPA through breast milk, the manufacturer recommends initiating DMPA at 6 weeks postpartum in women who are breast feeding.[43] DMPA is also safe in women with sickle-cell disease and may reduce the propensity of red blood cell sickling.[44] DMPA does not alter blood pressure nor increase the risk of thromboembolic disorders. DMPA may be used in women with seizure disorders and may even decrease the frequency of seizures.[45] Noncontraceptive benefits observed in women using DMPA include reducing the risk of anemia due to less menstrual blood loss and decreasing the incidence of menstrual cramps and pain at ovulation. The incidence of candida vulvovaginitis, ectopic pregnancy, and PID and the risk of endometrial and ovarian cancer are decreased in women using DMPA for contraception compared to women using no contraception.

Return of fertility may be delayed after discontinuation of DMPA. The median time to conception from the first omitted dose is 6 months.[3] Sixty-eight percent of women will be able to conceive within 12 months, 83% within 15 months, and 93% within 18 months of the last injection. Return to fertility does not appear to be affected by parity or duration of DMPA use.[43]

Menstrual irregularities, including irregular unpredictable spotting or, more rarely, continuous heavy bleeding, are the most frequent adverse effects from DMPA. In some cases, bleeding may be severe enough to cause significant drop in hemoglobin. Women who cannot tolerate prolonged bleeding may benefit from a short course of oral estrogen (i.e., 7 days of 2 mg estradiol or 1.25 mg conjugated estrogen).[16] The incidence of irregular bleeding decreases from 30% in the first year to 10% thereafter (such that most women are amenorrheic after the first year).[1] After 12 months of therapy, 57% of women report amenorrhea with the incidence increasing to 68% after 2 years.

Because estrogen concentrations may be lower than normal in women using DMPA, women can lose some bone density.[46,47] The clinical significance of this bone loss is unknown. Breast tenderness, weight gain, and depression are reported less commonly (<5%). Weight gain averages 1 kg annually and may not resolve until 6–8 months after the last injection.[16,46,48]

Minor elevations in serum total triglycerides and decreases in serum HDL cholesterol have been noted after DMPA exposure.[46] LDL cholesterol and total cholesterol concentrations have been increased in some studies with no change reported in others.[49,50] Carbohydrate metabolism and coagulation factors are not affected.[50,51] The clinical significance of these minor alterations in metabolism is unknown.

Although used in developing countries for decades, DMPA was not approved as a contraceptive in the U.S. market for many years because of a concern about a possible increased incidence of breast cancer.[1] Overall, the risk of breast cancer in women who have used DMPA is 1.0. However, two studies suggest that the risk may be increased in some groups. One study from the World Health Organization found a very slight increased risk in the first 4 years of use but the risk did not increase with longer duration of use.[52,53] Another study found a possible increased risk in women initiating use at an early age.[54] These studies suggest that if any effect exists at all, medroxyprogesterone may enhance the growth of already existing tumors. DMPA was approved for use in the United States as a contraceptive because worldwide data in millions of women showed benefit on maternal mortality and demonstrated other noncontraceptive benefits, outweighing any possible increased risk of breast cancer.

Other side effects are similar to those seen with progestogen-only oral contraceptives. Common side effects (>5%) include abdominal pain or discomfort, asthenia, dizziness, headache, and nervousness.

NORPLANT

The Norplant contraceptive system is a set of six implantable, nonbiodegradable, soft, silicone rubber capsules, each filled with 35 mg of crystalline levonorgestrel. These capsules are inserted just under the skin to provide continuous long-term contraception. Norplant, which was developed by the Population Council and approved for use in the United States in the early 1990s, is estimated to be in use in approximately 1.8 million women worldwide. During clinical trials, the rate of levonorgestrel release reached 85 μg/d and achieved plasma concentrations of 0.4–0.5 ng/d within 24 hours after insertion. The rate of release gradually declined to approximately 30 μg/d over 60 months. Both hard and soft Norplant capsules were used during the trials. The newer soft capsules allowed more levonorgestrel to be released into the blood. Cumulative failure rates were higher among women who used the hard capsules, particularly heavier women. Body weight inversely affected circulating concentrations of levonorgestrel with weight over 70 kg (154 pounds) having the most significant impact over time on lowering concentrations of levonorgestrel. Although Norplant is not recommended for use by women heavier than 154 pounds, the cumulative failure rates through the end of 5 years in heavy women (>154 pounds) using the currently available soft product (2.4%) was significantly less than in those that had the original hard capsules (9.3%).[55] Norplant may be less effective in heavy women in the fourth and fifth years of use.[1] Because the cumulative pregnancy rate in all groups of women significantly increases during the sixth year, Norplant should be replaced after 5 years. A new system can be inserted immediately after removal of the old system.

Similar to other progestin-only methods of contraception, the most common side effect of Norplant is irregular menstrual bleeding that occurs in approximately 60–70% of women during the first year after insertion. Prolonged bleeding can be treated with a short course of estrogen (i.e., 2 mg estradiol or 1.25 mg conjugated estrogen for 7 days).[16] Spotting and bleeding decrease in amount and duration with time. Unlike Depo-Provera, fertility returns quickly after removal of Norplant. Most women return to baseline ovulatory patterns within the first month after removal of the system. Other progesterone-related adverse effects that usually occur in the first year include, headache, depression, nervousness, breast discharge, mastalgia, dizziness, acne, hirsutism, hair loss, changes in appetite, and weight gain. Because of the extremely low concentrations of levonorgestrel released from Norplant system, drugs that significantly increase hepatic enzymes, including most antiseizure medications and rifampin, lower the efficacy of the contraceptive. Ovarian cysts may occur but usually regress spontaneously within 1 month of detection.[16]

Noncontraceptive benefits are similar to Depo-Provera and no clinically significant adverse effects have been observed on carbohydrate metabolism in nondiabetic women, blood coagulation, liver function, lipid metabolism, serum cortisol, renal function or electrolytes.

PERIODIC ABSTINENCE

The avoidance of sexual intercourse during the days of the menstrual cycle when conception is likely to occur may be used by highly motivated couples. Using the abstinence (rhythm) method, women rely on physiologic changes, such as basal body temperature and cervical mucus, during each cycle to determine the fertile period. The major reasons for lack of acceptance are the relatively high pregnancy rates among users and the need to avoid intercourse for several days during each menstrual cycle. To overcome these drawbacks, many women use barrier methods or spermicides during the fertile period.[2,56]

Barrier Techniques and Spermicides

The effectiveness of barrier methods and spermicides depends almost exclusively on a couple's motivation to use them consistently and correctly. These methods include the diaphragm, cervical cap, sponge, condom, and spermicide.[17] Besides contraception, an advantage to using these methods is that they can reduce the rate of transmission of sexually transmitted diseases.[2]

The diaphragm, a reusable dome-shaped rubber cap with a flexible rim, is inserted vaginally and fits over the cervix in order to decrease access to sperm. The diaphragm is available in 11 sizes and requires a prescription from a physician who has fitted the patient for the correct size.[16,57] The effectiveness of the diaphragm depends on its function as a barrier and the spermicidal cream or jelly placed in the diaphragm before insertion.[2] The diaphragm may be inserted as long as 6 hours before intercourse and must be left in place for at least 6 hours after intercourse.[17] If intercourse occurs more than once within 6 hours, the patient must not remove the diaphragm, but rather insert more spermicide and wear the diaphragm for 6 hours after subsequent acts of intercourse or use a condom.[3] Contraindications to the diaphragm are listed in Table 77.1. Users of diaphragms appear to have a lower incidence of cervical neoplasia, which may be attributed to the adjunctive spermicide and the diaphragm's barrier effect against the human papillomavirus.[4] Diaphragm use has also been associated with an increased incidence of urinary tract and yeast infections.[4]

The Prentif cervical cap is a soft, deep, rubber cup with a firm round rim smaller than a diaphragm that fits over the cervix like a thimble.[1,3] Spermicide, used to fill the cap one-third full prior to insertion, is held in place against the cervix until removed.[3] The cap remains effective for more than one episode (up to 48 hours) of intercourse without adding more spermicide and is less messy to use than a diaphragm; it may not be possible because of the limited number of sizes, however, to fit some women with this device.[1,3] It is recommended that women not wear the cap for longer than 48 hours, to reduce the possible risk of toxic shock syndrome.[3]

The vaginal contraceptive sponge (Today), which contains the spermicide nonoxynol-9, is no longer available in the United States because the only manufacturer discontinued production in early 1995.[1,17]

Condoms are devices that create a mechanical barrier, preventing direct contact with semen, genital lesions and discharges, and infectious secretions.[1,3] Most U.S. condoms are made of latex rubber, which is impermeable to viruses; a small proportion (5%), however, is made from young lamb intestine, which is not.[1,3] Condoms are used worldwide as protection from sexually transmitted diseases. When used in conjunction with any other barrier methods, their effectiveness theoretically approaches 95%.[3,17] Spillage of semen or perforation and tearing of the condom can occur, but can be minimized with proper use.[16,57,58] Mineral oil-based lotions or lubricants can decrease the barrier strength of latex by 90% in just 60 seconds; thus making water-soluble lubricants preferable.[1] A condom for women (Reality) was approved in April 1993, by the FDA and appears to be as effective as the diaphragm in preventing pregnancy.[59] The female condom is a prelubricated, soft, loose fitting polyurethane sheath, closed at one end, with flexible rings at both ends. Properly positioned, the ring at the closed end covers the cervix, and the sheath lines the walls of the vagina. The outer ring remains outside the vagina, covering the labia; this may make it more effective than the male condom in preventing transmission of diseases such as herpes because it protects the labia from coming in contact with the base of the penis.[59] The manufacturer reports a use-effective pregnancy rate of 26% per year, based on a 6-month follow-up study of 200 women.[4]

Spermicides, most of which contain nonoxynol-9, are chemical surfactants that destroy sperm cell walls and offer some protection against sexually transmitted diseases and cervical cancer.[1] Spermicides are available as foams, creams, suppositories, jellies, and film.[2] Use of spermicidal foam requires that the can be shaken well to disperse the spermicide before use. Spermicidal tablets or suppositories require 10–30 minutes to dissolve.[1] Spermicides can cause local irritation in both men and women. Additional spermicide must be used each time intercourse is repeated.[1]

Intrauterine Devices

Intrauterine devices (IUDs) create a hostile endometrium environment through low-grade intrauterine inflammation and increased prostaglandin formation. These effects interfere with the implantation of the fertilized ovum.[16,60] The IUD has several contraindications as listed in Table 77.1. The risk of PID among IUD users compared to nonusers ranges from 1–2.5%.[4] The increase in risk appears to be related to the introduction of bacteria into the genital tract during IUD insertion. Therefore, the risk of infection is highest during the first 20 days after the procedure.[1] Ideal patients for IUD use include parous, monogamous women, who are not at risk for PID.[4] Two IUDs are currently marketed in the United States; both are shaped like a "T" and are medicated, one with copper (ParaGard) and the other with progesterone (Progestasert). ParaGard provides better contraceptive effectiveness than previous copper devices and can be left in place for 10 years.[1,4] A disadvantage of Progestasert is that it must be replaced annually, but it has been associated with less blood loss during menstruation and less dysmenorrhea.[1]

An IUD containing levonorgestrel is available outside the United States. This IUD releases levonorgestrel at a constant rate of 20 μg/d for up to 5 years. At this dosage, systemic hormonal effects are decreased.[3]

THERAPEUTIC OUTCOME

If used correctly, the typical use failure rates for some of the commonly used methods of reversible contraception are as follows: OCs (3%), long-acting injectable (0.3%) or implantable (0.09%) progestins, male condoms (12%), spermicide alone (21%), diaphragm with spermicide (18%), periodic abstinence (20%), and the IUD (i.e., progesterone [0.2%] or copper [0.8%]).[1,3] These percentages reflect the percent of accidental pregnancy during the first year of use.

CONCLUSION

Choosing a contraceptive method most suited to the patient's needs will significantly reduce the chance of pregnancy. Information from a medical and sexual history and a thorough physical exam are essential when evaluating the various available methods. Understanding the risks and contraindications is essential for both the patient and prescriber. Table 77.1 compares and contrasts the available methods. Both verbal and written instructions concerning the chosen method should be given to the patient, and follow-up appointments can increase compliance and allow time for the patient to ask questions.[4]

REFERENCES

1. Anonymous. Choice of contraceptives. Med Lett Drug Ther 1995;37:9–12.
2. Mishell DR. Contraception. N Engl J Med 1989;320(12): 777–785.
3. Hatcher RA, Trussell J, Stewart F, et al. Contraceptive Technology, 16th ed. New York, Irvington, 1994.
4. Heath CB. Helping patients choose appropriate contraception. Am Fam Physician 1993;48:1115–1124.
5. Gearhart JG, Phillips DM. Choosing an oral contraceptive. Fam Pract Recert 1989;11(3):65–77.
6. Baird DT, Glasier AF. Hormonal contraception. N Engl J Med 1993;328:1543–1548.
7. Duchin SE, Ledger WJ, Schulze RJ, Speroff L. OCs: Risks, benefits, guidelines. Patient Care 1989;March 30:89–111.
8. ACOG Technical Bulletin. Oral contraception. 1987;106:1–6.
9. Kelley HW, Miles PA, Buster JE, Scragg WH. Adenocarcinoma of the endometrium in women taking sequential oral contraceptives. Obstet Gynecol 1976;47(2):200–202.
10. Smith MA, Youngkin EQ. Current perspectives on combination oral contraceptives. Clin Pharm 1984;3:485–496.
11. Connell EB. Oral contraception, in Kase NK, Weingold AB (eds): Principles and Practice of Clinical Gynecology. New York, John Wiley & Sons, 1983, p 1007.
12. Guillebaud J. The Pill, 3rd ed. Oxford, Oxford University Press, 1984.
13. Tayob Y, Adams J, Jacobs HS, Guillebaud J. Ultrasound demonstration of increased frequency of functional ovarian cysts in women using progestogen-only oral contraception. Br J Obstet Gynecol 1985;92(10):1003–1009.
14. Dickey RP. Managing Contraceptive Pill Patients, 7th ed. Durant, OK, Creative Informatics, 1993.
15. Ruggiero RJ. Contraception, in Applied Therapeutics. The Clinical Use of Drugs, 5th ed. Applied Therapeutics, 1992, p 67–3.
16. Speroff L, Darney P. A clinical guide for contraception. Baltimore, Williams & Wilkins, 1992.
17. Gearhart JG, Phillips DM. Choosing a method of contraception: Perceptions, risks and benefits. Fam Pract Recert 1989;11(2):24–36.
18. Wall DM, Roos MP. Update on combination oral contraceptives. Am Fam Physician 1990;42(4):1037–1048.
19. Check WA. Conference highlights trends and controversies in oral contraceptive use. Clin Pharm 1989;8:752–760.
20. Kalkhoff RK. Relative sensitivity of postpartum gestational diabetic women to oral contraceptive agents and other metabolic stress. Diabetes Care 1980;3:421–424.
21. Perlman JA, Russell-Briefel R, Ezzati T, Lieberknecht G. Oral glucose tolerance and the potency of contraceptive progestins. J Chronic Dis 1985;38:857–864.
22. Van der Vange N, Kloosterboer HJ, Haspels AA. Effect of seven low-dose combined oral contraceptive preparations on carbohydrate metabolism. Am J Obstet Gynecol 1987;156:918–922.
23. Kung AW, Ma JT, Wong VC, et al. Glucose and lipid metabolism with triphasic oral contraceptives in women with a history of gestational diabetes. Contraception 1987;35:257–269.
24. Skouby SO, Kuhl C, Molsted-Pedersen K, Christensen MS. Triphasic oral contraception: Metabolic effects in normal women and those with previous gestational diabetes. Am J Obstet Gynecol 1985;153:495–500.
25. Kloosterboer HJ, van Wayjen RG, van den Ende A. Comparative effects of monophasic desogestrel plus ethinyloestradiol and triphasic levonorgestrel plus ethinyloestradiol on lipid metabolism. Contraception 1986;34:135–144.
26. Percival-Smith RK, Morrison BJ, Sizto R, Abercrombie E. The effect of triphasic and biphasic oral contraceptive preparations on HDL-cholesterol and LDL-cholesterol in young women. Contraception 1987;35:179–187.
27. Kay CR. Progestogens and arterial disease—evidence from the Royal College of General Practitioners' study. Am J Obstet Gynecol 1982;142:762–765.
28. Connell EB. Oral contraceptives. The current risk–benefit ratio. J Reprod Med 1984;29(suppl 7):513–523.
29. Slone D, Shapiro S, Kaufman DW, et al. Risk of myocardial infarction in relation to current and discontinued use of oral contraceptives. N Engl J Med 1981;305(8):420–424.
30. Mishell DR. Oral contraception 1990: Taking stock. Dialog Contraception 1990;3(1)1–6.
31. Hulka BS. Oral contraceptive use and risk of endometrial, ovarian, and breast cancer. Centers for Disease Control cancer and steroid hormone study. JAMA 1983;249:1600.
32. Derman R. Oral contraceptives: Assessment of benefits. J Reprod Med 1986;31:879–886.

33. Gearhart JG, Phillips DM. The female reproductive system, in Taylor RD (ed). Family Medicine: Principles and Practice, 3rd ed. New York, Springer-Verlag, 1988.
34. D'Arcy PF. Drug interactions with oral contraceptives. Drug Intell Clin Pharm 1986;20:353–362.
35. Stoehr GP, White J. Managing drug interactions with oral contraceptives. J Obstet Gynecol Nurs 1983;12:327–332.
36. Vessey MP, Lawless M, McPherson K, Yeates D. Fertility after stopping use of intrauterine contraceptive device. Br Med J 1983;286:106.
37. Rothman KJ, Louik C. Oral contraceptives and birth defects. N Engl J Med 1978;299:522–524.
38. Janerich DT, Piper JM, Glebatis DM. Oral contraceptives and birth defects. Am J Epidemiol 1980;112:73–79.
39. Harlap S, Shiono PH, Ramcharan S. Congenital abnormalities in the offspring of women who use oral and other contraceptives around the time of conception. Int J Fertil 1985;30:39–47.
40. American Academy of Pediatrics Committee on Drugs. Transfer of drugs and other chemicals into human milk. 1989;84(5):924–936.
41. Anonymous. Ovral as a "morning-after" contraceptive. Med Lett Drug Ther 1989;31:93–94.
42. Depo-Provera Contraception Injection package information. Kalamazoo, MI, Upjohn, December 1992.
43. American Health Consultants Depo Provera Update: Not FDA-approved, but experts recommend Depo-Provera. Contracept Tech Update 1992;13:1–20.
44. Kaunitz AM. Injectable contraception. Clin Obstet Gynecol 1989;32(2):356–368.
45. Mattson RH, Rebar RN. Contraceptive methods for women with neurologic disorders. Am J Obstet Gynecol 1993;168:2027–2032.
46. Olin BR, ed. Drug Facts and Comparions. St. Louis, MO, JB Lippincott, 1993, pp 108n–108p.
47. Cundy T, Evans M, Roberts H, et al. Bone density in women receiving depot medroxyprogesterone acetate for contraception. Br Med J 1991;303:13–16.
48. Nash HA. Depo Provera: A review. Contraception 1975;12:377–393.
49. Garza-flores J, De la Cruz DL, Valles de Bouges V, et al. Long-term effects of depo-medroxyprogesterone acetate on lipoprotein metabolism. Contraception 1991;44:61–71.
50. Fahmy K, Khairy M, Allam G, et al. Effects of depo-medroxyprogesterone acetate on coagulation factors and serum lipids in Egyptian women. Contraception 1991;44:431.
51. Fahmy K, Abdel-Razik M, Shaaraway M, et al. Effects of long acting progestagen-only injectable contraceptives on carbohydrate metabolism and hormonal profile. Contraception 1991;44:419–430.
52. WHO Collaborative Study of Neoplasia and Steroid contraceptives. Breast-cancer and depot-medroxyprogesterone acetate: A multinational study. Lancet 1991;338:833–838.
53. Bonhomme MG, Potts DM, Fortnry JA, Allen MY. Safety of depot medroxyprogesterone acetate [letter]. Lancet 1991;338:942.
54. Paul C, Skegg DCG, Spears GFS. Depot medroxyprogesterone (Depo-Provera) and risk of breast cancer. Br Med J 1989;299:759–762.
55. Sivin I. International experience with Norplant and Norplant II. Contraception 1988;19:81–94.
56. Zinaman MJ. Why you should know about natural family planning. Contemp Ob/Gyn Special Issue: Fertility 1988;69–86.
57. Heaton CJ, Smith MA. The diaphragm. Am Fam Physician 1989;39(5):231–236.
58. Anonymous. Can you rely on condoms? Consumer Reports, March 1989.
59. Anonymous. The Female Condom. Med Lett 1993;35:123–124.
60. The intrauterine device. ACOG Technical Bulletin. May 1987.

Chapter 78

Premenstrual Syndrome

Martha P. Fankhauser, MS

Menstrual cycle-linked mood and physical symptoms are commonly experienced by women during their reproductive years.[1] *Dysmenorrhea* (painful or difficult menstruation) usually begins at menarche and is associated with painful cramps and backache at the onset of menses. *Premenstrual molimina* describes the common physical symptoms of breast tenderness and bloating.[2] Approximately 75% of women experience one or more physical symptoms just before or during menses.[3] Women with changes in mood have been described as having *premenstrual tension* or *premenstrual syndrome* (PMS). PMS is the cyclic recurrence (during the luteal phase of the menstrual cycle) of a combination of psychologic, behavior, and physical symptoms that cause dysfunctioning or interference with normal activities (Table 78.1).[1]

A subtype of PMS called *late luteal phase dysphoric disorder* (LLPDD) was recently renamed *premenstrual dysphoric disorder* (PMDD).[3] The essential features of PMDD include marked depression, anxiety, liability of mood, and irritability that are comparable to the severity of having a major depressive episode. The diagnosis requires at least five symptoms (including at least one of the mood/anxiety changes) to be present for most of the time during the past year. The symptoms must occur during the last week of the luteal phase, decline in severity within a few days after the onset of menses, and be absent in the week postmenses. The diagnosis of PMDD requires marked impairment in social or occupational functioning and is considered to be a severe subtype of PMS.

Prevalence and Clinical Course

Dysmenorrhea is one of the most common gynecologic problems in postpubescent women and occurs during ovulatory cycles. The prevalence of dysmenorrhea increases from early to late adolescence and decreases after age 30–35. Approximately 40–50% of women have painful menstrual cramps and up to 10% have impaired functioning for 1–3 days per month (missing work or school due to pain). Dysmenorrhea may be "primary" (or idiopathic), which occurs during ovulatory cycles, or "secondary" to some type of pelvic pathology (e.g., intrauterine devices, endometriosis, pelvic inflammatory disease [PID], ovarian cyst, endometrial cancer, adhesions, and benign uterine tumors). Symptoms of dysmenorrhea are similar to PID and ectopic pregnancy, which are serious or life-threatening conditions; thus, a physician should rule out the presence of secondary causes of dysmenorrhea.

Differences in premenstrual symptoms between age groups have been reported. The severity of symptoms has been correlated with parity, ovulation, length and regularity of the menstrual cycle, and the intensity and duration of menstrual flow.[3] Dysmenorrhea and irritability are more common in younger women, whereas edema, depression, and pain from endometriosis are more common in the later reproductive years.[1] As ovarian hormones decline during the perimenopausal phase and ovulation ceases, premenstrual symptoms will disappear. Premenstrual symptoms may continue after a hysterectomy if the ovaries are left intact, but should cease after a bilateral oophorectomy (removal of the ovaries), after the administration of ovulation-suppressing drugs, and during pregnancy.[1]

Depending on the criteria and population studied, approximately 20–50% of women experience moderate premenstrual symptoms with 3% to 5% having such severe symptoms (i.e., meeting the diagnostic criteria for PMDD) that functioning is significantly affected.[3] Women with recurrent major depressive disorder or bipolar I or II disorder (or a family history of mood disorders) have increased risk for premenstrual dysphoria. Postpartum depression, mania, or psychosis, and previous mood and/or anxiety disorders have been associated with PMDD.[3] Severe premenstrual behavior has resulted in marital discord, physical and verbal abuse of others, difficulties in parenting, criminal behavior, poor work or school performance, work absenteeism, social isolation, accidents, hospitalizations, suicide, and homicide.[1–4]

Pathophysiology

Several biologic, psychologic, cognitive, and social theories have been proposed for PMS, but there are no definite con-

TABLE 78.1. CHARACTERISTICS OF DYSMENORRHEA AND PREMENSTRUAL SYNDROME

Dysmenorrhea	Premenstrual Syndrome
40–50% occurrence	20–50% occurrence; 3–5% have severe type
Starts at menarche	May start at teens to late 20s
Occurs a few days before menses with peak intensity during menstrual flow	Occurs 4–14 days before menses and stops by 4 days into the menstrual phase
Decreases with parity	Increases with parity
Decreases with age	Increases with age and ceases at menopause
Physical symptoms: cramps, backache, headache	Multiple symptoms: emotional, behavioral, physical
Etiology: prostaglandins	Etiology: unknown, with multiple theories
Treated: NSAIDs	Treated: target symptom approach; antidepressants for PMDD

clusions regarding its etiology.[1,4–6] Premenstrual changes in behavior, eating habits, and sexual activity occur in other mammalian species that have cyclical changes in estrogen and progesterone levels. The occurrence of premenstrual physical and psychological symptoms is closely linked to the rise and fall of gonadotropin and ovarian hormones, neurotransmitters, and prostaglandins during the menstrual cycle.

The menstrual cycle is a complex and rapidly changing biological process that involves the hypothalamus, pituitary, and ovaries.[6,7] The hypothalamus produces gonadotropin-releasing hormone (GnRH), a neurohormone that regulates the release of luteinizing hormone (LH) and follicle-stimulating hormone (FSH) from the anterior pituitary. GnRH must be released in the correct amounts and at the right pulse rate to stimulate gonadotropin secretion and to cause ovulation.

Release of GnRH is regulated by positive and negative feedback effects from other neurotransmitters (e.g., norepinephrine [NE], dopamine [DA], serotonin [5-HT], and endorphins) and by LH, FSH, and ovarian hormones.[6,7] NE and 5-HT promote GnRH secretion, whereas DA inhibits it. Endogenous opiates (produced by the anterior pituitary) decrease FSH and LH by inhibiting GnRH in the hypothalamus. When opiate receptors are blocked (by opiate antagonists such as naltrexone), GnRH pulses occur more frequently and at higher amplitudes. Continuous activation of GnRH pituitary receptors may eventually cause a desensitization of the receptors, which decreases gonadotropin secretion and shuts down reproductive functioning. GnRH release is mediated by the amines (NE and 5-HT) and its pulsating pattern is modified by the endorphins and gonadal steroids.

Gonadotropin-releasing hormone agonists (GnRH-As) cause a dramatic decrease in both the physical and behavioral symptoms of PMS due to the down-regulation of FSH and LH.[7] GnRH-As have been used to inhibit ovulation in severe PMS (described as a medical ovariectomy or pseudo-menopausal state). Medications that suppress ovulation (e.g., estradiol implants, danazol) have been reported to be effective in PMS. Postmenopausal women who receive sequential estrogen and progesterone replacement therapy (e.g., estrogen for days 1–25 and progesterone from days 10–25) may have cyclical changes in their mood and physical symptoms that resemble PMS. Postmenopausal women receiving estrogen-only or continuous estrogen and progesterone therapy usually have fewer mood changes or physical complaints.

GONADAL HORMONES

The relationship between premenstrual symptoms and the absolute levels of ovarian steroid hormones and their metabolites during the luteal phase has yielded contradictory results.[7] Early PMS research focused on a progesterone-deficiency theory, but several studies have found no difference in progesterone levels during the menstrual cycle in women with or without PMS.[8,9] The beginning of premenstrual symptoms parallels the postovulatory rise in progesterone levels, but the highest severity of symptoms occur 5–6 days after the peak of progesterone levels.[7] When estrogen levels peak during the preovulatory phase, women feel better and have minimal symptoms.

The rate of decline in gonadal hormones during the late luteal phase has been proposed as being more important in causing symptoms than absolute basal values.[7,10] There is some evidence that perimenopausal declines in estrogen and progesterone may play an important role in the pathogenesis of PMS. The gradual progressive loss of ovarian function during the reproductive years until menopause may be responsible for the physical and psychologic symptoms observed with PMS.

NEUROTRANSMITTERS/NEUROPEPTIDES

Women have an increased susceptibility for mood disorders, thus, a biologic hypothesis has been proposed that there may be a link between the hypothalamic–pituitary–gonadal (HPG) axis, female sex hormones, and affective disorders.[11,12] The brain contains receptors for several steroid hormones (e.g., estrogen, progestins, androgens, glucocorticoids, mineralocorticoids) that regulate numerous biologic functions. The activity of neurotransmitters and peptides (e.g., 5-HT, melatonin, DA, endogenous opiates) parallels the gonadal hormonal fluctuations and is involved in the feedback regulation of the ovulatory cycle.[7] 5-HT, an inhibitory neurotransmitter, has a reciprocal relationship with the gonadal hormones and inhibits DA activity. DA, a direct inhibitor of prolactin secretion, may be involved in the regulation of prolactin, which peaks at midcycle and during the luteal phase if ovulation occurs. Changes in DA activity may cause psychotic symptoms (e.g., delusions, hallucinations) in some women prior to menses.[7]

A 5-HT deficiency theory has been proposed as causing depression and premenstrual dysphoria.[11] Decreased serotonergic activity has been associated with depressed mood, irritability, anxiety, impulsivity, aggression, and increased appetite.[13] Platelet uptake of 5-HT (a model for measuring serotonergic activity) has been reported to be decreased in patients with depression and during the week before menstruation among women with PMS. Lower platelet content of 5-HT, lower whole-blood 5-HT concentrations, and lower levels of melatonin (a metabolite of 5-HT) during the luteal phase have been reported in women with PMS compared to normal controls.[13] Deficiencies of the serotonergic system may help to explain the similarities in mood and behaviors for both depression and PMDD (e.g., feeling hopeless and helpless, decreased interest in activities, fatigue, sleep disturbances, appetite changes).

Changes in the monoamine turnover and metabolism during the menstrual cycle may influence behavior, mood, and physical well-being.[7] Monoamines such as 5-HT and NE are metabolized by monoamine oxidase (MAO) and by catechol-o-methyltransferase (COMT), which decreases the amount available for neural transmission. In animal models, the activity of MAO and COMT is decreased by estradiol and increased by progesterone; thus, there may be a link between monoamine activity and ovarian steroids.[7] MAO inhibitors (MAOIs) inhibit the MAO enzyme and prolong the activity of monamines. Tricyclic antidepressants (TCAs) block the reuptake of 5-HT and NE into the presynaptic neuron, which increases the amount available for neurotransmission. Both MAOIs and TCAs are effective agents for the treatment of depression. Selective serotonin reuptake inhibitors (SSRIs) inhibit the reuptake of 5-HT and show promise in the treatment of PMDD. The strong relationship between 5-HT deficiency, depression, and premenstrual dysphoria suggests that the serotonergic system plays an important role in the mood changes associated with PMDD.[13]

The hormonal feedback system that controls neuroendocrine balance is extremely complex and may be vulnerable to psychosocial and environmental stresses. The interaction between sex hormones, neurotransmitters, and other neuromodulators is no doubt involved in female-specific mood disorders such as postpartum depression, oral contraceptive-induced depression, and perimenopausal mood disorders.[11,12]

OTHER HORMONES/PEPTIDES

Several biologic markers (e.g., prolactin, melatonin, opiate peptides, cortisol response to dexamethasone, thyroid-stimulating hormone response to thyrotropin-releasing hormone, platelet MAO levels) fluctuate during the menstrual cycle, but so far none has definitively differentiated women with and without PMS. Interpretations of the absolute levels of hormones, neurotransmitters, and neuropeptides is difficult because of variations in sampling time, diurnal changes in levels, effect of stress on neuroendocrine functioning, and normal fluctuations during the menstrual cycle.[14,15]

DIAGNOSIS AND ASSESSMENT

More than 100 different symptoms have been associated with PMS.[5] Several PMS symptoms (e.g., anger, irritability, anxiety, tension, depression, or mood swings) overlap with psychiatric disorders, particularly anxiety and affective disorders.[16] Approximately 50% of women with PMS complaints may have an underlying mood disorder and meet the criteria for a concurrent PMDD diagnosis.[3] Premenstrual exacerbations of underlying disorders (anxiety, panic, depression, bulimia, drug and alcohol abuse, migraine headaches, seizures, and herpes) have been reported and should not be confused with PMS.[3]

PMS diagnosis can be difficult because core symptoms differ from woman to woman and may vary in type and intensity between menstrual cycles.[5] The most common pattern of PMS is a gradual increase in symptoms during the week prior to menses, a peak just before the onset of menses, and a rapid decline in symptoms over the first 4 days after the onset of menses. Other atypical pattern subtypes of PMS include (1) a gradual worsening of symptoms during the late luteal phase that persists into the early follicular phase of the next cycle, (2) a brief episode at ovulation followed by a symptom-free period and a recurrence of symptoms during the late luteal phase, and (3) continual PMS symptoms from ovulation until after menses ceases. Women with a normal 28-day menstrual cycle are usually symptom-free for 2–3 weeks; women with shorter menstrual cycles may be symptom-free for only 1 week during the cycle.[3]

Some women experience positive changes premenstrually such as increased energy and productivity. The majority of women have negative premenstrual changes, such as disrupted sleep, fatigue, and food cravings. Physical changes usually occur a few days before menstruation (back pain, breast tenderness, headaches, water retention, and bloating sensations in the abdomen), but are not as bothersome as the emotional and behavioral changes. The most distressing PMS symptoms include irritability, depression, fatigue, tension, and mood swings.[17] Women with PMS often complain of labile mood, anger attacks, feeling out of control, oversensitivity, crying episodes, difficulty concentrating, impaired reasoning, clumsiness, and a craving for sweet or salty foods.[1,2] In the climacteric phase preceding menopause (ages 35–50 years), women frequently report sleep disturbance, hot flashes, anxiety attacks, depression, and decreased short-term memory.

The evaluation of PMS should include the family history of PMS and affective disorders; an assessment of the patient's menstrual, obstetric, and gynecologic history; and a complete drug history (caffeine, alcohol, nicotine, drugs of abuse, prescription and nonprescription drugs).[17,18] Oral contraceptives and estrogen/progesterone sequential replacement therapy may cause the same symptoms as PMS. Self-medication with alcohol, marijuana, or caffeine can exacerbate or obscure the PMS symptoms.

No diagnostic laboratory tests are available for PMS. Depending on the patient's presenting complaints, laboratory tests and a physical examination (including a pelvic exam) may be necessary to rule out medical problems (e.g., hypoglycemia, hypothyroidism, anemia, endometriosis, ovarian cysts, hyperprolactinemia, infections).[19] Hormonal and vitamin level tests (e.g., vitamins B_6 and B_{12}, magnesium, estradiol, progesterone, prolactin, testosterone, FSH, LH) are expensive and are not helpful in establishing the diagnosis.[19] Women in their forties to fifties, may be perimenopausal, and a serum FSH level is recommended to rule out estrogen deficiency. Subclinical hypothyroidism or autoimmune thyroiditis should be ruled out because hypothalamic–pituitary–thyroid axis dysfunction has been associated with mood and behavioral changes that are similar to PMS.

The most important diagnostic approach is the prospective daily charting of PMS symptoms for a minimum of two menstrual cycles. The use of a standardized, reliable, and valid PMS rating scale is critical for an accurate diagnosis.[2] Several PMS self-rating scales are available and include the 47-item Menstrual Distress Questionnaire (MDQ),[20] the Premenstrual Distress Questionnaire (PDQ),[21] the 20-item Daily Rating Form (DRF) scale developed from the retrospective 95-item Premenstrual Assessment Form (PAF),[22] the Calendar of Premenstrual Experiences (COPE),[23] and the Prospective Record of the Impact and Severity of Menstrual Symptoms (PRISM) calendar.[1] Daily charting helps to identify symptoms and quantify their severity so that individualized treatment approaches can be selected. In addition, daily basal body temperatures are helpful to determine when ovulation occurs and morning/evening weights help to monitor fluid retention.

The diagnosis of PMS requires that symptoms (1) appear or change in severity during the luteal phase compared with the follicular phase of the menstrual cycle, and (2) disappear or return to baseline shortly after the onset of menses or during the full flow of menses. In 1983, the National Institute of Mental Health (NIMH) recommended that the diagnosis of PMS be made only when the severity scores for symptoms change by at least 30% during the luteal phase (6–7 days prior to the onset of menses) compared with the follicular phase (6–7 days after the cessation of menstruation) for at least two consecutive menstrual cycles.[24]

PMS Treatment Approaches

A wide variety of pharmacologic and nonpharmacologic treatments are available for PMS (Table 78.2).[15,16,18] Treatment approaches for PMS are usually tailored to the primary symptom complaints (or target symptoms) after a prospective 2- to 3-month menstrual cycle assessment. The goal of PMS treatment is to minimize symptoms and improve functioning and well-being without causing adverse effects.

FIRST-LINE APPROACHES

Education and Counseling

Education and supportive counseling are considered first-line approaches to help women cope with PMS symptoms. Individual and group psychotherapy, couples or family counseling, cognitive behavioral approaches, and PMS support groups are often beneficial.[17] Stress reduction techniques (biofeedback, relaxation therapy, meditation, yoga, body massages), learning to effectively recognize and handle stress, and assertiveness training are important tools women need for living with PMS.[25]

Nutrition and Exercise

An initial treatment approach for most women with PMS is a well-balanced diet (including the reduction of refined sugar, foods high in sodium, caffeine-containing beverages, and methylxanthine-containing foods such as chocolate) combined with a regimen of regular exercise.[26] Conditioning exercise (aerobics, running, swimming, and bicycling) has been shown to reduce premenstrual fluid retention and breast symptoms.[27] Eating smaller and more frequent meals high in complex carbohydrates and protein and low in simple sugars often helps "hypoglycemia-like" episodes and food cravings. Increased caffeine consumption is associated with higher PMS rates.[28] Caffeine may cause sleep disturbances, irritability, and nervousness and is associated with breast tenderness and swelling (or fibrocystic breast disease). Premenstrual craving of salty foods may be related to fluid retention, bloating, edema, and weight gain. Women should be encouraged to reduce or discontinue alcohol intake, nicotine use, and drugs of abuse because these contribute to unhealthy lifestyles and negatively impact physical and mental health.

Sleep Hygiene

Severe insomnia or fatigue can significantly affect daily functioning. A woman with PMS may wake up during the

TABLE 78.2. TREATMENT APPROACHES FOR PREMENSTRUAL SYNDROME

First-line Approaches
Nonpharmacologic
- Education and counseling
- Stress reduction
- Well-balanced diet with smaller and more frequent meals
- Dietary restriction (sugar, salt, caffeine)
- Limit/eliminate alcohol, nicotine, and drugs of abuse
- Regular exercise
- Good sleep hygiene

Vitamin/mineral
- Calcium 1.0 g/d
- Pyridoxine 50–100 mg qd-bid
- Magnesium 50–100 mg bid
- Multivitamin/mineral supplement

Weight gain/bloating
- Spironolactone 25 mg bid-qid
- Hydrochlorothiazide 25–50 mg qd-bid
- Triamterene 50–100 mg qd-bid

Mastodynia
- Caffeine restriction
- Vitamin E 200–600 IU qd
- Evening primrose oil 0.5–1.5 g bid

***Physical symptoms* (e.g., dysmenorrhea, cramps, headache)**
- Aspirin or acetaminophen 325–650 mg every 4–6 h (not to exceed 2.6 g/d)
- Ibuprofen 200–400 mg every 4–6 h (not to exceed 1.2 g/d)
- Mefenamic acid 500 mg followed by 250 mg every 6 h to 500 mg tid (not to exceed 7 days)
- Naproxen sodium 550 mg followed by 275 mg every 6–8 h to 550 mg bid (not to exceed 1.375 g/d)

Insomnia
- Caffeine restriction
- Diphenhydramine 25–50 mg hs
- Trazodone 25–150 mg hs
- Doxepin 10–75 mg hs
- Melatonin 0.1–2 mg hs

Second-line Approaches
Mastodynia
- Bromocriptine 2.5–7.5 mg bid from 10–14 days until menses
- Danazol 50–100 mg bid

Hormonal
- Progesterone (PO, sublingual, vaginal, or rectal suppository) 200 mg bid from 10–14 days before menses; PO or IM chronic therapy (questionable efficacy in PMS)
- Estradiol 1–2 mg/d (PO) ± intermittent progestin; 0.05–0.2 mg/24 h (transdermal) ± intermittent progestin
- Oral contraceptives (biphasic or triphasic)

Anxiety/depression/mood swings
- Alprazolam 0.25–0.5 mg bid-qid from 10–14 days before menses, then slowly tapered and discontinued
- Buspirone 5–20 mg tid or from 10–14 days before menses
- Nortriptyline 50–125 mg/d to 150 mg/d
- Clomipramine 25–75 mg/d to 250 mg/d
- Nefazodone 100–400 mg/d
- Fluoxetine 20–40 mg/d (during luteal phase or continuous treatment) (sertraline, paroxetine, fluvoxamine, or venlafaxine are alternative treatments)
- Lithium carbonate 300–600 mg bid for recurrent mood swings (valproate or carbamazepine are alternative treatments)

Third-line Approaches
Antiestrogen agents
- Danazol 200–400 mg/d for 3–6 months

Gonadotropin-releasing hormone agonists
- Leuprolide 3.75 mg IM monthly for 6 months

Bilateral ovariectomy

night with complaints of nervousness and that her mind is racing.[5] She may complain of restless sleep and feeling fatigued on arising. Good sleep hygiene (e.g., a regular sleep schedule, avoiding caffeinated beverages and alcohol, morning or afternoon exercise, relaxation therapy, and a light bedtime snack) should be recommended as first-line approaches.

Over-the-counter (OTC) antihistamines (e.g., diphenhydramine 25–50 mg at bedtime) can be tried for acute sleep disturbances but may cause anticholinergic side effects and daytime sedation. L-Tryptophan (the amino acid precursor to serotonin) was commonly used for insomnia and for PMS until it was withdrawn from the market because of its association with causing an eosinophilia-myalgia syndrome (e.g., muscle pain, fatigue, fever, rashes). Melatonin (a metabolite of serotonin that is produced by the pineal gland under the influence of darkness) is available as on OTC preparation and is becoming a popular sleep-aid for women with PMS. Chronic use of hypnotic agents (e.g., triazolam, temazepam, flurazepam, zolpidem) is not recommended for premenstrual insomnia because tolerance and physical dependence may result. Alternative treatments for insomnia include a low dose of a sedative antidepressant such as trazodone, amitriptyline, or doxepin taken 1–2 hours before bedtime. Antidepressants have the advantage of not causing physical dependence and may be beneficial in the treatment of premenstrual dysphoria.

Vitamins/Minerals

Pyridoxine

Pyridoxine (vitamin B_6) is a water-soluble B complex vitamin. Pyridoxal phosphate acts as a coenzyme in the metabolism of protein, carbohydrate, and fat; as a cofactor for the final steps of the biosynthesis of dopamine and serotonin; and in the production of prostaglandins from essential fatty acids. A deficiency of pyridoxine decreases the synthesis of dopamine (causing an increase in prolactin secretion) and reduces tryptophan metabolism (causing a deficiency of brain serotonin).[26] There is no evidence of pyridoxine deficiency in women with PMS, but it is commonly used as a vitamin treatment. Pyridoxine in doses of 100–800 mg/d was shown to improve PMS symptoms in some controlled studies, although other studies found no specific effects.[26] A review of 12 controlled studies revealed little support for the efficacy of pyridoxine in PMS.[29]

Pyridoxine supplement is recommended for women with PMS taking oral contraceptives and estrogen therapy since estrogenic substances may increase the demand for pyridoxine. Patients should be started on low daily doses (25–50 mg/d) that are increased gradually by 25 mg/d up to 100–200 mg/d until symptoms are relieved. Side effects of pyridoxine (nausea and headache) are rare at lower doses. Doses greater than 200 mg/d are not recommended because higher doses are associated with pyridoxine-induced peripheral neuropathy (numb feet, unstable gait, decreased sensation to touch).[30] When pyridoxine is discontinued, these symptoms will lessen, but it may take several months for sensations to return to normal.

Calcium and Magnesium

Few studies have investigated the use of single-mineral therapy (e.g., calcium, magnesium, zinc, or copper) in the treatment of PMS. Low blood levels of calcium during the luteal phase and low intracellular magnesium levels in women with PMS compared to controls have been reported.[26] Low magnesium levels may cause a depletion of dopamine, resulting in increased prolactin concentrations. Dairy products and calcium may interfere with gastrointestinal absorption of magnesium, but the significance of this is not known.

Both calcium and magnesium were reported to be effective in preliminary PMS trials and caused minimal adverse effects.[5] Elemental calcium in doses of 1000 mg/d reduced mood changes, fluid retention, and pain in two double-blind, placebo-controlled studies.[31,32] Magnesium supplementation (360 mg/d administered in divided doses from day 15 to the onset of menses) was shown to improve mood symptoms in a double-blind, placebo-controlled PMS study.[33] Calcium and magnesium supplementation are relatively inexpensive and may have less toxicity than megadose vitamin products.

Nutritional Supplements

Optivite, a combination of high-dose multiple vitamins and micronutrients, is promoted as a nutritional supplement for PMS. A placebo-controlled study with Optivite reported beneficial effects in PMS,[34] but further studies are needed to replicate the results in a larger population. The recommended dose of Optivite is 6–12 tablets per day and the product is relatively expensive. Optivite is high in pyridoxine (300 mg) and magnesium (250 mg), but contains only 125 mg of calcium per 6 tablets, which is significantly below the recommended daily allowance of calcium for women to prevent osteoporosis.

Weight Gain/Bloating

Bloating, swelling, and weight gain are common premenstrual complaints despite little evidence that women with PMS actually retain fluid.[5] Swelling of the breasts and bloating in the lower abdomen may be associated with local fluid shifts within the breast and bowel instead of fluid retention or an increase in total body water.[1] For some women, there is a marked fluid retention during the premenstrual week that presents as edema, bloating sensations, and weight gain.

Dietary salt restriction or reducing sodium intake should be the first-line treatment for fluid retention. If this approach is not effective and there is a documented weight gain of 5 pounds or more, then diuretic therapy may be indicated. Estrogen causes sodium and water retention by increasing aldosterone levels, which may be linked to fluid retention. Spironolactone, a synthetic steroid aldosterone antagonist with potassium-sparing properties, has been studied in the treatment of weight gain and bloating. In one double-blind placebo-controlled study, spironolactone (in doses of 25 mg four times daily [range of 25–200 mg/d] for 10 days before the onset of menses) reduced bloating and weight gain in approximately 60% of women with PMS.[35] Spironolactone has the advantage of not causing hypokalemia, but it may cause antiandrogenic effects and should not be used during pregnancy and lactation due to possible tumorigenic effects in rats.[15] Other diuretics (e.g., hydrochlorothiazide, chlorothiazide, hydroflumethiazide, benzthiazide, metolazone, chlorthalidone, triamterene) have been used in treating fluid retention, but few controlled PMS studies have been done.

Mastodynia

Vitamin E

Vitamin E (α-tocopherol), a fat-soluble vitamin, is used as an antioxidant in treating fibrocystic breast disease (cystic mastitis). Administration of vitamin E in doses from 150–600 U/d has been reported to decrease breast tenderness and swelling along with other symptoms (e.g., headache, fatigue, food cravings, depression, anxiety) in double-blind placebo-controlled studies by one research group.[15,36] Further studies are needed with vitamin E since some of the studies were not well controlled and some investigators have reported no change in breast tenderness.

Essential Fatty Acids/Evening Primrose Oil

A deficiency of prostaglandin E_1 (PGE_1) has been proposed as a cause of some PMS symptoms (e.g., low levels of PGE_1 may increase prolactin's effect on breast tissue and cause mastodynia).[26] *Cis*-linolenic acid, an essential fatty acid contained in vegetable oils, is converted to gamma-linolenic acid (the precursor to PGE_1). *Cis*-linolenic acid, magnesium, pyridoxine, zinc, and vitamin C are involved in the synthesis of PGE_1.

Evening primrose oil (which contains γ-linolenic acid) in doses of 500–3000 mg/d has been reported to reduce the severity of breast symptoms in PMS. However, controlled studies have reported no significant difference between evening primrose oil and placebo in treating anxiety and depression. Efamol (contains *cis*-linoleic acid and its metabolite γ-linoleic acid) was shown to decrease breast symptoms and depression in one study[37] but had no effect on mood or physical symptoms in other PMS trials.[33,39] To date, limited data support the use of evening primrose oil or essential fatty acids in the treatment of mastodynia.

Physical Symptoms (Dysmenorrhea, Cramps, Headache)

OTC PMS Products

Many women use nonprescription products to treat abdominal pain and cramping, headache, and fluid retention. Several PMS OTC products are available and commonly contain either acetaminophen or ibuprofen (for analgesia) in combination with caffeine, ammonium chloride or pamabrom (for diuresis), and diphenhydramine hydrochloride or pyrilamine maleate (an antihistamine for sedation).[15] Aspirin, acetaminophen, ibuprofen, or naproxen are often effective in relieving dysmenorrhea, headache, and muscle or joint pain. Mild PMS symptoms may respond to OTC products but severe symptoms rarely respond. There are no controlled studies reporting efficacy of OTC products in PMS, and some ingredients, such as caffeine, often worsen insomnia and irritability.

Prostaglandin Inhibitors

Nonsteroidal anti-inflammatory drugs (NSAIDs) inhibit prostaglandin synthesis and exhibit anti-inflammatory, analgesic, and antipyretic activity. NSAIDs are effective in treating pain syndromes such as dysmenorrhea and in menstrual migraines.[40,41] Dysmenorrhea is associated with the release of prostaglandins during the late luteal phase, which causes uterine contractions and pain. Increases in prostaglandins correlate with the premenstrual physical complaints (e.g., back and muscle aches, headache, breast tenderness, gastrointestinal [GI] discomfort, nausea, dizziness, irritability, depression, lethargy).[40,41]

Mefenamic acid has been reported to be effective in several double-blind, placebo-controlled trials by reducing menstrual pain, as well as breast tenderness, bloating, irritability, and depression.[15,41] Inconsistencies in the studies and differences in doses and regimens make comparisons of the findings difficult. The long-term intermittent use of mefenamic acid has not been studied and it is associated with several serious adverse effects (e.g., renal failure, GI bleeding). The usual recommended dose for mefenamic acid in primary dysmenorrhea is 500 mg, followed by 250 mg every 6 hours as necessary (preferably administered with food). Mefenamic acid should not be used in children younger than 14 years and should not be used for more than 2–3 days for primary dysmenorrhea due to increased risk of adverse effects.

Naproxen sodium (550 mg twice daily administered 1 week before menses) significantly reduced pain and some behavioral changes in a placebo-controlled PMS study.[42] Ibuprofen has been reported to be as effective as mefenamic acid and more effective than placebo, aspirin, or propoxyphene in relieving dysmenorrhea. Since both naproxen and ibuprofen are available OTC, many women self-medicate with these agents.

For the treatment of dysmenorrhea, NSAIDs therapy should be started with the earliest onset of pain. The usual adult dose of naproxen is 500 mg (550 mg of naproxen sodium), followed by 250 mg (275 mg of naproxen sodium) every 6–8 hours as necessary. The total daily dose of naproxen should not exceed 1.25 g/d (or 1.375 g/d of naproxen sodium). Initial adult dosing of ibuprofen is usually 200 mg every 4–6 hours; doses may be increased up to 400 mg every 4–6 hours if necessary, but doses should not exceed 1.2 g/d. To be most effective, NSAIDs should be started during the last week of the luteal phase before the onset of dysmenorrhea and continued through menstruation on a scheduled instead of an as-needed basis.[5] NSAIDs are effective in treating dysmenorrhea and menstrual migraine, but their role in treating other PMS symptoms remains unestablished. NSAIDs cause several side effects (e.g., upset stomach, heartburn, nausea, vomiting, diarrhea, constipation, anorexia, rash) and are contraindicated in patients with aspirin sensitivity, peptic ulcer disease, gastritis, bleeding disorders, and renal insufficiency.

If menstrual migraines do not respond to NSAIDs, other treatment approaches and combination drugs are available such as a beta-adrenergic blocker (propranolol 40–240 mg/d in divided doses) or a TCA (amitriptyline 25–100 mg/d). Low-dose estradiol therapy (oral or transdermal patch) starting on days 24–26 and continued for 7 days through menstruation may be helpful to decrease the "estrogen withdrawal" migraine.[5] Ovulation-suppressing agents (e.g., continuous estrogen therapy, oral contraceptives, danazol, GnRH-As) may be effective for menstrual migraines but should be reserved for second- or third-line treatments.

SECOND-LINE APPROACHES

Mastodynia

Bromocriptine

Bromocriptine, an ergot derivative with dopamine agonist activity, has been used to inhibit prolactin secretion and reduce breast swelling and tenderness. Prolactin suppression usually occurs at doses of 5 mg/d of bromocriptine. In double-blind studies, bromocriptine (1.25–2.5 mg twice daily administered from ovulation until the start of menses) improved breast engorgement and mastalgia.[43,44] Most women can be started on 2.5 mg/d and the dose can be adjusted up or down depending on symptom response and adverse effects. Higher doses are associated with an increased frequency of adverse effects (e.g., nausea, vomiting, dizziness, headache, fatigue, cardiovascular effects).

Danazol

Danazol, a synthetic steroid of ethisterone, is used to treat endometriosis and cystic mastitis. Danazol has antiestrogen and androgen effects and inhibits gonadotropin secretion, which causes anovulation and amenorrhea at higher doses.[15] The antiestrogen effect of danazol causes a "pseudomenopause" and may result in irregular bleeding, decreased breast size, hot flashes, depression/anxiety, and increased risk of cardiovascular disease due to elevated low density lipoprotein (LDL) cholesterol concentrations.

Several studies have reported positive effects with danazol in the treatment of mastalgia[45] and premenstrual dysphoria.[46] Because of significant antiestrogen and androgenic adverse effects, danazol should not be used as a first-line agent. At higher doses (>200 mg/d) an increased incidence and severity of adverse effects is seen (e.g., headache, irregular bleeding, weight gain, fluid retention, nausea and vomiting, oily skin, acne, hirsutism, changes in libido, lowering of the voice). When PMS coexists with endometriosis and cystic mastitis or if mastalgia is the primary complaint, danazol may be considered a first-line agent. Danazol should be reserved for short-term treatment for breast pain (starting with 50 mg twice daily and increased as tolerated). Doses of 200 mg twice daily for 3–6 months are used to suppress ovarian function prior to an ovariectomy. Further comparative studies are needed to evaluate the long-term effects of antiestrogen therapy.

Hormonal

The hormonal treatments of PMS can be classified into two categories: medications that supplement hormones during the menstrual cycle (e.g., luteal phase progesterone or estrogen therapy) or those that suppress the menstrual cycle by causing anovulation. Suppression of ovulation can effectively prevent PMS, but several of the treatments (estrogen and progesterone implants, GnRH-As, danazol) are still investigational and should only be used as third-line treatment options.

Progesterone

For many years, administration of progesterone by vaginal suppositories during the luteal phase was the most common hormonal treatment for PMS.[47] After several double-blind, placebo-controlled studies, it is now thought that progesterone is no better than placebo for treating PMS.[15,47] Part of the controversy with progesterone therapy surrounds the form (i.e., natural versus synthetic), length of treatment (i.e., luteal phase versus chronic therapy), and type of administration (oral, buccal/sublingual, vaginal, rectal, or implants). Only a few controlled PMS studies have used oral, sublingual, or nasally administered progesterone. Although synthetic progestins are considered to be less effective than natural progesterone, a placebo-controlled PMS study reported that orally administered medroxyprogesterone acetate was effective.[48] Oral medroxyprogesterone acetate (30 mg/d) has been used for suppression of ovulation but has the risk of causing depression, headaches, weight gain, and thromboembolic disorders. Natural progesterone is available in an injectable oil (50 mg/mL); 50–100 mg/d of intramuscular progesterone is used for women who cannot tolerate or absorb the drug from suppository formulations. Long-acting preparations of synthetic progestins (i.e., medroxyprogesterone acetate [Depo-Provera] administered every 1–3 months and levonorgestrel implants [Norplant] administered every 5 years) have been used for contraception, but little is known about their safety and efficacy in PMS. The long-term effects of progestin therapy on uterine, ovarian, pituitary, adrenal, and hepatic function has not been determined.

Adverse effects of progesterone include vaginal spotting, breakthrough bleeding, amenorrhea, monilial infection, anal or vaginal irritation, nausea, diarrhea, flatulence, weight change, edema, depression, and decreased libido.[49] Progesterone may make some PMS symptoms worse (e.g., fatigue, depression, fluid retention, irritability, acne, increase in appetite) and should be used with caution in certain medical conditions (e.g., migraine, seizure disorders, asthma, cardiac or renal disease). Progestins are contraindicated in patients with thrombophlebitis and thromboembolic disorders. Because of its questionable efficacy and risk of adverse effects, progesterone-only therapy is not recommended as a first-line treatment in PMS.

Estradiol

Estradiol, the active estrogen produced by the ovaries, is effective for menstrual migraines and for estrogen replacement therapy to control menopausal symptomatology. Initial placebo-controlled studies reported that estradiol implants and transdermal estradiol patches are beneficial in reducing some PMS symptoms.[50,51] Micronized estradiol may be administered orally, and is available as a parenteral oil injection and a transdermal patch. The transdermal estradiol patches may cause skin irritation and should be replaced at a new application site every 3–4 days.

So far, all estradiol studies have used intermittent progestin therapy (norethisterone 5 mg/d for 7 days each month to induce regular menses), which can cause PMS-like side effects.[47] Estrogen-progestin combinations have been associated with an increased risk of thrombophlebitis, pulmonary embolism, and cerebral thrombosis due to the progestin effects. Chronic estrogen-only therapy has certain risks (e.g., increasing endometrial, ovarian, and breast cancer, gallbladder disease) and should not be administered during pregnancy due to risks of causing adverse effects in the fetus. An oral or transdermal estradiol trial (combined with cyclical or continuous progestin replacement therapy if the uterus is present) may be appropriate for perimenopausal women after the age of 40 to treat the decline in ovarian function. Until further long-term studies are done, estrogen replacement therapy should be reserved for the management of moderate to severe vasomotor symptoms associated with menopause.

Oral Contraceptives

Oral contraceptives or OCs (estrogen–progestin combinations) cause anovulation and may be useful in reducing dysmenorrhea, depression, and irritability.[47] OCs may worsen PMS symptoms in approximately 30% of women, but some women may derive benefit.[15] Biphasic or triphasic products have been used in PMS, but some reports suggest that triphasic products may cause more mood changes.[52] OCs high in progestin content have been recommended for PMS but may be associated with breakthrough bleeding and/or spotting, amenorrhea, acne, hirsutism, fatigue, and depression. Pyridoxine replacement therapy, 50 mg/d, is recommended for women who become depressed while taking OCs.[53] Serious adverse effects of OCs include hypertension, increases in plasma triglyceride and LDLs, cholestatic jaundice, gallbladder disease, and myocardial infarction. OCs should be used with caution in women who smoke because of an increased risk of thromboembolism.

Anxiety/Depression/Mood Swings

Antianxiety Agents

Alprazolam, a triazolobenzodiazepine with γ-aminobutyric acid (GABA) augmenting effects, is marketed for the treatment of anxiety and panic disorder. Two placebo-controlled studies reported therapeutic effects with alprazolam in PMDD (e.g., improvement in anxiety, depression, mood swings, irritability, sleep disturbances)[54,55] when doses of 0.25–4 mg/d in divided doses were used (average of 0.75 and 2.25 mg/d per study). Alprazolam was started 8–12 days before menses, and the dose was slowly decreased by no more than 25% per day during menses to avoid withdrawal symptoms. Side effects were minimal with lower doses, but higher doses were associated with drowsiness. In a 3-month double-blind placebo-controlled study with a continuous dosing regimen of alprazolam (0.25 mg three times per day), subjects with PMDD had significant improvement in anxiety, irritability, tension, and feelings of being out of control in comparison to placebo.[56] The initial studies using alprazolam in PMDD showed efficacy compared with placebo treatment, but one placebo-controlled study has reported no observable differences in PMS ratings.[57] Other benzodiazepines may be effective to decrease anxiety, restlessness, and insomnia; however, there are no controlled studies in PMS. Benzodiazepines may cause dose-related drowsiness and impairment in motor and cognitive functioning and have the risk of causing withdrawal symptoms when doses are rapidly decreased. Because of dependency problems, benzodiazepines should be used with caution in dependency-prone patients or those with a history of alcohol and drug abuse.

Buspirone, a partial serotonin-1_A agonist, is marketed for the treatment of generalized anxiety disorder. An initial multicenter open trial with buspirone (5 mg three times a day and increased as needed up to 60 mg/d) reported an antianxiety effect in approximately 70% of women with PMS.[58] Buspirone is administered chronically for the treatment of anxiety, but some PMS studies only used buspirone during the luteal phase (or 12 days before menstruation). Further PMS studies are needed to determine if intermittent use of buspirone is as effective as chronic therapy. Side effects of buspirone include headache, dizziness, nausea, fatigue, and dry mouth during the initial titration phase. Buspirone has minimal side effects and has the advantage over benzodiazepines of not causing dependence or a withdrawal syndrome after abrupt discontinuation.

Antidepressants

Women with premenstrual dysphoria may have decreased serotonergic activity during the luteal phase as suggested by decreased platelet uptake of 5-HT, whole-blood 5-HT levels, and melatonin levels.[13,15] Initial studies using antidepressant agents in treating PMDD reported positive benefits. Nortriptyline, a secondary amine TCA that increases both 5-HT and NE activity, was effective in an open trial in women with PMDD.[59] Nortriptyline dosage ranged from 50–125 mg/d and side effects included dry mouth, constipation, drowsiness, insomnia, and overstimulation. Clomipramine, a tertiary amine TCA that blocks reuptake of 5-HT and NE, was found to significantly reduce irritability and dysphoria in doses of 25–75 mg/d taken either daily or from ovulation until the onset of menstruation in two placebo-controlled PMDD studies.[60,61] Nefazodone, an antidepressant related to trazodone that possesses both 5-HT_2 antagonism and weaker 5-HT reuptake inhibition effects, was investigated in an open-labeled study in women with PMDD.[62] In doses of 100–400 mg/d administered twice daily, nefazodone was reported to significantly improve PMS symptoms in two different PMDD groups defined as those with or without coexisting major depression or dysthymia. The most common adverse effects were experienced during the initial phase of the study (e.g., nausea, headache, and drowsiness) and most subjects developed tolerance to the adverse effects over the 8-week trial.

Serotonergic augmenting antidepressants appear to have considerable promise in treating a wide range of symptoms in women with PMDD. Fluoxetine, a selective serotonin uptake inhibitor (SSRI), has been reported to be beneficial in several case reports, in four placebo-controlled trials, and in a long-term open study lasting approximately

1.5 years.[63–69] Fluoxetine, in doses of 20–40 mg/d, was generally well tolerated and effective in diminishing mood symptoms, food craving, overeating, and weight gain. In the long-term study, women reported improvement in relationships along with a reduction in PMS symptoms; the most common adverse effect reported was sexual dysfunction (decreased libido and delayed orgasm).[69] SSRIs have the advantage of not causing significant weight gain, drowsiness, cardiovascular changes, and anticholinergic side effects common with TCAs. Other 5-HT augmenting antidepressants such as sertraline,[70] paroxetine,[71] and fluvoxamine may be effective in reducing the mood changes associated with PMS, but further controlled studies are needed. Venlafaxine, a 5-HT and NE reuptake inhibitor, has adverse effects similar to SSRIs but little is known about its efficacy in PMS. Side effects of SSRIs are mild (and dose related) and are usually worse during the first few weeks of starting therapy (e.g., nausea, headache, nervousness, insomnia, decreased appetite, decreased libido). For women with premenstrual exacerbation of an underlying depression or PMDD, an adequate trial for 6–12 months of standard doses of antidepressants is recommended.

Mood Stabilizers

Lithium carbonate (600–1800 mg/d) is primarily used in treating cyclothymia (low-grade mood swings) or bipolar mood disorder (manic depressive illness). Several case reports and uncontrolled trials with lithium reported benefit in PMS patients, but controlled trials failed to find a consistent therapeutic effect.[72] Lithium may be appropriate for women with predominant mood swings or those with a history of recurrent affective disorder. Lithium should be used with caution in women of childbearing age because of its potential teratogenic effects. Lithium has numerous adverse effects (e.g., hypothyroidism) and requires routine blood level monitoring.

Valproate, an anticonvulsant used in the treatment of bipolar disorder, was administered to eight women with PMS using low doses (range of 125–500 mg/d with mean serum levels of 32.5 μg/mL).[73] Only three of the eight women reported a decrease in both PMS and migraine headaches using low-dose valproate therapy. Further controlled studies using higher doses of valproate (that achieve serum levels of 50–100 μg/mL) are needed to determine valproate's effectiveness in women with prominent or rapid mood changes. Other mood stabilizers such as carbamazepine have not been adequately studied in the treatment of PMS.

THIRD-LINE APPROACHES

Gonadotropin-Releasing Hormone Agonists (GnRH-As)

GnRH-As, also called luteinizing hormone releasing hormone agonists, cause a down-regulation of pituitary gonadotropin secretion and result in anovulation and amenorrhea. GnRH-As (administered subcutaneously, intranasally, by implants, or by intramuscular depot injections) suppress estradiol and progesterone levels, thus causing pseudomenopause and significantly decreasing physical and behavioral PMS symptoms.[74,75] Initially, some women noted a "flare" in PMS symptoms during the first few weeks of GnRH-A treatment, which was followed by a reduction in the physical and behavioral symptoms of PMS.

Buserelin, an investigational GnRH-A, was shown to have beneficial effects in PMS when administered intranasally for six menstrual cycles in a small number of subjects.[75] Histrelin, another investigational GnRH-A, was administered by daily subcutaneous injections in eight women with severe PMS, resulting in a 75% improvement in luteal phase symptoms.[76] Sequential estrogen and progestin replacement therapy was then added to the GnRH-A therapy and there continued to be a 60% improvement in PMS symptoms. The use of a combination of GnRH-A plus an "add-back" of estrogen/progestin may help to reverse antiestrogenic and antiprogesterone effects without decreasing the effectiveness of GnRH-As in severe PMS.

Nafarelin acetate is approved as a nasal spray for the management of endometriosis, but little is known about its effectiveness in PMS. Regular use of nafarelin inhibits ovulation and causes hot flashes, decreased libido, vaginal dryness, headaches, mood swings, and insomnia. Other GnRH-As (gonadorelin, goserelin, leuprolide) are marketed for the treatment of endometriosis, breast and prostatic cancer, polycystic ovarian disease, and precocious puberty. Depot leuprolide (3.75 mg/month), when compared to placebo treatment, was found to reduce physical and behavioral symptoms in women without premenstrual depression but was not effective in women with severe premenstrual depression.[77] A double-blind study comparing depot goserelin (3.6 mg/month) with a placebo reported that the GnRH-A significantly improved physical symptoms of PMS (e.g., breast discomfort) but did not reduce the psychological symptoms (e.g., depression, anxiety, irritability).[78]

GnRH-As may improve cyclical mood changes during short-term therapy, but the chronic effects of suppressing ovarian hormone secretion could result in significant antiestrogen effects (e.g., osteoporosis and cardiovascular disease) and worsening of mood without low-dose hormone replacement therapy. Until the long-term safety of GnRH-A is established, it should be used as a third-line agent and reserved for the most severe cases of PMS.

Ovariectomy

Surgical ablation of the menstrual cycle (bilateral salpingo-oophorectomy and hysterectomy) has been performed to treat PMS and should be reserved as the last resort treatment for severe symptoms.[79,80] A 3- to 6-month trial of a GnRH-A or danazol is recommended before radical surgery to determine if anovulation is effective since the ovariectomy is not reversible.[5] A hysterectomy without an ovariectomy is not effective for PMS. If an ovariectomy is done without an hysterectomy, women need both estrogen and progestin replacement therapy. Unopposed estrogen therapy increases the risk for endometrial hyperplasia, therefore, intermittent or continuous progestin therapy for 7 or more days of a cycle is recommended. Women who have both the ovariectomy and hysterectomy can receive continuous estrogen replacement therapy without intermittent progestin therapy since there is no risk for endometrial cancer.[80]

Miscellaneous Therapies

Many other therapies have been tried for PMS (e.g., sleep deprivation, bright-light phototherapy, acupuncture, naltrexone, clonidine, verapamil, atenolol, L-tryptophan, melatonin, vitamin A, potassium, antihistamines, tamoxifen, fenfluramine, doxycycline, antifungal therapy).[2,5,15,16] Few controlled studies have been performed to determine clinical efficacy and safety of these alternative therapies in PMS.[81,82] Although most uncontrolled drug trials show positive effects, most controlled (drug versus placebo) studies generally report little difference between treatments. Women with PMS have a high placebo response rate, so clinical studies should be controlled and include a placebo washout phase.

Evaluation of Therapeutic Outcomes

In general, therapeutic strategies should be individualized, and medications should not be prescribed unless nonpharmacologic approaches have failed or unless PMS symptoms cause disruption in functioning. The weighing of risk versus benefit of pharmacologic interventions is important since some medications cause significant adverse effects.[82] Women with prominent mood or anxiety symptoms should receive a trial of an antidepressant (e.g., fluoxetine) or an antianxiety agent (e.g., alprazolam) since these medications have been found to be effective in PMDD in several well-designed studies.[16,81,82] A treatment trial of three menstrual cycles is recommended to adjust dosages based on adverse effects and efficacy. It may be necessary to try several different treatments before an acceptable therapy is identified. A stepwise approach is recommended so that the least toxic agent is used first before resorting to experimental treatments (GnRH agonists) or surgery (ovariectomy). Currently, there are no FDA-approved medications for PMS or treatment guidelines for selecting therapy. Further double-blind, placebo-controlled studies in larger populations are needed to determine the efficacy, safety, and long-term use for specific PMS treatments.

Conclusion

Premenstrual symptoms are common complaints in women during their reproductive years. The exact cause of PMS is unknown, but biologic, social, and psychologic factors appear to contribute to the variability and severity of the disorder. A correct diagnosis of PMS is essential. An evaluation and careful workup should be conducted over several menstrual cycles to rule out other possible causes and to identify target symptoms through daily charting. Education, supportive therapy, regular exercise, dietary changes (e.g., limiting caffeine, salt, and alcohol), and good sleep hygiene are extremely beneficial for most women. If more specific pharmacologic approaches are needed, then a target symptom approach is preferred. Because PMS symptoms often intensify with age, women may not seek treatment for PMS until their thirties or forties, when symptoms are more bothersome or distressing. Different treatment approaches and combination therapies may be needed over time depending on target symptoms identified during daily charting. After a 3-month trial of any PMS therapy, the risks versus benefits of each treatment should be evaluated.

References

1. Mortola JF. Issues in the diagnosis and research of premenstrual syndrome. Clin Obstet Gynecol 1992;35:587–598.
2. Reid RL. Premenstrual syndrome. Curr Prob Obstet Gynecol Fertil 1985;8:1–57.
3. American Psychiatric Association. Diagnostic and Statistical Manual of Mental Disorders, 4th ed. Washington, DC, American Psychiatric Press, 1994, pp 715–718.
4. Logue CM, Moos RH. Premenstrual symptoms: Prevalence and risk factors. Psychosom Med 1986;48:388–414.
5. Johnson SR. Clinician's approach to the diagnosis and management of premenstrual syndrome. Clin Obstet Gynecol 1992;80:637–657.
6. Severino SK, Moline ML. Premenstrual Syndrome: A Clinician's Guide. New York, Guilford Press, 1989, pp 1–141.
7. Backstrom T. Neuroendocrinology of premenstrual syndrome. Clin Obstet Gynecol 1992;35:612–628.
8. Rubinow DR, Hoban MC, Grover GN, et al. Changes in plasma hormones across the menstrual cycle in patients with menstrually related mood disorder and in control subjects. Am J Obstet Gynecol 1988;158:5–11.
9. Watts JF, Butt WR, Edwards RL, Holder G. Hormonal studies in women with premenstrual tension. Br J Obstet Gynecol 1985;92:247–255.
10. Halbreich U, Endicott J, Goldstein S, Nee J. Premenstrual changes and changes in gonadal hormones. Acta Psychiatr Scand 1986;74:576–586.
11. Steiner M. Female-specific mood disorders. Clin Obstet Gynecol 1992;35:599–611.
12. Severino SK, Moline ML. Premenstrual syndrome. Obstet Gynecol Clin North Am 1990;17:889–903.
13. Rapkin AJ. The role of serotonin in premenstrual syndrome. Clin Obstet Gynecol 1992;35:629–636.
14. Rubinow DR, Schmidt PJ. Models for the development and expression of symptoms in premenstrual syndrome. Psychiatr Clin North Am 1989;12:53–68.
15. Severino SK, Moline ML. Premenstrual Syndrome: A Clinician's Guide. New York, Guilford Press, 1989, pp 162–246.

16. Rausch JL, Weston S, Plouffe L. Role of psychotropic medication in the treatment of affective symptoms in premenstrual syndrome. Clin Obstet Gynecol 1992;35:667–678.
17. Keye WR. General evaluation of premenstrual symptoms. Clin Obstet Gynecol 1987;30:396–407.
18. Hamilton JA, Parry B, Alagna S, et al. Premenstrual mood changes: A guide to evaluation and treatment. Psychiatr Ann 1984;14:426–435.
19. Osofsky HJ, Keppel W, Kuczmierczyk AR. Evaluation and management of premenstrual syndrome in clinical psychiatric practice. J Clin Psychiatry 1988;49:494–498.
20. Moos RH. The development of a menstrual distress questionnaire. Psychosom Med 1968;30:853–867.
21. Magos AL. Premenstrual syndrome. Contemp Rev Obstet Gynaecol 1988;1:80–92.
22. Endicott J, Nee J, Cohen J, Halbreich U. Premenstrual changes: Pattern correlates of daily ratings. J Affective Disord 1986;10:127–135.
23. Mortola JF, Girton L, Beck L, Yen SSC. Diagnosis of premenstrual syndrome by a simple prospective and reliable instrument: The calendar of premenstrual experiences. Obstet Gynecol 1990;76:302–307.
24. Anderson M, Severino SK, Hurt SW, Williams NA. Premenstrual syndrome research: Using NIMH guidelines. J Clin Psychiatry 1988;49:484–486.
25. Keye WR. Premenstrual syndrome: Seven steps in management. Postgrad Med 1988;83:167–173.
26. Chuong CJ, Dawson EB. Critical evaluation of nutritional factors in the pathophysiology and treatment of premenstrual syndrome. Clin Obstet Gynecol 1992;35:679–692.
27. Prior JC, Vigna Y, Sciarretta D, et al. Conditioning exercise decreases premenstrual symptoms: A prospective, controlled 6-month trial. Fertil Steril 1987;47:402–408.
28. Rossignol AM, Bonnlander H. Caffeine-containing beverages, total fluid consumption and premenstrual syndrome. Am J Public Health 1990;80:1106–1110.
29. Kleignen J, Ter Riet G, Knipschild P. Vitamin B_6 in the treatment of the premenstrual syndrome: A review. Br J Obstet Gynaecol 1990;97:847–852.
30. Parry GJ, Bredensen DE. Sensory neuropathy with low-dose pyridoxine. Neurology 1985;35:1466–1468.
31. Thys-Jacobs S, Ceccarelli S, Bierman A, et al. Calcium supplementation in premenstrual syndrome: A randomized crossover trial. J Gen Intern Med 1989;4:183–189.
32. Alvir JMaJ, Thys-Jacobs S. Premenstrual and menstrual symptoms clusters and response to calcium treatment. Psychopharmacol Bull 1991;27:145–148.
33. Facchinetti F, Borela P, Sances G, et al. Oral magnesium successfully relieves premenstrual mood changes. Obstet Gynecol 1991;78:177–181.
34. Chakmakjian ZH, Higgins CE, Abraham GE. The effect of a nutritional supplement, Optivite for Women, on premenstrual tension syndromes: II. Effect on symptomatology, using a double blind cross-over design. J Appl Nutr 1985;37:12–17.
35. Vellacott ID, O'Brien PMS. Effect of spironolactone on premenstrual syndrome symptoms. J Reprod Med 1987;32:429–433.
36. London RS, Murphy L, Kitlowski KE, Reynolds MA. Efficacy of α-tocopherol in the treatment of PMS. J Reprod Med 1987;32:400–404.
37. Puolakka J, Makarainen L, Viinikka L, Ylikorkala O. Biochemical and clinical effects of treating the premenstrual syndrome with prostaglandin synthesis precursors. J Reprod Med 1985;30:149–153.
38. Khoo SK, Munro C, Battistatta D. Evening primrose oil and treatment of premenstrual syndrome. Med J Aust 1990;153:189–192.
39. Collins A, Cerin A, Coleman G, Landgren BM. Essential fatty acids in the treatment of premenstrual syndrome. Obstet Gynecol 1993;81:93–98.
40. Pickles VR. Prostaglandins and dysmenorrhea. Acta Obstet Gynecol Scand 1979;87(suppl):7–12.
41. Budoff PW. The use of prostaglandin inhibitors for the premenstrual syndrome. J Reprod Med 1983;28:465–468.
42. Facchinetti F, Fioroni L, Sances G, et al. Naproxen sodium in the treatment of premenstrual symptoms: A placebo-controlled study. Gynecol Obstet Invest 1989;28:205–208.
43. Ylostalo P. Cyclical or continuous treatment of the premenstrual syndrome (PMS) with bromocriptine. Eur J Obstet Gynecol Reprod Biol 1984;17:337–343.
44. Andersch B. Bromocriptine and premenstrual symptoms: A survey of double-blind trials. Obstet Gyn Surv 1983;38:643–646.
45. Derzko CM. Role of danazol in relieving the premenstrual syndrome. J Reprod Med 1990;35:97–102.
46. Halbreich U, Rojansky N, Palter S. Elimination of ovulation and menstrual cyclicity (with danazol) improves dysphoric premenstrual syndromes. Fertil Steril 1991;56:1066–1069.
47. Muse K. Hormonal manipulation in the treatment of premenstrual syndrome. Clin Obstet Gynecol 1992;35:658–666.
48. Hellberg D, Claesson B, Nilsson S. Premenstrual tension: A placebo-controlled efficacy study with spironolactone and medroxyprogesterone acetate. Int J Gynaecol Obstet 1991;34:243–248.
49. Maxon WS. The use of progesterone in the treatment of PMS. Clin Obstet Gynecol 1987;30:465–477.
50. Magos AL, Brincat M, Studd JW. Treatment of the premenstrual syndrome by subcutaneous oestradiol implants and cyclical oral norethisterone: Placebo-controlled study. Br Med J 1986;292:1629–1633.
51. Watson NR, Studd JWW, Savvas M, et al. Treatment of severe premenstrual syndrome with oestradiol patches and cyclical oral norethisterone. Lancet 1989;2:730–732.
52. Bancroft J, Sanders D, Warner P, Loudon N. The effects of oral contraceptives on mood and sexuality: A comparison of triphasic and combined preparations. J Psychosom Obstet Gynaecol 1987;7:1–8.
53. Parry BL, Rush AJ. Oral contraceptives and depressive symptomatology: Biological mechanisms. Compr Psychiatry 1979;20:347–358.
54. Harrison WM, Endicott J, Nee J. Treatment of premenstrual dysphoria with alprazolam. Arch Gen Psychiatry 1990;47:270–275.
55. Smith S, Rinehart JS, Ruddock VE, Schiff I. I. Treatment of premenstrual syndrome with alprazolam: Results of a double-blind, placebo-controlled, randomized crossover clinical trial. Obstet Gynecol 1987;70:37–43.
56. Berger CP, Presser B. Alprazolam in the treatment of two subsamples of patients with late luteal phase dysphoric dis-

order: A double-blind placebo-controlled crossover study. Obstet Gynecol 1994;84:379–385.
57. Schmidt PJ, Grover GN, Rubinow DR. Alprazolam in the treatment of premenstrual syndrome: A double-blind, placebo-controlled trial. Arch Gen Psychiatry 1993;50:467–473.
58. David D, Freeman A, Harrington TM, et al. Buspirone for anxious women in a primary care environment: A multicenter open evaluation. Adv Ther 1987;4:251–264.
59. Harrison WM, Endicott J, Nee J. Treatment of premenstrual depression with nortriptyline: A pilot study. J Clin Psychiatry 1989;50:136–139.
60. Sundblad C, Modigh K, Andersch B, Eriksson E. Clomipramine effectively reduces premenstrual irritability and dysphoria: A placebo-controlled trial. Acta Psychiatr Scand 1992;85:39–47.
61. Sundblad C, Hedberg MA, Eriksson E. Clomipramine administered during the luteal phase reduces the symptoms of premenstrual syndrome: A placebo controlled trial. Neuropsychopharmacology 1993;9:133–145.
62. Freeman EW, Rickels K, Sondheimer SJ, et al. Nefazodone in the treatment of premenstrual syndrome: A preliminary study. J Clin Psychopharmacol 1994;14:180–186.
63. Rickels K, Freeman EW, Sondheimer S, Albert J. Fluoxetine in the treatment of premenstrual syndrome. Curr Therapeutic Res 1990;48:161–166.
64. Stone AB, Pearlstein TB, Brown WA. Fluoxetine in the treatment of late luteal phase dysphoric disorder. J Clin Psychiatry 1991;52:290–293.
65. Menkes DB, Taghavi, Mason PA, et al. Fluoxetine treatment of severe premenstrual syndrome. Brit Med J 1992; 305:346–347.
66. Menkes DB, Taghavi, Mason PA, Howard RC. Fluoxetine's spectrum of action in premenstrual syndrome. Int Clin Psychopharmacol 1993;8:95–102.
67. Wood SH, Mortola JF, Chan YF, et al. Treatment of premenstrual syndrome with fluoxetine: A double-blind, placebo-controlled, crossover study. Obstet Gynecol 1992;80:339–344.
68. Pearlstein TB, Stone AB. Long-term fluoxetine treatment of late luteal phase dysphoric disorder. J Clin Psychiatry 1994;5:332–335.
69. Steiner M, Steinberg S, Stewart D, et al. Fluoxetine in the treatment of premenstrual dysphoria. N Engl J Med 1995; 332:1529–1534.
70. Freeman EW, Rickels K, Sondheimer SJ, Wittmaack FM. Sertraline versus desipramine in the treatment of premenstrual syndrome: An open-label trial. J Clin Psychiatry 1996;57:7–11.
71. Eriksson E, Hedberg MA, Andersch B, et al. The serotonin reuptake inhibitor paroxetine is superior to the noradrenaline reuptake inhibitor maprotiline in the treatment of premenstrual syndrome: A placebo-controlled trial. Neuropsychopharmacology 1995;12(2):167–176.
72. Steiner M, Haskett RF, Osmum NJ. Treatment of premenstrual tension with lithium carbonate. Acta Psychiatr Scand 1980;61:96–102.
73. Jacobsen FM. Low-dose valproate: A new treatment for cyclothymia, mild rapid cycling disorders, and premenstrual syndrome. J Clin Psychiatry 1993;54:229–234.
74. Muse KN, Cetel NS, Futterman LA, Yen SSC. The premenstrual syndrome: Effects of "medical ovariectomy." N Engl J Med 1984;311:1345–1349.
75. Hammarback S, Backstrom T. Induced anovulation as treatment of premenstrual tension syndrome: A double-blind cross-over study with GnRH-agonist versus placebo. Acta Obstet Gynecol Scand 1988;67:159–166.
76. Mortola JF, Girton L, Fischer U. Successful treatment of severe premenstrual syndrome by combined use of gonadotropin-releasing hormone agonist and estrogen/progestin. J Clin Endocrinol Metab 1991;72:252A–F.
77. Brown CS, Ling FW, Andersen RN, et al. Efficacy of depot leuprolide in premenstrual syndrome: Effect of symptom severity and type in a controlled trial. Obstet Gynecol 1994;84:779–786.
78. West CP, Hillier H. Ovarian suppression with the gonadotropin-releasing hormone agonist goserelin (Zoladex) in management of the premenstrual tension syndrome. Hum Reprod 1994;9(6):1058–1063.
79. Casson P, Hahn PM, Van Vugt DA, Reid RL. Lasting response to ovariectomy in severe intractable premenstrual syndrome. Am J Obstet Gynecol 1990;162:99–105.
80. Casper RH, Hearn MT. The effect of hysterectomy and bilateral oophorectomy in women with severe premenstrual syndrome. Am J Obstet Gynecol 1990;162:105–109.
81. Gise LH, Lebovits AH, Paddison PL, Strain JJ. Issues in the identification of premenstrual syndromes. J Nerv Ment Dis 1990;178:228–234.
82. Mortola JF. A risk–benefit appraisal of drugs used in the management of premenstrual syndrome. Drug Safety 1994;10:160–169.

Chapter 79

Hormone Replacement Therapy

Patricia Moynahan Mullins, PharmD, Mark C. Pugh, PharmD, and Andrea O. Moore, PharmD

MENOPAUSE

Menopause is simply defined as the loss of ovarian function leading to a state of permanent amenorrhea.[1,2] It is but one event in a series of physiologic, endocrinologic, and psychologic changes that signify the transition from reproductive to nonreproductive life, which are termed the *climacteric.*

The terms *menopause* and *climacteric* are not synonymous.[1] The main distinction between these two terms is that menopause is a discrete event while events of the climacteric span several years. The term *perimenopausal* is often used to refer to an arbitrarily defined time period of the climacteric including the first few years before and after menopause.[1,3]

Although menopause is usually thought of as a discrete event, in reality the change from regular menstruation to permanent amenorrhea is marked by a series of irregular cycles. Mean menstrual-cycle length is increased and the intermenstrual interval may vary widely. These irregular cycles continue until no more ovarian follicles capable of responding to gonadotropin stimulation exist. A period of amenorrhea lasting at least 1 year is used clinically to define the onset of menopause.[3]

HISTORY

The phase in a woman's life that in modern times is called the climacteric has been recognized at least from biblical times.[2] Until the twentieth century, the cause of events surrounding the menopause remained unknown. Endocrine research in 1920s led to the discovery and isolation of the hormonal compounds estrogen and progesterone, produced by the ovary. These discoveries fostered the medicinal use of estrogen to relieve menopausal symptoms, first reported by Mazer and Israel in 1935.[1]

The last few decades have been marked by extensive research into the physiology and treatment of menopausal symptoms. This research has been accompanied by a greater understanding of the hazards of estrogen therapy. In 1975, the first reports linking endometrial cancer with exogenous estrogen use were published.[4–6] These papers were followed by numerous scientific and lay publications examining the benefits and risks of hormone replacement therapy for the treatment of menopausal symptoms.[1]

EPIDEMIOLOGY

Based on both historical writings and modern data, the average age of onset of natural menopause has remained remarkably constant and is estimated to be 51.4 years.[1,7] Premature menopause, defined as a loss of ovarian function before the age of 35 years, is secondary to a variety of causes including ovarian surgery (surgical castration), endocrinologic, and autoimmune disorders (Table 79.1).[7] Age of onset appears to be unaffected by race, socioeconomic status, alcohol consumption, age of menarche, or age of last pregnancy. However, women who are cigarette smokers may undergo menopause up to 2 years earlier than nonsmokers possibly because of the gametotoxic effects of cigarette smoke constituents or effects on steroid hormone metabolism by the liver.[1,7]

Although the age of onset of natural menopause is constant, the proportion of women living a significant number of years beyond the age is increasing. Current data place the number of women over the age of 50 years in the United States at 40 million. Projections for the end of the twentieth century estimate this group will grow to 50 million.[8] Given the current life expectancies in the United States, by the end of the century women can expect to live one-third of their life span after the onset of menopause.[1]

PHYSIOLOGY

The underlying cause of the climacteric is an age-related loss of ovarian function that results in a decline in estrogen secretion by the ovarian follicular unit. Throughout life, the number of viable ovarian follicles declines. At birth, 1 to 2 million are present, but by the age of puberty this number

TABLE 79.1. POTENTIAL CAUSES OF PREMATURE MENOPAUSE

Idiopathic
Identifiable karyotypic abnormalities
Exposure to gametotoxic environmental agents
Viral oophoritis
Autoimmune oophoritis
Isolated ovarian failure
Associated with other autoimmune disease
Iatrogenic
Ovarian surgery (surgical castration)
Radiation therapy
Cytotoxic chemotherapy
Defective gonadotropin action
Congenital absence of the thymus
17-Hydroxylase deficiency
Galactosemia

(Compiled from Ref. 7.)

has declined to 300,000–400,000. By age 45 less than 10,000 ovarian follicles remain. Most follicles are lost due to follicular atresia, a normal physiologic process of degeneration of the oocyte and its surrounding stroma.[1] Fewer than 300–400 follicles are lost by ovulation over the woman's reproductive life span. The number of follicles present at puberty and the extent of follicular atresia over the subsequent years determine the age of menopause. Although some follicles remain in postmenopausal women, they are less sensitive to gonadotropin stimulation, implying that the more hormonally sensitive or functionally normal follicles are depleted earlier in life.[1]

The gradual but complete loss of functional follicles as a women ages results in alterations of endocrine function involving the gonadotropins and estrogens (Fig. 79.1).

Estrogens

The major circulating estrogen during the reproductive years is 17β-estradiol (E_2). Estradiol, in the premenopausal women, is produced primarily by the ovary with additional amounts being synthesized in the peripheral tissue by conversion from testosterone or estrone (BE_1). Once the functional follicles are exhausted after menopause, estradiol secretion from the ovary ceases and the primary circulating estrogen is estrone. Estrone has approximately one-third the estrogenic potency of estradiol. In postmenopausal women, the majority of estrone is derived by the peripheral conversion of androstenedione by an extraglandular aromatase found primarily in adipose tissue. Virtually all circulating estradiol in the postmenopausal period is derived from conversion of estrone. Estrone concentrations exceed estradiol by about fourfold after menopause. Unlike the cyclic fluctuations of estrogen in the reproductive years, the levels

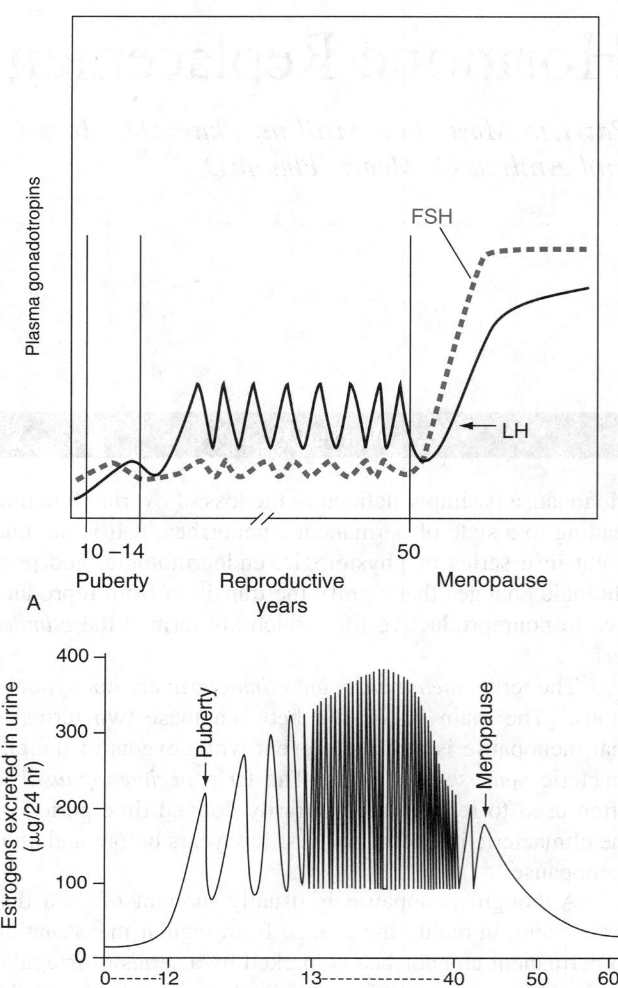

Figure 79.1. (A) Comparison of gonadotropin production at various ages. *(Reproduced from Carr BR, Wilson JD. Disorders of the ovary and female reproductive tract, in Petersdorf RG, Adams RD, Braunwald E, et al [eds]: Harrison's Principles of Internal Medicine, 10th ed. New York, McGraw-Hill, 1983, pp 700–720, with permission of the publisher.)* (B) Comparison of estrogen production at various ages in sexual life. *(Reproduced from Guyton AC. Female physiology before pregnancy, and the female hormones, in Textbook of Medical Physiology, 7th ed. Philadelphia, WB Saunders, 1986, pp 968–982, with permission.)*

of estrone and estradiol remain relatively constant after menopause.[1]

Gonadotropins

Postmenopausal decline in ovarian estradiol production causes diminished negative-feedback effects on the anterior pituitary gland, which results in a compensatory increase in secretion of the gonadotropins, follicle-stimulating hormone (FSH), and luteinizing hormone (LH).[2] Therefore, for the first time since puberty, the level of FSH exceeds LH (Fig. 79.1) and is the inverse of the ratio found in the premenopausal period. The peak levels of FSH and LH are reached 2–3 years after menopause and remain stable or decline slightly over the remaining years of life.[1]

Even though postmenopausal FSH and LH levels are substantially elevated compared to those during the premenopausal period, the remaining follicles generally do not respond to gonadotropin stimulation because of their relative gonadotropin insensitivity. However, occasionally a follicle will mature and release a burst of estradiol. Corpus luteum formation may follow, but progesterone secretion is limited. The result is unopposed estrogen stimulation without cyclic progesterone secretion. These events may be responsible for the occurrence of dysfunctional uterine bleeding during the perimenopausal period.[3]

DIAGNOSIS

The diagnosis of menopause should be approached with the idea of excluding physical or laboratory changes unrelated to decreasing estrogen. Many signs and symptoms observed during menopause can be attributed to aging. Body systems affected by aging include the cardiovascular system, respiratory system, nervous system, immune system, and skin and musculoskeletal system. With the exception of the gonads, the endocrine system undergoes very little change during aging. Specifically, the diagnosis of menopause should involve a comprehensive medical history and thorough physical exam with complete blood count and with measurement of serum FSH. Altered thyroid function, which may mimic menopausal symptoms, and pregnancy must be excluded. A breast exam and mammography should be performed. In the absence of other disease processes, an elevated FSH concentration of 30 pg/mL or greater indicates the woman is menopausal.[1,9] In symptomatic patients with either elevated or borderline (15–30 pg/mL) FSH concentrations, hormone replacement therapy (HRT) may be considered. Until recently, HRT was not usually recommended for asymptomatic women in the absence of other medical risk factors even though FSH is elevated.[9] A growing body of clinical data now supports the use of HRT for prevention or treatment of osteoporosis and for its cardioprotective benefits.

SYMPTOMS

Symptom complexes specifically related to estrogen deprivation include genitourinary atrophy, vasomotor instability, and osteoporosis. Other changes include blood lipid alterations and increased incidence of atherosclerotic cardiovascular diseases, insomnia, and psychosexual symptoms.

Genitourinary Atrophy

Large numbers of estrogen receptors are located in the vagina, vulva, urethra, and trigone of the bladder. Atrophy of these tissues begins with diminished estrogen concentrations and continues, at different rates for the specific tissues, over many years. The vulva undergoes atrophy, and there is thinning of hair of the mons and shrinkage of the labia minora. A decrease in subcutaneous fat and elasticity of the tissue causes the labia majora to flatten. Atrophic changes of the vulva (Kraurosis vulvae) lead to pruritus and pain.[1,10] Vaginal epithelium becomes pale and thin, leading to diminished distensibility and reduced secretion; the tissue is easily traumatized and may bleed. The vaginal pH rises to an alkaline range of pH 6–8 (usual premenopausal pH is 4.5–5) creating a favorable environment for bacterial colonization by various pathogens. The incidence of atrophic vaginitis increases during postmenopausal years, producing symptoms of itching, bleeding, or dyspareunia. Decreased estrogen is probably not the direct cause of uterine prolapse; hernias in the anterior (cystocele) and posterior (rectocele) vaginal wall, coupled with a decrease in tissue elasticity, could account for the higher incidence of these conditions in the climacteric.[1,10]

The urethra may become rigid and inelastic and undergo epithelial thinning. The urethral syndrome, a recurrent nonbacterial urethritis, is more common in postmenopausal women. Despite changes in the urethra and supporting pelvic tissue, there does not appear to be any increase in stress urinary incontinence in postmenopausal women compared with premenopausal women. Bacteriuria is found in 7–10% of postmenopausal women versus 4% of premenopausal women. Postmenopausal women may be more prone to bacteriuria due to mucosal atrophy and increased vaginal contamination caused by vaginal foreshortening.[1,10] Treatment with intravaginal or systemic estrogen reverses the thinning of the vaginal mucosa through epithelial proliferation and decreases vaginal pH to its more normal acidic state. Estrogen therapy often relieves symptoms of vaginitis and frictional dyspareunia and improves urinary frequency, dysuria, nocturia, urgency, postvoiding dribbling, and, to some extent, stress urinary incontinence.[1,10]

Vasomotor Instability

Vasomotor symptoms or hot flashes most often prompt the postmenopausal woman to seek medical care. The cause of these symptoms is estrogen deficiency, possibly leading to aberrant surges of LH or gonadotropin-releasing hormone (GnRH), which affect the hypothalamic neurons that control central thermoregulation centers. The rate of decrease in estrogen concentrations is directly related to the severity of vasomotor responses. Hot flushes (or flashes) are experienced by 75–85% of women following natural menopause and by 37–50% of premenopausal women who undergo bilateral oophorectomy. They are most common within 12–24 months after the last menstrual period, gradually subsiding thereafter. The hot flush is an acute, episodic event that initially occurs several times a day, often during sleep. Peripheral blood flow increases causing increased skin temperature. Perspiration occurs as a homeostatic response designed to dissipate heat; an increase in heart rate probably reflects a sympathetic response to change in skin temperature.[11] Hot flushes are frequently associated with nausea, dizziness, headache, palpitations, diaphoresis, and night sweats that interrupt sleep.[1,10] Estrogen has traditionally been the drug of choice for relieving hot flushes, but medroxyprogesterone in relatively high doses, some ergot alkaloids, or α-adrenergic agonists such as clonidine are also effective.[1,11] When prescribed to control vasomotor symptoms, estrogen should be started at the lowest dose that controls the hot flushes, and continued for 3–5 years, when it can be tapered and discontinued by most women, in the absence of other justification for HRT.[12]

Osteoporosis

Osteoporosis is a universal, gradual loss of bone mass that eventually compromises the skeleton and results in fractures after minimal trauma (see Chapter 83 for a more detailed discussion of osteoporosis.) Rather than a single pathologic condition, osteoporosis is a heterogeneous disease process involving multiple etiologies and affecting both men and women. Estrogen deficiency, as a factor in osteoporosis, was recognized in 1941 when Albright and associates described the association between estrogen deficiency, at surgical or natural menopause, and osteoporotic fractures. Recent long-term clinical trials have demonstrated that osteoporotic fractures can be prevented by estrogen replacement through modification of bone loss.[13]

The medical and socioeconomic considerations of managing postmenopausal osteoporosis is a major concern in the United States. Although the exact incidence is unknown, osteoporosis is thought to affect between 15 and 20 million individuals in this country. About 1.2 million fractures annually are related to osteoporosis. Vertebral crush fractures are most common, but hip fractures have the most serious sequelae. Annually, 150,000–200,000 hip fractures occur, and about 10% of patients who suffer a hip fracture die from surgical complications within 6 months. Another 100,000–150,000 patients require institutional rehabilitation and skilled care at a total estimated annual health cost of about $6 billion. By age 70, 15% of women will experience a wrist fracture, 25% will experience a vertebral fracture, and 15% will experience a hip fracture.[14] The greatest risk of postmenopausal osteoporosis occurs in slender, sedentary females of Caucasian or Asian descent. Social history (e.g., smoking, alcohol use), family/medical history, and chronic use of specific drugs (e.g., corticosteroids) are also risk factors.

The precise mechanism by which estrogen prevents bone loss is unknown. Exogenous estrogen administration reverses biochemical changes (decreases in serum calcium, phosphorus, alkaline phosphatase, and osteocalcin) and urinary output of calcium and hydroxyproline associated with estrogen withdrawal. Conflicting changes are seen in the regulatory hormones that control calcium homeostasis, particularly parathyroid hormone. Overall, the response of bone to estrogen therapy is a reduced rate of resorption with normal mineralization of the remodeling unit.[14]

For maximal benefit, estrogen replacement should begin as soon as possible after menopause. After 6–24 months, bone resorption and formation return to a state of equilibrium and bone mass stabilizes. Estrogen therapy should continue for at least the next 10–15 years. Despite their preventive effect, estrogens alone do not restore bone that has been lost. Fractures may still occur despite estrogen replacement if bone demineralization was severe before replacement therapy. It is uncertain if estrogen therapy should be initiated as late as 10–15 years after menopause when osteoporosis is the only indication. Progestins, in combination with estrogen, do not impair estrogen's bone-preserving actions. Some progestins used as single-agent therapy will protect against bone loss, but clarification of the overall role of progestins in osteoporosis awaits further study.[14]

Cardiovascular Disease

Coronary artery disease is a multifactoral problem associated with identifiable risk factors including hypertension, hyperlipidemia, diabetes, and cigarette smoking. After menopause the incidence of coronary artery disease rapidly increases; after surgical menopause the risk is more than 2.2-fold greater. Each year coronary artery disease is responsible for the deaths of approximately 500,000 women in the United States.[15]

In most studies, estrogen replacement produces a potentially beneficial effect on cardiovascular risk by favorably altering the serum lipid profile. Estrogens lower low-density lipoprotein (LDL) cholesterol and increase high-density lipoprotein (HDL) cholesterol. Other mechanisms, such as platelet effects and direct effects on vessel wall physiology, may also be cardioprotective. While triglycerides may be higher in estrogen users, blood pressure and fasting blood glucose levels are unchanged or lower.[16,17] In most studies, estrogen therapy has shown a 50% or greater reduction in cardiovascular disease and related mortality.[16] Recent evidence suggests that the beneficial cardiovascular effects of estrogen replacement after menopause are most pronounced in the presence of angiographically defined coronary artery disease.[17]

In contrast to the effects of estrogen on the lipid profile, progestins, unlike natural progesterone, may attenuate or eliminate the benefits on HDL cholesterol. To maximize cardiovascular protection, progestin therapy should be limited to low doses and reserved for those with an intact uterus.[16] A recently published 3-year placebo-controlled trial (Postmenopausal Estrogen/Progestin Interventions or PEPI) comparing estrogen alone with three estrogen/progestin combinations confirmed the cardiovascular benefits of combined treatment on HDL cholesterol, an encouraging finding for women who require the addition of progestin to an estrogen-containing regimen.[18]

Other Symptoms

Freud characterized the woman at menopause as "quarrelsome and obstinate, petty and stingy, sadistic and analerotic."[1] Others have popularized the notion that menopause is characterized by "an erratic disorientation of the woman's entire frame of mind."[1] However, there is very little objective evidence to support a causal role for decreased estrogen in most psychologic disorders or symptoms that are associated with menopause.[1]

Insomnia and fatigue, which affect 30–40% of postmenopausal women, may be related to estrogen deficiency. Some estrogen-deficient women suffer from chronic sleep deprivation, which can be verified by sleep polygraphs documenting a close temporal relationship between hot flushes and waking episodes.[1] Mood changes, such as irritability, depression, insomnia, impaired memory, and crying spells are usually regarded as "hormone-related" symptoms that precede and postdate menopause. Although many of these changes are estrogen dependent, depression and anxiety may be caused by numerous nonhormonal conditions.[12]

Estrogens may modify the metabolism of several central nervous system (CNS) neurotransmitters, thus accounting for their behavioral effects.[1] Response of some psychologic symptoms to estrogen have been attributed to a placebo response.[1] However, some prescribers use an estrogen trial for symptomatic patients with no other clinical evidence of a CNS problem.[12]

A decrease in any basic human activity, including sexual function, has an impact on the quality of life. Most women experience some change in sexual function in the years immediately before and after menopause. Sexual function is influenced by the interaction between complex hormonal factors and nonbiologic factors, including psychologic and sociocultural factors and interpersonal relationships. That estrogen deficiency may be a possible cause for a change in libido and sexual response rests on the hypothesis that sexual disinterest is a consequence of dyspareunia, resulting from atrophic changes of the genitourinary tract. However, dyspareunia occurs in less than 8% of postmenopausal patients, and oophorectomy before menopause does not affect libido unless the uterus is also removed.[1] In 1966, Masters and Johnson characterized the physiologic changes in menopause that are related to sexual function. These changes are classified into five disorder categories: desire phase; excitement phase (touch sensations impairment, clitoral sensation impairment, vaginal dryness, urinary incontinence); orgasmic phase (primary or secondary nonorgasmic responses); dyspareunia (including vaginismus, a conditioned response to painful penetration); and a dysfunctional male partner. The effects of decreased estrogen on the CNS, the peripheral nervous system, and the cardiovascular system, as well as on specific tissues, may account for most changes and may explain why estrogen therapy can markedly improve sexual function in some women. Counseling and referral to a specialist is not required in the majority of cases of sexual dysfunction associated with menopause.[19]

Nonhormonal Treatment for Menopause

Most clinical symptoms present in the menopausal period are associated directly with estrogen deficiency and thus nonpharmacologic measures are not generally helpful. Some of the problems in menopausal women including cardiovascular disease, obesity, muscle weakness, and osteoporosis are also related to aging. These symptoms may respond to aerobic exercise and resistance training. Behavioral symptoms may respond to psychiatric counseling.[8,20]

Response of vasomotor symptoms to various nonhormonal agents including clonidine, β blockers, veralapride, naloxone, methyldopa, clomifene, and androgens has been studied, but these investigations have generally not been well designed. In noncontrolled trials, clonidine increased LH and had peripheral vascular effects; both effects may improve hot flushes. Placebo-controlled studies have not demonstrated a significant reduction in hot flushes with clonidine. Veralapride, a dopaminergic agent similar to metoclopramide, eliminated hot flushes in 60–80% of women in several clinical studies. Patients remained free of symptoms for up to 3 months after discontinuing veralapride. Adverse effects included galactorrhea and breast tenderness. Clomifene, a weak estrogenic/antiestrogenic compound, may be beneficial in the treatment of some symptoms of menopause, but it is not effective in relieving hot flushes.[8]

Calcium supplementation and weight-bearing exercise are primary nonhormonal preventions and treatments for osteoporosis. Clomifene, which decreases urinary calcium loss and may block parathyroid hormone-induced bone resorption, may be particularly useful in the prevention of osteoporosis. Other agents, including calcitonin and etidronate, may also be beneficial in preventing osteoporosis.[8,21]

For the treatment of vaginal dryness and dyspareunia a mucoadherent compound, polycarbophil, is available on a nonprescription basis. This agent is a long-acting lubricant that lowers vaginal pH, and its development marks significant progress relative to previously available water-soluble lubricants.[8]

HRT produces a favorable alteration in the serum lipid profile, may have vasodilatory properties, and shows other properties thought to be cardioprotective. However, exercise and diet along with other lifestyle practices such as smoking abstinence and moderation in alcohol consumption form the primary approach to prevention of cardiovascular disease.[15,17]

Estrogen Replacement Therapy

Indications for estrogen replacement therapy include relief from vasomotor symptoms, genitourinary dysfunction, and certain psychologic changes and prevention or treatment of osteoporosis. Estrogen therapy is also effective in reducing cardiovascular morbidity and mortality.[12]

PHARMACOLOGY

The end product of estrogen synthesis from cholesterol in ovarian follicles is 17β-estradiol, the most potent estrogen. Estradiol is rapidly oxidized to estrone, which is then hydrated to the even weaker estriol. Estrogens attach to tissue-specific receptor proteins in the cytoplasm of target organs including the ovaries, uterus, fallopian tubes, vagina, bladder, urethra, and breast. Other target organs include the skin, adrenals, cardiovascular system, gastrointestinal tract (colon, pancreas, and liver), and the CNS (pituitary, hypothalamus, and spinal cord).[1,2,22] This estrogen–protein complex diffuses through the nuclear membrane and ultimately binds to materials in the cell nucleus. Synthesis of DNA, RNA, and other proteins increases, resulting in characteristic changes in the responsive tissues. Estrogen receptors have not been found in bone and the specific mechanism of action of hormonal therapy in osteoporosis is unclear.[23]

Any estrogen capable of binding to the estrogen receptors in target organs should alleviate menopausal symptoms. Exogenous estrogens administered orally, transdermally, or vaginally are the major useful forms of therapy (Table 79.2). Injectable estrogens are not generally used for treating menopausal symptoms because of poor patient acceptance and because of fluctuating plasma concentrations, with initial peaks and subsequent low estrogen levels.[13,22] Subcutaneous pellets of estradiol have been studied and used clinically. Because estradiol is not metabolized significantly in subcutaneous tissue, this dosage form results in a preferential increase in estradiol rather than in estrone and other metabolites. Although compliance is improved with this route of administration, it is not popular because implantation and removal require minor surgery.[13]

Several oral estrogen products are commercially available. Conjugated equine estrogens are purified from the urine of pregnant mares. Estrogens are metabolized and conjugated by the liver in preparation for excretion. The product obtained from horse urine is a mixture of estrogen compounds, mostly sulfates and glucuronides, some of which are not found in humans. The pharmacokinetics of orally administered equine estrogens is complex because of the many different estrogen compounds in the products.[22]

Absorption of oral estradiol tablets has become more reliable with micronized formulations, but estradiol is metabolized significantly on first pass through the liver to other less active metabolites. Oral estrone tablets also provide relief of symptoms at appropriate doses.[13,22]

Estrogen, in vaginal creams, is readily absorbed through the vaginal epithelium and is a feasible treatment not only for urogenital symptoms, but for other menopausal symptoms as well. Estradiol is metabolized very little as it is absorbed from the vagina, and this route of administration results primarily in increased estradiol serum concentrations. Unfortunately, these concentrations return to baseline in approximately 6 hours. Because of the short duration of increased serum concentrations and because vaginal creams are messy and dosage is difficult to control, they are not widely used.[22]

A transdermal patch containing estradiol is the newest commercially available dosage form. One patch is applied to the skin, usually on the lower trunk. This dosage form offers parenteral therapy with little metabolism of estradiol and convenient administration and precise dosing.[22] Transdermal patches containing the active ingredient in the adhesive and formulations containing estrogen and progestin are under study.

A complicating pharmacokinetic feature of exogenous estrogen replacement is the relatively high first-pass metabolism of orally administered estrogens. Approximately 60–90% of an orally administered dose of estrogen is converted to estrone or inactive metabolites. Consequently, high doses of exogenous estrogens need to be administered to compensate for this effect.[24] Transdermal administration of estrogens, such as 17β-estradiol, results in estradiol levels equivalent to those in the early to mid-follicular phase and an estrone-to-estradiol ratio of approximately 1:1, which closely resembles the premenopausal state.[25] Oral administration can also achieve similar estradiol levels, but only at the expense of a higher estrone-to-estradiol ratio.[26] Unlike oral estrogen replacement, transdermal estrogen delivery has no significant effect on production of certain hepatic proteins, renin substrate, sex-hormone-binding globulin, thyroxine-binding globulin, and cortisol-binding globulin. Elevations in these proteins may be associated with some of the adverse effects of oral estrogen therapy including hypertension, gallbladder disease, and thrombosis, although the clinical significance of this effect is not yet established.[13,27]

The effects of transdermal estrogen administration on the lipid profile appear to be less favorable than with orally administered estrogens, presumably because of the

TABLE 79.2. ESTROGEN PRODUCTS

Agent	Dosage Form	Dose	Indications
Estrone aqueous suspension	Injection	0.1–5 mg IM 2–3 times/week	A,B
Estrogenic substance or estrogen aqueous suspension (primarily estrone) injection	Injection	0.1–1.0 mg IM 2–3 times/week	A,B
Estradiol cypionate (in oil)	Injection	1–5 mg/d IM every 3–4 weeks	C
Estradiol valerate (in oil)	Injection	10–20 mg every 4 weeks	A,B,C
Conjugated estrogens	Oral	0.03–1.25 mg/d[a]	A,B,C,D
Conjugated estrogens/medroxyprogesterone acetate	Oral	0.625 mg/2.5 mg per day[b]	C,D
Conjugated estrogens/medroxyprogesterone acetate	Oral	0.625 mg per day for 14 days,[b] then 0.625 mg/5 mg per day for 14 days[b]	C,D
Micronized estradiol	Oral	0.5–2 mg/d[a]	A,B,C,D
Esterified estrogens (75–85% estrone sulfate and 6–15% sodium equilin)	Oral	0.3–1.25 mg/d[a]	A,B,C,D
Estropipate (piperazine estrone sulfate)	Oral	0.75–6 mg/d[a]	A,B,C
Ethinyl estradiol	Oral	0.02–1.5 mg/d[a]	A,C
Quinestrol	Oral	0.1 mg/d for 7 days, then 0.1 mg once weekly	A,B,C
Chlorotrianisene	Oral	12–25 mg/d for 21 days	A,B,C
Estropipate vaginal cream	Topical	3–6 mg daily for 3 weeks	B
Micronized estradiol vaginal cream	Topical	Daily[c]	B
Conjugated estrogens vaginal cream	Topical	1.25–2.5 mg daily for 3 weeks	B
Dienestrol vaginal cream	Topical	Once or twice daily[c]	B
Estrone vaginal cream	Topical	2–4 mg daily	B
Estradiol transdermal	Transdermal	0.05–0.1 mg system twice weekly	A,B,C,D

Key: A, replacement therapy of estrogen deficiency-associated conditions (i.e., female hypogonadism); B, senile vaginitis and Kraurosis vulvae; C, moderate to severe vasomotor symptoms associated with menopause; D, osteoporosis.

[a]May administer continuously or cyclically with 3 weeks of daily estrogen followed by 1 week off.

[b]Blister pack dosage cards used for single prescription convenience in continuous or cyclic combination regimens.

[c]Typical regimen: Initial therapy one dose daily for 2 weeks, followed by 2 additional weeks of daily therapy at one-half dose, followed by maintenance therapy of one dose 1–3 times/week for three weeks. Check drug information references for specific regimens. (Compiled from Ref. 22.)

lack of a first-pass effect on the liver. Short-term and some longer term (6 months or more) studies report no alteration in lipid profiles with transdermal administrations.[25] However, other long-term studies report increased HDL[28] and decreased LDL.[29]

The typical transdermal estrogen regimen involves the application of one patch twice weekly. Administration may be either continuous, or in 3-week cycles with 1 week estrogen free. As with oral estrogen therapy, the addition of a progestin is recommended for the last 10–13 days of the cycle in women receiving cyclic therapy who have an intact uterus.[30]

CLINICAL USE

Because the symptoms of menopause are primarily linked to declining endogenous estradiol, most therapeutic interventions replace estrogens and thereby relieve the symptoms associated with menopause. In general, the smallest dose of estrogen that alleviates symptoms or prevents disease is used for the shortest possible time period.

Vasomotor Instability

The symptoms of vasomotor instability respond to exogenous estrogen therapy.[31,32] In most women, the period of bothersome vasomotor symptoms lasts from 3–5 years, and therapy for these symptoms can be limited to that time span.[12] A variety of estrogens, including dosage forms and schemes for administration, exist (Table 79.2). A popular regimen is oral therapy with conjugated equine estrogens starting at doses of 0.3–0.625 mg/d given in 25-day cycles, with 5 estrogen-free days. Other estrogen agents include micronized estradiol 0.5–2 mg/d, ethinyl estradiol 0.02–0.05 mg/d, esterified estrogens 0.3–1.25 mg/d, or chlorotrianisene 12–25 mg/d. Quinestrol is given 0.1 mg/d for 7 days, then once weekly thereafter. These estrogens are prescribed in the same cyclic regimen as conjugated equine estrogens. The addition of a progestin is standard therapy in women with an intact uterus because of the adverse consequences of unopposed estrogen therapy, specifically the increased risk of endometrial cancer. One common regimen is the addition of medroxyprogesterone acetate 5–10 mg daily during the last 10–12 days of the cycle.[33] Other progestins used in cyclic therapy include norethindrone 2.5 mg, norgestrel 150 μg, or micronized oral progesterone 300 mg.[34] This cyclic regimen results in the return of regular menstrual periods, which some women find objectionable.

For women in whom cyclical bleeding is unacceptable, an alternative regimen involves the continuous administration of estrogens, with the addition of a progestin for 10–12 days during the calendar month. Advantages include a less complicated schedule and less likelihood of return of symptoms during the estrogen-free period.[34] Continuous combined estrogen–progestin therapy may be associated with a 40% incidence of breakthrough bleeding, especially during the first 6 months.[35] Some clinicians have advocated the continuous administration of estrogens and lower dose progestins (2.5–5 mg daily medroxyprogesterone acetate) as an effective alternative to cyclic therapy with the benefit of avoidance of withdrawal bleeding.[36–38] See Table 79.2 for combination product availability. The long-term effects of these treatments are unknown, especially their effects on cardiovascular morbidity and mortality, although using surrogate markers of cardiovascular disease and a follow-up period of 3 years showed effects comparable to estrogen alone.[18]

Dosing of estrogen must be individualized based on the severity and duration of symptoms. A periodic reassessment of therapy, with an attempt to reduce dose or withdraw therapy, should be conducted. Because vasomotor symptoms are self-limiting, estrogen treatment should be tapered and discontinued when the need no longer exists, if no other indication for estrogen therapy exists.

Urogenital Atrophy

Various vaginal preparations of estrogen are effective in the treatment of vaginal itching, dryness, burning, and other symptoms associated with changes in the vaginal epithelium caused by menopause. The goal of therapy is to restore the epithelium to its premenopausal state and thereby reduce these symptoms. Therapy is generally initiated with the smallest dose to restore the vaginal epithelium, usually 2–4 g of estradiol cream (0.1 mg estradiol/g) given once daily for 1–2 weeks initially. Therapy is tapered to half-doses for an additional 2 weeks. Maintenance therapy can be continued with 1 g given one to three times weekly in the usual cyclic manner.[39] Alternatives to estradiol cream include dienestrol (0.01 mg/g) 5–6 g/d, conjugated estrogens (0.625 mg/g) 2–4 g/d, or estropipate (1.5 mg/g) 2–4 g/d given in the same cyclic manner as estradiol. Oral or transdermal administration of estrogens may also be used to treat the symptoms of urogenital atrophy in the same doses and regimens discussed for use in vasomotor instability.

Osteoporosis

It is important to begin HRT soon after menopause (preferably within 3 years) to prevent loss of bone density and subsequent risk of hip, vertebral, and wrist fractures. In one study of hip fractures, there was a long-lasting protective benefit in the first 4 years after menopause; in older women, estrogen therapy within the previous 2 years was also protective. HRT should be used for at least 5 years to substantially decrease fracture rate. If HRT therapy is discontinued, bone loss begins immediately. The dose of estrogen required to prevent bone loss is 0.625 mg daily. Lower doses of conjugated estrogen, e.g., 0.312 mg/d, may prevent bone loss if used in conjunction with high daily doses of elemental calcium (at least 1500 mg/d).[34] Esterified estrogens at doses of 0.625 mg/d, oral ethinyl estradiol 0.02 mg/d, micronized 17β-estradiol 1 mg/d, and transdermal estrogen patches (delivering estradiol 0.05–0.10 mg/d, administered as one patch twice weekly) are alternative regimens. The addition of progestin is not detrimental to bone effects. Adequate intake of calcium and regular weight-bearing exercise are also important adjunctive treatments to be used in conjunction with HRT.

Cardiovascular Disease

Most studies investigating the use of estrogens in protecting the cardiovascular system have used oral estrogen in doses similar to those used for prevention of osteoporosis. The most effective regimen has not been established.[15,17]

PROGESTIN THERAPY

Progesterone, a secretory product of the corpus luteum, is the primary natural progestational substance. Progestins act on the endometrium to change proliferative endometrial tissue into secretory tissue. Progestins alone are as effective as estrogens for relief of vasomotor symptoms. These agents also are useful in the treatment and prevention of osteoporosis, by increasing the formation of new bone. Synthetic progestins appear to stimulate bone formation via androgenic or anabolic effects.[8]

The administration of a progestin for 10 days each month with estrogen replacement therapy serves three major purposes: to decrease the risk of estrogen-induced irregular bleeding, endometrial hyperplasia, and carcinoma; to protect against breast carcinoma; and to enhance estrogen prophylaxis of osteoporosis.[34]

Natural progesterone is poorly absorbed when administered orally and thus synthetic forms of 17α-hydroxy progesterone and 19-nortestosterone are used clinically. The 19-nortestosterone derivatives must be converted to norethisterone in order to be biologically active. Because the 19-nortestosterone derivatives possess androgenic activity, they tend to cause acne and increase oil production on the skin and scalp. These products are used primarily in oral contraceptives.[22,34] The 17-hydroxyprogesterone derivatives, used primarily in hormone replacement therapy, are less androgenic but are associated with depression and anxiety symptoms.[13,34] Micronized natural progesterone is used clinically; however, large doses are required due to significant first-pass metabolism. Medroxyprogesterone acetate is the progestin generally used in treating menopausal symptoms because it is relatively well absorbed orally and has a more acceptable side-effect profile.

CLINICAL USE

In addition to using a progestin in cyclic estrogen replacement therapy to prevent endometrial hyperplasia, progestins alone are used successfully to treat vasomotor instability. Medroxyprogesterone acetate 20 mg/d orally has been employed.[40] Depot medroxyprogesterone acetate 50–100 mg intramuscularly given every 2–3 months is as effective as conjugated estrogens in relieving vasomotor symptoms.[41] In women for whom estrogen therapy is contraindicated, progesterone may be a suitable alternative for treatment of osteoporosis. Recommended dosages are oral medroxyprogesterone acetate 5–10 mg/d or the depot injection form 100–200 mg every 2–3 months.[8]

ADVERSE EFFECTS

Progestins may cause certain dose-related physical, psychologic, and metabolic side effects. When used alone or during the progestin phase of a combination regimen, an iatrogenic premenstrual tension-like syndrome may occur. Breast tenderness or mastalgia, bloating, edema, and abdominal cramping, as well as anxiety, irritability, and depression, are frequent complaints. Weight gain, headache, and drowsiness may occur. Approximately 5% of patients are intolerant to all types of progestins, but others may benefit from a dosage reduction or change to another type of progestin. There are no convincing data to support the premise that continuous-combined HRT reduces progesterone-induced adverse effects relative to sequential HRT.[34]

Progestins alone or with estrogen cause monthly bleeding in 80–90% of women; unopposed estrogen causes monthly withdrawal bleeding in 25% of patients. For women with moderate to severe postmenopausal symptoms, the inconvenience of bleeding may be offset by symptom relief. However, for the asymptomatic woman receiving estrogen for its cardiovascular or bone effects, or for the woman who has been postmenopausal for a number of years, regular withdrawal bleeding may be unacceptable. Some women choose not to begin or to continue HRT because of bleeding.[34] Continuous therapy with an estrogen–progestin combination is an option for women who wish to avoid monthly bleeding.

Progestins, both the C-19 nortestosterone derivatives and the C-21 derivatives, cause a dose-related decrease in HDL cholesterol and an increase in LDL cholesterol levels. To minimize the possibility of negating the cardioprotective effects of estrogens, progestins should be used in the minimum dosage required for endometrial protection when prescribed with estrogen.[34] Some data exist that suggest this adverse effect of progestins on HDL cholesterol may be a short-term effect. Women using combined therapy and those using unopposed estrogens for more than 3 years had HDL levels 11% higher and LDL levels 10–14% lower than women not receiving hormonal therapy. Much research is currently being done to find a synthetic progestin without this adverse effect on lipids.[42] Although not yet available for clinical use as progestin replacement agents, three 19-nortestosterone derivatives or gonanes—gestodene, norgestimate, and desogestrel—with relatively fewer androgenic effects than the estranes (norethindrone and norethindrone acetate) are of interest.[35]

EVALUATION OF THERAPEUTIC OUTCOMES

Before initiating hormone replacement therapy (HRT), menopause should be verified. Because periods of amenorrhea are not sufficiently reliable to signal the beginning of menopause, other diagnostic means are necessary. An FSH level of 30 pg/mL or greater indicates the beginning of menopause. If FSH levels are unavailable, the progestin challenge test can be used for diagnosis. This method, whereby a progestin is given for 10 days, is relatively inexpensive and easy to administer. Absence of withdrawal bleeding indicates lack of significant estrogen secretion and endometrial stimulation. If withdrawal bleeding occurs, the progestin can be repeated in monthly cycles until withdrawal bleeding fails to occur.[13]

The presence of any estrogen-dependent cancer should be ruled out before the initiation of HRT. Mammography should be performed if the woman has not recently undergone this procedure. A complete physical exam including breast exam and lipid profile should be performed to establish a baseline. In women with an intact uterus, a periodic endometrial biopsy should be taken, generally every 2–3 years, to screen for the development of endometrial hyperplasia. Routine follow-up visits with breast and pelvic examinations are recommended at yearly intervals.[13]

RISKS AND BENEFITS

Patients who do not understand the purpose, risks, and side effects of HRT may refuse treatment, exhibit poor compliance, or discontinue therapy. Although acceptance of HRT is ultimately a decision for the patient and her physician, family and friends may offer opinions about what constitutes appropriate use, providing anecdotal details to support these opinions. HRT has also captured the attention of the media, and much of the patient's education, sometimes reflecting misinformation or misinterpretation of facts presented in an abbreviated format, may arise from lay publications or programs.[43]

Among the risks of therapy that may figure prominently in the patient's decisions about HRT are concerns about endometrial and breast cancer, coagulation and thrombosis, cardiovascular events, and neurologic effects.[12,43] Concerns about endometrial (uterine) and breast cancer are primary therapy considerations for many women. Although estrogen is not a carcinogen, it may act as an accelerative growth factor when cancer is present. Breast cancer is a contraindication to estrogen replacement therapy,[12,43] except in patients where powerful overriding indications exist and where careful follow-up can be assured.[44] Studies examining the risk of breast cancer in women receiving estrogen replacement at menopause have not shown a consistent pattern of increased risk, possibly due to methodologic deficiencies and flaws in study design. However, because disagreement exists regarding the possible association of estrogen replacement and breast cancer, all women receiving estrogen replacement should practice regular breast self-examination along with annual physician breast examinations and routine mammography.[12,44] The potential protective role for added progestins in breast cancer prevention is still not established.[12]

In contrast to the questionable association of HRT and breast cancer, the association between endometrial cancer and estrogen use has been recognized since 1975. Increased frequency of uterine cancer is related to endometrial hyperplasia, a predictable result of unopposed estrogen therapy (estrogen therapy without progestional agents).[44] Overall, estrogen users have a fourfold to eightfold increase (range 1.7- to 20-fold) in risk of developing endometrial cancer relative to the risk in the normal population of 100 cases per 100,000. Risk, which persists after discontinuation of estrogens, is related to various factors including duration of use, dosage, method of administration, drug-free interval, and concomitant progestin use.[14,44] The addition of progestin to estrogen therapy confers protection against hyperplasia and is generally recommended, either cyclically for at least 10 days per month or continuously in patients with an intact uterus.[12,44]

Because estrogens and progestins produce a complex variety of effects on coagulation, a history of thromboembolism is a relative contraindication to estrogen therapy.[44] Progestins may increase or reduce prostacyclin production, while synthetic estrogens specifically or preferentially increase prostacyclin activity. Platelet aggregation is generally unchanged by estrogens, although there are limited data to the contrary. Virtually all clotting factors, particularly factors II, VIII, IX, X, and XII and fibrinogen, are elevated by synthetic estrogens such as ethinyl estradiol and diethylstilbestrol. The effects on clotting factors are primarily related to estrogen potency. Elevations are relatively marked with ethinyl estradiol, but are either not observed or are not clinically significant after use of estrogen patches and ointment or natural estrogens.[12,44] In general, total estrogen potency in HRT is less than that received by most women taking oral contraceptives.

Despite producing increased amounts of clotting factors, estrogens do not produce a hypercoagulable state because the clotting proenzymes remain inactive until exposed to injured vascular endothelium. Also, antithrombin III is not reduced to a clinically significant degree by either oral or transdermal estrogens. Plasminogen, a major factor in the fibrinolytic pathway, and plasminogen activity are elevated by estrogens. These effects are enhanced by estrogen–progestin combination therapy. Plasminogen effects along with normal antithrombin III activity ensure against inappropriate venous thrombosis. Clinical trials have shown no increase in risk of thromboembolism in postmenopausal women receiving estrogen replacement.[12,44]

Most recent studies have demonstrated potential benefit of postmenopausal estrogen use on the risk of cardiovascular disease, including stroke, myocardial infarction, and cardiovascular death. The benefits of estrogen in cardiovascular disease are generally attributed to their favorable effects on lipids and lipoproteins. Enhanced prostacyclin production, resulting in vasodilation, is also beneficial. LDL cholesterol is reduced and HDL cholesterol is increased. These changes are seen with both oral and nonoral ethinyl estradiol and with oral, but not vaginal, conjugated estrogens. Transdermal estrogen patches do not appear to produce favorable effects on lipids and lipoproteins. In contrast, synthetic progestins have an effect on prostacyclin and on lipoproteins that is opposite that of estrogens, at least in the short term. At conventional doses of progestin, HDL cholesterol is decreased, an effect that may ameliorate or abolish estrogen's beneficial effects. In balancing the effects of unopposed estrogens on the intact uterus in the patient at high cardiovascular risk, some authorities recommend relatively high-dose estrogen (e.g., conjugated estrogens 1.25 mg) with cyclic progestin (e.g., medroxyprogesterone acetate 5 mg) for the first 2 weeks of the cycle, a regimen associated with a favorable lipid profile.[12] Most women do not need added progestins after a hysterectomy.[12]

The concern that hypertension may be caused or exacerbated by estrogens has contributed to the belief that hypertension is a contraindication to estrogen therapy.[12] The bulk of recent clinical evidence shows no causal relationship between estrogen replacement therapy and hypertension. Oral estrogen therapy, particularly potent synthetic products, but not transdermal estrogen, causes increased renin substrate and may increase angiotensin II and aldosterone, although the clinical significance of these changes is unknown.[44] Progestins, however, produce a dose-related elevation in blood pressure by causing sodium and water retention.[12]

Estrogen therapy may potentiate headaches, including migraine headache. Therefore, a history of migraine headache is a relative contraindication to estrogen replacement therapy. In some patients, the frequency of headache may be reduced over a period of about 4 weeks by a reduction in estrogen dosage. Parenteral testosterone has also been used to alleviate estrogen-induced headache.[12]

Conclusion

Menopause is caused by an age-related loss of ovarian function and the resultant decline in estrogen secretion by the ovarian follicles. Symptoms related to estrogen deprivation include genitourinary atrophy, vasomotor instability, and osteoporosis. Other symptoms experienced during menopause include insomnia and fatigue, behavioral changes, and changes in libido. Because most clinical symptoms present in the menopausal period are associated directly with the lack of estrogen, HRT is the most effective treatment modality. The most popular regimen for HRT is oral estrogen given cyclically, with the addition of a progestin in women with an intact uterus.

HRT is not free of adverse effects and the decision to treat menopausal symptoms must be weighed by both risks and benefits. Risks of therapy include concerns about breast and endometrial cancer, coagulation and thrombosis, cardiovascular events, and neurologic effects. The return of regular monthly bleeding, in response to cyclic HRT regimens, is unacceptable to many women; continuous therapy should be considered. Benefits of estrogen replacement therapy include relief of hot flushes and genitourinary symptoms, as well as long-term positive effects on bone and lipids. Future investigation is needed in several areas, particularly in determining the role of estrogens in breast cancer and in the development of synthetic progestins with no negative effects on lipids. HRT plays an important role in the preventive medical care of postmenopausal women and most postmenopausal women without an absolute contraindication should receive HRT.

References

1. London SN, Hammond CB. The climacteric, in Danforth DN, Scott JR (eds): Obstetrics and Gynecology, 5th ed. Philadelphia, JB Lippincott, 1986, p 905.
2. Utian WH. Biosynthesis and physiologic effects of estrogen and pathophysiologic effects of estrogen deficiency: A review. Am J Obstet Gynecol 1989;161:828–831.
3. Korenman SG. Menopausal endocrinology and management. Arch Intern Med 1982;142:1131–1136.
4. Smith DC, Prentice R, Thompson DJ, Herrmann WL. Association of exogenous estrogen and endometrial carcinoma. N Engl J Med 1975;293:1164.
5. Weiss NS. Risks and benefits of estrogen use. N Engl J Med 1975;293:1200.
6. Ziel HK, Finkle WD. Increased risk of endometrial carcinoma among users of conjugated estrogens. N Engl J Med 1975;293:1167.
7. Haney AF. The physiology of the climacterium. Clin Obstet Gynecol 1986;20:397–406.
8. Young RL, Kumar NS, Goldzieher JW. Management of menopause when estrogen cannot be used. Drugs 1990;40:220–230.
9. Wells RG. Hormone replacement before menopause. Is it a good idea? Postgraduate Med 1989;86:61–71.
10. Mishell DR. Estrogen replacement therapy: An overview. Am J Obstet Gynecol 1989;161:1825–1827.
11. Ravnikar V. Physiology and treatment of hot flushes. Obstet Gynecol 1990;75:3S–8S.
12. Notelovitz M. Estrogen replacement therapy: Indications, contraindications, and agent selection. Am J Obstet Gynecol 1989;161:1832–1841.
13. Sitruk-Ware R. Estrogen therapy during menopause: Practical treatment recommendations. Drugs 1990;39:203–217.
14. Genant HK, Baylink DJ, Gallagher JC. Estrogens in the prevention of osteoporosis in postmenopausal women. Am J Obstet Gynecol 1989;161:1842–1846.
15. Hammond CB. Estrogen replacement therapy: What the future holds. Am J Obstet Gynecol 1989;161:1864–1868.
16. Lobo RA. Cardiovascular implications of estrogen replacement therapy. Obstet Gynecol 1990;75:18S–25S.
17. Sullivan JM, Zwaag RV, Hughes JP, et al. Estrogen replacement and coronary artery disease. Arch Intern Med 1990;150:2557–2562.
18. PEPI Trial Group. Effects of estrogen or estrogen/progestin regimens on heart disease risk factors in postmenopausal women. JAMA 1995;273:199–208.
19. Sarrel PM. Sexuality and menopause. Obstet Gynecol 1990;75:26S–30S.
20. Shangold MM. Exercise in the menopausal woman. Obstet Gynecol 1990;75:53S–58S.
21. Watts NB, Harris ST, Genant HK, et al. Intermittent cyclical etidronate treatment of postmenopausal osteoporosis. N Engl J Med 1990;323:73–79.
22. Anon. Estrogens (systemic and vaginal), in Johnson KW (ed): USPDI 1994. Rockville, MD, U.S. Pharmacopoeial Convention, 1994, p 1304.
23. Bauwens SF. Osteomalacia and osteoporosis, in DiPiro JT, Talbert RL, Hayes PE, et al. (eds): Pharmacotherapy: A Pathophysiologic Approach. New York, Elsevier, 1989, p 865.
24. Lievertz RW. Pharmacology and pharmacokinetics of estrogens. Am J Obstet Gynecol 1987;156:1289–1293.
25. Chetkowski RJ, Meldrum DR, Steingold KA, et al. Biologic effects of transdermal estradiol. N Engl J Med 1986;314:1615–1620.
26. Powers MS, Schenkel L, Darley PE, et al. Pharmacokinetics and pharmacodynamics of transdermal dosage forms of 17-estradiol: Comparison with conventional oral estrogens used for hormone replacement. Am J Obstet Gynecol 1985;152:1099–1106.
27. Mashchak CA, Lobo RA, Dozono-Takano R, et al. Comparison of pharmacodynamic properties of various estrogen formulations. Am J Obstet Gynecol 1982;144:511–518.

28. Stanczyk FZ, Shoupe D, Nunez V, et al. A randomized comparison of nonoral estradiol delivery in postmenopausal women. Am J Obstet Gynecol 1988;159:1540–1546.
29. Jensen J, Riis BJ, Strom V, et al. Long-term effects of percutaneous estrogens and oral progesterone on serum lipoproteins in postmenopausal women. Am J Obstet Gynecol 1987;156:66–71.
30. Balfour JA, Heel RC. Transdermal estradiol: A review of its pharmacodynamic and pharmacokinetic properties, and therapeutic efficacy in the treatment of menopausal complaints. Drugs 1990;40:561–582.
31. Jensen J, Christiansen C. Dose response and withdrawal effects on climacteric symptoms after hormonal replacement therapy: A placebo-controlled therapeutic trial. Maturitas 1983;5:125–133.
32. Lauritzen CH. The female climacteric syndrome: Significance, problems and treatment. Acta Obstet Gynecol 1976;53(suppl):47–61.
33. Lufkin EG, Carpenter PC, Ory SJ, et al. Estrogen replacement therapy: Current recommendations. Mayo Clin Proc 1988;63:453–460.
34. Whitehead MI, Hillard TC, Crook D. The role and use of progestogens. Obstet Gynecol 1990;74(suppl):59S–76S.
35. Belchetz PE. Hormonal treatment of postmenopausal women. N Engl J Med 1994;330:1062–1071.
36. Staland B. Continuous treatment with natural oestrogens and progestogens: A method to avoid endometrial stimulation. Maturitas 1981;3:145–156.
37. Jensen J, Riis BJ, Strom V, Christiansen C. Continuous estrogen–progestogen treatment and serum lipoproteins in postmenopausal women. Br J Obstet Gynaecol 1987;94:130–135.
38. Sporrong T, Hellgren M, Samsioe G, Mattsson LA. Comparison of four continuously administered progestogen plus oestradiol combinations for climacteric complaints. Br J Obstet Gynaecol 1988;95:1042–1048.
39. Anon. in McEvoy GK (ed): AHFS Drug Information 95. Bethesda, MD, American Society of Health-System Pharmacists, 1995, p 2150.
40. Schiff I, Tulchinsky D, Cramer D, Ryan KJ. Oral medroxyprogesterone in the treatment of postmenopausal symptoms. JAMA 1980;244:1443–1445.
41. Lobo RA, McCormick W, Singer F, Roy S. Depo-medroxyprogesterone acetate compared with conjugated estrogens for the treatment of postmenopausal women. J Am Coll Obstet Gynecol 1984;63:105.
42. Nachtigall LE. Enhancing patient compliance with hormone replacement therapy at menopause. Obstet Gynecol 1990;75:77S–80S.
43. Barrett-Connor E, Winhard DL, Criqui MH. Postmenopausal estrogen use and heart disease risk factors in the 1980s. JAMA 1989;261:2095–2100.
44. Lufkin EG, Carpenter PC, Ory SJ, et al. Estrogen replacement therapy: Current recommendations. Mayo Clin Proc 1988;63:453–460.

Section 9
Immunologic Disorders

Chapter 80
Function and Evaluation of the Immune System

Philip D. Hall, PharmD, and Joseph A. Tami, PharmD

Knowledge of the immune system has rapidly expanded over the past few years, enabling an understanding of normal immune system function as well as identification of the role of the immune system dysfunction in a multitude of disease states. To analyze adequately the immune system in disease processes, it is vital to comprehend normal immune function and to recognize immune dysfunction. This chapter presents first an overview of the immune system then a discussion of the evaluation of immune function in the clinical setting. The term "immune system" encompasses a wide range of components including mechanical immunodefenses, soluble mediators as well as cellular and humoral immune processes. The section illustrating immune function also focuses on those laboratory examinations commonly available in clinical settings or likely to be available in the near future.

The immune system primarily serves to protect the body against infectious pathogens. To accomplish this task, the immune system exhibits specificity, memory, mobility, and replicability. Specificity refers to the ability of the immune system to distinguish between non-cross-reacting antigens. Memory allows a quicker and more vigorous response to pathogenic invasion. Because elements of the immune system are mobile, local reactions may provide systemic protection. All cellular components of the immune system can replicate, allowing the immune response to be amplified.[1] In addition, the immune response normally distinguishes "self" from "nonself," preventing damage to the host. This discrimination between "self" and "nonself" is done by the adaptive or specific arm of the immune response. The immune system is commonly separated into two functional divisions: innate (nonspecific) and adaptive (specific) (Table 80.1).[2] Despite this simple separation, both divisions heavily interact.

The innate arm provides the first line of defense against pathogens. One of the most frequently overlooked methods of host defense is the body's ability to provide a physical and chemical defense against invading pathogens. The skin, the largest organ of the body, has the primary role of providing this physical defense. Alterations in the skin, such as burns or abrasions, allow an easier route of entry for pathogens. The gastrointestinal (GI) tract also plays an important role in providing a physical defense against pathogenic invasion. The low pH of the stomach (pH 1–2) kills many organisms. The constant sloughing of intestinal cells also limits systemic infection because infected cells are frequently replaced. Drugs, such as cell-cycle-specific antineoplastics, which disrupt the sloughing process, leave the patient at an increased risk of infection. Likewise, the respiratory tract has its forms of physical defense, namely, the cilia lining the epithelium of the lungs, which generate the ability to remove organisms in that area. Mucus that coats the epithelial cells serves in part to prevent microorganisms from adhering to cell surfaces. The combination of cilia, mucus, and coughing provides a natural barrier to invasion via the respiratory tract. Other examples of mechanical or nonspecific defenses include lysozymes in tears and saliva, the normal flora of the lower GI tract, and normal urine

TABLE 80.1. FUNCTIONAL DIVISIONS OF THE IMMUNE SYSTEM

	Innate	Adaptive
Physical barriers	Skin and mucous membranes	None
Specificity	None	Yes
Memory	No	Yes
Soluble factors	Lysozymes, complement, acute phase proteins	Antibodies, lymphokines
Cells	Neutrophils, monocytes, macrophages, NK cells, eosinophils	B lymphocytes, T lymphocytes

(From Hall P. D. Immunomodulation with intravenous immunoglobulin. Pharmacotherapy 1993;13(6):565, with permission.)

flow. It is these physical and chemical defenses that often mount the first line of defense against antimicrobial infections. It is well known that conditions or devices that allow microorganisms to transgress these normal barriers predispose patients to infections. As such, patients with a substantial loss of the skin from a burn or those who require mechanical ventilation, bladder catheterization, or central venous access are at increased risk of infection.

THE IMMUNE RESPONSE

When an infectious pathogen eludes the physical defenses of the body, an immune response involving both soluble mediators and leukocytes is generated against the pathogen.

INNATE RESPONSE

Innate immunity is present from birth and involves the stimulation of cells that nonspecifically recognize foreign invaders and destroy them. The innate leukocytes are monocytes, macrophages, neutrophils, basophils, mast cells, and eosinophils. Monocytes, macrophages, neutrophils, and eosinophils act as phagocytes, while mast cells and basophils secrete inflammatory mediators when stimulated. The phagocytes recognize, internalize, and destroy invading pathogens. These cells utilize nonspecific recognition systems to identify the pathogen. On the surface of phagocytic cells exist receptors for complement and antibody (Fc receptors). Complement or antibodies coat infectious pathogens in a process termed *opsonization;* then the antibody or complement binds to the receptors on the innate leukocyte (Fig. 80.1), thereby activating the phagocytic process.

The granulocytic cells of the body include neutrophils, eosinophils, and basophils. The cytoplasmic granules of these cells often contain inflammatory mediators or digestive enzymes. Neutrophils are polymorphonuclear cells (often denoted as PMNs for this reason), which comprise the primary human defense against pathogenic bacteria and make up the majority of leukocytes in the bloodstream. Neutrophils respond to chemotactic factors, such as interleukin-8 and C3a and C5a, breakdown products of complement, that are released from infected or inflamed tissue. Neutrophils migrate to sites of infection in a process termed *chemotaxis,* whereupon they recognize, adhere to, and phagocytose pathogens. Neutrophils can only recognize pathogens coated with either complement or IgG (antibody) via the complement and antibody receptors located on the surface of the neutrophil. Once bound, the neutrophil then releases its granular contents into vacuoles and generates the release of oxidative metabolites, thereby killing engulfed pathogens.[3]

Eosinophils are also granulocytic cells, but they have a minor role in combatting bacterial infections. Patients with drug-induced neutropenia or other neutrophil deficiency states are not protected against microbial pathogens by eosinophils. However, eosinophils play a major role against nonphagocytable multicellular pathogens, such as parasites. With their cytoplasmic granules and ability to generate oxidative substances, the eosinophils are capable of destroying multicellular parasites even when the eosinophil is unable to phagocytose the parasite. Eosinophils recognize pathogens coated by complement or IgE (antibody). Because of their ability to bind IgE, eosinophils contribute to the pathogenesis of allergic disorders (i.e., asthma).[4]

Macrophages and monocytes are mononuclear cells capable of phagocytosis. These cells also have the ability to release soluble factors with inflammatory properties. Monocytes are found within the bloodstream while macrophages are found in the tissues. Tissue macrophages are believed to arise from the migration of monocytes. Macrophages differ from monocytes by possessing an increased number of Fc and complement receptors. Macrophages are found within specific tissues such as the liver, spleen, GI tract, lymph nodes, brain, and others. These specific types of macrophages are often called histiocytes or are referred to by a specialized name depending on the site where they are found (Kupffer's cells in the liver, Langerhans' cells in the skin, osteoclasts in the bone, microglial cells in the central nervous system, etc.). The term *reticuloendothelial system* (RES) was commonly used to refer to macrophages found in reticular connective tissue; however, the term *mononuclear phagocyte system* is now the preferred nomenclature.

In addition to phagocytosing pathogens, monocytes/macrophages act as antigen-presenting cells (APCs) to stimulate the adaptive (specific) system. Macrophages internalize the organism, digest it into small peptide fragments, and then place these antigenic fragments together

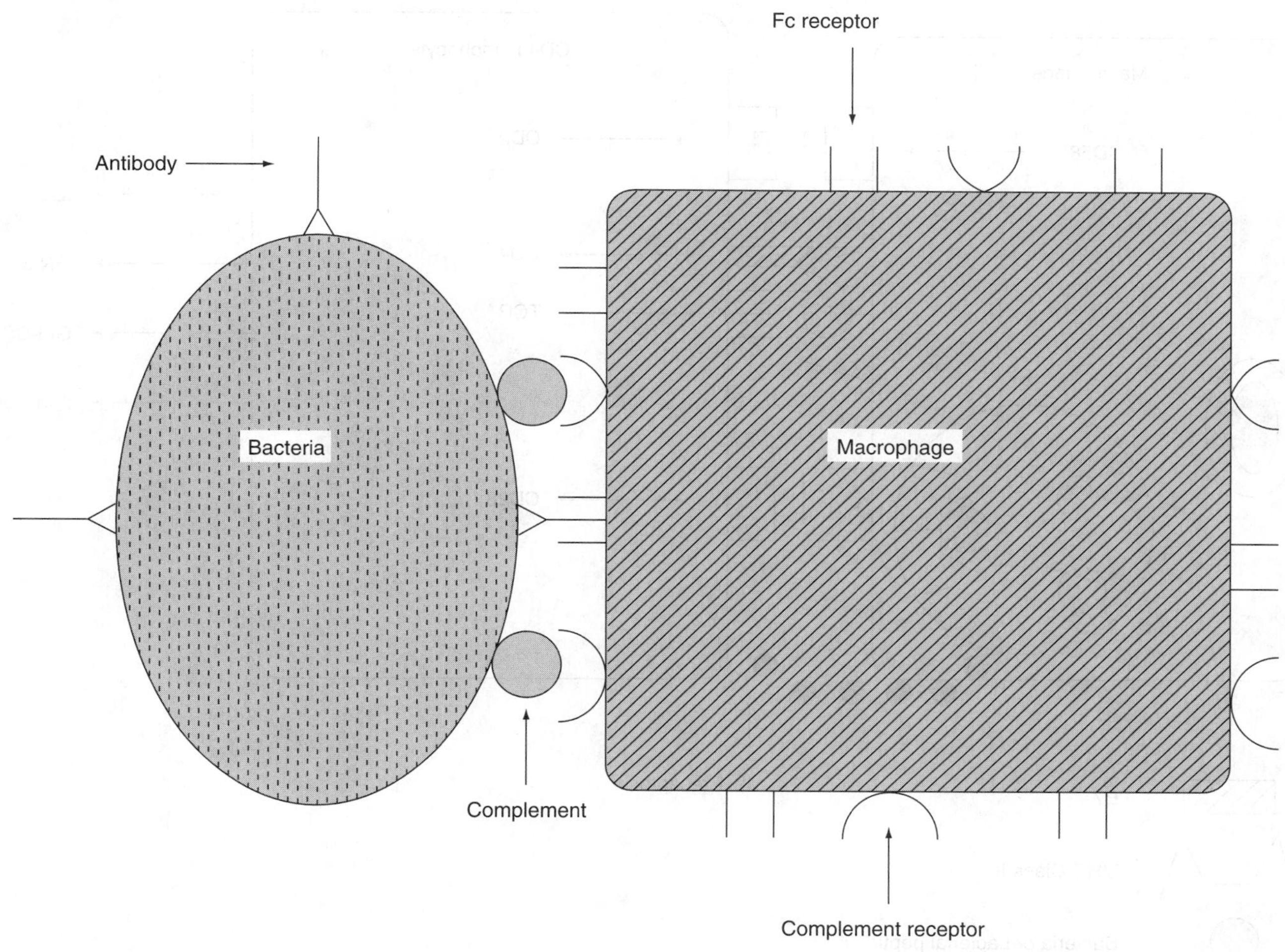

Figure 80.1. Phagocytosis of bacteria by macrophages. Macrophages recognize bacteria coated or opsonized with antibody or complement. On the surface of the macrophage reside receptors for the antibody (Fc receptor) and complement.

with major histocompatibility complex (MHC) proteins. Once the APC has formed the antigen/MHC complex, it places the complex on the surface of the APC. This complex is recognized by the T-cell receptor on the surface of T lymphocytes, which will activate the T lymphocyte (Fig. 80.2). Other cells, B lymphocytes and dendritic cells, can act as APCs.[2,5,6]

Cells that act primarily by releasing inflammatory mediators include mast cells and basophils. Mast cells are tissue cells predominantly associated with IgE-mediated inflammation. They are especially abundant in the skin, lungs, and nasal mucosa. Granules within the mast cells contain large amounts of histamine. Basophils are similar to mast cells because they contain granules filled with histamine; however, they are typically found circulating in the blood and are not found in connective tissue. Like mast cells, basophils also express high-affinity IgE Fc receptors. IgE-mediated anaphylaxis (Type I hypersensitivity) is caused by the stimulation of mast cell and/or basophil degranulation (release of histamine) by allergen binding to IgE bound on the surface of mast cells or basophils.[7]

Soluble mediators of innate immunity include complement and C-reactive protein (CRP). The complement system consists of 20 plasma proteins and 5 regulatory membrane proteins, which play a key role in immune defense. The three major functions of the complement system include (1) the ability to lyse certain microorganisms and cells, (2) the ability to stimulate the chemotaxis of phagocytic cells, and (3) the ability to coat or opsonize foreign pathogens, which allow phagocytosis of the pathogen by leukocytes expressing complement receptors. Complement factors (C3a, C5a) act as chemotaxis factors for phagocytic cells.

Two different pathways are utilized in stimulating the complement cascade. In the classic pathway, antibody binding to its target antigen or CRP binding to bacteria or fungi activates the first component of complement (C1), thereby initiating the complement cascade. The alternative complement pathway does not require the presence of a specific complement-fixing antibody but is stimulated directly by

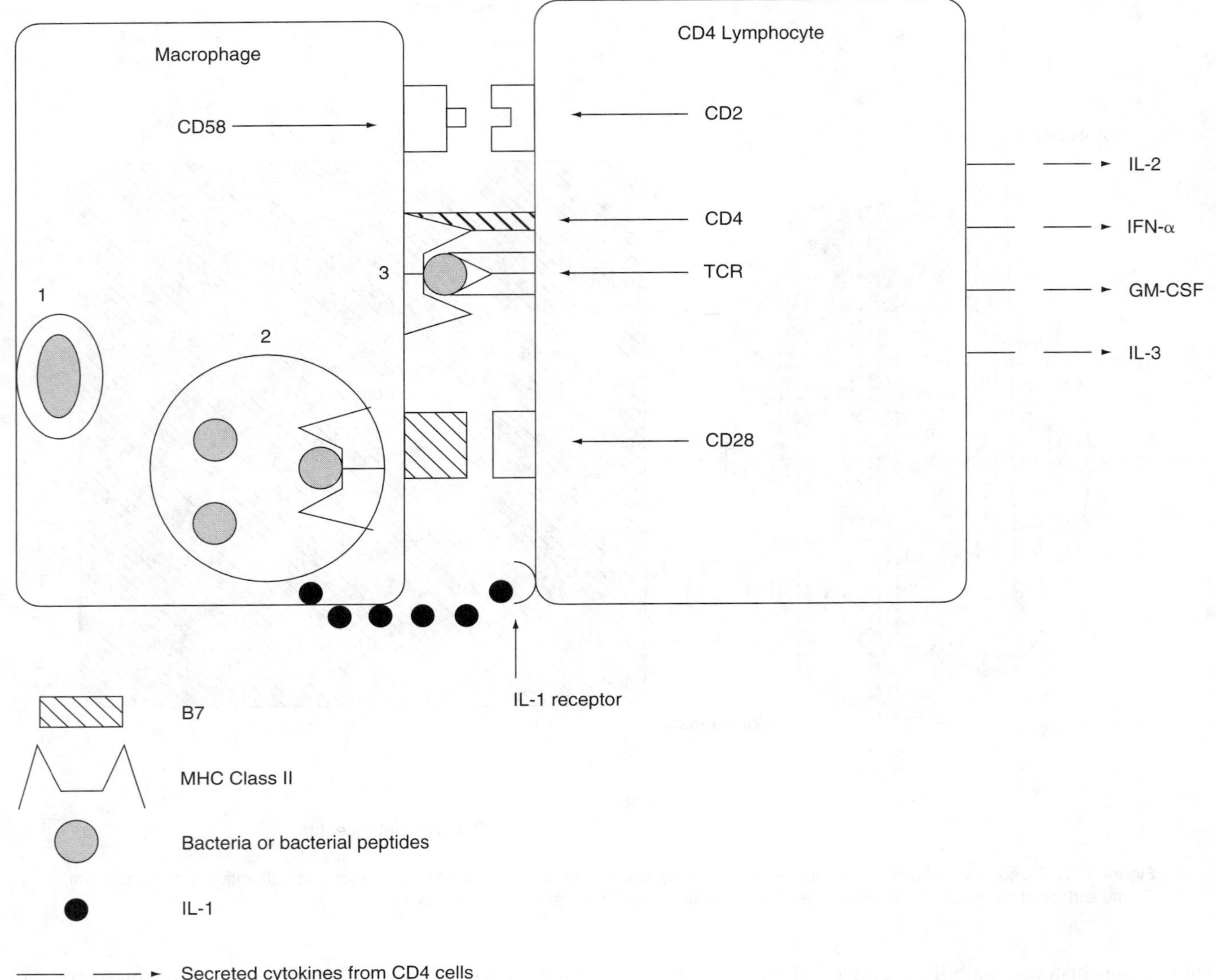

Figure 80.2. Macrophage presentation to CD4 T lymphocytes. After phagocytosis of the bacteria by the macrophage (1), the bacteria is digested into small peptides and becomes associated with MHC class II within the endosome (2). Finally the MHC class II plus antigen is expressed on the surface of the macrophage (3). CD4 T-lymphocyte activation requires the T-lymphocyte receptor (TCR) to recognize the antigenic peptide plus MHC class II as well as the B7–CD28 interaction. IL-1 secreted by macrophage also activates the T lymphocyte. The CD2–CD58 interaction allows for adherence between the T lymphocyte and macrophage. Upon activation, CD4 lymphocytes secrete numerous cytokines to up-regulate the immune response (IL-2, IFN-γ) and growth factors (IL-3, GM-CSF).

microorganisms. Mannose-binding protein, an acute-phase reactant, binds to mannose-rich glycoconjugates on microorganisms and can activate both the classic and alternative pathways. Patients with hereditary deficiencies of complement have recurrent bacterial infections.[2,8]

ADAPTIVE RESPONSE

To amplify the immune response, activation of the adaptive immune system is required. The adaptive immune response differs from the innate immune response in two critical areas: specificity and memory. Lymphocytes (T and B) comprise the cells of the adaptive-response. These cells have surface receptors specific for the invading organism. In a manner that utilizes genetic rearrangement of their DNA, it is estimated that lymphocytes have the ability to recognize more than 10^{16} different types of antigens. Generally, the body will utilize both the innate and adaptive immune responses to kill foreign pathogens. The adaptive immune response can be divided into two major arms: humoral or cell mediated. The B lymphocytes and activated B lymphocytes (plasma cells) that secrete antibody comprise the humoral arm of adaptive immune response. The humoral response is so denoted because it was found that the factors that provided the immune protection could be found in the humor or serum. The cell-mediated arm is controlled primarily by T lymphocytes. The immune protection provided by these cells could not be transferred by serum alone. Rather, it is essential to actually have T lymphocytes present, thus the term cell-mediated immunity. T lymphocytes are specially tailored to deal with infections that are intracellular, such as virally infected cells, whereas B lymphocytes secrete antibodies that can neutralize pathogens prior to their entry into host cells.

T lymphocytes do not recognize intact antigen. T lymphocytes recognize processed antigen in association with MHC. APCs (macrophages, dendritic cells, Kupffer's cells) phagocytose the pathogen then break down the pathogen and express peptide fragments (processed antigen) in association with MHC on their surface. T lymphocytes express a specific antigen receptor, T-cell receptor (TCR). The TCR is comprised of two chains with each chain having a variable and constant region. The variation of the amino acid sequence within the variable domain of TCR gives the cell its unique antigen specificity. Linked to the TCR is a complex of single chains known as the CD3 complex.

Two signals are required for T-lymphocyte activation. The first step of activation involves the T lymphocyte recognizing both the processed antigen and MHC molecule complex. The second signal involves the interaction of the B7 molecule on the APC with the CD28 molecule on the surface of T lymphocyte (Fig. 80.2). Without the second signal, the T lymphocyte becomes anergic or inactive.[9] After the two signals, a message is sent through the TCR to the CD3 complex into the cell. Then a calcium influx occurs with subsequent activation of the T lymphocyte. Soluble factors such as the interleukins are released from the activated T lymphocytes to stimulate other cells of the immune system.

T-lymphocyte populations can be classified by cell surface markers or functional activity. Typically, T lymphocytes are divided into helper cells ($CD4^+$), suppressor cells ($CD8^+$), and cytotoxic cells ($CD8^+$). Each of the subclasses appears to play a distinct role in the cell-mediated immune response.

The primary role of $CD4^+$ cells is to stimulate other cells in the immune response. Based on surface markers, two subgroups of $CD4^+$ T lymphocytes have been identified: helper/inducer ($CD4^+$, $CD29^+$) and helper/suppressor ($CD4^+$, $CD45RA^+$). The helper/inducer subtype amplifies the immune response and $CD8^+$ cytotoxic cells.[10] The helper/suppressor induces $CD8^+$ suppressor cells.[11] Functionally, $CD4^+$ cells can be divided into T_{H1} and T_{H2}. This functional system was first described in mice. T_{H1} cells secrete interleukin-2 (IL-2) and interferon (IFN-γ) and stimulate $CD8^+$ cytotoxic cells, whereas T_{H2} cells secrete IL-4, IL-5, and IL-10 and stimulate B-lymphocyte production of antibody.[12] This functional classification of $CD4^+$ T-lymphocytes is not fully confirmed in humans, but has been well described in individuals with human immunodeficiency virus (HIV). In HIV patients, a shift to T_{H2} from the normally predominant T_{H1} subclass has been demonstrated.[13]

$CD8^+$ suppressor cells down-regulate the immune response once the pathogen has been destroyed. Obviously, continued activation of the immune response may not be beneficial to the host. Down-regulation of autoreactive cells may also occur to prevent autoimmune disease. $CD8^+$ cytotoxic cells are instrumental in killing cells recognized as foreign, such as those that have become infected by a virus. These cells also play an important beneficial role in the eradication of tumor cells, but also are responsible for rejection of transplanted organs. $CD8^+$ T lymphocytes recognize antigen in association with MHC class I.

B lymphocytes recognize antigen via its associated antibody or immunoglobulin located on the surface of the cell. The antibody on the surface can recognize an intact pathogen, such as a bacteria, and present antigen to T lymphocytes (i.e., acting as APC). However, the major function of B lymphocytes is to produce antibody to bind to the invading pathogen, a process that first entails activation of the lymphocyte. The activation of B lymphocyte also requires two steps: (1) recognition of antigen by the surface immunoglobulin, and (2) the presence of B-lymphocyte growth factors (IL-4, -5, -6) secreted by activated $CD4^+$ T lymphocytes. Once activated, the B lymphocyte becomes a plasma cell, a differentiated cell capable of producing and secreting large quantities of antibody. A fraction of activated B lymphocytes does not differentiate into plasma cells, but rather it forms a pool of memory cells. The memory cells will respond to subsequent encounters with the pathogen and allow for a quicker and more vigorous response to the pathogen. Some B lymphocytes can become activated without help from T lymphocytes, but these responses are generally weak and do not invoke memory.

When binding of a specific antigen to the surface immunoglobulin receptor of B lymphocytes occurs, the B lymphocyte matures into a plasma cell and produces large quantities of antibody that have the ability to bind to the inciting antigen. The secreted antibodies may be of five different isotypes. On primary exposure to the pathogen, the plasma cell will secrete IgM, but there is a switch to predominantly IgG during the first exposure. On second exposure the memory B lymphocytes will predominately produce IgG. Isotype switching from IgM to IgG, IgA, or IgE is controlled by T lymphocytes. Table 80.2 illustrates normal serum concentrations for the five different isotypes.[14]

An antibody or immunoglobulin is a glycoprotein comprised of two different chains, heavy and light (Fig. 80.3). The basic structure of every immunoglobulin consists of four peptide chains: two identical heavy chains and two identical light chains held together by disulfide bonds. The basic structure of the antibody is a Y-shaped figure. Each arm of the Y is formed by the linkage of the end of the

TABLE 80.2. FIVE IMMUNOGLOBULIN CLASSES IN MAN AND THEIR CHARACTERISTICS

	IgG	IgM	IgA[a]	IgE[b]	IgD[c]
Serum conc. (mg/dL)	1000	120	250	0.05	3
Serum half-life (days)	23	5	6	2	3
Antibacterial lysis	+	+++	+	?	?
Antiviral activity	+	+	+++	?	?
Complement fixation	+	++++	0	0	0
Placental transfer	Yes	No	No	No	No

[a]IgA is involved in secretory response.
[b]IgE is involved in allergic response.
[c]IgD is a membrane receptor on B lymphocytes. (Adapted from Ref. 16, with permission.)

light chain to its heavy chain partner. These arms contain the portions described as the Fab fragments (fragments of antigen binding). The stem of the Y contains the heavy chains that comprise the Fc (crystallizable fragment) portion of the antibody. It is within the Fc portion that complement is activated once the antibody has bound its target. Likewise, it is the Fc portion of the antibody that is recognized by Fc receptors on the surface of phagocytes (Fig. 80.1). The amino acid composition of the same isotype is homogenous except in the variable regions of the light (VL) and heavy chains (VH). The variation in amino acid composition of the variable region gives the antibody its unique specificity (Fig. 80.3).

IgG, the most prevalent of the antibody classes, comprises approximately 80% of serum antibody. IgG is usually the second isotype of antibody to be produced in an initial humoral immune response. IgG is the only isotype of antibody that can cross the placenta. Therefore, maternal humoral protection of neonates is primarily due to maternal IgG that has crossed the placenta *in utero*.

Four different subclasses of IgG have been described: IgG1, IgG2, IgG3, and IgG4. These subclasses differ slightly in their constant amino acid sequences. IgG1 constitutes the majority (60%) of the subclasses. It appears that different subclasses recognize different types of antigen. IgG1 and IgG3 are principally responsible for recognition of protein antigens while IgG2 and IgG4 commonly bind to carbohydrate antigens.[15] Other differences in the subclasses are the ability to activate complement with IgG3 and IgG1 being the most efficient and IgG4 unable to activate complement.

IgM can be found on the surface of B lymphocytes as a monomeric Y-shaped structure. IgM, secreted from plasma cells, is a pentamer in which five of the monomers are joined by a joining chain (J chain). IgM is the first class of antibody to be produced on initial exposure to an antigen. Because the pentameric form of IgM has no Fc portions exposed, phagocytic cells cannot bind pathogens opsonized by IgM. However, IgM is an excellent activator of complement cascade (classic pathway).

IgA is found primarily in the fluid secretions of the body, tears, saliva, nasal fluids, and also in mucus of the GI tract. IgA functions by preventing pathogens from adhering

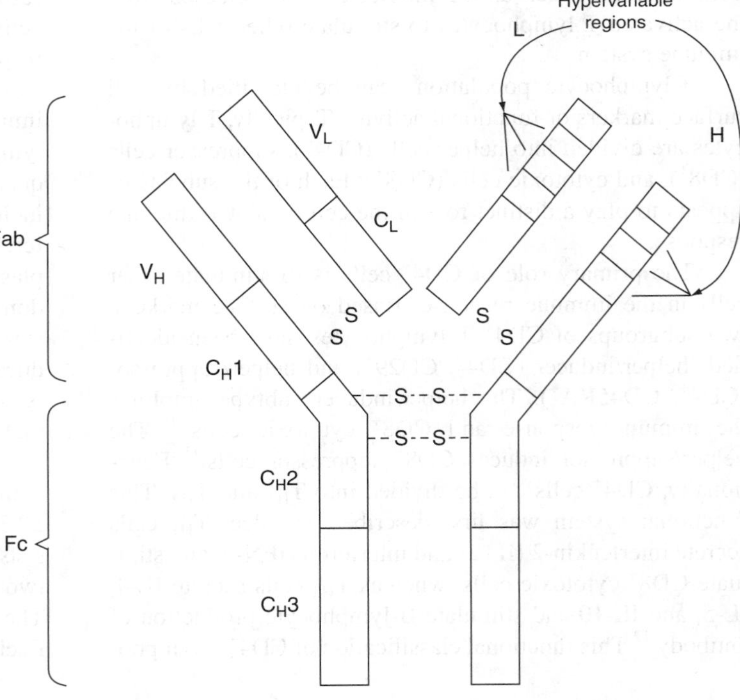

Figure 80.3. IgG molecule. Prototype of immunoglobulin molecule showing heavy (H) and light (L) chains, each with common (C) and variable (V) regions, each of which has hypervariable regions. Antigen combines with antibody in the cavity formed by hypervariable ends of H and L chains. These two chains are joined by disulfide bonds (S–S). Light chains have one variable (V_L) and one constant (C_L) region. Heavy chains have one variable (V_H) and three or four common regions (C_H1 through C_H3), but IgE has an additional CH_4 region. Light chains and V_H and C_H1 make up the Fab region. Other common regions of the H chain make up the Fc region. The COOH ends of the molecules are in the constant regions, and the NH_2 ends of the molecules are in the variable regions. *(Reprinted with permission from JAMA 1992;268(20):2790–2796. Copyright 1992, American Medical Association.)*

to and infecting the epithelial cells at these sites. IgA is also secreted in a nursing mother's breast milk as are IgG and IgM. In bodily secretions, IgA is in a dimeric form in which two monomers are held together by a J chain and secretory chain.

IgD is the least understood isotype. IgD is found on the surface of B lymphocytes at different stages of maturation and may be involved in the differentiation of these cells. The main function of IgD has not yet been determined.

IgE is the least common of the serum antibody isotypes. Most of the IgE in the body is bound to the IgE Fc receptors on mast cells. When antigen is bound by the IgE on the surface of mast cells, it causes the release of various inflammatory substances from the mast cell. The overall effect is the stimulation of inflammation. Asthma and hay fever are a few examples of allergic reactions primarily due to antigen binding to IgE.[16]

Natural killer (NK) cells, often referred to as large granular lymphocytes, are the third type of lymphocyte. NK cells do not express on their surface specific receptors like the TCR on T lymphocytes, and are not restricted by MHC, but they do express Fc receptors for IgG. NK cells were originally described and named because of their ability to lyse tumor cells without prior sensitization. Upon exposure to IL-2, NK cells exhibit greater cytotoxic activity against a wide variety of tumors. The majority of lymphokine-activated killer (LAK) cells used to treat melanoma and renal cell carcinoma are NK cells. NK cells play important roles in surveillance against tumors and virally infected host cells, and in the regulation of hematopoiesis.[17]

Major Histocompatibility Complex

The MHC, an association of genes found on chromosome 6 in humans, is also known as the human leukocyte antigen (HLA) complex. The genes from this complex encode for molecules that play a pivotal role in immune recognition and response. The MHC complex is divided into three different classes: I, II, and III. The molecules encoded by class I HLA genes include HLA-A, HLA-B, and HLA-C antigens. These molecules can be found on all nucleated cells within the body as well as on platelets. Class I antigens are not found on mature red blood cells. Molecules encoded by class II HLA genes include HLA-DP, HLA-DQ, and HLA-DR molecules. The expression of these molecules is more restricted and can be found primarily on APCs such as macrophages, B lymphocytes, and so on. The class III HLA antigens encode for soluble factors, complement, and tumor necrosis factor (TNF).

In order for a $CD4^+$ T lymphocyte to become activated, it must recognize the antigenic peptide in association with MHC class II (Fig. 80.2). $CD8^+$ T lymphocytes recognize antigenic peptide in association with class I molecules. Class I molecules generally contain endogenous peptides from within the cell such as viruses while class II molecules contain exogenous peptides from antigen that has been phagocytosized such as bacteria (Fig. 80.2). For it to destroy a virally infected cell, a $CD8^+$ cytotoxic T lymphocyte requires two steps. First, its TCR must recognize the antigenic fragment such as a viral protein in association with MHC class I. The second step involves the costimulatory step of B7–CD28 binding. Because any cell can become infected, it is advantageous for the $CD8^+$ cytotoxic T lymphocyte to recognize the MHC class I molecule, which is expressed on all cells except red blood cells. The ability of the MHC class I to present endogenous peptides allows the $CD8^+$ cytotoxic T lymphocytes to screen cells constantly for infections.[6]

Cytokines

Cytokines orchestrate the complex homeostasis of cells and tissues by acting in both an autocrine and paracrine fashion. For example, activated $CD4^+$ T lymphocytes secrete IL-2 to activate itself as well as $CD8^+$ T lymphocytes and NK cells. Cytokines, soluble factors released or secreted by cells, affect the activity of other cells or the secreting cell itself. Cytokines can also be membrane bound (e.g., IL-1 alpha). In the context of this chapter, cytokines that affect the immune response will be discussed. Cytokines may be divided into different categories such as interleukins, interferons, hematopoietic growth factors, tumor necrosis factors, and transforming growth factors (Table 80.3).[18–21] Research has shown that many of these factors have a broad spectrum of effects dependent on their concentration, the presence of other factors, and the target cell. It is important to remember that *in vivo* cytokines do not act alone but in combination with other cytokines. For example, activated $CD4^+$ T lymphocytes secrete both IL-2 and IL-12, which are synergistic in activating NK cells. As shown in Table 80.3, cytokines are broadly classified as regulatory or hematopoietic growth factors. Remember that their classification does not describe all their activities. Granulocyte-macrophage colony-stimulating factor (GM-CSF), released by activated T lymphocytes, acts as a hematopoietic growth factor, but also activates granulocytes and macrophages to phagocytize foreign pathogens.

The division of the immune system into the two functional groups does not imply that the divisions do not interact. As shown in Figs. 80.1 and 80.2, both systems heavily interact. To generate a vigorous immune response, both soluble mediators (complement, antibody, and cytokines) and cells (neutrophils, macrophages, T lymphocytes, and B lymphocytes) are needed. Generally, the innate system will respond first. Macrophages and neutrophils in the tissues will recognize the opsonized pathogen (Fig. 80.1). To amplify the immune response, the macrophages will present antigen to $CD4^+$ T lymphocytes. The activated $CD4^+$ T lymphocytes will then secrete cytokines to activate B lym-

TABLE 80.3. CYTOKINES

Cytokines	Sources	Principal Effects
Regulatory		
IL-1	Macrophages	Activation of T and B lymphocytes, hematopoietic growth factor
IL-2	CD4$^+$ T lymphs	Activation of T lymphs, B lymphs, and NK cells
IL-4	CD4$^+$ T lymphs, mast cells	B- and T-lymphocyte growth factor, activation of macrophages, promotes IgE production, proliferation of bone marrow precursors
IL-5	CD4$^+$ T lymphs, mast cells	Activation of B lymphs and eosinophils, promotes IgE production
IL-6	CD4$^+$ T lymphs, macrophages, mast cells, fibroblasts	T- and B-lymph growth factor, hematopoietic growth factor, augments inflammation
IL-8	T lymphs, monocytes, endothelial cells, fibroblasts	Neutrophil and T-lymph chemotaxis
IL-10	T and B lymphs, macrophages	Cytokine synthesis inhibitory factor, growth of mast cells
IL-12	T lymphs	Synergism with IL-2, activation of NK cells, induces T_{H1} cells
IL-13	Activated T lymphs	Proliferation of B lymphs, suppression of proinflammatory cytokines, directs IgE isotype switching
TNF-α	Macrophages, T lymphs	Activation of neutrophils, endothelial cells, lymphs, and liver cells to produce acute phase proteins
TNF-β	T lymphs	Tumoricidal
IFN-α	Monocytes, other cells	Antiviral, activation of NK cells and macrophages, up-regulation MHC class I
IFN-γ	T lymphs, NK cells	Activation of macrophages, NK cells; up-regulation of MHC classes I & II
Hematopoietic Growth Factors		
IL-3	T lymphs	Maturation and differentiation of hematopoietic and mast cells
IL-7	BM stromal cells	Lymphopoietin
IL-9	T lymphs	Maturation and proliferation of T lymphs and mast cells
IL-11	BM stromal cells	Maturation of B lymphs and megakaryocytes
G-CSF	Macrophages, endothelial cells, fibroblasts	Maturation and activation of neutrophils
GM-CSF	T lymphs, macrophages, endothelial cells, fibroblasts	Maturation and activation of granulocytes and monocytes/macrophages
M-CSF	Macrophages, endothelial cells, fibroblasts	Maturation and activation of monocytes/macrophages

phocytes, CD8$^+$ T lymphocytes, NK cells, macrophages, and neutrophils. The next section of the chapter will look at evaluating the immune system.

EVALUATION OF COMPONENTS OF THE IMMUNE SYSTEM

Assessment of a patient's immune function requires consideration of multiple components including mechanical defenses, cell phenotypes and numbers, and soluble components. Recent developments in biotechnology have allowed extraordinary progress in characterization of immune function. Despite the technological advances, careful patient evaluations are required to properly identify patients with compromised immune systems. Specific methods for assessment of patient immune status are discussed below.

MECHANICAL AND NONSPECIFIC IMMUNODEFENSES

As discussed earlier, the mechanical aspects of host defense are extremely important in protection from infection; therefore, assessment of mechanical defenses is critical. Much of the assessment of mechanical immunodefense is accomplished by recognition of situations where it is compromised. Careful patient examination usually reveals the extent of compromise, and laboratory tests are generally not necessary for evaluation of this component. To evaluate the extent of compromise in mechanical immunodefenses, the clinician should carefully examine the patient and identify the specific types of risks present. Specific examples of altered mechanical defenses are listed in Table 80.4.

CELLULAR ASPECTS OF IMMUNE FUNCTION

A major aspect of the assessment of immune function relates to the cells of the immune system. Assessment of cells in the clinical setting includes determination of cell number, cell type, and/or function. Generally, quantification of the cell types and numbers is performed first because of its rapid turnaround and correlation with clinical picture.

TABLE 80.4. EXAMPLES OF ALTERATION IN MECHANICAL IMMUNODEFENSES THAT RESULT IN IMPAIRED IMMUNE STATUS

Reduced gastric pH
- Achlorhydria
- Use of histamine-2 blockers
- Patients with acquired immunodeficiency syndrome (AIDS)

Break in skin barrier
- Burns
- Surgical incision
- Penetrating trauma
- Vascular access devices

Impaired mucociliary function of the lungs
- Smoking

Impaired esophageal or epiglottal function
- Endotracheal intubation
- Stroke
- Recumbent position

Altered urine flow
- Urinary stones
- Anatomic deformities obstructing flow
- Bladder catheter

Anatomic alterations of the heart resulting in turbulent blood flow and endocarditis

Indwelling catheters

Quantification

To screen cell numbers quickly, a complete blood count (CBC) with differential is performed. Normal cell counts are shown in Table 80.5.[22,23] This test often steers the differential diagnosis. In interpreting a CBC with differential, several factors must be considered. A normal cell count does not mean that a leukocyte disorder does not exist. For example, in chronic granulomatous disease, a child has a normal neutrophil count, but the neutrophils are unable to destroy the bacteria. Second, a differential comes back as percentage of the CBC; therefore, one must assess the absolute number as well as the percentage of white cell subtypes. For example, a patient admitted to the hospital with pneumonia has an elevated WBC (15,000 cells/mm^3) that is predominantly neutrophils (segs + bands × 100 = 80%). The percentage of lymphocytes appears low at 15%, but the absolute number of lymphocytes is actually normal (2250 cells/mm^3). A third factor to consider is that the majority of lymphocytes are in secondary lymphoid organs (lymph nodes, spleen), and changes in peripheral blood lymphocytes do not mirror changes in the secondary lymphoid organs.[24] In addition, the majority of granulocytes, macrophages, and mast cells are in the tissues, not the bloodstream.

Generally, the numbers of granulocytes (neutrophils, basophils, eosinophils) and monocytes are assessed by a

TABLE 80.5. LEUKOCYTES IN ADULTS

Cell	Absolute Count (Range)[a]	Percent (Range)
White blood cell	7.5 (4.5–11.0)	100
Neutrophils	4.5 (2.3–7.7)	60 (50–70)
Eosinophils	0.2 (0.0–0.45)	3 (0–5)
Basophils	0.04 (0.0–0.2)	1 (0–2)
Monocytes	0.3 (0.0–0.8)	4 (0–10)
Lymphocytes	2.1 (1.6–2.4)	32 (28–39)
T lymphs	1.4 (1.1–1.7)	72 (67–76)[b]
CD4$^+$	0.8 (0.7–1.1)	42 (38–46)[b]
CD8$^+$	0.7 (0.5–0.9)	35 (31–40)[b]
B lymphs	0.3 (0.2–0.4)	13 (11–16)[b]
NK cells	0.3 (0.2–0.4)	14 (10–19)[b]
CD4:CD8 ratio	1.2 (1.0–1.5)	

[a]×10^3 cells/mm^3.
[b]Percent of lymphocyte subpopulations expressed as percentage of total lymphocyte population.

CBC with differential. It long has been recognized that the lower the absolute neutrophil count, the greater the risk of infection. Drugs (e.g., chemotherapy) and diseases (e.g., collagen vascular disorders) may lower the neutrophil count and make the patient more susceptible to infections. Patients with a neutrophil count below 1500 cells/mm^3 are considered to have neutropenia. Functional analysis of these cell types is rarely done in routine clinical practice. Patients with functional deficits in these cell types are generally referred to tertiary medical centers for evaluation and treatment.

A count of lymphocytes may be performed for overall number by a routine CBC with differential. Total lymphocyte count has been used as a measure of nutritional status, because this rapidly changes with nutrient loss or repletion. This is a relatively gross measure of a patient's immune status although it has been correlated to patient outcome and risk of infection. Quantification of specific lymphocyte subsets is also important in some situations.

The availability of monoclonal antibodies against lymphocyte cell surface markers (CDs) and the invention of flow cytometry have allowed specific quantification of lymphocyte subsets. These evaluations are valuable for assessment of patients with immune deficiency states such as AIDS or leukemias, and for patients that have received organ transplants. They allow the detection of specific lymphocyte subsets such as CD4$^+$ and CD8$^+$ T lymphocytes. Quantification of CD3$^+$ and CD4$^+$ cells is used to monitor OKT3 immunosuppression and in the clinical management of AIDS patients, respectively. CD3$^+$ is a marker for all T lymphocytes (CD4$^+$ and CD8$^+$).

The principle underlying the determination of lymphocyte subsets is a characteristic cell surface marker (cluster designation or CD) that distinguishes one subset from another. The CD is usually a protein or glycoprotein on the surface of the cell. Cells can be detected by monoclonal antibodies that bind to the specific CDs such as CD4 or CD8. The monoclonal antibodies have been bound to substances such as fluorescein or phycoerythrin dyes, which fluoresce green or red, respectively, when exposed to light of a certain wavelength. This fluorescence then allows detection and enumeration of the lymphocyte subsets by a flow cytometer. The flow cytometer analyzes individual cells to determine their fluorescence (presence or absence of surface-bound antibody) as well as light scatter (to determine cell size). Flow cytometry can be used for leukocyte phenotyping, tumor cell phenotyping, and for some types of DNA analysis. Some of the most common CD antigens and their respective cells are listed in Table 80.6.[25]

FUNCTIONAL EVALUATION OF IMMUNE RESPONSE

IN VIVO

The most common *in vivo* assay of lymphocyte function is the delayed hypersensitivity skin test. This test specifically evaluates the presence of delayed-type hypersensitivity or memory T lymphocytes. By injecting a small amount of test material (antigen to which the patient has previously been exposed) into the patient's skin, a visual assessment can be made of the patient's ability to react to the antigen.

When an antigen to which a normal patient has previously been exposed is injected into the skin, the area of the injection becomes infiltrated with lymphocytes within a few hours. In the next stage, additional lymphocytes and phagocytes (macrophages, neutrophils) infiltrate. The maximal intensity of the inflammatory reaction is 24–72 hours. This reaction is often referred to as type IV hypersensitivity (cell mediated). In type I hypersensitivity, a positive skin reaction is usually evident within 15 minutes and always within 24 hours. Type I hypersensitivity involves the release of histamine from basophils and mast cells when antigen binds to the IgE on the surface of these cells.

TABLE 80.6. CLUSTER OF DIFFERENTIATION (CD) GUIDE: CHARACTERIZATION OF HUMAN LEUKOCYTE ANTIGENS

CD	Predominant Cellular Distribution
CD1	Thymocytes, Langerhans' cells
CD3	T lymphocytes
CD4	Helper T lymphocytes, monocytes, macrophages
CD5	T lymphocytes, B-lymphocyte subset
CD8	Cytotoxic/suppressor T lymphocytes, NK cells
CD14	Monocytes, neutrophils
CD19	B lymphocytes
CD25	Activated T lymphocytes, B lymphocytes; IL-2 receptor alpha chain (Tac)
CD29	$CD4^+$ T-lymphocyte subset (helper/inducer)
CD34	Lymphoid and myeloid precursors (stem cell)
CD45RA	$CD4^+$ T-lymphocyte subset (helper/suppressor), B lymphocytes, NK cells
CD56	NK cells

Key: NK, natural killer.

There are a number of reasons that a patient will not react to an antigen injected intradermally. Most commonly, the patient may not have had a previous exposure to the antigen. Nonresponsiveness may occur from anergy (dysfunction of cell-mediated immunity) due to immunosuppression from drugs (corticosteroids, cyclosporine, etc.) or disease (AIDS, cancer, etc.). A small subset of patients may be genetically unresponsive to the antigen.

A delayed hypersensitivity skin test can be performed by two methods. In one method, the patient can be administered a dose of antigen at a time sufficiently preceding the skin test so that the immune response can develop. Then the skin test with the same antigen is applied and the extent of reactivity measured. The most common method is to administer a panel of five or six recall antigens. The most common antigens are *Candida,* coccidiodin, mumps, *Trichophyton,* and purified protein derivative of tuberculin (PPD). More than 90% of the population will show a positive reaction to two or more of these antigens. After injection of the recall antigens, the patient should be carefully observed for the occurrence of immediate reactions. Measurements in millimeters of induration and erythema at the site of injection should be taken 24, 48, and 72 hours after injection. A reaction is considered positive if the diameter of induration and erythema is 5 mm or greater. Reaction to even a single antigen indicates a functioning cell-mediated immunity. The degree of sensitivity relates to the area of induration.[25]

The accepted indications for delayed hypersensitivity skin testing include evaluation of immune disorders and chronic diseases that cause cellular immune dysfunction (e.g., uremia, cancer, AIDs, etc.), exposure to infectious pathogens (e.g., *Mycobacterium tuberculosis*), evaluation of nutritional status because malnutrition can result in cellular immune deficit, and, in some cases, assessment of immune senescence.

In vivo assessment of B-lymphocyte function involves immunizing the patient with a protein (e.g., tetanus toxoid) and a polysaccharide (e.g., Pneumovax) antigen to quantitate antibody response after immunization. After 2–3 weeks, the patient's serum is tested for antibodies specific for the immunized antigen. This test measures B-lymphocyte responsiveness to the inoculated antigens. It is used to evaluate responsiveness to a vaccine but is reserved for patients who are suspected to have impaired B-lymphocyte function.[25]

IN VITRO

There are a number of specific lymphocyte functional assays, but most of these assays are used in the research setting. Many of these assays are performed at most tertiary care medical centers. One of these tests is the lymphocyte proliferation assay. In this assay, lymphocytes are obtained from a patient's peripheral blood and cultured *in vitro.* The cells are exposed to a nonspecific mitogen such as pokeweed mitogen, phytohemagglutin, or concanavalin A. Then the cells are incubated in growth media containing tritium-labeled (^{3}H) thymidine (a DNA precursor). In the presence of the mitogens, normal lymphocytes will be stimulated to proliferate. Proliferation results in incorporation of ^{3}H thymidine, which can be measured on a β counter. The patient sample would be compared to normal, healthy controls. Patients with immune deficiencies (AIDS, cancer, etc.) have fewer active or less active lymphocytes, as detected by this test.

A modification of the lymphocyte proliferation assay is used in allogeneic bone marrow transplantation to evaluate how closely a donor and host are "matched" in order to predict a patient's risk for graft-versus-host disease. A mixed lymphocyte culture (MLC) assesses the potential of the donor cells to attack the host cells, graft-versus-host disease (Chapter 129). In this test, donor cells and host cells are incubated *in vitro.* The host lymphocytes are irradiated prior to the incubation so that they cannot proliferate. *In vitro,* ^{3}H thymidine is provided to the cells and uptake is measured. The degree of uptake is related to proliferation of donor lymphocytes. If the cells are well matched, proliferation is minimal. If the cells are mismatched, proliferation will be noted with the level of proliferation predictive of the potential extent of graft-versus-host disease.

In addition to the test described previously, a number of other tests have been devised to evaluate the function of CD8$^+$ T lymphocytes, NK cells, and monocytes/macrophages. Although these evaluations are not commonly performed, they may be helpful in some specific diseases. A thorough discussion of these tests is available.[26]

Humoral Aspects of Immune Function

The humoral components of the immune system (immunoglobulins, complement, and cytokines) are often assessed. Assays of humoral components may be either quantitative to determine the absolute concentration of the factor or qualitative to determine the function of the component.

IMMUNOGLOBULINS

The most common evaluation of immunoglobulins is the estimation of total immunoglobulin. This is obtained by subtracting the albumin concentration from the total protein concentration. This difference gives a gross estimation of the total immunoglobulin concentration. Actual determination of the total immunoglobulin concentration is done by serum protein electrophoresis (SPEP). Five separate zones are detected by this method: albumin, α_1-globulin, α_2-globulin, β-globulin, and γ-globulin. The γ-globulin fraction contains the five isotypes of immunoglobulin (IgG, IgA, IgM, IgE, IgD). A normal total immunoglobulin or γ-globulin concentration ranges from 0.8–1.6 g/dL. This test is used to determine if patients have hypogammaglobulinemia (primary and secondary immunodeficiencies), a monoclonal peak (multiple myeloma, Waldenstrom's macroglobulinemia), or a polyclonal hypergammaglobulinemia (chronic inflammatory conditions such as systemic lupus erythematosus and chronic active hepatitis). Total immunoglobulin or γ-globulin concentrations cannot be used to measure antigen-specific antibodies or specific isotypes.

In a patient suspected of having humoral immune deficiency or B-lymphocyte failure (primary and secondary immunodeficiency), specific immunoglobulin isotypes in the plasma should be measured. These are usually determined by radial immunodiffusion or by rate nephelometry. Table 80.2 lists the normal concentrations of different isotypes.

There are many indications for the measurement of antigen-specific antibody. Some common indications are listed in Table 80.7. The most common methods to perform these measurements include enzyme-linked immunosorbent assay (ELISA), radioimmunoassay (RIA), Western blot, and radioallergosorbent test (RAST). The most common

TABLE 80.7. POTENTIAL INDICATIONS FOR MEASUREMENT OF ANTIGEN-SPECIFIC ANTIBODY

Environmental or drug allergy
Exposure to or infection with bacteria
Streptococci (ASO titer)
Staphylococcus aureus (teichoic acid antibody)
Neisseria gonorrhoeae
Legionella pneumophila
Exposure to or infection with viruses
Human immunodeficiency virus
Cytomegalovirus
Epstein–Barr virus
Hepatitis A, B, or C
Rubella
Exposure to or infection with other pathogens
Syphilis
Lyme disease
Typhoid
Chlamydia
Immune disorders
Rheumatoid arthritis
Systemic lupus erythematosus
Idiopathic thrombocytopenia
Blood typing and cross-matching
Transplantation
HLA antibodies

reason to measure antigen-specific antibody is to determine whether a patient has been exposed to an infectious agent. Generally, IgM antibodies directed against the pathogen indicates an active infection while IgG antibodies directed against the pathogen indicates prior exposure. For example, in hepatitis A and cytomegalovirus infections, the presence of the IgM antibody against the virus supports the diagnosis of an active infection while the presence of the IgG antibody signifies immunity to the virus. Initially, plasma cells produce IgM in response to an infection, but memory B lymphocytes produce IgG. Therefore, IgG concentrations will go up in a second exposure, but IgM antibodies will be present during an active infection and shortly after recovery from the infection. Other uses of antigen-specific antibody include determining if a patient has had exposure and is likely to be protected from further infection (e.g., Rubella virus) or to indicate adequate response to vaccination (e.g., hepatitis B).

Antigen-specific IgE is commonly measured in patients with allergies. Because the presence of antigen-specific IgE is related to clinical allergy, measurement of these antibodies can be helpful in diagnosing allergies and determining offending substances. A standard method for determination of allergen-specific IgE is the RAST. The basic technique involves adding the antigen of interest, which is bound to beads or disks, to the patient's serum. After precipitation and several washings, the antibody bound to the bead or disk is isolated. Finally, a radiolabeled antibody that binds to IgE is added. After further washings, the radiolabeled antibody bound to IgE which is bound to the antigen on the bead or disk is counted on a gamma counter.

Examination of serum for an antigen-specific IgE is not the only way to determine the presence of allergen-specific IgE. Another method is by antigen skin testing. When it is produced, IgE binds to high-affinity IgE Fc receptors on basophils or mast cells. Contact of an allergen with the specific IgE on the basophil or mast cell surface causes activation of these cells and the release of inflammatory mediators (e.g., histamine). When this occurs systemically, it can cause anaphylaxis. When it occurs in a confined area such as the skin, erythema and induration are observed within a few minutes of allergen injection. This is the principle used for detection of penicillin allergy as well as for environmental or food allergies. A positive skin reaction (5 mm or greater of induration) within 15–20 minutes is indicative of the presence of allergen-specific IgE.

IgG SUBCLASSES

The four subclasses of IgG are IgG1, IgG2, IgG3, and IgG4. They make up 65, 20, 10, and 5% of total plasma IgG, respectively. Concentrations of the subclasses are often measured in patients with primary and secondary immunodeficiencies. IgG2 and IgG4 deficiencies are associated with chronic infections. IgG4 deficiencies are also associated with autoimmune disorders. Measurement of the subclasses can be performed by ELISA.

COMPLEMENT SYSTEM

The complement system consists of a group of over 20 different plasma proteins involved in lysing and opsonizing invading pathogens as well as serving as chemotactic factors. The various proteins of the complement system are named by numbers following the letter C (C1, C2, etc.). A global assessment of the complement system is the CH_{50}. The CH_{50} (total hemolytic complement test) measures the ability of the patient's entire classic complement system to lyse sheep red blood cells opsonized with antibody. This test does not provide an indication of the function of any specific complement component but is used as a screening test for any complement system defects. If a defect is found, individual complement proteins can then be evaluated by functional or immunochemical methods. Assessment of the complement system is important in patients suspected of having humoral immune deficiencies (i.e., recurrent infections).

Several disease states can alter complement concentrations. SLE, rheumatoid arthritis with vasculitis, poststreptococcal glomerulonephritis, gram-negative infections, and subacute bacterial endocarditis are associated with a decrease in CH_{50} assay and various components of the complement system. The liver is the primary source of several components of the complement system (C2, C3, C4, factors B and D); therefore, in liver failure a decrease in complement levels is observed. Inherited complement deficiencies have been described in patients with SLE, recurrent gonococcal and meningococcal infections, Raynaud's phenomenon, and hereditary angioedema.[25]

CYTOKINES

Scientists have identified and cloned many of the various natural cytokines within the body that are responsible for altering immune function. Methods to detect levels of these cytokines within the blood have been developed. For nearly all the currently identified cytokines, commercial kits are available to measure endogenous and exogenously administered cytokines. Most of the commercial cytokine measurements are done by ELISA or RIA. ELISAs and RIAs are easy to run but measure immunoactivity, not biologic activity. Bioassays measure biologic activity, but are cumbersome and extremely variable. Therefore, most researchers prefer ELISAs and RIAs.[27,28]

We are still at the very early stages of interpreting endogenous cytokine concentrations. Not only is the immune system affected by cytokines such as IL-1, IL-6,

TNF-α, but other systems (skeletal, endocrine, central nervous system) also are affected. Measurement of cytokine concentrations may be important in the evaluation of the immune system as well as of other systems.

When we administer cytokines in therapeutic trials, we may change not only the concentration of that particular cytokine, but also the concentration of other cytokines. Several studies have demonstrated that the systemic administration of GM-CSF to patients not only increases concentrations of GM-CSF but also TNF-α, IL-6, macrophage colony-stimulating factor, and erythropoietin.[29,30] Secondary endogenous cytokine release should be taken into account when monitoring cytokine concentrations.

In the future, tissue concentrations as well as blood concentrations may be measured. For example, while many centers currently measure cyclosporine concentrations to estimate the potential for immunosuppressive effects, it may be more advantageous to monitor IL-2 concentrations. One of the primary actions of cyclosporine is the inhibition of IL-2 production. Furthermore, perhaps it may be beneficial to measure tissue concentrations of IL-2 in the transplanted organ to get a better estimate of the state of immunologic suppression.

SOLUBLE RECEPTORS AND RECEPTOR ANTAGONISTS

Two types of cytokine inhibitors have been described: (1) receptor-binding antagonists and (2) cytokine-binding inhibitors. The best characterized receptor-binding antagonist is the interleukin-1 receptor antagonist (IL-1RA), which inhibits binding of IL-1 to its receptor by competing for the same binding site.[31,32]

Cytokine-binding inhibitors bind the cytokine before it is able to reach its target receptor. The best characterized cytokine-binding inhibitors are soluble cytokine receptors. Several soluble cytokine receptors have been described both *in vitro* and *in vivo,* soluble IL-2 receptor (sIL-2R), sIL-4R, sIL-6R, sIL-7R, sIFN-gR, and sTNFR. The best characterized soluble cytokine receptor is the sIL-2R. While patients with normal immune systems have relatively low titers of sIL-2R, it has been demonstrated that patients with a wide variety of diseases exhibit an increase in sIL-2R. This may reflect an increase in the activity of the immune system. Because sIL-2R has the ability to bind free IL-2, it has been postulated that IL-2R is shed from the surface of cells to down-regulate the immune response. In hairy cell leukemia, the neoplastic cells secrete sIL-2R, and sIL-2R concentrations correlate with tumor burden. A reduction in sIL-2R closely parallels the clinical response of tumors to α-interferon therapy. Relapse is preceded by a rise in the sIL-2R concentrations.[33] sIL-2R concentrations have also been correlated with rejection of transplanted organs.[34] Our better understanding of soluble receptors and receptor antagonists may allow us to mimic natural mechanisms for minimizing the toxicity of administering cytokines (e.g., IL-2, TNF-α, IL-1, etc.) as well as immunomodulation of various diseases (e.g., solid organ transplant rejection, collagen vascular disorders, sepsis, etc.).

CONCLUSION

Our understanding of the immune system has increased dramatically during the last decade. An immune response encompasses dynamic events involving both immunologic cells (phagocytes, lymphocytes, etc.) and soluble mediators (complement, cytokines, antibodies, etc.). A better understanding of the normal immune response allows us to investigate the pathophysiology of diseases where the immune response is inappropriate. All clinicians need a basic understanding of the immune system and familiarity with parameters to monitor immune system function in order to refine the development of immunologic treatments for diseases ranging from diabetes mellitus to collagen vascular disorders to cancer.

REFERENCES

1. Claman HN. The biology of the immune response. JAMA 1992;268:2790–2796.
2. Male D, Roitt I. Introduction to the immune system, in Roitt I, Brostoff, Male D (eds): Immunology. London, Mosby, 1993, pp 1.1–1.12.
3. Lehrer RI, Ganz T, Selsted ME, et al. Neutrophils and host defense. Ann Intern Med 1988;109:127–142.
4. Weller PF. The immunobiology of eosinophils. N Engl J Med 1991;324:1110–1118.
5. Selijelid R, Eskeland T. The biology of macrophages. Eur J Haematol 1993;51:267–275.
6. Restifo NP. Antigen processing and presentation: An update, in DeVita VT, Hellman S, Rosenberg SA (eds): Biologic Therapy of Cancer Updates, Vol 2. Philadelphia, JB Lippincott, 1992, pp 1–10.
7. Galli SJ. New concepts about the mast cell. N Engl J Med 1993;328:257–265.
8. Johnston RB. The complement system in host defense and inflammation: The cutting edges of a double edged sword. Pediatr Infect Dis J 1993;12:933–941.
9. Chen L, Linsely PS, Hellstrom KE. Costimulation of T cells for tumor immunity. Immunol Today 1993;14:483–485.
10. Morimoto C, Letvin NL, Boyd W, et al. The isolation and characterization of human helper inducer T cell subset. J Immunol 1985;134:3762–3769.
11. Morimoto C, Letvin NL, Distaso JA, et al. The isolation and characterization of human suppressor inducer T cell subset. J Immunol 1985;134:1508–1515.
12. Romagnani S. Human TH_1 and TH_2 subsets: Regulation of differentiation and role in protection and immunopathology. Int Arch Allergy Immunol 1992;98:279–285.

13. Clerici M, Hakim F, Venzon DJ, et al. Changes in interleukin-2 and interleukin-4 production in asymptomatic, human immunodeficiency virus-seropositive individuals. J Clin Invest 1993;91:759–765.
14. Feldmann M. Cell cooperation in the antibody response, in Roitt I, Brostoff, Male D (eds): Immunology. London, Mosby, 1993, pp 7.1–7.16.
15. Heiner DC. IgG subclass composition of intravenous immunoglobulin preparations: Clinical relevance. Rev Infect Dis 1986;8(suppl 4):S391–S395.
16. Goodman JW. Immunoglobulin structure and function, In Stites DP, Terr AI (eds): Basic and Clinical Immunology. East Norwalk, CT, Appleton and Lange, 1991, pp 109–121.
17. Robertson MJ, Ritz J. Biology and clinical relevance of human natural killer cells. Blood 1990;76:2421–2438.
18. Basic components, in Chapel H, Haeney M (eds): Essentials of Clinical Immunology. London, Blackwell Scientific Publications, 1993, pp 1–32.
19. Oppenheim JJ, Ruscetti FW, Faltynek C. Cytokines, in Stites DP, Terr A (eds): Basic and Clinical Immunology. Norwalk, CT, Appleton and Lange, 1991, pp 78–100.
20. Du XX, Williams DA. Interleukin-11: A multifunctional growth factor derived from the hematopoietic microenvironment. Blood 1994;83:2023–2030.
21. Zurawski G, de Vries JE. Interleukin 13, an interleukin 4-like cytokine that acts on monocytes and B cells, but not on T cells. Immunol Today 1994;15:19–26.
22. Hannet I, Erkeller-Yuksel F, Lydyard P, et al. Developmental and maturational changes in human blood lymphocyte subpopulations. Immunol Today 1992;13:215–218.
23. White blood count and differential, in Bakerman S (ed): ABC's of Interpretive Laboratory Data. Greenville, NC, Interpretive Laboratory Data, Inc, 1984, pp 444–447.
24. Westermann J, Pabst R. Lymphocyte subsets in the blood: A diagnostic window on the lymphoid system? Immunol Today 1990;11:406–410.
25. Lopez M, Gleisher T, deShazo RD. Use and interpretation of diagnostic immunologic laboratory tests. JAMA 1992;268:2970–2990.
26. Rose NR, Friedman H, Fahey JL (eds). Manual of Clinical Laboratory Immunology, 3rd ed. Washington, DC, American Society of Microbiology, 1986, Chapters 43–46.
27. Van Brunt J. Assaying cytokines. Biotechnology 1991;9:439–441.
28. Rabinowitz J, Petros WP, Peters WP. Cytokine kinetics: Clinical pharmacology studies complementing recombinant growth factor trials. Cancer Bull 1994;46:40–47.
29. Rabinowitz J, Petros WP, Stuart A, Peters WP. Characterization of endogenous cytokine concentrations after high-dose chemotherapy with autologous bone marrow support. Blood 1993;81:2452–2459.
30. Stehle B, Weiss C, Ho A, Hunstein W. Serum levels of tumor necrosis factor alpha in patients treated with granulocyte-macrophage colony stimulating factor. Blood 1990;75:1895–1896.
31. Fernandez-Botran R. Soluble cytokine receptors: Their role in immunoregulation. FASEB J 1991;5:2567–2574.
32. Larrick JW, Wright SC. Native cytokine antagonists. Baillieres Clin Haematol 1992;5:681–702.
33. Ho AD, Grossman M, Knauf W, et al. Plasma levels of soluble CD8 antigen and interleukin-2 receptor antigen in patients with hairy cell leukemia, relationship with splenectomy and with clinical response to therapy. Leukemia 1989;3:718–723.
34. Lawrence EC, Holland VA, Young JB, et al. Dynamic changes in soluble interleukin-2 receptor levels after lung and heart–lung transplantation. Am Rev Respir Dis 1989;140:789–796.

Chapter 81

Systemic Lupus Erythematosus and Other Collagen Vascular Diseases

Mark B. Burlingame, PharmD, and Jeffrey C. Delafuente, MS

The collagen vascular diseases are a heterogeneous group of diseases that can involve the musculoskeletal system, integument, and blood vessels. Each collagen vascular disease has its own set of diagnostic criteria although diagnosis can be difficult because of overlapping and nonspecific clinical presentations. The etiology of the various collagen vascular diseases is often unknown although the immune system is usually involved in mediation of disease. Therefore, pharmacotherapy usually includes anti-inflammatory or immunosuppressive drugs.

Although the prevalence of other collagen vascular diseases may be greater than systemic lupus erythematosus (e.g., polymyalgia rheumatica), SLE is discussed most extensively in this chapter because it is a major collagen vascular disease with numerous clinical manifestations; its pharmacotherapy can be complex, and a plethora of data is available on the therapy of SLE. Since all of the diseases discussed in this chapter have an immune-mediated pathogenesis, the therapeutic principles of lupus can be applied to other autoimmune collagen vascular diseases. The collagen vascular diseases discussed include systemic sclerosis, polymyositis/dermatomyositis, polymyalgia rheumatica, and systemic vasculitis and were chosen because they are seen in general practice.

Systemic Lupus Erythematosus

Systemic lupus erythematosus (SLE) is a fluctuating, multisystem disease with a diversity of clinical presentations. Abnormal immunologic function and formation of antibodies against "self" antigens underlie the pathogenesis of SLE.

Lupus is the Latin word for wolf and was first used to describe erosive skin lesions that looked as though a wolf had eaten away the flesh. The term *lupus erythematosus* was first used in 1851 by Cazenave, a Frenchman who described an illness in a patient with manifestations occurring in the skin. It is not surprising that SLE was first recognized as a skin disorder, because cutaneous manifestations constitute one of the most common clinical features of the disease. Further descriptions by Kaposi in 1872 and Osler in 1895 led to the concept of a multisystem disease, as it became recognized that patients developed complications in other organ systems.[1]

Autoantibodies in this disease became apparent with the development of the lupus erythematosus (LE) cell test in 1948 and the fluorescent antinuclear antibody test in 1957.[1] Recognition of SLE as an autoimmune disease of multisystemic nature led the American Rheumatism Association (ARA) to develop criteria for identifying lupus patients (Table 81.1). These criteria were originally developed in 1971 and revised in 1982. The criteria do not include all the clinical manifestations of the disease and are used primarily for distinguishing SLE from other collagen vascular diseases and determining patients for clinical studies.[2] To classify a patient as having SLE, 4 or more of the 11 criteria must be present. Although these criteria may be helpful, diagnosis requires additional serologic, immunopathologic, and clinical evaluations.

EPIDEMIOLOGY

The incidence of SLE has been reported as 1.0–7.6 per 100,000 population per year with a prevalence of 5.8–51.0 per 100,000 population.[3,4] The disease occurs predominantly in women, with a reported female-to-male ratio approaching 10:1.[4,5] This predominance is considered most visible during reproductive years although some reports, particularly in Europe, have indicated a peak incidence in middle-aged women.[4] The reported incidence in blacks and some other races is usually higher than in whites.[4] Although the most typical SLE patient is a young adult woman, the disease can occur in people of any age, race, and sex.

TABLE 81.1. THE 1982 REVISED CRITERIA FOR CLASSIFICATION OF SYSTEMIC LUPUS ERYTHEMATOSUS[a]

Criterion	Definition
Malar rash	Fixed erythema, flat or raised, over the malar eminences, tending to spare the nasolabial folds
Discoid rash	Erythematous raised patches with adherent keratotic scaling and follicular plugging; atrophic scarring may occur in older lesions
Photosensitivity	Skin rash as a result of unusual reaction to sunlight, by patient history or physician observations
Oral ulcers	Oral or nasopharyngeal ulceration, usually painless, observed by a physician
Arthritis	Nonerosive arthritis involving two or more peripheral joints, characterized by tenderness, swelling, or effusion
Serositis	Pleuritis—convincing history of pleuritic pain or rub heard by a physician or evidence of pleural effusion *or* Pericarditis—documented by ECG or rub or evidence of pericardial effusion
Renal disorder	Persistent proteinuria greater than 0.5 g/d or greater than 3+ if quantitation not performed *or* Cellular casts—may be red cell, hemoglobin, granular, tubular, or mixed
Neurologic disorder	Seizures—in the absence of offending drugs or known metabolic derangements, e.g., uremia, ketoacidosis, or electrolyte imbalance *or* Psychosis—in the absence of offending drugs or known metabolic derangements, e.g., uremia, ketoacidosis, or electrolyte imbalance
Hematologic disorder	Hemolytic anemia—with reticulocytosis *or* Leukopenia—fewer than 4000/mm^3 total on two or more occasions *or* Lymphopenia—fewer than 1500/mm^3 on two or more occasions *or* Thrombocytopenia—fewer than 100,000/mm^3 in the absence of offending drugs
Immunologic disorder	Positive LE cell preparation *or* Anti-DNA; antibody to native DNA in abnormal titer *or* Anti-Sm; presence of antibody to Sm nuclear antigen *or* False-positive serologic test for syphilis known to be positive for at least 6 months and confirmed by *Treponema pallidum* immobilization or fluorescent treponemal antibody absorption test
Antinuclear antibody	An abnormal titer of antinuclear antibody by immunofluorescence or an equivalent assay at any point in time and in the absence of drugs known to be associated with "drug-induced lupus" syndrome

[a]The proposed classification is based on 11 criteria. For the purpose of identifying patients in clinical studies, a person shall be said to have systemic lupus erythematosus if any 4 or more of the 11 criteria are present, serially or simultaneously, during any interval of observation. (From Tan EM, Cohen AS, Fries JF, et al. The 1982 revised criteria for the classification of systemic lupus erythematosus. Arthritis Rheum 1982;25:1274, with permission.)

ETIOLOGY

The etiology of abnormal autoantibody production and development of SLE is still unknown. Genetic, environmental, and hormonal factors all may have a role in loss of self-tolerance and expression of disease.

Population, family, and twin studies suggest a genetic predisposition for the development of SLE. For example, studies in twins show a monozygotic concordance rate of between 30 and 60%; however, the risk in dizygotic twins is the same as that in first-degree relatives. Genetic analysis predicts that as many as four genes are involved in the expression of lupus in humans. Evidence indicates that major histocompatibility complex genes, such as the human leukocyte antigen (HLA) genes in humans, may be important in lupus. Environmental agents that may have a role in induction or activation of SLE include ultraviolet light, drugs, hair dyes, foods, and infection with viruses, bacteria, or parasites. Additionally, androgen may inhibit, and estrogen enhance, the expression of autoimmunity.[6]

PATHOPHYSIOLOGY

A major event in the development of SLE is excessive and abnormal autoantibody production. Many of these antibodies are directed against nuclear constituents of the cell and are called collectively *antinuclear antibodies.* A patient with SLE usually has more than one antigen-specific antinuclear antibody in his or her serum and tissues. These are antibodies against such nuclear constituents as double-stranded or native DNA (dsDNA), single-stranded or denatured DNA (ssDNA), and RNA. Four RNA-associated antigens frequently occurring in SLE are the Sm antigen, ribonuclear protein (RNP), Ro (SS-A) antigen, and La (SS-B) antigen. Antibodies may also be directed against the phospholipid moiety of the prothrombin activator complex (lupus anticoagulant) and against cardiolipin. The lupus anticoagulant and anticardiolipin antibody are cross-reactive and constitute the two main types in a group of autoantibodies called antiphospholipid antibodies.[7]

The abnormal and excessive production of autoantibodies may be related to a defect in lymphocyte regulation. Patients with active multisystem lupus have an increase in number or activity (or both) of B cells and subsequently an increase in antibody production. The increase in B-cell activity may result from decreased numbers and function of suppressor T cells and increased T-helper-cell activity.[6]

Cytokines are secreted molecules that are involved in the activation of lymphocytes. Several cytokines, such as interleukin-1 (IL-1), IL-2, IL-4, and IL-6 are important regulators of B-cell function in humans. Many cytokine abnormalities are found in patients with lupus and may be important in disease pathogenesis.[6]

The mechanism of tissue injury in SLE is thought to be related to immune complex formation and deposition in the kidney and other tissues, resulting in cell damage, complement fixation, and inflammation.[8]

CLINICAL PRESENTATION

As previously mentioned, SLE is a multisystem disease. Table 81.2 lists many of the signs and symptoms that may present in a patient with SLE. While certain of these may be more common than others, each patient presents differently and the course of the disease is highly unpredictable. Furthermore, SLE is not static, and most patients have fluctuations or "flare-ups" during the course of the disease.

Nonspecific signs and symptoms such as fatigue, fever, anorexia, and weight loss are frequently seen in patients with active disease. Musculoskeletal involvement (e.g., arthralgia, myalgia, arthritis) is very common in SLE. Up to 95% of patients will develop this type of manifestation at some time during the course of the disease.[9] Joint involvement tends to be symmetrical and may affect multiple sites. Objective evidence of musculoskeletal disease is often missing, although a few patients may present with deforming arthritis or subcutaneous nodules.

Manifestations in the skin and mucous membranes are seen in more than 80% of patients.[9] The most well known of these is the butterfly rash, which occurs over the bridge of the nose and the malar eminences. The classic butterfly rash is seen in approximately one-half of patients and is often observed after sun exposure. In fact, photosensitivity is common to many SLE patients that present with cutaneous manifestations. Patients should use sunscreens when outdoors for prolonged periods. Skin lesions characteristic of discoid lupus occur in up to 25% of patients with SLE and may occur without other clinical or serologic evidence of lupus.[9] Some individuals are said to develop subacute cutaneous lupus erythematosus, the nature of whose lesions falls between discoid and the butterfly rash. Other cutaneous manifestations include vasculitis (which may be ulcerative), levido reticularis, periungual erythema, Raynaud's phenomenon, and alopecia.

TABLE 81.2. CLINICAL SIGNS AND SYMPTOMS OF SLE

Common Features	Uncommon Features
Arthritis	Hepatomegaly
Arthralgias	Splenomegaly
Fever and constitutional symptoms	Retinopathy
Pleuritis	Myalgias
Mucocutaneous involvement	Raynaud's phenomenon
Nephritis	Abdominal pain
Pericarditis	
Libman–Sacks endocarditis	
Lymphadenopathy	
Neuropsychiatric disease	
Anemia	
Leukopenia	
Photosensitive rash (sun exposure)	

Another common source of symptomatology in SLE is the pulmonary system. Pleurisy, coughing, or dyspnea may be the first manifestation of SLE itself. Pleurisy may present as pleuritic pain, a pleural rub, or a pleural effusion that is usually exudative in nature. Lupus pneumonitis may present acutely with fever, dyspnea, tachypnea, cough, rales, and patchy infiltrates or chronically with interstitial fibrosis. Lupus pneumonitis is an uncommon manifestation of SLE and has a poor prognosis.[9,10]

Cardiac manifestations of SLE often present as pericarditis, myocarditis, or ECG changes. Coronary artery disease is occurring with increasing frequency in lupus patients, especially those with long-standing disease.[11] It is thought that corticosteroid therapy may contribute significantly to the development of heart disease in these patients.

Neuropsychiatric manifestations of SLE may present in a diversity of ways, from psychosis to seizure to peripheral neuropathy. This aspect of lupus is seen in 40–70% of patients and may be an important factor contributing to morbidity and mortality.[12]

Gastrointestinal manifestations occur in approximately 50% of SLE patients. Symptoms are often nonspecific for lupus and include dyspepsia, abdominal pain, and swallowing difficulty. Mesenteric vasculitis may be problematic, particularly if arterial perforations occur. Hepatomegaly may present in some patients although liver dysfunction is not characteristic of lupus. Pancreatitis may also be present in an occasional patient.[9]

Hematologic Manifestations

Anemia is found in many cases of SLE. It is usually an anemia of chronic inflammation, with a mild normochromic, normocytic smear and low serum iron but adequate iron stores. Some patients may develop a hemolytic anemia with a positive Coombs' test. Leukopenia, usually mild, is present in approximately half of SLE patients. Both granulocytes and lymphocytes may be affected but there is usually a larger decrease in the amount of circulating granulocytes. The absolute number of both T lymphocytes and B lymphocytes decreases. Thrombocytopenia may occur in SLE and is usually due to antiplatelet antibodies resulting in phagocytosis in the spleen.[9]

Another interesting finding associated with SLE is the presence of antiphospholipid antibodies such as the lupus anticoagulant (LA) and anticardiolipin antibodies. Although the LA is directed against the prothrombin activator complex and implies potential bleeding complications, this is not the case. In fact, the presence of LA and other antiphospholipid antibodies may be associated with thrombosis, neurologic disease, thrombocytopenia, and fetal loss, and is termed the *antiphospholipid syndrome.*[7,13]

Lupus Nephritis

Clinical evidence of renal involvement, such as a rising serum creatinine or proteinuria, is generally associated with a poorer outcome compared with patients without renal involvement.[14] Progression to end-stage renal disease is a major cause of morbidity and mortality in SLE. However, the extent and course of renal disease are quite variable and many lupus nephritis patients do very well. The World Health Organization (WHO) has classified lupus nephritis on the basis of histologic characteristics observed following renal biopsy. This system identifies lupus nephritis as mesangial, focal proliferative, diffuse proliferative, membranoproliferative, or membranous glomerulonephritis.[15] Many patients progress from one form of nephritis to another during the course of the disease. Renal biopsy findings such as diffuse proliferative glomerulonephritis and high activity and/or chronicity indices may be associated with a poor outcome, although the prognostic value of this information is uncertain.[15,16]

DIAGNOSIS

As mentioned earlier, the diagnostic criteria listed in Table 81.1 should not be the primary means for diagnosing SLE, although many of the criteria may be valuable in the diagnostic process. Epidemiologic characteristics, clinical signs and symptoms, and common laboratory abnormalities are all used in diagnosing SLE.

Once the disease is suspected, serologic tests may be helpful in making the diagnosis. A serologic test extensively used to aid in the diagnosis of SLE is the fluorescent antinuclear antibody (ANA) test. Nearly all SLE patients are ANA positive, but other disease states are also associated with a positive test (Table 81.3); however, in other diseases many of the positive ANA tests are of a lower titer. The pattern of immunofluorescence of the ANA test may also be of diagnostic value (Table 81.3) with a peripheral (also called rim) pattern being specific for SLE. Detecting antibodies to specific nuclear constituents may also be diagnostically useful. Antibodies to native (dsDNA) and to Sm antigen are quite specific for SLE.[17]

PROGNOSIS

In earlier years, SLE was associated with a poor prognosis. For example, one report of cases diagnosed between 1949 and 1953 showed a 4-year survival rate of 51%.[18] Today, probably as a result of improved treatment and improved diagnostic techniques that allow earlier diagnosis, the 10-year survival rate approaches 90%.[19]

An important prognostic sign is that of lupus nephritis. A 10-year survival rate of 87% in patients without evidence of nephritis compared with 65% in patients with nephritis has been reported.[14] However, infection has replaced renal disease as the most common cause of death from SLE.[19] Death is usually a result of kidney involvement, central nervous system (CNS) disease, or infection.[11,14] Cardiovascular disease has emerged as a prominent cause of death as lupus patients live longer.[11] In fact, hypertension has been reported as a risk factor for the development of renal deterioration and death in patients with SLE.[20]

TABLE 81.3. ANTINUCLEAR ANTIBODY TEST: PATTERNS, ANTIGENS, AND SPECIFICITIES

Pattern	Antigen	Disease
Peripheral	Double-stranded DNA	SLE
Speckled	Acidic nuclear protein	Rheumatoid arthritis
	Ribonucleoprotein	SLE
	Extractable nuclear antigen	Scleroderma
		Mixed connective tissue disease
Homogeneous	Deoxyribonucleoprotein	Rheumatoid arthritis
	Histone	SLE, drug-induced lupus
Nucleolar	Nucleolar RNA	Progressive systemic sclerosis

Pregnancy in SLE patients has been associated with exacerbation of disease during pregnancy, exacerbation during early postpartum, and a greater incidence of spontaneous abortion. Exacerbation of lupus during pregnancy seems to be less likely if the disease is in remission at conception.[21] Antiphospholipid antibodies may be associated with a greater likelihood of fetal loss. Corticosteroids, aspirin, and heparin, alone and in various combinations, have been used to try to improve fetal outcome.[22] However, the optimal treatment regimen for pregnant patients with antiphospholipid antibodies is yet to be determined.

PHARMACOTHERAPY

In general, drug therapy for SLE is designed to suppress the immune response and inflammation. Table 81.4 lists common agents and doses used to control SLE. In general, the choice of drug therapy depends on the extent and severity of disease.

Nonsteroidal Anti-Inflammatory Drugs

As discussed earlier, signs and symptoms such as fever, arthritis, skin rash, and serositis are among the most common in patients with active disease. Therefore, in many patients with mild disease, initial treatment with a nonsteroidal anti-inflammatory drug (NSAID) is a logical choice. The choice of NSAIDs in SLE is empiric. The dose used should be adequate to provide anti-inflammatory effects.

TABLE 81.4. DRUG TREATMENT OF SYSTEMIC LUPUS ERYTHEMATOSUS

Drug Class	Drug and Dose	Indication
NSAID	Various agents Anti-inflammatory dose	Mild disease: fever, arthritis, skin rash, serositis
Antimalarial	Hydroxychloroquine, 200–400 mg PO daily	Mild disease: arthritis, skin rash, serositis
	Chloroquine, 250–500 mg PO daily	
Corticosteroid	Prednisone 1–2 mg/kg/d PO (or equivalent)	Initial control of severe disease
	<1 mg/kg/d (or equivalent)	Control of mild disease or maintenance after disease suppression with higher doses
	Methylprednisolone, 500–1000 mg IV daily × 3–5 d	Life-threatening disease
Cytotoxic	Azathioprine, up to 4 mg/kg/d PO	Most commonly used in severe lupus nephritis
	Cyclophosphamide, up to 4 mg/kg/d PO	
	Cyclophosphamide, 0.5–1.0 g/m^2 IV every 1–3 months	

Patients with SLE taking NSAIDs may experience a decline in renal function because of drug effects and not the underlying disease. Prostaglandins may be important mediators of renal hemodynamics in patients with SLE, possibly increasing susceptibility to the renal sequelae from prostaglandin inhibition.[23] Awareness of this effect is important, because declining renal function might be mistakenly attributed to progression of lupus nephritis. There also exist reports of an association between aseptic meningitis in SLE patients and the use of ibuprofen, sulindac, diclofenac, and tolmetin.[12]

Antimalarial Drugs

Antimalarial agents such as chloroquine and hydroxychloroquine have been used successfully in the management of discoid lupus and SLE. A randomized trial of discontinuation of hydroxychloroquine treatment provided further evidence for the role of antimalarial therapy in controlling disease exacerbations.[24] In general, the manifestations of SLE that can be managed with antimalarials are cutaneous manifestations, arthralgia, pleuritis, mild pericardial inflammation, fatigue, cognitive dysfunction, and mild anemia and leukopenia.[25] Because these drugs are not effective immediately, they are best used in long-term management. Response to chloroquine occurs in 1 month while the maximal effect of hydroxychloroquine may not occur for 3–6 months.[25] Hydroxychloroquine is probably safer than chloroquine and is considered the antimalarial of first choice.

The mechanism of action of the antimalarial drugs is uncertain. It has been proposed that antimalarials interfere with antigen processing in macrophages and other cells.[26] Other effects of antimalarials that may benefit patients with SLE include inhibition of cytokines, decreased sensitivity to ultraviolet light, anti-inflammatory activity, antiplatelet effects, and antihyperlipidemic activity.[25]

Dosage and duration of therapy depend on patient response, tolerance of side effects, and development of retinal toxicity, which is a potentially irreversible adverse reaction associated with long-term therapy, especially with chloroquine. Current recommended doses of antimalarials in SLE are hydroxychloroquine 200–400 mg daily and chloroquine 250–500 mg daily. Side effects of these drugs include headache, nervousness, insomnia, dermatitis, pigmentary changes of the skin and hair, gastrointestinal disturbance (e.g., nausea), flu-like symptoms, and reversible cycloplegia resulting from deposition of the drug in the cornea. Retinal toxicity is uncommon when the currently recommended doses are used and is least common with hydroxychloroquine[25]; however, because of the possibility of permanent damage associated with the retinopathy, an ophthalmologic evaluation should be done every 3 months with chloroquine and every 6–12 months with hydroxychloroquine.[25] If retinal abnormalities are noted, antimalarial therapy should be discontinued.

Corticosteroids

Corticosteroid therapy is commonplace in therapeutic regimens for SLE. Although evidence for improved survival with corticosteroid therapy is inadequate, these agents are known to be effective for suppressing the clinical expression of disease and are considered by many to be a major factor in the improved prognosis of recent years. Although most controlled trials of corticosteroid therapy have been conducted in patients with severe lupus nephritis, evidence suggests that corticosteroids are also effective in the management of severe cases of CNS disease, pneumonitis, polyserositis, vasculitis, thrombocytopenia, and others.[27]

A patient with the diagnosis of SLE does not automatically require corticosteroid therapy. Mild disease with such manifestations as fever, arthralgia, pleuritis, or skin manifestations may respond adequately to NSAIDs or antimalarials, but patients with clinical manifestations that are more serious or unresponsive to other drugs may require corticosteroids.

The goal of treatment when using corticosteroids in SLE is to suppress and maintain suppression of active disease with the lowest dose possible. In patients with mild disease, low-dose therapy (e.g., prednisone 15–20 mg daily) is adequate; however, in patients with more severe disease (e.g., severe hemolytic anemia or cardiac involvement) higher doses, such as prednisone 1–2 mg/kg daily, may be required. Once adequate suppression of disease is achieved, the dose should be tapered to the minimum amount required for continued disease suppression. When analyzing the need to treat with corticosteroids, the clinician should consider other conditions that may increase the risk of corticosteroid therapy such as infection, hypertension, diabetes, obesity, osteoporosis, and psychiatric disease.[27]

Steroid pulse therapy is the administration of short-term, high-dose, intravenous corticosteroids with the goal of inducing remission in SLE patients with serious, life-threatening disease, such as diffuse proliferative glomerulonephritis, CNS involvement, or hemolytic disease. A standard pulse regimen consists of intravenous methylprednisolone 500–1000 mg for 3 to 5 consecutive days. Pulse therapy is usually followed by high-dose oral therapy that is rapidly tapered to low-dose maintenance therapy.[27] Potential advantages of pulse therapy over high-dose oral steroids include a quicker response and avoidance of side effects associated with the longer duration of therapy required with oral steroids. Methylprednisolone pulse therapy is not without adverse effects, including infection, gastrointestinal and taste disturbances, hyperglycemia, facial flushing, rapid increases in blood pressure, arrhythmias, seizures, and sudden death.[27,28] Thus, pulse therapy represents an alternative mode of treatment for patients with life-threatening disease and/or disease unresponsive to other pharmacotherapy.

Cytotoxic Drugs

Perhaps the most controversial issue concerning drug therapy for SLE is the role of cytotoxic (or immunosuppressive) drugs. Included in this category are the alkylating agent cyclophosphamide and the antimetabolite azathioprine. These agents, usually used in combination with corticosteroids, have been the mainstays of U.S. immunosuppressive therapy. Although both are known to suppress and stabilize extrarenal disease activity, evaluation has focused predominantly on lupus nephritis, the major factor associated with morbidity and mortality in SLE. Additionally, when reviewing studies of cytotoxic drug therapy for lupus nephritis, the clinician should be aware that more recent clinical trials define the endpoint "mortality" as the number of patient deaths plus the number of patients progressing to end-stage renal disease. This allows for comparison with earlier trials when chronic dialysis and renal transplantation were not readily available.

Both cyclophosphamide and azathioprine have been shown to delay the onset of nephritis and prolong survival in the New Zealand mouse, the animal model of SLE.[29] Results in human trials, however, have been inconclusive and contradictory, probably because of a paucity of adequately controlled trials, because of the variable presentation and course of disease, because trials were short and included few patients, and because subjects are usually studied late in the course of severe renal disease (e.g., diffuse proliferative glomerulonephritis).[16]

Azathioprine has not been shown to be clearly more effective than prednisone alone. Although some studies have shown azathioprine to be associated with improved survival and a steroid-sparing effect, other studies indicate no significant advantage.[16] Azathioprine is given orally in doses up to 4 mg/kg/d. Azathioprine is generally less toxic than cyclophosphamide, but adverse reactions may be serious and include suppression of hematopoiesis, opportunistic infection, cancer, hepatotoxicity, pulmonary fibrosis, pancreatitis, and teratogenesis.[16] Thus, it is not clear whether possible benefits outweigh risks to justify its role in the therapeutic management of lupus nephritis.

The case for cyclophosphamide is only slightly more convincing. As with azathioprine, not all controlled studies indicate a survival advantage in lupus nephritis patients receiving cyclophosphamide.[30] Controlled studies that indicate a possible advantage of cyclophosphamide are usually of longer duration, such as the series of clinical trials examining the role of various cytotoxic drug regimens in lupus nephritis reported from the National Institutes of Health (NIH).[16] Longer NIH trials have utilized a chronicity index based on renal biopsy information as a predictor of renal functional outcome. One report indicated a marginal advantage of oral cyclophosphamide over oral prednisone alone after a mean follow-up of 85 months.[31] In another NIH report, improved probability of survival, free of renal failure, has been reported for patients receiving intermittent (every 3 months), intravenous cyclophosphamide (0.5–1.0 g/m^2 of body surface area) plus low-dose prednisone compared to prednisone alone in patients with active glomerulonephritis.[32] The most significant benefit was observed in high-risk patients who were identified as having chronic histologic change based on the chronicity index. In the same cohort of NIH patients in which follow-up was extended for an additional 4 years, the probability of progression to end-stage renal disease was less in groups treated with intravenous cyclophosphamide, or oral cyclophosphamide, or combined oral cyclophosphamide and azathioprine.[33]

Of course, cyclophosphamide therapy is not without risk. Serious toxic effects include suppression of hematopoiesis, opportunistic infection, bladder complications (hemorrhagic cystitis and cancer), sterility, and teratogenesis.[16] Bladder complications may be minimized by administering cyclophosphamide in an intermittent, intravenous regimen,[32] or by concomitant use of mesna.[16]

The evidence supporting the usefulness of cytotoxic drugs for patients with SLE is questionable; however, there may be a role for these drugs in patients with serious disease such as severe lupus nephritis.

ALTERNATIVE AND EXPERIMENTAL TREATMENTS

Plasmapheresis

Another potential treatment for severe cases of SLE is removal of autoantibodies and immune complexes from serum using plasmapheresis (also called plasma exchange), a process where 3–4 liters of the patient's plasma is removed and replaced with a plasma substitute. In addition to removal of cytotoxic constituents from serum, plasmapheresis may also affect immunologic responses by improving reticuloendothelial phagocytic cell function and increasing antibody production.[34] Because of the potential for enhancing antibody production, it has been suggested that plasmapheresis be accompanied by corticosteroid and/or cytotoxic drug therapy.[34]

Clinical improvement after plasmapheresis has been reported in uncontrolled observations; however, a controlled trial of plasmapheresis combined with prednisone and cyclophosphamide in patients with severe lupus nephritis failed to show improved outcome over treatment with prednisone and cyclophosphamide alone.[35] Plasmapheresis is of questionable benefit and should be reserved for patients with disease refractory to conventional drug therapy.

Total Lymphoid Irradiation

In patients with severe lupus nephritis unresponsive to high-dose prednisone, treatment with total lymphoid irradiation (TLI) may improve proteinuria and enable a reduction in maintenance prednisone dosage.[36] However, TLI may cause complications such as neutropenia and serious bacterial and herpes zoster infections.[36,37]

Cyclosporine

Knowledge of the immunosuppressive activity of cyclosporine and its effect on T lymphocytes has provided the rationale for trials in humans with SLE.[38] Cyclosporine administered in average doses of 5 mg/kg/d has reportedly suppressed disease activity in patients with severe lupus, including those with nephritis unresponsive to corticosteroids.[38,39] Another trial using cyclosporine doses of 3 mg/kg/d reduced proteinuria in patients with lupus nephritis.[40] Adverse effects limiting cyclosporine use in patients with nephritis include nephrotoxicity and hypertension.

Immune Globulin

The effectiveness of intravenous immune globulin (IVIG) in patients with idiopathic thrombocytopenic purpura has resulted in an examination of its use in other autoimmune diseases. In doses of 0.4 g/kg/d for 5 days, IVIG has reportedly improved clinical and immunologic features of disease activity in patients with severe manifestations of lupus such as thrombocytopenia, nephritis, encephalitis, and pneumonitis.[41–44] The mechanism of action of IVIG is not clear but may be attributed to down-regulation of autoantibody production and solubilization and removal of immune complexes.

Prostaglandins

Prostaglandins and thromboxane, products of the cyclooxygenase pathway of arachidonic acid metabolism, are thought to affect renal hemodynamics in patients with lupus nephritis.[22,45] In addition, prostaglandins of the E series have favorable effects on T lymphocytes and immune complexes in murine models of lupus.[46]

Trials of intravenous prostaglandin E, 160 μg daily, for 3–4 weeks, have been reported in children and young adults with lupus nephritis unresponsive to high-dose corticosteroids with or without cytotoxic drugs.[46,47] Improvement occurred in clinical renal indices such as urinary protein and creatinine clearance as well as a reduction in glomerular immune deposits. Additionally, improved immunologic indices such as increased complement and decreased anti-

DNA antibody levels occurred. Improvement was maintained in some patients for 1 year or longer.

Continuous infusions of an antagonist of the vasoconstrictor thromboxane A_2 resulted in increases in renal blood flow and glomerular filtration rate in patients with lupus nephritis.[45] Further studies using long-acting thromboxane antagonists are needed to realize potential long-term benefits from these drugs.

DRUG-INDUCED LUPUS

A drug-induced SLE-like syndrome was first described in 1945 and was associated with the use of sulfadiazine.[48] Today, procainamide and hydralazine are most commonly associated with drug-induced lupus (DIL), although numerous other drugs have been implicated (Table 81.5).[48,49] A consensus on diagnostic criteria for DIL does not exist and many reported cases do not satisfy the 1982 revised ARA criteria for identification of SLE patients.[49] It has been suggested that DIL be suspected in patients with no history of idiopathic lupus, who develop antinuclear antibodies and at least one clinical feature of SLE, and whose symptoms resolve following drug discontinuation.[49]

The epidemiologic characteristics of DIL are different from those of idiopathic SLE. In general, patients with procainamide- or hydralazine-induced lupus develop the disease in their fifth and sixth decades of life.[48,49] This is much later compared with idiopathic SLE, probably because the majority of people that use these drugs are older. Other observations include a greater percentage of white patients and an absence of female predominance when compared with idiopathic SLE.[48,49] In addition, patients of the slow acetylator phenotype may have a greater risk for developing DIL, particularly with procainamide and hydralazine.[48–50]

TABLE 81.5. MEDICATIONS IMPLICATED IN DRUG-INDUCED LUPUS

Acebutolol	Leuprolide	Phenylbutazone
Aminoglutethimide	Levodopa	Phenytoin
Atenolol	Lithium	Prazosin
Captopril	Lovastatin	Primidone
Carbamazepine	Mephenytoin	**Procainamide**
Chlorpromazine[a]	Methimazole	Promethazine
Chlorprothixene	**Methyldopa**	Propylthiouracil
Clonidine	Methysergide	Psoralen
Danazol	Metrizamide	**Quinidine**
Diclofenac	Minoxidil	Spironolactone
Disopyramide	Nalidixic acid	Streptomycin
Ethosuximide	Nitrofurantoin	Sulindac
Gold salts	Nomifensine	Sulfasalazine
Griseofulvin	Oral contraceptives	Tetracycline
Hydralazine	Para-aminosalicylate	Thioridazine
Ibuprofen	**Penicillamine**	Timolol
Interferon (α, γ)	Penicillin	Tolazamide
Isoniazid	Perphenazine	Tolmetin
Labetalol	Phenelzine	Trimethadione

[a]Drugs in boldface represent those with best evidence of association. (Adapted from Yung RL, Richardson BC. Drug-induced lupus. Rheum Dis Clin North Am 1994;20:62, with permission.)

In DIL, the development of a positive ANA test occurs more rapidly and symptoms present more often with a slow acetylator phenotype.[50] Procainamide-induced lupus can present as early as 1 month or as late as 12 years after starting therapy. Hydralazine-induced lupus is related to dose and appears in patients receiving 100 mg/d or greater.[49]

Musculoskeletal symptoms are the most common clinical manifestations, while renal and CNS involvement is rare or absent in both procainamide- and hydralazine-induced lupus.[48] Pleuropulmonary manifestations are also common, particularly in procainamide-induced disease.[49]

A positive ANA test is found in nearly all cases of procainamide- or hydralazine-induced cases.[48,49] The immunofluorescence pattern is usually homogenous and antibodies are primarily against ssDNA and not dsDNA as in idiopathic SLE. Antihistone antibodies are associated with DIL but are not specific for DIL and are found in idiopathic SLE and other diseases (e.g., rheumatoid arthritis).[49]

If signs and symptoms of SLE appear in a patient and are thought to be drug related, the drug should be discontinued. If the lupus is drug induced, the clinical manifestations should disappear in days to weeks although it may take up to 1 year or longer for symptoms and serologic abnormalities to resolve completely.[48,49] A NSAID might be useful in treating musculoskeletal manifestations. Other, more aggressive drug therapy should not be necessary unless manifestations are deemed more serious.

SYSTEMIC SCLEROSIS

CLINICAL MANIFESTATIONS

Systemic sclerosis is characterized by alteration of the microvasculature and by massive deposition of collagen. This disease can present as a spectrum of differing manifestations depending on affected areas and the extent of disease. Sclerosis of the skin is a hallmark for this disease. There can be a proximal diffuse (truncal) sclerosis, with skin tightness and marked skin thickening involving most of the body. There can also be internal organ involvement, such as the gastrointestinal tract, lung, kidney, or heart, which can result in death. Scleroderma refers to patients with only skin involvement. Disease that affects only the fingers and toes is referred to as sclerodactyly.

Most patients with systemic sclerosis have Raynaud's phenomenon, where the digits turn white, followed by a bluish color, which is then followed by reddening in response to an appropriate stimulus. Usually the precipitating event is cold temperature or emotion. The pallor is due to vasospasm; the bluish color is from ischemia; and the reddish color is caused by a reactive hyperemia. Raynaud's phenomenon is a common manifestation of other syndromes and most patients with Raynaud's phenomenon do not have systemic sclerosis. Approximately 70% of patients with systemic sclerosis have symptoms of gastroesophageal reflux.[51]

In patients who have only sclerodactyly there is about an 80% incidence of survival at 5 years following diagnosis.[52] Patients with diffuse sclerosis have a 5-year survival rate of about 50%.[52] Elderly individuals and patients with poor renal function, anemia, or pulmonary involvement have a poorer prognosis.

ETIOLOGY AND PREVALENCE

The cause of systemic sclerosis is unknown. Ninety-five percent of patients have identifiable autoantibodies. Patients with limited cutaneous involvement often have the CREST syndrome (*C*alcinosis, *R*aynaud's, *E*sophageal dysmotility, *S*clerodactyly, *T*elangiectasias). Most of these patients have anticentromere antibodies.[51] The prevalence of the disease is estimated between 4–290 cases per million population.[52]

TREATMENT

There are no well-controlled trials evaluating and comparing various forms of therapy. The available data are difficult to interpret because of the heterogeneity of the disease and spontaneous remissions that can occur. There is also a lack of objective measures to assess changes in clinical status. D-penicillamine is most often used for skin involvement. This drug does seem to improve the skin manifestations and prolong survival.[52] The initial dose of D-penicillamine is 250 mg daily, with gradual increases in dose every 2–3 months, to an optimal dose of 750–1000 mg/d. Response occurs over many months and the drug is not always effective.[51] The high incidence of severe adverse events and dropout rates from D-penicillamine limits its usefulness. Anti-inflammatory agents and corticosteroids have not been effective in systemic sclerosis.

Angiotensin-converting enzyme (ACE) inhibitors have dramatically improved survival in patients with renal involvement. Patients with sclerosis of the kidneys develop hypertension leading to a renal crisis. In these patients plasma renin activity and angiotensin concentrations can be more than twice normal. Renal involvement should be anticipated in all systemic sclerosis patients who develop hypertension. Patients with systemic sclerosis and hypertension should be treated and maintained with an ACE inhibitor regardless of renal involvement. ACE inhibitors have allowed some dialysis-dependent systemic sclerosis patients to discontinue dialysis.[53] Prior to the use of ACE inhibitors in systemic sclerosis, renal disease was the major cause of death.[54]

Treatment of Raynaud's phenomenon requires patient education and sometimes drug therapy. Patients must maintain their peripheral extremity and core body temperatures. Wearing appropriate clothing in cold environments is essential. Reaching into a freezer with unprotected hands should be avoided. Smoking causes cutaneous vasoconstriction and should be eliminated, including passive smoke. When preventive measures are not sufficient, calcium channel blocking agents have become the agents of choice for Raynaud's phenomenon. Nifedipine, 10–20 mg TID or QID, decreases the frequency and duration of attacks.[53] Diltiazem, 60 mg TID or QID, can also be used. The sustained-release formulations of these agents may enhance patient compliance.

POLYMYOSITIS/DERMATOMYOSITIS

CLINICAL MANIFESTATIONS

Polymyositis and dermatomyositis (PM/DM) are chronic inflammatory diseases of skeletal muscle of unknown etiology. Dermatomyositis is distinguished from polymyositis by a typical rash, which is red, scaly, and plaque-like over the knuckles, wrists, elbows, and knees. In PM/DM there is proximal muscle weakness in the shoulder and hip girdles and trunk. The onset is insidious and patients usually notice lower extremity weakness and may complain of difficulty in rising from a chair or climbing stairs. There is an increase in serum creatine kinase concentration and electromyography abnormalities. The creatine kinase concentration may be as much as 50 times normal.[55] Muscle biopsies show a necrotizing inflammatory process. The skin lesions show a histology that is almost identical to that of SLE with immunoglobulins deposited along the dermal–epidermal border.[56] In fact, patients may develop features associated with other connective tissue diseases, such as arthritis, Raynaud's phenomenon, or overlap syndromes in which the patient has SLE, rheumatoid arthritis, Sjögren's syndrome, or scleroderma, in addition to the myositis.[57]

TREATMENT

Large controlled trials of drug therapy have not been conducted. The goal of therapy is to increase muscle strength so as to improve function in activities of daily living (bathing, dressing, feeding, toileting, etc.). Treatment consists of physical therapy during periods of remission and rest during periods of disease activity.[56] Corticosteroids are the first line of drug therapy for PM/DM. There is no consensus as to the optimal dose of corticosteroid to use. Most clinicians use prednisone at a starting dose of 40–100 mg/d or approximately 1 mg/kg/d.[55–57] Patients who do not have an initial response may benefit from higher prednisone doses of 1.5 mg/kg/d.[57] The initial dose of prednisone is continued for 1–2 months or until maximum benefit is achieved or a remission is induced. The full effect of prednisone may not be evident for several months. Approximately 90% of patients treated with prednisone will have some improvement.[58] The prednisone dose is tapered when muscle strength improves and serum creatine kinase concentrations decrease. If the prednisone is working and there are no serious side effects, then the drug is slowly tapered. Again, there is no consensus on how to accomplish this. One author advocates decreasing the daily dose at weekly intervals by 5 mg until reaching a dose of 30 mg/d, then slowing the taper by 2.5 mg/d at weekly intervals.[56] The dose that maintains a good clinical response can be used as maintenance. Tapering too quickly can cause an exacerbation of disease activity. Monitoring serum creatine kinase concentrations is useful because they tend to increase several weeks before clinical symptoms become apparent.[56] Although some have advocated tapering to an every-other-day regimen,[55] others have found QOD dosing not to be as good as daily dosing.[57] Patients with milder disease tend to have better results with QOD dosing than those patients with more severe disease. Some clinicians will treat patients with daily prednisone for 1 or more years, while others may use QOD therapy for many years.

One complication from corticosteroid use is the development of a myopathy. Based on symptoms it is difficult to know if increased muscle weakness is due to the corticosteroid or worsening disease status. Lowering the prednisone dose may be useful. If patients get better on a lower dose of prednisone, then most likely the muscle weakness was due to the drug. It may take 2–8 weeks for this to become clinically evident. Use of serum creatine kinase concentration may also be useful because this does not increase with steroid myopathy. It is possible that a steroid myopathy and worsening disease can coexist.

Although most patients with PM/DM improve with prednisone, some will not and some will develop corticosteroid resistance. In these patients azathioprine has been used at a dose of 1.5–3 mg/kg/d.[55] Clinical response may take 3–6 months. Another alternative is methotrexate at a dose of 7.5–20 mg once weekly. There are no large series of data available on clinical outcomes in patients on alternative therapies for PM/DM. These alternative therapies may also be beneficial in patients who cannot take corticosteroids because of serious adverse effects.

POLYMYALGIA RHEUMATICA

CLINICAL MANIFESTATIONS

Polymyalgia rheumatica (PMR) is characterized by aching and morning stiffness of the neck, shoulder, and pelvic girdle musculature and torso. Stiffness is greatest following periods of inactivity, such as sleeping. Pain and morning stiffness may last from 1–6 hours. Fatigue, anorexia, and low-grade fever are common signs and symptoms. The erythrocyte sedimentation rate (ESR) is generally more than 40 mm/h, and often is more than 100 mm/h. Some patients go from exhibiting no symptoms to overt clinical manifestations overnight, while others have a gradual onset of symptoms over a number of weeks. The etiology is unknown. There is a close association between PMR and temporal arteritis or giant cell arteritis. Some researchers suggest that these disease entities are variants of the same disorder. PMR occurs primarily in individuals older than 50 years of age, with a mean age onset of approximately 70 years.[59]

TREATMENT

The treatment of choice for PMR is prednisone at a dose of 10–20 mg/d. This therapy is so effective that if improvement does not occur within a week, another diagnosis should be considered. The ESR should decrease by 2 weeks and be normal after 4 weeks of therapy. The prednisone should be tapered beginning several weeks following control of symptoms. The rate of tapering is based on clinical response. A taper of 2.5 mg/d at monthly intervals to 10 mg/d followed by a slower tapering of 1 mg/d at monthly intervals has been suggested.[60,61] The lowest dose of prednisone that controls symptoms should be used for maintenance, which is usually between 7 and 15 mg/d.[60] Maintaining the ESR in the normal range is a good monitoring parameter. For elderly patients the normal ESR may be slightly higher than that usually given as a reference value by the clinical laboratory. PMR is a self-limited disease and patients usually continue maintenance therapy for 2–5 years.[59,60] Every-other-day prednisone has not been as successful as daily therapy.

PMR-associated temporal arteritis and giant cell arteritis require aggressive therapy with high-dose corticosteroids, such as prednisone at a dose of 40–60 mg/d or higher. These forms of arteritis can cause permanent loss of vision if not treated promptly. Patients should be educated to seek immediate medical care for possibly related symptoms such as jaw pain on chewing, temporal headache, visual changes, or mental status changes.

SYSTEMIC VASCULITIS

CLINICAL MANIFESTATIONS

Clinical manifestations of vasculitis are heterogeneous and are due to inflammation and damage to blood vessels. Vasculitis can be primary, as in Wegener's granulomatosis and polyarteritis nodosa, or secondary from other disease states, such as rheumatoid arthritis or SLE. Immune complexes can develop at the site of the vessel damage, or circulating immune complexes can be deposited in the vessel wall. The immune complexes can then activate the humoral immune system, leading to inflammation and damage. Cellular-mediated immunity may also be involved in some vasculitides.[62] There are numerous forms of vasculitis and there is currently no universally accepted scheme to classify them. Table 81.6 lists some systemic vasculitis syndromes.

TREATMENT

There are few controlled trials of pharmacologic treatments for the various forms of vasculitis. Treatment is guided by the severity, prognosis, and response of the vasculitis. For example, a drug-induced hypersensitivity vasculitis resulting in a rash may require only that the drug be discontinued. At the other end of the spectrum, Wegener's granulomatosis is a fatal vasculitis if not aggressively treated with corticosteroids often in combination with cyclophosphamide. Each type of vasculitis has its recommended therapeutic protocol, which usually includes the use of anti-inflammatory agents and immunosuppressive agents, either alone or in combination.

TABLE 81.6. CLASSIFICATION OF SYSTEMIC VASCULITIS SYNDROMES

Hypersensitivity Vasculitis
- Due to exogenous agents
  - Drugs
  - Infection
  - Henoch–Schönlein purpura
  - Serum sickness-like reactions
- Due to endogenous agents
  - Autoimmune disease
  - Malignancy
  - Systemic connective tissue diseases
  - Cryoglobulinemia

Systemic Necrotizing Vasculitis
- Polyarteritis nodosa
- Polyangiitis overlap syndrome
- Allergic granulomatosis

Wegener's Granulomatosis

Giant Cell Arteritis
- Temporal arteritis
- Takayasu's arteritis

Thromboangiitis Obliterans (Buerger's Disease)

EVALUATION OF THERAPEUTIC OUTCOMES

The diversity of clinical features and disease severity associated with the collagen vascular diseases leads to a number of possible clinical outcomes with a broad range of desired therapeutic outcomes. Achieving desired therapeutic outcomes for most of the collagen vascular diseases is highly variable. Currently, it is not possible to predict which patients will have a satisfactory therapeutic response and which patients will have unrelenting progressive disease. These diseases often have fluctuating courses necessitating frequent changes in drug therapy and drug doses.

Evaluation of drug therapy of several of the collagen vascular diseases often only requires monitoring for resolution of symptoms such as rash or muscle pain. However, patients with life-threatening disease receiving aggressive pharmacotherapy may require intensive monitoring and evaluation of therapy. For example, the patient receiving cytotoxic drug therapy for severe lupus nephritis requires close monitoring of laboratory indices of renal function as well as monitoring symptomatology and laboratory indices for possible bone marrow suppression, infection, cystitis, or other possible undesired therapeutic outcomes.

Evaluation of therapeutic outcomes should also include an awareness of the possibility of drug therapy mimicking signs and symptoms of disease such as the lupus patient receiving NSAID therapy and presenting with renal insufficiency or the patient with polymyositis receiving prednisone presenting with an exacerbation of muscle weakness.

CONCLUSION

SLE is a disease that affects multiple organ systems and consists of abnormal immunologic function and the development of autoantibodies. The disease is quite variable in clinical presentation and progression. The cause of lupus is unknown although several factors (e.g., genetics, environment, hormones) may predispose an individual to the development of the disease. Although SLE was once thought to be rapidly fatal, today more than 90% of patients survive 5 years.

Drug therapy is nonspecific and is aimed at suppressing the inflammation and abnormal immune response associated with active disease. Clinical trials with various agents have often been inadequate and contradictory, and the therapeutic management of lupus is not optimal. Nevertheless, drug therapy of recent years probably has contributed significantly to the improved survival of these patients. As the understanding of SLE progresses, we can expect to see the development of more specific and optimal treatment and further improvement in survival.

Each of the collagen vascular diseases has its own recommended form of therapy. For most of these diseases, there are few well-controlled clinical trials evaluating pharmacotherapy. Treatment of most of these diseases requires anti-inflammatory or immunosuppressive drugs. Monitoring therapeutic outcomes is essential since drugs and drug doses may need to be modified frequently.

REFERENCES

1. Blotzer JW. Systemic lupus erythematosus I: Historical aspects. Md Med J 1983;32:439–441.
2. Tan EM, Cohen AS, Fries JF, et al. The 1982 revised criteria for the classification of systemic lupus erythematosus. Arthritis Rheum 1982;25:1271–1277.
3. Michet CJ, McKenna CH, Elveback LR, et al. Epidemiology of systemic lupus erythematosus and other connective tissue diseases in Rochester, Minnesota, 1950 through 1979. Mayo Clin Proc 1985;60:105–113.
4. Hopkinson N. Epidemiology of systemic lupus erythematosus. Ann Rheum Dis 1992;51:1292–1294.
5. Vitali C, Bencivelli W, Isenberg DA, et al. Disease activity in systemic lupus erythematosus: Report of the Consensus Study Group of the European Workshop for Rheumatology Research. I. A descriptive analysis of 704 European lupus patients. Clin Exp Rheum 1992;10:527–539.
6. Steinberg AD, Gourley MF, Klinman DM, et al. Systemic lupus erythematosus. Ann Intern Med 1991;115:548–559.
7. Tomer Y, Buskila D, Shoenfeld Y. Pathogenic significance and diagnostic value of lupus autoantibodies. Int Arch Allergy Immunol 1993;100:293–306.
8. Condemi JJ. The autoimmune diseases. JAMA 1992;268:2882–2892.
9. Schur PH. Clinical features of SLE, in Kelley WM, Harris ED, Ruddy S, Sledge CB (eds): Textbook of Rheumatology, 4th ed. Philadelphia, WB Saunders, 1993, p 1017.
10. Segal AM, Calabrese LH, Ahmad M, et al. The pulmonary manifestations of systemic lupus erythematosus. Semin Arthritis Rheum 1985;14:202–224.
11. Rubin LA, Urowitz MB, Gladman DD. Mortality in systemic lupus erythematosus: The bimodal pattern revisited. Q J Med 1985;55:87–98.
12. Barr WG, Merchut MP. Systemic lupus erythematosus with central nervous system involvement. Psychiatr Clin North Am 1992;15:439–454.
13. Love PE, Santoro SA. Antiphospholipid antibodies: Anticardiolipin and the lupus anticoagulant in systemic lupus erythematosus (SLE) and in non-SLE disorders. Ann Intern Med 1990;112:682–698.
14. Wallace DJ, Podell T, Weiner J, et al. Systemic lupus erythematosus—survival patterns. Experience with 609 patients. JAMA 1981;245:934–938.
15. Austin HA, Muenz LR, Joyce KM, et al. Prognostic factors in lupus nephritis. Contribution of renal histologic data. Am J Med 1983;75:382–391.
16. Donadio JV, Glassock RJ. Immunosuppressive drug therapy in lupus nephritis. Am J Kidney Dis 1993;21:239–250.
17. Craft J, Hardin JA. Antinuclear antibodies, in Kelley WM, Harris ED, Ruddy S, Sledge CB (eds): Textbook of Rheumatology, 4th ed. Philadelphia, WB Saunders, 1993, p 164.
18. Merrell M, Shulman LE. Determination of prognosis in chronic disease, illustrated by systemic lupus erythematosus. J Chron Dis 1955;1:12–32.
19. Mills JA. Systemic lupus erythematosus. N Engl J Med 1994;330:1871–1879.
20. Ginzler EM, Felson DT, Anthony JM, Anderson JJ. Hypertension increases the risk of renal deterioration in systemic lupus erythematosus. J Rheumatol 1993;20:1694–1700.
21. Hayslett JP. The effect of systemic lupus erythematosus on pregnancy and pregnancy outcome. Am J Reprod Immunol 1992;28:199–204.
22. Petri M. Systemic lupus erythematosus and pregnancy. Rheum Dis Clin North Am 1994;20:87–118.
23. Ter Borg EJ, de Jong PE, Meijer S, Kallenberg CGM. Renal effects of indomethacin in patients with systemic lupus erythematosus. Nephron 1989;53:238–243.
24. The Canadian Hydroxychloroquine Study Group. A randomized study of the effect of withdrawing hydroxychloroquine sulfate in systemic lupus erythematosus. N Engl J Med 1991;324:150–154.
25. Wallace DJ. Antimalarial agents and lupus. Rheum Dis Clin North Am 1994;20:243–263.
26. Fox RI. Mechanism of action of hydroxychloroquine as an antirheumatic drug. Semin Arthritis Rheum 1993;23(2 suppl 1):82–91.
27. Hahn BH. Management of systemic lupus erythematosus, in Kelley WM, Harris ED, Ruddy S, Sledge CB (eds): Textbook of Rheumatology, 4th ed. Philadelphia, WB Saunders, 1993, p 1043.
28. Elenbaas J. Steroid pulse therapy in systemic lupus erythematosus. Drug Intell Clin Pharm 1983;17:342–343.
29. Stevens MB, Hahn BH. Management of systemic lupus erythematosus. Bull Rheum Dis 1982;32:35–42.
30. Donadio JV, Holley KE, Ilstrup DM. Cytotoxic drug treatment of lupus nephritis. Am J Kid Dis 1982;2(1 suppl 1):178–181.
31. Carette S, Klippel JH, Decker JL, et al. Controlled studies of oral immunosuppressive drugs in lupus nephritis. A long-term follow-up. Ann Intern Med 1983;99:1–8.
32. Austin HA, Klippel JH, Balow JE, et al. Therapy of lupus nephritis. Controlled trial of prednisone and cytotoxic drugs. N Engl J Med 1986;314:614–619.
33. Steinberg AD, Steinberg SC. Long-term preservation of renal function in patients with lupus nephritis receiving treatment that includes cyclophosphamide versus those treated with prednisone only. Arthritis Rheum 1991;34:945–950.
34. Lewis EJ. Plasmapheresis for the treatment of severe lupus nephritis: Uncontrolled observations. Am J Kid Dis 1982;2(suppl 1):182–187.
35. Lewis EJ, Hunsicker LG, Lan SP, et al. A controlled trial of plasmapheresis therapy in severe lupus nephritis. N Engl J Med 1992;326:1373–1379.
36. Strober S, Farinas ML, Field EH, et al. Treatment of lupus nephritis with total lymphoid irradiation. Observations during a 12-79-month followup. Arthritis Rheum 1988;31:850–858.

37. Ben-Chetrit E, Gross DJ, Braverman A, et al. Total lymphoid irradiation in refractory systemic lupus erythematosus. Ann Intern Med 1986;105:58–60.
38. Favre H, Miescher PA, Huang YP, et al. Cyclosporin in the treatment of lupus nephritis. Am J Nephrol 1989;9(suppl 1):57–60.
39. Feutren G, Querin S, Noel LH, Chatenoud L. Effects of cyclosporine in severe systemic lupus erythematosus. J Pediatr 1987;111:1063–1068.
40. Balletta M, Sabella D, Magri P, et al. Cyclosporin plus steroids versus steroids alone in the treatment of lupus nephritis. Contrib Nephrol 1992;99:129–130.
41. Winder A, Molad Y, Ostfeld I, et al. Treatment of systemic lupus erythematosus by prolonged administration of high dose intravenous immunoglobulin: Report of 2 cases. J Rheumatol 1993:20:495–498.
42. Maier WP, Gordon DS, Howard RF, et al. Intravenous immunoglobulin therapy in systemic lupus erythematosus-associated thrombocytopenia. Arthritis Rheum 1990;33:1233–1239.
43. Lin CY, Hsu HC, Chiang H. Improvement of histological and immunological change in steroid and immunosuppressive drug-resistant lupus nephritis by high-dose intravenous gamma globulin. Nephron 1989;53:303–310.
44. Corvetta A, Bitta RD, Gabrielli A, et al. Use of high-dose intravenous immunoglobulin in systemic lupus erythematosus: Report of three cases. Clin Exp Rheumatol 1989;7:295–299.
45. Pierucci A, Simonetti BM, Pecci G, et al. Improvement of renal function with selective thromboxane antagonism in lupus nephritis. N Engl J Med 1989;320:421–425.
46. Lin CY. Improvement in steroid and immunosuppressive drug resistant lupus nephritis by intravenous prostaglandin E_1 therapy. Nephron 1990;55:258–264.
47. Nagayama Y, Mamura Y, Tamura T, Muso R. Beneficial effect of prostaglandin E_1 in three cases of lupus nephritis with nephrotic syndrome. Ann Allergy 1988;61:289–295.
48. Stratton MA. Drug-induced systemic lupus erythematosus. Clin Pharm 1985;4:657–663.
49. Yung RL, Richardson BC. Drug-induced lupus. Rheum Dis Clin North Am 1994;20:61–86.
50. Hess E. Drug-related lupus [editorial]. N Engl J Med 1988;318:1460–1462.
51. Miller M. Scleroderma. Aust Fam Physician 1993;22:2112–2119.
52. Perez MI, Kohn SR. Systemic sclerosis. J Am Acad Dermatol 1993;28:525–547.
53. Yost JH, Spencer-Green G. Diagnosis and management of vascular disease in systemic sclerosis. Compr Ther 1993;19(2):53–59.
54. Black CM. Scleroderma—clinical aspects. J Intern Med 1993;234:115–118.
55. Dalakas MC. Clinical, immunopathologic, and therapeutic considerations of inflammatory myopathies. Clin Neuropharmacol 1992;15:327–351.
56. Strauss KW, Gonzalez-Buritica H, Khamashta MA, Hughes GRV. Polymyositis-dermatomyositis: A clinical review. Postgrad Med J 1989;65:437–443.
57. Targoff IN. Diagnosis and treatment of polymyositis and dermatomyositis. Compr Ther 1990;16(4):16–24.
58. Cronin ME. Treatment, pp 153–155, in Plotz PH (moderator): Current concepts in the idiopathic inflammatory myopathies: Polymyositis, dermatomyositis, and related disorders. Ann Intern Med 1989;111:143–157.
59. Stander PE. Polymyalgia rheumatica. Clinical features and management. Postgrad Med 1989;86(5):131–138.
60. Goodwin JS. Progress in gerontology: Polymyalgia rheumatica and temporal arteritis. J Am Geriatr Soc 1992;40:515–525.
61. Lestico MR, Boh LE, Schuna AA. Polymyalgia rheumatica. Clin Pharm 1993;12:571–580.
62. Fauci AS, Leavitt RY. Vasculitis, in McCarty DJ, Koopman WJ (eds): Arthritis and Allied Conditions, 12th ed. Philadelphia, Lea & Febiger, 1993, pp. 1301–1322.

Chapter 82

Allergic and Pseudoallergic Drug Reactions

Joseph T. DiPiro, PharmD, FCCP, and Chester T. Stafford, MD

The practice of pharmacotherapy requires selection of the most appropriate drug regimen to ensure maximal therapeutic efficacy with minimal risk of adverse drug reactions. Drugs may cause adverse effects by a variety of mechanisms, allergic and pseudoallergic reactions being among the most common. Allergic drug reaction refers to an adverse effect involving immunologic mechanisms. Adverse drug effects not proven to be immune mediated, but resembling allergic reactions in their clinical presentation, are referred to as "allergic-like" or "pseudoallergic" reactions.

Allergic drug reactions can be caused by a variety of drug classes, may result in a wide array of clinical syndromes, and can affect any tissue or organ. The molecular basis for some allergic drug reactions is well defined, whereas many common drug reactions, while believed to be immune mediated, are poorly understood.

Allergic reactions account for 5–10% of all adverse drug reactions[1] and are responsible for up to 5% of reactions to medications among hospitalized patients.[2–5] The true frequency of allergic drug reactions is difficult to determine, because many reactions may not be reported and others may be difficult to distinguish from nonallergic adverse events. Dermatologic reactions represent the most common form of allergic drug reactions. Cutaneous manifestations range from mild, localized pruritic rash to generalized urticaria and angioedema or severe vesiculobullous eruptions. Reactions to specific drugs are discussed later.

Clinical Manifestations of Allergic and Allergic-like Drug Reactions

ANAPHYLAXIS

Anaphylaxis is an acute, life-threatening allergic reaction involving multiple organ systems.[6,7] The manifestations of anaphylaxis may include signs and symptoms referable to the skin, gastrointestinal (GI) tract, respiratory tract, and cardiovascular system. Patients may experience adverse effects involving any combination of these systems. Common dermatologic manifestations include pruritus, urticaria, erythema, and angioedema. GI manifestations include nausea, abdominal pain, vomiting, and diarrhea. With respiratory tract involvement the patient may experience chest tightness, stridor, or bronchospasm. The major cardiovascular manifestations include hypotension, tachycardia, and dysrhythmias.

Anaphylactic reactions generally begin within 30 minutes, but almost always within 2 hours after exposure to the inciting allergen. The risk of fatal anaphylaxis is greatest within the first few hours. After apparent recovery, anaphylaxis may recur 6–8 hours after antigen exposure. Because of the possibility of recurrent "late-phase" reactions, patients should be observed for at least 12 hours after an anaphylactic reaction. Fatal anaphylaxis most often results from asphyxia due to laryngeal edema or from cardiovascular collapse.

SERUM SICKNESS

Serum sickness is a clinical syndrome resulting from the effects of soluble circulating immune complexes that form under conditions of antigen excess. The reaction commonly results from the use of heterologous antisera containing foreign (donor) antigens. It can occur when equine serum is administered in the form of antitoxins or antivenins. The onset of serum sickness usually occurs 7–14 days after antigen administration. Fever, malaise, and lymphadenopathy are the most common clinical manifestations. Arthralgias, urticaria, and morbilliform skin eruption may also be present. Although often associated with administration of heterologous antisera, serum sickness may also be caused by drugs including sulfonamides, hydantoins, penicillins, and cephalosporins (especially cefaclor). In addition, immune complex-mediated systemic lupus erythematosus-like syndrome has been attributed to reactions from drugs such as hydralazine, procainamide, isoniazid, and phenytoin.

DRUG FEVER

Fever may occur in response to an inflammatory process, or develop as a manifestation of a drug reaction, and it may pose a diagnostic and therapeutic dilemma for the clinician. A large number of drugs have been reported to cause fever including methyldopa, procainamide, phenytoin, barbiturates, quinidine, and a variety of antibiotics. These drugs may directly affect the central nervous system to alter temperature regulation, or stimulate the release of endogenous pyrogens (e.g., interleukin-1 and tumor necrosis factor) from white blood cells. Drugs may also cause fever as a result of their pharmacologic effects on tissues, for example, fever resulting from massive tumor cell destruction due to chemotherapy. However, the mechanism of drug fever remains unknown for agents such as amphotericin B and radiographic contrast agents.

The temperature pattern of drug-induced fever is quite variable. It may be low grade and continuous or spiking and intermittent. A temporal relationship between drug administration and occurrence of fever has been noted for some medications. Generally, withdrawal of the causative agent results in prompt defervescence as soon as the drug is completely metabolized. Fever usually recurs on readministration of the causative agent.

DRUG-INDUCED AUTOIMMUNITY

A number of autoimmune diseases have been associated with drugs. Autoimmune mechanisms may involve a variety of tissues and organs. A commonly recognized drug-related autoimmune disorder is systemic lupus erythematosus (SLE) induced by procainamide, hydralazine, or isoniazid. Twelve to 25% of patients taking procainamide and 7–13% of those taking hydralazine have been reported to have clinical manifestations of SLE.[8,9] The most common clinical manifestations include arthralgias, myalgias, and polyarthritis. Facial rash, ulcers, and alopecia occur less frequently. Renal or pulmonary involvement may also occur. These reactions typically develop several months after beginning the drug and generally resolve soon after it is discontinued.

Other syndromes believed to involve autoimmune mechanisms include drug-induced hemolytic anemia due to methyldopa, renal interstitial nephritis produced by methicillin, and hepatitis caused by phenytoin and halothane. Interstitial nephritis is characterized by fever, rash, and eosinophilia associated with proteinuria and hematuria. Hepatic damage due to drugs is generally manifested as either hepatocellular necrosis or cholestatic hepatitis. Drug-induced hepatitis has been associated with phenothiazines, sulfonamides, halothane, phenytoin, and isoniazid (see Chapter 38, Drug-Induced Liver Disease). Hepatocellular destruction is evidenced by elevations in serum transaminases. Hepatomegaly and jaundice may sometimes be evident. Cholestasis may be manifested by jaundice and elevations in serum alkaline phosphatase, and sometimes by rash, fever, and eosinophilia.

VASCULITIS

Vasculitis is a clinicopathologic process characterized by inflammation and necrosis of blood vessels. The vasculitic process may be limited to the skin or may involve multiple organs including the liver, kidney, joints, or central nervous system. Characteristically, cutaneous vasculitis is manifested by purpuric lesions that vary in size and number. Vasculitis may also be manifested as papules, nodules, ulcerations, or vesiculobullous lesions, generally occurring on the lower extremities, but the upper extremities, including the hands, may also be involved. Drugs associated with vasculitis include allopurinol, β-lactam antibiotics, sulfonamides, thiazide diuretics, and phenytoin.

DERMATOLOGIC REACTIONS

A wide variety of dermatologic drug reactions have been reported to have an immunologic basis.[10] As previously noted, cutaneous reactions are the most common manifestations of allergic drug reactions. Although most dermatologic reactions are mild and resolve promptly after discontinuing the drug, some may progress to serious or even life-threatening reactions (e.g., toxic epidermal necrolysis and Stevens–Johnson syndrome). Table 82.1 lists drugs and agents most commonly associated with cutaneous reactions.[11] Antimicrobials are implicated most frequently. The

TABLE 82.1. TOP 10 DRUGS OR AGENTS REPORTED TO CAUSE SKIN REACTIONS

	Reactions per 1000 Recipients
Amoxicillin	51.4
Trimethoprim/ sulfamethoxazole	33.8
Ampicillin	33.2
Iopodate	27.8
Blood	21.6
Cephalosporins	21.1
Erythromycin	20.4
Dihydralazine hydrochloride	19.1
Penicillin G	18.5
Cyanocobalamin	17.9

(From Bigby M, Jick S, Jick H, et al. Drug-induced cutaneous reactions. A report from the Boston Collaborative Drug Surveillance Program on 15,438 consecutive inpatients, 1975 to 1982. JAMA 1986;256:3358–3363, with permission. Copyright 1986, American Medical Association.)

clinical presentation of dermatologic drug reactions is discussed in more detail in Chapter 91.

RESPIRATORY REACTIONS

Drugs may also produce upper or lower respiratory tract reactions, including rhinitis and asthma. Respiratory tract manifestations may result from direct injury to the airway or may occur as a component of a systemic reaction (e.g., anaphylaxis). Asthma may be induced by aspirin and other nonsteroidal anti-inflammatory agents as discussed in the following paragraphs, or by sulfites used as preservatives in foods and medications. Other pulmonary drug reactions believed to be immunologic include acute infiltrative and chronic fibrotic pulmonary reactions. The latter is often caused by antineoplastics such as bleomycin. For a more detailed discussion of drug-induced pulmonary disease see Chapter 28.

HEMATOLOGIC REACTIONS

Most formed elements and soluble components of the hematopoietic system may be affected by immunologic drug reactions. Eosinophilia is a common manifestation of drug hypersensitivity and may be the only presenting sign. Hemolytic anemia may result from hypersensitivity to drugs. Other hematologic reactions include thrombocytopenia, granulocytopenia, and agranulocytosis. For a detailed discussion of hematologic reactions see Chapter 96.

MECHANISMS OF ALLERGIC DRUG REACTIONS

Drugs can cause allergic reactions by a variety of immunologic mechanisms. Although some reactions are relatively well defined, the majority are due to mechanisms that are either unknown or poorly understood.

The following criteria suggest that a drug reaction may be immunologically mediated[12]: (1) The reaction occurs in a small percentage of patients receiving the drug, (2) the observed reaction does not resemble the drug's pharmacologic effect, (3) the type of manifestation is similar to that seen with other allergic reactions (e.g., anaphylaxis, urticaria, serum sickness), (4) there is a lag time between first exposure of the drug and reaction, (5) the reaction is reproduced even by minute doses of the drug, (6) the reaction is reproduced by agents with similar chemical structures, (7) eosinophilia is present, and (8) the reaction resolves after the drug has been discontinued. Exceptions to each of these criteria are commonly observed.

Many allergic reactions can be classified into one of four immunopathologic categories, designated by Coombs and Gell[13] as types I, II, III, and IV (Table 82.2). Some drug reactions suspected of being immunologically mediated are considered possibly allergic. Examples include drug-associated skin eruptions, drug fever, drug-induced hepatitis, and interstitial nephritis. Other drug reactions can be classified as "pseudoallergic" or idiosyncratic. Examples include anaphylactoid (anaphylaxis-like) reactions to radiocontrast media, sulfite sensitivity, and reactions to local anesthetics.

TABLE 82.2. CLASSIFICATION OF ALLERGIC DRUG REACTIONS

Type	Descriptor	Characteristics	Typical Onset	Examples
I	Anaphylactic (IgE mediated)	Allergen binds to IgE on basophils or mast cells resulting in release of inflammatory mediators	Within 30 minutes	Immediate penicillin reaction Blood products Polypeptide hormones Vaccines Dextran
II	Cytotoxic	Cell destruction occurs because of cell-associated antigen that initiates cytolysis by antigen-specific antibody (IgG or IgM). Most often involves blood elements.	Typically 5–12 hours	Penicillin, quinidine, phenylbutazone, thiouracils, sulfonamides, methyldopa
III	Immune complex	Antigen–antibody complexes form and deposit on blood vessel walls and activate complement. Result is a serum-sickness-like syndrome.	3–8 hours	Serum sickness. May be caused by penicillins, sulfonamides, radiopaque dyes, hydantoins
IV	Cell mediated (delayed)	Antigens cause activation of lymphocytes, which release inflammatory mediators.	24–48 hours	Graft rejection Tuberculin reaction

DRUGS AS ANTIGENS

In general, small molecular weight (MW) compounds (less than 10,000 MW) are not immunogenic. Most drugs are less than 1000 MW. To become immunogenic, these small compounds must first combine with carrier proteins in plasma or tissue. Penicillin G (MW 356) is an example of a drug that binds covalently to serum proteins through amide or disulfide linkages. For drugs like sulfonamides, the parent compound must first be converted to a metabolite before it can combine with the macromolecule. The species that combines with the carrier macromolecule is referred to as a hapten or an incomplete antigen. Some macromolecular drugs such as insulin are referred to as complete antigens because they do not require binding with another molecule to evoke an immune response.

In some cases the inciting allergen may not actually be the drug itself but contaminants of the drug product. For example, frequent reactions to early penicillin preparations were attributed to impurities. In addition, drug additives may also cause allergic reactions. Dyes, preservatives, and a variety of excipients have been implicated.

EFFECTORS OF ALLERGIC DRUG REACTIONS

Allergic drug reactions can involve most of the major components of the immune system including the cellular elements, immunoglobulins, complement, and cytokines. Most immunoglobulin isotypes have been implicated in immunologically mediated drug reactions. Immunoglobulin E (IgE) bound to basophils or mast cells mediates immediate (anaphylactic) type reactions. IgG or IgM antibodies may also be involved in allergic reactions, resulting in destruction of cells and tissues.

Cellular Elements

A variety of leukocytes may be involved in immunologic drug reactions. Basophils, mast cells, eosinophils, and lymphocytes are most frequently involved. Platelets and vascular endothelial cells are also important because they can also release a number of inflammatory mediators. Most cells of the body including nerve cells can become directly or indirectly involved in allergic drug reactions.

Basophils and mast cells play prominent functional roles in immediate allergic reactions. Both cells are believed to originate from a common hematopoietic stem cell. They each have approximately 10^5 high-affinity cell surface receptors for IgE. Cross-linking of at least two cell surface IgE molecules by multivalent antigen is necessary to trigger mediator release. Bridging of cell surface IgE molecules and the resultant effect on histamine release is illustrated in the left upper quadrant of Fig. 82.1.

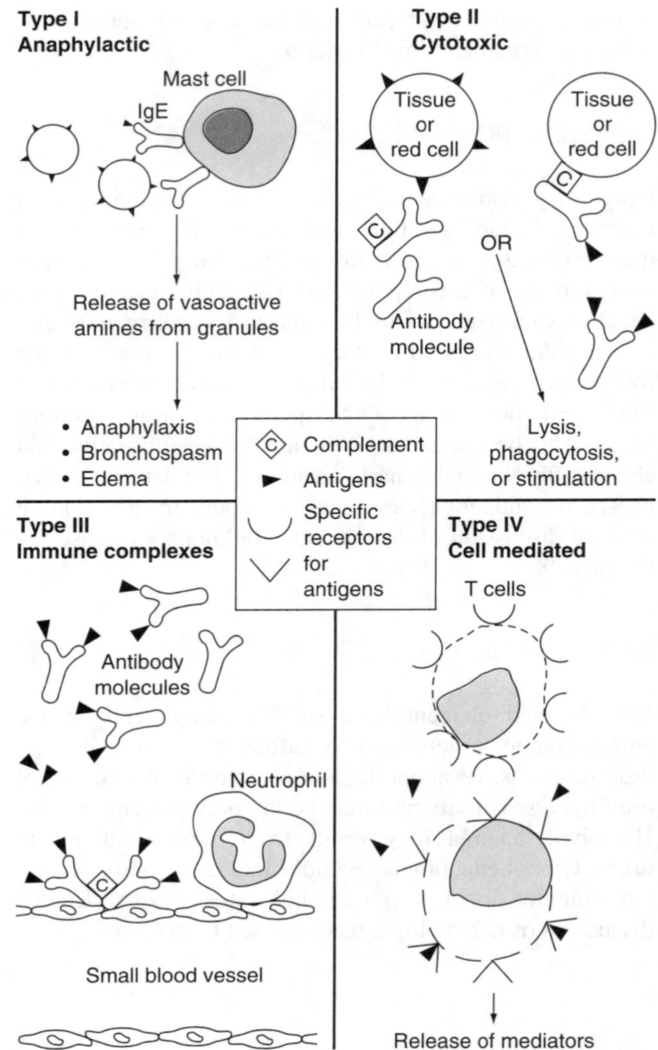

Figure 82.1. Hypersensitivity reactions. *(From Stites DP, Stobo JD, Fundenberg HH, et al. Basic and Clinical Immunology, 4th ed. Los Altos, CA, Lange Medical Publications, 1982, p 137, with permission.)*

Basophils account for 0.5–2% of all circulating leukocytes. Mast cells are morphologically and biochemically distinct cells that reside in a variety of tissues of the skin and respiratory and digestive tracts.[14]

Mediators of Allergic Reactions[15]

The release of a number of preformed, pharmacologically active chemical mediators is triggered by antigen cross-linking IgE molecules on the surface of circulating basophils and tissue mast cells. Preformed mediators include histamine, serotonin, eosinophil chemotactic factor (ECF-A), neutrophil chemotactic factor (NCF-A), and bradykinin generating factor, also known as basophil kalikrein of anaphylaxis (BK-A). Newly generated mediators include platelet-activating factor and arachidonic acid metabolites (e.g., prostaglandins, thromboxanes, leukotrienes). Each of these mediators is discussed in the following sections.

Histamine

Histamine is a low molecular weight amine compound formed by decarboxylation of histidine and stored in basophil and mast cell granules. The release of histamine from these sites is triggered by antigen cross-linking with IgE on surface membranes of mast cells and basophils. One function of histamine is believed to be as a host defense against invasion by parasites. The tissue effects of histamine are evident within 1–2 minutes, but it is rapidly metabolized within 10–15 minutes. The major effects of histamine on target tissues include increased capillary permeability, contraction of bronchial and vascular smooth muscle, and hypersecretion of mucous glands.

Serotonin

Serotonin is also a low molecular weight amine stored in and released from platelets and mast cells. Its effects are similar to histamine. It may cause vasoconstriction or vasodilatation in some animal species but has no proven role in human anaphylaxis.

Eosinophil Chemotactic Factor(s)

This group of preformed cellular tetrapeptides and dodecapeptides is released by stimulated mast cells. They attract eosinophils to inflammatory sites and participate in phagocytosis.

Neutrophil Chemotactic Factor

Neutrophil chemotactic factor is a high molecular weight protein that enhances neutrophil migration to areas of mast cell activation.

Bradykinin Generating Factor

Bradykinin generating factor is a series of proteases that activate Hageman factor, resulting in the production of kinins, including bradykinin, which is more potent than histamine on a molar basis in causing vascular permeability and contraction of smooth muscle.

Platelet-Activating Factor

Platelet-activating factor (PAF) is a glyceride-derived substance that is released by mast cells, alveolar macrophages, neutrophils, platelets, and other cells but not by basophils. It has potent bronchoconstrictor effects and also causes platelet aggregation and lysis. It attracts neutrophils and causes their activation. Also, PAF enhances vascular permeability and can cause pain, pruritus, and erythema.

Leukotrienes

The leukotrienes (LT) are metabolites of arachidonic acid produced through the 5-lipoxygenase pathway. They have potent effects on bronchial and vascular smooth muscle. Three important leukotrienes, LTC_4, LTD_4, and LTE_4, are produced by mast cells; however, LTC_4 is the major leukotriene produced by basophils and eosinophils. The leukotrienes have more potent bronchoconstrictor effects than histamine and can also increase vascular permeability and cause arteriolar vasoconstriction followed by vasodilatation. Their effects are slower in onset but longer lasting than those of histamine. They have previously been called the "slow-reacting substance of anaphylaxis" (SRS-A). Another product, leukotriene B_4 (LTB_4), is a potent chemoattractant, particularly for neutrophils. It is also produced by neutrophils, macrophages, and monocytes.

Prostaglandins and Thromboxanes

These are metabolites of arachidonic acid produced through the cyclooxygenase pathway. The actions of prostaglandins (PGs) vary considerably. Some have vasoconstrictive and/or bronchodilatory properties, whereas others are vasodilatory (e.g., PGD_2) and/or bronchoconstrictive (e.g., $PGF_{2\alpha}$). PGD_2 is the major prostaglandin product of mast cells. It is a potent inhibitor of platelet aggregation. Thromboxanes cause platelet aggregation and are important regulators of coagulation.

Immunoglobulins

As mentioned previously, immunoglobulins play an important role in allergic reactions. Immunoglobulin molecules can trigger activation of other components of the immune system by binding to antigen. For example, IgE bound to divalent antigen on the surface of mast cells results in mast cell activation and liberation of inflammatory mediators. In addition, IgG or IgM may cause cell destruction by activating the complement system or by enhancing phagocytosis. When antigen–antibody complexes bind to the cell surface Fc receptor of neutrophils, monocytes, or macrophages, complement may be activated, resulting in cell destruction, or the antibody-coated cell may be more easily engulfed by phagocytic cells. By either mechanism, essential host cells (e.g., platelets, red cells, or endothelial cells) may be destroyed to the detriment of the host. Complement and inflammatory cells may also be activated by antigen–antibody complexes. These complexes are aggregates of antibody and polyvalent antigen that form when appropriate proportions of each are present.

Complement

The complement system consists of approximately 20 plasma proteins. They are involved in a variety of immunologic responses, including enhancement of phagocytosis through opsonization of target cells, cell lysis, and generation of anaphylatoxins (C3a, C4a, and C5a), which can cause non–IgE-mediated activation of mast cells and release of inflammatory mediators.

CLASSIFICATION OF IMMUNOPATHOLOGIC DRUG REACTIONS

An immunologic mechanism has been identified for some drug reactions. Many can be classified into one of four immunopathologic reactions as described by Coombs and Gell.[13] These reactions are discussed as follows.

TYPE I

Type I reactions require the presence of IgE specific for the drug antigen or other allergen. It is assumed that on initial exposure to the antigen, predisposed individuals produce IgE specific for the drug allergen. IgE binds to basophils and mast cells. On repeat exposure to the antigen, two or more IgE molecules on the basophil or mast cell surface may be bound by one multivalent antigen molecule (referred to as cross-linking) (Fig. 82.1). This binding initiates a signal to the cell and the cell becomes activated. Activation causes the extracellular release of granules with preformed inflammatory mediators including histamine, serotonin, heparin, proteases (e.g., tryptase in the mast cell), bradykinin generating factor, eosinophil chemotactic factors, and neutrophil chemotactic factor, as well as generation of newly formed mediators as previously discussed. Substances in the latter category are mostly lipid metabolites from arachidonic acid, which is a major component of cell walls. Arachidonic acid metabolites include leukotrienes, prostaglandins, thromboxanes, and PAF among others. Most of these substances are produced by the activated mast cell; however, only one leukotriene (LTC_4) is produced by the basophil.

Generation of a type I reaction can be evident as an immediate hypersensitivity reaction, or anaphylaxis. Anaphylaxis can occur on a local basis, typically in the nasal mucosa, respiratory tract, skin, or GI tract; or anaphylaxis may be generalized. In the former case, localized symptoms such as rhinitis or asthma may be evident. In the latter, a severe systemic reaction can occur characterized by hypotension and bronchoconstriction. Other manifestations of generalized anaphylaxis include pruritus, urticaria, and angioedema.

A prototype of a type I reaction is the immediate reaction after benzylpenicillin exposure in sensitized individuals. It is assumed that a person has had an initial exposure to benzylpenicillin and then produces IgE specific for the benzylpenicilloate or other penicillin metabolites. On subsequent exposure the benzylpenicillin or metabolite bound to a macromolecule (e.g., albumin) cross-links IgE that is on the surface of basophils and mast cells. The result is an immediate hypersensitivity, or anaphylactic reaction. It is important to note that other allergic reactions caused by penicillin, particularly delayed dermatologic reactions, involve other mechanisms.

TYPE II

Type II immunopathologic reactions involve destruction of host cells (usually blood cells) through cytotoxic antibodies by one of two mechanisms (Fig. 82.1). First, the drug as antigen binds to the cell (e.g., the platelet or red blood cell). Antibodies (IgG or IgM) specific for the bound drug, or to a component of the cell surface that has been altered by the drug, then bind initiating a cytolytic reaction. The cell destruction may be mediated by complement or by phagocytic cells that have Fc receptors on their surface. Activation of complement near the cell surface can result in loss of cell membrane integrity and cell death. Alternately, neutrophils, monocytes, or macrophages may bind to the cell coated with antibody bound by IgG Fc receptors on the attacking cell surface. The result is phagocytosis of the target cell. The process of enhancement of phagocytosis by antibody-covered cell surface is referred to as opsonization. In addition, cell-bound IgG may direct the nonphagocytic action of T cells or natural killer cells, which results in cell destruction by a process called antibody-dependent cellular cytotoxicity (ADCC). This process can proceed in a nonspecific fashion, as T cells bind to the target cell through IgG Fc receptors on the T-cell surface. Contact is necessary between the target and effector cell.

Cells commonly affected by these types of reactions include erythrocytes, leukocytes, and platelets, resulting in hemolytic anemia, agranulocytosis, or thrombocytopenia, respectively. Other non–drug-related examples of type II reactions include erythroblastosis fetalis, Graves' disease, myasthenia gravis, and blood transfusion reactions. This process may be initiated by drugs such as penicillin, quinidine, quinine, phenacetin, cephalosporins, and sulfonamides, among others. For a complete discussion of this topic see Chapter 96, Drug-Induced Hematologic Disorders.

Another type of reaction that may affect the formed elements in blood is the "innocent bystander" reaction. With this type of reaction, antigen–antibody complexes formed in blood bind nonspecifically to cells. Complement is then activated, resulting in cell lysis.

Type II reactions may also involve antitissue antibodies in noncytolytic processes. An example of this mechanism is antibody binding to a cell surface receptor resulting in either receptor blockade or activation. Examples of these types of reactions include the autoimmune diseases, myasthenia gravis, and Graves' disease, respectively.

TYPE III

Type III immunologic reactions are caused by antigen–antibody complexes that are formed in blood. The complexes form with drug allergen and antibody in varying ratios, and may deposit in tissues, resulting in local or disseminated inflammatory reactions. Antigen–antibody complex formation can result in platelet aggregation, complement activation, or macrophage activation. When complement is activated, C3a, C4a, and C5a (anaphylatoxins) may be formed and can cause vascular permeability changes and mast cell activation. The latter leads to release and production of inflammatory mediators as discussed previously. Chemotactic substances such as C4b are also produced, and they cause the influx of neutrophils and result in the release of a number of toxic substances from the neutrophil (e.g., proteinases, collagenases, kinin-generating enzymes, and reactive oxygen and nitrogen substances), which can cause local tissue destruction.

Platelet aggregation may also occur as a result of immune complex formation. Activation of platelets may result in the formation of microthrombi and the release of vasoactive mediators. Also, insoluble complexes may be phagocytized by macrophages and activate these cells.

The formation of antigen–antibody complexes can lead to a number of clinical syndromes. The Arthus reaction is an example. In this model, a high level of preformed specific IgG antibody combines with antigen to produce a localized edematous, erythematous reaction within 5–8 hours. The reaction involves local formation of insoluble antigen–antibody complexes, complement activation with anaphylatoxin release, mast cell degranulation, and influx of polymorphonuclear cells.

TYPE IV

Type IV immunopathologic reactions are mediated by T cells and involve delayed hypersensitivity. Type IV reactions require memory T cells specific for the antigen in question. On exposure to the antigen the T cells become activated and produce an inflammatory response. Although these reactions may be associated with adverse effects (e.g., contact dermatitis), they may also be useful for diagnostic purposes. Examples of the latter include the use of the purified protein derivative (PPD) antigen from *Mycobacterium tuberculosis* used in the tuberculin skin test and other recall skin test antigens, such as mumps. After intradermal injection, these antigens produce a local reaction (erythema and induration) within 48–72 hours. Delayed contact hypersensitivity can also be caused by a wide variety of chemicals and drugs.

OTHER ALLERGIC REACTIONS

The mechanism of a number of allergic reactions is not known; however, they are believed to be immune mediated. Perhaps most common are the delayed dermatologic reactions that occur with a variety of drugs (especially penicillins and sulfonamides). These reactions may be evident as macropapular, morbilliform, or erythematous rashes; exfoliative dermatitis; photosensitivity reactions; or eczema. These reactions often cause pruritus, urticaria, and angioedema.

Other serious dermatologic syndromes may be the result of immunologic reactions. These include the Stevens–Johnson syndrome, characterized by rash, erythema multiforme with mucous membrane involvement, and toxic epidermal necrolysis (widespread blister formation in the epidermis), which are referred to as febrile mucocutaneous syndromes. Drugs commonly associated with these syndromes include the penicillin and sulfonamide antibiotics as well as a number of other agents. Drug-induced fever may also involve immunologic mechanisms; however, this is unclear. Other general types of reactions believed to be immune mediated include hepatic drug reactions (cholestatic or hepatocellular) and pulmonary reactions, for example, interstitial pneumonitis, which has been associated with nitrofurantoin.

ANAPHYLACTOID REACTIONS

A number of substances can produce an anaphylactoid (anaphylaxis-like) reaction that is similar to anaphylaxis in clinical signs and symptoms. The substances causing these reactions can produce the direct release of inflammatory mediators from cells, possibly by a pharmacologic effect, but this is not believed to occur through cell-bound IgE. These reactions are sometimes referred to as "pseudoallergic." Drugs that can produce anaphylactoid reactions include opiates, iodinated radiocontrast agents, vancomycin, amphotericin, and D-tubocurarine. A number of other agents may produce anaphylactoid reactions by altering the metabolism of inflammatory mediators such as prostaglandins or kinins.

FACTORS RELATED TO THE OCCURRENCE OR SEVERITY OF ALLERGIC DRUG REACTIONS

A number of factors influence the likelihood of allergic drug reactions. Among these are the dose of the allergen, the route of exposure, and the sensitivity of the individual. For many drugs, the severity of a reaction is determined by the dose and the duration of exposure. A relatively larger dose or longer duration of treatment encourages development of drug sensitivity. The route of administration also influences drug sensitivity. The topical route of drug administration appears to be the most likely to sensitize and predispose to drug reactions. It appears that the oral route is the safest and the parenteral route is the most hazardous for administration of drugs in sensitive individuals. In fact, there are relatively few reported cases of immediate hypersensitivity-associated deaths with oral β-lactam antimicrobials.[16] Although intravenous administration is more likely to result in severe immediate reactions in a sensitized individual, it may be the least likely route for inducing sensitivity. One possible explanation is that intravenous administration results in systemic drug exposure for the shortest period of time.

Individual host factors are also important in determining drug sensitivity. There may be a genetic predisposition for some types of allergic reactions. It is known that slow acetylators of procainamide and hydralazine are at increased risk for lupus erythematosus.

In general, the risk of drug allergy appears to be increased in patients who are atopic (history of allergic rhinitis, asthma, and/or atopic dermatitis). In addition, patients with a history of drug allergy appear to be at increased risk of adverse reaction to other pharmacologic agents. Age seems to be related to the risk of allergic reactions that occur less frequently in children. This may be related to immaturity of the immune system or decreased exposure. It is also well recognized that the presence of concurrent diseases predisposes to drug reactions. Examples include the morbilliform rash, which occurs after ampicillin administration to patients with infectious mononucleosis, the reactions that occur with trimethoprim/sulfamethoxazole in AIDS patients, and allergic reactions with blood products, which occur in patients with IgA deficiency.

DRUGS COMMONLY CAUSING ALLERGIC OR ALLERGIC-LIKE DRUG REACTIONS

β-LACTAM ANTIMICROBIALS

Allergic reactions to penicillin occur in 0.7–8% of treatment courses.[17] The most common reactions to penicillin include urticaria, pruritus, and angioedema. One in 10 allergic reactions is life-threatening and 10% of these are fatal. All four of the major types of hypersensitivity reactions have been reported with penicillin, as well as some reactions that do not fit into these categories. A wide variety of idiopathic reactions occur, for example, maculopapular eruptions, eosinophilia, Stevens–Johnson syndrome, and exfoliative dermatitis. Maculopapular rash occurs in about 2% of treatment courses of penicillin and in 5.2–9.5% with ampicillin. The incidence of ampicillin rash increases to 69–100% in patients with Epstein–Barr virus infection, cytomegalovirus infection, or acute lymphocytic leukemia.

Some aspects of the mechanism of penicillin immunogenicity have been determined. Because benzylpenicillin is a relatively small molecule (MW 356) it must combine with macromolecules (usually proteins) to elicit an immune response. Penicillin may covalently bind to the lysine residues of proteins such as albumin through an amide linkage involving the β-lactam ring (Fig. 82.2). This is the

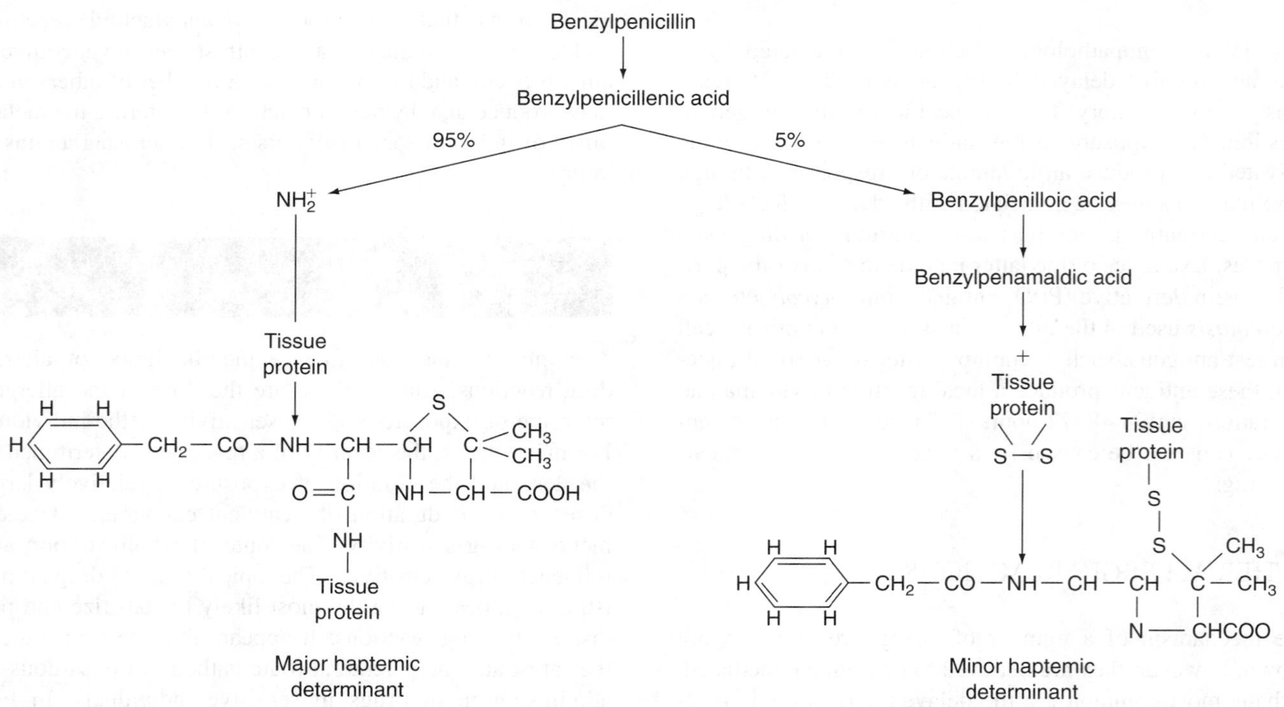

Figure 82.2. Formation of the benzl penicilloyl hapten–protein complex. *(From Stafford CT, Adverse drug reactions. Medical Times 1988;116:31–42, with permission.)*

penicilloyl–protein conjugate and is referred to as the "major antigenic determinant." In addition, a number of other penicillin metabolites may covalently bind to proteins. These are referred to as "minor antigenic determinants." The terms major and minor refer to the relative proportions of these conjugates that are formed and not to the clinical severity of the reactions generated. In fact, the minor antigenic determinants are more likely to cause anaphylactic reactions. The humoral immune response to penicillin has been well studied. From one report of 60 patients that received 3 or more grams per day of penicillin for at least 10 days, 38% had detectable IgG response to benzylpenicilloyl groups and 18% had detectable IgE response.[18] Immediate hypersensitivity reactions may be mediated by IgE for minor as well as major determinants.

Patients who are allergic to penicillins may also be sensitive to other β-lactams. For many β-lactam antimicrobials, the mechanism of reactivity is not fully understood. The exact incidence of cross-reactivity between cephalosporins and penicillins is not known; however, it is believed to be low. Although a history of penicillin allergy has been associated with an increased risk of reaction with cephalosporins,[19] it is not known if the cephalosporin reactions were immunologically mediated. Some investigators have administered cephalosporins to patients who had positive skin tests to penicillin and reactions were not evident.[20,21] Results of skin testing with cephalosporins may not be reliable because the mechanism of cephalosporin sensitivity has not been clearly defined. At present, patients with positive penicillin skin tests are advised not to receive cephalosporins if they can be avoided. Patients who have experienced only mild, cutaneous reactions, such as maculopapular rashes, may receive cephalosporins with caution.

Other new β-lactam derivatives (monobactams and carbapenems) have been studied for potential cross-reactivity with penicillins. *In vitro* and *in vivo* studies have demonstrated that the monobactam, aztreonam, only weakly cross-reacts with penicillin and that it may be safely administered to most patients who are penicillin allergic.[22] In contrast, there appears to be considerable cross-reactivity between the carbapenem, imipenem, and penicillin. Therefore, imipenem (and other carbapenems) should not be administered to patients who have positive penicillin skin tests.

RADIOCONTRAST MEDIA

Radiocontrast agents frequently cause allergic-like reactions as these agents are commonly used in medical practice. It has been reported that 5–10% of patients receiving radiocontrast agents experience some type of adverse reaction. Of the variety of reactions reported, approximately 1% are urticarial, 0.25% dyspnea, and fatal reactions occur as frequently as 0.01%. Also, angioedema, bronchospasm, and hypotension have been reported in less than 1% of patients receiving these agents.[23,24] In addition, radiocontrast agents may cause dose-dependent toxic reactions that can cause cardiovascular effects, arrhythmias, changes in renal blood flow, diuresis, or proteinuria.[23]

The mechanism of reactions to radiocontrast agents is not clearly understood. Allergic-like reactions are not IgE mediated. Potential mechanisms of reactivity include the activation of complement directly by the radiocontrast agents.[25] Also, the older radiocontrast agents have a high osmolarity and it is possible that they can directly activate mast cells and basophils (IgE independent mechanism), resulting in the release of inflammatory mediators.[26] Relatively new, low-osmolar contrast agents appear to result in fewer anaphylactoid reactions. In a report of 800 intravascular procedures, the frequency of immediate generalized reactions to high-osmolar radiocontrast agents was 9.1%. This contrasted with a frequency of 0.5% of 181 intravascular procedures, using low-osmolar agents in patients that had previously experienced an immediate generalized reaction with high-osmolar agents.[27] The relative risk of having a reaction to a lower osmolarity, nonionic agent is estimated to be at least five times lower than with conventional agents.[23]

It is difficult to identify patients at risk of reactions from radiocontrast agents. History is helpful, because a patient who has experienced previous reactions is more likely to experience subsequent reactions. The risk of allergic reactions to radiocontrast media is greater in patients with a history of atopy or asthma.[23] Despite a common misconception, a seafood allergy does not appear to predispose to radiocontrast media reactions. Skin testing or oral testing is not useful with these agents. Some regimens have been recommended to prevent reactions in patients who have previously experienced them. One pretreatment regimen includes the administration of prednisone 50 mg orally 13, 7, and 1 hour(s) before the procedure, diphenhydramine 50 mg orally or intramuscularly 1 hour before the procedure, and 25 mg ephedrine orally 1 hour before.[28] The ephedrine should be omitted if the patient has angina, dysrhythmia, or hypertension. Guidelines have been published for treatment of acute reactions to contrast media.[23]

INSULIN

Insulin is capable of producing a variety of allergic reactions. A protein molecule, insulin is a complete antigen. It may be of beef, pork, or human (recombinant) origin. Allergic reactions to insulin have been reported from all three sources. Reactions to insulin may involve the insulin molecule itself or other substances that have been added to insulin (e.g., protamine). Insulin may cause reactions through a variety of immunologic mechanisms. It is known that the majority of patients have anti-insulin antibodies after a few months of therapy.

Insulin reactions may be limited to the site of injection or they may produce systemic reactions. Local reactions most often present as a wheal and flare at the injection site and may occur immediately after injection or up to 8–12 hours later. Generally, these reactions are mild, do not require treatment, and resolve with continued insulin administration. If a patient does not tolerate the local reaction well, antihistamines may be given or a different insulin source (or product of higher purity) may be substituted. Rarely, systemic reactions to insulin (urticaria or anaphylaxis) occur. IgE-mediated reactions to insulin allergy appear to be declining with greater use of human insulins.[29] Skin testing with various products can aid in selecting the type of insulin least likely to cause a systemic reaction. Human insulin appears to be least allergenic but may occasionally cause reactions. In some patients, insulin desensitization may be indicated.

ASPIRIN AND NSAIDS

Aspirin and other nonsteroidal anti-inflammatory drugs (NSAIDs) produce characteristic reactions in susceptible patients.[30,31] The two general types of reactions to aspirin are urticaria/angioedema and rhinosinusitis/asthma. Approximately 1% of the population exposed to NSAIDs experiences urticaria or angioedema while about 0.5% experiences rhinosinusitis/asthma.[32,33]

The rhinosinusitis/asthma syndrome typically develops in middle-age patients who are nonatopic and have no history of aspirin intolerance. Generally, it progresses from rhinitis to sinusitis with nasal polyps and steroid-dependent asthma. It is uncommon in children and young adults. However, children with asthma may be aspirin sensitive. In retrospective studies 1.9–5.6% of asthmatics are aspirin sensitive,[34,35] while 16–44% of adults may be sensitive. In aspirin-sensitive asthmatics, administration of aspirin and NSAIDs may provoke an asthmatic attack. Ketorolac can cause severe, life-threatening bronchospasm in aspirin-sensitive asthmatics.[36] The mechanism of aspirin sensitivity is not completely understood. One suspected mechanism of aspirin and NSAID sensitivity is cyclooxygenase blockade, which may facilitate production of alternative arachidonic acid metabolites (e.g., leukotrienes). This is supported by the observation that the reaction occurs with other NSAIDs but infrequently with acetaminophen or salicylates. It is possible that aspirin and NSAIDs may directly stimulate mast cells to release inflammatory mediators. Also, subjects with aspirin-induced asthma have a marked increase in airway responsiveness to leukotrienes.[37]

In patients with asthma or those suspected of being sensitive to aspirin, an oral or inhalation challenge can be performed. This should be performed with great caution, in a hospital setting, with resuscitation equipment at hand. For patients known to be aspirin sensitive the major preventive measure is avoidance. Other agents reported to be cross-reactive with aspirin include tartrazine dye, indomethacin, and phenylbutazone.

NSAIDs have also been associated with pulmonary infiltrates and eosinophilia (PIE) syndrome. This syndrome is associated with fever, cough, dyspnea, infiltrates on chest roentgenogram, and a peripheral eosinophilia that develop 2–6 weeks after initiating treatment. PIE syndrome has been reported more frequently for naproxen compared with other NSAIDs and is noted to resolve rapidly after discontinuation of the offending agent.[38]

SULFONAMIDES

Sulfonamide drugs are a common cause of allergic reactions. These agents are included in a number of drug classes including antimicrobials, diuretics, oral hypoglycemics, and carbonic anhydrase inhibitors. Although immediate reactions can occur, sulfonamides typically cause delayed cutaneous reactions, often beginning with fever then followed by a rash (morbilliform eruptions, erythema multiforme, or, less frequently, toxic epidermal necrolysis).[39] Other reactions to sulfonamides may include mucocutaneous, GI, hepatic, renal, or hematologic complications, which may be fatal. It is believed that sulfonamide reactions are immune mediated and involve the production of reactive metabolites (hydroxylamines).[40]

Trimethoprim/sulfamethoxazole (TMX/sulfa) is frequently used for preventive or active treatment of *Pneumocystis carinii* pneumonia in patients with the acquired immunodeficiency syndrome (AIDS). Adverse reactions to TMX/sulfa have been observed to occur much more frequently in these patients compared to those without AIDS. Cutaneous eruptions have been reported to occur in 3.4% of hospitalized patients[11] and in 69% of patients with AIDS.[41] One study reported 32 of 37 AIDS patients experienced adverse reactions to therapeutic doses of TMX/sulfa.[42] In a study of 143 patients that received TMP/sulfa for treatment of *P. carinii* pneumonia, a CD4:CD8 ratio > 0.10 and a treatment course for less than 14 days were predictive of hypersensitivity.[43]

DETECTION AND MANAGEMENT OF ALLERGIC AND PSEUDOALLERGIC DRUG REACTIONS

Identification of patients at high risk for allergic drug reactions requires a careful history and, where appropriate, performance of specific tests to evaluate sensitivity. One of the most helpful tests to evaluate risk is the allergen skin test. For some drugs, skin testing can demonstrate the presence of drug-specific IgE and predict a relatively high risk of immediate hypersensitivity reactions. Note that skin testing does not predict the risk of delayed or dermatologic reactions.

It is evident that a higher proportion of patients report an "allergic reaction" to penicillin than actually experience a reaction. However, patients with a history of penicillin allergy are recognized to have a fourfold to sixfold greater risk of subsequent reactions.[17] In addition, a negative history of penicillin allergy does not eliminate the risk of immediate reactions, because many serious and even fatal allergic reactions to β-lactam antibiotics occur in patients who have no history of penicillin allergy.[17]

Skin testing can reduce the uncertainty of β-lactam sensitivity and should be performed in all patients who have a history of β-lactam allergy and require treatment with these agents. Testing for the major penicillin determinant is accomplished with penicilloyl-polylysine (PPL) (Pre-Pen, Kremers-Urban). If this agent alone is used, patients reacting only to minor determinants will be missed. At present, there is no commercially available product that can be used to test for most of the minor determinants. Benzylpenicillin (at a concentration of 10,000 U/mL) has been used; however, some reactive patients will still be missed. It is estimated that 93% of patients at risk for acute allergic reactions will be identified by skin testing with penicilloyl-polylysine and penicillin G.[44] The procedure for performing penicillin skin testing is presented in Table 82.3.

The National Institute of Allergy and Infectious Diseases reported a collaborative trial to test the predictive value of skin testing with major and minor penicillin derivatives.[45] The frequency of IgE-mediated reactions was 1.2 and 0% (568 patients) with positive and negative history of penicillin allergy, respectively, who were all skin test negative. Twenty-two percent of skin-test-positive patients who received penicillin experienced immediate or accelerated penicillin allergy. Eighty-four percent of skin-test-positive patients had dermal reactions to skin testing with the major determinant (benzyl penicilloyl-octalysine) while 16% reacted only to an experimental minor determinant mixture of benzylpenicillin, benzylpenicilloate, and benzylpenicilloyl-*N*-propylamine.

Immediate hypersensitivity reactions to penicillin are rare after a properly performed negative skin test. Dermatologic reactions occur in 1% of skin-test-negative patients.[17] A negative penicillin skin test indicates that the risk of life-threatening reactions is extremely low with administration of penicillin or other β-lactams. Occasionally, patients may experience systemic reactions after skin testing. Also, it is recognized that certain types of patients (e.g., those with dermatographism or taking antihistamines) may be unsuitable for skin testing because a false-positive or false-negative test may result. No reliable skin testing protocol or *in vitro* assay is presently available to predict a reaction to sulfonamides.

TABLE 82.3. PROCEDURE FOR PERFORMING PENICILLIN SKIN TESTING

A. Percutaneous (prick) skin testing

Materials	Volume
Pre-Pen 6×10^{-5} M	1 drop
Penicillin G 10,000 U/mL	1 drop
β-Lactam drug 3 mg/mL	1 drop
0.03% albumin-saline control	1 drop
Histamine control (1 mg/mL)	1 drop

1. Place a drop of each test material on the volar surface of the forearm.
2. Prick the skin with a sharp needle inserted through the drop at a 45° angle gently tenting the skin in an upward motion.
3. Interpret skin responses after 15 minutes.
4. A wheal at least 2 × 2 mm with erythema is considered positive.
5. If the prick test is nonreactive, proceed to the intradermal test.
6. If the histamine control is nonreactive, the test is considered uninterpretable.

B. Intradermal skin testing

Materials	Volume
Pre-Pen 6×10^{-5} M	0.02 mL
Penicillin G 10,000 U/mL	0.02 mL
β-Lactam drug 3 mg/mL	0.02 mL
0.03% albumin-saline control	0.02 mL
Histamine control (.1 mg/mL)	0.02 mL

1. Inject 0.02–0.03 mL of each test material intradermally (amount sufficient to produce a small bleb).
2. Interpret skin responses after 15 minutes.
3. A wheal at least 6 × 6 mm with erythema and at least 3 mm greater than the negative control is considered positive.
4. If the histamine control is nonreactive, the test is considered uninterpretable.

Antihistamines may blunt the response and cause false-negative reactions.

TREATMENT OF ANAPHYLAXIS

Anaphylaxis requires prompt treatment to minimize the risk of death or serious morbidity. On presentation, attention should first be given to restoration of respiratory and cardiovascular function. A protocol for the treatment of anaphylaxis is presented in Table 82.4. Epinephrine is administered as primary treatment to counteract bronchoconstriction and vasodilatation. Epinephrine should be administered subcutaneously or intramuscularly and at the site of antigen injection to delay absorption of the antigen. Crystalloids should be administered intravenously to restore intravascular volume. Typically, 1 L of 0.9% sodium chloride or lactated Ringer's solution will be administered over 10–15 minutes. This may be repeated if the patient is still believed to be volume depleted. Intravenous fluids should be given early in the course in an attempt to prevent shock. A maintenance intravenous fluid will then be initiated. An immediate priority is establishment and maintenance of an airway. This should be

TABLE 82.4. TREATMENT OF ANAPHYLAXIS

1. Place patient in recumbent position and elevate extremities.
2. Monitor vital signs often (or continuously if possible).
3. Apply tourniquet proximal to site of antigen injection; remove every 10–15 minutes.
4. Administer epinephrine 1:1000 into nonoccluded site: 0.3–0.5 mL subcutaneously or intramuscularly in adults and 0.01 mL/kg subcutaneously or intramuscularly in children.
5. Administer aqueous epinephrine 1:1000 into site of antigen injection; 0.15–0.25 mL subcutaneously in adults and 0.005 mL/kg subcutaneously in children.
6. Establish and maintain airway with oropharyngeal airway device, endotracheal intubation, transtracheal catheterization, or cricothyrotomy.
7. Administer oxygen at 6–10 L/min.
8. Institute rapid replacement with 0.9% sodium chloride, lactated Ringer's, or colloid solution (e.g., 5% albumin or 4% hetastarch).
9. For hypotension in adults, administer norepinephrine, 32 μg/min (use 8 mg in 500 mL dextrose 5%) with the rate adjusted to maintain low-normal blood pressure. Alternatively, administer dopamine at 2–10 μg/kg/min intravenously.
10. If refractory hypotension is present, administer cimetidine 300 mg or ranitidine 50 mg, intravenously over 3–5 minutes.
11. If bronchospasm is present, administer aminophylline 6 mg/kg intravenously over 20 minutes.
12. Administer hydrocortisone sodium succinate 100 mg intravenously (push) and 100 mg intravenously in saline every 2–4 hours to block the late-phase reaction.
13. Administer diphenhydramine 1–2 mg/kg intravenously (up to 50 mg) over 3 minutes to block histamine-1 receptors.
14. For adults taking a β-adrenergic blocker, administer atropine (0.5 mg intravenously) every 5 minutes until heart rate is greater than 60 beats/min, or isoproterenol 2–20 μg/min intravenously titrated to heart rate of 60 beats/min, or glucagon 0.5 mg/kg intravenously (push) followed by 0.07 mg/kg/h continuously intravenously.

achieved by the use of endotracheal intubation if necessary. When a patient with anaphylaxis is hypotensive, vasopressors will also be needed in addition to crystalloids. Norepinephrine is the vasoconstrictor agent of choice for treatment of anaphylactic shock, although dopamine may also be useful.

A number of other agents may be required for treatment of anaphylactic reactions. Corticosteroids (hydrocortisone sodium succinate intravenously) are recommended to prevent the late-phase reaction. Aminophylline may be used as adjunctive therapy for bronchospasm. Histamine-1 (H_1)-receptor blockers (e.g., diphenhydramine) may be administered to reduce some of the symptoms associated with anaphylaxis; however, these agents are not effective as primary therapy. H_2-receptor blockers such as cimetidine have been used for treatment of refractory hypotension[46] although routine use is controversial.

DESENSITIZATION

For some patients allergic to penicillin, no reasonable alternatives exist and penicillin therapy may be necessary for treatment of severe, life-threatening infection. In this situation, penicillin desensitization should be considered. Desensitization can reduce the risk of anaphylaxis, but does not influence the likelihood of other types of reactions such as exfoliative dermatitis or Stevens–Johnson syndrome.

Penicillin desensitization should be performed in a hospital setting where resuscitation equipment is readily available. Prior to initiating the protocol, the patient should be stabilized and fluid, pulmonary, and cardiovascular function optimized. The use of premedicants (e.g., antihistamines or corticosteroids) is controversial because these agents may mask the early signs of acute reactions and do not reliably reduce the severity of acute reactions. About one-third of patients who have undergone desensitization experienced mild, transient allergic reaction either during the desensitization procedure or during penicillin therapy.[17] Patients who can take oral medication should undergo desensitization with oral penicillin. Protocols for oral and intravenous penicillin desensitization are presented in Tables 82.5 and 82.6. It is important that once the desensi-

TABLE 82.5. PROTOCOL FOR ORAL PENICILLIN DESENSITIZATION

	Phenoxymethyl Penicillin			
Step[a]	Concentration (U/mL)	Volume (mL)	Dose (U)	Cumulative Dose (U)
1	1000	0.1	100	100
2	1000	0.2	200	300
3	1000	0.4	400	700
4	1000	0.8	800	1500
5	1000	1.6	1600	3100
6	1000	3.2	3200	6300
7	1000	6.4	6400	12,700
8	10,000	1.2	12,000	24,700
9	10,000	2.4	24,000	48,700
10	10,000	4.8	48,000	96,700
11	80,000	1.0	80,000	176,700
12	80,000	2.0	160,000	336,700
13	80,000	4.0	320,000	656,700
14	80,000	8.0	640,000	1,296,700
Observe for 30 minutes				
15	500,000	0.25	125,000	
16	500,000	0.5	250,000	
17	500,000	1.0	500,000	
18	500,000	2.25	1,125,000	

[a]The interval between steps is 15 minutes. (Reproduced from Sullivan TJ. Current Therapy in Allergy. St. Louis, MO, CV Mosby, 1985, pp 57–61, with permission.)

TABLE 82.6. PARENTERAL DESENSITIZATION PROTOCOL

Injection No.	Benzylpenicillin Concentration (U)	Volume (mL)	Route
1[a,b]	100	0.1	ID
2	100	0.2	SC
3	100	0.4	SC
4	100	0.8	SC
5[b]	1000	0.1	ID
6	1000	0.3	SC
7	1000	0.6	SC
8	10,000	0.1	ID
9	10,000	0.2	SC
10	10,000	0.4	SC
11	10,000	0.8	SC
12[b]	100,000	0.1	ID
13	100,000	0.3	SC
14	100,000	0.6	SC
15[b]	1,000,000	0.1	ID
16	1,000,000	0.2	SC
17	1,000,000	0.2	IM
18	1,000,000	0.4	IM
19	Continuous IV infusion at 1,000,000 U/h		

[a]Administer doses at intervals of not less than 20 minutes.
[b]Observe and record skin wheal-and-flare response. (From Weiss ME, Adkinson NF. Immediate hypersensitivity reaction to penicillin and related antibiotics. Clin Allergy 1988;18:515–540, with permission.)

tization protocol is begun it not be interrupted except for severe reactions. Antihistamines may be administered to treat reactions. Also, if the patient completes the desensitization regimen and then undergoes penicillin treatment, a lapse between doses of as little as 8 hours can allow for reemergence of sensitivity.

Skin tests often become negative during and shortly after desensitization. The mechanism by which desensitization is protective is unclear. It does not seem to be that penicillin-specific IgE is neutralized or that IgG as "blocking antibody" is produced. One possible explanation is that basophils and mast cells attain some degree of tolerance on exposure to the antigen.

Potential Future Therapies for Allergic Drug Reactions

Developments that may reduce the incidence of allergic drug reactions in the future include (1) the more general availability of *in vitro* and *in vivo* assays that detect patient sensitivity to drug exposure, (2) the elimination of unnecessary contaminants within drug products, (3) the deliberate synthesis of less immunogenic drugs, and (4) the use of univalent haptens to block allergen reactivity. Also, it is likely that clinicians will have many new agents in the future to prevent and treat allergic drug reactions. These include leukotriene antagonists, agents that block receptors of inflammatory mediators, antibodies that bind and inactivate inflammatory mediators, antibodies that bind IgE but prevent cross-linking, and a host of other agents having a variety of actions on the immune system.

Conclusion

Allergic reactions can occur with any type of drug substance and this risk must be weighed against the possible clinical benefit from the drug. Allergic drug reactions can take many forms, from relatively benign to life threatening. The risk of allergic and allergic-like drug reactions can be minimized by obtaining a careful patient history and, when possible, performing diagnostic tests (e.g., penicillin skin testing) that predict the likelihood of allergic reactions. Further investigation into the mechanisms of allergic and allergic-like drug reactions may lead to more effective therapeutic measures for prevention and treatment.

References

1. Anderson JA, Adkinson NF. Allergic reactions to drugs and biologic agents. JAMA 1987;258:2891–2899.
2. Parker CW. Drug allergy (a review in three parts). N Engl J Med 1975;292:511, 732, 957.
3. Jick H. Adverse drug reactions: The magnitude of the problem. J Allergy Clin Immunol 1984;74:555.
4. DeWeck AI. Drugs as allergens. J Allergy Clin Immunol 1986;78:1047.
5. Stafford CT. Adverse drug reactions. Medical Times 1988;116:31–42.
6. Stafford CT. Life-threatening allergic reactions. Postgrad Med 1989;86:235–241.
7. Bochner BS, Lichtenstein LM. Anaphylaxis. N Engl J Med 1991;324:1785–1790.
8. Perry HM, Tan EM, Carmody S, et al. Relationship of acetyltrans-serase activity to antinuclear antibodies and toxic symptoms in hypertensive patients treated with hydralazine. J Lab Clin Med 1970;76:114.
9. Blomgren SE, Condemi JJ, Vaughan JH. Procainamide-induced lupus erythematosus. Clinical and laboratory evaluations. Am J Med 1972;57:338.
10. Roujeau JC, Stern RS. Severe adverse cutaneous reactions to drugs. N Engl J Med 331;1994:1272–1285.
11. Bigby M, Jick S, Jick H, et al. Drug-induced cutaneous reactions. A report from the Boston Collaborative Drug Surveillance Program on 15,438 consecutive inpatients, 1975 to 1982. JAMA 1986;256:3359–3363.
12. DeSwarte RD. Drug allergy, in Patterson R (ed): Allergic Diseases, 3rd ed. Philadelphia, JB Lippincott, 1985.
13. Coombs RRA, Gell PGH. The classification of allergic reactions responsible for clinical hyposensitivity and disease, in

Gell PGH, Coombs RRA (eds): Clinical Aspects of Immunology, 2nd ed. Oxford, Blackwell Scientific Publications, 1968, p 190.
14. Schwartz LB, Austen KF. The mast cell and mediators of immediate hypersensitivity, in Samter M, Talmage DW, Frank MM, et al (eds): Immunologic Diseases, 4th ed. Boston, Little, Brown, 1988.
15. Serafin WF, Austen KF. Mediators of immediate hypersensitivity reactions. N Engl J Med 1987;317:30–34.
16. Sullivan TJ, Yecies LD, Shatz GS, et al. Desensitization of patients allergic to penicillin using orally administered β-lactam antibiotics. J Allergy Clin Immunol 1982;69:275–282.
17. Weiss ME, Adkinson NF. Immediate hypersensitivity reactions to penicillin and related antibiotics. Clin Allergy 1988;18:515–540.
18. Adkinson NF. Risk factors for drug allergy. J Allergy Clin Immunol 1984;74:567–572.
19. Anderson JA. Cross-reactivity to cephalosporins in patients allergic to penicillin. J Infect Dis 1986;5:557–561.
20. Saxon A. Immediate hypersensitivity reactions to β-lactam antibiotics. Rev Infect Dis 1983;5:S368.
21. Solley GO, Gleich GJ, Van Dellen RG. Penicillin allergy: A clinical experience with a battery of skin test reagents. J Allergy Clin Immunol 1982;69:238–244.
22. Saxon A, Beall GN, Rohr AS, et al. Immediate hypersensitivity reactions to β-lactam antibiotics. Ann Intern Med 1987;107:204–215.
23. Bush WH, Swanson DP. Acute reactions to intravascular contrast media: Types, risk factors, recognition, and specific treatment. Am J Radiol 1991;157:1153–1161.
24. Shehadi WH. Adverse reactions to intravenously administered contrast media. Am J Radiol 1975;124:145.
25. Lieberman. Radiocontrast reactions. Clin Rev Allergy 1986;4:229–245.
26. Lasser EC, Walter AJ, Lang JH. An experimental basis for histamine release in contrast material reactions. Radiology 1974;110:49–59.
27. Greenberger PA, Patterson R. The prevention of immediate generalized reactions to radiocontrast media in high-risk patients. J Allergy Clin Immunol 1991;87:867–872.
28. Greenberger PA. Contrast media reaction. J Allergy Clin Immunol 1984;74:600.
29. Patterson R, Roberts M. Grammer LC. Insulin allergy: Reevaluation after two decades. Ann Allergy 1990;64:459–462.
30. Samter M, Stevenson DD. Reactions to aspirin and aspirin-like drugs, in Samter M, Talmage DW, Frank MM, et al (eds): Immunologic Diseases, 4th ed. Boston, Little, Brown, 1988.
31. Stevenson DD. Diagnosis, prevention and treatment of adverse reactions to aspirin and non-steroidal antiinflammatory drugs. J Allergy Clin Immunol 1984;74:617.
32. Chafee FH, Settipane GA. Aspirin intolerance: I. Frequency in an allergic population. J Allergy Clin Immunol 1974;53:193.
33. MacDonald JR, Mathison DA, Stevenson DD. Aspirin intolerance in asthma, detection by oral challenge. J Allergy Clin Immunol 1972;50:198.
34. Falliers CJ. Aspirin and subtypes of asthma risk factor analysis. J Allergy Clin Immunol 1973;52:141.
35. Giraldo B, Blumenthal MN, Spink WW. Aspirin intolerance and asthma: A clinical and immunologic study. Ann Intern Med 1969;71:479.
36. Vicks SD, Dean JR, Tenholder MF. Ketorolac induced respiratory failure in an aspirin-sensitive asthmatic. Immunol Allergy Pract 1991;13:23–25.
37. Lee TH. Mechanisms of aspirin sensitivity. Am Rev Resp Dis 1992;145:S34–S36.
38. Goodwin SD, Glenny RW. Nonsteroidal anti-inflammatory drug-associated pulmonary infiltrates with eosinophilia. Arch Intern Med 1992;152:1521–1524.
39. Anonymous. Serious adverse reactions with sulfonamides [bulletin]. FDA Drug Bull 1984;14:5–6.
40. Reider MJ, Uetrecht J, Shear NH, et al. Diagnosis of sulfonamide hypersensitivity reactions by in vitro "rechallenge" with hydroxylamine metabolites. Ann Intern Med 1989;110:286–289.
41. Mitsurjasu R, Groopman J, Vallerding P. Cutaneous reaction to trimethoprim-sulfamethoxazole in patients with AIDS and Kaposi's sarcoma. N Engl J Med 1983;308:1535–1536.
42. Gordin SM, Simon GL, Wofsy CB, et al. Adverse reactions to trimethoprim/sulfamethoxazole in patients with the acquired immunodeficiency syndrome. Ann Intern Med 1984;100:495–499.
43. Carr A, Swanson C, Penny R, Cooper DA. Clinical and laboratory markers of hypersensitivity to trimethoprim-sulfamethoxazole in patients with *Pneumocystis carinii* pneumonia and AIDS. J Infect Dis 1993;167:180–185.
44. Sogn DD. Penicillin allergy. J Allergy Clin Immunol 1984;74:589–599.
45. Sogn DD, Evans R, Shepherd GM et al. Results of the National Institute of Allergy and Infectious Diseases collaborative clinical trial to test the predictive value of skin testing with major and minor penicillin derivatives in hospitalized patients. Arch Intern Med 1992;152:1025–1032.
46. Yarbrough JA, Moffitt JE, Brown DA, et al. Cimetidine in the treatment of refractory anaphylaxis. Ann Allergy 1989;63:235–238.

Section 10
Bone and Joint Disorders

Chapter 83

Osteoporosis and Osteomalacia

Mary Beth O'Connell, PharmD, BCPS, FASHP, FCCP, and Steven F. Bauwens, PharmD, FASCP

Disorders of bone metabolism constitute a major cause of disability in women, especially in women older than 50, and older men. Disability results from fractures, kyphosis, and pain. The underlying cause is usually osteopenia, osteoporosis, or osteomalacia. Osteopenia is a clinically important decrease in bone mass relative to expected values adjusted for age, race, and gender. The true definition of osteoporosis is a condition resulting from bone fractures in a person with low bone mass. In the literature and in lay and medical language, osteoporosis is used synonymously with osteopenia. Osteomalacia is characterized by deficient mineralization of bone, leading to increased unmineralized osteoid and decreased bone strength.

This chapter examines the physiology of normal bone and the pathophysiology of osteopenia, osteoporosis, and osteomalacia; describes different methods for assessing bone mass and integrity; and explores nonpharmacologic and pharmacologic treatment regimens to prevent or treat osteoporosis and osteomalacia.

Bone Physiology

NORMAL FUNCTION OF BONE

Bone has two basic functions in humans: (1) structural support, which allows locomotion and protection of vital organs; and (2) a depot for calcium, phosphorus, magnesium, sodium, and carbonate. The essential role of bone in maintaining normal ion and buffer concentrations in the extracellular fluid takes precedence over the supportive role. Bone will be destroyed to maintain homeostasis of these various elements. A substantial amount of bone loss leads to osteopenia and then to osteoporosis.

TYPES OF BONE

Adult bone comprises two distinct types and structures (Fig. 83.1). Cortical (compact) bone is found in the midshafts and outer surfaces of long bones and on the surfaces of flat bones. Trabecular (cancellous) bone is found in the inner aspects of the metaphyses of the long bones and between the cortical surfaces of the vertebrae, ribs, and pelvic bones. The composition of each type of bone varies (Table 83.1). The outer layer of the cortical bone is the periosteum and the inner aspects of cortical and trabecular bone compose the endosteum. Cortical bone is made up of organized Haversian systems, called osteons, which are lamellar arrays of dense bone organized around a central canal containing the microcirculation. Osteocytes are dispersed in deep lacunae throughout these systems. Trabecular bone is an avascular spongy meshwork of interlacing bony spicules, which lacks the organized Haversian systems. Osteocytes are scattered throughout the inner substance of trabecular bones. Because of a larger surface area and more abundant cell population, trabecular bone is more metabolically active than cortical bone and responds more quickly to hormonal stimuli.

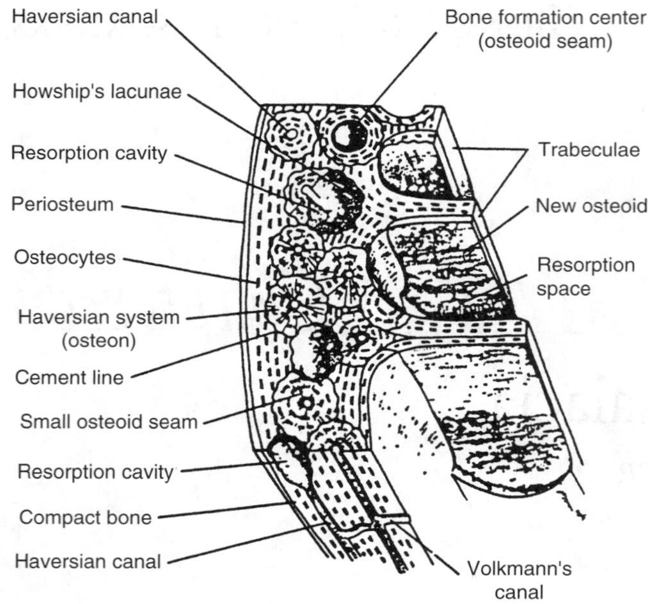

Figure 83.1. Cross and longitudinal section of bone showing remodeling units in cortical bone and on endosteal surfaces. *(From Parfitt AM, Duncan AH. Metabolic bone disease affecting the spine, in Rothman R, Simeone F [eds]: The Spine, 2nd ed. Philadelphia, WB Saunders, 1982, p 777, with permission.)*

COMPOSITION OF BONE

Bone is basically connective tissue that becomes mineralized. The three primary elements of bone are a protein matrix, a mineral phase, and bone cells. Approximately 95% of bone matrix, occupying about 50% of the total bone volume, is composed of fibrous protein collagen.[1] The remaining bone volume is primarily mucopolysaccharides. Osteonectin is a protein found only in bone that binds selectively to bone hydroxyapatite crystals and bone collagen. This protein appears to link bone mineral and collagen and may play a role in initiating the mineralization of bone matrix. Osteocalcin constitutes about 25% of the noncollagenous protein of bone and binds to hydroxyapatite. Osteocalcin is secreted exclusively by osteoblasts with serum concentrations reflective of osteoblastic activity.

The mineral phase accounts for most of the remaining half of bone volume and about two-thirds of the total bone weight. The primary mineral of mature bone is hydroxyapatite, a microcrystalline material with the formula $Ca_{10}(PO_4)_6(OH)_2$. The hydroxyapatite crystals are impure, containing substantial amounts of sodium, potassium, magnesium, and carbonate.

Bone cells occupy only about 3% of the total volume of bone (Fig. 83.2).[2] The surfaces of bone are covered by cells that are either actively producing or removing bone or are quiescent. The three primary bone cell types are osteoblasts, osteocytes, and osteoclasts. Osteoblasts are found in continuous layers on the surfaces of newly forming bone. Osteoblasts are cells that produce bone matrix and control its mineralization. Thereafter, the osteoblast either remains quiescent on the surface as a flattened resting cell or becomes an osteocyte buried in the newly formed bone.

Osteocytes are connected to each other by cytoplasmic extensions, which fill the canaliculi between them. This cellular network may permit control of the rate of ion transport into and out of bone and regulate the rate of mineralization of the newly formed bone matrix. Osteoclasts are large, usually multinucleate cells found on the resorbing surfaces of mineralized bone and are located in surface depressions referred to as resorption bays or Howship's lacunae. They are primarily responsible for the removal of bone matrix.

REMODELING AND COUPLING

Bone is in a state of dynamic equilibrium, constantly being resorbed and synthesized in a continual process of repair and regeneration called remodeling (Fig. 83.2).[3–8] The process of remodeling occurs on the bone surfaces in discrete packages called bone multicellular units (BMUs). Osteoclasts and osteoblasts are responsible for the remodeling process, working together in a synchronized fashion, called coupling. The linking of osteoblast to osteoclast activity is mediated by various chemical signals that are still being fully elucidated. In cancellous bone, resorption is usually limited to the surface along a relatively broad

TABLE 83.1. DISTRIBUTION OF CORTICAL AND TRABECULAR BONE AT VARIOUS SITES, AND ESTIMATED LIFETIME LOSSES FOR MEN AND WOMEN

Site	Cortical Bone (%)	Trabecular Bone (%)	Total Loss in Women (%)	Total Loss in Men (%)
Midradius	95	5	30	5
Distal radius	30–50	30–50	39	11
Neck of femur	75	25	58	36
Trochanteric	50	50	53	35
Lumbar vertebrae	40	60	45	13

(Adapted from Epidemiol Rev 1985;7:178–208; J Clin Invest 1981;67:324–329; and J Clin Invest 1982;70:716–723.)

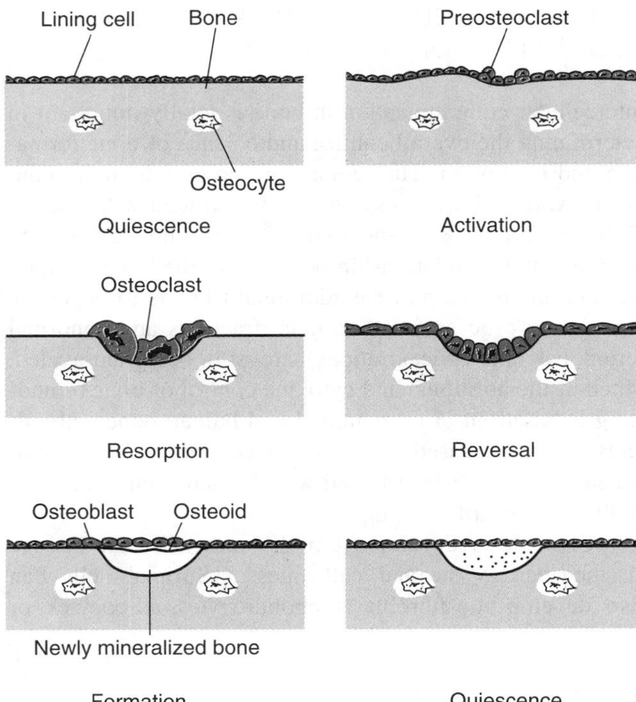

Figure 83.2. The remodeling sequence for cortical and trabecular bone. After activation, osteoclasts are mobilized on the bone surface. The osteoclasts resorb a pocket of bone, and osteoblasts lay down new bone filling the pocket. *(From Bauwens SF, Drinka PJ, Boh LB. Primary osteoporosis: Pathogenesis and management strategies. Clin Pharm 1986;5:642, with permission.)*

front, whereas in cortical bone, resorption progresses in a tunneling fashion behind a cutting cone of osteoclasts.

Initially, osteoblasts produce compounds that begin the recruitment, differentiation, and maturation of osteoclasts.[3–8] Other processes may also be involved.[3–8] Mature osteoclasts adhere to bone surface and create the ruffled border. Osteoclasts release substances that increase osteoblast formation.

Over the next 5–7 days, the osteoclasts release hydrogen ions and proteases to destroy the mineralized bone, creating a cavity or lacuna. The destroyed bone may release growth factors such as insulin-like growth factor I and II, platelet-derived growth factor, heparin-binding growth factor, transforming growth factor beta, and bone morphogenetic proteins, all of which increase osteoblast production and inhibit osteoclast activity.

Next the osteoblasts increase in number and mature. Over the next few weeks, osteoblasts begin producing the osteoid, the material filling in the lacuna. Osteoblasts also probably release compounds such as growth factors, which decrease osteoclast activity and control the composition and mineralization of the osteoid. Alkaline phosphatase, found within osteoblasts, may also control mineralization.

The osteoblasts lay down new layers of bone matrix (osteoid), oriented along lines of physical stress. The osteoid is composed of protein, glycoprotein, and polysaccharides. Osteoblasts secrete collagen in a soluble form that subsequently becomes cross-linked and insoluble, forming fibrils. The orientation of the major longitudinal axis of the collagen fibers is along the lines of maximal mechanical stress. After bone collagen is secreted, approximately 10 days pass before mineral becomes deposited along the unmineralized collagen matrix, called the osteoid seam. The type I collagen of bone osteoid calcifies. Calcitriol (1,25-vitamin D) promotes bone formation by providing adequate serum concentrations of minerals. Osteocalcin, osteonectin, and phosphoproteins may assist in controlling mineralization, which occurs over the next several months. Some of the osteoblasts that produce bone substances

TABLE 83.2. HORMONES AND LOCAL FACTORS INVOLVED IN BONE REMODELING AND THEIR EFFECT ON BONE CELL FUNCTION

	Action	
	Resorption	**Formation**
Hormones		
Steroid		
$1,25(OH)_2D_3$	↑	↓[a]
Sex steroids (estrogen, progesterone, androgen)	↓	↑–
Glucocorticoids	–	↓
Polypeptide		
PTH	↑	↓↑[b]
Calcitonin	↑	–
Growth hormone	–	↑
Thyroid hormone	↑	–
Local factors		
Produced by bone cells or bone tissue		
IGF-I, IGF-II	?	↑
TGF-β	↓	↑
FGFs	–	↑
PDGF	↑	↑
Granulocyte colony-stimulating factor (G-CSF)	↑	?
GM-CSF	↑	?
Bone morphogenetic protein (BMP)	?	↑
Osteoinductive factor (OIF)	↓	↑
Synthesized by bone-related tissue		
Cartilage-derived IGF-1, basic FGF, TGF-β	↓	↑
Blood-cell–derived		
IL-1	↑	?
TNF	↑	↓
Gamma interferon (γ-IFN)	↓	–
Other factors		
Prostaglandins	↑	↑↓
Binding proteins	?	?

[a]Decreases proliferation of osteoblast-like cells at high concentrations and stimulates proliferation at low concentrations; decreases collagen synthesis.
[b]Decreases collagen synthesis; intermittent administration promotes increased collagen synthesis and increased osteoblast number and activity. (From Ref. 5.)
Key: ↑, increase; ↓, decrease; –, no effect; ?, effect unknown.

around themselves turn into osteocytes and become a permanent part of the bone. The whole remodeling process on average takes approximately 100 days.

Trabecular bone undergoes more remodeling than cortical bone. Remodeling occurs in 25% of trabecular bone and 3% of cortical bone each year.[4] Trabecular bone has a greater surface area and greater exposure to bone marrow. Theoretically, coupling keeps bone resorption and formation equalized, which maintains the skeletal bone mass. However, because resorption is more rapid than formation, an empty volume of bone, called the remodeling space, temporarily exists, occupying about 0.5–1.0% of the skeleton at any given time. The balance between bone resorption and formation is called the remodeling balance. The balance usually exists until the third decade, when an age-related imbalance begins between resorption and formation. Some conditions such as hormonal deficiencies and certain medications and diseases can also cause a disproportionate shift in bone formation or resorption, resulting in bone mass loss and later osteoporosis.

HORMONES AND LOCAL FACTORS IN THE REGULATION OF REMODELING

Intercellular communication in bone is vitally important in determining the overall control and balance of bone formation and resorption. The remodeling process is under control by various hormones, cytokines, and feedback systems (Table 83.2, Figs. 83.3 and 83.4).[3–8] The complete feedback process, the interrelationship between all the bone stimulators and inhibitors, and the additional triggers to begin the remodeling process (such as microfractures and abnormal serum calcium concentrations) are still being unraveled. Much of the hormonal and cytokine control of bone remodeling is based on *in vitro* animal and human bone cell cultures or animal-based research. Concentrations of some of the substances are ascertained with human sampling, especially with regard to aging.

Osteoblasts develop from the mesenchymal lineage of the marrow stromal cell lines.[4,5] Stromal cells can also develop into fibroblasts, chondrocytes, adipocytes, or

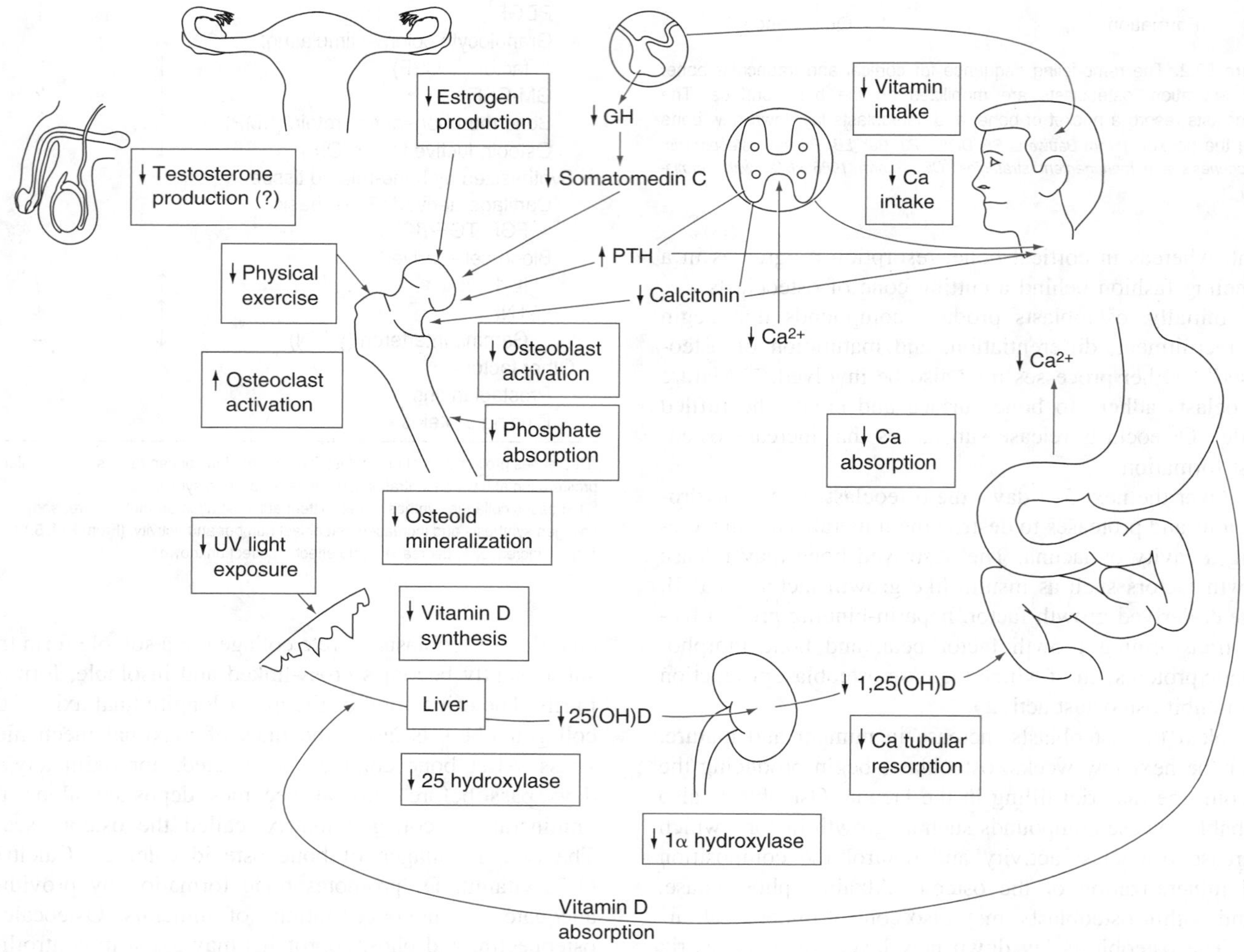

Figure 83.3. Simplified overview of the factors involved in the pathogenesis of osteopenia, osteoporosis, and osteomalacia. GH, growth hormone; PTH, parathyroid hormone.

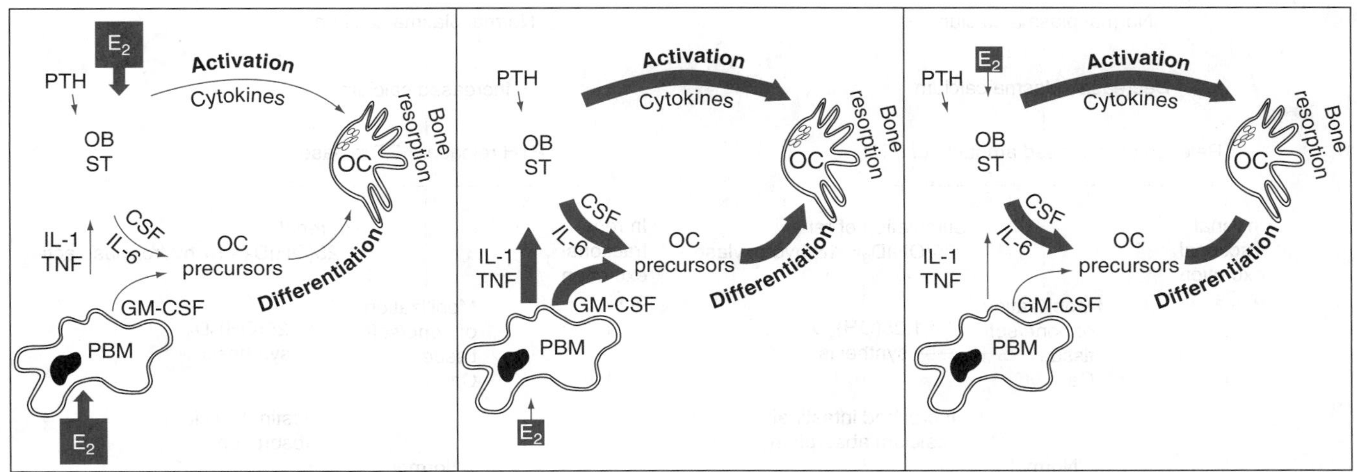

Figure 83.4. Estrogen regulates bone cell cytokines. ***(Left)*** Normal bone remodeling. With E_2 acting as an inhibitor, peripheral blood monocytes (PBM) serve as a source of limited quantities of IL-1, TNF, and GM-CSF; and the stromal cells or osteoblasts secrete small amounts of IL-6 and CSF. ***(Middle)*** Estrogen deficiency: the role of PBM. Absence of E_2 action on PBM causes increased secretion of IL-1, TNF, and GM-CSF; consequently, osteoclast differentiation and activation are increased. ***(Right)*** Estrogen deficiency: the role of stromal cells and osteoblasts. In the deficient situation, osteoblasts and stromal cells secrete more IL-6, causing increased osteoclast differentiation and also secrete more cytokines that directly activate osteoclasts. OB, osteoblasts; ST, stromal cells; OC, osteoclast; and CSF, colony stimulating factors. *(From Ref. 6.)*

muscle cells. Transforming growth factor beta increases chemotaxis, mitogenesis, and differentiation of osteoblasts.[3] Osteoblasts have receptors for parathyroid hormone (PTH), 1,25-vitamin D, estrogen, and other hormones.[5] Under the control of PTH, interleukin (IL)-1, and tumor necrosis factor alpha (TNF-α), osteoblasts synthesize or secrete compounds that mineralize the osteoid, control osteoclast differentiation and maturation, and control the remodeling cycle.[3,6] Bone morphogenetic proteins, members of the transforming growth factor beta family, may control osteocalcin and alkaline phophatase production by the osteoblasts.[3] Some of the compounds produced by the osteoblasts include type I collagen, noncollagenous matrix proteins, osteonectin, growth factors, prostaglandins, collagenase, and tissue plasminogen activator.[5] Osteoblasts can secrete IL-6, IL-11, granulocyte–macrophage colony-stimulating factor, and macrophage colony-stimulating factor.[3–8] These hormones and cytokines most likely have effects on other cell lines besides the osteoclasts and its precursors. Osteoblast production of IL-6, an agent augmenting osteoclast production, is under the control of PTH, PTH-related peptide, 1,25-vitamin D, transforming growth factor beta, IL-1, and TNF.

Osteoclasts are derived from granulocyte–macrophage colony-forming units. The differentiation and maturation of an osteoclast cannot begin without stromal osteoblastic cells.[4] Compounds such as IL-1, -3, -6, and -11, transforming growth factor alpha, 1,25-vitamin D, PTH, TNF, granulocyte–macrophage stimulating factor, leukemia inhibitory factor, and stem cell factor can influence differentiation and maturation of osteoclasts.[3–8] The formation of the granulocyte–macrophage colony-forming unit is under the control of IL-3 and -6. These interleukins may also influence osteoclast maturation further in the development process. The promonocyte either becomes a monocyte or a preosteoclast. The conversion to an osteoclast first begins with osteoclast-activating factors such as transforming growth factor alpha. The preosteoclast conversion to a late preosteoclast is controlled by PTH, 1,25-vitamin D, and IL-1. Further conversion to the osteoclast is controlled by IL-1 and 1,25-vitamin D.

All known hormonal and local simulators of osteoclastic bone resorption, including PTH, 1,25-vitamin D, IL-1, and TNF mediate their stimulatory effects on the osteoclast through an initial effect on the osteoblast.[3–8] Unlike osteoblasts, receptors for PTH and 1,25-vitamin D have not been found on osteoclasts. Calcitonin, which can bind to the osteoclast receptor, may be involved in decreasing its activity. Estrogens and androgens can inhibit IL-6 production and thereby inhibit osteoclast production.

SERUM CALCIUM AND PHOSPHATE REGULATION

The movement of calcium and phosphorus in and out of bone is under the control of three major hormones: PTH, 1,25-vitamin D, and calcitonin.[9] Figure 83.5 shows the interrelationships of these three hormones on mineral metabolism. When the serum calcium is low, PTH increases, resulting in increased bone resorption and vitamin D metabolism to its active form, 1,25-dihydroxyvitamin D. The 1,25-vitamin D metabolite increases calcium absorption from the gut and tubular reabsorption from the kidneys. When the calcium serum concentration returns

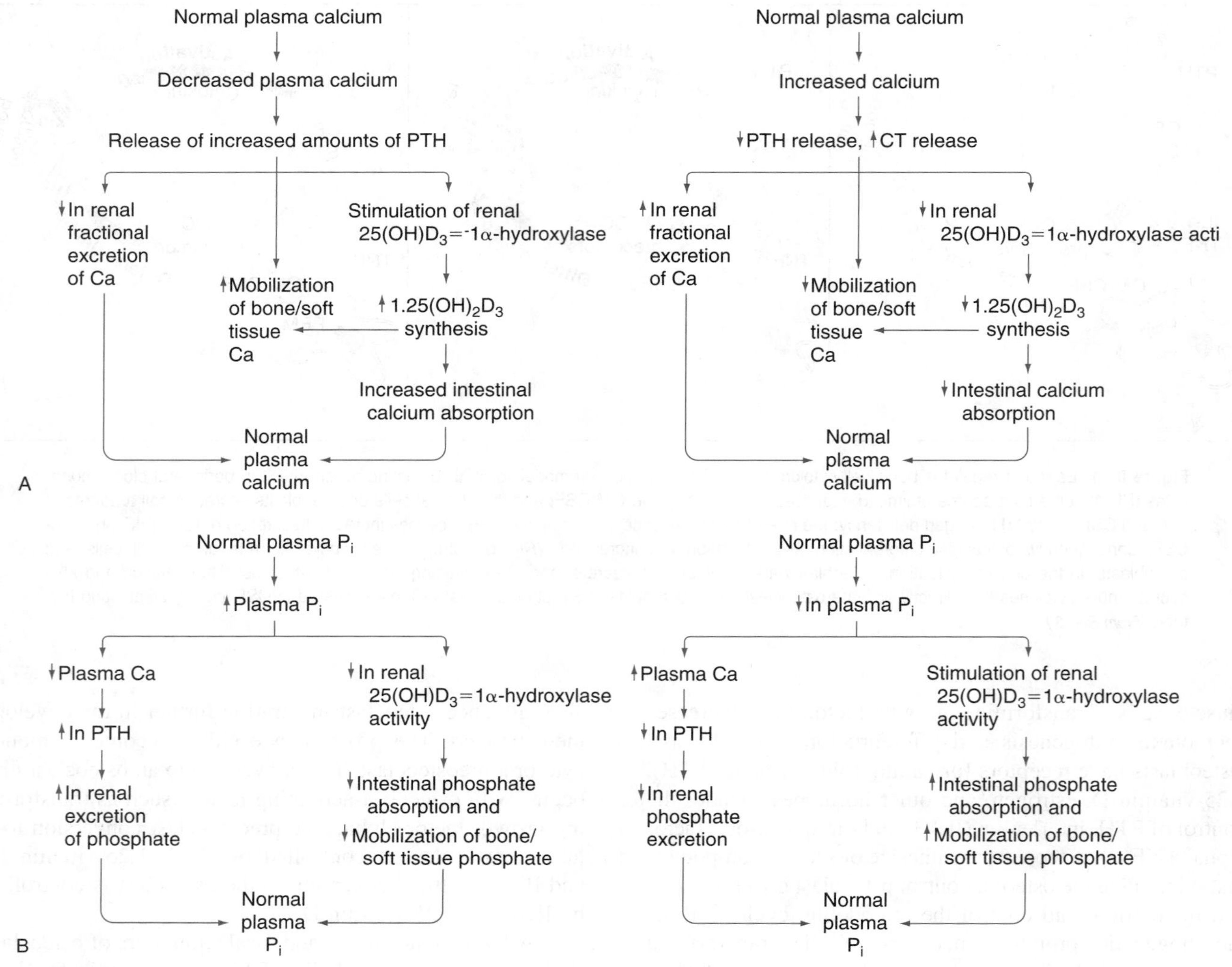

Figure 83.5. (A) Physiologic defenses in hypo- or hypercalcemic states. (B) Physiologic defenses in hypo- or hyperphosphatemic states. CT, calcitonin. *(From Ref. 9.)*

to normal, PTH production decreases and so does bone resorption.

Evaluation of Osteopenic Bone Disorders

HISTORY AND PHYSICAL EXAMINATION

The duration and severity of the disorder, age of onset, location, and frequency of fractures should be assessed during the initial physical examination. Attempts should be made to elicit the presence of osteoporotic risk factors (Table 83.3). Abnormalities of the bone-remodeling process play a critical role in the development of osteoporosis and osteomalacia. Both disorders have distinct clinicopathologic characteristics; however, differentiation between them in clinical practice is difficult.

RADIOLOGIC QUANTIFICATION

Bone can be quantified using several noninvasive techniques, including radiography, photon and x-ray absorptiometry, and computerized tomography scan.[10] Table 83.4 compares these techniques. Routine x-ray techniques are capable of detecting generalized osteopenia only after 20–50% of bone mass is lost. Single-photon absorptiometry (SPA) is recommended for measurement of the forearm (primarily cortical bone) and dual-energy x-ray absorptiometry (DEXA) for the spine (primarily trabecular bone) and hip (combination of trabecular and cortical bone). SPA does not distinguish between cortical and trabecular bone mass and cannot be used with soft tissue. DEXA can be used with soft tissue. Computerized tomography provides a three-dimensional picture and directly measures both trabecular and cortical bone densities. Ultrasound techniques are being explored.

TABLE 83.3. FACTORS COMMONLY ASSOCIATED WITH OSTEOPOROSIS

Genetic
White or Asiatic ethnicity
Positive family history
Small body frame (less than 58 kg)
Lifestyle
Smoking
Inactivity
Nulliparity
Excessive exercise (producing amenorrhoea)
Early natural menopause
Late menarche
Nutritional Factors
Milk intolerance
Lifelong low dietary calcium intake
Excessive alcohol intake
Consistently high animal protein intake
Medical Disorders
Anorexia nervosa
Thyrotoxicosis
Cushing's syndrome
Type I diabetes
Alterations in gastrointestinal and hepatobiliary function
Occult osteogenesis imperfecta
Mastocytosis
Rheumatoid arthritis
Long-term parenteral nutrition
Prolactinoma
Hemolytic anemia, hemochromatosis, and thalassaemia
Ankylosing spondylitis
Drugs
Thyroid replacement drugs
Glucocorticoid drugs
Anticoagulants (heparin)
Chronic lithium therapy
Chemotherapy
GnRH agonist or antagonist therapy
Anticonvulsant drugs
Extended tetracycline use[a]
Diuretics producing calciuria[a]
Phenothiazine derivatives[a]
Cyclosporin[a]
Aluminum-containing antacids[a]

[a]Not yet associated with decreased bone mass although identified as either toxic to bone in animals or inducing calciuria and/or calcium malabsorption in human beings. (From Ref. 7.)
Key: GnRH = gonadotropin releasing hormone.

The indications for radiologic quantification of bone mass have not definitively been established. In fact, if estrogen-replacement therapy is primarily prescribed for preventing cardiovascular disease, then knowledge of bone density would not influence the decision to use estrogens. Suggested indications for radiographic quantification of bone mass include characterizing bone loss as fast or slow, establishing fracture risk, determining the efficacy of preventive or treatment regimens, and assisting patients in prevention and treatment decisions. Women told that their bone density was less than normal were more likely to take measures to prevent further bone loss, begin hormones, and try to prevent falls.[11]

ILIAC CREST BIOPSY

The quality and quantity of bone, as well as the rate of turnover, can be studied by obtaining an intact core of cortical and trabecular bone from the iliac crest. From this sample, specific bone tissue volumes (osteoid, mineralized bone, and marrow space) and surface bone cell types (osteoclast, osteoblast, and inactive lining cells) are quantified. A tetracycline agent is administered for 3 days, and 12 days later a different tetracycline is given for another 3 days. The specific tetracycline used does not appear to make a difference. The distance between the two distinct tetracycline bands provides the basis for categorizing patients as fast (high turnover) or slow (slow turnover) mineralizers. Bone biopsy is useful for differentiating osteoporosis from osteomalacia.

BIOCHEMICAL EVALUATION

Advanced biochemical tests have somewhat improved the ability to diagnose specific types of metabolic bone disease. The pathogenesis of some diseases, however, such as osteoporosis, is multifactorial and as such is not well described by chemical abnormalities. Further, some of the newer tests are expensive, of variable reliability, and not widely available. Technical assay problems, diurnal variation, kinetics of the compound, and relationship to remodeling and disease pathology influence the usefulness of these tests.

The preferred tests to determine if bone formation is ongoing are the presence or rise in osteocalcin and total alkaline phosphatase.[12] Rises in alkaline phosphatase are not sensitive and specific to bone formation. Other tests being developed or used in research studies include procollagen I extension peptides, osteonectin, and sialoprotein II.

The preferred tests to determine if bone resorption is ongoing are fasting urinary hydroxyproline and calcium corrected for creatinine production and pyridinoline and deoxypyridinoline cross-links.[12] The hydroxyproline and calcium tests are not sensitive or specific. Other tests include serum tartrate-resistant alkaline phosphatase, type I collagen degradation products, hydroxylysine glycosides, and gamma carboxyglutamic acid.

Other tests that may be helpful to detect other causes of bone disease are serum calcium, phophorus, vitamin D, vitamin D metabolites, and PTH concentrations (Table 83.5).[13] In the future, concentrations of some of the other hormones and cytokines involved in bone resorption and formation may be employed.

TABLE 83.4. NONINVASIVE MEASUREMENTS OF BONE MINERAL DENSITY

Technique	Site	Precision[a] (%)	Accuracy[b] (%)	Examination Time (min)	Absorbed Dose of Radiation[c] (mrem)
Single-photon absorptiometry	Proximal and distal radius, calcaneus	1–3	5	15	10–20
Dual-energy photon absorptiometry	Spine, hip, total body	2–4	4–10	20–40	5
Dual-energy x-ray absorptiometry	Spine, hip, total body	0.5–2	3–5	3–7	1–3
Quantitative computed tomography	Spine	2–5	5–20	10–15	100–1000

[a]Precision is the coefficient of variation (standard deviation by the mean) for repeated measurements over a short period of time in young, healthy persons.
[b]Accuracy is the coefficient of variation for measurements in a specimen whose mineral content has been determined by other means (e.g., measurement of ashed weight).
[c]To convert millirems to millijoules per kilogram of body weight, multiply by 0.01. (From Johnston CC, Slemenda CW, Melton LJ. Current concepts: Clinical use of bone densitometry. N Engl J Med 1991;324:1105–1109, with permission.)

OSTEOPOROSIS

Osteoporosis is defined as a universal, gradual reduction in bone mass (osteopenia) to a point where the skeleton is compromised, resulting in fractures with minimal trauma. Since the term osteoporosis is routinely used in the literature and medical community to refer to both osteopenia and osteoporosis, osteoporois will refer to both in this chapter. Osteoporosis is not a single disease entity with a single cause, but rather a very heterogeneous disease process involving a number of contributing etiologic factors (Table 83.3).[7] Three categories of osteoporosis have been established: postmenopausal, senile, and secondary (Table 83.6).

EPIDEMIOLOGY

About 1.2 million fractures are reported each year in the United States. The annual hip fracture incidence alone is estimated to range from 147,000 to 250,000, with approxi-

TABLE 83.5. CHEMICAL FINDINGS IN THE FORMS OF RICKETS AND OSTEOMALACIA

Type of Rickets	[CA]	[P1]	Alk Phos	PTH	25 (OH) Vit D	1,25(OH) Vit D	TRP (%)	Urinary [CA]	Misc. Serum and Urine Findings
Vitamin D deficiency	Low/Nrml	Low	High	High	Low	Low	Low	Low	
Phosphate deficiency	Nrml	Low	High	Nrml	Nrml	Nrml	High	Nrml	
Gastrointestinal and enteric	Low	Low	High	High	Low/Nrml	Low/Nrml	Low	Low	
Vitamin D resistant									
Hypophosphatemic (Albright)	Nrml	Low	High	Nrml	Nrml	Nrml	Low	Nrml	Glycosuria, aminoaciduria, etc.
Type I Vitamin D dependent	Low	Low	High	High	Nrml	Low	Low	Low	
Type II Vitamin D dependent	Low	Low	High	High	High/Nrml	High/Nrml	Low	Low	
Renal tubular acidosis	Low	Low	High	High	High/Nrml	High/Nrml	Low	High	Low NA, K; High Cl acidosis/alk urine
Renal osteodystrophy	Low	High	High	High	Low	Low	?	Low	High BUN and creatinine

(From Ref. 13.)

TABLE 83.6. CLASSIFICATION OF OSTEOPOROTIC TYPES

	Type I Post-menopausal	Type II Senile	Type III Secondary
Age	55–70	75–90	Any age
Years past menopause	5–15	25–40	Any age
Sex ratio F:M	20:1	2:1	1:1
Fracture site	Spine	Hip, spine, pelvis, humerus	Spine, hip, peripheral
Bone loss			
Trabecular	+++	++	+++
Cortical	+	++	+++
Contributing factor			
Menopause	+++	++	++
Age	+	+++	++
Biochemistry			
PTH	↓	↑	↓↑
$1,25(OH)_2D_3$	↓	↓	↓↑
Calcium absorption	↓	↓	↓
1 α hydroxylase response to PTH	↑	→	?

(From Sem Nephrol 1992;12:109–115.)

mately 80% resulting from minor trauma. About 40% of women will have at least one vertebral fracture by the time they are 80 years of age. One-third of women and one-sixth of men will experience a hip fracture by their late 80s. Hip fracture is associated with a 5–20% decrease in expected survival the first year and an additional 13% mortality the next year.[14] One fourth to one half of hip fracture patients are unable to walk independently after the fracture heals. About one-half of the women and men 60 years or older hospitalized for a hip fracture will be discharged to a nursing home. About one fourth of them will still reside in the nursing home 1 year later. The number of persons experiencing a hip fracture will rise in the future because the population is rapidly growing older and the incidence of fractures increases with age. By the year 2040, the incidence of hip fractures will exceed 500,000.[14] The annual cost of osteoporotic hip fractures is about $10 billion and may rise to $240 billion by 2040.[14]

TYPES OF OSTEOPOROSIS

At least three types of osteoporosis exist (Table 83.6). Type I, most often referred to as postmenopausal osteoporosis, affects primarily trabecular bone in women within the first 15–20 years following menopause. The rate of trabecular bone loss is three times normal, while the rate of cortical loss is only slightly above normal. Consequently, fractures of the vertebrae and distal forearm are seen most frequently.

Type II or senile osteoporosis affects men and women older than age 70. Cortical and trabecular bone density values show a proportionate loss. The clinical manifestations of type II osteoporosis are multiple wedge, hip, and radius fractures.

Type III osteoporosis or osteoporosis secondary to other diseases or medications occurs in either sex at any age.

RISK FACTORS FOR OSTEOPOROSIS

Multiple genetic, environmental, medical, and social conditions can influence both a woman's,[7] and a man's[8] likelihood of developing osteoporosis (Table 83.3). Women with relatives, especially their mothers, who have experienced a fracture and with lean body stature, have a higher likelihood of osteoporosis. Women—because of the combination of lower peak bone mass, estrogen deficiency, and age-related bone loss—have lower bone density and more fractures than men. Age at menarche and menopause, chemical or surgical menopause, and nulliparity increase osteoporosis incidence. Racial factors—Caucasian and Asian—are associated with osteoporosis, but African-Americans can develop this condition. Environmental conditions such as sun exposure influence the production of vitamin D and thus bone density. Certain diseases, immobilization, and medications (see as follows) can develop type III, secondary osteoporosis. Social habits such as poor intake of calcium at any point in life, physical inactivity, excessive caffeine and alcohol use, and smoking influence bone density in women and men.

Risk factors for low bone density and hip fractures established in elderly and black women cohorts support the previously listed risk factors, but some differences have been noticed. Additional risk factors identified in elderly women include low muscle strength, falls, change in fat mass, poor depth perception, and poor contrast sensitivity.[15] Past calcium intake, past or current use of estrogens or thiazides, and alcohol ingestion were not consistently associated with low bone density or hip fractures.[15,16] Data from 362 black women indicated that risk factors for hip fracture were stroke, the need for ambulatory aids, lower limb dysfunction, lower body mass, and alcohol intake.[17]

BONE DENSITY AND OSTEOPOROTIC FRACTURE INCIDENCE

The World Health Organization (WHO) defines low bone mass as bone density that is 1–2.5 standard deviations less than the normal premenopausal value. Osteoporosis is listed when bone densities are greater than 2.5 standard deviations and severe osteoporosis labeled as bone densities greater than 2.5 standard deviations with fractures. Although fractures associated with osteoporosis are generally attributed to low bone mass at the fracture site, considerable overlap exists between the bone density measured in normal patients and those with osteoporosis. Many individuals with above-average bone densities fracture, while others with relatively low bone mineral density survive serious trauma without fracture. Decreased trabecular connectivity and microfracture repair and the association between cortical and trabecular bone loss could partially explain the variability in the relationship between bone density and fracture incidence.

As more studies are conducted, an association between bone density and fractures becomes apparent.[18] Vertebral fractures were increased 2- to 2.4-fold for each 1 standard deviation below baseline bone densities.[19] In the elderly, for every 1 standard deviation below normal of femoral bone density, the age-adjusted hip fracture incidence increased 2.6 times.[20] Low bone density at one site does not always predict fractures at another site. Although associations may exist, substantial variability in fracture incidence is still not explained.

PATHOPHYSIOLOGY

Postmenopausal Osteoporosis

Estrogen deficiency is associated with an increase in bone resorption without an increase in bone formation. Estrogen receptors have been identified on osteoblasts, osteoclasts, and macrophages. The secretion of cytokines and other compounds by the osteoblasts most likely is influenced by estrogens. Human and animal studies indicate that estrogen deficiency increases the release of IL-1, TNF, and granulocyte–macrophage colony-stimulating factor (GM-CSF) from peripheral blood monocytes and IG-6 and colony-stimulating factors from stromal cells and osteoblasts (Figure 83.4).[6] Interleukin-1 is a potent inducer of resorption. TNF-α induces osteoclast differentiation and maturation and bone resorption. Estrogen replacement decreases the cytokine production, leading to resorption, increased calcitonin concentrations, decreased prostaglandin E_2 (a stimulator of osteoblast collagen production and bone resorption), decreased insulin-like growth factor I secretion, and increased calcium absorption.[6,21]

Age-Related/Senile Osteoporosis

Maximal bone mineral content of cortical bone occurs in men and women in the second to fourth decade of life, followed by a slow decline. Women have less bone mass at skeletal maturity, requiring less bone to be lost before the threshold for fractures is reached. In women, cortical bone loss proceeds at a rate of 3% per decade until menopause, at which time it accelerates to about 9% per decade.[22] The rate returns to normal 10–20 years after menopause. Men lose bone at 3–4% per decade throughout life. Over a lifetime, women lose about 35% of their cortical bone, men about 23%. Lumbar spine decreases 6% per decade in women and 2% per decade in men throughout life.[23] A 1–10% per year decrease in vertebral bone mass occurs 3–10 years after menopause.

Four basic factors contribute to the onset of age-related bone loss: decreased osteoblast function, decreased calcium and vitamin D absorption, biochemical imbalances, and sex hormone deficiencies. After age 40, less bone is formed than is resorbed in any given BMU. This coupling imbalance appears to increase with age. This does not result from complete osteoblast senescence, because fracture repair in the elderly does not appear to be delayed. Therefore, the impairment in the regulation of the osteoblast may be the result of abnormalities of systemic or local factors. Calcium absorption decreases with age in both sexes, especially after the age of 70. Most elderly consume less than the recommended daily amounts of calcium and vitamin D. Along with decreased intake, decreased sun exposure (and thus decreased skin conversion), and impaired liver or kidney metabolism of vitamin D to 1,25-dihydroxyvitamin D also lead to decreased active vitamin D metabolite concentrations. Serum PTH concentrations are increased secondary to the decreased serum calcium and potentially secondary to aging. An increase in serum PTH would lead to increased bone turnover by increasing the number of BMUs and, when uncoupling occurred, to increased bone loss. In some studies, aging has been associated with decreased serum calcitonin concentrations.

Osteoporosis in Men

Osteoporosis occurs in men[8] but with a lower incidence than in women. The lower osteoporosis incidence in men may result from higher peak bone mass at skeletal maturity, shorter life expectancy, lower bone loss rate during aging, fewer falls, and/or a gradual (versus a distinct) cessation of hormone production. One-fourth to one-fifth of all hip fractures occur in men, causing substantial morbidity, mortality and health care expenditures. Vertebral fractures are common in men but forearm fractures are uncommon. The pathogenesis, risk factors, and clinical features of male osteoporosis are similar to those of postmenopausal osteoporosis. Decreased calcium, vitamin D, growth hormone, and insulin-like growth factor concentrations and increased PTH concentrations are seen in aging men as well as in aging women. In addition, aging and osteoporosis are associated with decreased testosterone levels. The contribution of male hormone deficiency toward bone loss, however, is less well defined than estrogen deficiency, as men do not go through a process equivalent to menopause. Gonadal function does decrease in older men, and overt male hypogonadism is associated with fractures. Frequently, secondary causes exist for men with osteoporosis.

Drug-Induced Osteoporosis

Heparin, excessive thyroid replacement, glucocorticoids, anticonvulsants, and cyclosporine have been associated with low bone density and fractures. Heparin therapy in excess of 15,000–30,000 units per day for greater than 3–6 months has been associated with vertebral fractures and decreased bone density in pregnant women. The mechanism is unknown. In one study about one third of the pregnant women had their proximal femur density decreased by greater than 10%.[24] Thyroid hormones can increase osteoclasts, decrease calcitonin concentrations, and increase bone resorption. Compared with no thyroid therapy in a cross-sectional study, current thyroid replacement therapy was associated with lower spine, hip, and radial bone densities.[25] Doses greater than 200 μg per day or at least 1.6 μg/kg were associated with decreased bone mass. Thyroid users with concomitant estrogen-replacement therapy had less bone loss. Glucocorticoids decreased bone formation and increased bone resorption with prednisone doses of 7.5 mg or greater; however, decreased bone density has been associated with lower oral doses and high-dose inhalation therapy.[26] This medication-induced disease is discussed further below.

Anticonvulsants increase vitamin D metabolism and produce osteomalacia. With long-standing disease, the decreased bone structure leads to osteoporosis and fractures. Transplant patients can develop osteoporosis as a function of glucocorticoid therapy, decreased renal function, increased parathyroid hormone concentrations, or potentially cyclosporine therapy.[27] Further exploration is required.

CLINICAL PRESENTATION

The usual presentation of osteoporosis is shortened stature, kyphosis, lordosis, or a fracture, most commonly of the vertebra, hip, or forearm. The fractures frequently occur after minor trauma, such as bending, lifting, jumping, and falling from the standing position. Recurrent fractures are common with the time frame unpredictable. Vertebral body collapse is the most frequently seen fracture, especially in early postmenopausal women. As a result, back pain of variable intensity and spine deformities occur. Some patients may have a fracture with no pain, with the fracture discovered on routine x-ray or in relationship to height reduction. Acute pain usually completely resolves in 2–3 months.

The acute phase may also be followed by chronic back pain, which manifests as a nagging, deep, dull pain localized to the general area of the fracture. Long-term pain management may be required. Nonsteroidal anti-inflammatory drugs (NSAIDs) provide benefit, but, for some patients unresponsive to NSAIDs, narcotics or calcitonin may be required. Multiple fractures with or without pain may lead to dorsal kyphosis and exaggerated cervical lordosis, frequently referred to as Dowager's or widow's hump. Chest wall changes can lead to pulmonary and cardiovascular complications. Collapsed vertebra rarely lead to spinal cord compression.

PREVENTION AND TREATMENT

Many factors limit the evaluation of possible therapeutic prevention and treatment interventions for osteoporosis. Not only are symptoms episodic and unrelated to the severity of the disease state, but also even when fractures have occurred, further fractures may continue even though further reduction of bone mass is stopped or significantly slowed. The only way to show true effectiveness of a given treatment is to demonstrate a significant decrease in the fracture rate, which requires many years of follow-up. Another approach has been to show that bone mass increased or bone loss slowed. The assumed expectation is that decreased bone loss will result in decreased fracture rate.

Osteoporosis prevention can be accomplished by increasing peak bone mass in women and men under the age of 35–40 years and eliminating or decreasing the bone loss in postmenopausal women and older men. Two therapeutic goals exist for existing osteoporosis: Prevent further bone loss and prevent subsequent fractures. Pain control may be an important issue for women and men with fractures.

NONPHARMACOLOGIC PREVENTION AND TREATMENT METHODS

Social Habit and Diet Changes

Caffeine ingestion should be decreased to less than 2–5 cups of caffeine per day in women and men.[28,29] Caffeine increases urinary calcium excretion. No adaption occurs with long-term ingestion. Older women are more prone to caffeine-induced calcium-excretion problems, especially if concomitant calcium supplementation is not taken.[29]

Women and men should stop smoking since smoking has been associated with lower bone mass and increased fracture rates.[30,31] Based on a comparison of twin pairs in which one twin either did not smoke or smoked less than the other, every 10 pack/year difference decreased spine bone density by 2% and femural bone density by 1%.[30] Smoking causes earlier menopause and increases metabolism of endogenous and exogenous sex hormones.[32]

An association between alcohol use and low bone density and fractures has been found in some but not all studies.[33] Alcohol may induce nutritional deficiencies in calcium, vitamin D, and magnesium. Liver disease may decrease metabolism of vitamin D to its active metabolite. PTH concentrations can be altered in alcoholics. Potentially, a direct effect exists on calcium absorption and bone remodeling through prostaglandins, granulocyte–macrophage progenitor cells, and mineralization rate. Reduced alcohol intake will improve the overall health of patients.

Exercise

Men and women can gain two benefits from increased aerobic and strengthening exercises: prevention of bone loss and fewer falls (since muscle tone is improved). The type, duration, and style of exercise to provide such benefits is still being determined. The data continue to be conflicting, with some studies showing an increase in bone mass, while others show no effect. Studies do seem to suggest that bones most directly stressed by exercise have the greatest benefit in affecting bone mineral density (BMD); in general, a positive effect is seen when BMD is simply maintained.

Originally, aerobic exercises were advocated for osteoporosis patients. However, a high-intensity strength training program produced increased femoral neck and lumbar spine bone density,[34] and walking more than 7.5 miles per week produced higher bone densities than walking less than 1 mile per week.[35] In contrast, a 1-year brisk walking program was not associated with significant bone density changes compared with nonwalkers.[36] Swimming improved bone density in men but not women.[37] Exercise programs designed to improve body mechanics and general conditioning may prevent falls and traumatic injuries, which would reduce the rate of fractures without any effect on bone density. Exercise cannot be recommended as sole therapy for osteoporosis prevention, but it should be incorporated into an overall health-maintenance regimen.

Of note, very vigorous exercise programs such as for elite athletes can produce amenorrhea, which leads to low bone density and fractures in women. Amenorrhea occurs in 35–40% of highly trained endurance women athletes and results from low gonadotropin concentrations. Oral contraceptives are being administered to amenorrheic athletes to overcome this estrogen-deficiency state.

Fall Prevention

In elderly patients, prevention of falls gains greater importance since currently no safe, effective, and approved regimens exist for building new strong bones. Since decreased muscle strength is associated with falls, exercises should be conducted to increase muscle strength. Home environments should be redesigned, eliminating opportunities for falls. Slip rugs and extension cords should be removed, hand rails should be placed on the bath tub, and nonslip tape should be placed inside tubs.

A patient's medication profile should be reviewed for psychotropic, antihypertensive, and diuretic medications associated with falls. Sedatives should be discontinued or switched to short-acting agents. Diuretics should be given during the day to prevent nocturnal voiding. Orthostatic blood pressure problems should be resolved through slow arousal from lying and sitting positions. Other psychotropic medications should also be eliminated or altered if altered balance or confusion result.

ANTIRESORPTIVE PREVENTION AND TREATMENT

Calcium

Almost all of the body's calcium content is stored in bone. An equilibrium exists between calcium requirements for the body and bone resorption. A feedback system between serum calcium concentration, parathyroid hormone, and vitamin D controls the destruction of bone to meet the body's calcium needs[9] (Figs. 83.3 and 83.5). On average, the American diet for all ages is insufficient for calcium.

Clinical Effectiveness

Most studies, especially recent placebo-controlled, randomized clinical trials, support supplemental calcium to decrease bone loss.[38,39] The prevention against bone loss appears to be better in bones with a greater cortical bone content since spine results are generally less favorable than hip and radius effects. A better effect of calcium supplementation may be experienced in women with the lowest dietary or life history of calcium intake. The epidemiologic studies find fewer fractures in women with greater calcium intakes. Only a few calcium studies have been conducted for a long enough time frame with sufficient sample sizes and study design to evaluate fracture incidence. These studies generally find fracture rates lower with calcium supplementation.

Comparison studies find calcium to be less beneficial than hormone-replacement therapy, especially for women in whom therapy is initiated within 5 years of menopause. Since most hormone-replacement studies included calcium supplementation, calcium should still be advocated in estrogen users. Of note, estrogen users require only 1 g of daily calcium (versus 1.5 g in nonestrogen users).[40] Exercise combined with calcium therapy also has a greater effect than does exercise alone.

Calcium Administration

All patients, regardless of age, should meet the NIH consensus conference recommendations for calcium (Table 83.7).[40] Women and men under 30–40 years of age may be able to increase their bone mass, while peri- and postmenopausal women and men older than 40 will decrease the rate of bone loss with calcium supplementation. In the United States, more than two-thirds of all women between the ages of 18 and 30 ingest less than the recommended daily allowance (RDA) for calcium, which is 800 mg elemental calcium daily. More than 75% of women older than 35 years have calcium intakes of less than the RDA. Approximately 60–70% of men between the ages of 15 and 35 maintain intakes above the RDA, and 75% of men throughout their

TABLE 83.7. OPTIMAL CALCIUM REQUIREMENTS RECOMMENDED BY THE NATIONAL INSTITUTES OF HEALTH CONSENSUS PANEL

Age Group	Optimal Daily Intake of Calcium (mg)
Infants	
Birth–6 mo	400
6 mo–1 yr	600
Children	
1–5 yr	800
6–10 yr	800–1200
Adolescents/young adults	
11–24 yr	1200–1500
Men	
25–65 yr	1000
Over 65 yr	1500
Women	
25–50 yr	1000
Over 50 yr (postmenopausal)	
On estrogens	1000
Not on estrogens	1500
Over 65 yr	1500
Pregnant and nursing	1200–1500

(From Ref. 40.)

life maintain intakes above 500 mg daily. Controversy surrounds calcium requirements for the elderly, primarily because the current RDA was established for any adult older than 51 years, leaving little margin of safety to compensate for the reduced absorption of calcium seen with aging. The NHANES II study showed that 50% of older adults consume less than 800 mg of calcium daily.[41]

Pharmacists should assist patients in selecting the appropriate calcium regimen to give them the NIH-recommended calcium requirements (Table 83.7).[40] Calcium may be ingested either in food or through oral supplementation. Table 83.8 lists foods with high calcium content, primarily dairy products. Calcium absorption from milk is about 25–35%.[42] Fruits and vegetables high in oxalate (spinach and rhubarb) and phylates (bran and whole cereals) have less calcium available for absorption because of binding.[42] When dietary intake is inadequate, oral calcium supplements are a convenient means of ensuring adequate calcium intake. The various preparations provide varying amounts of calcium. Table 83.9 lists some common forms of calcium and their calcium content. Calcium carbonate contains the most elemental calcium by weight (40%).

Calcium tablets should be ingested between meals to enhance absorption. Calcium carbonate has acid-dependent absorption, while calcium citrate has acid-independent absorption. Some elderly may have decreased acid secretion. To overcome this age-associated change, calcium carbonate can be taken with meals or calcium citrate used. The calcium absorption fraction decreases as tablet size increases. Therefore, divided doses of 500 mg or less should be ingested to enhance the amount absorbed.

Generally, calcium carbonate 500 mg twice daily is used because of its high content and lower cost. It is difficult to choose which calcium carbonate product to use because bioavailability data are not easily accessible for all products. Recent data have shown that many preparations have unacceptable dissolution or disintegration rates.[43] These parameters can change among products.

Since the goal of supplementation is to provide the amount of calcium the body needs, few side effects are experienced. The most common side effect is constipation, which can have a higher incidence in elderly patients. Calcium should not be administered with fiber laxatives. Calcium can decrease iron, tetracycline, ciprofloxacin, etidronate, phenytoin, and fluoride absorption when given concomitantly. Calcium channel blocker activity may be decreased if the serum calcium concentration is increased above normal values. Concurrent administration of calcium and phosphates needs to be monitored to prevent calcium phosphate precipitation and tissue calcification.

Diuretics

Thiazide diuretics promote a decrease in renal calcium excretion, while loop diuretics increase renal calcium excretion. Based on case-controlled studies, current thiazide diuretic use for at least 6–10 years[44,45] has been associated with increased hip, spine, radius, and heel bone density in women[44,46] and radius bone density in men.[46] Hip fractures either decreased in women and men[45] or did not change in women.[44] Past users had bone density and fracture rates similar to those who never used diuretics. Con-

TABLE 83.8. CALCIUM CONTENT OF VARIOUS FOODS

Food	Serving Size	Calcium Content (mg)
Milk (skim)	1 qt	1212
Milk (whole)	1 qt	1152
Sardines	8 medium	354
Yogurt (low-fat)	1 cup	345
Swiss cheese	1 oz	250
Red salmon	½ cup	250
Turnip greens, cooked	½ cup	245
Creamed cottage cheese	1 cup	211
Cheddar cheese	1 oz	211
Ice cream	1 cup	200
American processed cheese	1 oz	150
Spinach (frozen, chopped, cooked)	½ cup	113
Chocolate fudge	3½ oz	100

TABLE 83.9. ORAL CALCIUM SUPPLEMENTATION PRODUCTS

Preparation	Tablet Size: mg	Tablet Size: mg Elemental Calcium/Tablet	To Supply 1 g Elemental Calcium (tablets/d)
Calcium carbonate (40% elemental calcium)			
Generic	650	260	4
Cal-Sup (Riker Laboratories)	750	300	4
Caltrate (Lederle Laboratories)	1500	600	2
Os-Cal 500 (Marion Laboratories)	1250	500	2
Tums (Norcliff-Thayer)	500	200	5
Titralac (3M Company)	420	168	6
Generic calcium gluconate (9% elemental calcium)	650	58.5	17
Generic calcium lactate (13% elemental calcium)	650	84.5	12
Generic dibasic calcium phosphate (23% elemental calcium)	500	115	9

current thiazides and estrogens resulted in greater bone mineral density[46] than did estrogens alone and fewer side effects than did thiazides alone.[47] HDL increased; LDL, fasting glucose, and fasting insulin decreased; and the increased glucose and insulin concentrations after a glucose challenge were not blunted with the combination.

Vitamin D and Its Metabolites

Vitamin D is obtained by dietary intake and created by ultraviolet light's effect on 7-dehydrocholesterol conversion. Vitamin D is metabolized in the liver to 1-hydroxyvitamin D and then to the active metabolite, 1,25-dihydroxyvitamin D, in the kidney. 1,25-dihydroxyvitamin D (calcitriol) has multiple effects on bone metabolism. Calcium absorption is increased in the small intestine as a result of stimulating the active calcium transport system. The increased calcium concentration decreases PTH release and thereby decreases bone resorption. Vitamin D stimulates both osteoblasts and osteoclasts. Variable results on bone density and fractures have been documented.[48]

Clinical Effectiveness

Based on two large sample size clinical trials, vitamin D may have a role in osteoporosis prevention or treatment. In ambulatory nursing home residents, 800 IU of vitamin D_3 and 1.2 g calcium resulted in increased femur bone density and decreased hip and nonvertebral fractures compared with placebo.[49] Calcitriol 0.25 μg twice daily for 3 years decreased new vertebral fractures in women with less than five vertebral fractures at baseline, decreased peripheral fractures, and produced similar side effects to those of 1 g calcium.[50] However, many studies with smaller samples and less stringent study designs did not find important benefits with vitamin D_3 or calcitriol.

Vitamin D Administration

Vitamin D supplementation should be given to patients ingesting less than the vitamin D RDA of 400 IU for people 6 months to 24 years and 200 IU for those 25 years and older. Of note, many believe the current RDAs, especially for the elderly, are too low. Seasonal variations exist for serum vitamin D concentrations; thus seasonal differences in dosage requirements may also exist. Since most elderly have low vitamin D concentrations, they can be started on 200–800 IU vitamin D_3 or D_2. A 1,25-dihydroxyvitamin D metabolite concentration may be worth pursuing to determine if liver and kidney metabolism has occurred with vitamin D, especially in patients with advanced osteoporosis. Pharmacologic doses of vitamin D or its metabolites are not yet considered standard therapy for preventing osteoporosis but is sometimes used for treating patients with serious osteoporosis or low 1,25-dihydroxyvitamin D concentrations.

Vitamin D products can cause hypercalcemia and hypercalciuria. A higher incidence of both is seen with calcitriol. A decrease in dose or dietary calcium restriction may be required. These high calcium concentrations could aggravate verapamil and digoxin activity. Concomitant thiazides may increase the serum calcium concentrations. Cholestyramine, mineral oil, phenytoin, and barbiturates can decrease vitamin D concentrations.

Hormonal Therapy

The specific mechanisms by which estrogens protect against bone loss is still being unraveled (Fig. 83.4).[6,21] An estrogen receptor has been isolated on osteoblast, osteoclast, and macrophage cells. Estrogens produce a decrease in bone resorption, increase in calcitriol concentrations, and increase in intestinal calcium absorption and retention. Estrogens decrease cytokines and other bone-influencing compounds, which lead to decreased bone resorption.

Clinical Effectiveness

The osteoporosis consensus development conference in 1993 stated estrogen-replacement therapy (ERT) was the medication of choice for preventing osteoporosis.[51] The

Food and Drug Administration (FDA) has approved ERT for osteoporosis prevention.

Studies have shown that ERT consistently preserves both cortical and trabecular bone. The greatest positive effect is seen during the period of accelerated bone loss, immediately following menopause. A significant increase of 2–3% per year in bone mass may occur if estrogen therapy has been initiated within the first 3–6 years following menopause. This increase occurs because as an antiresorptive agent, estrogen produces a transient uncoupling of bone remodeling, slowing resorption and allowing formation to continue until a new equilibrium is established between the two.

If ERT initiation is delayed following menopause, bone mass will still be preserved but the women will have already lost substantial amount of bone secondary to the initial accelerated bone loss due to menopause. Continuous hormone replacement therapy (estrogens and progesterones, HRT) appears to be similar to cyclic HRT in preserving bone mass at cortical and trabecular bone sites.[52,53] Estradiol implants inserted every 6 months for 3 years resulted in an increase in spine and radial bone density.[54]

Women who began ERT between the ages of 61 and 70 years experienced less bone loss over 3 years than similarly aged women receiving placebo.[55] Elderly women younger than 75 years old with more than 7 years of ERT use had greater bone density than never-ERT users, but the women older than 75 years old only had significantly greater bone density of the radius.[56] Notedly, only 10% of this elderly cohort had ever used ERT.

ERT decreases osteoporotic fracture incidence.[57] Greater effects are seen with decreasing hip and spine fractures versus radius fractures. Case control studies yield a relative risk for hip fractures with ever-ERT use of 0.2–0.7.[57] Three of these studies evaluated prevention for greater than 5 years with relative risks of 0.2–0.5. Based on cohort studies, the relative risks of ever-ERT use were 0.4–1.0. In one study, which evaluated therapy for at least 15 years, the relative risk was 0.9. The preservation of this fracture prevention benefit has been concurrently evaluated in a prospective epidemiology study begun in 1986 of 9704 ambulatory, nonblack elderly women, 13% with current ERT/HRT use and 27% with past use.[58] Current users had significantly fewer wrist and nonspine fractures and a trend toward fewer hip fractures. Previous use did not influence fracture incidence. A significantly lower hip fracture incidence was seen in elderly women who had begun ERT/HRT before osteoporosis developed and were 75 years of age or older. Early onset for current users resulted in significantly fewer hip, wrist, and nonspine fractures. Late onset for current users and early and late onset for past users did not influence fracture incidence.

Clinical trials of long duration, such as the Women's Health Initiative (WHI), are required to determine the true effect of ERT/HRT in women who begin therapy around and after menopause. The WHI clinical trial enrolled women 50–79 years old in 1993–1994 into a 10-year study to evaluate the effect of low-fat diets, calcium and vitamin D supplementation, ERT/HRT, and counseling programs on the incidences of cardiovascular disease, cancer, and osteoporotic fractures.

The decision to use ERT/HRT for a woman to prevent bone loss and fractures must include the other potential benefits of ERT/HRT.[57,59] The major benefit may be the cardiovascular protective benefit, documented in numerous case control and cohort studies of early and late postmenopausal women.[57] The relative risk for cardiovascular disease calculated by a meta-analysis was 0.56 (0.5–0.61).[60] An estimated 5250 lives would be saved for every 100,000 women who use ERT.[61] The relative risk for ERT was 0.69 (0.47–1.02) and for HRT was 0.68 (0.38–1.22).[60] ERT decreases or maintains total cholesterol, decreases LDL, increases HDL, and decreases lipoprotein(a), all associated with decreasing cardiovascular risk. Of note, ERT does increase triglycerides, which increases cardiovascular risk in women.

Since transdermal ERT bypasses the liver, less positive lipid effects, which occur after about 6 months of therapy, are achieved compared with oral ERT. Combination therapy with progesterones and androgens can minimize or eliminate the positive lipid effect; however, the effect is still greater than placebo.[62] Based on the Postmenopausal Estrogen and Progesterone Intervention (PEPI) trial, a positive lipid effect was seen with continuous HRT therapy, but it was less than with cyclic ERT with micronized progesterone.[63] Other mechanisms for ERT/HRT prevention of cardiovascular disease include decreased fibrinogen and antithrombin III, increased factor VII and protein C, decreased fasting glucose and insulin, increased prostacyclin, increased blood flow, increased stroke volume, and antioxidant activity.

The other potential benefits of ERT have been validated to various degrees.[57] ERT can decrease urge and stress incontinence, vaginal atrophy, dyspareunia, and urinary tract infections. Many women experienced more energy and a positive mood, but the contrary also can be experienced, especially with HRT. Strokes may be decreased[57] and memory maintained or improved.[64] More research needs to be conducted in each of these areas.

ERT/HRT Administration

A dose–response relationship exists between bone mass and conjugated estrogens in doses of 0.3–2.5 mg, estradiol 0.05–2.0 mg, and transdermal estradiol 0.05–0.1 mg/d. The suggested doses for ERT for osteoporosis prevention are conjugated estrogens 0.625 mg, ethinyl estradiol 0.02 mg, estropipate 0.625 mg, esterified estrogens 0.625 mg, estradiol 0.5 mg, and transdermal estradiol 0.05 mg/day.

Since inexpensive, accurate techniques for assessing bone response are not available to determine the efficacy of lower doses, standard doses should be used. Vaginal administration results in significant systemic absorption. None of the ERT products are considered interchangeable. Each product produces different estradiol and estrone concentrations. Estradiol is the predominant estrogen before menopause, while estrone is the predominant estrogen after menopause.

No theories exist for the best estrogen compound for bone and cardiovascular protection. Oral estradiol is converted via the first-pass effect to estrone. The major and minor components of conjugated estrogens have some bone and cardiovascular protection effects. In the long-term epidemiology studies, the majority of patients used conjugated estrogens.

The most common regimens are continuous or cyclic. Continuous therapy is initiated first because 60–80% of women will be amenorrheic 6–12 months after starting therapy and fewer women will have hyperplasia.[65,66] However, until then, random spotting and bleeding will occur. For continuous therapy, conjugated estrogen 0.625 mg or equivalent is administered daily and medroxyprogesterone 10 mg is administered for 10–14 days at the beginning of the month or 2.5–5.0 mg is administered daily. For the cyclic regimen, conjugated estrogen 0.625 mg or equivalent is administered for 3 weeks, with medroxyprogesterone 10 mg administered for the last 10–14 days. Medroxyprogesterone for 12–14 days produces less endometrial hyperplasia than dosage for 10 days. Investigations with medroxyprogesterone 10 mg for 10–14 days every 3, 4, 6, or 12 months is ongoing. Preliminary results suggest quarterly progesterone may be of benefit.[67]

The duration of therapy is not known. Based on a cohort study with 68% of the women receiving ERT or HRT for more than 10 years, ERT/HRT was found to sustain a decrease in both cortical and trabecular bone loss compared to non-ERT/HRT users.[68] The effects of long-term therapy begun early after menopause may not yield the same results as long-term therapy begun later in life. Epidemiology data support conflicting views of the effect of short- and long-term ERT/HRT when measured in elderly women.[56,58] Long-term clinical trials such as the WHI provide information on the benefits and adverse reactions of long-term therapy.

With regard to duration, another concern with stopping ERT/HRT is the accelerated rate of bone loss experienced in both early and late postmenopausal women users on discontinuation. A group of women treated with estrogens for 4 years, followed by 4 years of no estrogen, showed the same degree of bone loss as a control group followed for 8 years.[69] All the bone loss in the former group occurred during the nondrug phase of the study. When elderly women stop ERT, accelerated late bone loss was also experienced but the amount of bone mass at the end of the study was still higher than the never-ERT users.[55] ERT/HRT therapy shifts the bone density curve to give women higher amounts of bone mass at later years in their life. Currently lifetime use of estrogens is being considered. This decision may be driven more by ERT/HRT cardiovascular protection and other proven and investigational benefits than osteoporosis fracture prevention. Of note, the positive lipid effect with ERT was maintained for at least 20 years.[70]

The risks of ERT/HRT must be considered when advocating these medications for osteoporosis prevention and treatment. Unopposed ERT for more than 6 months causes up to a tenfold increase in endometrial cancer.[57,71] Concomitant progesterone therapy for at least 10–14 days a month usually eliminates this risk, even to lower than that of nonusers. Progesterone therapy is not needed for women with a hysterectomy.

Meta-analysis of the ERT/breast cancer data yields composite relative risks around 1, supporting the fact that ERT does not increase breast cancer.[57] The relative risks do increase with duration of use, predominantly after 15–20 years of therapy. More data on ERT/HRT users for long-term durations need to be collected to assess the true risk. The WHI study will provide some of these answers. ERT/HRT is associated with benign increased breast density on mammography.

Of note, women who develop endometrial or breast cancer while on ERT generally have longer survival times. Proposed theories include better access to health care, earlier detection with better survival rates, and less cardiovascular disease. Cardiovascular deaths are the most common cause of death in cancer patients. In the past, ERT/HRT was absolutely contraindicated for breast cancer patients. Clinical trials have been published and are ongoing in this subset of women. Preliminary results in women in breast cancer remission are promising in terms of safety and efficacy of ERT.[72]

Common adverse reactions for HRT include vaginal spotting and bleeding; breast tenderness and breast enlargement, especially in older women; pedal edema; and weight gain. On the cyclic therapy, vaginal bleeding should be evaluated if bleeding occurs on days 1–9 or 16–31 if progestin is given for the first 10 days.[59] For the continuous regimen, vaginal bleeding needs to be evaluated if bleeding is heavier than premenopause periods, lasts for more than 10 days, occurs more than once a month, and persists after 10 months of therapy.[59] Uncommon adverse reactions are facial hair growth, bloating, nausea, vomiting, leg pain, headache/migraines, increase or decrease in sexual desire, dizziness, and mood changes. Rare events include skin darkening, acne, rash, loss of pubic hair, stomach pain, and jaundice. A 2.5-fold increase in cholelithiasis exists. Although the package insert states increased thromboembolic events, no thromboembolic events have been reported or *in vitro* alterations measured with ERT/HRT. ERT/HRT may decrease the metabolism of corticosteroids, oral anticoagulants, and tricyclic antidepressants, resulting in a return of the underlying disease. Enzyme inducers and smoking may increase estrogen metabolism.

Women with active estrogen-dependent cancers should not receive ERT/HRT. All abnormal genital bleeding needs an evaluation before starting HRT therapy. Current thromboembolic disease is considered a relative contraindication by some, whereas some consider thromboembolic disease during pregnancy or with past oral contraceptive use an absolute contraindication.

Based on the National Prescription Audit and the National Disease and Therapeutic Index, approximately one out of every four to six women received ERT/HRT in 1992.[73] Of the users, 62% were 40–59 years old. Women were more likely to use ERT if suggested by a physician.[74] Of prescriptions written for ERT/HRT in 1992, 50–60% came from gynecologists and 20% from family medicine or general practitioners.[73]

Compliance with ERT/HRT is an important issue for pharmacists to address. The two most common reasons women discontinue usage are vaginal bleeding and breast tenderness. Women need to be educated about vaginal bleeding and its suspected onset, frequency, and duration. Dosage manipulations may need to be done to control and eliminate vaginal bleeding. If amenorrhea does not develop after 1 year, predictable bleeding patterns with cyclic therapy may be preferred. Breast tenderness may decrease with time. The use of an exercise or more supportive bra and/or wearing the bra to bed may decrease tenderness. The benefits versus the adverse reactions must be continually reemphasized.

Pharmacoeconomic studies support ERT use for fracture prevention, especially when cardiovascular disease is included in the model. Assuming 90% of high-risk and 70% of moderate-risk women took HRT for 15 years beginning at age 50, $5.1 million dollars would be saved for every 100,000 women.[75] Based on a model with hip fractures, cardiovascular mortality, and endometrial and breast cancer predictions, 5 years of ERT would yield 1593 quality adjusted life years (QALY) and 25 years would yield 6314 QALY.[76]

Tamoxifen

Tamoxifen has been found to be both an estrogen antagonist, thus its breast cancer prevention effect, and an estrogen agonist, thus its osteoporosis and cardiovascular disease prevention effect. Tamoxifen 10 mg twice daily for 5 years was associated with an increase in lumbar bone density (0.8%) while the placebo group lost bone density (−0.7%, $p = 0.06$) even after adjusting for body mass index, exercise, and calcium intake.[77] Tamoxifen may also prevent cardiovascular disease but has been associated with an increase in endometrial cancer. Once FDA approved, tamoxifen may be an option for preventing osteoporosis in breast cancer patients.

Tibolone

Tibolone is a synthetic hormone being evaluated as an estrogen substitute. Preliminary data suggest that tibolone may not cause vaginal bleeding but will still be effective at decreasing bone loss.[78]

Oral Contraceptives

The association of past use of oral contraceptives on bone density in later life has been assessed with epidemiology studies.[79,80] A retrospective analysis of 2297 women revealed that past oral contraceptive use resulted in greater spine, distal radius and ulnar bone densities.[79] In contrast, data from the Royal College of General Practitioners Oral Contraceptive prospective epidemiology study of 23,000 women recruited in 1968–1969 showed no protective effect of ever use of oral contraceptives on fracture rate.[80]

Oral contraceptives have been explored to maintain bone mass in premenopausal,[81] elite athletes and anorexia nervosa patients[82] with amenorrhea, and in perimenopausal women.[83] Amenorrheic women due to hypothalmic or ovarian disorders responded to 0.03 mg ethinyl estradiol and 0.15 mg desogestrel for 12–24 months with an increase in lumbar spine and Ward's triangle bone densities compared to baseline values but not with femoral neck, tibial diaphysis, or tibial epiphysis bone densities.[81] In anorexia nervosa women with amenorrhea, oral contraceptive use resulted in higher lumbar spine but not femoral neck bone densities.[82] In perimenopausal women between 40 and 49 years old, 2 years of ethinyl estradiol and desogestrel resulted in increased vertebral bone density compared to the group receiving only calcium.[83] Since estrogen deficiency is associated with an accelerated rate of bone loss, in the future oral contraceptive use during the perimenopausal time frame may allow women to experience no periods of estrogen deficiency. However, the safety of oral contraceptives in older women still needs to be further established.

Progesterones

Progesterones have been shown to retard bone loss when administered alone. Medroxyprogesterone 20 mg daily for 2 years prevented loss of cortical bone, but not of trabecular bone in the spine.[84] The addition of progesterone to estrogen therapy does not seem to have any additional beneficial bone effects compared with estrogen alone. Progesterones minimize estrogen's positive HDL elevations but decrease estrogen's negative triglyceride elevations. Progesterones are also associated with most of the side effects of combination therapy such as withdrawal bleeding and mood changes. Consequently, progesterone use in women without an intact uterus is unwarranted.

Testosterone

Methyltestosterone is being coadministered with estrogen therapy when decreased libido, sexual function or energy level, depression, or headaches exist during ERT/HRT.[85] Testosterone implants given every 6 months are being investigated. Methyltestosterone may have virilizing adverse effects and potentially impact the lipid profile. In some of the osteoporosis and menopause studies, a significant negative lipid effect has not been measured.

Testosterone replacement therapy has been used in hypogonadal men but its use for prevention of bone loss in men has been minimally studied. Testosterone concentrations decrease with aging in men.[8] In testosterone-deficient men, 10–115 months of replacement therapy resulted in increased distal bone density[86] or spinal bone density.[87] A transdermal testosterone patch is being evaluated for replacement therapy. Testosterone is contraindicated in men with prostatic cancer and should be used cautiously in men with prostatic hypertrophy. Adverse reactions include liver toxicity, gynecomastia, and painful erections.

Calcitonin

Salmon calcitonin is approved by the FDA for prevention of postmenopausal osteoporosis and Paget's disease. Salmon calcitonin is 50 times more potent than human calcitonin. A feedback system exists between calcium, calcitonin, and parathyroid hormone with high serum calcium concentrations increasing serum calcitonin and thus decreasing resorption.[9] Receptors for calcitonin have been found on osteoclasts and renal cell membranes. Stimulation of these receptors results in a decrease in osteoclastic activity and a renal effect of decreasing tubular reabsorption of sodium and calcium. Calcitonin decreases osteoclast bone attachment, motility, life span, and numbers along with altering the cellular structure. Bone density is preserved because the mineral, matrix, and collagen material is not broken down and, potentially, by a positive effect on osteoblasts.

Clinical Effectiveness

Clinical trials have shown a stabilization or increase in bone mass, especially lumbar bone density.[88,89] Cortical bone either remains constant or has a slight increase. Most studies have had insufficient patient samples and short durations to assess fracture rate, especially hip fractures. However, a few studies show no change to protection against vertebral fractures.[87,89–91] Patients with high bone turnover respond better than those with normal or low bone turnover rates, however, elderly women, those assumed to have low bone turnover rate, have been shown to have decreased bone resorption with calcitonin.[90] Calcitonin also has a beneficial effect for steroid-induced osteoporosis, a high bone turnover state.

Calcitonin has gained additional interest for osteoporosis pain control.[92] Both subcutaneous and intranasal administration bring pain relief within 1–12 weeks to patients with osteoporotic or metastatic bone pain. Daily administration is initially used and then decreased to 50–100 IU two to three times a week. Potential mechanisms of action include decreased prostaglandin synthesis, altered intracellular calcium concentrations, increased beta endorphin synthesis, or a direct effect.

Calcitonin Administration

Some trials with continuous administration for 2 years have found the bone density effect to plateau or decrease after 12–18 months. Potentially, the neutralizing antibodies, which develop in 40–70% of patients treated with subcutaneous calcitonin, can minimize calcitonin's effect and may be partly responsible for the resistance sometimes observed with continuous long-term treatment. To overcome resistance, intermittent therapy such as 50 IU intranasally five times per week, 100 IU subcutaneously every day for 10 days each month, or 100 IU subcutaneously for 3 months and then no treatment for 1 month is being investigated. Intranasal calcitonin 50 IU/day for 5 days each week with 500 mg daily supplemental calcium for 5 years significantly increased lumbar bone density (1.8%) compared to calcium alone (–5.8%).[89] Concomitant calcium and, when needed, vitamin D should be used.

Compliance with subcutaneous calcitonin is often poor because of the need to administer calcitonin by injection and its expense. Intranasal calcitonin spray and rectal suppositories are being investigated. Calcitonin nasal absorption is 10–25%. Nasal administration produces fewer side effects. Side effects of subcutaneous administration are nausea, anorexia, diarrhea, stomach discomfort, abdominal pain, salty taste, injection site pain, and flushing. Most side effects decrease over time and may also decrease with nighttime administration.

Bisphosphonates

Bisphosphonates adsorb to bone hydroxyapatite, become a permanent part of bone structure, and are resistant to enzymatic hydrolysis. The estimated half-life of bisphosphonates is similar to the half-life of bone (1–10 years). When osteoclasts bind to the bisphosphonate bone surface, its structure and function are altered, preventing adherence. When osteoclasts phagocytize bone crystals containing these agents, their metabolic activity is inhibited and their ability to resorb additional bone is reduced. Etidronate also inhibits bone mineralization and osteomalacia may result.

Clinical Effectiveness

Initial studies with bisphosphonates were conducted in small samples with short durations while later studies were conducted with larger samples and placebo controlled, randomized, long duration study designs.[93] Only women with osteoporosis have been enrolled except for one study. Therefore, bisphosphonates are reserved for treatment versus prevention of osteoporosis. The effect of bisphosphonates is greater for lumbar bone than cortical, however, unlike fluoride, cortical bone is not weakened as a result of increasing lumbar bone density. Etidronate has been administered as an intermittent regimen with various other agents to create a coherence regimen. The additional agents have not augmented etidronate's activity. Intermittent single-agent etidronate decreased new vertebral fracture rate for the first 2 years, increased vertebral fracture rate in the third year, and decreased vertebral fractures in the fourth year in women at greatest risk, those with at least three vertebral fractures at baseline.[94] Daily low-dose pamidronate resulted in increased spine and trochanter bone density, no change in femoral neck and Ward's triangle, and a trend toward decreased vertebral fractures ($p = 0.07$).[95] Alendronate decreased lumbar but not femoral bone density.[96]

Bisphosphonate Administration

Intermittent etidronate is currently the only FDA-approved bisphosphonate regimen for osteoporosis treatment. Pamidronate is approved for Paget's disease and malignant hypercalcemia but not for osteoporosis treatment. Alendronate is pending FDA approval for osteoporosis treatment. Investigational bisphosphonates include clodronate, tiludronate, residronate, and many others. Calcium and, when needed, vitamin D should also be used but administered at different times. Bisphosphonates are poorly absorbed, 1–5%. Food significantly decreases their absorption. Nausea and diarrhea are the most common side effects.

Investigational Bone Antiresorption Therapy

Ipriflavone and strontium can decrease bone resorption.[48] Ipriflavone inhibits osteoclast production, inhibits PTH responsiveness, and increases osteoblast maturation. Clinical trials with ipriflavone have found an increase in radial bone density, no change in lumbar bone density, and a decrease in bone pain. Strontium can replace calcium in bone and uncouple resorption and formation; however, high doses may decrease bone strength. In one study, diclofenac sodium 150 mg/d for 4 weeks positively changed bone resorption biochemical markers in the subset of responding postmenopausal women.[97] Since prostaglandins may have a role in bone remodeling, NSAIDs through their decreased prostaglandin production effect could influence bone. Other antiresorptive investigational agents include echistatin and potassium bicarbonate to create a better acid–base balance in the body, thereby, minimizing bone destruction to correct acid imbalances.

BONE FORMATION TREATMENTS

Fluoride

Fluoride is approved in some countries for osteoporosis treatment, but not in the United States. Fluoride (sodium fluoride or monofluorophosphate) has a predominant effect of increasing bone formation in cancellous bone. Through a mitogenic effect, fluoride may increase osteoblasts. The fluoride ion serves as a hydroxy radical in the hydroxyapatite crystals, forming fluorapatite. Fluorapatite alters the size and structure of crystals resulting in increased bone crystallinity and a decrease in solubility. The net effect is a mineral system more resistant to resorption. Adequate calcium concentrations are required. Furthermore, fluoride also produces an uncoupling of the remodeling process, which favors formation over resorption. The remodeling cycle is prolonged because a longer time frame between matrix formation and mineralization exists. Bone density has been shown to increase with fluoride, but the bone formed may be somewhat disorganized, resulting in immature woven bone rather than lamellar bone. This type of bone appears to be more resistant to compressive forces but less to torsional strain, which is believed to be responsible for hip fractures. New bone forms on existing bone but does not build new bridges between old bone.

Clinical Effectiveness

The increase in bone mass with fluoride treatment may be related to dose and duration.[98] Fracture risk is not always decreased. Sustained release sodium fluoride 25 mg twice daily decreased the vertebral fracture rate,[99] whereas higher doses such as 90 and 60 mg on alternate days did not.[98] When first-year fractures are excluded, significant decreases in vertebral fracture rate can be seen. Twenty to 40% of fluoride users will be nonresponders. Intermittent fluoride regimens are currently being explored. Patients with the greatest bone density increases have fewer fractures.

Hip and peripheral fractures have been increased in some studies. Despite calcium supplementation, enough calcium may not be absorbed to mineralize the large amounts of newly formed matrix in the cancellous bone, resulting in the removal of mineral from cortical bone. Use of lower doses and sustained-release products with sufficient calcium and vitamin D may decrease the negative effect on cortical bone.

Fluoride Administration

Currently lower doses (10–20 mg fluoride), sustained-release products, and intermittent therapy are being investigated. The 1993 consensus on osteoporosis recommended low doses for less than 5 years.[98] The currently available product, sodium fluoride, contains 1.1 mg of elemental fluoride for every 2.2 mg. Disodium monofluorophosphate 200 mg is equivalent to 16.4 mg of elemental fluoride. At least 1–1.5 g of calcium and, when needed, vitamin D should also be prescribed. Calcium and fluoride should be given individually to prevent chemical binding, because about 25% less fluoride is absorbed when fluoride and calcium are administered concurrently. Of note, some of the monofluorophosphate products are being developed as combination products with calcium. Antacids can also decrease fluoride absorption. Since about 40–70% of a fluoride dose is cleared by the kidneys, dosage adjustments are required for patients with creatinine clearances less than 50 mL/min. The average half-life of fluoride is 3–7 hours in patients with normal renal function.

No established recommendations exist for monitoring fluoride. Some studies that allowed dosage alterations decreased the dose when the alkaline phosphatase, osteocalcin, or hydroxyproline excretion increased by 50% or more or increased the dose if no changes were seen.[98,99] Gastrointestinal and osteoarticular symptoms represent the most commonly seen adverse effects. Gastrointestinal symptoms include nausea, vomiting, diarrhea, abdominal pain, and occasional gastrointestinal bleeding. Osteoarticular symptoms include plantar facial pain, periarticular pain, synovitis, and arthritis. Symptoms disappear within 1–8 weeks after discontinuation and generally reappear if reinstituted, even at a lower dose. These symptoms have been shown to be reduced significantly with the use of lower doses and slow-release products.

Androgens and Anabolic Steroids

Androgens may enhance osteoblast activity. An androgen receptor has been isolated on osteoblast cells.[85] The effect on muscle mass and the relationship between muscle mass, strengthening, and weight-bearing exercise and increased bone mass may also explain androgen's effect. Nandrolone decanoate 50 mg IM every 2–4 weeks increased forearm[101] or vertebral bone density.[102] Stanozolol 2 mg three times per day for 21 days and then no medication for 7 days resulted in a lower parathyroid concentration, less calcium loss, and increased total body calcium, but no change in radial bone density.[103] Oxandrolone has not been shown to have a beneficial effect on bone mass. Methandrostenolone increases total body calcium in postmenopausal women, but clinical studies have been disappointing. Most women develop adverse reactions such as liver function alterations, negative lipid effects, hirsutism, hoarseness, acne, and other virilizing adverse effects, thus limiting androgen use.

INVESTIGATIONAL BONE FORMATION AGENTS

Recombinant growth hormone[104,105] and growth factors (IGF-I, IGF-II, TGF_B)[104] have been investigated for treating osteoporosis in small numbers of patients for short and long time frames. Growth hormone increases IGF-I production by the liver and osteoblasts. Growth hormone and IGF-I receptors exist on bone cells. Growth hormone and IGF have been associated with stimulating both bone formation and bone resorption, whereas TGF_B also increased bone formation but decreased bone resorption. Aging decreases both growth hormone and IFG-I. In the elderly, growth hormone increases IGF-I levels.

In growth hormone clinical trials, bone formation and bone resorption have been stimulated based on blood and urine indices but minimal to no changes occur in bone density. In children and adults, growth hormone has been associated with the following adverse reactions: glucose intolerance, hyperinsulinemia, hypertension, edema, and aggravated carpel tunnel syndrome. Side effects also occurred with growth factors. Means of delivering these agents to the site of action or determining the dosage required for bone but not systemic effects are being explored. Most likely these agents will not be given as single agents but may have a future role with combination therapy to stimulate and/or mimic the normal bone remodeling process. These agents have been used in coherence regimens.

PTH stimulates bone turnover, differentiation of new bone and remodeling units, and renal tubular reabsorption of calcium, but the few clinical studies reported do not show any significant benefit.[105]

COHERENCE THERAPY

Perhaps the most logical approach to management of osteoporosis is the theoretical model first described by Frost and now referred to as the activation-depression-free-repeat (ADFR) regimen, also called coherence therapy.[105] This model exploits the normal remodeling sequence as it is now understood. The first phase requires use of an agent that increases the activation of new BMUs; this could be achieved by administration of PTH, thyroid hormone, 1,25-vitamin D, or growth hormone. The second phase would shift the bone balance within the particular BMU with such agents as calcitonin and bisphosphonates, which would inhibit the activation of newly generated osteoblasts but not osteoclasts. The net result would be an overfilling of the BMUs with osteoblasts because of the absence of inhibiting factors; thus bone mass would increase.

GLUCOCORTICOID-INDUCED OSTEOPOROSIS

The true incidence of osteoporosis in patients receiving oral glucocorticoids is unknown. The available data have suggested a 30–50% incidence of atraumatic fractures.[26] Most of the incidence data is derived from cross-sectional, single-point measurements compared to nonsteroid users. From the few longitudinal studies and clinical trials of sufficient duration, bone loss began within the first 6–12 months of therapy. The bone loss rate has been reported faster during the initiation of therapy and decreased with long-term duration. Trabecular bone has a greater loss than cortical bone.

The true effect of inhaled steroids is still being evaluated. Short-term inhaled steroid studies relied predominantly on biochemical markers and suggested that high-dose inhaled steroids can decrease markers of formation and increase markers of resorption.[26] Most inhaler studies have been confounded by patients' previous oral steroid use and short-course oral burst therapies. In the only study with new asthmatics nieve to steroids, beclomethasone at doses of 200, 1000, and 2000 μg/d for 3 weeks each decreased osteocalcin but increased serum calcium.[106] Due to the very short study durations, long-term effects are still unknown but probably minimal with standard therapy.

Glucocorticoids decrease bone formation and increase bone resorption as a result of steroid effects on calcium balance, osteoclasts, osteoblasts and muscle strength.[26,107] Patients receiving glucocorticoids have decreased osteocalcin concentrations, a marker of decreased formation, and increased urinary hydroxyproline excretion, a marker of resorption. The amount of bone replaced during each remodeling cycle is reduced by 30%. The decrease in calcium gastrointestinal absorption and increase in renal excretion leads to a negative calcium balance and secondary hyperparathyroidism. Steroids seem to have a direct effect on intestinal calcium absorption since vitamin D concentrations are usually within normal ranges or elevated. As parathyroid hormone and vitamin D concentrations increase and calcitonin production decreases, osteoclast activity increases. A greater surface area of bone undergoes osteoclast resorption. A decrease in the replication, differentiation, and life span of osteoblasts occurs. Decreases in gonadal hormone secretion (ovarian, testicular, and adrenal) lead to decreased production of prostaglandin E_2 and IGF-I. The inhibition of IGF-I production and action results in increased sensitivity by bone to the effects of PTH and 1,25-hydroxyvitamin D.

Osteonecrosis, also called aseptic necrosis, and muscle wasting are serious complications of steroid therapy. Aseptic necrosis usually involves the femoral and humeral heads causing intense pain and decreased mobility. The metabolic effects induced by steroids cause a substantial loss of muscle strength, which can result in osteoporosis. Muscle weakness, resulting from myopathy, may contribute to bone loss by removing the normal forces on bone produced by strong muscle contraction and the immobility imposed by the weakness. Both situations could increase the rate of bone loss.

Men and women are equally susceptible to the effects of glucocorticoids on bone. Daily doses of 7.5 mg or more of prednisone cause substantial loss of trabecular bone in most patients. Smaller doses have fewer effects on premenopausal women; however, men and postmenopausal women may lose bone, even on low-dose therapy. Longer duration and total doses of greater than 10 g of prednisone are associated with osteoporosis development. Other risk factors include age older than 50 years, low bone density at the onset of therapy, high bone turnover rates, and family history. Risk factors for osteoporosis probably increase the likelihood of glucocorticoid-induced osteoporosis.

DETECTION

Monitoring schemes to assess glucocorticoid-induced osteoporosis have been suggested but not validated.[26,107] Measurement of urinary calcium excretion may be helpful in assessing calcium balance and susceptibility to secondary hyperparathyroidism. Serum osteocalcin levels and total urinary hydroxyproline excretion may be useful. Because vitamin D deficiency will augment the adverse effects of steroid therapy on bone, serum vitamin D or 1,25-vitamin D could be measured to assess vitamin D status.

X-ray examination may be useful in steroid-induced osteoporosis. Vertical and horizontal trabeculae tend to be equally thin, providing a uniformly translucent appearance of the vertebrae, ribs, and pelvis. Pseudocallus formations, cartilaginous callus that becomes highly mineralized in an amorphous fashion at the site of stress fractures, may occur in large numbers. They represent a hallmark finding since they are not seen in postmenopausal or senile osteoporosis.

PREVENTION AND TREATMENT

Although steroids have been used therapeutically for four decades, well-established prevention and treatment therapies for glucocorticoid-induced osteoporosis have not been determined.[26,107] The most common recommendation made is to discontinue therapy, however, alternative treatments may not be available for the underlying disease. Steroid exposure should be minimized by using the lowest possible dose for the shortest period of time. Alternate-day therapy, although effective for reducing other adverse effects, does not appear to lessen bone loss. Although not yet available in the United States, deflazacort, a derivative of prednisone, has been used in Europe with promising results of reduced catabolic effects, including steroid-induced bone loss.[108] Low-dose inhalation therapy may have less bone loss.

Some of the other medications used to prevent and treat regular osteoporosis may be of some benefit.[26,107] Most of the prevention and treatment studies were short term, had small sample sizes and measured calcium balance or biochemical markers versus bone density and fracture prevention. Supplemental calcium, thiazides, and vitamin D therapy may increase calcium absorption, decrease calcium urinary excretion, and/or reverse negative calcium balance. Estrogen replacement therapy (0.625 mg conjugated estrogens or equivalent daily), subcutaneous or intranasal calcitonin, etidronate (400 mg daily for 2 weeks and then off for 11 weeks), pamidronate 150 mg with 1 g calcium per day, or nandrolone decanoate have improved calcium balance and/or decreased vertebral bone loss. Vitamin D therapy may produce hypercalcemia and nandrolone decanoate can produce virilizing adverse reactions. Fluoride therapy did not significantly improve response in some of the studies.

OSTEOMALACIA

Osteomalacia results from abnormal mineralization of new bone matrix. In children and adolescents, osteomalacia is called rickets and affects their growth due to defective calcification of the epiphyseal cartilage. Since bone remodeling occurs in all bones and throughout life, unmineralized matrix accumulates in the whole skeleton and can produce abnormal and weak bone structure.

EPIDEMIOLOGY

The incidence of osteomalacia is not known. In the United States, the specific incidence is thought to be low due to vitamin D-supplemented foods and sun exposure. However, in the United States, 22% of patients with hip fractures had abnormally low 25-hydroxyvitamin D concentrations and 30% had hyperosteroidosis.[109] Further, almost 60% of elderly nursing home residents had serum vitamin D levels that were below normal during the summer and 81% had abnormal vitamin D levels during the winter.[110] In countries with vitamin D-deficient diets or decreased dermal exposure to sun such as women fully clad due to religious or cultural beliefs, osteomalacia can be found. Asian diets are also high in phytates, which bind calcium decreasing its absorption and lignins, which bind bile acids decreasing vitamin D absorption. The incidences may also be low due to a lack of detection and misdiagnosis. Many women with osteoporosis may have osteomalacia or both diseases.

PATHOPHYSIOLOGY

Numerous causes of osteomalacia exist (Table 83.10), each with its own special characteristics.[9,13,111] The main pathologic categories are vitamin D metabolism abnormalities, phosphate deficiency, mineralization defects, rapid bone formation, and miscellaneous causes. Defective matrix mineralization results from lack of calcium and phosphate substrate and/or osteoblast or cellular dysfunction. Osteoblast dysfunction is responsible for the increased thickness observed at the osteoid seams. Matrix synthesis continues at a normal rate while maturation and mineralization are defective. Osteoblast function may be normal with defective mineralization due to deficits of calcium, phosphorus, or both. These deficits may also influence osteoblast activity. The amount of calcium and phosphate in the body is controlled by a feedback system between calcium and phosphate serum concentrations, parathyroid hormone, 1,25-vitamin D and calcitonin (Fig. 83.5).[9] Nonmineralized or poorly mineralized osteoid occurs in both cortical and trabecular bone. As a result, less mineral than normal exists for a given bone volume, making it weak and potentially irregular in structure.

Aging can result in osteomalacia. Aging is associated with decreased sun exposure, thus decreasing dermal production of vitamin D; decreased kidney or liver function, which decreases the metabolism of vitamin D to its active moiety; decreased nutrition, leading to decreased calcium and vitamin D absorption; and decreased GI responsiveness to vitamin D.

DRUG-INDUCED OSTEOMALACIA

Induction of hepatic microsomal oxidase enzymes that accelerate the conversion of vitamin D and its metabolites to rapidly excreted inactive compounds is the most common drug-induced cause of osteomalacia. Phenytoin is frequently implicated because of its high usage pattern and, to a lesser extent, phenobarbital. Potentially any hepatic oxidase-inducing drug could reduce levels of vitamin D metabolites. Etidronate and fluoride can alter bone mineralization. Excessive aluminum-containing antacids and high-dose calcium supplementation ingestion can create a phosphate deficiency state due to phophorous/phosphate binding. Aluminum can also be absorbed and accumulate in patients with severe renal impairment or who are undergoing hemodialysis. Potential mechanisms for aluminum-induced osteomalacia include suppression of parathyroid hormone secretion, inhibition of osteoblasts, or interference with hydroxyapatite crystal formation.[111] Individuals at highest risk for developing drug-induced osteomalacia are those receiving high doses, having marginal daily intakes of vitamin D, and receiving inadequate exposure to sunlight.

CLINICAL PRESENTATION

Patients with osteomalacia generally complain of easy fatigability, malaise, and bone pain. The pain is diffuse, dull and aching, poorly localized, and accompanied by bone tenderness. Muscle strain, weight bearing, or pressure on a bone worsens the pain with pain greater at night. Long-standing osteomalacia with vague pain has been misdiagnosed as muscular rheumatism, arthritis, or herniated lumbar disks. Skeletal deformities are caused by softening of the bone and include bowing, gibbous, and pigeon chest. The spinal manifestations may lead to scoliosis, kyphosis, and shortening of the spine. Changes in height caused by vertebral collapse are not seen unless osteoporosis is also present. In fact, vertebral collapse may be prevented by osteomalacia, because it produces increased bone elasticity, which dissipates acute stress more easily. Growth retarda-

TABLE 83.10. PATHOGENESIS OF OSTEOMALACIA AND RICKETS

- Abnormalities in vitamin D metabolism
  - Vitamin D deficiency
    - Nutritional deficiency
    - Lack of exposure to sunlight
    - Malabsorption syndromes
  - Abnormal dermal production of vitamin D_3
    - Chronic renal failure
    - Aging
  - Abnormal hepatic synthesis of 25-hydroxyvitamin D
    - Primary biliary cirrhosis
    - Biliary atresia
    - Biliary fistula
  - Defective renal synthesis of 1,25-dihydroxyvitamin D
    - Hypoparathyroidism
    - Pseudohypoparathyroidism
    - Chronic renal failure
    - Vitamin D-dependent rickets type I
    - Hypophosphatemic rickets
    - Tumor-induced osteomalacia
    - Age-related osteomalacia
  - Defective end-organ response to 1,25-dihydroxyvitamin D
    - Vitamin D-dependent rickets type II
    - Anticonvulsant drugs
  - Renal loss of vitamin D-binding protein
    - Nephrotic syndrome
- Phosphate deficiency
  - Diminished intake
    - Neonatal rickets
    - Excess aluminum hydroxide ingestion
  - Impaired renal tubular reabsorption of phosphate
    - Primary renal tubular defects
      - X-linked hypophosphatemic osteomalacia
      - Adult onset hypophosphatemic osteomalacia
- Phosphate deficiency (cont.)
      - Sporadic acquired hypophosphatemic osteomalacia
      - Fanconi syndromes
        - Wilson's disease
        - Lowe's disease
        - Glycogen storage disease
        - Cystinosis
    - Secondary renal tubular "defects"
      - Primary hyperparathyroidism
      - Secondary hyperparathyroidism
      - Renal tubular acidosis
      - Tumor-induced osteomalacia
- Defects in mineralization
  - Enzyme deficiency
    - Hypophosphatasia
  - Circulating inhibitors of calcification
    - Chronic renal failure
    - Hypophosphatasia (increased pyrophosphate)
    - Drugs and ions
    - Diphosphonates
    - Fluoride
    - Aluminum or iron intoxication
  - Abnormal bone collagen or matrix
    - Chronic renal failure
    - Osteogenesis imperfecta
    - Fibrogenesis imperfecta ossium
- States of rapid bone formation
  - Postoperative primary hyperparathyroidism with florid osteitis fibrosa cystica
  - Osteopetrosis
- Miscellaneous
  - Parenteral alimentation (aluminum intoxication)

(From Ref. 111.)

tion, abnormal teeth, and changes in the skull bones occur in children with untreated rickets. Muscle weakness is frequently seen and proximal weakness in the lower extremities may lead to a waddling gait. Muscle wasting may also occur. Unwillingness to tense muscles because of increased pain may appear as muscle weakness. Severe hypocalcemia may cause paresthesias, muscle cramps, and tetany. Hypophosphatemia may explain some of the muscle weakness. Pseudofractures and fractures may occur later in the disease course. Especially in the elderly, fractures may be labeled erroneously secondary to osteoporosis rather than osteomalacia or a combination of the two.

BIOCHEMICAL AND ROENTGENOGRAPHIC CHANGES

Low serum calcium and phosphate and increased alkaline phosphatase and parathyroid hormone concentrations are common. In mild cases, these values may be normal even though the histologic evidence suggests osteomalacia. Urinary excretion of less than 100 mg of calcium over 24 hours is suggestive of osteomalacia and should warrant a workup. Various etiologies of osteomalacia offer a different biochemical picture and may help in identifying the underlying cause[13] (Table 83.5).

Skeletal x-ray films show a generalized picture of osteopenia in both cortical and trabecular bone.[13] These films show thin cortices and fuzzy trabeculae with a ground-glass appearance at the osteoid seams. Unmineralized osteoid produces ribbonlike transverse and incomplete zones of radiolucency. The most distinctive feature, however, is the occurrence of pseudofractures, which are also referred to as Looser's lines or Milkman's fractures. These represent stress fractures in which the normal process of healing is impaired by the mineralization defect of osteomalacia. They appear on x-ray films as symmetric radiolucent bands. Fractures and pseudofrac-

TABLE 83.11. USUAL RANGE OF ADULT VITAMIN D DOSES FOR TYPES OF OSTEOMALACIA CLASSIFIED BY MECHANISM

Disease	Vitamin D Dose[a] (mg/d)
Vitamin D deficiency	0.025–0.125
Vitamin D malabsorption	0.1–10.0[b,c]
Liver disease (impaired 25-OH-D formation)	0.25–1.0[c]
Anticonvulsants (increased 25-OH-D metabolism)	0.05–1.25
Impaired formation of 1,25-$(OH)_2D$ (vitamin D dependent, CRF[d])	0.25–7.5[b,c]
Vitamin D resistance	Varies

[a]Use of either ergocalciferol (D_2) or cholecalciferol (D_3), 10 μg = 400 IU.
[b]Exact dose depends on specific cause.
[c]May require a vitamin D metabolite to overcome conversion limitations.
[d]Chronic renal failure.

tures associated with osteomalacia usually show increased uptake of bone-seeking isotopes with external scanning, sometimes misinterpreted as a primary malignancy with metastases to bone.

TREATMENT

Management of the underlying disease state should be undertaken. For osteomalacia, vitamin D or one of its metabolites is usually required; the dose and duration differ markedly according to the specific etiology (Table 83.11). Supplemental phosphorus is administered when phosphorus depletion occurs and may need to be given alone or in combination with vitamin D. If osteoporosis existed concurrently, bone recovery is incomplete and the patient will still be at risk of sustaining a fracture.

Initial treatment restores vitamin D metabolite concentrations, normal osteoblastic function, and normal mineralization. The amount needed to replete the stores varies between disease states, between patients, and even within the same patient at various times. A vitamin D dose that is below the expected dose required to manage the specific type of osteomalacia, as outlined in Table 83.11, should be initiated. At a constant dose, steady-state equilibrium is reached in 4–6 weeks. If 1,25-vitamin D is used, a higher dose may be initiated because its half-life is shorter than other vitamin D preparations, permitting easier and safer titration. Steady state will be achieved sooner. At steady state, an additional 4 weeks of therapy is required for the clinical, biochemical, and radiologic effects to be seen. This process takes weeks to months, depending on the severity of the osseous changes. Patients debilitated by the disease can become asymptomatic within 2–3 months.

The dose of vitamin D may be monitored using serum alkaline phosphatase. When the serum concentration starts to fall, the dose of vitamin D should be reduced until the lowest possible dose is found. In most circumstances, the final maintenance dose is slightly lower than the dose needed to produce healing. Calcium concentrations should also be monitored.

Various vitamin D compounds and metabolites are available. Products and suggested doses to reverse resistant hypocalcemia and osteopenia are listed in Table 83.12.[112] Doses of 5000–100,000 units (125 μg–2.5 mg) of vitamin D_2 may be required for initial therapy.[111] Vitamin D_2 (ergocalciferol, a plant product) and vitamin D_3 (cholecalciferol) undergo the same metabolic conversion; 25 hydroxylation in the liver and then 1 hydroxylation in the kidney to the active moiety 1,25-hydroxyvitamin D_2 or D_3. Calcifediol, 25-hydroxyvitamin D, does not require liver metabolism and may be a preferred agent in patients with severe liver disease. The half-life is 2–3 weeks. Calcitriol, 1,25-hydroxyvitamin D, requires no metabolism, has a 6-hour half-life, and has a rapid onset of action. Dihydrotachysterol is a synthetic compound which undergoes liver but not kidney conversion to the active compound. Calcitriol and dihydrotachysterol could be used in renal failure patients.

TABLE 83.12. DRUGS USEFUL IN TREATING HYPOCALCEMIA AND OSTEOPENIA RESISTANT TO PHYSIOLOGIC DOSES OF VITAMIN D

Nonproprietary Name	Abbreviation	Commercial Name	Effective Daily Dose	Time for Reversal of Toxic Effects, (days)
Ergocalciferol	Vitamin D_2	Calciferol	1–10 mg	17–60
Calcifediol	$25(OH)D_3$	Calderol	0.05–0.5 mg	7–30
Dihydrotachysterol	—	Dihydrotachysterol	0.1–1 mg	3–14
Calcitriol	$1,25(OH)_2D_3$	Rocaltrol	0.5–1 μg	2–10

(From Ref. 113.)

Conclusion

Osteoporosis is a disease of decreased bone mass (osteopenia) and fractures. Postmenopausal estrogen deficiency, age-associated bone loss, and various diseases and medications can lead to osteoporosis. Currently with modern medicine, bone loss can only be prevented or decreased—new strong bone cannot be created. Prevention is, therefore, the key to controlling this disease. Prevention of osteoporosis primarily includes adequate calcium and vitamin D intake and exercise throughout life for women and men and estrogen replacement therapy after menopause for women. Treatment of established osteoporosis relies on preventing further bone loss, which can include calcium and vitamin D supplementation, estrogen replacement therapy, calcitonin, and bisphosphonates. For women with an intake uterus, concomitant progesterone therapy is needed with estrogen replacement therapy. Many medications are under investigation to build bone or prevent its loss.

Osteomalacia is a disease of decreased bone mineralization with multiple etiologies, all of which have some impairment of calcium, phosphorous, or vitamin D homeostasis. Bone pain, skeletal structure abnormalities, and muscle weakness develop. Vitamin D is the predominant therapy, with the dose, duration, and product variable according to the underlying etiology and liver and kidney function. The underlying disease and medication etiologies should also be resolved.

References

1. Robey PG. The biochemistry of bone. Endocrinol Metab Clin North Am 1989;18:859–902.
2. Bullough PG, Bansal M, DiCarlo EF. The tissue diagnosis of metabolic bone disease. Orthop Clin North Am 1990;21:65–79.
3. Mundy GR. Visions for the future in osteoporosis research. Osteoporosis Int 1993;suppl 2:S29–S34.
4. Manolagas SC, Jilka RL. Bone marrow, cytokines, and bone remodeling. Emerging insights into the pathophysiology of osteoporosis. N Engl J Med 1995;332:305–311.
5. Zerwekh J. Bone metabolism. Semin Nephrol 1992;12:79–90.
6. Horowitz M. Cytokines and estrogen in bone: Anti-osteoporotic effects. Science 1993;260:625–626.
7. Dempster D, Lindsay R. Pathogenesis of osteoporosis. Lancet 1993;341:797–801.
8. Seeman E. The dilemma of osteoporosis in men. Am J Med 1995;98(suppl 2A):S76–S88.
9. Kumar R. Vitamin D and calcium transport. Kid Int 1991;40:1177–1189.
10. Genant HK, Faulkner KG, Gluer CC. Measurement of bone mineral density: Current status. Am J Med 1991;91(suppl 5B):S49–S53.
11. Rubin SM, Cummings SR. Results of bone densitometry affect women's decisions about taking measures to prevent fractures. Ann Int Med 1992;116:990–995.
12. Delmas PD. Biochemical markers of bone turnover I: Theoretical considerations and clinical use in osteoporosis. Am J Med 1993;95(suppl 5A):S11–S6.
13. Mankin HJ. Rickets, osteomalacia, and renal osteodystrophy: An update. Ortho Clin North Am 1990;21:81–96.
14. Barrett-Connor E. The economic and human costs of osteoporotic fracture. Am J Med 1995;98(suppl 2A):S3–S8.
15. Cummings SR, Nevitt MC, Browner WS, et al. Risk factors for hip fractures in white women. N Engl J Med 1995;332:767–773.
16. Bauer DC, Browner WS, Cauley JA, et al. Factors associated with appendicular bone mass in older women. Ann Int Med 1993;118:657–665.
17. Grisso JA, Kelsey JL, Strom BL, et al. Risk factors for hip fracture in black women. N Engl J Med 1994;330:1555–1559.
18. Wasnich RD. Bone mass measurements in diagnosis and assessment of therapy. Am J Med 1991;91(suppl 5B):S54–S58.
19. Wasnich R. Bone mass measurement: Prediction of risk. Am J Med 1993;95(suppl 5A):S610.
20. Cummings SR, Black DM, Nevitt MC, et al. Bone density at various sites for prediction of hip fractures. Lancet 1993;41:72–75.
21. Duursma SA, Raymakers JA, Boereboom FTJ, Scheven BAA. Estrogen and bone metabolism. Obstet Gynecol Surv 1991;47:38–44.
22. Mazess RB. On aging bone loss. Clin Orthop 1982;165:239–252.
23. Riggs BL, Wahner HW, Dunn WL, et al. Differential changes in bone mineral density of the appendicular and axial skeleton with aging. J Clin Invest 1981;67:328–335.
24. Barbour LA, Kick SD, Steiner JF, et al. A prospective study of heparin-induced osteoporosis in pregnancy using bone densitometry. Am J Obstet Gynecol 1994;170:862–869.
25. Schneider DL, Barrett-Connor EL, Morton DJ. Thyroid hormone use and bone mineral density in elderly women. JAMA 1994;271:1245–1249.
26. Joseph JC, Corticosteroid-induced osteoporosis. Am J Hosp Pharm 1994;51:188–197.
27. Shane E, Rivas, MD, Silverberg SJ, et al. Osteoporosis after cardiac transplantation. Am J Med 1993;94:257–264.
28. Hasling C, Sondergaard K, Charles P, Mosekilde L. Calcium metabolism in postmenopausal osteoporotic women is determined by dietary calcium and coffee intake. J Nutr 1992;122:1119–1126.
29. Massey LK, Whiting SJ. Caffeine, urinary calcium, calcium metabolism and bone. J Nutr 1993;123:1611–1614.
30. Hopper JL, Seeman E. The bone density of female twins discordant for tobacco use. N Engl J Med 1994;330:387–392.
31. Hollenbach KA, Barrett-Connor E, Edelstein SL, Holbrook T. Cigarette smoking and bone mineral density in older men and women. Am J Public Health 1993;83:1265–1270.
32. Baron JA, LaVecchia CL, Levi F. The antiestrogenic effect of cigarette smoking in women. Am J Obstet Gynecol 1990;162:502–514.
33. Moniz C. Alcohol and bone. Br Med Bult 1994;50:67–75.
34. Nelson ME, Fiatarone MA, Morganti CM, et al. Effects of high-intensity strength training on multiple risk factors for osteoporotic fractures. JAMA 1994;272:1909–1914.

35. Krall EA, Dawson-Hughes B. Walking is related to bone density and rates of bone loss. Am J Med 1994;96: 20–26.
36. Cavanaugh DJ, Cann CE. Brisk walking does not stop bone loss in postmenopausal women. Bone 1988;9:201–204.
37. Orwoll ES, Ferar J, Oviatt SK, et al. The relationship of swimming exercise to bone mass in men and women. Arch Intern Med 1989;149:2197–2200.
38. Cumming RG. Calcium intake and bone mass: A quantitative review of the evidence. Calcif Tissue Int 1990;47:194–201.
39. Heaney RP. Bone mass, nutrition, and other lifestyle factors. Am J Med 1993;95(suppl 5A):S29–S33.
40. NIH Consensus Development Panel on Optimal Calcium Intake. Optimal calcium intake. JAMA 1994;272:1942–1948.
41. Barrett-Connor E. The RDA for calcium in the elderly: Too little, too late. Calcif Tissue Int 1989;44:303–307.
42. Weaver CM. Calcium bioavailability and its relation to osteoporosis. PEBM 1992;200:157–160.
43. Carr CJ, Shamgraw RF. Nutritional and pharmaceutical aspects of calcium supplementation. Am Pharm 1987;27:49–57.
44. Cauley JA, Cummings SR, Seeley DG, et al. Effects of thiazide diuretic therapy on bone mass, fractures, and falls. Ann Int Med 1993;118:666–673.
45. LaCroix AZ, Wienpahl J, White LR, et al. Thiazide diuretic agents and the incidence of hip fracture. N Engl J Med 1990;322:286–290.
46. Morton DJ, Barrett-Connor EL, Edelstein SL. Thiazides and bone mineral density in elderly men and women. Am J Epidemiol 1994;139:1107–1115.
47. Saxman KA, Barrett-Connor EL, Morton D. Thiazide-associated metabolic abnormalities and estrogen replacement therapy: An epidemiological analysis of postmenopausal women in Rancho Bernardo, California. J Clin Endocrinol Metab 1994;78:1059–1063.
48. Brandi ML. New treatment strategies: Ipriflavone, strontium, vitamin D metabolites and analogs. Am J Med 1993;95(suppl 5A):S69–S74.
49. Chapuy MC, Arlot ME, Duboeuf F, et al. Vitamin D_3 and calcium to prevent hip fractures in elderly women. N Engl J Med 1992;327:1637–1642.
50. Tilyard MW, Spears GFS, Thomson J, Dovey S. Treatment of postmenopausal osteoporosis with calcitriol or calcium. N Engl J Med 1992;326:357–362.
51. Consensus development conference: Diagnosis, prophylaxis, and treatment of osteoporosis. Am J Med 1993; 94:646–650.
52. Grey AB, Cundy TF, Reid IR. Continuous combined oestrogen/progestin therapy is well tolerated and increases bone density at the hip and spine in post-menopausal osteoporosis. Clin Endocrinol 1994;40:671–677.
53. Nielsen SP, Brenholdt O, Hermansen F, Munk-Jensen N. Magnitude and pattern of skeletal response to long term continuous and cyclic sequential oestrogen/progestin treatment. Br J Obstet Gynaecol 1994;101:319–324.
54. Ryde SJS, Bowen-Simpkins K, Bowen-Simpkins P, et al. The effect of oestradiol implants on regional and total bone mass: A three-year longitudinal study. Clinc Endocrinol 1994;40:33–38.
55. Quigley MET, Martin PL, Burnier AM, Brooks P. Estrogen therapy arrests bone loss in elderly women. Am J Obstet Gynecol 1987;156:1516–1523.
56. Felson DT, Zhang Y, Hannan MT, et al. The effect of postmenopausal estrogen therapy on bone density in elderly women. N Engl J Med 1993;329:1141–1146.
57. Grady D, Rubin SM, Petitti DB, et al. Hormone therapy to prevent disease and prolong life in postmenopausal women. Ann Int Med 1992;117:1016–1037.
58. Cauley JA, Seeley DG, Ensrud K, et al. Estrogen replacement therapy and fractures in older women. Ann Int Med 1995;122:9–16.
59. American College of Physicians. Guidelines for counseling postmenopausal women about preventive hormone therapy. Ann Int Med 1992;117:1038–1041.
60. Psaty BM, Heckbert SR, Atkins D, et al. A review of the association of estrogens and progestins with cardiovascular disease in postmenopausal women. Arch Intern Med 1993;153:1421–1427.
61. Henderson BE, Ross RK, Paganini-Hill A, Mack TM. Estrogen use and cardiovascular disease. Am J Obstet Gynecol 1986;154:1181–1186.
62. Nabulsi AA, Folsom AR, White A, et al. Association of hormone-replacement therapy with various cardiovascular risk factors in postmenopausal women. N Engl J Med 1993;328:1069–1075.
63. The Writing Group for the PEPI Trial. Effects of estrogen or estrogen/progestin regimens on heart disease risk factors in postmenopausal women. JAMA 1995;273:199–208.
64. Fillit H. Estrogens in the pathogenesis and treatment of Alzheimer's disease in postmenopausal women. Ann NY Acad Sci 233–239.
65. Archer DF, Pickar JH, Bottiglioni F, et al. Bleeding patterns in postmenopausal women taking continuous combined or sequential regimens of conjugated estrogens with medroxyprogesterone acetate. Obstet Gynecol 1994;83: 686–692.
66. Woodruff JD, Pickar JH, et al. Incidence of endometrial hyperplasia in postmenopausal women taking conjugated estrogens (Premarin) with medroxyprogesterone acetate or conjugated estrogens alone. Obstet Gynecol 1994;170:1213–1223.
67. Ettinger B, Selby J, Citron JT, et al. Cyclic hormone replacement therapy using quarterly progestin. Obstet Gynecol 1994;83:693–700.
68. Lafferty FW, Fiske ME. Postmenopausal estrogen replacement: A long-term cohort study. Am J Med 1994;97:66–77.
69. Lindsay R, Aitken JM, Anderson JB, et al. Long-term prevention of postmenopausal osteoporosis by estrogen. Lancet 1976;2:1038–1041.
70. Barrett-Connor E, Wingard DL, Criqui MH. Postmenopausal estrogen use and heart disease risk factors in the 1980s. Rancho Bernardo, Calif, revisited. JAMA 1989;261:2095–2100.
71. Grady D, Gebretsadik T, Kerlikowske K, et al. Hormone replacement therapy and endometrial cancer risk: A meta-analysis. Obstet Gynecol 1995;85:304–313.

72. Cobleigh MA, Berris RF, Bush T, et al. Estrogen replacement therapy in breast cancer survivors. JAMA 1994;272:540–544.
73. Wysowski DK, Golden L, Burke L. Use of menopausal estrogens and medroxyprogesterone in the United States, 1982–1992. Obstet Gynecol 1995;85:6–10.
74. Ferguson KJ, Hoegh C, Johnson S. Estrogen replacement therapy: A survey of women's knowledge and attitudes. Arch Intern Med 1989;149:133–136.
75. Clark AP, Schuttinga JA. Targeted estrogen/progestogen replacement therapy for osteoporosis: Calculation of health care cost savings. Osteoporosis Int 1992;2:195–200.
76. Gorsky RD, Koplan JP, Peterson HB, Thacker SB. Relative risks and benefits of long-term estrogen replacement therapy: A decision analysis. Obstet Gynecol 1994;83:161–166.
77. Love RR, Barden HS, Mazess RB, et al. Effect of tamoxifen on lumbar spine bone mineral density in postmenopausal women after 5 years. Arch Intern Med 1994;154:2585–2588.
78. Geusens P, Dequeker J, Gielen J, Schot LPC. Non-linear increase in vertebral density induced by a synthetic steroid (Org OD 14) in women with established osteoporosis. Maturitas 1991;13:155–162.
79. Kleerekoper M, Brienze RS, Schultz LR, et al. Oral contraceptive use may protect against low bone mass. Arch Intern Med 1991;151:1971–1976.
80. Cooper C, Hannaford P, Croft P, Kay CR. Oral contraceptive pill use and fractures in women: A prospective study. Bone 1993;14:41–45.
81. Haenggi W, Casez JP, Birkhaeuser H, et al. Bone mineral density in young women with long-standing amenorrhea: Limited effect of hormone replacement therapy with ethinylestradiol and desogestrel. Osteoporosis Int 1994;4:99–103.
82. Seeman E, Szmukler GI, Formica C, et al. Osteoporosis in anorexia nervosa: The influence of peak bone density, bone loss, oral contraceptive use, and exercise. J Bone Miner Res 1992;7:1467–1474.
83. Gambacciani M, Spinetti A, Taponeco F, et al. Longitudinal evaluation of premenopausal vertebral bone loss: Effects of a low-dose oral contraceptive preparation on bone mineral density and metabolism. Obstet Gynecol 1994;83:392–396.
84. Gallagher JC, Kable WT, Goldgar D. Effect of progestin therapy on cortical and trabecular bone: Comparison with estrogen. Am J Med 1991;90:171–178.
85. Sands R, Studd J. Exogenous androgens in postmenopausal women. Am J Med 1995;98(suppl 1A):S76–S79.
86. Devolgalear JP, deCooman S, deDeuxchaisnes CN. Low bone mass in hypogonadal males. Effect of testosterone substitution therapy, a densitometric study. Maturitas 1992;15:17–23.
87. Jackson JA, Kleerekoper M. Osteoporosis in men: Diagnosis, pathophysiology, and prevention. Medicine 1990;69:137–152.
88. Reginster JY. Calcitonin for prevention and treatment of osteoporosis. Am J Med 1993;95(suppl 5A):S44–S47.
89. Reginster JY, Meurmans L, Deroisy R, et al. A 5-year controlled randomized study of prevention of postmenopausal trabecular bone loss with nasal salmon calcitonin and calcium. Eur J Clin Invest 1994;24:565–569.
90. Overgaard K, Hansen MA, Jensen SB, Christiansen C. Effect of salcatonin given intranasally on bone mass and fracture rates in established osteoporosis: A dose-response study. BMJ 1992;305:556–561.
91. Burkhardt P, Burnand B. The effect of treatment with calcitonin on vertebral fracture rate in osteoporosis. Osteoporosis Int 1993;3:24–30.
92. Gennari C, Agnusdei D, Camporeale A. Use of calcitonin in the treatment of bone pain associated with osteoporosis. Calcif Tissue Int 1991;49(suppl 2):S9–S13.
93. Papapoulos SE, Landman JO, Bijvoet OLM, et al. The use of bisphosphonates in the treatment of osteoporosis. Bone 1992;13:S41–S49.
94. Harris ST, Watts NB, Jackson RD, et al. Four-year study of intermittent cyclic etidronate treatment of postmenopausal osteoporosis: Three years of blinded therapy followed by one year of open therapy. Am J Med 1993;95:557–567.
95. Reid IR, Wattie DJ, Evans MC, et al. Continuous therapy with pamidronate, a potent bisphosphonate, in postmenopausal osteoporosis. J Clin Endocrinol Metab 1994;79:1595–1599.
96. Rossini M, Gatti D, Zamberlan N, et al. Long-term effects of a treatment course with oral alendronate of postmenopausal osteoporosis. J Bone Miner Res 1994;9:1833–1837.
97. Bell NH, Hollis BW, Shary JR, et al. Diclofenac sodium inhibits bone resorption in postmenopausal women. Am J Med 1994;96:349–353.
98. Kanis JA. Treatment of symptomatic osteoporosis with fluoride. Am J Med 1993;95(suppl 5A):S53–S61.
99. Pak CYC, Sakhaee K, Piziak V, et al. Slow-release sodium fluoride in the management of postmenopausal osteoporosis. Ann Intern Med 1994;120:625–632.
100. Gutteridge DH, Kent GN, Prince RL, et al. Fluoride treatment of osteoporosis: Cyclical non-blinded or continuous blinded studies? Osteoporosis Int 1993;suppl 1:S215–S217.
101. Need AG, Nordin BEC, Chatterton BE. Double-blind placebo-controlled trial of treatment of osteoporosis with the anabolic nandrolone decanoate. Osteoporosis Int 1993;suppl 1:S218–S222.
102. Passeri M, Pedrazzoni M, Pioli G, et al. Effects of nandrolone decanoate on bone mass in established osteoporosis. Maturitas 1993;17:211–219.
103. Chestnut CH, Ivey JL, Gruber HE, et al. Stanozolol in postmenopausal osteoporosis: Therapeutic efficacy and possible mechanisms of action. Metabolism 1993;32:571–580.
104. Rubin CD, Southwestern internal medicine conference: Growth hormone-aging and osteoporosis. Am J Med Sci 1993;305:120–129.
105. Riggs BL. Formation-stimulating regimens other than sodium fluoride. Am J Med 1993;95(suppl 5A):S62–S68.
106. Puolijoki H, Liippo K, Herrala J, et al. Inhaled beclomethasone decreases serum osteocalcin in postmenopausal asthmatic women. Bone 1992;13:285–288.
107. Lukert BP, Raisz LG. Glucocorticoid-induced osteoporosis. Rheum Dis Clin North Am 1994;20:629–650.

108. Olgaard K, Storm T, vanWowern N, et al. Glucocorticoid-induced osteoporosis in the lumbar spine, forearm, and mandible of nephrotic patients: A double-blind study on the high-dose, long-term effects of prednisone versus deflazacort. Calcif Tissue Int 1992;50:490–497.
109. Doppelt SH. Vitamin D, rickets, and osteomalacia. Orthop Clin North Am 1984;15:671–686.
110. Webb AR, Pilbearn C, Hanafin N, et al. An evaluation of the relative contributions of exposure to sunlight and of diet to the circulating concentrations of 25-hydroxyvitamin D in an elderly nursing home population in Boston. Am J Nutr 1990;51:1075–1081.
111. Hutchinson FN, Bell NH. Osteomalacia and rickets. Semin Nephrol 1992;12:127–145.
112. Hassler MR, Cordy PE. Metabolites and analogues of Vitamin D. Which for what? JAMA 1982;247:841–844.

Chapter 84

Rheumatoid Arthritis and the Seronegative Spondyloarthropathies

Arthur A. Schuna, MS, FASHP, Michael J. Schmidt, PharmD, and Denise Walbrandt Pigarelli, PharmD

Rheumatoid Arthritis

Rheumatoid arthritis is the most common systemic inflammatory disease characterized by symmetrical joint involvement. Extra-articular involvement including rheumatoid nodules, vasculitis, eye inflammation, neurologic dysfunction, cardiopulmonary disease, lymphadenopathy, and splenomegaly are manifestations of the disease. Although the usual disease course is chronic, some patients will spontaneously enter a remission.

EPIDEMIOLOGY

Rheumatoid arthritis is estimated to have a prevalence of 2–3% and does not have any racial predilections. The disease is three times more common in women. In people age 15–45 years, women predominate by a ratio of 6:1; the sex ratio is approximately equal among patients in the first decade of life and in those more than 60 years old.

Epidemiologic data suggest that a genetic predisposition and exposure to unknown environmental factors may be necessary for expression of the disease. The major histocompatibility complex (MHC) molecules, located on T lymphocytes, appear to have an important role in most patients with rheumatoid arthritis. These molecules can be characterized using human lymphocyte antigen (HLA) typing. A majority of patients with rheumatoid arthritis have HLA-DR4, HLA-DR1, or both antigens found in the MHC region. Although the MHC region is important, it is not the sole determinant, as patients can have the disease without these HLA types. Rheumatoid arthritis is six times more common among dizygotic twins and nontwin children of parents with rheumatoid factor-positive, erosive rheumatoid arthritis when compared with children whose parents do not have the disease. If one of a pair of monozygotic twins is affected, the other twin has a 30 times greater risk of developing the disease.[1,2]

PATHOPHYSIOLOGY

Chronic inflammation of the synovial tissue lining the joint capsule results in the proliferation of this tissue. The inflamed, proliferating synovium characteristic of rheumatoid arthritis is called *pannus* (Fig. 84.1). This pannus invades the cartilage and eventually the bone surface, producing erosions of bone and cartilage, leading to destruction of the joint.

The factors that initiate the inflammatory process are unknown. Infectious agents have been postulated as a cause of rheumatoid arthritis. The evidence supporting this possibility includes the similarity between rheumatoid arthritis and acute inflammatory arthritides associated with known infectious agents (e.g., rheumatic fever following streptococcal infection, Lyme arthritis, postviral arthritis). Also, synovitis resembling rheumatoid arthritis can be produced experimentally in animals by injection of bacterial cell wall fragments. No specific infectious agent has been isolated from the joints of patients suffering from rheumatoid arthritis.

The immune system is a complex network of checks and balances designed to discriminate self from nonself (foreign) tissues. It helps rid the body of infectious agents, tumor cells, and products associated with the breakdown of cells. In rheumatoid arthritis this system no longer can differentiate self from nonself tissues and attacks the synovial tissue and other connective tissues.

The immune system has both humoral and cell-mediated functions. The humoral component is necessary for the formation of antibodies. These antibodies are produced by plasma cells. Most patients with rheumatoid arthritis form

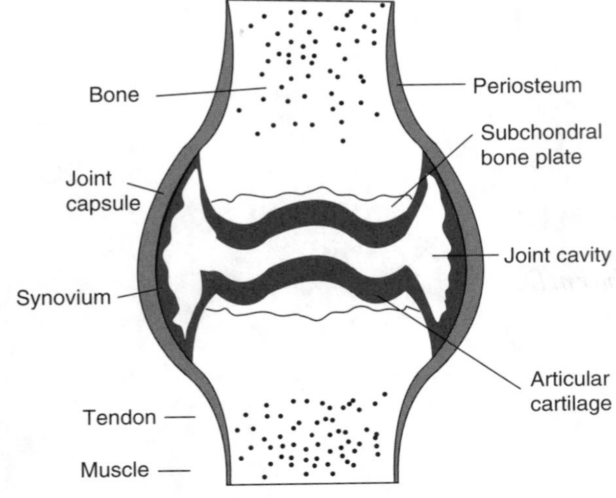

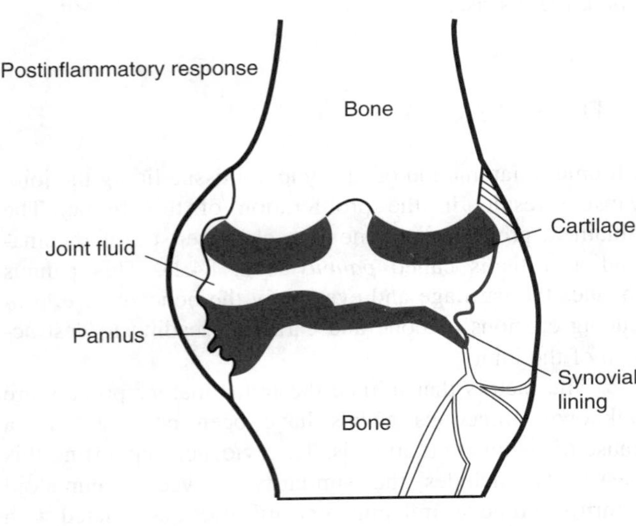

Figure 84.1. (A) Schematic diagram of a normal diarthrodial joint. (B) Schematic diagram of a knee joint with active rheumatoid arthritis showing pannus invading and destroying the cartilage and bone. *(Reproduced from the Arthritis Foundation Allied Health Professions Teaching Slide Collection, Copyright © 1980, with permission.)*

antibodies called rheumatoid factors. Rheumatoid factors have not been identified as pathogenic nor does the quantity of these circulating antibodies always correlate with disease activity. Seropositive patients tend to have a more aggressive course of their illness than do seronegative patients. Immunoglobulins can activate the complement system. The complement system amplifies the immune response by encouraging chemotaxis, phagocytosis, and the release of lymphokines by mononuclear cells.

The cellular component of the inflammatory process consists of polymorphonuclear cells, macrophages, and lymphocytes (Fig. 84.2). Antigen-presenting cells (including macrophages) engulf and process antigens, which are then presented to T lymphocytes. The processed antigen is recognized by MHC proteins on the lymphocyte, which activates it to stimulate the production of T and B cells. Lymphocytes may be either B cells (derived from bone marrow) or T cells (derived from thymus tissue). T cells may be either T-helper (which promote inflammation) or T-suppressor cells (which attenuate the inflammatory response). Activated T cells produce cytotoxins, which are directly toxic to tissues, and cytokines, which stimulate further activation of inflammatory processes and attract cells to areas of inflammation. Macrophages are stimulated to release prostaglandins and cytotoxins. Activated B cells produce plasma cells, which form antibodies. These antibodies in combination with complement result in the accumulation of polymorphonuclear leukocytes (PMNs). These PMNs release cytotoxins, free oxygen radicals, and hydroxyl radicals, which promote cellular damage to synovium and bone. Patients with rheumatoid arthritis appear to have an excessive amount of T-helper cell activity in synovial tissues.

Vasoactive substances also play a role in the inflammatory process. Histamine, kinins, and prostaglandins are released at the site of inflammation. These substances increase both blood flow to the site of inflammation and the permeability of blood vessels. These substances cause the edema, warmth, erythema, and pain associated with inflamed joints and also make it easier for granulocytes to pass from blood vessels to the site of inflammation.

The end results of the chronic inflammatory changes are variable. Loss of cartilage may result in a loss of the joint space. The formation of chronic granulation or scar tissue can lead to loss of joint motion or bony fusion (called ankylosis). Laxity of tendon structures can result in a loss of support to the affected joint, leading to instability or subluxation. Tendon contractures may also occur, leading to chronic deformity.[3–8]

CLINICAL PRESENTATION

The symptoms of rheumatoid arthritis usually develop insidiously over the course of several weeks to months. Prodromal symptoms include fatigue, weakness, low-grade fever, loss of appetite, and joint pain. Stiffness and muscle aches (myalgias) may precede the development of joint swelling (synovitis). Fatigue may be more of a problem in the afternoon. During disease flares, the onset of fatigue begins earlier in the day and subsides as disease activity lessens. Most commonly, joint involvement tends to be symmetric; however, early in the disease some patients present with an asymmetric pattern involving one or a few

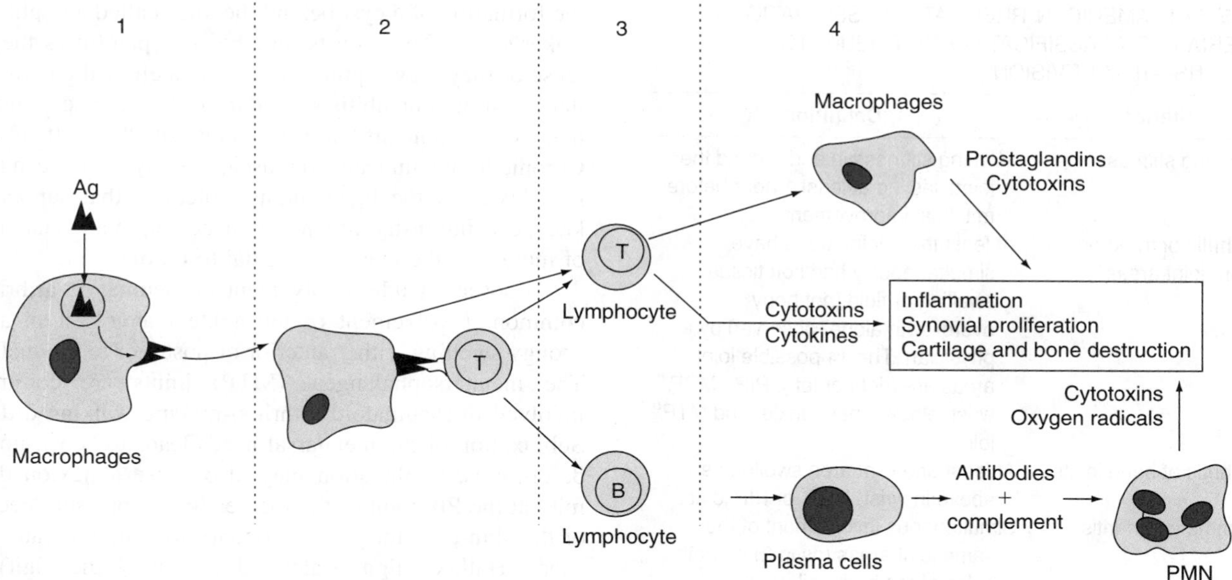

Figure 84.2. Pathogenesis of the inflammatory response. *Phase 1:* Antigen-presenting cells phagocytizes antigen. *Phase 2:* Antigen is presented to T lymphocyte. T lymphocyte attaches to antigen at MHC portion of cell wall causing activation. *Phase 3:* Activated T cell stimulates T and B lymphocyte production, promoting inflammation. *Phase 4:* Activated T cells and macrophages release factors that promote tissue destruction, increase blood flow, and result in cellular invasion of synovial tissue and joint fluid. Ag, antigen; PMN, polymorphonuclear leukocyte.

joints, which eventually develops into the more classic presentation. About 20% of patients develop an abrupt onset of their illness with fevers, polyarthritis, and constitutional symptoms (e.g., depression, anxiety, fatigue, anorexia, weight loss).[1,2] No single test or physical finding can be used to make the diagnosis of rheumatoid arthritis, but criteria have been developed to aid in its diagnosis (Table 84.1).

Joint Involvement

The joints most frequently affected by rheumatoid arthritis are the small joints of the hands, wrists, and feet (Fig. 84.3). In addition, elbows, shoulders, hips, knees, and ankles may be involved. Patients usually experience joint stiffness that is typically worse in the morning. The duration of stiffness tends to be directly correlated with disease activity, usually exceeds 30 minutes, and may persist all day. Chronic inflammation with lack of an adequate exercise program results in loss of range of motion, atrophy of muscles, weakness, and deformity. A functional classification scale to indicate a patient's degree of impairment is frequently used (Table 84.2).

On examination, the swelling of the joints may be visible or may be apparent only by palpation. The swelling feels soft and spongy, because it is caused by proliferation of soft tissues or fluid accumulation within the joint capsule. The swollen joint may appear erythematous and feel warmer than nearby skin surfaces, especially early in the course of the disease. In contrast, the swelling associated with osteoarthritis is usually bony (caused by osteophytes) and is infrequently associated with signs of inflammation.

Involvement of the hands and wrists is common in rheumatoid arthritis. Hand involvement is manifested by pain, swelling, tenderness, and grip weakness during the acute phase and by subluxation, instability, ulnar deviation, and muscle atrophy in the chronic phase of the disease. Functional difficulties with clasp, grasp, and pinch alter both strength and fine motor movement. These difficulties can affect the activities of daily living (ADL) necessary for self-care. Tenosynovitis involving the flexor tendons of the hands can result in restriction of motion or locking of digits in a flexed position. Tenosynovitis of the extensor tendons of the hand may result in pain, swelling, and spontaneous rupture with loss of function.

Deformity of the hand may be seen with chronic inflammation. Subluxations of the wrists and metacarpophalangeal (MCP) joints may be seen. The thumbs may develop flexion at the MCP joint and hyperextension of the interphalangeal (IP) joint, which may make pinch grip difficult. Involvement of tendons in the hands can result in either hyperextension at the proximal interphalangeal (PIP) joint and flexion of the distal interphalangeal (DIP) joint (called a swan-neck deformity; see Fig. 84.4) or flexion at PIP with hyperextension of the DIP (called a boutonniere deformity; see Fig. 84.5). Ulnar deviation of the fingers may also occur as a result of tendon abnormalities associated with rheumatoid arthritis (Fig. 84.6).

Wrist involvement can result in joint space narrowing, collapse, and subluxation leading to grip weakness.

TABLE 84.1. AMERICAN RHEUMATISM ASSOCIATION CRITERIA FOR CLASSIFICATION OF RHEUMATOID ARTHRITIS—1987 REVISION

Criteria[a]	Definition
1. Morning stiffness	Morning stiffness in and around the joints lasting at least 1 hour before maximal improvement
2. Arthritis of three or more joint areas	At least three joint areas have simultaneously had soft tissue swelling or fluid (not bony overgrowth alone) observed by a physician. The 14 possible joint areas are (right or left): PIP,[b] MCP,[b] wrist, elbow, knee, ankle, and MTP[b] joints
3. Arthritis of hand joints	At least one joint area swollen as above in wrist, MCP, or PIP joint
4. Symmetric arthritis	Simultaneous involvement of the same joint areas (as in 2) on both sides of the body (bilateral involvement of PIP, MCP, or MTP joints is acceptable without absolute symmetry)
5. Rheumatoid nodules	Subcutaneous nodules, over bony prominences, or extensor surfaces, or in juxta-articular regions, observed by a physician
6. Serum rheumatoid factor	Demonstration of abnormal amounts of serum "rheumatoid factor" by any method that has been positive in less than 5% of normal control subjects
7. Radiographic changes	Radiographic changes typical of RA on posterior–anterior hand and wrist x-rays, which must include erosions or unequivocal bony decalcification localized to or most marked adjacent to the involved joints (osteoarthritis changes alone do not qualify)

[a]For classification purposes, a patient is said to have rheumatoid arthritis (RA) if he or she has satisfied at least four of the above seven criteria. Criteria 1 through 4 must be present for at least 6 weeks. Patients with two clinical diagnoses are not excluded. Designation as classic, definite, or probable rheumatoid arthritis is *not* to be made.
[b]PIP, proximal interphalangeal; MCP, metacarpophalangeal; MTP, metatarsophalangeal.

Destruction of the cartilage at the radioulnar joint results in pain with rotational movement of the forearm. Carpal tunnel syndrome is caused by entrapment of the median nerve by inflamed synovium. This results in pain and tingling in the fingers and grip weakness.

Swelling at the elbow is most evident at the radial-humeral joint. Shoulder pain may result from involvement of the joint itself or from tendon inflammation (tendinitis) or inflammation of the bursa (bursitis) near the deltoid muscle.

The knee can also be involved, with loss of cartilage, instability, and joint pain. Synovitis of the knee may cause the formation of a cyst behind the knee called a popliteal or Baker's cyst. These cysts may become painful as they get tense or they may rupture, producing a clinical picture similar to thrombophlebitis secondary to the release of inflammatory components into the area of the calf muscle. Chronic joint pain leads to muscle atrophy, which can result in a laxity of the ligamentous structures that support the knee, causing instability. Maintenance of an adequate range of motion of the knee is essential to normal gait.

Foot and ankle involvement in rheumatoid arthritis is common. Involvement of the ankle may result in a soft spongy swelling, either anterior or posterior to the malleoli. The metatarsophalangeal (MTP) joints are commonly involved in rheumatoid arthritis, making walking difficult. Subluxation of the metatarsal heads leads to "cock-up" toe deformities. Subluxation may also cause a flexion deformity at the PIP joint of the toe, leading to pressure necrosis of the skin over the joint secondary to irritation caused by shoes. Hallux valgus (lateral deviation of the digit) and bunion or callus formation may occur at the great toe (Fig. 84.7). A widening of the foot commonly occurs with long-standing disease.

Involvement of the spine usually occurs in the cervical vertebrae; lumbar vertebral involvement is rare. Involvement of the first and second cervical vertebrae (C-1 to C-2) can lead to instability of this joint. Patients with this problem are at a greater risk for spinal cord compression, although this complication is rare.

The temporomandibular joint (jaw) can be affected, resulting in malocclusion and difficulty in chewing food. Inflammation of cartilage in the chest can lead to chest wall pain. Hip pain may occur as a result of destructive changes in the hip joint, soft tissue inflammation (e.g., bursitis), or referred pain from nerve entrapment at the lumbar vertebrae.

Extra-Articular Involvement

Rheumatoid Nodules

Rheumatoid nodules occur in 20% of patients with rheumatoid arthritis. These nodules are most commonly seen on the extensor surfaces of the elbows, forearms, and hands but may also be seen on the feet and at other pressure points. They may also develop in the lung or pleural lining of the lung and rarely in the meninges. Rheumatoid nodules are asymptomatic and do not require any special intervention. Nodules are more commonly observed in patients with erosive disease.[8]

Vasculitis

Vasculitis is usually seen in those patients with long-standing rheumatoid arthritis. Vasculitis may result in a wide variety of clinical presentations. Invasion of blood vessel walls by inflammatory cells results in an obliteration of the vessel, producing infarction of tissue distal to the area of

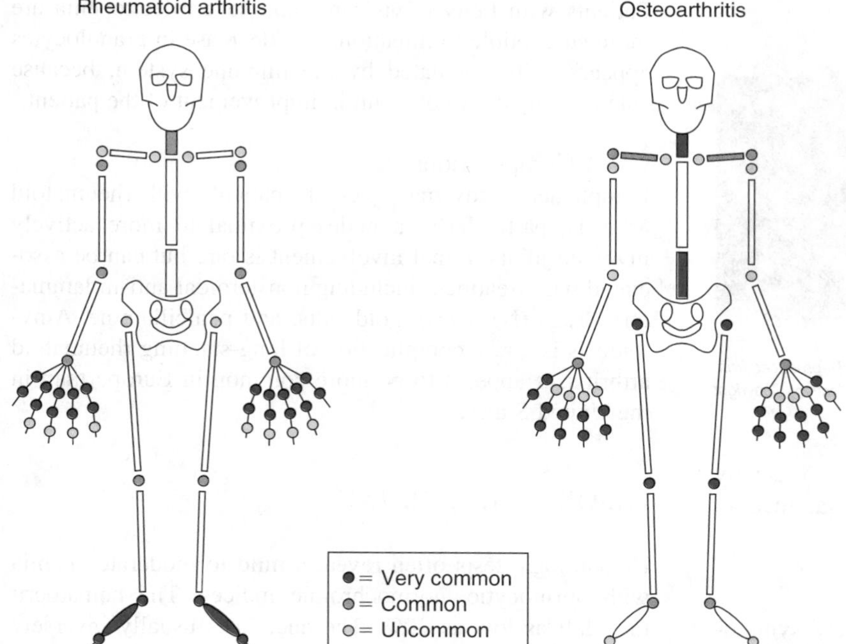

Figure 84.3. Patterns of joint involvement in rheumatoid arthritis and osteoarthritis.

involvement. Most commonly, small-vessel vasculitis produces infarcts near the ends of the fingers or toes, especially around the nail beds. These infarcts are usually of little consequence.

Vasculitis may also cause the breakdown of skin, especially in the lower extremities, producing ulcers that may be indistinguishable in appearance from stasis ulcers. However, these ulcers do not heal with the usual modes of treatment used for stasis ulcers. Involvement of larger vessels with vasculitis can result in life-threatening complications. Infarction of vessels supplying blood to nerves can cause irreversible motor deficits. Involvement of vessels supplying other organ systems can lead to visceral involvement and a polyarteritis nodosa-like illness. Aggressive treatment of the inflammatory process is necessary in these patients. Fortunately, the more serious vasculitic picture is rarely seen.

Pulmonary Complications

Rheumatoid arthritis may involve the pleura of the lung, which is often asymptomatic. Pleural fluid obtained from patients with effusion characteristically has a low glucose concentration (frequently 10–50 mg/dL). Pulmonary fibrosis may also develop as a result of rheumatoid involvement; smoking appears to increase the risk of this complication. Rheumatoid nodules may develop in lung tissue and appear similar to neoplasms on chest x-ray films. Interstitial pneumonitis and arteritis are rare, potentially life-threatening complications of rheumatoid arthritis.

TABLE 84.2. FUNCTIONAL CLASSIFICATIONS OF RHEUMATOID ARTHRITIS

Class I	Capable of all activities without handicap
Class II	Able to conduct normal activities despite handicap of discomfort or limited mobility of one or more joints
Class III	Functional capacity only adequate to perform a few of the normal duties of usual occupation
Class IV	Bed or confined to wheelchair, capable of little or no self-care

Ocular Manifestations

Ocular manifestations include keratoconjunctivitis sicca and inflammation of the sclera, episclera, and cornea. Atrophy of the lacrimal duct may result in a decrease in tear formation, causing dry and itchy eyes, termed keratoconjunctivitis sicca. When this is observed in association with rheumatoid arthritis, it is referred to as Sjögren's syndrome. Artificial tears may be used to relieve symptoms. Inflammation of the superficial layers of the sclera (episcleritis) is generally self-

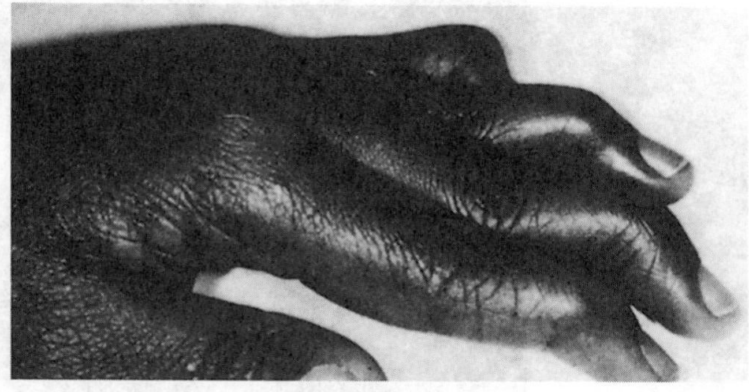

Figure 84.4. Swan-neck deformity in rheumatoid arthritis. *(Reproduced from the Arthritis Foundation Allied Health Professions Teaching Slide Collection, Copyright © 1980, with permission.)*

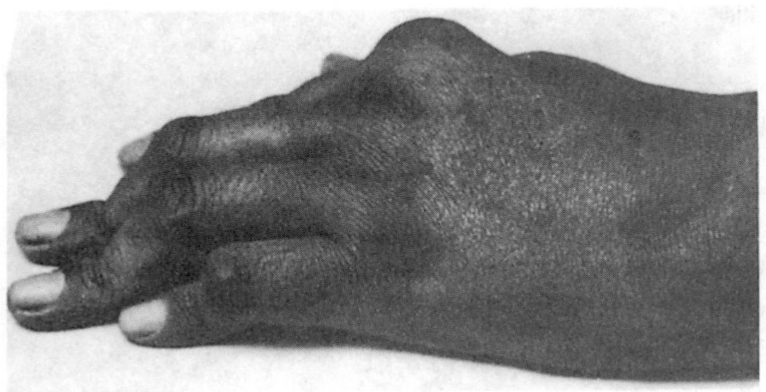

Figure 84.5. Boutonniere deformity in rheumatoid arthritis. *(Reproduced from the Arthritis Foundation Allied Health Professions Teaching Slide Collection, Copyright © 1980, with permission.)*

limiting. Involvement of deeper tissues (scleritis) usually results in a more serious, painful, and chronic inflammation. Rheumatoid nodules may develop on the sclera.

Cardiac Involvement

This occurs in rheumatoid arthritis but is rarely symptomatic. Pericarditis may occur, resulting in the accumulation of fluid. Although many patients show evidence of previous pericarditis at autopsy, the development of clinically evident pericarditis with tamponade is a rare complication. Cardiac conduction abnormalities and aortic valve incompetence, caused by aortic root dilatation, may occur. Myocarditis is a rare complication of rheumatoid arthritis.

Felty's Syndrome

Rheumatoid arthritis in association with splenomegaly and neutropenia is known as Felty's syndrome. Thrombocytopenia may also be a manifestation of the syndrome. Patients with Felty's syndrome and severe leukopenia are more susceptible to infection. The decrease in granulocytes appears to be mediated by the immune system, because splenectomy does not result in improvement of the patient.[9]

Other Complications

Lymphadenopathy may occur in patients with rheumatoid arthritis, particularly in nodes proximal to more actively involved joints. Renal involvement is rare but can be associated with treatment including nonsteroidal anti-inflammatory drugs (NSAIDs), gold salts, and penicillamine. Amyloidosis is a rare complication of long-standing rheumatoid arthritis. It appears to be more common in Europe than in the United States.

LABORATORY FINDINGS

Hematologic tests often reveal a mild to moderate anemia with normocytic, normochromic indices. The hematocrit may fall as low as 30%. The anemia is usually inversely related to inflammatory disease activity and is referred to as an anemia of chronic disease. This type of anemia does not respond to iron therapy and can present a diagnostic dilemma, because NSAIDs may induce gastritis and chronic blood loss leading to iron-deficiency anemia. Laboratory tests useful in differentiating these anemias include stool guaiac (or other stool tests for occult blood), serum iron/iron binding capacity ratio (decreased in iron deficiency), and mean corpuscular volume (more likely to be decreased in iron deficiency). Other causes of anemia must also be considered in the differential diagnosis (see Chapter 93, Anemias).

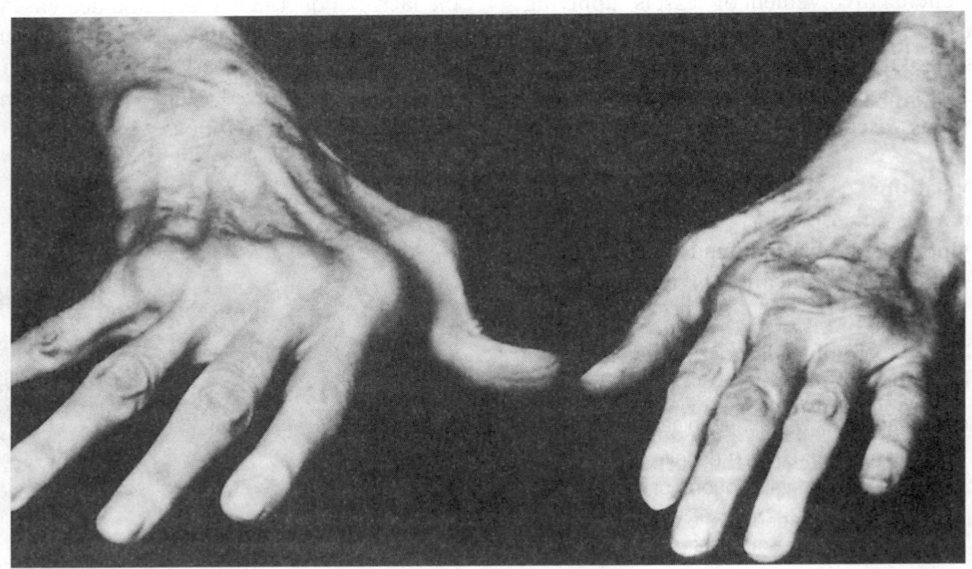

Figure 84.6. Ulnar deviation of the fingers of the right hand. *(Reproduced from the Arthritis Foundation Allied Health Professions Teaching Slide Collection, Copyright © 1980, with permission.)*

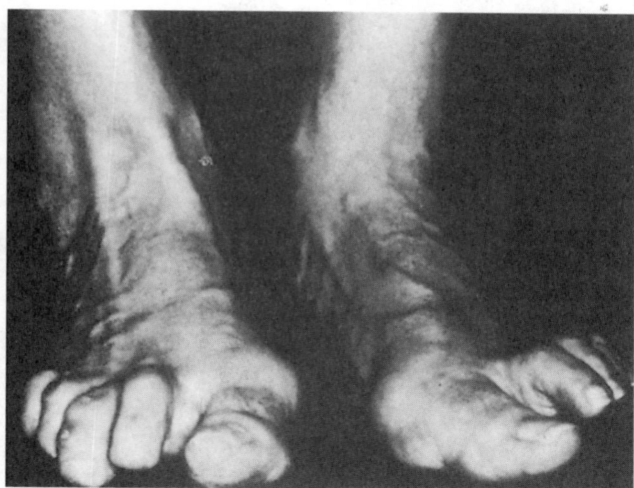

Figure 84.7. Foot involvement of rheumatoid arthritis with hallux valgus deformity of the first digit and hammer toe deformity of second through fifth digits bilaterally. *(Reproduced from the Arthritis Foundation Allied Health Professions Teaching Slide Collection, Copyright © 1980, with permission.)*

TABLE 84.3. DISEASES ASSOCIATED WITH A POSITIVE RHEUMATOID FACTOR

Rheumatic diseases
Rheumatoid arthritis
Sjögren's syndrome (with or without arthritis)
Systemic lupus erythematosus
Progressive systemic sclerosis
Polymyositis/dermatomyositis
Infectious diseases
Bacterial endocarditis
Tuberculosis
Syphilis
Infectious mononucleosis
Infectious hepatitis
Leprosy
Other causes
Aging
Interstitial pulmonary fibrosis
Cirrhosis of the liver
Chronic active hepatitis
Sarcoidosis

Thrombocytosis is another common hematologic finding with active rheumatoid arthritis. Platelet counts rise and fall in direct correlation with disease activity. Thrombocytopenia may result from toxicity of gold salts, penicillamine, or immunosuppressive therapy. Thrombocytopenia may also be observed in Felty's syndrome or vasculitis.

Although leukopenia is associated with Felty's syndrome, it may also result from toxicity of gold, penicillamine, and immunosuppressive drugs. Leukocytosis is commonly seen as a result of corticosteroid treatment.

The erythrocyte sedimentation rate (ESR) is usually elevated in patients with rheumatoid arthritis and other inflammatory diseases. This test is very nonspecific, and although the ESR usually falls as patients respond to therapy, there is a large variability among patients in response to treatment.

Rheumatoid factor is present in 60–70% of patients with rheumatoid arthritis. The usual laboratory test for rheumatoid factor is an antibody specific for IgM rheumatoid factor. Patients with rheumatoid arthritis and a negative test for rheumatoid factor may have IgG or IgA rheumatoid factors, but tests for these are not routinely available. Rheumatoid factor tests are usually reported positive at a specific serum dilution. Serum is diluted to a standard series of dilutions; the greatest dilution that yields a positive test result will be reported (e.g., rheumatoid factor positive at 1 : 640). Higher dilutional titers of rheumatoid factors usually indicate a more severe disease, but like the ESR, the large interpatient variability makes this test difficult to use as a means of assessing patient progress. Rheumatoid factor may be positive in patients without rheumatoid arthritis (Table 84.3).

Antinuclear antibodies (ANA) are detected in 25% of patients with rheumatoid arthritis. These antibodies usually have a diffuse pattern of immunofluorescence. Tests for antibodies to double-stranded DNA (usually positive in systemic lupus erythematosus, SLE) are negative. Serum complement is usually normal, although complement concentrations of joint fluid are often depressed from consumption secondary to the inflammatory process. In patients with vasculitis, serum complement concentrations may be low.

Synovial fluid usually is turbid because of the large number of leukocytes in inflammatory fluid. White cell counts of 5000–50,000/mm^3 are not uncommon in inflamed joints. The fluid is usually less viscous than that in normal joints or in fluid associated with osteoarthritis. Glucose concentrations of joint fluid are normal or low compared with those in serum drawn at the same time as synovial aspirates. The decrease is not as profound as the decrease associated with joint infection or SLE.

Radiologic manifestations of rheumatoid arthritis include soft tissue swelling and osteoporosis near the joint (periarticular osteoporosis). Erosions tend to occur later in the course of the disease and are usually seen first in the MCP and PIP joints of the hands and the MTP joints of the feet. Erosions are usually first seen at the margin of the joint near the interface of the head of the bone with the synovial tissue (Fig. 84.8).

GENERAL MANAGEMENT PRINCIPLES

The primary objective is to improve or maintain functional status, thereby improving quality of life. Treatment of rheumatoid arthritis is a multifaceted approach that includes pharmacologic and nonpharmacologic therapies. Recent emphasis has been placed on aggressive treatment early in

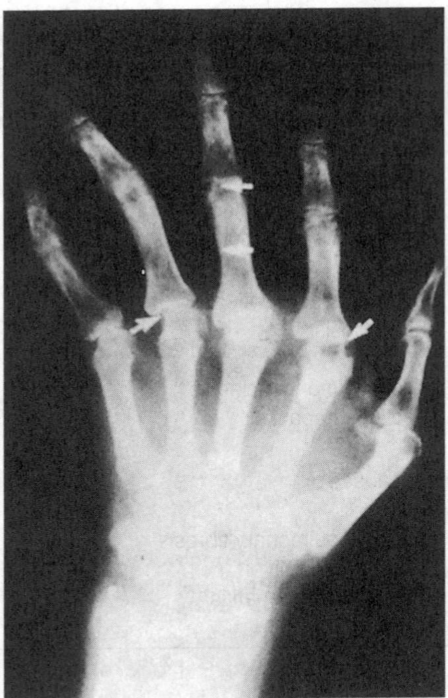

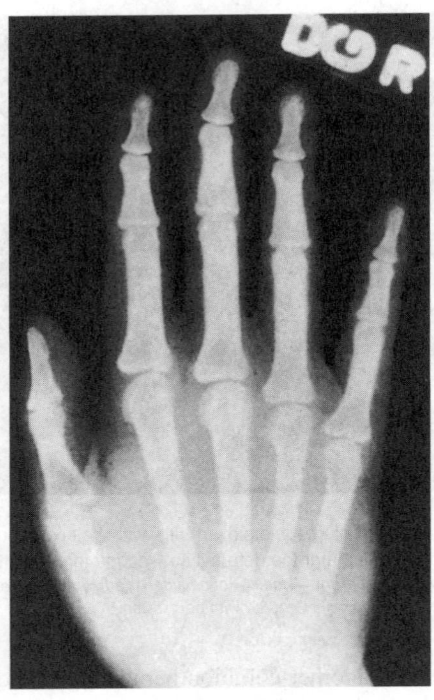

Figure 84.8. Radiograph of normal hand *(right)* and rheumatoid arthritis *(left)* with joint space narrowing, periarticular osteoporosis, and erosions *(see arrows)*. *(Reproduced from the Arthritis Foundation Allied Health Professions Teaching Slide Collection, Copyright © 1980, with permission.)*

the disease course. Goals of treatment include decreasing symptoms of morning stiffness and joint swelling and preserving range of motion. Since the majority of rheumatoid arthritis patients perceive pain as their biggest problem, control or minimization of pain is important. Additional goals include preventing joint destruction and systemic complications.

Evaluation of Therapeutic Outcome

The evaluation of therapeutic outcome is based primarily on improvements of clinical signs and symptoms of rheumatoid arthritis. Clinical signs of improvement include a reduction in joint swelling, decreased warmth over actively involved joints, and decreased tenderness to joint palpation. Improvement in RA symptoms includes reduction in perceived joint pain and morning stiffness, longer time to onset of afternoon fatigue, and improvement in ability to perform ADL. Joint radiographs may be of some benefit in assessing the progression of the disease, but are fraught with many problems.[10] Laboratory monitoring is of little value in monitoring individual patient response to therapy. Monitoring of therapeutic toxicity of drugs is indicated in Table 84.4. Routine monitoring of patients is essential to the safe use of these drugs. In addition, patients should be questioned about symptoms of the adverse effects outlined in the drug monograph section of this chapter.

Nondrug Therapy

Nondrug therapy consists of rest, occupational therapy, physical therapy, use of assistive devices, weight reduction, and surgery.

Rest is an essential component of a nonpharmacologic treatment plan. It relieves stress on inflamed joints and prevents further joint destruction. Rest also aids in alleviation of pain. Too much rest and immobility may lead to decreased range of motion and, ultimately, muscle atrophy and contractures.

Occupational and physical therapy can provide the patient with skills and exercises necessary to increase or maintain mobility. These disciplines may also provide patients with supportive and adaptive devices such as canes, walkers, and splints.

Other nondrug therapeutic options include weight loss and surgery. Weight reduction helps to alleviate inflamed joint stress. This should be instituted and monitored with close supervision of a health care professional. Tenosynovectomy, tendon repair, and joint replacements are surgical options for patients with rheumatoid arthritis. Such management is often reserved for patients with severe disease.[11,12]

Drug Therapy

Figure 84.9 presents a treatment algorithm for RA. This figure reflects a more aggressive treatment approach than has

TABLE 84.4. USUAL DOSES AND MONITORING PARAMETERS FOR ANTIRHEUMATIC DRUGS

Drug	Usual Dose	Monitoring Parameters	
		Initial	**Maintenance**
NSAIDs	Table 84.5	Scr or BUN, CBC q 2–4 weeks p starting therapy for 1–2 months salicylates: serum salicylate levels if therapeutic dose and no response	Same as initial plus stool guaiac q 6–12 months
Methotrexate	Oral or IM: 7.5–15 mg q week	Baseline: AST, ALT, alk phos, alb, t. bili, hep B & C studies, CBC w/plt, Scr	CBC w/plt, AST, alb q 1–2 months
Gold			
Auranofin	Oral: 3 mg daily to bid	Baseline: UA, CBC w/plt	Same as initial q 1–2 months
Gold sodium thiomalate or aurothioglucose	IM: 10-mg test dose, then weekly dosing 25–50 mg, after response may increase dosing interval	Baseline and until stable: UA, CBC w/plt preinjection	Same as initial every other dose
Hydroxychloroquine	Oral: 200–300 mg bid, after 1–2 months may decrease to 200 mg bid or daily	Baseline: color fundus photography and automated central perimetric analysis	Ophthalmoscopy q 9–12 months and Amsler grid at home q 2 weeks
Sulfasalazine	Oral: 500 mg bid, then increase to 1 g bid max	Baseline: CBC w/plt, then q week for 1 month	Same as initial q 1–2 months
Azathioprine	Oral: 50–150 mg daily	CBC w/plt, AST q 2 weeks for 1–2 months	Same as initial q 1–2 months
D-Penicillamine	Oral: 125–250 mg daily, may increase by 125–250 mg q 1–2 months, max: 750 mg daily	Baseline: UA, CBC w/plt, then q week for 1 month	Same as initial q 1–2 months, but q 2 weeks if dose change
Cyclophosphamide	Oral: 1–2 mg/kg/d	UA, CBC w/plt q week for 1 month	Same as initial q 2–4 weeks
Cyclosporine	Oral: 2.5 mg/kg/d	Scr, blood pressure q month	Same as initial
Corticosteroids	Oral, IV, IM, IA, and soft tissue injections: variable	Glucose, blood pressure q 3–6 months	Same as initial

Key: alb, albumin; alk phos, alkaline phosphatase; ALT, alanine aminotransferase; AST, aspartate aminotransferase; BUN, blood urea nitrogen; CBC, complete blood count; hep, hepatitis; IA, intra-articular; IM, intramuscular; IV, intravenous; p, after; plt, platelet; q, every; Scr, serum creatinine; t. bili, total bilirubin; UA, urinalysis.

been previously suggested. Prevention of destructive disease is the basis for this treatment strategy. Many rheumatologists believe early introduction of slow-acting antirheumatic drugs (SAARDs) results in a more favorable outcome. SAARDs include methotrexate, gold, hydroxychloroquine, sulfasalazine, penicillamine, azathioprine, and cyclophosphamide. Some factors identified as predictors for poor outcome include men <50 years, postmenopausal women, poor functional status at first visit, insidious onset, positive rheumatoid factor, radiographic bone erosions, intense clinical inflammation, and markedly elevated erythrocyte sedimentation rate.[13]

NSAIDs alone do not prevent the debilitating complications seen in RA, possibly because of the limited role prostaglandins play in the inflammatory cascade (Fig. 84.2). Used as primary therapy, NSAIDs should be given on a scheduled basis in anti-inflammatory doses. When in combination with SAARDs, NSAIDs may be used as adjunctive therapy for symptomatic control. In some patients, as-needed dosing may be adequate.

SAARDs should be used in all patients except those with limited disease or those with class IV disease in whom little reversibility of disease is expected. Of the SAARDs, methotrexate appears to have the best long-term outcome. It is less toxic and is less likely to be discontinued than other SAARDs. Gold or hydroxychloroquine should be considered in patients who have contraindications or are refractory to methotrexate. The other agents in Fig. 84.9 should be considered second- or third-line drugs in the treatment of RA.

Corticosteroids can be used in various ways. They are valuable in controlling symptoms during the initiation phase of SAARDs. A burst of corticosteroids can be used in acute flares. Continuous low doses may be adjuncts when SAARDs do not provide adequate disease control. Corticosteroids may be injected into joints and soft tissues to

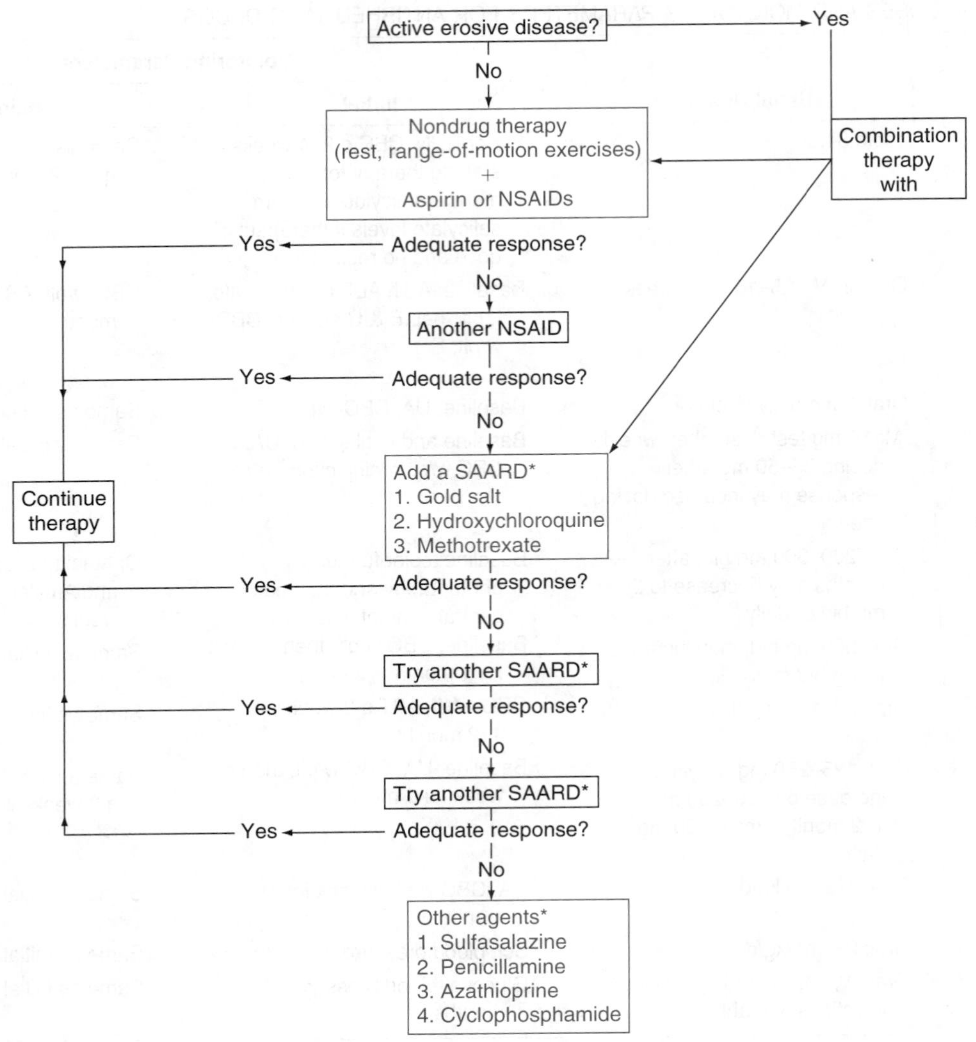

Figure 84.9. Algorithm for treatment of rheumatoid arthritis. *Corticosteroids may be necessary for patients with severe inflammatory disease in any of these phases to enable the patient to be more functional while awaiting the beneficial effects of therapy or in patients with partial responses to therapy.

control local inflammation. Steroids should seldom be used as monotherapy because of their high risk of toxicity. NSAIDs and SAARDs have steroid-sparing properties that permit reductions of steroid doses.

For monitoring parameters and dosing guidelines for SAARDs and NSAIDs used in rheumatoid arthritis, see Tables 84.4 and 84.5.

Nonsteroidal Anti-Inflammatory Drugs

NSAIDs are generally accepted as first-line therapy for the symptomatic treatment of mild RA. NSAIDs possess both analgesic and anti-inflammatory properties and reduce stiffness associated with RA. NSAIDs mainly inhibit prostaglandin synthesis, which is only a small portion of the inflammatory cascade (Fig. 84.2). NSAIDs alone will not prevent joint erosions, and some rheumatologists advocate early combination therapy with slow-acting agents. For discussion of the mechanism of action, adverse effects, and drug interactions, see the anti-inflammatory drugs section of the Osteoarthritis chapter in this text (Chapter 85).[14–16]

Methotrexate

Methotrexate (MTX) was first used to treat psoriatic arthritis and was approved by the FDA for RA in 1988. Use of MTX has slowly increased with time, and it is now the SAARD of choice. MTX is contraindicated in pregnant and nursing women. It is also contraindicated in patients with chronic liver disease, immunodeficiency, pleural or peritoneal effusions, leukopenia, thrombocytopenia, preexisting blood disorders, and creatinine clearance of less than 40 mL/min.

Absorption of MTX is variable and averages about 70% of an oral dose. MTX is 35–50% bound to albumin; it may be displaced by highly protein-bound drugs such as NSAIDs, but the clinical importance of this interaction is

TABLE 84.5. DOSAGE REGIMENS AND DURATIONS OF ANTIPLATELET EFFECT FOR NONSTEROIDAL ANTI-INFLAMMATORY DRUGS

Drug	Recommended Anti-Inflammatory Total Daily Dosage			Approximate Duration of Antiplatelet Effect
	Adult	Children	Dosing Schedule	
Aspirin	2.6–5.2 g	60–100 mg/kg	qid	14 days
Diclofenac	150–200 mg	—	tid to qid	5–10 hours
Diflunisal	0.5–1.5 g	—	bid	2–7 days
Etodolac	0.2–1.2 g (max 20 mg/kg)	—	tid to qid	36 hours
Fenoprofen	0.9–3.0 g	—	qid	15–24 hours
Flurbiprofen	200–300 mg	—	bid to qid	24–48 hours
Ibuprofen	1.2–3.2 g	20–40 mg/kg	tid to qid	5–10 hours
Indomethacin	50–200 mg	2–4 mg/kg (max 200 mg)	bid to qid	24–48 hours
Ketoprofen	150–300 mg	—	tid to qid	5–10 hours
Meclofenamate	200–400 mg	—	tid to qid	24–48 hours
Nabumetone	1–2 g	—	daily to bid	4–7 days
Naproxen	0.5–1.0 g	10 mg/kg	bid	4 days
Naproxen sodium	0.55–1.1 g	—	bid	4 days
Nonacetylated salicylates[a]	1.2–4.8 g	—	bid to 6×/day	None
Oxaprozin	0.6–1.8 g (max. 26 mg/kg)	—	daily to tid	8–10 days
Piroxicam	10–20 mg	—	Daily	7–20 days
Sulindac	300–400 mg	—	bid	4 days
Tolmetin	0.6–1.8 g	15–30 mg/kg	tid to qid	8–16 hours

[a]Choline salicylate, magnesium salicylate, salsalate, sodium salicylate, and sodium thiosalicylate.

not known. The highest concentrations of MTX are distributed into the kidney, liver, gallbladder, spleen, and skin. Increased concentrations are found in synovial fluid of inflamed joints. MTX is extensively metabolized intracellularly to polyglutamated derivatives. It is excreted renally, 80% unchanged, by glomerular filtration and active transport. Some MTX may be reabsorbed, but this transport process may be saturated even with low doses, resulting in increased renal clearance.

MTX has a fairly rapid onset of action; results may be seen as early as 2–3 weeks after starting therapy. Some 45–67% of patients remain on MTX therapy in studies ranging from 5–7 years.[17,18] Sustained efficacy is also reported in patients receiving MTX for up to 15 years.[19] MTX may be given intramuscularly or orally. Doses greater than 15 mg/week are generally given parenterally because of decreased oral bioavailability at larger doses.

The toxicities of MTX therapy are mainly gastrointestinal, hematologic, pulmonary, and hepatic. Stomatitis occurs in 3–10% of patients and may be painful or painless. Diarrhea, nausea, and vomiting may occur in up to 10% of patients. The most common hematologic toxicity is thrombocytopenia in 1–3% of patients. Leukopenia may also occur, but in a smaller number of patients. Although pulmonary fibrosis and pneumonitis are severe adverse effects, they are rare. Elevated liver enzymes may occur in up to 15% of patients; cirrhosis is rare. Guidelines for monitoring hepatotoxicity in patients taking MTX for rheumatoid arthritis have been established. Liver biopsy is now recommended before beginning MTX therapy only for patients with a history of excessive alcohol use, ongoing hepatitis B or C infection, or recurring elevation of aspartate aminotransferase. Biopsies during MTX therapy are recommended only for patients who develop consistently abnormal liver-function tests.[20]

Because it is a folic acid antagonist, MTX can induce a folic acid deficiency. This deficiency is thought partly responsible for MTX toxicity, and supplementation with folic acid 1 mg per day has been shown to alleviate some adverse effects. Addition of folic acid to an MTX regimen for rheumatoid arthritis does not compromise drug efficacy.[21]

Gold

Once thought to be the "gold standard" for treatment of rheumatoid arthritis, the popularity of gold therapy has declined in recent years. This reduction results from the limited efficacy and relatively high toxicity of these compounds. Gold is available as oral (auranofin) or intramuscular (aurothioglucose or gold sodium thiomalate) dosage forms. The antirheumatic effects of oral or injectable gold may be delayed 3–6 months.

Auranofin is poorly absorbed from the gastrointestinal tract, and the extent of distribution to various body compartments is unknown. Urinary excretion accounts for approximately 60% of the drug absorbed, fecal elimination the other 40%.

Aurothioglucose and gold sodium thiomalate are rapidly absorbed after intramuscular injection, although aurothioglucose may be absorbed more slowly because it is an oil suspension. Synovial fluid concentrations of these drugs are much greater than with auranofin. Injectable gold is 85–95% protein bound. Metabolism of parenteral gold is unknown, but the compounds are probably not degraded to elemental gold. Urinary elimination averages 70%. After cumulative dosing of 1 gram of these drugs, they may be detected in the urine 12–15 months after drug discontinuation.

Toxicities of gold compounds are similar, whether taken orally or parenterally. Metallic taste can be a harbinger of other adverse effects. Dermatologic effects such as skin rash and stomatitis require discontinuation of gold therapy; patients may be rechallenged with gold after resolution of these side effects. Renal toxicity manifests as proteinuria and hematuria; hematologic toxicity presents as anemia, leukopenia, or thrombocytopenia. These toxicities are reversible if the drug is discontinued. Gastrointestinal events such as nausea, vomiting, and diarrhea resolve with time or dosage decrease and are more common with auranofin. Injectable gold preparations, particularly gold sodium thiomalate, may cause nitrotoid reactions that may involve flushing, palpitations, hypotension, tachycardia, headache, or blurred vision. Such reactions are self-limiting and usually respond to change of gold salt. Patients may experience increased joint symptoms for 1–2 days after an injection. This is referred to as a postinjection disease flare. If the flare is severe, therapy must be changed.[22–24]

Hydroxychloroquine

The pharmacokinetics of hydroxychloroquine (HCQ) are poorly understood but are probably similar to chloroquine. It is well absorbed orally and widely distributed to body tissues. HCQ is partially metabolized in the liver and is excreted renally. The onset of action of HCQ may be delayed up to 6 weeks, but the drug cannot be considered a therapeutic failure until 6 months of therapy have elapsed.

The main advantage of HCQ is the lack of myelosuppressive, hepatic, and renal toxicities that may be seen with other slow-acting agents. Monitoring of HCQ toxicity is, therefore, simplified in comparison with other SAARDs. Short-term toxicities of HCQ include gastrointestinal effects such as nausea, vomiting, and diarrhea, which can be managed by taking doses with food. Ocular toxicity includes accommodation defects, benign corneal deposits, blurred vision, scotomas (small areas of decreased or absent vision in the visual field), and night blindness. Although the risk of true retinopathy with HCQ approaches zero, preretinopathy may occur in 2.7% of patients. All patients must understand the importance of adhering to HCQ monitoring guidelines as delineated in Table 84.9. Any visual change must be reported immediately. Dermatologic toxicities include rash, alopecia, and increased skin pigmentation; neurologic adverse effects such as headache, vertigo, and insomnia are usually mild.[25–27]

Sulfasalazine

Sulfasalazine, a prodrug, is cleaved by bacteria in the colon into sulfapyridine and 5-aminosalicylic acid (5-ASA). It is believed that the sulfapyradine moiety is responsible for the agent's antirheumatic properties, although the exact mechanism of action is not known. Once the colonic bacteria have cleaved sulfasalazine, sulfapyradine and 5-ASA are rapidly absorbed from the gastrointestinal tract. Sulfapyradine rapidly distributes throughout the body, but higher concentrations are found in certain tissues such as serous fluid, liver, and intestines. Both sulfasalazine and its metabolites are excreted in the urine. Antirheumatic effects should be seen in 1–2 months.

Use of sulfasalazine is often limited by its adverse effects. Gastrointestinal adverse effects such as nausea, vomiting, diarrhea, and anorexia are the most common. These can be minimized by initiating therapy with low doses and gradually titrating to higher doses, dividing the dose more evenly throughout the day, or using enteric-coated preparations. Rash, urticaria, and serum sickness-like reactions can be managed with antihistamines and, if indicated, corticosteroids. If a hypersensitivity reaction occurs, therapy should be stopped immediately and another SAARD substituted. Sulfasalazine has been associated with leukopenia, alopecia, stomatitis, and elevated hepatic enzymes. It may also cause the patient's urine and skin to turn a yellow-orange color.

Sulfasalazine's absorption can be decreased when antibiotics are used that destroy the colonic bacteria. Sulfasalazine also binds iron supplements in the gastrointestinal tract that can lead to a decreased absorption of sulfasalazine. The administration of these two agents should be temporally separated to avoid this interaction. Sulfasalazine can potentiate warfarin's effects by displacing it from protein-binding sites. Close monitoring of the patient's international normalized ratio (INR) is indicated.[28,29]

Azathioprine

Azathioprine is an alkylating agent that is generally considered safer but slower acting than cyclophosphamide. Azathioprine is a purine analogue that is biologically converted to 6-mercaptopurine and is believed to interfere with DNA and RNA synthesis.

Azathioprine is rapidly absorbed after oral dosing and is approximately 30% bound to plasma proteins. The major route of elimination is renal, and doses should be reduced by 25% for patients with creatinine clearances (Cr Cl) of 10–50 mL/min and by 50% for Cr Cl < 10 mL/min.

Antirheumatic effects can be seen within 3–4 weeks. If no response is seen after 12 weeks at maximal dosages, azathioprine should be discontinued.

The major adverse effect associated with azathioprine use is reversible bone-marrow suppression (e.g., leukopenia, macrocytic anemia, pancytopenia, thrombocytopenia) that appears to be dose related. When this occurs, it is common practice to stop the drug temporarily until the marrow recovers. Therapy may be reinstituted at a 25% dose reduction. Other adverse effects include gastrointestinal intolerance, oncogenic potential, stomatitis, infections, drug fever, and hepatotoxicity. Allopurinol inhibits xanthene oxidase, which decreases the metabolism of 6-mercaptopurine and increases the likelihood of myelosuppression. If the two agents must be used together, azathioprine should be reduced to approximately 30% of the usual dose.[30,31]

D-Penicillamine

The pharmacokinetics of this heavy metal chelating agent are not well known. The drug is quickly absorbed from the gastrointestinal tract, but food, antacids, and iron will decrease the amount absorbed. The extent of distribution to body tissues is unknown. D-Penicillamine (DP) is metabolized in the liver and excreted mainly as inactive disulfide metabolites in the urine and feces.

Therapeutic effects may be delayed 1–3 months after starting therapy. Most clinical responses are seen within 6 months.

Early adverse effects of DP include a pruritic, erythematous skin rash, metallic taste, and hypogeusia (decreased taste sensation). Hypogeusia may last 2–3 months and resolves without intervention. A rash or metallic taste occurring after 6 months of therapy with DP requires the drug to be decreased or withheld. It may be reinstituted at a lower dose. Stomatitis, which may be painful or painless, usually improves with a decrease in DP dose. Nausea, vomiting, anorexia, and dyspepsia may occur and are managed by dosage reduction. DP may induce glomerular nephritis, which manifests as proteinuria and hematuria. Other autoimmune diseases include polymyositis, Goodpasture's syndrome, myasthenia gravis, systemic lupus erythematosus, and pemphigus. If any of these develop, DP must be discontinued. Although autoimmune diseases are rare, they are the primary reason most clinicians reserve DP for patients with RA resistant to other therapies.[32,33]

Cyclophosphamide

Cyclophosphamide is derived from nitrogen mustard. It has been shown to be fairly toxic and is reserved for severe, refractory cases of RA. The mechanism of action of cyclophosphamide is not fully known. It appears to be toxic to resting and rapidly dividing cells by cross-linking DNA and damaging DNA repair mechanisms. Cyclophosphamide is rapidly absorbed from the gastrointestinal tract. It is primarily metabolized by the liver into active metabolites; the parent compound is not biologically active.

The adverse effects associated with cyclophosphamide therapy often outweigh its benefits. Adverse effects include oncogenic potential, gastrointestinal intolerance, alopecia, hemorrhagic cystitis, immune system suppression, and gonadal failure. To minimize cyclophosphamide's oncogenic potential, it is often given as intermittent pulse therapy rather than daily since this regimen lowers the total amount of drug ingested. Cyclophosphamide is reserved for life-threatening RA complications.[30,31]

Cyclosporine

Until recently, cyclosporine (CSA) was considered experimental for treating rheumatoid arthritis. Its absorption is variable and incomplete, and the drug has a large volume of distribution (about 13 L/kg). CSA undergoes hepatic metabolism and has many metabolites; one or more of these may have pharmacologic action. The principal route of elimination is biliary; less than 10% is excreted in the urine.

The onset of action of CSA appears to be 1–3 months. Clinically important toxicities of CSA 1–10 mg/kg/d include hypertension, hyperglycemia, nephrotoxicity, tremor, gastrointestinal intolerance, hirsutism, and gingival hyperplasia. Hypertension and nephrotoxicity appear to be reversible after CSA is discontinued.

Because drug therapy for rheumatoid arthritis is long term (perhaps lifelong) and is commonly administered to older adults, the current recommendation is to reserve CSA for patients refractory to or intolerant of other disease-modifying antirheumatic drugs. The drug should be avoided or used cautiously in patients 60 years or older, hypertensives, or patients with serum creatinine greater than 1.0 mg/dL.[34,35]

Corticosteroids

Corticosteroids are used in RA for their anti-inflammatory and immunosuppressive properties. Despite their effects on the immune system, they do not appear to alter the course of disease. They interfere with antigen presentation to T lymphocytes, inhibit prostaglandin and leukotriene synthesis, and inhibit neutrophil and monocyte superoxide radical generation. Corticosteroids also impair migration and cause redistribution of monocytes, lymphocytes, and neutrophils, thus blunting the inflammatory and autoimmune responses.

Oral corticosteroids are rapidly and completely absorbed from the gastrointestinal tract. They are primarily metabolized and inactivated by the liver and excreted in the urine. The elimination half-life of most corticosteroids is sufficiently long that once-daily dosing is possible.

Oral corticosteroids can be used in several ways. They can be used in "bridging" therapy, continuous low-dose therapy, and short-term high-dose bursts to control flares of RA. Oral steroids (e.g., prednisone, methylprednisolone) can be used to control pain and synovitis while SAARDs are taking effect. This is termed "bridging" therapy and is often used in patients with debilitating symptoms when SAARD therapy is initiated. Patients with difficult-to-control disease may be placed on low-dose, long-term corticosteroid therapy to control their symptoms. Prednisone doses below 7.5 mg daily are well tolerated but are not devoid of the long-term adverse effects associated with corticosteroids. The lowest dose of corticosteroid that controls symptoms should be used to reduce adverse effects. Alternate-day dosing of low-dose oral corticosteroids is usually ineffective in RA; symptoms usually flare on days without medication. High-dose corticosteroid bursts are often used to suppress flares of the disease. High doses are sustained for several days until symptoms are controlled, followed by a taper to the lowest effective dose.

Corticosteroids may also be delivered by injection. The intramuscular route is preferable in patients with compliance problems, since a depot effect is achieved. Depot forms of corticosteroids include triamcinolone acetonide, triamcinolone hexacetonide, and methylprednisolone acetate. This provides the patient with 2–8 weeks of symptomatic control. The depot effect provides a physiologic taper, avoiding hypothalamic–pituitary axis (HPA) suppression. It should be noted that the onset of effect via this route may be delayed by several days. Intravenous corticosteroids may be used to provide the patient with large amounts of drug during a steroid burst to control severe symptoms of RA. Intra-articular injections of depot forms of corticosteroids can be useful in treating synovitis and pain when a small number of joints are affected. The onset and duration of symptomatic relief is similar to those of intramuscular injection. The intra-articular route is often preferred because it is associated with the fewest number of systemic adverse effects. If efficacious, intra-articular injections may be repeated every 3 months. No one joint should be injected more than two to three times per year, because of the risk of accelerated joint destruction and atrophy of tendons. Soft tissues such as tendons and bursa may also be injected. This may help control the pain and inflammation associated with these structures. The onset and duration of symptomatic relief is similar to those of intramuscular and intra-articular injections.

Adverse effects are the major limitations to the long-term use of corticosteroids. They include HPA suppression, Cushing's syndrome, osteoporosis, myopathies, glaucoma, cataracts, gastritis, hypertension, hirsutism, electrolyte imbalances, glucose intolerance, skin atrophy, and increased susceptibility to infections. To minimize these effects, use the lowest effective corticosteroid dose and limit the duration of use. Patients on long-term therapy should be given calcium and vitamin D (and estrogen supplements for postmenopausal women) to minimize bone loss. Etidronate or calcitonin may be necessary in patients with evidence of clinically important bone loss. There is no evidence that corticosteroids alone increase the risk of gastrointestinal ulcerations, even though they have been often implicated. Therefore, gastrointestinal protective measures are not usually indicated.[36–38]

Innovative Therapy

As our understanding of the immunopathology of rheumatoid arthritis improves, better ways of suppressing the immune response will be developed. Inhibitors of the cytokines interleukin-1 and tumor necrosis factor are currently under investigation. Monoclonal antibodies directed against the T-cell receptor may help to turn off the inflammatory process. T-cell "vaccination," which down-regulates the immune response, has been successful in treating experimental arthritis in mice. Monoclonal antibodies against adhesion molecules, which prevent the migration of immune cells to the synovium, have been tried with some success in humans. Finally, type II collagen, minocycline and omega III fatty acids have been reported to be of some benefit in treating RA.

SERONEGATIVE SPONDYLOARTHROPATHIES

The seronegative spondyloarthropathies are a group of rheumatic diseases characterized by spinal involvement and negative rheumatoid factors. Peripheral joint involvement, when it exists, tends to be asymmetrical and often involves fewer joints than does rheumatoid arthritis. Psoriatic arthritis, ankylosing spondylitis, Reiter's syndrome, and arthropathy associated with inflammatory bowel disease are some of these disorders. The long-term outcome of patients with these diseases is usually a lesser degree of functional disability compared with that of rheumatoid arthritis. The clinical presentation of these diseases, especially early in their course, may be difficult to distinguish from that of seronegative rheumatoid arthritis. The distinction is important because of the differences in the approach to treatment and clinical outcomes.[2]

There is a genetic predisposition for these diseases. HLA-B27 histocompatibility antigen is positive in a much higher proportion of patients with these disorders than in the general population. Environmental factors play a role in some of these disorders. Reiter's syndrome has occurred in epidemics following outbreaks of *Salmonella* and *Shigella* gastroenteritis and may also be associated with *Chlamydia* infections.

PSORIATIC ARTHRITIS

Psoriatic arthritis occurs in 7% of patients with psoriasis. There are four major patterns of joint involvement:

(1) the classical presentation predominantly involving the distal interphalangeal joints of the hands;
(2) arthritis mutilans, in which severe destructive changes, with resorption of bone, results in "telescoping" (shortening) of digits;
(3) the oligoarticular pattern, in which a few joints are involved; and
(4) symmetric polyarthropathy, which mimics seronegative rheumatoid arthritis.

There is no relationship between the clinical course of the skin disease and the course of the joint activity. There is a relationship between psoriatic nail changes, pitting and onycholysis (lifting of the distal portion of the nail from the nail bed), and joint involvement. Digits often develop a characteristic "sausage-like" appearance with diffuse swelling of the finger, as opposed to the articular swelling observed in rheumatoid arthritis. Inflammation of tendon insertion sites is commonly seen. Involvement of the sacroiliac joints is seen in 20% of patients. There are no specific laboratory tests to help identify this disorder.

Most patients respond well to NSAIDs. Most clinicians believe indomethacin is particularly effective. Methotrexate may be considered the SAARD of choice in patients who need more than NSAIDs because it treats both the arthritis and skin disease. Gold salts, azathioprine, and sulfasalazine have been effective in psoriatic arthritis. Etretinate, used to treat the skin manifestations, has also been suggested to have anti-inflammatory properties useful in treating the joint symptoms. Hydroxychloroquine may also be useful, but exacerbations of the patient's skin disease can occur. Prednisone may be useful in treating both skin and joint disease; however, the complications of long-term treatment with corticosteroids make their use in chronic management less desirable.[39,40]

ANKYLOSING SPONDYLITIS

This disease primarily involves the axial skeleton. Inflammation of the spinal column and sacroiliac joints can eventually lead to fusion of these joints with a resultant loss of motion. The disease is more often diagnosed in men. HLA-B27 is positive in 90% of patients with ankylosing spondylitis (compared with 6–8% of the normal population). Enthesopathy (inflammation of tendinous attachments to bone) is the predominant pathologic finding in patients with ankylosing spondylitis. Asymmetric peripheral arthritis may be seen in one-third of the patients. Involvement of the lower extremities is more common than upper extremity arthritis. Inflammation of rib articulations can result in bony fusion and a decrease in the ability to expand the chest with breathing. Iritis occurs in 25% of patients. Topical corticosteroids may be required to relieve the inflammation. Involvement of the aortic root can lead to cardiac murmurs and, rarely, to serious cardiac disease. Involvement of the cardiac conduction system can lead to electrocardiographic abnormalities and arrhythmias.

Patients usually present with back pain and stiffness that typically improves with activity. NSAIDs are the primary mode of treatment. Indomethacin is particularly effective for most patients. Although these drugs provide symptomatic relief, nothing appears to alter the clinical course of the disease. Sulfasalazine has been shown to be of benefit in treating the peripheral arthritis, but has not been shown to alter the spinal disease. Other SAARDs may be tried but there is limited documentation of their efficacy. In severe cases, the end result of the chronic inflammation is bony fusion of the spine (radiographically giving the spine the classic bamboo appearance). Physical therapy is essential to help prevent spinal flexion deformities.[41,42]

REITER'S SYNDROME

Reiter's syndrome is an inflammatory disease with the classic triad of symptoms of arthritis, urethritis, and conjunctivitis. Some patients do not demonstrate all three symptoms seen in the classic presentation.

The arthritis is typically asymmetrical in distribution. Enthesopathy is a common feature in Reiter's syndrome; heel pain and calcification of the plantar fascial insertion (calcaneal spur) are common findings. Urethritis may occur episodically during the course of the disease. Conjunctivitis may be asymptomatic; other serious inflammatory eye diseases have also been reported. Characteristic skin rashes associated with Reiter's syndrome include circinate balanitis (a scaly erythematous rash surrounding the head of the penis) and keratoderma blennorhagicum (a dry scaly rash on the soles of the feet and the palmar surface of the hands, accompanied by vesicles). Painless mucosal ulcers of the mouth and genitalia may occur. The usual course of Reiter's disease is characterized by acute exacerbations and asymptomatic intervals, although chronic arthritis may also be seen. Some patients may have a single episode of illness lasting weeks to months. There is a strong association between Reiter's syndrome and bacterial dysentery or venereal infections.

Treatment is symptomatic, with NSAIDs being the primary form of therapy. Injections of corticosteroids into inflamed tendon insertion sites may be of value in isolated inflamed tendonitis. Sulfasalazine may be tried in those patients with clinically important peripheral joint involvement. Because of the association with infectious diseases, antimicrobial treatment has been tried with variable results. The value of gold, penicillamine, hydroxychloroquine, and immunosuppressive agents has not been proven in controlled studies.

ARTHRITIS ASSOCIATED WITH INFLAMMATORY BOWEL DISEASE

Arthritis occurs in 11% of patients with ulcerative colitis and 21% of patients with Crohn's disease. Joint distribution is usually asymmetrical and often involves only a few joints. An ankylosing spondylitis-like picture may be seen. The synovitis usually is not chronic in nature and does not result in deformity. Colectomy usually results in resolution of the arthritis associated with ulcerative colitis. Analgesics and NSAIDs may be used for symptomatic treatment.[2]

CONCLUSION

Rheumatoid arthritis is the most common inflammatory arthritis, affecting approximately 3% of the population. The disease is characterized by symmetric swelling and stiffness of the involved joints. The stiffness is usually more prominent in the morning. Extra-articular features of rheumatoid arthritis include rheumatoid nodules, vasculitis, and ocular, cardiac, and pulmonary complications. The course of the disease is highly variable. Treatment is aimed at relieving pain and inflammation and maintaining and preserving joint function. The initial drug treatment in patients with mild disease is either aspirin or NSAIDs. Nondrug therapy, including exercise and adequate rest periods, should be used early in the course of treatment. One of the SAARDs such as methotrexate, gold, or hydroxychloroquine may be added to NSAID therapy in patients with inadequate response to initial treatment or those with more active disease. Sulfasalazine, penicillamine, azathioprine, and cyclophosphamide may be effective in patients failing to respond to or having serious toxicity to other SAARDs. The use of cyclophosphamide must be weighed against the potential for long-term toxicity. Corticosteroids are a useful adjunct for treatment, but because of adverse effects should be used in the lowest possible dose for the shortest possible treatment interval.

The seronegative spondyloarthropathies are a cluster of inflammatory rheumatic diseases that include psoriatic arthritis, ankylosing spondylitis, Reiter's syndrome, and the arthropathy associated with inflammatory bowel disease. These diseases have many of the features of rheumatoid arthritis but are distinctly different, with a greater tendency for asymmetric peripheral joint inflammation and involvement of the axial spine. Psoriatic arthritis may be treated in much the same way as rheumatoid arthritis. The efficacy of SAARDs in the management of the other seronegative diseases is not as well documented.

REFERENCES

1. Harris ED. The clinical features of rheumatoid arthritis, in Kelly WN, Harris ED, Ruddy S, Sledge CB (eds): Textbook of Rheumatology, 4th ed. Philadelphia, WB Saunders, 1993, p 943.
2. Schumacher HR, Klippel JH, Koopman WJ (eds). Primer of the Rheumatic Diseases, 10th ed. Atlanta, GA, The Arthritis Foundation, 1993.
3. Claman HN. The biology of the immune response. JAMA 1992;268:2790–2796.
4. Condemi JJ. The autoimmune diseases. JAMA 1992;268:2882–2892.
5. Harris ED. Pathogenesis of rheumatoid arthritis, in Kelley WN, Harris ED, Ruddy S, Sledge CB (eds): Textbook of Rheumatology, 4th ed. Philadelphia, WB Saunders, 1993, p 833.
6. Harris ED. Rheumatoid arthritis: Pathophysiology and implications for therapy. N Engl J Med 1990;322:1277–1289.
7. Sewell KL, Trentham DE. Pathogenesis of rheumatoid arthritis. Lancet 1993;341:283–290.
8. Snyderman R. Mechanisms of inflammation and leukocyte chemotaxis in the rheumatic diseases. Med Clin North Am 1986;70:217–235.
9. Hard ER. Extraarticular manifestations of rheumatoid arthritis. Semin Arthr Rheum 1979;8:151–176.
10. Brower AC. Use of the radiograph to measure the course of rheumatoid arthritis: The gold standard of fool's gold. Arthr Rheumatol 1990;33:316–324.
11. St. Clair EW, Polisson RP. Therapeutic approaches to the treatment of rheumatoid arthritis. Med Clin North Am 1986;70:285–304.
12. Harris ED. The management of rheumatoid arthritis, in Kelley WN, Harris ED, Ruddy S, Sledge CB (eds): Textbook of Rheumatology, 4th ed. Philadelphia, WB Saunders, 1993, p 912.
13. Vikingsson A, Graziano FM. Rheumatoid arthritis. Importance of early diagnosis in long-term outcome. Postgrad Med 1993;94(8):165–180.
14. Green JM, Winickoff RN. Cost-conscious prescribing of non-steroidal anti-inflammatory drugs for adults with arthritis. Arch Intern Med 1992;152:1995–2002.
15. Brooks PM, Day RO. Nonsteroidal antiinflammatory drugs—differences and similarities. N Engl J Med 1991;324:1716–1725.
16. Paulus HE. Current medicinal approaches to the treatment of rheumatoid arthritis. Clin Orthop 1991;265:96–102.
17. Pincus T, Marcum SB, Callahan LF. Long-term drug therapy for rheumatoid arthritis in seven rheumatology private practices: II. second line drugs and prednisone. J Rheumatol 1992;19:1885–1894.
18. Wolfe F, Hawley DJ, Cathey MA. Termination of slow acting antirheumatic therapy in rheumatoid arthritis: A 14-year prospective evaluation of 1017 consecutive starts. J Rheumatol 1990;17:994–1002.
19. Weinblatt ME, Maier AL. Long-term experience with low dose weekly methotrexate in rheumatoid arthritis. J Rheumatol 1990;17(suppl 22):33–38.
20. Kremer JM, Alarcon GS, Lightfoot RW Jr, et al. Methotrexate for rheumatoid arthritis. Suggested guidelines for monitoring liver toxicity. Arthr Rheumatol 1994;37(3):316–328.
21. Morgan SL, Baggott JE, Vaughn WH, et al. The effect of folic acid supplementation on the toxicity of low-dose

methotrexate in patients with rheumatoid arthritis. Arthr Rheumatol 1990;33(1):9–18.
22. Furst DE. Mechanism of action, pharmacology, clinical efficacy and side effects of auranofin. An orally administered organic gold compound for the treatment of rheumatoid arthritis. Pharmacotherapy 1983;3:284–298.
23. Champion GD, Cairns DR, Bieri D, et al. Dose response studies and long-term evaluation of auranofin in rheumatoid arthritis. J Rheumatol 1988;15:28–34.
24. Gibbons RB. Complications of chrysotherapy. A review of recent studies. Arch Intern Med 1979;139:343–346.
25. Ruiz RS, Saatci OA. Chloroquine and hydroxychloroquine retinopathy: How to follow affected patients. Ann Ophthalmol 1991;23:290–291.
26. Finbloom DS, Silver K, Newsome DA, Gunkel R. Comparison of hydroxychloroquine and chloroquine use and the development of retinal toxicity. J Rheumatol 1985;12:692–694.
27. Mackenzie AH. Antimalarial drugs for rheumatoid arthritis. Am J Med 1983(Dec 30);(suppl):48–58.
28. McConkey B. Disease-modifying antirheumatic drugs: Gold, penicillamine, antimalarials, and sulfasalazine. Curr Opin Rheumatol 1991;3:348–354.
29. Neumann VC, Taggart AJ, LeGallez P, et al. A study to determine the active moiety of sulfasalazine in rheumatoid arthritis. J Rheumatol 1986;13:285–287.
30. Luqmani RA, Palmer RG, Bacon PA. Azathioprine, cyclophosphamide and chlorambucil. Baillieres Clin Rheumatol 1990;4:595–619.
31. Brooks PM. Clinical management of rheumatoid arthritis. Lancet 1993;341:286–290.
32. Jaffe IA. Penicillamine: An anti-rheumatoid drug. Am J Med 1983(Dec 30);(suppl):63–68.
33. Muijsers AO, Van de Stadt RJ, Henrichs AMA, et al. D-penicillamine in patients with rheumatoid arthritis. Serum levels, pharmacokinetic aspects, and correlation with clinical course and side effects. Arthr Rheumatol 1984;27(12):1362–1369.
34. Horton S, Resman-Targoff BH, Thompson DF. Use of cyclosporine in rheumatoid arthritis. Ann Pharmacother 1993;27:44–46.
35. Tugwell P. Cyclosporine in rheumatoid arthritis: Documented efficacy and safety. Semin Arthr Rheumatol 1992;21(6 suppl 3):30–38.
36. Moeser PJ. Corticosteroid therapy for rheumatoid arthritis: Benefits and limitations. Postgrad Med 1991;90:175–182.
37. Weiss MM. Corticosteroids in rheumatoid arthritis. Semin Arthr Rheumatol 1989;19:9–21.
38. Caldwell JR, Furst DE. The efficacy and safety of low-dose corticosteroids for rheumatoid arthritis. Semin Arthr Rheumatol 1991;21:1–11.
39. Gladman DD. Psoriatic arthritis: Recent advances in pathogenesis and treatment. Rheum Dis Clin North Am 1992;18:247–256.
40. Goupille P, Soutif D, Valet J-P. Treatment of psoriatic arthritis. Seminars Arthr Rheumatol 1992;21:355–367.
41. Buxbaum J. Therapy for seronegative spondyloarthropathies. Curr Opin Rheumatol 1992;4:500–506.
42. Laurent R. Are there any antirheumatic drugs that modify the course of ankylosing spondylitis? Bailliere's Clin Rheumatol 1990;4:387–400.

Chapter 85

Osteoarthritis

Larry E. Boh, MS, RPh

Osteoarthritis (OA), the most common form of joint disease, affects nearly 10% of the population older than the age of 60 and remains an important public health problem. It ranks second only to cardiovascular diseases in producing severe chronic disability.[1,2] Because of the costs associated with the care of individuals and the progress in understanding of this disease, we have seen a renewed interest in its etiology and treatment.

OA affects primarily the weight-bearing joints of the peripheral and axial skeleton, causing pain, limitation of motion, deformity, and progressive disability. Throughout the literature, terms such as osteoarthrosis, degenerative joint disease (DJD), or hypertrophic arthritis are used to describe this disease, although none of these terms is truly adequate. Osteoarthrosis, a term used primarily in Europe, implies a general lack of inflammation and excess materials in the joint. DJD suggests a wearing out, deterioration, or breakdown of the joint. Hypertrophic arthritis, the earliest historic designation, describes only one aspect of the disease, the overgrowth of bone and cartilage.

Thus, there exists no consensus on the definition of this disease.[2,3] Because articular cartilage is a very anabolic, synthetic, and reparative tissue, and inflammation may be present in up to 75% of osteoarthritic joints,[2–6] the most commonly used designation "osteoarthritis" will probably continue to be used. With this term, it remains important to remember that osteoarthritis is not a single disorder but a sequence of events or a pattern of reactions that lead to joint injury. It is generally characterized as a noninflammatory disorder of the joints whereby deterioration and changes to the articular cartilage result in formation of new bone at the surfaces of the joint.

Historical Perspective

OA occurs not only in humans, but in many other animal species as well. In some of these species such as dogs or horses, it is considered a major health problem. Historically, it has been observed in all vertebrates with bony skeletons, from reptiles, birds, and mammals to the prehistoric dinosaurs. Interestingly, OA has not been observed in animals with cartilaginous skeletons such as sharks but has been seen in whales, dolphins, and fish.[7,8] These findings are contrary to the "wear-and-tear" theory historically described in the literature, because these species are constantly supported by water.

It was not until 1907 that OA was identified as a separate clinical entity by Garrod.[7] This occurred despite numerous clinical and pathologic descriptions dating back to the early 1800s when Heberden first described the presence of nodes or nodules on the distal hand joints. Between 1907 and 1910, the differentiation between rheumatoid arthritis (RA) and OA was made in terms of clinical and pathologic presentation. This has led to the present attempts to define the heterogeneity of OA into various subsets based on classification of joints involved, presence of specific features or causative factors, primary (idiopathic) or secondary (result of previous joint damage).

Epidemiology

Osteoarthritis remains the most prevalent of the rheumatic diseases and a common cause of decreased worker productivity and disability.[2,9–11] The disease prevalence increases with age. Radiographic data confirm the presence of OA at some site in the body in the majority of individuals older than 65 years of age and in more than 80% of those ages 75 and older. Although numerous epidemiologic studies have reported on the prevalence of OA, estimates of the true prevalence remain imprecise because of a lack of a clear diagnostic definition and variations in the reporting mechanisms.[12] Further, many patients with radiographic evidence of OA do not have symptoms or disabilities for which they seek health care, thus making estimates of disease extent and severity difficult without large-scale controlled population data.

PREVALENCE BY AGE, SEX, AND RACE

In the United States, the most frequently cited series of prevalence data are reported by the National Centers for

Health Statistics (NCHS). These data, referred to as the National Health Interview Survey (NHIS) and the National Health and Nutrition Examination Survey (NHANES), are based on probability samples of the U.S. civilian, noninstitutionalized population more than 20–30 years ago. Using this information, an estimated 15.8 million adults, or 12% of those between 25–74 years of age, have signs and symptoms of OA. As anticipated, the proportion of moderate to severe cases also increases with age. In the less than 45-year-old group, 19.3% of hands and 23.9% of feet were categorized as mild to severe. By comparison, in the 75- to 79-year-old group, 85% and 51% have this degree of changes in the hands and feet, respectively. OA of the knee also increased from less than 0.1% in people between the ages of 25–34 to 10–20% for those 65–74 years old. Likewise, the proportion of individuals with OA classified as moderate to severe increased with age, reaching 33% of knees and about 50% of hips for individuals between 65 and 74 years of age.

In the United States, both sexes tend to be equally affected by OA. However, older women are about twice as likely as men to be affected with OA of the knee and hands.[2,11,13] In Europe, a report of a Dutch village of 6585 randomly selected individuals, also confirms this observation of increased prevalence in women and severity.[14] In women ages 65–70 years, 75% had OA of their distal interphalangeal joint (DIP), also known as Heberden's nodes, in contrast to less than 60% of men in that same age group (Fig. 85.1).

Racial, ethnic, and urban–rural differences in the prevalence of OA are often difficult to establish because of the variations in sampling procedures and diagnostic criteria. OA of the knee has been reported to be twice as prevalent in black than white women.[13] The Chinese, East Indians, and Native Americans have a lower prevalence of hip OA than do Caucasians.[2] These differences, whether related to lifestyles, occupations, or genetic differences further underscore the importance of a variety of factors that must be considered when evaluating the prevalence data.

INCIDENCE

Only recently has information become available addressing the issue of incidence of OA in a population.[15] The overall incidence of newly diagnosed OA of the hip or knee was about 200/100,000 person–years in this population-based study in 1985 of 98 individuals. The incidence of hip OA was greater in women than in men while the rate for knee disease was similar in both sexes. Rates at both the knee and hip increase with age in men but plateau after menopause in women. With this population-based data, it is estimated that approximately 500,000 new symptomatic cases of idiopathic OA occur annually in the white population of the United States.

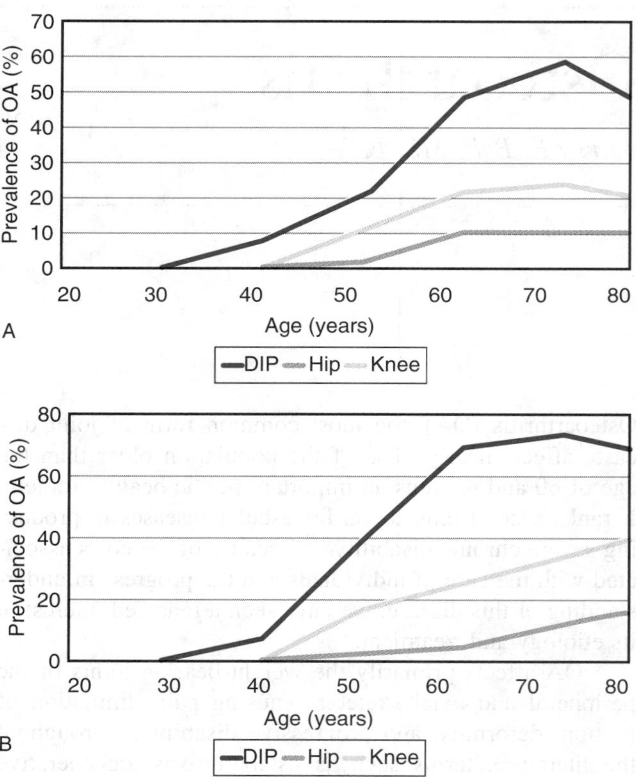

Figure 85.1. Prevalence of radiographic osteoarthritis of the hip, knee, and distal interphalangeal (DIP) joints. (A) Men; (B) women. *(Adapted from Van Saase JL, Van Romunde LK, Cats A, et al. Epidemiology of osteoarthritis: Zoetermeer survey. Comparison of radiological osteoarthritis in a Dutch population with that in 10 other populations. Ann Rheum Dis 1989;48:271–280, with permission.)*

RISK FACTORS—OBESITY

Increased body mass has been closely associated with OA at the knee and less strongly with hip OA.[2,11,16] Historically, until the Framingham data, it was difficult to establish whether obesity preceded or even caused OA, or whether the obesity occurred as a result of the sedentary lifestyle in patient's with OA. From this report, individuals who were in the highest quintile for body mass, at the beginning of this 36-year follow-up study, demonstrated a relative risk for developing knee OA of 1.5 for men and 2.1 for women. The relative risk for developing severe knee OA, increased further to 1.9 for men and 3.2 for women. A subsequent report demonstrated that, in obese individuals, a weight loss of as little as 5 kg could further reduce the risk by up to 50% of developing symptomatic knee OA.[16]

OCCUPATION, SPORTS, AND TRAUMA

The role of repetitive use either through work or leisure activities has been implicated in causing OA. In certain workers that perform repetitive activities such as dock workers, basket weavers, cotton mill workers, or jackhammer operators, a higher incidence of OA of the hand has been observed.[2,17,18] In professional sports, such as football, there appears to be a higher incidence in the development of lower extremity OA. However, in those individuals engaged in long-distance running the development of OA does not occur with increased frequency.[19,20] This increased occurrence of developing OA in certain types of occupations or activities is believed to be related to the repeated exposures throughout the day. Thus duration and intensity of the activity appear to play a major role. Further, trauma to the joint, loss of ligament integrity, or damage of the meniscus can lead to the development of knee OA. This model of joint instability, used to study the development of OA in dogs, may also account for the higher incidence of OA in football players who have trauma-associated knee injuries.

GENETIC FACTORS

Heredity is a determinant with certain types of osteoarthritis. Heberden's nodes are 10 times more prevalent in women than men and their occurrence about twice as likely if a woman's mother has these findings. Other types of osteoarthritis associated with genetic links include involvement of the first metatarsophalangeal joints, generalized osteoarthritis, and the recently described genetic defect in type II procollagen.[21,22] This discovery—of a genetic link that alters the cartilage matrix and leads to premature development of osteoarthritis—enhances understanding of the disease and may ultimately lead to screening at-risk patients and the targeting of therapeutic modalities in selected patients.

OSTEOPOROSIS

In individuals with osteoporosis, several reports have been made of an inverse relationship associated with osteoarthritis of either the knee or hip, although this remains a controversial issue.[2,23,24] Less dense bone in osteoporosis may be better able to distribute the load across the joint thus slowing the development of OA. However, a confounding variable is that obesity—common in OA—is often associated with increased bone mass in almost all skeletal sites.[2,24,25]

PATHOPHYSIOLOGY

The major changes associated with osteoarthritis involve cartilage and the associated joint. Over the past several years, considerable interest has led to advances in the understanding of articular cartilage function and physiology. This knowledge has dispelled the wear-and-tear theory and focused attention on the dynamic changes occurring within the joint as normal functioning is sought to be maintained.[2,4–6,26] Thus the pathogenesis of OA involves not only the biomechanical forces but other factors such as inflammatory, biochemical, and immunologic.

Before discussing these factors, it is useful to classify OA clinically. Based on proceedings of a workshop on the etiopathogenesis of osteoarthritis, the two major categories are defined as *idiopathic* (primary) and *secondary* (Table 85.1).[26] Idiopathic OA is further defined as *localized,* which refers to involvement at a specific joint, or *generalized,* in which three or more sites of OA exhibit extensive involvement. Secondary refers to the development of OA that occurs because of other reasons such as trauma, metabolic or endocrine disorders, or congenital factors. To assist in uniform reporting of rheumatic diseases, a classification scheme and criteria for OA of the hip, knee, and hand have been reported by the American College of Rheumatology (ACR).[27] These criteria include both subjective and objective factors such as pain, bony changes on examination, sedimentation rate, and radiographic features consistent with OA.

To assist the reader in understanding the relationships and changes associated with osteoarthritis, normal cartilage function, biochemistry, and mechanics of a diarthroidal joint are reviewed. More detailed discussions of cartilage biochemistry and function can be found elsewhere.[2,4–6,26,28,29]

TABLE 85.1. CLASSIFICATION OF OSTEOARTHRITIS

Primary	Secondary
Idiopathic	Trauma—acute/chronic
Generalized	Underlying joint disorder
	Local (fracture/infection)
	Diffuse (rheumatoid arthritis)
Erosive	Systemic metabolic or endocrine disorders
	Wilson's disease
	Acromegaly
	Hyperparathyroidism
	Hemochromatosis
	Paget's disease
	Diabetes mellitus
	Obesity
	Crystal deposition disease
	Basic calcium phosphate crystal disease
	Calcium pyrophosphate dihydrate
	Hydroxyapatite
	Other calcium-containing crystals
	Monosodium urate monohydrate
	Neuropathic disorders
	Intra-articular corticosteroid overuse
	Avascular necrosis
	Bone dysplasia

(Compiled from Refs. 27 and 32.)

NORMAL CARTILAGE

Function

In the free-moving diarthrodial joint (Fig. 85.2) cartilage provides a low-friction surface covering the concave and convex ends of the bone. Its major features are to (1) provide for movement within the required range of motion, (2) distribute load across the joint tissues thereby preventing damage, and (3) promote stability during use. It is avascular, aneural, and alymphatic with a calcified base covering a thin layer of cortical bone known as the subchondral plate. Because of its frictionless surface, cartilage provides a smooth gliding surface during movement of the joint and serves as a shock absorber or load support. Upon compression from weight loading, it is easily deformed; up to 40% of its height can be compressed. As a result, when a load is applied, cartilage can provide a large contact area and disperse this force more uniformly to the underlying bone. Despite these characteristics, cartilage is relatively thin (2–5 mm thick), so that loading energy is not taken up there but actually transmitted directly to the bone. Therefore, the greatest share of loading energy is taken up within the tendons, ligaments, and surrounding muscles of that joint.

Structure and Biochemical Composition of Cartilage

Histologically, articular cartilage is a hydrated (75–80% water by weight) extensive extracellular matrix (ECM) comprising a small number of chondrocytes (<5%). The remainder (20–25%) of the cartilage matrix consists of two types of macromolecules: type II collagen and large aggregates of proteoglycans or aggrecans. Cartilage can be divided into four zones: a superficial or tangential zone, an intermediate or transitional zone, the deep or radial zone, and the calcified cartilage zone located below the tidemark and above the subchondral bone. These zones typically reflect the changes between composition of chondrocytes, distribution of collagen, and heterogeneity of proteoglycan components in the cartilage matrix (Fig. 85.3). At the basal zone, the type II collagen fibers are perpendicular and serve to anchor cartilage to the subchondral bone. At the superficial zone, these collagen fibers are densely packed and are parallel to the motion of the surface.

Chondrocytes

Chondrocytes control the synthesis and degradation of this matrix by affecting the production of collagen and proteoglycans. Since adult articular cartilage is avascular, the chondrocytes must receive their nutrition from the synovial fluid. With the cyclic movement and loading of joints, nutrients flow into the cartilage, while immobilization reduces nutrient supply.

Recently, considerable interest has developed in the role peptide growth factors play in regulating chondrocyte function.[4,5,29] Some of these growth factors—such as low concentrations of insulin-like growth factor, epidermal growth factor, or fibroblast growth factor—cause an enhanced proliferation of chondrocytes and synthesis of proteoglycans. At the same time, the cytokines such as interleukin-1 (IL-1) and tumor necrosis factor (TNF-α) have been shown to induce chondrocytes to release major matrix metalloproteases (MMP) such as collagenase (MMP-1) and stromelysin (MMP-2), which have the ability to degrade most if not all of the matrix proteins. These cytokines also have the ability to suppress the synthesis of proteoglycans and collagen within the ECM.[4,5,29]

This role of growth factors has raised considerable interest in how these factors may ultimately interact to regulate chondrocyte function and enhance articular cartilage repair. Despite enthusiasm in reviewing these effects, it is

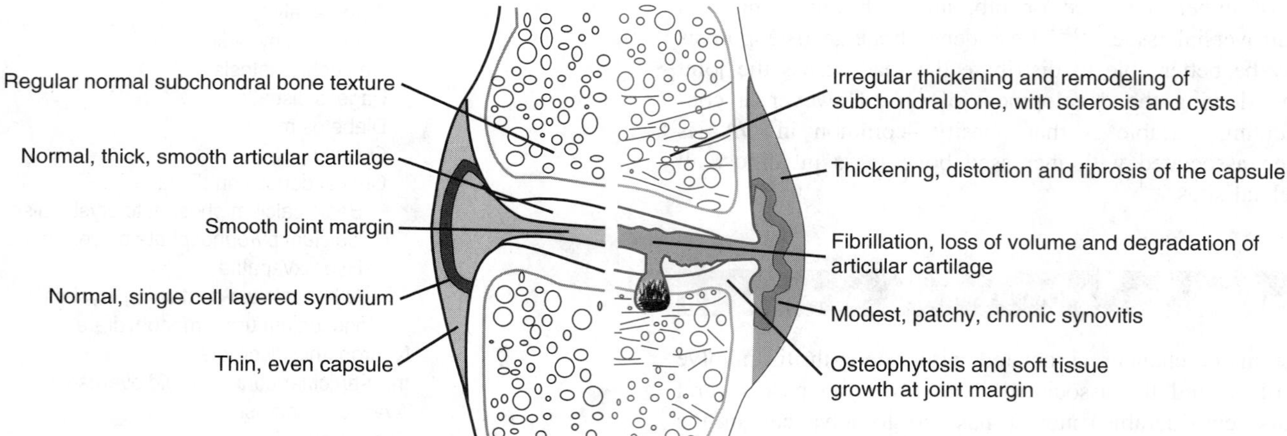

Figure 85.2. Characteristics of osteoarthritis in the diarthrodial joint.

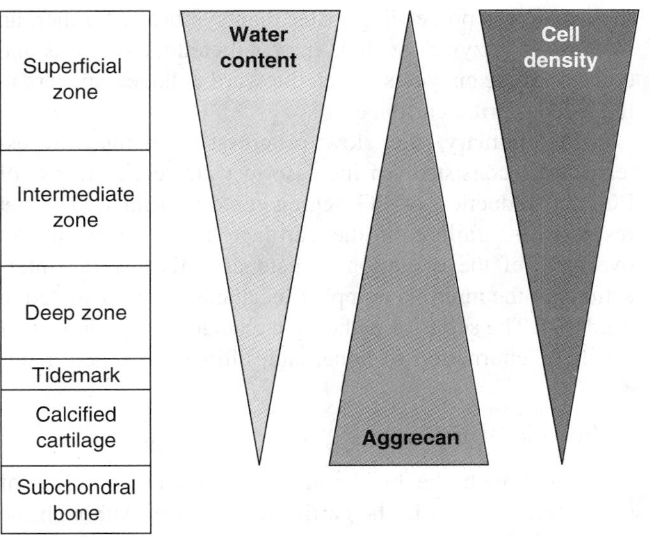

Figure 85.3. Structure and composition of articular cartilage by zone.

important to use caution in applying findings from one type of tissue to another, extrapolating *in vitro* to *in vivo* data, and developing therapeutic agents that may affect a particular factor. Since the actions of growth factors and cytokines have multiple complex roles in the regulation of articular cartilage, they should be viewed more as messengers, effectors, or signaling agents.[5]

The role of biomechanical factors such as defined loads and strains also appears to affect how chondrocytes alter the production of proteoglycans. In some studies, joint loading has markedly improved the production of proteoglycans.[5] Therefore, this area of biochemical and biomechanical study appears to hold considerable promise for improving understanding about osteoarthritis.

Collagen

Of the approximately 14 distinct types of collagen, five types (type II, IX, X, XI, and VI) are primarily located in cartilage. The most predominant type (about 80–95%) of collagen found in articular cartilage is type II.[4,5,30] The other types of collagen are found in reduced amounts and their exact function has not been clearly defined.[5] It does appear that type IX may play a role in linking to other matrix molecules; interestingly, this molecule is also a proteoglycan.[2,3] The network of type II collagen fibrils and their cross-linking among collagen molecules and other ECM proteins provides the tensile strength and maintenance of the tissue's volume and shape. This is accomplished by the ordering of the collagen fibers. Near the surface, the fibers remain in a direction parallel to the surface thereby providing the ability to dissipate forces. In contrast, collagen fibers located near the basal layer are perpendicular to the surface. This allows the collagen fibers to assume a role in anchoring of the uncalcified cartilage to the calcified zone or subchondral bony endplate.

Proteoglycans

The large aggregates of proteoglycans (PGs) provide the "stuffing material" for the matrix. The predominant type of proteoglycan in cartilage is called *aggrecan.* Each aggregate consists of a linear protein linked to repeating chains of disaccharides called glycosaminoglycans (GAGs). The GAGs include negatively charged chondroitin 4-sulfate, chondroitin 6-sulfate (CS) chains, and keratan sulfate (KS). By covalently binding to the protein core, these molecules form a proteoglycan subunit. The subunits then combine with long hyaluronate molecules to form aggregates. The aggregates retain and maintain the water content of the cartilage because of their highly hydrophilic and anionic properties. These characteristics give cartilage its resilience and load-bearing properties.

Under pressure, these compounds release water and enhance solute flux and chondrocyte nutrition; then, on removal of pressure, the compounds regain their water content. It is also this property that renders the PG molecular structure vulnerable to degradation by the matrix metalloproteases; cleavage of only one or two peptide bonds can totally alter the properties of this molecule. Thus PG turnover occurs at a faster rate than does collagen turnover. When protease degradation of proteoglycans has been experimentally induced, cartilage has maintained its shape but lost its elastic properties.[4,5]

With the degradation of the ECM there is a release of collagen and proteoglycan fragments into the synovial fluid. This liberation of contents eventually reaches the blood and urine. Various experimental assays have been created to identify and measure these compounds to assist with diagnosis or as monitoring tools. Although experimental, these tools provide additional approaches to aid understanding of the metabolic changes within the joint.[2]

OSTEOARTHRITIC CARTILAGE

Biochemical Changes

Several changes have been reported in the composition of osteoarthritic cartilage (Table 85.2). An initial biochemical change in cartilage appears to be an increase in water content of the cartilage matrix despite a reduction in the hydrophilic proteoglycans. This initial change results in a thickened articular cartilage but one less able to withstand mechanical forces. Although the reason for this change is not clearly understood, it may relate to damage of the collagen fiber network, which is no longer able to restrain the PGs. This allows the molecules to increase hydration and expand.[4,5,25] The decrease in proteoglycan content appears to correlate with the severity of the disease and may relate to the release of the many matrix metalloproteases.

Soon after these changes in water content occur, the GAG composition changes, reflecting changes in keratan

TABLE 85.2. CHANGES IN OSTEOARTHRITIC CARTILAGE

Increase in water content
Increase in chondroitin sulfate 4 to chondroitin sulfate 6 ratio
Increase in proteases, especially neutral metalloproteinases
Decrease in glycosaminoglycans—chondroitin sulfate and keratan sulfate
Decrease in proteoglycan aggregation
Decrease in proteoglycan monomer size
Minimal change in collagen content

(Compiled from Refs. 27 and 32.)

sulfate and the ratio of chondroitin 4-sulfate to chondroitin 6-sulfate. These changes may result in decreased PG–collagen interaction in the cartilage. The collagen content does not appear to change until severe disease is present. Increases in collagen synthesis and in the distribution and diameter of the fibers have been noted.[4–6,25]

Originally, researchers believed that cartilage passively eroded away. However, cellular activity actually increases, suggesting that the articular cartilage is responding with a reparative process.[4,12,25] This increase in activity appears to continue only until the disease is advanced and may suggest a possible failure of the chondrocytes.

Despite the increase in matrix synthesis controlled by the chondrocytes, there continues to be a loss of proteoglycan and an increase in water content. This implies that

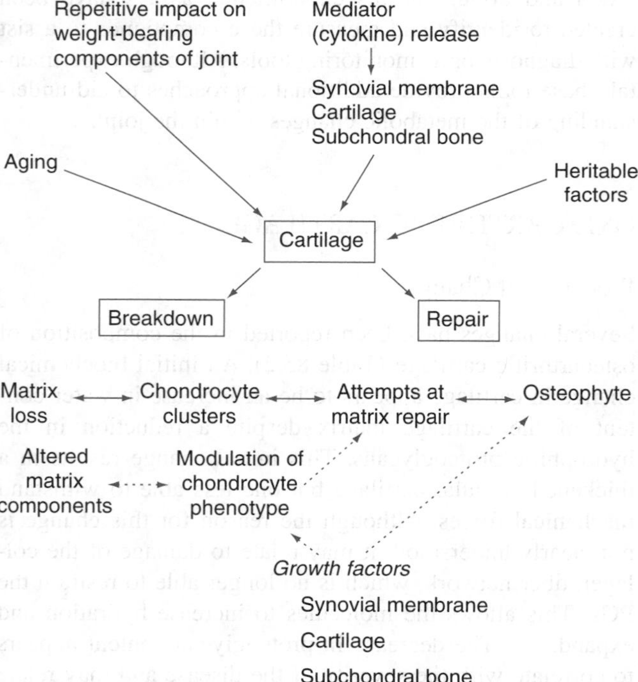

Figure 85.4. Factors contributing to the evolution of osteoarthritis. *(From Hamerman D. The biology of osteoarthritis. N Engl J Med 1989;320(2):1322–1330, with permission.)*

degradation is proceeding faster than synthesis. Further, an increase in enzymes such as matrix metalloproteinases and collagenolytic enzymes directed toward collagen appears in the osteoarthritic cartilage.

In summary, the slow progressive changes in osteoarthritis consist of an increase in water content, loss of PG, and reduction of PG aggregates of cartilage. The net result is the failure of the cartilage to repair itself. An overview of the evolution of osteoarthritis and the interactions of the multiple complex mechanisms are depicted in Fig. 85.4. The series of pathologic changes results in loss of cartilage, eburnation of bone, and, ultimately, severe pain.

Pathologic Changes

Coexistent with the biochemical changes are a series of pathologic changes in the cartilage and bone. Although the early pathologic changes are not well defined in humans, the intermediate- and late-stage changes in osteoarthritis are well characterized. To address the early changes, two animal models, the canine cruciate-deficient and the rabbit meniscectomy models, have provided useful information. Further, changes are similar for weight-bearing and non-weight-bearing joints and for idiopathic OA and secondary osteoarthritis. Specifically, the following are observed in cartilage:

1. An initial thickening of the articular cartilage occurs. This reflects the damage to the collagen network and increase of water content.
2. Joint synovial lining may show moderate degrees of inflammation.
3. Fibrillation, a splitting of the noncalcified cartilage believed to be related to the biochemical changes described earlier. This exposes the underlying bone, which may ultimately lead to microfractures of the subchondral bone.
4. Horizontal splitting of cartilage between the calcified and uncalcified layers secondary to shearing damage.
5. Cartilage thinning and erosions progressing to focal exposure of the calcified cartilage and underlying bone as a result of grinding damage or abrasive wear.

As destruction of the cartilage progresses, pathologic changes in subchondral bone occur. The appearance varies considerably depending on the site of cartilage loss; areas lacking the protective layer of cartilage demonstrate the most changes. The superficial portion of subchondral bone contains necrotic osteocytes. Increased osteoblastic and osteoclastic activity with osteolytic foci or cysts is observed below the superficial layer. The exposed area of bone may contain fibrous or chondroid tissue, presumably reflecting reactive bone resorption and vascular changes. With continued progression, the cartilaginous layer is completely eroded, leaving denuded subchondral bone that becomes dense, smooth, and glistening (eburnation). This alters the physical properties of the bone and results in a brittle, stiffer bone less able to resist the stress of bearing weight.[4,5,25] The subchondral bone then develops sclerosis and microfractures. Microfractures result in the production of callus and increased amounts of osteoid. New bone formation at the joint margins, away from the area of cartilage destruction, is referred to as *osteophytes.* An interesting observation is that osteophytes can occur in the absence of cartilage destruction and, conversely, cartilage destruction can occur in the absence of osteophytes. Osteophytes may be an attempt to stabilize the joints and may not be part of the destructive aspects of osteoarthritis.

The joint capsule and synovium also show a variety of pathologic changes secondary to OA. Inflammation, such as synovitis, is seen and may result from the release of inflammatory mediators such as prostaglandins secreted by the chondrocytes.[25]

CLINICAL PRESENTATION

SIGNS/SYMPTOMS

The clinical presentation (Table 85.3) depends on the duration of disease, the joints affected, and the severity of joint involvement. The predominant symptom is a localized deep, aching pain associated with the affected joint. If more than one joint is involved or if systemic symptoms are present, another form of arthritis or connective tissue disease should be considered. However, many patients with documented OA (either pathologically or radiographically) remain asymptomatic.

Early in the course of the disease, pain occurs when the joint is first used and becomes relieved by rest or removal of weight from the affected joint. Later, the pain occurs with minimal motion or activity and may be present even during rest. The pain is not related to the destruction of cartilage, because cartilage is aneural (Fig. 85.5). Rather, the pain arises from the activation of nociceptive nerve endings by the mechanical and chemical irritants related to joint pathology.[31] Pain caused by a bursitis, tendinitis, or muscular pain can also confuse the patient's presentation and require an accurate diagnosis. Weather or changes in the barometric pressure also seem to aggravate the pain associated with OA.

The joints most commonly affected in primary OA are the distal and proximal interphalangeal (DIP and PIP) joints of the hand, the first carpometacarpal joint, knees, hips, cervical and lumbar spine, and the first metatarsophalangeal (MTP) joint of the toe. In addition to pain in the affected joint, limitation of motion, stiffness, crepitus,

TABLE 85.3. CLINICAL PRESENTATION OF OSTEOARTHRITIS

Age
- Usually elderly

Sex
- Age <45 more common in men
  - >45 more common in women (hands)

Symptoms
- Pain
- Deep, aching
- Pain on motion
- Early in disease—pain with use
- Late in disease—pain at rest
- Stiffness
  - Rarely exceeds 15 min; related to weather
  - Localized to involved joints
- Limited joint motion
- Instability of weight-bearing joints
- Crepitus, crackling

Signs/Physical Examination
- Monoarticular or oligoarticular; asymmetrical involvement
- Joints frequently involved
  - Hands—DIP, PIP, first carpometacarpal joint
  - Foot—first metatarsophalangeal
  - Hips, knees, cervical spine, lumbar spine
- Observations on joint examination
  - Bony proliferation or occasional synovitis
  - Local tenderness
  - Crepitus
  - Muscle atrophy
  - Limited motion with passive/active movement
  - Effusions
- Characteristics of synovial fluid
  - High viscocity
  - Mild leukocytosis (<2000 WBC/mm^3)

Laboratory Values
- No specific test
- ESR, hematologic survey, chemistry survey are normal
- No systemic manifestations

Key: DIP, distal interphalangeal; PIP, proximal interphalangeal; ESR, erythrocyte sedimentation rate. (Compiled from Refs. 27, 32, and 78.)

and deformities may be present. The limitation of motion that develops as the disease progresses is related to the loss of articular surfaces, muscle spasms, capsular contracture, and mechanical blockage secondary to osteophytosis. Patients may also notice a decreased range of motion (ROM) of an affected joint by describing limitations in performing normal activities of daily living (ADLs). A sense of weakness or instability (described by patients as the joint "gives way") is yet another feature associated with this limitation of motion observed in patient's with lower extremity involvement.

Joint stiffness is often another complaint expressed by patients with OA. The joint stiffness is of a relatively short duration, unlike that described by patients with rheumatoid arthritis. Most important, the stiffness lasts less than 30

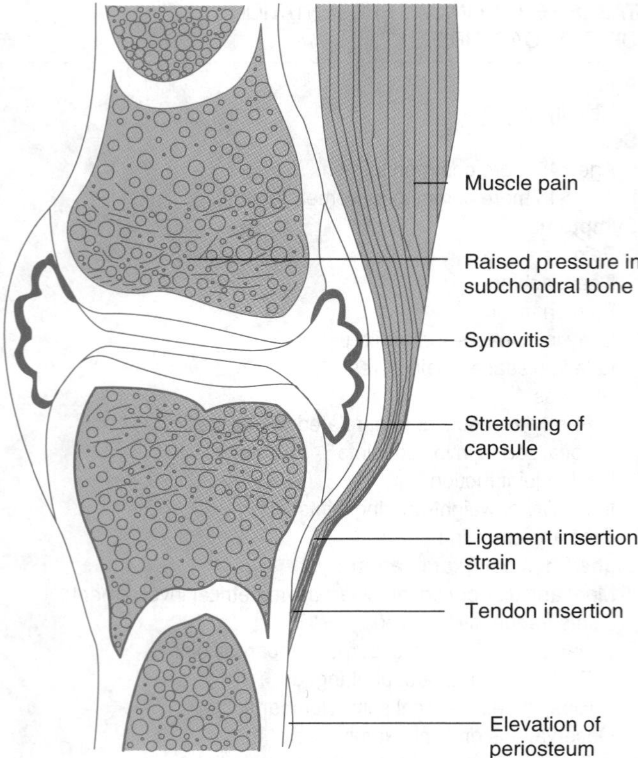

Figure 85.5. Possible causes of pain in osteoarthritis.

minutes and often occurs after sitting or resting for some time. However, after movement it seems to resolve, leading some to describe this as a "gelling phenomenon." Crepitation, or the crackling-grating sound heard as the joint moves, is related to irregularity of the joint surface and loss of cartilage. Joint enlargement is typically related to bony proliferation or in some cases thickening of the synovium and joint capsule. The presence of a warm, red, tender joint may suggest an inflammatory type of synovitis.

Joint deformity may be present in the later stages of OA and is the result of subluxation, collapse of subchondral bone, formation of bone cysts, or bony overgrowths. Patient descriptions of joint swelling require close clinical inspection to separate synovial thickening (inflammation) from the bony proliferation observed in OA.

PHYSICAL EXAMINATION

Physical examination of the affected joint or joints reveals pain, tenderness, crepitus, and possible joint enlargement.[27,32] The specific findings reported on physical examination of the commonly affected joints in OA in contrast to RA are shown in Fig. 84.3 in the Rheumatoid Arthritis chapter.

Hands

Hand involvement in OA primarily involves the DIP, PIP, and first carpometacarpal (Fig. 85.6). Heberden's and Bouchard's nodes are bony enlargements (osteophytes) of the DIP and PIP joints, respectively. Heberden's nodes usually develop slowly, are nonpainful, occur on both lateral and medial aspects of the joint, and are approximately 10 times more common on women than men.[27] Occasionally, these nodes become red, warm, swollen, and painful, usually as a result of trauma or use. A strong female hereditary predominance is demonstrated on questioning of the patient.

In patients with first carpometacarpal joint involvement, pain and tenderness are common. The increase in osteophytosis gives the radial aspect of the hand the characteristic square appearance termed the *shelf sign.* Difficulty pinching and opening the tops of bottles or jars is a frequent concern.

Knees

The knee is one of the most commonly affected joints. It is important to localize the symptoms because the joint has three separate articulations: the patellofemoral and the medial and lateral compartments (Fig. 85.7). Pain related to climbing stairs is typically associated with patellofemoral joint involvement. Presentation with a bowlegged deformity (genu varum) is caused by medial compartment involvement; knock-knee deformity (genu valgum) results from lateral compartment involvement. The symptoms include pain, tenderness, crepitation, limited extension with passive or active motion, and joint instability. These symptoms may cause the patient to limit the use of this joint, thereby causing muscle atrophy. Transient joint effusions may also occur. The synovial fluid is typically noninflammatory (white blood cell [WBC] count $<2000/mm^3$ with normal protein).

Hips

The symptoms of OA of the hip frequently appear in older individuals and can be described by the three patterns of hip joint involvement: superolateral, medial pole, and concentric (Fig. 85.8). Hip osteoarthritis is associated with buttock or groin pain exacerbated when the patient is bearing weight, standing up, or walking. Pain located on the outside of the hip is typically bursitis and should not be confused with hip disease. Stiffness is common, especially after inactivity, and joint motion may be limited.

Spine

Degenerative changes result from involvement of the intervertebral disks, vertebral bodies, or posterior apophyseal articulations. In the lumbar spine area L3–4 involvement is most common. The resulting nerve root compression can cause pain, paresthesias, loss of reflexes, and muscle weakness in the distribution of the affected nerve root.

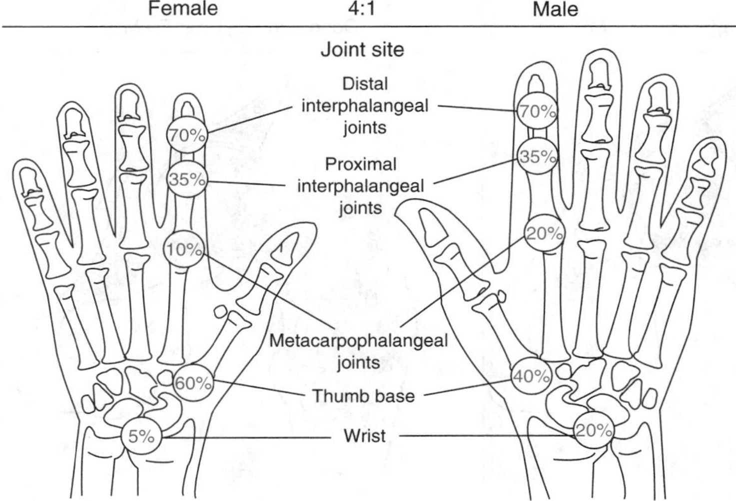

Figure 85.6. Distribution of osteoarthritis of the hands. *(Adapted from Dieppe P. Osteoarthritis: Clinical features and diagnostic problems, in Klippel JH, Dieppe PA (eds): Rheumatology. London, Mosby-Year Book Europe Limited, 1994, sec. 7, chap. 4, pp 1–16)*

Feet

The involvement in the feet is limited primarily to the first metatarsophalangeal joint. Pain, tenderness, and stiffness are the predominant symptoms.

Other joints not commonly involved include the shoulder, elbow, acromioclavicular, sternoclavicular, and temporomandibular joint. (For a more detailed discussion, see Ref. 32.)

LABORATORY FINDINGS

No specific clinical laboratory abnormalities occur in primary OA. Erythrocyte sedimentation rate (ESR), routine chemistry studies, complete hematologic surveys, and urinalysis are generally normal. However, the ESR may be slightly elevated in patients with generalized or erosive inflammatory OA. The rheumatoid factor test is negative. Analysis of the synovial fluid reveals fluid with high viscosity. This fluid demonstrates a mild leukocytosis (<2000 WBC/mm^3) with predominantly mononuclear cells. In the case of secondary osteoarthritis associated with an underlying metabolic disorder or endocrinopathy, specific laboratory tests are indicated to identify the cause.

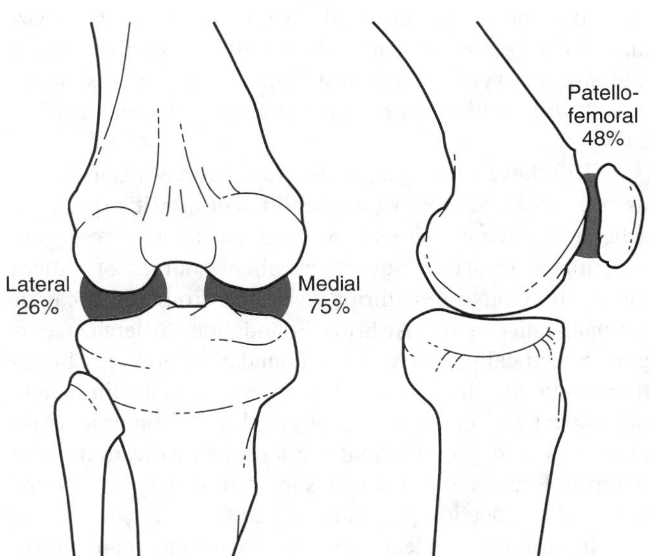

Figure 85.7. Distribution of osteoarthritis of the knees. *(Adapted from Dieppe P. Osteoarthritis: Clinical features and diagnostic problems, in Klipel JH, Dieppe PA (eds): Rheumatology. London, Mosby-Year Book Europe Limited, 1994, sec. 7, chap. 4, pp 1–16)*

RADIOLOGIC EVALUATION

Radiologic evaluation is an absolute necessity in the diagnosis of OA. In early, mild OA, radiographic changes may be normal. With the progression of degenerative changes in cartilage, the joint space may begin to narrow, subchondral bony sclerosis occurs, and marginal osteophyte and cyst formation may develop. Late in the disease process, subluxation and deformity sometimes occur. In general, osteoporosis and joint erosions are not seen, but they do occur in a subset of patients with erosive OA.

Technetium-99*m* bone imaging has also been used to demonstrate the appearance of OA and may actually precede the development seen on plain radiographs of the affected joint. Specifically, weight-bearing radiographs at the knee provide better definition of the joint space. Newer imaging techniques such as computed tomography (CT) scans and magnetic resonance imaging (MRI) or ultrasonographic techniques are also used but often provide limited useful information in routine examination of OA joints.[27] Joint arthroscopic examination can also confirm the diagnosis or extent of OA present in a particular joint; however, few clinical situations require this procedure to establish a diagnosis of OA.

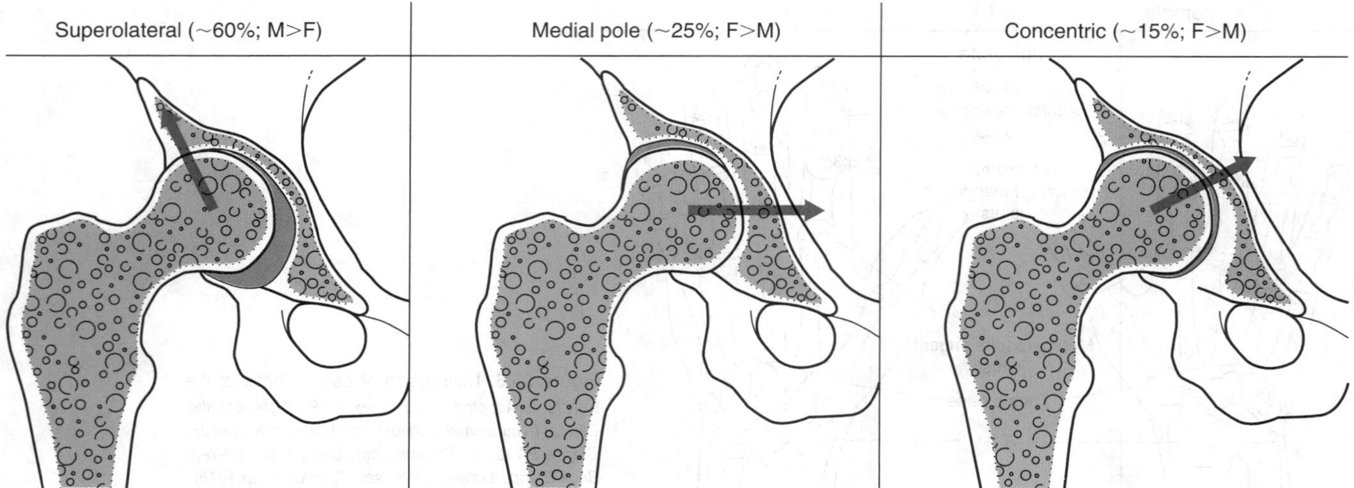

Figure 85.8. Distribution of osteoarthritis of the hip joint. *(Adapted from Dieppe P. Osteoarthritis: Clinical features and diagnostic problems, in Klippel JH, Dieppe PA (eds): Rheumatology. London, Mosby-Year Book Europe Limited, 1994, sec. 7, chap. 4, pp 1–16)*

DIAGNOSIS

The diagnosis of osteoarthritis is strongly dependent on an evaluation of the patient's history, clinical examination of the affected joint(s), and radiologic findings. Awareness of other connective tissue diseases that may exhibit DIP joint involvement such as with psoriatic arthritis or Reiter's syndrome (discussed in Chapter 84, Rheumatoid Arthritis) can sometimes result in confusion. Although the diagnosis is relatively straightforward, a complete examination of all clinical information is required and not until all components are evaluated can an accurate diagnosis be made.

PROGNOSIS

The prognosis for patients with primary OA is variable and depends on the joint involved. If a weight-bearing joint or the spine is involved, considerable morbidity and disability are possible. In the case of secondary OA, the prognosis depends on the underlying cause of osteoarthritis. Treatment of the cause may prevent further progression but does not reverse joint changes already present.

TREATMENT

Successful therapeutic management of the patient with OA depends on accurate diagnosis of the degree and extent of joint involvement. Because many patients are commonly asymptomatic, radiologic diagnosis and clinical examination and history are paramount. Further, the optimal treatment approach must be individualized to include, as appropriate, physical therapy, occupational therapy, dietary considerations, drug therapy, surgery, and patient education. The major goals are to (1) educate the patient, caregivers, and relatives; (2) relieve symptoms such as pain and stiffness; (3) preserve the joint motion and function by limiting disease progression; and (4) minimize the disability.

NONDRUG THERAPY

An effective management plan requires more than drug therapy. The first step is to educate the patient about the extent, degree of involvement, prognosis, and management approach. OA is often thought of by both the public and some within the medical community as a "wear-and-tear" disease. Patients often will accept that belief, and attribute symptoms to just "one of those things" associated with getting older and therefore not seek medical care.

To relieve their symptoms, patients may resort to the use of various alternative medications or arthritis-quackery schemes. Patients should be warned about these and encouraged to access several excellent sources of patient information on osteoarthritis available from the local or national units of the Arthritis Foundation (Atlanta, Georgia). Specifically, the Arthritis Foundation provides literature about the disease and information about clinics and other local agencies offering physical and economic assistance and information about the various medications. The Arthritis Foundation also sponsors various support groups and public education programs.

In addition, contact between OA patients and trained lay personnel to review self-care status has demonstrated a beneficial effect in reducing pain and improving physical function in individuals at high risk of morbidity.[33] This approach again highlights the importance of personal contact and interventions as a way to influence patient outcomes positively.

Diet

For the overweight patient, dietary counseling is an important recommendation. The excess weight can contribute not only to the progression of the disease but also to the contraction of the muscles that span and stabilize the joint. Further, obese patients scheduled to undergo total joint replacement of the hips or knees generally have a poorer surgical outcome and postoperative prognosis than patients of normal weight. Weight reduction requires a motivated patient and participation in a supervised program.

Physical/Occupational Therapy

Physical therapy—with heat or cold treatments and an exercise program—helps to maintain and regain joint range of motion, relieve pain, and reduce muscle spasms. Such simple measures as a warm bath or warm water soaks may be effective in reducing pain and diminishing stiffness. With heat application, patients should be cautioned to avoid lying on the heat source for longer than 30 minutes to minimize the risk of burns. Other heat-application techniques consist of diathermy or ultrasound to the affected joints (but not in patients with artificial metal joints because the potential for deep thermal burns exists). These techniques are reserved primarily for deep-seated joints (hips/spine) and are more costly than simpler forms of heat application. Transcutaneous electrical nerve stimulation (TENS), the transmission of an electrical current from the skin to a peripheral nerve, may provide some pain relief primarily for acute pain; however, it is cumbersome and expensive.[34]

Exercise programs using isometric techniques are designed to strengthen the muscles and improve joint function and motion. The program should favor isometric over isotonic exercises because the latter can aggravate the affected joint. Typical exercises for knee involvement consist of quadriceps-setting exercises and straight leg raises designed to strengthen knee and leg muscles. Each exercise should be taught and then observed before the patient is allowed to exercise at home. The exercises should be performed three to four times daily. If severe pain develops during exercise, the patient should be instructed to decrease the number of exercises.

Supervised fitness walking has also been shown to improve a patient's functional status and should be encouraged in selected patients.[35] To assist with walking, various assistive devices—including splints, canes, walkers, and braces—can be used during exercise or daily activities. These devices should be carefully selected to meet each patient's functional abilities and limitations. Patients should then be carefully instructed and their understanding evaluated on the use of the various devices. Other orthotic devices such as heel cups or insoles may also be tried to help relieve pain and improve a patient's ability to walk.

Surgery

Surgical procedures are indicated for patients with severe disease or with substantial pain or marked functional disabilities and in whom conservative therapy has not been effective.[36,37] Often the main indication for surgery in OA is pain of the degree and extent that it hinders a patient's lifestyle. For patients with mild disease of the knee, an osteotomy will correct the malalignment seen with genu varum or genu valgum. Joint debridement may also be indicated to remove free cartilage fragments, eliminate locking, and reduce pain. If osteophytes are large, removal may be attempted to increase joint range of motion. For severe, advanced disease a partial or total arthroplasty is performed primarily to relieve pain, although improvement of motion is also possible. The increased motion occurs more commonly with hip than with knee joint replacements. An arthrodesis or joint fusion can also be performed to reduce the pain associated with degenerative changes, but it will restrict motion of that joint.

DRUG THERAPY

Drug therapy in OA is directed at the symptomatic relief of pain and inflammation when present. Since OA is a disease often occurring in an older aged individual who may also have other preexisting medical conditions, a conservative approach to the use of medications is warranted (Fig. 85.9). This does not imply that patients should not use medications for pain relief, but that the regimen of choice requires a very individualistic approach. Some patients with mild symptoms may require simple topical or oral analgesics; those receiving no relief from the analgesics or those with signs of active inflammation may benefit from the use of an anti-inflammatory medication.

Analgesics

The pain in OA is not related to the degenerating cartilage because cartilage is aneural. Rather, pain occurs primarily at three local sites: synovium, soft tissue around the joint, and bone.[9,34]

The major oral analgesics of choice are acetaminophen and aspirin in doses of 325–650 mg four times daily. To achieve anti-inflammatory activity, aspirin in doses greater than 3.6 g/d is necessary. The zero-order kinetics of anti-inflammatory doses of aspirin has been well described[38]; monitoring of serum salicylate concentrations for efficacy or toxicity is required when anti-inflammatory doses are being administered or if toxicity is suspected. The use of serum salicylate levels is not routine in the treatment of OA. The serum half-life of salicylates ranges from 2 hours for anal-

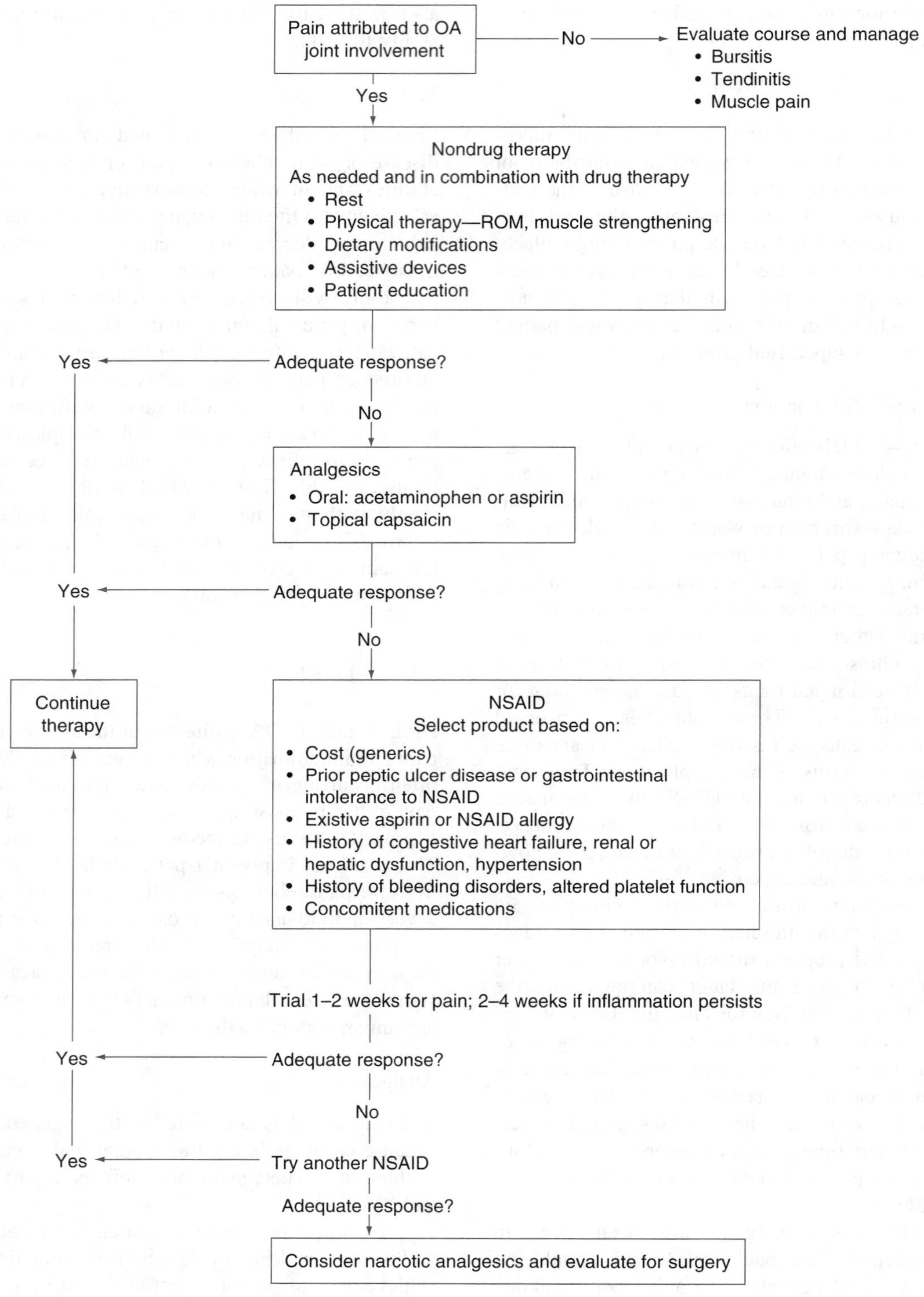

Figure 85.9. Treatment for osteoarthritis.

gesic doses to more than 20 hours for anti-inflammatory doses. Serum concentrations should be measured after five half-lives. The relationship of serum salicylate concentrations to clinical response or toxicity has been described.[38] Therapeutic anti-inflammatory levels are 15–30 mg/dL. Plasma concentrations greater than 30 mg/dL generally correlate with the onset of tinnitus, except in children or in the elderly patient with preexisting hearing loss.

Aspirin is also highly protein bound; increasing doses result in an increase in the apparent volume of distribution as protein-binding site saturation occurs. Low albumin concentrations, increasing age, and highly protein-bound drugs can increase the toxic effects from salicylates.[38] Urinary pH changes can affect the excretion of salicylates several-fold, because an alkaline urine increases the excretion of salicylates. In the choice of a particular aspirin product, several factors related to toxicity should be considered; a large variety of acetylated and nonacetylated salicylate products exist (Table 85.4).

First, salicylates can cause adverse gastrointestinal effects ranging from mild discomfort to gastric ulcers.[39–41] To minimize these effects, the salicylates should be taken with food or milk. Also, enteric-coated products cause less gastric mucosal injury compared with buffered or plain aspirin.[39] However, caution should be used if the enteric products are taken with antacids or milk since the coating can be destroyed, resulting in an increase in abdominal symptoms in susceptible individuals. The nonacetylated salicylate products also produce less gastrointestinal irritation and bleeding than plain aspirin.[42]

Second, the decreased platelet aggregation observed with aspirin is not seen with the nonacetylated salicylate products.[38] These nonacetylated salicylates are a safer alternative in the patient with a bleeding disorder or in those

TABLE 85.4. MEDICATIONS COMMONLY USED IN TREATMENT OF OSTEOARTHRITIS

Medication	Dosage and Frequency	Maximum Dosage (mg/d)
Oral analgesics		
Acetaminophen	325–650 mg every 4–6 hours or 1 g 3–4 times per day	4000
Tramadol	50–100 mg every 4–6 hours	400
Topical analgesics		
Capsaicin 0.025% or 0.075%	Apply to affected joint 3–4 times per day	—
Nonsteroidal anti-inflammatory drugs (NSAIDs)		
Carboxylic Acids		
Acetylated salicylates		
Aspirin, plain, buffered or enteric coated	325–650 mg every 4–6 hours pain. Anti-inflammatory doses start at 3600 mg/d in divided doses	3600[a]
Nonacetylated salicylates		
Salsalate	500–1000 mg 2–3 times per day	3000[a]
Diflunisal	500–1000 mg 2 times per day	
Choline salicylate[b]	500–1000 mg 2–3 times per day	3000[a]
Choline magnesium salicylate	500–1000 mg 2–3 times per day	3000[a]
Acetic acids		
Etodolac	800–1200 mg/d in divided doses	120–1200
Diclofenac	100–150 mg/d in divided doses	200
Indomethacin	25 mg 2–3 times a day; 75 mg SR once daily	200; 150
Ketorolac[c]	10 mg every 4–6 hours	40
Nabumetone[d]	500–1000 mg 1–2 times a day	2000
Propionic acids		
Fenoprofen	300–600 mg 3–4 times per day	3200
Flurbiprofen	200–300 mg/d in 2–4 divided doses	300
Ibuprofen	1200–3200 mg/d in 3–4 divided doses	3200
Ketoprofen	150–300 mg/d in 3–4 divided doses	300
Naproxen	250–500 mg twice per day	1500
Naproxen sodium	275–550 mg twice per day	1375
Oxaprozin	1200 mg daily	1800
Fenamates		
Meclofenamate	200–400 mg/d in 3–4 divided doses	400
Mefenamic acid[e]	250 mg every 6 hours	1000
Pyrazoles		
Phenylbutazone[f]	100–200 mg twice per day	400
Oxicams		
Piroxicam	20 mg daily	20

[a]Monitor serum salicylate levels over 3–3.6 g/d.
[b]Only available as a liquid; 870 mg salicylate/5 mL.
[c]Not approved for treatment of OA or more than 5 days.
[d]Nonorganic acid but metabolite is an acetic acid.
[e]Not approved for treatment of OA.
[f]Not to exceed 1 week in patients greater than 60 years old.

patients scheduled to undergo a surgical procedure. Third, a clinically important syndrome of aspirin intolerance exists in some patients. Administration of aspirin can result in two kinds of reactions: type A—bronchoconstriction, vasomotor rhinitis, and nasal polyps or laryngeal edema; type B—urticaria and angioedema. Type A occurs in 2–4% of asthmatics with cross-sensitivity to other nonsteroidal anti-inflammatory drugs (NSAIDs) (although a nonacetylated salicylate may be tolerated). The postulated mechanism for this reaction was inhibition of prostaglandin synthesis, but other potential mechanisms may exist, as described in a recent review.[43]

Type B reactions generally occur with other salicylates.[43,44] Other toxic responses to aspirin products include impaired renal function and increases in serum transaminases. Another factor to consider in selection of a product is cost. Nonacetylated products are considerably more expensive than plain aspirin.

For patients who need only analgesic therapy, acetaminophen 650 mg four times daily provides analgesia comparable with that provided by aspirin 650 mg four times daily without the associated gastrointestinal toxicity of aspirin. The lack of anti-inflammatory properties of acetaminophen limits its usefulness in patients with evidence of inflammation. However, several recent reports have demonstrated the comparable efficacy of acetaminophen (2.6–4 g/d) to either ibuprofen at doses of 1200 or 2400 mg/d or naproxen 750 mg/d in relieving the pain symptoms associated with OA of the knee.[45,46] This has lead some clinicians to recommend the use of acetaminophen in doses less than 4 g/d as first-line therapy for the short-term symptomatic relief of OA pain.[45–47]

Generally, acetaminophen is well tolerated by patients, but when taken in excess, for prolonged periods of time, or by at-risk populations, hepatic or renal toxicity have been reported.[48–50] Likewise, a potential increase in acetaminophen toxicity can occur when nonprescription acetaminophen products (especially extra-strength ones) are used concurrently with prescription acetaminophen-containing products.

To avoid the systemic effects associated with various medications, the use of topical products may also be tried either alone or as an adjunct to oral analgesics or NSAIDs. Topical administration of capsaicin, an extract of red peppers that produces release of and ultimately depletion of substance P, has been beneficial in providing pain relief in OA. The depletion of substance P, a principal transmitter of nociceptive impulses from the periphery to central nervous system, was first used for temporary relief of neuralgia associated with herpes zoster infections or in patients with diabetic neuropathy.[51–53] This product is administered either two to four times a day by gently rubbing the cream around the affected joint. Pain relief often takes several weeks of consistent application before maximal pain relief is noted. It is generally well tolerated by most patients, though some will report a burning or stinging sensation when it is first applied.

Other analgesics include the newly approved tramadol, a centrally acting analgesic, or propoxyphene or stronger narcotics such as codeine. These agents are often reserved for patients who have failed single- or multiple-agent therapy with simple analgesics, topical agents, or NSAIDs. Patients should be instructed to use these products primarily for severe pain and for the shortest duration possible. Ideally, prescriptions should be written for a limited quantity with only one or two refills to minimize the abuse potential associated with these agents and to assist with assessing the degree of patient discomfort experienced. If the pain becomes unbearable and limits a patient's ADLs, then surgery is indicated rather than using more or stronger narcotics.

Nonsteroidal Anti-Inflammatory Drugs

NSAIDs provide analgesic effects at lower doses and anti-inflammatory activity at higher doses. Several NSAIDs from a variety of chemical classes are available (Table 85.4); more products are in various phases of clinical testing in Europe and the United States.[54,55]

As a class of compounds, the NSAIDs are all comparably effective in reducing pain and modifying or diminishing the inflammatory process. Although the exact mechanism of action is unknown, a major component of the activity of all NSAIDs is believed to be related to a reduction of prostaglandin biosynthesis by inhibition of cyclooxygenase (PGHS-1 and PGHS-2) (Fig. 85.10).[54,56–59] PGHS-1 concentrations within the body are relatively constant, being present in vascular endothelial cells, platelets, and kidney collecting tubules. PGHS-2 concentrations are relatively low but increase during the inflammatory response. Recently, attention has focused on which isoenzyme is inhibited by the various NSAIDs, because selective inhibition of PGHS-2 may result in less toxicity (gastrointestinal, antiplatelet, renal) while still maintaining anti-

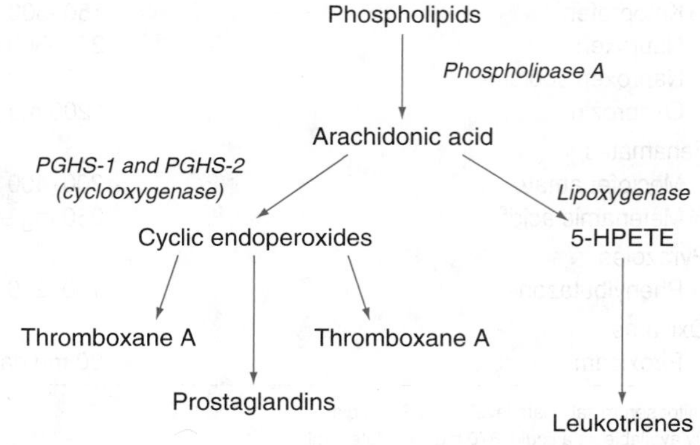

Figure 85.10. Pathway of synthesis of prostaglandins and leukotreine. PGHS-1 and PGHS-2 are prostaglandin H_1 and H_2 synthetases.

inflammatory effects. Although this appears to be an interesting observation in some models, it has not been consistently observed and further study is warranted.[59]

Other actions of the NSAIDs at various dose ranges include inhibiting a variety of enzymes, proteoglycan synthesis, transmembrane ion fluxes, cell–cell binding, and the immune system.[54,56,59]

The choice of a particular NSAID is frequently a matter of prescriber preference based on past treatment, cost, patient preference, toxic effects, and compliance. In general, the NSAIDs are indicated after simple analgesics have failed to relieve pain, toxic effects have developed, or inflammation is present. All NSAIDs are as effective as aspirin in terms of analgesia or anti-inflammatory properties and cause fewer gastrointestinal complaints than does aspirin.[40,54,58–60] These characteristics have encouraged many clinicians to select the NSAIDs before aspirin; however, often the NSAIDs are considerably more expensive, unless generic products are available (e.g., ibuprofen, naproxen).

The pharmacokinetics of the individual NSAIDs are generally similar except for serum half-lives.[54,58,61] All are well absorbed after oral administration, are highly protein bound (greater than 90%), and have a low volume of distribution (<0.2 L/kg). Elimination is via hepatic biotransformation to inactive metabolites (except sulindac or nabumetone, which are metabolized to an active form), with renal excretion of less than 5% of unchanged drug. Total body clearance is low (for most NSAIDs, less than 200 mL/min). They readily penetrate the joint fluid in concentrations approximately 60% of the mean plasma concentration, regardless of the elimination half-life of the drug. This may account for a portion of the relatively prolonged biologic effects of NSAIDs with short half-life.[54,58] Therapeutic monitoring of serum and synovial drug concentrations has not been successfully applied.[54,58] The anti-inflammatory effect generally peaks after 2–3 weeks, irrespective of the half-life. Analgesic effectiveness usually occurs 1–2 hours after taking the NSAID and lasts up to 24 hours. The most variable property appears to be the serum half-life, which ranges from 1 hour for tolmetin to 60–90 hours for phenylbutazone.

Patient response to the NSAIDs is typically variable and highly individual.[54,58] A patient may respond well to one drug in a particular chemical class but experience little or no benefit from another NSAID in the same class. Therefore, other NSAIDs may be used in a selective manner after an adequate trial (2–3 weeks) at an adequate dose (either anti-inflammatory or analgesic) of other NSAIDs in a chemical class. Patients should always be instructed that a trial with more than one product may be necessary and compliance with the scheduled regimen is important in evaluating effectiveness. Combination of NSAIDs with other NSAIDs or aspirin increases toxic effects while providing no added benefit.[40]

Gastrointestinal complaints are the most common adverse effects observed with NSAIDs and account for many treatment failures.[40,54,58,61] To minimize adverse effects, administration with food or milk should be encouraged, except for the enteric-coated products, (milk or antacids may destroy the enteric coating and cause increased gastrointestinal symptoms in selected patients). Diarrhea can occur but is more commonly observed with meclofenamate than the other NSAIDs.

All NSAIDs have the potential to cause gastrointestinal bleeding through a variety of mechanisms related to direct topical or systemic effects of the NSAIDs.[40,54,58,62] As organic acids, most NSAIDs are weak acids (except nabumetone), which allows the compounds to become nonionized at a pH of <3.5 in the stomach. This results in the transport across the cell membrane and "ion trapping" within the cell, thereby causing cell death. The systemic manifestations of the NSAIDs are related to inhibition of prostaglandins responsible for providing gastric mucosal protection.

No patient or subgroup of patients is completely free from the risk of NSAID-associated complications or ulcers. Patient symptoms correlate poorly with the endoscopic appearance and severity of mucosal injury. Up to 50% of patients with dyspepsia have mucosa with normal appearance, while approximately 40% of asymptomatic patients have endoscopic evidence of erosive gastritis.[40] However, several factors definitely increase the risk of ulcers and complications related to NSAIDs. These include age >65 years; prior ulcer disease or complications; therapy with high-dose or multiple NSAIDs; concomitant corticosteroid therapy; and NSAID therapy duration less than 3 months. Although testing for fecal occult blood has been recommended as a way to predict NSAID-induced ulcers, it has not been proven reliable. Instead, other pathologic processes that may cause gastrointestinal bleeding may be present and require further investigation.[40]

The location of the mucosal injury secondary to NSAIDs is important when reviewing trials of therapies designed to prevent this injury. The most common site of mucosal injury is to the gastric mucosa, although duodenal damage also occurs in a similar percentage of patients. However, ulcer complications associated with NSAIDs occur with equal frequency at these two sites. H_2-receptor antagonists can prevent NSAID-induced *duodenal* mucosal lesions but not *gastric* ones.[40] Only misoprostil has been demonstrated to unequivocally protect the gastric and duodenal mucosa from the effects of NSAIDs.[63,64] Furthermore, misoprostil did not interfere with the anti-inflammatory effects of the NSAIDs.

Sucralfate has been demonstrated to be less effective than misoprostil in preventing gastric ulcers in patients on NSAIDs.[63] No comparative controlled trials on the use of proton-pump inhibitors have been published to date in full text form.

Despite these trials, there remains no clear protocols outlining use of misoprostil in preventing mucosal injury.[65] In part, the questions of whether misoprostil prevents ulcer complications as opposed to endoscopic changes and concerns of cost effectiveness about use of misoprostil for all versus certain high-risk individuals remain unanswered.

NSAIDs cause a variety of renal complications, including peripheral edema, transient acute renal insufficiency, tubulointerstitial nephropathy, hyperkalemia, and renal papillary necrosis.[54,58,66–69] Many of these complications may be mediated by inhibition of prostaglandins, which have an important role in the regulation of intrarenal blood flow in vasoconstricted states. Highly prone to developing renal insufficiency are patients with congestive heart failure, cirrhosis/ascites, volume contraction (from any cause), and advanced age. Clinical findings associated with NSAID-induced renal syndromes include an increased serum creatinine, blood urea nitrogen (BUN), serum potassium, peripheral edema, and weight gain. Prostaglandin-mediated renal effects are reversible upon discontinuance of therapy. Most data suggest that sulindac and possibly the nonacetylated salicylates are less likely to cause renal insufficiency. However, sulindac can decrease renal function in patients with underlying renal disease or in cirrhosis.[54,58,59] Thus, close monitoring of the serum creatinine for this complication is required and should be based on the drugs' half-lives.[68] After a baseline creatinine determination, agents with a short half-life should have a follow-up creatinine determination within several days, while those with longer half-lives may require a follow-up creatinine level after 5–7 days.

All NSAIDs can cause drug-induced hepatitis. Fortunately, this adverse effect is relatively uncommon. The NSAIDs used in the treatment of OA most frequently implicated include diclofenac and sulindac.[58,70–72] Patient monitoring should include baseline liver studies consisting of the transaminases, AST, and ALT, with therapy stopped if these values exceed two to three times normal.

Other toxic effects include hypersensitivity reactions, rash, or central nervous system complaints such as drowsiness, dizziness, headaches, depression, confusion, and tinnitus.[54,58] Additionally, all the agents that inhibit PGH_1 synthetase affect platelet function to some extent. Aspirin inhibition is irreversible, and platelet function returns to normal only after 5–7 days, whereas the other NSAIDs cause a reversible inhibition that allows platelet function to return to normal sooner (1–3 days) after discontinuance. In either case, the nonacetylated salicylate products and nabumetone—which appear to affect only PGH_2 synthetase—may be preferable for the patient with a bleeding disorder or as a temporary treatment before elective surgical procedures.[54,57,58] Finally, NSAIDs should be used cautiously during pregnancy because of risk to the fetus.[73]

Important drug interactions with the NSAIDs are frequently related to either pharmacokinetic or pharmacologic interactions. These interactions have been described in several excellent reviews.[54,58,74–76] The most potentially serious interactions include the concomitant use of NSAIDs with lithium, warfarin, oral hypoglycemics, methotrexate, lithium, antihypertensives, angiotensin-converting enzyme (ACE) inhibitors, β blockers, and diuretics. Although these effects are variable and often only have been reported with certain NSAIDs, anticipation and careful monitoring can prevent serious adverse effects. Patient monitoring should also include the use of over-the-counter (OTC) NSAIDs and the H_2-receptor antagonist famotidine because a combination of NSAIDs may increase the risk of gastrointestinal toxicity leading to self-medication with an OTC H_2 antagonist product.

A continuing controversy in the treatment of OA with NSAIDs is whether these agents actually help or hinder the progression of osteoarthritis.[47,54,77] Experimental data in animals have demonstrated the ability of salicylates and some NSAIDs to suppress proteoglycan biosynthesis in articular cartilage, while tiaprofenic acid, diclofenac, and piroxicam have been shown to stimulate proteoglycan synthesis. Although the final verdict is not in and further clinical trial data are needed in humans, the findings clearly raise some interesting issues concerning selection of NSAIDs and duration of therapy.

Corticosteroids

Systemic corticosteroid therapy is not recommended in the treatment of osteoarthritis.[27] The side effects associated with prolonged use outweigh any potential benefits of therapy. The use of intra-articular corticosteroids (IAC) may temporarily be helpful, but their long-term benefit remains controversial.[78] If used, IAC should be administered infrequently at intervals of 4–6 months for any given joint. If no improvement occurs from one or two injections, then further treatment is not likely to succeed. After injection, the patient should be instructed to minimize joint activity and the joint stress load for several days. The use of injection of corticosteroids into the ligaments or pericapsular areas can be beneficial and is associated with reduced risks relative to IAC administration.

Other Drugs

A variety of experimental strategies have been used in attempts to target the biochemical changes observed in articular cartilage.[78–81] Glycosaminoglycans (GAG) compounds such as Rumalon, Arteparon (a GAG polysulphate), or Cartrophen (a polysulphated polysaccharide) have been used in some countries and are of considerable interest. These compounds appear to stimulate the synthesis of cartilage but may also play a role in inhibiting the degradative enzyme reactions of articular cartilage.

Other attempts to inhibit the degradative MMPs have included the use of tetracycline or doxycycline, which has markedly reduced the severity of OA in dogs.[81] Still other approaches have centered on affecting the chondrocytes controlling the articular cartilage through the use of various inhibitors of cytokines, such as IL-1 and TNF, which may produce cartilage degradation. Hyaluronic acid (HA), which provides the backbone structure for the large proteoglycan complexes, has been administered via intra-articular injections in an attempt to provide lubrication for the joint surfaces.

Despite the renewed interest in these various regimens, the majority of approaches have undergone limited controlled trials in humans and should be considered experimental.

Evaluation of Therapeutic Outcomes

Pharmacotherapy monitoring is patient specific, focusing on the degree and extent of joint involvement, patient age, concomitant medications and disease states, and the nondrug and drug therapy selected. Generally, the monitoring plan for assessing therapeutic efficacy consists of establishing the patient's baseline pain through the use of a pain visual analogue scale (VAS) and identifying the range of motion for the affected joint (flexion, extension, abduction, or adduction). Depending on the joint affected, measurement of grip strength and 50-foot walking time may aid in the assessment of hand or hip/knee OA, respectively. Baseline radiographs of the respective joint are often performed to assist with establishing the degree and/or extent of joint involvement and may be repeated when the clinical course indicates a worsening of patient symptoms. Other measures include the clinician's global assessment based on the patient's history of activities and limitations caused by the OA as well as documentation of analgesic or NSAID use. Lastly, the use of disease-specific quality of life (QOL) questionnaires for arthritis provide yet another valuable tool in assessing a patient's clinical response to various therapeutic interventions.[82–84]

Establishment of monitoring parameters for adverse effects depends on the therapeutic regimen chosen. Often, the most effective approach is through direct patient questioning. Patients should be questioned directly to establish if they are having any "problems" with their medications rather than first just listing a series of adverse effects. This approach is quite useful and can be followed up with more direct questions relating to the most common adverse effects associated with the respective medication. With most NSAIDs, symptoms of abdominal pain, heartburn, nausea, or change in stool color are often valuable questions to identify gastrointestinal complaints. Patients should also be monitored for any signs of skin rash, headaches, drowsiness, weight gain, or alterations in blood pressure. Baseline serum creatinine determinations, hematology profiles, and serum transaminases with repeat levels as needed are useful in identifying specific toxicities to the kidney, liver, gastrointestinal tract, or bone marrow.

Conclusion

Osteoarthritis is a very common, slowly progressive disorder that affects diarthrodial joints. It is characterized by a progressive deterioration of articular cartilage resulting in loss of articular cartilage and osteophyte formation. Clinically, the manifestations occur later in life and consist of gradual onset of joint pain, stiffness, and limitation of motion. The primary treatment goal is to reduce pain, maintain function, and prevent further destruction. An individualized approach consisting of nondrug therapy such as rest/exercise regimens and drug therapy can be successful in attaining these goals. Currently, the mainstay of therapy consists of oral or topical analgesics and NSAIDs. Experimental therapy aimed at preventing the progression of OA requires further clinical investigations before becoming widely accepted.

References

1. Peyron JG. Osteoarthritis: The epidemiologic viewpoint. Clin Orthop 1986;213:13–19.
2. Brandt KD, Slemenda CW. Osteoarthritis: Epidemiology, pathology, and pathogenesis, in Schumacher HR (ed): Primer on the Rheumatic Diseases, 10th ed. Atlanta, GA, Arthritis Foundation, 1993, pp 184–187.
3. Dougalos M. Clinical assessment of osteoarthritis in clinical trials. Curr Opin Rheumatol 1995;7:87–91.
4. Hamerman D. The biology of osteoarthritis. N Engl J Med 1989;320:1322–1330.
5. Trippel SB. Articular cartilage research. Curr Opin Rheumatol 1990;2:777–782.
6. Ratcliffe A, Seibel MJ. Biochemical markers of osteoarthritis. Curr Opin Rheumatol 1990;2:770–776.
7. Dieppe P. Osteoarthritis: Introduction, in Klippel JH, Dieppe PA (eds): Rheumatology. London, Mosby–Year Book Europe Limited, 1994, sec 7, chap 2, pp 1–2.
8. Peyron J. Inflammation in osteoarthritis (OA): A review of its role in clinical picture, disease progress, subsets and pathophysiology. Semin Arthr Rheumatol 1981;11:115S–116S.
9. Hutton CW. Treatment, pain, and epidemiology of osteoarthritis. Curr Opin Rheumatol 1990;2:765–769.
10. Lawrence RC, Hochberg MC, Kelsey JL, et al. Estimates of the prevalence of selected arthritic and musculoskeletal diseases in the United States. J Rheumatol 1989;16:427–441.
11. Felson DT, Anderson JJ, Naimark A, et al. The prevalence of chondrocalcinosis in the elderly and its association with knee osteoarthritis: The Framingham study. J Rheumatol 1989;16:1241–1245.
12. Spector TD, Hochberg MC. Methodological problems in the epidemiological study of osteoarthritis. Ann Rheum Dis 1994;53:143–146.

13. Davis MA, Ettinger WH, Neuhaus JM, et al. Knee osteoarthritis and physical functioning: Evidence from the NHANEWSI epidemiologic follow-up study. J Rheumatol 1991;18:591–598.
14. Van Saase JL, Van Romunde LK, Cats A, et al. Epidemiology of osteoarthritis: Zoetermeer survey. Comparison of radiological osteoarthritis in a Dutch population with that in 10 other populations. Ann Rheum Dis 1989;48:271–280.
15. Wilson MG, Michet CJ, Strup DM, Melton IJ. Idiopathic symptomatic osteoarthritis of the hip and knee: A population-based incidence study. Mayo Clin Proc 1990;60:1214–1221.
16. Felson DT, Zhang Y, Anthony JM, et al. Weight loss reduces the risk for symptomatic knee osteoarthritis in women. Ann Intern Med 1992;117:535–539.
17. Lindberg H, Montgomery F. Heavy labor and the occurrence of gonarthrosis. Clin Orthop 1987;214:235–236.
18. Bergenudd H, Lindgarde F, Nilsson B. Prevalence and co-incidence of degenerative changes of the hands and feet in middle age and their relationship to occupational workload, intelligence and social background. Clin Orthop 1989;239:306–310.
19. Lane NE, Bloch DA, Hubert HB, et al. Running, osteoarthritis, and bone density: Initial 2-year longitudinal study. Am J Med 1990;88:453–459.
20. Panush RS, Schmidt C, Caldwell Jr, et al. Is running associated with degenerative joint disease? JAMA 1986;255:1152–1154.
21. Eye DR, Weis MA, Moskowitz RW. Cartilage expression of a type II collagen mutation in an inherited form of osteoarthritis associated with a mild chondrodysplasia. J Clin Invest 1991;87:357–361.
22. Vikkula M, Palotie A, Ritvaniemi P. Early onset osteoarthritis linked to the type II procollagen gene. Arthr Rheumatol 1993;36:401–409.
23. Knight SM, Ring EFJ, Bhalla AK. Bone mineral density and osteoarthritis. Ann Rheum Dis 1992;51:1025.
24. Hannan MT, Anderson JJ, Zhang Y, et al. Bone mineral density and knee osteoarthritis in elderly men and women: The Framingham study. Arthr Rheumatol 1993;12:1671–1680.
25. Brandt KD, Mankin HJ. Pathogenesis of osteoarthritis, in Kelly WN, Harris ED, Ruddy S, Sledge CB (eds): Textbook of Rheumatology, 4th ed. Philadelphia, WB Saunders, 1993, pp 1355–1373.
26. Mankin HJ, Brandt KD, Shulman LE. Workshop on etiopathogenesis of osteoarthritis. J Rheumatol 1986;13:1130.
27. Moskowitz RW, Goldberg VM. Osteoarthritis: Clinical features and treatment, in Schumacher HR (ed): Primer on the Rheumatic Diseases, 10th ed. Atlanta, GA, Arthritis Foundation, 1993, pp 188–190, 331–332.
28. Williams CJ, Jimenez SA. Heredity, genes and osteoarthritis. Rheum Dis Clin North Am 1993;190:523–543.
29. Pelletier JP, DiBattista JA, Roughley P, et al. Cytokines and inflammation in cartilage degradation. Rheum Dis Clin North Am 1993;190:545–568.
30. Mayne R. Cartilage collagens. Arthr Rheumatol 1989;32(3):241–246.
31. Zimmermann M. Pain mechanism and mediators in osteoarthritis. Semin Arthr Rheumatol 1989;18(4):22S–29S.
32. Dieppe P. Osteoarthritis: Clinical features and diagnostic problems, in Klippel JH, Dieppe PA (eds): Rheumatology. London, Mosby-Year Book Europe Limited, 1994, sec 7, chap 4, pp 1–16.
33. Rene J, Weinberger M, Mazzuca SA, et al. Reduction of joint pain in patients with knee osteoarthritis who have received monthly telephone calls from lay personnel and whose medical treatment regimens have remained stable. Arthr Rheumatol 1992;35:511–515.
34. Kantor TG. Concepts in pain control. Semin Arthr Rheumatol 1989;18(4):94S–99S.
35. Kovar PA, Allegrante JP, MacKenzie CR, et al. Supervised fitness walking in patients with osteoarthritis of the knee. Ann Intern Med 1992;116:529–534.
36. Harris WH, Sledge CB. Total hip and total knee replacement (part I). N Engl J Med 1990;323(11):725–731.
37. Harris WH, Sledge CB. Total hip and total knee replacement (part II). N Engl J Med 1990;323(12):801–807.
38. Dromgoole SH, Furst DE, Paulus HE. Rational approaches to the use of salicylates in the treatment of rheumatoid arthritis. Semin Arthr Rheumatol 1981;11:257–283.
39. Graham DY, Smith JL. Aspirin and the stomach. Ann Intern Med 1986;104:390–398.
40. Lichtenstein DR, Syngal S, Wolfe MM. Nonsteroidal anti-inflammatory drugs and the gastrointestinal tract. Arthr Rheumatol 1995;1:5–18.
41. Hollander D. Gastrointestinal complications of nonsteroidal anti-inflammatory drugs: Prophylactic and therapeutic strategies. Am J Med 1994;96:274–281.
42. Morassut P, Yang W, Karsh J. Aspirin intolerance. Semin Arthr Rheumatol 1989;19(1):22–30.
43. Szczeklik A, Gryglewski RJ, Czerniawska-Mysik G. Clinical patterns of hypersensitivity to nonsteroidal anti-inflammatory drugs and their pathogenesis. J Allergy Clin Immunol 1977;60:276–284.
44. Abrishami MA, Thomas J. Aspirin intolerance—a review. Ann Allergy 1977;39:28–37.
45. Bradley JD, Brandt KD, Katz BP, et al. Comparison of an anti-inflammatory dose of ibuprofen, an analgesic dose of ibuprofen, and acetaminophen in the treatment of patients with osteoarthritis of the knee. N Engl J Med 1991;325:87–91.
46. Williams HJ, Ward JR, Egger MJ, et al. Comparison of naproxen and acetaminophen in a two-year study of treatment of osteoarthritis of the knee. Arthr Rheumatol 1993;36:1196–1206.
47. Brandt KD. NSAIDs in the treatment of osteoarthritis. Friends or foes? Bull Rheum Dis 1993;42:1–3.
48. Black M, Raucy J. Acetaminophen, alcohol and cytochrome P-450 [editorial]. Ann Intern Med 1986;104:427–429.
49. Whitcomb DC, Block GD. Association of acetaminophen hepatotoxicity with fasting and ethanol use. JAMA 1994;272:1845–1850.
50. Perneger TU, Whelton PK, Klag MJ. Risk of kidney failure associated with the use of acetaminophen, aspirin and nonsteroidal anti-inflammatory drugs. N Engl J Med 1994;331:1675–1679.
51. Rumsfield JA, West DP. Topical capsaicin in dermatologic and peripheral pain disorders. DICP Ann Pharmacother 1991;25:381–387.
52. Mapp P, Kidd B. The role of substance P in rheumatic disease. Semin Arthr Rheumatol 1994;23:(6, suppl 3):3–9.

53. Altman RD, Aven A, Holmburg CE, et al. Capsaicin cream 0.025% as monotherapy for osteoarthritis: A double-blind study. Semin Arthr Rheumatol 1994;23:(6, suppl 3):25–39.
54. Brooks PM, Day RO. Nonsteroidal anti-inflammatory drugs—differences and similarities. N Engl J Med 1991;324(24):1716–1725.
55. Mossinghoff GJ. In: Development of New Medicines for Arthritis. Washington, Pharmaceutical Manufacturers Association, 1991.
56. Abramson SB, Weissmann G. The mechanisms of action of nonsteroidal antiinflammatory drugs. Arthr Rheumatol 1989;32(1):1–9.
57. DeWitt DL, Meade EA, Smith WL. PGH synthase isoenzyme selectivity: The potential for safer nonsteroidal anti-inflammatory drugs. Am J Med 1993;95(suppl 2A):2A–40S.
58. Furst DE. Are there differences among nonsteroidal anti-inflammatory drugs? Arthr Rheumatol 1994;1:1–9.
59. Simon LS. Actions and toxicity of the nonsteroidal anti-inflammatory drugs. Curr Opin Rheumatol 1995;7:159–166.
60. Abramson SB. Treatment of gout and crystal arthropathies and uses and mechanism of action of nonsteroidal anti-inflammatory drugs. Curr Opin Rheumatol 1992;4:295–300.
61. Verbeeck RK, Blackburn JL, Loewen GR. Clinical pharmacokinetics of nonsteroidal anti-inflammatory drugs. Clin Pharmacokinet 1983;8:397–331.
62. Schoen RE, Vender RJ. Mechanisms of nonsteroidal anti-inflammatory drug-induced gastric damage. Am J Med 1989;86:449–458.
63. Agrawal NM, Roth S, Graham DY, et al. Misoprostol compared with sucralfate in the prevention of nonsteroidal anti-inflammatory drug-induced gastric ulcer: A randomized, controlled trial. Ann Intern Med 1991;115:195–200.
64. Graham DY, White RH, Moreland LW, et al. Duodenal and gastric ulcer prevention with misoprostol in arthritis patients taking NSAIDs. Ann Intern Med 1993;119:257–262.
65. Walt RP. Drug therapy: Misoprostol for the treatment of peptic ulcer and anti-inflammatory drug-induced gastroduodenal ulcerations. N Engl J Med 1994;327:1575–1580.
66. Murray MD, Brater DC. Renal toxicity of the nonsteroidal anti-inflammatory drugs. Ann Rev Pharmacol Toxicol 1993;32:435–465.
67. Garella S, Matarese RA. Renal effects of prostaglandins and clinical adverse effects of nonsteroidal anti-inflammatory agents. Medicine 1984;63:165–181.
68. Murray MD, Brater DC. Adverse effects of nonsteroidal anti-inflammatory drugs on renal function. Ann Intern Med 1990;112:559–560.
69. Murray KM, Keane WR. Review of drug-induced acute interstitial nephritis. Pharmacotherapy 1992;12:462–467.
70. Rodriguez LA, Williams R, Derby LE, et al. Acute liver injury associated with nonsteroidal anti-inflammatory drugs and the role of risk factors. Arch Intern Med 1994;154:311–316.
71. Rabinovitz M, Van Thiel DH. Hepatotoxicity of non-steroidal anti-inflammatory drugs. Am J Gastroenterol 1992;87:1696–1704.
72. Furst DE, Anderson W. Differential effects of diclofenac and aspirin on serum glutamic oxaloacetic transaminase elevations in patients with rheumatoid arthritis and osteoarthritis. Arthr Rheumatol 1993;36:804–810.
73. Roubenoff R, Hoyt J, Petri M, et al. Effects of anti-inflammatory and immunosuppressive drugs on pregnancy and fertility. Semin Arthr Rheumatol 1988;18(2):88–110.
74. Furst DE. Clinically important interactions of nonsteroidal anti-inflammatory drugs with other medications. J Rheumatol 1988;15(suppl 17):58–62.
75. Hansen P, Horn JR, eds. All NSAID are not alike with regard to drug interactions. Drug Int Newsl 1987;7:7–11.
76. Johnson AG, Nguyen TV, Day RO. Do nonsteroidal anti-inflammatory drugs affect blood pressure. Ann Intern Med 1994;121:289–300.
77. Brandt KD. Should nonsteroidal anti-inflammatory drugs be used to treat osteoarthritis? Rheum Dis Clin North Am 1993;19:29–45.
78. Brandt KD. Management of osteoarthritis, in Kelly WN, Harris ED, Ruddy S, Sledge CB (eds): Textbook of Rheumatology, 4th ed. Philadelphia, WB Saunders, 1993, pp 1385–1399.
79. Creamer P, Dieppe PA. Novel drug treatment strategies for osteoarthritis. J Rheumatol 1993;20:1461–1463.
80. Ghosh P. Osteoarthritis and hyaluronan. Palliative or disease-modifying treatment? Semin Arthr Rheumatol 1993;22(suppl 1):1–3.
81. Yu LP, Smith GN, Brandt KD, et al. Reduction of the severity of canine osteoarthritis by prophylactic treatment with oral doxycycline. Arthr Rheumatol 1992;35:1150–1159.
82. Dougados M. Clinical assessment of osteoarthritis in clinical trials. Curr Opin Rheumatol 1995;7:87–91.
83. Gill TM, Geinstein AR. A critical appraisal of the quality of quality-of-life measurements. JAMA 1994;272:619–626.
84. Wilson IB, Cleary PD. Linking clinical variables with health-related quality of life: A conceptual model of patient outcomes. JAMA 1995;273:59–65.

Chapter 86

Gout and Hyperuricemia

David W. Hawkins, PharmD, and Daniel W. Rahn, MD

The term *gout* describes a disease spectrum including hyperuricemia, recurrent attacks of acute arthritis associated with monosodium urate crystals in leukocytes found in synovial fluid, deposits of monosodium urate crystals in tissues (tophi), interstitial renal disease, and uric acid nephrolithiasis.[1]

Hyperuricemia may be an asymptomatic condition, with an increased serum uric acid as the only apparent abnormality. Statistically, hyperuricemia is defined as a serum urate concentration greater than two standard deviations above the population mean. But for determination of the risk for gout, hyperuricemia is defined as a supersaturated urate concentration.[2] By this definition, a urate concentration greater than 7.0 mg/dL is abnormal and is associated with an increased risk for gout. This corresponds to a measured value greater than 7.5 mg/dL by most autoanalyzers. Population studies have shown that urate concentration (and consequently the risk of gout) correlates with age, serum creatinine, blood urea nitrogen, male sex, blood pressure, body weight, and alcohol intake. Men are affected by gout approximately 10 times more often than women; the mean age of first attack is 47 years.

PATHOPHYSIOLOGY

In humans, uric acid is the end product of the degradation of purines. It serves no known physiologic purpose and therefore is regarded as a waste product. In lower animals, the enzyme uricase breaks down uric acid to the more soluble allantoin, and thus uric acid does not accumulate. Gout occurs exclusively in humans in whom a miscible pool of uric acid exists. Under normal conditions, the amount of cumulated uric acid is about 1200 mg in men and about 600 mg in women. The size of the urate pool is increased severalfold in individuals with gout. This excess accumulation may result from either overproduction or underexcretion.

OVERPRODUCTION OF URIC ACID

The purines from which uric acid is produced originate from three sources: dietary purine, conversion of tissue nucleic acid to purine nucleotides, and *de novo* synthesis of purine bases. The purines derived from these three sources enter a common metabolic pathway, leading to the production of either nucleic acid or uric acid. Under normal circumstances, uric acid may accumulate excessively if production exceeds excretion. The average human produces about 600–800 mg of uric acid each day.

Several enzyme systems regulate purine metabolism. Abnormalities in these regulatory systems could result in overproduction of uric acid. Uric acid may also be overproduced as a consequence of increased breakdown of tissue nucleic acids such as occurs with myeloproliferative and lymphoproliferative disorders. Dietary purines play an unimportant role in the generation of hyperuricemia in the absence of some derangement in purine metabolism or elimination.

Two enzyme abnormalities resulting in an overproduction of uric acid have been well described (Fig. 86.1). The first is an increase in the activity of phosphoribosyl pyrophosphate (PRPP) synthetase, which leads to an increased concentration of PRPP. PRPP is a key determinant of purine synthesis and thus uric acid production. The second is a deficiency of hypoxanthine-guanine phosphoribosyl transferase (HGPRT).

HGPRT is responsible for the conversion of guanine to guanylic acid and hypoxanthine to inosinic acid. These two conversions require PRPP as the cosubstrate and are important reutilization reactions involved in the synthesis of nucleic acids. A deficiency in the HGPRT enzyme leads to increased metabolism of guanine and hypoxanthine to uric acid and more PRPP to interact with glutamine in the first step of the purine pathway.[3] Complete absence of HGPRT results in the childhood Lesch–Nyhan syndrome, characterized by choreoathetosis, spasticity, mental retardation, and markedly excessive production of uric acid. A partial deficiency of the enzyme may be responsible for marked hyperuricemia in otherwise normal healthy individuals.

UNDEREXCRETION OF URIC ACID

Uric acid does not accumulate as long as a balance exists between uric acid production and elimination. Uric acid is eliminated in two ways. About two-thirds of the uric acid

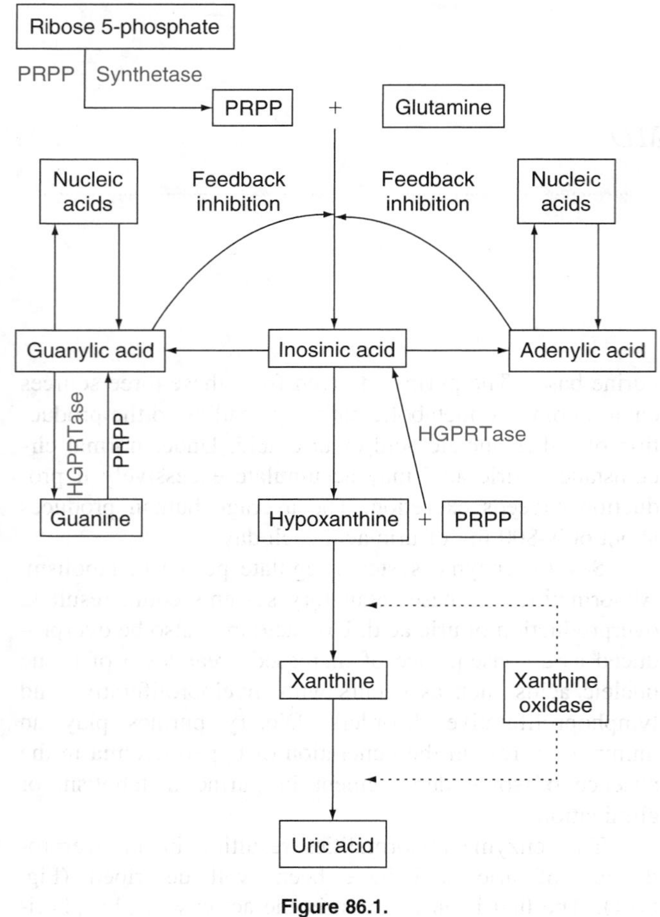

Figure 86.1.

produced each day is excreted in the urine. The rest is eliminated through the gastrointestinal tract, after enzymatic degradation by colonic bacteria.

A decline in the urinary excretion of uric acid to a level below the rate of production leads to hyperuricemia and an increased miscible pool of sodium urate. Almost all the urate in plasma is freely filtered across the glomerulus.

TABLE 86.1. CONDITIONS ASSOCIATED WITH HYPERURICEMIA

Primary gout	Diabetic ketoacidosis
Myeloproliferative disorders	Lactic acidosis
Lymphoproliferative disorders	Starvation
Chronic hemolytic anemia	Toxemia of pregnancy
Pernicious anemia	Glycogen storage disease type 1
Psoriasis	Obesity
Sarcoidosis	Congestive heart failure
Renal dysfunction	Down syndrome
Lead toxicity	Hyperparathyroidism
Acute alcoholism	Hypoparathyroidism
Acromegaly	Hypothyroidism

TABLE 86.2. DRUGS CAPABLE OF INDUCING HYPERURICEMIA AND GOUT

Diuretics	Nicotinic acid
Salicylates (<2 g/d)	Ethanol
Pyrazinamide	L-Dopa
Ethambutol	Cytotoxic drugs

The concentration of uric acid appearing in the urine is determined by multiple renal tubular transport processes in addition to the filtered load. Evidence at present favors a four-component model including glomerular filtration, tubular reabsorption, tubular secretion, and postsecretory reabsorption.

Approximately 90% of filtered uric acid is reabsorbed in the proximal tubule, probably by both active and passive transport mechanisms. There is a close linkage between proximal tubular sodium reabsorption and uric acid reabsorption; so states that enhance sodium reabsorption (e.g., dehydration) also lead to increased uric acid reabsorption. The exact site of tubular secretion of uric acid has not been determined; this too appears to involve an active transport process. Postsecretory reabsorption occurs somewhere distal to the secretory site.

Factors that decrease uric acid clearance or increase its production will result in an increase in serum urate concentration. Some of these factors are listed in Table 86.1. Drugs that decrease renal clearance of uric acid through modification of filtered load or one of the tubular transport processes are listed in Table 86.2.

The pathophysiologic approach to the evaluation of hyperuricemia requires determining whether the patient is overproducing or underexcreting uric acid. This can be accomplished by placing the patient on a purine-free diet for 3–5 days and then measuring the amount of uric acid excreted in the urine in 24 hours. Normal individuals produce 600–800 mg of uric acid daily and excrete less than 600 mg in urine. Individuals who excrete more than 600 mg on a purine-free diet may be considered overproducers. Hyperuricemic individuals who excrete less than 600 mg of uric acid per 24 hours on a purine-free diet may be defined as underexcretors of uric acid. It is very difficult in clinical practice, however, to maintain someone on a purine-free diet for several days. On a regular diet, excretion of greater than 1000 mg per 24 hours reflects overproduction; less than this is probably normal.

Clinical Characteristics of Gout

Gout is a disease manifested by acute attacks of arthritis, nephrolithiasis, gouty nephropathy, and aggregated deposits of sodium urate (tophi) in cartilage, tendons, synovial membranes, and elsewhere.[4]

ACUTE GOUTY ARTHRITIS

Acute attacks of gouty arthritis are characterized by rapid onset of excruciating pain, swelling, and inflammation. The attack is typically monoarticular at first, most often affecting the first metatarsophalangeal (MTP) joint and then, in order of frequency, the insteps, ankles, heels, knees, wrist, fingers, and elbows. In one-half of initial attacks, the first MTP joint is affected. Of gouty patients, 90% experience attacks in the great toe at some point in their disease.

The predilection of acute gout for peripheral joints of the lower extremity is probably related to the low temperature of these joints combined with high intra-articular urate concentration. Synovial effusions are postulated to occur transiently in weight-bearing joints during the day in the course of routine activity. At night, water is reabsorbed from the joint space leaving behind a supersaturated solution of monosodium urate, which can precipitate attacks of acute arthritis. Attacks begin at night with the patient awakening from sleep with excruciating pain.

The development of crystal-induced inflammation involves a number of chemical mediators causing vasodilation, increased vascular permeability, and chemotactic activity for polymorphonuclear leukocytes.[5] Phagocytosis of urate crystals by the leukocytes results in rapid lysis of cells and a discharge of proteolytic enzymes into the cytoplasm. The inflammatory reaction that ensues is associated with intense joint pain, erythema, warmth, and swelling. Fever is common as is leukocytosis. Untreated attacks may last from 3–14 days before spontaneous recovery.

Although acute attacks of gouty arthritis may occur without apparent provocation, a number of conditions may precipitate an attack. These include stress, trauma, alcohol ingestion, infection, surgery, rapid lowering of serum uric acid by ingestion of uric acid-lowering agents, and ingestion of certain drugs known to elevate serum uric acid concentrations. The diagnosis is best accomplished by aspiration of synovial fluid from the affected joint and identification of intracellular crystals of monosodium urate monohydrate in synovial fluid leukocytes.

URIC ACID NEPHROLITHIASIS

Nephrolithiasis occurs in 10–25% of patients with gout.[6] Factors that predispose individuals to uric acid nephrolithiasis include excessive urinary excretion of uric acid, an acidic urine, and a highly concentrated urine. The risk of renal calculi approaches 50% in individuals whose renal excretion of uric acid exceeds 1100 mg/d. In addition to pure uric acid stones, hyperuricosuric individuals are at increased risk for mixed uric acid–calcium oxalate stones, and pure calcium oxalate stones. Uric acid stones are usually small, round, and radiolucent. Uric acid stones containing calcium are radiopaque.[6]

Uric acid has a pK_a of 5.5. Therefore, when the urine is acidic, uric acid exists primarily in the un-ionized, less soluble form. At a urine pH of 5.0, for example, only 6–8 mg of uric acid may be dissolved in 100 mL of urine. When the urine pH is 7.0, the solubility of uric acid in urine is increased to 124–160 mg per 100 mL of urine. In patients with uric acid nephrolithiasis, urinary pH is typically less than 6.0 and frequently less than 5.5. When an acidic urine is saturated with uric acid, spontaneous precipitation of stones may occur.

GOUTY NEPHROPATHY

There are two types of gouty nephropathy: acute uric acid nephropathy and chronic urate nephropathy.[7] In acute uric acid nephropathy, acute renal failure occurs as a result of blockage of urine flow secondary to massive precipitation of uric acid crystals in the collecting ducts and ureters. This syndrome is a well-recognized complication in patients with myeloproliferative or lymphoproliferative disorders and is a result of massive malignant cell turnover, particularly after initiation of chemotherapy.

Chronic urate nephropathy is caused by the long-term deposition of urate crystals in the renal parenchyma. Microtophi may form, with a surrounding giant cell inflammatory reaction. A decrease in the kidney's ability to concentrate urine and the presence of proteinuria may be the earliest pathophysiologic disturbances. Hypertension and nephrosclerosis are common associated findings. Although renal failure occurs in a higher percentage of gouty patients than expected, it is not clear that hyperuricemia per se has a harmful effect on the kidney. The chronic renal impairment seen in individuals with gout may result largely from the co-occurrence of hypertension, diabetes mellitus, and atherosclerosis.

TOPHACEOUS GOUT

Tophi (urate deposits) are uncommon in the general population of gouty subjects and are a late complication of hyperuricemia. The most common sites of tophaceous deposits in patients with recurrent acute gouty arthritis are the base of the great toe, the helix of the ear, olecranon bursae, Achilles tendon, knees, wrists, and hands. Eventually even the hips, shoulders, and spine may be affected. In addition to causing obvious deformities, tophi may damage surrounding soft tissue, cause joint destruction and pain, and even lead to nerve compression syndromes including carpal tunnel syndrome.

TREATMENT

The goals in the treatment of gout are to terminate the acute attack, prevent recurrent attacks of gouty arthritis, and prevent complications associated with chronic deposition of urate crystals in tissues.[8] Distinction must be made between the goals of therapy for the acute attack and the chronic management of hyperuricemia.

ACUTE GOUTY ARTHRITIS

Acute attacks of gouty arthritis may be treated successfully with colchicine or any of a variety of nonsteroidal anti-inflammatory drugs (NSAIDs).[9] Colchicine can be given orally or parenterally. The usual oral dose is 0.5 or 0.6 mg at hourly intervals until the joint symptoms subside; the patient develops nausea, vomiting, or diarrhea; or the patient has taken a maximum of 12 tablets. About 75–95% of patients with acute gouty arthritis respond favorably to colchicine when ingestion of the drug is begun within 12 hours of the onset of joint symptoms. If the initiation of colchicine is delayed longer than 24 hours after the onset of acute symptoms, the probability of success with the drug diminishes substantially.[10]

The major problem associated with the use of oral colchicine is that gastrointestinal toxicity occurs in 50–80% of patients before the relief of the attack. The elderly patient is likely to become severely dehydrated and may incur serious electrolyte losses.

This high incidence of GI toxicity may be circumvented by administering colchicine intravenously. The initial intravenous dose of colchicine is 2 mg. If relief is not obtained, an additional 1-mg dose may be given at 6 and 12 hours to a total dose of 4 mg for a specific attack. The colchicine should be diluted with 20 mL of normal saline before administration to minimize sclerosis of the vein. The intravenous administration of colchicine eliminates most of the gastrointestinal symptoms associated with the oral dose but subjects the patient to the risk of local extravasation, which can cause inflammation in and necrosis of the surrounding tissue. Very small difficult-to-inject veins and renal impairment represent relative contraindications to intravenous colchicine therapy.

No additional colchicine should be given for 7 days and oral colchicine should be temporarily discontinued, primarily because of the risk of bone marrow toxicity. Colchicine should not be used intravenously in individuals who are neutropenic, have severe renal impairment (creatinine clearance less than 10 mL/min), or have combined renal and hepatic insufficiency. The dose should be reduced in individuals who have been on colchicine chronically.

Indomethacin is as effective as colchicine in the treatment of acute gouty arthritis.[11] Because acute gastrointestinal toxicity occurs far less frequently with indomethacin than with colchicine, it is preferred. Side effects unique to indomethacin include headache and dizziness. All NSAIDs have been implicated in the cause of gastric ulceration and bleeding, but with short-term therapy this is not likely.

When indomethacin is used in the treatment of acute gouty arthritis, it is customary to start with a relatively large dose for the first 24–48 hours and then taper the therapy over 3–4 days to minimize the risk of recurrent attacks. For example, 75 mg of indomethacin should be given initially, followed by 50 mg every 6 hours for 2 days, then 50 mg every 8 hours for 1 or 2 days.

A number of other NSAIDs (e.g., naproxen, fenoprofen, ibuprofen, piroxicam) are also effective in relieving the inflammation of acute gout.[12] If further testing and clinical experience indicate a lower incidence of adverse reactions to these agents, these agents are likely to become the drugs of choice in the treatment of gouty arthritis. All NSAIDs should be used with caution in individuals with a history of acid peptic disease, congestive heart failure, chronic renal failure, or coronary artery disease.

Corticosteroids may be used to treat acute attacks of gouty arthritis, but they are reserved primarily for resistant cases. Doses of 40–80 USP units of ACTH gel are given intramuscularly every 6–8 hours for 2–3 days and then the doses are reduced in stepwise fashion and discontinued. Intra-articular administration of triamcinolone hexacetonide in a dose of 20–40 mg may be useful in treating acute gout limited to a single joint. Prednisone may be administered orally in doses of 30–60 mg daily in patients with multiple-joint involvement. Because rebound attacks may occur upon steroid withdrawal, colchicine 0.6 mg should be given two or three times daily during and several days after steroid therapy.

NEPHROLITHIASIS

The medical management of uric acid nephrolithiasis includes hydration sufficient to maintain a urine volume of 2–3 L/d, alkalinization of urine, avoidance of purine-rich foods, moderation of protein intake, and reduction of urinary uric acid excretion.

Maintenance of a 24-hour urine volume of 2–3 L with an adequate intake of fluids is desirable for all gouty patients, but especially for those with excessive (>1.0 g/d) uric acid excretion. Alkalinizing agents should be used with the objective of making the urine less acid. Urine pH should be maintained at 6.0–6.5. In this pH range, up to 85% of uric acid will be in the form of the soluble urate ion.

Reduction of urine acidity can be accomplished by the administration of sodium bicarbonate or Shohl's solution (40 g citric acid and 98 g sodium citrate per liter). With the former, 2–6 g/d is given in equally divided doses at 6- to 8-hour intervals. A dose of 20–60 mL of Shohl's solution per day, given in three or four divided doses, provides an equivalent amount of alkali. If use of a sodium salt is contraindicated, potassium citrate may be used instead.

One must keep in mind that the older patient with uric acid kidney stones may also have hypertension, congestive heart failure, or renal insufficiency and obviously should not be exposed to overload with alkalinizing sodium salts or unlimited fluid intake. Acetazolamide, a carbonic anhydrase inhibitor, produces rapid and effective urinary alkalinization and is sometimes used in conjunction with alkali therapy. When a 250-mg dose of acetazolamide is given at bedtime, the excretion of an acidic urine in the early morning hours is avoided. The usual tachyphylaxis (rapid tolerance) to this drug is obviated by a daily repletion dose of bicarbonate.

Since the advent of allopurinol, a low-purine, low-protein diet in the patient with uric acid lithiasis is no longer as critical as it once was; however, it is still advisable to instruct the patient to avoid foods rich in purine and to limit the protein to not more than 90 g/d. Such a diet is still palatable and reduces appreciably the amount of uric acid in the urine.

The mainstay of drug therapy for recurrent uric acid lithiasis is allopurinol. It is effective in reducing both serum and urinary uric acid levels, thus preventing the formation of calculi. Allopurinol is also recommended as prophylactic treatment in the patient who will receive cytotoxic agents for the treatment of lymphoma or leukemia. The marked increase in uric acid production associated with cytolysis of a neoplasm predisposes a patient to the development of uric acid nephrolithiasis.

PROPHYLACTIC THERAPY

After the first attack of acute gouty arthritis or after the passage of the first renal stone, a decision to institute prophylactic therapy must be entertained. If the first episode was mild and responded promptly to treatment, the patient's serum urate concentration was only minimally elevated and the 24-hour urinary uric acid excretion was not excessive (<1000 mg/24 hours on a regular diet), then prophylactic treatment can be withheld. Some patients never have a second attack or a second stone. Others may not experience a second gouty episode for 5–10 years. A wait-and-see attitude, therefore, seems justified in patients who meet these conditions.

On the other hand, if the patient had a severe attack of gouty arthritis, a complicated course of uric acid lithiasis, a substantially elevated serum uric acid (>10.0 mg/dL), or a 24-hour urinary excretion of uric acid of more than 1000 mg, then prophylactic treatment should be instituted immediately after resolution of the acute episode. Prophylactic therapy is also appropriate for patients with frequent (i.e., more than two or three per year) attacks of gouty arthritis even if the serum uric acid concentration is normal or only minimally elevated.

Recurrences of acute gouty arthritis may be prevented with continuous low-dose daily oral colchicine or by uric acid lowering therapy with either uricosuric agent or inhibition of xanthine oxidase with allopurinol. Combination therapy consisting of colchicine plus a uricosuric agent or allopurinol may be employed in resistant cases. The choice of treatment depends on the serum urate concentration, the amount of uric acid excreted in a 24-hour period, and the renal function status of the patient.[13]

Prophylactic therapy with low-dose oral colchicine, 0.5–0.6 mg twice daily, may be effective in preventing recurrent arthritis in patients with no evidence of visible tophi and a normal or slightly elevated serum urate concentration. Patients do not become resistant to or tolerant of daily colchicine, and, if they sense the beginning of an acute attack, they should increase the dose to 1 mg every 2 hours; in most instances the attack will abort after 1 or 2 mg of colchicine. If the serum urate concentration is within the normal range, and the patient has been symptom free for a period of a year, maintenance colchicine may be discontinued. The patient should be advised, however, that discontinuation of the treatment program may be followed by an exacerbation of acute gouty arthritis.

Patients with a history of recurrent acute gouty arthritis and a significantly elevated serum uric acid concentration are probably best managed with uric acid lowering therapy. Colchicine at a dose of 0.5 mg twice daily should be administered during the first 6–12 months of antihyperuricemic therapy to minimize the risk of acute attacks that may occur during initiation of uric acid lowering therapy. The therapeutic objective of antihyperuricemic therapy is to reduce the serum urate concentration below 6 mg/dL, well below the saturation point.

Reduction of the serum urate concentration can be accomplished pharmacologically by increasing the renal excretion of uric acid or by decreasing its synthesis. The drugs most widely used to increase uric acid excretion are probenecid and sulfinpyrazone. Several other uricosuric drugs are available in Europe, but they have not been approved for use in the United States.

Uricosuric Drugs

Uricosuric drugs increase the renal clearance of uric acid by inhibiting the renal tubular reabsorption of uric acid. Therapy with uricosuric drugs should be started at a low dose to avoid marked uricosuria and possible stone formation. The maintenance of adequate urine flow and alkalinization of the urine with sodium bicarbonate or Shohl's solution during the first several days of uricosuric therapy further diminish the possibility of uric acid stone formation. Probenecid is given initially at a dose of 250 mg twice a day for 1–2 weeks, then 500 mg twice a day for 2 weeks.

Thereafter, the daily dose is increased by 500-mg increments every 1–2 weeks until satisfactory control is achieved or a maximum dose of 3.0 g is reached. The initial dose of sulfinpyrazone is 50 mg twice a day for 3–4 days, then 100 mg twice a day, increasing the daily dose by 100-mg increments each week until the serum urate concentration is in the desired range.

The major side effects associated with uricosuric therapy are gastrointestinal irritation, rash and hypersensitivity, precipitation of acute gouty arthritis, and stone formation. These drugs are contraindicated in patients who are allergic to them and in patients with impaired renal function (i.e., creatinine clearance below 50 mL/min).

Xanthine Oxidase Inhibitor

Currently, allopurinol is the only approved drug used for inhibiting uric acid synthesis.[14] Both allopurinol and its major metabolite, oxypurinol, are xanthine oxidase inhibitors, and thus impair the conversion of hypoxanthine to xanthine and xanthine to uric acid. Allopurinol also lowers the intracellular concentration of PRPP. Because of the long half-life of its metabolite, allopurinol can be given once daily. An oral daily dose of 300 mg is usually sufficient. Occasionally, as much as 600–800 mg/d may be necessary.

Allopurinol is the antihyperuricemic drug of choice in patients with a history of urinary stones or impaired renal function, in patients who have lymphoproliferative or myeloproliferative disorders and need pretreatment with a xanthine oxidase inhibitor before initiation of cytotoxic therapy to protect against acute uric acid nephropathy, and in patients with gout who are overproducers of uric acid. The major side effects of allopurinol are skin rash, leukopenia, occasional gastrointestinal toxicity, and increased frequency of acute gouty attacks with the initiation of therapy.

ASYMPTOMATIC HYPERURICEMIA

Questions are often raised regarding the indications for drug therapy for asymptomatic hyperuricemia. The purported benefits from treatment include prevention of acute gouty arthritis, tophi formation, nephrolithiasis, and chronic urate nephropathy. The first three complications are easily controlled should they develop; therefore, antihyperuricemic therapy is not warranted to prevent these conditions. The prevention of urate nephropathy might be a stronger indication because it is irreversible even with proper treatment. Available data indicate, however, that gouty nephropathy is extremely rare in the absence of clinical gout, and evidence that elevation of uric acid by itself may cause renal disease is weak and inconclusive.[15,16] As previously discussed, renal impairment is very rare in the absence of concurrent hypertension and atherosclerosis. In addition, it is unclear whether uric-acid-lowering therapy protects renal function in such individuals.

The risk of gouty arthritis or nephrolithiasis rises with increasing serum urate and urinary acid concentration. Epidemiologic data show that patients with serum urate concentrations greater than 10 mg/dL have a greater than 50% chance of developing gouty arthritis. This risk runs even higher in elderly patients. Moreover, it has been shown that the risk of nephrolithiasis is about 20% when urinary uric acid excretion is less than 700 mg/d, but 50% when the value exceeds 1100 mg/d. Close observation is essential, therefore, in individuals with severe hyperuricemia and overproduction of uric acid with uric-acid-lowering therapy instituted if necessary for occurrence of clinical gout or deterioration in renal function.

CONCLUSION

Hyperuricemia may lead to acute arthritis, chronic gout, or kidney stones or remain asymptomatic. Asymptomatic hyperuricemia need not be treated, especially if the serum urate concentration remains below 10 mg/dL.

Acute gouty arthritis requires either colchicine or a nonsteroidal anti-inflammatory drug to treat the underlying inflammatory condition. The management of uric acid kidney stones includes hydration and alkalinization of the urine. Prevention of recurrent gouty arthritis or recurrent nephrolithiasis and treatment of chronic gout all require hypouricemic therapy with either a uricosuric drug or allopurinol. Allopurinol is the hypouricemic drug of choice in patients with a history of uric acid stones or renal insufficiency and in patients known to be overproducers of uric acid.

REFERENCES

1. Wyngaarden JB, Kelley WN. Gout and Hyperuricemia. New York, Grune and Stratton, 1976.
2. Levinson DJ, Becker MA. Clinical gout and the pathogenesis of hyperuricemia, in McCarty DJ, Koopman WJ (eds): Arthritis and Allied Conditions, 12th ed. Philadelphia, Lea & Febiger, 1993, pp 1773–1805.
3. Wilson JM, Young AB, Kelley WN. Hypoxanthine-guanine phosphoribosyltransferase deficiency. N Engl J Med 1983;309:900–910.
4. Boss GR, Seegmiller JE. Hyperuricemia and gout: Classification, complications, and management. N Engl J Med 1979;300:1459–1468.
5. Beutler A, Schumacher HR. Gout and "pseudogout": When are arthritis symptoms caused by crystal deposition? Postgrad Med 1994;95:103–116.
6. Yu T. Nephrolithiasis in patients with gout. Postgrad Med 1978;63:164–170.

7. Klineberg JR. Role of the kidneys in the pathogenesis of gout. Postgrad Med 1978;63:45–150.
8. Star VL, Hochberg MC. Prevention and management of gout. Drugs 1993;45:212–222.
9. Wallace SL, Singer JZ. Therapy in gout. Rheum Dis Clin North Am 1988;14:441–457.
10. Wisner DE, Simkin PA. Management of gout and hyperuricemia. Primary Care 1984;11:283–294.
11. Simkin PA. Management of gout. Ann Intern Med 1979;90:812–816.
12. German DC, Holmes EW. Hyperuricemia and gout. Med Clin North Am 1986;70:419–436.
13. Edwards NL. The diagnosis and management of gouty arthritis. Compr Ther 1983;9(9):14–19.
14. Rundles RW. The development of allopurinol. Arch Intern Med 1985;145:1492–1503.
15. Fessel WJ. Renal outcomes of gout and hyperuricemia. Am J Med 1979;67:74–82.
16. Dykman D, Simon EE, Avioli W. Hyperuricemia and uric acid nephropathy. Arch Intern Med 1987;147:1341–1345.

Section 11

Disorders of the Eyes, Ears, Nose, and Throat

Chapter 87

Drug-Induced Ear and Eye Toxicity

Timothy S. Lesar, PharmD

A large number of medications have been identified as toxic to the ears or eyes. These adverse reactions vary from minor, reversible effects to serious, permanent impairment of hearing, vestibular function, or vision. Knowledge of the potential toxic effects of drugs and of methods limiting toxicity will minimize these adverse effects. The major drugs associated with ocular or ototoxic effects as well as mechanisms and characteristics of the toxic effects, risk factors, monitoring parameters, and management of adverse effects are reviewed in this chapter.

Drug-Induced Ototoxicity

Toxic effects on the structures of the inner ear and its neural pathways include temporary or permanent ototoxicity resulting from adverse effects on the cochlea, producing hearing loss, and/or the vestibular apparatus, producing vertigo, ataxia, lightheadedness, and other symptoms. The overall incidence of drug-induced ototoxicity is unknown; however, drug-induced deafness has been estimated to occur in 1.6 to 3 per 1000 medical patients.[1,2]

MANIFESTATIONS AND RISK FACTORS

The primary symptoms of drug-induced ototoxicity are the cochlear signs of tinnitus and hearing loss and the vestibular signs of lightheadedness, nystagmus, ataxia, vertigo, nausea, and vomiting. Tinnitus is a subjective ringing, buzzing, ticking, clicking, screaming, or roaring noise. It may be quite distressing to patients, and in some cases may mask concomitant hearing loss. Drug-induced tinnitus may precede or occur concomitantly with hearing impairment, although several drugs produce tinnitus without hearing loss. Patients with drug-induced hearing impairment may notice muffling of speech, fullness of the ear, and hearing loss affecting selected or all frequencies depending on the responsible agent or severity of toxicity. Raising of the patient's voice may alert the clinician to possible hearing loss.

Hearing ability is measured by audiometry. In pure-tone audiometry, the "threshold" of hearing pure tones at frequencies as low as 250 Hz is measured. The threshold is defined as the minimum effective sound pressure capable of evoking a hearing sensation 50% of the time. Hearing thresholds are measured in decibels (dB)—a measure of the intensity of sound, with the level 0 dB defined as the normal hearing threshold in healthy young adults. An increase of 10–20 dB in auditory threshold is considered mild, 21–40 dB moderate, and more than 40 dB severe hearing loss. Hearing loss at frequencies of 500–3000 Hz (speech range) will produce the most clinically noticeable deafness. Most patients do not detect or complain of hearing loss unless impairment exceeds 30 dB at frequencies less than 3000–4000 Hz; however, most humans can hear frequencies up to 20,000 Hz. Evaluation of drugs for ototoxicity typically involves audiograms performed at 250–8000 Hz, with ototoxicity commonly defined as an increase in auditory threshold of 15–20 dB at two or more frequencies. However, changes in threshold occur in normal individuals and evaluation of ototoxicity requires use of baseline evaluations, serial measurements, and the use of other appropriate controls.

Drug-induced hearing loss at high frequencies may not be detected, thereby underestimating the true incidence of ototoxicity.[3–5] It is important to detect subclinical hearing loss at high frequencies (>4000 Hz) and less than 30 dB. Early, minor hearing loss may be reversible with dosage reduction or drug discontinuation, whereas more severe toxic effects may be irreversible. Minor degrees of impairment are caused by degeneration of sensory hair cells, and the subsequent use of additional ototoxic drugs may result in a similar minor degree of toxicity; however, because of the preexisting damage, the additional hearing loss may be clinically important.[6] Clinicians should be aware of the ototoxic potential of medications or combinations of medications and watch for hearing loss. No standard recommendations for audiometric monitoring of patients receiving ototoxic drugs exist, but the decision process usually involves the selection of high-risk patients, establishment of baseline hearing levels, serial audiometry during therapy, and audiometry testing after drug discontinuation. The clinical usefulness of audiometric monitoring is limited by the need for patient cooperation, the inability to perform sensitive testing, and the need to continue lifesaving medications despite toxic effects. The decision to alter drug therapy if a patient is experiencing ototoxicity should be based on careful assessment of the risk-to-benefit ratio.[3–5,7–12]

When damage to the vestibular apparatus (i.e., labyrinth hair cells) and related innervation occurs, the patient may complain of lightheadedness, headache, giddiness, whirling sensations, a bouncing, spinning, or lurching of the room or objects, inability to focus or fixate on ocular images, nausea, vomiting, and cold sweats. These symptoms occur primarily when the patient is in motion. The patient may display nystagmus, ataxia, and unsteady gait and posture. The symptoms of vestibular toxicity tend to improve gradually with time because of increased reliance on visual and proprioceptive inputs and central compensatory mechanisms for equilibrium. If these abilities are limited or impaired, compensation does not occur and vestibular toxicity may severely disrupt the patient's ability to function.[8]

Risk factors associated with an increased incidence of drug-induced ototoxicity include increased drug concentrations and/or prolonged exposure of the inner ear to the drug, concomitant use of more than one ototoxic drug, dehydration, fever, noise exposure, preexisting hearing loss, bacteremia, heredity, prior exposure to ototoxic agents, and possibly advanced age.[7–18]

MECHANISMS OF OTOTOXICITY

Organ-specific drug toxicity such as ototoxicity may result from a unique susceptibility of the injured tissue to the drug, accumulation of the drug within the organ, or more likely a combination of both factors. Inner ear injury may result from reversible alteration of normal physiologic functions, such as loop diuretic inhibition of endolymph formation by the stria vascularis. Alteration of physiologic functions for prolonged periods of time may result in a degeneration of tissue dependent on the particular physiologic function. Direct toxic effects on the sensory end organs, such as hair cells of the organ of Corti or crista ampularis of the vestibular apparatus as seen with aminoglycosides or cisplatin, result in cell death and irreversible toxicities.[6–18]

ANTIMICROBIAL AGENTS

Aminoglycoside Antibiotics

Because of the frequency, severity, irreversibility, and cumulative effects of their toxicity, these drugs are among the most ototoxic of all drugs. All aminoglycosides are thought to produce ototoxicity, although the individual agents differ in severity, frequency, and site (cochlear versus vestibular) of damage. Aminoglycoside ototoxicity may occur after parenteral administration, aerosolization, oral use, topical use, bladder, wound or cavity irrigation, or possibly topical otic administration. Auditory toxicity (cochlear damage) is generally irreversible and usually occurs after 2–5 days or more of therapy; onset may occur after drug discontinuation; hearing loss may regress or progress after drug discontinuation. Tinnitus frequently precedes or coincides with the development of ototoxicity. The tinnitus is usually high pitched or ringing, possibly intermittent initially and subsequently becoming constant. Tinnitus may continue for several days to 2 weeks after discontinuation of therapy. Hearing loss is typically bilateral and symmetric but may occur unilaterally, particularly with amikacin, kanamycin, and netilmicin. Some reversible decrease in hearing may occur after single doses. High-frequency (>3000–4000 Hz) hearing loss is evident first, and loss may progress to all frequencies. Clinically, the patient may initially notice loss of sound discrimination ("muffled voices") rather than decreased sensitivity and complain of fullness of the ears.

The degree of hearing impairment ranges from minor loss of sensitivity or discrimination at high frequencies to complete deafness. While damage to the hair cells of the cochlea by aminoglycosides is thought to be irreversible, up to 50% of patients show partial or complete recovery of hearing within 2 weeks of drug discontinuation.[19–22]

Aminoglycoside-induced vestibular toxicity may occur with or without concomitant hearing loss, but is more likely to occur alone or concurrently with hearing loss during gentamicin, streptomycin, and tobramycin therapy (i.e., these are more vestibulotoxic) than with netilmicin, kanamycin, or amikacin therapy. Streptomycin is primarily vestibulotoxic. Vestibular toxicity may initially present as headache, nausea and vomiting, trouble with ocular fixation or focus, dizziness, or lightheadedness. These symptoms may coexist with more severe vestibular symptoms such as vertigo, nystagmus, ataxia, and gait instability. Symptoms are minimal or absent when the patient is bedridden and are exacerbated upon sitting, standing, or eye closure. The vestibular symptoms may persist for 1–2 weeks, followed by 2 weeks to 2 months of adaption. During this period symptoms decrease, and may be present only when the patient ambulates, makes quick movements, or closes the eyelids. The compensation period may be lengthened or less complete in patients with visual impairment or proprioceptive deficits. After adaption to vestibular damage, symptoms usually occur only during eyelid closure.[8–11,19–22]

The reported incidence of aminoglycoside ototoxicity ranges from 0.6–30% for auditory toxicity (usually defined as a loss of 15–20 dB at 250–8000 Hz) and 0–75% for vestibular toxicity, with an overall average of 7.5% for both. The frequency reported depends on the drug, as well as study design and definition of ototoxicity.[7,9–11,22–27] Neomycin is thought to be the most auditory (cochlear) toxic aminoglycoside and for this reason, as well as because of nephrotoxicity, it is never administered parenterally; however, neomycin-induced ototoxicity has been reported after topical, bladder, aerosolized, intrawound, intracavity, and oral administration.[28,29] Vestibular toxicity from neomycin occurs less frequently. Streptomycin is the most vestibular toxic aminoglycoside, producing this adverse effect in 20–75% of patients depending on dose. Streptomycin is associated with a 4–15% incidence of hearing impairment.

Of the commonly used parenteral aminoglycosides (gentamicin, tobramycin, amikacin, and netilmicin), clinical differences in ototoxic potential are less clearly defined. Gentamicin is somewhat more vestibulotoxic than cochleotoxic, whereas kanamycin, amikacin, and netilmicin are more cochleotoxic than vestibulotoxic; tobramycin is more equally cochleotoxic and vestibulotoxic. Significant differences in ototoxic potential of aminoglycosides have been demonstrated in studies in animals; however, clinical studies demonstrate a similar incidence of auditory toxicity with gentamicin, amikacin, and tobramycin, whereas netilmicin has been reported to have similar or less auditory toxicity than the other aminoglycosides. The ranges of reported incidence of auditory toxicity for individual agents are 10–60% for kanamycin, 2–24% for gentamicin, 0.4–22% for tobramycin, 3–24% for amikacin, and 0.5–10% for netilmicin. Most studies report an overall incidence of 3–10% for aminoglycoside toxicity; however, the risk for an individual patient depends on the presence of risk factors. Vestibular toxicity occurs most frequently with gentamicin (up to 30%), then tobramycin (up to 4.6%), and less commonly with amikacin and netilmicin (1.3%). Because of the lack of comparative trials, the true relative frequency of vestibular toxicity has not been well established.[7–11,21–27]

The mechanism for the ototoxicity produced by aminoglycosides is most likely due to the entry of drug into the perilymph and endolymph and the unique sensitivity of various cells within the inner ear to the toxic effects of these antibiotics. Aminoglycosides enter relatively quickly (peak 3 hours after a dose) and leave the inner ear fluids slowly, but the association between drug concentrations in cochlear and vestibular fluids and tissues is unclear. It is likely that toxicity is both a function of total exposure (related to area under the concentration–time curve) and concentrations achieved.[10–12,28,30–34] The pathologic findings in animals demonstrate that the earliest sign of aminoglycoside toxicity is degeneration of the outer hair cells of the organ of Corti at the basal turn of the cochlea. The site specificity of the damage at the basal turn corresponds with the clinical finding of early high-frequency hearing loss. With continued exposure to aminoglycosides, hair cell death progresses toward the apex of the cochlea (to affect lower frequency hearing). Eventually, inner hair cells, other organ of Corti cells, the stria vascularis, and Reissner's membrane may degenerate. After death of the hair cells, retrograde degeneration of the auditory nerve occurs. Vestibular toxicity is characterized by damage to hair cells of the ampullary cristae, utricle maculae, and saccule maculae. The exact mechanism by which sensory hair cell damage occurs remains controversial, but may involve direct toxicity to the hair cells, alteration of endolymph electrolyte composition, or both. The toxicity of aminoglycosides has been related to binding of hair cell membrane phosphoinositides, resulting in membrane disruption, loss of magnesium with resultant block of enzyme function, and inhibition of protein synthesis. Susceptibility to aminoglycoside ototoxicity appears to be genetically linked. The site specificity of ototoxicity (cochlear versus vestibular) may result from differences in endolymph production mechanisms or in hair cell membrane lipid characteristics between the two sites.[9,20,22,32,33]

A number of risk factors have been associated with the development of aminoglycoside ototoxicity; whether these represent independent risk factors is uncertain (Table 87.1). Controlling serum concentrations of the aminoglycosides may minimize the incidence of ototoxicity, although the relationship between serum concentration and ototoxicity has not been well established.[35] Serum concentrations should be monitored and dosage adjustments made to maintain "peak" (gentamicin, tobramycin, netilmicin <10–12 μg/mL; kanamycin, amikacin < 32 μg/mL) and "trough" (gentamicin, tobramycin, netilmicin < 2 μg/mL; kanamycin, amikacin < 10 μg/mL) concentrations within recommended

TABLE 87.1. RISK FACTORS ASSOCIATED WITH AMINOGLYCOSIDE OTOTOXICITY

Total Dose	Total Daily Dose
Exposure to high-intensity noise	Impaired renal function
Intrinsic ototoxic potential of drug	Multiorgan failure
Concomitant ototoxic drug	Bacteremia
Elevated serum concentrations	Fever
Dehydration	Prior aminoglycoside therapy
Advanced age	Concomitant ear infection
Hereditary susceptibility	Concomitant ototoxic drug

ranges. Many patients exhibit ototoxicity despite appropriate serum concentrations because of the presence of the additional risk factors listed in Table 87.1. The frequency of ototoxicity with the use of extended dosage interval (once-daily) aminoglycosides appears to be at least equivalent, if not lower than traditional dosing methods.[36]

The concurrent use of other ototoxic drugs, particularly loop diuretics and vancomycin, has been associated with increased ototoxicity.[9,22,37,38] Ethacrynic acid appears to result in clinically important increases in ototoxicity, whereas the increase in incidence is much less with furosemide and bumetanide; however, diuretic-induced dehydration may potentiate aminoglycoside toxicity. Evidence in animals suggests vancomycin potentiates aminoglycoside toxicity.[39] High noise levels produce ototoxic lesions similar to those produced by aminoglycosides, and studies in animals suggest an additive effect. Previous aminoglycoside or other ototoxic drug therapy may produce subclinical toxicity, with subsequent courses of aminoglycoside producing clinically important toxicity.

The potential for ototoxicity should be considered in all patients receiving aminoglycosides. An assessment for the presence of risk factors should be performed. Serum concentrations should be monitored early in therapy and doses adjusted appropriately. Additional ototoxic agents should be avoided or used sparingly if possible. Symptoms indicating ototoxicity should be noted and follow-up audiometry or vestibular function tests used if appropriate. Fluid status should be monitored and dehydration avoided. Noise exposure should be kept to a minimum. If ototoxicity occurs, the drug should be discontinued, if possible, and replaced with a nonototoxic agent.

Erythromycin and Analogues

Cases of fully reversible and partially reversible ototoxicity after oral, intravenous, and intraperitoneal administration of erythromycin have been reported.[40–47] The incidence of ototoxicity has been reported to be as high as 20–30% depending on the patient population studied.[42,46] Both base and salt forms of erythromycin have been associated with ototoxicity, suggesting that any form of the drug may produce toxicity. Typical ototoxicity is characterized by a bilateral, sensorineural impairment (caused by nerve damage) of hearing at all frequencies, occasionally associated with slurred speech, double vision, and confusion.[41] Tinnitus may be present and has been described as "blowing." Signs of vestibular toxicity and central nervous system toxicity may be present in some patients. Erythromycin ototoxicity is associated with the administration of large doses (>4 g/d); however, smaller (>2 g/d) daily doses may produce toxic effects in patients with impaired hepatic or renal function. Concentrations above 12 μg/mL have been associated with a high frequency of ototoxicity.[42] Doses of less than 2 g/d are infrequently associated with toxic effects except when administered intraperitoneally to peritoneal dialysis patients. Ototoxicity usually occurs within 4–8 days of starting the ototoxic dose, and may occur as little as 12 hours to as long as 32 days after initiation of therapy. Onset of recovery from hearing loss may begin within 24 hours to 3 days, and partial or complete recovery occurs 2–30 days after dose reduction or discontinuation. Cases of permanent hearing loss, tinnitus, and vestibular abnormalities have been reported.[9,46] Risk factors include high dose (more than 2–4 g) combined with renal impairment, prolonged therapy, hepatic failure, intravenous administration, increased age, use with other ototoxic agents, and use with inhibitors of erythromycin metabolism.

The mechanism of erythromycin ototoxicity is unknown, but may involve both peripheral and CNS auditory pathways.[45] Cochlear hair cell damage has been demonstrated after instillation of erythromycin into the middle ear. The risk for erythromycin ototoxicity may be minimized by limiting doses to 2 g/d or less in patients with renal or hepatic failure and those of extreme age. In patients treated with >2 g/d, dose reduction should be considered once clinical improvement occurs. The erythromycin analogues azithromycin[47] and clarithromycin[48,49] have also been associated with ototoxicity when used in high doses for prolonged courses of therapy.

Vancomycin and Analogues

Previously, auditory toxicity was considered an important adverse neurotoxic effect of vancomycin.[12,13,19,50,51] Ototoxicity characterized by initial high-frequency hearing loss and tinnitus, progressing to permanent impairment of hearing at all frequencies, was associated with vancomycin. Ototoxicity was thought to occur with increased frequency when peak serum concentrations exceeded 45–60 μg/mL; however, the relationship between drug levels and ototoxicity is unclear and based primarily on case reports. Recent reviews of the literature cast doubt on the ototoxic potential of vancomycin when used alone.[41,51,52,53] The drug is not ototoxic in animals and reported cases of ototoxicity usually involved the coadministration of other ototoxic agents such as erythromycin and aminoglycosides. Ototoxicity from appropriately dosed vancomycin used alone appears to be relatively infrequent. Use of vancomycin concomitantly with other ototoxic agents or in patients with risk factors may increase the frequency of this adverse effect.[27,51] The vancomycin analogues teicoplanin and daptomycin have not been associated with ototoxicity.[52]

Minocycline

The tetracycline antibiotic minocycline is associated with a high frequency of reversible ototoxicity manifested by vestibular symptoms.[54,55] Common symptoms include dizziness, vertigo, ataxia, lightheadedness, and a "spaced out" feeling frequently accompanied by nausea, vomiting, and tinnitus. The frequency, onset, and severity of vestibular toxicity appear to be related to dosage regimen and possibly female sex. Minocycline administered as 50 mg orally every 12 hours produces toxic effects in 11–14%, 75 mg every 12 hours in 53%, 100 mg every 12 hours in 60–77%, and with higher doses in up to 97%. The onset of symptoms occurs earlier (within 24 hours) with loading doses or high-dose regimens. Onset of symptoms occurs between 1 and 3 days in patients receiving 100 mg every 12 hours. Symptoms are often severe enough to require drug discontinuation or greatly impair daily activities in 5–52% of patients, and they appear to be dose related. The risk of developing vestibular side effects is two to three times higher for females than for males given the same dose. This sex difference may be related to the higher serum concentrations found in females compared with males administered the same dose.

Patients prescribed minocycline, particularly those on long-term therapy for rheumatoid arthritis should be informed of the vestibular effects and their impact on ability to perform tasks requiring motor coordination, such as driving. Because of the vestibular toxicity, minocycline is no longer considered the drug of choice for *Neisseria meningitidis* prophylaxis. Vestibular effects abate within 48 hours of discontinuation of minocycline in three-fourths of affected patients; however, 15% may have symptoms persisting 72 hours or longer.

ANTIMALARIAL AGENTS

Quinine and chloroquine have been associated with reversible and irreversible ototoxicity.[9,12,56–58] Quinine in small doses frequently produces tinnitus, and in therapeutic doses (greater than 200–300 mg/d) produces reversible hearing loss, tinnitus, and dizziness in 20% of patients. Even the small amounts in tonic water have been associated with altered vestibular function, which is significant enough to restrict the use of tonic water by pilots.[56] Severe sensorineural deafness may occur with prolonged therapy at high doses or in overdose. Hearing loss typically affects lower frequencies. Ototoxicity of quinine is closely related to serum concentrations.[56] Profound hearing loss has been reported in infants whose mothers took chloroquine during pregnancy.

The mechanism by which quinine produces ototoxicity is unclear; however, cystic degeneration of the stria vascularis, degeneration of cochlear neurons, and loss of hair cells occur. Injury may be caused by spasm of cochlear blood vessels, producing anoxia and subsequent cellular damage. Reversible hearing loss may result from altered hair cell motility. Hearing loss usually occurs after prolonged use or when administered intravenously. Chloroquine has also been associated with tinnitus, ataxia, and imbalance upon rapid head turning. Severe, irreversible sensorineural deafness has been reported with as little as 1 g. Deafness may develop or progress after drug discontinuation. Chloroquine has been shown to accumulate in the pigmented cells of the stria vascularis, producing cell death and disruption of endolymph production. Similar to quinine, chloroquine may produce cochlear vascular spasm or altered hair cell motility. Hydroxychloroquine and primaquine are associated with tinnitus.[56–58]

NONSTEROIDAL ANTI-INFLAMMATORY DRUGS

Salicylates and other nonsteroidal anti-inflammatory drugs (NSAIDs) may produce reversible ototoxicity. Aspirin and other salicylates produce dose- and concentration-related auditory toxicity. Tinnitus has been used in the past as a guide to dosing; however, there is considerable variability in the relationship between serum concentration and tinnitus. Tinnitus is characterized as a high-pitched ringing or hissing noise that frequently precedes and/or occurs concomitantly with hearing loss. Hearing loss may occur equally at all frequencies or predominantly at high frequencies. Deafness is typically bilateral and symmetrical; however, cases of unilateral hearing loss have been reported. Rare cases of vertigo have been reported with aspirin. The ototoxic effects of aspirin occur in 0.3–1.7% of patients. The frequency of toxicity is clearly dose and/or concentration related, with daily doses above 2.7 g or total serum concentrations above 25–30 mg/dL associated with increased incidence of ototoxicity. Unbound serum salicylate concentrations may be more closely associated with ototoxicity. Doses above 4 g/d produce tinnitus in approximately 50% and hearing loss (usually 20–40 dB) in 25% of patients. The elderly may be at a higher risk for salicylate toxicity. Ototoxicity has been reported after oral, intravenous, and topical salicylate administration.[10,12–14,56,59–61]

Salicylate ototoxicity is considered fully reversible, with recovery occurring within 24–72 hours regardless of the degree of hearing loss. Rare cases of irreversible hearing loss have been reported with aspirin.

The mechanism by which salicylates produce ototoxic symptoms is unclear, because no inner ear morphologic changes have been demonstrated in studies in animals. Proposed mechanisms include altered neural action potential of the cochlea, sensory cell function, or secondary changes because of the production of vasoconstriction of inner ear blood vessels resulting in tissue ischemia. Salicylates as well as other NSAIDs may produce decreased prostaglandin and increased leukotriene concentrations in the perilymph. Salicylates may also affect eighth cranial nerve function. Vasoconstriction results from inhibition of vasodilating prostaglandins.[10,56,61] Other NSAIDs have been associated with a lower incidence (1–3%) of similar ototoxic symptoms. Indomethacin produces vertigo and/or dizziness in 3–9% of patients.

LOOP DIURETICS

The potent "loop" diuretics, ethacrynic acid, furosemide, bumetanide, and torsemide, produce a similar dose-related ototoxicity, but differ in the individual frequency and severity. Ethacrynic acid is associated with significantly greater ototoxicity than are furosemide and bumetanide. Ototoxicity usually manifests as a rapid onset of bilateral hearing loss (within minutes of a large rapidly administered intravenous dose), often accompanied by tinnitus and symptoms of vestibular toxicity. Toxicity of ethacrynic acid may result from a cysteine adduct metabolite and is related to dose and rate of administration. Doses as little as 50–100 mg intravenously may cause ototoxicity. Risk of toxicity increases with high doses and prolonged use. Hearing loss occurs typically at middle and high frequencies, although occasional loss of discrimination at all frequencies may occur. Hearing loss is usually reversible within 1–24 hours of drug discontinuation, although a number of cases of permanent hearing loss have been reported.

Furosemide produces similar ototoxic symptoms; however, the frequency and severity of toxicity are less. Like ethacrynic acid, rapid infusions of furosemide produce dramatic, reversible hearing loss. Moderate to high doses (120–2000 mg) administered at rates of 4 mg/min or less are unlikely to produce ototoxicity, whereas high doses (1–2 g) given at rates of 25 and 67 mg/min produce toxicity in 50% and 100% of patients, respectively. The majority of cases of furosemide ototoxicity have occurred with doses greater than 240 mg, although doses as low as 40 mg have been associated with toxicity. Ototoxicity has been reported after oral administration of furosemide 160–800 mg/d. Most patients recover from furosemide ototoxicity within several hours of drug discontinuation; however, permanent hearing impairment can occur.[10,62,63]

Bumetanide is five to six times more ototoxic than furosemide on a milligram-to-milligram basis; however, the diuretic potency of bumetanide is 40 times that of furosemide. Data in animals suggest that bumetanide produces two to seven times less ototoxicity than furosemide. Large clinical studies report that bumetanide produces ototoxicity effects in 1.1–1.7% of patients, whereas furosemide produces toxic effects in 3–6.5%; however, these studies were not designed to compare ototoxicity of these two drugs, and clear clinical differences have not been demonstrated. Limited data on torsemide ototoxicity are available, but animal studies demonstrate ototoxicity similar to that of furosemide and bumetanide.[10,63–65]

Loop diuretic-induced ototoxicity appears to result from inhibition of enzymes in the stria vascularis. This results in a loss of endocochlear potential because of reduction in the endolymph–perilymph potassium and sodium concentration differences and corresponds to the rapid onset and recovery of hearing loss encountered clinically. Morphologic changes in the organ of Corti and outer sensory hair cells have been demonstrated with ethacrynic acid, and the degeneration of hair cells corresponds to the permanent ototoxicity encountered clinically. Risk factors for development of loop diuretic ototoxicity include rapid infusion rate of large doses, large doses, renal failure, hepatic failure, cardiac failure, the specific diuretic administered, previous ototoxic drugs, and concomitant use of ototoxic (particularly aminoglycosides) agents.[10,12–16,63]

ANTITUMOR AGENTS: CISPLATIN AND OTHERS

Cisplatin, a potent antineoplastic agent, produces a high incidence of ototoxicity. The primary manifestation of cisplatin ototoxicity is hearing loss, although vestibular toxicity has also been reported. Hearing loss is commonly noted 2–5 days after the first or second dose.[12,66–69] The hearing loss produced by cisplatin occurs in 30–70% of patients receiving a cumulative dose of 50–100 mg/m^2. Hearing frequencies above 2000–3000 Hz (usually 4000–8000 Hz) are most commonly affected; however, lower frequencies may be affected particularly in severe toxicity. Hearing loss is usually bilateral (less commonly unilateral) and symmetrical and characterized initially by degeneration of the outer hair cells near the base of the organ of Corti. With continued therapy, hair cell loss progresses apically, then to the inner hair cells. Hearing loss tends to occur early in therapy (after one or two treatments), may occur suddenly, and is usually irreversible, although some recovery may occur. Tinnitus accompanies hearing loss in up to 30% of patients; it occurs intermittently but is not predictive of impending ototoxicity.

Ototoxicity may be more frequent in children and older patients, those with preexisting hearing loss, low serum albumin, and low hematocrit/hemoglobin.[70] Other chemotherapeutic agents—including carboplatin, bleomycin, dactinomycin, mechlorethamine, vincristine, fludarabine and cytarabine—have been reported to cause hearing loss and tinnitus. Methotrexate has been reported to produce tinnitus.[66]

DEFEROXAMINE

The chelating agent deferoxamine produces a high-frequency sensorineural hearing loss. Toxicity is characterized by a generally reversible loss of high-frequency hearing. Permanent hearing loss requiring the use of hearing aids may occur. Tinnitus may occur. The incidence of auditory toxicity appears to be dose related, with doses above 35–50 mg/kg/d for 3 months producing toxicity in 25–75% of patients. Greater risk for toxicity has been associated with minimal iron overload (serum ferritin <2000 g/L). This may result in increased nonchelated deferoxamine available to bind metaloenzymes found in the cochlea. Routine use of audiograms is recommended to help guide dosing of deferoxamine and monitoring of toxicity.[71–73] Dose reduction results in stabilization of hearing loss and possible improvement in some patients. Patients with mild auditory toxicity should receive no more than 30–40 mg/kg/d, while those with moderate toxicity or clinical signs of ototoxicity should be limited to 10–25 mg/kg/d. Patients with clinical ototoxicity may demonstrate improvement in hearing following a 2- to 4-week drug-free interval.[10,71–73]

TOPICALLY APPLIED DRUGS

Several drugs may be ototoxic when applied to the middle ear (or into the external auditory canal in patients with perforated tympanic membranes). The clinical importance of the ototoxic potential of topical agents in humans remains controversial. Despite widespread use of topical agents, few studies of ototoxicity exist. Studies in animals have demonstrated the ototoxic effects of topically applied aminoglycosides, chloramphenicol, polymyxin, erythromycin, and tetracycline. However, extrapolation of animal data to humans may not be appropriate based on anatomic differences.

Use of these antimicrobials in patients with otitis media with perforated tympanic membrane or during ear surgery may possibly result in ototoxicity. Drugs and other substances diffuse readily from the middle ear to the inner ear through the round window membrane.

Other ototoxic compounds include lidocaine and the antiseptics *m*-cresyl acetate in isopropanol and castor oil (Cresylate), chlorhexidine, acetic acid, and povidone–iodine. High concentrations of propylene glycol have been found to be toxic in animals. For these reasons, ototopical medications must be used carefully during ear surgery or in patients with perforated tympanic membranes.[10,12,74–76]

DEVELOPMENTAL OTOTOXICITY

The administration of ototoxic agents is frequently required in the care of pregnant patients and in neonates. The administration of aminoglycosides (studies primarily involving streptomycin for tuberculosis) during pregnancy has been associated with cases of vestibular and cochlear toxicity. However, a number of studies have demonstrated a low risk of ototoxicity to the fetus of mothers treated with aminoglycosides. Factors related to risk may include stage of development, dose, and duration of therapy. The ototoxic loop diuretic furosemide crosses the placenta, and with prolonged therapy may result in the accumulation of ototoxic concentrations. Both aminoglycosides and loop diuretics are commonly used in the care of premature infants. The incidence of ototoxicity with the use of aminoglycosides in neonates has been reported to range from 0–36%. Factors related to the incidence of toxicity may include dose, treatment duration, use of loop diuretics, noise level, and the presence of medical complications. The use of furosemide in neonates can result in ototoxicity. Reduced renal excretion and furosemide metabolism producing high and prolonged serum concentrations combined with increased permeability of the cochlea increase the potential for toxicity. All ototoxic agents should be used with care during pregnancy and in newborns.[9,10,77]

OTHER MEDICATIONS

Several other medications are associated with ototoxicity. A complete listing is beyond the scope of this chapter and comprehensive listings are available.[9,10,78–81] Commonly used medications and associated ototoxic effects are listed in Table 87.2.

DRUG-INDUCED OCULOTOXICITY

Drugs administered both systemically and nonsystemically may produce adverse effects on the eye and surrounding tissues. Adverse effects of drugs may involve external ocular functions and structures—oculomotor function, eyelids, lacrimation, conjunctiva, and cornea—or internal structures—trabecular meshwork, ciliary body, iris, lens, uveal tract, retina, and optic nerve. This section reviews the major types of drug-induced ocular toxicity and discusses the medications most commonly associated with specific adverse effects. Nonspecific alterations of visual functions as an extension of pharmacologic effects are not addressed in detail and the reader is referred to available comprehensive texts, and compilations of drugs producing ocular effects and toxicity are available.[82–86]

EXTERNAL OCULAR STRUCTURES

Eyelids and Periorbital Structures

The primary toxic effects of drugs on the eyelids are discoloration, edema, and altered eyelid position. Discoloration or pigmentation of the periorbital skin may occur

TABLE 87.2. OTOTOXIC DRUGS

Drug	Comment
Antimicrobials	
Aminoglycoside	See text
Ampicillin	Reversible hearing loss
Antimalarials	See text
Capreomycin	Reversible hearing loss, tinnitus
Chloramphenicol	Reversible hearing loss
Clindamycin	Tinnitus
Colistin	Hearing loss
Cotrimoxazole	Reversible hearing loss
Doxycycline	Tinnitus
Erythromycin derivatives	See text
Furazolidone	Hearing loss, tinnitus
Metronidazole	Tinnitus
Minocycline	See text
Paromomycin	Auditory/vestibular toxicity
Polymixin B	Reversible hearing loss
Rifampin	Reversible hearing loss
Sulfonamides	Tinnitus and vertigo
Tetracycline	Tinnitus
Thiabendazole	Tinnitus
Vancomycin	See text
Salicylates and NSAIDs	See text
Loop Diuretics	See text
Antineoplastic Agents	See text
Miscellaneous	
Aminophylline	Tinnitus
Antihistamines	Tinnitus
Caffeine	Tinnitus
Carbamazepine	Tinnitus
Contraceptive steroids	Reversible hearing loss
Deferoxamine	See text
Diazoxide	Reversible hearing loss
Haloperidol	Tinnitus
Interferons	Hearing loss
Levodopa	Tinnitus
Lidocaine	Tinnitus, ototoxic with topical use
Metaproterenol	Tinnitus
Molindone	Tinnitus
Monoamine oxidase inhibitors	Tinnitus
Morphine	Tinnitus
Penicillamine	Tinnitus
Pentazocine	Tinnitus
Propranolol	Tinnitus
Propoxyphene	Hearing loss, tinnitus
Prophylthiouracil	Hearing loss, tinnitus
Quinidine	Reversible hearing loss, tinnitus, vertigo
Tocainide	Tinnitus
Tricyclic antidepressants	Hearing loss, tinnitus
Verapamil	Tinnitus

concomitantly with drug-induced discoloration of other skin areas or occur solely or most prominently in the periorbital area. Drugs associated with periorbital pigmentation of the skin include the antiarrhythmic amiodarone and the antipsychotic agents chlorpromazine and other phenothiazines.

The thin, loosely attached skin of the eyelids and periorbital area allows substantial swelling to occur. Edema of the eyelids and periorbital area may occur secondary to direct effects of drugs or secondarily to drug-induced thyroid disorder or hypersensitivity reactions. Drugs associated with directly producing periorbital or eyelid edema include nifedipine, chlorthalidone, leuprolide, sulfonamides, and primidone.

Drug-induced ptosis (drooping of upper eyelid) occurs secondary to direct effects on lid musculature or innervation or as part of myasthenia gravis-related reactions. Drugs associated with ptosis include barbiturates, guanethidine, bretylium, phenytoin, chloroquine, penicillamine, chloral hydrate, trimethadione, polymyxin B, and vinca alkaloids.

Oculomotor Function

Alteration of the control of external ocular muscles produces oculomotor dysfunction and results in nystagmus, oculogyric crisis, strabismus, and ocular weakness and paralysis (ophthalmoplegia). The external ocular muscles are innervated by cranial nerves III, IV, and VI and serve to place an object on the fovea rapidly, maintain the object near the fovea, maintain eye position with respect to changes in head and body movement, align visual axis to maintain bifoveal fixation, and maintain eye position with respect to target.

The drugs most commonly associated with oculomotor dysfunction are the anticonvulsants (e.g., phenytoin, phenobarbital), which produce broken pursuit movements and nystagmus, and dopamine blocking agents such as the antipsychotic drugs (phenothiazines and butyrophenones), which produce oculogyric crisis. Nalidixic acid, corticosteroids, ethanol, and vincristine may produce cranial nerve palsies. Complete listings of medications associated with altered oculomotor dysfunction are available (Table 87.3).[82,83]

Lacrimation

The tear film serves a number of purposes in maintaining ocular function. Tears maintain an optically uniform corneal surface, provide a mechanism for flushing debris from the eye, act as lubricants, provide nutrition to the corneal epithelium, and provide an antibacterial function. The tear film consists of three layers: the superficial oily layer, the aqueous layer, the mucoid layer. Medications have been associated with both hyposecretion and hypersecretion of tears (Table 87.3).

Secretion of tears by the lacrimal gland is under both sympathetic and parasympathetic control. Drugs with anticholinergic properties such as antihistamines and tricyclic antidepressants are the most frequent cause of decreased tear secretion. Sedative–hypnotic drugs (e.g., barbiturates) reduce tear production when ingested for a prolonged period.[85,86] Thiazide diuretics, amiodarone, some beta-blocking agents, and isotretinoin may produce decreased tear secretion. Isotretinoin also appears to alter tear components so as to decrease tear film break-up time. Busulfan and cyclophosphamide have been reported to produce a dry-eye syndrome with an extreme decrease in tear production.[87,88] Drug-induced hypersecretion of tears is most commonly produced by cholinergic drugs or is secondary to external ocular irritation caused by drug secretion into the tears. The increased tear production associated with doxorubicin, methotrexate, and 5-fluorouracil (5-FU) appears to result from ocular irritation.[87–92] Increased tearing is frequently associated with drug-induced conjunctival and corneal inflammation and irritation (see below). After severe inflammation, as might occur in the Stevens–Johnson syndrome, scarring of the conjunctiva may result in a dry eye from damage to tear component-producing cells and glands.

Conjunctiva and Cornea

The major drug-induced toxic effects involving the conjunctiva and cornea are inflammation of the conjunctiva (conjunctivitis), cornea (keratitis), or both (keratoconjunctivitis), and formation of deposits or pigmentation in the conjunctiva and/or the cornea.

Inflammation of the conjunctiva and/or cornea may be a result of drug hypersensitivity or a direct toxic effect.[93] External ocular inflammation secondary to drug hypersensitivity may be a local reaction or part of a systemic hypersensitivity reaction. Severe inflammation of the eyelids, conjunctiva, and cornea, such as that occurring with Stevens–Johnson syndrome, may result in symblepharon (adhesions between the bulbar and palpebral conjunctiva) and subsequently corneal scarring.

Commonly used medications associated with allergic conjunctivitis and keratoconjunctivitis include chloral hydrate, sulfa drugs, phenytoin, allopurinol, salicylates and other NSAIDs, and quinidine.[82–86,88,93] Nonallergic inflammation of the conjunctiva and/or cornea results from a direct irritant or toxic effect on the involved tissues. Severe conjunctivitis and keratitis may be produced by antineoplastic agents (e.g., doxorubicin, cytarabine, busulfan, cyclophosphamide, ifosfamide, 5-fluorouracil, chlorambucil, and methotrexate) as a result of the secretion of the antineoplastics into the tears.[88,91–95] Isotretinoin produces or exacerbates preexisting blepharoconjunctivitis in approximately 40–50% of patients. The blepharoconjunctivitis is dose related and may be transient, improving without dose reduction. A fine epithelial keratitis occurs in one-third of patients taking isotretinoin.[91,96] The biphosphonate agent pamidronate may also produce conjunctivitis 16–48 hours following a dose. Auranofin and injectable gold salts produce conjunctivitis in 3–10% of patients and may rarely produce corneal ulcers.[82,84,89] Other systemic medications have been associated with external ocular inflammation, although rarely. Almost any topical ophthalmic medication—including artificial tears and contact lens solutions—may produce inflammation or keratopathy of either the allergic or the nonallergic type.[82–86,88–90,96–98] Systemic and topical medications must be considered as possible etiologies in patients presenting with external ocular inflammation.

Prolonged therapy with certain medications may result in the formation of deposits or opacities within the conjunctiva or cornea. Such deposits may result when a drug or drug metabolite accumulates in tissues to produce visible deposits, or photosensitive drug deposits combined with light exposure produce such pigmentation. Conjunctival deposits have been reported after prolonged therapy (longer than 10 years) with tetracyclines for acne vulgaris.[88,99] These deposits are located in conjunctival cysts and range from unpigmented to black in color. Topical epinephrine may produce similar brown to black conjunctival deposits as a result of collections of adrenochrome within the conjunctiva, primarily within the light-exposed palpebral fissure.[82] Long-term, high-dose therapy with a phenothiazine, particularly chlorpromazine, may produce a brownish discoloration of the conjunctiva.[88–90,100,101] Such changes may be caused by the photosensitizing actions of chlorpromazine, resulting in protein complexation and denaturization or deposition of chlorpromazine derivatives followed by excess melanin production. Phenothiazine conjunctival discoloration occurs in patients with concomitant marked corneal and lens deposits. Clearing of the conjunctival pigmentation occurs once chlorpromazine is discontinued.

Other medications have been associated with conjunctival deposits or discoloration, including amiodarone, mitoxanthrone, gold salts, iron supplements, quinoline derivatives, and penicillamine.[82–84,88–90] The conjunctival deposit/discoloration is usually of minimal clinical importance other than for cosmetic reasons.

Drug-induced corneal deposits are also of little clinical relevance because the deposits are usually reversible and rarely cause intolerable symptoms. The quinoline antimalarial agents, for example, chloroquine and hydroxychloroquine (less commonly amiodaquine and quinacrine), produce dose-related corneal deposits.[82–85,88–90,102–108] The deposits, which are either diffuse or subsequently coalesce to form a whorl-like pattern, are usually gray to golden in color when found in the superficial corneal epithelium and may be more yellowish when found in the stroma. Corneal deposits may appear within weeks to months of initiation of therapy at doses greater than 250 mg/d chloroquine or 400

TABLE 87.3. DRUG-INDUCED OCULOTOXIC EFFECTS

Drug	Adverse Ocular Effects
Anti-Inflammatory Agents	
Corticosteroids	Glaucoma, cataracts, pseudotumor cerebri, exophthalmos, ptosis, chemosis, retinopathy
Cyclosporine	Decreased visual acuity, optic disk edema, eyelash hypertrichosis
Gold salts, auranofin	Conjunctivitis, corneal deposits, cataracts
Ibuprofen	Blurred vision, color vision disturbance, optic neuritis, amblyopia
Indomethacin	Corneal deposits, retinopathy (both rare)
Ketoprofen	Pseudotumor cerebri
Phenylbutazone	Conjunctivitis, blurred vision, corneal deposits
Piroxicam	Burning eyes, blurred vision
Salicylates	Conjunctivitis
Antimicrobial Agents	
Amiodaquine	Corneal deposits, retinopathy
Clarithromycin	Corneal opacities
Clofazamine	Conjunctival deposits, corneal deposits, pigmentary retinopathy
Chloramphenicol	Optic neuritis
Chloroquine/hydroxychloroquine	Conjunctival deposits, corneal deposits, pigmentary retinopathy, accommodative changes
Didanosine	Retinopathy, optic disk edema
Diethylcarbamazine	Ocular inflammation
Ethambutol	Optic neuritis, retinal changes, color vision changes
Gentamicin	Pseudotumor cerebri
Griseofulvin	Corneal deposits, pseudotumor cerebri
Hepatitis vaccine	Retinopathy
Influenza vaccine	Retinopathy
Isoniazid	Optic neuritis
Minocycline	Conjunctival deposits, scleral pigmentation
Metronidazole	Myopia, oculogyric crisis, photophobia, optic neuritis
Nalidixic acid	Altered color vision, visual disturbance, optic neuritis, pseudotumor cerebri
Nitrofurantoin	Extraocular muscle paralysis, pseudotumor cerebri
Quinine	Retinal ischemia (in overdose)
Rifabutin	Uveitis, contact lens staining
Rifampin	Keratoconjunctivitis, contact lens staining
Streptomycin	Nystagmus
Sulfonamides	Conjunctivitis, optic atrophy, uveitis
Suramin	Keratoconjunctivitis, optic atrophy
Tetracyclines	Conjunctival pigmentation, pseudomotor cerebri, myopia
Vaccinations	Optic atrophy
Antineoplastic Agents	
BCNU/CCNU/MeCCNU	Optic neuritis, optic atrophy, retinopathy
Busulfan	Keratoconjunctivitis sicca, cataracts
Carmustine	Retinopathy, retinal infarcts/hemorrhage
Chlorambucil	Keratitis, retinal hemorrhage, papilledema, cataracts
Cisplatin	Retinopathy, optic neuritis, papilledema
Cyclophosphamide	Keratoconjunctivitis sicca, blurred vision
Cytosine arabinoside	Corneal opacities, keratoconjunctivitis, ophthalmoplegia
Doxorubicin	Lacrimation, conjunctivitis, ophthalmoplegia
5-Fluorouracil	Lacrimation, keratoconjunctivitis, tear duct fibrosis, optic neuritis
Fludarabine	Blurred vision, photophobia, optic nerve damage
Ifosfamide	Keratoconjunctivitis
Interferons	Retinopathy
Interleukins	Uveitis
Leuprolide	Lide edema, retinopathy, retinal hemorrhage
Methotrexate	Conjunctivitis, optic neuropathy
Mitotane	Cataracts, retinopathy
Mitoxanthrone	Scleral discoloration
Nitrogen mustard	Uveitis

TABLE 87.3. DRUG-INDUCED OCULOTOXIC EFFECTS *(Continued)*

Drug	Adverse Ocular Effects
Procarbazine	Nystagmus, diplopia, retinal hemorrhage, papilledema
Tamoxifen	Corneal opacity, optic neuropathy
Vinca alkaloids	Optic neuropathy, ophthalmoplegia
Cardiovascular Agents	
Amiodarone	Corneal opacities, transient blurred vision with large doses, retinal toxicity, optic neuritis, cataracts
Diazoxide	Lacrimation
Digitalis glycosides	Blurred vision, halos around objects, color vision disturbance
Ergot alkaloids	Central retinal artery occlusion
Flecainide	Corneal deposits
Guanethidine	Conjunctival hyperemia, ptosis
Methyldopa	Cystoid macular edema
Metoprolol	Dry eyes
Mexilitine	Blurred vision, nystagmus
Minoxidil	Optic neuritis
Nicotinic acid	Cystoid macular edema
Nifedipine	Transient retinal ischemia, eye pain, blurred vision
Pindolol	Dry eyes
Propranolol	Dry eyes, conjunctivitis, inflammatory pseudotumor
Quinidine	Dry eyes, keratopathy, blurred vision, corneal deposits, retinopathy
Reserpine	Conjunctival hyperemia
Streptokinase	Uveitis
Central Nervous System	
Amantadine	Transient blurred vision
Barbiturates	Nystagmus, ptosis
Bromocriptine	Myopia
Carbamazepine	Nystagmus, cataracts
Ethchlorvynol	Optic neuritis
Lithium	Blurred vision, exophthalmos, pseudomotor cerebri
Narcotic analgesics	Miosis
Phenothiazine	Conjunctival deposits, corneal deposits, cataracts, retinopathy, oculogyric crisis
Phenytoin	Nystagmus, cataracts, ptosis
Propofol	Conjunctivitis
Protriptyline	Rare corneal deposits
Sertraline	Anisocoria
Trimethadione	Glare, photophobia, blurred vision, altered color vision
Miscellaneous Agents	
Acetazolamide	Myopia, cystoid macular edema
Allopurinol	Cataracts
Amantidine	Corneal deposits, blurred vision
Clomiphene	Blurred vision
Contraceptives (oral)	Occlusion of retinal vasculature, retinal edema, optic neuritis, corneal edema
Dantrolene	Lacrimation
Deferoxamine	Cataracts, optic neuritis, retinopathy
Diphenhydramine	Filamentary keratitis, myopia
Disulfiram	Optic neuritis
Gallium nitrate	Optic neuritis
Ipratropium (inhaled)	Mydriasis, precipitation of angle-closure glaucoma
Isotretinoin/oral retinoids	Conjunctivitis, dry eyes, corneal opacities, myopia, optic neuritis, keratitis, double vision, uveitis, impaired color vision
Metipranolol (ocular)	Uveitis
Muromonab CD3 (OKT3)	Retinopathy
Pamidronate	Uveitis
Penicillamine	Rare retinopathy, ocular myasthenia gravis
Thiazide diuretics	Myopia, decreased tear production, cystoid macular edema
Warfarin	Intraocular hemorrhage

mg hydroxychloroquine (hydroxychloroquine is thought to be less oculotoxic than chloroquine). At these doses, 30–70% of patients will develop opacities, whereas the incidence is only 0–4% at lower doses unless used for prolonged periods of time.[104] Symptoms produced by corneal deposits include decreased corneal sensation, blurred vision, glare, and photophobia; however, these symptoms are seldom intolerable and infrequently require drug discontinuation. The corneal deposits that develop in response to the quinolines are unrelated to the retinopathy associated with these agents.[102] Opacities generally disappear within 6–8 weeks of drug discontinuation.[88,104]

Amiodarone causes corneal deposits similar to those produced by chloroquine.[82,88–90,109] The development of amiodarone-induced cornea verticillata is dose and duration related. At doses less than 200 mg/d, only minor or no deposits develop. At doses above 400 mg/d, more than 90% of patients develop deposits. At doses of 400 mg or greater, deposits develop within 10 days in some patients and by 1–2 months in almost all patients. The deposits are clinically indistinguishable from those produced by chloroquine. The deposits develop to a point and do not progress despite continued constant administration, and produce symptoms in only 4–6% of patients. The major patient complaints are blurred vision, glare, photophobia, and halos around lights. Like chloroquine, corneal deposits result from deposition of drug–phospholipid complexes. The drug apparently reaches the cornea primarily by secretion into the tears. Use of artificial tears has been reported to possibly decrease the incidence/severity of the deposits, probably as a result of drug dilution. The lack of deposits in children is most likely a result of the more rapid tear turnover rate in this population. The corneal deposits typically clear 3–18 months after drug discontinuation, disappearing slowly at first and then more rapidly.

Chlorpromazine produces two types of corneal deposit: (1) cornea verticillata, similar to that produced by chloroquine and amiodarone; and (2) a fine, diffuse, brownish granular deposit. The cornea verticillata occurs only with prolonged use of high doses (>2000 mg/d) and is similar to that described with chloroquine. The mechanism of chlorpromazine-induced cornea verticillata is assumed to be identical to that for the disease induced by chloroquine and amiodarone. The diffuse granular deposits produced by chlorpromazine are thought to be similar to those found in the conjunctiva, being located primarily within the palpebral fissure. The incidence of corneal deposits has been associated with the total dose of chlorpromazine administered. In patients receiving less than a 0.5-kg total dose, deposits are rare, whereas patients receiving greater than 1–2.5 kg demonstrate higher frequencies of corneal deposits. Others have suggested that the daily dosage rate rather than total dose is important, with doses less than 300 mg/d rarely producing deposits. Corneal deposits are rarely seen in patients without chlorpromazine-induced lens deposits (see below). Corneal deposits occur in 20–50% of patients with lens deposits. The corneal deposits rarely cause clinical symptoms and are sometimes slowly reversible upon drug discontinuation. Other antipsychotics (e.g., loxapine, dibenzoxazepine, trifluoperazine, fluphenazine, prochlorperazine, chlorprothixine, perphenazine, thiothixene, and possibly thioridazine) have occasionally been associated with corneal deposits.[110,111]

Other medications associated with the development of corneal opacities include indomethacin, gold salts, iron salts, vitamin D, cytarabine, isotretinoin, clarithromycin, phenylbutazone, protriptyline, tamoxifen, silver protein (argyrol), vinblastine, and quinidine.[82–84,88–90,96,111–114]

INTERNAL OCULAR STRUCTURES

Medications may alter the function of, or be toxic to, internal structures of the eye, resulting in drug-induced glaucoma (see Chapter 88), lens opacities (cataracts), uveitis, retinopathy, and optic neuritis. Unlike many of the adverse effects on the external ocular structures, adverse effects on internal structures may produce serious irreversible impairment of vision.

Lens

Other than reversible pharmacologic changes in accommodation (most commonly with parasympathetic acting agents) caused by ciliary body constriction/relaxation, the major adverse drug effects on the lens are cataracts (lens opacities) and myopia. Commonly used medications that produce cataracts with significant frequency include the phenothiazines, corticosteroids, amiodarone, gold salts, and topical parasympathomimetic agents used in the treatment of glaucoma. Other medications associated with cataracts are listed in Table 87.3.

Cataracts caused by phenothiazines, like the conjunctival and corneal deposits, are most common with chlorpromazine. The mechanism of phenothiazine-induced cataracts is thought to be a photosensitivity reaction similar to that which produces the conjunctival and corneal deposits. The phenothiazine lens opacities often start as fine dot-like deposits that eventually form larger granules with continued therapy. Phenothiazine lens opacities are thought to result when these agents combine with melanin to form a photosensitive product. The incidence of chlorpromazine-induced cataracts is greater than that of corneal or conjunctival deposits and is dose and duration related. Epidemiologic studies have found the use of phenothiazines to increase the risk of cataracts by 3.5-fold. Fifty percent of patients given a total dose of 0.5 kg and 90% of patients given a total dose of 2.5 kg demonstrate deposits. Deposits are rare with doses less than 0.5 kg. Dosage rate also appears to play an important role, with higher rates (>2 g/d) producing deposits within months of initiation of therapy and rates less than 300 mg/d infrequently producing cataracts unless therapy is prolonged. Lenticular opacities almost universally appear before corneal and conjunctival deposits. Phenothiazine-induced cataracts rarely produce symptoms and are typically slowly reversible upon drug discontinuation or switching to an alternative antipsychotic agent.[88–90,114]

Corticosteroids administered systemically or topically to the eye have been identified as cataractogenic.[88–90,115–122] Cataracts have been clearly demonstrated after nasal or inhalation therapy use. Systemic absorption from the skin may also result in cataracts following prolonged use, and such patients should be considered at risk. The cataracts are usually bilateral and symmetric, although 10% of patients may demonstrate asymmetric opacities. The reported incidence of cataracts in patients receiving corticosteroid therapy ranges from 5–96%. Diabetics and children appear to be more susceptible, and genetic predisposition may explain the variation in reported incidence rates. Dose and duration were previously thought to be closely related to incidence of cataracts, but there appears now to be no relation between dosage rate, total dose, duration of therapy, or age of patient and cataracts, and development of cataracts appears to be a function of individual susceptibility. Corticosteroid-induced cataracts rarely produce symptoms; however, cataracts caused by corticosteroids accounted for 9% of all presenile cataracts requiring removal in one study.[85] Alterations of lens capsule permeability, decreased lens ATPase, altered lens electrolyte concentrations, decreased aqueous humor potassium and ascorbic acid, and increased aqueous humor pH are possible etiologies of corticosteroid cataracts. Lens opacities produced by corticosteroids are thought to be largely irreversible; however, cases of progression after discontinuation and regression (primarily in children) during therapy and after discontinuation have been reported.

Myopia has been reported during therapy with a number of medications.[82–85,88] The primary mechanisms include ciliary muscle contraction, producing accommodation, and hydration of the lens, increasing the refractive power. Parasympathomimetics and narcotics produce myopia because of ciliary muscle contraction. Drugs that produce myopia as a result of lens hydration include corticosteroids; metronidazole; tetracyclines; bromocriptine; sulfonamide antibiotics; sulfa derivatives such as thiazide diuretics, spironolactone, and acetazolamide; and antihistamines. Myopia is typically transient, disappearing with discontinuation or, in many cases, with continued dosing.

Uveal Tract

The uvea, or middle coat of the eye, consists of the iris, ciliary body, and choroid. A large number of medications alter the function of the iris (i.e., mydriasis or miosis) and ciliary body (alteration of accommodation) through direct pharmacologic effects. Such agents include anticholinergics, cholinergics, opiates, and adrenergic agents. Medications have also been reported to produce inflammatory reactions of the uvea, or "uveitis." Uveitis is a term used to describe these inflammatory conditions, which may also involve other ocular structures such as the sclera (scleritis, episcleritis), vitreous, and retina. Uveitis may be further defined as involving anterior, intermediate, or posterior ocular structures, and as being acute or chronic in nature.[123]

Symptoms of uveitis will depend on the site of inflammation. Drug-induced uveitis most commonly involves the anterior structures of the eye (anterior uveitis). Signs and symptoms may include, a red (or "injected" eye), eye pain, decreased vision, photophobia, synechiae, cells in the anterior chamber, hypopyon, and cells in the anterior vitreous. Drug-induced uveitis may be misdiagnosed as endophthalmitis because of their similar presentations. The mechanism by which drugs produce uveitis is unknown, but it may involve direct or indirect toxicity or inflammatory reactions or triggering of an autoimmune reaction. Drug-induced uveitis is commonly bilateral but may be unilateral.

Rifabutin produces a high frequency (up to 35% of patients) of anterior uveitis when used at high doses (>300 mg/d) or at lower doses when combined with agents known to reduce the clearance of rifabutin such as clarithromycin and fluconazole. The onset of uveitis is usually at 8–30 weeks of therapy, and tends to occur earlier at higher doses. Most cases of rifabutin uveitis may be treated with topical corticosteroids and the drug continued or administered at a lower dose. Some patients require complete drug discontinuation for resolution. The mechanism by which rifabutin produces uveitis is unknown; a site-specific Jarisch–Herxheimer type reaction or local toxic effects have been proposed.[124–129]

Medication-related uveitis suggesting an immune reaction or alteration of the immune system has been reported with pamidronate, sulfonamides (primarily trimethoprim–sulfamethoxazole), ibuprofen, interleukins, and streptokinase.[130–134] The antiglaucoma topical beta-blocking agent metipranolol produces anterior uveitis, particularly at higher concentrations (0.6%). Uveitis has been reported with the formulation marketed in the United States (0.3%). Metipranolol-related uveitis may be accompanied by an increased intraocular pressure, a troubling occurrence in glaucoma patients.[135]

Retina and Optic Nerve

Toxic effects on the sensory retina and optic nerve are the most important organ-specific adverse effects of drugs on the eye. These effects may impair vision significantly and occasionally are irreversible. Monitoring for drug-induced retinal and optic nerve toxicity is essential for early recognition. The mechanisms of drug-induced retinal toxicity are variable and may involve direct toxic effects, accumulation of drug in retinal structures, ischemia secondary to effects on retinal vasculature or immune reactions. Commonly used medications producing significant retinal toxicity include the phenothiazines, 4-aminoquinoline antimalarials, tamoxifen, other antineoplastic agents, and deferoxamine.

The phenothiazine-type antipsychotic agent thioridazine produces a toxic pigmentary retinopathy. The development of retinopathy is clearly dose dependent, with doses above 800–1200 mg/d associated with a high frequency of retinopathy.[82–85,88–90,136,137] Doses less than 800 mg/d are generally considered safe; however, cases of retinopathy have occurred with doses less than 800 mg/d. Symptoms of toxic retinopathy often occur within 2 weeks to 3 months of initiation of high-dose thioridazine. Patients may complain of blurred vision, brown-colored vision, or other abnormalities of color vision, decreased night vision, and scotomas (blind spots) around the area of central vision. Some patients may retain normal central visual acuity. These early symptoms may be associated with retinal edema or optic disk hyperemia, or the fundus may appear normal. Within weeks to months, funduscopic evaluation may detect diffuse, fine, deep retinal pigment deposits in the pole posterior to the equator of the globe. The macula may be spared in some cases.

With continued therapy, the pigment granules begin to coalesce and may form plaques of pigment. Eventually, multiple large areas of depigmentation appear associated with atrophy of the retinal pigment epithelium, choriocapillaris, and retina. Retinal arteriole attenuation may occur. Vision testing will demonstrate normal to decreased central acuity, constricted visual field and paracentral scotomas, and altered color vision. Thioridazine produces retinopathy after binding to the melanin of the retinal pigmented epithelium (RPE) and choroid, inhibiting oxidative phosphorylation within the retina and producing outer rod segment degeneration. Cellular debris from rod degeneration accumulates, producing the characteristic pigmentary changes in the retina. Upon discontinuation of thioridazine, visual acuity, night vision, and color vision generally improve; however, some patients show no improvement in vision and even progression of retinopathy. Early pigmentary changes generally clear with discontinuation; however, later changes may be permanent.

All patients starting on high-dose, long-term thioridazine therapy should have an ophthalmologic exam and be routinely examined for vision and funduscopic changes. Patients complaining of blurred vision, altered color vision, decreased night vision, or blind spots must be carefully examined. If retinopathy occurs, thioridazine should be discontinued and an alternative drug chosen.

Chlorpromazine has been rarely associated with the development of retinal pigmentation. Doses of 800–2400 mg/d for approximately 2 years are required to produce retinopathy. The chlorpromazine-induced retinopathy is less severe than that produced by thioridazine and is reversible upon drug discontinuation.

The 4-aminoquinoline antimalarial agents chloroquine and hydroxychloroquine produce a dose-dependent toxic retinopathy.[104–108,138,139] These agents are used in the long-term therapy of patients with rheumatoid arthritis, systemic lupus erythematosus, and other autoimmune conditions. With this long-term use, the potential for retinal toxicity needs to be considered. Although most cases of toxicity have been reported with chloroquine, hydroxychloroquine is also toxic, though considered safer than chloroquine with a lower frequency and severity of toxicity. Daily doses of less than 250 mg chloroquine or 400 mg hydroxychloroquine are only rarely (<5%) associated with the development of retinal damage. Larger doses produce retinopathy in up to 15% of patients continuing therapy for more than 1 year and may be more toxic in patients with systemic lupus erythematosus. Older studies suggested that total dosage consumption was important; however, recent data suggest that the dosage rate is the most important determinant of risk, with daily doses of chloroquine less than 4.5 mg/kg and of hydroxychloroquine less than 6.5 mg/kg less commonly associated with toxicity.[104,137]

Retinopathy produced by quinoline derivatives is unrelated to the development of corneal deposits. Early changes are similar to retinal changes seen with age and are difficult to identify without a baseline evaluation. Symptoms are frequently absent at this stage, or the patient may complain of blurred vision. With continued chloroquine use, the classic retinal findings of increased macula granular pigmentation surrounded by alternating concentric rings of hypopigmented and hyperpigmented retinal epithelium ("bull's-eye retinopathy") develop. At this stage, symptoms of blurred vision, reading difficulties with missing words or letters (caused by paracentral scotomas), photophobia, decreased night vision, flashes or streaks of light, large visual field defects, and altered color vision are present. Symptoms do not always parallel the retinal findings.

Advanced retinopathy is characterized by a generalized retinopathy; disruption of the retinal pigmented epithelium, attenuated retinal arterioles, optic disk pallor, and severe visual impairment may occur. Retinopathy is thought to occur as a result of the binding and accumulation of these cationic amphophilic compounds to the phospholipids of lysosomes and melanin of the retinal pigmented epithelium and the choroid and decreasing retinal protection from toxic free radicals and resulting in injury and death of inner retinal cell layers (rods and cones). Early retinal toxicity with absent or minimal symptoms is usually reversible with drug discontinuation; however, when the bull's-eye lesion and significant symptoms are present, retinopathy remains stable when the drug is stopped, although some improvement in vision may occur. Occasionally, retinopathy may progress despite drug discontinuation; such "progressive" retinopathy is more likely to occur when more severe retinal damage has occurred during therapy. Rare cases of retinopathy appearing and progressing after drug discontinuation have been reported.

Because of the irreversible nature of all but early retinopathy, close monitoring for ocular toxicity is required during chloroquine therapy. A baseline examination is mandatory, with follow-up monitoring every 6 months during therapy. Useful monitoring parameters include ophthalmoscopic exam, visual fields with white and red targets, visual acuity, and retinal electrophysiologic studies. Patient self-testing for scotomas using Amsler's grid monthly is also suggested. Chloroquine and hydroxychloroquine retinopathy may be limited by administering doses less than 4.5 mg/kg/d (chloroquine) or 6.5 mg/kg/d (hydroxychloroquine), a careful, conscientious monitoring program, and discontinuation at first signs of retinopathy. Drug holidays during the summer months and use of dark sunglasses to decrease sun exposure may be of value in limiting toxic effects. Infrequent cases of retinal abnormalities after therapy with amiodaquine, quinine, mepacrine, and quinacrine have also been reported.[102–108,138,139]

Retinal toxicity occurs with the use of a number of other medications. Long-term use of oral contraceptives has been rarely associated with retinal abnormalities including retinal vein occlusion, retinal arteriole occlusion, retinal hemorrhage, altered macula function, retinal edema, abnormal color vision, and possible accelerated progression of retinitis pigmentosa.[140] Deferoxamine therapy has been associated with the development of pigmentary retinopathy after administration of 12–96 g of deferoxamine over 4–17 days. Symptoms of blurred vision and color vision abnormalities occurred concomitantly with the bilateral retinopathy. After drug discontinuation, some regression of retinopathy occurred; however, baseline vision was not regained.[72,141,142]

Tamoxifen therapy has been reported to produce a retinopathy characterized by fine, white refractile retinal opacities, cystoid macular edema, and occasional depigmentation of retinal pigmented epithelium. Tamoxifen is a cationic amphophilic compound as is chloroquine, and a similar mechanism of binding to lysosomal phospholipid may be the mechanism of retinal toxicity. High-dose tamoxifen therapy (90–180 mg/d and cumulative doses of >90 g) is associated with a more frequent and more severe—and possibly irreversible—retinal toxicity. However, retinal toxicity may also occur with low-dose (10–40 mg/d) therapy. The frequency of retinal toxicity with low-dose therapy has been reported to be 1.5–6%. The toxicity with low-dose therapy appears mild and reversible. Routine ophthalmologic monitoring for low-dose patients is not generally recommended unless visual symptoms occur. Tamoxifen therapy has also been associated with optic neuritis and optic disk edema.[143–147]

The calcium channel blocker nifedipine may produce transient retinal ischemia, purportedly because of a "steal" phenomenon with resultant transient decreased acuity and visual field defects.[148] Cardiac glycoside toxicity frequently produces disturbance of vision (particularly color vision) because of inhibition of Na/K-ATPase in the sensory retina cells. Prolonged cardiac glycoside therapy may rarely produce irreversible retinopathy.[149]

Didanosine (ddl) use in children with HIV infection has been associated with the development of peripheral atrophy of the retinal pigmented epithelium. Toxicity appears to occur in approximately 7% of patients and may be more frequent at higher doses. The retinopathy occurred after 36 weeks of therapy and may continue to progress despite dose reduction. Progression of retinopathy stops with drug discontinuation and may be at least partially reversible. Children receiving ddl for more than 4–6 months should be monitored for retinal toxicity.[150] Didanosine has also been associated with optic neuritis in an adult patient.[151]

Another agent commonly used in AIDs patients, clofazamine, an antimycobacterial, has been reported to cause a bulls-eye retinopathy similar to that of chloroquine.[152] Interferon alfa use is associated with the development of retinal ischemia with resultant retinal nerve fiber layer damage, hemorrhage, and retinal edema. Most patients are asymptomatic and the ischemia is reversible with drug discontinuation. Regular ophthalmologic exams should be considered for patients receiving interferon alfa to avoid progression to irreversible toxicity.[153] Vaccination with hepatitis B vaccine and influenza vaccine has resulted in acute lesions of the pigmented epithelium. It is possible that these vaccines trigger an autoimmune response to antigens in the pigmented epithelium.[154] Administration of muromonab-CD3 (OKT3) has produced substantial visual loss after two to three doses. This visual loss appeared to be secondary to retinal ischemia secondary to arteriolar constriction.[155] Quinine overdose is also associated with acute visual loss secondary to ischemia. The visual loss associated with quinine has been reversed with nitrate therapy.[156] Chemotherapeutic agents administered intracarotid have been associated with retinal toxicity secondary to vaso-occlusive effects as well as an apparent direct toxic effect on the retina.[157] Other examples of toxic retinal drug reactions have included hemorrhage after epidural corticosteroid injection or leuprolide, cystoid macular edema with methyldopa, topical epinephrine, thiazide diuretics, acetazolamide, and nicotinic acid, and decreased night vision or night blindness with isotretinoin.[96,158,159] Other medications associated with retinopathy are listed in Table 87.3.

Adverse effects of drugs on the optic nerve and visual tracts include optic neuropathy, optic atrophy, retrobulbar neuropathy, and papilledema. Optic neuropathy, an inflammation of the optic nerve, produces symptoms including blurred vision, scotomas, constricted visual fields, altered color vision, and occasionally edema or hyperemia of the optic disk. Ethambutol produces two types of dose-dependent optic neuropathy (either axial or periaxial) after 1–3 months of therapy.[159–161] Axial (or central) neuropathy is more common than periaxial neuropathy and is characterized by decreased visual acuity, central scotomata, and disturbance and red–green color vision. Subtle swelling of the optic disk and splinter hemorrhages may be present when symptoms occur suddenly. The less common periaxial optic neuropathy is characterized by the presence of paracentral scotomata without significant decreases in visual function or color vision disturbance.

Cases of possibly idiosyncratic, rapid onset, irreversible vision loss have been reported. The incidence of optic neuropathy is rare (0.8–1.7%) at doses of 15 mg/kg/d or less; 1–8% for 15–25 mg/kg/d and doses greater than 25 and 50 mg/kg/d produce optic neuritis in 5% and 10% of patients, respectively. Optic neuropathy may be preceded by peripheral neuropathy. The mechanism of toxicity is thought to be an ethambutol metabolite-induced chelation and subsequent decrease in zinc content of the retina and optic nerve. Ethambutol-induced optic neuropathy is generally slowly reversible within 3 months of drug discontinuation; more severely affected patients recover more slowly or less completely. Some experts recommend administration of 100–250 mg zinc sulfate three times daily in patients with optic neuropathy.

Patients failing to recover after drug discontinuation may show regression of visual loss when given high-dose hydroxycobalamin (40 mg/d). Continued therapy with ethambutol in patients with optic neuropathy may produce optic atrophy and irreversible visual loss. Patients receiving ethambutol should undergo a basic visual examination, including visual acuity, visual field, and color vision tests. Patients should be warned of possible ocular toxicity and should be counseled to report immediately decreased visual acuity, trouble in reading, blind spots, and abnormal color vision. Only in patients receiving doses greater than 15 mg/kg/d should routine visual examinations during therapy be considered. Isoniazid, an agent often used in combination with ethambutol, also produces optic neuropathy, particularly in malnourished patients, and presents with symptoms similar to those seen with ethambutol. The optic neuropathy usually responds to therapy with pyridoxine.

Deferoxamine produces a bilateral optic neuropathy with symptoms similar to those observed with ethambutol. The mechanism of toxic optic neuropathy may be similar to that of ethambutol-induced disease, with chelation and a subsequent decrease in retinal zinc and/or copper. Deferoxamine-induced optic neuropathy may occur within 4 days to 3 months. Long-term or high-dose therapy with chloramphenicol is associated with optic neuropathy when total doses exceed 75–100 g.[162] Optic neuropathy with chloramphenicol is characterized by sudden decrease in visual acuity, halos around objects, scotomata, altered color vision, and orbital pain with onset of neuropathy. A funduscopic exam may demonstrate papilledema, disk hyperemia, flame hemorrhage, and exudates. Discontinuation of chloramphenicol produces total regression of symptoms. Continuation of therapy may result in optic nerve atrophy.

Other agents reported to produce optic neuropathy or optic atrophy include minoxidil, propoxyphene (in overdose), carmustine, vincristine, cisplatin, ethchlorvynol, sulfonylurea hypoglycemics and other sulfa derivatives, leuprolide, tamoxifen, metronidazole, amiodarone, corticosteroids, barbiturates, and possibly oral contraceptives and isotretinoin. Optic neuropathy has also been reported after vaccination for measles/mumps/rubella, influenza, and swine flu.

Papilledema, or swelling of the optic disk secondary to a benign increase in intracranial pressure (pseudotumor cerebri), may be produced by a number of medications. The primary symptoms are headache and enlarged blind spot, with swelling of the optic disk upon funduscopy. Drugs associated with papilledema include corticosteroids (also corticosteroid withdrawal), cyclosporin, tetracyclines, oral contraceptives, isotretinoin, aminoglycosides, and nalidixic acid. Drug discontinuation commonly results in regression of all symptoms; however, total or partial visual loss may occur in some patients.[82,88–90,163]

DRUG-INDUCED CONTACT LENS PROBLEMS

The use of medications may also interfere with the use of contact lenses. Interactions may occur between drugs and the contact lens (i.e., staining of the lens by rifampin, rifabutin, sulfasalazine, or topical epinephrine) or lens solutions (i.e., reactions caused by use of tetracyclines and thimerosol-preserved solutions). Medications may interfere with contact lens wear through decreased lacrimation (i.e., anticholinergics), increased lacrimation (i.e., reserpine), corneal edema resulting in poor lens fit (i.e., estrogens), and decreased acuity secondary to a change in refraction (i.e., myopia produced by thiazide diuretics). The physical properties of ophthalmic medications such as ointments, suspensions, and gels may also affect the use of contact lenses. Additionally, important symptoms may be masked when patients self-administer ocular antihistamines, decongestants, or astringents in response to ocular irritation secondary to the contact lens.

Adverse ocular effects of medications may be falsely associated with the contact lens. Contact lens wearers should be counseled to avoid applying topical medications while wearing lenses unless the product is specifically designed for concurrent use or ordered to do so by an ophthalmologist. Drug absorbed into a soft contact lens will result in prolonged corneal exposure to high drug concentrations, potentially increasing the risk for toxicity. The drug or drug vehicle may be incompatible with the lens or lens care solution.

Remember that nonprescription ophthalmics may mask symptoms and that both topical and systemic medication could interfere with contact lens fit and tolerance.[164]

Conclusion

Adverse drug reactions involving the ears and eyes are relatively uncommon. However, because of the delicate and complicated structure and function of these organs, serious irreversible damage may be produced when toxicity occurs. Awareness of potential ototoxic and oculotoxic drugs and of factors increasing the risk of toxicity allows the clinician to minimize the frequency and consequences of toxicity.

References

1. The Boston Collaborative Surveillance Program. Drug-induced deafness. JAMA 1973;224:515–516.
2. Porter J, Jick M. Drug induced anaphylaxis, convulsions, deafness and extrapyramidal symptoms. Lancet 1978;1:581–588.
3. Nadol JB. Hearing loss. New Engl J Med 1993;329:1092–1102.
4. Meyerhoff WL, Yellin W, Maale GE, et al. Audiologic threshold monitoring of patients receiving ototoxic drugs. Ann Otol Rhinol Laryngol 1989;98:950–954.
5. Campbell KCM, Durrant J. Audiologic monitoring for ototoxicity. Otolaryngol Clin North Am 1993;26:903–914.
6. Gendeh BS, Said H, Gibb AG, et al. Gentamicin ototoxicity in continuous ambulatory peritoneal dialysis. J Otolaryngol Otol 1993;107:681–685.
7. Brummet RE, Morrison RB. The incidence of aminoglycoside antibiotic induced hearing loss. Arch Otolaryngol Head Neck Surg 1990;116:406–410.
8. Black FO, Pesznecker SC. Vestibular ototoxicity. Clinical considerations. Otolaryngol Clin North Am 1993;26:713–736.
9. Chiodo AA, Alberti PW. Experimental, clinical and preventive aspects of ototoxicity. Eur Arch Otorhinolaryngol 1994;251:375–392.
10. Scott PMJ, Griffiths MV. A clinical review of ototoxicity. Clin Otolaryngol 1994;19:3–8.
11. Brummet RE, Fox KE. Aminoglycoside induced hearing loss in humans. Antimicrobial Agents Chemother 1989;33:797–800.
12. Griffin JP. Drug induced ototoxicity. Br J Audiol 1988;22:195–210.
13. Walker EM, Fazekas-May MA, Bowen WR. Nephrotoxic and ototoxic agents. Clin Lab Med 1990;10:323–354.
14. Huang MY, Schacht J. Drug induced ototoxicity pathogenesis and prevention. Med Tox Adv Drug Exp 1989;4:452–467.
15. Matz GJ. Clinical perspectives on ototoxic drugs. Ann Otol Rhinol Laryngol 1990;99:39–41.
16. Rybak LP. Drug ototoxicity. Ann Rev Pharmacol Toxicol 1986;26:79–99.
17. Norris CH. Drugs affecting the inner ear. Drugs 1988;36:754–772.
18. Manian FA, Stone WJ, Alford RH. Adverse antibiotic effects associated with renal insufficiencies. Rev Infect Dis 1990;12:236–244.
19. Bergstrom L, Thompson PL. Ototoxicity, in Northern JL (ed): Hearing Disorders, 2nd ed. Boston, Little Brown, 1984, pp 253–266.
20. Bendush CL. Ototoxicity: Clinical considerations and comparative information, in Whelton A, Neu HC (eds): The Aminoglycosides. Microbiology, Clinical Use and Toxicology. New York, Marcel Dekker, 1982.
21. Govaerts PJ, Claes J, Van DeHeyning PH, et al. Aminoglycoside induced ototoxicity. Toxicol Lett 1990;52:227–251.
22. Matz GJ. Aminoglycoside cochlear toxicity. Otolaryngol Clin North Am 1993;26:705–712.
23. Buring JE, Evans DA, Mayrent SL, et al. Randomized trials of aminoglycoside antibiotics: Quantitative overview. Rev Infect Dis 1988;10:951–957.
24. Mattie H, Craig WA, Pechere JC. Determinants of efficacy and toxicity of aminoglycosides. J Antimicrobial Chemother 1989;24:281–293.
25. Tron BA, Huy P, Deffrennes D. Aminoglycoside ototoxicity: Influence of dosage regimen on drug uptake and correlation between membrane binding and some clinical features. Acta Otolaryngol 1988;105:511–515.
26. Kitasato I, Yokota M, Inouge S, et al. Comparative ototoxicity of ribostamycin, dactimicin, dibekacin, kanamycin, amikacin, tobramycin, gentamicin, sizomicin and netilmicin in the inner ear of guinea pigs. Chemotherapy 1990;36:155–168.
27. Moore RD, Smith CR, Lietman PS. Risk factors for the development of auditory toxicity in patients receiving aminoglycosides. J Infect Dis 1984;149:23–30.
28. Garrison L, Dutro M. Ototoxicity from topical neomycin [letter]. Clin Pharm 1982;1:301.
29. Johnson CA. Hearing loss following the application of topical neomycin. J Burn Care Rehab 1988;9:162–164.
30. Matz GJ, Lerner SA. Prospective studies of aminoglycoside ototoxicity in adults, in Lerner SA, Matz GJ, Hawkins JE (eds): Aminoglycoside Ototoxicity. Boston, Little, Brown, 1981.
31. Wersall J. Recent otological evaluation of aminoglycoside antibiotics. J Antimicrob Chemother 1984;13(suppl A):31–36.
32. Schacht J. Biochemical basis of aminoglycoside ototoxicity. Otolaryngol Clin North Am 1993;26:845–856.
33. Hutchin T, Cortopassi G. Proposed molecular and cellular mechanisms for aminoglycoside ototoxicity. Antimicrob Agents Chemother 1994;38:2517–2520.
34. Beaubien AR, Ormsby E, Bayne A, et al. Evidence that amikacin ototoxicity is related to total perilymph area under the concentration-time curve regardless of concentration. Antimicrob Agents Chemother 1991;35:1070–1074.
35. Beaubien AR, Desjardens S, Ormsby E, et al. Incidence of amikacin ototoxicity: A sigmoid function of total drug exposure independent of plasma levels. Am J Otolaryngol 1989;10:234–243.
36. Bates RD, Nahata MC. Once-daily administration of aminoglycosides. Ann Pharmacother 1994;28:757–766.

37. Smith CR, Leitman PS. Effect of furosemide on aminoglycoside-induced nephrotoxicity and auditory toxicity in humans. Antimicrob Agents Chemother 1983;23:133–137.
38. Yamare H, Nakai Y, Konishi. Furosemide-induced alteration of drug pathway to cochlea. Acta Otolaryngol (Stokhh) 1988;(suppl 44):28–35.
39. Brummett RE, Fox KE, Jacobs F, et al. Augmented gentamicin ototoxicity induced by vancomycin in guinea pigs. Arch Otolaryngol Head Neck Surg 1990;116:61–64.
40. Haydon RC, Thelin JW, Davis WE. Erythromycin ototoxicity: Analysis and conclusions based on 22 case reports. Otolaryngol Head Neck Surg 1984;92:678–684.
41. Brummett RE, Fox KE. Vancomycin and erythromycin induced hearing loss in humans. Antimicrob Agents Chemother 1989;33:791–796.
42. Swanson DJ, RJ Sung, Fine MJ, et al. Erythromycin ototoxicity: Prospective assessment with serum concentrations and audiograms in a study of patients with pneumonia. Am J Med 1992;92:61–68.
43. Cramer R. Erythromycin ototoxicity. Drug Intel Clin Pharm 1986;20:764–765.
44. Brummett RE. Ototoxicity liability of erythromycin and analogues. Otolaryngol Clin North Am 1993;26:811–819.
45. Sacristan JA, Soto JA, de Cos MA. Erythromycin induced hypoacusis in 11 new cases and literature review. Ann Pharmacother 1993;27:950–955.
46. Vasquez EM, Maddux MS, Sanchez J, Pollak R. Clinically significant hearing loss in renal allograft recipients treated with intravenous erythromycin. Arch Int Med 1993;153:879–882.
47. Wallace MR, Miller LK, Nguyen M-T, Shields AR. Ototoxicity with azithromycin. Lancet 1994;343:241.
48. Fernandez-Martin J, Leport C, Morlat P, et al. Pyrimethamine–clarithromycin combination for acute toxoplasma encephalitis in patients with AIDS. Antimicrob Agents Chemother 1991;35:2049–2052.
49. Dautzenberg B, Saint Marc T, Meyohas C, et al. Clarithromycin and other antimicrobial agents in the treatment of disseminated mycobacterium avium infections in patients with acquired immunodeficiency syndrome. Arch Int Med 1993;153:368–372.
50. Farber BF, Moellering RC. Retrospective study of the preparations of vancomycin from 1974 to 1981. Antimicrob Agents Chemother 1984;23:138–141.
51. Bailie GR, Neel D. Vancomycin ototoxicity and nephrotoxicity. Med Toxicol 1988;3:376–386.
52. Brummett RE. Ototoxicity of vancomycin and analogues. Otolaryngol Clin North Am 1993;26:821–828.
53. Cantu TG, Yamanaka-Yuen NA, Lietman PS. Serum vancomycin concentrations: Reappraisal of their clinical value. Clin Infect Dis 1994;18:533–543.
54. Gump GW, Ashikaga T, Fink T, et al. Side effects of minocycline: Different dosage regimens. Antimicrob Agents Chemother 1977;12:642–646.
55. Drew TM, Altman R, Black K, et al. Minocycline for prophylaxis of infection in *Neisseria meningitidis:* High rate of side effects in recipients. J Infec Dis 1976;133:194–198.
56. Jung TTK, Rhee C-K, Lee CS, et al. Ototoxicity of salicylate, nonsteroidal anti-inflammatory drugs, and quinine. Otolaryngol Clin North Am 1993;26:781–810.
57. Alvan G, Kalrsson KK, Hellgren U, Villen T. Hearing impairment related to plasma quinine concentration in healthy volunteers. Br J Clin Pharmacol 1991;31:409–412.
58. Dwivedi GS, Mehra YN. Ototoxicity of chloroquine phosphate. A case report. J Laryngol Otol 1978;92:701–703.
59. Miller RR, Jick H. Acute toxicity of aspirin in hospitalized medical patients. Am J Med Sci 1977;274:271–279.
60. Miller RR. Deafness due to plain and long acting aspirin tablets. J Clin Pharmacol 1978;18:468–471.
61. Brien J. Ototoxicity associated with salicylates. A brief review. Drug Safety 1993;9:143–148.
62. Gallagher KL, Jones JR. Furosemide-induced ototoxicity. Ann Intern Med 1979;91:744–745.
63. Rybak LP. Ototoxicity of diuretics. Otolaryngol Clin North Am 1993;26:829–844.
64. Tuzel IH. Comparison of adverse reactions to bumetanide and furosemide. J Clin Pharmacol 1981;21:615–619.
65. Brummett RE, Bendrick T, Himes D. Comparative ototoxicity of bumetanide and furosemide when used in combination with kanamycin. J Clin Pharmacol 1981;21:628–636.
66. Schweitzer VG. Ototoxicity of chemotherapeutic agents. Otolaryngol Clin North Am 1993;26:759–789.
67. Moroso MJ, Blair R. A review of cisplatin ototoxicity. J Otolaryngol 1983;12:365–369.
68. Melamed LB, Selin MA, Schuchiman D. Cisplatin ototoxicity in gynecologic cancer patients. Cancer 1985;55:41–43.
69. Schaeffer SD, Wright FG, Post JD, et al. Cisplatin vestibular toxicity. Cancer 1981;47:857–859.
70. Blakely BW, Gupta AK, Myers SF, Schwan S. Risk factors for ototoxicity due to cisplatin. Arch Otolaryngol Head Neck Surg 1994:120:541–546.
71. Gallant T, Boyden MH, Gallant LA, et al. Serial studies of auditory neurotoxicity in patients receiving deferoxamine therapy. Am J Med 1987;83:1085–1090.
72. Olivieri NF, Buncic JR, Chew E, et al. Visual and auditory neurotoxicity in patients receiving subcutaneous deferoxamine infusions. N Engl J Med 1986;314:869.
73. Porter JB, Jaswon MS, Huehns ER, et al. Desferrioxamine ototoxicity: Evaluation of risk factors in thalassemic patients and guidelines for safe dosage. Br J Haematol 1989;73:403–409.
74. Podishin L, Fradis M, David JB. Ototoxicity of ear drops in patients suffering from chronic otitis media. J Laryngol Otol 1989;103:46–50.
75. Rohn GN, Meyerhoff WL, Wright CG. Ototoxicity of topical agents. Otolaryngol Clin North Am 1993;26:747–758.
76. Roland PS. Clinical ototoxicity of topical antibiotic drops. Otolaryngol Head Neck Surg 1994;110:598–602.
77. Henley CM, Rybak LP. Developmental ototoxicity. Otolaryngol Clin North Am 1993;26:857–871.
78. Davies DM. Drug-induced deafness. Adv Drug React Bull 1978;69:244–277.
79. Worthington EL, Lunin LF, Heath M, et al. Index-Handbook of Ototoxic Agents, 1966–1971. Baltimore, MD, Johns Hopkins University, 1973.
80. Drucker T. Drugs that can cause tinnitus. ATA Newslett 1979;4:3–5.
81. Miller JJ. Handbook of Ototoxicity. Boca Raton, FL, CRC Press, 1980.

82. Fraunfelder FT, Meyer SM. Drug Induced Ocular Side Effects and Drug Interactions, 3rd ed. Philadelphia, Lea and Febiger, 1987.
83. Grant WM. Toxicity of the Eye, 3rd ed. Springfield, IL, Charles C Thomas, 1986.
84. Crombie AL. Eye disorders, in Davies DM (ed): Textbook of Adverse Drug Reactions, 3rd ed. Oxford, Oxford University Press, 1985, pp 515–529.
85. Spiteri MA, James DG. Adverse ocular reactions to drugs. Postgrad Med J 1983;59:343–349.
86. Miller D. Systemic medications. Int Ophthalmol Clin 1981;21:177–183.
87. Imperia PS, Lazarus HM, Lass JH. Ocular complications of systemic cancer chemotherapy. Surv Ophthalmol 1989;34:209–230.
88. Jaanus SD. Ocular side effects of selected systemic drugs. Optometry Clin 1992;2:73–96.
89. Anon. Ocular adversae effects of systemic therapy: Minimising the risks. Drug Ther Perspect 1994;3(8):14–16.
90. Rennie IG. Clinically important ocular reactions to systemic drug therapy. Drug Safety 1993;9:196–211.
91. Sugar J. Ocular side effects of systemic therapy of cutaneous diseases. Int Ophthalmol Clin 1985;21:173–183.
92. Vizel M, Oster MW. Ocular side effects of cancer chemotherapy. Cancer 1982;49:1999–2002.
93. Perry HD. Drugs and toxins. Int Ophthalmol Clin 1982;18:97–108.
94. Griffen JD, Garnick MB. Eye toxicity of cancer chemotherapy: A review of the literature. Cancer 1981;48:1539–1549.
95. Ritch PS, Hansen RM, Hever OK. Ocular toxicity from high dose cytosine arabinoside. Cancer 1983;51:430–432.
96. Gold JA, Shupack JL, Nemec A. Ocular side effects of retinoids. Int J Dermatol 1989;28:218–225.
97. Schwab I, Abbott L. Toxic ulcerative keratopathy; an unrecognized problem. Ophthalmology 1989;46:1181–1193.
98. Rosenwasser GOD, Holland S, Pflugfelder SC, et al. Topical anesthetic abuse. Ophthalmology 1990;97:967–972.
99. Font RL, Sheldon G, et al. Pigmented conjunctival cysts following tetracycline/minocycline therapy. Ophthalmology 1983;90:1462–1468.
100. Gowdey CW, Coleman LM, Crawford EM. Ocular changes and phenothiazine derivatives in long-term residents of a mental retardation center. Psych J Univ Ottawa 1985;10:248–253.
101. Bond WS, Yee GC. Ocular and cutaneous effects of chronic phenothiazine therapy. Am J Hosp Pharm 1980;37:74–78.
102. Portnoy JZ, Callen JP. Ophthalmologic aspects of chloroquine and hydroxy-chloroquine therapy. Int J Dermatol 1983;22:273–278.
103. Zeuhlke RL, Lillis PJ, Tice A. Antimalarial therapy for lupus erythematosus: An apparent advantage of quinacrine. Int J Dermatol 1981;20:57–61.
104. Lozier JR, Friedlander MH. Complications of antimalarial therapy. Int Ophthalmal Clin 1989;29:172–178.
105. Tobin DR, Kruhel GB, Rynes RI. Hydroxychloroquine. Seven-year experience. Arch Ophthalmol 1982;100:81–83.
106. Cox NH, Paterson WD. Ocular toxicity of antimalarials in dermatology: A survey of current practice. Br J Dermatol 1994;131:878–882.
107. Mazzuca SA, Yung R, Brandt KD, et al. Current practices for monitoring ocular toxicity related to hydroxychloroquine (Plaquenil) therapy. J Rheumatol 1994;21:59–63.
108. Bernstein HN. Ocular safety of hydroxychloroquine. Ann Ophthalmol 1991;23:292–295.
109. Ingram DV, Jaggarao NSV, Chamberlain DA. Ocular changes resulting from therapy with amiodarone. Br J Ophthalmol 1982;66:676–679.
110. Gaultieri T, Lefler H, Guimond, et al. Corneal and lenticular opacities in mentally retarded young adults treated with thioridazine and chlorpromazine. Am J Psychiatry 1982;139:1178–1180.
111. Rasmussen K, Kirk L, Faurby A. Deposits in the lens and cornea of the eye during long-term chlorpromazine medication. Acta Psychiatr Scand 1980;53:1–4.
112. Bron AJ, McLendon BF, Camp AV. Epithelial deposition of gold in the cornea in patients receiving systemic therapy. Am J Ophthalmol 1979;88:354–360.
113. Beck M, Mills PV. Ocular assessment of patients treated with tamoxifen. Cancer Treat Rep 1979;63:1833–1834.
114. Isaac NE, Walker AM, Jick H, Gorman M. Exposure to phenothiazine drugs and risk of cataract. Arch Ophthalmol 1991;109:256–260.
115. Urban RC, Cottier E. Corticosteroid-induced cataracts. Surv Ophthalmal 1986;31:102–110.
116. Leske MC, Chylak LT, Wu S-Y, et al. The lens opacity case control study. Risk factors for cataract. Arch Ophthalmol 1992;109:244–251.
117. Allen MB, Ray SG, Leitch AG, et al. Steroid aerosols and cataract formation. Br Med J 1989;299:432–433.
118. Santamaria J. Steroidal agents: Their systemic and ocular complications. Ocular Inflamm Ther 1983;1:19–26.
119. Ghanchi F. Young patients on inhaled corticosteroids and cataract. Lancet 1993;342:1306–1307.
120. Sammartino JP. Ocular toxicity of systemic drugs. Am Fam Phys 1985;31:226–229.
121. Rubin B, Palestine AG. Complications of corticosteroids and immunosuppressive drugs. Int Ophthalmol Clin 1989;159–171.
122. Mishra AV, Ramsey MS, Orr AC. Causes of presenile cataracts extracted at the Halifax Infirmary Hospital, 1976–85. Can J Ophthalmol 1989;24:117–119.
123. Anglade E, Whitcup SM. The diagnosis and management of uveitis. Drugs 1995;49:213–223.
124. Rosenbaum JT. Drug-induced uveitis: Reporting inflammation while avoiding inflaming reports. Am J Ophthalmol 1994;118:805–806.
125. Jacobs DDS, Piliero PJ, Kuperwaser MG, et al. Acute uveitis with rifabutin use in patients with human immunodeficiency virus infection. Am J Ophthalmol 1994;118:716–722.
126. Saran BS, Maguire AM, Nichols C, et al. Hypopyon uveitis in patients with acquired immunodeficiency syndrome treated for systemic *Mycobacterium avium* complex infection with rifabutin. Arch Ophthalmol 1994;112:1159–1165.
127. Havlir D, Torriani F, Dube M. Uveitis associated with rifabutin. Ann Int Med 1994;121:510–512.

128. Shafran SD, Deschenes J, Miller M, et al. Uveitis and pseudojaundice during a regimen of clarithromycin, rifabutin, and ethambutol. N Engl J Med 1994;330:438–439.
129. Frank MO, Graham MB. Rifabutin and uveitis. N Engl J Med 1994;330:868.
130. Macarol V, Fraunfelder. Pamidronate disodium and possible ocular adverse reactions. Am J Ophthalmol 1994;118:220–224.
131. Tilden ME, Rosenbaum JT, Fraunfelder FT. Systemic sulfonamides as a cause of bilateral, anterior uveitis. Arch Ophthalmol 1991;109:67–69.
132. Kaplan BH, Nevitt MP, Pach JM, Herman DC. Aseptic meningitis and iridocyclitis related to ibuprofen. Am J Ophthalmol 1994;117:119–120.
133. Wu W C-S, Mannion B, Stone RM. Uveitis associated with interleukin-3 and interleukin 6 therapy. Arch Ophthalmol 1995;330:408–409.
134. Proctor BD, Joondeph BC. Bilateral anterior uveitis: A feature of streptokinase induced serum sickness. N Engl J Med 1994;330:576–577.
135. Melles RB, Wong IG. Metipranolol-associated granulomatous iritis. Am J Ophthalmol 1994;118:712–715.
136. Fishman GA. Toxic retinopathies. Contemp Ophthalmol 1980;1:1–5.
137. Ball WA, Caroff SN. Retinopathy, tardive dyskinesia, and low-dose thioridazine. Am J Psychiatry 1986;143:256–257.
138. Olansky AJ. Antimalarials and ophthalmologic safety. Am Acad Dermatol 1982;6:19–23.
139. Marks JS. Chloroquine retinopathy: Is there a safe daily dose? Ann Rheum Dis 1982;41:52–58.
140. Petursson GS, Fraunfelder FT, Meyer M. Oral contraceptives. Ophthalmology 1981;88:368–371.
141. Lakhanpal V, Shocket SS, Jiji R. Deferoxamine (Desferal) induced toxic retinal pigmentary degeneration and presumed optic neuropathy. Ophthalmology 1984;91:443–451.
142. Mehta AM, Engstrom RE, Kreiger AE. Deferoxamine-associated retinopathy after subcutaneous injection. Am J Ophthalmol 1994;118:260–261.
143. Mihm LM, Barton TL. Tamoxifen-induced ocular toxicity. Ann Pharmacother 1994;28:740–741.
144. Pavlidis NA, Petris C, Briassoulis E, et al. Clear evidence that long term low dose tamoxifen treatment can induce ocular toxicity. Cancer 1992;69:2961–2964.
145. Chern S, Danis RP. Retinopathy associated with low-dose tamoxifen. Am J Ophthalmol 1993;116:372–373.
146. Heier JS, Dragoo RA, Enzenauer RW, Waterhouse WJ. Screening for ocular toxicity in asymptomatic patients treated with tamoxifen. Am J Ophthalmol 1994;117:772–775.
147. Kaiser-Kupfer M, Kupfer C, Rodrigues MM. Tamoxifen retinopathy. A clinicopathologic report. Ophthalmology 1981;88:89–93.
148. Pitlik S, Manor R, Lipshitz I, et al. Transient retinal ischemia induced by nifedipine. Br Med J 1983;287:1845–1846.
149. Weleber RG, Shults WT. Digoxin retinal toxicity. Clinical and electrophysiologic evaluation of cone dysfunction syndrome. Arch Ophthalmol 1981;99:1568–1572.
150. Whitcup SM, Butler KM, Caruso R, et al. Retinal toxicity in human immunodeficiency virus infected children treated with 2′,3′-dideoxyinosine. Am J Ophthalmol 1992;113:1–7.
151. Fafeiuillade A, Aubert L, Chaffanjon P, Quilichini R. Optic neuritis associated with dideoxyinosine. Lancet 1991;337:615–616.
152. Forster DJ, Causey DM, Rao NA. Bull's eye retinopathy and clofazamine. Ann Int Med 1992;116:876–877.
153. Guyer DR, Tiedeman J, Yannuzzi LA, et al. Interferon-associated retinopathy. Arch Ophthalmol 1993;111:350–356.
154. Brezin AP, Massin-Korobelnik P, Boudin M, et al. Acute posterior multifocal placoid pigment epitheliopathy after hepatitis B vaccine. Arch Ophthalmol 1995;113:297–300.
155. Dukar O, Barr CC. Visual loss complicating OKT3 monoclonal antibody therapy. Am J Ophthalmol 1993;115:781–785.
156. Moore D, Marshall J, Henry JA. Research into quinine ocular toxicity. Br J Ophthalmol 1992;76:703.
157. Kupersmith MJ, Seiple WH, Holopigian K, et al. Maculopathy caused by intra-arterially administered cisplatin and intravenously administered carmustine. Am J Ophthalmol 1992;113:435–438.
157. Kushner FH, Olson JC. Retinal hemorrhage as a consequence of epidural steroid injection. Arch Ophthalmol 1995;113:309–313.
158. Fraunfelder FT, Edwards R. Possible ocular adverse effects associated with leuprolide injections. JAMA 1995;273:773.
159. Karmon G, Savir H, Zevin D, et al. Bilateral optic neuropathy due to combined ethambutol and isoniazid therapy. Ann Ophthalmol 1979;11:1013–1017.
160. Alvarez KL, Krop L. Ethambutol-induced ocular toxicity revisited. Ann Pharmacother 1993;27:102–103.
161. Nasemann J, Zrenner E, Riedel KG. Recovery after severe ethambutol intoxication—psychophysical and electrophysiologic correlations. Doc Ophthalmol 1989;279–292.
162. Godel V, Nemet P, Lazar M. Chloramphenicol optic neuropathy. Arch Ophthalmol 1980;98:1417–1421.
163. Avery R, Jabs DA, Wingard JR, et al. Optic disc edema after bone marrow transplantation. Possible role of cyclosporine toxicity. Ophthalmology 1991;98:1294–1301.
164. Engle J. Contact lens products, in Covington T (ed): Handbook of Nonprescription Drugs, 10th Ed. Washington, DC, Am Pharmaceutical Association, 1993.

Chapter 88

Glaucoma

Timothy S. Lesar, PharmD

The glaucomas are a group of ocular diseases, characterized by changes in the optic nerve head (optic disk), and loss of visual sensitivity and field. Increased intraocular pressure (IOP), a traditional diagnostic criterion, is no longer part of the definition of glaucoma because many patients with high IOP never develop glaucoma and many patients with characteristic glaucomatous disk changes and visual loss have normal IOP. Two major types of glaucoma have been identified: open angle and closed angle. Open-angle glaucoma accounts for the great majority of cases. Either type may be a primary, inherited disorder; secondary to disease, trauma, or drugs; or congenital. Both primary and secondary glaucomas may be caused by a combination of open-angle and closed-angle mechanisms (Table 88.1). (See Fig. 88.1 for a diagram of the eye.) Glaucoma affects up to 15 million Americans with 1.5–2.5 million individuals having resultant visual field damage. The prevalence rate varies with age, race, diagnostic criteria and other factors. In the United States, open-angle glaucoma occurs in 1–2% of the population over the age of 40; the incidence increases with age, and it is responsible for 12–15% of the blindness in the United States. The incidence of glaucoma varies by ethnic group, with blacks having a higher incidence (over 11% in those over the age of 80 years) than Caucasians.[1–3] In this chapter, the pathophysiology, clinical findings, and drug therapy of glaucoma are reviewed.

Visual Loss, Intraocular Pressure, and Aqueous Humor

The specific cause of glaucomatous optic disk changes, retinal nerve fiber damage, and visual loss are unknown. Previously, increased IOP was considered to be the sole cause of the visual damage; however, it is now recognized that IOP is only one of many factors associated with the development and progression of glaucoma. Retinal ischemia, caused by either increased IOP or a reduced or dysregulated retinal and choroidal blood flow (or both), is likely to be a primary factor. Indeed, open-angle glaucoma may represent a number of distinct diseases or conditions that simply manifest the same symptoms. Susceptibility to visual loss at a given IOP varies considerably; some patients do not demonstrate damage at high IOPs, whereas other patients have progressive visual field loss despite an IOP in the "normal" range. Although IOP poorly predicts which patients will have visual field loss, the risk of visual field loss clearly increases with increasing IOP. Despite control of IOP, progression of visual field and optic disk changes occurs in some, but not all patients. "IOP sensitive" and "IOP insensitive" types of glaucoma may exist. Presently, the drug therapy of glaucoma is designed to reduce IOP, thereby reducing the risk for progression of visual loss. Future therapies for glaucoma may also involve the use of "neuroprotectants" that will protect the retinal nerve in ischemia or agents that alter retinal and choroidal blood flow. An understanding of IOP and aqueous humor will assist the reader in understanding the drug therapy of glaucoma.[1,2,4–6]

The mean normal population IOP is 15.5 ± 2.5 mm Hg, with frequency distribution skewed toward higher pressures. Intraocular pressures consistently greater than 21 mm Hg are found in 5–7% of the general population. The incidence increases with age such that abnormal IOP is found in 15% of those 70–75 years old. Intermittently very high IOP is found in patients with angle-closure glaucoma. Constant inflow of aqueous humor from the ciliary body (Fig. 88.2) and resistance to outflow result in an IOP great enough to produce an outflow rate equal to the inflow rate. Despite considerable research, the physiologic and pharmacologic controls of aqueous inflow and outflow and, therefore, of IOP have not been completely defined. Aqueous humor is formed in the ciliary body through both filtration and secretion. Fluid-pressure gradients produce an ultrafiltrate of the blood in the stroma of the ciliary process. Because ultrafiltration depends on pressure gradients, blood pressure and IOP changes influence aqueous formation. Osmotic gradients produced by active secretion of sodium and bicarbonate—and possibly other solutes such as ascorbate—from the ciliary body epithelial cells into the aqueous humor result in movement of water from the pool of stromal ultrafiltrate into the posterior chamber, forming the aqueous humor.

Carbonic anhydrase appears to be involved in this secretion of the solutes sodium and bicarbonate and may

TABLE 88.1. CLASSIFICATION OF GLAUCOMA

- I. Primary glaucoma
  - A. Open angle
  - B. Angle closure
    1. With pupillary block
    2. Without pupillary block
- II. Secondary glaucoma
  - A. Open angle
    1. Pretrabecular
    2. Trabecular
    3. Post-trabecular
  - B. Angle closure
    1. With pupillary block
    2. Without pupillary block
- III. Congenital glaucoma

explain the IOP-lowering effects of carbonic anhydrase inhibitors. Receptor systems controlling aqueous inflow have not been fully elucidated, but pharmacologic studies suggest that β-adrenergic agents increase inflow whereas α_2-adrenergic, α-adrenergic blocking, β-adrenergic blocking, dopamine blocking, and adenylate cyclase stimulating agents decrease aqueous inflow. Aqueous humor produced by the ciliary body is secreted into the posterior chamber at a rate of approximately 2–3 µL/min. The pressure in the posterior chamber produced by the constant inflow pushes the aqueous humor between the iris and lens and through the pupil into the anterior chamber of the eye (Fig. 88.3).[7–11]

Aqueous humor in the anterior chamber leaves the eye by two routes: (1) filtration through the trabecular meshwork to Schlemm's canal and (2) traversal of the anterior face of the iris and absorption into iris blood vessels (uveoscleral outflow). Outflow via the trabecular meshwork accounts for drainage from the eye of 1.5–2.5 µL/min of aqueous humor. Uveoscleral outflow occurs at a rate of 0.2–0.5 µL/min. Cholinergic agents such as pilocarpine increase outflow by physically pulling open the meshwork pores through ciliary muscle contraction. The outflow of aqueous is also increased by β-adrenergic agonists such as epinephrine and albuterol. The net effect of β-adrenergic agents and epinephrine is a decrease in IOP. Prostaglandin F2-alpha and analogues as well as α_2-agonist agents increase uveoscleral outflow, and cholinergic agents such as pilocarpine may decrease uveoscleral outflow; however, the net effect of cholinergic agents is a decrease in IOP. The increased IOP in open-angle glaucoma results from the decreased facility for aqueous outflow through the trabecu-

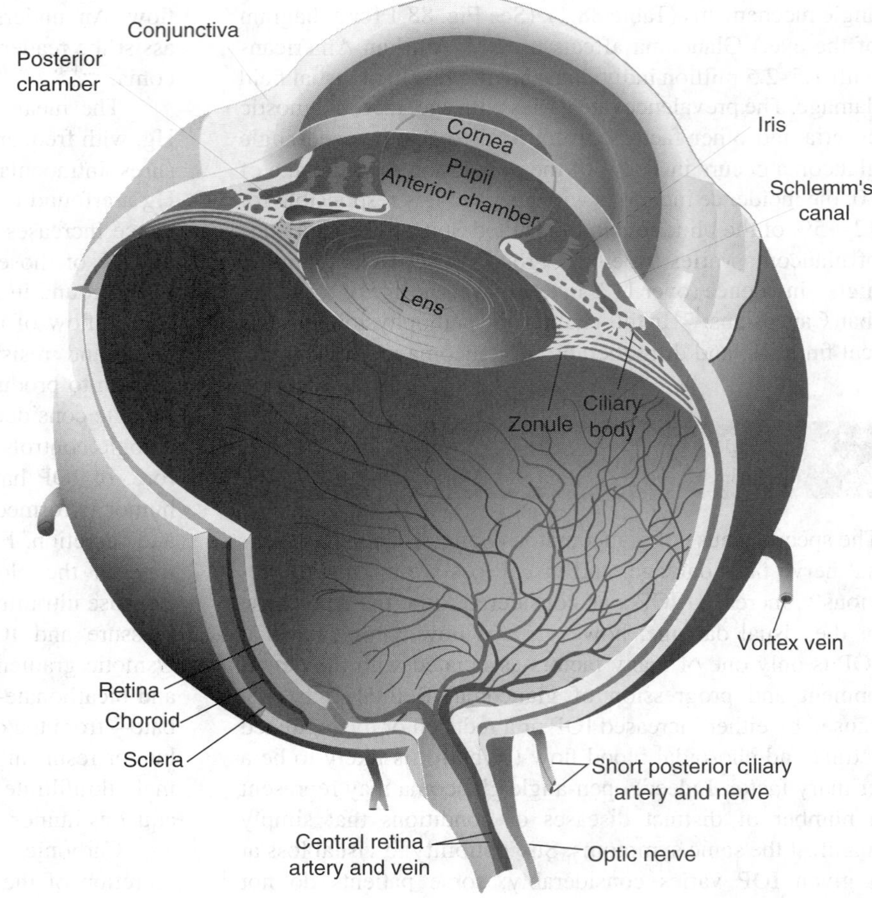

Figure 88.1. The human eye. *(From Newell FW. Ophthalmology: Principles and Concepts, 5th ed. St Louis, MO, CV Mosby, 1982, with permission.)*

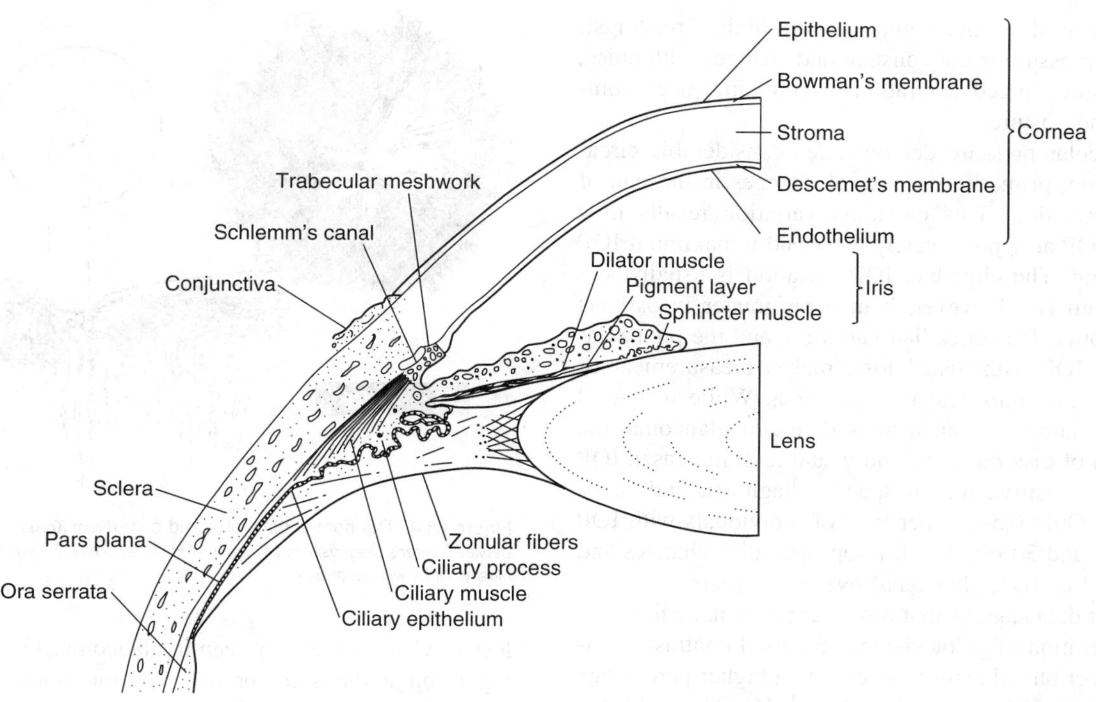

Figure 88.2. The anterior chamber angle and surrounding structures. *(From Vaughn D, Asbury T. General Ophthalmology, 10th ed. Los Altos, CA, Lange Medical Publications, 1983, with permission.)*

lar meshwork. Aqueous production in primary open-angle glaucoma is normal.[8–15]

The balance between the inflow and outflow of aqueous humor in the eye determines the intraocular pressure (Fig. 88.3). The IOP is measured by tonometry—either indentation tonometry, applanation tonometry, or a noncontact method using an air pulse. The noncontact applanation tonometer measures the pressure required to flatten the cornea with a steadily increasing stream of air. These methods may result in slightly different pressure readings. The average IOP measured in large populations is 15.5 ± 2.5 mm Hg; however, the distribution of pressures around the

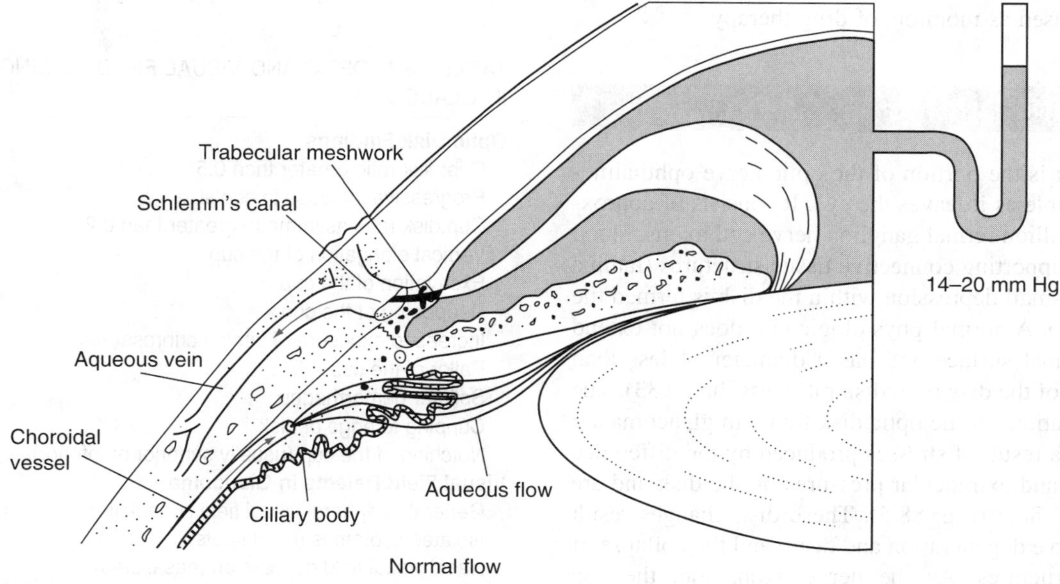

Figure 88.3. Cross section of anterior segment of the eye, demonstrating aqueous humor formation and flow and outflow pathways. *(From Kolker A, Hetherington S. Becker-Shaffer's Diagnosis and Therapy of the Glaucomas, 5th ed. St. Louis, MO, CV Mosby, 1983, with permission.)*

mean is skewed to the right (toward higher readings). Intraocular pressure is not constant and changes with pulse, blood pressure, forced expiration or coughing, neck compression, and posture.

Intraocular pressure demonstrates considerable circadian variation, primarily because of changes in the rate of aqueous formation. This circadian variation results in a minimum IOP at approximately 6 PM and a maximum IOP at awakening. The circadian IOP variation is usually less than 3–4 mm Hg; however, it may be greater in patients with glaucoma. This circadian variation, and the poor relationship of IOP with visual loss, makes measurement of IOP a poor screening test for glaucoma. While increased IOP is associated with an increased risk of glaucoma, the progression of disk changes, and visual loss, increased IOP is both an insensitive and nonspecific diagnostic and monitoring tool. Only 0.5–1% per year of individuals with IOP between 21 and 30 mm Hg develop optic disk changes and visual field loss (i.e., glaucoma) over 5–15 years.

Recent data suggest that more subtle retinal damage—such as alteration of color vision, decreased contrast sensitivity, and peripheral acuity—occurs in a higher percentage of patients with IOP greater than 21 mm Hg. The incidence of visual field defects increases to as high as 28% in individuals with IOP above 30 mm Hg. For a given abnormal IOP, the incidence of glaucoma increases with age. In patients with preexisting optic nerve damage, the worse the existing damage, the more sensitive the eye is to a given IOP. On the other hand, about 35–50% of patients with glaucomatous visual field loss have an IOP of less than 21 mm Hg (i.e., "normal" IOP). Thus, the IOP is a poor predictor of optic nerve damage and therefore outcome of drug therapy. More direct measurements of therapeutic outcome such as optic disk examination and visual field evaluation must also be used as monitors of drug therapy.[1,2,4,5,16]

Optic Disk and Visual Fields

The optic disk is the portion of the optic nerve ophthalmoscopically visible as it leaves the eye. It consists of approximately one million retinal ganglion nerve cell axons, blood vessels, and supporting connective tissue structures (lamina cribosa). The small depression within the disk is termed the cup (Fig. 88.4). A normal physiologic cup does not extend below the retinal surface and has a diameter of less than one-third that of the disk (cup:disk ratio less than 0.33). The common alterations of the optic disk found in glaucoma are thought to be a result of stresses produced by the difference in intraocular and extraocular pressures on the disk and are listed in Table 88.2 (Fig. 88.5). These disk changes result from optic nerve degeneration and death and the collapse of supporting structures. As the nerve axons die, the cup becomes larger in relation to the whole disk. The pattern of optic disk changes is consistent with visual field losses and

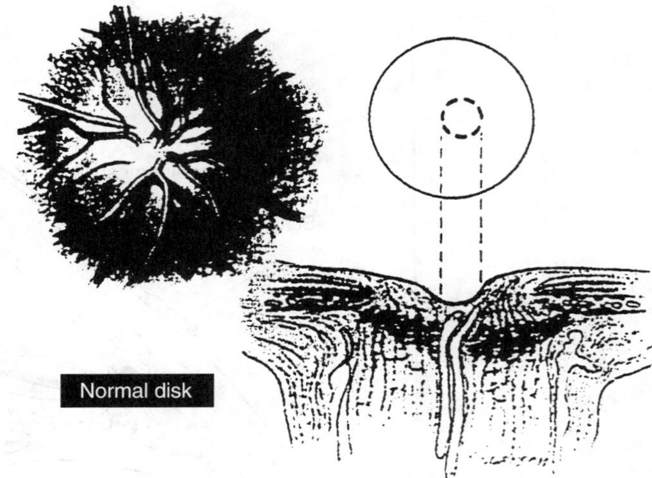

Figure 88.4. The normal optic disk and cup. *(From Kolker A, Hetherington S. Becker-Shaffer's Diagnosis and Therapy of the Glaucomas, 5th ed. St Louis, MO, CV Mosby, 1983, with permission.)*

loss of visual sensitivity seen in glaucoma. The axons passing through the superior and inferior poles of the disk, which are the axons serving the arcuate areas—areas of the retinas most commonly susceptible to visual loss in glaucoma, have thinner supporting structures, and are more susceptible to damage. These anatomic losses correspond to the typical arcuate visual field losses of glaucoma. These axons are also larger and serve retinal cells responsible for night vision, and correspond to the loss of light sensitivity seen early in glaucoma patients. A loss of retinal nerve fiber layer visibility is seen in the majority of glaucoma patients with detectable visual field loss.[1,2,17,18]

Determination of visual field allows assessment of optic nerve damage and is a primary monitoring parameter

TABLE 88.2. OPTIC AND VISUAL FIELD FINDINGS IN GLAUCOMA

Optic Disk Findings
Cup:disk ratio greater than 0.5
Progressive increase in cup size
Cup:disk ratio asymmetry greater than 0.2
Vertical elongation of the cup
Excavation of the cup
Deepening of the cup
Increased exposure of lamina cribrosa
Pallor of the cup
Splinter hemorrhages
Cupping to edge of disk
Notching of the cup (usually superior or inferior)
Visual Field Defects in Glaucoma
General peripheral visual field constriction
Isolated scotomas (blind spots)
Nasal visual field depression (nasal step)
Enlargement of the blind spot
Large arclike scotomas

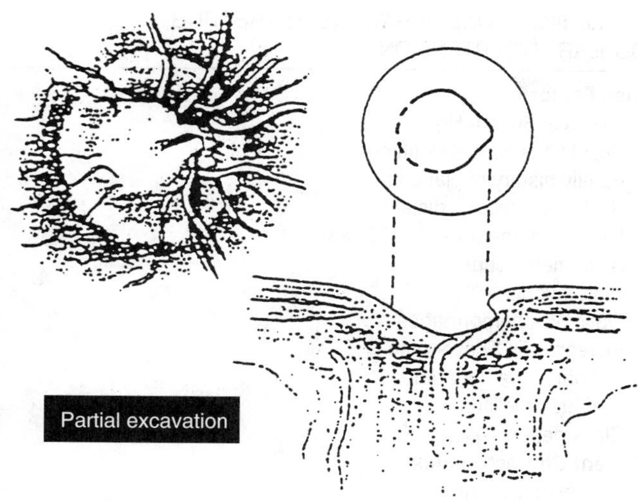

Figure 88.5. Early optic disk and cup changes in glaucoma. *(From Kolker A, Hetherington S. Becker-Shaffer's Diagnosis and Therapy of the Glaucomas, 5th ed. St Louis, MO, CV Mosby, 1983, with permission.)*

in treatment. However, visual field changes lag behind optic disk changes and a loss of 20% of axons is usually required before detectable visual field defects are noted. The peripheral visual field is measured using an automated visual field instrument called a *perimeter.* Characteristic visual field loss occurs in glaucoma (Fig. 88.6 and Table 88.2), but loss of central visual acuity does not occur until late in the disease. Therefore, IOP, optic disk changes, and perimetry are the primary diagnostic and monitoring parameters. Other indicators such as color vision changes and contrast sensitivity may allow earlier and more sensitive detection of glaucomatous changes.[1,2]

The mechanism by which increased IOP produces optic nerve damage remains controversial. Vasogenic theories suggests that optic nerve damage results from insufficient blood flow to the retina secondary to the high perfusion pressure required in the eye with high IOP, dysregulated perfusion, or vessel wall abnormalities. The insufficient blood flow produces ischemia and results in degeneration of axonal (axoplasmal) fibers of the retina. A second theory suggests that the increased IOP may disrupt axoplasmal flow directly or by "arching" of the lamina cribrosa. Both mechanisms, as well as others, could be operative in producing the optic nerve damage observed in glaucoma.[1,2,4–6,18]

Primary Open-Angle Glaucoma

DIAGNOSIS AND MONITORING PARAMETERS

Primary open-angle glaucoma (POAG) is a bilateral, genetically determined disorder constituting 60–70% of all glaucomas and 90–95% of primary glaucomas. POAG manifests as optic nerve degeneration characterized by disk changes and visual field loss (Table 88.2). An increased IOP is not required for diagnosis of POAG. POAG is a chronic, slowly progressive disease found primarily in individuals older than 50 years, although it may occur earlier. Symptoms do not present until substantial visual field constriction occurs. Central visual acuity is typically maintained, even in the late stages of the disease. POAG is a bilateral disease; however, one eye may have greater progression of disease than the other. Detection and diagnosis involve evaluation of the optic disk and retinal nerve fiber layer, assessment of the visual fields, and measurement of IOP. The presence of characteristic disk changes and visual field loss with or without increased IOP confirms the diagnosis of glaucoma. Typical disk changes and field loss occurring at an IOP of less than 21 mm Hg accounts for 35–50% of patients and is sometimes referred to as "low-tension" glaucoma. Elevated IOP (greater than 21 mm Hg) without disk changes or visual field loss with increased IOP is observed in 5–7% of individuals and is known as ocular hypertension.[1,2,11,19]

The basic, underlying disorder producing the retinal nerve damage of POAG is unknown. Retinal nerve ischemia secondary to increased IOP and/or vascular abnormalities appears to play a key role. The increased IOP seen in patients with POAG is caused by a decreased aqueous outflow facility, resulting in an imbalance between aqueous production and aqueous outflow. A number of factors altering blood flow to the choroid and retina such as regulation of blood flow, and vessel wall disease may be important

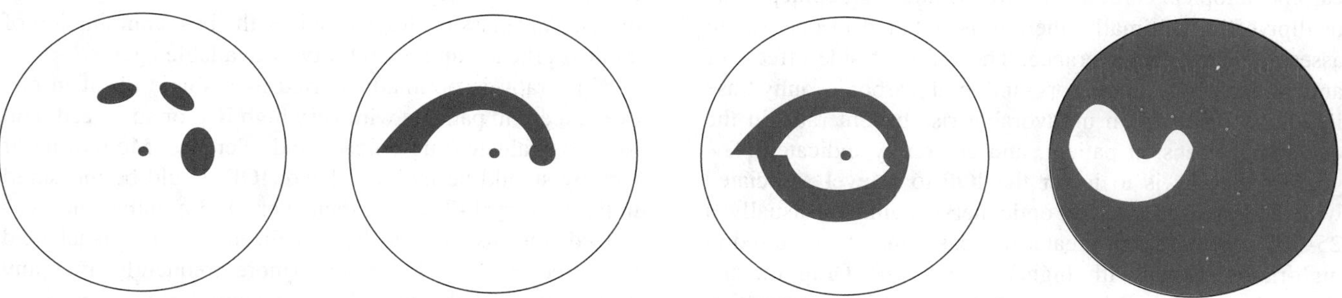

Figure 88.6. Schematic representation of the progression of visual field loss (darkened areas) in glaucoma.

additive or independent factors in producing retinal nerve ischemia and cell loss. The rate of ciliary body aqueous production and the aqueous flow from the posterior chamber to the trabecular meshwork are normal; however, histologic changes in the meshwork or Schlemm's canal in glaucomatous eyes appear to produce an increase in resistance to aqueous outflow.

Secondary open-angle glaucoma has many causes, including systemic diseases, trauma, surgery, rubeosis, lens changes, ocular inflammatory diseases, and medications. A system for classifying secondary glaucomas into pretrabecular, trabecular, and post-trabecular forms has been proposed. This classification allows drug therapy to be chosen on the basis of the pathogenic mechanism involved. In pretrabecular forms, a membrane overlies the meshwork and does not permit aqueous outflow. The membrane may be fibrovascular, such as neovascular growth in diabetics, fibrous ingrowth, or the result of inflammation. Trabecular forms of secondary glaucoma result from either an alteration of meshwork or an accumulation of material in the intertrabecular spaces. This type of glaucoma may result from accumulation of cells, pigment or protein in the meshwork, or alteration of the meshwork secondary to trauma, corticosteroids, edema, inflammation, and trauma. The post-trabecular forms result primarily from disorders causing increased visceral venous blood pressure. Examples of such conditions include Sturge–Weber syndrome, retrobulbar tumors, and carotid-cavernous fistulas.[1]

TREATMENT APPROACH AND GOALS

All patients with characteristic optic disk changes or visual field defects (i.e., glaucoma by definition) should be treated. Treatment of the patient with ocular hypertension remains controversial, because only 0.5–1% per year develop visual field loss. Treatment of the ocular hypertension in these patients is based on the presence or absence of risk factors known to increase the chance of developing visual field loss and on the presence of certain individual traits (Table 88.3). Persons with ocular hypertension with additional risk factors usually will be treated with a well-tolerated topical agent such as a β-blocking agent, pilocarpine, a topical carbonic anhydrase inhibitor, epinephrine, or dipivefrin. Optimally, therapy is initiated in one eye to assess efficacy and tolerance. The frequent side effects of anticholinesterase inhibitors and oral carbonic anhydrase inhibitors result in an unfavorable risk:benefit ratio in the ocular hypertension patient, and are rarely indicated. The goal of therapy is to lower the IOP to a level associated with a decreased risk of optic nerve damage—usually a 25–30% decrease, but greater decreases may be required in high-risk patients with higher initial IOP. Drug therapy should be monitored by measurement of IOP, examination of the optic disk, assessment of the visual fields, and evaluation of the patient for drug side effects and compliance with therapy. Patients who are unresponsive to, or intolerant of, a drug should be switched to an alternative agent rather than given an additional drug. Patients failing to respond adequately to simple topical therapy may require multiple topical drugs, cholinesterase inhibitors, or oral carbonic anhydrase inhibitors; however, some clinicians prefer to discontinue all medications in such patients and closely monitor for development of disk changes or visual field loss and treat when this occurs.[1,2,18]

TABLE 88.3. CONSIDERATIONS IN TREATING OCULAR HYPERTENSION

Risk Factors
- IOP over 30 mm Hg
- Suspicious optic disk fittings
- Family history of glaucoma
- Systemic vascular disease
- Increased age (over 65–70 years)
- Asymmetric cups
- High myopia
- Optic disk hemorrhages
- Increasing IOP over time
- Retinal nerve fiber defects
- Diabetes mellitus
- Black patients

Patient Characteristics
- One-eyed patients
- Young patients (longer exposure to high IOP)
- Unreliable patients
- Unreliable visual fields
- Optic disk not visualized
- Patient desires treatment
- Patient with retinal vascular occlusion

Controversy exists as to whether the initial therapy of glaucoma should be surgical trabeculectomy (filtering procedure), argon laser trabeculectomy, or medical therapy.[1,2,20] Drug therapy of patients with documented glaucomatous change is initiated in a stepwise manner, starting with lower concentrations of a single well-tolerated topical agent (e.g., β blocker, pilocarpine, carbonic anhydrase inhibitor, dipivefrin, or epinephrine). The choice of initial drug depends on individual patient characteristics and concurrent disease states, as well as physician preference. Generally, a β-blocking agent is chosen if no contraindication exists. This class of drugs provides the best combination of clinical efficacy and tolerability of available agents.

Therapy is optimally started as a single agent in one eye (except in patients with very high IOP or advanced field loss) to evaluate drug efficacy and tolerance. Monitoring of therapy should be individualized: IOP should be measured initially every 1–2 weeks, then every 1–3 months when stabilized; the disk should be visualized and the visual field measured every 6–12 months (more frequently after any change in drug therapy). Patients should always be questioned regarding compliance with prescribed therapy. Initial

IOP response does not predict long-term IOP control, requiring continuous regular monitoring of IOP. In patients who fail therapy, the drug concentration and/or frequency (depending on agent being used) should be increased. Generally, more than one drop per dose does not improve response, but increases the likelihood of side effects and cost of therapy. When using more than one medication, apply drops at least 5–10 minutes apart to provide optimal ocular contact for each agent.

The value of an agent to which the patient has shown a loss of IOP control following an initial response can be measured by discontinuing the medication completely and determining if an increase in IOP occurs. Patients responding to, but intolerant of, initial therapy may be switched to another drug or an alternative dosage form of the same medication. For patients failing to respond to high concentrations of an initial drug, a switch to an alternative agent after 1 day of concurrent therapy or, if only a partial response occurs, addition of another topical drug to be used in combination should be considered.

The need to use combination therapy should be documented by therapeutic trial. Patients prescribed combinations that include timolol or epinephrine should be instructed to instill these agents first because they improve ocular absorption of subsequently instilled agents. Because of the frequency of side effects, topical cholinesterase inhibitors and oral carbonic anhydrase inhibitors are considered second-line agents to be used in patients who fail less toxic therapy. A number of drugs or drug combinations may need to be tried before an effective and well-tolerated regimen is identified.

The ultimate goal of drug therapy in the glaucoma patient is to preserve visual function through the reduction of the IOP to a level at which no further optic nerve damage occurs. Because of the poor relationship between IOP and optic nerve damage, no specific target IOP exists. Indeed, drugs used to treat glaucoma such as the β-blocking agents may act to halt visual loss through mechanisms separate from, or in addition to, IOP reduction such as improvements in retinal or choroidal blood flow. Typically, a 25–30% reduction is desired, but greater reductions may be desired in patients with initially high IOP or those with substantial visual field loss. In patients with early visual field loss or optic disk changes, reduction of the IOP below 21 mm Hg is usually desired; in patients with more advanced disease, reduction below 15–19 mm Hg is usually desired. Even lower IOP (i.e., low to midteens) is required in patients with very advanced disease, those showing continued damage at higher IOP, and those patients with low-tension glaucoma. Drug therapy is monitored by measurement of IOP, but optic disk and visual field findings consistent with no disease progression are the primary therapeutic endpoints of therapy. Medications may fail to control progression of visual field loss despite attainment of an IOP of less than 20 mm Hg. Such patients may be particularly sensitive to even "normal" IOP; they frequently have advanced field loss and may require lowering of IOP to the midteens. Large circadian fluctuations may also contribute to progressive nerve damage in the face of normal IOP.

When drug therapy fails, is not tolerated, or is excessively complicated, surgical procedures such as laser trabeculoplasty or a surgical trabeculectomy (filtering procedure) to produce aqueous drainage paths may be performed to improve aqueous outflow. Surgical trabeculectomy is successful in controlling IOP in 75% of patients over a 5-year period of time; however, a number of complications may occur postsurgically. Filtering procedures involving placement of draining tubes or destruction of the ciliary body may be required when other methods fail; however these procedures have a high complication rate.[1,2,18,19]

Treatment of secondary glaucomas is similar to that of POAG; however, the choice of drug should be based more on the underlying cause of the IOP. Miotics are effective if the drugs improve aqueous outflow through the meshwork; however, if most of the meshwork is covered, blocked, or damaged so that the action of miotics to open the trabecular meshwork has limited effect, the drug will be ineffective. In addition, patients with inflammation should not be treated with miotics, because increased pain and possible inflammation may result. Depending on the effect of the underlying disease on the outflow routes, epinephrine may or may not be useful. Drugs such as β blockers, α_2-adrenergic agonists and carbonic anhydrase inhibitors may be the most useful agents in the treatment of secondary open-angle glaucoma, because these drugs decrease aqueous production and do not rely on improving damaged outflow pathways. Beta-blockers, α_2 agonists, and carbonic anhydrase inhibitors (CAIs) are also the primary agents used in the prevention and treatment of increased IOP in the postoperative period.[1]

PATIENT EDUCATION

An important consideration in patients failing to respond to drug therapy is compliance. Poor compliance or noncompliance occurs in 25–60% of glaucoma patients. A large percentage of patients fail to use topical ophthalmic drugs correctly. The patient should be taught the following procedure:

- Wash and dry the hands.
- With a forefinger, pull down the outer portion of the lower lid to form a "pocket" to receive the drop.
- Grasp the dropper bottle between the thumb and fingers with the hand braced against the cheek or nose with the head upward.
- Place the dropper over the eye while looking at the tip of the bottle; then, look up and place a single drop in the eye.
- The lids should be closed but not squeezed or rubbed for 1–3 minutes after instillation. This increases the ocular availability of the drug.

Preferably, nasolacrimal occlusion (NLO) should be used to improve ocular bioavailability and reduce systemic absorption.[1] The patient induces nasolacrimal occlusion for 1–3 minutes by closing the eyes and placing the index finger over the nasolacrimal drainage system in the inner corner of the eye. This maneuver as well as eyelid closure itself decreases punctal drainage of drug, thereby decreasing the amount of drug available for systemic absorption from the nasopharyngeal mucosa. The use of NLO may significantly improve drug response, reduce side effects, and allow less frequent dose intervals and the use of lower drug concentrations. Use of more than one drop per dose does not significantly improve response but may increase side effects. When two drugs are to be administered, instillations should be separated by at least 3–5 minutes (preferably 10 minutes) to prevent the drug administered first from being washed out. The patient should be taught not to touch the dropper bottle tip with eye, hands, or any surface.

Compliance with glaucoma therapy is commonly inadequate, and should always be considered a possible cause of drug therapy failure. Assessment of compliance by health care providers is generally poor, so that all patients should be continually encouraged to diligently administer prescribed therapy as instructed. To improve compliance, the patient should be fully informed of the expectations of therapy and the need to continue therapy despite a lack of symptoms. Possible side effects of the medication and ways of reducing them should be discussed. Compliance will be improved by good communication, close monitoring, and use of well-tolerated and convenient drug regimens. For example, the use of once-a-day timolol gel-forming solution or pilocarpine gel may greatly improve compliance over the use of standard solutions multiple times daily.[1,18]

PROGNOSIS

In most cases of POAG the overall prognosis is excellent. Progression to severe visual loss is rare when POAG is discovered early and adequately treated. Patients with advanced visual field loss rarely have continued field loss if the IOP is maintained at less than 15–18 mm Hg; however, of patients with IOP greater than 22 mm Hg, 30% have visual loss. Thus, the keys to medical treatment of POAG are an effective, well-tolerated drug regimen, close monitoring of therapy, and compliance. Medications will successfully control IOP in 60–80% of patients over a 5-year period. Patients failing or intolerant of medical therapy are candidates for laser or surgical trabeculectomy.[1,2,18,20]

DRUGS USED TO TREAT GLAUCOMA

β-Blocking Drugs

The topical β-blocking agents are the most commonly used type of antiglaucoma medications. Beta blockers lower intraocular pressure by 20–30% with a minimum of local ocular side effects. These agents are commonly the agents of choice in treating POAG if no contraindications exist. The β-blocking agents produce ocular hypotensive effects by decreasing the production of aqueous by the ciliary body, without producing substantial effects on aqueous outflow facility. The mechanism by which β blockers decrease aqueous inflow remains controversial, but it is most frequently attributed to β_2-adrenergic receptor blockade in the ciliary body.

Five ophthalmic β blockers are presently available: timolol, levobunolol, metipranolol, carteolol, and betaxolol. Timolol, levobunolol, and metipranolol are nonspecific β-blocking agents, whereas betaxolol is a β_1-adrenergic-selective agent. Carteolol is a nonspecific β blocker with intrinsic sympathomimetic activity (ISA). Despite differences in potency, selectivity, lipophilicity, and ISA, the five agents reduce IOP to a similar degree, though betaxolol has been reported to produce somewhat less lowering of IOP than timolol and levobunolol. Levobunolol has been reported to be more effective than timolol and betaxolol in reducing postcataract surgery IOP increases. Levobunolol solution is more effective in controlling IOP than other agents when given as aqueous solutions on a once-daily schedule. Timolol in the form of a gel-forming solution (Timolol XER Merck, West Point, PA) provides equivalent IOP control with once-daily administration when compared with an equal concentration of the aqueous solution administered twice daily.

Despite the poor relationship between IOP control and reduction in visual loss, patients in whom IOP is better controlled are associated with a better outcome. Limited data suggest that long-term IOP control and visual outcomes are better with β-blocking agents than with pilocarpine. Differences in effects of the various β-blocking agents on retinal and choroidal blood flow theoretically could result in differences in visual outcome independent of IOP control. The more specific β_1-blocking agent betaxolol and the ISA carteolol produce fewer deleterious changes to, or actually improved, blood flow to the retina compared with nonspecific blocking agents. Data comparing outcomes with timolol and betaxolol suggest better visual function outcomes with betaxolol despite equivalent IOP control. Additional data are required to determine definitively the long-term equivalency of the various β-blocking agents on visual outcome. The choice of a specific β-blocking agent is generally based on differences in side-effect potential and individual patient response.[1,18,21–25]

Local side effects with β blockers are usually minimal, though stinging upon application, particularly with betaxolol solution (less with betaxolol suspension) and metipranolol, occurs commonly. Other local effects include dry eyes, corneal anesthesia, blepharitis, blurred vision, and rarely conjunctivitis, uveitis, and keratitis. Metipranolol is most clearly associated with uveitis, particularly at higher concentrations. Loss of IOP control has been associated with metipranolol local ocular adverse effects. Carteolol has generally been tolerated as well or better than other agents. Some local reactions may be a result of preservatives used in the commercially available products. Switching from one β blocker to another, or switching the type of formulation, may improve local tolerance in patients experiencing local side effects.

Systemic effects are the most important adverse affects of β blockers. Drug absorbed systemically may produce decreased heart rate, reduced blood pressure, negative inotropic effects, conduction defects, bronchospasm, block symptoms of hypoglycemia, central nervous system (CNS) effects, and alteration of serum lipids. The β_1-specific agent betaxolol and possibly carteolol (due to ISA) are less likely to produce the systemic side effects caused by β-adrenergic blockade, such as the cardiac effects and bronchospasm, but a real risk still exists. The use of Timoptic as a gel-forming liquid, or betaxolol as a suspension allows administration of less drug per day, and therefore reduces the chance for systemic side effects compared with the aqueous solutions.

Because of their systemic side effects, ophthalmic β blockers should be used with caution in patients with pulmonary diseases, sinus bradycardia, second- or third-degree heart block, congestive heart failure, atherosclerosis, diabetes, and myasthenia gravis, and in patients receiving oral β-blocker therapy. The use of NLO will reduce the risk or severity of systemic side effects as well as optimize response. Overall, β-adrenergic blocking agents are well tolerated by patients and most potential problems can be avoided by appropriate patient evaluation, drug choice, and monitoring of drug therapy.

In patients failing or having an inadequate response to single drug therapy with a β-blocking agent, the addition of a parasympathomimetic agent (i.e., pilocarpine), an α_2 agonist, or carbonic anhydrase inhibitor (topical or oral) will usually result in additional IOP reduction. Epinephrine or dipivefrin added to nonselective β-blocking agents results in minimum if any additional IOP reduction, but addition to the β_1 specific agent betaxolol generally will provide additional IOP reduction.[1,18,21–24]

Parasympathomimetic Agonists

The parasympathomimetic (cholinergic) agents reduce IOP by increasing aqueous humor trabecular outflow. The increase in outflow is a result of physically pulling open the trabecular meshwork secondary to ciliary muscle contraction, thereby reducing resistance to outflow. These agents reduce uveoscleral outflow. Pilocarpine, the parasympathomimetic agent of choice in POAG, is available as an ophthalmic solution, an ocular insert, and a hydrophilic polymer gel (Table 88.4). Pilocarpine produces similar (20–30%) reductions in IOP as seen with β-blocking agents, but effects on visual outcome may be poorer.[24] Pilocarpine in POAG or ocular hypertension is initiated as 0.5–1% solution, one drop three to four times daily. The use of NLO improves response and reduces the need for an every-6-hour dosing frequency.

Use of one drop of 2% pilocarpine every 12 hours and NLO provides optimal response in many patients. Both drug concentration and frequency may be increased if IOP reduction is inadequate. Patients with darkly pigmented eyes frequently require higher concentrations of pilocarpine than patients with lightly pigmented eyes. Concentrations of pilocarpine above 4% rarely improve IOP control in patients other than those with darkly pigmented eyes. Increasing the concentration of pilocarpine may not result in a greater IOP reduction but may increase the duration of action.[25] Administration more often than every 3–4 hours is inconvenient and exposes the patient to a higher risk of side effects. Instead, such patients should be switched to an alternative form of pilocarpine or to an alternative agent.

Pilocarpine gel (Pilocarpine HS) is a product containing 4% pilocarpine in a hydrophilic polymer gel. The slow dissolution of the gel and increased ocular contact time, which improve ocular absorption, result in control of IOP for a 24-hour period. Treatment with pilocarpine gel 4% is equivalent to treatment with pilocarpine solution 4% four times daily or timolol 0.5% twice daily. When using every-24-hour dosing of pilocarpine gel, the adequacy of IOP control late in the dosing interval should be confirmed. Pilocarpine gel has been associated with the development of a fine corneal haze after 8 weeks of use. The pilocarpine Ocusert is a solid, elliptical, sustained-release device designed for placement in the conjunctival sac and delivery of pilocarpine over a 7-day period. The Ocusert should be placed in the eye at bedtime so early side effects occur during sleep. The advantages of the Ocusert are convenience of weekly placement, possibly improved control of diurnal IOP increases, and decreased frequency of side effects. The disadvantages include a "burst" release of drug upon insertion, increased cost, discomfort, undetected loss of the device, and increased dexterity required for unit placement.

Ocular side effects of pilocarpine include miosis, which decreases night vision and vision in patients with central cataracts. Constriction of the visual field occurs secondary to miosis and should be considered when evaluating visual field changes in a glaucoma patient. Pilocarpine ciliary muscle contraction produces accommodative spasm, particularly in young patients still able to accommodate (pre-presbyopic). Pilocarpine also may produce frontal headache, browache, periorbital pain, eyelid twitching, and conjunctival irritation or injection early in therapy, which tends to decrease in severity over 3–5 weeks of continued therapy. Cholinergics produce a breakdown of the blood–aqueous barrier and may result in a worsening of an ocular inflammatory reaction or condition. Systemic cholinergic side effects of pilocarpine such as diaphoresis, nausea, vomiting, diarrhea, cramping, urinary frequency, bronchospasm, and heart block are rare, but may be seen in patients using high concentrations (6–8%) or with overzealous use in treatment of acute angle closure. Other side

TABLE 88.4. TOPICAL AGENTS USED IN THE TREATMENT OF GLAUCOMA

Drug	Form	Strength%[a]	Brand Name	Dose Frequency[a]	Mechanism of IOP Reduction
β-Adrenergic Blockers					Decreased aqueous flow
Betaxolol	Solution	0.5	Betoptic	q 12 h	
	Suspension	0.25	Betoptic S	q 12 h	
Carteolol	Solution	1	Ocupress	q 12 h	
Levobunolol	Solution	0.25, 0.5	Betagan	q 12–24 h	
Metipranolol	Solution	0.3	OptiPranolol	q 12 h	
Timolol	Solution	0.25, 0.5	Timoptic	q 12–24 h	
	Gelling soln.	0.25	Timoptic XE	q 24 h	
Adrenergic Agents					
α/β agonist					
Epinephrine HCl	Solution	0.25, 0.5, 1, 2	Epifrin, Glaucon	q 12 h	Increased aqueous outflow
Epinephrine bitartrate	Solution	2		q 12 h	
Epinephrine borate	Solution	0.5, 1, 2	Epinal	q 12 h	
Dipivefrin	Solution	0.1	Propine	q 12 h	Increased aqueous outflow
α_1 agonist					Decreased aqueous inflow
Apraclonidine	Solution	1	Iopidine	pre- and post-op	
	Solution	0.5	Iopidine	q 8–12 h	
Parasympathomimetics					
Direct acting					Increased aqueous outflow
Pilocarpine	Solution	0.25–10	Numerous	q 4–12 h	
Pilocarpine	Gel	4	Pilopine HS	q 24 h	
Carbachol	Solution	0.75, 1.5, 2.25	IsoptoCarbachol	q 8–12 h	
Cholinesterase inhibitors					Increased aqueous outflow
Physostigmine	Solution	0.25, 0.5	Isopto Eserine	q 8–12 h	
Demecarium	Solution	0.125	Humorsol	q 8–72 h	
Echothiophate	Solution	0.03–0.25	Phospholine Iodide	q 12–24 h	
Isoflurophate	Ointment	0.25	Floropryl	q 8–72 h	
Carbonic Anhydrase Inhibitors					
Dorzolamide	Solution	2	Trusopt	q 8–12 h	Decreased aqueous inflow
Prostaglandin Analogues					
Latanoprost	Solution	0.005	Xalatan	q 24 h	Increased uveoscular outflow

[a]Use of nasolacrimal occlusion (NLO) may allow use of lower concentrations at longer intervals.

effects associated with direct-acting miotics include retinal tears or detachment, allergic reaction, permanent miosis, cataracts, precipitation of angle-closure glaucoma, and, rarely, miotic cysts of the pupillary margin.

Carbachol is a potent, direct-acting miotic agent; its duration of action is longer than that of pilocarpine (8–10 hours) because of resistance to hydrolysis by cholinesterases. This drug may also act as a weak inhibitor of cholinesterase. Patients with an inadequate response to, or intolerance of, pilocarpine as a result of ocular irritation or allergy frequently do well on carbachol. Some patients may have adverse reactions to the benzalkonium chloride used in carbachol solutions to improve ocular bioavailability. The usual dose is 1 drop of 0.75–1.5% carbachol three times daily. Use of higher concentrations may be used in those failing lower concentrations. Use of NLO may allow use of lower concentrations at longer intervals (every 12 hours). The ocular and systemic side effects of carbachol are similar but more frequent, constant, and severe than those of pilocarpine.[1,10,19,25–29]

The cholinesterase inhibitors used in the treatment of POAG include the shorter acting reversible inhibitor physostigmine, the longer acting relatively irreversible agents demecarium, and the long-acting relatively irreversible inhibitors echothiophate and isofluorophate (Table 88.4). These agents are potent inhibitors of pseudocholinesterase, but also inhibit true cholinesterase. Because of the serious ocular and systemic toxic effects of these agents, the cholinesterase inhibitors are reserved primarily for patients not responding to or intolerant of other therapy. Because of their cataractogenic properties, many ophthalmologists will use these agents only in patients without lenses (aphakia) or those with artificial lenses (pseudophakia). The ocular and periocular parasympathomimetic side effects are more common and more severe than with pilocarpine or carbachol. In addition to the parasympathomimetic effects, the cholinesterase inhibitors may produce severe fibrinous iritis (particularly with the irreversible inhibitors), synechiae, iritic cysts, conjunctival thickening, and occlusion of the nasolacrimal ducts.

Cataracts occur at high frequency with the use of cholinesterase inhibitors, particularly echothiophate, after about 10–18 months of therapy. The incidence of cataracts appears to increase with increasing concentration, with up to 60% of patients developing cataracts at higher concentrations. The inhibition of systemic pseudocholinesterase by these agents decreases the rate of succinylcholine hydrolysis, resulting in prolonged muscle paralysis. Cholinesterase inhibitors should be discontinued at least 2 weeks before procedures in which succinylcholine is to be used.

The role of cholinesterase inhibitors in glaucoma is limited by the frequency and potential toxicity of these agents. In phakic patients, cholinesterase inhibitors should be administered only if intolerance or failure results with use of other antiglaucoma medications. Cholinesterase inhibitors have been shown to provide additional IOP lowering effects when used with β blockers, carbonic anhydrase inhibitors, and sympathomimetic (adrenergic) agents. Like all agents for glaucoma, therapy should be initiated with lower concentrations of these agents. A once-daily administration frequency should be used in most patients unless very high IOP is present. Use of NLO will likely improve response and reduce systemic side effects and should be used for all patients using cholinesterase inhibitors. The cholinesterase inhibitors should be used with caution in patients with asthma, retinal detachments, narrow angles, bradycardia, hypotension, heart failure, Down's syndrome, epilepsy, parkinsonism, peptic ulcer, and ocular inflammation and in those receiving cholinesterase inhibitor therapy for myasthenia gravis or exposure to carbamate or organophosphate insecticides and pesticides.[1,10,18,19,26–30]

Adrenergic Agents

The sympathomimetic agents used to treat glaucoma include epinephrine, the epinephrine prodrug dipivefrin (dipivaloyl epinephrine), and the α_2-adrenergic agonist apraclonidine. The mechanism of action by which epinephrine lowers IOP has not been fully elucidated; however, an increase in outflow facility through the trabecular meshwork appears to be the primary mechanism. Compared with β blockers or miotics, epinephrine and dipivefrin reduce IOP less. For this reason epinephrine is generally used as initial therapy in patients with mild to moderate increases in IOP or in combination with other agents. Epinephrine is available as epinephrine hydrochloride, epinephrine bitartrate, and epinephryl borate solutions. Epinephryl borate and epinephrine hydrochloride are labeled as the concentration of epinephrine base; however, epinephrine bitartrate 2% is equivalent to epinephrine base 1.1%.

The various salts of epinephrine produce equivalent IOP-lowering effects and adverse reactions. Patients with minor ocular irritation from one salt of epinephrine may occasionally benefit from use of another salt because of differences in pH of the commercial solutions. The borate salt is available as a neutral solution while the hydrochloride and bitartrate are acidic. Epinephrine used in combination with parasympathetic agents or CAIs result in additive IOP lowering. Epinephrine plus betaxolol may result in greater IOP reduction than in combination with nonspecific β blockers. When used in combination with β blockers, the two drugs should be given at least 3 hours apart.

A factor limiting the usefulness of epinephrine is the high frequency of local ocular side effects. Tearing, burning, ocular discomfort, browache, conjunctival hyperemia, punctate keratopathy, allergic blepharoconjunctivitis, rare loss of eyelashes, stenosis of the nasolacrimal duct, and blurred vision may occur. Prolonged use (over 1 year) may result in deposition of pigment (adrenochrome) in the conjunctiva and cornea. Pigment may also deposit in soft contact lenses, turning them black. These side effects occur less frequently with dipivefrin. Epinephrine may produce mydriasis (particularly when combined with a β blocker) and may precipitate acute angle-closure glaucoma in patients with narrow anterior chambers. A transient increase in IOP may occur with initial therapy, particularly in patients not using other antiglaucoma medications.

A relative contraindication to the use of epinephrine (and dipivefrin) is aphakia (i.e., after cataract removal) or lens dislocation because of the development of degeneration of the macular portion of the retina. This cystoid macular edema occurs in 20–30% of aphakic eyes treated with epinephrine and may result from increased prostaglandin production. The edema is dose dependent and disappears with drug discontinuation. Decreased blood flow to the macula is of concern in aphakic patients as well. Systemic side effects of epinephrine include headache, faintness, increased blood pressure, tachycardia, arrhythmias, tremor, pallor, anxiety, and increased perspiration. Epinephrine should be used with caution in patients with cardiovascular diseases, cerebrovascular diseases, aphakia, angle-closure glaucoma, hyperthyroidism, and diabetes mellitus and in patients undergoing anesthesia with halogenated hydrocarbon anesthetics. Use of the prodrug dipivefrin allows use of lower concentrations secondary to improved intraocular absorption (10–15 fold). The 0.1% dipivefrin produces equivalent IOP reduction as 1–2% epinephrine. Dipivefrin may therefore be tolerated by patients unable to tolerate epinephrine solutions. Using NLO with epinephrine and dipivefrin will improve therapeutic response and reduce risk of systemic side effects.[1,10,18,29–32]

Apraclonidine, a relatively selective α_2-adrenergic agonist structurally similar to clonidine, is available as an ophthalmic solution indicated for prevention or control of postsurgical increases in IOP and as an adjunctive agent in the treatment of open-angle glaucoma. Apraclonidine reduces IOP by decreasing the rate of aqueous humor production (some increase in uveoscleral outflow may also occur). A number of studies have investigated the potential role of apraclonidine in ocular hypertension or glaucoma. The drug reduces IOP by 18–27% at peak (2–5 hours) and by 10% at 8–12 hours. Comparative trials demonstrate a reduction of IOP similar to that obtained with 0.5% timolol. Use of apraclonidine 0.5% every 8 hours appears to provide the maximum IOP lowering effects in long-term use.

Use of NLO may improve response and allow longer dosing frequency (i.e., every 12 hours). Some patients have demonstrated a loss of IOP control with use of apraclonidine for periods greater than 1–2 months; however, many patients demonstrate long-term IOP control. Confirmation of continuing IOP-lowering effects with apraclonidine is required for all patients using the agent for prolonged periods. Combinations of apraclonidine with β blockers *or* CAIs produces additional IOP reduction. Addition of apraclonidine to maximum medical therapy for glaucoma will frequently produce additional IOP reduction. This may allow delaying the need to undergo filtering surgery.

Local adverse effects occur frequently with apraclonidine. An allergic type reaction characterized by lid edema, eye discomfort, foreign object sensation, itching, and hyperemia occurs in approximately 14% of patients and commonly necessitates drug discontinuation. Systemic side effects include dizziness and somnolence, dry mouth, and a reduction in blood pressure and pulse. Apraclonidine should be used with caution in patients with cardiovascular diseases, renal compromise, cerebrovascular disease, and diabetes, and in those taking antihypertensives and other cardiovascular drugs, monoamine oxidase inhibitors, and tricyclic antidepressants.

The role of α_2-adrenergic agonists in the treatment of POAG is primarily as an adjunctive therapy in patients not responding adequately to other drugs, as an alternative to miotics or epinephrine when adding a drug to β-blocker therapy, patients not tolerating other therapies, and for postlaser or postsurgical IOP elevation. Preliminary data suggest the agent may be useful in acute angle-closure glaucoma. Brimonidine is an additional α_2-adrenergic agonist under investigation for the treatment of glaucoma.[1,13,14,18,33–36]

Carbonic Anhydrase Inhibitors

CAIs reduce IOP by decreasing ciliary body aqueous humor secretion by up to 40–60%. The exact mechanism by which CAIs inhibit aqueous production is not known, because the role carbonic anhydrase plays in aqueous production is undefined. Active secretion of sodium and bicarbonate ions may produce an osmotic gradient resulting in transfer of water from the ciliary body to the aqueous humor. The enzyme may also maintain tissue pH for the optimal functioning of ciliary body enzyme systems involved in the formation of the aqueous flow.[1,10]

Topical CAIs such as dorzolamide are well tolerated and indicated for monotherapy or adjunctive therapy of glaucoma and ocular hypertension. Dorzolamide, a relatively specific inhibitor of carbonic anhydrase enzyme II, is the most potent topical CAI and reduces IOP by 15–26%. Dorzolamide 2% administered every 8 hours provides maximal IOP reduction; however, this topical agent is not as effective as topical β blockers in reducing IOP, nor as effective as oral CAIs. Tolerance to the IOP-lowering effects of dorzolamide over time does not appear to occur. Topical CAIs commonly provide additional IOP reductions when combined with other classes of antiglaucoma agents such as β blockers and cholinergic agents. The drug may provide additional IOP lowering in patients on maximal medical therapy for glaucoma. Dorzolamide is generally well tolerated. Local side effects encountered with dorzolamide include frequent transient burning and stinging, ocular discomfort and transient blurred vision, tearing, conjunctivitis, lid reactions, and photophobia. A superficial punctate keratitis occurs in 10–15% of patients. Systemic side effects are unusual despite the accumulation of dorzolamide in red blood cells (RBCs). Steady-state RBC levels are obtained at 8 weeks. Despite the systemic accumulation of drug, the percent of systemic carbonic anhydrase inhibited is less than that required to produce renal or respiratory effects.

Because of their favorable side-effect profile, topical CAIs provide an alternative to epinephrine and cholinergics as monotherapy or adjunctive therapy in patients with inadequate response to, or those unable to use, a β-blocking agent. The drug may add additional IOP reduction in patients using other single or multiple topical agents. The usual dose of dorzolamide is one drop of 2% solution every 8–12 hours. Administration every 12 hours produces less IOP reduction than administration every 8 hours. Use of NLO should optimize response to dorzolamide given at any interval.[13,14,37]

Systemic CAIs are indicated in patients failing to respond to or tolerate maximum topical therapy. Systemic and topical CAIs should not be used in combination because no data exist concerning improved IOP reduction, and the risk for systemic side effects is increased. Oral CAIs reduce aqueous inflow by 40–60% and IOP by 25–40%. The available systemic CAIs (Table 88.5) produce equivalent IOP reduction but differ in potency, side effects, dosage forms, and duration of action. Despite their excellent effects on elevated IOP of any etiology, the systemic CAIs frequently produce intolerable side effects. As a result, CAIs are considered second- or third-line agents in the treatment of POAG.

On average, only 30–60% of patients are able to tolerate CAI therapy for prolonged periods. Intolerance to CAI therapy most commonly results from a symptom complex thought to result from systemic acidosis that includes malaise, fatigue, anorexia, nausea, weight loss, altered taste, depression, and decreased libido. Other side effects include renal calculi, increased uric acid, blood dyscrasias, diuresis, and myopia. Elderly patients do not tolerate CAIs as well as younger patients. The three available CAIs produce the same spectrum of side effects; however, the drugs differ in the frequency and severity of the side effects listed. Acetazolamide, standard or sustained-release cap-

TABLE 88.5. CARBONIC ANHYDRASE INHIBITORS

Drug	Form	Strength (mg)	Brand Name	Dose	IOP Reduction (h)		
					Onset	Peak	Duration
Acetazolamide	Injection	500	Diamox	500 mg IV or IM	2 min	0.25–0.5	2–5
	Tablets	125, 250	Diamox	125–250 mg bid–qid	1–1.5	2–4	8–12
	Capsules	500	Diamox Sequels[a]	500 mg bid	2	8–12	12–24
Dichlorphenamide	Tablets	50	Daranide	25–50 mg bid–qid	0.5–1	2–4	6–12
Methazolamide	Tablets	50	Neptazane	25–100 mg bid–tid	2–4	6–8	10–12

[a]Sustained-release capsule.

sules (Diamox Sequels), and methazolamide (Neptazane) are commonly considered the best-tolerated CAIs.

CAIs should be used with caution in patients with sulfa allergies, sickle cell disease, respiratory acidosis, pulmonary disorders, renal calculi, electrolyte imbalance, hepatic disease, renal disease, diabetes mellitus, or Addison's disease. Concurrent use of a CAI and a diuretic may rapidly produce hypokalemia. High-dose salicylate therapy may increase the acidosis produced by CAIs, while the acidosis produced by CAIs may increase the toxicity of salicylates.[1,10,18,38–43]

Prostaglandin F2-alpha Analogues

Analogues of prostaglandin F2-alpha reduce IOP by increasing the uveoscleral outflow of aqueous humor. Reduction in IOP with one drop of 0.005% latanoprost is similar to or greater than that seen with timolol 0.5% twice daily. In addition, nocturnal control of IOP is improved compared to timolol. Latanoprost produces fewer systemic side effects than timolol, but an increase in the frequency of punctate corneal erosions and conjunctival hyperemia was noted with latanoprost. Iris pigmentation increases in 7–16% of patients, particularly those with green–brown or blue–brown eyes, which become more blue in color. The frequency of iris pigmentation changes increases with corresponding increases in the duration of treatment. Latanoprost can be used in combination with other antiglaucoma agents for additional IOP control due to its unique mechanism of action. Given its excellent efficacy and side-effect profile, latanoprost provides an alternative to patients not responding to or tolerating other agents. Studies of long-term tolerance, efficacy, and the implications of iris pigmentation changes are needed to clearly define the place of latanoprost in glaucoma therapy.[1,13,14,45,46]

Future Drug Therapies

New approaches to the reduction of IOP and other methods of prevention of glaucomatous visual field loss will hopefully provide more effective and better tolerated therapies. A number of new drug classes have been shown to reduce IOP including cannabinoids, dopamine blocking agents, angiotensin-converting enzyme (ACE) inhibitors, and calcium channel blockers.[1] Oral calcium channel blockers also may improve or maintain visual fields in patients with glaucoma. Ethacrynic acid improves aqueous outflow through the trabecular meshwork by making the meshwork more permeable. Local reactions, including keratitis with ethacrynic acid solutions, appear to be reduced by the use of an ointment formulation.[46]

ANTIPROLIFERATIVES USED IN GLAUCOMA SURGERY

Surgical methods for reduction of IOP involve the creation of a channel through which aqueous humor can flow from the anterior chamber to the subconjunctival space ("filtering bleb") where it is reabsorbed by the vasculature. A major reason for failure of the procedure is healing and scarring of the sight. Modification of the healing process to maintain patency is possible with the use of antiproliferative agents.

The antiproliferative agents 5-fluorouracil (5-FU) and mitomycin are used in patients undergoing glaucoma filtering surgery to improve success rates by reducing the inflammatory response and fibroblast proliferation. While most commonly used in patients with increased risk for suboptimal surgical outcome (postcataract and previous failed filtering procedure), use of these agents also improves success in low-risk patients. 5-FU is administered subconjunctively in 5-mg doses as either a 10 mg/mL or 50 mg/mL solution. The injection site is 90–180 degrees from the surgical site.

Regimens commonly used include twice-daily injections for 1 week followed by once-daily injections for a second week, or as a once-daily injection for 1 week, then one injection every other day for 1 week. Use of 5-FU in this manner has been associated with serious corneal toxicities. Mitomycin is used topically in a concentration of 0.2–0.5 mg/mL and placed on the surgical site using a soaked cotton swab or Gelfoam for 2.5–5 minutes, then rinsed away. Mitomycin use is associated with less corneal toxicity than 5-FU. With the use of either agent, the risks of postoperative infection, wound leaks, and prolonged ocular hypotony are increased.[47]

ANGLE-CLOSURE GLAUCOMA

Primary angle-closure glaucoma accounts for only 5% or less of primary glaucomas; however, when acute angle closure occurs, it must be treated as an emergency to avoid visual loss. Angle-closure glaucoma results from mechanical blockage of the trabecular meshwork by the iris. Blockage of the meshwork occurs intermittently, resulting in extremely high IOP and symptoms of acute angle-closure glaucoma. Between attacks of angle-closure glaucoma, the IOP is usually normal unless the patient has concomitant POAG. Primary angle-closure glaucoma occurs in patients with inherited shallow anterior chambers, which produce a narrow angle between the cornea and iris or tight contact between the iris and lens ("pupillary block") (Figs. 88.7 and 88.8). Secondary angle-closure glaucoma results from any cause (i.e., synechiae) of trabecular meshwork blockade by the iris. The presence of a narrow angle is determined by visualization of the angle by gonioscopy. Other tests for angle-closure glaucoma involve provocation of an angle-closure-induced IOP increase. These tests attempt to produce angle closure through mydriasis (dark room test, mydriasis test) or by gravity (prone test) and measure any increase in IOP resulting from the provocative test.

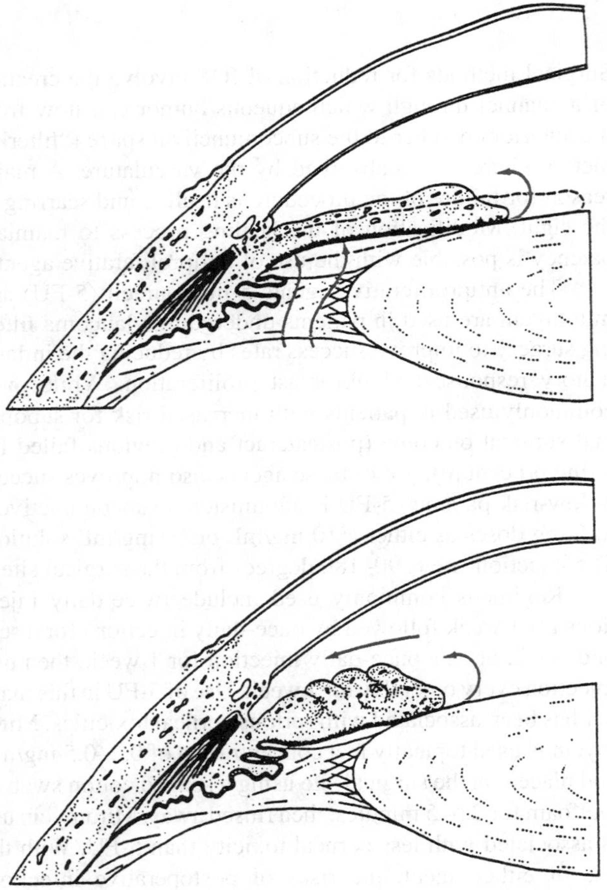

Figure 88.7. In the narrow-angle eye, the lens is displaced anteriorly in relation to the ciliary body and the iris root. When the eye is miotic (dotted line), the iris lies firmly against the lens, producing pupillary block, but the iris root is pulled away from the trabecular meshwork. In mid-dilation, pupillary block is present but the lax iris bows forward to block the meshwork. With further dilation, pupillary block is broken and the iris does not bow forward, allowing aqueous to flow to the meshwork. *(From Kolker A, Hetherington S. Becker-Shaffer's Diagnosis and Therapy of the Glaucomas, 5th ed. St Louis, MO, CV Mosby, 1983, with permission.)*

Two major types of primary angle-closure glaucoma have been described: angle closure with pupillary block and angle closure without pupillary block. Angle closure with pupillary block (Fig. 88.7) results when the iris is in firm contact with the lens. This produces a relative block of aqueous flow through the pupil to the anterior chamber, resulting in a bowing forward of the iris, which blocks the trabecular meshwork. Angle closure with pupillary block (Fig. 88.8) most commonly occurs when the pupil is in mid-dilation. In this position the combination of pupillary block and relaxed iris allows the greatest bowing of the iris; however, angle closure may occur during miosis or mydriasis.

Angle-closure glaucoma without pupillary block occurs in patients with an abnormality called a plateau iris. The iris root of these patients is inserted anteriorly, very close to the trabecular meshwork. Mydriasis causes the peripheral iris to bunch up and block the meshwork. The mydriasis produced by anticholinergic drugs or any other drug results in precipitation of both types of angle-closure glaucoma, whereas drug-induced miosis may produce pupillary block.

Patients with untreated angle-closure glaucoma typically experience intermittent prodromal symptoms brought on by precipitating events. The symptoms include blurred or hazy vision with halos around lights, caused by a hazy, edematous cornea, and occasionally headache.

Increased IOP during such prodromal episodes is not great enough or long enough to produce the other symptoms of a full-blown attack. Such prodromal attacks last 1–2 hours, at which time pupillary block is broken by further mydriasis or miosis, or miosis occurs in patients

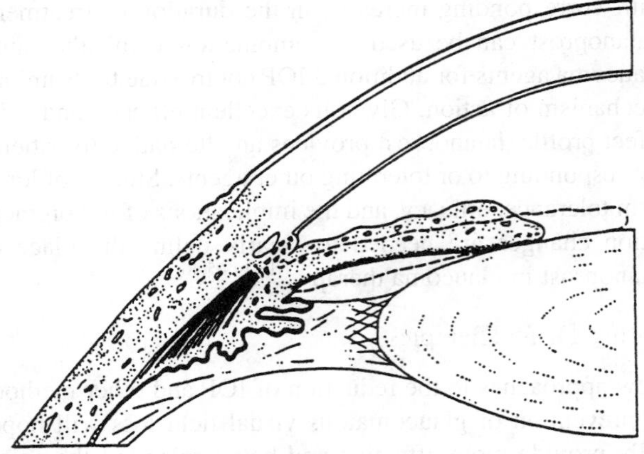

Figure 88.8. In an eye with plateau iris, the iris is attached anteriorly on the ciliary body. In miosis (dotted line), the root of the iris is pulled away from the meshwork and pupillary block is minimal. In mydriasis, the root of the iris bunches up, blocking the meshwork and producing angle closure. *(From Kolker A, Hetherington S. Becker-Shaffer's Diagnosis and Therapy of the Glaucomas, 5th ed. St Louis, MO, CV Mosby, 1983, with permission.)*

TABLE 88.6. OSMOTIC AGENTS USED IN GLAUCOMA

Drug	Molecular Weight	Strength (%)	Dose	Route	Distribution[a]	Ocular Penetration[b]	IOP Reduction (h)		
							Onset	Peak	Duration
Mannitol	182	5, 10, 15, 20, 25	1–2 g/kg	IV	Extracellular	Poor	0.25	0.5–1	6–9
Urea	60	30	1–1.5 g/kg	IV	Total	Good	0.25	1–2	5–6
Sodium ascorbate	198	20	0.5–1 g/kg	IV	Total	Good	0.5	1–2	8–12
Glycerin	92	50, 75	1–1.5 g/kg	PO	Extracellular	Moderate	0.25	0.5–1.5	4–6
Isosorbide	146	45	1–2 g/kg	PO	Total	Good	0.25	0.5–1.5	4–6
Ethanol	46	40–50	2–3 mL/kg	PO	Total	Good	0.5	1–2	8

[a]Distribution in body water.
[b]Prefer poor intraocular penetration for IOP reduction.

with plateau iris. Acute angle closure produces the symptoms associated with a cloudy, edematous cornea, ocular pain or discomfort, nausea, vomiting, abdominal pain, and diaphoresis. On examination, the patient is found to have a closed angle, narrow anterior chamber, hyperemic conjunctiva, and an edematous and hyperemic optic disk. The rate at which IOP increases may be a determinant of when full-blown symptoms occur. Visual fields demonstrate generalized constriction. In prolonged attacks, total loss of vision may occur if the IOP is high enough. Tonometry reveals IOPs as high as 40–90 mm Hg.

The goal of initial therapy for angle-closure glaucoma is rapid reduction of the IOP to preserve vision and to avoid surgical or laser iridectomy on a hypertensive, congested eye. Iridectomy is the definitive treatment of angle-closure glaucoma; it produces a hole in the iris that permits an aqueous flow to move directly from the posterior chamber to the anterior chamber. Drug therapy of an acute attack typically involves administration of pilocarpine, hyperosmotic agents, and a secretory inhibitor (CAI and/or β blocker). With miosis produced by pilocarpine, the peripheral iris is pulled away from the meshwork. Though traditionally the drug of choice, the use of pilocarpine as initial therapy is controversial. Miotics may worsen angle closure by increasing pupillary block and producing anterior movement of the lens because of drug-induced accommodation.

At IOPs greater than 60 mm Hg, the iris may be ischemic and unresponsive to miotics; as the pressure drops and the iris responds, miosis occurs. During this period of time, the tendency to use excessive amounts of pilocarpine must be avoided. The dose of pilocarpine traditionally used was a 1–2% solution instilled every 5 minutes for three doses, then every 15–30 minutes until the angle opens. However, many practitioners hold application of pilocarpine until IOP has been reduced by other agents, then apply a single drop of 1–2% pilocarpine to produce miosis. In either case, the unaffected contralateral eye should be treated with the miotic every 6 hours to prevent development of angle closure.

IOP in acute angle-closure glaucoma can be effectively reduced by decreasing aqueous humor production by application of a topical β blocker and a CAI agent orally or intravenously. Preliminary evidence suggests apraclonidine may be useful in the management of elevated IOP of angle-closure glaucoma.[1,10,48–50] An osmotic agent is also commonly administered because these drugs produce the most rapid decrease in IOP (Table 88.6). Oral glycerin or isosorbide can be used if an oral agent is tolerated; if not, intravenous mannitol should be used. Osmotic agents reduce IOP by withdrawing water from the eye secondary to the osmotic gradient between the blood and the eyes. These drugs are among the first-line agents in the treatment of angle-closure glaucoma or other forms of acute IOP elevations.

Osmotic agents are also used to reduce IOP perioperatively in patients undergoing ocular surgery. These agents are used only for short periods of time because of eventual dimunition of effects over time and adverse effects. Oral administration is preferred, but intolerance to oral osmotic agents is common, because of high frequency of nausea and vomiting. Of the two available oral agents, isosorbide and glycerin are equally effective, but isosorbide may be slightly better tolerated than glycerin. Isosorbide, unlike glycerin, will not produce hyperglycemia in diabetics. Mannitol is the preferred parenteral osmotic agent. Side effects other than nausea and vomiting include headache, confusion, and volume overload.[1,10]

Once the IOP is controlled, pilocarpine should be given every 6 hours until iridectomy is performed. Patients failing all other medical therapies may respond to retrobulbar anesthesia and external pressure to the eye. Retrobulbar anesthesia blocks ciliary body aqueous production and ocular congestion and relieves pain. Patients failing therapy altogether will require an emergency iridectomy. Because peripheral iridectomy essentially "cures" primary angle-closure glaucoma, long-term drug therapy is not used.

Medications of Potential Hazard in Glaucoma

A number of medications have been associated with increased IOP or carry labeling that cautions against use of the medication in glaucoma patients. The potential for a medication to produce or worsen glaucoma depends on the type of glaucoma and whether or not the patient is adequately treated.

Patients with treated, controlled POAG are at minimal risk of induction of an increase in IOP by systemic medications with anticholinergic properties or vasodilators; however, in the patient with untreated glaucoma or uncontrolled POAG, the potential of these medications to increase IOP should be considered. Topical anticholinergic agents used to produce mydriasis may result in an increase in IOP. Potent anticholinergic agents such as atropine or homatropine are most likely to increase the IOP. Weaker anticholinergics such as tropicamide that produce less cycloplegia are less likely to increase the IOP and are favored, along with phenylephrine, when mydriasis is desired in the POAG patient. Inhaled, nasal, topical, or systemic glucocorticoids may produce increased IOP in both normal individuals and patients with POAG.

Patients with POAG appear to be particularly susceptible to glucocorticoid-induced increases in IOP. Glucocorticoids reduce the facility of aqueous outflow through the trabecular meshwork. The decreased facility of outflow appears to result from the accumulation of extracellular material blocking the trabecular channels. The potential of a glucocorticoid to increase IOP is related to its anti-inflammatory potency and intraocular penetration. The increase in IOP induced by glucocorticoids appears to be an inherited trait. Within the general population, 66.2% have an IOP increase of 1.6 mm Hg after 4 weeks of 0.1% dexamethasone, 28.8% have an increase of 10 mm Hg, and 5% have an increase of 16 mm Hg or more. Thus, patients should be treated with the lowest potency and dose and for the shortest time possible when steroids are indicated.

In patients predisposed to angle-closure glaucoma (i.e., narrow anterior chambers), angle closure may be produced by any drug that produces mydriasis. The topical use of anticholinergics or sympathomimetic agents is most likely to result in angle closure. Systemic anticholinergic and sympathomimetic agents must also be used with caution in such patients. Inhaled anticholinergics such a ipratropium have precipitated angle closure. The patient should be instructed to avoid the use of nonprescription agents such as cold remedies, appetite suppressants, and antimotion sickness and sleep aids, which contain anticholinergic or sympathomimetic ingredients. As previously discussed, potent miotic agents such as echothiophate may produce angle closure by increasing pupillary block. Drugs associated with potentiation of glaucoma are listed in Table 88.7.[1,10,51,52]

TABLE 88.7. DRUGS THAT MAY INDUCE OR POTENTIATE GLAUCOMA

Open-Angle Glaucoma	Angle-Closure Glaucoma
Corticosteroids (high risk)	Topical anticholinergics (high risk)
Topical anticholinergics	Topical sympathomimetics (high risk)
Systematic anticholinergics (low risk)	Antihistamines
Heterocyclic antidepressants (low risk)	Systemic anticholinergics
Phenothiazines (low risk)	Heterocyclic antidepressants
Vasodilators (low risk)	Antihistamines
Cimetidine (low risk)	Phenothiazines
	Ipratropium
	Benzodiazepines
	Theophylline (low risk)
	Vasodilators (low risk)
	Systemic sympathomimetics (low risk)
	CNS stimulants (low risk)
	Tetracyclines (low risk)
	Carbonic anhydrase inhibitors (low risk)
	Monoamine oxidase inhibitors (low risk)
	Topical cholinergics (low risk)

CONCLUSION

Glaucoma is a group of primary and secondary diseases, management of which presents a considerable challenge to the pharmacotherapist. Successful therapy requires rational use of antiglaucoma medications by the clinician and patient compliance with the selected regimen, combined with conscientious monitoring for side effects and disease progression. The reward for successful therapy is considerable: the maintenance of vision. The overview of the clinical findings, pathology, and drug therapy presented in this chapter provides the clinician with the fundamentals necessary to understand and treat glaucoma.

REFERENCES

1. Shields MB. Textbook of Glaucoma, 3rd ed. Baltimore, Williams and Wilkins, 1992.
2. Quigley HA. Open angle glaucoma. N Engl J Med 1993;328:1097–1106.
3. Tielsch JM, Sommer A, Katz J, et al. Racial variations in the prevalence of primary open angle glaucoma. JAMA 1991;266:369–374.
4. Schumer RA, Podos SM. The nerve of glaucoma. Arch Ophthalmol 1994;112:37–44.
5. Fechtner RD, Weinreb RN. Mechanisms of optic nerve damage in primary open angle glaucoma. Surv Ophthalmol 1994;39:23–42.
6. Langham ME. Ocular blood flow and vision in healthy and glaucomatous eyes. Surv Ophthalmol 1994 (May);38:(suppl):S161–S168.
7. Mao LK, Stewart WC, Shields MB. Correlation between intraocular pressure control and progressive damage in

primary open angle glaucoma. Am J Ophthalmol 1991;111:51–55.

8. Newell FW. Ophthalmology: Principles and Concepts, 7th ed. St Louis, MO, CV Mosby 1991.
9. Vaughn D, Asbury T, Riordan-Eva P. General Ophthalmology, 13th ed. Los Altos, CA, Appleton Lange, 1992.
10. Havener WH. Ocular Pharmacology, 5th ed. St Louis, MO, CV Mosby, 1983.
11. Caprioli J. The aqueous, in Hart WM (ed): Adler's Physiology of the Eye: Clinical Applications, 9th ed. St Louis, MO, CV Mosby, 1992.
12. Brubaker RF. Flow of aqueous in humans. Invest Ophthal Vis Sci 1991;32:3145–3166.
13. Hurvitz LM, Kaufman PL, Robin AL, et al. New development in the drug treatment of glaucoma. Drugs 1991;41:514–532.
14. Serle JB. Pharmacologic advances in the treatment of glaucoma. Drugs Ageing 1994;5:156–170.
15. Novack GD, Robin AL, Derick RJ. New medical treatments for glaucoma. Int Ophthalm Clin 1993:33:183–202.
16. Hart WM. Intraocular pressure, in Hart WM (ed): Adler's Physiology of the Eye: Clinical Applications, 9th ed. St. Louis, MO, CV Mosby, 1992.
17. Caprioli J. Automated perimetry in glaucoma. Am J Ophthalmol 1991;111:235–239.
18. Taniguchi T, Kitazawa Y. A risk-benefit assessment of drugs used in the management of glaucoma. Drug Safety 1994;11:68–74.
19. Migdahl C. Primary open angle glaucoma, in Tasman W, Jaeger E (eds): Duanes Clinical Ophthalmology, revised. Philadelphia, JB Lippincott, 1994, pp 1–32.
20. Sherwood MB, Migdal CS, Hitchings RA, et al. Initial treatment of glaucoma: Surgery or medications. Surv Ophthalm 1993:37:293–305.
21. Zimmerman TJ. Topical ophthalmic beta blockers: A comparative review. J Ocular Pharmacol 1993;9:373–384.
22. Frishman WH, Fuksbrumer MS, Tannenbaum M. Topical ophthalmic beta-adrenergic blockade for the treatment of glaucoma and ocular hypertension. J Clin Pharmacol 1994;34:795–803.
23. Brooks AMV, Gilies WE. Ocular beta-blockers in glaucoma management. Drugs Aging 1992;2:208–221.
24. Kaiser H, Flammer J, Stumpfig D, Hendrickson P. Long term visual field follow up of glaucoma patients treated with beta-blockers. Surv Ophthalmol 1994 (May);38(suppl):S156–S160.
25. Zimmerman TJ, Sharir M, Nardin GF, Fuqua M. Therapeutic index of pilocarpine, carbachol, and timolol with nasolacrimal occlusion. Am J Opthalmol 1992;114:1–7.
26. Zimmerman TJ. Pilocarpine. Ophthalmology 1981;88:85–88.
27. Zimmerman TJ, Wheeler TM. Miotics, side effects and ways to avoid them. Ophthalmology 1982;89:76–80.
28. Vogel R, Crick RP, Mills KB, et al. Effect of timolol versus pilocarpine on visual field progression in patients with primary open angle glaucoma. Ophthalmology 1992;99:1505–1511.
29. Everitt DE, Avorn J. Systemic effects of medications used to treat glaucoma. Ann Intern Med 1990;112:120–125.
30. Gerber SL, Cantor LB, Brater DC. Systemic drug interactions with topical glaucoma medications. Surv Ophthalmol 1990;35:205–218.
31. Fraunfelder FT, Mayer SM. Systemic adverse reactions to glaucoma medications. Int Ophthalmol Clin 1990;30:143–146.
32. Podos SM. Epinephrine. Ophthalmology 1980;87:721–723.
33. Toris CD, Tafoya ME, Camras CB, Yablonski ME. Effects of apraclonidine on aqueous humor dynamics in human eyes. Ophthalmology 1995;102:456–461.
34. Butler P, Mannschreck M, Lin S, et al. Clinical experience with long term use of 1% apraclonidine. Arch Ophthalmol 1995;113:293–296.
35. Nagasubramanian S, Hitchings RA, Demailly P, et al. Comparison of apraclonidine in chronic open angle glaucoma. Ophthalmology 1993;100:1318–1323.
36. Stewart WC, Ritch R, Shin DH, et al. The efficacy of apraclonidine as an adjunct as timolol therapy. Arch Opthalmol 1995;113:287–292.
37. Wikerson M, Cyrlin M, Lippa EA, et al. Four-week safety and efficacy study of dorzolamide, a novel, active topical carbonic anhydrase inhibitor. Arch Ophthalmol 1993;111:1343–1350.
38. Lichter PR, Newman LP, Wheeler NC, et al. Patient tolerance to carbonic anhydrase inhibitors. Am J Ophthalmol 1978;85:495–502.
39. Shrader CE, Thomas JV, Simmons RJ. Relationship of patient age and tolerance to carbonic anhydrase inhibitors. Am J Ophthalmol 1983;96:730–733.
40. Kooner KS, Zimmerman T. Pearls in glaucoma management. Ann Ophthalmol 1985;16:507–508.
41. Joyce PW, Mills KB, Richardson T, et al. Equivalence of conventional and sustained-release oral dosage formulations of acetazolamide in primary open-angle glaucoma. Br J Clin Pharmacol 1989;597–606.
42. Fraunfelder FT, Meyer SM, Bagby GC, et al. Hematologic reactions to carbonic anhydrase inhibitors. Am J Ophthalmol 1985;100:79–81.
43. Anderson CJ, Kaufman PL, Sturm RJ. Toxicity of combined therapy with carbonic anhydrase inhibitors and aspirin. Am J Ophthalmol 1978;86:516–519.
44. Camras CB. Comparison of latanoprost and timolol in patients with ocular hypertension and glaucoma. Ophthalmol 1996;103:138–147.
45. Watson P, Stjernschantz J. A six-month, randomized, double masked study comparing latanoprost with timolol in open angle glaucoma and ocular hypertension. Opthalmol 1996;103:126–137.
46. Wang R-F, Podos SM, Serle JB, et al. Effects of topical ethacrynic acid ointment vs timolol on intraocular pressure in glaucomatous monkey eyes. Arch Opthalmol 1994;112:390–394.
47. Skuta GL. Antifibrotic agents in glaucoma filtering surgery. Int Ophthalmol Clin 1993;33:165–182.
48. Greenidge KC. Angle closure glaucoma. Int Ophthalmol Clin 1990;30:177–186.
49. Kooner KS, Zimmerman TJ. Management of acute elevated intraocular pressure: Part II. Treatment. Ann Ophthalmol 1988;20:87–88.
50. Kramer P, Ritch R. The treatment of acute angle closure glaucoma revisited. Ann Ophthalmol 1984;16:1101–1103.
51. Francois J. Corticosteroid glaucoma. Ophthalmologica 1984;188:76–81.
52. Abel SR. Drug-induced potentiation of glaucoma. US Pharm 1981;Dec:76–81.

Chapter 89

Allergic Rhinitis

J. Russell May, PharmD, Timothy A. Feger, MD, and Margaret F. Guill, MD

Rhinitis is inflammation of the nasal mucous membrane. Allergic rhinitis is caused by mucous membrane exposure to inhaled allergenic materials that elicit a specific immunologic response. It is characterized by sneezing, nasal itching and watery rhinorrhea, often associated with nasal congestion. Itching of the throat, eyes, and ears frequently accompanies allergic rhinitis.

There are two types of allergic rhinitis. Seasonal allergic rhinitis, commonly known as hay fever, occurs in response to specific allergens present seasonally—in the spring or fall. Seasonal allergens include pollen from trees, grasses, and weeds and typically cause more acute symptoms. Perennial allergic rhinitis is a year-round disease caused by nonseasonal allergens such as house dust mites, animal dander, and molds, typically resulting in subtle, chronic symptoms. Unfortunately, some patients have a combination of these two types of allergic rhinitis, suffering all year with seasonal exacerbations.

Magnitude of Problem

Allergic rhinitis is one of the most common medical disorders found in humans. It affects 20% of the American population and ranks as the sixth most prevalent chronic illness in the United States.[1] Patients are limited in their ability to do normal daily functions, concentration is impaired, sleep is disturbed, social interaction is limited, and emotional well-being is affected.[2] In addition potentially serious complications may occur, such as those related to the paranasal sinuses, eustachian tube, olfaction, and possibly lower airways.

The economic impact of allergic rhinitis is enormous. Millions of dollars are spent each year on physician services and medication for treatment of this chronic illness. In 1980, it was estimated that allergic rhinitis accounted for 2 million lost school days and 3.5 million lost work days, resulting in an approximate cost of more than 150 million dollars in lost wages.[3] Because many patients self-medicate allergic symptoms with nonprescription medications, a full understanding of the pathophysiology of allergic rhinitis and treatment options is necessary to give patients the most appropriate advice.

Epidemiology

PREDISPOSING FACTORS

There is a strong genetic predisposition to allergic rhinitis. A family history of allergic rhinitis, atopic dermatitis, or asthma suggests that rhinitis is allergic. Likewise, a personal history of other atopic diseases (e.g., atopic dermatitis as an infant) predisposes to the development of allergic rhinitis later in life.[4,5] The risk of developing allergic rhinitis is approximately 30% for children with one atopic parent and approaches 50% for those with two allergic parents.[6] Peak incidence occurs in childhood and adolescence, with approximately 70% of patients developing symptoms by the age of 30 years.[7]

Allergen exposure is another predisposing factor. For allergic rhinitis to occur, an individual must be exposed to a protein that elicits the allergic response in that individual. Many potential sufferers never develop symptoms because they never come into contact with the appropriate allergen.

For reasons that are unclear, positive skin tests indicating allergen sensitization have been observed more frequently in people in higher socioeconomic classes and in people who live in suburban areas compared with those living in more crowded and polluted inner city areas.[8,9] Further epidemiologic studies are needed to confirm and explain these findings. Once symptoms have started, they can be exacerbated by various nonspecific irritants, such as cigarette smoke, strong odors, air pollution, and climatic changes.

ALLERGENS

Allergens that produce seasonal rhinitis are the protein components of airborne pollen grains from a variety of trees, grasses, and weeds. Ragweed and grass pollen are the most common offenders in the United States; however, this changes with the geographic region. In general, tree pollens cause symptoms in the spring, grass pollens cause symptoms in the late spring to summer, and weed pollens are the culprits in the late summer to early fall. Patients who are hypersensitive to all three may have overlapping problem periods that can lead to a misdiagnosis of perennial rhinitis. Flowering plants that depend on insect pollination do not usually cause allergic rhinitis.

To complicate matters further, the antigenic components of many grasses are similar, resulting in cross-allergenicity. These include fescue, Kentucky bluegrass, orchard, redtop, and timothy. Fortunately, the trees that produce many of the offending airborne pollens produce pollens that are antigenically distinct. These trees include ash, beech, birch, cedar, hickory, maple, oak, poplar, and sycamore.

Mold spores are also significant allergens, with *Alternaria* and *Cladosporium* being the major outdoor molds. Spores are present year-round; however, there are seasonal increases because of mold growth on decaying vegetation. Thus mold spores can be responsible for both perennial and seasonal allergies.[10]

Indoor allergens are usually present perennially; most important among these are house dust mites and animal dander, with cockroaches and certain mold species being relevant in some areas.[11,12] Food allergen-induced rhinitis may be present in children; however, this is controversial. Food allergies are commonly characterized by urticaria and angioedema, but some patients may experience respiratory symptoms.

PATHOPHYSIOLOGY

NASAL PHYSIOLOGY

Knowledge of nasal physiology aids in the understanding of allergic rhinitis. The nose performs three air-conditioning functions to prepare the air for the lungs. During the fraction of a second air is in the nose, it is heated, humidified, and cleaned. The cleaning process plays a role in the development of allergic rhinitis. As the air passes through the nose, the turbulence throws particulate matter against a mucous blanket. The rhythmic movements of the nasal cilia cause the mucous blanket to move posteriorly at approximately 9 mm/min, where it is eventually swallowed[13]; therefore, foreign particles are removed via the gastrointestinal tract and do not reach the lungs.

The vascular tissue in the nose is erectile. Stimulation of sympathetic fibers causes vasoconstriction, reduction in erectile tissue size, and airway widening. Parasympathetic stimulation causes vasodilatation, increase in erectile tissue size, and airway narrowing.[14]

Located in the nasal mucosa are the mast cells, which participate in the regulation of nasal patency by releasing mediators such as histamine.[15] Histamine has a direct effect on H_1 vascular receptors, causing increased airway resistance. Histamine increases epithelial permeability; thus, allergens penetrate the submucosa, where mast cell density is greater.[16]

THE IMMUNE RESPONSE

Allergic reactions in the nose are mediated by antigen–antibody responses involving allergens interacting with specific IgE molecules bound to nasal mast cells and basophils. In allergic subjects these cells are increased in both number and reactivity. During inhalation, airborne allergens enter the nose and are processed by lymphocytes, which produce antigen-specific IgE, thereby sensitizing genetically predisposed hosts. Upon nasal reexposure, IgE bound to mast cells interacts with the airborne allergen triggering release of inflammatory mediators (Fig. 89.1).[17]

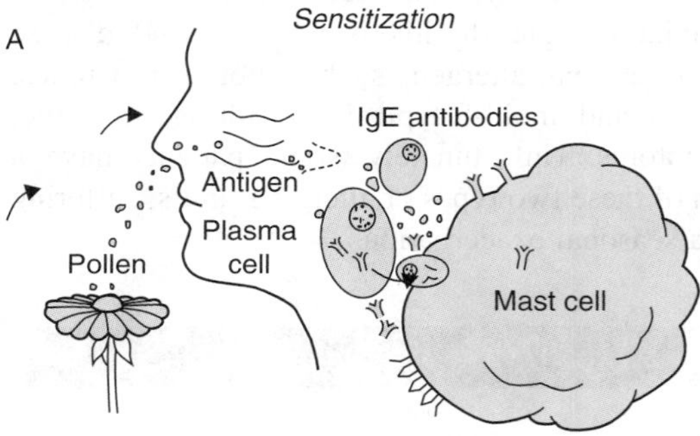

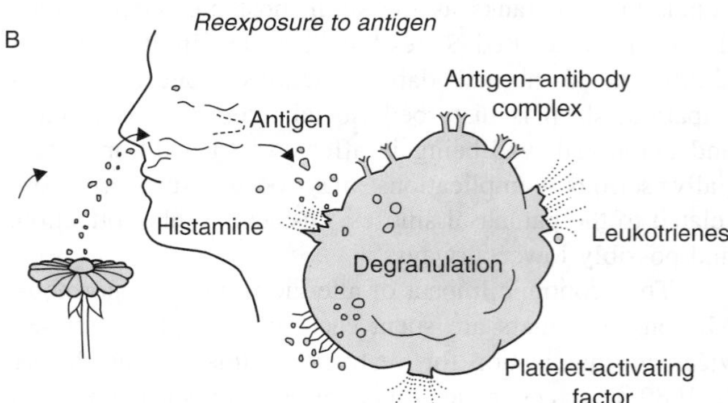

Figure 89.1. Allergen sensitization and the allergic response. (A) Exposure to antigen stimulates IgE production and sensitization of mast cells with antigen-specific IgE antibodies. (B) Subsequent exposure to the same antigen produces an allergic reaction when mast cell mediators are released.

Both immediate and late phase reactions are observed after allergen exposure. The immediate reaction occurs within minutes, resulting in the rapid release of preformed mediators and newly generated mediators from the arachidonic acid cascade as the mast cell membrane is disturbed (Table 89.1).[18] These mediators of immediate hypersensitivity include histamine, leukotrienes C4, LTD4, LTE4, prostaglandin D_2, tryptase, and kinins.[14,19] In addition the mast cell has been found to be a source of several cytokines that are probably relevant to the chronicity of the mucosal inflammation that characterizes allergic rhinitis.[20] The physiologic responses to these inflammatory mediators include vasodilatation, increased vascular permeability, and the production of nasal secretions.[14,21] Histamine, probably the most important mediator,[18] causes vascular engorgement leading to nasal congestion, directly stimulates secretion of mucus, and increases glandular secretion.

Several hours after the initial exposure to an allergen, a late-phase reaction may occur. This reaction involves an influx of inflammatory cells (e.g., eosinophils, monocytes, macrophages, basophils) and activation of the rich lymphocyte population.[22,23] The patient experiences renewed allergic symptoms without additional allergen exposure. With repeated allergen exposure this late-phase reaction may become virtually continuous, resulting in persistent nasal inflammation.[24,25] The inflamed mucosa becomes hyperresponsive characterized by exacerbation of nasal symptoms when the patient is exposed to nonspecific or irritant triggers. Subsequent exposure to lower doses of the same allergen produces repeated or persistent nasal symptoms in the "primed" host.

TABLE 89.1. MAST CELL MEDIATORS

Mediator	Effect
Performed and Rapidly Released	
Histamine	Stimulates irritant receptors
	Pruritis
	Vascular permeability
	Mucosal permeability
	Smooth muscle contraction
Neutrophil chemotactic factor	Influx of inflammatory cells
Eosinophil chemotactic factor	Influx of inflammatory cells
Kinins	Vascular permeability
N-α-tosyl L-arginine methyl esterase	Vascular permeability
Newly Generated	
Leukotrienes	Smooth muscle contraction
	Vascular permeability
	Mucus secretion
Prostaglandins	Pruritis
	Vascular permeability
	Mucus secretion
	Chemotaxis
	Mucus secretion
	Neutrophil chemotaxis
Thromboxanes	Smooth muscle spasm
Platelet-activating factor	Mucus secretion
	Airway permeability
	Chemotaxis
	Vascular permeability
Granule Matrix Contents	
Heparin	Anti-inflammatory
Tryptase	Protein hydrolysis
Kallekrein	Protein hydrolysis

CLINICAL PRESENTATION

SYMPTOMS

The patient with allergic rhinitis typically complains of clear rhinorrhea, paroxysms of sneezing, nasal congestion, postnasal drip and puritic eyes, ears, nose, or palate. Symptoms of allergic conjunctivitis are more frequently associated with seasonal than perennial allergic rhinitis. A majority of the perennial allergens, such as dust mites and molds, are indoors where air velocity is too low for substantial deposition of allergenic particles on the conjunctiva.

Symptoms secondary to the late-phase reaction, predominantly nasal congestion, begin 3–5 hours after antigen exposure and peak at 12–24 hours. Subsequent symptoms, both allergic and irritant, are more easily elicited because of the "priming effect." For instance, a ragweed-sensitive patient, when exposed to ragweed pollen out of season, responds with modest symptoms and may be very tolerant of irritants such as air pollution or tobacco smoke. During the ragweed season, however, when the nasal mucosa is already inflamed, exposure to small doses of pollen or to irritants to which the patient is usually tolerant elicits a more severe response.

COMPLICATIONS

Not only is allergic rhinitis aggravating, it frequently leads to further complications, particularly if the patient does not receive adequate treatment. Untreated rhinitis symptoms may lead to inability to sleep, chronic malaise, fatigue, and poor work or school efficiency. Patients are often plagued by loss of smell or taste, with sinusitis or polyps underlying many cases of allergy-related hyposmia.[26,27] Postnasal drip with cough can also be bothersome.

The role of allergic rhinitis in the development of acute otitis media or chronic middle ear effusion remains controversial.[28,29] However, some studies have suggested allergy as a predisposing factor in up to 80% of recurrent or chronic otitis media.[30] Hearing problems in children related to middle ear effusion may lead to delayed development of language in young children or school problems in older children.[31]

Structural facial and dental problems can result from chronic allergic rhinitis.[32,33] The chronic edema and venous stasis may contribute to the development of a high-arched, V-shaped palate. Mouth breathing caused by nasal obstruction can be responsible for dental malocclusion and orthodontic problems.[32,33] Constant upward rubbing of the nose *(allergic salute)* can cause a permanent transverse crease across the lower nose; nasal congestion leads to venous pooling and dark circles under the eyes known as *allergic shiners.*

Allergic rhinitis is clearly a risk factor for asthma, with approximately 90% of asthmatics younger than 16 years having allergies.[34] Asthma is more common in those with perennial than seasonal allergic rhinitis and it is less likely to be "outgrown" when associated with allergic rhinitis.[35–37]

Acute and chronic sinusitis are relatively common complications of allergic rhinitis.[38] Nasal polyps are less common but nonetheless bothersome; they require specific therapy but may improve with management of the underlying allergic state. Epistaxis can also be a problem; it is related to mucosal hyperemia and inflammation.

DIAGNOSIS

Allergic rhinitis is differentiated from other causes of rhinitis by a thorough history, physical examination, and certain diagnostic tests. The medical history consists of a careful description of symptoms, environmental factors and exposures, results of previous therapy, use of other medications, previous nasal injuries, previous nasal or sinus surgery, family history, and the presence of other medical problems. Identification of specific causative allergens may be difficult. For example, a reaction induced by mowing the yard may not be caused by grass pollens, but by the disturbance of various weeds, molds, or other plants in the lawn. With perennial allergic rhinitis the cause-and-effect relationship is less clear, making the diagnosis more difficult.[39] This is especially true with such covert allergens as house dust mites and molds.

Physical examination may reveal allergic shiners, a transverse nasal crease caused by repeated rubbing of the nose, and adenoidal breathing. Pale, bluish, edematous nasal turbinates coated with thin, clear secretions are characteristic. Tearing, conjunctival injection and edema, and periorbital swelling may be present.

Nasal scrapings will provide a representative sample of cells infiltrating the nasal mucosa and can be helpful in supporting the diagnosis.[40] Microscopic examination of the nasal smear from an allergic individual will typically show numerous eosinophils. The peripheral eosinophil count may be elevated in allergic rhinitis, but it is nonspecific and has limited usefulness.[34]

The above diagnostic evaluation is supported by determination of the presence or absence of specific IgE by allergen skin testing or *in vitro* assays (e.g., radioallergosorbent test [RAST]). Two different methods of skin testing are available. The epicutaneous test, also known as the scratch or prick test, is performed by making a superficial wound in the outermost layer of skin. A drop of antigen is placed in the wound and allowed to diffuse into the underlying skin. The intradermal test is performed by injecting 0.01–0.05 mL of diluted allergen between the layers of skin. With both procedures, a positive test produces a wheal and flare reaction within 15–30 minutes. The epicutaneous-prick test is the fastest and least expensive screening tool; intradermal tests should be reserved for patients who give negative prick tests but in whom there is a high degree of suspicion of an allergic etiology.[41]

The variability in potency and stability of skin testing extracts has led to a movement for the development of standardized extracts, which have a defined potency and are labeled with a common unit, the Bioequivalent Allergy Unit (BAU).[42] This provides the allergist with guidance in selecting common safe and effective doses for diagnosis and treatment. Skin test results may vary depending on the anatomic site, method of skin testing, or even time of day at which the test is performed.[41,43] Also, the concurrent use of antihistamines or sympathomimetics may alter the test response. The allergens available for testing are numerous and include extracts of tree, grass, and weed pollens, and molds, foods, and other miscellaneous inhalants. Selection should be based on patient history.

RAST is an *in vitro* assay for measurement of specific IgE that is rarely justified in clinical practice because it is more expensive and less sensitive than skin tests.[44] Such *in vitro* testing may be useful when appropriate specific skin test extracts are not available, when negative controls produce a wheal reaction, when antihistamine therapy cannot be discontinued, or in the presence of dermatographia.[9] Total IgE levels are elevated in only 30–40% of allergic rhinitis patients, and it is also elevated in some nonallergic conditions, thus limiting its diagnostic usefulness.[9,34]

TREATMENT

AVOIDANCE

Avoidance of offending allergens is the most direct method of preventing allergic rhinitis but is often the most difficult to accomplish. Mold growth can be reduced by maintaining household humidity below 50% and removing obvious growth with bleach or disinfectant. Patients sensitive to animals will benefit most by removing pets from the home[45]; however, cat allergen may remain in the house for several months after removal of the pet.[46] Commercial spraying is the only measure shown to reduce cockroach exposure.

Efforts to eliminate dust mites should be rigorous, particularly in the bedroom. Exposure to dust mites can be reduced by encasing mattresses and pillows with impermeable covers and washing bed linens in hot water.[45,47] Washable area rugs are preferable to wall-to-wall carpeting. Acaricide treatment of carpets has been shown to denature the dust mite allergen. It has been shown that atopic infants who are exposed to high levels of dust mites are at increased risk for developing asthma.[48] Environmental control of these allergens may be helpful in forestalling further rhinitis and preventing later asthma.

Older central air-filtration systems for houses were expensive and minimally effective.[49] High-efficiency particulate air (HEPA) filters have minimal effect on the heavy mite allergens, but are effective in removing lightweight particulates including pollens, mold spores, and cat allergen, thus reducing allergic respiratory symptoms.[50]

Patients with seasonal allergic rhinitis should keep windows closed and minimize time spent outdoors during pollen seasons. Filter masks can be worn while gardening or mowing the lawn. When avoidance is impractical or produces only a partial response, several pharmacologic approaches can be used to treat allergic rhinitis.

TREATMENT/PREVENTION OF SYMPTOMS

Common therapeutic modalities for treating allergic rhinitis are directed at relief of symptoms. This group includes antihistamines and decongestants (both oral and topical). Knowledge of pathophysiology and the inflammatory state has led to prophylactic therapy for more severe disease with cromolyn and topical steroids. One may have difficulty interpreting the medical literature for a variety of reasons, including lack of uniformity in the research methodologies and failure to identify types of rhinitis (allergic versus nonallergic).[51] Also, allergic rhinitis is one of several conditions that shows a response to placebo.[52]

Antihistamines

Histamine H_1-receptor antagonists are antihistamines that prevent the binding of histamine from the receptor sites. This prevents the histamine response (increased airway resistance) in sensory nerve endings and blood vessels. It is likely, although still unproven, that the histamine-induced increase in epithelial permeability is inhibited.[16] Newer agents in this pharmacologic class offer potential advantages over some of the traditionally used agents, as described in the following paragraphs.

Antihistamines are more effective in preventing the actions of histamine than in reversing these actions once they have taken place. Reversal of symptoms is, at least in part, caused by the anticholinergic properties of these drugs. This activity is responsible for the drying effect of antihistamines, which reduces the problem of nasal, salivary, and lacrimal gland hypersecretion. Antihistamines antagonize capillary permeability, wheal-and-flare formation, and itching.

Histamine H_2-receptor antagonists, such as cimetidine and ranitidine, may have some effect on histamine-induced nasal blockage but not on sensory nerves.[9] Combining one of these agents with an H_1 antagonist may result in synergism when treating various urticarial syndromes.[53] The H_2 antagonists have no role in treating allergic rhinitis.

In general, the antihistamines are well absorbed, have a large volume of distribution, and are metabolized by the liver. There appears to be considerable interpatient variation in mean serum half-life.[54] Also, the therapeutic effects of these agents are more prolonged than might be predicted by their half-lives.

Sustained-release products have been available for several years. Although published data to support their use are lacking, many patients claim they are beneficial. In some patients, the duration of action is similar to that of the traditional tablet forms.[55]

Drowsiness is usually the chief complaint of patients who take antihistamines. Drowsiness can interfere with a patient's ability to drive a car or operate machinery and may interfere with a patient's ability to function adequately at the workplace. The sedative effects of antihistamines vary from class to class. Table 89.2 lists common antihistamines and their relative potential for causing sedation.

The sedative effects of antihistamines can be useful in patients who suffer from sleeplessness caused by the symptoms of allergic rhinitis. In these patients, a bedtime dose may prove beneficial. Tolerance occurs within 24 hours of the first dose.[56] The mechanism for sedation is not well understood, but its central effect depends on the drug's ability to cross the blood–brain barrier.[57] Most antihistamines are lipid soluble and cross this barrier easily.

A major advance in antihistamine therapy occurred with the development of the peripherally acting antihistamines, first terfenadine, followed by astemizole and loratidine. These agents are highly selective peripheral histamine H_1-receptor antagonists with little or no central or autonomic nervous system effects. Determining advantages of one of the agents over the other, particularly differences in efficacy, is difficult because of previously mentioned study design problems. Clinical important drug interactions with these nonsedating agents are described in Chapter 7.

One clear difference between these nonsedating agents is their elimination half-lives. Loratidine's half-life is the shortest, ranging from 7.8–15 hours, followed by terfenadine (16–23 hours) and astemizole (20–60 hours).[58] The clinical relevance of these differences is yet to be determined.

The new nonsedating agents should not be automatically substituted for older agents. Many patients respond to and tolerate the older agents quite well. Because many of the older agents are generically available, they are much less expensive. Average wholesale price of many of the generically available agents is less than $1 for a 2-week

TABLE 89.2. RELATIVE SIDE-EFFECT PROFILE OF ANTIHISTAMINES

Agent	Relative Sedative Effect	Relative Anticholinergic Effect
Alkylamine class		
Brompheniramine maleate	Low	Moderate
Chlorpheniramine maleate	Low	Moderate
Dexchlorpheniramine maleate	Low	Moderate
Ethanolamine class		
Carbinoxamine maleate	High	High
Clemastine fumarate	Moderate	High
Diphenhydramine hydrochloride	Low	High
Ethylenediamine class		
Pyrilamine maleate	Low	Low to none
Tripelennamine hydrochloride	Moderate	Low to none
Phenothiazine class		
Methdilazine hydrochloride	Low	High
Promethazine hydrochloride	High	High
Trimeprazine	Moderate	High
Piperadine class		
Azatadine maleate	Moderate	Moderate
Cyproheptadine hydrochloride	Low	Moderate
Diphenylpyraline hydrochloride	Low	Moderate
Phenindamine tartrate	Low to none	Moderate
Miscellaneous		
Astemizole	Low to none	Low to none
Terfenadine	Low to none	Low to none
Loratadine	Low to none	Low to none

supply, compared with more than $15 for some of the nonsedating agents.

Anticholinergic (drying) effects lend to the agents' therapeutic efficacy. Dry mouth, difficulty in voiding urine, constipation, and potential cardiovascular effects may be troublesome. Table 89.2 lists several antihistamines and their relative anticholinergic effects. Keep in mind that the differences may be small. Patients with a predisposition to urinary retention (e.g., elderly men, those on concurrent anticholinergic therapy) should use antihistamines with caution. Caution should also be used in patients with increased intraocular pressure, hyperthyroidism, and cardiovascular disease.

Other side effects of antihistamines include loss of appetite, nausea, vomiting, epigastric distress, constipation, and diarrhea.

Antihistamines are more effective when taken approximately 1–2 hours before the anticipated exposure to the offending allergen. If tolerance develops to the therapeutic effect, change to an agent in a different chemical class may be effective.[59]

Patients should be counseled about the proper use of antihistamines. Side effects, especially drowsiness, should be emphasized. Patients should be warned against taking other central nervous system depressants, including alcohol. Patients should be told not to take a double dose when a dose is missed. Taking the antihistamine with meals or at least a full glass of water will help prevent the gastrointestinal side effects (e.g., nausea, vomiting, epigastric distress). Patients should check with their pharmacists and read labels before taking nonprescription medications. Many cold products and sleep aids contain antihistamines. Patients should be instructed not to use more than one antihistamine at a time. Table 89.3 lists the recommended dosages of the commonly prescribed agents.

Allergic conjunctivitis, often associated with allergic rhinitis, can be treated with an ophthalmic antihistamine such as levocabastine. A nasal spray form of levocabastine is under investigation for allergic rhinitis.

Decongestants

Topical and systemic decongestants are sympathomimetic agents that act on adrenergic receptors in the nasal mucosa, producing vasoconstriction. Decongestants shrink swollen mucosa and improve ventilation.

Topical Decongestants

Topical decongestants are applied directly to swollen nasal mucosa via drugs or sprays. Table 89.4 lists some of the com-

TABLE 89.3. ORAL DOSAGES OF COMMONLY PRESCRIBED ANTIHISTAMINES AND DECONGESTANTS

Drug	Dosage and Interval: Adults	Dosage and Interval: Children
Antihistamines		
Chlorpheniramine maleate, plain	4 mg every 6 h	6–12 yr: 2 mg every 6 h 2–6 yr: 1 mg every 6 h
Chlorpheniramine maleate, sustained release	8–12 mg at bedtime or 8–12 mg every 8 h	6–12 yr: 8 mg at bedtime <6 yr: not recommended
Diphenhydramine hydrochloride	25–50 mg every 8 h	5 mg/kg/d divided every 8 h (up to 25 mg per dose)
Clemastine fumerate	1.34 mg twice daily to 2.68 mg three times daily	Not recommended
Astemizole	30 mg on day 1, 20 mg on day 2, then 10 mg daily	Not recommended
Loratidine	10 mg daily	Not recommended
Terfenadine	60 mg twice daily	6–12 yr: 30–60 mg twice daily 3–6 yr: 15 mg twice daily
Decongestants		
Pseudoephedrine	60 mg every 4–6 h 120 mg every 12 h for sustained release	6–12 yr: 30 mg every 4–6 h 2–5 yr: 15 mg every 4–6 h
Ephedrine sulfate	25–50 mg every 4 h	2–3 mg/kg/d divided every 4 h (up to 25 mg every 4 h)
Phenylpropranolamine	25 mg every 4 h or 50 mg every 8 h for sustained release	6–12 yr: 12.5 mg every 4 h 2–5 yr: 6.25 mg every 4 h

mon topical decongestants and their duration of action. The use of these agents results in little or no systemic absorption.

Because these agents are extremely effective and available to patients over the counter (OTC), they are widely used. Prolonged use of these agents results in a condition known as rhinitis medicamentosa or "status asthmaticus of the nose." This condition is thought to be caused by severe nasal edema and reduced receptor sensitivity.[60] Patients who develop this condition use more spray more often with less response. While the methods used to treat this "addiction" have not been formally studied, several are commonly used. Abrupt cessation works, but it is difficult because of rebound congestion that may leave the patient congested for several days or weeks. Sleeping may become difficult. Nasal steroids have been used successfully, but they take several days to work. Weaning the patient off topical decongestants can be accomplished by decreasing the dosing interval or the concentration over several weeks. Combining the weaning process with nasal steroids may prove useful.

TABLE 89.4. DURATION OF ACTION OF TOPICAL DECONGESTANTS

Drug	Duration (h)
Short-acting	Up to 4
Phenylephrine hydrochloride	
Intermediate-acting	4–6
Naphazoline hydrochloride	
Tetrahydralazine hydrochloride	
Long-acting	Up to 12
Oxymetazoline hydrochloride	
Xylometazoline hydrochloride	

Other side effects of topical decongestants include burning, stinging, sneezing, and dryness of the nasal mucosa.

Patients should be counseled on the use of topical decongestants to prevent rhinitis medicamentosa. Patients should be instructed to use as small a dose as possible as infrequently as possible and only when absolutely necessary (e.g., at bedtime to aid in falling asleep). Duration of therapy should always be limited to 3–5 days.

Systemic Decongestants

Oral decongestants are not as effective on an immediate basis as the topical agents but they may last longer and cause less local irritation. Also, rhinitis medicamentosa is not a problem. The most commonly used agents are pseudoephedrine, phenylpropanolamine, and ephedrine.

The pharmacokinetic variables for pseudoephedrine, phenylpropanolamine, and ephedrine are summarized in Table 89.5.

The therapeutic index for phenylpropanolamine is very low. It can produce severe or life-threatening hypertension at less than three times the usual OTC dose of 37.5 mg.[61,62] The therapeutic index for ephedrine is also low; doses exceeding two to three times the therapeutic dose can cause clinically important hypertension.[61]

TABLE 89.5. PHARMACOKINETIC VARIABLES OF SYSTEMIC DECONGESTANTS

Drug	Half-Life (h)	Mechanism of Metabolism or Elimination
Pseudoephedrine	3–8	Partially metabolized; majority excreted unchanged in urine
Ephedrine	3–6	Majority excreted unchanged in urine
Phenylpropanolamine	3–4	Majority excreted unchanged in urine

Pseudoephedrine appears to be the safest of the three. Doses of 180 mg have been shown to produce no measurable change in blood pressure or heart rate.[63] In higher doses (210–240 mg), pseudoephedrine has raised both blood pressure and heart rate.[64] All three systemic decongestants can cause mild central nervous system stimulation, even at therapeutic doses.

Table 89.3 lists the usual doses for pseudoephedrine, phenylpropanolamine, and ephedrine. Because most of the studies on the effect of decongestants on blood pressure were performed in normotensive patients, hypertensive patients should, unless absolutely necessary, avoid these drugs, especially phenylpropanolamine and ephedrine. Severe antihypertensive reactions can occur with any of these agents when given with monoamine oxidase inhibitors.[65]

As with antihistamines, patients should be encouraged to read product labels to avoid therapeutic duplications. Because most OTC appetite suppressants contain phenylpropanolamine, they should not be taken in combination with decongestants.

Combination Products

Numerous products combining an antihistamine with a decongestant are available. The combination seems rational because of the different mechanisms of action. Two well-controlled studies have documented the efficacy of pseudoephedrine in combination with triprolidine.[66,67] On the basis of these two studies, the Food and Drug Administration upgraded this product's designation to "effective." Studies with some of the nonsedating antihistamines combined with pseudoephedrine look promising.[68,69] As previously mentioned, patients should read labels to avoid therapeutic duplication. The therapeutic benefit of products containing more than one antihistamine has not been demonstrated. Specific symptoms should be treated with a single drug when possible.

Topical Steroids

The desired benefits of corticosteroids must be weighed against the potential risks. While corticosteroids are universally accepted to be effective in allergic rhinitis, concern over side effects has limited their systemic use. Topical steroids appear to be effective with minimal side effects. Systemic corticosteroids are known to inhibit the symptoms of the late-phase response (occurring several hours after antigen challenge) but not the early-phase or immediate response.[70] Topical therapy may inhibit early- as well as late-phase response.[71]

In vivo studies have shown several effects of topical steroids on the nasal mucosa: a decrease in the number of epithelial mediator cells,[72] reduction in epithelial permeability,[73] reduction of the secretory response to stimulation of nasal cholinergic receptors,[74] and partial inhibition of the immediate allergen-induced nasal symptoms.[75] One study suggests that topical corticosteroids inhibit the increase in mast cell density that occurs in the nasal mucosa during pollen season.[76] The effects of nasal steroids appear to be local rather than systemic. After nasal administration of steroids, nasal symptoms improve; however, eye symptoms remain.[77] Although combining topical nasal steroids with antihistamines prophylactically has resulted in little additive or synergistic effect in the nose, better control of eye symptoms has been demonstrated.[78]

Topical steroids produce only minor side effects, the most common being sneezing, stinging, and epistaxis. Suppression of the hypothalamic–pituitary–adrenal axis has not been a problem with therapeutic doses.[79] Local infections with *Candida albicans* have occurred rarely. Aqueous corticosteroid nasal sprays have proven to be equally effective to older Freon-propelled delivery systems but with much less nasal bleeding and drying.[80] Table 89.6 lists the available topical steroids and their usual doses.

The therapeutic benefits of topical steroids are not immediate. Patients need to understand this to ensure cooperation and continuation of therapy. Some patients notice improvement in a few days, but peak responses may not be observed for 2–3 weeks. Once a response is achieved the dosage may be reduced. Blocked nasal passages should be cleared with a decongestant before administration to ensure adequate penetration of the spray. Topical steroids should not be used in patients with nasal septum ulcers or recent nasal surgery or trauma.

Cromolyn Sodium

Cromolyn sodium is a mast cell stabilizer. This is a local effect seen in lung mucosa, nasal mucosa, and eyes. A nasal solution is used for the symptomatic prevention and treatment of allergic rhinitis.

Cromolyn sodium has the unique property of preventing antigen-triggered mast cell degranulation and release of the mediators of allergic reactions, including histamine.[81] One hypothesis on the mechanism is that the drug interferes with calcium transport across the mast cell membrane. Cromolyn sodium has no direct antihistaminic, anticholinergic, or anti-inflammatory properties.

TABLE 89.6. DOSAGES OF TOPICAL STEROIDS

Drug	Dosage and Interval
Beclomethasone diproprionate	>12 yr: 1 inhalation (42 μg) per nostril 2–4 times a day (maximum, 336 μg/d) 6–12 yr: 1 inhalation per nostril 3 times per day
Budesonide	>6 yr: 2 sprays (64 μg) per nostril in AM and PM or 4 sprays per nostril in the AM (maximum, 256 μg)
Flunisolide	Adults: 2 sprays (50 μg) per nostril twice daily (maximum, 400 μg) Children: 1 spray per nostril 3 times a day
Triamcinolone acetonide	>12 yr: 2 sprays (110 μg) per nostril once daily (maximum, 440 μg/d)

Similar to topical steroids, the most common side effects result from local irritation—sneezing and nasal stinging.

The dose in adults and children older than 6 years is one spray in each nostril three to four times per day at regular intervals.

For seasonal rhinitis, treatment should be initiated just before the usual start of the offending allergen's season. Treatment should continue throughout this season. In perennial rhinitis, the effects may not be seen for 2–4 weeks; therefore, antihistamines or decongestants may be needed during this initial phase of therapy. As the cromolyn sodium begins to work, the need for these medications should decrease.

Cromolyn sodium must come into contact with the entire nasal lining; therefore, patients should be instructed to clear nasal passages before administration. Inhaling through the nose during administration aids in this process. One author has theorized that if 90% of the nasal lining is reached by the spray, allergic reactions in the remaining 10% can evoke symptoms in the entire mucous membrane.[16]

Future Drug Therapy

Several new agents will soon be available for the treatment of allergic rhinitis. How these agents compare with those just described remains to be seen. Table 89.7 lists and describes some of the drugs currently under investigation.

IMMUNOTHERAPY

History

The first report of the successful use of grass pollen extract injections to treat allergic rhinitis was published in 1911 by Noon.[82] The therapy was first called desensitization; however, this did not seem appropriate because skin reactivity remained. The name was changed to hyposensitization. While the term *hyposensitization* is still used today, immunotherapy has become the most accepted term.

Immunotherapy was widely used for many years without the benefit of controlled clinical trials. In 1954, Franklin and Augustin[83] reported 80% improvement in patients receiving grass pollen extract compared with 33% improvement in a placebo group. Numerous studies are available today documenting the effectiveness of immunotherapy for seasonal pollen-related rhinitis as well as for perennial allergic rhinitis caused by house dust mites and animal dander.[84–88] Opponents have argued that most of the benefit is caused by placebo effect and patient bias. The use of immunotherapy remains somewhat controversial, even in light of the increase in documentation of benefit.

Mechanism of Action

The mechanisms explaining the improvement from allergen immunotherapy remain unclear. Numerous immuno-

TABLE 89.7. FUTURE DRUG THERAPY FOR TREATING ALLERGIC RHINITIS

Drug Name	Class	Comments
Acrivastine	Nonsedating antihistamine	Will probably be combined commercially with pseudoephedrine
Azelastine	Antihistamine	May block the synthesis and release of mediators
Cetirizine	Antihistamine	Metabolite of hydroxyzine, minimal sedation
Fluocortin butyl	Topical corticosteroid	May have higher ratio of local anti-inflammatory activity to systemic activity
Ipratropium	Anticholinergic	Nasal spray dosage form reduces nasal secretions
Ketotifen	Mast cell stabilizer Antihistamine	Orally effective
Mequitazine	Antihistamine	Peripherally acting, nonsedating similar to terfenadine
Oxatomide	Mast cell stabilizer Antihistamine	Orally effective
Zileuton	Leukotriene antagonist	New drug class being investigated for ulcerative colitis, arthritis, asthma, and allergic rhinitis

logic changes have been documented, including suppression of seasonal rises of IgE antibodies,[89] decreased basophil reactivity and sensitivity to allergens,[90] generation of antigen-specific suppressor cells,[91] and production of IgG antibodies that block the allergen–IgE interaction.[92,93]

Adverse Reactions

Adverse reactions can occur with immunotherapy and range from mild to life threatening. Among the most common are mild local reactions consisting of induration and swelling at the site of the injection. Other more serious reactions (e.g., generalized urticaria, bronchospasm, laryngospasm, vascular collapse) occur rarely; however, deaths from anaphylactic reactions to allergen immunotherapy have been reported.[94]

Severe reactions are treated with epinephrine, antihistamines, and systemic corticosteroids. Patients receiving β-adrenergic blocking agents by any route (oral or topical) are at risk for severe, life-threatening anaphylaxis from immunotherapy injections.[95] Many physicians will not prescribe immunotherapy for patients who require these drugs.[96] In general, however, immunotherapy with inhalant allergens conducted by experienced personnel is a safe mode of therapy for resistant rhinitis symptoms. Immunotherapy is safe in pregnancy and does not appear to affect the development of asthma or rhinitis in offsprings.[97] Recent studies have failed to demonstrate any consequences of long-term administration of allergen immunotherapy, such as induction of circulating immune complexes or immune complex-like disorders.[98]

Therapeutic Use

Certain patients are more likely to benefit from immunotherapy. Those whose symptoms are uncontrolled by medication and are unable to avoid the offending allergen should be considered candidates for allergen immunotherapy. Patients with intolerable side effects (e.g., drowsiness, nervousness, urinary retention) or those who become resistant to medication should consider immunotherapy. Patients with coexisting disease states that limit the use of medication (e.g., hypertension, diabetes) may also benefit from this approach to treatment.

The selection of antigens should be based on patient history and skin test results. Numerous regimens for administration of selected allergens have been suggested. In general, very dilute solutions (1:100,000 to 1:1,000,000,000 wt/vol) are given one to two times per week. The concentration is increased until the maximum tolerated dose is achieved. This maintenance dose is continued every 2–6 weeks, depending on clinical response. Best results are usually obtained when injections are given year-round rather than seasonally.[99]

FUTURE DEVELOPMENTS

Future therapeutic strategies might include the use of specific anticytokine antibodies such as IL-4 and IL-5. Topical interferon-γ may also be a future treatment modality.[9] Future research efforts should not focus solely on acquiring additional symptomatic therapies but also on altering the natural course of the illness.

Treatment of allergens with formaldehyde has resulted in products with substantially less allergenicity but only slightly less immunogenicity. This means a higher therapeutic-to-toxic ratio. Thus, maintenance doses are achieved much faster and patients may need booster shots only every 3 months. Polymerized extracts have advantages similar to those of allergoids. The pollen allergen extracts are treated with glutaraldehyde.

EVALUATION OF THERAPEUTIC OUTCOMES

The therapeutic goal for patients with allergic rhinitis is to minimize or prevent symptoms. Evaluation of success is primarily accomplished through discussions with the patient. Both relief of symptoms and tolerance of drug therapy must be discussed. As previously mentioned, many of the pharmacotherapeutic options are used to prevent symptoms. Patients must be thoroughly knowledgeable about the proper timing and administration of prophylactic regimens. If the patient cannot tolerate or is unable to remain compliant with the chosen drug regimen, alternatives should be discussed and mutually selected.

CONCLUSION

Allergic rhinitis is one of the most common diseases in man. Treatment is justified in most cases because of the potential for complications. Therapeutic modalities include avoidance of allergens and pharmacologic management with antihistamines, topical and systemic decongestants, topical steroids, cromolyn sodium, and immunotherapy. Patient counseling regarding the proper selection and use of available drug therapy is crucial to successful management of allergic rhinitis. Future developments in these treatment modalities look promising.

REFERENCES

1. Naclerio R. Allergic rhinitis. N Engl J Med 1991;325(12):860–869.
2. Juniper E, Guyatt G, Andersson B, Ferrie P. Comparison of powder and aerosolized budesonide in perennial rhinitis: Validation of rhinitis quality of life questionaire. Ann Allergy 1993;70:225–230.

3. US Department of Health and Human Services. Asthma and allergies: An optimistic future. Bethesda, MD, Dept of Health and Human Services, 1980, pp 380–388.
4. Weeke E. Epidemiology of allergic diseases in children. Rhinology 1992;13(suppl):5–12.
5. Sibbald B, Rink E. Epidemiology of seasonal and perennial rhinitis: Clinical presentation and medical history. Thorax 1991;46(12):895–901.
6. Smith J. The epidemiology of allergic rhinitis, in Settipane GA (ed): Rhinitis. Allergy Proc 1982:86–91.
7. Evans R. Epidemiology and natural history of asthma, allergic rhinitis, and atopic dermatitis. In Middleton E Jr, Reed CE, Ellis EF, et al (eds): Allergy: Principles and Practice, 4th ed. St Louis, MO Mosby–Year Book, 1993, pp 1109–1136.
8. Sibbald B. Epidemiology of allergic rhinitis, in Burr ML (ed): Epidemiology of Clinical Allergy, Monographs in Allergy. Basel, Karger, 1993, pp 61–79.
9. International Rhinitis Management Working Group. International consensus report on the diagnosis and management of rhinitis. Allergy 1994;49(19):1–34.
10. Platts-Mills T, Hayden M, Chapman M, Wilkins S. Seasonal variation in dust mite and grass pollen allergens in dust from the houses of patients with asthma. J Allergy Clin Immunol 1987;79:781–791.
11. Jacobs R. Non-allergic chronic rhinitis syndromes. Immunol Allergy Clin North Am 1987;7:93.
12. Kivity S, Struhar D, Greif J, Schwartz Y, Topilsky M. Cockroach allergen: An important cause of perennial rhinitis. Allergy 1989;44(4):291–293.
13. Connel J. Nasal disease: Mechanisms and classifications. Ann Allergy 1983;50:227–235.
14. Raphael G, Baraniuk J, Kaliner M. How and why the nose runs. J Allergy Clin Immunol 1991;87(2):457–467.
15. Ballow M. Allergic rhinitis and conjuctivitis. Postgrad Med 1984;76:197–206.
16. Mygind N. Mediators of nasal allergy. J Allergy Clin Immunol 1982;70:149–159.
17. Gomez E, Corrado O, Baldwin D, et al. Direct *in vivo* evidence for mast cell degranulation during allergen-induced reactions in man. J Allergy Clin Immunol 1986;78:637–645.
18. Naclerio R, Togias A. The nasal allergic reaction: Observations on the role of histamine. Clin Exp Allergy 1991;21(suppl 2):13–19.
19. White M, Kaliner M. Mediators of allergic rhinitis. J Allergy Clin Immunol 1992;90(4):699–704.
20. Bradding P, Iain H, Wilson S, et al. Immunolocalization of cytokines in the nasal mucosa of normal and perennial rhinitic subjects. J Immunol 1993;151:3853–3865.
21. Mygind N. Glucocorticosteroids and rhinitis. Allergy 1993;48:476–490.
22. Naclerio R. Inflammation in allergic rhinitis. Res Clin Forums 1992;14:49–55.
23. Lozewicz S, Davies R. Inflammatory cells in allergic rhinitis. Resp Med 1991;85:259–261.
24. Naclaerio R, Proud D, Togias A, et al. Inflammatory mediators in late antigen-induced rhinitis. N Engl J Med 1985;313:65–70.
25. Bentley A. Immunohistology of the nasal mucosa in seasonal allergic rhinitis: Increases in activated eosinophils and epithelial mast cells. J Allergy Clin Immunol 1992;89:877–883.
26. Cowart B, Flynn-Rodden K, McGeady S, Lowry L. Hyposmia in allergic rhinitis. J Allergy Clin Immunol 1993;91(3):747–751.
27. Apter A, Mott A, Cain W, et al. Olfactory loss and allergic rhinitis (clinical conference). J Allergy Clin Immunol 1992;90(4):670–680.
28. Fireman P. Nasal allergy: A risk factor for middle ear disease. Ann Allergy 1987;58:395–400.
29. Todd N. Allergy as a cause of otitis media. Immunol Allergy Clin North Am 1987;7:371–381.
30. Bernstein J. Otitis media with effusion: An allergic disease? Compr Ther 1980;6:15–21.
31. Nuss R, Berman S. Medical management of persistent middle ear effusion. Am J Asthma Allergy Pediatr 1990;4:17–22.
32. Trask G, Shapiro G, Shapiro P. The effects of perennial allergic rhinitis on dental and skeletal development: A comparison of sibling pairs. Am J Orthodont Dentofac Orthoped 1987;92(4):286–293.
33. Shapiro G, Shapiro P. Nasal airway obstruction and facial development. Clin Rev Allergy 1984;2:225–236.
34. Kalliner M, Lemanske R. Rhinitis and asthma. JAMA 1992;268(20):2807–2829.
35. Linna O, Kokkonen J, Lukin M. A 10-year prognosis for childhood allergic rhinitis. Acta Paediatrica 1992;81(2):100–102.
36. Aberg N, Engstrom I. Natural history of allergic diseases in children. Acta Paediatr Scand 1990;79(2):206–211.
37. Verdiani P, Di C S, Baronti A. Different prevalence and degree of nonspecific bronchial hyperreactivity between seasonal and perennial rhinitis. J Allergy Clin Immunol 1990;86(4):576–582.
38. Shapiro G. Role of allergy in sinusitis. Ped Infect Dis 1985;4(suppl 6):S55–S59.
39. Sibbald B, Rink E. Labeling of rhinitis and hayfever by doctors. Thorax 1991;46(5):378–381.
40. Romero J, Scadding G. Eosinophilia in nasal secretions compared to skin prick and nasal challenge in the diagnosis of nasal allergy. Rhinology 1992;30(3):169–175.
41. Turkeltaub P. Skin testing, in Creticos PS (ed): Immunotherapy: A Practical Guide to Current Procedures. Milwaukee, American Academy of Allergy and Immunology, 1994, vol 2, p 2–11.
42. Turkeltaub P. Standardized extracts in practice, in Creticos PS (ed): Immunotherapy: A Practical Guide to Current Procedures. Milwaukee, American Academy of Allergy and Immunology, 1994, vol 4, p 4-4.
43. Lee R, Smolensky M, Leach C. Circadium rhythms in the cutaneous reactivity to histamine and selected antigens, including phase relationship to urinary cortisol excretion. Ann Allergy 1977;38:231–236.
44. Badhwar A, Druce H. Allergic rhinitis. Med Clin North Am 1992;76(4):789–803.
45. Colloff M, Ayres J, Carswell F, et al. The control of allergens of dust mites and domestic pets: A position paper. Clin Exp Allergy 1992;22(suppl. 2):1–28.
46. Wood R, Chapman M, Adkinson N. The effect of cat removal on allergen content in household dust samples. J Allergy Clin Immunol 1989;83:730.
47. Andersen A, Roesen J. House dust mite, *Dermatophagoides pteronyssinus,* and its allergens: Effects of washing. Allergy 1989;44(6):396–400.

48. Sporik S, Holgate S, Platts-Mills T. Exposure to house dust mite allergen and the development of asthma in childhood: A prospective study. N Engl J Med 1990;323:502.
49. Kooistra J, Pasch R, Reed C. The effects of air cleaners on hay fever symptoms in air conditioned homes. J Allergy Clin Immunol 1978;61:315–319.
50. Reisman R, Mauriello P, Davis G, et al. A double-blind study of the effectiveness of a high efficiency particulate air (HEPA) filter in the treatment of patients with perennial allergic rhinitis and asthma. J Allergy Clin Immunol 1990;85(6):1050–1057.
51. Delafuente JC, Davis TA, Davis JA. Pharmacotherapy of allergic rhinitis. Clin Pharm 1989;8:474–485.
52. Shevchuk YM, Plosker GL. A medical marvel. Can Pharm J 1987:597–601.
53. Delafuente JC. Use of H_2 histamine antagonists in allergic disorders. Clin Pharm 1988;7:422.
54. Simons FER, Simon KJ. H_1 receptor antagonists. Clinical pharmacology and use in allergic disease. Pediatr Clin North Am 1983;30:899–914.
55. Fowle ASE, Hughes DTD, Knight GJ. The evaluation of histamine antagonists in man. Eur J Clin Pharmacol 1971;3:215–220.
56. Bye CE, Claridge R, Peck AW, et al. Evidence for tolerance to central nervous effects of the histamine antagonist, triprolidine, in man. Eur J Clin Pharmacol 1977;12:181–186.
57. Garrison JC. Histamine, bradykinin, 5-hydroxytryptamine and their antagonists, in Gilman AG, Rall TW, Nies AS, et al (eds): The Pharmacological Basis of Therapeutics, 8th ed. New York, Macmillan, 1990, pp 575–599.
58. Mann KV, Crowe JP, Tietze KJ. Nonsedating histamine H_1-receptor antagonists. Clin Pharm 1989;8:331–344.
59. Cooper JW. Antihistamines and decongestants in the treatment of chronic rhinitis, in Settipane GA (ed): Rhinitis. Providence, RI, New England and Regional Allergy Proceedings, 1982, pp 103–107.
60. Mygind N. Clinical investigations of allergic rhinitis and allied conditions. Allergy 1979;34:195–208.
61. Pentel P. Toxicity of over-the-counter stimulants. JAMA 1984;252:1898–1903.
62. Horowitz JD, Lang WJ, Howes LG, et al. Hypertensive response induced by phenylpropanolamine in anorectic and decongestant preparations. Lancet 1980;1:60–61.
63. Empey DE, Young GA, Letley E, et al. Dose response study of the nasal decongestant and cardiovascular effects of pseudoephedrine. Br J Clin Pharmacol 1980;9:351–358.
64. Drew CDM, Knight GT, Hughes DTD, et al. Comparison of the effects of D-(−)ephedrine and L-(+)-pseudoephedrine on the cardiovascular and respiratory systems in man. Br J Clin Pharmacol 1978;6:221–225.
65. Hansten PD. Monoamine oxidase inhibitor interactions, in Drug Interactions, 5th ed. Philadelphia, Lea and Febiger, 1985.
66. Diamond L, Gerson K, Cato A, et al. An evaluation of triprolidine and pseudoephedrine in the treatment of allergic rhinitis. Ann Allergy 1981;47:87–91.
67. Connell JT, Williams BO, Allen S, et al. A double-blind controlled evaluation of Actifed and its individual constituents in allergic rhinitis. J Intern Med Res 1982;10:341–347.
68. Hebert J, Bedard PM, Carpio JD, et al. Loratadine and pseudoephedrine sulfate: A double-blind placebo-controlled comparison of a combination tablet (SCH 434) and its individual components in seasonal allergic rhinitis. Am J Rhinol 1988;2:71–75.
69. Dockhorn RJ, Shellenberger MK, Moore KS, et al. Evaluation of acrivastine and pseudoephedrine in seasonal allergic rhinitis [abstract]. Ann Allergy 1985;55:393.
70. Pauwels R. Mode of action of corticosteroids in asthma and rhinitis. Clin Allergy 1986;16:281–288.
71. Pipkorn V, Proud D, Lichtenstein LM, et al. Inhibition of mediator release in allergic rhinitis by pretreatment with topical glucocorticosteroids. N Engl J Med 1987;316:1506–1510.
72. Holmes TH, Treuting T, Wolff HG. Life situations, emotions, and nasal disease. Evidence on summative effects inhibited in patients with hay fever. Psychosom Med 1951;13:71–82.
73. Sorenson H, Mygind N, Pedersen CB, et al. Long-term treatment of nasal polyps with beclomethasone dipropionate aerosol. III. Morphological studies and conclusions. Acta Otolaryngol 1976;82:260–263.
74. Molm L, Wihl JA, Lamm CJ, et al. Reduction of metacholine-induced nasal secretion by treatment with a new topical steroid in perennial non-allergic rhinitis. Allergy 1981;36:209–214.
75. Okuda M, Senba O. Effects of beclomethasone dipropionate spray on subjective and objective findings in perennial allergic rhinitis. Clin Otolaryngol 1980;5:315–321.
76. Gomez E, Clague JE, Gatland D, et al. Effect of topical corticosteroids on seasonally induced increases in nasal mast cell. Br Med J 1988;296:572–573.
77. Mygind N. Local effects of intranasal betamethasone dipropionate aerosol in hay fever. Br Med J 1973;4:464–466.
78. Juniper EF, Kline PA, Hargreave FE, et al. Comparison of beclomethasone dipropionate aqueous nasal spray, astemizole, and the combination in the prophylactic treatment of ragweed pollen-induced rhinoconjunctivitis. J Allergy Clin Immunol 1989;83:627–633.
79. Small P, Black M, Frenkiel S, et al. Beclomethasone dipropionate in the management of rhinitis—a review. Ann Allergy 1982;49:127–130.
80. Dunn AM, Wilson RSE, Baggott PJ. A comparison of beclomethasone diproprionate aqueous nasal spray and beclomethasone dipropionate pressurized nasal spray in the management of seasonal rhinitis. Postgrad Med J 1984;60:404–406.
81. Foreman JC, Garland LG. Cromoglycate and other antiallergic drugs: A possible mode of action. Br Med J 1976;1:820–821.
82. Noon L. Prophylactic inoculation against hayfever. Lancet 1911;1:1572–1573.
83. Franklin A, Augustin R. Prophylaxis of summer hayfever and asthma: Controlled trial comparing crude grass pollen extracts and isolated main protein component. Lancet 1954;1:1055–1057.
84. Johnstone D. Immunotherapy in the prevention of allergic disease. Pediatr Asthma Allergy Immunol 1987;1:15–30.
85. Varney V, Gaga M, Frew A, et al. Usefulness of immunotherapy in patients with severe summer hay fever uncontrolled by antiallergic drugs. BMJ 1991;302:265–269.

86. Corrado O, Pastorello E, Ollier S. A double-blind study of hyposensitization with an alginate conjugate extract of *Dermatophagoides pteronyssinus* (Conjuvac®) in patients with perennial rhinitis. Allergy 1989;44:108–115.
87. Ewan P, Alexander M, Snape C, et al. Effective hyposensitization in allergic rhinitis using a partially purified extract of house dust mite. Clin Allergy 1988;18:501–508.
88. Lofkvist T, Agrell B, Dreborg S, Svensson G. Effects of immunotherapy with a purified standardized allergen preparation of *Dermatophagoides farinae* in adults with perennial allergic rhinoconjuctivitis. Allergy 1994;49(2):100–107.
89. Lichtenstein L, Ishizaka K, Norman P, et al. IgE antibody measurements in ragweed hay fever: Relationship to clinical severity and the results of immunotherapy. J Clin Invest 1973;52:472–482.
90. Pruzansky J, Patterson R. Histamine release of leukocytes of hypersensitive patients. II. Reduced sensitivity of leukocytes after injection therapy. J Allergy 1967;39:44–50.
91. Rocklin R, Sheffer A, Greindar D, et al. Generation of antigen-specific suppressor cells during allergy desensitization. N Engl J Med 1980;302:1213–1219.
92. Pecquet C, Murrieta M, Michelen V, et al. Blocking activity of mite-specific IgG antibodies studied by skin tests. Allergy 1989;44(6):427–431.
93. Darcy M, Wilson A, Wheeler A. The IgG subclass of antibodies to grass pollen allergens produced in hay fever patients during hyposensitization. Clin Allergy 1976;6:227–236.
94. Lockey R, Benedict L, Turkeltahb P, et al. Fatalities from immunotherapy and skin testing. J Allergy Clin Immunol 1987;79:660–677.
95. Togood J. Risk of anaphylaxis in patients receiving β-blocker drugs. J Allergy Clin Immunol 1988;81:1–5.
96. Executive Committee of the American Academy of Allergy and Immunology. Position statement: β-Adrenergic blockers, immunotherapy, and skin testing. J Allergy Clin Immunol 1989;84:129–130.
97. Settipane R, Chafee F, Settipane G. Pollen immunotherapy in pregnancy: Long-term follow-up of offsprings. Allergy Proceed 1988;9(5):555–561.
98. Katelaris C, Walls R. A study of possible ill effects from prolonged immunotherapy in treatment of allergic disease. Ann Allergy 1984;53:257–261.
99. Rocklin R. Clinical and immunologic aspects of allergen specific immunotherapy in patients with seasonal allergic rhinitis and/or asthma. J Allergy Clin Immunol 1983;72:323–334.

Section 12
Dermatologic Disorders

Chapter 90

Common Skin Disorders: Acne and Psoriasis

Phillip A. Nowakowski, PharmD, Jean A. Rumsfield, PharmD, and Dennis P. West, PhD, FCCP

Nearly 2000 skin disorders are readily visible and brought to the attention of health care practitioners daily. Skin rash is a frequent reason for visits to physicians.[1] The pharmacist's role in dermatology can be quite varied and depends on the particular cutaneous abnormality. A pharmacist may screen patients to identify dermatologic disorders, identify drug-induced causes of dermatoses, initiate drug therapy (considering vehicle and active ingredients), and monitor for therapeutic effect, adverse reactions, and patient compliance.

The clinical approach to solving dermatologic problems involves analysis, assessment, establishment, and initiation of a treatment plan followed by careful drug monitoring (Table 90.1). This algorithm is similar to problem-solving approaches in other specialties, but major differences include the development of an objective database by physical examination of the integument and lesions as well as description of the dermatoses in specific, brief, concise, and uniform terminology. Important aspects of the physical examination of skin and definitions of lesion types are presented. This is designed to assist the pharmacist in identifying common dermatologic disorders and appropriate treatment regimens. Examination of the skin should include observations on color and consistency of lesions, anatomic localization and distribution, configuration, size, border, and other superficial characteristics.

Lesion Morphology

COLOR

Lesion color, attributed to a variety of causes, is of major diagnostic importance. The consistency of color should also be noted. Some lesions have consistent color throughout, while others may vary in color from the border to an area of central clearing (see Table 90.2).

DISTRIBUTION

The distribution of lesions may be helpful in determining a diagnosis (Figs. 90.1 and 90.2). Lesions may be localized to an anatomic area or generalized over the surface of the body. Lesions involving only exposed areas or body-fold areas (intertriginous) should be differentiated.

CONFIGURATION

Configuration is also essential to diagnosis and may be defined as the relationship of one lesion to another or how lesions are grouped (see Table 90.3).

Lesion size can be approximated in centimeters or using familiar objects (e.g., 5 cm or the size of a dime); bor-

TABLE 90.1. AN APPROACH TO SOLVING THE DERMATOLOGIC PROBLEMS OF PATIENTS[a]

Knowledge Base	Action	Patient Data Base
Dermatologic manifestations	Analyze the problem	Subjective data Objective data
Therapeutic endpoints	Assess the problem	
Risk versus benefit	Establish optimal treatment plan for the patient	
Pharmaceutic and pharmacokinetic considerations		
Drug/disease/lab interactions		
Monitoring parameters	Monitor the patient Therapeutic effect Adverse effects Compliance	

[a]The approach to any dermatologic problem is basically the same; however, the distribution of responsibilities between physician and pharmacist varies, depending on the diagnosis and whom the patient approaches first.

ders should be categorized as demarcated (sharply circumscribed) or diffuse (ill defined). Superficial characteristics such as elevations or depressions in skin, changes in texture, presence of moisture or dried exudate, and firmness should also be noted. Usually, the characteristics of a lesion are communicated in a few singular terms describing the morphologic "type" of lesion. Description of lesion type, along with color, distribution, size, and configuration, is the most accepted method of communicating what is noted by physical assessment. Use of uniform terminology aids in diagnosis and allows others to visualize the lesions. The glossary at the end of the chapter defines the most common lesion types.

ACNE

Acne is a common, self-limiting, multifactorial disease involving the sebaceous follicles of the face and upper trunk. Acne affects 80% of the population between the ages of 12 and 25.[2] In the United States, at least 350,000 patients have acne severe enough to require treatment. Although acne is generally self-limiting and non-life-threatening, the psychologic effect on patients is profound. This is reflected in the amount of money spent on acne therapy in the United States each year. Sales of nonprescription acne medications exceed $100 million; an equivalent amount is spent on antiacne prescription drugs.[2] The pharmacist plays a major role in educating patients on causes of acne, recommending treatment regimens, and counseling on proper drug use.

PATHOPHYSIOLOGY

The causes of acne are multifactorial and not completely understood (Fig. 90.3). Etiologic theories of acne include the role of androgens, *Propionibacterium acnes,* sebum production, and follicle growth.

Sebaceous follicles, which normally produce substances to moisturize the skin, are found on the face, chest, back, and shoulders. A cross-sectional view of the sebaceous follicle (Fig. 90.4) illustrates the opening to the skin (orifice or pore) and a long narrow canal extending into the dermis. Sebaceous glands develop at puberty in response to androgen stimulation and are attached to the follicle canal by sebaceous ducts. Sebum produced in sebaceous glands is transported through ducts to the canal and onto the surface of the skin. The follicular canal may also contain fine vellus hair, keratinous material (similar to skin surface cells), and bacteria (usually *P. acnes*). Acne is believed to be caused by a derangement in the structure or function of the normal sebaceous follicle.

Formation of the primary lesion, the comedo (or comedone), may be simplistically thought of as plugging of the sebaceous follicle. Histologically, a widening of the fol-

TABLE 90.2. EXAMPLES OF LESIONAL COLOR VARIATION

Lesion Description	Color	Pathophysiologic Mechanism	Precipitating Factor(s)
Hyperpigmented	Darkened areas	Melanin deposition	Pregnancy, sunlight, oral contraceptives
Hypopigmented	Lightened	Lack of melanin	Autoimmune phenomena
Jaundiced	Yellowish	Increased bilirubin or carotene	Hepatitis
Cyanotic	Bluish	Excess reduced hemoglobin	Hypoxia
	Reddish blue	Capillary stasis	Increased red blood cells
Erythematous	Red	Dilation of blood vessels	Inflammation, sunburn
Violaceous	Purple	Aging lesion, formerly erythematous	Bruising trauma

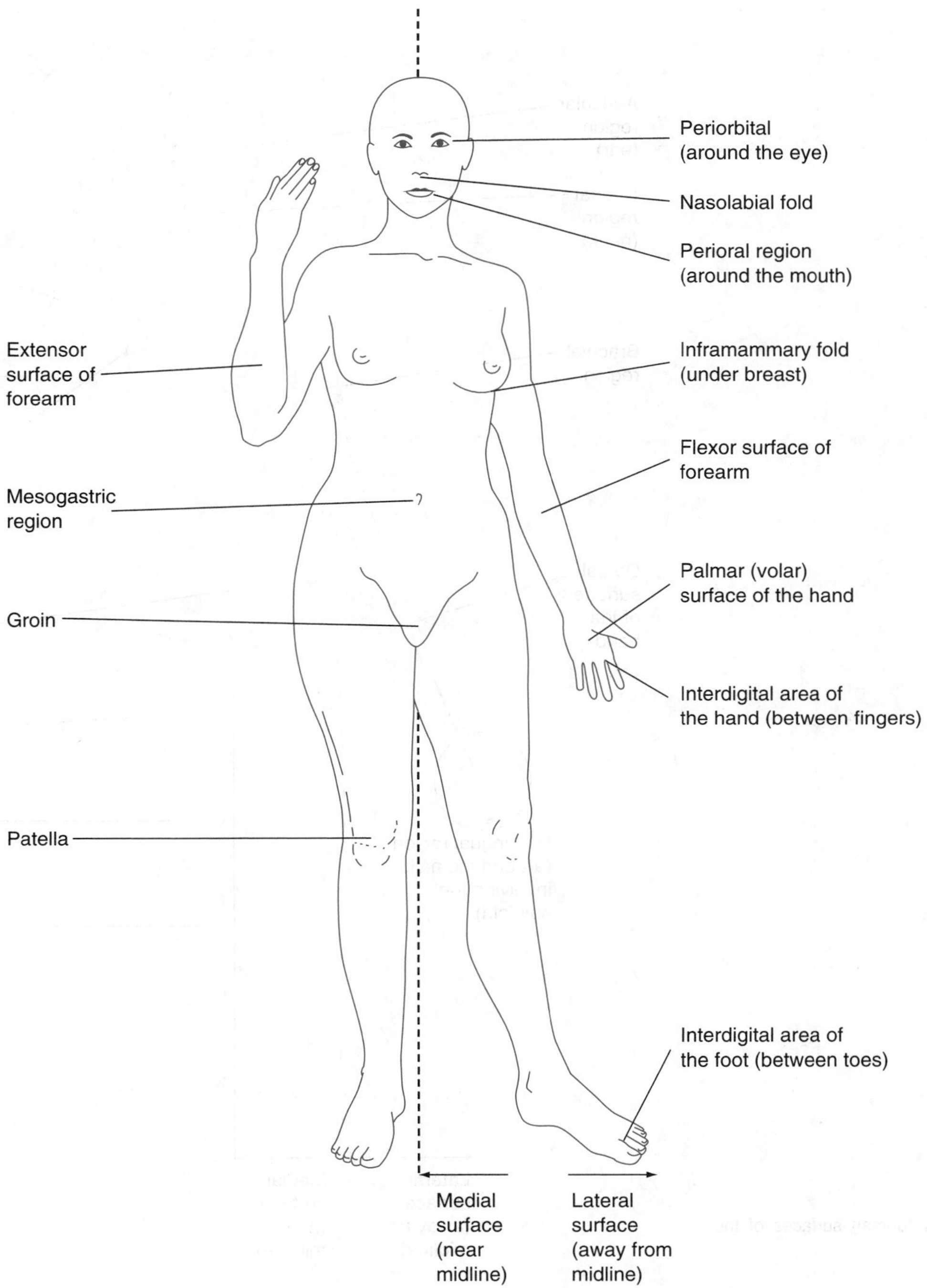

Figure 90.1. Anterior (ventral) surfaces of the body.

licular canal along with an increase in cell production is seen.[3] Sebaceous glands atrophy and sebum mixes with excess loose cells in the follicular canal to form a keratinous plug. This lesion clinically appears as a "blackhead," or open comedo. Trauma or inflammatory changes in the primary lesion may lead to formation of a "whitehead," or closed comedo. If the follicular wall is damaged or ruptured by trauma or irritation, the contents of the follicle may extrude into dermis and initiate an inflammatory reaction clinically seen as a pustule. Factors that induce or transform acne lesions are unknown.

Androgens

Androgens stimulate growth of sebaceous follicles and enhance production of sebum. During the second decade of

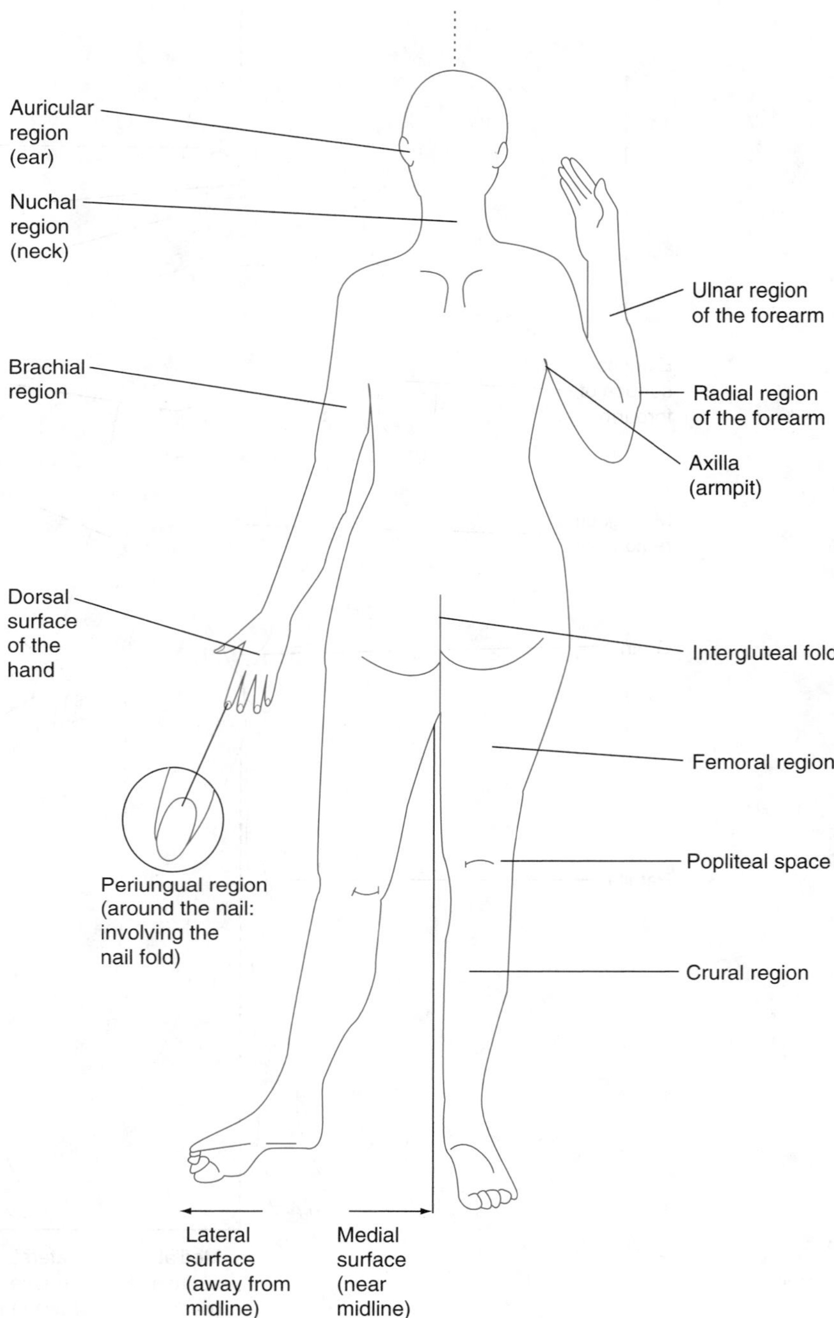

Figure 90.2. Posterior (dorsal) surfaces of the body.

life, sebum production closely parallels both androgen production and the presence of acne. Although testosterone is the most potent androgen, its metabolites and weaker androgens (e.g., androstenedione, dehydroepiandrosterone, dehydroepiandrosterone sulfate) are increased in acne patients and may stimulate sebaceous gland activity.[3] Skin, hair follicles, and sebaceous glands can metabolize androgens to active dihydrostestosterone, and acne-prone skin may demonstrate increased increased metabolic activity.[3]

TABLE 90.3. EXAMPLES OF LESIONAL CONFIGURATION

Type	Description
Clustered	Grouped lesions
Linear	Straight line
Annular	Circular
Polycyclic	Two or more adjacent, circular lesions
Serpiginous	Snakelike with wavy borders
Geographic	Irregular maplike borders

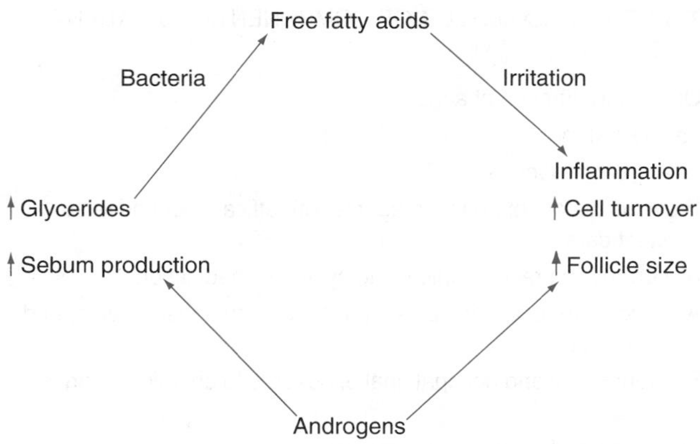

Figure 90.3. Acne pathogenesis.

These abnormalities are not, however, found in all acne patients, and more specific diagnostic tools are being developed to assess endocrine abnormalities in acne.

Sebum Production

Sebum is produced in the sebaceous glands and consists of glycerides, wax esters, squalene, and cholesterol. At times, a relationship between increased sebum secretion and severity of acne is present.[4] The glyceride component of sebum is converted to free fatty acids and glycerol by lipases, products of *P. acnes.*[5] Free fatty acids may irritate the follicular wall and cause increased cell turnover and inflammation.[4] More recently this has been considered an oversimplification; glycerol has been identified as a substrate for *P. acnes,* while free fatty acids may function as a measure of *P. acnes* activity and viability.

Follicle Growth

Abnormal alterations in the follicle wall and its cell growth (keratinization) have been noted histologically in association with acne.[4] The increased production of loosely adherent keratin cells has been correlated with obstruction of the follicles seen in comedo formation. Whether this abnormality is inherent or secondary to irritation or other factors is uncertain. Steroid acne has been recognized with common use of corticosteroids in organ transplant and oncologic treatment regimens. Although the precise pathogenesis of steroid acne is still controversial, folliculitis has been reported to be a common denominator between acne vulgaris and steroid acne.[6]

Bacteria

P. acnes is part of the normal flora in the sebaceous follicle and plays an important role in the initial development and maintenance of the inflammatory response present in acne. Although *P. acnes* counts are typically higher in patients with acne, and antibiotic therapy reduces these counts, the pathogenic role of *P. acnes* is not that of simple infection. *P. acnes* may be considered antigenic and capable of causing increased antibody formation (IgG, IgM), leading to an inflammatory response.[5] Immune complex-mediated complement activation as a result of *P. acnes* may lead to vascular leakage, mast cell degranulation, and leukocyte chemotaxis.[5] Levels of antibodies to *P. acnes* are higher in patients with severe forms of acne than in normal controls. *P. acnes* may activate the complement cascade via both classic and alternate pathways and produce direct tissue damage.[5] Also, chemotactic factors may be secreted by *P. acnes,* diffuse through the follicle wall, and activate neutrophil chemotaxis and complement.[2] Hydrolytic enzymes released by complement activation may damage the follicle wall and lead to more severe, inflammatory acne. Neutrophils are an important factor in severe inflammatory acne and patients may demonstrate neutrophil defects of either very high or low chemotaxis as well as impaired phagocytosis. *P. acnes* may also evoke a cell-mediated immune

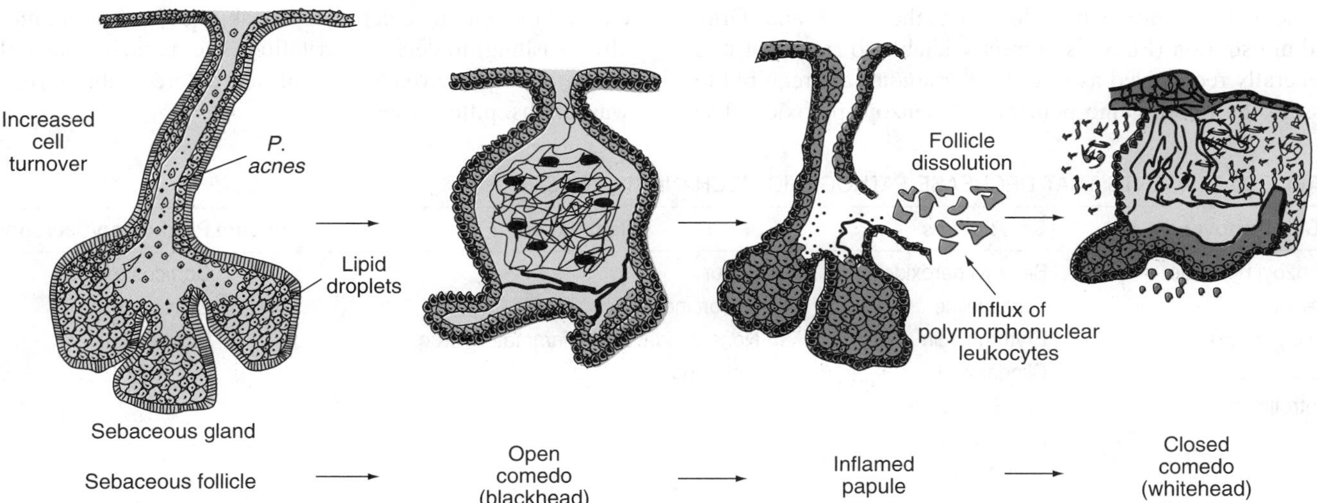

Figure 90.4. Cross-sectional view of the sebaceous follicle.

response, but this is yet to be clarified.[5] Although the exact cause of acne is unclear, its pathogenesis involves many factors that are interrelated (Figs. 90.3 and 90.4).

CLINICAL PRESENTATION

Clinically, acne ranges from mild (few open comedones) to severe (multiple inflamed papules, pustules, and nodule-sized lesions). Acne lesions may take as long as a month to develop and several months to heal completely. Fibrosis associated with healing may lead to permanent scarring. Most forms of adolescent acne are self-limiting, but more severe forms may be persistent and require advanced treatment.

ASSESSMENT

An in-depth drug and medical history should be obtained to determine what, if any, acne exacerbating factors can be eliminated (see Table 90.4).

TABLE 90.4. EXAMPLES OF COMPONENTS TO PATIENT HISTORY FOR ACNE

Onset and duration of acne
Family history
Exacerbating factors
Previous history of antiacne agents with efficacy and adverse effect data
All current and recent topical and systemic medications
All topical products such as soaps, moisturizers, astringents, and cosmetics
Environmental and occupational exposures to chemicals and toxins
Allergies (food, drug, environmental)

TOPICAL TREATMENT

Aggressive therapy may be required to modify or inhibit inflammatory acne. An important goal of therapy is to prevent or minimize scarring, and the treatment of choice depends on severity and individual patient tolerance. Because acne is a multifactorial process, multiple treatment approaches may be required for control. Medications may be grouped according to their proposed mechanism of action on acne (Table 90.5). Tables 90.6 and 90.7 summarize treatment guidelines.

Benzoyl Peroxide

Benzoyl peroxide is an effective treatment for mild and moderately severe acne. However, the Food and Drug Administration (FDA) is currently unable to state that it is generally recognized as safe; further studies are required to assess the tumorigenic potential of benzoyl peroxide. The mechanism of action is uncertain, although benzoyl peroxide is decomposed on the skin by cysteine, liberating free oxygen radicals that oxidize bacterial proteins.[7] Daily application of 10% benzoyl peroxide for 2 weeks can reduce free fatty acid levels by 50% and *P. acnes* levels by 98%.[7] Benzoyl peroxide is also a primary irritant that increases the sloughing rate of epithelial cells, loosens the follicular plug structure, and thus is comedolytic.[8]

Dryness and irritation from benzoyl peroxide may limit therapy in some patients and contact dermatitis may occur in 1–3% of patients.[9] To limit irritation and increase patient tolerance to benzoyl peroxide, one may initiate therapy with a low potency (2.5%) and increase strength (5–10%) or slowly increase application frequency (every other day, each day, then twice a day).

Benzoyl peroxide is available in soaps, lotions, creams, and gels. Gel formulations are usually most potent, while the lotions and soaps are of weaker potency. Gels are usually alcohol, propylene glycol, or water based; the alcohol-based preparations generally cause more dryness and irritation. Fair or moist skin is usually more sensitive to irritation from benzoyl peroxide; thus, patients should be advised to apply medication to dry skin (at least 30 minutes after washing) to decrease irritation. The oxidizing capability of benzoyl peroxide may bleach colored fabrics (e.g., washcloths, pillowcases).

TABLE 90.5. AGENTS THAT DECREASE PATHOGENIC MECHANISMS IN ACNE

Cell Turnover	*P. acnes*	Inflammation	Sebum Production/Secretion
Benzoyl peroxide	Benzoyl peroxide	Sulfur	Corticosteroids
Tretinoin	Tetracycline	Resorcinol	Estrogens
Salicylic acid	Erythromycin	Nonsteroidal anti-inflammatory drugs	Isotretinoin
Abrasives	Clindamycin	Isotretinoin	
Isotretinoin	Co-trimoxazole		
	Minocycline		
	Isotretinoin		
	Azelaic acid		

TABLE 90.6. TOPICAL TREATMENT GUIDELINES

Active Ingredient	Formulation	Strength	Regimen	Potential Side Effects
Benzoyl peroxide	Soaps, lotions, creams, gels	2.5–10%	Initially every other day or daily, then twice daily	Irritation based on form and strength
Tretinoin	Cream, gel, solution	0.025–0.05%	Initially every other day or daily	Excessive drying, erythema Concomitant use of other irritants increases adverse effects
Sulfur/resorcinol/salicylic acid	Creams, lotions, gels, soaps	0.5–10% in various combinations	Daily	
Clindamycin	Solution, gel, lotion	1%	Twice daily	Drying, gastrointestinal effects
Tetracycline	Solution	2.2%	Twice daily	Burning and stinging following application, skin discoloration
Erythromycin	Solution, powder; gel as a combination product	1.5–2%	Twice daily	Drying, erythema

Azelaic Acid

Topical azelaic acid apparently interfers with DNA synthesis in some of the bacteria associated with acne vulgaris. Inhibition of thioredoxin reductase by azelaic acid provides a rationale for this property.[10] In a series of investigations using 20% azelaic acid cream as a therapy for acne, it was found that the treatment, compared with its placebo, significantly reduced inflamed lesions after 1 month and noninflamed lesions after 2 months.[11] In an open study of 100 unselected patients of either gender, the rates of improvement obtained indicate that topical 20% azelaic acid cream can be considered an effective therapy chiefly for papulopustular acne and with a good patient tolerance.[12]

Tretinoin

Tretinoin (topical vitamin A acid) is unique in its effect on the follicular epithelium. Tretinoin increases cell turnover in the follicular wall and decreases cohesiveness of cells, leading to extrusion of existing comedones and inhibition of the formation of new comedones.[13] Tretinoin also decreases the number of cell layers in the stratum corneum from 14 to 5.[7] A "flare" of acne may suddenly appear after 3–6 weeks of treatment followed by clinical clearing by 8–12 weeks.[13] Irritation, erythema, and peeling often limit successful therapy and allergic contact dermatitis has been reported in a few cases, although not as frequently as with benzoyl peroxide.[13] Tolerance to irritation may be managed by titrating strength and frequency of application. Tretinoin is currently available in 0.05% solution (most irritating), 0.01% and 0.025% gel, and 0.025%, 0.05%, and 0.1% cream (least irritating). Treatment initiation with 0.025% cream is usually recommended for mild acne in people with fair complexions, 0.01% gel for moderate acne in fair skin with oily complexion, and 0.025% gel for severe acne with oily skin.

Patients should be advised to apply the medication to dry skin approximately 30 minutes after washing to minimize erythema and irritation. Slowly increasing application frequency from every other day to daily, then twice daily over a few weeks to months may increase tolerance to tretinoin. Increased sensitivity to sun exposure, wind, cold, and other irritants has also been evident in patients using tretinoin. A combination of benzoyl peroxide each morning and tretinoin at bedtime may enhance efficacy and be less irritating than either agent used alone.[14]

Sulfur/Resorcinol/Salicylic Acid

These topical agents are keratolytic and mildly antibacterial. The term *keratolytic* refers to the effect of solubilization of the intracellular cement of keratin cells in the stratum corneum. Although evidence for efficacy in treatment of acne is conflicting, each agent has been classified as effective by an advisory review panel of the FDA. Combinations of these agents are often considered synergistic (e.g., sulfur and resorcinol, salicylic acid and benzoyl peroxide). These products may be less irritating than benzoyl peroxide and tretinoin; however, they are not considered effective comedolytic agents as are benzoyl peroxide and tretinoin. Disadvantages of these agents include the odor created by hydrogen sulfide upon reaction of sulfur with the skin, the brown scale from use of resorcinol, and salicylism from long-term use of high concentrations of salicylic acid on permeable (inflamed and/or abraded) skin.

Topical Antibacterial Products

Topical antibacterials (e.g., clindamycin, erythromycin, tetracycline) have been used effectively to treat acne by concentrating medication to the affected area and subsequently decreasing the risk of systemic toxicity. Clinical tri-

TABLE 90.7. ORAL TREATMENT GUIDELINES

Active Ingredient	Formulation	Strength	Regimen	Potential Side Effects
Tetracycline	Tablets, capsules	250–500 mg	1 g/d initial; if no response in 2–3 weeks or severe acne, 2–3 g/d Maintenance 125–500 mg/d	Gastrointestinal upset, hypersensitivity syndromes Photosensitivity Drug and food interactions
Erythromycin	Tablets as various salts	250–500 mg	1 g/d as base; if no response in 2–3 weeks or severe acne, 2–3 g/d Maintenance 250–500 mg/d	Gastrointestinal upset, rashes Drug interactions
Clindamycin	Capsules	75–150–300 mg	300–450 mg/d	Diarrhea, pseudomembranous colitis
Isotretinoin	Capsules	10–20–40 mg	0.5–1 mg/kg/d in two divided doses Maximum of 2 mg/kg/d	Cheilitis, erythema, dryness Gastrointestinal effects Teratogenicity

als that compare the efficacy of topical versus systemic antibacterials are difficult to evaluate because early formulations were often prepared extemporaneously or different vehicles were used.[15,16]

Clindamycin is considered the most effective topical antibacterial agent for acne, although no well-controlled trials have been conducted. In one study, *in vivo* topical clindamycin significantly reduced the numbers of *P. acnes,* while topical erythromycin and tetracycline did not[17]; however, reduction of the percentage of free fatty acids in sebum has been noted with the use of topical tetracycline and erythromycin.[17]

A topical preparation of erythromycin plus zinc has been reported to be significantly better than 500 mg/d oral tetracycline in reducing overall acne severity and papule lesion counts.[18] In a randomized, double-blind study of 122 patients with acne vulgaris, a 4% erythromycin and zinc combination lotion was more effective than 2% erythromycin lotion. The higher concentration of erythromycin may have been more effective, or the zinc acetate complex may enhance the penetration of erythromycin into the skin.[19]

Disadvantages of topical antibiotic dosage forms include occasional irritation and stinging upon application. Although tetracycline is the most frequently prescribed oral antibiotic for acne, it is the least frequently prescribed topical antibiotic. On the skin, tetracycline photo-oxidizes to produce a visible yellow tinting with a relative lack of efficacy.[17] Diarrhea and pseudomembranous colitis may occur from the use of topical clindamycin.[20,21] Antimicrobial resistance from widespread use of topical antibiotics for acne has been postulated but not substantiated as a serious clinical problem.[17]

Oral Antibacterial Agents

Few well-controlled, double-blind studies have been conducted on the efficacy of oral antibiotics in acne. Nevertheless, oral antibiotics are considered effective and relatively safe for inflammatory types of acne.[17,22] Tetracycline (and derivatives), erythromycin, clindamycin, and trimethoprim/sulfamethoxazole can significantly decrease the percentage of free fatty acids in skin surface lipids and also decrease numbers of *P. acnes.*[17] Tetracycline exhibits additional activity by reducing the amount of keratin in sebaceous follicles and by inhibiting chemotaxis, phagocytosis, complement activation (by the alternate pathway), and cell-mediated immunity.[17] Tetracycline also appears to have an affinity for inflammatory cells and bacteria, resulting in higher drug concentrations in areas of inflamed skin.[17] Drawbacks to the use of tetracycline include a drug–food interaction with dairy products, photosensitivity, gastrointestinal disturbances, and predisposition to superinfections (i.e., vaginal candidiasis).

Clindamycin use for acne is limited by diarrhea and risk of pseudomembranous colitis. Erythromycin may have a safer adverse effect profile when compared with tetracycline; efficacy profiles are similar.[17,23] In refractory cases, minocycline or doxycycline may be effective because of greater lipid solubility and enhanced penetration into tissue and sebaceous follicles.[8,24] Disadvantages of minocycline include a high incidence of vestibular toxicity and discoloration of skin and teeth.[24]

Although trimethoprim/sulfamethoxazole may be effective in tetracycline-resistant acne, it should perhaps be reserved for refractory cases to minimize the risk of resistance.[17,25]

Another consideration in the use of oral antibiotics for acne is a potential interaction with oral contraceptives. Ampicillin and tetracycline apparently decrease the intestinal flora needed to hydrolyze conjugated ethinyl estradiol excreted into the bile; thus, enterohepatic recirculation is interrupted and the amount of active estrogen is reduced.[26] The clinical importance of this interaction is not well established, but several pregnancies have been reported with concurrent use of ampicillin or tetracycline and oral contraceptives.[26] Women taking oral contraceptives (especially agents containing less than 50 g estrogen) should be informed of the potential for this interaction, especially before initiation of long-term oral antibiotics.

Isotretinoin

Isotretinoin is indicated for patients with severe recalcitrant comedonal acne unresponsive to conventional therapies. It has multiple actions against comedonal acne, including (1) decreased sebum production and change in sebum composition, (2) inhibition of *P. acnes* growth within follicles, (3) inhibition of inflammation, and (4) altered patterns of keratinization within follicles (decreased size and increased differentiation).[27] After a 16-week course of therapy, isotretinoin produces a greater than 70% success rate followed by a prolonged remission of more than 20 months.[28]

Adverse effects from isotretinoin are numerous, frequent, and often dose related.[29,30] At least 90% of patients receiving isotretinoin experience dry lips, and 30% may show dryness and desquamation of the face. Hypertriglyceridemia may be found in more than 25% of patients. Conjunctivitis and eye irritation may be noted by patients, especially those using contact lenses. Muscle and joint pain, including complaints of backache, are common and may be attributed to catabolic effects on mesenchymal tissues of cartilage, connective tissue, and bone. Skeletal hyperostosis was first noted in patients taking high-dose, long-term isotretinoin for disorders of keratinization, but more recently asymptomatic hyperostosis has occurred in patients on short-course regimens for acne. The relative risk and clinical importance of these skeletal changes are undetermined.

An increase in creatinine phosphokinase and blood glucose, as well as photosensitivity, pseudotumor cerebri, and excess granulation tissue, has occurred during use of isotretinoin.[28] The incidence of teratogenicity in babies of mothers exposed to isotretinoin is high and well documented. Of 16 case reports of adverse pregnancy outcomes in women exposed to isotretinoin, 9 were spontaneous abortions and 7 were babies with major birth defects (e.g., hydrocephalus, small or partially occluded external auditory canals, and cardiac abnormalities).[31] In addition, five normal pregnancies were reported, but timing of exposure to isotretinoin was uncertain.[31]

Other oral agents investigated for the treatment of acne include ibuprofen, zinc, spironolactone, prednisone, dexamethasone, and oral contraceptives.

EVALUATION OF THERAPEUTIC OUTCOMES

Acne is a common self-limiting disease for which there are several effective therapeutic modalities. Recognition of the pathogenic factors associated with acne, selection of an appropriate treatment regimen, and monitoring for adverse effects often lead to a successful outcome. Concepts of therapy should be conveyed to the patient and the importance of compliance should be emphasized. Achievement of clinical effectiveness by any given therapeutic regimen may require 6–8 weeks. Patients may also notice an "exacerbation" of acne after initiation of therapy. Inflammatory acne lesions may take approximately 4 weeks to surface; therefore, new follicular plugging should be well controlled after 2 months of effective therapy. For topical agents, all acne-prone areas should be treated, because the purpose of therapy is to prevent or minimize the formation of new lesions[8] and to minimize the risk of scarring, a permanent endpoint for moderate to severe disease.

PSORIASIS

Psoriasis is a common chronic disease characterized by recurrent exacerbations and remissions of thickened, erythematous, and scaling lesions. Statistics indicate that approximately 1% of the U.S. population has psoriasis.[32] There is no known cure for psoriasis, and the annual cost of chronic care is estimated to be at least 5% of the individual U.S. median income.[32]

This debilitating disease occurs in all racial groups and has equal distribution between men and women.[5,33] The mean age of onset is 27 years, with approximately 35% of cases occurring before age 20[34]; however, the age of onset is widely variable from infancy to old age.

PATHOPHYSIOLOGY

The cause of psoriasis is unknown and the lack of an adequate animal model has impeded research. There are several hypotheses regarding the pathophysiology of psoriasis (see Table 90.8).

DEFECTS IN EPIDERMAL CELL CYCLE

The search for an inherent skin defect as a pathogenic mechanism for psoriasis has provided much information and numerous hypotheses. Psoriatic epidermal cells proliferate at a rate sevenfold faster than normal epidermal cells.[35,36] The germinative cell population increases in psoriatic skin, and duration of the cell cycle is calculated at

TABLE 90.8. POSSIBLE ETIOLOGIC FACTORS OF PSORIASIS

Defects in epidermal cell cycle
Disruption in arachidonic acid metabolism
Genetics
Exogenous trigger factors
Climate
Stress
Infection
Trauma
Drugs
Immunologic mechanisms

37.5 hours (versus 300 hours in normal skin).[36] Lesion-free skin in psoriatic patients is generally considered to be involved, as epidermal proliferation is elevated in apparently normal skin.[37]

DISRUPTION IN ARACHIDONIC ACID METABOLISM

Other abnormalities found in psoriatic skin include evidence of increased metabolic activity and increased cGMP, DNA, RNA, IgG, and C3.[36,37] In psoriatic lesions, arachidonic acid levels are 30 times normal, 12-L-hydroxy-5,8,10,14-eicosatetraenoic acid (HETE) levels are 80 times normal, and prostaglandin E_2 levels are 50% higher than normal. Glucocorticoids normalize levels of arachidonic acid and HETE by inhibition of phospholipase A and may be partly responsible for regression of psoriatic lesions.[36]

GENETICS

There is a significant genetic component in psoriasis, but the exact mode of inheritance is uncertain.[38] Approximately 36% of patients with psoriasis have at least one immediate relative with the disorder.[34] Monozygotic twins have a higher concordance for psoriasis than dizygotic twins.[34] Studies of histocompatibility antigens in psoriatics indicate statistically significant associations on the B, C, and D loci, more specifically, HLA-B13, HLA-B17, and HLA-B37.[33,39] The most significant risk is with HLA-CW6, where the relative likelihood for developing psoriasis is 9 to 15 times normal.[8] In addition, the B13 and B17 loci appear to be linked with the gene that expresses CW6.[37]

EXOGENOUS TRIGGER FACTORS

Factors such as climate, stress, infection, trauma, and drugs may aggravate psoriasis. Warm seasons and sunlight reportedly improved psoriasis in 80% of patients, while 90% reported worsening in cold weather. Also, stress worsened psoriasis in 30–40% of patients; however, the exact role stress plays in exacerbation of psoriasis is uncertain.

Infection has been identified retrospectively as a common precipitating factor in psoriasis. A review of 245 cases of psoriatic children indicates that 25% had initial onset of the disease after clinically documented infections, while 54% had exacerbation during a 2- to 3-week interval after an upper respiratory infection.[40] Another study indicates that exacerbation of psoriasis is common 1–2 weeks after acute streptococcal infection.[41]

Psoriasis may also occur at the site of injury to normal-appearing skin (Koebner response). The incidence is variable, ranging up to 76% in retrospective studies and 51% in prospective studies.[37] The Koebner response may be induced by a variety of causes including rubbing, venipuncture, bites, surgery, and pressure. The mechanism for development of the Koebner response is unknown and is not unique to psoriasis. The length of time between injury and lesion development, although variable, is usually a few days to weeks.

Lithium carbonate and β-adrenergic blocking agents are among the most commonly noted drugs to exacerbate psoriasis.[42,43]

CLINICAL PRESENTATION

The clinical appearance of psoriatic lesions, although not scarring, may almost be categorized as disfiguring, especially for patients with severe disease in cosmetic areas.

In general, psoriatic lesions are characterized by sharply demarcated, erythematous papules and plaques often covered with silver-white fine scales. Initial lesions are usually small papules that enlarge over time and coalesce into large plaques, sometimes as serpiginous or geographic forms. If the fine scale is removed, a salmon-pink lesion is exposed, perhaps with punctate bleeding from prominent dermal capillaries (Auspitz sign).

The appearance of psoriatic lesions also varies depending on the area of the body affected and the type of psoriasis. Scalp psoriasis ranges from diffuse scaling on an erythematous scalp to thickened plaques with exudation, microabscesses, and fissures. Trunk, back, arm, and leg lesions may be generalized, scattered, discrete, guttate (droplike) lesions, or large plaques. Palms, soles, face, and genitalia may be involved as well. Affected nails are often pitted with collections of subungual keratotic material. Yellow spots under the nail plate may also be seen.

Patients with pustular psoriasis have lesions with a mixture of brown and white noninfected pustules associated with erythema and scaling. Usually, pustular psoriasis affects the palms and soles symmetrically, but infrequently more severe forms of generalized pustular psoriasis (von Zumbusch variety) may occur with erythroderma, "lakes" of coalescent pustules, fever, malaise, and leukocytosis.

Psoriatic arthritis is a distinct clinical entity in which both psoriatic lesions and inflammatory "arthritis" occur. Classically, distal interphalangeal joints and adjacent nails are involved, but knees, elbows, wrists, and ankles may also be involved. Skin lesions usually precede joint involvement, although the reverse may occur, or skin lesions and joint disease may occur simultaneously. The clinical appearance of psoriasis may sometimes be confused with numerous other dermatologic diseases; thus, the differential diagnosis is extensive and histopathology may be helpful.

TABLE 90.9. PSORIATIC PATIENT ASSESSMENT

Onset and duration of psoriasis
Family history
Exacerbating factors
Previous history of antipsoriasis agents with efficacy and side effect data
All current and recent topical and systemic medications
Environmental and occupational exposure to chemicals and toxins
Allergies (food, drug, environmental)

ASSESSMENT

The pharmacist is in a unique position to evaluate and educate the psoriatic patient because of the myriad drug therapy options available as nonprescription and prescription products (see Table 90.9).

TREATMENT

Although the exact cause of psoriasis is unknown, treatment approaches are reliable and offer good control of the disorder. Psoriasis is often a lifelong relapsing and remitting disease, so modes of therapy should be selected with long-term consequences in mind. Major factors for consideration include the extent and site of disease involvement and the age of the patient. The goal of therapy is to achieve complete clearing of lesions, but partial clearing is acceptable at times, using regimens with decreased toxicity and increased patient acceptability. Drug treatments for psoriasis are listed in Table 90.10. Treatment guidelines are listed in Tables 90.11 and 90.12.

Emollients/Keratolytics

Moisturizers or emollients hydrate the stratum corneum (after application of an occlusive oily film) and minimize evaporation of water from the stratum corneum.[44] Hydration causes the stratum corneum to swell and flatten the surface contour. Moisturizers may decrease the binding forces within the horny layer, enhance desquamation, and eliminate scaling.[44] Moisturizers may also increase pliability of the skin, have antipruritic activity, and possess mild vasoconstrictor activity. Moisturizers often need to be applied three times a day to achieve a beneficial response. Adverse effects include folliculitis or allergic contact dermatitis.

Keratolytics are used to remove scale, smooth the skin, and decrease hyperkeratosis.[44] Salicylic acid, the most frequently used keratolytic agent, is generally applied in concentrations of 2–10% or higher. A possible mechanism of salicylic acid keratolysis is that it causes a decrease in corneocyte-to-corneocyte cohesion in the abnormal horny layer of psoriatic skin. Lower concentrations of salicylic acid exhibit a keratin-dispersing effect, while concentrations of 5% or higher have a corneolytic (exfoliative) action.[45] Although salicylic acid may enhance percutaneous penetration of some drugs, it also produces local irritation.[44] Application of salicylic acid to large areas of skin may induce salicylism with symptoms of nausea, vomiting, tinnitus, or hyperventilation.[46]

TABLE 90.10. EXAMPLES OF DRUG TREATMENTS FOR PSORIASIS

Topical	Systemic
Emollients and keratolytics	Ultraviolet-A and oral psoralens (systemic PUVA)
Coal tar	Methotrexate
Anthralin	Retinoids
Calcipotriene	Sulfasalazine
Methotrexate (under investigation)	Cyclosporine
UVA and topical psoralens (topical PUVA)	Tacrolimus

Coal Tar

Although tar derivatives have been used to treat skin diseases for two millennia, relatively little is known about their composition or mechanism of action.[47] Tars are derived from wood such as pine or juniper, shale (ichthammol), and bituminous coal (coal tar). In recent years, wood and shale tars have fallen out of use because they possess relatively less efficacy than coal tar.[48] Coal tar contains thousands of hydrocarbon compounds formed from distillation of bituminous coal.[47] When applied to normal skin, coal tar causes predominantly transient epidermal hyperplasia during the first 2 weeks of therapy followed by a cytostatic effect with epidermal thinning.[49] There is additional evidence that coal tar can cross-link with DNA, and in combination with ultraviolet light, may increase prostaglandin synthesis in the skin. Suppression of DNA synthesis in the epidermis may be measured via the hairless mouse model used to predict the antipsoriatic effectiveness of coal tar derivatives.[50]

Coal tar is an effective treatment for psoriasis; however, its disadvantages include unpleasant odor, ability to stain skin and clothing, ability to reversibly darken or alter light hair colors, and ability to tarnish silver in jewelry. Coal tar is usually applied topically to lesions (often at bedtime), but may also be used in bath water and as a shampoo.

Concern with the long-term use of coal tar is risk of carcinogenicity. Crude coal tar contains many polynuclear aromatic hydrocarbons that are known carcinogens. Retrospective studies of psoriatic patients treated with crude coal tar have not indicated any increase in cancer cases compared with controls[47]; however, there are cases indicating a

TABLE 90.11. TOPICAL TREATMENT GUIDELINES

Active Ingredient	Formulation	Strength	Regimen	Potential Side Effects
Emollients	Lotions, creams, ointments	N/A	Three to four times daily	Folliculitis Contact dermatitis
Salicylic acid (keratolytic)	Gels, lotions	2–10%	Two to three times daily	Can be irritating Has resulted in salicylism
Coal tar	Creams, gels, lotions, ointments, solutions	1–48.5%	Apply in the evening, allowing to remain through the night	Messy and burdensome Can be irritating, photoreactions
Anthralin	Creams, ointments	0.1–1%	Usually in the evening, allowing to remain through the night. Short contact regimens also have been used	Stains skin and clothing Can be irritating
Calcipotriene	Ointment	50 μg/g	Twice daily, no more than 100 g/week, for up to 8 days	Burning and stinging in 10% of patients
Corticosteroids	Creams, lotions, ointments, solutions	Variable potency	Two to four times daily for maintenance; may use occlusion at night	Local tissue atrophy, striae, epidermal thinning, glucocorticoid systemic effects
Methoxsalen	Lotion	1%	Apply to area prior to UVA therapy	Photoreaction, exaggerated burning

higher rate of cutaneous carcinoma in patients exposed to tar and ultraviolet light. Controlled studies are needed to determine the carcinogenicity risk associated with the clinical use of crude and refined coal tars.

Anthralin

Anthralin, an anthrone derivative of chrysarobin (from the South American araroba tree), is used topically to treat psoriasis.[51] Although anthralin (under the name dithranol) has been used for 70 years in Great Britain, it has only recently been extensively used in the United States. Anthralin appears to inhibit DNA synthesis by intercalation between DNA strands.[52] Another possible mechanism is that anthralin may decrease epidermal proliferation by mitochondrial inhibition. Irritation and inflammation are common with anthralin therapy and, to a point, correlate with clinical efficacy.[51,53] Other hypotheses support the role of anthralin-generated free radicals in producing both antipsoriatic effects and irritation.[54]

Inflammation, irritation, and staining of skin and clothing (via oxidation and binding to keratins) are often therapy-limiting effects. Fortunately, anthralin exerts its clinical effects at low cellular concentrations; therefore, short-contact therapy regimens (application for 20 minutes) have been found effective with decreased side effects.[55] Titrating the strength of anthralin slowly from a low concentration (0.1–0.25%) to a higher concentration (0.5–1%) may minimize irritation.

Anthralin was traditionally formulated in stiff paste bases to provide adherence to plaques. More recently, cream formulations have been developed that are more cosmetically appealing and appear to be as clinically effective. The patient must apply anthralin products only to affected areas of skin, because contact with uninvolved skin may result in excessive and unwanted irritation and staining, which usually disappears within 1–2 weeks of discontinuation. Staining of affected plaques is a sign of resolution, however, as cell turnover has been slowed enough to take up the stain.[52] Despite the demonstrated efficacy of anthralin, some patients will not tolerate local irritation and staining.

Calcipotriene

Calcipotriene, a synthetic vitamin D analogue, is approved as a topical agent for the treatment of moderate plaque psoriasis. Calcipotriene binds to receptors in epidermal keratinocytes, resulting in the inhibition of cell proliferation and induction of cell differentiation.[56] Calcipotriene may also exert effects on immunocompetent cells. Calcium metabolism is minimally affected by the application of calcipotriene when used as directed. Calcipotriene has been evaluated in several open label or randomized, double-blind controlled studies and has been shown to be effective in improving or clearing psoriatic plaques.[57–60] On average, improvement was seen within 2 weeks of treatment, with approximately 70% of the patients demonstrating marked improvement after 8 weeks of treatment.

Maintenance therapy may be required for long-term control of the condition. Lesional and perilesional irritation occurred in approximately 10% of treated patients and consisted of a mild burning and stinging sensation. The facial area is sensitive to calcipotriene and facial irritation has been reported following local application, as well as sec-

TABLE 90.12. ORAL TREATMENT GUIDELINES

Active Ingredient	Formulation	Strength	Regimen	Potential Side Effects
Sulfasalazine	Suspension, tablets	250 mg/5 mL, 500 mg	3–4 g/d	Gastrointestinal upset
Methoxsalen	Capsules	10 mg	Dosed on a mg/kg basis, 2 hours before UVA exposure	Burns, erythema, gastrointestinal upset, CNS effects, ocular damage, skin cancer
Methotrexate	Tablets, injection	2.5 mg, 20–25 mg/mL	2.5–5 mg every 12 hours for three doses every week	Anemia, leukopenia, thrombocytopenia, gastrointestinal upset
Etretinate	Capsules	10 mg, 25 mg	0.75–1 mg/kg/d in divided doses	Dry mouth and lips, eye irritation, gastrointestinal upset hematologic and hepatic effects
Cyclosporine	Capsules, solution	25 mg, 100 mg, 100 mg/mL	3–4 mg/kg/d in two divided doses; may increase to 5 mg/kg/d (ideal body weight), in 1 month if no response. Do not exceed	Nephrotoxicity, gastrointestinal upset, hypertension, tremor, monitor liver function tests
Tacrolimus	Capsules	1 mg, 5 mg	0.15 mg/kg twice daily; titrate based on side effects	Nephrotoxicity, gastrointestinal upset, hypertension, tremor, monitor liver function tests

ondary exposure. Dry skin, peeling, rash, and worsening of psoriasis have also been reported. Hypercalcemia is rare, but has occurred when excessive amounts of calcipotriene were applied.[60,61]

Whether calcipotriene will be used as first-line therapy or as an adjunctive remains to be seen.

Topical Corticosteroids

Topical corticosteroids may play an important adjunctive role in the treatment of psoriasis by decreasing erythema, pruritus, and scaling. The mechanism of topical steroid efficacy in psoriasis is uncertain. Steroid receptors have been identified in the skin, and synthesis and mitosis of DNA in epidermal cells have been halted by topical steroids in hairless mice.[62,63] Topical corticosteroids appear to inhibit phospholipase A, lowering the amounts of arachidonic acid, prostaglandins, and leukotrienes in the skin.[64]

A wide variety of topical steroids are available in different potencies and vehicles as described in USP-DI, 1995. Products with a low-potency ranking have a modest anti-inflammatory effect and are safest for long-term application. These products are also the safest products for use on the face and intertriginous areas, with occlusion, and in infants and young children.[65]

Products with a medium-potency ranking are used in moderate inflammatory dermatoses. Examples of conditions for which these products are frequently used include chronic eczematous dermatoses such as hand eczema and atopic eczema. Medium-potency preparations may be used on the face and intertriginous areas for a limited duration.[65]

High-potency preparations are used in more severe inflammatory dermatoses. Examples of conditions for which these products are frequently used include more severe eczematous dermatoses, lichen simplex chronicus, and psoriasis. They may be used for an intermediate duration, or for longer periods in areas with thickened skin secondary to chronic conditions. High-potency preparations may also be used on the face and intertriginous areas but only for a short treatment duration.[65]

Very high potency products are used primarily as an alternative to systemic adrenocorticoid therapy when local areas are involved. Examples of conditions for which very high potency products are frequently used include thick, chronic lesions caused by psoriasis, lichen simplex chronicus, and discoid lupus erythematosus. There is a high likelihood of skin atrophy with the use of very high potency preparations. They may be used for only a short duration of therapy and on small surface areas. Occlusive dressings should not be used with these products.[65]

The choice of steroid and vehicle depends on the severity and extent of involvement, the area of the body to be treated, and the anticipated duration of treatment. Topical steroids are available in ointments, creams, lotions, gels, and sprays.

Ointments are considered the most clinically effective in psoriasis because of their hydrating effect and ability to enhance penetration of the steroid into the skin by lipophilicity.[66] Ointments are not suited for use in areas such as the axilla, groin, or other intertriginous areas where maceration and folliculitis may develop secondary to the occlusive effect. Creams are often preferred by patients and may be used in intertriginous areas even though their water content makes them more drying than ointments.

In severe, acute forms of psoriasis, and other inflammatory dermatoses, a patient may be instructed to apply a high-potency topical steroid every 2 hours for 24–48 hours, followed by application three or four times a day. For maintenance, application two to four times a day is adequate. Adverse reactions are of several types and common. Local tissue atrophy, degeneration, and striae are manifestations of steroid effect on collagen synthesis and fibroblast growth. If detected early, atrophy and striae may be reversible upon drug discontinuation, but in many cases of prolonged therapy with high-potency agents these changes may be permanent. Thinning of the epidermis may result in visible distended capillaries (telangiectasias) and purpura. Acneform eruptions and masking of symptoms of bacterial or fungal skin infections have been reported.

Systemic consequences of topical corticosteroid use include risk of suppression of the hypothalamic–pituitary–adrenal axis, hyperglycemia, and development of cushingoid features. Avoidance of prolonged therapy with high-potency agents minimizes the risk of these side effects. Tachyphylaxis and rebound flare of psoriasis after abrupt cessation of topical corticosteroid therapy can also occur. With proper monitoring, topical corticosteroids are a safe and effective adjunct to psoriasis treatment.

Sulfasalazine

Oral sulfasalazine (3–4 g/d for 8 weeks) has been reported to be an effective therapy for plaque-type psoriasis in some patients.[67] When used as a single agent in the treatment of psoriasis, it is not as effective as is therapy with methotrexate, psoralen plus ultraviolet-A light (UVA), or etretinate. One distinct advantage of sulfasalazine therapy compared with these other treatments is its lower incidence of severe side effects.[67]

Systemic Therapy–Photochemotherapy: Oral and Topical Psoralen and Long-Wave Ultraviolet A Light

The use of psoralens with UVA (PUVA) has been studied since the early 1970s and was approved by the FDA in 1982. Efficacy studies indicated that control of psoriasis occurred in nearly 90% of patients.[68]

Psoralens react with nucleic acids and intercalate between base pairs. When DNA is irradiated with long-wave ultraviolet light (320–400 nm, UVA), the psoralens covalently bind to pyrimidine bases, forming a cross-link.[69] PUVA may also affect immune responses in the skin and circulating lymphocytes, as demonstrated by a decreased ability to mount delayed hypersensitivity responses to contact sensitizers and increased risk of cutaneous cancer in treated patients.[70,71]

Candidates for PUVA therapy usually have severe incapacitating psoriasis unresponsive to topical therapies without history of photosensitivity, skin cancers, cataracts, or x-ray therapy of the skin. Methoxsalen (8-methoxypsoralen or 8-MOP) is usually dosed at 0.6–0.8 mg/kg and is given 2 hours before exposure to UVA. Serum methoxsalen concentrations usually peak within 0.5–2 hours of ingestion; however, a large interindividual and intraindividual variation in absorption may complicate titration of effective therapy.[72] Dosing of UVA is determined by patient skin type and history of previous response to ultraviolet radiation.

Topical Psoralens

Trioxsalen baths and UV light have been proven to be beneficial for psoriasis.[73–76] More recent studies confirm low 8-MOP levels after 8-MOP bath water treatments, which may be responsible for the absence of systemic side effects.[77,78]

Methotrexate

Oral methotrexate is indicated in the treatment of severe forms of psoriasis (e.g., psoriatic arthritis, erythrodermic psoriasis, pustular psoriasis, and extensive psoriasis) refractory to other therapy.[79] Methotrexate appears to act directly on the proliferating epidermal cells of psoriasis.[80] Through inhibition of the synthesis of thymidylate, one of the precursors to the DNA base pairs, cell division is halted. Biochemical inhibition by methotrexate is somewhat specific for cells in the S phase of the cell cycle; thus, its action is targeted against the majority of psoriatic cells found in this phase (six times normal).[80] Psoriatic cells may be more dependent on the thymidylate pathway and may further target the action of methotrexate to diseased skin.

Several dosage and administration regimens for methotrexate have been used in the treatment of psoriasis, but the "triple-dose" regimen is probably the most common.[80] This regimen involves oral methotrexate administration at 12-hour intervals for three doses to provide inhibition for the 36-hour cell cycle period in psoriasis. After a test dose of 2.5–5 mg, the patient is usually given 2.5 mg every 12 hours for three doses per week. This dose is increased by 2.5 mg per week to maximum effect and minimum toxicity.

Because therapy is often prolonged, a baseline liver biopsy is recommended before treatment and at intervals of 1.0–1.5 g cumulative dose of methotrexate.[79] Leukocyte and platelet counts should be monitored every 4 weeks with hemoglobin, serum creatinine, aspartate and alanine transaminases, alkaline phosphatase, and urinalysis performed every 3–4 months.[79] A yearly chest x-ray film is also recommended.

The use of any drug in addition to methotrexate should be carefully evaluated. Potentially interacting drugs are salicylates, many NSAIDs, ethanol, sulfonamides, barbiturates, retinoids, and others.[81] Topical methotrexate therapy for psoriasis is under investigation. Laurocapram-containing methotrexate formulations provide effective local inhibition of epidermal DNA synthesis in the *in vivo* hairless mouse and minipig models, providing the biochemical rationale for topical use in the treatment of psoriasis.[82] Careful patient selection to exclude those with serious risk factors allows highly effective treatment of psoriasis with relatively low risk of toxicity.

Etretinate

Etretinate is a vitamin A derivative (retinol) effective in treating severe pustular and erythrodermic forms of psoriasis. Summaries of preliminary testing in the United States indicate that, of 642 psoriatic patients treated with etretinate, 15% had clearing, 37% had greater than 75% clearing, 31% had 50–75% clearing, and 17% had unsatisfactory response.[83]

The mechanism of etretinate's effect on psoriasis is unknown. An antikeratinizing effect and an alteration of cell proliferation have been noted with decreased levels of polyamines.[84] Phosphorylation of proteins within erythrocyte membranes is altered in psoriatic patients and normalized with etretinate therapy. Doses of 1 mg/kg/d are used and are titrated to the lowest effective dose. Although the half-life of etretinate is approximately 12 hours, it appears to be stored in adipose tissue and may be detected in serum for at least 1 year after discontinuation.[84] The predominant active metabolite of etretinate, acitretin, is minimally stored in fat and, therefore, much more rapidly excreted; however, it has a side effect profile similar to that of the parent compound.[85,86]

Etretinate as monotherapy does not achieve total clearing in all patients, but may be important adjuvant therapy for PUVA by reducing the carcinogenic risks of that modality.[87]

Peeling of palms and soles, softening of the nails, diffuse hair loss, and dryness of mucous membranes occur in patients taking etretinate. As with isotretinoin, etretinate therapy often results in an increase in serum triglycerides and cholesterol, with a lowering of high-density lipoprotein.

Transient increases in aspartate and alanine transaminases and lactate dehydrogenase have been reported from etretinate therapy along with a few documented cases of hepatitis.[88,89] Careful patient selection and monitoring are essential for optimum results with etretinate therapy.

Acitretin

Compared with the antipsoriatic retinoid etretinate, the aromatic retinoid acitretin represents an active compound with improved elimination kinetics. Acitretin plus UVB combination treatment represents a possible therapeutic regimen in severe psoriasis.[86] A major drawback is that acitretin apparently metabolizes in some degree to etretinate, which in turn poses the original hazards identified with etretinate use (e.g., prolonged retention in the host).

Cyclosporine

Systemically administered cyclosporine has been used increasingly during the past 5 years in the treatment of severe psoriasis because of its remarkable efficacy coupled with its immunosuppressive properties. Combination of cyclosporine with PUVA or intensive UVB therapy is not recommended in view of the increased risk incurred by the use of an immunosuppressive drug with a potential skin carcinogen.[90] Side effects of cyclosporine include renal dysfunction, hypertension, paresthesia, hypertrichosis, gingival hyperplasia, and gastrointestinal disorders. Skin malignancies almost exclusively develop in patients previously treated with PUVA and/or methotrexate.[91] Intralesional cyclosporine has been clinically effective in psoriasis. A suitable topical preparation could serve as monotherapy or as a dose-sparing modality in conjunction with systemically administered cyclosporine.[92]

Tacrolimus

Tacrolimus, an immunosuppressant indicated to prevent organ allograft rejection, has also been found to be useful in treating recalcitrant psoriasis.[93,94] Four psoriatic patients received systemic tacrolimus to prevent solid organ graft rejection and three patients received systemic tacrolimus on a trial basis for severe recalcitrant psoriasis.[94] All seven patients experienced a marked reduction in erythema and scale at the end of 1 week and complete remission within 4 weeks. Remission continued following the reduction or discontinuation of corticosteroids in the transplant recipients. Toxicity secondary to tacrolimus included increases in serum creatinine and urea nitrogen, which remained higher than pretreatment levels despite dosage reductions. Hypertension, trembling, paresthesia, and insomnia were also experienced by the patients. Whether systemic tacrolimus can be safely used in psoriasis remains to be seen; however, topical formulations are being investigated as an alternative approach.[95]

EVALUATION OF THERAPEUTIC OUTCOMES

Psoriasis is a common hyperproliferative epidermal disorder for which several effective therapeutic modalities control rather than cure the condition. Recognition of the pathogenic factors associated with psoriasis, selection of an appropriate treatment regimen, and monitoring for adverse effects as well as disease progression often lead to a satisfactory outcome. Concepts of therapy should be adequately conveyed to the patient and the importance of compliance should be emphasized.

Achievement of clinical efficacy by any given therapeutic regimen requires days to weeks. Initial dramatic response may be achieved with some agents such as corticosteroids; however, sustained benefit with pharmacologically specific antipsoriatic therapy usually requires a range of about 2–4 weeks for noticeable response. Positive response to therapy is noted as normalization of involved areas of skin as measured by reduced erythema and scaling as well as flattening of plaques.

As with most pharmacotherapy choices, risk–benefit issues are of great importance in treating an epidermal-based disorder that may be seriously debilitating to the patient. The purpose of pharmacotherapy in this disorder is often an effort to keep or establish the patient as functional in his or her social and job environments as well as to preserve emotional and physical health.

CONCLUSION

Rational dermatologic therapy must be principled in the pathogenesis of the disorder. Major advances in recent years have allowed a better understanding of disease mechanisms and have produced a high level of interest in the field of dermatopharmacology.

Common skin disorders such as acne and psoriasis are excellent clinical models for demonstrating broad areas of potential pharmacologic intervention and therapeutic benefit. For many other common dermatologic disorders, these same principles apply.

GLOSSARY: SKIN LESION TYPES

Atrophy. Usually denotes decrease in thickness of the skin, a depression (hypotrophic), or a nodular scarring reaction (hypertrophic). Repeated insulin injections may cause lipoatrophy.

Bulla. An elevated fluid-filled lesion greater than 1 cm. These large blisters may be tense or flaccid to palpation.

Crust. Dried exudate on top of a lesion. Exudate may be thin or thick and red, yellow, or brown in color.

Cyst. Similar to a tumor or nodule but saclike, containing either fluid or solid material. A cyst is usually not transparent as is a vesicle or bulla.

Erosion. A superficial denuded area of skin. Unlike an ulcer, an erosion usually damages the epidermis only.

Excoriation. A mechanical abrasion of the skin. Excoriations may be caused by trauma from fingernails, which may result in exudate and crusting.

Fissure. A linear break in the skin to the depth of the dermis.

Lichenification. A raised flat-topped lesion, often with transverse ridges and leatherlike texture from long-term rubbing or scratching. Lichenification is a common sign in several forms of dermatitis.

Macule. A flat lesion (in the plane of the skin) denoted by a change in normal skin color. Usually well circumscribed with distinct outline and no elevation or depression of skin (e.g., a "freckle" is a macule).

Nodule. An elevated, rounded lesion like a papule but larger than 1 cm in diameter.

Papule. An elevated solid lesion less than 1 cm in diameter (pea-sized). Like a pea, the surface may be smooth or rough, soft or firm. Papules may consist of superficial skin debris and may range in color from red and yellow to black.

Patch. May be macular but usually implies an area larger than 1 cm.

Plaque. An elevated patch usually larger than 1 cm in diameter and with a flat top. Plaques may sometimes consist of many papules grouped together.

Purpura. Extravasation of blood through vessel walls (e.g., bruise). Purpuric lesions the size of pinpoints are known as petechiae. Lesions greater than 2 cm in diameter are called ecchymoses.

Pustule. An elevated, round, well-circumscribed lesion filled with pus. It may be used to describe an inflamed papule. Pustules contain cellular debris of yellow, green, or white color and may occur around follicles.

Scale. Overaccumulation of loose epidermal cells. Scale may be white, yellow, or brown, shiny or dull, and dry or greasy.

Telangiectasia. A permanent enlargement in the caliber (and usually an increase in the number) of capillaries near the surface of the skin. Telangiectasias appear as distended vessels visible through the skin and usually blanch (turn white) under application of pressure.

Tumor. A description used to define size and not malignancy. A tumor is usually an elevated, often round, lesion greater than 2–3 cm in diameter.

Ulcer. Destruction of the skin down to the dermis or subcutaneous tissue and often with irregular but well-demarcated borders. Ulcers may be any size or shape, but depth is an important criterion.

Vesicle. An elevated lesion that is less than 1 cm in diameter, filled with clear, red, or yellow fluid, and well circumscribed. An example of a vesicle is a blister formed via the cleavage between epidermis and dermis.

Wheal. Similar to a plaque (elevated, round, or flat topped, red or pink) but edematous and pruritic and evanescent. Urticaria (hives) is an example of wheal formation.

REFERENCES

1. Johnson M-L, Johnson KG, Engel A. Prevalence, morbidity, and cost of dermatologic diseases. J Am Acad Dermatol 1984;11:930–936.
2. Shalita AR, Freinkel RK. Acne. J Am Acad Dermatol 1984;11:957–959.
3. Pochi PE. Hormonal therapy of acne. Dermatol Clin 1983;1:377–384.
4. Shalita AR. Acne vulgaris: Current concepts in pathogenesis and treatment. Int J Dermatol 1976;15:182–187.

5. Solomon JA, Pochi PE. Acne vulgaris, in Stone J (ed): Dermatologic Immunology and Allergy. St. Louis, MO, CV Mosby, 1985, pp 649–660.
6. Hurwitz RM. Steroid acne. J Am Acad Dermatol 1989;21:1179–1181.
7. Arndt KA. Acne, in Manual of Dermatologic Therapeutics, 5th ed. Boston, Little, Brown, 1995, pp 3–15.
8. Melski JW, Arndt KA. Topical therapy for acne. N Engl J Med 1980;302:503–506.
9. Eaglstein WH. Allergic contact dermatitis to benzoyl peroxide. Arch Dermatol 1968;97:527.
10. Schallreuter KU, Wood JW. A possible mechanism of action for azelaic acid in the human epidermis. Arch Dermatol Res 1989;202:168–171.
11. Cunliffe WJ, Holland KT. Clinical and laboratory studies on treatment with 20% azelaic acid cream for acne. Acta Derm Venereol (Stockh) 1989;(suppl 143):31–34.
12. Cavicchini S, Caputo R. Long-term treatment of acne with 20% azelaic acid cream. Acta Derm Venereol (Stockh) 1989;(suppl 143):40–44.
13. Thomas JR III, Doya JA. The therapeutic uses of topical vitamin A acid. J Am Acad Dermatol 1981;4:505–513.
14. Hurwitz S. The combined effect of vitamin A acid and benzoyl peroxide in the treatment of acne. Cutis 1976;17:585–590.
15. Franz TJ. On the bioavailability of topical formulations of clindamycin hydrochloride. J Am Acad Dermatol 1983;9:66–73.
16. Eady EA, Holland KT, Cunliffe NJ. Should topical antibiotics be used for the treatment of acne vulgaris? Br J Dermatol 1982;107:235–246.
17. Eady EA, Holland KT, Cunliffe WJ. The use of antibiotics in acne therapy: Oral or topical administration? J Antimicrob Chemother 1982;10:89–115.
18. Schachner L, Eaglstein W, Kittles C, Mertz P. Topical erythromycin and zinc therapy for acne. J Am Acad Dermatol 1990;22:253–260.
19. Habbema L, Koopmans B, Menke HE, et al. A 4% erythromycin and zinc combination (Zineryt) versus 2% erythromycin (Eryderm) in acne vulgaris: A randomized double-blind comparative study. Br J Dermatol 1989;121:497–502.
20. Becker LE, Bergstresser PR, Whiting DA, et al. Topical clindamycin therapy for acne vulgaris. Arch Dermatol 1981;117:482–485.
21. Parry MF, Rha CK. Pseudomembranous colitis caused by topical clindamycin phosphate. Arch Dermatol 1986;122:583–594.
22. Ad Hoc Committee on the Use of Antibiotics in Dermatology. Systemic antibiotics for treatment of acne vulgaris, efficacy and safety. Arch Dermatol 1975;111:1630–1636.
23. Gammon WR, Meyer C, Lantis S, et al. Comparative efficacy of oral erythromycin versus oral tetracycline in the treatment of acne vulgaris. J Am Acad Dermatol 1986;14:183–186.
24. Jonas M, Cunha BA. Minocycline. Ther Drug Monit 1982;4:137–145.
25. Nordin K, Hallander H, Fredriksson T, Rylander C. A clinical and bacteriological evaluation of the effect of sulphamethoxazole-trimethoprim in acne vulgaris, resistant to prior therapy with tetracyclines. Dermatologica 1978;157:245–253.
26. Hansten PD, Horn JR. Inhibition of oral contraceptive efficacy. Drug Interactions Newslett 1985;5(2):7–10.
27. Rumsfield JA, West DP, Tse CST, et al. Isotretinoin in severe, recalcitrant cystic acne: A review. Drug Intell Clin Pharm 1983;17:329–333.
28. Shalita AR, Cunningham WJ, Leyden JJ, et al. Isotretinoin treatment of acne and related disorders: An update. J Am Acad Dermatol 1983;9:629–638.
29. Gilchrest BA. Retinoid pharmacology and skin, in Mukhtar H (ed): Pharmacology of the Skin. Boca Raton, FL, CRC Press, 1995, pp 167–181.
30. Goulden V, Cunliffe WJ. The long-term experience with isotretinoin treatment of acne, in Dahl MV, Lynch PJ (eds): Current Opinion in Dermatology. Philadelphia, Current Science, 1995, pp 231–234.
31. Anonymous. Adverse effects with isotretinoin. FDA Drug Bull 1983;13:21–23.
32. Krueger GG, Bergstresser PR, Lowe NJ, et al. Psoriasis. J Am Acad Dermatol 1984;11:937–947.
33. Watson W. Psoriasis: Epidemiology and genetics. Dermatol Clin 1984;2:363–371.
34. Farber EM, Nail ML. The natural history of psoriasis in 5,600 patients. Dermatologica 1974;148:1–18.
35. Weinstein GD, McCullough JL, Ross PA. Cell kinetic basis for pathophysiology of psoriasis. J Invest Dermatol 1985;85:579–583.
36. Baden HP. Biology of the epidermis and pathophysiology of psoriasis and certain ichthyosiform dermatoses, in Soter NA, Baden HP (eds): Pathophysiology of Dermatologic Diseases. New York, McGraw-Hill, 1984, pp 101–126.
37. Krueger GG. Psoriasis: Current concepts of its etiology and pathogenesis, in Dobson RL, Thiers BH (eds): Yearbook of Dermatology, Chicago, Year Book Medical Publishers, 1981.
38. Elder JT. Cytokine and genetic regulation of psoriasis, in Callen JP (ed): Advances in Dermatology, vol 10. St. Louis, MO, Mosby–Year Book, 1995, pp 99–134.
39. Russell TJ, Schultes LM, Kuban DJ. Histocompatibility (HL-A) antigens associated with psoriasis. N Engl J Med 1972;287:738–740.
40. Nyfors A, Lemholt K. Psoriasis in children: A short review and a survey of 245 cases. Br J Dermatol 1975;92:437–442.
41. Whyte HJ, Baughman RD. Acute guttate psoriasis and streptococcal infection. Arch Dermatol 1964;89:350–356.
42. Skoven I, Thormann J. Lithium compound treatment and psoriasis. Arch Dermatol 1979;115:1185–1187.
43. Neumann HAM, van Joost T. Adverse reactions of the skin to metoprolol and other beta-adrenoreceptor-blocking agents. Dermatologica 1981;162:330–335.
44. Marks R. Topical therapy for psoriasis: General principles. Dermatol Clin 1984;2:383–388.
45. Weirich EG. Dermatopharmacology of salicylic acid. I: Range of dermatotherapeutic effects of salicylic acid. Dermatologica 1975;151:268–273.
46. Davies MG, Briffa DV, Greaves MW. Systemic toxicity from topically applied salicylic acid. Br Med J 1979;1:661.
47. Lin AN, Moses K. Tar revisited. Int J Dermatol 1985;24:216–218.

48. Polano MK. Topical Skin Therapeutics. London, Churchill Livingstone, 1984, p 95.
49. Lavker RM, Grove GL, Kligman AM. The atrophogenic effect of crude coal tar on human epidermis. Br J Dermatol 1981;105:77–82.
50. Lowe NJ, Breeding J, Wortzman MS. The pharmacological variability of crude coal tar. Br J Dermatol 1982;107:475–479.
51. Ashton RE, Andre P, Lowe NJ, Whitefield M. Anthralin: Historical and current perspectives. J Am Acad Dermatol 1983;9:173–192.
52. Swanbeck G, Thyresson N. Interaction between dithranol and nucleic acids. Acta Derm Venereol (Stockh) 1965;45:344–348.
53. Barr RM, Misch KJ, Hensby CN, et al. Arachidonic acid and prostaglandin levels in dithranol erythema: Time course study. Br J Clin Pharmacol 1983;16:715–717.
54. Finnen MJ, Lawrence CM, Shuster S. Inhibition of dithranol inflammation by free-radical scavengers. Lancet 1984;2:1129–1130.
55. Gorsulowsky DC, Voorhees JJ, Ellis CN. Anthralin therapy for psoriasis: A new look at an old compound. Arch Dermatol 1985;121:1509–1511.
56. Berth-Jones J, Fletcher A, Hutchinson PE. Epidermal cytokeratin and immunocyte responses during treatment of psoriasis with calcipotriol, in Norma AW, Bouillon R, Thomasset M (eds): Vitamin D: Gene Regulation, Structure-Function Analysis and Clinical Application. Berlin, de Gruyter, 1991, p 424.
57. Kragballe K, Fogh K. Treatment of psoriasis by the topical application of the novel cholecalciferol analogue calcipotriol (MC 903). Arch Dermatol 1989;125:1647–1652.
58. Kragballe K, Gjertsen BT, DeHoope D, et al. Double-blind, right/left comparison of calcipotriol and betamethasone valerate in treatment of psoriasis vulgaris. Lancet 1991;337:193–196.
59. Berth-Jones J, Chu AC, Dodd WAH, et al. A multicenter parallel-group comparison of calcipotriol ointment and short contact dithranol therapy in chronic plaque psoriasis. Br J Dermatol 1992;127:266–271.
60. Cunliffe WJ, Claudy A, Faiross G, et al. A multicenter comparative study of calcipotriol and betamethasone 17-valerate in patients with psoriasis vulgaris. J Am Acad Dermatol 1992;26:736–743.
61. de Jong EM, van de Kerkhof PM. Simultaneous assessment of inflammation and epidermal proliferation in psoriatic plaques during long-term treatment with the vitamin D analogue MC 903: Modulations and interrelations. Br J Dermatol 1991;124:221–229.
62. Cornell RC, Stoughton RB. The use of topical steroids in psoriasis. Dermatol Clin 1984;2:397–409.
63. Cornell RC. Topical glucocorticoids in dermatology, in Dahl MV, Lynch PJ (eds): Current Opinion in Dermatology, 2nd ed. Philadelphia, Current Science, 1995, pp 193–197.
64. Hammarstrom S, Hamberg M, Duell EA, et al. Glucocorticoid in inflammatory proliferative skin disease reduces arachidonic and hydroxyeicosatetraenoic acids. Science 1977;197:994–996.
65. Anonymous. Corticosteroids (topical), in USP-DI, 15th ed, vol 1. Rockville, MD, Rand McNally, 1995, pp 858–876.
66. Burdick KH, Haleblian JK, Poulsen BJ, Cobner SE. Corticosteroid ointments: Comparison by two human bioassays. Curr Ther Res 1973;15:233–242.
67. Gupta AK, Ellis CN, Siegel MT, et al. Sulfasalazine improves psoriasis. Arch Dermatol 1990;126:487–493.
68. Bickers DR. Position paper—PUVA therapy. J Am Acad Dermatol 1983;8:265–270.
69. Cole RS. Light-induced crosslinking of DNA in the presence of a furocoumarin (psoralen). Biochem Biophys Acta 1970;217:30–39.
70. Thorvaldsen J, Volden G. PUVA-induced diminution of contact allergic and irritant skin reactions. Clin Exp Dermatol 1980;5:43–46.
71. Elmets CA, Bergstresser PR. Ultraviolet radiation effects on immune processes. Photochem Photobiol 1982;36:715–719.
72. Goldstein DP, Carter DM, Ljunggren B, Burkholder J. Minimal phototoxic doses and 8-MOP plasma levels in PUVA patients. J Invest Dermatol 1982;78:429–433.
73. Fischer T, Alsins J. Treatment of psoriasis with trioxsalen baths and dysprosium lamps. Acta Derm Venereol (Stockh) 1976;56:383–390.
74. Salo OP, Lassus A, Taskinen J. Trioxsalen bath plus UVA treatment of psoriasis. Acta Derm Venereol (Stockh) 1981;61:551–554.
75. Berne B, Fischer T, Michealsson G, Noren P. An 8-year follow-up of 149 psoriasis patients. Photodermatol 1984;1:18–22.
76. Turjanma K, Salo H, Reunala T. Comparison of trioxsalen bath and oral methoxsalen PUVA in psoriasis. Acta Derm Venereol (Stockh) 1985;86–88.
77. Lowe NJ, Weingarten D, Bourget T, Moy LS. PUVA therapy for psoriasis: Comparison of oral and bath water delivery of 8-methoxypsoralen. J Am Acad Dermatol 1986;14:754–760.
78. David M, Lowe NJ, Halder RM, Borok M. Serum 8-methoxypsoralen (8-MOP) concentrations after bath water delivery of 8-MOP plus UVA. J Am Acad Dermatol 1990;23:931–932.
79. Roenigk HH, Auerbauch R, Maibach HI, Weinstein GD. Methotrexate guidelines revised. J Am Acad Dermatol 1982;6:145–155.
80. Weinstein GD. Chemotherapy for psoriasis. Dermatol Clin 1984;2:431–438.
81. Roenigk HH, Auerbach R, Maibach HI, Weinstein GD. Methotrexate in psoriasis: Revised guidelines. J Am Acad Dermatol 1988;19:145–156.
82. Weinstein GD, McCullough JL, Olsen E. Topical methotrexate therapy for psoriasis. Arch Dermatol 1989;125:227–230.
83. Dicken CH. Retinoids: A review. J Am Acad Dermatol 1984;11:541–552.
84. Ellis CN, Grekin RC, Kragtalle K, et al. Retinoids, in Stone J (ed): Dermatologic Immunology and Allergy. St. Louis, MO, CV Mosby, 1985, pp 851–876.
85. Kingston TP, Matt LH, Lowe NJ. Etretin therapy for severe psoriasis. Arch Dermatol 1987;123:55–58.
86. Ruzicka T, Sommerburg C, Braun-Falco O, et al. Efficiency of acitretin in combination with UV-B in the treatment of severe psoriasis. Arch Dermatol 1990;126:482–486.
87. Halioua B, Saurat J-H. Risk : benefit ratio in the treatment of psoriasis with systemic retinoids. Br J Dermatol 1990;122:(suppl 36):135–150.

88. Weiss VC, Layden T, Spinowitz A, et al. Chronic active hepatitis associated with etretinate therapy. Br J Dermatol 1985;112:591–597.
89. Weiss VC, West DP, Ackerman R, Robinson LA. Hepatotoxic reactions in a patient treated with etretinate. Arch Dermatol 1984;120:104–106.
90. Griffiths CEM, Voorhees JJ. Cyclosporin A in the treatment of psoriasis: A clinical and mechanistic perspective. J Invest Dermatol 1990;95:53S–55S.
91. Krupp P, Monka C. Side-effect profile of cyclosporin A in patients treated for psoriasis. Br J Dermatol 1990;122 (suppl 36):47–56.
92. Griffiths CEM. Systemic and local administration of cyclosporine in the treatment of psoriasis. J Am Acad Dermatol 1990;23:1242–1247.
93. Thompson AW, Carroll PB, McCauley J, et al. FK 506: A novel immunosuppressant for treatment of autoimmune disease. Springer Semin Immunopathol 1993;14:323–344.
94. Jegasothy BV, Ackerman CD, Todo S, et al. Tacrolimus (FK 506)—a new therapeutic agent for severe recalcitrant psoriasis. Arch Dermatol 1992;128:781–785.
95. Lauerma AI, Maibach HI. Topical FK 506—Clinical potential or laboratory curiosity? Dermatol 1994;188:173–176.

Chapter 91

Drug-Induced Skin Disorders

Phillip A. Nowakowski, PharmD, Jean A. Rumsfield, PharmD, and Dennis P. West, PhD, FCCP

Cutaneous reactions to drugs occur in approximately 2–3% of medical inpatients.[1] Skin rash is a frequent reason for patient visits to physicians.[2] Establishment of a relationship between medication use and subsequent development of cutaneous reactions, however, is often difficult. Unfortunately, mechanisms underlying adverse drug reactions are poorly understood and few diagnostic tests are available to properly establish cause and effect. Patients with drug-induced reactions are often taking more than one drug, making detection of the causative agent difficult. The picture is further complicated because small doses of a drug may evoke severe reactions even if that agent was previously well tolerated.[3]

Drug History

A thorough and organized approach is essential to proper diagnosis of a drug-induced skin reaction. Patient evaluation should include (1) a comprehensive drug history, (2) awareness of various clinical manifestations of drug allergy and cutaneous reactions, (3) awareness of factors that favor development of allergic reactions to drugs, and (4) awareness of the immunologic and nonimmunologic mechanisms involved in cutaneous reactions to drugs.[4–6]

A patient may experience a skin reaction while on multiple drugs. Most authorities advise that the first drug(s) to consider is that initiated within the week preceding the reaction. This short temporal relationship does not hold for all drugs (e.g., onset perhaps 2 weeks after discontinuation of semisynthetic penicillins, onset perhaps 6 months for β-blocker-induced psoriasiform eruptions, onset of 2 months to perhaps 5 years for drug-induced systemic lupus erythematosus).[7] Each drug should be individually considered as a potential cause.

A Guide to Drug Eruptions,[8] is updated at 4- to 5-year intervals and is a useful source of confirmed and tabulated information on drug-induced skin reactions. With an increased number of drugs undergoing shorter premarketing phases, a greater number of skin reactions are expected to occur during postmarketing surveillance. The pharmacist plays an important role in identifying and reporting possible drug-induced skin reactions and in monitoring or preventing recurrence.

Diagnosis

Although several *in vitro* and *in vivo* tests have been used to diagnose drug allergy, the availability and reliability of these tests are limited.[9–11] The *in vitro* radioallergosorbent test (RAST) may be used to detect IgE or IgG antibodies and has produced the most reliable results in detecting penicillin allergy.[8] The modified Coombs test and bacteriophage inhibition test have even higher sensitivity for detecting IgG and IgE antibodies, although more elaborate laboratory resources are required.[8] The lymphocyte transformation test is considered the most reliable *in vitro* test for diagnosis of both immediate and delayed drug reactions, but results appear to depend on the type of drug or type of skin eruption.[8]

Patch testing, useful in determining contact dermatitis, has limited applications in drug allergy, particularly in delayed hypersensitivity reactions, fixed-drug eruptions, and toxic epidermal necrolysis.[8] Scratch or prick testing with drugs and/or metabolites may be useful in type I reactions (i.e., penicillin allergy) although there are practical limitations to this method. Dechallenge/rechallenge continues to be regarded as the most definitive method for ascertaining drug-induced reactions. However, it is often not an option if a patient has experienced a potentially life-threatening reaction or if the suspected agent cannot be discontinued. In some cases, rechallenge may not result in the same reaction, which further clouds the picture.

Clinical Presentation

It is important to recognize the clinical manifestations of a drug allergy. Symptoms of an allergic drug reaction usually have an acute onset, may last several minutes to months, or may occur periodically throughout an exposure period. An accurate description of the characteristics of a cutaneous drug reaction should be obtained. Although drug hypersensitivity is impossible to predict, certain drug and host factors increase the likelihood of a reaction.

Drug allergy is more frequent in older individuals[12] and may be related to the development of the immune response and to increased exposure to drugs. Individual genetic factors may also predispose an individual to drug allergy: differences in drug metabolism, differences in immune response, differences in tissue receptor sites, and differences in elaboration of immunologic mediators may all play a role.[13] In addition, a previous history of allergic reactions may increase the risk of development of an allergic reaction. Hepatic and renal disorders may alter drug metabolism and provoke an allergic response.[14]

To induce an immune response (i.e., hypersensitivity reaction), the drug or its metabolite must act as, or form, a complete antigen. For example, proteins contained in sera, vaccines, biologicals, and allergens may act as complete antigens; however, most drugs are small molecules and must bind with larger molecules to create a complete antigen. Haptens are often drugs capable of such binding. Once a complete antigen is formed, the immune system reacts to neutralize, destroy, or eliminate it from the host.

The route of administration may influence drug allergy. For example, topical application of drugs has the greatest propensity to induce allergy, followed by the intravenous route and the oral route. Although not strictly dose related, such factors as the number of drugs, the dose of drug, and the duration of therapy may influence the likelihood of developing a hypersensitivity reaction.

The host's ability to react to antigenic material is the basis for specific immune reactions. The ultimate physiologic role of the immune system is to differentiate "self" from "nonself" and eliminate foreign materials from the body. The type of immunologic mediation of hypersensitivity may determine the category of reaction and thus the clinical presentation of drug-induced skin disorders.

For a discussion of allergic drug reaction mechanisms, see Chapter 82, Allergic and Pseudoallergic Drug Reactions.

PATTERNS OF CUTANEOUS REACTIONS

Because any drug may induce cutaneous reactivity, a complete review of drug-induced skin reactions is not practical; however, for common cutaneous drug reactions, their clinical course, possible mechanisms, etiologies, and management are described in the following sections. Maculopapular reactions and urticaria occur most often. The clinical type and frequency of cutaneous reactions to drugs for a series of 225 patients are listed in Table 91.1.[14]

TABLE 91.1. TYPE AND FREQUENCY OF CUTANEOUS DRUG REACTIONS

	No. Patients (%) with Drug Reactions	
Eruption Type	**Total (%)**	**Verified by Provocation (%)**
Fixed-drug eruption	77 (34.2)	51 (66.2)
Exanthematous eruption	71 (31.6)	47 (66.2)
Urticaria/angioedema	45 (20.0)	26 (57.8)
Gold dermatitis	15 (6.7)	0 (0)
Purpuric eruption	5 (2.2)	0 (0)
Erythema multiforme	4 (1.8)	2 (50.0)
Toxic epidermal necrolysis	3 (1.3)	0 (0)
Stevens–Johnson syndrome	2 (0.9)	1 (50.0)
Exfoliative dermatitis	2 (0.9)	1 (50.0)
Systemic lupus erythematosus-like eruption	1 (0.4)	0 (0)
Total	225 (100.0)	128 (56.9)

(Compiled from Ref. 14.)

MACULOPAPULAR ERUPTIONS

Clinical Presentation

Macular or maculopapular skin reactions are common drug-induced skin eruptions. Morbilliform, exanthematous, scarlatiniform, and rubellaform are common morphologic descriptions of maculopapular eruptions. Such reactions often start on the trunk or in areas of pressure or trauma and are frequently symmetrical. Flat or raised, reddened lesions, varying from a few millimeters to confluent large areas, are characteristic, but vesicles may be present. Involvement of mucous membranes or palms and soles is variable and infrequent; mild fever may also accompany the reaction.[15]

The course of a maculopapular eruption is variable and may be classified as an "early" or "late" reaction.[8] In an early reaction, the eruption appears within 2–3 days of drug administration in previously sensitized patients. Sensitization may occur without symptoms or rash because drug fever (or elevated temperature), for example, often goes unnoticed. Also, fever may be a symptom of the disease for which the drug is being prescribed.[8] The "late" reaction appears approximately 9 days after drug exposure, although with previous sensitization the onset may be quicker. Because of individual patient differences, reactions may occur any time from the first day of exposure to 2 weeks after therapy. A maculopapular rash usually fades a few days after discontinuation of the causative agent. Occasionally, eruptions decrease or disappear even with continued medication use and may not always recur with drug rechallenge.[15]

Pathogenesis

The variable and unpredictable course of maculopapular eruptions makes identification of the mechanism or pathogenesis difficult. A hypersensitivity reaction, possibly secondary to cell-mediated allergy, has been suggested by skin testing, lymphocyte transformation, and macrophage-migration inhibition tests.[10] That these tests are positive in a small portion of patients with maculopapular eruptions suggests the likelihood of a different mechanism. Immune complex reactions have also been suggested.[10] Although definitive cause-and-effect relationships have been established for the penicillins, many other drugs have been associated with maculopapular eruptions (see Table 91.2).

Diagnosis

Serologic tests rarely establish a diagnosis of drug-induced delayed hypersensitivity; thus, patient history may often be the only diagnostic clue. Maculopapular rashes generally do not persist for prolonged periods, although recurrence may present as more serious and extensive exfoliative skin reactions.[10]

Management

Conservative measures using lukewarm water baths or cool water compresses are recommended for mild to moderate involvement. Systemic antihistamines may be added for itching. Severe reactions may be treated with a short-term course of a systemic corticosteroid.[6]

TABLE 91.2. DRUGS ASSOCIATED WITH MACULOPAPULAR ERUPTIONS

Allopurinol	Penicillamine
Barbiturates	Penicillins
Benzodiazepines	Phenothiazines
Carbamazepine	Phenylbutazone
Chloramphenicol	Piroxicam
Erythromycin	Pyrazolon derivatives
Ethionamide	Rifampin
Gold salts	Streptomycin
Hydantoin derivatives	Sulfonamides (including sulfonylureas and thiazide diuretics)
Ibuprofen	Sulindac
Indomethacin	Tetracyclines
Isoniazid	Tolmetin
Nitrofurantoin	

(Compiled from Ref. 8.)

URTICARIA

Clinical Presentation

Urticarial lesions consist of raised, pruritic erythematous wheals (hives) ranging in size from a few millimeters to geographic lesions extending over the chest or trunk. The raised edematous and plaque-like features of these lesions may result from localized vasodilation and transudation of fluid from small cutaneous blood vessels. This edematous response is induced by degranulation of mast cells in the dermis, causing release of histamine and other mediators of inflammation. The causes of mast cell degranulation are numerous and not limited to drugs (e.g., foods, allergens, infection, heat, cold). Drugs frequently associated with urticaria are listed in Table 91.3.

Pathogenesis

Drug-induced urticaria may be caused by IgE-dependent, circulating immune complexes or by nonimmunologic activation of effector pathways.[15] In IgE-dependent reactions the drug (antigen) forms a bridge between the IgE molecule and the surface of the mast cell, resulting in degranulation and liberation of histamine. Clinically, urticarial lesions may appear within minutes to hours of drug exposure in a sensitized patient; this is termed an immediate reaction. Reactions that occur within 12–36 hours of drug exposure are called accelerated reactions. In some cases, urticarial lesions may be the first manifestation of anaphylaxis; thus, close monitoring is indicated.

Hypersensitivity that is established during administration of the drug with symptoms not appearing until 8–21 days after exposure is termed a late reaction. Other symptoms that may accompany urticaria in late reactions include fever, lymphadenopathy, joint swelling, and arthralgias.

Some drugs do not require an allergic mechanism to induce urticaria. Certain amines may displace histamine from intracellular storage sites, while other drugs directly degranulate mast cells through complement or arachidonic acid-dependent pathways.[8] Examples include acetylsalicylic acid, atropine, opiates, quinine, thiamine, pilocarpine, iodinated radiocontrast dyes, and nonsteroidal anti-inflammatory

TABLE 91.3. DRUGS ASSOCIATED WITH URTICARIA

Acetylsalicylic acid	Opiates
Gold	Penicillins
Heparin	Sulfonamides
Ibuprofen	Sulindac
Indomethacin	Tartrazine
Iodinated radiocontrast media	Tolmetin
Naproxen	

(Compiled from Ref. 8.)

agents. Drug concentrations may play a role in the appearance of these reactions.

The course of acute urticaria is variable, but the condition usually resolves within 1–3 days. Chronic urticaria has a more prolonged, sometimes indefinite course. For example, it may be stimulated from penicillin found in dairy products or by molds within the environment.[10]

Identification of the causative agent in urticaria may be difficult when multiple drugs and exposures to foodstuffs and environmental allergens are present.

Diagnosis

Urticaria presents as wheals that are usually well defined, erythematous, and plaque-like. These edematous and pruritic lesions are unique in that a particular lesion is often evanescent (i.e., transient—disappearing in a matter of hours).

Management

Appropriate management depends on the severity of symptoms and the ability to identify and remove the offending agent. Recent reports indicate that the tricyclic antidepressant doxepin may block H_1 and H_2 receptors and may be effective in patients with chronic urticaria.[16] Topical agents other than mild antipruritic agents are not necessary, and topical antihistamines (used for local anesthetic effect) are best avoided because of their high incidence of contact sensitization.[17] Ketotifen is an oral H_1-receptor blocker with antiallergenic and antiasthmatic properties. It appears to be a worthwhile agent for difficult cases of urticaria that are resistant to conventional antihistamines, but it is available only on a compassionate-use basis in the United States.[18]

FIXED-DRUG ERUPTIONS

Clinical Presentation

A fixed-drug eruption consists of an erythematous round or oval lesion ranging from a few millimeters to 20 cm in diameter.[8] Initially, one lesion appears; other lesions may subsequently occur. With time the color turns to a dusky-red or violaceous hue. The lesion may also be edematous with formation of vesicles or bullae. The patient may complain of itching in the affected area, but sensations of warmth or burning are more common without additional systemic symptoms. Lesions may appear on any part of the skin or mucous membranes, although the lips and genitalia are more commonly affected.[19] Healing occurs over 7–10 days after discontinuation of the offending agent and often leaves a dark hyperpigmented patch. Reexposure to the offending drug results in recurrence of the eruption (within 30 minutes to 8 hours) in the exact location as the previous reaction.[19] The recurrence after rechallenge in the same site led to the label "fixed-drug eruption."

Pathogenesis

The fixed-drug eruption is the only cutaneous reaction for which drugs or chemicals are considered the sole cause (see Table 91.4). The pathogenesis of fixed-drug eruption is not well understood. In some cases, topical application of the drug to the affected area will again exacerbate the reaction.[19]

Usually, a single drug is responsible for a fixed-drug eruption, although some patients react to multiple agents (especially when the compounds are chemically related).[19] Diagnosis may be established by biopsy. The drug should not be readministered because extensive bullous lesions may occur.[8]

Management

Systemic corticosteroids and antihistamines are often used, but they typically have minimal or no apparent effect on the course of fixed-drug eruptions.[19] Removal of the offending agent and conservative measures with cool water compresses during the acute phase, and bleaching creams for hyperpigmented areas of involvement during chronic phases, are generally recommended.

PHOTOSENSITIVITY

Clinical Presentation

Sun- and drug-induced cutaneous photoreactions are increasingly more common, not only because of increased use of tanning booths and emphasis on tanning, but also because of the increased number of photosensitizing chemicals used in cosmetics and drugs. Clinically, photosensitivity reactions appear very similar to a sunburn; these may include erythema, edema, papules, and plaque-like perhaps urticarial, lesions, sometimes with vesicle formation. The hallmark of photosensitivity eruptions is their appearance

TABLE 91.4. DRUGS THAT PRODUCE FIXED-DRUG ERUPTIONS

Barbiturates	Ibuprofen
Dapsone	Ipecac
Digitalis compounds	Metronidazole
Diphenhydramine	Phenolphthalein
Disulfiram	Phenothiazines
Epinephrine	Phenylbutazone
Erythromycin	Quinidine
Gold	Sulfonamides
Griseofulvin	Sulindac
Hydralazine	Tetracyclines
Hydroxyurea	Trimethoprim

(Compiled from Refs. 8 and 19.)

on areas of skin receiving the greatest exposure to sunlight (e.g., the tops of the ears, nose, cheeks, lateral and lower posterior surfaces of the neck, extensor surfaces of the forearms, and dorsa of the hands).[8] In some cases, the eruption may extend to non–sun-exposed areas and generalize over the body.[20] Chronically, reactions may become hyperpigmented or hypopigmented, perhaps atrophic and with yellowish papules as well as telangiectasias.

Pathogenesis

Phototoxic and photoallergic reactions are two different types of photosensitivity conditions often difficult to differentiate. Phototoxic reactions are the most common and depend on the dose of drug and the amount of sunlight. A phototoxic reaction occurs in 100% of those exposed to adequate amounts of drug and sunlight on first exposure to such stimuli. The drug or metabolite is thought to act as a chromophore, absorbing ultraviolet light (usually long wave). The ultraviolet light activates the drug or metabolite to emit energy that may damage adjacent tissue. The wavelength of light needed to produce a reaction depends on the absorption spectrum of the drug.[8] The resulting damage appears as an intensified sunburn with desquamation and peeling.

A photoallergic reaction is less common and, by definition, depends on an antigen–antibody or cell-mediated hypersensitivity phenomenon.[20] Photoallergic reactions do not generally occur on first exposure and require a sensitization period to the drug or metabolite. It is postulated that ultraviolet light reacts with the drug or metabolite in the skin to produce a hapten. The hapten combines with a tissue antigen to form a complete antigen that elicits an allergic response on subsequent exposure. Once sensitization is achieved, minimal amounts of drug are usually needed to produce a reaction.[8] Topically applied drugs or chemicals and airborne allergens may also produce photosensitivity reactions at their point of contact with the skin. Ingredients found in perfumes, deodorants, and aftershave lotions are examples of photocontactants. See Table 91.5 for drugs that frequently produce photosensitivity reactions.

Diagnosis

Diagnosis of photosensitivity reactions is usually based on history and clinical presentation, although histology or patch testing may be helpful.[20] Discontinuation of the offending agent should result in slow regression of the eruption, although 10–20% of patients may have a persistent photosensitivity for prolonged periods.[10,21]

Management

Management for acute reactions includes avoidance of sunlight, topical remedies (e.g., cool wet dressings, soothing shake-lotions, corticosteroids), and topical or systemic antipruritic agents.[20]

TABLE 91.5. DRUGS THAT PRODUCE PHOTOSENSITIVITY REACTIONS

Amiodarone	Piroxicam
Carbamazepine	Protriptyline
Dacarbazine	Quinidine
Furosemide	Sulfonamides
Ketoprofen	Sulfonylureas
Naproxen	Sulindac
Oral contraceptives	Tetracyclines
Phenothiazines/chlorpromazine	Thiazides
Phenylbutazone	

(Compiled from Refs. 8, 10, and 21.)

Identification and removal of the inciting agent are ideal. For cases in which this is not possible, sunscreens or psoralen ultraviolet light treatment (PUVA) have been used.[21] The use of sunscreens to prevent photoreactions may be problematic. Most sunscreens do not block the entire spectrum of ultraviolet light that may be responsible for mediating many photoreactions. Paradoxically, sunscreens may also produce a photocontact eruption in sensitized patients.[8,10,22] *para*-Aminobenzoic acid, a common ultraviolet-β-blocking ingredient in sunscreens, is chemically similar to thiazides, sulfonylureas, furosemide, and carbonic anhydrase inhibitors. Patients allergic to such agents should use alternative sunscreens containing oxybenzone or cinoxate to avoid cross-reactivity.

ALOPECIA

Many drugs have been associated with partial or total hair loss, either as an extension of their pharmacologic effect or as an adverse reaction with an unknown mechanism[23] (see Table 91.6).

Antimitotics/Cytostatics

Hair loss from cytostatic agents is well recognized and occurs because of a direct effect of the drug on the hair follicle. The incidence of alopecia in patients receiving high-dose cyclophosphamide has ranged from 21–48%.[24]

Cyclophosphamide inhibits mitosis of actively growing hair follicles, resulting in a thinned and weakened hair

TABLE 91.6. DRUGS ASSOCIATED WITH ALOPECIA

Carbamazepine	Hydantoin derivatives
Clofibrate	Isotretinoin
Colchicine	Propranolol
Ethionamide	Valproate sodium
Etretinate	Vitamin A (high dose)

(Compiled from Refs. 8 and 23.)

shaft susceptible to damage with minor trauma.[24] The extent of alopecia appears to be dose dependent and may often occur within 4–6 days of the first dose.[25] Regrowth usually occurs after discontinuation of the drug, although shedding of normal mature hairs may continue for a prolonged period.[25]

Anticoagulants

Heparin and warfarin may sometimes induce alopecia 2–3 months after initiation of therapy.[25] The exact mechanism is unknown, although it is postulated that actively growing hairs are prematurely entered into the telogen (resting phase) and shed.[8] Higher doses (and not duration of exposure) are thought to influence primarily the degree of hair loss, which may be diffuse and/or extensive. Regrowth occurs after discontinuation of the drug.[25]

Thioamides

Agents used to treat hyperthyroidism may not only cause a dose-dependent hair loss, but may change the texture of the remaining hair to dry, brittle, and lusterless.[8] This may be an extension of thioamide pharmacologic effect, because hypothyroidism presents with a similar picture.

Oral Contraceptives

Two types of alopecia are associated with oral contraceptive use. First, a diffuse hair loss sometimes occurs within 1–4 months of discontinuation of oral contraceptives.[25] This is analogous to postpartum alopecia (pregnancy slows the conversion of actively growing hair to mature hair). Second, during oral contraceptive therapy, a more diffuse alopecia, similar to the male pattern, may occur.[26] Progesterone stimulation via the androgenic effects of oral contraceptives may cause this type of alopecia.

VASCULITIS

Clinical Presentation

Vasculitis is characterized by inflammation and damage of blood vessels that may affect various organ systems. It commonly appears on the lower extremities or pressure-dependent areas of the skin as red or purple (purpuric) lesions. These lesions range in size from a pinpoint to several centimeters. Early lesions are often macular, although they are commonly raised (palpable) and may have hemorrhagic bullae.[27] Lesions may persist 1–4 weeks or longer and in some cases become yellow to brown upon healing.[27] Systemic symptoms such as burning, stinging, malaise, arthralgias, and fever may be present. Other organ systems, including the liver, kidney, brain, and joints, may also be affected. Table 91.7 lists drugs that frequently cause vasculitis.

TABLE 91.7. DRUGS ASSOCIATED WITH VASCULITIS

Allopurinol	Phenylbutazone
Anticoagulants	Phenytoin
Cimetidine	Piroxicam
Fluoxetine	Propylthiouracil
Hydralazine	Quinine
Ibuprofen	Sulfonamides
Indomethacin	Thiazides
Penicillins	

(Compiled from Refs. 8, 10, and 15.)

Pathogenesis

It is often difficult to distinguish among various types of vasculitis and to identify a cause. Although skin tests or *in vitro* testing assists in the diagnosis, identification of a causative source is difficult.

Management

Management includes removal of the offending or suspected agent.[27] Bedrest and compression of lesions may promote healing. Although their efficacy is not well documented, oral corticosteroids have been used by some clinicians to inhibit cell-mediated immunity, decrease inflammation, and suppress immunoglobulin synthesis.[27] Cyclophosphamide, plasmapheresis, indomethacin, sulfones, colchicine, and aspirin have been tried with variable success.[27] Interestingly, some therapeutic modalities are listed as causative agents, suggesting that further research is needed to identify the pathogenic processes involved in vasculitis.

HYPERPIGMENTATION

Drugs may produce color changes in the skin by a variety of mechanisms, including deposition of melanin in the dermis and stimulation of melanin formation. Appearance, location, mechanism, and course of hyperpigmentation induced by commonly used drugs vary by pharmacologic grouping. Drugs known to induce pigmentary changes include hydantoins, metals (see Table 91.8), antimalarials, phenothiazines, oral contraceptives, tetracyclines, chemotherapeutic agents (see Table 91.9), and amiodarone.

HYDANTOIN DERIVATIVES

Approximately 10% of patients taking phenytoin or related agents develop a brown patchy hyperpigmentation on light-exposed areas.[8] Although the hyperpigmentation deepens with light exposure, it usually does not disappear during

TABLE 91.8. HEAVY METAL-INDUCED HYPERPIGMENTATION

Agent	Color	Region Involved	Special Features
Mercury	Gray brown, slate green	Skin folds (topical), gingival pigmentation (systemic)	Caused by deposition of metallic granules and increased melanin production; formerly used in bleaching agents
Silver	Slate gray, blue gray	Sun-exposed areas, mucosa sclerae, nails	Silver granule deposition that activates melanin production; occurs months to years after ingestion
Bismuth	Blue gray	Skin, conjunctiva, oral and vaginal mucosa, black line along gingival margin	Deposition of metallic granules or interaction with bacteria in mouth; more common with parenteral use
Arsenic	Brown, bronze	Trunk, "raindrop"-shaped hyperkeratotic papulonodular lesions; palms, soles	Activates enzymes that form melanin and deposit in skin; used systemically for psoriasis and as a health tonic; pigmentation appears 1–20 years after exposure
Gold	Blue gray	Periorbital, generalized chrysiasis, sun-exposed areas	Caused by deposition of metallic particles in epidermis, occurs months to years after exposure and is permanent

(Compiled from Refs. 8 and 29.)

winter months.[28] Hydantoin derivatives appear to cause an increase in melanin of the basal layer and induce dispersion of melanin granules in an animal model.[28] Women appear to be affected more than men, suggesting a hormonal origin with light as a triggering factor.[28]

ANTIMALARIAL AGENTS

Approximately 25% of patients taking antimalarials for more than 3 or 4 months develop pigmentation changes.[29] The pigmentation patterns vary and include patchy, irregular blue-black or gray lesions on pretibial areas or diffuse facial hyperpigmentation. A transverse band in the middle of the nail has also been reported.[29] The onset of pigmentation changes has ranged from 4–20 months, with discontinuation of therapy resulting in lightening but persistence of lesions.[29] Quinacrine causes a diffuse lemon-yellow skin discoloration that gives the patient a jaundiced appearance. Scleral coloration is slight and pigmentation returns to normal 1–4 months after therapy.[29]

PHENOTHIAZINES

Pigmentation changes induced by phenothiazines (e.g., chlorpromazine, thioridazine) range from a bronze color in sun-exposed areas to a violet, purplish gray with long-term exposure.[29] Forehead, cheeks, nose, hands, and upper extremities are most commonly affected. An increased deposition of melanin occurs in the dermis and phenothiazine-melanin complexes are believed responsible for color changes. Pigmentation is not usually totally reversible but may fade slowly in winter months or upon discontinuation of therapy.[29]

ORAL CONTRACEPTIVES

Melasma, characterized by irregular brown macules on the cheeks, forehead, or upper lip, is a frequent cutaneous reaction to oral contraceptives.[26] Estrogen, progesterone, or sun exposure may be responsible for the increased melanin deposition in the dermis and epidermis.[29] Onset usually occurs within 1–20 months, but hyperpigmentation may persist after discontinuation.[26] Sunscreens may be helpful in minimizing the extent of hyperpigmentation.

TETRACYCLINES

Bluish pigmentation of previously inflamed skin may result from tetracycline deposition after prolonged high-dose therapy.[8,29] Several types of pigmentation changes have been reported with the use of minocycline. Blue-black coloration in areas of active scarring, generalized blue-gray pigmentation on sun-exposed areas, generalized muddy hue, and discoloration of teeth have been noted.[29] Coloration commonly fades after cessation of therapy.[30]

CLOFAZIMINE

Clofazimine has been used extensively to treat lepromatous leprosy.[31] It has also been found to be effective in the treatment of mycobacterial infections in patients with AIDS,[32] discoid lupus erythematosus,[33] and pyoderma gangrenosum.[34] A frequent side effect of clofazimine is deep brown pigmentation, which may especially affect areas of skin with leprosy lesions.[31]

TABLE 91.9. CHEMOTHERAPEUTIC AGENTS ASSOCIATED WITH HYPERPIGMENTATION

Agent	Color	Region Involved	Special Features
Busulfan	Brown	Face, forearms, chest, trunk, hands	Accelerates melanin formation by enzymes; incidence more frequent in dark-skinned patients; resolves on discontinuation
Bleomycin	Brown	Linear bands on chest, back	Incidence 8%–20%; reversible on discontinuation
Doxorubicin	Black-brown	Tongue, palms, soles, nails	Increased incidence in dark-skinned patients; reversible on discontinuation
Mechlorethamine (topical)	Brown	Areas of contact	Toxic effect on keratinocytes; increased melanocytes; some aggregation

(Compiled from Ref. 29.)

AMIODARONE

A gray-blue coloration in sun-exposed areas has been reported in up to 10% of patients receiving amiodarone.[35] The discoloration may be caused by the incorporation of amiodarone into lysosomes, causing an accumulation of polar lipids.[36] Symptom onset has ranged from 6–39 months after initiation of therapy and discontinuation may cause slow fading of the lesion.[29]

ERYTHEMA MULTIFORME/ STEVENS–JOHNSON SYNDROME

CLINICAL PRESENTATION

Erythema multiforme is a cutaneous reaction of variable morphology that evolves and changes over time. Initially, a round, 1- to 10-cm, erythematous macule may appear, which becomes edematous and papular over time.[36] These lesions may enlarge into plaques or form concentric rings of erythema and clearing with a central vesicular or necrotic area. Lesions with zones of concentric color change are termed "iris" or "target" lesions and may enlarge and coalesce into polycyclic configurations. Hands, feet, limbs, mucous membranes, and face are the sites most commonly affected, with an acute onset often preceded by mild upper respiratory symptoms. Lesions begin to resolve in 4–5 days, with complete healing in 2–4 weeks, although new lesions can appear during this period.[36] Postinflammatory hyperpigmentation may occur after healing.

Stevens–Johnson syndrome (SJS) is considered a severe variant of erythema multiforme with extensive mucosal and conjunctival edema, erosions, high fever, myalgias, vomiting, diarrhea, and arthralgias. Skin lesions may be severe with large bullae and areas of denudation. The onset of these lesions is variable, but healing usually occurs within 6 weeks. Complications include keratitis, conjunctival scarring, blindness, pneumonia, dehydration, and esophagitis.[36]

PATHOGENESIS

The pathogenesis of erythema multiforme and SJS is not completely elucidated. Evidence indicates that both an immune complex mechanism and cell-mediated immune reactivity may be involved.[10] Identification of the etiologic factor is also difficult, because erythema multiforme may be precipitated by totally unconnected factors. Drugs are frequently implicated (see Table 91.10), but viruses, bacteria, fungi, vaccines, and other diseases have been associated with erythema multiforme.[36]

Diagnosis of erythema multiforme is based largely on history, clinical appearance, and histology. Often, prodromal symptoms are treated with antibiotics; thus, etiology (e.g., virus, bacteria, or drug) is difficult to clarify.

MANAGEMENT

Because mild forms of erythema multiforme are self-limiting, usually only symptomatic treatment is instituted, for example, tap water compresses for blisters and necrosis, antihistamines for pruritus, and one-half–strength hydrogen peroxide gargle for oral lesions. Patients should be carefully monitored for progression to more severe forms or development of complications. The efficacy of using systemic corticosteroids for severe erythema multiforme and SJS is not clearly defined.[37,38] Systemic corticosteroids per-

TABLE 91.10. DRUGS ASSOCIATED WITH ERYTHEMA MULTIFORME

Barbiturates	Propranolol
Carbamazepine	Quinine
Diflunisal	Salicylates
Hydantoins	Sulfonamides
Ibuprofen	Sulfonylureas
Penicillins	Sulindac
Phenolphthalein	Thiazides
Phenylbutazone	

(Compiled from Refs. 8, 10, and 36.)

haps have greatest utility when used in high doses early in the reaction (first few days) versus late in the reaction when diminishing benefit is obtained and morbidity and mortality may actually increase in association with corticosteroid use.

Toxic Epidermal Necrolysis

CLINICAL PRESENTATION

Although toxic epidermal necrolysis (TEN) is considered common, its true incidence may not be correctly estimated because of misdiagnosis and confusion with similar severe skin reactions. In many cases, there is a prodromal state of malaise, sore throat, pyrexia, headache, and myalgias, followed by an acute onset of cutaneous manifestations within hours or days.[8,10,39] The eruption may present in various forms, often as a macular lesion with a burning sensation that enlarges over the body. The lesions may form large flaccid bullae within the erythema or directly progress to massive detachment of the epidermis. At this point, the epidermis is easily rubbed off by light pressure with outer coverings of ruptured bullae clinging to underlying tissue. Because lesions may appear on any area of skin (e.g., palms, soles, mouth, throat, nose, trachea, eyelids, conjunctiva, cornea, and vagina), the picture may be similar to a second-degree burn or scald. Hairy areas are less commonly involved.

Complications are numerous and include fluid and electrolyte imbalance from loss of epidermis; septicemia; erosion of the mucous membranes of the mouth, nose, urethra, vagina, or rectum; corneal ulceration; and conjunctivitis. Internal organs may also be involved in severe cases, with possible manifestation of pneumonia, hepatocellular damage, gastrointestinal ulceration, nephritis, and myocardial damage.[10]

PATHOGENESIS

The pathogenic mechanisms responsible for TEN are unknown. The onset of TEN after drug exposure suggests a hypersensitivity-immunologic reaction, although there is little supporting evidence.[40] A TEN-like eruption has occurred in patients with a graft-versus-host reaction after bone marrow transplant or blood transfusion.[41]

Normocytic anemia, leukopenia, granulocytopenia, and neutropenia are commonly present in TEN with no readily accountable cause.[40,41] Drugs are often implicated as precipitating factors, but this is also difficult to verify because many patients receive multiple drugs (see Table 91.11). Other factors associated with TEN include vaccinations; viral, bacterial, and fungal infections; and neoplasia.[39]

The prognosis for TEN depends on the patient's age, extent of skin involvement, concurrent diseases, and complications.[10] Mortality is about 3% within the first 3 or 4 days of the acute episode.[8,10] After the acute episode, the epidermis may regenerate within 2–3 weeks, with complete healing in 6 weeks.[8]

TABLE 91.11. DRUGS ASSOCIATED WITH TOXIC EPIDERMAL NECROLYSIS

Allopurinol	Penicillins
Barbiturates	Phenylbutazone
Chloramphenicol	Quinine
Hydantoin derivatives	Sulfonamides
Ibuprofen	Sulindac
Indomethacin	Tolmetin

(Compiled from Ref. 8.)

MANAGEMENT

Management includes identification and withdrawal of the inciting factor, fluid and electrolyte maintenance, treatment or prevention of bacterial involvement, and prevention of ocular complications.[42] Management should be tailored to the individual case; some clinicians prefer referral to a burn unit.

Although the empiric use of systemic corticosteroid therapy is well documented, it is controversial because of a lack of well-controlled studies.[37,38] Some clinicians advocate corticosteroid use only within the first 48–72 hours of onset to prevent progression of complications[39]; others attribute delayed morbidity to systemic steroid use.[40] Without a definitive cause or known pathogenesis, supportive care is necessary to minimize mortality from TEN.

Conclusion

Unfortunately, no methods currently exist to determine unequivocally if a given medication is the cause of a particular skin eruption. Diagnosis is based largely on clinical appearance and morphology of lesions, dermatohistopathology, history, and in some cases *in vitro* tests or rechallenge.[43] A thorough history of drug and chemical exposure must be obtained, including the use of nonprescription medications and topical medications that may alter the morphologic appearance of the original lesion. The clinician should also consider the possibility of reaction to excipients or dyes contained in the drug formulation.

References

1. Shapiro S, Slone D, Siskind V, et al. Drug rash with ampicillin and other penicillins. Lancet 1969;2:969–972.

2. Johnson M, Johnson KG, Engel A. Prevalence, morbidity, and cost of dermatologic diseases. J Am Acad Dermatol 1984;11:930–936.
3. Baer RL, Witten VM. Drug eruptions, in Yearbook of Dermatology 1960–1961 Series. Chicago, Year Book Medical Publishers, 1961, pp 9–37.
4. Witte K, West DP. Immunology of adverse reactions to drugs. Pharmacother 1982;2:54–65.
5. Witte KW, West DP. Immunology of adverse reactions to antimicrobial agents, in Jeljaszewicz J, Pulverer G (eds): Antimicrobial Agents and Immunity. London, Academic, 1986, pp 217–249.
6. Arndt KA. Drug eruptions, allergic, in Arndt KA (ed): Manual of Dermatologic Therapeutics, 5th ed. Boston, Little, Brown, 1995, pp 60–63.
7. Bruinsma W. Drug monitoring in dermatology. Int J Dermatol 1986;25:166–168.
8. Bruinsma W. A Guide to Drug Eruptions, 6th ed. Oosthuizen, The Netherlands, De Zwaluw, 1995.
9. Merk HF, Mukhtar H, Hertl M. Drug-induced skin disorders, in Mukhtar H (ed): Pharmacology of the Skin. Boca Raton, FL, CRC Press, 1992, pp 151–166.
10. Schulz KH. Cutaneous manifestations of drug allergy, in De Weck AL, Bundgaard H (eds): Allergic Reactions to Drugs. Berlin, Springer-Verlag, 1983, pp 135–162.
11. Roujeau JC, Stern RS. Severe adverse cutaneous reactions to drugs. N Engl J Med 1994;331:1272–1285.
12. Nelson HS. Allergic reactions to drugs. Adv Asthma Allergy 1976;3:18–35.
13. Sullivan TJ. Drug allergy, in Middleton E Jr, Reed CE, Ellis EF, et al. (eds): Allergy Principles and Practice. St. Louis, MO, Mosby, 1993, pp 1726–1746.
14. Alanko K, Stubb S, Kauppinen K. Cutaneous drug reactions: Clinical types and causative agents. Acta Derm Venereol (Stockh) 1989;69:223–226.
15. Wintroub BU, Stern R. Cutaneous drug reactions: Pathogenesis and clinical classification. J Am Acad Dermatol 1985;13:167–179.
16. Greene SL, Reed CE, Schroeter AL. Double-blind crossover study comparing doxepin with diphenhydramine for the treatment of chronic urticaria. J Am Acad Dermatol 1985;12:669–675.
17. Yaffe SJ, Bierman CW, Cann HM, et al. Antihistamines in topical preparations. Pediatrics 1973;51:299–301.
18. Jay GT, Chow MSS. Focus on ketotifen: A long acting, H_1-receptor blocker with mast cell stabilizing properties. Hosp Formul 1989;24:632–645.
19. Korkij W, Soltani K. Fixed drug eruption. Arch Dermatol 1984;120:520–524.
20. Epstein JH, Wintroub BU. Photosensitivity due to drugs. Drugs 1985;30:42–57.
21. Robinson HN, Morison WL, Hood AF. Thiazide diuretic therapy and chronic photosensitivity. Arch Dermatol 1985;121:522–524.
22. Anonymous. Drugs that cause photosensitivity. Med Lett 1986;28:51–52.
23. Brodin MB. Drug-related alopecia. Dermatol Clin 1987;5:571–579.
24. Hood AF. Cutaneous complications of immunosuppressive agents. Dermatol Clin 1983;1:591–606.
25. Dawber RBR, Ebling FJG, Wojnarowska FT. Disorders of hair, alopecia of chemical origin, in Champion RH, Burton JL, Ebling FJG (eds): Textbook of Dermatology, 5th ed. Oxford, Blackwell, 1992, pp 2582–2584.
26. Jelinek JE. Cutaneous side effects of oral contraceptives. Arch Dermatol 1970;101:181–186.
27. Mackel SE. Treatment of vasculitis. Med Clin North Am 1982;66:941–954.
28. Moller H. Pigmentary disturbances due to drugs. Acta Derm Venereol (Stockh) 1966;46:423–431.
29. Granstein RD, Sober AJ. Drug and heavy metal-induced hyperpigmentation. J Am Acad Dermatol 1981;5:1–18.
30. Basler RSW. Minocycline-related hyperpigmentation. Arch Dermatol 1985;121:606–608.
31. Job CK, Yoder L, Jacobson RR, Hastings RC. Skin pigmentation from clofazimine therapy in leprosy patients: A reappraisal. J Am Acad Dermatol 1990;23:236–241.
32. Masur H, Tuazon C, Gill V, et al. Effect of combined clofazimine and ansamycin therapy on *Mycobacterium avium–Mycobacterium intracellulare* bacteremia in patients with AIDS. J Infect Dis 1987;155:127–129.
33. Crovato F, Levi L. Clofazimine in the treatment of annular lupus erythematosus. Arch Dermatol 1981;117:249–250.
34. Michaelson G, Molin L, Ohman S, et al. Clofazimine, a new agent for the treatment of pyoderma gangrenosum. Arch Dermatol 1976;112:344–349.
35. Trimble JW, Mendelson DS, Fetter BF, et al. Cutaneous pigmentation secondary to amiodarone therapy. Arch Dermatol 1983;119:914–918.
36. Huff JC, Weston WL, Tonnesen MG. Erythema multiforme: A critical review of characteristics, diagnostic criteria, and causes. J Am Acad Dermatol 1983;8:763–775.
37. Barton P, Flowers F. Controversies in the management of erythema multiforme and toxic epidermal necrolysis, in Dahl MV, Lynch PJ (eds): Current Opinion in Dermatology, 2nd ed. Philadelphia, Current Science, 1995, pp 27–31.
38. Duarte AM, Pruksachatkunakorn C, Schachner LA. Life-threatening dermatoses in pediatric dermatology, in Callen JP (ed): Advances in Dermatology, vol 10. St. Louis, MO, Mosby–Year Book, 1995, pp 329–371.
39. Parsons JM. Management of toxic epidermal necrolysis. Cutis 1985;36:305–311.
40. Westly ED, Wechsler HL. Toxic epidermal necrolysis. Arch Dermatol 1984;120:721–726.
41. Goeens J, Song M, Fondu P. Haematological disturbances and immune mechanisms in toxic epidermal necrolysis. Br J Dermatol 1986;114:255–259.
42. Brady WJ, DeBehnke D, Crosby DL. Dermatological emergencies. Am J Emerg Med 1994;12:217–237.
43. Kalish RS. Drug eruptions: A review of clinical and immunologic findings. Adv Dermatol 1991;6:221–238.

Section 12

HEMATOLOGIC DISORDERS

Chapter 92

Hematopoiesis

William P. Petros, PharmD, and Maha A. Elkordy, MD

Hematopoiesis is defined as the formation and maturation of blood cells and their derivatives. There is a tremendous daily turnover rate of cells in this system with more than 6 billion cells produced per kilogram of body weight every 24 hours.[1] These accelerated processes result in vastly exaggerated and rapid responses to the slightest perturbation.

In humans, hematopoiesis takes place primarily in the bone marrow. Hematopoietic cells were among the first to be evaluated for their biologic functions and pattern of maturation; however, recent identification of the protein molecules (cytokines) that seem to regulate this system has yielded an extraordinary amount of new information regarding its control. The process of continual hematopoietic cell production is complicated, involving interactions between immature cells, the surrounding microenvironment, and cytokines.

This chapter discusses the regulation, proliferation, and some functions of hematopoietic cells. This information is essential to understanding the pathophysiologic and therapy-related hematopoietic effects covered elsewhere in the text. Directly related chapters include Chapter 80, Function and Evaluation of the Immune System; Chapter 93, Anemias; Chapter 96, Drug-Induced Hematologic Disorders; and Chapter 119, Basic Principles of Cancer Treatment and Cancer Chemotherapy.

FUNCTIONS OF MATURE HEMATOPOIETIC CELLS

The hematopoietic system consists of three primary cell components: erythrocytes, platelets, and leukocytes. The latter term encompasses a functionally diverse group of cells that includes neutrophils, lymphocytes, monocytes/macrophages, eosinophils, plasma cells, and basophils. Typical concentrations of mature hematopoietic cells found in the peripheral blood of adults are shown in Table 92.1.

LEUKOCYTES

Neutrophils (Segs and Bands)

The major functions of neutrophils (also known as polymorphonuclear leukocytes) are to prevent pathogenic microorganism invasion and to localize and kill these microorganisms. These effects are mediated by a series of events, including migration to the site (chemotaxis), recognition/attachment to the invader, phagocytosis, lysosomal fusion, degranulation, and local generation of oxidants (respiratory burst) and degrading enzymes (Fig. 92.1).[2] A neutrophil is attracted to the site of infection by chemotactic factors. Once migration to the site has occurred, the neutrophil ingests the opsonized microorganism (opsonization is the process whereby antibody and complement coat the microorganism, allowing for increased neutrophil recognition). Following ingestion or phagocytosis, the cytoplasmic granules within the neutrophil fuse with the phagosome or phagocytosed macrophage, thereby initiating degranulation and release of enzymes. These degrading enzymes kill the microorganism through oxygen reduction. Secretion of these enzymes may also result in localized host tissue injury. Neutrophil activity may be intensified by the actions of cytokines such as granulocyte colony-stimulating factor

TABLE 92.1. AVERAGE (NORMAL RANGE) ADULT BLOOD CELL CONCENTRATIONS

White cell count ($\times 10^9$/L)	7.8 (4.4–11.3)	
Red cell count ($\times 10^{12}$/L)	Male	5.21 (4.52–5.90)
	Female	4.60 (4.10–5.10)
Hemoglobin[a] (mg/dL)	Male	15.7 (14.0–17.5)
	Female	13.8 (12.3–15.3)
Hematocrit	Male	0.46 (0.42–0.50)
	Female	0.40 (0.36–0.45)
Mean corpuscular volume (fL/red cell)	88.0 (80.0–96.1)	
Platelet count ($\times 10^9$/L)	311 (172–450)	

[a]May be 0.5–1.0 mg/dL lower in black patients.

(G-CSF) and granulocyte–macrophage colony-stimulating factor (GM-CSF).[3]

Eosinophils

Effector functions similar to those of neutrophils are elicited by eosinophils; however, it is done with less efficiency. Eosinophil activity is primarily directed against large invaders such as helminths and other parasites that cannot be phagocytized. During an allergic reaction, activated mast cells secrete chemicals that attract and stimulate eosinophils, which in turn produce substances that neutralize or degrade the reaction products of mast cells. Unfortunately, the eosinophil constituents may also damage normal tissue and cause secondary histamine release. High concentrations of eosinophils for prolonged periods may result in damage to the cardiac and central nervous systems, with possible pulmonary and dermatologic involvement.[4]

Basophils and Mast Cells

These cells function as mediators of inflammatory processes via massive release of their granule contents upon stimulation. The released chemicals include heparin, histamine, and other substances. The mediator may be vasoactive, bronchoconstrictive, and/or chemotactic (attractive) for eosinophils.[5,6]

Monocytes/Macrophages

Monocytes are derived from the granulocyte–monocyte colony-forming unit. They are peripheral cells in transit from the bone marrow to tissues. Once in the tissues, under

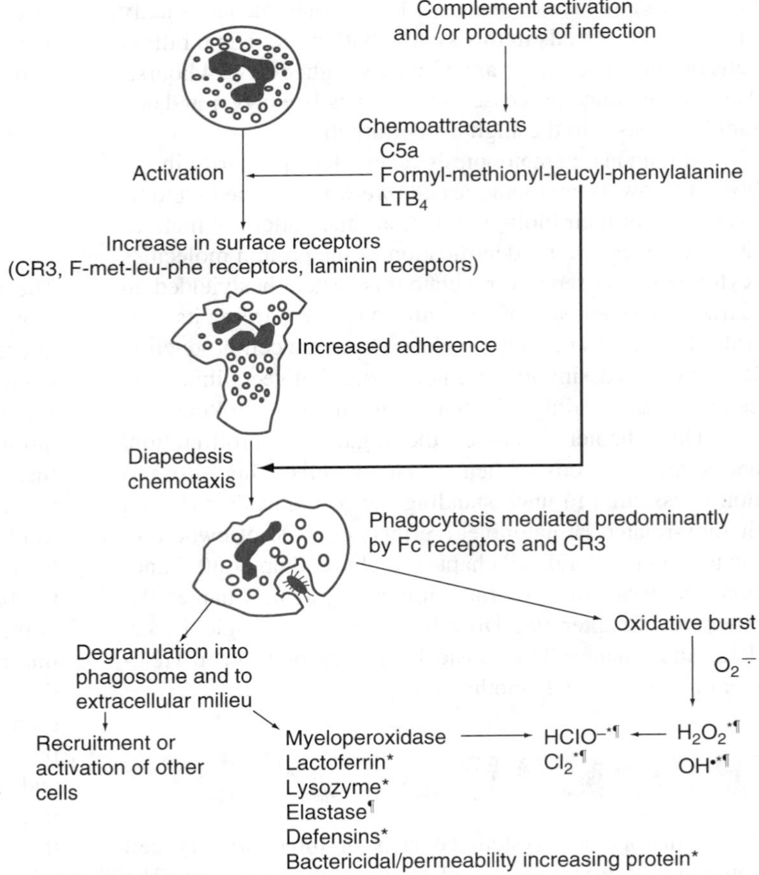

Figure 92.1. Neutrophil responses to infection or inflammation. *(Reprinted by permission of The New England Journal of Medicine, vol 317; p 688, 1987.)*

the influence of local factors, monocytes are transformed to macrophages.

Macrophages exist in the liver (Kupffer's cells), spleen, lymph nodes, microglial (CNS) cells, skin (Langerhans' cells), and bone. A variety of functions are performed by monocytes and macrophages, including initiation of immune responses for recognition by lymphocytes, regulation of immune response intensity, phagocytosis of foreign invaders, tumor cytotoxicity, degradation of cellular debris, and secretion of peptide molecules called monokines (a subclassification of cytokines).[7] Examples of monokines include interferons, tumor necrosis factor, and interleukin-1. Monokines and other cytokines regulate the activity of these cells.

Lymphocytes

The primary functions of lymphocytes are to control and be the effector cells for the immune system. Many of these cells also are important synthetic sites for various cytokines. Lymphocytes can be functionally divided into cells that display cell-mediated immunity (T cells) and those that are responsible for humoral immunity (B cells) (Table 92.2). B lymphocytes ultimately become plasma cells, which produce immunoglobulin specific for an antigen attached to the cell's surface. Several different T-cell subtypes are found in peripheral blood. These include the cytotoxic suppressor T cells (CD8), which attack intracellular pathogens and regulate the size and duration of the immune response, as well as helper T cells (CD4). The latter cells are responsible for delayed hypersensitivity, stimulation of B-cell differentiation (maturation), and antibody production, in addition to regulation of inflammatory reactions. Null cells are a separate subset of lymphocytes that lacks surface markers of B or T origin. These cells, also referred to as LGL or large granular lymphocytes, are thought to perform functions such as direct cytotoxicity to foreign entities, and they act either alone (natural killer cells) or in concert with immunoglobulin (antibody-dependent cellular cytotoxicity).[8,9] Further details regarding lymphocytes are found in Chapter 80, Function and Evaluation of the Immune System.

TABLE 92.2. LYMPHOCYTE-MEDIATED IMMUNE FUNCTION

Cellular Immunity (T Cells)
1. Provides resistance against intracellular pathogens such as viruses, protozoa, fungi, and bacteria
2. Mediates allogeneic transplant rejection
3. Responsible for contact dermatitis
4. Provides autologous reaction to tumor cells

Humoral Immunity (B Cells)
1. Major component of allergic reactions and other autoimmune diseases
2. Aids in eradication of encapsulated bacteria
3. Inactivates circulating toxins
4. May play role in antitumor reactions

PLATELETS

Platelets (thrombocytes) interact to facilitate blood coagulation by several mechanisms. These include localization of the thrombus; providing a specific receptor site for clotting factors as well as the necessary phospholipid surface for the conversion of prothrombin to thrombin; and protection of thrombin from antithrombin. The process is initiated with a vascular injury that causes platelets to adhere to the exposed collagen fibers of the damaged wall as blood flows out. These events require the presence of other plasma proteins, namely, von Willebrand factor. Platelets then aggregate through a process that is calcium dependent. Following aggregation, various platelet mediators are released (thromboxane, serotonin, platelet factor V), resulting in the formation of an irreversible platelet aggregate with subsequent formation of a stable fibrin cross-linked clot.[10,11]

ERYTHROCYTES

The primary function of the erythrocyte is to carry oxygen from the lungs to the peripheral tissues. Its optimal design enables efficient oxygen transport via the hemoglobin molecule. Oxygen release is controlled by the general metabolic state of the patient and local factors.

Hematopoietic Structure and Compartments

Embryonic development of hematopoietic tissue occurs in the yolk sac mesenchyme, with fetal transition occurring in the liver and spleen. Very immature hematopoietic cells can also be found in umbilical cord blood, but not many are evident in the peripheral blood of adults.[12] The ultimate location of immature hematopoietic cells is in the bone marrow. The average adult has approximately 1.7 liters of bone marrow, which provides an optimal environment for the development and proliferation of hematopoietic cells. The hematopoietic bone marrow is primarily located in the central portion of the pelvis, ribs, vertebrae, skull, and femora/humeri epiphyses. The anatomic structure of the bone marrow is characterized by the central venous marrow sinus, which is linked by course vascular sinusoids that intertwine a reticulin mesh where the cells are suspended. Thus hematopoiesis occurs in the extravascular marrow spaces, which also contain endothelial cells, fibroblasts, macrophages, and adipocytes, collectively termed bone marrow stroma.[13] Stromal cells are thought to be important hematopoietic components, providing growth factors, collagen, and cell-adhesion proteins.[14] When these cells are

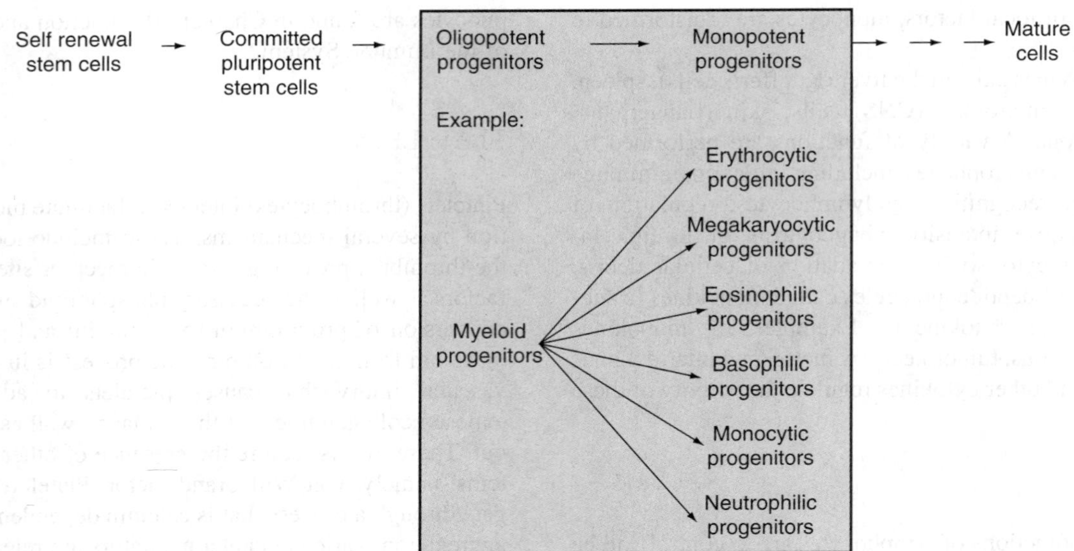

Figure 92.2. This rudimentary model of hematopoiesis displays the basic steps a cell may take from its inception as a stem cell in the bone marrow, through stages in which it can become multiple (oligopotent) or only one specific (monopotent) type of mature blood cell.

combined with accessory cells (lymphocytes/monocytes) and cytokines, the mixture is referred to as the hematopoietic microenvironment. Egress of more mature cells from the bone marrow occurs through the endothelial cell barrier. Release of cells such as neutrophils may be stimulated by complement, steroids, or endotoxin. Immature cells that may ultimately become any one of the blood cellular components can be transiently mobilized from the bone marrow into peripheral blood by administration of a cytotoxic chemotherapy drug (e.g., cyclophosphamide)[15] or a colony-stimulating factor (e.g., G-CSF or GM-CSF).[16] This process is commonly referred to as "priming" the bone marrow for peripheral blood progenitor or stem cells.

The least mature hematopoietic cell, accounting for only a fraction of a percent of bone marrow cells, is referred to as the stem cell. These cells have the unique potential to ultimately become any of the mature hematopoietic cells, thus they are termed *pluripotent* and, importantly, have self-renewal capacity (Fig. 92.2).[17] Extensive research has been conducted describing the morphologic and immunologic characteristics indicative of the earliest stem cell; however, investigators have yet to arrive at a consensus model. Only a small percentage of these cells is likely to be dividing at any one time, thus most are dormant in the cell cycle. Stem cell renewal and differentiation occur within the bone marrow under the influence of the marrow microenvironment. Stromal endothelial cells, fibroblasts, and fat cells (adipocytes) are necessary to support stem cell proliferation and division by providing anchorage for adhesion and secreting various hematopoietic growth factors necessary for differentiation. It is the characteristics of the local microenvironment (cellular matrix and growth factor concentrations) that influence the differentiation of a particular hematopoietic lineage, favoring it over another.

The next step in hematopoietic cell differentiation is thought to be represented by committed pluripotent stem cells that can still differentiate into any cell line (red blood cells [RBCs], white blood cells [WBCs], platelet); however, they have a limited capacity for self-renewal (Fig. 92.2).

Cells that choose to differentiate can proceed to either myeloid or lymphoid cell precursors (oligopotent progenitors). These cells may ultimately become B or T lymphocytes in the case of lymphoid cells. Myeloid progenitors may become granulocytes, erythrocytes, macrophages, or megakaryocytes as outlined in the following and displayed in Fig. 92.2. Nomenclature for immature hematopoietic cells often uses terms developed during *in vitro* experiments of cell proliferation. Thus the term burst-forming unit (BFU) or colony-forming unit (CFU) is added to the suffix of the cell lines ultimately produced by the specific cell.

Leukocytes found in the peripheral blood can generally be classified into neutrophils (most frequently occurring blood leukocyte subdivided into the more mature segs and less mature bands), lymphocytes, monocytes, eosinophils, basophils, and the tissue derivative of the latter, the mast cell. Immature neutrophils such as metamyelocytes are rarely seen in peripheral blood. Strictly speaking, the group of cells referred to as granulocytes includes neutrophils, eosinophils, and basophils; however, common use tends to include only the former cell type. The terminally differentiated leukocytes, which are usually not seen in blood, include the macrophage or histiocyte (derived from monocytes) and plasma cells (derived from B lymphocytes).

Most of the body's neutrophils and neutrophilic precursors reside in the bone marrow (approximately 9 billion

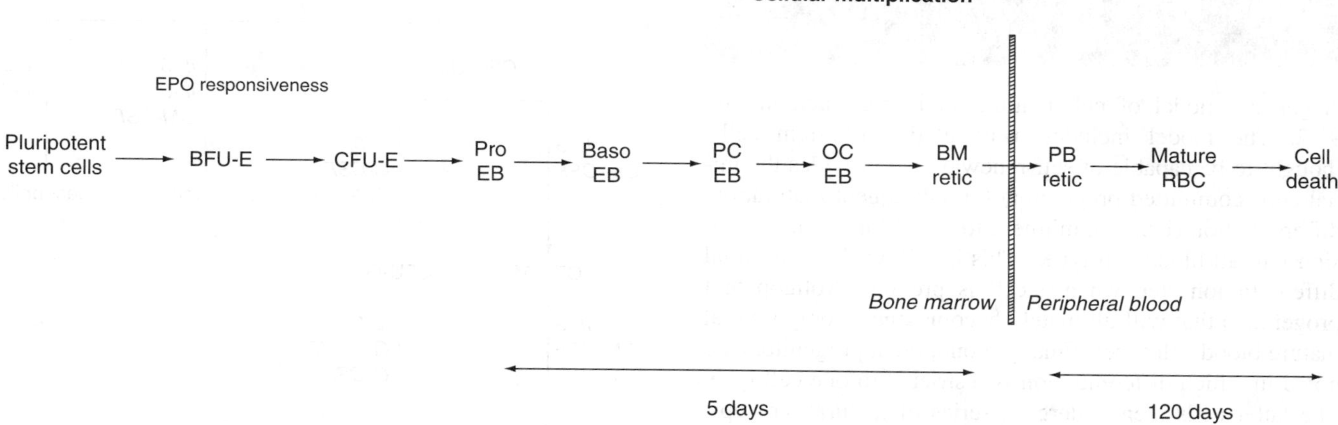

Figure 92.3. The suspected differentiation pattern of cells into mature erythrocytes is shown including the various immature cell types that have been identified. In addition, the cells that may be stimulated by the cytokine erythropoietin are identified. BFU, burst-forming unit; E, erythroid; CFU, colony-forming unit; EB, erythroblast; PC, polychromatophilic; OC, orthochromatophilic; BM, bone marrow; retic, reticulocyte; EPO, erythropoietin.

cells) in contrast to the circulation (approximately 700 million). Similarly, only 1% of the eosinophils in the body are found in peripheral blood, whereas the skin, lungs, and gastrointestinal tract are the preferred sites of residence.[4] There is no marrow reserve pool of monocytes. Neutrophil development in the bone marrow initiates with the stem cell and proceeds through intermediate precursors such as the myeloblast, promyelocyte, myelocyte, and metamyelocyte.

Only a small fraction of the total body pool of lymphocytes resides in the blood. Mature B lymphocytes express surface immunoglobulin, which functions as an antigen receptor. Most of these cells migrate from the bone marrow to areas such as the lymph nodes (dense collections of lymphocytes, plasma cells, and macrophages that are supplied by postcapillary venules and drained by a system of efferent lymphatics) and spleen where antigenic stimulation results in specific immunoglobulin production.[13] Immature T cells are found in the circulation on their way to full maturation in the thymus. Approximately 75% of blood lymphocytes are T cells, 15% null cells, and 10% B cells. Various antigens are expressed on the T-cell surface depending on the degree of cell maturity and function termed clusters of differentiation (CD).

Progenitor cells, which give rise to platelets, are referred to as CFU-MK (colony-forming unit megakaryocyte). Megakaryocytes account for only 0.05–0.02% of marrow cells. Maturation of megakaryocytes is accompanied by morphologic changes in both the cytoplasm and nucleus. At differing stages of maturation one can therefore see granules, organelles, and increasing segmentation of the nucleus. Cells in this lineage progress through three stages of development: commitment, proliferation, and differentiation, similar to that of leukocytes.[18,19]

The term *erythron* has been used to describe collectively the erythropoietic cellular structure, composed of all cells that lie along this pathway starting with the earliest committed erythroid progenitor and ending with the mature circulating RBC. The earliest cell committed to the erythroid lineage is known as a BFU-E (erythroid). One BFU-E can proliferate into several hundred progeny using *in vitro* culture systems. These cells follow in differentiation by the CFU-E cell and subsequently to the nucleated normoblast and the immediate RBC precursor, the circulating anuclear reticulocyte as outlined in Fig. 92.3. The remaining RNA is typically lost from the RBC within 2 days of its appearance in the peripheral blood, thus the mature cell does not synthesize new proteins such as enzymes.[20]

The erythrocyte precursor cell types display a continuum of changes in shape, hemoglobin concentration, Rh antigen, and erythropoietin (EPO) receptor expression with maturity. However, mature erythrocytes express significantly lower EPO receptor density than that of proerythroblasts.[21]

Neonatal RBCs primarily contain fetal hemoglobin (HbF), which is replaced within a few months by adult hemoglobin (HbA), 85% of which is synthesized in the erythropoietic marrow. Heme synthesizing cells must have a mitochondria; therefore, its synthesis cannot occur in the mature erythrocyte. Genetic alterations in hemoglobin structure may dramatically alter the stability or solubility of the hemoglobin and also cell confirmation. The characteristic biconcave disk shape of the normal RBC is approximately 8×2 μm. Pathologic alterations in plasma lipids may affect the outer phospholipid membrane of the RBC thus changing the cell's shape and survival. Blood types are characterized by the antigenic structure of the external surface of the cell membrane. Membrane function, integrity, and phagocytosis of the cells are affected by interactions of antibodies with RBC surface antigens.

Normal Regulation of Cell Proliferation and Differentiation

A generic model of cell maturation is presented in Fig. 92.2. The model includes a population of stem cells, thought to be capable of self-renewal, that provides the initial cell (committed progenitor) for subsequent maturation, differentiation (i.e., commitment to a cell line), and expansion into all blood cell types. This is followed by an initial differentiation step when a cell is produced (oligopotent progenitor) that will ultimately become one of only several mature blood cell types. Finally monopotent progenitors are noted in which differentiation is restricted to one cell type. The latter cells then undergo a series of maturation steps, ultimately resulting in a mature cell.

THE STEM CELL

The decision of a stem cell to self-renew versus differentiate and the selection of lineage by a multipotential progenitor cell during the differentiation process are thought to be stochastic (random) events. Conversely, survival and proliferation of the subsequent progenitor cells is thought to be regulated by the group of cytokines referred to as colony-stimulating factors (also known as CSFs, hematopoietins, hematopoietic cytokines, or hematopoietic growth factors).[22] Receptors for a variety of CSFs are present on the surface of stem cells, which agrees with *in vitro* studies demonstrating stimulatory activity for cytokines such as stem cell factor (SCF), IL-6, G-CSF, IL-11, IL-12, and leukemia inhibitory factor when present in combinations. Whether or not therapeutic use of a CSF that is thought to primarily act on more mature cells will result in exhaustion (depletion) of the stem cell pool over the course of multiple cycles of therapy is under active debate and study.[23] Proposed "cascades" of hematopoiesis are represented in Figs. 92.3 through 92.6. Inserted within some figures are the suspected sites in the process where CSFs are thought to interact by promoting the production, prolifera-

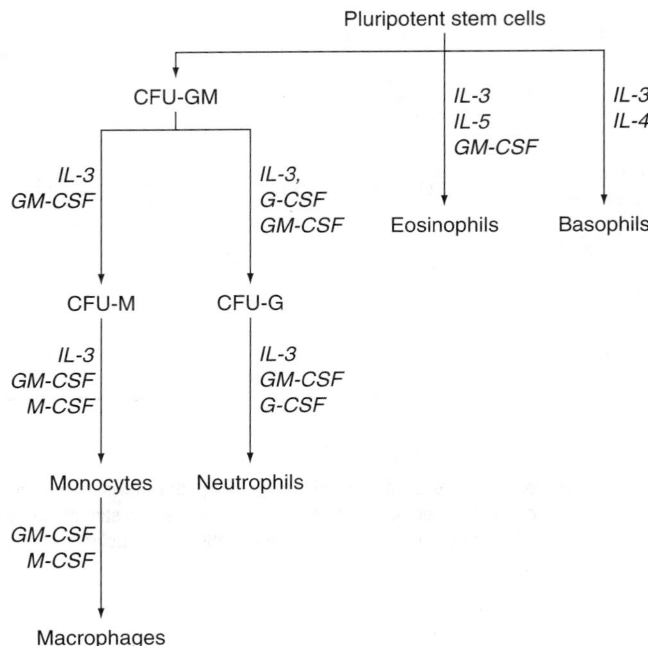

Figure 92.5. Maturation of precursor cells into granulocytes and macrophages, including some intermediate precursor cells (CFU-GM, G, and M) is depicted. The CSFs that affect the more terminal (mature) pathways are also shown. (CSFs that regulate immature cell types are not displayed.) CFU, colony-forming unit; G, granulocyte; M, monocyte.

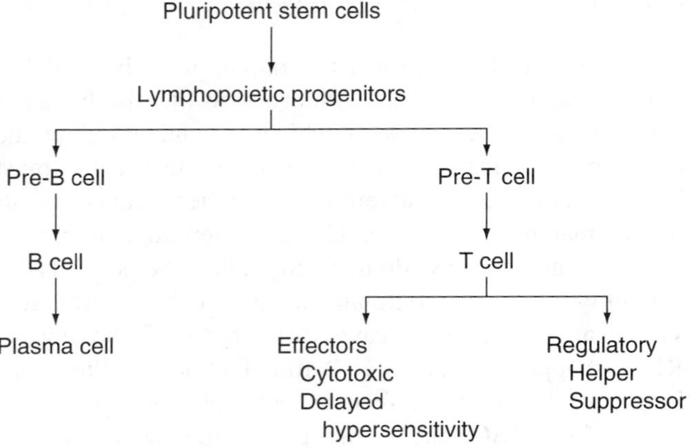

Figure 92.4. The pattern of lymphocyte maturation and differentiation into T and B cells is displayed. The plasma cell is a factory for antibodies whereas the T cells have both effector and regulatory functions on the immune system.

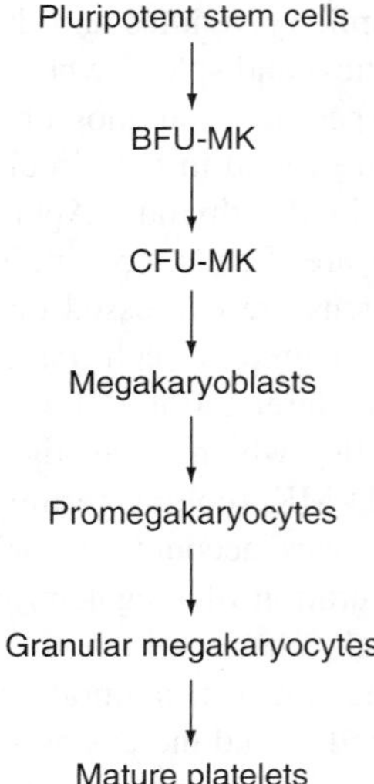

Figure 92.6. Megakaryocyte precursors undergo several maturation steps prior to becoming mature platelets as outlined in this figure. BFU, burst-forming unit; MK, megakaryocyte; CFU, colony-forming unit.

tion, and survival of hematopoietic cells. These schema are simple representations of a system of complex interactions between stimulatory and inhibitory cytokines that may not be adequately described by the *in vitro* models used thus far to define them. Details regarding the clinical pharmacology of individual CSFs are presented in Chapter 119.

Immature bone marrow precursor cells such as the myeloblast (first recognizable cell of granulocytic differentiation), promyelocyte, myelocyte, and erythroblast are thought to be capable of replication. This is in contrast to most mature hematopoietic cells, which are incapable of division. Exceptions to the latter statement include monocytes, macrophages, and tissue mast cells. Evaluation of reasons for a change in hematopoietic cellular concentration over time must be conducted with a thorough knowledge of the mechanisms of both cellular production and destruction.

NEUTROPHILS

Blood neutrophils are in constant exchange with an equal number of "marginated" cells. The latter are stuck to the walls of vessels in the peripheral blood, liver, lungs, and spleen. Demargination or the converse, increased adhesion, can therefore dramatically change the peripheral neutrophil concentration even though cell production remains constant. A variety of stimuli can result in demargination including exercise, epinephrine, corticosteroids, and sickle-cell anemia.[24] Conversely, transient neutropenia can occur via stimulation of margination by conditions such as malaria, some viral infections, and onset of hemodialysis.[25]

Normally it takes 14 days for neutrophil production and differentiation in the bone marrow. G-CSF, GM-CSF, and IL-3 are thought to be important regulatory molecules of neutrophil production (Fig. 92.5). A healthy adult will produce approximately 1.6 billion neutrophils per kilogram body weight per day.[26] Blood neutrophils are totally replaced at least twice in each 24-hour period, thus the average circulation time for any one cell is approximately 6–12 hours. Most of this transgression is thought to be for effector functions in the tissues and not simply an elimination process. The total amount of noncirculating (i.e., storage) neutrophils is more than 15 times the amount in blood. Absolute storage cell numbers are subject to alteration by prior exposure to chemotherapy or deficiency in cofactors required for their synthesis (e.g., folate). When conditions call for an acute increase in blood neutrophils the pattern of cells thus changes to one more similar to that in the marrow (i.e., band concentration increases relative to seg concentration; normal ratio <0.1 to 0.3).[27] This phenomenon, often referred to as a "shift to the left," denotes a circulating neutrophil population made of less mature cells. Infectious processes are often accompanied by such a shift as well as increased outflow of cells from storage forms in the bone marrow; however, extreme cases may require so many granulocytes at the infection site that marrow pools are depleted, resulting in neutropenia. Cytokine expression, and thus hematopoiesis, may be impaired in the elderly, resulting in a reduced ability to tolerate myelosuppressive chemotherapy.[28]

EOSINOPHILS

The typical blood circulation time for an eosinophil is approximately 6 hours but may survive weeks within tissues. Cytokines thought important in eosinophil production or function include IL-1, IL-3, GM-CSF, G-CSF, and, perhaps most important, IL-5. Corticosteroids cause a transient margination of eosinophils and inhibit release of mature cells from the bone marrow.[4]

MONOCYTES/MACROPHAGES

Both macrophages and T lymphocytes secrete cytokines, which stimulate monocytopoiesis.[29] Examples of cytokines that act on relatively mature monocytes include M-CSF and GM-CSF. Blood monocytes have a shorter marrow transit time than neutrophils (6 versus 13 days, respectively); however, there is no monocyte reserve in the marrow.[27] The peripheral blood turnover of these cells is at a much slower rate (circulation half-life 3 days) than neutrophils; similarly, tissue macrophages are thought to be very long-lived. Macrophages may be able to produce their own progeny as well as attract additional monocytes for differentiation in the local environment.

LYMPHOCYTES

Immature T cells produced in the bone marrow ultimately migrate to the thymus where they both expand and mature into immunologically competent cells (Fig. 92.4). Lymphopoiesis is facilitated by a variety of cytokines including IL-2, IL-4, and IL-7, while others such as transforming growth factor-β may decelerate this process.[30] T lymphocytes are probably the longest lived hematopoietic cell since experimental evidence exists for the life span of some to be greater than 10 years. The term *lymphokine* is used to describe cytokines secreted by T cells. Lymphokines such as interleukin-2 are important in both activation and proliferation of the immune response; however, monokines are also important regulators of lymphocyte development. T and B lymphocytes have important interactions with each other in both lymphocyte development and activation, which seem necessary for immunocompetence. There is some evidence for age-associated reductions in circulating helper and suppressor T cells and B cells.[31]

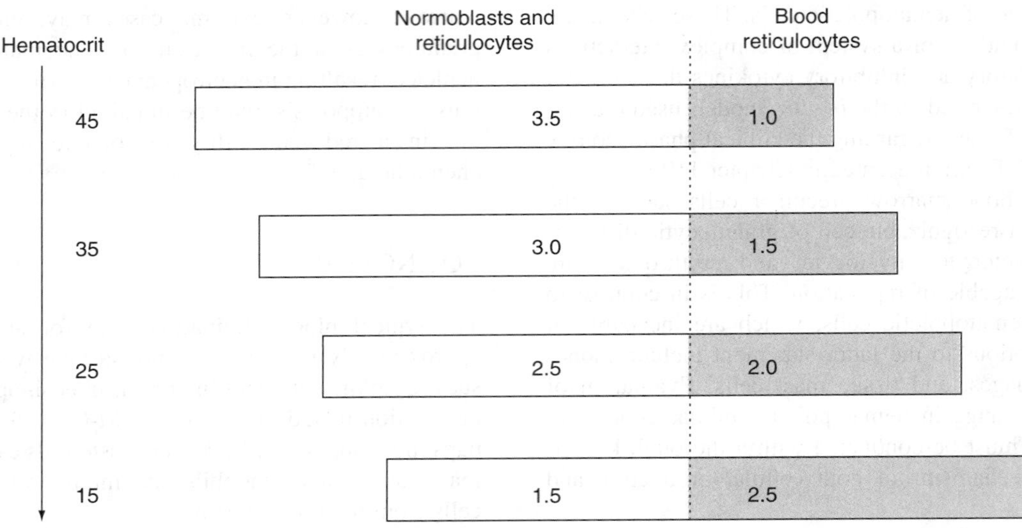

Figure 92.7. Correction of hematocrit with the marrow and blood reticulocyte maturation times. With a hematocrit of 45 the blood reticulocytes circulate for 1 day, whereas reduction in hematocrit to 15 results in a 2.5-day circulation time. The numbers found under the blood reticulocyte column can be used as a correction factor in evaluation of reticulocyte concentrations as described in the text. *(From Hillman RS, Finch CA. Red Cell Manual. Philadelphia, FA Davis, 1992, p 59. Reprinted with permission.)*

PLATELETS

Thrombopoiesis is the term used to describe the process of platelet production. The bone marrow manufactures 40,000 platelets/mL blood each day. Proliferation and differentiation of platelet precursors are thought to be primarily influenced by cytokines such as IL-6, IL-11, leukemia inhibitory factor, and perhaps most specifically by the recently described thrombopoietin (Fig. 92.6).[32,33] Other hematopoietins that may act in concert producing synergistic effects include: IL-3, IL-1, GM-CSF, EPO, and SCF.[34] The platelet survival time is a clinical test that can estimate the rate of platelet turnover.[35] In normal individuals this time is 9.5 ± 0.6 days.[36]

The normal life span of an RBC is approximately 100–120 days with a circulating cell turnover rate of 1% per day. This translates into a typical adult producing approximately 200 billion reticulocytes every day. Conditions such as anemia or hypoxemia primarily stimulate the renal peritubular interstitial cells to produce EPO by interaction with the renal oxygen sensor. The degree of elevation in blood EPO concentrations is dependent on the severity of anemia or hypoxemia. This in turn recruits RBC precursors and shortens the normal time for differentiation if adequate cofactors such as iron, folate, and B_{12} are present. While the overall time for differentiation is shortened (as is the duration of time a reticulocyte spends in the marrow), the blood maturation time is lengthened. The increase in EPO concentrations are relatively quick (within hours), but the effects on marrow transpire over several days. The ultimate increase in RBC mass occurs at an even slower pace, generally over weeks to months (Fig. 92.3). Multiple other endogenous cytokines are also thought to play a role in either stimulating or inhibiting erythropoiesis by acting on the early progenitors. These include GM-CSF, G-CSF, IL-1, IL-3, IL-6, IL-9, SCF, and some stromal proteins.[21]

Adequate production of RBCs for a degree of anemia is best assessed by evaluation of the number of circulating reticulocytes. The normal range is approximately 0.4–1.7% of the RBCs; however, this would obviously be higher in anemic patients with adequate productive capacity. A corrected reticulocyte count is calculated by multiplying this value by the hemoglobin and dividing by the normal hemoglobin expected for a healthy patient with similar characteristics. Additional correction accounts for the increased life span of reticulocytes in the peripheral blood of patients depending directly on their degree of anemia. Figure 92.7 displays correction factors that can be used to accommodate for these changes.[37] Direct assessment of erythropoiesis in the bone marrow can be performed by estimating the myeloid to erythroid (M/E) cell ratio from a marrow aspirate. The normal adult ratio is 3:1 to 5:1 but can obviously be influenced by changes in erythroid or myeloid production. RBCs lose flexibility with age and eventually undergo lysis or are phagocytized and removed by the monocyte–macrophage system (primarily via the spleen). Accelerated red cell destruction can be grossly quantitated by increases in plasma concentrations of bilirubin and LDH.[37]

Clinical laboratories measure RBC concentrations with excellent accuracy; however, the most useful tool for assessment of the blood's oxygen-carrying capacity is the hemoglobin. This is due to variability in RBC size. The average RBC and hemoglobin concentrations in healthy adult male and female patients are approximately 5.21, 4.60 × $10^6/mm^3$, and 15.7, 13.8 g/dL, respectively. Variations in normal concentrations will also be evident depending on age, menstruation status, race, environmental factors, and pregnancy.[38]

Disease-Associated Hematopoietic Changes

NEUTROPHILS

The usual definition of neutropenia is an absolute neutrophil count below 1800/mm^3 in white patients, 1400/mm^3 in black patients, and 1500/mm^3 for children 1 month to 10 years old. Clinical manifestations of neutropenia (i.e., infection) are not typically evident without other cofactors until the concentration drops below 1000/mm^3.[39] Accompanying factors that may influence the risk of infection for a particular patient include skin and mucous membrane integrity; vascular tissue supply; nutritional status; and lymphocytopenia, monocytopenia, or hypogammaglobinemia. Persistent agranulocytosis (less than 500/mm^3 or no measurable neutrophils) is almost uniformly fatal without use of supportive antibiotics. Disorders resulting in defective granulopoiesis can be subdivided into those that result in marrow aplasia or diseases that replace the normal neutrophilic component. (See Chapter 96 for drug-induced neutropenia.) Diseases associated with granulopoietic suppression include viral infection, tuberculosis, anorexia, autoimmune diseases (e.g., systemic lupus erythematosus), Felty's syndrome (rheumatoid arthritis/splenomegaly/leukopenia), myelodysplastic syndromes, and leukemias.[39,40] A congenital form of severely defective neutrophil production (Kostmann syndrome) has been described that is possibly a result of defective regulation of the late-acting hemopoietin G-CSF.[41] Patients with the rare disorder of cyclic neutropenia display periodic wide fluctuations in the WBCs at approximately 3-week intervals that last for 3–6 days. Other forms of chronic neutropenias may occur with adequate marrow stores and can be relatively benign in symptomatology.

Neutrophilia is typically defined as an absolute neutrophil count greater than 7.5×10^9 cells/L blood, and is sometimes referred to as a leukemoid reaction, if extreme.[24] Acute neutrophilia may be a result of emotional or physical stimuli (e.g., exercise, seizures, labor, pain, temperature changes), infections, inflammation/tissue necrosis, or drugs/toxins (e.g., CSFs, epinephrine, corticosteroids, lithium, vaccines, endotoxin). Chronic causes of increased neutrophils include persistent infections, inflammation, malignancies, drugs, metabolic/endocrine disorders, cigarette smoking, hereditary/congenital abnormalities, and myeloproliferative diseases such as polycythemia vera.[24]

EOSINOPHILS

Eosinophilia (absolute count greater than 700/mm^3) may result from neoplastic processes, parasitic or fungal infections, gastrointestinal disorders, malignancies, dermatitis, granulomatous disorders (e.g., sarcoidosis, Wegener's disease), or collagen-vascular diseases in addition to the more typical cause, allergic reactions.[42] One mechanism that may be common to several of these etiologic factors has been postulated to be from antigenic stimulation of T cells, which produce a cytokine (e.g., IL-5) that mediates eosinophil proliferation.[43] Infections may cause eosinopenia; however, its significance is not thought to be of concern in that setting.

BASOPHILS

Basophilia may be seen frequently in patients with myeloproliferative disorders and in association with inflammatory reactions/diseases. Viral infections, iron deficiency, or lung cancer can sometimes increase basophil counts. Mastocytosis is usually evident only on analysis of tissue or bone marrow mast cells. Causes include hypersensitivity reactions, malignancy, osteoporosis, and chronic liver or renal disease.

MONOCYTES

Monocytosis ($>0.8 \times 10^9$ cells/L) occurs with some infections (e.g., tuberculosis, histoplasmosis, toxoplasmosis, bacterial endocarditis, and salmonellosis), collagen vascular diseases (rheumatoid arthritis, systemic lupus erythematosus), gastrointestinal disorders (ulcerative colitis, alcoholic liver disease), leukemias, and up to 60% of nonhematologic malignancies; however, abnormally low monocyte concentrations occur in patients with hairy cell leukemia or aplastic anemia.[44]

LYMPHOCYTES

Significant reductions in lymphocyte concentration ($<1 \times 10^9$ cells/L) can be evident without apparent cause or in a variety of diseases, including: acute inflammatory disorders, severe uremia, immune deficiency diseases such as systemic lupus erythematosus, chronic infections such as tuberculosis or human immunodeficiency virus infection, malignancies, and connective tissue diseases.[45] Lymphocytosis ($>4 \times 10^9$ cells/L) may occur with mononucleosis, pertussis, measles, chicken pox, and in lymphoid malignancies. A progressive increase in mature lymphocytes may be indicative of chronic lymphocytic leukemia. Increased atypical lymphocytes may be demonstrated in patients with infections (mononucleosis, hepatitis, cytomegalovirus, etc.), allergic reactions, or lymphomas.[46]

PLATELETS

Both qualitative and quantitative platelet disorders have important pathophysiologic consequences. Thrombocytopenia, defined as a platelet count <150,000 cells/mm^3, may result from a defect in production, increased sequestration, or accelerated destruction.[47]

Certain stimuli may cause injury to the marrow by reducing the number of megakaryocytes available. Drugs, chemicals, radiation, and infection are among the potential causes of marrow injury. Diseases producing general bone marrow failure or those that invade the bone marrow may result in thrombocytopenia. Examples of the latter include cancers such as leukemia, lymphoma, myelofibrosis, myelodysplastic metastatic solid tumors (breast and prostate cancer), and infections such as those caused by mycobacterium. Suboptimal platelet production may also result from defects in maturation seen with vitamin B_{12} and/or folate deficiency, or in congenital syndromes.[48]

Alteration in platelet distribution may also result in thrombocytopenia. Splenomegaly is the most frequent cause of increased platelet sequestration.

Idiopathic thrombocytopenic purpura (ITP) is a common cause of thrombocytopenia due to accelerated destruction of platelets. Antiplatelet antibodies combine with platelets in ITP, which sensitizes them to removal by the immune system. Accelerated platelet destruction can also be seen in patients with connective tissue disorders. Approximately 14% of patients with systemic lupus erythematosus experience thrombocytopenia similar to ITP.

ERYTHROCYTES

Suboptimal erythropoiesis can be classified by changes in the size of RBCs noted on exam of the peripheral blood. The excretory and endocrine functions of the kidney usually mirror each other, thus renal dysfunction can result in anemia by reduction in EPO production, resulting in a normochromic, normocytic pattern. Other causes of insufficient erythropoiesis include replacement of bone marrow by fibrosis, solid tumors, or leukemia as well as defects in erythroid maturation. Relative deficiencies in the cofactors required for heme/RBC synthesis such as iron, folate, and B_{12} may also be important contributors. Structurally, RBC macrocytosis denotes defects in the maturation of the nucleus, whereas microcytosis is indicative of cytoplasmic defects (reduced hemoglobin synthesis). A detailed description regarding the pathogenesis and treatment of anemic disorders is found in Chapter 93.

Exaggerated erythropoiesis with increased RBC mass (polycythemia) can be mistaken for a reduction in plasma volume. Symptoms are not always immediately evident but may progress to reduced tissue oxygenation, thrombosis, and congestive heart failure. The most common etiology is hypoxia; however, alternative causes can be subdivided based on their ability to stimulate EPO production. EPO (or a similar cytokine) may be produced in response to genetic alterations or a variety of malignancies including angioblastoma, hepatomas, and hypernephroma.[49] Polycythemia vera, a malignancy of the bone marrow stem cells, results in an increased sensitivity of RBC precursors to stimulation by EPO and is accompanied in many patients by thrombocytosis and leukocytosis.

Clinical Uses of Hematopoietic Cells

BONE MARROW

The treatment of a number of malignancies and some nonmalignant diseases can benefit from the use of very high doses of chemotherapy or irradiation; however, these doses are of such magnitude that many, if not all, of the normal hematopoietic cells are severely damaged. The patient experiences a prolonged period of time with few, if any, granulocytes following such therapy, and therefore is at a very high risk of developing serious infections. The infusion (transplantation) of bone marrow following the anticancer therapy helps to decrease the period of absolute neutropenia and thereby risk of infection or marrow failure to repopulate (re-engraft). Bone marrow transplantation involves the removal of bone marrow from a donor, administration of intensive doses of chemotherapy, and reinfusion of the bone marrow to the recipient. If the donor and recipient are the same individual, this is termed autologous bone marrow transplantation. If the donor and recipient are different individuals, this is termed allogeneic transplantation.

Allogeneic transplantation is more complicated than autologous transplantation because of the potential reaction of donor T lymphocytes against the host tissues, termed graft-versus-host disease (GVHD). This type of transplant is most commonly used in acute leukemias, chronic myelogenous leukemia, aplastic anemia, thalassemia, sickle cell anemia, and severe combined immunodeficiency. Autologous transplantation is most commonly used in malignancies such as breast cancer and Hodgkins and non-Hodgkins lymphoma.

A number of laboratory techniques are evolving to allow the harvested bone marrow to grow in the laboratory prior to infusion and to cleanse the marrow of malignant cell contaminants in the autologous transplant setting.

PERIPHERAL BLOOD PROGENITOR CELLS

Hematopoiesis may also be augmented following intensive chemotherapy with reinfusion of autologous peripheral blood progenitor cells (PBPCs).[50] The PBPCs are less mature hematopoietic cells that circulate in the peripheral blood. Comparatively high numbers of these cells appear in the peripheral blood following administration of cytokines such as G-CSF or GM-CSF, but also following the administration of some chemotherapy agents (e.g., cyclophosphamide).[51,52] These cells may subsequently be collected or harvested through a process termed apheresis or leukopheresis, stored in the lab and readministered following chemotherapy. Some centers use PBPC exclusively, while others combine these with bone marrow.

CORD BLOOD TRANSPLANTATION

It has been shown that human umbilical cord blood contains hematopoietic stem cells capable of reconstituting bone marrow.[53] A phenomenal number of cord blood donors is one advantage to this strategy since the cord and its associated blood are commonly discarded following delivery. This technology is very early in its development; however, optimization of methods to help these cells reproduce in the laboratory will produce a tremendous potential alternative to BMT. Cord blood stem cell (CBSC) reinfusions have largely been performed from HLA-identical siblings; although, the greatest utility may be for HLA-mismatched, unrelated transplants. CBSC transplants are thought to be associated with less chance for GVHD, thereby providing adequate hematopoietic reconstitution with less toxicity.

REFERENCES

1. Erslev AJ, Lichtman MA. Structure and function of the marrow, in Williams WJ, Beutler E, Erslev AJ, Lichtman MA (eds): Hematology, 4th ed. New York, McGraw-Hill, 1990, p 37.
2. Lehrer RI, Ganz T, Selsted ME, et al. Neutrophils in human diseases. N Engl J Med 1987;317:687–694.
3. Lieschke GJ, Burgess AW. Granulocyte colony-stimulating factor and granulocyte-macrophage colony-stimulating factor. N Engl J Med 1992;327:28–35.
4. Weller PF. The immunobiology of eosinophils. N Engl J Med 1991;324:1110–1118.
5. Kitamura Y, Kasugai T, Arizono N, Matsuda H. Development of mast cells and basophils: Processes and regulation mechanisms. Am J Med Sci 1993;306:185–191.
6. Galli SJ, Dvorak AM, Dvorak HF. Morphology, biochemistry, and function of basophils and mast cells, in Williams WJ, Beutler E, Erslev AJ, Lichtman MA (eds): Hematology, 4th ed. New York, McGraw-Hill, 1990, p 840.
7. Johnston RB. Monocytes and macrophages. N Engl J Med 1988;318:747–752.
8. Kipps TJ, Carson DA. Functions of B lymphocytes and plasma cells in immunoglobulin production, in Williams WJ, Beutler E, Erslev AJ, Lichtman MA (eds): Hematology, 4th ed. New York, McGraw-Hill, 1990, p 932.
9. Kipps TJ, Carson DA. Functions of T lymphocytes: T-cell receptors for antigen, in Williams WJ, Beutler E, Erslev AJ, Lichtman MA (eds): Hematology, 4th ed. New York, McGraw-Hill, 1990, p 939.
10. Thompson AR, Harker LA. Manual of Hemostasis and Thrombosis, 3rd ed. Philadelphia, FA Davis, 1983, p 47.
11. Mustard JF, Packham MA, Kinlough-Rathbone RL. Platelets, blood flow, and the vessel wall. Circulation 1990;81(suppl 1):I40–I41.
12. Gordon MY. Physiological mechanisms in BMT and haematopoiesis-revisited. Bone Marrow Transplant 1993;11:193–197.
13. Weiss LP. Functional organization of the hematopoietic tissues, in Hoffman R, Benz EJ, Shattil SJ et al (eds): Hematology—Basic Principles and Practice. New York, Churchill Livingstone, 1991, p 82.
14. Greenberger J. The hematopoietic microenvironment. Crit Rev Oncol/Hematol 1991;11:65–84.
15. To LB, Shepperd KM, Haylock DN, et al. Single high doses of cyclophosphamide enable the collection of high numbers of hematopoietic stem cells from the peripheral blood. Exp Hematol 1990;18:442–447.
16. Peters WP, Rosner G, Ross M, et al. Comparative effects of granulocyte-macrophage colony-stimulating factor and granulocyte colony-stimulating factor on priming peripheral blood progenitor cells for use with autologous bone marrow after high-dose chemotherapy. Blood 1993;81:1709–1719.
17. Spangrude GJ, Heimfeld S, Wessman IL. Purification and characterization of mouse hematopoietic stem cells. Science 1988;241:58–62.
18. Williams N, Levine RF. The origin, development and regulation of megakaryocytes. Br J Hematol 1982;52:173–180.
19. Hoffman R. Regulation of megakaryocytopoiesis. Blood 1989;74:1196–1112.
20. Papayannopoulou T, Abkowitz J. Biology of erythropoiesis, erythroid differentiation, and maturation, in Hoffman R, Benz EJ, Shattil SJ et al (eds): Hematology—Basic Principles and Practice. New York, Churchill Livingstone, 1991, p 252.
21. McGuire MJ, Spivak JL. Erythropoiesis, in Anderson KC, Ness PM (eds): Scientific Basis of Transfusion Medicine—Implications for Clinical Practice. Philadelphia, PA, WB Saunders, 1994, p 1.
22. Ogawa M. Differentiation and proliferation of hematopoietic stem cells. Blood 1993;81:2844–2853.
23. Moore MAS. Does stem cell exhaustion result from combining hematopoietic growth factors with chemotherapy? If so, how do we prevent it? Blood 1992;80:3–7.
24. Dale DC. Neutrophilia, in Williams WJ, Beutler E, Erslev AJ, Lichtman MA (eds): Hematology, 4th ed. New York, McGraw-Hill, 1990, p 816.
25. Coates T, Baehner R. Leukocytosis and leukopenia, in Hoffman R, Benz EJ, Shattil SJ et al (eds): Hematology—Basic Principles and Practice. New York, Churchill Livingstone, 1991, p 552.
26. Gabrilove J. Granulopoiesis, in Anderson KC, Ness PM (eds): Scientific Basis of Transfusion Medicine—Implications for Clinical Practice. Philadelphia, WB Saunders, 1994, p 17.
27. Boggs DR, Winkelstein A. White Cell Manual. Philadelphia, FA Davis, 1983, p 29.
28. Rothstein G. Hematopoiesis in the aged: A model of hematopoietic dysregulation? Blood 1993;82:2601–2604.
29. Bagby GC, Segal GM. Growth factors and the control of hematopoiesis, in Hoffman R, Benz EJ, Shattil SJ et al (eds):

Hematology—Basic Principles and Practice. New York, Churchill Livingstone, 1991, p 97.
30. Jordan SC. Cytokines and lymphocytes, in Kunkel SL and Remick DG (eds): Cytokines in Health and Disease. New York, Marcel Dekker, 1992, p 309.
31. Yamashiki M, Nishimura A, Kosaka Y, James SP. Two-color analysis of peripheral lymphocyte surface antigens in inherently healthy adults. J Clin Lab Anal 1994;8:22–26.
32. Du, Williams DA. Interleukin-11: A multifunctional growth factor derived from the hematopoietic microenvironment. Blood 1994;83:2023–2030.
33. Metcalf D. Thrombopoietin—at last. Nature 1994; 369:519–520.
34. Gordon MS, Hoffman R. Growth factors affecting human thrombocytopoiesis: Potential agents for the treatment of thrombocytopenia. Blood 1992;80:302–307.
35. Shulman NR, Jordan JV Jr. Platelet kinetics, in Colman RW, Hirsh J, Marder VJ, Saltzman EW (eds): Hemostasis and Thrombosis. Basic Principles and Clinical Practice, 2nd ed. Philadelphia, JB Lippincott, 1987, pp 341–351.
36. Harker LA, Finch CA. Thrombokinetics in man. J Clin Invest 1969;48:963–974.
37. Hillman RS, Finch CA. Red Cell Manual. Philadelphia, FA Davis, 1992, p 59.
38. Glassman AB. Anemia: Diagnosis and clinical considerations, in Harmening DM (ed): Clinical Hematology and Fundamentals of Hemostasis, 2nd ed. Philadelphia, FA Davis, 1992, p 54.
39. Lichtman MA. Classification and clinical manifestations of neutrophil disorders, in Williams WJ, Beutler E, Erslev AJ, Lichtman MA (eds): Hematology, 4th ed. New York, McGraw-Hill, 1990, p 802.
40. Malech HL, Gallin JI. Neutrophils in human disease. N Engl J Med 1987;317:687–694.
41. Dong F, Hoefsloot LH, Schelen AM, et al. Identification of a nonsense mutation in the G-CSF receptor in severe congenital neutropenia. Proc Natl Acad Sci 1994;91:4480–4484.
42. Boggs DR, Winkelstein A. White Cell Manual, 4th ed. Philadelphia, FA Davis, 1983, p 54.
43. Sanderson CJ. Interleukin-5, eosinophils and disease. Blood 1992;79:3101–3109.
44. Lichtman MA. Classification and clinical manifestations of disorders of monocytes and macrophages, in Williams WJ, Beutler E, Erslev AJ, Lichtman MA (eds): Hematology, 4th ed. New York, McGraw-Hill, 1990, p 879.
45. Williams WJ. Lymphocytopenia, in Williams WJ, Beutler E, Erslev AJ, Lichtman MA (eds): Hematology, 4th ed. New York, McGraw-Hill, 1990, p 964.
46. Williams WJ. Lymphocytosis, in Williams WJ, Beutler E, Erslev AJ, Lichtman MA (eds): Hematology, 4th ed. New York, McGraw-Hill, 1990, p 963.
47. Rutherford CJ, Frenkel EP. Thrombocytopenia. Issues in diagnosis and therapy. Med Clin North Am 1994;78:555–575.
48. Williams WJ. Classification and clinical manifestations of disorders of hemostasis, in Williams WJ, Beutler E, Erslev AJ, Lichtman MA (eds): Hematology, 4th ed. New York, McGraw-Hill, 1990, p 1338.
49. Tabbara IA. Erythropoietin biology and clinical applications. Arch Intern Med 1993;153:298–304.
50. Kessinger A, Armitage JO, Landmark JD, et al. Autologous peripheral hematopoietic stem cell transplantation restores hematopoietic function following marrow ablative therapy. Blood 1988;71:723–727.
51. Peters WP, Rosner G, Ross M, et al. Comparative effects of granulocyte-macrophage colony-stimulating factor (GM-CSF) and granulocyte colony-stimulating factor (G-CSF) on priming peripheral blood progenitor cells for use with autologous bone marrow after high-dose chemotherapy. Blood 1993;81:1709–1719.
52. To LB, Shepperd KM, Haylock DN, et al. Single high doses of cyclophosphamide enable the collection of high numbers of hematopoietic cells from the peripheral blood. Exp Hematol 1990;18:442–447.
53. Auerbach AD, Liu Q, Ghosh R, et al. Prenatal identification of potential donors for umbilical cord blood transplantation for Fanconi anemia. Transfusion 1990;30:682–687.

Chapter 93

Anemias

William J. Spruill, PharmD, and William E. Wade, PharmD, FASHP

Anemias are a group of diseases characterized by a decrease in either hemoglobin (HgB) or red blood cells (RBCs), which results in a decrease in the oxygen-carrying capacity of blood. They are often a sign of underlying disease and can be characterized in laboratory terms as a decrease in the oxygen-carrying pigment, hemoglobin, or a decreased hematocrit below the normal range.

The goals of this chapter are to review the maturation and development cycle of RBCs, classification systems, definitions, pathophysiology, and laboratory tests and procedures used in the diagnosis and treatment of anemias.

Anemias can be classified on the basis of morphology of the RBCs, etiology, or pathophysiology. Table 93.1 gives some examples of each of these classifications.

Iron deficiency anemia, anemia of chronic disease, and anemias associated with acute bleeding account for roughly 75% of all anemias.[1] The remaining 25% consist of anemias resulting from such conditions as bone marrow damage, decreased erythropoiesis, and hemolysis.

Maturation and Development

In the normal adult, RBCs are formed in the marrow of the vertebrae, ribs, sternum, clavicle, pelvic (iliac) crest, and the proximal epiphyses of the long bones such as the upper ends of the femur and humerus. In a child, most bone marrow space is hematopoietically active in order to meet increased RBC requirements. With increasing age, available bone space exceeds blood cell production requirements and much marrow space is filled with inactive fatty reserve marrow. This reserve space can be reactivated in the event that other hematopoietic marrow fails or RBC life span decreases.

Like all blood cells, RBCs originate from undifferentiated mesenchymal stem cells in the bone marrow. These stem cells have the property of self-renewal and, through cell division and differentiation, can form populations of progenitor cells that are now committed to production of specific cell lines. Hematopoietic growth factors participate in the differentiation of the stem cell into a committed progenitor cell that then undergoes mitosis; one cell remains in the stem cell pool and the other committed stem cell serves as the initial precursor for erythrocyte formation. In this manner, all blood cells can develop from a similar stem cell population, which is normally self-sustaining.

In normal RBC formation (normoblastic erythropoiesis), the committed stem cell undergoes a dynamic maturation process involving multiple mitotic divisions, with folate and vitamin B_{12}-dependent synthesis and splitting of RNA and DNA (Table 93.2). This process is accompanied by the ongoing incorporation of hemoglobin and iron into the gradually maturing RBC, which is then released from the marrow into the circulating blood as a reticulocyte. This maturation process takes about 1 week. Over the next several days the reticulocyte loses its nucleus, shrinks slightly, and develops into a mature enucleated RBC called an *erythrocyte*.

Two abnormal forms of erythropoiesis, microcytic and megaloblastic, result in mature microcytes and macrocytes, respectively. Megaloblasts are larger nucleated precursors that proceed through stages of development similar to those of normoblastic erythropoiesis. Megaloblasts are typically seen with folic acid and B_{12} deficiency anemias. Microcytes are cells that are smaller than normal; they can contain a normal hemoglobin concentration (normochromic), or they can have a decreased concentration of hemoglobin (hypochromic). Microcytosis commonly accompanies iron deficiency anemia.

STIMULATION OF ERYTHROPOIESIS

Production of RBCs is initiated by the hormone EPO, which is produced mainly (90%) by the kidneys in response to a decrease in tissue oxygen caused by a decreased hemoglobin. In the healthy individual, 10–30 mU/mL (IU/L) EPO are required to maintain normal hemoglobin and hematocrit concentrations. If an anemia develops, especially severe anemia, concentrations as high as 10,000 mU/mL may be seen. Decreased tissue oxygen signals the kidneys to increase production and release of EPO into the plasma, which (1) stimulates stem cells to differentiate into rubriblasts, (2) increases the rate of mitosis, (3) increases the release of reticulocytes from the marrow, and (4) induces hemoglobin formation. When hemoglobin synthesis is

TABLE 93.1. CLASSIFICATION SYSTEMS FOR ANEMIAS

I. Morphology. Classifies anemias based on the red blood cell's size (microcytic, normocytic, macrocytic) and hemoglobin content (hypochromic, normochromic, hyperchromic)
- Macrocytic
  - Megaloblastic anemias
    - Vitamin B_{12} deficiency
    - Folic acid deficiency anemia
- Hypochromic, microcytic
  - Iron deficiency anemia
  - Genetic anomaly
    - Sickle cell anemia
    - Thalassemia
    - Other hemoglobinopathies (abnormal hemoglobins)
- Normocytic anemias
  - Recent blood loss
  - Hemolysis
  - Bone marrow failure
  - Anemias of chronic disease
  - Renal failure
  - Endocrine disorders
  - Myeloplastic anemias

II. Etiology. Classifies anemias on the basis of three fundamental mechanisms
- Deficiency
  - Iron
    - Vitamin B_{12}
    - Folic acid
    - Pyridoxine
- Central—caused by impaired bone marrow function
  - Anemia of chronic disease
  - Anemia of the elderly
  - Malignant bone marrow disorders
- Peripheral
  - Bleeding (hemorrhage)
  - Hemolysis (hemolytic anemias)

III. Pathophysiology. Classifies anemias based on an evaluation of the pathophysiologic etiology
- Excessive blood loss
  - Recent hemorrhage
    - Trauma

Excessive blood loss (cont.)
- Recent hemorrhage (cont.)
  - Peptic ulcer
  - Gastritis
  - Hemorrhoids
- Chronic hemorrhage
  - Vaginal bleeding
  - Peptic ulcer
  - Intestinal parasites
  - Aspirin and other nonsteroidal anti-inflammatory agents
- Excessive red cell destruction
  - Extracorpuscular (i.e., outside the cell) factors
    - RBC antibodies
    - Drugs
    - Physical trauma to RBC (artificial valves)
    - Excessive sequestration in the spleen
- Intracorpuscular factors
  - Heredity
  - Disorders of hemoglobin synthesis
- Inadequate production of mature RBCs
  - Deficiency of nutrients (B_{12}, folic acid, iron, protein)
  - Deficiency of erythroblasts
    - Aplastic anemia
    - Isolated (often transient) erythroblastopenia
    - Folic acid antagonists
    - Antibodies
  - Conditions with infiltration of bone marrow
    - Lymphoma
    - Leukemia
  - Myelofibrosis
    - Carcinoma
  - Endocrine abnormalities
    - Hypothyroid
    - Adrenal insufficiency
    - Pituitary insufficiency
  - Chronic renal disease
  - Chronic inflammatory disease
    - Granulomatous diseases
    - Collagen-vascular diseases
  - Hepatic disease

accelerated, the critical hemoglobin concentration necessary for maturity is reached more rapidly and a feedback mechanism stops further RBC nucleic acid synthesis such that the last mitotic division is skipped, causing an earlier release of reticulocytes. Early appearance of reticulocytes, in larger quantities, in the peripheral circulation (reticulocytosis) is another indication that RBC production is being stimulated.

SYNTHESIS OF HEMOGLOBIN

Hemoglobin is composed of two identical half molecules, and its synthesis within RBCs is under genetic control. Hemoglobin is a tetrahedron, that is, a four-sided crystal geometric-shaped molecule consisting of a protein (globin) component comprised of two α and two β chains; each chain is linked to a heme group consisting of a porphyrin ring structure with an iron atom chelated at its center, which is capable of binding oxygen. The globin portion of hemoglobin consists of two pairs of polypeptide chains containing from 141 to 146 amino acids, depending on the type of hemoglobin being formed. The hemoglobin formed in an adult is composed of 96% hemoglobin A, 3% hemoglobin A_2, and 1% fetal hemoglobin (Hb F). These polypeptide chains are attached to and folded around each heme structure giving hemoglobin its unique tetrahedron shape.

The initial step in the synthesis of heme from the substrate succinyl CoA and glycine requires the presence

TABLE 93.2. ERYTHROCYTE MATURATION SEQUENCE

Least mature form	Rubriblast (proerythroblast)
Second cell formed	Prorubricyte (basophilic erythroblast)
Third cell formed	Rubricyte (last mitotic stage) (polychromatic erythroblast)
Fourth cell formed	Metarubricyte (pyknotic erythroblast)
Fifth cell formed	Reticulocyte
Most mature form	Erythrocyte (non-nucleated)

of pyridoxine phosphate (vitamin B_6) as a catalyst. Following heme's synthesis in the cytoplasmic mitochondria of the RBC, it diffuses into the extramitochondrial space to combine with the completed α and β chains forming hemoglobin.

A defect or block in hemoglobin synthesis can lead to RBCs that appear abnormal and are usually hypochromic. These RBCs reflect a lack of hemoglobinization. Because the cell remains in the marrow longer while waiting for proper hemoglobin synthesis to occur, an increased number of cell divisions may occur, resulting in a final mature erythrocyte that is smaller than normal—a microcyte.

Under normal conditions the body produces approximately 6.25 g of hemoglobin per day. The maximal output of hemoglobin in the event of a hemolytic disease has been calculated at about 40 g/d. Consequently, the normal RBC survival time of 120 days can be decreased to 18–20 days before occurrence of an anemia if the bone marrow functions at maximal capacity. When the hemolytic destruction of RBCs exceeds marrow production capacity, anemia will develop, causing the hemoglobin value to decrease to a steady-state level such that production is equal to destruction. Hemoglobin values in these hemolytic anemias, such as sickle cell anemia, will remain stable unless other factors further shorten RBC life span.

TOTAL BODY IRON

The average adult body contains about 4 g of iron, approximately two-thirds of which exists in the form of hemoglobin. Another 13% exists as myoglobin, while the same percentage exists as a combination of ferritin and hemosiderin. Because inorganic iron is quite toxic, the body has an intricate system for iron absorption, transport, storage, assimilation, and elimination.

INCORPORATION OF IRON INTO HEME

The delivery of iron to the bone marrow for incorporation into the RBC hemoglobin molecule is carried out by a specific plasma transport protein (globulin) called *transferrin*. Transferrin flow into body cells is accomplished by its binding to transferrin receptors, which circulate and then attach to cells needing iron. Likewise, there is a reduction in transferrin receptors on the surface of cells not currently needing iron, thus preventing iron-rich cells from receiving excess iron.[2]

Circulating transferrin is normally only about 30% saturated with iron. Calculation of transferrin saturation and total iron binding capacity (TIBC) are explained later in this chapter in the section on Laboratory Evaluation. Transferrin delivers extra iron to other body storage sites such as the liver, marrow, and spleen for later use. This iron is stored within macrophages of the reticuloendothelial system as either ferritin or hemosiderin. Ferritin consists of a ferric hydroxyphosphate core surrounded by a protein shell called *apoferritin.* Hemosiderin can be described as compacted ferritin molecules with an even greater iron-to-protein shell ratio; physiologically it is a more stable but less available form of storage iron.

ABSORPTION OF IRON

The normal daily Western diet contains approximately 12–15 mg of iron mainly in the ferric (Fe^{3+}) nonabsorbed form. This is first ionized by stomach acid and then reduced to the ferrous state (Fe^{3+}) and absorbed primarily in the duodenum and to a smaller extent in the jejunum via intestinal mucosal cell uptake and subsequent transfer across the cell into the plasma.[3] The average intake of iron from this diet is about 6 mg per 1000 calories (about 10–30 mg of iron per day).[4]

Daily losses, and thus requirements for iron, are 1 mg in adult males and postmenopausal females, and 1.5–3 mg in menstruating females. Children and pregnant women have increased iron demands. Children require more iron due to growth-related increases in blood volume, while pregnant women have an increased iron demand from fetal development. Iron overload is prevented because only the amount of iron lost per day is absorbed. This represents about 5–10% (1 mg) of daily dietary intake. However, up to 8–12 mg/d can be absorbed if iron requirements increase.

Heme and nonheme iron are absorbed by distinct pathways. Dietary heme, iron from hemoglobin and other heme proteins found in meat, is cleaved by gastric acids and proteases to free heme, which is oxidized to its ferric state, forming hemin, and is then absorbed. Nonheme iron may first be converted to the ferrous form in order to be absorbed. The absorption of nonheme iron is increased by gastric acid and by other dietary components such as most meats and ascorbic acid. Absorption is decreased by dietary components that form insoluble complexes or chelates with iron (phytates, tannates, and phosphates).[5] Phytates, a natural component of grains, brans and some other vegetables, form stable, poorly absorbed complexes and partially explain the increased prevalence of iron deficiency anemia in poorer countries where grains and vegetables compose a disproportionate part of the normal diet, while the more readily absorbed heme iron is lacking in their diet. Last, because gastric acid improves iron absorption, patients who have undergone a gastrectomy or have achlorhydria will have decreased iron absorption.

NORMAL DESTRUCTION OF RBCs

Older blood cells are destroyed in the marrow by a phagocytic breakdown (Fig. 93.1). The amino acids from the globin chains return to an amino acid pool; the porphyrin heme structure splits forming biliverdin and releasing its iron. Iron returns to the iron pool for reuse while biliverdin is further enzymatically reduced to bilirubin. This bilirubin is released from the marrow into the plasma where it binds to albumin and is transported to the liver for glucuronide conjugation and excretion via the bile. If the liver is unable to carry on this conjugation in the normal manner, as seen with intrinsic liver disease or oversaturation of conjugation enzymes by excessive cell hemolysis, the result would be an elevated indirect (unconjugated) bilirubin laboratory value. Should there be an obstruction in the biliary excretion pathway for the already conjugated bilirubin, an elevated direct bilirubin would result. Comparison of direct and indirect bilirubin values helps determine if the defect in bilirubin clearance occurs before or after bilirubin enters the liver.

The hemoglobin in RBCs, which is destroyed by intravascular hemolysis, becomes attached to a haptoglobin and is carried back to the marrow for processing in the normal manner. The spleen is also capable of RBC destruction.

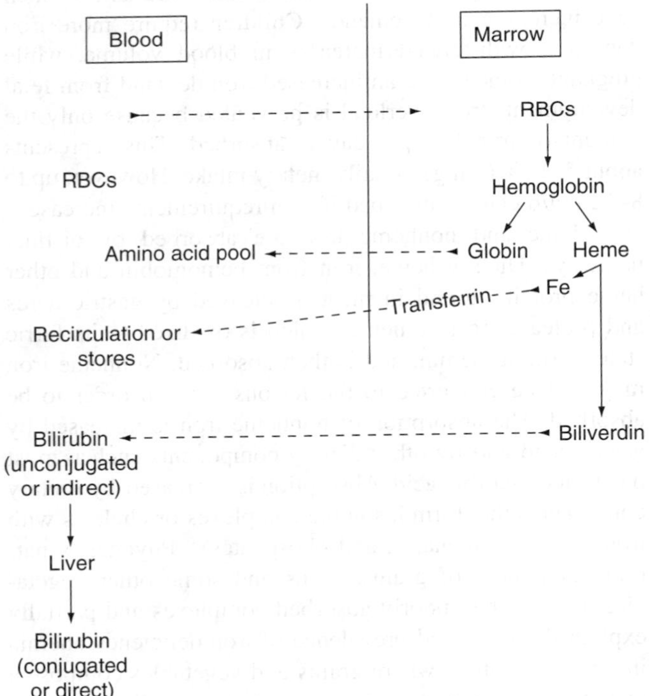

Figure 93.1. Destruction of RBCs.

DIAGNOSIS OF ANEMIA

GENERAL PRESENTATION OF ANEMIAS

Presenting signs and symptoms of anemias depend on the rate of development of the anemia. Anemia of recent onset is most likely to present with cardiorespiratory symptoms such as tachycardia, light-headedness, and breathlessness, whereas if onset is more chronic in nature the presenting symptoms may include fatigue, headache, vertigo, faintness, sensitivity to cold, pallor, and loss of skin tone. These symptoms represent the manifestation of an illness, not a specific disease. More specific symptoms of the various anemias are discussed later, in order to attempt to determine definitively the cause of the anemia.

LABORATORY EVALUATION

Evaluation of anemia involves a complete blood count including RBC indices, a reticulocyte index, examination of the peripheral blood smear, and a stool for occult blood. Mild anemias will usually have normal RBC indices. Elevated reticulocytes often indicate bleeding or hemolysis. Low reticulocyte counts indicate anemia due to inadequate bone marrow production. Iron deficiency can be easily detected with a serum ferritin level. Table 93.3 shows normal hematologic values while the laboratory tests used to evaluate anemias are discussed as follows.

Hemoglobin

The higher values seen in males are due to stimulation of RBC production by androgenic steroids. Hemoglobin can be reduced because of a decreased quantity of hemoglobin per RBC or because of a decreased actual number of RBCs.

Hematocrit

Hematocrit is the actual volume of RBCs in a unit volume expressed as a percent. A low hematocrit indicates a reduction in either number or size of RBCs or an increased plasma volume.

RBC Count

RBC count is an indirect estimate of the hemoglobin content of the blood.

RBC Indices

Wintrobe indices were introduced in 1934 by Maxwell Wintrobe to describe certain morphologic characteristics of the RBCs.

Mean Corpuscular Volume

Mean corpuscular volume (MCV) indicates macrocytic, normocytic, or microcytic morphology as it represents the average volume, measured with a Coulter counter, of the RBCs.

TABLE 93.3. NORMAL HEMATOLOGIC VALUES

Test	Reference Range (yr)			
	2–6	**6–12**	**12–18**	**18–49**
Hemoglobin (g/dL)	11.5–11.5	11.5–15.5	M 13.0–16.0 F 12.0–16.0	M 13.5–17.5 F 12.0–16.0
Hematocrit (%)	34.0–40.0	35.0–45.0	M 37.0–49.0 F 36.0–46.0	M 41.0–53.0 F 36.0–46.0
MCV (μm^3)	75–87	77–95	M 78–98 F 78–102	80–100
MCHC (%)	—	31–37	31–37	31–37
MCH (pg)	24–30	25–33	25–35	26–34
RBC (million/mm^3)	3.9–5.3	4.0–5.2	M 4.5–5.3	M 4.5–5.9
Reticulocyte count, absolute (%)				0.5–1.5
Serum iron (μg/dL)		50–120	50–120	M 50–160 F 40–150
TIBC (μg/dL)	250–400	250–400	250–400	250–400
Ferritin (ng/mL)	7–140	7–140	7–140	M 15–200 F 12–150
Folate (ng/mL)				1.8–16[a]
Vitamin B_{12} (pg/mL)				100–900[a]
Erythropoietin (U/mL)				0.01–0.03

[a]Varies by assay method.

It is based on the relationship of RBC size to hematocrit. For example, if the average size of the RBC is increased, then the same number of RBCs will have a slightly larger total cell mass and an increased hematocrit, while a decreased RBC size will give a decreased hematocrit. Folic acid and vitamin B_{12} deficiency anemias are macrocytic.

Mean Corpuscular Hemoglobin

Mean corpuscular hemoglobin (MCH) is the average weight of hemoglobin in an RBC. Two morphologic changes, microcytosis or hypochromia, can reduce MCH. A microcytic cell contains less hemoglobin because it is a smaller cell, whereas a hypochromic cell has a low MCH because of the decreased amount of hemoglobin present in a normocytic cell. Cells commonly are both microcytic and hypochromic. MCH alone cannot distinguish between microcytosis and hypochromia. The most common cause of an elevated MCH is macrocytosis.

Mean Corpuscular Hemoglobin Concentration

MCH concentration (MCHC) is the weight of hemoglobin per volume of cells (i.e., concentration). MCHC is independent of cell size and, therefore, is more useful than the MCH in distinguishing between microcytosis and hypochromia. A low MCHC always indicates hypochromia; a microcyte with a normal hemoglobin concentration will have a low MCH but a normal MCHC.

Total Reticulocyte Count

Determination of the reticulocyte count in normocytic anemia differentiates hypoproliferative marrow from a compensatory marrow response to an anemia. Occasionally, a patient's hematocrit decreases while their absolute number of reticulocytes remains the same. This results in a falsely elevated reticulocyte percentage. For example, if a patient's hematocrit decreases by 50% (from 50 to 25%) the corresponding reticulocyte percentage doubles. This problem is corrected by expressing the reticulocyte count as an absolute number; to do this, the percentage of reticulocytes (expressed as a decimal) is multiplied by the total RBC count. A corrected percentage of reticulocytes can also be calculated by multiplying the reticulocyte percent by the patient's hematocrit and then dividing the product by an average normal hematocrit (for men or women).

$$\text{Corrected reticulocyte count (\%)} = \text{observed \%} \times \frac{\text{patient's Hct}}{\text{normal Hct}}$$

Serum Iron

Serum iron is the concentration of iron bound to transferrin. Normally transferrin is about one-third bound (saturated) to iron. Unfortunately, the serum iron level of many patients with iron deficiency anemia (IDA) remains within the lower limits of normal, giving a false-negative test. There is also a 20–30% diurnal variation in serum iron levels (it is best to draw blood levels in the morning) and a 20–25% day-to-day variation among individuals.[6] Consequently, as a diagnostic tool, serum iron levels are best interpreted in conjunction with the total iron-binding capacity. Serum iron is decreased with IDA and ACD and is increased with hemolytic anemias and iron overload.

Total Iron-Binding Capacity

TIBC is an indirect measurement of serum transferrin, performed by adding an excess of iron to plasma to saturate all transferrin with iron. The excess (unbound) iron is then removed and the serum iron concentration is determined. Unlike the serum iron level, the TIBC is remarkably constant. The finding of a low serum iron and a high TIBC indicates IDA.

Percent Transferrin Saturation

Transferrin saturation is the ratio of the serum iron to the TIBC expressed as a percentage, that is, transferrin saturation = (serum iron/TIBC) × 100. In IDA, the serum iron decreases and the TIBC increases, making the percent saturation of the iron-binding capacity less than 13%. This is a common measure of IDA.

Serum Ferritin

The concentration of ferritin (storage iron) in the serum is proportional to total iron stores and, consequently, is a reliable indicator of body iron stores. Low serum ferritin levels are virtually diagnostic of IDA as they are decreased only in IDA, whereas serum iron may be decreased in IDA and anemia of chronic disease.

Folic Acid Level

Folic acid values may vary depending on assay method used. Decreased levels indicate a folate deficiency megaloblastic anemia that may exist with a vitamin B_{12} deficiency anemia.

Vitamin B_{12} Level

Vitamin B_{12} levels may vary depending on assay method used. Low levels indicate vitamin B_{12} deficiency anemia.

The Schilling Test

This test is used to diagnose vitamin B_{12} deficiency anemia caused by a B_{12} absorption defect resulting from lack of intrinsic factor (pernicious anemia). An oral dose of cobalt-labeled vitamin B_{12} is administered. If sufficient GI intrinsic factor is being produced gastrointestinally, the B_{12} will be absorbed. Concomitantly, a large intramuscular dose of nonlabeled vitamin B_{12} is given to saturate tissue-binding sites and flush the radiolabeled B_{12} into the urine. Normally, approximately 33% of the absorbed radiolabeled B_{12} appears in the urine over 24 hours. Patients with pernicious anemia excrete less than 8% of the original oral radiolabeled dose. After several days, this test is repeated, except that the oral radiolabeled B_{12} is administered along with a sufficient amount of intrinsic factor. Results within the normal range indicate that the defect is in intrinsic factor production as opposed to dietary lack of vitamin B_{12}.

Erythropoietin

Endogenous EPO levels can increase up to 100- to 1000-fold during hypoxia or anemia. This marked increase is not seen in patients with end-stage renal disease, patients on chemotherapy, and AIDS patients, especially those taking AZT. These patients will have an erythropoietin response that is insufficient to correct their anemia.

PATHOPHYSIOLOGY AND TREATMENT OF ANEMIAS

ANEMIAS DUE TO ABNORMAL HEMOGLOBIN SYNTHESIS

A defect in hemoglobin synthesis as well as certain acquired defects in EPO precursor cell metabolism may cause changes in iron incorporation, producing a cell with an excess of nonheme iron within the cytoplasm. These cells, called sideroblasts, cause sideroblastic anemia, which is usually macrocytic.

Sideroblastic anemia can be congenital (hereditary-sex linked in males) or acquired. The acquired forms can be either primary or secondary to drugs, toxins (lead, alcohol), or other disease states. Hypocupremia has long been associated with sideroblastosis. Excess zinc intake will also cause sideroblastic anemia by binding preferentially to copper, causing impaired copper absorption and hypocupremia.[7] Primary acquired sideroblastic anemia is usually classified as a myelodysplastic syndrome and may eventually transform into acute myeloblastic leukemia in a proportion of patients.

Other hereditary defects in heme synthesis can lead to an overproduction of heme precursors, causing the disease porphyria. The most common porphyria, acute intermittent porphyria (AIP), results from a hereditary (autosomal dominant) partial deficiency in the enzyme uroporphyrinogen I synthetase, responsible for converting porphobilinogen to uroporphyrinogen. This in turn causes an inhibition of the normal feedback mechanism of porphyrin synthesis, leading to an excess production of the heme intermediate pigments uroporphyrin I and coproporphyrin I, which can then be detected in abnormal amounts in urine and feces to confirm the diagnosis of AIP.

AIP is characterized by neuropsychiatric, neuromuscular, and autonomic dysfunction, and intense abdominal pain. In the liver, this enzyme deficiency results in increased inducibility of abnormal heme intermediates by certain drugs. Drugs and agents known to induce hepatic cytochrome P-450 or to increase hepatic heme turnover are theoretically capable of precipitating porphyria. Barbiturates,[8] estrogens,[9] alcohol,[10] heavy metals such as lead, and certain other chemicals have been documented to induce porphyria in genetically susceptible people.

Genetic expression of an abnormal amino acid substitution in either the α- or β-globin chains can lead to a variety of hemoglobinopathies causing such hemolytic diseases as sickle cell anemia and thalassemia (see Chapter 95, Sickle Cell Anemia). Hundreds of these abnormal hemoglobin diseases exist, and are best diagnosed by hemoglobin electrophoresis. Factors that decrease production and those that further shorten RBC life span will alter the stable hemoglobin level in chronic hemolytic diseases.

HEMOCHROMATOSIS (IRON OVERLOAD)

A hereditary gastrointestinal (GI) disease, hemochromatosis, results from a loss of regulation of iron absorption; the resultant iron deposition in various tissues causes multiple organ system failure including cirrhosis and various forms of heart disease. Primary or hereditary hemochromatosis results from a genetic defect in iron metabolism that increases the intestinal absorption of iron from a normal diet. It is inherited as an autosomal recessive trait and is more common in men than women. Secondary or acquired hemochromatosis results from some abnormality other than a primary increase in intestinal iron absorption. Possible causes of secondary hemochromatosis include excess medicinal or dietary iron or repeated blood transfusions.[11] Marked increases in transferrin saturation (>60%) are suggestive of this disease and warrant further evaluation of ferritin levels and liver biopsy. This disease is rare, with a prevalence of less than 0.1%.[12] Early diagnosis with periodic prophylactic phlebotomy employed early in the disease can lessen late-stage disease complications.

IRON DEFICIENCY ANEMIA

Pathophysiology

In IDA, iron stores are depleted prior to development of anemia; therefore, the earliest change observed is a decrease in serum ferritin relative to baseline. Unfortunately IDA is not usually detected at this level. With continuing iron depletion, the hemoglobin drops slightly and serum ferritin falls below 12. The TIBC increases and serum iron concentration decreases. The hemoglobin, hematocrit, and RBC indices usually remain normal. In the later stages of IDA, the hemoglobin and hematocrit fall below normal values and a microcytic, hypochromic anemia develops. Microcytosis may precede hypochromia as erythropoiesis is programmed to maintain normal hemoglobin concentration in deference to cell size. As a consequence, even slightly abnormal hemoglobin and hematocrit levels may indicate significant depletion of iron stores and should not be ignored. Conversely, with treatment of IDA, these monitoring parameters return to normal in reverse order of their development.

As previously discussed, IDA is usually microcytic and hypochromic. It is believed to occur in approximately 25% of patients with anemia. The most commonly cited causes of IDA include inadequate dietary intake, inadequate absorption from the GI tract, increased iron demands, blood loss, and certain diseases. Dietary deficiencies most frequently result from decreased consumption of animal protein and ascorbic acid[13] as a consequence of chronic alcoholism, food faddism, prolonged illness with anorexia, or poor nutrition. Inadequate absorption from the GI tract is usually a sequel to such disorders as malabsorption syndromes, postgastrectomy states, the presence of certain foods or drugs, or unrelenting diarrhea. Demands for iron may increase during infancy, pregnancy, adolescence, or old age. Blood loss may occur as a result of many disorders, including trauma, hemorrhoids, peptic ulcers, gastritis, GI carcinoma, diverticular disease, copious menstrual flow, nose bleeds, or postpartum bleeding.[14] Occult blood loss from a single GI lesion has been shown to be a frequent cause of "idiopathic" IDA.[15]

Diseases contributing to the development of IDA include rheumatoid arthritis (with chronic aspirin ingestion), various carcinomas, and renal disease. With IDA, the possibility of multifactorial etiology must always be kept in mind. Other causes of hypochromic microcytic anemia that must be considered include thalassemia (especially thalassemia minor) and heavy metal poisoning (mostly lead).

Signs and Symptoms

Manifestations of IDA include koilonychia (spooning of the nails), angular stomatitis and glossitis, and craving for substances low in iron (i.e., pica), such as clay, ice, or cornstarch. These symptoms usually do not appear until the hemoglobin concentration falls below 8 or 9 g/100 mL.

Laboratory Manifestations

Abnormal laboratory findings in patients with IDA include low serum iron and ferritin levels, and a high TIBC. Serum ferritin is the first parameter to decrease in iron deficiency. It is considered the indirect measurement of choice for evaluating iron stores. Levels lower than 15 g/L indicate deficient iron stores for the general population. The major disadvantage of using this parameter in evaluating iron stores is the same as that for serum iron and TIBC: In patients with renal or liver disease, carcinoma, infection, or inflammatory processes, the measured values may be elevated to greater than 50 g/L and may not correlate with iron stores in the bone marrow.[16] Hemoglobin concentrations below 11 g/100 mL and hematocrits less than 38% usually indicate a decrease in RBC mass that may be caused by iron deficiency. Low concentrations of ferritin (less than 10–12 g/L) are indicative of iron deficiency. In patients with inflammatory disorders, however, these values may be within normal limits despite the presence of iron deficiency. Liver disease causes an elevation in serum ferritin; thus ferritin should not be used for diagnostic purposes in patients with even mild hepatic pathology. Transferrin saturation is also used to assess IDA. One major disadvantage of this test is the large biologic variation in serum iron levels. Iron concentrations are highest in the morning and lowest at night. Therefore, it is generally recommended that blood for transferrin saturation testing be drawn in the morning or early afternoon hours. Low values (below 15%) during these times will likely indicate iron deficiency anemia; however, as mentioned before, low serum transferrin saturation values may also be present in inflammatory disorders. Fortunately, the TIBC usually helps to differentiate the diagnosis in these patients; a TIBC greater than 400 g% suggests IDA, whereas values below 200 g% usually represent inflammatory disease.

Free erythrocyte protoporphyrin can also be used in the diagnosis of IDA. Iron normally binds with protoporphyrin to form heme. When iron levels are low, the serum concentration of protoporphyrin not bound to iron is elevated. This test is very helpful in distinguishing between iron deficiency and thalassemia minor, because values are normal in the latter and elevated in the former. Unfortunately, free erythrocyte protoporphyrin is also elevated in inflammatory disorders and lead poisoning and, thus, is less effective in distinguishing iron deficiency in patients in whom these other two conditions are also present.

Therapy

Treatment of IDA usually consists of dietary supplementation and the administration of therapeutic iron preparations. Food substances play a significant role in the prevention as well as the treatment of IDA. Iron absorption varies greatly with different foods. Iron is poorly absorbed from vegetables, grain products, dairy products, and eggs; it is best absorbed from meat, fish, and poultry. Substitution of meat for eggs, milk, or cheese in a mixed meal has been shown to quadruple the absorption of iron from the entire meal.[17] Beverages have also been shown to affect iron absorption. For example, orange juice doubles the absorption of iron from an entire meal, whereas tea or milk will reduce absorption to less than one-half.[18,19] It is thus recommended that meat, orange juice, and other ascorbic acid-rich foods be included in meals and that if milk and tea are used, they be consumed in moderation between meals.

In most cases of IDA, oral iron therapy with soluble ferrous iron salts is the recommended treatment. Iron is best absorbed in the reduced ferrous form with maximal absorption occurring in the duodenum, primarily due to the iron being maintained in a soluble form by the acid medium of the stomach and by mucopolysaccharide chelator substances that prevent the iron from precipitating. In the alkaline environment of the small intestines, iron tends to form insoluble complexes that are unavailable for absorption. Thus, the preferred iron preparation is nonenteric-coated ferrous salts. Slow-release or sustained-release iron preparations do not undergo sufficient dissolution until reaching the small intestines and consequently iron absorption is significantly reduced,[20,21] which can cause an attenuation in the hematinic effects. The dose of iron to be administered depends on the patient's ability to tolerate the administered iron. In patients with iron deficiency, it is generally recommended that approximately 200 mg elemental iron be administered each day, in two to three divided doses.[22] Table 93.4 shows the percent elemental iron of commonly available iron salts. Note that ferrous sulfate is also available as an exsiccated (dried) form that contains approximately 30% elemental iron as opposed to the nonexsiccated form that is only 20% elemental iron. The percentage of iron absorbed progressively decreases as the dose increases, but the absolute amount absorbed increases. Food interferes with the absorption of iron; therefore, iron should preferably be administered one or more hours before meals, if possible. But many patients experience nausea and diarrhea when iron is administered on an empty stomach, thus necessitating administration with food. However, these effects may be offset by giving smaller amounts of iron with each administration. Although some forms of iron are combined with ascorbic acid or antacids, previous studies have shown that addition of ascorbic acid or other ingredients does not enhance absorption from oral iron preparations when given on an empty stomach. Approximately 60–65 mg elemental iron is provided per 300- to 325-mg sulfate salt tablet, approximately 37–39 mg elemental iron per 300- to 325-mg gluconate tablet, and 33 mg elemental iron per 100-mg fumerate tablet.

Evaluation of Therapeutic Outcomes

In the evaluation of therapeutic outcomes, one would expect therapeutic doses of iron to raise the hemoglobin value by 1–2 g% per week. As the hemoglobin level approaches nor-

TABLE 93.4. IRON PRODUCTS

Salt	Elemental Iron (%)
Ferrous sulfate	20
Ferrous sulfate, exsiccated	30
Ferrous gluconate	12
Ferrous fumarate	33
Ferric pyrophosphate	12
Ferrous carbonate	48

mal, the rate of increase slows progressively. A hemoglobin response of less than 2 g/100 mL over a 3-week period is unacceptable and should be further evaluated. In addition, reticulocytosis occurs within 7–10 days after initiation of iron therapy. If the patient does not develop reticulocytosis, the diagnosis or therapy needs to be reevaluated.

Iron therapy should continue for a period sufficient for complete restoration of iron stores to normal. The time interval required to accomplish this goal varies from patient to patient, but in general, at least 3–6 months of therapy is necessary.[26] Patients with negative iron balances caused by bleeding may require iron replacement therapy for only a month after correction of the underlying lesion, whereas patients with recurrent negative balances may require long-term treatment. This latter group may require as little as 30–60 mg of elemental iron daily.

Adverse reactions to therapeutic doses of iron are primarily gastrointestinal in nature and consist of discoloration of feces (dark), constipation or diarrhea, nausea, and vomiting. Failure to develop at least some of these symptoms, even mildly, may indicate noncompliance. Should these side effects be intolerable, the dose may be taken with meals or the total daily dose may be decreased to 110–120 mg elemental iron. Administration of iron with meals, however, reduces the amount of iron absorbed by more than one-half.

Failure to respond to the preceding treatment regimen necessitates reevaluation of the situation. Common causes of treatment failures include noncompliance with therapy, misdiagnosis (e.g., inflammation), malabsorption, and blood loss equal to the rate of production. Malabsorption can be ruled out by the iron test in which plasma iron levels are determined at half-hour intervals for 2 hours following the administration of 50 mg elemental iron as liquid ferrous sulfate. If plasma iron levels increase by more than 50 ng% during this time, absorption is satisfactory.

Parenteral Iron Therapy

Parenteral iron therapy may be necessary when there is evidence of iron malabsorption, when intolerance of orally administered iron exists, and when noncompliance is a problem. Other conditions that may warrant parenteral iron therapy include patients with a high intake of antacids or other substances that bind to iron and inhibit its absorption, and patients with significant blood loss who refuse transfusions and in whom oral iron therapy is not possible.

Parenteral iron is commonly given with EPO to patients receiving chronic hemodialysis and chronic ambulatory peritoneal dialysis. Iron dextran, a complex of ferric hydroxide and dextran containing 50 mg of iron per milliliter, may be given intramuscularly (by Z-tract administration) or intravenously in these situations. Methods of intravenous administration include multiple slow injections of the undiluted iron dextran solution or as an infusion of a diluted preparation. This latter method is often referred to as total dose infusion. Intramuscular iron dextran is given via Z-tract administration in order to minimize staining of the skin. Because each intramuscular dose is limited to 2 mL (containing only 100 mg iron), multiple injections are often required. Problems with this administration route include patient discomfort, sterile abscesses, tissue necrosis, or atrophy. In addition, up to 30% of an administered dose remains physiologically unavailable. These disadvantages make the intravenous route the preferred route of administration.

Iron dextran must be processed in the reticuloendothelial cells for the iron to be biologically available. The absorption and metabolism characteristics vary with the route and amount of drug given.

Absorption of an intramuscular dose of iron dextran occurs in two phases. During the first 72 hours, iron dextran is absorbed primarily through the lymphatics into the left superior vena cava. A smaller amount is absorbed directly through the intramuscular capillary network into the blood.[26] A second, slower phase involves uptake of the iron dextran complex by macrophages, with subsequent transport through the lymphatics into the blood. About 60% of an intramuscular dose of iron dextran is absorbed after 3 days and up to 90% is absorbed within 3 weeks.[27] The remainder is absorbed slowly over several months or longer.

Intravenous doses of iron dextran are taken up immediately by the reticuloendothelial system.[28] Small to intermediate intravenous doses (50–500 mg of elemental iron) can be cleared from the plasma within 3 days of administration. In contrast, larger intravenous doses of iron dextran (greater than 500 mg of elemental iron) are processed by the reticuloendothelial system at a constant rate of 10–20 mg/h.[29] Doses this large are associated with increased plasma concentrations of iron dextran for as long as 3 weeks.

Once iron is absorbed into the blood, cells of the reticuloendothelial system phagocytize the iron dextran complex and cleave the dextran moiety, making free iron available to the body as circulating iron, transferrin-bound iron, or storage iron (ferritin and hemosiderin). Iron dextran can remain within the reticuloendothelial cells for many months. Equations for calculating the dose in patients with IDA and patients with anemia secondary to blood loss can be found in Table 93.5. When given by intermittent intravenous administration, the dose should not exceed 50 mg iron per minute (1 mL/min). The manufacturer suggests no more than 100 mg of iron dextran be administered daily. However, numerous reports have been made in which the total dose of iron dextran needed was administered as a single dose by IV infusion.[30,31] Although not FDA approved, this method is efficacious and convenient. If the total dose required to correct the anemia is given in a single dose, one must be aware of the increased possibility of adverse reactions such as arthralgia, myalgia, flushing, malaise, and fever. Other adverse reactions, which may occur with iron

TABLE 93.5. EQUATIONS FOR CALCULATING DOSES OF IRON DEXTRAN

In patients with iron deficiency anemia:

$$\text{mg of iron} = W \times (100 - \%\text{Hb}) \times 0.3$$

where *W* is the patient's weight in pounds and %Hb is the patient's observed hemoglobin expressed as a percentage of the normal hemoglobin concentration (assuming 14.8 g of hemoglobin per 100 mL is equivalent to 100% concentration).

If the patient weighs 13.6 kg (30 lb) or less, the dose is 80% of the calculated amount.

In patients with anemia secondary to blood loss (hemorrhagic diathesis or long-term dialysis):

$$\text{mg of iron} = \text{blood loss} \times \text{hematocrit}$$

where blood loss is in milliliters and hematocrit is expressed as a decimal fraction.

dextran, include staining of the skin, pain at the injection site, allergic reactions, and possible anaphylaxis (rare). Patients most likely to experience adverse effects with iron dextran include individuals with a history of allergies, asthma, or an inflammatory disease. Patients with preexisting immune-mediated diseases such as active rheumatoid arthritis or systemic lupus erythematosus are considered high risk because of their hyperreactive immune response capabilities. It is suggested that all patients receiving iron dextran injection receive a test dose of 25 mg intramuscularly or intravenously, or a 5- to 10-minute infusion of the diluted solution. Patients should then be observed for more than 1 hour for untoward reactions. Should none be experienced, the remainder of the dose can then be administered. Patients receiving total dose infusions can have the remaining solution infused during the next 2–6 hours.

Evaluation of Therapeutic Outcomes of Parenteral Iron Therapy

When large amounts of parenteral iron are administered, either by total dose infusion or by multiple IM or IV doses, iron status should be closely monitored. Hemoglobin and hematocrit should be measured weekly and serum iron and ferritin levels should be measured at least every month.

Another form of treatment of IDA is blood transfusions. However, this form of therapy should be avoided when cardiovascular compromise exists. Once the hematocrit value falls below 30, the oxygen-carrying capacity in older patients drops precipitously, thus predisposing them to ischemia. Tachycardia, angina, ischemic patterns on ECG, cerebrovascular insufficiency, postural hypotension, and prerenal azotemia are clear-cut indications for transfusions to maintain the hematocrit above 30. An exception to this treatment modality is the occasional patient encountered who has developed low hematocrit values over extended time periods. These patients often demonstrate cardiac compromise despite hematocrits in the 20s. Therapy in these patients should consist of iron therapy, followed by transfusion only if necessary.

MEGALOBLASTIC ANEMIAS

Megaloblastosis results from interference in folic acid and vitamin B_{12} interdependent nucleic acid synthesis in the immature erythrocyte. Because DNA and RNA synthesis is retarded, one or more mitotic cell divisions are skipped, resulting in an abnormally large cell. Synthesis of the RNA and DNA necessary for cell division depends on a series of reactions catalyzed by vitamin B_{12} and folic acid (Fig. 93.2). In this process, dietary folates are absorbed and converted (A) to 5-methyl tetrahydrofolate (5-MTHF), which is then converted via a B_{12}-dependent (B) reaction to tetrahydrofolate (THF) (C). After gaining a carbon, THF is converted to a folate cofactor (D), 5,10-methylene tetrahydrofolate (5,10-METHF), used by thymidylate synthetase enzyme (E) in the biosynthesis of nucleic acids. The 5,10-METHF cofactor is converted to dihydrofolate (DHF) (F) during biosynthesis. Normally, dihydrofolate reductase enzyme reduces DHF back to tetrahydrofolate (C), which can again pick up a carbon and be recycled to produce more 5,10-METHF (D).

VITAMIN B_{12} DEFICIENCY ANEMIA

Etiology and Pathophysiology

The etiology of vitamin B_{12} deficiency anemia due to lack of GI intrinsic factor was elucidated in a 1936 experiment by Castle and Ham. Their study has since been republished as a "landmark article" by JAMA.[32] Patients with pernicious anemia were fed beef muscle simultaneously with recovered gastric juices from normal subjects and responded appropriately as evidenced by a reticulocytosis and increased RBC count. This lead to the isolation (from liver), chemical identification, and eventual synthesis of vitamin B_{12} (the extrinsic factor) in the 1940s and 1950s.

Adult onset pernicious anemia has an estimated annual incidence of new cases of 100/1 million population, and it is slightly more common in women. There is a sharp increase in incidence with increasing age, suggesting that it is a consequence of gastric epithelial aging.

The three major causes of vitamin B_{12} deficiency are inadequate intake, decreased absorption, and inadequate utilization. Vitamin B_{12} is a water-soluble vitamin that humans obtain by ingestion of animal foodstuffs containing B_{12}, primarily meat and dairy products. Body stores of vitamin B_{12} range from 2–5 mg, with the daily requirement

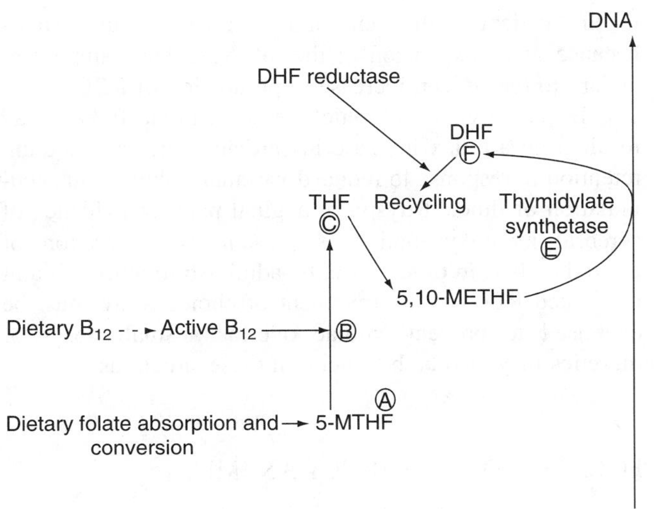

Figure 93.2. Drug-induced megaloblastosis. DHF, dihydrofolate; THF, tetrahydrofolate; 5-MTHF, 5 methyl THF; 5,10-METHF, 5,10-methylene THF.

being approximately 1–5 g. The average daily diet contains more than 20 g of B_{12} such that it would take 1360 days (3–4 years) to become B_{12} deficient in a person deprived of vitamin B_{12}. As previously stated, vitamin B_{12} is necessary for DNA synthesis; it is also important in metabolic reactions involving folic acid and in maintaining the integrity of the neurologic system.

Inadequate dietary consumption of vitamin B_{12} is rare. It is usually only seen in patients who are strict vegetarians, because body stores are large and meats and vegetables are a readily available source.

Decreased absorption of vitamin B_{12} occurs in patients with a deficiency of *intrinsic factor* and can be diagnosed with the Schilling test. A decrease in the production of intrinsic factor results in acquired pernicious anemia, while dysfunction of the intrinsic factor causes congenital pernicious anemia. Vitamin B_{12} deficiency may also result from overgrowth of bacteria in the bowel that utilize B_{12} or from injury or removal of ileal receptor sites where vitamin B_{12} and the intrinsic factor complex. Blind-loop syndrome, fish tapeworm infestations, intestinal resections, tropical sprue, regional enteritis, and Crohn's disease may all contribute to the development of vitamin B_{12} deficiency.[33]

In the portal blood, vitamin B_{12} is bound to the transport protein, transcobolamin II, which rapidly delivers the vitamin to sites of utilization and storage. In persons with a transcobolamin II deficiency, B_{12} cannot be transported from the blood to utilization and storage sites. Consequently, the patient has a normal B_{12} level but evidence of frank B_{12} deficiency.

Signs and Symptoms

As is true in most forms of anemia, certain symptoms are cardiovascular in origin and result when the body can no longer tolerate the increased cardiac output stimulated by the anemia. Clinically, vitamin B_{12} deficiency presents as a megaloblastic anemia (with hypersegmented neutrophils), with gastric mucosal atrophy, followed by neuropsychiatric abnormalities as a result of combined degeneration of the spinal cord and brain.

The most frequently reported neurologic symptoms are paresthesias and ataxia. Other reported symptoms include glossitis, diminished vibratory sensation in the lower extremities, muscle weakness, dysphagia, anorexia, irritability, dementia, and psychosis.[34]

Laboratory Findings

Once anemia has been confirmed with a low RBC count and low hemoglobin/hematocrit, the RBC indices must be examined. In macrocytic anemias, MCV is usually elevated above 100 m^3. Leukopenia and thrombocytopenia may be present, although these usually are not severe. A peripheral blood smear demonstrates macrocytosis accompanied by hypersegmented polymorphonuclear leukocytes (one of the earliest and most specific indications of this disease) and oval macrocytes. Serum lactate dehydrogenase and bilirubin levels are elevated as a result of hemolysis or ineffective erythropoiesis. Serum iron and transferrin saturation are usually elevated; however, iron levels may be low in 21–33% of patients with pernicious anemia. The reticulocyte count is low and serum B_{12} levels are usually low.[35]

Recommendations with regard to vitamin B_{12} deficiency include a screening of all suspected patients with a low B_{12} level. Vitamin B_{12} values below 150 pmol/L in a patient with macrocytosis, hypersegmented polymorphonuclear leukocytes, peripheral neuropathy, or dementia is diagnostic of B_{12} deficiency, even though the Schilling test may be normal. Approximately one-third of patients with pernicious anemia will not demonstrate macrocytosis if complicated by iron deficiency, thalassemia, or a predominant neurologic involvement.

Vitamin B_{12} values of 200–300 pg/mL are suggestive and should be repeated in 1–3 months. If this value is less than 200 pg/mL, a Shilling test should be performed. In patients with a normal Schilling test, oral B_{12} should be initiated and continued until the B_{12} level is greater than 300 pg/mL. With an abnormal Schilling test, or in patients who do not respond to oral therapy, the patient must receive intramuscular vitamin B_{12}.[36]

When evaluating low serum B_{12} levels, it is important to rule out other causes besides dietary deprivation and malabsorption. For example, falsely low levels may be seen in patients receiving antibiotics, anticonvulsants, cytotoxic agents, oral contraceptives, and high-dose vitamin C. In addition, conditions that can result in falsely low B_{12} levels include multiple myeloma, malignancy, aplastic anemia, transcobalamin I deficiency, gastrectomy, the third trimester of pregnancy, and radioisotope diagnostic studies.

Additional laboratory abnormalities, which may be present in patients with vitamin B_{12} deficiency, include parietal cell antibodies, serum intrinsic factor blocking antibody, and elevated serum levels of both homocysteine and methylmalonic acid.

Treatment

All patients with B_{12} deficiency probably demonstrate some hematologic response to treatment with either folic acid or vitamin B_{12}. However, conversion of the bone marrow to normoblastic morphology would probably not be complete with the administration of folic acid alone. In the rare cases of nutritional deficiency, oral administration of vitamin B_{12} may be given.

Oral vitamin B_{12} (cobalamin) can also be used effectively to treat pernicious anemia but in much larger doses than that used to treat B_{12} deficiency. Cobalamin can be absorbed by both an intrinsic factor dependent and independent route. The independent route is less effective and requires large B_{12} doses in order to provide adequate absorption.[37] Observed clinical response to oral doses of 1000 mg daily has been confirmed by cyanocobalamin absorption rate studies. The mean absorption rate in patients with pernicious anemia is 1.2% across a wide range of doses.[38]

A commonly used parenteral vitamin B_{12} regimen consists of initiation with daily injections of 800–1000 μg of cyanocobalamin or hydroxycobalamin for 1–2 weeks. This initial 2 weeks of therapy should saturate B_{12} stores in the body and resolve clinical manifestations of the deficiency. At that time, the dose can be decreased to 100–1000 μg once weekly until normalization of the hemoglobin and hematocrit occurs. Thereafter, monthly injections of 100–1000 μg for life should be administered.[33]

Evaluation of Therapeutic Outcomes

A rapid response to vitamin B_{12} therapy is observed in most patients. Bone marrow becomes normoblastic after 24 hours, reticulocytosis is noted within 2–3 days, the hemoglobin begins to rise after the first week, and the leukocyte count and platelet count normalize after about 7 days. A failure to observe these findings usually indicates an incorrect diagnosis or other factors contributing to the anemia, such as iron deficiency or thalassemia trait. The demands for iron may be greater during initiation of therapy as a result of increased erythropoiesis.[39]

Potential adverse effects that may be associated with B_{12}-induced reticulocytosis include hyperuricemia and hypokalemia. Rebound thrombocytosis may precipitate thrombotic events. Another side effect of vitamin B_{12} therapy is sodium retention. This effect is more likely to occur in the patient with compromised cardiovascular status because of an expansion of the intravascular volume secondary to the sudden increase in production of RBCs.

In patients with chronic anemia, cardiac failure may result from a reflex increase in cardiac output and sodium retention in response to reduced vascular volume and accumulation of fluid. If dyspnea, anginal pain, or evidence of cerebral hypooxygenation is present, administration of packed cells is in order. Usually, administration of one unit of packed RBCs is the treatment of choice. Care must be exercised to prevent cardiac overload. Small doses of diuretics may also be beneficial in these situations.

FOLIC ACID DEFICIENCY ANEMIA

Etiology and Pathophysiology

Folic acid is a heat-labile vitamin that is necessary for the production of nucleic acids, proteins, amino acids, purines, and thymine and hence DNA and RNA. Because humans are unable to synthesize the total daily folate requirements, they must depend on a dietary source of this vitamin. Major dietary sources of folate include fresh vegetables and fruits, yeast, mushrooms, and such animal organs as liver and kidney. Even though body demands for folate are high (because of high RBC synthesis and turnover), the minimum daily requirement is 50–100 mg. The body stores approximately 10–20 mg folate; thus, cessation of dietary folate intake would result in depletion of all body stores within a few months. Folic acid deficiency results in the development of large functionally immature erythrocytes termed megaloblasts.

The major causes of folic acid deficiency include inadequate intake, decreased absorption, hyperutilization, and inadequate utilization. Folic acid deficiency is associated with poor eating habits seen in elderly patients, alcoholics, food faddists, the poverty stricken, and those who are chronically ill or in demented states. Decreased absorption of folic acid may occur in patients with malabsorption syndromes such as nontropical and tropical sprue, or after the administration of certain drugs. Celiac disease is the most common cause of malabsorption of folate, but other conditions such as Crohn's disease and extensive small bowel resection can also reduce absorption.[40]

Hyperutilization of folic acid may occur in states in which the rate of cellular division is increased. Examples include pregnancy, hemolytic anemia, myelofibrosis, malignancy, chronic inflammatory disorders such as Crohn's disease, rheumatoid arthritis or psoriasis, long-term dialysis, and the growth spurts seen in adolescence and infancy. This is primarily of importance when the daily intake of folate is borderline, resulting in inadequate replacement of folate stores.

Several drugs (Table 93.6) have been reported to cause a folic-acid-deficiency megaloblastic anemia by either interfering with folate absorption or inhibiting the dihydrofolate reductase enzyme necessary for conversion of DHF to its active tetrahydrofolate form.

Although phenytoin may induce a megaloblastic anemia, folic acid supplementation in these patients may decrease phenytoin's anticonvulsant activity by increasing the metabolism of phenytoin.[64] Routine supplementation is therefore not recommended; however, close monitoring for this potential interaction is advised.

Signs and Symptoms

For the most part the symptoms associated with folate deficiency are similar to those seen in patients with B_{12} deficiency. The major difference between these two disease entities is the relative absence of neurologic manifestations in folate-deficient megaloblastic anemia. Symptoms have an insidious onset that often precludes early identification of the etiology.

Laboratory Findings

Laboratory changes associated with folate deficiency megaloblastic anemia are similar to those seen in vitamin B_{12} deficiency anemia with the exception of a decreased serum and RBC folate level. Because serum folate levels are quite sensitive to short-term changes in folate balance, the erythrocyte folate level is a better predictor of true tissue folate stores. Erythrocyte folate levels are established during erythrocyte formation and persist throughout the life span of the cell, making this test less sensitive to daily folate variations.

TABLE 93.6. DRUG-INDUCED MEGALOBLASTOSIS[a]

Impaired absorption or folate inactivation
Phenytoin[41–43]
Phenobarbital[5,44]
Primadone[5,45]
Alcohol[47,48]
Oral contraceptives[48–52]
Sulfasalazine[53,54]
Inhibition of dihydrofolate reductase necessary for conversion of DHF to THF, the metabolically active folate cofactor for nucleic acid synthesis
Methotrexate[55]
Trimethoprim[56–59]
Triamterene[60–61]
Inadequate or inactive vitamin B_{12}
Neomycin[62]
Colchicine[63]

[a]Only phenytoin, phenobarbital, primidone, and methotrexate have a frequent incidence of reported megaloblastosis.

Treatment

Folic acid deficiency is treated by administration of exogenous folic acid. For replenishment of folate stores, it is recommended that therapy be initiated with 50 µg/d orally for 2 days, followed by 2 mg orally twice a week or 0.5–1 mg daily. Therapy should be continued for approximately 4 months, which is a sufficient amount of time for all folate-deficient RBCs to be cleared from the circulation. Once the cause of the deficiency is corrected, therapy can usually be discontinued. Long-term folate administration may be necessary in chronic hemolytic states, refractory malabsorption, and myelofibrosis. It is also recommended that patients with a folic acid deficiency be placed on diets containing foods high in folates. For patients with cardiovascular problems, the approach is the same as that for B_{12} deficiency anemia. Low-dose folate therapy (500 µg/d) may be administered when anticonvulsant drugs produce a megaloblastic anemia. Such therapy will obviate the need to remove the anticonvulsant.

Although megaloblastic anemia during pregnancy is rare, the most common cause is folate deficiency. This usually manifests itself as underweight, premature infants and suboptimal health for the mother. Prophylactic folate therapy during pregnancy in women with poor diets, multiple pregnancies, and thalassemia minor may be a useful preventive measure. The recommended dose is 200–300 µg/d.

Evaluation of Therapeutic Outcomes

Symptomatic improvement as evidenced by increased alertness, appetite, and cooperation are often noted early during a course of treatment. Reticulocytosis again occurs within 2–3 days and peaks within 5–8 days after beginning therapy. Hematocrit begins to rise within 2 weeks of beginning therapy and should reach normal levels within 2 months. Last, the MCV will initially increase due to an increase in reticulocytes, but will then gradually decrease to normal thereafter.

ANEMIA OF CHRONIC DISEASE

Pathophysiology

Anemia of chronic disease (ACD) is a hypoproliferative anemia that has traditionally been associated with infectious, inflammatory, or neoplastic diseases lasting more than 1 or 2 months.[65,66] Pathologically, the RBC life span is shortened and the bone marrow's capacity to respond to erythropoietin is inadequate to maintain normal hemoglobin concentration. The cause of this defect is still not certain but appears to involve a block in the release of iron from the reticuloendothelial cells of the marrow. It is thought that various cytokines released during these illnesses inhibit the production or action of erythropoietin or inhibit RBC production.[67]

Laboratory Findings

Examination of the bone marrow reveals an abundance of iron, so it appears that the release mechanism for this iron is the central defect. Serum iron is usually decreased, but, unlike IDA, serum ferritin is normal or increased and iron-binding capacity is decreased. The anemia of chronic disease is usually normocytic; hematocrits as low as 25% have been reported in 20% of patients with ACD.[68] The diagnosis is usually one of exclusion, with particular emphasis on evaluation of possible IDA as the primary anemia or coexistent with ACD due to chronic disease-associated conditions such as GI blood loss from aspirin, other nonsteroidal anti-inflammatory agents, or steroids, or malignancy-associated bleeding. Although usually referred to as anemia of chronic disease, it can occur in conditions with fairly rapid onset of several weeks, such as a pneumonia. It can also often coexist with anemia of renal disease and IDA. Table 93.7 shows diseases associated with ACD.

Treatment

The treatment of ACD is somewhat less specific than treatment of other anemias. Usually, recovery from the anemia occurs with recovery of the inflammatory process. During inflammation, iron therapy is ineffective by either the oral or parenteral route. Red cell transfusions are effective, but should be limited to situations where oxygen transport is inadequate due to other medical problems.

TABLE 93.7. DISEASES CAUSING ANEMIA OF CHRONIC DISEASE

- **Common Causes**
  - Chronic infections
    - Tuberculosis
    - Other chronic lung infections
    - Subacute bacterial endocarditis
    - Osteomyelitis
    - Chronic urinary tract infections
  - Chronic inflammation
    - Rheumatoid arthritis
    - Systemic lupus erythematosus
    - Rheumatoid (collagen-vascular) diseases
    - Inflammatory osteoarthritis
    - Gout
    - Chronic inflammatory liver diseases
  - Malignancies
    - Carcinoma
    - Hodgkin's disease
    - Leukemia
    - Multiple myeloma
- **Less Common Causes**
  - Alcoholic liver disease
  - Congestive heart failure
  - Thrombophlebitis
  - Chronic obstructive lung disease
  - Ischemic heart disease

Last, erythropoietin (EPO) has been used to stimulate erythropoiesis in patients with chronic diseases. These patients have a relative erythropoietin deficiency, that is, EPO levels are not as elevated as they should be for the degree of anemia they have. They also have a relatively impaired response to erythropoietin. Consequently, ACD has been successfully treated with recombinant human erythropoietin in several studies using rheumatoid arthritis patients,[69] yet other studies have found no role for erythropoietin in treatment of ACD.[70]

ANEMIA OF RENAL FAILURE

Pathophysiology

Patients with chronic renal failure (CRF) have several reasons to be anemic. Decreased erythropoietin (EPO) production by the kidneys is the primary mechanism of severe anemia associated with end-stage renal disease.[71] The uremic environment of CRF decreases RBC life span, requiring an increased demand for RBCs that often cannot be supplied with decreased serum erythropoietin levels.[72] An increased demand for folic acid for new RBC production coupled with the body's limited folic acid stores can cause a folic acid deficiency anemia. Last, many CRF patients become iron deficient due to blood and iron loss from hemodialysis[76] (see Chapter 43, Acute Renal Failure).

Patients with end-stage renal failure experience anemia that is largely caused by the kidneys' diminished ability to produce EPO, the hormone that stimulates the production and differentiation of bone marrow erythroid progenitor cells. Specifically, EPO binds to erythroid cells in the bone marrow, resulting in the production of messenger RNA coded for erythrostimulatory responses.

Treatment and Therapeutic Outcomes

Patients with CRF are unable to produce appropriate levels of EPO, and many of these patients are transfusion dependent. Due to the inherent risks associated with repeated transfusions (i.e., febrile reactions, iron overload, hepatitis, AIDS, rejection of future transplants), alternative therapy is desirable; recombinant human EPO, or epoietin alfa, is an efficacious alternative, reversing the anemia of CRF in essentially all patients in whom it has been administered. Epoietin has become the mainstay in the management of anemia associated with renal failure.

The goal of epoietin therapy is to raise the patient's hematocrit value to a target range up to 36%. Starting doses of epoietin are 50–100 U/kg, administered three times a week. Doses should be reduced as the hematocrit approaches 36%. The dose of epoietin should then be individualized to maintain the hematocrit within the suggested target range of 30–36%. It is important to remember that considerable interpatient half-life variations exist for this product and administration may require individual regimens for optimum therapeutic value.

Epoietin may be administered intravenously or subcutaneously. The subcutaneous route may provide more sustained epoietin concentrations, which are more advantageous than the peak and trough levels achieved with intravenous bolus administration. This suggests that the amount of time the levels remain above baseline EPO concentrations may be most important in determining hematopoietic response.[73]

The major side effect encountered with epoietin therapy is an elevation of diastolic blood pressure. Approximately 30–47% of patients receiving this product experience this effect, which is thought to occur as a consequence of an increase in peripheral vascular resistance. It is estimated that approximately 25% of these patients will experience an increase of greater than 10 mm Hg, thus producing or aggravating existing hypertension, which often requires adjustments in the patient's blood pressure medications.[79] No evidence exists that this blood pressure change is related to a direct pressor effect of epoietin. It appears that the major risk factor for the development of hypertension is severe anemia and not the rate of rise of hematocrit with therapy.

One major reason for failure to respond with epoietin therapy is the development of iron depletion. Iron deficiency arises during epoietin therapy primarily because raising of hematocrit levels requires a massive transfer of iron from storage areas to RBCs for manufacturing new hemoglobin. Other causes of iron deficiency include blood loss secondary to bleeding, retention of blood in dialyzer and tubing, or laboratory test phlebotomy. Chronic renal failure patients with transferrin saturations of at least 20% and serum ferritin levels below 100 ng/mL are probably candidates for concurrent iron therapy.[75] The agent of choice for prevention of iron storage deficiency is ferrous sulfate, 325 mg at bedtime. As with any IDA, if a patient does not respond to oral iron supplementation, parenteral iron therapy is indicated. Fortunately, many patients respond appropriately to oral iron.

ANEMIA IN THE ELDERLY

One of the most common clinical problems observed in the elderly is anemia.[77] Although it is often assumed that anemia is an inevitable part of the aging process, studies in normal healthy elderly populations demonstrate that this is not true.[78] What is observed in these patients is a progressive decrease in bone marrow reserve with age, and a decrease in hormonal response to hematologic stress.[79] Although hemoglobin levels usually remain normal, the diminished marrow reserve leaves the elderly patient more susceptible to other causes of anemia. Such causes may include the presence of multiple minor and often unrecognized diseases that negatively affect erythropoiesis.[80] One major factor often overlooked that may contribute to the presence of anemia in the older population is nutritional status. Anemia is rarely encountered in affluent and healthy elderly communities.[81] On the other hand, cross-sectional studies demonstrate a higher prevalence of anemia in low socioeconomic populations, which also have been shown to have a high prevalence of other nutritional deficiencies. Thus, nutritional deficiencies not usually severe enough to affect the hematopoietic system in the younger population may account for anemia in the aged. In addition, it is possible that marginal deficiencies of one or more nutrients acting alone or in combination over prolonged time periods may cause anemia in the elderly. Therefore, one might conclude that anemia is never a normal consequence of aging; however, the aging hematopoietic system is more susceptible to minor stresses so that anemia (as well as other diseases) may develop more readily in older individuals as compared to their younger counterparts.

Surveys have demonstrated the prevalence of anemia in elderly men to range from 6–30% and 10–22% in older women.[80] Specific deficiencies resulting in anemia in these patients include iron deficiency and vitamin B_{12} or folic acid (megaloblastic anemia). Other causes for anemia in this population include anemia of chronic disease, anemia associated with malignancy, or a premalignant condition.[82] Some patients will have a combination of these causes as the etiology of their anemia.

Geriatric patients can be classified as having a low, moderate, or high risk of anemia with a given hemoglobin value. Men are considered at high risk with a hemoglobin level under 12 g/dL, moderate risk if the value is 12–14 g/dL and low risk at values greater than 14 g/dL. Elderly women are high risks with levels less than 10 g/dL, moderate risk with values of 10–12 g/dL and low risk at values greater than 12 g/dL.[83] Iron-binding capacity decreases with aging due to factors such as malnutrition and chronic disease. Serum ferritin levels increase in the older patient population and this increase may be attributable to acute and chronic inflammatory conditions.

Some authorities are of the opinion that the usual ranges for laboratory values used to assess for anemia should be lowered in the elderly. These investigators are of the opinion that a significant number of elderly do not have an identifiable cause of anemia. Their argument for lowering the "normal" values is that by doing so, one reduces the need for extensive, and often invasive, workups of the patient, which may not lead to definitive etiologies that explain an apparent anemia. Obviously, the downside to this argument is the possibility of missing an underlying disease process in a patient population at risk. Even though a definitive cause may not be identified, the presence of low hemoglobin and hematocrit values may aggravate existing diseases. Elderly patients often have a decline in functional reserve of most organ systems. Even mild to moderate anemia may cause confusion or worsen a dementia; precipitate or aggravate congestive heart failure or angina; cause syncope and falls secondary to postural hypotension; intensify functional disability and fatigue in arthritis, parkinsonism, or stroke; and dampen motivation for rehabilitation.[84]

Iron Deficiency Anemia in the Elderly

Iron deficiency is the most commonly seen anemia in the elderly. The most reliable laboratory test for diagnosing IDA is the serum ferritin value. Patients with values greater than 100 μg/L have an 8–16% probability of having IDA, whereas those with values less than 18 μg/L have a probability of greater than 97% of having the disease. Values between 45 and 100 μg/L have a 24–41% chance of having the disease. This suggests that bone marrow studies for a definitive diagnosis are only necessary in patients with ferritin values of less than 45 μg/L.

Preferred therapy for IDA in the elderly is ferrous sulfate. The usual dose is 200 mg elemental iron three times a day, with most patients requiring treatment for 6 months to replace marrow stores.[85] A pediatric elixir is available for those who have difficulty swallowing tablets; however, the iron content of these preparations is low and they may stain teeth and dentures. Parenteral iron therapy should be utilized in geriatric patients when indicated. In cachectic patients with little muscle mass, the intravenous route of administration may be preferred.

Occasionally, iron-deficient patients will require transfusion therapy. Whenever this treatment modality is used, it is important to monitor this therapy closely in order to avoid precipitating heart failure as a result of restoring extravascular volume too rapidly. An infusion of one-half unit packed RBCs over 2 hours is usually well tolerated.[86]

Macrocytic Anemia in the Elderly

The second most common form of anemia in the elderly is macrocytic anemia. Specifically, deficiencies in vitamin B_{12} and folic acid are the primary etiologies of this form of anemia. Laboratory findings that suggest a megaloblastic anemia include pancytopenia, macrocytosis, hypersegmented polymorphonuclear leukocytes on peripheral smear, decreased reticulocyte index, increased lactic dehydrogenase, and indirect hyperbilirubinemia. The diagnosis for B_{12} deficiency is a serum concentration of less than 100 pg/mL, whereas serum folate levels of less than 2 ng/mL or red cell folate levels less than 100 ng/mL are indicative of folic acid deficiency.

Evidence exists that suggests cobalamine deficiency is more common in older individuals than generally perceived.[87] Pernicious anemia is the major cause of B_{12} deficiencies, because this condition increases significantly with advancing age. Vitamin B_{12} fails to be adequately absorbed as a result of atrophic gastritis and decreased secretion of intrinsic factor. Manifestations of pernicious anemia in the elderly consist of weakness, fatigue, anorexia, reduced drive, sore tongue and mouth, and a lemon-yellow discoloration of the skin. Neurologic manifestations include ataxia, loss of position sense, peripheral neuropathy, urinary incontinence, impotence, paresthesias, and visual disturbances. Neuropsychiatric symptomatology does not correlate well with the presence of hematologic abnormalities, because up to 28% of patients with B_{12}-deficiency-induced neuropsychiatric problems do not have macrocytosis or anemia.[88] A study by Carmel and associates[87] found a 29% prevalence of low B_{12} levels in a group of patients with primary degenerative dementia. Consequently, slightly low B_{12} levels should not be ignored in the evaluation of dementia and other neurologic and psychiatric abnormalities. Five to 8% of patients diagnosed with pernicious anemia develop gastric carcinoma in 15–20 years.

Treatment of vitamin B_{12} deficiency consists of 100 μg injections of cyanocobolamin weekly until stores are replenished. At this point, monthly or every-three-months injections of 1000 μg will usually be adequate. The therapeutic endpoint is maintaining normal serum B_{12} levels and reversing other laboratory abnormalities encountered with this disease.

Megaloblastic anemia secondary to folic acid deficiency is less common in the elderly. Patients in whom this disorder is most likely to occur include those with protein-calorie malnutrition and excessive alcohol consumption, because alcohol impairs folic acid absorption from the GI tract. Therapy in the older patient for folic acid deficiency is the same as in the younger population.

HEMOLYTIC ANEMIA

Pathophysiology

Hemolytic anemia is one of the least common forms of anemia encountered in clinical practice. The mechanisms responsible for decreasing the survival time of RBCs are

TABLE 93.8. COMMON CLASSES OF HEMOLYTIC ANEMIAS

Intrinsic (intracorpuscular; are usually genetically inherited)
Membrane defect
Spherocytosis and elliptocytosis
Hemoglobin defect
Sickle cell anemia
Thalassemia syndrome
Metabolic defect
Glucose-6-phosphate dehydrogenase (G6PD) deficiency
Many other enzyme deficiencies
Extrinsic
Membrane defect
Autoimmune hemolytic anemias
Oxidants, may cause unstable hemoglobin to clump

numerous. The severity of hemolytic anemia varies with the mechanism. Hemolysis may be mild, chronic, compensated, and lifelong or acute, severe, and life threatening.

The normal 120-day life span of an RBC comes from its inherent flexibility in passage through the microvasculature and spleen without disruption of the cell membrane or sequestration and phagocytosis by reticuloendothelial cells. Hemolysis, as defined by an RBC life span of less than 120 days, results from one of three primary defects: (1) membrane defects, (2) alterations in hemoglobin solubility or stability, and (3) changes in intracellular metabolic processes. These changes in membrane integrity, hemoglobin stability, and cell metabolism can be from intrinsic or extrinsic origin. These changes may be caused by intrinsic or extrinsic mechanisms. Intrinsic defects are intracorpuscular changes and are often genetically determined; extrinsic defects, or extracorpuscular changes, are usually the cause of acquired hemolytic anemia. Acquired disorders result mainly from a direct effect on the membrane and less often from alterations in hemoglobin or metabolism. Table 93.8 lists examples of the different classes of hemolytic anemias.

Causes of hemolytic anemia vary in the younger patient compared to the elderly patient. Most younger patients exhibit congenital disease, while older patients most often experience autoimmune hemolytic anemia. A positive Coombs' test is diagnostic in the latter group.

Defects in one of the three main components of the RBC can cause a decreased RBC life span leading to a hemolytic anemia. Membrane defects causing swollen or shrunken cells, cause an alteration of cell shape leading to spherocytes or even cell fragments.

Hereditary spherocytosis is the most common inherited disorder of the RBC membrane. In this disorder, RBCs lose their flexible biconcave characteristics and become tight spheres. These altered cells can still deliver oxygen to body cells; however, when these rigid cells enter the splenic microcirculation, they cannot pass through the pores lining the sinusoids of the spleen and consequently become trapped in the splenic pulp where they are eventually destroyed by the reticuloendothelial cells. These patients are at risk of developing cholelithiasis or cholecystitis, pigment bile stones, mild jaundice, and splenomegaly. The treatment of choice for hereditary spherocytosis is splenectomy. Although the spherocytosis persists, the hemolysis is no longer a problem once the spleen has been removed.

Alterations in hemoglobin's solubility or stability, as seen with sickle cell anemia and the thallasemias, cause cell deformations leading to hemolysis. See Chapter 95, Sickle Cell Anemia, for a further discussion of these diseases.

Last, alterations in cell metabolism (enzymopathies) lead to hemolytic disease by causing an alteration in cell dimensions and hemoglobin solubility. The two major metabolic pathways necessary for normal RBC metabolism are the hexose monophosphate shunt, with its associated enzyme systems, and the Embden–Myerhof pathway of anaerobic glycolysis. The former is responsible primarily for maintaining hemoglobin in the reduced state and thus preventing the formation of methemoglobin; the later metabolizes glucose to lactic acid, which leads to ATP formation.

The most common metabolic abnormality resulting in a hemolytic syndrome is glucose-6-phosphate dehydrogenase (G6PD) deficiency in the hexose monophosphate shunt pathway. Hemoglobin is oxidized to methemoglobin and then to sulfhemoglobin. Heinz bodies of denatured hemoglobin form, resulting in damage to the RBC membrane. Hemolysis results from the action of the spleen and reticuloendothelial system on these damaged cells. The disease more typically presents in whites of Mediterranean descent upon exposure to oxidant drugs and chemicals or with infection.

Treatment

Therapy of this condition consists of avoidance of oxidant medications and chemicals. Currently, there is no specific therapy that compensates for the enzyme deficiency.

References

1. Bergin JJ. Evaluation of anemia. Postgrad Med J 1985;77(3):253–269.
2. Cook JD, Skikne BS, Baynes RD. Serum transferrin receptor. Ann Rev Med 1993;44:63–74.
3. Charlton RW, Bothwell TH. Iron absorption. Ann Rev Med 1983;34:55–68.
4. Committee on Iron Deficiency of the AMA Council on Foods and Nutrition. Iron deficiency in the United States. JAMA 1968;203:407.
5. Hallberg L, Rossander L, Skanberg A-B. Phytates and the inhibitory effort of bran on iron absorption in man. Am J Clin Nutr 1987;45:988–965.
6. Long R. Diurnal variation of serum iron in normal individuals. Clin Chem 1978;24:842–847.
7. Ramadurai J, Shapiro C, Kozloff M, Telfer M. Zinc abuse and sideroblastic anemia. Am J Hematol 1993;42:227–228.
8. Hryhorczuk DO, Hogan MM. Variegate porphyria and heavy metal poisoning from ingestion of moonshine. South Med J 1983;76:1027–1031.
9. McKenzie AW, Acharya U. Oestrogen-induced familial porphyria. Br J Dermatol 1975;92:707–709.
10. Doss M, Baumann H, Sixel F. Alcohol in acute porphyria [letter]. Lancet 1982;1:1307.
11. Kirking MH. Treatment of chronic iron overload. Clin Pharm 1991;10:775–783.
12. Edwards CQ, Griffen LM, Goldgar D, et al. Prevalence of hemochromatosis among 11,065 presumably healthy blood donors. N Engl J Med 1988;318:1355–1362.
13. English EC, Finch CA. Iron deficiency: A systematic approach. Drug Therapy 1984(April);19–20, 25–27.

14. Stucky WJ. Common anemias: A practical guide to diagnosis and management. Geriatrics 1983;38:42–48.
15. Rockey DC, Cello JP. Evaluation of the gastrointestinal tract in patients with iron-deficiency anemia. N Engl J Med 1993;329:1691–1695.
16. Beissner RS, Trowbridge AA. Clinical assessment of anemia. Postgrad Med 1986;80:83–95.
17. Cok JD. Food iron absorption in human subjects—III. Comparison of the effect of animal proteins on non-heme iron absorption. Am J Clin Nutr 1976;29:859–867.
18. Dallman PR, Siimes MA, Stekel A. Iron deficiency in infancy and childhood. Am J Clin Nutr 1980;6:86–118.
19. Monsen ER, Hallberg L, Layrisse M. Estimation of available dietary iron. Am J Clin Nutr 1978;31:134–141.
20. McGrath K. Treatment of anaemia caused by iron, vitamin B_{12} or folate deficiency. Med J Aust 1989;151:693–697.
21. Beutler E. The common anemias. JAMA 1988;259:2433–2437.
22. Dallman PR. Iron deficiency: Diagnosis and treatment. West J Med 1981;134:496–505.
23. Hobbs J, Rodriguez AR. Megaloblastic anemias. Am Fam Phys 1980;22:128–136.
24. Freedman ML. Common hematologic problems: Diagnosis and treatment. Geriatrics 1983;38:119–123, 127–130, 134.
25. Cooper BA. Megaloblastic anemia: When to suspect it, how to treat it. Drug Ther Hosp 1984 (April);55–57, 61–62, 67–69.
26. Beresford CR, Goldberg L, Smith JP. Local effects and mechanism of absorption of iron preparations administered intramuscularly. Br J Pharmacol 1957;12:107–114.
27. Will G. The absorption, distribution and utilization of intramuscularly administered iron-dextran: A radioisotopy study. Br J Haematol 1968;14:395–406.
28. Grime AJ, Hutt MSR. Metabolism of ^{59}Fe-dextran complex in human subjects. Br J Med 1957;2:1074–1077.
29. Henderson PA, Hillman RS. Characteristics of iron dextran utilization in man. Blood 1969;34:357–375.
30. Auerbach M, Witt D, Toler W, et al. Clinical use of the total dose intravenous infusion of iron dextran. J Lab Clin Med 1988;111:566–570.
31. Halpin TC, Bertino JS, Rothstein FC. Iron-deficiency anemia in childhood inflammatory bowel disease: Treatment with intravenous iron-dextran. JPEN 1982;6:9–11.
32. Castle WB, Ham TH. Observations on the etiologic relationship of achylia gastrica to pernicious anemia. JAMA 1936;107:1456–1463. (Reprinted in JAMA 1984;251:522.)
33. Clementz GL, Schade SG. The spectrum of vitamin B_{12} deficiency. Am Fam Phys 1990;41:150–162.
34. Healton EB, Savage DG, Brust JC. Neurologic aspects of cobalamin deficiency. Medicine 1991;70(4):229–245.
35. Christensen DJ. Diagnosis of anemia: Clues to greater precision. Postgrad Med J 1983;73:293–297, 300.
36. McRae TD, Freedman ML. Why vitamin B_{12} deficiency should be managed aggressively. Geriatrics 1989;44:70–79.
37. Doscherholmer A, Hager PS, Liu M. A dual mechanism of vitamin B_{12} plasma absorption. J Clin Invest 1957;36:1551–1557.
38. Berlin H, Berlin R, Brante G. Oral treatment of pernicious anemia with high doses of vitamin B_{12} without intrinsic factor. Acta Med Scand 1968;184:247–258.
39. Carmel R, Weiner JM, Johnson CS. Iron deficiency occurs frequently in patients with pernicious anemia. JAMA 1987;257:1081–1083.
40. McGrath K. Treatment of anaemia caused by iron, vitamin B_{12} or folate deficiency. Med J Aust 1989;151:693–697.
41. Blair JA, Matty AJ. Acid microclimate in intestinal absorption. Clin Gastroenterol 1974;3(1):183–197.
42. Hoffbrand A, et al. Mechanism of folate deficiency in patients receiving phenytoin. Lancet 1968;2:528–530.
43. Wickramasinghe SN, Williams G, Saunders J, Durston JH. Megaloblastic erythropoiesis and macrocytosis in patients on anticonvulsants. Br Med J 1975;4:136–137.
44. Klipstein FA. Subnormal serum folate and macrocytosis associated with anticonvulsant drug therapy. Blood 1964;23:68–86.
45. Dallman PR, Yip R, Johnson C. Prevalence and causes of anemia in the United States, 1976–1980. Am J Nutr 1984;39:437–445.
46. Eichner ER. The hematologic disorders of alcoholism. Am J Med 1973;54:621–630.
47. Wu A, Chanarin I, Slavin G, Levi AJ. Folate deficiency in the alcoholic—its relationship to clinical and hematological abnormalities, liver disease and folate stores. Br J Haematol 1975;29:469–478.
48. Necheles TF, Snyder LM. Malabsorption of folate polyglutamates associated with oral contraceptive therapy. N Engl J Med 1970;282:858–859.
49. Paton A. Oral contraceptives and folate deficiency. Lancet 1969;1:418.
50. Shojania AM, Hornady G, Barnes PH. Oral contraceptives and serum folate levels. Lancet 1968;1:1376–1377.
51. Shojania AM, Hornady G, Barnes PH. Oral contraceptives and folate metabolism. Lancet 1969;1:886.
52. Streiff RR. Folate deficiency and oral contraceptives. JAMA 1970;214:105–108.
53. Halsted CH, Gandhi G, Tamerra T. Sulfasalazine inhibits the absorption of folates. N Engl J Med 1981;305:1513–1517.
54. Franklin JL, Rosenberg IH. Impaired folic acid absorption in inflammatory bowel disease: Effects of salicylazosulfapyridine (Azulfidine). Gastroenterology 1973;64:517–525.
55. Douglas IDC, Price LA. Bone marrow toxicity of methotrexate: A reassessment. Br J Haematol 1973;24:625–631.
56. Chanarin I, England JM. Toxicity of trimethoprim sulphamethoxazole in patients with megaloblastic haemopoiesis. Br J Med 1972;1:651–653.
57. Tamtamy SE. Co-trimoxazole and the blood. Lancet 1974;1:929–930.
58. Jewkes RF, Edwards MS, Grant BJG. Haematological changes in patient on long term treatment with trimethoprim-sulphonamide combination. Postgrad Med J 1970;46:723–726.
59. Kahn SB, Fein SA, Brodsky I. Effects of trimethoprim on folate metabolism in man. Clin Pharmaco Ther 1968;9:550–560.
60. Lieberman FL, Bateman JR. Megaloblastic anemia possibly induced by triamterene in patients with alcoholic cirrhosis: Two case reports. Ann Intern Med 1968;68:168–173.
61. Corcino J, Waxman S, Herbert V. Mechanism of triamterene induced megaloblastosis. Ann Intern Med 1970;73:419–424.

62. Jacobson E. An experimental malabsorption syndrome induced by neomycin. Am J Med 1960;28:524.
63. Webb DI, Chodos RB, Mahar CQ, Faloon WW. Mechanism of vitamin B_{12} malabsorption in patients receiving colchicine. N Engl J Med 1968;279:845–850.
64. MacCosbe PE, Toomey K. Interaction of phenytoin and folic acid. Clin Pharm 1983;2:362–369.
65. Lee GR. The anemia of chronic disease. Semin Hematol 1983;20:465–479.
66. Samson D. The anaemia of chronic disorders. Postgrad Med J 1983;59:543–550.
67. Means RT, Krantz SB. Progress in understanding the pathogenesis of the anemia of chronic disease. Blood 1992;80(7);1639–1647.
68. Cash JM, Sears DA. The anemia of chronic disease: Spectrum of associated diseases in a series of unselected hospitalized patients. Am J Med 1989;87:638–644.
69. Pincus T, Olsen NJ, Russell IJ. Multicenter study of recombinant human erythropoietin in correction of anemia in rheumatoid arthritis. Am J Med 1990;89:161–166.
70. Nielsen OJ, Anderson LS, Ludwigsen E. Anaemia of rheumatoid arthritis: Erythropoietin concentrations and red cell distribution width in relation to iron status. Ann Rheum Dis 1990;49(6):349–353.
71. Paganini EP. Overview of anemia associated with chronic renal disease: Primary and secondary mechanisms. Semin Nephrol 1989;9(1):3–8.
72. Shaw AB. Haemolysis in chronic renal failure. Br Med J 1967;2:213–216.
73. Eschbach JW, Adamson JW. Recombinant human erythropoietin: Implications for nephrology. Am J Kidney Dis 1988;11:203–209.
74. Flaharty KK. Clinical pharmacology of recombinant human erythropoietin (r-HuEPO). Pharmacotherapy 1990;10:9S–14S.
75. Adamson JW, Eschback JW. Treatment of the anemia of chronic renal failure with recombinant human erythropoietin. Ann Rev Med 1990;41:349–360.
76. Van Wyck DB. Iron deficiency in patients with dialysis-associated anemia during erythropoietin replacement therapy: Strategies for assessment and management. Semin Nephrol 1989;9:21–24.
77. Guyatt GH, Patterson C, Ali M. Diagnosis of iron deficiency anemia in the elderly. Am J Med 1990;88:205–209.
78. Baldwin JG, Lichtenstein LS. Longitudinal study of hemoglobin and hematocrit in the elderly. Blood 1986;68(5, suppl 1):52a.
79. Lipschitz DA, Udupa KB, Milton KY, Thompson CO. Effect of age on hematopoiesis in man. Blood 1984;63:502–509.
80. Mansouri A, Lipschitz DA. Anemia in the elderly patient. Med Clin North Am 1992;76:619–630.
81. Gary PJ, Goodwin JS, Hunt WE. Iron status and anemia in the elderly: New findings and a review of previous studies. J Am Geriatr Soc 1983;31:389–399.
82. Howe RB. Anemia in the elderly: Common causes and suggested diagnostic approach. Postgrad Med J 1983;73:153–160.
83. Daly MP. Anemia in the elderly. Am Fam Phys 1989;39:129–136.
84. Walsh JR. Equivocal anemia in the elderly. J Fam Pract 1989;28:521–523.
85. Scott RB. Common blood disorders: A primary care approach. Geriatrics 1993;48:72–80.
86. Babitz LE, Freedman ML. Anemia in the aged. Compr Ther 1988;14:55–64.
87. Carmel RO. Pernicious anemia. Report of patients without the expected finding of very low serum cobalamin levels, anemia and macrocytosis. Arch Intern Med 1988;148:1705–1707.
88. Lindenbaum J, Healton EB, Savage DG. Neuropsychiatric disorders caused by cobalamin deficiency in the absence of anemia or macrocytosis. N Engl J Med 1988;318:1720–1728.
89. Lipschitz DA, Mitchell CO, Thompson C. The anemia of senescence. Am J Hematol 1981;11:47–54.
90. Hobbs J, Rodrigquez AR. Megaloblastic anemias. Am Fam Phys 1980;22:128–136.
91. Oski FA. The nonhematologic manifestations of iron deficiency. Am J Dis Child 1979;133:315–321.
92. Freedman ML. Common hematologic problems: Diagnosis and treatment. Geriatrics. 1983;38:119–123, 127–130, 134.

Chapter 94

Coagulation Disorders

Mariela Diaz-Linares, PharmD, Keith A. Rodvold, PharmD, FCCP, BCPS, and William R. Friedenberg, MD

This chapter describes a pathophysiologic approach to diagnosis and management of patients with common coagulation disorders. The chapter is divided into two sections: fundamental concepts of hemostasis and thrombosis, and clinical application of these fundamentals with regard to hemostatic disorders and thrombotic disorders. The general categories of disorders contrast congenital bleeding illnesses with acquired disorders of coagulation. Treatment of each coagulation disorder is discussed.

Regulation of Hemostasis

Hemostasis is the spontaneous arrest of bleeding from damaged blood vessels. Hemostasis and thrombosis are regulated by a series of complex actions and reactions of procoagulant and anticoagulant events.[1,2] The exact mechanisms that precisely regulate the balance between clot formation and lysis are not completely understood. The following is a brief description of the physiologic interaction and regulation of four major components of the normal hemostatic system: (1) the vessel wall, (2) platelets, (3) the coagulation system, and (4) the fibrinolytic system.

VESSEL WALL AND PLATELETS

The blood vessel and circulating platelets play central roles in primary hemostasis. The involvement of vessel wall includes vasoconstriction, formation of platelet plugs, and regulation of coagulation and fibrinolysis (Fig. 94.1). Platelet function in response to vascular injury includes four phases: (1) adhesion, (2) aggregation, (3) secretion, and (4) elaboration of procoagulant activity. Formation of a platelet plug proceeds through the sequence of platelet adhesion to exposed subendothelial connective tissue structures; platelet aggregation by adenosine diphosphate, thromboxane A_2, and thrombin recruitment; contribution of platelet coagulant activity to the coagulation process, which stabilizes the plug with a fibrin mesh; and retraction of the platelet mass to provide a dense thrombus.

The endothelial cell, and especially its surface, is intimately involved in the balance between clotting and bleeding. Procoagulant molecules, such as von Willebrand's factor, and anticoagulant proteins, such as tissue plasminogen activator, are secreted by these cells. Prostaglandins, such as prostacyclin, inhibit platelet aggregation, whereas thromboxane A_2, released by platelets, promotes aggregation. Thrombomodulin on the surface of the cell reacts with thrombin to activate proteins C and S, which inhibit the plasma cascade of coagulation factors. There is a dynamic balance of fibrinolysis and fibrin formation, both of which interact with platelets at the cell surface to keep the blood in fluid phase and prevent bleeding at the same time.[3]

COAGULATION SYSTEM

The coagulation and fibrinolytic systems serve two interrelated and opposing functions. The formation of a fibrin clot occurs as a result of the coagulation system, while the fibrinolytic system dissolves the polymerized clot and restores blood flow. To generate fibrin for the formation of the clot, fibrinogen is cleaved by thrombin. Thrombin, generated by the intrinsic or extrinsic pathways, plays a key role in the hemostatic system (Fig. 94.1); it is involved in platelet aggregation, fibrin formation, and the modulation of fibrinolysis.

Twelve plasma proteins are considered coagulation factors (Table 94.1). It is convenient to divide the coagulation factors into three groups on the basis of biochemical properties. These groups include vitamin K-dependent factors (II, VII, IX, and X), contact activation factors (XI and XII, prekallikrein, high molecular weight kininogen), and thrombin-sensitive factors (V, VIII, XIII, and fibrinogen).

Coagulation factors and enzymes of the fibrinolytic system circulate as inactive precursors (zymogens). Coagulation of blood entails a cascading series of proteolytic reactions. At each step a clotting factor undergoes limited proteolysis and becomes an active protease (designated by a lowercase "a," as in Xa). This clotting factor enzyme activates the next clotting factor until ultimately an insoluble fibrin clot is formed.

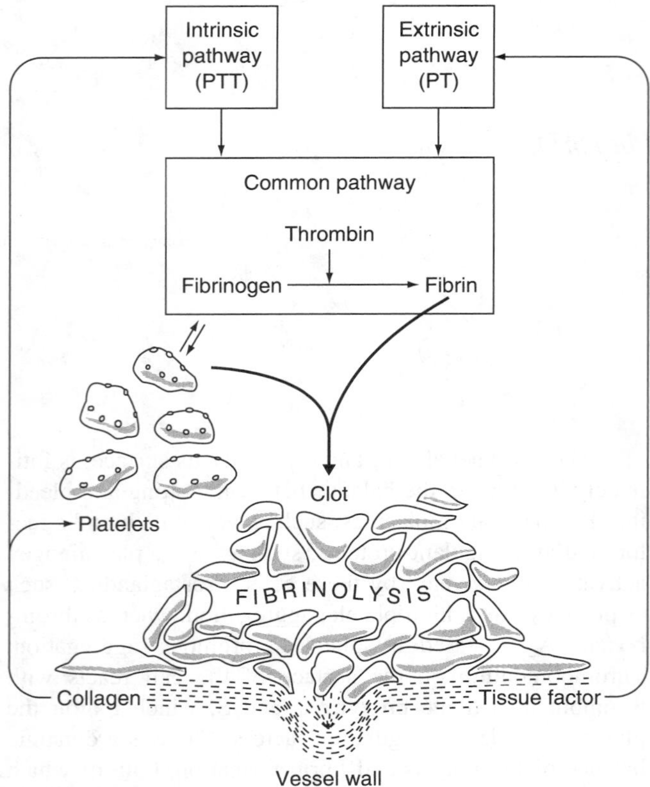

Figure 94.1. Simplified scheme of the hemostatic system, showing interaction of vessel wall, platelets, coagulation pathways, and fibrinolytic system. Not shown are regulatory and inhibitory mechanisms. *(From Stead RB. Regulation of hemostasis, in Goldhaber SZ (ed): Pulmonary Embolism and Deep Vein Thrombosis. Philadelphia, WB Saunders, 1985, p 28, with permission.)*

Clotting is initiated by either an intrinsic or an extrinsic pathway, with subsequent factor interactions that converge at the common pathway (Fig. 94.2). Both pathways can be activated when normal components of the vascular endothelium come into contact with blood. Tissue factor catalyzes factor VII. Tissue factor is found in many organs (brain, lungs, kidneys, and liver) extrinsic to blood; therefore, it initiates the extrinsic clotting pathway by catalyzing factor VII. In the extrinsic system, factor VII undergoes proteolytic activation by tissue factor. Factor VIIa, calcium, tissue thromboplastin, and factor X form a lipoprotein complex that results in activation of factor X. After this step, the extrinsic system is identical to the intrinsic system.

In the intrinsic pathway, all the protein factors necessary for coagulation are present in the circulating blood. Contact by circulating factor XII with subendothelial membrane initiates the intrinsic pathway. This activation phase includes several other factors including high molecular weight kininogen and prekallikrein. Factor XIIa, with cofactor high molecular weight kininogen, activates factor IX to factor IXa. Factor VIII, factor IXa, calcium, and platelet phospholipid form a lipoprotein complex with prothrombin and activate it to thrombin. A fibrin clot is formed after thrombin converts fibrinogen to fibrin.

Because thrombin has a central role in coagulation, its generation is the focus of two important regulatory systems. Antithrombin III complexes to thrombin and inactivates thrombin as well as several other serine proteases (IXa, Xa, XIa, XIIa). Patients with a hereditary or acquired deficiency of antithrombin III have a high incidence of recurrent thromboembolic disease. Heparin enhances the inhibitory capacity of antithrombin III and is present on the surface of endothelial cells. The second system involves thrombin exerting an inhibitory influence on clot formation by activating protein C.[4] Protein C and its cofactor, protein S, are vitamin K-dependent proteins that inactivate factors V and VIII of the coagulation cascade (Fig. 94.2).

FIBRINOLYSIS

The fibrinolytic system is part of the localized repair of damaged endothelium as a regulatory mechanism in clot formation. Plasminogen is incorporated into the clot formation by binding to fibrin. Plasminogen activators (tissue-type plasminogen activator and urokinase-like plasminogen activator) are released in response to thrombin or venous stasis. Plasmin, converted from zymogen plasminogen, enzymatically digests fibrin, dissolves the clot, and releases a number of fibrin degradation products (fibrin split products). The interaction between plasminogen activators, plasminogen, and fibrin restricts the fibrinolytic activity to the site of the clot. Plasminogen activator inhibitor and α_2-plasmin inhibitor inactivate plasmin to prevent systemic fibrinolysis.

LABORATORY TESTS

The initial diagnosis of coagulation disorders can be established from a detailed clinical history, a physical examination, and the results of a few laboratory tests.[5–8] The most common screening tests include bleeding time, prothrombin time, activated partial thromboplastin time, thrombin time, and platelet count. The results of these standard laboratory procedures can distinguish bleeding disorders due to defects in the intrinsic, extrinsic, and common coagulation pathways (Fig. 94.2) or from alterations in the number of functioning platelets. Specific assays of individual coagulation factors and platelet function tests can be determined after abnormalities are identified by initial screening tests. The following is a brief review of simple tests that are available in most hospital or clinical settings. These tests are summarized in Table 94.2.

Bleeding Time[9]

In conjunction with the platelet count, determination of the bleeding time allows the examiner to make funda-

TABLE 94.1. BLOOD COAGULATION FACTORS

Factor[a]	Synonym	Role
I	Fibrinogen	Terminal substrate of the coagulation system, polymerizes into fibrin fibers upon proteolysis by thrombin
II	Prothrombin	Vitamin K-dependent zymogen of the serine protease thrombin
V	Proaccelerin labile factor	Nonenzymatic procofactor for factor Xa in the prothrombinase complex
VII	Proconvertin	Vitamin K-dependent zymogen of factor VIIa that activates factor X via the extrinsic pathway and factor IX via the alternate pathway
VIII	Antihemophilic factor A	Nonenzymatic procofactor of factor IXa in the factor X activation complex
IX	Antihemophilic factor B, Christmas factor	Vitamin K-dependent zymogen of factor IXa that activates factor X
X	Stuart–Power factor	Vitamin K-dependent zymogen of factor Xa, the protease of the prothrombinase complex
XI	Plasma thromboplastin antecedent	Zymogen of protease factor XIa that converts factor IX to factor IXa
XII	Hageman factor	Zymogen of factor XIIa that activates factor XI and prekallikrein
XIII	Fibrin-stabilizing factor	Zymogen of a transglutaminase that covalently cross-links fibrin monomers with each other
Prekallikrein	Fletcher factor	Zymogen of kallikrein that activates factor XII and cleaves high molecular weight kininogen to liberate bradykinin
High molecular weight kininogen	Flaujeac's, Fitzgerald's, or Williams' factor	Nonenzymatic contact activation cofactor of factor XIIa and kallikrein

[a]Coagulation factors are numbered with Roman numerals in order of their discovery. The most frequent synonyms are listed. Factor III (tissue factor) and factor IV (calcium ions) have been omitted from the table. (From Lammle B, Griffin JH. Formation of the fibrin clot: The balance of procoagulant and inhibitory factors, in Rugger ZM (ed): Clinics in Haematology. Philadelphia, WB Saunders, 1985, p 282, with permission.)

mental decisions regarding abnormalities of primary hemostasis. Patients with an abnormal bleeding time but a normal platelet count are arbitrarily designated as having qualitative abnormalities of platelet function (thrombocytopathy). Such patients include those with von Willebrand's disease, those who have recently ingested various antiplatelet drugs (i.e., aspirin), and those with uremia or dysproteinemia.

Prothrombin Time[10]

The prothrombin time (PT) assesses the function of the extrinsic system and common pathway of the coagulation system. In particular, the test measures the activity of the vitamin K-dependent factor, factor VII. PT reflects the time required for fibrin strands to appear after the addition of tissue thromboplastin and calcium to a patient's plasma. Thus, the PT yields evidence about the current synthetic capacity of the liver, the adequacy of vitamin K absorption, and the inhibition of clotting factor synthesis by warfarin.

Activated Partial Thromboplastin Time[11]

The activated partial thromboplastin time (APTT) measures the activity of the intrinsic system and common pathway. APTT reflects the time required for a fibrin clot to form after calcium and an activating agent are added to the patient's plasma. APTT is widely used for monitoring heparin therapy.

Thrombin Time[12]

The thrombin time (TT) assesses the clotting of plasma by thrombin and is affected by quantitative and qualitative abnormalities of fibrinogen. The TT measures the time required for the formation and the appearance of the fibrin clot. The test bypasses all earlier steps of the coagulation pathway. It is commonly used to monitor the effect of systemic fibrinolytic therapy and can be modified for monitoring heparin therapy.

Congenital Disorders

HEMOPHILIA

Inherited plasma coagulation disorders result from rare defects in single coagulation proteins. The two X-linked disorders, hemophilia A (factor VIII deficiency), and hemophilia B (factor IX deficiency), account for almost all known congenital coagulation defects.

Hemophilia A is also called classic hemophilia and is the oldest known congenital coagulopathy.[13] The writers of

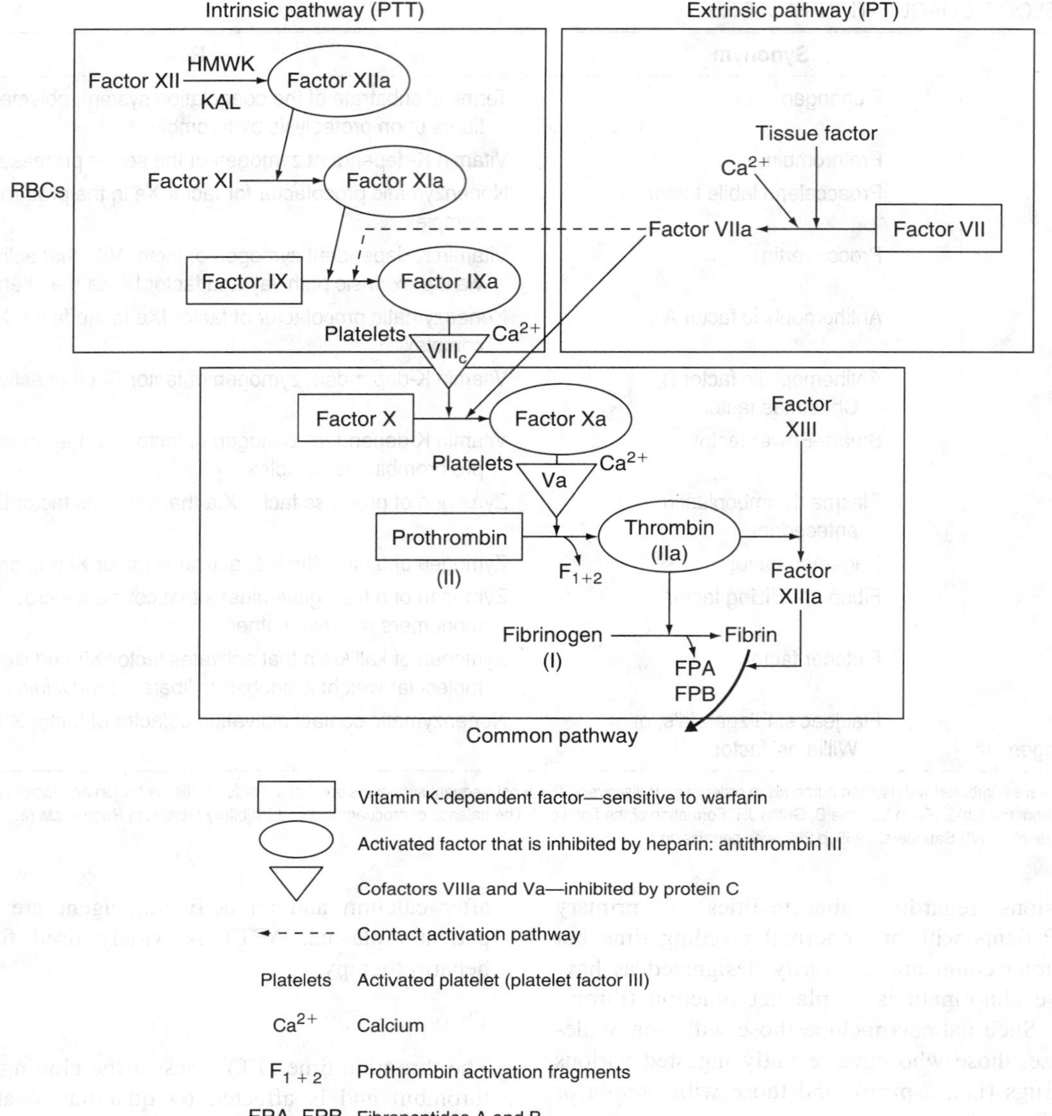

Figure 94.2. The coagulation pathways. Important features include the contact activation phase, vitamin K-dependent factors (affected by warfarin), the activated serine proteases that are inhibited by heparin: antithrombin III, and the role of platelets and calcium. Factors VIIIc and Va are nonenzymatic cofactors that are inactivated by protein C. The protime (PT) measures the function of the extrinsic and common pathways; the partial thromboplastin time (PTT or APTT) measures the function of the intrinsic and common pathways. HMWK, high molecular weight kininogen; KAL, kallikrein. *(From Stead RB. Regulation of hemostasis, in SZ Goldhaber (ed): Pulmonary Embolism and Deep Vein Thrombosis. Philadelphia, WB Saunders, 1985; p 32, with permission.)*

the Talmud decreed that boys whose older brothers or cousins had bled to death after circumcision need not undergo the procedure. In general, only males are affected by the disease, but females are carriers. The incidence of hemophilia A in the overall population is approximately 1 or 2 per 10,000 males.[14] The National Heart and Lung Institute estimates the frequency to be 25 per 100,000 males in the United States. Approximately 85% of those affected have hemophilia A (factor VIII deficiency); the remaining have hemophilia B (factor IX deficiency). Both hemophilia A and hemophilia B are recessive sex-linked diseases; the defective gene is located on the X chromosome. Affected males have the abnormal allele on their X chromosome and no matching allele on their Y chromosome; thus, their sons would be normal (assuming the mother is not a carrier), and their daughters would be obligatory carriers. Female carriers have one normal allele and, therefore, do not have a hemorrhagic tendency. Sons of a female carrier and a normal male have a 50% chance of being hemophiliacs, whereas daughters have a 50% chance of being carriers. This mode of inheritance with a "skipped generation"—the female carriers who are chil-

TABLE 94.2. LABORATORY PROCEDURES

Procedure	Reagent Content	Normal Range	System Tested	Disease Detected and Therapy Monitored
Template bleeding time	None	1–8 min	Platelets and capillaries	Thrombocytopathy, von Willebrand's disease, and thrombocytopenia
Activated partial thromboplastin time (APTT)	Phospholipid contact activator	<42 s	Intrinsic	Mild (40–50%) deficiencies of factors VIII, IX, and XI (hemophilias); deficiency of factor XII; von Willebrand's disease; disseminated intravascular coagulation; inhibitors; heparin therapy
Prothrombin time (PT)	Tissue thromboplastin	10–12 s	Extrinsic	Factor VII deficiency (acquired or hereditary); vitamin K deficiency; DIC; inhibitors; warfarin therapy
Thrombin time (TT)	Thrombin	20–24 s	Conversion of fibrinogen to fibrin	Hypofibrinogenemia and dysfibrinogenemia; fibrin split products; presence of heparin

(Modified from Triplett DA. Hemostasis: A Case Oriented Approach. New York, Igaku-Shoin, 1985, p 66, with permission.)

dren of the hemophiliacs do not express the disease but pass it on to the next male generation—was first described accurately early in the nineteenth century. The most celebrated carrier was Queen Victoria. One of her sons was a hemophiliac and at least two of her daughters were carriers. Victoria's daughters spread hemophilia throughout the royal families of Europe.

Hemophilia has been observed in few females.[14] This can occur if a hemophiliac marries a female carrier or if the normal X chromosome in the carrier female undergoes extreme lyonization. Lyonization is the process by which one of the X chromosomes in a female degenerates and does not produce effective gene products. There have been extremely rare cases where patients have had either one X chromosome or an autosomal dominant mode of transmission. In the older literature, many of these cases of female hemophilia were thought to be von Willebrand's disease.

Before 1947, it was thought that all patients with sex-linked, hereditary bleeding disorders had classic hemophilia resulting from factor VIII (antihemophilic factor) deficiency.[15] In 1947, blood from one patient with presumed classic hemophilia was found to correct the clotting abnormality in another patient. Subsequent investigators showed that both of these disorders were inherited as sex-linked recessive disorders with identical means of inheritance, but one was due to a deficiency of factor IX (plasma thromboplastin component, or Christmas factor).

Modern techniques of molecular biology have been successful in cloning the gene for factor VIII production.[13] The gene is 186,000 bases long. The coagulant material encoded by the gene originates from liver cells, although other tissues such as the kidney, spleen, and lymph glands have also been found to be sources of the coagulant material (factor VIII). This protein cofactor is missing in hemophilia A. The entire factor VIII molecule consists of this factor VIII coagulant material, along with a larger molecule, von Willebrand's factor, which is the protein that mediates adhesion of platelets to the subendothelium.[14,16,17] The larger part of the molecule is absent, decreased, or defective in von Willebrand's disease. Von Willebrand's factor circulates as a complex with factor VIII in normal plasma and appears to stabilize the latter. Antibodies have been produced to both the factor VIII coagulant material and the von Willebrand's factor and are called factor VIII antigen and von Willebrand's factor antigen, respectively.

At least 500 hemophiliac factor genes have been examined and many different mutations have been pinpointed. The kind of mutations that can affect the factor VIII gene include deletions and missense and nonsense mutations. Deletions and nonsense mutations are associated with the more severe forms of hemophilia A. A wider range of clinical conditions has been associated with more than 80 missense mutations.[18] Classic hemophilia A is caused by a deficiency of factor VIII coagulant material, with the degree of deficiency depending on the degree of genetic defect. In patients with classic hemophilia, there is a deficiency of factor VIII coagulant material but not of von Willebrand's factor, which appears to be synthesized in endothelial cells.

All patients with hemophilia B have decreased factor IX clotting activity.[15] The molecular basis for this decrease varies; some patients have decreased synthesis of a normal molecule, whereas others appear to have normal amounts of factor IX antigen with markedly decreased coagulant activity and thus are thought to have an abnormal protein with retained antigenic characteristics. There are several variants of factor IX deficiency, one of which is hemophilia B_m.[15,19] This disorder is characterized by a prolonged PT, whereas in most patients with hemophilia B this test is normal. The subscript "m" refers to the family name of the original patient. These patients have been shown to have the factor IX molecule by the presence of cross-reactive material, but the protein does not have normal coagulant activity. The specific protein abnormality has been identified in several different types of these variants. It is this abnormal protein that is believed to interfere with a factor VII–tissue factor activation of factor X, thereby prolonging the PT. The mechanism of this interference is unknown. About 5% of hemophilia B patients are hemophilia B_m variants. There are several other variants of hemophilia B, but they all have similar clinical manifestations.

The complete amino acid sequence for the circulating factor IX molecule has been delineated, and the gene for factor IX has been cloned. The entire gene is 35,000 nucleotides long.[19]

Molecular biologists use various techniques to detect carriers of either hemophilia A or B. In addition, prenatal diagnosis can be carried out if sufficient fetal DNA is obtained by cell culture of amniotic fluid or by biopsy of the chorionic villi.[13,19]

Hemophilia has been cured following liver transplantation.[18] Three patients that underwent liver transplant secondary to end-stage liver disease normalized their factor VIII levels. However, the need for lifelong immunosuppression and the risks associated with the surgical procedure preclude this option for most patients. It should be possible to cure hemophiliacs by introducing the appropriate gene into their cells.[20] Gene therapy for hemophilia is currently in the developmental stages and holds promise of a cure for this disease.[20]

Clinical Presentation

Hemophilia A

Clinical bleeding is usually correlated with the degree of deficiency of factor VIII. Patients with less than 1% factor VIII are classified as severe hemophiliacs; those with 1–5% are moderate hemophiliacs; and those with greater than 5% are mild hemophiliacs.[21] Most bleeding episodes are characterized by joint and muscle hemorrhage, with prolonged bleeding after trauma or surgery. Minor trauma and abrasions, which are frequently controlled with platelet plugs, do not pose clinical problems in patients with hemophilia.

Joint hemorrhages frequently involve the large joints, especially the weight-bearing ones. These episodes are frequently spontaneous, begin in childhood, and can lead to disabling arthropathies.

Muscle hematomas, especially psoas hematomas, can lead to false diagnoses, including appendicitis, and can also compress nerves leading to weakness or paralysis. Bleeding into vital organs can cause significant dysfunction: Retroperitoneal bleeding can obstruct one or both kidneys or bleeding into the oral cavity can obstruct the airway. Occasionally, bleeding into the subperiosteum after trauma can cause pseudotumors with bone necrosis.

Although mucous membrane bleeding is more common in disorders affecting platelet function, genitourinary, gastrointestinal, and intracranial bleeding may occur.

Hemophilia B

Hemophilia B (factor IX deficiency) is similar in all of its clinical manifestations to hemophilia A, with the severity of the disorder paralleling the degree of factor deficiency.[15]

Diagnosis

Patients who have spontaneous bleeding or bleeding out of proportion to what is expected clinically from an injury or surgical procedure may have a coagulopathy. Screening tests to detect coagulopathies include platelet count, bleeding time, PT, and APTT (Table 94.3).[12,22] TT can provide rapid information on the later stages of the coagulation mechanism and may also be useful. Depending on the results of these tests, additional tests including specific factor assays may be utilized to establish the specific diagnosis.

The APTT is an excellent test for screening deficiencies in the pathways of coagulation and has been reported to detect 99–100% of hemophilia A patients.[12,22] The sensitivity of the test is therefore excellent. If clinically normal patients are screened, there is an approximately 2% false-positive rate; this rate is approximately 11% for patients being evaluated for abnormal bleeding. Normal APTT and PT essentially rule out a significant plasma coagulation defect. Preoperative screening for coagulation disorders with the APTT shows that the incidence of clinically inapparent coagulopathies is so low that false-positive results greatly outnumber true-positive results and make screening pointless. The most critical piece of information is an adequate clinical assessment, including a medical history related to any prior history of bleeding problems. In patients for whom a clinical assessment is not possible, patients who have clinical evidence to suggest a bleeding disorder, such as liver disease and malabsorption, or patients undergoing procedures that may interrupt normal coagulation, such as extracorporeal circulation, screening tests are recommended.

Ideally, the APTT is sensitive to factor deficiency states of less than 30% activity. Patients with a normal PT but an abnormal APTT typically have deficiencies of factors that are unique to the intrinsic system (i.e., factors VIII, IX, XII, and XI). The specific factor assay for factor VIII or IX will reveal the appropriate defect. The exception to this is

TABLE 94.3. TESTS IN PATIENTS WITH HEMOPHILIA A, HEMOPHILIA B, AND VON WILLEBRAND'S DISEASE

	Hemophilia[a]		von Willebrand's Disease			
	A	B	I	II-A	II-B	III
APTT	A	A	A	A/N	A/N	A
PT	N	N/A[b]	N	N	N	N
Factor VIII	A	N	A	A/N	A/N	A
vWF:Ag	N	N	A	A/N	A/N	A
vWF:R	N	N	A/N	A	A	A
RIPA	N	N	A/N	A	A[c]	A
vWF multimers						
In plasma	N	N	Reduced, absent	Largest absent	Largest absent	None
In platelets	N	N	N	Largest absent	All present	None
Factor IX	N	A	N	N	N	N
TT	N	N	N	N	N	N
Bleeding time	N	N	A	A	A	A
Platelet adhesion	N	N	A	A	A	A
Other factors	N	N	N	N	N	N

[a]A, abnormal; N, normal.
[b]Prothrombin time is abnormal in hemophilia B_m.
[c]Platelet aggregation with ristocetin is increased.

the deficiency of factor IX in hemophilia B_m in which case the PT as well as the APTT is prolonged.

In addition, any patient with factor VIII deficiency should undergo the laboratory tests necessary to define von Willebrand's disease to be sure that the patient does not have this disorder or a variant thereof (Table 94.3).

Treatment

The total care of hemophilia requires a multitude of medical and paramedical personnel.[18] In the United States and the United Kingdom, the treatment of hemophilia has become centralized because of federally funded regional comprehensive hemophilia programs. In addition to centralizing the treatment, the federal government has supported the high cost of hemophilia treatment, thus decreasing the difficulty of providing care to both the institution and the patient. These patients frequently require primary care physicians, hematologists, orthopedic surgeons, nurses, physical medicine specialists, dentists, genetic counselors, psychologists, social workers, and vocational counselors along with pharmaceutical services and inpatient and outpatient treatment facilities associated with adequate coagulation testing.

In addition to some of the previously mentioned preventive medicine aspects necessary from birth, children need to be educated about physical protection during usual play. Passenger restraints in automobiles are especially important to children with hemophilia. Physical exercise is encouraged along with a daily program to improve muscle and joint function.

Newborn male infants who may be hemophiliacs should not be circumcised until the diagnosis is excluded. Blood should be obtained from a peripheral vein and not from a femoral or jugular vein puncture because of the danger of hematoma formation. Babies with hemophilia should receive routine immunizations, including immunization against hepatitis B. These small-gauge needles do not usually cause hematomas.

Genetic counseling with a neutral attitude should be offered and female relatives who may be carriers should be tested. Female relatives who are carriers may have a mild to moderate bleeding diathesis and can be forewarned of any difficulty with either trauma or surgery.

As children grow they may be taught to administer their own factor concentrate so that they may achieve independence. Concurrent illnesses can complicate hemophilia. Minor infections are frequently associated with bleeding into the site of inflammation and need to be followed closely.

Hemophilia A

The degree of severity determines the choice of treatment among these patients. Those with severe or moderate disease are treated with either cryoprecipitate or factor VIII concentrate.[14,19] Lyophilized factor VIII concentrate is easy to store, reconstitute, and administer. In addition these products are subject to various purification processes, decreasing the chances of transmitting blood-borne viruses.[23] Recombinant DNA technology has made it possible to have two products with structural and functional characteristics similar to plasma-derived factor VIII. The safety and efficacy of these products have been demonstrated in large-scale trials.[24,25]

Opinions of which factor concentrate to use vary widely among physicians. These physician opinions can be grouped into four general categories: (1) those who use plasma-derived products on all their patients because they are satisfied with viral-inactivation methods and do not think that plasma-derived products would have any degree of immunosuppression; (2) those who are concerned for the previously mentioned reasons advocate only recombinant products; (3) those who are worried about the potential immunosuppressant effects of plasma-derived products choose recombinant products for patients who have the human immunodeficiency virus (HIV positive) and plasma-derived products for patients without the human immunodeficiency virus (HIV negative); and (4) those who choose recombinant products for patients previously untreated and plasma-derived products for the rest of their patients.

Table 94.4 summarizes the factor VIII products currently available in the United States. All products are equally effective with similar rates of antibody development. However, plasma-derived products carry the potential for transmission of blood-borne viruses other than HIV and hepatitis, although the implications of this small chance are unknown at this time. The main factors that influence choice are cost and the preferences of the physician and/or patient; however, there is no solid evidence to support the preference of one product.

The factor is quantitated in units, where 1 unit of factor VIII is the amount found in 1 mL of pooled plasma. By definition, 1 unit of factor VIII per milliliter is 100% of normal. Dosing factor VIII will depend on several factors including the severity of the bleeding episode, desired plasma level, half-life of the infused factor, body weight, and plasma volume.[21,26,27] The usual half-life of factor VIII is 8–12 hours; thus, in order to maintain a specific factor level, it is necessary to infuse the factor at least twice daily or as a continuous infusion. Administration via continuous infusion has been shown to be safe and effective and may be more convenient than bolus therapy for inpatients.[28] One way of calculating the appropriate initial dose is based on the observation that each unit of factor VIII infused per kilogram of body weight yields a 2% rise in plasma factor VIII levels. The following equation may also be used to calculate an initial dose of factor VIII:

$$\text{Factor VIII (units)} = (\text{desired level} - \text{actual level}) \times 0.5\ (\text{weight})$$

This equation assumes a plasma volume of 5% of the patient's body weight in kilograms. It is usually necessary to administer half the loading dose every 12 hours in order to sustain a desired level of factor VIII. As previously mentioned, dosing factor VIII depends on several variables and the approach to replacement therapy is generally empiric. Each case must be considered individually. Table 94.5 is designed to provide general guidelines for dosing factor VIII based on the site and severity of the bleeding episode.[27] Mild bleeding episodes are not included in the table because they should be managed without the use of blood products. The general goal is to achieve a factor VIII level of 30–50% to maintain hemostasis. To achieve this in 8–12 hours, it is necessary to have twice this level immediately after the infusion to allow for the decay with time. This level of factor is satisfactory for joint or muscle hemorrhage, but with severe bleeding or major surgical procedures the level should be raised to and maintained at 75–100% for up to a week.

TABLE 94.4. FACTOR VIII PREPARATIONS

Manufacturer	Brand Name	Viral Inactivation or Exclusion Method	Annual Cost[a] ($)
Alpha	Profilate-OSD[b]	Solvent-detergent	72,000
American Red Cross	AHF-M[b]	Solvent-detergent	28,000
Armour	Humate-P[b]	Pasteurized	104,000
	Monoclate-P[b]	Pasteurized/ monoclonal antibody	
Baxter	Hemophil M[b]	Solvent-detergent/ monoclonal antibody	72,000
	Recombinate[c]	Affinity chromatography	94,000
Miles/Bayer	Koate HP[b]	Solvent-detergent	72,000
	Kogenate[d]	Affinity chromatography	94,000

[a]Based on 1994 average wholesale price *(Red Book)*, and consumption of 80,000 units/yr.
[b]Plasma derived.
[c]Hamster ovary cell derived.
[d]Hamster kidney cell derived. (Adapted from Anonymous. Recombinant antihemophilic factor. Med Lett Drugs Ther 1993;35(898):51.)

Cryoprecipitate is rich in factor VIII, fibrinogen, and von Willebrand factor, and still in use in some hemophiliac centers, although it has been replaced for the most part by factor VIII concentrates. In general, each bag of cryoprecipitate contains approximately 70–100 units of factor VIII activity per 10- to 20-mL bag. The potency of cryoprecipitate will vary from bag to bag; therefore, the dose can only be estimated. The number of bags necessary to achieve a desired level of factor VIII may be estimated by calculating the amount of factor VIII in units required as previously discussed.[27]

Mild factor VIII deficiency may be treated with 1-desamino-8-D-arginine vasopressin (desmopressin acetate, DDAVP), which transiently increases factor VIII and von Willebrand factor levels and shortens prolonged bleeding time.[30,31] DDAVP is a synthetic analog of the antidiuretic hormone vasopressin. If the patient has a mild bleeding

TABLE 94.5. FACTOR VIII REPLACEMENT THERAPY FOR SEVERELY AFFECTED HEMOPHILIACS[a]

Site of Hemorrhage	Desired Factor VIII Level (% of normal)	Factor VIII Dose (units/kg body weight[b])	Frequency of Dose[c] (interval in hours)	Duration (days)
Hemarthroses	30–50	≈25	24	1–2
Superficial intramuscular hematoma	30–50	≈25	24	1–2
Gastrointestinal tract	50–100	≈25–50	12	7–10
Epistaxis	30–50	≈25	12	Until resolved
Oral mucosa	30–50	≈25	12	Until resolved
Hematuria	30–100	≈25–50	12	Until resolved
Central nervous system	75–100	50	8–12	7–10 days or until healing occurs
Retropharyngeal	75–100	50	8–12	7–10 days or until healing occurs
Retroperitoneal	75–100	50	8–12	7–10 days or until healing occurs

[a]Mild or moderately affected patients may respond to DDAVP, which should be used in lieu of blood or blood products whenever possible.
[b]The factor VIII may be administered in a continuous infusion if the patient is hospitalized. After initial bolus, about 150 units factor VIII per h is usually sufficient in an average-sized adult.
[c]Both the frequency of dosing and duration of therapy may be adjusted in keeping with the severity and duration of each patient's bleeding episode. (From Roberts HR, Jones MR. Hemophilia and related conditions: Congenital deficiencies of prothrombin (factor II), factor V, and factors VII to XII, in Williams WJ, Beutler E, Erslev AJ, Lichtman MA (eds): Hematology. New York, McGraw-Hill, 1990, p 1460, with permission.)

episode, such as a hemarthrosis, DDAVP 0.3–0.4 μg/kg IV infused over 15–30 minutes may be given. Factor levels should be measured to ensure that an adequate response has been achieved.[29] DDAVP can result in a fourfold to sixfold rise in factor VIII levels, with maximum levels occurring at about 90–120 minutes postinfusion with persistent activity for greater than 6 hours. The injection can be repeated within 12–24 hours depending on the severity of the bleeding episode and the clinical response. It is important to realize that the factor increments become attenuated with frequent dosages. Subcutaneous DDAVP in the same doses recommended above for IV has been shown to be as effective as the IV form and is more practical for self-administration.[32,33]

Intranasal administration of DDAVP via a concentrated nasal spray (Stimate) has become available in the United States. It effectively increases factor VIII levels but to a lesser extent than that of parenteral DDAVP. The nasal spray may serve as an alternative to the parenteral formulation, especially in patients with mild bleeding episodes who need to self-administer DDAVP. Before starting intranasal DDAVP, a test dose should be performed to assure adequate response to this particular formulation.[34]

Very few adverse effects are associated with DDAVP. Most side effects are probably secondary to mild vasodilation.[30] The most commonly observed side effect is facial flushing. Side effects less frequently reported include mild headaches, increased heart rate, and decreased blood pressure. Although rarely seen DDAVP has the potential to cause water retention, which may lead to severe hyponatremia secondary to its potent antidiuretic effects. Since DDAVP can also increase plasminogen activator, some experts suggest the concomitant use of aminocaproic acid (EACA) in order to inhibit the potential fibrinolysis that may occur. Use of DDAVP reduces exposure to blood-borne viruses. Caution should be exercised when administering DDAVP to patients with a history of recurrent thrombosis.

The prophylactic use of factor VIII concentrates in severe hemophilia has been explored.[35] The rationale comes from observations where patients with moderate disease rarely develop arthropathy. The goal of prophylactic replacement is to maintain a level of factor VIII of at least 1% in these patients. Infusion of the factors at least three times a week in a dose range between 24–40 IU factor VIII/kg can maintain this goal. Patients that have received this approach since age one have almost no bleeding episodes, and have had completely normal joints during follow-up.[35] Cost considerations are a concern with the prophylactic regimens. Pharmacokinetic dosing models have been proposed as a cost-saving approach to prophylaxis.[36]

Hemophilia B

High purity factor IX plasma concentrate is currently considered the treatment of choice for hemophilia B.[37] These products have rapidly replaced the older products, known as prothrombin complex concentrate (PCC). PCC, in addition to factor IX, contains vitamin K-dependent factors responsible for the thromboembolic complications observed with their administration.[23] Available high purity factors include Alphanine and Alphanine-SD (Alpha Therapeutic), and Mononine (Armour). The first two products contain 50 units of factor IX activity per milligram of protein and Mononine contains at least 150 units per milligram of protein. No thromboembolic complications have been reported with either product, and excellent hemostasis during bleeding episodes is observed.[38]

The half-life of factor IX is approximately 24 hours, with normal hemostasis being achieved when plasma levels are approximately 10–25%. Each unit of factor IX infused per kilogram body weight yields a 1% rise in the level of factor IX. As with factor VIII, the success of infusion depends on achievement of appropriate factor IX levels, which requires monitoring with factor IX assays. Although hemostasis is usually achieved between 10 and 25%, plasma levels of 40% have been recommended for severe muscle and joint bleeding, with levels of 60% recommended for major surgery. With major surgery, replacement therapy should be continued for at least a week.

Treatment of Inhibitors in Hemophilia

Antibodies to factor VIII and IX, also known as inhibitors, develop in a group of patients with hemophilia, challenging the management of these patients. The incidence of inhibitors was thought to be around 15%; however, prospective studies with more intensive screening surveillance reports the incidence to be as high as 52%.[39–41] The type of product that the patient receives (plasma-derived versus recombinant) does not seem to affect the development of inhibitors.[42]

These inhibitors are usually IgG immunoglobulin. They do not precipitate human factor VIII or IX and do not fix complement. They are directed against the factor coagulant portion of the complex. Advances in the characterization of these antibodies have allowed differentiation between alloantibodies and autoantibodies.[43,44] These antibodies may be recognized when a calculated dose of factor does not produce the expected plasma level. In such cases inhibitor levels should be determined in order to help guide therapy in these patients. Inhibitor titers are reported in Bethesda units (BU) in the United States. Patients with inhibitors to factor VIII/IX are divided into two groups: low responders who have low levels of inhibitors (2–5 BU/mL) with little or no rise in antibody titers after exposure to the factor, and high responders who have an anamnestic response after exposure to factor VIII/IX and usually have higher inhibitor levels (>10 BU/mL). Approximately 20% of this population are low responders and 50–60% are high responders.

The treatment of patients with factor inhibitors will depend on the titer of the inhibitor and can be approached in two ways. First, one may attempt to reduce inhibitor levels prophylactically with immunosuppressive agents (i.e., cyclophosphamide), gamma globulin infusions, plasmapheresis, or by production of immune tolerance using high-dose or frequent regular infusions of the factor.[45] The second method is used to achieve hemostasis in acute bleeding episodes or for surgery. If the patient has low inhibitor titers (<5 BU/mL) an anamnestic response is unlikely, and hemostasis may be achieved with a high dose of factor (usually twice the dose ordinarily indicated). These patients should have an inhibitor level 7–10 days after therapy to assure that inhibitor titers did not rise. Patients with high inhibitor titers (>10 BU/mL), however, usually have an anamnestic response to the factor. Hemostasis can usually be achieved in these patients with PCC, activated prothrombin complex concentrate (APCC), or porcine factor VIII.[45–47] The dose of PCC required is usually at least twice the dose of factor VIII/IX used in noninhibitor patients. Initial doses are usually in the range of 50–75 units/kg every 12 hours depending on the severity of the bleeding episode.

The patients must be clinically monitored since there are no laboratory tests to measure effectiveness of therapy. If the patient does not appear to be responding to PCC infusions, then APCC should be used in similarly high doses. Porcine factor VIII concentrate is intended for use in patients who have developed inhibitors against factor VIII. The neutralizing activity of these inhibitors is usually absent or weaker against nonhuman as opposed to human factor VIII. The dose of porcine factor VIII may be estimated using the same criteria that is used for human factor VIII. Response to therapy may be monitored with factor VIII levels. Tolerance may be induced by the use of porcine factor VIII, and the inhibitor may not recur.

Recombinant factor VIIa (rFVIIa) seems to offer an alternative treatment for patients with inhibitors.[46] In a series of 57 patients, none developed antibodies to factor VII. Hemostasis was achieved for hemophilia A and B using doses of 70–100 μg/kg every 2–3 hours and prolonging the interval of administration as clinical improvement occurred. Prothrombin time has been suggested as a monitoring parameter for rFVIIa response.[48]

Figure 94.3 summarizes the therapeutic options in the management of hemophilia A patients with inhibitors.[45] The same algorithm can be applied to the management of hemophilia B patients, except that factor IX should be substituted for factor VIII. The use of porcine factor VIII is not indicated for the inhibitors in hemophilia B.

Surgery in Hemophilia

Surgical procedures in hemophilic patients must be accompanied by several steps in order to avoid potentially life-threatening hemorrhage. Table 94.6 provides general guidelines for management of hemophilic patients who require surgery.[49]

In general, all hemophiliacs undergoing surgery—whether it is minor or major—require a factor VIII level of 100% 1 hour prior to the procedure. Maintenance factor VIII levels, however, will depend on the type of surgical procedure performed. Antifibrinolytic agents such as EACA and tranexamic acid have been shown to be effective as adjunctive therapy in the control of bleeding after some surgical procedures, including dental extractions.[50,51] These agents inhibit fibrinolysis by inhibiting plasminogen activators resulting in clot preservation. The recommended doses and duration of therapy are listed in Table 94.6. Since tranexamic acid is 7 to 10 times more potent than EACA, lower

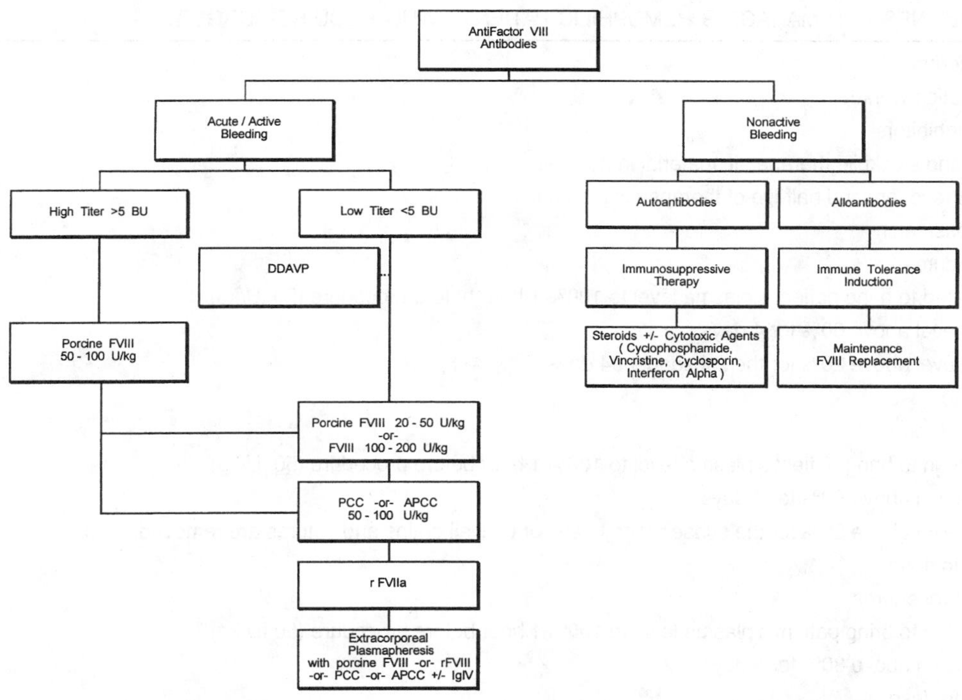

Figure 94.3. Treatment algorithm for the management of patients with hemophilia and factor VIII antibodies. *(Adapted from: Kessler CM. Factor VIII inhibitors: An algorithmic approach to treatment. Semin Hematol 1994;31:33–36, with permission.)*

doses can be used. EACA has a half-life of 1–2 hours with peak plasma levels occurring at 2 hours. Tranexamic acid has a half-life of 80 minutes and peak plasma concentrations occur at 3 hours. Both drugs are mainly renally excreted. Side effects are rare and mostly limited to nausea, vomiting, and diarrhea.[50] EACA is contraindicated in patients with hematuria because of the potential for ureteral or intrarenal obstruction by blood clots.

Pain Management in Hemophilia

Pain can be a common occurrence in this population. Pain can be either acute or chronic. Acute pain is due to pressure from hemorrhage into joints, muscle, or other tissues.[18] Chronic pain usually occurs secondary to permanent changes in the anatomy of joints. Acute pain should always be assumed to be due to bleeding. Control of the bleeding episode should control the pain. Pain that persists days after correction of the coagulation problem should be evaluated on the basis of the possibility of permanent joint changes. The relief of the chronic pain may require nonpharmacologic interventions such as surgery and the use of narcotic analgesics in addition to acetaminophen.[21]

Hemophilic patients, as well as other patients with coagulation disorders, should avoid the use of drugs that affect platelet aggregation such as aspirin and nonsteroidal anti-inflammatory drugs (NSAIDs). Pharmacists have an important role in the education of these patients. It is important to make the patient aware of the various aspirin-containing and NSAIDs available over the counter.

Evaluation of Therapeutic Outcome

Pharmacists can assume an active role in the management of patients with hemophilia as members of the multidisciplinary team taking care of these patients. Understanding that the main goal in the treatment of hemophilia is to control and prevent bleeding episodes and their long-term sequelae, like arthropathies, pharmacologic and nonpharmacologic interventions should be aimed at achieving this goal. Appropriate selection of product according to the type and site of bleeding (e.g., factor concentrates versus DDAVP), an adequate dose corresponding to the desired level and patient weight, and the optimal duration of therapy is required to be established for each particular episode. The institution of home therapy for the administration of factor concentrates is frequent in these patients, especially since it can lead to the early establishment of therapy and more independence to the patient. Assuring compliance with the regimen and that it is instituted as soon as the onset of bleeding symptoms, along with adequate education regarding proper storage, handling, and administration of these products, are integral components for a successful home program. In addition, the patient should become familiar with common side effects and how

TABLE 94.6. GUIDELINES FOR MANAGING HEMOPHILIC PATIENTS WHO REQUIRE SURGERY

Before surgical procedure
1. Complete coagulation workup
2. Incubate test for inhibitors
3. Calculate needs and stockpile therapeutic material in hospital
4. Survival study for recovery and half-life of therapeutic material
5. Red cell type, crossmatch

Minor surgical procedures
1. Give dose calculated to bring patient's plasma level to 100% 1 hour before procedure (50 IU/kg)
2. Maintain plasma level above 60% for 4 days
3. Maintain plasma level above 20% for the subsequent 4 days
4. Assay daily prior to dose

Major surgical procedures
1. Give dose calculated to bring patient's plasma level to 100% 1 hour before procedure (50 IU/kg)
2. Maintain plasma level above 60% for 4 days
3. Maintain plasma level above 20% for the subsequent 4 days or until all drains and sutures are removed
4. Assay daily prior to dose

Orthopedic surgical procedures
1. Give dose calculated to bring patient's plasma level to 100% 1 hour before procedure (50 IU/kg)
2. Maintain plasma level above 80% for 4 days
3. Assay daily prior to dose
4. Maintain plasma level above 40% for the subsequent 4 days
5. If patient is casted, discontinue replacement until rehabilitation program is begun
6. If not casted, maintain above 20% for ambulation
7. For rehabilitation program, maintain above 10% for 3 weeks

Dental procedures
1. Give EACA 100 mg/kg IV 4 hours before surgery or tranexamic acid 10 mg/kg
2. Give factor replacement dose calculated to bring patient's plasma level to 100% 1 hour before procedure
3. Continue EACA 100 mg/kg orally q6h for 7 days or tranexamic acid for 7 days (adults, 2 g three times a day for 7 days)
4. Repeat one dose of replacement therapy in 3 days if procedure is extensive

(From Hilgartner MW. Factor replacement therapy, in Hilgartner MW, Pochedly C (eds): Hemophilia in the Child and Adult. New York, Raven Press, 1989, p 14, with permission.)

to react to them. Fear of acquiring viral infections, in particular HIV, through plasma-derived products can lead to poor compliance with therapy or to delayed medical attention during a bleeding episode. Patient counseling can serve as a tool to overcome these fears.

Surveillance for the development of inhibitors, especially in patients with severe disease and high usage of factor concentrates, should be part of the pharmaceutical interventions, so that the discovery of the presence of inhibitors when the patient fails to respond to therapy is avoided. Development of inhibitors challenges the management and control of bleeding episodes. A full understanding of the clinical situation and the titer of the inhibitor is mandatory in order to address treatment options for each patient. Dose and frequency of administration for the product selected (e.g., porcine factor VIII or rFVIIa) vary from patient to patient. Since there is no laboratory test to measure effectiveness of therapy in this scenario, close clinical monitoring for worsening or resolution of the symptoms is required to optimize the outcome.

Preparation for any surgical intervention and assurance of the required levels of factor VIII or XI depending on the type of procedure are maintained through surgery and afterward are vital for a successful surgery with minimal or no complications. The previously mentioned scenarios are examples of different areas were management interventions can have a positive impact on the overall quality of the care and outcome of hemophiliacs.

VON WILLEBRAND'S DISEASE

Von Willebrand's disease is probably the most common inheritable coagulopathy.[14,16,17] The first clinical description of the disease was made by von Willebrand in 1926. Von Willebrand's disease is caused by an abnormality, quantitative or qualitative, of von Willebrand's factor and results both in abnormal platelet function and defective plasma clotting. Von Willebrand's factor (vWF) is a glycoprotein that can be found in classic hemophiliac plasma and normal plasma. At first, it was called factor VIII-related antigen or protein, as antibodies had been raised against protein fractions containing factor VIII coagulant activity. It is now known that factor VIII is distinct from vWF, but forms a dissociable complex with it.[51] Von Willebrand's factor can normally be detected in plasma, vessel walls, and platelets. Almost all of the vWF in platelets is located in the alpha granules. Within endothelial cells, vWF has been located on the plasma membrane and in the endoplasmic reticulum of the cytoplasm, as well as in cell-specific organelles.

Von Willebrand's factor has a dual role in hemostasis, facilitating platelet adhesion to injured vessel walls and binding the antihemophilic factor (factor VIII) in a complex, thus serving as a carrier of factor VIII in plasma.

The basic subunit of vWF is a protein chain with a molecular weight of approximately 230,000. The subunits are held together in a very complex way by disulfide bonds, forming proteins that vary widely in molecular weight. Von Willebrand's factor consists of a series of multimers ranging from 800,000 to 14,000,000 in molecular weight. The large multimers are thought to be the most hemostatically efficient with a greater potential for interaction with platelets and binding to the subendothelium. Von Willebrand's factor must join the platelets with the subendothelium to cause effective platelet function.

In 1973, Howard[53] showed that the antibiotic ristocetin causes platelet aggregation dependent on vWF. Platelet aggregation with ristocetin became a model system in the study of platelet-vWF interactions. Von Willebrand's factor activity was measured on the basis of platelet aggregation and expressed as ristocetin cofactor activity. Since ristocetin and vWF agglutinate platelets fixed with paraformaldehyde or formalin, formalin-fixed platelets are now used to measure this activity.

High molecular weight forms of vWF seem to have the highest ristocetin cofactor activity and appear to be the most efficient in promoting adhesion in these systems. Some commercial factor VIII concentrates contain only low molecular weight multimers of vWF and are less efficient in promoting platelet adhesion.

Von Willebrand's factor appears to be the carrier protein for factor VIII as it circulates in normal blood. Although the site of factor VIII has not been established, factor VIII antigen has been demonstrated in the endothelial cells lining liver sinusoid, but not in other types of endothelium. Von Willebrand's factor also seems to be a stimulator of factor VIII production, because when vWF is given to a patient who lacks the complete complex, the factor VIII activity in the patient's blood increases more than can be explained by the factor VIII activity in the infused material.

Clinical Presentation

Von Willebrand's disease is usually inherited in the heterozygous form as an autosomal dominant disorder.[14,16,17] Genetic variants are defined according to the qualitative and quantitative abnormalities of vWF, which run true in affected kindreds. One affected person may be markedly different from another within a kindred with respect to the amount of factor deficiency but not the type of deficiency. Types I, II-A, II-B, and II-D are inherited as autosomal dominant characteristics, whereas types II-C and III are inherited as autosomal recessive disorders. These genetic variants are described in the Diagnosis section.

Patients with von Willebrand's disease frequently present with mucosal bleeding such as epistaxis, gingival bleeding, easy bruising, menorrhagia, and postsurgical bleeding, especially after operations on mucosal surfaces such as tonsillectomy, vaginal surgery, and dental surgery. In the most severe forms of the disease the bleeding starts in early childhood and tends to decrease with age or with pregnancy. In milder forms the disease may not be discovered until an episode of trauma or surgery when the patient is an adult. The bleeding into joints and muscles characteristic of hemophilia is rare in von Willebrand's disease.

Diagnosis

Von Willebrand's disease and its variants are defined by the type of abnormality in vWF: quantitative, qualitative, or both (Table 94.3).[14,16,17] Von Willebrand's factor activity is measured as the bleeding time and by the ristocetin cofactor test. The bleeding time has been shown to be reasonably reproducible and accurate when obtained by the template technique. The ristocetin cofactor test measures the ability of the patient's plasma to agglutinate normal washed, fresh, or formalin-fixed platelets in the presence of ristocetin. Ristocetin-induced platelet aggregation (RIPA) is measured on platelet-rich plasma with an aggregometer.

Von Willebrand's factor is also measured by quantitation of von Willebrand's antigen, usually by electrophoresis with precipitating antibody to von Willebrand's factor or by radioimmunoassay.

The multimeric structure of von Willebrand's factor is demonstrated by electrophoresis in sodium dodecyl sulfate agarose or acrylamide gels. The multimers are then identified with radiolabeled antibody to vWF and autoradiography. The bands separate on the basis of their molecular size, and the relative proportions of large and small multimers can be demonstrated. Genetic variants are defined by the results of these tests. Factor VIII coagulant activity is usually low and commensurate with the degree of vWF deficiency. In some patients, however, factor VIII levels may approach normal.

Recent advances in the genetic analysis of patients with von Willebrand's disease have improved the understanding of the genetic and biochemical differences among this heterogeneous group of patients. An increasing number of subtypes have been described, and this pattern is expected to continue as genetic analysis becomes of widespread use in clinical practice.[52,54] In addition, a new and revised classification for vWD is being considered for future use. In the following section, the more clinically significant types of von Willebrand's disease are described with respect to the preceding tests and the pattern of inheritance.

Type I

The most common form of von Willebrand's disease is inherited as an autosomal dominant disorder and is expressed as a decrease in von Willebrand's antigen and vWF; multimers of all sizes are found in plasma and platelets. Although the amount of vWF is usually proportional to the level of von Willebrand's antigen, the amount of factor VIII may be higher. RIPA is normal or decreased. The bleeding time is usually prolonged. Type I von Willebrand's disease appears to result from production of decreased amounts of structurally normal vWF.

Rare variants of von Willebrand type I have been identified (types B and C). Quantitative differences in multimers in plasma characterize each subtype.

Type II

Type II von Willebrand's disease was originally described as a normal concentration of von Willebrand's antigen with a qualitative defect in von Willebrand's protein. Ristocetin cofactor activity (vWF) is low compared with the concentration of von Willebrand's antigen. The differentiation between the various subtypes is based on the multimeric pattern of vWF in plasma and platelets. The response of platelets to ristocetin is also an important characteristic.

Type II-A von Willebrand's disease is inherited as an autosomal dominant disorder and is characterized by the absence from plasma of large- and medium-size von Willebrand's multimers and the absence from platelets of large multimers. There is marked reduction in ristocetin cofactor and the response to ristocetin of platelet aggregation. Factor VIII antigen and coagulant material may be decreased or normal. DDAVP increases the numbers of small multimers in plasma but does not increase large multimers.

Type II-B is inherited as an autosomal dominant disorder and is characterized by the absence from plasma of large multimers. They are present in platelets. Plasma levels of von Willebrand's antigen, factor VIII coagulant material, and vWF may be decreased or normal. Aggregation of platelets in response to ristocetin is increased, with strong agglutination in the presence of ristocetin too weak to agglutinate normal platelets. DDAVP may cause a sudden release of large multimers, causing widespread platelet aggregation with marked thrombocytopenia. This disorder appears to result from a qualitative defect in the formation of large multimers, causing enhanced affinity to cellular binding sites. These patients may be mildly thrombocytopenic.

Type III

A few patients have been found to have a severe plasma deficiency of vWF, with essentially no protein being found in either plasma or platelets. Factor VIII activity is low in proportion to the markedly reduced vWF and von Willebrand's antigen. Type III is inherited as an autosomal recessive disorder; heterozygotes appear normal. The bleeding time is severely prolonged.

Pseudo von Willebrand's Disease

This is also known as platelet-type von Willebrand's disease because it results from an abnormality in the platelet instead of in vWF. It is inherited as an autosomal dominant disorder; the platelets bind normal vWF at concentrations of ristocetin lower than those needed for normal platelets to bind. RIPA is enhanced. Von Willebrand's factor alone without ristocetin may aggregate platelets. Multimeric analysis may show depletion of the large multimers of vWF and may resemble type II-B disease. Some patients have chronic thrombocytopenia. DDAVP and cryoprecipitate may result in platelet aggregation and worsen the thrombocytopenia.

Acquired von Willebrand's Disease

Patients with altered immune status or polycythemia rubra vera have been reported to develop a disorder resembling von Willebrand's disease, with prolonged bleeding times and reduced levels of factor VIII-related activities.[54] Patients with systemic lupus erythematosus and other connective tissue diseases, monoclonal gammopathies, lymphoproliferative disease, and Wilms' tumor have been reported to have this disease. In some cases, inhibitors (antibodies) develop been detected in the plasma that are capable of binding to factor VIII–von Willebrand factor complex, removing it at an accelerated rate.

Treatment

The goals of therapy are to improve factor VIII level and to improve the bleeding time. No standard method to determine the adequate concentration of ristocentin cofactor needed to achieve hemostasis is available.[51] Diagnosis of von Willebrand's disease and the type is important to guide therapy. However, during serious trauma or other acute situations presenting with severe bleeding this information may not be available. In this scenario replacement therapy should be the treatment of choice. The use of cryoprecipitate carries the risk of transmitting blood-borne viruses; different strategies have been attempted to reduce the size of the donor pool. Repetitive plasmapheresis of a single donor to extract cryoprecipitate or pretreatment with DDAVP to augment the donor's preexisting factor VIII and vWF levels are examples of these strategies.[56,57]

Cryoprecipitate administered in amounts of approximately 1 bag/10 kg every 12 hours is usually sufficient.[27,29,58] Once again it is difficult to determine specific dosages due to the variability of disease that exists from case to case. Thus, the doses recommended in this chapter are meant as a guide on which clinicians can build. Despite adequate correction of the factor VIII level with appropriate amounts of cryoprecipitate calculated to achieve a factor VIII level appropriate for the clinical condition, the bleeding time is frequently corrected for only 6–12 hours. There is usually a discrepancy between vWF activity and factor VIII level 24 hours after the infusion if more cryoprecipitate is not given. It is difficult to monitor the effect of replacement therapy in von Willebrand's disease because it does not correlate with any laboratory values. The bleeding time can be unreliable because it may only be transiently shortened. Another approach in the treatment of severe von Willebrand's disease is to follow the cryoprecipitate infusion with a DDAVP infusion. This seems to improve bleeding time in patients with a persistent abnormal bleeding time after cryoprecipitate infusion.[59]

The majority of the commercial concentrates used for the treatment of hemophilia A are not suitable because they lack high molecular weight multimers and, therefore, fail to correct the bleeding time.[23,60] Humate-P is a commercial concentrate that contains sufficient large vWF multimers to provide adequate hemostasis. Many physicians have advocated the use of Humate-P for replacement therapy instead of cryoprecipitate.[21,58] Koate-HS and Koate-HP have been reported to achieve clinical hemostasis prior to surgery.[61] A vWF concentrate has been developed in Europe. *In vitro* characterization of this concentrate has shown a multimer pattern and composition similar to that of plasma.[57]

In mild von Willebrand's disease, DDAVP should be used because any plasma product carries the risk of transmitting hepatitis.[30,57] Intravenous DDAVP, at 0.3–0.4 μg/kg over 15–30 minutes, usually induces a dose-dependent increase in all factor VIII-related activities, with both factor VIII and vWF increasing fourfold to sixfold. This usually lasts 4–8 hours and is effective in mild or moderate type I disease and in type II-A disease. The dose may be repeated in 8–12 hours, but the response diminishes with repeated treatment. Laboratory monitoring should be initiated if treatment is extended. Intranasal DDAVP also can be considered. The side effects of DDAVP were described in the discussion of treatment of hemophilia A.

Patients with mild hemophilia A may also be treated with DDAVP, but patients with either severe type I von Willebrand's disease or severe hemophiliacs do not respond well. In type II-A, DDAVP increases plasma vWF, but the qualitative abnormality is not corrected and the bleeding time may be shortened but not normalized.[57] DDAVP should not be used before the type of von Willebrand's disease is defined by multimeric analysis, because in type II-B, *in vivo* platelet aggregation and severe thrombocytopenia may occur.[61] In addition, DDAVP is not beneficial in either type II-C or type II-D.

Menorrhagia is a frequent problem in women with von Willebrand's disease. Oral contraceptives may be very effective in controlling this symptom. Inhibitors of the fibrinolytic system may be of special value in those tissues rich in fibrinolytic activity such as the ear, nose, and throat region and especially with tooth extractions. Patients with von Willebrand's disease should be encouraged to avoid aspirin and nonsteroidal anti-inflammatory drugs (NSAIDs) because of their effects on platelet function.

Inhibitors can develop in severe type III von Willebrand's disease. In severe bleeding situations PCC has been used with favorable results. Plasmapheresis is another approach used in these situations.[56]

Evaluation of Therapeutic Outcome

Hemorrhagic manifestations will depend on the type and severity of the disease; thus it is instrumental in order to provide optimal management to know the subtype of von Willebrand's disease and the patient's prior response to therapy if available. Currently, the goal in the treatment of von Willebrand's disease is to improve factor VIII and bleeding time. The choice of cryoprecipitate, Humate-P, or DDAVP will depend on the von Willebrand's disease subtype and the severity of the bleeding episode. Awareness of common side effects and how to respond to them must be part of the treatment plan. Patient education is needed regarding self-management of superficial bleeding with pressure maneuvers or topical hemostatic agents. If DDAVP is indicated proper storage and adequate subcutaneous administration techniques must also be covered. Good oral hygiene can prevent mucosal bleeding. Patients should avoid activities that can predispose them to bleeding. Risks of complications during surgery will depend on the type of procedure and the subtype of von Willebrand's disease; these factors will also determine the replacement product to use and duration of therapy. Awareness of aspirin-containing products and over-the-counter NSAIDs would ensure patient avoidance of these products and prevention of bleeding episodes.

OTHER CONGENITAL FACTOR DEFICIENCIES

In addition to deficiencies in factors VIII and IX, congenital deficiencies in fibrinogen, in factors II, V, VII, X, XI, XII, XIII, contact factors, and combinations of factor deficiencies have been reported to form multiple defects.[62] Contract factor abnormalities, including deficiencies in factor XII (the Hageman factor) and prekallikrein (Fletcher factor), prolong the APTT but do not lead to any bleeding diathesis. The only contact factor deficiency that causes bleeding diathesis is factor XI deficiency. Most other deficiencies are inherited as autosomal recessive disorders and are rare. Some patients with abnormal molecules, such as fibrinogen, may have an increased tendency to develop thromboembolic disease. The usual treatment for these

TABLE 94.7. REPLACEMENT THERAPY FOR COAGULATION FACTOR DEFICIENCY

Factor	Desired Hemostatic Level in Bleeding Surgical Patients	*In Vivo* Recovery	Biologic Half-Life	Therapeutic Dose	Component or Derivative
Fibrinogen	50–100 mg/dL	50–70%	72–144 hours	1 unit cryoprecipitate per 5 kg body weight	Cryoprecipitate (100–250 mg fibrinogen/bag)
Prothrombin	10–25%	50%	48–120 hours	10–20 mL plasma per kg body weight	Plasma or PCC
Factor V	10–30%	~80%	4.5–36 hours (avg: 12 hours)	20 mL fresh-frozen plasma per kg body weight, then 2–6 mL fresh-frozen plasma per kg body weight every 12 hours × 5–10 days	Fresh-frozen plasma
Factor VII	>10%	100%	2–5 hours	10–20 mL plasma per kg body weight every 12 hours	Plasma or PCC
Factor X	10–40%	50–95%	20–42 hours	10–20 mL plasma per kg body weight, then 3–6 mL plasma per kg body weight every 12 hours	Plasma or PCC
Factor XI	20–30%	90%	40–80 hours	10–20 mL plasma per kg body weight, then 5 mL/kg body weight daily	Plasma
Factor XIII	<5%	50–100%	12 days	4–6 bags cryoprecipitate or 500 mL plasma every 3 weeks	Cryoprecipitate or plasma

(Modified from Menitove JE. Preparation and clinical use of plasma derived fractions, in Williams WJ, Beutler E, Erslev AJ, Lichtman MA (eds): Hematology. New York, McGraw-Hill, 1990, p 1666, with permission.)

deficiencies is fresh-frozen plasma, although there may be instances in which PCC is necessary to treat factor II, VII, or X deficiencies. Cryoprecipitate may be used to treat a fibrinogen deficiency (see Table 94.7).[29,58]

Complications of Replacement Therapy

Transmission of blood-borne viruses is always a concern when blood and blood-derived products are used. The infection of a large number of hemophiliac patients with hepatitis viruses and HIV during the 1980s prompted the development of virucidal methods to inactivate infectious agents.[23] All currently available factor concentrates under-go donor screening and viral inactivation methods in an effort to minimize donor exposure in patients who do require large amounts of factor. The most common method of inactivation is heat treatment, which includes dry and wet heat. Wet heat is done while the concentrate is in suspension or in solution (pasteurization) and appears to be more effective than dry heat. Other methods of viral inactivation include chemical (solvent/detergent) and affinity chromatography with monoclonal antibodies. These methods effectively eliminate lipid-coated viruses such as HIV and hepatitis B; however, there is still some risk of acquiring blood-borne viruses.[63] Hepatitis A virus has been transmitted in Europe. Protein-coated viruses such as B19 parvovirus are not inactivated by current methods.[23] This last one can be a concern for the HIV-positive hemophiliac, because of the potential for chronic anemia in patients with immune deficiency.

Other complications associated with factor administration include allergic reactions, fever, chills, urticaria, and nausea. Factor concentrates also contain blood group isoagglutinins (anti-A or anti-B) and, when administered in large amounts to patients with blood group A or B, hemolysis can occur.

In addition to the complications listed previously, PCC also has the potential for causing thromboembolic phenomenon (e.g., deep vein thrombosis, pulmonary embolism, disseminated intravascular coagulation) thought to be secondary to the presence of activated vitamin K-dependent factors. Antifibrinolytics such as EACA and tranexamic acid should be avoided in patients receiving PCC in order to avoid thrombotic complications.

Porcine factor VIII, used in patients with inhibitors to factor VIII, is not known to transmit hepatitis or HIV. However, allergic-type reactions including fever, chills, skin rashes, nausea, and headaches have been reported. Patients who experience these reactions may be treated with hydrocortisone and/or diphenhydramine.[64]

Recombinant factor VIII lacks the risk of transfusion-transmitted diseases associated with human factor VIII. Newly diagnosed hemophiliacs or those who are HIV seronegative would benefit most from this product. Adverse effects with these products include metallic taste, mild dizziness, mild rash, burning at the infusion site, and a small drop in blood pressure.[25,26]

ACQUIRED COAGULATION DISORDERS

DISSEMINATED INTRAVASCULAR COAGULATION

Consumptive coagulopathy or defibrination syndrome were some of the terms used in the past to describe the phenomena known today as disseminated intravascular coagulation (DIC).[65] This is a serious complication of several clinical disorders, and can be acute or chronic. Some known clinical settings in which acute and chronic DIC occur are listed in Table 94.8.

Although the causes for DIC can be diverse, once the triggering event is provided the pathophysiology leading to DIC is the same. An overwhelming insult will lead to the formation of thrombin and plasmin beyond the control of the regulatory systems. This process is summarized in Fig. 94.4. Once thrombin is formed it leads to the cleavage of fibrinopeptide A and B from fibrinogen, leaving a fibrin monomer. The monomer polymerizes into a clot leading to microvascular and macrovascular thrombosis. Thrombosis will ultimately decrease blood flow to multiple organs leading to organ damage. Plasmin, also circulating systemically, cleaves fibrinogen into fibrinogen degradation products (FDPs). FDPs can combine with the fibrin monomer before polymerization and the monomer becomes solubilized (also known as soluble fibrin monomer), impairing hemostasis and leading to hemorrhage. Also, some of the FDP may adhere to platelets, causing platelet disfunction that may contribute to clinically significant hemorrhage. In addition plasmin is a proteolytic enzyme that can degrade factors V, VIII, IX, XI, and other plasma proteins. Circulation of plasmin can activate the complement system leading to red cell and platelet lysis. The activated complement system also increases vascular permeability that can cause hypotension and shock.[65,66]

Acute DIC is characterized by a rapid and extensive depletion of coagulation factors and inhibitors as well as evidence of excessive fibrinolysis, which presumably is an attempt to compensate for microvascular clotting. Normally, a constant, balanced dynamic process of clotting and fibrinolysis operates to prevent organ dysfunction, bleeding, or clotting. In acute DIC, this process is disrupted by some sort of injury that causes excessive intravascular coagulation, overcoming normal inhibitory processes. In subacute or chronic DIC, the balance between depletion and synthesis of coagulation factors in the circulation may make diagnosis difficult.

In summary, bleeding problems observed during DIC can be the product of consumption of coagulation factors during clotting, depletion or dysfunction of platelets, interference in fibrin formation by FDP, and lysis of clots by plasmin. It is important to remember that in parallel with the bleeding process thrombosis is occurring and the extent of microvascular obstruction will determine the degree of organ damage.

TABLE 94.8. CONDITIONS ASSOCIATED WITH DISSEMINATED INTRAVASCULAR COAGULATION

Infectious	**Intravascular Hemolysis**
Bacterial	Hemolytic transfusion reaction
Gram-negative	Minor hemolysis
Gram-positive	Massive transfusion
Mycoplasmal	**Cardiovascular**
Rickettsial	Postcardiac arrest
Rocky Mountain Spotted Fever	Aortic aneurysm
Viral	Prosthetic device (aortic balloon)
Cytomegalovirus	Giant hemangiomas
Hepatitis	Acute myocardial infarction
Varicella	Peripheral vascular disease
Chlamydial	**Pulmonary**
Psittacosis	Adult respiratory distress syndrome
Fungal	Pulmonary embolism
Aspergillosis	Pulmonary infarction
Candidiasis	Hyaline membrane disease
Histoplasmosis	**Miscellaneous**
Mycobacterial	Snake bite
Protozoal	Heat stroke
Malaria (falciparum)	Hypothermia/hyperthermia
Tissue Injury	Organic solvent poisoning
Burns	Aspirin poisoning
Extensive surgery	Fat embolism
Crush injuries	Severe anoxia
Multiple trauma	Liver disease
Head trauma	Hematologic
Obstetrics	Sickle cell crisis
Amniotic fluid embolism	Paroxysmal nocturnal hemoglobinuria
Placental abruption	Collagen vascular disease
Missed abortion	Immune complex
Eclampsia	Anaphylaxis
Malignancy	Systemic lupus
Leukemia	
Most carcinomas	
Other	
Pheochromocytoma	
Myeloma	
Sarcomas	
Neuroblastoma	
Histiocytosis X	
Polycythemia vera	

(From Gilbert JA, Scalzi RP. Disseminated intravascular coagulation. Emerg Med Clin North Am 1993;11:475, with permission.)

Clinical Presentation

Acute DIC occurs secondary to many clinical conditions as listed Table 94.8.[65,67] Sepsis is one of the more common causes and, although more frequently linked to gram-nega-

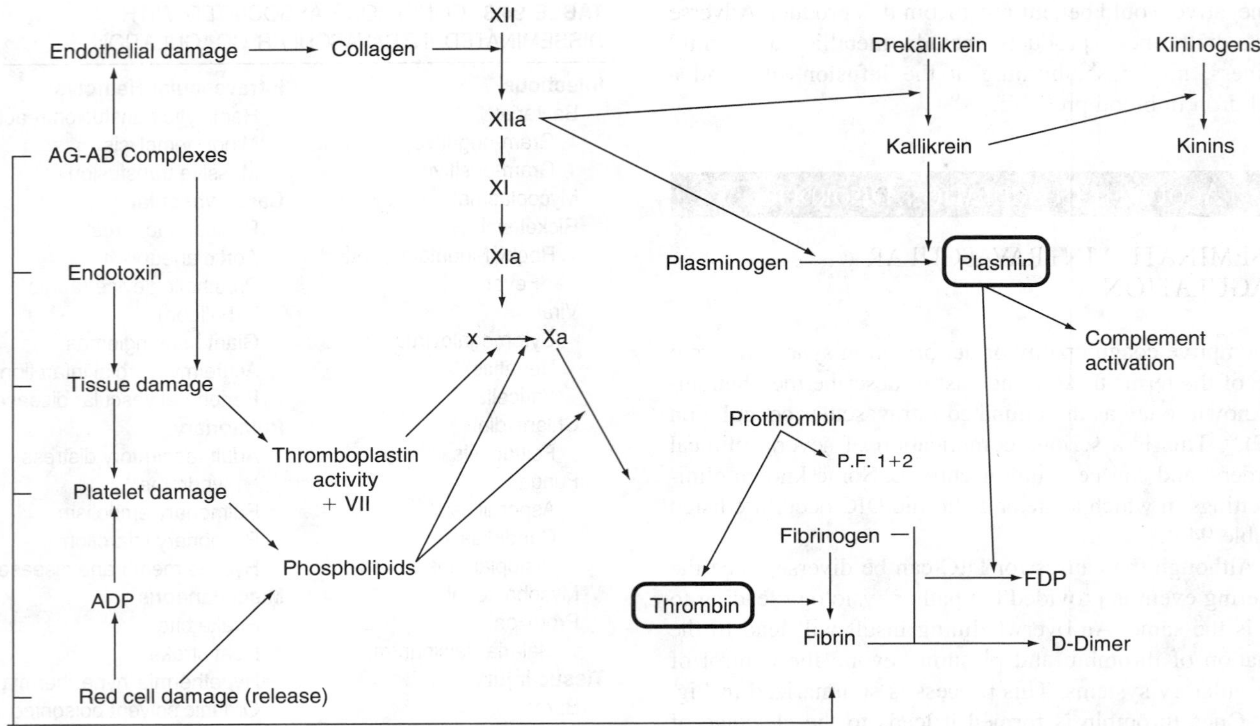

Figure 94.4. Triggering mechanisms of disseminated intravascular. *(Adapted from: Bick RL. Disseminated intravascular coagulation. Objective criteria for diagnosis and management. Med Clin North Am 1994;78:511–543, with permission.)*

tive bacteria, it may occur with gram-positive organisms, fungi, and viruses. Acute DIC may be seen in late pregnancy associated with either abruptio placentae and placenta previa or with a dead fetus or amniotic fluid embolism. Patients who have severe hypotension, who require prolonged surgery, or who suffer tissue injury such as burns or heat stroke may experience DIC.

Subacute and chronic DIC is more commonly associated with malignancies, especially solid tumors. Mucin-producing adenocarcinomas, especially those originating in the gastrointestinal tract or the prostate and sometimes in other organs such as the lung or breast, may be associated with smoldering DIC. Promyelocytic leukemia is almost always associated with DIC to the point that prophylactic treatment has been recommended. In addition, vascular disorders (such as giant hemangiomas) and chronic liver disease have been associated with smoldering DIC.

Diagnosis

Disseminated intravascular coagulation should be suspected on clinical grounds in any of the previously mentioned clinical situations. It should also be considered if the patient develops bleeding from many sites, including oozing from intravenous lines or from invasive procedures. DIC should be suspected with multiple-organ-system failure. Massive bleeding from the gastrointestinal tract or genitourinary system, peripheral cyanosis of the extremities, renal and/or cardiopulmonary failure, or purpura fulminans may dominate the clinical picture.

The laboratory diagnosis of DIC is based on a complete battery of laboratory tests.[65–67] A single laboratory abnormality is insufficient for a diagnosis of DIC. The relative importance of any particular laboratory test is controversial. Routine tests of blood coagulation including PT, APTT, and TT should be done. The PT is usually prolonged, while the APTT is more variable and frequently normal. Occasionally, both tests may be decreased rather than increased. The TT is usually prolonged, because of the absolute decrease in fibrinogen as well as the presence of fibrin split products, which inhibit the conversion of fibrinogen to fibrin. D-dimer is a neoantigen formed as a result of plasmin digestion of cross-linked fibrin; thus, D-dimer is a more specific measure of fibrin degradation products. Because liver disease frequently causes abnormalities in these tests, it can be difficult to separate patients who have decreased synthesis of coagulation factors secondary to liver disease from those with DIC.

Fibrinogen levels below 150 mg/dL and platelet counts below 150,000/mm^3 are seen in 95% of all DIC patients. In addition, 75% of patients have schistocytes (red blood cell fragments). Unfortunately, these findings may also be observed in severe liver disease and hypersplenism. Depressed antithrombin III, protein C, and protein S levels are seen in most patients. Severe initial decreases in antithrombin III levels is a constant finding in septic DIC, and the degree of suppression correlates with mortality in this group. Fibrin split products are not usually greater than 100 μg/dL in chronic liver disease but are quite elevated in patients with DIC; thus, this finding is more specific. Mild elevations in fibrin split products may be seen in many other inflammatory diseases and in association with hematomas and deep vein thrombosis, but these are usually less than 40 μg/dL.

Paracoagulation tests, such as the ethanol gelation or the protamine sulfate precipitation test, measure fibrin monomers and should be specific for DIC but are of low specificity in most series. Factor VIII and V levels should be decreased in DIC; however, these tests may be quite variable. The most specific findings are a low platelet count associated with elevated fibrin split products and depressed antithrombin III and fibrinogen levels. Because the generation of thrombin is the sine qua non of DIC, it would be useful to measure thrombin in plasma. Thrombin cleaves fibrinopeptides A and B from fibrinogen; thus, fibrinopeptides A and B should be elevated in patients with DIC. Initial studies of fibrinopeptide A in patients suspected of having DIC have shown a good correlation, but other inflammatory conditions such as systemic lupus erythematosus, infections, and thrombosis may also result in elevated levels, thus decreasing the specificity of this test.

Treatment (Table 94.9)

The diagnosis of DIC is very difficult, and if left unrecognized it may lead to death as a result of hemorrhage and/or thrombosis. Because of the different mechanisms and clinical manifestations that can occur with DIC, controversy regarding optimal treatment exists. However, there is a consensus that the most important step in the treatment of DIC is treatment of the underlying disease.[65–67] In patients in whom the disease is self-limited, such as a pregnant woman with abruptio placentae or retained placenta, delivery of the fetus with the products of conception usually returns hemostasis to normal. In those patients who have overwhelming sepsis or shock, antibiotics and treatment of hypotension are the mainstays of therapy. In patients who are receiving maximum treatment for the underlying condition, but in whom the process is worsening or in whom bleeding develops, either replacement of deficient factors or the use of anticoagulants has been tried. Fresh-frozen plasma provides volume to expand intravascular space and replaces clotting factors including fibrinogen. If hypofibrinogenemia is severe, cryoprecipitate may be useful, because in addition to the factor VIII in each unit there is a significant amount of fibrinogen. Although it has been argued that replacement of coagulation factors "adds fuel to the fire," in practice this does not appear to make the situation worse, and frequently hemostasis is improved. Antithrombin III (which should remove thrombin from the circulation) is present in fresh-frozen plasma and may be beneficial.

TABLE 94.9. SEQUENTIAL THERAPY FOR DISSEMINATED INTRAVASCULAR COAGULATION

Individualize therapy
Site(s) and severity of hemorrhage
Site(s) and severity of thrombosis
Hemodynamic status
Age
Treat or remove triggering process
Component therapy as indicated
Fresh-frozen plasma
Antithrombin concentrate
Platelet concentrates
Packed red cells
Cryoprecipitate
Stop intravascular clotting problem
Subcutaneous or intravenous heparin
Antithrombin concentrate
Antiplatelet agents?
Inhibit residual fibrino(geno)lysis
EACA
Tranexamic acid

(Adapted from Bick RL. Disseminated intravascular coagulation. Objective criteria for diagnosis and management. Med Clin North Am 1994;78:531, with permission.)

The use of purified antithrombin III has been evaluated in septic shock with DIC.[68] Administration of antithrombin III did not have a significant impact on mortality although, a trend toward improved mortality was observed. Doses used in this trial were higher than doses recommended for replacement: 90–120 IU/kg was the loading dose followed by a continuous infusion of 100 IU/kg. Based on this only trial and anecdotal experiences, the routine use of antithrombin III for all patients with DIC is not recommended at this time.

Anticoagulation is controversial in patients with DIC and specific guidelines are not available.[65,66,69] The main pathogenic factor of DIC is considered to be the generation of intravascular thrombin. Interference of thrombin activity with an agent such as heparin appears to be a logical therapeutic step. The main advantage of heparin is to prevent further consumption of hemostatic factors, since it has no influence on already established microthrombis within the vasculature. Since the major complication of heparin therapy is bleeding, some experts argue against the anticoagulation of patients with an already existing bleeding disorder. Anecdotal reports of improvement in individual patients abound, but controlled clinical studies are lacking. Heparin has not been shown to reduce morbidity or mortality in uncontrolled series. Heparin rarely restores the coagulopathy to normal, although both the deficiency of coagulation factors and the thrombocytopenia may improve. If the patient does not respond to the replacement of coagulation factos, heparin followed by factor replacement may improve the coagulopathy. If the patient has an underlying condition that can be brought under control, improvement of the coagulopathy may provide sufficient time for the DIC to abate. Heparin may be given either as an intravenous bolus (every 4 hours) or as a continuous intravenous infusion via pump. The dose of heparin in DIC is controversial, ranging anywhere from full-dose to low-dose heparin.[65] Full-dose heparin requires that 5000 units as intravenous bolus be administered followed by a continuous infusion at 1000 U/h. Some experts advocate the use of low-dose heparin such as 500 U/h and adjusting the dose based on clinical and laboratory data. Low-dose subcutaneous heparin of 80–100 U/kg every 4–6 hours has been used with success.[65] It is difficult to monitor the APTT, because oftentimes it is elevated before initiation of heparin therapy. Therefore, it is best to follow fibrin degradation products and fibrinogen levels.

Clinical situations in which heparin may be useful have been identified. These include patients who have progressive organ dysfunction, evidence of dermal necrosis or ischemia, retained dead fetus syndrome, aortic aneurysms, hemangiomas, and in patients who require replacement of hemostatic factors. Anticoagulation is contraindicated in patients who have evidence of bleeding into a closed space (e.g., intracranial, intraperitoneal, pericardial).[69]

Heparin with replacement of coagulation factors, including fresh-frozen plasma, cryoprecipitate, and platelets, has been recommended routinely for patients with acute progranulocytic leukemia. In those patients with metastatic carcinoma of the prostate, in whom hormonal therapy may be very efficacious, prophylactic anticoagulation prior to hormonal therapy may be life saving if the patient has DIC.[69]

Antifibrinolytics, such as EACA, have been used in patients in whom the dominant clinical picture is one of excessive fibrinolysis.[56,57,59] It is important that an accurate distinction between defibrination and fibrinolysis be made prior to institution of antifibrinolytic agents. Because EACA can increase fibrin deposition, many experts believe that it is contraindicated more often than not. Most clinicians prefer to use EACA only in conjunction with heparin, unless the patient has recently had cardiopulmonary bypass surgery or has carcinoma of the prostate, the two clinical conditions in which isolated fibrinolysis without generation of thrombin has been well documented. In patients with chronic liver disease, who manifest dominant fibrinolysis, inhibition of the fibrinolytic system has been attempted but is generally unsuccessful.

The procoagulant role of tumor necrosis factor-α (TNF-α) has been proposed as a cause of DIC in sepsis.[69] Treatment against TNF-α such as monoclonal antibodies may prove to be helpful against DIC in the future. Other treatment modalities may include infusion of protein C, the use of protease inhibitors such as gabexate mesylate (FOY), or the use of thrombin inhibitors such as dermatan sulphate.[71–73]

Evaluation of Therapeutic Outcome

The management of DIC is surrounded with controversy and the optimal approach to these patients is still to be determined. Diagnosis and treatment of the underlying disease should be the goal in all cases. Determination of the dominant process between hemorrhage or thrombosis if possible can help focus the treatment approach toward the dominant process. This is often impossible, however, leading to the institution of replacement therapy of the deficient clotting factors and an attempt to control the clotting problems with agents such as heparin. Table 94.9 delineates a sequential approach for DIC, although it is important to remember that treatment for each patient must be individualized.

Risk versus benefit should be considered at the start of any given therapy along with contraindications of the therapy for each patient. Monitoring therapy with laboratory tests can be difficult because the underlying process can cause a variety of laboratory abnormalities. For example, monitoring heparin using APTT can be a complex task especially when the patient has a baseline abnormal APTT; in this case, monitoring fibrinogen and D-dimer to adjust therapy may be more useful. In addition, it is important to combine laboratory parameters with clinical assessment in order to make rational treatment adjustments. Aggressive hemodynamic stabilization and other supportive measures to prevent development of organ failure are also important in the overall management and outcome of these patients, especially since the development of organ failure carries a poor prognosis.

VITAMIN K DEFICIENCY

Vitamin K_1 is necessary for carboxylation of factors II, VII, IX, and X to make complete γ-carboxyglutamic acid molecules from glutamic acid residues.[73] When vitamin K deficiency occurs, the inactive precursors of these coagulation factors, which do not bind calcium, accumulate in the plasma and act as vitamin K antagonists. These have been called protein induced by vitamin K antagonists. Vitamin K is also necessary for the active form of protein C, which inhibits the activated factor V and VIII molecules. In most clinical situations, vitamin K deficiency causes a bleeding diathesis as a result of the marked deficiency of factors II, VII, IX, and X.

Vitamin K is found in green vegetables and is synthesized by bacteria in the large intestine. Naturally occurring vitamin K_1 is fat soluble, but the synthetic analogues are water soluble so that they may be administered parenterally.

Hemorrhagic Disease of the Newborn

Infants may become deficient in vitamin K because of the absence of this vitamin in human milk and because their gut has not had sufficient time to be colonized by bacteria. In addition, some infants may be too immature ability to synthesize vitamin K-dependent clotting factors from the liver. These infants may bleed from the umbilical cord, from the gastrointestinal tract, or occasionally into the brain after birth.

The risk for bleeding was originally thought to be during the first week of life, but it can occur up to the twelfth week of life.[35] Risk factors identified for late hemorrhagic diseases of the newborn include exclusive breast feeding and failure to give vitamin K. The use of oral vitamin K_1 in Japan and Europe is associated with a higher incidence of late hemorrhagic diseases of the newborn.

Although the normal neonate has a mild deficiency of coagulation factors, if vitamin K deficiency exists, the vitamin K-dependent factors are usually less than 25% of normal. In this situation the PT and APTT are prolonged, but TT, fibrinogen, and platelet count are normal. Levels of vitamin K-dependent factors will substantiate the diagnosis.

Infants usually respond to 1 mg of vitamin K_1 parenterally on the first day, which can be repeated every 8 hours until the clotting tests have returned to normal. If there is life-threatening hemorrhage, fresh-frozen plasma should correct the defect immediately. In the United States, it is a common practice to use prophylactic parenteral vitamin K_1 among obstetrical units.

Malabsorption

Patients may become vitamin K deficient because of poor nutrition or malabsorption.[75] A careful dietary history is important in this regard. Patients with a poor diet may have other manifestations of malabsorption, such as vitamin deficiencies and anemia. Broad-spectrum antibiotics may sterilize the large intestine postoperatively, and if vitamin K_1 is not administered, the patient may become vitamin K deficient even more quickly.

Malabsorption resulting from diseases of the small intestine such as celiac disease, amyloidosis, Whipple's disease, and short-bowel syndrome may cause abnormal development in children, weight loss, muscle wasting, and steatorrhea, as well as other manifestations of malnutrition such as vitamin deficiencies and anemia. Significant malabsorption can occur even without symptoms of diarrhea or steatorrhea, requiring quantitation of fat excretion to confirm the presence of malabsorption.

Severe vitamin K deficiency is also seen in obstructive jaundice where bile salts do not reach the small intestine and therefore vitamin K cannot be absorbed. Patients with malabsorption from small-bowel disease or obstructive jaundice require parenteral administration of vitamin K. Vitamin K_1 10 mg weekly is usually sufficient.

Treatment

The treatment of vitamin K deficiency is vitamin K_1. The dose, frequency, and duration of vitamin K_1 depend on the severity of the deficiency and the patient's response.[75] The dose of vitamin K_1 ranges from 2–25 mg and may be administered orally, intramuscularly, subcutaneously, or intravenously. After an oral dose of vitamin K_1 one can expect an increase in blood coagulation factors 6–12 hours later. Even when administered parenterally, the prothrombin time will take 24–48 hours to normalize. Close monitoring of PT in these patients can help to guide therapy. Failure to correct PT after 48 hours should raise suspicion about the etiology of the coagulation abnormality (e.g., liver disease).

The route of administration is dependent on the severity as well as the etiology of prothrombin deficiency. For instance, in patients with severe hypoprothrombinemia it is best to avoid the intramuscular route due to the risk of forming a hematoma. Because of the rare anaphylactic reaction associated with the intravenous route of administration, this route is often restricted to patients who are thrombocytopenic and unable to absorb the drug via the gastrointestinal tract. Vitamin K_1 can be administered subcutaneously to those patients without an intravenous site or postoperatively. In cases of severe hemorrhage, patients should receive fresh-frozen plasma as a source of vitamin K-dependent factors in order to assure immediate correction. Because patients on long-term total parenteral nutrition (TPN) can become vitamin K deficient, it is good practice to prophylactically add 10 mg of vitamin K_1 to the TPN solution weekly.

Identification of patients at risk for vitamin K deficiency and institution of treatment are key components in pharmaceutical care. Selection of the best route of administration and dose are decisive elements for an optimal outcome.

LIVER DISEASE

Clinical Presentation

Liver disease can be associated with bleeding disorders. The degree of coagulopathy correlates with the degree of hepatocellular disease. The liver synthesizes the majority of blood coagulation factors including fibrinogen (factor I) and factors II, VII, IX, X, XII, XIII, and V. In addition, clotting inhibitors of the fibrinolytic system like plasminogen, α_2-antiplasmin, and α_2-macroglobulin are regulated by the hepatic cells. Furthermore, the clearance of activated clotting or fibrinolytic factors, and end products of the fibrinogen–fibrin conversion can be impaired, leading to a fibrinolytic state. Decreased platelet count and function are fairly common findings in liver disease. In addition to the defect in synthesis of these coagulation factors, DIC may occur. The development of DIC can potentially have an additive effect to the coagulopathy observed. Patients have a poor prognosis if hepatocellular disease is so severe that a coagulopathy occurs.[76]

PT, APTT, and TT are useful in screening for a deficiency of liver-dependent factors. The PT is sensitive to deficiencies in the vitamin K-dependent factors (factors II, VII, IX, and X). The APTT helps to determine deficiencies in factor IX as well as some other factors. The TT is helpful in detecting hypofibrinogenemia and dysfibrinogenemia as well as the presence of fibrin degradation products that interfere with fibrin polymerization. Another test that is sometimes useful in hepatic disease is the measurement of clotting time using snake venom, which is not affected by heparin. This test indicates the degree of dysfibrinogenemia. Because defects in polymerization may occur before severe hypofibrinogemia, this may be an indication of the degree of liver dysfunction.

Factor V is synthesized by hepatic cells but is not dependent on vitamin K. Therefore, it may be useful in distinguishing vitamin K deficiency from liver disease. The deficiency of antithrombin III occurs with severe hepatocellular disease and may contribute to the development of DIC. Tests of the lytic system, such as an euglobulin clot lysis time, may show increased activity, either because of decreased clearance of fibrinolytic factors or because of DIC. In acute hepatic failure, plasminogen may be low, reflecting both decreased synthesis and increased catabolism associated with DIC.

Treatment

Treatment of the coagulopathy may occur under two different scenarios: overt bleeding or the correction of the coagulation parameters (e.g., PT, APTT) prior to an invasive procedure. In addition, treatment for other conditions may be necessary (e.g., encephalopathy).

Patients with liver disease should be evaluated with a PT, APTT, TT, and platelet count.[76,77] Although patients can have severe abnormalities in these tests, bleeding may not occur. Patients who are not bleeding should not be treated. Conversely, major bleeding may occur with normal tests secondary to esophageal varices or peptic ulcer disease. To be sure that a vitamin K deficiency is not contributing to the abnormalities, most clinicians administer 10–25 mg of vitamin K_1 for one or several days to be sure that the liver is synthesizing to its capacity.

When a patient bleeds in association with a coagulopathy, replacement therapy may decrease bleeding tendency. Overt bleeding requires aggressive management with blood products. Fresh-frozen plasma supplies all the missing coagulation factors, but fluid overload may be a serious problem. Intensive monitoring to determine frequency of administration is needed for each patient, and to evaluate signs and symptoms of fluid overload. Usually 1–2 units (250–500 mL) of fresh-frozen plasma is necessary every 6 hours in a seriously ill patient. Repeated PT or APTT after completion of infusion can be used to determine if extra units are needed. Additional fresh-frozen plasma may be required if the PT or APTT is greater than 1.5 times the upper limits of the control value.[58] If the patient has ascites, the half-life of many of these factors is decreased, and it is difficult to correct the coagulopathy. Prothrombin complex concentrates can be given, but there is an increased risk of precipitating intravascular coagulation and causing DIC if it is not already present. In general, the use of these concentrates is not recommended. Only when the administration of fresh-frozen plasma does not correct the coagulopathy and the patient continues to have serious bleeding should PCCs be considered.

The use of heparin and antifibrinolytic drugs (EACA) is controversial. EACA has been tried and may be successful, especially with mucosal bleeding from the genitourinary tract; however, acute renal failure may occur. Heparin has not been demonstrated to improve survival and may exacerbate the underlying coagulopathy even if DIC is present. In the few clinical studies that have been done, both controlled and uncontrolled trials have not shown any definite benefit with heparin in severe acute hepatic necrosis. Platelet transfusions may also be necessary if thrombocytopenia occurs secondary to hepatocellular disease and/or hypersplenism.

REFERENCES

1. Bick RL, Murano G. Physiology of hemostasis. Clin Lab Med 1994;14:677–707.
2. Lammle B, Griffin JH. Formation of the fibrin clot: The balance of procoagulant and inhibitory factors. Clin Haematol 1985;14:281–342.
3. Fenton JW, Ofosu FA, Brezniak DV, et al. Understanding thrombin and hemostasis. Hematol Oncol Clin North Am 1993;7:1107–1119.
4. Clouse LH, Comp PC. The regulation of hemostasis: The protein C system. N Engl J Med 1986;314:1298–1304.
5. Lowe GDO. Laboratory support in the diagnosis of coagulation disorders. Clin Haematol 1985;14:571–595.
6. Hassouna HI. Laboratory evaluation of hemostatic disorders. Hematol Oncol Clin North Am 1993;7:1161–1236.
7. Suchman AL, Griner PF. Diagnostic uses of activated partial thromboplastin time and prothrombin time. Ann Intern Med 1986;104:810–816.
8. Santoro SA. Laboratory evaluation of hemostatic disorders, in Hoffman R, Benz EJ, Shattil SJ, et al. (eds): Hematology—Basic Principles and Practice. New York, Churchill Livingstone, 1991, pp 1266–1276.
9. Hougie C. Bleeding time, in Williams WJ, Beutler E, Erslev AJ, Lichtman MA (eds): Hematology. New York, McGraw-Hill, 1990, pp 1775–1776.

10. Hougie C. One-stage prothrombin time, in Williams WJ, Beutler E, Erslev AJ, Lichtman MA (eds): Hematology. New York, McGraw-Hill, 1990, pp 1768–1770.
11. Hougie C. Partial thromboplastin time (PTT) and activated partial thromboplastin time tests, in Williams WJ, Beutler E, Erslev AJ, Lichtman MA (eds): Hematology. New York, McGraw-Hill, 1990, pp 1766–1768.
12. Hougie C. Methods for estimating fibrinogen concentration, in Williams WJ, Beutler E, Erslev AJ, Lichtman MA (eds): Hematology. New York, McGraw-Hill, 1990, pp 1770–1771.
13. Lawn RM, Vehar GA. The molecular genetics of hemophilia. Sci Am 1986;254:48–54.
14. Mammen EF. Factor VII abnormalities. Semin Thromb Hemost 1983;9:22–27.
15. Mammen EF. Factor IX abnormalities. Semin Thromb Hemost 1983;9:28–30.
16. Zimmerman TS, Ruggeri ZM, Fulcher CA. Factor VII/von Willebrand factor. Prog Hematol 1983;13:279–309.
17. Holmeberg L, Nilsson IM. Von Willebrand disease. Clin Haematol 1985;14:461–488.
18. Hoyer LW. Hemophilia A. N Engl J Med 1994;330:38–47.
19. Thompson AR. Structure, function, and molecular defects of factor IX. Blood 1986;67:565–572.
20. Lozier JN, Brinkhous KM. Gene therapy and the hemophilias. JAMA 1994;271:47–51.
21. Lusher JM, Warrier I. Hemophilia A. Hematol Oncol Clin North Am 1992;6:1021–1033.
22. Bowie EJW, Owen CA. The significance of abnormal preoperative hemostatic tests. Prog Hemost Thromb 1980;5:179–209.
23. Kasper CK, Lusher JM, and the Transfusion Practices Committee. Recent evolution of clotting factor concentrates for hemophilia A and B. Transfusion 1993;33:422–434.
24. Lusher JM, Arkin S, Abildaard CF, Schawartz RS, and the Kogenate Previously Untreated Patient Study Group. Recombinant factor VIII for the treatment of previously untreated patients with hemophilia A. N Engl J Med 1993;328:453–459.
25. Bray GL, Gomperts ED, Courter S, et al. A multicenter study of recombinant factor VIII (Recombinate): Safety, efficacy, and inhibitor risk in previously untreated patients with hemophilia A. Blood 1994;83:2428–2435.
26. Anonymous. Recombinant antihemophilic factor. Med Lett Drugs Ther 1993;35(898):51–52.
27. Roberts HR, Jones MR. Hemophilia and related conditions: Congenital deficiencies of prothrombin (factor II), factor V, and factors VII to XII, in Williams WJ, Beutler E, Erslev AJ, Lichtman MA (eds): Hematology. New York, McGraw-Hill, 1990, pp 1453–1473.
28. Bona RD, Weinstein RA, Weisman SJ, et al. The use of continuous infusion of factor concentrates in the treatment of hemophilia. Am J Hematol 1989;32:8–13.
29. Menitove JE. Preparation and clinical use of plasma derived fractions, in Williams WJ, Beutler E, Erslev AJ, Lichtman MA (eds): Hematology. New York, McGraw-Hill, 1990, pp 1659–1673.
30. Richardson DW, Robinson AG. Desmopressin. Ann Intern Med 1985;103:228–239.
31. Rodeghiero F, Castaman G, DiBona E, Ruggeri M. Consistency of responses to repeated DDAVP infusions in patients with von Willebrand's disease and hemophilia A. Blood 1989;74:1997–2000.
32. Ghirardini A, Chistolini A, Trindelli MC, et al. Clinical evaluation of subcutaneously administered DDAVP. Thromb Res 1988;49:363–372.
33. Mannucci PM, Vicente V, Alberca I, et al. Intravenous and subcutaneous administration of desmopressin (DDAVP) to hemophiliacs: Pharmacokinetics and factor VIII responses. Thromb Hemostas 1987;58:1037–1039.
34. Package insert. Stimate (desmopressin acetate) nasal spray. Rhône-Poulenc Rorer. Collegeville, PA. 1994.
35. Nilsson IM, Berntorp E, Löfquist, Petersson H. Twenty-five years' experience of prophylactic treatment in severe haemophilia A and B. J Intern Med 1992;232:25–32.
36. Berntorp CM, Björrkman S, Lindvall K. Pharmacokinetic dosing in prophylactic treatment of hemophilia A. Eur J Haematol 1993;51:247–252.
37. Roberts HR, Eberst ME. Current management of hemophilia B. Hematol Oncol Clin North Am 1993;7:1269–1279.
38. Kim HC, McMilan CW, White GC, et al. Purified factor IX using monoclonal immunoaffinity technique: Clinical trials in hemophilia B and comparison to prothrombin complex concentrates. Blood 1992;79:568–575.
39. Bray G. Inhibitor questions: Plasma-derived factor VIII and recombinant factor VIII. Ann Hematol 1994;68:S29–S34.
40. Ehrenforth S, Kreuz W, Scharrer I, et al. Incidence of development of factor VIII and factor IX inhibitors in haemophiliacs. Lancet 1992;339:594–598.
41. Rosendal FR, Nieuwenhuis HM, Berg VD, et al. A sudden increase in factor VIII inhibitor development in multitransfused hemophilia A patients in the Netherlands. Blood 1993;81:2180–2186.
42. Addiego J, Kasper C, Abildgaard C, et al. Frequency of inhibitor development in haemophiliacs treated with low-purity factor VIII. Lancet 1993;342:462–464.
43. Hoyer LW, Scandella D. Factor VIII inhibitors: Structure and function in autoantibody and hemophilia A patients. Semin Hematol 1994;31:1–5.
44. Ludlam CA, Morrison AE, Kessler C. Treatment of acquired hemophilia. Semin Hematol 1994;31:16–19.
45. Kessler CM. Factor VIII inhibitors: An Algorithmic approach to treatment. Semin Hematol 1994;31:33–36.
46. Hedner U, Glazer S. Management of hemophilia patients with inhibitors. Hematol Oncol Clin North Am 1992;6:1035–1045.
47. Kasper CK. The therapy of factor VIII inhibitors, in Zimmerman TS, Rugerri ZM (eds): Coagulation and Bleeding Disorders: The Role of Factor VIII and von Willebrand Factor. New York, Marcel Dekker, 1989, pp 59–75.
48. Lindley CM, Sawyer WT, Macik BG, et al. Pharmacokinetics and pharmacodynamics of recombinant factor VIIa. Clin Pharmacol Ther 1994;55:638–648.
49. Hilgartner MW. Factor replacement therapy, in Hilgartner MW, Pochedly C (eds): Hemophilia in the Child and Adult. New York, Raven Press, 1989, pp 1–26.
50. Verstraete M. Clinical application of inhibitors of fibrinolysis. Drugs 1985;29:236–261.
51. Walsh LN, Rizza CR, Mathews JM, et al. Epsilon-aminocaproic acid therapy for dental extractions in hemophilia and Christmas disease: A double blind controlled trial. Br J Haematol 1971;20:463–475.

52. Ruggeri ZM. Structure and function of von Willebrand factor: Relationship to von Willebrand disease. Mayo Clin Proc 1991;66:847–861.
53. Howard MA, Sawers RJ, Kirkin BG. Ristocetin: A means of differentiating von Willebrand's disease into two groups. Blood 1973;41:687–690.
54. Bloom AL. Von Willebrand factor: Clinical features of inherited and acquired disorders. Mayo Clin Proc 1991;66:743–751.
55. Sadler JE, Gralnick HR. Commentary: A new classification for von Willebrand Disease. Blood 1994;84:676–679.
56. Aledort LM. Treatment of von Willebrand's disease. Mayo Clin Proc 1991;66:841–846.
57. Scott JP, Montgomery RR. Therapy of von Willebrand disease. Semin Thromb Hemost 1993;19:37–47.
58. Fresh-Frozen Plasma, Cryoprecipitate, and Platelets Administration Practice Guidelines Development Task Force of the College of American Pathologists. Practice parameters for the use of fresh-frozen plasma, cryoprecipitate, and platelets. JAMA 1994;271:777–781.
59. Cattaneo M, Moia M, Della Valle P, et al. DDAVP shortens the prolonged bleeding times of patients with severe von Willebrand disease treated with cryoprecipitate. Evidence for a mechanism of action independent of released von Willebrand factor. Blood 1989;74:1972–1975.
60. Mannucci PM, Tenconi PM, Castarman G, Rodeghiero F. Comparison of four virus-inactivated plasma concentrates for treatment of severe von Willebrand disease: A cross-over randomized trial. Blood 1992;79:3130–3137.
61. Hanna WT, Bonna RD, Zimmerman CE, et al. The use of intermediate and high purity factor VIII products in the treatment of von Willebrand disease. Thromb Haemost 1994;71:173–179.
62. Mammen EF. Congenital coagulation disorders. Semin Thromb Hemost 1983;9:1–72.
63. Shapiro CN. Transmission of hepatitis viruses. Ann Intern Med 1994;120:82–84.
64. Hay CRM, Lozier JN, Lee CA, et al. Porcine factor VIII therapy in patients with congenital hemophilia and inhibitors: Efficacy, patient selection, and side effects. Semin Hematol 1994;31:20–25.
65. Bick RL. Disseminated intravascular coagulation. Objective criteria for diagnosis and management. Med Clin North Am 1994;78:511–543.
66. Risberg B, Andreasson S, Erickson E. Disseminated intravascular coagulation. Acta Anaesthesiol Scand 1991;35:S60–S71.
67. Gilbert JA, Scalzi RP. Disseminated intravascular coagulation. Emerg Med Clin North Am 1993;11:465–480.
68. Fourrier F, Chopin C, Huart JJ, et al. Double-blind, placebo-controlled trial of antithrombin III concentrates in septic shock with disseminated intravascular coagulation. Chest 1993;104:883–888.
69. Feinstein DI. Treatment of disseminated intravascular coagulation. Semin Thromb Hemostas 1988;14:351–362.
70. Levi M, ten Cate H, van der Poll T, van Deventer SJH. Pathogenesis of disseminated intravascular coagulation in sepsis. JAMA 1993;270:975–979.
71. Okajima K, Imamura H, Koga S, et al. Treatment of patients with disseminated intravascular coagulation by protein C. Am J Hematol 1990;33:277–278.
72. Cofrancesco E, Boschetti C, Leonardi P, et al. Dermatan sulphate for the treatment of disseminated intravascular coagulation (DIC) in acute leukaemia: A randomized, heparin-controlled pilot study. Thromb Res 1994;74:65–75.
73. Okamura T, Niho Y, Itoga T, et al. Treatment of disseminated intravascular coagulation and its prodromal stage with gabexate mesilate (FOY): A multicenter trial. Acta Haematol 1993;90:120–124.
74. Shearer MJ. Vitamin K. Lancet 1995;345:229–234.
75. Marcus R, Coulston AM. Fat-soluble vitamins: Vitamins A, K, and E, in Gilman AG, Rall TW, Nies AS, Palmer T (eds): The Pharmacological Basis of Therapeutics. New York, Pergamon Press, 1990, pp 1563–1566.
76. O'Grady JG, Langley PC, Isola LM, et al. Coagulopathy of fulminant hepatic failure. Semin Liver Dis 1986;6:159–163.
77. Violi F, Ferro D, Quintarelli, et al. Clotting abnormalities in chronic liver disease. Dig Dis 1992;10:162–172.

Chapter 95

Sickle Cell Anemia

Clarence E. Curry, Jr., PharmD, and Eula D. Beasley, PharmD

Although Herrick[1] has generally been credited with the discovery of sickle cell anemia (SCA), Konotey-Ahulu[2] has presented evidence that the problem had been recognized in Africa by Ghanians long before the earliest description offered in the medical literature after the turn of the twentieth century. Such information suggests that SCA is not a distinctly modern problem, as once thought.

After Herrick's case report of a 20-year-old black male West Indian student observed in 1904, but unreported until 1910, many investigators became interested in this disorder and subsequently made contributions to the literature. In 1917, Emmel[3] offered pertinent information regarding the familial nature of the disease. He also suggested that sickling of red blood cells (RBCs) might occur because of a decreased oxygen supply. Huck[4] later showed that the sickling characteristic was contained in the RBCs as opposed to the plasma. He also suggested that the sickling process was reversible. The reversibility of the sickle shape was subsequently demonstrated by Hahn and Gillespie,[5] who showed that the process depended on the degree of oxygenation of plasma hemoglobin. A state of reduced oxygen tension results in the sickle form. In 1930, Scriver and Waugh[6] confirmed, *in vivo,* the reversibility of the sickling process. In 1940, Ham and Castle[7] discussed the pathogenesis of *in vivo* sickling. They suggested that sickling results in an increase in blood viscosity and decreased blood circulation, leading to increased deoxygenation and greater sickling.

Neel[8] and Beet,[9] working independently, provided evidence that SCA and sickle cell trait were inheritable. In a 1948 paper, Watson et al.[10] speculated that sickling occurred in adult patients due to a different type of adult hemoglobin. Their speculation was based on observations of infants who did not show sickling until they were about 4 months old. In 1949, Nobel laureate Linus Pauling and his coworkers,[11] using moving boundary electrophoresis, reported that hemoglobin from a patient with SCA had a mobility different from that of hemoglobin from a normal adult. As a result, the hemoglobin of SCA patients was referred to as sickle hemoglobin or hemoglobin S (Hb-S) and the hemoglobin of normal individuals, hemoglobin A (Hb-A).

Etiology

The biochemical defect that leads to the development of hemoglobin S involves the substitution of valine for glutamic acid as the sixth amino acid in the β polypeptide chain. Hemoglobin C, another abnormal hemoglobin commonly included in the sickle cell disease group, is produced by the substitution of lysine for glutamic acid as the sixth amino acid in the β chain (Fig. 95.1).

The α chains of Hb-S, Hb-A, and Hb-C are structurally identical. Therefore, sickling and the related sequelae can be explained on the basis of the chemical difference in the β chain. When deoxygenated, both Hb-S and Hb-A have similar physical properties in dilute solutions; however, in concentrated solutions, deoxygenated Hb-S is insoluble and forms a gel, whereas deoxygenated Hb-A remains soluble. This solubility difference represents the physiochemical basis for sickling.

Incidence

A common misconception is that sickle hemoglobin is found only in people of African heritage. However, it also occurs in a wide area including the Mediterranean region, parts of Greece and Italy, as well as India, Iran, and Turkey. Serjeant[12] has noted that sickle hemoglobin is becoming more common in the United Kingdom, France, the Netherlands, Belgium, and Germany. Central America and South America also are affected.

Hemoglobin S is the most frequently found sickle gene among the black population in the United States, where the frequency of sickle cell trait is about 8% and that of sickle cell disease is 1 in 400.

Hemoglobin C is found chiefly in west and northern Africa or in descendants of people from this area, with the highest frequency in northern Ghana.[13] Hb-C has a frequency of about 3% in the U.S. population. Other abnormal hemoglobins seen in various areas are hemoglobin E (Sri Lanka, Malaysia, Thailand, Cambodia, Laos, Burma, Indonesia, Vietnam, and the Philippines) and hemoglobin D

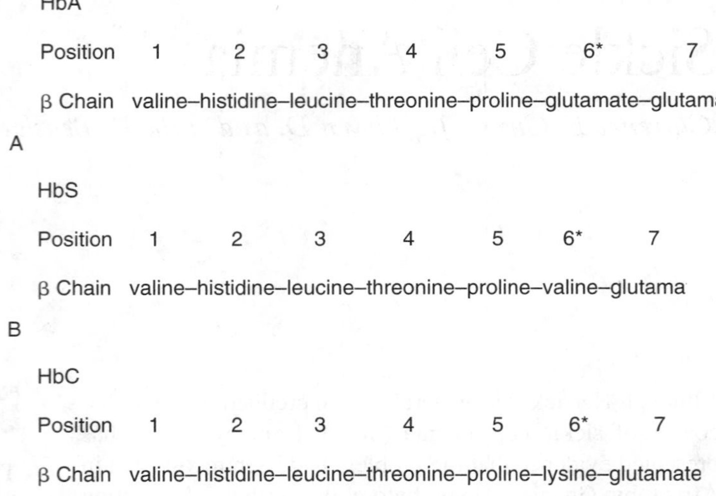

Figure 95.1. The sixth-position (*) amino acid in the β chain differentiates (A) Hb-A from (B) Hb-S and (C) Hb-C.

(India, Pakistan, Afghanistan, and Iran). Of all the sickle hemoglobin genes, Hb-S is the most common.

For years it has appeared that sickle cell trait offered a degree of protection against malarial infection. Abnormal RBCs are less easily parasitized by *Plasmodium falciparum* than are normal RBCs. Consequently, reports have suggested that persons who are heterozygous for the sickle gene (trait) have a selective advantage in regions (tropical areas) where malaria is hyperendemic.[14] However, later observations have shown that adults with the trait, unlike children, were sick more often from this infection than adults with Hb-C or normal homozygotes.[15] It now appears that the advantage of individuals carrying the trait over those with normal hemoglobin is a limited one, occurring especially during the early childhood years before the child has developed a substantial degree of acquired immunity owing to their own antibody production.[16]

Hemoglobinopathies are inherited in an autosomal dominant manner. Patients having SCA must inherit two genes for the S hemoglobin. Figure 95.2 illustrates the genetic profiles possible for offspring of parents with normal hemoglobin, sickle cell trait, and SCA. A person with entirely normal hemoglobin is designated AA. A person with the sickle cell trait is designated AS. Sickle cell anemia is represented as SS.

When one parent has normal hemoglobin and the other carries the sickle cell trait (Example One), the children may have either normal hemoglobin or sickle cell trait. No child from this union would have SCA.

When both parents carry the trait (Example Two), there is a 50% chance a child will carry sickle cell trait, a 25% chance a child will have SCA, and a 25% chance the child will have normal hemoglobin.

If one parent has SCA and the other parent has normal hemoglobin (Example Three), all children will carry the trait. Again, no child from this union will have SCA.

Offspring from the union of one parent with SCA and the other with sickle cell trait have a 50% chance of having SCA and a 50% chance of carrying sickle cell trait (Example Four).

The union of two persons with SCA, if able to produce offspring, would produce only children with SCA.[17]

Pathophysiology

In the pathogenesis of sickle cell disease, three known problems appear to constitute the basis of the various clinical manifestations: impaired circulation, destruction of RBCs, and stasis of blood flow. These three problems probably relate directly to two major disturbances involving RBCs. The first involves damage to the membrane of the RBCs containing hemoglobin S. These cells may lose potassium and water, leading to a dehydrated state that enhances the formation of sickled forms. After continually repeating this process, the RBC membrane probably retains greater quantities of calcium and develops a more rigid form, that of an irreversibly sickled cell (ISC).

When the blood of patients with sickle cell disease is deoxygenated, blood viscosity increases. This second disturbance has been related to an alteration of the flow properties of RBCs containing polymerized hemoglobin S. The polymerization process is a manifestation of the β-chain substitution of valine for glutamic acid.[15] Polymerization allows deoxygenated hemoglobin molecules to exist as a semisolid gel. This process is affected by small changes in mean corpuscular hemoglobin concentration (MCHC). Temperature, pH, and the oxygen affinity of the RBCs all contribute to the deoxygenation process. These cells have more difficulty deforming themselves than normal cells and, as a result, remain more rigid, retarding their flow, particularly through the microcirculation. Evidence suggests that significant amounts of intracellular polymerized Hb-S, enough to bring about a change in normal erythrocyte flow, may exist at oxygen saturation levels as high as 80–90%[18]; however, such a

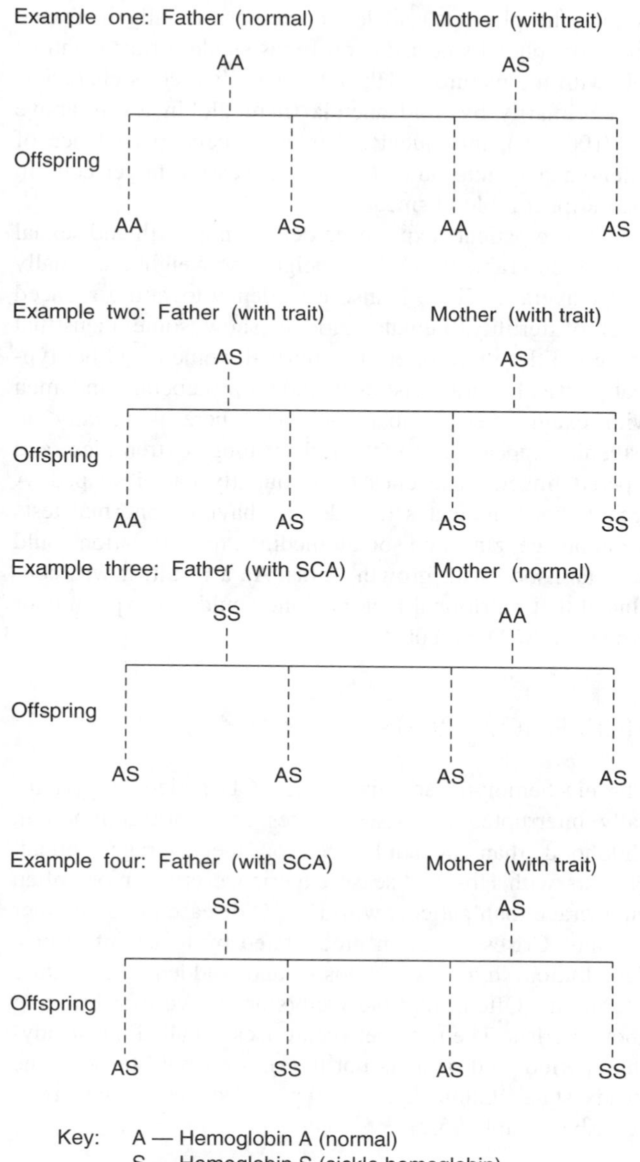

Figure 95.2. Inheritance scheme for the sickle gene.

finding has yet to be specifically related to the actual clinical events in a SCA patient. The presence of sickled RBCs increases blood viscosity and encourages sludging in the capillaries and small venous vessels. Such obstructive events lead to local tissue hypoxia, which tends to accentuate the pathologic process. Other events, such as the elevation of fibrinogen or globulin level, or both, also increase blood viscosity and, thus, would aggravate the hematologic environs in the sickle cell patient (e.g., during infections).[19] The cycle of sickling and unsickling that occurs in response to variations in oxygen tension results in loss of the cell membrane containing hemoglobin. This sickle–unsickle cycle leads to loss of the membrane and to production of the ISC. Membranes of ISCs are permanently deformed regardless of the oxygenation state of the hemoglobin within the cell.

Intravascular destruction of sickle cells may occur at an accelerated rate in this disease. In view of the various stresses of circulation, including rigid deoxygenated cells and repetitive sickle–unsickle cycles, cell fragmentation is a likely result.[20]

It has been known for a number of years that some cells of patients with sickle cell disease contain increased amounts of hemoglobin F (Hb-F) and that Hb-F does not appear to participate in the gelling of deoxygenated Hb-S. Red blood cells containing Hb-F sickle less readily than cells with Hb-S. In contrast, ISCs exhibit a lower concentration of Hb-F and a higher MCHC. ISCs are also smaller than other red cells of patients with SCA. Increased levels of fetal hemoglobin moderate or even ameliorate the disease in some patients, thereby producing more benign forms of SCA.

The pathogenesis of a number of clinical manifestations associated with sickle cell disease is not easily attributed directly to the sickling phenomenon. Other factors may be responsible. For example, impairment in reticuloendothelial function in SCA may be noted early in the sickle cell disease patient due to functional asplenia, loss of splenic function with an intact spleen. This defect may be related to the increased susceptibility of many of these patients to infection (particularly pneumococcal disease) and to disseminated intravascular coagulation (DIC).[19] Patients with SCA have a deficient pneumococcal opsonization, although the exact nature of the defect is debatable.[21,22]

Clinical Presentation

In the patient who is homogyzous for Hb-S, the anemia usually appears from 4–6 months after birth. Symptoms are delayed because the infant's RBCs contain mainly fetal hemoglobin (Hb-F). Fetal hemoglobin's oxygen carrying ability and its lesser propensity to engage in sickling prevents the development of early clinical symptoms. Still, sufficient quantities of Hb-S are present at birth to allow a diagnosis to be made by hemoglobin electrophoresis. As RBC turnover occurs during those early months, RBCs containing Hb-F are replaced by cells containing Hb-S. This replacement process typically leads to attacks of pain frequently accompanied by fever. Pneumonia is often a common initial symptom and splenomegaly a common finding. Many cases initially present with pain and swelling of the hands and feet. This condition is commonly referred to as "hand-and-foot syndrome" or dactylitis. Many states have established newborn screening programs for SCA and other hemoglobinopathies along the lines of the long-standing PKU screening.[23]

The term *sickle cell disease* (SCD) does not exclusively imply that the patient is homozygous for hemoglobin S (Hb-SS). Sickle cell anemia is a form of SCD in which both abnormal genes code for formation of hemoglobin S; however, varying degrees of anemia may be present in other variants of SCD.

As previously noted, a person who carries sickle cell trait has one normal gene (A) and one abnormal gene (S, C, D, etc.). Such a person would not belong in the SCD group. A person with a genotype of AS is often referred to as a heterozygote; however, caution must be exercised because the heterozygous states can be pathologic, especially sickle–C and sickle–thalassemia.[3] Beta thalassemia is often found in conjunction with Hb-S. Beta^{+} thalassemia usually leads to a milder course than the homozygous SS state. Beta^{0} thalassemia leads to a course similar to that of the homozygous SS patient. In addition, several haplotypes characterize the beta^{s} gene resulting in differing clinical and hematologic courses. Included among these types are the three most commonly found in the United States: the Central Africa Republic (CAR) haplotype, characterized by severe disease; the Atlantic West African Senegal (SEN) haplotype, characterized by mild disease; and the Central West African Benin (BEN) haplotype, characterized by a course intermediate to the preceding two. Although there are a number of other haplotypes seen around the world, the remaining major types include Saudi Arabian (Saudi) and Cameroon (CAM). Both of these types usually result in milder courses.[24]

Hemoglobin disorders can be screened by hemoglobin electrophoresis on cellulose acetate, followed by solubility testing for sickling in all blood samples showing anything other than the usual Hb-A. If such tests suggest the presence of abnormal hemoglobin patterns, confirmation should be sought using such methods as citrate agar electrophoresis, quantitation of hemoglobin fractions, alkali denaturation, and family studies.[25]

Persons with sickle cell trait are usually asymptomatic, although some clinical signs and symptoms have occasionally been associated with sickle cell trait. An impairment of renal function, which probably arises from the sickling of RBCs, tends to promote a more dilute urine. Such patients may be at some risk of dehydration during periods in which the body normally conserves water, such as hot and dry weather. Hematuria has also been noted and probably also relates to sickling within the kidney.

Castro and Scott[26] have shown that a group of persons with sickle cell trait had a small but statistically significant decrease in RBC size and in MCHC; however, the decreases did not affect the blood hemoglobin or hematocrit levels. The cause is unknown. Although some persons with sickle cell trait may experience abnormalities under certain conditions, these instances are not routine and trait carriers are not considered to have clinical disease.

The usual clinical signs and symptoms associated with Hb-SS disease include chronic anemia, fever and pallor, arthralgia, scleral icterus, abdominal pain, weakness, anorexia, fatigue, liver, and heart, and hematuria. Infants may show enlargement of the spleen. The typical Hb-SS patient exhibits reduced Hgb and increased reticulocyte count. The platelets and leukocytes are usually increased and a peripheral smear demonstrates sickle forms. Contrast this with the picture of Hb-SC disease, which is characterized primarily by mild anemia (hemoglobin levels above 9 g/100 mL), infrequent episodes of pain, persistence of splenomegaly into adult life, and excessive target cells in the peripheral blood smear.

These patients experience delays in growth and sexual maturation (Table 95.1). Both height and weight are usually below average. There is also a tendency toward a reduced level of fertility. Female patients show some menstrual abnormalities more often than normal women.[27] Other typical physical characteristics include a protuberant abdomen with exaggerated lumbar lordosis. There is usually an asthenic appearance with rather long extremities and tapered fingers. The chest is frequently barrel shaped. A recent report indicates that despite having abnormal tests for bone age, zinc, and somatomedin c, no correlation could be established with growth status. As a result, it was concluded that nutritional factors alone could not explain poor growth in SCD patients.[28]

SICKLE CELL CRISIS

Chronic hemolytic anemia in the SCD patient is periodically interrupted by crises. Crises are more common in childhood than in adulthood for the average patient. Patients with Hb-SS disease experience crises more often on average than patients with Hb-SC disease or some other variants. Crises are often precipitated by fever, infections, dehydration, hypoxia, acidosis, and sudden temperature alterations. Often, multiple factors are at work in bringing about a crisis. The time between crises is called the steady-state period, and patients not in crisis are said to be in the steady state.[2] Clinically, four types of crises are generally described (Table 95.2).

TABLE 95.1. DELAYED GROWTH AND SEXUAL MATURATION IN SICKLE CELL DISEASE

Growth is delayed in both sexes; in variant as well as homozygous SCA.

Weight is more affected than height; delays are more significant in children >7 years.

Adolescents with homozygous disease, on the average, experience a 2-year delay in sexual maturation.

No pituitary–hypothalamic axis abnormalities have been demonstrated.

The degree of anemia correlates positively with a delay in growth.

Nutritional factors (intake, requirements, absorption, and utilization) are thought to be important in the delayed growth process. Mechanisms are yet undetermined.

(Adapted from Wethers DL. Delayed growth and sexual maturation in SCD. Ann NY Acad Sci 1989;565:137–142.)

TABLE 95.2. MANIFESTATIONS OF SICKLE CELL DISEASE: CRISES AND COMPLICATIONS

Crisis	Characteristic
Vaso-occlusive	Infarction/pain
Hemolytic	Massive hemolysis
Splenic sequestration	Sequestration of red blood cells
Aplastic	Bone marrow failure
Organ system	Complication
Pulmonary	Acute chest syndrome
Neurologic	Various, including cerebrovascular accident
Dermatologic	Chronic ulcers
Cardiovascular	Hypertrophy
Genitourinary	Priapism, hematuria, hyposthenuria
Skeletal	Aseptic necrosis, osteomyelitis
Ocular	Retinal problems
Hepatic	Cholelithiasis

Aplastic (Hypoplastic) Crisis

The bone marrow becomes hypoplastic. There may be associated pain. There is a definite drop in reticulocytes accompanied by a rapidly developing severe anemia. The crises is often thought to be caused by a viral infection. The presenting patient is most often under the age of 18.

Hemolytic Crisis

The patient affected shows a rate of hemolysis even greater than that usually present. Hemoglobin and RBC levels fall, often without a change in the number of reticulocytes and with a hyperplastic bone marrow. This crisis may be accompanied by pain and fever. An increase in the icteric state is usually observed. This condition may be confused with glucose-6-phosphate dehydrogenase (G6PD) deficiency particularly during a febrile episode when antipyretics are used.[29]

Splenic Sequestration Crisis

This crisis is described as a sudden massive enlargement of the spleen and liver resulting from the sequestration by these organs of blood from the reticuloendothelial system. There is a dramatic fall in hematocrit and hemoglobin concentration, with no evidence of marrow failure and accelerated hemolysis. The trapping of the sickled red cells by the spleen also leads to a drop in circulating blood volume resulting in hypotension and shock. The condition is most often seen in infants and children because they have intact spleens that have not undergone multiple infarctions and fibrosis. Because repeated infarctions lead to autosplenectomy as the disease progresses, the incidence of this type of crisis declines as adolescence approaches. These crises are a cause of sudden death in young children. It is rarely seen in adult Hb-SS patients but may be seen in adult Hb-SC or sickle cell thalassemia patients.[30]

Vaso-Occlusive (Infarctive) Crisis

This most common type of crisis has a number of clinical manifestations. Pain usually occurs over the involved areas, but there may be no change in hemoglobin or other laboratory values. Laboratory changes that may be seen include leukocytosis, increased serum fibrinogen, and decreased serum pH and bicarbonate. A recent study of pain in SCD has concluded that early death is associated with the number of pain episodes in patients older than 20 years. Adult patients with three or more episodes of pain per year had a higher death rate than those with fewer than three episodes per year.[31] Painful crisis may have numerous possible precipitating factors including dehydration, muscular exertion, emotional upset, and changes in climate. The following are the usually observed manifestations:

Sickle cell dactylitis (hand-and-foot syndrome). A condition that occurs in infancy and early childhood, in which the dorsal aspects of the hands and feet, as well as the fingers and toes, swell. The episodes are painful and accompanied by erythema. There usually is no permanent damage.

Involvement in joints and extremities. This form of crisis may be caused by areas of infarction over long bones or of periarticular tissues of the larger joints. Often, the pain mimics that of rheumatic fever. Pain may migrate from one site to another. Mild temperature elevations may be noted.

Abdominal involvement. These crises may simulate an acute abdominal process suggesting surgical intervention. The episodes are usually due to areas of infarction in abdominal structures. The pain may be severe and episodic in nature. Although the usual duration is about 3 or 4 days, protracted courses are occasionally encountered. Low-grade fever is often present.

Hepatic involvement. This type of crisis is characterized by a rise in the serum bilirubin level well beyond the steady-state value, as some degree of hyperbilirubinemia is common in SCD. It is associated with right upper-quadrant pain. Widespread intrahepatic sickling may occur, leading to hepatocellular necrosis and swelling. Such an extensive occurrence could be fatal. These severe obstructive jaundice processes, as well as episodes of cholelithiasis, must be distinguished early in affected patients. Hepatic crises are seen more often in the older sickle cell patient.

Pulmonary involvement. Lung infarctions occur in both children and adults. Children seem to have pulmonary episodes most often as a result of infection. It may sometimes be very difficult to distinguish between infection and infarction and, indeed, both may be present. Infection is usually due to the pneumococcus; infarction is often related to embolization from sickled RBCs or pieces of necrotic bone marrow tissue.

COMPLICATIONS

Acute chest syndrome is the pulmonary illness that occurs in SCD patients and is characterized by cough, dyspnea, chest pain, fever, pulmonary infiltration, and an equivocal response to antibiotic therapy.[32] Pulmonary infarcts seem more often to involve the lower lobes of the lungs and are a frequent cause of pleural effusions. Pneumonia appears to occur most often in the middle and upper lobes. These pulmonary manifestations can and do occur in the absence of bone, joint, or abdominal pain. There is some degree of disagreement over the predominant cause of acute chest syndrome. Oppenheimer and Esterly[33] reviewed autopsy findings on 36 patients with sickle cell anemia; intimal proliferation and pulmonary infarcts had occurred in more than one-fifth of the cases. Sprinkle and associates[32] recently reviewed 100 cases in children and found little evidence of bacterial infection to support the clinical picture seen. These data contrast dramatically with those of Barrett-Conner,[34] who showed pulmonary infarction in only 5% of 66 cases. Furthermore, intravascular fluid overload with pulmonary edema can occasionally simulate sickle cell lung disease in the sickle cell patient hospitalized for other causes.[35] Sudden death can occur after the occlusion of large vessels in the absence of infarction. Pulmonary edema has been a common finding in patients who have died suddenly, the pulmonary capillaries of such patients being overly distended from packed sickled cells.[36]

Neurologic abnormalities can occur in both adults and children. Vaso-occlusive processes occasionally lead to cerebral vascular occlusion in which patients show signs and symptoms similar to those of stroke. These include drowsiness, paralysis, transitory or permanent blindness, aphasia, visual disturbances, spinal cord infarction, and convulsions. The onset is usually sudden, but occasionally may be gradual. Milder symptoms may occur as a result of vascular stasis. Some patients recover rapidly and completely. Others are left with permanent neurologic deficits.

Chronic leg ulcers are a difficult problem and a common finding in many young adults with Hb-SS disease. The inner aspect of the lower leg just above the ankle seems to be the site most often affected. Ulcers are often seen after trauma or infection. They are usually slow to heal (several weeks to a year).

Cholelithiasis is a common occurrence in the SCD patient. It is seen more frequently and at a younger age than in the general population. It is the result of the chronic hemolysis that occurs in increased bilirubin production. Cholecystitis, exemplified by pain in the right iliac fossa, can be confused with abdominal pain crises.[37]

As with any anemia, cardiovascular abnormalities, including cardiac enlargement and various murmurs, occur. Patients complain of various degrees of exertional dyspnea, tachycardia, and palpitation owing to the decreased oxygen-carrying capacity of the system. Effects are most prominent in Hb-SS disease.

Priapism is a very painful complication that develops in certain male patients. It is caused by sickling in the sinusoids of the penis. This produces a sustained painful erection that might last several hours or several days. Impotence has been reported after repeated episodes. A recent report[38] discussed a syndrome that has been seen in some priapism patients. Called ASPEN (Association of Sickle Cell Disease, Priapism, Exchange Transfusion and Neurological Events), it occurs after partial exchange transfusion to treat priapism and is characterized by severe headache and other neurologic symptoms ranging from seizures to obtundation that requires ventilation.

Destructive bone and joint problems are frequently seen. Aseptic necrosis, particularly of the femoral or humeral heads, causes permanent damage and disability. This problem is seen both in patients with Hb-SS disease and in heterozygous patients. Patients are also susceptible to an increased incidence of osteomyelitis. The organism most often responsible is *Salmonella.*

Ocular problems occur in the form of transient monocular blindness, visual field defects from retinal hemorrhage, retinal detachment, vitreous hemorrhage, venous microaneurysms, and neovascularization in the adult. Patients with Hb-SC disease are most likely to suffer from these disorders.

Renal complications include unilateral hematuria and hyposthenuria. Death from renal disease is unusual except in long-term survivors.

GENERAL MANAGEMENT

Although management techniques have improved the general health and life prospects of the typical patient with SCA, the therapeutic management of this problem continues to be largely centered around supportive care.

FOLIC ACID

Folic acid demands are increased in sickle cell patients because there is accelerated erythropoiesis. Low serum folate levels are common and megaloblastic changes have been reported.[39–41] The incidence of megaloblastic anemia in association with SCD, however, is unknown. Although folic acid supplementation has become standard, there is little controlled data evaluating this therapy. A double-blind controlled study of folate supplementation in 117 Jamaican children ages 6 months to 4 years did not support the need for routine folate supplementation. Folic acid 5 mg/d did not result in significant improvement in hemoglobin levels, growth characteristics, or occurrence of infections. In addition, folic acid supplementation did not affect painful episodes. The mean corpuscular volume, however, was significantly lower in the folate-treated group, suggesting the existence of a marginal folate deficiency in patients receiving placebo. As the authors caution, however, the results of this study may not be applicable elsewhere due to dietary differences. In general, patients who are at increased risk of folate deficiency include infants, pregnant women, and adolescents.[42]

Although it is not clear that folic acid supplementation is essential, there exists at least a theoretical argument for prescribing folate supplementation in all sickle cell patients due to increased demands. A dose of 1 mg/d is most commonly used and is more than adequate for supplementation.[39–41]

PROPHYLAXIS OF PNEUMOCOCCAL INFECTIONS

Administration of the pneumococcal vaccine alone or in combination with prophylactic penicillin may be of benefit in sickle cell patients. Sickle cell patients are more susceptible to infection due to encapsulated organisms than the general population due mainly to impairment of splenic function. There is an especially high risk of pneumococcal infections with sickle cell patients being 300 to 400 times more likely to develop pneumococcal septicemia or meningitis.[43] Several studies have been conducted to evaluate the efficacy of immunization against pneumococcal infections. Results have varied greatly. Prior to 1983, however, the available pneumococcal vaccine was a 14-valent product. It now contains 23 capsular polysaccharide types. Although there are no controlled studies demonstrating decreased morbidity and mortality from pneumococcal infection with the use of the 23-valent product, it is recommended that all patients with sickle cell disease receive the vaccine at 24 months of age or shortly thereafter.[23]

The use of prophylactic penicillin has been shown to decrease the risk of pneumococcal septicemia and meningitis. Early administration of prophylactic penicillin, with therapy preferably begun before the age of 4 months, is suggested in children with sickle cell anemia. It has not been determined how long prophylactic penicillin therapy should be continued. In patients in whom penicillin therapy is begun in infancy it is recommended that it be continued indefinitely until a safe discontinuation time is determined by clinical studies. The initiation of therapy in children older than age 5 who have not received previous prophylaxis is probably not required.[23] Regimens that have been utilized are shown in Table 95.3.[44–46]

TABLE 95.3. PNEUMOCOCCAL PROPHYLAXIS REGIMENS

Benzathine penicillin	600,000 U IM q month	Ref. 44
Benzathine penicillin	600,000 U IM q 4 weeks for age 6 months–6 yr; 1.2 mU q 4 weeks for age >6 yr	Ref. 45
Penicillin V potassium	125 mg bid orally	Ref. 46

Potential noncompliance is a concern with long-term oral penicillin use. The occurrence of pneumococcal septicemia with some subsequent deaths has been reported in patients who were prescribed penicillin, but were noncompliant.[47]

Another concern in the attempt to decrease pneumococcal infections is the increase in the number of penicillin-resistant pneumococcal strains. Drug-resistant strains are far more common now than they were in the past.[48] This will present new challenges in the sickle cell population.

HEMOPHILUS INFLUENZA VACCINE

Routine pediatric immunization should include administration of the hemophilus b conjugate vaccine. This is of particular importance in the sickle cell patient due to increased susceptibility to hemophilus influenza infections. It is currently recommended that an immunization series be initiated at 2 months of age when possible with an appropriate vaccine. For children age 15 months to 5 years who have not received prior immunization against hemophilus influenza a single dose should be administered.

TRANSFUSION/EXCHANGE TRANSFUSIONS

Transfusion therapy has been used to treat life-threatening complications of SCD. Transfusions have yielded favorable results after central nervous system (CNS) infarction. Transfusions have been used prior to surgery to theoretically reduce the risk associated with anesthesia. They have also been given prior to childbirth.[49] In addition, aggressive transfusion therapy has shown favorable results in cases of acute multiorgan failure associated with sickle cell pain episodes.[50]

Blood transfusion after a stroke is a common practice today. Chronic transfusion in these patients has been shown to decrease the chance of further strokes and halt clinical progression. Although it is not certain whether transfusion therapy improves the arteriogram, it does prevent the recurrence of cerebrovascular accidents.[51]

Sarnaik et al.[52] described a prophylactic transfusion program in 27 children who had experienced at least one episode of CNS infarction. Transfusions were given on an outpatient basis initially at 3-week intervals. The frequency was later adjusted to maintain a hemoglobin level of

10–12 g/d, a hemoglobin S quantitation of 25% or less, and a peripheral smear with little or no sickling. Twenty-five patients had no recurrence of CNS events. The other two patients had only transient recurrences. Twelve of the 27 completely recovered neurologic function and an additional 12 showed definite improvement. Although the remaining 3 patients showed no improvement, they had nonprogressive neurologic deficits. A decrease in hospitalizations for sickle cell-related complications was also noted. In this study the duration of therapy ranged from 1–9 years.

When transfusion therapy is used in stroke victims, the questions of whether and when transfusion may be safely stopped remain unresolved because strokes have occurred after cessation of therapy.[53] It has been suggested that transfusion regimens be maintained for more than 2 years.[51]

Transfusion therapy has also been used prior to childbirth. The use of prophylactic transfusions during pregnancy has been shown to decrease the number of painful crises. However, medical and obstetrical complications remained otherwise unchanged. In light of the possible risks associated with blood transfusions, their routine use for prevention of vaso-occlusion in pregnancy appears unjustified.[54]

It is the risks of transfusion therapy that must be weighed against possible benefits in the general sickle cell population. Chronic transfusions reduce the proportion of circulating sickle cells. This approach may, at the least, prevent many serious complications and improve the quality of life.[51] One case report of a patient with severe SCD, who received continuous transfusions over a 13-year period, records eradication of the symptoms of the disease.[49]

Limitations of transfusion therapy include iron overload, transfusion-related infection such as hepatitis or AIDS, and sensitization to the blood received. In one study, 30% of SCA patients who received blood transfusions became alloimmunized.[55] The risk of alloimmunization has been estimated to be 8–36%. Development of alloantibodies makes it difficult to find compatible blood and places the patient at increased risk of having a delayed hemolytic transfusion reaction in the future.[56]

Progress is being made in reducing the risks associated with transfusion therapy. Desferoxamine, an iron chelator, is used to combat transfusional iron overload. Conventional therapy consists of daily subcutaneous infusions of 1–2 grams over 10–12 hours. Higher doses, for example, 6 g/d, have been administered intravenously at a rate of 15 mg/kg/h in patients who have large iron stores or who have been poorly compliant to subcutaneous regimens. Patients should receive regular auditory assessments and eye examinations during therapy because the drug may produce otic and ocular side effects.[57,58]

The risk of transfusion therapy may be further limited by administration of the hepatitis vaccine, which reduces the risk of hepatitis B. The vaccine, however, offers no protection against hepatitis C. Blood screening tests are now available that detect the presence of antibodies to the hepatitis virus. Routine blood screening may also protect against exposure to the AIDS virus. Finally, the use of compatible donor blood decreases the risk of sensitization.

Exchange transfusion is an alternative to the transfusion of whole blood. Exchange transfusion has been used to treat several complications of SCA including cerebrovascular accidents, acute chest syndrome, priapism, and intractable leg ulcers. Standard exchange transfusion involves the exchange of RBCs only. The goal is to remove Hb-S and replace it with Hb-A. The sickle erythrocytes are consequently diluted with normal cells. During this process the patient's plasma is returned to the patient.[59] Exchange transfusion results in increased oxygen-carrying capacity with minimal change in blood volume.[39] There have, however, been reports of neurologic events following the use of exchange transfusion in the treatment of priapism.[38]

Whole-blood exchange has also been performed, although only in a limited number of patients. In this procedure, not only are the patient's red cells replaced with normal red cells, but also the patient's plasma is replaced with albumin or an albumin–saline combination. The interest in performing such an exchange was prompted by suggestions that plasma factors may contribute to abnormal adherence of sickled cells to the vascular endothelium. Whole-blood exchange produced good clinical outcome, but it has yet to be determined whether it is superior to standard red cell exchange.[59]

GELATION INHIBITORS

A nonstandard therapeutic approach that continues to be investigated in the sickle cell population is the use of gelation inhibitors. The goal with these agents is to inhibit the gelation of deoxyhemoglobin S. This inhibition can be affected by alteration of the sickle hemoglobin. In addition, because gelation is concentration dependent, decreasing the sickle hemoglobin concentration (e.g., by increasing the concentration of fetal hemoglobin) may markedly delay gelation. Many drugs have been considered as possible gelation inhibitors. Among them, hydroxyurea, azacytidine, and butyrate are receiving the most consideration. Although cyanates have been studied, the toxicity associated with the agent has limited its appeal.

Hydroxyurea administration has produced beneficial effects in several small studies. Platt[60] found that 5-day courses of hydroxyurea 50 mg/kg/d orally in three divided doses resulted in increases in fetal reticulocytes and fetal hemoglobin. Reticulocytes increased within 48–72 hours, peaked in 7–11 days, and decreased by 18–21 days. Veith et al.[61] also reported increases in fetal hemoglobin after 3-day courses of hydroxyurea. Doses ranged from 36–50 mg/kg/d. Charache et al.[62] reported improvement after long-term therapy. The hydroxyurea regimen was not uniform, but instead was tailored to patient response and tolerance. More recent data has also been promising with hydroxyurea administration producing a twofold to 10-fold increase in fetal hemoglobin.[63] An additional study reported a threefold to 25-fold increase in hemoglobin F-containing reticulocytes accompanied by a 2.3- to 16-fold increase in the percentage of hemoglobin F.[64] These increases were seen with doses producing tolerable marrow toxicity. Although bone marrow suppression was noted, with decreases in reticulocytes and white cell counts, the degree of suppression did not merit reduction of the hydroxyurea dose. The more promising picture is apparently attributable to a new approach in dosing. Whereas earlier studies used a standard initial hydroxyurea dose of 50 mg/kg/d, later studies have started more conservatively. For example, Rodgers et al.[63] used initial doses of 10–20 mg/kg/d and slowly titrated the dose upward as needed and tolerated. In the Goldberg study,[64] final doses ranged from 9–23 mg/kg/d. In one small study administration of erythropoietin and iron alternated with hydroxyurea administration resulted in an increase in hemoglobin levels beyond that achieved with hydroxyurea alone.[65] This is in contrast to a prior study that utilized daily hydroxyurea doses and showed no further increase in fetal hemoglobin with the addition of erythropoietin.[64] Hydroxyurea is believed to cause stimulation of fetal hemoglobin as a result of the erythroid regeneration that follows cytoreduction. In one earlier study, however, where therapy produced marrow suppression that was substantial, minimal therapeutic benefit was seen.[66] With the exception of possible bone marrow suppression, no other toxicities definitively related to the drug have been noted in the studies.

Azacytidine has also been shown to cause significant increases in fetal hemoglobin and a decrease in ISCs. Hemolysis is also decreased with azacytidine therapy. The effect of azacytidine on fetal hemoglobin synthesis, however, is transient. Repeated courses would be needed unless methods of prolonging the effect are found. Minimal side effects have been noted during treatment. The most common side effects have been gastrointestinal. There is also the potential for development of bone marrow toxicity. Thus far, marrow toxicity has not been a common problem in studies involving sickle cell patients, although it has occurred. This side effect was accompanied by a slowed response to azacytidine therapy.[67–69]

Cytarabine also stimulates fetal reticulocyte production. The increase in fetal reticulocytes is preceded by a marked decrease in absolute reticulocyte count.[62] In a pilot trial, IV administration of arginine butyrate resulted in an increase in fetal-globin production. Minimal side effects were seen. Further studies of this agent are warranted.[70]

CETIEDIL

Cetiedil citrate, an agent not currently available commercially in the United States, is a prototype of agents that affect primarily RBC membranes. An iminoester developed from 3-thienylacid, this vasodilator is used in Europe to treat intermittent claudication and other vascular diseases. In a double-blind randomized study, cetiedil was superior to placebo in decreasing the duration of crises and reducing the number of painful sites. Cetiedil use, however, did not reduce parenteral analgesic requirements. No serious adverse effects occurred. The most common side effects were nausea, vomiting, headache, and dry mouth. The incidence of these side effects was similar to that in the group receiving placebo. The exact mechanism of action is not known; however, the beneficial effects may result from its ability to produce peripheral vasodilation, to reduce plasma fibrinogen concentration and blood viscosity, to inhibit platelet aggregation, and to inhibit calmodulin. Calmodulin is a protein important in the activation of calcium-dependent enzymes in RBC membranes.[71]

PENTOXIFYLLINE

Researchers have reported a significant decrease in the number of painful crises in patients who received pentoxifylline. For example, one study that utilized a pentoxifylline regimen of 400 mg orally three times per day showed a significant decrease in the number and severity of painful crises. Not all studies, however, have yielded positive results. Although pentoxifylline may find a place in preventive therapy of sickle cell crises, it does not appear to have a role in the actual treatment of a crisis that is already in process.[72]

BONE MARROW TRANSPLANTATION

Bone marrow transplantation (BMT) has yielded remarkable results in the treatment of sickle cell anemia. Allogenic BMT from a matched sibling donor who does not have the disease has resulted in cure of the disease. There have been more than 50 successful transplants in children and young adults. These transplants were performed with preoperative administration of busulfan, cyclophosphamide, and sometimes antithymocyte globulin. Bone marrow transplantation, however, has several limitations. There are a limited number of patients for whom there is an HLA-matched sibling without the disease. In addition, there is a 10% transplant-related mortality rate. Graft rejection and graft-versus-host disease is also a concern, with a reported incidence of up to 20%. The cost of such a procedure may also be prohibitive.[23]

PROPHYLACTIC HEPARIN

The use of low-dose heparin (5000 units subcutaneously every 12 hours) was examined in four patients with SCD and frequent severe painful crises. Heparin administration reduced the severity and duration of pain in these patients.

Emergency room and hospital admissions were greatly reduced. No significant toxicity was noted. The major complaint was minimal discomfort at the injection site. The mechanism of the beneficial effect of heparin is unknown, but may be due to altering of membrane properties of platelets, RBCs, and/or endothelial cells.[73]

PRIAPISM

Most therapeutic approaches may be ineffective in treating priapism in sickle cell patients. Therapy has included hot baths, ice packs, alkalinization, transfusions, anticoagulants, beta blockers, estrogens, and gonadotropin-releasing hormone analogues.[40,74] Stilbestrol has been used to help prevent attacks of priapism. The effective dose varied not only among patients, but also within patients, with requirements sometimes fluctuating with time.[74] Successful use of pentoxifylline in a sickle cell patient also has been reported.[75] Another treatment option may be terbutaline, which has been successfully used to treat intraoperative penile erection and priapism induced by erectogenic pharmacologic agents. For persistent penile erection, a subcutaneous dose of 0.25–0.5 mg has been given every 4–6 hours. An oral regimen of 2.5–5 mg every 4–6 hours is another option suggested by the investigators.[76,77] More recently, Levine and Guss[78] reported the successful use of monthly injections of a gonadotropin-releasing hormone analogue in a patient who experienced recurrent episodes of painful erections. Resolution of priapism persisted for more than a year with continued therapy. More invasive approaches to the treatment of priapism include aspiration of the corpora cavernosa and more extensive surgery.

IDIOPATHIC UNILATERAL RENAL HEMATURIA

In cases of idiopathic unilateral renal hematuria, a high fluid intake should be maintained to prevent clotting and urethral colic. Iron therapy may be needed if blood loss continues.[39] If blood loss is brisk, transfusions may be necessary.[43] Nephrectomy should be considered only in cases involving massive hemorrhaging.[39]

MANAGEMENT OF CRISES

VASO-OCCLUSIVE CRISIS

Hydration and analgesia are the mainstays of treatment for vaso-occlusive (painful) crises; however, there is no consensus on specific guidelines for their use. In hospitalized patients, infusion of 4 L or more fluid per day in adults and 2500 mL/m^2 in children has been recommended. Glucose-in-saline solutions, for example, 5% glucose in one-half normal saline or 5% glucose in one-quarter normal saline, are appropriate in this setting. The superiority of a given intravenous fluid has not been established. Outpatients may be managed through oral consumption of 2–3 L of fluid per day.[53] Overhydration should be avoided, however, because vigorous intravenous fluid therapy has been associated with the development of pulmonary edema in some hospitalized patients.[32]

Despite the common and frequent use of analgesics in sickle cell patients, controlled studies to determine the optimal regimen are lacking. Although meperidine has frequently been used in sickle cell crises, morphine is now considered by many practitioners to be the drug of choice. Morphine has the advantage of having a longer duration of action than meperidine. Its use also avoids the possible problems resulting from accumulation of the meperidine metabolite, a potential toxicity to which sickle cell patients are especially prone. Various analgesic regimens have been employed and the search for better regimens continues.

There is at present no consensus regarding whether analgesics in sickle cell crisis should be administered on a scheduled rather than an as-needed basis. A scheduled regimen does produce more consistent serum levels. It has been argued that administration on a scheduled basis before severe pain ensues, results in the need for less medication.[79] More institutions are moving toward the use of continuous intravenous infusions of narcotics and the use of patient-controlled analgesia. Patient-controlled analgesia combines the advantages of providing steady analgesic blood concentrations with the ability to administer additional bolus doses instantaneously when needed at the touch of a button.

Cole et al.[80] reported their 5 years of experience with intravenous narcotic therapy in pediatric patients in severe sickle cell pain crisis. Patients receiving morphine received a 0.15 mg/kg bolus followed by an infusion of 0.07–0.10 mg/kg/h. The meperidine regimen consisted of a 1 mg/kg bolus followed by a 0.50–0.7 mg/kg/h infusion. Doses were then titrated every 3–4 hours until satisfactory analgesia was obtained. Patients who during earlier episodes had received only bolus narcotic injections preferred the continuous infusion. Side effects including nausea, vomiting, lethargy, and abdominal distension occurred more frequently with the continuous infusion than with bolus administration. This was probably due to the use of higher doses, because infusions were reserved for patients with more severe pain.

Patient-controlled analgesia is also being used in the treatment of crisis-related pain. Although optimum regimens have not been developed, this treatment approach may play an increasing role in the management of the SCA patient. McPherson and associates[81] evaluated the use of patient-controlled analgesia (PCA), using meperidine in 16 adult patients. Baseline infusions were initiated at 20 mg/h and escalated to 30 mg/h. One to two bolus doses of 2.5–5 mg were allowed each hour. The latter patients to be entered into the study also received hydroxyzine 50 mg given orally every 6 hours. This regimen produced only a 30% reduction in patient pain scores. Despite the quantitatively modest results, 10 of 16 patients rated the PCA regimen as very good or excellent. No adverse effects were noted during the study. The authors believed, consequently, that PCA when optimized will be a safe, effective alternative for pain control in vaso-occlusive crises. Morphine has also been evaluated. In a two-phase study of sickle cell patients who were treated in the emergency department, morphine administered by PCA was as effective as aggressive fixed-schedule intermittent administration of morphine.[82] Successful use of PCA morphine therapy in pediatric patients has also been reported.[83]

Although published data on the use of PCA specifically in SCA is limited, the general effectiveness of PCA is becoming more well established. PCA dosing guidelines for treating acute pain in a cross-section of patients is shown in Table 95.4 and is a reasonable regimen for use in sickle cell pain crisis. Patient monitoring with this PCA regimen includes checking of vital signs 5 minutes after the loading dose and at 15-minute intervals for two checks. This is followed by four checks at 30-minute intervals, four checks at 2-hour intervals, and thereafter checks every 4 hours for the duration of patient-controlled analgesia if the patient is stable.[84] This regimen allows for titration of the dose with close monitoring to minimize side effects. Hydromorphone also may be used in PCA. In addition to intravenous administration, hydromorphone can be administered subcutaneously in PCA, therefore avoiding the problems of venous access.[85] In addition to the pharmacokinetic advantages of PCA, the avoidance of wide variation in opioid blood concentrations, and avoidance of the pain–analgesia cycle, PCA instills in the patient a greater sense of control.[86]

Although its use is declining, intermittent meperidine is still sometimes utilized in treating hospitalized patients in sickle cell crisis. Intramuscular meperidine is generally prescribed at dosages ranging from 75–125 mg every 3–4 hours.[53] Concern regarding meperidine-induced seizures has prompted some clinicians to limit the use of this agent. However, prudent use can minimize this side effect. Seizures are a concern when high doses of meperidine are used. They probably result from the accumulation of normeperidine, a meperidine metabolite. Factors that may predispose a patient to development of seizures include doses greater than 100 mg every 2 hours for more than 24 hours, renal failure, alkaline urine, concurrent use of enzyme inducers, and coadministration of phenothiazines.[79,87]

TABLE 95.4. REPRESENTATIVE PROTOCOL FOR PCA

	Morphine	Meperidine
Suggested concentration	1–5 mg/mL	10 mg/mL
PCA bolus dose	0.5–1 mg	5–10 mg
Lock-out interval	10–20 min	10–20 min
Loading dose	1–2 mg	5–10 mg
Continuous rate/hour	1–2 mg/h	10–20 mg/h
Titration	10–20% increase or decrease/h	

(From Barbaccia JB. Pharmacy and Therapeutics Committee monograph: Patient controlled analgesia. Washington, DC, Washington Hospital Center, 1989, with permission.)

Although oxygen is still utilized in the treatment of sickle cell crisis, controlled clinical studies of the intervention are lacking. Oxygen administration is, of course, widely recommended for events that produce hypoxemia. In an attempt to elucidate the effects of oxygen on erythropoiesis and sickled erythrocytes, Embury et al.[88] administered oxygen continuously for 5 days to patients who were not in crisis. This resulted in an increase in arterial oxygen tension and a decrease in irreversibly sickled cells. However, there was a decline in erythropoietin levels and in the number of reticulocytes. The decline was a delayed effect, occurring after the first 2 days of therapy. After oxygen inhalation was discontinued, erythropoietin and reticulocyte levels increased, as did levels of ISCs, which reached levels higher than those before oxygen therapy in two of the three patients. Acute painful episodes occurred in these patients. It is suggested that, when indicated, oxygen inhalation be administered on an intermittent rather than a continuous basis. Solanski[89] reported one case in which overzealous use of oxygen resulted in an excessive partial pressure and is believed to have caused an acute suppression of erythropoiesis. In addition, the usefulness of oxygen administration is limited because the occlusion prevents the oxygen from reaching the areas where it is most needed. Consequently, it does not correct the poor oxygen in occluded areas that is causing the pain.

Because crises may be precipitated by infection, an infectious etiology should be ruled out in presenting patients. Appropriate empiric therapy should be initiated in patients with high fever or patients who appear critically ill. Sickle cell patients are particularly prone to infection caused by pneumococcus, haemophilus influenza, and salmonella species.

Dextran use has also been advocated in the treatment of vaso-occlusive crises. Dextran decreases erythrocyte aggregation and blood viscosity and thus improves microcirculation. Despite early positive results in a limited number of patients, the benefit of dextran has not been established in controlled trials.[90,91]

Although hospitalization is necessary for severe crisis, milder cases may be treated on an outpatient basis with rest, hydration, warmth, and oral analgesics.[83] Oral analgesic options include nonsteroidal anti-inflammatory drugs (NSAIDs) or acetaminophen generally in combination with codeine or a codeine derivative. Ketorolac, a newer NSAID, is receiving particular attention due to its potency, which has been compared to that of narcotic analgesics.[23]

SPLENIC SEQUESTRATION CRISIS

Splenic sequestration crisis is a major cause of mortality in young sickle cell patients. The sequestration of red cells in the spleen may result in a rapid drop of hematocrit leading to hypovolemia, shock, and death. Acute treatment includes whole-blood transfusion to correct hypovolemia. Broad-spectrum antibiotic therapy, which includes coverage for pneumococcus and haemophilus influenza, may also be warranted since infection may precipitate crises. The indications for splenectomy are controversial. Splenic sequestration crises tend to recur, however, and prompt splenectomy remains a treatment option. Splenectomy is probably merited, even after a single sequestration crisis, if that event is life threatening. Repetitive episodes, even if less serious, also may merit a splenectomy. For children less than 2 years of age, chronic blood transfusions have been recommended to prevent sequestration and allow delay of splenectomy until the age of 2 when risk of postsplenectomy septicemia becomes less.[23,92]

APLASTIC CRISIS

Treatment of aplastic crisis is primarily supportive. Blood transfusions may be needed if the anemia that develops is severe. The patient should also be receiving folic acid supplementation since folic acid deficiency has been implicated as a cause of aplastic crisis. Although it is possible that a bacterial infection may precipitate aplastic crisis, it is more likely that a virus, probably a parvovirus, is the precipitating factor.[43,92] Consequently, antibiotic therapy generally is not warranted with aplastic crisis.

HEMOLYTIC CRISIS

There is no specific treatment for hemolytic crises. Treatment is supportive and may include blood transfusions.

EVALUATION OF THERAPEUTIC OUTCOMES

In the long-term management of the patient with sickle cell anemia, administration of folic acid is aimed at preventing folate deficiency and megaloblastic changes. Folate levels and MCV values should be monitored. The efficacy of still nonstandard interventions such as administration of pentoxifylline and gelation inhibitors can best be assessed in terms of the decrease in number, severity, and duration of sickle cell pain crises. When painful crises do occur, the evaluation of effectiveness of analgesics depends mainly on the subjective assessments made by the patient and health care practitioners. Adequate hydration is important in the resolution of painful crisis. However, caution should be exercised to avoid overhydration, especially in patients predisposed to complications from this therapy such as renal failure patients and patients with cardiac dysfunction. Evaluation of the efficacy of prophylactic immunizations and antibiotics involves monitoring for the occurrence of pneumococcal or haemophilus infections. When infections do occur, appropriate antibiotic therapy should be initiated and the patient monitored for laboratory and clinical improvement. The success of blood transfusions poststroke can be assessed through monitoring for clinical progression or the occurrence of subsequent strokes.

CONCLUSION

The standard approach to the treatment of SCA has remained unchanged over the past few years. Treatment still consists primarily of supportive care. When vaso-occlusive crises occur, hydration and administration of analgesics remain the core interventions. In the general management of SCA, the goal is to decrease the number of sickle cell crises, to decrease the complications arising from the disease, and to improve the overall quality of life. The interventions that are commonly employed today may help to decrease the complications of SCA; however, they do not affect the underlying pathophysiology. Folate administration is still standard. In addition, administration of the pneumococcal vaccine with or without prophylactic penicillin may help decrease the number of infections in this population. For children less than 5 years of age, immunization against haemophilus influenza is also recommended. More attention is now being given to attempts to decrease gelation of sickle cells, primarily by increasing fetal hemoglobin. In this area, several agents are being studied; hydroxyurea, butyrate, and azacytidine, perhaps, look most promising.

REFERENCES

1. Herrick JB. Peculiar elongated and sickle-shaped red blood corpuscles in case of severe anemia. Arch Intern Med 1910;6:517–521.
2. Konotey-Ahulu FID. The sickle cell diseases: Clinical manifestations including the "sickle cell." Arch Intern Med 1974;133:611–619.
3. Emmel VE. A study of the erythrocytes in a case of severe anemia with elongated and sickle-shaped red blood corpuscles. Arch Intern Med 1917;20:586–598.
4. Huck JG. Sickle cell anemia. Bull Johns Hopkins Hosp 1923;34:335–344.
5. Hahn EV, Gillespie EB. Sickle cell anemia: Report of case greatly improved by splenectomy; experimental study of sickle cell formation. Arch Intern Med 1927;39:233.
6. Scriver JB, Waugh TR. Studies on a case of sickle-cell anemia. Can Med Assoc J 1930;23:375–380.

7. Ham TH, Castle WB. Relation of increased hypotonic fragility and of erythrostasis to the mechanism of hemolysis in certain anemias. Trans Assoc Physicians 1940;55:127–132.
8. Neel JV. The inheritance of sickle cell anemia. Science 1949;110:64–66.
9. Beet EA. The genetics of the sickle cell trait in a Bantu tribe. Ann Eugenics 1949;14:279–284.
10. Watson J, Stahman AW, Bilello EP. Significance of the paucity of sickle cells in newborn negro infants. Am J Med Sci 1948;215:419–423.
11. Pauling L, Itano HA, Singer SJ, et al. Sickle cell anemia: A molecular disease. Science 1949;110:543–548.
12. Serjeant GR. Geography and the clinical picture of sickle cell disease: An overview. Ann NY Acad Sci 1989;565:109–119.
13. Cerami A, Washington E. Sickle Cell Anemia. New York, Third Press, 1974.
14. Allison AC. Protection afforded by sickle cell trait against subtertian malarial infections. Br Med J 1954;1:290.
15. Thompson GR. Significance of hemoglobins S and C in Ghana. Br Med J 1962;1:682.
16. Edelstein SJ. The Sickled Cell: From Myths to Molecules. Cambridge, MA, Harvard University Press, 1986.
17. Ferguson AD, Carrington HT, Scott RB. Studies in sickle cell anemia—a clinical review. Med Ann DC 1955;24:517–532.
18. Rodgers GP, Noguchi CT, Schechter AN. Noninvasive techniques to evaluate the vaso-occlusive manifestations of sickle cell disease. Am J Pediatr Hematol Oncol 1985;7:245–253.
19. Rickles F, O'Leary DS. Role of coagulation system in pathophysiology of sickle cell disease. Arch Intern Med 1974;133:635–641.
20. Bensinger TA, Gillete PN. Hemolysis in sickle cell disease. Arch Intern Med 1974;133:624–631.
21. Winkelstein JA. Pneumococcal infections in sickle cell disease. J Pediatr 1977;91:521.
22. Winkelstein JA. The role of complement in the host's defense against *Streptococcus pneumoniae.* Rev Infect Dis 1981;3:289.
23. Buchanan GR. Sickle cell disease: Recent advances. Curr Probl Pediatr 1993;23:219–229.
24. Powars DR. Bs-Gene-cluster haplotypes in sickle cell. Hem Onc Clin North Am 1991;5(3):476–447, 485–486.
25. Scott RB, Castro O. Sickle cell thalassemia: Interpretation of test results. JAMA 1981;246:81.
26. Castro O, Scott RB. Red blood cell counts and indices in sickle cell trait in a black American population. Hemoglobin 1985;9:65–67.
27. Samuels-Reid J, Scott RB. Characteristics of menstruation in sickle cell disease. Fertil Steril 1985;43:139–141.
28. Finan AC, Elmer MA, Sasanow SR, et al. Nutritional factors and growth in children with sickle cell disease. Am J Dis Child 1988;142(2):237–240.
29. Scott RB, Samuels-Reid JH. Sickle cell disease, in Gellis SS, Kagan BM (eds): Current Pediatric Therapy. Philadelphia, WB Saunders, 1990, p 241.
30. Githers JH, Gross GP, Eife RF, et al. Splenic sequestration syndrome at mountain altitudes in sickle/hemoglobin C disease. J Pediatr 1977;90:203–206.
31. Platt OS, Thorington BD, Brambilla DJ, et al. Pain in sickle cell disease: Rates and risk factors. N Engl J Med 1994;325:11–16.
32. Sprinkle RH, Cole T, Smith S, et al. Acute chest syndrome in children with sickle cell disease. Am J Pediatr Hematol Oncol 1986;8:105–110.
33. Oppenheimer EH, Esterly J. Pulmonary changes in sickle disease. Am Rev Respir Dis 1971;103:853–859.
34. Barrett-Conner E. Acute pulmonary disease in sickle cell anemia. Am Rev Respir Dis 1971;104:159–165.
35. Young RC, Castro O, Baxter RP, et al. The lung in sickle cell disease: A clinical overview of common vascular, infectious and other problems. J Natl Med Assoc 1981;73:19–26.
36. Bromberg PH. Pulmonary aspects of sickle cell disease. Arch Intern Med 1974;133:652–657.
37. Lachman BS, Lazerson J, Starshak RJ, et al. The prevalence of cholelithiasis in sickle cell disease as diagnosed by ultrasound and cholecystography. Pediatrics 1979;64:601–603.
38. Siegel JF, Rich MA, Brock WA. Association of sickle cell disease, priapism, exchange transfusion, and neurological events: ASPEN syndrome. J Urol 1993;150:1480–1482.
39. Charache S. The treatment of sickle cell anemia. Arch Intern Med 1974;133:698–705.
40. Maclver JE, Went NL. Sickle cell anemia complicated by megaloblastic anemia of infancy. Br Med J 1960;1:775–779.
41. Alperin JB. Folic acid deficiency complicating sickle cell anemia. Arch Intern Med 1967;120:298–306.
42. Rabb LM, Grandison Y, Mason K, et al. A trial of folate supplementation in children with homozygous sickle cell disease. Br J Haematol 1983;54:589–594.
43. Galloway SJ, Harwood-Nuss AL. Sickle-cell anemia—a review. J Emerg Med 1988;6:213–226.
44. John AB, Ramlal A, Jackson H, et al. Prevention of pneumococcal infection in children with homozygous sickle cell disease. Br Med J 1984;288:1567–1570.
45. El-Hazmi MAF, Bahakim HM, Al-Swailem AM, et al. Symptom-free intervals in sicklers: Does pneumococcal vaccination and penicillin prophylaxis have a role? J Trop Pediatr 1990;36:56–62.
46. Gaston MH, Vertu JL, Woods G, et al. Prophylaxis with oral penicillin in children with sickle cell anemia. N Engl J Med 1986;314:1593–1599.
47. Buchanan GR, Siegel JD, Smith SJ, DePasse BM. Oral penicillin prophylaxis in children with impaired splenic function: A study of compliance. Pediatrics 1982;70:926–930.
48. Breiman RF, Butler JC, Tenover FC, et al. Emergence of drug-resistant pneumococcal infections in the United States. JAMA 1994;271:1831–1835.
49. Finch C, Lee MY, Leonard JM. Continuous RBC transfusions in a patient with sickle cell disease. Arch Intern Med 1982;142:279–282.
50. Hassell KL, Eckman JR, Lane PA. Acute multiorgan failure syndrome: A potentially catastrophic complication of severe sickle cell pain episodes. Am J Med 1994;96:155–162.
51. Piomelli S. Chronic transfusions in patients with sickle cell disease. Am J Pediatr Hematol Oncol 1985;7:51–55.
52. Sarnaik S, Soorya D, Kim J, et al. Periodic transfusions for sickle cell anemia and CNS infarction. Am J Dis Child 1979;133:1254–1257.

53. Smith JA. Management of sickle cell disease: Progress during the past 10 years. Am J Pediatr Hematol Oncol 1983;5:360–366.
54. Koshy M, Burd L, Wallace D, et al. Prophylactic red-cell transfusion in pregnant patients with sickle cell disease. N Engl J Med 1988;319:1447–1452.
55. Vichinsky EP, Earles A, Johnson RA, et al. Alloimmunization in sickle cell anemia and transfusion of racially unmatched blood. N Engl J Med 1990;322:1617–1621.
56. Cox JV, Stean E, Cunningham G, Frenkel EP. Risk of alloimmunization and delayed hemolytic transfusion reactions in patients with sickle cell disease. Arch Intern Med 1988;148:2485–2489.
57. Cohen A, Mizanin J, Schwartz E. High-dose intravenous chelation therapy with deferoxamine. Prog Clin Biol Res 1989;309:125–131.
58. Cohen A, Martin M, Mizanin J, et al. Vision and hearing during deferoxamine therapy. J Pediatr 1990;117:326–330.
59. Talacki CA, Ballas SK. Modified method of exchange transfusion in sickle cell disease. J Clin Apheresis 1990;5:183–187.
60. Platt OS, Orkin SH, Dover G, et al. Hydroxyurea enhances fetal hemoglobin production in sickle cell anemia. J Clin Invest 1984;74:652–656.
61. Veith R, Galanello R, Papayannopoulou T, Stamatoyannopoulos G. Stimulation of F-cell production in patients with sickle cell anemia treated with cytarabine or hydroxyurea. N Engl J Med 1985;313:1571–1575.
62. Charache S, Dover GJ, Moyer MA, Moore JW. Hydroxyurea-induced augmentation of fetal hemoglobin production in patients with sickle cell anemia. Blood 1987;69:109–116.
63. Rodgers GP, Dover GJ, Noguchi CT, et al. Hematologic responses of patients with sickle cell disease to treatment with hydroxyurea. N Engl J Med 1990;322:1037–1045.
64. Goldberg MA, Brugnara C, Dover GJ, et al. Treatment of sickle cell anemia with hydroxyurea and erythropoietin. N Engl J Med 1990;323:366–372.
65. Rodgers GP, Dover GJ, Uyesaka N, et al. Augmentation by erythropoietin of the fetal-hemoglobin response to hydroxyurea in sickle cell disease. N Engl J Med 1993;328:73–80.
66. Dover GJ, Humphries RK, Moore TG. Hydroxyurea induction of hemoglobin F production in sickle cell disease: Relationship between cytotoxicity and F cell production. Blood 1986;67:735–738.
67. Ley TJ, DeSimone J, Noguchi CT, et al. 5-Azacytidine increases gamma-globulin synthesis and reduces the portion of dense cells in patients with sickle cell anemia. Blood 1983;62:370–380.
68. Dover GJ, Charache S, Boyer SH, et al. 5-Azacytidine increases HbF production and reduces anemia in sickle cell disease: Dose-response analysis of subcutaneous and oral dosage regimens. Blood 1985;66:527–532.
69. Humphries RK, Dover G, Young NS, et al. 5-Azacytidine acts directly on both erythroid precursors and progenitors to increase production of fetal hemoglobin. J Clin Invest 1985;75:547–557.
70. Perrine SP, Ginder GD, Faller DV, et al. A short-term trial of butyrate to stimulate fetal-globin-gene expression in the beta-globin disorders. N Engl J Med 1993;328:81.
71. Benjamin LT, Berkowitz LR, Orringer E, et al. A collaborative double-blind randomized study of cetiedil citrate in sickle cell crisis. Blood 1986;67:1442–1447.
72. Ambrus JL. Stiff red cell syndrome. A review of the treatment of sickle cell disease with pentoxifylline. J Med 1993;24:1–9.
73. Chaplin H Jr, Monroe MC, Malecek AC, et al. Preliminary trial of minidose heparin prophylaxis for painful sickle cell crises. East Afr Med J 1989;66(9):574–584.
74. Serjeant GR, DeCeular K, Maude GH. Stilbestrol and stuttering priapism in homozygous sickle-cell disease. Lancet 1985;2:1274–1276.
75. Rardin KB, Washington TG, Beasley EB. Use of pentoxifylline in treating priapism in two patients with sickle cell anemia. Paper presented to 21st Annual ASHP Midyear Clinical Meeting, Las Vegas, NV, December 9, 1986.
76. Shanta TR. Intraoperative management of penile erection by using terbulatine. Anesthesiology 1989;70:707–709.
77. Shanta TR, Finnerty DP, Rodriquez AL. Treatment of persistent penile erection and priapism using terbulatine. J Urol 1989;141:1427–1429.
78. Levine LA, Guss SP. Gonadotropin-releasing hormone analogues in the treatment of sickle cell anemia-associated priapism. J Urol 1993;150:475–477.
79. Shimomura SK, Harris S. Pain management of patients with sickle cell anemia. Hosp Pharm 1979;14:332–336.
80. Cole TB, Sprinkle RH, Smith SJ, Buchanan GR. Intravenous narcotic therapy for children with severe sickle cell pain crisis. Am J Dis Child 1986;140:1255–1259.
81. McPherson E, Perlin E, Finke H, et al. Patient-controlled analgesia in patients with sickle-cell vaso-occlusive crisis. Am J Med Sci 1990;299(1):10–12.
82. Gonzalez ER, Bahal N, Hansen LA, et al. Intermittent injection vs patient-controlled analgesia for sickle cell crisis pain. Arch Intern Med 1991;151:1373–1378.
83. Grundy R, Howard R, Evans J. Practical management of pain in sickling disorders. Arch Dis Child 1993;69:256–259.
84. Barbaccia JB. Pharmacy and Therapeutics Committee monograph: Patient controlled analgesia. Washington, DC, Washington Hospital Center, 1989.
85. Ballas SK. Treatment of pain in adults with sickle cell disease. Am J Hematol 1990;34:49–54.
86. Patient controlled analgesia. Med Lett 1989;31:104.
87. Shapiro BS. The management of pain in sickle cell disease. Pediatr Clin North Am 1989;36:1029–1045.
88. Embury SH, Garcia JF, Mohandas N, et al. Effects of oxygen inhalation on endogenous erythropoietin kinetics, erythropoiesis and properties of blood cells in sickle cell anemia. N Engl J Med 1984;311:291–295.
89. Solanski DL. Sickle cell anemia, oxygen treatment and anaemic crisis. Br Med J 1983;287:725–726.
90. Oski FA, Viner ED, Purugganan H, et al. Low molecular weight dextran in sickle cell crisis. JAMA 1965;191:43.
91. Watson-Williams EJ. Sickle cell crisis treated with rheomacrodex. Lancet 1963;1:1053.
92. Evans, JPM. Practical management of sickle cell disease. Arch Dis Child 1989;64:1748–1751.

Chapter 96

Drug-Induced Hematologic Disorders

Michael D. Parr, PharmD, and Michael Doukas, MD

Although drug-induced hematologic disorders are an expected complication of therapy in most patients who are treated with antineoplastic agents, the appearance of drug-induced hematologic disorders in patients receiving other types of drug therapy is an uncommon side effect. The development of drug-induced hematologic disorders in patients receiving medications is often an idiosyncratic reaction and can be life threatening. The incidence of drug-induced hematologic disorders depends on a number of factors including the cell line affected, the specific drug, dose of the drug, and possibly genetic predisposition. The exact incidence of drug-induced hematologic disorders is difficult to estimate but studies in Sweden reported an incidence of approximately 0.01% of drug-induced agranulocytosis in the general population.[1–3] Mortality has decreased in recent years but still ranges from 11–48% for drug-induced hematologic disorders.[1–3] The Swedish studies demonstrated a higher incidence of agranulocytosis in the elderly population and a greater risk in females as opposed to males. The mortality rates appear to be highest with aplastic anemia followed by drug-induced thrombocytopenia, then agranulocytopenia, and finally hemolytic anemia.[4]

The diagnosis of drug-induced hematologic disorders is often difficult since a number of different disease states may cause symptoms and laboratory abnormalities similar to aplastic anemia, agranulocytosis, and so on. In addition, patients can be taking a number of different medications at the time the blood disorder first appears. Therefore, a process of exclusion must be developed to determine which drug is the culprit in a patient with drug-induced hematologic disorders. Before a drug can be implicated, it must be determined if the patient was actually taking the drug in question. Next a temporal relationship to the initiation of the drug and the onset of symptoms must be established.

Depending on the results of the investigation, a drug can be placed into one of five categories relating to probability that a drug caused the hematologic disorders (Table 96.1).[5] Category 1 is a causative reaction where the drug is regarded as the actual cause of the drug-induced hematologic disorder by meeting the relationships previously stated and where the reaction has been reported in the literature before. The second category is classified as a probable reaction. Drugs in this category are related temporally to the drug-induced hematologic disorders and are reported in the literature to cause blood abnormalities but lack reproducibility of laboratory data. The next category is a possible reaction caused by the drug. The main medications that fall into this class are new drugs, for which insufficient data exist in the literature to document this type of reaction. There is, however, a temporal relationship between the drug and the disorder. Category 4 is a coincident reaction where the drug exposure occurred but another cause for the disorder is found (i.e., a disease). The final category is a negative relationship in which no temporal relationship exists.

Due to the severity of these disorders, rechallenge of the patient with the suspected drug is in most cases unethical. The testing of a medication *in vitro* to determine if the suspected drug is the actual culprit would therefore be advantageous. Unfortunately, *in vitro* testing is expensive and frequently does not yield conclusive results due to the wide variety of possible mechanisms that can cause drug-induced hematologic disorders. One study demonstrated that only 19% of the cases with suspected drug-induced agranulocytosis could be documented by *in vitro* testing.[6] Clinicians often never know the exact cause of the blood disorder in a given patient.

The mechanisms by which drugs induce blood disorders differ due to the wide variety of chemical structures involved. In addition, a particular drug may cause a drug-induced hematologic disorder by several different mechanisms (i.e., quinidine). The types of drug-induced hematologic disorders can be separated into four classifications (Table 96.2).[5] One case report demonstrated two types of immune-mediated hemolysis occurring in a patient simultaneously.[7] Other mechanisms may also be involved. Drugs such as the antiviral agent zidovudine may cause severe anemia (frequently requiring blood transfusions) and agranulocytosis by inhibition of DNA synthesis.[8,9] Amphotericin B may cause anemia by oxidative damage to the red blood cells.[10] Investigators have also hypothe-

TABLE 96.1. CATEGORIES RELATING TO THE PROBABILITY OF DRUG-INDUCED HEMATOLOGIC DISORDERS

1. Causative
2. Probable
3. Possible
4. Coincidental
5. Negative

TABLE 96.2. TYPES OF DRUG-INDUCED HEMATOLOGIC DISORDER

1. An abnormal sensitivity to the drug or one of the drug's metabolites by a stem cell population
2. Genetic predisposition (i.e., oxidative hemolytic anemia)
3. Abnormal metabolism of the drug causing formation of a toxic metabolite
4. An immune-mediated effect on a mature cellular component of the blood or on the stem cell population

sized that certain drugs may cause changes in the microenvironment of the bone marrow, resulting in drug-induced hematologic disorders.[11] Viral infections have been speculated to have an additive effect when a patient has been exposed to a virus and to a drug that may cause drug-induced hematologic disorders affecting T-cell lymphocytes and stem cells.[12] Currently, however, neither changes in the microenvironment nor concomitant viral infection have been documented to cause drug-induced hematologic disorders.

For the reader to understand a more detailed explanation of the mechanisms previously discussed, a basic knowledge of hematopoiesis and immunology is needed. Some investigators believe that the earlier the drug-induced hematologic disorders occur in the differentiation process, the more severe the disorder will become.[13] Figure 96.1 shows the differentiation of a neutrophil from a stem cell and the arrows indicate several possible sites where drugs can induce agranulocytosis.

Any cell lines can be affected in drug-induced hematologic disorders including the white blood cells (WBCs), red blood cells (RBCs), and platelets. When a drug causes decreases in all three cell lines accompanied by a hypoplastic bone marrow, the result is termed drug-induced aplastic anemia. The decrease in WBC count alone by a medication is termed drug-induced agranulocytosis. Drugs can affect RBCs by causing a number of different anemias including drug-induced immune hemolytic anemia, drug-induced oxidative hemolytic anemia, or drug-induced megaloblastic anemia. A medication-induced decrease in platelet count is called drug-induced thrombocytopenia. The rest of this chapter discusses specific aspects of drug-induced hematologic disorders with particular emphasis on the dyscrasias previously stated.

DRUG-INDUCED APLASTIC ANEMIA

Drug-induced aplastic anemia can be defined as a pancytopenia (a decrease in all of the cellular components of peripheral blood) with a hypocellular bone marrow (a bone marrow demonstrating a decreased production of blood cells), and no gross evidence of increased peripheral blood cell destruction. A diagnosis of aplastic anemia can be made if the patient meets two of the following criteria: a WBC count of 3500/mm^3 or less, a platelet

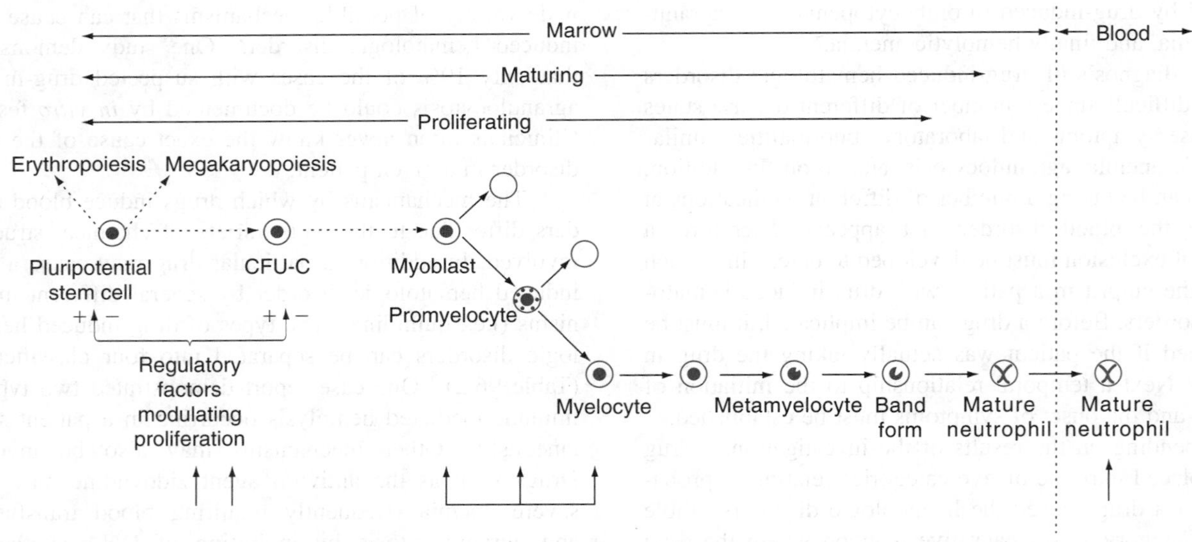

Figure 96.1. Differentiation of the stem cell to the mature neutrophil. The arrows indicate possible sites of drug-induced agranulocytosis. *(From Ref. 36, with permission.)*

count of 55,000/mm^3 or less, or a hemoglobin value of 10.0 g/dL or less with a reticulocyte count of 30,000/mm^3 or less.[14] The bone marrow must be free of neoplastic infiltration or significant myelofibrosis.[15] There also must be no history of exposure to antineoplastic agents or to intensive radiation. The onset of drug-induced aplastic anemia is insidious with symptoms usually appearing on the average about 6.5 weeks after initiation of the offending agent.[16] The disease often appears after the drug has been discontinued. Symptoms include fatigue, weakness, stomatitis, easy bruisability, petechiae, and purpura. Less common manifestations are infection related to a decrease in the WBC count and bleeding, which is seen later due to thrombocytopenia. The incidence of drug-induced aplastic anemia in patients taking medications is approximately 2.2:1,000,000[17] and is higher in patients taking such drugs as indomethacin and phenylbutazone.[14] Table 96.3 lists a number of drugs that have been associated with drug-induced aplastic anemia.

The etiology of drug-induced aplastic anemia is felt to be due to damage to the hematopoietic stem cell. The earlier the stem cell is affected in the maturation process, the greater the likelihood that the drug-induced aplastic anemia will be long term.[13] There is no evidence that drug-induced aplastic anemia occurs due to the destruction of the microenvironment of the bone marrow.[15] Three mechanisms have been proposed as causes of damage to the stem cell line.[16] First, there may be a dose-dependent toxic effect on hematopoiesis. The second mechanism is idiosyncratic. Idiosyncratic mechanisms include individual variations in the pharmacokinetics of the suspected drug or a hypersensitivity of the stem cells to the bone marrow destructive effects of the implicated drug. The third mechanism is a drug- or metabolite-induced immune reaction that is specific to the stem cell population.

The dose-dependent mechanism for development of aplastic anemia can best be illustrated by the antineoplastic agents. This type of toxicity can be beneficial in particular situations such as bone marrow transplantation. In bone marrow transplantation, large doses of chemotherapeutic drugs are given to prepare patients for infusion of the donor marrow. Patients who develop drug-induced aplastic anemia in doses that are tolerated by the large majority of patients receiving the drug would fall into the category of an idiosyncratic reaction. Drugs that cause drug-induced aplastic anemia in a minority of patients can imply abnormal metabolism or excretion of a drug.

TABLE 96.3. DRUGS ASSOCIATED WITH APLASTIC ANEMIA

Acetazolamide	Oral antidiabetics
Antihistamines	Oxyphenbutazone
Carbamazepine	Penicillamine
Chloramphenicol	Pentoxifylline
Chloroquine	Phenobarbital
Chlorothiazide	Phenothiazines
Felbamate	Phenytoin
Furosemide	Propylthiouracil
Gold salts	Quinidine
Indomethacin	Sulfonamides
Interferon (alpha)	Ticlopidine
Methimazole	

A possible example of this is chloramphenicol-induced aplastic anemia. Investigators have hypothesized that this cause of chloramphenicol-induced aplastic anemia is the result of abnormal metabolism of chloramphenicol. The nitrobenzene ring present on chloramphenicol is thought to be reduced to form a nitroso group on the chloramphenicol molecule.[18] The nitroso group then could interact with DNA in the stem cell to cause damage to the chromosomes and eventually cell death. Other investigators have hypothesized that bacteria from the gastrointestinal (GI) tract may metabolize chloramphenicol to marrow toxic metabolites.[19] A second type of chloramphenicol bone marrow depression can also be seen. This reaction is dose dependent and reversible. In this reaction chloramphenicol affects primarily the erythroid cell line due to injury of the mitrochondria.[18] Overall, the incidence of chloramphenicol-induced aplastic anemia has fallen due to decreased use of the agent.[20] Other drugs thought to induce aplastic anemia include phenytoin and carbamazepine. Metabolites from phenytoin and carbamazepine are theorized to bind covalently to macromolecules in the cell and then cause cell death by either direct toxicity to the stem cell or by causing the death of lymphocytes involved in regulating hematopoiesis.[21]

Phenylbutazone-induced aplastic anemia is thought by some to result from low phenylbutazone clearance.[15,16] It is suggested that the drug accumulates to toxic concentration and kills the stem cell population. Researchers have demonstrated a decreased clearance of phenylbutazone in patients with phenylbutazone-induced aplastic anemia. However, the drug has never been shown to be toxic to stem cells even in high concentrations. The exact mechanism of phenylbutazone-induced aplastic anemia is therefore still unclear.

Genetic predisposition may also influence the development of drug-induced aplastic anemia. Studies in animals and a case report of chloramphenicol-induced aplastic anemia in identical twins suggest a genetic predisposition to development of drug-induced aplastic anemia.[15,18]

Drug-induced aplastic anemia due to the development of an immune reaction has also been speculated. The mechanism could be similar to drug-induced immune agranulocytosis or drug-induced immune hemolytic anemia (discussed later in the chapter). The appearance of antibodies to chloroquine and subsequent bone marrow suppression supports the previous hypothesis.[16] Drugs could also affect the function of suppressor T cells, which in turn could initiate the inhibition of stem cell production.[16] The clinical success of antithymocyte globulin in the treatment of possible drug-induced aplastic anemia may also indicate a drug effect on suppressor T-cell function in drug-induced aplastic anemia.[22]

TREATMENT

The 2-year survival rate for a patient who develops drug-induced aplastic anemia is approximately 62%.[16] As with all cases of drug-induced hematologic disorders, the suspected offending agent must be removed. Early withdrawal of the agent may allow for reversal of the aplastic anemia.[16] Patients with drug-induced aplastic anemia need to be treated symptomatically for infection and bleeding. Antithymocyte globulin has been employed to reverse aplastic anemia in doses of 20 mg per kilogram of body weight per day by intravenous infusion for 8 consecutive days.[23]

Corticosteroids have been used in drug-induced aplastic anemia but their efficacy is questionable.[16] Several investigators have employed cyclosporine for the treatment of aplastic anemia with beneficial results,[24,25] but one prospective study in 12 patients showed no response to cyclosporine.[26] Granulocyte-macrophage colony-stimulating factor (GM-CSF)[27,28] and interleukin-1[29] have also been investigated in the treatment of aplastic anemia with some success. An additional case report described the use of cyclosporine and filgrastim (G-CSF) in combination in the treatment of aplastic anemia.[30] If long-term bone marrow supression continues after initial treatment with the previous agents, the only viable option at present is bone marrow transplantation. Some experts believe bone marrow transplantation is the treatment of choice if the patient has a matched donor.

DRUG-INDUCED AGRANULOCYTOSIS

Drug-induced agranulocytosis can be defined as a drug-mediated reduction in the mature myeloid cells in the blood (granulocytes and immature granulocytes [bands]) to a total count of 2000 cells/mm^3 or less. Symptoms of agranulocytosis include sore throat, fever, malaise, weakness, and chills. It occurs more frequently in females than males.[31] The overall mortality rate in agranulocytosis is 16%.[32] Mortality in patients with agranulocytosis increases when the patient develops bacteremia or renal failure.[32] The symptoms can appear rapidly, within 7–14 days after initiation of the offending agent, or in the case of phenothiazine-induced agranulocytosis, patients can be asymptomatic at the time of diagnosis probably due to a milder form of the disorder.[5] In the large majority of cases the drug-induced agranulocytosis will resolve over time.[5] Table 96.4 provides a list of medications that have been reported to cause drug-induced agranulocytosis.

A number of different mechanisms may produce drug-induced agranulocytosis. Initially, it was thought that drugs affected only the mature granulocytes, causing a "maturation arrest." In recent years, however, studies have demonstrated a possible toxic effect of drugs on the myeloid colony-forming unit in the bone marrow (either a direct toxic effect or antibody mediated)[33,34]; this may be the most frequent mechanism of drug-induced agranulocytosis.[31] Drug-induced agranulocytosis can be classified into three types.[35] The type I reaction is immune mediated and involves the drug or drug metabolite, antibodies, and neutrophils. A type II reaction is associated with accumulated drug toxicity in hypersensitive individuals. The final type,

TABLE 96.4. DRUGS ASSOCIATED WITH AGRANULOCYTOSIS

Acetaminophen	Indomethicin
Acetazolamide	Isoniazid
Acetylsalicylic acid	Levamisole
Alloporinol	Levodopa
p-Aminosalicylic acid	Lincomycin
Benzodiazepines	Meprobamate
Beta-lactam antibiotics	Methazolamide
Brompheniramine	Methimazole
Captopril	Methyldopa
Carbamazepine	Metronidazole
Ceftriaxone	Nitrofurantoin
Chloramphenicol	Oxyphenbutazone
Chloroproamide	Penicillamine
Cimetidine	Phenothiazines
Clindamycin	Phenylbutazone
Clomipramine	Phenytoin
Clozapine	Phetazocine
Dapsone	Primidone
Desipramine	Procainamide
Doxycycline	Propranolol
Ethacrynic acid	Propylthiouracil
Ethosuximide	Pyrimethamine
Fenoprofen	Quinine
Flucytosine	Rifampin
Ganciclovir	Streptomycin
Gentamicin	Sulfa antibiotics
Gold salts	Thiazide diuretics
Griseofulvin	Tocainide
Hydralazine	Tolbutamide
Hydroxychloroquine	Vancomycin
Ibuprofen	Zidovudine
Imipramine	

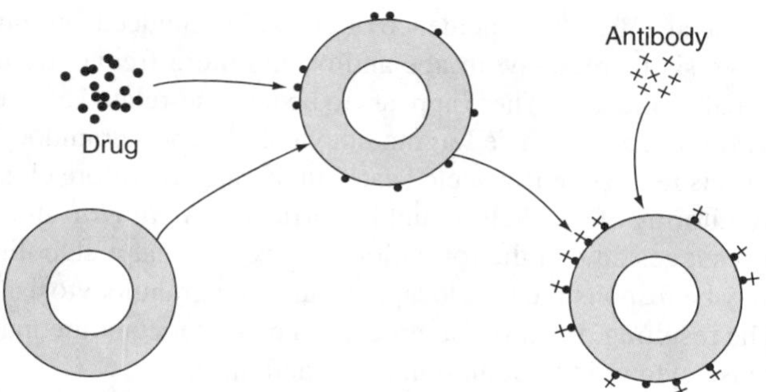

Figure 96.2. The drug absorption mechanism. The drug binds to the membrane of the blood cell. Antibodies are formed to the drug-membrane complex (a hapten). The antibodies then attach to the complex and cell toxicity occurs. *(From Ref. 57, with permission.)*

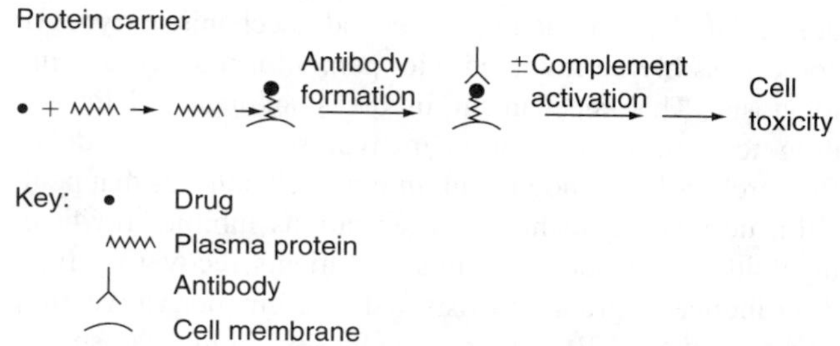

Figure 96.4. The protein carrier mechanism. The drug combines with a plasma protein. The complex then attaches to the cell membrane, and antibody formation is stimulated. Antibodies later attach to the complex and activate complement. The cell is lysed then by the complement. *(From Ref. 36, with permission.)*

type III, represents other etiologies induced by a combination of both immune and toxic mechanisms.

Drug-induced immune agranulocytosis (type I) has been theorized to develop by one of four different mechanisms.[36] The first type involves drug absorption on the membrane of the neutrophil. The drug membrane complex then acts as a hapten to stimulate antibody formation. The antibodies produced attach to the drug-membrane complex causing WBC destruction through complement activation and removal by the phagocytic system (Fig. 96.2). This hapten-type reaction is often seen when drugs are given in large doses. The penicillin derivatives are frequently associated with this type of agranulocytosis. The dose at which this immune-mediated reaction occurs is usually higher than 150 mg/kg/d with the majority of penicillin derivatives but has occurred at lower doses.[34,37,38]

The second type of immune-mediated agranulocytosis is called the "innocent bystander phenomenon." In this reaction, the drug combines with a drug-specific antibody. The complex is nonspecifically absorbed to the neutrophil membrane, resulting in complement in activation. The activated complement then destroys the cell (Fig. 96.3). Quinidine has been associated with this type of reaction.

A similar type of immune response involves a protein carrier that combines with the drug and then attaches to the cell membrane. This in turn causes antibody formation. The antibodies attach to the drug protein carrier–membrane complex and activate complement. The cells are then cleared by the phagocytic system (Fig. 96.4).

The final mechanism for an immune-mediated reaction is the production of autoantibodies to a "spoiled membrane" caused by the offending drug. The mechanism involves the drug producing an alteration in the neutrophil membrane, which induces the formation of autoantibodies (antibodies that attach directly to the neutrophil). These antibodies attach to the neutrophil, causing cellular destruction by the phagocytic system (Fig. 96.5).

The onset of symptoms due to immune-mediated mechanisms is rapid, occurring in 7–15 days. In the case of penicillin-induced agranulocytosis, the patient can often be restarted on a lower dose of penicillin after the neutropenia has resolved without any relapse of drug-induced agranulocytosis.[37,38] Due to the rapid onset of symptoms and the

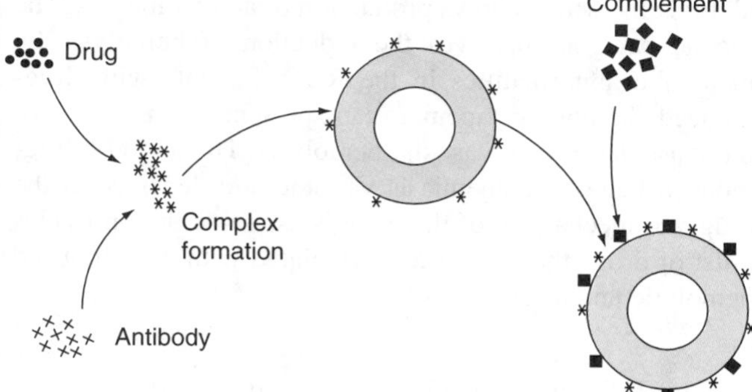

Figure 96.3. The innocent bystander mechanism. The drug induces antibody formation. The antibodies and drug form a complex in the serum, and the complex nonspecifically binds to the cell membrane. Complement is activated and the cell is lysed. *(From Ref. 57, with permission.)*

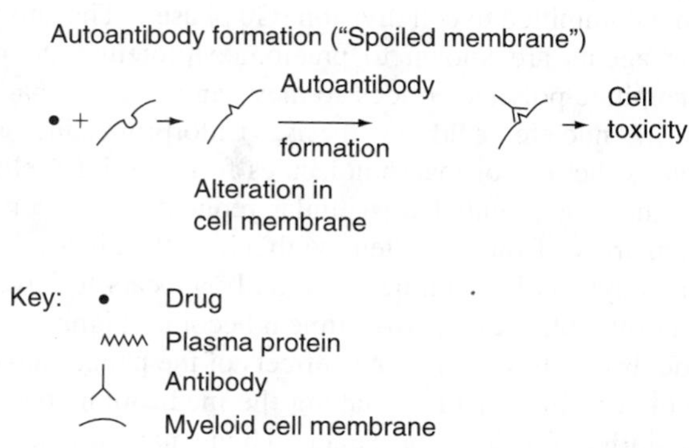

Figure 96.5. The autoantibody mechanism. A drug induces an alteration in the cells membrane. Autoantibodies are formed to the altered cell membrane and cell toxicity occurs. *(From Ref. 36, with permission.)*

dose-related phenomenon, a second mechanism (type II) could possibly be involved with penicillin-induced agranulocytosis. This mechanism involves an accumulation of drug to toxic concentration in hypersensitive individuals. Researchers have shown with *in vitro* cell cultures that penicillin derivatives in high concentrations inhibit growth of myeloid colony-forming units in patients recovering from drug-induced agranulocytosis.[39] Penicillin derivative may therefore exert WBC suppression by several mechanisms.

Antithyroid medications such as propylthiouracil and methimazole produce agranulocytosis in about 0.3–0.6% of patients.[40,41] The mechanism by which antithyroid agents cause agranulocytosis is unknown, but antibodies to granulocytes have been demonstrated.[42,43] In a study by Cooper et al.[40] agranulocytosis occurred more frequently in older patients (>40 years old) and occurred within 2 months after initiation of therapy. The investigators also reported a possible dose relationship with methimazole.[40] For patients receiving less than 30 mg/d of methimazole no agranulocytosis occurred but in patients receiving higher doses, neutropenia was seen.[40] There appeared to be no dose relationship with conventional doses of propylthiouracil. However, another study demonstrated no relationship between age or dose in the incidence of thioamide-induced agranulocytosis.[44]

The phenothiazines as a group are known to cause a type II drug-induced agranulocytosis. The onset of phenothiazine-induced agranulocytosis is approximately 2–15 weeks after initiating therapy.[36] Short-term toxicity is not usually seen in patients taking phenothiazines on a chronic basis, although there is one report of acute agranulocytosis in a child who accidentally ingested a large quantity of chlorpromazine.[33] Usually patients have ingested 10–20 grams of a phenothiazine before the onset of neutropenia. Phenothiazine-induced agranulocytosis occurs most frequently in females older than 50 years of age.[5] The mechanism by which phenothiazines cause the drug-induced agranulocytosis has been primarily studied with chlorpromazine.[5] Chlorpromazine is thought to affect cells in the cell cycle that are in the phase that manufactures enzymes needed for DNA synthesis (G1 phase) or the phase in which cells are resting and not committed to cell division (G0 phase).[5] The antipsychotic agents are known to precipitate proteins and may coprecipitate polynucleotides so they can no longer participate in nucleic acid synthesis. Chlorpromazine also increases the loss of macromolecules from the intracellular pools that are essential for cellular replication.[5] When the bone marrow from a patient with phenothiazine-induced agranulocytosis is examined it initially appears to have no cellularity (aplastic), but over time it becomes highly hyperplastic. It is believed that toxic effects of the phenothiazines are not seen in all patients taking the medications because the majority of patients have enough bone marrow reserve to overcome the toxic effects.[5] A recently released antipsychotic clozapine has demonstrated approximately a 10 times higher incidence of agranulocytosis than the other antipsychotic agents.[45] The incidence of clozapine-induced agranulocytosis increases with age and occurs more frequently in female patients.[46] There appears to be no dose-related effects with clozapine-induced agranulocytosis.[46] The agranulocytosis is reversible if detected early in therapy, therefore close monitoring of the WBC count is warranted. An *in vitro* study has suggested that the formation of a free radical metabolite may be responsible for clozapine-induced agranulocytosis.[47] The resulting oxidative stress caused by this metabolite may cause cytotoxicity or an immune reaction.[47]

TREATMENT

The primary treatment of drug-induced agranulocytosis is the removal of the offending drug. Following discontinuation of the drug most cases of neutropenia will resolve over time and only symptomatic treatment (i.e., antimicrobials for infections, etc.) is necessary. In severe cases, a course of intravenous immune globulin at 400 mg/kg/d four to five times day has demonstrated efficacy in autoimmune neutropenia.[48] Sargramostim (GM-CSF) and filgrastim (G-CSF) have been be used to decrease the time period of neutropenia with varying degrees of success.[49–55] The dose for both sargramostim and filgrastim in the literature for the treatment of drug-induced agranulocytosis was 10 μg per kilogram of body weight.[52–54] However, it is recommended that according to package insert instructions (250 mg/m^2 for sargramostim and 5 μg/kg for filgrastim). The time to recovery of the granulocyte count ranged from 3–15 days.[52–55]

DRUG-INDUCED HEMOLYTIC ANEMIA

Drug-induced hemolytic anemia is a disorder that affects RBCs in which the cells are damaged or destroyed (hemolyzed). The causes of drug-induced hemolytic anemia can be divided into two categories: immune or metabolic. The first category can be similar to immune-regulated agranulocytosis or it may be due to the suppression of regulator cells, which allows production of autoantibodies. The second category involves the induction of hemolysis by metabolic abnormalities in the RBC. Patients with drug-induced hemolytic anemia can present with signs of intravascular or extravascular hemolysis. The onset of drug-induced hemolytic anemia is variable and depends on the drug and mechanism of the hemolysis. Table 96.5 provides a list of drugs that have been associated with drug-induced hemolytic anemia.

DRUG-INDUCED IMMUNE HEMOLYTIC ANEMIA

As stated earlier, the proposed mechanisms by which drugs can cause drug-induced immune hemolytic anemia are sim-

TABLE 96.5. DRUGS ASSOCIATED WITH HEMOLYTIC ANEMIA

Acetaminophen	Methysergide
p-Aminosalicylic acid	Nomifensine
Cephalosporins	Omeprazole
Chlopropamide	Penicillins
Chlorpromazine	Probenecid
Diclofenac	Procainamide
Hydralazine	Quinidine
Hydrochlorothiazide	Quinine
Ibuprofen	Rifampin
Isoniazid	Sulfonamides
Levodopa	Streptomycin
Mefenamic acid	Tetracycline
Melphalan	Tolbutamide
Methadone	Triameterene
Methyldopa	

ilar to the mechanisms that produce drug-induced agranulocytosis. The first mechanism is the adsorption of the drug to the RBC membrane to form a hapten and subsequent antibody formation. A study by Yust et al.[56] demonstrated that once the RBCs were coated with the antibodies, the cells were destroyed by either phagocytosis or cell-mediated cytotoxicity. The effector cells in both processes were mononuclear phagocytes.[56] The penicillin and cephalosporin derivatives given in high doses are mainly associated with this type of immune reaction.[57] Other drugs that have been reported to cause drug-induced immune hemolytic anemia by this process include tetracycline and certain antineoplastic agents (i.e., cyclophosphamide, cisplatin, and melphalan).[57]

Drug-induced immune hemolytic anemia has also been described as occurring due to the innocent bystander phenomenon. Quinidine and phenacetin are the prototype drugs of this reaction. Drugs that induce this reaction form complexes with drug-specific antibodies that adhere to the RBC membrane. Complement then lyses the RBC membrane.[57] This type of mechanism is associated with acute intravascular hemolysis. A third type of immune-mediated mechanism has been seen with cephalosporin derivatives. The cephalosporins can combine with nonspecific proteins including albumin, IgG, IgA, and fibrinogen and adhere to the RBC. The binding is not immunologic in origin and hemolytic anemia has not been associated with this reaction (Fig. 96.6). However, the reaction can cause difficulties in cross-matching patients for blood transfusions, due to the nonspecific binding of antibodies to the RBC membrane.[57]

Typically, patients with a positive direct Coombs' test caused by systemic disease will have antibodies attached to their RBC membranes. These antibody-coated cells are then removed by the phagocytic system, which in turn causes an extravascular hemolysis. Methyldopa has long been known

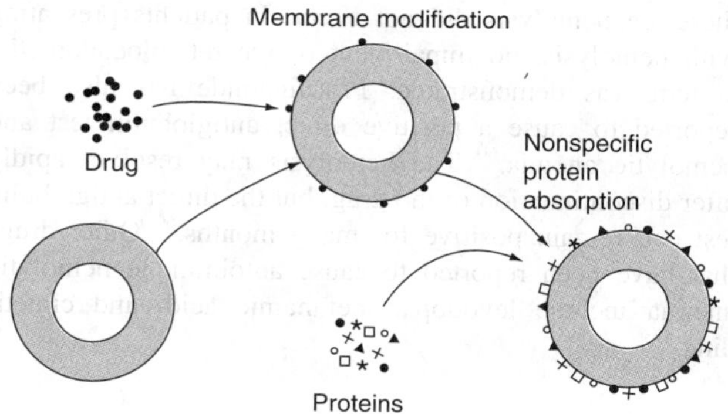

Figure 96.6. The nonspecific binding of proteins mechanism. The drug combines with the cell membrane, which in turn causes a nonspecific binding of serum protein. This reaction is seen primarily with the cephalosporins and no cell lysis or toxicity occurs. *(From Ref. 57, with permission.)*

to produce a Coombs' positive hemolytic anemia but the clinical course of the anemia does not follow the typical presentation of an immune hemolytic anemia. The first difference is that the majority of patients who develop a positive direct Coombs' test due to causes other than methyldopa will develop extravascular hemolysis. However, of the 15–20% of patients who develop a positive direct Coombs' test (also called direct antiglobulin test) after taking methyldopa, only 0.8% will develop hemolysis.[57] Second, the time between the development of a hemolytic anemia and a positive direct antiglobulin test is usually short. Patients with methyldopa-induced hemolytic anemia will present from 18 months to 4 years after initiation of the drug, but most patients will develop a direct positive antiglobulin test much earlier (3–6 months) after therapy is initiated.[57] Another differentiating factor in the development of hemolysis due to methyldopa is that although hemolysis may subside promptly after discontinuation of the drug, the antiglobulin test may remain positive from 7–20 months.[57] Patients who are antiglobulin test positive but are not hemolyzing can receive blood transfusions without any adverse effects.

Due to the many contradictions seen in methyldopa-induced hemolytic anemia and our past misunderstanding of the immune system, a number of mechanisms for the cause of this disorder have been proposed over the years. The most plausible mechanism is one in which researchers demonstrated that methyldopa inhibited the proliferation of nonspecific suppressor T cells.[58] This inhibition of suppressor T cells allows unregulated production of autoantibodies by plasma cells. The increase in autoantibodies causes the antiglobulin test to turn positive. However, this mechanism still does not explain why only a small number of patients with a positive direct Coombs' test develop hemolytic anemia. Kelton et al.[59] demonstrated that methyldopa impairs reticuloendothelial cell function. In Coombs' positive patients receiving methyldopa, patients with impairment of the reticuloendothelial system could not clear the RBCs coated with autoantibodies from their bloodstream, therefore hemolysis did not occur. In patients presenting with hemolysis, no impairment of the reticuloendothelial system was demonstrated. Procainamide has also been reported to cause a positive direct antiglobulin test and hemolytic anemia.[60] The hemolysis may resolve rapidly after discontinuation of the drug, but the direct antiglobulin test can remain positive for many months.[60] Other drugs that have been reported to cause autoimmune hemolytic anemia include levodopa, mefanamic acid, and cimetidine.[57]

TREATMENT

The treatment of drug-induced immune hemolytic anemia includes the removal of the offending agent and supportive care. As in agranulocytosis intravenous immune globulins have been used in severe cases of immune hemolytic anemia.[61]

Drug-Induced Oxidative Hemolytic Anemia

Drug-induced oxidative hemolytic anemia is a hereditary condition most often associated with a glucose-6-phosphate dehydrogenase (G6PD) enzyme deficiency but can occur because of other enzyme defects (i.e., NADH methemoglobin reductase or GSH peroxidase). The concentration of the G6PD enzyme is decreased in 13% of American black males, 3% of American black females, and in some other ethnic groups (e.g., Greek, Sardinians, Sephardics Jews).[62]

Drug-induced oxidative hemolytic anemia occurs under these conditions[63]:

1. An abnormal increase in oxidative stress exceeds the normal sources of reducing power.
2. Structural abnormalities of the RBC hemoglobulin molecule render the cells more susceptible to oxidant stress despite normal reducing sources.
3. There is a deficiency of reducing power in the RBC; therefore, the cell cannot react appropriately to normal increases in oxidative stress.

Excessive oxidative stress can denature the hemoglobulin molecule and increase the RBC membrane rigidity, resulting in cell lysis. The degree of hemolysis depends on the severity of the enzyme deficiency and the amount of oxidative stress. However, the dose required for hemolysis to occur is often less than prescribed quantities of the suspected agent.[63] Any drug that places oxidative stress on the RBC will cause drug-induced oxidative hemolytic anemia, but severe hemolysis is rare.[63] An interesting case of drug-induced oxidative hemolytic anemia occurred in a child when dapsone (an oxidizing agent) was transferred through the breast milk of the mother, who was taking the drug.[64] For a list of agents that can cause drug-induced oxidative hemolytic anemia refer to Table 96.6.

TABLE 96.6. DRUGS ASSOCIATED WITH OXIDATIVE HEMOLYSIS

Ascorbic acid	Menadiol
Aspirin	Methylene blue
Benzocaine	Nitrofurantoin
Chloramphenicol	Nitrofurazone
Chloraquine	Phenazopyridine
Dapsone	Salazosulphapyridine
Diazoxide	

TREATMENT

The treatment for drug-induced oxidative hemolytic anemia is removal of the drug. No other therapy is usually necessary since most cases of drug-induced oxidative hemolytic anemia are mild in severity. Patients should be advised to avoid medication capable of inducing the hemolysis.

Drug-Induced Megaloblastic Anemia

Drug-induced megaloblastic anemia is the result of abnormal development of RBC precursors called megaloblasts in the bone marrow. Examination of peripheral blood will show a rise in the mean corpuscular hemoglobin. These megaloblastic changes are due to the direct or indirect effects of the drug on DNA synthesis. The abnormality can be seen in any portion of the replication process including DNA assembly, base precursor metabolism, or RNA synthesis.[65] The antineoplastic agents because of their pharmacologic action on DNA replication are most frequently associated with drug-induced megaloblastic anemia. However, other drugs such as cotrimoxazole, phenytoin, or the barbiturates have also been implicated. Cotrimoxazole has been reported to cause drug-induced megaloblastic anemia with both low and high doses.[66,67] The drug-induced megaloblastic anemia produced by cotrimoxazole is thought to occur most frequently in patients with a partial B_{12} or folate deficiency.[65] Because the drug's affinity for human dihydrofolate reductase is low, patients with adequate stores of these vitamins are probably at low risk of developing drug-induced megaloblastic anemia. Phenytoin, primidone, and phenobarbital have been postulated to cause drug-induced megaloblastic anemia by either inhibiting folate absorption or by increasing the folate catabolism. In both instances, relative deficiency of folate is produced. Table 96.7 provides a list of drugs that have been suggested to produce drug-induced megaloblastic anemia.

TABLE 96.7. DRUGS ASSOCIATED WITH MEGALOBLASTIC ANEMIA

p-Aminosalicylate	Neomycin
Azathioprine	Nitrofurantoin
Chloramphenicol	Oral contraceptives
Cochicine	Phenobarbital
Cyclophosphamide	Phenytoin
Cytarabine	Primidone
5-Fluorodeoxyuridine	Pyrimethamine
5-Fluorouracil	Sulphasalazine
Hydroxyurea	Triamterene
6-Mercaptopurine	Trimethoprim
Methotrexate	Vinblastine

TREATMENT

When drug-induced megaloblastic anemia is related to chemotherapy, no real therapeutic option is available and drug-induced megaloblastic anemia is an accepted side effect of therapy. If drug-induced megaloblastic anemia occurs due to cotrimoxazole, a trial course of folinic acid 5–10 mg up to four times a day may correct the anemia.[66,67] Folic acid supplementation of 1 mg every day will often correct the drug-induced megaloblastic anemia produced by either phenytoin or phenobarbital, but some clinicians suggest that supplementation of folic acid may decrease the effectiveness of the antiepileptic medications.

Drug-Induced Thrombocytopenia

The mechanism of drug-induced thrombocytopenia is similar to that of drug-induced agranulocytosis and drug-induced hemolytic anemia: either a toxic or an immune-mediated reaction. If the effect from the drug is a direct toxicity, there will be a decrease in megakaryocytes in the bone marrow. This differs from an immune reaction where there is increased peripheral destruction of platelets and an increased number of megakaryocytes. Early symptoms of drug-induced thrombocytopenia include increased bruising, petechiae, ecchymosis, and epistaxis. Bleeding from mucous membranes and severe purpura can appear later in the disorder. Patients who develop drug-induced thrombocytopenia must be transfused when their platelet count drops to less than 20,000 platelets/mm^3.

Drugs that induce thrombocytopenia by their toxic effects are primarily cancer chemotherapy agents, but organic solvents, pesticides, and amrinone have also been implicated. Amrinone has been shown to cause thrombocytopenia in up to 18.6% of the patients taking the drug.[68] The thrombocytopenia is mild in severity and can occur from 24 hours to 2 weeks after initiation of the drug orally. Although investigators have demonstrated an amrinone-dependent antibody, it is believed that because of the rapid onset, the dose-related response, and the absence of anamestic effect, the disorder is indicative of a reaction other than immune mediated, probably toxic.[68] Amphotericin B has also been implicated in a case of thrombocytopenia. The mechanism proposed by the author was a toxic effect on the bone marrow since no peripheral destruction of the patient's platelets occurred.[69]

In the majority of patients, drug-induced thrombocytopenia is caused by an immune reaction. The mechanisms are similar to those described earlier in the chapter. The formation of a hapten between the drug and a molecule on the platelet membrane is seen with penicillin derivatives, trimethoprim, and heparin. A complete list of medications known to cause drug-induced thrombocytopenia can be found in Table 96.8. Hapten-mediated thrombocytopenia occurs 7–15 days after initiation of the drug and is seen frequently in patients receiving large doses of the medication (i.e., penicillin derivatives > 150 mg/kg).[70,71] The recovery period is often short in duration.[72]

Heparin can cause at least two types of thrombocytopenia.[73] The first is mild and occurs 2–4 days after initiation of therapy. The platelet count then slowly returns to normal following the initial drop. The patients develop no major sequelae from the thrombocytopenia. The mechanism for this type of reaction may be sequestration of platelets.[73]

The second type of heparin-induced thrombocytopenia is the severe form of the reaction and may be associated with thrombosis.[73,74] The platelet count generally begins to drop 6–12 days after starting heparin therapy. Patients can develop thrombocytopenia and thrombosis even on low-dose heparin[73,75] or with heparin-coated catheters.[76] The reaction is mediated by the formation of antibodies to the platelet–heparin complex. The antibodies attach to the complex and fix complement, allowing the activation of archi-

TABLE 96.8. DRUGS ASSOCIATED WITH THROMBOCYTOPENIA

Acetazolamide	Hydroxychloroquine
Acetylsalicylic acid	Interferon
Allopurinol	Isoniazid
Aminoglutethimide	Meclofenamate
Aminosalicylic acid	Morphine
Amrinone	Penicillin
Cephalothin	Phenylbutazone
Chlorothiazide	Phenytoin
Cimetidine	Procainamide
Desipramine	Quinidine
Diazepam	Quinine
Digitoxin	Rifampin
Furosemide	Sulfisoxazole
Hydrochlorothiazide	Trimethoprim

donic acid and endoperoxide by the platelets.[77] The platelets subsequently aggregate and form a thrombus. Recently, investigators have shown that antibodies formed to heparin may also attach to endothelial cells on the wall of arteries. The binding of the antibodies then helps to promote the formation of the thrombus.[78] The incidence of heparin-induced thrombocytopenia with thrombosis has been reported to be three to four times higher with bovine sources of heparin compared to porcine[79,80] but several studies have demonstrated no differences between animal sources of heparin.[80–83] In one patient, changing from a bovine source to a porcine source in the face of active heparin-induced thrombocytopenia and thrombosis did not eliminate the disorder.[84] Drug manufacturers are looking at low molecular weight heparin products to determine if they can decrease the incidence of heparin-induced thrombocytopenia.[85] Investigators are also studying these products to determine if they can be used as an anticoagulant in patients who have developed thrombocytopenia due to heparin.[85] One study has demonstrated that antibodies to heparin can interact with low molecular weight heparin, but they established that there was no binding to heparin-like drugs called "heparinoid."[86]

The thrombocytopenia induced by gold salts is also related to antibody formation to platelets.[87,88] The incidence of gold-induced thrombocytopenia is from 1–3% and often has a abrupt and severe onset.[87] The autoantibody formed to the platelet appears to be associated with the human leukocyte antigens (HLA), which are located on the platelet membrane and on a number of other different cells in the body.[87,88] The HLA antigens are specific antigens that allow the body to determine between antigens (i.e., tissue, platelets, etc.) that are part of a particular individual genetic make-up (self-antigens) or genetically dissimilar antigens (non–self-antigens). The recognition of HLA antigens controls the immunologic response of an individual to a particular antigenic stimulus. In some types of autoimmune diseases, HLA antigens are associated with development of the disease. The recognition of these HLA antigens in combination with antigenic determinants causes the patients own immune system to attack the patient's own body. In gold-induced thrombocytopenia, a similar reaction occurs. An interaction between the gold salts and the HLA antigens occurs, causing the platelets to be recognized as non-self, thus inducing destruction of the platelets. The most commonly reported HLA antigen associated with induction of the autoantibodies is DR-3, but DR-4 may also interact with the antibodies.[87–89] The exact mechanism by which gold causes the formation of the autoantibody to regulated DR-3 and DR-4 antigens has not been elucidated.

The third mechanism described for drug-induced thrombocytopenia is the innocent bystander immune response. The most commonly implicated drug is quinidine and the drug-induced thrombocytopenia is frequently related to high doses of quinidine.[90] Quinidine may also form a hapten with the platelet membrane to produce thrombocytopenia.[91]

TREATMENT

The primary treatment of drug-induced thrombocytopenia is removal of the offending drug and symptomatic treatment of the patient. In the case of heparin-induced thrombocytopenia with thrombosis, some clinicians recommend the administration of antiplatelet drugs[92] or low molecular weight heparin products.[85] At the present time, however, no studies have been performed to demonstrate the efficacy of the antiplatelet agents. In addition, it appears that large doses of steroids have no effect.[93] In gold salt-induced thrombocytopenia, however, some investigators believe prednisone in a dose of 60 mg daily is beneficial in correcting the thrombocytopenia.[87]

CONCLUSION

The occurrence of a drug-induced blood disorder is rare. The mechanisms of the disorders often involve either an immune or toxic effect on the affected blood cell line. The primary treatment is removal of the drug in question and symptomatic support of the patient.

REFERENCES

1. Arneborn P, Palmblad J. Drug-induced neutropenia—a survey for Stockholm 1973–1978. Acta Med Scand 1982;212:289–292.
2. Arneborn P, Palmblad J. Drug-induced neutropenia in the Stockholm region 1973–1975; Frequency and causes. Acta Med Scand 1978;204:283–286.
3. Arneborn P, Palmblad J. Drug-induced neutropenias in the Stockholm region 1976–1977. Acta Med Scand 1979;206:241–243.
4. Hine LK, Gerstman BB, Wise RP, et al. Mortality resulting from blood dyscrasias in the United States: 1984. Am J Med 1990;88:151–153.
5. Pisciotta V. Drug-induced agranulocytosis. Drugs 1978;15:132–143.
6. Claas FHJ. Drug-induced immune granulocytopenia. Baillieres Clin Immunol Allergy 1987;1:357–368.
7. Ehmann WC. Cephalosporin-induced hemolysis: A case report and review of the literature. Am J Hematol 1992;40:121–125.
8. Richman DD, Fischl MA, Grieco MH, et al. The toxicity of azidothymidine (AZT) in the treatment of patients with AIDS and AIDS-related complex. N Engl J Med 1987;317:192–197.
9. Furman P, Fyle JA, St Clair MH, et al. Phosphorylation of 3′-azido-3′-deoxythymidine and selective interaction of the 5′-triphosphate with human immunodeficiency virus reverse transcriptase. Proc Natl Acad Sci USA 1986;83:8333–8337.

10. Brajtburg J, Elberg S, Schwartz DR, et al. Involvement of oxidative damage in erythrocyte lysis induced by amphotericin B. Antimicrob Agents Chemother 1985;27:172–176.
11. Haak HL. Experimental drug-induced aplastic anemia. Clin Haematol 1980;9:621–639.
12. Levy M. The combined effect of viruses and drugs in drug-induced diseases. Med Hypoth 1984;14:293–296.
13. Niewg HO. Aplastic anemia (panmyelopathy), in Girdwood RH (ed): Blood Disorders Due to Drugs and Other Agents. Amsterdam, Excerpta Media, 1974.
14. The International Agranulocytosis and Aplastic Anemia Study. Risk of agranulocytosis and aplastic anemia. A first report of their relation to drug use with special reference to analgesics. JAMA 1986;256:1749–1757.
15. Vincent PC. In vitro evidence of drug action in aplastic anemia. Blut 1984;49:3–12.
16. Heimpel H, Heit W. Drug-induced aplastic anemia: Clinical aspects. Clin Haematol 1980;9:641–662.
17. Lubran MM. Hematologic side effects of drugs. Ann Clin Lab Sci 1989;19:114–121.
18. Yunis AA, Miller AM, Salem Z, et al. Chloramphenicol toxicity: Pathogenetic mechanisms and the role of the p-NO_2 in aplastic anemia. Clin Tox 1980;17:359–373.
19. Jimenez JJ, Arimura GK, Abou-Khalil WH, et al. Chloramphenicol-induced bone marrow injury: Possible role of bacterial metabolites of chloramphenicol. Blood 1987;70:1180–1185.
20. Malkin D, Koren G, Saunders EF. Drug-induced aplastic anemia pathogenesis and clinical aspects. Am J Pediatr Hematol Oncol 1990;12:402–410.
21. Gerson WT, Fine DG, Spielberg SP, et al. Anticonvulsant-induced aplastic anemia: Increased susceptibility to toxic drug metabolites *in vitro.* Blood 1983;61:889–893.
22. Thomas ED, Storb R. Acquired severe aplastic anemia: Progress and perplexity. Blood 1984;64:325–328.
23. Champlin R, Ho W, Gale RP. Antithymocyte globulin treatment in patients with aplastic anemia. N Engl J Med 1983;308:113–118.
24. Litzow MR, Kyle RA. Multiple responses of aplastic anemia to low-dose cyclosporine therapy despite development of a myelodysplastic syndrome. Am J Hematol 1989;32:226–229.
25. Bridges R, Pineo G, Blahey W. Cyclosporin A for the treatment of aplastic anemia refractory to antithymocyte globulin. Am J Hematol 1987;26:83–87.
26. Jacobs P, Wood L, Martell RW. Cyclosporin A in the treatment of severe acute aplastic anaemia. Br J Haematol 1985;61:267–272.
27. Antin JH, Smith BR, Holmes W, et al. Phase I/II study of recombinant human granulocyte-macrophage colony stimulating factor in aplastic anemia and myelodysplastic syndrome. Blood 1988;72:705–713.
28. Vadhan-Raj S, Buescher S, Broxmeyer HE, et al. Stimulation of myelopoiesis in patients with aplastic anemia by recombinant human granulocyte-macrophage colony-stimulating factor. N Engl J Med 1988;319:1628–1634.
29. Walsh CE, Liu JM, Anderson SM, et al. A trial of recombinant human interleukin I in patients with severe refractory aplastic anaemia. Br J Haematol 1992;80:106–110.
30. Bertrand Y, Amri F, Capdeville R, et al. The successful treatment of two cases of severe aplastic anaemia with granulocyte-colony stimulating factor and cyclosporine A. Br J Haematol 1991;79:648–652.
31. Heit W, Heimpel H, Fischer A, et al. Drug-induced agranulocytosis: Evidence for the commitment of bone marrow haematopoiesis. Scand J Haematol 1985;35:459–468.
32. Julia A, Olona M, Bueno J, et al. Drug-induced agranulocytosis: Prognostic factors in a series of 168 episodes. Br J Haematol 1991;79:366–371.
33. Burckart GJ, Snidow J, Bruce W. Neutropenia following acute chlorpromazine ingestion. Clin Tox 1981;18:797–801.
34. Neftel KA, Muller MR, Hauser SD, et al. More on penicillin-induced leukopenia. N Engl J Med 1983;308:901.
35. Heit WF. Hematologic effects of antipyretic analgesics: Drug-induced agranulocytosis. Am J Med 1983;75:65–68.
36. Young GA, Vincent PC. Drug-induced agranulocytosis. Baillieres Clin Haematol 1980;9:483–504.
37. Kirkwood CF, Smith LL, Rustagi PK, et al. Neutropenia associated with B-lactam antibiotics. Clin Pharm 1983; 2:569–578.
38. Homayouni H, Gross PA, Setia V, et al. Leukopenia due to penicillin and cephalosporin homologues. Arch Intern Med 1979;139:827–828.
39. Neftel KA, Hauser SP, Muller MR. Inhibition of granulopoiesis *in vivo* and *in vitro* by β-lactam antibiotics. J Infect Dis 1985;152:90–98.
40. Cooper DS, Goldmiriz D, Lewin AA, et al. Agranulocytosis associated with antithyroid drug. Ann Intern Med 1983;98:26–29.
41. Tajiri J, Noguchi S, Murakami T, et al. Antithyroid drug-induced agranulocytosis. The usefulness of routine white blood cell count monitoring. Arch Intern Med 1990;150:621–624.
42. Toth AL, Mant MJ, Shivji S, et al. Propylthiouracil-induced agranulocytosis: An unusual presentation and a possible mechanism. Am J Med 1988;85:725–727.
43. McIntyre PA, Laleli YR, Hodkinson BA, et al. Evidence for antileukocyte antibodies as a mechanism for drug-induced agranulocytosis. Trans Assoc Am Phys 1971;84:217–225.
44. Werner MC, Romaldini JH, Bromberg N, et al. Adverse effects related to thionamide drugs regimen. Am J Med Sci 1989;297:216–219.
45. Clozaril new drug application. vols 28–31, 36, 39, 48, 50, 52, 84, 98, 99, 100, 103. East Hanover, NJ, Sandoz, Inc., 1987 August 10, 1987.
46. Alvir JM, Lieberman JA, Safferman AZ, et al. Clozapine-induced agranulocytosis. Incidence and risk factors in the United States. N Engl J Med 1993;329:162–167.
47. Fischer V, Haar JA, Greiner L, et al. Possible role of free radical formation in clozapine (Clozaril) induced agranulocytosis. Molecular Pharmacol 1991;40:846–853.
48. Lakos A, Timar L. Treatment of idiopathic chronic neutropenia with high-dose intravenous immunoglobulin. Am J Dis Child 1987;141:12–13.
49. Willfort A, Lorber C, Kapiotis S, et al. Treatment of drug-induced agranulocytosis with recombinant granulocyte colony-stimulating factor (rh G-CSF). Ann Hematol 1993;66:241–244.
50. Delannoy A. GM-CSF therapy for drug-induced agranulocytosis. J Intern Med 1992;231:269–271.

51. MacDonald AG, Capell HA, Murphy J. Gold-induced aplastic anemia unresponsive to G-CSF. Annal Rheum Dis 1993;52:488.
52. Teitelbaum AH, Bell AJ, Brown SL. Filgrastim (r-metHuG-CSF) reversal of drug-induced agranulocytosis. Am J Med 1993;95:245–246.
53. Nielsen H. Recombinant human granulocyte colony-stimulating factor (rhG-CSF): Filgrastim treatment of clozapine-induced agranulocytosis. J Intern Med 1993;234:529–531.
54. Bjorkholm M, Pisa P, Arver S, Beran M. Haematologic effects of granulocyte-macrophage colony stimulating in a patient with thiamazole-induced agranulocytosis. J Intern Med 1992;232:443–445.
55. Nand S, Bayer R, Prinz R. Granulocyte-macrophage colony stimulating factor for the treatment of drug induced agranulocytosis. Am J Hematol 1991;37:267–269.
56. Yust I, Frisch B, Goldsher N. Simultaneous detection of two mechanisms of immune destruction of penicillin-treated human red blood cells. Am J Hematol 1982;13:53–62.
57. Petz LD. Drug-induced immune haemolytic anaemia. Baillieres Clin Haematol 1980;91:455–482.
58. Kirtland HH, Mohler DN, Horwitz DA. Methyldopa inhibition of suppressor-lymphocyte function. A proposed cause of auto immune hemolytic anemia. N Engl J Med 1980;302:825–832.
59. Kelton JG. Impaired reticulonendothelial function in patients treated with methyldopa. N Engl J Med 1985;313:596–600.
60. Kleinman S, Nelson R, Smith L, et al. Positive direct antiglobulin tests and immune hemolytic anemia in patients receiving procainamide. N Engl J Med 1984; 311:809–812.
61. Hilgartner MW, Bussel J. Use of intravenous gamma globulin for the treatment of autoimmune neutropenia of childhood and autoimmune hemolytic anemia. Am J Med 1987;83(suppl 4A):25–29.
62. Wallach J. Ed. Interpretation of Diagnostic Tests: A Handbook Synopsis of Laboratory Medicine, 3rd ed. Boston, Little, Brown, 1978.
63. Gordan-Smith EC. Drug-induced oxidative haemolysis. Clin Haematol 1980;9:557–586.
64. Sanders SW, Zone JJ, Foltz RL, et al. Hemolytic anemia induced by dapsone transmitted through breast milk. Ann Intern Med 1982;96:465–466.
65. Scott JM, Weir DG. Drug-induced megaloblastic change. Clin Haematol 1980;9:587–605.
66. Magee F, O'Sullivan H, McCann SR. Megaloblastosis and low-dose trimethoprim-sulfamethoxazole. Ann Intern Med 1981;95:657.
67. Kobrinsky NL, Ramsay NK. Acute megaloblastic anemia induced by high-dose trimethoprim-sulfamethoxazole. Ann Intern Med 1981;94:780–781.
68. Ansell J, Tiarks C, McCue J, et al. Amrinone-induced thrombocytopenia. Arch Intern Med 1984;144:949–952.
69. Chan CP, Tuazon CU, Lessin LS. Amphotericin-B-induced thrombocytopenia. Ann Intern Med 1982;96:332–333.
70. Murphy MF, Riordant T, Minchinton RM, et al. Demonstration of an immune-mediated mechanism of penicillin-induced neutropenia and thrombocytopenia. Br J Haematol 1983;55:155–160.
71. Salamon DJ, Nusbacher J, Stroupe T, et al. Red cell and platelet-bound IgG penicillin antibodies in a patient with thrombocytopenia. Transfusion 1984;24:395–398.
72. Miescher PA, Graf J. Drug-induced thrombocytopenia. Clin Haematol 1980;9:505–519.
73. Johnson RA, Lazarus KH, Henry DH. Heparin-induced thrombocytopenia prospective study. Am J Hematol 1984;17:349–353.
74. Cines DB, Kaywin P, Bina M, et al. Heparin-associated thrombocytopenia. N Engl Med 1980;303:788–795.
75. Cheng TC. Thrombocytopenia associated with minidose heparin therapy. Post Grad Med 1981;70:73–78.
76. Laster JL, Nichols WK, Silver D. Thrombocytopenia associated with heparin-coated catheters in patients with heparin-associated antiplatelet antibodies. Arch Intern Med 1989;149:2285–2287.
77. Arthur CK, Isbister JP, Aspery EM. The heparin-induced thrombosis–thrombocytopenia syndrome (HITTS): A review. Pathology 1985;17:82–86.
78. Cines DB, Tomaski A, Tannenbaum S. Immune endothelial cell injury in heparin-associated thrombocytopenia. N Engl J Med 1987;316:581–589.
79. King DJ and Kelton JG. Heparin-associated thrombocytopenia. Ann Intern Med 1984;100:535–540.
80. Bell WR, Royall RM. Heparin-associated thrombocytopenia: A comparison of three heparin preparations. N Engl J Med 1980;303:902–907.
81. Green D, Martin GJ, Shoichet SH, et al. Thrombocytopenia in a prospective, randomized, double-blind trial of bovine and porcine heparin. Am J Med Sci 1984;288(2):60–64.
82. Rao AK, White GC, Sherman L, et al. Low incidence of thrombocytopenia with porcine mucosal heparin. A prospective multicenter study. Arch Intern Med 1989;149:1285–1288.
83. Bailey RT, Ursick JA, Heim KL, et al. Heparin-associated thrombocytopenia: A prospective comparison of bovine lung heparin, manufactured by a new process, and porcine intestinal heparin. Drug Intell Clin Pharm 1986;20:374–378.
84. Guay DR, Richard A. Heparin-induced thrombocytopenia—association with a platelet aggregating factor and cross-sensitivity to bovine and porcine heparin. Drug Intell Clin Pharm 1984;18:398–401.
85. Chong BH, Ismdil F, Cade J, et al. Heparin-induced thrombocytopenia: Studies with a new low molecular weight heparinoid, Org 10172. Blood 1989;73:1592–1596.
86. Kikta MJ, Keller MP, Humphrey PV, et al. Can low molecular weight heparins and heparinoids be safely given to patients with heparin-induced thromocytopenia syndrome? Surgery 1993;114:705–710.
87. Armstrong RD, Faith A, Panayi GS, et al. Gold-induced thrombocytopenia: Detection of anti-platelet antibody. Clin Rheumatol 1983;2:183–188.
88. Adachi JD, Bensen WG, Singal DP, et al. Gold induced thrombocytopenia: Platelet associated IgG and HLA typing in three patients. J Rheumatol 1984;11:355–357.
89. Coblyn JS, Weinblatt M, Holdsworth D, et al. Gold-induced thrombocytopenia. A clinical and immunogenic study of twenty-three patients. Ann Intern Med 1981;95:178–181.

90. Kelton JG, Meltzer D, Moore J, et al. Drug-induced thrombocytopenia is associated with increased binding of IgG to platelets both *in vivo* and *in vitro.* Blood 1981;58:524–529.
91. Chong BH, Berndt MC, Koutts J, et al. Quinidine-induced thrombocytopenia and leukopenia: Demonstration and characterization of distinct antiplatelets and antileukocyte antibodies. Blood 1983;62:1218–1223.
92. Matsuo T, Yamada T, Chikahira Y, et al. Effect of aspirin on heparin-induced thrombocytopenia (HIT) in a patient requiring hemodialysis. Blut 1989;59:393–395.
93. Rector TS, Cipolle RJ, Seifert RD, et al. Characteristics of heparin-associated thrombocytopenia. Am J Hosp Pharm 1979;36:1561–1565.

PART THREE

Diseases of Infectious Origin

Chapter 97

Use of Laboratory Tests in Infectious Diseases

Michael N. Dudley, PharmD, FCCP

The treatment of infectious diseases provides a unique opportunity for the clinician to individualize drug therapy. No other group of diseases is more amenable to *ex vivo* study of drug effects—one can indeed study the etiology of a disease in the absence of a host. This possibility has resulted in the development and utilization of many tests of antimicrobial activity to guide the clinician in the selection and monitoring of patient response to therapy. However, although clinicians have an impressive array of tests to guide them, considerable controversy remains regarding the appropriate, cost-efficient use of even some of the most fundamental measures of antimicrobial activity.[1] This chapter reviews the basic tests available to the clinician in the clinical laboratory that are useful in the diagnosis and treatment of infectious diseases.

Laboratory Tests Confirming the Presence of Infection

NONSPECIFIC TESTS

Several tests are routinely used to detect the presence of infection. Their usefulness lies in that they are "sensitive" in detecting the presence of an infection (i.e., give a positive result when there is truly an infection). A positive result with these tests usually prompts a more directed search for specific pathogens in body sites using some of the techniques for identification of a pathogen described later in this chapter.

White Blood Cell Count and Differential

Moderate to high elevation of the total white blood cell (WBC) count often indicates the presence of systemic infection. In bacterial infections, the total WBC count usually rises above the normal range (5–10,000/mm^3). The leukocytosis may be mild, particularly in elderly patients or in less serious infections, or it may exceed 50,000 cells/mm^3 in overwhelming sepsis; however, the absolute WBC count remains a nonspecific test as elevations may be observed in noninfectious diseases (e.g., leukemia, rheumatoid arthritis) or during drug therapy (e.g., corticosteroids, lithium).

The differential count may be of further use in defining the cause of the leukocytosis and occasionally the etiology of infection. Table 97.1 displays the normal differential of the WBC count for an adult. Bacterial infections generally result in an increase in neutrophils (polymorphonuclear leukocytes, PMNs, "segs"). This is the principal cell type involved in cell-mediated host response to bacterial infection. Microscopic examination of a peripheral blood smear may disclose morphological changes in the cytoplasm of these cells (e.g., toxic granulations, vacuolization) that are suggestive of bacterial infection. Immature cells ("bands," "stabs") are often released from the bone marrow into the peripheral circulation during acute infection. This so-called "shift-to-the-left" (so named because of the location of these cells in diagrams depicting neutrophil maturation in basic immunology texts) may exceed 10–20% of the total number of WBCs.

Leukocytosis secondary to bacterial infection does not occur in all hosts. For example, bacterial infections are frequently a complication of neutropenia from cancer chemotherapy; these patients are incapable of developing a leukocytosis in response to bacterial infection. Indeed, the outcome of infection in these patients is highly dependent on a rise in WBC count. In the elderly, leukocytosis is frequently absent during an acute bacterial infection and overwhelming sepsis may also produce a low WBC count.

Lymphocytosis is most frequently associated with viral infection. For example, acute Epstein–Barr virus infection (mononucleosis) produces an absolute leukocytosis with a lymphocytic predominance. These lymphocytes are frequently described as being "atypical" because of their morphologic appearance on microscopic examination. Lymphopenia, particularly with the helper (i.e., CD-4) sub-

TABLE 97.1. NORMAL WHITE BLOOD CELL DIFFERENTIAL IN AN ADULT

Cell Type	Percent (%)
Neutrophils (PMNs[a])	50–70
Immature neutrophils (bands, stabs)	3–5
Metamyelocytes	0–1
Lymphocytes	20–40
Monocytes	0–7
Eosinophils	0–5
Basophils	0–1

[a]PMNs, polymorphonuclear leukocytes.

set of T-cell lymphocytes, is characteristic of human immunodeficiency virus (HIV) infection.

Monocytosis is less frequently associated with acute bacterial infection, although its presence has been associated with the response of certain infections (e.g., tuberculosis) to chemotherapy. Eosinophilia may result from parasitic infection.

Other Tests

Other nonspecific laboratory tests may be useful in diagnosing infection. Large elevations of the erythrocyte sedimentation rate (ESR, "sed" rate) are associated with acute or chronic infection, particularly endocarditis, chronic osteomyelitis, and intra-abdominal infection. Unfortunately, a normal ESR does not exclude the possibility of infection. The ESR is frequently elevated due to noninfectious causes such as collagen vascular disease.[2] Serum complement concentrations, particularly the C3 component, are often reduced in serious infections because of consumption during the host defense process. Acute phase reactants such as C-reactive proteins may be elevated in acute infection and may support a clinical diagnosis of infection. Certain cytokines (e.g., interleukin-1, interleukin-6, tumor necrosis factor-alpha) are elevated in certain stages of infection and may be useful in identifying patients with serious infections such as sepsis.[3]

Laboratory Identification of Pathogens

COLONIZATION VERSUS INFECTION

One of the most difficult tasks confronting the clinician is the differentiation between infection and colonization with potential pathogens in certain body sites. *Colonization* may be defined as the presence of an organism at a body site *without* production of disease in a host. *Infection* implies the presence of an organism within tissues with invasiveness that often results in a *response* by the host's immune defenses.

The body is not a sterile arena. Many body sites are colonized with bacteria such that they are regarded as "normal" flora. Table 97.2 lists bacteria commonly found in several body sites. While these bacteria are considered normal flora, they become pathogenic when introduced into other body sites or fluids through trauma or breakdown of host defenses. For example, while *Staphylococcus epidermidis* is considered normal flora on skin, it is a pathogen if found in cerebrospinal fluid, particularly following a surgical procedure such as placement of a cerebrospinal shunt.

DIRECT EXAMINATION

One of the most rapid and readily available methods for the laboratory diagnosis and identification of pathogens is direct examination of body fluids or tissues believed to be infected. Gram stain characteristics (positive, negative, or variable) and morphologic appearance (e.g., coccus or bacillus) provide rapid, often definitive identification of bacteria and may be of great use in selecting empiric antimicrobial therapy. Table 97.3 lists some common infecting pathogens grouped according to Gram stain and other characteristics. Certain other bacterial (e.g., mycobacteria) and fungal pathogens may be best identified microscopically using special reagents or stains. Other pathogens may be identified through special stains, wet mounts, fixed slides, or specimens treated with fluorescent antibody specific for an antigen associated with a pathogen. Newer DNA hybridization techniques (described in the following section) allow for direct examination of tissues with signal-emitting probes that are specific for the nucleic acids of pathogens.[4]

TABLE 97.2. ORGANISMS FREQUENTLY REGARDED AS NORMAL, COLONIZING FLORA

Skin	**Upper Respiratory Tract**
Diphtheroids (e.g., *Corynebacterium* sp.)	*Bacteroides* sp.
Propionibacteria	*Haemophilus* sp.
Staphylococci (esp. coagulase-negative strains)	*Neisseria* sp.
Streptococci	Streptococci
Gastrointestinal Tract	**Genital Tract**
Bacteroides sp.	*Corynebacterium* sp.
Clostridium sp.	*Enterobacteriaceae*
Diphtheroids	*Lactobacillus* sp.
Enterobacteriaceae (e.g., *Escherichia coli, Klebsiella* sp.)	*Mycoplasma* sp.
Fusobacterium sp.	Staphylococci
Streptococci (anaerobic)	Streptococci

TABLE 97.3. EXAMPLES OF IMPORTANT BACTERIAL PATHOGENS CLASSIFIED ACCORDING TO STAINING CHARACTERISTICS, MORPHOLOGY, AND OTHER SALIENT FEATURES

Gram-Positive Cocci
- Staphylococci
  - Coagulase-positive
    - *Staphylococcus aureus*
  - Coagulase-negative
    - *Staphylococcus epidermidis*
- Streptococci
  - Anaerobes
    - *Peptostreptococcus*
- *Streptococcus pneumoniae* (diplococcus, pneumococcus)
- Group A, β-hemolytic
  - *Streptococcus pyogenes*
- Group B
  - *Streptococcus agalactiae*
- Group D
  - Enterococcal species
    - *Enterococcus rafinosus*
    - *Enterococcus faecalis*
    - *Enterococcus durans*
    - *Enterococcus faecium*
  - Nonenterococcal species
    - *Streptococcus bovis*
    - *Streptococcus equinus*
  - Viridans group
    - *Streptococcus sanguis*
    - *Streptococcus mitior*
    - *Streptococcus mutans*
    - *Streptococcus milleri*

Gram-Positive Bacilli
- *Bacillus* sp.
  - *Bacillus cereus*
- *Clostridium* sp.
  - *Clostridium difficile*
  - *Clostridium perfringens*
  - *Clostridium tetani*
- Diphtheroids
  - *Corynebacterium diphtheriae*
  - JK group *Corynebacterium*
  - *Listeria monocytogenes*

Gram-Negative Bacilli
- Anaerobes
  - *Bacteroides fragilis*
  - *Bacteroides* sp.
- Enterobacteriaceae
  - *Citrobacter* sp.
  - *Enterobacter* sp.
  - *Escherichia coli*
  - *Klebsiella* sp.
  - *Serratia* sp.
  - *Morganella* sp.
  - *Proteus*
    - Indole-negative—*P. mirabilis*
    - Indole-positive—*P. vulgaris*
  - *Providencia* sp.
  - *Salmonella* sp.
  - *Serratia* sp.
  - *Shigella* sp.
- *Pseudomonas* sp.
  - *Pseudomonas aeruginosa*
  - *Pseudomonas cepacia*
- ***Xanthomonas maltophilia***

Gram-Negative Cocci
- *Moraxella catarrhalis*
- *Neisseria gonorrhoeae*
- *Neisseria meningitidis*

Mycobacteria (acid-fast bacilli)
- *Mycobacterium avium–intracellulare complex*
- *Mycobacterium bovis*
- *Mycobacterium fortuitum*
- *Mycobacterium tuberculosis*

Fungi
- Yeasts
  - *Candida* sp. *(C. albicans, C. krusei, C. tropicalis)*
  - *Cryptococcus neoformans*
- *Aspergillus* sp.
  - *Aspergillus fumigatus*

CULTURES

Growth and subsequent identification of etiologic agents from body fluids or tissues believed to be infected remain the most frequently utilized method of determining the etiology of infection. Most clinical laboratories are capable of cultivating aerobic and anaerobic gram-positive and gram-negative bacteria and certain fungi. Cultures of more fastidious bacteria, which may require special media or conditions (e.g., mycobacteria, chlamydia, *Legionella* sp.), and viral cultures are often only performed in larger hospitals or reference laboratories because of the expense of equipment, need for specialized personnel, and time involved in processing samples.

Assurance of proper collection and handling of specimens greatly enhances the correct interpretation and usefulness of culture of infected material. Careful collection of certain specimens (e.g., urine, sputum) to avoid contamination with commensal organisms is necessary to obtain meaningful results. When more fastidious organisms are suspected to be present in a sample, rapid transport of the specimen in appropriate transport medium and containers to the microbiology laboratory for processing is necessary to ensure recovery of a pathogen. For example, anaerobic bacteria from an abscess are best recovered when fluid for culture is collected by needle aspiration into a syringe and transported directly to the laboratory for inoculation rather than on a cotton swab.

Recent technological advances have enabled the rapid detection of growth of bacteria or fungi present in certain specimens within hours after collection. Several automated blood culturing systems (e.g., Bactec®) use bottles of growth media containing ^{14}C-labeled carbohydrates and amino acids. Aseptically collected blood samples submitted for culture are inoculated into these bottles and incubated. Early growth of bacteria is detected through determination of radiolabeled CO_2 produced by bacterial growth in bottles. Other similar systems detect production of CO_2 through nonradiometric methods or through oxygen consumption. Use of lysis centrifugation where blood is collected in tubes containing a reagent that lyses cells is extremely useful in detecting certain pathogens, such as *Mycobacterium avium–intracellulare* complex in acquired immunodeficiency syndrome.[5]

Once growth of a pathogen is established, bacteria are identified by fermentation properties, Gram staining characteristics, morphology, and growth characteristics on selective media. Biochemical profiling has become the basis for identification of bacteria. Classification of bacteria into certain groups based on sugar fermentation properties can broadly define a group of pathogens; for example, classification of aerobic gram-negative rods into lactose versus nonlactose fermenting bacteria has been useful for preliminary diagnosis of diarrheal pathogens. Other tests can be more specific; for example, *Pseudomonas aeruginosa* can be readily differentiated from other hospital-acquired gram-negative aerobic bacilli by the oxidase test, which takes only a few minutes to perform. This information may be of great value in the selection of empiric antibiotic therapy.

Definitive identification of bacteria may be accomplished by analysis of all the fermentation properties of an organism using commercially available biochemical testing panels. A suspension of the organism is inoculated into several small chambers containing various sugars or other reagents. Automated, "walkaway" systems are able to inoculate test panels and photometrically "read" the results of cuvettes containing various sugars and other reagents. The results are then compared with a library to give definitive identification of the organism.

A limited number of laboratories are capable of growing and isolating more fastidious microorganisms, including viral pathogens. Properly collected specimens are inoculated into tissue culture, and the virus type is identified by changes in culture cell morphology (e.g., cytopathic effect, syncytia formation) or detecting viral antigens (e.g., p24 antigen for HIV) in culture medium. However, the introduction of techniques in molecular biology has obviated the need for cultivation of many of these pathogens in the clinical laboratory.

Growth of organisms in specimens collected from patients receiving antimicrobial therapy may be slowed or inhibited by the antibiotic present in the specimen; this is particularly true in blood cultures where more fastidious organisms are present. This problem is partially remedied by the presence of certain components of culture medium, such as sodium polyanetholesulfonate (a polyanionic compound added to most blood culture media for its anticoagulant properties) and thiol broth. Some laboratories routinely add β-lactamase to all blood culture bottles. Commercial sources of bottled blood culture media containing antibiotic-binding resins (e.g., Bactec® 16B) are available.

DIAGNOSIS OF INFECTION USING IMMUNOLOGIC AND MOLECULAR METHODS

ANTIBODY AND ANTIGEN DETECTION

For many bacterial, fungal, and viral infections, culture of pathogens is neither feasible nor possible. Immunologic methods that detect the presence of patient antibody directed against a pathogen or an antigenic component are used in the definitive diagnosis of infection. A single antibody titer may be useful (e.g., antibody against surface proteins of HIV as measured in the widely used screening tests for HIV infection) for diagnosis of an infection. However, past or asymptomatic infection may result in low levels of unprotective antibody titers; in this case, an increasing antibody titer measured in specimens collected during the acute and convalescing stages of infection may be useful in confirming a diagnosis.

Similar principles are also utilized in detection of bacterial, fungal, and viral antigens in clinical specimens or culture. These methods have the advantages of usually being rapid and having acceptable sensitivity (i.e., the ability to detect a true positive test) and specificity (i.e., the ability of a test to give a negative result in the absence of disease). Many tests (e.g., identification of group A streptococci) can be performed in an office setting during regular hours.

Antibody or antigen may be detected by several techniques, including agglutination, immunodiffusion, immunoelectrophoresis, immunofluorescence, radioimmunoassay, immunoprecipitation, complement fixation, and immunoassay (e.g., enzyme-linked immunosorbent assay [ELISA]).

TECHNIQUES BASED ON MOLECULAR BIOLOGY

Use of Probes Specific for a Pathogen's Nucleotides

The recent development of methods for amplification of RNA and DNA sequences specific for pathogens has allowed for rapid, sensitive, and specific methods for identification of pathogens in clinical samples or cultures. Probe-based techniques utilize an oligonucleotide sequence that binds ("hybridizes") with a complementary nucleotide sequence from the microorganism. The probe is also labeled with a signal-emitting molecule (e.g., autoradiography) or a nonisotopic colorimetic or chemoluminescent antibody is directed against the probe. This technique may be applied in culture or tissue specimens *in situ,* which allows for a more definitive pathological diagnosis.[6]

Nucleic Acid Amplification

Polymerase Chain Reaction

Polymerase chain reaction (PCR) has become an enormously important tool in the detection of specific DNA or RNA from pathogens present in very low numbers. Its principle lies in the ability to produce copies of low amounts of pathogen-specific DNA (or RNA if initial reverse-transcription is employed) in the laboratory without the need for probes. In many cases, PCR may be capable of detecting fewer than 10 copies of DNA in a clinical sample. The technique involves serial cycles of heat-induced separation of double-stranded DNA and addition of specific "primers" that are synthetic oligonucleotides that correspond to the flanking areas of the section of DNA to be amplified (Fig. 97.1). Addition of a heat-stable DNA polymerase elongates the primers and results in a twofold increase in the number of DNA fragments. The process is repeated for several cycles to result in an exponential expansion of copies of targeted DNA.[7]

While sensitive for detecting low levels of DNA, PCR is not without problems. The major drawback is the occurrence of false-positives due to contamination of instruments and work areas with amplified DNA from previous runs.

Branched DNA

Recently, an additional technique for specific amplification of DNA has been developed. This approach differs from

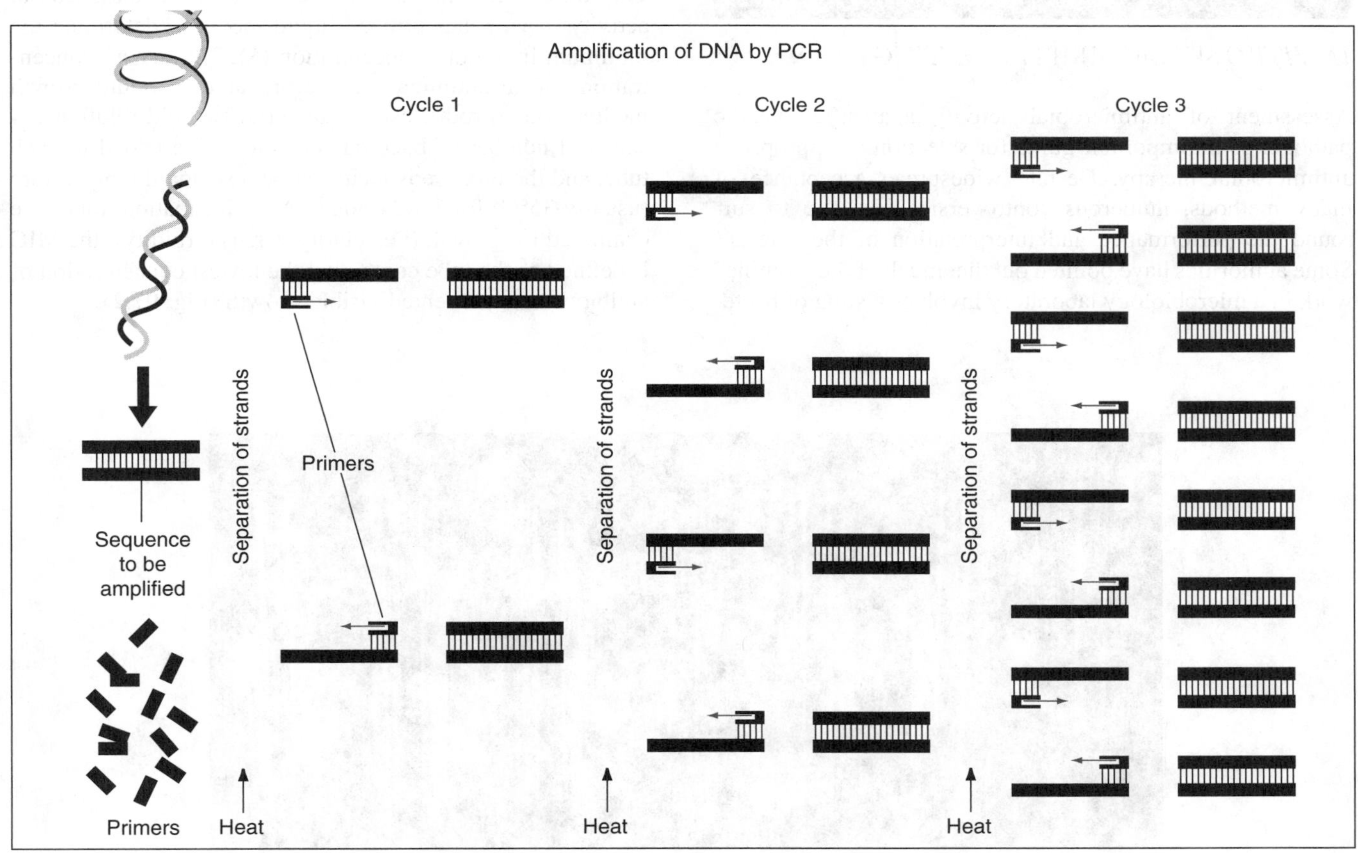

Figure 97.1. Amplification of DNA using PCR. The DNA sequence to be amplified is selected by primers, which are short synthetic oligonucleotides that correspond to sequences adjacent to the DNA to be expanded. After an excess of primers is added to the DNA, together with heat-stable DNA polymerase, the strands of both the genomic DNA and the primers are separated by heating and allowed to cool. The heat-stable polymerase elongates the primers on both strands, thus generating two new identical double-stranded DNA molecules. Several additional cycles are introduced, each doubling the amount of DNA. *(From Rosenthal N. Tools of the trade—recombinant DNA. N Engl J Med 1994;331:315–317. Reprinted by permission of* The New England Journal of Medicine. *Copyright 1994, Massachusetts Medical Society.)*

PCR in that it involves tethering a target nucleic acid to a solid support through a series of hybridizations with synthetic oligonucleotides. These oligonucleotides include probes that capture or bind to a branched DNA-amplified molecule.

The use of these DNA amplification systems in clinical samples has generated considerable enthusiasm, and many clinical laboratories are beginning to use these techniques. Reverse-transcription has further enabled extension of the technology to RNA-containing viruses, such as HIV, hepatitis C, and rotavirus. Detection of bacteria such as *Mycobacterium tuberculosis, Borrelia burgdorferi* (Lyme disease), and other organisms present in low numbers in patients may become a highly useful technique for diagnosis and monitoring of the response to therapy. Approaches using "universal primers" for PCR have enabled detection of newer sequences of nucleosides in clinical samples and resulted in the identification of newer pathogens.[6]

Evaluation of the Pharmacodynamic Properties of Antimicrobials

IN VITRO SUSCEPTIBILITY TESTING

Assessment of antimicrobial activity against a specific pathogen is an important guide for selection of appropriate antimicrobial therapy. Despite widespread acceptance of many methods, numerous controversies continue to surround the performance and interpretation of these tests.[1] Some authorities have pointed out that much of the "routine" work in a microbiology laboratory involves testing of bacteria with a high probability of susceptibility to most drugs, and that a more directed effort toward a detailed workup of organisms in more serious infections should be undertaken. Nevertheless, *in vitro* antibiotic susceptibility testing remains an important means of individualizing patient pharmacotherapy of infectious diseases. However, recent studies show that treatment of infections with drugs shown to be susceptible *in vitro* is associated with clinical improvement, whereas treatment with antibacterial agents to which the bacteria are resistant is associated with failure to improve.[8]

Drug resistance has now become an important consideration in the use of antifungal and antiviral therapy. Although experience in the clinical application of information on drug resistance is limited, procedures for susceptibility testing of yeasts against antifungal agents have been standardized.[9] Some standardized methods for testing for antiviral drug resistance have recently been developed, but testing remains limited to research facilities.

Minimum Inhibitory Concentration

The time-tested method for evaluation of antibacterial activity *in vitro* has utilized liquid media to determine the minimum inhibitory concentration (MIC). Varying concentrations of an antimicrobial are prepared in liquid growth medium (i.e., broth), usually in serial twofold dilutions. A standard number of bacteria (inoculum) are added to each tube, and the mixture is incubated at a standard temperature (usually 35°C) for 18–24 hours. After incubation, tubes are examined for growth (i.e., clarity versus turbidity); the MIC is defined as the tube containing the lowest concentration of antibiotic that prevented visible growth (Fig. 97.2).

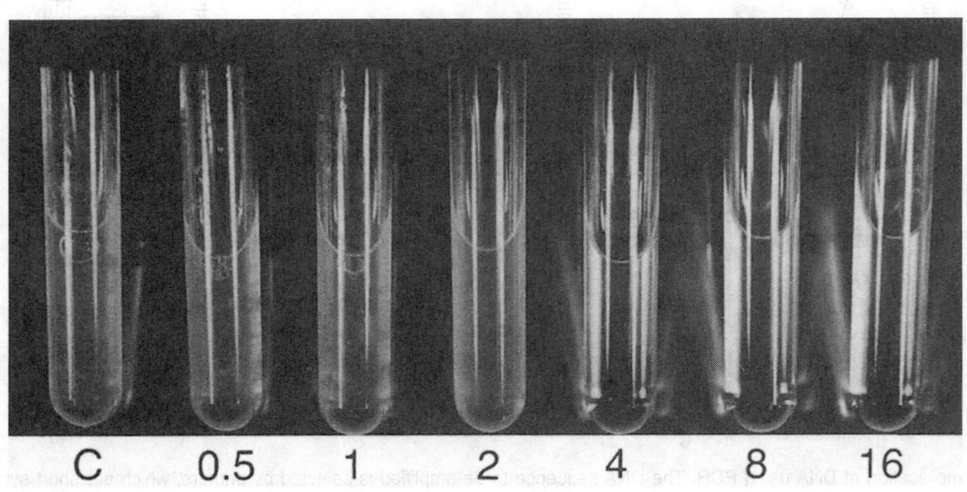

Figure 97.2. Tube dilution MIC determination for gentamicin against a strain of *P. aeruginosa*. The gentamicin concentrations in each tube (from left to right) are 0 (C), 0.5, 1, 2, 4, 8, and 16 mg/L. Tubes are shown following a 20-hour incubation at 37°C. Turbidity is seen in the control tube containing no drug (C), and in those containing 0.5, 1, and 2 mg/L of gentamicin. The tubes with 4, 8, and 16 mg/L of drug are clear. Thus, the MIC of this organism for gentamicin is 4 mg/L.

Several factors influence the value of the MIC. Bacterial growth medium and cation content can significantly affect the activity of many drugs. For example, aminoglycoside and quinolone antibiotics are less active against *P. aeruginosa* in medium supplemented with physiologic concentrations of magnesium and calcium cations than in medium without these additions. The MICs of many antibiotics that are highly bound to plasma proteins are significantly higher in medium containing human serum than in unsupplemented medium; however, testing of certain drugs in serum-supplemented medium has not gained widespread acceptance. The inoculum size (the amount of bacteria tested) significantly affects the MIC of some drugs against certain organisms. This is particularly true for most β-lactam antibiotics and gram-negative bacilli, where a 100-fold increase in the size of the inoculum increases the MIC to an extent that organisms might be considered susceptible at a lower inoculum but resistant at a larger one. Fortunately, standardized guidelines for testing and quality assurance procedures have been largely adopted by most clinical and research laboratories.[10]

The MIC may also be determined on solid medium using an agar-dilution method. Susceptibility testing of certain more fastidious bacteria may be best accomplished only on solid medium; until recently, susceptibility testing of *Mycobacterium tuberculosis* was done exclusively by this method. With this method, the drug to be tested is diluted in molten agar to make known concentrations of drug. Molten agar is then poured into petri dishes and allowed to harden. After the agar has hardened, bacterial inocula are applied to the surface of the agar in drops or with calibrated multi-tip prongs (Steers replicator). Hence, several strains of bacteria may be tested simultaneously on the plate. Plates are then incubated and inspected for growth. As with the tube-dilution method, the MIC is the plate with the lowest drug concentration on which no growth of the organism is observed.

Interpretation

The MIC serves as a quantitative measure of drug activity against bacteria. Several studies in animal models of infection and humans have demonstrated a relation between MIC values and the dosage regimen or drug exposure required for clinical efficacy.[11] However, the clinical application of MIC values is largely facilitated through interpretative guidelines for categories familiar to most clinicians. On the basis of the MIC an organism is classified as "susceptible," "intermediate," or "resistant" to the agent tested.

Pathogens classified as susceptible to an antibiotic are those with the lowest MICs and thus are the organisms most likely eradicated during therapy of human infection using "usual" drug doses. Conversely, resistant organisms are bacteria with higher MICs, suggesting that less than optimal clinical results might be anticipated if the tested drug was used for the treatment of an infection, even at the highest doses. Organisms that are moderately susceptible to the drug are classified as having intermediate susceptibility and appear to be less likely to be effectively treated than a strain in the susceptible range. Treatment of organisms in this range may be successful when maximum doses of drug are used, or the drug is known to be concentrated in the infected body site. In some cases, the intermediate classification exists because the number of strains with MICs in that range is small and their susceptibility is really indeterminate (i.e., the organism may be either susceptible or resistant). The intermediate classification also serves as a buffer zone to avoid major changes in the interpretation of the MIC value (i.e., susceptible versus resistant due to the twofold dilution step).

Organisms may also be termed "conditionally susceptible" to a drug. This classification has been applied in those instances in which organisms are inhibited by high drug concentrations achievable only in certain body fluids (e.g., urine). This classification has been deleted from recently approved standards for susceptibility testing (and is included in the intermediate category as previously described), but some laboratories may continue to use it.

Table 97.4 lists interpretative categories and their respective MIC breakpoints for the susceptible, intermediate, and resistant categories for frequently used antimicrobials as recommended by the National Committee for Clinical Laboratory Standards (NCCLS).[10] Breakpoint concentrations are determined using several criteria. First, the pharmacokinetic properties of the drug in humans are of obvious importance. Serum and tissue concentrations following usual doses should normally exceed the MIC of an organism; however, the magnitude and duration of time that these concentrations should exceed the MIC will vary according to the drug class and bacterial species. However, some principles related to drug area under the concentration versus time curve (AUC) may be applicable across several drug classes and serve as the most precise method to incorporate this information.[11] Second, the distribution of MICs for a group of bacteria for a drug is considered. Figure 97.3 depicts the distribution of MICs for cefotetan, a cephalosporin antibiotic.[12] Breakpoints for susceptibility or resistance set in the areas of a "peak" are less desirable because interpretive classification of a large number of organisms would be affected by the usual twofold dilution variability of the test; for example, a large number of organisms could fluctuate between the classifications of susceptible and resistant. Finally, the clinical efficacy of an agent against bacteria with given MIC values is considered. Although the clinical response of patients cannot always be correlated with the MIC of an infecting pathogen, observations on the response of a large number of patients with infec-

TABLE 97.4. INTERPRETIVE BREAKPOINTS FOR BROTH-DILUTION MIC TESTING OF AEROBIC BACTERIA

Drug	Susceptible (μg/mL)	Moderately Susceptible (μg/mL)	Resistant (μg/mL)
Aminoglycosides			
Amikacin, kanamycin	≤16	32	≥64
Gentamicin,[a] tobramycin	≤4	8	≥16
Netilmicin	≤8	16	≥32
Cephalosporins, cephems, and monobactams			
Cefazolin, cephalothin, cefamandole, ceforanide, cefuroxime, ceftazidime, cefarazil, cefoxitin, loracarbef, aztreonam	≤8	16	≥32
Cefotaxime, ceftizoxime, ceftriaxone, moxalactam	≤8	16–32	≥64
Cefoperazone, cefotetan, cefmetazole	≤16	32	≥64
Clindamycin	≤0.5	1–2	>4
Glycopeptides			
Teicoplanin	≤8	16	≥32
Vancomycin	≤4	8–16	≥32
Imipenem	≤4	8	≥16
Macrolides			
Azithromycin	≤2	4	≥8
Clarithromycin	≤2	4	≥8
Erythromycin	≤0.5	1–4	≥8
Penicillins			
Amoxicillin/clavulanate			
For *Haemophilus* sp., *S. aureus*	≤4/2	—	≥8/4
Others	≤8/4	16/8	≥32/16
Ampicillin			
For *Haemophilus* sp.	≤2	—	≥4
For Enterobacteriaceae	≤8	16	≥32
Mezlocillin, piperacillin (with or without 4 mg/L of tazobactam), and ticarcillin (with or without 2 mg/L of clavulanate)	≤16	32–64	≥128
For *Pseudomonas aeruginosa*	≤64	—	≥128
For other gram-negative bacilli	≤16	32–64	≥128
Nafcillin, oxacillin[b]	≤2	—	≥4
Penicillin G			
For streptococci	≤0.12	0.25–2	≥4
For enterococci	<8	—	≥16
For pneumococci, *N. gonorrhoeae*	≤0.06	0.1–1	≥2
Quinolones			
Ciprofloxacin	≤1	2	≥4
Ofloxacin, lomefloxacin, floroxacin	≤2	4	≥4
Norfloxacin	≤4	8	≥16
Tetracyclines	4	8	≥16
Trimethoprim-sulfamethoxazole	≤2/38	—	≥4/76

[a]For testing enterococci: susceptible ≤500 mg/L; resistant >500 mg/L.
[b]For testing staphylococci. *(Compiled from Ref. 10.)*

tions (particularly those in a borderline range) and previous experience with other similar agents may be useful in selecting final breakpoints.

Similarities between many antimicrobial agents have enabled development of "class" testing and predictor panels. For example, cephalothin may be tested and the results extrapolated to cefazolin or other "first-generation" cephalosporins. Although this was formerly possible with late-generation cephalosporins and some gram-negative bacteria, recent elucidation of extended-spectrum β-lactamases with specific inactivation profiles for certain cephalosporins have eliminated this approach. In other cases, testing of some agents may allow for prediction of results with other drugs; for example, susceptibility to the least active mem-

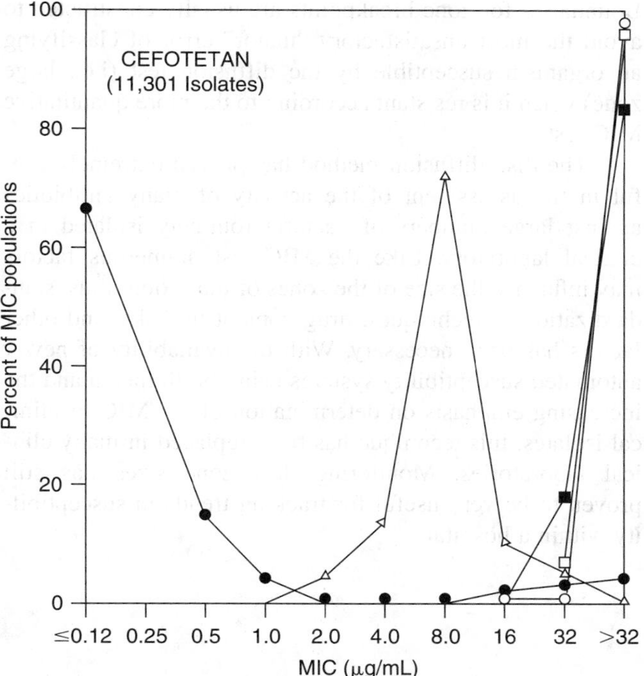

Figure 97.3. Frequency distribution of MICs for cefotetan of *P. aeruginosa* (■), *Acinetobacter* sp. (_), *S. aureus* (△), enterococci (m), and Enterobacteriaceae (●) Almost all *Enterobacteriaceae* have MICs less than the susceptibility breakpoint of 8 mg/L; in contrast, most of the MICs for *S. aureus* fall on this breakpoint, which will result in most of these strains reading either susceptible or intermediate to the drug. Most of the other strains are resistant to cefotetan. *(From Ayers LW, Jones RN, Barry AL, et al. Cefotetan, a new cephamycin: Comparison of in vitro antimicrobial activity with other cephems, β-lactamase stability, and preliminary recommendations for disk diffusion testing. Antimicrob Agents Chemother 1982;22:875, with permission.)*

ber of a group often means that other more potent agents will be active as well.

Limitations

While the MIC is regarded as the most standardized quantitative measure of antimicrobial activity, it is not without some limitations. Preparation of several serial twofold drug dilutions and inoculation with bacteria are both time consuming and expensive and, thus, not feasible in most clinical laboratories. This disadvantage has been largely bypassed by the development of techniques using smaller volumes of liquid medium and automation (see as follows).

The MIC should not be regarded as an "all-or-none" phenomenon, as numerous effects of subinhibitory antibiotic concentrations on bacteria have been described. Moreover, subpopulations of bacteria within an inoculum may be inhibited by drug concentrations below the MIC, while others may require concentrations much higher than the measured MIC. Exposure to drug through chemotherapy *in vivo* may select for these bacteria, which may be important determinants of clinical response to antimicrobial therapy.

It is emphasized that while these interpretative classes are of great value in selecting antimicrobial therapy, they are not always accurate predictors of success or failure of drug therapy. Drug therapy of infectious diseases caused by organisms susceptible to the agent used is not an assurance of a clinical cure, because numerous other factors may be important in achieving a good clinical result. For example, methicillin-resistant *S. aureus* may appear susceptible to certain cephalosporins (e.g., cefazolin) *in vitro,* but the clinical efficacy of many of these agents in infections due to these bacteria has not been established. The results of drug susceptibility testing must be applied in the context of the site of infection, the pharmacodynamic and pharmacokinetic properties of the drug, and the clinical status of the patient.

Disk Diffusion Assay

In view of the impracticality of performing MIC testing on a large number of organisms against numerous drugs in a clinical hospital laboratory, Bauer et al.[13] developed a rapid, convenient method of determining the susceptibility of bacteria to several antibiotics in the 1950s. Paper disks impregnated with a fixed amount of antibiotic are placed onto an agar surface with a "lawn" of the strain of bacteria to be tested (Fig. 97.4). Drug diffuses from the disk into the

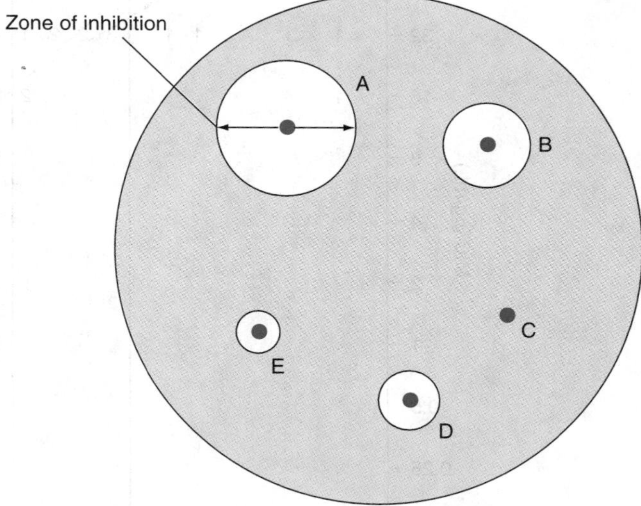

Figure 97.4. Disk diffusion susceptibility test. Five disks (A–E) for different drugs were placed on the surface of a seeded agar plate of a test organism and incubated for 18 hours. Antibiotic has diffused from the disk into the agar and is in decreasing concentration with increasing distance from the disk. Antibiotic in the agar inhibited growth of bacteria on the surface according to the susceptibility to the drug. A large zone of inhibition is observed for drug A, indicating that the organism is susceptible to this agent. In contrast, small or nonexistent zones are observed for drugs E and C, respectively, suggesting the organism is resistant to these drugs. Depending on the established breakpoints for zones of inhibition, the results for B and D indicate that the organism may be susceptible or intermediate to these drugs.

medium, with drug concentrations in the agar decreasing at greater distances from the disk. The plate is incubated and bacteria grow on the surface of the agar, except in areas where the drug concentration in the agar exceeds a critical valve. These zones of inhibition are measured using calipers or scanning devices.

Interpretation of the zone size is facilitated by the log–linear relationship between the MIC and the zone of inhibition produced by a disk containing a fixed amount of drug. The zone sizes of organisms with higher MICs tend to be small, whereas those for more susceptible organisms tend to be large. "Scattergrams" are constructed using the MICs and zones of inhibitions measured on agar from studies of a large number of bacteria (Fig. 97.5). Using MIC breakpoints (i.e., susceptible, resistant), the corresponding zone breakpoints are constructed. As shown in Fig. 97.5, this relationship is not perfect in that some organisms with higher MICs occasionally have large zones and vice versa. Boundaries for zone breakpoints are usually constructed to avoid the most unsatisfactory "major" error of classifying an organism susceptible by the diffusion test (i.e., large zone) when it is resistant according to the more quantitative MIC test.

The disk diffusion method has proved extremely useful in the assessment of the activity of many antibiotics against large numbers of bacteria routinely isolated in a clinical laboratory. Like the MIC test, numerous factors may influence the size of the zones of inhibition; thus, standardization of techniques, drug content in disks, and other factors has been necessary. With the availability of newer automated susceptibility systems using broth media and the increasing emphasis on determination of the MIC of clinical isolates, this technique has been replaced in many clinical laboratories. Monitoring disk zone sizes has still proven to be very useful for tracking trends in susceptibility within a hospital.

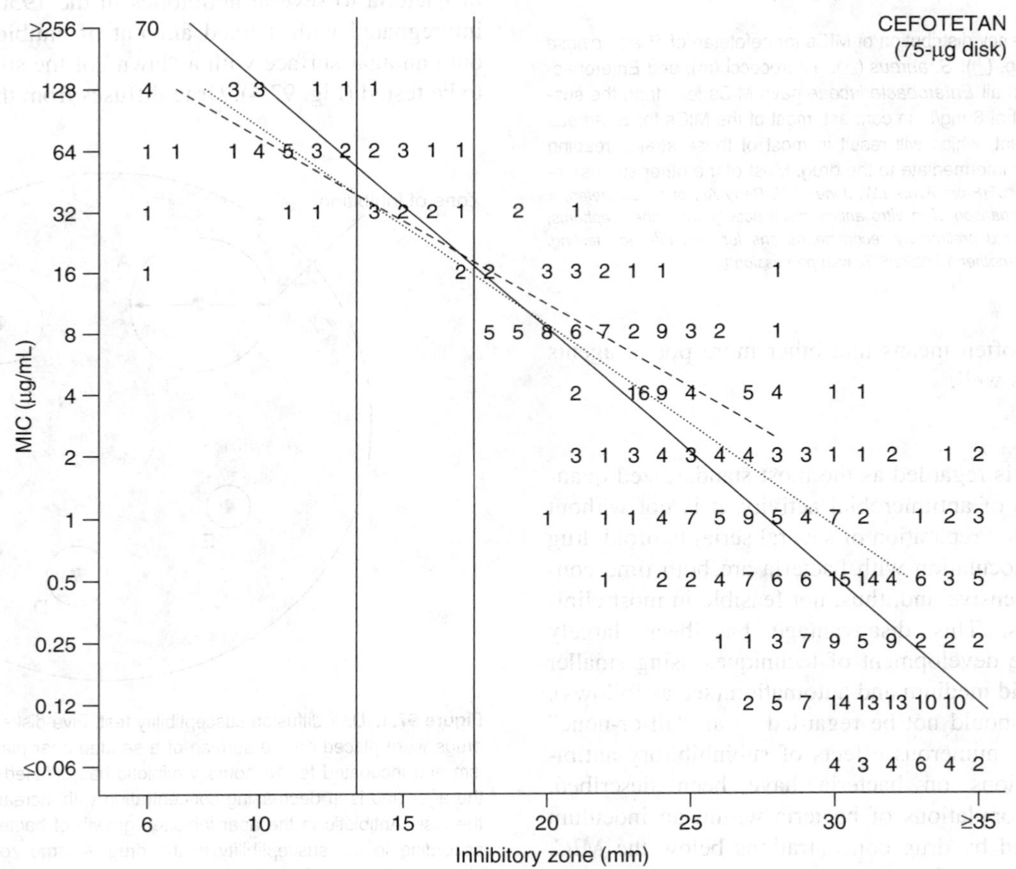

Figure 97.5. Scattergram showing the relation between the MIC and the zone of inhibition for isolates tested against cefotetan using broth dilution and disk diffusion methods using a disk containing 75 µg of cefotetan. Regression lines for MICs from 0.01–256 (—), 0.5–256 (...), and 2–256 (--) mg/L are drawn. Vertical lines indicate the corresponding proposed breakpoints for resistant (≤14 mm) and susceptible (≥17 mm). *(From Ayers LW, Jones RN, Barry AL, et al. Cefotetan, a new cephamycin: Comparison of in vitro antimicrobial activity with other cephems, β-lactamase stability, and preliminary recommendations for disk diffusion testing. Antimicrob Agents Chemother 1982;22:875, with permission.)*

Etest

A recently developed proprietary device called the Etest (AB Biodisk, Solna, Sweden) combines the principles of disk diffusion susceptibility testing with the quantitative nature of MIC testing. The device consists of a plastic strip impregnated with a gradient of antibiotic concentrations. The strip is placed directly on the surface of an agar plate seeded with the organism to be tested and the plate incubated as with disk diffusion testing. A "tear-shaped" zone of inhibition is formed (Fig. 97.6) and the point of intersection between the zone of inhibition and the scale is read as the MIC. This method has been tested for determination of the susceptibility of several strains of bacteria, including many fastidious strains, and has been found to be a highly reproducible and acceptable alternative to MIC testing.[14]

Detection of Resistance Factors

Understanding of the mechanisms for antibiotic resistance has allowed for direct testing of clinical isolates for specific enzymes or genes conferring drug resistance. This technique has obvious advantages in that cultivation of an organism may not be necessary for purposes of drug testing. Many bacteria could be screened for drug resistance, and certain drugs excluded for use in a patient.

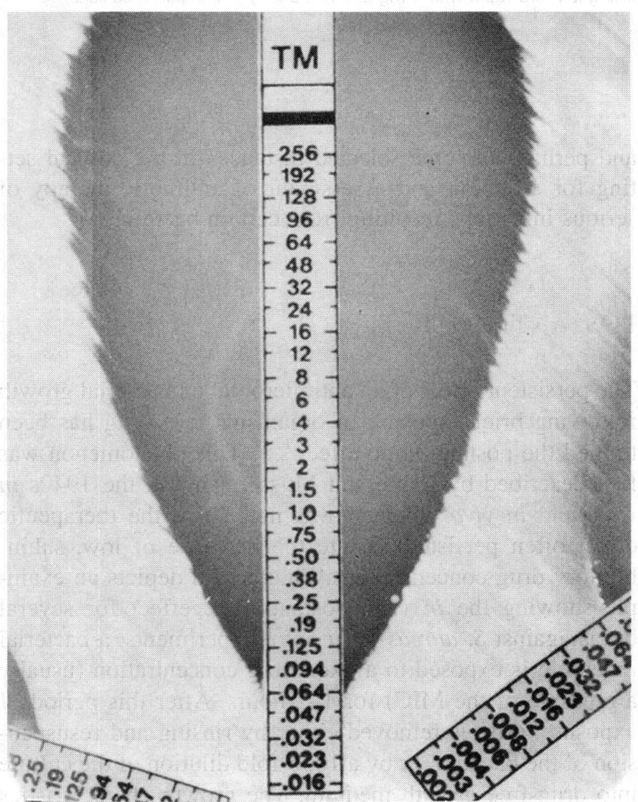

Figure 97.6. Photograph of surface of agar plate showing inhibition of bacterial growth surrounding the Etest strip. MIC is read at the point where the zone of inhibition intersects the printed scale. *(Photograph courtesy of AB Biodisk, Solna, Sweden.)*

Beta-lactamase production by bacteria may be rapidly detected by use of a chromogenic cephalosporin, nitrocephin. Colonies of growing cultures of bacteria can be "touched" to a disk or paper containing nitrocephin that changes color when hydrolyzed, thus indicating the presence of β-lactamase. This test has been shown to be a rapid, reliable method for detecting β-lactamase production by *Haemophilus* spp., *N. gonorrhoeae, Moraxella catarrhalis,* staphylococci, and enterococci.

Techniques using DNA hybridization have also been extended for use in detecting drug resistance. Probes for specific β-lactamases have been developed and proved useful for detecting resistance to cephalosporins. PCR has been used to screen for antibiotic resistance genes, such as the *mec* determinant in staphylococci.

AUTOMATED ANTIMICROBIAL SUSCEPTIBILITY TESTING

The availability of many new antimicrobials, as well as the greater demand for rapid quantitative susceptibility testing of clinical isolates, has led to the development of several automated "walkaway" systems for determining antimicrobial susceptibility.[15] Most of these systems test drugs and bacteria in very small volumes of broth as is done with the tube dilution method. Transmission or scattering of light through cuvettes or microdilution wells containing drug and bacteria is periodically or continuously monitored and recorded in a computer. In many systems, incubation for as little as 3 hours is all that is required to obtain results. Studies comparing many of these newer systems with standard techniques of broth or agar dilution have documented good agreement between methods. However, resistance to certain drugs (e.g., *Enterobacter* sp. and cephalosporins) may not be adequately detected by some systems.

An obvious advantage in automation is the reduction in turnaround time for results of antimicrobial susceptibility testing to allow for modification of therapy. Many systems reduce the amount of time by an entire day or more, and such systems have been associated in some studies with a reduction in the cost of antimicrobial therapy.[16] Information concerning susceptibility may be "autofiled" to the patient-care area. However, in many cases, the newly generated information is not acted on by physicians because of rounding practices, and so on; several investigators have shown that the use of bacteriologic data had not changed significantly compared with conventional overnight approaches.[16]

SPECIAL *IN VITRO* TESTS OF ANTIMICROBIAL ACTIVITY

In addition to the tests previously described, several special tests of antimicrobial pharmacodynamics have been developed. Although they are not usually performed in the clinical laboratory setting, these tests are frequently used in the assessment of antimicrobials and may be integrated with other pharmacologic properties to determine optimal dosage schedules in patients.

MINIMUM BACTERICIDAL CONCENTRATION

While the MIC is useful in determining the lowest concentration of drug capable of inhibiting an organism's growth, it may also be of value to determine if an antimicrobial will kill the organism (i.e., if it is bactericidal). The ability of an antibiotic to exert a bactericidal effect at clinically achievable drug concentrations may be assessed by determination of the minimum bactericidal concentration (MBC). The test is performed using the results from broth-dilution MIC testing. An aliquot of broth from each dilution without visual evidence of bacterial growth is inoculated onto antibiotic-free agar and incubated for 24 hours. The MBC is defined as the lowest concentration of drug that results in a 99.9% reduction in the initial bacterial density (3 log drop). For example, if 1×10^5 colony-forming units (CFUs) of bacteria per milliliter was originally inoculated into broth medium, then only 10^2 CFUs of bacteria per milliliter must remain after exposure in liquid medium to meet the criteria for bactericidal activity.

Bactericidal activity of an antimicrobial agent alone or in combination may be crucial for certain infections, such as bacterial endocarditis and meningitis. Some strains of bacteria normally killed by certain antibiotics are sometimes only inhibited by them; these strains are often termed "tolerant." Antimicrobial tolerance has been defined as the situation where the MBC:MIC ratio is greater than or equal to 32.

TIMED-KILL CURVE

Although the MBC test yields information on the net reduction in bacteria over a 24-hour period, it may be desirable to characterize the *rate* of killing of bacteria during exposure to antimicrobials alone or in combination. Figure 97.7 depicts an example of a timed-kill curve for varying concentrations of ciprofloxacin, a fluoroquinolone antibiotic, against *P. aeruginosa.* As shown in this example, the rate of bacterial killing is concentration dependent. The timed-kill curve analysis appears to be most useful in research studies evaluating antimicrobial activity alone or in combination,

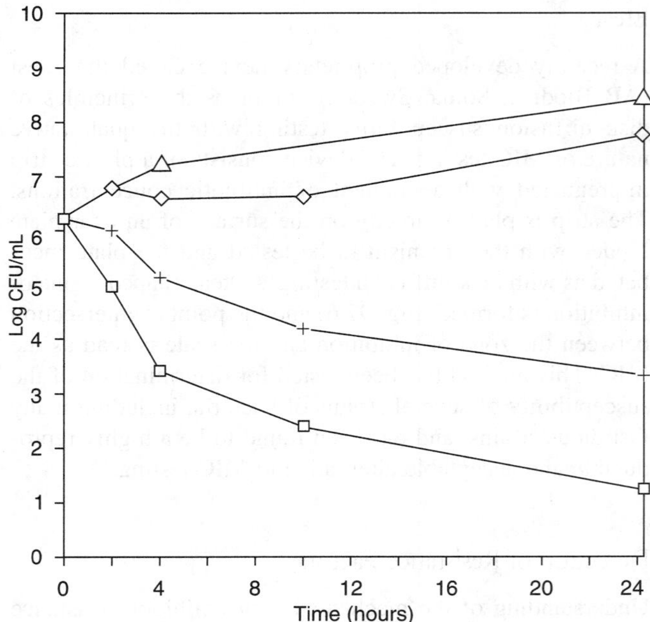

Figure 97.7. Timed-kill curve showing the effect of no drug (control, △), 0.4 mg/L (◇), 2 mg/L (+), and 4 mg/L (□) of ciprofloxacin on a strain of *P. aeruginosa in vitro.* Two and 4 mg/L of ciprofloxacin meet the criteria for a bactericidal effect (99.9% reduction in the starting inoculum), but bacterial killing is more rapid with 4 mg/L. *(From Dudley MN. Unpublished data.)*

and perhaps in some selected instances in the clinical setting for selection and assessment of antibiotic therapy of serious infections resulting from certain bacteria.

POSTANTIBIOTIC EFFECT

The persistent effect of an antimicrobial on bacterial growth following brief exposure of organisms to a drug has been termed the postantibiotic effect.[17,18] This phenomenon was first described by Eagle and Musselman[19] in the 1940s *in vitro* and *in vivo* where it was noted that the therapeutic effect often persisted despite the presence of low, subinhibitory drug concentrations. Figure 97.8 depicts an example showing the *in vitro* postantibiotic effect for several drugs against *S. aureus.* In *in vitro* experiments, a bacterial inoculum is exposed to a fixed drug concentration (usually a multiple of the MIC) for 1–2 hours. After this period of exposure, drug is removed either by rinsing and resuspension of the bacteria, or by a 1000-fold dilution of the culture into drug-free growth medium. The growth characteristics of exposed bacteria are compared with a control (i.e., unexposed) culture processed in the same way and the difference in time required for exposed and control cultures to increase 10-fold (i.e., one-log growth) is the *in vitro* postan-

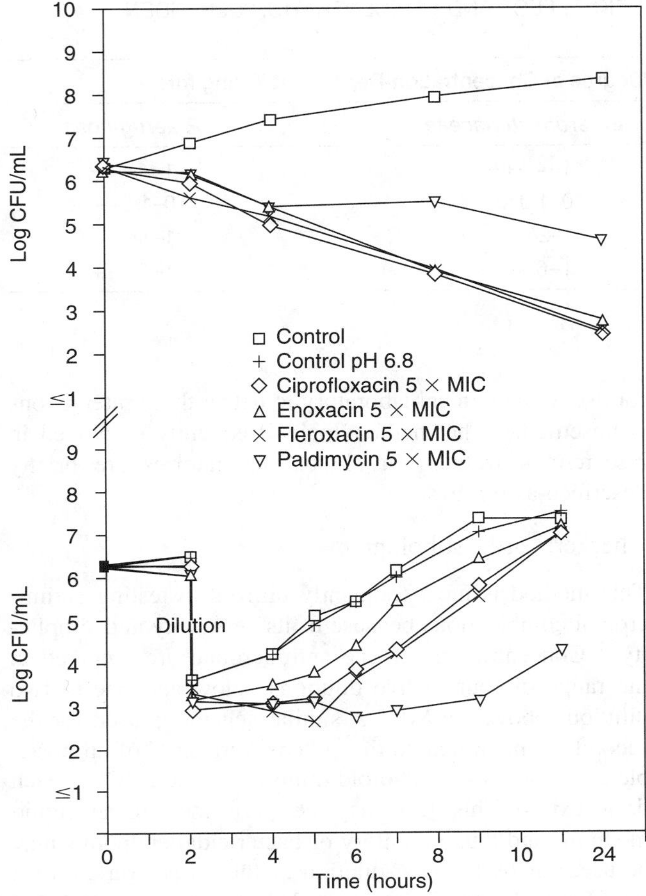

Figure 97.8. *In vitro* bactericidal effects (top panel) and postantibiotic effect (bottom panel) of three fluoroquinolones (ciprofloxacin, fleroxacin, and enoxacin) and paldimycin against a strain of *S. aureus.* All drugs except paldimycin met criteria for a bactericidal effect by 24 hours. For determination of the postantibiotic effect, the bacteria was incubated with the drugs in Mueller–Hinton broth for 2 hours and then the drug "removed" by a 1:1000 dilution of cultures with fresh, drug-free prewarmed broth. The PAE was about 1 hour for enoxacin, 2 hours for fleroxacin and ciprofloxacin, and 9 hours for paldimycin. *(From Dudley MN. Unpublished data.)*

tibiotic effect. Studies *in vitro* and in animal models of infection have confirmed the existence of a postantibiotic effect with exposure to higher and often more sustained drug concentrations[20]; it may be difficult to distinguish this effect from that of subinhibitory concentrations. However, these concepts have led to the development of antimicrobial dosage regimens that exploit this phenomenon. For example, the presence of a postantibiotic effect *in vitro* and *in vivo* has led to intensive studies of novel dosage regimens of aminoglycosides such as administration of the entire daily dose at once.

Although the postantibiotic effect (PAE) is often cited as a desirable characteristic of antimicrobials, considerable controversy exists concerning its clinical relevance and application in development of drug dosage regimens. Factors such as drug concentration tested, duration and number of exposures to drug, pH, inoculum size, medium, and growth phase influence the results. While this phenomenon has spurred interest in development of novel dosage regimens in patients, more study is needed to determine if a detectable PAE *in vitro* is associated with therapeutic effects in patients receiving antimicrobials with short half-lives at prolonged dosing intervals.

Table 97.5 summarizes available data on the *in vitro* PAE and degree of concentration dependence on bacterial killing for selected major groups of bacteria and drug classes.

TESTING OF ANTIMICROBIAL COMBINATIONS

It is occasionally desirable to assess the effect of various combinations of antibiotics against a bacterial pathogen. Antimicrobial *synergism* is defined as an interaction between two or more agents that results in an effect greater than that expected from the sum of their independent effects. Conversely, combinations may be considered *antagonistic* if a combination of antimicrobials exerts an effect less than that observed when each agent is considered independently. Combinations of antimicrobials that are neither synergistic nor antagonistic may be termed *indifferent* if the agents appear to work similarly alone or in combination, or *additive* if the effects of a combination simply reflect addition of each of their respective activities.

The clinical significance of antimicrobial synergism and antagonism has undergone considerable debate.[21,22] Some studies suggest that the presence of antimicrobial synergism may enhance the clinical response in neutropenic patients with infection. This appears to be particularly true in bacteremia or infections resulting from *P. aeruginosa.*[23] Other studies have disputed the significance of *in vitro* synergy in the treatment of even the most serious infections, particularly when highly potent β-lactams are used.[24,25] Studies in enterococcal endocarditis, particularly in animal models, have stressed the importance of antimicrobial combinations resulting in a synergistic bactericidal effect for optimal cure of infection.[26]

In vivo antagonism between antimicrobials and correlation with *in vitro* observations have been observed less frequently. The most often cited example of *in vivo* antagonism is from the study of Lepper and Dowling.[27] They demonstrated a higher fatality rate in adults with pneumococcal meningitis treated with penicillin plus tetracycline (an antagonistic combination *in vitro*) than in those treated with penicillin alone.

TABLE 97.5. COMPARISON OF DEGREE OF *IN VITRO* POSTANTIBIOTIC EFFECT AND CONCENTRATION-DEPENDENT BACTERIAL KILLING FOR MAJOR DRUG CLASSES AND BACTERIA

	In Vitro PAE (h)/Degree of Concentration-Dependent Killing for:		
Drug Class	***S. aureus***	***Enterobacteriaceae***	***P. aeruginosa***
Aminoglycosides	1–2/++[a]	1–4/+++	1–4/+++
β-Lactams	2–6/0 to ++	0–1/0 to +	0–1/0–+
Carbapenems	1–3/++	1–2/++	1–4/+
Fluoroquinolones	1–3[b]/+++	1–6/+++	1–6/+++

[a]No (0), slight (+), moderate (++), or high (+++) degree of concentration-dependent killing.
[b]*S. aureus* only. (Adapted from Refs. 17, 18, and 20.)

Table 97.6 lists several examples of drug combinations frequently associated with synergism or antagonism *in vitro.* Occasionally two antimicrobials of the same class may be antagonistic. For example, certain β-lactam antimicrobials may induce (through interaction with a complex system of regulatory genes) production of chromosomal β-lactamase. If one uses combination β-lactam therapy against *Enterobacter* sp. with a strong inducing compound (e.g., imipenem, cefoxitin) in combination with a labile compound (e.g., piperacillin), one can see antagonism *in vitro* and in animal models of infection.[28,29] Use of combinations of weak and strong inducer compounds should be discouraged.

While the definitions just introduced appear straightforward in description, the most appropriate methodology for use in the clinical laboratory to detect these interactions is unsettled.[30] The methodologies frequently employed in research as well as in clinical laboratories are briefly described as follows.

TABLE 97.6. EXAMPLES OF DRUG COMBINATIONS FREQUENTLY SYNERGISTIC OR ANTAGONISTIC *IN VITRO* AGAINST BACTERIA AND FUNGI

Drug Combinations	**Examples of Organisms**
Synergistic	
Aminoglycosides	
+ A broad-spectrum penicillin[a]	Gram-negative bacilli
+ A cephalosporin	Gram-negative bacilli
+ Ampicillin or penicillin G	Enterococci
+ Antistaphylococcal penicillin	Staphylococci
Penicillins	
Nafcillin or oxacillin + rifampin	Staphylococci
Broad-spectrum penicillin[a] + a third-generation cephalosporin	Gram-negative bacilli
Antifungals	
Amphotericin B + flucytosine	*Cryptococcus neoformans*
Antivirals	Human immunodeficiency virus (HIV)
Zidovudine + α-interferon	HIV
Antagonistic	
Broad-spectrum penicillin	
+ Imipenem	*Enterobacter cloacae, Pseudomonas aeruginosa, Citrobacter* sp.
+ Chloramphenicol	*Streptococcus pneumoniae*
Aminoglycoside + chloramphenicol	Enterobacteriaceae

[a]Mezlocillin, piperacillin, ticarcillin, or azlocillin.

Checkerboard/Isobologram

This method is most frequently utilized in testing antimicrobial combinations because of its versatility and simplicity.[21] Concentrations of one antimicrobial are prepared in the range of four to five dilutions below and one to two dilutions above the MIC. A similar scheme is used for the second antimicrobial so that a "checkerboard" of all possible combinations (in twofold dilutions of the MIC) of each drug exists. This test may be performed using liquid medium (and thus inhibitory or bactericidal endpoints may be used) or by the agar-dilution method. Bacteria are then added and the results are recorded as with MIC or MBC testing. The lowest concentration of drug within each respective row or column that inhibits growth (or is bactericidal) is plotted on x and y axes to form an isobologram (Fig. 97.9). The line connecting the respective MICs for each drug is the line of additivity. An inward bowing of the plotted line indicates an additivity or synergism; an outward bowing denotes antagonism.

Alternatively, an isobologram may be expressed mathematically by calculation of the fractional inhibitory concentration index (FIC index). The FIC index is calculated as

$$FIC = \frac{A}{MIC_A} + \frac{B}{MIC_B}$$

where A or B is the lowest concentration of drug that is inhibitory in the presence of the second drug, and the MIC is the minimum inhibitory concentration of the drug when tested alone. With this method, synergy is defined as an FIC index less than or equal to 0.5, additivity is an FIC index equal to 1, and antagonism corresponds to an FIC index greater than or equal to 2. As described previously, bactericidal endpoints may alternatively be used in this equation. Other mathematical expressions that incorporate concepts related to mutually exclusive and nonexclusive inhibitors and drug concentration are available for more detailed analysis in the research setting.[30–32]

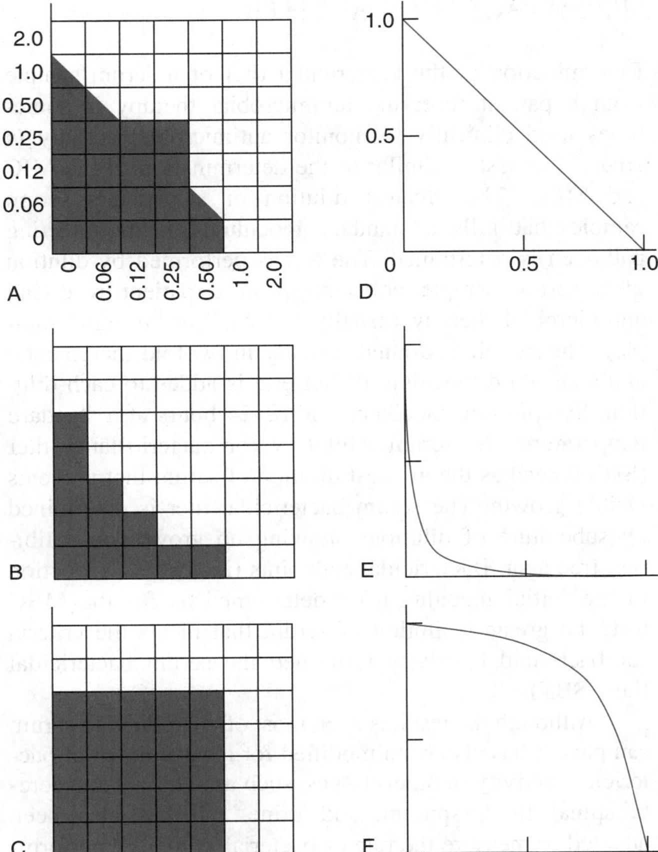

Figure 97.9. (A–C) Checkerboard dilution technique for assessment of antimicrobial concentrations. Increasing concentrations of each drug are placed in each of the cells (tubes or wells) as one moves from the lower left corner upwards (first drug) or to the right (second drug). Shaded areas depict areas of visible growth after inoculation with test organisms and incubation. The corresponding results are plotted on isobolograms, plotted as fractions of the MIC for each drug. Panels A and D, B and E, and C and F depict additivity, synergism, and antagonism, respectively. *(Adapted from Krogstad DJ, Moellering RC Jr. Antimicrobial combinations, in Lorian V (ed): Antibiotics in Laboratory Medicine, 2nd ed. Baltimore, MD, Williams and Wilkins, 1986, p 548, with permission. Copyright © by Williams & Wilkins, 1978.)*

Timed-Kill Curves

Combinations of two antimicrobials may increase or decrease the rate of killing relative to that observed with either antibiotic alone. To detect this interaction, the timed kill is performed as described earlier, except that two antibiotics at fixed concentrations are incubated with bacteria over a given period of time. Synergism with this method is defined as a greater than or equal to 100-fold increase in killing of bacteria with the combination as compared to the most active drug alone when tested at the same concentration (Fig. 97.10).

Other Methods

Other less frequently used qualitative methods of evaluating antimicrobials include the double-disk diffusion test. This test is performed by placing two disks containing one of each of the antibiotics to be tested on solid medium in such proximity that their zones of inhibition would not be expected to overlap. A synergistic or additive interaction is observed when there is an extension of these zones of inhibition between the two drugs.

Other more elaborate methods of evaluating antimicrobial combinations include use of *in vitro* kinetic models. *In vitro* kinetic models expose bacteria to changing concentrations of two drugs as would occur *in vivo.* The number of viable organisms surviving exposure to both drugs as a function of time with the combination regimen is compared with the results of single-drug experiments. This technique has been limited to use in the research laboratory.[33]

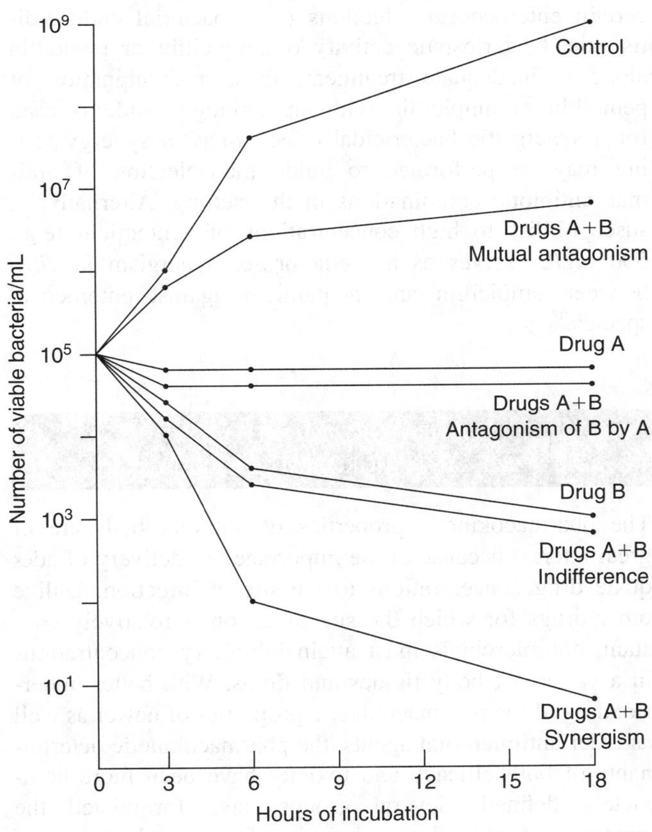

Figure 97.10. Timed-kill curve illustrating synergistic, antagonistic, and indifferent effects of two antibiotics tested on fixed concentrations. *(From Rahal JJ. Antibiotic combinations: The clinical relevance of synergy and antagonism. Medicine 1978;57:181, with permission.)*

Interpretation and Use

It is still unsettled as to which *in vitro* method best predicts clinical outcome, because there often is a discrepancy between the conclusions obtained using different tests. In some cases, synergism between two drugs against an organism reflects increased killing of bacteria; in others, a synergistic effect may simply reflect the prevention by the second drug of the growth (and thus "emergence") of resistant subpopulations of bacteria that would normally grow to detectable numbers during a 24-hour incubation with a single drug.[34]

Testing of antimicrobial combinations in the clinical laboratory appears to be useful in certain situations. It is often necessary to assess the activity of certain antibiotic combinations against antibiotic-resistant bacteria isolated from a patient (e.g., gram-negative bacilli). In this setting, it is hoped that the strain that is resistant to one or both of the single drugs might become "susceptible" to the combination through a synergistic interaction. In other cases, a synergistic combination may be desired when either of the drugs alone is only bacteriostatic against an organism. For example, most enterococci (e.g., *Enterococcus faecalis*) are inhibited but not killed by clinically achievable concentrations of penicillin derivatives. In certain enterococcal infections (e.g., bacterial endocarditis), the bacteriostatic activity of ampicillin or penicillin alone is inadequate treatment; thus, a combination of penicillin or ampicillin with an aminoglycoside is used for a synergistic bactericidal effect. *In vitro* synergy testing may be performed to guide the selection of optimal antibiotic combinations in this setting. Alternatively, susceptibility to high concentrations of gentamicin (e.g., 500 mg/L) serves as a predictor for synergism *in vitro* between ampicillin and gentamicin against enterococci species.[11]

Laboratory Monitoring of Antimicrobial Therapy

The pharmacokinetic properties of antimicrobials are of great interest because of the importance of delivery of adequate drug concentrations to the site of infection. Unlike other drugs for which the site of action is relatively constant, antimicrobials must attain inhibitory concentrations in a variety of body tissues and fluids. With better understanding of the pharmacokinetic properties of newer as well as older antimicrobial agents, the pharmacokinetic determinants of both efficacy and toxicity have been more completely defined. Several groups have formulated the approach of individualized dosing for several classes of antimicrobials, which considers both pharmacokinetic as well as pharmacodynamic characteristics.

SERUM BACTERICIDAL TITER

Determination of the bactericidal titer of a serum sample from a patient receiving antimicrobial therapy is sometimes used clinically to monitor antimicrobial activity *in vivo*.[35] The test is similar to the determination of the MIC and MBC. The greatest dilution of a patient's serum sample that kills a standard inoculum of the infecting pathogen is determined. The test is performed by dilution of a serum sample collected from a patient receiving antimicrobial therapy (usually a "peak" or "trough" sample). The sample is diluted (usually in twofold increments) and a standard inoculum of bacteria is added to each dilution. Samples are incubated for 18–24 hours at a standard temperature; the serum inhibitory (or bacteriostatic) titer (SIT) is read as the greatest dilution of serum that prevents visible growth. The serum bactericidal titer is determined by subculture of dilutions showing no growth on antibiotic-free agar. Bactericidal endpoints (i.e., 99.9% reduction in the initial inoculum) are determined as for the MBC test; the greatest dilution of serum that meets the criteria for bactericidal activity is termed the serum bactericidal titer (SBT).

Although the test has been most often applied to serum samples, it has also been modified for measurement of bactericidal activity in other tissues, such as synovial and cerebrospinal fluid, sputum, and urine.[35] It has also been adapted to measure the rate of bacterial killing by performing a timed-kill curve analysis on one or several dilutions of serum.[36,37]

Interpretation

The SBT is theoretically useful for monitoring antibiotic therapy because it integrates information regarding the antibiotic susceptibility of the infecting pathogen and the *in vivo* pharmacology of the antibiotic in a given patient. Indeed, the serum bactericidal titer for most drugs may be estimated mathematically by dividing the serum drug concentration by the MBC.

As described previously, some bacteria may be considered tolerant to certain antimicrobials. Because the MBC is seldom determined in clinical laboratories, tolerant strains of bacteria may be detected by comparison of the serum inhibitory and bactericidal titers. For example, a serum inhibitory titer of 1:64 with a bactericidal titer of 1:2 would be indicative of a tolerant organism.

The SBT is probably most useful in assessing the activity of antimicrobial combinations against a pathogen. Several studies have noted enhancement of the serum bactericidal activity observed with a single drug by addition of a second agent. The serum bactericidal assay has been utilized as a means of investigating synergism between drugs *in vivo*.[38]

Limitations

The same technical factors that influence the results of MIC and MBC tests are applicable to the serum bacteriostatic and bactericidal assays. In particular, the use of serum versus broth for making dilutions of the sample may be important, particularly for highly protein-bound drugs. Binding of drugs to serum proteins may be decreased when the sample is diluted in growth medium rather than serum because of dilution of proteins in the original sample. Thus, large dilutions would result in a greater free fraction of bioactive drug because of dilutions of proteins. These and other issues surrounding the performance and interpretation of the SBT necessitate standardization to make the test of greater clinical value.[36]

Use

The serum bactericidal assay has been utilized in the management of patients with bacterial endocarditis, osteomyelitis, pneumonia, bacteremia, urinary tract infections, septic arthritis, and meningitis.[35,36,37] Despite widespread use of the test, there are no definitive data defining the optimal titer associated with cure of these infections. On the basis of studies on endocarditis, infection in the immunocompromised host, and osteomyelitis, most studies suggest that dosage regimens should achieve a peak bactericidal titer of 1:8 or greater.[35]

The SBT has also been used as a guide for changing from parenteral to oral antibiotic therapy of endocarditis or bone and joint infection. Use of the test in this setting provides confirmation of adequate oral absorption of antibiotics to allow for prolonged therapy in the outpatient setting.

More recently, serial measurements of the SIT or SBT have been employed in the evaluation of antimicrobial regimens. The reciprocal of the titer is plotted over time and the area under the bactericidal titer versus time curve is calculated. This area could also be calculated by comparison of the AUC for the drug compared with the MIC or MBC of a pathogen of interest. This approach seems most useful in studying the combined effects of combination antimicrobial regimens or of drugs with active metabolites.[38]

ANTIBIOTIC ASSAY

Monitoring of serum concentrations of antibiotics remains the most widespread method for individualization of anti-infective therapy. For most drugs, the therapeutic window (toxic versus therapeutic antimicrobial concentration) is large; moreover, both toxic and efficacious concentrations *in vivo* are not defined for many agents, particularly β-lactam antibiotics. Therefore, serum concentration monitoring is not warranted for most agents in the clinical setting because of unproved clinical value; however, judicious use of serum level monitoring with appropriate interpretation and dosage adjustment may be useful for some agents.

Assay Methodology

Microbiological Assay

Bioassay of antimicrobial agents is performed by several methods. The most commonly employed method is a modification of the disk diffusion technique used for determining antibiotic susceptibility. Paper disks are placed onto, or wells are punched into the surface of, agar containing bacteria known to be highly susceptible to the agent to be assayed. A fixed volume (usually 10 μL) of known concentration of the drug to be assayed or sampled is placed on the disks or in the wells. The measured zone of inhibition and the logarithm of drug concentration are plotted; the drug concentration in unknown samples is determined from measurement of the zone site surrounding disks spotted with unknown concentrations of drug and the plotted standards.

Advantages of this method include its relative ease of performance and low cost for equipment. Disadvantages include possible interference by other antibiotics present in the sample, lack of precision, and slow turnaround time.

Fluorescence Polarization Immunoassay (FPIA)

This technique involves application of the principles of fluorescence when molecules are exposed to light. Fluorescein-labeled drug and antibody directed against the drug are added in constant amounts to samples or standards. The antibody–fluorescein-labeled drug complex results in a change in the fluorescence polarization. Changes in fluorescence polarization occur because of competition for antibody between drug present in the sample and fluorescein-labeled drug added to the sample; therefore, high drug concentrations in the sample reduce the extent of binding of fluorescein-labeled drug to antibody and, thus, the extent of reduction in fluorescence polarization.

Advantages of this technique include automation through the use of the TDX system (Abbott Laboratories, North Chicago, IL). Disadvantages include the expense for reagents and cost for purchase of the automated system.

Radioimmunoassay (RIA)

This technique involves the interaction among radiolabeled drug, unlabeled antibiotic, and antibody directed against the drug. Equilibrium between antibody and the sources of antigen-radiolabeled drug and drug sample is allowed to occur, and the amount of bound or free radiolabeled drug is determined using standard radiometric methods of detection. Advantages of the system include good precision; disadvantages include the expense of the disposal of radioactive wastes.

High-Pressure Liquid Chromatography (HPLC)

In this technique, the principles of separation of different molecular species are used by passing a mobile solvent phase over a stationary phase. Drugs with a polarity similar to that of the stationary phase will be retained for a time on the column and then released. These temporarily retained substances are detected using ultraviolet, fluorescence, electrochemical, or radiometric methods. The detector response is proportional to the amount of molecules seen; standard curves containing known drug concentrations are related to the detector response, usually recorded as peak area or peak height. Advantages include rapid turnaround time, precision, and ability to detect metabolites. Disadvantages include the cost of instruments and the expertise required.

Timing of Collection of Serum Samples

Generally, peak and trough samples are collected to assess maximum and minimum antimicrobial concentrations. Samples for determination of the trough drug concentration should be collected just prior to the next dose. Timing the collection of samples to obtain meaningful peak concentration data appears to be critical. Generally, it is desirable to allow for the distribution phase of the drug to have been completed to more closely characterize extravascular concentrations. Moreover, most interpretive methods use the simplified one-compartment pharmacokinetic model. Therefore, samples for determining the peak concentration are generally collected 1 hour after the start of a 15- to 45-minute intravenous infusion, but there are some exceptions. Serum concentrations of orally administered drugs also tend to peak 1 hour after the dose. Clinicians should ensure that the proper dosing history and sample collection times are recorded to facilitate proper interpretation of serum concentration data.

It is often recommended that one should wait for steady-state pharmacokinetic conditions (approximately four half-lives) before determining serum antibiotic levels. Although this approach might simplify pharmacokinetic interpretation and adjustment of drug doses to some extent, it may be clinically unsound in the treatment of certain infectious diseases. For many infections, achievement of therapeutic serum concentrations early during the course of antibiotic therapy may be an important determinant of survival from an infection. One should ensure that adequate serum concentrations of certain agents have been achieved in critically ill patients and not delay collection of samples simply because steady-state pharmacokinetic conditions do not exist. Indeed, one can apply appropriate methods for the analysis of drug concentration data at non–steady-state conditions to aid in pharmacokinetic parameter estimation and dosage adjustment.

Specific Agents

Target "therapeutic" ranges for agents where serum level monitoring has been employed for treatment of infection are listed in Table 97.7. Serum level monitoring of aminoglycosides and vancomycin has been extensively studied, although this practice has been recently challenged.

Aminoglycosides

The influence of serum aminoglycoside levels on clinical response in gram-negative infection has been reported in several studies.[39–43] However, a recent review concluded that the widely disseminated therapeutic ranges for serum levels were poorly supported by the data.[42] Although the clinical benefit of specific levels still remains unproved, the ranges listed in Table 97.7 can be applied based on controlled studies.

New regimens of aminoglycosides where the daily dose is administered as a single dose have gained some acceptance for use in humans.[50,51] The impetus for these regimens has been to exploit the pharmacodynamics of these agents (e.g., concentration-dependent bacterial killing and a postantibiotic effect), and minimize drug toxicity. Traditional methods of serum level monitoring using trough concentrations would be expected to be uninformative for once-daily dosing, since concentrations 24 hours after a dose should be undetectable in most patients, even those with mild renal dysfunction. Thus, newer monitoring strategies using peak levels, with a second level 6–12 hours after a dose, should be considered, particularly in children. Alternatively, single point methods with serum levels collected between 2–8 hours after a dose can be employed.[43] Additional prospective studies linking serum levels with outcome from single daily dosage regimens with these agents are needed.

Controversy surrounding the influence of serum aminoglycoside concentrations on the development of nephrotoxicity and ototoxicity has existed for several years. Early studies have suggested that trough concentrations exceeding 2–4 mg/L for gentamicin and tobramycin and 10 mg/L for amikacin predisposed patients to nephrotoxicity. More recent analyses of several patient variables have concluded that other patient factors may be more important and that development of ototoxicity and nephrotoxicity is more closely related to total dose and duration of therapy.[42] In many of the studies evaluating nephrotoxicity, high serum concentrations were most likely the *result,* not the *cause,* of the reduction in glomerular filtration rate.

Vancomycin

There are no definitive data correlating peak or trough serum concentrations with efficacy[48]; however, most dosage regimens used in clinical studies and dosing nomograms provide peak concentrations between 20 and 50 mg/L and trough concentrations of less than 10 mg/L.[47–49]

TABLE 97.7. "THERAPEUTIC" SERUM CONCENTRATIONS FOR SELECTED ANTIMICROBIAL AGENTS

Drug	Time of Collection	Target Concentrations (mg/L)	Comments
Aminoglycosides[39–42]	Peak (1 h after the start of a 15- to 45-min infusion)	<5	Urinary tract infections
Traditional dosage regimens			
Gentamicin		>5	Bacteremia
Tobramycin		>6	Bacterial pneumonia
		>12	Endocarditis caused by *Pseudomonas aeruginosa*
	Trough	<2–3	High trough concentrations are most likely a *result* and not a *cause* of nephrotoxicity
Amikacin	Peak	>15	Urinary tract infections
		>20	Bacteremia
		>24	Bacterial pneumonia, other serious infections
	Trough	<9–10	See comments regarding trough gentamicin/ tobramycin concentrations
Single Daily Dosage Regimens[43]			
Gentamicin	8 h postdose	1.5–6	Concentrations above this range associated with nephrotoxicity in one study with netilmicin
Netilmicin			
Tobramycin			
Chloramphenicol[44]	Peak (0.5–1.5 h after 0.5-h IV infusion of succinate salt, or 1.5–3.0 h after oral dose of palmitate)	10–25	Serum concentrations exceeding 25 may be, but are not always, associated with toxicity
Flucytosine[45,46]	Peak (1–2 h postdose)	<100	Levels consistently exceeding this concentration are associated with hematological toxicity 5-Fluorouracil concentrations associated with toxicity have been detected in some patients receiving flucytosine
Vancomycin[47–49]	Peak (1–2 h after a 30- to 60-min infusion)	20–50	Recommendations should be considered tentative, as definitive data are not available
	Trough	<10	

Although intravenous administration of vancomycin (particularly early formulations) has been associated with the development of ototoxicity and nephrotoxicity, recent studies in animals show that it is not ototoxic and minimally nephrotoxic.[48] Further, there are no definitive relationships between concentrations and rare episodes of toxicity. The "red man" syndrome reported with IV infusions of vancomycin has not been correlated with serum levels, but may occur more frequently with infusions of less than 2 hours.[53]

INTEGRATION OF MIC AND SERUM LEVEL DATA

There has been considerable progress in the advance of our understanding of the role of drug pharmacokinetics in the effective treatment of infectious disease. Dosage regimens have been designed to exploit pharmacodynamic characteristics elucidated in the laboratory and ultimately tested in the clinic.[20,34,54,55]

As described previously, organisms with lower MICs to a drug are more likely to respond to treatment with that agent. Similarly, larger daily doses (exposures) of the drug would also be expected to improve the probability of clinical response. Hence, the difference or ratio between the exposure to drug (defined *in vivo* as the area under the plasma concentration versus time curve, or AUC) and its level of susceptibility would be expected to express the likelihood of response. Further, the drug AUC captures information concerning all facets of exposure that actually do determine response. For example, both the peak drug concentration and the duration of time drug concentrations remain above an index for intrinsic activity (e.g., the MIC increases with an increase in AUC). These interrelationships between plasma drug concentrations and MIC are shown in Fig. 97.11.

Within a range of AUC values over a fixed period (e.g., 24 hours), the type of exposure profile may be important. For example, for a given daily dose (AUC), is it best to give the entire dosage as a large single dose, or should it be divided into smaller doses and given more fre-

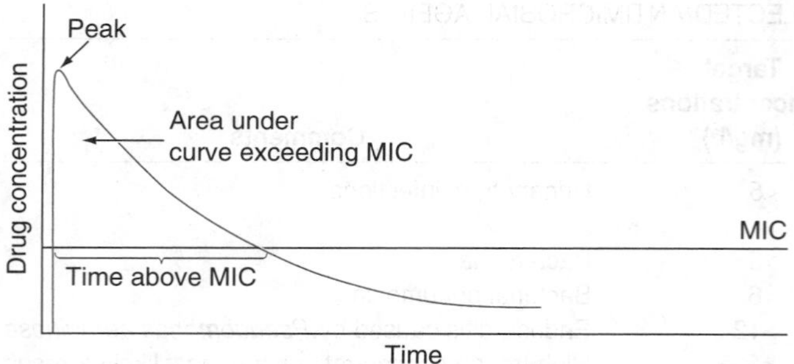

Figure 97.11. Pharmacokinetic parameters related to the MIC. As one increases the AUC, the time above the MIC, peak:MIC and AUC:MIC ratios all increase as well. *(Reprinted by permission from* Applied Pharmacokinetics: Principles of Therapeutic Drug Monitoring, *third edition, by William E. Evans, Jerome J. Schentag, and William J. Jusko, published by Applied Therapeutics, Inc., Vancouver, Washington, © 1992.)*

quently, or even as a continuous infusion? As described previously, currently approved daily doses of aminoglycosides may be most efficacious and least toxic when given as a single daily dose. In contrast, the efficacy of a given level of exposure (AUC) for β-lactams seem best when small doses are given more frequently or as a continuous infusion.[20,34,54,55]

The capability to integrate MIC information with pharmacokinetic data has resulted in considerable interest in development of stochastic control of antibiotic dosage to achieve target levels of exposure relative to the MIC. Although initial studies have developed relationships for some drugs, prospective studies will be required to determine if optimizing exposure relative to susceptibility data will improve outcomes.[34,54]

Conclusion

Molecular biology, automation, and computerization have led to considerable advances in the type and application of data available to the clinician in the management of infectious diseases. Combined with rapid, definitive diagnosis and drug susceptibility data, the incorporation of pharmacologic characteristics of anti-infectives can improve the outcome of many infectious diseases.[55] Although in the past most practitioners tended to discount the importance of antimicrobial dosage, increasingly serious nosocomial infections with antibiotic-resistant bacteria, particularly in immunocompromised patients, warrant application of these concepts. In particular, the availability of newer, more site-nonspecific agents such as antivirals and immune-based therapies will require development of newer strategies, which utilize information developed in the clinical laboratory.

References

1. Sanders CC. A problem with antimicrobial susceptibility tests. ASM News 1991;57:187–190.
2. Sox HC, Liang MH. The erythrocyte sedimentation rate: Guidelines for rational use. Ann Intern Med 1986;104:515–523.
3. Casey LC, Balk RA, Bone RC. Plasma cytokine levels correlate with survival in patients with the sepsis syndrome. Ann Intern Med 1993;15:771–778.
4. Naber SP. Molecular pathology—diagnosis of infectious diseases. N Engl J Med 1994;331:1212–1215.
5. Smith-Elekes S, Weinstein MP. Blood cultures. Infect Dis Clin North Am 1993;7:221–234.
6. Tenover F. DNA hybridization techniques and their application to the diagnosis of infectious diseases. Infect Dis Clin North Am 1993;7:171–181.
7. Rosenthal N. Tools of the trade-recombinant DNA. N Engl J Med 1994;331:315–317.
8. Lorian V, Burns L. Predictive value of susceptibility tests for the outcome of antibacterial therapy. J Antimicrob Chemother 1990;25:175–181.
9. Pfaller MA, Rinaldi MG. Antifungal susceptibility testing. Current state of technology, limitations, and standardization. Infect Dis Clin North Am 1993;7:435–444.
10. National Committee for Clinical Laboratory Standards (NCCLS). Methods for Dilution Antimicrobial Susceptibility Tests for Bacteria that Grow Aerobically, 3rd ed, approved standard. NCCLS document M7-A3 (ISBN 1-56238-209-8). NCCLS, 771 East Lancaster Avenue, Villanova, PA, 19085, 1993.
11. Craig WA. Qualitative susceptibility tests versus quantitative MIC tests. Diag Microbiol Infect Dis 1993;16:231–236.
12. Ayers LW, Jones RN, Barry AL, et al. Cefotetan, a new cephamycin: Comparison of *in vitro* antimicrobial activity with other cephems, β-lactamase stability, and preliminary recommendations for disk diffusion testing. Antimicrob Agents Chemother 1982;22:859–877.
13. Bauer AW, Kirby MM, Sherris JC, et al. Antibiotic susceptibility testing by a standardized, single-disk method. Am J Clin Pathol 1966;45:493–496.
14. Thornsberry C. Foreword to ETEST symposium. Diag Microbiol Infect Dis 1992;15:459–463.
15. Tilton RC. Automation and mechanization in antimicrobial susceptibility testing, in Lorian V (ed): Antibiotics in Laboratory Medicine, 3rd ed. Baltimore, Williams and Wilkins, 1991, pp 106–119.
16. Granato PA. The impact of same-day tests versus traditional overnight testing. Diag Microbiol Infect Dis 1993;16:237–243.
17. Bundtzen RW, Gerber AU, Cohn DL, et al. Postantibiotic suppression of growth. Rev Infect Dis 1981;3:28–37.
18. Zhanel GG, Hoban DJ, Harding GKM. The postantibiotic effect: A review of *in vitro* and *in vivo* data. Ann Pharmacother 1991;25:153–163.
19. Eagle H, Musselman AD. The slow recovery of bacteria from the toxic effects of penicillin. J Bacteriol 1949;58:475–490.
20. Ebert SC, Craig WA. Pharmacodynamic properties of antibiotics: Application to drug monitoring and dosage regimen design. Infect Control Hosp Epidemiol 1990;11:319–326.

21. LaForce FM. Systemic antimicrobial therapy of nosocomial pneumonia: Monotherapy vs combination therapy. Eur J Clin Microbiol Infect Dis 1989;8:61–68.
22. Barriere SL. Monotherapy versus combination antimicrobial therapy: A review. Pharmacotherapy 1991;11(2 Part 2):64S–71S.
23. Dejongh CA, Joshi JH, Newman KA, et al. Antibiotic synergism and response in gram-negative bacteremia in granulocytopenic cancer patients. Am J Med 1986;80(suppl 5C):96–100.
24. Bodey GP. Synergism: Should it determine antibiotic selection in neutropenic patients? Arch Intern Med 1985;145:1964–1966.
25. Hilf M, Yu VL, Sharp J, et al. Antibiotic therapy for *Pseudomonas aeruginosa* bacteremia: Outcome correlations in a prospective study of 200 patients. Am J Med 1989;87:540–546.
26. Herman DJ, Gerding DN. Screening and treatment of infections caused by resistant enterococci. Antimicrob Agents Chemother 1991;35:215–219.
27. Lepper MM, Dowling HF. Treatment of pneumococcic meningitis with penicillin compared with penicillin plus aureomycin. Arch Intern Med 1951;88:489–494.
28. Dudley MN. Bacterial resistance to beta-lactam antibiotics: Assessment of management strategies. Pharmacother 1995;15:1S–38S.
29. Blaser J. Interactions of antimicrobial combinations *in vitro:* The relativity of synergism. Scand J Infect Dis 1991;74(suppl):71–79.
30. Chou T-C, Talalay P. Analysis of combined drug effects: A new look at a very old problem. Trends Pharmacol Sci 1983;4:450–454.
31. Bunow B, Weinstein JN. COMBO: A new approach to the analysis of drug combinations *in vitro.* Ann NY Acad Sci 1990;616:490–494.
32. Pritchard MN, Shipman C Jr. A three-dimensional model to analyze drug–drug interactions. Antiviral Res 1990;14:181–206.
33. Zinner SH, Dudley MN, Blaser J. *In vitro* models for the study of combination antibiotic therapy in neutropenic patients. Am J Med 1986;80(suppl 6B):156–159.
34. Dudley MN. Commentary on dual individualization with antibiotics, in Evans WE, Schentag JJ, Jusko WJ (eds): Applied Pharmacokinetics—Principles of Therapeutic Drug Monitoring, 3d ed. Vancouver, WA, Applied Therapeutics, 1992, pp. 18-1–18-13.
35. Wolfson JS, Swartz MN. Serum bactericidal activity as a monitor of antibiotic therapy. N Engl J Med 1985;312:968–975.
36. Reller LB. The serum bactericidal test. Rev Infect Dis 1986;8:803–808.
37. Van der Auwera P, Klastersky J. Bactericidal activity and killing rate of serum in volunteers receiving ciprofloxacin alone or in combination with vancomycin. Antimicrob Agents Chemother 1986;30:892–895.
38. Barriere SL, Kapusnik JE, Ely E, et al. Analysis of a new method for assessing activity of combinations of antimicrobials. Area under the bactericidal activity curve. J Antimicrob Chemother 1985;16:49–59.
39. Zaske D. Aminoglycosides, in Evans WE, Schentag JJ, Jusko WJ (eds): Applied Pharmacokinetics, 3rd ed. Vancouver, WA, Applied Therapeutics, 1992, pp 14-1–14-47.
40. Moore RD, Smith CR, Lietman PS. The association of aminoglycoside plasma levels with mortality in patients with gram-negative bacteremia. J Infect Dis 1984;149:443–448.
41. Moore RD, Smith CR, Lietman PS. Association of aminoglycoside plasma levels with therapeutic outcome in gram-negative pneumonia. Am J Med 1984;77:657–662.
42. McCormack JP, Jewesson PJ. A critical reevaluation of the "therapeutic range" of aminoglycosides. Clin Infect Dis 1992;14:320–339.
43. Blaser J, Konig C, Simmen H-P, Thurnheer U. Monitoring serum concentrations for once-daily netilmicin dosing regimens. J Antimicrob Chemother 1994;33:341–348.
44. Nahata MC. Chloramphenicol, in Evans WE, Schentag JJ, Jusko WJ (eds): Applied Pharmacokinetics, 3rd ed. Vancouver, WA, Applied Therapeutics, 1992, pp 16-1–16-24.
45. Barriere SL. Pharmacology and pharmacokinetics of traditional systemic antifungal agents. Pharmacotherapy 1990;10(suppl):134S–140S.
46. Stamm AM, Diasio RB, Dismukes WE, et al. Toxicity of amphotericin B plus flucytosine in 194 patients with cryptococcal meningitis. Am J Med 1987;83:236–242.
47. Matzke GR. Vancomycin, in Evans WE, Schentag JJ, Jusko WJ (eds): Applied Pharmacokinetics: Principles of Therapeutic Drug Monitoring, 3rd ed. Vancouver, WA, Applied Therapeutics, 1992, pp 15-1–15-31.
48. Cantu TG, Yamanaka-Yuen NA, Lietman PS. Serum vancomycin concentrations: Reappraisal of their clinical value. Clin Infect Dis 1994;18:533–543.
49. Moellering RC Jr. Monitoring serum vancomycin levels: Climbing the mountain because it is there? [editorial] Clin Infect Dis 1994;18:544–546.
50. Bates RD, Nahata MC. Once-daily administration of aminoglycosides. Ann Pharmacother 1994;28:757–766.
51. Rotschager JC, Rybak MJ. Single daily dosing of aminoglycosides: A commentary. Ann Pharmacother 1994;28:797–801.
52. Viscoli C, Dudley MN, Ferrea G, et al. Serum concentrations and safety of single daily dosing of amikacin in children undergoing bone marrow transplantation. J Antimicrob Chemother 1991;27(suppl C):113–120.
53. Healy DP, Sahai JV, Fuller SH, et al. Vancomycin-induced histamine release and "red man syndrome": Comparison of 1- and 2-hour infusions. Antimicrob Agents Chemother 1990;34:550–554.
54. Schentag JJ, Ballow CH, Paladino JA, et al. Dual individualization with antibiotics: Integrated antibiotic management strategies for use in hospitals, in Evans WE, Schentag JJ, Jusko WJ (eds): Applied Pharmacokinetics: Principles of Therapeutic Drug Monitoring, 3rd ed. Vancouver, WA, Applied Therapeutics, 1992, pp 17-1–17-20.
55. Drusano GL. Human pharmacodynamics of beta-lactams, aminoglycosides, and their combination. Scand J Infect Dis 1991;74(suppl):235–248.

Chapter 98

Selection of Antimicrobial Regimens

Steven L. Barriere, PharmD, FCCP

Choosing an antimicrobial agent to treat or prevent an infection is far more complicated than simply matching a drug to a known or suspected pathogen. There is, however, a generally accepted systematic approach to the selection and evaluation of an antimicrobial regimen (Table 98.1). Unfortunately, all too often we are tempted to ignore the systematic approach to designing an optimum regimen in favor of broad-spectrum therapy that will "cover everything." This approach is not only unsystematic, but it is expensive, potentially more toxic, and will lead to widespread resistance and difficult-to-treat superinfections.

Another abuse of antimicrobial agents is their application when, in fact, they are not needed. The best example of this is the well-recognized and widespread practice of prescribing antibacterials for self-limited, clinical conditions that are most likely viral in origin.

Initial selection of antimicrobial therapy is nearly always "empiric." That is, therapy begins before the offending organism is identified. Infectious diseases are generally acute, and a delay in beginning antimicrobial therapy may result in serious morbidity or even mortality. An example is the rapidly lethal nature of various forms of meningitis. Thus, antimicrobial therapy selection is based on information gathered from the patient's history and physical examination and from the results of Gram stains or rapidly performed tests on clinical specimens. This information coupled with knowledge of the most likely offending organism(s) and an institution's local susceptibility patterns allows for a rational selection of drugs to treat the patient.

This chapter outlines, in some detail, the systematic approach for selection of antimicrobial therapeutic regimens. The principles for selection of antimicrobial prophylactic regimens are discussed in Chapter 115.

Confirming the Presence of Infection

FEVER

The presence of a temperature greater than the expected 98.6°F (37°C) "normal" body temperature is considered a hallmark of infectious diseases, but may be caused by several other factors. Body temperature is controlled in the hypothalamus.[1] The thermoregulatory center of the hypothalamus contains neurons whose function is affected by the temperature of the blood supply via direct connections with temperature receptors in skin and muscle. In addition, the circadian rhythm, a built-in temperature cycle, is also operational. The daily rhythm is particular for each individual. Temperature readings in the hypothalamic structures result in signals sent along various neuronal pathways that result in peripheral heat conservation or loss (vasoconstriction or vasodilation). In a healthy person, the internal thermostat is set between the morning low temperature and the afternoon peak as controlled by the circadian rhythm. During fever, the hypothalamus is reset at a higher level and all of the above functions of the hypothalamus operate normally.[1]

Fever is defined as a controlled elevation of body temperature above the normal range. The normal range for most humans is 36–37.8°C. Substances that cause fever are called pyrogens. In the case of infection-produced fever, various microbial antigens stimulate macrophages, which release so-called endogenous pyrogens, now recognized to be interleukins (ILs, particularly IL-1) and tumor necrosis factor. IL-1 acts on hypothalamic endothelial tissues to produce release of prostaglandins and other arachidonic acid metabolites. These substances act on thermoregulatory neurons to elevate the internal thermostat. Consequently, the vasomotor center and various peripheral efferents produce and conserve heat.[1] This all results in elevated body temperature or fever. Note that this is a highly simplified summary of a very complex series of events. However, the fundamental concepts are outlined.

The development of fever is common to all vertebrate species and has been demonstrated to be an important host defense, even in cold-blooded animals such as fish and lizards. When these animals are injected with exogenous pyrogen (e.g., endotoxin) they modify their behavior to elevate body temperature, such as swimming close to the surface and basking in the sun. The elevation of body temperature results in increased survival from infection. The

TABLE 98.1. SYSTEMATIC APPROACH FOR SELECTION OF ANTIMICROBIALS

A. Confirm the presence of infection
   1. Fever
   2. Signs and symptoms
   3. Predisposing factors
B. Identification of the pathogen (Chapter 97)
   1. Collection of infected material
   2. Stains
   3. Serologies
   4. Culture
C. Selection of presumptive therapy
   1. Host factors
   2. Drug factors
D. Monitor therapeutic response
   1. Clinical assessment
   2. Laboratory tests
   3. Assessment of therapeutic failure

mechanisms for this are enhanced leukocyte migration, augmented lymphocyte function, and reduced microbial replication.

Of course, fever is a manifestation of many disease states other than infection. In particular, many collagen vascular (autoimmune) disorders and several malignancies may have fever as a manifestation. A patient with fever and no other, or nonspecific, complaints may have an infection as well as many other diseases. Fever of unknown or undetermined origin is a diagnostic dilemma and has been reviewed extensively elsewhere.[2]

In addition, many drugs have been identified as causes of fever.[3] Drug-induced fever is defined as persistent fever in the absence of infection or other underlying condition. The fever must coincide temporally with the administration of the offending agent and disappear promptly upon its withdrawal, after which it remains normal.[3]

The mechanism of drug-induced fever is believed to be due to either a hypersensitivity reaction or development of an antigen (drug)–antibody complex that results in the stimulation of macrophages and release of IL-1. Although this is not a common drug effect, accounting for no more than 5% of all drug reactions, it should be suspected under the correct circumstances. Almost any medication can produce drug-induced fever but certain ones appear to be more often responsible than others. These include β-lactam antibiotics, anticonvulsants, and a variety of other medications including allopurinol, hydralazine, nitrofurantoin, sulfonamides and related compounds, phenothiazines, and methyldopa.[3]

Noninfectious etiologies of fever may be referred to as "false-positives." Although these certainly may confuse the clinician, even more troublesome are "false-negatives": the absence of fever in a patient with signs and symptoms consistent with an infectious disease. Some types of minor infection do not produce fever (e.g., uncomplicated cystitis), but more important are true false-negatives induced by antipyretics, undetected antimicrobial therapy, or overwhelming infection. A careful questioning of the patient or family should be done to assess the ingestion of any medication that can mask fever. These include aspirin, acetaminophen, nonsteroidal anti-inflammatory agents, and corticosteroids. Similarly, treatment of a disease state with only partially effective therapy may also temporarily reduce fever and other signs of infection. A good example of this is the use of bacteriostatic drugs in a patient with infective endocarditis.

The use of antipyretics should be discouraged during the treatment of infection unless absolutely necessary. The common practice of administering an antipyretic during the treatment of infection may mask a poor therapeutic response. Moreover, elevated body temperature, unless very high (>105°F), is not harmful and may be beneficial as previously noted.[1] Artificial means of reducing elevated body temperature (e.g., cooling blankets) are generally unnecessary and may even be dangerous. Fever patterns are believed by some to be helpful in establishing the etiology of the increased temperature. For example, high-spiking fevers are believed to be more consistent with an infectious process, whereas sustained fevers are associated with collagen vascular disease or malignancy. Although these guidelines may be generally true, there are reports of high-spiking fever due to drugs. In addition, many subacute infectious processes may produce relatively modest but sustained elevations in temperature. Overall, characterization of the fever pattern probably offers little in the general assessment of the patient.[4]

SIGNS AND SYMPTOMS

Most infections result in elevated white blood cell (WBC) counts (leukocytosis) because of the mobilization of granulocytes and/or lymphocytes to ingest and destroy invading microbes. The generally accepted range of normal values for WBC counts is between 4000 and 10,000/mm^3. Values above or below this range hold important prognostic and diagnostic value.

Classically, bacterial infections are associated with elevated granulocyte counts (neutrophils, basophils), often with immature forms (band neutrophils) seen in peripheral blood smears ("left-shift"). The presence of immature forms is an indication of increased bone marrow response to the infection. With infection, peripheral leukocyte counts may be very high, but are rarely higher than 30,000 to 40,000/mm^3. Since leukocytosis indicates the normal host response to infection, low leukocyte counts after the onset of infection indicate an abnormal response and are generally associated with a poor prognosis of bacterial infection.[5] Relative lymphocytosis, even with normal or slightly elevated total WBC counts, is generally associated with viral or fungal infections. Many types of infections, however, may be accompanied by a completely normal WBC count and differential.

The classic signs of pain and inflammation may be manifested by swelling, erythema, tenderness, and purulent drainage. Unfortunately, these are only visibly apparent if the infection is superficial or in a bone or joint. The manifestations of inflammation in deep-seated infections such as meningitis, pneumonia, endocarditis, and urinary tract infection must be ascertained by examining tissues or fluids. For example, the presence of polymorphonuclearleukocytes (neutrophils) in spinal fluid, lung secretions (sputum), and urine is highly suggestive of bacterial infection.

Symptoms referable to an organ system must be carefully sought out, for they not only help in establishing the presence of infection, but also aid in narrowing the list of potential pathogens. For example, a febrile patient with complaints of flank pain and dysuria may well have pyelonephritis. In this situation, enteric gram-negative bacilli, especially *Escherichia coli,* are the predominant pathogens. However, if a febrile patient has no symptoms referable to an organ system, but only constitutional complaints, the list of possible infectious diseases is quite long.[2] A febrile individual with cough and sputum production probably has a pulmonary infection. What is not so evident, however, is the etiologic organism in this situation, because it may be due to bacteria, mycobacteria, viruses, or mycoplasmas.[6] In this situation, attention to the patient's history and background disease states is important. Even more important is careful examination of infected material (in this case sputum) to try and ascertain the identity of the pathogen.

Table 98.2 lists factors that predispose patients to infection. Generally, immunosuppressive disease states lead to a wide variety of infections (e.g., acquired immune deficiency syndrome), while other diseases may predispose the patient to a certain type of infectious disease (e.g., recurrent meningococcal infection with complement deficiency). Information from the patient's history regarding underlying disease is vitally important, since the presence of an underlying condition may not only predispose patients to infection, but also may modify the likely offending pathogen. For example, purulent meningitis in an otherwise healthy adult is almost invariably caused by meningococci or pneumococci, whereas this same infection in a patient with a lymphoma may be caused by *Listeria monocytogenes,* which will infect an immunocompetent patient in only one-third of cases.[7] For a thorough discussion on infection in immunocompromised patients, see Chapters 114 and 117.

Many factors predisposing to infection are related to disruption of the host's integumentary barriers. For example, trauma, burns, and iatrogenic wounds induced in surgery may lead to a substantial risk of infection depending on the severity and location of the injury or disruption. For a complete discussion of the various risks involved in surgical procedures, see Chapter 115.

Controversy remains over the exact role that certain risk factors play. For example, the more frequent incidence of urinary tract infections in diabetic patients may simply be the result of frequent manipulation of the urinary tract (catheterizations) but is probably more frequent only in diabetics with neurologic complications affecting bladder emptying.[8] In addition, there is some doubt over the immunosuppressive role of pregnancy in dissemination of chronic granulomatous diseases such as tuberculosis.

TABLE 98.2. FACTORS PREDISPOSING TO INFECTION

Alterations in normal flora of the host
Disruption of natural barriers
Skin/mucous membranes
Cilia of respiratory tract
pH and motility of bowel
Age
Immunosuppression secondary to:
Malnutrition
Underlying disease (hereditary or acquired)
Hormones (e.g., pregnancy, corticosteroids)
Drugs (e.g., cytotoxic agents)

IDENTIFICATION OF THE PATHOGEN

Infected body materials must be sampled, if at all possible or practical, before institution of any antimicrobial therapy for two reasons. First, Gram stain of the material may rapidly reveal bacteria, or acid-fast stain may detect mycobacteria or actinomycetes. Second, delay in obtaining infected fluids or tissues until after therapy is started may result in false-negative culture results or alterations in the cellular and chemical composition of infected fluids. This is particularly true in patients with urinary tract infections, meningitis, and septic arthritis.[9]

In addition to the potentially infected materials produced by the patient (sputum, urine, stool, wound, or sinus drainage), other less accessible fluids or tissues must be obtained based on localized signs or symptoms (e.g., spinal fluid in meningitis, joint fluid in arthritis). Abscesses and cellulitic areas should also be aspirated. Finally, blood cultures should nearly always be performed in the acutely ill, febrile patient. Blood culture collection is usually timed to sharp elevations in temperature, suggesting the possibility of microorganisms (or microbial antigens) in the bloodstream. However, in selected diseases, especially endocarditis, the bacteremia is qualitatively continuous, so cultures may be obtained at any time.[10]

Once positive Gram stain and/or culture results are obtained, the clinician must be cautious in determining whether the organism recovered is a true pathogen, a contaminant, or is part of the normally expected flora from the site of specimen collection. This latter consideration is especially problematic with cultures obtained from the skin, oropharynx, nose, ears, eyes, throat, and perineum. These surfaces are heavily colonized with a wide variety of bacteria, some of which may be pathogenic in certain settings. For example, coagulase-negative staphylococci are found in cultures of all the aforementioned sites, yet are seldom regarded as pathogens unless recovered from blood, venous access catheters, or prosthetic devices.

Importantly, cultures of specimens from purportedly infected sites, which are obtained by sampling from or through one of these contaminated areas, may contain significant numbers of the normal flora.

Particularly problematic are expectorated sputum specimens that must be carefully evaluated by determination of the presence of squamous epithelial cells and leukocytes.[6] A predominance of epithelial cells in sputum specimens casts doubt on the pathogenic role of any bacteria recovered, especially when multiple types of organisms are seen on Gram stain. In contrast, the discovery of leukocytes in large numbers with one predominant type of organism is a more reliable indicator. In general, however, sputum evaluation has poor sensitivity and specificity as a diagnostic test.[6]

Caution must also be taken in the evaluation of positive culture results from normally sterile sites (e.g., blood, cerebrospinal fluid, joint fluid). The recovery of bacteria normally found on the skin in large quantities (e.g., coagulase-negative staphylococci, diphtheroids) from one of these sites may be a result of contamination of the specimen rather than true infection. However, these organisms may be pathogenic in certain settings. For example, as noted previously, coagulase-negative staphylococci are common infecting organisms of prosthetic devices, indwelling intravenous catheters, and cerebrospinal fluid shunts.

Gram-staining techniques, culture methods, and serologic identification, as well as susceptibility testing, are covered in detail in Chapter 97. Emphasis must be placed on the proper collection and handling of specimens and careful assessment of Gram stain or other test results, in guiding the clinician toward appropriate selection of initial antimicrobial therapy.

Selection of Presumptive Therapy

To select rational antimicrobial therapy for a given clinical situation, a variety of factors must be considered. These include the severity and acuity of the disease, host factors, factors related to the drugs used, and the necessity for use of multiple agents. In addition, there are generally accepted "drugs of choice" for the treatment of most pathogens (see Appendix 98.1).

The drugs of choice are compiled from a variety of sources and are intended as guidelines rather than specific rules for antimicrobial use. Relevant to this is the consideration of local susceptibility data whenever possible rather than information published by other institutions or national compilations. External susceptibility data for either formulary considerations or drug selection in the individual patient may be misleading. Because of antimicrobial usage patterns, the types of patients cared for, and the surgical procedures performed, the susceptibility of bacteria in any given hospital or community may differ substantially from another.

For example, the prevalence of methicillin-resistant *Staphylococcus aureus* (MRSA) in some centers is quite high, whereas in others the problem may be nonexistent. This particular situation will influence the selection of therapy for possible *S. aureus* infection where either a β-lactam compound or vancomycin would be the choices. The problem of differing susceptibilities is not only limited to gram-positive bacteria but also gram-negative organisms and all drug classes are affected.

The severity and/or acuity of the infectious process dictates the necessity for use of so-called "empiric" antimicrobial therapy. In most cases, therapy is started before results of culture and susceptibility testing are available, because a delay of 24–48 hours would be incurred. This delay would, obviously, compromise the health of the patient if the infection were rapidly progressive. Moreover, a great deal of antibiotic use is in ambulatory patients, who are unlikely to return for treatment after having been seen by a physician. Thus, therapy is often begun "empirically" or without knowledge of the exact infecting organism(s). Empiric therapies are directed at organisms that are frequently known to cause the infection in question. These organisms are discussed in Chapters 99–118.

To define the most likely infecting organisms, a careful history and physical examination must be performed. In addition, a variety of host factors should be considered to help identify the likely etiologic agent as well as to assist in the selection of the best initial or empiric therapy for the patient.

HOST FACTORS

In evaluating a patient for initial or empiric therapy, the factors listed in Table 98.3 should be considered. Allergy to the antimicrobial agents being considered for therapy would seem to preclude their use. However, a very careful assessment of allergic histories must be performed since many patients may confuse common adverse drug effects, such as gastrointestinal (GI) disturbance, with true allergic

TABLE 98.3. HOST FACTORS IN SELECTION OF ANTIMICROBIAL THERAPY

Allergy or history of adverse drug reactions
Age of patient
Pregnancy
Genetic or metabolic abnormalities
Renal and hepatic function
Site of the infection
Concomitant drug therapy
Underlying disease state(s)

reactions.[11] Among the most commonly cited antimicrobial allergies are those to penicillin and/or related compounds. One can find many authoritative sources that recommend other β-lactam compounds, especially cephalosporins, in this setting, because of suggestive evidence that few patients with penicillin allergy will react to a cephalosporin. Therefore, the true cross-reactivity between these two β-lactam classes may be lower than suspected. Regardless, in the absence of complete penicillin skin-testing capabilities, a rule of thumb for giving cephalosporins to penicillin-allergic patients is to avoid them in patients who give a good history for immediate or accelerated reactions (anaphylaxis, laryngospasm) and to give them cautiously in patients with a history of delayed reaction such as rash.[12] If gram-negative infection is suspected or documented, therapy with a monobactam may be appropriate, since cross-reactivity with other β-lactams is virtually nil.[13]

The patient's age is an important factor, both in trying to identify the likely etiologic agent and in assessing the patient's ability to detoxify or eliminate the drug(s) to be used. The best example of age determinant of organisms is in bacterial meningitis where the pathogens differ as the patient grows from the neonatal period, to infancy and childhood, and into adulthood.[14] A neonate's hepatic and liver function is not well developed, but becomes extremely efficient during infancy and childhood, and slowly wanes with increasing age. Thus, both drug selection and drug dosage must be adjusted based on the age of the patient.

Specific patient groups require additional considerations when using antimicrobials. For example, neonates (especially when premature) may develop kernicterus when given sulfonamides. This results from displacement of bilirubin from serum albumin.[15] Chloramphenicol as a cause of the "gray baby" syndrome is well established. The mechanism of this effect is an inability of the newborn's liver to metabolize (and detoxify) the drug leading to shock and cardiovascular collapse.[16] Thus, serum concentrations of chloramphenicol must be monitored to ensure that concentrations of the drug do not exceed 20–25 μg/mL.

Although it is generally believed that the elderly are more predisposed to adverse drug effects, there are no clear-cut explanations for this.[17] An important example is that hepatotoxicity from the antimicrobial agent isoniazid has been documented to increase in frequency with age.[18]

During pregnancy, not only is the fetus at risk for drug teratogenicity, but also the pharmacokinetic disposition of certain drugs may be altered.[19] Penicillins, cephalosporins, and aminoglycosides are cleared from the peripheral circulation more rapidly during pregnancy. This is probably due to the marked increases in intravascular volume, glomerular filtration rate, and hepatic/metabolic activities, especially during late pregnancy. The net result is that maternal serum antimicrobial concentrations may be as much as 50% lower during this period than in the nonpregnant state. Increased dosage of certain compounds may be necessary to achieve therapeutic levels during late pregnancy.

Inherited or acquired metabolic abnormalities will influence the therapy of infectious diseases in a variety of ways. For example, patients with impaired peripheral vascular flow may not absorb drugs given by intramuscular injection. In addition, certain metabolic states may predispose patients to enhanced drug toxicity. For example, patients who are phenotypically slow acetylators of isoniazid are at greater risk for development of peripheral neuropathy.[20] Patients with severe deficiency of glucose-6-phosphate dehydrogenase (G6PD) may develop significant hemolysis when exposed to drugs such as sulfonamides, nitrofurantoin, nalidixic acid, antimalarials, dapsone, and perhaps chloramphenicol.[21] Although mild deficiencies are found in blacks, the more severe forms of the disease are generally confined to persons of Eastern Mediterranean origin.

Patients with diminished renal and/or hepatic function will accumulate certain drugs unless dosage is adjusted. Although many antimicrobial reactions are idiosyncratic, there are significant dose-related toxicities associated with a number of agents. Table 98.4 lists drugs by antimicrobial class, identifies their route of elimination, and the dose-related toxicity to be avoided.

Clear-cut identification of the site of the infection or the likely source of a bacteremia can aid in defining the most likely organisms. For example, the overwhelming majority of urinary tract infections are caused by enteric gram-negative bacilli, especially *E. coli.*[22] In contrast, bone and joint infections in children are nearly always due to *S. aureus.*[23] Bacterial pneumonia in an adult, acquired in the community, is very likely caused by *Streptococcus pneumoniae,* whereas this same infection, acquired in the hospital, is more likely due to enteric gram-negative bacilli such as *Enterobacter* or opportunists such as *Pseudomonas aeruginosa.*[24]

The most common source of bacteremias is the urinary tract, and the majority of the bacteremias from this site are caused by enteric gram-negative bacilli.[22] In contrast, bacteremia from an intravenous catheter site is very likely caused by staphylococci.[25]

TABLE 98.4. ROUTES OF ANTIMICROBIAL ELIMINATION AND DOSE-RELATED TOXICITIES

Drugs	Primary Route of Elimination	Degree of Accumulation[a]	Dose-Related Toxic Effect(s)
Penicillins			
Ampicillin	Renal	Significant	CNS (seizures, etc.)
Carbenicillin	Renal	Significant	Platelet dysfunction, CNS toxicity, sodium overload
Methicillin	Renal	Moderate	?Nephritis
Mezlocillin	Renal/hepatic[b]	Moderate	?Platelet dysfunction
Nafcillin	Renal/hepatic[b]	Insignificant	?Neutropenia
Oxacillin	Renal/hepatic[b]	Insignificant	?Neutropenia
Penicillin G	Renal	Significant	CNS toxicity; hyperkalemia (with K^+ salt)
Piperacillin	Renal/hepatic[b]	Moderate	?Platelet dysfunction
Ticarcillin	Renal	Significant	CNS toxicity, platelet dysfunction
Cephalosporins			
Cefamandole	Renal	Significant	Hypoprothrombinemia
Cefepime	Renal	Significant	None
Cefazolin	Renal	Significant	CNS toxicity
Cefmetazole	Renal	Significant	Hypoprothrombinemia
Cefonicid	Renal	Significant	None
Cefoperazone	Hepatic/renal[b]	Moderate	Hypoprothrombinemia
Cefotaxime	Renal/hepatic[b]	Moderate	None
Cefotetan	Renal	Significant	Hypoprothrombinemia
Cefoxitin	Renal	Significant	None
Ceftazidime	Renal	Significant	None
Cefizoxime	Renal	Significant	None
Ceftriaxone	Renal/hepatic[b]	Insignificant	None
Cefuroxime	Renal	Significant	None
Aminoglycosides	Renal	Significant	Nephrotoxicity, ototoxicity
Tetracyclines	Renal (except doxycycline)	Significant	Exacerbation of azotemia, possible hepatotoxicity
Miscellaneous			
Aztreonam	Renal	Moderate	None
Chloramphenicol	Hepatic	Moderate	Gray baby syndrome, marrow suppression
Ciprofloxacin	Renal/hepatic	Moderate	CNS toxicity
Clindamycin	Hepatic	Moderate	None

Any concomitant therapy the patient is receiving may influence both the selection of drug therapy, the dosage, and monitoring. For example, administration of isoniazid to a patient who is also receiving phenytoin may result in phenytoin toxicity. This is caused by an inhibition of phenytoin metabolism by isoniazid. In addition, the selected antimicrobial therapy itself may adversely affect the management of another disease. A list of selected drug interactions involving antimicrobials and antimicrobial interference with laboratory tests is provided in Table 98.5.

Concomitant disease states may influence the selection of therapy. Certain diseases will predispose patients to a particular infectious disease or will alter the type of infecting organism. For example, patients with diabetes mellitus and resulting peripheral vascular disease often develop lower extremity soft tissue infections. Patients with chronic lung disease or cystic fibrosis develop frequent pulmonary infections, which may be caused by somewhat different microorganisms than are found in otherwise normal hosts.

Patients with immunosuppressive diseases such as malignancies or acquired immunologic deficiencies are highly predisposed to infections, and the types of organisms may be vastly different from what would be expected. For example, patients undergoing chemotherapy for acute forms of leukemia are often profoundly granulocytopenic and are predisposed to infections caused by staphylococci, enteric gram-negative bacilli, and fungi.[26] In contrast, patients with the acquired immune deficiency syndrome (AIDS) often become infected with an enormous variety of organisms[27] (Chapter 117). Complicating this assessment is the possibility that the immunosuppressed patient may have been taking prophylactic or suppressive antimicrobial agents such as trimethoprim–sulfamethoxazole for *Pneumocystis carinii* pneumonia, fluconazole for fungal infection, or acyclovir for viral disease.

TABLE 98.4. ROUTES OF ANTIMICROBIAL ELIMINATION AND DOSE-RELATED TOXICITIES (*Continued*)

Drugs	Primary Route of Elimination	Degree of Accumulation[a]	Dose-Related Toxic Effect(s)
Miscellaneous *(cont.)*			
Erythromycin	Hepatic	Insignificant	Ototoxicity
Fleroxacin	Renal	Moderate	CNS toxicity
Imipenem	Renal	Significant	CNS toxicity
Lomefloxacin	Renal	Moderate	CNS toxicity
Metronidazole	Hepatic/renal	Moderate	Encephalopathy, neuropathy
Ofloxacin	Renal	Significant	CNS toxicity
Polymyxins	Renal	Significant	Nephrotoxicity, neuropathy, neuromuscular blockade
Sulfonamides	Renal/hepatic[b]	Moderate	Kernicterus
Trimethoprim	Renal	Moderate	Megaloblastic anemia
Antifungal Agents			
Amphotericin B	Unknown	Insignificant	Most adverse effects increase in frequency with cumulative dose, not individual dosage size
Fluconazole	Renal	Significant	?Hepatotoxicity
Flucytosine	Renal	Significant	Marrow suppression, ?hepatoxicity
Itraconazole	Hepatic	Insignificant	?None
Miconazole	Hepatic	Insignificant	?Hepatoxicity
Ketoconazole	Hepatic	Insignificant	None
Antiviral Agents			
Acyclovir	Renal	Significant	CNS toxicity, nephrotoxicity
Foscarnet	Renal	Significant	Nephrotoxicity, CNS toxicity
Ganciclovir	Renal	Significant	Marrow suppression
Vidarabine	Hepatic/renal[b]	Insignificant	?CNS toxicity
Ribavirin	Hepatic	Insignificant	?
Antitubercular Agents			
Isoniazid	Hepatic	Insignificant	Neuropathy
Ethambutol	Renal	Moderate	Optic neuritis
Pyrazinamide	Hepatic	Moderate	?None
Rifampin	Hepatic	Insignificant	?None

[a]Accumulation of parent compound and/or active/toxic metabolites in patients with decreased capacity of primary route of elimination.
[b]Accumulation is probably significant in combined hepatic and renal failure, but data are sparse.

DRUG FACTORS

Pharmacokinetics

In selecting an antimicrobial agent for empiric therapy, the kinetic disposition of the agent is an important consideration. This is partly because of cost considerations (less frequent dosing is less costly) and also because drugs should be selected that are best suited for the patient's elimination capacity.

As described previously, chronic renal and hepatic dysfunction predispose patients to certain types of infections, thereby dictating the type of therapy. In addition, it would be desirable, whenever possible, to select agents that either will not worsen the underlying dysfunction or will not be dependent on the compromised organ system for detoxification or removal from the body. This is certainly not always possible and drugs are often selected that will accumulate to a significant extent in renal and/or hepatic failure.

Finally, in the present era of cost containment, giving unnecessarily large doses of expensive drugs is not cost effective. An excellent example is administration of "full" doses of a drug like cefazolin to a patient with poor renal function. Not only is this potentially toxic to the central nervous system, but also doses as small as 250–500 mg once daily would be adequate rather than the standard dosage of 1 gram every 8 hours.

Tissue Penetration

The relevance of tissue concentrations of antimicrobials has long been disputed. Since methods to measure the concentrations of antimicrobial agents have become widely used as research tools, a great deal of data have been generated in this area. Some of the difficulties with interpreting these data include a lack of correlation with clinical outcomes and poor understanding of whether the antimicrobial agents are present in a biologically active

TABLE 98.5. ANTIMICROBIAL INTERACTIONS

Antimicrobial	Other Agent(s)	Results of Interaction
Aminoglycosides	Neuromuscular blocking drugs	Increased neuromuscular blockade
	Other nephrotoxins or ototoxins (e.g., cisplatin amphotericin B, ethacrynic acid, vancomycin, cyclosporine)	Increased nephrotoxicity or ototoxicity
	Penicillins	Inactivation of both drugs (a particular problem in renal failure and when obtaining drug levels)
Sulfonamides	Sufonylureas	Hypoglycemia
	Phenytoin	Increased serum concentration of phenytoin leading to toxicity
	Oral anticoagulants (warfarin derivatives)	Enhanced hypoprothrombinemia
Chloramphenicol	Phenytoin, tolbutamide, ethanol	Increased serum concentration of other agents and enhanced pharmacologic effect or increased toxicity
Metronidazole (also cefamandole, moxalactam, cefoperazone)	Ethanol (including ethanol-containing medications)	Disulfiram-like reaction
Macrolides, azalides	Theophylline	Increased serum theophylline concentration
	Terfenadine, astemizole	Cardiac arrhythmias
Fluconazole	Phenytoin, warfarin	Inhibits metabolism of these drugs
	Rifampin	Enhances metabolism of fluconazole
Itraconazole	Astemizole, terfenadine	Cardiac arrhythmias
	Phenytoin, warfarin	Inhibits metabolism of these drugs
	Rifampin	Enhances metabolism of itraconazole
Quinolones (norfloxacin, ciprofloxacin, ofloxacin, lomefloxacin, enoxacin)	Multivalent cations (antacids, iron, sucralfate, zinc)	Decreased absorption of quinolone
	Theophylline	Inhibits metabolism of theophylline (ciprofloxacin and enoxacin)
Rifampin	Coumarin anticoagulants	Decreased anticoagulant effect (increased metabolism of drug)
	Quinidine	Decreased effect of quinidine
	Digoxin	Decreased effect of digoxin
	Methadone	Narcotic withdrawal
	Propranolol	Decreased effect of propranolol
	Oral contraceptives	Decreased effect (pregnancy)
	Fluconazole; ketoconazole	Decreased antifungal effect
Tetracyclines	Antacids, iron, calcium	Inhibit intestinal absorption of tetracycline
Penicillins and cephalosporins	Uricosuric agents (probenecid, high-dose aspirin, etc.)	Block excretion of β-lactams, causing higher serum levels
	Copper reduction test for glycosuria (Clinitest tablets)	False-positive test for glycosuria (not seen with glucose oxidase method)
Isoniazid	Phenytoin	Increased serum concentrations of both

form.[28] An example of the former problem is the recognized efficacy of drugs with low biliary fluid concentrations in the treatment of cholecystitis and/or cholangitis, and the absence of enhanced efficacy of drugs whose primary route of elimination is biliary excretion of active drug. An example of the latter difficulty is with penetration to deep infections (e.g., abscesses), where various factors such as acid pH, WBC products, and various enzymes may inactivate even high concentrations of certain drugs.

The central nervous system (CNS) is one body site where antimicrobial penetration is relatively well defined and correlations with clinical outcomes are established.[29] Cerebrospinal fluid (CSF) concentrations of antimicrobial agents necessary to eradicate bacterial meningitis have been defined, and drugs that do not reach significant concentrations in CSF should be avoided in treating meningitis. Apart from the bloodstream, other body fluids where drug concentration data are clinically relevant include urine, synovial fluid, and peritoneal fluid.

Caution must be taken in selecting an antimicrobial agent for clinical use on the basis of tissue/fluid penetration. Apart from CNS penetration data, more attention should be paid to clinical efficacy, antimicrobial spectrum, toxicity, and cost than to comparative data on penetration into a given body site.

Pharmacodynamic Considerations

A great deal of research has been devoted recently to the study of antimicrobial pharmacodynamics—that is, the relationship between drug concentration and the effects on microorganisms. Emerging from these efforts has come a better understanding of the concentration–effect relationships between classes of antimicrobials and selected bacteria.[30] For example, it has been demonstrated that certain basic pharmacokinetic parameters such as area under the concentration-vs-time curve (AUC) and maximal plasma concentration (C_{max}) can be predictive of treatment outcome when specific ratios of AUC or C_{max} to the minimum inhibitory concentration (MIC) are achieved. This is relevant for those antimicrobials that produce concentration-dependent bactericidal effects, for example, aminoglycosides and fluoroquinolones. When such concentration-dependent killing is coupled with a prolonged postantibiotic effect (PAE) (a prolonged lag period of growth following a brief exposure to an antimicrobial),[31] it may be possible to modify dosage regimens to take advantage of these effects. An example is the increasing use of single daily dosed aminoglycosides. For these regimens the drug is given as a single large daily dose (rather than two to three smaller ones). Such regimens may be more effective and less toxic than standard dosages.[30]

In contrast, antimicrobials that affect cell wall synthesis (e.g., β-lactams) do not produce concentration-dependent killing nor do they produce prolonged PAE, but rather time-dependent bactericidal effects.[30] Therefore, the most important pharmacodynamic relationship for these antimicrobials is the duration that drug concentrations exceed the MIC. For example, frequent small doses or a continuous infusion of β-lactams appear to be correlated with good outcome.[32] These findings for β-lactams have been largely confined to experiments in neutropenic animal models. There are very limited clinical data to support this relationship, but research is ongoing.[32]

Drug Toxicity

It is incumbent on health professionals to avoid toxic drugs whenever possible. Certainly, if one has the choice of two drugs that are equally efficacious yet one is less toxic, then the decision is clear. The less toxic drug, even if more costly, should be selected. Unfortunately, all too often we are faced with much more difficult decisions, not only in selection of one drug regimen over another but whether or not to use drugs at all in a given clinical situation. In making these choices, we must assess the risk–benefit ratio for the use of each drug.

An example of the risk–benefit analysis in deciding to use a drug is the indication for administering isoniazid prophylactically to prevent tuberculosis. Because the hepatotoxicity of isoniazid increases in frequency with age, older persons who are candidates for isoniazid prophylaxis (positive skin test) must have additional risk factors for tuberculosis to balance the potential toxic effects. These include evidence of recent skin test conversion, immunosuppression, or previous gastrectomy. Older patients without additional risk factors are more likely to suffer toxicity from isoniazid than derive benefit from its use.[33]

Cost

The costs of drug therapy are increasing dramatically especially as new products, derived from biotechnology, are introduced. Hence, drug therapy (always a target for cost reductions) is becoming more important to manage as the health care system becomes more sophisticated. Greater attention is being paid to the pharmacoeconomics of drug therapy, where patient outcomes are valued and the costs to arrive at those outcomes are estimated. With increasing numbers of patients enrolled in managed-care organizations, understanding the true cost of antimicrobial therapy is more important than ever. The total cost of antimicrobial therapy includes much more than just the acquisition cost of the drugs.[34]

The total economic impact of antimicrobial therapy is detailed in Table 98.6. Many ancillary costs affect the true cost of therapy. These include factors such as storage, preparation, and administration, as well as all of the costs incurred from adverse effects, and factors such as length of hospitalization, readmissions, and all directly provided

TABLE 98.6. TOTAL ECONOMIC IMPACT OF ANTIMICROBIAL THERAPY

Drug acquisition cost
Storage/inventory cost
Preparation
Distribution
Administration
Monitoring
Adverse effects
Impact on length of stay
Cost of control systems

health care goods and services. More difficult to value, but equally as important, are indirect costs such as patient quality of life issues. Pharmacoeconomic analysis is becoming more widely applied and utilized, in order to derive values such as cost–benefit ratios and the cost-effectiveness of various products compared to one another. A detailed review of pharmacoeconomic analyses is beyond the scope of this chapter, but excellent reviews of the subject are available.

Until the present, cost containment in drug therapy has largely been devoted to identifying expensive or high-cost products and attempting to minimize their use. It is increasingly appreciated that use of the most effective treatment, *regardless* of its cost, may be the most *cost effective* because this treatment may result in the desirable outcome at the lowest total cost (as defined previously).[35] For example, despite the high daily cost of imipenem compared to other antimicrobials, the total costs associated with other regimens providing comparable outcomes may be greater due to toxicity, drug delivery, convenience for the nurse and/or patient, and other issues. A great deal more research in this area is needed and multidisciplinary, collaborative efforts with the involvement of pharmacy, medicine, nursing, and microbiology are essential.[36]

COMBINATION ANTIMICROBIAL THERAPY

In selecting a drug regimen for a given patient, consideration must be given to the necessity for using more than one drug. Combinations of antimicrobials are generally used for the following reasons: (1) to broaden the spectrum of coverage for empiric therapy, (2) to achieve synergistic activity against the infecting organism, and (3) to prevent the emergence of resistance.

Broadening the Spectrum of Coverage

Increasing the "coverage" of antimicrobial therapy is generally necessary in mixed infections where multiple organisms are likely to be present. This is the case in intraabdominal and female pelvic infections in which a variety of aerobic and anaerobic bacteria may produce disease.[37] Traditionally, a combination of a drug active against aerobic gram-negative bacilli, such as an aminoglycoside, and a drug active against anaerobic bacteria, such as metronidazole or clindamycin, is selected. Newer β-lactam compounds, which possess good activity against both of these types of organisms, such as the cephamycins, imipenem, or the β-lactam/β-lactamase inhibitor combinations may be adequate to replace the combination and, thereby, reduce the cost of therapy.

The other clinical situation in which increased spectrum of activity is desirable is in nosocomial infection. Hospital-acquired infections, except as previously noted, are generally only caused by one organism, but many different organisms may be possible. Therefore, broad-spectrum therapy is generally prescribed at least initially.[24] Again, newer β-lactam agents such as the third-generation cephalosporins may be adequate in certain situations in lieu of various combinations. However, the enhanced gram-negative spectrum of these compounds has been achieved at the expense of gram-positive activity. Thus, most infectious disease consultants would add a drug with good antistaphylococcol activity to the regimen, such as a penicillinase-resistant penicillin or vancomycin. This is especially true in immunosuppressed patients in whom such broad-spectrum coverage is dictated by the likelihood of streptococci, staphylococci, and enteric gram-negative bacilli.[26]

The concept of broad-spectrum coverage in immunosuppressed patients takes on new meaning when pulmonary infection is present. In this setting, especially in patients with lymphoproliferative disorders, the possible causative organisms include fungi, protozoa *(P. carinii),* viruses (cytomegalovirus), and bacteria (*Legionella* spp. and others).[26] Thus, empiric regimens escalate in size beyond antibacterial regimens consisting of two or three agents; regimens in immunocompromised patients may include trimethoprim–sulfamethoxazole, amphotericin B, erythromycin, and possibly acyclovir. Such an approach should be avoided whenever possible, and every attempt made to establish the diagnosis by means of bronchoscopy or other minimally invasive procedure. However, in a critically ill, immunosuppressed patient, it may not be possible, for a variety of reasons, to perform an invasive diagnostic test. In such a circumstance, combinations of antiviral, antifungal, antimycobacterial, and/or antibacterial drugs may be necessary to keep the patient alive until such time when more diagnostic testing is possible or information is available. One must be cautious, however, not to fall into the trap of "spiraling empiricism" or unjustifiable escalation of the treatment of infection.[38]

Synergism

The achievement of synergistic antimicrobial activity is advantageous for infections caused by enteric gram-negative bacilli in immunosuppressed patients. Traditionally, combinations of aminoglycosides and β-lactams have been used since these drugs together generally act synergistically against a wide variety of bacteria. However, the data supporting superior efficacy of synergistic over nonsynergistic combinations is weak. At best, it would appear that synergistic combinations produce better results in infections caused by *Pseudomonas aeruginosa,* in certain infections caused by *Enterococcus* sp. and, perhaps, in patients with profound, persistent neutropenia.[26,39] Older data in the literature strongly support superior efficacy of combinations in immunosuppressed patients in which both drugs are active against the infecting pathogen. However, these data were generated using drugs less potent than those currently available. Evidence against the necessity for synergistic combinations is provided by the efficacy of newer β-lactams such as imipenem and third-generation cephalosporins in this setting.[40]

The most obvious example of the use of synergy is the treatment of enterococcal endocarditis. The causative organism is usually only inhibited by penicillins, but is rapidly killed by the addition of streptomycin or gentamicin to a penicillin.[39] The necessity for bactericidal activity in the treatment of endocarditis underscores the need for these synergistic combinations.

Preventing Resistance

The use of combinations to prevent the emergence of resistance is widely applied but not often realized. The only circumstance where this has been clearly effective is in the treatment of tuberculosis. The prevalence of resistance to a first-line drug such as isoniazid or rifampin in a population of organisms may be as high as 1 in 10^6 to 10^8. Since the bacterial load in a patient with active tuberculosis often exceeds this, two drugs are given to reduce the likelihood of encountering resistance to less than 1 in 10^{10}.[33] There is ample evidence from *in vitro* data and experimental bacterial infections that combinations of drugs with different mechanisms are effective in prevention of the emergence of resistance. However, data from clinical trials are either conflicting or do not convincingly support this concept.[41]

Disadvantages of Combination Therapy

Although there are potentially beneficial effects from combining drugs, there also are potentially serious liabilities. Examples include additive nephrotoxicity from drugs such as aminoglycosides, amphotericin, and possibly vancomycin.[42] Inactivation of aminoglycosides by penicillins may be clinically significant when excessive doses of penicillin are given to a patient in renal failure.[43] Accumulation of penicillin has resulted in decreased serum concentrations of aminoglycosides *in vivo.* This same reaction can falsely lower aminoglycoside concentrations even in properly dosed patients if serum samples containing both drugs are not properly handled (frozen until assayed or promptly assayed).

Finally, one must be concerned with the use of potentially antagonistic combinations. Antagonism has been demonstrated experimentally when a bacteriostatic drug (chloramphenicol) diminished the bactericidal and curative effects of gentamicin.[44] However, there are few clinical data that demonstrate this antagonism in humans. The most frequently cited example is the study of the treatment of pneumococcal meningitis in which a group of patients who received chlortetracycline in addition to penicillin G had a higher mortality rate from the infection.[45] Such combinations should probably be avoided, whenever possible, unless the clinical situation warrants the use of both drugs for different pathogens. For example, the use of a tetracycline in combination with a β-lactam is appropriate for pelvic inflammatory disease due to the likely presence of *Chlamydia* as well as the usual bacterial pathogens.[37]

Of more current relevance is the increasing use of β-lactam antimicrobials in combination. Agents that are capable of inducing β-lactamase production in bacteria such as *Enterobacter cloacae* and *P. aeruginosa* (e.g., imipenem, cephamycins) may antagonize the effects of enzyme-labile drugs such as penicillins.[46] This mechanism of antagonism is clearly demonstrable *in vitro* and in experimental models of infection. Although clinical failures of such combinations have not yet been found to result from this mechanism, the laboratory data are highly supportive of avoiding these combinations.

MONITORING THERAPEUTIC RESPONSE

Once antimicrobial therapy has been instituted, the patient must be monitored carefully for a therapeutic response. Clinical assessment of the patient on a daily basis, or more or less often as needed, is clearly the most effective. Subjective findings in addition to an objective assessment (physical examination) are very valuable.

Serum bactericidal titers are occasionally used in the management of selected infections. Although the data to support their use are weak, many clinicians will test the ability of the patient's serum to kill the infecting organism in bacterial endocarditis.[47] The goal is to achieve peak levels of activity of ≥1:16 dilutions. That is, serum obtained from the patient while receiving antimicrobial therapy can be diluted at least 16-fold and still contain enough of the antimicrobial agent to kill the infecting organism. Another clinical situation in which these titers have been used includes acute osteomyelitis in children, for whom oral antimicrobial therapy may be used for most of the duration of therapy.[47]

Determinations of serum (or other fluid) levels of antimicrobials may be useful in assuring outcome and/or preventing toxicity. There are only a few antimicrobials that require serum concentration monitoring, and then only in selected situations. These include the aminoglycosides, flucytosine, and chloramphenicol. Achievement of adequate aminoglycoside concentrations within the first few days of therapy of gram-negative infection has been correlated with better therapeutic outcome.[48] In addition, assuring that excessive concentrations of flucytosine or chloramphenicol (in neonates) are avoided will prevent toxicity.

Various methods are available to individualize drug dosages. The purpose of individualization is to tailor the dose of a drug administered to the patient's infectious process (e.g., urinary tract infection versus meningitis), as well as the patient's excretory and metabolic capacity. The rationale has been, in part, discussed previously, but the complete individualization analysis involves more than the simple recognition that a drug dosage should be adjusted. Reliance on simple formulas or nomograms may be hazardous since these methods of dosage adjustment seldom, if ever, consider all of the possible factors that may affect kinetic disposition.[49] For example, although there are several nomograms available to adjust aminoglycoside dosage, none of the easier, more popular methods allows for abnormally low or high volumes of distribution.

Changes in the distribution volume may have significant impact on the efficacy and/or safety of therapy. An unexpectedly low volume of distribution (such as in the dehydrated patient) will result in higher, potentially toxic concentrations, whereas a larger than expected volume (such as in patients with edema or ascites) will result in low, potentially subtherapeutic concentrations. There are various methods to individualize dosage regimens for the specific patient at hand. All are reasonably effective as long as careful attention is paid to the factors that have been outlined previously. The most effective methods use measured serum concentrations of the drugs rather than estimations from renal function tests to assess true drug clearance from the body.[50]

FAILURE OF ANTIMICROBIAL THERAPY

A variety of factors may be responsible for apparent lack of response to therapy. Factors include those directly related to the host, those related to the pathogen, and, although unlikely, laboratory error in identification and/or susceptibility testing. Factors directly related to the antimicrobial agents being utilized are only a small proportion of the possibilities.

Failures Caused by Drug Selection

Factors directly related to the drug selection include an inappropriate drug selection or dosage or route of administration. For example, selection of a bacteriostatic drug for endocarditis, or administration of a drug by intramuscular injection to a patient with compromised peripheral circulation (e.g., shock) may result in inadequate therapy. Malabsorption of a drug product because of GI disease (e.g., short-bowel syndrome) or a drug interaction (e.g., complexation of fluoroquinolones with multivalent cations resulting in reduced absorption) may lead to potentially subtherapeutic serum concentrations.

Accelerated drug elimination is also possible. This may occur in patients with cystic fibrosis or during pregnancy, when more rapid clearance or larger volumes of distribution may result in low serum concentrations, particularly for aminoglycosides.

Inactivation of antimicrobial agents by other drugs may occur, as in the case of aminoglycoside inactivation by penicillins. Finally, a common cause of failure of therapy is due to poor penetration into the site of infection. This is especially true for the so-called "privileged" sites such as the central nervous system, the eye, and the prostate gland.

Failures Caused by Host Factors

Host defenses must be considered in evaluating a patient who is not responding to antimicrobial therapy. Patients who are immunosuppressed (e.g., granulocytopenia from chemotherapy, AIDS) may respond poorly to therapy because their own defenses are inadequate to eradicate the infection despite seemingly adequate drug regimens. A good example is the poor response of infection in granulocytopenic patients that is seen when their WBC counts remain low during therapy. This is in contrast to a much better response when granulocyte counts rise during therapy.[26]

Other host factors are related to the necessity for surgical drainage of abscesses or removal of foreign bodies and/or necrotic tissue. If these situations are not corrected, they result in persistent infection and, occasionally, bacteremia, despite adequate antimicrobial therapy.

Failures Caused by Microorganisms

Factors related to the pathogen include the development of drug resistance during therapy. Primary resistance refers to the intrinsic resistance of the pathogens producing the infection. However, acquisition of resistance during treatment has become a major problem as well (see as follows).[51] It has become increasingly obvious that, despite the development and introduction of numerous new antimicrobial agents, bacterial resistance has continued to increase, both within and across different bacterial genera.

All of the newer antibacterial agents developed and licensed in the past 5 years are targeted toward improved activity against gram-negative bacteria. This list includes fluoroquinolones, carbapenems, β-lactam/β-lactamase inhibitor combinations, and newer "fourth-generation" cephalosporins. Although these new antimicrobials have addressed the majority of resistance issues among gram-negative organisms, resistance among gram-positive bacteria and mycobacteria have become particularly problematic.[52] Among these, the organisms where resistance has increased most dramatically include enterococci, pneumococci, and *Mycobacterium tuberculosis.* Enterococci have been isolated recently with multiple resistance patterns. They may be resistant to β-lactams (by virtue of β-lactamase production, and/or altered penicillin-binding proteins [PBP]), vancomycin (via alterations in peptidoglycan synthesis), and high levels of aminoglycosides (via enzymatic degradation). For infections due to organisms with multiple resistance, the available treatment is suboptimal

mal and may include various combinations of the previously named medications to attack multiple sites of action.[39]

Pneumococci resistant to penicillins, certain cephalosporins, and macrolides are increasingly common. These organisms are generally susceptible to vancomycin and cefotaxime or ceftriaxone. *M. tuberculosis* resistant to one or more first line antitubercular agents (INH, rifampin, ethambutol, streptomycin, and pyrazinamide) have increased in frequency as well. This has been observed principally in populations of prison inmates and patients with AIDS. Lack of effective, well-tolerated treatment has resulted in a very high mortality rate in patients infected with multiply resistant strains.[53]

The increase in resistance among these organisms is believed to be due, in large part, to continued overuse of antimicrobials in the community, as well as in hospitals, and the increasing prevalence of immunosuppressed patients receiving long-term suppressive antimicrobials for the prevention of infections. Note that these resistance patterns are regionally variable, and susceptibility patterns in the community (or hospital) should be monitored closely to promote rational antimicrobial selection.[52]

The emergence of resistance during antimicrobial therapy has been reviewed in detail elsewhere.[51] The situation where this is reported most frequently is pulmonary or other deep-seated infection due to *P. aeruginosa.* This occurs in 20–30% of cases and with all available antibacterial agents including imipenem. This organism and a group of enteric gram-negative bacilli (*Enterobacter aerogenes, E. cloacae, Citrobacter freundii, Serratia marcescens,* and a few others) can produce a β-lactamase that is capable of hydrolyzing broad-spectrum cephalosporins and, to a lesser extent, penicillins.[52] These enzymes are categorized as Richmond–Sykes type I and their genetic code is found on the chromosome. Resistant mutants of these aforementioned organisms that produce large quantities of these enzymes may be present within an infection, and may be responsible for the emergence of resistance during therapy. The mutants occur at a frequency of 1 in 10^6 to 1 in 10^8 bacteria, the numbers of bacteria commonly encountered in clinical infections.[52] However, because only 10^4 to 10^5 bacteria are tested for susceptibility in the microbiology laboratory, this potential resistance may not be detected. Treatment of infection due to *Enterobacter, Citrobacter, Serratia,* or *P. aeruginosa* with a third-generation cephalosporin or aztreonam may produce an initial clinical response by eradicating all of the susceptible bacteria in the population. Within a few days, however, the highly resistant subpopulations have a selective advantage and may overgrow the infection site to produce a relapse.[52] These bacteria usually retain susceptibility to aminoglycosides, imipenem, and fluoroquinolones but are resistant to all other β-lactams. It should be obvious that host defenses are extremely important in this scenario. Patients who are not immunosuppressed and whose infections are not deep seated or carry a small burden of organisms may do very well with third-generation cephalosporin or aztreonam monotherapy.[52] However, debilitated patients with pulmonary infections, abscesses, or osteomyelitis are at high risk for drug failure. In these situations a combination regimen to prevent the emergence of resistance or the use of imipenem or a fluoroquinolone may be warranted for empiric therapy.

Host abnormalities may be responsible for predisposition to or persistence of infection, including cardiac or pulmonary disease, immunosuppressive disorders, and structural abnormalities of various organ systems. (For complete discussions of these factors, the reader is referred to the chapters on the individual disease states.) Administration of various adjunctive measures such as colony-stimulating factors, immunoglobulins, antibodies, antitoxins, and immunostimulatory agents may be beneficial depending on the circumstances. Obviously, prevention of infection is more desirable than treating an established disease. Therefore, active or passive immunization is often used to either prevent or abort many infectious diseases (Table 98.7). Finally, there has been a great increase in the use of colony-stimulating factors (e.g., G-CSF, GM-CSF). These products have been shown to be very effective in reducing the incidence and severity of infection in patients with chemotherapy-induced granulocytopenia,[54] and they are being evaluated as adjunctive therapy for the treatment of selected infections.

TABLE 98.7. AGENTS USED FOR ACTIVE OR PASSIVE IMMUNIZATION

Passive	Active
Antitoxins	**Bacterial**
Botulism	Cholera
Diphtheria	Diphtheria
Tetanus	Hemophilus
Immunoglobulins	Meningococci
Hepatitis A or B	Pertussis
Pertussis	Pneumococci
Poliomyelitis	Tetanus
Rabies	Tuberculosis (BCG)
RSV	Typhoid
Rubella	**Viral**
Tetanus	Hepatitis B
Vaccinia	Influenza
Varicella	Measles
CMV	Mumps
	Poliomyelitis
	Rabies
	Rubella
	Smallpox
	Yellow fever

The number of cases of sepsis and septic shock have increased dramatically over the past decade and, despite advances in antimicrobial therapy and intensive care support, the mortality rates have not decreased appreciably.[55] The rationale behind the development of new adjunctive therapies for sepsis is to inhibit the effects of the various endogenous mediators, or to prevent their activation by blocking the effect of exogenous microbial products (e.g., endotoxin). To these ends, several agents have been developed that are in various stages of clinical or preclinical testing. These include antiendotoxin monoclonal antibodies, bactericidal permeability-increasing protein (binds endotoxin and affects cell wall permeability), anti-TNF monoclonal antibodies and TNF soluble receptors, IL-1 receptor antagonist and an IL-1 soluble receptor, and antagonists to platelet activating factor, bradykinin, and leukocyte adhesion proteins.[56]

The rationale for the use of these agents is based on sound and encouraging preclinical research. Initial clinical results appeared promising for several of these agents, but recent clinical trial results have been disappointing. A few, however, may become commercially available within the next few years.[57]

Attention must be paid to the literature on antimicrobials to assist in the selection of therapy. The results from prospective, controlled, randomized clinical trials should be evaluated whenever possible when considering appropriate antimicrobial therapy. Results from prelicensing "open" trials offer only limited information that may be useful in this regard, as patients in these trials are generally not seriously ill, are not infected with multiply resistant bacteria, and other confounding factors found in most clinical situations are excluded by virtue of study design. Therefore, comparative data in more seriously ill patients is essential for appropriate application of new agents.[58]

In addition, postmarketing trials may be important if their results demonstrate superiority of one regimen over another, either in efficacy, safety, or cost effectiveness. It must be remembered that appropriate antimicrobial therapy may change as new organisms are discovered, susceptibility patterns change, and new drugs become available, and as new clinical trial results are published.

REFERENCES

1. Dinarello CA, Cannon JG, Wolff SM. New concepts on the pathogenesis of fever. Rev Infect Dis 1988;10:168–189.
2. Dinarello CA, Wolff SM. Fever of unknown origin, in Mandell GL, Douglas RG, Bennett JE (eds): Principles and Practice of Infectious Diseases, 3rd ed. New York, Churchill Livingstone, 1990, pp 468–479.
3. Young EJ, Fainstein V, Musher DM. Drug-induced fever: Cases seen in the evaluation of unexplained fever in a general hospital population. Rev Infect Dis 1982;4:69–77.
4. Musher DM, Fainstein V, Young EJ, et al. Fever patterns. Their lack of clinical significance. Arch Intern Med 1979;139:1225–1228.
5. McCue JD. Improved mortality in gram-negative bacillary bacteremia. Arch Intern Med 1985;145:1212–1216.
6. Niederman MS, Bass JB, Campbell GD, et al. Official ATS statement: Guidelines for the initial management of adults with community-acquired pneumonia—diagnosis, assessment of severity, and initial antimicrobial therapy. Am Rev Resp Dis 1993;148:1418–1426.
7. Wispelwey B, Tunkel AR, Scheld WM. Bacterial meningitis in adults. Infect Dis Clin North Am 1990;4:645–660.
8. Sobel JD. Pathogenesis of urinary tract infections: Host defenses. Infect Dis Clin North Am 1987;1:751–772.
9. Greenlee JE. Approach to diagnosis of meningitis. Infect Dis Clin North Am 1990;4:583–598.
10. Washington JA. The microbiological diagnosis of infective endocarditis. J Antimicrob Chemother 1987;20(suppl A):29–36.
11. Weiss ME. Drug allergy. Med Clin North Am 1992;76:857–882.
12. Saxon A. Immediate hypersensitivity reactions to beta-lactam antibiotics. Rev Infect Dis 1983;5(suppl 2):S368–S378.
13. Saxon A, Swabb EA, Adkinson NF. Investigation into the immunologic cross-reactivity of aztreonam with other beta-lactam antibiotics. Am J Med 1985;78(suppl 2A):19–26.
14. Saez-Llorens X, McCraken GH. Bacterial meningitis in neonates and children. Infect Dis Clin North Am 1990;4:623–644.
15. Kantor HI, Sutherland DA, Leonard JT, et al. Effect of bilirubin metabolism in the newborn of sulfisoxazole administered to the mother. Obstet Gynecol 1961;17:494–500.
16. Powell DA, Nahata MC. Chloramphenicol: New perspectives on an old drug. Drug Intell Clin Pharm 1982;16:295–300.
17. Gardner ID. The effect of aging on susceptibility to infection. Rev Infect Dis 1980;2:801–810.
18. Kopanoff DE, Snider DE Jr, Caras GJ. Isoniazid-related hepatitis. A US public health cooperative surveillance study. Am Rev Respir Dis 1978;117:991–1001.
19. Chow AW, Jewesson PJ. Pharmacokinetics and safety of antimicrobial agents during pregnancy. Rev Infect Dis 1985;7:287–313.
20. Relling MV. Polymorphic drug metabolism. Clin Pharm 1989;8:852–863.
21. Tabbara IA. Hemolytic anemias: Diagnosis and management. Med Clin North Am 1992;76:649–668.
22. Johnson JR, Stamm WE. Urinary tract infections in women: Diagnosis and treatment. Ann Intern Med 1989;111:906–917.
23. Nelson JD. Acute osteomyelitis in children. Infect Dis Clin North Am 1990;4:513–522.
24. Craven DE, Steger KA. Nosocomial pneumonia in the intubated patient—new concepts on pathogenesis and prevention. Infect Dis Clin North Am 1989;4:843–866.
25. Richet H, Hubert B, Nitemberg G, et al. Prospective multicenter study of vascular catheter-related complications and risk factors for positive central catheter cultures in ICU patients. J Clin Microbiol 1990;28:2520–2525.
26. Pizzo PA. Management of fever in patients with cancer and treatment-induced neutropenia. N Engl J Med 1993;328:1323–1332.

27. Smith GH. Treatment of infections in the patient with the acquired immunodeficiency syndrome. Arch Intern Med 1994;154:949–973.
28. Nix DE, Goodwin SD, Peloquin CA, et al. Antibiotic tissue penetration and its relevance: Impact of tissue penetration on infection response. Antimicrob Agents Chemother 1991;35:1953–1959.
29. Scheld WM. Theoretical and practical considerations of antibiotic therapy for bacterial meningitis. Pediatr Infect Dis 1985;4:74–83.
30. Drusano GL. Human pharmacodynamics of beta-lactams, aminoglycosides and their combinations. Scand J Infect Dis 1991(suppl);74:235–248.
31. Spivey JM. The post-antibiotic effect. Clin Pharm 1992;11:865–875.
32. Craig WA, Ebert SC. Continuous infusion of beta-lactam antibiotics. Antimicrob Agents Chemother 1992;36:2577–2583.
33. American Thoracic Society. Treatment of tuberculosis and tuberculosis infection in adults and children. Am Rev Resp Dis 1986;134:355–363.
34. Guglielmo BJ, Brooks GF. Antimicrobial therapy—cost benefit considerations. Drugs 1989;38:473–480.
35. McGhan WF. Pharmacoeconomics and the evaluation of drugs and services. Hosp Formul 1993;28:365–378.
36. Marr JJ, Moffet HL, Kunin CM. Guidelines for improving the use of antimicrobial agents in hospitals: A statement by the Infectious Diseases Society of America. J Infect Dis 1988;157:869–876.
37. Landers DV, Wolner-Hanssen P, Paavonen J, et al. Combination antimicrobial therapy in the treatment of acute pelvic inflammatory disease. Am J Ob Gyn 1991;164:849–858.
38. Kim JH, Gallis HA. Observations on spiraling empiricism: Its causes, allure, and perils, with particular reference to antibiotic therapy. Am J Med 1989;87:201–206.
39. Eliopoulos GM. The ten most commonly asked questions about resistant enterococcal infections. Infect Dis Clin Pract 1994;3:125–129.
40. DePauw BE, Deresinski SC, Feld R, et al. Ceftazidime compared with piperacillin–tobramycin for the empiric treatment of fever in neutropenic patients with cancer. Ann Intern Med 1994;120:834–844.
41. Barriere SL. Bacterial resistance to beta-lactams and its prevention with combination antimicrobial therapy. Pharmacotherapy 1992;12:391–396.
42. Rybak MJ, Albrecht LM, Boike SC, et al. Nephrotoxicity of vancomycin, alone and with aminoglycoside. J Antimicrob Chemother 1990;25:679–687.
43. Manian FA, Stone WJ, Alford RH. Adverse antibiotic effects associated with renal insufficiency. Rev Infect Dis 1989;10:43–55.
44. Sande MA, Overton JW. *In vivo* antagonism between gentamicin and chloramphenicol in neutropenic mice. J Infect Dis 1973;128:247–250.
45. Lepper MH, Dowling HF. Treatment of pneumooccic meningitis with penicillin compared with penicillin plus aureomycin. Arch Intern Med 1951;88:489–494.
46. Barriere SL. Therapeutic considerations in using combinations of newer beta-lactam antibiotics. Clin Pharm 1986;5:24–33.
47. Vosti K. The serum bactericidal test: past, present, and future use in the management of patients with infections. Curr Clin Top Infect Dis 1989;10:43–55.
48. Moore RD, Smith CR, Lietman PS. Association of aminoglycoside plasma levels with therapeutic outcome in gram-negative pneumonia. Am J Med 1984;77:657–662.
49. Lesar TS, Rotschafer JC, Strand LM, et al. Gentamicin dosing errors with four commonly used nomograms. JAMA 1982;248:1190–1193.
50. Goldman MP, Fuller MA. A practical alternative to conventional aminoglycoside dosing methods. Ann Pharmacother 1993;27:1333–1339.
51. Milatovic D, Braveny I. Development of resistance during antibiotic therapy. Eur J Clin Microbiol 1987;6:234–244.
52. Murray BE. The problems and dilemma of antimicrobial resistance. Pharmacotherapy 1992;12(6 Part 2):86s–93s.
53. Neu HC. The crisis in antibiotic resistance. Science 1992;257:1064–1073.
54. Klastersky J. Febrile neutropenia. Curr Opin Oncol 1993;5:625–632.
55. Bone RC, Balk RA, Cerra FB, et al. Definitions for sepsis and organ failure and guidelines for use of innovative therapies in sepsis. Chest 1992;101:1644–1655.
56. Barron RL. Pathophysiology of septic shock and implications for therapy. Clin Pharm 1993;12:829–845.
57. Dinarello CA, Gelfand JA, Wolff SM. Anticytokine strategies in the treatment of the systemic inflammatory response syndrome. JAMA 1993;269:1829–1835.
58. Gilbert DN. Guidelines for evaluating new antimicrobial agents. J Infect Dis 1987;156:934–941.

Drugs of Choice

First choice
Alternative(s)

Gram-Positive Cocci

Streptococcus (groups A, B, C, G, and *S. bovis*)
Penicillin G[a] or V[b] or ampicillin
Erythromycin, FGC,[c,d] vancomycin

Streptococcus pneumoniae
Penicillin G or V or ampicillin
Erythromycin, FGC,[c,d] cefotaxime or ceftriaxone,[d,e] chloramphenicol[e]

***Streptococcus*, viridans group**
Penicillin G ± gentamicin[f]
Vancomycin ± gentamicin

Enterococcus
Ampicillin (or penicillin G) + gentamicin[g] (in serious infection)
Vancomycin and gentamicin (UTI: nitrofurantoin, tetracycline, or fluoroquinolone) ampicillin–sulbactam (for β-lactamase-producing strains)

Staphylococcus aureus
Penicillinase-negative
Penicillin G or V
FGC,[c,d] clindamycin, vancomycin
Penicillinase-positive
PRP[h]
FGC,[c,d] vancomycin, clindamycin,[i] BLIC[j]
Methicillin-resistant
Vancomycin ± rifampin or gentamicin
Trimethoprim–sulfamethoxazole or fluoroquinolone,[k] both ± rifampin

Gram-Negative Cocci

Moraxella catarrhalis
Trimethoprim–sulfamethoxazole
Amoxicillin/clavulanate, erythromycin, tetracycline, TGC

Neisseria gonorrhoeae
Uncomplicated infection
Ceftriaxone or fluoroquinolone[k]
APPG,[l] cephamycin,[m] tetracycline, amoxicillin/probenecid
DGI[n]
Ceftriaxone + doxycycline
TGC,[o] cephamycin

Neisseria meningitidis
Penicillin G
TGC,[o] chloramphenicol

Gram-Positive Bacilli

Clostridium perfringens
Penicillin G
Clindamycin, metronidazole

Clostridium tetani
TIG[p]
Penicillin, tetracycline

Clostridium difficile
Metronidazole or vancomycin[q]
Bacitracin

Corynebacterium diphtheriae
Antitoxin + erythromycin
Penicillin G

Listeria monocytogenes
Ampicillin ± gentamicin
Trimethoprim–sulfamethoxazole

Gram-Negative Bacilli

Acinetobacter spp.
Imipenem
Aminoglycoside, ESP,[r] fluoroquinolone, trimethoprim–sulfamethoxazole, ampicillin/sulbactam

Aeromonas hydrophila
Trimethoprim–sulfamethoxazole
Gentamicin, fluoroquinolone, imipenem

Bacteroides fragilis **(and others)**
Metronidazole
BLIC,[s] clindamycin, cephamycin,[m] imipenem, ESP[r]

Bordetella pertussis
Erythromycin
Trimethoprim–sulfamethoxazole

Campylobacter **sp.**
Fluoroquinolone or erythromycin
Tetracycline, gentamicin

Enterobacter **sp.**
Fluoroquinolone, imipenem, or cefepime
Gentamicin + ESP,[r] trimethoprim–sulfamethoxazole, TGC[o]

Escherichia coli
FGC[c]
Gentamicin, TGC,[o] ampicillin, fluoroquinolone

Gardnerella vaginalis
Metronidazole
Ampicillin

Haemophilus influenzae
TGC,[o,t] trimethoprim–sulfamethoxazole
BLIC,[j] cefuroxime, chloramphenicol, ampicillin/amoxicillin, sulfa/erythromycin

Klebsiella pneumoniae
FGC,[c,d] aminoglycoside
TGC,[o,t] trimethoprim–sulfamethoxazole, fluoroquinolone[k]

Legionella **sp.**
Erythromycin ± rifampin
Trimethoprim–sulfamethoxazole, ciprofloxacin, clarithromycin

Pasteurella multocida
Penicillin G
Tetracycline, BLIC[j]

Proteus mirabilis
Ampicillin
FGC,[c,d] gentamicin, trimethoprim–sulfamethoxazole, fluoroquinolone

Proteus **(indole-positive) (including *Providencia rettgeri, Morganella morganii, Proteus vulgaris*)**
TGC[o]
Aminoglycoside, trimethoprim–sulfamethoxazole, fluoroquinolone,[k] imipenem, ESP

Providencia stuartii
TGC[o]
Aminoglycoside, trimethoprim–sulfamethoxazole, fluoroquinolone,[k] imipenem, ESP

Pseudomonas aeruginosa
Aminoglycoside + ESP[r] or ceftazidime
Ciprofloxacin, aztreonam + aminoglycoside, imipenem

Pseudomonas cepacia
Trimethoprim–sulfamethoxazole
Ceftazidime, chloramphenicol

Salmonella typhi
Fluoroquinolone[k] or TGC[o]
Trimethoprim–sulfamethoxazole, ampicillin, chloramphenicol

Salmonella **(non-typhi)**
TGC[o,u]
Trimethoprim–sulfamethoxazole, fluoroquinolone[k]

Serratia marcescens
TGC[o]
Aminoglycoside, trimethoprim–sulfamethoxazole, fluoroquinolone,[k] imipenem, ESP
Shigella
Fluoroquinolone[k]
Trimethoprim–sulfamethoxazole, ampicillin, ceftriaxone
Xanthomonas maltophilia
Trimethoprim–sulfamethoxazole
Minocycline, ceftazidime, fluoroquinolone

Miscellaneous Organisms
Actinomyces israelii
Penicillin G
Tetracycline
***Afipia felis* (cat scratch fever)**
Ciprofloxacin
Trimethoprim–sulfamethoxazole
Nocardia
Trimethoprim–sulfamethoxazole
Sulfonamide,[v] amikacin, minocycline, imipenem
Chlamydiae
Tetracycline or erythromycin
Sulfonamide, ofloxacin, clarithromycin
Mycoplasma pneumoniae
Erythromycin
Tetracycline, clarithromycin
Rickettsia
Tetracycline
Chloramphenicol, fluoroquinolone
***Rochalimaea henselae* (bacillary angiomatosis)**
Erythromycin
Tetracycline
Treponema pallidum
Penicillin G
Tetracycline, ceftriaxone
Borrelia burgdorferii
Doxycycline
Ceftriaxone, azithromycin, clarithromycin

Fungi
***Aspergillus* sp.**
Amphotericin B
Itraconazole
Blastomycosis
Itraconazole or amphotericin B
Ketoconazole
***Candida* sp.**
Amphotericin B or fluconazole
Ketoconazole,[w] flucytosine[x]
Coccidioides immitis
Amphotericin B
Fluconazole, ketoconazole, itraconazole
Cryptococcus neoformans
Amphotericin B ± flucytosine
Fluconazole, itraconazole
Histoplasma capsulatum
Amphotericin B or itraconazole
Ketoconazole
Mucormycosis
Amphotericin B
None
Sporothrix schenkii
Itraconazole, Iodides[y]
Amphotericin B

Viruses
Cytomegalovirus
Ganciclovir
Foscarnet
Herpes simplex
Tri-fluridine,[z] acyclovir,[aa] or famciclovir
Vidarabine, idoxuridine,[z] foscarnet
***Human immunodeficiency virus* (HIV)**
Zidovudine
Didanosine, zalcitabine, stavudine, saguinavir, ritonavir, indinavir
Influenza A
Amantadine
Rimantadine, ribavirin
Respiratory syncitial virus
Ribavirin
None
Varicella-zoster
Acyclovir
Vidarabine

---

[a] Either aqueous penicillin G or benzathine penicillin G (pharyngitis only).
[b] Only for soft tissue infections or upper respiratory infections (pharyngitis, otitis media).
[c] First-generation cephalosporins—cefazolin, cephalexin, cephradine, or cefadroxil.
[d] Some penicillin-allergic patients may react to cephalosporins.
[e] For the treatment of meningitis.
[f] Gentamicin should be added if tolerance or "moderately susceptible" (MIC ≥ 0.1 g/mL) organisms are encountered; streptomycin is used but may be more toxic.
[g] Must be added for synergy in cases of endocarditis, meningitis, and perhaps bacteremic pyelonephritis.
[h] Penicillinase-resistant penicillin: nafcillin or oxacillin; methicillin is probably more nephrotoxic.
[i] Not reliably bactericidal, so should not be used for endocarditis.
[j] β-Lactamase inhibitor combination: ampicillin/sulbactam, amoxicillin/clavulanate.
[k] Ciprofloxacin, ofloxacin, fleroxacin.
[l] Aqueous procaine penicillin G.
[m] Cefoxitin, cefotetan, cefmetazole.
[n] Disseminated gonococcal infection.
[o] Third-generation cephalosporins—cefotaxime, ceftizoxime, ceftriaxone.
[p] Tetanus immune globulin.
[q] Oral administration only.
[r] Extended-spectrum penicillin—ticarcillin, mezlocillin, or piperacillin.
[s] β-lactamase inhibitor combination: ampicillin/sulbactam, ticarcillin/clavulanate, piperacillin/tazobactam
[t] Should only be used in serious infections.
[u] Antibiotics should not be given for gastroenteritis, because the carrier state may be prolonged without significant clinical benefit.
[v] Sulfisoxazole, sulfadiazine (preferred for CNS disease), trisulfapyrimidines.
[w] Mucocutaneous disease only.
[x] May be added to amphotericin for potential synergy, but only if *in vitro* susceptibility is documented. Resistance develops frequently if used alone.
[y] Lymphocutaneous disease only.
[z] Keratitis only.
[aa] Topical form for primary genital disease only; oral form to treat severe genital disease and to prevent recurrence of genital infections; IV form for severe mucocutaneous, disseminated, or meningoencephalitic disease.

Chapter 99

Central Nervous System Infections

Karl J. Madaras-Kelly, PharmD, Beth E. Ostergaard, PharmD, and John C. Rotschafer, PharmD, FCCP

Central nervous system (CNS) infections include a wide variety of clinical conditions and etiologies. Meningitis, meningoencephalitis, encephalitis, brain and meningeal abscesses, and shunt infections are all included under this heading.

CNS infections are frequently associated with adverse neurologic sequelae and mortality. Although mortality rates for CNS infections have declined since the advent of modern antimicrobial therapy, overall mortality rates for patients with meningitis, the most common CNS infection, are still high (3–33%).[1–5] In addition, approximately 10% of patients who survive meningitis may develop persistant neurologic disabilities such as seizures, sensorineural hearing loss, and hydrocephalus.[1,3] Sixty percent of patients with gram-negative bacilliary meningitis may experience complications as a result of their infection.[1–5] Despite the availability of antimicrobial therapy against the most common CNS pathogens, the adequate treatment of CNS infections continues to be problematic.

In the past, CNS infections were primarily community based. Presently, an increasing number of CNS infections are nosocomial.[3,4] CNS infections may be caused by a variety of bacteria, fungi, viruses, and parasites. Significant and concerning changes in antimicrobial susceptibility have been occurring with the most common bacterial organisms associated with meningitis; *Streptococcus pneumoniae, Haemophilus influenzae,* and *Neisseria meningitidis.* Undoubtedly, these changes will continue to affect antibiotic management of these bacterial pathogens. The last national surveillance study of bacterial meningitis performed in the United States was conducted in 1986 by the Centers for Disease Control (CDC).[6] At that time, *H. influenzae* was the most commonly identified etiology of bacterial meningitis overall (45%), followed by *S. pneumoniae* (18%), and *N. meningitidis* (14%). However, recently the CDC reported an 82% decrease in the incidence of *H. influenzae* type B between 1985 and 1991 for children less than 5 years old, which coincides with the increased distribution of Hib vaccine in this age group.[1,7]

In addition, significant and concerning changes in antimicrobial susceptibility have been occurring with the most common bacterial organisms associated with meningitis. Approximately 30–40% of *H. influenzae* and 5–10% of *S. pneumoniae* are resistant to ampicillin and penicillin, respectively. Undoubtedly, these changes will continue to affect antibiotic management of these bacterial pathogens.

CNS infections are divided into two categories: septic and aseptic. Septic or bacterial infections are the result of hematogenous spread from a primary site of infection, parameningeal seeding from a localized infection, or trauma or congenital defects in the CNS. Aseptic infection is a term broadly used to describe chemical irritants, viral, fungal, parasitic, tuberculous, sarcoid, neoplastic, and syphilitic processes of the CNS.

Signs and symptoms of CNS infection have clinical features similar to those of a variety of infectious diseases. Fever, peripheral leukocytosis with a left shift, and malaise are common observations. Symptoms in the elderly may be uniquely different in that they may resemble stroke or endocarditis. Signs and symptoms in the neonate may be limited to just fever and irritability. Usually the cerebrospinal fluid (CSF) pattern of pleocytosis (an increasing number of leukocytes, especially lymphocytes, in the CSF), increased protein concentration, and decreased glucose concentration with respect to time can be used to help differentiate viral, fungal, and bacterial etiologies.[2,4,8,9] The ability to diagnose and institute effective therapy rapidly is paramount to patient survival without sequelae.

Several additional factors are important in the diagnosis of CNS infections. The clinical setting (hospital, community, or long-term care center) may give some clue as to the etiology of infection. Whether the CNS is anatomically intact or has recently been traumatized is of key importance in the proper diagnosis. The age of the patient (discussed later) and the season of the year may also assist in identifying likely pathogens. Integration of clinical, demographic, and laboratory data is crucial to the proper diagnosis and the selection of appropriate antimicrobial agents. This chapter presents relevant aspects of the pathogenesis, pathophysiology, and antimicrobial therapy of CNS infections.

Anatomy and Physiology of the CNS

MENINGES[8,10]

The skull and vertebrae protect the CNS from blunt or penetrating trauma (Fig. 99.1). The brain is suspended in these structures by CSF and is surrounded by the meninges. The meninges are made up of three separate membranes. The dura mater, or pachymeninges, lies directly beneath and is adherent to the skull. The other two membranes are referred to collectively as the leptomeninges. The pia mater lies directly over the brain tissue itself; the arachnoid is the middle layer between the dura mater and pia mater. Between the pia mater and arachnoid is the subarachnoid space, which serves as the conduit for CSF. By definition, meningitis is an infection of the subarachnoid space.

CEREBROSPINAL FLUID[10]

Approximately 85% of CSF is produced within the fourth and lateral ventricles by the choroid plexus (Fig. 99.1). CSF volume in the CNS is related to patient age. Infants have approximately 40–60 mL of CSF, whereas older children have approximately 60–100 mL and adults have approximately 110–160 mL. Normally, CSF is produced at the rate of approximately 0.5 mL/min and flows unidirectionally downward through the spinal cord. CSF is removed by the arachnoid villi (Fig. 99.1) and vertebral venus plexus located in the spinal cord and does not recommunicate with the point of production.

CSF (Table 99.1) is normally clear, has a protein content of <50 mg/dL, has a glucose concentration of approximately 50–66% of the simultaneous peripheral concentration, has a pH approximately that of blood, and usually contains fewer than ten white blood cells (WBCs) per mm^3, all of which should be mononuclear.

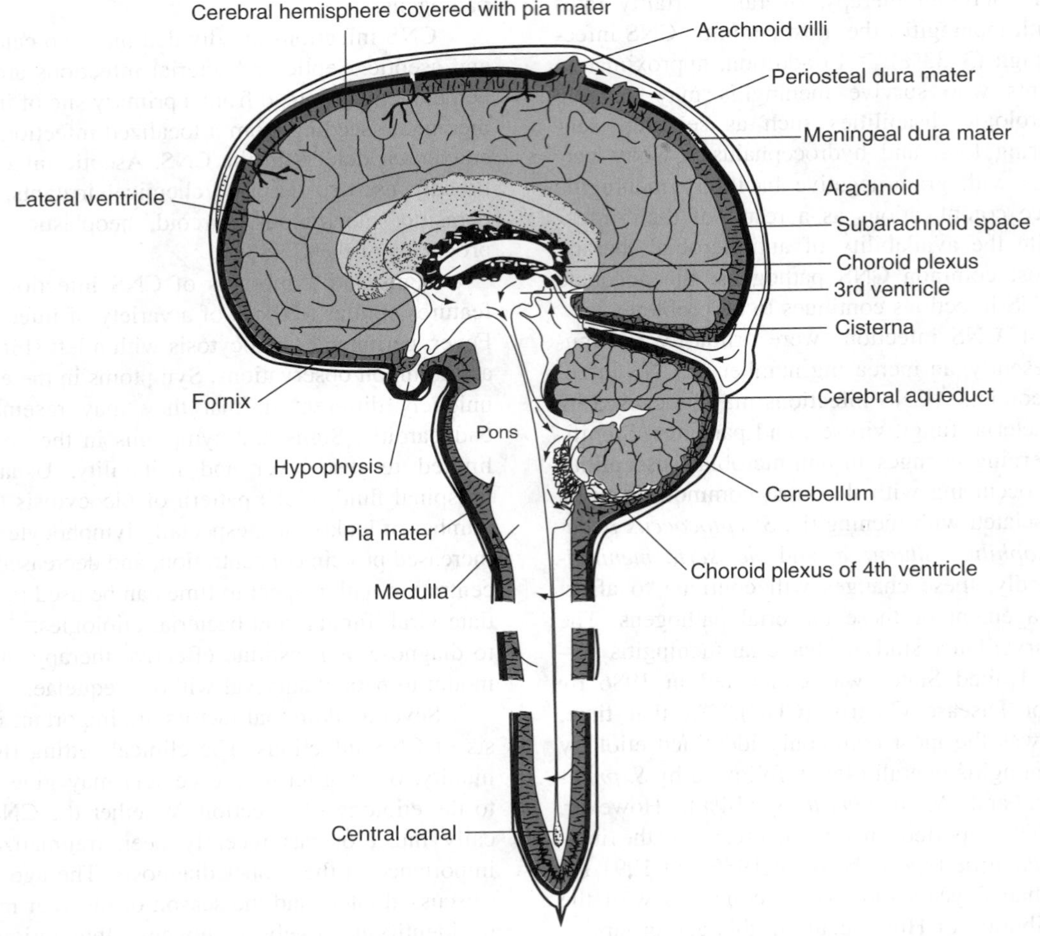

Figure 99.1. Diagram of the central nervous system.

TABLE 99.1. TYPICAL COMPONENTS OF NORMAL AND ABNORMAL CEREBROSPINAL FLUID

Type	Normal	Bacterial	Viral	Fungal	Tuberculosis
WBC (mm^3)	<10[a]	400–100,000	5–500	40–400	100–1000
Differential	>90%[a]	>90 PMN[b]	50[c,d]	>50[c]	>80[c,d]
Protein (mg/dL)	<50	80–500	30–150	40–150	≥40–150
Glucose (mg/dL)	½–⅔ serum	<½ serum	<30–70	<30–70	<30–70

[a]Monocytes.
[b]PMN = polymorphonuclear cells.
[c]Lymphocytes.
[d]Initial CSF WBC may reveal a predominance of PMNs. (Adapted from Maxson S, Jacobs RF. Viral meningitis. Tips to rapidly diagnose treatable causes, Postgrad Med 1993;93(8): 153–166, with permission.)

BLOOD–BRAIN BARRIER/ BLOOD–CSF BARRIER[10]

The CNS has natural barriers to the exchange of drugs and endogenous compounds among the blood, brain, and CSF. The blood–brain barrier consists of tightly joined capillary endothelial cells (Fig. 99.2). Drug entry into brain tissue is accomplished by direct passage through the capillary endothelial cell. Having traversed this barrier, the drug must then penetrate the glial cells that envelop the capillary structure.

Passage of chemical substances into the CSF is controlled by the blood–CSF barrier (Fig. 99.2). This barrier is created by the ependymal cells of the choroid plexus, which function similarly to renal tubular epithelial cells. Like the active transport system in the kidney, the secretion of substances out of the choroid plexus can be inhibited by the administration of probenecid. The active transport system

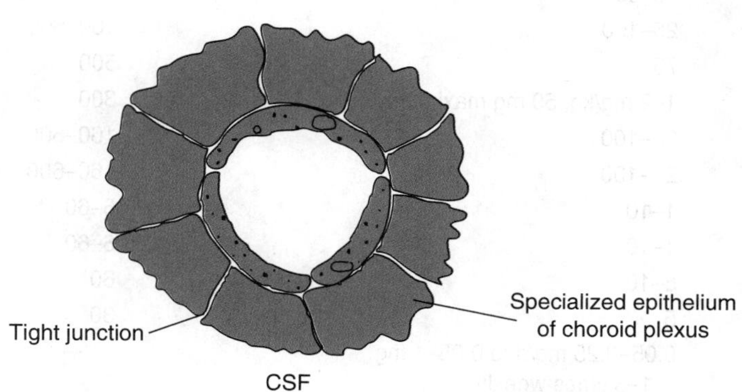

Figure 99.2. Schematic representation of a brain tissue capillary, normal tissue capillary, and blood cerebrospinal fluid barrier capillary. *(From Zabinski RA, Vance-Bryan K, Rotschafer JC. The management of central nervous system infection. J Pharm Pract 1991;4(3):170–191, with permission.)*

TABLE 99.2. PENETRATION OF ANTIMICROBIAL AGENTS INTO THE CEREBROSPINAL FLUID

Therapeutic Levels in CSF with or without Inflammation	
Sulfonamides	Trimethoprim
Chloramphenicol	Isoniazid
Rifampin	Pyrazinamide
Ethionamide	Cycloserine
Metronidazole	
Therapeutic Levels in CSF with Inflammation of Meninges	
Penicillin G	Ampicillin ± sulbactam
Carbenicillin	Ticarcillin ± clavulanic acid
Nafcillin	Mezlocillin
Piperacillin	Cefuroxime
Cefotaxime	Ceftizoxime
Ceftriaxone	Ceftazidime
Imipenem	Aztreonam
Vancomycin	Ciprofloxacin
Ofloxacin	Ethambutol
Flucytosine	Fluconazole
Pyrimethamine	Ganciclovir
Acyclovir	Foscarnet
Vidarabine	
Nontherapeutic Levels in CSF with or without Inflammation	
Aminoglycosides	First-generation cephalosporins
Cefoperozone	Second-generation cephalosporins[a]
Clindamycin[b]	Ketoconazole
Amphotericin B[c]	Itraconazole[c]

[a]Cefuroxime is an exception.
[b]Achieves therapeutic brain tissue concentrations.
[c]Achieves therapeutic concentrations for *C. neoformans* therapy.

of the choroid plexus is also inhibited by the inflammatory process associated with meningitis.

Several factors influence the transfer of antibiotic from capillary blood into the CNS. With increased meningeal inflammation, there will be greater antibiotic penetration (Table 99.2). Antibiotics having a low molecular weight are more easily passed through biological barriers than compounds of high molecular weight. Only antibiotics that are un-ionized at the physiologic or pathologic pH are capable of diffusion. Compounds that are highly lipid soluble penetrate more readily than water-soluble compounds. Antibiotics that are not extensively protein bound in the serum provide a larger free fraction of drug capable of passing into the CSF. Passage of large, polar antibiotics into the CSF may be assisted by a carrier transport system.

Problems of CSF penetration may also be overcome by direct instillation of antibiotics by intrathecal, intracisternal, or intraventricular routes of administration.[11–16] (Table 99.3). The advantages of direct instillation, however, must be weighed against the risks of invasive CNS procedures. Intrathecal administration of antibiotics is unlikely to produce therapeutic concentrations in the ventricles because of the unidirectional flow of CSF.[12] Although intraventricular administration from a therapeutic standpoint may be preferred over intrathecal administration, the former requires neurosurgical placement of an Ommaya or Rickham reservoir.[13] The use of intraventricular antibiotic therapy is seldom necessary given currently available systemic antibiotic therapy. Prins et al.,[17] in a recent review of antibiotic-induced endotoxin release, stated that children receiving both parenteral antibiotics and intrathecal gentamicin had higher CSF endotoxin levels, higher CSF interleukin-1 beta levels, and higher mortality than children just receiving parenteral antibiotics. These differences were attributed to the direct CSF administration of gentamicin, which is interesting given that gentamicin is generally thought to blunt endotoxin release caused by β-lactam antibiotics.[17]

Another option to maintain therapeutic antibiotic concentrations within the CSF is to limit drug clearance by interfering with antibiotic transport out of the CNS. With

TABLE 99.3. INTRAVENTRICULAR AND INTRATHECAL ANTIBIOTIC DOSAGE RECOMMENDATIONS

Antibiotic	Adult Dose (mg)	Expected CSF Concentration[a] (mg/L)	References
Ampicillin	10–50	60–300	109–111
Methicillin	25–100	160–600	109–111
Nafcillin	75	500	111
Cefazolin	1–2 mg/kg, 50 mg maximum	300	112
Cephalothin	25–100	160–600	109–111
Chloramphenicol	25–100	160–600	109, 110, 113
Gentamicin	1–10	6–60	12, 109–111, 113
Tobramycin	1–10	6–60	12
Amikacin	5–10	60	114, 115
Vancomycin	5	30	116–118
Amphotericin B	0.05–0.25 mg/d to 0.05–1 mg 1–3 times weekly	—	14

[a]Assumes adult CSF volume = 150 mL.

most β-lactam antibiotics, the use of probenecid will reduce the rate of antibiotic clearance from the CSF, but it may also increase the incidence of adverse drug reactions.

Pathophysiology of the Central Nervous System (Fig. 99.3)

The development of newer, more active antimicrobial agents during the past two decades has not significantly reduced the mortality and neurologic sequelae of acute bacterial meningitis as was originally hoped. However, using experimental animal models, significant advances have been made in recent years toward an understanding of the pathophysiologic mechanisms of brain injury caused by CNS infections. This improved understanding has led to the development of new treatment modalities, which may have a significant impact on the morbidity and mortality with infections of the CNS.

The critical first step in the acquisition of acute bacterial meningitis is nasopharyngeal colonization of the host by the bacterial pathogen. The bacteria must first attach themselves to nasopharyngeal epithelial cells with bacterial surface structures called lectins.[18] The bacteria are then phagocytized across nonciliated columnar nasopharyngeal cells into the host's bloodstream.[18] Antibodies such as secretory IgA are found in high concentrations within nasopharyngeal secretions and work to inhibit bacterial colonization.[18]

After bacteria access the patient's bloodstream, the bacteria must overcome host defense mechanisms. A common characteristic of most CNS bacterial pathogens is the presence of an extensive polysaccharide capsule that is resistant to neutrophil phagocytosis and complement opsonization. Studies with *H. influenzae, Eschericia coli,* and *N. meningitidis* have found that strains of bacteria that lack polysaccharide capsules are unable to cause meningitis. The host, however, possesses other defense mechanisms that can effectively counteract the encapsulated bacteria.[18,19] Capsular polysaccharides activate the alternate complement pathway and cleave C3 with subsequent attachment of C3b to bacterial surfaces. C3b promotes phagocytosis and clearance of infecting pathogens. Patients (e.g., splenectomized and sickle cell patients) who cannot activate the alternative complement pathway are predisposed to bacterial infections by encapsulated microorganisms and to meningitis.

The mechanism and exact site of bacterial invasion into the CNS are currently unknown, but recent studies sug-

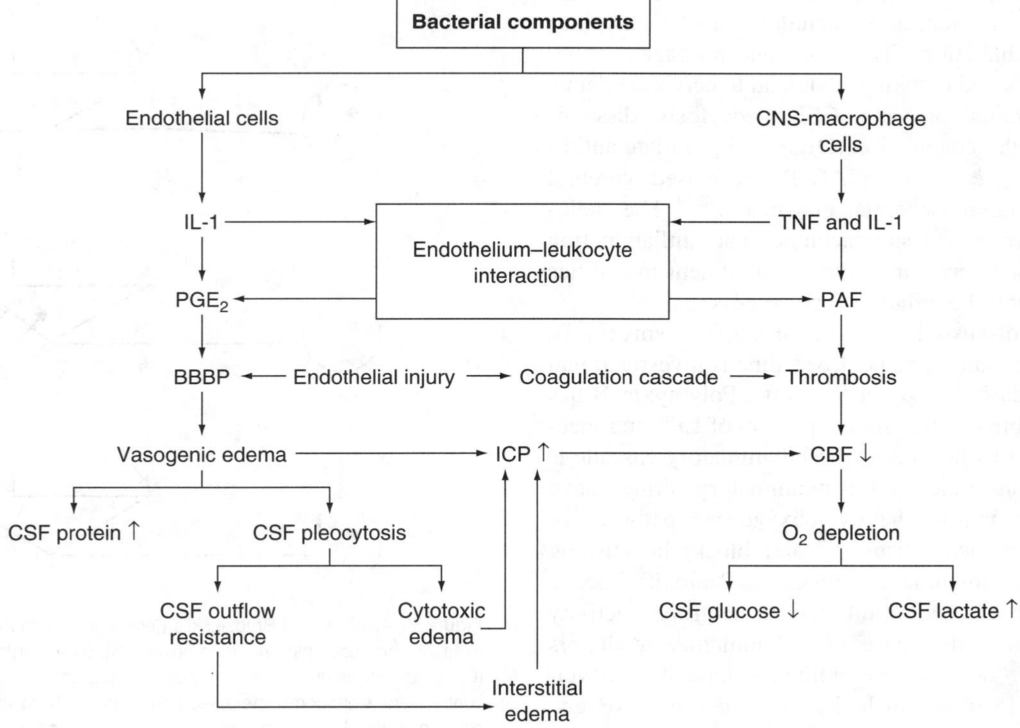

Figure 99.3. Hypothetical schema of pathophysiologic events that occur during bacterial meningitis. IL-1, interleukin-1; TNF, tumor necrosis factor; PAF, platelet-activating factor; CBF, cerebral blood flow; CSF, cerebrospinal fluid; PGE_2, prostaglandin E_2; ICP, intracranial pressure; BBBP, blood–brain barrier permeability. *(From Sáez-Llorens X, Ramilo O, Mustafa MM, et al. Molecular pathophysiology of bacterial meningitis: Current concepts and therapeutic implications. J Pediatr 1990;116(5):677, with permission.)*

gest that invasion into the subarachnoid space is accomplished by continuously exposing the CNS to large bacterial inocula. Bacteremia with inoculum densities of at least 10^3 colony-forming units/mL appear to be essential for subarachnoid space invasion.[18] Although several sites of bacterial invasion have been theorized, the most plausible are those sites that are most highly perfused. The choroid plexus sustains exceptional blood flow rates (approximately 200 mL/g/min) and, consequently, is the most likely site of CNS bacterial invasion. In addition, cells of the choroid plexus possess receptors that facilitate bacterial adherence and allow bacterial transport into the subarachnoid space.[18] Host defense mechanisms within the subarachnoid space are inadequate to combat bacterial pathogens, and bacteria replicate freely within the CSF until either bacterial overgrowth occurs or an effective antibiotic regimen is administered that terminates the process.

Bacterial cell death causes the release of cell wall components such as lipopolysaccharide (LPS), lipid A (endotoxin), lipoteichoic acid, teichoic acid, and peptidoglycan depending on whether the pathogen is gram positive or gram negative. These cell wall components cause capillary endothelial cells and CNS macrophages to release cytokines (interleukin-1 [IL-1] and tumor necrosis factor [TNF]). These cytokines interact with capillary endothelial cells and CNS leukocytes to release products of the cyclooxygenase–arachidonic acid pathway (prostaglandins and thromboxanes) and platelet activating factor (PAF). PAF activates the coagulation cascade, and arachidonic acid metabolites stimulate vasodilatation. These events propagate other sequential events and cytokines that lead to cerebral edema, elevated intracranial pressure, CSF pleocytosis, disseminated intravascular coagulation (DIC), inappropriate antidiuretic hormone secretion (SIADH), decreased cerebral blood flow, cerebral ischemia, and death.[18,19] The delineation of the process of subarachnoid space inflammation has kindled new interest in exploring treatment modalities designed to inhibit the inflammatory process.

Although discussed here, the use of polymyxin B, monoclonal antibodies, and pentoxifylline is investigational and is not standard therapy at this time. Polymyxin B has been shown to bind to the lipid A portion of LPS and inactivate it so that this portion of the inflammatory cascade is interrupted. Nonsteroidal anti-inflammatory drugs have been shown to inhibit the cyclooxygenase pathway of arachidonic acid metabolism,[18,19] and block the ensuing events of this inflammatory process. Pentoxifylline, a methylxanthine, indirectly inhibits CNS neutrophil activity and limits neutrophil release of inflammatory mediators such as TNF.[18–20] Monoclonal antibodies have been developed to the CD18 family of leukocyte receptors, TNF, and the lipid A portion of LPS. However, during the last 5 years, clinical trials for systemic gram-negative sepsis have raised questions as to the efficacy and safety of these products, leaving their current role in mediating the septic cascade in CNS infections undefined.[18,19]

CLINICAL PRESENTATION AND DIAGNOSIS

On initial presentation, differentiation of patients with bacterial, viral, or fungal meningitis is virtually impossible. The clinical signs and symptoms of meningitis are variable and dependent on the age of the patient. Adult patients will present with variable complaints of fever, stiffness of the

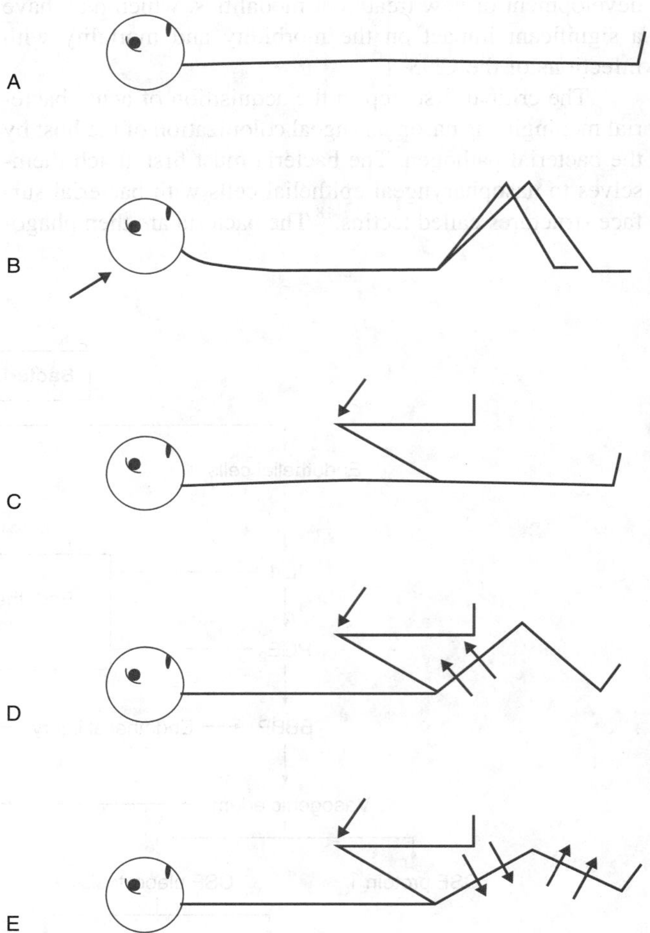

Figure 99.4. (A and B) Brudzinski's neck sign. Flexion of the neck by the examiner produces hip and knee flexion (B). (C–E) Brudzinski's leg signs. (C) Examiner passively flexes patient's leg (arrow). (D) The identical contralateral sign: contralateral leg begins to flex (arrows). (E) The reciprocal contralateral sign: the same leg that exhibited the active flexion begins to extend spontaneously, a reflex resembling a little kick (double arrows). *(From Verghese A, Gallemore G. Kernig's and Brudzinski's signs revisited. Rev Infect Dis 1987;9(6):1190, with permission.)*

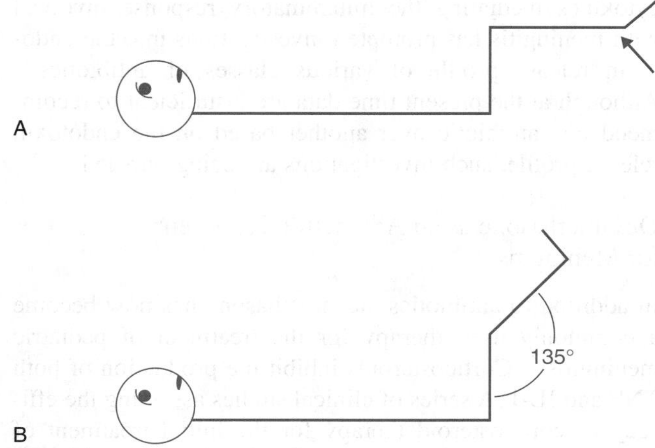

Figure 99.5. Kernig's sign. (A) Examiner flexes hip 90° to the trunk, and attempts to extend the knees. (B) "Contracture" or extensor spasm at the knee 135°. *(From Verghese A, Gallemore G. Kernig's and Brudzinski's signs revisited. Rev Infect Dis 1987;9(6):1190, with permission.)*

neck and/or back, nuchal rigidity, positive Brudzinski's sign (Fig. 99.4) and/or positive Kernig's sign (Fig. 99.5).[21] Later in the course of the disease, the patient may experience seizures, focal neurologic deficits, and hydrocephalus. Conversely, young infants infected with bacterial meningitis may reveal only nonspecific symptoms such as irritability, altered sleep patterns, vomiting, high-pitched crying, decreased oral intake, or seizures.[22] As a child ages, a more CNS-specific clinical presentation becomes prevalent; changes in activity level, somnolence, confusion, or lethargy are frequently reported.[22] Generally, children less than 2 years of age do not present with the classical meningitis characteristics such as photophobia, headache, stiff neck, Kernig's or Brudzinski's sign.[22] Up to 50% of patients diagnosed with meningitis have received prior antibiotic therapy.[2] These patients may present less frequently with fever or mental status changes and may have a longer duration of symptoms.[23]

The diagnosis of bacterial meningitis is usually made on the basis of examination of CSF collected soon after the diagnosis is suspected. Typically, three tubes of CSF are collected via lumbar puncture for laboratory analysis and culture. The CSF in tubes 1, 2, and 3 are most often examined for chemistry, microbiology, and hematology tests, respectively.[2] Any contamination with skin flora and disinfectant should be minimal after the first tube of CSF is collected. In addition to CSF examination, blood cultures should be performed because meningitis can frequently arise via hematogenous dissemination.

Analysis of CSF chemistries typically includes measurement of glucose and total protein concentrations. Elevated CSF protein ≥50 mg/dL and a CSF glucose concentration less than 50% of the simultaneously obtained peripheral value suggest bacterial meningitis (Table 99.1).

Hematologic examination of WBC count and accompanying differential will characteristically reveal the presence of 200–10,000 WBC/mm^3 (≥95% polymorphonuclear cells) in bacterial meningitis. However, in some cases of viral meningitis the initial examination of CSF may reveal a predominance of polymorphonuclear cells.[8,9] In addition, the values for CSF glucose, protein, and WBC concentrations found with bacterial meningitis overlap significantly with those for viral, tuberculous, and fungal meningitis.[24] Therefore, CSF WBC counts and glucose and protein concentrations cannot always be relied on to establish or rule out bacterial meningitis. Typical laboratory findings for bacterial, viral, tuberculous, and fungal meningitis are summarized in Table 99.1.[24]

The lack of specificity and sensitivity associated with traditional CSF chemistries as predictive indicators has preempted the search for additional diagnostic entities. CSF pH, CSF lactate, and CSF C-reactive protein concentrations have been suggested as adjunctive diagnostic indicators to distinguish between bacterial and viral meningitis.[22] Because CSF pH and C-reactive protein lack specificity in patients with partially treated or slightly abnormal CSF, they are of questionable diagnostic value.[22,25] TNF-α has also been identified as a CSF marker for bacterial meningitis.[26] In the case of gram-negative meningitis where CSF may contain measurable concentrations of endotoxin, the limulus lysate assay may be of value. At this time, neither TNF-α nor endotoxin assays are approved for diagnostic use.

Gram stain and aerobic culture of the CSF are the most important laboratory tests performed when attempting to diagnose bacterial meningitis. Recovery of bacterial pathogens from both culture and Gram stain can be greatly influenced by the quantity of CSF available for culture and the prior use of antimicrobial therapy.[2] When performed before antibiotic therapy is initiated, Gram stain is both rapid and sensitive and can confirm the diagnosis of bacterial meningitis in 60–90% of cases.[8,9] The sensitivity of Gram stain decreases to 40–60% in patients receiving prior antibiotic therapy.[2]

Several rapid diagnostic methods are available for identifying potential bacterial pathogens from CSF.[8,9,27,28] Latex fixation, latex coagglutination, and enzyme immunoassay (EIA) tests provide for the rapid identification of *S. pneumoniae,* Group B *Streptococci, N. meningitidis,* type B *H. influenzae,* and *E. coli* (K1).[8,9] The rapid identification latex tests work on the principle of bringing potential capsular antigens of the pathogen-causing meningitis in contact with a specific antibody, causing an antigen–antibody reaction. This capsular antigen–antibody reaction can be observed visually and can be accomplished quickly without waiting for culture results. In recent years, the widespread introduction of more sensitive latex fixation and coagglutination tests have made counterimmunoelectrophoresis virtually obsolete.[2] Although the sensitivity and specificity of latex fixation and coagglutination tests vary with the manufacturer of the antibody, density of antigen present in the CSF, and the pathogen being tested, overall no specific product appears to be superior in identification of all antigens.[8,9]

TREATMENT

Mortality associated with bacterial meningitis usually occurs within 24–48 hours of onset, and the importance of supportive care cannot be emphasized enough, particularly early in the course of treatment. The administration of fluids, electrolytes, antipyretics, analgesia, and other supportive measures are indicated as needed for patients presenting with acute bacterial meningitis. Although supportive care is important initially, appropriate antibiotic therapy (empiric or definitive) should be started as soon as possible. Isolation and identification of the causative agent can direct the selection of the most appropriate antimicrobial therapy for the patient (Tables 99.4–99.6).

Because of compromised phagocytosis in the CSF caused by impaired opsonic activity and reduced levels of complement and immunoglobulin,[18,19,29,30] peak CSF antibiotic concentrations should be approximately 10 times the minimum bactericidal concentration (MBC) of the microorganism causing bacterial meningitis.[31,32] Recent interest in gram-negative endotoxin and the various cytokines mediating the inflammatory response involved with meningitis has prompted investigations into the endotoxin release profile of various classes of antibiotics.[17] Although at the present time data are insufficient to recommend one antibiotic over another based on the endotoxin release profile, such investigations are being pursued.

Dexamethasone as an Adjunctive Treatment for Meningitis

In addition to antibiotics, dexamethasone has now become a commonly used therapy for the treatment of pediatric meningitis.[33] Corticosteroids inhibit the production of both TNF and IL-1. A series of clinical studies assessing the efficacy of corticosteroid therapy for the initial treatment of bacterial meningitis have reported conflicting results.[34–38] The majority of trials were conducted on small sample populations, each with different pathogenic bacterial causes and treatment modalities. Several meta-analyses have summarized the use of corticosteroids as adjunctive therapy for the treatment of meningitis.[39,40] In general, the trials have shown a significant improvement in markers of active infection such as CSF glucose concentrations, as well as CSF protein and lactate concentrations, when corticosteroids are administered as adjunctive treatment.

Consistently, the trials have detected a significantly lower incidence of neurologic sequelae commonly associated with bacterial meningitis. In trials that measured inflammatory mediators, lower levels of TNF, PAF, or IL-1 were detected in patients treated with dexamethasone.[34,36,37] How-

TABLE 99.4. BACTERIAL MENINGITIS: MOST LIKELY BACTERIA AND EMPIRIC THERAPY BY AGE GROUP

Age Commonly Affected	Most Likely Organisms	Empiric Therapy	Risk Factors for All Age Groups
Newborn–1 month	Gram negative enterics[a] Group B streptococcus *Listeria monocytogenes*	Ampicillin + CTX or CRT or CZ[b] or AG[c]	Respiratory tract infection Otitis media Mastoiditis Head trauma Alcoholism
1 month–4 years	*Haemophilus influenzae* *Neisseria meningitidis* *Streptococcus pneumoniae*	CTX or CRT or CZ or ampicillin + chloramphenicol	High-dose steroids Splenectomy Sickle cell disease Immunoglobulin deficiency
5–29 years	*N. meningitidis* *S. pneumoniae* *H. influenzae*	CTX or CRT or CZ or ampicillin + chloramphenicol	Immunosuppression
30–60 years	*S. pneumoniae* *N. meningitidiis*	CTX or CRT or CZ	
>60 years	*S. pneumoniae* Gram-negative enterics *Listeria monocytogenes*	Ampicillin + CTX or CRT or CZ or AG[c]	

[a] *E. coli, Klebsiella* spp., *Enterobacter* spp. common.
[b] CTX, cefotaxime; CRT, ceftriaxone, CZ, ceftizoxime.
[c] Aminoglycoside—gentamicin used most frequently.

TABLE 99.5. ANTIMICROBIAL AGENTS OF FIRST CHOICE AND ALTERNATIVE CHOICE IN TREATMENT OF MENINGITIS CAUSED BY GRAM-POSITIVE MICROORGANISMS

Organism	Antibiotic of First Choice[a]	Alternative Antibiotics[a]
Streptococcus pneumoniae		
Penicillin susceptible	Penicillin G 200,000–300,000 units/kg/d, every 4 h IV max: 4 million units every 4 h IV	Chloramphenicol 100 mg/kg/d, every 6 h max: 1.5 g IV every 6 h Cefotaxime 200 mg/kg/d every 4 h max: 2 g IV every 4 h Ceftriaxone 100 mg/kg/d every 24 h max: adults 2 g IV every 12 Ceftizoxime 200 mg/kg/d every 6–8 h max: 3–4 g IV every 8 h
Low-level penicillin resistance[c]	Cefotaxime or ceftriaxone	Vancomycin 30–40 mg/kg/d IV
High-level penicillin resistance[d]	Vancomycin ± ceftriaxone	Imipenem 80 mg/kg/d max: 1 g IV every 6 h
Group B *Streptococcus*	Penicillin	Cefotaxime Ceftriaxone Ceftizoxime Chloramphenicol
Staphylococcus aureus		
Penicillin resistant	Nafcillin 200 mg/kg/d every 4 h max: 2 g every 4 h IV	Vancomycin
Methicillin resistant	Vancomycin	—
Staphylococcus epidermidis		
Penicillin resistant	Nafcillin	Vancomycin
Methicillin resistant	Vancomycin	
Listeria monocytogenes	Ampicillin 200–400 mg/kg/d, every 6 h IV or Pen G max: 2 g every 4 h IV plus aminoglycoside IV—usually gentamicin	Trimethoprim 10 mg/kg/d and sulfamethoxazole 50 mg/kg/day, every 6 h

[a]Recommended doses for adults and pediatric patients with normal renal and/or hepatic function.
[b]Pediatrics.
[c]Incidence of low-level resistance is 10–20%.
[d]Incidence of high-level resistance is 1–2%; therapeutic recommendations for this infection have not been clearly defined.

ever, no study has detected a significant difference in time to bacterial eradication and only one study detected a significant difference in mortality between patients treated with dexamethasone plus antibiotics or antibiotic therapy alone.[35] Based on these investigations, some authors have advocated that all infants (>2 months) and children with suspected bacterial meningitis receive dexamethasone.[1,34,36–38,41]

However, routine use of dexamethasone in meningitis is not without controversy and several authors have outlined shortcomings regarding the current clinical evidence supporting the use of dexamethasone in pediatric bacterial meningitis.[1,42] A potential concern is that adjunctive dexamethasone therapy might reduce the penetration of antibiotics into the CSF by inhibiting meningeal inflammation. In experimental models of meningitis, steroids have been shown to decrease the CSF concentrations of ampicillin, rifampin, vancomycin, and gentamicin.[38,43] Recently, ceftriaxone penetration into CSF has been shown to be unaffected by concurrent dexamethasone administration in pediatric patients.[44]

A fundamental problem with corticosteroid investigations to date is that the majority of patients in comparative dexamethasone trials had *H. influenzae* meningitis. While *H. influenzae* was the most commonly identified causative pathogen responsible for bacterial meningitis in the United States in 1986, the incidence of *H. influenzae* meningitis has decreased dramatically due to the introduction of polysaccharide conjugate vaccines.[1,7] At this time, it is unclear whether steroids are beneficial in meningitis caused by *S. pneumoniae, N. meningitidis,* group B *Streptococci,* and so on. A retrospective analysis of pediatric patients with pneumococcal meningitis and one unblinded, noncontrolled trial suggest that adjunctive steroids may decrease the neurologic sequelae and mortality associated with *S. pneumoniae* meningitis.[37,45]

Currently, the American Academy of Pediatrics suggests that the use of dexamethasone be considered for infants and children 2 months of age or older with proven or strongly suspected bacterial meningitis.[41] If dexamethasone is used, the commonly utilized intravenous dose is 0.15 mg/kg every 6 hours for 4 days. Alternatively, prospective randomized, double-blind studies have found dexamethasone 0.15 mg/kg every 6 hours for 2 days or dexa-

TABLE 99.6. ANTIMICROBIAL AGENTS OF FIRST CHOICE AND ALTERNATIVE CHOICE IN TREATMENT OF MENINGITIS CAUSED BY GRAM-NEGATIVE ORGANISMS

Organism	Antibiotic of First Choice[a]	Alternative Antibiotics[a]
Neisseria meningitidis (meningococcal)	Penicillin G 200,000–300,000 u/kg/d IV	Cefotaxime 200 mg/kg/d every 4 h max: 2 g IV every 4 h Ceftriaxone 100 mg/kg/d every 24 h[b] max: adults 2 g IV every 12 h Ceftizoxime 200 mg/kg/d every 6–8 h max: 3–4 g IV every 8 h Chloramphenicol 100 mg/kg/d max: 1.5 g IV every 6 h
Escherichia coli	Cefotaxime	Ceftriaxone Ceftizoxime Chloramphenicol
Haemophilus influenzae		
β-Lactamase positive	Cefotaxime	Ceftriaxone Ceftizoxime
β-Lactamase negative	Ampicillin	Cefotaxime Ceftriaxone Ceftizoxime
Pseudomonas aeruginosa	Ceftazidime 85 mg/kg/d max: 2 g IV every 6 h plus tobramycin 5–7.5 mg/kg/d IV[c]	Imipenem 80 mg/kg/d max: 1 g IV every 6 h Piperacillin 200–300 mg/kg/d max: 3 g every 4 h IV plus Tobramycin
Enterobacteriaceae	Cefotaxime	Ceftriaxone Ceftizoxime Piperacillin plus aminoglycoside Imipenem

[a]Recommended doses for adults and pediatric patients with normal renal and/or hepatic function.
[b]Pediatrics.
[c]Direct CNS administration may be added; see Table 99.3 for dosage.

methasone 0.4 mg/kg every 12 hours for 2 days to be equally effective and potentially less toxic regimens as well.[38,46] Dexamethasone should be administered prior to the first antibiotic dose and serum hemoglobin and stool guaiac should be monitored for evidence of GI bleeding.[34,36,42,45,46]

CAUSATIVE AGENTS

Neisseria Meningitidis (Meningococcus)

Neisseria meningitidis meningitis is most commonly found in children and young adults. The source of the infection is usually an asymptomatic carrier. Most cases usually occur in the winter or spring at a time when viral meningitis is relatively uncommon. Five serogroups of *N. meningitidis* (A, B, C, Y, and W-135) are primarily responsible for this type of meningitis. Serogroups A and C are usually associated with epidemics of meningitis, while serogroup B is the primary cause of isolated cases of meningitis. Serogroup Y is more frequently associated with pneumonia and is rarely associated with meningitis.

Patients are initially colonized and at some point develop a bacteremia, which likely occurs prior to the patient's hospital admission. As a result of the bacteremia, there is metastatic seeding; the meninges are the most common site.[18,19] After the acute phase of meningitis has resolved, there is a unique immune reaction that distinguishes meningococcal meningitis from other bacterial causes. Approximately 10–14 days after the onset of the disease and despite successful treatment, the patient develops a characteristic immunologic reaction of fever, arthritis (usually involving large joints), and pericarditis.[47] At this time, examination of synovial fluid will reveal a large number of polymorphonuclear cells, elevated protein concentrations, and normal glucose concentration. Cultures of synovial fluid at this time will be sterile. The reaction may last a week or longer and no additional antibiotic therapy is required.[47] However, the patient may benefit from nonsteroidal anti-inflammatory agents.

Approximately 50% of patients die within the first 24 hours as a result of an acute fulminant course associated with meningococcemia. Other patients develop a picture of chronic meningococcemia that is characterized by episodes of fever, arthritis, and a morbilliform rash that recurs every 48–72 hours.[47]

Seizures and coma are uncommon with meningococcal meningitis. However, patients may behave aggressively and are often maniacal. Patients may develop VIth, VIIth, and VIIIth cranial nerve dysfunction noted by deafness and transiently impaired ocular movements. Deafness unilaterally, or more commonly bilaterally, may develop early or late in the disease course.[47] Sensorineural hearing loss is usually permanent, whereas conductive hearing impairment is often reversible. The incidence of sensorineural hearing loss varies with the etiologic organism (*S. pneumoniae,* 31%; *N. meningitidis,* 10.5%; and *H. influenzae,* 6%).[48] Pomeroy et al.[49] found that many of the neurologic deficits are transient and resolve within 1 year following meningitis.

The presence of petechiae may be the primary clue that the underlying pathogen is *N. meningitidis.* Approximately 50% of patients with meningococcal meningitis have purpuric lesions, petechiae, or both. Patients may have an obvious or subclinical picture of disseminated intravascular coagulation (DIC), which may progress to infarction of the adrenal glands and renal cortex and cause widespread thrombosis.

Aggressive, early intervention with high-dose intravenous crystalline penicillin G, 50,000 units/kg every 4 hours intravenously, is usually recommended for treatment of *N. meningitidis* meningitis. Chloramphenicol is bactericidal for *N. meningitidis* and may be used in place of penicillin G. Several third-generation cephalosporins (e.g., cefotaxime) approved for the treatment of meningitis are acceptable alternatives to penicillin G (Table 99.6).

Cases of meningitis caused by relatively and completely penicillin-resistant meningococci have been reported.[50] The clinical significance of this resistance is unknown since it has not been correlated with any treatment failures. However, absolutely penicillin-resistant meningococci have been identified. Absolutely resistant strains produce β-lactamase, whereas the strains that are only relatively resistant have an alteration of penicillin-binding protein. These resistance patterns may necessitate a future change away from penicillin as the antibiotic treatment of choice for meningococcal meningitis.

Close contacts of patients contracting *N. meningitidis* meningitis are at an increased risk of developing meningitis. Secondary cases of meningitis usually develop within the first week following exposure, but may take up to 60 days after contact with the index case.[51] Risk factors in these contacts have been estimated at 200 to 1000 times that of the general population.[52,53] Young children are at the greatest risk of contracting *N. meningitidis;* however, all ages are at risk, especially close contacts exposed via household, day-care, or military contact.

Prophylaxis of contacts should be started without delay and, therefore, without the aid of culture and sensitivity studies, because most secondary cases occur within the first week of the index case contact. Adult patients should receive 600 mg of rifampin orally every 12 hours for four doses. Children 1 month to 12 years of age should receive 10 mg/kg of rifampin orally every 12 hours for four doses, and children younger than 1 month should receive 5 mg/kg orally every 12 hours for four doses.[52]

Rifampin can eliminate pharyngeal colonization of meningococci although it is not 100% effective.[51] A single dose of ciprofloxacin has been used successfully for meningococcal chemoprophylaxis,[29,54] but carries a relative contraindication in children because of its potential to cause cartilage damage. A single intramuscular dose of ceftriaxone 125–250 mg is a viable alternative to rifampin and may be particularly useful in instances where rifampin should not be used (e.g., pregnancy).[51,52,55]

Vaccination is of limited value in the sporadic cases of meningococcal meningitis, which are caused primarily by serogroup B and vaccines are available only for serogroups A, C, Y, and W-135.[52] Close contacts who are being vaccinated should also receive rifampin because there may be a 2-week delay in achieving protective antibody titers after vaccination.[52] Patients receiving rifampin should be counseled as to the expected red-to-orange color change in urine and other body secretions.

Streptococcus Pneumoniae (Pneumococcus or Diplococcus)

Pneumococcal meningitis occurs in the very young (1–4 months) and the very old. It is the most common cause of meningitis in adults and accounts for 12% of meningitis episodes in children 2 months to 10 years. Approximately 50% of cases are secondary to primary infections involving parameningeal foci such as the ear or paranasal sinuses. Pneumonia, endocarditis, CSF leak secondary to head trauma, splenectomy, alcoholism, sickle cell disease, and bone marrow transplantation may all predispose the patient to the development of pneumococcal meningitis. Failure to develop a pleocytosis in CSF is a poor prognostic sign. Case fatality rates in children are highest with this organism and approach 20%.

Bacteremia tends to be less common with *S. pneumoniae* than *N. meningitidis.* Neurologic complications such as coma and seizures are common with pneumococcal meningitis.[47] Traumatic tears of the dura, fracture of the cribriform plate or paranasal sinuses, nasal meningoceles, repeated episodes of otitis media, and osteomyelitis of the skull floor are risk factors for recurrent pneumococcal meningitis.

Treatment with intravenous crystalline penicillin G (50,000 units/kg every 4 hours) in adult patients with normal renal function usually results in a favorable outcome, although there have been increasing reports of intermediate and completely penicillin resistant *S. pneumoniae* in the United States and worldwide.[56–60] These resistant strains are becoming an increasing problem and meticulous testing of all CSF isolates for penicillin resistance has been recommended. Chloramphenicol represents a useful alternative to penicillin G and is bactericidal for *S. pneumoniae.* Several third-generation cephalosporins may also serve as alternatives to penicillin in the treatment of penicillin-sensitive and penicillin-resistant pneumococcal meningitis; however, third-generation cephalosporins containing a 3-methylthiotetrazole substitution (e.g., cefoperazone, moxalactam) should be avoided as the ratio of achievable antibiotic concentrations in CSF to MBC of the *S. pneumoniae* is too low to be considered curative. Drugs such as cefotaxime and ceftriaxone may prove useful as alternatives to penicillin G for relatively resistant strains (penicillin MIC of 0.1–1.0 mg/L). However, treatment failures in the management of meningitis with third-generation cephalosporins for pencillin-resistant pneumococci have been reported.[61,62] The combination of vancomycin and ceftriaxone has been shown to be synergistic for penicillin-resistant pneumococci and has been suggested for initial management until the results of antimicrobial susceptibility testing are available.[63]

Optimal therapy for highly resistant strains of pneumococci (penicillin MIC ≥ 2 mg/L) has not yet been clearly defined.[60] Outcome may depend on the serotype of the microorganism (especially type 3), whether the infection is primary or secondary, and the number of WBCs in CSF.[47] While cefotaxime, ceftriaxone, vancomycin, and imipenem are potentially useful for penicillin-sensitive and relatively resistant strains of pneumococcus, clear guidelines need to be established for completely penicillin-resistant strains. Some concern would also seem warranted with the use of imipenem for CNS infections due to the possibility of drug-induced seizures. Vancomycin alone or possibly in combination with ceftriaxone would probably be the most effective option at the present time.[56,57,63] Some authors have suggested that to achieve therapeutic CSF concentrations of vancomycin direct administration may be necessary.[64]

Virtually all serotypes of *S. pneumoniae* exhibiting intermediate or complete resistance to penicillin are found in the current 23 serotype pneumococcal vaccine and clinicians need to universally immunize appropriate patients.[57,60] Unfortunately, the efficacy of this product in children less than 2 years and compromised adults limits this strategy as a solution to the problem of penicillin-resistant pneumococci.[65]

Chemoprophylaxis and vaccination for close contacts of an index case with *S. pneumoniae* meningitis are generally not recommended because the risk of acquiring secondary pneumococcal disease is similar to the infection rate in the general population.[52,53] However, vaccination and chemoprophylaxis with oral penicillin reduce the incidence of pneumococcal septicemia and meningitis in young patients with sickle cell disease.[52]

Gram-Negative Meningitis

During the last 20 years, the incidence of gram-negative bacillary meningitis, excluding *H. influenzae* has been increasing in both children and adults. Currently, enteric gram-negative organisms are the fourth leading cause of meningitis, with only *S. pneumoniae, H. influenzae,* and *N. meningitidis* having a higher incidence.

There are several predisposing factors to the development of gram-negative meningitis. Congenital defects, accidental cranial trauma, and neurosurgery alter the anatomic defenses and may predispose the patient to this form of meningitis. The use of antimicrobial agents with exclusive gram-positive activity preoperatively in neurosurgery may also predispose the patient to development of a gram-negative infection. Any form of communication between the skin and subarachoid space, such as a dermal sinus, greatly increases the risk of gram-negative meningitis. Gram-negative bacteremia by itself is an infrequent cause of meningitis without some form of CNS trauma. Other risk factors for the development of gram-negative meningitis include diabetes, malignancy, urinary tract infection in neonates, cirrhosis, parameningeal infection, strongyloidiasis, spinal anesthesia, and hospitalization in general.

Elderly debilitated patients may also be at increased risk of gram-negative meningitis but usually lack classic signs and symptoms of the disease. Nuchal rigidity may be difficult to detect because of the presence of cervical arthritis in the elderly. The presence of a low-grade fever and changes in mental status, without other obvious cause, should prompt consideration of lumbar puncture. In the postneonatal period, the two most common organisms causing gram-negative meningitis are *E. coli* and *K. pneumoniae* together, which are responsible for 60–70% of cases.

The optimal antimicrobial agent(s), route of administration, and duration of therapy for gram-negative bacillary meningitis have yet to be fully defined.

The treatment of meningitis due to *P. aeruginosa* remains a special problem since antibiotics such as antipseudomonal penicillins and aminoglycosides, which show good antibacterial activity against *P. aeruginosa,* penetrate the CSF poorly. Initially, cases of *P. aeruginosa* meningitis should be treated with ceftazidime or piperacillin plus an aminoglycoside, usually tobramycin.[66–68] Since aminoglycosides penetrate CSF poorly, their inclusion is predominantly to aid in the treatment of extracerebral infection(s). If the pseudomonad is initially suspected to be antibiotic resistant or becomes resistant during therapy, an intraventricular aminoglycoside should be considered along with intravenous aminoglycoside. Preservative-free forms of gentamicin and tobramycin are available and should be used for direct administration into the CSF. Intraventricular aminoglycoside dosages should be adjusted to the estimated CSF volume (0.03 mg of tobramycin or gentamicin/mL of CSF and 0.1 mg of amikacin/mL of CSF every 24 hours). CSF flows unidirectionally with gravity and most data suggest that intraventricular aminoglycoside administration is more likely to produce therapeutic concentrations throughout the CSF than intrathecal administration.[12,68] Ventricular levels of aminoglycoside should be monitored every 2 or 3 days, just prior to the next intraventricular dose, and "trough levels" should approximate 2–10 mg/L. Technically such determinations are often contaminated with residual aminoglycoside from the previous dose, making interpretation difficult.

Gram-negative organisms, other than *P. aeruginosa,* causing meningitis can likely be treated with a third-generation cephalosporin such as cefotaxime, ceftizoxime, ceftriaxone, or ceftazidime. In situations where the offending organism is not initially known, ceftazidime may not reliably produce CSF antibiotic concentrations greater than 10 times the MBC for gram-positive organisms. Cefoperazone produces unreliable antibiotic concentrations in the CSF because of its high protein binding and should not be a drug of first choice for gram-negative meningitis. In adults, daily doses of 8–12 g/d of these third-generation cephalosporins or 2 g of ceftriaxone should produce CSF concentrations of 5–20 mg/L.

Limitations to the use of third-generation cephalosporins with a 3-methylthiotetrazole substitution such as cefoperazone in gram-negative meningitis may include such adverse reactions as bleeding diathesis, resistance caused by inducible type 1 β-lactamases, and superinfection resulting from the broad spectrum of antimicrobial activity. None of the third-generation cephalosporins are effective for *Listeria monocytogenes* and perhaps only ceftazidime would be effective in treating *P. aeruginosa* meningitis. Although chloramphenicol is a bactericidal antibiotic for *H. influenzae, N. meningitidis,* and *S. pneumoniae,* the antibiotic produces only a bacteriostatic effect for most gram-negative organisms.

Trimethoprim–sulfamethoxazole (TMP/SMX) produces CSF levels of 1.9–5.7 mg/L for the former and 20–63 mg/L for the latter when given parenterally in doses of 10 mg/kg/d (trimethoprim) and 50 mg/kg/d (sulfamethoxazole). In addition to several of the Enterobacteriaceae, TMP/SMX may be useful for *Acinetobacter* spp., *Serratia* spp. and *L. monocytogenes* meningitis.[69] One additional advantage of TMP/SMX is that antibiotic penetration into the CSF is not dependent on meningeal inflammation. However, TMP/SMX is not bactericidal.

Clinical experience with fluoroquinolones in the treatment of gram-negative meningitis is minimal and should only be considered when bacterial meningitis is caused by multiply resistant gram-negative rods.[70] Fluoroquinolones are not approved for the treatment of bacterial meningitis. Therapy for gram-negative meningitis should be continued for 10 days after cultures of CSF become sterile. CSF cultures may remain positive for 10 days or more on a regimen that will eventually be curative. Therapeutic efficacy can be monitored through bacterial colony counts every 2 or 3 days and colony counts should progressively decrease over the period of therapy.

Haemophilus Influenzae

In the past, *H. influenzae* was the most common cause of meningitis in children 6 months to 3 years. *Haemophilus influenzae* meningitis in older individuals may indicate a parameningeal focus of infection, middle ear infection, or CSF leakage. The disease is often a complication of primary infectious involvement of the middle ear, paranasal sinuses, or lungs. Spread of the organism may then occur either via the veins draining these areas or via bacteremia originating from the local focus of infection.[19,71]

Coma and seizures commonly occur early in the course of the disease. Morbiliform and petechial rashes are very uncommon but may resemble the rash seen with meningococcal infection. Sterile, subdural effusions are common with *H. influenzae* but not with other forms of meningitis.[47] These effusions may provoke a fever after an initial defervescence, seizures, or vomiting, any of which may necessitate repeated subdural paracentesis.

Approximately 30–40% of *H. influenzae* are ampicillin resistant. For this reason, many clinicians use chloramphenicol with ampicillin or a third-generation cephalosporin for initial antimicrobial therapy. Once bacterial susceptibilities are available, chloramphenicol can be discontinued if the organism proves ampicillin sensitive. However, chloramphenicol requires serum concentration monitoring in order to avoid toxic or subtherapeutic levels. Most clinicians consider the third-generation cephalosporins to be the drugs of choice for meningitis caused by *H. influenzae.* The third-generation cephalosporins (such as cefotaxime and ceftriaxone) are very active against β-lactamase-producing and non-β-lactamase-producing strains of *H. influenzae,* are relatively free of toxicity, and do not require serum concentration monitoring.

Because cases of *H. influenzae* meningitis occur in clusters, treatment of close contacts of patients is usually recommended.[52] Secondary cases resulting from close contact with the index case occur within 30 days of the onset of disease. As with meningococcal meningitis, close contacts may be at 200 to 1000 times the risk of the general population for acquiring *H. influenzae* meningitis.[52]

Close contacts are usually defined as household members, individuals sharing sleeping quarters, crowded confined populations, day care attendees, and nursing home residents.[52] The disease may also be transmitted in the laboratory setting, sexually, or nosocomially. Without intimate contact with the index patient's respiratory secretions, the risk of acquiring *H. influenzae* meningitis is low.[52]

The goal of prophylaxis is to protect close contacts from the index case by eliminating nasopharyngeal and oropharyngeal carriage of *H. influenzae*. Cultures are of no immediate value and may cause a delay in starting effective prophylaxis.

Prophylaxis for *H. influenzae* is no longer recommended when at least one member of the same household as the index case is less than 4 years of age if all contacts <4 years old are fully immunized.[41,52,72] For this purpose, a "household contact" is anyone (including adults) who has spent 4 hours or more with the index case for at least 5 of the 7 previous days prior to the initiation of therapy. Households with children <12 months (regardless of vaccination status) or with children ages 1–3 years who are not adequately vaccinated should all receive rifampin prophylaxis[72] in order to eliminate nasopharyngeal carriage and the subsequent spread of disease to others. Because the risk is greatest within the first week of exposure, chemoprophylaxis should be initiated as soon as possible after exposure.[41,52] Prophylaxis is not indicated for persons having casual contact with the index case at work or school, nor is it indicated for most hospital employees. The index case should also receive chemoprophylaxis prior to discharge from the hospital because there have been reports of recolonization after successful antibiotic therapy.[41,52]

Studies conflict regarding recommendations for chemoprophylaxis of day-care center contacts. The American Academy of Pediatrics[41] suggests that chemoprophylaxis is indicated if two cases are identified within a 60-day period. In addition, if day-care contacts are less than 2 years of age or if the number of day-care attendees is small, prophylaxis should be given if only one case is identified. Finally, chemoprophylaxis should only be attempted if all children participate or if treated contacts are excluded from attending the center.

It is important to remember that the incidence of secondary acquisition of *H. influenzae* meningitis is low and that secondary infection accounts for only 2% of all cases.[52]

Adults should receive 600 mg of rifampin daily for 4 days.[52] Children 1 month to 12 years should receive 20 mg/kg (maximum 600 mg) per day for 4 days, and children less than 1 month should receive 10 mg/kg/d for 4 days.[52] Minocycline is an alternative to rifampin chemoprophylaxis; however, there is a high incidence of drug-induced vestibular dysfunction. Patients receiving *H. influenzae* prophylaxis should be carefully monitored because failures do occur and patients may go on to develop meningitis.

Since the introduction of effective vaccines, the incidence of *H. influenzae* type b disease in the United States has declined.[7] Currently, there are five *H. influenzae* type b (HIB) conjugate vaccines available in the United States (see Vaccines, Toxoids, and other Immunobiologics, Chapter 116). The Food and Drug Administration (FDA) has recently approved the use of four of these vaccines for use in children who are 2 months of age or older (HbOC [HibTITER, TETRAMUNE], PRP-OMP [PedvaxHIB], and PRP-T [ActHIB, OmniHIB]).[72,73] The diphtheria conjugate vaccine (ProHIBIT) has not demonstrated suitable clinical efficacy (i.e., antibody response) in controlled trials of children younger than 15 months of age. Although the other conjugate vaccines have proven efficacy in Caucasians, only the PedvaxHIB vaccine has proven efficacy in Native American children.[72]

Recently the CDC set out new guidelines regarding the use of HIB conjugate vaccines: (1) Any of the conjugate vaccines, with the exception of ProHIBIT, are indicated for the primary vaccination series in infants older than 2 months of age. (2) Three doses of HbOC or PRP-T and two doses of PRP-OMP should be administered to infants younger than 6 months; ideally at 2, 4, and 6 months. (3) Two doses of the previously mentioned vaccines should be given to infants first seen between 7 and 11 months of age. (4) One dose of these vaccines should be administered to infants first seen between 12 and 14 months of age. (5) All infants should receive a booster dose at 15 months of age or 2 months after their last vaccination. Any of the currently licensed conjugate vaccines (HbOC, PRP-T, PRP-OMP, PRP-D) can be used for the dose at 15 months, because they all appear to be effective at that age. The CDC recommends completion of the primary series with the same Hib conjugate vaccine, if possible. If different vaccines are administered, a total of three doses is necessary to assure adequate response.[72] Because Alaskan Natives are at increased risk for disease during early infancy, it may be advantageous to administer the PRP-OMP Hib vaccine in this population due to the substantial antibody response elicited after just one dose.[72,73]

Listeria Monocytogenes

Listeria monocytogenes is a gram-positive diphtheroid-like organism and is responsible for 3% of all reported cases of meningitis. The disease affects primarily neonates, immunocompromised adults, and the elderly. In the immunocompromised patient, the CSF resembles that found in bacterial meningitis.

Usually, the patient's GI tract becomes colonized with the organisms, which then penetrate the gut lumen. If there is not a sufficient cell-mediated response (T lymphocyte, macrophages), bacteremia, meningitis, meningoencephalitis, or cerebritis may develop.[74] Infection of the brain may be diffuse or localized, possibly involving the cerebral hemispheres, thalamus, and brain stem. Approximately 75% of *L. monocytogenes* infections in immunocompromised hosts result in CNS seeding.[74]

The incidence of *L. monocytogenes* meningitis tends to peak in the summer and early fall. As with gram-negative meningitis, the presentation may be subtle and insidious. Clinical suspicion should prompt lumbar puncture. *Listeria monocytogenes* produces primarily a mononuclear CSF response.[74] One common laboratory error seen with *L. monocytogenes* is the tendency to misidentify the organism on Gram stain as a diphtheroid or streptococcus.

Treatment of *L. monocytogenes* meningitis with penicillin G or ampicillin may result in only a bacteriostatic effect and possible persistence of the infection. Usually the combination of penicillin G or ampicillin with an aminoglycoside results in a bactericidal effect. Patients should be treated for 2–3 weeks after defervescence to prevent the possibility of relapse.[74] Usually combination therapy is employed for at least 10 days and the remaining course of therapy is completed with penicillin G or ampicillin alone. Trimethoprim–sulfamethoxazole may be an effective alternative, because adequate CSF penetration is achieved with these agents.

Mycobacterium Tuberculosis

Mycobacterium tuberculosis var. *hominis* is the primary cause of tuberculous meningitis. Tuberculous meningitis is difficult to diagnose in a timely manner and is associated with significant morbidity and mortality.[75] The most useful, although unelicited, diagnostic clue is a history of known contact with an index case of tuberculosis or a prior history of tuberculosis. Up to 40% of patients may present with evidence of pulmonary involvement with hilar adenopathy; however, tuberculous meningitis may exist in the absence of disease in the lung or extrapulmonary sites. The tuberculin skin test (purified protein derivative [PPD]) is negative in 5–50% of cases.[75]

Upon initial examination, CSF usually contains from 100–1000 WBC/mm^3, which may be 75–80% polymorphonuclear cells.[24,75,76] Over time, the pattern of WBC in the CSF will shift to lymphocytes and monocytes. CSF glucose may initially be normal, but gradually decreases as the disease progresses.[75,76] Protein concentration within the CSF may be normal or elevated with high protein levels shown to correlate with advanced disease.[75–77]

One potentially useful diagnostic sign unique to tuberculous meningitis is paralysis of the VIth cranial nerve, which initially may be unilateral and then progress to become bilateral.[47] The sensitivity of the acid fast bacilli (AFB) smear is enhanced by the examination of multiple CSF specimens collected on consecutive days. Initial AFB smears are approximately 37% sensitive and as high as 87% sensitive following subsequent smears. Cultures of CSF may be positive in 45–90% of cases depending on the quantity of CSF used in the culture, pathogen density, and the experience in the laboratory culturing *M. tuberculosis*. Positive culture results may take up to 8 weeks, providing little help with initial diagnosis.[75,76]

Isoniazid is the mainstay in virtually any regimen to treat *M. tuberculosis*.[75,76] Unfortunately, the incidence of multiple antibiotic-resistant strains of *M. tuberculosis* has dramatically increased, necessitating the use of four and five antibiotics at a time.[78,79] Isoniazid penetrates CSF with or without meningeal inflammation and achieves concentrations >30 times the MIC of *M. tuberculosis* (MICs of 0.05–0.2 mg/L).[74] Rifampin's penetration of CSF approximates only 20% of serum concentrations in the presence of meningeal inflammation. However, *M. tuberculosis* is so exquisitely sensitive to rifampin that its low penetration ratio is of little clinical significance.[75,76,80] Like isoniazid, the incidence of *M. tuberculosis* resistance to rifampin has increased, necessitating empiric multiple antibiotic regimens.

Pyrazinamide is a small molecule and penetrates CSF well even in the absence of meningeal inflammation. Streptomycin, an aminoglycoside, penetrates CSF poorly even in the presence of meningeal inflammation. Ethambutol is a weak antitubercular agent and reaches the CSF in moderate concentrations. Ethambutol's use is also limited by a high incidence of dose-related optic neuritis. Ethionamide and cycloserine are two other agents that are sometimes used to treat tuberculous meningitis. These agents both penetrate CSF well even in the absence of meningeal inflammation.[75,76]

In children, the usual dose of isoniazid is 10–20 mg/kg/d (maximum 300 mg/d). Adults usually receive 5–10 mg/kg/d or a daily dose of 300 mg. Supplemental doses of pyridoxine hydrochloride (vitamin B_6) 50 mg/d are recommended to prevent the peripheral neuropathy associated with isoniazid administration.[75,76,79] Concurrent administration of rifampin is recommended at doses of 10–20 mg/kg/d (maximum 600 mg/d) for children and 600 mg/d for adults.[75,76] The addition of pyrazinamide (children and adults 15–30 mg/kg/d; maximum in both 2 g/d) to the regimen of isoniazid and rifampin is now recommended.[75,76] The duration of concomitant pyrazinamide therapy should be limited to 2 months in order to avoid hepatotoxicity. As of 1993, the CDC recommends a regimen of four drugs for empiric treatment of *M. tuberculosis,* unless resistance to isoniazid in the area is <4%.[79] This regimen should consist of isoniazid, rifampin, pyrazinamide, and ethambutol 15–25 mg/kg/d (maximum 2.5 g/d) or streptomycin 15–30 mg/kg/d (maximum 1 g/d) for the first 2 months, generally followed by isoniazid plus rifampin for the duration of therapy. Therapy after the first 2 months should be individualized based on susceptibility patterns.[79] Patients with *M. tuberculosis* meningitis should be treated for a duration of 9 months or longer with multiple drug therapy.

The use of steroids for tuberculous meningitis remains controversial. In some cases administration of steroids as oral prednisone 40–60 mg/d or 0.2 mg/kg/d of IV dexamethasone has resulted in a dramatic clearing of sensorium, remission of CSF abnormalities, reduction in fever, and elimination of headaches.[75,76,80] Concerns regarding the use of steroids include their possible interference with CSF chemistry studies and penetration of antitubercular agents.

Despite the controversy, the trend toward improved outcome when steroids are administered generally supports their use for tuberculous meningitis.[81]

Despite early diagnosis and treatment, tuberculous meningitis has a mortality rate of 10–50%.[75,76] The most useful prognostic indicator is the level of patient consciousness at the start of therapy. Patients who are comatose at the start of therapy have a mortality rate of approximately 75%.[76] Other negative prognostic factors include old age, poor nutrition, evidence of miliary disease, high initial CSF protein concentrations, presence of hydrocephalus, and evidence of elevated intracranial pressure.[76] Ten to 30% of patients surviving the disease have physical or mental sequelae including deafness, vertigo, and short-term memory loss.[75,76]

Cryptococcus Neoformans

In the United States, cryptococcal meningitis is the most common form of fungal meningitis and is a major cause of morbidity and mortality in immunosuppressed patients. Patients with HIV are at a 5–10% risk of developing cryptococcus during their lifetime.[82] *Cryptococcus neoformans* is a soil fungus acquired by inhalation of spores from the environment. In immunocompromised hosts, especially neoplastic patients or AIDS patients, the organisms often disseminate from the lungs. The primary site of dissemination is the meninges, although the skin, prostate, bone, kidneys, eyes, liver, spleen, adrenals, and lymph nodes may also be infected.[83]

The symptoms of cryptococcus meningitis are insidious and may be present for months before the correct diagnosis is made. Fever and a history of headaches are the most common symptoms, although altered mentation and evidence of focal neurologic deficits may be present. Examination of CSF usually reveals small numbers of WBCs ($<150/mm^3$), which are primarily lymphocytes. Diagnosis is based on the presence of a positive CSF, blood, sputum, or urine culture for *C. neoformans.* CSF cultures are positive in more than 90% of cases. The organism can be seen microscopically when stained with India ink. An additional rapid test helpful in diagnosis is latex agglutination, which detects the presence of cryptococcal antigens.[83] This test is positive in >90% of culture positive cases. The cryptococcal antigen test can be used to follow the prognosis of non-AIDS patients but cryptococcal antigen titers do not correlate well with treatment efficacy in AIDS patients.[84] Risk factors predictive of a poor outcome include lethargy at presentation, a high CSF cryptococcal antigen titer, and low CSF WBC count.[85]

Despite poor penetration into the CSF, amphotericin B has long been the drug of choice for treatment of acute *C. neoformans* meningitis. Amphotericin B 0.5–1 mg/kg/d combined with flucytosine 100 mg/kg/d is more effective than amphotericin alone with successful outcomes in 75% of non-AIDS patients and 50% in AIDS patients.[86] Unfortunately, in the AIDS population, flucytosine is often poorly tolerated causing bone marrow suppression and GI distress.

Due to the high acute mortality rate of up to 40% and the 50% relapse rate in AIDS patients receiving therapy, many new agents and regimens are being investigated in this population.[85] Amphotericin B alone, although less effective, has been used in AIDS patients with preexisting granulocytopenia.[86,87] Intraventricular amphotericin B in addition to intravenous amphotericin B plus flucytosine has been suggested as initial therapy, but intraventricular amphotericin is generally reserved for patients who fail to respond to systemic therapy.[83] A small, noncomparative open study evaluating the safety and efficacy of liposomal amphotericin B (AmBisome) found the product to be well tolerated and moderately effective.[88]

Azole therapy is the most studied alternative regimen for the treatment of *C. neoformans* meningitis in AIDS patients. Fluconazole at doses of 200 mg/d was compared to amphotericin B alone with no significant difference in overall mortality between groups.[89] The group of patients who received fluconazole did have a higher 2-week mortality rate and time to CSF conversion.[89] High-dose fluconazole therapy (800 mg/d) was tried with limited results as salvage therapy in eight AIDS patients who had failed previous antifungal therapy.[90] Itraconazole 200 mg orally twice daily was less effective than amphotericin B plus flucytosine in a small nonblinded study.[91] Jones and colleagues[92] conducted a pilot study of flucytosine 150 mg/kg/d plus fluconazole 400 mg/d in a small group of AIDS patients. Efficacy was similar to that seen in studies using fluconazole alone, and serious toxicity from flucytosine occurred in one-fourth of the patients.[92]

Due to the high relapse rate following acute therapy for *C. neoformans,* AIDS patients require lifelong maintenance or suppressive therapy.[82] A large multicenter controlled trial compared fluconazole (200 mg/d) and amphotericin B (1 mg/kg/week) in the prevention of relapse.[93] Two percent of patients receiving fluconazole versus 18% of patients on amphotericin B relapsed. In addition, the amphotericin B group had significantly more frequent bacterial infections, bacteremias, and drug-related toxicity.[93] Therefore, the standard of care for AIDS-associated cryptococcal meningitis is primary therapy, generally using amphotericin B with or without flucytosine or fluconazole alone, followed by maintenance therapy with fluconazole, for the life of the patient.[82]

Viral Meningitis

Meningitis typically is characterized as being either “purulent” or “aseptic.” While purulent meningitis refers to a bacterial etiology, aseptic meningitis historically was defined by diagnosis of exclusion. Aseptic meningitis has been defined as an acute meningeal irritation, usually benign and self-limiting, with complete recovery and sterile pleocytic CSF.[24] At least 70% of aseptic meningitis cases are caused by viruses; however, unusual bacterial organisms such as *M. tuberculosis, Brucella* spp., and *Borrelia burgdorferi* can cause aseptic meningitis.[24,94,95] In addition, fungal pathogens, certain drugs, vaccines, and systemic diseases or malignancies have been associated with aseptic meningitis syndrome.[24,94,96]

The epidemiology of viral meningitis in the United States has changed dramatically since the mid-1960s due to the introduction of large-scale polio and mumps immunization programs. Worldwide, mumps and polio are still responsible for a significant percentage of viral meningitis cases. However, in the United States, the incidence of poliomyelitis has decreased from 17.6 cases per 100,000 in 1955 to 0.01 cases per 100,000 in 1972. Similarly, the incidence of mumps has decreased 98% between 1967 and 1985. The low incidence of meningitis associated with these entities (1–3% for mumps; 4–8% poliomyelitis) and their decreased prevalence now make mumps and polio infrequent causes of viral meningitis in the United States today. Eighty-five percent of all viral meningitis cases are currently caused by nonpolio enteroviruses such as coxsackie B virus, echoviruses, and enteroviruses.[24] Arboviruses such as St. Louis, Eastern equine, Western equine, and California arboviruses were responsible for 78 cases of viral meningitis/encephalitis in 20 states in 1993.[58] The remaining 10% of viral meningitis cases are caused by a variety of pathogens such as adenoviruses, influenzae virus A and B, rotavirus, corona virus, cytomegalovirus, varicella-zoster, herpes simplex, Epstein–Barr virus, and lymphocytic choriomeningitis.[24,94,97] Although aseptic meningitis is responsible for a substantial portion of meningitis cases, because aseptic meningitis is frequently a diagnosis of exclusion, the actual incidence of aseptic meningitis may be much higher. The incidence of aseptic meningitis peaks in late summer and continues into fall.

The pathogen of viral meningitis is acquired primarily by hematogenous spread or alternatively by neuronal spread.[97] After entry to the host, primary viral replication occurs, eventually resulting in dissemination through the reticuloendothelial system or vasculature. The choroid plexus or infection of the capillary endothelial cells may provide a conduit for CNS infection.[97] Viruses such as polio, herpes, and varicella-zoster may gain access to the CNS by axonal retrograde transmission from peripheral nerve endings.[97] Once a particular virus gains access to the CNS, the course is dependent on the virulence of the particular virus and the host immune response. In a manner similar to purulent meningitis, host response to CNS infections is mediated by a complex cascade of inflammatory cytokines. In contrast to purulent meningitis, host response to viral meningitis is primarily mediated through cytotoxic T lymphocytes. Although TNF is a prominent mediator in purulent bacterial meningitis, TNF concentrations are not increased in viral meningitis whereas both IL-1 and interferon (INF) alpha and gamma concentrations are.[98] TNF concentrations have been suggested as a diagnostic tool for differentiating between purulent and viral meningitis.[98] While cytokine assays are available for investigational use, they are not routinely used in the clinical diagnosis of viral meningitis.

The clinical syndrome seen with viral meningitis is generally independent of the particular viral etiology and may vary depending on the patient's age. Common signs in adults include headache, mild fever (<40°C), nuchal rigidity, malaise, drowsiness, nausea, vomiting, and photophobia. Only fever and irritability may be evident in the infant, and meningitis must be ruled out as a cause of fever when no other localized findings are observed in a child. The duration of symptoms generally lasts 1 to 2 weeks and specific manifestations outside of the meninges can also occur depending on the particular viral etiology.

Laboratory examination of CSF usually reveals a pleocytosis with 10–1000 WBCs/mm^3, which are primarily lymphocytic; however, 20–75% of patients with viral meningitis may have a predominance of polymorphonuclear cells on initial examination of the CSF, especially in enteroviral meningitis.[24] Upon repeat lumbar puncture, 90% of patients initially presenting with a predominance of neutrophils experience a shift to a predominance of mononuclear cells. Other laboratory findings include normal to mildly elevated protein concentrations and normal or mildly reduced glucose concentrations[24] (Table 99.1).

Historically, the pathogen responsible for aseptic meningitis was not identified.[99] Poor laboratory recovery of viral pathogens, the generally benign course of the disease, and the limited treatment options for aseptic meningitis made the need for specific identification of pathogens questionable. However, recent advances in diagnostic laboratory techniques and the potential for decreased costs associated with longer duration of hospitalization for patients with unconfirmed viral meningitis have led to a reevaluation of the need for confirmatory pathogen diagnosis.[95,99] When clinical signs warrant pathogen identification, appropriate laboratory diagnostic techniques should be undertaken.

Although there are numerous pathogenic causes of viral meningitis, much of the clinical presentation, diagnosis, and treatment is similar for different viral pathogens. The most commonly isolated viral etiologies are discussed as follows.

Nonpolio enteroviruses are unenveloped single-strand RNA viruses. Commonly, the incidence of enteroviral meningitis peaks in late summer and continues into early fall. Enteroviruses are transmitted in the host via the fecal–oral route. The clinical presentation of enteroviral infection is frequently nonspecific and characterized by fever, nausea, vomiting, and malaise; however, GI symptoms may not present at all. Following a prodrome of 1–2 days, headache, photophobia, and neck stiffness develop.

Diagnosis is confirmed by cell culture from the CSF where the incidence of successful isolation has ranges from 40–80%.[98] In addition, enterovirus can be isolated from throat swabs (60%) and stool cultures (80%), but are not necessarily diagnostic because the virus is shed in the stool for 1–2 weeks following infection.[99] Treatment for enteroviral meningitis consists of supportive care, fluids, antipyretics, and analgesics. Generally, the disease progression is self-limiting, and the patient fully recovers without long-term neurologic complications. However, a recent assessment of the potential for long-term neurologic abnormalities in children <1 year old with enteroviral meningitis has suggested that enteroviral meningitis may not be a completely benign disease.

Although up to 10% of viral meningitis cases are caused by arboviruses, these viruses are most commonly associated with encephalitis.[97] The four most common pathogens are the St. Louis virus, the California virus, and the Eastern and Western equine viruses. These viruses are transmitted by the bites of ticks and mosquitoes. Typically an incubation period of 2–14 days precedes the onset of clinical symptoms. Infection of the brain tissue results in fever, headache, paralysis, and coma. While many patients have a benign presentation, symptomatic cases are associated with a higher degree of mortality. Mortality rates of 50–75% have been reported for Eastern equine virus while mortality rates for Western equine and St. Louis virus are 10–20%.[97] Treatment is supportive and in the majority of cases the disease is self-limiting.[97]

Human immunodeficiency virus (HIV) encephalitis is the most common CNS complication associated with AIDS. Frequently, patients may complain of headache, photophobia, or stiff neck at the time of presumed seroconversion. However, as the disease progresses, neurologic symptoms are frequently reported due to other opportunistic infections as well. The diagnosis of viral meningitis is difficult because mental status and neurologic exams are not sensitive enough to detect early changes. Direct evidence of HIV meningitis can be obtained through CSF culture on p24 antigen testing. Diagnostic workup of other potential more treatable copathogens, such as HSV, *Toxoplasma gondii, M. tuberculosis,* cryptococcus, and so on, should be performed as well.

Both types 1 and 2 of herpes simplex virus have been associated with infections of the CNS.[100] Herpes simplex type 1 (HSV1) is associated with meningoencephalitis, whereas herpes simplex type 2 (HSV2) is associated predominantly with meningitis. HSV2 infection of the meninges is most likely hematogenously spread from an initial site of infection. Sexually active adults acquire herpes simplex meningitis during or after an attack of genital or rectal herpes. While HSV2 can frequently be cultured from CSF, HSV1 cannot. The diagnosis is usually made by culture or by a fourfold rise in complement-fixing antibody to the virus. It is paramount that diagnosis be established as early as possible because without treatment the mortality rate is between 50–85%, and unlike other viral encephalitides, specific and effective therapy is available. The definitive diagnosis can be established only with a brain biopsy. Although a herpes simplex etiology may be strongly suspected on the basis of local findings after clinical evaluation, in only half of these patients will the clinical diagnosis be confirmed by brain biopsy.[100]

Acyclovir has replaced vidarabine as the drug of choice for herpes simplex encephalitis. In patients with normal renal function, acyclovir is usually administered as 10 mg/kg every 8 hours. Herpes virus resistance to acyclovir has been reported with increasing incidence, particularly from immunocompromised patients with prior or chronic exposures to acyclovir.[101] The alternative treatment for acyclovir-resistant herpes simplex virus is vidarabine. Vidarabine is used intravenously in a dose of 15 mg/kg/d. Because of its poor solubility in water, the drug must be mixed in large volumes of parenteral fluid and infused over a 12-hour period. In addition, patients receiving vidarabine should be monitored for leukopenia, megaloblastic anemia, thrombocytopenia, and a parkinsonian-like neurologic syndrome.

Shunt Infections

Surgical shunting procedures are used in patients with hydrocephalus to produce a decompression of the two lateral ventricles by diverting CSF from the ventricles into another body compartment.[102] The two most popular techniques are ventriculoatrial (VA) and ventriculoperitoneal (VP) shunts. In the VP shunts, fluid is diverted into the peritoneal cavity; the VA shunt diverts CSF into the right atrium.

Inevitably a surgical procedure leaving a foreign device in place is associated with a high risk of infection. Shunt infections have a lifetime incidence of infection of 1.5–39%, with most studies reporting a rate of 10–15%.[102,103] In the last 15 years, the incidence of shunt infections has decreased by 50%, which is most likely due to improved surgical technique. There appears to be no difference in infectious risk whether the surgical procedure is the initial placement or a revision.[102,103] Children requiring shunt replacement prior to 3 months of age, elderly patients requiring shunt procedures, lengthy surgical procedures, surgical emergencies, and, possibly, the type of shunt are all potential risk factors for infection. If a VA shunt is used and the distal catheter tip is at or below T7 in children, the risk of infection seems to increase. Optimal placement of the VA distal catheter tip in adults is between T5 and T7. Children with VA shunts require further revision with growth.

Staphylococcus epidermidis is the primary cause of VA and VP shunt infections. *Staphylococcus aureus* is the second leading cause of shunt infection with an estimated incidence of 25%.[102,103] Collectively, *Klebsiella* sp., *E. coli,* and *Proteus* sp. cause approximately 5–10% of shunt infections.[102] *Haemophilus influenzae, S. pneumoniae,* and *N. meningitidis* cause 5% of all shunt infections.[102] Approximately 70% of all shunt infections are clinically apparent within 2 months of the shunting procedure.[102] Eighty percent are evident within 6 months of surgery. A variety of etiologies have been postulated for shunt infections. One obvious possibility is site contamination at the time of surgery. A second possibility is hematogenous spread of organisms that contaminate the shunt. Organisms may migrate in a retrograde fashion from a contaminated distal catheter tip. The former observation reinforces the impression that most infections of CSF prostheses occur as a result of implantation of the organism at the time of surgery or of contamination of the device by ward personnel during manipulation. This is supported by the fact that most infections of CSF prostheses are caused by skin flora.[102]

Several factors are involved in the infectious process: the magnitude of pathogen contamination, the intrinsic virulence of the offending organism, and the presence or absence of functioning host defense mechanisms. With *S. epidermidis,* there may be "slime" (mucin, glycocalyx) production that allows the organism to colonize and adhere to the shunt, which protects the organism from phagocytosis.[102]

Tenderness along the path of the catheter across the rib margin is suggestive of a VP shunt infection. Approximately one-third of patients with VP shunt infections will present with abdominal symptoms. Several complications can arise from both VA and VP shunt infections. Chronic bacteremia, glomerular nephritis (shunt nephritis), hypocomplementemia, and septic pulmonary embolization may result from VA shunts. Complications from VP shunts include infectious peritonitis, bowel obstruction secondary to adhesions, bowel perforation, and peritoneal cysts.

CLINICAL PRESENTATIONS

Diagnosis is usually based on clinical suspicion. In patients with shunts, every febrile episode should be evaluated as a possible shunt infection. Blood cultures are positive in about 95% of patients with VA shunts but in only 20% of patients with VP shunts. Culturing of CSF obtained percutaneously from the shunt reservoir or tubing is the most useful diagnostic procedure. These cultures are usually positive in more than 95% of patients not receiving antibiotics. Although shunt cultures of CSF may be positive, CSF obtained by lumbar puncture may be culture negative. As a rule, CSF is not as reactive in shunt infections as in other CNS infections. CSF WBC counts average $<100/mm^3$. Presence of WBCs in CSF correlates well with culture results. When more than 100 WBC are seen per cubic millimeter of CSF, the cultures are positive in more than 90% of cases. When CSF contains fewer than 20 $WBCs/mm^3$, less than 50% of the cultures are positive. If cultures are negative but the CSF white count remains elevated, the patient should be evaluated for an anaerobic or fungal infection. Hypoglycorrhachia (low glucose concentrations in CSF) is usually not severe.

TREATMENT

Treatment usually involves the use of parenteral antibiotics, externalization of the infected shunt, and, possibly, intraventricular antibiotic administration. Systemic antibiotic therapy should be started based on the suspected initial pathogen and the usual antimicrobial patterns of susceptibility. Serious consideration should be given to the possibility of methicillin-resistant strains of both *S. aureus* and in particular *S. epidermidis.* Depending on the organism, various combinations of systemic antibiotic therapy may be used. When methicillin-resistant strains are suspected, patients with normal renal function should receive vancomycin, gentamicin, and rifampin (600 mg every 12 hours).[11,14,16,102,103] Vancomycin and gentamicin doses should be adjusted as guided by patient renal function and follow-up serum and possibly CSF concentrations.

Both VA and VP shunts have percutaneous ports that allow direct instillation of antibiotics into the ventricles. Treatment with parenteral and intraventricular antibiotics will result in 35–55% of patients being successfully treated without removal of the shunt. An external ventricular drainage device, established by exteriorizing the infected shunt or by placing a ventricular catheter, is preferred over immediate replacement with a new shunt. Shunt exteriorization with appropriate antibiotic therapy will result in greater than 95% of patients being successfully treated.

Several factors should be evaluated when direct methods are used for instillation of antibiotics into the CNS. Consideration should be given to total CSF volume sensitivity of the offending pathogen, desired antibiotic concentration in CSF, and variability in pharmacokinetics of antibiotics in CSF. As previously discussed, CSF volume varies with age. If antibiotic is delivered to one ventricle, or into the intralumbar space, only a fraction of CSF volume is available for drug distribution. Over the next several hours, the antibiotic begins to equilibrate. With intrathecal administration, distribution of antibiotic throughout the CSF is unlikely. For these reasons, the initial antibiotic concentration in CSF at the point of injection may be several thousand micrograms per milliliter. These extremely high antibiotic concentrations may be potentially irritating and toxic to sensitive neurologic tissue. The sensitivity of the bacterial pathogen and an estimate of CSF volume can be used to arrive at a dose that will produce the desired ratio between the CSF antibiotic concentration and the MBC of the pathogen.

BRAIN ABSCESSES

Brain abscesses are relatively uncommon, with an estimated incidence of 4 per 1,000,000 population.[104–107] Brain abscesses may be caused by a parameningeal focus, extension from a skull fracture, penetrating wound, craniofacial osteomyelitis, dental sepsis, bacterial meningitis, or as a complication of neurosurgery.[104–107] Infections outside the CNS having a bacteremic component (e.g., pneumonia) can result in seeding of the brain with microorganisms and abscess formation. Parameningeal infections (e.g., middle ear or sinuses) cause a brain lesion by direct extension or through vascular channels. The two most likely groups of patients are young males in their thirties and children between 4 and 7 years of age (often with a history of congenital heart disease).[104,105,108]

A prerequisite for the development of a brain abscess is an area of focal ischemia or necrosis. Polycythemic thromboses, hypoxia, or septic emboli can cause ischemia, which can create a microaerophilic environment ideal for anaerobic organisms. Abscesses tend to localize in the white matter, which is more poorly vascularized than the gray matter or the junction between white and gray matter. The inflammation related to the abscess may be associated with cerebral edema and increased intracranial pressure. This further interferes with blood flow to an already ischemic area.[104,105,108]

CLINICAL PRESENTATION

Most patients have a history of symptoms of less than 2 weeks. The primary symptom is headache, which occurs in approximately 75% of patients.[104] Approximately 50% of patients complain of nausea and vomiting, and one-third of patients may have seizures.[104] Fever may or may not be present. Altered states of consciousness with lethargy, confusion, irritability, and coma are common. An underlying history of congenital heart disease, otitis, sinusitis, or pulmonary infection accompanied by this constellation of symptoms should heighten the suspicion of a possible brain abscess.[104,108]

As the abscess begins to enlarge, symptoms become consistent with those of a space-occupying lesion. Most patients at this stage begin to experience significant neurologic sequelae such as hemiplegia, focal or generalized seizures, papilledema, and nuchal rigidity.[104,105,108] Attempts to obtain CSF by lumbar puncture should be approached cautiously, because elevated intracranial pressure may precipitate herniation of the brainstem because of the sudden release in pressure once the needle is inserted into the intrathecal space. Evidence of papilledema may indicate the presence of elevated intracranial pressure; however, computed tomography (CT) has shown evidence of intracranial pressure in patients without evidence of papilledema. CSF is also of little diagnostic value for brain abscess. Usually, patients have an elevated opening pressure on lumbar puncture, pleocytosis with several hundred WBCs (primarily lymphocytes), elevated CSF protein concentration, and normal CSF glucose concentration.[104,105,108] X-rays demonstrate an abnormality in approximately 50% of patients.[104] Perhaps the most useful diagnostic tool is CT with and without contrast. Radionuclide brain scan and arteriography may also be of some help in making the diagnosis.[104,105,108]

During the past several years, several improvements have been made in the isolation and identification of bacteria responsible for causing brain abscesses. Use of anaerobic transport media and expeditious processing on the part of the microbiology laboratory have greatly improved the yield of bacteria from clinical specimens. In most cases, at least two or more species of bacteria are isolated from a bacterial abscess in the CNS. Often, these bacteria tend to be a mixture of aerobes and anaerobes.[104–107] The most common bacterial causes of abscess are streptococci; most notably *Streptococcus milleri, Streptococcus viridans,* nonhemolytic streptococci, enterococcus, β-hemolytic streptococcus, *Peptostreptococcus* spp., and *Bacteroides* spp., which are found in 25–60% of such patients.[104,105,108] The Enterobacteriaceae and *S. aureus* are also associated with brain abscesses. Opportunistic organisms should also be considered when dealing with the immunosuppressed patient.[104,105,108]

TREATMENT

Treatment of brain abscesses is usually accomplished with parenteral antibiotics and surgical removal of purulent material. As in meningitis, antibiotic selection should be guided by the likelihood that the antibiotic selected will produce satisfactory concentrations in the brain tissue. Because meningitis may not be present with brain abscesses, antibiotic selection should be based on the ability of the antibiotic to enter the CNS independent of meningeal inflammation. Some consideration should also be given to the change in environment caused by the abscess. Differences in pH, oxygen tension, presence of WBCs, and presence of purulent material may adversely affect antibiotic performance. Studies done to date demonstrate that penicillin G, chloramphenicol, and clindamycin produce satisfactory but sometimes inconsistent levels in brain tissue.[108] Ampicillin, nafcillin, and cloxacillin have been shown to produce poor concentrations in brain tissue, whereas metronidazole has been shown to produce therapeutic concentrations, even after oral administration.[108] Usually, initial antibiotic regimens include combinations of penicillin G, chloramphenicol, or metronidazole with cefotaxime. These regimens are aimed at streptococci, anaerobes including *Bacteroides fragilis,* enteric bacilli, and *Haemophilus* spp. Patients are usually treated for 6–8 weeks. Very aggressive antibiotic regimens are used (penicillin G 20–40 million units/d, ampicillin 12–18 g/d, cefotaxime 12 g/d, and metronidazole 30 mg/kg/d), with dosages adjusted for age, renal function, and hepatic function.[104,105,108]

Once the abscess lesion has been localized, and if the lesion is operable, neurosurgery may be indicated if the patient has continuous increases in intracranial pressure, continued reduced levels of consciousness, or an increase in neurologic deficits. Aspiration, marsupialization, and excision of the abscess represent standard therapeutic alternatives. Patients who are at increased surgical risk because of underlying medical conditions, multiple abscesses, inoperable lesions, concomitant meningitis/ependymitis, or concomitant hydrocephalus may not be candidates for neurosurgery. Bartlett has shown that with relatively small abscesses, parenteral antibiotics by themselves may effectively reduce and eliminate the abscess.

Approximately 50% of patients with brain abscesses recover without neurologic sequelae. Of the remaining patients, 25% have sequelae but likely can lead a normal life. The other 25% have substantial sequelae that compromise their quality of life. Approximately 10% of patients are severely retarded or cannot be cared for at home. The condition of the patient at the time of presentation to the hospital is a major determining factor in clinical outcome. Patients who are herniating or rupturing or who have substantial underlying diseases are unlikely to have a favorable clinical prognosis.[104,105,108]

Conclusion

The morbidity and mortality of acute bacterial meningitis remains significant despite advances in antimicrobial therapy and supportive care. Through the use of animal models, we are beginning to understand the role of chemical mediators in the pathophysiology of bacterial meningitis. Bacteria initiate an infection, invade the CNS, and induce meningeal inflammation. Rapid CSF sterilization remains a therapeutic goal and the use of dexamethasone as well as other treatment modalities that disrupt the inflammatory process may reduce the morbidity of bacterial meningitis.

The development of rapid diagnostic tests has also improved the clinician's ability to treat CNS infections. Latex agglutination assays are available for each of the major meningeal pathogens. CT and magnetic resonance imaging (MRI) are other diagnostic tools that assist the clinician's ability in treating brain abscesses, as well as fungal and parasitic CNS infections.

The development of more potent, less toxic antimicrobial agents that enter the CNS in therapeutic concentrations should further the therapy of bacterial CNS infections. The third-generation cephalosporins have become the standard of care for many CNS infections, and the triazole antifungals (e.g., fluconazole) have been shown to be effective treatment alternatives to amphotericin B in the management of fungal meningitis.

Routine vaccination of young infants may have an important impact on the future incidence of meningitis in infants and young children. Universal immunization programs are already drastically reducing the incidence of type B *H. influenzae* meningitis in children. Routine vaccination programs may also prove to be an effective strategy in combating penicillin resistant pneumococcal disease. To prevent disease caused by other pathogens, an effective vaccine against group B meningococci must be developed, and the immunogenicity of the pneumococcal and quadravalent meningococcal vaccines must be improved.

Undoubtedly, these advances will have a therapeutic impact on the morbidity and mortality caused by CNS infections.

References

1. Quagliarello VJ, Scheld WM. New perspectives on bacterial meningitis. Clin Infect Dis 1993;17:603–610.
2. Gray LD, Fedorko DP. Laboratory diagnosis of bacterial meningitis. Clin Microbiol Rev 1992;5:130–145.
3. Durand ML, Calderwood SB, Weber DJ, et al. Acute bacterial meningitis in adults. A review of 493 episodes. N Engl J Med 1993;328:21–28.
4. Roos KL, Scheld WM. The management of fulminant meningitis in the intensive care unit. Infect Dis Clin North Am 1989;3:137–155.
5. Tunkel A, Wispelwey B, Scheld W. Pathogenesis and pathophysiology of meningitis. Infect Dis Clin North Am 1990;4:555–581.
6. Wenger J, Hightower A, Group tBMS. Bacterial meningitis in the United States. 1986. Report of a multistate surveillance study. J Infect Dis 1990;162:1316–1323.
7. Adams WG, Deaver KA, Cochi SL, et al. Decline of childhood *Haemophilus influenzae* type b (Hib) disease in the Hib vaccine era. JAMA 1993;269:221–226.
8. Greenlee J. Approach to diagnosis of meningitis, cerebrospinal fluid evaluation. Infect Dis Clin North Am 1990;4:583–598.
9. Robinson R, Robert H. Acute bacterial meningitis I: Diagnosis. Dev Med Child Neurol 1990;32:79–86.
10. Greenlee J. Anatomic considerations in central nervous system infections, in Mandell G, Douglas R, Bennett J (eds): Principles and Practice of Infectious Diseases, 3rd ed. New York, Churchill Livingstone, 1990, pp 732–741.
11. Klein O, Neu HC. Use of antimicrobial agents to treat central nervous system infection. Neurosurg Clin North Am 1992;3:323–341.
12. Kaiser A, McGee Z. Aminoglycoside therapy of gram-negative bacillary meningitis. N Engl J Med 1975;293:1215–1220.
13. Ratcheson R, Ommaya A. Experience with the subcutaneous cerebrospinal fluid reservoir. N Engl J Med 1968;279:1026–1031.

14. Wen DY, Bottini AG, Hall WA, Haines SJ. The intraventricular use of antibiotics. Neurosurg Clin North Am 1992;3:343–355.
15. Wright P, Kaiser A, Bowmann C. The pharmacokinetics and efficacy of an aminoglycoside administered into the cerebral ventricles in neonates: Implications for further evaluation of this route of therapy in meningitis. J Infect Dis 1981;143:141–147.
16. Thea D, Barza M. Use of antibacterial agents in infections of the central nervous system. Infect Dis Clin North Am 1989;3:553–571.
17. Prins J, van Deventer S, Kuijper E, Speelman P. Clinical relevance of antibiotic induced endotoxin release. Antimicrob Agents Chemother 1994;38:1211–1218.
18. Tunkel A, Scheld M. Pathogenesis and pathophysiology of bacterial meningitis. Clin Microbiol Rev 1993;6:118–136.
19. Saez-Llorens X, Ramilo O, Mustafa M. Molecular pathophysiology of bacterial meningitis: Current concepts and therapeutic implications. J Pediatr 1990;116:671–684.
20. Sullivan G, Carper H, Novick WJ. Inhibition of the inflammatory action of interleukin-1 and tumor necrosis factor (alpha) on neutrophil function by pentoxifylline. Infect Immun 1988;56:1722.
21. Verghese A, Gallemore G. Kernig's and Brudzinski's signs revisited. Rev Infect Dis 1987;9:1187–1192.
22. Lipton JD, Schafermeyer RW. Evolving concepts in pediatric bacterial meningitis—Part I: Pathophysiology and diagnosis. Ann Emerg Med 1993;22:1602–1612.
23. Rothrock SG, Green SM, Wren J, et al. Pediatric bacterial meningitis: Is prior antibiotic therapy associated with an altered clinical presentation? Ann Emerg Med 1992;21:146–152.
24. Maxson S, Jacobs RF. Viral meningitis. Tips to rapidly diagnose treatable causes. Postgrad Med 1993;93:153–166.
25. Hansson LO, Axelsson G, Linne T, et al. Serum C-reactive protein in the differential diagnosis of acute meningitis. Scand J Infect Dis 1993;25:625–630.
26. Glimaker M, Kragsbjerg P, Forsgren M, Olcen P. Tumor necrosis factor-alpha (TNFα) in cerebrospinal fluid from patients with meningitis of different etiologies: High levels of TNFα indicate bacterial meningitis. J Infect Dis 1993;167:882–889.
27. Case M, Ryther S, Novitsky T. Detection of endotoxin in antibiotic solutions with limulus amoebocyte lysate. Antimicrob Agents Chemother 1983;23:649–652.
28. Provine H, Gardner P. The Gram-stained smear and its interpretation. Hosp Pract 1974;9:85–91.
29. Gaunt P, Lambert B. Single dose ciprofloxacin for the eradication of pharyngeal carriage of *Neisseria meningitidis.* J Antimicrob Chemother 1988;21:489.
30. Fijen CAP, Kuijper EJ, Tjia HG, et al. Complement deficiency predisposes for meningitis due to nongroupable meningococci and *Neisseria*-related bacteria. Clin Infect Dis 1994;18:780–784.
31. Tauber M, Sande M. General principles of therapy of pyogenic meningitis. Infect Dis Clin North Am 1990;4:661–676.
32. Levison M, Bush L. Pharmacodynamics of antimicrobial agents: Bactericidal and post antibiotic effects. Infect Dis Clin North Am 1990;4:645–659.
33. Lebel MH. Dexamethasone therapy of bacterial meningitis. Antibiot Chemother 1992;45:169–183.
34. Lebel M, Freij BJ, Syrogiannopoulos G. Dexamethasone therapy for bacterial meningitis. Results of two double-blind, placebo-controlled trials. N Engl J Med 1988;319:964–971.
35. Lebel MH, Hoyt J, Waagner DC, et al. Magnetic resonance imaging and dexamethasone therapy for bacterial meningitis. Am J Dis Child 1989;143:301–306.
36. Odio CM, Faingezicht I, Paris M, et al. The beneficial effects of early dexamethasone administration in infants and children with bacterial meningitis. N Engl J Med 1991;324:1527–1531.
37. Girgis NI, Farid Z, Mikhail IA, et al. Dexamethasone treatment for bacterial meningitis in children and adults. Pediatr Infect Dis J 1989;8:848–851.
38. Schaad UB, Lips U, Gnehm HE, et al. Dexamethasone therapy for bacterial meningitis in children. Lancet 1993;342:457–461.
39. Yurkowski PJ, Plaisance KI. Prevention of auditory sequelae in pediatric bacterial meningitis: A meta-analysis. Pharmacother 1993;13:494–499.
40. Havens PL, Wendelberger KJ, Hoffman GM, et al. Corticosteroids as adjunctive therapy in bacterial meningitis. Am J Dis Child 1989;143:1051–1055.
41. Committee on Infectious Diseases. In A. A. O. Pediatrics, (ed): The 1988 Redbook. Elk Grove Village, IL, American Academy of Pediatrics, 1988, pp 204–210.
42. The Meningitis Working Party of the British Paediatric Immunology and Infectious Diseases Group. Should we use dexamethasone in meningitis? Arch Dis Childhood 1992;67:1398–1401.
43. Paris MM, Hickey SM, Uscher MI, et al. Effect of dexamethasone on therapy of experimental penicillin- and cephalosporin-resistant pneumococcal meningitis. Antimicrob Agents Chemother 1994;38:1320–1324.
44. Gaillard JL, Abadie V, Cheron G, et al. Concentrations of ceftriaxone in cerebrospinal fluid of children with meningitis receiving dexamethasone therapy. Antimicrob Agents Chemother 1994;38:1209–1210.
45. Kennedy WA, Hoyt MJ, McCracken GHJ. The role of corticosteroid therapy in children with pneumococcal meningitis. Am J Dis Child 1991;145:1374–1378.
46. Syrogiannopoulos GA, Lourida AN, Theodoridou MC, et al. Dexamethasone therapy for bacterial meningitis in children: 2- versus 4-day regimen. J Infect Dis 1994;169:853–858.
47. Weinstein L. Bacterial meningitis. Med Clin North Am 1985;69:219–229.
48. Dodge P, Davis H, Feigin R. Prospective evaluation of hearing impairment as a sequela of acute bacterial meningitis. N Engl J Med 1984;311:869–874.
49. Pomeroy SL, Holmes SJ, Dodge PR, Feigin RD. Seizures and other neurologic sequelae of bacterial meningitis in children. N Engl J Med 1990;323:1651–1656.
50. Van Esso D, Fortanals D, Uriz S. *Neisseria meningitidis* strains with decreased susceptibility to penicillin. Pediatr Infect Dis J 1987;6:483.
51. Schwartz B. Chemoprophylaxis for bacterial infections: Principles of and application to meningococcal infections. Rev Infect Dis 1991;13:S170–S173.
52. Lieberman J, Greenberg D, Ward J. Prevention of bacterial meningitis. Vaccines and chemoprophylaxis. Infect Dis Clin North Am 1990;4:703–729.

53. Cuevas LE, Hart CA. Chemoprophylaxis of bacterial meningitis. J Antimicrob Chemother 1993;31:79–91.
54. Pugsley M, Sworzack D, Horowitz E. Efficacy of ciprofloxacin in the treatment of nasopharyngeal carriers of *Neisseria meningitidis.* J Infect Dis 1987;156:211–213.
55. Schwartz B, Al-Ruwais A, As'Ashi J. Comparative efficacy of ceftriaxone and rifampicin in eradicating pharyngeal carriage of group A *Neisseria meningitidis.* Lancet 1988;1:1239–1242.
56. Appelbaum PC. Antimicrobial resistance in *Streptococcus pneumoniae:* An overview. Clin Infect Dis 1992;15:77–83.
57. Caputo GM, Appelbaum PC, Liu HH. Infections due to penicillin-resistant pneumococci. Clinical, epidemiologic, and microbiologic features. Arch Intern Med 1993;153:1301–1310.
58. Anonymous. Prevalence of penicillin-resistant *Streptococcus pneumoniae*—Connecticut, 1992–1993. Morb Mortal Wkly Rep 1994;43:216–217, 223.
59. Cherubin C, Eng R, Norrby R. Penetration of newer cephalosporins into cerebrospinal fluid. Rev Infect Dis 1989;11:526–548.
60. Jacobs MR. Treatment and diagnosis of infections caused by drug-resistant *Streptococcus pneumoniae.* Clin Infect Dis 1992;15:119–127.
61. Jose Catalan M, Fernandez JM, Vazquez A, et al. Failure of cefotaxime in the treatment of meningitis due to relatively resistant *Streptococcus pneumoniae.* Clin Infect Dis 1994;18:766–769.
62. John CC. Treatment failure with use of a third-generation cephalosporin for penicillin-resistant pneumococcal meningitis: Case report and review. Clin Infect Dis 1994;18:188–193.
63. Friedland IR, Paris M, Ehrett S, et al. Evaluation of antimicrobial regimens for treatment of experimental penicillin- and cephalosporin-resistant pneumococcal meningitis. Antimicrob Agents Chemother 1993;37:1630–1636.
64. Luer M, Hatton J. Vancomycin administration into the cerebrospinal fluid: A review. Ann Pharmacother 1993;27:912–921.
65. Butler JC, Breiman RF, Campbell JF. Pneumococcal polysaccharide vaccine efficacy. JAMA 1993;270:1826–1831.
66. Zabinski R, Vance-Bryan K, Rotschafer J. The management of central nervous system infections. J Pharm Practice 1991;4:170–191.
67. Korvick JA, Yu VL. Antimicrobial agent therapy for pseudomonas aeruginosa. Antimicrob Agents Chemother 1991;35:2167–2172.
68. Rodriguez W, Khan W, Cocchetto D. Treatment of *Pseudomonas* meningitis with ceftazidime with or without concurrent therapy. Pediatr Infect Dis J 1990;9:83–87.
69. Wolff MA, Young CL, Ramphal R. Antibiotic therapy for enterobacter meningitis: A retrospective review of 13 episodes and review of the literature. Clin Infect Dis 1993;16:772–777.
70. Wolff M, Boutron L, Singlas E. Penetration of ciprofloxacin into cerebrospinal fluid of patients with bacterial meningitis. Antimicrob Agents Chemother 1987;31:899–902.
71. Tunkel A, Scheld M. Pathogenesis and pathophysiology of bacterial meningitis. Clin Microbiol Rev 1993;6:118–136.
72. Centers for Disease Control. Recommendations for use of *Haemophilus* b conjugate vaccines and a combined diphtheria, tetanus, pertussis, and *Haemophilus* b vaccine. Morb Mortal Wkly Rep 1993;42:1–15.
73. American Academy of Pediatrics. AAP formulates provisional recommendations for use of HIB vaccine in younger infants. AAP News Release, 1990.
74. Rubin R, Hooper D. Central nervous system infection in the compromised host. Med Clin North Am 1985;69:281–296.
75. Leonard J, Dez Prez R. Tuberculous meningitis. Infect Dis Clin North Am 1990;4:769–787.
76. Holdiness M. Management of tuberculosis meningitis. Drugs 1990;39:224–233.
77. Kent SJ, Crowe SM, Yung A, et al. Tuberculous meningitis: A 30-year review. Clin Infect Dis 1993;17:987–994.
78. Block AB, Cauthen GM, Onorato IM. Nationwide survey of drug-resistant tuberculosis in the United States. JAMA 1994;271:665–671.
79. Centers for Disease Control. Initial therapy for tuberculosis in the era of multidrug resistance. Recommendations of the Advisory Council for the Elimination of Tuberculosis. Morb Mortal Wkly Rep 1993;42:1–8.
80. Ellard GA, Humphries MJ, Allen BW. Cerebrospinal fluid drug concentrations and the treatment of tuberculous meningitis. Am Rev Resp Dis 1993;148:650–655.
81. Alzeer AH, FitzGerald JM. Corticosteroids and tuberculosis: Risks and use as adjunct therapy. Tubercle Lung Dis 1993;74:6–11.
82. Dismukes WE. Management of cryptococcus. Clin Infect Dis 1993;17:S507–S512.
83. Sugar A, Stern J, Dupont B. Overview: Treatment of cryptococcal meningitis. Rev Infect Dis 1990;12:S338–S348.
84. Powderly WG, Cloud GA, Dismukes WE, Saag MS. Measurement of cryptococcal antigen in serum and cerebrospinal fluid: Value in the management of AIDS-associated cryptococcal meningitis. Clin Infect Dis 1994;18:789–792.
85. Powderly WG. Therapy for cryptococcal meningitis in patients with AIDS. Clin Infect Dis 1992;14:S54–S59.
86. Bennett JE, Dismukes W, Duma R. A comparison of amphotericin B alone and combined with flucytosine in the treatment of cryptococcal meningitis. N Engl J Med 1979;301:126–131.
87. Chuck SL, Sande MA. Infections with *Cryptococcus neoformans* in the acquired immunodeficiency syndrome. N Engl J Med 1989;321:794–799.
88. Coker RJ, Viviani M, Gazzard BG. Treatment of Cryptococcosis with liposomal amphotericin B (AmBisome) in 23 patients with AIDS. AIDS 1993;7:829–835.
89. Saag MS, Powderly WG, Cloud GA, et al. Comparison of amphotericin B with fluconazole in the treatment of acute AIDS-associated cryptococcal meningitis. N Engl J Med 1992;326:83–89.
90. Berry AJ, Finaldi MG, Graybill JR. Use of high-dose fluconazole as salvage therapy for cryptococcal meningitis in patients with AIDS. Antimicrob Agents Chemother 1992;36:690–692.
91. de Gans J, Portegies P, Tiessens G. Itraconazole compared with amphotericin B plus flucytosine in AIDS patients with cryptococcal meningitis. AIDS 1992;6:185–190.

92. Jones BE, Larsen RA, Bozzette S, et al. A phase II trial of fluconazole plus flucytosine for cryptococcal meningitis [abstract], in Abstracts of the VII International Conference on AIDS. Rome, Instituto Superiore di Sanita, 1991.
93. Powderly WG, Saag MS, Cloud GA. A controlled trial of fluconazole or amphotericin B to prevent relapse of cryptococcal meningitis in patients with the acquired immunodeficiency syndrome. N Engl J Med 1992;326:793–798.
94. Nelsen S, Sealy DP, Schneider EF. The aseptic meningitis syndrome. Am Fam Phys 1993;48:809–815.
95. Dalton M, Newton RW. Aseptic meningitis. Develop Med Child Neurol 1991;33:446–458.
96. Marinac JS. Drug- and chemical-induced aseptic meningitis: A review of the literature. Ann Pharmaco 1992;26:813–821.
97. Rubeiz H, Roos RP. Viral meningitis and encephalitis. Sem Neurology 1992;12:165–177.
98. Glimaker M. Enteroviral meningitis. Diagnostic methods and aspects on the distinction from bacterial meningitis. Scand J Infect Dis 1992;85:1–64.
99. Overall JCJ. Is it bacterial or viral? Laboratory differentiation. Pediatr Rev 1993;14:251–261.
100. Connolly K, Hammer S. The acute aseptic meningitis syndrome. Infect Dis Clin North Am 1990;4:599–622.
101. Gateley A, Gander R, Johnson P. Herpes simplex virus type 2 meningoencephalitis resistant to acyclovir in a patient with AIDS. J Infect Dis 1990;161:711.
102. Kaufman B, Tunkel A, Pryor J. Meningitis in the neurosurgical patient. Infect Dis Clin North Am 1990;4:677–701.
103. Walters BC. Cerebrospinal fluid shunt infection. Neurosurg Clin North Am 1992;3:387–401.
104. Wispelwey B, Scheld W. Brain abscess, in Mandell G, Douglas R, Bennett J (eds): Principles and Practice of Infectious Diseases, 3rd ed. New York, Churchill Livingstone, 1990, pp 777–788.
105. Saez-Llorens X, Unana M, Odio C. Brain abscess in infants and children. Pediatr Infect Dis 1989;8:449–458.
106. Carpenter JL. Brain stem abscesses: Cure with medical therapy, case report, and review. Clin Infect Dis 1994;18:219–226.
107. Osenbach RK, Loftus CM. Diagnosis and management of brain abscess. Neurosurg Clin North Am 1992;3:403–421.
108. Donald F. Treatment of brain abscess. J Antimicrob Chemother 1990;25:310–312.
109. Salmon J. Ventriculitis complicating meningitis. Am J Dis Child 1972;124:35–40.
110. McLaurin R. Infected cerebrospinal fluid shunts. Surg Neurol 1973;1:191–195.
111. Wald S, McLaurin R. Cerebrospinal fluid antibiotic levels during treatment of shunt infections. J Neurosurg 1980;S2:41–46.
112. Gardner P, Leipzig T, Phillips P. Infections of central nervous system shunts. Med Clin North Am 1985;69:297–314.
113. Sells C, Shurtleff D, Loeser J. Gram-negative cerebrospinal fluid shunt associated infections. Pediatrics 1977;59:613–619.
114. Sklaver A, Greenman R, Hoffman T. Amikacin therapy of gram-negative bacteremia and meningitis. Arch Intern Med 1978;138:713–716.
115. Wirt T, McGee Z, Oldfield E, Meecham W. Intraventricular administration of amikacin for complicated gram-negative meningitis and ventriculitis. J Neurosurg 1979;50:95–99.
116. Congeni B, Tan J, Salstrom S. Kinetics of vancomycin after intraventricular and intravenous administration. Pediatr Res 1979;13:459–463.
117. Visconti E, Peter G. Vancomycin cerebrospinal fluid shunt infections. J Neurosurg 1979;51:245–246.
118. Pau A, Samego R, Fisher M. Intraventricular vancomycin: Observation of tolerance and pharmacokinetics in two infants with ventricular shunt infections. Pediatr Infect Dis 1986;5:93–96.

Chapter 100

Lower Respiratory Tract Infections

Philip Toltzis, MD, Madolin K. Witte, MD, and Michael D. Reed, PharmD

The treatment of infections arising within the respiratory tract continues to be a common yet therapeutically challenging clinical concern. Respiratory infections remain the major cause of morbidity from acute illness in the United States, and most likely represent the single most common reason patients seek medical attention. These demographic data have far-reaching implications when considering the dramatic changes occurring in methods of health care reimbursement within the United States today. This chapter focuses on bacterial and viral infections involving the lower respiratory tract, which includes the tracheobronchial tree and lung parenchyma.

Lung Defenses

A description of lower respiratory tract infections would be incomplete without a brief discussion of the physiologic mechanisms by which lungs normally resist infection (for greater detail please see Refs. 1–4). The respiratory tract has an elaborate system of host defenses, including humoral mechanisms, cellular mechanisms, and important mechanical mechanisms such as the mucociliary transport system.[1–4] When functioning properly, the host defenses of the respiratory tract are markedly effective in protecting against pathogen invasion and in removing potentially infectious agents from the lungs.[2–4] For the most part, infections in the lower respiratory tract occur only when these defense mechanisms are impaired. Examples of impaired defenses would include dysgammaglobulinemia or compromised ciliary function caused by the chronic inflammation that accompanies cigarette smoking. In addition, local defenses may be overwhelmed when a particularly virulent microorganism or excessive inoculum invades lung parenchyma. The majority of pulmonary infections follow colonization of the upper respiratory tract with potential pathogens, which, after achieving sufficiently high concentrations, gain access to the lung via aspiration of oropharyngeal secretions. Less commonly, microbes enter the lung via the blood from an extrapulmonary source or by the inhalation of infected aerosolized particles. The specific type of pulmonary infection caused by an invading microorganism is determined by a variety of host factors, including age, the anatomic features of the airway, and specific characteristics of the infecting agent. The most common infections involving the lower respiratory tract include bronchitis, bronchiolitis, pneumonia, and lung abscess.

General Approach to Diagnosis

Lower respiratory tract infections in both children and adults are most commonly a result of either viral or bacterial invasion of lung parenchyma. The diagnosis of viral infections rests primarily on the recognition of a characteristic constellation of clinical signs and symptoms. Since treatment is largely supportive, only occasionally does the diagnosis require laboratory confirmation; this is achieved through serologic tests or the identification of the organism by culture or antigen detection in respiratory secretions. In contrast, since bacterial pneumonia usually necessitates expedient, effective, and specific antibiotic therapy, its management depends, in large part, on isolation of the etiologic agent by culture from lung tissue or secretions. The pharynx is colonized with many organisms that can potentially cause pneumonia; therefore, culture of expectorated sputum can be misleading unless the specimen is examined to ensure that it has originated from the lower respiratory tract.[5,6] The Gram stain provides the easiest method to distinguish lower from upper respiratory tract secretions; moreover, through determination of the shape and color of the bacteria, the Gram stain frequently narrows the microbiological differential diagnosis sufficiently to allow accurate initial therapy. Scanned under low power (10×) microscopy, Gram-stained expectorated upper respiratory tract secretions contain many irregularly shaped epithelial cells with little evidence of

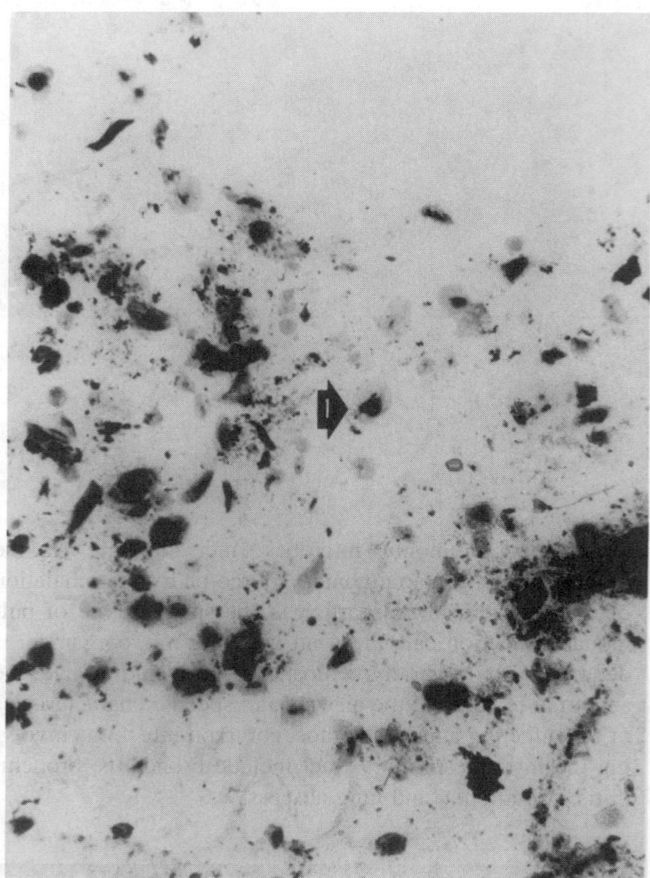

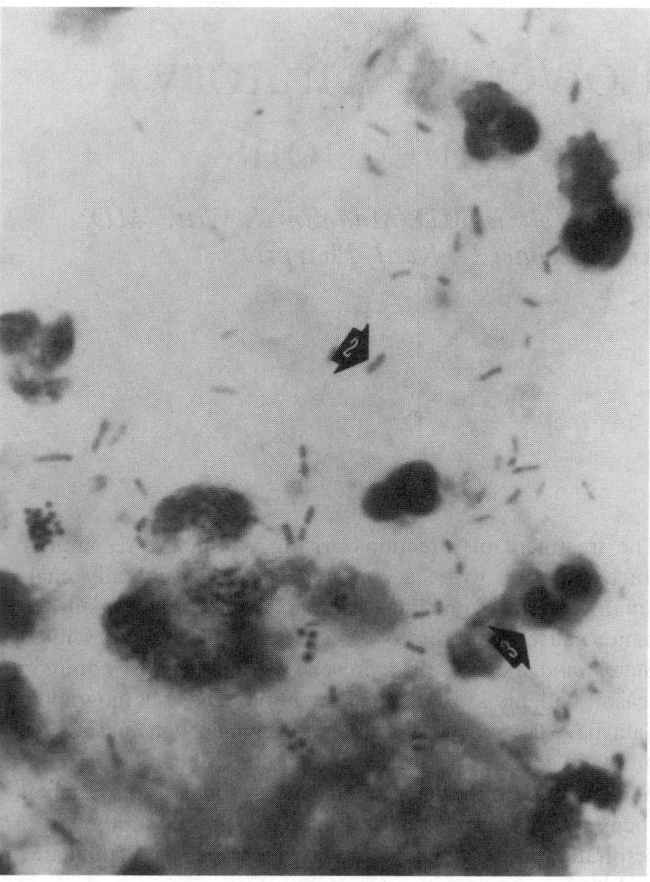

Figure 100.1. Gram stain of sputum. *Left panel.* Scanned under low power (10×), this sample contains many irregularly shaped epithelial cells (arrow 1) and no inflammatory cells, indicating that the specimen was derived from the upper respiratory tract. *Right panel.* Under oil emersion (100×), this specimen contains a predominance of gram-negative rods (arrow 2) and many polymorphonuclear cells (arrow 3) per high power field, confirming that this specimen was derived from the lower respiratory tract. The sample grew *Klebsiella pneumoniae.*

inflammation and microorganisms of a variety of morphologies are present (Fig. 100.1). In contrast, a lower tract specimen from a patient with bacterial pneumonia usually contains multiple neutrophils per high-powered field and a single, predominant bacterial species. Culture of specimens confirmed to originate from the lower tract by Gram stain provide valuable diagnostic information in the majority of patients with bacterial pneumonia.[7,8]

An accurate treatment regimen for the patient with uncomplicated lower respiratory tract infection can usually be established by the history, physical examination, chest radiograph, and properly collected sputum cultures interpreted in light of current knowledge of the most common lung pathogens and their antibiotic sensitivity patterns within one's community. More invasive diagnostic methods (e.g., transtracheal aspiration, lung biopsy, etc.) should be reserved for very ill patients who are unable to expectorate sputum or are not responding to empiric therapy, or for pulmonary infections occurring in the immunocompromised patient. Although expensive, sophisticated radiographic evaluations may be useful in selected patients in defining or confirming a diagnosis of specific lung infection.[9]

Transtracheal aspiration is a safe technique for sampling lower respiratory tract secretions and yields bacteriologic results more reliable than those obtained from routine sputum collection.[10] Lower tract specimens also can be obtained through flexible bronchoscopy, using either a protected brush to avoid contamination from organisms in the upper respiratory tract, or through bronchoalveolar lavage.[11] Transbronchial and open lung biopsy offer a high diagnostic yield but carry a substantially increased risk of morbidity including pneumothorax and bleeding.[9]

BRONCHITIS

The bronchiolitides (i.e., bronchitis and bronchiolitis) refer to an inflammatory condition of the tracheobronchial tree that is usually associated with a generalized respiratory infection. The infectious agents are usually of viral origin, and the inflammatory process does not extend to include the alveoli. The diagnosis of bronchitis or bronchiolitis is based primarily on clinical considerations. In an attempt to more specifically describe bronchitis, the disease entity is frequently classified as either acute or chronic. Acute bronchitis most commonly occurs in the young and old, whereas bronchiolitis is a disease of infancy. Chronic bronchitis primarily affects adults.

ACUTE BRONCHITIS

Epidemiology

Acute bronchitis most commonly occurs during the winter months, following a pattern very similar to those of other acute respiratory tract infections. Cold, damp climates and/or the presence of high concentrations of irritating substances such as air pollution or cigarette smoke may precipitate attacks.[12,13]

Etiology

Respiratory viruses are by far the most common infectious agents associated with acute bronchitis. The common cold viruses, rhinovirus and coronavirus, and lower respiratory tract pathogens, including influenza virus, adenovirus, and respiratory syncytial virus, account for the majority of cases. In children, similar pathogens are observed with the addition of the parainfluenza viruses. While the true incidence remains to be defined, *Mycoplasma pneumonia* also appears to be a frequent cause of acute bronchitis. More recently, a new *Chlamydia psittaci* strain, often denoted as TWAR or *Chlamydia pneumoniae,* has been associated with acute respiratory tract infections.[14] Although a variety of bacteria including *Streptococcus pneumonia, Streptococcus* spp., *Staphylococcus* spp., and *Haemophilus* spp. may be isolated from throat or sputum culture, it is probable that these organisms represent contamination by normal flora of the upper respiratory tract rather than true pathogens. While a primary bacterial etiology for acute bronchitis appears rare, secondary bacterial infection may be involved; however, the exact significance of a secondary bacterial infection is not well established.

Pathogenesis

Because acute bronchitis is primarily a self-limiting illness and rarely a cause of death, limited data are available to describe the actual pathology or pathophysiology. In general, infection of the trachea and bronchi yields hyperemic and edematous mucous membranes with an increase in bronchial secretions. Destruction of respiratory epithelium can range from mild to extensive and may affect bronchial mucociliary function.[15] In addition, the increase in bronchial secretions, which can become thick and tenacious, further impairs mucociliary activity. The probability of permanent damage to the airways as a result of acute bronchitis remains unclear; however, epidemiologic evaluations support the belief that recurrent acute respiratory infections may be associated with increased airway hyperreactivity and possibly the pathogenesis of chronic obstructive lung disease.[13,16,17]

Clinical Presentation

The initial manifestations of acute bronchitis are primarily upper respiratory in nature. Depending on the etiologic agent, symptoms may be predominantly nasal as with the common cold or may involve the pharynx as in nasopharyngitis. Nonspecific complaints including malaise and headache frequently accompany the coryza and sore throat. Cough is the hallmark of acute bronchitis and occurs early. The onset of cough may be insidious or abrupt and will persist despite the resolution of nasal or nasopharyngeal complaints. Frequently, the cough is initially nonproductive but progresses, yielding mucopurulent sputum. In older children and adults, the sputum is raised and expectorated; in the young child, sputum is often swallowed and can result in gagging and vomiting. Substantial discomfort may result from the coughing. Dyspnea, cyanosis, or signs of airway obstruction are rarely observed unless the patient has underlying pulmonary disease (e.g., emphysema, chronic obstructive pulmonary disease). Fever, when present, rarely exceeds 39°C and appears most commonly with adenovirus, influenza virus, and *M. pneumonia* infections.

Initial physical examination is generally unimpressive, usually revealing a variable degree of rhinitis. Chest examination may reveal rhonchi and coarse, moist rales bilaterally. Chest radiographs, when performed, are usually normal. The diagnosis is usually made on the basis of a typical history and physical examination without the need for microbiological confirmation. Bacterial cultures of expectorated sputum are generally of limited utility due to the inability to avoid normal nasopharyngeal flora by the sampling technique. In routine cases, viral cultures are unnecessary and frequently unavailable. Viral antigen detection tests, developed to rapidly identify respiratory viral antigens from nasal secretions, can be obtained in many hospital laboratories and in some practice settings when a specific diagnosis is necessary for clinical or epidemiological reasons.[18] Cultures or serologic diagnosis of *M. pneumonia* and culture or direct fluorescent antibody detection for *Bordetella pertussis* should be obtained in prolonged or severe cases when epidemiologic considerations would suggest their involvement.[19] The white blood cell (WBC) count is usually normal or slightly elevated (>10,000/mm^3) with a predominance of neutrophils in approximately one-third of the cases.

Treatment

The treatment of acute bronchitis is symptomatic and supportive in nature. Bed rest and mild analgesic–antipyretic therapy are often helpful in relieving the associated lethargy, malaise, and fever. Aspirin or acetaminophen (650 mg in adults or 10–15 mg/kg per dose in children) or ibuprofen (200–400 mg in adults or 10 mg/kg per dose in children) should be administered every 4–6 hours. In children, aspirin should be avoided and acetaminophen used as the preferred agent because of the possible association between aspirin use and the development of Reye's syndrome.[20] More recently, the use of ibuprofen as an antipyretic has increased. The drug's antipyretic efficacy appears identical to that of aspirin or acetaminophen although its duration of antipyretic effect may be slightly longer (e.g., 3–4 hours for aspirin and acetaminophen versus 5–6 hours for ibuprofen). Caution should be exercised in the administration of ibuprofen in very young and elderly patients and in individuals with poor renal function. Aspirin and ibuprofen inhibit prostaglandin synthesis and may adversely influence renal function in these predisposed patient populations.

Patients suffering from acute bronchitis frequently medicate themselves with over-the-counter cough and cold remedies containing various combinations of antihistamines, sympathomimetics, and antitussives despite the lack of definitive evidence supporting their effectiveness. In fact, the tendency of these agents to dehydrate bronchial secretions could potentially aggravate and prolong the recovery process. Patients should be encouraged to drink fluids to prevent dehydration and possibly decrease the viscosity of respiratory secretions. Mist therapy and/or the use of a vaporizer may further promote the thinning and loosening of respiratory secretions.[21] Persistent, mild cough, which may be bothersome, may be treated with dextromethorphan; more severe coughs may require intermittent codeine or other similar agents.[22] In severe cases, cough may be persistent enough to disrupt sleep, and the use of a mild sedative–hypnotic, concomitantly with a cough suppressant, may be desirable; however, antitussives should be used cautiously when the cough is productive. The primary or supplemental use of expectorants is questionable because their clinical effectiveness has not been well established.[22]

Routine use of antibiotics in the treatment of acute bronchitis should be discouraged; however, in patients who exhibit persistent fever or respiratory symptomatology for more than 4–6 days, the possibility of a concurrent bacterial infection should be suspected. When possible, antibiotic therapy should be directed toward anticipated respiratory pathogen(s) (i.e., *Streptococcus pneumonia, Haemophilus influenzae*) and/or those demonstrating a predominant growth upon throat culture. *Mycoplasma pneumonia,* if suspected by history or positive cold agglutinins (titers ≥ 1:32), or if confirmed by culture or serology, may be treated with erythromycin or its analogues. During known epidemics involving the influenza A virus, amantadine or rimantadine may be effective in minimizing associated symptomatology if administered early in the course of the disease.[23] In severe cases occurring in debilitated patients or patients with underlying cardiac or pulmonary disease, aerosolized ribavirin therapy may be beneficial. At present, however, the exact role of ribavirin therapy remains to be defined (see section on Bronchiolitis).

CHRONIC BRONCHITIS

Epidemiology

Chronic bronchitis is a nonspecific disease that affects primarily adults. Current estimates suggest that between 10% and 25% of the adult population 40 or older suffer from chronic bronchitis. Despite prevailing confusion surrounding the diagnosis and treatment of chronic bronchitis, it is clear from these figures that this disease entity is responsible for substantial health care dollar expenditures and lost wages.[24] Similar to acute bronchitis, cold, damp climates and the presence of elevated airborne concentrations of irritating substances may favor this disease.[24,25] Chronic bronchitis occurs more commonly in men than in women.

Etiology

Despite the recognition for decades of chronic bronchitis as a specific disease entity, the exact cause of this disease (or syndrome?) remains unidentified. Current data and experience suggest that chronic bronchitis is a result of several contributing factors; the most prominent of these include cigarette smoking, exposure to occupational dusts, fumes, and environmental pollution, and bacterial (and possibly viral) infection. The influence that each of these factors and others, either alone or in combination, contributes to the etiology and prevalence of chronic bronchitis is unknown. Cigarette smoke is a well-known airway irritant and is believed by many to be the predominant factor in the etiology of chronic bronchitis. Studies of lungs from smoking and nonsmoking individuals have clearly demonstrated a substantial increase in the number of alveolar macrophages,[25] as well as the presence of bronchial inflammation, in individuals who smoke cigarettes. Although the majority of patients who suffer from chronic bronchitis have a positive smoking history, no history of smoking can be identified in as many as 10% of cases. These findings suggest that additional airway irritants, either alone or more probably in combination, are responsible for the pathogenesis of chronic bronchitis.

In addition to the preceding, the influence of recurrent respiratory tract infections during childhood or young adult life on the later development of chronic bronchitis remains obscure. The available data suggest that recurrent respiratory infections at a young age predispose individuals to the development of chronic bronchitis;[17] however, it is unclear whether these recurrent respiratory tract infections are a result of unrecognized anatomic abnormalities of the airways or impaired pulmonary defense mechanisms.

Pathogenesis

As discussed previously, the chronic inhalation of an irritating noxious substance compromises the normal secretory and mucociliary function of bronchial mucosa. In chronic bronchitis, the bronchial wall is thickened and the number of mucus-secreting goblet cells in the surface epithelium of both larger and smaller bronchi is markedly increased.[26] In contrast, goblet cells are generally absent from the smaller bronchi of normal individuals. In addition to the increased number of goblet cells, hypertrophy of the mucus glands and dilatation of the mucus gland ducts are also observed.[26] As a result of these changes, chronic bronchitics have substantially more mucus in their peripheral airways, further impairing normal lung defenses. This increased quantity of tenacious secretions within the bronchial tree frequently causes mucus plugging of the smaller airways. Accompanying these changes are squamous cell metaplasia of the surface epithelium, edema and increased vascularity of the basement membrane of larger airways, and variable chronic inflammatory cell infiltration.[26] Continued progression of this pathology can result in residual scarring of small bronchi, augmenting airway obstruction and the weakening of bronchial walls.

Clinical Presentation

The hallmark of chronic bronchitis is cough that, depending on the severity of the disease, may range from a mild "smoker's" cough to severe incessant coughing productive of purulent sputum. Coughing may be precipitated by multiple stimuli including simple, normal conversation. Expectoration of the largest quantity of sputum usually occurs upon arising in the morning, although many patients expectorate sputum throughout the day. The expectorated sputum is usually tenacious and can vary in color from white to yellow-green. As a result, many patients complain of a frequent bad taste in their mouth and halitosis. In the absence of an acute pulmonary exacerbation of chronic bronchitis or another concurrent or underlying illness, most chronic bronchitics remain professionally and socially active.

The diagnosis of chronic bronchitis is based primarily on clinical assessment and history. By definition, any patient who reports the coughing up of sputum on most days for at least 3 consecutive months each year for 2 consecutive years suffers from chronic bronchitis.[27] The diagnosis of chronic bronchitis is made only when the possibilities of bronchiectasis, cardiac failure, cystic fibrosis, and lung carcinoma have been effectively excluded. In an attempt to be more specific in the diagnosis, some investigators have added lost wages for 3 or more weeks to the criteria. In addition, many clinicians attempt to subdivide their patients into one of three subgroups: (1) those patients with "simple" chronic bronchitis, (2) those with chronic or recurrent mucopurulent bronchitis (based on the presence of mucopurulent sputum confirmed by microscopic analysis), and (3) those with chronic obstructive bronchitis (based on the clinical history and the presence of airway obstruction documented by pulmonary function testing). Much of the confusion and controversy surrounding the diagnosis, clinical assessment, and evaluation of therapeutic intervention in chronic bronchitis results from inconsistencies in the definition and application of diagnostic criteria.

With the exception of pulmonary findings, the physical examination of patients with mild to moderate chronic bronchitis is usually unremarkable. Chest auscultation usually reveals inspiratory and expiratory rales, rhonchi, and mild wheezing with an expiratory phase that is frequently prolonged. Normal vesicular breathing sounds are diminished. Depending on the severity of the disease, an increase in the anteroposterior diameter of the thoracic cage (observed as a "barrel chest"), hyperresonance on percussion with obliteration of the area of cardiac dullness, and depressed diaphragms with limited mobility are often observed. In more advanced stages, cyanosis is common and may be accompanied by a compensatory erythrocytosis. Clubbing of the digits is infrequent, but when observed is usually reflective of advanced disease. In more advanced stages of chronic bronchitis, physical findings associated with cor pulmonale including cardiac enlargement, hepatomegaly, and edema of the lower extremities may be observed. In general, chronic bronchitics tend to maintain at least normal body weight and are commonly obese. Radiographic studies are of limited value either in the diagnosis or as a means of sequentially following a patient. A decrease in vital capacity and a prolongation of expiratory flow are usually found from pulmonary function studies.

Although the results may infrequently be difficult to interpret, the microscopic and laboratory assessment of sputum is considered an important component in the overall evaluation of patients with chronic bronchitis. When performed, a fresh sputum specimen obtained as an early morning sample is preferred. Comparison of the cellular constituents of chronic bronchitic sputum with those of normal sputum can provide insight into the degree of activity of the disease processes.[24,28] An increased number of polymorphonuclear granulocytes often suggests continual bronchial irritation, whereas an increased number of eosinophils may suggest an allergic component that should be further investigated. Ciliated epithelial cells may also be identified and appear to correlate with the amount of coughing the patient has undergone to produce the sputum. Gram staining of the sputum often reveals a mixture of both gram-positive and gram-negative bacteria, reflecting normal oropharyngeal flora and tracheal colonization by *S. pneumonia* and *H. influenzae.* The role of sputum culture in the assessment of lung infection in chronic bronchitis remains controversial and is discussed in further detail later. The most common bacterial isolates identified from sputum culture in patients experiencing an acute exacerbation of chronic bronchitis are outlined in Table 100.1

Treatment

The approach to the treatment of chronic bronchitis must be multifactorial. A complete occupational/environmental history for the determination of exposure to noxious, irritating gases, as well as preference toward cigarette smoking must be assessed. Often easier discussed than accomplished, honest yet reasonable attempts should be made with the patient to reduce either their exposure to (i.e., "second-hand" smoke) or reduce or eliminate completely the number of cigarettes smoked daily. In an organized, coordinated cessation program (e.g., counseling, hypnotherapy), the adjunctive use of nicotine substitutes (e.g., nicotine gum) may promote reduction or complete withdrawal from cigarette smoking. Often just as difficult is the modification of exposure to irritating substances within the home and the workplace.

During acute pulmonary exacerbations of the disease, a patient's ability to mobilize and expectorate sputum may be dramatically reduced. In these instances, attempts at postural drainage techniques, with instruction and/or active participation from a respiratory therapist, may assist in promoting clearance of pulmonary secretions. In addition, humidification of inspired air may promote the hydration (liquefaction) of tenacious secretions allowing for more productive removal. The use of mucolytic aerosols (e.g., *N*-acetylcysteine; DNAse) is of questionable therapeutic value, particularly considering their propensity to induce bronchospasm and excessive cost. Similarly, the value of prepostural and postpostural drainage bronchodilator aerosols remains to be defined. In contrast, oral or aerosolized bronchodilators may be of benefit to some patients during acute pulmonary exacerbations. For those patients that consistently demonstrate clinical limitation in airflow, a therapeutic challenge of bronchodilators (e.g., albuterol aerosol) should be considered. Although chronic theophylline administration has been extensively used in the past, this therapy is being used with decreasing frequency in favor of aerosolized β_2-receptor agonists. Albuterol is most commonly used, 1 to 2 puffs of the metered dose inhaler 3 to 4 times daily. The role, if any, of the long-acting β_2-receptor agonist, salmeterol, in these patients is unknown.

TABLE 100.1. COMMON BACTERIAL PATHOGENS ISOLATED FROM THE SPUTUM OF PATIENTS WITH AN ACUTE EXACERBATION OF CHRONIC BRONCHITIS

Pathogen	Estimated Incidence[a]
Haemophilus influenzae[b]	24–26
Haemophilus parainfluenzae	20
Streptococcus pneumoniae	15
Moraxella catarrhalis[b]	15
Klebsiella pneumoniae	4
Serratia marcescens	2
Neisseria meningitidis[b]	2
Pseudomonas aeruginosa	2

[a]Expressed as percent of cultures.
[b]Often β-lactamase positive.

In contrast to the preceding, further treatment recommendations are less clear. Determination of an optimal therapy is hampered by a lack of uniformity in definition of chronic bronchitis and by a lack of consensus as to what constitutes an acute pulmonary exacerbation. In the most simple terms, an acute pulmonary exacerbation of chronic bronchitis is characterized by an increased cough, dyspnea, and alterations in appearance and amount of sputum produced. As previously discussed, some clinicians have added to these clinical findings a change in a patient's "normal" quiescent state, as well as lost wages. Substantial confusion relative to treatment guidelines has resulted from these less than critical and often conflicting opinions in our understanding of what establishes an acute pulmonary exacerbation of chronic bronchitis. Furthermore, this confusion has dramatically limited our understanding of the therapeutic impact of antimicrobial therapy. To better assess the occurrence of an infectious cause of an acute exacerbation, some investigators[24] suggest careful examination of sputum for increased numbers of bacteria and neutrophils over baseline values when the patient is clinically stable.

A plethora of studies have attempted to describe a beneficial effect of antibiotic administration upon the acute and chronic treatment of chronic bronchitics (see Tables 100.2 and 100.3 for selected citations). Numerous comparative evaluations including placebo-controlled studies have suggested definite clinical benefit, whereas other similar studies have not. The antibiotics most frequently selected (e.g., ampicillin, tetracycline, chloramphenicol, trimethoprim–sulfamethoxazole) possess variable *in vitro* activity against the common sputum isolates *H. influenzae, S. pneumonia,* and *M. pneumonia* (e.g., tetracycline, erythromycin, chloramphenicol). In general, these conflicting results appear independent of which antibiotic was used or regimen compared. Thus, the wide disparity that exists in the results from these studies, combined with the difficulties in recognition and lack of standardized diagnostic criteria noted previously, serves as the basis for the enormous controversy surrounding the use of antibiotics in chronic bronchitis. These issues have been expertly reviewed by Tager

TABLE 100.2. COMPARATIVE STUDIES OF ANTIBIOTIC THERAPY FOR ACUTE EXACERBATIONS OF CHRONIC BRONCHITIS

Study	Drug Regimen	Therapeutic Outcome
Elmes PC et al. Br Med J 1957;2:1272–1275	Oxytetracycline versus placebo	Treatment reduced time lost from work
Berry DG et al. Lancet 1960;1:137–139	Oxytetracycline versus placebo	Treatment group demonstrated more rapid improvement
DeKock MA et al. South Afr Med J 1970;44:1064–1065	Tetracycline versus trimethoprim–sulfamethoxazole	No difference
Pines A et al. Br J Dis Chest 1972;66:107–115	Tetracycline versus chloramphenicol versus placebo	⅔ patients improved with treatment; ½ with placebo
British Thoracic Association Br J Dis Chest 1972;66:199–206	Tetracycline versus trimethoprim–sulfamethoxazole	No difference
Nictora MB et al. Ann Intern Med 1982;97:18–21	Tetracycline versus placebo	No difference
Anthonisen NR et al. Ann Intern Med 1987;106:196–204	Various antibiotics versus placebo	Treatment promoted earlier resolution of symptoms

(Adapted from Sachs FL. Chronic bronchitis, in Pennington JE (ed): Respiratory Infections: Diagnosis and Management. New York, Raven Press, 1983, with permission.)

and Speizer[29] and Chodosh,[24] who provide insight into this problem and clinically relevant "consensus" recommendations. Further, the need to use newer oral antibiotics (e.g., cefuroxime, cefixime, amoxicillin–clavulanate, quinolones, or azilides), which possess more potent *in vitro* activity against sputum isolates, appears limited as clinical response often appears independent of pathogens' *in vitro* sensitivity. Nevertheless, these therapeutic data require careful and cautious interpretation, recognizing that chronic bronchitis represents a continuum; most studies evaluate the efficacy of drug therapy over a specific finite period. For this reason, some investigators are encouraging clinicians to assess the "infection-free period" when chronic bronchitics are off antibiotics as an important clinical outcome variable directing future drug selection and criteria for beginning antibiotics in individual patients. The length of the infection-free time period with a particular antibiotic regimen is important. The longest infection-free period defines that antibiotic regimen as the "regimen of choice" for the specific patient for future acute exacerbations of their disease. Despite this experience, it is important to note that the impact such therapy may have on the disease or its progression if incorporated as an aggressive targeted strategy over time is less well characterized.

The primary goal of the treatment of acute exacerbations of chronic bronchitis is to foster prompt resolution of symptoms and positively influence the duration of the patient's symptom-free post-treatment time period. Antibiotics are an important component of treatment, and agents should be selected that are effective against responsible pathogens, demonstrate the least susceptibility to drug interactions (e.g., erythromycin/ciprofloxacin and theophylline), and can be administered in a manner that promotes compliance. Antibiotics commonly used in the treatment of these patients and their respective adult starting doses are outlined in Table 100.4. It is important to note that doses of antibiotics should be adjusted as needed to the desired clinical effect and the lowest incidence of acceptable side effects. A frequent, successful clinical strategy to enhance the duration of symptom-free periods incorporates

TABLE 100.3. COMPARATIVE STUDIES OF ADMINISTRATION OF PROPHYLACTIC ANTIBIOTICS TO PATIENTS WITH CHRONIC BRONCHITIS

Study	Drug Regimen	Therapeutic Outcome
Buchanan J et al. Lancet 1958;719–722	Tetracycline versus control	Fewer exacerbations/patient/year with therapy
Murdoch JM et al. Br Med J 1959;2:1277–1285	Tetracycline versus control	Fewer exacerbations with therapy
Datta N et al. Lancet 1960;2:723–727	Oxytetracycline versus penicillin and sulfa versus control	No significant differences
Fletcher CM et al. Br Med J 1966;1:1317–1322	Oxytetracycline versus control	Less time lost from work; no difference in exacerbations

(Adapted from Sachs FL. Chronic bronchitis, in Pennington JE (ed): Respiratory Infections: Diagnosis and Management. New York, Raven Press, 1983, with permission.)

TABLE 100.4. ORAL ANTIBIOTICS COMMONLY USED FOR THE TREATMENT OF ACUTE RESPIRATORY EXACERBATIONS IN CHRONIC BRONCHITIS

Antibiotic	Usual Adult Dose (g)	Dose Schedule (doses/d)
Preferred Drugs		
Ampicillin	0.5–1	4
Amoxicillin	0.5–1	3
Ciprofloxacin	0.5–0.75	2
Ofloxacin	0.2–0.4	2
Doxycycline	0.1	2
Minocycline	0.1	2
Tetracycline HCl	0.5	4
Amoxicillin–clavulanate	0.5	3
Trimethoprim–sulfamethoxazole	1 DS[a]	2
Lomefloxacin	0.4	1
Supplemental Drugs		
Erythomycin	0.5	4
Clarithromycin	0.25–0.5	2
Cephalexin	0.5	4
Cefaclor	0.25–0.5	3

[a]DS, double strength tablet (160 trimethoprim/800 mg sulfamethoxazole).

higher dose antibiotic regimens using the upper limit of the recommended daily antibiotic dose for a period of 10–14 days.

Ampicillin is often considered the drug of choice for the treatment of acute exacerbations of chronic bronchitis. Unfortunately, the need for multiple repeat daily doses (four times daily) and the increasing incidence of penicillin-resistant β-lactamase-producing strains of bacteria (Table 100.1) have limited the usefulness of this safe and very cost-effective antibiotic. Similarly, variable susceptibility patterns of important bacterial pathogens to some cephalosporins (cephalexin, cefaclor), tetracyclines (tetracycline HCl), and erythromycin salts have severely limited their usefulness as first-line drugs in the treatment of these patients. The value of the erythromycins when mycoplasma is involved is unquestionable whereas the value, if any, of the newer erythromycin analogues, azithromycin or clarithromycin, in the treatment of these patients is not known. Current experience suggests that azithromycin and clarithromycin should be considered as second-line therapy. In contrast, the fluoroquinolones have emerged as effective alternative agents, particularly when gram-negative pathogens are involved. The increased cost of fluoroquinolones compared with doxycycline and minocycline must be carefully weighted against the possible superiority of quinolones in their apparent initial success rate and more prolonged infection-free time period.[24]

It is apparent that it is extremely difficult to assess when an acute pulmonary exacerbation of chronic bronchitis has occurred. Attempts at sequential following of serum antibody titers to a large number of microorganisms (bacteria and viruses), as well as using sputum colony counts as an indicator of an acute exacerbation, have met with limited success.[24] Furthermore, and just as confusing, is the issue of prophylaxis against acute pulmonary exacerbations by the continuous administration of antimicrobial agents (Table 100.3). Clinical opinion and the currently available data suggest that the decision to use antibiotics for the prevention and/or treatment of an acute exacerbation of chronic bronchitis should be made on an individual patient-specific basis. In those patients whose history suggests recurrent exacerbations of their disease that might be attributable to certain specific events (i.e., seasonal-winter months), a trial of prophylactic antibiotics might be beneficial. If no clinical improvement is noted over an appropriate period (e.g., 2–3 months per year for 2–3 years), one might elect to discontinue further attempts at prophylactic therapy. Similarly, such patient-specific trials could be performed in individuals experiencing acute exacerbations, focusing on defining the "infection-free period." Although less than desirable, this method of clinical assessment might distinguish that subset of patients who will benefit from prophylactic antibiotic therapy from those who will not.

BRONCHIOLITIS

Epidemiology

Bronchiolitis is an acute viral infection of the lower respiratory tract of infants that shows a definite seasonal pattern. The disease most commonly affects infants during the first year of life, with peak attack rates occurring in children between the ages of 2 and 10 months. Infectious bronchiolitis is unusual in children older than 2 years of age. The occurrence of bronchiolitis peaks during the winter months and persists through early spring. This pattern of occurrence reflects that of the primary etiologic agent, respiratory syncytial virus. Bronchiolitis remains one of the major reasons infants under 6 months require hospitalization. Current estimates suggest that the hospitalization rate for infants younger than 6 months for bronchiolitis approximates 6 per 1000 children per year.[13,30] The incidence of bronchiolitis appears to be more common in males than females.

Etiology

Respiratory syncytial virus is the most common cause of bronchiolitis, accounting for 45–60% of all cases. During epidemic periods, the incidence of respiratory syncytial virus-induced bronchiolitis can exceed 80% of cases. Parainfluenza viruses type 3 (10–15%), type 1 (5–10%), and type 2 (1–5%) are the second most common etiologic pathogens, constituting as a group nearly 25% of cases. Bacteria serve as secondary pathogens in only a small minority of cases.

Clinical Presentation

A prodromal period usually lasting from 2–7 days precedes the onset of clinical symptoms. These symptoms usually occur after a 4- to 6-day incubation period after exposure to adults or older children with the common cold or other viral respiratory infections. During this prodromal period, infants may be irritable and restless and have a mild fever. The most common clinical signs of bronchiolitis are cough and coryza. As symptoms progress, infants may experience vomiting, diarrhea, noisy breathing, and an increase in respiratory rate. For those infants presenting to a hospital, examination reveals a rapid pulse and a respiratory rate between 40 and 80 breaths per minute. Breathing is labored with retractions of the chest wall, nasal flaring, and grunting. Chest auscultation reveals wheezing and inspiratory rales. Mild conjunctivitis may be observed in up to one-third of infants, whereas 5–10% may have a concurrent otitis media. As a result of limited oral intake due to coughing combined with vomiting and diarrhea, infants are frequently dehydrated. The increased work of breathing and tachypnea most likely further increases fluid loss. In most cases, this clinical picture persists between 3 and 7 days. Although the hospital course of bronchiolitic children is often variable, substantial clinical improvement is usually observed within the first 2 days, with gradual improvement and resolution over the next 7–21 days.

The diagnosis of bronchiolitis is based primarily on history and clinical findings. It is important for the clinician to attempt to differentiate between bronchiolitis and a host of other clinical entities affecting infants, which may produce a similar picture of dyspnea and wheezing. Asthma, congestive heart failure, anatomic airway abnormalities, cystic fibrosis, foreign bodies, gastroesophageal reflux, and salicylism are the primary disease entities that may present with wheezing on physical examination in children. The isolation of a viral pathogen in the respiratory secretions of a wheezing child establishes a presumptive diagnosis of infectious bronchiolitis. However, the ability to identify specific viral pathogens is often hindered by the limited availability of special virology laboratories. The proliferation of commercial enzyme-linked immunosorbent assays (ELISA) and fluorescent antibody staining techniques of nasopharyngeal secretions has increased the ability to identify viral antigens within several hours.[30]

Multiple clinical laboratory determinations have been used to assist in the management of cases of bronchiolitis. Roentgenographic evaluation of the chest in children with bronchiolitis yields variable findings but may help to distinguish this illness from other entities characterized by wheezing. The peripheral WBC count is usually normal or only slightly elevated. In those children requiring hospitalization, abnormalities in blood gas tensions are frequent and appear to relate to disease severity. Hypoxemia is common and acts to increase the respiratory drive, whereas hypercarbia is seen only in the most severe cases. Despite the presence of moderate degrees of hypoxemia, clinical cyanosis is unusual.

Treatment

Bronchiolitis is a self-limiting illness and usually requires no therapy unless the infant is hypoxic or dehydrated. In severely affected children, the mainstays of therapy for bronchiolitis are oxygen therapy and intravenous fluids. Reversal of hypoxemia is usually achieved by the administration of 40% oxygen. Adequate fluids should be provided to prevent or correct dehydration. Clinical assessment combined with blood gas determinations is used to monitor the adequacy of therapy. Aerosolized β-adrenergic therapy appears to offer little benefit for the majority of patients, and may even be detrimental.[31,32] However, they may offer some benefit to the child with a predisposition toward bronchospasm. In hospitalized patients, bronchodilator therapy may be offered initially but should not be pursued in the absence of clear-cut clinical benefit. Similarly, controlled trials of corticosteroids have failed to reveal any therapeutic benefit (or harmful effect) when administered to bronchiolitic infants.[33] As a result, the routine use of systemically administered corticosteroids is discouraged. Although it has been common practice to place children with bronchiolitis in mist tents, there are no data to document the effectiveness of this practice. Because bacteria do not represent primary pathogens in the etiology of bronchiolitis, antibiotics should not be routinely administered. Despite this, many clinicians frequently administer antibiotics initially while awaiting culture results, because the clinical and radiographic findings in bronchiolitis are often suggestive of a possible bacterial pneumonia.

Ribavirin may offer an effective therapy for bronchiolitis. Although ribavirin, a synthetic nucleoside, possesses *in vitro* antiviral properties against a variety of RNA and DNA viruses, including influenza A, influenza B, and parainfluenza,[34] it is approved only in aerosolized form against respiratory syncytial virus.[35,36] Use of the drug requires special equipment (small-particle aerosol generator) and specifically trained personnel for administration via oxygen hood or mist tent. Special care must be taken to avoid drug particle deposition and the resultant clogging of respiratory tubing and valves in mechanical ventilators. The potential for mechanical ventilator malfunction can be easily prevented by following simple precautionary procedures.

When administered as a small particle aerosol, ribavirin has been shown to diminish systemic and respiratory symptoms, fever, and viral shedding associated with respiratory syncytial virus infections in infants. However, the effectiveness of this agent in routine respiratory syncytial virus bronchiolitis is moderate at best. Because of the requirement for special aerosolization equipment and the cost of the drug itself, most experts recommend reserving use of ribavirin for more severely ill patients, including those with chronic lung disease (particularly bronchopulmonary dysplasia), congenital heart disease, prematurity, and immunodeficiency (especially severe combined immunodeficiency and HIV infection); ribavirin also should be considered in any patient requiring mechanical ventilation.[37,38]

PNEUMONIA

Epidemiology

Prior to the antibiotic era, pneumonia was referred to as "the captain of the men of death" and bore a mortality rate in excess of 50%.[39] While the availability of antimicrobial therapy has significantly improved the outcome in this disease, pneumonia remains the most common infectious cause of death in the United States. Pneumonia occurs throughout the year, with the relative prevalence of disease resulting from different etiologic agents varying with the seasons. It occurs in persons of all ages, although the clinical manifestations are most severe in the very young, the elderly, and the chronically ill.

Pathogenesis

Microorganisms gain access to the lower respiratory tract by three routes. They may be inhaled as aerosolized particles or may enter the lung via the bloodstream from an extrapulmonary site of infection; however, aspiration of oropharyngeal contents, a common occurrence in both healthy and ill persons during sleep, is the major mechanism by which pulmonary pathogens gain access to the normally sterile lower airways and alveoli. When pulmonary defense mechanisms are functioning optimally, aspirated microorganisms are cleared from the region before infection can become established; however, aspiration of potential pathogens from the oropharynx can result in pneumonia if lung defenses are impaired. Factors that promote aspiration, such as altered sensorium and neuromuscular disease, may result in an increase in the size of the inoculum delivered to the lower respiratory tract, thereby overwhelming local defense mechanisms. Lung infections with viruses suppress the antibacterial activity of the lung by impairing alveolar macrophage function and mucociliary clearance, thus setting the stage for secondary bacterial pneumonia. Mucociliary transport is also depressed by ethanol and narcotics and by obstruction of a bronchus by mucus, tumor, or extrinsic compression. All of these factors can severely impair the pulmonary clearance of aspirated bacteria.

In addition to the myriad factors that promote the development of pneumonia by impairing lung defenses, characteristics of bacterial colonization of the upper airway can influence the development of lower respiratory tract infections. The high carriage rate of *S. pneumonia* in the pharynx of normal persons (60% infants, 25% children and their parents) accounts for this organism being the most common cause of acute bacterial pneumonia. The demonstrated resistance of normal respiratory epithelial cells to colonization with aerobic gram-negative rods is reflected in the low incidence of pneumonia caused by this group of bacteria in otherwise healthy adults. In contrast, the high prevalence of oropharyngeal colonization by gram-negative bacilli in elderly and seriously ill patients is associated with increased attachment and adherence of these organisms to upper airway epithelial cells[40] and a high incidence of gram-negative bacillary pneumonia in this patient population. Thus, it is clear that host factors are extremely important in determining whether pneumonia will develop after endogenous aspiration. Likewise, the causative agent in most cases of pneumonia is determined by the host factors of age and underlying health status, as well as by the clinical setting in which the infection occurs.

The vast majority of pneumonia cases acquired in the community by otherwise healthy adults are due to one of two organisms: *S. pneumonia* (pneumococcus) and *M. pneumonia.* Pneumococcus is the most common cause of bacterial pneumonia in all age groups and accounts for approximately 70% of all acute bacterial pneumonias in the United States. *Mycoplasma pneumonia* is believed to account for 10–20% of cases. Community-acquired pneumonias caused by *Staphylococcus aureus* and gram-negative rods are observed primarily in the elderly, especially those residing in nursing homes, and in association with alcoholism and other debilitating conditions.[41,42] Gram-negative aerobic bacilli and *S. aureus* are also the leading causative agents in hospital-acquired pneumonia.[43] Anaerobic bacteria are the most common etiologic agents in pneumonia that follows the gross aspiration of gastric or oropharyngeal contents. Pneumonia in infants and children is caused by a wider range of microorganisms and, unlike adults, nonbacterial pathogens predominate.[44] Most pneumonias in the pediatric age group are due to viruses, especially respiratory syncytial virus, parainfluenza, and adenovirus. *Mycoplasma pneumonia* is an important pathogen in older children, and other nonbacterial pathogens such as *Chlamydia trachomatous, Ureaplasma urealyticum, Pneumocystis carinii,* and cytomegalovirus are frequent causes of pneumonia during the first 3 months of life. Beyond the neonatal period, the pneumococcus is the major bacterial pathogen in childhood pneumonia followed by group A streptococcus and *S. aureus. Haemophilus influenza* type B, once a major childhood pathogen, has become an infrequent cause of pneumonia since the introduction of active vaccination against this organism in the late 1980s.[45]

Clinical Presentation

Bacterial Pneumonia

Bacterial pneumonia is most commonly caused by the gram-positive streptococci and staphylococci and gram-negative organisms that normally inhabit the gastrointestinal tract ("enterics") and soil and water ("nonenterics"). In addition, *Legionella multiphilia,* itself a weakly staining gram-negative nonenteric organism, accounts for a small percentage of community- and hospital-acquired bacterial pneumonia. Finally, *Mycobacterium tuberculosis,* an acid-fast staining bacillus, is reemerging as an important cause of pneumonia in urban centers throughout the United States.

Gram-Positive and Gram-Negative Bacterial Pneumonia

Although a wide array of gram-positive and gram-negative organisms can cause pneumonia, they usually present a similar clinical appearance. Typically the onset of illness is abrupt or subacute, with fever, chills, dyspnea, and productive cough predominating. Pneumococcus, staphylococcus, the enteric gram-negative rods, and occasionally other organisms may produce local irritation or destruction of blood vessels leading to rust-colored sputum or hemoptysis. On physical examination the patient is tachypneic and tachycardiac, frequently with chest wall retractions and grunting respirations. Consolidation of the underlying lung is reflected in diminished breath sounds on auscultation over the affected area accompanied by inspiratory crackles as pus-filled alveoli open during lung expansion. Other signs of localized lung consolidation include dullness to percussion, increased tactile fremitus, whisper pectoriloquy, and egophony. Pleural effusions, both sterile and empyematous, may be associated with many of these entities, evidenced by distant breath sounds and a wide area of dulled percussion.

The chest radiograph and sputum examination and culture are the most useful diagnostic tests in gram-positive and gram-negative bacterial pneumonia. Typically the chest radiograph reveals a dense lobar or segmental infiltrate. However, patchy consolidation occasionally may be seen with virtually all these pathogens. Occasionally, pneumonia resulting from hematogenous spread of the organisms results in a diffuse, alveolar pattern on chest radiograph. Gram stain of the expectorated sputum demonstrates many polymorphonuclear cells per high-powered field in the presence of a predominant organism, which is reflected in heavy growth of a single species on culture. Other laboratory tests are less sensitive or specific. Blood cultures may be helpful in identifying the offending organism but are positive in only a minority of cases. The complete blood count usually reflects a leukocytosis with a predominance of polymorphonuclear cells; in some instances, particularly pneumococcus, the elevation of the WBC count may be pronounced. However, normal or mildly elevated WBC counts do not exclude bacterial pneumonic disease. The patient may also be hypoxic as reflected by low oxygen saturation on arterial blood gas or pulse oximetry.

Although clinical appearance of the gram-positive and gram-negative pneumonias are similar, there are epidemiologic and clinical clues that render one more likely than the others.

Gram-Positive Bacteria. Pneumococcus is the most common community-acquired bacterial pneumonia, accounting for 25–60% of cases. It is particularly prevalent and severe in patients with splenic dysfunction, diabetes mellitus, chronic cardiopulmonary or renal disease, or HIV infection. *Staphylococcus aureus* pneumonia occurs in both the community and hospital setting.[43] Community-acquired disease is identified most frequently in young infants, patients with early cystic fibrosis, and those recovering from an antecedent respiratory viral infection. *Staphylococcus aureus* is a prominent cause of nosocomial pneumonia and may result from hematogenous spread from a distant source. In both settings it is characteristically severe and accompanied by the formation of pneumatoceles (i.e., air-containing cavities within the lung). Group B streptococcus, while rare in adults, is the most common cause of bacterial pneumonia among neonates, where it typically causes a clinical and radiographic picture nearly indistinguishable from hyaline membrane disease.[46] Group A streptococcus is an uncommon cause of community-acquired pneumonia. It most frequently occurs after a viral respiratory tract infection and only occasionally is associated with streptococcal pharyngitis. The organism is very pyogenic and the presentation can be severe.

Enteric Gram-Negative Bacteria. Community-acquired enteric gram-negative pneumonia is identified most frequently among patients with chronic illness, especially alcoholism and diabetes mellitus. The enteric gram-negative bacteria are also leading causes of nosocomial pneumonia, since the upper respiratory tract becomes rapidly colonized with gram-negative organisms after hospitalization, particularly among critically ill patients and those receiving antibiotics or H_2-receptor antagonists. Outbreaks of nosocomial disease occasionally maybe caused by contaminated respiratory therapy equipment.[42,43,47] *Klebsiella pneumoniae* is the most frequently encountered pathogen among the gram-negative enteric bacteria, although the relative prominence of these organisms varies from hospital to hospital. The gram-negative bacilli are associated with high mortality, sometimes exceeding 50%[42]; their potential to produce significant morbidity and mortality has recently been enhanced by the emergence of highly antibiotic-resistant organisms in some hospital settings.[48,49]

Nonenteric Gram-Negative Bacteria. The most prominent nonenteric gram-negative rods associated with pneumonia include pseudomonas, haemophilus, and moraxella. Like the enteric gram-negative organisms, *Pseudomonas aeruginosa* is a frequent cause of hospital-acquired pneumonia and is particularly prominent among neutropenic and burn patients. In addition, cystic fibrosis patients suffer from chronic, multilobar infections with *P. aeruginosa* as well as other pseudomonas species; these infections are punctuated with acute exacerbations. *Haemophilus influenza* type B historically has been a prominent pathogen in childhood pneumonia. However, since the introduction of the conjugated haemophilus vaccines in the late 1980s, there has been a dramatic drop in the incidence of all invasive disease due to this organism in the pediatric age group. However, two different clinical presentations of *H. influenza* pneumonia are still seen in adults. The most common by far is the bronchopneumonia form, which develops most frequently in patients with underlying chronic lung disease and is believed to represent, in most patients, an exacerbation of chronic bronchitis. Because asymptomatic colonization of the lower respiratory tract with *H. influenza* occurs in patients with chronic lung disease, culture of sputum or transtracheal aspirates may not be reliable in this population, and the diagnosis rests on antigen detection or isolation of the bacteria from pleural fluid. In the second form of *H. influenza* pneumonia, segmental or lobar involvement predominates. The course of this illness is more acute, with sudden onset of cough, fever, and pleuritic chest pain. Finally, *Moraxella catarrhalis*, an important cause of otitis media and sinusitis, has been found to be an increasingly important cause of lower respiratory tract infections in immunoincompetent and hospitalized patients.[50]

Legionella pneumophilia

Of the several *Legionella* species known to cause pneumonia in humans, *L. pneumophilia* is by far the most important. After the organism was identified as the cause of the outbreak at the American Legion convention in Philadelphia in 1976, retrospective immunologic and bacteriologic analyses identified it as being the etiologic agent in outbreaks of illness occurring prior to the 1970s.[51] *Legionella pneumophilia* is a fastidious, poorly staining gram-negative bacillus that elaborates exotoxin and endotoxin. It is a water and soil organism and is most probably transmitted by air, aerosol, or water. Outbreaks of illness caused by *L. pneumophilia* have been linked to excavation sites and contaminated water from air conditioners and showers. Person-to-person transmission has not been demonstrated. In addition to epidemics, *L. pneumophilia* causes sporadic illness that peaks in summer and fall. Individuals who are male, middle-age or older, immunocompromised, chronic bronchitics, or cigarette smokers are at increased risk. The incidence of sporadic cases of *L. pneumophilia* pneumonia in children is similar to that in adults, accounting for 1–5% of community-acquired pneumonias that require hospitalization.[52]

Infection with *L. pneumophilia* is characterized by multisystem involvement, including rapidly progressive pneumonia. It has a gradual onset, with prominent constitutional symptoms such as malaise, lethargy, weakness, and anorexia occurring early in the course of the illness. A dry, nonproductive cough is initially present, which over several days becomes productive of mucoid or purulent sputum. Fevers exceeding 40°C develop in over half of patients and are typically unremitting and associated with a relative bradycardia. Pleuritic chest pain and progressive dyspnea may be seen, and fine rales are found on lung exam, progressing to signs of frank consolidation later in the course of the illness. Large pleural effusions, empyema, and lung abscess are uncommon in this disease. Extrapulmonary manifestations remain evident throughout the course of the illness and include diarrhea, nausea, vomiting, myalgias, and arthralgias. Substantial changes in a patient's mental status, often out of proportion to the degree of fever, are seen in approximately one-fourth of patients. Obtundation, hallucinations, grand mal seizures, and focal neurologic findings have also been associated with this illness. Although abnormalities in hepatic and renal function may be noted on laboratory assessment, these are usually of limited clinical significance. Chest roentgenograms initially reveal patchy alveolar infiltrates that may be bilateral. Progression to lobar or multilobar consolidation is frequent, as are small pleural effusions.

Laboratory findings include leukocytosis with predominance of mature and immature granulocytes in 50–75% of patients. Urinalysis may reveal proteinuria, hematuria, and casts; liver function tests (e.g., serum glutamic–oxaloacetic transaminase, serum glutamic–pyruvic transaminase, bilirubin) may be abnormal. Hyponatremia and hypophosphatemia have also been frequently reported. Because *L. pneumophilia* stains poorly with commonly used stains, routine microscopic examination of sputum is of little diagnostic value. While it exhibits slow growth and has highly selective growth requirements, *L. pneumophilia* has been successfully isolated from tissue using specialized medium. In addition to diagnosis by culture, fluorescent antibody testing can be performed to diagnose Legionnaire's disease. Direct fluorescent antibody examination of respiratory tract secretions, lung tissue, or pleural fluid is the most rapid means of establishing the diagnosis. The sensitivity of this method approaches 70% for sputum and 90% for lung tissue, and diagnostic specificity is high for both.[53] Because this diagnostic test is complex and difficult to perform, it is unavailable in most clinical laboratories. As such, the diagnosis of Legionnaire's disease is often initially presumptive, based on a suggestive clinical presentation.

Anaerobic Pneumonia

Anaerobic pneumonitis is most likely to occur in individuals predisposed to aspiration by impaired consciousness and may be more prevalent in those with periodontal disease or dysphagia. In addition, bronchogenic carcinoma is an associated underlying condition that should be suspected in patients with anaerobic pneumonia who do not appear predisposed to aspiration. A variety of gram-positive and gram-negative anaerobic bacteria indigenous to the upper airway may cause pneumonitis when large quantities of oropharyngeal secretions are aspirated into the lower airways. The organisms most frequently implicated are *Peptostreptococcus* spp., *Fusobacteria, Bacteroides melaninogenicus, Bacteroides fragilis,* and *Peptococcus* spp.; polymicrobial infections with anaerobes and aerobes such as *S. aureus, S. pneumonia,* and gram-negative bacilli are common.[54]

The course of illness is typically indolent with cough, low-grade fever, and weight loss, although an acute presentation may occur. Rigors are notably absent and bacteremia is rare. Putrid sputum, when present, is highly suggestive of the diagnosis. Chest radiographs reveal infiltrates typically located in dependent lung segments, and lung abscesses develop in 20% of patients 1–2 weeks into the course of the illness.[54]

Tuberculosis

Tuberculosis is caused by the acid-fast bacillus *M. tuberculosis.* After years of steady decline, the number of cases of pneumonia caused by *M. tuberculosis* in the United States has progressively increased since the mid-1980s. The new epidemic is most prominent in urban neighborhoods afflicted with crowded conditions and poor access to health care. Unlike previous eras in which tuberculosis was most frequently seen in elderly men, infection currently is identified in increasing numbers of young minority adults.[55] The reason for the resurgence of tuberculosis is at least partially related to coinfection with human immunodeficiency virus (HIV); HIV-infected patients are more likely to develop symptomatic disease with its associated fits of coughing than their immunocompetent counterparts, and this enables further spread of infection.[56] Other groups prone to tuberculosis include the homeless, patients in chronic care facilities and homes for the elderly, and recent immigrants from areas of the world in which tuberculosis remains endemic. The reemergence of tuberculosis in the United States has been accompanied by the development of multiple-drug resistance, that is, of mycobacteria that are resistant to two or more of the first-line antituberculous drugs. Infection caused by these organisms is poorly responsive to alternative therapy and is associated with mortality rates exceeding 50%.[57,58]

Tuberculosis is spread person to person through the inhalation of droplet nuclei generated by vigorous coughing. The majority of patients who become infected with *M. tuberculosis* remain asymptomatic despite life-long infection and have a normal chest radiograph. Infection in these patients is detected only through routine skin testing. Less frequently, particularly in those with poor immunity, the infection cannot be contained by local macrophages and the tuberculous burden grows sufficiently such that it causes clinical manifestations. Adult disease (from adolescence onward) begins with constitutional complaints followed by a prominent chronic, troublesome cough productive of mucopurulent material. The infection initially appears in the lung apices with little or no hilar adenopathy and, in advanced disease, results in lung necrosis, producing a cavity containing enormous numbers of organisms. With sufficient cough, the cavitary contents are mobilized and aspirated into other areas of the lung, where additional cavities may be formed. In contrast, pediatric tuberculosis commonly is associated with little cough even in the presence of extensive pulmonary infection. Instead, the child presents with a subacute course of poor appetite, weight loss, lethargy, fever, and sweats. The chest radiograph reveals a widened mediastinum representing enlarged hilar lymph nodes reacting to the tuberculin inoculum. In progressive cases, the nodes impinge upon or erode through a large bronchus, resulting in a dense consolidation of the segment distal to the lesion. Cavitary disease is uncommon.

Nonbacterial Pneumonia

Viruses, mycoplasma species, chlamydial species, and parasites are recognized causes of pneumonia syndromes in all age groups. The designation "atypical pneumonia," distinct from the "typical" bacterial pneumonia most commonly seen in adults, has been used to describe the illness caused by many of these agents.

Mycoplasma pneumoniae

Taxonomically the mycoplasmas are included in their own class labeled Mollicutes. Although their small size and filterability are similar to viruses, the structure of their ribosomal RNA indicates that they have evolved from bacteria and, unlike any virus, they contain cytoplasm and can replicate in an extracellular environment. They are distinguished from eubacteria by their low genetic content; in addition, the mycoplasmas lack a cell wall and are surrounded instead by a lipid membrane.

Mycoplasma pneumoniae causes human disease throughout the year, with a slightly increased incidence in fall and early winter. During summer months when other causes of pneumonia are less common, *M. pneumoniae* is responsible for a greater proportion of cases. Both infection and disease from *M. pneumoniae* are common, with two-thirds of children ages 2–5 years and 97% of persons older than 17 years of age having detectable serum antibody to the organism.[59] Overall, *M. pneumoniae* is responsible for approximately 20% of pneumonia cases, although in enclosed populations such as military recruits and college dormitory residents it may cause more than 50% of pneumonia cases. Infection is spread by close person-to-person contact, and the incubation period is 2–3 weeks. *Mycoplasma pneumoniae* infections are unusual in children under 5 years of age and show a peak incidence in older children and young adults. Only 3–10% of persons infected with *M. pneumoniae* develop pneumonia, with the majority of respiratory tract involvement being manifested as pharyngitis and tracheobronchitis. Asymptomatic infection is apparently common.

Mycoplasma pneumoniae presents with a gradual onset of fever, headache, and malaise, with the appearance 3–5 days after the onset of illness of a persistent, hacking cough that initially is nonproductive. Sore throat, ear pain, and rhinorrhea are often present. Chills are only occasionally seen, and pleuritic pain is uncommon. Lung findings are generally limited to rales and rhonchi; findings of consolidation are rarely present. Nonpulmonary manifestations are extremely common and include nausea, vomiting, diarrhea, myalgias, arthralgias, polyarticular arthritis, skin rashes, myocarditis and pericarditis, hemolytic anemia, meningoencephalitis, cranial neuropathies, and Guillain–Barré syndrome. Systemic symptoms generally clear in 1–2 weeks, while respiratory symptoms may persist up to 4 weeks. Although the course of mycoplasmal pneumonia is usually benign and self-limited, severe respiratory disease may develop in patients with sickle cell disease, agammaglobulinemia, and chronic obstructive lung disease.

Radiographic findings are generally more impressive than the patient's physical findings, and include patchy or interstitial infiltrates, which are most commonly seen in the lower lobes. Small unilateral, transient pleural effusions are common but large effusions and empyema are rare. Roentgenographic abnormalities resolve slowly, and 4–6 weeks may be required for complete resolution.

Sputum Gram strain may reveal mononuclear or polymorphonuclear leukocytes, with no predominant organism. While *M. pneumoniae* can be cultured from respiratory secretions using specialized medium, its growth is slow and 2–3 weeks may be necessary for culture identification. Indirect evidence of infection by *M. pneumoniae* is the presence of elevated levels of serum cold hemagglutinins. These IgM antibodies develop in approximately half of patients with mycoplasmal pneumonia and can be elevated in other illnesses, especially viral infection.[59] A definitive diagnosis can also be made by demonstrating a fourfold or greater rise in serum antibodies to *M. pneumoniae;* however, because this test also requires 2–4 weeks for results, the diagnosis of mycoplasmal pneumonia during the acute phase of the illness must be based on the characteristic history, the appropriate clinical setting, and typical physical findings.

Viral Pneumonia

Viruses are not a common cause of pneumonia in adults except in the immunosuppressed. Influenza virus, usually type A, is the most common cause of pneumonia in the adult civilian population, whereas adenoviruses cause most cases in military trainees. In contrast, viruses are by far the most common agents producing pneumonia in infants and young children, with respiratory syncytial virus, parainfluenza, and adenovirus producing most cases.[44]

All viral respiratory tract infections occur more commonly in the winter, and rapid person-to-person spread through susceptible populations is typical. Underlying cardiac or pulmonary disease predisposes to increased incidence and severity of viral lower respiratory tract infection, especially with influenza virus in adults and respiratory syncytial virus in children. Radiographic findings are nonspecific and include bronchial wall thickening and perihilar and diffuse interstitial infiltrates. Pleural effusions may be seen especially in adenovirus and parainfluenza pneumonia.

The clinical pictures produced by respiratory viruses are sufficiently variable and overlap to such a degree that an etiologic diagnosis cannot confidently be made on clinical grounds alone. Although virus isolation in tissue culture is possible, 7 or more days is often required for virus identification; thus, this method usually cannot be relied on for definitive diagnosis during the acute phase of illness. Serologic tests for virus-specific antibodies are often used in the diagnosis of viral infections. The diagnostic fourfold rise in titer between acute and convalescent phase sera may require 2–3 weeks to develop; however, same-day diagnosis of viral infections is now possible through the use of indirect immunofluorescence tests on exfoliated cells from the respiratory tract. The immunofluorescence technique frequently employs a battery of monoclonal antibodies, including those against influenza A and B, respiratory syncytial virus, parainfluenza, and adenovirus to provide rapid diagnosis of a range of viral infections.

Pneumonia in Special Clinical Circumstances

Pneumonia in the HIV-Infected Patient

HIV infects and destroys helper T lymphocytes bearing the CD4 surface molecule; these cells are critical for orchestrating a wide variety of immunological responses. Their depletion consequently results in the dysfunction of both cell-mediated and humoral immunity. As a result, a broad range of pathogens can cause pneumonia in HIV infection (Table 100.5).[60] The HIV-infected patient may be afflicted with pneumonia multiple times in his or her lifetime, particularly in the advanced stages of the disease, and a given episode may be caused by more than one species.[61]

The clinical presentation of pneumonia in HIV-infected persons is frequently not helpful in distinguishing one pathogen from another. The pneumonia usually is subacute in onset and consists of fever, nonproductive cough, and dyspnea.[60,61] Radiographically, most of these entities produce a multilobular or diffuse pattern.[62] Some practitioners initially treat the HIV-treated patient with pneumonia empirically, covering the most common entities (bacteria and *P. carinii*). More frequently, however, given the wide array of possible pathogens, a specific microbiologic diagnosis is aggressively pursued early in the patient's course through sputum induction or bronchoalveolar lavage to allow a rational choice of an antimicrobial regimen.

TABLE 100.5. PULMONARY COMPLICATIONS OF HIV INFECTION

Infections
- *Viruses*
  - Cytomegalovirus
  - Herpes simplex virus
  - Varicella-zoster virus
  - Respiratory syncytial virus and other common respiratory pathogens (parainfluenza virus, adenovirus)
  - Measles virus
- *Bacteria*
  - Pyogenic organisms (especially *Streptococcus pneumoniae, Haemophilus influenzae*)
  - *Mycobacterium tuberculosis*
  - *Mycobacterium avium* complex and other nontuberculous mycobacteria
- *Fungi*
  - *Histoplasma capsulatum*
  - *Coccidioides immitus*
  - *Cryptococcus neoformans*
  - *Candida* species
  - *Aspergillus* species
- *Parasites*
  - *Pneumocystis carinii*
  - *Toxoplasma gondii*
  - Cryptosporidia
  - *Strongyloides stercoralis*

Malignancies
- Kaposi's sarcoma
- Non-Hodgkin's lymphoma
- Smooth muscle tumors

Lymphocytic Interstitial Pneumonitis
Nonspecific Interstitial Pneumonitis
Drug-Induced Pneumonitis

(Adapted from Murray JF, Mills J. Pulmonary infectious complications of human immunodeficiency virus infection. Am Rev Respir Dis 1990;141:1357, with permission.)

Pneumonia in the Neutropenic Host

Neutropenia in the cancer patient is a common complication of aggressive chemotherapy but occasionally can result from the cancer itself. The risk of infection in the cytopenic patient is significantly increased when the absolute neutrophil count falls below 500 cell/mm^3 and the neutropenia persists for longer than 7 days.[63] The regular administration of recombinant colony-stimulating factors to cytopenic cancer patients, to shorten the duration of neutropenia, has decreased the incidence of serious complicating infections.[64] Nevertheless, when such infections do occur they frequently affect the lungs.

The range of organisms that can cause pneumonia in the cytopenic cancer patient includes a broad range of bacteria and fungi. Prominent among these are enteric and nonenteric (particularly pseudomonas) gram-negative rods, streptococci, and staphylococci, as well as the fungi candida, aspergillus, and mucor.[63] The chest radiograph may reveal the lobar pattern atypical of bacterial infection in the normal host or it may exhibit a diffuse pattern; sometimes the pneumonia remains invisible by chest radiograph until the neutropenia resolves. Noninfectious entities may also cause pulmonary symptoms; these include toxicity from radiation or chemotherapy, or infiltration of the lung parenchyma by the tumor itself.

Nosocomial Pneumonia

After the urinary tract and the bloodstream, the lungs are the most frequent site of infection acquired in the hospital.[65,66] Nosocomial pneumonia is seen most commonly in critically ill patients. Several factors have been identified that predispose to the development of nosocomial pneumonia, including the severity of illness, the duration of hospitalization, and prior antibiotic exposure.[65–67] However, the strongest predisposing factor is mechanical ventilation (intubation), which bypasses the natural airway defenses against the migration of upper respiratory tract organisms into the lower tract.[68] This situation is exacerbated by the wide use of H_2-receptor blocking agents in the intensive care unit.[69,70] Such use increases the pH of gastric secretions and may promote the proliferation of microorganisms in the upper gastrointestinal tract. Subclinical microaspirations are events that occur routinely in intubated patients resulting in the inoculation of bacteria-contaminated gastric contents into the lung and a higher incidence of nosocomial pneumonia.

The organisms most commonly associated with nosocomial pneumonia are *S. aureus* and enteric and nonenteric gram-negative bacilli, the organisms that colonize the pharynx of the hospitalized, critically ill patient.[68] The diagnosis of nosocomial pneumonia is usually established by the presence of a new infiltrate on chest radiograph, fever, worsening respiratory status, and the appearance of thick, neutrophil-laden respiratory secretions. In actuality, the diagnosis is often difficult to make in the intensively ill patient with underlying lung pathology that can itself be associated with an abnormal, changing radiograph, such as congestive heart failure or chronic lung disease. Broad-spectrum antibiotics frequently are started empirically even in equivocal circumstances, with bronchoscopy reserved for poorly responsive cases.

Since the organisms that cause nosocomial pneumonia are derived from the pharynx and gastrointestinal tract, there has been recent interest in decontaminating both sites with a broad-spectrum regimen of nonabsorbable antibiotics to prevent the development of pneumonia.[71,72] The success of this strategy has been variable, and its effectiveness requires further investigation before its routine can be recommended.

TREATMENT OF BACTERIAL PNEUMONIA

The treatment of bacterial pneumonia, like the treatment of most infectious diseases, initially involves the empiric institution of a relatively broad-spectrum antibiotic that is effective against probable pathogens after appropriate cultures and specimens for laboratory evaluation have been obtained. Therapy should be narrowed to cover specific pathogens once the results of cultures are known. Multiple factors that help define the potential pathogens involved include patient age, previous and current medication history, underlying disease(s), major organ function, and present clinical status. These factors must be evaluated to select properly an effective empiric antibiotic regimen, as well as the most appropriate route for drug administration (e.g., oral, parenteral). For a more detailed discussion on the principles of antibiotic selection, please see Chapter 98.

Numerous antibiotics are available and the majority have been shown to be effective in the treatment of bacterial pneumonia. Superiority of one compound over another when both demonstrate similar *in vitro* activity and tissue distribution characteristics is difficult to define. Our opinions on appropriate empiric choices for the treatment of bacterial pneumonias relative to a patient's underlying disease are shown in Table 100.6 for adults and Table 100.7 for children. As mentioned before, once the causative pathogen is identified, the empiric antibiotic regimen should be changed to an effective therapeutic agent with a more narrow antimicrobial spectrum. A complete listing of antimicrobial agents for specifically directed therapy is beyond the scope of this chapter and is presented in Chapter 98, Selection of Antimicrobial Regimens.

The plethora of commercially available antimicrobial agents with documented bacterial and clinical effectiveness in the treatment of pneumonia often appears endless. These large numbers of often expensive drugs mandate our critical evaluation for formulary selection and clinical use. Similarities in *in vitro* activity, resistance to bacterial-inactivating enzymes, and overall effectiveness often make rational therapeutic decisions difficult and potentially even appear random. However, some general principles may be applied to guide

TABLE 100.6. EMPIRIC ANTIMICROBIAL THERAPY FOR PNEUMONIA IN ADULTS[a]

Clinical Setting	Usual Pathogen(s)	Presumptive Therapy
Previously healthy, ambulatory patient	Pneumococcus, *Mycoplasma pneumoniae*	Erythromycin, tetracycline
Elderly (nursing home residence)[b]	Pneumococcus, *Klebsiella pneumoniae, Staphylococcus aureus, Haemophilus influenzae*	Semisynthetic penicillin[c] plus aminoglycoside; or ticarcillin/clavulanate; cephalosporin[d]; imipenem
Chronic bronchitis	Pneumococcus, *H. influenzae*	Ampicillin, tetracycline, TMP-SMZ,[e] cefuroxime, amoxicillin/clavulanate
Alcoholism[b]	Pneumococcus, *K. pneumoniae, S. aureus, H. influenzae*	Semisynthetic penicillin[c] or ticarcillin/clavulanate plus aminoglycoside; cephalosporin[d]; imipenem
Aspiration		
Community	Mouth anaerobes	Penicillin or clindamycin
Hospital/residential care	Mouth anaerobes, *S. aureus*, gram-negative enterics	Penicillin or clindamycin plus aminoglycoside
Nosocomial pneumonia[b]	*K. pneumoniae, Enterobacter* spp., *Pseudomonas aeruginosa, S. aureus, Escherichia coli*	Ticarcillin, piperacillin, mezlocillin, aztreonam, or imipenem plus aminoglycoside, or ceftazidime

[a]See section on Treatment of Bacterial Pneumonia.
[b]Systemically effective quinolone may prove to be a viable alternative for initial therapy in these patients.
[c]Semisynthetic penicillin (e.g., nafcillin, oxacillin).
[d]Second- or third-generation cephalosporin (e.g., cefuroxime, ceftriaxone, cefotaxime, ceftazidime).
[e]TMP-SMZ, trimethoprim–sulfamethoxazole. (Adapted from Pennington JE. Community-acquired pneumonia and acute bronchitis, in Pennington JE (ed): Respiratory Infection: Diagnosis and Management. New York, Raven Press, 1983, with permission.)

TABLE 100.7. EMPIRIC ANTIMICROBIAL THERAPY FOR PNEUMONIA IN PEDIATRIC PATIENTS

Age	Usual Pathogen(s)	Presumptive Therapy
1 month	Group B streptococcus, *Haemophilus influenzae* (nontypable), *Escherichia coli, Staphylococcus aureus*	Ampicillin/sulbactam, aminoglycoside, or cephalosporin[a]; imipenem
	CMV, RSV, adenovirus	Ribavirin for RSV
1–3 months	*Chlamydia, Ureaplasma,* CMV, *Pneumocystis carinii* (afebrile pneumonia syndrome)	Erythromycin, TMP–SMZ
	RSV	Ribavirin
	Pneumococcus, S. aureus	Semisynthetic penicillin[b] or cephalosporin[a]
3 months–6 years	Pneumococcus, *H. influenzae,* RSV, adenovirus, parainfluenza	Ampicillin or cephalosporin[c] Ampicillin/sulbactam Ribavirin for RSV
>6 years	Pneumococcus, *Mycoplasma pneumoniae,* adenovirus	Erythromycin

Key: CMV, cytomegalovirus; RSV, respiratory syncytial virus; TMP–SMZ, trimethoprim–sulfamethoxazole.
[a]Third-generation cephalosporin (e.g., ceftriaxone, cefotaxime).
[b]Semisynthetic penicillin (e.g., nafcillin, oxacillin).
[c]Second-generation cephalosporin (e.g., cefuroxime, cefprozil).

rational antibiotic choice. First, in community-acquired pneumonia the bacterial causes are relatively constant, even across geographic areas and patient populations. In many circumstances, the emergence of organisms resistant to traditional antibiotics has not been a prominent problem. Initial therapy should consist of older, less expensive agents, with newer antibiotics reserved for unresponsive illness or special circumstances. The indiscriminate use of recently introduced agents increases health care cost and, in some instances (such as with the recent widespread use of quinolones), induces resistance among a significant percentage of community-acquired organisms.[73] It must be emphasized, however, that the rapidly evolving epidemiology of bacterial resistance, including the increasing emergence of penicillin-resistant pneumococcus in many areas of the United States and Europe,[74] forces the clinician to be vigilant and knowledgeable about antibiotic sensitivity patterns in each community.

In contrast, antibiotic selection within the hospital environment demands greater care because of constant changes in antibiotic resistance patterns *in vitro* and *in vivo.* Ironically, some β-lactam antibiotics, which were developed to treat multiple-antibiotic–resistant hospital-acquired organisms, can themselves induce broad-spectrum bacterial β-lactamases and thereby lead to even greater problems with resistance.[75] These facts underscore the importance of sequentially documenting the epidemiology of pathogens and infectious diseases within a specific practice or institution. As a result, an antimicrobial agent for a specific infectious disease favored in one practice site may not be the most desirable selection in another, despite similarities in size and patient profile. Strict and careful control and, possibly, rotation of empiric antibiotics in the hospital environment may help to limit the emergence of resistant organisms. However, newer antibiotics developed to treat resistant, hospital-acquired pathogens are costly; therefore, their use must be moderated to some extent in an era where capitated hospital costs and mandated budget cuts will not tolerate careless antibiotic use (see Chapter 98).

The *in vitro* spectrum of antibacterial activity of systemically absorbed fluoroquinolone antibiotics (e.g., ciprofloxacin, enoxacin, ofloxacin, pefloxacin) would suggest that these drugs have an important role in the treatment of bacterial infections of the lower respiratory tract. Numerous clinical studies available in the literature describe the efficacy of these drugs for the treatment of purulent bronchitis, acute exacerbations of chronic bronchitis, pneumonia, and cystic fibrosis. However, their widespread use by primary care physicians has led to pathogen resistance and treatment failures, including, perhaps most important, isolates of *S. pneumonia.* Although newer quinolones are more active against common respiratory tract pathogens than older agents, this experience renders it difficult to recommend their indiscriminate use for routine community-acquired pneumonia. Nevertheless, these drugs may be effective alternative agents for the treatment of nosocomial pneumonia for hospitalized patients and patients residing in extended-care facilities. At present, quinolone use in pediatrics remains restricted and limited due to possible fluoroquinolone-induced destructive lesions of growing cartilage. However, the need for quinolones for the treatment of selected infections arising in pediatric patients continues, and their safety in these patients has served as the foundation for ongoing controlled, clinical efficacy and safety trials in pediatric patients.

Among the more recently introduced classes of oral antibiotics, the newer macrolides possess excellent activity against most *S. pneumonia* and mycoplasma. Azithromycin and clarithromycin appear to offer highly viable alternative agents to erythromycin, particularly in those patients who are intolerant to erythromycin analogues (e.g., gastrointestinal upset) and, for azithromycin, are taking medications that may result in a clinically significant drug–drug interaction with erythromycin (e.g., astemizole, carbamazepine).

Thus, until more specific drug interaction data are available, patients who receive clarithromycin should receive drugs known to interact with erythromycin cautiously and be monitored closely for any possible side effects from a drug interaction (see Chapter 98).

Numerous investigators have demonstrated that antibiotic concentrations in respiratory secretions in excess of the pathogen minimum inhibitory concentration (MIC) are necessary for successful treatment of pulmonary infections.[76,77] The concept of a blood–bronchus barrier, analogous but dissimilar to the blood–brain barrier, has been used to assess the characteristics of drug penetration into pulmonary secretions. The ability of a drug to penetrate respiratory secretions depends on multiple physicochemical factors, including molecular size, lipid solubility, and degree of ionization at serum and biologic fluid pH. Studies performed in animals and cystic fibrosis patients suggest that larger molecular size favors the accumulation of drugs in bronchial secretions. This finding contrasts with data on drug penetration of other physiologic compartments, such as the cerebrospinal fluid, and may be a result of the trapping of lower molecular weight compounds in mucin pores. The importance of this finding cannot be overemphasized; however, the rate at which a drug may accumulate in certain respiratory secretions would appear to remain an important factor relative to the drug's clinical efficacy in treating pulmonary infections. The un-ionized form of a drug and lipid solubility also appear to favor drug penetration. It should be noted that the pH of infected bronchi is often more acidic than that of normal tissue and blood.[78] Fewer data are available assessing the influence of drug protein binding on the rate and amount of respiratory secretion penetration. As the degree of protein binding has been shown to influence a drug's ability to traverse membranes, a similar relationship would be expected within the lung. Thus, it is prudent to assess the pharmacokinetic–pharmacodynamic correlates of drug binding to serum proteins, tissue distribution, and *in vitro* potency when selecting an antimicrobial regimen. These concepts relating to overall drug penetration of respiratory secretions, and others, have led to the clinical practice of administering certain antibiotics (e.g., aminoglycosides) to achieve high peak serum concentrations on the assumption that higher (and possibly more effective) biologic fluid concentrations of the drug will be achieved. Substantial clinical experience supports this practice for treating pulmonary infections with certain antibiotics, although more data are needed to describe the relationships between these variables and clinical response.

Prior to the availability of newer β-lactam and quinolone antibiotics possessing consistently potent activity against multiple gram-negative pathogens, the administration of antibiotics or direct endotracheal instillation was promoted by some investigators.[79,80] This method of drug administration is an attempt to provide increased "topical" concentrations of antibiotics that do not appear to penetrate respiratory secretions effectively while reducing the likelihood of systemic toxicity. In addition, greater local concentrations of antibiotics, particularly for the polymyxins and aminoglycosides, are believed to partially overcome the substantial decrease in antibiotic bioactivity observed when these agents interact with the purulent material present in infectious foci.[81,82] Despite these potential theoretical advantages, the role of antibiotic aerosols or direct endotracheal instillation in clinical practice remains ill defined.

Sputum is frequently assessed as possibly representing the pharmacodynamic interface for pulmonary infections. It should be noted that sputum represents only one of many pulmonary fluids and secretions, although sputum may serve as a reservoir for pathogen growth.[76,77] These beliefs have led many investigators to assess antibiotic concentrations in sputum, frequently describing sputum drug concentrations as a ratio of serum to sputum drug concentration. Although sputum drug concentrations provide us with some insight into the characteristics of drug penetration of respiratory secretions, caution should be exercised in the interpretation of these data. Current data describing sputum drug concentrations are often difficult to interpret because of differences in analytical techniques, method of sputum sampling, and the random nature of sampling times relative to drug dose. Moreover, representation of sputum drug concentrations as a ratio of serum drug concentration can be misleading and most probably should be described relative to absolute drug concentration or apparent area under the drug-concentration curve in sputum. To more accurately describe the distribution characteristics of antimicrobial agents in sputum, research studies should be designed to allow sequential repeated sputum sampling over a dosage interval under both first-dose and steady-state conditions.[83,84]

Prevention of some cases of pneumonia is possible through the use of vaccines against selected infectious agents. Inactivated influenza virus vaccines formulated annually to contain antigens representative of expected prevalent strains are widely available and generally well tolerated. Immunization is recommended for individuals likely to experience serious complications from influenza infection, such as patients with underlying heart or lung disease, chronic renal disease, and the elderly. Although it should not replace active immunization, amantadine may be administered for prevention of influenza A infection, beginning as soon as possible after exposure and continuing for at least 10 days. The recommended dose is 5 mg/kg/d in two to three divided doses not to exceed 150 mg/d in children 1–9 years old, and 200 mg/d in two divided doses in patients 9 or older. In addition, polyvalent polysaccharide vaccines are available for two of the leading causes of bacterial pneumonia, pneumococcus and *H. influenzae* type B. For a detailed description of the use of these vaccines the reader is referred to Chapter 116, Vaccines, Toxoids, and other Immunobiologics.

The supportive care of the patient with pneumonia includes the use of humidified oxygen for hypoxemia, administration of bronchodilators when bronchospasm is present, and chest physiotherapy with postural drainage if there is evidence of retained secretions. Additional therapeutic adjuncts include adequate hydration, optimal nutritional support, and fever control.

Lung Abscess

A lung abscess is a localized area of suppuration within pulmonary parenchyma accompanied by necrosis of lung tissue. While a multitude of factors may predispose to the development of lung abscess, the majority are due to aspiration of infected oropharyngeal secretions.[85] Periodontal disease, oropharyngeal infections, depressed sensorium, decreased cough reflex resulting from alcoholism, anesthesia, or neurologic disorders, and esophageal disease causing impaired swallowing all predispose to the development of lung abscess. Endobronchial obstruction caused by foreign body or tumor, septic emboli, and bland or septic pulmonary infarction may also lead to abscess formation. Secondary lung abscesses complicating bacterial pneumonia account for approximately 20% of cases, and most commonly follow infections with *S. aureus* and *K. pneumonia.*[86]

PATHOGENESIS

The bacteriology of primary lung abscess reflects that of the oropharyngeal flora and, as such, is characteristically anaerobic and polymicrobial. Using transtracheal aspiration to obtain specimens for microbiologic studies, Bartlett et al.[85] recovered anaerobic bacteria from 93% of patients with primary lung abscess, with the most common isolates being *Bacteroides melanogenicus, Fusobacterium nucleatum,* and anaerobic or microaerophilic gram-positive cocci. Mixed infections with anaerobes and aerobes were seen in nearly half. *Staphylococcus aureus* and enteric gram-negative bacilli are more common isolates in patients whose disease developed in the hospital/residential home setting rather than in community-acquired cases.[87] The microbiology of lung abscess in pediatric patients is similar to that reported for adults.[88]

The most common sites for the development of lung abscess are the portions of the lung that are dependent in the supine position. These include the posterior segments of the upper lobes and the apical segments of the lower lobes, with the right lung being involved far more frequently than the left. The infection begins as a pneumonitis, with alveolar edema and an inflammatory infiltrate; it progresses to necrotizing pneumonia, characterized by multiple small cavitations. If treatment is delayed or inadequate, further progression of the infection and necrosis results in the formation of a single large abscess cavity that becomes bound by fibrosing inflammatory tissue that limits its further expansion. The abscess cavity may communicate with a bronchus or with the pleural space.

CLINICAL PRESENTATION

The course of primary lung abscess is gradually progressive, with most patients having symptoms for several weeks prior to diagnosis.[87] General malaise, low-grade fever, weight loss, night sweats, and pleuritic chest pain are frequent complaints. Patients commonly exhibit a cough productive of copious amounts of sputum, which in approximately half of the cases is putrid. Physical findings may include signs of frank consolidation, localized rales, or, in late cases, cavernous breath sounds.

The chest radiograph is diagnostic of lung abscess and typically reveals a single, thin-walled cavity, which may contain an air–fluid level. Etiologic diagnosis depends on bacteriologic studies on lower airway secretions. Because the normal inhabitants of the oropharynx are the leading pathogens in lung abscess, cultures of expectorated sputum specimens are of little value in diagnosis of this disease entity. Transtracheal aspiration is 80–90% accurate in establishing an etiologic diagnosis in anaerobic and aerobic lung abscess and is a safe and useful diagnostic adjunct when a specific bacteriologic diagnosis is necessary. Specimens for laboratory evaluation may also be obtained by fiber optic bronchoscopy.

TREATMENT

Antimicrobial therapy is the keystone of treatment of lung abscess. Prolonged treatment may be necessary to achieve cure without relapse. Initial treatment with parenteral antibiotics until defervescence and clinical improvement are achieved is generally recommended. Thereafter, oral therapy may be instituted and continued until satisfactory radiographic clearing has occurred, a process that may take several months. The choice of antimicrobial agents should be based on results of bacteriologic studies when available or on the clinical setting in which the infection occurred. In the past, lung abscesses acquired in the community were nearly always caused by anaerobic organisms (i.e., mouth anaerobes) susceptible to penicillin G, previously the drug of choice for primary lung abscess in this setting. However, the increasing prevalence of penicillin-resistant, β-lactamase–producing bacteria, most notably *Bacteroides* spp.,[89] has led many experts to recommend alternative agents. For abscesses resulting from aspiration events, most authorities recommend clindamycin (10 mg/kg/dose, up to 600 mg, IV every 6–8 hours). Alternative therapies includes cefoxitin (30–40 mg/kg/dose, up to 2 g, IV every 6 hours) or one of the β-lactam/β-lactamase inhibitor combinations, such as ampicillin–sulbactam (50 mg of ampicillin/kg/dose, up to 2.0 g, IV every 6 hours) or ticarcillin–clavulanate (50 mg ticarcillin/kg/dose, up to 3.0 g, IV every 6 hours). Some experts continue to use high dose penicillin G (25–50,000 units/kg/dose, up to 2 million units, IV every 4–6 hours) in combination with either clindamycin or metronidazole (7.5 mg/kg/dose, up to 500 mg, IV every 6 hours). When *S. aureus* and gram-negative bacilli, as well as anaerobes, are implicated in lung abscesses, combination antibiotic therapy is recommended. Clindamycin and the β-lactam/β-lactamase inhibitors both possess activity against *S. aureus* as well as anaerobes, and a combination of clindamycin plus a broad-spectrum cephalosporin, or a β-lactam/β-lactamase inhibitor plus an aminoglycoside, provides effective coverage in this circumstance.

The time course of resolution of primary lung abscess treated with appropriate antimicrobial agents depends on the size and location of the abscess cavity. In a review of 60 patients with primary lung abscess, Weiss[90] noted 80% radiographic resolution within 1 month of therapy for cavitations less than 3 cm in diameter, whereas in larger abscesses, resolution occurred in only 30% by 1 month. By 3 months, 70% showed complete radiographic resolution. Abscesses involving the right upper lobe resolved more slowly than those in other locations. Because of the eminent success of properly chosen antimicrobial therapy in the treatment of these infections, surgical drainage of primary lung abscess is rarely indicated. Bronchoscopy should be strongly considered to exclude foreign body and malignancy as predisposing conditions and, if the cavity of the abscess communicates with a bronchus, to aid in drainage. The mortality rate for primary lung abscess is 5–10%[87]; however, the prognosis for patients with severe underlying disease, such as malignancy and immunosuppression, is much more guarded.

References

1. Reynolds HY. Normal and defective respiratory host defenses, in Pennington JE (ed): Respiratory Infections: Diagnosis and Management. New York, Raven Press, 1983, pp 1–23.
2. Sibille Y, Reynolds HY. Macrophages and polymorphonuclear neutrophils in lung defense and injury. Am Rev Respir Dis 1990;141:471–501.
3. Kolls JK, Nelson S, Summer WR. Recombinant cytokines and pulmonary host defense. Am J Med Sci 1993;306:330–335.
4. Mason CM, Nelson S. Normal host defenses and impairments associated with the delayed resolution of pneumonia. Sem Resp Infect 1192;7:243–255.
5. Todd JK. Bacteriology and clinical relevance of nasopharyngeal and oropharyngeal cultures. Pediatr Infect Dis 1984;3:159–163.
6. Davidson M, Tempest B, Palmer DL. Bacteriologic diagnosis of acute pneumonia. Comparison of sputum, transtracheal aspirates and lung aspirates. JAMA 1976;235:158–163.
7. Griffen JJ, Meduri GU. New approaches in the diagnosis of noscocomial pneumonia. Med Clin North Am 1994;78:1091–1122.
8. Cook DJ, Brun-Buisson C, Guyatt GH, et al. Evaluation of new diagnostic technologies: Bronchoalveolar lavage and the diagnosis of ventilator associated pneumonia. Crit Care Med 1994;22:1314–1322.
9. Galvin JR, Gingrich RD, Hoffman E, et al. Ultrafast computed tomography of the chest. Radiol Clin North Am 1994;32:775–793.
10. Bartlett JG. Diagnostic accuracy of transtracheal aspiration bacteriologic studies. Am Rev Respir Dis 1977;115: 777–782.
11. Jimenez P, Saldias F, Meneses M, et al. Diagnostic bronchoscopy in patients with community-acquired pneumonia. Comparison between bronchoalveolar lavage and telescoping plugged catheter cultures. Chest 1993; 103:1023–1027.
12. Monto AS, Ross HW. The Tecumseh study of respiratory illness. X. Relation of acute infections to smoking, lung function and chronic symptoms. Am J Epidemiol 1978;107:57–64.
13. Stark JM. Lung infections in children. Curr Opinion Pediatr 1993;5:273–280.
14. Aldous MB, Grayston JT, Wang SP, et al. Seroepidemiology of *Chlamydia pneumoniae* TWAR infection in Seattle families, 1966–1979. J Infect Dis 1992;166:646–649.
15. Reed SE, Bayde A. Organ cultures of respiratory epithelium infected with rhinovirus and parainfluenza virus studied by scanning electron microscope. Infect Immunol 1972;6:68–76.
16. Stark JM, Busse WW. Respiratory virus infection and airway hyperreactivity in children. Pediatr Allergy Immunol 1991;2:95–110.
17. Lebowitz MD, Burrows B. The relationship of acute respiratory illness history to the prevalence and incidence of obstructive lung disorders. Am J Epidemiol 1977; 105:544–554.
18. Krasinski K, LaCouture R, Holzman RS. Screening for respiratory syncytial virus and assignment to a cohort at admission to reduce nosocomial transmission. J Pediatr 1990;116:894–898.
19. Farizo KM, Cochi SL, Zell ER, et al. Epidemiological features of Pertussis in the United States, 1980–1989. Clin Infect Dis 1992;14:708–719.
20. Hurwitz ES, Barrett MJ, Bregman D, et al. Public health service study of Reye's syndrome and medications. Report of the main study. JAMA 1987;257:1905–1911.
21. Dulfano MJ, Adler K, Wooten O. Physical properties of sputum. IV. Effects of 100 percent humidity and water mist. Am Rev Respir Dis 1973;107:130–132.
22. Irwin RS, Curley FJ, Bennett FM. Appropriate use of antitussives and protussives. A practical review. Drugs 1993;46:80–91.
23. Hayden FG, Monto AS. Oral rimantadine hydrochloride therapy of influenza A virus H3N2 subtype infection in adults. Antimicrob Agents Chemother 1986;29:339–341.
24. Chodosh S. Treatment of acute exacerbations of chronic bronchitis: State of the art. Am J Med 1991;91(suppl 6A):87S–92S.

25. Reynolds HY, Merrill WW. Airway changes in young smokers that may antedate chronic obstructive lung disease. Med Clin North Am 1981;65:667–689.
26. Heard BE, Khatchatourov V, Otto H, et al. The morphology of emphysema, chronic bronchitis and bronchiectasis: Definition, nomenclature and classification. J Clin Pathol 1979;32:882–892.
27. Definition and classification of chronic bronchitis for clinical and epidemiologic purposes. A report to the Medical Research Council by their Committee on the Aetiology of Chronic Bronchitis. Lancet 1965;1:775–779.
28. Murray PR. Macroscopic and microscopic evaluation of respiratory specimens. Clin Lab Med 1982;2:259–267.
29. Tager I, Speizer FE. Role of infection in chronic bronchitis. N Engl J Med 1975;292:563–571.
30. Sarkkinen HK, Halonen PE, Arstila PP, et al. Detection of respiratory syncytial, parainfluenza type 2, and adenovirus antigens by radioimmunoassay and enzyme immunoassay on nasopharyngeal specimens from children with acute respiratory disease. J Clin Microbiol 1981;13:258–265.
31. Hughes DM, Lesouef PN, Landau LI. Effect of salbutamol on respiratory mechanics in bronchiolitis. Pediatr Res 1987; 22:83–86.
32. Wang EE, Milner R, Allen U, et al. Bronchodilators for treatment of mild bronchitis: A factorial randomized trial. Arch Dis Child 1992;67:289–293.
33. Stecenko MA. Treatment of viral bronchiolitis: Do steroids make sense? Contemp Pediatr 1987;(April):121–130.
34. Patterson JL, Fernandez-Larsson R. Molecular mechanisms of action of ribavirin. Rev Infect Dis 1990;12:1139–1146.
35. Rodriquez WJ, Kim HW, Brandt CD, et al. Aerosolized ribavirin in the treatment of patients with respiratory syncytial virus disease. Pediatr Infect Dis J 1987;6:159–163.
36. Janai HK, Stuttman HR, Zaleska M, et al. Ribavirin effect on pulmonary function in young infants with respiratory syncytial virus bronchiolitis. Pediatr Infect Dis J 1993; 12:214–218.
37. 1994 Redbook: Report of the Committee on Infectious Diseases, 23rd ed., Committee on Infectious Diseases, American Academy of Pediatrics. 1994, pp 570–574.
38. Meert KL, Sarnaik AP, Gelmini MJ, et al. Aerosolized ribavirin in mechanically ventilated children with respiratory syncytial virus lower respiratory tract disease: A prospective, double-blind, randomized trial. Crit Care Med 1994;22:566–572.
39. Osler W. The Principles and Practice of Medicine, 4th ed. New York, Appleton-Century-Crofts, 1901, p 108.
40. Johanson WG Jr, Woods DE, Chadhuri TR. Association of respiratory tract colonization with adherence of gram-negative bacilli to epithelial cells. J Infect Dis 1979;139:667–673.
41. Gleckman RA, Roth RM. Community-acquired bacterial pneumonia in the elderly. Pharmacotherapy 1984;4:81–88.
42. Carden DL, Gibb KA. Pneumonia and lung abscess. Emerg Med Clin North Am 1983;1:345–370.
43. Toews GB. Nosocomial pneumonia. Clin Chest Med 1987;8:467–479.
44. Klein JO. Emerging perspectives in management and prevention of infections of the respiratory tract in infants and children. Am J Med 1985;78:38–44.
45. Vadheim CM, Greenberg DP, Eriksen E, et al. Protection provided by *Haemophilus influenzae* type b conjugate vaccines in Los Angeles county: A case-control study. Pediatr Infect Dis J 1994;13:274–280.
46. Baker CJ, Edwards MS. Group B streptococcal infections, in Remington JS, Klein JO (eds): Infectious Disease of the Fetus and Newborn Infant, 3rd ed. Philadelphia, WB Saunders, 1990, pp 742–811.
47. Pierce AK, Sandord JP. State of the art: Aerobic gram-negative bacillary pneumonias. Am Rev Resp Dis 1974; 110:647–658.
48. Chow JW, Fine MJ, Shlaes DM, et al. *Enterobacter bacteremia:* Clinical features and emergence of antibiotic resistance during therapy. Ann Intern Med 1991;115:585–590.
49. Meyer KS, Urban C, Eagan JA, et al. Nosocomial outbreak of *Klebsiella* infection resistant to late-generation cephalosporins. Ann Intern Med 1993;119:353–358.
50. Hager H, Verghese A, Alvarez S, et al. *Branhamella catarrhalis* respiratory infections. Rev Infect Dis 1987;9:1140–1149.
51. Meyer RD, Finegold SM. Legionnaire's disease. Ann Rev Med 1980;31:219–232.
52. Orenstein WA, Overturf GD, Leedom JM, et al. The frequency of *Legionella* infection prospectively determined in children hospitalized with pneumonia. J Pediatr 1981;99:403–406.
53. Zuravleff JJ, Yu VL, Shonnard J, et al. Diagnosis of Legionnaire's disease: An update of laboratory methods with new emphasis on isolation by culture. JAMA 1983;250:1982–1985.
54. Bartlett JG. Anaerobic bacterial pneumonitis. Am Rev Respir Dis 1979;119:19–23.
55. Rieder HL, Cauthen GM, Kelly GD, et al. Tuberculosis in the United States. JAMA 1989;262:385–389.
56. Sunderman G, McDonald RJ, Maniatis T, et al. Tuberculosis as a manifestation of the acquired immunodeficiency syndrome (AIDS). JAMA 1986;256:362–366.
57. Goble M, Iseman MD, Madsen LA, et al. Treatment of 171 patients with pulmonary tuberculosis resistant to isoniazid and rifampin. N Engl J Med 1993;328:527–532.
58. Edlin BR, Tokars JI, Grieco MH, et al. An outbreak of multidrug-resistant tuberculosis among hospitalized patients with the acquired immunodeficiency syndrome. N Engl J Med 1992;326:1514–1521.
59. Broughton RA. Infections due to *Mycoplasma pneumoniae* in childhood. Pediatr Infect Dis 1986;5:71–85.
60. Murray JF, Mills J. Pulmonary infectious complications of human immunodeficiency virus infection. Am Rev Resp Dis 1990;141:1356–1372 (part I); 1582–1598 (part II).
61. Meduri GU, Stein DS. Pulmonary manifestations of acquired immunodeficiency syndrome. Clin Infect Dis 1992;14:98–113.
62. Naidich DP, McGuinness G. Pulmonary manifestations of AIDS. CT and radiographic correlations. Radiol Clin North Am 1991;29:999–1017.
63. Pizzo PA. Management of fever in patients with cancer and treatment-induced neutropenia. N Engl J Med 1993;328:1323–1332.
64. Lieschke GJ, Burgess AW. Granulocyte colony stimulating factor and granulocyte macrophage stimulating factor. N Engl J Med 1992;327:28–35.

65. Brown RB, Hosmer D, Chen HC, et al. A comparison of infections in different ICU's within the same hospital. Crit Care Med 1985;13:472–476.
66. Martin MA. Nosocomial infections in intensive care units: an overview of their epidemiology, outcome, and prevention. New Horizons 1993;1:162–171.
67. Jarvis WR, Edwards JR, Culver DH, et al. Nosocomial infection rates in adult and pediatric intensive care units in the United States. Am J Med 1991;91(suppl 3B):185S–91S.
68. Craven DE, Steger KA, Barber TW. Preventing nosocomial pneumonia: State of the art and perspectives for the 1990's. Am J Med 1991;91(suppl 3B):44S–53S.
69. Driks MR, Craven DE, Celli BR, et al. Nosocomial pneumonia in intubated patients given sucralfate as compared to antacids or histamine type 2 blockers. N Engl J Med 1987;317:1376–1382.
70. Craven DE, Kunches LM, Kilinsky V, et al. Risk factors for pneumonia and fatality in patients receiving continuous mechanical ventilation. Am Rev Resp Dis 1986;133:792–796.
71. Ledingham IM, Alcock SR, Eastaway AT, et al. Triple regimen of selective decontamination of the digestive tract, systemic cefotaxime, and microbiological surveillance for prevention of acquired infection in intensive care. Lancet 1988;1:785–790.
72. Brun-Buisson C, Legrand P, Rauss A, et al. Intestinal decontamination for control of nosocomial multiresistant gram-negative bacilli: Study of an outbreak in an intensive care unit. Ann Intern Med 1989;110:873–881.
73. Jacoby GA. Prevalence and resistance mechanisms of common bacterial respiratory pathogens. Clin Infect Dis 1994;18:951–957.
74. Friedland IR, McCracken GH Jr. Management of infections caused by antibiotic-resistant *Streptococcus pneumoniae.* N Engl J Med 1994;331:377–382.
75. Jacoby GA, Archer GA. New mechanisms of bacterial resistance to antimicrobial agents. N Engl J Med 1991;324:601–612.
76. Honeybourne D, Baldwin DR. The site concentrations of antimicrobial agents in the lung. J Antimicrob Chemother 1992;30:249–260.
77. Cunha BA. Antibiotic pharmacokinetic considerations in pulmonary infections. Sem Resp Infect 1991;6:168–182.
78. Bodem CR, Lampton LM, Miller DP, et al. Endobronchial pH. Relevance to aminoglycoside activity in gram-negative bacillary pneumonia. Am Rev Resp Dis 1983; 127:39–41.
79. Gough PA, Jordan NS. A review of the therapeutic efficacy of aerosolized and endotracheally instilled antibiotics. Pharmacotherapy 1982;2:367–377.
80. Stout SA, Derendorf H. Local treatment of respiratory infections with antibiotics. Drug Intell Clin Pharm 1987;21:322–329.
81. Bryant RE, Hammond D. Interaction of purulent material with antibiotics used to treat pseudomonas infections. Antimicrob Agents Chemother 1974;6:702–707.
82. Levy J, Smith AL, Kenny MA, et al. Bioactivity of gentamicin in purulent sputum from patients with cystic fibrosis or bronchiectasis: Comparison with activity in sputum. J Infect Dis 1983;148:1069–1076.
83. Blumer JL, Stern RC, Klinger JD, et al. Ceftazidime therapy in patients with cystic fibrosis and multiply-drug-resistant pseudomonas. Am J Med 1985;79(suppl 2A):37–46.
84. Mendelman PM, Smith AL, Levy J, et al. Aminoglycoside penetration, inactivation, and efficacy in cystic fibrosis sputum. Am Rev Resp Dis 1985;132:761–765.
85. Bartlett JG, Gorbach SL, Tally FP. Bacteriology and treatment of primary lung abscess. Am Rev Respir Dis 1974;109:510–518.
86. Bartlett JG. Anaerobic infection of the lung and pleural space. Am Rev Respir Dis 1974;110:56–77.
87. Bartlett JG, Gorbach SL, Finegold SM. The bacteriology of aspiration pneumonia. Am J Med 1974;56:202–207.
88. Brook I, Finegold SM. Bacteriology and therapy of lung abscess in children. J Pediatr 1979;94:10–12.
89. Levison ME, Mangura CT, Lorber B, et al. Clindamycin compared with penicillin for the treatment of anaerobic lung abscess. Ann Intern Med 1983;98:466–471.
90. Weiss W. Cavity behavior in acute primary nonspecific lung abscess. Am Rev Resp Dis 1973;198:1273–1275.

Chapter 101

Upper Respiratory Tract Infections

Monique Richer, PharmD, BCPS,
and Marc LeBel, PharmD, FCCP, FCSHP

Otitis media, pharyngitis, and sinusitis are the most common acute upper respiratory tract infections of early childhood. Inadequate understanding of the underlying microbiology, pathophysiology, and predisposing factors can compromise their management. Treatment failures and the development of resistant pathogens may lead to severe secondary outcomes, such as irreversible deafness, speech and learning impairments, rheumatic fever, acute glomerulonephritis, and meningitis. With a better understanding of the disease process and the advent of an armamentarium of new antimicrobial agents, management and outcome can now be improved.

OTITIS MEDIA

When discussing otitis media, misinterpretation can occur as a result of the indifferent use of descriptive terms. Table 101.1 lists the recommended terminology.[1] *Otitis media* is a nonspecific term describing an inflammation of the middle ear.[1] It is classified according to clinical presentation. *Acute otitis media* involves the rapid onset of signs and symptoms of inflammation in the middle ear that manifests clinically as one or more of the following: otalgia (denoted by pulling of the ear in some infants), hearing loss, fever, or irritability. Clinical presentation may include nonspecific symptoms such as lethargy, anorexia, vomiting, or diarrhea. The tympanic membrane is opaque, bulging, and has limited or no mobility to pneumatic otoscopy, all indicative of a middle ear effusion. Otorrhea (purulent discharge) through perforation of the tympanic membrane or through tympanostomy tubes, accompanied by otalgia and fever, is also indicative of acute otitis media. Redness of the tympanic membrane is not pathognomonic since it can result from sneezing, coughing, crying, or fever.

Otitis media with effusion (accumulation of liquid in the middle ear cavity) differs from acute otitis media in that signs and symptoms of an acute infection are absent. The opacity of the tympanic membrane makes the type of effusion, serous, mucus, or purulent, difficult to determine. Otitis media with effusion is classified according to the duration of the effusion: acute, less than 3 weeks; subacute, 3 weeks to 3 months; chronic, longer than 3 months. Middle ear effusion declines exponentially over a period of weeks to months. It is expected that 36–77% of episodes will resolve within 1 month and that 9–32% of children will have had an episode lasting more than 3 months.[2] This indicates that otitis media with effusion may be a complication of acute otitis media, making it difficult to distinguish between the two.

Chronic purulent otitis media is characterized by a chronic inflammation of the middle ear and the mastoid, with purulent otorrhea, in the presence of a perforated tympanic membrane or of tympanostomy tubes.

Otitis media without effusion (also called myringitis) is a rare condition characterized by redness and opacity of the eardrum. Mobility is unaltered and there is absence of a middle ear effusion.

EPIDEMIOLOGY

Acute otitis media is the most frequent diagnosis in infants and children who visit physicians because of illness.[2] Acute episodes are more frequent during the first 3 years of life, with the peak incidence occurring between 9 and 12 months.[2] A marked decrease in incidence has been demonstrated after the age of 6. Studies in the United States have shown that by the age of 1 year, more than 60% of the children will have had one or more episodes of otitis media, and 17% will have had at least three episodes. By the age of 7, it is estimated that more than 93% of the children will have experienced otitis media, and more than 40% will have had over three episodes.[2,3] Although considered uncommon in adults, U.S. surveys identified approximately 4 million visits to physicians per year by adults for middle ear infection.[1]

TABLE 101.1. RECOMMENDED CLASSIFICATION OF OTITIS MEDIA AND COMMONLY USED SYNONYMS

Acute Otitis Media	Otitis Media with Effusion
Suppurative	Serous
Purulent	Nonsuppurative
Bacterial	Mucoid
	"Glue ear"

ETIOLOGY

Several risk factors[1,2] contribute to the higher incidence and increased frequency of otitis media.

Age at first episode. The earlier children experience their first episode of otitis media, the greater the risk of developing more severe, persistent, and recurrent episodes. Infants with a first episode before the age of 6 months have a relative risk of 1.5 of acute otitis media in the next 24 months compared with children with a first episode at an age older than 6 months.[2]

Environmental factors. A history of recurrent acute otitis media or respiratory tract infections in a sibling doubles the risk of developing acute otitis media. Parental smoking may increase the risk of otitis media.[2,4] Children who attend day-care centers are at a greater risk for acute otitis media, recurrent episodes, and also otitis media with effusion.[2,4,5]

Season. The frequency of otitis media is greater in winter months and appears to parallel the outbreaks of viral infections of the respiratory tract, in particular infections with respiratory syncytial virus, influenza A and B, adenovirus, and rhinovirus.[2,6]

Gender. Males are more prone to episodes of acute otitis media and are at a greater risk for recurrent disease.

Race. The incidence of acute otitis media is more predominant in Caucasians than in the American black population.[2] Native Americans and Inuit represent a population in which this disease is severe, widespread, and recurrent.[2,7] Children in underdeveloped areas frequently present with a necrotizing process of the middle ear.[1] The differences observed among races are attributed to factors such as anatomic differences of the eustachian tube, living conditions, availability of medical care, and the small sample sizes of the study groups.

Malformations. Infants with anatomic problems such as Down syndrome, submucous cleft, and/or a cleft palate are particularly at risk for the development of acute otitis media and recurrences.

Nutrition. Breast-feeding appears in most studies as a significant protective factor in the development of otitis media.[2] Exclusive breast-feeding for 4 months or more resulted in a decreased risk for single and recurrent episodes of otitis media during the first year of life.[4,8] This protection proved to be independent of risk factors such as maternal smoking, gender, siblings, and day-care attendance.[8] This protective effect could be attributed to the infant being held in an upright position during breast-feeding or to the presence of secretory IgA or prostaglandin E_1 in breast milk.[4,8]

Immunity. Several studies have suggested that children with allergies, atopy, and immunoglobulin G (in particular IgG_2) deficiencies exhibit a higher risk of acute otitis media.[2,9] However, in children with no known immunodeficiency, total serum immunobglobulin G concentrations were found to be of the same magnitude in both children with recurrent acute otitis media and those without.[10]

Socioeconomic status. A correlation between poor social conditions and middle ear disease has been noted.[1,2] Crowded living and poor sanitary conditions may explain the high prevalence of acute otitis media in underprivileged children.

COMPLICATIONS

Complications and sequelae of otitis media are categorized as intracranial and intratemporal. The intracranial complications, meningitis and brain abscess, are infrequent.[2] Intratemporal sequelae, eardrum diseases, are more frequent and can result in hearing loss.[2] The hearing loss can affect speech and language development, cognitive and academic performance, and behavior.[2]

ANATOMY AND PATHOPHYSIOLOGY

The middle ear is best described as an air-filled cavity that begins at the tympanic membrane and extends to the nasopharynx via the eustachian tube (Fig. 101.1) It is contiguous with air-filled cells of the mastoid, but also shares the same respiratory mucosa as the nose, nasopharynx, and eustachian tubes. Signs and effects of inflammation, infection, or obstruction in one area are therefore likely to be reflected throughout the respiratory tract. This is the basis of one theory of the pathogenesis of middle ear disease: The patient has an antecedent event that results in congestion of the respiratory mucosa, causing secretions to accumulate in the middle ear; bacteria present in the middle ear proliferate in the secretions resulting in acute otitis media. In recurrent episodes of acute otitis media or otitis media with effusion, anatomic or physiologic abnormalities of the eustachian tube are the most important factors. Abnormal function of the eustachian tube represents the second theory of otitis media pathogenesis.

The eustachian tube lies at a 45° angle to the horizontal plane in adults, and at a 10° angle in infants (Fig. 101.1). Its primary functions with respect to the middle ear are three-

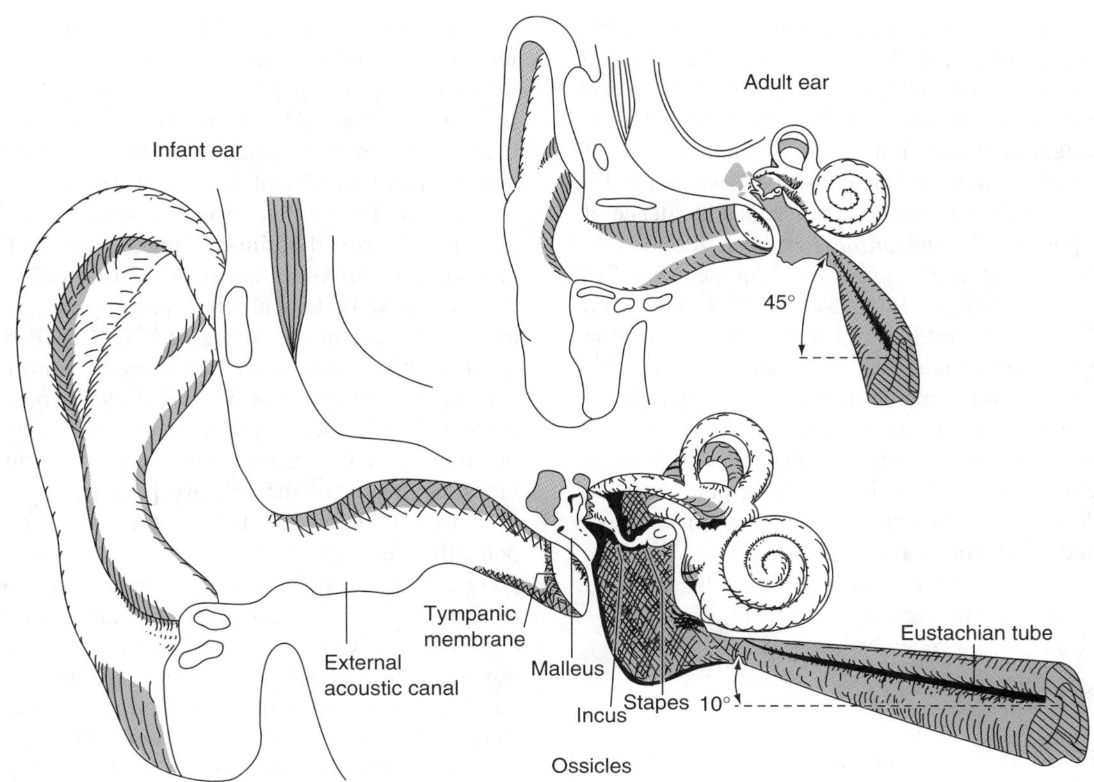

Figure 101.1. Anatomic differences between the angle of the eustachian tube of the infant and adult. *(From Bluestone CD, Klein JO. Otitis media with effusion, atelectasis, and eustachian tube dysfunction, in Bluestone CD, Stool SE, Scheetz MD (eds): Pediatric Otolaryngology. Philadelphia, PA, WB Saunders, 1983, p 366, with permission.)*

fold: regulation of atmospheric pressure between both sides of the tympanic membrane; protection from nasopharyngeal secretions; and draining secretions from the middle ear into the nasopharynx.[11] In infants, this difference in angulation may cause improper drainage of the middle ear as a result of decreased gravitational effects on the eustachian tube. It has also been noted that the eustachian tubes are shorter than those of adults. This can impair the capillary action needed to prevent nasopharyngeal reflux.[11] In addition, the muscle responsible for eustachian tube opening, the tensor veli palatini, is less efficient. Thus the abnormal function of the eustachian tube can cause reflux, aspiration, or insufflation of nasopharyngeal bacteria up to the middle ear.

CLINICAL PRESENTATION

The presence of otalgia, partial deafness (secondary to effusion), fever, and a sudden onset of irritability are symptoms that characterize acute otitis media. This usually occurs in a child who has had an upper respiratory tract infection for several days. However, otitis media may be present in the absence of the aforementioned characteristics and reinforces the need for regular otoscopic examination.[1]

The diagnosis of otitis media is based on examination of the tympanic membrane. Inflammation or opacity of the tympanic membrane, the presence or absence of light reflection and bulging of the tympanic membrane are all suggestive of otitis media. Insufflation with a pneumatic otoscope allows for assessment of tympanic membrane mobility and is currently considered essential to the proper diagnosis of acute otitis media.

Mobility of the tympanic membrane can also be determined with a tympanometer. This instrument uses the reflection of sounds by the eardrum to detect the presence of liquid in the middle ear cavity. In difficult cases, the use of tympanocentesis provides a definitive diagnosis of otitis media and yields identification and susceptibility patterns of the pathogens.

MICROBIOLOGY

Bacterial cultures from the middle ear effusion of children over 1 month of age with acute, symptomatic otitis media have yielded strains of *Streptococcus pneumonia* (30%), predominantly nontypable strains of *Haemophilus influenzae* (21%), *Moxarella catarrhalis* (12%), and to a lesser extent, group A β-hemolytic *Streptococcus pyogenes* (3%) and *Staphylococcus aureus* (2%). In infants younger than 1 month, *Staphylococcus* are found in higher frequency. *Escherichia coli, Pseudomonas aeruginosa,* and group B streptococci have also been cultured from middle ear aspirates. The bacteriology of middle ear effusion has changed little since the mid-1970s, with the exception of the emergence of ampicillin resistance in *H. influenzae.*[12] Prevalence of β-lactamase production (the most frequent type of resistance) by *H. influenzae* (for non–type-B strains only) varies from one medical center to another. The incidence of β-lactamase positive *H. influenzae* has been reported to range from 30–40% of all *H. influenzae.*[13] An increased frequency of *M. catarrhalis* from 5% to 23% has been reported.[12,14] A high rate of β-lactamase production (70–90%) by *M. catarrhalis* has been documented.[13,15,16] The bacteriology of otitis media in adults is comparable.[17] Reported incidences for *H. influenzae* and *S. pneumonia* were 26% and 21%, respectively. The incidence of β-lactamase-producing isolates was lower. Anaerobic bacteria such as *Chlamydia trachomatis* as well as viruses have been suspected of playing a role in otitis media.[14,18] Their contribution to the disease process is obscured by the difficulty in isolating these pathogens.

TREATMENT

Although otitis media occurs commonly, there is no universally accepted method of management. A panoply of clinical studies compares the use of antibiotics, decongestants, antihistamines, or adjuvant steroid administration and adenenoidectomy. Oral antibiotics are still the mainstay of therapy. However, the common practice of antibiotic administration for otitis media has been questioned. European investigators evaluated the use of nasal drops and analgesics over the traditional treatment with antibiotics in episodes of acute otitis media. In approximately 5000 children evaluated, it was estimated that 90% had their acute episode of otitis media cured within 3–4 days with symptomatic treatment only.[19] Persistent symptoms for more than 4 days justified a course of antibiotics with or without myringotomy (incision of the tympanic membrane). Deficiencies in the selection of the study population, methodology, and data analysis prevent these studies from being conclusive. The sharp decrease in suppurative complications of acute otitis media observed with the advent of antibiotic therapy constitutes in itself a sufficient reason for using antibiotics. In addition, it is difficult to identify those who would or would not benefit from initiation of antimicrobial treatment.

Antibiotic Therapy

The selection of the appropriate antibiotic is based on antimicrobial susceptibility, penetration into the middle ear, clinical efficacy, compliance factors, adverse effects profile, and cost.

Antimicrobial Activity (Table 101.2)

Amoxicillin and ampicillin, with excellent *in vitro* activity against *S. pneumoniae* and most *H. influenzae* isolates from the middle ear, are still the first choice in the treatment of acute otitis media in areas where the emergence of β-lactamase-producing *H. influenzae* and *M. catarrhalis* is limited.[1,13] The addition of the β-lactamase inhibitor clavulanic acid to amoxicillin increases its activity against aminopenicillin-resistant strains of *H. influenzae* and *M. catarrhalis.* Drugs that evade the action of β-lactamase also include trimethoprim–sulfamethoxazole (TMP–SMX), cefixime, cefuroxime axetil, cefaclor, cefprozil, cefpodoxime proxetil, loracarbef, azithromycin, clarithromycin and erythromycin–sulfisoxazole.[1,20–24] TMP–SMX offers good activity against *H. influenzae.* Unfortunately, its activity against group A *Streptococcus* is poor and pneumococcal resistance appears to be increasing. The combination of sulfisoxazole with erythromycin also provides coverage for the primary pathogens. In addition, it is a useful alternative for patients who are allergic to penicillin and cephalosporins. Cefaclor has demonstrated good activity against most pathogens. However, resistant strains of *H. influenzae* and *M. catarrhalis* have been reported.[12,20] Cefuroxime axetil, cefixime, cefprozil, cefpodoxime, and loracarbef are active against most microorganisms isolated in middle ear fluid, notably against all β-lactamase–producing strains.[20] Loracarbef and cefixime are less potent than amoxicillin against group A streptococci. The *in vitro* spectrum of activity of azithromycin and clarithromycin includes most pathogens that cause otitis media. Streptococci that are resistant to erythromycin can exhibit cross-resistance to azithromycin.[21] The combination of clarithromycin and its active metabolite has been demonstrated to have synergistic or additive activity against *H. influenzae.*[21]

Penetration into the Middle Ear Fluid

In addition to having adequate *in vitro* antimicrobial activity, bactericidal concentrations of the antimicrobial agent need to be present in the middle ear fluid. Table 101.3 presents the available data in terms of ratio between middle ear fluid concentrations (MEFC) of antimicrobials to minimal inhibitory concentrations (MIC_{90}), the lowest MIC required to inhibit 90% of the bacterial strains tested, of the three primary pathogens. This ratio allows for a better interpretation of antibiotic penetration in the middle ear and can serve to explain the lesser efficacy observed in certain clinical trials. Amoxicillin and ampicillin achieve concentrations that are two to six times higher than the MIC_{90} for the primary non–β-lactamase–producing pathogens of otitis media. Middle ear fluid penetration of cefaclor is low with concentrations being equal to the MIC_{90}. Erythromycin ethylsuccinate does not achieve appreciable concentrations in the middle ear, whereas the estolate salt demonstrates excellent penetration. None of the first-generation cephalosporins attains appreciable ratios for the β-lactamase–producing microorganisms (not shown in Table 101.3). The ratio of MEFC to MIC_{90} with respect to *S. pneumoniae* is high with cefprozil, cefuroxime, and clar-

TABLE 101.2. *IN VITRO* SPECTRUM OF ACTIVITY OF ANTIBIOTICS USED IN UPPER RESPIRATORY TRACT INFECTIONS

	Streptococcus pneumoniae	*Haemophilus influenzae* β-Lactamase Negative	β-Lactamase Positive	*Moxarella catarrhalis* β-Lactamase Negative	β-Lactamase Positive	Group A β-Hemolytic Streptococci
Ampicillin or amoxicillin	+	+	–	+	–	+
Azithromycin	+	+	+	+	+	+
Clarithromycin/14-hydroxyclarithromycin	+	+	+	+	+	+
Erythromycin	+	–	–	+	+	+
Erythromycin–sulfisoxazole	+	+	+	+	+	+
Trimethoprim–sulfamethoxazole	+	+	+	+	+	–
Amoxicillin–clavulanate	+	+	+	+	+	+
Cefaclor	+	+	±	+	+	+
Cefixime	+	+	+	+	+	+
Cefpodoxime proxetil	+	+	+	+	+	+
Cefprozil	+	+	+	+	+	+
Cefuroxime axetil	+	+	+	+	+	+
Loracarbef	+	+	+	+	+	+

Key: +, highly susceptible; ±, moderately susceptible; –, nonsusceptible.

ithromycin and its 14-hydroxy metabolite. The ratio is low for second- and third-generation cephalosporins with respect to β-lactamase–producing *H. influenzae* and *M. catarrhalis.* Clarithromycin and its primary metabolite attain excellent ratios of MEFC to the MIC_{90} of *M. catarrhalis.* However, its use resulted in reports of therapeutic failures when *H. influenzae* was the causative agent.[27]

Clinical Efficacy

Evaluating the efficacies of the antibiotics used in the treatment of otitis media is not straightforward. The majority of clinical trials of antibiotic therapy are comparative and often determine both clinical and bacteriological outcomes. More than 90% clinical success rates, generally defined as absence of all presenting signs and symptoms of acute otitis media, can be achieved in the presence of bacteriologi-

TABLE 101.3. RELATIONSHIP BETWEEN THE CONCENTRATION OF ANTIMICROBIALS USED IN OTITIS MEDIA AND THE MIC_{90} OF THE THREE PRIMARY MICROORGANISMS

	Streptococcus pneumoniae	*Haemophilus influenzae* β-Lactamase Negative	β-Lactamase Positive	*Moxarella catarrhalis* β-Lactamase Negative	β-Lactamase Positive
Amoxicillin	>+++++[a]	++	0	>+++++	0
Ampicillin	>+++++	++	0	+++	0
Cefaclor	+	+	+	+	+
Cefixime	+	>+++++	+	>+++++	+
Cefprozil	>+++++	++	++	0	0
Cefuroxime axetil	>+++++	>+++++	ND[b]	>+++++	ND
Clarithromycin/14-hydroxy-	>+++++	0	0	++++	++++
clarithromycin	>+++++	0	0	>+++++	>+++++
Erythromycin					
-estolate	+++	0	0	++	++
-ethylsuccinate	+	0	0	++	++
Loracarbef	+++	+	+	>+++++	+
Trimethoprim	+	++	+++	0	0
Sufamethoxazole	+	++++	++	ND	ND

[a]Relationship between the antimicrobial maximum concentration in middle ear fluid and the MIC_{90}; each + indicates that the antimicrobial concentration is onefold above the MIC_{90}; >+++++ indicates that the concentrations exceed the MIC_{90} fivefold; 0 indicates that the antimicrobial concentration is less than onefold the MIC_{90}.
[b]ND, no data available. (From Refs. 1, 20, 22, and 25–27.)

cal cure (sterile middle ear fluid culture) and 62% clinical cure can be observed with bacteriological failure.[28] An 80% clinical success rate was demonstrated in nonbacterial otitis media. It is also important to consider that symptomatic improvement can be observed without antibacterial therapy. A meta-analysis evaluating the complete clinical resolution of otitis media (exclusive of middle ear effusion) reported that the spontaneous rate of resolution without antibiotics or tympanocentesis was 81%.[29] The use of antibiotics increased resolution by 13.7%. Albeit modest, the impact of antibiotic use on clinical resolution was significant. Conversely, symptoms can persist despite effective antibacterial therapy, especially in the presence of viral infections.

Compliance Factors

Most children with otitis media become asymptomatic within 24–72 hours of the initiation of therapy. It is therefore not surprising that less than 50% of the children treated for otitis media complete the full course of antimicrobials.[30] The number of daily doses to be administered has an impact on the compliance to a therapeutic regimen. Table 101.4 summarizes the recommended doses and dosing schedules of the primary antimicrobials utilized in the treatment of upper respiratory tract infections. Short dosing intervals and the recommended 10-day course of antimicrobial therapy for acute otitis media certainly represent contributory factors to noncompliance. A shortened therapy duration of 5 days with amoxicillin has shown comparable efficacy for children whose disease responds rapidly. This regimen may improve antibiotic compliance as well as decrease therapy cost and risk of side effects.[31] It should be noted that in this study, tympanocentesis was performed in every patient and may have had an impact on outcome. In a randomized, double-blind clinical trial, rates of improvement, failure, relapse, and reinfection with a single dose of ceftriaxone (50 mg/kg, intramuscularly) were comparable to a 10-day course of oral amoxicillin (40 mg/kg/d) in children with acute otitis media.[32]

Although liquid formulations of antimicrobials offer flexibility in dosage adjustment for children, palatability of these preparations impacts on compliance. Fortunately, the majority of the antimicrobial suspensions on the market for children are flavored.

Adverse Effects

The most frequent adverse reactions associated with the use of antimicrobials in the treatment of acute otitis media are gastrointestinal and cutaneous. The incidence of diarrhea is highest with ampicillin (>20%). The addition of clavulanic acid to amoxicillin increases, in a dose-related matter, the incidence of diarrhea, nausea, and vomiting when compared to amoxicillin alone. Cefixime is reported to cause diarrhea more often than cefaclor and the other cephalosporins (11–20%). The incidences of rashes and diarrhea with the newer cephalosporins cefpodoxime proxetil, cefprozil, and loracarbef range from 1–3% and are similar to that of other cephalosporins and penicillins. Erythromycin–sulfisoxazole has been associated with abdominal cramping as well as diarrhea when the erythromycin component exceeded 40 mg/kg/d. Gastrointestinal disturbances were reported less frequently with azithromycin and clarithromycin than with erythromycin.

The potential for hypersensitivity reactions with β-lactams and with sulfonamide containing antimicrobials is well recognized. The nonallergic rash, well described with aminopenicillins, is reported in approximately 10% of treated patients. Agents containing sulfonamides (TMP–SMX, erythromycin–sulfisoxazole) are known

TABLE 101.4. PEDIATRIC DOSING REGIMEN AND COST OF ANTIBIOTICS USED IN UPPER RESPIRATORY TRACT INFECTIONS

Antibiotic(s)	Total Daily Dose and Regimen	Cost ($)[a]	Liquid Formulation (mg/5 mL)
Penicillin V	50 mg/kg (every 6 h)	3.36[b]	125–250
Amoxicillin	30–40 mg/kg (every 8 h)	4.08[b]	125–250
Pivampicillin	40–50 mg/kg (every 12 h)	18.00[c]	175
Amoxicillin–clavulanate (4:1)	30 mg/kg of amoxicillin (every 8 h)	38.48	125/31.25–250/62.5
TMP–SMX (1:5)	8–10 mg/kg TMP (every 12 h)	6.05[b]	40/200
Cefaclor	40 mg/kg (every 8–12 h)	55.23	125–250
Cefixime	8 mg/kg (every 12–24 h)	46.06	100
Cefpodoxime proxetil	10 mg/kg (every 12 h)	54.00	50–100
Cefprozil	30 mg/kg (every 12 h)	60.36	125–250
Loracarbef	30 mg/kg (every 12 h)	70.20	100
Erythromycin–sulfisoxazole (1:3)	40 mg/kg of erythromycin (every 8 h)	16.12	200/600
Erythromycin ethylsuccinate	30 mg/kg (every 6–8 h)	7.86[b]	200–400
Erythromycin estolate	30 mg/kg (every 6–8 h)	13.99[b]	125–250

[a]Cost based on average wholesale price (Redbook, 1994).
[b]Cost based on generic price.
[c]Cost based on Canadian availability.

to cause rare hematologic effects and cutaneous reactions that could be as severe as exfoliative dermatitis or Stevens–Johnson syndrome. Cefaclor has been linked to the development of a serum–sickness-like illness associated with multiform erythema (1.1%), which is reversible with discontinuation of treatment.

Cost of Treatment

Since the efficacy, antimicrobial activity, and adverse effect profiles of many of the treatment regimens are comparable, cost of treatment becomes the issue. Table 101.4 lists the average wholesale price for different antimicrobial agents for the 10-day regimen for a 20-kg child. Amoxicillin has the lower cost. Amoxicillin–clavulanate and the newer cephalosporin offer broader bacterial coverage but are by far more expensive. Cefuroxime axetil, clarithromycin, and azithromycin were not included in this list because of the unavailability of a liquid formulation.

Antibiotic Selection

Amoxicillin remains the antibiotic of choice for the treatment of acute otitis media despite the concerns about increasing incidence of β-lactamase production among *H. influenzae* and *M. cattarhalis.*[12,33] The extension of antimicrobial coverage to include β-lactamase–producing organisms does not significantly increase the rate of clinical resolution or resolution of middle ear effusion.[29] But in the setting of increased resistance to β-lactam agents, TMP–SMX and amoxicillin–clavulanate are appropriate choices. TMP–SMX may not be effective when *Streptococcus pyogenes* (group A hemolytic streptococcus) is the causative organism.[12] Cefaclor offers adequate coverage of β-lactamase–producing organisms except some strains of *H. influenzae* and *M. catarrhalis.*[20] Cefixime, cefpodoxime proxetil, cefuroxime axetil, and loracarbef are effective as second-line agents in the treatment for acute otitis media caused by resistant strains of *H. influenzae* and *M. cattarhalis.* Azithromycin and clarithromycin are not approved in children and, like cefuroxime axetil, are not available in liquid form. In the treatment of childhood episodes of acute otitis media, evaluation of the comparative efficacies of the various antimicrobial agents has not yielded significant differences.[29] Amoxicillin is appropriate as a first-line agent in the treatment of adult otitis media.[17] In all other respects, the pharmacologic management of adult otitis media is similar to its management in children.

Supportive Treatment

In addition to antimicrobial therapy, supportive therapy with analgesics, antipyretics, and local heat have been shown to be beneficial in the comfort of the child. Although antihistamines and decongestants have been used for the symptomatic relief of acute otitis media, studies have not shown them to be efficacious in the resolution of effusion or relief of symptoms. Until studies can support their efficacy, the use of oral decongestants such as pseudoephedrine or phenylpropanolamine should be limited to 1 or 2 days of treatment, if any.

EVALUATION OF THERAPEUTIC OUTCOMES

With proper treatment, symptoms of acute otitis media in most children will abate within 24–72 hours. When otalgia or fever persists or recurs during therapy, a β-lactamase–producing microorganism should be suspected and an agent with β-lactamase activity should be used (Fig. 101.2). If treatment with the second-line agent fails, tympanocentesis to identify the pathogen may be indicated, particularly if the child is symptomatic or has an underlying disease.

All children should be reexamined at the end of the 10-day antibiotic therapy. Even with an efficacious antibiotic treatment, effusion of the middle ear may be present in 50% of children following treatment with antibiotics[2,12] and may persist for up to 3 months.[2] If the middle ear effusion persists

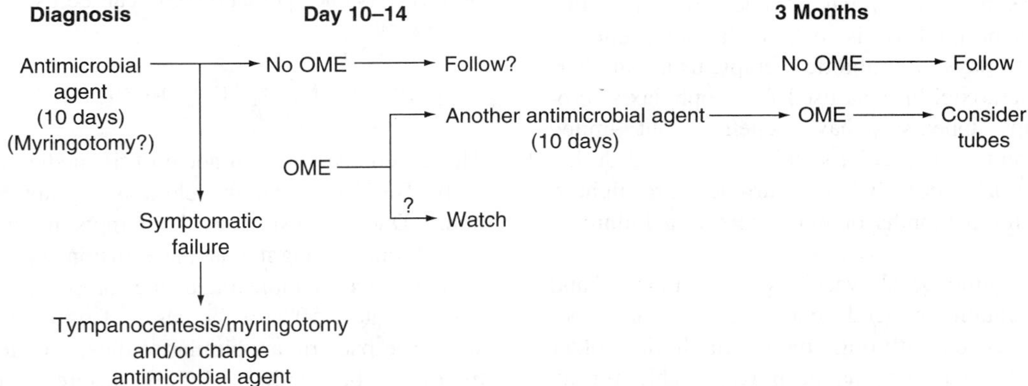

Figure 101.2. Recommended management plan for children with acute otitis media. OME, otitis media with effusion. *(From Bluestone CD. Management of otitis media in infants and children: Current role of old and new antimicrobial agents. Pediatr Infect Dis J 1988;7:S129–136, with permission.)*

beyond the initial 10 days of antimicrobial therapy several options can be considered: (1) another course of drug therapy using the same agent or an alternative antibiotic; one with β-lactamase activity is preferable if resistant strains are prevalent in the community; (2) topical or systemic decongestants, antihistamines, or a combination of these; or (3) systemic corticosteroids or eustachian tube–middle ear inflation. Unfortunately, none of these methods has been shown to be effective in randomized, controlled trials.[12] If the effusion persists beyond 2–3 months, it is termed otitis media with effusion and should be treated as described in the section on Otitis Media with Effusion.

Recurrent Acute Otitis Media

If the signs and symptoms of acute otitis media occur within 1 month of the initial episode, it is assumed that the same microorganism caused the infection. Emergence of resistance may be suspected. This new episode should be treated with a different antibiotic, preferably one with β-lactamase activity. If the new episode occurs over 1 month after the initial infection in a child who was completely free of signs and symptoms between episodes, the management of the recurrent episodes is the same as the first episode. If children exhibit more than four episodes in a 6-month period or six episodes in a 12-month period, these patients can be managed by chemoprophylaxis with antimicrobials, and/or myringotomy and insertion of tympanostomy tubes.[12]

Chemoprophylaxis

Several studies have demonstrated the effectiveness of chemoprophylaxis, but the indications, duration, and the most effective agent are still controversial.[34] The following regimens have been advocated: (1) amoxicillin (20–30 mg/kg/d) in one dose at bedtime or in two divided doses every 12 hours; (2) sulfisoxazole (80–100 mg/kg/d) every 24 hours; and (3) TMP–SMX (equivalent of 4 mg/kg/d of TMP) every 24 hours. It should be noted that TMP–SMX is not approved by the FDA for this indication. The appropriate course of treatment in patients who develop acute otitis media while on prophylaxis is to treat the acute episode with the usual 10 days of antibiotic therapy, using an alternative agent if amoxicillin was used for prophylaxis. Prophylactic therapy appears to have beneficial but limited effect on recurrent otitis media, should be initiated during the winter and early spring when recurrences are highest, and continued for 3 months or until there is a failure of therapy.

The antipneumococcal vaccines, Pnu-Imune® and Pneumovax®, contain frequently encountered pneumococcal antigens associated with otitis media. In children older than 2 years, this vaccine has been responsible for an approximately 10–20% reduction of acute otitis media (33% in day-care centers).[35] Unfortunately, children less than 2 years of age respond poorly to most polysaccharide vaccines. At this time, data are inadequate to evaluate the vaccine's effectiveness in routine prevention of otitis media in children older than 2 years.[35] The *Haemophilus* type B polysaccharide vaccine is not useful in the prevention of acute otitis media since nontypable strains of *H. influenzae* are most frequently implicated.

Myringotomy and Insertion of Tympanostomy Tubes

The most popular surgical approach to the treatment of recurrent episodes of otitis media is myringotomy and insertion of tympanostomy tubes (Fig. 101.3). Studies have shown that the insertion of tympanostomy tubes reduces recurrent episodes of otitis media by 50% with an infection-free period of 3 months for most.[36] The insertion of tympanostomy tubes interrupts the cycle of recurrent infections, rapidly restores essential hearing for a short period, and relieves the discomfort that causes irritability in children. The advantages associated with tube placement are not reached without potential risks, primarily, exposure to general anesthesia and permanent scarring of the tympanic membrane. The category of patients who can benefit most from tympanostomy tube placement, as well as the optimal duration of therapy, needs to be determined.[34]

Placement of tympanostomy tubes should be performed when the effusion of the middle ear is sterile. If acute otitis media occurs while the patient has tympanostomy tubes, an antimicrobial treatment such as amoxicillin should be instituted. Identification of the microorganism can also be attempted. If infection persists during antimicrobial therapy, the tympanostomy tubes themselves may be the cause, and their removal should be considered. *Pseudomonas aeruginosa* should be considered in this setting.

The following treatment options should be offered to parents of children or to patients experiencing recurrent otitis media and in whom the effusion appears to clear between bouts: (1) adequate and appropriate antimicrobial therapy of each episode; (2) antimicrobial prophylaxis; or (3) tympanostomy tube placement.[12] In recalcitrant cases, prophylaxis and tympanostomy can be used together.

OTITIS MEDIA WITH EFFUSION

The difference between acute otitis media and otitis media with effusion is that the child is asymptomatic with the latter. Due to unsuccessful attempts to culture bacteria, it was once thought that the effusion was sterile. Recent studies have demonstrated the presence of bacteria in approximately 50% of the cases of otitis media with effusion. The bacteria are similar to those isolated in acute otitis media but with a slightly different distribution: *H. influenzae,* 12–50%; *S. pneumoniae,* 3–40%; and *Staphylococcus epidermidis,* 19–37%. *Staphylococcus aureus* and *M. catarrhalis* are encountered less frequently.[1]

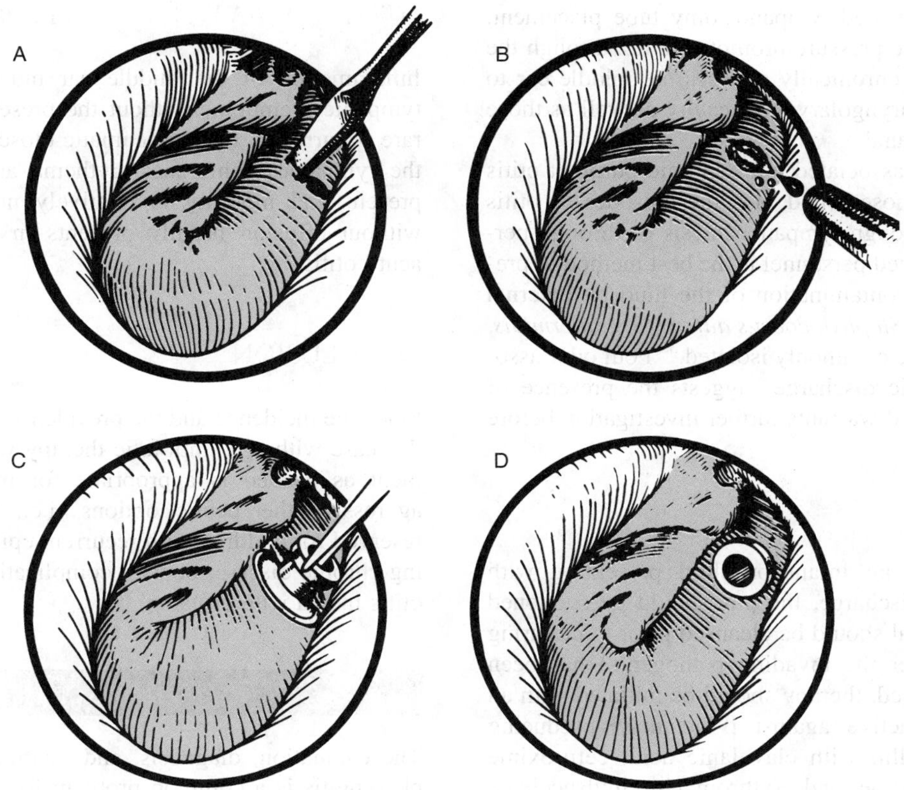

Figure 101.3. Insertion of tympanostomy tube. (A) Radical incision of the tympanic membrane, (B) aspiration of middle ear effusion, (C) insertion of short biflanged tympanostomy tube, (D) appearance of tube in the anterosuperior portion of tympanic membrane. *(From Bluestone CD, Klein JO. Otitis media with effusion, atelectasis, and eustachian tube dysfunction, in Bluestone CD, Stool SE, Scheetz MD (eds): Pediatric Otolaryngology. Philadelphia, PA, WB Saunders, 1983, p 484, with permission.)*

Chronic otitis media with effusion, described as an effusion lasting more than 3 months, requires antibiotic treatment. A short course of antibiotics appears to be effective in the short-term clearance of the effusion.[34] However, the effect is limited and is of relatively short duration.[34] Decongestants alone or in combination with antihistamines as well as systemic or intranasal corticosteroids have not been shown to be efficacious or to speed the resolution of the effusion. Improvement of effusion is best seen with insertion of tympanostomy tubes. Tonsillectomy with or without adenoidectomy remains controversial in the management of chronic effusion. It is indicated in children with nasopharyngeal obstruction secondary to adenoid tissue hypertrophy and presenting with more than four tonsillopharyngitis episodes per year. This surgical procedure is not presently indicated in patients with chronic otitis media with effusion.

Treatment of chronic otitis media with effusion is also indicated to prevent hearing loss, due to the presence of middle ear effusion, which can lead to an impairment of cognitive and language function resulting in disturbances in psychosocial adjustment.[37] In addition to hearing loss, treatment should be undertaken in the following instances: (1) occurrence in young infants, due to their inability to communicate symptoms; (2) concurrence of an acute purulent upper respiratory tract infection; (3) the presence of permanent conductive-sensorineural hearing loss; (4) vertigo or tinnitus; (5) the presence of severe atelectasis; (6) changes of the middle ear, such as adhesive otitis or ossicular involvement; (7) presence of effusion for 2–3 months or longer; or (8) frequent episodes of effusion, resulting in the accumulation of time of effusion during a period of 6 out of 12 months.[12]

CHRONIC PURULENT OTITIS MEDIA

Chronic purulent otitis media is described as an inflammation of the middle ear and mastoid with otorrhea of at least 3 months' duration. This condition is prevalent in Native Americans, Inuit, and children with cleft palate. The chronic otorrhea may be associated with a perforation or rupture of the central portion of the tympanic membrane and commonly accompanies an episode of otitis media with effusion or a complicated tympanostomy tube placement. The resulting positive pressure promotes reflux through the eustachian tube and chronically exposes the middle ear to pathogens of the pharyngolaryngeal cavity as well as those of the external ear canal.

The pathogens associated with chronic purulent otitis media differ from those found in acute episodes of otitis media. Sampling through tympanocentesis or through perforation by experienced personnel is the best method to prevent the accidental contamination of the fluid by external ear canal pathogens. *Staphylococcus aureus, S. epidermidis,* and *P. aeruginosa* are commonly isolated.[38] Foul odor associated with otorrhetic discharge suggests the presence of anaerobic bacteria and warrants further investigation before initiation of therapy.

Treatment

On examination of an infant or child presenting with chronic otorrhetic discharge, the pus should be suctioned and the external canal should be cleansed prior to culturing the middle ear. After the invading pathogen(s) has been identified or speculated, therapy should be initiated with an oral drug that is active against β-lactamase–producing organisms. Amoxicillin with clavulanic acid, cefuroxime axetil, cefaclor, cefixime, and erythromycin ethylsuccinate with sulfisoxazole are first-line agents. Topical treatment with a suspension containing polymyxin B, neomycin, and hydrocortisone (Cortisporin) or one composed of neomycin, polymyxin E, and hydrocortisone (Colymycin) has been advocated but is not commonly used because of the potential for ototoxicity.[38] If *Pseudomonas* is found or suspected, it may be necessary to admit the patient to the hospital for the administration of parenteral antipseudomonal antimicrobials such as ceftazidime, ticarcillin, or aztreonam (not available in Canada). The use of fluoroquinolones, such as ciprofloxacin, can be considered in adults.

Daily aural hygiene is useful in preventing reinfection and aiding in the healing process of the tympanic membrane. In approximately 88% of patients treated, the combination of antimicrobials and aural hygiene has demonstrated a cessation of otorrhetic discharge within 5–7 days.[38] Cleansing agents such as carbamide peroxyde (Debrox) and solutions containing propylene glycol should be used cautiously when perforation or transtympanic tubes are present. Hydrogen peroxide solution (3%) diluted as 1:1 or 1:3 with sterile water is a valuable aural cleanser for pus and debris removal. No data are available with respect to toxicity in the presence of perforation or transtympanic tubes.

In recalcitrant cases, the presence of a cholesteatoma should be considered. For those patients with persistent discharge or presenting with a recurrent episode, a referral to a otolaryngologist for further evaluation and long-term management is indicated.

OTITIS MEDIA WITHOUT EFFUSION

Inflammation of the middle ear mucous membrane and tympanic membrane without the presence of effusion is a rare occurrence. Upon pneumatic otoscopic examination of the tympanic membrane, erythema and opacification are present and mobility is relatively normal. Otitis media without effusion usually presents in the early stages of acute otitis.

CONCLUSION

Since the incidence and the prevalence of acute otitis media decrease with age, antibiotic therapy with supportive treatment as needed is appropriate for most children. More aggressive therapeutic options (i.e., surgery) should be reserved for children with recurrent episodes, with underlying chronic disease, or with complications and sequelae of otitis media with effusion.

Pharyngitis

The evaluation, diagnosis, and treatment of patients with pharyngitis is a common problem for all providers of primary health care. In 1975, it was estimated that 15.3 million patients sought care for the relief of sore throat symptoms in the United States.

Pharyngitis is an inflammation of the pharynx and surrounding lymphoid tissue that may be of viral or bacterial origin. Viruses appear to be the cause of the majority of episodes, often as constituents of the common cold. However, a significant number are of bacterial origin, with group A β-hemolytic streptococci *(Streptococcus pyogenes)* being the most prevalent microorganism. It is important to differentiate viral from streptococcal tonsillopharyngitis because of the sequelae of group A β-hemolytic *Streptococcus* (GAβHS) pharyngitis and its favorable response to antibiotic treatment.

ETIOLOGY AND PATHOPHYSIOLOGY

Age plays an important role in the microbiologic etiology of acute pharyngitis. In children less than 3 years of age, the etiology is usually viral; the peak incidence of GAβHS is between 5 and 10 years of age.[39] Adenoviruses (types 1, 2, 3, and 5), parainfluenza, respiratory syncytial viruses, rhinoviruses, coxsackieviruses, and influenza A and B are common causes of viral pharyngitis in children and adolescents.[40] In adults, the most common viruses in pharyngitis are rhinoviruses, influenza A and B, and parainfluenza. Viral sore throats attributed to rhinoviruses and coronaviruses are associated with mild episodes. Adenoviruses (types 4 and 7) and herpes simplex viruses, though less prevalent, are attributed to the more severe episodes of pharyngitis.[40]

Epstein–Barr (infectious mononucleosis), influenza, measles, and varicella viruses are capable of producing symptoms of pharyngitis as part of their viradrome. The incidence of mononucleosis and measles is highest in late childhood to adolescence, whereas influenza and varicella viruses are common throughout the age groups. Enterovirus infections such as coxsackieviruses and echoviruses may be complicated by herpangina (posterior stomatitis pharyngitis).

Bacterial pathogens constitute 5–30% of all pharyngitis and the symptomatology generally overlaps that of viral pharyngitis. The normal bacterial flora of the pharynx is host to gram-positive and gram-negative cocci and rods, both aerobic and anaerobic in nature. Normal flora is constituted by *Staphylococcus, Streptococcus,* diphtheroids, *Neisseria,* and *Bacteroides* of low pathogenicity. The pathogenic pneumococci, GAβHS, *Corynebacterium diphtheriae,* and *H. influenzae* are present in accountable numbers as well. GAβHS is the most prevalent bacterial pathogen in symptomatic pharyngitis (25–50%). An increasing number of reports indicate synergistic infection with *S. aureus, M. catarrhalis, H. influenzae,* and anaerobic organism.[39] The prompt diagnosis and treatment of GAβHS pharyngitis has decreased the incidence of its nonsuppurative sequelae: rheumatic fever and acute poststreptococcal glomerulonephritis. The endemic incidence of rheumatic fever is 0.3% and can increase to 3% following a streptococcal pharyngitis epidemic. The United States has seen a precipitous fall in the incidence of rheumatic fever during the past 20–30 years as a result of early diagnosis and treatment of GAβHS, improved living conditions, and possible changes in the rheumatogenicity of streptococcal strains. Antibiotic treatment of GAβHS pharyngitis decreases the incidence of rheumatic fever, but has yet to be proven effective in the prevention of poststreptococcal glomerulonephritis.[41] The nephrogenicity of the streptococcal strain appears to be the determining factor in the development of this complication.

Transmission of GAβHS is mediated by the respiratory route via droplet, and it is readily spread among children, adults, and possibly pets within a household. The transmission may be mediated through close contact with symptomatic or asymptomatic individuals who are colonized in the oronasopharynx, skin, vagina, or rectum. The incubation period of GAβHS is 2–5 days and, like acute otitis media, occurs in a seasonal pattern, with a majority of cases presenting in winter and early spring.[35] Groups C and G streptococci have been associated with acute episodes of pharyngitis, but are not associated with the development of rheumatic fever or poststreptococcal glomerulonephritis.[35]

Four frequently used terms to describe streptococcal throat infections must be defined. *Streptococcal pharyngitis* describes the symptomatic disease with a positive culture and a host antibody response to the infection. *Possible streptococcal pharyngitis* is similar to streptococcal pharyngitis in that the patient is symptomatic and has a positive culture but lacks antibody formation. *Streptococcal carriage* differs from the aforementioned conditions in that the patient may or may not be symptomatic, has no host response, has a positive culture despite treatment, but is not likely to transmit the bacteria. *Streptococcal colonization* is characteristic of an asymptomatic patient with positive cultures.[42]

Other bacteria have been implicated in the etiology of pharyngitis. *Staphylococcus aureus, S. pneumoniae, H. influenzae,* and *M. catarrhalis* have been cultured from throat swabs and surface or core tonsillar samples.[39] Culturing and sampling techniques play an important role in the estimates of the incidence of these organisms. The variations in technologies over the past decades complicate the estimations of prevalence and incidence of these microorganisms.

Toxigenic strains of *C. diphtheriae* can cause pharyngitis and lead to diphtheria. Like GAβHS, diphtheria is spread through respiratory secretions and has an incubation period of 2–5 days. Fortunately, as a result of immunization programs, diphtheria is rare in North America.

When there is a difficulty in establishing a diagnosis, noninfectious causes of pharyngitis should be considered. Allergies, sinusitis, and certain malignancies affect the upper respiratory tract or pharynx directly and should be evaluated before initiation of antibiotic therapy. The exposure to irritating substances (e.g., cigarette smoke, environmental pollutants, ingestion of caustic substances, ingestion of hot foods or liquids) or direct trauma to the pharynx may cause pharyngitis and should not be excluded as primary causes.

CLINICAL PRESENTATION

In the majority of cases of acute pharyngitis, it is not possible to differentiate, on a clinical basis, between viral and bacterial etiology.[39] Epidemiologic factors such as family history, physical examination, history of contact with patients having a cold or influenza, and time of the year can provide information necessary to establish the appropriate diagnosis. In addition, certain viral and bacterial pathogens have specific presenting signs and symptoms. Rhinovirus and coronavirus pharyngitis are accompanied by cough and coryza. Pharyngitis caused by adenoviruses will present with erythema or follicular hyperplasia with or without a tonsillar exudate. Adenovirus pharyngitis, a syndrome more severe than the common cold, is characterized by conjunctivitis. Pharyngitis caused by the Epstein–Barr virus manifests as erythema, edema, white-gray tonsillar exudates, and palatal petechiae. Fever, cervical lymphadenopathy, malaise, and splenomegaly are clinical features that are also associated with mononucleosis. The herpangina caused by enteroviruses may present as painful gray-white papulovesicular lesions 1–2 centimeters in diameter, surrounded by ulcerated erythema on the soft palate, anterior tonsillar pillars, or uvula.

Age of the patient provides helpful insights into the diagnosis of GAβHS. Patients between the ages of 2 and 14 are more susceptible to GAβHS pharyngitis. The rarity of this disease in infants and children younger than 3 years of age has been attributed to the low adherence of GAβHS to buccal epithelial cells. Fever, sore throat, anterior cervical adenopathies, headache, abdominal pain, erythema of the pharynx, tonsillar exudate, lymphatic hyperplasia, and scarlatiniform rash are suggestive of GAβHS pharyngitis. Scarlet fever, rash, impetigo, and infected ulcers around the nostrils and the mouth are indicative of a streptococcal infection.

The question of "to culture or not" is currently still debated. The primary purpose of obtaining a throat culture in a patient who presents with signs and symptoms of pharyngitis is to identify the GAβHS, to initiate treatment, and to avoid sequelae. Table 101.5 lists the criteria for the identification of individuals with pharyngitis in whom a culture is currently recommended.

A throat culture obtained from the surface of the tonsils and the posterior pharyngeal wall is the most commonly used test for the identification of GAβHS. The time necessary to obtain results (24–48 hours) is the major disadvantage of this method. Rapid streptococcal tests are available for the identification of GAβHS. These tests detect the GAβHS antigen directly from a throat swab in 7–70 minutes for completion (depending on the test). This allows patients to be treated earlier, thus lowering the risk of transmission of GAβHS. Even though these rapid test kits provide a faster diagnosis than does the aerobic culture, they are less sensitive. The current recommendation is to perform a throat culture if a negative result is obtained with the rapid test kits. It is important to note that a rapid diagnosis for the prevention of acute rheumatic fever is not essential, since antibiotic therapy can be initiated as late as 9 days after the onset of streptococcal pharyngitis and still be effective.[35]

Test for antibodies such as antistreptolysin O (ASO) and antideoxyribonuclease B (anti-DNase B) are useful in confirming a recent GAβHS infection. These tests can aid in the diagnosis of patients with acute rheumatic fever or acute glomerulonephritis. However, they are of no immediate value in the diagnosis and management of acute streptococcal infection.[35]

The incidence of *C. diphtheriae* pharyngitis is rare in North America but the complications associated with this pathogen warrant accurate diagnosis and immediate treatment. The clinical characteristics of diphtheria are a grayish membrane overlaying the tonsils, cervical adenopathy with edema, and a toxic appearance.

TABLE 101.5. CONDITIONS WHERE A THROAT CULTURE IS RECOMMENDED IN PHARYNGITIS

Children aged 3–15 years, with an elevated temperature and sore throat as the primary complaint

Close contact with a person with streptococcal pharyngitis

Individuals with a history of rheumatic fever or heart disease

Epidemic of the following pathogens:
- Group A β-hemolytic streptococcus
- *Corynebacterium diphtheriae*

Individuals presenting with pharyngitis and one or more of the following signs and symptoms:
- Fever
- Anterior cervical adenopathy
- Tonsillar exudate
- Beefy red color of pharynx
- Lymphatic hyperplasia
- Scarlatiniform rash

TREATMENT

The treatment of viral pharyngitis is symptomatic. Appropriate antibiotic therapy for GAβHS infection prevents acute rheumatic fever, reduces the period of contagion, limits the spread of infection, and reduces the incidence of suppurative complications.[39] When deciding on an optimal antibiotic regimen, the etiology of the infection and the antibiotic concentrations achieved above the MIC in tonsillar tissue are important considerations. Penicillins and erythromycin attain varying degrees of concentration in the tonsillar tissue; however, since tonsillar tissue samples were generally contaminated with blood and sampling techniques are not standardized, the accuracy of tonsillar concentrations has yet to be determined.[43] Early initiation of antibiotic therapy decreases the duration of symptoms; however, when penicillin treatment was delayed, a lower incidence of subsequent GAβHS pharyngitis was observed.[39]

Many antimicrobial agents are appropriate choices in the treatment of GAβHS pharyngitis. These agents include penicillin, amoxicillin, ampicillin, several cephalosporins, erythromycin, and erythromycin–sulfisoxazole. Antibiotic selection should take into account treatment failures, the presence of copathogens, and cost (Table 101.4). Penicillin remains the mainstay of therapy for patients infected with GAβHS. All strains of GAβHS are very susceptible to penicillin ($MIC_{90} \leq 0.005$ g/mL). Resistance of GAβHS to penicillin has not been documented. Children with GAβHS pharyngitis should receive penicillin V 25–50 mg/kg/d in two to four divided doses given orally for 10 days, or benzathine penicillin 25,000–50,000 U/kg intramuscularly as a single dose. The use of the injectable form of penicillin favors compliance but is painful and increases the risk of allergic reactions.

For the penicillin-allergic patient, erythromycin estolate 20–30 mg/kg/d in two to four divided doses or erythromycin ethylsuccinate 40–50 mg/kg/d in two to four divided doses for 10 days are suitable alternatives.[35] However, resistance of GAβHS to erythromycin has been observed in the United States in approximately 5% of the strains isolated. Ampicillin and amoxicillin offer no advantages over penicillin. Cephalexin, taken three to four times daily, and cefadroxil, in a once-daily administration, have been demonstrated to be more effective in eradicating GAβHS than penicillin. However, penicillin V is the only agent prospectively shown to reduce the incidence of rheumatic fever due to GAβHS. Cefuroxime axetil and cefaclor are acceptable alternatives. The former can be given twice daily but is not available in liquid form. Clinical trials have also evaluated the newer cephalosporins cefpodoxime proxetil and loracarbef as well as azithromycin in the treatment of GAβHS pharyngitis. In adults, azithromycin administered daily for 5 days and loracarbef administered twice daily for 10 days were comparable to a 10-day regimen of penicillin V in terms of clinical cure, eradication, and recurrence.[44,45] Strains resistant to azithromycin were isolated. In children and adults, cefpodoxime proxetil given twice daily for 5 days was comparable to penicillin V in the treatment of GAβHS pharyngitis.[46] The newer cephalosporins offer the advantages of prolonged dosing intervals and shorter durations of therapy. Unfortunately, these benefits are outweighed by their costs (Table 101.4).

The antimicrobial therapy of choice for *C. diphtheriae* pharyngitis is penicillin G 150,000 U/kg/d intravenously every 6 hours, or erythromycin 50 mg/kg/d given orally for 7–10 days. The coadministration of diphtheria antitoxin is advised, as well as isolation of the patient until 3 consecutive days of negative nose and throat cultures are obtained.

EVALUATION OF THERAPEUTIC OUTCOMES

An important issue in the antimicrobial treatment of GAβHS is the incidence of bacteriologic and clinical failure rates that occurs on completion of therapy. Bacteriologic treatment failure rates with 10 days of oral penicillin V approximate 30–35%.[39] A shorter course of therapy can increase the failure rate. Intramuscular benzathine penicillin G has demonstrated a failure rate of approximately 19–25%. Patients who fail to respond to penicillin may harbor a greater number of penicillin-resistant, β-lactamase–producing microorganisms.[39] Other causes besides copathogenicity include lack of compliance and recurrent exposure. A recurrent episode of pharyngitis should be classified as either a relapse (due to the same bacterial strain) or as a reinfection (due to a new strain). For a relapse, it is appropriate to change the antimicrobial agent. Cephalosporins with β-lactamase activity are good alternatives. If a new strain is present, the initial antimicrobial can be reinstated. With persistent recurrent episodes, penicillin for 10 days with rifampin for the last 4 days is suggested.[39]

Tonsillectomy and adenoidectomy in children with recurrent pharyngitis do not significantly decrease the number of GAβHS infections when compared with controls who did not undergo surgery. The recommended approach in children with severe and recurrent pharyngitis is to delay the surgery hoping for an eventual improvement. If no improvement is seen, tonsillectomy can be considered.

It is important to control the spread of GAβHS infection. The risk of spreading to close contacts is maximal during the acute phase of the infection. During the incubation period and the first weeks of the carrier state, the communicability of GAβHS infection is minimal. Twenty-four hours following efficacious antibiotic treatment, the individual is no longer at risk for contagion.

SINUSITIS

Sinusitis is a common condition affecting children and adults and is associated with both bacterial and viral infections of the upper respiratory tract. Children have between six and eight common colds per year depending on age, number of siblings, and type of day-care services. Adults experience approximately two to three common colds per year, and incidence may increase while parenting or working with young children. Of these upper respiratory infections, 1–5% will be complicated by acute sinusitis.

ANATOMY AND PATHOPHYSIOLOGY

The sinuses are four-paired, air-filled cavities, which are situated around the nasal cavity and adjoin the orbits and anterior cranial fossa (Fig. 101.4). The maxillary, sphenoid, and ethmoid sinuses are well developed at birth, whereas the frontal sinuses originate from the ethmoid sinuses and are not fully developed until 10 years of age. The sinuses are contiguous with mucosa of the upper respiratory tract and are lined with ciliated pseudocolumnar epithelium. Small tubular openings, sinus ostia, connect the sinus cavities and facilitate drainage of the sinuses into the nasal cavity through the activity of the ciliated cells.[47]

Conditions that affect patency of the sinus ostia, normal function of the mucociliary sinus epithelium, normal immune defenses of the upper respiratory tract, or events that introduce microorganisms into the sinuses predispose to sinus infections.[48] Bacterial and viral infections of the respiratory tract and allergic inflammation are conditions that cause sinus ostia obstruction, and lead to retention of secretions. Alterations in the mucosa due to debilitating diseases such as cystic fibrosis or by direct cytotoxic effects on the cilia due to viruses predispose the nasal cavity and the

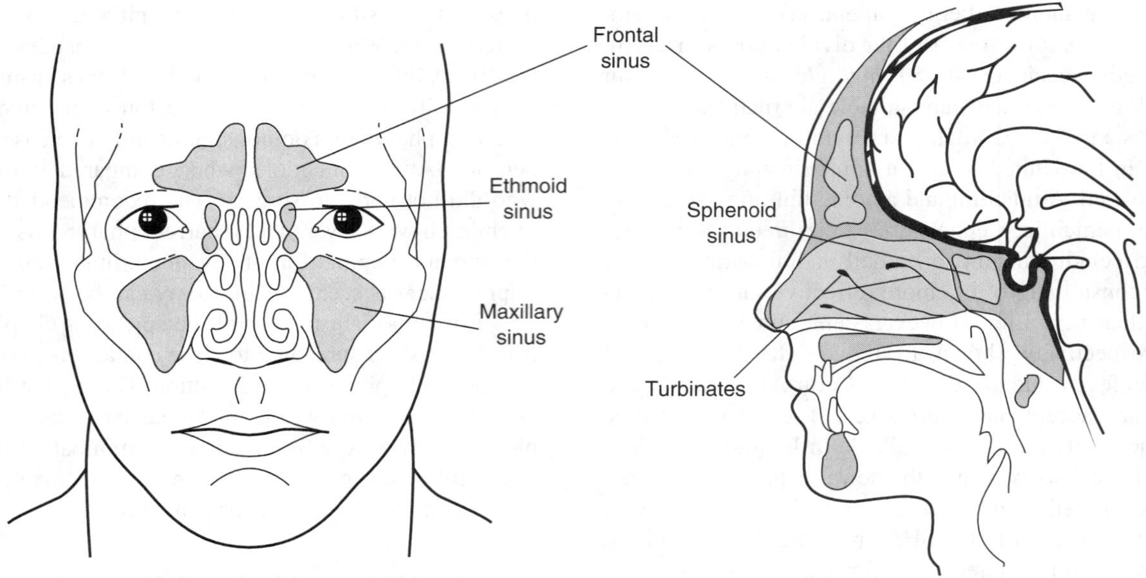

Figure 101.4. Anatomy of the sinus cavities.

paranasal sinuses to bacterial invasion. Alterations in the immune status by diseases or drugs allow bacteria with low pathogenicity to become pathogenic. The indirect introduction of microorganisms through dental extractions and infections of the maxillary molar teeth predisposes to maxillary and chronic sinusitis.[48]

ETIOLOGY

The clinical presentation of sinusitis is dependent on the acuteness or chronicity of the infection as well as the patient's age. When children present with acute sinusitis, the differentiation between the common cold or allergic rhinitis is often difficult. The most commonly encountered symptoms in all cases include mucopurulent nasal discharge, nasal congestion, tenderness over the involved sinus, and fever.[48]

Sinusitis should be suspected if a patient has a history of common cold with persistent rhinitis and failure of symptoms to resolve. The persistence of nasal discharge and a daytime cough for more than 10 days following a viral infection of the upper respiratory tract is indicative of sinusitis. The previously clear, thin nasal discharge associated with viral infections may become mucoid or purulent with an increase in both viscosity and quantity. Progression of the daytime cough is the symptom for which parents seek medical attention, even though the child may not appear ill despite a low-grade fever.[49] In children, the presence of malodorous breath in the absence of pharyngitis and poor dental hygiene or morning periorbital swelling with or without pain may be signs of a sinus infection.[49]

An usually severe cold characterized by high fever (greater than 39.0°C), purulent and viscous nasal discharge, hyposmia (abnormal decrease in sensitivity to odors), facial pain over the affected sinuses that worsens with movement, and periorbital swelling with or without headache may also be indicative of bacterial sinusitis.[49] The periorbital swelling is worse on awakening and may decrease with severity as the day progresses. Headaches caused by sinusitis respond poorly to analgesics. The pain corresponds to the sinuses affected and is described as a feeling of fullness or a dull ache. The incidence of this type of headache in children under 5 years of age is rare, the frontal sinuses not being fully developed.

CLINICAL PRESENTATION

In addition to history and physical examination, the diagnosis of sinusitis may require cytologic examination of nasal aspirates, transillumination of maxillary and frontal sinuses for patients older than 10 years of age, radiography, ultrasonography, computed tomography, and magnetic resonance imaging.

An interesting and useful but rarely used laboratory tool is the cytological examination of fresh nasal secretions. On microscopic examination, a high concentration of polymorphonuclear cells with intracellular bacteria is often observed. Polymorphonucleocytes generally predominate during viral infections but when present in high numbers in a chronic and profuse rhinorrhea, they are suggestive of sinusitis. A differentiation between chronic sinusitis and allergic rhinitis can be made when eosinophils predominate. If the smear is devoid of eosinophils, chronic sinusitis can be suspected.

Transillumination is helpful in the diagnosis of maxillary and frontal sinusitis. Both the patient and the examiner must be in a darkened room. The maxillary sinuses are transilluminated when a high-intensity light source, shielded from the examiner, is placed over the midpoint of the inferior orbital rim. Light transmission through the hard palate is assessed by the examiner with the patient's mouth open. To transilluminate the frontal sinuses, the high-intensity light source is placed beneath the medial border of the supraorbital ridge. Assessment of the symmetry of the blush bilaterally provides clues to the diagnosis. Due to the increased thickness of the soft tissue and bony vault in children 10 years of age and younger, the clinical diagnosis of sinusitis with transillumination is not helpful.

Radiography can confirm the diagnosis of bacterial sinusitis. Diagnostic findings suggestive of bacterial sinusitis are air-liquid levels in sinus cavities, mucosal thickening, and partial or complete opacification of the sinus cavities. When a patient presents with signs and symptoms suggesting sinusitis and abnormal maxillary sinus radiographs, bacteria will be present 75% of the time. However, a normal radiograph in a patient with clinical signs and symptoms of sinusitis does not suggest that the patient is free of disease.

Ultrasonography has the advantage of using nonionizing radiation and better distinguishes between mucosal thickening and the presence of sinus secretions. The use of ultrasound has been shown to be highly specific, but not very sensitive.

Computed tomography and magnetic resonance imagery are useful in cases of sinusitis that are complicated by intracranial or intraorbital suppuration. Due to the expense of these diagnostic aids, their use is reserved for complicated cases of sinusitis.

MICROBIOLOGY

The bacteriology of sinus secretions in children is similar to that found in adults.[49] The dominant organisms are *S. pneumoniae* (31–36%), nontypable *H. influenzae* (21–23%), and *M. catarrhalis* (2–19%).[49] Infrequently encountered bacteria include *S. pyogenes, S. aureus,* and anaerobic bacteria such as *Peptostreptococcus, Fusobacterium,* and *Bacteroides melaninogenicus.* Concurrent abundant growth of two species is rare. Viruses such as rhinovirus, influenza virus, adenovirus, and the parainfluenza virus are isolated in 15% of antral aspirates and are generally remnants of upper respiratory tract viral infections.

Currently, the microbial etiology of patients presenting with sinusitis can only be determined by direct sinus aspiration. This procedure is recommended in the following situations: (1) patients with sinusitis who fail conventional therapy, (2) immunosuppressed patients with sinusitis, (3) severe headache and facial pain, and (4) in the presence of life-threatening complications such as intraorbital or intracranial suppuration.

TREATMENT

Many symptoms of sinusitis will resolve without medical therapy within 48 hours. When they persist, pharmacotherapy should be directed toward symptomatic relief, restoring and improving sinus function, preventing intracranial complications, and eradicating the causative pathogen(s). Antibiotics are the mainstay of therapy of sinusitis, and selection of the appropriate agent is directed against the most likely pathogens. Amoxicillin is an appropriate agent for most uncomplicated cases of sinusitis. If β-lactamase–resistant strains are suspected, the patient is allergic to penicillin, the presentation is accompanied by mild periorbital edema, or if there is an apparent antibiotic failure, alternative regimens can be used.[49] Trimethoprim–sulfamethoxazole is efficacious in adults but may be ineffective in group A streptococcal infections. Cefaclor, erythromycin–sulfisoxazole, and amoxicillin–clavulanate are appropriate alternatives. Loracarbef and azithromycin favorably compared to doxycycline and amoxicillin, respectively, in the treatment of acute maxillary sinusitis in adults.[50,51] Acute sinusitis is treated for 10–14 days but duration can be extended to 30 days in protracted cases.

Vasoconstrictor sprays or drops such as xylometazoline or oxymetazoline may facilitate drainage. The use of such agents should not exceed more than 72 hours due to a tolerance effect and possible rebound congestion. Purulent secretions present in the nose should be removed before administration. Topical decongestants should be used with caution in the pediatric population.

EPIGLOTTITIS AND CROUP

Epiglottitis and croup are two distinct entities, both resulting from infections of the laryngeal area (Table 101.6).[52] Noisy breathing is characteristic of these two clinical diseases. As shown in Fig. 101.5, they both cause airway obstruction but at different anatomic sites.

EPIGLOTTITIS

Epiglottitis is a true airway emergency in which acute airway obstruction can occur. It is caused primarily by *H. influenzae* type B. Epiglottitis is more prevalent in children ages 2–6.[52] The onset of the disease is rapid and the evolution is often brisk. Fever, sore throat, dysphagia, dysphonia, and sialorrhea (excessive secretion of saliva) are acute signs and symptoms of the disease. Airway obstruction evolves rapidly and manifests by respiratory distress,

TABLE 101.6. DIFFERENTIATING CLINICAL FEATURES OF EPIGLOTTITIS AND CROUP

Feature	Epiglottitis	Croup
Age	3–7 years	>3 years
Gender	Male = Female	Male > Female
Season	All seasons	Late spring and late fall
Pathogens(s)	Bacterial: *H. influenzae* B	Viral: parainfluenzae (type 1, 2 and 3)
Progression	Rapid	Slow (generally at night)
Clinical presentation	Sitting, toxic, typical posture	Supine, nontoxic, barking cough
Dysphagia	Marked, occasional drooling	None
Fever	>39.4°C (103°F)	<39.4°C (103°F)
Stridor	Rare	Frequent
WBC	>18,000 mm^3	Normal
Treatment	Parenteral antibiotics, intubation	Cool mist, racemic epinephrine
Recurrence	Rare	Common

irritability, fatigue, and anxiety. The typical posture of the child (tripod), with arms at the side, upper body set forward, neck extended with the chin thrust forward, and mouth wide open maximizes the size of the supraglottic airway. A severe respiratory stridor can be heard, drooling is present, and spontaneous cough is absent. Once epiglottis is suspected, the diagnosis should be confirmed by a person who is prepared for immediate airway intervention. When obtainable, the lateral neck roentgenogram will show an edematous epiglottis along with edema of prevertebral soft tissue.[52] When the child has been stabilized, blood and nasopharyngeal cultures can be obtained to assess microorganisms' susceptibility.

Treatment

The primary concern in the management of epiglottitis is establishing and maintaining the airway. Initial therapy may involve the use of a moist oxygen tent to help facilitate the breathing. In severe cases, endotracheal intubation or a tracheostomy may be required.

Antibiotic therapy should be instituted if epiglottitis is suspected and empirically directed against *H. influenzae* type B. The combination of ampicillin 200 mg/kg/d and chloramphenicol 100 mg/kg/d (maximum 4 g/d) provides coverage of ampicillin-resistant microorganisms until sensitivities are known. The second- or third-generation cephalosporins cefuroxime (100–150 mg/kg/d given every 8 hours), cefotaxime (50–100 mg/kg/d given every 6 hours), or ceftriaxone (50–75 mg/kg/d given every 12 hours) are appropriate and often preferred. Recommended duration of treatment is 7–10 days. The optimum course of therapy needs to be further investigated.[52,53] The use of corticosteroids and inhalation therapy (nebulization or IPPB [intermittent positive-pressure breathing]) with or without epinephrine is controversial for the treatment of epiglottitis.

Isolation of the hospitalized patient is indicated until 24 hours after initiation of effective therapy. Household contacts, defined as individuals residing in the home of the index patient or nonresidents who spent 4 or more hours with the index patient for at least 5 of the 7 days preceding the day of hospitalization, should receive chemoprophylaxis with rifampin (20 mg/kg/d for 4 days given once a day, maximum 600 mg/d). Management of day-care and nursery school contact groups should be individualized.[35]

CROUP

In contrast to epiglottitis, croup is often preceded by a prodrome (e.g., a common cold), and its onset and progression are less rapid. Viral croup (acute laryngotracheobronchitis) is caused primarily by parainfluenzae (type 1 and 2).[52] Typically, children less than 3 years of age are affected, with a majority of the cases appearing during the cold and flu season. Young children are predisposed to complications of the laryngeal region due to their small upper airway. Signs of laryngeal obstruction in the presence of a moderate fever (100°F), appear 2–3 days after the onset of a cold. Persistent spontaneous cough, stridor, hoarseness of the voice, and a barking cough are suggestive of croup. A benign nocturnal waxing and waning pattern, which occurs over 2–3 days, is characteristic of croup. In the majority of episodes, the child will fully recover without any specific treatment.

On examination of the oral cavity a slight pharyngitis with a normal epiglottis can be seen. Although rarely indicated, neck radiography may reveal a narrowing of the subglottic region (Fig. 101.5). Indirect laryngoscopic examination may show edema and exudate formation in this region.[52]

Bacterial tracheitis, or pseudomembranous croup, is a rare but life-threatening type of croup. Unlike acute laryngotracheobronchitis, *S. aureus,* streptococci, and *H. influenzae* can be isolated from the tracheal mucosa. In bacterial croup, the patient appears toxic and is at risk for upper respiratory tract obstruction. Often confused with epiglottitis, the characteristic barking cough and absence of drooling help to differentiate bacterial tracheitis. Spasmotic croup, or recurrent croup, is thought to be a variant of acute laryngotracheobronchitis and is characterized by a sudden nocturnal onset.

Treatment

Each episode of croup should be considered individually because some patients may benefit from simple therapy, whereas others may require a more complex approach. Ambient air humidification and ingestion of liquids can prevent the drying and crusting of the inflamed mucosa, and help to liquefy exudates.[52] In minor cases, these treat-

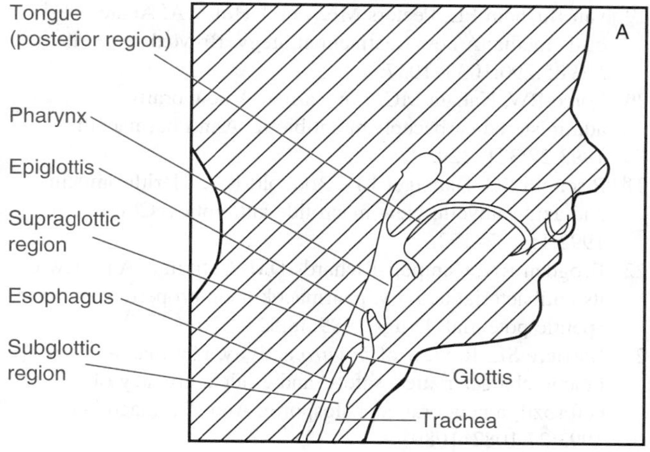

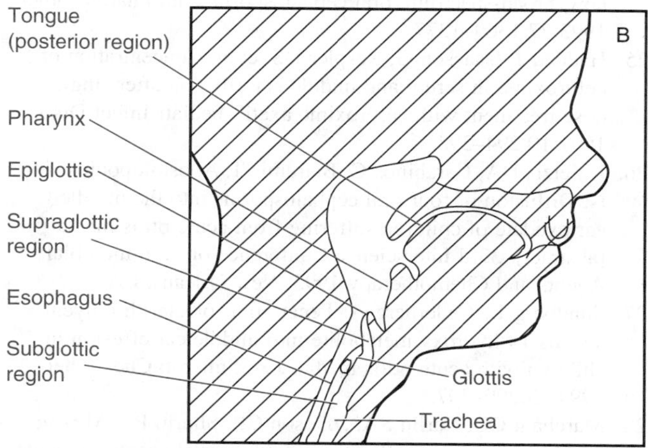

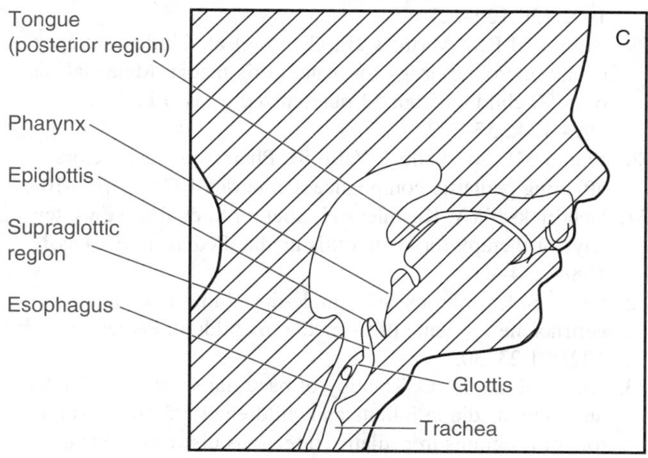

Figure 101.5. Schematic representation of the upper respiratory tract. (A) normal, (B) epiglottitis, (C) croup.

ments can be performed at home (the child is placed in the bathroom with a warm running shower).

Because of its drying effect, oxygen therapy should be reserved for cyanotic children. The use of an oxygen tent allows the combination of oxygen and humidity and provides a comfortable breathing environment for the child. In most serious cases, racemic epinephrine inhalation may provide relief. The mechanism of action involves vasoconstriction of the edematous subglottic area by the alpha agonist activity. It may provide additional relief by β_2 stimulation leading to bronchial smooth muscle relaxation.[52] The recommended doses are 0.25 mL of a 2.25% solution of racemic epinephrine for children less than 6 months old and 0.5 mL for older children.[52] Any child that receives treatment should be admitted to the hospital because the duration of action of racemic epinephrine is less than 2 hours and a relapse may occur. The use of corticosteroids in the treatment of croup is controversial. The use of dexamethasone may reduce the need for subsequent administration of racemic epinephrine.

Since croup is almost exclusively viral in nature, antibiotic therapy is not indicated. Children with persistent fever (more than 4 days) and those showing a deterioration of their condition should be empirically treated with antibiotic to prevent possible subsequent bacterial superinfection.

LARYNGITIS

Laryngitis is an acute self-limited affliction often seen in school-age children and in adults. This inflammation of the larynx is frequently associated with a viral infection of the upper respiratory tract. The microorganisms most often encountered are influenzae A and B virus and adenovirus.[35] Laryngitis may, on occasion, be associated with concurrent bacterial infections (e.g., GAβHS, *S. pneumoniae*) and symptoms of certain diseases (e.g., bronchitis, pneumonia, pertussis, measles, diphtheria).[54] Consequently, it may be accompanied by cough, dysphagia, dyspnea, rhinorrhea, or fever.

The prominent symptom of this disease is an unnatural change in the voice. Hoarseness and aphonia may occur and may be accompanied by a tickling sensation of the throat and a constant desire to clear the throat. In contrast to epiglottitis and croup, respiratory distress is not present. Severity varies according to the pathogens and the history of previous episodes. Adenoviruses cause a more severe disease with fever, sore throat, and systemic signs such as headache, myalgia, and prostration.

TREATMENT

Treatment of laryngitis is symptomatic. The voice should be rested; steam inhalation treatment and the ingestion of large quantities of water provide symptomatic relief and help to liquefy respiratory secretions.[52] Respiratory irritants such as cigarette smoke and known allergens should be avoided. If a bacterial pathogen has been isolated, antimicrobial treatment may be in order.

REFERENCES

1. Bluestone CD, Klein JO. Otitis media, atelectasis, and eustachian tube dysfunction, in Bluestone CD, Stool SE, Scheetz MD (eds): Pediatric Otolaryngology. Philadelphia, WB Saunders, 1990, pp 322–334.
2. Infante-Rivard C, Fernandez A. Otitis media in children: Frequency, risk factors, and research avenues. Epidemiol Rev 1993;15:444–465.
3. Teele DW, Klein JO. The greater Boston otitis media study group. Epidemiology of otitis media during the first seven years of life in children in greater Boston: A prospective, cohort study. J Infect Dis 1989;160:83–94.
4. Owen MJ, Baldwin CD, Swank PR, et al. Relation of infant feeding practices, cigarette smoke exposure, and group child care to the onset and duration of otitis media with effusion in the first two years of life. J Pediatr 1993;123:702–711.
5. Henderson FW, Giebink GS. Otitis media among children in day care: Epidemiology and pathogenesis. Rev Infect Dis 1986;8:533–538.
6. Henderson FW, Collier AM, Sanyal MA, et al. A longitudinal study of respiratory viruses and bacteria in the etiology of acute otitis media with effusion. N Engl J Med 1982;306:1377–1383.
7. Wiet RJ, DeBlanc GB, Stewart J, Weider DJ. Natural history of otitis media in the American native. Ann Otol Rhinol Laryngol 1980;68(suppl):14–19.
8. Duncan B, Ey J, Holberg CJ, et al. Exclusive breast-feeding for at least 4 months protects against otitis media. Pediatrics 1993;91:867–872.
9. Bernstein JM. Recent advances in immunologic reactivity in otitis media with effusion. J Allergy Clin Immunol 1988;81:1004–1009.
10. Branefors-Helander P, Dahlberg T, Nylén. Acute otitis media. A clinical, bacteriological and serological study of children with frequent episodes of acute otitis media. Acta Otolaryngol 1975;80:399–409.
11. Bluestone CD, Doyle WJ. The ears: Anatomy and physiology of eustachian tube and middle ear related to otitis media. J Allergy Clin Immunol 1988;81:997–1003.
12. Bluestone CD. Management of otitis media in infants and children: Current role of old and new antimicrobial agents. Pediatr Infect Dis J 1988;7:S129–S136.
13. Anonyme. Médicaments pour le traitement de l'otite moyenne aiguë chez les enfants. La lettre médicale 1994;17:119–121.
14. Del Beccaro MA, Mendelman PM, Inglis AF, et al. Bacteriology of acute otitis media: A new perspective. J Pediatr 1992;120:81–84.
15. Kovatch A, Wald E, Michaels R. Beta-lactamase-producing *Branhamella catarrhalis* causing otitis media in children. J Pediatr 1983;102:261–264.
16. Carlin SA, Marchant CD, Shurin PA, et al. Host factors and early therapeutic response in acute otitis media. J Pediatr 1991;118:178–183.
17. Celin SE, Bluestone CD, Stephenson J, et al. Bacteriology of acute otitis media in adults. JAMA 1991;266:2249–2252.
18. Ruuskanen O, Arola M, Heikkinen T, Ziegler T. Viruses in acute otitis media: Increasing evidence for clinical significance. Pediatr Infect Dis J 1991;10:425–427.
19. van Buchem FL, Peeters MF, van'T Hof MA. Acute otitis media: A new treatment strategy. Br Med J 1985;290:1033–1037.
20. Force RW, Nahata MC. Loracarbef: A new orally administered carbacephem antibiotic. Ann Pharmacother 1993;27:321–329.
21. Piscitelli SC, Danziger LH, Rodvold KA. Clarithromycin and azithromycin: New macrolide antibiotics. Clin Pharm 1992;11:137–152.
22. Brogden RN, Campoli-Richards DM. Cefixime. A review of its antibacterial activity, pharmacokinetic properties and therapeutic potential. Drugs 1989;38:524–550.
23. Barrière SL. Review of *in vitro* activity, pharmacokinetic characteristics, safety, and clinical efficacy of cefprozil, a new oral cephalosporin. Ann Pharmacother 1993;27:1082–1089.
24. Chocas EC, Paap CM, Godley PJ. Cefpodoxime proxetil: A new, broad-spectrum, oral cephalosporin. Ann Pharmacother 1993;27:1369–1377.
25. Haddad J, Isaacson G, Respler DS, et al. Concentration of cefuroxime in serum and middle ear effusion after single dose treatment with cefuroxime axetil. Pediatr Infect Dis J 1991;10:294–298.
26. Kafetzis DA, Carabinos C, Bairamis T, Apostolopoulos N. Diffusion of four oral cephalosporins into the middle ear exudate of children suffering from acute otitis media [abstract]. 33rd Interscience Conference on Antimicrobial Agents and Chemotherapy 1993, New Orleans, LA.
27. Sundberg L, Cederberg A. Penetration of clarithromycin and its 14-hydroxy metabolite into middle ear effusion in children with acute otitis media. J Antimicrob Chemother 1994;33:299–307.
28. Marchant CD, Carlin SA, Johnson CE, Shurin PA. Measuring the comparative efficacy of antibacterial agents for acute otitis media: The "Pollyanna phenomenon." J Pediatr 1992;120:120–127.
29. Rosenfeld RM, Vertrees JE, Carr J, et al. Clinical efficacy of antimicrobial drugs for acute otitis media. Metaanalysis of 5400 children from 33 randomized trials. J Pediatr 1994;124:355–367.
30. Mattar ME, Markello J, Yaffe SJ. Pharmaceutical factors affecting pediatric compliance. Pediatrics 1975;55:101–108.
31. Hendrickse WA, Kusmiesz H, Shelton S, et al. Five vs. ten days of therapy for acute otitis media. Pediatr Infect Dis J 1988;7:14–23.
32. Green SM, Rothrock SG. Single-dose intramuscular ceftriaxone for acute otitis media in children. Pediatrics 1993;91:23–30.
33. Klass PE, Klein JO. Therapy of bacterial sepsis, meningitis and otitis media in infants and children: 1992 poll of directors of programs in pediatric infectious diseases. Pediatr Infect Dis J 1992;11:702–705.
34. Williams RL, Chalmers TC, Stange KC, Chalmers FT, Bowlin SJ. Use of antibiotics in preventing recurrent acute otitis media and in treating otitis media with effusion. A meta-analytic attempt to resolve the brouhaha. JAMA 1993;270:1344–1351.
35. American Academy of Pediatrics. Report of the Committee on Infectious Diseases. Evanston, IL, American Academy of Pediatrics, 1994.

36. Gebhart DE. Tympanostomy tubes in otitis media prone child. Laryngoscope 1981;91:849–866.
37. Teele DW, Klein JO, Chase C, et al. Otitis media in infancy and intellectual ability, school achievement, speech, and language at age 7 years. J Infect Dis 1990;162:685–694.
38. Bluestone CD. Current management of chronic suppurative otitis media in infants and children. Pediatr Infect Dis J 1988;7(suppl):S137–S140.
39. Pichichero ME. Controversies in the treatment of streptococcal pharyngitis. Fam Phys 1990;42:1567–1576.
40. Van Cauwenberge PB, Vander Mijnsbrugge A-M. Pharyngitis: A survey of the microbiologic etiology. Pediatr Infect Dis J 1991;10(suppl):S30–S42.
41. Quinn RW. Comprehensive review of morbidity and mortality trends for rheumatic fever, streptococcal disease, and scarlet fever: The decline of rheumatic fever. Rev Infect Dis 1989;11:928–953.
42. Centor RM, Meier FA, Dalton HP. Throat cultures and rapid tests for diagnosis of group A streptococcal pharyngitis. Ann Intern Med 1986;105:892–899.
43. Neu HC. Contemporary antibiotic therapy in otolaryngology. Otolaryngol Clin North Am 1984;17:745–760.
44. Hooton TM. A comparison of azithromycin and penicillin V for the treatment of streptococcal pharyngitis. Am J Med 1991;91(suppl 3A):23S–26S.
45. McCarty J. Loracarbef versus Penicillin VK in the treatment of streptococcal pharyngitis and tonsillitis in an adult population. Am J Med 1992;92(suppl 6A):74S–79S.
46. Portier H, Chavanet P, Waldner-Combernoux A, et al. Five versus ten days treatment of streptococcal pharyngotonsillitis: A randomized controlled trial comparing cefpodoxime proxetil and phenoxymethyl penicillin. Scan J Infect Dis 1994;26:59–66.
47. Wald ER. Rhinitis and Acute Chronic Sinusitis, in Bluestone CD, Stool SE, Scheetz MD (eds): Pediatric Otolaryngology. Philadelphia, WB Saunders, 1990, pp 729–744.
48. Sullivan Baker A. Sinusitis. Medical Grand Rounds 1984;3:154–165.
49. Wald ER. Sinusitis in children. Pediatr Infect Dis J 1988;7(suppl):S150–S153.
50. Nord CE, the Scandinavian Study Group. Loracarbef versus doxycycline in the treatment of acute bacterial maxillary sinusitis. J Antimicrob Chemother 1993;31:949–961.
51. Casiano RR. Azithromycin and amoxicillin in the treatment of acute maxillary sinusitis. Am J Med 1991;(suppl 3A):27S–30S.
52. Cressman WR, Myer CW. Diagnosis and management of croup and epiglottitis. Pediatr Clin North Am 1994;41:265–276.
53. Sawyer SM, Johnson PDR, Robertson CF, et al. Successful treatment of epiglottitis with two doses of ceftriaxone. Arch Dis Child 1994;70:129–132.
54. Cherry JD. Acute epiglottitis, laryngitis, and croup, in Remington JS, Swartz MN (eds): Current Clinical Topics in Infectious Diseases, vol 2. New York, McGraw-Hill, 1982, pp 1–32.

Chapter 102

Ophthalmic Infections

Richard Fiscella, RPh, MPH

This chapter describes infective processes involving periocular and ocular structures. It also reviews antimicrobial therapy and presents current clinical aspects of ophthalmic treatment. Vision can be decreased or lost through ocular infections. Bacterial corneal ulcers may cause permanent scarring even if the infectious process is stopped. Endophthalmitis may cause destruction of delicate intraocular structures even though the eye may be "sterilized." Although some ocular infections may be self-limiting, most should be treated appropriately to prevent permanent ocular damage.

The eye presents a unique treatment situation unlike any other part of the body (Fig. 102.1). Therapy may vary from the use of topical medication for a bacterial conjunctivitis to topical, periocular, intraocular, and intravenous therapy for the treatment of endophthalmitis. The route of administration used depends on the availability of the drug at the site of infection in inhibitory concentrations. As mentioned earlier, an external ocular infection may be treated with an antimicrobial agent that is only applied topically in ointment or drop form. When the infectious processes involve deeper ocular structures, effective treatment modalities must incorporate other routes of administration to achieve adequate tissue levels. In some severe corneal ulcers and infections of the inner layers of the eye (endophthalmitis), subconjunctival injections are employed. In addition, endophthalmitis usually requires direct injections into the vitreous (intravitreal) to achieve therapeutic tissue levels. Drugs must penetrate in effective concentrations and yet be nontoxic to ocular structures.

For background discussion on ocular anatomy please see Chapter 88, Glaucoma. Alteration of normal defense mechanisms subjects the eye to microbial infection. Major external defense mechanisms include the repetitive movement of the eyelid and the tears. The tears provide a media for the flow of antibacterial substances and a constant mechanical washing of the cornea. Specific antibacterial agents found in the tears include lysozyme, lactoferrin, β-lysine, and immunoglobins A and G. The acute inflammatory reaction and development of specific bacterial, fungal, and viral immunity also play an essential role in the external defenses of the eye.

Ocular infections can be divided into periocular, conjunctivitis, keratitis (corneal), and endophthalmitis (infections of the inner eye contents)/panophthalmitis (infections of the inner and outer eye structures).

Periocular Infections

Periocular infections encompass infections of the eyelids, the lacrimal system, the orbits, and surrounding sinuses.

INFECTIONS OF THE EYELIDS

Infections of the eyelids, hordeolum (stye), chalazion, and blepharitis, are among the most common ocular problems and can range from the very mild to quite severe.

Hordeolum externum is usually a staphylococcal infection of an eyelash follicle and Moll's (sweat) or Zeis (sebaceous) glands. Internal hordeolums are infections of the meibomian glands, which are modified sebaceous glands located within the lid.[1] Most infections are usually self-limited and respond well to treatment. Rarely are they of a chronic nature. Both internal and external hordeolums are usually associated with staphylococcal infections.

Chalazions are chronic granulomatous inflammations of the meibomian glands on the upper and lower lids. They seldom subside on their own and recurrence can suggest a possible malignancy and should be ruled out.[2] Chalazia are one of the most common eyelid masses and can be mistaken for or may conceal a neoplasm (a basal cell or sebaceous carcinoma).

Blepharitis is an inflammation of the lid margins. The lids help to maintain an even flow of tear film over the cornea, provide mechanical protection for the eye, and supply the lipid component of the tear film. Blepharitis is usually considered a bilateral and chronic condition. Many cases of blepharitis may be accompanied by a secondary bacterial infection. Blepharitis is sometimes considered to consist of two main types, staphylococcal and seborrheic.[3] Other clinicians have further subdivided these, but that is beyond the discussion of this chapter.[4–6] Other rare types

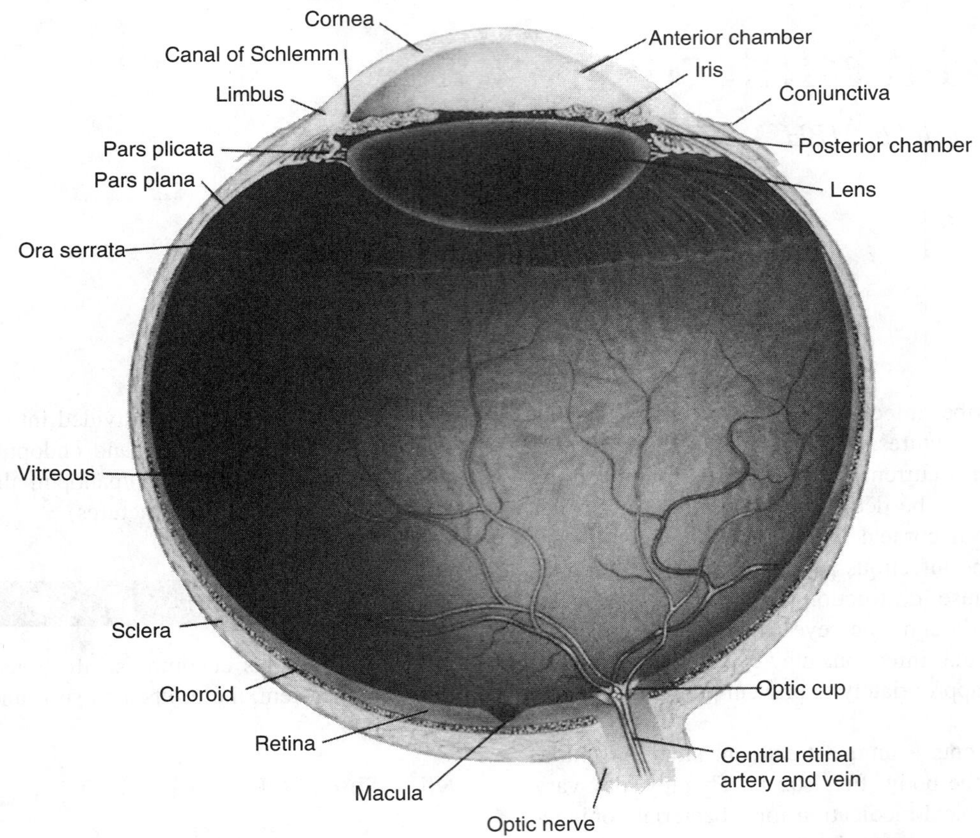

Figure 102.1. Diagrammatic representation of horizontal (meridional) section through left human eye.

have also been reported including viral, atopic, psoriatic, and fungal. The most common form is the seborrheic type with the accompanying staphylococcal infection, although other organisms have been isolated including *Staphylococcus epidermidis, Propionibacterium acnes,* and *Corynebacterium* sp.[4] Investigators have reported that the patients with various seborrheic blepharitis varieties usually have a seborrheic dermatitis present also.[5] Patients with only staphylococcal blepharitis have no significant dermatologic disease reported compared to the normal population.

Chronic blepharitis is one of the most typical complaints of an eye patient. *Staphylococcus aureus* and *S. epidermidis* are reported to be the major organisms isolated in clinical staphylococcal and seborrheic/staphylococcal blepharitis. These organisms probably do not play a primary role in the other types of blepharitis, although they may play a secondary role.

Meibomianitis is an uncommon and chronic inflammation of the meibomian glands that is usually bilateral. It is seen most commonly during the middle years of life and is usually associated with seborrheic blepharitis. Patients with primary meibomianitis, in contrast to the patients with staphylococcal blepharitis, have associated seborrheic dermatitis or acne rosacea.[4,5]

Impetigo of the eyelids has been reported when there is a combination of bacteria staphylococcus and/or streptococcus, which have spread from facial areas and appear as a vesiculopustular eruption.

Clinical Presentation

Hordeolums generally present with pain, redness, and some swelling of the lid. There is stretching of the tissues, and the pain fibers in the lid margins are very sensitive. On diagnosis, an internal hordeolum may point to the conjunctival surface or skin and an external hordeolum always points to the skin. The internal hordeolum may have a more prolonged course, while the external hordeolum will usually subside within 3–4 days after becoming apparent.

Chalazia may present with an initial painless swelling over a period of weeks. Most progress, rather than regress, as in a hordeolum. They may become cosmetically disfiguring, with increasing size and redness and some may become large enough to distort vision.

Blepharitis is usually characterized by a redness and irritation of the eye lids. The signs and symptoms, ranging from mild to severe, are crusting, discharge, scaling, ocular discomfort, itching, foreign body sensation, and photophobia. Staphylococcal blepharitis is usually involved in the waxing and waning stages that may occur in conjunction with conjunctivitis and a punctate keratitis. In staphylococcal blepharitis the patient typically complains of local irritation and burning and often has complaints of dry eyes. Adults with primary meibomianitis often have concomitant rosacea and/or seborrheic blepharitis and may have an underlying dermatologic disorder.[5–7] If treated inadequately, staphylococcal blepharitis frequently lasts for years, producing chronically red eyelid margins and possible scarring. The longer the disease has been present the more difficult it is to treat effectively.

Treatment (Table 102.1)

Hordeolums, in general, are treated with warm compresses three to four times daily until the lid appears less swollen and red and feels better. In most cases, antibiotics are not required, especially for the single, rare stye. Surgical drainage is not indicated, and treatment with systemic and topical antibiotics is not usually warranted. Topical use of antibacterials may be warranted if the hordeolum recurs (Table 102.2). In cases of severe internal hordeolum, systemic antistaphylococcal therapy is beneficial. Most styes are usually isolated instances, and therefore, patients usually require minimal follow-up.

Chalazia, unlike hordeolums, do not subside on their own in the majority of cases. Many require excision, although they usually decrease in size over time. Some clinicians suggest that the use of local corticosteroid injections may be helpful in relieving the associated inflammation accompanying chalazia. An intralesional injection of triamcinolone acetonide, 0.5–3 mg, may be effective for controlling or eliminating the lesion.[8]

Treatment of blepharitis is usually a long and tedious process and requires that the patient comply with the therapeutic regimen as closely as possible. Local hygiene and, in some cases, topical antimicrobial therapy are the basic treatment choices. The therapeutic endpoint is to reduce the symptoms as much as possible and prevent further eyelid complications.

Local hygiene is very important if the patient wishes to enjoy some relief. Patients are instructed to use warm compresses for 5–10 minutes two to four times daily on the closed lids. Because it has been thought to be associated with little ocular irritation, patients should then apply diluted baby shampoo from a dampened and clean washcloth to the brows and lids. Some patients have complained of redness and irritation with the use of baby shampoo. Other ophthalmic cleansers (OcuSoft) have been developed that are less irritating than baby shampoo in the eye and are effective in cleansing away oily debris, lipids, and crusting that produce some of the problems seen in blepharitis. The prior application of warm compresses helps to loosen and melt some of the lipid debris prior to the use of the shampoo or cleanser.

In mild bacterial infections or in patients with staphylococcal and seborrheic blepharitis, topical ophthalmic antibiotic therapy is used, in addition to hot compresses and lid hygiene. Staphylococcal or ulcerative blepharitis is best treated with topical antibiotic ophthalmic ointments, such as bacitracin 500 U/g or erythromycin 5 mg/g. Erythromycin, bacitracin, tetracycline, chloramphenicol, and sulfonamides have all been used to treat blepharitis, as *S. aureus* and *S. epidermidis* are the most frequently isolated organisms.[4] However, the sulfonamides and tetracycline have been reported to be less effective against *S. aureus* and *S. epidermidis*.

Bacitracin and erythromycin are not available in ophthalmic drop form. Ointments are reasonable vehicles if the patient applies them at bedtime to reduce the accompanying blurred vision. Chloramphenicol use has fallen dramatically because of the reported systemic toxicity from topical administration.[9] The aminoglycosides, gentamicin and tobramycin, appear to be effective agents and are available as ointments and drops. Use of neomycin is limited, as previous authors have noted, because of its hypersensitivity reactions.[4,5] Some investigators have utilized a topical preparation of vancomycin, 50 mg/mL, if culture and sensitivity have shown that the organism is resistant to methicillin.[10,11] In recurrent cases, the utilization of a systemic antibiotic may be considered; dicloxacillin or cephalexin (especially in impetigo) or erythromycin 250–500 mg four times a day may be employed. Although tetracyclines are not very effective against staphylococci, there is evidence that they have a salutary effect on the ocular components of rosacea[12] and are also reported to be most helpful in patients with recalcitrant secondary meibomianitis.[3,4] Although most patients can be discontinued from the systemic tetracycline after 4 or more weeks, some patients may require chronic tetracycline once daily to maintain control. Antibiotic ophthalmic ointment may be applied four times a day for 1–2 weeks, then reduced to twice a day. Once the eyelid appears normal, application may be reduced to daily at bedtime. If a seborrheic condition is present, then the scalp should be shampooed with an antiseborrheic agent, such as selenium sulfide. In refractory cases, mild corticosteroid solutions may be applied to the scalp or mild corticosteroid cream may be applied to the forehead, although many clinicians discourage the use of any topical corticosteroids because of the ocular side effects.

In general, it is best to instruct patients that this disease can be a chronic condition and if flare-ups occur, aggressive use of warm compresses, cleansers, and, if appropriate, topical and systemic antibiotics may help to reduce the acute stage of blepharitis. Because blepharitis is usually considered a chronic condition, occasional warm compresses and lid scrubs are probably also helpful in reducing recurrences of the disease.

TABLE 102.1. THERAPEUTIC RECOMMENDATIONS FOR THE TREATMENT OF PERIOCULAR INFECTIONS

Periocular Infection	Treatment Recommendations[a]	Dose and Duration of Treatment
Hordeolum (stye)	Warm compresses to lid	3–4 times daily until resolution
	Add antibacterial (for recurring external disease erythromycin ophthalmic ointment	Apply 2–3 times daily to lids for 2–3 weeks
	Add oral antistaphylococcal antibiotics for recurring internal disease (dicloxacillin or cephalexin)	250–500 mg orally every 6 hours for 1–2 weeks
Chalazion	May require intralesional steroid injection—triamcinolone acetonide	0.5–3 mg single intralesional injection
Blepharitis (meibomianitis)	Warm compresses to lids	2–4 times daily for 5–10 minutes; may require continual therapy
	And lid scrubs with baby shampoo or nonirritating ophthalmic cleaner	1–2 times daily
	Add for secondary bacterial infections (staphylococcal) (ophthalmic bacitracin or erythromycin ointment)	Apply 1–2 times daily after compresses and lid scrubs Vancomycin 50 mg/mL eyedrops for MRSA[b]
	May massage eyelid margin if meibomian gland obstruction	
	Rosacea is often treated with oral tetracycline plus lid scrubs and topical antibacterial agents	250 mg four times daily reduced to once daily after inflammation lessened
Impetigo	Oral antistaphylococcal agents such as dicloxacillin or cephalexin	250–500 mg orally four times daily for 1–2 weeks
Pediculosis	Ophthalmic lubricating ointment	Apply 4 times daily until eradicated
Dacryoadenitis (lacrimal gland)	**(Acute)** warm compresses	3–4 times daily for 1 week
	And antistaphylococcal agents dicloxacillin or cephalexin	250–500 mg orally four times daily
Canaliculitis (nasolacrimal passages)	Irrigation of canaliculi with antibiotic solution such as penicillin 160,000 U/mL	One time irrigation, if at all Surgery may be definitive treatment
	Add local antibiotic if susceptible to organism isolated	
Dacryocystitis (lacrimal sac)	**(Acute dacryocystitis)** systemic antibiotics active against *Streptococcus pneumoniae* and *S. aureus* (e.g., cephalexin or dicloxacillin) possible gram-negative rods, anaerobes, and fungi	Cover for 7–10 days 250–500 mg orally four times daily Treatment depends on organism isolated (see Stamford reference[34])
	(Chronic dacryocystitis) local irrigation of antibiotics to site	Single use irrigation
Cellulitis[c] (preseptal/orbital)	**(Adults; Preseptal)** cefuroxime or amoxicillin–clavulanate	250–500 mg orally every 12 hours 250–500 mg orally every 8 hours
	(Adults; Orbital) clindamycin and cefotaxime intravenously	60 mg every 8 hours (clindamycin)/1–2 g every 8 hours (cefotaxime)
	(Children; Preseptal) cefaclor or amoxicillin–clavulanate or cefuroxime axetil	40 mg/kg/d (cefaclor) or 250–500 mg every 8 hours or 125–500 mg every 12 hours (cefuroxime) all given orally
	(Children; Orbital) intravenous antibiotics such as cefuroxime	100 mg/kg/d every 6 hours intravenously
	or ceftriaxone **and** nafcillin	50–75 mg/kg/d in divided doses every 12 hours (ceftriaxone) 150 mg/kg/d 1–2 grams every 4–6 hours (nafcillin) intravenously
	and then follow-up with oral antibiotics from preseptal above	May continue intravenous antibiotics for days to week depending on patient response, then switch to PO antibiotics

[a]For further information see Reynolds LA, Closson RG. Extemporaneous Ophthalmic Preparations. Vancouver, WA, Applied Therapeutics, Inc, 1993.
[b]MRSA, methicillin resistant *Staphylococcus aureus.*
[c]Antibiotic recommendations may have to be amended if chronic condition or etiology of cellulitis is known.

TABLE 102.2. INSTILLATION OF OPHTHALMIC OINTMENTS AND DROPS

How to Instill Eyedrops
1. Wash hands.
2. Remove cap from plastic bottle.
3. Tilt head slightly back.
4. Gently pull down lower lid.
5. Hold bottle vertically with dropper pointed downward close to front of eye.
6. Instill drops into pocket between eye and lid.
7. Close eyes gently for approximately 3 minutes.[a]

How to Use Eye Ointment (Salve)
1. Wash hands.
2. Remove cap from tube.[b]
3. With one hand, gently pull lower lid down.
4. While looking up, squeeze a small amount of ointment (about an inch) inside lower lid. Be careful not to touch tip of tube to eye or fingers.
5. Close eye gently and, keeping it closed, roll eyeball in all directions. Temporary blurriness may occur.
6. Replace cap on tube.

[a]Gentle eyelid closure or occlusion of punctum reduces the incidence of systemic side effects. This is more significant with some ophthalmic medications (e.g., β blockers and phenylephrine).
[b]When opening tube for the first time, squeeze out the first inch and discard; it may be too dry.

Pediculosis (lice infestation) is a lid infection in which the adult lice thrive in the cilia, and their eggs (nits) cling to the eyelashes. Infestation of the eyelid is rare and almost always secondary to pubic infestation of the patient or through sexual contact. Mechanical removal of the lice and the nits should be attempted, and treatment with an ophthalmic lubricating ointment, which blocks the oxygen needed for the organism to survive, is recommended.[13] Permethrin 1% is reportedly less toxic than lindane when applied to the eyelid; however, both of these products must be kept out of the eye.[14]

Evaluation of Therapeutic Outcomes

Generally, follow-up for hordeolums is not required. The goal of treatment with chalazia is usually related to acute treatment of the plugged gland, possibly requiring localized steroid injection or surgical removal. Control of concurrent blepharitis is helpful in reducing the occurrence of chalazia. However, blepharitis is a chronic condition that lends itself well to patient education on prevention and treatment. Proper lid hygiene and lid soaks are essential and this fact must be reinforced. Treatment success or failure is determined by visual inspection of the eye and patient symptoms.

INFECTIONS OF THE LACRIMAL APPARATUS

Infections of the lacrimal apparatus may involve the major and minor lacrimal glands (dacryoadenitis), the upper and or lower canaliculi (canaliculitis), and the lacrimal sac (dacryocystitis). Tears are secreted by the lacrimal glands and the accessory lacrimal glands of Krause and Wolfring. The conjunctiva and meibomian glands contain goblet cells, which also make up part of the tear secretion. Tears drain into the canaliculi, the lacrimal sac, the nasolacrimal duct, and then into the inferior turbinate. Patients with disorders of the lacrimal apparatus complain of tearing or dry eyes. The symptoms are investigated by irrigation to test the patency of the canaliculi and the nasolacrimal ducts and by palpitation of the nasolacrimal gland. If the complaint is dry eyes, the quantity of tear production should be assessed (Schirmer test) and the appearance of the tear film studied with the aid of a slit-lamp.

Etiology

There are many causes of tearing, such as conjunctivitis, keratitis, iritis, and foreign bodies. However, if tearing is the only symptom, the cause in the great majority of cases will be found in the lacrimal drainage apparatus. Dacryocystitis or infection of the lacrimal sac, may occur in any age group and is a common acute or chronic disease. It is most often unilateral and is always secondary to obstruction of the nasolacrimal duct.[15] In acute dacryocystitis the usual infectious agent is *S. aureus* or, occasionally, β-hemolytic streptococcus. In chronic dacryocystitis, *Streptococcus pneumoniae* is the predominant organism, although gram-negative bacteria, anaerobic bacteria, fungi, and so on, may also be found.[16] *Haemophilus influenzae* may be the preliminary pathogen in children. Cultures are usually difficult to obtain.

Canaliculitis is an uncommon chronic unilateral condition caused by infection with mixed aerobic and anaerobic bacterial, fungal, or even viral organisms. *Actinomyces israelii, Candida albicans,* or *Aspergillus* species have all been isolated as infectious agents.[16–18] Dacryoadenitis, or inflammation of the lacrimal gland, is a rare unilateral condition that may be seen in children as a complication of mumps, measles, or influenza, and in adults in association with gonorrhea. It also may develop following an injury to the lacrimal gland or as a retrograde infection from a bacterial conjunctivitis. There are two types of chronic dacryoadenitis and it may sometimes be seen bilaterally as a manifestation of sarcoidosis. It usually occurs in blacks and is self-limited. Chronic dacryoadenitis may also occur in lymphosarcoma, tuberculosis, and lymphatic leukemia.

Clinical Presentation

In the event of tearing without associated symptoms, the disorder is usually in the lacrimal drainage system or, rarely, the result of hypersecretion. In chronic dacryocystitis most patients have minor complaints, with some tearing and redness. Some patients may have recurrent bouts of conjunctivitis. Acute dacryocystitis presents with more severe and sudden complaints of pain, redness, and tenderness over the lacrimal sac. Canaliculitis is usually unilateral, is seen more often in females, and usually presents with tearing, swelling, pain, and tenderness of the inner corner of the eye. Dacryoadenitis presents with pain and swelling of the upper eyelid. Patients also complain of tenderness in the lacrimal area and possibly some localized periorbital edema. Infections from certain organisms such as *Neisseria gonorrhoeae* or streptococci may also produce a purulent discharge.

Treatment (Table 102.1)

In adults, therapy for acute dacryocystitis should consist of warm compresses and a systemically administered cephalosporin or penicillin that is active against penicillinase-producing staphylococci. Cephalexin, 250–500 mg four times daily, would be effective. Obstruction of the nasolacrimal duct is the basic cause of dacryocystitis, and the disease is usually persistent until the obstruction is relieved, even if medical treatment is given. Because probing is usually unsuccessful in adults, dacryocystorhinostomy (surgical procedure that creates an opening in the nasal bone to allow the lacrimal sac to drain directly into the nose) is usually necessary if symptoms are severe. In canaliculitis, curettage of the necrotic material in the involved canaliculus followed by forceful irrigation is usually effective. Irrigation of the canaliculi with an antibiotic solution and then use of topical antibiotic drops has been advocated by some clinicians. For instance, in the treatment of *Arachnia* and *Actinomyces,* penicillin 160,000 U/mL for irrigant and penicillin drops 60,000 U/mL may be helpful. Amphotericin B in a concentration of 1–5 mg/mL is used against *Candida* and *Aspergillus.*[16] If herpetic canaliculitis is diagnosed, no specific antiviral agent is recommended for treatment, although biweekly irrigation is suggested.[17] A short course of antibiotics is generally given for 7 days or so after the canaliculi is cleared of debris. If bacterial infection is present, usually staphylococci, then appropriate systemic antibiotic therapy should be employed. Incision may be necessary if the pus collects in the gland under tension. Acute dacryoadenitis is treated with a short course of antibiotics effective against the most common organisms, primarily staphylococci, but also may include *Chlamydia trachomatis* and occasionally *N. gonorrhoeae.*[18]

Evaluation of Therapeutic Outcomes

The goal of therapy is to reduce the acute flare-up and/or infection, since many of these conditions may respond to surgery with or without antibacterial treatment. In most of these situations, especially with canaliculitis and dacryocystitis, removal of the obstruction may be considered curative itself. Antimicrobial therapy is usually instituted after the surgical procedure. Susceptibility of the organism should be determined and topical therapy instituted for 1–2 weeks. Chronic conjunctivitis on the affected side should warn the patient that this may signal reinfection. Because recurrence can happen in most of these conditions, the patient must always be vigilant for the signs and symptoms of reinfection such as swelling, tenderness, irritation, and conjunctival redness.

PRESEPTAL CELLULITIS, ORBITAL CELLULITIS, AND INFECTIONS OF THE SINUSES

Preseptal cellulitis is an ocular infection of the soft tissue of the eyelids and the periocular area prior to the orbital septum. Orbital cellulitis is a soft tissue infection that involves the entire orbit. It may evolve from preseptal cellulitis and is considered a more severe infection that, if not properly treated, could result in loss of vision, meningitis, and possibly death. Spread of a sinusitis to the surrounding areas may produce secondary complications including orbital cellulitis.

Etiology

The most common microbial agents in orbital cellulitis associated with sinusitis are *S. aureus, S. epidermidis,* streptococci, *Escherichia coli, H. influenzae* (especially in children), diphtheroids, *Pseudomonas* spp., and polymicrobial anaerobes and aerobes.[19,20] Preseptal and orbital cellulitis occur more frequently in the winter months probably secondary to the increased incidence of respiratory and sinus infections. These infections are more prevalent in children and young people, with preseptal cellulitis (87%) being reported much more commonly than orbital cellulitis (13%).[21,22] Orbital cellulitis in adults is usually related to some predisposing factor such as sinusitis, trauma, polyps, allergy, and dental extraction.[19] Adults have a higher incidence of polymicrobial and anaerobic organisms as offending agents versus children who predominantly have aerobic organisms. Sinusitis is one of the most common causes of orbital cellulitis, occurring in up to 85% of cases according to some investigators.[19,22] Sinus infection orbital complications have been classified into various stages that help the clinician to determine the prognosis and length of treatment.[23]

Clinical Presentation

The presenting signs and symptoms of preseptal cellulitis may be difficult to distinguish from orbital cellulitis. In general, most patients with preseptal cellulitis have some lid swelling, normal vision, normal ocular motility, mild fever, normal pupillary reaction, and little proptosis (anterior displacement of the globe) or pain on motion of the eye. Moderate to severe swelling of the lids, proptosis, chemosis, pain, fever, injection of lid, malaise, and increasing intraocular pressure may all be seen in patients with orbital cellulitis. Progressive loss of consciousness and facial weakness may suggest fungal involvement. In patients with a sinusitis that has progressed to an orbital cellulitis, it is important for the clinical diagnosis to be supplemented with orbital imaging, because routine sinus radiographs may fail to demonstrate early cellulitis and sinusitis.

Treatment (Table 102.1)

Careful diagnosis and staging of preseptal and orbital cellulitis is essential in monitoring the effectiveness of treatment. The site or origin of the infection and a careful patient history will help in selection of the most appropriate therapy. Aspiration of abscesses where appropriate (rarely in children), and/or culture and sensitivity, is essential for adequate treatment. Proper selection of empiric antibiotics until such information is available is the most important pharmacologic intervention. In general, preseptal cellulitis may be treated with oral antibiotics on an outpatient basis. Daily monitoring of patients must be undertaken to preclude any extension of this infection. Orbital cellulitis requires immediate treatment with intravenous antibiotics and careful assessment of the patient's orbital involvement. In adults, preseptal cellulitis may be treated with systemic antibiotics such as dicloxacillin or cephalexin 250–500 mg orally every 6 hours, unless some predisposing consideration suggests another etiology of the pathogenic organism. As an example, spread from the sinus may require more complete coverage against *H. influenzae,* with agents such as cefuroxime axetil 250–500 mg every 12 hours. In more serious cases, adults should generally be covered for penicillin-resistant, gram-negative, and anaerobic organisms. Empiric antibiotics may include the use of clindamycin 600 mg intravenously every 8 hours and cefotaxime 1–2 g every 8 hours. Consideration for regional epidemiologic variations should be taken into account when selecting the appropriate antibiotic regimen.

In children, the risk of *H. influenzae* infection is even greater and therefore an agent that is effective against both *H. influenzae* and *S. aureus* and *S. epidermidis* would be best. Oral cefaclor 40 mg/kg/d, amoxicillin–clavulanate potassium 250–500 mg in three divided doses, or cefuroxime axetil tablets 125–500 mg twice per day would be acceptable. Amoxicillin–clavulanate potassium and cefuroxime are the antibiotics of first choice in children because of their effective coverage against *S. aureus,* pneumococcus, and *H. influenzae* including many β-lactamase–producing strains. Amoxicillin–clavulanate is also available in suspension and chewable tablets for children. Cefuroxime is available in both intravenous and oral forms (although the oral form is not a suspension, only tablets). The parenteral form is dosed at 100 mg/kg/d in four divided doses. Because of its good soft tissue, bone, and cerebrospinal fluid penetration, intravenous cefuroxime may be indicated if more serious involvement such as an orbital abscess or cavernous sinus thrombosis is suspected.[19,23] Antibiotic selection may be changed depending on results of the culture and sensitivity.

Sinus decongestion with nasal sprays such as oxymetolazone used twice daily may be helpful to clear up the sinus conditions. In some instances, surgical drainage of an abscess may be required.

Evaluation of Therapeutic Outcomes

In most cases, preseptal or orbital cellulitis should respond to proper antibacterial treatment, and recurrence should not be a problem. The goal of therapy is to ascertain that proper antibacterial coverage is utilized and the regimen is for a sufficient time course. Patients are monitored for a decrease in signs and symptoms including eye pain, lid edema and swelling, hyperemia, proptosis, and an improvement in ocular motility. A decrease in the white blood cell count, if initially elevated, may also be helpful in noting improvement. In cases where sinusitis was an initiating factor, careful observation of future episodes of sinusitis should be monitored closely.

CONJUNCTIVITIS

Inflammation and/or infection of the conjunctiva (conjunctivitis) is the most common eye disease in the Western Hemisphere. This chapter stresses infectious causes, although there are many other less common causes of conjunctivitis including toxic, mechanical, allergic, atopic, and systemic lupus erythematosus. Infectious conjunctivitis includes viral, bacterial, rickettsial, and fungal organisms. It may vary in severity from a mild hyperemia with tearing (hay fever conjunctivitis) to a severe necrotic process (membranous conjunctivitis).

ETIOLOGY

Bacterial conjunctival infections may be either acute or chronic. Bacterial conjunctivitis may, in most instances, be a self-limiting disease. The organisms most commonly causing acute conjunctivitis are staphylococci, streptococci, pneumococci, moraxella, or haemophilus. Anaerobic organisms have been recovered but their role remains in doubt.[24,25] Most organisms exude a purulent or mucopurulent discharge. *Neisseria gonorrhoeae* causes a severe and purulent discharge. Pseudomembranes, which are rare components of bacterial conjunctivitis, suggest an infection with *Streptococcus pyogenes* or *Corynebacterium diphtheriae.*[25]

Trachoma, caused by *Chlamydia trachomatis,* is rare in the United States except among Native Americans of the southwestern states, where it is mild and relatively uncomplicated. However, with more than 400 million of the world's population afflicted, it is one of the most common of all chronic human diseases. It may eventually produce corneal scarring and is a leading cause of blindness in the world. Inclusion conjunctivitis, caused by *Chlamydia oculogenitalis,* usually bilateral, is a common disease, especially in sexually active young people.

Viral conjunctivitis is a very common type of infectious conjunctivitis and, with few exceptions, there is no definitive treatment. Most cases produce mild symptoms, are follicular type, contagious, and usually self-limited. The actual virus is not often identified by examination and requires specific serologic and culture testing. The adenoviruses are most often found in epidemics and, rarely, some of these viruses may lead to keratitis and produce vision reduction.

Ophthalmia neonatorum is an acute conjunctivitis of the newborn infant caused by a multitude of agents, which has been reported to have an incidence of up to 12%.[26,27] It usually presents as a purulent discharge from the eyes occurring during the first month of life. The pathogenic organisms are transmitted from contamination of the baby's eye as it passes through the birth canal, a nosocomial infection during the first few weeks of life, or a mild chemical irritation from the silver nitrate solution.[28,29] Chlamydial infections of infants are found in the first 3–10 days of life and have been increasing in incidence in the last few years. The bacterial causes of conjunctivitis most commonly include *S. aureus, S. pneumoniae,* and *H. influenzae.* Occasionally, these infections have been reported to appear as early as 1 day after birth, although the majority occur between days 3 and 5. *Neisseria* conjunctivitis is very serious and must be treated immediately. It is essential to differentiate between *N. meningitidis* and *N. gonorrhoeae* conjunctivitis, since the former may represent a possible metastatic meningitis.

CLINICAL PRESENTATION

The important symptoms of conjunctivitis are a foreign body sensation, a scratching or burning sensation, a sensation of fullness around the eyes, itching, and, when the cornea is affected, photophobia. Many patients come into the pharmacy with general eye complaints and would like the pharmacist to suggest an eyedrop that would be effective. It is important for the pharmacist to be able to distinguish the common or benign ocular complaints from more serious eye disease. Keratitis, iritis, and acute glaucoma are usually included in the differential diagnosis of conjunctivitis (Table 102.3). Of course, if there is any doubt, it is prudent to have the patient see an ophthalmologist at once to prevent a possible vision-threatening disease.

Foreign body sensation and scratching or burning are often associated with swelling and papillary hypertrophy, which normally accompany conjunctival hyperemia. If there is pain, the cornea is probably also affected. Pain that is more severe on waking and improves during the day suggests staphylococcal infection versus pain that is severe during the day and better on waking, which suggests keratoconjunctivitis sicca (dry eye). Itching, if complained of

TABLE 102.3. DIFFERENTIAL DIAGNOSIS OF THE RED EYE

	Conjunctivitis			Keratitis			
	Bacterial	Viral	Allergic	Bacterial	Viral	Iritis	Glaucoma (Acute)
Blurred vision	0	0	0	+++	0 to ++	+ to ++	++ to +++
Pain	0	0	0	++	0 to +	++	++ to ++++
Photophobia	0	0	0	++	++	+++	– to ++
Discharge	Purulent + to +++	Watery + to ++	White, ropy +	Purulent +++	Watery +	0	0
Injection	+++	++	+	+++	+	0 to + (Limbal)	+ to ++ (Limbal)
Corneal haze	0	0	0	+++	+ to ++	0	+ to +++
Ciliary flush	0	0	0	+++	+	++ to +++	+ to ++
Pupil	Normal	Normal	Normal	Normal or miotic (iritis)	Normal	Miotic	Mid-dilated nonreactive
Intraocular pressure	Normal	Normal	Normal	Normal	Normal	Normal, low or high	High
Preauricular nodes	Rare	Usual	0	0	0	0	0
Smear	Bacterial PMNs	Lymph	Eos	Bacteria PMNs	0	0	0

Key: 0, absent or none; +, mild; ++, moderate; +++, severe; PMNs, polymorphonucleocytes; Eos, eosinophils. (Adapted from Syed NA, Hyndiuk RA. Infectious conjunctivitis. Infect Dis Clin North Am 1992;6(4):789–805, with permission.)

spontaneously rather than in response to questioning, usually indicates that the patient has an allergic conjunctivitis.

The signs of conjunctivitis may include hyperemia (redness), tearing, exudation, pseudoptosis, papillary hypertrophy, chemosis, follicles, pseudomembranes, and membranes on the conjunctiva, granulomas, and preauricular adenopathy. Papillary conjunctivitis is a nonspecific inflammatory response due to the infiltration of the papillae with lymphocytes, eosinophils, plasma cells, and polymorphonuclear leukocytes. It produces a velvety appearance and is seen in conjunction with allergic and bacterial conjunctivitis. A follicular conjunctivitis is derived from lymphoid tissue and the follicles contain lymphocytes and macrophages and produce lobular projections. It is most commonly associated with viral infections.

In bacterial conjunctivitis, causal organisms can then be identified by microscopic examination of the stained conjunctival material. The acute types of bacterial conjunctivitis occasionally become chronic but are usually self-limited, lasting a maximum of 2 weeks if untreated. Hyperacute bacterial conjunctivitis, such as that caused by *N. gonorrhoeae,* must be treated immediately, because it may penetrate the intact corneal epithelium and is not considered a self-limiting process. This infection is most often acquired through sexual contact with an infected partner or by autoinoculation. The inflammatory reaction may be relatively mild. As with most forms of hyperacute conjunctivitis, there is an accompanying copious purulent discharge, lid swelling, preauricular lymphadenopathy, throbbing globe pain, and foreign body sensation. Chronic forms of conjunctivitis may be caused by staphylococci and coliforms and usually consist of mild eye irritation, redness, and conjunctival thickening.

In chlamydial conjunctivitis, the chlamydial agent initially infects the urethra of the male and the cervix of the female. Transmission to the eyes in adults is generally from the genitourinary tract to the eyes. Indirect transmission in inadequately chlorinated swimming pools can also occur. Chlamydial (inclusion) disease in adults produces a chronic follicular conjunctivitis with minimal redness and irritation.

In ophthalmia neonatorum, if silver nitrate is still utilized for prophylaxis, the conjunctivitis presents as a mild chemical irritation, which is usually self-limited. Neonatal chlamydial conjunctivitis is usually seen in a week or more and may be in association with chlamydial otitis media or pneumonia.[26,29] Gonococcal conjunctivitis is seen shortly after birth and is one of the few organisms that produces a fulminant course within hours, which may progress to corneal perforation if not treated adequately.

TREATMENT (TABLE 102.4)

Although many cases of conjunctivitis are self-limiting, treatment is often initiated to shorten the course of the disease, prevent patient discomfort, reduce the spread to others, and possibly diminish the chance of chronic disease. Cultures and antibiotic sensitivity tests should be performed before treatment, especially in neonates, in children with suspected *H. influenzae,* and in any patient with hyperacute conjunctivitis, since these require systemic treatment. Gram stain and culture are recommended for all cases and are mandatory if the disease is purulent, membranous, or pseudomembranous. Antibiotic sensitivity studies are also highly desirable, so that an appropriate drug can be substituted if the organism was not sensitive to the initial antimicrobial agent. It is important to culture both eyes even though the patient may exhibit symptoms in only one. In this way the "normal" flora of the uninvolved eye can be differentiated from the flora of the inflamed involved eye. Hot compresses may provide desirable symptomatic relief in the early stages of the disease. Antibiotics should be continued 4 or 5 days after all symptoms have subsided. Topical preparations of neomycin with gramicidin and polymyxin B sulfate are generally good combinations due to their broad antibacterial spectrum and because they are seldom used systemically. However, neomycin produces allergic reactions in 5–10% of the patients if therapy is continued for longer than a week. In addition, it may also produce punctate epithelial erosions of the cornea. Sulfacetamide or sulfasoxazole ophthalmic preparations cause fewer side effects but are less effective. Erythromycin as a 0.5% ointment is also a useful ophthalmic preparation against gram-positive cocci, but staphylococci rapidly develop a resistance to this antibiotic. Chloramphenicol 0.5% ophthalmic solution is nonirritating and penetrates the cornea and conjunctiva well. A few cases of idiosyncratic aplastic anemia have been reported with the use of chloramphenicol eye drops, although the incidence is very low. Topical gentamicin or tobramycin should be reserved for more serious infections caused by sensitive organisms. Conjunctivitis caused by *S. aureus* should be treated with bacitracin ophthalmic ointment 500 U/g, five to six times a day, decreasing the frequency of application as the condition improves. Since this organism causes a chronic conjunctivitis, treatment should continue daily at bedtime for 1 month after all signs of the infection have vanished. Trimethoprim–polymixin B is effective for the treatment of bacterial conjunctivitis and is said to cause fewer topical side effects than neomycin or sulfacetamide.[30] The quinolone antibiotics, ciprofloxacin 0.3%, ofloxacin 0.3%, and norfloxacin 0.3%, are all safe and effective in treating bacterial conjunctivitis.[31] They are usually administered every 2 hours while awake for 1–2 days, then every 4 hours thereafter for up to 1 week.

Systemic antibiotics are required for the treatment of gonococcal, diphtheritic, tularemic, and granulomatous, and possibly *H. influenzae*, conjunctivitis. Gonorrheal conjunctivitis should be treated vigorously to prevent serious involvement of the cornea. Recommended therapy for adult

TABLE 102.4. PHARMACOTHERAPEUTIC RECOMMENDATIONS FOR THE TREATMENT OF CONJUNCTIVITIS

Type of Conjunctivitis	Agent(s) for Treatment	Dose and Duration
Viral	Vasoconstrictors (naphazoline 0.1%)	May be useful for short-term local application but of limited value and overuse may produce rebound congestion
	and artificial tear and cold compresses	As needed for patient comfort
Bacterial[a]	**Any** of the various antibacterial drops (check sensitivity)	Dosing may vary; but usually initially may be as often as every 2–4 hours for 1–2 days; then reduce to 4 times daily usually up to a week
	Sulfacetamide	
	Polymyxin B/trimethoprim	
	Quinolones (noroxin, ofloxacin, ciprofloxacin)	
	Aminoglycosides (gentamicin, tobramycin)	
Allergic	**May use one or combination of agents**	Combination therapy requires further study
	Vasoconstrictor/antihistamine (e.g., naphazoline 0.05%/antazoline 0.5%)	Use 4–6 times daily
	H_1-receptor antagonists (levocabastine)	Four times daily for 2 weeks
	NSAIDs (ketorolac)	Four times daily
	Mast cell stabilizers (lodoxamide)	Four times daily (not approved indication yet; used up to 3 months in vernal conjunctivitis)
Chlamydial	**Topical "adjunctive" therapy** erythromycin ophthalmic ointment **or** tetracycline ointment	Two to three times daily
	Required "systemic" therapy	
	Tetracycline	Tetracycline 500 mg orally three times daily
	or doxycycline	Doxycycline 100 mg orally twice daily
	or erythromycin	Erythromycin 250 mg orally four times daily
		Any of the above for minimum of 3 weeks; recommended for 4–6 weeks

[a]*H. influenzae, N. gonorrhoeae,* and *N. meningitidis* require systemic and topical antibiotic treatment.

gonococcal keratoconjunctivitis is ceftriaxone 1 g daily intramuscularly for 5 days, especially in light of the reported penicillinase-producing strains of *N. gonorrhoeae*.[25,32] This regimen is more cost effective than hospitalization and treatment with aqueous penicillin G 10 million units intravenously daily for 5 days. A single dose of ceftriaxone 125 mg intramuscularly has been found to have a cure rate of 100% in gonococcal ophthalmia neonatorum.[33] Adjunctive topical therapy was not required. Alternate therapy could consist of spectinomycin 2–4 g in one intramuscular injection, especially in penicillin-allergic patients, with ophthalmic tetracycline ointment as an optional adjunct. Gonococcal infection caused by penicillinase-producing organisms usually responds to spectinomycin. Adults with gonorrhea should be treated for presumed chlamydial infection with doxycycline 100 mg twice daily for 7 days or tetracycline 500 mg four times daily for 3 weeks.[34]

The current recommended treatment for chlamydial conjunctivitis is a 4- to 6-week course of oral tetracycline 1–1.5 g/d orally in four divided doses or doxycycline 100 mg twice daily. Erythromycin 1–1.5 g/d orally can be used for pregnant women or children less than 9 years old in four divided doses. Several courses are sometimes necessary for an actual cure.[35] Topical sulfonamide therapy may be added. In children less than 9 years old or in pregnant women, oral sulfonamides or erythromycin should be substituted because of the side effects caused by tetracyclines on developing teeth. Ofloxacin or azithromycin may be reasonable substitutes in adults, although the duration of therapy and FDA approval have not been established.

Although topical treatment alone probably can cure trachoma, it requires a much longer treatment than therapy with systemically administered antibiotics. Tetracycline 1% ophthalmic ointment applied twice per day, 6 days per week, for 10 weeks is the recommended therapy. Systemic therapy consists of oral tetracycline 1–1.5 g daily in four divided doses, doxycycline 100 mg twice daily, or erythromycin 1–1.5 g/d in four divided doses. In some cases, several courses of antibiotics may be required for effective treatment.

The goal of treatment in most cases of viral conjunctivitis is to prevent complications, relieve symptoms, and prevent secondary bacterial conjunctivitis. Topical vasoconstrictors such as naphazoline 0.02–0.1%, with or without topical antihistamines such as antazoline 0.5% or pheniramine 0.3%, may be helpful in relieving some of the symptoms of irritation. Some clinicians will empirically prescribe an antibacterial agent such as sulfacetamide 10% or gentamicin 0.3% topically three to four times daily to prevent secondary bacterial infection. However, there is little study data to support this indication.

Prophylaxis for ophthalmia neonatorum has shifted from the use of silver nitrate 1% solution to agents that would also be effective against chlamydial organisms. Tetracycline 1% and erythromycin 0.5% sterile ophthalmic ointments are now commonly used for the prophylaxis of newborns because of effectiveness against both gonococcus and chlamydia.[26]

Among the viral diseases of the conjunctiva for which there is no specific treatment are Newcastle virus disease, adenovirus infections, Echo virus disease, epidemic keratoconjunctivitis, and rubeola. Herpes simplex conjunctivitis has been treated with trifluridine ophthalmic drops every 2 hours for 7 days and has met with some success, although treatment may not be indicated.

EVALUATION OF THERAPEUTIC OUTCOMES

Since most cases of conjunctivitis are self-limiting, the goal of therapy is to provide supportive care and to reduce signs and symptoms of the disease as much as possible. Hyperacute cases (e.g., gonococcal) require a full course of systemic antibiotics in addition to local ocular therapy. In most cases of both viral and allergic conjunctivitis, reduction of pain, irritation, redness, itching, and congestion are the main considerations. In bacterial conjunctivitis, reduction of ocular symptoms should occur within a few days with antibacterial treatment versus up to 2 weeks without. Prophylaxis against the initial signs of allergic conjunctivitis may be possible with topical mast cell stabilizers such as lodoxamide. More immediate relief may be realized with potent H_1 blockers, such as levocabastine or nonsteroidal anti-inflammatory agents such as ketorolac. The potential for relapse with *Chlamydial* conjunctivitis is a concern, and reinforcement about taking the full course of systemic antibiotics is essential.

KERATITIS

The corneal epithelium, tears, movement of the lids, and so on, all help prevent the normal cornea from becoming infected. More than half of corneal ulcers were associated with prior topical corticosteroid administration, corneal transplant, contact lens use, and trauma.[36] In fact, contact lens wear accounts for approximately 52% of corneal ulcers in recent years and is considered the most significant risk factor for ulcerative keratitis.[37] Overnight wear of either extended wear or disposable contact lenses appear to have the highest incidence of contact lens associated corneal ulceration.[38,39] Other major predisposing factors to keratitis cases include diabetes mellitus, systemic corticosteroids, dementia, rheumatoid arthritis, immunosuppression (not steroids), cocaine abuse, and alcoholism. Only a very few organisms can penetrate an intact corneal epithelium unless the patient is immunocompromised. Aggressive and early treatment is important in preventing a potentially blinding condition.

ETIOLOGY

The most common organisms causing bacterial keratitis include *Pseudomonas aeruginosa, S. aureus, S. pneumoniae,* and *S. epidermidis.*[38] Organisms usually thought to be nonpathogenic such as *S. epidermidis, Corynebacterium,* and *P. acnes* can also cause keratitis. Less common bacterial agents are *Proteus, Serratia, E. coli, H. influenzae, Neisseria,* and *Klebsiella.* Fungal infections with *Candida, Fusarium,* or *Aspergillus* normally follow trauma to the cornea from vegetative matter.[38,40] Although the incidence of herpes simplex keratitis is much lower than that of bacterial or fungal, recurrence is common since the viruses remain dormant in adjacent ganglion and are shed in response to physical or psychological stress.

Acanthamoeba, a protozoan, has been found to produce a keratitis that has been associated with wearing of soft contact lenses, and minor corneal trauma. The incidence has increased in the United States and Britain, and is usually associated with contact lens wear, and probably in conjunction with swimming or hot tub use.[39]

The dominance of pathogens changes with geography.[38,40] Gram-positive cocci have the highest incidence among microorganisms responsible for corneal ulceration and have their greatest prevalence in the northern and eastern United States. Gram-negative bacilli, especially *P. aeruginosa,* rank one of the highest nationwide; fungi are rare in the North but occur in significant numbers in the southern and western portions of the United States.

CLINICAL PRESENTATION

Microbial infections of the cornea are characterized by epithelial defects surrounded by edema. Many patients present with foreign body sensations, blurred or reduced vision, iritis, and pain. Stromal involvement is often present and, with continued progression, corneal neovascularization, hypopyon, and corneal thinning may appear.

In general, the clinical appearance of most corneal ulcers does not provide a definitive diagnosis. It is often difficult to differentiate by clinical appearance alone a bacterial keratitis from a fungal keratitis from a sterile soft-contact-lens-induced corneal infiltrate. Cultures of bacterial corneal ulcers may not have organisms isolated because of prior antibacterial treatment or because of mixed infections with other bacterial or viral organisms. *Neisseria gonorrhoeae, Listeria, Haemophilis aegypticus,* and *C. diphtheriae,* and possibly *P. aeruginosa,* can all invade an intact corneal epithelium. The resulting keratitis, especially that seen with *Neisseria,* may be associated with a purulent discharge. *Pseudomonas* causes rapid necrosis and characteristic mucopurulent discharge and may cause corneal perforation within 1–2 days if not treated promptly. Filamentous fungi *(Fusarium, Aspergillus)* display as a gray or dirty-white rough, textured surface with elevated margins.[41] Branching lines radiate from the fungal ulcer and satellite lesions may appear. Yeast fungi *(Candida)* appear as oval outlines with a plaquelike surface. Fungal infections can also be very destructive with ulceration that may thin the cornea to the point of perforation.

Herpes simplex keratitis is identified by characteristic dendritic figures. The deeper stromal infections display blotchy, cheesy-white infiltrates that may lie under the ulcer.[42] Herpes simplex virus can also be responsible for secondarily infected bacterial ulcers.

The initial signs and symptoms of *Acanthamoeba* keratitis are somewhat nonspecific and subtle, and have been mistreated as bacterial and/or herpes simplex infections. Initial presenting signs may include a limbitis (inflammation around the limbus), perineural infiltrates, a low-grade anterior uveitis, lid edema, and epithelial irregularity.[39,43,44] A ring-shaped stromal infiltrate is considered pathognomonic for the infections. Improved staining techniques such as calcifluour white and indirect fluorescent antibody have more quickly identified this organism.[43] More recently, clinicians have found that careful and prompt diagnosis and initiation of immediate treatment within 1 month of onset have improved the prognosis and visual outcome.[44]

TREATMENT (TABLE 102.5)

The corneal epithelium consists of cells that have tight intercellular junctions that normally present quite a barrier to penetration of drug into the anterior chamber. This epithelial barrier is basically a lipid wall, which prevents a drug that is too water soluble from penetrating through it into the stroma, which is considered to be the more water-soluble medium. If the epithelium is compromised or missing, as it is in keratitis, penetration of drug from topical or subconjunctival injection into the cornea and anterior chamber is greater.

The initial antibiotic regimen for bacterial keratitis should be chosen empirically based on the prevalence of pathogens known to be producing this disease in the community. Because of the difficulty in determining the etiology of the ulcer, most clinicians initiate therapy with an aggressive antibacterial regimen. The most frequently prescribed first-line regimen consists of an aminoglycoside in a "fortified" ophthalmic solution and a first-generation cephalosporin alternating every 15–30 minutes.[45] Gentamicin (or tobramycin) 9–15 mg/mL is commonly used, alternating with cefazolin in a concentration of 50–133 mg/mL. These ophthalmic solutions are not commercially available and must be compounded. Some centers have begun to replace cefazolin with vancomycin 50 mg/mL, especially if there is concern about resistant *Staphylococcus*. Topical vancomycin is reported to be irritating though because of the low pH.[46] Ciprofloxacin 0.3% has been found effective for single-agent empiric corneal ulcer treatment, with a shorter average time to healing and a reduced duration of therapy than conventional therapy.[47] Others caution the use of ciprofloxacin as single agent because of the concerns of possible resistant organisms.[48] The results of a Gram stain and the gross morphology of the bacterium may be somewhat helpful in guiding the clinician; however, a single-agent regimen should be used cautiously until the culture results are definite. Following a decrease in purulence and a reduction in ulcer size, the intervals between antimicrobial instillation and/or frequency of instillation should be prolonged to reduce the inhibition of corneal regeneration caused by concentrated antimicrobial solutions. In most cases, one of the antibiotics is discontinued when a definite organism has been identified and sensitivity noted. Studies have shown that topical loading doses consisting of an initial drop of gentamicin-fortified solution every minute for 5 minutes produced higher corneal levels. These investigators[49] also showed that extended dosing intervals of three drops every 2 hours maintained aqueous fluid peak and trough levels equal to those produced by the one drop per hour regimen. Although an initial loading dose is recommended with the fortified aminoglycoside preparations, a multiple drop, extended-interval dosing regimen must be used with caution until further clinical studies are done.

Antibiotics may also be administered by subconjunctival injection. Although individually both subconjunctivally and topically administered antibiotics are effective, one may choose the subconjunctival route if there is question of compliance or for the treatment of infants and children when diminished effectiveness of drops may be due to tear washout. When used concomitantly, subconjunctival injections yield temporarily high aqueous fluid concentrations to supplement the moderate but sustained drug levels provided by topically administered drops.[38] Cefazolin 100 mg and gentamicin 20–40 mg may be given subconjunctivally at 12- to 24-hour intervals. Subconjunctival volumes should be between 0.2 and 0.5 mL, although occasionally up to 1 mL may be injected. Subconjunctival administration of two different antibiotics should be given 180 degrees away to avoid any inactivation of antibacterial agents. Intravenous administration of antibiotics is used when corneal perforation threatens infection of intraocular processes or if there may be scleral extension.[38]

Routine *in vitro* bacterial susceptibility testing assumes attainment of usual plasma levels of antibiotics. Such tests do not accurately reflect the activity of the high concentrations achieved by topical instillation and therefore may not accurately predict clinical response. Ten cases of "resistant" pseudomonal keratitis, as defined by standard criteria,

TABLE 102.5. PHARMACOTHERAPEUTIC RECOMMENDATIONS FOR THE TREATMENT OF KERATITIS

Keratitis	Agents for Treatment[a]	Dose and Duration
Bacterial	Cefazolin 10% **and** aminoglycoside 1–1.5%	Alternate every 15–30 minutes × 1–2 days; reduce frequency; treatment may last for 3 weeks
	or ciprofloxacin 0.3%	Initially every 15 minutes × 6 hours, then every 30 minutes up to 24 hours, reducing to every hour day 2, then every 4 hours days 3–14
Viral	Trifluridine	9 times daily × 14 days, then every 4 hours × 7 days
	or idoxuridine 0.1% solution	Every hour during day, every 2 hours at night decrease to 2 and 4 hours, respectively, up to 21 days
	or vidarabine	Apply 5 times daily up to 21 days
Acanthamoeba	Neomycin **and/or** propamidine drops (or possibly ointment) **and/or** imidazoles (clotrimazole, miconazole)	May start off drops every 1–2 hours alternating these agents and reducing frequency depending on patient response
	and/or polyhexamethylene biguanide (PHMB)	Patients may require treatment for weeks to months
Fungal	Natamycin **or** amphotericin B (compounded) **or** imidazoles (compounded)	May start every hour and reduce frequency depending on patient response for any of these agents Treatment may continue for weeks to months depending on patient response

[a]For further information see Reynolds L, Closson R. Extemporaneous Ophthalmic Preparations. Vancouver, WA, Applied Therapeutics, Inc, 1993.

responded satisfactorily to treatment with fortified (14 mg/mL) gentamicin.[50] Initial therapy should not be changed if there is evidence of improvement. Only if the ulcer has failed to respond to initial treatment should therapy be changed. If corneal scrapings fail to identify specific bacteria, broad-spectrum treatment is continued. If the ulcer still fails to improve, the clinician should investigate other possible causative etiologies such as resistant bacteria, or possibly fungal, viral, or *Acanthamoeba* organisms.

Generally, ophthalmic ointments are not utilized in keratitis except in some special instances such as dry eye syndrome. Ophthalmic ointments create a physical barrier for subsequent antibiotic solutions, are not easily prepared by the pharmacist, and would be needed in higher concentrations than the current commercial preparations.[51]

Natamycin is the first-line treatment in fungal infections of the cornea. This drug provides broad-spectrum antifungal action with minimal pain and corneal irritation. It is the only commercially available ophthalmic antifungal suspension. Other available alternatives include amphotericin B, miconazole, fluconazole, and ketoconazole; however, the topical applications of these drugs are somewhat limited since they must be compounded. *Candida* infections refractory to natamycin may respond to the alternative agents. Good clinical data to support adjunctive oral therapy is sparse and most regimens are based on anecdotal case reports.

Therapy of viral infections begins with mechanical debridement of the involved rim along with a rim of normal epithelium. This is followed by topical instillation of vidarabine, or idoxuridine five times daily for 2–3 weeks; or trifluridine may be used every hour while awake and every 2 hours at night (nine times daily) for 2–3 weeks.[42] Trifluridine penetrates stromal areas well, is probably best tolerated, and has generally become the drug of first choice for herpes simplex keratitis. Antiviral drug resistance in ocular herpes simplex virus type 1 infections by any of the currently available ophthalmic antivirals has not been reported to be much of a problem.[52] Acyclovir ophthalmic solution or ointment is not available in the United States, although it is found in many other countries.

In addition to antimicrobials, adjunctive drug treatment is required for conditions secondary to the ulcer. Anterior chamber reaction is often associated with corneal ulcers. The resulting decreased motility of the iris allows synechiae formation (adhesions between the iris and lens or cornea). Treatment with topical atropine 1% or scopolamine 0.25% drops two to three times daily will help prevent synechiae formation.

Topical corticosteroid use is still somewhat controversial. The use of topical corticosteroids in stromal keratitis may aid in preventing corneal scarring and perforation.[42,53] Some clinicians recommend their use especially when the visual axis is involved or when the inflammatory reaction is severe. One group of investigators found that the use of topical corticosteroids did not increase the rate of complications and that no delay in healing rate was noted with topical corticosteroid treatment. However, they also noted that there was no difference in visual outcome in either group.[54] Corticosteroids must be tapered with ophthalmic use as with other routes of administration, to prevent rebound inflammation. Topical corticosteroid use in epithelial viral keratitis is relatively contraindicated. Some clinicians will also use systemic prednisone in doses of 40–100 mg daily for 1–2 weeks in a decreasing dose to augment topical corticosteroid or if topical steroids are contraindicated.

If transient increases of intraocular pressure result from the keratitis, reduction can be achieved with hyperosmotics (e.g., glycerin 50%), carbonic anhydrase inhibitors (e.g., acetazolamide), or β-blockers (e.g., timolol). Miotics (e.g., pilocarpine) should be avoided. If corneal perforation occurs or is imminent despite antimicrobial treatment, penetrating keratoplasty or corneal transplant may be indicated.

Successful medical management of *Acanthamoeba* keratitis has been attempted by many clinicians with variable results. Antimicrobial agents are usually not effective against the cystic form of the organism and may be toxic to the surrounding tissue because of the concentrations of antimicrobial agents required for achieving inhibitory levels. Currently, one of the most effective regimens appears to be intensive treatment with neomycin/polymyxin-B/gramicidin, propamidine isethionate 0.1%, polyhexamethylene biguanide (PHMB) 0.02%, and either miconazole 1% or clotrimazole 1% eyedrops.[55] Propamidine isethionate 0.1% (Brolene) is not available in the United States but can be bought over the counter in the United Kingdom. Miconazole injectable has been used directly in the eye from the ampule or in a 1:1 dilution with saline. PHMB 0.02%, an environmental biocide in swimming pools, has been reported to be effective in combination with neomycin and propamidine, in treating *Acanthamoeba* keratitis.[44,56]

No specific eyedrop regimen has been established, although most clinicians start treatment with these drops in alternating fashion every 1–2 hours. Reduction of therapy is dependent on the patient's response, date of diagnosis, and so on. Patients may be treated for periods of months to years. The role of topical corticosteroids has not been established and their use remains controversial. Epithelial debridement appears to be helpful as an adjunct to treatment. The physician's prompt diagnosis of keratitis is important for adequate treatment. Proper education of the contact lens user is essential in reducing the incidence of corneal ulcers. Utilization of sterile saline solution, proper contact lens sterilization techniques, and avoidance of ocular predisposing conditions, such as swimming with soft contact lenses, will help to prevent cases of infectious keratitis.

EVALUATION OF THERAPEUTIC OUTCOMES

Bacterial corneal ulcers require long-term follow-up and treatment. Therapy is in many cases individualized, depending on the organism isolated, patient response, size of the ulcer and the rate of epithelial healing, reduction of the underlying corneal infiltrate, and so on. Therefore, it is essential that patients be educated about the importance of continuing their therapy as prescribed. Patients may be continued on antibacterial and anti-inflammatory therapy at decreased intervals for weeks to months depending on their response. Even though healing of the epithelial defect is essential, this may be only one consideration. Recurrence, reinfections, corneal scarring, and so on, are all concerns for possible further treatment. Of course, *Acanthamoeba* infections may require topical treatment for many months before the signs and symptoms of the patient are significantly reduced to discontinue therapy.

Many cases of viral keratitis may be benign and self-limiting, while others can produce severe corneal scarring and vascularization. These more severe cases may require chronic treatment for the rest of the patient's life for recurrence and complications associated with viral keratitis.

Although the initial treatment for most infectious corneal ulcers may be appropriate, patients may still require a corneal transplant for visual rehabilitation from severe corneal scarring, vascularization, and so forth.

ENDOPHTHALMITIS

Endophthalmitis is an intraocular infection and/or inflammation of either exogenous or endogenous origin. In many instances, it is commonly of bacterial origin, although the incidence of fungal and viral endophthalmitis is on the increase. Prognosis is guarded especially in the acute onset and traumatic cases of endophthalmitis, and it should be treated as an ocular emergency. The chance of residual useful vision is highly dependent on many factors, which are discussed later. Panophthalmitis is similar to endophthalmitis but involves all layers of the eye, including external structures.

ETIOLOGY

Endophthalmitis occurs as a complication of ocular surgery, penetrating ocular trauma, or metastatic ocular involvement. The incidence of endophthalmitis varies depending on multiple factors. The geographic location, the type of surgical procedure performed, the use of preoperative antibiotics, and the type of penetrating injury may all have some bearing on the incidence of endophthalmitis. For instance, in some countries the incidence of endophthalmitis following cataract surgery is more than 1%. In the United States, reported incidence in most studies is less than 0.1%.

The type of surgical procedure performed has some influence on the incidence of endophthalmitis. Keratoplasty and glaucoma procedures have very low incidences of endophthalmitis in the immediate postoperative period. However, the infection rate for filtering bleb surgery in glaucoma, for an extended period of time, jumps dramatically. Rates from 1–18% have been reported.[57,58]

Postoperative bacterial endophthalmitis typically is characterized by pain and a virulent and destructive course. A low-grade indolent chronic form of endophthalmitis is caused mainly by an anaerobic opportunistic bacterial organism, *P. acnes.*[57,58] Postoperative indolent endophthalmitis is characterized by a delayed onset of a few weeks to several months after surgery, may demonstrate transient steroid responsiveness, and is seen most commonly after extracapsular cataract extraction with intraocular lens implantation.

The bacteria isolated from *acute onset* postoperative endophthalmitis include *S. epidermidis* and *S. aureus, Streptococcus* species, gram-negative organisms including *P. aeruginosa,* and *Proteus mirabilis.*[58,59] In *delayed onset* postoperative endophthalmitis, *P. acnes* is most commonly reported along with *S. epidermidis* and fungi as the infecting organisms.[58–60] *Bleb-associated* postoperative endophthalmitis, is usually seen months to years after the glaucoma surgical procedure. The common offending organisms include *H. influenzae* (including adults), *Streptococcus* species, *S. aureus,* and *P. aeruginosa.*[60,61]

Post-traumatic sources of endophthalmitis include mainly penetrating trauma and the offending organism may vary including Streptococcal isolates,[62,63] *S. epidermidis* and *S. aureus,* gram-negative organisms, *Bacillus* species, and fungi. *Bacillus* species are responsible for causing a very virulent and devastating endophthalmitis.[63,64]

Endogenous endophthalmitis usually arises from embolic phenomena. The most common sources of emboli include infected heart valves, metastatic systemic infections including various cancers, and from injection site abscesses or direct introduction of microorganisms into the bloodstream in intravenous drug abusers.[60] Fungal organisms have been isolated in both traumatic and postoperative endophthalmitis, although the majority of cases of mycotic infection occur from endogenous sources.[60,65,66] Fungal infections with *Candida* are the most common form of endogenous endophthalmitis[60,67,68] and are generally believed to be associated with the use of broad-spectrum antibiotics, indwelling catheters, hyperalimentation, antineoplastic agents, immunosuppressive therapy, parental drug abuse, low birth weight infants, and surgery (especially abdominal).[65–67] Bacterial organisms associated most commonly with endogenous endophthalmitis include Streptococcal species, staphylococci, *Neisseria meningitidis,* occasional gram-negative organisms, and *Bacillus cereus* often isolated from intravenous drug abusers.[60,67]

Viral endophthalmitis is believed to occur most commonly from an endogenous source and is usually diagnosed as a retinitis. It may exhibit many of the signs and symptoms of an endogenous endophthalmitis and therefore may be treated as aggressively. Patients with viral retinitis have had various viruses isolated from systemic and ocular aspirates including herpes simplex type I, herpes zoster, and cytomegalovirus.[69,70] Many cases of viral endophthalmitis or retinitis have been found in immune compromised hosts. Cytomegalovirus retinitis and other posterior segment opportunistic infections associated with acquired immunodeficiency syndrome patients has been on the increase and are discussed in Chapter 117.

CLINICAL PRESENTATION

The clinical picture of endophthalmitis varies depending on the pathogenic organisms identified, the extent of intraocular involvement, and the cause of the infection. Many patients with *acute postoperative* or *traumatic* endophthalmitis present with pain in the eye, diminished red reflex (light reflects back in clear media as a red reflection), hypopyon (white blood cells in the anterior chamber), and decreased visual acuity. A slight leukocytosis in the peripheral blood may be seen. Some variation in clinical presentation may exist, and case reports of painless endophthalmitis[71] or no hypopyon have been reported. Systemic signs and symptoms may or may not be present at all. On the other extreme, *B. cereus* causes a virulent form of endophthalmitis with accompanying ocular proptosis and lymphadenopathy.[64,68] In *chronic* or *delayed onset* postoperative endophthalmitis, the patient may present with low-grade ocular inflammation of weeks to months duration.[61] Bleb-associated delayed onset usually presents with signs and symptoms of acute postoperative endophthalmitis.[60]

In *endogenous* or *metastatic* endophthalmitis, a thorough physical examination with internal medicine or an infectious disease evaluation is important since up to 78% of patients with *C. albicans* endophthalmitis (ECE) will at some point have disseminated candidiasis.[72] Ocular examinations are important in all patients with candidiasis, especially if the patient has complaints of blurred vision or pain, since it may provide the first evidence of systemic involvement.[73]

Occasionally, an acute inflammatory response arises, especially in a postoperative patient, that is indistinguishable from a bacterial or fungal endophthalmitis. Such cases of sterile endophthalmitis are treated as bacterial infections, if any doubt exists. Culture information is very important in determining the pathogenicity and prognosis in endophthalmitis. It is still recommended to obtain culture and sensitivities of the site of entry (if applicable) and of the aqueous and vitreous fluids. Samples should be cultured for aerobic, anaerobic, and fungal growth.[60]

The best final visual acuities are usually achieved in those that have less virulent organisms isolated, prompt and aggressive treatment, and a normal host immune response.

TREATMENT (TABLE 102.6)

Patients with suspected endophthalmitis require aqueous and vitreous fluid aspirations to obtain sample material for culture and sensitivity. Aqueous fluid taps have been negative in many cases of endophthalmitis, while vitreous cultures have in turn been positive. Rapid identification of the organism responsible for endophthalmitis is essential. Prompt treatment may help to reduce visual morbidity and complications associated with endophthalmitis. Culture methods are indispensable because of their specificity, especially in identifying the causative pathogen in infectious endophthalmitis; however, 48 hours to 14 days are required to identify offending agents.[74] Direct examination of vitreous specimens can provide a more rapid way to identify the sensitive organism. Conventional methods include Gram, Giemsa, or potassium hydroxide (KOH) stains, or newer techniques including fluorescein antibody staining and lectins.

The treatment of endophthalmitis remains controversial. Randomized studies to determine the most appropriate therapy have not been reported. For instance, studies comparing the results in eyes treated with or without vitrectomy (a procedure to withdraw the vitreous fluid; similar to draining an abscess) are usually biased because the more severe cases undergo vitrectomy.[75] Treatment of endophthalmitis is determined by a variety of factors including the pathogenic organisms, the extent of intraocular involvement, and the course of the infection. The goal of treatment is to attain inhibitory and nontoxic levels of antimicrobial and/or anti-inflammatory agent(s) inside the eye while preserving intraocular tissue function. Treatment of acute endophthalmitis should be aggressive and include empiric wide-spectrum antibacterial coverage, until culture and sensitivity results are known (Table 102.6). Treatment of chronic or low-grade endophthalmitis usually does not present with the immediate urgency of acute endophthalmitis.

TABLE 102.6. PHARMACOTHERAPEUTIC RECOMMENDATIONS FOR ENDOPHTHALMITIS

Endophthalmitis	Agents for Treatment[a]	Dose and Duration
Traumatic endophthalmitis	**Intravitreal**—vancomycin 1 mg and amikacin 400 μg **or** ceftazidime 2 mg	Usually one time only
	and/or subconjunctival—ceftazidime 100 mg and vancomycin 25 mg	Usually only once or twice; some clinicians do not advocate use
	and topical—gentamicin 1.5% and cefazolin 10% or vancomycin 5% and amikacin 2% or ceftazidime 5%	Initially every 1 hour alternating and reduce over next few days
	and systemic—gentamicin or ceftazidime and cefazolin or clindamycin or vancomycin	Given intravenously × 7–14 days
Postop endophthalmitis	**Intravitreal**—same as for traumatic	As above
	Subconjunctival—vancomycin 25 mg and gentamicin 20 mg	As above
	Topical—same as for traumatic	As above
	Systemic—gentamicin and clindamycin or cefazolin, possibly ciprofloxacin and/or cefazolin	Clindamycin in "dirty" injuries
Bleb associated endophthalmitis	Aggressive **topical**	Topical every 30 minutes alternating
	and intravitreal	As for traumatic above
	and systemic antibiotic	Systemic for approximately 7 days
	and/or periocular vancomycin and ceftriaxone or ceftazidime drugs of choice	Periocular injection(s) × 1
Chronic endophthalmitis	Partial excision of lens capsule abscess	Some surgical treatment may be required
	and intravitreal vancomycin 1 mg **or** clindamycin 360 μg	May repeat weeks later if no response
Endogenous endophthalmitis	**Intravenous** amphotericin B if fungal etiology suspected (fluconazole may offer some benefit, but further study is needed)	Most treatment will last 7–14 days depending on severity
	Intravitreal amphotericin 5 μg	Intravitreal injection rarely repeated
	If gram negative, *S. pneumoniae,* or bacterial agent suspected, aggressive systemic antibiotics and intravitreal agents as above for traumatic	

[a]For further information, see Reynolds L, Closson R. Extemporaneous Ophthalmic Preparations. Vancouver, WA, Applied Therapeutics, Inc, 1993.

The inflammatory and/or infectious process involves most inner structures of the eye including the vitreous cavity and retina. Drug concentrations in the eye are dependent on whether the drug crosses the blood–ocular barrier (blood/retinal and blood/aqueous), the drug clearance from the eye, and the concentration of free drug in the blood. Aggressive therapy of endophthalmitis may therefore be required and may consist of topical, intravenous, intraocular, and, possibly, periocular administration of anti-infectives and/or corticosteroids.[76] Intraocular penetration from systemic, periocular, and topical routes of administration have generally been thought to be poor or slow to reach therapeutic levels. This is due in part to restrictions of drug penetration by the blood–ocular barrier. The blood–ocular barrier is somewhat analogous to the blood–brain barrier. It is a lipoidal barrier and drug usually crosses in proportion to its lipid solubility.

The blood–retinal barrier (BRB) is much harder to traverse than the blood–aqueous barrier. Penetration into the vitreous or through the BRB is more difficult, even during inflammation. Organic acids, such as penicillin or cefazolin, may be actively transported out of the vitreous by the ciliary body and retinal pigment epithelium. All compounds are removed to some extent by diffusion into the anterior chamber and out by the normal aqueous outflow mechanism. Therefore, to achieve therapeutic vitreous levels, many clinicians have supported the use of intravitreal antibiotics or antifungals for the treatment of endophthalmitis.[60,62,64,76]

Specific treatment recommendations can be found in Table 102.6 depending on the type of endophthalmitis treated. Specific advantages of various agents are discussed in the following paragraphs.

Most *topical* antibiotics penetrate into the aqueous fluid, and in vitrectomized patients may reach inhibitory concentrations in the posterior segment of the eye. Some clinicians use fortified eyedrops to increase the aqueous levels of antibiotics. Cefazolin 100 mg/mL (or possibly vancomycin 50 mg/mL) and fortified gentamicin 13.6 mg/mL (or amikacin 20 mg/mL) ophthalmic solutions alternating every 15–30 minutes are advocated for empiric treatment for bacterial keratitis. Because higher aqueous levels are achieved, the logical extension of this regimen has been for the treatment of endophthalmitis. No clinical study has proven fortified antibiotic drops to be more efficacious in endophthalmitis than commercial strength ophthalmic solutions, except in possibly blebitis, considered a possible precursor of endophthalmitis.[77] Others have found vancomycin and amikacin ophthalmic solutions to be an effective combination although vancomycin topically is irritating to the eye because of the low pH.[46] Some clinicians believe that topical ciprofloxacin is a reasonable alternative single agent.

Systemic antibiotics are of uncertain value in endophthalmitis. One study found that systemic administration of intravenous antibiotics may not be indicated in less virulent cases of endophthalmitis.[78] However, systemic administration of cefazolin,[79,80] imipenem,[81,82] ciprofloxacin,[83] and probably ceftriaxone and ceftazadime[81] may achieve inhibitory levels against many organisms in the vitreous fluid, especially during inflammatory conditions and with repeat administration. More studies need to be done in human patients to determine if systemic antibiotic administration is of real benefit in the treatment of endophthalmitis.

Broad-spectrum coverage with an intravenous aminoglycoside (gentamicin or amikacin) and cephalosporin would be appropriate. Cefazolin must be used with caution in a patient with a true penicillin allergy. Intravenous cefazolin is indicated because of its potential to achieve effective intravitreal drug levels against *S. epidermidis* in inflamed eyes after repeat injections.[77–80] In a patient with a penicillin allergy, an alternative may be the use of clindamycin or vancomycin and gentamicin. Clindamycin or vancomycin and gentamicin by the intravenous route are also indicated if the patient is suspected of having a *B. cereus* endophthalmitis, because of a reported synergy against that organism. Ceftriaxone, because of its good ocular penetration and activity against streptococcus and *H. influenzae*, may be an effective agent for systemic administration in cases of bleb-associated endophthalmitis where those organisms are considered major pathogens.[84] Therapy with parenteral cefazolin instead of vancomycin may be initiated because of the possibility of developing nephrotoxicity and ototoxicity when vancomycin is combined with an aminoglycoside. However, systemic vancomycin administration may be of limited value since it probably does not penetrate the eye in therapeutic concentrations.[85]

Intraocular antibiotics in acute endophthalmitis are given immediately upon the patient's diagnosis. A normal intravitreal cocktail consists of amikacin 400 μg and vancomycin 1 mg, both per 0.1 mL. Vancomycin has been utilized as standard therapy within the last few years because of reported concerns of resistant *S. epidermidis*.[58,86] Amikacin is used for gram-negative coverage because it is believed to be less toxic to the retina than gentamicin and more effective in cases of gentamicin-resistant organisms and more effective in the treatment of Mycobacterium.[76,87,88] Other clinicians recommend empiric treatment of vancomycin 1 mg and ceftazidime 2 mg to avoid concerns of potential macular toxicity from intravitreal aminoglycosides.[89] However, because of limited clinical experience with ceftazidime, reported synergy against many organisms (specifically streptococci, staphylococci, and enterococci) with vancomycin and amikacin, better concentration-dependent killing effectiveness, reduced susceptibility to inoculum effects with aminoglycosides, and potential incompatibility of vancomycin and ceftazidime, amikacin is still recommended by some clinicians.[90–92]

If vitrectomy is indicated, some investigators may add antibiotics and steroids to the vitrectomy solution, although many clinicians do not advocate this because of scant information on potential retinal toxicity. Intravenous, topical, and intravitreal antibiotics may be changed as the results of culture and sensitivity become available.

Subconjunctival antimicrobial injections may be used as adjunctive therapy and possibly produce enhanced aqueous and vitreous drug levels. These injections may be very irritating and painful to the patient who presents with a highly inflamed eye; therefore, repeat injections are usually not often given.

Postoperative endophthalmitis has been treated with varying approaches. Preoperative antimicrobial prophylaxis is an important consideration. An exhaustive review of prophylactic antibiotics for ophthalmic surgery was conducted by Starr.[93] His conclusions were that properly selected antibiotics over a 1- to 2-day course were effective in reducing the postoperative incidence of endophthalmitis. Ocular flora bacterial counts are decreased or eradicated and, therefore, one of the main sources for endophthalmitis is considerably reduced. Povidone iodine 5% eyedrops have been found effective in reducing the perilimbal flora after instillation prior to intraocular surgery.[94]

Propionibacterium acnes is sensitive to clindamycin and vancomycin and either may be given for intraocular administration. However, chronic endophthalmitis may require removal of the entire capsular bag (the remaining part of the "capsule" after cataract extraction), since organisms tend to localize around the posterior chamber lens in the capsular bag.[95–97] Despite these measures, some individuals will also require vitrectomy to lessen the intraocular load of this organism.[97]

In contrast to postsurgical endophthalmitis where the visual prognosis is improved with earlier diagnosis, intravitreal antibiotics, and microsurgical techniques, the visual prognosis in post-traumatic endophthalmitis is usually poor. The possible causative organisms must be considered in determining the initial antibiotic treatment prior to the availability of culture results. In treating traumatic endophthalmitis, especially cases occurring in a rural setting where vegetative or "dirty" injuries are more common, an intravitreal injection of gentamicin or amikacin combined with either clindamycin or vancomycin is recommended because *Bacillus* species are the causative organisms in many cases. Similar systemic, topical, and subconjunctival coverage is advised as adjunct therapy. Gentamicin and clindamycin may show synergistic activity against *Bacillu*s species.[62] Vancomycin and gentamicin are also effective against *Bacillus* species and in cases of methicillin-resistant strains of *S. epidermidis*.

In contrast to other forms of endophthalmitis, metastatic bacterial endophthalmitis is rare and patients usually have another focus of infection.[81] Despite the introduction of new antimicrobials and advances in microsurgical instrumentation and technology, only 10% of eyes with endogenous bacterial endophthalmitis retain good vision.[67] Subsequently, the management of endogenous bacterial endophthalmitis remains controversial.[60,67]

Fungal organisms have been isolated in traumatic, endogenous, and postoperative endophthalmitis.[58,60,62,64] If fungal metastatic endophthalmitis is suspected, an intravitreal injection of 5 μg/0.1 mL of amphotericin is recommended. Intravenous amphotericin along with oral administration of 5-fluorocytosine (50–150 mg/kg) may also be indicated. A vitrectomy may be performed with an intravitreal injection of amphotericin B given after the procedure. Amphotericin B is only compatible in D_5W and should not be diluted in balanced salt solution or normal saline.

Intravenous amphotericin B may be required to treat eyes where a high suspicion for *C. albicans* endophthalmitis exists.[98] The use of systemic antifungal therapy is based on the presence of disseminated candidiasis in a large percentage of these patients with the need to treat the disseminated infection. Fluconazole, a water-soluble and better tolerated antifungal agent, may produce high intravitreal levels in both the inflamed and uninflamed rabbit eye.[99] Topical natamycin is indicated for fungal keratitis but its use is of questionable value because of poor anterior chamber penetration.

Corticosteroids are used in bacterial endophthalmitis by many clinicians since this overwhelming inflammatory condition threatens to destroy the sensitive intraocular structures.[99] They are not recommended in fungal endophthalmitis, although there is some evidence they may be beneficial.[99] Corticosteroids are usually given for endophthalmitis concomitantly with antimicrobial agents. Corticosteroids may be given by periocular, subconjunctival, topical, or intraocular routes.

Intravitreal injections of corticosteroids are given by some clinicians together with antibiotics when bacterial endophthalmitis is suspected. Others recommend intraocular dexamethasone with any suspected case of bacterial endophthalmitis.[61,67] In some instances, topical prednisolone acetate to quiet anterior segment inflammation or oral prednisone in high doses (1–2 mg/kg) is employed for short-term use should posterior inflammation or membrane formation continue or increase. Judicious use of a corticosteroid may be effective in reducing the ocular inflammatory process and preventing further destruction of delicate intraocular tissues.

EVALUATION OF THERAPEUTIC OUTCOMES

Broad-spectrum empiric drug therapy is indicated for the treatment of acute infectious endophthalmitis. Antimicrobial regimens consisting of intravenous, intraocular, and topical anti-infectives are administered to achieve effective intraocular and periocular drug concentrations. It is essential that the pharmacist be aware of the proper dosage ranges of intravitreal and subconjunctival injections to prevent preparation errors. Proper calculation and dilution of intravitreal injections is critical and an error may cause retinal toxicity (Table 102.6). Serum levels of systemic antimicrobial agents should be monitored when appropriate.

In acute postoperative and traumatic endophthalmitis, treatment with aggressive intravenous and topical therapy may be given for up to 2 weeks, especially if a virulent organism was isolated. Many clinicians believe that after initial intravitreal antibiotics, administration of systemic and topical antibiotics, and a possible vitrectomy, the acute infectious process has been halted. Generally, further treatment with systemic or periocular/intraocular antibiotics is not required. In chronic postoperative endophthalmitis, the low-grade infectious and inflammatory process may continue for weeks to months. Patients may require repeat intraocular antibiotics and possibly further surgical procedures depending on the patient's visual rehabilitation.

Glossary

Blepharitis. Inflammation of the eyelids.
Chalazion. Meibomian gland granulomatous inflammation.
Chemosis. Swelling of the conjunctiva.
Dacryocystitis. Infection of the lacrimal sac.
Dendrites. Branching-like process seen with herpes simplex infections.
Endophthalmitis. Intraocular inflammation or infection, may be acute or low grade and chronic.
Filtering bleb surgery. Surgical procedure that allows aqueous fluid to percolate under the conjunctiva, thereby reducing intraocular pressure.
Fornix. Conjunctival cul-de-sac.
Fortified eyedrops. Higher concentration compounded drops than those commercially available.
Giemsa stain. Differential staining of blood smears.
Hordeolum (stye). Infection of the glands of the eye.
Hyperemia. Redness of the conjunctiva.
Hypopyon. Collection of white blood cells in the anterior chamber.
Injection. Congestion of conjunctival blood vessels.
Iridocylitis. Inflammation of the iris and ciliary body.
Keratoconjunctivitis sicca. Dry eye.
Limbus. Junction between cornea and sclera.
Orbital septum. A fibrous membrane extending from the orbit onto the lids.
Proptosis. Displacement outward of the globe.
Pseudoptosis. A condition resembling ptosis.
Ptosis. Drooping eyelid.
Rosacea. Vascular and follicular dilation involving the nose and cheeks.
Seborrheic blepharitis. Blepharitis related to overactivity of the sebaceous glands.

References

1. Bullen CL, Liesegang TJ, McDonald TJ, et al. Ocular complications of Wegener's granulomatosis. Ophthalmology 1983;90:279–290.
2. Harvey JT, Anderson RL. The management of meibomian gland carcinoma. Ophthalmic Surg 1982;13:56–60.
3. Freeman LN, Green WR. Periocular infections, in Mandel GL, Douglas RG, Bennett JE (eds): Principles and Practice of Infectious Diseases, 3rd ed. New York, Churchill Livingstone, 1990, p 995.
4. Dougherty JM, McCulley JP, Deneau DG. Comparative bacteriology of chronic blepharitis. Br J Ophthalmol 1984;68:524–528.
5. McCulley JP, Dougherty J. Clinical impressions on the diagnosis, pathophysiology and treatment of blepharitis. Fort Worth, TX, Alcon Pharmaceutical, October 1983.
6. Raskin EM, Speaker MG, Laibson PR. Blepharitis. Infec Dis Clin North Am 1992;6:4:777–787.
7. Lempert SL, Jenkins MS, Brown SI. Chalazia and rosacea. Arch Ophthalmol 1979;97:1652–1655.
8. Bartlett JD. Diseases of the eyelids, in Bartlett JD, Jaanus SD (eds): Clinical Ocular Pharmacology, 2nd ed. Boston, Butterworths; 1989, p 460.
9. Fraunfelder FT, Bagby GC Jr, Kelly DJ. Fatal aplastic anemia following topical administration of ophthalmic chloramphenicol. Am J Ophthalmol 1982;93:356.
10. Kahn J, Hoover D, Ide CH. Methicillin-resistant *Staphylococcus epidermidis* blepharitis. Am J Ophthalmol 1984;98:562–565.
11. Fleischer AB, Hoover DL, Kahn JA, et al. Topical vancomycin formulation for methicillin-resistant *Staphylococcus epidermidis* blepharoconjunctivitis. Am J Ophthalmic 1986;101:283–287.
12. Brown SI, Shahinian L. Diagnosis and treatment of ocular rosacea. Ophthalmology 1978;85:779–786.
13. Couch JM, Green WR, Hirst LW, et al. Diagnosing and treating phthirus pubic palpebrarum. Surv Ophthalmic 1982;26:219–225.
14. Permethrin for scabies. Med Lett Drugs Ther 1990;32:21–22.
15. Welham R. The lacrimal drainage apparatus, in Miller S (ed): Clinical Ophthalmology. Bristol, Wright, 1987, pp 391–394.
16. Starr M. Lacrimal drainage system infections, in Smith's Ophthalmic Plastic and Reconstructive Surgery. St. Louis, CV Mosby, 1987, p 975.
17. Semes L, Clopus RJ. Diseases of the lacrimal system, in Bartlett J, Jaanus S (eds): Clinical Ocular Pharmacology, 2nd ed. Boston, Butterworths, 1989, pp 510–511.
18. Boruchoff AS, Boruchoff SE. Infections of the lacrimal system. Infect Dis Clin North Am 1992;6;4:925–932.
19. Rootman J, Robertson W, Lapointe J. Inflammatory diseases, in Rootman J (ed): Diseases of the Orbit. Philadelphia, JB Lippincott, 1988, pp 143–155.
20. Jones D. Microbial preseptal and orbital cellulitis, in Duane TD (ed): Clinical Ophthalmology. Philadelphia, JB Lippincott, 1989, pp 1–22.
21. Weiss A, Friendly D, Eglin K, et al. Bacterial periorbital and orbital cellulitis in childhood. Ophthalmology 1983;90:195.

22. Gray W, Blanchard C. Sinusitis and its complications. Am Fam Phys 1987;35:232–243.
23. Lessner A. and Stern GA. Preseptal and orbital cellulitis. Infec Dis Clin North Am 1992;6;4:933–952.
24. Antonios S, Tabbara K. Bacterial conjunctivitis, in Tabbara K, Hyndiuk R (eds): Infections of the Eye. Boston, Little, Brown, 1986, pp 413–420.
25. Syed NA and Hyndiuk RA. Infectious conjunctivitis. Infec Dis Clin North Am 1992;6:4:789–805.
26. deToldedo AR and Chandler JW. Conjunctivitis of the newborn. Infec Dis Clin North Am 1992;6(4):807–813.
27. Ridgway GL. A fresh look at ophthalmia neonatorum. Trans Ophthalmol Soc UK 1986;105:41–42.
28. Isenberg SJ, Apt L, Yoshimori R, et al. Source of the conjunctival bacterial flora at birth and implications for ophthalmia neonatorum prophylaxis. Am J Ophthalmol 1988;106:458–462.
29. McDonnell P, Green RW. Conjunctivitis, in Mandels GL, Douglas RG, Bennett JE (eds): Principles and Practices of Infectious Diseases, 3rd ed. New York, Churchill Livingstone, 1990, p 978.
30. Anonymous. Trimethoprim–polymyxin B for bacterial conjunctivitis. Med Lett Drugs Ther 1990;32:71–72.
31. Ogawa GSH, Hyndiuk RA. The fluoroquinolones: New antibiotics in ophthalmology. Inter Ophthal Clin 1993;33;4:59–68.
32. Wan WL, Farkas GC, May WN, Robin J. The clinical characteristics and course of adult gonococcal conjunctivitis. Am J Ophthalmol 1986;102:575–583.
33. Laga M, Naamara W, Brunham RC, et al. Single-dose therapy of gonococcal ophthalmia neonatorum with ceftriaxone. N Engl J Med 1986;315:1382–1385.
34. Samford JP. Guide to Antimicrobial Therapy 1993. Dallas, TX, Antimicrobial Therapy, Inc, 1993, p 12.
35. Tarantino PA, Barron BA. Sexually transmitted disease of the eye. Ocular Infect Dis 1993;1:3:60–90.
36. Gudmundsson OG, Ormerod LD, Kenyon KR, et al. Factors influencing predilection and outcome in bacterial keratitis. Cornea 1989;2:115–121.
37. Sugar J. Contact lenses and corneal ulcers. Arch Ophthalmol 1994;112:173–174.
38. Liesegang TL. Bacterial keratitis. Infec Dis Clin North Am 1992;6(4):815–829.
39. Palmer ML, Hyndiuk RA. Contact lens-related infectious keratitis. Inter Ophthalmol Clin 1993;33(1):23–49.
40. Liesegang TJ, Forster RF. Spectrum of microbial keratitis in South Florida. Am J Ophthalmol 1980;90:38–41.
41. Terry JE. Disease of the cornea, in Bartlett JD, Jaanus SD (eds): Clinical Ocular Pharmacology, 2nd ed. Boston, Butterworths, 1989, p 577.
42. Foulks G, Pavan D. Cornea and external disease, in Pavan-Lanston D (ed): Manual of Ocular Diagnosis and Therapy, 2nd ed. Boston, Little, Brown, 1985, pp 76–97, 434–347.
43. Fiscella R. New eye infection: Difficult to detect, easier to prevent. US Pharm 1989:75–81.
44. Bacon AS, Dart JK, Ficker LA, et al. *Acanthamoeba* keratitis, the value of early diagnosis. Ophthalmology 1993;100:1238–1243.
45. Treatment of bacterial keratitis, in Gardner S (ed): Ocular Therapeutics and Management. Atlanta, Ocular Therapeutics and Management, Inc, 1990, pp 1–10.
46. Baron B. Corneal toxicity from acidic vancomycin solution. Arch Ophthalmol 1993;111:18.
47. Parks DJ, Abrams DA, Sarfarazi FA, et al. Comparison of topical ciprofloxacin to conventional antibiotic therapy in the treatment of ulcerative keratitis. Am J Ophthalmol 1993;115:471–477.
48. Snyder ME, Katz HR. Ciprofloxacin-resistant bacterial keratitis. Am J Ophthalmol 1992;114:336–338.
49. Glasser DB, Gardner S, Ellis JG, Pettit TH. Loading doses and extended dosing intervals in topical gentamicin therapy. Am J Ophthalmol 1985;99:329–332.
50. Ormerod DL, Heseltine PR, Alfonso E, et al. Gentamicin-resistant pseudomonal infection; rationale for a redefinition of ophthalmic antimicrobial sensitivities. Cornea 1989;8:195–199.
51. Hyndiuk RA, Skorich DN, Davis SD, et al. Fortified antibiotic ointment in bacterial keratitis. Am J Ophthalmol 1988;105:239–243.
52. Menage MJ, de Clercq E, van Lierde A, et al. Antiviral drug sensitivity in ocular herpes simplex virus infection. Br J Ophthalmol 1990;74:532–535.
53. Mader TH, Stulting RD. Viral keratitis. Infect Dis Clin North Am 1992;6;4:831–847.
54. Carmichael TR, Gelfand Y, Welsh NH. Topical steroids in the treatment of central and paracentral corneal ulcers. Br J Ophthalmol 1990;74:528–531.
55. Berger S, Mondino B, Hoft R, et al. Successful medical management of acanthamoeba keratitis. Am J Ophthalmol 1990;110:395–403.
56. Yee E, Fiscella R, Winarko T. Topical polyhexamethylene biguanide (pool cleaner) for treatment of *Acanthamoeba* keratitis. Am J Hosp Pharm 1993;50:2522–2523.
57. Bohigian G, Olk R. Factors associated with a poor visual result in endophthalmitis. Am J Ophthalmol 1986;101:332–341.
58. Speaker MG, Menikoff JA. Postoperative endophthalmitis: Pathogenesis, prophylaxis, and management. Inter Ophthal Clin 1993;1:51–70.
59. Stern G, Engel H, Driebe W. The treatment of postoperative endophthalmitis: Results of differing approaches to treatment. Ophthalmology 1989;96:62–67.
60. Pflugfelder SC, Flynn HW Jr. Infectious endophthalmitis. Infec Dis Clin North Am 1992;6:4:859–873.
61. Mandelbaum S, Meisler DM. Postoperative chronic microbial endophthalmitis. Inter Ophthal Clin 1993;33:71–79.
62. Boldt HC, Pulido JS, Blodi CF, et al. Rural endophthalmitis. Ophthalmology 1989;96:1722–1726.
63. Affeldt JC, Flynn HW, Forster RK, et al. Microbial endophthalmitis resulting from ocular trauma. Ophthalmology 1987;94:407–413.
64. Brinton G, Topping T, Hyndiuk R. Posttraumatic endophthalmitis. Arch Ophthalmol 1984;102:547–550.
65. Elliott J, O'Day D. Mycotic endophthalmitis in drug abusers. Am J Ophthalmol 1979;88:66–72.
66. Clinch TE, Duker JS, Eagle RC Jr, et al. Infantile endogenous candida endophthalmitis presenting as a cataract. Surv Ophthalmol 1989;34:107–112.
67. Peyman GA, Schulman J. Intravitreal drug therapy, in Peyman G, Schulman J (eds): Intravitreal Surgery: Principles and Practice. Norwalk, CT, Appleton-Century-Crofts, 1986, pp 407–410.

68. Brod RD, Flynn HW, Clarkson JG, et al. Endogenous candida endophthalmitis: Management without intravenous amphotericin B. Ophthalmology 1990;97:666–674.
69. Schulman J, Peyman G. Management of viral retinitis. Ophthalmic Surg 1989;19:876–884.
70. Pepose JS, Holland G, et al. Acquired immune deficiency syndrome: Pathogenic mechanisms of ocular disease. Ophthalmology 1985;92:472–484.
71. Deutsch T, Goldberg MF. Painless endophthalmitis after cataract surgery. Ophthalmic Surg 1984;15:837–840.
72. Parke DW, Jones DB, Gentry LO. Endogenous endophthalmitis among patients with candidemia. Ophthalmology 1982;89:789–795.
73. Deutsch D, Adler S, Teller J, Savir H. Endogenous candida endophthalmitis. Ann Ophthalmol 1989;21:260–268.
74. Rao NA. A laboratory approach to rapid diagnosis of ocular infections and prospects for the future. Am J Ophthalmol 1989;107:283–291.
75. Stern G, Engel H, Driebe W. The treatment of postoperative endophthalmitis; results of differing approaches to treatment. Ophthalmology 1989;96:62–67.
76. Schulman J, Fiscella R, Peyman G, et al. Infectious endophthalmitis. Curr Opin Ophthalmol 1990;1:389–395.
77. Brown RH, Yang LH, Walker SD, et al. Treatment of bleb infection after glaucoma surgery. Arch Ophthalmol 1994;112:57–61.
78. Pavan PR, Brinser JH. Exogenous bacterial endophthalmitis treated without systemic antibiotics. Am J Ophthalmol 1987;104:121–126.
79. Martin DF, Ficker LA, Aguilar HA, et al. Vitreous cefazolin levels after intravenous injection; effects of inflammation, repeated antibiotic doses, and surgery. Arch Ophthalmol 1990;108:411–414.
80. Alfaro VH, Pince K, Park J, et al. Systemic antibiotic prophylaxis in penetrating ocular injuries. Retina 1992;12:S3–S6.
81. Barza M. Antibacterial agents in the treatment of ocular infections. Infect Dis Clin North Am 1989;13:533–551.
82. Axelrod JL, Newton JC, Klein RM, et al. Penetration of imipenem into human aqueous and vitreous humor. Am J Ophthalmol 1987;104:649–653.
83. Luthy R, Joos B, Gassmann F. Penetration of ciprofloxacin into the human eye. First International Ciprofloxacin Workshop. Amsterdam, Excerpta Medica, 1986, pp 192–196.
84. Mandelbaum S, Forster R, Gelender H, Culbertson A. Late onset endophthalmitis associated with filtering blebs. Ophthalmology 1985;92:964–972.
85. Doft BH, Barza M. Endophthalmitis vitrectomy study. Arch Ophthalmol 1991;109:1060–1061.
86. Davis JL, Koidou-Tsiligianni A, Pflugfelder SC, et al. Coagulase-negative staphylococcal endophthalmitis: Increase in antimicrobial resistance. Ophthalmology 1988;95:1404–1410.
87. Oum BS, D'Amico DJ, Wong KW. Intravitreal antibiotic therapy with vancomycin and aminoglycoside: An experimental study of combination and repetitive injections. Arch Ophthalmol 1989;107:1055–1060.
88. Roussel TJ, Stern WH, Goodman DF, Whitcher JP. Postoperative mycobacterial endophthalmitis. Arch Ophthalmol 1987;105:1199–1201.
89. Campochiaro PA, Lim JI. Aminoglycoside toxicity in the treatment of endophthalmitis. Arch Ophthalmol 1994;112:48–53.
90. Doft BH, Barza M. Ceftazidime or amikacin: Choice of intravitreal antimicrobials in the treatment of postoperative endophthalmitis. Arch Ophthalmol 1994;112:17–18.
91. Aaberg TM, Flynn HW, Murray TG. Intraocular ceftazidime as an alternative to the aminoglycosides in the treatment of endophthalmitis. Arch Ophthalmol 1994;112:18–19.
92. Fiscella R. Physical incompatibility of vancomycin and ceftazidime for intravitreal injection. Arch Ophthalmol 1993;113:730.
93. Starr M. Prophylatic antibiotics for ophthalmic surgery. Surv Ophthalmol 1983;27:353–373.
94. Boes DA, Lindquist TD, Fritsche TR, et al. Effects of povidone-iodine chemical preparation and saline irrigation on the perilimbal flora. Ophthalmology 1992;99:1569–1574.
95. Meisler DM, Mandelbaum S. *Propionibacterium*-associated endophthalmitis after extracapsular cataract extraction. Review of reported cases. Ophthalmology 1989;96:54–61.
96. Semel J, Nobe J, Bowe B, et al. *Propionibacterium acnes* isolated from explanted intraocular lens in pseudophakic bullous keratopathy. Cornea 1989;8:259–262.
97. Sawusch MR, Michels RG, Stark WJ, et al. Endophthalmitis due to *Propionibacterium acnes* sequestered between IOL optic and posterior capsule. Ophthalmic Surg 1989;20:90–92.
98. Holland GN. Discussion: Treatment of endogenous candida endophthalmitis. Ophthalmology 1989;96:672–674.
99. Schulman JA, Peyman GA. Intravitreal corticosteroids as an adjunct in the treatment of bacterial and fungal endophthalmitis. Retina 1992;12:336–340.

Chapter 103

Skin and Soft Tissue Infections

Larry H. Danziger, PharmD, Douglas Fish, PharmD, and Erkan Hassan, PharmD

Infections of the skin and soft tissues are some of the most common infections seen both in and out of the hospital setting. These infections may involve any or all layers of the skin, fascia, and muscle. They may also spread far from the initial site of infection leading to more severe infectious complications such as gram-negative sepsis or glomerulonephritis as a sequela of streptococcal infection.

The treatment of skin and soft tissue infections may at times necessitate both medical and surgical management. This chapter presents details of the pathogenesis and management of some of the more important infections involving the skin and soft tissues.

Pathophysiology of Skin and Soft Tissue Infections

Under normal circumstances the skin and subcutaneous tissues are extremely resistant to infection. Even when high concentrations of bacteria are applied topically or injected into the soft tissue a resultant infectious process is rare.[1,2] Conditions that may predispose to development of skin infections include (1) a high concentration of bacteria (>10^5 microorganisms), (2) occlusion of the blood supply to the affected area, (3) availability of proper bacterial nutrients, and (4) damage of the corneal layer allowing for bacterial penetration.[3]

The majority of infectious processes of the skin and soft tissues result from the disruption of normal host defenses such as skin puncture, abrasion, or introduction of some foreign body. The nature and severity of the infection depends on both the type of microorganism present and the site of inoculation. A large percentage of these infections is caused by the normal skin flora (Table 103.1). Exposed areas of the body (face, neck, etc.) generally have the highest bacterial density and *Staphylococcus epidermidis* is the most common microorganism, whereas the axillary and groin areas (moister areas) are most frequently colonized with gram-negative bacilli.[4] Because most bacterial inoculations of skin occur with intact skin or intact local host defense mechanisms, infections are usually aborted or very limited in nature.

Bacterial infections of the skin can be classified as primary (pyodermas/cellulitis) or secondary (invasion of the wound) (Table 103.2). Primary bacterial infections are usually caused by a single bacterial species and involve areas of generally normal skin (e.g., impetigo, erysipelas). Secondary infections, however, develop in areas of previously damaged skin and are frequently polymicrobic in nature.

Cellulitis

Cellulitis is generally an acute, spreading infectious process that initially affects the epidermis and dermis and may subsequently spread within the superficial fascia. This process is characterized by inflammation, but with little or no necrosis or suppuration of soft tissue. A variety of bacteria are responsible for the several types of cellulitis most commonly encountered (Table 103.2).

Classical cellulitis is caused by group A β-hemolytic streptococci (most commonly *Streptococcus pyogenes*) or by *Staphylococcus aureus*. Occasionally, other gram-positive cocci such as *Streptococcus pneumoniae* or, in the newborn, group B streptococci can be etiologic agents.

Clinical Presentation

Cellulitis is characterized by erythema and edema of the skin; the lesion, which may be extensive, is nonelevated and has poorly defined margins. Tender lymphadenopathy associated with lymphatic involvement is common. Malaise, fever, and chills are also commonly present. There is usually a history of an antecedent wound from minor trauma, an ulcer, or surgery.

Cellulitis of an incised wound may be caused by any microorganism, but the most aggressively spreading lesions are caused by group A streptococci or *Clostridium perfringens*. Group A streptococcus can produce a rapidly evolv-

TABLE 103.1. PREDOMINANT MICROORGANISMS OF NORMAL SKIN

Bacteria
- Gram positives
- *Staphylococcus epidermidis*
- Diphtheroids
  - *Corynebacterium* spp.
  - *Proprionibacterium*
- *Staphylococcus aureus*
- *Streptococcal* species
- Anaerobic micrococci
- *Bacillus* spp. (soil organism)
- Gram negatives
- Enterobacteriaceae

Fungii

Yeast
- *Pityrosporon ovale*
- *Candida* spp.

ing cellulitis over a very short period of time. It is often impossible to differentiate streptococcal and staphylococcal cellulitis. A Gram stain of a smear obtained by injection and aspiration of 0.5 mL of saline (using a small-gauge needle) into the advancing edge of the erythematous lesion may help in making the microbiologic diagnosis but often yields negative results.[5] Generally, the diagnosis is made on clinical grounds, that is, the appearance of the lesion.

Cellulitis is considered a serious disease because of the propensity of the infection to spread through lymphatic tissue and to the bloodstream. Bacteremia may be present in up to 30% of cases of cellulitis. In older patients, cellulitis of the lower extremities may also be complicated by thrombophlebitis.

Gram-negative cellulitis can be caused by a wide variety of organisms, such as *Escherichia coli, Proteus* spp., *Klebsiella* spp., and anaerobes (especially *Bacteroides* spp.). These infections are often polymicrobic in nature (see section on Bacterial Diabetic Foot Infections) and involve *Peptostreptococcus* or other anaerobic microorganisms. Acute cellulitis with mixed flora generally occurs in diabetics where the skin is adjacent to some site of trauma, at sites of surgical incisions to the abdomen or perineum, or where host defenses have been compromised (vascular insufficiency or venous insufficiency ulcers). As with other types of cellulitis, warmth, redness, and induration are observed, and there may also be gas formation (crepitus). If the cellulitis progresses it can lead to areas of gangrene. Because these infections often occur in poorly controlled diabetics and patients with alterations in host defense mechanisms and/or with poor nutrition, generalized systemic findings such as hypotension, dehydration, and altered mental status are common. Often, needle aspiration of the leading edge of the lesion and subsequent Gram staining and culture are helpful in making a diagnosis. A leukocytosis of greater than 20,000/cm^3 is not uncommon.

Haemophilus influenzae cellulitis occurs most often in young children between 1 and 5 years of age. Most adults have bactericidal antibody and/or anticapsular antibodies to *H. influenzae* and so are less often infected. *Haemophilus influenzae* is carried in the oropharynx and nasopharynx as part of the normal flora, and cellulitis frequently occurs in close association with an upper respiratory tract infection.[6]

Haemophilus influenzae cellulitis characteristically causes a purple-red cellulitis of the face, neck, or upper extremities. In young children the lesion has margins that are indistinct, blue-red to purple-red in color, and surrounded by an area of edema and induration. Regional lymphadenopathy is rarely present. In adults, the distinctive discolorations may not be present.[7]

Fever (in the range of 39–40°C) and leukocytosis (≥20,000/cm^3) are common. Blood cultures are positive for *H. influenzae* in roughly 80% of patients. Aspiration, Gram

TABLE 103.2. BACTERIAL CLASSIFICATION OF IMPORTANT SKIN AND SOFT TISSUE INFECTIONS

Primary Infections	
Cellulitis	Group A streptococcus, *S. aureus, Haemophilus influenzae* (children); occasionally other streptococci or gram-negative bacilli
Gangrenous	Group A streptococcus, anaerobic streptococci plus a second organism, cellulitis (*Staphylococcus* sp. or gram-negative bacilli, e.g., *Proteus*)
Crepitant cellulitis	*Clostridia* sp., *Bacteroides* sp., anaerobic streptococci, gram-negative bacilli *(Klebsiella, E. coli)*
Impetigo	Group A streptococcus, *S. aureus*
Erysipelas	Group A streptococcus
Secondary Infections	
Bite wounds	*Pasteurella multocida, S. aureus, Eikenella corrodens,* anaerobic streptococci, *Fusobacterium* sp., *Bacteroides* sp.
Burn wounds	*Pseudomonas aeruginosa, Enterobacter* sp., other gram-negative bacilli, *S. aureus, Streptococcus* sp.
Diabetic foot infections	*Proteus* sp., *E. coli, S. aureus, Bacteroides fragilis,* anaerobic streptococci
Infections in intravenous drug abusers	*S. aureus, Streptococcus* sp., gram-negative bacilli, *Bacteroides* sp.
Decubitus ulcers	Gram-negative bacilli, *Pseudomonas aeruginosa,* various gram-positive and -negative anaerobes
Lymphangitis (acute)	Group A streptococcus, *S. aureus. Pasteurella multocida*

stain, and culture of the margin of the cellulitis are positive in approximately 50% of all cases.[7]

TREATMENT

Antimicrobial therapy of bacterial cellulitis depends on the type of bacteria either documented to be present or suspected based on the clinical presentation. In some instances the rapid identification and treatment are imperative (i.e., group A streptococci). Local care of cellulitis includes elevation and immobilization of the involved area to decrease local swelling. Such care often aids in the rapid resolution of symptoms. Cool sterile saline dressings can decrease the local pain and can be followed later with moist heat to aid in localization of the cellulitis. Surgical intervention (incision and drainage) as a mode of therapy is rarely indicated in the treatment of cellulitis.

As streptococcal cellulitis is indistinguishable clinically from staphylococcal cellulitis, administration of a semisynthetic penicillin (nafcillin or oxacillin) is recommended until a definitive diagnosis, by skin or blood cultures, can be made (Table 103.3).[7,8] If documented to be a mild cellulitis secondary to streptococci, oral penicillin VK 250–500 mg four times daily or intramuscular procaine penicillin for 10–14 days is adequate. For more severe streptococcal infections aqueous penicillin G should be used intravenously.[7,8] Mild to moderate staphylococcal infections may be treated orally with dicloxacillin 250–500 mg four times daily.

In penicillin-allergic patients, oral or parenteral erythromycin may be used.[7,8] Alternatively, a first-generation cephalosporin such as cefazolin (500 mg every 8 hours for mild infections or 1–2 g every 6–8 hours for serious infections) may be used cautiously for patients who have not experienced immediate or anaphylactic penicillin reactions and are penicillin skin test negative. In cases where an oral cephalosporin can be used, cefadroxil 500 mg twice daily or cephalexin 250–500 mg four times daily is recommended. Clarithromycin and azithromycin, newer oral derivatives of erythromycin, have been shown to be effective in the treatment of cellulitis due to gram-positive organisms but are considerably more expensive.[9] When erythromycin or cephalosporins cannot be used due to methicillin-resistant staphylococci or severe allergic reactions to β-lactam antibiotics, intravenous vancomycin

TABLE 103.3. INITIAL PARENTERAL TREATMENT REGIMENS FOR CELLULITIS DUE TO VARIOUS PATHOGENS

Pathogen	Regimen
Staphylococcal or unknown gram-positive infection	Nafcillin or oxacillin 1–2 g every 4–6 h[a,b]
Streptococcal (documented)	Procaine penicillin G 600,000 units intramuscularly every 8–12 h[a] *or* Aqueous penicillin G 1–2 million units intravenously every 4–6 h[a]
Haemophilus influenzae	*Children:* Ampicillin 50–100 mg/kg/d in four divided doses[c] *or* Cefuroxime 75 mg/kg/d in three divided doses or a third-generation cephalosporin (i.e., ceftriaxone 75–100 mg/kg once or twice daily, or cefotaxime 200 mg/kg/d in three or four divided doses)[d]
	Adults: Ampicillin 0.5–1 g every 6 h[c] *or* Cefuroxime 0.75–1.5 g every 8 h or a third-generation cephalosporin (i.e., ceftriaxone 1 g once daily, or cefotaxime 1–2 g every 6–8 h)[e]
Other single gram-negative aerobes	Aminoglycoside[f] or cephalosporin (first- or second-generation depending on severity of infection or susceptibility pattern)[10]
Polymicrobic infection without gram-positive anaerobes	Aminoglycoside[f] + penicillin G 0.6–1.0 million units every 4–6 h or a semisynthetic penicillin (i.e., nafcillin 1–2 g every 4–6 h depending on isolation of staphylococci or streptococci)
Polymicrobic infection with anaerobes	Aminoglycoside[f] + clindamycin 0.9 g every 8 h[10,11] or metronidazole 0.5–0.75 g every 8 h *or* Single-drug therapy with second- or third-generation cephalosporin[112,121,122] (i.e., cefoxitin 1–2 g every 6 h or ceftizoxime 1–2 every 8 h) *or* Single-drug therapy with imipenem/cilistatin 0.5 g every 6–8 h[148]

[a]For penicillin-allergic patients, use erythromycin 0.5–1 g every 6 h.
[b]For methicillin-resistant staphylococci, use vancomycin 0.5–1.0 g every 6–8 h with dosage adjustments made for renal dysfunction.
[c]In areas with high incidence of b-lactamase-producing strains, a third-generation cephalosporin should be used until sensitivities are available.
[d]For penicillin-allergic children, use trimethoprim–sulfamethoxazole (4 mg/kg twice daily) or chloramphenicol 50–100 mg/kg/d in four divided doses.
[e]For penicillin-allergic adults, use trimethoprim–sulfamethoxazole (4–5 mg/kg twice daily) or a fluoroquinolone (ciprofloxacin: 200–300 mg IV or 750 mg PO twice daily; ofloxacin 400 mg IV or PO twice daily).
[f]Gentamicin or tobramycin, 2 mg/kg loading dose, then maintenance dose determined by serum concentrations.

should be administered. Therapy should be given for 10–14 days. Ceftriaxone 50–100 mg/kg as a single daily dose has been reported to be efficacious in the treatment of cellulitis in pediatric patients.[10] Studies have also shown imipenem and the β-lactamase inhibitor combination antibiotics (ampicillin/sulbactam, ticarcillin/clavulanic acid, and piperacillin/tazobactam) to be equivalent to standard therapies in adults.[11–13] However, the cost of these newer agents without increased efficacy compared to other reliable regimens makes them less desirable. Ciprofloxacin and ofloxacin, given orally, have also demonstrated efficacy similar to parenteral cephalosporins in the treatment of soft tissue infections caused by gram-positive organisms.[14–16] The use of fluoroquinolones is of concern because of increasing reports of resistance among gram-positive bacteria, particularly staphylococci. Sensitivity testing is recommended when a fluoroquinolone is to be used. Also the fluoroquinolones are not approved for use in children.

When treated promptly with appropriate antibiotics, the majority of patients with cellulitis are cured rapidly. Failure to respond to therapy may be indicative of an underlying local or systemic problem, or misdiagnosis.

For cellulitis caused by gram-negative bacilli or a mixture of microorganisms, immediate antimicrobial chemotherapy as determined by Gram stain is essential, along with appropriate surgical excision of necrotic tissue and drainage. If there is no obvious focus for the infection some internal source should be sought (i.e., perforated viscus or rectal tear) and repaired if possible. As this type of infectious process is often polymicrobic in nature, specific antibiotic therapy is directed toward not only gram-negative enteric bacilli but also anaerobic gram-negative organisms (e.g., *Bacteroides*) and anaerobic streptococci. Many different treatment regimens are possible depending on the bacteriology of the lesion (Table 103.3). Usually an aminoglycoside combined with an antianaerobic cephalosporin, extended spectrum penicillin, or clindamycin will be used. Second- or third-generation cephalosporins have been suggested as single-agent therapy in certain instances.[17,18] Therapy should be 10–14 days in duration.

Ceftazidime has been found to be effective in the treatment of cellulitis caused by both gram-negative and gram-positive bacteria.[19,20] The fluoroquinolones have excellent coverage against most gram-negative bacteria and moderate activity against *Pseudomonas aeruginosa.* Both oral and intravenous fluoroquinolones (ciprofloxacin and ofloxacin) have been evaluated in the treatment of gram-negative cellulitis and have been shown to be safe and effective.[14–16,19,21] When there is suspicion of a mixed infection or, more specifically, anaerobes present, the treatment regimen should be broadened to include agents with good activity against anaerobes. Because gram-negative cellulitis can progress quickly to serious tissue invasion, therapeutic intervention should be immediate. If treated early, a quick response can be seen. Unfortunately, because this infection often occurs in patients with compromised immune defenses, the disease process may still progress even with therapeutic intervention. If the infectious process is secondary to a systemic cause (e.g., diabetes), the treatment course can be prolonged and may be associated with high morbidity and mortality.

In mild *H. influenzae* infections in children, either ampicillin 50–100 mg/kg/d in four divided oral doses or amoxicillin (not recommended for use in infants 4 weeks of age or less) 20–40 mg/kg/d in three divided oral doses (maximum 1500 mg/d) may be used. Treatment should be given for 7–10 days. Alternative treatments for penicillin-allergic patients include oral cephalosporins (cefaclor or cefuroxime) or trimethoprim–sulfamethoxazole (TMP–SMX). If the *H. influenzae* is a β-lactamase producer or the patient is allergic to penicillin, then either a cephalosporin or TMP–SMX should be used as first-line therapy.

For severe *H. influenzae* infections in young children the drug of choice was previously intravenous ampicillin. However, due to the increasing incidence of β-lactamase–producing strains resistant to ampicillin, it may be advisable to use a third-generation cephalosporin (ceftriaxone or cefotaxime) until results of culture and sensitivity tests are known. Cefuroxime may also be used as an alternative agent at institutions where cefuroxime-resistant *H. influenzae* are not common. For children with severe allergic reactions to penicillin, chloramphenicol or TMP–SMX should be used.

Dosing of chloramphenicol should be determined by use of serum concentrations, as the pharmacokinetics of the drug may change in critically ill children and adults when given either intravenously or orally.[22,23] Data are now available supporting the concept of dosage alterations in patients with underlying liver, renal, or gastrointestinal dysfunction.[24–26] In general, for severe infections, maintenance of serum concentrations of chloramphenicol in the range of 10–20 μg/mL is associated with successful outcome and a low incidence of toxicity.[27]

Treatment of *H. influenzae* infections in adults is similar to that in children. Ampicillin 0.5–1 g every 6 hours or amoxicillin 0.5–1 g every 8 hours may be used orally for mild infections. In severe infections, a second- or third-generation cephalosporin should be used in areas where β-lactamase–producing strains are common. Fluoroquinolones (ciprofloxacin or ofloxacin) or TMP–SMX may be used in patients with severe penicillin allergy.

ERYSIPELAS

Erysipelas (Saint Anthony's fire) is a distinct type of superficial cellulitis with extensive lymphatic involvement. It is almost always due to *S. pyogenes* (group A streptococci). Other streptococci (in the newborn) and rarely *S. aureus* can cause similar skin lesions.

Erysipelas most commonly occurs in infants, young children, and the elderly, and frequently in patients with nephrotic syndrome. This infection also occurs in areas of preexisting lymphatic obstruction or edema. Erysipelas manifests as a warm, painful, edematous, indurated lesion sharply circumscribed by an elevated border. In adults it occurs most commonly on the skin of the face and involves the bridge of the nose and cheeks. Fever and leukocytosis are common.

The causative organism usually cannot be cultured from the surface skin lesion but may sometimes be aspirated from the edge of the advancing lesion.[5,28] The microorganism most likely gains access via some small break in the skin (i.e., accidental injury, ulcer, or surgical wound). Approximately one-third of patients have had a preceding streptococcal respiratory infection.

Mild to moderate cases of erysipelas in adults are treated with procaine penicillin G 600,000 units intramuscularly twice daily or penicillin VK 250–500 mg orally four times daily for 7–10 days.[29] Dramatic improvement is generally expected 24–48 hours after treatment has begun. Penicillin-allergic patients can be treated with erythromycin 250–500 mg orally every 6 hours for 7–10 days. Strains resistant to erythromycin have been documented so some caution is warranted.[29] For more serious infections aqueous penicillin G 2–8 million units daily should be administered intravenously and the patient should be hospitalized.[7,30]

Impetigo

Impetigo is another distinctive type of superficial cellulitis caused by group A streptococci (known as streptococcal impetigo or impetigo contagiosa). *Staphylococcus aureus* may be the causative agent in approximately 10% of patients. Impetigo is most common during hot, humid weather, which facilitates colonization of the skin with microorganisms. Minor trauma such as scratches or insect bites then allows entry of organisms into the superficial layers of skin and infection ensues. Impetigo occurs most commonly in children. It is also highly communicable and infections are readily spread through close contact, especially among siblings, day-care centers, and schools.[7]

Impetigo manifests initially as small, fluid-filled vesicles. These lesions then rapidly develop into pus-filled blisters that readily rupture. The purulent discharges of these lesions dry to form golden-yellow crusts that are quite characteristic of impetigo. Pruritus is common, and scratching of the lesions may further spread infection through excoriation of the skin. Other systemic signs of infection are minimal.

The drug of choice for treatment of impetigo is penicillin. It may be administered as either a single intramuscular dose of benzathine penicillin G (300,000–600,000 units in children, 1.2 million units in adults) or as oral penicillin VK (25,000–90,000 units/kg/day divided in four doses in children, 250–500 mg orally four times daily in adults) given for 7–10 days. Penicillin-allergic patients can be treated with oral erythromycin (30–50 mg/kg/d divided in four doses in children, 250–500 mg every 6 hours in adults) for 7–10 days. With proper treatment, healing of skin lesions is generally rapid and occurs without residual scarring. Removal of crusts by soaking in soap and warm water may also be helpful in providing symptomatic relief.[7,31]

Lymphangitis

Acute lymphangitis refers to an inflammation involving lymphatic subcutaneous channels. This acute process is secondary to bacterial pathogens, most frequently group A streptococci, but may occasionally be caused by *S. aureus* or *Pasteurella multocida*.[1,32,33] Chronic lymphangitis is not generally associated with pain or systemic signs of infection and is most commonly caused by sporotrichoids (a type of fungus).[33] Lymphadenitis (acute or chronic inflammation of the lymph nodes) may also occur when bacteria or other microorganisms reach the lymph nodes and elicit an inflammatory response. The remainder of this discussion pertains only to acute lymphangitis. Further information regarding the pathogenesis and treatment of chronic lymphangitis or lymphadenitis may be found in other published sources.[32,33]

Acute lymphangitis is not contained locally but spreads along the lymphatic channels. Systemic manifestations of infection often develop rapidly before any sign of infection at the initial site of inoculation is evident, or even after the initial lesion has subsided. The systemic symptoms are often more profound than would be expected from examination of the cutaneous lesion. Acute lymphangitis is characterized by the rapid development of fine red linear streaks extending proximally from the extremities. These linear streaks may be a few to several centimeters wide and extend from the initial site of infection toward the regional lymph nodes, which are usually enlarged and tender. Peripheral edema of the involved extremity may often be present.[1,33]

Systemic symptoms are often prominent and include fever, chills, malaise, and headache. A peripheral leukocytosis is generally noted. Cultures of the affected lesions often yield negative results, as the infection resides within the lymphatic channels; however, the offending pathogen can often be identified by Gram stain of the initial lesion if done early in the course of the disease.

Identification of a peripheral lesion associated with proximal red linear streaks directed toward the regional lymph nodes is diagnostic of acute lymphangitis. At times, thrombophlebitis and acute lymphangitis in the lower extremities may be confused, because both are associated with red linear streaking and tender areas; however, in thrombophlebitis no portal of entry is identifiable.

Penicillin is the treatment of choice for acute lymphangitis. For mild cases 600,000 units of intramuscular procaine penicillin G once or twice daily is used initially; the patient may then (over 24–48 hours) be converted to oral penicillin VK 250–500 mg four times daily for a total of 10 days.[33] In more severely ill patients with bacteremia, aqueous penicillin G 600,000 to 2 million units is given intravenously every 4–6 hours.

If the suspicion is high that *S. aureus* is the causative pathogen, a semisynthetic penicillinase-resistant penicillin should be used (i.e., nafcillin 1–2 g every 4–6 hours depending on the severity of the infection). For penicillin-allergic patients, erythromycin 250–500 mg four times daily for 10–14 days may be used.

Pressure Sores

The terms *decubitus ulcer, bed sore,* and *pressure sore* are used interchangeably. The decubitus ulcer and the bed sore are types of pressure sores. The term *decubitus ulcer* is derived from the Latin word *decumbere,* meaning "lying down." Pressure sores, however, can develop regardless of a patient's position. Pressure sores are most frequently seen in chronically debilitated persons, in the elderly, and in persons with serious spinal cord injury. Generally, those patients who are at risk for pressure sores are elderly or chronically ill young patients who are immobilized either to bed or wheelchair and who may have altered mental status often associated with incontinence.

PATHOPHYSIOLOGY

Many factors are thought to predispose patients to the formation of pressure sores: paralysis, paresis, immobilization, malnutrition, anemia, infection, and advanced age. Four factors thought to be most critical to their formation are pressure, shearing forces, friction, and moisture; however, there is still debate as to the exact pathophysiology of pressure sore formation.

It is widely believed that pressure is the essential element in the formation of pressure sores. The areas of highest pressure are most often generated over the bony prominences. Studies have shown that when the pressure is relieved intermittently within a 2-hour period, only minimal changes occur in soft tissue and skin structures.[34] Therefore, both the degree of pressure and the length of time that the pressure is applied are of importance.

Shearing forces are caused by the sliding of adjacent parallel surfaces of soft tissues in an unequal fashion. This situation can occur when the head of a bed is raised, causing the upper torso to slide downward, transmitting pressure to the sacrum and other areas. This effect results in occlusion or distortion of vessels, leading to compromise of the dermis. At the same time, shearing forces are created by sitting and gravity; the posterior sacral skin area can become fixed secondary to friction with the bed. The effects of friction and shearing forces combine, resulting in transmission of force to the deep portion of the superficial fascia and leading to further damage of soft tissue structures.

Compounding the problems of shearing and friction forces are the macerating effects of excessive moisture in the local environment, resulting from incontinence and/or perspiration. This factor is of critical importance, because when combined with the other forces, it increases the risk of pressure sore formation fivefold.[35]

CLINICAL PRESENTATION

The persistence of the causative factors as discussed previously often results in pressure sore formation. Without treatment an initial small localized area of ulceration can rapidly progress to 5–6 cm within days. The visible ulcer is just a small portion of the actual wound; up to 70% of the total wound is below the skin. A pressure gradient phenomenon is created by which the wound takes on a conical nature; the smallest point is at the skin surface and the largest portion of the defect is at the base of the ulcer (Fig. 103.1).

Pressure sores can occur anywhere on the body. More than 95% of all pressure sores are located on the lower part of the body (65% in the region of the pelvis and 3.4% on the lower extremities) (Fig. 103.2). The most common sites on the lower portion of the body are the sacral and coccygeal areas, ischial tuberosities, and greater trochanter.

Pressure sores vary greatly in their severity, ranging from an abrasion to large lesions that can penetrate into the deep fascia involving both bone and muscle. Numerous sys-

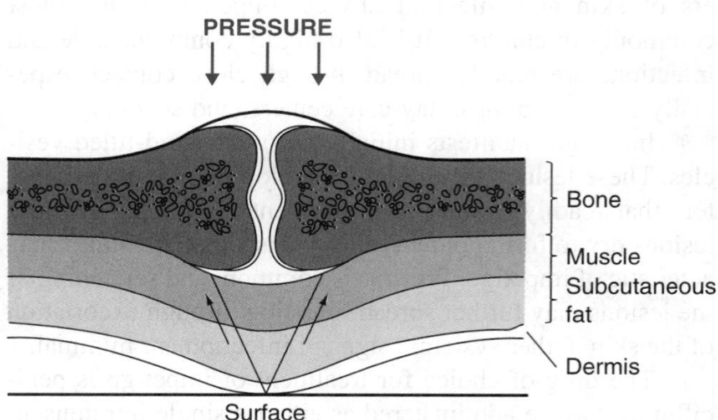

Figure 103.1. Distribution of forces involved with sore formation in a conical fashion. *(From Reuler JB, Cooney TG. The pressure sore: Pathophysiology and principles of management. Ann Intern Med 1981;94:661–666, with permission.)*

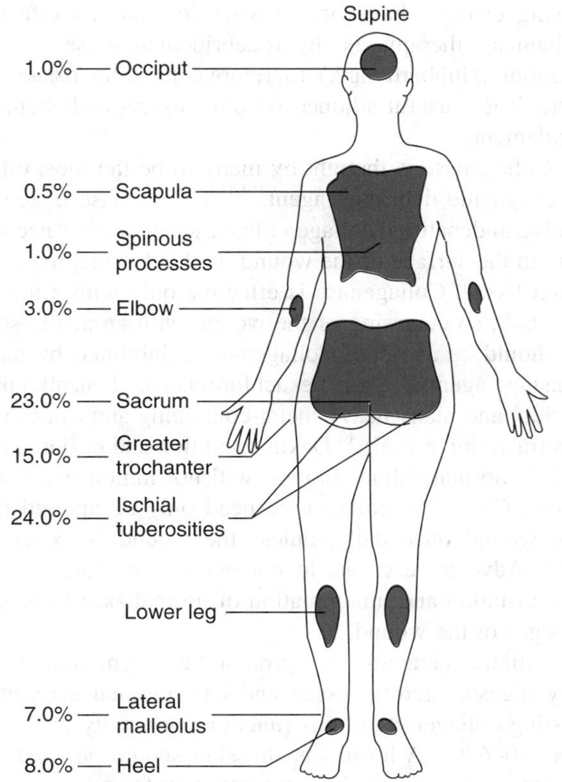

Figure 103.2. Supine view of areas where pressure sore formation tends to occur. *(Adapted from Reuler JB, Cooney TG. The pressure sore: Pathophysiology and principles of management. Ann Intern Med 1981;94:661–666, with permission.)*

tems for classification of pressure sores have been described; the two most frequently used systems are those of Shea[36] and the 1989 National Pressure Ulcer Advisory Panel.[37] These classification systems define the various stages of progression a pressure sore may advance through (Table 103.4).

Complications of pressure sores are not uncommon and may be life threatening. The most frequently encountered complications are infectious in nature. Pressure sores are routinely colonized by a wide variety of microorganisms; gram-negative aerobes and anaerobes are most often associated with the infections.[38] Systemic infections are not infrequent, with the most common organisms being gram-negative aerobes and anaerobes. Extension to the bone can occur and can lead to osteomyelitis and pyarthroses.

MANAGEMENT

Prevention

Prevention is the single most important aspect in the management of pressure sores. Prevention is far easier and less costly than the intensive care necessary for the healing and

TABLE 103.4. PRESSURE SORE CLASSIFICATION

Stage 1	Pressure sore is generally reversible, is limited to the epidermis, and resembles an abrasion. It is best described as an irregularly shaped area of soft tissue swelling, with induration and heat.
Stage 2	A stage 2 sore may also be reversible; it extends through the dermis to the subcutaneous fat along with extensive undermining.
Stage 3[a]	In this instance the sore or ulcer extends further into subcutaneous fat along with extensive undermining.
Stage 4[a]	The sore or ulcer is characterized by penetration into deep fascia involving both muscle and bone.

[a]Stage 3 and 4 lesions are unlikely to resolve on their own and often require surgical intervention. (From Ref. 36.)

eventual closure of pressure sores. Of primary importance then is the ability to identify those patients who are at high risk so that preventive measures may be instituted.

Friction and shearing forces can be minimized by proper positioning. Skin care and prevention of soilage are important, with the intent being to keep the surface relatively free from moisture. Patients with problems of incontinence should be frequently cleaned, and efforts should be made to keep the involved areas dry. Natural sheepskin is believed to be useful in minimizing the effects of moisture, shearing forces, and friction. Relief of pressure is probably the single most important factor in preventing pressure sore formation. Relief even for 5 minutes once every 2 hours is believed to give protection against pressure sore formation.[34] A variety of pressure relief devices are available and are used in attempts to prevent pressure sore formation. The principal objective is to disperse pressure over a greater surface area or change the location of pressure contact points, preventing pressure sores from progressing to a critical level.

Medical Management

The medical approach to the treatment of pressure sores depends on the stage of the disease. Medical management is generally indicated for lesions that are of moderate size and of relatively shallow depth (stage 1 or 2 lesions) and are not located over a bony prominence. Depending on their location and severity, from 30–80% of these ulcers will heal without an operation. Generally, medical treatment is not indicated for the management of those ulcers that extend through superficial fascia or into bone (stage 3 and 4). When the disease becomes this severe, surgical intervention is almost always necessary.

Management of pressure sores differs little from that of other wounds; the basic principles of wound care still apply. The process of wound healing can be characterized by three phases. First, in response to necrosis and soft tissue destruction, an inflammatory reaction occurs. Second, usually 4–5 days after the injury, cellular proliferation occurs. In this stage granulation tissue forms and collagen is deposited, reducing the effective size of the wound. Third, in the final phase, reepithelialization and contraction of the wound occur. Therefore, wound closure is the result of granulation, contraction, and epithelialization. This reparative process can be retarded by necrotic tissue, local infection, continued pressure on the wound, or various systemic factors (anemia, edema, diabetes mellitus, malnutrition). These concomitant secondary factors should be corrected to allow for maximal healing of the wound, in this case the pressure sore.

The goal of topical therapy is to clean and decontaminate the ulcer, to promote wound healing by permitting the formation of healthy granulation tissue, or to prepare the wound for an operative procedure. The main factors to be considered for successful topical therapy (local care) are (1) relief of pressure, (2) cleaning measures (debridement), (3) disinfection, and (4) stimulation of granulation tissue. Before any topical agents can be employed effectively, good wound care is necessary.

Debridement

The goals of debridement and cleansing measures are removal of devitalized tissue and reduction of bacterial contamination, which can slow granulation time and therefore impede healing. Debridement can be accomplished by surgical, mechanical (wet-to-dry dressing changes, which refers to application of saline-soaked gauze to the wound; after drying, the gauze is removed and with it any adherent necrotic tissue), or chemical means. Chemical debridement is time consuming and is an extremely controversial issue (Table 103.5). None of the currently available debriding agents has been documented to be superior to wet-to-dry dressings.[39] Surgical debridement rapidly removes necrotic material from the wound, but the associated risks include destruction of surrounding viable tissue, inadvertent enlargement of the ulcer, and possible extension of any existing infection. Mechanical debridement routinely uses the wet-to-dry dressing technique, which can be very painful and may possibly disrupt newly formed granulation tissue. To avoid these problems wet-to-moist or wet-to-wet dressing changes have been suggested. Another effective mechanical therapy is hydrodebridement—use of the whirlpool (Hubbard tank) to remove necrotic tissue and debris. It is a useful adjunct to both surgical and chemical debridement.

TABLE 103.5. CHEMICAL DEBRIDING AGENTS

Enzymes
Sutilains (Travase)
Collagenase (Santyl/Biozyme-C)
Fibrinolysin and desoxyribonuclease (Elase)
Trypsin (Granulex)
Papin (Panafil)
Streptokinase/streptodornase (not commercially available)
Elements
Dextranomer (Debrisan)
Hydrogen peroxide
Silver nitrate

Collagenase is thought by many to be the most effective enzymatic debriding agent.[40,41] Collagenase is able to dissolve undenatured collagen fibers, which anchor necrotic tissue to the surface of the wound, without damaging granulation tissue. Collagenase is effective only within the pH range 6–8, so cleansing of the wound with an acidic solution should be avoided. Collagenase is inhibited by many cleansing agents (e.g., hexachlorophene, benzalkonium chloride) and many heavy metal-containing antiseptics (silver nitrate, thimerosal).[40] Dakin's solution and buffered (pH 7.0–7.5) normal saline solution will not inhibit enzymatic activity. Generally, collagenase need only be applied to a clean wound once daily, unless the wound is extremely soiled. Adverse reactions to collagenase are rare. It may cause irritation and inflammation of normal skin located at the edges of the wound.

Sutilains (Travase) is a proteolytic enzyme that selectively digests necrotic tissue and has minimal activity in digesting collagen. Sutilains functions optimally in the pH range 6.0–6.8.[42] A loose wet dressing should be used and kept moist to allow the best environment for release of the enzyme. The entire dressing process should be repeated every 6–8 hours.[40] Sutilains is inactivated by the same agents as is collagenase. Adverse reactions reported with the use of sutilains include burning pain, paresthesias, transient dermatitis at the site of application, and occasional bleeding.[40] Sutilains has been documented to improve healing rates in studies in both animals and humans. Other enzymatic debriding agents such as Elase and trypsin are also available but not as commonly used. To date no specific enzymatic preparation has been shown to be more effective than any other product and use depends on user preference. These agents are an aid, not a substitute, in the debridement process.

Dextranomer (Debrisan) is purported to both clean and debride wounds. It consists of beads composed of hydrophilic dextran molecules crosslinked with *O*-glycerylene groups. The material is chemically inert and is believed to work by molecular and capillary absorption of fluid from the wound. Dextranomer appears to be effective in cleansing exudative venous stasis and decubitus ulcers. It also appears to increase tissue granulation, decrease wound inflammation, and decrease pus and debris; however, its cost and application techniques limit its usefulness. Few controlled trials are available with which to gauge accurately this drug's efficacy. Application of dextranomer should be preceded by cleansing of the wound, with the site left moist. The site is then packed with dry beads to a depth of 1/8 to 1/4 inch and covered with gauze. Two to three times daily the material should be removed and the application repeated. No major adverse reactions have been reported with the use of dextranomer, although application and removal of the beads may cause intermittent pain, bleeding, blistering, and erythema in some patients.

Disinfection

A number of agents have been used to disinfect pressure sores (Table 103.6) as well as other types of open wounds; however, objective clinical trials evaluating their efficacy are lacking. The agents used for disinfection and wound cleansing are classified as soaps, astringents, disinfectants, and topical antibiotics. These agents are used to reduce the bacterial content of open wounds. Most pressure sores are infected with both aerobic and anaerobic microorganisms; however, disinfectants have not been shown to penetrate tissue effectively to completely eradicate these organisms.[43] Therefore, use of these agents does not produce sterile wounds, but may decrease the number of bacteria present to fewer than 100,000 organisms per gram of tissue. This is important since infecting organisms can retard wound healing by depriving cells of oxygen.[43]

Paradoxically, there is debate as to whether disinfectants help or interfere with wound healing. Branemark and associates[44] reported that many disinfecting agents microscopically cause tissue damage within already existing wounds and therefore may delay wound healing. Studies of the effects of various topical antimicrobials and povidone-iodine on wound healing have yielded inconsistent results.[45,46] The role of topical antibiotics (Table 103.6) is still unclear. These products do not penetrate deeper tissue and have not been documented to reduce bacterial counts by significant amounts. Problems with resistance, systemic toxicity, and sensitization further cloud any potential benefit.[43]

Although disinfectants do not sterilize a wound and may interfere with wound healing, they may be a potential benefit. These agents can be used to help clean the wound (by decreasing the bacterial counts), but should be stopped when the wound is clean and granulation appears to be occurring.

TABLE 103.6. DISINFECTING AGENTS

Acetic acid	Topical antibiotics
Sodium hypochlorite (Dakin's)	Mupirocin ointment
Sodium oxychlorosene	Neomycin
Hydrogen peroxide	Gentamicin
Povidone-iodine	Chloramphenicol
Hexachlorophene	Bacitracin
	Polymyxin B
	Metronidazole

Granulation/Epithelialization

After the pressure sore has been adequately debrided and disinfected, and pressure, friction, and moisture have been kept to a minimum, granulation and reepithelialization begin. An agent that promotes and hastens this process would obviously be desirable. Many agents (Table 103.7) have been suggested, but hardly any evidence of a supportive nature exists.

Karaya has been used successfully in the treatment of excoriated skin sites around ostomies. This probably led to its use in the treatment of pressure sores to hasten granulation[47]; however, the data and number of patients evaluated are too small to draw any conclusion of possible benefit. Some researchers have cautioned against its use because it is a potential irritant and/or it may disrupt the overlying fragile epithelial tissue present on the healing wound. Sugar—either powdered, granulated, or a paste—has been claimed to be an effective granulating agent for wounds for two reasons. First, sugar is thought to work by attracting the bacteria to a growth site more hospitable than the diseased tissue (the new site is then removed with dressing changes).[48] Second, the hypertonicity of the sugar may

TABLE 103.7. AGENTS USED TO PROMOTE GRANULATION AND EPITHELIALIZATION[a]

Pharmacologic Agents	**Polyurethane Film Dressings**
Sugar	Op-Site
Karaya	Tegaderm
Insulin	Acu-Derm
Powdered gelatin	Bioclusive
Gelatin sponge (Gelfoam)	Opraflex
Benzoyl peroxide	**Hydrogel Dressings**
Dextranomer	Vigilon
Scarlet red	Geliperm
Mercurochrome	**Synthetic Barrier Dressings**
Occlusive Dressings	Hydron
Hydrocolloid occlusive dressing	Silicone spray
DuoDerm	Silicone foam
Comfeel ulcer care	
Intact	
Restore wound care	

[a]Partial listing of wound care products.

directly stimulate wound healing.[48] The only randomized study done to date compared a sugar–egg white mixture with collagenase and dextranomer.[49] Although only 17 patients were evaluated, none of the 5 patients randomized to the sugar–egg white protocol responded. Caution should be used if sugar is selected because bacterial contamination (with *Bacillus* spp.) and other excipients present in the commercial product (cornstarch, tricalcium phosphate) may lead to problems.

Some other agents that have been used but found to be effective in only a small number of patients include insulin, Gelfoam, benzoyl peroxide, phenytoin, and ketaserin. The objective evidence available to support the use of these products is poor due either to poor study design or to the small number of patients studied.

A different approach to decreasing the time needed for wound healing is aimed at wound dressing materials (Table 103.7). Wound dressing materials should keep the wound moist, allow free exchange of air, act as a physical barrier to bacteria, and prevent physical damage. Two representative types of products are of some interest. They are represented by DuoDerm and Op-Site (Table 103.7). Hydrocolloid occlusive dressings (DuoDerm) are opaque and impermeable to water and oxygen.[43] This type of dressing absorbs moisture from the wound exudate and forms a gel-like covering over the wound. Op-Site is representative of the polyurethane film class of product. This group is semipermeable, allowing evaporation. One study compared Op-Site, DuoDerm, wet-to-dry dressing, and a control in pigs.[50] Significantly faster reepithelialization and greater collagen synthesis were noted in the wounds covered with Op-Site and DuoDerm. Both wet-to-dry gauze dressing changes and DuoDerm lead to damaged epithelium during removal. The major appeal of these occlusive-type dressings is that they need to be changed only once every several days versus several times daily for the traditional wet-to-dry dressing technique.

Two other product categories are the hydrogel dressings and the synthetic barrier dressings. Hydrogel dressings are nonadhesive and oxygen permeable unless covered by a nonpermeable barrier, and they will maintain a moist environment. Synthetic barrier dressings consist of an inert powder and a liquid solvent. When mixed together a paste is formed that when applied will adhere to the wound, maintaining a moist surface. This dressing allows the wound exudate to pass through and then be absorbed by a secondary dressing.

Other nonpharmacologic approaches to shortening the healing time have included the use of oxygen,[51] hydrotherapy,[52] high-frequency, high-intensity sound waves,[53] and electrotherapy.[54] Unfortunately, although as previously stated more than 2000 agents have either been studied or used in the treatment of pressure sores, few controlled trials have been done that show any single agent to be efficacious. Whichever agent is selected, it must be evaluated on its own merits by the clinician, as limited scientific data are available.

RECOMMENDATIONS

The goal of treatment is to enhance or assist the body's own repair process. The practitioner should not only assess the wound but also the patient's underlying immune status (diabetes mellitus or cancer) and nutritional status. Initially, an attempt should be made to identify the causative or contributing factors that have lead to the development of the pressure sore and either eradicate them or substantially lessen their presence. These factors may include pressure, friction, or moisture (excessive seating or incontinence).

Next the patient should be evaluated for pain or tenderness at the wound or surrounding tissues. An attempt should be made to alleviate the patient's pain either via drug therapy or by mechanical intervention.

During the initial phase of the evaluation, the wound should be evaluated for the presence or absence of local or systemic infection. The absence or presence of purulent discharge with or without a foul odor may give clues as to the presence of infection.

Treatment of the wound begins with the removal of necrotic tissue via either debridement or surgery, along with elimination of any infection. The goal of therapy is to maintain a "clean and moist" environment. This process may take from days to weeks and include either topical or systemic therapy. Those patients with superficial wounds may require only 2–3 days of therapy while those with severely infected wounds will require a full 10- to 14-day treatment course of antimicrobials.

Unfortunately, there is no one right way to treat patients with pressure sores. Therefore, the patient needs to be continually reassessed and treatment changed accordingly. Some broad major guidelines can be recommended for the treatment of pressure sores (stages 1 and 2):

1. Relieve pressure.
2. Avoid unnecessary friction and shearing forces.
3. Prevent patient from lying in a moist environment.
4. Use debridement, either pharmacologic or via minor surgical approach.
5. Keep the wound clean by pharmacologic means or through use of a physical barrier.
6. Use occlusive dressing (may also lead to increased healing and simplify the nursing care routine) if possible.

For stage 3 and 4 pressure sores, surgical management is most likely the major approach, with follow-up according to guidelines 1 through 6.

Infections in Intravenous Drug Abusers

Intravenous drug abuse remains an important health problem with estimates of at least 1.2 million people addicted to just heroin alone in the United States. Infectious complications are the most frequent cause of illness and hospitalization of intravenous drug abusers.[55] Intravenous drug abusers are predisposed to a number of infectious complications including endocarditis, septic arthritis, osteomyelitis, pneumonia, and a variety of skin and soft tissue infections. Abscess formation and cellulitis at the site of injection are the most common infectious complications encountered in this population.[55] These skin and soft tissue infections are most frequently located on the upper extremities.

Soft tissue infections of the intravenous drug abuser are generally polymicrobic in nature, and usually more than two types of bacteria are isolated per patient.[56–58] *Staphylococcus aureus* or streptococcal species are believed to account for the majority of organisms isolated in these patients (range 37.5–60.6%). The role of anaerobic bacteria in these infections is unclear. Investigators have reported the presence of anaerobic bacteria in 6–67% of patients with soft tissue infections.[56–58] Recently fungal infections (primarily candida) have been noted to be on the increase as a cause of skin and soft tissue infections in intravenous heroin users.[59]

Why differences exist among researchers with respect to the bacteriology of these types of infections is unknown. It is possible that the bacteriology of infections in intravenous drug abusers may be different depending on geographic location.[57]

Data from various researchers support the belief that the source of organisms causing infectious complications in intravenous drug abusers is the patient and not the drug of abuse or drug use paraphernalia[57,58,60]; however, "street heroin" has been reported to be contaminated by a number of organisms. Organisms causing infection are believed to originate from multiple sources, including the mouth, the crushing of drug prior to injection, saliva (to moisten the cotton used to filter materials prior to injection), the blowing of clots from needles and syringes, or the use of poor injection technique, which introduces bacteria into the skin.[57] Fungal infections of the skin or soft tissues have been associated with the use of contaminated lemon juice, as a diluent, and not due to any contamination of the heroin itself.[59]

Generally, those patients with mild infections present with typical signs and symptoms of localized cellulitis and lymphangitis (see sections on Cellulitis and Lymphangitis). The lesion will be erythematous, with swelling, increased skin temperature, and almost always lymphadenitis. Occasionally cellulitis presents as a necrotizing cellulitis, which is associated with a high mortality rate. It is characterized by signs of systemic illness, severe pain, swelling, a turbid watery pus, and occasionally soft tissue crepitus.

Nondrug treatment modalities for soft tissue infections in intravenous drug abusers include rest and immobilization of the involved extremity. When indicated, incision and drainage are of extreme importance. All available material should be aspirated and cultured for both aerobes and anaerobes, and examined by Gram stain. Blood cultures should be obtained, because between 25% and 35% of patients may be bacteremic.[57,61]

Very little attention has been focused on the antibiotic regimens for this patient population. A well-localized cutaneous infection in a non–toxic-appearing patient can be treated with local incision and drainage followed by appropriate dressing change techniques with or without an oral antibiotic. In this case, in which gram-positive microorganisms are most frequently involved, a semisynthetic penicillin would be appropriate.[61,62] Also, the clinician should be aware that a growing number of resistant gram-positive stains are being reported and, if isolated, treatment should be modified accordingly.

The more seriously ill-appearing patient or a patient with extensive cellulitis or deep-seated infections requires the above nondrug treatment modalities in addition to parenteral antibiotics. In these patients a penicillinase-resistant penicillin (nafcillin 9–12 g/d) and an aminoglycoside (gentamicin 2 mg/kg loading dose followed by a maintenance dose based on renal function) should be initiated. Intravenous drug abusers have been reported to have a more rapid rate of aminoglycoside elimination and a larger-than-normal volume of distribution; therefore, these patients require close monitoring of serum concentrations.[63]

If the patient presents with a soft tissue infection associated with systemic toxicity, and watery, foul-smelling exudate, the suspicion should be high that anaerobes are present. In this case the combination of an aminoglycoside and an antianaerobic agent (clindamycin 900 mg intravenously every 8 hours or metronidazole 500–750 mg every 8–12 hours) should be instituted. Use of either clindamycin or metronidazole is warranted considering the increasing trend of *Bacteroides fragilis* and *Bacteroides melaninogenicus* resistance to penicillin.[64] Monotherapy in the seriously ill patient with ticarcillin/clavulanic acid, piperacillin/tazobactam, or imipenem may also be appropriate. If *Candida albicans* is identified then appropriate treatment with either amphotericin B or fluconazole is warranted.[59]

The antibiotic regimen should be modified on the basis of the final culture results. Many intravenous drug abusers have been documented to self-medicate themselves with antibiotics, which may account for the noted changes in patterns of susceptibility.[57]

Infected Bite Wounds

One of the common problems seen in emergency rooms in the United States is the bite wound. If left untreated, complications including soft tissue infection or osteomyelitis may occur, possibly requiring extensive debridement or amputation. Approximately 1–2 million people in this country are bitten by dogs annually. The incidence of other bites (cats, humans, snakes) remains undetermined. Most of the data currently available derive from anecdotal case reports, making therapeutic decisions often controversial.

DOG BITES

Dog bites account for 80–90% of all animal bite wounds requiring medical attention. Dog bites commonly occur in individuals less than 20 years of age (52.2% of reported cases) who are most often male (57.8%). More than 70% of bites are to the extremities.[65] Occasionally, facial bites may occur, seen most often in children under 15, and can be a lethal event via exsanguination.

Health care providers see two distinct groups of patients seeking medical attention for dog bites.[65] The first group of patients presents 8–12 hours after the injury. These patients require general wound care, repair of tear wounds, or rabies and/or tetanus therapy. The second group of patients presents more than 12 hours after the injury has occurred. These patients usually have clinical signs of infection and seek medical attention for infection-related complaints (i.e., pain, purulent discharge, swelling). Those patients at greatest risk of acquiring an infection after a bite have had a puncture wound (usually the hand), have not sought medical attention within 12 hours of the injury, and are older than 50.[66,67]

The infected dog bite is usually characterized by a localized cellulitis and pain at the site of injury. The cellulitis usually spreads proximally from the initial site of injury. If *Pasteurella multocida* is present, a rapidly progressing cellulitis with a gray malodorous discharge may be encountered. Fewer than 20% of patients have a concomitant adenopathy or lymphangitis. Fever is uncommon. Wounds close to bones or joints may lead to infections of these structures.

Infections from dog bite wounds are due predominantly to organisms documented to be from the dog's oral flora.[68] Studies examining the normal flora of the dog frequently isolate *P. multocida, S. aureus,* coagulase-negative staphylococci, and various unnamed organisms.[69,70] Wound site cultures in both infected and noninfected patients have similar bacteria present, with aerobic organisms (including facultative bacteria) isolated from 74% and anaerobic organisms isolated from 41%. The most frequently isolated organisms from infected and noninfected wounds are *S. aureus,* α-hemolytic streptococci, *Streptococcus intermedius, P. multocida, Eikenella corrodens, Capnocytophaga canimursus, Bacteroides* sp., and *Fusobacterium* sp.[71] Cultures obtained from noninfected bite wounds unfortunately have not been of value in predicting the subsequent development of infection. Documentation of the mechanism of injury is important; if possible, an immunization history of the animal should be obtained. It is also important for the patient's tetanus immune status to be determined.

Wounds should be thoroughly irrigated with a sterile saline solution or a chlorhexidine scrub solution. Proper irrigation significantly decreases the rate of subsequent infection.[66] Several management techniques used in the treatment of bite wounds remain controversial; these include the extent and type of debridement,[66] the use of primary closure within 24 hours of the injury,[71,72] and indications for the use of antibiotics.

Data on the role of prophylactic antimicrobial therapy for the early noninfected bite wound are controversial.[73,74] Until recently, most suggestions concerning the use of prophylactic antibiotics were based on retrospective studies or on observations of complicated cases. Callaham[66] demonstrated that patients treated with penicillin VK 40,000 IU/kg four times a day for 5 days had an infection rate of 10% compared with a 25% infection rate for those patients treated with placebo. Although a trend toward benefit with the use of prophylactic antibiotics was noted, there was no significant difference in infection rates between groups. Elenbass et al.[75] reported that prophylactic administration of oxacillin 500 mg four times a day for 5 days in a similar number of patients did not improve outcome compared with administration of placebo in adult patients with noninfected full-thickness wounds presenting within 24 hours of injury.

Because controlled studies have not definitively shown any benefit to the prophylactic use of antibiotics for noninfected bites, they are not routinely recommended; however, a semisynthetic penicillinase-resistant penicillin orally or amoxicillin/clavulanic acid should be used for puncture wounds, wounds to the hands, and wounds in compromised hosts.[76,77] Tetracycline or TMP–SMX is recommended as an alternative form of therapy for those patients allergic to penicillins. Erythromycin may be considered an alternative for tetracycline in growing children or pregnant women. If erythromycin is selected then sensitivities should be obtained, because *P. multocida* isolates will be resistant in up to 50% of cases. Prophylactic therapy should be given for 5 days. In addition to irrigation and antibiotics, when indicated, the injured area should be immobilized and elevated.

Infections developing within the first 24 hours of a bite are most often caused by *P. multocida* and should be treated with penicillin or amoxicillin/clavulanic acid (tetracycline is an alternative for nonpregnant adult penicillin-allergic patients).[76,77] For severe infections, intravenous penicillin therapy should be started and followed by oral therapy when the signs of cellulitis have subsided. Treatment should be given for 10–14 days. Semisynthetic penicillinase-resistant penicillins should be avoided in these cases because of their poor activity against *P. multocida.* Activity of certain oral cephalosporins (e.g., cephalexin, cefaclor, cefadroxil) against this organism *in vitro* has been conflicting.[78,79] Susceptibilities should be done before prescribing a first- or second-generation cephalosporin where *P. multocida* is considered to be a potential pathogen.

For those infections developing more than 36–48 hours after the bite, the risk of *P. multocida* being involved dramatically decreases in likelihood. Therapy in this instance includes a penicillinase-resistant penicillin (e.g., dicloxacillin) or a cephalosporin (e.g., cefuroxime axetil) and should be given for a full 10–14 days.[76] Results of a Gram stain should be used to confirm the appropriateness of therapy.

The fluoroquinolones are highly active *in vitro* against the aerobic isolates found in these bite wounds; however, in general they have very little activity against the anaerobes isolated in these infections. Their role in the therapy of bite wounds has yet to be defined.

Tetanus does not commonly occur after dog bites; however, it is a theoretical possibility. If the immunization history of a patient with anything other than a clean minor wound is not known, tetanus/diphtheria toxoids (Td) and tetanus immune globulin (TIG) should be administered. Patients with wounds that do not require immunization with tetanus/diphtheria toxoid are those who have had three or more immunization doses of TIG within the past 5 years. Patients who have received three or more doses of TIG within the last 10 years or patients who received two doses of TIG within the first 24 hours of injury do not require additional TIG therapy.[80] Because the rabies virus can be transmitted via saliva, rabies may be a potential complication of a bite. When the symptoms of rabies develop after a bite the prognosis for survival is poor. Roughly 3% of rabies cases documented in animals were in dogs (the most frequent vectors are skunks, raccoons, and bats).

Once a patient has been exposed to rabies the treatment objectives consist of thorough irrigation of the wound, tetanus prophylaxis, antibiotic prophylaxis, if indicated, and immunization. Postexposure prophylaxis immunization consists of *both* passive antibody administration and vaccine administration. The only exceptions to antibody administration are patients who have been previously immunized and have the appropriate degree of documented rabies antibody titers.

CAT BITES

Cats are probably the second most common cause of animal bite wounds in the United States, but unfortunately very few data are available on the incidence and infection rate of these bites.[68] The major problems associated with cat bites are puncture wounds and scratches usually located on the lower extremities. Approximately 40% of cat bites and scratches become infected. These infections are frequently caused by *P. multocida,* which has been isolated in the oropharynx of 50–70% of healthy cats.[67] Both tularemia *(Pasteurella tularensis)* and rabies have also been transmitted by cat bites.[67] The management of cat bites is similar to that discussed for dog bites. Antibiotic therapy with penicillin is the mainstay and therapy is as described for dog bites.

HUMAN BITES

Infected human bites can occur as bites from the teeth or from blows to the teeth (clenched-fist injuries). Human bites are generally more serious than animal bites and carry a higher likelihood of infection. Infections can occur in up to 50% of patients with human bites.[81]

Self-inflicted bites most commonly occur on the lips or around the fingernails (from sucking or biting the nails). Bites by others can occur to any part of the body but most often involve the hands. Bites to the hand are most serious and more frequently become infected. The clenched-fist injury is a traumatic laceration caused by one person hitting another in the mouth and is one of the most serious of bite wounds. The areas most commonly affected by this injury are the third and fourth metacarpophalangeal joints.

Patients with infected bites to the hand may develop a painful, throbbing, swollen extremity. The wound often has a purulent discharge and the patient complains of a decreased range of motion. In addition to a cellulitis, other complications such as osteomyelitis, septic arthritis, and tenosynovitis can occur. Loss of a digit or hand has been reported.

Infections caused by these injuries are similar and most often caused by the normal oral flora, which include both aerobic and anaerobic microorganisms. The most frequent aerobic organisms are streptococcal species, *S. aureus, Haemophilus parainfluenzae, Klebsiella pneumoniae,* and *Eikenella corrodens.*[82,83] The most common anaerobic organisms are *Bacteroides* sp., *Fusobacterium* sp., *Peptostreptococcus* sp., and *Peptococcus* sp.[82,83] Anaerobic microorganisms have been isolated in the range of 40% of human bite and 55% of clenched-fist injuries.

Management of bite wounds consists of aggressive irrigation, surgical debridement, and immobilization of the affected area. Primary closure for human bites is not generally recommended. If damage to a bone or joint is suspected, radiographic evaluation should be undertaken. Tetanus toxoid and antitoxin may be indicated.

Patients with noninfected bite injuries should be given prophylactic antibiotic therapy. Initial therapy should consist of a penicillinase-resistant penicillin (e.g., dicloxacillin) in combination with penicillin. Prophylactic therapy should be given for 3–5 days as for dog bites. A first-generation cephalosporin is not recommended, as the sensitivity to *E.*

corrodens is variable.[84] For infected bite wounds, penicillin and a penicillinase-resistant penicillin or amoxicillin/clavulonic acid should be empirically started and changed pending the culture results. Hospitalization for minor wounds is not necessary if surgical repair of vital structures has not been performed. Those patients suffering serious injuries should be started on intravenous antibiotics. Duration of therapy for infected bite injuries should be 7–14 days.

Antibiotic therapy should always be used in clenched-fist injuries. Therapy should include penicillin (or ampicillin) plus a penicillinase-resistant penicillin until the final cultures are available. Therapeutic failures have been documented when either first-generation cephalosporins or penicillinase-resistant penicillins have been used alone, most likely because of their poor and variable activity against *E. corrodens.*[85,86] Therapy should be continued from 7–14 days.

BACTERIAL DIABETIC FOOT INFECTIONS

With the development of insulin (1923) the patterns of morbidity and mortality for diabetic patients changed dramatically. Diabetes mellitus is estimated to affect approximately 11 million people in the United States.[87] Disorders of the foot are the most common complication of diabetes, accounting for approximately 20% of all hospitalizations in diabetic patients at an annual cost estimated at 200–350 million dollars.[87] Approximately 25% of diabetic patients will experience a significant soft tissue infection at some time during the course of their illness. Infection of the lower extremities is also the most common septic problem leading to hospitalization of diabetics.

Three key factors are involved in the causation of diabetic foot problems: neuropathy, angiopathy and ischemia, and immunologic defects. Any of these disorders can occur in isolation; however, they frequently occur together.

Diabetic involvement of the autonomic nervous system plays an important role in the pathogenesis of foot lesions. Experimental findings indicate that diabetic neuropathy may be at least partially caused by nerve swelling resulting from increased polyalcohol sorbitol accumulation secondary to hyperglycemia.[88a] This neuropathy may affect the motor nerve supply of small intrinsic muscles of the foot, may cause diminished sensory perception (absence of pain), or may damage the sympathetic nerve supply, which can result in an absence of sweating. This leads to dry cracked skin, which can become secondarily infected. Sensory neuropathies may also predispose to repetitive minor injuries, which eventually result in skin breakdown and formation of lesions.[87]

Atherosclerosis is more common in the diabetic than in the nondiabetic; it appears at a younger age and progresses more rapidly. Diabetics and nondiabetics also differ in regard to which blood vessels are involved and the extent of the involvement. Diabetics may have problems with both small vessels (microangiopathy) and large vessels (macroangiopathy) that can result in varying degrees of ischemia, ultimately leading to infections.

Diabetic patients typically have normal humoral immunity, normal levels of immunoglobulins, and a normal antibody response. However, the defect in host defense mechanisms appears to be at the cellular level.[88a] Patients with diabetes have been documented to have impaired phagocytosis and intracellular microbicidal function compared with nondiabetics, perhaps related to angiopathy and low tissue levels of oxygen.[87] The exact defects in the host defense system of diabetics are not completely understood.

Although the bacteriology of diabetic foot infections has long been known to be polymicrobic (an average of 2.5–5.8 isolates per culture), the true spectrum of microorganisms present has only recently come to be appreciated. Previously, the emphasis was on the importance of *S. aureus,* streptococci, and aerobic gram-negative bacilli in causing infections of the lower extremities of diabetics. With the advent of more sophisticated culture techniques, obligate anaerobes have also been shown to have a significant part in the bacterial flora of these infections.[88b,89] The most common aerobic isolates are *Proteus mirabilis,* group D streptococci, *E. coli,* and *S. aureus.* The principal anaerobic isolate is *B. fragilis,* followed by *Peptococcus* and *Peptostreptococcus.*

Superficial cultures from the infected wound are often not very reliable. The correlation between superficial culturing techniques and a true deep culture (via biopsy or needle aspiration of drainage or abscess fluid) is poor.[89] Therefore, cultures and sensitivity tests should be done, preferably with specimens obtained from deep culture.

Clinical signs and symptoms of infection of the diabetic foot may not be present secondary to the angiopathy and neuropathy. Often when the infection is noticed it is even more extensive than it appears. Certain lesions are typical of diabetic foot infections; these include paronychia (infection of the soft tissue adjacent to the nail), infections of the middle foot secondary to painless trauma, toe web space infections, or a mal perforans puncture wound (infection of the sole of the foot over the head of the metatarsals). Diabetic foot infections may be further complicated by necrotizing skin and soft tissue infections and/or osteomyelitis. Osteomyelitis is one of the most serious complications of foot problems in diabetic patients and may occur in 30–40% of infections.[87] In one review, roughly one-third of 247 patients with osteomyelitis were diabetic.[90]

In the treatment of diabetic foot infections the use of intravenous antibiotics alone often is not adequate. In addition to the need for local wound care, immobilization of the extremity in question, control of hyperglycemia (maintaining serum glucose below 200 mg/dL may alleviate impairment of phagocytosis), drainage, debridement, and amputation are often necessary.

Knowledge of the polymicrobic flora involved in these infections is useful in determining the most appropriate approach to antibiotic therapy. Considering that an average of 2.5–5.8 organisms per specimen are present, various antibiotic regimens have been advocated by many researchers. Suggested therapy has included such regimens as gentamicin plus ampicillin,[89] cloxacillin plus kanamycin,[90] gentamicin plus clindamycin,[88] or a penicillinase-resistant penicillin (e.g., nafcillin, dicloxacillin) alone.[87] Some of these regimens are inadequate, because they evolved prior to newer culture techniques that demonstrated the importance of anaerobes; others may place the patient at greater risk for toxicity. Because these patients may already have an underlying component of diabetic nephropathy that places them at higher risk of nephrotoxicity, recent recommendations have strongly advocated the avoidance of aminoglycoside antibiotics unless no alternative agents are available.[87] When an aminoglycoside is used, care must be taken to avoid further compromising renal function.

Monotherapy with broad-spectrum parenteral antimicrobials along with appropriate medical and/or surgical management is often effective in treating moderate to severe infections (including those in which osteomyelitis is present). Monotherapy is particularly attractive due to the potential advantages of convenience, cost, and avoidance of toxicities. The use of cefoxitin has been evaluated in two studies,[91,92] one of which is the only existing randomized, double-blind study[92] in these infections. These studies have shown that cefoxitin therapy may result in microbiologic or clinical cure rates ranging from 60–90%.

Initial (empiric) therapy for diabetics requiring hospitalization for lower extremity infections is similar to that for polymicrobic cellulitis with anaerobes (Table 103.3). The drug of choice should be cefoxitin or cefotetan, as determined by cost. Alternatives such as ticarcillin/clavulanate 3.1 g every 4–6 hours, ampicillin/sulbactam 1.5 to 3 g every 6 hours, or piperacillin/tazobactam 3.375 g every 6 hours may also be useful,[13,93,94] although relatively little data are available and these agents may be more costly. Imipenem/cilastatin may also be an acceptable alternative,[95] although again relatively few studies are available. In patients with penicillin allergies, clindamycin plus either gentamicin or a fluoroquinolone (either parenteral or oral) may be effective alternative regimens.[96,97] Many additional antimicrobials may safely be used in patients with diabetic foot infections; vancomycin is frequently used due to its excellent activity against gram-positive pathogens. All antibiotic regimens should be adjusted as necessary for renal dysfunction.

As information from deep wound tissue culture becomes available and the clinical condition of the patient is assessed, drug therapy should be modified accordingly. Treatment of soft tissue infections in diabetic patients should generally be 10–14 days in duration. However, in cases of underlying osteomyelitis treatment should continue for 6–12 weeks.[87]

Outpatient therapy with oral antimicrobials such as cefaclor, ciprofloxacin, ofloxacin, or amoxicillin/clavulanic acid may be appropriate in those diabetics with mild uncomplicated cellulitis.[98,99] However, clinical trials evaluating the treatment of skin and soft tissue infections utilizing these agents have included relatively few diabetic patients. Significant failure and/or relapse rates have been reported by several investigators in the treatment of skin and soft tissue infections with the use of oral agents, and the development of resistance was problematic in some infections involving *P. aeruginosa*.[100,101] Therefore, the use of oral antimicrobials in serious infections, especially those complicated by osteomyelitis, extensive ulceration, and/or areas of necrosis should be used cautiously. Treatment with a parenteral agent should also be considered if a mild infection being treated with an oral agent has failed to show improvement within 48–72 hours of beginning therapy.

Recommendations for the management of the infected diabetic foot:

1. Initially assess the extent of the lesion.
2. Culture wound for both anaerobes and aerobes. It is crucial to obtain deep tissue cultures to ensure the most reliable results.
3. Debride necrotic tissue and keep wound clean with dressing changes as needed (generally two to three times daily).
4. Maximize diabetic control to ensure optimal healing.
5. Restrict the patient initially to bedrest, leg elevation, and control of edema, if present.
6. Rule out possibility of osteomyelitis via x-ray and/or bone scan.
7. Mild uncomplicated infections can be treated in the outpatient setting with an oral antimicrobial regimen as previously described. Treatment should last at least 10–14 days.
8. For more severe cases or those complicated by the presence of osteomyelitis, parenteral antimicrobial therapy should be used. In severely infected cases, therapy should be continued until healing of the wound can be documented. If improvement is seen in 7–14 days the regimen may be converted to an oral regimen. Therapy should continue for at least 6–12 weeks.
9. After healing of the infected ulcer has occurred, a program for prevention should be designed.

Burn Wound Infections

Of the approximately 1.45 million burn injuries that occur in the United States each year, a surprisingly low percentage

(4%) results in a visit to the emergency department.[102] Of these approximately half-million emergency department visits, about 100,000 are classified as severe burns and 6000 result in death on an annual basis. Devastating as this may be, the number of yearly burn injuries has been decreasing over time.[103] The major determinants of death in order of importance for burn patients are cardiovascular/renal failure; pulmonary failure; extent of burn injury; age; and sex (women>men).[104] Multiorgan system failure has also been associated with a high (98%) mortality rate, with infection being the major cause of death in 75% of all burn injury deaths.[105,106]

There are several alterations in the normal host defense mechanisms of the burn patient that predispose the patient to infection. First, thermal injury disrupts the protective membrane barrier of the skin. Less obvious membrane damage may occur to the pharyngeal, nasal, and tracheal mucosa due to inhalation injury. The formation of coagulated skin and exudate (the eschar) provides for an ideal growth medium for microorganisms which is inaccessible to systemic antibiotics due to its avascular nature. Second, alterations in cell-mediated and humoral immunity occur which result in a decrease in circulating IgG concentrations and alterations in T-suppressor, T-helper, and interleukin-2-producing cell activity. T cells are responsible for recognizing antigens (i.e., bacteria) preventing an overzealous immunologic response, and stimulating B-cell lymphocytes to differentiate and promote antibody formation. Therefore, T-cell depression may impair nearly all immune functions. Third, nonspecific changes occur in the microvascular system, impaired white blood cell margination, impaired chemotaxis of phagocytic cells and macrophages, increased prostaglandins, leukotrienes, thromboxane, and endotoxin release. The resulting impairment in polymorphonuclear leukocyte chemotactic function is directly related to burn size and the patient's prognosis due to an inability to phagocytize and destroy the opportunistic organism.[107,108]

The typical clinical features following burn injury are visible swelling with blister formation, loss of the protective epithelium resulting in wet and weeping surfaces. Due to the fluid shifts associated with these changes, major burns may result in hypovolemic shock without adequate fluid resuscitation. Overhydration of tissues may aggravate the edema formation, increasing the risk of infection and ischemia.

Edema formation in humans is maximal around 6 hours postinjury, starts to resolve by 24 hours, and is usually resolved in 6–7 days. The magnitude of the fluid shifts appears to be linearly related to the time of heat exposure and temperature of the exposure.[109] Although a partial thickness burn and a deep full thickness burn will result in coagulation necrosis, the deep burn eliminates microcirculation and limits edema formation. This has led investigators to report that the typical full thickness burn results in less edema and blister formation than the less severe partial thickness burns.[110]

Most burn wounds are initially sterile, because the heat encountered destroys not only the cutaneous elements but also the surface microorganisms. Normally, the burn wound becomes colonized with gram-positive organisms within 48 hours after injury. These organisms are found within the sweat glands and hair follicles. After the first 3 days and up to 3 weeks after the injury, gram-negative bacteria proliferate within the burn wound. The source of these gram-negative organisms is typically from the patient's gastrointestinal tract, upper respiratory tract, or from the physical environment. Protecting the burn wound with topical agents as well as excising the eschar will prevent the microorganisms from migrating along hair follicles and sweat glands to viable tissue.[111] The staging of the microbial status of burn wounds has been suggested as shown in Table 103.8. The mortality from burn wounds increases as the staging increases.[111]

Prior to the availability of penicillin, gram-positive bacteria were the most frequently isolated microorganism. However, the majority of burn wound infections are now caused primarily by gram-negative bacteria. Initially, *P. aeruginosa* was the most common bacteria identified; however, the use of potent antibiotics has reduced its overall incidence. No single microorganism is responsible for the majority of burn wound infections. Some other commonly isolated gram-negative bacteria include *Enterocbacter cloacae, Providencia stuartii, Serratia marcescens,* and *Klebsiella* sp.

If the bacterial concentration at the burn site exceeds 10^6 microorganisms per gram of tissue, then spread to viable tissue and bacteremia usually occurs.[112] The process of seeding the systemic circulation with organisms from the burn site is termed *burn wound sepsis.* Burn wound sepsis is characterized by deterioration of the burn wound and, subsequently, signs of systemic sepsis.

TREATMENT

Following thermal injury, a variety of measures may be initiated to resuscitate the patient. Initially, all foreign material should be lavaged from the burn site. Patients should receive tetanus prophylaxis. Aseptic technique should be observed by all personnel caring for the patient in addition to wearing a cap, gown, mask, and gloves whenever burn wounds are exposed. Intravenous catheters should be changed frequently with the tip of the catheter cultured. Aggressive nutritional replacement should be instituted to meet the patient's hypermetabolic needs.

Fluid resuscitation is the prime objective of initial burn therapy.[113] Swift and appropriate fluid resuscitation can greatly decrease morbidity and mortality from this type of injury. The most commonly used guidelines for fluid

TABLE 103.8. STAGING THE STATUS OF BURN WOUNDS

Stage I: Colonization	
A. Superficial	Limited microbes on surface of the burn wound
B. Penetration	Organisms found in variable thickness of eschar
C. Proliferation	Densely populated areas of organisms at the nonviable/viable tissue interface
Stage II: Invasion	
A. Microinvasion	Organisms in viable tissue immediately adjacent to subeschar
B. Generalized	Extensive penetration of organisms deep into viable tissue
C. Microvascular	Involvement of lymphatics and microvascular

(Adapted from Ref. 111.)

resuscitation for burn shock consist of fluid administered through two large-bore intravenous lines at a rate adequate to produce a urine output of 30 mL/h. Known as the Parkland formula, Ringer's lactate is administered at a dose of 4 mL per percent of total burn surface area burn per kilogram of body weight. Fifty percent of the fluid replacement need is administered in the first 8 hours from the time of burn. The remaining 50% is administered over the next 16 hours based on clinical evaluation. After the first 24 hours, maintenance fluid administration is then administered in amounts to account for normal basal fluid needs plus calculated evaporated water loss from the wound. This is usually achieved via a combination of colloid and crystalloid solutions. Recently a "burn calculator" circular card has been described that may help in rapidly determining fluid needs in burn patients.[114]

Another major goal of burn wound therapy is to prevent the wound from becoming infected. Therapy includes prompt removal of necrotic tissue from the burn injury and immediate closure of the wound with skin grafts. One of the main methods of controlling burn wound sepsis is prevention of local burn infection via the use of topical antibiotics. The use of topical antibiotics is aimed at controlling the rate of bacterial proliferation in the burn to allow the injury to heal (form granulation tissue) without leading to systemic sepsis. The use of topical antimicrobial agents has led to a decreased incidence of conversion of partial thickness wounds to full thickness wounds by local infection.

AVAILABLE AGENTS

Ideal Characteristics of Topical Agents

Topical antimicrobials used prophylactically should have activity against a broad range of gram-positive, gram-negative, and fungal organisms. Although the ideal agent should be able to penetrate the eschar, systemic absorption should be nonexistent or minimal. The ideal agent should be easy to apply, be painless upon application, and have a long duration of action.

Several topical antibiotics have been used effectively in preventing bacterial proliferation within the burn wound. The three most commonly used products are described here.

Silver Sulfadiazine

One of the most commonly used topical agents, silver sulfadiazine has demonstrated *in vitro* activity against a wide range of gram-positive and gram-negative bacteria including *S. aureus, E. Coli, Proteus* sp., Enterobacteriaceae, and *C. albicans.*[115] It is not clear if the compound or the separate moieties acting individually are responsible for the antimicrobial effects of the drug. After removal of the serous discharge and as much of the eschar as possible, 3 mm of silver sulfadiazine is applied to the burn area once or twice a day. The area may be either covered with a light dressing or left uncovered (this allows for free range of motion).

Silver sulfadiazine is effective in the prevention of wound colonization by gram-negative bacteria for up to 2 weeks in extensively injured patients.[116] This agent does not penetrate deep extensive burns, resulting in treatment failures as wound size exceeds 50–60% total body surface area. Those involved with routine application of this drug should wear protective clothing.

Systemic sulfadiazine absorption and toxicity may occur, however it is generally minimal and even with extensive burns is rare. Allergic skin reactions have been reported in the form of a macular rash. These reactions occur in 1–5% of patients and are usually well tolerated.[115,116] Neutropenia associated with thrombocytopenia may occur early in therapy (within 5 days of treatment), occurring in approximately 5% of patients. These effects are usually reversible and may resolve with continued use of the drug. Bacterial resistance to silver sulfadiazine has been reported to occur, most commonly to gram-negative organisms and with protracted use.[117,118] Silver sulfadiazine is most useful as a prophylactic agent, prior to major bacterial colonization of the burn site, because of its poor ability to penetrate the eschar.

Sodium Mafenide

This agent was introduced more than 20 years ago and currently maintains activity against most gram-positive and gram-negative organisms including anaerobes with few reports of resistance. One of the unique features of this agent is its rapid and almost total ability to penetrate the eschar.[119] Mafenide is metabolized to an inactive salt, which is then eliminated renally. After the burn wound is cleaned, this agent should be applied to a depth of 3 mm; the site may be left uncovered or may be covered with a light dressing. The rapid absorption and inactivation of mafenide results in subtherapeutic antibacterial concentrations after 8–10 hours.[120] Therefore, to maintain therapeutic wound concentrations, mafenide should be applied every 12 hours. More frequent administration may result in toxicity. To avoid possible fungal overgrowth, mafenide may be used in combination with topical nystatin.[121]

Upon application, mafenide usually causes pain at the wound site; this has been attributed to its high osmolarity. The pain usually resolves within 60 minutes. In addition, approximately 5% of patients will develop a mild maculopapular rash[119] (although some have reported the incidence of the maculopapular rash to be as high as 50%). Of greater concern is the alkaline diuresis induced by mafenide and its metabolite via carbonic anhydrase inhibition and osmotic diuresis, respectively. Systemic metabolic acidosis and hyperventilation may occur when mafenide is used in patients with burns covering greater than 20% of body surface area.[117] In addition, methemoglobinemia has also been associated with mafenide use.[122] The use of mafenide may be limited due to its toxicity profile and an increased incidence of superinfections caused by resistant *P. stuartii* and fungi.[117] However, mafenide remains a useful agent for short-term use in the control of established invasive burn wound infections particularly due to its ability to penetrate the eschar.

Silver-Nitrate Solution (5%)

Silver nitrate 5% has been used since the mid-1960s in the treatment of the burn patient and is active against most gram-positive and gram-negative microorganisms including some *Pseudomonas* strains.[123] Silver nitrate is an effective prophylactic agent in the prevention of wound colonization. However, as with the other agents, its efficacy diminishes as burn size increases and exceeds 50–60% of total body surface area. In addition, silver nitrate is inadequate for the treatment of deep tissue infections due to its poor tissue absorption characteristics.

Silver nitrate should be administered by applying it to 6–8 layers of gauze, which then covers the wound as a wet dressing. The solution is then applied every 2 hours to maintain adequate concentrations at the wound site. The dressings are changed two to three times a day.

Although silver nitrate is painless and does not cause local allergic reactions, hyponatremia may occur due to the hyponatremic nature of the solution leaching sodium from open wounds.[123] Silver nitrate discolors surrounding tissue, sheets, and hospital supplies a brown or black color upon contact. A rare complication of silver nitrate is methemoglobinemia, resulting from the absorption of nitrite produced by the reduction of nitrate from bacteria. The need for bulky wet dressings and side effects limits silver nitrate's role in the therapy of burn patients.

Systemic Fungal Infection

Burn patients may also encounter difficulty with fungal infections. Wound discoloration to a dark infected-appearing tissue should raise the suspicion of a fungal infection. Common organisms causing fungal infections include *Aspergillus, Mucor, Candida,* and *Geotrichum* species. The treatment of choice for fungal infection is extensive surgical excision and debridement to noninfected tissues. Systemic or topical therapy is directed at the offending pathogen but plays only a secondary role. If the clinical picture is consistent with systemic fungal infection, appropriate intravenous fungal therapy is required.

Recommendations for the management of burn wound infections:

1. The burn wound should be kept clean and free of infection.
2. Wash and debride loose eschar twice daily.
3. A great deal of effort in the management of burn injuries is aimed at the prevention and treatment of infections. To control wound surface bacteria, topical antibiotics should be applied twice daily.
4. Infections in the burn patient may be either at the site of the injury or at other sites. The patient should be watched closely for signs of systemic infection.
5. If signs of systemic infection are present, then parenteral antibiotics should be used. Serum concentrations of drugs should be monitored closely (if possible) since the hyperdynamic state of the burn patient has been documented to alter the pharmacokinetics of drugs. Careless and indiscriminate use of antimicrobials in this setting is a problem but should be avoided to minimize the potential for the emergence of resistant strains of bacteria.

References

1. Simmons RL, Ahrenholz DH. Infections of skin and soft tissues, in Simmons RL, Howard RJ (eds): Surgical Infections. New York, Appleton-Century-Crofts, 1982, pp 507–683.
2. Roetinger W, Edgerton MT, Kurtz LD, et al. Role of inoculation site as a determinant of infection in soft tissue wounds. Am J Surg 1973;126:354–358.
3. Ducan WC, McBride ME, Knox JM. Experimental production of infection in humans. J Invest Dermatol 1970;54:319–323.
4. Noble WC, Somerville DA. Microbiology of the Human Skin. Philadelphia, WB Saunders, 1974.
5. Hook EW, Hooton TM, Horton C, et al. Microbiologic evaluation of cutaneous cellulitis in adults. Arch Intern Med 1986;146:295–297.

6. Granoff C, Nankerves G. Cellulitis due to HF type B antigemia and antibody responses. Am J Dis Child 1976;130:1211–1214.
7. Swartz MN. Cellulitis and superficial infections, in Mandell GL, Douglas RG, Bennett JE (eds): Principles and Practice of Infectious Diseases, 3rd ed. New York, Churchill Livingstone, 1990, pp 796–807.
8. Magnussen CR. Skin and soft tissue infections, in Reese R, Douglas G (eds): A Practical Approach to Infectious Diseases, 2nd ed. Boston, Little, Brown, 1983, pp 239–265.
9. Piscitelli SC, Danziger LH, Rodvold KA. Clarithromycin and azithromycin: New macrolide antibiotics. Clin Pharm 1992;11:137–152.
10. Dagan R, Moshe P, Watemberg N, et al. Outpatient treatment of serious community-acquired pediatric infections using once daily intramuscular ceftriaxone. Pediatr Infect Dis J 1987;6:1080–1084.
11. Gould IM, Hudson M, Morris J, et al. Imipenem versus standard therapy in the treatment of serious soft tissue infection. Drugs Exp Clin Res 1988;14(8):555–558.
12. Kulhanjian J, Dunphy M, Hamstra S, et al. Randomized comparative study of ampicillin/sulbactam vs. ceftriaxone for treatment of soft tissue and skeletal infections in children. Pediatr Infect Dis J 1989;8:605–610.
13. Tan JS, Wishnow RM, Talan DA, et al. Treatment of hospitalized patients with complicated skin and skin structure infections: Double-blind, randomized, multicenter study of piperacillin–tazobactam versus ticarcillin–clavulanate. Antimicrob Agents Chemother 1993;37:1580–1586.
14. Gentry LO, Ramirez-Ronda CH, Rodriquez-Noriega E, et al. Oral ciprofloxacin vs. parenteral cefotaxime in the treatment of difficult skin and skin structure infections. Arch Intern Med 1989;148:2579–2583.
15. Gentry LO. Therapy with newer oral β-lactam and quinolone agents for infections of the skin and skin structures: A review. Clin Infect Dis 1992;14:285–297.
16. Gentry LO, Rodriguez-Gomez G, Zeluff BJ, et al. A comparative evaluation of oral ofloxacin versus intravenous cefotaxime therapy for serious skin and skin structure infections. Am J Med 1989;87(suppl 6C):57S–60S.
17. LeFrock J, Blais F, Schell, et al. Cefoxitin in the treatment of diabetic patients with lower extremity infections. Infect Surg 1983;2:361–374.
18. Hughes C, Johnson C, Bamberger D, et al. Treatment and long-term follow-up of foot infections in patients with diabetes or ischemia: A randomized, prospective, double-blind comparison of cefoxitin and ceftizoxime. Clin Ther 1987;10(suppl A):36–49.
19. Thadepalli H, Mathai D, Chuah SK, et al. Ciprofloxacin versus ceftazidime in skin and soft tissue infections. J Chemother 1989;1(1):30–34.
20. Solomkin JS, Cocchetto DM. Ceftazidime versus tobramycin plus ticarcillin in the treatment of soft-tissue infections. Clin Ther 1986;9(1):123–134.
21. Dominquez J, Palma F, Vega ME, et al. Brief report: Prospective, controlled, randomized non-blind comparison of intravenous/oral ciprofloxacin with intravenous ceftazidime in the treatment of skin or soft-tissue infections. Am J Med 1989;87(suppl 5A)13:136S–137S.
22. Slaughter R, Pieper J, Cerra F, et al. Chloramphenicol sodium succinate kinetics in the critically ill patient. Clin Pharmacol Ther 1982;28:69–77.
23. Kauffman R, Tirumoosthi M, Buckley J, et al. Relative bioavailability of intravenous chloramphenicol succinate and oral chloramphenicol palmitate in infants and children. J Pediatr 1981;99:963–967.
24. Marks M, LaFerriere C. Chloramphenicol: Recent developments and clinical indications. Clin Pharm 1982;1:315–320.
25. Brasfield J, Record K, Griffen W, et al. Chloramphenicol and chloramphenicol succinate concentration in patients with renal impairment. Clin Pharm 1983;2:355–358.
26. Azzollini F, Gazzanega A, Lodola E, et al. Elimination of chloramphenicol and thiamphenicol in subjects with cirrhosis of the liver. Int J Clin Pharmacol 1976;6:130–143.
27. Feder HM, Osier C, Madefazo EG. Chloramphenicol: A review of its use in clinical practice. Rev Infect Dis 1981;3:479–491.
28. Uman SJ, Kunin CM. Needle aspiration in the diagnosis of soft tissue infections. Arch Intern Med 1975;135:959–961.
29. Peter G, Smith A. Group A streptococcal infections of the skin and pharynx. N Engl J Med 1977;297:311–317.
30. Goepel JR, Richards DG, Harris DM, et al. Fulminant *Streptococcus pyogenes* infection. Br Med J 1980;281:1412.
31. Baltimore RS. Treatment of impetigo: A review. Pediatr Infect Dis 1985;4:597–601.
32. Swartz M. Lymphadenitis and lymphangitis, in Mandell GL, Douglas RG, Bennett JE (eds): Principles and Practice of Infectious Diseases, 3rd ed. New York, Churchill Livingstone, 1990, pp 818–825.
33. Dajani AS, Garcia RE, Wolinski E. Etiology of lymphadenitis in children. N Engl J Med 1963;268:1329–1341.
34. Kosiak M. Etiology of decubitus ulcers. Arch Phys Med Rehabil 1961;42:19–29.
35. Reuler JB, Cooney TG. The pressure sore: Pathophysiology and principles of management. Ann Intern Med 1981;94:661–666.
36. Shea JD. Pressure sores—classification and management. Clin Orthop 1975;112:89–100.
37. National Pressure Ulcer Advisory Panel. Pressure ulcers: Incidence, economics, risk. Consensus Development Conference statement. West Dundee, IL, 1989.
38. Galpen JE, Chow AW, Bayer AS, et al. Sepsis associated with decubitus ulcers. Am J Med 1976;61:346–350.
39. Antypas PG. Management of pressure sores. Curr Probl Surg 1980;17:229–244.
40. Nierman MM. Treatment of dermal and decubitis ulcers. Drugs 1978;15:226–230.
41. Varma AO, Burgatch E, German FM. Debridement of dermal ulcers with collagenase. Surg Gynecol Obstet 1973;136:281–282.
42. Coopwood TB. Evaluation of a topical enzymatic debridement agent—sutilains ointment. South Med J 1976;69:834.
43. Longe RL. Current concepts in clinical therapeutics: Pressure sores. Clin Pharm 1986;5:669–681.
44. Branemark PI, Ekholm R, Albrektsaen B, et al. Tissue injury caused by wound disinfectants. J Bone Joint Surg 1967;49A:48–62.

45. Geronemus R, Mertz P, Eaglstein W. Wound healing. The effects of topical antimicrobial agents. Arch Dermatol 1979;115:1311–1314.
46. Dennis D, Luterman A, Ramenofsky F, et al. Does PVP-iodine interfere with wound healing? Infect Surg 1983;4:371–374.
47. Wallace G, Hayter J. Karaya for chronic skin ulcers. Am J Nurs 1974;74:1094–1098.
48. Verkonick PJ. A preliminary report of decubitus care. Am J Nurs 1961;61:68–69.
49. Parish LC, Collins E. Decubitus ulcers: A comparative study. Cutis 1979;23:106–110.
50. Alvarez OM, Mertz AM, Englstein WH. The effect of occlusive dressings on collagen synthesis and re-epithellialization in superficial wounds. J Surg Res 1983;35:142–148.
51. Olenjniczaks S, Zrelinski A. Topical oxygen promotes healing of leg ulcers. Resident Staff Phys 1977;23:165–242.
52. Knight AL. Medical management of pressure sores. J Fam Prac 1988;27:95–100.
53. Paul BJ, Lafratta CW, Dawson AR, et al. Use of ultrasound in the treatment of pressure sores in patients with spinal cord injuries. Arch Phys Med Rehabil 1960;41:438.
54. Wolcott LE, Wheeler PC, Hardwicke HM, et al. Accelerated healing of skin ulcers by electrotherapy: Preliminary clinical results. South Med J 1969;62:795–801.
55. White AG. Medical disorders in drug addicts. JAMA 1973;223:1469–1471.
56. Webb D, Thadepalli H. Skin and soft-tissue polymicrobial infections from intravenous abuse of drugs. West J Med 1979;130:200–204.
57. Orangio GR, Pitlick SD, Latta PD, et al. Soft-tissue infections in parenteral drug abusers. Ann Surg 1984;199:97–100.
58. Moustoukas N, Nichols R, Smith J, et al. Contaminated street heroin. Relationship to clinical infections. Arch Surg 1983;118:746–749.
59. Bisbe J, Miro J, Latorre, et al. Disseminated candidiasis in addicts who use brown heroin: Report of 83 cases and review. Clin Infec Dis 1992;15:910–923.
60. Tuazon CV, Hill R, Sheayren JN. Microbiologic study of street heroin and injection paraphernalia. J Infect Dis 1974;1299:327–329.
61. Crane L, Levine D, Aervos M, et al. Bacteremia in narcotic addicts at Detroit Medical Center. Microbiology, epidemiology, risk factors, and empiric therapy. Rev Infect Dis 1986;8:364–373.
62. Markowitz N, Pohlod D, Saravolatz L, et al. *In vitro* susceptibility patterns of methicillin-resistant and susceptible *Staphylococcus aureus* strains in a population of parenteral drug abusers from 1972 to 1981. Antimicrob Agents Chemother 1983;23:450–457.
63. King CH, Creger RJ, Ellner JJ. Pharmacokinetics of tobramycin and gentamicin in abusers of intravenous drugs. Antimicrob Agents Chemother 1985;27:285–290.
64. Louria D. Surgical infections in drug addicts [invited commentary]. World J Surg 1980;4:412–413.
65. Goldstein E. Bite wounds and infection. Clin Infec Dis. 1992;14:633–640.
66. Callaham ML. Treatment of common dog bites: Infection risk factors. J Am Coll Emerg Phys 1978;7:83–87.
67. Rest JG, Goldstein EJC. Management of human and animal bite wounds. Emerg Med Clin North Am 1985;3:117–126.
68. Goldstein EJC, Citron DM, Finegold SM. Role of anaerobic bacteria in bite wound infections. Rev Infect Dis 1984;6(suppl 1):S177–S183.
69. Baile WE, Stowe EC, Schmitt AM. Aerobic bacterial flora of oral and nasal fluids of canines with reference to bacteria associated with bites. J Clin Microbiol 1978;7:223–231.
70. Saphir DA, Carter GR. Gingival flora of the dog with special reference to bacteria associated with bites. J Clin Microbiol 1976;3:344–349.
71. Goldstein EJC, Citron DM, Finegold SM. Dog bite wounds and infection: A prospective clinical study. Ann Emerg Med 1980;9:508–512.
72. Lee M, Buhr A. Dog bites and local infections with *Pasteurella septica.* Br Med J 1960;1:169–171.
73. Callaham ML. Prophylactic antibiotics in common dog bite wounds: A controlled study. Ann Emerg Med 1980;9:410–414.
74. Goldstein EJC. Bites, in Mandell GL, Douglas RG, Bennett JE (eds): Principles and Practice of Infectious Diseases. New York, John Wiley and Sons, 1985, pp 632–635.
75. Elenbass RM, McNaoney WK, Robinson WA. Prophylactic oxacillin in dog bite wounds. Ann Emerg Med 1982;11:248–251.
76. Elliot DL, Tolle SW, Goldberg L, et al. Pet-associated illness. N Engl J Med 1985;313:985–995.
77. Feder HM, Shanley JD, Barbera JA. Review of 59 patients hospitalized with animal bites. Pediatr Infect Dis J 1987;6:24–28.
78. Goldstein E, Citron DM, Richwals GA. Lack of *in vitro* efficacy of oral forms of certain cephalosporins, erythromycin, and oxacillin against *Pasteurella multocida.* Antimicrob Agents Chemother 1988;32(2):213–215.
79. Holst E, Rollof J, Miorner H. *In vitro* activities of cefcanel and some other cephalosporins against *Pasteurella multocida.* Antimicrob Agents Chemother 1989;33(12):2142–2143.
80. Goldstein EJ, Reinhardt JF, Murray PM, et al. Outpatient therapy of bite wounds. Demographic data, bacteriology, and a prospective, randomized trial of amoxicillin/clavulanic acid versus pencillin ± dicloxacillin. Int J Derm 1987;26(2):123–127.
81. Mann RJ, Hoffield TA, Farmer CB. Human bites of the hand: Twenty years of experience. J Hand Surg 1977;2:97–99.
82. Goldstein EJC, Citron DM, Wield B, et al. Bacteriology of human and animal bite wounds. J Clin Microbiol 1978;8:667–672.
83. Peeples E, Boswick JA, Scott FA. Wounds of the hand contaminated by human and animal saliva. J Trauma 1980;20:383–389.
84. Goldstein E, Gombert M, Agyare E. Susceptibility of *Eikenella corrodens* to newer beta-lactam antibiotics. Antimicrob Agents Chemother 1980;18:832–833.
85. Goldstein E, Miller T, Citron D, et al. Infections following clenched-fist injury: A new perspective. J Hand Surg 1978;3:455–459.
86. Goldstein E, Barene M, Miller TA. *Eikenella corrodens* in hand infections. J Hand Surg 1983;8:563–566.

87. Lipsky BA, Pecoraro RE, Wheat LJ. The diabetic foot: Soft tissue and bone infection. Infect Dis Clin North Am 1990;4:409–432.
88a. LeFrock JL, Joseph WS. Lower extremity infections in diabetics. Infect Surg 1986;5:135–145.
88b. Louis JT, Bartlet JG, Tally FP, et al. Aerobic and anaerobic bacteria in diabetic foot ulcers. Ann Intern Med 1976;85:461–463.
89. Sharp CS, Bessman AN, Wagner FW, et al. Microbiology of deep and superficial tissues in infected diabetic gangrene. Surg Gynecol Obstet 1979;149:217–219.
90. Waldvogel FA, McDoff G, Swartz MN. Osteomyelitis: A review of clinical features, therapeutic considerations and unusual aspects. N Engl J Med 1970;282:198–216.
91. LeFrock J, Blais F, Schell RF, et al. Cefoxitin in the treatment of diabetic patients with lower extremity infections. Infect Surg 1983;2:361–374.
92. Hughes C, Johnson C, Bamberger D, et al. A randomized double-blind trial of ceftizoxime vs. cefoxitin for therapy of lower extremity infections in patients with diabetes mellitus and/or peripheral vascular disease. Clin Ther 1987;10(suppl A):36–41.
93. Rao B, See RC, Chuah SK, et al. Ticarcillin plus clavulanic acid versus moxalactam in the treatment of skin and soft tissue infections. Am J Med 1985;79(suppl 5B):126–129.
94. Johnson CC, Reinhardt JF, Wallace SL. Safety and efficacy of ticarcillin plus clavulanic acid in the treatment of infections of soft tissue, bone, and joint. Am J Med 1985;79(suppl 5B):136–140.
95. Calandra GB, Raupp W, Brown KR. Imipenem/cilastatin treatment of lower extremity skin and soft tissue infections in diabetics. Scand J Infect Dis 1987;52(suppl):15–19.
96. Sesin PG, Paszko A, O'Keefe E. Oral clindamycin and ciprofloxacin therapy for diabetic foot infections. Pharmacother 1990;10:154–156.
97. Gentry LO, Rodriugez-Gomez G, Zeluff BJ, et al. A comparative evaluation of oral ofloxacin versus intravenous cefotaxime therapy for serious skin and skin structure infections. Am J Med 1989;87(suppl 6C):57–60S.
98. Gentry LO, Ramirez-Ronda CH, Rodriguez-Noriega E, et al. Oral ciprofloxacin vs parenteral cefotaxime in the treatment of difficult skin and skin structure infections. Arch Intern Med 1989;149:2579–2583.
99. Parish LC, Aten EM. Treatment of skin and skin structure infections: A comparative study of Augmentin and cefaclor. Cutis 1984;34:567–570.
100. Eron LJ, Harvey L, Hixon DL, et al. Ciprofloxacin therapy of infections caused by *Pseudomonas aeruginosa* and other resistant bacteria. Antimicrob Agents Chemother 1985;28:308–310.
101. Valainis GT, Pankey GA, Katner HP, et al. Ciprofloxacin in the treatment of bacterial skin infections. Am J Med 1987;82(suppl 4A):230–232.
102. American Burn Association. Hospital and prehospital resources for optimal care of patients with burn injury: Guidelines for development and operation of burn centers. J Burn Care Rehab 1990;11:97–104.
103. Elberg JJ, Scroder HA, Glent-Madsen L, et al. Burns: Epidemiology and the effect of a prevention programme. Burns, Including Thermal Injury 1987;13:391–393.
104. Bonate PL. Pathophysiology and pharmacokinetics following burn injury. Clin Pharmacokinet 1990;18:118–130.
105. Polk HC. Consensus summary on infection. Trauma 1979;19:894.
106. Marshall WG, Dimick AR. The natural history of major burns with multiple system failure. Trauma 1983;23:102–105.
107. Moran K, Munster AM. Alterations of the host defense mechanism in burned patients. Surg Clin North Am 1987;67:47–56.
108. Ninnerman JL. Clinical and immune status of burn patients. Antibiot Chemother 1987;39:16–25.
109. Arturson G, Jakobsson OP. Oedema measurements in a standard burn model. Burns 1985;12:1–7.
110. Demling RH, Mazess RB, Witt RM, et al. The study of burn wound edema using dicromatic absorptiometry. J Trauma 1978;18:124.
111. Pruitt BA, McManus AT. The changing epidemiology of infection in burn patients. World J Surg 1992;16:57–67.
112. Lindberg RB, Moncreif JA, Mason AD. Control of experimental and clinical wound sepsis by topical application of sulfamylon compounds. Ann NY Acad Sci 1986;150:950–960.
113. Demling R. Fluid resuscitation, in Boswick J (ed): The Art and Science of Burn Care. Rockville, Maryland, Aspen, 1982, p 189.
114. Milner SM, Hodgetts TJ, Rylah LT. The burns calculator: A simple proposed guide for fluid resuscitation. Lancet 1993;342:1089–1091.
115. Pegg SP. The role of drugs in the management of burns. Drugs 1982;24:256–260.
116. Monafo WW, Freedman B. Topical therapy for burns. Surg Clin North Am 1987;67:133–145.
117. Bridges K, Lowbury EJ. Drug resistance in relation to use of silver sulphadiazine cream in a burn unit. J Clin Pathol 1977;30:160–167.
118. McManus AT, Denton CL, Mason AD. Mechanisms of *in vitro* sensitivity to sulfadiazine silver. Arch Surg 1983;118:161–166.
119. Moyer CA, Brentano L, Gravens DL, et al. Treatment of large human burns with 0.5 per-cent silver nitrate solution. Arch Surg 1965;90:812–867.
120. Harrison H, Blackmore W, Bales H, et al. The absorption of ^{14}C labelled sulfamylon acetate through burned skin. J Trauma 1972;12:986–993.
121. Heggers JP, Robson MC, Herndon, DN, et al. The efficacy of nystatin combined with topical microbial agents in the treatment of burn wound sepsis. J Burn Care Rehabil 1989;10:508–511.
122. Ohlgisser M, Adler M. Ben-Dov D, et al. Methaemoglobinemia induced by mafenide acetate in children. Br J Anaesth 1978;50:299–301.
123. Ryna CM, Tomplkins RG. Topical Therapy II: Burns, in Chernow B (ed): The Pharmacologic Approach to the Critically Ill Patient, 3rd ed. Baltimore, MD, William & Wilkins 1994.

Chapter 104

Infective Endocarditis

Ron E. Polk, PharmD

Endocarditis is an inflammation of the endocardium, the membrane lining the chambers of the heart and covering the cusps of the heart valves.[1,2] More commonly, endocarditis refers to infection of the heart valves by various microorganisms. If untreated, endocarditis is usually fatal. With treatment, the average mortality is approximately 20%, although the range in mortality is wide depending on the presence or absence or various risk factors discussed as follows.[3]

Endocarditis is often referred to as either acute or subacute depending on the clinical presentation. Acute bacterial endocarditis is a fulminating infection associated with high fevers, systemic toxicity, and death within a few days to weeks if untreated. This syndrome most frequently follows infection of previously normal valves by virulent bacteria such as *Staphylococcus aureus*. Subacute bacterial endocarditis (SBE) is a more indolent infection caused by less invasive organisms such as viridans streptococci, usually occurring in a setting of prior valvular heart disease. Infection may also follow surgical insertion of a prosthetic heart valve, resulting in prosthetic valve endocarditis (PVE).[4]

Although endocarditis is caused primarily by bacteria, the clinical presentation does not reliably predict the causative organism. In addition, endocarditis caused by fungi and other atypical microorganisms has become more common. Therefore, the more encompassing term *infective endocarditis* (IE) is preferred.

Epidemiology and Etiology

Infective endocarditis is an uncommon infection, accounting for approximately 1 of every 1000 hospital admissions.[1] The male-to-female ratio is 2:1. Overall, the mean age of patients with IE exceeds 50 years and it is an unusual illness in children.[5] As the population ages, and as valve replacement surgery becomes more common, the mean age of patients with IE is increasing. However, an exception is the intravenous (IV) drug abuser, who tends to be a younger male.

Most persons with IE have evidence of preexisting cardiac valvular abnormalities or other risk factors, although a predisposing factor may be absent in up to 25% of cases.[6] Most types of structural heart disease resulting in turbulence of blood flow will increase the risk for IE. Some of the most important include:

- Congenital heart disease accompanied by cyanosis (such as patent ductus arteriosus and ventricular septal defects)
- Rheumatic heart disease following rheumatic fever
- Mitral valve prolapse with regurgitation
- Degenerative valvular lesions in the elderly, such as valvular stenosis and regurgitation
- Presence of a prosthetic valve
- IV drug abuse

The prevalence of these risk factors within the community will influence the type of IE observed locally. Historically, rheumatic heart disease was the most prevalent risk factor of IE, although this has become less common as the overall frequency of acute rheumatic fever has declined. Recent outbreaks of rheumatic heart disease in different geographic areas of the United States suggest that this may once again become a common risk factor for IE.[2] The risk of IE in persons with mitral valve prolapse and regurgitation is small, but because the condition is prevalent, it is an important contributor to the overall number of cases. PVE occurs in 1–4% of patients who have undergone valve replacement surgery.[4] Other predispositions for IE include arteriovenous fistulae (including access for hemodialysis), and various intravascular devices, such as central venous catheters, which are associated with nosocomial IE in patients with a prosthetic valve.[7]

Nearly every organism causing human disease has been reported to cause IE (Table 104.1). Three groups of organisms cause most cases of IE: streptococci (50–60%), staphylococci (25%), and enterococci (10%).[1,8] In general, streptococci cause IE in patients with underlying cardiac

TABLE 104.1. ETIOLOGIC AGENTS IN INFECTIVE ENDOCARDITIS

Agent	Percentage of Cases
Streptococci	60–80
Viridans streptococci	30–40
Other	15–25
Enterococci	5–18
Staphylococci	20–35
Coagulase-positive	10–27
Coagulase-negative	1–3
Gram-negative aerobic bacilli	1.5–13
Fungi	2–4
Miscellaneous	<5
Culture-negative	<5–24

(From Scheld WM, Sande MA. Endocarditis and intravascular infections, in Mandell GL, Douglas RG, Bennett JE (eds): Principles and Practice of Infectious Diseases, 4th ed. New York, Churchill Livingstone, 1995, p 681, with permission.)

abnormalities, such as mitral valve prolapse or rheumatic heart disease. PVE within 1 year of valve surgery (early PVE) is most commonly caused by staphylococci (*S. aureus* and coagulase-negative staphylococci) implanted at the time of surgery, whereas PVE occurring after 1 year has a microbial etiology similar to that of native valve endocarditis.[3] *Staphylococcus aureus* is the most common cause of IE in IV drug abusers. However, there are many exceptions to the preceding generalizations and isolation of the causative pathogen and determination of its antimicrobial susceptibilities offer the best chance for successful therapy.

PATHOPHYSIOLOGY

The development of IE via hematogenous spread, the most common route, requires the sequential occurrence of several factors[1]:

1. The endothelial surface of the heart must be damaged. This occurs with turbulent blood flow associated with the valvular lesions previously described.
2. Platelet and fibrin deposition occurs on the abnormal epithelial surface. These deposits are referred to as nonbacterial thrombotic endocarditis (NBTE).
3. Bacteremia results in colonization of the endocardial surface. Most often, bacteremia is the result of trauma to a mucosal surface having a high concentration of resident bacteria, such as the oral cavity and gastrointestinal tract. Transient bacteremia commonly follows certain dental and gastrointestinal procedures.
4. Staphylococci, viridans streptococci, and enterococci are most likely to adhere to NBTE, probably because of production of specific adherence factors, such as dextran production by some oral streptococci.[9] Gram-negative bacteria have a low propensity to adhere to heart valves and are uncommon causes of IE.
5. After colonization of the endothelial surface, fibrin, platelets, and bacteria continue to aggregate and a "vegetation" forms. The protective cover of fibrin and platelets allows unimpeded bacterial growth to concentrations as high as 10^9–10^{10} organisms per gram of tissue. The vegetations that form may be single or multiple and vary in size from a few millimeters to centimeters. Bacteria within the vegetation grow slowly and are protected from antibiotics and host defenses.

Turbulent flow and eddy currents set up by abnormal valvular function injure the endocardium and promote IE "downstream" from the abnormal flow (e.g., on the atrial side of mitral regurgitant flow and on the ventricular surface of incompetent aortic valves). The mitral valve tends to be more commonly infected in subacute cases, whereas acute infections more commonly involve the aortic valve. With the formation of vegetations, valvular tissue may be destroyed. Continuing destruction may lead to acute heart failure via perforation of the valve leaflet or rupture of the chordae tendineae, papillary muscle, or in the patient with PVE, valve dehiscence. Occasionally, valvular stenosis may occur. Abscesses may develop in the valve ring or in myocardial tissue itself. Even with resolution of the process, fibrosis of tissue with some dysfunction may result.

Because of the friability of some vegetations, fragments may be released downstream. These infected particles are referred to as septic emboli. Septic emboli from right-sided endocarditis commonly lodge in the lung, causing pulmonary abscesses. Emboli from left-sided vegetations commonly affect organs with high blood flow, such as kidneys, spleen, and brain, but may involve any organ resulting in abscess or infarction.

Circulating immune complexes consisting of antigen, antibody, and complement may be deposited in organs such as the kidney, producing local inflammation and damage (glomerulonephritis). Other potential pathologic changes that result from immune complex deposition or septic emboli include the development of "mycotic" aneurysms (although the aneurysm is usually bacterial in origin, not fungal), cerebral infarction, splenic infarctions and abscesses, and skin manifestations such as petechiae, Osler nodes, and Janeway lesions (as follows).

The pathogenesis of early PVE differs from the hematogenous route already discussed, because bacteria from the skin of the patient or operating room personnel may be directly inoculated during surgery. The recently placed, nonendothelialized valve is much more susceptible to bacterial colonization than are native valves. Bacteria may also colonize the new valve from a contaminated bypass pump, cannulas, and pacemakers, or from a nosocomial bacteremia subsequent to an intravascular catheter.[4,7,10] With late PVE the mechanism of bacterial colonization and pathogenesis is similar to that which occurs in native valve endocarditis.[4,10,11]

CLINICAL PRESENTATION

The clinical presentation of patients with IE is highly variable (Table 104.2). Fever is the most common finding and is often accompanied by other nonspecific symptoms. The fever may be relatively low grade, particularly in subacute cases. Heart murmurs are found in 85% of patients at presentation, with a much lower percentage documented as new or changing murmurs. In patients with SBE, evidence of long-standing infection may include embolic phenomena, such as splenic or renal infarction and skin lesions (vide infra). In the majority of patients, the disease begins insidiously and gradually worsens. The patient may present with nonspecific findings such as fatigue, weakness, and low-grade fever accompanied by anorexia and weight loss. Arthralgias and myalgias are also common. In contrast, patients with the acute form, such as an IV drug abuser with IE caused by *S. aureus,* may appear with classic signs of sepsis.

Other important clinical signs, especially prevalent in subacute illness, may include the following peripheral manifestations ("stigmata") of endocarditis:

- *Osler nodes:* Purplish or erythematous subcutaneous papules or nodules that may appear on the pads of the fingers and toes. These lesions may be 2–15 mm in size and are painful and tender. These are not specific for IE and may be the result of embolic and/or immunologic phenomena.
- *Janeway lesions:* Hemorrhagic, painless plaques that may develop on the palms of the hands or soles of the feet. These lesions are also believed to be embolic in origin.
- *Splinter hemorrhages:* Thin, linear hemorrhages found under the nail beds of the fingers or toes. These lesions are not specific for IE and are actually more commonly the result of traumatic injuries.
- *Petechiae:* Small (usually 1–2 mm in diameter), erythematous, hemorrhagic lesions that are not painful or tender. These lesions may appear anywhere on the skin but are more evident on the anterior trunk, the buccal mucosa and palate, and conjunctivae. They are nonblanching and resolve after a few days.

TABLE 104.2. CLINICAL MANIFESTATIONS OF INFECTIVE ENDOCARDITIS

Symptoms	Percentage	Physical Findings	Percentage
Fever	80	Fever	90
Chills	40	Heart murmur	85
Weakness	40	Changing murmur	5–10
Dyspnea	40	New murmur	3–5
Sweats	25	Embolic phenomenon	>50
Anorexia	25	Skin manifestations	18–50
Weight loss	25	Osler nodes	10–23
Malaise	25	Splinter hemorrhages	15
Cough	25	Petechiae	20–40
Skin lesions	20	Janeway lesion	<10
Stroke	20	Splenomegaly	20–57
Nausea/vomiting	20	Septic complications (pneumonia, meningitis, etc.)	20
Headache	15		
Myalgia/arthralgia	15	Mycotic aneurysms	20
Edema	15	Clubbing	12–52
Chest pain	15	Retinal lesion	2–10
Abdominal pain	15	Signs of renal failure	10–15
Delirium/coma	10		
Hemoptysis	10		
Back pain	10		

(From Scheld WM, Sande MA. Endocarditis and intravascular infections, in Mandell GL, Bennett JE, Dolin R (eds): Principles and Practices of Infectious Diseases, 4th ed. New York. Churchill Livingstone, 1995, p 748, with permission.)

- *Clubbing of the fingers:* Proliferative change in the soft tissues about the terminal phalanges that may be observed in long-standing bacterial endocarditis.
- *Roth spot:* Retinal infarct with central pallor and surrounding hemorrhage.
- *Emboli:* Embolic phenomena may occur in up to one-third of cases and may result in significant complications. Left-sided endocarditis can result in renal artery emboli causing flank pain with hematuria, splenic artery emboli causing abdominal pain, and cerebral emboli, which may result in hemiplegia or alteration in mental status. Right-sided endocarditis, most often seen in IV drug abusers, may result in pulmonary emboli, causing pleuritic pain with hemoptysis and pneumonia. Splenomegaly is also a frequent finding and is more common in patients with endocarditis of prolonged duration.

LABORATORY FINDINGS

Patients with IE virtually always have some laboratory abnormalities; however, none is specific for endocarditis.[12] A normocytic, normochromic anemia with a low serum iron and low iron-binding capacity is common in subacute endocarditis. In subacute endocarditis the white blood cell count is usually normal or only slightly elevated, sometimes with a mild left shift. The erythrocyte sedimentation rate is usually elevated.

BLOOD CULTURES

The hallmark of IE is a continuous bacteremia caused by shedding of bacteria from the vegetation into the bloodstream.[1,2,12] More than 95% of patients with IE should have a positive blood culture when three samples are obtained over 24 hours. If there is evidence of cardiac decompensation, several blood cultures should be collected at once and empiric treatment begun immediately. Blood cultures should be held for up to a month to detect growth of fastidious organisms, or in patients who received prior antibiotics. In contrast to bacterial valvular infections, only about one-half of patients with fungal endocarditis have positive blood cultures. "Culture-negative" endocarditis describes the patient in whom a clinical diagnosis of IE is likely, but blood cultures have failed to yield a pathogen.[12] This condition is most often a consequence of previous antibiotic therapy.

ECHOCARDIOGRAPHY

Two-dimensional echocardiography, using either the transthoracic (TTE) or transesophageal (TEE) technique, is increasingly important in identifying and localizing valvular lesions in patients suspected of having IE.[1,2,13] TEE is more sensitive for detecting vegetations (≥90%), compared to TTE (~50%) (Fig. 104.1). TEE is also helpful for diagnosing IE when blood cultures are negative or in planning for surgical intervention. Although a negative echocardiogram does not completely exclude endocarditis, a positive test may reveal an unsuspected large vegetation (e.g., >1 cm), ring abscess, or intracardiac fistula, alerting the physician to the need for aggressive monitoring for septic emboli and heart failure or urgent surgical intervention.[11,13]

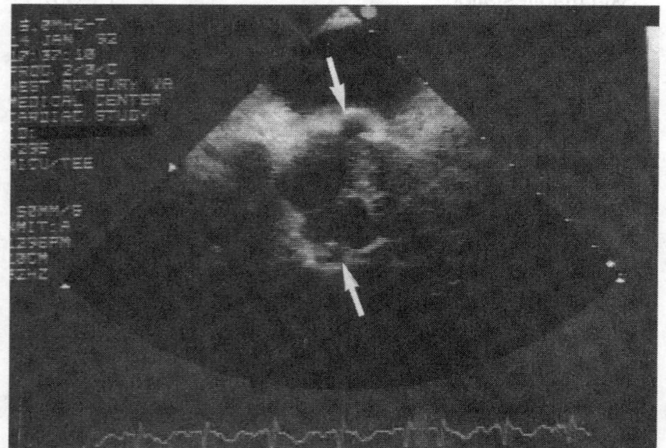

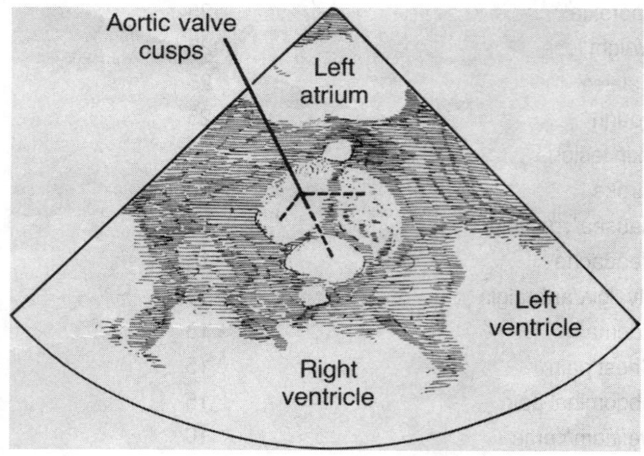

Figure 104.1. *Left.* Transesophageal echocardiogram of the aortic valve in a patient with IE caused by *S. aureus* showing two localized abscesses *(arrows)*. *Right.* Line drawing of left panel. *(Reprinted by permission of* The New England Journal of Medicine. *From Jay ME, Silver MT. Images in clinical medicine. N Engl J Med, vol 327, p 1734. Copyright 1992, Massachusetts Medical Society.)*

Diagnosis

The preceding list of signs and symptoms in the patient with IE are not specific, and the diagnosis is oftentimes not straightforward.[14,15] New criteria have recently been proposed that include major criteria (typical blood culture and positive echocardiogram) and minor criteria (predisposition, fever, vascular phenomena, immunologic phenomena, suggestive echocardiogram, and suggestive microbiologic findings).[16] These criteria increase the number of patients with a diagnosis of definite IE.

Prognosis

Without appropriate antimicrobial therapy and surgery if required, IE is usually fatal. With proper management, recovery can be expected in most patients. Factors associated with increased mortality include (1) congestive heart failure, (2) culture-negative endocarditis, (3) endocarditis caused by resistant organisms such as fungi and gram-negative bacteria, (4) left-sided endocarditis caused by *S. aureus,* and (5) prosthetic valve endocarditis.[1,3]

Treatment

GENERAL PRINCIPLES OF ANTIMICROBIAL THERAPY

The most important approach to treatment of IE includes isolation of the pathogen followed by high-dose, bactericidal antibiotics for an extended period.[17,18] Large doses of parenteral antimicrobials are usually necessary to provide the greatest chance of achieving bactericidal concentrations within the vegetations. For some pathogens, such as enterococci, the use of synergistic antimicrobial combinations is essential to obtain a bactericidal effect. Combination antibiotics are also used to decrease the probability of resistant organisms emerging during treatment (e.g., PVE caused by coagulase-negative staphylococci), or to hasten the pace of clinical and microbiologic response (e.g., some streptococcal and staphylococcal infections).

A long duration of therapy is ordinarily required for adequate treatment of IE, even for very susceptible pathogens. Microorganisms in the vegetations are enclosed in an area where host defenses are impaired and where organized fibrin deposits protect the microbes from phagocytic cells. In addition, the concentrations of bacteria in these vegetations may be very high, and the resulting inoculum effect may further resist killing. Moreover, many bacteria are not actively dividing, further limiting the rate at which bacteria are killed. For most patients, 4–6 weeks of therapy are required. Specific recommendations from the American Heart Association for treating IE caused by the most common organisms are discussed here and are summarized in Tables 104.3 through 104.7.[19]

Pharmacodynamic investigations in the animal model of IE allow quantitation of bacterial densities within vegetations over time as a function of antibiotic concentration and these have confirmed many of the treatment principles of IE observed empirically.[20,21] The effective antibiotic concentrations in serum may be many times the MBC of the infecting pathogen, depending on additional characteristics. The most effective antibiotics are those that have a rapid and homogeneous distribution into the vegetation and those that kill bacteria most rapidly and are least susceptible to a large inoculum. Among the clinically useful antibiotics, aminoglycosides have the most favorable characteristics, followed by β-lactams and then glycopeptides.[21]

SURGERY

Surgery is an important adjunct to management of endocarditis in certain patients.[22] The major causes of death in patients with IE are heart failure and infection of vital organs from septic embolization. In most cases, valvectomy and valve replacement are performed to remove infected tissues and restore hemodynamic function. The most important indications for surgery include the following[4,21]:

- Moderate to severe congestive heart failure
- Valvular obstruction
- Local suppurative complications such as a myocardial abscess
- Endocarditis caused by resistant organisms (e.g., most cases of endocarditis caused by Enterobacteriaceae, *Pseudomonas,* or fungi)
- Almost all cases of early PVE
- Persistent bacteremia or other evidence of failure of appropriate medical therapy

Replacement of an infected valve for the conditions listed is recommended even in the presence of active and uncontrolled infection. If valvular dysfunction requires surgery, early valve replacement is preferable to waiting for the completion of antimicrobial therapy. When valve replacement surgery is performed in the face of active infection the frequency of reinfection is surprisingly low. The aggressive use of early surgical intervention is particularly important in PVE. Early studies reported mortality with surgery in patients with early and late PVE to be 74% and 43%, respectively,[4] although more recent trials have found mortality to be 20–30%.[10]

TABLE 104.3. SUGGESTED REGIMENS FOR THERAPY FOR ENDOCARDITIS DUE TO PENICILLIN-SUSCEPTIBLE VIRIDANS STREPTOCOCCI AND *STREPTOCOCCUS BOVIS* (MIC ≤ 0.1 μg/mL)

Antibiotic	Adult Dose and Route	Pediatric Dose and Route	Duration (wk)
1. Aqueous crystalline penicillin G[a]	12–18 million U/24 h IV either continuously or in 6 equally divided doses	150,000–200,000 U/kg per 24 h IV (not to exceed 20 million U/24 h) either continuously or in 6 equally divided doses	4
or			
ceftriaxone	2 g once daily IV or IM		4
2. Aqueous crystalline penicillin G	12–18 million U/24 h IV either continuously or in 6 equally divided doses	150,000–200,000 U/kg per 24 h IV (not to exceed 20 million U/24 h) either continuously or in 6 equally divided doses	2
With gentamicin[b]	1 mg/kg IM or IV (not to exeed 80 mg) every 8 h	2–2.5 mg/kg IV (not to exceed 80 mg) every 8 h	2
3. Vancomycin[c]	30 mg/kg per 24 h IV in 2 equally divided doses, not to exceed 2g/24 h unless serum levels are monitored		4

[a]Preferred in most patients older than 65 years of age and in those with impairment of the eighth nerve or of renal function.
[b]When obtained 1 h after a 20–30 minute IV infusion or IM injection, serum concentration of gentamicin of approximately 3 μg/mL is desirable; trough concentration should be <1μg/mL.
[c]Vancomycin dosages should be reduced in patients with impaired renal function. In obese patients, dosing should be based on ideal body weight. Dosing of aminoglycosides on a milligram per kilogram basis will produce higher serum concentrations in obese than in lean patients. Therefore, in obese patients, dosing should be based on ideal body weight. Relative contraindications to use of aminoglycosides are age greater than 65 years or renal or eighth nerve impairment. (From Bisno AL, Dismukes WE, Durack DT, et al. Antimicrobial treatment of infective endocarditis due to viridans streptococci, enterococci, and staphylococci. JAMA 1989;261:1471–1477, with permission. Copyright 1989, American Medical Association.)

TABLE 104.4. THERAPY FOR ENDOCARDITIS DUE TO STRAINS OF VIRIDANS STREPTOCOCCI AND *STREPTOCOCCUS BOVIS* RELATIVELY RESISTANT TO PENICILLIN G (MIC > 0.1 μg/mL AND < 0.5 μg/mL)[a]

Antibiotic	Adult Dose and Route	Pediatric Dose and Route	Duration (wk)
1. Aqueous crystalline penicillin G[a]	18 million U/24 h IV either continuously or in 6 equally divided doses	200,000–300,000 U/kg per 24 h IV (not to exceed 20 million U/24 h) given continuously or in 6 equally divided doses	4
With gentamicin[b]	1 mg/kg IM or IV (not to exceed 80 mg) every 8 h	2–2.5 mg/kg IM or IV (not to exceed 80 mg) every 8 h	2
2. Vancomycin[c]	30 mg/kg per 24 h IV in 2 equally divided doses, not to exceed 2g/24 h unless serum levels are monitored		4

[a]Cephalothin or cefazolin (with an aminoglycoside for the first 2 weeks) can be used in patients whose penicillin hypersensitivity is not of the immediate type. Antibiotic doses should be modified appropriately for patients with impaired renal function.
[b]Gentamicin should be given in addition to penicillin for the first 2 weeks. Aminoglycosides given on a milligram per kilogram basis will produce higher serum concentrations in obese than in lean patients. Therefore, in obese patients, dosing should be based on ideal body weight. (From Bisno AL, Dismukes WE, Durack DT, et al. Antimicrobial treatment of infective endocarditis due to viridans streptococci, enterococci, and staphylococci. JAMA 1989;261:1471–1477, with permission. Copyright 1989, American Medical Association.)
[c]Vancomycin dosages should be reduced in patients with impaired renal function. In obese patients, dosing should be based on ideal body weight.

TREATMENT OF SPECIFIC ORGANISMS

VIRIDANS STREPTOCOCCAL ENDOCARDITIS

The term viridans streptococcus refers to a large number of different species, such as *S. mutans, S. sanguis,* and *S. mitior* and are the most common cause of IE, especially in cases involving native valves.[18,23] These bacteria are usually α-hemolytic and are common inhabitants of the human mouth and gingiva. During dental surgery, and even when brushing the teeth, these organisms can cause a transient bacteremia, which in the susceptible individual can result in IE. "Alpha-strep" endocarditis is typically subacute and the response to medical treatment is usually good. *Streptococcus bovis* is not a viridans streptococcus, but is included here because it is penicillin sensitive and treatment regimens are the same as for viridans streptococci. It is a group D streptococcus and resides in the gastrointestinal tract. IE caused by *S. bovis* is associated with gastrointestinal pathology, especially colon carcinoma.[1]

Antimicrobial regimens for viridans streptococci have been well studied and response rates exceed 95% in uncomplicated cases. Viridans streptococci are penicillin susceptible, although some are more susceptible than others. Most are "exquisitely" sensitive to penicillin G and have minimum inhibitory concentrations (MIC) ≤0.1 μg/mL.[19,23] Approximately 10–20% are "moderately" susceptible, MIC = 0.1–0.5 μg/mL. This difference in *in vitro* susceptibility has led to recommendations that the MIC should be determined for all viridans streptococci, and the results be used to guide therapy. Although some streptococci are "tolerant" to the killing effects of penicillin (vide infra), this has not been demonstrated to be clinically important, and treatment is the same as for nontolerant organisms.[18,19]

Recommended therapy in the uncomplicated case caused by fully susceptible strains is 2 weeks of combined therapy with penicillin G and gentamicin[19,23] (Table 104.3). Gentamicin is now preferred because serum concentrations are more easily obtained, clinicians are more experienced with its use, and the few strains of streptococci that are resistant to the synergistic effects of streptomycin–penicillin (vide infra) remain susceptible to gentamicin–penicillin. Other aminoglycosides are not recommended. An alternate regimen, 4 weeks of high-dose parenteral penicillin G alone, is equally effective (Table 104.3).[19,23] A 2-week course of penicillin alone is associated with an unacceptably high relapse rate.[24] The decision as to which of the two regimens should be used depends on the perceived risk versus benefit. For example, a 2-week course of an aminoglycoside in an elderly patient with renal impairment may be associated with ototoxicity and worsening renal impairment (in the case of gentamicin). On the other hand, a 4-week course of penicillin alone generally entails greater expense. For patients with complicated infection (e.g., shock or intracardiac abscesses), or when the streptococcus has an MIC of 0.1–0.5 μg/mL, combination therapy with gentamicin and penicillin for the first 2 weeks, followed by penicillin alone for an additional 2 weeks is recommended (Table 104.4).[19,23]

The rationale for combination therapy for penicillin–susceptible viridans streptococci is that synergy against these organisms is usually observed when cell wall active agents are combined with aminoglycosides *in vitro* and *in vivo.*[17–19,23] Synergy results in more rapid sterilization of vegetations in animal models of endocarditis[20] and probably explains the high response rates observed in patients treated for a total of 2 weeks.[19,25] In contrast, for IE caused by streptococci relatively resistant to penicillin (MIC = 0.1–0.5 μg/mL), combination therapy for 2 weeks is recommended, followed by penicillin alone for 2 additional weeks.[19,23] Some authors question the need for combination therapy for such relatively resistant streptococci, pointing out that there are few human data to suggest that patients with endocarditis caused by these organisms respond less well to penicillin alone.[26]

Therapy for the patient with penicillin allergy is relatively straightforward. Vancomycin is effective and is the drug of choice. First-generation and some third-generation (e.g., ceftriaxone) cephalosporins are also effective and may be cost effective.[27,28] Cephalosporins should be avoided in patients who have immediate hypersensitivity to penicillin. It is important to remember that the majority of patients who report an "allergy" to penicillin will have a negative result to penicillin skin testing, and are consequently at very low risk of anaphylaxis.[29] Since the published experience with penicillin is more extensive than that with the alternative regimens, it is necessary to obtain a thorough history of the purported allergy to penicillin before using second-line therapy.

STAPHYLOCOCCAL ENDOCARDITIS

Endocarditis caused by staphylococci is becoming more prevalent, in part because of increasing IV drug abuse, more frequent employment of peripheral and central venous catheters, and more valve replacement surgery.[2,4,7,10,30,31] *Staphylococcus aureus* is the most common organism causing IE both among IV drug abusers and in persons with venous catheters. Coagulase-negative staphylococci (CNST, usually *S. epidermidis*) are prominent causes of PVE. Staphylococcal endocarditis is not a homogeneous disease and appropriate management requires consideration of several factors: (1) Is the organism methicillin resistant? (2) Should combination therapy be used? (3) Is the infection on a native valve or a prosthetic valve? (4) Is the patient an intravenous drug abuser? (5) Is the infection on the left or right side of the heart?

TABLE 104.5. THERAPY FOR ENDOCARDITIS DUE TO *STAPHYLOCOCCUS* IN THE ABSENCE OF PROSTHETIC MATERIAL[a]

Antibiotic	Adult Dose and Route	Pediatric Dose and Route	Duration
Methicillin-Susceptible Staphylococci			
Regimen for non–penicillin-allergic patients			
Nafcillin	2 g IV every 4 h	150–200 mg/kg per 24 h IV (not to exceed 12 g/24 h) in 4 to 6 equally divided doses	4–6 wk
or			
Oxacillin	2 g IV every 4 h	150–200 mg/kg per 24 h IV (not to exceed 12 g/24 h) in 4 to 6 equally divided doses	4–6 wk
With optional addition of gentamicin[b,c]	1 mg/kg IM or IV (not to exceed 80 mg) every 8h	2–2.5 mg/kg IV (not to exceed 80 mg) every 8 h	3–5 d
Regimen for penicillin-allergic patients			
Cefazolin[d] (or other first generation cephalosporin in equivalent dosages)	2 g IV every 8 h	80–100 mg/kg per 24 h IV (not to exceed 6 g/24 h) in equally divided doses every 8 h	4–6 wk
With optional addition of gentamicin[b]	Same as for non–penicillin-allergic patient	Same as for non–penicillin-allergic patient	3–5 d
Vancomycin[b,e]	30 mg/kg per 24 h IV in 2 equally divided doses, not to exceed 2 g/24 h unless serum levels are monitored	40 mg/kg per 24 h IV in 2 or 4 equally divided doses, not to exceed 2 g/24 h unless serum levels are monitored	4–6 wk
Methicillin-Resistant Staphylococci			
Vancomycin[b,e]	30 mg/kg per 24 h IV in 2 equally divided doses, not to exceed 2 g/24 h unless serum levels are monitored	40 mg/kg per 24 h IV in 2 or 4 equally divided doses, not to exceed 2 g/24 h unless serum levels are monitored	4–6 wk

[a]Antibiotic doses should be modified appropriately for patients with impaired renal function. For treatment of endocarditis due to penicillin-susceptible staphylococci (MIC <0.1 μg/mL), aqueous crystalline penicillin G (Table 104.3, first regimen) should be used for 4–6 weeks instead of nafcillin or oxacillin. Shorter antibiotic courses have been effective in some drug addicts with right-sided endocarditis due to *Staphylococcus aureus*.
[b]Dosing of aminoglycosides and vancomycin on a milligram per kilogram basis will give higher serum concentrations in obese than in lean patients.
[c]Benefit of additional aminoglycoside has not been established. Risk of toxic reactions due to these agents is increased in patients who are older than age 65 years or who have renal or eighth nerve impairment.
[d]There is potential cross-allergenicity between penicillins and cephalosporins. Cephalosporins should be avoided in patients with immediate-type hypersensitivity to penicillin.
[e]Peak serum concentration of vancomycin should be obtained 1 h after infusion and should be in the range of 30–45 μg/mL for twice daily dosing. Each dose of vancomycin should be infused over 1 h. See text for consideration of optional addition of gentamicin. (From Bisno AL, Dismukes WE, Durack DT, et al. Antimicrobial treatment of infective endocarditis due to viridans streptococci, enterococci, and staphylococci. JAMA 1989;261:1471–1477, with permission. Copyright 1989, American Medical Association.)

Any patient who develops staphylococcal bacteremia is at risk for endocarditis, and many investigators have attempted to develop criteria that identify the bacteremic patient who is also likely to have IE.[31] Hospitalized patients with *S. aureus* bacteremia in whom a focus of infection can be identified, such as a vascular catheter, have less than a 10% incidence of endocarditis after appropriate antimicrobial treatment for 2 weeks, as long as the patient does not have a prosthetic valve or additional clinical evidence for endocarditis.[30,31] In contrast, patients with outpatient-acquired *S. aureus* bacteremia and no known focus of infection are more likely to have IE, and prolonged treatment may be warranted. These general distinctions are most helpful when applied to IV drug abusers but may be less accurate in patients with diabetes.[31]

The recommended therapy for patients with left-sided IE caused by methicillin-sensitive *S. aureus* (MSSA) is 4–6 weeks of oxacillin or nafcillin, often combined with a short course of an aminoglycoside (Table 104.5). From *in vitro* studies, aminoglycoside antibiotics and penicillinase-resistant penicillins or vancomycin are synergistic for most MSSA, and in animal models of endocarditis combinations of a penicillin with an aminoglycoside eradicate organisms from vegetations more rapidly than penicillins alone.[30,31] In

TABLE 104.6. TREATMENT OF STAPHYLOCOCCAL ENDOCARDITIS IN THE PRESENCE OF A PROSTHETIC VALVE OR OTHER PROSTHETIC MATERIAL[a]

Antibiotic	Adult Dose and Route	Pediatric Dose and Route	Duration (wk)
Regimen for Methicillin-Resistant Staphylococci			
Vancomycin[b,c]	30 mg/kg per 24 h IV in 2 equally divided doses, not to exceed 2 g/24 h unless serum levels are monitored	40 mg/kg per 24 h IV in 2 or 4 equally divided doses, not to exceed 2 g/24 h unless serum levels are monitored	≥6
With rifampin[d]	300 mg PO every 8 h	20 mg/kg per 24 h PO (not to exceed 900 mg/24 h) in 2 equally divided doses	≥6
and			
With gentamicin[c,e,f]	1.0 mg/kg IM or IV (not to exceed 80 mg) every 8 h	2–2.5 mg/kg per 24 h IV (not to exceed 80 mg) every 8 h	2
Regimen for Methicillin-Susceptible Staphylococci			
Nafcillin or oxacillin[g]	2 g IV every 4 h	150–200 mg/kg per 24 h IV (not to exceed 12 g/24 h) in 4 to 6 equally divided doses	≥6
With rifampin[d]	300 mg PO every 8 h	20 mg/kg per 24 h PO (not to exceed 900 mg/24 h) in 2 equally divided doses	≥6
and			
With gentamicin[c,e,f]	1.0 mg/kg IM or IV (not to exceed 80 mg) every 8 h	2–2.5 mg/kg IV (not to exceed 80 mg) every 8 h	2

[a]Vancomycin and gentamicin doses must be modified appropriately in patients with renal failure.
[b]Peak serum concentrations of vancomycin should be obtained 1 h after infusion and should be in the range of 30–45 μg/mL for twice daily dosing. Each dose should be infused over 1 h.
[c]Aminoglycosides or vancomycin given on a milligram per kilogram basis will produce higher serum concentrations in obese than in lean patients.
[d]Rifampin is recommended for therapy of infections due to coagulase-negative staphylococci. Its use in coagulase-positive staphylococcal infections is controversial. Rifampin increases the amount of warfarin sodium required for antithrombotic therapy.
[e]Serum concentration of gentamicin should be monitored and dose should be adjusted to obtain a peak level of approximately 3 μg/mL.
[f]Use during initial 2 weeks. See text on alternative aminoglycoside therapy for organisms resistant to gentamicin.
[g]First-generation cephalosporins or vancomycin should be used in penicillin-allergic patients. Cephalosporins should be avoided in patients with immediate-type hypersensitivity to penicillin and in patients infected with methicillin-resistant staphylococci. (From Bisno AL, Dismukes WE, Durack DT, et al. Antimicrobial treatment of infective endocarditis due to viridans streptococci, enterococci, and staphylococci. JAMA 1989;261:1471–1477, with permission. Copyright 1989, American Medical Association.)

human studies, addition of an aminoglycoside for the first week of therapy to nafcillin hastens the resolution of fever and bacteremia, although no effect on survival or relapse rates has been found.[32]

If a patient has a mild allergy to penicillin, first-generation cephalosporins have also been effective (Table 104.6). The use of cephalosporins, particularly cefazolin, has been somewhat controversial for MSSA endocarditis. In the majority of studies these agents appear effective; however, there are reports of failures with cephalosporins despite *in vitro* susceptibility.[33] It has been suggested that cefazolin is more labile to staphylococcal β-lactamase than other cephalosporins accounting for some reported cefazolin failures.[34] Other agents such as clindamycin or rifampin should not be used alone because of high relapse rates with either compound. Moreover, resistance of staphylococci to rifampin given as a single agent develops rapidly.[35] If there is a history of immediate hypersensitivity to penicillin, vancomycin is the agent of choice. Vancomycin, however, only slowly kills *S. aureus* and is generally regarded as inferior therapy to penicillinase-resistant penicillins for MSSA. The use of rifampin as an adjunctive therapy is controversial. Rifampin may be added to vancomycin in refractory or complicated infections in patients with left-sided IE and, in some cases, addition of rifampin appeared to result in dramatic patient improvement.[30,31,36] Generally, antibiotic therapy should be continued for 4–6 weeks. Unfortunately, left-sided IE caused by *S. aureus* continues to have a poor prognosis with a mortality rate of 25–40%.[3,30,31] For reasons discussed in the following section, intravenous drug abusers have a more favorable response to therapy.

TABLE 104.7. THERAPY FOR ENDOCARDITIS DUE TO ENTEROCOCCI (OR TO VIRIDANS STREPTOCOCCI WITH A MIC ≥0.5 μg/mL)[a]

Antibiotic	Adult Dose and Route	Pediatric Dose and Route	Duration (wk)
Regimen for Non–Penicillin-Allergic Patients			
Aqueous crystalline penicillin G	18–30 million U/24 h IV given continuously or in 6 equally divided doses	200,000–300,000 U/kg per 24 h IV (not to exceed 30 million U/24 h) given continuously or in 6 equally divided doses	4–6
With gentamicin[b,c,d]	1 mg/kg IM or IV (not to exceed 80 mg) every 8 h	2–2.5 mg/kg IM or IV (not to exceed 80 mg) every 8 h	4–6
Ampicillin	12 g/24 h IV given continuously or in 6 equally divided doses	300 mg/kg per 24 h IV (not to exceed 12 g/24 h) in 4 to 6 equally divided doses	4–6
With gentamicin[b,c,d]	1 mg/kg IM or IV (not to exceed 80 mg) every 8 h	2–2.5 mg/kg IM or IV (not to exceed 80 mg) every 8 h	4–6
Regimen for Penicillin-Allergic Patients (desensitization should be considered; cephalosporins are not satisfactory alternatives)			
Vancomycin[e]	30 mg/kg per 24 h IV in 2 equally divided doses, not to exceed 2 g/24 h unless serum levels are monitored	40 mg/kg per 24 h IV in 2 equally divided doses, not to exceed 2 g/24 h unless serum levels are monitored	4–6
With gentamicin[b,c,d]	1 mg/kg IM or IV (not to exceed 80 mg) every 8 h	2–2.5 mg/kg IM or IV (not to exceed 80 mg) every 8 h	4–6

[a]Antibiotic doses should be modified appropriately in patients with impaired renal function.
[b]Choice of aminoglycoside depends on resistance level of infecting strain (see text). Enterococci should be tested for high-level resistance (MIC ≥2000 μg/mL).
[c]Serum concentration of gentamicin should be monitored and dose adjusted to obtain a peak level of approximately 3 μg/mL.
[d]Dosing of aminoglycosides and vancomycin on a milligram per kilogram basis will give higher serum concentrations in obese than in lean patients.
[e]Peak serum concentrations of vancomycin should be obtained 1 h after infusion and should be in the range of 30–45 μg/mL for twice daily dosing and 20–35 μg/mL for four times daily dosing. Each dose should be infused over 1 h. (From Bisno AL, Dismukes WE, Durack DT, et al. Antimicrobial treatment of infective endocarditis due to viridans streptococci, enterococci, and staphylococci. JAMA 1989;261:1471–1477, with permission. Copyright 1989, American Medical Association.)

Treatment of Methicillin-Resistant Staphylococcal Endocarditis

During the past decade, greater numbers of staphylococci have become resistant to methicillin and isoxazolyl penicillins.[37] At tertiary care hospitals, up to 50% of *S. aureus* and 80% of CNST are methicillin resistant. Vancomycin is the drug of choice for these organisms since all methicillin-resistant *S. aureus* (MRSA) and most CNST are susceptible (Table 104.6). Addition of rifampin to vancomycin in a prospective trial in 42 addicts with IE caused by MRSA did not result in a more rapid rate of sterile blood cultures, and there was a suggestion that rifampin antagonized the effects of vancomycin.[38] In contrast, patients with PVE caused by methicillin-resistant staphylococci, especially coagulase-negative strains, should receive combination antimicrobial therapy (vide infra).

Treatment of Staphylococcus Endocarditis in the Intravenous Drug Abuser

IE in the IV drug abuser is most frequently (60–80%) caused by *S. aureus,* although other organisms may be more common in certain geographic locations.[39] In this setting the tricuspid valve is most frequently infected, resulting in right-sided IE. Most patients have no history of valve abnormalities, are usually otherwise healthy, and their response to medical treatment is usually good. Nonetheless, surgery may be required in up to 25% of cases.

Standard treatment for MSSA consists of 4 weeks of therapy with a penicillinase-resistant penicillin (Table 104.6), and the clinical response in patients with right-sided IE is generally excellent. In contrast to treatment of left-sided IE, addition of an aminoglycoside to penicillin did not improve outcome in *S. aureus* IE in addicts with right-sided disease.[40]

While 4 weeks of monotherapy with a β-lactamase–stable penicillin is considered optimal therapy, an uncontrolled study found that a select group of addicts with uncomplicated right-sided endocarditis caused by MSSA could be successfully treated with 2 weeks of combination therapy.[41] Forty-seven of 50 patients (94%) were cured after treatment with IV nafcillin (1.5 g every 4 hours) and tobramycin (1.0 mg/kg every 8 hours). A provocative finding was that 2 of the 3 patients treated with vancomycin relapsed, resulting in early termination of this arm of study. In a follow-up investigation, these workers reviewed their experience in 13 IV drug users with IE caused by MSSA who were treated with vancomycin.[42] Five patients (38%) demonstrated an unsatisfactory response to treatment, which is considerably poorer in comparison to results with penicillinase-resistant penicillins. This finding may be related to a slower rate of *in vitro* kill of *S. aureus* by vancomycin compared with nafcillin.[42] These data are consistent with a prospective study in 47 patients with MRSA IE in which patients treated with vancomycin remained bacteremic for a median duration of 7 days, which is substantially longer than has been found in other studies with β-lactam therapy. Although vancomycin historically has been regarded as therapeutically equivalent to penicillins for MSSA infections, these data suggest that careful documentation of the nature of the penicillin allergy should be undertaken before using vancomycin. If vancomycin is selected, a full 4 weeks of therapy is recommended.[43] A second reason to select a penicillin over vancomycin for MSSA infection is the increasing prevalence of vancomycin-resistant enterococci (VRE). Vancomycin is often used inappropriately which contributes to selection of VRE.[44,45] Recent recommendations severely limit the approved uses of vancomycin.

A preliminary report found a predominantly oral regimen to be effective in ten addicts with uncomplicated right-sided endocarditis caused by MSSA.[43,46] Patients received oral ciprofloxacin for 3 weeks (750 mg every 12 hours) and rifampin (300 mg every 12 hours) for the first 7 days. These findings require confirmation in randomized trials before this therapy can be recommended, especially since antibiotic resistance and therapeutic failures in staphylococcal disease have emerged when ciprofloxacin has been given.[47] Nevertheless, in selected cases, oral therapy, abbreviated therapy, and outpatient therapy may be appropriate because costs of hospitalization may be appreciably reduced.[46]

TOLERANCE

Another consideration is that some staphylococci exhibit a phenomenon called "tolerance." A tolerant organism is one which is inhibited, but not killed, by an antibiotic normally considered to be bactericidal.[18,49] One definition of a tolerant strain is the minimum bactericidal concentration (MBC) is greater than 32 times the MIC. In contrast, for most non-tolerant staphylococci, the MIC and MBC are almost the same. Because bactericidal activity is required for successful treatment of IE, there has been concern that infection with a tolerant organism may relapse after treatment. When stringent and consistent criteria are used to detect tolerance among *S. aureus,* the frequency is actually very low, suggesting that tolerance may be primarily a laboratory phenomenon with little clinical significance.[50] Nevertheless, some animal studies of endocarditis suggest that tolerant strains do not respond as readily to β-lactam therapy.[20,51] However, the clinical importance of tolerance has not been clearly demonstrated, and the most recent American Heart Association guidelines for treatment of IE state that concern for tolerance among staphylococci should not affect antibiotic selection.[19]

PROSTHETIC VALVE ENDOCARDITIS

PVE that occurs within 1 year of surgery is usually caused by staphylococci implanted at the time of surgery.[4,10,51] Since this is a nosocomial infection, methicillin-resistant organisms are common and vancomycin is the cornerstone of therapy. PVE responds poorly to medical treatment and has a higher mortality compared to native valve endocarditis, in part because the sewing ring is often infected in addition to the valve leading to valve dehiscence and incompetence and resulting in acute heart failure, which may be fatal.[11] Surgery is often a more essential component of management than are antibiotics. Because of the high morbidity and mortality associated with PVE and refractoriness to therapy, combinations of antimicrobials are usually recommended.[4,10,51,52] For methicillin-resistant staphylococci (both MRSA and CNST), vancomycin is used with rifampin for 6–8 weeks (Table 104.6). An aminoglycoside is added for the first 2 weeks if the organism is susceptible. For methicillin-susceptible staphylococci, a penicillinase-stable penicillin is used in place of vancomycin. Another reason for combination therapy is to prevent the emergence of resistance to rifampin, which frequently occurs when it is used alone. While vancomycin is active *in vitro* for all MRSA, some coagulase-negative staphylococci are resistant to vancomycin.[53] Optimum therapy for these unusual organisms is unknown.

ENTEROCOCCAL ENDOCARDITIS

Enterococci are gram-positive cocci that are normal inhabitants of the human gastrointestinal tract and are ordinarily of low virulence.[54] Historically, they were considered group D streptococci, but have been reclassified into the genus *Enterococcus (E. faecalis* and *E. faecium). Enterococcus faecalis* is the most common (~90%) clinical isolate of the two species. Enterococci cause 5–18% of endocarditis cases and are noteworthy for the following reasons: (1) no single antibiotic is bactericidal; (2) MICs to penicillin are relatively high (1–25 μg/mL); (3) they are intrinsically resistant to all cephalosporins and relatively resistant to aminoglycosides (i.e., "low-level" aminoglycoside resistance); (4) they are killed only by a combination of a cell wall active agent, such as a penicillin or vancomycin, plus an aminoglycoside; and (5) resistance to all available drugs is increasing.[55,56]

Monotherapy with penicillin for IE caused by enterococci results in relapse rates of 50–80%, and combination therapy is always recommended for susceptible strains.[55] The relapse rate following penicillin–gentamicin therapy for susceptible strains is <15%.[3] The killing of enterococci by an aminoglycoside–penicillin combination is the best clinical example of antibiotic synergy. Because the aminoglycoside cannot penetrate the bacterial cell in the absence of the penicillin, enterococci will usually appear to be "resistant" to aminoglycosides by routine susceptibility testing (e.g., low-level resistance). However, in the presence of an agent that disrupts the cell wall, such as penicillin or vancomycin, the aminoglycoside can gain entry, attach to bacterial ribosomes, and cause rapid cell death. An aminoglycoside–vancomycin combination is also synergistic against enterococci and is appropriate therapy for the penicillin-allergic patient.[55]

Enterococcal endocarditis ordinarily requires 4–6 weeks of high-dose penicillin G or ampicillin, plus an aminoglycoside for cure (Table 104.7). A 6-week course is recommended for patients with symptoms longer than 3 months, recurrent cases, and patients with mitral valve involvement. Ampicillin has greater *in vitro* activity, although there are no clinical data to document differences in efficacy compared to penicillin G. Historically, streptomycin has been the most extensively studied aminoglycoside, although gentamicin is presently favored. In the treatment of enterococcal endocarditis, relatively low serum concentrations of the aminoglycoside appear adequate for successful therapy, such as a gentamicin peak concentration of approximately 3 g/mL,[55] although this is a matter of active debate.[57] This treatment does not have the uniformly high success rate seen with IE caused by viridans streptococci, presumably because the organism is more resistant to killing.

Resistance among enterococci to the preceding drugs is increasing.[54,56] Enterococci which exhibit "high-level" resistance to streptomycin (MIC > 2000 μg/mL) are not synergistically killed by penicillin and streptomycin because the aminoglycoside either no longer binds to the ribosome or is inactivated by an aminoglycoside-modifying enzyme, streptomycin adenylase.[56] Since enterococci will appear resistant to aminoglycosides on routine susceptibility testing, the only way to distinguish high-level from low-level resistance is by performing special susceptibility tests using 500–2000 μg/mL of the aminoglycoside. High-level streptomycin-resistant enterococci occur with a frequency of 40–50%, and high-level resistance to gentamicin is now found in 10–50% of isolates. Although most gentamicin-resistant enterococci are resistant to all aminoglycosides (including amikacin), 30–50% remain susceptible to streptomycin.[56] High-level gentamicin resistance is mediated by a bifunctional aminoglycoside-modifying enzyme, 6′-acetyltransferase/2″-phosphotransferase, and most strains also possess streptomycin adenylase. These organisms have not commonly caused IE, data on appropriate therapy are sparse, and therapeutic options are few. Case reports indicate that some patients will respond to very high doses of ampicillin as observed in the early trials of penicillin monotherapy.[58]

In addition to isolates with high-level aminoglycoside resistance, β-lactamase-producing enterococci (especially *E. faecium*) are increasingly reported.[54,59,60] Therapy with vancomycin is usually recommended, although penicillin-β-lactamase inhibitor combinations appear effective.[59] Vancomycin and resistant enterococci are increasingly reported, especially for *E. faecium* (VREF). Vancomycin resistance occurs when the bacterium replaces the normal vancomycin target, D-alananine, D-alananine, with a peptidoglycan precursor that does not bind vancomycin, D-alanine, D-lactate.[60] Some isolates remain susceptible *in vitro* to tetracyclines, and novobiocin but these cannot be regarded as optimum therapy. An experimental streptogramin, quinupristin/dalfopristin (syncercid®) appears to be most promising. Of great concern is that these multiply-resistant enterococci will transmit resistance traits to *S. aureus*.

GRAM-NEGATIVE BACILLI

Endocarditis caused by gram-negative bacilli is relatively uncommon; although the incidence may be increasing.[61] Patients at higher risk include IV drug abusers and those with prosthetic valves. The organism most commonly associated with gram-negative rod endocarditis in IV drug abusers is *Pseudomonas aeruginosa.* Other gram-negative bacilli causing IE include other pseudomonads, *Serratia marcescens, Escherichia coli, Enterobacter, Salmonella,* and *Haemophilus.* Generally, these infections have a poor prognosis with mortality rates as high as 60–80%.[3]

Overall, there is very little clinical information on which to base solid recommendations for treatment. For most cases of IE due to *P. aeruginosa* and Enterobacteriaceae, antibiotics and valve replacement are necessary. Antimicrobial therapy includes the combination of an aminoglycoside and an extended-spectrum β-lactam.[61] One group of investigators reviewed the therapeutic outcome of patients with *Pseudomonas* endocarditis and compared the benefit of combining varying doses of aminoglycosides with or without valve replacement.[62,63] When patients were treated with "low-dose" aminoglycosides (<5 mg/kg/d gentamicin) with or without surgery, the survival rates were 50% and 25%, respectively. When higher doses were used (at least 8 mg/kg/d gentamicin), the survival rate was 65%, and when high-dose therapy was combined with surgery, survival was 86%. Even at the higher dosage, the frequency of aminoglycoside toxicity was low.

The appropriate regimen for the treatment of gram-negative bacillary endocarditis caused by Enterobacteriaceae depends on the results of *in vitro* susceptibility testing. For *Klebsiella pneumoniae, E. coli,* and *Proteus mirabilis,* a third-generation cephalosporin is frequently combined with an aminoglycoside. Treatment should generally be continued for 6 weeks. In light of the recalcitrant nature of many valvular gram-negative bacillary infections to medical therapy alone, consultation with a cardiac surgeon on confirmation of the diagnosis is an essential component of care for these patients.

FUNGAL ENDOCARDITIS

Fungi cause fewer than 3% of cases of endocarditis and most patients have undergone recent cardiovascular surgery, are IV drug abusers, have received prolonged treatment with IV catheters or antibiotics, or are immunocompromised.[1,8,64] *Candida* sp. and *Aspergillus* sp. are most commonly involved, and the underlying mortality is high for the following reasons: (1) the large, bulky vegetations that often form, (2) the systemic septic embolization that often occurs, (3) the tendency for fungi to invade the myocardium, (4) the poor penetration of vegetations by antifungals, (5) the low toxic/therapeutic ratio of agents such as amphotericin B, and (6) the lack of consistent fungicidal activity of available antifungal agents.

Since these infections occur infrequently, there are scant clinical data from which solid treatment recommendations may be made. Amphotericin B, with or without flucytosine, along with valve replacement is recommended for *Candida* and *Aspergillus* endocarditis.[64] The usefulness of fluconazole and itraconazole is unknown at this time, although their lack of fungicidal activity would suggest a limited role. For almost all cases of PVE caused by fungi, combined antifungal and surgical therapy is required.

LESS COMMON CAUSES OF INFECTIVE ENDOCARDITIS

HACEK GROUP

Gram-negative bacteria from the HACEK group (*Haemophilus* sp., *Actinobacillus actinomycetemcomitans, Cardiobacterium hominis, Eikenella corrodens, Kingella* sp.) are unusual causes of IE, and typically present as a subacute illness with large vegetations and emboli.[61] These oropharyngeal organisms are typically slow growing and fastidious, and should be considered as possible causes of "culture-negative" endocarditis. High-doses of a third-generation cephalosporin for 4 weeks is recommended therapy, and valve replacement is often required.[19]

EVALUATION OF THERAPEUTIC OUTCOMES

The evaluation of patients treated for IE includes assessment of signs and symptoms, reculture of blood, *in vitro* microbiologic tests (e.g., MIC, MBC, or serum bactericidal titers), antimicrobial serum concentration determinations, and other tests that may be necessary in the evaluation of organ function.[65]

SIGNS AND SYMPTOMS

With successful treatment, fever usually subsides within a week of initiating therapy.[65] Persistence of fever may indicate ineffective antimicrobial therapy, emboli, infections of intravascular catheters that have been in place for long periods of time, or a drug reaction. In some patients, low-grade fever may persist even with appropriate antimicrobial therapy. With defervescence the patient should begin to feel better and other symptoms, such as lethargy or weakness, should subside.

BLOOD CULTURES AND BACTERIAL SUSCEPTIBILITY

With effective therapy, blood cultures should be negative within a few days, although microbiological response to vancomycin may be unusually slow.[65] If bacteria continue to be isolated from blood beyond the first few days of therapy, it may indicate that the antimicrobials are inactive against the pathogen, or that the doses used are not producing adequate concentrations at the site of infection. After the initiation of therapy, blood cultures should be rechecked, possibly daily, until they are found negative. During the remainder of therapy, frequent blood culturing is not necessary.

For all isolates from blood cultures, MICs and possibly MBCs should be determined.[19,66] The antimicrobials tested should include those being used and alternatives that may be required as a result of intolerance, allergy, or resistance. Occasionally, it may be useful to determine if synergy exists for antimicrobial combinations, although synergistic regimens can usually be predicted from literature sources. Methods for *in vitro* determinations of synergy are summarized in Chapter 97.

SERUM BACTERICIDAL TITER

Serum bactericidal titers (SBTs) (also called "Schlicter tests") have been used for many years and in association with a number of infectious diseases.[66,67] The SBT is the greatest dilution of a patient's serum sample, obtained while receiving antimicrobial treatment, that kills greater than 99.9% of an inoculum of the infecting pathogen *in vitro* over 18–24 hours. Because the antibiotic in serum accounts for the vast majority of the bactericidal activity, knowledge of the serum concentration and the MBC for the organism will reliably predict the SBT. SBTs are a rudimentary form of pharmacodynamic modeling since the titer incorporates both the pharmacokinetics of the antibiotic and the MBC.

In animal models of endocarditis, studies suggest that an SBT of 1:8 is predictive of response.[20] In humans with endocarditis, however, the correlation with SBTs and outcome is less clear. A multicenter study found peak and trough SBTs of ≥1:64 and ≥1:32 were associated with 100% response, respectively, although a lower titer did not predict failure.[68] For most streptococci causing endocarditis it is easy to achieve an SBT ≥1:32 because the MBC is low relative to achievable concentrations of penicillin. However, for enterococci, methicillin-resistant staphylococci, and gram-negative bacilli, it may be difficult to achieve high SBTs. Thus SBTs are of little use in IE caused by streptococci and in MSSA (where serum concentrations are high and MBCs are low), but may be of value for more unusual organisms where the treatment experience is more limited.

The reasons that SBTs have not always predicted outcome include the failure to consider variables that are likely to be important determinants of response, such as size of the vegetation, host defenses, rates of kill, and location of the infection (left or right side of the heart). Lack of test standardization has been another problem, and is addressed in greater detail in Chapter 97. Primary variables include method of diluting serum (using broth or serum), bacterial inoculum size, timing of collection of the blood sample (peak or trough), and measurement of the test endpoint.

At present, SBTs have little value in monitoring common types of IE. This test may be useful when the causative organisms are only moderately susceptible to antimicrobials, when less well-established regimens are used, or when response to therapy is suboptimal and dosage escalation is considered. In addition, an extremely high SBT may suggest that a decrease in antimicrobial dose is acceptable when the patient is at high risk of drug toxicity.

SERUM DRUG CONCENTRATION

Of the agents commonly used for IE, serum concentration determinations are routinely available for aminoglycosides (except streptomycin) and vancomycin.[65] However, few data exist to support the necessity of attaining any specific serum concentrations in patients with IE. While it is true that serum concentrations of the antimicrobial should generally exceed the MBC of the organism, in practice this principle is usually not helpful in monitoring patients with endocarditis. This is because aminoglycoside concentrations rarely exceed the MBC for certain organisms, such as streptococci and enterococci, or because concentrations have not been correlated to response, such as aminoglycosides and vancomycin for staphylococci.[69,70] However, in IE caused by *P. aeruginosa,* clinical trials previously discussed suggest that higher aminoglycoside concentrations (e.g., 15–20 μg/mL) improve the outcome to therapy.[62,63] These higher concentrations are justified because of the high mortality associated with IE caused by *P. aeruginosa.* In contrast, when aminoglycosides are given in combination for IE caused by gram-positive cocci, peak serum concentrations are recommended to be on the low side of the traditional ranges (3 μg/mL for gentamicin and tobramycin). Some animal models of endocarditis suggest greater efficacy with single large doses of aminoglycosides at infrequent intervals compared to more frequent administration,[71] and limited human trials have reported success.[28] However, most clinicians would not use single daily doses of aminoglycosides in IE until more human data are available.

ANTICOAGULATION

The use of anticoagulants for patients with native valve endocarditis is ordinarily contraindicated because of increased frequency of subarachnoid hemorrhage or other bleeding complications, possibly from areas of embolic infarction or from mycotic aneurysms. With prosthetic valve endocarditis the use of anticoagulants is controversial; however, it is probably best that patients who require anticoagulants for prosthetic valves be continued on them during endocarditis therapy.[72,73]

PREVENTION OF ENDOCARDITIS

Antimicrobial prophylaxis is used to prevent IE in patients believed to be at high risk.[74,75] The use of antimicrobials for this purpose requires consideration of (1) the types of patients who are at risk; (2) procedures causing bacteremia; (3) the organisms that are likely to cause endocarditis; and (4) the pharmacokinetics, spectrum, cost, and ease of administration of available agents. The objective of prophylaxis is to diminish the likelihood of IE in high-risk individuals who are undergoing procedures that cause transient bacteremia (Table 104.8). Although there are no prospective human trials to demonstrate a benefit of prophylaxis, animal studies have shown benefit, and retrospective studies in humans suggest a reduction of endocarditis in selected cases following dental surgery when prophylaxis is employed.[76] The mechanism of a beneficial effect in humans is unclear, but antibiotics may decrease the number of bacteria at the surgical site, kill bacteria once introduced into the blood, and/or prevent adhesion to the valve. A recent trial found that prophylaxis did not reduce the frequency of bacteremia immediately following tooth extraction compared to a control group, suggesting a reduction in adhesion as a more likely mechanism.[77]

PATIENTS AT RISK

Patients with certain cardiac lesions, particularly those with a history of rheumatic heart disease and prosthetic heart valves, are at risk for developing endocarditis (Table 104.9). However, only 15–25% of patients who develop IE are in a definable high-risk category and only a small proportion of high-risk patients (estimated to be 1 of 53–115,500 persons) will develop IE if prophylaxis is not given.[74,75,78] Thus even if prophylaxis were 100% effective, and all high-risk subjects received prophylaxis prior to a procedure known to result in bacteremia, the overall incidence of IE would decrease by less than 10%. Despite the low probability that IE will develop, prophylaxis for dental surgery and some gastrointestinal procedures is recommended because of the significant morbidity associated with IE. Patients undergoing valve implant surgery are at a much greater risk for IE than for dental surgery. Such patients should receive parenteral prophylaxis, although the most appropriate agent is a matter of debate.

PROCEDURES CAUSING BACTEREMIA

Bacteremia accompanies many everyday events, such as brushing teeth (~25%) and chewing (~38%), although certain medical and surgical procedures are more likely to cause a transient bacteremia.[79] For dental procedures of the gums and oral structures which causes bleeding, viridans streptococci frequently (~40%) cause bacteremia, whereas instrumentation and surgery of the gastrointestinal and genitourinary tracts more often result in enterococcal bacteremia.

TABLE 104.8. DENTAL OR SURGICAL PROCEDURES FOR WHICH ENDOCARDITIS PROPHYLAXIS IS RECOMMENDED[a]

- Dental procedures known to induce gingival or mucosal bleeding, including professional cleaning
- Tonsillectomy and/or adenoidectomy
- Surgical operations that involve intestinal or respiratory mucosa
- Bronchoscopy with a rigid bronchoscope
- Sclerotherapy for esophageal varices
- Esophageal dilatation
- Gallbladder surgery
- Cystoscopy
- Urethral dilatation
- Urethral catheterization if urinary tract infection is present
- Urinary tract surgery if urinary tract infection is present
- Prostatic surgery
- Incision and drainage of infected tissue
- Vaginal hysterectomy
- Vaginal delivery in the presence of infection

[a]This table lists selected procedures but is not meant to be all inclusive. (From Dajani AS, Bisno AL, Chung KJ. Prevention of bacterial endocarditis: Recommendations by the American Heart Association. JAMA 1990;264:2919–2922, with permission. Copyright 1990, American Medical Association.)

TABLE 104.9. CARDIAC CONDITIONS[a]

Endocarditis Prophylaxis Recommended
- Prosthetic cardiac valves, including bioprosthetic and homograft valves
- Previous bacterial endocarditis, even in the absence of heart disease
- Most congenital cardiac malformations
- Rheumatic and other acquired valvular dysfunction, even after valvular surgery
- Hypertrophic cardiomyopathy
- Mitral valve prolapse with valvular regurgitation

Endocarditis Prophylaxis Not Recommended
- Isolated secundum atrial septal defect
- Surgical repair without residua beyond 6 mo of secundum atrial septal defect, ventricular septal defect, or patent ductus arteriosus
- Previous coronary artery bypass graft surgery
- Mitral valve prolapse without valvular regurgitation[b]
- Physiologic, functional, or innocent heart murmurs
- Previous Kawasaki disease without valvular dysfunction
- Previous rheumatic fever without valvular dysfunction
- Cardiac pacemakers and implanted defibrillators

[a]This table lists selected conditions but is not meant to be all inclusive.
[b]Individuals who have a mitral valve prolapse associated with thickening and/or redundancy of the valve leaflets may be at increased risk for bacterial endocarditis, particularly men who are 45 years of age or older. (From Dajani AS, Bisno AL, Chung KJ. Prevention of bacterial endocarditis: Recommendations by the American Heart Association. JAMA 1990;264:2919–2922, with permission. Copyright 1990, American Medical Association.)

TABLE 104.10. RECOMMENDED STANDARD PROPHYLACTIC REGIMEN FOR DENTAL, ORAL, OR UPPER RESPIRATORY TRACT PROCEDURES IN PATIENTS WHO ARE AT RISK[a]

Drug	Dosing Regimen[b]
Standard regimen	
Amoxicillin	3 g orally 1 h before procedure; then 1.5 g 6 h after initial dose
Amoxicillin/penicillin-allergic patients	
Erythromycin	Erythromycin ethylsuccinate, 800 mg, or erythromycin stearate, 1 g, orally 2 h before procedure; then half the dose 6 h after initial dose
or	
Clindamycin	300 mg orally 1 h before procedure and 150 mg 6 h after initial dose

[a]Includes those with prosthetic heart valves and other high-risk patients.
[b]Initial pediatric doses are as follows: amoxicillin, 50 mg/kg; erythromycin ethylsuccinate or erythromycin stearate, 20 mg/kg; and clindamycin, 10 mg/kg. Follow-up doses should be one half the initial dose. Total pediatric dose should not exceed total adult dose. The following weight ranges may also be used for the initial pediatric dose of amoxicillin: <15 kg, 750 mg; 15 to 30 kg, 1500 mg; and >30 kg, 3000 mg (full adult dose). (From Dajani AS, Bisno AL, Chung KJ. Prevention of bacterial endocarditis: Recommendations by the American Heart Association. JAMA 1990;264:2919–2922, with permission. Copyright 1990, American Medical Association.)

TABLE 104.11. ALTERNATE PROPHYLACTIC REGIMENS FOR DENTAL, ORAL, OR UPPER RESPIRATORY TRACT PROCEDURES IN PATIENTS WHO ARE AT RISK

Drug	Dosing Regimen[a]
Patients unable to take oral medication	
Ampicillin	Intravenous or intramuscular administration of ampicillin, 2 g, 30 min before procedure; then intravenous or intramuscular administration of ampicillin, 1 g, or oral administration of amoxicillin, 1.5 g, 6 h after initial dose
Ampicillin/amoxicillin/penicillin-allergic patients unable to take oral medications	
Clindamycin	Intravenous administration of 300 mg 30 min before procedure and an intravenous or oral administration of 150 mg 6 h after initial dose
Patients considered high risk and not candidates for standard regimen	
Ampicillin, gentamicin, and amoxicillin	Intravenous or intramuscular administration of ampicillin, 2 g, plus gentamicin, 1.5 mg/kg (not to exceed 80 mg), 30 min before procedure; followed by amoxicillin, 1.5 g, orally 6 h after initial dose; alternatively, the parenteral regimen may be repeated 8 h after initial dose
Ampicillin/amoxicillin/penicillin-allergic patients considered high risk	
Vancomycin	Intravenous administration of 1 g over 1 h, starting 1 h before procedure; no repeated dose necessary

[a]Initial pediatric doses are as follows: ampicillin, 50 mg/kg; clindamycin, 10 mg/kg; gentamicin, 2.0 mg/kg; and vancomycin, 20 mg/kg. Follow-up doses should be one half the initial dose. Total pediatric dose should not exceed total adult dose. No initial dose is recommended in this table for amoxicillin (25 mg/kg is the follow-up dose). (From Dajani AS, Bisno AL, Chung KJ. Prevention of bacterial endocarditis: Recommendations by the American Heart Association. JAMA 1990;264:2919–2922, with permission. Copyright 1990, American Medical Association.)

TABLE 104.12. REGIMENS FOR GENITOURINARY/GASTROINTESTINAL PROCEDURES

Drug	Dosage Regimen[a]
Standard regimen	
Ampicillin, gentamicin, and amoxicillin	Intravenous or intramuscular administration of ampicillin, 2 g, plus gentamicin, 1.5 mg/kg (not to exceed 80 mg), 30 min before procedure; followed by amoxicillin, 1.5 g, orally 6 h after initial dose; alternatively, the parenteral regimen may be repeated once 8 h after initial dose
Ampicillin/amoxicillin/penicillin-allergic patient regimen	
Vancomycin and gentamicin	Intravenous administration of vancomycin, 1 g, over 1 h plus intravenous or intramuscular administration of gentamicin, 1.5 mg/kg (not to exceed 80 mg), 1 h before procedure; may be repeated once 8 h after initial dose
Alternate low-risk patient regimen	
Amoxicillin	3 g orally 1 h before procedure; then 1.5 g 6 h after initial dose

[a]Initial pediatric doses are as follows: ampicillin, 50 mg/kg; amoxicillin, 50 mg/kg; gentamicin 2 mg/kg; and vancomycin, 20 mg/kg. Follow-up doses should be half the initial dose. Total pediatric dose should not exceed total adult dose. (From Dajani AS, Bisno AL, Chung KJ. Prevention of bacterial endocarditis: Recommendations by the American Heart Association. JAMA 1990;264:2919–2922, with permission. Copyright 1990, American Medical Association.)

ANTIBIOTIC REGIMENS

A 3-g dose of amoxicillin is recommended for adult patients at risk, given 60 minutes prior to undergoing procedures associated with bacteremia.[79,80] This is to be followed by 1.5 g 6 hours later (Table 104.10). For penicillin-allergic patients or those undergoing gastrointestinal surgery, alternative prophylaxis is recommended (Tables 104.11 and 104.12). The appropriate duration of antimicrobial prophylaxis is not precisely known, but is believed to be relatively short. It appears that these newer guidelines are often not adhered to, at least not for dental surgery.[81,82]

REFERENCES

1. Scheld WM, Sande MA. Endocarditis and intravascular infections, in Mandell GL, Dolin R, Bennett JE (eds): Principles and Practice of Infectious Diseases, 4th ed. New York, Churchill Livingstone, 1995, pp 740–783.
2. Bayer A S. Infective endocarditis. Clin Infect Dis 1993;173:313–320.
3. Gold MJ. Cure rates and long-term prognosis, in Kaye D (ed): Infective Endocarditis, 2nd ed. New York, Raven Press, 1992, pp 455–464.
4. Threlkel MG, Cobbs CG. Infectious disorders of prosthetic valves and intravascular devices, in Mandell GL, Dolin R, Bennett JE (eds): Principles and Practice of Infectious Diseases, 4th ed. New York, Churchill Livingstone, 1995, pp 783–793.
5. Saiman L, Prince A, Gersony WM. Pediatric infective endocarditis in the modern era. J Pediatr 1993;122:847–853.
6. Steckelberg JM, Wilson WR. Risk factors for infective endocarditis. Infect Dis Clin North Am 1993;7:9–19.
7. Fang G, Keys TF, Gentry LO, et al. Prosthetic valve endocarditis resulting from nosocomial bacteremia. A prospective, multicenter study. Ann Intern Med 1993;119:560–567.
8. Tunkel AR. Infecting microorganisms, in Kaye D (ed): Infective Endocarditis, 2nd ed. New York, Raven Press, 1992, pp 85–97.
9. Johnson CM. Adherence events in the pathogenesis of infective endocarditis. Infect Dis Clin North Am 1993;7:21–36.
10. Whitener C, Caputo GM, Weitekamp MR, Karchmer AW. Endocarditis due to coagulase-negative staphylococci: Microbiologic, epidemiologic, and clinical considerations. Infect Dis Clin North Am 1993;7:81–96.
11. Murphy JG, Foster-Smith K. Management of complications of infective endocarditis with emphasis on echocardiographic findings. Infect Dis Clin North Am 1993;7:153–165.
12. Kaye KM, Kaye D. Laboratory findings including blood cultures, in Kaye D (ed): Infectious Endocarditis, 2nd ed. New York, Raven Press, 1992, pp 117–124.
13. Mugge A. Echocardiographic detection of cardiac valve vegetations and prognostic implications. Infect Dis Clin North Am 1993;7:877–898.
14. Lukes AS, Bright DK, Durack DT. Diagnosis of infective endocarditis. Infect Dis Clin North Am 1993;7:1–8.
15. Bush LM, Johnson CC. Clinical syndrome and diagnosis, in Kaye D (ed): Infectious Endocarditis, 2nd ed. New York, Raven Press, 1992, pp 99–115.
16. Durack DT, Lukes AS, Bright DK. New criteria for diagnosis of infective endocarditis: Utilization of specific echocardiographic findings. Am J Med 1994;96:200–209.
17. Baldassarre JS, Kaye D. Principles and overview of antibiotic therapy, in Kaye D (ed): Infectious Endocarditis, 2nd ed. New York, Raven Press, 1992, pp 169–190.
18. Levison ME. In vitro assays, in Kaye D (ed): Infectious Endocarditis, 2nd ed. New York, Raven Press, 1992, pp 151–167.
19. Wilson WR, Karchmer AW, Dajani AS, et al. Antibiotic treatment of adults with infective endocarditis due to streptococci, enterococci, staphylococci, and HACEK microorganisms. JAMA 1995;274:1706–1713.
20. Tunkel AR, Scheld WM. Experimental models of endocarditis, in Kaye D (ed): Infectious Endocarditis, 2nd ed. New York, Raven Press, 1992, pp 37–56.
21. Carbon C, Cremieux A-C, Fantin B. Pharmacokinetics and pharmacodynamic aspects of therapy of experimental endocarditis. Infect Dis Clin North Am 1993;7:37–51.
22. Douglas JL, Dismukes WE. Surgical therapy of infective endocarditis on natural valves, in Kaye D (ed): Infectious Endocarditis, 2nd ed. New York, Raven Press, 1992, pp 397–411.
23. Roberts RB. Streptococcal endocarditis: the viridans and beta hemolytic streptococci, in Kaye D (ed): Infectious Endocarditis, 2nd ed. New York, Raven Press, 1992, pp 191–208.
24. Tompsett R, Robbins WC, Berntsen C Jr. Short-term penicillin and dihydrostreptomycin therapy of streptococcal endocarditis. Results of the treatment of thirty-five patients. Am J Med 1958;24:57–67.
25. Wilson WR, Thompson RL, Wilkowsky CJ, et al. Short-term therapy for streptococcal infective endocarditis. Combined intramuscular administration of penicillin and streptomycin. JAMA 1981;245:360–363.
26. DiNubile MJ. Treatment of endocarditis caused by relatively resistant nonenterococcal streptococci: Is penicillin enough? Rev Infect Dis 1990;12:112–115.
27. Francioli PB. Ceftriaxone and outpatient treatment of infective endocarditis. Infect Dis Clin North Am 1993;7:97–116.
28. Francioli P, Ruch W, Stamboulian D, et al. Treatment of streptococcal endocarditis with a single daily dose of ceftriaxone and netilmicin for 14 days: a prospective multicenter study. Clin Inf Dis 1995;21:1406–10.
29. Weiss ME, Adkinson NF. Beta-lactam allergy, in Mandell GL, Bennett JE, Dolin R (eds): Principles and Practice of Infectious Diseases, 4th ed. New York, Churchill Livingstone, 1995, pp 272–278.
30. Karchmer A. Staphylococcal endocarditis. In Kaye D (ed): Infectious Endocarditis, 2nd ed. New York, Raven Press, 1992, pp 225–249.
31. Mortara LA, Bayer AS. Staphylococcus aureus bacteremia and endocarditis: New diagnostic and therapeutic concepts. Infect Dis Clin North Am 1993;7:53–68.
32. Korzeniowski O, Sande MA. The National Collaborative Endocarditis Study Group. Combination antimicrobial ther-

apy for *Staphylococcus aureus* endocarditis in patients addicted to parenteral drugs and in non-addicts. Ann Intern Med 1982;97:496–503.

33. Bryant RE, Alford RH. Unsuccessful treatment of staphylococcal endocarditis with cefazolin. JAMA 1977;237:569–570.
34. Sabath LD. Reappraisal of the antistaphylococcal activities of first-generation (narrow spectrum) and second-generation (expanded spectrum) cephalosporins. Antimicrob Agents Chemother 1989;33:407–411.
35. Mandell GL, Moorman DR. Therapy of experimental staphylococcal infections: Effect of rifampin alone and in combination on development of resistance. Antimicrob Agents Chemother 1980;17:658–662.
36. Faville RJ, Zaske DE, Kaplan EL, et al. *Staphylococcus aureus* endocarditis: Combined therapy with vancomycin and rifampin. JAMA 1978;240:1963–1965.
37. Chambers HF. Methicillin-resistant staphylococci. Clin Microbiol Rev 1988;1:173–186.
38. Levine DP, Fromm BS, Reddy BR. Slow response to vancomycin or vancomycin plus rifampin in methicillin-resistant *Staphylococcus aureus* endocarditis. Ann Intern Med 1991;115:674–680.
39. Sande MA, Lee B, Mills J, Chambers HF. Endocarditis in intravenous drug abusers, In Kaye D (ed): Infectious Endocarditis, 2nd ed. New York, Raven Press, 1992, pp 345–357.
40. Ahrams B, Sklaver A, Hoffman T, et al. Single or combination therapy of staphylococcal endocarditis in intravenous drug abusers. Ann Intern Med 1979;90:789–791.
41. Chambers HF, et al. Right-sided endocarditis in intravenous drug abusers: Two-week combination therapy. Ann Intern Med 1988;104:619–624.
42. Small PM, Chambers HF. Vancomycin for *Staphylococcus aureus* endocarditis in intravenous drug users. Antimicrob Agents Chemother 1990;34:1227–1231.
43. Chambers H. Short-course combination and oral therapies of *Staphylococcus aureus* endocarditis. Infect Dis Clin North Am 1993;7:69–80.
44. Ena J, Dich R, Jones R, et al. The epidemiology of intravenous vancomycin usage in a university hospital. JAMA 1993;269:598–602.
45. Hospital Infection Control Practices Advisory Committee (HIC PAC). Recommendations for preventing the spread of vancomycin resistance. Infection Control and Hosp Epidemiol 1995;16:105–113.
46. Dworkin RJ, et al. Treatment of right-sided *Staphylococcus aureus* endocarditis in intravenous drug abusers with ciprofloxacin and rifampin. Lancet 1989;2:1071–1073.
47. Tebas P, Martinez Ruiz R, Roman F, et al. Early resistance to rifampin and ciprofloxacin in the treatment of right-sided *Staphylococcus aureus* endocarditis [letter]. J Infect Dis 1991;163:204–205.
48. Patton JP. Infective endocarditis: Economic considerations, in Kaye D (ed): Infective Endocarditis, 2nd ed. New York, Raven Press, 1992, pp 413–422.
49. Douglas JL, Cobbs CG. Prosthetic valve endocarditis, in Kaye D (ed): Infective Endocarditis, 2nd ed. New York, Raven Press, 1992, pp 375–396.
50. Sherris J. Problems in in vitro determination of antibiotic tolerance in clinical isolates. Antimicrob Agents Chemother 1986;30:633–637.
51. Voorne GP, Thompson J, Goessens WHF, et al. Role of tolerance in cloxacillin treatment of experimental *Staphylococcus aureus* endocarditis. J Infect Dis 1991;163:640–643.
52. Karchmer AW, Archer GL. The endocarditis study group. Methicillin-resistant *Staphylococcus epidermidis* prosthetic valve endocarditis. 24th Interscience Conference on Antimicrobial Agents and Chemotherapy, October 1984, abstract 476.
53. Johnson AP, Uttey AH, Woodford N, George RC. Resistance to vancomycin and teicoplanin: An emerging clinical problem. Clin Microbiol Rev 1990;3:280–291.
54. Murray BE. The life and times of the enterococcus. Clin Microbiol Rev 1990;3:46–65.
55. Eliopolis GM. Enterococcal endocarditis, in Kaye D (ed): Infective Endocarditis, 2nd ed. New York, Raven Press, 1992, pp 209–223.
56. Eliopolis GM. Aminoglycoside resistant enterococcal endocarditis. Infect Dis Clin North Am 1993;7:117–133.
57. Fantin B, Carbon C. Importance of the aminoglycoside dosing regimen in the penicillin-netilmicin combination for treatment of *Enterococcus faecalis*-induced experimental endocarditis. Antimicrob Agents Chemother 1990;34:2387–2391.
58. Lipman ML, Silva J. Endocarditis due to *Streptococcus faecalis* with high-level resistance to gentamicin. Rev Infect Dis 1989;11:325–328.
59. Wells VD, Wong ES, Murray BE, et al. Infections due to beta-lactamase-producing, high-level gentamicin-resistant *Enterococcus faecalis*. Ann Intern Med 1992;116:285–292.
60. Tailor SA, Bailey EM, Rybak MJ. Enterococcus, an emerging pathogen. Ann Pharmacother 1993;27:1231–1242.
61. Hessen MT, Abrutyn E. Gram-negative bacterial endocarditis, in Kaye D (ed): Infective Endocarditis, 2nd ed. New York, Raven Press, 1992, pp 251–264.
62. Reyes MP, Brown WJ, Lerner AM. Treatment of patients with *Pseudomonas* endocarditis with high dose aminoglycoside and carbenicillin therapy. Medicine 1978;57:57–67.
63. Reyes MP, Lerner AM. Current problems in the treatment of infective endocarditis due to *Pseudomonas aeruginosa.* Rev Infect Dis 1983;5:314–321.
64. Moyer DV, Edwards JE. Fungal endocarditis, in Kaye D (ed): Infective Endocarditis, 2nd ed. New York, Raven Press, 1992, pp 299–312.
65. Santoro J, Ingerman M. Response to therapy: Relapse and reinfections, in Kaye D (ed): Infective Endocarditis, 2nd ed. New York, Raven Press, 1992, pp 423–433.
66. Levinson ME. *In vitro* assays, in Kaye D (ed): Infective Endocarditis, 2nd ed. New York, Raven Press, 1992, pp 151–167.
67. MacLowery JD. Perspective: The serum dilution test. J Infect Dis 1989;160:624–629.
68. Weinstein MP, Stratton CW, Ackley A, et al. Multicenter collaborative evaluation of a standardized serum bactericidal test as a prognostic indicator in infective endocarditis. Am J Med 1985;78:262–269.

69. McCormack JP, Jewesson PJ. A critical reevaluation of the "therapeutic range" of aminoglycosides. Clin Infect Dis 1992;14:320–339.
70. Cantu TG, Yamnanaka-Yuen NA, Lietman PS. Serum vancomycin concentrations: A reappraisal of their clinical value. Clinical Infect Dis 1994;18:533–543.
71. Blatter M, Fluckiger U, Entenza J, et al. Simulated human serum profiles of one daily dose of ceftriaxone plus netilmicin in treatment of experimental streptococcal endocarditis. Antimicrob Agents Chemother 1993;37:1971–1976.
72. Wilson WR, Geraci JE, Danielson GK, et al. Anticoagulant therapy and central nervous system complications in patients with prosthetic valve endocarditis. Circulation 1978;57:1004–1007.
73. Davenport J, Hart RG. Prosthetic valve endocarditis 1976–1987. Antibiotics, anticoagulation and stroke. Stroke 1990;21:993–999.
74. Durack DT. Prevention of infective endocarditis. NEJM 1995;332:38–44.
75. Greenman RL, Bisno AL. Prevention of bacterial endocarditis, in Kaye D (ed): Infective Endocarditis, 2nd ed. New York, Raven Press, 1992, pp 465–481.
76. Van der Meer JT, Van Wijk W, Thompson J, et al. Efficacy of antibiotic prophylaxis for prevention of native-valve endocarditis. Lancet 1992;339:135–139.
77. Hall G, Hedstrom SA, Heimdahl A, Nord CE. Prophylactic administration of penicillins for endocarditis does not reduce the incidence of postextraction bacteremia. Clin Infect Dis 1993;17:188–194.
78. Freedman LR. To prevent or not to prevent bacterial endocarditis—that is the question! Clin Infect Dis 1993;17:195–197.
79. Guntheroth WG. How important are dental procedures as a cause of infective endocarditis? Am J Cardiol 1984;54:797–801.
80. Dajani AS, Bisno AL, Chung KJ. Prevention of bacterial endocarditis: Recommendations by the American Heart Association. JAMA 1990;264:2919–2922.
81. Wahl MJ. Myths of dental-induced endocarditis. Arch Intern Med 1994;154(2):137–144.
82. Wehrmacher WH. Myths: Endocarditis. Arch Intern Med 1994;154:129–130.

Chapter 105

Tuberculosis

Steven C. Ebert, PharmD

Despite the fact that *Mycobacterium tuberculosis* colonizes few hosts other than humans and survives only briefly when isolated in the environment, efforts in the United States to eliminate tuberculosis disease have failed. Through shifts in the population considered endemic for tuberculosis, changes in health care policies, an increase in the number of immunocompromised individuals, and the development of drug resistance, tuberculosis has indeed staged a "comeback" in the United States. This chapter discusses the epidemiology of tuberculosis, alterations in the host–parasite relationship, drug resistance and its implications, new methods for diagnosis, and new treatment strategies for tuberculosis. In addition, the responsibilities pharmacists may assume to manage this disease successfully and reduce its overall incidence are addressed.

History/Incidence in the United States

Tuberculosis has afflicted man since the beginning of recorded history. It was originally termed "phthisis" because of the emaciated features of patients with the disease. Mummies from Egyptian tombs, as well as preserved corpses from Incan and Mayan burial sites, have shown evidence of tuberculous infection. Tuberculosis has been most prevalent in cultures that built cities, placing individuals in proximity. In Europe and the United States, tuberculosis did not become a major public health problem until the Industrial Revolution brought people together to work and live. During the eighteenth and nineteenth centuries, as many as 25% of recorded adult deaths could be attributed to tuberculosis.[1] Paradoxically, the threat of tuberculosis has prompted many advances in the prevention of infection, such as pasteurization of milk and isolation of infected persons.

Today, tuberculosis remains the leading cause of infectious deaths in the world. It is estimated that one in every three patients in the world is infected with *M. tuberculosis.* Approximately 3 million people worldwide die from tuberculosis annually. In the United States, approximately 13 million people are infected, with 23,000–25,000 new cases each year, resulting in an annual death rate of about 2000 patients. Prior to 1984, the annual incidence of tuberculosis had declined steadily by about 5% per year (Fig. 105.1). However, in 1984, this decline slowed, and the incidence of tuberculosis in the United States actually increased during 1988–1992 from 9.3 to 10.5/100,000. Since then, implementation of more stringent screening criteria, infection control practices, and treatment protocols have resulted in a downturn in incidence (case rate in 1994 was approximately 8.5/100,000), but the likelihood of eradication of this disease in this country appears very bleak.

Tuberculosis is now concentrated in patients who are the most difficult to treat: underprivileged patients without access to health care and who live in crowded conditions; recalcitrant patients who are noncompliant with treatment protocols; and immune-compromised patients, who are unable to ward off the disease.

Pathogenesis and Natural History

The genus *Mycobacterium* consists of more than 20 species of aerobic, non-spore-forming rod-shaped bacteria that, after staining with carbol-fuchsin, retain a red pigment despite attempts at decolorization with acid-alcohol. This feature is of importance in identifying mycobacteria and is the source for the common term *acid-fast bacilli* (AFB). Numerous tests are performed to distinguish different species of mycobacteria, including niacin production, catalase production, pigment production and its influence by light (Runyon class), and growth rate.[2] Only *Mycobacterium tuberculosis, M. bovis,* and *M. africanum* have been shown to be pathogenic to normal human hosts, with *M. tuberculosis* being the most prevalent by far. Most strains of *M. tuberculosis* are slow growing (generation time 15–20 hours), produce niacin and heat-sensitive catalase, and lack pigment production.

Certain mycobacteria other than tuberculosis (MOTT), or "atypical mycobacteria," such as *M. kansasii, M. fortuitum,* and *M. avium-intracellulare* have been shown to be pathogenic in immunocompromised patients, most notably those with acquired immunodeficiency syndrome (AIDS). Treatment of these pathogens is discussed in the chapter on AIDS (Chapter 117).

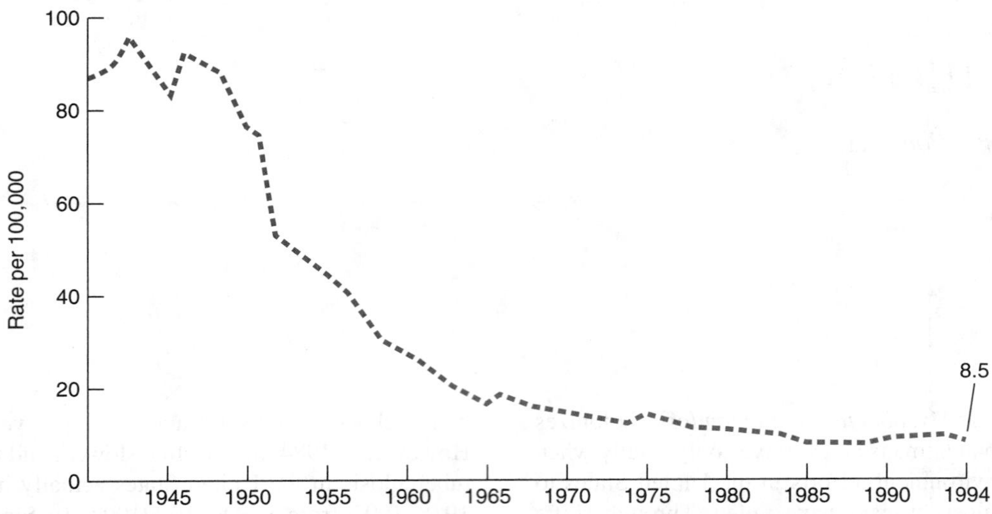

Figure 105.1. Case rate per 100,000 population in the United States from 1942–1994.

TRANSMISSION

The pathophysiology of tuberculosis involves a complex interplay between pathogen and host. Depending on the host immune status and load of tubercle bacilli, tuberculous infection may range in scope from a single granuloma that is clinically undetectable to widely disseminated disease involving nearly all organ systems.

Tuberculosis is invariably transmitted from person to person via microsize droplet nuclei that are dispersed by either coughing or sneezing.[3] The classic studies of Riley and colleagues in the late 1950s[4] demonstrated the ability of air circulated from a hospital ward of patients with tuberculosis to cause disease in guinea pigs. When the air was filtered or exposed to ultraviolet radiation, the animals were not infected.[4] It is estimated that 30% of individuals who experience a "significant" length of direct contact with a person with pulmonary tuberculosis will develop tuberculous infection.

Although many specifics are lacking, the process by which the immune system recognizes and suppresses mycobacterial proliferation is now being elucidated. The cell lines responsible for immunity to mycobacteria are the macrophage and T lymphocytes. T lymphocytes with an αβ MHC receptor compose 95% of lymphocytes and are capable of processing both whole-cell and soluble antigens. The αβ T lymphocytes are further divided into CD4 (helper) and CD8 (cytotoxic/suppressor) lymphocytes. One subset of these CD4 lymphocytes appears to act against mycobacteria. This subset receives antigen from macrophages, is activated by IL-12, and is suppressed by IL-4 and IL-10. These lymphocytes secrete IFN-γ, which activates macrophages to destroy mycobacteria. Later, these lymphocytes transform into cytolytic cells, which destroy cells harboring mycobacteria.[5]

A second group of T lymphocytes possesses a γδ MHC receptor. These cells process only whole cell antigen and are important in arresting the primary infection.[5]

PRIMARY INFECTION

Primary infection is initiated by the alveolar implantation of organisms in droplet nuclei that are small enough (1–5 μm) to escape the ciliary epithelial cells of the upper respiratory tract. The degree of subsequent progression of infection to clinical disease depends on the initial inoculum size as well as the state of the host's cell-mediated immune system.[3,6,7] Once implanted, the organisms multiply and are ingested by pulmonary macrophages where they continue to multiply, albeit more slowly. Intracellular organisms then spread to involve regional lymph nodes in the hilar, mediastinal, and retroperitoneal areas. At this point (days 5–15), αβ CD4 lymphocytes are presented with antigen, activate, and secrete IFN-γ, which stimulates macrophages to become bactericidal. Depending on the concentration of antigen present and the inflammatory response evoked, tissue necrosis and calcification of the originally infected site and regional lymph nodes may occur, resulting in the formation of a radiodense area referred to as a *Ghon complex.*

After this stage of lymph node involvement, organisms may be held in check or, more frequently, spread via the bloodstream to a variety of organ systems. These include other lymph nodes, bone and bone marrow, the liver, kidneys, central nervous system, and most commonly the posterior apical region of the lungs. Seeding of these sites probably occurs because of their relatively high blood flow but limited lymphatic drainage.[6] Nodular infiltrates that may arise in the apices of the lung secondary to this hematogenous spread are referred to as *Simon foci.* By this time (days 15–25), macrophages have begun to form granulomas to contain the organisms. In addition, $\gamma\delta$ lymphocytes now begin to destroy AFB-containing macrophages. This acts to reduce the number of bacteria, but also probably prevents "overstimulation" of the immune system, which could result in autoimmunity.[5]

Concurrent with the proliferation of organisms is the development of delayed hypersensitivity via activation and multiplication of CD4 lymphocytes. When activated lymphocytes reach an adequate number (usually 1–3 months after infection), tissue hypersensitivity results as evidenced by the presence of a positive tuberculin skin test, and any remaining viable organisms within the body will be contained. It should be noted, however, that the immune-mediated cessation of dissemination and the development of cutaneous hypersensitivity are two separate events. This will have implications in the use of the tuberculin skin test to determine the existence of infection.

Finally, by days 20–40, some CD4 lymphocytes transform into cytolytic forms, which also destroy macrophages containing AFB. Dissemination is halted, and remaining mycobacteria reside within granulomas or macrophages that have avoided detection and lysis.[5]

The arrest of mycobacterial proliferation is characterized pathologically by formation of granulomas of two types: *proliferative* granulomas, which are stable and can effectively limit the spread of the organism, and *caseating* granulomas, so named for their cheese-like appearance, which have a necrotic center, are relatively unstable, and permit the limited growth of *M. tuberculosis* within them.[3,6,7]

The size of the inoculum of organisms delivered, the integrity of the host's cell-mediated immune system, the rate at which it arrests the proliferation of organisms, and the presence or absence of other underlying factors influence the subsequent clinical course of the disease. Approximately 90% of patients who experience primary disease have no further clinical manifestations other than a positive skin test either alone (70%) or in combination with radiographic evidence of stable granulomas (15–20%).[6,8] Approximately 3–5% of patients (usually children, the elderly, or the immunocompromised) experience "progressive primary" disease, which occurs before skin test conversion. This form of the disease is characterized by progressive pneumonia originating at the site of the primary infection (usually the lower lobes) and frequently by dissemination, leading to meningitis and often to involvement of the upper lobes of the lung as well.

The remaining 7–10% of patients develop "reactivation disease," which arises subsequent to the hematogenous spread of the organism.[6,8] The vast majority of those who experience reactivation do so within 1 year of the primary infection, and nearly all will experience it within 2 years. The apical areas of the lung have been the most common sites for reactivation (85% of cases). For reasons that are not entirely known (waning cellular immunity, loss of specific T-cell clones, blocking antibody),[9] organisms within granulomas emerge and begin multiplying extracellularly. This typically originates as a small lesion that is visualized as an alveolar infiltrate. The resultant inflammatory response produces caseating granulomas, which will eventually liquify and cavitate as a result of the inflammatory process. Because the host has prior immunity at the time of reactivating disease, the immune response may in fact contribute to the severity of the infection. For example, cavitary pulmonary tuberculosis, caused largely by invasion of neutrophils into lung parenchyma, is seen almost exclusively in previously sensitized individuals. The aerobic environment of a cavity enhances growth of the organism; bacterial counts within the cavity may be as high as 10^8 organisms per milliliter of sputum. Fluid within the cavity is easily aerosolized by coughing, which results in the spread of the organism to other areas within the upper and lower respiratory tracts as well as into the surrounding environment. Partial healing may result from fibrosis of cavities and other infected sites, but the potential exists for breakdown of these areas and subsequent reactivation.[3,6] If left untreated, pulmonary tuberculosis will eventually spread to involve the entire respiratory tract, resulting in hypoxia, respiratory acidosis, and death.

In some cases, a caseating granuloma at an extrapulmonary site will undergo liquefaction and release tubercle bacilli resulting in symptomatic disease. Although the number of cases of pulmonary tuberculosis in the United States reported per year has increased only slightly, the number of extrapulmonary cases has increased, currently accounting for approximately 15–20% of all new cases.[10,11] Organs and systems most commonly involved include the central nervous system (meningitis and cranial tuberculomas), peritoneum, genitourinary tract, lymphatic system, skeletal system, pericardium, adrenal glands, and liver.[7,11] As with the pulmonary form, extrapulmonary tuberculosis left untreated may result in mortality.

Occasionally, a massive inoculum of organisms may be introduced into the bloodstream, causing widely disseminated disease and granuloma formation known as *miliary tuberculosis*. While primary miliary tuberculosis (occurring at the time of initial bacillemia) is most common, some patients may develop miliary tuberculosis from a second bacillemia occurring during reactivation. This form of the disease acquired its name from the millet seed-like appearance of the small granulomas viewed on chest x-ray as well as in films of other soft tissues.[6,8]

Occasionally, patients experience the reactivation form of the disease more than 2 years after primary infection. In the United States, development of tuberculosis in patients with a positive skin test is statistically more likely to be caused by reactivation rather than reinfection.[12] Reinfection is uncommon because of the low rate of exposure in this country and because previously sensitized individuals possess some degree of immunity to reinfection.

The various forms of tuberculosis infection occur at different degrees of frequency in different populations (Table 105.1). These different presentations make diagnosis of tuberculosis through recognition of "classic" signs and symptoms very difficult, especially as the percentage of patients who develop "atypical" forms of the disease continues to increase.

Prior to 1984, low infection transmission rates (<10 other individuals on average) and low reactivation rates (approximately 10% of the newly infected persons) resulted in a decline of new cases in each "generation." In addition, the index case patient was likely to be successfully treated with chemotherapeutic agents.

Beginning in the 1980s and continuing into the 1990s this scenario changed. Because of the shifting epidemiology of tuberculosis, it is now common for an index case to transmit the disease to more than 10 other persons. Likewise, due to immunocompromise, the newly infected persons often have a greater than 10% chance to develop active disease. Finally, because many "new" tuberculosis patients have less access to health care, it is less likely that the patient will complete a successful course of chemotherapy. All these features contribute to the increase in the number of cases of tuberculosis in the United States, and all must be addressed and corrected.

INFLUENCE OF HIV INFECTION ON PATHOGENESIS

As antimycobacterial $\alpha\beta$ CD4 lymphocytes multiply in response to tuberculous infection, HIV multiplies within these cells and selectively destroys them. This results in a relative overabundance of CD8 lymphocytes and, more important, other CD4 lymphocytes. These cells are without mycobactericidal activity and suppress mycobactericidal activity of other lymphocytes and macrophages through production of IL-4 and IL-10. The impairment of CD4 lymphocyte activity increases the rate and extent of tuberculous infection.[5]

HIV infection thereby increases the risk that a patient infected with *M. tuberculosis* will develop active disease. While the *lifetime* risk for an immunocompetent patient with tuberculous infection to develop active disease is about 10%, HIV-infected patients coinfected with *M. tuberculosis* have about a 10% *annual* risk of developing tuberculosis.[13] The Centers for Disease Control and Prevention (CDC) estimates an HIV-infected individual with tuberculous infection to be 113–170 times more likely to develop active diseases than an HIV seronegative patient.

Without a doubt, the concurrence of HIV infection in patients with tuberculosis has shifted the frequency with which progressive primary infection, as opposed to reactivation disease, occurs in the United States. Historically, about 90% of all cases of tuberculosis in this country have been reactivation disease from previous infection. Based on sophisticated epidemiologic studies using DNA fingerprinting, investigators now estimate that 40–50% of all new cases of tuberculosis arise from recent infection. The presence of HIV infection has been established as a major risk factor for rapid-onset disease.[14–16]

As suggested, evidence exists that the immune response associated with tuberculous infection may increase HIV replication in both lymphocytes and macrophages, and subsequently accelerate progression of HIV disease. Markers of HIV progression such as serum β_2 microglobulin concentration are higher in HIV-infected patients with tuberculous infection.[17] In addition, HIV-infected patients with tuberculous infection who are not treated progress to AIDS more rapidly than those without infection, or those who receive prophylactic antimycobacterial chemotherapy.[18] This has prompted widespread screening for tuberculous infection in HIV-infected patients, and empiric chemoprophylaxis for those in whom infection cannot be ruled out.

TABLE 105.1. LIKELIHOOD OF VARIOUS CLINICAL PRESENTATIONS OF TUBERCULOUS INFECTION IN DIFFERENT PATIENT GROUPS

Status at Exposure	Asymptomatic Infection	Progressive Primary Infection	Reactivation Pulmonary	Extrapulmonary Disease	Miliary Tuberculosis
<1 yr old	++	+++	+/–	++	+
1–5 yr	++	++	+/–	++	+
6–10 yr	++	+	+	+	+
11–15 yr	+++	+/–	+	+	+/–
HIV (–) adult	+++	+/–	+	+	+/–
HIV (+) adult	+	++	+	++	+

Key: +++, predominant feature; ++, common; +, occasional; +/–, rare.

EPIDEMIOLOGY

RISK FACTORS FOR INFECTION

Because tuberculosis is transmitted directly from human to human via aerosolized particles, individuals who are exposed to active cases of pulmonary tuberculosis in relatively closed environments are at highest risk for becoming infected.[19] As such, close contacts (greater than 40 h/week) of patients with pulmonary tuberculosis are at particularly high risk, with an estimated infection rate of 25–30%.[3,19] Even exposure to patients with extrapulmonary tuberculosis poses a risk, however, if the infected site is exposed to the environment.

The increase in tuberculosis in the United States results from the spreading of the disease into the population that is least capable of defending itself against it: the poor and the homeless, who have no access to health care; those living in crowded conditions (residents of hospitals, nursing homes, prisons, crack houses, homeless shelters) who are in proximity to other infected individuals; and the immunocompromised, who are not able to ward off the disease once infection develops.

From 1985 to 1992, the frequency of tuberculosis cases in the United States increased from 9.3 to 10.5 per 100,000, up 12.9%. This increase was not, however, a result of an increase in the rate of disease in all demographic groups. In fact, over the same period, the incidence of tuberculosis in Caucasians decreased by 11.1%. Tuberculosis has become a disease of the underprivileged, which unfortunately often translates into ethnic minorities. From 1985 to 1992, the incidence of tuberculosis in Hispanic Americans increased by 4.7%; in Asian-Pacific Islanders, by 12%; and in non-Hispanic blacks, by nearly 38%. Much of this may be attributed to the influx of immigrants from countries with high rates of tuberculosis. From 1986 to 1993, the proportion of tuberculosis cases in the United States that occurred in foreign-born individuals increased from 21.6% to 29.6%, with most cases occurring within 5 years of immigration. Forty-four percent of foreign-born patients with tuberculosis were Hispanic, and 35% were Southeast Asian.[20]

Crowded living conditions have also contributed to the rise in tuberculosis case rates. The frequency of tuberculosis in rural populations has remained essentially unchanged, but has increased by 29% in urban populations since 1985. In some urban areas such as central Harlem, the rate of tuberculosis approximates that seen in some Third World countries.

Tuberculosis has traditionally been considered a disease of the elderly. The elderly (older than 65 years) comprise the age group with the largest number of infected persons.[10,19,21] This group accounts for 12% of the total population, but for 27% of tuberculosis cases reported in 1987, this is a case rate of 20.6 per 100,000.[21] The higher prevalence rate in this population may in part reflect reactivation of disease acquired in the early 1900s. However, a substantial number of elderly patients are infected *de novo*, especially those residing in nursing homes. The rate of tuberculous infection in nursing home residents is twice that of the elderly population as a whole, with the risk increasing proportionately with the length of stay.[21]

Despite the high prevalence rate in the elderly, the greatest increase in case rates has occurred in the 25- to 44-year-old age bracket.[10,19] This can be attributed to the increased rates in minority populations, where the highest case rate occurs in individuals 30–34 years of age (Fig. 105.2).[22] This age group also reflects persons of child-bearing age. Ominously, the rate of tuberculosis in children is also on the rise. The differences between whites and nonwhites is even more pronounced at younger ages; currently, 80% of new cases of tuberculosis in the United States that occur in persons less than 15 years of age occur in ethnic minorities.[19] It appears, therefore, that the upswing in tuberculosis case rates has occurred due to an increased infection rate in certain younger populations, especially those in crowded living conditions with reduced access to health care.

Males have a twofold higher rate for tuberculosis than do females.[19] Finally, health care workers in hospitals and long-term care facilities appear to be at risk, especially those involved in respiratory care such as respiratory therapists and pulmonologists.[23–26]

No discussion of tuberculosis would be complete without describing the interplay between tuberculosis disease and HIV infection. Many individuals attribute the rise in tuberculosis either directly or indirectly to the HIV epidemic. In 1990, in excess of 5% of HIV-infected patients had been diagnosed with tuberculosis, and 39% of patients with tuberculosis had concurrent HIV infection. When asymptomatic tuberculous infection is considered, the numbers are likely much greater.[27] Overlaps exist between

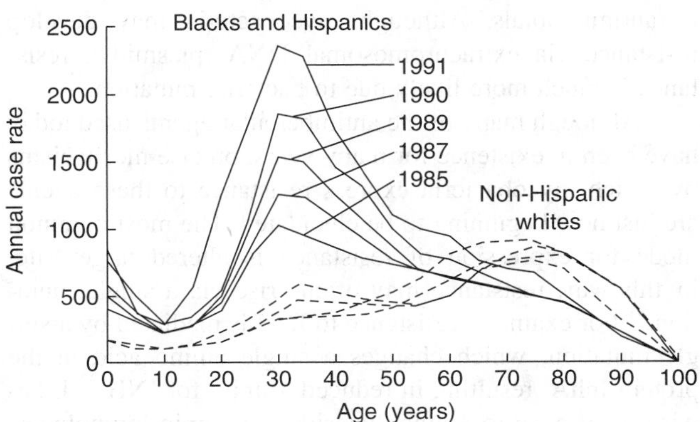

Figure 105.2. Tuberculosis rates by age group, for whites and nonwhite minorities, United States, 1985–1991.

patients at risk for HIV infection and for tuberculosis. Disproportionately high numbers of tuberculosis patients are intravenous (IV) drug abusers, reside in larger cities such as New York City, have been imprisoned, are less than 44 years of age, or have been hospitalized on wards designated for HIV-infected patients. While it does not appear that HIV disease itself increases the risk of tuberculous infection, many of the habits and experiences associated with HIV-infected patients increase their risk for infection.[28,29]

RISK FACTORS FOR DISEASE

In addition to risks for infection, the risk that infection will progress to clinical disease must be considered. Compared to a person with no risk factors and tuberculous infection for an undetermined period of time, individuals who have developed infection within the previous 2 years are at 10-fold greatest risk for either progressive primary infection or reactivation disease. Infected children <2 years of age and the elderly are considered to have a two to five times greater risk for developing clinical tuberculosis. For persons with underlying immune suppression (renal failure, cancer, immunosuppressive drug treatment), the risk is estimated at 4- to 16-fold. Finally, the CDC estimate HIV-infected patients with tuberculous infection are 113 times more likely to develop active tuberculosis and, with AIDS patients, the risk increases to 170-fold.[30] These patients must therefore be monitored closely and/or offered chemoprophylactic therapy. All patients with HIV infection should be screened for tuberculous infection, and vice versa.

DRUG RESISTANCE

MECHANISMS

Mycobacterium tuberculosis is remarkably capable of modifying its genetic makeup to adapt to its surroundings. Part of this adaptability includes its ability to develop resistance to antimicrobials. Although mycobacteria may develop resistance via extrachromosomal DNA (plasmids), resistance is much more likely due to bacterial mutation.[31]

Although many of the antitubercular agents used today have been in existence for many years, precise mechanisms by which mycobacteria express resistance to these agents are just now beginning to be elucidated. The most common mode for expression of resistance is altered target site; in this way, resistance may often arise via a single mutation.[31] For example, resistance to INH is mediated by a single mutation, which changes a single amino acid in the protein InhA, resulting in reduced affinity for INH.[32] Likewise, resistance to aminoglycosides, rifampin, quinolones, ethambutol, and pyrazinamide are via altered target site affinity.[31,33] The inducible production of β-lactamase constitutes the only clinically relevant means of resistance not mediated through alteration of the binding site.[34] The development of resistance by *M. tuberculosis* exerts a profound negative impact on the success of chemotherapy.

EPIDEMIOLOGY OF RESISTANCE

The resurgence of tuberculosis in the United States has been accompanied by an increase in the number of drug-resistant isolates. Since 1985, the fraction of strains resistant to isoniazid has more than doubled; the same may be said for strains resistant to rifampin. Approximately 1 strain in 7 is resistant to at least one antitubercular agent, and 1 in 30 is resistant to both isoniazid and rifampin (i.e., multidrug-resistant *M. tuberculosis,* or MDR-TB). The increase in drug-resistant isolates is particularly dramatic in New York City: Residents are 50 times more likely to be infected with a strain of MDR-TB than those living outside New York City.[35]

The most "newsworthy" means by which MDR-TB occurs is through infection from another individual with MDR-TB. Residents of hospital wards, prisons, homeless shelters, and other institutions who are likely to come into close contact with MDR-TB patients are at greatest risk. In addition, health care workers, guards, caregivers, and so on are at risk, as it appears these resistant strains retain their virulence properties. Transmission of drug-resistant strains from person to person has been documented in studies involving DNA fingerprinting.[28,36]

Despite the concern regarding transmission of MDR-TB, this method of acquisition only accounts for about 10% of cases. In the remaining 90%, MDR-TB arises from an infection with a bacterial strain that is initially sensitive to all antituberculosis drugs or perhaps resistant to only one drug. Not surprisingly, a history of previous drug therapy is associated with a marked increase in the likelihood of drug resistance, particularly to rifampin and/or multiple drugs.[37] One study noted the frequency of MDR-TB to be twice as high in previously treated patients compared to patients without previous treatment.[37] Unfortunately, the incidence of drug resistance ultimately extends to untreated patients as well.

Inappropriate management (noncompliance, incorrect drug selection, reduced bioavailability) results in the emergence of MDR-TB mutants.[38,39] This has become increasingly common because most individuals with tuberculosis are either unable or unwilling to complete a course of chemotherapy. In one hospital in Harlem, more than 80% of patients discharged with tuberculosis failed to complete their therapy![40] On a national average, it is estimated that one in three patients treated for tuberculosis will be noncompliant. Because many noncompliant patients who harbor drug-resistant strains may live in proximity to a large number of other individuals (e.g., homeless shelters), direct transmission of resistant strains becomes a possibility and, in this country, an increasing menace.[38] Thus, the establishment of programs that improve/ensure patient compliance is essential in reducing the incidence of MDR-TB.

CLINICAL PRESENTATION

NON-HIV-INFECTED PATIENTS

The clinical presentation of pulmonary tuberculosis is nonspecific, indicative only of a slowly evolving infectious process. A patient with subclinical or early disease may be completely asymptomatic. When the population of organisms increases to a certain point, however, the patient begins to complain of generalized malaise, anorexia, weight loss, and fatigue as well as intermittent fevers with alternating chills and night sweats. Subsequently, a cough with increasing sputum production develops. Often insidious in onset, the cough is frequently attributed to other causes, such as viral syndrome or exacerbation of chronic bronchitis. Pleuritic chest pain may or may not be a concurrent complaint. Hemoptysis and shortness of breath may also occur and are usually indicative of advanced disease.

Expectoration and/or swallowing of sputum containing large numbers of organisms may result in extension of disease involving the upper respiratory or gastrointestinal tract. Ulceration of the pharynx, larynx, tongue, and oral mucosa as well as otitis media, gastric ulceration, and perirectal abscess may occur.[3,7]

Physical exam is nonspecific, suggestive of progressive pulmonary disease. Dullness to chest percussion suggests consolidation in involved areas of the lung. Rales and increased vocal fremitus are frequently observed upon auscultation. In patients in whom impaired oxygenation has developed, cyanosis and clubbing of the digits may be seen.

Abnormal laboratory data are usually limited to moderate elevations in the white blood cell count with a lymphocyte predominance. Other abnormal values may occasionally be observed, but are too infrequent to be useful diagnostically.[3]

Clinical features associated with extrapulmonary tuberculosis vary depending on the organ system(s) involved, but typically consist of slowly progressive compromise of organ function with low-grade fever and other constitutional symptoms, as mentioned previously. Patients with genitourinary tuberculosis may present with sterile pyuria or culture-negative urinary tract infection, hematuria, abnormal intravenous pyelogram, epididymitis, irregular menses, or infertility. Lymphadenitis often involves the cervical and supraclavicular nodes, and may appear as a neck mass with spontaneous drainage. Tuberculous arthritis and osteomyelitis most commonly occur in the elderly, and usually affect the lower spine and weight-bearing joints. Abnormal behavior, headaches, or convulsions are suggestive of tuberculous meningitis, often without pulmonary involvement. Involvement of the peritoneum, pericardium, larynx, and adrenal glands also occurs.[7]

The clinical presentation of tuberculosis in the elderly is often atypical in nature, mimicking other respiratory diseases. Many clinical findings are muted or absent altogether. Compared with younger patients, tuberculosis in the elderly is associated with fevers and/or positive skin tests 50% less often, sputum production and/or hemoptysis 60% less often, and night sweats 80% less often.[41,42] Weight loss appears to be equally prevalent in both groups. In contrast, mental status changes are twice as common in the elderly, and mortality due to tuberculosis in the elderly is sixfold more common than in younger patients.[41] Tuberculosis is a preventable cause of death in the elderly which should not be overlooked.

Tuberculosis in children is more apt to present in a manner similar to a typical bacterial pneumonia, termed *progressive primary tuberculosis.* Clinical disease often begins with 1–2 months after exposure, preceding cutaneous hypersensitivity. In contrast to that seen in adults, pulmonary tuberculosis in children often involves the lower and middle lobes of the lung.[3,43,44] In addition, dissemination to sites such as lymph nodes, gastrointestinal and genitourinary tracts, bone marrow, and meninges is not uncommon. Due to the delay in recruitment of cellular immunity, cavitary disease is observed infrequently in pulmonary disease of children. This results in a much smaller number of resident tubercle bacilli in a child with tuberculosis than in an adult with cavitary disease. This may be of significance when determining the intensity and duration of antituberculous chemotherapy.[44]

HIV-INFECTED PATIENTS

The clinical features of patients with HIV infection who develop tuberculosis may be markedly different from those classically observed in immunocompetent individuals (Table 105.2). The degree to which the clinical presentation of tuberculosis differs in HIV-infected patients depends on the extent of HIV infection.[45] In AIDS patients, tuberculosis is much more likely to present as the progressive primary form, to involve extrapulmonary sites, and to involve multiple lobes of the lung.

Tuberculosis in AIDS patients is less likely to involve cavitary disease, be associated with a positive skin test, or be associated with fever. Nonspecific findings of tuberculosis such as malaise, weight loss, weakness, and fever are in fact the norm in AIDS patients. Needless to say, this makes diagnosis based on clinical findings extremely difficult.

Because of their superimposed social and physical compromise, HIV-infected patients with tuberculosis require particularly aggressive therapy to account for issues such as noncompliance, more rapid progression, and drug resistance.

TABLE 105.2. CLINICAL FEATURES OF TUBERCULOSIS IN HIV-POSITIVE VERSUS -NEGATIVE PATIENTS

	HIV-Negative (Immunocompetent)	HIV-Positive (AIDS)
Onset	Gradual	Abrupt
Presentation	Reactivation	Progressive primary
PPD Result	Usually positive	Usually negative
Chest radiograph	Apical infiltrate	Diffuse, lower lobes
Extrapulmonary forms	Occasional	Common
Other pathogens present	Occasional	Common
AFB-positive sputum	Usually	Usually
Response to therapy	Excellent	Fair–good

DIAGNOSIS/SCREENING

Antimycobacterial therapy is indicated in two groups of individuals: those with asymptomatic infection, in whom the likelihood of disease progression outweighs that of drug toxicity; and those with symptomatic disease (tuberculosis). Although diagnostic tests exist to identify both groups, all have their limitations, and newer techniques (to be discussed) are necessary.

IDENTIFICATION OF INDIVIDUALS WITH ASYMPTOMATIC INFECTION

Screening of individuals at risk for tuberculous infection is achieved through the use of the tuberculin skin test, most often employing purified protein derivative (PPD). The types of individuals who should be screened with PPD are shown in Table 105.3.

The CDC recommends that the following individuals be screened for tuberculous infection and/or tuberculosis: HIV-infected persons[46]; close contacts of known or suspected cases of active tuberculosis; patients with medical risk factors such as silicosis, gastrectomy, jejunoileal bypass, weight less than 90% of ideal body weight, chronic renal failure, diabetes mellitus, use of high-dose corticosteroids or other immunosuppressive drugs, and hematologic or other malignancies; patients with chest radiographs showing fibrotic lesions consistent with old tuberculosis; medically underserved low-income groups, especially racial minorities[47]; immigrants and other foreign-born individuals[48]; alcoholics and intravenous drug users[49]; residents and employees of long-term care facilities such as nursing homes, prisons, and mental institutions[50,51]; and health care workers and trainees.[52] It is probably unnecessary to screen asymptomatic individuals without at least one of the above risk factors. However, one author proposes that a one-time screening of low-risk individuals at age 50 would be cost effective.[53]

The most widely used screening method for tuberculous infection is the tuberculin skin test, which uses PPD.[54,55] It may be used for identifying patients with subclinical infection as well as active disease. PPD as it exists today was developed in 1941 and consists of proteins derived from a single strain of *M. tuberculosis.* To distinguish it from skin tests for other mycobacteria, it is designated PPD-S, in recognition of its developer, Florence Seibert. One test unit (1 TU) of PPD-S contains 0.00002 mg of protein.[54] Current preparations of PPD-S contain Tween 80 as a stabilizer, which prevents the protein from adhering to the inside of the container or syringe, which would result in loss of potency.[54,55]

Three test strengths of PPD-S are available: first strength (1 TU), intermediate strength (5 TU), and second strength (250 TU). The intermediate-strength form is almost invariably used for routine screening and diagnostic purposes. First-strength PPD-S is sometimes used for testing patients in whom a severe reaction may be expected (i.e., patients with known prior positive test), although few data exist to support this practice.[55,56] Second-strength PPD-S may be used in testing patients with depressed cell-mediated immunity who have had a negative result with the intermediate-strength test, but appear likely to have tuberculosis on the basis of clinical criteria.

The basis for use of the tuberculin skin test is the fact that the majority of persons infected with *M. tuberculosis* manifest cutaneous hypersensitivity to the PPD antigen because of the recruitment of T lymphocytes that were sensitized during the primary infection. This results in the development of erythema and induration (swelling) at the test site, which are maximal at 48 hours after test administration. Even after effective chemotherapy has been given, cutaneous hypersensitivity persists, albeit to a gradually decreasing extent.[55,57]

The Mantoux method of PPD administration, which is the most reliable technique, consists of the intradermal injection of 0.1 mL of PPD containing 5 TU into the volar or dorsal surface of the forearm using a 27-gauge needle, keeping the bevel upward. A small wheal should be visible at the site to confirm intradermal disposition of the PPD. The test is read 48–72 hours after injection by measuring the diameter of the zone of induration. It is important that the size of the induration, not erythema, be measured. Although 48 hours is usually considered the best time for reading test results, a positive reaction remains for at least 5 days after the test has been administered.[55,56]

In the early 1980s, two commercially available products, Aplisol® and Tubersol®, were standardized to be immunologically equivalent to CDCs "gold standard" product, PPD-S. Since that time, these two products have enjoyed widespread use. However, in the late 1980s the original lots of Aplisol® were depleted, and new lots were generated. This led to some concerns that the Aplisol® product is now excessively immunogenic, and may result

TABLE 105.3. CANDIDATES FOR SCREENING WITH PPD SKIN TEST

Individuals	Initial Screening	Retest Periodically	Test If Local Outbreak
HIV-infected	×	If possible	N/A
Hospital employees	×	Annually–semiannually	Yes, if exposed
Nursing home staff	×	Annually	Yes, if exposed
Nursing home residents	×	Probably not	Yes, if exposed
Workers at prisons, homeless shelters, clinics, etc.	×	Annually	Yes, if exposed
Immigrants	×	If possible	N/A
Health care students	×	Annually–biannually	Yes, if exposed
General population	No	No	Yes, if exposed

in false-positive reactions in some individuals.[58] This phenomenon has been described in a number of case reports. Based on this, many institutions have now switched entirely to Tubersol® for screening and diagnostic purposes. Although Tubersol® is four times as expensive as Aplisol®, the additional expense resulting from retesting (and possibly unnecessarily treating) patients with positive reactions to Aplisol® more than outweighs the additional test costs.

While the tuberculin skin test alone cannot induce cutaneous hypersensitivity *de novo,* it may sufficiently enhance the low-level reactivity present in some patients so that conversion of a "negative" test result to a "positive" result could occur after repeat testing. This "booster effect" usually occurs in patients with past tuberculous infection, immunization with BCG, or from infection with MOTT.[7,59–61]

In individuals who will be skin tested periodically (e.g., annually, semiannually), it is recommended that the initial testing involve a "two-stage" method (i.e., PPD tests are placed twice within a 1- to 2-week period) to detect boosters.[62] Newer ATS criteria for a positive test result have greatly reduced the number of false-positive boosted tests. All individuals who initially boost should be further examined for evidence of tuberculosis. At best, a boosted skin test (>5–10 mm, depending on the group tested[63]) has a 50% positive predictive value for infection, as evidenced by current or future active disease.[61] Concurrent skin testing with other mycobacterial antigens may improve specificity, but this is not usually done.[61] If factor(s) other than infection with *M. tuberculosis* may be identified as the cause for the boosted reaction, subsequent skin tests should be viewed as positive only if they are significantly larger (>5 mm) than the boosted result. In any event, the clinician should also consider other factors (history of exposure, signs/symptoms) when determining whether a subsequent skin test result is "positive," and should not base the decision to treat or not to treat solely on this result. Some individuals will, with repeated tests administered weekly, boost only after the third or fourth test; these individuals are much less likely to exhibit a reaction to PPD after 1 year.[62] Therefore, two-stage PPD testing appears sufficient.

Nonboosters are considered to be without infection, and any subsequent "positive" skin test should be viewed as indicative of recent infection requiring treatment.[7,59]

As mentioned previously, the size of reaction to a PPD skin test considered "positive" (i.e., meriting further testing and/or treatment) must be defined in the context of the clinical situation, taking into account the time frame since infection and the immune status of the patient. Different cutoff points for the size of induration are used for different patient populations, which take into account the following criteria:

Time proximity of skin test application to documented exposure to an active case of tuberculosis
Degree of patient immune suppression that could result in a false-negative test and/or result in progression of latent disease
Time frame elapsed since last negative test
Likelihood of a false-positive reaction due to "boosting"
Likelihood of toxicity to chemotherapy

For patients with AIDS or young children with recent exposure to an index case, any extent of induration might be read as "positive." For HIV-infected patients or those suspected of having HIV infection but who refuse HIV testing, as well as all others with documented recent exposure, a cutoff of 5 mm is used to initiate treatment. For individuals who were recently (≤2 years ago) skin test negative, as well as those with a reaction of unknown duration and radiographic signs of old tuberculosis, or a history of diabetes, gastrectomy, cancer, immunosuppressive therapy, or renal failure, reactions >10 mm are considered positive. Finally, for those with a reaction of unknown duration and with no other risk factors, a reaction size of 15 mm is considered necessary to initiate treatment.

Skin testing with PPD results in a 30% false-negative rate overall. False-negative results may result from faulty test material, poor administration technique, observer error, or impairment of the host's immune system (Table 105.4).[55,56] For example, the false-negative rate to PPD in AIDS patients approaches 70%.[45,64] To minimize the inci-

TABLE 105.4. REASONS FOR FALSE-NEGATIVE TUBERCULIN SKIN TESTS

Faulty testing material
- Outdated material
- Improper storage
- Bacterial contamination
- Adsorption onto container (not Tween stabilized)

Improper administration
- Dose too small
- Injection made too deeply

Improper interpretation
- Delay in interpretation
- Bias by interpreter
- Faulty technique

Depression of tuberculin sensitivity
- Noninfectious diseases that impair the immune system
  - Sarcoidosis
  - Amyloidosis
  - Lymphomas
  - Leukemias
  - AIDS
- Viral infections
  - Rubeola
  - Influenza
  - Epstein–Barr virus
  - Hepatitis A or B
  - Varicella zoster virus
  - Polio
  - Cytomegalovirus
- Live attenuated viral vaccines
- Drug therapy
  - Topical or systemic corticosteroids
  - Immunosuppressive or cytotoxic drugs
- Miscellaneous
  - Elderly (>60 years)
  - Crohns' disease
  - Solid tumors
  - Radiation therapy
  - Systemic lupus erythematosus
  - Miliary tuberculosis
  - Uremia

dence of false-negative results, proper storage and administration techniques for tuberculin should be observed.

Many individuals promote the use of other skin tests as "controls" to ensure that the patient does not exhibit cutaneous anergy. These control tests should probably be used in two situations[65]:

when screening HIV-infected patients for tuberculous infection

OR

when attempting to diagnose active tuberculosis in a patient who may be immunocompromised (elderly, immunosuppressive therapy, malnourished, overwhelming infection).

In other words, use of a control skin test battery in individuals undergoing routine screening is unnecessary. The two or (three) skin tests advocated by the CDC as controls are mumps and tetanus (and candida).

Since HIV-infected patients are frequently anergic, a negative PPD test result cannot be taken literally.[66–70] Nevertheless, both PPD and control tests should be used, as anergic patients may occasionally demonstrate a reactive PPD result.[63,69] In some studies, HIV-infected individuals who were anergic and were in a high-risk category (homeless, IV drug abuser, prisoners, migrant laborers, immigrants) were as likely to develop tuberculosis as those with a positive tuberculin test.[68,70] This has led the CDC to recommend that empiric preventive therapy be strongly considered for any HIV-infected patient who is anergic and in whom the incidence of new infection is 1%/year or cumulative infection prevalence is 10% or greater (see high-risk groups previously listed). For individuals suspected of having active tuberculosis, skin testing with PPD and controls should also be performed.

SYMPTOMATIC DISEASE

Patients who are diagnosed as having tuberculous infection by skin testing as well as those who present with clinical findings consistent with tuberculosis should undergo diagnostic testing to rule out active disease. Confirmatory diagnosis of a clinical suspicion of tuberculosis must be made via chest x-ray and microbiological examination of sputum or other infected material. A positive result from one or more of these procedures must be observed to initiate treatment. Whether one or more of these tests is positive depends on the site and extent of infection as well as the underlying physical status of the patient.

Radiologic Diagnosis

A chest x-ray should be routinely ordered in patients suspected of having tuberculosis to assist in the initial diagnosis and to assess the extent of disease in those previously diagnosed. Although no pathognomonic pattern exists, a number of radiographic findings occur that are characteristic of tuberculosis. In the reactivation form of the disease, ongoing infection is characterized by patchy infiltrates of the upper segments or apices of the lung with ipsilateral lymph node involvement.[3,7] In advanced cases, cavitation is commonly observed. Granulomas in various stages of development are also seen frequently. In quiescent disease, calcification of granulomas often occurs. Thickening of the pleura and apical scarring are also seen in patients with past history of active disease.

Early primary tuberculosis in children or in AIDS patients is often characterized by a discrete lower lobe lesion with enlarged hilar lymph nodes. Subsequent active disease in the lower lobes of the lung, however, is radiographically indistinct from other pneumonias.[3] In fact, the finding of an apical infiltrate on chest x-ray, felt to be pathognomonic of tuberculosis in an immunocompetent individual, is more likely to be *Pneumocystis carinii* in a patient with advanced HIV infection.[71]

Microbiologic Diagnosis

In addition, every attempt should be made to isolate *M. tuberculosis* from the site of infection. Examination of sputum is important in providing microbiologic evidence of pulmonary tuberculosis.[7] Acid-fast bacilli may be detected by sputum fluorochrome fluorescent stain in 50–80% of all patients with active pulmonary tuberculosis.[1] To detect AFB by staining, 10,000 AFB/mL of specimen is necessary.[1] Cultures result in a higher yield (90%), but are time and labor consuming.[1,7] Sputum collected in the morning is considered to have the highest number of organisms per volume and hence the highest yield.[72] Multiple sputum collections over 3 consecutive days are recommended. For patients unable to expectorate sputum, sputum induction with aerosolized hypertonic saline or aspiration of gastric fluid may be attempted. Alternatively, bronchoscopy or aspiration of gastric fluid may be attempted, although these should probably be avoided in the elderly due to the risks for aspiration.[7,73] For patients with suspected extrapulmonary tuberculosis, sampling of fluid and/or biopsy of the infected site may be attempted, although the likelihood of a positive AFB smear or culture is low (with the exception of liver and bone marrow biopsies). Sputum or other specimens (urine, tissue, other fluids) should be digested with acid to remove proteinaceous material and other bacteria before being sent for acid-fast stain and culture, although some AFB may be lost as well. Blood cultures are also unlikely to be positive, although bacteremia is relatively common in AIDS patients.[74]

Cultures are generally performed using both solid (Lowenstein–Jensen and/or Middlebrook agars) and liquid (conventional and radiometric broth) media. Identification of *M. tuberculosis* has been simplified since the advent of DNA probes, which distinguish *M. tuberculosis* from other mycobacteria. Cultures using newer broth-based media with radioactive isotope detectors (BACTEC) have considerably shortened the time to positive cultures and, subsequently, susceptibility results. Drug susceptibility tests should also be performed routinely. In the past, agar-based susceptibility testing required at least 4–6 weeks to complete. The BACTEC system detects microbial metabolism in a mycobacteria-specific medium containing ^{14}C. It detects organisms in an average of 9 days and determines identification in 5 days and drug susceptibility in 6 additional days.[7,75] Rapid susceptibility testing is now strongly advocated for all isolates of *M. tuberculosis* in patients who are to begin therapy, and again if therapy does not appear to be successful.

Due to the relatively low sensitivity of staining techniques and long turnaround time for cultures, other diagnostic methods are being investigated. Of these, polymerase chain reaction (PCR) testing for mycobacterial DNA appears promising. While some false positive results may occur, the negative predictive value is quite high (85–95%). Other methods being tested for even more sensitive and rapid detection and identification include use of genetic probes, immunoassays (RIA, ELISA) for mycobacterial antigens and antibodies, and detection of by-products of mycobacteria such as tuberculostearic acid.[75,76]

TREATMENT

FACTORS TO CONSIDER WHEN SELECTING THERAPY

The selection of a chemotherapeutic regimen for tuberculosis has traditionally been based on the severity of illness (i.e., more clinically severe forms of disease require treatment with more antimicrobials for a longer period of time, and vice versa). However, it has been proposed that a more important basis for chemotherapy is the total number of tubercle bacilli present within the body.[44,77] Asymptomatic patients with tuberculous infection have a bacillary load of approximately 10^3–10^4 organisms, compared with 10^{11} bacteria in a patient with cavitary pulmonary tuberculosis.[3,44,77] As the number of organisms increases, the likelihood of resistance developing to a single antimicrobial also increases. It is estimated that, for a strain of isoniazid-susceptible mycobacteria, 1 in 10^6 organisms will be resistant to the drug. For treatment of asymptomatic disease, it would appear that the risk of resistance to isoniazid (INH) as monotherapy would be quite low; this has been substantiated in the literature.[78] In contrast, resistance would be very likely to occur if INH alone were used to treat cavitary tuberculosis. By adding another drug such as rifampin, to which 1 in 10^7 organisms is resistant, the likelihood of resistance is reduced, as only 1 in 10^{13} ($10^6 \times 10^7$) organisms would be resistant to both drugs. In general, INH and rifampin are the antimycobacterial agents most capable of preventing resistance, followed by ethambutol, streptomycin, and pyrazinamide (PZA).[44]

Three subpopulations of mycobacteria are postulated to exist within the body, each of which may be eliminated best with certain antituberculous agents.[44,77] Most numerous (10^7–10^9) are the extracellular, rapidly dividing bacteria, often within cavities. These are killed most readily by INH, streptomycin, quinolones, penicillin β-lactamase inhibitor combinations, and ethambutol (when used in doses of 25 mg/kg/d). A second group (10^5–10^7) is comprised of those organisms residing within caseating granulomas; these organisms are usually in a dormant metabolic state but on occasion will increase their activity for short periods of time. PZA is converted to pyrazinoic acid in the region of the granuloma where the pH reaches 5.5. Pyrazinoic acid is effective at killing those organisms within the granuloma. INH and rifampin are also likely to be active against this subpopulation. The final subset is the intracellular mycobacteria present within macrophages (10^4–10^6). The acidic environment within macrophages inhibits the activity of most agents, but agents such as INH, rifampin, and PZA are effective for this purpose in killing intracellular bacteria.

In summary, INH alone appears sufficient for treatment of asymptomatic infection due to sensitive organisms, whereas combination chemotherapy is used for active disease to reduce resistance and eradicate all three subpopulations of organisms. The regimen of INH and streptomycin that was used in the 1950s had to be continued for 18–24 months to be effective; this regimen killed only extracellular organisms and required that other bacterial populations, or "persisters," migrate to extracellular sites where they would be more susceptible to, or could be destroyed by, the host's immune system.[77] Today, by combining antituberculous agents directed at all populations of bacteria, one can effect eradication of mycobacteria in the lung in a much shorter period of time. The elimination of the slowly growing bacteria that exist intracellularly and within granulomas is imperative for the success of short-course (6–9 months) chemotherapy. Use of shorter courses of therapy allows less time for adverse effects to occur and is less costly as well.[79]

Selection of a treatment plan (e.g., which drugs, how many, how long) depends on a number of patient- and disease-related factors. These are listed in Table 105.5. The number of antimicrobials used in therapy depends on the estimated number of acid-fast bacilli in the body, the likelihood of resistance, and the desired duration of therapy. For example, it is generally assumed that asymptomatic patients harbor fewer bacteria than do symptomatic patients; therefore, monotherapy is generally considered adequate for chemoprophylaxis. For symptomatic patients, cavitary disease is associated with a higher number of bacteria, which implies a higher likelihood of primary resistance to single- or double-drug therapy. A greater number of drugs will be chosen for therapy in a patient suspected of being infected with a drug-resistant strain, in order to assure that at least three active agents are being used. Although debatable, more drugs are usually employed in HIV-infected patients and patients with extrapulmonary tuberculosis, regardless of susceptibility. Finally, if short-course therapy is desired, a greater number of drugs are used, ideally including agents with activity against each of the three subtypes of mycobacteria (extracellular, intracellular, granuloma).

TABLE 105.5. FACTORS TO CONSIDER WHEN CHOOSING THE NUMBER OF DRUGS FOR THERAPY OF TUBERCULOUS INFECTION

Use Fewer Drugs	Use More Drugs
Asymptomatic disease	Symptomatic disease
Longer course of therapy	Shorter course of therapy
No cavitary disease	Cavitary disease
Pulmonary disease only	Extrapulmonary disease
HIV-negative patient	HIV-positive patient
Doubt resistance	Suspect resistance
INH- or rifampin-susceptible	INH- and rifampin-resistant

PHARMACOLOGY OF ANTITUBERCULAR AGENTS

Isoniazid

Isoniazid remains the mainstay for treatment of patients with both asymptomatic and symptomatic infection. It exhibits bactericidal activity against mycobacteria in all environments *in vivo*. In 1991, 9% of all clinical isolates of *M. tuberculosis* tested were resistant to INH.[35]

Therapy with INH results in development of adverse effects in approximately 5.5% of patients. A transient elevation in serum transaminases occurs in 12–15% of patients and usually occurs within the first 8–12 weeks of therapy.[80] Overt hepatotoxicity, however, occurs in only 1% of cases. Destruction of hepatocytes by accumulation of reactive hydrazine metabolites is most frequently cited as the cause. Risk factors for hepatotoxicity include patient age (Table 105.6), preexisting liver disease, and pregnancy/postpartum state.[80,81] Moderate consumption of alcohol is probably not a risk factor if it has not resulted in preexisting liver disease.

Isoniazid also may result in neurotoxicity, most frequently presenting as peripheral neuropathy or, in overdose, seizures and coma.[80,82] Central nervous system effects such as ataxia, mental status changes, or exacerbation of preexisting convulsive disorders are also occasionally observed. Isoniazid exerts its neurotoxic effect through enhanced elimination of pyridoxine and/or competitive inhibition

TABLE 105.6. EFFECT OF AGE ON INCIDENCE OF HEPATITIS FROM ISONIAZID

Age (yr)	Frequency (%)
0–19	0.3–0.6
20–34	0.3–2.2
35–49	1.2–3.2
50–64	2.3–3.4
>65	2.3–4.2

(Adapted from Refs. 132 and 133.)

with pyridoxine in its action as a cofactor in the synthesis of synaptic neurotransmitters.[80] Patients with pyridoxine deficiency such as alcoholics, children, and the malnourished are at increased risk, as are patients who are slow acetylators of INH and those predisposed to neuropathy such as diabetics. Coadministration of as little as 6 mg of pyridoxine daily will reduce the incidence of these neurotoxic effects from 20% to less than 1%.[80] Isoniazid has been reported to inhibit the metabolism of phenytoin, carbamazepine, primidone, and warfarin.[83] Patients who are being treated with these agents should be monitored closely and appropriate dose adjustments should be made when necessary.

Rifampin

The clinical use of rifampin to treat tuberculosis has allowed substantial shortening of the duration of chemotherapeutic regimens and reduced the frequency of failure due to resistance. In fact, drug resistance to rifampin is the one of the most ominous prognostic factors influencing the outcome of therapy. In 1991, 4% of all clinical isolates of *M. tuberculosis* tested were resistant to rifampin.[35]

Adverse effects associated with rifampin are infrequent and rarely necessitate withdrawal of drug. Elevations in hepatic enzymes have been attributed to rifampin in 10–15% of patients, with overt hepatotoxicity occurring in less than 1%. Rifampin has the potential to augment the hepatotoxicity of INH by increasing microsomal enzyme activity, which is the enzyme system responsible for converting monoacetyl hydrazine into a hepatotoxic intermediate. When INH and rifampin are used together, elevations in serum transaminases occur in 20–30% of patients, usually within the first 8 weeks of therapy.[80] In most cases this is transient in nature. More frequent adverse effects of rifampin include rash, fever, and gastrointestinal distress.

Allergic reactions to rifampin have been reported, and occur mainly in patients receiving therapy at twice-weekly intervals. Sensitization of the immune system and development of antirifampin antibodies are postulated to occur, with subsequent rechallenge resulting in symptoms.[80] These reactions may take the form of a flulike syndrome, with development of fever, chills, headache, arthralgias, and, rarely, hypotension and shock. Alternatively, hemolytic anemia or acute renal failure may occur.[84]

Rifampin's induction of hepatic enzymes may enhance the elimination of a number of drugs including theophylline, steroids, narcotics, oral hypoglycemics, zidovudine, and warfarin.[85] In addition, an increase in vitamin D metabolism has been reported with rifampin, with development of osteomalacia in some cases.[80]

Females who use oral contraceptives should be advised to use another form of contraception during therapy. The colorizing effects of rifampin on urine, other secretions, and contact lenses should be discussed with the patient.

Pyrazinamide

Incorporation of pyrazinamide into the early stage of chemotherapy results in more rapid reduction in counts of acid-fast bacilli, enabling success with 6-month short-course chemotherapy. In 1991, 6% of all clinical isolates of *M. tuberculosis* tested were resistant to PZA.[35]

Hepatotoxicity is the major limiting adverse effect seen with PZA therapy. Results of early studies that used doses of 2 g daily reported a 15% incidence of hepatitis.[80] The incidence is much lower when daily doses of 1–2 g are used. Patients at risk are primarily those with preexisting impairment in hepatic function.

Pyrazinamide's primary metabolite, pyrazinoic acid, may compete with uric acid for elimination via the kidney, resulting in exacerbation of gout in susceptible individuals. Interestingly, this effect may be diminished when rifampin is administered concurrently.[86] Pyrazinamide also frequently causes gastrointestinal irritation with nausea and vomiting.

Ethambutol

Ethambutol remains a useful orally administered antitubercular agent to be used in situations of suspected or documented resistance. In 1991, 2–3% of all clinical isolates of *M. tuberculosis* tested were resistant to ethambutol.[35]

Retrobulbar neuritis is the major adverse effect noted in patients treated with ethambutol. Incidence is dose related, with occurrence rates of 5% in patients receiving daily doses of 25 mg/kg but less than 1% in those treated with 15 mg/kg daily.[80] Patients usually complain of a change in visual acuity and/or inability to see the color green. Risk factors for toxicity include high (25 mg/kg/d) doses of drug and decreased renal function leading to drug accumulation. Avoidance of ethambutol use in children is recommended because of the difficulty in monitoring visual acuity in this group. Other adverse effects that may be observed include rash, fever, arthralgias, and gastrointestinal irritation.

Ethambutol should probably not be used in children who are too young to undergo testing for color blindness. Patients should have baseline tests of renal function and visual acuity, with follow-up tests of vision every 1–2 months.

Streptomycin

Streptomycin was released in 1947 and was the first antibiotic to be used in the treatment of tuberculosis. It is one of three aminoglycoside antibiotics (along with amikacin and kanamycin) that are active against mycobacteria. Streptomycin is now available only on special order from Pfizer and is used exclusively for the treatment of tuberculosis. In 1991, 6% of all clinical isolates of *M. tuberculosis* tested were resistant to streptomycin.[35]

Impairment of eighth cranial nerve function is the most important adverse effect of streptomycin. Vestibular function is most frequently affected, but hearing may also be impaired. If treatment with streptomycin continues despite the occurrence of toxicity, damage may not be completely reversible.[80] Pain on injection and sterile abscess formation may also occur during therapy with streptomycin. Streptomycin is the least nephrotoxic of the aminoglycosides, with an estimated incidence of renal toxicity of less than 1%. Neuromuscular blockade has been reported to occur rarely.

Quinolones

Ofloxacin and ciprofloxacin have been used in the treatment of tuberculosis. Both agents are bactericidal against extracellular *M. tuberculosis* and achieve good intracellular concentrations, although their intracellular bactericidal activity has not been established. These agents are also useful because they are available in both oral and intravenous dosage forms. Ofloxacin has generally been favored over ciprofloxacin because of its higher serum concentrations in relationship to *in vitro* activity.

Ofloxacin is usually used in combination with other agents in the treatment of documented MDR-TB. In addition, it is recommended for chemoprophylaxis (together with PZA) for patients with asymptomatic infection due to MDR-TB. Patients receiving full doses of PZA (15 mg/kg/d) and ofloxacin (800 mg daily) frequently experience adverse effects including headache, dizziness, confusion, joint pain, gastrointestinal distress, and/or dysuria. These may be due in part to a reduction in the urinary excretion of ofloxacin and/or pyrazinoic acid by the other agent. It is suggested that the dose of one or both agents be reduced by 25–50% if adverse effects develop.

Penicillin-β-Lactamase Inhibitors

M. tuberculosis produces a penicillinase similar to that of Enterobacteriaceae. This enzyme is inhibited by β-lactamase inhibitors such as sulbactam, clavulanic acid, and tazobactam. Studies in animals demonstrated the efficacy of ampicillin–sulbactam and amoxicillin–clavulanate against *M. tuberculosis.* Reports in humans have been anecdotal, with some successes noted. However, their hydrophilic characteristics suggest their penetration into granulomas and intracellular fluid is limited. Amoxicillin–clavulanic acid may be considered a third or fourth-line agent for treating tuberculosis, in combination with other more lipophilic antitubercular drugs. Its utility is likely to be restricted to MDR-TB. Ampicillin–sulbactam again possesses the advantage of being available as an intravenous agent. It may be considered part of a therapeutic regimen for treatment of drug-resistant tuberculosis, but only in a patient with MDR-TB who is unable to take oral medications.

Rifabutin

Rifabutin (ansamycin) is an analogue of rifampin with greater activity than rifampin against *M. avium* complex. It does not, however, demonstrate any advantage over rifampin against *M. tuberculosis.* AIDS patients who are receiving prophylactic rifabutin and develop tuberculosis are more likely to be infected with a rifampin-resistant strain. Because rifabutin (like rifampin) will increase the metabolism of many drugs, dose modifications of these other drugs will likely be necessary. This is of particular importance in the HIV-infected patient, where the interaction between the rifamycins and either zidovudine or azole antifungals may result in reduced efficacy.

Macrolides/Azalides

The new macrolide, clarithromycin, and azalide, azithromycin, represent substantial advances in the treatment of *M. avium* complex, but demonstrate limited activity against *M. tuberculosis,* and are not considered to be viable therapeutic alternatives.

In summary, few new antimycobacterial agents have been introduced to help combat drug-resistant strains. Of these, the quinolones appear most useful, but they are not a panacea, because adverse effects and drug resistance are also associated with their use. For the most part, the clinician must continue to utilize conventional chemotherapy, but must do so in the most efficient and conscientious manner possible.

PROGNOSIS

The success of chemotherapy for tuberculosis depends on three factors. The most important factor is the susceptibility of the isolate, particularly its susceptibility to rifampin. For patients infected with pan-sensitive strains or strains resistant to only one drug (excluding rifampin), the success rate of chemotherapy approaches 100%. In contrast, for rifampin-resistant (usually MDR-TB) strains, treatment is much more difficult.[87,88] It is estimated that the failure rate for MDR-TB is 80 times greater than that for susceptible strains.[87] This reflects the relatively poor activity of second- and third-line antitubercular agents, compared with rifampin and isoniazid.

As stated previously, a second important factor affecting prognosis is patient compliance. To achieve at least a 75% success rate, it is important that patients receive antitubercular therapy for at least 4 months, regardless of the regimen used. Ideally, therapy should continue for 4–6 months after sputum cultures have converted to negative. In noncompliant patients, relapse and failure rates of 15–25% are not uncommon.

A final factor influencing the prognosis is the immune status of the patient at the time of infection. In particular, HIV-infected patients with tuberculosis tend to experience worse outcomes than do seronegative individuals. In HIV-infected patients, it is important to distinguish death due to tuberculosis from death due to other causes. In studies that have examined the response to chemotherapy of HIV-infected patients with drug-susceptible tuberculosis, the risk for failure has been two to three times greater than for seronegative patients.[89,90] Because HIV-infected patients often possess other factors that worsen their prognosis (noncompliance, resistant strains), the overall prognosis is poorer, with failure rates of 50–70%.[89,90]

DRUG REGIMENS/FOLLOW-UP

Asymptomatic Infection

For patients with asymptomatic infection, the goal of therapy is to minimize disease progression. For the most part, this translates into "chemoprophylaxis" of all patients with a "positive" tuberculin skin test, as well as those HIV-seropositive anergic patients who are at high risk of infection, such as the homeless, IV drug abusers, and institutionalized patients. In all cases, the likelihood of morbidity and mortality due to the disease must be weighed against the likelihood of drug toxicity. Individuals who qualify for chemoprophylaxis and the appropriate drug regimens are listed in Table 105.7.

Chemoprophylaxis should be initiated in patients who are asymptomatic and have sufficient objective evidence of infection (history of recent exposure, skin test result, underlying disease state[s]) to merit therapy, *or* are infected with HIV, are anergic, and possess other risk factors for tuberculous infection (IV drug abuser, history of recent institutionalization/incarceration, exposure to others with tuberculosis).

Children who are close contacts of active cases of tuberculosis but are initially PPD negative should nonetheless be started on INH and retested after 3 months have elapsed.[91,92] Therapy may be discontinued if the repeat skin test is also negative, or continued for a total of 12 months if the test is positive.

Most clinicians now believe that a 6-month course of INH administered daily is sufficient in most asymptomatic patients.[93,94] Children, HIV-positive patients (or high-risk patients who refuse testing), and patients with stable abnormal chest films should still remain on therapy for 12 months. Although a regimen of daily INH 5 mg/kg (children: 10 mg/kg) to a maximum of 300 mg is recommended, individuals likely to be noncompliant may be treated with a regimen of 15 mg/kg (to a maximum of 900 mg) twice weekly with observation.

TABLE 105.7. ANTIMICROBIAL REGIMENS FOR CHEMOPROPHYLAXIS OF TUBERCULOSIS IN ASYMPTOMATIC PATIENTS

Patient Type/Situation	Drug and Regimen
Child with documented recent exposure to an index case of pulmonary tuberculosis	Skin test and INH for three months; continue for 12 months if skin test positive
Adult with "positive" PPD skin test and no other confounding factors	INH for 6 months
HIV-infected patient with "positive" PPD skin test, or anergic with risk factors for tuberculosis	INH for 12 months
Positive skin test and documented exposure to INH-resistant TB	PZA/rifampin or PZA/ethambutol for 12 months
Positive skin test and documented exposure to INH- and rifampin-resistant TB	PZA/ofloxacin for 12 months

Some physicians are hesitant to treat asymptomatic patients, even with positive skin tests, for fear of toxicity due to INH. It has been documented repeatedly that the risk of infection outweighs the risk for drug toxicity in patients eligible for treatment. In fact, recent reports suggest that this may even be the case in elderly patients and patients at lower risk for developing tuberculosis.[93,95]

When initiating chemoprophylaxis, the likelihood of infection with a drug-resistant strain should be determined. This will be difficult to confirm, because isolation of *M. tuberculosis* in asymptomatic patients is rarely successful. Some objective evidence of exposure to an index patient with drug-resistant tuberculosis should be obtained before using alternatives to INH (i.e., life-style of the exposed patient is insufficient evidence for suspecting drug resistance). If the individual has been exposed to a patient with INH-resistant *M. tuberculosis* or a patient who has failed chemotherapy, chemoprophylaxis with rifampin alone or in combination with pyrazinamide or ethambutol should be initiated and continued for 12 months. If the index case has documented MDR-TB, combination therapy with pyrazinamide and ofloxacin is recommended. All other patients should receive INH alone for 6 months (12 months for HIV-infected patients and children). As in the past, all patients treated with INH should receive pyridoxine 25–50 mg daily. All patients who receive chemoprophylaxis or empiric therapy for AFB-negative, symptomatic pulmonary tuberculosis should be monitored monthly for improvement/worsening of symptoms. Any worsening of the clinical condition should prompt a chest radiograph and sputum analysis for AFB.

Symptomatic Disease, Culture-Positive, Resistance Unlikely

For patients infected with *M. tuberculosis* who have clinically active disease, the goals of chemotherapy are to arrest progression of the disease, to eliminate all abnormal physical and laboratory tests, and, through eradication of nearly all (if not all) acid-fast bacilli, prevent relapse of the disease. In addition, it is important to isolate patients who are likely to transmit the disease to other individuals (i.e., those with pulmonary tuberculosis). Finally, persons who have come in contact with an infected patient must be located and examined for the presence of tuberculous infection. Tables 105.8 and 105.9 list drug regimen options and doses for treatment of symptomatic infection.

Short-course (6 months) chemotherapy with multiple antimicrobial agents is now the standard for treating drug-susceptible tuberculosis, because it results in equal or better efficacy, less toxicity, and better compliance than longer courses.[88,96–98] Patients who complete only 4 months of the 6-month short-course regimens are less likely to experience relapse than those who complete 4 months of a standard two-drug 9-month regimen.[96–98]

Current practices of chemotherapy for tuberculosis utilize combinations of two classes of agents: those that rapidly eliminate extracellular organisms from the sputum and decrease infectivity ("early bactericidal" drugs such as INH and streptomycin), and those that destroy slowly dividing organisms within granulomas and macrophages ("sterilizing" drugs such as rifampin and PZA).[44,96] As mentioned previously, this allows courses of therapy as short as 6 months to be used while preventing resistance from occurring. Bacteriostatic drugs such as ethambutol are of use in present-day regimens only when resistance to one or more bactericidal agents is suspected.[44]

Two distinct phases of this short-course form of chemotherapy are employed. The initial or "induction" phase is usually 2 months in duration. The goal of this phase is to rapidly destroy extracellular bacteria and thereby render the sputum noninfectious. Daily dosing of drugs is required because of the relatively rapid growth of this target population of bacteria. INH and rifampin constitute the core regimen for this phase. They are used in combination with pyrazinamide ± streptomycin or ethambutol when resistance is suspected and/or more rapid killing is desired.

The second or "continuation" phase is of longer duration and is designed to eliminate "persisters" from the body. Combined therapy with INH and rifampin is again used here; addition of other agents appears to offer no benefit.[96–101] During the continuation phase INH and rifampin may be dosed twice weekly rather than daily.[102] The organisms remaining at this point reside mainly within macrophages of granulomas and grow more slowly, allowing a longer dosing interval to be used. In addition, because rifampin is most active against organisms with intermittent spurts of growth activity, twice-weekly dosing theoretically may potentiate its action. Twice-weekly dosing is also less expensive and usually results in better patient compliance.

Initial antimycobacterial therapy should be selected based on the suspected susceptibility of the isolate. All patients should receive initial therapy with daily INH/rifampin/pyrazinamide.[88] In patients who have been treated previously and/or who may have been exposed to patients with drug-resistant strains, drug resistance should be suspected, and a fourth drug (either ethambutol or streptomycin) should be added.[30] In patients who are documented failures to conventional (three-drug) therapy or are considered likely to be infected with multidrug-resistant strains (e.g., part of a localized outbreak), both streptomycin and ethambutol should be added.[30]

When one or more of the above-mentioned "first-line" agents cannot be used (intolerance, drug resistance), the clinician must substitute a greater number of alternative agents to achieve the same degree of efficacy. In some cases older, more toxic agents such as ethionamide, para-aminosalicylic acid, cycloserine, or capreomycin must be used. The search continues for new agents that may serve as alternatives for first-line agents without the toxicity of older drugs.

Patients with pulmonary tuberculosis should be placed in strict respiratory isolation. The 1992 guidelines issued by

TABLE 105.8. TREATMENT REGIMEN OPTIONS FOR SYMPTOMATIC TUBERCULOSIS

Option 1—Reliably Compliant Patient, Drug Resistance Unlikely	Option 2—Less Reliable Patient and/or Drug Resistance Suspected	Option 3—Unreliable Patient; Drug Resistance Likely
INH/Rif/PZA +/– EMB or STR *daily* for 2 *months,* followed by INH/RIF 2–3 times weekly for 4 months	INH/RIF/PZA/EMB or STR *daily* for 2 *weeks,* followed by same drugs 2–3 times weekly for 6 *weeks,* followed by INH/RIF 2–3 times weekly for 4 months	INH/RIF/PZA/EMB or STR 2–3 times weekly for entire 6 months

For regimens utilizing 2–3 times weekly dosing, treatment should be via directly observed therapy (DOT). While a 6-month duration of therapy is noted, therapy should continue for 3 months after culture conversion to negative. HIV-infected patients should routinely be treated for 9 months total (6 months after culture conversion) by extending the maintenance period to 7 months.

Key: INH, isoniazid; RIF, rifampin; PZA, pyrazinamide; EMB, ethambutol; STR, streptomycin.

TABLE 105.9. DOSING REGIMENS FOR COMMON ANTITUBERCULAR AGENTS IN ADULTS AND CHILDREN, ASSUMING NORMAL RENAL AND/OR HEPATIC FUNCTION

Drug	Doses in Adults (Maximum)	Doses in Children (Maximum)
Isoniazid	5 mg/kg (300 mg) daily, or 15 mg/kg (900 mg) 2–3 times weekly	10–20 mg/kg (300 mg) daily, or 20–40 mg/kg (900 mg) 2–3 times weekly
Rifampin	10 mg/kg (600 mg) daily or 2–3 times weekly	10–20 mg/kg (600 mg) daily or 2–3 times weekly
Pyrazinamide	15–30 mg/kg (2000 mg) daily, 50–70 mg/kg (4000 mg) 2 times weekly, or 50–70 mg/kg (3000 mg) 3 times weekly	Same as for adults
Ethambutol	15–25 mg/kg (2500 mg) daily, 50 mg/kg (2500 mg) 2 times weekly, or 25–30 mg/kg (2500 mg) 3 times weekly	Same as for adult; avoid use in children less than 6 years of age
Streptomycin	15 mg/kg (1000 mg) daily, 25–30 mg/kg (1500 mg) 2 times weekly, or 25–30 mg/kg (1000 mg) 3 times weekly	20–30 mg/kg (1000 mg) daily; same as for adults 2–3 times weekly

the National Institute for Occupational Safety and Health (NIOSH) state that all health care workers who must come in contact with the patient while in respiratory isolation should wear a powered, half-mask respirator equipped with a high efficiency particulate air (HEPA) filter, which will filter particles of 1 μm. Whether this drastic approach is feasible and necessary, however, has been hotly debated. Nonpowered HEPA filters have also been advocated by the Occupational Safety and Health Administration (OSHA) at a cost of $7.50 to $9.00 each.[103] Other alternatives that are slightly less efficient, yet less expensive and easier to use, include dust/mist and dust/mist/fume respirators at a cost of approximately $1.00 each. Final recommendations from OSHA are still pending. In the meantime, some institutions have been fined for not adhering to these preliminary recommendations. One published study concluded that, at the authors' institution, switching from dust/mist masks to HEPA filters would prevent one case of occupationally acquired tuberculosis every 41 years, at an additional cost of $1.3 million to $18.5 million. The use of these more expensive respirators would result in an additional cost of $7 million per case of tuberculosis and $100 million per life saved.[104] Clearly, this issue has not been resolved, and the more conservative approach to protection stated by NIOSH has not been met with enthusiasm by many.

A fixed combination product (Rifater, Marion Merrell-Dow) of rifampin 120 mg, isoniazid 50 mg, and pyrazinamide 300 mg is now available in the United States. It is anticipated that the use of this product will enhance compliance. However, the typical daily dose for this product will be five to six tablets daily, which is a similar number of doses required for the drugs taken separately. In addition, the ratio of dose strengths reflects the doses administered on a daily basis; these ratios change when drug therapy is changed to a twice-weekly regimen. For example, while the twice-weekly dose of isoniazid in an adult is three times the daily dose, the dose of rifampin is unchanged (Table 105.9).

Patients should have sputum samples sent for AFB stains every 1–2 days, until a consistent downward trend in the number of AFB observed in sputum is realized. This may typically take 10–14 days. After that time, the patient may be removed from isolation and, if symptomatically improved, discharged from the hospital.[78] The remainder of the course of therapy may be completed on an outpatient basis. However, the schedule of administration will depend on the reliability of the patient to comply with therapy (Table 105.8).[30,78] Once on maintenance therapy, patients should have sputum collected for AFB stain every 2 weeks until negative, and sputum cultures performed monthly until negative. It is anticipated that cultures will convert to negative within 2 months. If sputum cultures continue to be positive after 4 months, drug resistance should be suspected.

THERAPEUTIC ENDPOINTS

The following time line would constitute an "ideal" approach to/response to short-course chemotherapy:

Day 0	Isolate sent for susceptibility tests; respiratory isolation initiated.
Day 5	Symptomatic improvement (fever, malaise, cough) noted.
Day 14	Substantial reduction in AFB in sputum; stable chest radiograph; remove from isolation, discharge.
2 months	Sputum is AFB negative; susceptibility results allow modification of therapy.
4 months	Last sputum culture was negative.
6 months	Discontinue drug therapy.

EFFICACY/EFFECTIVENESS

For patients infected with drug-susceptible strains who are treated with appropriate therapy and are compliant and/or treated with directly observed therapy (DOT), efficacy approaches 100%. Noncompliance, drug resistance, extrapulmonary disease, and concomitant disease states reduce the overall effectiveness of chemotherapy of tuberculosis to about 75%.

MONITORING

Microbiological monitoring is as outlined previously. In addition, patients should have serum chemistries performed for AST/ALT periodically, depending on the presence of other factors that may increase the likelihood of hepatotoxicity (advanced age, alcohol abuse, and possibly pregnancy). Hepatotoxicity should be suspected in patients whose transaminases exceed 350 u/mL or whose total bilirubin exceeds 3 mg/dL. At this point, the offending agent(s) should be discontinued, and alternatives selected. Audiometric testing should be performed in patients who must receive streptomycin for more than 2 months. Vision testing should be performed on all patients who must receive ethambutol for more than 2 months. All patients diagnosed with tuberculosis should be tested for HIV infection.

OTHER THERAPEUTIC ISSUES/SITUATIONS

Smear and/or Culture Negative

In some instances, patients who present with signs and symptoms of pulmonary tuberculosis along with some evidence of infection of *M. tuberculosis* (i.e., a positive skin test) will not have acid-fast bacilli isolated. These patients may have very low numbers of organisms, and empiric therapy with INH and rifampin for 6 months appears warranted. Patients with smear-negative tuberculosis have been shown to achieve more rapid sterilization of sputum than smear-positive patients. Six months of therapy with INH and rifampin appears to be adequate for smear-negative, culture-positive patients.[105,106] Many clinicians opt to discontinue empiric antitubercular therapy in PPD-positive patients with clinical findings consistent with tuberculosis who are both sputum smear- and culture-negative. However, some studies have demonstrated a 75% rate of progression in these individuals.[107] Investigators in Arkansas[108] have reported that for patients in whom sputum smears and cultures have been consistently negative throughout therapy, treatment with only 4 months of combined INH and rifampin is adequate. In foreign countries or areas where resistance to INH or rifampin may occur, therapy with four drugs (INH, rifampin, PZA, and ethambutol) should be used.[105]

Drug Resistance Likely or Suspected

Patients in whom relapse of disease occurs despite adequate treatment usually present within 6 months after completion of therapy. Relapse is usually due to organisms that are susceptible to the antituberculous drugs used initially.[30,31,109–113] In contrast, failure during therapy is frequently associated with resistance. Noncompliance is the major cause of therapeutic failure. Drug resistance should be suspected in the following situations:

- Patients who have received prior therapy for tuberculosis
- Patients from geographic areas with a high prevalence of resistance (New York, Mexico, Southeast Asia)
- Patients who are homeless, institutionalized, IV drug abusers, and/or infected with HIV
- Patients who still have AFB-positive sputum smears after 2 months of therapy
- Patients who still have positive cultures after 4 months of therapy

Patients who require retreatment (along with those in whom therapy is failing and those with a documented exposure to drug-resistant organisms) should be considered to be infected with resistant organisms until proven otherwise. In patients with prior treatment, therapy should be modified to include two additional drugs that have not been used previously. For initial therapy in suspected drug-resistant tuberculosis, a four-drug regimen should be used (Table 105.8). These regimens may be altered when the susceptibility pattern becomes known.

Drug Resistance Proven

Therapy may need to be modified if drug resistance is detected from the initial susceptibility report. Specific therapy will depend on the susceptibility pattern observed and is outlined in Table 105.10.[114] When resistance to rifampin is documented, the duration of therapy required increases markedly.

Surgical intervention including lobectomy was once a common mode of treatment for tuberculosis. Today, indications for surgery are limited to removal of necrotic tissue, drainage of abscesses and other sites of fluid collection, and as a last resort for infection due to organisms resistant to multiple agents.[3,115]

"Unreliable" Patient

The CDC has modified its recommended therapeutic regimens to account for trends in drug resistance and noncompliance. For patients in whom there is no question about compliance, medications may continue to be given daily on a self-administered basis. However, for those in whom compliance may be a problem (and any patient receiving streptomycin), subsequent therapy should be administered on a twice- or three-times-weekly basis, using DOT.[113] DOT may be performed by having the patient come to a clinic or through home visits. This form of therapy improves compliance and, secondarily, the frequency of

TABLE 105.10. SUGGESTED DRUG REGIMENS FOR DOCUMENTED DRUG-RESISTANT TUBERCULOSIS

Documented Resistance to:	Change Therapy to (X):								Duration (months)
	Rif	PZA	EMB	Amik	Quin	Ethio	CyS	PAS	
INH,PZA,S	X	X	X	X					6–9
INH,EMB,S	X	X		X	X				6–12
INH,RIF,S		X	X	X	X				18–24
INH,RIF,EMB,S		X		X	X	X±	X±	X±	24+
INH,RIF,PZA,S			X	X	X	X±	X±	X±	24+
INH,RIF,PZA,EMB,S				X	X	X±	X±	X±	24+

Key: INH, isoniazid; RIF, rifampin; PZA, pyrazinamide; EMB, ethambutol; S, streptomycin; Amik, amikacin 15–20 mg/kg/d; Quin, quinolone such as ofloxacin 800 mg/d; Ethio, ethionamide 500–1000 mg/d; CyS, cycloserine 500–1000 mg/d; PAS, *p*-aminosalicylate 10–12 g/d. For isolates resistant to four drugs, surgical intervention (lobectomy) should be considered. (Adapted from Ref. 11.)

favorable outcomes. In addition, DOT reduces the incidence of both primary and secondary drug resistance within a community.[116]

It is generally considered that the homeless and other underprivileged individuals constitute the group of patients considered "unreliable," and that DOT should be reserved for them. However, "responsible" patients cared for by private physicians may be treated with daily, unsupervised therapy. A study conducted in Baltimore, Maryland, compared outcomes (sputum culture conversion to negative at 3 months) in patients with pulmonary tuberculosis who were treated by private physicians with outcomes in patients treated via DOT in a city-run clinic. Surprisingly, 3-month culture conversion occurred in only 40% of the private-care patients, compared with 90% in the city clinic-care patients![117] Clearly, expansion of the use of DOT to nearly all patients with tuberculosis may be of benefit.

Pregnancy

Women with tuberculosis should be cautioned against becoming pregnant, as the disease poses a risk to the fetus as well as to the mother. Treatment regimens for tuberculosis in pregnant patients should involve agents with minimal teratogenic potential. Studies that have examined the incidence of birth defects resulting from various antituberculous drugs concluded that the risk to infants born to mothers treated with INH or ethambutol was equal to that in normal populations.[78,118–120] Rifampin therapy was also associated with a low complication rate.[120] However, treatment with streptomycin resulted in a higher than normal rate of infant malformations, mainly in the form of ototoxicity.[119,120] The teratogenic potential of PZA is unknown, and its use should therefore be avoided.

Pregnant women with active tuberculosis should probably receive INH and rifampin for a period of 9 months. If a third drug is necessary, ethambutol may be added. Therapy with INH for asymptomatic tuberculous infection may be delayed until after pregnancy or, if recent skin test conversion has occurred, started during the second trimester of pregnancy.[120] Although most antituberculous drugs are excreted in breast milk, the amount of drug received by the infant through nursing is insufficient to cause toxicity.[120]

Children

Tuberculosis in children may be treated with regimens similar to those used in adults. A regimen of both INH and rifampin given daily for 1–2 months followed by rifampin and INH daily or twice weekly for 8 months has been shown to be highly effective.[44,121] Alternatively, short-course therapy using 6-month regimens similar to those observed in adults may be used.[44,78,122,123] Doses of INH and rifampin on a milligram per kilogram basis are higher than those used in adults (Table 105.9).[44]

HIV Infected

Tuberculosis in AIDS patients and other immunocompromised hosts may be managed with chemotherapeutic regimens similar to those used in immunocompetent individuals. Differentiation must be made between infection with *M. tuberculosis* and MOTT such as *M. avium* complex, because therapy for the latter requires a greater number of antimicrobials and is associated with more treatment failures.[64] While short-course therapy of tuberculosis may be used,[89,124] some failures have been reported.[125] Therefore, a longer course of therapy (INH, rifampin, and PZA for 2–3 months followed by INH and rifampin for 6–7 months) is generally recommended. As was noted previously, prognosis is particularly poor for HIV-infected patients infected with MDR-TB.[89]

INH and/or rifampin may interact with other medications frequently administered to AIDS patients (e.g., fluconazole, ketoconazole, zidovudine), so dose adjustments of these drugs may be necessary.[64,85]

Extrapulmonary tuberculosis has traditionally been considered to be a more severe form of the disease, and recommendations for treatment usually include three or more drugs given for an extended period of time. From a theoretical standpoint, patients with only extrapulmonary disease probably harbor fewer organisms than do those with pulmonary tuberculosis. Considering the fact that the extravascular penetration of most antituberculous agents is excellent, it would appear that short-course therapy would be adequate for treatment. Studies have confirmed this theory, demonstrating greater than 95% success rates for 6- and 9-month treatment regimens.[121,126] Adjunctive therapy with corticosteroids may be of benefit in some patients with tuberculous meningitis.[127] Most antituberculous agents pass easily into the cerebrospinal fluid, and the use of steroids will have little impact on their penetration into cerebrospinal fluid.[128]

BCG VACCINATION

The bacille Calmette–Guérin (BCG) is an attenuated, hybridized strain of *M. bovis.* It was originally developed in 1921 and is used as a prophylactic vaccine against tuberculosis. Administration of BCG vaccine is compulsory in 64 countries and is officially recommended in 118 others.[129]

Vaccination with BCG produces a subclinical infection resulting in sensitization of T lymphocytes and cross-immunity to *M. tuberculosis,* as well as cutaneous hypersensitivity and a positive tuberculin skin test.[129,130] BCG vaccination should be used only in geographic areas where tuberculosis infection rates are sufficiently high to preclude the use of the PPD skin test as a screening tool and where health programs are inadequate to detect newly infected individuals.[78] Such areas include underdeveloped countries in Asia, Africa, and South America as well as certain metropolitan areas within the United States and other developed countries where large immigrant populations exist.

BCG has been used to immunize infants in undeveloped countries to protect against active tuberculosis. Use of the vaccine precludes the ability to detect asymptomatic tuberculous infection through skin testing and may lead to boosting in later life. Although estimates of BCG's efficacy to prevent tuberculosis have ranged from 0–80%, a recently published meta-analysis estimated the success rate at 50% (i.e., reducing the infection rate by one-half).[131] Nearly all studies with BCG have been performed in countries with very high (1%) annual case rates for TB. None have been performed in the United States. Based on this lack of information, widespread use of BCG in the United States cannot be recommended. However, in certain situations, such as in health care workers who are constantly exposed to infected patients, other high-risk individuals (estimated annual rate of infection > 1%) who cannot take INH, or close contacts (i.e., family members) of individuals who are noncompliant with therapy and/or are infected with drug-resistant strains, BCG may become a viable alternative for prevention of tuberculosis.

PATIENT COOPERATION

As stated previously, good patient compliance is the cornerstone to effective antimycobacterial chemotherapy. Pharmacists should educate patients on the importance of continuing their chemotherapy, despite symptomatic improvement. Many patients with tuberculosis have little insight into the cause of their disease, and fail to take their medication because they view the disease as a social malady, not an infectious disease. Pharmacy-based centers for patients in DOT programs could be developed. Alternatively, the pharmacist should become part of a multidisciplinary clinic (with nurses, physicians, social workers) devoted to successful outpatient chemotherapy of tuberculosis patients and their families.

REFERENCES

1. Sepkowitz KA, Raffalli J, Riley L, et al. Tuberculosis in the AIDS era. Clin Microbiol Rev 1995;8:180–199.
2. Boyars MC. The microbiology, chemotherapy, and surgical treatment of tuberculosis. J Thorac Imag 1990;5:1–7.
3. Haas DW, Des Prez RM. *Mycobacterium tuberculosis,* in Mandell GL, Bennett JE, Dolin R (eds): Principles and Practice of Infectious Diseases, 4th ed. New York, John Wiley and Sons, 1995, pp 2213–2243.
4. Riley RL, Mills CC, Nyka W, et al. Aerial dissemination of pulmonary tuberculosis; a two-year study of contagion in a tuberculosis ward. Am J Hygiene 1959;70:185–196.
5. Orme IM, Andersen P, Boom WH. T cell response to *Mycobacterium tuberculosis.* J Infect Dis 1993;167:1481–1497.
6. Haque AK. The pathology and pathophysiology of mycobacterial infections. J Thorac Imag 1990;5:8–16.
7. American Thoracic Society. Diagnostic standards and classification of tuberculosis. Am Rev Respir Dis 1990;142:725–735.
8. Geppert EF, Leff A. The pathogenesis of pulmonary and miliary tuberculosis. Arch Intern Med 1979;139:1381–1383.
9. Kleinhenz ME, Ellner JJ. Antigen responsiveness during tuberculosis: Regulatory interactions of T cell subpopulations and adherent cells. J Lab Clin Med 1987;110:31–40.
10. Rieder HL, Cauthen GM, Kelley GD, et al. Tuberculosis in the United States. JAMA 1989;262:385–389.
11. Alvarez S, McCabe WR. Extrapulmonary tuberculosis revisited: A review of experience at Boston City and other hospitals. Medicine 1984;63:25–55.
12. Stead WW. Pathogenesis of a first episode of chronic pulmonary tuberculosis in man: Recrudescence of residuals of the primary infection or exogenous reinfection? Am Rev Respir Dis 1967;95:729–745.
13. Markowitz N, Hansen NI, Wilcosky TC, et al. Tuberculin and anergy testing in HIV-seropositive and HIV-seronegative persons. Ann Intern Med 1993;119:185–193.
14. Alland D, Kalkut GE, Moss AR, et al. Transmission of tuberculosis in New York City: An analysis of DNA finger-

printing and conventional epidemiologic methods. N Engl J Med 1994;330:1710–1716.

15. Small PM, Hopewell PC, Singh SP, et al. The epidemiology of tuberculosis in San Francisco: A population-based study using conventional and molecular methods. N Engl J Med 1994;330:1703–1709.
16. Daley CL, Small PM, Schecter GF, et al. An outbreak of tuberculosis with accelerated progression among persons infected with the human immunodeficiency virus: An analysis using restricted-fragment-length polymorphisms. N Engl J Med 1992;326:231–235.
17. Wallis RS, Vjecha M, Amir-Tahmasseb M, et al. Influence of tuberculosis on human immunodeficiency virus (HIV-1): Enhanced cytokine expression and elevated β_2-microglobulin in HIV-1-associated tuberculosis. J Infect Dis 1993;167:43–48.
18. Pape JW, Jean SS, Ho JL, et al. Effect of isoniazid prophylaxis on incidence of active tuberculosis and progression of HIV infection. Lancet 1993;342:268–272.
19. Bloch AB, Rieder HL, Kelley GD, et al. The epidemiology of tuberculosis in the United States. Semin Respir Infect 1989;4:157–170.
20. McKenna MT, McCray E, Onorato I. The epidemiology of tuberculosis among foreign-born persons in the United States, 1986 to 1993. N Engl J Med 1995;332:1071–1076.
21. Bentley DW. Tuberculosis in long-term care facilities. Infect Control Hosp Epidemiol 1990;11:42–46.
22. Centers for Disease Control. Cases of specified notable diseases, United States, weeks ending December 29, 1990, and December 30, 1989. MMWR 1991;39:944.
23. Malasky C, Jordan T, Potulski F, et al. Occupational tuberculous infections among pulmonary physicians in training. Am Rev Respir Dis 1990;142:505–507.
24. Kantor HS, Poblete R, Pusateri SL. Nosocomial transmission of tuberculosis from unsuspected disease. Am J Med 1988;84:833–838.
25. Sepkowitz KA. Tuberculosis and the health care worker: A historical perspective. Ann Intern Med 1994;120:71–79.
26. Pearson ML, Jereb JA, Frieden TR, et al. Nosocomial transmission of multidrug-resistant *Mycobacterium tuberculosis:* A risk to patients and health care workers. Ann Intern Med 1992;117:191–196.
27. Rosenblum LS, Castro KG, Dooley S, Morgan M. Effect of HIV infection and tuberculosis on hospitalizations and cost of care for young adults in the United States, 1985 to 1990. Ann Intern Med 1994;121:786–792.
28. Small PM, Shafer RW, Hopewell PC, et al. Exogenous reinfection with multidrug-resistant *Mycobacterium tuberculosis* in patients with advanced HIV infection. N Engl J Med 1993;328:1137–1144.
29. Beck-Sague C, Dooley SW, Hutton MD, et al. Hospital outbreak of multidrug-resistant *Mycobacterium tuberculosis* infections: Factors in transmission to staff and HIV-infected patients. JAMA 1992;268:1280–1286.
30. Centers for Disease Control. Meeting the challenge of multidrug-resistant tuberculosis: Summary of a conference. MMWR 1992;41(RR-11):51–71.
31. Jacobs RF. Multiple-drug-resistant tuberculosis. Clin Infect Dis 1994;19:1–10.
32. Dessen A, Quemard A, Blanchard JS, et al. Crystal structure and function of the isoniazid target of *Mycobacterium tuberculosis.* Science 1995;267:1638–1641.
33. Bloom BR, Murray CJL. Tuberculosis: Commentary on a reemergent killer. Science 1992;257:1055–1064.
34. Zhang Y, Steingrube VA, Wallace RJ. Beta-lactamase inhibitors and the inducibility of the beta-lactamase of *Mycobacterium tuberculosis.* Am Rev Resp Dis 1992;145:657–660.
35. Bloch AB, Cauthen GM, Onorato IM, et al. Nationwide survey of drug-resistant tuberculosis in the United States. JAMA 1994;271:665–671.
36. Fischl MA, Uttamchandam RB, Daikos GL, et al. An outbreak of tuberculosis caused by multiple-drug-resistant tubercle bacilli among patients with HIV infection. Ann Intern Med 1992;117:177–183.
37. Chawla PK, Klapper PJ, Kamholz SL, et al. Drug-resistant tuberculosis in an urban hospital including patients at risk for human immunodeficiency virus infection. Am Rev Resp Dis 1992;146:280–284.
38. Frieden TR, Sterling T, Pablos-Mendez A, et al. The emergence of drug-resistant tuberculosis in New York City. N Engl J Med 1993;328:521–526.
39. Mahmoudi A, Iseman MD. Pitfalls in the care of patients with tuberculosis: Common errors and their association with the acquisition of drug resistance. JAMA 1993;270:65–68.
40. Brudney K, Dobkin J. Resurgent tuberculosis in New York City: Human immunodeficiency virus, homelessness, and the decline of tuberculosis control programs. Am Rev Resp Dis 1991;144:745–749.
41. Alvarez S, Shell C, Berk SL. Pulmonary tuberculosis in elderly men. Am J Med 1987;82:602–606.
42. Umeki S. Comparison of younger and elderly patients with pulmonary tuberculosis. Respiration 1989;55:75–83.
43. Snider DE, Rieder HL, Combs D, et al. Tuberculosis in children. Pediatr Infect Dis J 1988;7:271–278.
44. Starke JR. Multidrug therapy for tuberculosis in children. Pediatr Infect Dis J 1990;9:785–793.
45. Jones BE, Young SMM, Antoniskis D, et al. Relationship of the manifestations of tuberculosis to CD4 cell counts in patients with human immunodeficiency virus infection. Am Rev Resp Dis 1993;148:1292–1297.
46. Centers for Disease Control. Tuberculosis and human immunodeficiency virus infection: Recommendations of the advisory committee for the elimination of tuberculosis (ACET). MMWR 1989;38:236–249.
47. Centers for Disease Control. Tuberculosis control among homeless populations. MMWR 1987;36:257–260.
48. Centers for Disease Control. Tuberculosis among foreign-born persons entering the United States. MMWR 1990;38(RR-18):1–21.
49. Friedman LN, Sullivan GM, Bevilaqua RP, et al. Tuberculosis screening in alcoholics and drug addicts. Am Rev Respir Dis 1987;136:1188–1192.
50. Centers for Disease Control. Prevention and control of tuberculosis in facilities providing long-term care to the elderly. MMWR 1990;39(RR-10):7–20.
51. Centers for Disease Control. Prevention and control of tuberculosis in correctional institutions. MMWR 1989;38:313–325.

52. Stead WW. Annual tuberculosis screening of hospital employees—an idea whose time has not passed. Am Rev Respir Dis 1987;136:803–804.
53. Schecter CB, Rose DN, Fahs MC, et al. Tuberculin screening: Cost-effectiveness analysis of various testing schedules. Am J Prev Med 1990;6:167–175.
54. Snider DE. The tuberculin skin test. Am Rev Respir Dis 1982;125(suppl):108–118.
55. Sbarbaro JA. Skin testing in the diagnosis of tuberculosis. Semin Respir Infect 1986;1:234–238.
56. Reichman LB. Tuberculin skin testing: The state of the art. Chest 1979;76(suppl):764–770.
57. Burstin SJ, Muspratt JA, Rossing TH. The tuberculin test: Studies of the dynamics of reactivity to tuberculin and candida antigen in institutionalized patients. Am Rev Respir Dis 1986;134:1072–1074.
58. Lifson AR, Watters JK, Thompson S, et al. Discrepancies in tuberculin skin test results with two commercial products in a population of intravenous drug users. J Infect Dis 1993;168:1048–1051.
59. Thompson NJ, Glassroth JL, Snider DE, et al. The booster phenomenon in serial tuberculin testing. Am Rev Respir Dis 1979;119:587–597.
60. Cauthen GM, Snider DE. Delayed tuberculin boosting in the older population. Am Rev Respir Dis 1986;134:857–858.
61. Menzies R, Vissandjee B, Rocher I, St. Germain Y. The booster effect in two-step tuberculin testing among young adults in Montreal. Ann Intern Med 1994;120:190–198.
62. Rosenberg T, Manfreda J, Hershfield ES. Two-step tuberculin testing in staff and residents of a nursing home. Am Rev Resp Dis 1993;148:1537–1540.
63. Webster CT, Gordin FM, Matts JP, et al. Two-stage tuberculin skin testing in individuals with human immunodeficiency virus infection. Am J Respir Crit Care Med 1995;151:805–808.
64. Barnes PF, Bloch AB, Davidson PT, et al. Tuberculosis in patients with human immunodeficiency virus infection. N Engl J Med 1991;324:1644–1650.
65. Centers for Disease Control. Purified protein derivative (PPD)-tuberculin anergy and HIV infection: Guidelines for anergy testing and management of anergic persons at risk of tuberculosis. MMWR 1991;40(RR-5):27–33.
66. Graham NMH, Nelson KE, Solomon L, et al. Prevalence of tuberculin positivity and skin test anergy in HIV-1-seropositive and -seronegative intravenous drug users. JAMA 1992;267:369–373.
67. Huebner RE, Schein MF, Hall CA, Barnes SA. Delayed-type hypersensitivity anergy in human immunodeficiency virus-infected persons screened for infection with *Mycobacterium tuberculosis.* Clin Infect Dis 1994;19:26–32.
68. Moreno S, Baraia-Etxaburu J, Bouza E, et al. Risk for developing tuberculosis among anergic patients infected with HIV. Ann Intern Med 1993;119:194–198.
69. Pesanti EL. The negative tuberculin test: Tuberculin, HIV, and anergy panels. Am J Respir Crit Care Med 1994;149:1699–1709.
70. Selwyn PA, Sckell BM, Alcabes P, et al. High risk of active tuberculosis in HIV-infected drug users with cutaneous anergy. JAMA 1992;268:504–509.
71. Barnes PE, Steele MA, Young SMM, Vachon LA. Tuberculosis in patients with human immunodeficiency virus infection: How often does it mimic *Pneumocystis carinii* pneumonia? Chest 1992;102:428–432.
72. Schluger NW, Rom WN. Current approaches to the diagnosis of active pulmonary tuberculosis. Am J Resp Crit Care Med 1994;149:264–267.
73. Mehta J, Krish G, Berro E, et al. Fiberoptic bronchoscopy in the diagnosis of pulmonary tuberculosis. South Med J 1990;83:753–755.
74. Bouza E, Diaz-Lopez MD, Moreno S, et al. *Mycobacterium tuberculosis* bacteremia in patients with and without human immunodeficiency virus infection. Arch Intern Med 1993;153:496–500.
75. Daniel TM. The rapid diagnosis of tuberculosis: A selective review. J Lab Clin Med 1990;116:277–282.
76. Wilkins EGL, Ivanyi J. Potential value of serology for diagnosis of extrapulmonary tuberculosis. Lancet 1990;2:641–644.
77. Mitchison DA. Basic mechanisms of chemotherapy. Chest 1979;76(suppl):771–781.
78. American Thoracic Society. Treatment of tuberculosis and tuberculosis infection in adults and children. Am J Respir Crit Care Med 1994;149:1359–1374.
79. O'Brien RJ. Present chemotherapy of tuberculosis. Semin Respir Infect 1989;4:216–224.
80. Girling DJ. Adverse effects of antituberculous drugs. Drugs 1982;23:56–74.
81. Snider DE, Caras GJ. Isoniazid-associated hepatitis deaths: A review of available information. Am Rev Resp Dis 1992;145:494–497.
82. Brent J, Vo N, Kulig K, et al. Reversal of prolonged isoniazid-induced coma by pyridoxine. Arch Intern Med 1990;150:1751–1753.
83. Holdiness MR. Clinical pharmacokinetics of the antituberculosis drugs. Clin Pharmacokinet 1984;9:511–544.
84. Davis CE, Carpenter JL, Ognibene AJ, et al. Rifampin-induced acute renal failure. South Med J 1986;79:1012–1015.
85. Burger DM, Meenhorst PL, Koks CHW, Beijnen JH. Pharmacokinetic interaction between rifampin and zidovudine. Antimicrob Agents Chemother 1993;37:1426–1431.
86. Steele MA, Des Prez RM. The role of pyrazinamide in tuberculosis chemotherapy. Chest 1988;94:845–850.
87. Goble M, Iseman MD, Madsen LA, et al. Treatment of 171 patients with pulmonary tuberculosis resistant to isoniazid and rifampin. Engl J Med 1993;328:527–532.
88. Hong Kong Chest Service/British Medical Research Council. Controlled trial of 2, 4, and 6 months of pyrazinamide in 6-month, three-times-weekly regimens for smear-positive pulmonary tuberculosis, including an assessment of a combined preparation of isoniazid, rifampin, and pyrazinamide. Am Rev Resp Dis 1991;143:700–706.
89. Busillo CP, Lessmau KD, Sanjana V, et al. Multidrug resistant *Mycobacterium tuberculosis* in patients with human immunodeficiency virus infection. Chest 1992;102:797–801.
90. Fischl MA, Daikos GL, Uttamchandani RB, et al. Clinical presentation and outcome of patients with HIV infection and tuberculosis caused by multiple-drug-resistant bacilli. Ann Intern Med 1992;117:184–190.

91. Starke JR. Current chemotherapy for tuberculosis in children. Infect Dis Clin North Am 1992;6:215–238.
92. Grossman M, Hopewell PC, Jacobs RF, et al. Consensus: Management of tuberculin-positive children without evidence of disease. Pediatr Infect Dis J 1988;7:243–246.
93. Rose DN, Schecter CB, Silver AL. The age threshold for isoniazid prophylaxis: A decision analysis for low-risk tuberculin reactors. JAMA 1986;256:2709–2713.
94. International Union Against Tuberculosis, Committee on Prophylaxis. Efficacy of various durations of isoniazid preventive therapy for tuberculosis: Five years of follow-up in the IUAT trial. Bull WHO 1982;60:555–564.
95. Stead WW, To T, Harrison RW, et al. Benefit–risk considerations in preventive treatment for tuberculosis in elderly persons. Ann Intern Med 1987;107:843–845.
96. Stratton MA, Reed MD. Short-course drug therapy for tuberculosis. Clin Pharm 1986;5:977–987.
97. Combs DL, O'Brien RJ, Geiter LJ. USPHS tuberculosis short-course chemotherapy trial 21: Effectiveness, toxicity, and acceptability. Ann Intern Med 1990;112:397–406.
98. Hong Kong Chest Service/British Medical Research Council. Five-year follow-up of a controlled trial of five six-month regimens of chemotherapy for pulmonary tuberculosis. Am Rev Resp Dis 1987;136:1339–1342.
99. East and Central African/British Medical Research Council. Controlled clinical trial of 4 short-course regimens of chemotherapy (three 6-month and one 8-month) for pulmonary tuberculosis: Final report. Tubercle 1986;67:5–15.
100. Castelo A, Jardim JRB, Goihman S, et al. Comparison of daily and twice-weekly regimens to treat pulmonary tuberculosis. Lancet 1989;2:1173–1176.
101. Cohn DL, Catlin BJ, Peterson KL, et al. A 62-dose, 6-month therapy for pulmonary and extrapulmonary tuberculosis: A twice-weekly, directly-observed, and cost-effective regimen. Ann Intern Med 1990;112:407–415.
102. Singapore Tuberculosis Service/British Medical Research Council. Five-year follow-up of a clinical trial of three 6-month regimens of chemotherapy given intermittently in the continuation phase in the treatment of pulmonary tuberculosis. Am Rev Resp Dis 1988;137:1147–1150.
103. Decker MD. OSHA enforcement policy for occupational exposure to tuberculosis. Infect Control Hosp Epidemiol 1993;14:689–693.
104. Adal KA, Anglim AM, Palumbo L, et al. The use of high efficiency particulate air filter respirators to protect hospital workers from tuberculosis: A cost-effectiveness analysis. N Engl J Med 1994;331:169–173.
105. Hong Kong Chest Service/Tuberculosis Research Center, Madras/British Medical Research Council. A controlled trial of 3-month, 4-month, and 6-month regimens of chemotherapy for sputum-smear-negative pulmonary tuberculosis. Am Rev Respir Dis 1989;139:871–876.
106. Dutt AK, Moers D, Stead WW. Smear-negative, culture-positive pulmonary tuberculosis: Six-month chemotherapy with isoniazid and rifampin. Am Rev Respir Dis 1990; 141:1232–1235.
107. Hong Kong Chest Service/British Medical Research Council. A controlled trial of 2-month, 3-month, and 12-month regimens of chemotherapy for sputum-smear-negative pulmonary tuberculosis. Am Rev Respir Dis 1984;130:23–28.
108. Dutt AK, Moers D, Stead WW. Smear- and culture-negative pulmonary tuberculosis: Four-month short-course chemotherapy. Am Rev Respir Dis 1989;139:867–870.
109. Suwanogool S, Smith SM, Smith LG, et al. Drug resistance encountered in the retreatment of *Mycobacterium tuberculosis* infections. J Chron Dis 1984;37:925–931.
110. Iseman MD, Madsen LA. Drug-resistant tuberculosis. Clin Chest Med 1989;10:341–353.
111. Mitchison DA, Nunn AJ. Influence of initial drug resistance on the response to short-course chemotherapy of pulmonary tuberculosis. Am Rev Respir Dis 1986;133:423–430.
112. Swai OB, Aluoch JA, Githui WA, et al. Controlled clinical trial of a regimen of two durations for the treatment of isoniazid-resistant pulmonary tuberculosis. Tubercle 1988;69:5–14.
113. Centers for Disease Control. Initial therapy for tuberculosis in the era of multidrug resistance: Recommendations of the advisory council for the elimination of tuberculosis. MMWR 1993;42(RR-7):1–8.
114. Iseman MD. Treatment of multidrug-resistant tuberculosis. N Engl J Med 1993;329:784–791.
115. Iseman MD, Madsen L, Goble M, et al. Surgical intervention in the treatment of pulmonary disease caused by drug-resistant *Mycobacterium tuberculosis*. Am Rev Respir Dis 1990;141:623–625.
116. Weis SE, Slocum PC, Blais FX, et al. The effect of directly observed therapy on the rates of drug resistance and relapse in tuberculosis. N Engl J Med 1994;330:1179–1184.
117. Chaulk CP, Bartlett JG, Chaisson RE. 15 years of directly observed therapy for TB. Program and Abstracts, 32nd Annual Meeting, Infectious Diseases Society of America, Orlando, FL, October 7–9, 1994, abstract 181.
118. Hamadeh MA, Glassroth J. Tuberculosis and pregnancy. Chest 1992;101:1114–1120.
119. Snider DM, Layde PM, Johnson MW, et al. Treatment of tuberculosis during pregnancy. Am J Respir Dis 1980;122:65–79.
120. Jacobs RF, Abernathy RS. Management of tuberculosis in pregnancy and the newborn. Clin Perinatol 1988;15:305–319.
121. Kendig EL. Evolution of short-course antimicrobial treatment of tuberculosis in children, 1951–1984. Pediatrics 1985;75:684–686.
122. Biddulph J. Short course chemotherapy of childhood tuberculosis. Pediatr Infect Dis J 1990;9:794–801.
123. Kumar L, Dhand R, Singhi PD, et al. A randomized trial of fully intermittent vs. daily followed by intermittent short course chemotherapy for childhood tuberculosis. Pediatr Infect Dis J 1990;9:802–806.
124. Small PM, Schecter GF, Goodman PC, et al. Treatment of tuberculosis in patients with advanced human immunodeficiency virus infection. N Engl J Med 1991;324:289–294.
125. Sunderam G, Mangura BT, Lombardo JM, et al. Failure of "optimal" four-drug short-course tuberculosis chemotherapy in a compliant patient with human immunodeficiency virus. Am Rev Respir Dis 1987;136:145–1478.
126. Dutt AK, Moers D, Stead WW. Short-course chemotherapy for extrapulmonary tuberculosis: Nine years' experience. Ann Intern Med 1986;104:7–12.

127. Holdiness MR. Management of tuberculous meningitis. Drugs 1990;39:224–233.

128. Kaojarern S, Supmonchai K, Phuapradit P, et al. Effect of steroids on cerebrospinal fluid penetration of antituberculous agents in tuberculous meningitis. Clin Pharmacol Ther 1991;49:6–12.

129. Grange JM, Gibson J, Osborn TW, et al. What is BCG? Tubercle 1983;64:129–139.

130. Centers for Disease Control. Use of BCG vaccines in the control of tuberculosis. MMWR 1988;37:663–675.

131. Colditz GA, Brewer TF, Berkey CS, et al. Efficacy of BCG vaccine in the prevention of tuberculosis: Meta-analysis of the published literature. JAMA 1994;271:698–702.

132. Comstock GW. Prevention of tuberculosis among tuberculin reactors: Maximizing benefits, minimizing risks. JAMA 1986;256:2729–2730.

133. Dash LA, Constock GW, Flynn JPG. Isoniazid preventive therapy: Retrospect and prospect. Am Rev Resp Dis 1980;121:1039–1044.

Chapter 106

Gastrointestinal Infections and Enterotoxigenic Poisonings

Tom A. Larson, PharmD, and Russell E. Seay, PharmD

Collectively, gastrointestinal infections are among the more common causes of morbidity and mortality around the world. In underdeveloped and developing countries, acute gastroenteritis involving diarrhea is the leading cause of mortality in infants and young children under 4 years of age.[1] Estimates range from 3–5 billion cases of diarrhea per year resulting in 5–10 million deaths annually.[2] As a result of the high turnover of body fluid proportional to body weight, especially extracellular fluid, the infant is more susceptible to dehydration and the associated sequelae resulting from diarrhea. Effects from negative fluid balance can be seen with as little as 5% dehydration.[3] In the United States, more than 210,000 children per year are hospitalized for gastroenteritis.[4] National mortality records from 1973 to 1983 revealed an average of 504 children, 1 month to 4 years of age, died each year in the United States with diarrhea as a primary diagnosis. Approximately 50% of the deaths due to diarrhea were in infants less than 3 months of age, with 80% occurring before 1 year of age. Half of the deaths occurred after arriving at medical facilities.[5] These figures underscore the severity of diarrhea in children and the urgency for timely reversal of progressive dehydration. Acute diarrhea is much less common among elderly patients. However, because the elderly are more likely to develop dehydration than younger adults, complications may be especially debilitating.

Because of the self-limited nature of infectious diarrhea after appropriate rehydration and the economic burden of identification, the infectious agents often go unidentified. Bacteria, viruses, and protozoans account for the vast majority of infectious diarrhea. This chapter focuses on the bacterial and viral etiologies of gastrointestinal infections and their treatment.

Rehydration Therapy

Although infection may require specific antimicrobial therapy based on etiology (Table 106.1), the mainstay of therapy is rehydration. Initial assessment of fluid loss is essential for rehydration. Weight loss is the most reliable means of determining the extent of water loss. If the degree of weight loss is not available, clinical signs such as changes in skin turgor, sunken eyes, dry mucous membranes, decreased tearing, decreased urine output, altered mentation, and changes in vital signs can be helpful in determining approximate deficits[6] (Table 106.2). Physical assessment is generally more reliable in young children and infants than in adults.

When losses are mild to moderate, oral rehydration therapy (ORT) is often successful. Fluid loss greater than 10% body water is considered severe. Although ORT may be successful in reversing severe dehydration, parenteral replacement is indicated as initial treatment for the patient in shock or a comatose state, the patient unable to tolerate oral fluids, the patient with ileus, and the patient with persistent vomiting or stool output greater than 100 mL/kg/h.[7]

The necessary components of ORT solutions include glucose, sodium, potassium, chloride, and water (Table 106.3). Glucose in concentrations of 2–3% enhances the absorption of sodium from the intestine, and water is passively absorbed with the sodium.[8] Glucose concentrations greater than 5% may produce an osmotic diarrhea, worsening the dehydration. Glycine and lysine will improve glucose absorption.[9] Glutamine has also been proposed as an additive because of its function as a metabolic fuel for enterocytes.[10] Boiled rice gruel, although more laborious to prepare, has been suggested as a rehydration agent because it is easily digested and is hydrolyzed to glucose, glycine, lysine, leucine, isoleucine, and oligopeptides. Slow rice hydrolysis allows some rice absorption to take place before hydrolysis occurs. Therefore, a larger carbohydrate load can be given with rice solutions, resulting in a greater nutritional advantage without an increased osmotic load in the gut.[11–13] Mung bean (lentils), cow's milk, glycine, and cereal preparations have been used successfully as rehydration substrates.[12–16]

Sodium content should be between 75 and 90 mEq/L for initial rehydration. Maintenance rehydration requires

TABLE 106.1. ANTIBIOTIC SELECTION

Organism	First Choice	Alternatives
Clostridium difficile	Metronidazole	Vancomycin, bacitracin, cholestyramine
Campylobacter	Fluoroquinolone[a]	Erythromycin, clindamycin, aminoglycoside, doxycycline
Escherichia coli	Fluoroquinolone	TMP–SMX,[b] aminoglycoside chloramphenicol, ampicillin
Salmonella	Ciprofloxacin, ceftriaxone, cefoperazone, TMP–SMX	
Shigella	Fluoroquinolone, norfloxacin	TMP–SMX, ampicillin
Vibrio cholerae	Fluoroquinolone, doxycycline	TMP–SMX
Yersinia enterocolitica	Ciprofloxacin, norfloxacin, ofloxacin	TMP–SMX, antipseudomonal aminoglycoside

Dosing Guidelines

Drug	Children[c]	Adults[d]
Amikacin (IV)	15–22.5 mg/kg/d every 8 h	15 mg/kg/d divided every 8–12 h
Ampicillin (IV)	100–200 mg/kg/d divided every 6 h	150–200 mg/kg/d divided every 6 h
(PO)	50 mg/kg/d divided every 6 h	250–500 mg every 6 h
Bacitracin (PO)	800–1200 units/kg/d every 8 h	25,000 units every 6 h
Cefoperazone (IV)	100–150 mg/kg/d divided every 8–12 h	4–16 g/d divided every 6–12 h
Ceftriaxone (IV)	50–100 mg/kg/d divided every 12–24 h	1–2 g/d divided every 12–24 h
Chloramphenicol (PO)	50–75 mg/kg/d divided every 6 h	50 mg/kg/dose every 6 h
Ciprofloxacin (IV)	NR	200–400 mg every 12 h
(PO)		500–750 mg every 12 h
Clindamycin (PO)	20–30 mg/kg/d divided every 6 h	150–450 mg every 6 h
(IV)	25–40 mg/kg/d divided every 6–8 h	150–900 mg every 8 h
Doxycycline (PO)	NR	100 mg every 12–24 h
Enoxacin (PO)	NR	600–800 mg/d divided every 12–24 h
Erythromycin (PO)	30–40 mg/kg/d divided every 6–8 h	250–500 mg every 6 h
Gentamicin (IV)	3–7.5 mg/kg/d divided every 8 h	3–5 mg/kg/d divided every 8 h
Lomefloxacin (PO)	NR	400 mg every 24 h
Metronidazole (PO)	15–35 mg/kg/d divided every 8 h	500 mg every 6 h
Netilmicin (IV)	3–7.5 mg/kg/d divided every 8 h	4–6.5 mg/kg/d divided every 8 h
Norfloxacin (PO)	NR	400 mg every 12 h
Ofloxacin (PO)	NR	200–400 mg every 12 h
TMP–SMX (PO)	8–12 mg/kg/d divided every 12 h	160 mg every 12 h
Tobramycin (IV)	3–6 mg/kg/d divided every 8 h	3–5 mg/kg/d divided every 8 h
Vancomycin (PO)	10–50 mg/kg/d divided every 6 h, max 125 mg per dose	125 mg every 6 h

Key: NR, not recommended.
[a]Fluoroquinolone: ciprofloxacin, ofloxacin, lomefloxacin, enoxacin (fluoroquinolones are not approved for children).
[b]TMP–SMX, trimethoprim–sulfamethoxazole.
[c]Adapted from Ref. 28.
[d]Adapted from Ref. 27.

sodium concentrations between 40 and 60 mEq/L. The American Academy of Pediatrics recommends rehydration with a more electrolyte-concentrated rehydration phase and a subsequent maintenance phase using the more dilute solutions and larger volume. The rehydration phase should provide replacement of estimated fluid deficits in 4–6 hours. Volume goals are usually 50–75 mL/kg. The maintenance phase should not exceed 150 mL/kg/d and is generally adjusted to equal stool output and insensible water loss.[17] Infants may have significant insensible water loss and often require additional free water if solutions with higher sodium concentration, such as the World Health Organization (WHO) solution, are used for maintenance therapy. Soft drinks that have been decarbonated (by stirring vigorously), liquid gelatin desserts with twice the water content, and fruit juices have been used but have less desirable electrolyte and carbohydrate content, and are usually hyperosmolar. With mild to moderate dehydration, fluid loss should be replaced within 24 hours, with half of the deficit being given in the first 8 hours if possible. Severe dehydration is generally classified by disturbance in serum sodium concentrations. Isonatremic dehydration accounts for the majority of cases, while hyponatremia and hypernatremia account for 15% and 5% of cases, respectively.[3] Guidelines for parenteral fluid replacement of severe fluid loss are shown in Table 106.4.

TABLE 106.2. SIGNS OF DEHYDRATION

% body weight loss as water	Clinical signs
Adults and Older Children	
<4 (mild)	Decreased tearing, thirsty, alert, restless
4–8 (moderate)	Decreased skin turgor, sunken eyes, tachycardia, reduced urine flow, postural hypotension, dry mucous membranes, thirsty
>8 (severe)	Hypotension, muscle cramps, variable alertness, cold, sweaty, cyanotic, wrinkled skin, usually conscious
Infants and Young Children	
<5 (mild)	Thirsty, alert, restless, moist mucous membranes, normal urine flow, tearing
5–10 (moderate)	Thirsty, restless, lethargic, irritable, tachycardia, hypotension, deep respirations, sunken fontanel, sunken eyes, absent tearing, dry mucous membranes, reduced and dark urine
>10 (severe)	Drowsy, limp, cold, sweaty, cyanotic, comatose, tachycardia, tachypnea, very sunken fontanels, hypotension, sunken eyes, absent tears, dry mucous membranes, no urine production

(Adapted from Refs. 3 and 110.)

Recommendations regarding feeding have shifted from withholding for 12–24 hours to feeding as tolerated. Breast milk and soy formula and cow's milk-based formulas can be continued although recommendations exist for dilution of the milk-based formulas to half-strength. It has been found that early initiation of feeding has shortened the course of diarrhea. Initially, easily digested foods, such as bananas, applesauce, and cereal, may be added as tolerated. Foods high in fiber, sodium, and sugar should be avoided. Lactase deficiency may be exacerbated among known lactase-deficient patients and may persist up to 10 days. After starting rehydration therapy, parents should be instructed to observe the child for a reversal of the signs of dehydration, increased stool consistency, and decreased stool frequency. If ORT is not improving the fluid status, the patient will continue to produce frequent large volume, watery stools. These children should be closely supervised by medical support.[18,19]

BACTERIAL INFECTIONS

The bacterial species most commonly associated with gastrointestinal infection and infectious diarrhea in the United States are *Shigella* sp., *Salmonella* sp., *Campylobacter* sp., *Yersinia* sp., *Escherichia* sp., *Clostridium* sp., and *Staphylococcus* sp. Although not a leading cause in North America, *Vibrio* sp. is a leading cause on a global scale. Bacterial-induced infectious diarrhea is classified according to the mechanism by which disease is produced. The two most commonly recognized mechanisms involve enterotoxin-stimulated hypersecretion (secretory diarrhea) and mucosal invasion (invasive diarrhea). *Vibrio cholerae* is the classic example of an enterotoxin-producing organism. These organisms colonize and adhere to the gastrointestinal mucosa and produce an enterotoxin that may be associated with disruption or dissolution of the brush border mem-

TABLE 106.3. COMPARISON OF SOLUTIONS USED IN ORAL REHYDRATION AND MAINTENANCE

	Electrolytes (mEq/L)						
Product	Na	K	Cl	Base	Other Cations	Carbohydrate (g/L)	Osmolarity (mOsm/L)
Infalyte (Penwalt)	50	20	40	30	—	20	251
Lytren (Mead Johnson)	50	25	45	30	—	20	583
Pedialyte (Ross)	45	20	35	30	—	25	388
Pedialyte RS (Ross)	75	20	65	30	—	25	314
Ricelyte (Mead Johnson)	50	25	45	34	—	30	200
WHO (Unicef)	90	20	80	30	—	20	333
Resol (Wyeth)	50	20	50	34	4 Ca, 4 Mg, 5 PO4	20	
Rehydraltye (Ross)	75	20	65	30		25	
EquaLYTE (Ross)	78.2	22.3	67.6	30.1		25	305
Less Desirable Alternatives							
Cola	0–6.5	0–4	—	13	—	100–120	390–750
Gatorade	20–24	3	17	30	—	46–58	305
Grape juice	3	31–34	—	32	—	156	1180
Jell-O (½ strength)	6–17	0.2	0–5			70–80	600
Kool-Aid	1	1	—		—	102	250–590
7-Up	5–7	2	—		—	74–102	535

(Adapted from package information and Ref. 109.)

TABLE 106.4. PARENTERAL REPLACEMENT OF FLUID DEFICIT FOR SEVERELY DEHYDRATED (>10% OF BODY WEIGHT) CHILDREN

Type of Dehydration	Replacement Solution	% Replaced During Noted Period		
		0–12 h	12–24 h	24–48 h
Isonatremic (130–150 mEq/L)	D_5 ⅓ NS	50	50	—
Hyponatremic (<130 mEq/L)	D_5 ½ NS	75	25	—
Hypernatremic (>150 mEq/L)	D_5 ¼ NS	25	25	50

Key: D_5, dextrose 5%; NS, normal saline (0.9% sodium chloride). (Adapted from Ref. 3.)

brane and/or cytotoxic activity resulting in inflammation and hemorrhage of intestinal tissue. Enterotoxigenic *E. coli* and *Clostridium difficile* also cause diarrhea secondary to enterotoxin release. Actual mucosal invasion resulting in diarrhea may occur with gastrointestinal infection by *Shigella* sp., *Salmonella* sp., *Yersinia* sp., and enteroinvasive *E. coli.* These groups actually invade the distal intestinal mucosa with occasional penetration into the lamina propria, lymph nodes, or blood. After invading the mucosal cells, these bacteria produce diarrhea by different proposed mechanisms including toxin production, hormone release, ulceration, and prostaglandin release.[20]

ENTEROTOXIGENIC (CHOLERA-LIKE) DIARRHEA

CHOLERA *(VIBRIO CHOLERAE)*

Vibrios are aerobic, curved, gram-negative bacilli commonly found in surface water. The two species most often causing human illness are *Vibrio cholerae* and *Vibrio parahemolyticus.* Although the disease caused by each species is strikingly different, only *V. cholerae* is discussed because it best characterizes the secretory-type diarrheas.

Epidemiology and Etiology

Cholera has been endemic in the Ganges delta, West Bengal, Bangladesh, and southern Asia (including Southeast Asia) since at least 1817. Three different biotypes have produced seven pandemic episodes since then: classic, El Tor, and a new classic variant. The last documented epidemic in the United States occurred in 1911.

Four mechanisms for transmission have been proposed, including animal reservoirs, chronic carriers, asymptomatic or mild disease victims, or water reservoirs. A relatively large inoculum (10^8 organisms) is required to produce clinical disease. The ratio of symptomatic to asymptomatic infections is about 1:30 (or less) for the El Tor biotype versus 1:2–4 for the "classic" biotype. Excreted bacteria may remain viable for up to a week in water, with El Tor variants surviving slightly longer than classic biotypes. There appears to be an inverse relationship between attack rate and age. After clinical disease, about 90–100% protection from recurrence is seen for several years.[21–24]

Pathophysiology

Most pathology of cholera is thought to result from an enterotoxin (cholera toxin) produced by the bacteria. The toxin contains six subunits of two types: one subunit A (activating moiety) and five B subunits (binding moiety). Subunit B binds to a GM_1 monosialosyl ganglioside of the intestinal epithelial cell wall, allowing subunit A to enter the cell. Subunit A stimulation of intracellular adenylate cyclase activity increases cyclic AMP-mediated secretion of chloride ion into the intestinal lumen. The toxin likely acts along the entire intestinal tract; however, most fluid loss occurs in the duodenum where secretory capacity is greatest. The effects of the toxin persist for many hours.[22] Cholera toxin does not appear to affect the glucose-facilitated sodium resorptive capacity of the gut. The net effect of cholera toxin is isotonic secretion (primarily in the small intestine), which exceeds the absorptive capacity of the intestinal tract (primarily the colon).

Clinical Presentation

The incubation period of *V. cholerae* is 6–48 hours. The clinical presentation is characterized by a spectrum from the asymptomatic state to the most severe typical cholera syndrome. In the most severe state, this disease can progress to death in a matter of 2–4 hours if not treated. More typically, however, progression from the first watery stool to shock takes two to three times longer, with death delayed up to several days. Some patients may experience a prodrome, a sense of fullness and borborygmus, prior to the first watery stool. Initial stools generally do not have the "rice water" appearance that is classically seen with cholera.

Most signs and symptoms are a direct result of fluid and electrolyte loss. These frequently include poor skin turgor, sunken eyes, cyanosis, shallow or absent pulses, tachycardia, hypotension, and tachypnea. The presentation generally correlates well with the severity of fluid loss from diarrhea. Fluid collection within the intestines may cause further intravascular depletion without diarrhea.

Surprisingly, despite the profound intravascular fluid loss, even in cases where peripheral pulses are absent, patients are generally easily aroused and give appropriate responses to questioning. In children, however, altered consciousness and even convulsions may be the first sign of hypoglycemia.[25] Hypokalemia is often seen in children, perhaps as a reflection of a greater potassium loss with diarrhea than seen with adults. Altered consciousness, muscle weakness and cramping, cardiac arrhythmias, and ileus may be manifestations of electrolyte losses. Other complications include acidosis, renal failure secondary to volume depletion, iatrogenic water intoxication from overrehydration, and aspiration pneumonia.

Treatment

The mainstay of treatment for cholera consists of fluid and electrolyte replacement. Current clinical data suggest that rice-based oral rehydration significantly reduces the rate of stool output as compared to glucose-based rehydration solutions. Meta-analyses of general studies indicate that rice-based rehydration formulations are the preferred ORT for cholera patients.[13,18] Volume loss can be dramatic, with a few patients losing a liter or more of isotonic fluid every hour. The amounts of water and salts given are dictated by those that are lost. Intravenous therapy is usually required only in severe cases because most cases of hypovolemia can be managed with ORT.

Antibiotics have been shown to shorten the duration of diarrhea, decrease the volume of fluid lost, and shorten the duration of the carrier state.[26] The tetracyclines or fluoroquinolones are selected most often.[27,28] When the tetracyclines are not available or desirable, as in pregnancy or young children, cotrimoxazole is an appropriate alternative. Other agents such as chloramphenicol and furazolidone have also been effective.[29] Increasing multiple-antibiotic resistance may dictate regional antibiotic selection. Antibiotics need only be given for 3–5 days in most cases. Lindebaum et al.[26] found a 20% relapse with antibiotic therapy of less than 48 hours. Preliminary use of cholera vaccines have exhibited only 50% efficacy and a short, 6-month duration. Newer vaccines using purified cholera toxin, or live attenuated, recombinant strains have been well tolerated and highly immunogenic.[30] In early clinical trials these vaccines have shown potential as prophylactic agents.[31,32]

ESCHERICHIA COLI

Escherichia coli is a gram-negative bacillus belonging to the family Enterobacteraceae. It is divided into five groups based on mechanisms of diarrheal disease and toxin production: enterotoxigenic *E. coli* (ETEC), enteroinvasive *E. coli* (EIEC), enteropathogenic *E. coli* (EPEC), enteroadhesive *E. coli* (EAEC), and enterohemorrhagic *E. coli* (EHEC).

The most common group is ETEC, which closely resembles *V. cholerae*. Although not recognized as a significant cause of diarrhea until the second half of this century, ETEC is now incriminated as being the most common cause of traveler's diarrhea, the most common cause of diarrhea in children in certain areas of the world, and a common cause of food- and/or water-associated outbreaks.[33,34]

Pathophysiology

ETEC are capable of producing two plasmid-mediated enterotoxins: heat-labile toxin (HLT) and heat-stable toxin (HST). HLT, a cholera-like toxin, has two subunits (A and B) that have similar antigenic properties and action on the gut mucosa. The net effect of this toxin on the mucosa is production of a cholera-like secretory diarrhea. HST has a rapid onset of action, is nonantigenic, has a low molecular weight, and probably acts only on the small intestine.[35]

Clinical Presentation

Diarrhea caused by ETEC is often characterized by abrupt onset of watery diarrhea, with or without abdominal cramping. Severe cases may be indistinguishable from cholera. Usually, there is no blood or pus in the stool. Signs and symptoms are directly dependent on the extent of fluid loss, which in most cases is subclinical. Most ETEC diarrhea resolves within 24–48 hours without complication.

Treatment

Most patients do not require specific therapy, although some will have loss of fluid and electrolytes requiring replacement therapy. Most cases respond readily to ORT and although antibiotic therapy is seldom necessary, prophylaxis has been shown to effectively prevent the development of ETEC diarrhea.[36] Effective prophylactic agents include tetracycline, cotrimoxazole, neomycin, furazolidone,[37] norfloxacin, and ciprofloxacin.[27] Because multiple-antibiotic resistance among ETEC has developed in many countries, many prescribers prefer to reserve antibiotics for treatment of symptomatic patients.[36,38–41] Nonantibiotic regimens, including bismuth subsalicylate and cholestyramine, have also been recommended as effective prevention or treatment regimens.[42–46]

PSEUDOMEMBRANOUS COLITIS (*CLOSTRIDIUM DIFFICILE*)

Pseudomembranous colitis (PMC) was first reported in 1883 and first associated with antibiotic therapy in 1955. Although described in the preantibiotic era, the incidence has increasingly been associated with antibiotic administration. Recent evidence suggests that PMC is the result of toxins produced by *Clostridium difficile*.[47]

Epidemiology and Etiology

Clostridium difficile is a spore-forming, gram-positive, obligate anaerobic bacillus. The incidence of intestinal colonization is variable ranging from over 70% in infants to 3% in healthy adults.[48] With antibiotic-altered flora, reports of colonization among adults increase to 20–46%. The relation between the colonized state and active disease is poorly understood. Newborn infants may be colonized with toxin-producing strains yet have no clinical disease. This colonization is reduced to adult levels by 2 years of age.

The exact incidence of PMC within the United States is not known. It occurs most often in epidemic fashion and affects high-risk groups such as the elderly, debilitated patients, cancer patients, surgical patients, or any patient receiving antibiotics. PMC has been associated most often with broad-spectrum antimicrobials, including clindamycin, ampicillin, or cephalosporins. As many as 10% of selected patients receiving clindamycin may acquire PMC.[49]

Pathophysiology

Pseudomembranous colitis is thought to be caused by toxins produced by strains of *C. difficile.* Two toxins (A and B) have been described.[48] Toxin A has been characterized as an enterotoxin and toxin B has been described as a nonenterotoxic cytotoxin.[20] The exact mechanism by which these toxins produce human disease remains to be elucidated. The toxins appear to act on mucosal membranes, causing necrosis, inflammation, increased peristalsis, and loss of fluid and electrolytes.

Clinical Presentation

Symptoms can occur from several days after the start of antibiotic therapy to several weeks after antibiotics are discontinued. The onset of illness is often abrupt. PMC is characterized by vomiting, fever, cramping, abdominal pain and tenderness, and profuse greenish diarrhea (watery or mucoid), either during or after antibiotic therapy. Fevers of 103–105°F, marked leukocytosis, and hypoalbuminemia are also common.[48] Pseudomembranous lesions, which look like whitish-yellow raised plaques, can be found anywhere in the colon. Diagnosis is made by colonoscopic visualization of pseudomembranes. A diagnostic dilemma exists if a patient has positive stool cultures and/or positive cytotoxin assays and no demonstrable pseudomembranes. This group of patients has been classified as having *C. difficile*-associated diarrhea. Evidence suggests that approximately 23% of these cases resolve spontaneously within 48–72 hours.[50] Because the cytotoxins can be demonstrated within 24 hours of stool collection, some of these patients may receive inappropriate antibiotic therapy. Gramstain of stools is not helpful; however, leukocytes are present in about half of patients with PMC. Most pseudomembranous plaques are distal and are easily seen with sigmoidoscopy. However, plaques may occur anywhere in the colon or rectum. Therefore, when sigmoidoscopy and proctoscopy are negative, PMC cannot be ruled out.

Treatment

As with all types of diarrhea, supportive care is of primary concern. Fluid and electrolyte losses may be significant. If possible, it is ideal to stop the offending antibiotic. Teasley et al.[51] showed that 23% of patients with *C. difficile*-associated diarrhea had resolution within 72 hours simply by discontinuing the inducing agent. If the patient has not improved within 72 hours, has severe disease, requires continuation of the inducing antibiotic, or is a high-risk patient (pediatric, elderly, debilitated), antibiotic therapy should be promptly initiated. *Clostridium difficile* is usually susceptible *in vitro* to vancomycin, metronidazole, bacitracin, rifampin, ampicillin, and cephalosporins. Clinically, however, resistance to rifampin develops quickly, and β-lactamase produced by intestinal flora inactivates ampicillin and cephalosporins making these antibiotics ineffective. Many isolates are resistant to tetracyclines or erythromycin.

Vancomycin 500–2000 mg/d orally for 10 days has historically been suggested as the treatment of choice. The well-documented efficacy of vancomycin is very likely a result of excellent activity against *C. difficile* and poor absorption from the gastrointestinal tract. Oral doses of 125 mg four times daily have resulted in fecal concentrations greater than 300 mg/mL, far exceeding the minimum inhibitory concentration (MIC) breakpoint of susceptibility.[48,50] Because clinical response to vancomycin 125 mg every 6 hours or 500 mg every 6 hours has been shown to be similar, the lower dose is preferred unless the patient is critically ill or has impending ileus.[48] Clinical response is generally observed within the first 4 days of therapy. Pediatric dosage recommendations range from 10–40 mg/kg/d orally, divided into four doses for 7–10 days.[52,53] Vancomycin therapy for PMC is given orally because gastrointestinal concentrations after parenteral administration are very low and unpredictable.

Relapse after discontinuation of vancomycin may occur in 12–39% of patients. This is thought to be caused by residual spores and/or failure to restore normal flora. Retreatment with vancomycin is often successful. Some investigators have found prophylaxis with *Lactobacillus* sp. or *Saccharomyces* sp. to be helpful in small numbers of patients. Further trials should help determine the role of flora replacement prophylaxis.[54,55]

Although vancomycin has been the drug of choice for several years, some authors now suggest that in many cases metronidazole may be the agent of choice.[27,51] A large prospective study comparing metronidazole (1 g/d) and vancomycin (2 g/d) among 101 veterans with antibiotic-associated diarrhea and stool cultures positive for *C. difficile* showed no significant difference in efficacy, toxicity, or relapse rate.[50] These results are somewhat surprising in light of extensive metronidazole absorption and reports implicating metronidazole as a PMC-inducing agent. The number of study patients with PMC was not large and although metronidazole and vancomycin appear to be equally effective, more experience is required. Because of its mutagenic and tumorigenic potential in laboratory animal experiments, metronidazole should not be used indiscriminately in pregnant women.

A second alternative agent for treatment of *C. difficile*-associated diarrhea and colitis is bacitracin. Bacitracin is poorly absorbed from the gastrointestinal tract, resulting in high fecal concentrations. Young et al.[56] recently reported that bacitracin 80,000 U/d given orally was less effective than oral vancomycin 500 mg/d in clearing *C. difficile* from stools. Agents were comparable in control of colitis symptoms. The number of reported cases is far too few to suggest bacitracin as more than an alternative agent. Further studies are required.

Anion exchange resins have been used with variable success in mild cases. The usual adult dose of cholestyramine is 4 g orally three to four times daily for 3–19 days. Cholestyramine has been shown to bind vancomycin; however, *in vitro* data suggest that there is no loss of antibiotic activity.[57] Concomitant administration should be avoided, or administration of antibiotics and exchange resins should be separated by several hours. Asymptomatic patients with positive fecal cultures may outnumber symptomatic patients. Treatment of asymptomatic patients, either with metronidazole, which is not effective, or vancomycin, which may be associated with a prolonged carrier state, is not recommended.[58]

Drugs that inhibit peristalsis, such as diphenoxylate, are contraindicated. Some patients have become worse after use of these drugs. They may be particularly dangerous to use in infants. Slowing of fecal transit time is thought to result in extended toxin-associated damage.[59]

INVASIVE (DYSENTERY-LIKE) DIARRHEA

BACILLARY DYSENTERY (SHIGELLOSIS)

Bacillary dysentery, a self-limited intestinal infection caused by *Shigella* sp., is characterized by fever and abdominal pain with small volumes of feces often containing blood and mucus. The shigellae are gram-negative bacilli belonging to the family Enterobacteriaceae. Four species most often associated with disease are *S. dysenteriae* type I, *S. flexneri, S. bovdii,* and *S. sonnei.* In a similar fashion, enteroinvasive (EIEC) and enterotoxigenic (ETEC) *E. coli* may also cause an intestinal disorder that is difficult to differentiate from shigellosis based on symptoms alone.[60]

Epidemiology and Etiology

The shigellae have worldwide distribution, with regional differences in prevalence of subgroups responsible for disease. For example, in the United States the common causes of shigellosis are *S. sonnei,* responsible for four out of five cases, and *S. flexneri.* Cases caused by other shigellae are most often acquired during travel to other countries, specifically developing countries. Epidemics are uncommon in areas of the world where sanitation standards are high. Poor sanitation, poor personal hygiene, inadequate water supply, malnutrition, and increased population density are associated with increased risk of shigella gastroenteritis epidemics, even in developed countries.

The majority of cases are thought to result from fecal–oral transmission. A few well-documented food- and water-associated outbreaks have been reported. In the tropics, peak incidence of shigellosis correlates well with peak infestation of flies, suggesting that flies may be an important vector of transmission. Peak incidence in the United States is in late summer.

Shigellosis is primarily a disease of children, with the highest incidence between ages 6 months and 5 years. Infection among infants is uncommon and only one-third of all cases occur in adults. The reported incidence in the United States ranges from 15,000–20,000 cases per year.[61]

Pathogenesis

Ingestion of as few as 10–200 viable organisms of the shigella species has been shown to cause disease in healthy adults, explaining the ease with which the disease is transmitted from person to person. This is contrasted by the comparatively large inoculum of *E. coli* required to initiate infection (>10^8 bacteria). Shigella species and enteroinvasive *E. coli* cause dysentery upon penetrating the epithelial cells lining the colon.[62] The bacteria multiply and spread within the submucosa, but rarely extend beyond the mucosa. Penetration of the mucosa is coded by large "invasion plasmids" and results in distortion of the crypts, death to gastric epithelium causing focal ulceration, sloughing of mucosal cells, bloody mucoid exudate into the gut lumen, and submucosal accumulation of inflammatory cells with microabscess formation. Microabscesses may eventually coalesce, forming larger abscesses. Infection frequently involves the entire colon. Some shigella species produce a cytotoxin, or shigatoxin, the pathogenic role of which is unclear although it is thought to damage endothelial cells of the lamina propria, resulting in microangiopathic changes that can progress to hemolytic uremic syndrome. Watery diarrhea commonly precedes the dysentery and may be a result of these toxins.[63]

Clinical Presentation

Signs and symptoms are initially nonspecific: nausea, fever, malaise, abdominal tenderness of the lower quadrants, and hyperactive bowel sounds. Frequent watery stools, 10–25 per day, appear within 48 hours, and are followed by bloody diarrhea and dysentery within a few days. Stools are greenish in color and often contain mucus and/or blood,[64] as well as many leukocytes. Proctoscopic exam reveals hyperemic mucosa, increased mucus secretion, and multiple superficial bleeding ulcers.

Laboratory findings are *quite* variable. White blood cell counts are inconsistent and range from a leukopenia to a pronounced leukocytosis with a "left shift." Fluid and electrolyte loss may be significant, particularly in infants and elderly patients. Stool culture will establish shigella species as the causative agent. Immunofluorescent-labeled antiserum will give rapid and precise diagnosis; however, it is not readily available. Shigella-specific "invasion plasmids" are now detectable directly from stool without cultivation by amplification of DNA by the polymerase chain reaction allowing same day, sensitive test results.[65]

If untreated, bacillary dysentery usually lasts about 1 week (range 1–30 days). Complications are unusual but may include severe dehydration, generalized seizures, septicemia, toxic megacolon, perforated colon, arthritis, protein-losing enteropathy, and hemolytic-uremic syndrome. Mortality is rare, but it may be more likely with *S. dysenteriae* type I.[63]

Treatment

Shigellosis is generally a self-limiting disease. Patients most often become afebrile and completely recover within 4–7 days. Approximately 10% experience a recurrence. Treatment of bacillary dysentery generally includes correction of fluid and electrolyte disturbances and occasionally antimicrobials in the very young and elderly. Fluid and electrolyte losses can generally be replaced with oral therapy, as dysentery is generally not associated with significant fluid loss. Intravenous replacement is necessary only for those patients with severe illness.

Because shigellosis is usually a self-limiting disease and antibiotic resistance is an increasing concern, some clinicians feel antibiotics should be reserved for the severely ill. However, because antibiotic therapy has been shown to shorten the period of fecal shedding (usually 1–4 weeks in patients not receiving antimicrobials) and attenuate the clinical illness, many clinicians prefer to treat with antibiotics.[38] Cotrimoxazole and ampicillin have been shown to be equivalent for treatment of shigellosis caused by susceptible strains. With an increasing incidence of ampicillin-resistant strains in much of the world, cotrimoxazole has become the treatment of choice.[66] Bicozamycin, a nonabsorbable agent, has been shown to be as effective as cotrimoxazole. This is surprising because the disease is invasive by nature and systemic absorption was once thought to be required for therapeutic effect.[67] Other antibiotics shown to have activity include sulfamethoxazole, nalidixic acid, the quinolones, and furazolidone. Recent studies would suggest that severe shigellosis in children may respond to short-course intravenous therapy with newer cephalosporins.[68] Antispasmodics and agents that inhibit intestinal peristalsis should not be used because they may prolong fever and diarrhea, worsen the dysentery, and possibly contribute to development of toxic megacolon.[69] Oral vaccines directed against *S. flexneri* 2a, *S. sonnei,* and both *S. typhi* and *S. flexneri* 2a are under development. These vaccines contain avirulent live organisms, which colonize the gut and stimulate local immune response to the shigella antigen. Preliminary results are encouraging, although an ideal vaccine has not yet been developed.[30,70,71]

SALMONELLOSIS

Salmonella sp. are gram-negative bacilli belonging to the family Enterobacteriaceae. The genus *Salmonella* has three species *(S. typhi, S. enteritidis,* and *S. choleraesuis)* of which there are more than 1700 different stereotypes. Reports to the Centers for Disease Control (CDC) show serotype *S. typhimurium* as the most common isolate. The 10 most commonly isolated serotypes accounted for 71% of all isolates. The number of reported isolates increased from 19,659 in 1968 to 38,881 in 1983.[72]

Human disease caused by salmonella generally falls into four categories: acute gastroenteritis, bacteremia, extraintestinal localized infection, and enteric fever (typhoid and paratyphoid fever).

Epidemiology

Salmonellosis is a disease primarily of infants, children, and adolescents. One-third of all cases reported to the CDC were in persons less than 1 year of age, and most cases were children under 10 years of age. As with shigellosis, there is a seasonal pattern with greatest frequency in the summer months.[73]

Contaminated food or water has been implicated in the majority of cases. Direct fecal–oral transmission occurs less frequently but is particularly important in children. Foods most often implicated in human salmonellosis are poultry, poultry products, beef, pork, and dairy products. Pets, particularly reptiles, have been shown to be a common source of infection.

Most reports of outbreaks occur sporadically within households and institutions. It is quite common for family contacts to acquire infection. Person-to-person contact and use of common fomites are likely responsible for outbreaks in neonatal and pediatric wards.[74] While the incidence of salmonella infection overall has increased over the past decade, that attributed to *S. typhi* has declined.

Pathophysiology

Salmonellae are much more sensitive to lower gastric pH than shigellae. Therefore, a relatively larger inoculum is required to cause infection (10^5–10^{12} bacteria) although inoculums of approximately 1000 organisms have been known to cause gastroenteritis. Agents or disease states that decrease gastric acidity or decrease gastric emptying time may predispose patients to infection. Other predisposing conditions include previous antibiotics, which alter the protective normal flora, lack of previous exposure to salmonellae, and immunodeficient states.

Salmonellae enterocolitis appears to occur secondary to mucosal invasion of microorganisms. The different serotypes have a broad range of invasive potential. Some salmonellae like *S. choleraesuis,* the most invasive, are frequently associated with bacteremia and metastatic localization, whereas others seldom cause disease. Mucosal invasion, however, does not appear to explain completely the extensive fluid loss of some patients. Some investigators have suggested enterotoxin production, or local inflammatory exudates as possible mechanisms of pathology; however, these require further study.[75]

Organisms that invade beyond the mucosa enter the mesenteric lymphatics, causing a local hyperplasia and monocytic infiltrates. Lymphatic flow then carries bacteria to the general circulation via the thoracic duct. Most circulating bacteria are cleared by the reticuloendothelial system. Bacteria not cleared may cause metastatic infection in various organs.

Symptoms such as headache, fever, chills, malaise, nausea, vomiting, and abdominal pain are apparently caused by endotoxins. Other as-yet unclear mechanisms may also play a role.

Clinical Presentation

Enterocolitis

Most patients experience symptoms within 24 hours of ingestion. Patients often complain of nausea and vomiting followed by crampy abdominal pain, fever, and diarrhea, although the actual presentation is quite variable. Some patients do not have increased stool frequency, while others have more than one stool per hour. Stools are generally loose, and may be mucoid and/or bloody (dysentery-like). Temperatures usually range between 100 and 102°F, but may be higher. Some evidence suggests that higher fever, greater than or equal to 104°F, is associated with shorter bacterial excretion.[76] Diarrhea and fever usually spontaneously resolve within 1–5 days, but may last 2 weeks. Cases lasting longer should suggest other pathology.[77]

Stool cultures inevitably yield the causative organism if obtained early. However, recovery of organisms continues to decrease with time so that by 3–4 weeks, only 5–15% of adult patients are passing salmonella. Infants and children tend to pass bacteria for longer periods than adults. Some patients may continue to shed salmonella for a year or longer. These "chronic carrier" states are rare for serotypes other than *S. typhi.*

Bacteremia

Salmonellae can produce bacteremia without classic enterocolitis or enteric fever. The clinical syndrome is characterized by persistent bacteremia and prolonged intermittent fever with chills. Stool cultures are frequently negative. This is most frequent, and highly likely, with serotype *S. choleraesuis* infections (50%). Leukocyte counts are often within the normal range.

Localized Infections

Extraluminal infection and/or abscess formation can occur at any site. They may follow any of the other syndromes, or may be the primary presentation. Metastatic infections have been reported to involve bone, cysts, heart, kidney, liver, lungs, pericardium, spleen, and tumors. The clinical presentation is usually determined by the organ systems involved. Polymorphonuclear leukocyte counts are often elevated.

Enteric Fever (Typhoid and Paratyphoid)

Enteric fever caused by *S. typhi* is called typhoid fever. If caused by any other serotype, it is referred to as paratyphoid fever. The clinical presentations of typhoid fever and paratyphoid fever are generally indistinguishable, although in retrospect, paratyphoid fever tends not to be as severe as typhoid fever. Time to onset of symptoms is inversely related to the inoculum size. The onset of symptoms is gradual. Nonspecific symptoms of fever, dull headache, malaise, anorexia, and myalgias are most common. Initially, fever tends to be remittent, but gradually progresses over the first week to temperatures that are often sustained over 104°F. Many patients have vague abdominal discomfort with constipation or diarrhea. Other frequently encountered symptoms include chills, nausea, vomiting, cough, weakness, and sore throat. Symptoms slowly subside within 4 weeks, although without treatment, illness may be prolonged, lasting 2 months or longer.[78]

Physical examination generally reveals an acutely ill patient. An erythematous maculopapular rash, known as rose spots, appears primarily on the abdomen in 15–50% of patients. The abdomen may also be tender, particularly in the lower quadrants. Hepatomegaly and/or splenomegaly may also be present in 50% of the cases, and cervical lymph nodes may be enlarged. Auscultation of the chest will often reveal moist rales. In 5–10% of patients, an altered state of consciousness may be observed.[78]

A normochromic anemia may develop rapidly without evidence of gastrointestinal blood loss, although intestinal bleeding may be contributory. Leukopenia may be caused by a relative decrease in polymorphonuclear leukocytes. White cell counts may range from 1200–20,000 per cubic millimeter. As many as one-third of the patients have elevated levels of the liver enzymes glutamic-oxaloacetic transaminase and alkaline phosphatase. Transient proteinuria with normal creatinine clearance can occur early.[75,77,78] About 80% of patients have positive blood cultures. Bacteremia persists in about one-third for several weeks if not treated. Diagnostic tests other than culture are unreliable.

Intestinal perforation, thrombophlebitis, toxemia with circulatory collapse, intestinal hemorrhage, and pneumonia all contribute to a fatality rate of 1–2%. Without treatment, mortality may be 10%.

Treatment

Enterocolitis

Most patients require no therapeutic intervention. Fever generally resolves in approximately 2 days and diarrhea should resolve in approximately 1 week. When required, the most important part of therapy for salmonella enterocolitis is fluid and electrolyte replacement. The vast majority of patients respond well to ORT. If vomiting prevents ORT, or the patient presents with severe hypovolemia, intravenous solutions may be necessary. Antimicrobials are not indicated as part of the therapy of uncomplicated enterocolitis because they have not been shown to shorten the course of this self-limiting disorder. In addition, antibiotics may prolong the excretion of organisms in the stool.[79] One reason for prolonged excretion of salmonella with antibiotics may be related to altered intestinal flora. Antibiotic therapy should be considered if there is suspected transition to one of the other salmonella syndromes (bacteremia, localized infection, or enteric fever) or if underlying conditions predispose to systemic spread. Both cotrimoxazole and ciprofloxacin have been used to treat salmonella enterocolitis.[80]

Bacteremia and Localized Infections

Chloramphenicol or ampicillin is most frequently used for the treatment of these syndromes. Cotrimoxazole, which has been shown to be effective in treatment of localized salmonella infections, should be considered when the organism is resistant to both chloramphenicol and ampicillin. When bactericidal activity is desired, as with endocarditis or other intravascular infections, ampicillin is the preferred agent, although floroquinolones and third-generation cephalosporins have also been used. The duration of antibiotic therapy should be dictated by the site; for example, osteomyelitis should be treated for 4–6 weeks or longer.

Enteric Fever (Typhoid and Paratyphoid)

Chloramphenicol has been the mainstay of therapy in most areas of the world. Although a number of antibiotics have demonstrated activity against salmonella, chloramphenicol has been shown to attenuate the disease course more consistently. Chloramphenicol resistance is often encountered in Mexico, Southeast Asia, and India because of an R factor, which also transfers resistance to sulfonamides, tetracycline, and streptomycin. Ampicillin, amoxicillin, and cotrimoxazole are also effective, although response is not as predictable as with chloramphenicol. These agents should be considered alternatives and used when chloramphenicol is contraindicated or chloramphenicol resistance is suspected.[81,82] Therapy should be continued for at least 2 weeks. Clinical response to antibiotics is often seen within 2 days; however, temperatures slowly normalize within 3–5 days.

Although not a currently recommended standard of practice, some clinicians feel that severely ill patients may have a beneficial response to a short course of corticosteroids. One study using large doses of dexamethasone given intravenously during the first 48 hours supports this opinion.[83] Antidiarrheal agents or laxatives should not be used because they may prolong illness or precipitate perforation. Live oral attenuated vaccine Ty21a and parenteral v: polysaccharida vaccine have been shown to confer 60–90% efficacy for a duration of 2 and 3 years, respectively.[30] Newer genetically engineered mutants may confer similar efficacy with greater efficiency, however further clinical evidence is pending.

CAMPYLOBACTERIOSIS

The *Campylobacter* species are non-spore-forming, flagellated, curved, gram-negative bacilli. Of the 13 recognized species, *C. jejuni, C. fetus,* and *C. pylori,* now known as *Helicobacter pylori,* are considered the major pathogens for humans. Although recognized for their ability to cause disease in the late 1940s, the routine isolation techniques required for speciation of *Campylobacter* were not readily available until the 1970s.[84]

Epidemiology

Campylobacter species are now thought to be a major cause of diarrhea, comparable to *Salmonella* and *Shigella.* Although occurring in all age groups, approximately 80% of cases reported to the CDC surveillance program were in persons less than 35 years old.[85,86] Prevalence of infection increases with age resulting in 40–50% of the population becoming seropositive by 60 years of age.[84] Most reported cases occur during the summer months.

Mammals, such as livestock, dogs, cats, and birds, including poultry, are believed to be the primary reservoir of *Campylobacter.* Transmission of infection appears to be by the fecal–oral route or by ingestion of contaminated food or water.

Pathophysiology

Campylobacter sp. is susceptible to acid, much like salmonella. Therefore, a larger inoculum of approximately 500 organisms is required to initiate infection. This inoculum is thought to be lower when the bacteria are ingested along with foods, antacids, or histamine (H_2) blocking agents.

Conditions in the upper small intestine are favorable for multiplication. Flagella-mediated adherence and tissue invasion by bacteria have been demonstrated in the jejunum, ileum, and colon. In addition to the invasive mechanism, extracellular toxins and heat-stable enterotoxins may mediate the inflammatory response and induce complement activation.[84]

Clinical Presentation

Incubation usually ranges from 1–12 days with an average of 2–4 days. The most common symptoms include diarrhea of varying consistency and severity, abdominal pain, and fever. Nausea, vomiting, headache, myalgias, and malaise may also occur. Bowel movements may be numerous, bloody (dysentery-like), foul smelling, melenic, and range from loose to watery (cholera-like). Cramping and abdominal pain are usually relieved by defecation. Generalized abdominal pain with tenderness and fever may mimic appendicitis.[85]

The disease is self-limiting and signs and symptoms usually resolve in about a week, but may persist longer in 10–20% of patients. A reactive arthritis, which usually disappears within 6 months, may be seen in as many as 5% of cases. Complications of campylobacteriosis, including thrombophlebitis, abscess, septicemia, peritonitis, empyema, urinary tract infection, and cholecystitis are relatively uncommon, but occur more frequently in those who are immunocompromised.

Treatment

As with other acute diarrheal illnesses, fluid and electrolyte support is a mainstay of therapy. The majority of *Campylobacter*-induced fluid loss can be managed with ORT. Antibiotic therapy is not necessary in the majority of cases.[87] Antibiotics should be considered in the very young and the very old and when the patient has severe bloody diarrhea, continued fever (>102°F), persistence of symptoms beyond 7 days, worsening symptoms, or a compromised immune system. *Campylobacter* sp. are susceptible to erythromycin, tetracycline, chloramphenicol, clindamycin, ciprofloxacin, and the aminoglycosides. A plasmid-coding tetracycline resistance does exist in *C. jejuni* and may transfer within the genus.[84] Currently, erythromycin is the agent of choice[27]; however, two studies were unable to demonstrate the superiority of erythromycin therapy in altering the clinical course when compared to placebo.[87,88] The self-limiting nature of the disease is suggested as a possible explanation. Both studies were able to show that erythromycin hastens the bacteriological cure, which may be of epidemiological benefit. Antimotility drugs may impede the resolution of infection.[87] A complete discussion of the treatment of *H. pylori* has been included in Chapter 32.

YERSINIOSIS

The genus *Yersinia* includes six species known to cause disease in humans. Of these, *Y. enterocolitica* and *Y. pseudotuberculosis* are more likely to be associated with intestinal infection. There are marked geographic differences in the predominant serotypes causing infection. *Yersinia enterocolitica* and *Y. pseudotuberculosis* gastroenteritis most commonly occurs in children and young adults with over 75% of reported cases in persons less than 20 years of age.[89,90] The incidence of cases appears to be on the increase, perhaps reflecting an increased awareness and improved isolation techniques. Peak incidence occurs during the winter months.

The organisms have been isolated from a variety of food sources, including raw goat and cow milk. Refrigeration does not deter the development of adherence and invasive virulence factors. Also, *Y. enterocolitica* has been isolated from a number of mammals; however, the transmission of disease from these reservoirs to humans is poorly understood.[20]

Pathophysiology

The pathophysiology of yersiniosis in humans is not clearly understood. It appears that the bacteria spread from the intestinal epithelium to the lamina propria and the muscularis mucosae. Bacterial proliferation begins in the reticuloendothelial cells causing local necrotic lesions, and may spread to local lymph nodes producing a purulent lymphadenitis. With septicemia, localized purulent lesions may develop in various organs.[20]

Clinical Presentation

These bacteria cause a wide spectrum of clinical syndromes. The majority of cases present with enterocolitis that is mild and self-limiting. Symptoms, generally lasting 1–3 weeks, include vomiting, abdominal pain, diarrhea, and fever. A clinical syndrome seen in older children and adolescents presenting with mesenteric adenitis, fever, right lower quadrant pain, and leukocytosis may be clinically indistinguishable from appendicitis.[89] Development of chronic abdominal pain following yersinia enteritis has been reported.

As many as one-third of adults with *Y. enterocolitica* may have an immunologically mediated polyarthritis within 1 month of the onset of diarrhea. Joints involved frequently include the fingers, wrists, toes, ankles, and knees. Symptoms often resolve spontaneously, but may persist for several months.[91] Other syndromes that frequently occur are erythema nodosum and exudative pharyngitis. Septicemia caused by either *Y. enterocolitica* or *Y. pseudotuberculosis* is uncommon and is most often reported in patients with underlying disease. Signs and symptoms are similar to those seen with other gram-negative bacteremias. Other organ systems may be infected secondarily. The mortality rate of bacteremia may be as high as 50–75%, despite antibiotic therapy.

Treatment

The utility of antimicrobials for treating yersinia-associated enterocolitis and mesenteric adenitis is difficult to evaluate, because these diseases are generally self-limiting and are easily managed with oral rehydration solutions (Table 106.3). As a result, controlled trials with cotrimoxazole have failed to demonstrate beneficial effects[90]; however, in severe disease, bacteremia, or localizing forms of the disease, antibiotic treatment is indicated. *Yersinia enterocolitica* is generally susceptible to third-generation cephalosporins, aminoglycosides, chloramphenicol, tetracycline, and cotrimoxazole. It is frequently resistant to penicillin G, ampicillin, and first-generation cephalosporins. Suggested antibiotics of choice[27] are shown in Table 106.1. *Yersinia pseudotuberculosis* is generally susceptible to antibiotics active against *Y. enterocolitica* as well as ampicillin.

ACUTE VIRAL GASTROENTERITIS

Acute viral gastroenteritis was unknown until the 1970s. Although the exact incidence is unknown, gastroenteritis is second in frequency only to viral respiratory illness. In half of these cases, a pathogen is not identified. As methods of detection improve, more accurate estimates of viral and/or bacterial etiology can be determined. Viruses that have been recovered from the stools of patients with gastroenteritis include rotavirus, enteric adenovirus, Norwalk virus, calicivirus, astrovirus, and coronavirus. Rotavirus accounts for the majority of morbidity and even mortality among children with gastroenteritis, while Norwalk and Norwalk-like viruses account for the majority of adult cases.[7,92,93]

ROTAVIRUSES

Epidemiology and Etiology

Rotaviruses, also called infantile gastroenteritis virus, reovirus-like, or orbivirus-like, are double-stranded wheel-shaped RNA viruses 70 nm in diameter found worldwide. Although rotaviruses have been isolated from a variety of mammals and birds, the exact mechanism of transfer or principal vectors of infection are poorly understood. Water, food, or inspired droplets have been suspected; however, it is generally thought that the primary route is fecal–oral. Although infection is most often seen in children, adults can be infected and may act as a potential reservoir for transmission. Outbreaks are not thought to be common among infants; however, this age group may be more susceptible to complications as evidenced by a higher hospitalization rate.

Rotaviruses have been associated with up to 50% of enteritis in hospitalized children.[92] The highest frequency of rotavirus-associated diarrhea appears between ages 6 and 24 months. After 2 years of age, antirotavirus antibodies have been demonstrated. The incidence of rotavirus infections in the United States peaks in January and February. Incubation and duration of viral shedding are thought to range from 1–4 days and 6–10 days, respectively. The exact mechanism by which the rotaviruses cause diarrhea is not known. Limited human histologic studies show mild intestinal villous shortening, reticular cell enlargement, shortened columnar epithelial cells, mononuclear infiltration of the lamina propria, and decreased microvillae. Rotavirus infection may cause altered sugar absorption.

Clinical Presentation

Clinical manifestations of rotavirus infections vary from asymptomatic (which is common in adults) to severe nausea, vomiting, and diarrhea with dehydration. Symptoms are characterized initially by nausea and vomiting. Diarrhea occurs in most patients and lasts from 1–9 days, but some patients experience only loose stool with no increase in frequency.[93] Other signs and symptoms include fever, respiratory symptoms, irritability, lethargy, pharyngeal erythema, rhinitis, red tympanic membranes, and palpable cervical lymph nodes. Dehydration and electrolyte disturbances occur more frequently in children. Although uncommon, severe cases may result in death as soon as 24 hours after initial symptoms. Reye's syndrome has also been reported following rotavirus infection. Neonates may have asymptomatic rotavirus particles in their stool. Some evidence suggests that institutionalized infants are more susceptible to spread than those taken care of at home.[93]

Exposure may result in immunologic protection for several years. Human milk containing rotavirus antibodies appears to have a passive protective effect and may be an effective form of treatment among immunodeficient patients.

Laboratory findings reflect the degree of vomiting and/or diarrhea. Dehydration may result in elevated blood urea nitrogen and urine specific gravity. Electron microscopy, fluorescent virus precipitin test, radioimmunoassay, enzyme-linked immunosorbent assay (ELISA), and latex agglutination are reliable ways to detect rotavirus, with the latter three most practical for general use.

Treatment

Treatment of rotavirus-associated vomiting and/or diarrhea is directed at prevention or correction of dehydration. Studies are being conducted to explore active and passive immunity as viable means of prevention or treatment. These include administration of human or bovine milk containing rotavirus antibodies, oral immune globulin, or vaccines and antibodies.[71] A live-attenuated vaccine and a quadrivalent vaccine active against the four serotypes of rotavirus are currently in field trials.[30,94]

NORWALK AND NORWALK-LIKE AGENTS

Epidemiology

Parvovirus-like agents constitute a group of viruses 25–32 nm in diameter that can cause acute gastroenteritis. The Norwalk agent was the first of these agents to be described. Agents of this group are named according to the location of the outbreak of illness or contaminated source such as: Norwalk, Hawaii, Montgomery County, W, Ditchling, Cockle, Paramatta, Snow Mountain, and Marin County.

As with most viruses, the epidemiology of the Norwalk-like agents is poorly understood. The disease can affect all age groups and is nonseasonal. Studies of prevalence of antibody production have shown the incidence to increase from about 10% in 3–4 year olds to more than 50% by age 50. The exact vectors of transmission are not known; however, the fecal–oral route is believed to be important, as is contaminated food or water. A common food source is generally implicated.

Pathophysiology

The pathophysiology of this disease is similar to that caused by the rotavirus agents. Human volunteer studies have shown histopathologic changes appear within 24 hours of viral challenge, and clinical manifestations appear within 48 hours. Brush border enzyme activity may be decreased resulting in lactose intolerance, but it generally returns to preinfection levels within 2 weeks. The exact mechanisms of virus-induced vomiting or diarrhea are unknown.

Clinical Presentation

Norwalk-like viral gastroenteritis is characterized by sudden onset of abdominal cramps with nausea and/or vomiting. Although adults frequently experience nonbloody diarrhea, children experience vomiting more often. Other frequent complaints are myalgias, headache, and malaise, which are accompanied by fever in about 50% of cases. Signs and symptoms generally last only 12–60 hours.

Treatment

The disease is generally self-limiting and does not require therapy. On occasion, oral rehydration may be required. Rarely is parenteral hydration necessary.

ENTERIC ADENOVIRUS

Epidemiology

Adenovirus is a 70- to 75-nm icosahedral virus previously associated with respiratory, ocular, and genitourinary infections; however, serotypes 31, 40, and 41 have been identified as gastrointestinal pathogens. Estimated incidence ranges from 5–20% of hospitalizations for childhood diarrheal episodes in developed countries. Peak incidence is in children less than 2 years of age, and infections occur year-round although reports suggest a predominance of cases in the warmer months. Transmission is primarily person to person and fecal–oral, and shedding from the gut may be long term.[7,95] The incubation period ranges from 3–10 days. The main symptom is diarrhea, although vomiting, fever, and respiratory symptoms also occur. Symptoms often continue for 1–2 weeks, however, with less intensity than those produced by rotaviruses.[7,95]

OTHER POTENTIAL VIRAL PATHOGENS

Although less commonly associated with severe gastrointestinal disease, calicivirus, astrovirus, pestivirus, torovirus, and coronavirus-like particles have been recovered from diarrheal stools. In HIV-infected patients, the presence of diarrhea has been associated with virus in 35% of stool specimens. Astrovirus, picobirnavirus, calicivirus, and adenovirus appear to be the most commonly isolated viral pathogens.[96] More specific characteristics of these agents are presented in Table 106.5.

Bacterial Food Poisoning

Food poisoning results from the ingestion of food containing pathogenic microorganisms, preformed toxins that were produced by microorganisms, or other toxic compounds. An average of 18,335 cases from 479 outbreaks are reported annually to the CDC, although estimates for actual cases are approximately 12.6 million consuming approximately 8.4 billion dollars in health care expenditures.[97] Although a number of bacteria can cause food poisoning (Table 106.6),[98] this discussion is limited to the most common causes of bacterial food poisoning, *Salmonella* sp. (57%), *Shigella* (18%), *Staphylococcus aureus* (6%), and the potentially lethal *Clostridium* sp. (5%). Classification of food poisoning based on clinical symptoms has been proposed. Some suggested categories are nausea and vomiting, noninflammatory diarrhea, inflammatory diarrhea, neurologic symptoms, and systemic or miscellaneous symptoms.[97]

STAPHYLOCOCCAL FOOD POISONING

Staphylococcal food poisoning results from the ingestion of food contaminated by a preformed enterotoxin produced by certain strains of *S. aureus* growing within the food.[99] During 1983–1987, 3181 cases were reported to the CDC, making it the third most common form of food-borne illness. Infections are usually mild and of short duration, allowing it to go unrecognized and unreported.

TABLE 106.5. AGENTS RESPONSIBLE FOR ACUTE VIRAL GASTROENTERITIS AND DIARRHEA

Virus	Peak Age of Onset	Time of Year	Incubation	Duration	Detection[a]	Mode of Transmission	Symptoms
Rotavirus	6 months to 2 years	October to April	1–4 days	3–8 days	EM, RIA, EIA, culture, LA	Fecal/oral, aerosol?	Vomiting, watery diarrhea, fever, abdominal pain, lactose intolerance
Enteric adenovirus	<2 years	Year around	3–10 days	7–9 days	EM, EIA, RIA, culture	NR[b]	Diarrhea, respiratory symptoms, vomiting, fever
Calicivirus	3 months to 6 years	Year around with peak in winter	1–3 days	4 days	EM, RIA	NR	Vomiting, diarrhea
Astrovirus	<7 years	Winter	24–36 hours	1–4 days	EM, IEM	NR	Nonspecific vomiting, diarrhea, fever, abdominal pain
Pestivirus	<2 years	NR	NR	3 days	NR	NR	Mild
Coronavirus-like particles	<2 years	Fall and early winter	NR	7 days	EM	NR	Respiratory disease
Enterovirus	NR	NR	NR	NR	NR	NR	Mild diarrhea, secondary organ damage
Norwalk	School age and older	Variable	1–2 days	12–24 hours	IEM, RIA	Fecal/oral, food, aerosol?	Nausea, vomiting (younger patients), diarrhea (older patients), abdominal cramps, headache, fever, chills, myalgias

[a]EM, electron microscopy; EIA, enzyme immunoassay; IEM, immune electron microscopy; RIA, radioimmunoassay; LA, latex agglutination.
[b]NR, not reported. (Adapted from Refs. 7, 92, 107, and 108.)

TABLE 106.6. FOOD POISONINGS

Organism	Time to Symptoms (h)	Principal Foods	Peak Incidence (USA)	Principal Mechanism of Pathophysiology	Duration	Treatment
Staphylococcus aureus	1–6	Salad, pastries, ham, poultry	Summer	Preformed toxins A–E (heat stable)	12 h	Supportive
Bacillus cereus	1–6	Meats, vegetables, fried rice	None	Preformed toxins	12 h	Supportive
	8–16			Toxin production *(in vivo)*	24 h	Supportive
Clostridium perfringens (type A)	6–24	Meats, poultry	Fall, winter, spring	Toxin production *(in vivo)*	24 h	Supportive
Vibrio parahemolyticus	16–72	Shellfish	Spring, summer, fall	Toxin production and tissue invasion	2–7 d	Supportive
Salmonella spp.	16–48	Beef, poultry, water, eggs, dairy products	Summer	Tissue invasion	2–7 d	Supportive
Shigella spp.	16–48	Salad, water	Summer	Tissue invasion	2–7 d	Supportive
Enteropathogenic *Escherichia coli*	16–48	Water	None	Tissue invasion	2–7 d	Supportive
Campylobacter	16–48	Poultry, dairy products, clams, water	Spring, summer	Tissue invasion	2–7 d	Supportive
Enterotoxigenic *E. coli*	16–72	Water	None	Toxin production *(in vivo)*	1–7 d	Supportive
Vibrio cholerae	16–72	Water	—	Toxin production *(in vivo)*	2–12 d	Supportive, antibiotics
Yersinia enterocolitica	16–48	Dairy products		Toxin production and/or tissue invasion	1–30 d	Supportive
Clostridium botulinum	12–72	Canned fruits, vegetables, meats, honey	None	Preformed toxins A, B, and E (children and adults) Toxin production *(in vivo)* (infants)		Supportive (including mechanically assisted ventilation) Trivalent antitoxin

Toxigenic *S. aureus* is a common component of the normal skin flora of humans. Often the offending organism can be recovered from the person preparing the contaminated food. Commonly, foods rich in protein, salt, and sugar are reported to be contaminated such as potato and macaroni salads, custard-filled pastries, ham, sausages, poultry, and dairy products. Enterotoxin production generally results from leaving foods at room temperature, allowing the staphylococci to grow. At least five heat-stable toxins, A through E, exist, although A is responsible for approximately 55% of staphylococcal food-borne illness. These toxins have little or no local effect on the digestive tract. The exact mechanism by which the toxins produce disease is unknown, but emesis probably results from stimulation of the vomiting center in the brain.

Symptoms are rapid in onset, generally occurring within 1–6 hours of ingestion of toxin-containing foods. The condition is most often characterized by nausea and vomiting (75%), although abdominal cramps and diarrhea (68%) may also be present, usually lasting less than 12 hours. Myalgias, headache, sweating, chills, and fever (16%) may also be present. Complications are rare and most often related to dehydration.[100,101] Rehydration therapy is generally required only in severe cases. Antibiotics have not been shown to be beneficial.

SALMONELLA FOOD POISONING

Worldwide, salmonellosis resulting from contaminated food represents 60–80% of reported cases of food-borne illness. Nearly 40,000 cases are reported annually in the United States, and estimates for actual infection incidence are as high as 4 million cases annually.

Raw animal foods, such as eggs, unpasteurized milk, and hamburger, as well as contaminated vegetable foods are the major vectors of salmonella food poisoning. Most cases occur from July through November.

Prevention of salmonella food poisoning can be accomplished by proper importation and exportation control of vector products, decontamination of animal feed, animal vaccination, and good animal husbandry practices.[101] Proper preparation and handling of potential food vectors is essential in reducing the incidence of illness. Eggs should be stored only short term, held no longer than 2 hours at room temperature, prepared in small batches, thoroughly cooked before serving, and consumed immediately after preparation.[102] Further information regarding gastrointestinal salmonella infection is presented under "Salmonellosis."

SHIGELLA FOOD POISONING

Like salmonella, food-borne shigella disease usually manifests as inflammatory diarrhea. From 1983–1987, 9971 cases from 44 outbreaks were documented by the CDC making shigella the second most common food-borne pathogen. *Shigella sonnei* is the most common isolate in the United States, whereas *Shigella flexneri* has been noted overseas and *Shigella dysenteriae* is common in Third World countries.[97]

Shigella is common in the summer and fall and is spread from person to person via fecal–oral contamination, most commonly in vegetables, eggs, and cheese. The clinical syndrome resulting from the production of a shiga toxin was described in the shigellosis section. Diagnosis is made by culturing shigella from the stool. Treatment is best accomplished with cotrimoxazole, a floroquinolone, or a third-generation cephalosporin.[97]

CLOSTRIDIUM FOOD POISONING

Food-borne clostridium infections are related to *Clostridium perfringens,* which manifests with a noninflammatory diarrhea, and *Clostridium botulinum,* which is characterized by neurologic symptoms.

Clostridium perfringens

Clostridium perfringens was associated with 2743 cases from 24 outbreaks of food-borne illness in the United States during 1983–1987. Two distinct syndromes are possible. Type A organisms are seen in western nations and result in a 24-hour illness. It most often results after ingestion of cooked meat or poultry that has not been consumed within 2–3 hours. Spores in the meat multiply rapidly and produce a heat-labile enterotoxin. Symptoms, such as watery diarrhea (92%) and epigastric pain (81%), often occur within 8–24 hours and generally resolve within 12–24 hours. Other symptoms can include nausea (25%), vomiting (9%), and fever (24%). Type C organisms can be found in undercooked pork and occur in underdeveloped tropical regions. Type C can produce a toxin-related syndrome called enteritis necroticans, which is a coagulative, transmural necrosis of the intestinal wall. This syndrome can result in intestinal perforation leading to sepsis and mortality in approximately 40% of victims.[97]

Clostridium botulinum

Food-borne botulism results from the ingestion of food contaminated with preformed toxins or toxin-producing spores from *C. botulinum,* an anaerobic, spore-forming, gram-positive bacillus. During 1983–1987, 212 cases were reported from 24 outbreaks in the United States. Clostridia are commonly found in a variety of environmental sources. Most commonly associated food vectors include alkaline fruit and vegetable preparations, seafood, domestic canning products, and honey. Although clostridia are strict anaerobes, the spores are resistant to a variety of environmental conditions including freezing. Botulism is almost always associated with improper preparation and/or storage of food, which allows the spores to germinate.

Seven distinct toxins (A–G) divided into four groups have been described. A, B, and E produce most of the human disease and appear to be geographically distributed. The toxins, which are produced by the bacteria and released upon lysis, are the most potent biologic or chemical toxins known to man. The toxin is internalized and prevents the release of the neurotransmitter acetylcholine at the peripheral cholinergic nerve terminal. Blockade is most evident in cranial nerves and at the neuromuscular junction. Toxin activity has prompted the use of minute locally injected doses to treat select spastic disorders.[103,104]

Food-borne botulism presents as a symmetric descending paralysis without sensory or central nervous system involvement. Symptoms usually begin to occur 18–24 hours after ingestion and progress over days to weeks. Other symptoms can include blurred vision, photophobia (90%), dysphagia (76%), generalized weakness (58%), nausea and vomiting (56%), and dysphonia (55%).[97]

Infant botulism begins with ingestion of clostridium spores, which leads to gastrointestinal colonization. The colonizing organism produces *C. botulinum* toxin *in vivo,* which can result in weakness, hypotonia, constipation, anorexia, decreased gag or suck reflex, and respiratory failure.[97]

Diagnosis is made by culturing *C. botulinum* from the stool. Treatment of botulism consists primarily of respiratory support and use of botulinum antitoxin. Respiratory failure may occur prior to involvement of other upper muscle groups. Respiratory support should be provided as needed. If evaluation is performed within several hours of ingestion, gastric lavage or induction of vomiting is suggested. Cathartics and enemas can also be used to remove residual toxin from the bowel, but are contraindicated in cases of ileus.

Although the effectiveness of antitoxins is unknown, patients diagnosed with botulism should receive botulinum antitoxin. Limited data comparing preantitoxin and postantitoxin eras suggest that patients with toxin type E botulism may benefit from antitoxin.[105] A retrospective review of 132 cases of type A botulism reported to the CDC between 1973 and 1980 suggested trivalent antitoxin to be beneficial.[106] After controlling for age and incubation period, patients treated with antitoxin were reported to have a lower fatality rate and a shorter clinical course than those who did not receive antitoxin. Patients receiving antitoxin within the first 24 hours of onset of symptoms had a shorter clinical course but about the same mortality rate as those receiving antitoxin late.

Botulinum antitoxin is a concentrated preparation of equine globulins obtained from horses immunized with toxins A, B, and E. Each 10-mL vial of trivalent antitoxin contains 7500 IU of type A, 5500 IU of type B, and 8500 IU of type E antitoxin. Data on the pharmacokinetics of the individual antitoxins are limited.[107] Because trivalent antitoxin is equine in origin, patients should be tested for hypersensitivity before receiving the product intravenously. After hypersensitivity testing, the current dosing recommendation is (as outlined in package insert) one vial given intravenously and one vial given intramuscularly. After 4 hours, if signs and symptoms worsen, one vial should be given intravenously. Another vial may be given intravenously after 12–24 hours. Antitoxin may be obtained from the Centers for Disease Control and Prevention, Atlanta, Georgia, (404)639-3670.

Other agents used experimentally as adjunctive therapy are guanidine and 4-aminopyridine, which have been shown to increase acetylcholine release. Data are limited yet promising.[108]

Prevention should always be stressed. Botulinum toxins are heat labile and readily destroyed by 10 minutes of boiling. All home-canned foods should be processed according to directions and boiled, not just warmed, prior to consumption.

REFERENCES

1. Tolia VK, Dubois RS. Update on oral rehydration: Its place in treatment of acute gastroenteritis. Pediatr Ann 1985;14:295–303.
2. Walsh JA, Warren KS. Selective primary health care: An interim strategy for disease control in developing countries. N Engl J Med 1979;301:967–974.
3. Kallen RJ. The management of diarrheal dehydration in infants using parenteral fluids. Pediatr Clin North Am 1990;37(2):265–286.
4. Ho M, Glass RI, Pinsky PF, et al. Rotavirus as a cause of diarrheal morbidity and mortality in the United States. J Infect Dis 1988;158:1112–1116.
5. Ho M, Glass RI, Pinsky PF, et al. Diarrheal deaths in American children: Are they preventable. JAMA 1988;260(22):3281–3285.
6. Williams EK, Lohr JA, Guerrant RL. Acute infectious diarrhea. II. Diagnosis treatment and prevention. Pediatr Infect Dis J 1986;5:458–465.
7. Christensen ML. Human viral gastroenteritis. Clin Microbiol Rev 1989;2(1):51–89.
8. Pizarro D, Castillo B, Posada G, et al. Efficacy comparison of oral rehydration solutions containing either 90 or 75 millimoles of sodium per liter. Pediatrics 1987;79:190–195.
9. Davies A and Jenkins HR. Management of gastroenteritis in early childhood. Drugs 1992;44:57–64.
10. Powell DW, Szauter KE. Nonantibiotic therapy and pharmacotherapy of acute infectious diarrhea. Gastroenterol Clin North Am 1993;22:683–707.
11. Mohan M, Sethi JS, Daral TS, et al. Controlled trial of rice powder and glucose rehydration solutions as oral therapy for acute dehydrating diarrhea in infants. J Pediatr Gastroenterol Nutr 1986;5(3):423–427.
12. Bhan MK, Ghai OP, Khoshoo V, et al. Efficacy of mung bean (lentil) and pop rice based rehydration solutions in comparison with the standard glucose electrolyte solution. J Pediatr Gastroenterol Nutr 1987;6:392–399.

13. Santosham M, Fayad IM, Hashem M, et al. A comparison of rice-based oral rehydration and "early feeding" for the treatment of acute diarrhea in infants. J Pediatr 1990;16:868–875.
14. Goepp JG, Katz SA. Oral rehydration therapy. Am Fam Phys 1993;47:843–848.
15. Gore SM, Fontaine O, Pierce NF. Impact of rice-based oral rehydration solution on stool output and duration of diarrhoea: Meta-analysis of 13 clinical trials. BMJ 1992;304:287–91.
16. Santosham M, Burns BA, Reid R, et al. Glycine-based oral rehydration solution: Reassessment of safety and efficacy. J Pediatr 1986;109:795–801.
17. American Academy of Pediatrics, Committee on Nutrition. Use of oral fluid therapy and post-treatment feeding following enteritis in children in a developed country. Pediatrics 1985;75(2):358–361.
18. Alam NH, Ahmed T, Khatun M, Molla AM. Effects of food with two oral rehydration therapies: A randomized, controlled clinical trial. Gut 1992;33:560–562.
19. Faruque ASG, Mahalanabis D, Islam A, et al. Breast feeding and oral rehydration at home during diarrhoea to prevent dehydration. Arch Dis Childhood 1992;67:1027–1029.
20. Gracey M. Bacterial diarrhoea. Clin Gastroenterol 1986;15(1):21–37.
21. Anonymous. Cholera in a tourist returning from Cancun, Mexico. New Jersey MMWR 1983;32:357.
22. Gill DM. The mechanism of action of cholera toxin. Adv Cyclic Nucleotide Res 1977;8:85.
23. Svennerholm A, Jeriborn M, Gothefors L, et al. Mucosal antitoxin and antibacterial immunity after cholera disease and after immunization with a combined B subunit-whole cell vaccine. J Infect Dis 1984;149:884–893.
24. Hug MI, Sanyal SC, Samadi AR, et al. Comparative behavior of classical and El Tor biotypes of *Vibrio cholerae* 01 isolated in Bangladesh during 1982. Diar Dis Res 1983;1:5–9.
25. Hirschorn N, Lindenbaum J, Greenough WC, et al. Hypoglycemia in children with acute diarrhea. Lancet 1966;2:128–132.
26. Lindebaum J, Greenough WB, Islam MR. Antibiotic therapy of cholera in children. Bull WHO 1967;37:529.
27. Sanford JP. Guide to Antimicrobial Therapy 1993. Bethesda, MD, Antimicrobial Therapy, 1993, pp 10–11, 39–41.
28. Nelson JD. Pocketbook of Pediatric Antimicrobial Therapy, 1993–4, 10th ed. Baltimore, Williams and Wilkins, 1993, pp 66–81.
29. Karchmer AW, Curlin GT, Hug MJ, et al. Furazolidone in paediatric cholera. Bull WHO 1970;43:373–378.
30. Levine MM, Noriega F. Vaccines to prevent enteric infections. Baillieres Clin Gastroenterol 1993;7:501–517.
31. Tacket CO, Losonsky G, Nafaro JP, et al. Onset and duration of protective immunity in challenged volunteers after vaccination with live oral cholera vaccine CVD 103-hgR. J Infect Dis 1992;166:837–841.
32. Clemens JD, Sack DA, Rao MR, et al. Evidence that inactivated oral cholera vaccine both prevent and mitigate *Vibrio cholerae* 01 infections in a cholera-endemic area. J Infect Dis 1992;166:1029–1034.
33. Guerrant RL, Moore RA, Kirschenfeld PM, et al. Role of toxigenic and invasive bacteria in acute diarrhea of childhood. N Engl J Med 1975;293:567–573.
34. Levine MM. *Escherichia coli* that cause diarrhea: Enterotoxigenic, enteropathogenic, enteroinvasive, enterohemorrhagic, and enteroadherent. J Infect Dis 1987;155(3):377–389.
35. Brook MG, Bannister BA. Diarrhoea-causing *Escherichia coli*. Dig Dis 1993;11:288–297.
36. Hart CA, Batt RM, Saunders JR. Diarrhoea caused by *Escherichia coli*. Ann Trop Paediatr 1993;13:121–131.
37. Gracey M. Travelers' diarrhea: Is drug therapy for prophylaxis and treatment of real benefit? Drugs 1984; 27:1–5.
38. DuPont HL, Reves RR, Galindo E, et al. Treatment of travelers' diarrhea with trimethoprim/sulfamethoxazole and with trimethoprim alone. N Engl J Med 1982;307:841–844.
39. DuPont HL, Ericsson CD, Reves RR, et al. Antimicrobial therapy for travelers' diarrhea. Rev Infect Dis 1986;8(S2):S217–222.
40. Sack RB. Antimicrobial prophylaxis of travelers' diarrhea: A selected summary. Rev Infect Dis 1986;8(S2):S160–S166.
41. DuPont HL, Ericsson CD, Johnson PC, et al. Antimicrobial agents in the prevention of travelers' diarrhea. Rev Infect Dis 1986;8(S2):S167–S171.
42. Steffen R, Heusser R, DuPont HL. Prevention of travelers' diarrhea by nonantibiotic drugs. Rev Infect Dis 1986;8(S2):S151–S159.
43. Ericsson CD, DuPont HL, Johnson PC. Nonantibiotic therapy for travelers' diarrhea. Rev Infect Dis 1986;8(S2):S202–S206.
44. Soriano-Brucher HE, Avendano P, O'Ryan M, et al. Use of bismuth subsalicylate in acute diarrhea in children. Rev Infect Dis 1990;12(S1):S51–S56.
45. DuPont HL, Ericsson DC, Johnson PC, et al. Use of bismuth subsalicylate for the prevention of travelers' diarrhea. Rev Infect Dis 1990;12(S1):S64–S67.
46. Steffen R. Worldwide efficacy of bismuth subsalicylate in the treatment of travelers' diarrhea. Rev Infect Dis 1990;12(S1):S80–S86.
47. Bartlett JG, Chang TW, Gurwith M, et al. Antibiotic-associated pseudomembranous colitis due to toxin-producing clostridia. N Engl J Med 1978;298:531–534.
48. Fekety R, Shah AB. Diagnosis and treatment of *Clostridium difficile* colitis. JAMA 1993;269:71–75.
49. Fekety R, Kim KH, Brown D, et al. Epidemiology of antibiotic-associated colitis. Isolation of *Clostridium difficile* from the hospital environment. Am J Med 1981;70:906–908.
50. Peterson LR, Kelly PJ. The role of the clinical microbiology laboratory in the management of *Clostridium difficile* associated diarrhea. Infect Dis Clin North Am 1993;7:277–293.
51. Teasley DG, Olson MM, Gerding DN, et al. Prospective randomized study of metronidazole versus vancomycin for clostridium-associated diarrhea and colitis. Lancet 1983;2:1043–1046.
52. Greenfield MD, Smith AL. Vancomycin in pediatrics. Pediatrics Rev 1983;5(6):185–189.

53. Leung AKC, Robson WLM. Acute diarrhea in children: What to do and what not to do. Postgrad Med 1989;86(8):161–174.
54. Gorbach SL, Chang TW, Goldin B. Successful treatment of relapsing *Clostridium difficile* colitis with *Lactobacillus* GG. Lancet 1987;2:1519.
55. Surawicz CM, McFarland LV, Elmer G, et al. Treatment of recurrent *Clostridium difficile* colitis with vancomycin and *Saccharomyces boulardii.* Am J Gastroenterol 1989;84:1285–1287.
56. Young GP, Ward P, McDonald M, et al. Comparison of oral bacitracin with vancomycin in therapy of antibiotic-associated colitis. Gastroenterology 1984;86:1306.
57. King C, Barrier SL. Analysis of *in vitro* interaction between vancomycin and cholestyramine. Antimicrob Agents Chemother 1981;19:326–329.
58. Johnson S, Homann SR, Bettin KM, et al. Treatment of asymptomatic *Clostridium difficile* carriers (fecal excretors) with vancomycin or metronidazole. A randomized, placebo-controlled trial. Ann Intern Med 1992;117:297–302.
59. Novak E, Lee DG, Seckman CE, et al. Unfavorable effect of atropine–diphenoxylate therapy in lincomycin-caused diarrhea. JAMA 1976;235:1451–1454.
60. Taylor DN, Echeverria P, Sethabutr O, et al. Clinical and microbiologic features of *Shigella* and enteroinvasive *Escherichia coli* infections detected by DNA hybridization. J Clin Microbiol 1988;26(7):1362–1366.
61. Anonymous. Shigellosis—United States, 1983. MMWR 1984;33(43):616.
62. LaBrec E, Schneider H, Magnani T. Epithelial cell penetration as an essential step in the pathogenesis of bacillary dysentery. J Bacteriol 1964;88:1503–1518.
63. Keusch GT, Bennish ML. Shigellosis: Recent progress, persisting problems and research issues. Pediatric Infect Dis J 1989;8:713–719.
64. DuPont HL, Hornick R, Dawkins A. The response of man to virulent *Shigella flexneri* 2a. J Infect Dis 1969;119:296–299.
65. Frankel G, Riley L, Giron JA, et al. Detection of shigella in feces using DNA amplification. J Infect Dis 1990;161:1252–1256.
66. DuPont HL. Nonfluid therapy and selected chemoprophylaxis of acute diarrhea. Am J Med 1985;78(suppl 6B): 81–90.
67. Ericsson CD, DuPont HL, Sullivan P, et al. Bicozamycin, a poorly absorbable antibiotic, effectively treats travelers' diarrhea. Ann Intern Med 1983;98:20–25.
68. Eidlitz-Marcus T, Cohen YH, Nussinovitch M, et al. Clinical and laboratory observations. Comparative efficacy of two- and five-day courses of ceftriaxone in treatment of severe shigellosis. J Pediatr 1993;123:822–824.
69. DuPont HL, Hornick R. Adverse effects of Lomotil therapy in shigellosis. JAMA 1973;226:1525–1528.
70. Brahmbhatt HN, Lindberg AA, Timmis KN. Shigella lipopolysaccharide: Structure, genetics, and vaccine development. Curr Top Microbiol Immunol 1992;180:45–63.
71. Edelman R. Prevention and treatment of infectious diarrhea: Speculations on the next ten years. Am J Med 1985;78(suppl 6B):99–106.
72. Anonymous. Human salmonella isolates—United States, 1983. MMWR 1984;33(49):693.
73. Anonymous. Salmonella Surveillance Summary for 1980. Atlanta, Centers for Disease Control, 1982.
74. Baine WB, Gangarosa EJ, Bennett JV. Institutional salmonellosis. J Infect Dis 1973;128:357–360.
75. Hook EW. Salmonella species (including typhoid fever), in Mandell GL, Douglas RG, Bennett JE (eds): Principles and Practice of Infectious Diseases. New York, John Wiley and Sons, 1985, pp 1256–1269.
76. El-Radhi AS, Rostila T, Vesikari T. Association of high fever and short bacterial excretion after salmonellosis. Arch Dis Child 1992;67:531–532.
77. Rubin RH, Weinstein L. Salmonellosis: Microbiologic, Pathologic, and Clinical Features. New York, Stratton Intercontinental Medical Book Corporation, 1977.
78. Hoffman TA, Ruiz CJ, Counts GW, et al. Waterborne typhoid fever in Dade County, Florida: Clinical and therapeutic evaluation of 105 bacteremic patients. Am J Med 1975;59:481–487.
79. Aserkoff B, Bennett JV. Effect of antibiotic therapy in acute salmonellosis on the fecal excretion of salmonellae. N Engl J Med 1969;281:636–640.
80. Sanchez C, Garcia-Restoy E, Garau J, et al. Ciprofloxacin and trimethoprim–sulfamethoxazole versus placebo in acute uncomplicated salmonella enteritis; a double-blind trial. J Infect Dis 1993;168:1304–1307.
81. Butler T, Rumans L, Arnold K. Response of typhoid fever caused by chloramphenicol-susceptible and chloramphenicol-resistant strains of *Salmonella typhi* to treatment with trimethoprim–sulfamethoxazole. Rev Infect Dis 1982;4:551–561.
82. Pillay N, Adams EB, Coombes DN. Comparative trial of amoxicillin and chloramphenicol in treatment of typhoid fever in adults. Lancet 1975;2:333–337.
83. Hoffman SL, Punjab NH, Kumala S, et al. Reduction of mortality in chloramphenicol-treated severe typhoid fever by high-dose dexamethasone. N Engl J Med 1984;310:8–88.
84. Cover TL, Blaser MJ. The pathobiology of *Campylobacter* infections in humans. Ann Rev Med 1989;40:269–285.
85. Pitkanen T, Ponka A, Pettersson T, et al. *Campylobacter* enteritis in 188 hospitalized patients. Arch Intern Med 1983;143:215–219.
86. Finch MJ, Riley LW. *Campylobacter* infections in the United States—results of an 11-state surveillance. Arch Intern Med 1984;144:1610–1612.
87. Nolan CM, Johnson KE, Coyle MB, et al. *Campylobacter jejuni* enteritis: Efficacy of antimicrobial and antimotility drugs. Am J Gastroenterol 1983;78:621–626.
88. Anders BJ, Lauer BA, Paisley JW, et al. Double-blind placebo controlled trial of erythromycin for treatment of campylobacter enteritis. Lancet 1982;1:131–132.
89. Marks MI, Pai C, Lafleur L, et al. *Yersinia enterocolitica* gastroenteritis: A retrospective study of clinical bacteriologic and epidemiologic features. J Pediatr 1980;96:26–31.
90. Pai C, Gillis F, Tuomanen E, et al. Clinical and laboratory observations: Placebo controlled double-blind evaluation of trimethoprim-sulfamethoxazole treatment of *Yersinia enterocolitica* gastroenteritis. J Pediatr 1984;104:308–311.

91. Winblad S. Arthritis associated with *Yersinia enterocolitica* infections. Scand J Infect Dis 1975;7:191–195.
92. Brandt CD, Kim HW, Rodriguez WJ, et al. Pediatric viral gastroenteritis during eight years of study. J Clin Microbiol 1983;18:71–78.
93. Hjelt K, Krasilnikoff PA, Gravballe PC, et al. Clinical features in hospitalized children with acute gastroenteritis. Acta Paediatric Scand 1985;74:96–101.
94. Schwab KS, Shaw RD. Viruses. Baillieres Clin Gastroenterol 1993;7:307–31.
95. Anonymous. Viral agents of gastroenteritis: Public health importance and outbreak management. MMWR 1990;39(RR-5):1–24.
96. Grohmann GS, Glass RI, Pereira HG, et al. Enteric viruses and diarrhea in HIV-infected patients. N Engl J Med 1993;329:14–20.
97. Bishai WR, Sears CL. Food poisoning syndromes. Gastroenterol Clin North Am 1993;22:579–608.
98. Archer DL, Young RE. Contemporary issues: Diseases with a food vector. Clin Microbiol Rev 1988;1(4): 377–398.
99. Feig M. Staphylococcal food poisoning. A report of two related outbreaks, and a discussion of the data presented. Am J Public Health 1950;40:279.
100. Holmberg SD, Blake PA. Staphylococcal food poisoning in the United States: New facts and old misconceptions. JAMA 1984;251:487–489.
101. Anonymous. Prevention of foodborne diseases. PAHO Bulletin 1988;22(2):207–208.
102. Anonymous. Update: *Salmonella enteritidis* infections and grade A shell eggs—United States 1989. MMWR 1990;38(51–52):877–880.
103. Gunderson CB. The effects of botulinum toxin on the synthesis, storage, and release of acetylcholine. Prog Neurobiol 1980;14:99.
104. Hatheway CL. Toxigenic *Clostridia.* Clin Microbiol Rev 1990;3(1):66–98.
105. Whittaker RL, Gilbertson RB, Garrutt AS. Botulism, type E: Report of eight simultaneous cases. Ann Intern Med 1964;61:448–454.
106. Tacket CO, Shandera WX, Mann JM, et al. Equine antitoxin use and other factors that predict outcome in type A foodborne botulism. Am J Med 1984;76:794–798.
107. Hatheway CH, Snyder JD, Seals JE, et al. Antitoxin levels in botulism patients treated with trivalent equine botulism antitoxin to toxin types A, B, and E. J Infect Dis 1984;150:407–412.
108. Sellin LC. Botulism—an update. Military Med 1984;149:12–16.
109. Facts and Comparisons, St. Louis, JB Lippincott, updated monthly, p 17a.
110. Feld LG, Kaskel FJ, Schoeneman MJ. The approach to fluid and electrolyte therapy in pediatrics. Adv Pediatr 1988;35:497–536.

Chapter 107

Intra-Abdominal Infections

Joseph T. DiPiro, PharmD, FCCP, and David A. Rogers, MD

Despite the introduction of many new antimicrobials and advances in diagnostic and therapeutic techniques, the treatment of intra-abdominal infection continues to pose many challenges. The nature of these infections varies considerably depending on the site of infection, the size of the bacterial inoculum, the underlying disease process, and the status of the patient's own defense mechanisms. Optimal therapeutic management usually requires a combination of drainage procedures, antimicrobials, and other measures that maintain vital organ function.

Intra-abdominal infections are those contained within the peritoneum or retroperitoneal space. The peritoneal cavity extends from the undersurface of the diaphragm to the floor of the pelvis and contains the stomach, most of the small bowel, the large bowel, liver and gallbladder, and spleen. The duodenum, pancreas, kidneys, adrenals, great vessels (aorta and vena cava), and most mesenteric vascular structures reside in the posterior retroperitoneum. These infections may be generalized or localized. They may be contained within visceral structures such as the liver, spleen, pancreas, or the female reproductive organs. Two general types of intra-abdominal infection are discussed throughout this chapter: peritonitis and abscess. Peritonitis is defined as the acute, inflammatory response of peritoneal lining to microorganisms, chemicals, irradiation, or foreign body injury. This chapter deals only with peritonitis of infectious origin. An abscess is a purulent collection of fluid separated by a more or less well-defined wall from surrounding tissue. It usually contains necrotic debris, bacteria, and inflammatory cells. These processes differ considerably in their presentation and the required approach to treatment.

ETIOLOGY

Peritonitis may be classified as either "primary" or "secondary." With primary peritonitis an intra-abdominal focus of disease may not be evident. Bacteria may be transported from the bloodstream to the peritoneal cavity where the inflammatory process begins. In secondary peritonitis a focal disease process is evident within the abdomen. In most cases this involves perforation of a hollow structure of the gastrointestinal tract and subsequent escape of intestinal contents.

Primary peritonitis is relatively uncommon. It has been reported to occur infrequently in adults as well as in normal infants and children. It occurs in 10–20% of patients with cirrhotic ascites, in other immunocompromised patients, and in patients undergoing peritoneal dialysis. In fact, it is estimated that 60% of all patients on chronic ambulatory peritoneal dialysis (CAPD) will have at least one episode of peritonitis during the first year.[1]

Recent paracentesis, upper gastrointestinal endoscopy, portacaval anastomosis, arterial or umbilical vein catheterization, and barium enema or sigmoidoscopy appear to increase the risk of primary peritonitis.

Table 107.1 summarizes many of the potential causes of bacterial peritonitis. These include inflammatory processes of the gastrointestinal tract or abdominal organs, mechanical problems such as bowel obstruction, vascular occlusions that may lead to gangrene of the intestines, and neoplasias that may cause intestinal perforation or obstruction. Other possible causes include those resulting from traumatic injuries or postoperative infections.

Abscesses are the result of chronic inflammation and most often occur without preceding generalized peritonitis. They may be located within one of the spaces of the peritoneal cavity or within one of the visceral organs. These collections often have a fibrinous capsule and may take from a few days to years to form.

The causes of intra-abdominal abscess somewhat overlap those of peritonitis and, in fact, both may occur sequentially or simultaneously. Appendicitis is the most frequent cause of abscess followed by pancreatitis and lesions of the genitourinary tract (particularly in women). Other potential causes of intra-abdominal abscesses include diverticulitis, lesions of the biliary tract, osteomyelitis of the spine, perforating tumors in the abdomen, trauma, and leaking intestinal anastomosis. For certain diseases, such as

TABLE 107.1. CAUSES OF BACTERIAL PERITONITIS

Primary Bacterial Peritonitis
Peritoneal dialysis
Cirrhosis with ascites
Secondary Bacterial Peritonitis
Miscellaneous causes
Diverticulitis with perforation
Appendicitis
Inflammatory bowel diseases
Salpingitis
Biliary tract infections
Necrotizing pancreatitis
Neoplasms
Intestinal obstruction
Perforation
Mechanical gastrointestinal problems
Any cause of small bowel obstruction
Vascular causes
Mesenteric arterial or venous occlusion
Mesenteric ischemia without occlusion
Trauma
Blunt abdominal trauma with rupture of intestine
Penetrating abdominal trauma
Iatrogenic intestinal perforation
Intraoperative events
Peritoneal contamination during abdominal operation
Leakage from gastrointestinal anastomosis

appendicitis and diverticulitis, abscesses occur much more frequently than does generalized peritonitis.

MICROFLORA OF GASTROINTESTINAL TRACT AND FEMALE GENITAL TRACT

A full appreciation of the nature of these processes requires an understanding of the normal microflora within the gastrointestinal tract. There are striking differences in gastrointestinal flora contained within the various segments of the gastrointestinal tract (Table 107.2), and this bacterial environment usually determines the severity of infectious processes in the abdomen.[2] Generally, the low gastric pH eradicates bacteria that enter the stomach. With achlorhydria, bacterial counts may rise to 10^5–10^7/mL. The normally low bacterial count also changes with gastric outlet obstruction and gastric cancer, in patients that have been on histamine-2 (H_2) receptor antagonists or antacids, or in the presence of blood.[3] In each of these situations the concentration of bacteria may increase by 1000- or 10,000-fold.

The biliary tract (gallbladder and bile ducts) is sterile in most healthy individuals but in certain groups it is likely to be colonized by aerobic gram-negative bacilli (particularly *Escherichia coli* and *Klebsiella* spp.) and enterococci.[4] Groups more likely to be colonized include those older than the age of 70, or those with acute cholecystitis, jaundice, or common bile duct stones.[5] Because these groups have a biliary tract that is more frequently colonized they are at greater risk of intra-abdominal infection.

At the distal ileum, particularly just before the ileocecal junction, bacterial counts of aerobes and anaerobes are quite high. In the colon there may be 400 to 500 different types of bacteria with bacterial concentrations often reaching 10^{11}/mL, and anaerobic bacteria outnumber aerobic bacteria by more than 1000 to 1. In fact, up to 50% of the dry mass of stool is bacteria. Fortunately, most colonic bacteria are not pathogens, because they cannot survive in environments outside the colon. Perforation of the colon results in the release of very large numbers of anaerobic and aerobic bacteria into the peritoneum.[6] The colonic flora are generally stable unless broad-spectrum antimicrobials have been in use, in which case increases in *Candida* or resistant bacteria are noted.

The lower female genital tract is generally colonized by a large number of aerobic and anaerobic bacteria. Anaerobes may number 10^9/mL and often include lactobacilli, eubacteria, clostridia, anaerobic streptococci, and, less frequently, *Bacteroides fragilis.* Aerobic bacteria are most often streptococci and *Staphylococcus epidermidis,* and these may number 10^8/mL.

PATHOPHYSIOLOGY

Intra-abdominal infection results from entry of bacteria into the peritoneal or retroperitoneal spaces or from bacterial collections within intra-abdominal organs. In primary peritonitis the route of bacterial spread is often not apparent. Bacteria may enter the abdomen via the bloodstream or the lymphatic system by transmigration through the bowel wall or via the fallopian tubes in females. Hematogenous bacterial spread (through the bloodstream) occurs more frequently with tubercular peritonitis or peritonitis associated with cirrhotic ascites.[7] When peritonitis results from peritoneal dialysis, skin surface flora are introduced via the peritoneal catheter.[8] In secondary peritonitis, bacteria most often enter the peritoneum or retroperitoneum as a result of disruption of the integrity of the gastrointestinal tract caused by diseases or traumatic injuries. Also, peritonitis or abscess may result from contamination of the peritoneum during a surgical procedure, or from lesions of the female genital tract.

The physiologic characteristics of the peritoneal cavity determine the nature of the response to infection or inflammation within it. The peritoneum is lined by a highly permeable, serous membrane with a surface area approximately that of skin. The normal peritoneal cavity contains about 50 mL of a serous fluid that is normally sterile, is low in protein and leukocytes, and contains no fibrinogen. These conditions change drastically with peritoneal infection or inflammation as will be described later.

After bacteria are introduced into the peritoneal cavity there is an immediate response to contain the insult.[8]

TABLE 107.2. USUAL MICROFLORA OF THE GASTROINTESTINAL TRACT

Site	Commonly Found Bacteria	Approximate Concentration (Log No. Organisms/mL)	
		Aerobes	Anaerobes
Stomach[a]	*Streptococcus, Lactobacillus*	10^0–10^2	Rare
Biliary tract	Normally sterile (*Escherichia coli, Klebsiella,* or enterococci in some patients)	0	0
Proximal small bowel	*Streptococcus* (including enterococci), *E. coli, Klebsiella, Lactobacillus,* diphtheroids	10^2	Few
Distal ileum	*E. coli, Klebsiella, Enterobacter,* enterococci, *Bacteroides fragilis, Clostridium,* peptostreptococci	10^4–10^6	10^5–10^7
Colon	*Bacteroides* spp., peptostreptococci, *Clostridium, E. coli, Klebsiella,* enterococci, *Enterobacter,* and many others	10^5–10^8	10^9–10^{11}

[a]With achlorhydria, H_2-antagonist therapy, gastric cancer, or gastric outlet obstruction, bacterial counts may rise to 10^5/mL.

Humoral and cellular defenses respond first; then the omentum migrates to the affected area. A limited bacterial inoculum is rapidly handled by defense mechanisms. Under certain conditions the bacterial insult is not contained and bacteria disseminate throughout the peritoneal cavity, resulting in peritonitis. This is more likely to occur in the presence of a foreign body or where there is (1) a large bacterial inoculum, (2) continuing bacterial contamination, and (3) contamination involving a mixture of organisms that by synergistic action are particularly virulent.

When bacteria become dispersed throughout the peritoneum the inflammatory process involves the majority of the peritoneal lining. There is an outpouring into the peritoneum of serous fluid containing leukocytes, fibrin, and other proteins which form exudates on the inflamed peritoneal surfaces and begin to form adhesions between peritoneal structures. This process, combined with a paralysis of the intestines ("ileus"), may result in confinement of the contamination to one or more locations within the peritoneum. Fluid also begins to collect in the bowel and distention may result. The fluid and protein shift into the abdomen ("third-spacing") may be so dramatic that circulating blood volume is decreased, which causes decreased cardiac output and possibly hypotension. The fluid imbalance may be worsened by accompanying fever, vomiting, or diarrhea. A reflex sympathetic response, manifested by sweating, tachycardia, and vasoconstriction may be evident. With an inflamed peritoneum, bacteria and the endotoxins are easily absorbed into the bloodstream (translocation) and this may result in septic shock. Other foreign substances that may be present in the peritoneal cavity potentiate peritonitis. These adjuvants, notably feces, dead tissues, barium, mucus, bile, and blood, have detrimental effects on host defense mechanisms, particularly on bacterial phagocytosis.

Peritonitis often results in mortality because of the effects on multiple organ systems. As mentioned before, fluid shifts and endotoxins may cause hypotension and shock. Fluid loss from the vasculature with generalized peritonitis is similar to that which occurs after a 50% second-degree burn. Hypoalbuminemia may result from protein loss into the peritoneum. Pulmonary function may be compromised because the inflamed peritoneum causes splinting (muscle rigidity caused by pain) which inhibits proper ventilation. Then, atelectasis and pulmonary shunting of blood may result in respiratory distress syndrome and hypoxemia. With fluid loss and hypotension or sepsis, renal perfusion may be compromised and acute renal failure is a potential threat. In addition, endotoxin is hepatotoxic and exposure during sepsis may lead to hepatic dysfunction.

If the body is successful in localizing peritoneal contamination but fails to completely eliminate bacteria, an abscess results. This collection of necrotic tissue, bacteria, and white blood cells may be at single or multiple sites and may be within one of the spaces of the peritoneal cavity or in one of the visceral organs. The location of the abscess is often related to the site of primary disease.[9] For example, abscesses resulting from appendicitis tend to appear in the right lower quadrant or the pelvis; those resulting from diverticulitis tend to appear in the left lower quadrant or pelvis.

An abscess begins by the combined action of inflammatory cells (such as neutrophils), bacteria, fibrin, and other inflammatory components. Bacteria may release heparinases which cause local thrombosis and tissue necrosis or fibrinolysins, collagenases, or other enzymes that allow extension of the process into surrounding tissues.

Neutrophils that have gathered in the abscess cavity die in 3–5 days, releasing lysosomal enzymes that liquefy the core of the abscess. A mature abscess may have a fibrinous capsule that isolates bacteria and the liquid core from antimicrobials and immunologic defenses.

In this environment the oxygen tension is low, anaerobic bacteria thrive, and the size of the abscess may increase. Also, abscesses are hypertonic, resulting in additional influx of fluid. Hypertonicity promotes the formation of bacterial L forms, which are resistant to antimicrobial agents that disrupt cell walls. This process may continue and stabilize for long periods of time and not be readily evident to patient or physician. In some instances the abscess may resolve, and infrequently it may erode into adjacent organs or it may rupture and cause diffuse peritonitis. If the abscess erodes through the skin it may result in a fistula, which connects the bowel to the skin, or a noncommunicating sinus tract.

Microbiology of Intra-Abdominal Infection

Primary bacterial peritonitis is often caused by a single organism. In children, the pathogen is usually *Streptococcus pneumoniae* or a group A streptococcus.[10] When peritonitis occurs in association with cirrhotic ascites, enteric organisms are usually responsible.[7] *Escherichia coli* is isolated most frequently, followed by streptococcal species (including pneumococcus), *Klebsiella, Bacteroides* spp., *Pseudomonas aeruginosa,* and numerous other organisms. Occasionally, primary peritonitis may be caused by *Mycobacterium tuberculosis.* Peritonitis in patients undergoing peritoneal dialysis is most often caused by common skin organisms: *S. epidermidis, Staphylococcus aureus,* streptococci, and diphtheroids.[8] Occasionally, aerobic gram-negative bacilli may cause infections, particularly in patients undergoing dialysis during hospitalization.

Because of the diverse bacteria present in the gastrointestinal tract, secondary intra-abdominal infections are often polymicrobial.[11] The mean number of isolates of microorganisms from infected intra-abdominal sites has ranged from 2.5 to 5.0, including an average of 1.4 to 2.0 aerobes and 2.4 to 3.0 anaerobes.[6,12] With proper anaerobic specimen collection, anaerobic organisms are isolated in most patients. In one report of patients with gangrenous and perforated appendicitis, an average of 10.2 different organisms was isolated from each patient, including 2.7 aerobes and 7.5 anaerobes. Purely aerobic or anaerobic infections are uncommon, as are infections caused by fungi. The frequencies with which specific bacteria were isolated in intra-abdominal infections are given in Table 107.3.[13] *Escherichia coli* and *Bacteroides* spp. were most often isolated from the infection site as well as from blood cultures. This pattern of infecting bacteria is similar to that seen in intra-abdominal abscesses. With patients that have severe infections the pattern of bacterial isolates may change and more commonly include *Candida, Enterococci, Enterobacter,* and *S. epidermidis.*[13]

Some visceral abscesses differ in character from most intra-abdominal abscesses. Hepatic abscesses may be polymicrobial (involving *E. coli* and anaerobes) or occasionally may be caused by amoeba. Pancreatic abscesses are often polymicrobial, involving enteric bacteria that ascend through the biliary system. Splenic abscesses usually result from hematogenous dissemination of bacteria such as *S. aureus,* streptococci, and occasionally *Salmonella* or anaerobic organisms.

Bacterial Synergism

There is much variation in infectious consequences after the introduction of bacteria into the peritoneal cavity. These differences are partially attributed to the competence of patient immune defenses against infection as well as factors related to the infecting bacteria. The size of the bacterial inoculum and the number and types of bacterial species present significantly affect patient outcome. The combination of aerobic and anaerobic organisms appears to greatly increase the risk of infection. In animal studies, combinations of aerobic and anaerobic bacteria were much more lethal than infections caused by the aerobes or anaerobes alone. Altemeier[14] noted a direct correlation between peri-

TABLE 107.3. PATHOGENS ISOLATED FROM 900 PATIENTS WITH INTRA-ABDOMINAL INFECTIONS FROM SIX INDEPENDENT STUDIES

Aerobic Bacteria	Percent of Patients	Anaerobic Bacteria	Percent of Patients
E. coli	51	*Bacteroides* sp.	72
Klebsiella sp.	14	Fusobacteria	7
Enterobacter sp.	6	Veillonela	2
Proteus sp.	16	Propionbacteria	5
Pseudomonas sp.	7	Clostridiae	23
Streptococci	12	Peptostreptococci	13
Enterococci	17	Peptococci	8
Staphylococci	5	Others	21
Others	8		

(Reprinted from Wittmar DH. Intra-Abdominal Infections: Pathophysiology and Treatment. New York, Marcel Dekker, 1991, p 69, by courtesy of Marcel Dekker Inc.)

tonitis mortality rates and the number of bacterial species cultivated from peritoneal fluid.

In intra-abdominal infections, facultative bacteria may provide an environment conducive to the growth of anaerobic bacteria.[15] Although many bacteria isolated in mixed infections are nonpathogenic by themselves, their presence may be essential for the pathogenicity of the bacterial mixture. The role of facultative bacteria in mixed infections may include (1) promotion of an appropriate environment for anaerobic growth through oxygen consumption, (2) production of nutrients necessary for anaerobes, or (3) production of extracellular enzymes that promote tissue invasion by anaerobes.

Animal models of intra-abdominal infection demonstrate that aerobic and anaerobic bacteria are important participants in abscess formation. In one series of experiments, gelatin capsules containing a mixture of 22 aerobic and anaerobic bacteria were implanted intraperitoneally into rats.[15] After implantation of the capsules, a two-stage disease process was apparent. During the first 5 days, acute generalized peritonitis was observed and the mortality rate was 39%. After 5 days, mortality from intra-abdominal infection was not observed; however, almost all surviving animals had intra-abdominal abscesses when sacrificed at 2 weeks. During the peritonitis stages, *E. coli* was noted in the bloodstream of most animals, and *E. coli, B. fragilis,* and enterococci were isolated from peritoneal exudates. Bacteremia could not be demonstrated during the abscess stage, but abscesses were found to contain predominantly anaerobic bacteria (*B. fragilis* and *Fusobacterium varium*). *Escherichia coli* and enterococcus were also isolated from the abscess cavity.

In further experiments, defined inocula of *E. coli,* enterococci, and *B. fragilis* were placed in the gelatin capsule implants alone or in varying combinations.[15] *Escherichia coli* was shown to produce peritonitis reliably in a significant percentage of animals whether or not it was introduced in combination with the other bacteria, and *B. fragilis* reliably produced abscesses, whether or not it was given in combination with other bacteria. The combination of *E. coli* with *B. fragilis* resulted in a 65% early mortality and abscesses in 100% of survivors. Enterococci or *F. varium* introduced alone did not result in mortality or abscesses.

These experiments support the concept that aerobic enteric bacteria and anaerobic bacteria are pathogens in intra-abdominal infection. Aerobic bacteria, particularly *E. coli,* appear responsible for the early mortality from peritonitis, whereas anaerobic bacteria are major pathogens in abscesses, with *B. fragilis* predominating. The role of enterococcus as a pathogen was not clear, because it failed to produce peritonitis or abscesses when given alone, but it may still participate in infectious processes by creating an environment favorable to other pathogens. The extension of this model is relatively limited because it simulates untreated intra-abdominal infection after free perforation of the colon.

Enterococcus can be isolated from many intra-abdominal infections in humans, but its role as a pathogen is not clear.[16] Antimicrobial regimens that are not effective against enterococcus *in vitro* have been successful in treating intra-abdominal infections. Antibiotics ineffective against enterococcus *in vitro,* such as cephalosporins, have been successfully used alone to treat intra-abdominal infections. Others have noted that enterococcal infection occurs in the presence of factors indicating failure of the host's defenses (e.g., immunocompromised patients).

Clinical Presentation

Intra-abdominal infections have a wide spectrum of manifestations, often depending on the specific disease process, its location and the magnitude of bacterial contamination, and concurrent host factors. Peritonitis is usually easily recognized but intra-abdominal abscesses may often continue for considerable periods of time, either going unrecognized or attributed to an unrelated disease process.

Generalized bacterial peritonitis usually commands the immediate attention of the physician, because the patient most often presents in acute distress. The patient lies still, usually on his or her back, possibly with hips slightly flexed. Any movement of the patient, including deep breaths, worsens the generalized abdominal pain, so the patient exhibits voluntary guarding of the abdomen and respirations are shallow and frequent. There is generalized abdominal tenderness on examination and after a short period of time the abdominal muscles become rigid, a product of involuntary guarding; this is called a "board-like abdomen." Bowel sounds are at first faint, then become absent as peristalsis ceases and abdominal distention ensues. Sometimes the patient has nausea often accompanied by vomiting. The secretion of serous fluid into the peritoneal cavity causes the vascular volume to contract. This, as well as the physiologic response to stress, causes a reflex tachycardia. Initially the patient's temperature is normal but increases to 100–102°F within the first few hours and rises to 103°F within 6–8 hours. Because of the fluid loss into the peritoneum and vomiting, the patient may appear dehydrated, and a decreased urine output is noted.

If peritonitis continues untreated the patient may go into hypovolemic shock from fluid loss into the peritoneum. This may be accompanied by generalized sepsis because the inflamed peritoneum absorbs bacteria and toxins from the suppurative process into mesenteric blood vessels. Dehydration with hypovolemic shock is the major factor for mortality in the early stage of peritonitis.

Laboratory evaluations usually demonstrate leukocytosis (15,000–20,000 WBC/mm^3), with neutrophils predominating and an elevated count of immature neutrophils (bands). The hematocrit and the blood urea nitrogen may be elevated because of the dehydration. Early after the insult the patient is usually alkalotic because of hyperventilation and vomiting. As the process progresses the patient may become acidotic from hypovolemia or presence of devitalized tissue, which leads to anaerobic metabolism. At this stage serum lactic acid will probably be elevated. Abdominal radiographs may be useful, as free air in the abdomen (indicating intestinal perforation) or distention of the small or large bowel is often evident.

The presentation of primary peritonitis can be quite different from that of secondary peritonitis. Primary peritonitis can develop over a period of days to weeks, evident as an acute febrile illness. Usually the patient has nausea, vomiting (sometimes with diarrhea), abdominal tenderness, and hypoactive bowel sounds although the abdominal signs are variable. The patient's temperature or WBC count may be only mildly elevated. The cirrhotic patient may have worsening encephalopathy.

Patients with peritonitis related to chronic peritoneal dialysis usually have abdominal pain and tenderness, possibly with nausea and vomiting, but fever is not a consistent finding. In these patients a cloudy dialysate drainage is often noted as a first sign of peritonitis indicating the presence of bacteria and inflammatory cells.

With primary peritonitis, routine evaluative procedures should be performed (e.g., serum chemistries, complete blood count, abdominal radiographs, blood cultures), and, if possible, ascitic fluid collected by paracentesis or peritoneal dialysate should be examined. In the presence of peritonitis, ascitic fluid usually contains greater than 300 leukocytes/mm^3 and bacteria may be evident on Gram stain of a centrifuged specimen; however, in 60–80% of patients with cirrhotic ascites, the Gram stain is negative.

Intra-abdominal abscesses pose a more difficult diagnostic challenge because the symptoms are often neither specific nor dramatic. The patient may complain of abdominal pain or discomfort but these symptoms are not reliable. Fever is usually present; often it is low grade, but it can have a high, spiking pattern. The patient may have paralytic ileus and abdominal distention. The abdominal examination is unreliable; tenderness and pain may be present, and a mass may be palpated.

Peritonitis may result from an abscess that ruptures, spreading bacteria and toxins throughout the peritoneum. In other patients, the entry of bacterial toxins into the systemic circulation from the abscess may lead to progressive multisystem organ failure (renal, hepatic, or cardiac).

Laboratory studies are generally not helpful in the diagnosis of intra-abdominal abscess although most patients will have leukocytosis. Some patients may have positive blood cultures, whereas others, particularly diabetics, may have hyperglycemia. The finding of *Bacteroides* or any two enteric bacteria in the bloodstream is often indicative of an intra-abdominal infectious process.

A number of radiographic methods are used to make the diagnosis of an intra-abdominal abscess. Plain radiographs may show air–fluid levels or may demonstrate the shift of normal intra-abdominal contents by the abscess mass. Gastrointestinal contrast studies may also demonstrate this displacement of abdominal structures. Both of these modalities provide indirect evidence of the abscess presence but are not generally helpful in precisely locating the abscess. Ultrasound is frequently the first radiographic modality used when the presence of an intra-abdominal abscess is suspected. It offers the advantage of portability, so the procedure may be done at the bedside. This is particularly helpful in the patient in the intensive care unit. The other advantage of this procedure is that it involves no radiation exposure. Limitations of ultrasound include the fact that it is often difficult to distinguish between an early abscess and loops of the intestine. In some patients, particularly the obese, it is technically impossible to perform the exam.[17] Computed tomography (CT) scan is frequently used to evaluate the abdomen for the presence of an abscess. Oral radiocontrast agents may be given to allow differentiation of the abscess from the bowel. Intravenous radiocontrast agents will be taken up preferentially in the wall of the abscess creating a unique radiographic appearance. Magnetic resonance imaging might be used to locate some intra-abdominal abscesses, particularly in the retroperitoneum but this modality offers no advantage when compared to CT scan and is infrequently used. The final diagnostic imaging modality is radioactive isotope imaging. Specific techniques include the use of gallium-67 citrate and indium-111-labeled leukocytes.[18] These studies require a long period of imaging and are not routinely employed.

Intra-abdominal infection caused by disease processes at specific sites often produces characteristic manifestations that are helpful in diagnosis. For example, a patient with diverticulitis may exhibit stabbing left lower quadrant abdominal pain and constipation. Fever and leukocytosis are often present and a tender mass is sometimes palpable. With appendicitis, the findings may be inconsistent but many patients have a sudden onset of periumbilical or epigastric pain, which is usually colicky and shifts to the right lower quadrant. The location of pain may vary, as the appendix can be in many locations in the abdomen. A mass may be palpable on abdominal or rectal examination. The patient's temperature is generally mildly elevated early and then increases. If perforation and diffuse peritonitis were to occur, the manifestations just described would apply. More frequently, however, appendiceal perforation results in a local abscess.

Abscesses in specific locations may produce clues to their existence. Pelvic abscesses may be palpable by pelvic examination. A subdiaphragmatic abscess may result in pleural effusion or dyspnea. Retroperitoneal abscesses may cause lumbar or psoas muscle spasm resulting in lower back pain and may cause the patient to flex the legs at the hip.

Intra-abdominal infections associated with the biliary tract may coincide with symptoms of acute cholecystitis. These include right upper quadrant abdominal pain and tenderness, sometimes radiating to the back, nausea and vomiting, and often a low-grade fever and leukocytosis. If there are stones present in the common bile duct, the patient is usually jaundiced and serum alkaline phosphatase may be elevated. In the infrequent but serious event of infected bile with common bile duct obstruction (cholangitis), the patient will usually have a high spiking fever, chills, and jaundice.

The presentation and outcome of any intra-abdominal infection are significantly influenced by the status of the patient. Those who are malnourished, have undergone multiple traumatic injuries, or are at the extremes of age are more likely to succumb to intra-abdominal infection or require an extended period for recovery. In addition to these factors, those with associated diseases such as diabetes mellitus, malignancies, renal failure, and cirrhosis are recognized to be immunocompromised and at greater risk for most infectious processes, including intra-abdominal infections. Other risk factors often related to intra-abdominal infection are the use of corticosteroids, particularly in patients with Crohn's disease, and radiation therapy for tumors. Also, use of antimicrobial agents may prevent the prompt diagnosis of abscesses, particularly subphrenic. In some instances acute intra-abdominal infectious processes may become chronic with the initiation of antimicrobial agents.

TREATMENT

GENERAL APPROACH

The treatment of intra-abdominal infection most often requires the coordinated use of a combination of modalities. The three major modalities are (1) prompt drainage, (2) support of vital functions, and (3) appropriate antimicrobial therapy.

The goals of treatment are the correction of intra-abdominal disease processes or injuries that have caused infection and the drainage of collections of purulent material (e.g., abscess). Antimicrobials are an important adjunct to surgical procedures in the treatment of intra-abdominal infections; however, the use of antimicrobial agents without surgical intervention is usually inadequate. For some specific situations (e.g., most cases of primary peritonitis), drainage procedures may not be required, and antimicrobial agents become the mainstay of therapy.

In the early phase of serious intra-abdominal infections much attention should be paid to maintenance of body organ system functions. With generalized peritonitis, large volumes of intravenous fluids are required to restore vascular volume and improve cardiovascular function. Adequate urine output should be maintained to ensure proper renal function. This is done by correcting hypovolemia and restoring cardiac output. The use of diuretics to improve urine output once these factors are corrected is controversial because they may worsen fluid deficits. Respiratory function can be assisted by a variety of methods including ventilatory support in severely ill patients. Often, the critically ill patient with intra-abdominal infection will require intensive care monitoring, particularly if there is cardiovascular or respiratory instability. Also, isolation procedures may be required if the infectious process poses a threat to other hospitalized patients.

An additional important component of therapy is parenteral nutrition. Intra-abdominal infections often directly involve the gastrointestinal tract or disrupt its function (i.e., paralytic ileus). The return of gastrointestinal motility may take days, weeks, and occasionally months. In the interim, parenteral nutrition allows patient recovery and wound healing while maintaining nutritional status.

DRAINAGE PROCEDURES

Primary peritonitis is treated with antimicrobials and does not require drainage. Secondary peritonitis requires surgical correction of the underlying pathology. The drainage of the purulent material is the critical element in the management of an intra-abdominal abscess. Without adequate drainage of the abscess, antimicrobial therapy and fluid resuscitation can be expected to fail.

Secondary peritonitis is treated surgically. At the time of laparotomy, attempts are made to correct the cause of the peritonitis. This may include patching a perforated ulcer with omentum, resection of a segment of perforated colon, or resection of a portion of gangrenous small intestine. The goal of all of these procedures is to remove the inflamed or gangrenous viscous and prevent further bacterial contamination. The presence of active inflammation increases the difficulty of the surgical procedure. This results in a higher morbidity and mortality rate than if the same procedures were performed in an elective setting without inflammation. Additionally, the presence of active inflammation may make it technically impossible to perform the definitive surgical procedure. In this situation, attempts are made to provide drainage of the infected or gangrenous structures. An example of this situation is empyema of the gallbladder. If it is unsafe or impossible to perform the cholecystectomy, then a tube is placed into the gallbladder. This procedure, cholecystostomy, provides for drainage of the purulent material present in the gallbladder. The gallbladder would then be removed at a subsequent operation. If an intra-abdominal abscess, separate from any intra-abdominal organ, is discovered during an exploratory laparotomy then it may be debrided, excised, or drained. If the intra-abdominal abscess involves an abdominal structure, then a resection of part or all of that organ may be required. An example of this situation is an abscess associated with diverticular disease of the colon. Management may include drainage of the abscess and resection of the involved colon. All foreign material, necrotic tissue, feces, blood, or pus should be removed from the operative field and the peritoneum should be copiously irrigated with 0.9% sodium chloride to decrease the concentrations of bacteria or other noxious substances.

Once an abscess is located, it must be drained. Traditionally, this would have been performed surgically. More recently, abscesses have been drained percutaneously using specially designed catheters.[19] The drainage is guided using ultrasound or computerized tomography. The initial studies using this technology were limited to single abscesses that were easily accessible and did not communicate with enteric structures. Based on good results with this group of patients, this technique has been applied to more complex abscesses or those that do communicate with enteric structures. The management of intra-abdominal abscess with percutaneous catheter drainage may represent the definitive procedure or the patient may require a subsequent procedure to treat the underlying conditions. In this latter circumstance, a significant advantage is obtained by first draining the abscess percutaneously. This allows the surgical procedure to be performed on a patient who is no longer suffering the systemic manifestations of uncontrolled infections.

A number of drainage techniques have been recently described using endoscopy and laparoscopy. These "minimal access techniques" may offer some advantages when compared to traditional surgery but will probably be used less often than radiologic assisted percutaneous drainage techniques.

The most valuable microbiologic information may be obtained at the time of operation or percutaneous abscess drainage. If pus or fluids are found that are believed infected, it is best to aspirate 2–3 mL into a syringe, remove any air, and tightly cap the syringe. The specimen should be taken promptly to the microbiology lab where a Gram stain should be performed immediately and cultures prepared for identification of aerobic bacteria and anaerobic bacteria. If there is no fluid available for collection, culture swab devices may be applied to the infected area. A swab transported under anaerobic conditions is required, and it should be analyzed as just described.

FLUID THERAPY

Aggressive fluid repletion and management are required for successful treatment of intra-abdominal infections. Fluid therapy is instituted for the purposes of achieving or maintaining proper intravascular volumes and adequate urine output and correcting acidosis. Intravascular volume is often decreased in patients with severe intra-abdominal infections because fluids accumulate in the abdomen; they collect in a "third space" at the expense of the plasma volume. Loss of fluid through vomiting, diarrhea, or a nasogastric suction tube contributes to dehydration. Intravascular volume can be assessed by blood pressure and heart rate but more accurately by measurement of central venous pressure or pulmonary capillary wedge pressure. When a contracted vascular volume is accompanied by hemorrhage, the hematocrit initially is about normal, but if there is no hemorrhage the hematocrit is usually elevated as an indication of hemoconcentration. Urine output should be continuously monitored in severely ill patients by use of a transurethral bladder catheter, quantitated hourly, and it should equal or exceed 1 mL/kg body weight per hour.

In patients with peritonitis, hypovolemia is often accompanied by acidosis, so a reasonable intravenous fluid would be lactated Ringer's, which contains the bicarbonate precursor, lactate, as well as sodium, potassium, and calcium. In the initial hour of treatment a large volume of solution may need to be administered to restore intravascular volume. Although this volume may frequently approach 4 L, much more fluid may be required to restore vital functions. For a few hours thereafter fluids may be required at a rate of 1 L/h. Maintenance fluids should be instituted (after intravascular volume is restored) with 0.9% sodium chloride and potassium chloride (20 mEq/L) or 5% dextrose and 0.45% sodium chloride with potassium chloride (20 mEq/L). The administration rate should be based on estimated daily fluid loss through urine and nasogastric suction, including 0.5–1.0 L for insensible fluid loss. Potassium would not routinely be included if the patient is hyperkalemic or has renal failure.

In patients with significant blood loss, blood should be given. This is generally in the form of packed red blood cells. The criteria for blood transfusion are controversial but a hematocrit of 25% is generally accepted. In the individual patient, the decision is often determined by the overall clinical status and the ability of the patient to compensate for the reduction in oxygen-carrying capacity associated with an acute anemia. Additional blood component therapy with clotting factors or platelets is also based on the needs of the individual patient. Aggressive fluid therapy must often be continued in the postoperative period as fluid will continue to sequester into the peritoneal cavity causing hypovolemia.

ANTIMICROBIAL THERAPY

The approach to antimicrobial therapy of intra-abdominal infection, in particular, the choice of antimicrobials used and the route of administration, has been the subject of much debate in recent years. Whatever agents are chosen and by whatever route they are administered, the goals of antimicrobial therapy remain the same: (1) to control bacteremia and the establishment of metastatic foci of infection, (2) to reduce suppurative complications after bacterial contamination, and (3) to prevent local spread of existing infection. Once suppuration has occurred (e.g., an abscess has formed), a cure by antibiotic alone is very difficult to achieve; antimicrobials may serve to improve the results that would have been attained with surgery alone.

An empiric antimicrobial regimen should be started as soon as the presence of intra-abdominal infection is suspected. Therefore, they are usually begun before identification of infecting bacteria is complete. Therapy must be initiated based on the likely pathogens. Predominant pathogens, as discussed in the previous section, vary depending on the site of intra-abdominal infection and the underlying disease process. Likely pathogens, those against which antimicrobial agents should be directed, are listed in Table 107.4.

The importance of providing antimicrobial coverage for aerobic and anaerobic pathogens was demonstrated with the previously described rat model of intra-abdominal contamination.[15] When gentamicin, an agent with excellent activity against aerobic gram-negative bacilli but no activity against anaerobic bacteria, was administered alone to the animals, most of the peritonitis was prevented and the mortality rate was reduced from 40% to 4%; however, most surviving animals still had intra-abdominal abscesses when sacrificed at 12 days. When clindamycin, an agent with excellent activity against anaerobic bacteria but no activity against aerobic gram-negative bacilli, was administered alone, the frequency of peritonitis and mortality remained about 40% while abscess formation was prevented in most survivors. As expected, when gentamicin and clindamycin were administered concurrently, mortality rates (from peritonitis) and abscess formation were both significantly reduced.

Using this same rat model, selected single-drug therapies, such as carbenicillin, moxalactam, cefoxitin, and cefotaxime, have also resulted in a significant reduction in the frequency of peritonitis *and* intra-abdominal abscesses.[20] Antimicrobial agents with good activity against aerobic gram-negative, enteric bacilli successfully reduced mortality rates from peritonitis, while agents active against *B. fragilis* and other anaerobes reduced the incidence of intra-abdominal abscesses.

Clinical Assessment

Many studies have been conducted evaluating or comparing the effectiveness of antimicrobials for treatment of intra-abdominal infections. Substantial differences in patient outcomes from treatment with a variety of agents have not been demonstrated. Solomkin et al.[21] noted that trials of antimicrobial therapy for intra-abdominal infection often had serious defects in design, and these defects usually prevented the detection of differences between agents.

In recent years, single agents (most often second-generation cephalosporins, extended-spectrum penicillins, or carbapenems) have been compared with combination drug regimens containing aminoglycosides. In almost all trials, the single-agent regimen has fared as well as the combination therapy; however, many of these trials included patients at relatively low risk. Often, the definition of intra-abdominal infection was extended to include patients with acute intra-abdominal bacterial contamination, such as after penetrating traumatic injuries, or "peritonitis" was extended to include patients with cholecystitis and diverticulitis. In fact, many of the reported trials with intra-abdominal infections were primarily conducted with patients who had bacterial contamination of the abdomen as a result of traumatic injuries or appendicitis. If most patients with traumatic abdominal injury are treated a few hours after injury, bacterial infection (peritonitis or abscess) is not established and

TABLE 107.4. LIKELY INTRA-ABDOMINAL PATHOGENS

Type of Infection	Aerobes	Anaerobes
Primary Bacterial Peritonitis		
Children (spontaneous)	Pneumococci, group A *Streptococcus*	—
Cirrhosis	*E. coli, Klebsiella,* pneumococci (many others)	—
Peritoneal dialysis	*Staphylococcus, Streptococcus*	—
Secondary Bacterial Peritonitis		
Gastroduodenal	*Streptococcus, E. coli*	
Biliary tract	*E. coli, Klebsiella,* enterococci	*Clostridium* or *Bacteroides* (infrequent)
Small or large bowel	*E. coli, Klebsiella,* spp., *Proteus* spp.	*Bacteroides fragilis* and other *Bacteroides, Clostridium*
Appendicitis	*E. coli, Pseudomonas*	*Bacteroides* spp.
Abscesses	*E. coli, Klebsiella,* enterococci	*B. fragilis* and other *Bacteroides, Clostridium,* anaerobic cocci
Liver	*E. coli, Klebsiella,* enterococci, staphylococci, amoeba	*Bacteroides* (infrequent)
Spleen	*Staphylococcus, Streptococcus*	

most infectious complications are avoided. In this group, antimicrobial agents are used to prevent infection rather than treat it.

Comparative trials of antimicrobials in patients who have sustained intraperitoneal bacterial contamination from traumatic injuries have most often included a combination of aminoglycoside with clindamycin or metronidazole versus a cephalosporin or extended-spectrum penicillin. The overwhelming weight of evidence supports that single-agent regimens with β-lactams that have antianaerobic activity perform as well as combination regimens with aminoglycosides plus clindamycin or metronidazole.[22]

With penetrating abdominal trauma, some investigators have examined key questions related to antimicrobials used to prevent infection, namely, the necessary duration and timing of antimicrobial therapy. Oresovich et al.[23] and Stone et al.[24] demonstrated that a short course of antimicrobial agents (12–24 hours) was as valuable in preventing infection after abdominal trauma as a course lasting 5–7 days.

A number of studies have been conducted in patients with established intra-abdominal infections. A compilation of the more notable studies is provided in Table 107.5. Generally, these studies do not demonstrate clinical differences between agents, although it is doubtful that many of the studies would have detected clinically significant differences in patient outcome, because the numbers of patients studied were often too few.

Comparative trials of antimicrobials for intra-abdominal infection have either compared one of the components of two combination drug regimens or compared single-drug regimens with combination regimens. In a few trials the anaerobic components of combination drug regimens have been compared.[31–33] These studies indicate that either clindamycin or metronidazole is effective against anaerobic bacteria involved in intra-abdominal infections.

Other studies have compared single-agent regimens (using cephalosporins, carbapenems, or penicillins) with combination regimens, and in these studies the β-lactams have produced results similar to those for the combination regimens. In a recent trial of 162 patients, imipenem/cilistatin was demonstrated to be more effective than the combination of tobramycin and clindamycin for intra-abdominal infections when acute trauma was excluded.[29]

Intra-abdominal infection presents in many different ways and with a wide spectrum of severity. The regimen employed and duration of treatment depend on the specific clinical circumstances (i.e., the nature of the underlying disease process and the condition of the patient). Compromised patients require more aggressive therapies than otherwise healthy patients who experience the same intra-abdominal infection.

Recommendations

For most intra-abdominal infections, the antimicrobial regimen should be effective against both aerobic and anaerobic bacteria.[34] Although it is impossible to provide antimicrobial activity against every possible pathogen, agents with activity against enteric gram-negative bacilli, such as *E. coli* and *Klebsiella,* and anaerobes such as *B. fragilis* and *Clostridia* spp., should be administered. If most of the organisms can be eliminated, the synergistic effect may be removed and the patient's defenses may be able to eradicate the remaining organisms.

Table 107.6 presents recommended and alternative regimens for selected situations. These are general guidelines, not rules, because there are many factors that cannot be incorporated into such a table.

Most patients with severe intra-abdominal infections (where there is generalized peritonitis or septic shock or where the patient has a high fever and shaking chills) should be placed on an aminoglycoside in combination with an antianaerobic agent or an agent demonstrated to be effective in this category of patients (e.g., imipenem/cilistatin). Gen-

TABLE 107.5. SOME COMPARATIVE STUDIES OF INTRA-ABDOMINAL INFECTION

Investigators	Agent(s) Tested	Number of Patients Studied	Percent of Patients with Satisfactory Outcome
Stone et al., 1982[25]	Cefotaxime	56	82
	Clindamycin/gentamicin	56	82
Malangoni et al., 1985[26]	Cefoxitin	59	83
	Tobramycin/clindamycin	53	79
Kager et al., 1986[27]	Ampicillin/sulbactam	46	87
	Clindamycin/gentamicin	37	97
Berne et al., 1987[28]	Aztreonam/clindamycin	56	95
	Gentamicin/clindamycin	28	100
Solomkin et al., 1990[29]	Imipenem/cilistatin	81	83
	Tobramycin/clindamycin	81	70
Brismar et al., 1992[30]	Imipenem/cilistatin	58	69
	Piperacillin/tazobactam	55	93

TABLE 107.6. RECOMMENDATIONS FOR INITIAL ANTIMICROBIAL AGENTS FOR INTRA-ABDOMINAL INFECTIONS

Primary Bacterial Peritonitis		
Cirrhosis	Aminoglycoside plus penicillin or antistaphylococcal cephalosporin	1. Add clindamycin or metronidazole if anaerobes are suspected 2. Third-generation cephalosporins, extended-spectrum penicillins, aztreonam, and imipenem as alternatives
Peritoneal dialysis	Regimen based on organism isolated 1. *Staphylococcus:* penicillinase-resistant penicillin or first-generation cephalosporin 2. *Streptococcus:* penicillin G 3. Aerobic gram-negative bacilli: aminoglycoside plus an antipseudomonal penicillin or ceftazidime 4. *Pseudomonas aeruginosa:* aminoglycoside plus antipseudomonal penicillin or ceftazidime	1. Alternative for resistant staphylococci is vancomycin 2. Alternative for *Streptococcus* is a first-generation cephalosporin 3. Alternatives for gram-negative bacilli are third-generation cephalosporins, aztreonam, and extended-spectrum penicillins with β-lactamase inhibitors
Secondary Bacterial Peritonitis		
Perforated peptic ulcer	First-generation cephalosporins	1. Antianaerobic cephalosporins[a] 2. Possibly add aminoglycoside if patient condition is poor
Other	Aminoglycoside with clindamycin or metronidazole	1. Add ampicillin if patient is immunocompromised or if biliary tract origin of infection 2. Aztreonam with clindamycin or imipenem/cilistatin alone 3. Antianaerobic cephalosporins,[a] extended-spectrum penicillins with β-lactamase inhibitor
Abscess		
General	Aminoglycoside with clindamycin or metronidazole	1. Aztreonam with clindamycin, imipenem alone, or extended-spectrum penicillins with β-lactamase inhibitor, as alternatives
Liver	As above but add a first-generation cephalosporin	2. Use metronidazole if amoebic liver abscess is suspected
Spleen	Aminoglycoside plus penicillinase-resistant penicillin	3. Alternatives for penicillinase-resistant penicillin are first-generation cephalosporins or vancomycin
Appendicitis		
Normal or inflamed	Antianaerobic cephalosporins[a] (discontinued immediately postoperation)	1. Aminoglycoside with clindamycin or metronidazole
Gangrenous or perforated	Aminoglycoside with clindamycin or metronidazole	1. Aztreonam with clindamycin, or imipenem alone 2. Antianaerobic cephalosporins[a] or extended-spectrum penicillins with β-lactamase inhibitor
Acute Cholecystitis	First-generation cephalosporin	Aminoglycoside plus ampicillin if severe infection
Cholangitis	Aminoglycoside with ampicillin with or without clindamycin or metronidazole	Use vancomycin for ampicillin if patient is allergic to penicillin
Acute Contamination from Abdominal Trauma	Antianaerobic cephalosporinsa or extended-spectrum penicillins	Aminoglycoside with one of the following: clindamycin, metronidazole, or antianaerobic cephalosporinsa

[a]Cefoxitin, cefotetan, ceftizoxime, and cefmetazole.

tamicin is the aminoglycoside of choice, based on its lower cost. Other aminoglycosides such as tobramycin, amikacin, and netilmicin have no advantages in intra-abdominal infections and are generally not drugs of first choice. Aztreonam may be used as an alternative to aminoglycosides.

The dosage for aminoglycosides should be adjusted on the basis of a patient's age, weight, and renal function. Because the enteric gram-negative bacilli are usually very susceptible to aminoglycosides and because aminoglycosides are well distributed into peritoneal fluid,[35] high serum aminoglycoside concentrations are generally not required. Unless relatively resistant bacteria are suspected, a gentamicin or tobramycin peak concentration of 5–6 μg/mL will usually be effective. Also, trough concentrations should not be allowed to decrease below 1 μg/mL for a substantial portion of the dosage interval. To achieve these serum concentrations, gentamicin or tobramycin dosage may range from 1–3 mg/kg per dose given as often as every 6 hours, or as infrequently as every 48 hours if the patient has renal failure. Once-daily aminoglycoside administration appears to be equivalent to multiple daily dosing.

When used for intra-abdominal infection, aminoglycosides should be combined with agents that are effective against the majority of *B. fragilis.* Clindamycin or metronidazole would be the agents of first choice but others such as antianaerobic cephalosporins (cefoxitin, cefotetan, ceftizoxime, or cefmetazole), piperacillin, mezlocillin, combinations of extended-spectrum penicillins with β-lactamase inhibitors, and even chloramphenicol would be suitable alternatives. Clindamycin should be administered intravenously in a dosage of 600 or 900 mg every 8 hours. Patients receiving multiple, broad-spectrum antimicrobial agents, particularly those who are immunocompromised, should receive an oral antifungal agent for prevention of fungal overgrowth in the mouth and gastrointestinal tract. The benefits of systemic antifungal prophylaxis (e.g., with fluconazole) have not been established and should not routinely be used.

With intra-abdominal contamination from the upper gastrointestinal tract (e.g., perforation of a peptic ulcer or biliary tract disease), *B. fragilis* is an uncommon pathogen and other agents may therefore be substituted for clindamycin or metronidazole. Alternatives would include ampicillin, penicillin, or first-generation cephalosporins.

Most studies of intra-abdominal infection have included agents with activity against both colonic aerobes and anaerobes and, presently, most clinicians would use an antimicrobial regimen that is active against both groups of bacteria. Because *B. fragilis* and *Clostridia* are regularly cultured from intra-abdominal infections, isolated in the bloodstream, and believed to be important participants in mixed bacterial infections, antimicrobial agents effective against them are usually recommended.

Ampicillin may be added to assure antimicrobial coverage for enterococci although this is controversial.[16] Regimens without activity against enterococci (e.g., gentamicin with clindamycin or cephalosporins) are generally effective in treating these infections; however, there are numerous reports of enterococcal superinfection in immunocompromised patients, particularly after cephalosporin use. Studies of human intra-abdominal infections have shown enterococci to be the most common gram-positive isolate.[36]

The failure of host defenses may be a critical factor in the pathogenicity of enterococci. In immunocompromised patients or in patients with valvular heart disease or a prosthetic heart valve,[37] there is more justification to provide specific antimicrobial activity against enterococci. Ampicillin or other penicillins that are active against enterococci (i.e., penicillin, piperacillin, mezlocillin) should be used in patients at high risk, patients with persistent or recurrent intra-abdominal infection, patients in shock, or patients who are immunosuppressed, such as after organ transplantation. Ampicillin remains the drug of choice for this purpose because it is most active *in vitro* against enterococci and is relatively inexpensive. Vancomycin is active against most enterococci; however, resistance is increasing and this agent should be reserved for established infections.

With peritonitis that occurs from chronic peritoneal dialysis, the antimicrobial regimen used should be tailored to the isolated organism. The selection of a specific agent or combination should be based on culture and susceptibility data. If microbiologic data are unavailable, empiric therapy with a first-generation cephalosporin plus an aminoglycoside is recommended. In less severe infections, a first-generation cephalosporin alone given intraperitoneally may suffice. Infection with staphylococci may be treated with a penicillinase-resistant penicillin (methicillin, nafcillin, oxacillin), first-generation cephalosporins, or vancomycin if the patient is allergic to penicillin or the isolate is resistant to methicillin. For streptococcal infections, penicillin or ampicillin would be preferable to penicillinase-resistant penicillins. Most aerobic gram-negative bacilli may be effectively treated with an aminoglycoside. For infections caused by *P. aeruginosa,* an antipseudomonal penicillin (ticarcillin, piperacillin, mezlocillin, or azlocillin) or ceftazidime may be added.

Patients with peritonitis who are undergoing chronic peritoneal dialysis (CPD) may receive parenteral as well as intraperitoneal antimicrobial agents. Intraperitoneal antimicrobial agents alone are often sufficient, unless severe infection is present. A number of agents may be instilled through peritoneal catheters. Recommended concentrations of antimicrobial agents for intraperitoneal irrigation solutions are 8 mg/L for gentamicin and tobramycin, 1–3 mg/L for clindamycin, 50,000 U/L for penicillin G, 125 mg/L for cephalosporins, 100–150 mg/L for ticarcillin or carbenicillin, 50 mg/L for ampicillin, 100 mg/L for methicillin, 30 mg/L for vancomycin, and 3 mg/L for amphotericin B.[38]

The usual duration of therapy for peritonitis associated with CPD is 10–14 days but may extend to 3 weeks.

Antimicrobial therapy should be continued until dialysate fluid is clear, cultures are negative for 2–3 days, and the patient is asymptomatic. When parenteral agents are administered, the initial dose would be the same as that for patients with normal renal function, while subsequent doses should be much less or given less frequently for renally excreted agents and should account for possible loss through peritoneal dialysis. Serum concentrations should be performed for aminoglycosides and vancomycin.

After acute bacterial contamination, such as with abdominal trauma where gastrointestinal contents enter the peritoneum, combination antimicrobial regimens are not required. If the patient is seen soon after injury (within 2 hours) and surgical measures are instituted promptly, single-agent regimens such as antianaerobic cephalosporins or extended-spectrum penicillins are effective in preventing most infectious complications. It is important though that antimicrobials be begun as soon as possible after injury.

For appendicitis, the antimicrobial regimen used should depend on the appearance of the appendix at the time of operation, which may be normal, inflamed, gangrenous, or perforated. Because the condition of the appendix is unknown preoperatively, it is advisable to begin antimicrobial agents before the appendectomy is performed. Reasonable regimens would be antianaerobic cephalosporins or, if the patient is seriously ill, a combination of aminoglycoside with clindamycin or metronidazole. If at operation the appendix is found to be normal or inflamed, postoperative antimicrobials would not be required. If the appendix is gangrenous or perforated, a treatment course of 7–10 days with the agents listed in Table 107.6 would be appropriate.

The necessary duration of treatment for intra-abdominal infections is not clearly defined. Acute intra-abdominal contamination, such as after a traumatic injury, may be treated with a very short course (24 hours). For established infections (peritonitis or intra-abdominal abscess) an antimicrobial course of at least 7 days is justified. This allows eradication of bacteria that may remain in the peritoneum after a surgical procedure or bacteria that may enter the peritoneum through healing suture lines. Comparative studies examining shorter courses of therapy (i.e., 2 or 3 days) have not been conducted to verify that longer courses are essential. Under certain conditions, therapy for longer than 7 days would be justified; for example, if the patient remains febrile or is in poor general condition, when relatively resistant bacteria are isolated, or when a focus of infection in the abdomen may still be present. For some abscesses, such as pyogenic liver abscess, antimicrobials may be required for a month or longer.

Intraperitoneal irrigation of antimicrobial agents for treatment of intra-abdominal infection has often been studied with somewhat conflicting results.[39] Intraoperative antimicrobial irrigation has not been shown to improve patient outcomes in comparison with copious intraoperative irrigation with normal saline. Possibly the most important aspect of peritoneal irrigation is the dilutional effect on bacteria and adjuvants or substances that promote infection (i.e., intestinal contents and hemoglobin). As discussed before, investigators have shown that most systemically administered antimicrobials easily cross the peritoneal membrane so that peritoneal fluid concentrations are similar to serum.[35,40] Confined areas, such as abscess, could be expected to attain much lower antimicrobial concentrations.

Evaluation of Therapeutic Outcomes

Whichever antimicrobial regimen is chosen, the patient should be continually reassessed to determine the success or failure of therapies. The clinician should recognize that there are many reasons for poor outcome of patients with intra-abdominal infection; improper antimicrobial administration is only one. The patient may be immunocompromised, which decreases the likelihood of successful outcome with any regimen. It is impossible for antimicrobials to compensate totally for a nonfunctioning immune system. There may be surgical reasons for poor patient outcome. Failure to identify all intra-abdominal foci of infection or leaks from a gastrointestinal anastomosis may cause continued intra-abdominal infection. Even when intra-abdominal infection is controlled, accompanying organ system failure, most often renal or respiratory, but possibly hepatic or cardiac, may lead to patient demise.

The outcome from intra-abdominal infection is not determined solely by what transpires in the abdomen. Unsatisfactory outcomes in patients with intra-abdominal infections may result from complications that arise in other organ systems. A complication commonly associated with mortality after intra-abdominal infection is pneumonia.[41,42] In fact, one investigator found that the cause of death in patients with intra-abdominal infection was more likely related to the lower respiratory tract than the abdomen.[41] A recent report found that a high APACHE II score, low serum albumin, and high New York Heart Association cardiac function status were significantly and independently associated with mortality.[43]

Once antimicrobials are initiated and other important therapies described before are used, most patients should show improvement within 2–3 days. Usually, temperature will return to near normal, vital signs should stabilize, and the patient should not appear in distress with the exception of recognized discomfort and pain from incisions, drains, and nasogastric tube. At 24–48 hours, aerobic bacterial culture results should return. If a suspected pathogen is not sensitive to the antimicrobial agents being given, the regimen should be changed if the patient has not shown sufficient progress. If the isolated pathogen is extremely sensitive to one antimicrobial, and the patient is progressing well, concurrent antimicrobial therapy may often be discontinued.

With present anaerobic culturing techniques and the slow growth of these organisms, anaerobes are often not identified until 4–7 days after culture, and sensitivity information is difficult to obtain. For this reason there are usually few data with which to alter the antianaerobic component of the antimicrobial regimen. A report indicating that anaerobes were not isolated should not be the sole justification for discontinuing antianaerobic drugs, because anaerobic bacteria that were present in the infectious process may not have been properly transported to the microbiology laboratory or other problems may have led to cell death *in vitro.*

Reasons for antimicrobial failure may not always be apparent. Even when antimicrobial susceptibility tests indicate that an organism is susceptible to the antimicrobial *in vitro,* therapeutic failures may occur. Possibly there is poor penetration of the antimicrobial into the focus of infection, or, after initiation of antimicrobial therapy, bacterial resistance may develop. Also, it is possible that an antimicrobial regimen may encourage the development of infection by organisms not susceptible to the regimen being used. Superinfection in patients being treated for intra-abdominal infection is often due to *Candida,* but enterococci or opportunistic gram-negative bacilli such as *Pseudomonas* or *Serratia* may be involved.

Treatment regimens for intra-abdominal infection can be judged successful if the patient recovers from the infection without recurrent peritonitis or intra-abdominal abscess and without the need for additional antimicrobials. A regimen can be considered unsuccessful if a significant adverse drug reaction occurs, if reoperation is necessary, or if patient improvement is delayed beyond 1 or 2 weeks.

Conclusion

The term *intra-abdominal infection* refers to many widely differing processes which require varying therapeutic approaches. The general approach to this problem includes adequate resuscitation, appropriate antibiotics, drainage of abscesses, and surgical correction of the underlying problem when appropriate. The microbiology of intra-abdominal infection is complex and agents with activity against aerobic gram-negative bacilli and anaerobes (particularly *B. fragilis*) will be most effective.

The use of newly introduced antimicrobial agents alone will not dramatically improve outcome of patients with intra-abdominal infection. Perhaps the greatest potential for improving patient outcome with these infections will come from treatments that improve patient immune function as well as from improved diagnostic techniques for abscesses, more rapid bacterial identification and determination of susceptibility, and better coordination of currently available technologies and procedures.

ACKNOWLEDGMENTS

Portions of this chapter were originally published in DiPiro JT, Mansberger JA, Davis JB. Current concepts in clinical therapeutics: Intraabdominal infections. Clin Pharm 1986; 5:34–50.

References

1. Saklayen MG. CAPD peritonitis. Incidence, pathogens, diagnosis, and management. Med Clin North Am 1990;74:997–1010.
2. Finegold SM. Microflora of the gastrointestinal tract, in Wilson SE, Finegold SM, Williams RA (eds): Intraabdominal Infection. New York, McGraw-Hill, 1982, pp 1–21.
3. Ruddell WSF, Axon ATR, Findlay JM, et al. The effect of cimetidine on gastric bacterial flora. Lancet 1980;1:672–674.
4. Lou MA, Mandal AK, Alexander JL, et al. Bacteriology of the human biliary tract and duodenum. Arch Surg 1977;112:965–967.
5. Keighley MRB. Infection and the biliary tree, in Blumgart LH (ed): The Biliary Tract. New York, Churchill Livingstone, 1982, pp 219–235.
6. Lorber B, Swenson RM. The bacteriology of intra-abdominal infections. Surg Clin North Am 1975;55:1249–1355.
7. Conn HO, Fessel JM. Spontaneous bacterial peritonitis in cirrhosis: Variations on a theme. Medicine 1971;50:161–197.
8. Rubin J, Rogers WA, Taylor HM, et al. Peritonitis during continuous ambulatory peritoneal dialysis. Ann Intern Med 1980;92:7–13.
9. Altemeier WA, Culbertson WR, Fullen WD, et al. Intra-abdominal abscesses. Am J Surg 1973;125:70–79.
10. Golden GT, Shaw A. Primary peritonitis. Surg Gynecol Obstet 1972;135:513–516.
11. Hau T, Ahrenholz DH, Simmons RL. Secondary bacterial peritonitis: The biologic basis of treatment. Curr Probl Surg 1979;16:1–65.
12. Nichols RL. Empiric antibiotic therapy of intraabdominal infections. Rev Infect Dis 1983;5(suppl):590–597.
13. Sawyer RG, Rosenlof LK, Adams RB, et al. Peritonitis into the 1990's: Changing pathogens and changing strategies in the critically ill. Am Surgeon 1992;58:82–87.
14. Altemeier WA. Bacterial flora of acute perforated appendicitis with peritonitis. Ann Surg 1938;107:517–528.
15. Bartlett JG. Pathogenesis of intra-abdominal sepsis, in Wilson SE, Finegold SM, Williams RA (eds): Intra-abdominal Infection. New York, McGraw-Hill, 1982, pp 36–51.
16. Dougherty SH. Role of enterococcus in intraabdominal sepsis. Am J Surg 1984;148:308–312.
17. Gazelle GS, Mueller PR. Abdominal abscess. Imaging and intervention. Radiol Clin North Am 1994;32:913–932.
18. Fry DE. Noninvasive imaging tests in the diagnosis and treatment of intra-abdominal abscesses in the postoperative patient. Surg Clin North Am 1994;74:693–709.

19. Pruett TL, Simmons RL. Status of catheter drainage of abscesses. Surg Clin North Am 1988;68:89–105.
20. Bartlett JG, Marien GJR, Dezfulian M, et al. Relative efficacy of β-lactam antimicrobial agents in two animal models of infections involving *Bacteroides fragilis*. Rev Infect Dis 1983;5(suppl):S338–S344.
21. Solomkin JS, Meakins JL, Allo MD, et al. Antibiotic trials in intra-abdominal infections: A critical evaluation of study design and outcome reporting. Ann Surg 1984;200:29–39.
22. Hooker KD, DiPiro JT, Wynn JJ. Aminoglycoside combinations versus single β-lactams for penetrating abdominal trauma: A meta analysis. J Trauma 1991;31:1155–1160.
23. Oresovich MR, Dellinger EP, Lennard ES, et al. Duration of preventive antibiotic administration for penetrating abdominal trauma. Arch Surg 1982;117:200–205.
24. Stone HH, Haney BB, Kolb LD, et al. Prophylactic and preventive antibiotic therapy: Timing, duration and economics. Ann Surg 1979;189:691–699.
25. Stone HH, Geheber CE, Kolb LD, et al. Clinical comparison of cefotaxime versus the combination of gentamicin plus clindamycin in the treatment of peritonitis and similar polymicrobial soft-tissue surgical sepsis. Clin Ther 1981;4(suppl A):67–80.
26. Malangoni MA, Condon RE, Spiegel CA. Treatment of intra-abdominal infections is appropriate with single-agent or combination antibiotic therapy. Surgery 1985;98:648–655.
27. Kager L, Malmborg AS, Nord CE, et al. A randomized, controlled trial of ampicillin plus sulbactams vs gentamicin plus clindamycin in the treatment of intra-abdominal infections: A preliminary report. Rev Infect Dis 1986;8(suppl 5):5583–5585.
28. Berne TV, Appleman MD, Chenella FC, et al. Surgically treated gangrenous or perforated appendicitis: A comparison of aztreonam and clindamycin versus gentamicin and clindamycin. Ann Surg 1987;205:133–137.
29. Solomkin JS, Dellinger EP, Christou NV, et al. Results of a multicenter trial comparing imipenem/cilistatin to tobramycin/clindamycin for intra-abdominal infections. Ann Surg 1990;212:581–591.
30. Brismar B, Malmborg AS, Tunevall G et al. Piperacillin-tazobactam versus imipenem-cilistatin for treatment of intra-abdominal infections. Antimicrob Agents Chemother 1992;36:2766–2773.
31. Smith JA, Skidmore AG, Forward AD, et al. Prospective, randomized, double-blind comparison of metronidazole and tobramycin with clindamycin and tobramycin in the treatment of intra-abdominal sepsis. Ann Surg 1980;190:213–220.
32. Canadian Metronidazole-Clindamycin Study Group. Prospective, randomized comparison of metronidazole and clindamycin, each with gentamicin, for the treatment of serious intra-abdominal infection. Surgery 1983;93:221–229.
33. Lennard ES, Minshew BH, Dellinger EP, et al. Stratified outcome comparison of clindamycin-gentamicin vs chloramphenicol-gentamicin for treatment of intra-abdominal sepsis. Arch Surg 1985;120:889–898.
34. Bohnen JMA, Solomkin JS, Dellinger EP, Bjornson HS, Page CP. Guidelines for clinical care: Anti-infective agents for intra-abdominal infection. Arch Surg 1992;127:83–89.
35. Gerding DN, Hall WH. The penetration of antibiotics into peritoneal fluid. Bull NY Acad Med 1975;51:1016–1019.
36. Jones RC. Antibiotics in trauma. J Surg Pract 1977;26–30.
37. Barrie PS, Christou NV, Dellinger EP, et al. Pathogenicity of the enterococcus in surgical infections. Ann Surg 1990;212:155–159.
38. Levison ME, Pontzer RE. Peritonitis and other intra-abdominal infections, in Mardell GL, Douglas RG, Bennett JE (eds): Principles and Practice of Infectious Diseases. New York, John Wiley and Sons, 1985, p 488.
39. Schein M, Gecelter G, Freinkel W, et al. Peritoneal lavage in abdominal sepsis: A controlled clinical study. Arch Surg 1990;125:1132–1135.
40. Wittman DH, Schassan HH. Penetration of eight β-lactam antibiotics into peritoneal fluid. Arch Surg 1983;118:205–213.
41. Mustard RA, Bohnen JMA, Rosati C, Schouten D. Pneumonia complicating abdominal sepsis. Arch Surg 1991;126:170–175.
42. Richardson JD, DeCamp MM, Garrison RN, Fry DE. Pulmonary infection complicating intra-abdominal sepsis. Ann Surg 1982;195:732–737.
43. Christou NV, Barie PS, Dellinger EP, et al. Surgical infection society intra-abdominal infection study. Arch Surg 1993;128:193–199.

Chapter 108

Parasitic Diseases

J. V. Anandan, PharmD

Once considered "exotic," parasitic diseases are now nearer to home because of the increased mobility of large segments of the population and the speed of international travel. Environmental changes in the world have increased the incidence of parasitic diseases among the local population. The construction of the Aswan Dam and the creation of Lake Nasser resulted in increased incidence of schistosomiasis in Egypt by creating new habitats for the intermediate snail host, while the construction of the TransAmazon Highway in Brazil exposed large numbers of workers to leishmaniasis.[1,2] To appreciate the prevalence of parasitic infections one should review Table 108.1, which was adapted from World Health Organization data.[3]

This chapter covers the major parasitic diseases including protozoan diseases (amebiasis, malaria, etc.), helminthic infections (ascariasis, enterobiasis, etc.), and ectoparasitic infestations (head and body lice). Emphasis is placed on diseases more frequently seen in the United States. World distribution of parasites is dependent on the presence of suitable hosts, habitats, and environmental conditions.[3] A human parasite that does not utilize an intermediate host is likely to be found in any inhabited region of the world as long as the environmental conditions are suitable. Ascaris (the round worm) and trichuris (the whip worm) require carelessness of habits for transfer. They are limited as they require time outside the body to reach the infective stage and are exposed to heat and dryness. The distribution of the hookworm is more limited, because the free-living forms are unprotected by resistant shells or cysts. African trypanosomiasis never occurs outside the range of the tsetse flies, malaria beyond the range of the infective *Anopheles,* and schistosomiasis in the absence of a specific water snail. The prevalence of clonorchiasis (Chinese liver fluke) is an example of the impact of both environmental and geographic factors. Clonorchiasis not only requires simultaneous presence of humans, specific snail species, and certain fish, but also unsanitary conditions that make the eggs accessible to the snails, an association of the snail and fish, and the established local habit of eating raw fish. The ability of some parasites to infect hosts other than humans may perpetuate an infection, even when human habits preclude the possibility of more than occasional access to the human body. In North America, the broad tapeworm *(Diphyllobothrium latus)* would perish if not for the fact that dogs and other carnivores, such as the brown bear, serve as reservoir hosts.

TABLE 108.1. WORLDWIDE PREVALENCE OF PARASITIC INFECTIONS

Disease	Number of Infections per Year (million)
Amebiasis	400
Malaria	800
African trypanosomiasis	1
American trypanosomiasis	12
Schistosomiasis	200
Onchocerciasis	30
Filariasis	250
Ascariasis	800
Hookworm	700
Trichuriasis	500
Giardiasis	200

HOST–PARASITE RELATIONSHIP

The association of two species for the purpose of obtaining food for either one or the other is called *symbiosis. Parasitism* is defined as a symbiotic relationship in which one species, the host, is injured through the activities of the other. Through evolution, parasites have made specific morphologic adaptations. Adaptation to the host has taken a number of forms: loss of locomotor organelles in the protozoan Sporozoa; partial and complete lack of digestive systems in the trematodes and cestodes, respectively; elaboration of proteolytic enzymes to penetrate the host intestinal mucosa by *Entamoeba histolytica,* the cercariae of the blood fluke that penetrate the skin of the host by elaborate enzymes; and finally, the ability to infect an intermediate host to increase reproductive capacity as seen among the cestodes and trematodes.[1,2]

Parasites normally inflict some degree of injury to the host, the extent of which is dependent on such factors as parasite load, nutritional status, and immunologic competence of the host. *Entamoeba coli* is considered commensal because it subsists on the bacterial flora of the gut and does not cause any harm to the host. Unlike *Entamoeba coli, Fasciolopsi buski,* the giant intestinal fluke, and *Entamoeba histolytica* can produce severe local damage to the intestinal wall. *Ascaris,* the round worm, can perforate the bowel wall, cause intestinal obstruction, and invade the appendix and bile duct. Malarial parasites destroy red cells by multiplying inside them. *Diphyllobothrium latum,* or the broad fishworm, removes vitamin B_{12} from the gastrointestinal tract, resulting in megaloblastic anemia.[1,2]

PROTOZOAN DISEASES

AMEBIASIS

Because of its worldwide distribution and serious gastrointestinal manifestations, amebiasis is one of the most important parasitic diseases of humans.[2–6] The major causative organism in amebiasis is *E. histolytica,* which inhabits the colon, and must be differentiated from the smaller *E. hartmanni,* which is considered nonpathogenic.[5] It is estimated that 50 million cases of invasive disease result each year worldwide, leading to an excess of 100,000 deaths.[5] In the United States, the incidence of amebiasis is estimated at about 4% in the general population.[5] The highest incidence is found in institutionalized mentally retarded patients, sexually active homosexuals, patients with acquired immune deficiency syndrome (AIDS), the Native American population, and new immigrants from endemic areas (e.g., Mexico, India, West and South Africa, and portions of Central and South America).[4,5]

Pathology

Entamoeba histolytica invades mucosal cells of colonic epithelium, producing the classic flask-shaped ulcer in the submucosa.[4,5] The trophozoite has a cytolethal effect on cells through a toxin. If the trophozoite gets into the portal circulation, it will be carried to the liver where it produces abscess and periportal fibrosis. Amebic ulcerations can affect the perineum and genitalia, and abscesses may occur in the lung and brain.

Clinical Presentation

The most frequent clinical manifestations of the disease are gastrointestinal, with vague complaints of abdominal discomfort and malaise to severe abdominal cramps, flatulence, and bloody diarrhea with mucus (heme-positive in 100%).[4,5]

Right upper quadrant pain, hepatomegaly, and liver tenderness, with referred pain to the left or right shoulder, usually suggest an amebic liver abscess. Liver abscesses that are located in the right lobe can spread to the lungs and pleura.[4,6–9] Pericardial infection, although rare, may be associated with extension of the amebic abscess from the left lobe of the liver.[4,6–9] Erosion of liver abscesses also presents as peritonitis.[4,5]

Eosinophilia is usually absent, although mild leukocytosis is not unusual in intestinal amebiasis.[4,5] A patient with liver abscess, however, will usually present with high fever, significant leukocytosis with left shift, elevated alkaline phosphatase, and liver tenderness on palpation.[4,5]

Review of the patient's history and recent travel cannot be overemphasized. Intestinal amebiasis is diagnosed by demonstrating *E. histolytica* cysts or trophozoites in fresh stool or from a specimen obtained by sigmoidoscopy. Stool examinations should include permanent trichrome stains.[4] Three stool samples obtained 24 hours apart will produce a 80–90% yield for *E. histolytica.*[4]

When amebic liver abscess is suspected from initial physical examination and history, confirmatory diagnostic procedures will include serology and liver scans (utilizing isotopes by ultrasound or computed tomography).[4,5,8,10] In rare instances, needle aspiration of the hepatic abscess may be attempted using ultrasound guidance.[4,5,8]

Treatment

In amebiasis, the goals of therapy are initially to eradicate the parasite by use of specific amebicides and then to render supportive therapy. A number of different regimens have been suggested, depending on the category of amebiasis: asymptomatic cyst passers, intestinal amebiasis, and amebic liver abscess.[4–6] Electrolyte replacement and nutritional support are essential adjunctive treatment modalities. Large hepatic abscess or amebic pericarditis may require needle aspiration or surgery before drug therapy.[4–10] Most regimens require a combination of drugs administered concurrently or sequentially.[11]

Careful history should be taken when one of the differential diagnoses is ulcerative colitis, because corticosteroid administration has the potential to unmask amebiasis and produce toxic megacolon.[4,5]All patients diagnosed as having inflammatory bowel disease should have a serologic test for amebiasis to avoid the serious consequence that results from administration of corticosteroids.[5]

Metronidazole (Flagyl), tetracycline, dehydroemetine, and chloroquine (Aralen) are tissue-acting agents, whereas iodoquinol (Yodaxin), diloxanide furoate (Furamide), and paramomycin (Humatin) are luminal amebicides.[4–6,9,11] A tissue-acting agent may be so well absorbed that only small amounts of the drug stay in the bowel and as such may prove ineffective as a luminal agent.[4–6] A luminal-acting agent, however, may be too poorly absorbed to be effective in the tissue. In the asymtomatic cyst passer, it is necessary to eradicate the causative agent from lumen to prevent intestinal amebiasis or the development of amebic liver abscess. Drug effectiveness must be monitored by stool examination, that is, three or more negative specimens from 1–3 months after treatment.

Asymptomatic cyst passers and patients with mild intestinal amebiasis should receive one of the following luminal agents: paromomycin 25–30 mg/kg/d three times daily for 7 days or iodoquinol 650 mg three times daily for 20 days or diloxanide furoate 500 mg three times daily for 10 days. Diloxanide furoate is only available from the Centers for Disease Control and Prevention in Atlanta.[3–6,11] The pediatric dose for paromomycin is the same as in adults, while the dose of iodoquinol is 30–40 mg/kg/d in three doses for 20 days, and diloxanide furoate is 20 mg/kg/d in three doses for 10 days.[11] Paromomycin is the preferred luminal agent in pregnant patients.[4]

Patients with severe intestinal disease or liver abscess should receive metronidazole 750 mg three times daily for 10 days, followed by a course of one of the luminal agents previously indicated.[9–14] In the pediatric patient the dose of oral metronidazole is 50 mg/kg/d in divided doses to be followed by a luminal agent.[11]

Patients who are too ill to take oral metronidazole should receive the drug in equivalent doses by the intravenous route.[5] Dehydroemetine 1–1.5 mg/kg/d for 5 days has been suggested as an alternative for metronidazole.[11]

Evaluation of Therapeutic Outcomes

Followup in patients with amebiasis should include repeat stool examination, serology, colonoscopy (in colitis) or computed tomography (CT) (in liver abscess) between days 5–7, at the end of the course of therapy, and monthly for 3 months.[4,5] Most patients with either intestinal amebiasis or colitis will respond in 3–5 days with amelioration of symptoms. Patients with liver abscesses may take 7–10 days to respond; patients not responding during this period may require aspiration of abscesses or exploratory laparotomy.

Sanitation and Preventive Measures

Travelers and tourists visiting an epidemic area should avoid local tap water, ice, salad, and unpeeled fruits. Water can be disinfected by use of iodine (tincture of iodine or commercial sources: Potable Aqua tablet, Wisconsin Pharmacal; or Globaline, Wallace & Trernain) or strong chlorine (laundry bleach) solution, but boiled water is probably the safest. An alternative or additional measure may be to carry a portable water purifier (Walbro Water Purifier). Because food handlers in Asia and Latin America may be a source of amebiasis, travelers should avoid eating at food stalls and open markets.

MALARIA

Malaria represents the most devastating disease in terms of human suffering and economic implications, affecting the largest number of people in the world, with deaths in excess of 1 million in tropical Africa.[15]

Malaria is transmitted by the bite of an infected *Anopheles* mosquito, which introduces the sporozoites (tissue parasites) of the plasmodia (i.e., *Plasmodium falciparum, P. vivax, P. malariae,* and *P. ovale*) into the bloodstream. The asexual reproduction stage develops in humans, while the sexual stage occurs in the mosquito.[16,17] The sporozoites invade parenchymal hepatocytes, multiply in stages referred to as exoerythrocytic stages, and become hepatic vegetative forms or schizonts. Schizonts rupture to release daughter cells or merozoites, which then infect erythrocytes.

Plasmodium falciparum and *P. malariae* remain in the primary exoerythrocytic stage in the liver for about 4 weeks before invading erythrocytes, while *P. vivax* and *P. ovale* can exist in the liver in the latent exoerythrocytic form for extended periods, and therefore infected subjects can experience relapses. The merozoites that invade the erythrocytes develop sequentially into ring forms, trophozoites, schizonts, and finally into merozoites, which can invade other erythrocytes, or develop into gametocytes, which undergo the sexual stage in the *Anopheles* vector. Erythrocytic forms never reinvade the liver without developing into sporozoites in the vector and, therefore, malaria infections from transfusion never result in the exoerythrocytic or "liver" form.[16,17] *Plasmodium falciparum* can result in high levels of parasitemia because of its ability to invade erythrocytes of all ages, unlike *P. vivax* and *P. ovale,* which only invade young cells.[17]

Epidemiology

The exact geographic distribution of the various species is not well documented; however, it is reported that *P. vivax* is more prevalent in India, Pakistan, Bangladesh, Sri Lanka, and Central America, while *P. falciparum* is predominantly in Africa, Haiti, and New Guinea. Both *P. falciparum* and *P. vivax* are prevalent in all of Southeast Asia, South America, the Middle East, North Africa, Ethopia, Somalia, and Sudan.[16,17] Most of the infections with *P. ovale* occur in Africa and the distribution of *P. malariae* is considered worldwide.

In the United States, most cases of malaria are reported in immigrants from endemic areas and in American travelers. Blood transfusion has also been cited as a cause of malarial infection.[17] The transmission of malaria from recent immigrants from endemic areas is a real threat because of the presence of two mosquito vectors, *Anopheles quadrimaculatus* and *A. freeborni,* in the United States.[17]

Pathology

The hallmark of the erythrocytic phase of malaria is fever; however, the reason for this is obscure.[17] The malarial paroxysm characterized by fever, chills, and rigor can cause vasodilation and orthostatic hypotension. The high fever, marked diaphoresis, and vomiting can lead to serious fluid and electrolyte abnormalities. The erythrocytic phase causes extensive hemolysis, which results in anemia and splenomegaly. The most serious complications are usually associated with *P. falciparum* infections, and include acute renal failure, pulmonary edema, thrombocytopenia, high-output heart failure, and cerebral congestion and hemorrhage.[16–25] It has been postulated that these complications are due to tissue hypoxia from anemia and alterations in the microcirculation. Hypoxia may be responsible for the loss of capillary endothelial integrity, leading to increased capillary permeability and interstitial edema. *Plasmodium malariae* has been implicated in immune-mediated glomerulonephritis and nephrotic syndrome.[17]

Clinical Presentation

The erythrocytic phase of malaria is preceded by a prodrome that includes headache, anorexia, malaise, fatigue, and myalgias. Patients may also have nonspecific complaints such as abdominal pain, chest pain, and arthralgias. The prodromal period is followed by the paroxysm, manifested as high fever, chills, and rigor.[17] The typical malarial paroxysm is usually followed by a "cold phase," severe pallor, cyanosis of the lips and nail bed, and cutis anserina ("goose flesh").[17,20] These symptoms are replaced by a "hot phase" in which the patient's fever may be between 40.5 and 41°C. Other symptoms during this phase will include warm dry skin, tachycardia, cough, severe headache, nausea, vomiting, abdominal pain, and delirium. Lactic acidosis and hypoglycemia have been reported as a complication of falciparum malaria during pregnancy.[16–23] Patients are usually asymptomatic between the malarial paroxysms.

To ensure a positive diagnosis, blood smears should be obtained every 12 to 24 hours for 3 consecutive days.[16,17] The presence of parasites in the blood 3–5 days after initiation of therapy suggests drug resistance. Although serologic tests for detection of indirect fluorescent antibodies to malaria are available, these are not useful. Recent advances for detecting malaria parasite have included *P. falciparum*-specific DNA probe after polymerase chain reaction amplification of target DNA sequences of the parasite.[16]

Treatment

In an adult, the chemoprophylaxis for all species of *Plasmodia* is chloroquine phosphate 300 mg (base) once weekly, beginning 1 week prior to departure and continued for 4 weeks after leaving an endemic area. The pediatric dose of chloroquine phosphate is 5 mg (base)/kg (maximum 300 mg).[11] When visiting or leaving an area endemic for *P. vivax* or *P. ovale,* primaquine phosphate (Primaquine) 15 mg (base) daily for 14 days beginning the last 2 weeks of chloroquine prophylaxis should be added to the regimen.[11,16] The pediatric dose of primaquine is 0.3 mg (base)/kg/d for 14 days. Pediatric doses of chloroquine can be calculated based on body weight. Tablets are then pulverized and placed in gelatin capsules. Parents can be instructed to suspend the dose in food, simple syrup, or drink.

In areas where chloroquine-resistant *P. falciparum* strains exist, travelers should receive mefloquine (Lariam) for prophylaxis.[26] The adult dose of mefloquine is 250 mg once weekly, beginning 1 week prior to departure and continuing for the full period of exposure, followed by 250 mg for 4 weeks after last exposure.[11] The pediatric dose of mefloquine for prophylaxis is as follows:

Body weight (kg)	Dose
15–19	¼ tablet
20–30	½ tablet
31–45	¾ tablet
>45	1 tablet

An alternative regimen for prophylaxis in chloroquine-resistant areas for those who cannot tolerate mefloquine is to take doxycycline 100 mg daily starting 2 days prior to departure, during exposure period, and continuing for 4 weeks after leaving the endemic area.[11,17,27] Children older than 8 years should receive 2 mg/kg/d (up to 100 mg) of doxycycline. Children younger than 8 years should not be given doxycycline.[11]

In an uncomplicated attack of malaria (for all plasmodia except chloroquine-resistant *P. falciparum*), chloroquine 600 mg (base) initially, followed by 300 mg (base) 6 hours later, and then 300 mg (base) daily for 2 days is the recommended regimen. In severe illness or when oral therapy is not tolerated, quinidine gluconate 10 mg/kg as a loading dose (maximum 600 mg) in 250 mL normal saline should be administered slowly over 1 to 2 hours followed by continuous intravenous infusion of 0.02 mg/kg/min until oral therapy can be started.[11,23,24] Oral quinine (300 mg every 8 hours) should follow the intravenous dose to complete 3 days for all infections, except for *P. falciparum* acquired in Thailand where a full 7-day course should be given.[11,17] The pediatric dose of intravenous quinidine gluconate is the same as in adults.[11] The pediatric dose of quinine is 25 mg/kg/d in three divided doses for 3 or 7 days.[11]

In *P. falciparum* (chloroquine-resistant) infections, a single dose of mefloquine 1250 mg should be used. The pediatric dose of mefloquine is 25 mg/kg as a single dose.[11,28] Intravenous quinidine gluconate followed by oral quinine should be administered for severe illness as indicated previously.[11,17,21–23] A second drug needs to be administered in chloroquine-resistant *P. falciparum* and this should follow the oral quinidine regimen: either a single dose of 3 tablets of pyrimethamine–sulfdoxime (Fansidar®) on the last day of intravenous quinidine, or tetracycline 250 mg four times daily for 7 days, or clindamycin 900 mg three times daily for 3 days.[11,22] Oral tetracycline should overlap oral quinine for 2–3 days.[11,17] The intravenous quinidine regimen requires close monitoring of the electrocardiogram and other vital signs.[23,24] Because *P. falciparum* malaria is associated with serious complications including pulmonary edema, hypoglycemia, jaundice, renal failure, coma, and death, careful monitoring of fluid status and hemodynamic parameters is mandatory. Exchange transfusion may be required in patients with *P. falciparum* malaria where parasitemia is >10%; this may manifest as mental status changes, pulmonary edema, or renal failure.[24] Either peritoneal or hemodialysis may be indicated in renal failure.

An active research program has been initiated to develop a malaria vaccine.[29–31] A vaccine that blocks the entry of sporozoites into the liver cells will prevent malaria at this stage. However, immunity to sporozoites does not protect the host against parasites in the erythrocytic cycle. Research has demonstrated that infective sporozoites of *P. falciparum* are covered by a polypeptide, circumsporozoite protein.[29] Isolation and identification of the gene encoding for this circumsporozoite protein has led to the development of a monoclonal antibody by recombinant DNA technology. This *P. falciparum* sporozoite vaccine, R32tet,[32] is now under investigation.

Evaluation of Therapeutic Outcomes

When advising potential travelers on prophylaxis for malaria one needs to be aware of the incidence of chloroquine-resistant *P. falciparum* malaria and the countries where this is prevalent.[11,17,28] Detailed recommendations for prevention of malaria may be obtained by calling the Centers for Disease Control and Prevention (CDC) Hotline, (404)332-4555, while alternatives for prophylaxis failure can be obtained from CDC at (404)488-4046. A number of newer drugs are under active study and include Halofantrine (Halfan) and Artemether.[11,21,28]

Acute *P. falciparum* malaria resistant to chloroquine should be treated with intravenous quinidine. These patients should have a central venous catheter to follow fluid status and the ECG should be closely monitored. Quinidine infusion should be temporarily slowed or stopped if the QT interval >0.6 seconds, an increase in QRS complex of >50% is observed, or hypotension unresponsive to fluid challenge results. The suggested quinidine levels should be maintained at 3–7 mg/L.[16,24] Blood smears should be checked every 12 hours until parasitemia is <1%. Resolution of fever should take place 36–48 hours after initiation of the intravenous quinidine therapy and the blood should be clear of parasites in 5 days.[17]

Travelers to endemic areas for malaria should be advised to remain in well-screened areas, wear clothes that cover most of the body, and sleep in mosquito nets. It is prudent to carry the insect repellent DEET (*N,N*-diethylmetatoluamide) or other insect sprays containing DEET for use in mosquito-infested areas. Readers are urged to check publications from the CDC for the list of countries where chloroquine-resistant *P. falciparum* exists.[28]

GIARDIASIS

Giardia lamblia, a protozoan, is responsible for a significant number of cases of traveler's diarrhea, though the most common cause still remains the enterotoxigenic-producing bacteria *Escherichia coli.*[32–35] Giardia is the most frequently identified intestinal parasite in the United States.[32–39]

The life cycle of *G. lamblia* includes two stages: the trophozoite and the cyst. Found in the small intestine, the gallbladder, and in the biliary drainage, *G. lamblia,* is a pear-shaped trophozoite with four pairs of flagella. Two nuclei that lie in the area of the sucking disk give the protozoan a characteristic facelike image.

The distribution of giardiasis is worldwide and the prevalence rate has been reported to be as high as 16% in some parts of the United States. Children seem to be more frequently affected than adults.[35,39]

Pathology

Giardiasis results from ingestion of *G. lamblia* cysts in fecally contaminated water or food. The protozoan excysts under the stimulus of low gastric pH to release the trophozoite.[35] Colonization and multiplication of the trophozoite leads to mucosal invasion, localized edema, and flattening of the villi, resulting in malabsorption states in the host.[35,39]

Lactose intolerance precipitated by giardiasis can persist even after eradication of the protozoan.[35] Achlorhydria, hypogammaglobulinemia, or deficiency in secretory immunoglobulin A (IgA) are predispositions for giardiasis.[35–37]

Clinical Presentation

Following an incubation period of 1–2 weeks after ingestion of the *G. lamblia* cysts, symptomatic giardiasis is marked by acute onset of diarrhea, cramplike abdominal pains, bloating, and flatulence.[35] Complaints from patients include malaise, nausea, anorexia, and belching. Chronic diarrhea may continue with foul-smelling, copious, light-colored fatty stools and weight loss.[35,39] Periods of diarrhea may alternate with constipation. Patients will complain of malaise, headache, and abdominal and epigastric discomfort frequently exacerbated by eating. Giardiasis can cause steatorrhea and vitamin B_{12} and fat-soluble vitamin deficiencies if left untreated.[35,38]

Diagnosis of giardiasis is made by examination of fresh stool or a preserved specimen during the acute diarrheal phase. Fresh stool specimens may show the trophozoites whereas preserved specimens usually yield the cysts. The alternative method is to use the string or Entero-Test (Hedeco, Palo Alto, CA). The Entero-Test consists of a weighted gelatin capsule secured to a nylon string, the free end of which is secured at the mouth while the capsule is swallowed. The string is removed in 4 to 6 hours and the end, which normally is located in the jejunum, is checked for trophozoites under a microscope.[35] If both the stool exam and string test prove unsuccessful, it may be necessary to attempt duodenal aspiration and biopsy to confirm the diagnosis; this may be more important in AIDS patients or in patients with hypogammaglobulinemia.[39] Most clinicians would advocate a clinical trial of the standard therapy before undertaking invasive diagnostic tests.[35,39–40] An indirect fluorescent antibody (IFA) that utilizes a monoclonal antibody to a protein in *Giardia* cyst is commercially available for detection of the *Giardia* antigen (Meridan Diagnostics Inc., Cincinnati, OH).[39]

Treatment

All symptomatic adults and children older than 8 years of age should be treated with oral metronidazole 250 mg three times daily for 7 days. The alternative oral drugs include furazolidone 100 mg four times or paromomycin 25–30 mg/kg/d in divided doses daily for 1 week.[11,39,40] The pediatric dose for metronidazole is 15 mg/kg/d three times daily for 7 days.[11] Furazolidone suspension (50 mg per 15 mL) is an alternative drug for pediatrics.[41] Quinacrine, which had been the drug of choice in giardiasis, has been discontinued by the manufacturer in the United States.

Evaluation of Therapeutic Outcomes

Patients with symptomatic giardiasis, positive stool samples, or detection of *Giardia* antigen by IFA or enzyme-linked immunoabsorbent assay (ELISA) should be treated with metronidazole for 7 days. Metronidazole produces cure rates between 85–95%.[39,40] Diarrhea will stop within a few days, although in some patients it may take 1–2 weeks. Cyst excretion will cease within days; however, intestinal dysfunction manifested as increased transit time and radiological changes (e.g., irregular thickening of the folds in the upper small intestine) may take a few months to resolve. Patients who fail initial therapy with metronidazole should receive a second course of therapy. Pregnant patients can receive paromomycin 25–30 mg/kg/d in divided doses for 7 days.[14,39]

Giardiasis can be prevented by good personal hygiene and caution in food and drink consumption. Preventive measures are similar to those discussed in amebiasis (see section on "Sanitation and Preventive Measures").

AMERICAN TRYPANOSOMIASIS

Two distinct forms of the genus *Trypanosoma* occur in humans, one associated with African trypanosomiasis (sleeping sickness) and the other with American trypanosomiasis (Chagas' disease).[42–44] *Trypanosoma brucei gambiense* and *T. brucei rhodesiense* are the causative organisms for African trypanosomiasis. In African trypanosomiasis, the parasite occurs as a long slender flagellated form called a trypomastigote in the blood and spinal fluid. In Chagas' disease, the trypomastigote is found in the bloodstream and an ovoid unflagellated intracellular form is found in cardiac and other tissues.[43,44]

Trypanosoma cruzi is the agent that causes American trypanosomiasis. American trypanosomiasis is transmitted by a number of species of a reduviid bug *(Triatoma infestans, Rhodrium prolixus)* that lives in wall cracks of houses in rural areas of North, Central, and South America. The reduviid bug is infected by sucking blood from animals (e.g., opossums, dogs, cats) or humans infected with circulating trypomastigotes.

Clinical Presentation

Acute infection is frequently seen in children, although Chagas' disease in adults can also be present with the acute phase. Unilateral orbital edema (Romana's sign) due to local inflammation produced by the multiplying parasite may be seen. A local inoculation granuloma or chagoma appearing on the skin as a dusty erythematous lesion may be present, indicating the site of entry of the parasite. Fever, hepatosplenomegaly, and lymphadenopathy may also be present. In chronic disease, patients will present with cardiomyopathy and congestive heart failure. Electrocardiograms will usually be abnormal, demonstrating extrasystoles, first-degree heart block, right bundle branch block, and other serious conduction disturbances.[44,45] Degeneration of the autonomic ganglia in the smooth muscle of the esophagus and colon lead to uncoordinated peristalsis. The end result has been reported to be "mega syndromes" or severe dilation of affected organs, primarily the esophagus (megaesophagus) and the colon (megacolon).[42]

A history to verify possible exposure to *T. cruzi* should be an important initial diagnostic workup. Recovery of *T. cruzi* would be definitive; however, this is not always possible, especially in chronic disease. Positive serologic tests using indirect hemagglutination test, ELISA, and a complement fixation test are utilized. False-positive reactions are seen especially in those exposed to leishmaniasis, syphilis, or malaria.[44]

Treatment

The oral drugs that have been used to treat *T. cruzi* infections are nifurtimox (Lampit, Bayer 2502, available from the Centers for Disease Control and Prevention) and benznidazole (Rochagan, available only in Brazil). The adult dose of nifurtimox is 8–10 mg/kg/d in divided doses for 120 days. Because pediatric patients tolerate the drug better than adults, the dose for children age 1 to 10 years is 15–20 mg/kg/d and age 11 to 16 years is 12.5–15 mg/kg/d in divided doses.[11] Symptomatic treatment for heart failure includes digitalis and diuretics, while the gastrointestinal complications require surgical revisions and reconstruction.

Evaluation of Therapeutic Outcomes

American trypanosomiasis (Chagas' disease), which is endemic in all Latin American countries, can be transmitted congenitally and by blood transfusion and organ transplantation.[44] Treatment with nifurtimox of the acute phase (fever, malaise, edema of face, generalized lymphadenopathy and heptosplenomegaly, etc.) produces only about a 50% curative rate.[44] Treatment of chronic infection with nifurtimox is not recommended. It is essential to identify *T. cruzi*-infected patients by serology and monitor the cardiovascular status of these patients by ECG periodically as part of routine follow-up, irrespective of therapy. The congestive failure of cardiomyopathic Chagas' disease is treated the same way as cardiomyopathies due to other causes.[45]

HELMINTHIC DISEASES

The majority of intestinal helminthic infections may not be associated with clearly defined manifestation of disease, but they can cause significant pathology. One of the factors that determines the pathogenicity of helminths is their population density. Light infections may be fairly well tolerated, while high populations of intestinal helminths can result in predictable disease presentations.[46–51] In the United States these infections are most frequently seen in recent immigrants from Southeast Asia, the Caribbean, Mexico, and Central America.[51] There is a higher incidence of helminthic infections in the southern states. Other populations that have a high risk of infestation include institutionalized patients (both young and elderly), preschool children in day-care centers, residents of Indian reservations, and homosexual individuals.[46,47] Certain conditions and drugs (fever, corticosteroids, and anesthesia) can cause atypical localization of worms.[50] Immunocompromised hosts can be overwhelmed by some helminthic infections, such as strongyloidiasis.[50,51]

NEMATODES

Hookworm Disease

This is an infection of the small intestine caused by either *Ancylostoma duodenale* or *Necator americanus*. *Necator americanus* is found in the southeastern United States where the temperature and humidity provide the proper environment. *Ancylostoma* is rarely seen in the United States.

The life cycles of both species of hookworm are similar. The adult worms live in the small intestine attached to the mucosa. The females liberate eggs, which are eliminated in the feces and develop into larvae. Infective larva enter the host in contaminated food or water or penetrate the skin, where a papular eruption with localized edema and erythema can result.

In the small intestine where the adult worm lives attached to the mucosa, injury is usually due to mechanical and lytic destruction of tissue. The loss of blood can lead to anemia and hypoproteinemia.[1,2,47,51]

Stool should be examined for eggs and the rhabditiform larvae. Eosinophilia (30–60% of peripheral white blood cells) is present in patients with chronic infection.

Treatment

Mebendazole (Vermox), an oral synthetic benzimidazole, is the agent of first choice. It is also effective against ascariasis, enterobiasis, and trichuriasis.[11,40,47,48–52] The adult dose for treatment of hookworm infestation is 100 mg twice daily for 3 days. Pediatric patients older than 2 years of age should receive the same dose as adults.[11]

Ascariasis

Ascariasis is caused by the giant roundworm, *Ascaris lumbricoides*. Female worms range from 20–35 cm in length. The worm is found worldwide, but more commonly in areas where sanitation is poor. In the United States, endemic areas include southeastern parts of the Appalachian range and the Gulf Coast states.[46,49] It is estimated that about 4 million people in the United States have ascariasis.[47]

Clinical Manifestations

During the migration of the larvae through the lungs, patients can present with pneumonitis, fever, cough, eosinophilia, and pulmonary infiltrates.[47] Other symptoms of ascariasis include abdominal discomfort, vomiting, and appendicitis.[49] Diagnosis is made by demonstrating the characteristic egg in the stool.

Treatment

In both adults and pediatric patients older than 2 years of age, the treatment for ascariasis is oral mebendazole (Vermox) 100 mg twice daily for 3 days. An alternative drug for ascariasis is pyrantel pamoate (Antiminth).[11]

Enterobiasis

Enterobiasis or pinworm infection is caused by *Enterobius vermicularis*. The pinworm is a small threadlike spindle-shaped worm about 1 cm long. It is the most widely distributed helminthic infection in the world. There are estimated to be 42 million cases in the United States.[46] The majority of those infected are children.

There are no significant pathologic changes with the infection. The most common problem is cutaneous irritation in the perianal region, made by the migrating females or presence of eggs. The intense pruritus and scratching can cause dermatitis and secondary bacterial infections. In children, the itching can cause loss of sleep and restlessness.

The most effective method of diagnosing pinworm infections is by the use of perianal swab using clear adhesive tape. The adhesive tape, which is applied to the perianal region with a tongue depressor, is microscopically examined for eggs.[46,51]

Treatment

The common agents for treatment include pyrantel pamoate, mebendazole, or albendazole (Zentel). The dose of pyrantel pamoate is 11 mg/kg (maximum 1 g) as a single oral dose, which can be repeated in 2 weeks. The dose of mebendazole for adults and children older than 2 years of age is 100 mg as a single oral dose; this may be repeated in 2 weeks.[11] Following treatment, all bedding and underclothes should be sterilized by steaming or boiling to eradicate the eggs. Bathroom rugs and toilet accessories should also be sterilized.

Evaluation of Therapeutic Outcomes for Nematodes

Morbidity and disease with intestinal nematodes is related to the intensity of infection or worm burden; subjects with transient exposure have less severe disease. The major adverse effects of intestinal nematodes is malnutrition, fatigue, and diminished work capacity. Treatment with antihelmintic agents results in complete eradication and significant change in the well-being of subjects. Unlike other nematodes, strongyloidiasis can perpetuate itself by autoinfection and, under immunosuppression, the filariform can invade various organs (e.g., lungs, central nervous system, etc.) to provide disseminated infection that can be fatal.[50]

ECTOPARASITES

A parasite that lives on the outside of the body of the host is called an *ectoparasite.* It is estimated that there are 3 million cases of pediculosis in the United States.[53–55] Pediculosis is usually associated with poor personal hygiene, and infections are passed from person to person through social and sexual contact. The three types of human lice belong to two genera: *Pediculus,* including the head and body lice, and *Phthirus,* with only one species, the crab louse.[1,2] The human louse is detectable to the human naked eye and measures about 2–3 mm long.

LICE

The two species that belong to this group include *Pediculus humanus capitis* (head louse) and *P. humanus corporis* (body louse). Female lice deposit eggs on the hair. The eggs (or nits) remain firmly attached to the hair and in about 10 days the lice hatch to form nymphs, which mature in 2 weeks. Using both their piercing mouth parts and pumping device, the larvae and adults feed on the blood of the host. The body louse and head louse are essentially identical, although they live on different parts of the body. Unlike the head louse, which lives on the hair, the body louse may more frequently be found on clothing of the infected host.

The pubic or crab louse is found on the hairs around the genitals, although they can occur in other areas of the body (e.g., eyelashes, beards, axillae).

Clinical Presentation

Patients usually complain of severe pruritus from papular lesions produced by the bite of the louse. Hypersensitivity to foreign material injected by the lice can produce macular swellings and occasionally lead to secondary bacterial infections. As a result of long-standing pediculosis and secondary infections, hyperpigmentation and thickening of the skin can take place, a condition referred to as "vagabond's" disease.[53,55]

Treatment

The agent of choice for all three infections—body, head, and crab lice—is 1% permethrin (Nix), which is applied topically.[14,54–56] Permethrin is a derivative of the flowers of the plant *Chrysanthemum cinerariaefolium.* The term "pyrethrin" is usually applied to several esters of chrysanthemic acid and pyrethric acid.[57] Permethrin has both pediculicidal and ovicidal activity against *P. humanus capitis.* The cure rate has been reported to be in the range of 97–99%.[54,57–60] Individuals who have a history of ragweed or chrysanthemum allergy should use this compound with caution. The side effects reported with permethrin products include itching, burning, stinging, and tingling.[54] Permethrin 1% is applied to the scalp after the hair has been dried following a shampooing. The scalp should be saturated with permethrin liquid and a towel should be wrapped around the scalp to allow the application to stay on for 10 minutes. The hair should then be rinsed off. A cream rinse of permethrin 1% (Nix-Creme Rinse) is also available and has been shown to be as effective as lindane.[58] Either of these two preparations may also be used for *Phthirus pubis* and *P. humanus* infestations.[11] Other members of the family or sexual partners should also be treated. All bedding and clothes should be sterilized by boiling or steaming to avoid reinfections. Seams of clothes should be examined to verify that all organisms are eradicated. A 1% yellow oxide of mercury ophthalmic ointment should be used twice daily for 7 days for crab louse infections of the eyelids. To minimize absorption and sensitivity to mercurial compounds, this topical preparation should be used sparingly.

Another alternative for pediculosis is pyrethrin 0.3% combined with 3% piperonyl butoxide and 1.2% petroleum distillate (R&C, RID).[53,54] The same directions for permethrin should be followed when applying this preparation. For the relief of pruritus, a soothing lotion of calamine liniment or lotion with 0.1% menthol may be used.

SCABIES

Scabies is caused by the itch mite *Sarcoptes scabiei,* which affects humans and animals. Mange in domestic animals is caused by the same organism. Infection usually affects the interdigital and popliteal folds, axillary folds, the umbilicus, and scrotum.[58,59]

Clinical Presentation

Patients complain of severe itching, inability to sleep, and may have excoriations in the interdigital web spaces, wrists, elbows, buttocks, groin, and scalp. Excoriations may lead to secondary bacterial infections. The diagnosis is made by looking for burrows formed by the mite and taking skin scrapings, which will demonstrate the mite on a wet mount.

Treatment

The treatment of choice is permethrin 5% (Elimite) cream.[11,58–60] To initiate the treatment, the skin should be scrubbed thoroughly in a warm soapy bath, using a soft brush to remove all scabs. The lotion is then applied to the whole body, avoiding the face, mucous membranes, and eyes. The application should be left on for 8–14 hours before bathing.[11] A single application has been demonstrated to eradicate 91% of scabies in subjects.[55,60] All close contacts should be checked and treated appropriately.[59]

Other agents used to treat scabies are γ-benzene hexachloride 1% lotion (Kwell, Lindane) and Crotamiton 10% (Eurax). These should be used in patients who have hypersensitivity to permethrin preparations. Topical corticosteroids and antihistamines may be used to decrease pruritus.

Evaluation of Therapeutic Outcomes

Permethrin (1–5%) for pediculosis and scabies is the preferred agent and remains the safest agent especially in infants and children.[58–60] One application of permethrin is consistently effective in eradicating more than 90% of all infections. However, pruritus may persist for a week or two because of the remnants of mite parts in the skin.

REFERENCES

1. Beaver PC, Jung RC, Cupp EW. Clinical Parasitology. Philadelphia, Lea and Febiger, 1984.
2. Markell EK, Voge M. Medical Parasitology. Philadelphia, WB Saunders, 1991.
3. Warren KS. Tropical medicine or tropical health: The Heath Clark lectures, 1988. Rev Infect Dis 1990;12:142–156.
4. Aucott JN, Ravdin JI. Amebiasis and nonpathogenic intestinal protozoa. Infect Dis Clin North Am 1993;7:467–485.
5. Ravadin JI, Petri WA. *Entamoeba histolytica* (amebiasis), in Mandell GL, Douglas Jr RG, Bennett JE (eds): Principles and Practice of Infectious Diseases, 3rd ed. New York, Churchill Livingstone, 1990, p 2036.
6. Irusen EM, Jackson TFHG, Simjee AE. Asymptomatic intestinal colonization by pathogenic *Entamoeba histolytica* in amebic liver abscess. Prevalence, response to therapy and pathogenic potential. Clin Infect Dis 1992;14:889–893.
7. Greenstein AJ, Bartu J, Dicker A, et al. Amebic liver abscess: A study of 11 cases compared with a series of 38 patients with pyogenic liver abscess. Am J Gastroenterol 1985;80:472–478.
8. Barnes PF, De Cock KM, Reynolds TN, et al. A comparison of amebic and pyogenic abscess of the liver. Medicine 1987;66:472–483.
9. Wolfe M. Intestinal and genital infections. Amebiasis, in Strickland GT (ed): Hunter's Tropical Medicine, 7th ed. Philadelphia, WB Saunders, 1991, p 550.
10. Filice C, Di-Perri G, Strosselli M, et al. Outcome of hepatic amebic abscesses managed with three different therapeutic strategies. Dig Dis Sci 1992;37:240–247.
11. Drugs for parasitic infections. Med Lett 1993;35:111–122.
12. Eli Zondo G, Weissleder R, Stark DD, et al. Amebic liver abscess: Diagnosis and treatment evaluation with MR imaging. Radiology 1987;165:795–800.
13. Thompson JE Jr, Forlenza S, Verma R. Amebic liver abscess: A therapeutic approach. Rev Infect Dis 1985;7:171–179.
14. Rosenblatt JE. Antiparasitic agents. Mayo Clin Proc 1992;67:276–287.
15. Wyler DJ. Malaria: Resurgence, resistance and research. N Engl J Med 1983;308:875–878,934–939.
16. Zucker JR, Campbell CC. Malaria: Principles of prevention and treatment. Infect Dis Clin North Am 1993;7:547–567.
17. Wyler DJ. Plasmodium species (malaria), in Mandell GL, Douglas Jr RG, Bennett JE (eds): Principles and Practice of Infectious Diseases, 3rd ed. New York, Churchill Livingstone, 1990, p 2056.
18. James MFM. Pulmonary damage associated with falciparum malaria: A report of ten cases: Pulmonary edema with features of ARDS seen in a patient. Ann Trop Med Parasit 1985;79:123–138.
19. Looareesuwan S, Ho M, Wattanagoon Y, et al. Dynamic alteration in splenic function during acute falciparum malaria. N Engl J Med 1987;317:675–679.
20. Gopdeuk V, Thuma P, Brittenham G, et al. Effect of iron chelation therapy on recovery from deep coma in children with cerebral malaria. N Engl J Med 1992;327:1473–1477.
21. Looareesuwan S, Kyle DE, Viravan C, et al. Treatment of patients with recrudescent falciparum malaria with sequential

combination of artesunate and mefloquine. Am J Trop Med Hyp 1992;47:794–799.
22. Kremsner PG, Winkler S, Brants C, et al. Curing of chloroquine-resistant malaria with clindamycin. Am J Trop Med Hyg 1993;49:650–654.
23. Phillips RE, Warrell DA, White NJ, et al. Intravenous quinidine for the treatment of severe falciparum malaria. N Engl J Med 1985;312:1273–1278.
24. Miller KD, Greenberg AE, Campbell CC. Treatment of severe malaria in the United States with continuous infusion of quinidine gluconate and exchange transfusion. N Engl J Med 1989;321:65–70.
25. Looareesuwan S, Charoenpan P, Ho M, et al. Fatal *Plasmodium falciparum* malaria after inadequate response to quinine treatment. J Infect Dis 1990;161:577–580.
26. Recommendations for the prevention of malaria among travellers. MMWR 1990;39(RR-3):1–10.
27. Pang LW, Boudreau EF, Limsomwong N, et al. Doxycycline prophylaxis for falciparum malaria. Lancet 1987;1:1161–1164.
28. Wyler DJ. Malaria chemoprophylaxis for the traveller. N Engl J Med 1993; 329:31–37.
29. Hoffman SL, Wistar R, Ballon WR, et al. Immunity to malaria and naturally acquired antibodies to the circumsporozoite protein or *Plasmodium falciparum.* N Engl J Med 1986;315:601–605.
30. Cook GC. Prevention and treatment of malaria. Lancet 1988;1:32–37.
31. Ballou WR, Sherwood JA, Chulay JD, et al. Safety and efficacy of a recombinant DNA *Plasmodium falciparum* sporozoite vaccine. Lancet 1987;1:1277–1281.
32. Mutz ED, Hudson-Wragg M, Mshar P, et al. Foodborne giardiasis in a corporate setting. J Infect Dis 1993;167:250–253.
33. Kent GP, Greenspan JR, Herdon JL, et al. Epidemic giardiasis caused by a contaminated public water supply. Am J Public Health 1988;78:139–143.
34. Quick R, Paugh K, Addiss D, et al. Restaurant-associated outbreak of giardiasis. J Infect Dis 1992;166:673–676.
35. Hill DR. *Giardia lamblia,* in Mandell GL, Douglas Jr RG, Bennett JE (eds): Principles and Practice of Infectious Diseases, 3rd ed. New York, Churchill Livingstone, 1990, p 2110.
36. Nayak N, Ganguly NK, Walia BNS, et al. Specific secretory IgA in milk of *Giardia lamblia*-infected and uninfected women. J Infect Dis 1987;155:724–727.
37. Janoff EN, Smith PD, Blaser MJ. Acute antibody responses to *Giardia lamblia.* J Infect Dis 1988;157:798–804.
38. Solomons NW. Giardiasis: Nutritional implications. Rev Infect Dis 1982;4:859–869.
39. Hill DR. Giardiasis. Issues in diagnosis and management. Inf Dis Clin North Am 1993;7:503–525.
40. Van Reken DE, Pearson RD. Antiparasitic agents, in Mandell GL, Douglas Jr RG, Bennett JE (eds): Principles and Practice of Infectious Diseases, 3rd ed. New York, Churchill Livingstone, 1990, p 398.
41. Quiros-Buelna E. Furozolidine and metronidazole for treatment of giardiasis in children. Scan J Gastroenterol 1989;169(suppl):65–69.
42. Garcia-Zapata MTA, McGreevy PB, Marsden PD. American trypanosomiasis, in Strickland GT (ed): Hunter's Tropical Medicine, 7th ed. Philadelphia, WB Saunders, 1991, p 628.
43. Kirchhoff LV. Chagas' disease: American trypanosomiasis. Infect Dis Clin North Am 1993;7:487–502.
44. Kirchhoff LV. American trypanosomiasis (Chagas' disease). A tropical disease now in the United States. N Engl J Med 1993;329:639–644.
45. Hager JM, Rahimtoola SH. Chagas' heart disease in the United States. N Engl J Med 1991;325:763–768.
46. Warren KS. Diseases due to Helminths. Introduction, in Mandell GL, Douglas Jr RG, Bennett JE (eds): Principles and Practice of Infectious Diseases, 3rd ed. New York, Churchill Livingstone, 1990, p 2134.
47. Mahmoud AF. Intestinal nematodes (roundworms), in Mandell GL, Douglas Jr RG, Bennett JE (eds): Principles and Practice of Infectious Diseases, 3rd ed. New York, Churchill Livingstone, 1990, p 2135.
48. Abadi K. Single dose mebendazole therapy for soil-transmitted nematodes. Am J Trop Med Hyg 1985;34:129–133.
49. Schwartzman JD. Intestinal nematodes that migrate through lungs (Ascariasis), in Strickland GT (ed): Hunter's Tropical Medicine, 7th ed. Philadelphia, WB Saunders, 1991, p 696.
50. Liu LX, Weller PF. Strongyloidiasis and other intestinal nematode infections. Infect Dis Clin North Am 1993;7:655–682.
51. Pearson RD, Guerrant RL. Intestinal nematodes that migrate through skin and lung, in Strickland GT (ed): Hunter's Tropical Medicine, 7th ed. Philadelphia, WB Saunders, 1991, p 700.
52. Ciesielski SD, Seed JR, Ortiz JC, Metts J. Intestinal parasites among North Carolina farm workers. Am J Public Health 1992;82:1258–1262.
53. Wilson BB, Weary PE. Lice (Pediculosis), in Mandell GL, Douglas Jr RG, Bennett JE (eds): Principles and Practice of Infectious Diseases, 3rd ed. New York, Churchill Livingstone, 1990, p 2163.
54. Facts and Comparisons Publication. St. Louis, MO, JB Lippincott, 1994, p 584a.
55. Hogan DJ, Schachner L, Tanglertsampan C. Diagnosis and treatment of childhood scabies and pediculosis. Pediat Clin North Am 1991;38:941–957.
56. Brandenburg K, Deinard A, Di Napoli J, et al. 1% Permethrin cream rinse vs lindane shampoo in treating pediculosis capitis. Am J Dis Child 1986;140:894–896.
57. Taplin D, Meinking TL. Pyrethrins and pyrethroids in dermatology. Arch Dermatol 1990;126:213–221.
58. Schultz MW, Gomez M, Hansen RC, et al. Comparative study of 5% permethrin cream and 1% lindane lotion for treatment of scabies. Arch Dermatol 1990;126:167–170.
59. Orkin M, Maibach HI. Scabies therapy—1993. Semin Dermol 1993;12:22–25.
60. Permethtrin for scabies. Med Lett 1990;32:21–22.
61. Goldsmith RS. Antiprotozoal drugs, in Katzung BG (ed): Basic and Clinical Pharmacology, 4th ed. Los Altos, CA, Appleton and Lange, 1989, p 645.
62. Goldsmith RS. Clinical pharmacology of antihelmintic drugs, in Katzung BG (ed): Basic and Clinical Pharmacology, 4th ed. Los Altos, CA, Appleton and Lange, 1989, p 666.
63. Webster LT Jr. Drugs used in the chemotherapy of helminthiasis, in Gilman AG, Rall TW, Nies AS, Taylor P (eds): The Pharmacological Basis of Therapeutics, 8th ed. New York, Pergamon Press, 1990, p 959.
64. Webster LT Jr. Drugs used in the chemotherapy of protozoal infections, in Gilman AG, Rall TW, Nies AS, Taylor P (eds): The Pharmacological Basis of Therapeutics, 8th ed. New York, Pergamon Press, 1990, pp. 979, 999, 1008.

Antiparasitic Drugs

Drug	Indications	Side Effects	Comments	References
Chloroquine phosphate (Aralen, Nivaquine) 250- and 500-mg tablets; 50 mg/mL (as HCl); 5-mL ampules	Malaria	GI: nausea, vomiting, diarrhea CNS: dizziness, headache, blurring of vision, confusion, fatigue Derm: pruritus	Administer oral dose after meals IV route: recommend EKG monitoring *Contraindication:* patients with psoriasis or porphyria	11, 16, 17, 28, 40, 61, 64
Dehydroemetine dihydrochloride[a] 30 mg/mL; 2-mL ampule	Amebiasis	GI: nausea, vomiting, diarrhea Card: hypotension, arrhythmias, cardiac failure Other: muscular pains, paralysis, death Cumulative toxicity: doses > 650 mg	Prolongation: QT, PR, QRS, ST segment on EKG (may be indication to stop therapy) *Contraindication:* cardiac and renal disease	4, 6, 9, 11, 40, 61, 64
Diloxanide furoate[a] (Furamide) 500-mg tablet	Amebiasis	GI: nausea, flatulence Derm: pruritis		9, 11, 40, 61, 64
Furazolidone (furoxone) 100-mg tablet Suspension: 50 mg/5 mL	Giardiasis Alternative to metronidazole	GI: nausea, vomiting Hypersensitivity: hypotension, fever, arthralgia, urticaria Other: headache	Disulfiram-like reaction with alcohol; avoid in G6PD[b] deficiency; may cause hemolysis; changes color of urine to brown	11, 35, 40, 41
Iodoquinol (Yodoxin) 210-mg tablet	Amebiasis	GI: abdominal pain, diarrhea Derm: rash	May interfere with thyroid function test *Contraindication:* patients with iodine intolerance	4, 5, 9, 11, 40, 64
Mebendazole (Vermox) 100-mg chewable tablet	Ascariasis Trichuriasis Hookworm Pinworm	GI: abdominal pain, diarrhea CNS: headache, dizziness Other: pyrexia, neutropenia	Drug should be taken with meals *Contraindication:* pregnancy *Drug interaction:* can increase serum levels of theophylline	11, 40, 47–49, 62, 63
Mefloquine 250-mg tablet	*P. falciparum* malaria	Incidence 17% GI: nausea, vomiting, abdominal pain, diarrhea Card: sinus bradycardia CNS: vertigo, dizziness, confusion, hallucinations, psychosis, convulsions Derm: itching, skin rash	Patients given doses in excess of 12 mg/kg should be carefully monitored because the side effects are dose related	11, 14, 16, 21, 27, 28
Metronidazole (Flagyl) Oral: 250 mg, 500-mg tablets IV	Amebiasis Giardiasis	GI: nausea, anorexia, vomiting, diarrhea, abdominal cramping, glossitis, metallic taste CNS: dizziness, vertigo, headache, paresthesias	Avoid alcohol; alcohol ingestion will cause the disulfiram reaction: abdominal distress, vomiting, hypotension *Contraindication:* first trimester of pregnancy	4–6, 9, 11, 40, 61, 64

(continued)

Drug	Indications	Side Effects	Comments	References
Nifurtimox[a] (Lampit, Bayer 2502)	South American trypanosomiasis	GI: anorexia, nausea CNS: peripheral neuritis, psychosis Hemat: Hemolysis in G6PD[b] deficiency patients	Monitor pulmonary function and hematologic parameters	11, 40, 43
Primaquine phosphate 26.3-mg tablet	Malaria *(P. vivax)* *(P. ovale)*	GI: nausea, abdominal pain CNS: mental depression	In G6PD[b] deficiency can cause hemolysis	11, 16, 17, 28, 40, 61
Pyrantel pamoate (Antiminth) 50-mg/mL suspension	Pinworm Hookworm	GI: anorexia, nausea, abdominal cramps, diarrhea CNS: headache, dizziness		11, 40, 48, 62, 63
Pyrimethamine (Daraprim) 25-mg tablet	Malaria (see pyrimethamine–sulfadoxime)	GI: abdominal pain, vomiting, glossitis Hemat: megaloblastic anemia, hemolytic anemia	Recommended that folinic acid 1–5 mg/d be concurrently administered; can cause hemolysis in patients with G6PD[b] deficiency	11, 40, 61, 64
Pyrimethamine 25 mg *plus* sulfadoxime 500 mg (Fansidar)	*P. falciparum*-resistant malaria	For pyrimethamine, see above GI: nausea, abdominal pain, stomatitis Hemat: agranulocytosis, aplastic anemia, leukopenia	Combination has recently been reported to cause the Stevens–Johnson syndrome; patients should be advised to call their physician/pharmacist if a skin rash or other reactions are seen	11, 16, 17, 28, 40, 61, 64
Quinidine gluconate 500 mg base/mL; 10 mL	Acute malaria	GI: nausea, vomiting, diarrhea Card: hypotension, widening of QRS and QT on EKG, heart block	Administration of IV quinidine requires close monitoring; should normally monitor EKG and all vital signs	11, 16, 23, 24, 40
Quinine sulfate 325 mg, 650-mg tablets	Acute malaria	Cinchonism: flushing, dizziness, nausea, vomiting, diarrhea (levels over 10 µg/mL) Card: hypotension, widening of QRS complex Hemat: hemolysis, leukopenia, thrombocytopenia	When drug is administered IV it should be administered by slow infusion (600 mg over 8 h); close monitoring of vitals and EKG *Avoid use:* IM administration	11, 16, 23, 24, 40

[a]Investigational drugs obtained from the Centers for Disease Control and Prevention Parasitic Disease Drug Service, Atlanta, GA 30333; (404)639-3670 (business hours: 8:00 AM–4:30 PM EST), (404)639-2888 (night, weekend, or holiday—for emergency calls only). Readers may also call local state health offices for specific information on travel information and parasitic diseases.
[b]G6PD, glucose-6-phosphate dehydrogenase.

Chapter 109

Urinary Tract Infections and Prostatitis

Timothy A. Mullenix, PharmD, MS, and Randall A. Prince, PharmD

Infections of the urinary tract represent a wide variety of clinical syndromes including urethritis, cystitis, prostatitis, and pyelonephritis and are the most commonly occurring bacterial infections encountered in medicine today. It is estimated that these infections account for 7 million physician visits annually. Also, they constitute the most commonly occurring nosocomial infection.[1] At least 20% of all females will suffer a symptomatic urinary tract infection (UTI) at some time in their lives, with many having multiple recurrences.[2] Infections in males occur much less frequently, but a higher proportion of these infections are associated with complications, such as septicemia and pyelonephritis.

A UTI may be defined as the presence of microorganisms in the urine that cannot be accounted for by contamination, which have the potential to invade the tissues of the urinary tract and adjacent structures. The infection may be confined to the growth of bacteria in the urine, which may or may not produce symptoms. UTI may present as several syndromes that are associated with an inflammatory response to microbial invasion and can range from asymptomatic bacteriuria to pyelonephritis with gram-negative septicemia.

In general, UTIs may be classified by several methods. Classically, they have been described by anatomic site of infection. Lower tract infections, such as cystitis, involve the bladder and manifest with symptoms of dysuria, frequency, urgency, and occasionally suprapubic tenderness. Upper tract infections involve the kidney and are referred to as pyelonephritis. Pyelonephritis is generally associated with more systemic symptoms such as fever, flank pain, and tenderness, but lower tract symptoms are frequently present also. The absence of systemic symptoms does not exclude upper tract infection.

Urinary tract infections may also be designated as uncomplicated or complicated. Uncomplicated infections are not associated with structural or neurologic abnormalities that may interfere with the normal flow of urine or the voiding mechanism. These infections usually occur in females of childbearing age who are otherwise normal, healthy individuals. Males are generally not classified as having uncomplicated UTIs because these infections are rare and most often represent a structural or neurologic abnormality.

Complicated UTIs are the result of a predisposing lesion of the urinary tract such as a congenital abnormality or distortion of the urinary tract, a stone, indwelling catheter, prostatic hypertrophy, obstruction, or neurologic deficit that interferes with the normal flow of urine and urinary tract defenses. Complicated infections occur in males and females and may involve both the upper and lower urinary tract.

Recurrent UTIs are characterized by multiple symptomatic episodes with asymptomatic periods occurring between these episodes. These infections are either due to reinfection or to relapse. Reinfections are caused by a new organism and account for the majority of recurrent UTIs. Relapse represents the development of repeated infections caused by the same initial organism.

Asymptomatic bacteriuria is a common finding, particularly among the elderly, when there is significant bacteriuria ($>10^5$ bacteria/mL of urine) in the absence of symptoms. Symptomatic abacteriuria or acute urethral syndrome consists of symptoms of frequency and dysuria in the absence of significant bacteriuria. This syndrome has been commonly associated with chlamydial infections.

Significant bacteriuria is a term introduced to distinguish the presence of microorganisms that represent true infection from those organisms that can contaminate the urine via passage through the distal urethra, prior to urine collection. Historically, bacterial counts equal to or more than 100,000 organisms per milliliter of urine in a clean-catch morning specimen were taken to indicate true infection.[3] Counts less than 100,000 may represent true infection in certain situations, for example, concurrent with antibacterial drug administration, rapid urine flow, low urinary pH, or upper tract obstruction.[4,5] Table 109.1 describes current clinical definitions of significant bacteriuria that depend on the clinical setting and method of specimen collection.[6] These criteria allow for more appropriate specificity and

TABLE 109.1. CRITERIA FOR DEFINING SIGNIFICANT BACTERIURIA

≥10^2 CFU coliforms/mL or ≥10^5 noncoliforms/mL in a symptomatic female
≥10^3 CFU bacteria/mL in a symptomatic male
≥10^5 CFU bacteria/mL in asymptomatic individuals on two consecutive specimens
Any growth of bacteria on suprapubic catheterization in a symptomatic patient
≥10^2 CFU bacteria/mL in a catheterized patient

(From Johnson CC. Definitions, classification, and clinical presentation of urinary tract infections. Med Clin North Am 1991;75:242.)

sensitivity in documenting infection under differing clinical circumstances.

EPIDEMIOLOGY

The prevalence of urinary tract infections varies with age and gender. In newborns and infants up to 6 months of age, the prevalence of bacteriuria is about 1% and is more common in boys.[7] Most of these infections are associated with structural or functional abnormalities of the urinary tract. Between the ages of 1 to 5, the incidence of urinary tract infection in females rises with infections in males declining significantly. The prevalence of bacteriuria in females and males is 4.5% and 0.5%, respectively, in this age group.[8] Infections occurring in preschool boys usually are associated with congenital abnormalities of the urinary tract. These infections are difficult to recognize due to the age of the patient, but often are symptomatic. In addition, it is believed that the majority of renal damage associated with UTI develops at this age.[9]

Through grade school and before puberty, the prevalence of UTI is about 1% with 5% of females reported to have significant bacteriuria prior to leaving high school.[10] Bacteriuria in males is rare with a prevalence of 0.03%. The prevalence of bacteriuria increases dramatically to 1–4% after puberty in nonpregnant females.[11] It is estimated that 20% of women suffer a symptomatic UTI at some point in their lives. Many women have recurrent infections with a significant proportion of these women having a history of childhood infections. In contrast, the prevalence of bacteriuria in adult men is very low (<0.1%).[12]

In the elderly, the ratio of bacteriuria in women and men is altered dramatically and is approximately equal in persons older than the age of 65.[13] The overall incidence of UTI increases substantially in this population with the majority of these infections being asymptomatic. This incidence increases further for those elderly residing in nursing homes and who are frequently hospitalized. This increase in infection rate is probably due to a number of factors including obstruction from prostatic hypertrophy in males, poor bladder emptying due to prolapse in females, fecal incontinence in demented patients, neuromuscular disease including strokes, and increased urinary instrumentation (catheterization).

PATHOGENESIS

ROUTE OF INFECTION

In general, urinary tract infections can be acquired via three possible routes: the ascending, hematogenous, and lymphatic pathways. The female urethra is usually colonized with bacteria believed to originate from the rectal flora.[14] The short length of the female urethra and proximity to the perirectal area make colonization of the urethra likely. Other factors that affect colonization of the urethra include diaphragm and spermicide use. Although there is evidence in females that bladder infections follow the colonization of the urethra, the mode of ascent of the microorganisms is incompletely understood. Sexual intercourse and massage of the urethra have been shown to allow bacteria to reach the bladder.[15,16] Once in the bladder, the organisms multiply quickly and can ascend the ureters to the kidney. This event is more likely to occur if vesicoureteral reflux is present. The fact that urinary tract infections are more common in females than males because of the anatomical differences in location and length of the urethra lends support to the ascending route of infection as the primary route of infection acquisition.

Infection of the kidney by hematogenous spread of organisms usually can occur as the result of dissemination of organisms from a distant primary infection in the body. Infections via the descending route are uncommon and involve a relatively small number of pathogens including *Staphylococcus aureus, Candida* spp., *Salmonella* spp., *Mycobacterium tuberculosis,* and *Enterococcus* spp. Of particular interest is the fact that it is difficult to produce experimental pyelonephritis by intravenously administering common gram-negative organisms, such as *Escherichia coli* and *Pseudomonas aeruginosa* in animal models.

There appears to be little evidence supporting a significant role for renal lymphatics in the pathogenesis of urinary tract infections. It is known that there are lymphatic communications between the bowel and the kidney, as well as the bladder and the kidney. However, there is no evidence that microorganisms are transferred to the kidney.[17] Thus, it appears the ascending route of infection is currently the most important.

Once bacteria reach the urinary tract, three factors determine the development of infection: the size of the inoculum, the virulence of the microorganism, and the competency of the natural host defense mechanisms. The majority of urinary tract infections reflect a failure in the host defense mechanisms.

HOST DEFENSE MECHANISMS

The normal urinary tract is generally resistant to invasion by bacteria and is very efficient in rapidly eliminating microorganisms that reach the bladder. The urine under normal circumstances is capable of inhibiting and killing microorganisms. The factors thought to be responsible include a low pH, extremes in osmolality, high urea concentration, and high organic acid concentration.[18] Bacterial growth is further inhibited in males because of the addition of prostatic secretions.[19]

The introduction of bacteria into the bladder stimulates micturition with increased diuresis and efficient emptying of the bladder. These factors are critical in preventing the initiation and maintenance of bladder infections. It is clear that patients who are unable to void urine completely are at greater risk of developing urinary tract infections and frequently have recurrent infections. It is also evident that patients with even small residual amounts of urine respond less favorably to treatment than patients who are able to completely empty their bladders.[20]

An important virulence factor of bacteria is their ability to adhere to urinary epithelial cells, resulting in colonization of the urinary tract, bladder infections, and pyelonephritis.[21] Various factors are present in the bladder that act as antiadherence mechanisms and thus prevent bacterial colonization and infection. The epithelial cells of the bladder are coated with a urinary mucus or slime called uromucoid. This thin layer of mucopolysaccharide is hydrophilic and strongly negatively charged. When bound to the uroepithelium, it attracts water molecules and forms a layer between the bladder and urine. The antiadherence characteristics of this uromucoid are nonspecific and when removed by dilute acid solutions result in rapid bacterial adherence.[22]

In addition, Tamm–Horsfall protein is a glycoprotein produced by the ascending limb of Henle and distal tubule, which is excreted into the urine and contains mannose residues. These mannose residues bind *E. coli* that contain type 1 fimbriae and prevent them from binding to these receptors on the mucosal surface of the bladder.[23] Other factors that possibly prevent adherence of bacteria include immunoglobulins IgG and IgA. Investigators have documented both systemic and local kidney immunoglobulin synthesis in upper urinary tract infections. The role of immunoglobulins in preventing bladder infection is less clear. However, it has been observed that patients with reduced urinary levels of secretory IgA are at increased risk of urinary tract infections.[24]

Once bacteria have actually invaded the bladder mucosa, an inflammatory response is stimulated with the mobilization of polymorphonuclear leukocytes (PMNs) and resulting phagocytosis. PMNs are primarily responsible for limiting the tissue invasion and controlling the spread of infection in the bladder and kidney. They do not play a role in preventing bladder colonization or infections and actually have been implicated in contributing to renal tissue damage.[25]

BACTERIAL VIRULENCE FACTORS

The virulence of an organism represents its ability to cause disease and is very important in determining the development and severity of infection. Bacteria that adhere to the epithelium of the urinary tract are associated with colonization and cause infection. The mechanism of adhesion of gram-negative bacteria, particularly *E. coli,* is related to bacterial fimbriae that are rigid hairlike appendages of the cell wall.[26] These fimbriae adhere to specific glycolipid components on epithelial cells. The most common type of fimbriae is type 1, which binds to mannose residues present in glycoproteins. Uromucoid and Tamm–Horsfall protein are rich in mannose residues. Organisms containing type 1 fimbriae are readily trapped and washed out of the bladder.[23] Other fimbriae are mannose resistant and are more frequently associated with pyelonephritis, such as *P. fimbriae*, which bind avidly to specific glycolipid receptors on uroepithelial cells.[27] These bacteria are resistant to washout or removal by uromucoid and are able to multiply and invade tissue, especially the kidney. In addition, polymorphonuclear leukocytes contain receptors for type 1 fimbriae, which facilitate phagocytosis, but they lack receptors for *P. fimbriae*.[28]

Other virulence factors include hemolysin and aerobactin. Hemolysin is a cytotoxic protein produced by bacteria that lyses a wide range of cells including erythrocytes, polymorphonuclear leukocytes, and monocytes. *Escherichia coli* and other gram-negative bacteria require iron for aerobic metabolism and multiplication. Aerobactin facilitates the binding and uptake of iron by *E. coli;* however, the significance of this property in the pathogenesis of urinary tract infections remains unknown.[29]

PREDISPOSING FACTORS TO INFECTION

In patients with underlying structural abnormalities of the urinary tract, the typical virulence factors previously discussed are usually lacking.[30] There are several known abnormalities of the urinary tract system that interfere with its natural defense mechanisms, the most important of which is obstruction. Obstruction can inhibit the normal flow of urine, disrupting the natural flushing and voiding effect in removing bacteria from the bladder, and resulting in incomplete emptying. Common conditions that result in residual urine volumes include prostatic hypertrophy, urethral strictures, calculi, tumors, bladder diverticula, and drugs such as anticholinergic agents. Additional causes of incomplete bladder emptying include neurologic malfunctions associated with stroke, diabetes, spinal cord injuries, tabes dorsalis, and other neuropathies.

Vesicoureteral reflux represents a condition in which urine is forced up the ureter to the kidney. Urinary reflux is not only associated with an increased incidence of UTIs and pyelonephritis, but also with producing renal damage.[31] Reflux may be the result of a congenital abnormality or more frequently the result of bladder overdistension from obstruction.

Other risk factors include urinary catheterization, mechanical instrumentation, pregnancy, and the use of diaphragms.

Etiology

The microbiological etiology of urinary tract infection is related to the UTI classification (i.e., complicated versus uncomplicated). The most common cause of uncomplicated urinary tract infections is *E. coli,* accounting for more than 80% of community-acquired infections followed by *Staphylococcus saprophyticus* (coagulase-negative staphylococcus), accounting for 5–15%. Other causes include *Klebsiella pneumoniae, Proteus* spp., *P. aeruginosa,* and *Enterococcus faecalis,* which occur rarely in uncomplicated, community-acquired infections (5–10%).[32]

Staphylococcus epidermidis is frequently isolated from the urinary tract, but it is usually considered a contaminant. Repeat cultures should be performed to help confirm the organism as a pathogen.

The urinary pathogens are quite different in complicated or nosocomial infections. There is a dramatic increase in the isolation of *Proteus* spp., *Klebsiella* spp., *Enterobacter* spp., *Pseudomonas* spp., staphylococci, and enterococci as causative organisms, whereas *E. coli* accounts for less than 50% of these infections. Recently, infections due to *E. faecalis* have increased and represent the second most frequently isolated organism in the hospitalized patient.[33] In part, this finding may be related to the extensive use of third-generation cephalosporin antibiotics, which are not active against the enterococci. *Staphylococcus aureus* infections may arise from the urinary tract, but are more commonly a result of bacteremia, producing metastatic abscesses in the kidney. *Candida* spp. have become common causes of urinary infection in the critically ill and chronically catheterized patient.

The majority of urinary tract infections are caused by a single organism; however, in patients with stones, indwelling urinary catheters, or chronic renal abscesses, multiple organisms may be isolated. Depending on the clinical situation, the recovery of multiple organisms may represent contamination and a repeat specimen should be obtained.

Clinical Presentation

The presenting signs and symptoms of urinary tract infections in adults are easily recognized. Unfortunately, a large portion of patients with significant bacteriuria are asymptomatic. These include normal healthy patients, elderly patients, children, pregnant patients, and patients with indwelling catheters. The typical symptoms of lower tract infections include dysuria, urgency, frequency, nocturia, and suprapubic heaviness or pain. Fever is uncommonly associated with lower tract infections.

The manifestations of upper tract infections classically include flank pain, costovertebral tenderness, or abdominal pain, and systemic symptoms such as fever, rigors, headache, nausea, vomiting, and malaise. Lower tract symptoms may or may not precede upper tract infections, but often occur 1–2 days prior to systemic symptoms. Attempts at differentiating upper tract from lower tract infections on the basis of symptoms alone are not reliable. Elderly patients frequently do not experience specific urinary symptoms, but will present with altered mental status, change in eating habits, or gastrointestinal symptoms. In addition, in patients with indwelling catheters or neurologic disorders, lower tract symptoms are usually absent, while flank pain and fever are common. Note, however, that many of these patients frequently develop upper tract infections with bacteremia with no or minimal urinary tract symptoms.

Diagnosis

Symptoms alone are unreliable for the diagnosis of bacterial urinary tract infections. The key to the diagnosis of UTI is the ability to demonstrate significant numbers of microorganisms present in an appropriate urine specimen to distinguish contamination from infection. The type and extent of laboratory examination required depends on the clinical situation.

There are three acceptable methods of urine collection. The first is the midstream clean-catch method. After cleaning the urethral opening area in both men and women, 20–30 mL of urine is voided and discarded. The next part of the urine flow is collected and should be processed immediately. Urine specimens that are allowed to sit at room temperature for several hours will result it falsely elevated colony counts. The midstream clean catch is the preferred method for the routine collection of urine for culture. The two other acceptable methods of urine collection include catheterization and suprapubic bladder aspiration. In patients who are uncooperative or are unable to void urine, catheterization may be necessary. If catheterization is performed carefully with aseptic technique, the method yields reliable results. Note, however, that the introduction of bacteria into the bladder may result and the procedure is associated with infection in 1–2% of patients.[34] Suprapubic bladder aspiration is a safe and painless procedure and is the procedure of choice in newborns, paraplegics, seriously ill patients, and adults when infection is suspected and routine procedures have provided confusing or equivocal results. Suprapubic aspiration bypasses the contaminating organisms present in the urethra and any bacteria found using this technique are generally considered to represent significant bacteriuria.

A standard urinalysis should be obtained in the initial assessment of a patient and includes a description of the color, specific gravity, pH of the urine, and the concentration determination of glucose, protein, ketones, blood, and bilirubin. These determinations can be performed by a dipstick method. An easy to perform and reliable method for the presumptive diagnosis of bacteriuria is the microscopic examination of the urine. This may be done by preparation of a Gram stain of unspun or centrifuged urine. The presence of at least one organism per oil-immersion field in a properly collected uncentrifuged specimen correlates with greater than or equal to 100,000 bacteria/mL of urine. For recognizing smaller numbers of organisms, a centrifuged specimen is more sensitive. Such examinations detect greater than or equal to 100,000 bacteria/mL with a sensitivity of greater than 90% and a specificity of more than 70%.[35] Counts of less than 30,000, however, are usually not reliably recognized by these methods.

Microscopic examination of the urine for leukocytes is also utilized to determine the presence of urinary tract infections. A count of 5–10 white blood cells (WBCs) per high power field in a centrifuged specimen is accepted as the upper limit of normal. The presence of greater than 10 WBCs/mm^3 is almost always present in symptomatic bacteriuria, but is absent in up to 30% of patients with asymptomatic bacteriuria.[36] It should be emphasized that pyuria is nonspecific and signifies only the presence of inflammation and not necessarily infection.[37] Thus, patients with pyuria may or may not have infection. Sterile pyuria has long been associated with urinary tuberculosis, as well as chlamydial and fungal infections.

Several biochemical tests have been developed for screening urine for the presence of bacteria. The most common is the Griess nitrate reduction test.[38] This dipstick test detects the presence of nitrite in the urine produced by the reduction of normally excreted nitrate by gram-negative bacteria. False-negative results of the nitrite tests are caused by the presence of gram-positive organisms and *Pseudomonas* sp., which do not reduce nitrate, a low urine pH, frequent voiding, and a dilute urine. The leukocyte esterase (LE) dipstick test detects the enzyme LE, which is found in primary neutrophil granules and indicates the presence of WBCs. When these tests are used together, the range of reported sensitivity and specificity is 70–100% and 60–98%, respectively, for the detection of bacteriuria.[39]

The most reliable method of diagnosing urinary tract infections is by quantitative urine culture. Urine in the bladder is normally sterile; therefore, it is statistically possible to differentiate contamination of the urine from infection by quantifying the number of bacteria present. This criterion is based on a properly collected midstream clean-catch urine specimen. Patients with infection usually have greater than 10^5 bacteria/mL of urine.[40] It should be emphasized that as many as one-third of women with symptomatic infection have less than 10^5 bacteria/mL.[41] It is likely that a significant portion of patients with urinary tract infections, either symptomatic or asymptomatic, also has less than 10^5 bacterial/mL of urine.

Several laboratory methods are utilized to quantitate bacteria present in the urine. The most accurate method is the pour-plate technique, in which a small volume of urine in combination with a diluent is pipetted on a petri dish followed by molten agar. This method is unsuitable for a high-volume laboratory because of its expense and time consumption. The streak-plate method is an alternative that involves using a calibrated loop technique to streak a fixed amount of urine on an agar plate. This method is used most commonly in diagnostic laboratories because it is simple to perform and less costly.

Once identification and quantification have been completed, the next step is to determine the susceptibility of the organism. There are several methods by which bacterial susceptibility testing in the laboratory may be performed. The two most commonly utilized methods are the Kirby–Bauer method and the tube-dilution method.[42] More recently, microdilution techniques, such as Vitek and Microscan, have been introduced that can rapidly and efficiently provide susceptibility information. Knowing the susceptibility and achievable urine concentration of the antibiotics puts the clinician in a better position to select an appropriate agent to treat the UTI.

Several methods have been used to determine the location of infection within the urinary system and to differentiate upper tract involvement from lower tract. The most direct method is the procedure of ureteral catheterization described by Stamey et al.[43] The method involves the passage of a catheter into the bladder and then into each ureter where quantitative cultures are obtained. It was found that, by utilizing this method, history and physical examination were of little value in predicting the site of infection. Although this method provides direct quantitative evidence, it is invasive, technically difficult, and expensive. The Fairley bladder washout technique is a modification of the Stamey procedure, which involves Foley catheterization only.[44] After the catheter is passed, bladder samples are obtained after which the bladder is washed out and cultures are taken at 10, 20, and 30 minutes. The procedure has shown that up to 50% of patients have renal involvement, regardless of signs and symptoms. Others have found 10–20% of tests to be equivocal.[45]

Noninvasive methods of localization may be more acceptable for routine use; however, they may be of limited clinical value. A number of studies have reported that patients with pyelonephritis have a defect in urinary concentrating ability.[46] However, the use of concentrating ability for localization of urinary tract infections is associated with a high false-positive and false-negative response and

TABLE 109.2. COMMONLY USED ANTIMICROBIAL AGENTS IN THE TREATMENT OF URINARY TRACT INFECTIONS

Agents	Comments
Oral Therapy	
Sulfonamides	These agents are useful for the first episodes of infection. They have generally been replaced by more active agents due to resistance formation. Only current advantage is low cost.
Trimethoprim–sulfamethoxazole	This combination is highly effective against most aerobic enteric bacteria, except *Pseudomonas aeruginosa.* High urinary tract tissue levels and urine levels are achieved, which may be important in complicated infection treatment. Also effective as prophylaxis for recurrent infections.
Penicillins Ampicillin Amoxicillin Amoxicillin–clavulanic acid Carbenicillin indanyl	Ampicillin is the standard penicillin that has broad-spectrum activity, including most enteric bacteria causing urinary tract infections. There have been increasing reports of areas of *E. coli* resistance. Amoxicillin is better absorbed and has fewer side effects. Amoxicillin–clavulanate therapy is preferred for resistance problems. Carbenicillin indanyl is only indicated for the treatment of urinary tract infections and is active against *Pseudomonas aeruginosa.*
Cephalosporins Cephalexin Cephradine Cefaclor Cefadroxil Cefuroxime Cefixime	There are no major advantages of these agents over other agents in the treatment of urinary tract infections and they are more expensive. They may be useful in cases of resistance to amoxicillin and trimethoprim–sulfamethoxazole. These drugs are not as effective for single-dose therapy.
Tetracyclines Tetracycline Doxycycline Oxytetracycline Minocycline	These agents are effective for initial episodes of urinary tract infections. Resistance, however, develops rapidly and their use should be guided by sensitivity testing. These agents also lead to candidal overgrowth. They are primarily useful for chlamydial infections.
Quinolones Nalidixic acid Oxolinic acid Cinoxacin Ciprofloxacin	Nalidixic acid, oxalinic acid, and cinoxacin are effective for initial episodes of infection due to *E. coli* and other Enterobacteriaceae, but not *Pseudomonas aeruginosa.* The newer quinolones have a greater spectrum of activity, including *Pseudomonas aeruginosa.* Ciprofloxacin and ofloxacin are indicated for systemic therapy, as well.

is not useful clinically. The most promising method is the antibody-coated bacteria (ACB) test, an immunofluorescent method that detects bacteria coated with immunoglobulin in freshly voided urine. The sensitivity and specificity of the test to detect upper tract infection has been reported to average 88% and 76%, respectively.[47] The test appears to be reliable and sensitive in detecting renal bacteriuria; however, several studies have reported high false-positive and false-negative results. False-positive rates of 20–30% have been reported in lower tract infections. These have primarily been related to the presence of prostatitis, yeasts, proteinuria, hemorrhagic cystitis, bladder tumors, and bladder stones. False-negative results occur in 20% of patients, primarily in early pyelonephritis when antibody titers are low. At present, ACB testing is primarily used as a research tool to study the pathogenesis, treatment, and epidemiology of urinary tract infections.

Some clinicians have observed that therapeutic outcome may be useful in separating patients with upper and lower tract infection. This statement is based on the assumption that virtually all patients with uncomplicated lower tract infections can be cured with a short course of antibiotic therapy and those who do not respond or relapse do so because of upper tract involvement. Presently, it is rarely necessary to localize the site of infection to direct the clinical management of the patient.

Management

The management of a patient with a UTI includes initial evaluation, selection of an antibacterial agent and duration of therapy, and follow-up evaluation. The initial selection of an antimicrobial agent for the treatment of UTI is primarily based on the severity of the presenting signs and symptoms, the site of infection, and whether the infection is determined to be complicated or uncomplicated. Other considerations include side-effect potential, cost, and the comparative inconvenience of different therapies.

Various pharmacologic factors may affect the action of antibacterial agents. Certainly the ability of the agent to reach the urine is of utmost importance. Factors that affect the rate of excretion include the patient's glomerular filtration rate and whether the agent is actively secreted. Filtration depends on the molecular size and degree of protein binding of the agent. Agents such as the sulfonamides,

TABLE 109.2. COMMONLY USED ANTIMICROBIAL AGENTS IN THE TREATMENT OF URINARY TRACT INFECTIONS *(Continued)*

Agents	Comments
Norfloxacin	
Ofloxacin	
Nitrofurantoin	This agent is effective as both a therapeutic and prophylactic agent in patients with recurrent urinary tract infections. Main advantage is the lack of resistance even after long courses of therapy. Adverse effects may limit its usefulness (e.g., GI intolerance, neuropathies, pulmonary reactions).
Azithromycin	Useful as single-dose therapy in chlamydial infections.
Methanamine hippurate Methenamine mandalate	These agents are reserved for prophylactic therapy or suppressive use between episodes of infection.
Parenteral Therapy	
Aminoglycosides Gentamicin Tobramycin Amikacin Netilmicin	Gentamicin and tobramycin are equally effective and gentamicin is less expensive. Tobramycin has greater pseudomonal activity which may be important in serious systemic infections. Amikacin is generally reserved for multiresistant bacteria.
Penicillins Ampicillin Carbenicillin Ticarcillin Mezlocillin Pipercillin	These agents are generally equally effective for susceptible bacteria. The extended-spectrum penicillins are more active against *Pseudomonas aeruginosa* and enterococci and are often preferred over cephalosporins. They are very useful in renally impaired patients or when an aminoglycoside is to be avoided.
Cephalosporins First, second, and third generation	Second- and third-generation cephalosporins have a broad spectrum of activity against gram-negative bacteria, but are not active against enterococci and have limited activity against *Pseudomonas aeruginosa* (ceftazidime active *P. aeruginosa*). They are useful for nosocomial infections and urosepsis due to susceptible pathogens.
Imipenem/cilastatin	Has a very broad spectrum of activity including gram-positive, gram-negative, and anaerobic bacteria. It is active against enterococci and *Pseudomonas aeruginosa* but may be associated with candidal superinfections.
Aztreonam	This monobactam is active only against gram-negative bacteria, including *Pseudomonas aeruginosa*. Generally useful for nosocomial infections when aminoglycosides are to be avoided and in penicillin-sensitive patients.

tetracyclines, and aminoglycosides enter the urine by filtration. As the glomerular filtration rate is reduced, the amount of drug entering the urine is reduced. Most β-lactams and quinolones are not only filtered, but also are actively secreted into the urine. For this reason, they achieve high urinary concentrations, regardless of their protein-binding characteristics or the presence of severe renal dysfunction.

Also, urine flow and the kinetics of voiding have been found to affect the treatment of UTIs. Diuresis induced by furosemide appears to protect the kidney from infection and augment the effect of antimicrobial agents. This augmentation occurs by improving leukocyte concentrations in the renal medulla and by diluting solutes that are known to inhibit phagocytic activity.[48] Paradoxically, diuresis also augments susceptibility in ascending infections by diluting the normal antibacterial properties of the urine. In clinical practice, the concentrations of antimicrobial agents in the urine are so high that dilution has little effect on efficacy.

In addition, diuresis causes an increase in voiding frequency, which reduces the inoculum size of the bacterial population. It appears that the critical factor is the amount of residual volume remaining after voiding. Shand et al.[20] reported that as little as 10 mL of residual urine can significantly inhibit the eradication of infection.

The ability to eradicate bacteria from the urinary tract is directly related to the sensitivity of the organism and the achievable concentration of the antimicrobial agent in the urine. Unfortunately, most susceptibility testing is directed at achievable concentrations in the blood. It is clear that there is a poor correlation between achievable blood levels of antimicrobial agents and eradication of bacteria from the urine.[49] In the treatment of lower tract infections, blood levels may not be important; however, achieving appropriate blood levels appears critical in patients with bacteremia and renal abscesses.

Ideally, any agent chosen should be well tolerated, well absorbed, achieve high urinary concentrations, and have a spectrum of activity limited to the known or suspected pathogen(s). Table 109.2 lists the most common agents used in the treatment of urinary tract infections along with comments concerning their general use. Table 109.3 presents an overview of various therapeutic options for outpatient therapy for UTI. Table 109.4 describes empiric treatment regimens for selected clinical situations.

TABLE 109.3. OVERVIEW OF OUTPATIENT ANTIMICROBIAL THERAPY FOR LOWER TRACT INFECTIONS IN ADULTS

Indication	Antibiotic	Dose	Interval[a]	Duration
Lower tract infection	Trimethoprim–sulfamethoxazole double-strength tablet	2 tablets	Single dose	1 d
		1 tablet	12 h	3 d
		1 tablet	12 h	7–14 d
	Amoxicillin	6 × 500 mg	Single dose	1 d
		1 × 250 mg	8 h	7–14 d
	Amoxicillin–clavulanate	1 × 500 mg	8 h	7–14 d
	Sulfisoxazole	4 × 500 mg	Single dose	1 d
		2 × 500 mg	6 h	7–14 d
	Trimethoprim	1 × 100 mg	12 h	7–14 d
	Norfloxacin	1 × 400 mg	12 h	3 d
		1 × 400 mg	12 h	7–14 d
	Ciprofloxacin	1 × 250–500 mg	12 h	3 d
	Ofloxacin	1 × 250–500 mg	12 h	7–14 d
		1 × 200 mg	12 h	7–14 d
Acute urethral syndrome				
Initial therapy	Trimethoprim–sulfamethoxazole double-strength tablet	2 tablets	Single dose	1 d
		1 tablet	12 h	3 d
		100 mg	12 h	10–14 d
After failure	Doxycycline	1 g	Single dose	1 d
	Azithromycin			
Long-term prophylaxis	Trimethoprim–sulfamethoxazole single strength	½ tablet	24 h	6 mo
Recurrent infections	Nitrofurantoin	50 mg	24 h	6 mo
	Trimethoprim	100 mg	24 h	6 mo

[a]Dosing interval for normal renal function.

UNCOMPLICATED URINARY TRACT INFECTIONS IN FEMALES

Acute, uncomplicated lower urinary tract infection is the most common form of urinary infection. These infections typically occur in women of childbearing age and are often related to sexual activity. Although the presence of dysuria, frequency, urgency, and suprapubic discomfort are frequently associated with lower tract infection, a significant number of patients have upper tract involvement as well.[50] These infections are predominantly caused by *E. coli,* and antimicrobial therapy should be directed against this organism initially. Other causes include *S. saprophyticus* and occasionally *Klebsiella* and *Proteus* species. Because the causative organisms and their susceptibilities are generally known, many advocate a cost-effective approach to their management. This includes a urinalysis and initiation of empiric therapy without a urine culture (see Fig. 109.1).[50]

Conventional therapy has consisted of an effective oral antibiotic administered for 7–14 days.[51] However, it is now apparent that acute cystitis is a superficial mucosal infection that can be eradicated with much shorter courses of therapy. Single-dose therapy provides high urinary concentrations for 12–24 hours and is highly effective in treating many women with acute cystitis. Cure rates have ranged from 82–100% using single doses of sulfisoxazole (2 grams), trimethoprim–sulfamethoxazole (two double-strength [DS] tablets), and amoxicillin (3 grams).[52–54] Advantages of single-dose therapy include less expense, greater compliance, fewer side effects, and less potential for the development of resistance. It should not be assumed that all antimicrobial agents are effective as single-dose agents. For example, a 2-gram oral dose of cefaclor produced a 57% failure rate in lower tract infections.[55] Recent data suggest that trimethoprim–sulfamethoxazole is the most efficacious agent as single-dose therapy and is comparable to multiple-dose regimens.[50] This finding may be related to the recent observations that *E. coli* causing community-acquired urinary tract infections are increasingly resistant to ampicillin, amoxicillin, and sulfonamides. In addition, oral β-lactams are eliminated more rapidly and do not achieve high renal tissue concentrations as compared to trimethoprim–sulfamethoxazole.

The failure to eradicate a urinary tract infection after single-dose therapy may indicate possible upper tract infection and correlates well with the ACB test in localizing infection.[56] Single-dose therapy should not be considered when symptoms of upper tract infection are present or suspected, stones or other urologic abnormalities are present, there is a previous history of antibiotic resistance, or in males. In other words, single-dose therapy

TABLE 109.4. EMPIRIC TREATMENT OF URINARY TRACT INFECTIONS/PROSTATITIS

Diagnosis	Pathogens	Treatment	Comments
Acute uncomplicated infection	*E. coli* *S. saprophyticus*	1. TMP–SMX × 3 days 2. Quinolone × 3 days	More effective than single-dose therapy
Pregnancy	As above	1. Amp/clav × 7 days 2. Cephalosporin × 7 days 3. TMP–SMX × 7 days	Avoid TMP–SMX during last trimester
Acute pyelonephritis			
Uncomplicated	*E. coli*	1. TMP–SMX × 14 days 2. Quinolone × 14 days	Can be managed as outpatient
Complicated	*E. coli, P. mirabilis, K. pneumoniae, Pseudomonas aeruginosa, E. faecalis*	1. Quinolone × 14 days 2. Amp/sulb or piperacillin plus an aminoglycoside	Severity of illness will determine duration of IV therapy. Culture results should direct treatment and an oral agent may complete 14 days of therapy
Prostatitis	*E. coli, Klebsiella pneumoniae, Proteus* spp., *Pseudomonas aeruginosa*	1. TMP–SMX × 4 weeks 2. Quinolone × 4 weeks	Acute prostatitis may require IV therapy initially. Chronic prostatitis may require longer treatment periods or surgery

should not be used in cases of complicated urinary tract infections.

Recently, reviews of single-dose therapy have questioned the efficacy of this treatment modality based on results from adequately controlled trials.[57,58] The conclusion from these reviews was that short-course (3-day therapy) may be superior to single-dose therapy and should be the treatment of choice. Three-day courses of amoxicillin, trimethoprim, trimethoprim–sulfamethoxazole, fluoroquinolones, or doxycycline have cure rates comparable to those with longer courses and the incidence of adverse events was no greater than with single-dose therapy. Other agents that have been suggested for short-course therapy include cephalexin, and amoxicillin–clavulanic acid. Short-course therapy should be reserved for those female patients with infection limited to the bladder and with no underlying complicating factors. Those patients with complicated infections should receive full-course therapy with an effective agent. Presently, empiric 3-day therapy with trimethoprim–sulfamethoxazole is recommended as optimal therapy.[32] Although the fluoroquinolones are equally effective and well tolerated, they are generally reserved for patients with treatment failures, allergies, or infections caused by some resistant organisms.

Follow-up urine cultures are not necessary in those patients who respond. However, in those women who do not respond to therapy or symptoms return within 2 weeks, urine culture and susceptibility should be performed. These patients should receive specific antimicrobial therapy for 10–14 days as directed by the susceptibility report.

SYMPTOMATIC ABACTERIURIA

Symptomatic abacteriuria, or acute urethral syndrome, represents a clinical syndrome in which females present with dysuria and pyuria but do not to have significant bacteriuria, using the criterion of 10^5 bacteria/mL of urine. Acute urethral syndrome is estimated to account for more than half of the complaints of dysuria seen in the community today. These women are most likely to be infected with small numbers of *E. coli* and other coliform bacteria, staphylococci, or *Chlamydia trachomatis.*[41] Additional causes include *Neisseria gonorrhoeae, Gardnerella vaginalis,* and *Ureaplasma urealyticum.*

Most patients presenting with pyuria will, in fact, have infection that requires treatment. Fihn et al.[59] examined 255 college women with acute dysuria and compared singly dosed trimethoprim–sulfamethoxazole (two DS tablets) with a 10-day course of one DS tablet twice per day. Of these women, 85% were found to have bacteriuria with greater than 10,000 bacteria/mL, 5% had *C. trachomatis* infection, 20% had vaginal candidiasis, two patients had genital herpes, and one patient had gonorrhea. There was no significant difference in the rate of resolution of symptoms and cure rates at 13 days were 76% for the single-dose treatment and 96% for the 10-day course. However, at 6 weeks, cure rates were 68% versus 79%, respectively. The authors concluded that treatment periods of intermediate duration may be optimal. In patients who present for the first time, cultures should be obtained for gonorrhea before treatment is started. Single-dose or short-course therapy with trimethoprim–sulfamethoxazole has been uti-

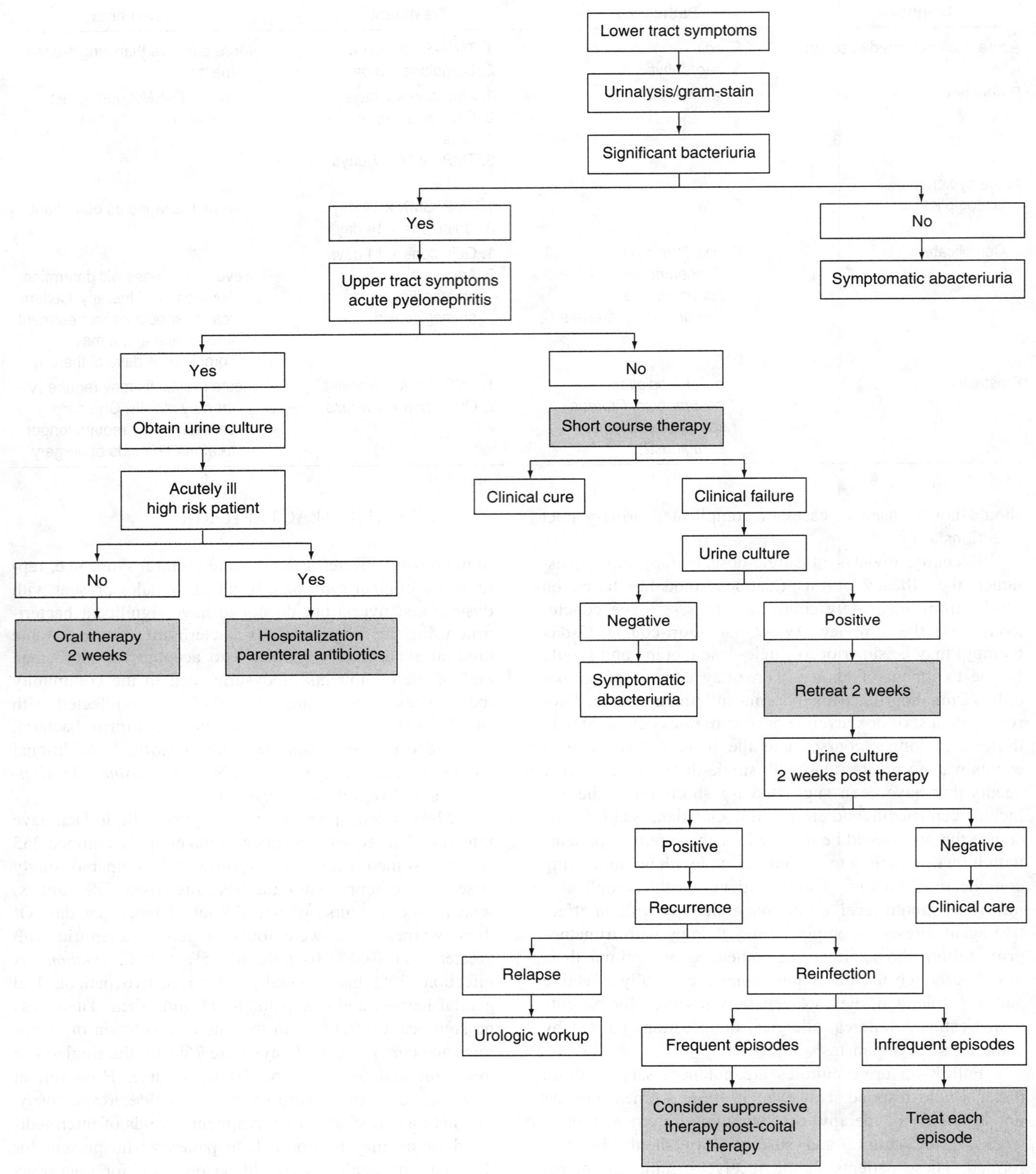

Figure 109.1. Management of urinary tract infections in females.

lized effectively and prolonged courses of therapy are not necessary for the majority of patients. If single-dose or short-course therapy is ineffective or if *Chlamydia* infection is suspected, treatment should consist of doxycycline for 7–10 days or a single 1-gram dose of azithromycin. Often concomitant treatment of all sexual partners is required to cure *Chlamydia* infections and prevent reacquisition.

ASYMPTOMATIC BACTERIURIA

Asymptomatic bacteriuria represents those patients who, in the absence of urinary symptoms, are found to have two consecutive urine cultures with $>10^5$ of the same organism. The majority of patients with asymptomatic bacteriuria are elderly and female. Another group of patients frequently having asymptomatic bacteriuria is pregnant women. Although this group of patients typically will respond to treatment, relapse and reinfection are very common and chronic asymptomatic bacteriuria is difficult to eradicate.

The management of asymptomatic bacteriuria depends on the age of the patient and whether they are pregnant. In children, because they have a greater risk of developing renal scarring and long-standing renal damage, treatment should consist of conventional courses of therapy, as described for symptomatic infections. It appears that the greatest risk of renal damage occurs during the first 5 years of life.[60] In the nonpregnant female, therapy is controversial; however, it appears that treatment has little effect on the natural course of infections.[61]

Asymptomatic bacteriuria in the elderly is characterized by two groups: those with persistent bacteriuria and those with intermittent bacteriuria. Most clinicians feel that asymptomatic bacteriuria in the elderly is a benign disease and may not warrant treatment because most data indicate that the patient without urinary tract obstruction is not destined to develop progressive renal damage.[62] However, some investigators who have demonstrated an association between bacteriuria and decreased survival have questioned this conclusion.[63,64] In this setting, there is no urgency in initiating therapy and two cultures should be obtained to confirm the presence of bacteriuria. There is evidence that treatment in ambulatory, nonhospitalized elderly women is effective in eliminating bacteria for at least 6 months and may protect against the development of symptomatic bacteriuria; however, only 50% of patients remained free of bacteria after 1 year.[65,66] Several studies in hospitalized elderly subjects, however, have not found antimicrobial therapy to be efficacious.[67,68] A number of questions remain unanswered, including the effect of eradication of bacteriuria on life expectancy, the cost effectiveness and risk–benefit ratio of therapy, and the effect on morbidity. Certainly with the current information and the high adverse reaction rate in this population, vigorous treatment and screening programs cannot be advocated.

COMPLICATED URINARY TRACT INFECTIONS

Acute Pyelonephritis

The presentation of high-grade fever and severe flank pain should be treated as acute pyelonephritis and aggressive management is warranted. Severely ill patients with pyelonephritis should be hospitalized and intravenous drugs administered initially. Although more mild cases may be managed with orally administered antibiotics in an outpatient setting, symptoms of nausea and vomiting and dehydration may require hospitalization.

At the time of presentation, a Gram stain of the urine should be performed, along with urinalysis, culture, and sensitivities. The Gram stain should indicate the morphology of the infecting organism(s) and direct the selection of an appropriate antibiotic. The precise identity and sensitivity of the infecting organism(s) will be unknown with the selection of an antimicrobial agent being empiric. In the mild to moderately symptomatic patient in which oral therapy is considered, an effective agent should be administered for at least a 2-week period. Although the sulfonamides and ampicillin or amoxicillin have been the primary choices for the treatment of gram-negative bacillary infections, they are no longer considered reliable agents in this setting. Reports that 25–35% of *E. coli* may be resistant have tempered their use.[69] In addition, treatment with trimethoprim–sulfamethoxazole (one DS tablet twice a day) for 2 weeks has been found to be superior to ampicillin even when the organisms were susceptible to both agents.[70] Oral antibiotics that have shown efficacy in this setting include trimethoprim, trimethoprim–sulfamethoxazole, amoxicillin–clavulanic acid, norfloxacin, and ciprofloxacin. If a Gram stain reveals streptococci, *E. faecalis* should be considered and ampicillin or amoxicillin is probably the agent of choice. Close follow-up of outpatient treatment is mandatory to assure success. In the seriously ill patient, the initial antibiotic regimen should be given parenterally, should provide a broad spectrum of coverage, and should be directed toward bacteremia or sepsis, if present. A number of antimicrobial agents have been used as empiric therapy. The traditional initial therapy has included an aminoglycoside in combination with ampicillin. Because of the increased incidence of ampicillin resistance in the community, other agents have been proposed. These include parenteral trimethoprim–sulfamethoxazole, aztreonam, piperacillin, ampicillin–sulbactam or ticarcillin–clavulanic acid, and the third-generation cephalosporins (cefotaxime, ceftriaxone, etc.). If the patient has been hospitalized in the last 6 months, has a urinary catheter, or is in a nursing home, the possibility of *Pseudomonas* and enterococcus infection, as well as resistant organisms, should be considered. In this setting, ceftazidime, ticarcillin–clavulanic acid, aztreonam, imipenem, or piperacillin in combination with an aminoglycoside is recommended. The rationale for combination therapy is that in experimental animals 3 days of aminoglycoside combination therapy followed by nonaminoglycoside single-agent therapy for 7 days resulted in a 100% cure rate.[71] If the patient responds to initial combination therapy, the aminoglycoside may be discontinued after 3 days. Although the aminoglycoside therapy is stopped, renal tissue concentrations of the aminoglycoside will persist for days. Based on sensitivity data, the patient can then be maintained or switched to a less expensive single agent and ultimately an appropriate oral agent may be used.

Effective therapy should stabilize the patient within 12–24 hours. A significant reduction in urine bacterial concentrations should occur in 48 hours. If bacteriologic response has not occurred, an alternative agent should be considered based on susceptibility testing. If the patient fails to respond clinically within 3–4 days or has persistently positive blood or urine cultures, further investigation is needed to exclude bacterial resistance, possible obstruction, papillary necrosis, intrarenal or perinephric abscess, or some other disease process. Usually by the third day of therapy, the patient is afebrile and much less symptomatic and the urine should be clear of bacteria. In general, parenteral therapy should be continued until the patient has become afebrile for at least 24 hours. In uncomplicated pyelonephritis, those female patients with no structural or functional urinary tract abnormalities, oral therapy can be initiated and continued to complete a 14-day course.[32] When upper tract infection is complicated by abscesses, more prolonged therapy (2–3 weeks) and drainage may be necessary. Follow-up urine cultures should be obtained 2 weeks after the completion of therapy to ensure a satisfactory response and to detect possible relapse.

Urinary Tract Infections in Males

The management of urinary tract infections in males is distinctly different and often more difficult than in females. Infections in male patients are considered to be complicated because they are caused by endogenous bacteria in the presence of an abnormality that disrupts the normal defense mechanisms of the urinary tract.[48] The incidence of infections in males less than 60 years of age is much less than that in females. During the adult years, the occurrence of infection can be directly related to some manipulation of the urinary tract. The most common causes are instrumentation of the urinary tract, catheterization, and renal and urinary stones. Uncomplicated infections are rare, but may occur in young males as a result of homosexual activity, lack of circumcision, and having sex with partners who are colonized with uropathogenic bacteria.[32] As the patient ages, the most common cause of infection is related to bladder outlet obstruction due to prostatic hypertrophy. In addition, the prostate gland may become infected and provide a source of recurrent infection in males.

The conventional view is that therapy in males requires prolonged treatment (Fig. 109.2). A urine culture should be obtained before treatment because the cause of infection in men is not as predictable as in women. Single-dose therapy is not recommended in this setting. Considerably less data are available comparing various antimicrobial agents in males as compared to females. If gram-negative bacteria are presumed, trimethoprim–sulfamethoxazole or trimethoprim is a preferred agent due to its ability to achieve high renal tissue and prostatic concentrations. If a resistant organism is suspected, a fluoroquinolone such as ciprofloxacin or norfloxacin should be considered. Initial therapy should be for 10–14 days. Factors associated with treatment success are isolation of a single organism, the absence of significant obstruction or anatomic abnormalities, a normally functioning urinary tract, and the absence of prostatic involvement. Parenteral therapy may be required in certain situations, such as severely ill patients, presence of acute prostatitis or epididymitis, and patients who cannot tolerate oral medications. Comparison of 2-week therapy versus 6-week therapy with trimethoprim–sulfamethoxazole in recurrent infections in males found cure rates to be 29% and 62%, respectively.[72] Others have advocated longer treatment periods in males, as well.[73] Follow-up cultures at 4–6 weeks after treatment are important in males to ensure bacteriologic cure. Many patients will require longer periods of treatment and possible alterations in antibiotics depending on culture and sensitivity results and clinical response.

RECURRENT INFECTIONS

Recurrent episodes of urinary tract infection account for a significant portion of all UTIs. Of those patients suffering from recurrent infections, 80% can be considered reinfections, that is, recurrence of infection by an organism different than that isolated from the preceding infection. These patients are most commonly females and can be divided into two groups: (1) those with less than two or three episodes per year and (2) those who develop more frequent infections.

Management strategies depend on the predisposing factors, number of episodes per year, and the patient's preference. Therapeutic options include self-administered therapy, postcoital therapy, and continuous low-dose prophylaxis. In those patients with infrequent infections, less than three infections per year, each episode should be treated as a separately occurring infection. Single-dose or short-course therapy should be used in symptomatic female patients with lower tract infection. Many women have been successfully treated with self-administered short-course therapy at the onset of symptoms.[74] Factors that have been commonly associated with recurrent infections include sexual intercourse and diaphragm use for birth control.

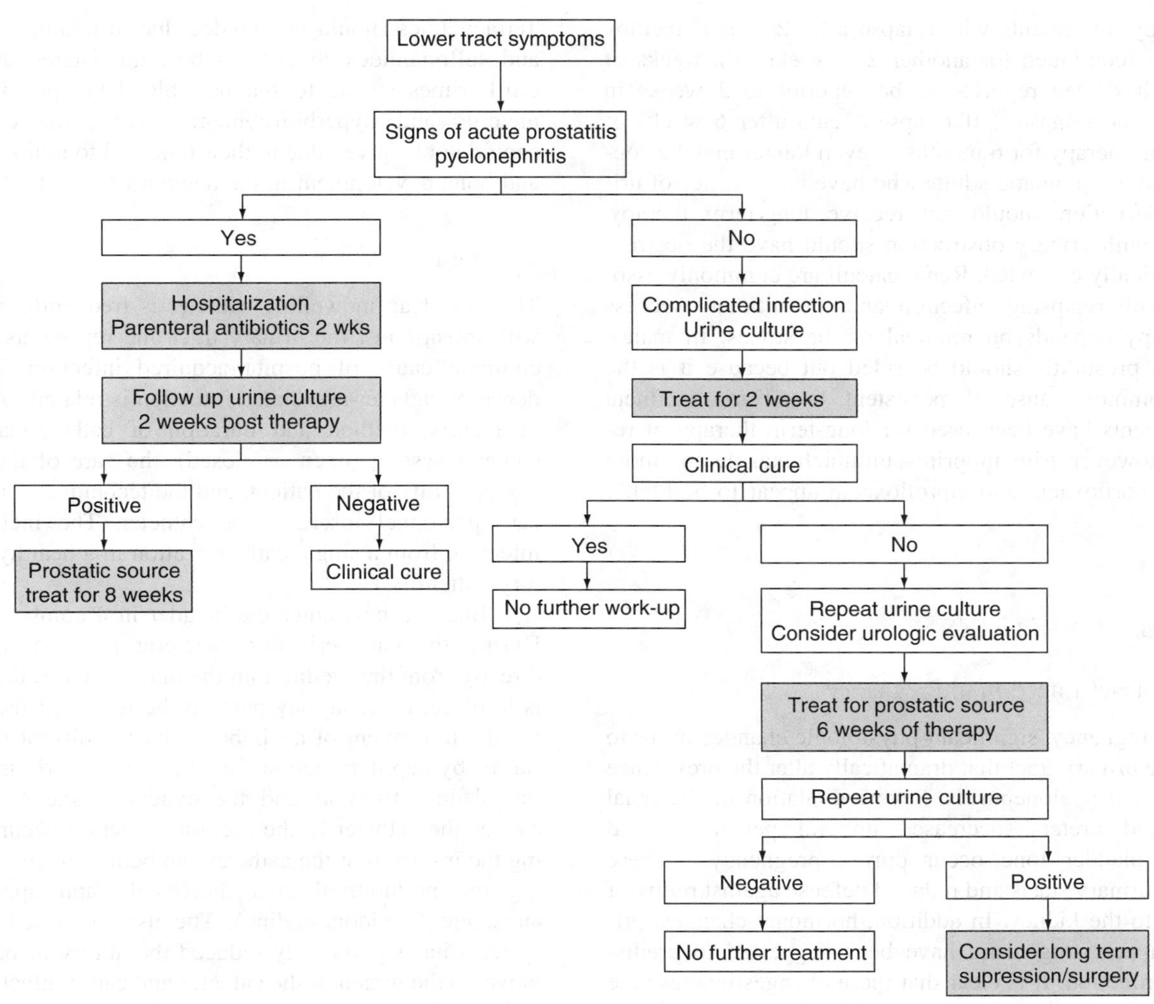

Figure 109.2. Management of urinary tract infections in males.

In those patients who have frequent symptomatic infections, long-term prophylactic antimicrobial therapy may be instituted. Prophylactic therapy has been found to reduce the frequency of symptomatic infections in elderly men, women, and children.[75] In women, most studies have shown a reinfection rate of 2 to 3 per patient year reduced to 0.1 to 0.2 per patient year with treatment.[76] Trimethoprim (100 mg daily), trimethoprim–sulfamethoxazole (40 mg/200 mg daily), norfloxacin (200 mg daily), and nitrofurantoin (50 or 100 mg daily) have all been found to reduce successfully the rate of reinfection as single-agent therapy.[48] Full-dose therapy with these agents is unnecessary and single daily doses can be utilized. Therapy is generally given for 6–12 months with urine cultures followed periodically. If symptomatic episodes develop, the patient should receive a full course of therapy with an effective agent and be restarted on prophylactic therapy.

In those women who experience symptomatic reinfections in association with sexual activity, voiding after intercourse may help prevent infection. Also, single-dose prophylactic therapy with trimethoprim–sulfamethoxazole taken after intercourse has been found to reduce significantly the incidence of recurrent infection in these patients.[77]

In postmenopausal women with recurrent infections, the lack of estrogen results in changes of the bacterial flora of the vagina, resulting in increased colonization by uropathogenic *E. coli.* Topically administered estrogen cream has been reported to reduce the incidence of infections in this population.[78]

The remaining 20% of recurrent urinary tract infections are relapses, that is, persistence of infection with the same organism after therapy for an isolated UTI. The recurrence of symptomatic or asymptomatic bacteriuria after therapy usually indicates that the patient has renal involvement, a structural abnormality of the urinary tract, or chronic bacterial prostatitis. In the absence of structural abnormalities, relapse is often related to renal infection and requires a longer duration of treatment. Women who relapse after short-course therapy should receive a 2-week course of therapy. In patients who relapse after 2 weeks, therapy should be continued for another 2–4 weeks. Six weeks of therapy has been reported to be superior to 2 weeks in patients who relapse.[79] If relapse occurs after 6 weeks of treatment, therapy for 6 months or even longer may be considered. Asymptomatic adults who have no evidence of urinary obstruction should not receive long-term therapy. Patients with urinary obstruction should have the obstruction surgically corrected. Renal calculi are commonly associated with relapsing infection and the ultimate success of therapy depends on removal of the stones. In males, bacterial prostatitis should be ruled out because it is the most common cause of persistent bacteriuria in men. Many agents have been used for long-term therapy of relapses; however, trimethoprim–sulfamethoxazole and more recently norfloxacin and ciprofloxacin appear to be highly effective.

SPECIAL CONDITIONS

Urinary Tract Infection in Pregnancy

During pregnancy, significant physiologic changes occur to the entire urinary tract that dramatically alter the prevalence of UTIs and pyelonephritis. Severe dilatation of the renal pelvis and ureters, decreased ureteral peristalsis, and reduced bladder tone occur during pregnancy.[80] These result in urinary stasis and reduced defense against reflux of bacteria to the kidney. In addition, hormonal changes, primarily hyperestrogenism, have been suggested to predispose to infection. It is clear that these changes increase the incidence of bacteriuria that can result in symptomatic infections, especially during the third trimester.

It is estimated that asymptomatic bacteriuria occurs in 4–7% of pregnant patients. Of these, 20–40% will develop acute asymptomatic pyelonephritis during pregnancy, while only 1% of patients who are not infected early in pregnancy develop pyelonephritis.[81] An association between UTI in pregnancy and prematurity has been suggested.[80] One study found an increase in the incidence of prematurity and low birth weight in pregnancies complicated by UTI versus those without infection.[82] This study appears to confirm the aforementioned association. In general, although the data that correlate bacteriuria to prematurity are believed to be "soft" by some authors, the association between asymptomatic bacteriuria and the development of pyelonephritis is indisputable. For this reason, quantitative urine cultures should be routinely monitored, especially early in pregnancy. In those patients with significant bacteriuria, symptomatic or asymptomatic, treatment is recommended in order to avoid possible complications during the pregnancy. Therapy should consist of an agent with a relatively low adverse effect potential (a sulfonamide, cephalexin, ampicillin, amoxicillin, nitrofurantoin) administered for 7 days. Tetracyclines should be avoided due to teratogenic effects and sulfonamides should not be administered during the third trimester due to the possible development of kernicterus and hyperbilirubinemia. Also, the quinolones should not be given due to their potential to inhibit cartilage and bone development in the newborn.

Catheterized Patients

The use of an indwelling catheter is frequently associated with infection of the urinary tract and represents the most common cause of hospital-acquired infection. The incidence of catheter-associated infection is related to a variety of factors: method and duration of catheterization, the catheter system (open or closed), the care of the system, susceptibility of the patient, and the technique of the health care personnel inserting the catheter. The incidence of infection from a single catheterization in a healthy ambulatory patient is 1%.[34]

Bacteria may enter the bladder in a number of ways. During the catheterization, bacteria may be introduced directly from the urethra into the bladder. Once the catheter is in place, bacteria may pass up the lumen of the catheter via the movement of air bubbles, by motility of the bacteria, or by capillary action. In addition, bacteria may reach the bladder from around the exudative sheath that surrounds the catheter in the urethra. Infection occurring during the insertion of the catheter can be minimized by cleaning the periurethral area thoroughly and applying an antiseptic (povidone-iodine). The use of closed drainage systems has significantly reduced the ability of bacteria to move up the lumen of the catheter and cause infection. Bacteria passing around the catheter sheath in the urethra is probably the most important pathway for infection. This path of acquisition can be minimized by avoiding manipulation of the catheter and trauma to the urethra and urethral meatus.

The use of an open drainage system, where the urine is collected in an unenclosed receptacle, causes infection in virtually all patients in 4 days.[83] This system has been replaced by the closed drainage system, which has the catheter leading into an enclosed sterile collection receptacle (Fig. 109.3). The closed system is capable of preventing bacteriuria in most patients for up to 10 days.[84] After 30 days of catheterization, however, there is a 78–95% incidence of bacteriuria even with the closed system. When bacteriuria occurs in the asymptomatic, short-term catheterized patient (less than 30 days), the use of systemic antibiotic therapy should be withheld and the catheter removed as soon as possible. If the patient becomes symptomatic, the catheter should again be removed and treatment as described for complicated infections should be started. The optimal duration of therapy has not been elucidated. In the long-term catheterized patient (more than 30 days), bacteriuria is inevitable. The administration of systemic antibiotic

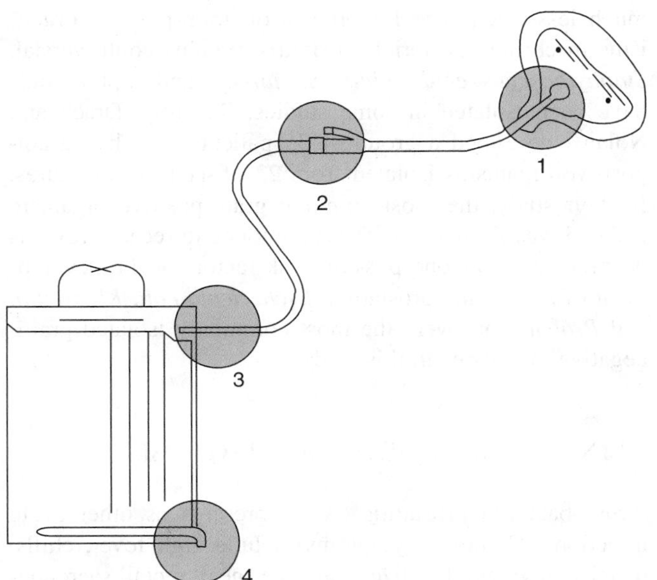

Figure 109.3. Entry points for bacteria. (1) Urethral meatus and around catheter; (2) junction between catheter and collection tube; (3) connection to drainage bag and reflux from bag to tubing; and (4) mouth of the spigot. *(From Kunin CM. Urinary tract infections. Med Clin North Am 1980;60:228, with permission.)*

therapy effective against the infecting organism will sterilize the urine; however, reinfection occurs rapidly in over 50% of patients and often results in the recolonization of the urine with resistant organisms. Symptomatic patients must be treated because they are at risk of developing pyelonephritis and bacteremia. Bacteria have been found to adhere to the catheter and produce a biofilm consisting of bacterial glycocalices, Tamm–Horsfall protein, and apatite and struvite salts which protect the bacteria from antibiotics. Recatheterization with a new, sterile unit should be performed if the existing catheter has been in place for more than 2 weeks.

Various methods have been proposed to prevent the development of bacteriuria and infection in the patient with an indwelling catheter. The success of these methods depends on the type of catheter and the length of time it is in place. The use of constant bladder irrigation with antiseptic or antibacterial solutions has been investigated.[83] The use of these irrigation solutions has been found to reduce the incidence of infection in the open drainage system; however, prospective comparisons in the closed drainage system have not shown any advantage. The use of prophylactic systemic antibiotics in these patients is not recommended. The use of antibiotics in patients with short-term catheterization has been found to reduce the incidence of infection over the first 4–7 days.[83] In long-term catheterized patients, the use of antibiotics only postpones the development of bacteriuria and leads to the emergence of resistance.[85] There is no evidence that antibiotic administration prevents the development of fever or acute pyelonephritis in long-term catheterized patients.

PROSTATITIS

Prostatitis can be defined as any inflammation of the prostate and surrounding tissue. This definition, however, is inadequate because prostatitis constitutes a spectrum of illnesses. It rarely occurs in young males, but is commonly associated with recurrent infections in persons older than 30 years. As many as 50% of all males develop some form of prostatitis at some period in their life.[86] The major difficulty with the management of prostatitis is the long duration of therapy and subsequent failure rates of 30–40%.

In 1978, Drach and colleagues[87] proposed a classification system based on the microscopic examination and culture of prostatic secretions and urine. Their classification scheme divided prostatitis into three main groups: bacterial prostatitis (subclassified as acute or chronic), nonbacterial prostatitis, and prostatodynia. Each of these syndromes is characterized by symptoms, but they differ as to the presence of bacterial growth in prostatic fluid (present in acute and chronic prostatitis), prostatic fluid leukocytosis and fat bodies (all syndromes except prostatodynia) and whether the prostate exam is abnormal (only in acute bacterial prostatitis).

By definition, pathogenic bacteria and significant inflammatory cells must be present in prostatic secretions and urine to make the diagnosis of bacterial prostatitis. The acute form is typically a severe illness characterized by a sudden onset of fever and urinary and constitutional symptoms. Chronic bacterial prostatitis represents a recurring infection with the same organism (relapse) that is the result of the incomplete eradication of bacteria within the prostate gland.

The second syndrome, nonbacterial prostatitis, is typified by the presence of signs and symptoms of infection including excessive inflammatory cells, but where pathogenic bacteria cannot be isolated. These patients typically have no history of previous UTI and have negative prostatic fluid cultures. Finally, prostatodynia is a syndrome in which patients present with the subjective constitutional symptoms of prostatitis, but lack all objective evidence of infection. Prostatic fluid leukocytosis, bacterial growth, and an abnormal prostate exam are absent.

PATHOGENESIS/ETIOLOGY

The exact mechanism of bacterial infection of the prostate is not well understood. The possible routes of infection include (1) ascending infection of the urethra, (2) reflux of infected urine into prostatic ducts, (3) invasion by rectal bacteria through direct extension or lymphatic spread, and (4) by hematogenous spread.

Blacklock[88] initially suggested that some men develop bacterial prostatitis when bacteria ascend the urethra during sexual intercourse. His comparisons of prostatic secretions of men with chronic bacterial prostatitis and the vaginal cultures of their sexual partners revealed that sexual partners grew identical organisms. Recent studies suggest that intraprostatic reflux of urine occurs commonly. This reflux results in direct inoculation of infected urine into the prostate and currently is regarded as the primary pathogenic mechanism of bacterial prostatitis.[89] In addition, intraprostatic reflux of sterile urine can result in a "chemical" prostatitis and may be the cause of nonbacterial prostatitis.[90]

Other known causes of bacterial prostatitis include indwelling urethral and condom catheterization, urethral instrumentation, and transurethral prostatectomy in patients with infected urine.

A number of physiologic factors are believed to contribute to the development of prostatitis. Functional abnormalities found in bacterial prostatitis include altered prostate secretory functions. Prostatic fluid obtained from normal males contains prostatic antibacterial factor (PAF). This heat-stable, low molecular weight cation is a zinc-complexed polypeptide that is bactericidal to most urinary tract pathogens.[91] The antibacterial activity of PAF is directly related to the zinc content of prostatic fluid. Prostate fluid zinc levels and PAF activity also appear diminished in patients with prostatitis as well as the elderly. Whether these changes are a cause or effect of prostatitis remains to be determined.

The pH of prostatic secretions in patients with prostatitis has also been reported to be altered.[92] Normal prostatic secretions have a pH in the range of 6.6–7.6. With increasing age, the pH tends to become more alkaline. In patients with inflammation of the prostate, prostatic secretions have been reported to have an alkaline pH in the range of 7–9. These changes suggest a generalized secretory dysfunction of the prostate, which not only may affect the pathogenesis of prostatitis, but also may influence the mode of therapy.[93]

Although the signs of inflammation are present in nonbacterial prostatitis, urinary pathogens are not found. Several sexually transmitted organisms, including *Chlamydia, Ureaplasma,* and *Trichomonas* have been implicated as nonbacterial pathogens.[94] It is unclear, however, if the isolation of these organisms represents urethral colonization or true prostatic infection.

Gram-negative, enteric organisms are the most frequent pathogens in bacterial prostatitis. *Escherichia coli* is the predominate organism, occurring in 75% of cases. Other gram-negative organisms, including *K. pneumoniae, Proteus mirabilis,* and species of *Pseudomonas, Enterobacter,* and *Serratia* are commonly isolated. Occasionally, cases of gonococcal and staphylococcal prostatitis occur, but are unusual.

Chronic bacterial prostatitis is most commonly caused by *E. coli* with other gram-negative organisms isolated much less often. The importance of gram-positive organisms in chronic bacterial prostatitis remains controversial. *Staphylococcus epidermidis, S. aureus,* and diphtheroids have been isolated in some studies. Recently, Drach and Nolan[95] described a group of 35 patients who had gram-positive organisms isolated from 23 of 41 (56%) cultures. In their study, the most common gram-positive organism isolated was *E. faecalis.* These authors cite recent previous hospitalization as one possible risk factor for the development of *E. faecalis* prostatitis. *Escherichia coli, Klebsiella,* and *Proteus* spp. were the most commonly isolated gram-negative organisms in this study.

CLINICAL PRESENTATION/DIAGNOSIS

Acute bacterial prostatitis (ABP) presents as other acute infections. Common symptoms include high fever, chills, malaise, myalgia, localized pain (perineal, rectal, sacrococcygeal), and other urinary tract symptoms (frequency, urgency, dysuria, nocturia, retention). Digital palpation of the prostate via the rectum may reveal a swollen, tender, warm, tense, or indurated prostate. Massage of the prostate will express a purulent discharge, which will readily grow the pathogenic organism. However, prostatic massage is contraindicated in ABP because of a risk of inducing bacteremia and associated pain.[95] For this reason, quantitative lower tract localization studies involving prostatic massage, like those performed in chronic bacterial prostatitis, are not performed. Instead, the diagnosis of ABP is easily made from the patient's clinical presentation and the presence of significant bacteriuria. As with other urinary tract infections, the infecting pathogen can be isolated from a midstream specimen.

In contrast to acute bacterial prostatitis, chronic bacterial prostatitis (CBP) is more difficult to diagnose and treat. Typically, CBP is characterized by recurrent urinary tract infections with the same pathogen. In fact, CBP is the most common cause of recurrent UTI in males. Although examination of prostate often reveals a normal gland, the patient's clinical presentation can vary widely. Presenting symptoms include the vague description of voiding difficulties such as frequency, urgency, and dysuria, along with low back pain and perineal and suprapubic discomfort. Many patients may be asymptomatic.

Because physical examination of the prostate is often normal, urinary tract localization studies are critical to the diagnosis of CBP. The method of quantitative localization culture, as described by Meares and Stamey,[96] remains the diagnostic standard (Fig. 109.4) Their method clearly aids the clinician in differentiating urethral from true prostatic infection. These localization studies revolve around the comparison of bacterial growth in sequential urine and prostatic fluid cultures obtained during micturition. The first 10 mL of voided urine is collected (voided bladder 1 or VB_1)

and constitutes urethral urine. After approximately 200 mL of urine has been voided, a 10-mL midstream urine sample is collected (VB_2). This specimen represents bladder urine. After the patient voids, the prostate is massaged and expressed prostatic secretions (EPS) are collected. After massage, the patient voids again and the first 10 mL of urine is collected (VB_3).

The unequivocal diagnosis of bacterial prostatitis is made when the number of bacteria in EPS is 10 times that of the urethral sample (VB_1) and the midstream sample (VB_2). If no EPS is available, the urine sample following massage (VB_3) should contain a bacterial count tenfold greater than that of VB_1 or VB_2.

If the bladder urine is infected with greater than 100,000 bacteria per milliliter, the site of infection cannot be localized. The urine should be sterilized with an appropriate antimicrobial agent that does not diffuse into the prostate (e.g., nitrofurantoin 100 mg orally every 8 hours or penicillin G 500 mg orally every 6 hours). After 4–5 days, the localization study should be repeated.

Both acute and chronic bacterial prostatitis are characterized by the presence of numerous WBC and lipid-containing macrophages (oval fat bodies) on microscopic exam of expressed prostatic secretions. The finding of greater than 15 WBCs per high-power field is diagnostic of prostatic inflammation.[97] Oval fat bodies are also indicative of prostatitis, because they are seldom found in healthy men or in men with UTIs from other causes. These findings, however, do not discriminate between bacterial versus nonbacterial causes of prostatitis.

The diagnosis of CBP is made by an accurately performed lower tract localization study as previously described. Histologic changes occurring in CBP are often focal in nature. Therefore, needle biopsy of the prostate gland is unreliable.[98]

TREATMENT

ABP responds well to appropriate antimicrobial therapy. Most antibiotics diffuse well into the acutely inflamed prostate. Prostatic penetration of antimicrobials occurs because the acute inflammatory reaction alters the cellular membrane barrier between the bloodstream and the prostate.

Most patients with ABP respond to empiric therapy with antibiotics specifically directed at the most commonly isolated organisms. If a presumptive diagnosis of ABP is made, a traditional regimen includes a combination of an aminoglycoside with a β-lactam antibiotic (e.g., gentamicin plus ampicillin). Oral or parenteral therapy with trimethoprim–sulfamethoxazole (TMP–SMX) has been advocated by others as initial therapy.[90] If patients are unable to tolerate TMP–SMX, then IV to oral sequential therapy with a fluoroquinolone, such as ciprofloxacin or ofloxacin, would be appropriate. As with other serious infections, the use of a single-drug regimen should be weighed against the severity of clinical presentation, the presence of drug allergies, and the individual risk for aminoglycoside toxicity. To date, well-designed comparative studies of various antibiotic regimens in the treatment of ABP are lacking. For this reason, therapy is often empiric and should be refined as the results of culture and sensitivity studies are known. Parenteral therapy should be maintained until the patient is afebrile and less symptomatic. The conversion to an oral antibiotic can be considered if the patient has responded to 5–7 days of intravenous therapy. The total course of antibiotic therapy should be 4 weeks in order to reduce the risk of development of chronic prostatitis.

Chronic bacterial prostatitis often presents a more vexing situation because cures are rarely obtained. In the past, it was recognized that despite high serum concentrations of

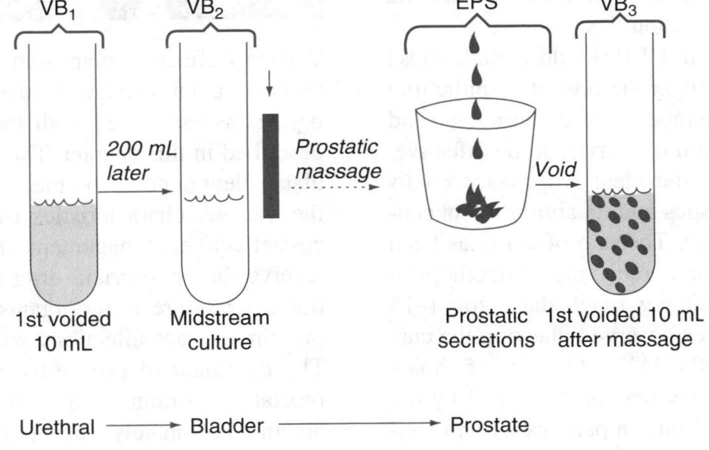

Figure 109.4. Segmented cultures of the lower urinary tract in men. *(From Meares EM Jr, Stamey TA. Bacteriologic localization patterns in bacterial prostatitis and urethritis. Invest Urol 1968;5:492, with permission.)*

bacterial drugs in excess of the minimal inhibitory concentrations (MICs) of the infecting organisms, bacteria (sensitive to the administered antibiotic) persisted in prostatic fluid. The failure to eradicate sensitive bacteria was thought to be related to the inability of antibiotics to reach sufficient concentrations in the prostatic fluid and cross the prostatic epithelium.

In a series of experiments in dogs, Winningham and colleagues[99] assessed the characteristics of diffusion of various antibiotics from plasma into canine prostatic fluid. The results showed that most antibiotics commonly used in the treatment of UTIs did not achieve effective concentrations in the prostatic fluid, even when plasma levels were exceedingly elevated. The only group of antibiotics found to concentrate in prostatic fluid was the macrolides (erythromycin, oleandomycin, rosamicin), trimethoprim, and clindamycin. The concentrations of these antibiotics were found to be several times that in the plasma. From these experiments, it was apparent that most antibiotics could not cross the prostatic epithelium.

Several factors that determine antibiotic diffusion into prostatic secretions were delineated from the canine model. Lipid solubility is a major determinant because only lipid-soluble drugs can diffuse from plasma across epithelial membranes. The degree of ionization in plasma also affects diffusion of drugs. Only un-ionized molecules can cross the lipid barrier of prostatic cells, and the drug's pK_a directly determines the fraction of unchanged drug.

The pH gradient across the membrane has an influence on tissue penetration as well. A pH gradient of at least one pH unit between separate compartments allows for ion trapping. As un-ionized drug crosses the epithelial barrier into prostatic fluid, it becomes ionized, thus allowing less drug to diffuse back across the lipid barrier. In early studies with the canine model, the prostatic pH was reported to be acidic, 6.4. More recent studies in man, however, have reported that the pH of prostatic secretions from the inflamed prostate is actually basic, 8.1–8.3.[92] This is dramatically different from that found in the canine model and affects the diffusing ability of antibiotics.

The choice of antibiotics in CBP should include those agents that are capable of crossing the prostatic epithelium into the prostatic fluid in therapeutic concentrations and which also possess the spectrum of activity to be effective. Trimethoprim was considered the ideal drug based on its favorable chemical characteristics and its ability to concentrate well in the canine prostate. The rate of cure has been only 32–71% among patients receiving trimethoprim 160 mg/sulfamethoxazole 800 mg twice daily for 4–16 weeks.[100–103] The low cure rates observed question the current recommendation that TMP–SMX is the drug of choice for CBP. The low cure rates may best be explained by the finding that the pH of prostatic fluid in patients with prostatitis is actually alkaline. This pH difference may impede the passage of trimethoprim across the prostatic epithelium. The sulfonamide portion of TMP–SMX probably contributes very little to the activity of trimethoprim in CBP.

Carbenicillin indanyl sodium has been reported to have limited efficacy in the treatment of CBP, even though carbenicillin was found not to concentrate in canine prostate. It has been demonstrated, however, that the esterified form of carbenicillin diffuses well into prostatic interstitial fluid and prostatic tissue.[104] Cure rates have been reported to be 60–74% in small, noncomparative clinical trials.[105,106] Carbenicillin is quite costly and currently is recommended only for those patients who have failed therapy with TMP–SMX or a fluoroquinolone.

Although other agents, including clindamycin, erythromycin, and tetracycline, penetrate well into prostatic tissues, they are of limited value in the treatment of CBP because of their inactivity against gram-negative organisms. The one exception may be erythromycin. The activity of erythromycin has been shown to be greatly enhanced against gram-negative organisms in an alkaline environment. Because the inflamed prostatic fluid has an alkaline pH, erythromycin was examined in patients with culture-proven gram-negative CBP. A cure rate of 88% was achieved.[107] Further investigation is required to delineate the role erythromycin may play in the treatment of CBP.

The introduction of the fluoroquinolones represents a major therapeutic advance in the management of bacterial prostatitis. These agents offer several advantages, such as a class-specific mechanism of action (inhibition of DNA gyrase), good prostatic tissue penetrability, and a relative lack of bacterial cross-resistance development. The fluoroquinolones can be used in the β-lactam or sulfonamide allergic or intolerant patient and where the avoidance of an aminoglycoside is desired. Some evidence suggests that the fluoroquinolones may be more effective than TMP–SMX with reported cure rates ranging from 50–90%.[108]

CONCLUSION

The cost-effective management of urinary tract infections requires a knowledge of the pathogenesis and causative organisms associated with the various clinical syndromes described in this chapter. The specific treatment of a particular patient depends on the various host factors present and the various characteristics of the antibiotics. Ultimately, cost-effective management requires that a given patient receive the appropriate drug for his or her clinical condition. As more resistant organisms develop, the management of urinary tract infections will become more challenging. The treatment of prostatitis, particularly chronic bacterial prostatitis, continues to be a clinical problem for the clinician. Fortunately, acute bacterial prostatitis is very amenable to therapy. A main issue for future research is the continued need to assess the comparative efficacy of various antimicrobial regimens in the management of chronic infections and those due to resistant organisms.

References

1. Patton JP, Nash DB, Abrutyn E. Urinary tract infections: Economic considerations. Med Clin North Am 1991;75:495–513.
2. Sanford JP. Urinary tract symptoms and infection. Ann Rev Med 1975;26:485–498.
3. Sanford JP, Favour CB, Mao FH, et al. Evaluation of the positive urine culture. Am J Med 1956;20:88–93.
4. Kass EH. Bacteriuria and the diagnosis of infection of the urinary tract. Arch Intern Med 1957;100:709–714.
5. Platt R. Quantitative definition of bacteriuria. Am J Med 1983;75:44–52.
6. Bartlett RC, Galan RS. Predictive value of urine culture. Am J Clin Pathol 1983;79:756–757.
7. McCracken GH. Diagnosis and management of acute urinary tract infection in infants and children. Pediatr Infect Dis 1987;6:107–112.
8. Randolph MF, Greenfield M. The incidence of asymptomatic bacteriuria and pyuria in infancy. J Pediatr 1964;65:57–66.
9. Huland H, Busch R. Pyelonephritis scarring in 213 patients with upper and lower tract infection: Long-term follow-up. J Urol 1984;132:936–939.
10. Kunin CM. The natural history of recurrent bacteriuria in school girls. N Engl J Med 1970;282:1443–1448.
11. Freedman LR. Natural history of urinary infections in adults. Kidney Int 1975;8(suppl 4):S96–S100.
12. Sobel JD, Kaye D. Urinary tract infection, in Mandell GL, Douglas RG, Bennett JE (eds): Principles and Practice of Infectious Diseases, 3rd ed. New York, Churchill Livingstone, 1990, pp 582–611.
13. Boscia JA, Kobasa WD, Knight RA, et al. Epidemiology of bacteriuria in an elderly ambulatory population. Am J Med 1986;80:208–214.
14. Stamey TA, Timothy M, Millar M, et al. Recurrent urinary infections in adult women: The role of introital enterobacteria. Calif Med 1971;115:1–19.
15. Bran JL, Levison ME, Kaye D. Entrance of bacteria into the female urinary bladder. N Engl J Med 1972;286:626–629.
16. Nicolle LE, Harding GKM, Preiksaitis J, et al. The association of urinary tract infection with sexual intercourse. J Infect Dis 1982;146:579–583.
17. Murphy JJ, Schoenberg HW. The role of the lymphatic system in pyelonephritis. Surg Forum 1960;10:880–883.
18. Kaye D. Antibacterial activity of human urine. J Clin Invest 1968;47:2374–2390.
19. Stamey TA, Fair WR, Timothy MM, et al. Antibacterial nature of prostatic fluid. Nature 1968;218:444–447.
20. Shand DG, Nimmon CC, O'Grady F, et al. Relation between residual urine volume and response to treatment of urinary infection. Lancet 1970;1:1305–1306.
21. Mulholland SG. Lower urinary tract antibacterial defense mechanisms. Invest Med 1979;17:93–97.
22. Parsons CL, Schrom SH, Hanno P, et al. Bladder surface mucin: Examination of possible mechanisms for its antibacterial effect. Invest Urol 1978;6:196–200.
23. Orskov I, Ferencz A, Orskov F. Tamm-Horsfall protein or uromucoid is the normal urinary slime that traps type-1 fimbriated *Escherichia coli.* Lancet 1980;1:887.
24. Riedasch G, Heck P, Rauterberg E, et al. Does low urinary sIgA predispose to urinary tract infection? Kidney Int 1983;23:759–763.
25. Sobel JD. Pathogenesis of urinary tract infections. Infect Dis Clin North Am 1987;1:751–772.
26. Leffler H, Svanborg-Eden C. Glycolipid receptors for uropathogenic *Echerichia coli* binding to human erythrocytes and uroepithelial cells. Infect Immun 1981;34:920–929.
27. Kallenius G, Mollby R, Svenson SB, et al. Occurrence of P-fimbriated *Escherichia coli* in urinary tract infections. Lancet 1981;2:1369–1372.
28. Perry A, Ofek I, Silverblatt FJ. Enhancement of mannose-mediated stimulation of human granulocytes by type-1 fimbriae aggregated with antibodies on *Escherichia coli* surfaces. Infect Immun 1983;39:1334–1335.
29. Svanborg-Eden C, de Man P. Bacterial virulence in urinary tract infection. Infect Dis Clin North Am 1987;1:731–750.
30. Svanborg-Eden C, Gotschlich EC, Korhonen TK, et al. Aspects of structure and function of pili on uropathogenic *E. coli.* Prog Allergy 1983;33:189–202.
31. Smellie JM, Normand KS. Bacteriuria, reflux and renal scarring. Arch Dis Child 1975;50:581–585.
32. Stamm WE, Horton TM. Management of urinary tract infections in adults. N Engl J Med 1993;329:1328–1334.
33. Pezzlo MT. Detection of bacteriuria by automated methods. Lab Med 1984;15:539–543.
34. Turck M, Goffe B, Petersdorf RG. The urethral catheter and urinary tract infections. J Urol 1962;88:834–837.
35. Schaberg DR, Culver DH, Gaynes RP. Major trends in the microbial etiology of nosocomial infection. Am J Med 1991;91(3B):72s–75s.
36. Stamm WE. Measurement of pyuria and its relation to bacteriuria. Am J Med 1983;75:53–58.
37. Thysell H. Evaluation of chemical and microscopical methods for mass detection of bacteriuria. Acta Med Scand 1969;185:393–400.
38. James GP, Paul KL, Fuller JB. Urinary nitrite and urinary tract infection. Am J Pathol 1978;70:671–678.
39. Pels RJ, Bor DH, Woolhandler S, et al. Dipstick urinalysis screening of asymptomatic adults for urinary tract disorders: II. Bacteriuria. JAMA 1989;262:1221–1224.
40. Kass EH. Asymptomatic infections of the urinary tract. Trans Assoc Am Physicians 1956;69:56–64.
41. Stamm WE, Wagner KF, Amsel R, et al. Causes of the acute urethral syndrome in women. N Engl J Med 1980;303:409–415.
42. Kunin CM. Diagnostic methods, in Kunin CM (ed): Detection, Prevention and Management of Urinary Tract Infections, 4th ed. Philadelphia, Lea and Febiger, 1987, pp 195–244.
43. Stamey TA, Govan DE, Palmer JM. The localization and treatment of urinary tract infections: The role of bacterici-

dal urine levels as opposed to serum levels. Medicine 1965;44:1–36.
44. Fairley KF, Bond AG, Brown RB, et al. Simple test to determine the site of urinary tract infection. Lancet 1967;2:427–428.
45. Fairley KF, Carson NE, Gutch RC, et al. Site of infection in acute urinary tract infection in general practice. Lancet 1971;2:615–618.
46. Ronald AR, Cutler RE, Turck M. Effect of bacteriuria on renal concentrating mechanisms. Ann Intern Med 1969;70:723–730.
47. Thomas VC, Forland M. Antibody-coated bacteria in urinary tract infection. Kidney Int 1982;21:1–7.
48. Kunin CM. Management of urinary tract infections, in Kunin CM (ed): Detection, Prevention, and Management of Urinary Tract Infections, 4th ed. Philadelphia, Lea and Febiger, 1987, pp 325–374.
49. Stamey TA, Fair WR, Timothy MM, et al. Serum versus urinary antimicrobial concentrations in cure of urinary tract infections. N Engl J Med 1974;291:1159–1163.
50. Johnson JR, Stamm WE. Urinary tract infections in women: Diagnosis and treatment. Ann Intern Med 1989;111:906–917.
51. Tolkoff-Rubin NE, Rubin RH. Urinary tract infection: Significance and management. Bull NY Acad Med 1986;62:131–148.
52. Fang LT, Tolkoff-Rubin NE, Rubin RH. Efficacy of single dose and conventional amoxicillin therapy in urinary tract infection localized by the antibody-coated bacteria technique. N Engl J Med 1978;298:413–416.
53. Souney P, Polk BF. Single dose antimicrobial therapy for urinary tract infection in women. Rev Infect Dis 1982;4:29–34.
54. Gruneberg RN, Brumfitt W. Single dose treatment of acute urinary tract infection: A controlled trial. Br Med J 1967;3:649–651.
55. Greenberg RN, Sanders CV, Lewis AC, et al. Single dose therapy for urinary tract infection with cefaclor. Am J Med 1981;71:841–845.
56. Stamm WE. Single dose treatment of cystitis. JAMA 1980;244:591–592.
57. Philbrick JT, Bracikowski JP. Single dose antibiotic treatment for uncomplicated urinary infection: Less for less? Arch Intern Med 1985;145:1672–1678.
58. Stamey TA. Recurrent urinary tract infections in female patients: An overview of management and treatment. Rev Infect Dis 1987;9(suppl 2):s195–s208.
59. Fihn SD, Johnson C, Roberts PL, et al. Trimethoprim/sulfamethoxazole for acute dysuria in women: A double-blind, randomized trial of single dose versus 10 day treatment. Ann Intern Med 1988;108:350–357.
60. Sherbotie JR, Cornfield D. Management of urinary tract infections in children. Med Clin North Am 1991;75:327–338.
61. Zhanel GG, Harding GKM, Guay DRP. Asymptomatic bacteriuria. Arch Int Med 1990;150:1389–1396.
62. Platt R. Adverse consequences of symptomatic urinary tract infection in adults. Am J Med 1987;82(suppl 6B):47–52.
63. Dontas AS, Kasviki-Charvati P, Papanayiotou PL, et al. Bacteriuria and survival in old age. N Engl J Med 1981;304:939–943.
64. Evans DA, Kass EH, Hennekens CH, et al. Bacteriuria and subsequent mortality in women. Lancet 1982;1:156–158.
65. Asscher AW, Sussman M, Waters WE, et al. Asymptomatic bacteriuria in the non-pregnant women. II: Response to treatment and follow-up. Br Med J 1969;1:804–806.
66. Boscia JA, Kobasa WD, Knight RA, et al. Therapy versus no therapy for bacteriuria in elderly ambulatory non-hospitalized women. JAMA 1987;257:1067–1071.
67. Nicolle LE, Bjornson J, Harding GKM, et al. Bacteriuria in elderly institutionalized men. N Engl J Med 1983;309:1420–1425.
68. Nicolle LE, Mayhew WJ, Bryan L. Prospective, randomized comparison of therapy and no therapy for asymptomatic bacteriuria in institutionalized women. Am J Med 1987;83:27–33.
69. Gruneberg RN. Antibiotic sensitivities of urinary pathogens, 1971–1982. J Antimicrob Chemother 1984;14:17–23.
70. Stamm WE, McKevitt M, Counts GW. Acute renal infection in women: Treatment with trimethoprim/sulfamethoxazole or ampicillin for 2 or 6 weeks. Ann Intern Med 1987;106:341–345.
71. Bergeron MG, Beauchamp D, Poirier A, et al. Continuous vs. intermittent administration of antimicrobial agents: Tissue penetration and efficacy *in vivo*. Rev Infect Dis 1985;3:84–97.
72. Gleckman R, Crowley M, Natsios GA. Therapy of recurrent invasive urinary tract infection in men. N Engl J Med 1979;301:878–880.
73. Smith JW, Jones SR, Reed WP, et al. Recurrent urinary tract infections in men: Characteristics and response to therapy. Ann Intern Med 1979;91:544–548.
74. Wong ES, McKevitt M, Running K, et al. Management of recurrent urinary tract infection with patient administered single-dose therapy. Ann Intern Med 1985;102:302–307.
75. Freeman RB, Smith WM, Richardson JA, et al. Long-term therapy for chronic bacteriuria in men: U.S. Public Health Service Cooperative Study. Ann Intern Med 1975;83:133–147.
76. Nicolle LE, Ronald AR. Recurrent urinary tract infections in adult women: Diagnosis and treatment. Infect Dis Clin North Am 1987;1:793–806.
77. Vosti K. Recurrent urinary tract infection: Prevention by prophylactic antibiotics after sexual intercourse. JAMA 1975;231:934–940.
78. Raz R, Stamm WE. A controlled trial of intravaginal estriol in postmenopausal women with recurrent urinary tract infections. N Engl J Med 1993;329:753–756.
79. Turck M, Ronald AR, Petersdorf RG. Relapse and reinfection in chronic bacteriuria. II: The correlation between site of infection and pattern of recurrence in chronic bacteriuria. N Engl J Med 1968;278:422–427.
80. Patterson TF, Andriole VT. Bacteriuria in pregnancy. Infect Dis Clin North Am 1987;1:807–822.
81. Krieger JN. Complications and treatment of urinary tract infections during pregnancy. Urol Clin North Am 1986;13:685–693.

82. McGrady GA, Daling JR, Peterson DR. Maternal urinary tract infection and adverse fetal outcomes. Am J Epidemiol 1985;121:377–381.
83. Warren JW. Catheter-associated urinary tract infection. Infect Dis Clin North Am 1987;1:823–854.
84. Schaeffer AJ. Catheter-associated bacteriuria. Urol Clin North Am 1986;13:735–747.
85. Butler HK, Kunin CM. Evaluation of specific antimicrobial therapy in patients while on closed catheter drainage. J Urol 1968;100:567–572.
86. Stamey TA. Pathogenesis and Treatment of Urinary Tract Infections. Baltimore, Williams & Wilkins, 1980.
87. Drach GW, Fair WR, Mears EM, et al. Classification of benign diseases associated with prostatic pain: Prostatitis or prostatodynia? J Urol 1978;120:266.
88. Blacklock NJ. Anatomical factors in prostatitis. Br J Urol 1974;147:807.
89. Kirby RS, Lowe D, Bultitude MI, et al. Intra-prostatic urinary reflux: An aetiological factor in abacterial prostatitis. Br J Urol 1982;54:729.
90. Meares EM. Prostatitis. Med Clin North Am 1991;75:405–424.
91. Fair WR, Couch J, Wehner N. Prostatic antibacterial factor: Identity and significance. Urology 1976;7: 169–177.
92. Pfau A, Perlberg S, Shapiro A. The pH of prostatic fluid in health and disease: Implications of treatment in chronic bacterial prostatitis. J Urol 1978;119:384–387.
93. Fair WR, Crane DB, Schiller N, et al. A reappraisal of treatment in chronic bacterial prostatitis. J Urol 1979;121:437–441.
94. Drach GW. Sexuality and prostatitis: A hypothesis. J Am Vener Dis Assoc 1976;3:87–88.
95. Drach GW, Nolan PE. Chronic bacterial prostatitis: Problems in diagnosis and therapy. Urology 1986;27(suppl):26–30.
96. Meares EM, Stamey TA. Bacteriologic localization patterns in bacterial prostatitis and urethritis. Invest Urol 1968;5:492–518.
97. Schaeffer AJ, Wendel EF, Dunn JK, et al. Prevalence and significance of prostatic inflammation. J Urol 1981;125:215–219.
98. Schmidt JD, Patterson MC. Needle biopsy study of chronic prostatitis. J Urol 1966;96:519–533.
99. Winningham DC, Nemoy NJ, Stamey TA. Diffusion of antibiotics from plasma into prostatic fluid. Nature 1968;219:139–143.
100. Paulson DF, White RD. Trimethoprim–sulfamethoxazole and minocycline hydrochloride in the treatment of culture-proved bacterial prostatitis. J Urol 1978;120:184–185.
101. Meares EM. Long-term therapy of chronic bacterial prostatitis with trimethoprim–sulfamethoxazole. Can Med Assoc J 1975;112(suppl):22s–25s.
102. Drach GW. Trimethoprim/sulfamethoxazole therapy of chronic bacterial prostatitis. J Urol 1974;111:637–639.
103. McGuire EJ, Lytton B. Bacterial prostatitis: Treatment with trimethoprim–sulfamethoxazole therapy of chronic bacterial prostatitis. Urology 1976;7:499–500.
104. Madsen PO, Baumueller A, Hoyme U. Experimental models for determination of antimicrobials in prostatic tissue, interstitial fluid and secretion. Scan J Infect Dis 1978;14(suppl):145–150.
105. Oliveri RA, Sachs RM, Caste PG. Clinical experience with geocillin in the treatment of bacterial prostatitis. Curr Ther Res 1979;25:415–421.
106. Mobley DF. Bacterial prostatitis: Treatment with carbenicillin indanyl sodium. Invest Urol 1981;19:31–33.
107. Mobley DF. Erythromycin plus sodium bicarbonate in chronic bacterial prostatitis. Urology 1974;2:60–62.
108. Naber KG. Use of quinolones in urinary tract infections and prostatitis. Rev Infect Dis 1989;2(suppl 5):s1321–s1337.

Chapter 110

Sexually Transmitted Diseases

Leroy C. Knodel, PharmD, and Maura A. Kraynak, PharmD

Over the years the spectrum of sexually transmitted diseases (STDs) has broadened from the classic venereal diseases—gonorrhea, syphilis, chancroid, lymphogranuloma venereum, and granuloma inguinale—to include a variety of pathogens known to be spread by sexual contact (Table 110.1).[1,2] *Chlamydial trachomatis* infections, genital herpes, cytomegalovirus infections, genital mycoplasmas, group B streptococcal infections, hepatitis, nonspecific vaginitis, enteric infections, genital warts, ectoparasitic diseases, and the acquired immune deficiency syndrome (AIDS) are now recognized as diseases for which sexual contact is epidemiologically important. Although most of these conditions have probably existed since antiquity, improvement in diagnostic capabilities and epidemiologic investigations have increased their recognition. Because of the large number of infected individuals, the diversity of clinical manifestations, and the high frequency of multiple STDs occurring simultaneously in infected individuals, the diagnosis and management of patients with STDs are much more complex than even a decade ago. Unfortunately, no single-dose antibiotic is available for eradicating more than one STD at a time. As a result, patients often require multiple antibiotics during a treatment course.

Despite a higher reported incidence of all major STDs in men, the complications of STDs generally are more frequent and severe in women. In particular, serious effects on maternal and infant health during pregnancy are well documented. Damage to reproductive organs, increased risk of cancer, complications associated with pregnancy, and transmission of disease to the fetus or newborn are associated with several STDs. As a result of the physiologic, psychosocial, and economic consequences of STDs, and because of the increasing incidence of STDs such as AIDS and genital herpes for which curative therapy is not available, there has been a resurgence of interest in STD research and the primary prevention of these diseases.[3]

With the exception of AIDS, which is reviewed in detail in Chapter 117, the most frequently occurring STDs in the United States are discussed in this chapter. For other less common STDs, only recommended treatment regimens are presented.

Epidemiology

Numerous interrelated factors contribute to the epidemic nature of sexually transmitted diseases. Sociocultural, demographic, and economic factors together with patterns of sexual behavior, host susceptibility to infection, changing properties of the causative pathogens, and environmental factors are important determinants of the frequency and distribution of STDs in the United States and worldwide. In the United States, accurate data on the incidence and distribution of STDs are incomplete because many of these diseases are not reportable. Even for those that are required to be reported, such as gonorrhea and syphilis, surveys indicate that gross underreporting occurs.[2,3]

Because of the heterogeneous nature of STDs, factors influencing their incidence or spread are not always consistent among the individual diseases; however, some uniformity occurs with the major STDs when various demographic factors are evaluated. Age is one of the most important demographic determinants of STD incidence. Overall, two-thirds of STD cases each year occur in persons in their teens and twenties, the peak years of sexual activity. With increasing age, the incidence of most STDs decreases exponentially. In sexually active teenagers, STD rates are highest in the youngest, suggesting that physiologic differences may contribute to their susceptibility. For some STDs such as gonorrhea, changing age demographics in the United States appear to have contributed to recent declines in their incidence.[2,4]

Age-specific rates of STDs are higher in men than in women; however, reported rates may not represent true gender differences, but rather may reflect greater ease of detection in men. For many STDs the clinical manifestations are more obvious in men, resulting in a greater percentage seeking confirmatory diagnosis and treatment. In recent years, the ratio of male to female cases for most

TABLE 110.1. SEXUALLY TRANSMITTED DISEASES

Disease	Pathogen
Bacterial	
Gonorrhea	*Neisseria gonorrhoeae*
Syphilis	*Treponema pallidum*
Chancroid	*Haemophilus ducreyi*
Granuloma inguinale (donovanosis)	*Calymmatobacterium granulomatis*
Salmonellosis	*Salmonella* sp.
Shigellosis	*Shigella* sp.
Campylobacter infection	*Campylobacter jejuni*
Nonspecific vaginitis	*Trichomonas vaginalis, Gardnerella vaginalis*
Group B streptococcal infections	Group B streptococcus
Chlamydial	
Nongonococcal urethritis	*Chlamydia trachomatis*
Lymphogranuloma venereum	*C. trachomatis*
Viral	
Herpes genitalis	Herpes simplex virus
Hepatitis B	Hepatitis B virus
Condylomata acuminata	Human papilloma virus
Molluscum contagiosum	Poxvirus
Cytomegalovirus infection	Cytomegalovirus
Mycoplasmal	
Nongonococcal urethritis	*Ureaplasma urealyticum*
Protozoal	
Trichomoniasis	*T. vaginalis*
Amebiasis	*Entamoeba histolytica*
Giardiasis	*Giardia lamblia*
Fungal	
Candidiasis	*Candida albicans*
Parasitic	
Scabies	*Sarcoptes scabiei*
Pediculosis	*Pediculus pubis*
Enterobiasis	*Enterobius vermicularis*

STDs has declined. Major reasons proposed for this change appear to be improvement in diagnosis of STDs in asymptomatic women and changes in female sexual behavior following the availability of improved methods of contraception. Interestingly, STDs rarely occur in lesbian women, despite the use of inanimate objects for sexual arousal.[2,4]

Rates for many STDs are higher in blacks and Hispanics than whites, and are lowest in Orientals; however, genital herpes is a common STD that has a disproportionately higher incidence in whites than blacks. Although not well studied, it is possible that race/ethnic disparities are related to socioeconomic differences.[2,4]

Sexual preference also plays a major role in the transmission of STDs. For all major STDs, rates are disproportionately greater in homosexual men than in heterosexuals. Also, a number of less common STDs, including several caused by enteric protozoans and bacterial pathogens, occur primarily in homosexual men. The major risk factors for homosexual men appear to be related to the greater number of sexual partners and the sexual practices of unprotected anal–genital and oral–anal intercourse.[2,4]

Marital status, socioeconomic status, and place of residence also are epidemiologically important when considering STDs. Sexually transmitted diseases are more common among single, separated, and divorced persons than among married individuals. Also, morbidity rates are highest among individuals of the lowest socioeconomic status and among urban populations.[2,4]

Some of the most serious sequelae of STDs are associated with congenital or perinatal infections. The majority of neonatal infections are acquired at birth, after infant passage through an infected cervix or vagina. Neonatal *C. trachomatis, Neisseria gonorrhoeae,* and herpes simplex virus (HSV) infections are associated with this type of spread. For pregnant women with syphilis, infection is usually transmitted transplacentally, producing a congenital infection. Depending on the organism, neonatal infections can manifest in a variety of ways. Ophthalmia neonatorum can result from chlamydial or gonorrheal infections, while syphilis and herpes infections can produce more severe complications including neurologic impairment. Neonatal herpes infections also are associated with a high mortality.

Prevention and Control Guidelines

Educating persons at risk of acquiring an STD and attempting to reduce transmission rates is a responsibility of all health professionals. By detecting disease in asymptomatic individuals and in people unlikely to seek treatment, transmission rates can decrease significantly. Another important area of prevention and control of STDs is through the evaluation, treatment, and counseling of sexual partners of persons diagnosed with an STD. It is important to remember to target prevention programs at all populations—adolescents, pregnant women, homosexuals, and heterosexuals.

Other than complete abstinence, the most effective way to prevent STD transmission is by using condoms with each act of sexual intercourse. When used correctly and consistently, latex condoms with or without spermicide are more effective in protecting against STD transmission than other condoms. Recently marketed, the female condom is a lubricated polyurethane sheath with a diaphragm-like ring on each end. When inserted into the vagina, it can act as a mechanical barrier to viruses, including the human immunodeficiency virus (HIV). The female condom may provide an alternative protective device for women with male sexual partners who do not desire to use a condom, although only prevention of trichomoniasis transmission is currently documented. Vaginal spermicides can reduce the risk for cervical chlamydia and gonorrhea, and some evidence exists that diaphragms may protect against cervical gonorrheal, chlamydial, and trichomonal infections. While vaginal spermicides and diaphragms may confer some protection to women, their effect on preventing transmission of disease to men has not been evaluated.[4]

Partners of individuals diagnosed with an STD should be notified, examined, and treated if necessary, regardless of the appearance of symptoms. Reporting syphilis, gonorrhea, and AIDS cases to local health departments not only fulfills statutory requirements, but assists in the identification of sexual partners of STD-diagnosed patients.

The varied spectrum of clinical syndromes produced by common STDs is determined not only by the etiologic pathogen(s), but also by differences in male and female anatomy and reproductive physiology. For many STDs the signs and symptoms overlap sufficiently to prevent accurate diagnosis without microbiologic confirmation. Frequently, symptoms are minimal or absent despite the presence of infection.[4] Common clinical syndromes associated with STDs are listed in Table 110.2.[4]

Gonorrhea

Neisseria gonorrhoeae is a gram-negative diplococcus responsible for an estimated 1 million infections per year in the United States.[5] Humans are the only known natural host of this intracellular parasite.[6–9] Because of its rapid incubation period and the large number of infected individuals with asymptomatic disease, gonorrhea is difficult to control. It is estimated that reported cases may represent only half of all cases diagnosed and treated.[6–10] The incidence of gonorrheal infections changes seasonally, with a higher reported number of cases occurring in the summer than in the winter or spring.

Gonorrheal infections occur 10 times more frequently in nonwhites than whites. Other risk factors characteristic of patients with *N. gonorrhoeae* include low socioeconomic status, urban residence, unmarried marital status, and a previous history of gonorrheal infection. In addition, prostitution and illicit drug use continue to be associated with a higher incidence of gonorrhea as well as other STDs.[10]

The risk of a male acquiring a urethral infection after a single episode of vaginal intercourse with an infected female is approximately 20–35% and increases dramatically with multiple exposure. It is believed that the risk of transmission is greater from males to females than females to males. No data are available on the risk of transmission after other types of sexual contact.[6–9]

On contact with a mucosal surface lined by columnar, cuboidal, or noncornified squamous epithelial cells, the gonococci attach to cell membranes by means of surface pili and are then pinocytosed. The virulence of the organism is mediated primarily by the presence of pili and other outer membrane proteins. Once mucosal damage is established, polymorphonuclear leukocytes invade the tissue, submucosal abscesses form, and purulent exudates are secreted.[10,11]

CLINICAL PRESENTATION

The clinical presentation of gonorrheal infections is varied. Infected individuals may be symptomatic or asymptomatic, have complicated or uncomplicated infections, and have infections involving several anatomic sites. Urethritis is the most common presenting manifestation in males, and usually develops within 2–8 days of exposure. Dysuria and urinary frequency are seen initially, followed in 1–2 days by a profuse, purulent urethral discharge. In approximately 25% of cases, the discharge is scant and only minimally purulent, making it almost indistinguishable from nongonococcal urethritis. Because most men seek treatment from discomforting symptoms, complications resulting from extension of the infection in males, such as epididymitis, prostatitis, inguinal lymphadenopathy, and urethral stricture, rarely are seen today. The majority of symptomatic patients who are not treated become asymptomatic within 6 months, with only a few becoming asymptomatic carriers of the disease.[6–9]

The most common site of gonococcal infection in women is the endocervical canal. Anterior spread of infected vaginal secretions produces urethritis. The incuba-

TABLE 110.2. SELECTED SYNDROMES ASSOCIATED WITH COMMON SEXUALLY TRANSMITTED PATHOGENS

Syndrome	Commonly Implicated Pathogens	Common Clinical Manifestations[a]
Urethritis	*Chlamydia trachomatis,* herpes simplex virus, *Neisseria gonorrhoeae, Trichomonas vaginalis, Ureaplasma urealyticum*	Urethral discharge, dysuria
Epididymitis	*C. trachomatis, N. gonorrhoeae*	Scrotal pain, inguinal pain, flank pain, urethral discharge
Cervicitis/vulvovaginitis	*C. trachomatis, Gardnerella vaginalis,* herpes simplex virus, human papilloma virus, *N. gonorrhoeae, T. vaginalis*	Abnormal vaginal discharge, vulvar itching/irritation, dysuria, dyspareunia
Genital ulcers (painful)	*Haemophilus ducreyi,* herpes simplex virus	Usually multiple vesicular/pustular (herpes) or papular/pustular *(H. ducreyi)* lesions that may coalesce; painful, tender lymphadenopathy[b]
Genital ulcers (painless)	*Treponema pallidum*	Usually single papular lesion
Genital warts	Human papilloma virus	Multiple lesions ranging in size from small papular warts to large exophytic condylomas
Pharyngitis	*C. trachomatis* (?), herpes simplex virus, *N. gonorrhoeae*	Symptoms of acute pharyngitis, cervical lymphadenopathy, fever[c]
Proctitis	*C. trachomatis,* herpes simplex virus, *N. gonorrhoeae, T. pallidum*	Constipation, anorectal discomfort, tenesmus, mucopurulent rectal discharge
Salpingitis	*C. trachomatis, N. gonorrhoeae*	Lower abdominal pain, purulent cervical or vaginal discharge, adnexal swelling, fever[d]

[a]For some syndromes, clinical manifestations may be minimal or absent.
[b]Recurrent herpes infection may manifest as a single lesion.
[c]Most cases of pharyngeal gonococcal infection are asymptomatic.
[d]Salpingitis increases the risk of subsequent ectopic pregnancy and infertility.

tion period is more variable in females but symptoms typically appear within 10 days following exposure. Symptoms are relatively nonspecific and include dysuria, urinary frequency, abnormal vaginal discharge, and abnormal uterine bleeding. Diagnosis based on symptoms alone is confounded because infection with other organisms may produce similar manifestations. The majority of gonococcal urethral or cervical infections in females are either asymptomatic or produce minimal symptoms.[6–10]

Other sites of gonococcal infection include the rectum, oropharynx, and eye. Anorectal gonococcal infections are common in females and in homosexual males. In homosexuals rectal intercourse is the primary cause, whereas most infections in women are due to perineal contamination with vaginal discharge. Many patients with anorectal gonorrhea have minimal if any symptoms. When present, symptoms range from mild pruritis to severe rectal pain, tenesmus, and a mucopurulent rectal discharge.[6–9]

Like rectal infections, pharyngeal infections are more common in females and homosexual males. Symptoms can mimic pharyngitis or tonsillitis, although patients are typically asymptomatic. Gonococcal conjunctivitis is rare and usually results from autoinoculation via the fingers from an anogenital infection.[6–9] As a result of the nonspecific signs and symptoms, many women do not seek treatment until after the development of serious complications such as pelvic inflammatory disease (PID). Approximately 15% of women with gonorrhea develop PID. Left untreated, PID can be an indirect cause of infertility and ectopic pregnancies. In 0.5–3.0% of patients with gonorrhea, the gonococci invade the bloodstream and produce disseminated disease. Disseminated gonorrhea infection (DGI) is three times more common in women than in men. The usual clinical manifestations of DGI are tender necrotic skin lesions, tenosynovitis, and monoarticular arthritis. Occasionally, mild hepatitis, myocarditis, and endocarditis occur; very rarely, gonococcal meningitis is reported. A third-generation cephalosporin such as ceftriaxone, ceftizoxime, or cefotaxime should initially be used for all DGI cases until results of sensitivity testing are available.[4,6–12]

DIAGNOSIS

Diagnosis of gonococcal infections can be made by Gram-stained smears, culture, or newer methods based on the detection of cellular components of the gonococcus (e.g., enzymes, antigens, DNA, or lipopolysaccharide) in clinical specimens. Various stains have been used to identify gonococci microscopically, with the Gram stain most widely used in clinical practice. Gram-stained smears are positive for gonococci when gram-negative diplococci of typical kidney bean morphology are identified within polymorphonuclear leukocytes. In the presence of equivocal smears (e.g., extracellular gonococcal forms that can be nonpathogenic, commensal *Neisseria,* or gram-negative diplococci of atypical morphology), a culture is mandatory. In urethral smears from men with symptomatic urethritis, the smear is highly sensitive and specific, and culture is considered optional. Gram-stained smears are specific but insensitive for endocervical, rectal, cutaneous, and asymptomatic male urethral infections. In these situations, culture is the most reliable means of diagnosis. Because of the presence of nonpathogenic *Neisseria* in the pharynx of most people, the Gram stain is not useful in the diagnosis of pharyngeal infection.[6–9]

Culture is considered the most reliable means of diagnosing gonococcal infections. Anatomic sites to be cultured depend on the individual's sexual preferences and body areas exposed. In women, because the urethra and other sites are rarely the sole locus of infection, cervical cultures produce the highest yield and are frequently performed in conjunction with rectal cultures. Urethral cultures are recommended in women who have had hysterectomies and in heterosexual men. In homosexual males, anorectal cultures generally produce the highest yields, and pharyngeal and urethral cultures are considered optional.[6–9]

Because technical constraints and cost preclude the use of culture techniques in most office settings and clinics, alternative methods of diagnosis have been developed that do not require convenient accessibility to a microbiology laboratory. These rapid diagnostic tests, which can be performed easily in an office, are based on detection of gonococcal antigens, enzymes, DNA, endotoxin, or lipopolysaccharide in clinical specimens. In most cases the tests do not have increased sensitivity or specificity over either Gram stain for symptomatic gonococcal urethritis in men or culture in women with endocervical infections. For gonococcal infections other than symptomatic urethritis in males, these tests may prove a more rapid means of diagnosis than culture. Various serologic tests detect antibody to *N. gonorrhoeae* or its components, but most are not sufficiently sensitive or specific to be clinically useful at present. In areas where penicillinase-producing strains of *N. gonorrhoeae* are prevalent, β-lactamase testing is an important consideration once the diagnosis of gonococcal infection is established. Testing usually is done using iodometric, acidometric, or chromogenic cephalosporin disk testing.[6–9]

TREATMENT

Penicillins, cephalosporins, tetracyclines, macrolides, rifampin, and the fluoroquinolones exhibit good activity *in vitro* against most strains of *N. gonorrhoeae.* Although sulfonamides and penicillin have been used in the treatment of gonorrhea, widespread resistance has developed during the past 30 years. Initially, chromosomally mediated resistant *N. gonorrhoeae* (CMRNG) strains exhibiting low-level penicillin resistance were isolated; subsequently, similar trends were noted with tetracyclines, spectinomycin, and other antibiotics. To circumvent this low-level resistance, higher doses of antibiotics and the concomitant use of probenecid with penicillin became standard.[6–8,13]

In the 1970s, penicillinase-producing strains of *N. gonorrhoeae* (PPNG) that demonstrated absolute resistance to penicillins secondary to plasmid-mediated production of β-lactamase were isolated. Today, penicillinase-producing strains are widespread throughout the world and constitute a significant percentage of all strains. Subsequently an increasing number of tetracycline-resistant strains of *N. gonorrhoeae* (TRNG) were identified and by the late 1980s these strains accounted for up to 15–20% of isolates in some parts of the United States.[5–7,9–12]

Many antimicrobial regimens are effective in treating uncomplicated gonorrhea; however, no single therapeutic regimen can be recommended as optimal because of regional differences in susceptibility and the high incidence of coexistent infections (particularly *C. trachomatis*) in certain populations. Since 1989 the Centers for Disease Control and Prevention (CDC) recommendations no longer include penicillins or tetracyclines in either the regimens of choice or alternative regimens for gonorrhea treatment. All currently recommended regimens are single-dose treatments with various oral or parenteral cephalosporins and fluoroquinolones (Table 110.3). Each of these agents has demonstrated efficacy in infections caused by CMRNG, PPNG, and TRNG strains.

Coexisting chlamydial infection, which is documented in up to 45% of individuals with gonorrhea, constitutes the major cause of postgonococcal urethritis, cervicitis, and salpingitis in patients treated for gonorrhea. As a result concomitant treatment with doxycycline or azithromycin is recommended in all patients treated for gonorrhea. Alone, none of the single-dose regimens recommended for gonorrhea is effective against chlamydia. Although previous CDC guidelines recommended the use of 250 mg of ceftriaxone, clinical experience indicates that 125 mg effectively eliminates *N. gonorrhoeae* and does not increase the risk for ceftriaxone-resistant strains.[6,12–15] The lower dosage regimen is less expensive and allows for a smaller volume to be injected into the deltoid muscle. However, vials containing less than 250 mg are unavailable at this time, and ceftriaxone remains an expensive alternative to oral antibiotic therapy.

Although oral therapy offers a promising alternative to the expense and pain associated with parenteral therapy, it may not be preferred for all cases of gonorrhea. Of the regimens of choice, only ceftriaxone is effective in eradicating both gonorrhea and incubating syphilis. Although no strains resistant to cefixime or the fluoroquinolones have been reported in the United States, ciprofloxacin-resistant strains of *N. gonorrhoeae* have been isolated in Asia and North America. Both ciprofloxacin 250 mg and 500 mg are safe

TABLE 110.3. TREATMENT OF GONORRHEA

Type of Infection	Recommended Regimen[a]	Alternative Regimen
Uncomplicated urethral, endocervical, rectal, proctitis, or epididymitis infection in adults[b,c]	Ceftriaxone 125 mg IM once; or ciprofloxacin 500 mg PO once; or cefixime 400 mg PO once; or ofloxacin 400 mg PO once plus A treatment regimen for presumptive *C. trachomatis* coinfection (see Table 110.5)	Spectinomycin 2 g IM once; or ceftizoxime 500 mg IM once; or cefotetan 1 g IM once; or cefoxitin 2 g IM once; or cefuroxime axetil 1 g PO once; or cefpodoxime proxetil 200 mg PO once; or lomefloxacin 400 mg PO once; or enoxacin 400 mg PO once; or norfloxacin 800 mg PO once plus A treatment regimen for presumptive *C. trachomatis* coinfection (see Table 110.5)
Gonococcal infections in pregnancy	Ceftriaxone 125 mg IM once[d,e] plus Erythromycin base 500 mg PO 4 times daily for 7 days	Spectinomycin 2.0 g IM once plus A treatment regimen for presumptive *C. trachomatis* coinfection (see Table 110.5)
Disseminated gonococcal infection in adults (>45 kg)[e,f,g,h]	Ceftriaxone 1 g IM or IV every 24 hours	Ceftizoxime 1 g IV every 8 hours or Cefotaxime 1 g IV every 8 hours until all symptoms resolve or Spectinomycin 2 g IM every 12 hours
Disseminated gonococcal infection in infants[i]	Ceftriaxone 25–50 mg/kg IV or IM once daily for 7 days or Cefotaxime 25 mg/kg IV or IM twice daily for 7 days	
Uncomplicated urethritis, vulvovaginitis, cervicitis, pharyngitis, or proctitis infection in children (<45 kg)	Ceftriaxone 125 mg IM once[j]	Spectinomycin 40 mg/kg IM once (not to exceed 2 g)
Gonococcal conjunctivitis	Ceftriaxone 1 g IM once[k]	
Ophthalmia neonatorum	Ceftriaxone 25–50 mg/kg IV or IM once (not to exceed 125 mg)	
Infants born to mothers with gonococcal infection (prophylaxis)	Ceftriaxone 25–50 mg/kg IV or IM (not to exceed 125 mg)	

[a] Recommendations are those of the CDC.
[b] Treatment failures are usually due to reinfection and necessitate patient education and sex-partner referral; additional treatment regimens for gonorrhea and chlamydia infections should be administered. Epididymitis should be treated for 10 days (see Table 110.5).
[c] Patients allergic to β-lactams should receive a quinolone. Persons unable to tolerate a β-lactam (penicillin or cephalosporin) or a quinolone should receive spectinomycin.
[d] Another recommended IM or PO cephalosporin also may be used.
[e] The fluoroquinolones, doxycycline, and erythromycin ethyl succinate are contraindicated during pregnancy.
[f] Patients treated with one of the recommended regimens should be treated with doxycycline or azithromycin for possible coexistent chlamydial infection.
[g] Patients with gonococcal meningitis should be treated for 10–14 days and those with endocarditis for at least 4 weeks with ceftriaxone 1–2 g IV every 12 hours.
[h] Treatment regimen should be continued for 24–48 hours after improvement begins and switched to cefixime 400 mg PO twice daily or ciprofloxacin 500 mg 2 times a day to complete a week of therapy.
[i] Treatment for 10–14 days is required if meningitis is present.
[j] Patients with bacteremia or arthritis should receive ceftriaxone 50 mg/kg (maximum 1 g) IM or IV once daily for 7 days. Patients with meningitis should be treated for 10–14 days, with a daily dose of ceftriaxone not to exceed 2 g.
[k] The eye should be lavaged one time with saline solution.

and effective for gonorrhea at all sites, but the 500 mg dose is recommended to minimize development of quinolone resistance. Ofloxacin is useful in eradicating both *N. gonorrhoeae* and *C. trachomatis;* however, different dosage regimens are required for each pathogen and it is unknown if the lower, multiple daily dosing regimen used in chlamydial infections is effective in eradicating gonorrheal infections.

Spectinomycin is still the preferred alternative for patients unable to tolerate the recommended cephalosporin or fluoroquinolone regimens. Some strains of PPNG resistant to spectinomycin have been reported. This resistance appears to be chromosomally mediated rather than plasmid mediated, and can be overcome with higher doses. Unlike ceftriaxone, spectinomycin is ineffective in pharyngeal gonorrhea. Pregnant women infected with *N. gonorrhoeae* should be treated with either a cephalosporin or spectinomycin since fluoroquinolones are contraindicated. Although not extensively studied, other effective alternative treatment regimens against PPNG and against PPNG resistant to spectinomycin include single doses of the cephalosporins cefoxitin, cefotaxime, cefotetan, or ceftizoxime, and several fluoroquinolones. Other cephalosporin alternatives include the oral agents cefuroxime axetil and cefpodoxime proxetil, but their antigonococcal activity is less than that of cefixime. Other antibiotics of proven efficacy in gonococcal infections are carbenicillin, rifampin, chloramphenicol, and some aminoglycosides; however, none of the antibiotics offers important advantages over other more commonly used agents.[6,12–14]

Ceftriaxone is the recommended therapy for DGI, gonococcal meningitis, endocarditis, and for any type of gonococcal infection in children. Parenteral therapy is suggested for children primarily because oral regimens have not been adequately studied. Ceftriaxone is preferred in homosexual males because of its efficacy in rectal, pharyngeal, and urethral gonorrhea. In cases of DGI, patients should be hospitalized and treated initially with either ceftriaxone, ceftizoxime, or cefotaxime. Although marked improvement is usually noted within 48 hours of initiating therapy, treatment should be continued as an outpatient with a 7-day course of either cefixime or ciprofloxacin. Children and pregnant or lactating women should not receive ciprofloxacin due to the concern for bone and joint disorders. Analgesics may be necessary in patients with joint involvement.[6,13,14]

Gonococcal ophthalmia is highly contagious in adults and neonates and requires intramuscular ceftriaxone therapy. Single-dose therapy is adequate for gonococcal conjunctivitis. Topical antibiotics are not sufficiently effective when used alone for ocular infections and are not necessary with appropriate systemic therapy. Infants with either type of ophthalmologic infection should be evaluated for signs of DGI.[6,13,14]

Treatment of gonorrhea during pregnancy is essential to prevent ophthalmia neonatorum. Gonococcal infections in newborns result primarily from passage through an infected birth canal, but also can be transmitted *in utero.* Ophthalmia neonatorum is the most common ophthalmic infection in newborns (1.6–12%), although membranes of the vagina, pharynx, or rectum also can become colonized. Conjunctival involvement usually develops within 7 days of delivery and is characterized by intense, bilateral conjunctival inflammation with chemosis. If not promptly treated, corneal ulceration and blindness can develop. Because neonatal prophylaxis with topical ocular antimicrobials is required by law in most states, gonococcal ophthalmia neonatorum is rare in the United States. The American Academy of Pediatrics recommends that either silver nitrate (1%), tetracycline (1%), or erythromycin (0.5%) be instilled in each conjunctival sac immediately postpartum. Approximately 2% of infants at risk of infection fail treatment with recommended ophthalmic antibiotics. As a result, infants born to infected mothers should also receive an intramuscular or intravenous injection of ceftriaxone 50 mg/kg for 7 days. Of the three topical agents, tetracycline and erythromycin are used most frequently because of their activity against chlamydia, another important cause of ophthalmia neonatorum. Silver nitrate produces a chemical conjunctivitis that may make assessment of therapeutic efficacy difficult, although the chemical reaction usually disappears within 3–5 days.[6,13,14,16,17]

Sulfamethoxazole–trimethoprim in doses of 6–10 tablets once daily for 3–5 days has demonstrated efficacy in the treatment of gonococcal infections and produces acceptable cure rates for coexisting *C. trachomatis;* however, these regimens have been associated with a high incidence of neurologic adverse effects. In preliminary trials the β-lactamase inhibitors sodium clavulanate and sulbactam in combination with penicillin, ampicillin, or amoxicillin have been used successfully in treating gonorrhea. Aztreonam and imipenem also are effective in gonococcal infections. However, they are not used routinely due to their cost and requirements for parenteral administration, as well as concerns regarding the development of resistance.[12–14]

Initial trials using vaccines prepared from gonococcal pili have been disappointing. Because of the heterogenicity of gonococcal pili it is unlikely that vaccines of this type will ever be clinically useful; however, other cell surface antigens common to all gonococci offer some hope that an effective vaccine can be developed in the future.[3,6,11,13]

EVALUATION OF THERAPEUTIC OUTCOME

Although it had been suggested that follow-up cultures should be obtained at least 3 days after treatment, combination gonorrhea/chlamydia therapy rarely results in treatment failures, and routine follow-up of patients treated with a regimen included in the CDC guidelines is not recommended. Patients receiving treatment with medications other than ceftriaxone should have follow-up cultures performed 4–7 days following therapy completion.[6,14] Persistence of symptoms following any treatment requires culture of the site(s) of gonorrheal infection, as well as susceptibility testing if gonococci are isolated. In most cases, the presence of gonococci indicates reinfection rather than treatment failure and reflects the need for improved patient education and sex partner referral. Persistence of symptoms can also be due to other infectious causes such as *C. trachomatis.*

SYPHILIS

Among diseases for which reporting to the U.S. Public Health Service CDC is required, syphilis is the fourth most frequently reported communicable disease in the United States. From 1986 to 1990, the incidence of all stages of syphilis in the United States increased dramatically, followed by a marked and steady decline. However, the incidence of syphilis remains disproportionately higher among blacks and Hispanics in comparison to whites. While primary and secondary syphilis were diagnosed in a much larger number of males than females for the 30-year period from 1960 to 1990, recent data indicate only a marginally greater occurrence in males today.[18] In addition to being highly contagious, syphilis is of major concern because, if left untreated, it can progress to a chronic systemic disease that can be fatal or seriously disabling.[19–21]

Syphilis is usually acquired by sexual contact with infected mucous membranes or cutaneous lesions, although on rare occasions it can be acquired by nonsexual personal contact, accidental inoculation, or blood transfusion. The causative organism of syphilis is *Treponema pallidum,* a spirochete. The risk of acquiring syphilis from an infected individual after a single exposure is approximately 30%. After sexual contact the organism penetrates the intact mucous membrane or a break in the cornified epithelium and spirochetemia occurs.[19–21]

Recently, a strong association between syphilis and HIV infection has been proposed. While complex and incompletely understood, it appears that syphilis, similar to other sexually transmitted genital ulcer diseases, may increase the risk of acquiring HIV in exposed individuals. Also, immunologic defects in HIV-infected individuals can modify the serologic response to syphilis, complicating the diagnosis as well as the assessment of the efficacy of antibiotic therapy. Further, anecdotal evidence suggests compromised immune function may result in an accelerated progression of syphilis requiring more aggressive antibiotic therapy in comparison to an immunocompetent host.[21–25]

CLINICAL PRESENTATION

Primary Syphilis

After exposure and an incubation period of 10–90 days (average, 21 days), a painless lesion or chancre appears at the site of treponemal penetrance. If several spirochetes penetrate simultaneously, multiple lesions can develop. Classically the chancre is single and begins as a dull red macule. Subsequently it develops into a papule that erodes and ulcerates. Although chancres vary markedly in appearance, most are rounded or oval in shape, indurated, and well marginated. Oral and anorectal chancres are common in homosexual males and frequently have an atypical appearance. All chancres are highly infectious, although they are generally painless lesions unless secondarily infected or located at extragenital sites. Even without treatment, chancres persist only for 1–8 weeks before spontaneously disappearing. Because syphilitic chancres can be confused with other infectious etiologies, appropriate diagnostic testing is important.[19,20,22]

Secondary Syphilis

The secondary stage of syphilis develops 2–6 weeks after the onset of the primary stage in untreated or inadequately treated patients. This stage is characterized by a variety of mucocutaneous eruptions, resulting from widespread hematogenous and lymphatic spread of *T. pallidum.* Skin lesions can either be generalized or localized to a small portion of the body and, with the exception of follicular lesions, are nonpruritic. Often lesions appear on the palms of the hands and the soles of the feet. Because few dermatologic conditions are characterized by palm and sole manifestations, involvement of these areas is highly suggestive of syphilis. In addition to the skin lesions, mild and transitory malaise, fever, pharyngitis, headache, anorexia, and arthralgia are common. Generalized lymphadenopathy also is seen in the majority of patients. With or without treatment, signs and symptoms of secondary syphilis disappear in 4–10 weeks; however, in untreated patients, lesions may recur at any time within 4 years.[19,20,22]

Latent Syphilis

By definition, persons with a positive serologic test for syphilis but with no other evidence of disease have latent syphilis. Latent syphilis is further divided into early and late latency. During early latency the patient is considered potentially infectious because of the risk of spontaneous mucocutaneous relapses. The U.S. Public Health Service defines early latency as 1 year from the onset of infection, although a longer interval such as 2–4 years is proposed by others. With the exception of pregnancy where the mother may pass the disease to the fetus, late latency is considered noninfectious, although the patient remains a host.[19,20]

A large percentage of untreated patients with late latent syphilis have no further sequelae; however, approximately 25–30% progress to late or tertiary syphilis. Treatment of all patients with latent syphilis is essential, because there is no way to predict which patients will develop tertiary disease.[19,20,22]

Tertiary (Late) Syphilis

Tertiary syphilis is a slowly progressing, inflammatory manifestation of the disease that can affect any organ in the body. The principal morbidity and mortality of syphilis relate to organ system involvement that can develop 2–30 years after the onset of syphilis.[19,20,22]

The most common manifestations of tertiary syphilis are benign gumma, neurosyphilis, and cardiovascular syphilis. The gumma, a nonspecific granulomatous lesion, is the classic lesion of late benign syphilis and develops in 50% of patients with tertiary syphilis. These chronic, destructive lesions characteristically involve the skin, bone, and upper respiratory tract, but can be found in any organ or tissue. Gummas of critical organs such as the heart or brain can be fatal.[19,20,22]

Neurosyphilis, found in approximately 20% of patients with tertiary disease, can produce general paresis, eighth cranial nerve deafness, optic atrophy and blindness, progressive dementia, meningovascular complications, and tabes dorsalis. Thirty percent of patients with tertiary disease develop cardiovascular syphilis, characterized by aortitis and aortic insufficiency. Syphilitic aortic aneurysms also are common.[19,20,22]

Congenital Syphilis

In pregnant women with syphilis, *T. pallidum* can cross the placenta at any time during pregnancy. However, fetal infection is not likely to occur if exposure takes place during the first 20 weeks of pregnancy. After this period, transplacental infections can occur resulting in fetal death, prematurity, or congenital syphilis. Symptoms can be seen during the first months of life (early congenital syphilis) or later in childhood or adolescence (late congenital syphilis). Manifestations of early congenital syphilis resemble those of secondary syphilis, while those of late congenital syphilis correspond to the tertiary stage in adults.[19,20,26]

DIAGNOSIS

Because *T. pallidum* is difficult to culture *in vitro,* diagnosis is based primarily on microscopic examination of serous material from a suspected syphilitic lesion or on results from serologic testing. In primary syphilis, diagnosis is established by the presence of *T. pallidum* on dark-field microscopic examination. Motile treponemes also can be found in cutaneous lesions and enlarged lymph nodes in patients with secondary syphilis. In incubating syphilis, confirmation is frequently by dark-field microscopic examination, because serologic tests can be unreactive early in the disease.[19,20,25,27–29] Another method of direct microscopic examination, the direct fluorescent antibody test (DFA-TP) using monoclonal or polyclonal antibodies specific for *T. pallidum,* has been used in the diagnosis of syphilis. The DFA-TP has greater specificity than dark-field examination and does not require the immediate examination of fresh specimens. However, it is more labor intensive and expensive than dark-field microscopy.[27]

Serologic tests used in the diagnosis of syphilis are categorized as nontreponemal or treponemal. Commonly used nontreponemal tests include the Venereal Disease Research Laboratory (VDRL) slide test, rapid plasma reagin (RPR) card test, reagin screen test (RST), unheated serum reagin (USR) test, automated reagin test (ART), or the toluidine red unheated serum test (TRUST). Nontreponemal tests rely on the detection of reagin, a heterogeneous group of antibodies. Most laboratories perform either the RPR card test or the VDRL slide test. These tests are inexpensive and easily performed. A positive nontreponemal test can indicate the presence of any stage of syphilis or congenital syphilis, although incubating syphilis and very early primary syphilis produce a negative reaction; however, because they are nonspecific tests, false-positive reactions occur, making them inappropriate alone to confirm the diagnosis. Transiently positive results can be seen in patients with acute febrile illnesses, after immunizations, and during pregnancy. Chronic false-positive results are commonly associated with heroin addiction, aging, chronic infections, connective tissue diseases, and malignant disease. In some cases false-positive reactions are familial and are related to abnormal serum globulin levels.[19,20–25,27–29]

Nontreponemal tests are used primarily as screening tests; however, because reaginic antibody titers also can be quantitated by testing serial dilutions of the patient's serum for reactivity, they are useful in following progression of the disease, recovery after therapy, and possible reinfection. Because antibody titers vary to some extent between tests, it is important that sequential serologic testing be performed using the same method each time. In patients successfully treated for primary and secondary syphilis, nontreponemal tests will almost always return to seronegativity. If these tests are going to return to negative in patients with early latent syphilis, they will do so within the first 4 years after adequate therapy. Patients treated for late latent syphilis or tertiary syphilis usually remain seropositive for life. Nontreponemal tests also can return to seronegativity in untreated patients, although this is uncommon and occurs more slowly than following adequate treatment.[19,20,27–29]

In some patients with secondary syphilis, a prozone phenomenon occurs that produces a negative VDRL despite the presence of high reaginic antibody titers. Because the agglutination reaction occurs only within fixed concentrations of antibody and antigen, a relative excess of antibody results in a nonreactive or weakly reactive test. This is corrected by diluting the patient's serum prior to testing.[19,20,27–29] For HIV-positive individuals with syphilis, the reactivity of nontreponemal tests can vary depending on the stage of the HIV infection. In the early stages, reaginic titers higher than in non–HIV-infected patients have been seen, resulting in the prozone phenomenon. However, during the later stages of HIV infection as immune function deteriorates, serologic responses can be reduced or delayed. As a result, the diagnosis of syphilis in HIV-infected individuals can be more difficult.[30]

In diagnosing all stages of syphilis, treponemal tests are more sensitive than nontreponemal tests. The fluorescent treponemal antibody absorption (FTAABS) test is the most frequently used treponemal test. In the FTAABS test, *T. pallidum* antigen is used to detect specific antibodies to treponemal organisms; however, because it requires fluorescence microscopy and is relatively difficult and expensive to perform, the FTAABS test is used primarily as a confirmatory rather than a screening test. The FTAABS test becomes positive earlier than nontreponemal tests in primary syphilis. After adequate antibiotic therapy for any stage of syphilis, the FTAABS test usually remains reactive for life, and therefore is not useful in assessing serologic response to therapy, relapse, or reinfection. False-positive reactions are reported in 1–2% of healthy persons. These reactions are usually transitory and the cause is unknown. In persons with Lyme disease, weakly positive tests are seen in up to 22% of subjects. Although the FTAABS test measures treponemal antibodies, it does not differentiate between syphilis and other nonvenereal treponemal diseases such as yaws and pinta. Other specific treponemal antibody tests are the *T. pallidum* hemagglutination assay (TPHA) and the microhemagglutination assay for antibodies to *T. pallidum* (MHATP).[19,20,27–29] The TPHA and the MHATP tests are easier to perform, less expensive, and slightly more specific than the FTAABS, but also are less sensitive in diagnosing the earliest stages of syphilis.[27–29]

TREATMENT

Treatment recommendations from the CDC are presented in Table 110.4.[14] Parenteral penicillin G is the treatment of choice for all stages of syphilis. Because *T. pallidum* multiplies slowly, single doses of short- or intermediate-acting penicillins do not provide the prolonged, low-level exposure to penicillin required for eradication of the treponeme. As a result benzathine penicillin G is the only penicillin effective for single-dose therapy.[14,19–22,25,31] The recommended treatment for syphilis of less than 1 year's duration is benzathine penicillin G 2.4 million units as a single dose. Although the relapse rate for this regimen is less than 3%, some advocate that 2.4 million units be administered once a week for 2 consecutive weeks. However, comparative studies of the two dosage regimens have not been conducted. In patients with syphilis of greater than 1 year's duration and normal cerebrospinal fluid (CSF) examination, benzathine penicillin G is administered weekly for three successive doses. Patients with abnormal CSF findings should be treated as having neurosyphilis. Preferred regimens for neurosyphilis provide treatment over a 31- to 35-day period with parenteral penicillin G. Benzathine penicillin G alone in standard weekly doses or procaine penicillin G in doses under 2.4 million units do not consistently provide treponemicidal levels in the CSF and have resulted in treatment failures.[14,19–22,31]

Since *T. pallidum* resistance to penicillin has not emerged, the primary need for alternative drugs in treating syphilis is for penicillin-allergic patients. Alternative regimens recommended for penicillin-allergic patients are doxycycline 100 mg orally twice daily, or tetracycline or erythromycin (stearate, ethyl succinate, or base) 500 mg orally four times daily for 2–4 weeks, depending on the duration of syphilis. Although neither the tetracyclines nor erythromycin have been evaluated as extensively as penicillin G in the treatment of syphilis, some evidence suggests higher treatment failure rates in erythromycin-treated patients. Alternative treatment regimens only should be used in cases of documented penicillin allergy and, given concerns regarding patient compliance with these regimens, follow-up serologic testing is of particular importance.[14,19,20,31]

Other antibiotics used successfully in treating syphilis include chloramphenicol, amoxicillin, and various cephalosporins such as ceftriaxone, cephalexin, and cephalothin; however, because they are either more expensive or potentially more toxic, and require administration of multiple doses, none offers significant advantages over benzathine penicillin G. While ceftriaxone is considered effective in eradicating incubating syphilis when given as a single 125-mg dose, higher doses and more frequent administration appear necessary for more advanced syphilis.[14,19–22,25,31]

For pregnant patients, penicillin is the treatment of choice at the dosage recommended for that particular stage of syphilis. To assure treatment success and prevent transmission to the fetus, some experts advocate an additional intramuscular dose of benzathine penicillin G 2.4 million units 1 week after completion of the recommended regimen. This may be particularly beneficial in women diagnosed and treated during the third trimester or those with secondary syphilis. In women allergic to penicillin, safe and effective alternatives are not available; therefore, skin testing should be performed to confirm a penicillin allergy. It is recommended that women with positive skin tests undergo penicillin desensitization and receive the appropriate treatment regimen for their stage of disease.[14]

TABLE 110.4. DRUG THERAPY AND FOLLOW-UP OF SYPHILIS

Stage/Type of Syphilis	Recommended Regimen[a]	Follow-up Serology
Primary, secondary, or latent syphilis of less than 1 year's duration (early latent syphilis)	Benzathine penicillin G 2.4 million units IM in a single dose[b]	Quantitative nontreponemal tests at 3 and 6 months for primary and secondary syphilis; at 6 and 12 months for early latent syphilis[c]
Syphilis of more than 1 year's duration (includes late latent syphilis of unknown duration and late or tertiary syphilis; excludes neurosyphilis)	Benzathine penicillin G 2.4 million units IM once a week for 3 successive weeks	Quantitative nontreponemal tests at 6 and 12 months for late latent syphilis[d]
Neurosyphilis	Aqueous crystalline penicillin G 12–24 million units IV (2–4 million units every 4 hours) for 10–14 days,[f] or Aqueous procaine penicillin G 2.4 million units IM daily plus probenecid 500 mg PO four times daily, both for 10–14 days[f]	CSF[e] examination every 6 months until the cell count is normal; if it has not decreased at 6 months or is not normal by 2 years, retreatment is suggested
Congenital syphilis	Aqueous crystalline penicillin G 50,000 units/kg IV every 12 hours during the first 7 days of life and every 8 hours thereafter for 10–14 days or Procaine penicillin G 50,000 units/kg IM daily for 10–14 days	Quantitative nontreponemal tests every 2–3 months until nonreactive (6–12 months)
Penicillin-allergic patients[g]		
Primary, secondary, or latent syphilis of less than 1 year's duration	Doxycycline 100 mg PO two times daily for 2 weeks or Tetracycline 500 mg PO four times daily for 2 weeks or Erythromycin 500 mg PO four times daily for 2 weeks	Same as for non-penicillin-allergic patients
Syphilis of more than 1 year's duration (except neurosyphilis)	Doxycycline 100 mg PO two times a day for 4 weeks or Tetracycline 500 mg PO four times daily for 4 weeks	Same as for non-penicillin-allergic patients

[a]Recommendations are those of the CDC.
[b]Some experts recommend multiple doses of benzathine penicillin G or other supplemental antibiotics in addition to benzathine penicillin G in HIV-infected patients with primary or secondary syphilis; HIV-infected patients with early latent syphilis should be treated with the recommended regimen for syphilis of more than 1 year's duration.
[c]More frequent follow-up (i.e., 1, 2, 3, 6, 9, and 12 months) recommended for HIV-infected patients.
[d]Minimal data exist on which to base specific follow-up recommendations for late syphilis.
[e]CSF, cerebral spinal fluid.
[f]Some experts administer benzathine penicillin G 2.4 million units IM after completion of the neurosyphilis regimens to provide a total duration of therapy comparable to that used for late syphilis in the absence of neurosyphilis.
[g]For nonpregnant patients; pregnant patients should be treated with penicillin after desensitization.

The majority of patients treated for primary and secondary syphilis experience the Jarisch–Herxheimer reaction after treatment. This benign, self-limiting reaction is characterized by flu-like symptoms such as transient headache, fever, chills, malaise, arthralgia, myalgia, tachypnea, peripheral vasodilation, and aggravation of syphilitic lesions. The exact mechanism of the reaction is unknown although proposed etiologies, including immunologic mechanisms and release of endotoxin or other toxic treponemal products, are not substantiated.[19,20] The Jarisch–Herxheimer reaction is independent of the drug and dose used and should not be confused with penicillin allergy. It usually begins within 2–4 hours of initiating therapy, peaks at 8 hours, and is complete within 12–24 hours. Most reactions can be managed symptomatically with analgesics, antipyretics, and rest. Steroids and antihistamines have been administered prior to initiation of syphilitic therapy but are of limited value.[14,19,20]

EVALUATION OF THERAPEUTIC OUTCOME

CDC recommendations for serologic follow-up of patients treated for syphilis are given in Table 110.4. Quantitative nontreponemal tests should be performed at 3 and 6 months in all patients treated for primary and secondary syphilis and at 6 and 12 months for early and late latent disease.[14] In general the time to reach seronegativity is proportional to the duration of the disease. Specific testing recommended for other stages of syphilis is included in Table 110.4.[14,21,27,29] Despite adequate therapy, some patients may remain seropositive based on nontreponemal test results. In these cases stabilization of low reaginic titers is indicative of adequate therapy. For women treated during pregnancy, monthly quantitative nontreponemal tests are recommended until the adequacy of therapy is established. Women who do not demonstrate a fourfold decrease in titer over a 3-month period or who show a fourfold increase in titer between tests should be retreated.[19–21]

CHLAMYDIA

Infections caused by *C. trachomatis* are believed to be the most common STD in the United States and the most common cause of nongonococcal urethritis (NGU). However, reporting is not required officially and microbiologic confirmation is frequently not performed in the United States. Despite these limitations, it is estimated that more than 4 million Americans contract chlamydial infections each year at a cost of greater than $2.4 billion dollars.[32] Precise diagnosis of chlamydia infections has been hampered because of the high percentage of infected individuals who have asymptomatic disease and because culture of the organism is both difficult and expensive.[14,33]

Chlamydia trachomatis is an obligate intracellular parasite that shares properties of both viruses and bacteria. Like viruses, chlamydiae require cellular material from host cells for replication; however, unlike viruses, chlamydiae maintain their cellular identity throughout development. Although *C. trachomatis* lacks a cell wall peptidoglycan, its major outer membrane is similar to gram-negative bacteria. Fifteen serovars (subspecies) of *C. trachomatis* exist, of which only the lymphogranuloma venereum strains produce potentially invasive infections. The remaining serovars are involved primarily with superficial infection of epithelial cells.[34–37]

Specific data on the risk of transmissibility of chlamydia after exposure are not available. It is estimated that coinfection with chlamydia occurs in up to 45% of individuals with gonorrhea. As a result, chlamydia is the most common cause of postgonococcal urethritis in heterosexuals.[12] All individuals diagnosed with *N. gonorrhoeae* should be assumed to have *C. trachomatis* present also.[38] Specific risk factors responsible for a woman contracting a cervical chlamydia infection are unclear, although single young women, those receiving oral contraceptives, and women who have had more than one sexual partner in the past 3 months are at a potentially greater risk of acquiring *C. trachomatis* infections.[32,38] An increased prevalence of chlamydia infections is reported among blacks, persons of low socioeconomic status, and persons residing in inner cities.[14] In addition to genital infections, ocular and pharyngeal infections occur. Such infections occur most frequently secondary to vaginal delivery through an infected birth canal and from orogenital contact, respectively.

CLINICAL PRESENTATION

In males, the most common symptoms of chlamydial genital tract infections are dysuria, urinary frequency, and a mucoid urethral discharge occurring 7–21 days after exposure. The discharge is usually less profuse and more mucoid or watery than the urethral discharge associated with gonorrhea. Typically, it is more obvious in the morning. In many cases the discharge is not noticeable, and crusting of the meatus or staining of undergarments may be the only sign. In approximately 25% of men with chlamydial infections, no signs or symptoms are present. *Chlamydia trachomatis* is responsible for approximately 50% of all cases of acute epididymitis reported in the United States annually.[34–37] Rectal infections occur in men practicing receptive anal intercourse, and while these infections are usually asymptomatic, they can produce complications such as proctitis or proctocolitis.[32]

The majority of women with chlamydial infections are asymptomatic. In women with urethral infections, dysuria and frequency are uncommon. When symptomatic, the most common manifestation of infection is endocervicitis with a mucopurulent discharge. On exam, the cervix tends to be friable and ectopic. In recent years, chlamydia has been recognized as a major cause of PID and its associated complications.[32] It also is suggested that women with active chlamydial infections or antichlamydial antibodies in their serum have an increased risk of cervical dysplasia.[34–37]

Similar to gonorrhea, chlamydia may be transmitted to an infant during contact with infected cervicovaginal secretions. Up to 70% of infants acquire chlamydial infection after endocervical exposure, with the primary morbidity associated with seeding of the infant's eyes, nasopharynx, rectum, or vagina. Neonatal conjunctivitis and pneumonia develop in up to 50% and 10–16% of exposed infants, respectively.[39] Inclusion conjunctivitis in newborns is usually self-limited, but can result in scarring and micropanus of the cornea. Interstitial pneumonitis occurring secondary to carriage in the nasopharynx is typically mild, but can be severe and require hospitalization.[11,34–37,39,40]

DIAGNOSIS

Because of the high rate of asymptomatic disease and the relative lack of specificity of symptoms when present, laboratory confirmation of chlamydial infection is important. Specific guidelines for diagnosing *C. trachomatis* infections are available from the CDC.[32] Prior to the availability of antigen-detection methods, diagnosis commonly was based on the presence of greater than four polymorphonuclear leukocytes per high-power field in a smear of urethral secretions and the exclusion of gonorrhea. This indirect means of diagnosis is neither sensitive nor specific.[33–37]

Cytologic techniques are of little practical value in the diagnosis of chlamydial genital tract infections because of their poor sensitivity. Because chlamydiae are obligate intracellular parasites, Giemsa-stained smears must be prepared from epithelial cell scrapings from the endocervix (women) or urethra (men) rather than from urine or urethral discharges. Such evaluation is most useful in screening patients to eliminate the possibility of gonorrhea. Although tissue culture techniques have close to a 100% specificity, they are not widely used for diagnostic purposes because they are time consuming, technically demanding, and expensive.[33–36] In addition, if treatment is withheld until culture results are available and the patient returns for treatment, a small percentage of patients may have progression to clinically evident PID. Also important, many infected individuals will not return for culture results and treatment and thus will remain infectious to others.[41]

Serologic tests also are of limited benefit in diagnosing chlamydial infections and are used primarily as a research tool. The presence of antibody in a blood sample does not differentiate an active infection from previous exposure, and the baseline prevalence of antibody in populations that are sexually active and at greatest risk is high.[32–36,38]

Two tests that allow rapid identification of chlamydial antigens in genital secretions are the direct fluorescent antibody (DFA) test and the enzyme-linked immunoabsorbent assay (ELISA). The DFA test utilizes fluorescein-conjugated monoclonal antibody that is incubated with specimen material on a slide and examined under a fluorescent microscope. The ELISA measures antigen–antibody reactions using a spectrophotometer. Based on limited comparative data, both tests have similar mean sensitivities and specificities in the range of 90–100% when properly performed. However, some ELISA methods are not specific for *C. trachomatis* and detect all three chlamydia species. A blocking assay can verify positive results.[32] Unlike the DFA test, which can be performed in less than 1 hour, the ELISA requires approximately 4 hours to perform. However, the ELISA is less complicated and can be used to test large numbers of specimens at the same time.[14,33,42] In populations with a low prevalence rate, the positive predictive value for each antigen detection method is 33–80% (DFA) and 44% (ELISA).

Rapid office tests for diagnosing chlamydial infections that use an enzyme immunoassay similar to home pregnancy tests are now available. Although the sensitivity and specificity of these tests are reported to be greater than 90%, lower sensitivities in the range of 48.5–77% are reported also.[38,41,43–45]

Several studies have been conducted using the leukocyte esterase test (LET), a urine dipstick test for detecting pyuria, in screening sexually active men for chlamydia and gonorrhea. Reported sensitivities and specificities are greatest in men less than 26 years of age with urethritis, although preliminary data suggest that the sensitivity and specificity of the test also may be acceptable in asymptomatic men considered at high risk of infection. Further study is necessary to determine the role of the LET and other noninvasive tests in screening large numbers of individuals at high risk for chlamydial infections.[46]

Other diagnostic tests, such as a nucleic acid hybridization test (DNA Probe), the polymerase chain reaction (CPCR), and ligase chain reaction (LCR), are currently under investigation. However, their use is primarily for research purposes at this time.[32,47,48]

TREATMENT

Rifampin, tetracyclines, macrolides, and sulfonamides display good *in vitro* and *in vivo* activity against *C. trachomatis.* Although penicillin, ampicillin, amoxicillin, piperacillin, azlocillin, mezlocillin, cefoperazone, ceftriaxone, and clindamycin possess some activity against chlamydia *in vitro,* they have demonstrated only marginal clinical efficacy. Variable *in vitro* activity has been demonstrated by the fluoroquinolones; in order of decreasing susceptibility, the most active agents are ofloxacin, ciprofloxacin, and lomefloxacin. In contrast to the tetracyclines and macrolides, the fluoroquinolones are bactericidal against *C. trachomatis.* Aminoglycosides, metronidazole, aztreonam, and most cephalosporins are not active *in vitro* against chlamydia.[14,33–37,40,49–52]

In clinical trials, tetracycline, minocycline, erythromycin, and trimethoprim–sulfamethoxazole have produced comparable cure rates of 85–95% in men with chlamydial urethritis. Although fewer studies have been conducted to assess the effectiveness of antibiotic therapy of uncomplicated cervical or urethral infection in women, cure rates appear similar to those reported in males; however, sulfonamides have no significant activity against *Ureaplasma urealyticum* and are not useful in the treatment of *C. trachomatis*-negative NGU. In limited testing, high-dose amoxicillin therapy (750 mg three times daily for 7 days) also has been effective in the treatment of chlamydial urethral infections in men. *In vitro* resistance has been reported for sulfonamides and rifampin. Recently, a relative resistance to both erythromycin and tetracycline has been reported.[53] Because of their effectiveness, low cost, and limited adverse effects, tetracycline and doxycycline have been most extensively evaluated and, until recently, were the two treatments of choice recommended by the CDC.[14,34–37,40,42,45,50–52]

In 1993, the CDC removed tetracycline and added the macrolide azithromycin to its recommended regimens and added the fluoroquinolone ofloxacin to its alternative regimens for genital chlamydial infections (Table 110.5). Azithromycin's safety and efficacy in persons less than 15 years of age is unknown. While azithromycin offers the advantage of single-dose therapy to ensure compliance, it is an expensive alternative to doxycycline.[14] The recommended doxycycline dosage for chlamydial infections is 100 mg twice daily for 7 days. However, longer regimens can be useful in patients experiencing relapses or for whom compliance is a concern. Single-dose studies using doxycycline have produced high failure rates. Similar to doxycycline, minocycline offers a convenient twice-daily dosage regimen, but is more expensive and is associated with a high incidence of dizziness and lightheadedness.[12,33–37,40,42,50–52]

Ofloxacin is the only fluoroquinolone with established efficacy in *C. trachomatis* infections. It is equally as effective as doxycycline, with efficacy rates ranging from 82–100%.[33,54] However, it should not be used during pregnancy or in persons less than 17 years of age. Ofloxacin is dosed twice daily for 7 days like doxycycline, but is more expensive. Although ciprofloxacin has activity against *C. trachomatis, N. gonorrhoeae,* and *U. urealyticum,* dosages as high as 2 grams per day have not consistently eradicated chlamydial infections. Chlamydia recurrence rates of up to 70% are reported with ciprofloxacin regimens of 500–1000 mg twice a day.[52]

For pregnant women with chlamydial urogenital infections, treatment can significantly reduce the risk of pregnancy complications and transmission to the newborn.[35,55,56] Since the use of doxycycline and ofloxacin are contraindicated during pregnancy, erythromycin base or erythromycin ethyl succinate are the recommended treatments (Table 110.5). Erythromycin stearate is probably

TABLE 110.5. TREATMENT OF CHLAMYDIAL INFECTIONS

Infection	Recommended Regimen[a]	Alternative Regimen
Uncomplicated urethral, endocervical, or rectal infection in adults	Doxycycline 100 mg PO 2 times daily for 7 days or Azithromycin 1 g once[b]	Ofloxacin 300 mg PO 2 times daily for 7 days[c] or Erythromycin base 500 mg PO 4 times daily for 7 days or Erythromycin ethyl succinate 800 mg PO 4 times daily for 7 days or Sulfasoxazole 500 mg 4 times daily for 10 days
Urogenital infections during pregnancy	Erythromycin base 500 mg 4 times PO daily for 7 days	Erythromycin base 250 mg PO 4 times daily for 14 days or Erythromycin ethyl succinate 800 mg PO 4 times daily for 7 days (or 400 mg PO 4 times daily for 14 days) or Amoxicillin 500 mg PO 3 times daily for 7 days[d]
Conjunctivitis of the newborn	Erythromycin suspension 50 mg/kg/d PO in 4 divided doses for 10–14 days	
Pneumonia in infants	Erythromycin suspension 50 mg/kg/d PO in 4 divided doses for 10–14 days	
Acute epididymo-orchitis	Ceftriaxone 250 mg IM[e] plus Doxycycline 100 mg PO 2 times daily for 10 days	

[a]Recommendations are those of the CDC.
[b]Data regarding the use of azithromycin in children ≤15 years old are not established.
[c]Ofloxacin is contraindicated during pregnancy and should not be used in patients ≤17 years old.
[d]Only if GI intolerance to erythromycin; limited data exist for efficacy.
[e]The efficacy of ceftriaxone 125 mg or azithromycin has not been studied and is unknown.

effective also, although it has not been adequately evaluated. Patients intolerant of the recommended erythromycin dosage should be treated with half of the daily dose for 2 weeks instead of 1 week. Amoxicillin 1.5 grams daily for 7–10 days appears to be as effective as erythromycin and is associated with a lower incidence of adverse effects; however, it is uncertain whether infections are actually eradicated or just suppressed.[12,33–37,40,42,50–52] Patients treated with azithromycin 1 gram orally have achieved a 100% cure rate without adverse effects to the fetus or infant.[57,58] Like erythromycin, azithromycin is in pregnancy category B and is probably an acceptable agent for use during pregnancy. Pregnant patients treated for chlamydial infections should undergo post-treatment cultures to ensure eradication of the infection.

Chlamydia trachomatis transmission during perinatal exposure can result in infections of the eye, oropharynx, lungs, urogenital tract, and rectum of the neonate or infant. For prophylaxis of ophthalmia neonatorum, various groups have proposed the use of erythromycin (0.5%) or tetracycline (1%) ophthalmic ointment in lieu of silver nitrate. Although silver nitrate and antibiotic ointments are effective against gonococcal ophthalmia neonatorum, silver nitrate is not effective for chlamydial disease and may cause a chemical conjunctivitis; however, neither topical erythromycin nor tetracycline has any effect on nasal carriage of chlamydia, so the potential for pneumonitis remains. The only acceptable treatment for chlamydial ophthalmia neonatorum is systemic therapy with oral erythromycin 50 mg/kg/d in four divided doses for 10–14 days. Topical sulfonamide, tetracycline, or erythromycin is no longer acceptable because of a high percentage of treatment failures.[14,16,17,33–37,40]

EVALUATION OF THERAPEUTIC OUTCOME

Treatment of chlamydial infections with the recommended regimens is highly effective, therefore, post-treatment cultures are not routinely recommended. However, if a clinician so chooses, post-treatment cultures should be obtained a minimum of 3 weeks after the completion of therapy. When positive, post-treatment cultures usually represent noncompliance, failure to treat sexual partners, or laboratory error, rather than inadequate therapy. Infants with pneumonitis should receive follow-up testing, since erythromycin is only 80% effective. A second course of therapy may be necessary in some patients.[14,16,17,32–37,40]

GENITAL HERPES

Genital herpes infections represent the most common cause of genital ulceration seen in the United States. It is estimated that approximately 31 million Americans have genital herpes, and this number is increasing yearly.[5] Whether these figures represent increased prevalence or greater recognition as a result of improved diagnostic capabilities is uncertain. Because of its morbidity, recurrent nature, and potential for complications, as well as its ability to be transmitted asymptomatically, genital herpes has received increasing attention in recent years.[59–62]

Herpes comes from the Greek "to creep" and is used to describe two distinct but antigenically related serotypes of herpes simplex virus. Herpes simplex virus type 1 (HSV-1) is most commonly associated with oropharyngeal disease and herpes simplex virus type 2 (HSV-2) is most closely associated with genital disease; however, each virus is capable of causing infections clinically indistinguishable in both anatomic areas.[25,59–61]

Humans are the sole known reservoir for HSV. Infection is transmitted via inoculation of virus from infected secretions onto mucosal surfaces (e.g., urethra, oropharynx, cervix, conjunctivae) or through abraded skin. On the basis of a retrospective study, the risk of developing genital herpes after sexual exposure to a person with an active infection is estimated to be 60%. Evidence that the virus survives for a limited time on environmental surfaces suggests the possibility of fomitic transfer as a nonvenereal route of transmission.[59,60,63]

The cycle of HSV infection occurs in five stages: primary mucocutaneous infection, infection of the ganglia, establishment of latency, reactivation, and recurrent infection. After viral inoculation, HSV infection is associated with cytoplasmic granulation, ballooning degeneration of cells, and production of mononucleated giant cells. Initially, the cellular response is predominantly polymorphonuclear, followed by a lymphocytic response. Replication occurs with viral spread to contiguous cells and peripheral sensory nerves. Latency then is established in sensory or autonomic nerve root ganglia. Latency appears to be lifelong, interrupted only by reactivation of the viral infection. It is unclear what factors are important in maintaining latency, but immune responses and emotional and physical stresses appear important in reactivating latent virus.[25,59,60,63–66]

CLINICAL PRESENTATION

The clinical manifestations of first episodes of genital herpes usually appear within 2–14 days after exposure. The signs and symptoms are influenced by many factors including previous exposure to HSV, previous genital herpes infection, viral type, and host factors such as age and site of infection. On the basis of retrospective studies, it is estimated that up to 50% of HSV-2 infections are asymptomatic, and these infections may represent the most common source of transmission of genital and neonatal herpes infections. As a result, identification of asymptomatic individuals with HSV-2 antibody may prove beneficial in the control of genital herpes transmission.[59,60,64–66]

In terms of the natural history of genital herpes infection and its treatment, it is important to distinguish between first-episode primary, first-episode nonprimary, and recurrent infections. Primary infections are classified as infections occurring in persons lacking antibody to either type of HSV. These infections are characterized by a prolonged duration of systemic and local symptoms, sometimes requiring hospitalization. More than 50% of patients with primary infections experience flu-like symptoms of fever, headache, malaise, and myalgias. Systemic symptoms gradually resolve over the course of a week. Local symptoms include development of pustular or ulcerative lesions on the external genitalia. Lesions usually begin as papules or vesicles that rapidly spread over the genitalia. Clusters of the lesions coalesce into large areas of ulceration, which over 2–3 weeks, crust and/or reepithelialize. Genital lesions are described as painful by more than 90% of infected men and women. Development of new lesions is fairly common during the first 10 days of a primary infection. Pain from the lesions tends to be most intense during the first 7–11 days of their appearance and gradually recedes. Other local symptoms can include itching, dysuria, vaginal or urethral discharge, and tender inguinal adenopathy; the latter is usually the last symptom to resolve. Viral shedding lasts approximately 11–12 days.[59,60,64,65,67,68]

First-episode nonprimary genital herpes is defined as an infection in individuals who have clinical or serologic evidence of prior HSV (usually HSV-1) infection at another body site. These infections tend to be milder than true primary infections, with a lower incidence of constitutional symptoms and a shorter duration of disease reported. Viral shedding usually lasts about 7 days.[60,64,65] Some data suggest that immunity produced by a prior HSV-1 infection also may reduce the risk of acquiring infection due to HSV-2.

In contrast to first-episode primary and first-episode nonprimary infections, recurrent infections are infrequently associated with systemic manifestations. Recurrent infection is localized to the genital area and is milder and of a shorter duration (e.g., 8–12 days). Viral shedding lasts approximately 4 days. Approximately 50% of patients with genital herpes experience a prodrome prior to the appearance of recurrent lesions. This typically consists of a mild tingling or itching sensation hours to a few days prior to the appearance of vesicles. In a few patients symptoms of sacral neuralgia are seen.[60,64,65,67–69]

As with a first-episode infection, symptoms of recurrent infection tend to be more severe in women, primarily as a result of the greater genital surface area involved. About 80% of patients with a first-episode HSV-2 genital infection experience a recurrence within 12 months compared with approximately 50% infected with HSV-1. The median number of recurrences is estimated at four per year when infection is caused by HSV-2 versus only one per year for HSV-1 infections. Symptoms of first-episode and recurrent infections tend to be more severe and prolonged in immunocompromised patients than in immunocompetent patients. In addition, immunocompromised patients are more susceptible to initial genital infection and subsequent recurrences, as well as generalized systemic infection.[25,60,64,65,67,68,70]

Complications from genital herpes infections result from both genital spread and autoinoculation of the virus and occur most commonly with primary first episodes. Lesions at extragenital sites such as the eye, rectum, pharynx, and fingers are not uncommon. Central nervous system involvement is occasionally seen and may take several forms including an aseptic meningitis, transverse myelitis, or a sacral radiculopathy syndrome.[60,64,65]

A major concern is the effect of genital herpes on neonates exposed during pregnancy. Neonatal herpes is associated with a high mortality and significant morbidity. It is transmitted to the newborn primarily through exposure to HSV in the birth canal but in rare cases also is transmitted transplacentally. The risk of transmission during birth appears much greater for first-episode primary infections than for recurrent infections. Neonatal herpes infection has a case-fatality rate of approximately 50%, with a large proportion of surviving infants experiencing significant morbidity.[25,60,63–65,71]

DIAGNOSIS

Confirmation of a genital herpes infection can be made only with laboratory testing. The nonspecific systemic symptoms seen with primary infection and even the lesions of genital herpes may be difficult to differentiate from other infectious and noninfectious etiologies. Typically, however, genital herpes lesions are painful to touch, in contrast to syphilitic chancres.

Tissue culture is the most specific (100%) and sensitive method (80–90%) of confirming the diagnosis of first-episode genital herpes; however, culture is relatively insensitive in recurrent infections due, in part, to the reduced viral concentration in recurrent lesions. Viral culture is expensive and time consuming, and improper collection or transport of specimens can result in false-negative results. In most situations, HSV isolation on tissue culture takes 24–96 hours. Following isolation, it is recommended that typing of the virus be performed because of prognostic implications (e.g., HSV-1 is associated with a lower rate of asymptomatic and symptomatic recurrence). In instances in which rapid detection is necessary, such as an impending birth, other detection methods may be more useful. Amplified culture techniques that combine cell culture for 24 hours and HSV-specific antibodies have sensitivities and specificities only slightly less than those of culture.[45,60–62,64,65,72]

The Tzanck test is a rapid detection method in which cells from suspected lesions are stained and examined for the presence of characteristic multinucleated giant cells.

While easy to perform and inexpensive, the specificity and sensitivity are low. Other detection methods with acceptable specificities and sensitivities that provide more rapid results than tissue culture also have been evaluated. Antigen-detection methods such as direct immunofluorescence, immunoperoxidase staining, and enzyme-linked immunosorbent assay have sensitivities of 70–90% compared with viral culture; however, sensitivities are significantly lower when assessing asymptomatic viral shedding. Diagnosis by either antigen-detection or tissue culture is difficult if suspected lesions are crusted or healed. In the case of subclinical or asymptomatic infections, such methods are even more unreliable in diagnosing genital herpes.[25,61–63]

The majority of patients infected with either HSV-1 or HSV-2 develop circulating antibodies to HSV antigens; however, current commercially available serologic assays for detection of HSV antibodies are often overutilized and have only limited utility in the diagnosis of genital herpes. The cross-reactivity of antibodies to HSV-1 and HSV-2 in most assays, coupled with the high prevalence of HSV-1 antibody in the adult population, makes it difficult to interpret the results. A negative antibody titer early in the course of a herpes infection followed by a fourfold or greater rise in the titer after the episode is diagnostic of a primary infection. A rise in antibody titer also can be seen after a first-episode nonprimary infection, but changes in antibody titer are uncommon during recurrent episodes or asymptomatic viral shedding.[45,60,64,65,72]

Serologic tests specific for identifying and differentiating HSV-1 and HSV-2 are increasingly being used in the research setting. Western blot assays and an immunoblot assay have been shown to be highly sensitive and specific. Also under study is the detection of HSV DNA by polymerase chain reaction. Preliminary data suggest that this test may be useful in detecting asymptomatic HSV in the genitourinary tract.[25,61,62]

While the diagnosis of genital herpes can be confirmed only by laboratory tests such as cell culture, less stringent diagnostic criteria (e.g., characteristic physical findings or clinical history) frequently are used in clinical practice. A presumptive diagnosis of genital herpes commonly is made based on the presence of dark-field-negative, vesicular, or ulcerative genital lesions. A prior history of similar lesions or recent sexual contact with an individual with similar lesions also is useful in making the diagnosis. Other STDs including chancroid, lymphogranuloma venereum, and granuloma inguinale, and causes such as trauma, allergic reactions, and bacterial or fungal infections are considered in the differential diagnosis.

TREATMENT

Palliative and supportive measures are the cornerstone of therapy for patients with genital herpes. To prevent bacterial superinfection, lesions must be kept clean and dry. The use of analgesics, antipyretics, and antipruritics may be warranted based on symptomatology. The goals of therapy in genital herpes infection are to shorten the clinical course, prevent complications, prevent the development of latency and/or subsequent recurrences, decrease disease transmission, and eliminate established latency. Current research has focused primarily on the treatment of first-episode infections, recurrences, and the suppression of recurrences.[25,62,64–74]

Specific chemotherapeutic approaches to treating genital herpes fall into six major areas: antiviral compounds, topical surfactants, photodynamic dyes, immune modulators, vaccines, and interferons (Table 110.6). However, few have undergone extensive evaluation and even fewer have demonstrated any significant clinical effects. Antiviral agents, in particular acyclovir, have been the most successful in promoting healing and resolution of symptoms.[25,62,64–74]

Acyclovir, a guanosine analogue available in intravenous, oral, and topical dosage forms, was the first antiviral agent to demonstrate significant efficacy in the treatment of genital herpes and the prophylaxis of recurrent infections. Currently it is the only antiviral agent in the United States with a labeled indication for genital herpes. Specific dosage recommendations are given in Table 110.7.[14] Selective phosphorylation of acyclovir in HSV-infected cells by HSV-specific thymidine kinase is the first step in the conversion to acyclovir triphosphate, the active moiety. Acyclovir triphosphate is a selective substrate and inhibitor of herpes virus DNA polymerase. As acyclovir is preferentially taken up and converted to its active form by HSV-infected cells, it has a low potential for toxicity in normal, uninfected cells.[75,76]

Oral and intravenous formulations of acyclovir have demonstrated efficacy in reducing viral shedding, duration of symptoms, and time to healing of first-episode genital herpes infections. In some studies, new lesion formation has been reduced and local symptoms improved with use of topical acyclovir; however, these effects are not as pronounced as with oral and intravenous therapy and systemic symptoms are not affected. Therefore, topical therapy is considered of little or no benefit in most patients. Combined use of topical acyclovir with oral therapy does not appear to offer any additional benefit over oral therapy alone. In humans no acyclovir regimen is known to prevent latency or alter the subsequent frequency and severity of recurrences. Oral acyclovir 200 mg five times daily for 7–10 days or when clinical resolution occurs is the treatment of choice for outpatients with first-episode genital herpes. Some evidence suggests that larger doses given less frequently (e.g., 400 mg three times daily) also may be efficacious. In patients with severe symptoms or complications necessitating hospitalization, parenteral acyclovir may be beneficial; however, the intravenous regimen has been asso-

TABLE 110.6. AGENTS STUDIED IN THE TREATMENT OF HERPES GENITALIS

Antiviral Compounds	Immune Modulators
Acyclovir	Inosiplex
Famciclovir	Levamisole
Valaciclovir	Transfer factor
Foscarnet	**Vaccines**
Vidarabine	BCG
Idoxuridine	Influenza
2-Deoxy-D-glucose	Polio
Lithium	Small pox
L-Lysine	**Interferons**
Phosphonoformate	Leukocyte interferon
Ribavirin	**Photodynamic Dyes**
(E)-5-(2-Bromovinyl)-2′-deoxyuridine (BVdU)	Neutral red
2′-Fluoro-5-iodoarabinosylcytosine	Acridine red
1-(2′-Fluoro-2′-deoxy-β-D-arabinofuranosyl)-thymidine	Proflavine
Topical Surfactants	**Others**
Chloroform	Butylated hydroxytoluene (BHT)
Ether	
Nonoxynol-9	
Povidone-iodine	
Intervir-A	

ciated with renal, gastrointestinal, bone marrow, and central nervous system toxicity, especially in patients with renal dysfunction.[60,64,65,67,68,70,72–77]

The role of acyclovir in the treatment of recurrent genital herpes episodes is controversial. Because of the self-limiting nature of recurrent infection in normal hosts, demonstration of therapeutic effects is difficult. There is no evidence that shortening the duration of recurrent episodes has any effect on the subsequent recurrence rate. In most instances, treatment with topical acyclovir, whether physician initiated (within 48 hours of onset) or patient initiated (at prodrome or earliest sign of recurrence), has shown no significant effects on symptomology, duration of viral shedding, or time to healing. When initiated early during the course of recurrence, oral acyclovir reduces the duration of viral shedding by approximately 1 day and diminishes the time to healing of lesions by 1–2 days. Appreciable effects on symptomology are not seen. Patients with prolonged episodes of recurrent infection are most likely to benefit from oral therapy instituted at the earliest sign of recur-

TABLE 110.7. TREATMENT OF GENITAL HERPES

Type of Infection	Recommended Regimen[a,b]	Alternative Regimen
First clinical episode of genital herpes[c]	Acyclovir 200 mg PO five times daily for 7–10 days, or until clinical resolution occurs	Acyclovir 5–10 mg/kg IV every 8 hours for 5–7 days or until clinical resolution occurs[d]
First clinical episode of herpes proctitis	Acyclovir 400 mg PO five times daily for 10 days, or until clinical resolution occurs	Acyclovir 5–10 mg/kg IV every 8 hours for 5–7 days or until clinical resolution occurs[d]
Recurrent infection		
Treatment	Acyclovir 200 mg PO five times daily, *or* 400 mg PO three times daily, *or* 800 mg PO twice daily for 5 days, initiated within 48 hours of onset of lesions[e]	
Suppression	Acyclovir 400 mg PO twice daily[f]	Acyclovir 200 mg PO 3–5 times daily

[a]Recommendations are those of the CDC.
[b]HIV-infected patients may require more aggressive therapy.
[c]Primary or nonprimary first episode.
[d]Only for patients with severe symptoms or complications that necessitate hospitalization.
[e]Treatment should be limited to patients with severe symptoms. Treatment is most beneficial when instituted at the earliest sign of recurrence (i.e., prodrome); therapy initiated 48 hours or more after the onset of symptoms has no effect.
[f]Indicated only for patients with frequent and/or severe recurrences; although safety and efficacy are documented in patients receiving daily therapy for as long as 5 years, it is recommended that therapy be discontinued after 1 year of continuous suppressive therapy to assess the patient's rate of recurrent episodes.

rence. Initial data demonstrating the efficacy of oral acyclovir in treating recurrent genital herpes were based on a recommended dose of 200 mg five times daily for 5 days; recent evidence indicates comparable efficacy with a regimen of either 800 mg twice daily or 400 mg three times daily. Both regimens are well tolerated and offer greater patient convenience. Because of the relative mildness and brevity of recurrent infections, parenteral administration of acyclovir is not justifiable.[60,64,65,67,68,70,72–77]

Acyclovir treatment of first-episode genital herpes does not prevent later recurrences; however, chronic oral therapy reduces the frequency and the severity of recurrences in 70–90% of patients experiencing frequent recurrences. In some patients experiencing breakthrough recurrences, HSV isolates resistant to acyclovir have been identified. Consideration must be given to the adverse effects of long-term administration of acyclovir to healthy young adults and the possibility of acyclovir-resistant HSV strains developing during suppressive therapy; however, clinical trials have found no evidence of cumulative toxicity or significant resistance in patients with frequent recurrences who were treated continuously for up to 6 years. Results from several controlled trials indicate the superiority of continuous acyclovir suppression for 1 year versus intermittent or weekend suppressive therapy.[25,60,64,65,67,70,72–78]

Patients with frequent (i.e., greater than 6 per year) and physically or psychologically distressing recurrences are candidates for suppressive therapy with multiple daily doses of oral acyclovir. Large single daily doses of acyclovir are associated with a greater risk of breakthrough recurrences than multiple daily doses. When recurrences are less severe or cost is a primary factor, consideration should be given to physician- or patient-initiated therapy at the earliest sign of recurrence (200 mg five times a day for 5 days). Because of its cost and potential for adverse effects, oral acyclovir is not recommended for routine use in all patients with recurrent genital herpes. Topical acyclovir has no role in either the treatment or prophylaxis of recurrent infections in most patients.[60,62,63,69–71]

Immunocompromised patients are at greatest risk for severe and recurrent HSV infections and have been shown to benefit from therapy with all three formulations of acyclovir. As with the immunocompetent host, effects are more pronounced with the intravenous and oral dosage forms. Both intravenous and oral acyclovir have been used to prevent reactivation of infection in patients seropositive for HSV who undergo transplantation procedures or induction chemotherapy for acute leukemia. Immunocompromised individuals such as patients with AIDS who fail treatment or prophylaxis with recommended doses of acyclovir, frequently demonstrate improved response with higher doses.[60,65,70,75,76]

The safety of acyclovir therapy during pregnancy is not established, although there is no evidence of teratogenic effects in humans. Because of the high maternal and infant morbidity associated with first-episode primary genital infections at or near term, the use of systemic acyclovir has been advocated as being appropriate; however, the effectiveness of such therapy is unknown. Use of acyclovir to treat or suppress recurrent episodes near term is more controversial, primarily due to the lack of data demonstrating significant benefits in this situation.[60,62,64,70,71,79–81]

With the increasing prevalence of genital herpes worldwide, the potential exists for widespread use and misuse of acyclovir, resulting in development of acyclovir-resistant HSV. *In vitro* resistance to acyclovir is shown to be mediated by alterations in either viral thymidine kinase or viral DNA polymerase. Clinically, the majority of resistant isolates have been thymidine kinase deficient. Studies in animals suggest that these mutants have reduced virulence and have greater difficulty in establishing latency than parent strains. Since the thymidine kinase-deficient mutants rapidly disappear with or without continued therapy, it is likely they are eliminated by normal host defense mechanisms. Although less common than thymidine kinase-deficient mutants, other resistant strains maintain virulency and can establish latency. The incidence and clinical implications of acyclovir resistance require further study, particularly with respect to immunocompromised hosts in whom resistance may develop with greater frequency and be of greater clinical importance.[60,63,75,76]

Numerous agents for the prophylaxis and treatment of genital herpes infections are being studied. Advances in antiviral research have stimulated the development and testing of several antiviral compounds. The antiviral agents foscarnet (intravenous and topical) and vidarabine (intravenous) are currently being evaluated in the treatment of genital herpes. Unlike acyclovir, neither of these agents requires activation by viral thymidine kinase. As a result, their use is of particular interest in immunocompromised patients with acyclovir-resistant HSV isolates. Famciclovir, a guanosine analogue similar to acyclovir, and the acyclovir prodrug valaciclovir are undergoing extensive evaluation in the management of genital herpes. When compared to acyclovir, both agents have better oral bioavailability and require less frequent dosing.

Topical and systemic interferons have not demonstrated consistent, clinically significant benefits in first-episode and recurrent genital herpes. Some reductions in pain and time to healing of lesions have been reported with an interferon preparation incorporated into nonoxynol-9-containing gel.[60,70] The immune modulators levamisole and transfer factor also are being evaluated, but data are too preliminary to draw any conclusions concerning their efficacy and safety.

Agents that can eliminate ganglionic latency and prevent recurrent HSV infections are not expected to be available in the near future. Therefore, several HSV vaccines currently in clinical trials hold the most promise in the prevention of infection and establishment of latency. However, stimulation of the immune response by repeated injection of heterologous vaccines (e.g., BCG and influenza vaccines) in patients with recurrent genital herpes is of no benefit in reducing the recurrence rate.[60,64,65,70]

EVALUATION OF THERAPEUTIC OUTCOME

At best, antiviral compounds such as acyclovir provide effective symptomatic and prophylactic therapy; however, antivirals are not curative. Patients receiving suppressive therapy should be monitored closely for adverse drug effects. Also, therapy should be withdrawn periodically to observe any changes in the patient's intrinsic pattern of recurrence. Presently there is no evidence that suppressive therapy has any effect on ganglionic latency. As a result, recurrence rates after discontinuation of acyclovir are similar to pretreatment rates in the majority of published studies. Although not yet demonstrated, it is possible that acyclovir prophylaxis may decrease or eliminate periods of asymptomatic viral shedding and reduce transmission of genital herpes.

TRICHOMONIASIS

Trichomoniasis is caused by *Trichomonas vaginalis,* a flagellated, motile protozoan. Humans are host to two other *Trichomonas* species, *T. tenax* and *T. hominis,* but *T. vaginalis* is the only species thought to be pathogenic. *Trichomonas* species are highly site specific, and *T. vaginalis* is not known to infect either the oropharynx or rectum.[82–84]

It is estimated that 2.5 to 3 million cases of vaginal trichomoniasis occur annually in the United States. The peak incidence in women occurs between the ages of 16 and 35, although there is a high prevalence between ages 35 and 45. Trichomoniasis is less common in women using barrier contraceptive methods or oral contraceptives. The contraceptive foams are believed to have some activity against *T. vaginalis,* although the clinical significance of this is unknown.[84] Age-incidence figures in men are less clear because of the difficulty in diagnosis, the high incidence of asymptomatic disease, and the high spontaneous cure rate.[82,84,85] However, it is believed that 30–40% of the male partners of *T. vaginalis*-infected women develop a trichomonas infection.[84]

Although infection by nonsexual contact is reported, it is uncommon. *Trichomonas vaginalis* can survive for short periods on moist surfaces, so the possibility of contamination of inanimate objects by body discharges exists. Infections can be spread by communal bathing or contact with infected bath or toilet articles. Neonatal infections also represent nonvenereal transmission of the disease.[82–85]

Trichomonads are isolated from the vagina, the urethra, and the Skene's gland in 90–95% of infected women. Infrequently they are recovered from the endocervix. Extragenital sites are epidemiologically important, because infection can persist and result in reinfection of the vagina if local therapy alone is used. This may account for the higher relapse rates reported for local versus systemic therapy. After attachment to the vaginal or urethral mucosa, trichomonads usually elicit an inflammatory response that manifests as a discharge containing large numbers of polymorphonuclear leukocytes.[82–84]

CLINICAL PRESENTATION

Trichomonal infections are much more common in women than in men. The incubation period of trichomoniasis is 4–20 days, with as many as 50% of infected women remaining asymptomatic. When symptomatic, females can present with mild to severe vaginal discharge, vulvar pruritis, and dysuria. Symptoms frequently worsen during menstruation when the pH of the vagina is optimal for growth of trichomonads. Vaginal discharge is noted in approximately 50–75% of infected women and classically has been described as malodorous, foamy, and greenish yellow in color; however, more typically the discharge is grayish and only mildly odoriferous. In up to 50% of women, severe pruritis is noted.[82–85]

On examination of symptomatic women, the vulva and surrounding areas may be diffusely erythematous and excoriated as a result of scratching. Secondary infection of excoriated areas is not uncommon. The vagina is often erythematous; surface erosions of the cervix are seen in up to 90% of women. Tender inguinal lymphadenopathy and lower abdominal pain occur infrequently. In a small percentage of patients there may be no abnormal findings on vaginal examination. There is no evidence that trichomonads spread beyond the cervix to cause PID or disseminated disease; however, it is suggested that cervical erosion secondary to trichomoniasis may contribute to malignant transformation.[82–85]

Trichomoniasis may be responsible for causing premature rupture of the membranes and preterm delivery. It can be transmitted to neonates after passage through an infected birth canal. The risk is low (5%) and most cases of neonatal infections are self-limited; however, persistent vaginal or urethral infections should be treated.[14,82,85]

In men, the majority of trichomonal infections are asymptomatic. The most common site of infection is the urethra. It is likely that differences in pathogenicity of trichomonads in men and women are dependent on differences in the microenvironment of the vagina and urethra. In symptomatic males, urethral discharge is seen most commonly, followed by pruritis and dysuria. The discharge may range from mucoid to purulent. *Trichomonas vaginalis* has been established as one cause of treatment failure in patients with presumed nongonococcal urethritis treated with tetracycline or erythromycin. For most men, trichomonal urethritis is apparently self-limited. *Trichomonas vaginalis* has been implicated in some cases of prostatitis and epididymitis.[82–85]

Patients presenting with signs and symptoms of a trichomoniasis should also be examined for other STDs. Women diagnosed with *T. vaginalis* have up to a three times greater risk of having gonorrhea also, while approximately 16–20% of men with gonococcal urethritis also have trichomoniasis.[84]

DIAGNOSIS

Because *T. vaginalis* produces nonspecific symptoms consistent with other causes of bacterial vaginosis, laboratory diagnosis is required. The diagnosis of *T. vaginalis* may be complicated because approximately 97% of symptomatic women are concomitantly colonized with yeast. Because *T. vaginalis* requires a pH range of 4.9–7.5 for survival, a vaginal discharge pH of greater than 5.0 usually indicates the presence of either *T. vaginalis* or *Gardnerella vaginalis* (bacterial vaginosis). The simplest and most reliable means of diagnosis is a wet-mount examination of the vaginal discharge. Trichomoniasis is confirmed if characteristic pear-shaped, flagellating organisms are observed. Because the wet mount is only about 75–80% sensitive, other means of diagnosis are necessary if no organisms are observed microscopically.[45,82–85]

Although the presence of trichomonads may be reported on a Papanicolaou (PAP) smear, the sensitivity of this cytologic technique is less than for wet mount and also is associated with a number of false-positive results. Stained smears of cervical specimens have been used in diagnosis, but appear less sensitive and more time consuming than the wet mount and, therefore, are not recommended. Culture techniques for trichomonads are highly specific and more sensitive than the wet mount; however, because up to 48 hours or longer may be necessary for growth, cultures are not useful in rapid diagnosis.[45,82–85]

In males, demonstration of trichomonads in urethral specimens by wet mount is difficult, and diagnosis depends largely on culture. Specimens from males should be taken prior to first voiding, as the small number of trichomonads in males may be reduced by micturation.[45,82–85]

TREATMENT

Metronidazole is the only antimicrobial agent available in the United States that is consistently effective in *T. vaginalis* infections. In only a few cases have *T. vaginalis* isolates been resistant to standard metronidazole doses. In these instances, doses higher than those routinely recommended may be necessary to achieve a cure.[14,82–86]

Treatment recommendations for *Trichomonas* infections are given in Table 110.8.[14] The standard therapy for trichomoniasis is metronidazole 2 grams orally as a single dose. When sexual partners are treated simultaneously, cure rates greater than 95% are reported. If sexual partners are not treated concurrently, cure rates are in the range of 80–90%. In limited clinical testing, single 1- and 1.5-gram doses of metronidazole also have been shown to produce high cure rates.[14,82–86]

Advantages of single-dose therapy over the multidose alternative regimen include better patient compliance, lower total dose, lower cost, and shorter exposure of the patient's gastrointestinal and urogenital anaerobic bacterial flora to the drug. As a result of the latter, the likelihood of developing pseudomembranous colitis or symptomatic candidal vulvovaginitis is decreased. Because high doses of metronidazole have mutagenic effects in bacteria and oncogenic effects in mice, a reduced time of exposure in humans may be beneficial. At present there is no conclusive clinical

TABLE 110.8. TREATMENT OF TRICHOMONIASIS

Type	Recommended Regimen[a]	Alternative Regimen
Symptomatic and asymptomatic infections	Metronidazole 2.0 g PO in a single dose[b]	Metronidazole 500 mg PO 2 times daily for 7 days[c]
Treatment in pregnancy	No treatment recommended unless symptoms are severe[d]	
Neonatal infections[e]	Metronidazole 10–30 mg/kg daily for 5–8 days	

[a]Recommendations are those of the CDC.

[b]Treatment failures should be treated with metronidazole 500 mg PO 2 times daily for 7 days. Persistent failures should be managed in consultation with an expert. Metronidazole 2 g PO daily for 3–5 days has been effective in patients infected with *T. vaginalis* strains mildly resistant to metronidazole, but experience is limited; higher doses also have been used.

[c]Recently the Anti-Infective Advisory Committee of the FDA recommended approval of a 375 mg twice daily for 7 days dosage regimen. This would be an alternative regimen to the 250 mg three times daily for 7 days regimen currently approved in the product labeling for metronidazole. Neither regimen is currently included in the CDC recommendations for the treatment of trichomoniasis.

[d]Metronidazole is contraindicated in the first trimester of pregnancy and generally should be avoided throughout pregnancy. A single 2-g dose may be used after the first trimester.

[e]Only infants with symptomatic trichomoniasis or with urogenital trichomonal colonization that persists beyond the fourth week of life.

evidence for either of these effects in humans after short-term, low-dose metronidazole therapy. Gastrointestinal complaints (e.g., anorexia, nausea, vomiting, diarrhea) are more common with the single 2-gram dose, occurring in 5–10% of treated patients. Some patients complain of a bitter metallic taste in the mouth. Patients intolerant of the single 2-gram dose because of gastrointestinal adverse effects can be treated with a 7-day course of 500 mg twice daily.[84]

To achieve maximal cure rates and prevent relapse with the single 2-gram dose of metronidazole, simultaneous treatment of infected sexual partners is necessary. However, in women treated with the alternative 7-day course, relapse rates are not appreciably different regardless of whether or not sexual partners are treated. It is speculated that in men spontaneous resolution of trichomonal infection or a reduction in the number of trichomonads below the inoculum necessary to transmit disease may occur during the 7 days of a female's therapy.[82–86]

Patients who fail to respond to an initial course usually respond to a second course of metronidazole therapy. In these cases sexual partners also should be retreated. For some *T. vaginalis* strains, higher dosages (2–7.5 grams daily for 3–5 days) are effective. Good response rates also are reported for metronidazole 2–3 grams orally plus a single 500-mg tablet administered intravaginally for 7–14 days. Use of intravenous metronidazole may be warranted for rare cases of intolerance to oral medication.[84,86]

Patients taking metronidazole should be instructed to avoid alcohol ingestion during therapy and for 1–2 days after completion of therapy because of a possible disulfiram-like effect. Metronidazole can potentiate the hypoprothrombinemic effects of warfarin, but a clinically significant effect is unlikely with single-dose regimens. Because metronidazole is secreted in breast milk, it is recommended that breast-feeding be interrupted for at least 24 hours after maternal ingestion of a single 2-gram dose.[14,82–86]

At present, no satisfactory treatment is available for pregnant women with *Trichomonas* infections. Metronidazole is contraindicated during the first trimester of pregnancy and many experts recommend avoiding its use throughout pregnancy. Metronidazole easily crosses the placenta and fetal blood levels are comparable to maternal levels. A clear association between teratogenic effects and maternal ingestion during pregnancy has not been shown; on the basis of limited data, short courses of metronidazole administered during the second and third trimesters do not appear to increase the incidence of teratogenicity, prematurity, or fetal death. In pregnant patients with severe symptoms who do not respond to local palliative treatment, a single 2-gram dose of metronidazole may be required.[14,82–86]

Various local therapies for trichomoniasis also have been proposed for pregnant patients. Clotrimazole vaginal suppositories, 100 mg at bedtime for 6–8 days, relieve symptoms in many women and produce cure rates of 50% or greater.[82] An alternative therapy is gentle douching with 2 tablespoons of vinegar in a quart of warm water once or twice daily until symptoms improve, then less frequently thereafter. This therapy generally provides some symptomatic improvement but few cures. Although once recommended, povidone-iodine douches should be avoided during pregnancy because of the risk of fetal thyroid suppression.[82–86]

Several 5-nitroimidazole antibiotics related to metronidazole (tinidazole, nimorazole, ornidazole, and carnidazole) are being investigated worldwide for the treatment of trichomoniasis. None appears superior to metronidazole in treating susceptible strains of *T. vaginalis*. Some of these antibiotics, however, may prove beneficial in infections exhibiting resistance to metronidazole.[82–86]

EVALUATION OF THERAPEUTIC OUTCOME

Follow-up is considered unnecessary in patients who become asymptomatic after treatment with metronidazole. When patients remain symptomatic, it is important to determine if reinfection has occurred. In these cases a repeat course of therapy, as well as identification and treatment or retreatment of infected sexual partners, is recommended. In situations where reinfection can be excluded, a relative resistance to metronidazole should be assumed and an alternative, multidose metronidazole regimen should be prescribed. Culture and sensitivity are warranted for infections unresponsive to alternative metronidazole regimens.

OTHER SEXUALLY TRANSMITTED DISEASES

Several STDs other than those previously discussed occur with varying frequency in the United States and throughout the world. While an in-depth discussion of these diseases is beyond the scope of this chapter, recommended treatment regimens are given in Table 110.9.[14]

CONCLUSION

More than 20 different diseases for which sexual transmission is epidemiologically important are identified. In the United States gonorrhea and chlamydia have reached epidemic proportions and the incidence of several other STDs, such as genital herpes, is on the rise. For most STDs effective drug therapies are available; however, current therapeutic approaches to genital herpes and AIDS are not curative and, for herpes infections, provide only palliation and suppression of symptoms. Technologic advances in laboratory medicine during the past 10 years have resulted in improved and more rapid diagnostic capabilities for many STDs. For STDs such as gonorrhea and chlamydia, which are associated with a high incidence of asymptomatic cases, these new diagnostic tests may hold particular significance. Asymp-

TABLE 110.9. TREATMENT REGIMENS FOR MISCELLANEOUS SEXUALLY TRANSMITTED DISEASES

Infection	Recommended Regimen[a]	Alternative Regimen
Chancroid *(Haemophilus ducreyi)*	Azithromycin 1 g PO in a single dose or Ceftriaxone 250 mg IM in a single dose or Erythromycin 500 mg PO four times daily for 7 days	Amoxicillin 500 mg plus clavulanic acid 125 mg three times daily for 7 days or Ciprofloxacin 500 mg PO two times daily for 3 days
Lymphogranuloma venereum	Doxycycline 100 mg PO two times daily for 21 days	Erythromycin 500 mg PO four times daily for 21 days or Sulfisoxazole 500 mg PO four times daily for 21 days or equivalent sulfonamide course
Condylomata acuminata		
External genital/perianal warts	Cryotherapy (e.g., liquid nitrogen or cryoprobe) or Podofilox 0.5% solution applied twice daily for 3 days, followed by 4 days of no therapy; cycle is repeated as necessary for a total of four cycles[b] or Podophyllin 10–25% in compound tincture of benzoin applied to lesions and washed off in 1–4 hours; repeat weekly for up to six applications[c] or Trichloroacetic acid 80–90% applied to warts; repeat weekly for up to six applications or Electrodesiccation[d] or electrocautery	
Vaginal warts	Cryotherapy with liquid nitrogen or Trichloroacetic acid 50–90% as for external warts or Podophyllin 10–25% in compound tincture of benzoin applied at weekly intervals[e]	

[a]Recommendations are those of the CDC.
[b]Genital warts only.
[c]Because podophyllin is systemically absorbed and toxic, use of large amounts should be avoided. Use of podophyllin is contraindicated in pregnancy.
[d]Electrodessication is contraindicated in patients with cardiac pacemakers or for lesions proximal to the anal verge.
[e]Some experts caution against vaginal use; care must be taken to ensure that the treated area is dry before removing the speculum.

tomatic patients constitute a large reservoir for transmission of disease and also are potential candidates for development of long-term complications of untreated disease.

As a result of the increasing problem of STDs, greater emphasis today is being placed on primary prevention of STDs. Sexually active persons can minimize their risk of transmitting or acquiring some STDs by avoidance of certain sexual practices and through the proper use of physical and chemical barriers during intercourse. In the future, vaccines providing protection from gonorrhea, genital herpes, and AIDS also may have a significant effect on reducing the incidence of these infections.

REFERENCES

1. Krieger JN. Biology of sexually transmitted diseases. Urol Clin North Am 1984;11:15–25.
2. Holmes KK, Bell TA, Berger RE. Epidemiology of sexually transmitted diseases. Urol Clin North Am 1984;11:3–13.

3. Stone KM, Grimes DA, Magder LS. Primary prevention of sexually transmitted diseases. JAMA 1986;255:1763–1766.
4. Adimora AA, Hamilton H, Holmes KK, Sparling PF. Sexually Transmitted Diseases, 2nd ed, Companion Handbook. New York, McGraw-Hill, 1994, pp 1–9.
5. Donovan P. Testing Positive: Sexually Transmitted Disease and the Public Health Response. New York, Alan Guttmacher Institute, 1993, pp 10–17.
6. Hook EW III, Holmes KK. Gonococcal infections. Ann Intern Med 1985;102:229–243.
7. Duncan WC. Gonorrhea 1983. Dermatol Clin 1983;1:43–51.
8. Harrison WO. Gonococcal urethritis. Urol Clin North Am 1984;11:45–53.
9. Carmen JC. Gonorrhea. US Pharmacist 1983;8(7):53–63.
10. Adimora AA, Hamilton H, Holmes KK, Sparling PF. Sexually Transmitted Diseases, 2nd ed, Companion Handbook. New York, McGraw-Hill, 1994, pp 25–40.
11. Britigan BE, Cohen MS, Sparling PF. Gonococcal infection: Model of molecular pathogenesis. N Engl J Med 1985;312:1683–1694.
12. Moran JS, Zenilman JM. Therapy for gonococcal infections: Options in 1989. Rev Infect Dis 1990;12(suppl 6):S633–S642.
13. Rice RJ, Thompson SE. Treatment of uncomplicated infections due to *Neisseria gonorrhoeae.* JAMA 1986;255:1739–1746.
14. Anonymous. 1993 sexually transmitted diseases treatment guidelines. Centers for Disease Control and Prevention. MMWR 1993;42(RR-14):1–102.
15. Freedman LD. Reduced dosage of ceftriaxone for uncomplicated gonorrhea in women. J Fam Pract 1990;31:201–205.
16. Hammerschlag MR. Neonatal conjunctivitis. Pediatr Ann 1993;22:346–351.
17. O'Hara MA. Ophthalmia neonatorum. Pediatr Clin North Am 1993;40:715–725.
18. Anonymous. Summary of notifiable diseases, United States. 1993. MMWR 1994;42:1–73.
19. Hutchinson CM, Hook EW III. Syphilis in adults. Med Clin North Am 1990;74:1389–1416.
20. Wendel GD Jr. Early and congenital syphilis. Obstet Gynecol Clin North Am 1989;16:479–494.
21. Hook EW III, Marra CM. Acquired syphilis in adults. N Engl J Med 1992;326:1060–1069.
22. Goens JL, Janniger CK, de Wolf K. Dermatologic and systemic manifestations of syphilis. Am Fam Physician 1994;50:1013–1020.
23. Marra CM. Syphilis and human immunodeficiency virus infection. Semin Neurol 1992;12:43–50.
24. Hook EW III. Management of syphilis in human immunodeficiency virus-infected patients [editorial]. Am J Med 1992;93:477–479.
25. Quinn TC, Zenilman J, Rompalo A. Sexually transmitted diseases: Advances in diagnosis and treatment. Adv Intern Med 1994;39:149–196.
26. Evans HE, Frenkel LD. Congenital syphilis. Clin Perinatol 1994;21:149–162.
27. Johnson PC, Farnie MA. Testing for syphilis. Dermatol Clin 1994;12:9–17.
28. Larsen SA. Syphilis. Clin Lab Med 1989;9:545–557.
29. Farnes SW, Setness PA. Serologic tests for syphilis. Postgrad Med 1990;87:37–46.
30. Jurado RL, Campbell J, Martin PD. Prozone phenomenon in secondary syphilis: Has its time arrived? Arch Intern Med 1993;153:2406–2407.
31. Hook III EW. Treatment of syphilis: Current recommendations, alternatives, and continuing problems. Rev Infect Dis 1989;11(suppl 6):S1511–S1517.
32. Anonymous. Recommendations for the prevention and management of *Chlamydia trachomatis* infections, 1993. Centers for Disease Control and Prevention. MMWR 1993; 42(RR-12):1–39.
33. Toomey KE, Barnes RC. Treatment of *Chlamydia trachomatis* genital infection. Rev Infect Dis 1990;12(suppl 6):S645–S651.
34. Bowie WR. Nongonococcal urethritis. Urol Clin North Am 1984;11:55–64.
35. Bowie WR. Epidemiology and therapy of *Chlamydia trachomatis* infections. Drugs 1984;27:459–468.
36. Martin DH. Chlamydial infections. Med Clin North Am 1990;74:1367–1388.
37. McGregor JA. Chlamydial infection in women. Obstet Gynecol Clin North Am 1989;16:565–592.
38. Majeroni BA. Chlamydial cervicitis: Complications and new treatment options. Am Fam Physician 1994;49:1825–1829.
39. Bell TA, Stamm WE, Wang SP, et al. Chronic *Chlamydia trachomatis* infections in infants. JAMA 1992;267:400–402 [Erratum, JAMA 1992;267:2188].
40. Schachter J, Grossman M, Sweet RL, et al. Prospective study of perinatal transmission of *Chlamydia trachomatis.* JAMA 1986;255:3374–3377.
41. Hook EW, Spitters C, Reichart CA, et al. Use of cell culture and rapid diagnostic assay for *Chlamydia trachomatis* screening. JAMA 1994;272:867–870.
42. Rapoza PA, Quinn TC, Kiessling LA, et al. Assessment of neonatal conjunctivitis with a direct immunofluorescent monoclonal antibody stain for *Chlamydia.* JAMA 1986;255:3369–3373.
43. Coleman P, Varitek V, Mushahwar IK, et al. Testpack chlamydia, a new rapid assay for the direct detection of *Chlamydia trachomatis.* J Clin Microbiol 1989;27:2811–2814.
44. Reichart CA, Gaydos CA, Brady WE, et al. Evaluation of Abbott Testpack Chlamydia for detection of *Chlamydia trachomatis* in patients attending sexually transmitted disease clinics. Sex Transm Dis 1990;17:147–151.
45. Martens MG. Office diagnosis of sexually transmitted diseases. Obstet Gynecol Clin North Am 1989;16:659–677.
46. Shafer M, Schachter J, Moscioki AB, et al. Urinary leukocyte esterase screening test for symptomatic chlamydial and gonococcal infections in males. JAMA 1989;262:2562–2566.
47. Shafer MA, Schachter J, Moncada J, et al. Evaluation of urine-based screening strategies to detect *Chlamydia trachomatis* among sexually active asymptomatic young males. JAMA 1993;270:2065–2070.
48. Jaschek G, Gaydos CA, Welsh LE, Quinn TC. Direct detection of *Chlamydia trachomatis* in urine specimens from symptomatic and asymptomatic men by using a rapid polymerase chain reaction assay. J Clin Microbiol 1993;31:1209–1212.

49. Tartaglione TA, Hooton TM. The role of fluoroquinolones in sexually transmitted disease. Pharmacother 1993;13:189–201.
50. Jaffe HW. Nongonococcal urethritis: Treatment of men and their sexual partners. Rev Infect Dis 1982;4(suppl):S772–S777.
51. Schachter J, Sweet RL, Grossman M, et al. Experience with the routine use of erythromycin for chlamydial infections in pregnancy. N Engl J Med 1986;276–279.
52. Hooten TM, Rogers ME, Medina TG, et al. Ciprofloxacin compared with doxycycline for nongonococcal urethritis: Ineffectiveness against *Chlamydia trachomatis* due to relapsing infection. JAMA 1990;264:1418–1421.
53. Jones RB, Van der Pol B, Martin DH, Shepard MK. Partial characterization of *Chlamydia trachomatis* isolates resistant to multiple antibiotics. J Infect Dis 1990;162:1309–1315.
54. Batteiger BE, Jones RB, White A. Efficacy and safety of ofloxacin in the treatment of nongonococcal sexually transmitted disease. Am J Med 1989;87(suppl 6C):755–775.
55. Chow JM, Yonekura L, Richwald GA, et al. The association between *Chlamydia trachomatis* and ectopic pregnancy: A matched-pair, case-control study. JAMA 1990;263:3164–3167.
56. Cohen I, Veille J-C, Calkins BM. Improved pregnancy outcome following successful treatment of chlamydial infection. JAMA 1990;263:3160–3163.
57. Bush MR, Rosa C. Azithromycin and erythromycin in the treatment of cervical chlamydial infection during pregnancy. Ob Gynecol 1994;84:61–63.
58. Stamm WE. Azithromycin in the treatment of uncomplicated genital chlamydial infections. Am J Med 1991;91(suppl 3A):19S–26S.
59. Kinghorn GR. Genital herpes: Natural history and treatment of acute episodes. J Med Virol 1993;suppl 1:33–38.
60. Mertz GJ. Herpes simplex virus infections. Med Clin North Am 1990;74:1433–1454.
61. Corey L. The current trends in genital herpes: Progress in prevention. Sex Transm Dis 1994;21(suppl 2):S38–S44.
62. Mertz GJ. Epidemiology of genital herpes infections. Infect Dis Clin North Am 1993;7:825–839.
63. Maccato M, Kaufman RH. Herpes genitalis. Dermatol Clin 1992;10:415–422.
64. Prober CG. Herpetic vaginitis in 1993. Clin Obstet Gynecol 1993;36:177–187.
65. de Ruiter A, Thin RN. Genital herpes: A guide to pharmacologic therapy. Drugs 1994;47:297–304.
66. Corey L, Spear PG. Infections with herpes simplex viruses (first of two parts). N Engl J Med 1986;314:686–691.
67. Dawkins BJ. Genital herpes simplex infections. Primary Care 1990;17:95–114.
68. Landy HJ, Grossman JH III. Herpes simplex virus. Obstet Gynecol Clin North Am 1989;16:495–515.
69. Mindel A. Long-term clinical and psychological management of genital herpes. J Med Virol 1993;suppl 1:39–44.
70. Stone KM, Whittington WL. Treatment of genital herpes. Rev Infect Dis 1990;12(suppl 6):S610–S619.
71. Blanchier H, Huraux J-M, Huraux-Rendu C, Sainte-Croix le Baleur A. Genital herpes and pregnancy—preventive measures. Eur J Obstet Gynecol Reprod Biol 1994;53:33–38.
72. Ashley RL. Genital herpes infections. Clin Lab Med 1989;9:405–420.
73. Kroon S. Genital herpes—when and how to treat. Semin Dermatol 1990;9:133–140.
74. Gold D, Corey L. Treatment of herpes simplex virus infections. Clin Lab Med 1987;7:815–829.
75. O'Brien JJ, Campoli-Richards DM. Acyclovir. An updated review of its antiviral activity, pharmacokinetic properties, and therapeutic efficacy. Drugs 1989;37:233–309.
76. Dorsky DI, Crumpacker CS. Drugs 5 years later: Acyclovir. Ann Intern Med 1987;107:859–874.
77. Corey L. First-episode, recurrent, and asymptomatic herpes simplex infections. J Am Acad Dermatol 1988;18(1, part 2):169–172.
78. Fife KH, Crumpacker CS, Mertz GJ, et al. Recurrence and resistance patterns of herpes simplex virus following cessation of ≤6 years of chronic suppression with acyclovir. J Infect Dis 1994;169:1338–1341.
79. Baker DA. Herpes and pregnancy: New Management. Clin Obstet Gynecol 1990;33:253–257.
80. Prober CG, Arvin AM. Genital herpes and the pregnant woman. Curr Clin Top Infect Dis 1989;10:1–26.
81. Whitley RJ. Neonatal herpes simplex virus infections. J Med Virol 1993;suppl 1:13–21.
82. Thomason JL, Gelbart SM. *Trichomonas vaginalis.* Obstet Gynecol 1989;74:536–541.
83. Hammill HA. *Trichomonas vaginalis.* Obstet Gynecol Clin North Am 1989;16:531–540.
84. Adimora AA, Hamilton H, Holmes KK, Sparling PF. Sexually Transmitted Diseases, 2nd ed, Companion Handbook. New York, McGraw-Hill, 1994, pp 212–222.
85. Sobel JD. Vaginal infections in adult women. Med Clin North Am 1990;74:1573–1602.
86. Lossick JG. Treatment of *Trichomonas vaginalis* infections. Rev Infect Dis 1982;4(suppl):S801–S818.

Chapter 111

Bone and Joint Infections

Edward P. Armstrong, PharmD, BCPS, and Victor A. Elsberry, PharmD, BCNSP

Bone and joint infections are comprised of two disease processes known respectively as osteomyelitis and septic or infectious arthritis. As such, they are unique and separate infectious entities, with different signs and symptoms and infecting organisms. Introduction of oral antibiotic therapy has had a dramatic impact on antibiotic regimens used to treat these diseases. However, in spite of advances in therapy, these infections continue to cause significant morbidity from residual damage and chronic recurring infections. Both infectious processes continue to be a serious problem from a diagnostic as well as a management viewpoint. Emphasis on initiating antibiotic therapy as soon as possible is important in reducing long-term complications.

EPIDEMIOLOGY

OSTEOMYELITIS

The most common method of classifying osteomyelitis is based on the route in which the infecting organism reaches the bone. Infection that results from spread through the bloodstream is termed *hematogenous osteomyelitis.* When the organism reaches the bone from an adjoining soft tissue infection, it is termed contiguous osteomyelitis. Osteomyelitis that results from direct inoculation such as from trauma, puncture wounds, or surgery generally is also classified under the contiguous osteomyelitis category. Patients with peripheral vascular disease are at risk for development of osteomyelitis, and these patients are often separated into a third distinct category due to their unique management features.

Osteomyelitis may also be classified based on the duration of the disease. Acute osteomyelitis describes infections of recent onset, usually several days to 1 week, while chronic infections are those of a longer duration. Some authors describe chronic infections as those with symptoms for more than 1 month before therapy and other authors define chronic infections as relapse of an initial infection. Yet a third system sometimes used to classify osteomyelitis has been developed by Cierney and Mader.[1] It is a staging system based on the anatomic location of the infection (e.g., medullary or superficial) and the physiologic status of the patient (e.g., otherwise healthy, systemic immunologic compromise, local immunologic compromise). This classification system may be useful when comparing patients between different studies and attempting to categorize the severity of infection.

Osteomyelitis is generally an uncommon disease. One classic publication reported that 247 patients had osteomyelitis in a prominent American teaching hospital during a 4-year period.[2] Acute hematogenous osteomyelitis has an estimated annual incidence of 4.5 per 100,000 population.[3] Osteomyelitis caused by contiguous spread, including postoperative, direct puncture, and that associated with adjacent soft tissue infections, comprises 47% of infections. Hematogenous osteomyelitis comprises 19% of infections, and osteomyelitis occurring in patients with significant peripheral vascular disease comprises 47% of infections. Reviewing osteomyelitis cases based on duration of disease, it is observed that acute disease constitutes 56% of patients and that chronic osteomyelitis, defined as having a previous hospitalization for the same infection, constitutes 44% of patients.

INFECTIOUS ARTHRITIS

Infectious or septic arthritis is an inflammatory reaction within the joint space. Distinct from osteomyelitis, septic arthritis is a more common disease and is known to be one of the most common causes of new cases of arthritis.[4] One series in children from a referral hospital reported 30.8 cases per year for 5 years.[5] Another study reported 97 cases of nongonococcal infections during an 18-year period and noted a slightly higher incidence of gonococcal infections.[6] Infectious arthritis may occur from many different types of microorganisms. Most infecting organisms are known to produce an infection in a single joint, termed *monarticular infections;* however, infections also may involve two or more joints. As with osteomyelitis, joint infections also may be classified according to the mechanisms by which the infecting organism reaches the joint. Infectious arthritis may result from the spread of an adjacent bone infection, from direct contamination of the joint space, or from hematogenous dissemination. Hematogenous spread of the disease comprises the majority of infections; spread from osteomyelitis and direct inoculation are much less frequent.[7] Infectious arthritis most commonly occurs in patients older than age 30; 20% of cases occur in children.[8]

PATHOPHYSIOLOGY

HEMATOGENOUS OSTEOMYELITIS

Hematogenous osteomyelitis is classically described as a disease of children because most cases occur in patients less than 16 years of age.[9] Table 111.1 summarizes the primary characteristics of osteomyelitis. Less commonly, these infections occur in older patients. One exception, vertebral osteomyelitis, involves the vertebrae and occurs most frequently in patients older than 50 years of age.

Unique features of the anatomy and physiology of some bones appears to predispose them to become infected.[10] The vascular structure within the long bones appears to predispose the bone for hematogenous infections to begin within the metaphyses (Fig. 111.1). The nutrient arteries of the long bones divide within the medullary canal of the bone into small arterioles. These end in hairpin turns near the growth plate and flow into veins, of much wider diameter, that drain the medullary cavity. An infection in hematogenous disease is initiated within the bend of the arterioles. There is considerable slowing of blood flow passing through the hairpin turns within the arterioles and then into the wider venous structures. This sludging of blood flow allows bacteria present within the bloodstream to settle and initiate an inflammatory response. In addition to these structural features, there also appears to be less active phagocytosis within the metaphysis. A lack of reticuloendothelial cells within this area of the bone may allow bacteria to settle and establish an infection. After the bacteria settle in the bone, avascular necrosis may occur from occlusion of the nutrient vessels and release of bacterial enzymes.

In addition to these anatomic and functional features, there is some evidence that trauma is associated with developing an infection in specific bones. Children who develop hematogenous osteomyelitis may report some type of trauma as an etiologic event. Animal data also indicate that traumatized bone is more likely to become infected than normal bone.

Once the infection is initiated, exudate begins to form within the bone, which produces increased pressure. The age of the patient largely determines the next stage in the pathophysiology. In children older than 12–18 months, the infection that started in the metaphysis of a long bone will be prevented from spreading into the joint because of the growth plate; however, the exudate will often expand laterally through the thin outer cortex of the bone and raise the loose periosteum. The periosteum is thick and not easily broken and the resulting pus usually remains subperiosteal. If there is significant periosteal damage, a soft tissue abscess may develop. Impairment of blood flow to the outer portion of the cortical bone may occur, producing dead bone that separates from healthy bone, termed *sequestra.* The elevated periosteum remains viable because its blood supply, derived from the overlying muscle, is unaffected. The raised periosteum will continue to produce bone; however, this new bone is now separated from the cortex because the periosteum has been raised from the infection. This new bone is termed *involucrum.*

In adults, the periosteum is tightly bound and the cortex is thick. These anatomic features generally cause the infections to remain intramedullary. As expected, subperiosteal abscess formations are less common in this population. The infection may spread to adjacent bone structures through the Haversian and Volkmann canals. Chronic osteomyelitis is more likely to occur if large segments of bone become avascular and necrotic.

Neonatal patients also have unique characteristics. In these patients there are blood vessels that spread through the cortex of the metaphyses and up into the epiphyses. This allows an infection that may have started within the

TABLE 111.1. TYPES OF OSTEOMYELITIS, AGE DISTRIBUTION, COMMON SITES, AND RISK FACTORS

Type of Osteomyelitis	Typical Age (yr)	Site(s) Involved	Risk Factors
Hematogenous	Less than 1	Long bones and joints	Prematurity, umbilical catheter or venous cutdown, respiratory distress syndrome, perinatal asphyxia
	1–20	Long bones (femur, tibia, humerus)	Infection (pharyngitis, cellulitis, respiratory infections), sickle cell disease, puncture wounds to feet
	Older than 50	Vertebrae	Diabetes mellitus, blunt trauma to spine, urinary tract infection
Contiguous	Older than 50	Femur, tibia, mandible	Hip fractures, open fractures
Vascular insufficiency	Older than 50	Feet, toes	Diabetes mellitus, peripheral vascular disease, pressure sores

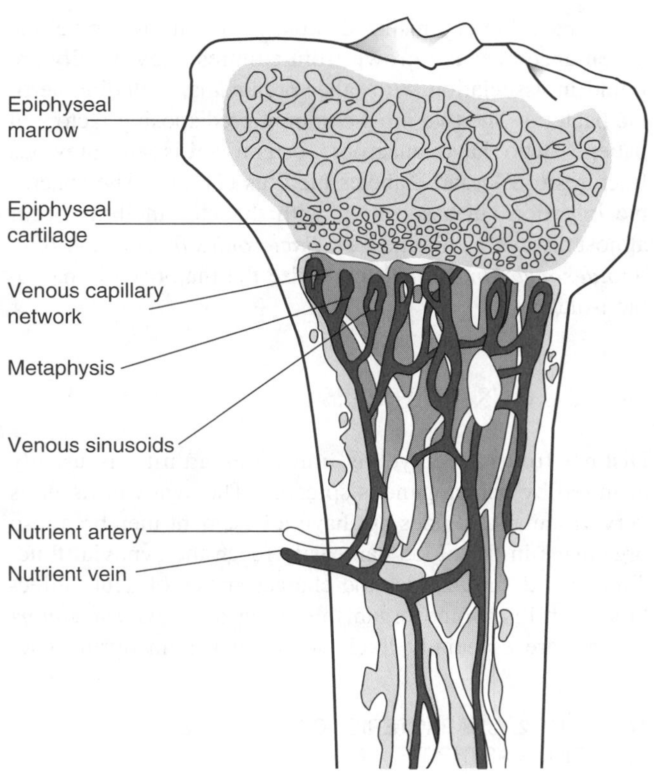

Figure 111.1. Cross section of normal bone.

metaphyseal area to spread easily to involve the epiphyses and then into the joint. Therefore, in infants, not only can the infection spread to involve the periosteum and the shaft as in children, but the infection also may spread to involve the joint.

Hematogenous osteomyelitis also is known to have a predilection for certain bones. The specific bones most likely to be involved also depend on the age of the patient. Children most commonly develop infections within the femur, tibia, humerus, and fibula. Vertebral infections are more common in patients older than 50 years of age. Neonatal infections commonly involve multiple bones.

The bacteriology of hematogenous osteomyelitis is unique compared with osteomyelitis caused by other routes of infection. A single organism is responsible for the vast majority of hematogenous infections. *Staphylococcus aureus* is isolated from 60–90% of the hematogenous infections in children. In one report of children with acute osteomyelitis during a 7-year period, *S. aureus, Haemophilus influenzae* type b, and *Pseudomonas aeruginosa* were responsible for 45%, 21%, and 10%, respectively, of the 75 cases for which organisms were identified.[11] Neonatal osteomyelitis has a wider spectrum in infecting organisms. The three most common etiologic agents are *S. aureus,* group B streptococcus, and *Escherichia coli.* The infections from *S. aureus* and *E. coli* have been linked to complications occurring during pregnancy or delivery, and they are most frequently involved in multiple bone infections.

Vertebral osteomyelitis has several unique features. Vertebral osteomyelitis most commonly occurs in adults. The highest incidence is noted in patients in their 50s and 60s. The lumbar and thoracic regions are the locations of the majority of infections. Hematogenous infections are most likely to develop in the vascular areas near the subchondral plate region of the vertebral body. Staphylococci cause approximately 60% of these infections; however, gram-negative organisms now play a significant role. It is presumed that these gram-negative organisms, particularly *E. coli,* most likely originate within the urinary tract. *Escherichia coli* vertebral infections have been associated with urinary tract infections, positive urine cultures, and bacteremias. *Mycobacterium tuberculosis* also is known to cause infections in the spine.[12] Skin and respiratory tract infections are other foci of infections known to lead to vertebral infections.

A unique category of osteomyelitis patients are those individuals with a history of intravenous (IV) drug abuse. More than 50% of the osteomyelitis infections in this group of patients are found in the vertebral column. Less than 20% of infections are located in either the sternoarticular or pelvic girdle. Infections are much less frequent within the extremities. A very unusual feature of osteomyelitis in the IV drug-abuser population is the spectrum of organisms. Gram-negative organisms are responsible for 88% of infections. *Pseudomonas aeruginosa,* either singly or in combination with other organisms, is cultured in 78% of all infections. *Klebsiella, Enterobacter,* and *Serratia* also may be found, but less commonly. In addition, staphylococcal and streptococcal organisms may be cultured.

Patients with sickle cell anemia and related hemoglobinopathies have a much higher rate of infection with *Salmonella* compared with other populations. *Salmonella* species are responsible for two-thirds of the infections in these patients. It is believed that bowel infarctions from the sickle cell disease may facilitate salmonellae entry into the bloodstream from the colon and spread hematogenously to the bone. Osteomyelitis in patients with sickle cell disease may occur in any bone, but it is observed to be most common in the medullary cavity of long or tubular bones. Because of the difficulty in separating bone pain during a sickle cell crisis from that of an infection, osteomyelitis may be relatively advanced in these patients when the diagnosis is made. Although salmonellae are cultured most frequently, staphylococci and other gram-negative organisms also may be isolated.

CONTIGUOUS-SPREAD OSTEOMYELITIS

This category of osteomyelitis includes those infections caused by direct entrance of organisms from a source outside of the body or by progressive spread of an infection from tissue adjacent to the bone. Penetrating wounds (e.g., trauma), open fractures, or various invasive orthopedic procedures may result in direct inoculation of organisms into the bone. More than 80% of cases of postoperative osteomyelitis are known to occur following open reductions of fractures. Specifically, these infections occur most commonly after internal fixation of a hip fracture or a femoral or tibial shaft fracture. Although less common, osteomyelitis also may occur following craniotomies, disk surgery, and repair of degenerative arthritis.

Osteomyelitis secondary to an adjoining soft tissue infection comprises another very important group of contiguous infections and most often involves the fingers and toes. Less commonly, infections may spread from infected teeth to involve the mandible or occur secondary to sinus infections by spreading through the mucosal lining of the sinuses into the vascular system surrounding the bone.

In contrast to hematogenous osteomyelitis, which most commonly occurs in children, contiguous-spread osteomyelitis most commonly occurs in patients older than age 50. Most likely this is due to the fact that important predisposing factors, such as hip fractures, are more common in this age group.

Contiguous-spread disease has several important differences compared with hematogenous osteomyelitis. Although *S. aureus* is still the most common organism isolated, infections with multiple organisms, including gram-negative bacilli, frequently occur. *Pseudomonas aeruginosa, Proteus, Streptococcus, E. coli, Staphylococcus epidermidis,* and anaerobes all may be isolated. One important exception to this wide range of organisms is puncture wounds of the feet. There is a strong correlation between puncture wounds of the feet and gram-negative osteomyelitis, especially infections caused by *P. aeruginosa.*

Patients with osteomyelitis in association with severe vascular insufficiency are extremely difficult to manage. As anticipated, most of these patients have diabetes mellitus or severe atherosclerosis, and develop their infections from contiguous-spread mechanisms. Generally these patients are between the ages of 50 and 70 years when they develop osteomyelitis. Frequently, patients with vascular disease develop osteomyelitis in their toes and fingers, and there is usually an adjacent area of infection such as cellulitis or dermal ulcers. Many diabetic patients who develop osteomyelitis also have other complications such as neuropathy and nephropathy.

Another important characteristic of osteomyelitis in association with vascular insufficiency is the spectrum of infecting organisms. Infections in these patients almost always include multiple organisms. The mixed floral infections often include *Staphylococcus* and *Streptococcus,* or the combination of *Staphylococcus, Streptococcus,* and Enterobacteriaceae. Enterococcus and anaerobic organisms also may be seen.

Anaerobic organisms also play a role in osteomyelitis. When anaerobes are grown from cultures, they usually are found in association with other organisms, including aerobic bacteria. The two most common predisposing factors in patients who have anaerobic osteomyelitis are previous fractures (48%) and diabetes mellitus (11%).[13] The anaerobic infections in association with diabetes mellitus occur almost always within the feet. *Bacteroides fragilis* and *Bacteroides melaninogenicus* comprise the majority of anaerobic isolates.

INFECTIOUS ARTHRITIS

Distinct from osteomyelitis, infectious arthritis is usually acquired by hematogenous spread.[14] The synovial tissue is very vascular and does not have a basement membrane, so organisms in the blood can easily reach the synovial fluid. Table 111.2 summarizes the characteristics of acute infectious arthritis. Some organisms, such as *Neisseria gonorrhoeae,* are especially likely to infect a joint during bac-

TABLE 111.2. CHARACTERISTICS OF ACUTE INFECTIOUS ARTHRITIS

Feature	Finding
Peak incidence	Children less than 16 years Adults greater than 50
Clinical findings	Fever of 38–40° in children; painful swollen joint in the absence of trauma Physical exam: effusion, restriction of joint motion, tenderness and warmth of joint
Most commonly affected joints	Knee, hip, ankle, elbow, wrist, and shoulder
Laboratory findings:	
Erythrocyte sedimentation rate	Elevated in 90% of cases
White blood cell count	Elevated in 30–60% of cases
Left shift	Seen in 2/3 of patients
Blood culture	Positive in 40% of cases
Needle aspiration of joint	Gram-stain diagnostic in 30–50% of cases. Synovial fluid cultures are positive in 60–80% of cases. Synovial fluid differential reveals 90% polymorphonuclear leukocytes. Synovial fluid glucose decreased relative to serum glucose. Lactic acid levels elevated in nongonococcal infectious arthritis, but not in gonococcal infectious arthritis

teremia. In addition, organisms also may gain access to the joint from a deep penetrating wound, an intra-articular steroid injection, arthroscopy, prosthetic-joint surgery, and contiguous osteomyelitis expansion into the joint. Table 111.3 summarizes the risk factors associated with adult infectious arthritis. Trauma also appears to be a risk factor in facilitating microorganism entry into the synovial space. Unlike children, adults often have significant systemic diseases that predispose them to infectious arthritis, such as diabetes mellitus, immunosuppressive states (cancer, liver disease), or preexisting arthritis.[15] IV drug abusers also are prone to develop septic arthritis. Arthritis, joint trauma, and surgery are other important risk factors, because chronic inflammation or trauma makes the joint more susceptible to infection. In addition, rheumatoid arthritis patients may be prone to bacterial infection because of an inherent phagocytic defect as well as concomitant corticosteroid therapy. Hormonal factors appear to play a role in *N. gonorrhoeae* infectious arthritis. Women are more prone to develop disseminated gonococcal infections than men. The second and third trimesters of pregnancy and during menstruation appear to be the times of greatest risk of developing gonococcal bacteremia.

After bacteria gain access to the joint, the organisms begin to multiply and produce a persistent purulent effusion within the joint. If this joint effusion is present beyond 7 days, chronic and sometimes irreversible damage may occur. Purulent effusions may promote cartilage destruction by increasing leukocyte enzyme activity. In conjunction with the development of the effusion, almost all patients will develop a hot, swollen, painful joint. The proteolytic enzymes within the effusion and pressure necrosis may lead to cartilage and bone damage.

Staphylococcus aureus is the single most common infecting organism; it is found in 40% of cases of nongonococcal bacterial arthritis. Streptococcal infections account for 33% of cases and gram-negative organisms comprise 23% of infections. Overall, *E. coli* is the most common of the gram-negative organisms; however, *P. aeruginosa* is the most frequent organism in IV drug abusers.[16]

Infants under 1 month of age may have infectious arthritis due to a broad range of organisms, with *S. aureus, Streptococcus,* and gram-negative organisms being most common. *Staphylococcus aureus, H. influenzae* type b, and *Streptococcus* are the most common pathogens in children less than 5 years of age. Within the adult population, *S. aureus* is responsible for the vast majority of nongonococcal infections. The most common cause of bacterial arthritis in adults less than 30 years of age is *N. gonorrhoeae,* which are the most common infections in women.

TABLE 111.3. RISK FACTORS FOR ADULT INFECTIOUS ARTHRITIS (MORE THAN ONE FACTOR MAY BE PRESENT)

Systemic corticosteroid use
Preexisting arthritis
Arthrocentesis
Distant infection
Diabetes mellitus
Trauma
Other diseases

(Adapted from Ref. 62.)

CLINICAL PRESENTATION

SIGNS AND SYMPTOMS

The specific signs and symptoms seen in osteomyelitis vary depending on the route by which the organism reached the bone and the age of the patient. Most patients with hematogenous osteomyelitis complain of significant tenderness of the infected area, pain, swelling, fever, chills, decreased motion, and malaise. Although this presentation is classic, some patients with hematogenous disease may only have mild tenderness and a low-grade fever. Although hematogenous neonatal osteomyelitis infections may rapidly spread to involve the joint, often there are few systemic symptoms present. A joint effusion, present in 60–70% of neonatal infections, decreased limb motion, and edema over the affected area may be the only signs from which to make a diagnosis.

A commonly described diagnostic dilemma is pyogenic vertebral osteomyelitis. Many patients complain of nonspecific symptoms such as severe back pain, fever or night sweats, and weight loss. Other patients may note a gradual onset in symptoms with a possible low-grade back pain and complaints of continuous back pain. The pain is typically described as being present at rest and increasing in severity with movement. Of great concern is that if the infection extends and compresses the spinal cord, neurologic symptoms may develop.[17]

Signs and symptoms of osteomyelitis caused by spread of infection from a contiguous focus depend on the precipitating cause. If the infection follows surgery or bone trauma, the symptoms of the infection are usually noted within 1 month. The most frequent symptom is simply pain in the area of infection. Less commonly, patients also may develop a fever and elevated white blood cell (WBC) count. On physical examination, a patient with contiguous-spread osteomyelitis may have an area of localized tenderness, warmth, edema, and erythema over the infected site. Patients with significant vascular insufficiency usually have local symptoms such as pain, swelling, and redness. Less commonly, patients with vascular disease also may have a fever and elevated WBC count.

Because the differences in the clinical presentation and microbiologic characteristics of infectious arthritis are major, it is useful to separate this disease into nongonococcal and gonococcal bacterial arthritis. Patients with nongonococcal bacterial arthritis almost always present with a fever, and 50% of the patients will have an elevated WBC count. The average initial synovial WBC count is 100,000/mm^3 or greater in nongonococcal bacterial disease.

Nongonococcal bacterial arthritis almost always involves only a single joint.[18] The knee is the most commonly involved joint, but infections also may occur in the shoulder, wrist, hip, ankle, interphalangeal, and elbow joints. Usually, the initial focus of infection that acted as the source for bacterial or microbial entrance can be identified. Common routes for bacterial entrance include infections of the respiratory tract, skin, and urinary tract. Blood cultures are important in these patients as they may be positive in 50% of patients.

In contrast to the other forms of infectious arthritis, the most frequent initial sign of disseminated gonococcal infections is a migratory polyarthralgia. In addition, two-thirds of patients also will complain of fever, dermatitis, and tenosynovitis (inflammation of the tendon sheath). Unique to gonococcal disease, 50% of these patients will have polyarthritis. Small papules on the trunk or extremities are the most frequent skin lesions seen in these infections, but only 30–40% of patients with disseminated gonococcal infection present with the classic hot, swollen, purulent joint. The mean synovial WBC count in gonococcal arthritis is usually 50,000/mm^3 or more.

Another type of infectious arthritis occurs following prosthetic joint surgery. Because joint operations are being performed more frequently, more cases are now occurring. Fortunately, the risk of developing a joint infection following surgery is low. Because these are clean operations, the risk of developing a postoperative infection is estimated to be less than 5%. However, infections are observed more commonly after surgical revision of prosthetic joints. As anticipated, the candidates for this surgical procedure are usually elderly and have a history of either osteoarthritis or rheumatoid arthritis. When patients develop infectious arthritis following joint surgery, they often state that they have experienced some pain in the area. With an infection present, their erythrocyte sedimentation rate is usually elevated, although a leukocytosis often is absent. Infections that result from postoperative contamination usually become apparent within 1 year of surgery. If an infection occurs after this period, it is usually the result of hematogenous spread rather than from the surgery itself. Staphylococci continue to comprise the most common infecting organisms. *Staphylococcus epidermidis* is responsible for 40% of prosthetic-joint infections, and *S. aureus* is responsible for 20% of infections.[19] However, multiple organisms and anaerobic bacteria also may be seen in some infections.

RADIOLOGIC AND LABORATORY TESTS

The evaluation of a patient who may potentially have osteomyelitis has several unusual aspects. Radiographs of the involved area should be obtained; however, bone changes characteristic of osteomyelitis are not seen for at least 10–14 days after the onset of the infection. Radiologists may note soft tissue swelling before any bone changes become obvious. Bone lesions do not appear on roentgenogram films until 10 days after infection because more than 50% of the bone matrix must be removed before the lesions can be detected. As an aide to improve the diagnosis, bone scanning is commonly used. Technetium and gallium scanning may be positive as early as 1 day after the onset of symptoms, well before any radiographic changes may be seen. The development of technetium bone scanning improves the ability to evaluate abnormal bone in a patient. Technetium is taken up in areas of rapid bone formation or in areas of increased blood supply. Unfortunately, bone scanning may be positive in only about 80% of patients who have acute hematogenous osteomyelitis. Tumor, bone repair, and other inflammatory processes may produce false-positive scans. If there is a major infection present, the bone may have become avascular, and thus a "hot spot" will not be detected. If a lesion is located with the bone scan, it may be useful in locating the infection more accurately for bone aspiration. It also may be helpful in patients with sickle cell disease when determining whether the patient has acute bone infarctions from a sickle cell crisis or acute hematogenous osteomyelitis.

As gallium concentrates in white blood cells, it also may be useful in making a diagnosis. Gallium may be more specific than technetium; however, sensitivity is not improved. If the technetium scan was "cold," the gallium scan will probably also be "cold." Another concern is that gallium scans require 24–36 hours for an appropriate study. Gallium also has been recommended as an aid in distinguishing between sickle cell bone infarction and osteomyelitis.

Despite the seriousness of osteomyelitis, often there are few laboratory abnormalities. Often, the erythrocyte sedimentation rate and the WBC count are the only laboratory abnormalities. The degree of abnormality of these two laboratory findings does not correlate with disease outcome.

Once a clinical assessment of osteomyelitis is suspected, it is important to establish a bacteriologic diagnosis by culture of the infected bone. Accurate culture information is especially important as a guide for treatment of osteomyelitis. Bone aspiration is valuable in determining an accurate bacteriologic diagnosis. In addition, performing a bone aspiration will determine whether there is an abscess present. The bone aspiration is performed with a large-bore needle in the area of maximum swelling and tenderness. An inner stylet is used to prevent bone from clogging the end of the needle. The needle is initially placed just to the outer cortex of the bone and the subperiosteal space is aspirated. If an abscess is located, the pus is cultured and a Gram stain is performed. If an abscess is found, drainage will be needed and the fluid cultured. If no abscess is found, the needle is then advanced into the bone through the cortex. Once the needle is within the medullary cavity of the bone, the marrow is aspirated. The aspirated material also will be sent for culture. Aspirates of subperiosteal pus or metaphyseal fluid yield a pathogen in 70% of cases. Cultures should be done for both aerobic and anaerobic bacteria. A Gram stain of the aspirate may be useful in initiating empiric antibiotic therapy. This allows a more appropriate choice of antibiotics from the first day of therapy, rather than waiting several days while culture results are pending.

If a specimen is obtained from a previously undrained or unopened wound abscess, the pathogen usually can be identified. In chronic osteomyelitis, however, identification can be more difficult. Open wounds and draining sinuses frequently are contaminated with other organisms and thus provide inaccurate culture information. A comparison between sinus-tract cultures and cultures obtained during surgery from 40 patients with chronic osteomyelitis demonstrated that less than half the sinus-tract cultures contained the operative pathogen.[20] Therefore, because of the inaccuracies with sinus-tract cultures, they cannot be relied on to reflect the pathogen. However, cultures of loculated pus aspirates in the area of orthopedic devices removed from infected bone can be trusted to identify the infecting organism. The preferable time to obtain culture material in a patient with chronic draining sinus is at the time of open surgical debridement.

In addition to performing cultures from the involved bone, it also is important to obtain cultures from any site believed to be the source of a bacteremia. In addition, it is important to obtain blood cultures. Approximately 50% of patients with hematogenous osteomyelitis will have positive blood cultures.

When evaluating the possibility of a patient having infectious arthritis, immediate joint aspiration with subsequent analysis of the synovial fluid is extremely important. The presence of purulent fluid usually indicates the presence of a septic joint. The synovial fluid WBC count is usually 50,000 to 200,000/mm^3 when an infection is present. Approximately half of the patients with an infected joint will have a low synovial glucose level, usually less than 40 mg/dL.

Gram stains of joint fluid demonstrate bacteria in 50% of patients with septic arthritis; however, such stains may be positive in only 25% of patients with gonococcal arthritis infections. Synovial fluid cultures usually are positive in patients with nongonococcal infections. Both blood and joint fluid should be cultured aerobically and anaerobically in a patient suspected of having an infected joint. Blood cultures are positive in one-half of patients with nongonococcal infections, but in only 20% of those with gonococcal infections. Pharyngeal, rectal, cervical, or urethral smears and cultures should be performed if a disseminated gonococcal infection is considered. As with osteomyelitis, most patients will have an elevated erythrocyte sedimentation rate.

Roentgenograms of infected joints often reveal distention of the joint capsule with soft tissue swelling in the adjacent space. Magnetic resonance imaging may be helpful in identifying an infected hip. In patients who have developed an infected prosthetic joint, loosening of the prosthesis may be seen radiographically.

PROGNOSIS

The prognosis, or ultimate outcome, of osteomyelitis depends on the acute or chronic nature of the disease and how rapidly appropriate therapy is initiated. Patients with acute osteomyelitis have the best prognosis. One study of 58 patients with acute osteomyelitis who had surgery as indicated and received injectable antibiotics for a median duration of 12 weeks had a cure rate of 83%.[21] Similar studies have shown cure rates of 80–94.7%.[22,23] In evaluating the cure rate, it is important to determine how recently a patient completed antibiotic therapy. Many clinicians consider a patient cured if there is no relapse within 1 year after completing antibiotic therapy.

In contrast, patients with chronic osteomyelitis have a much poorer prognosis.[24] Dead bone and other necrotic material from the infection act as a bacterial reservoir and make the infection very difficult to eliminate. Adequate surgical debridement to remove all the dead bone and necrotic material combined with prolonged administration of antibiotics provide the best chance to obtain a cure. The inability to remove all the dead bone may allow residual infection and require suppressive antibiotics to control infection.

In comparison, many patients who develop infectious arthritis recover with no long-term sequelae. Gonococcal arthritis usually resolves rapidly with antibiotics; however, patients with staphylococcal arthritis have a higher incidence of joint damage. Individuals at greatest risk for long-term sequelae are those patients who have symptoms present for more than 7 days before starting therapy, infections occurring within the hip joint, and infections caused by gram-negative organisms. Common, long-term residual effects following infectious arthritis are limited joint motion and persistent pain. Shortening of the affected extremity is another well-known complication. One study noted that more than half the children who subsequently developed residual joint damage were believed normal at the time of hospital discharge.[25]

TREATMENT

Following completion of the steps needed to determine the infecting organism, the most important treatment modality of acute osteomyelitis is the administration of appropriate antibiotics in adequate doses for a sufficient length of time. It is important to stress that early antibiotic therapy may avoid the need for surgery. A delay in treatment may allow bone necrosis to occur and make eradication of the infection much more difficult. In these patients, recurrent exacerbations of the infection may result if all necrotic tissue is not removed surgically and all microorganisms eliminated.

Following the initiation of adequate antibiotic therapy in a patient with hematogenous osteomyelitis, if the patient does not respond by having a decrease in fever, local swelling, redness, and pain, the patient should undergo surgical debridement of the infected area. It is important to emphasize the priority of starting antibiotics after the cultures have been obtained. One study reported no treatment failures in eliminating the infection if injectable antibiotics were started within 48 hours from the onset of symptoms in children with osteomyelitis.[26]

ANTIBIOTIC BONE CONCENTRATIONS

Antibiotics used in the management of acute osteomyelitis are generally given in high doses (adjusted for weight and renal and/or hepatic function) so that adequate antimicrobial concentrations are reached within the infected bone. Empirically, 8–12 g/d of a penicillinase-resistant penicillin (e.g., nafcillin or oxacillin), ampicillin, or cephalosporin, or a similar large dose of another parenteral antibiotic is used in the initial management of adults with osteomyelitis. However, these dosing recommendations are empiric; the relationship between a specific dose of a given antibiotic and its resultant concentration within the infected bone is largely unknown.

Semisynthetic penicillins, cephalosporins, clindamycin, and the aminoglycosides can be detected in bone homogenates soon after their administration.[27] Studies of bone concentrations of antibiotics often have shown a wide range of measured concentrations. It is believed that antibiotics most likely enter bone by passive diffusion from the blood supply into the infected tissue. Therefore, the blood supply to the infected tissue is believed to have a major impact on the resultant antibiotic concentration.

A great deal of the variability in antibiotic bone concentration data results from varied techniques of sampling and measuring bone antibiotic concentrations. Much of the data providing bone concentration information have been determined in patients who did not have infections, but instead were undergoing some type of orthopedic procedure such as a total hip replacement. In these studies, after the patient received the antibiotic, bone biopsies were obtained. The bone fragments are typically washed, allowed to dry, pulverized, and mixed with buffer. The supernatant fluid next undergoes assay procedures to determine the amount of drug present. The measured antibiotic concentration is then related back to the weight of the original bone sample. This technique does not separate the different bone layers nor does it estimate the concentrations within the infected bone. Newer techniques with animal models of osteomyelitis are attempting to provide more meaningful results.[28]

DURATION OF ANTIBIOTIC THERAPY

The specific length of antibiotic therapy needed in the management of osteomyelitis is not clearly defined. Dich et al.[29] observed a failure rate of 19% in children treated with injectable antibiotics for 3 weeks or less. For those patients treated for more than 3 weeks there was only 1 failure in 48 children. This study also found that the same results are achieved in patients treated for longer than 3 weeks with parenteral antibiotic therapy regardless of whether they receive subsequent oral antibiotics. Another trial in children with acute osteomyelitis also supported the minimum 3-week duration.[30] Thus, with the data indicating a minimum of 3 weeks of antibiotic therapy, the standard treatment for osteomyelitis has been parenteral antibiotics for 4–6 weeks. Although these data were determined in children, the duration of therapy recommendations are used in adults as well.

A modification of this recommendation has been used in some patients. Children receiving an appropriate oral antibiotic therapy regimen and adults receiving an oral fluoroquinolone antibiotic, such as ciprofloxacin, often require antibiotic therapy for a duration of 6 weeks. Monitoring the patient's clinical signs and symptoms and their erythrocyte sedimentation rate are important parameters in order to assess therapy. If signs or symptoms are still present at 6 weeks, therapy should be extended.

Glover et al.[21] conducted a retrospective evaluation of 58 patients who had acute osteomyelitis. Clinical symptoms of bone pain and tenderness were present for less than 7 days in 30 patients (52%) and for 8–14 days in another 8 patients (14%). Forty-four of the patients required surgical drainage. Following appropriate antimicrobial therapy for a median duration of 12 weeks, 48 patients were cured, 9 patients developed chronic osteomyelitis, and 1 patient died from unclear causes.

ORAL ANTIBIOTIC THERAPY

One of the most significant changes in the management of osteomyelitis is the use of oral antibiotics. Table 111.4 identifies requirements for the use of oral outpatient antibiotic therapy for osteomyelitis. Two primary populations have

TABLE 111.4. REQUIREMENTS FOR ORAL OUTPATIENT THERAPY FOR OSTEOMYELITIS

Confirmed osteomyelitis
Organism identified
Antibiotic sensitivity determined
Suitable oral agent available
Compliance assured
Suitable candidates:
Children with good clinical response to IV therapy
Adults without diabetes mellitus or peripheral vascular disease

benefited from oral treatment. Children responding to initial parenteral therapy may be excellent candidates to receive follow-up oral therapy with an agent such as dicloxacillin, cephalexin, or ampicillin, depending on their culture and sensitivity results. The other major population to benefit from oral therapy is adults with an infecting organism sensitive to a fluoroquinolone. The availability of ciprofloxacin has had a significant impact on the treatment of osteomyelitis in adults. These two populations now no longer routinely require expensive and complicated courses of long-term parenteral antibiotics.

The use of oral antibiotics has been well studied in children. Two studies documenting the effectiveness of oral therapy used injectable antibiotics initially and then switched to oral antibiotics when there was a decrease in the signs of inflammation and the erythrocyte sedimentation rate, or when the patient was afebrile for 3 days.[31,32] If pus was obtained on the initial needle aspirate or if a reduction in fever, local swelling, and tenderness did not occur despite adequate rest, immobilization, and intensive antibiotic therapy, the patients underwent surgical drainage.

A major issue in conducting these trials has been close monitoring of the patients. In addition to following the clinical and radiographic course of the patients, some studies included the measurement of serum antibiotic concentrations and others included serum bactericidal titers.[33–35] One study adjusted the oral antibiotic doses and added probenecid to regimens to raise the peak serum bactericidal titer to greater than 1:16 and to maintain a trough serum bactericidal titer greater than 1:2.[36] In another study, the target peak serum bactericidal titer was greater than 1:8.[37] Although somewhat controversial, serum bactericidal titers may be helpful in verifying the likelihood of success with an antibiotic, as well as in determining the adequacy of oral therapy.[38,39]

In addition, other studies also have supported the use of oral antibiotics in children with osteomyelitis.[40–42] A recent trial comparing oral and parenteral antibiotics in children with osteomyelitis noted that the incidence of chronic infections depended more on the time interval between the presentation of symptoms and the initiation of antibiotic therapy than whether the patients received oral or parenteral antibiotics.[43]

The patients enrolled in these trials generally had disease of recent onset, identification of the infecting organism, enforced compliance, and surgery as indicated. Many studies used microbiologic titers in monitoring the antibiotic regimens. In patients who meet these criteria, oral antibiotics appear to offer a great advantage in the treatment of osteomyelitis. Patients not meeting these criteria are more likely to develop chronic osteomyelitis with resultant recurrent exacerbations of the infection.

Ciprofloxacin is effective in the treatment of osteomyelitis caused by gram-negative strains such as *Enterobacter cloacae, Serratia marcescens,* and *P. aeruginosa.* Many strains of streptococci are relatively resistant. Its activity against gram-negative bacilli allows patients to be treated orally and avoids the potential toxic complications of 4–6 weeks of aminoglycoside therapy. Another benefit with this agent is that it may be administered on an every-12-hour schedule. However, an important limitation of the drug is that it should not be used in children younger than 16–18 years of age or in pregnant women because of its potential to cause cartilage damage. Other limitations of ciprofloxacin are that it has poor coverage against anaerobic organisms and Staphylococci may develop resistance.

Two trials have compared ciprofloxacin with standard parenteral antibiotic therapy in the treatment of osteomyelitis. Gentry and Rodriguez[44] conducted a prospective, randomized comparison of oral ciprofloxacin 750 mg twice a day with either a broad-spectrum cephalosporin or a nafcillin–aminoglycoside combination parenterally in 59 adult patients with chronic osteomyelitis. The clinical success rate was 24 of 31 (77%) for the ciprofloxacin group and 22 of 28 (79%) for the parenteral group. The most difficult organism to treat was polymicrobial osteomyelitis involving *P. aeruginosa,* in which five of the six treatment regimens failed. In addition, 5 of 15 (33%) courses of osteomyelitis due to a single gram-negative organism also failed. Overall, both treatment regimens were well tolerated. The results of this study indicate that oral ciprofloxacin monotherapy is as safe and effective as conventional parenteral therapy in cases of chronic osteomyelitis caused by susceptible organisms.

A second comparative trial was conducted in 26 patients who had post-traumatic chronic osteomyelitis.[45] Patients received 750 mg of ciprofloxacin orally every 12 hours or either nafcillin, clindamycin, or gentamicin alone or in combination. Both groups received their respective antibiotic courses for at least 4 weeks. Eleven of 14 (79%) patients in the ciprofloxacin group were cured versus 10 of 12 patients (83%) in the parenteral therapy group. The authors emphasize that since ciprofloxacin may have variable sensitivity against gram-positive organisms, sensitivity studies should be available before therapy is initiated. In another trial, ofloxacin given orally 400 mg twice daily produced no significant difference in cures compared to standard parenteral therapy in 33 patients with chronic osteomyelitis.[46] Long-term response was curative in 14 of 19 (74%) with ofloxacin and 12 of 14 (86%) who received standard parenteral therapy. However, concern was noted in that three of four *P. aeruginosa* patients treated with ofloxacin and one of two treated with ceftazidime did not achieve a cure. An uncontrolled trial found that ciprofloxacin 750 mg orally twice daily was curative in 19 of 20 *P. aeruginosa* osteomyelitis cases.[47]

Based on these studies, if an accurate diagnosis of the infecting organism is made in conjunction with thorough debridement, oral antibiotics are equally effective as parenteral antibiotics, except in patients with diabetes mellitus or severe peripheral vascular disease.[48] However, recently there has been concern raised with Staphylococci resistance to fluoroquinolones.[49] It has been known that methicillin-resistant *S. aureus* infections do not respond well to ciprofloxacin; however, resistance may also be troublesome for methicillin-sensitive strains. It is now recommended that when ciprofloxacin is to be used to treat osteomyelitis with mixed etiologies including *S. aureus,* ciprofloxacin should be combined with an antistaphylococcal drug.[50]

SELECTION OF ANTIBIOTICS

A critical component in the management of osteomyelitis is the selection of appropriate antibiotics. Empiric therapy must be selected on the basis of the most likely infecting organism while the results of culture and sensitivity data are pending. Empiric therapy recommendations are summarized in Table 111.5. Dosages expressed in terms of mg/kg/d are generally given in divided doses every 6–8 hours (i.e., three to four times a day).

Because *S. aureus,* streptococci, and *E. coli* are the most common infecting organisms in newborns, an IV dosage of 100 mg/kg/d (given in four divided doses) of cefazolin is appropriate. For children 5 years of age or younger, *S. aureus, H. influenzae* type b, and streptococci are the most common infecting organisms. Appropriate therapy in this age group is cefuroxime IV 100 mg/kg/d. For children older than five years of age, *S. aureus* is the most likely infecting organism and either nafcillin 40 mg/kg/d IV or cefazolin 100 mg/kg/d IV are recommended. If patients are allergic to penicillins or cephalosporins, vancomycin or clindamycin may be used for *S. aureus* coverage. Children with osteomyelitis usually can be successfully treated with 4 weeks of parenteral therapy.

An oral regimen may be an alternative to the previous recommendation in many cases of osteomyelitis in children. Children in whom the infecting organism is identified, who have undergone surgery if needed, and have had a good clinical response to IV therapy may be candidates for the alternate oral antibiotic regimen. It is currently recommended that parenteral antibiotic therapy be initiated and continued until there has been a resolution in the erythema, swelling, tenderness, and until the patient is afebrile. Dicloxacillin, cloxacillin, and cephalexin (100 mg/kg/d) are effective oral agents. Although controversial, if peak serum bactericidal titers are used in monitoring oral therapy, the antibiotic dose may be increased or probenecid may be added if the titer is not at least 1:8. Patients should be monitored with periodic WBC counts, erythrocyte sedimentation rates, and radiographic findings. When oral antibiotics are used, the total duration of oral and injectable therapy is usually at least 4–6 weeks. As previously stated, due to the risk of cartilage damage, fluoroquinolones should not be used in children.

Hematogenous osteomyelitis in adults is most frequently caused by *S. aureus* and thus is appropriately treated with 8–12 g/d of a penicillinase-resistant penicillin such as nafcillin. A similar dose of a first-generation cephalosporin, clindamycin 2.4 g/d or vancomycin 2 g/d

TABLE 111.5. EMPIRIC TREATMENT OF OSTEOMYELITIS

Patient Subtype	Likely Infecting Organism	Antibiotic[a]
Newborn	*S. aureus,* streptococci, *E. coli*	Cefazolin 100 mg/kg/d IV
Children 5 years of age or younger	*S. aureus, H. influenzae* type b, streptococci	Cefuroxime 100 mg/kg/d IV
Children older than 5 years of age	*S. aureus*	Nafcillin 40 mg/kg/d IV or cefazolin 100 mg/kg/d IV
Adults	*S. aureus*	Nafcillin 2 g IV every 4 hours or cefazolin 2 g IV every 8 hours
Intravenous drug abusers	*Pseudomonas*	Ciprofloxacin 750 mg PO twice daily or ceftazidime 2 g IV every 8 hours plus tobramycin 5 mg/kg/d IV
Postoperative or post-trauma patients	Gram-positive and gram-negative organisms	Nafcillin 2 g IV every 4 hours plus ceftazidime 2 g IV every 8 hours or ticarcillin–clavulanate 3.1 g IV every 4 hours
Patients with vascular insufficiency	Gram-positive and gram-negative organisms	Nafcillin 2 g IV every 4 hours or cefazolin 2 g IV every 8 hours plus ceftazidime 2 g IV every 8 hours
	If anaerobes suspected	Cefotetan 2 g IV every 12 hours or clindamycin 900 mg IV every 8 hours plus ceftazidime 2 g IV every 8 hours

[a]Dosage should be adjusted for some agents in patients with renal and/or hepatic dysfunction.

(with normal renal function) may be used in those individuals allergic to penicillin; however, if the infection is located within the vertebrae, *E. coli* must be considered and, thus, depending on the culture and sensitivity data, a switch to a cephalosporin may be needed. After institution of appropriate antibiotic therapy, the antimicrobial agent should be continued for at least 4–6 weeks total (parenteral plus oral).

Osteomyelitis in a patient with a hemoglobinopathy, such as sickle cell anemia, are commonly due to either *Salmonella* or *S. aureus*. Thus, empiric antibiotics of first choice are a penicillinase-resistant penicillin plus ampicillin. Alternatives to ampicillin are a third-generation cephalosporin, chloramphenicol, or ciprofloxacin (in adults).

Bone infections in patients with a history of IV drug abuse require coverage for gram-negative organisms; therefore, empiric treatment with ceftazidime 2 grams IV every 8 hours plus an aminoglycoside is indicated. If compliance can be assured, these patients are excellent candidates to receive oral ciprofloxacin 750 mg twice daily. Antibiotic therapy in these patients should be continued for at least 4–6 weeks.

As previously discussed, bone infections occurring after surgery or from contiguous spread of an adjacent soft tissue infection may be caused by several microorganisms. *Staphylococcus aureus* is the single most common organism, but multiple organisms may be involved. To provide the required broad-spectrum coverage, nafcillin 2 grams IV every 4 hours plus ceftazidime 2 grams IV every 8 hours should be used as initial therapy. An alternative single agent is ticarcillin–clavulanate potassium 3.1 grams IV every 4 hours; however, there is currently less experience with this agent. The antibiotic regimen may require modification after culture and sensitivity information is evaluated. Based on the culture and sensitivity data, ciprofloxacin may be an appropriate oral alternative for these patients. Frequently, the antibiotics must be continued for 6 weeks to obtain a cure and surgery often is required to remove any infected or devitalized tissue.

Patients with established vascular insufficiency who subsequently develop osteomyelitis are extremely difficult to manage. Impaired blood flow to the extremities impedes the healing process. Infections in these patients include a wide range of organisms including *S. aureus, Streptococcus,* anaerobes, and gram-negative organisms. Broad-spectrum therapy with a penicillinase-resistant penicillin in combination with ceftazidime is the preferred initial therapy. If anaerobes are suspected, an antianaerobic cephalosporin or clindamycin plus ceftazidime may be substituted. Ampicillin may need to be added to the regimen to provide coverage against enterococcus. However, in spite of aggressive antibiotic therapy along with surgical debridement, these patients continue to have very low cure rates. Amputation of the involved area may be required to obtain a cure of the infection. Uncontrolled data claim improved outcome with local antibiotic injections combined with end-diastolic pneumatic compression boots[51]; however, additional studies are needed.

Controversies in Therapy

Because the management of bone and joint infections frequently requires prolonged parenteral antibiotics, newer antibiotic regimens are currently being evaluated. Administration of antibiotics in the home environment and the use of antibiotics with extended elimination half-lives are being studied.

ACUTE OSTEOMYELITIS

Although acute osteomyelitis is one of the more common infectious diseases that may be treated with home IV antibiotics, not all patients are acceptable candidates for home administration. Patients must be screened to include those patients who are receiving a stable treatment program, who are interested in participating and are motivated, with good venous access, who have support from family members or neighbors, and who have home facilities for storage and refrigeration.[52] Young, otherwise healthy patients may be able to use a peripheral IV catheter; however, a central IV catheter may be required if venous access difficulties occur. Certain exclusion criteria also must be considered. Complications of other preexisting diseases such as diabetic retinopathy, intention tremor, disabling inflammation or degenerative joint disease, coagulopathies, or various neurologic disorders may prevent individuals from receiving home antibiotics.[53] Histories of alcoholism and IV drug abuse also are important exclusion criteria. Patients fluent in only a foreign language, or those who are illiterate or hard of hearing may have to be excluded if a qualified guardian is unavailable. In addition to meeting these initial screening criteria, patients must successfully complete a thorough training program before hospital discharge. Aseptic technique, proper catheter care, and correct administration techniques must be documented. Once a patient is receiving therapy in the home environment, continued monitoring of their antimicrobial therapy is important. It is vital to ensure compliance with the antimicrobial regimen.

In addition, the specific antibiotic regimen characteristics must be considered in evaluating a patient for home antibiotics. Some features that may be important include microbiologic culture and sensitivity data, the number of required daily antimicrobial doses, antibiotic stability data, and requirements for unique monitoring for the specific antimicrobial regimen, such as serum creatinine and peak and trough level measurements with aminoglycosides.[54] Although an organism may be sensitive to several antimicrobial agents, one antibiotic may provide practical benefits over the other agents.

Some cephalosporins have received a great deal of attention for use in patients with osteomyelitis. Benefits emphasized include their safety spectrum and less frequent dosing requirements with some agents. For example, an every-4-hour dosing regimen of nafcillin may be very effective within a hospital environment; however, this regimen may be difficult to follow on an outpatient basis. Long-acting cephalosporins such as cefonicid or ceftriaxone, although more expensive, may allow patients to receive a regimen that is easier to administer.

Ceftriaxone was studied in a group of 76 patients with either their first or recurrent episode of osteomyelitis.[55] Patients received either single- or twice-daily doses of ceftriaxone for an average of 37 days. Of the 85 causative organisms, 76 were eradicated in 68 of the 76 patients. Cure was achieved in 39 of 76 patients; improvement was observed in 27 patients. Two isolates of *E. cloacae* and one isolate of *P. aeruginosa* developed resistance to ceftriaxone during therapy. In addition, there were two cases of superinfection, one with *B. fragilis* and one with *Streptococcus faecalis*.

Thus, patients who have an infecting organism sensitive to one of the longer acting (less frequently dosed) cephalosporins and resistant to less expensive agents (e.g., cefazolin) may benefit from the newer antibiotics.[56] However, it is important to monitor for the development of resistant strains and superinfections.

CHRONIC OSTEOMYELITIS

Uncontrolled data also have been published with high-dose oral antibiotics (cloxacillin or penicillin V) for extended time periods. One study of 41 patients found that 29 patients had no further recurrences.[57] Another trial noted that 90 of 136 patients were symptom free after surgical removal of bone abscesses and sequestra along with oral antibiotic therapy for 6–12 months.[58]

One trial of home IV antibiotics in the management of 10 patients with chronic osteomyelitis has been published.[59] The patients had symptoms of their disease for 3 months to 58 years. There was an average of 2.7 organisms per patient obtained on bone biopsy with *P. aeruginosa, S. aureus,* and *S. faecalis* being the most common organisms. Surgery was performed on all but two patients. Intravenous antibiotics were administered on an inpatient basis for an average of 33 days and followed by outpatient therapy for an average of 111 days. Eight of the 10 patients were cured of their infections.

Developing treatment guidelines for chronic osteomyelitis based on such a wide variety of data is difficult. The importance of surgery and appropriate antibiotic therapy must be emphasized. Parenteral antibiotics probably should be used while the patient is hospitalized for surgical debridement. Following adequate surgery, if the infecting organism is sensitive, ciprofloxacin appears to be the preferred therapy. Its efficacy appears to match parenteral therapy, it is easy to administer, and it is much less expensive than a course of parenteral antibiotics. However, *S. aureus* resistance to ciprofloxacin must be kept in mind.

If the organism is not sensitive to ciprofloxacin, parenteral antibiotics for 4–6 weeks are needed. In individuals unable to have all the dead bone surgically removed, long-term suppressive therapy may control the infection.

INFECTIOUS ARTHRITIS

The three most important therapeutic maneuvers in the management of infectious arthritis are appropriate antibiotics, joint drainage, and joint rest. As previously mentioned, initial smears of the synovial fluid may be useful in initially selecting appropriate antibiotic therapy. If bacteria are not observed on the Gram stain in a patient who has a purulent joint effusion, antibiotics should still be initiated because of the high risk of an infection being present. A delay in initiating antibiotics significantly increases the likelihood for long-term complications.

The specific antibiotic selected depends on the most likely infecting organism. In infants less than 1 month old, the infecting organisms vary widely and empiric therapy must thus provide broad-spectrum coverage. A penicillinase-resistant penicillin, such as nafcillin or oxacillin (150 mg/kg/d), plus an aminoglycoside is appropriate. Children less than 5 years of age may be infected with *H. influenzae,* for which ampicillin therapy is indicated. The substitution of cefuroxime or addition of chloramphenicol may be required if the patient is located in a geographic area with a high level of ampicillin resistance.

In children older than 5 years of age and in adults, initial therapy with a penicillinase-resistant penicillin is appropriate to provide the necessary coverage against *S. aureus.* Therapy should be changed to vancomycin if the *S. aureus* is resistant to methicillin. As with osteomyelitis, IV drug abusers require *P. aeruginosa* coverage and, therefore, combination therapy with an aminoglycoside is needed. The antibiotics selected are usually administered parenterally. Antibiotics administered by this route achieve sufficient concentrations within the synovial fluid, and thus intra-articular antibiotic injections are not necessary.[60] Although studies to define clearly the appropriate length of therapy have not been conducted, 2–3 weeks of antibiotic therapy is generally adequate in nongonococcal infections. Joint fluid cultures are usually no longer positive after 7 days of antibiotics.

Disseminated gonococcal infections often respond quickly to antibiotics. Ceftriaxone 1 g/d for 7–10 days is the treatment of choice. After culture and sensitivity results are available, if the organism is sensitive, therapy can be switched on the fourth day to either oral amoxicillin, doxycycline, or tetracycline to complete the 7- to 10-day course of antibiotic therapy. Clinical resolution of signs and symptoms is usually rapid.

Closed-needle aspiration is recommended for all infected joints except the hip. Joint drainage may be repeated daily for 5–7 days until effusions no longer reaccumulate. Open drainage is required in hip infections since closed-needle aspiration is difficult.[61] During the initial phase of the infection, weight bearing, such as walking, on the joint should be avoided. Passive range-of-motion exercises should be initiated when the pain begins to subside in order to maintain joint mobility.

Evaluation of Therapeutic Regimens

Patients with bone and joint infections must be monitored closely. Table 111.6 summarizes a monitoring protocol. An assessment of a therapy's success or failure is based on the patient's clinical findings and laboratory values. The clinical signs of inflammation such as swelling, tenderness, pain, redness, and fever should resolve with appropriate therapy. Initially the clinical signs are assessed daily until improvement, then periodically thereafter. Elevations in WBC count also should gradually decline. The WBC count is usually obtained once or twice per week until it returns to the normal range. The erythrocyte sedimentation rate is usually determined weekly. Elevations in the erythrocyte sedimentation rate may not return to normal for several weeks of therapy. If by the end of the 4- to 6-week antibiotic course the clinical findings of osteomyelitis are no longer present and the erythrocyte sedimentation rate is within normal limits, the patient may be considered a clinical cure. However, keep in mind that patients may relapse after initially appearing cured. No relapse for 1 year is generally considered a complete cure.

TABLE 111.6. MONITORING PROTOCOL

Parameter	Frequency	Notes
Culture and sensitivity	At initiation of treatment	
White blood cell count	1–2 times/week until within normal range	
Erythrocyte sedimentation rate	Weekly	May not decrease to normal range until several weeks of therapy
Clinical signs of inflammation (redness, pain, swelling, tenderness, fever)	Daily during initiation of therapy	
Compliance of outpatient therapy	Reinforce before starting oral therapy and with each health care visit	Compliance is critical if treatment is to be successful

However, if a patient fails to resolve the clinical signs and symptoms of inflammation after appropriate empiric antibiotics, surgical debridement may be needed. In addition, the patient may have a resistant infecting organism that may require a modification of the antibiotic therapy. It is especially important to note the infecting organism and its sensitivity pattern. Follow-up cultures at subsequent debridements may be useful to assess the antibiotic therapy.

Despite apparently adequate surgery and antibiotics, some patients may fail therapy and have recurrent relapses in their infection. This scenario is more common in the population with chronic osteomyelitis. These patients may require long-term oral antibiotics in order to keep the infection under control.

Conclusion

Osteomyelitis and infectious arthritis are two infections that require special attention. Because the infecting organisms may vary, careful attention must be placed on adequate culture collection. Because of the difficulty in eliminating these infections, patients must receive antibiotics for an extended period of time and may require surgical drainage. Prolonged injectable antibiotics are commonly needed to cure the infections. Many children with acute osteomyelitis may be treated effectively with a carefully monitored oral regimen. The use of oral ciprofloxacin has had a major impact on the treatment of acute and chronic osteomyelitis in adults. Many patients with susceptible infecting organisms may be cured with prolonged ciprofloxacin therapy provided they have adequate surgical debridement, if needed. It is important to emphasize that osteomyelitis and septic arthritis are infections that require rapid initiation of therapy to prevent extensive tissue damage and obtain the best chance of cure.

References

1. Cierney G, Mader JT. Adult chronic osteomyelitis. Orthopedics 1984;7:1557–1564.
2. Waldvogel FA, Medoff G, Swartz MN. Osteomyelitis: A review of clinical features, therapeutic considerations and unusual aspects. N Engl J Med 1970;282:198–206,260–266,316–322.
3. Peltola H, Vahuanen V. A comparative study of osteomyelitis and purulent arthritis with special reference to aetiology and recovery. Infection 1984;12:75–79.

4. Sharp JT, Lidsky MD, Duffy J, et al. Infectious arthritis. Arch Intern Med 1979;139:1125–1130.
5. Fink CW, Nelson JD. Septic arthritis and osteomyelitis in children. Clin Rheum Dis 1986;12:423–435.
6. Goldenberg DL, Reed JI. Bacterial arthritis. N Engl J Med 1985;312:764–771.
7. Schmid FR. Routine treatment of septic arthritis. Clin Rheum Dis 1984;10:293–311.
8. Goldenberg DK, Cohen AS. Acute infectious arthritis: A review of patients with nongonococcal joint infections (with emphasis on therapy and prognosis). Am J Med 1976;60:369–377.
9. Dirschl DR, Almekinders LC. Osteomyelitis: Common causes and treatment recommendations. Drugs 1993;45:29–43.
10. Green NE, Edwards K. Bone and joint infections in children. Orthop Clin North Am 1987;18:555–576.
11. Faden H, Grossi M. Acute osteomyelitis in children: Reassessment of etiologic agents and their clinical characteristics. Am J Dis Child 1991;145:65–69.
12. Abbey DM, Hosea SW. Diagnosis of vertebral osteomyelitis in a community hospital by using computed tomography. Arch Intern Med 1989;149:2029–2035.
13. Raff MJ, Melo JC. Anaerobic osteomyelitis. Medicine 1978;57:83–103.
14. Ward JR, Atcheson SG. Infectious arthritis. Med Clin North Am 1977;61:313–329.
15. Roca RP, Yoshikawa TT. Primary skeletal infections in heroin users: A clinical characterization, diagnosis and therapy. Clin Orthop 1979;144:238–248.
16. Gifford DB, Patzakis M, Ivler D, et al. Septic arthritis due to pseudomonas in heroin addicts. J Bone Joint Surg (Am) 1975;57:631–635.
17. Osenbach RK, Hitchon PW, Menezes AH. Diagnosis and management of pyogenic vertebral osteomyelitis. Surg Neurol 1990;33:266–275.
18. Ho G, Su EY. Therapy for septic arthritis. JAMA 1982;247:797–800.
19. Inman RD, Gallegos RV, Brause BD, et al. Clinical and microbial features of prosthetic joint infection. Am J Med 1984;77:47–53.
20. Mackowiak PA, Jones SR, Smith JW. Diagnosis value of sinus tract cultures in chronic osteomyelitis. JAMA 1978;239:2772–2775.
21. Glover SL, McKendrick MW, Padfield C, et al. Acute osteomyelitis in a district general hospital. Lancet 1982;1:609–611.
22. Gillespie WJ, Mayo KM. The management of acute haematogenous osteomyelitis in the antibiotic era: A study of the outcome. J Bone Joint Surg (Br) 1981;63:126–131.
23. Khazenifar M, Weighill FH, Stanley JK. The management of childhood osteomyelitis. Postgrad Med J 1978;54:541–544.
24. Ingram C, Eron LJ, Goldenberg RI, et al. Antibiotic therapy of osteomyelitis in outpatients. Med Clin North Am 1988;72:723–738.
25. Howard JB, Highgenboten CL, Nelson JD. Residual effects of septic arthritis in infancy and childhood. JAMA 1976;236:932–935.
26. Jacobs JC. Acute osteomyelitis medical management in children. NY State J Med 1978;78:1273–1278.
27. Waldvogel FA, Vasey H. Osteomyelitis: The past decade. N Engl J Med 1980;303:360–370.
28. Mader JT, Adams K, Morrison L. Comparative evaluation of cefazolin and clindamycin in the treatment of experimental *Staphylococcus aureus* osteomyelitis in rabbits. Antimicrob Agents Chemother 1989;33:1760–1764.
29. Dich VQ, Nelson JD, Haltalin KC. Osteomyelitis in infants and children. Am J Dis Child 1975;129:1273–1278.
30. Syrogiannopoulos GA, Nelson JD. Duration of antimicrobial therapy for acute suppurative osteoarticular infections. Lancet 1988;1:37–40.
31. Tetzlaff TR, McCracken GH, Nelson JD. Oral antibiotic therapy for skeletal infections of children. J Pediatr 1978;92:485–490.
32. Bryson YJ, Connor JD, LeClerc M, et al. High-dose oral dicloxacillin treatment of acute staphylococcal osteomyelitis in children. J Pediatr 1979;94:673–675.
33. Rodriquez W, Ross S, Khan W, et al. Clindamycin in the treatment of osteomyelitis in children: A report of 29 cases. Am J Dis Child 1977;131:1088–1093.
34. Feigin RD, Pickering LR, Anderson D, et al. Clindamycin treatment of osteomyelitis and septic arthritis in children. Pediatrics 1975;55:213–223.
35. Kaplan SL, Mason EO, Feigin RD. Clindamycin versus nafcillin or methicillin in the treatment of *Staphylococcus aureus* osteomyelitis in children. South Med J 1982;75:138–142.
36. Prober CG, Yeager AS. Use of the serum bactericidal titer to assess the adequacy of oral antibiotic therapy in the treatment of acute hematogenous osteomyelitis. J Pediatr 1979;95:131–135.
37. Jordan GW, Kawachi MM. Analysis of serum bactericidal activity in endocarditis, osteomyelitis, and other bacterial infections. Medicine 1981;60:49–61.
38. Nelson JD, Bucholz RW, Kusmiesz H, et al. Benefits and risks of sequential parenteral-oral cephalosporin therapy for suppurative bone and joint infections. J Pediatr Orthop 1982;2:255–262.
39. Weinstein MP, Stratton CW, Hawley HB, et al. Multicenter collaborative evaluation of a standardized serum bactericidal test as a predictor of therapeutic efficacy in acute and chronic osteomyelitis. Am J Med 1987;83:218–222.
40. Anderson Jr, Scobie WG, Watt B. The treatment of acute osteomyelitis in children: A 10-year experience. J Antimicrob Chemother 1981;7(suppl A):43–50.
41. Jimenez-Shehab M, Barragan A. Oral cefadroxil in the treatment of bone and joint infections in children and adults. J Antimicrob Chemother 1982;10(suppl B):149–152.
42. Kolyvas E, Ahronheim G, Marks MI, et al. Oral antibiotic therapy of skeletal infections in children. Pediatrics 1980;65:867–871.
43. Vaughan PA, Newman NM, Rosman MA. Acute hematogenous osteomyelitis in children. J Pediatr Orthop 1987;7:652–655.
44. Gentry LO, Rodriguez GG. Oral ciprofloxacin compared with parenteral antibiotics in the treatment of osteomyelitis. Antimicrob Agents Chemother 1990;34:40–43.
45. Mader JT, Cantrell JS, Calhoun J. Oral ciprofloxacin compared with standard parenteral antibiotic therapy for chronic osteomyelitis in adults. J Bone Joint Surg (Am) 1990;72:104–110.

46. Gentry LO, Rodriguez-Gomez G. Ofloxacin versus parenteral therapy for chronic osteomyelitis. Antimicrob Agents Chemother 1991;35:538–541.
47. Dan M, Siegman-Igra Y, Pitlik S, Raz R. Oral ciprofloxacin treatment of *Pseudomonas aeruginosa* osteomyelitis. Antimicrob Agents Chemother 1990;34:849–852.
48. Gentry LO. Oral antimicrobial therapy for osteomyelitis. Ann Intern Med 1991;114:986–987.
49. Trucksis M, Hooper DC, Wolfson JS. Emerging resistance to fluoroquinolones in Staphylococci: An alert. Ann Intern Med 1991;114:424–426.
50. Wispelwey B, Scheld WM. Ciprofloxacin in the treatment of *Staphylococcus aureus* osteomyelitis: A review. Diag Microbiol Infect Dis 1990;13:169–171.
51. Dillon RS. Successful treatment of osteomyelitis and soft tissue infections in ischemic diabetic legs by local antibiotic injections and the end-diastolic pneumatic compression boot. Ann Surg 1986;204:643–649.
52. McAllister JC. The role of the pharmacist in home health care. Drug Intell Clin Pharm 1985;19:282–284.
53. Goldenberg RI. Pitfalls in the delivery of outpatient intravenous therapy. Drug Intell Clin Pharm 1985;19:293–296.
54. Reed MD. Evaluation of antibiotics for home care programs. Drug Intell Clin Pharm 1985;19:288–290.
55. Eron LJ, Goldenberg RI, Poretz DM. Combined ceftriaxone and surgical therapy for osteomyelitis in hospital and outpatient settings. Am J Surg 1984;148(4A):1–4.
56. Gentry LO. Antibiotic therapy for osteomyelitis. Infect Dis Clin North Am 1990;4:485–499.
57. Hedstrom SA. The prognosis of chronic staphyloccal osteomyelitis after long-term antibiotic treatment. Scand J Infect Dis 1974;6:33–38.
58. Bell SM. Further observations on the value of oral penicillins in chronic staphylococcal osteomyelitis. Med J Aust 1976;2:591–593.
59. Wagner DR, Collier D, Rytel MW. Long-term intravenous antibiotic therapy in chronic osteomyelitis. Arch Intern Med 1985;145:1073–1078.
60. Nelson JD. Antibiotic concentrations in septic joint effusions. N Engl J Med 1971;284:349–353.
61. Broy SB, Schmid FR. A comparison of medical drainage (needle aspiration) and surgical drainage (arthrotomy or arthroscopy) in the initial treatment of infected joints. Clin Rheum Dis 1986;12:501–522.
62. Esterhai JL, Gelb I. Adult septic arthritis. Orthop Clin North Am 1991;22:504.

Chapter 112

Gram-Negative Sepsis and Septic Shock

Steven B. Johnson, MD,
Kenneth E. Record, PharmD, and Joseph T. DiPiro, PharmD

"Sepsis" is an imprecise term suggesting a bloodstream invasion by bacteria or the toxic materials produced by bacteria resulting in overt and severe clinical signs and symptoms characteristic of systemic toxicity. Virtually any microorganism is capable of producing "sepsis," including gram-positive and gram-negative organisms, fungi, rickettsia, and viruses, and this presents a significant diagnostic challenge. The association of severe infection with circulatory failure, hypotension, and poor tissue perfusion is most frequently the manifestation of the Enterobacteriaceae and Pseudomonadaceae.

In the early 1950s, a number of uniformly fatal infectious diseases were on the decline, presumably due to the modern antibiotic era, but a fourfold increase in the frequency of gram-negative infections occurred in 1947 compared with 1941.[1] Concurrent with this increase in frequency, it became sufficiently clear that gram-negative bacilli were capable of producing fatal systemic complications as a result of bacteremia extending from infected body sites.[2,3] In addition, gram-negative sepsis (GNS) could occur when natural endogenous microbial flora demonstrated "opportunism" during periods of depressed defense mechanisms.

By 1972, Boston City Hospital reported nearly a 10-fold increase in the frequency of gram-negative infections since 1941. Although this is probably an overestimation of the true frequency of gram-negative bacteremias, considering community hospitals probably have a lesser rate, the magnitude of the problem generated considerable concern. The increasing incidence of gram-negative infection is particularly worrisome in light of reports demonstrating a 20–32% mortality associated with gram-negative bacteremias.[4–6]

Despite the advances in antimicrobial therapy and cardiovascular and respiratory support, the mortality rate from gram-negative bacteremia has not significantly changed. This may be expected if we consider that the hemodynamic and metabolic changes associated with septic shock occur as a result of cellular injury. Thus, the associated circulatory abnormalities of septic shock are late findings when injury is difficult to reverse. Clearly, early recognition and aggressive intervention to prevent the development of septic shock is of paramount importance if mortality rates are to be reduced.

A joint committee of the American College of Chest Physicians and the Society of Critical Care Medicine has standardized the terminology related to sepsis (Table 112.1).[7] These criteria provide specific physiologic variables that can be used to categorize a patient as having systemic inflammatory response syndrome, sepsis, severe sepsis, or septic shock, as well as hypotension or multiple organ dysfunction syndrome. The term "sepsis syndrome" should no longer be used. These definitions suggest a continuum of severity from systemic inflammatory response syndrome (SIRS) to sepsis, severe sepsis, and septic shock. Bacteremia, hypotension, and organ dysfunction can occur as a part of these processes. Bacteremia may occur in the absence of sepsis, and patients with sepsis may not have bacteremia.

Epidemiology and Etiology

The incidence of gram-negative sepsis in the United States is difficult to quantify. It has been estimated that more than 200,000 episodes of gram-negative sepsis occur annually, resulting in nearly 100,000 deaths.[8] Data from the Centers for Disease Control and Prevention reported that the incidence of septicemia from all microorganisms (defined as systemic disease associated with the presence and persistence of pathogenic microorganisms or their toxins in the blood) increased 139% between 1979 and 1987, from 73.6 to 175.9 cases per 100,000 persons.[9] A recent multicenter study of 1754 hospitalized patients at risk for sepsis demonstrated that 26% experienced sepsis syndrome (defined as hyperthermia or hypothermia, tachycardia, tachypnea with evidence of decreased organ perfusion).[10] The mortality rate for those with sepsis syndrome was 38%. Forty-seven

TABLE 112.1. DEFINITIONS RELATED TO SEPSIS

Condition	Definition
Bacteremia	The presence of viable bacteria in the blood.
Systemic inflammatory response syndrome (SIRS)	The systemic inflammatory response to a variety of severe clinical insults. The response is manifested by two or more of the following conditions: Temperature >38°C or <36°C Heart rate >90 beats/min Respiratory rate >20 breaths/min or $Paco_2$ <32 torr (<4.3 kPa) WBC > 12,000 cells/mm^3, <4000 cells/mm^3, or >10% immature (band) forms.
Sepsis	The systemic response to infection. This systemic response is manifested by two or more of the following conditions as a result of infection: Temperature >38°C or <36°C Heart rate >90 beats/min Respiratory rate >20 breaths/min or $Paco_2$ <32 torr (<4.3 kPa) WBC >12,000 cells/mm^3, <4000 cells/mm^3, or >10% immature (band) forms.
Severe sepsis	Sepsis associated with organ dysfunction, hypoperfusion, or hypotension. Hypoperfusion and perfusion abnormalities may include, but are not limited to, lactic acidosis, oliguria, or an acute alteration in mental status.
Septic shock	Sepsis with hypotension, despite adequate fluid resuscitation, along with the presence of perfusion abnormalities that may include, but are not limited to, lactic acidosis, oliguria, or an acute alteration in mental status. Patients who are on inotropic or vasopressor agents may not be hypotensive at the time perfusion abnormalities are measured.
Hypotension	A systolic blood pressure of <90 mm Hg or a reduction of >40 mm Hg from baseline in the absence of other causes for hypotension.
Multiple organ dysfunction syndrome	Presence of altered organ function in an acutely ill patient such that homeostasis cannot be maintained without intervention.

(From Ref. 7.)

percent of patients with sepsis syndrome experienced refractory shock, which had a mortality rate of 54%. Another recent multicenter study of 3708 patients at risk for sepsis (presence of at least two of the criteria for SIRS) found that SIRS occurred in 68%.[11] Among those with SIRS, 26% developed sepsis, 18% developed severe sepsis, and 4% developed septic shock. Mortality rates for SIRS, sepsis, severe sepsis, and septic shock were 7, 16, 20, and 46%, respectively.

The major offenders in gram-negative sepsis are the members of the families Enterobacteriaceae *(Escherichia, Klebsiella, Enterobacter, Serratia,* and *Proteus)* and Pseudomonadaceae. The pseudomonads, along with other gram-negative organisms, are ubiquitous in the environment. The enteric or coliform bacteria are part of the normal endogenous flora within the gastrointestinal tract, which represents the largest reservoir of gram-negative organisms. Thus, the integrity of gastrointestinal mucosa as a mechanical barrier is critical. The infectious implications of trauma, penetrating wounds, small surface ulcerations, mechanical obstructions, and ischemic necrosis of the bowel carry a high risk of infection with gram-negative organisms.

Escherichia coli is the most abundant gram-negative aerobic bacillus and in "community-acquired" infections is usually sensitive to most penicillins and cephalosporins. However, a less predictable pattern of antimicrobial resistance is encountered in "hospital-acquired" gram-negative infections. A distinction must be made based on the circumstances by which infection is acquired and treated. The recognition of the widespread presence of β-lactamase–producing organisms with hospital-acquired infection has certainly had a major impact on the search for enzyme-stable and nontoxic antimicrobials.[12]

A factor important to the epidemiology of gram-negative infection is the host's loss of colonization resistance. That is, normal host flora inhibits overgrowth of potentially pathogenic organisms. Loss of colonization resistance increases the risk of gram-negative infection, and a number of factors have augmented this phenomenon. The administration of antimicrobial agents presumably decreases the protective flora and allows for overgrowth of other virulent species. The severity of illness and loss of natural protective barriers such as skin, intestinal mucosa, the cough reflex, or neutropenia all contribute to an increased gram-negative burden for the host to combat.[13,14]

Community-acquired gram-negative infection usually arises from the endogenous flora in the biliary, urinary, or genital tracts. Environmental or exogenous aerobic gram-negative bacilli, which are comprised of coliforms and pseudomonads, represent a serious threat to the institutionalized patient. These organisms have the ability to colonize and invade directly through devices intended for supportive care of the patient (e.g., respiratory equipment, urinary catheters, feeding tubes).

The outcome of gram-negative infection corresponds to organism virulence and host susceptibility. The effect of differences in organism virulence has been outlined by Young[15] and is demonstrated in Table 112.2 for single bloodstream isolates and their corresponding frequency and mortality. Bryan and associates[6] noted that in patients with nonfatal disease, mortality was higher in hospital-acquired bacteremia. This was largely attributed to the observation that *E. coli* bacteremia was associated with a mortality of 13%, while *Pseudomonas aeruginosa* was associated with a mortality of 39%. A part of this disparity may be reflective of underlying disease.

The most important determinant of host susceptibility is the severity of such underlying disease. McCabe and Jackson[16] outlined a useful classification of disease severity and corresponding gram-negative bacteremia mortality based on the time sequence to a fatal event. A "rapidly fatal" disease such as acute leukemia, blastic relapses of chronic leukemia, aplastic anemias, and burns greater than 70% demonstrated a 91% mortality rate from gram-negative bacteremia. "Ultimately fatal" diseases (expected death within 4 years) showed the death rate due to bacteremia at 66%. Examples of such diseases included chronic leukemia, lymphoma, metastatic carcinoma, cirrhosis with hepatic coma or bleeding varices, and chronic renal disease with blood urea nitrogen levels greater than 70 mg%. Finally, "nonfatal" diseases such as diabetes mellitus and various obstetric conditions were associated with an 11% fatality rate due to bacteremias. Age or bacterial species was not a significant independent determinant of bacteremic fatality.

Other important studies have refined our understanding of the relationship between host, organism, and therapeutic interventions. "Appropriate antimicrobial therapy" (in which the organism was sensitive to the regimen) when compared with inappropriate or no therapy results in a significant reduction of the mortality rate due to bacteremia. As expected, this was more important in the ultimately fatal and nonfatal groups. The problem of gram-negative bacteremia leading to septic shock and the inherently high mortality (i.e., gram-negative bacteremias had a fatality rate eight times greater than gram-positive bacteremias) stimulated the Subcommittee on Health of the U.S. Senate to appoint a Special Study Group on Gram-Negative Rod Bacteremia. The role of antibiotic overuse in the increased incidence of gram-negative infections was a major focus. It was concluded that antibiotics were an important factor but quantitative assessment of the relationship between overuse and incidence was impossible.[6]

TABLE 112.2. GRAM-NEGATIVE BACTEREMIA

Frequency	Mortality
Escherichia coli	*Pseudomonas aeruginosa*
Klebsiella pneumoniae	*Klebsiella* sp.
Serratia[a]	*Proteus* sp.[a]
Enterobacter[a]	*E. coli*[a]
Proteus sp.[a]	*Enterobacter*[a]

[a]Rank order not significant.

Pathophysiology/Presentation

The pathophysiologic sequelae resulting from the interaction of the gram-negative bacillus and the human host are diverse, complex, and poorly understood. In human studies, it is difficult to demonstrate definitive relationships between infection and septic shock. Furthermore, clinical and histopathologic changes are difficult to attribute to intervening infection or underlying disease that may have similar effects. Finally, much of the work in animals has been difficult to adapt to humans due to marked differences in response to gram-negative stimuli. Figure 112.1 depicts a schematic representation of the pathogenesis of gram-negative sepsis and septic shock.

The pathophysiologic focus of gram-negative sepsis has been on the lipopolysaccharide component of the gram-negative cell wall. Commonly referred to as endotoxin, this substance is unique to the outer membrane of the gram-negative cell wall and is generally released when bacterial lysis occurs. The lipopolysaccharide molecule consists of three distinct regions. The outermost components, referred to as the *o-antigen,* has diverse antigenicity depending on species. The middle region, referred to as the *core,* has less antigenic diversity. *Lipid A* is the innermost region and is found in both aerobic and anaerobic gram-negative bacilli. Lipid A is highly immunoreactive and is responsible for most of the toxic effects. Although lipid A may affect tissues directly, its predominant effect is to activate macrophages and trigger the cascade of inflammatory mediators important to progression of sepsis and septic shock.[15] The mechanism by which endotoxin initiates the inflammatory process has become better understood. After gram-negative bacteria release endotoxin, the endotoxin must associate with a protein called lipopolysaccharide binding protein. This complex then engages a specific receptor (CD14) on the surface of the macrophage. The major role endotoxin maintains in the inflammatory progression of sepsis and the similarity of lipid A among bacterial species has allowed for the development of specific therapeutic modalities directed at lipid A as adjuncts to the management of sepsis.

The inflammatory process initiated with sepsis involves a complex interaction of pro- and anti-inflammatory mediators and the activation of a variety of cells. Some of the mediators involved include tumor necrosis factor α (TNF-α), interleukin 1 (IL-1), interleukin 6 (IL-6), which are produced by macrophages, as well as interleukin 8 (IL-8), platelet activating factor (PAF), leukotrienes, and thromboxane A_2. Also, there are mediators that down-regulate the inflammatory response, such as interleukin 1 receptor

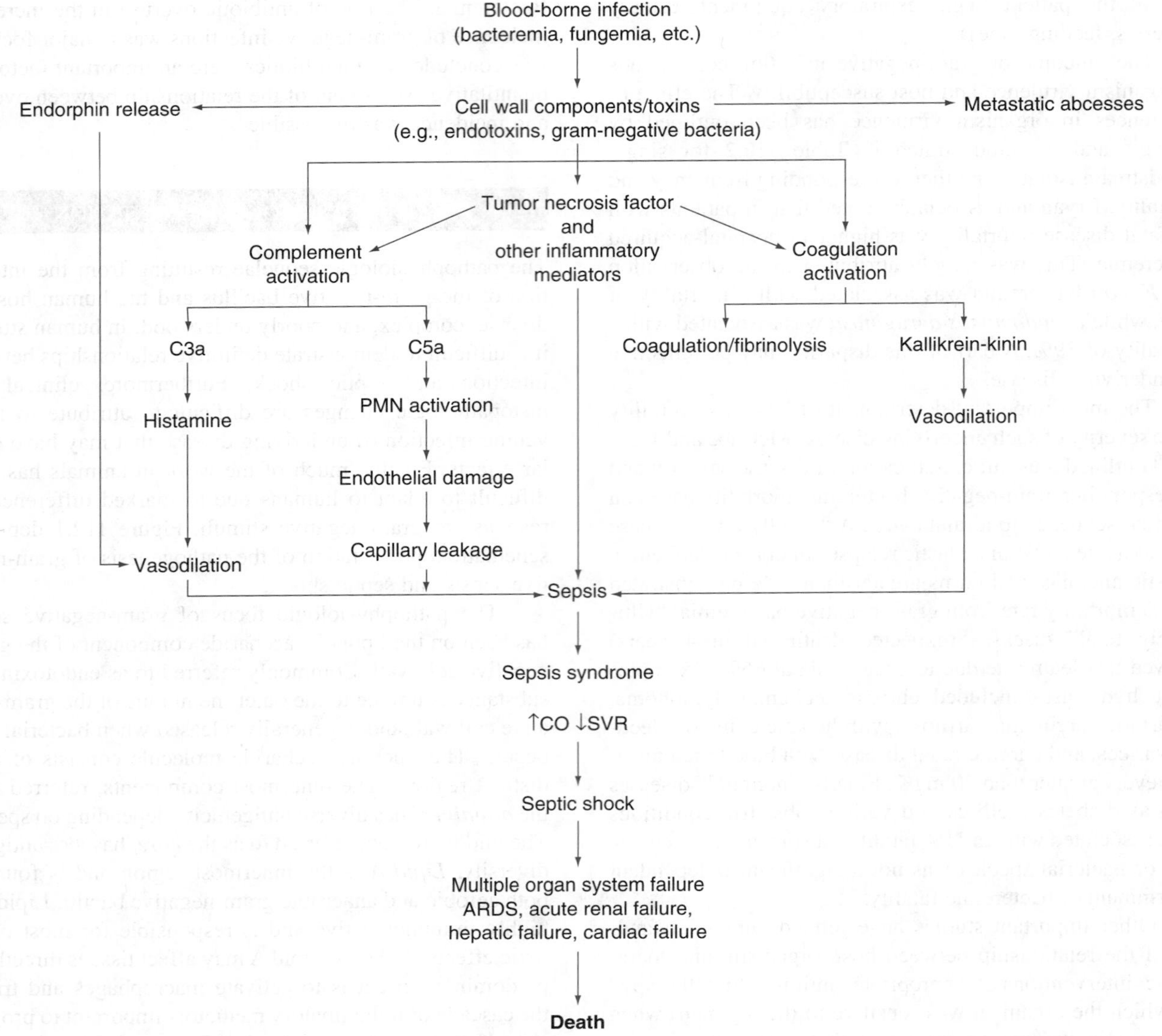

Figure 112.1. Pathogenesis of septic shock. PMN, polymorphonuclear leukocyte; ARDS, adult respiratory distress syndrome; SVR, systemic vascular resistance; CO, cardiac output.

antagonist (IL-1RA), interleukin 4 (IL-4), and interleukin 10 (IL-10).[17–19] The net effect of a given mediator may vary depending on the state of activation of the target cell, the nearby presence of other mediators, and the ability of the target cell to release other mediators that augment or inhibit the primary mediator.[17] TNF-α has been proposed as a central mediator of sepsis, although this is probably not an accurate picture since sepsis involves the action of many cytokines and cells. Evidence that supports an important role for TNF-α has been summarized by Young[15] and includes the following:

1. A mouse model known to be unresponsive to endotoxin failed to produce TNF-α from their macrophages.[20]
2. Endotoxin injected in healthy humans resulted in the detection of free TNF-α in plasma and many symptoms of gram-negative infections were observed.[21]
3. In meningococcemia, increased morbidity and mortality are associated with high levels of TNF-α.[22]
4. Purified TNF-α given to animals and humans produces the clinical symptomatology of gram-negative sepsis and septic shock.
5. Anti-TNF-α monoclonal antibodies injected into animals had a protective effect, particularly when the antibody was administered prior to the endotoxin challenge.[23]

Other studies provide evidence that TNF-α is the central mediator of the effect of endotoxin and works in conjunction with other cytokines (e.g., IL-1 and IL-6) to cause cellular damage.[24,25] In addition, TNF-α stimulates the release of cyclooxygenase-derived arachidonic acid metabolites (i.e., thromboxane A_2 and prostaglandins) causing vascular endothelial damage. Significant tissue damage can occur if the immune response to endotoxin is greatly exaggerated. The release of TNF-α is not specific for gram-negative organisms. Elevated levels of TNF-α have been described in certain parasitic infections.[26]

Through the actions of the mediators mentioned in the previous paragraphs, a variety of cells may become activated. With sepsis, the degree of cellular activation is believed to be detrimental to the host. Initially, macrophages become activated and produce inflammatory cytokines. These cytokines then influence a wide range of cells including endothelial cells, lymphocytes, hepatocytes, neutrophils, and platelets. A primary mechanism of injury with sepsis is through endothelial cells. These cells respond to and produce a variety of cytokines. When injured, endothelial cells allow circulating cells (e.g., granulocytes) and plasma constituents to enter inflamed tissues, which may result in organ damage. In addition, endothelial cells may cause vasodilatation through the action of nitric oxide on vascular smooth muscle. Pulmonary dysfunction may result from the destructive mechanisms (proteolytic enzymes and reactive oxygen species) of neutrophils that are attracted to lung tissue through the action of IL-8 (and other chemoattractants).

Measurement of endotoxin and cytokine levels in plasma has been proposed to detect sepsis in early stages or quantify the severity of sepsis. Many investigators have measured cytokine levels in the plasma or serum of patients experiencing sepsis to determine their utility as predictors for outcome or in attempts to determine the mechanisms of sepsis.

TNF-α has received much attention because it is elevated in the plasma of most patients with sepsis. However, septic patients are not the only ones who have elevated TNF-α levels. TNF-α levels may be increased in patients with a variety of diseases and in many healthy people.[27] TNF-α levels have been correlated with severity of sepsis. There is a correlation of TNF-α levels with severity of sepsis, and high TNF-α levels are found in patients with septic shock.[28–30] In contrast, IL-1 levels have been inconsistently associated with sepsis.[28]

Some investigators have suggested that IL-6 may be a more consistent predictor of sepsis since it remains elevated for a longer period of time than TNF-α. IL-6 levels have been related to severity of sepsis.[29] High IL-6 levels have also been related to mortality with sepsis.[31–34] Other cytokines, such as IL-8, have also been related to severity of sepsis and mortality.[35,36] Plasma endotoxin does not predict gram-negative infection or outcome from infection.[37]

The other clinical signs and symptoms of the endotoxin occur through the activation of complement and direct activation of Hageman factor. Hageman factor then activates coagulation and fibrinolysis and release of vasoactive peptides. Hypotension appears to be due, in part, to the release of vasoactive peptides such as the kinins (bradykinin and serotonin). Activation of complement can occur by the classic (antigen–antibody activation) pathway but, more important, by the alternate pathway. The pathophysiologic consequence of activated components of complement results in the generation of granulocyte chemotactic factors, anaphylatoxins, and other substances that augment or exaggerate the inflammatory response. This ultimately results in further deleterious effects on cell membranes.

Disseminated intravascular coagulation (DIC), a frequent complication of gram-negative sepsis, is mostly attributed to the activation of factor XII (Hageman factor) by endotoxin. The subsequent activation and use of coagulation factors II, V, VIII, and platelets far exceed the rate of synthesis resulting in inadequate levels to maintain hemostasis. Paradoxical bleeding may occur due to the consumption of clotting factors. As plasminogen (fibrinolytic system) is activated simultaneously, newly formed clots undergo rapid lysis. Fibrin breakdown results in circulating soluble peptides called fibrin degradation products. This may explain why autopsies fail to uncover thrombi when thrombosis has been clinically evident in the septic patient. Complications of DIC are varied and depend on the target organ affected and the severity of the coagulopathy. Severe clinical bleeding, thrombosis, tissue ischemia and necrosis, hemolysis, and major organ failure may result from disturbances induced by gram-negative bacteria on the coagulation systems.

Shock is the most ominous complication associated with gram-negative sepsis. In 1951, Waisbren's[2] classic description of a "shock-like picture" associated with gram-negative bacteremia suggested two clinically distinct syndromes. Approximately one-half of the patients evaluated exhibited hypotension with cold, clammy skin and lethargy (i.e., a low cardiac output, peripheral vasoconstrictive state). This condition was referred to as "cold shock," occurring late in the progression of sepsis and associated with a poor prognosis. In contrast, the other group exhibited manifestations of acute bacterial infections (e.g., fever, bounding rapid pulses, wide pulse pressure, warm flushed skin, hypotension). This state is characterized by a high cardiac output and peripheral vasodilation. This condition was referred to as "warm shock," occurring earlier in the progression of sepsis and associated with a better prognosis.

Another important complication of sepsis is acute respiratory distress syndrome (ARDS). This is a functional lung injury, characterized by diffuse alveolar damage, where the alveolocapillary membrane is injured, leading to noncardiogenic pulmonary edema through increased vascular permeability.[38] The result is that air spaces fill with fluid, and there is deterioration of gas exchange of the lung, impaired compliance, and refractory hypoxemia. This has been defined as acute lung injury with detection of bilateral pulmonary infiltrates on the frontal chest radiograph, a pulmonary-artery wedge occlusion pressure of ≤18 mm Hg (or no clinical evidence of elevated left atrial pressure on the basis on chest radiograph and other clinical data), and a ratio of PaO_2 to FiO_2 ≤200 (regardless of the level of positive end-expiratory pressure).[39] Approximately one-fourth of patients with gram-negative sepsis develop ARDS and this carries a mortality rate of 60–90%.[40]

To understand the management of sepsis, one must have an appreciation of the cardiovascular response in humans. The hallmark of the hemodynamic effect of sepsis is the hyperdynamic state characterized by high cardiac output and an abnormally low systemic vascular resistance (SVR). A low cardiac output appears to reflect inadequate maintenance of circulating volume. Recent evidence suggests that the myocardium is impaired by the endotoxic insult characterized by an impairment of ventricular performance. Parker et al.[41] observed a marked decrease in the left ventricular ejection fraction (EF) in 20 patients suffering from hypotension, hyperthermia, and documented infection.

In a dramatic study involving normal volunteers, Suffredini et al.[42] injected small doses of endotoxin from *E. coli* to study the cardiovascular effects with controls receiving saline. In subjects receiving endotoxin and before volume loading, the cardiac index increased by 53% and the heart rate by 36%. The SVR decreased by 46%. After volume loading, the ejection fraction decreased by 1% of the baseline value in subjects receiving endotoxin but increased by 14% in controls. Left ventricular end-diastolic and end-systolic indexes increased by 14 and 24%, respectively. Finally, left ventricular performance as measured by the ratio of the peak systolic pressure to end-systolic volume index was depressed in subjects receiving endotoxin and increased in the control group. The conclusions drawn from these data suggest that endotoxin depresses left ventricular function that is independent of changes in left ventricular volume or vascular resistance. These findings are consistent with those seen in septic shock and suggest that endotoxin or secondary mediators depress cardiovascular function.

Hypotension associated with sepsis raises the concern of oxygen delivery to the tissues (DO_2) and oxygen consumption by the tissues (VO_2). Sepsis results in distributive shock characterized by inappropriately increased blood flow to selected tissue at the expense of other tissue independent of oxygen needs. This perfusion defect is accentuated by an increased precapillary AV shunt. If perfusion decreases, oxygen extraction increases and the arteriovenous oxygen gradient widens. Cellular DO_2 is decreased but VO_2 remains unaffected. When increased oxygen demand occurs without increased blood flow, the increased VO_2 is compensated by increased oxygen extraction. If perfusion decreases sufficiently in the face of high metabolic demands, then the reserve DO_2 can be exceeded and tissue ischemia results. The aim of therapy is to prevent tissue ischemia and subsequent organ failure through supportive maintenance of the cardiovasculature with adequate fluid volume, inotropic agents, and pressor support as needed.

Principles of Therapy

The pathophysiologic spectrum of sepsis is an exaggerated inflammatory response to the presence of bacteria or endotoxin in the bloodstream. Epidemiologic and pathophysiologic information stresses the importance of early recognition and aggressive therapeutic intervention if mortality is to be avoided. The detection and elimination of all septic sources, appropriate antimicrobial therapy, and comprehensive supportive care (including hemodynamic monitoring, adequate volume, pressor, and metabolic support) are the cornerstones in the management of sepsis and septic shock. Recently, much interest has been focused on the potential ameliorative effects on inflammation by monoclonal antibodies against endotoxin and TNF, and IL-1 receptor antagonists. An algorithmic approach to the management of sepsis is shown in Fig. 112.2.

ANTIMICROBIAL THERAPY

Assuming one has done all he or she can to identify and eliminate the septic source, antimicrobial therapy becomes a major priority. Because of the inherent problems in the timely identification of the offending organism or organisms and the similar pathophysiologic picture of gram-positive as well as gram-negative organisms (aerobic and anaerobic) present in established sepsis, empiric regimens are directed at likely organisms from various body sites. The resistance patterns of one's hospital is of benefit in selecting specific regimens.

The following principles are useful guides in initiating antimicrobial therapy. Empiric therapy must be comprehensive. An attempt should be made to cover all likely pathogens in the context of the clinical setting. Therapy should be initiated rapidly. Clearing the bloodstream before the development of the complications of sepsis is a widely accepted mandate. A seriously ill patient or one who is in shock should only be treated with intravenous antibiotics. Absorption from intramuscular and oral sites may be erratic due to changes in regional blood flow. For empiric therapy or treatment of the immunocompromised patient, antimicrobial combinations likely to be synergistic are encouraged. Loading doses, particularly with aminoglycosides, should be given to maximize initial effect. Monitor patients carefully and, in particular, their renal function for potential aminoglycoside nephrotoxicity. Adjust aminoglycoside doses according to serum levels and the functional state of

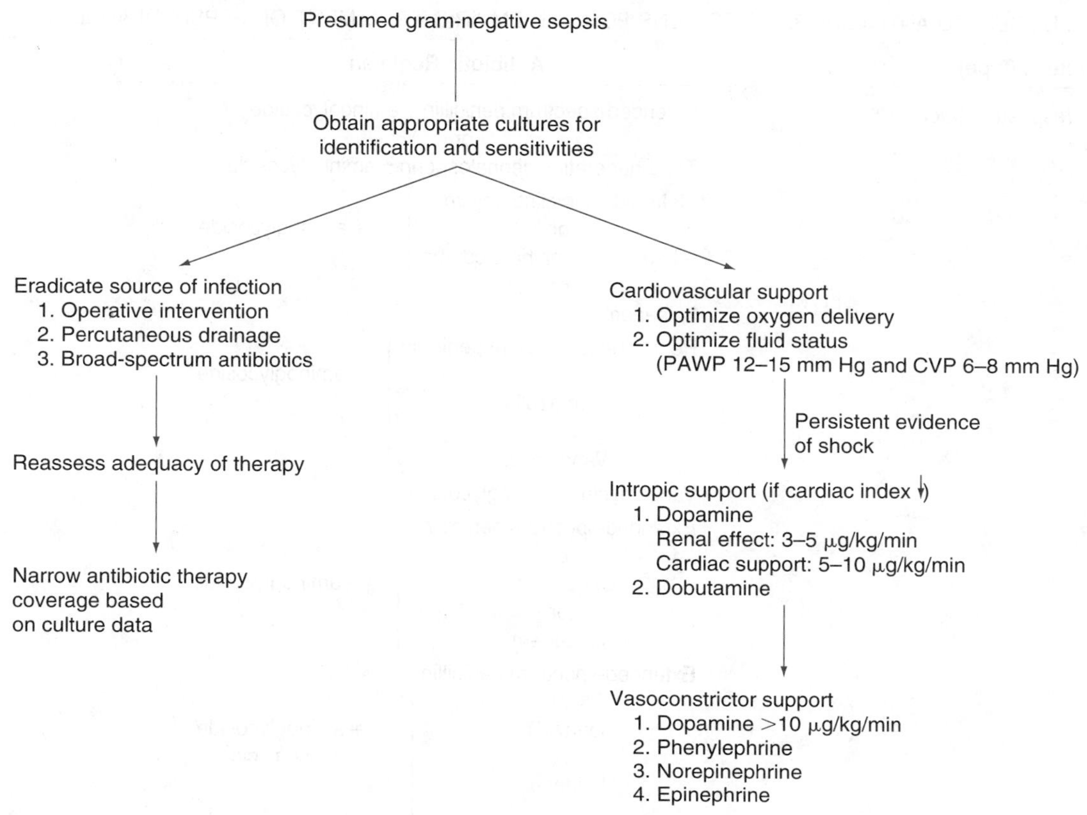

Figure 112.2. Treatment algorithm for the management of gram-negative sepsis. PAWP, pulmonary artery wedge pressure.

the kidneys. When the patient stabilizes, and if the pathogen is known, specific therapy considering safety and cost should become a primary concern.[43]

The choice of antimicrobial agents has been the subject of considerable debate over the last several years due to the availability of new antibiotics with expanded and enhanced activities *in vitro*. In the case of sepsis, well-defined comparative trials addressing efficacy of antibiotic regimens are lacking. The use of antibiotic combinations is usually recommended for the treatment of serious gram-negative bacillary infections for the following reasons:

1. To cover a broad range of organisms
2. To cover polymicrobial infections
3. To prevent the emergence of resistance from bacterial subpopulations that may be resistant to one of the antibiotic components
4. To provide an additive or synergistic effect

A few studies comparing monotherapy with standard combination regimens in selected clinical situations have demonstrated equal efficacy. Pizzo et al.[43] found equal efficacy in terms of preventing mortality when comparing ceftazidime alone against an aminoglycoside and an extended-spectrum penicillin in febrile neutropenic patients. One must pay particular attention to resistance patterns, particularly with *P. aeruginosa,* when considering monotherapy. Monotherapy is more likely to be successful in the non-neutropenic patient, in patients who are not immunocompromised, and against highly susceptible microorganisms. Most clinicians still empirically start critically ill patients on combination therapies and adjust treatment when organisms and sensitivities are known.

Table 112.3 provides suggestions for the selection of antimicrobial regimens in the empiric treatment of sepsis. Selection of specific agents should be considered on the basis of individual institution sensitivity patterns. In the non-neutropenic patient with a community-acquired urinary tract infection, a first- or second-generation cephalosporin may be appropriate because *E. coli* and *Klebsiella* are the major concerns. In the same patient where the source of infection is nonurinary, a combination of a penicillinase-resistant penicillin or a cephalosporin plus an aminoglycoside provides excellent coverage of *E. coli, Klebsiella,* and *Proteus* as well as gram-positive coverage (pneumococcus, *Staphylococcus aureus*). The traditional regimen for the patient acquiring a nosocomial infection consists of an aminoglycoside and a β-lactam agent. If the patient is non-neutropenic, a first- or second-generation cephalosporin is preferred because *Klebsiella* is much more likely to be present than *P. aeruginosa.* Finally, the combination of an

TABLE 112.3. SUGGESTED ANTIMICROBIAL REGIMENS FOR THE EMPIRIC TREATMENT OF SEPSIS IN ADULTS

Infection (Site or Type)	Antibiotic Regimen
Urinary tract or respiratory tract	Extended-spectrum penicillin + aminoglycoside or Third-generation cephalosporin ± aminoglycoside
Intra-abdominal	(Metronidazole/clindamycin or β-Lactamase inhibitor combo) + aminoglycoside or Imipenem
Soft tissue	(Penicillinase-resistant penicillin or Cefazolin or Vancomycin) + aminoglycoside
Central line	Vancomycin + aminoglycoside
Pseudomonas	(Extended-spectrum penicillin or Ceftazidime or Imipenem) + aminoglycoside
Unknown	(Extended-spectrum penicillin or Ceftazidime or Imipenem) + aminoglycoside + vancomycin

aminoglycoside and an antipseudomonal penicillin or an antipseudomonal cephalosporin is preferred in the neutropenic patient, the patient receiving assisted ventilation, or the patient with major thermal injury.

Amikacin is less susceptible than gentamicin and tobramycin to plasmid-mediated enzyme inactivation and has proven a valuable alternative in situations of suspected or established resistance to gentamicin and tobramycin. A few differences with respect to microbiologic activity exist between gentamicin, tobramycin, and amikacin. Tobramycin appears somewhat more active (based on an achievable serum level) than gentamicin against *P. aeruginosa*. However, gentamicin is more active than tobramycin against *Serratia*. Using an inhibitory index that accounts for the higher blood levels achieved with amikacin compared with minimum inhibitory concentrations, this drug appears more active against the *Klebsiella–Enterobacter–Serratia* group. It is not clear whether these differences have clinical significance.

The average duration of therapy in the normal host with gram-negative sepsis is 10–14 days.[44] Treatment may go considerably longer if the infection is persistent. The importance of identifying and employing appropriate measures to eliminate the source of infection is underscored here. In the neutropenic patient the duration of therapy is usually longer. These patients should be afebrile for 4–7 days, show signs of resolving infection at the source, and have rising neutrophil counts in excess of 500/μL. In the patient with marrow failure, clinical defervescence is generally sufficient in determining duration.

The clinical pharmacist has the opportunity to impact significantly the effectiveness of aminoglycoside therapy in gram-negative sepsis. These agents have narrow therapeutic windows, and there is a marked variability in individual peak serum levels. Some studies suggest that breakthrough bacteremias are associated with subtherapeutic aminoglycoside serum levels.[45] Thus, the frequent monitoring of aminoglycoside serum levels becomes imperative. Gentamicin and also tobramycin peak levels in the range of 5.0–10.0 μg/mL are generally associated with optimal response.[46] Amikacin peak levels of 20–40 μg/mL are likewise considered optimal. Monitoring serum concentrations may avert some toxicity by alerting the clinician to changes in renal function earlier than serum creatinine and overdosing errors.

An interesting controversy in the dosing of aminoglycosides is the use of single daily dosing. This is believed efficacious because higher peak concentrations result in a longer postantibiotic effect.[47] Another important feature of this concept is that in animal studies evaluating toxicity, the development of renal toxicity was delayed in the animals receiving equivalent single daily doses when compared with every-8-hour closing.[48] Two studies of gram-negative bacteremias comparing single, large daily doses of aminoglycosides (3.9 and 6 mg/kg/d) versus standard therapy (1.3 and 2 mg/kg every 8 hours), respectively, reported no differences in efficacy, and one report suggested a delay in the onset of nephrotoxicity with once-daily dosing. The single-daily-dose regimens achieved peak levels in the 15–24 μg/mL range and the standard dosing regimens achieved peak levels of approximately 8 μg/mL.[49,50] In the context of patients with gram-negative sepsis and the fluid resuscitation required, it is difficult to achieve therapeutic peak levels rapidly with standard dosing regimens. A single, large daily dose would help to alleviate this problem. However, more information is needed with regard to single daily doses and changes in volume of distribution.

The carboxy and ureidopenicillins make up the group of penicillins collectively known as antipseudomonal penicillins. Although there are major enhancements in activity of the ureidopenicillins (azlocillin, mezlocillin, piperacillin) over the carboxypenicillins (carbenicillin and ticarcillin), their major role in antimicrobial therapy is in combination with an aminoglycoside for potential infection caused by *P. aeruginosa.* Azlocillin and piperacillin are the most active against *Pseudomonas,* whereas ticarcillin and mezlocillin are comparably less active, and carbenicillin is least active. Unfortunately, no conclusive evidence from clinical trials suggests that the more active agents are any more effective than the less active agents when combined with an aminoglycoside against *P. aeruginosa.* The enhanced activity of the more recently introduced antipseudomonal penicillins is due to an increase in cell wall permeability and affinity for penicillin-binding proteins. They are very susceptible to inactivation by β-lactamases. It appears that all of these agents would benefit in combination with the β-lactamase inhibitors.

The development of new cephalosporins (third-generation), the carbapenems (imipenem), and the monobactams (aztreonam) has added tremendously active agents to the antimicrobial arsenal. These agents have exceptional *in vitro* activity against the Enterobacteriaceae but highly variable activity against *P. aeruginosa.* Agents such as cefotaxime, ceftizoxime, and ceftriaxone easily achieve serum levels 100 times greater than their minimum inhibitory concentrations against *E. coli* and *Klebsiella,* and suggest that monotherapy directed against those bacteria may be successful. However, resistance among *Pseudomonas, Serratia,* and *Enterobacter* is a concern and has limited their singular use.

The first studies reporting the efficacy of monotherapy compared with combination therapy employed cefoperazone and moxalactam.[51,52] Both agents demonstrated antipseudomonal activity in addition to an enhanced activity against the Enterobacteriaceae. Both studies suggested similar efficacy of monotherapy when compared with conventional regimens but the numbers of neutropenic patients were small and very few patients had *P. aeruginosa* bacteremias. Evidence is available that shows that the antipseudomonal third-generation cephalosporins plus aminoglycosides are similarly efficacious to antipseudomonal penicillin plus aminoglycoside combinations.[53] There is no convincing evidence that the combination of an aminoglycoside, penicillin, and cephalosporin regimen is superior to an aminoglycoside–β-lactam combination.

FLUID THERAPY AND PULMONARY SUPPORT

Eradication of the septic source is the most important consideration in the care of the patient with septic shock. Maintenance of adequate tissue oxygenation during and subsequent to eradication is an additional important consideration. Tissue oxygenation is dependent on adequate perfusion and adequate oxygenation of the blood. Rapid restoration of intravascular fluid volume and expansion of the extravascular space is an essential therapeutic intervention in the initial management of septic shock. The goal of fluid replacement is to maintain a systolic blood pressure greater than 90 mm Hg and prevent hypoperfusion to tissues and vital organs.[54] In its early stages, sepsis and septic shock are responsive to volume replacement, and several liters of fluid may be required to keep pace with capillary leakage to maintain an adequate intravascular volume. One must be aggressive but extremely careful with fluid loading during sepsis. The bacterial toxins and the host's own defense mediators can damage the capillaries of the lungs, resulting in significant fluid accumulation into the interstitial pulmonary space. As more fluid is accrued in the lungs, the transport of oxygen from the alveoli to the pulmonary vascular beds becomes more difficult. Thus, a ventilation–perfusion mismatch due to an increased pulmonary shunt may result in profound hypoxemia. The $Pa{CO_2}$ should be maintained at greater than 65 mm Hg with oxygen saturation greater than 90%. Determination of the pulmonary artery wedge pressure (PAWP), central venous pressure (CVP), cardiac output (CO), and systemic vascular resistance (SVR) through invasive monitoring is sometimes necessary and valuable to define the limits of fluid therapy.

Aggressive volume resuscitation is critical in patients with gram-negative sepsis although controversy exists regarding the optimal type of fluid (crystalloid versus colloid). Isotonic crystalloids distribute into the interstitial and intravascular spaces. They effectively restore volume loss and are less expensive than colloids. Large volumes are required (approximately 25% stays in the intravascular space) and expansion of the interstitial space results.[55] This expansion is desirable because it aids vascular capacitance but overexpansion results in excessive edema and compromised gas exchange in the lungs and peripheral tissues. An increase in pulmonary edema has been demonstrated during crystalloid volume expansion when compared with expan-

TABLE 112.4. CARDIOVASCULAR DRUGS USED IN SEPSIS

Agent	Dose (μg/kg/min)	Receptor	MAP	CI	SVRI	HR	PAWP
Dobutamine	2.5–40	$3\beta_1$, $1\beta_2$	NC	I	D	NC/I	D
Dopamine	2–3	3d, $1\beta_1$	NC	NC	NC	NC	NC
	5–10	$3\beta_1$, $2\beta_2$	NC/I	I	NC	NC	NC
	>10	$3\beta_1$, $3\alpha_{1,2}$	I	I	I	I	I
Epinephrine	0.005–0.05	$3\beta_1$, $3\beta_2$	NC	NC/I	NC/D	I	NC
	>0.05	$3\alpha_1$, $3\alpha_2$	I	I	I	I	I
Phenylephrine	0.03–2	$3\alpha_1$, $3\alpha_2$	II	NC/D	II	D	I
Norepinephrine	>0.05	3α, 2β	II	NC/I	II	D	I
Amrinone	5–30	N/A	NC/D	I	D	NC	D

Key: HR = heart rate; I = increased; MAP = mean arterial pressure; NC = no change; NC/D = no change or slight decrease; PAWP = pulmonary artery wedge pressure.

sion with colloids, but the effects are transitory and it is not known whether there are any long-term adverse effects.[56]

Iso-oncotic colloid solutions (plasma and plasma protein fractions), such as 5% albumin and 6% hetastarch, offer the advantage of more rapid restoration of intravascular volume with less volume infused. They improve tissue oxygenation increasing flow through the microcirculation.[2] Some drawbacks to the use of colloids are the lack of expansion of the interstitial space and high cost. Another disadvantage is the leakage of oncotically active particles into the interstitial space and the possibility of prolonging tissue edema. This is a concern during acute phases of inflammation and when capillary permeability to oncotically active solutes is increased.

Successful fluid resuscitation in sepsis usually requires a combination of crystalloid and colloid. Sepsis presents a complicated picture of capillary leak and multiple organ deterioration. Invasive hemodynamic monitoring is frequently necessary and the measurement of serum lactate can provide excellent assessment of tissue perfusion. An increased serum lactate indicates inadequate tissue perfusion, resulting in cellular anaerobic metabolism and lactate production.

Crystalloids are generally employed first with Ringer's lactate or normal saline for resuscitation purposes. Dextrose-containing solution should be reserved for maintenance fluids only. Colloids should be employed when crystalloids produce adverse effects such as pulmonary and peripheral edema or they do not achieve adequate tissue oxygenation.

Fluid resuscitation in sepsis usually requires hemodynamic monitoring. An acceptable PAWP is usually 12–15 mm Hg, but cardiac disease can affect this greatly. The stroke volume is calculated to more precisely evaluate ventricular function. The endpoint of fluid administration occurs when increases in the PAWP no longer result in an increase in the stroke volume.

Other factors to consider in adequate tissue oxygenation are hemoglobin and hematocrit. Blood transfusions often are necessary. The optimal hematocrit is not known and may differ from organ to organ.[57] Hematocrits should not exceed 35–40% because of a significant increase in blood viscosity. Czer and Shoemaker[58] suggest an optimal hematocrit of 30–32%.

INOTROPE AND VASOACTIVE DRUG SUPPORT

When fluid resuscitation is insufficient to maintain tissue perfusion, the use of inotropes and vasoactive drugs is necessary. Although there is no universally accepted protocol for cardiovascular support of the septic patient, selection and dosage are based on the pharmacologic properties of various catecholamines and how they influence hemodynamic parameters (Table 112.4). The following is a suggested protocol for the use of inotropes and vasoactive agents.

1. In the patient without marked hypotension, an inotrope without significant peripheral vascular effects is employed. The goal is to maintain blood pressure by supporting cardiac output. This strategy often is successful and reduces the possibility of impaired organ perfusion through pharmacologic peripheral vasoconstrictive effects. Dopamine in moderate doses (5–10 μg/kg/min) is used as a first-line agent for its selective effect on increasing cardiac output with minimal effect on the systemic vascular resistance. Dobutamine (5–30 μg/kg/min) has been suggested by some investigators to be superior to dopamine for maintaining tissue perfusion and oxygen consumption in critically ill, but the effect may not be significant in the septic patient.[59] Amrinone administered in 1 mg/kg bolus and 10 mg/kg/min continuous infusion is an alternative.
2. In the patient with significant hypotension (mean arterial pressure [MAP] <60 mm Hg) and a low systemic vascular resistance index (SVRI) (<500 dyne/s/cm^5/m^2) that cannot be overcome by inotropic agents, an α-adrenergic agent can be useful. In sepsis, the most

experience has been with norepinephrine. It often is combined with an inotrope such as dobutamine. Dopamine in higher doses, 5–20 μg/kg/min, is an alternative, but the dopaminergic effects are lost to the α-adrenergic effects.

3. Dopamine is widely used in low doses (2–3 μg/kg/min) to increase renal and mesenteric perfusion. Renal blood flow is enhanced even when used with norepinephrine.[60]
4. Pure α agonists such as phenylphrine can be employed either with other drugs or as single-agent therapy when SVR is markedly decreased. The goal of phenylephrine therapy is to increase SVR and MAP by increasing vasoconstriction. Prior to administering vasoactive agents, aggressive appropriate fluid resuscitation should occur. Vasoactive agents should not be considered an acceptable alternative to volume resuscitation.

INVESTIGATIONAL THERAPIES

The treatment of sepsis has been one of the most active areas of clinical investigation over the past few years. A wide variety of strategies have been used to attempt to reverse or control the inflammatory process initiated with sepsis (Table 112.5). One of the first general mechanisms to gain attention is direct inhibition of the effects of endotoxin from gram-negative bacteria. Studies have been conducted primarily with monoclonal antibodies that bind to the lipid A portion of the endotoxin molecule or with other binding substances such as bactericidal/permeability increasing protein or high density lipoprotein. Although this approach has not demonstrated consistent benefits for clinical treatment of sepsis, sepsis syndrome, or septic shock, clinical trials are continuing. A second general approach is inhibition of inflammatory cytokines through antibodies that bind the cytokines, competitive inhibitors for cytokine receptor binding, or through soluble receptors that bind the cytokine but do not activate the target cells. One of the primary approaches in this category is the use of antibodies that bind to TNF-α. Another general approach is the administration of anti-inflammatory cytokines or other substances. Substances under consideration for this purpose include IL-10, IL-4, as well as drugs such as pentoxiphylline. Although at the time of publication none of these strategies is clearly effective for treatment of sepsis, it is clear that an effective strategy will emerge of the many being investigated. A combination of approaches may be required to fully control and reverse this process.

CONTROVERSIES IN THE PHARMACOLOGIC MANAGEMENT OF SEPTIC SHOCK

The corticosteroids have been the subject of controversy in the management of the septic process. Because of their suppressive effect on the activation of polymorphonuclear leukocytes, complement activation, release of TNF, and the activation of the coagulation system, the administration of a

TABLE 112.5. SELECTED CLINICAL TRIALS FOR TREATMENT OF SEPSIS

Investigators	Agent Studied	Patients	Results/Comments
Zeigler et al.[61]	HA-1A (antilipid A antibody)	Gram-negative sepsis	Overall not effective for gram-negative sepsis, but appeared effective in patients with gram-negative bacteremia
Greenman et al.[62]	E5 (antilipid A antibody)	Gram-negative infection with systemic response	Overall not effective for gram-negative sepsis, but appeared effective in nonshock patients
Fisher et al.[63]	Interleukin-1 receptor antagonist	Sepsis syndrome or septic shock	Overall, not effective but modest reduction in mortality among high-risk patients
Dhainaut et al.[64]	Platelet-activating factor antagonist (BN 52021)	Severe sepsis	No significant effect overall, reduction in mortality for patients with gram-negative sepsis
Fisher et al.[65]	Anti-TNF antibody	Sepsis	Not effective for sepsis
Schedel et al.[66]	Polyclonal immunoglobulin (Pentaglobulin)	Gram-negative septic shock	Significantly lower mortality rate associated with immunoglobulin
Abraham et al.[67]	Anti-TNF antibody	Sepsis syndrome	Overall not effective for sepsis syndrome

single high dose of corticosteroids would appear useful in preventing the cascading complication of septic shock. When this is counterbalanced by well-known adverse effects on the host immune system, the decision to use steroids becomes more difficult.

A randomized prospective study evaluating the efficacy of steroids in gram-negative sepsis demonstrated no significant benefit over placebo therapy.[68] In this study, steroids resulted in an increased mortality rate among patients with elevated serum creatinine levels and in patients developing secondary infections. The same group subsequently reported that the use of methylprednisolone did not prevent sepsis-induced ARDS, a common complication of sepsis. Even though the incidence of ARDS was similar in the treatment versus placebo group, 69% of the treatment group failed to reverse their ARDS compared with 39% in the control group. Also, mortality at 14 days was 52% in the treatment group versus 22% in the placebo group.[68]

Heparinization for the treatment of DIC has been recommended because the paradoxical bleeding is caused by a "hypercoagulable state." Heparin has been shown to control this coagulopathy. However, there is little clinical evidence that heparin prolongs survival. It also is unclear whether abolishing the "consumption" of coagulation factors has any direct clinical benefits. Heparin therapy for DIC is discouraged by most clinicians. Hemorrhage is usually managed with the replacement of clotting factor, platelets, and appropriate supportive care.

Naloxone, through its antagonist effect on opiates and β endorphins, has been shown to raise and sustain systolic blood pressure in animals. Human trials are not available and are unlikely, because most patients with septic shock are managed with narcotic analgesics for pain, and the high doses of naloxone required to maintain blood pressure would surely abate the beneficial effects of the opiates.

Diuretics are widely used in sepsis, particularly when renal function appears to be failing. It is not clear whether the aggressive use of diuretics in the early oliguric phase of acute renal failure avoids the failure or makes the ensuing failure less severe. It appears that most clinicians have abandoned the use of large doses of loop diuretics because of fear of causing deafness. Prudent doses of diuretics are beneficial when volume expansion fails to maintain adequate urine output.

Conclusion

Gram-negative sepsis remains a serious problem. We have witnessed the development of an impressive array of treatment modalities and technologies that allows for the more precise management of sepsis. More developments are on the way. The apparent optimal success of all these advancements is still dictated by the early recognition of the septic process. The challenge to the clinician in the near future will be to understand how to apply these adjuncts in the most judicious way.

References

1. McGowan JE Jr, Barnes MW, Finland M. Bacteremia at Boston City Hospital: Occurrence and mortality during 12 selected years (1925–1972) with special reference to hospital acquired cases. J Infect Dis 1975;132:316.
2. Waisbren BA. Bacteremia due to gram-negative bacilli other than the *Salmonella.* Arch Intern Med 1951; 88:467.
3. Braude AI, Siemienski J, Williams D, et al. Overwhelming bacteremic shock produced by gram-negative bacilli: Report of 4 cases with 1 recovery. Univ Mich Med Bull 1953;19:23.
4. Wolff SM, Bennett JV. Gram negative-rod bacteremia. N Engl J Med 1974;291:733.
5. Scheckler WE. Septicemia and nosocomial infections in a community hospital. Ann Intern Med 1978;89(part 2):754.
6. Bryan CS, Reynolds KL, Brenner ER. Analysis of 1186 episodes of gram-negative bacteremia in nonuniversity hospitals: The effect of antimicrobial therapy. Rev Infect Dis 1983;5:629.
7. Bone RC, Balk RA, Cerra F, et al. American College of Chest Physicians/Society of Critical Care Medicine Consensus Conference: Definitions for sepsis and organ failure and guidelines for the use of innovative therapies in sepsis. Crit Care Med 992;20:864–874.
8. Parillo JE. Septic shock in humans: Clinical evaluation, pathophysiology, and therapeutic approach, in Shoemaker WC, Thompson WL, Holbrook P, et al (eds): Textbook of Critical Care, 2nd ed. Philadelphia, WB Saunders, 1989, pp 1006–1023.
9. Centers for Disease Control. Increase in national hospital discharge survey cases for septicemia. MMWR 1990;39:31–34.
10. Conboy K, Welage LS, Walawander MA, et al. Sepsis syndrome associated sequelae in patients at high risk for gram-negative sepsis. Pharmacotherapy 1995;15:66–77.
11. Rangel-Frausto MS, Pittet D, Costigan M, et al. The natural history of systemic inflammatory response syndrome (SIRS). A prospective study. JAMA 1995;273:117–123.
12. Jacoby GA, Archer GL. New mechanisms of bacterial resistance to antimicrobial agents. N Engl J Med 1991;324:601–612.
13. Johnson WG, Pierce AK, Sanford JP. Changing pharyngeal bacterial flora of hospitalized patients: Emergence of gram-negative bacilli. N Engl J Med 1969;281:1137.
14. Johnson WG, Pierce AK, Snadford JP. Nosocomial respiratory infections with gram-negative bacilli. Ann Intern Med 1972;77:701.
15. Young LS. Gram-negative sepsis, in Mandell GL, Douglas RG Jr, Bennett JE (eds): Principles and Practice of Infectious Diseases. New York, Churchhill Livingstone, 1990, pp 611–636.
16. McCabe WR, Jackson GG. Gram-negative bacteremia. I. Etiology and ecology. Arch Intern Med 1962;110:847.
17. Bone RC. The pathogenesis of sepsis. Ann Intern Med 1991;115:457–469.

18. Shapiro L, Gelfand JA. Cytokines and sepsis: Pathophysiology and therapy. New Horizons 1993;1:13–22.
19. Dinarello CA. The proinflammatory cytokines interleukin-1 and tumor necrosis factor and the treatment of septic shock syndrome. J Infect Dis 1991;163:1177–1184.
20. Beutler B, Krochin N, Milsark W, et al. Control of cachectin (tumor necrosis factor) synthesis: Mechanisms of endotoxin resistance. Science 1986;232:997–980.
21. Michie HR, Manogue KR, Spriggs DR, et al. Detection of circulating tumor necrosis factor after endotoxin administration. N Engl J Med 318:1481–1486.
22. Waage A, Halstensen A, Espevik T. Association between tumor necrosis factor in serum and fatal outcome in patients with meningococcal disease. Lancet 1987;1:355–357.
23. Buetler B, Milsark IW, Cerami A. Passive immunization with cachetin/tumor necrosis factor (TNF) protects mice from the lethal effects of endotoxin. Nature 229:869–871.
24. Tracey KJ, Beutler B, Lowry SF, et al. Shock and tissue injury induced by recombinant human cachetin. Science 1986;234:470–474.
25. Dinarello CA, Cannon JG, Solff SM, et al. Tumor necrosis factor (cachectin) is an endogenous pyrogen and induces production of interleukin-1. J Exp Med 1986;163:1433–1450.
26. Scuderi P, Sterling KE, Lam KS, et al. Raised serum levels of tumor necrosis factor in parasitic infections. Lancet 1986;2:1364–1365.
27. Bone RC. The pathogenesis of sepsis. Ann Intern Med 1991;115:457–469.
28. Damas P, Reuter A, Gysen P, et al. Tumor necrosis factor and interleukin-1 serum levels during severe sepsis in humans. Crit Care Med 1989;17:975–978.
29. Damas P, Ledoux D, Nys M, et al. Cytokine serum level during sepsis in human IL-6 as a marker of severity. Ann Surg 1992;215:356–362.
30. Cannon JG, Tompkins RG, Gelfand JA, et al. Circulating interleukin-1 tumor necrosis factor in septic shock and experimental endotoxin fever. J Infect Dis 1990;161:79–84.
31. Casey LC, Balk RA, Bone RC. Plasma cytokine and endotoxin levels correlate with survival in patients with sepsis syndrome. Ann Intern Med 1993;119:771–778.
32. Steinmetz HT, Herbertz A, Bertram M, Diehl V. Increase in interleukin-6 serum level preceding fever in granulocytopenia and correlation with death from sepsis. J Infect Dis 1995;171:225–228.
33. Calandra T, Gerain J, Heumann D, et al. High circulating levels of interleukin-6 in patients with septic shock: Evolution during sepsis, prognostic value, and interplay with other cytokines. Am J Med 1991;91:23–29.
34. Hack CE, DeGroot ER, Richelle JF, et al. Increased plasma levels of interleukin-6 in sepsis. Blood 1989;74:1704–1710.
35. Hack CE, Hart M, Strack RJM, et al. Interleukin-8 in sepsis: Relation to shock and inflammatory mediators. Infect Immun 1992;60:2835–2842.
36. Marty C, Misset B, Tamion F, et al. Circulating interleukin-8 concentrations in patients with multiple organ failure of septic and nonseptic origin. Crit Care Med 1994;22:673–679.
37. Guidet B, Barakett V, Vassal T, et al. Endotoxemia and bacteremia in patients with sepsis syndrome in the intensive care unit. Chest 1994;106:1194–1201.
38. Kollef MH, Schuster DP. The acute respiratory distress syndrome. N Engl J Med 1995;332:27–37.
39. Bernard GR, Artgas A, Brigham KL, et al. The American–European Consensus Conference on ARDS; definitions, mechanisms, relevant outcomes and clinical coordination. Am J Resp Crit Care Med 1994;149:818–824.
40. Martin MA, Silverman HJ. Gram-negative sepsis and the adult respiratory distress syndrome. Clin Infect Dis 1992;14:1213–1228.
41. Parker MM, Shelhamer JH, Bacharach SL. Profound but reversible myocardial depression in patients with septic shock. Ann Intern Med 1984;100:483.
42. Suffredini AF, Fromm RE, Parker MM, et al. The cardiovascular response of normal humans to the administration of endotoxin. N Engl J Med 1990;321:280–287.
43. Pizzo PA, Hathorn JW, Hiemenz J, et al. A randomized trial comparing ceftazidime alone with combination antibiotic therapy in cancer patients with fever and neutropenia. N Engl J Med 1986;315:552.
44. Morrison DC, Ryan JL. Endotoxin and disease mechanisms. Ann Rev Med 1987;38:417–432.
45. Moore RD, Lietman PS, Smith CR. The association of aminoglycoside plasma levels with mortality in patients with gram-negative bacteremia. J Infect Dis 1984;149:443–448.
46. Moore RD, Lietman PS, Smith CR. Clinical response to aminoglycoside therapy: Importance of the ratio of peak concentration to minimum inhibitory concentration. J Infect Dis 1987;155:93–97.
47. Kapusnik JE, Hackbarth CJ, Chambers HF, et al. Single, large, daily dosing versus intermittent dosing of tobramycin for treating experimental *Pseudomonas* pneumonia. J Infect Dis 1988;158:7–12.
48. Bennett WM, Plamp CE, Gilbert RA, et al. The influence of dosing regimen on experimental gentamicin nephrotoxicity: Dissociation of peak serum levels from renal failure. J Infect Dis 1979;140:546–580.
49. Sturm AW. Netilmicin in the treatment of gram-negative bacteremia: Single daily versus multiple daily dosage. J Infect Dis 1989;159:931–937.
50. Ter Braak EW, de Vries PJ, Bouter KP, et al. Once-daily dosing regimen for aminoglycoside plus β-lactam combination therapy of serious infections: Comparative trial with netilmicin plus ceftriaxone. Am J Med 1990;89:58–66.
51. Young LS. Empirical antimicrobial therapy in the neutropenic host. N Engl J Med 1986;315:580.
52. Oblinger MJ, Bowers JT, Sande MA, et al. Moxalactam therapy versus standard therapy for selected infections. Rev Infect Dis 1983;4(suppl):S181.
53. Bolivar R, Fainstein V, Elting L, et al. Cefoperazone for treatment of infections in patients with cancer. Rev Infect Dis 1983;5(suppl 2):S181.
54. Parillo JE, Parker MM, Natanson C. Septic shock in humans. Advances in the understanding of pathogenesis, cardiovascular dysfunction, and therapy. NIH conference report. Ann Intern Med 1991;113:227–242.
55. Weil MH, Rockow EE. A guide to volume repletion. Emerg Med 1984;16:101.
56. Rackow EC, Falk JL, Fein IZ, et al. Fluid resuscitation in circulatory shock: A comparison of the cardiorespiratory effects of albumin, hetastarch, and saline solutions in

patients with hypovolemic and septic shock. Crit Care Med 1983;11:839–850.

57. Conrad SA, Finkelstein FL, Madden MR, et al. Cardiovascular dysfunction in multiple organ failure, in Deitach EA (ed): Multiple Organ Failure, 1st ed. New York, Thieme Medical Publishers, 1990.
58. Czer LS, Shoemaker WC. Optimal hematocrits value in critically ill postoperative patients. Surg Gynecol Obstet 1978;126:778–783.
59. Shoemaker WC, Appel PL, Kram HB, et al. Comparison of hemodynamic and oxygen transport effects of dopamine and dobutamine in critically ill surgical patients. Chest 1989;96:120–126.
60. Schaer GL, Fink MP, Parilto JE. Norepi alone versus norepi plus low-dose dopamine: Enhanced renal blood flow with combination pressor therapy. Crit Care Med 1985;13:492–496.
61. Ziegler EJ, Fisher CJ Jr, Spring CL, et al. Treatment of gram-negative bacteremia and septic shock with HAIA monoclonal antibody against endotoxin. N Engl J Med 1991;324:429–436.
62. Greenman RL, Schein RMH, Martin MA, et al. A controlled clinical trial of E5 murine monoclonal IgM antibody to endotoxin in the treatment of gram-negative sepsis. JAMA 1991;266:1097–1102.
63. Fisher CJ, Dhainault JF, Pribble JP, et al. Recombinant human interleukin 1 receptor antagonist in the treatment of patients with sepsis syndrome. Results of a randomized, double-blind, placebo-controlled trial. Phase III rhIL-1ra Sepsis Study Group. JAMA 1994;27:1836–1843.
64. Dhainaut JFA, Tenaillon A, Tulzo YL, et al. Platelet-activating factor receptor antagonist BN 52021 in the treatment of severe sepsis: A randomized, double-blind, placebo-controlled, multicenter clinical trial. Crit Care Med 1994;22:1720–1728.
65. Fisher CJ, Opal SM, Dhainaut JF, et al. Influence of an anti-tumor necrosis factor monoclonal antibody on cytokine levels in patients with sepsis. The CB0006 Sepsis Syndrome Study Group. Crit Care Med 1993;21:318–327.
66. Schedel I, Dreikhausen U, Nentwig B, et al. Treatment of gram-negative septic shock with an immunoglobulin preparation: A prospective randomized clinical trial. Crit Care Med 1991;19:1104–1113.
67. Abraham E, Wunderink R, Silverman H, et al. Efficacy and safety of monoclonal antibody to human tumor necrosis factor alpha in patients with sepsis syndrome. A randomized, controlled, double-blind, multicenter clinical trial. JAMA 1995;273:934–941.
68. Bone RC, Fisher CJ Jr, Clemmer TP, et al. Early methylprednisolone treatment for septic syndrome and the adult respiratory distress syndrome. Chest 1987;92:1032–1036.

Chapter 113

Invasive Fungal Infections

Peggy L. Carver, PharmD

For many years, fungal infections were classified as either superficial "nuisance diseases," such as athlete's foot or vulvovaginal candidiasis, or as relatively rare infections confined primarily to endemic areas of the United States. When invasive fungal infections were encountered, amphotericin B was the only consistently effective, systemically active agent available for the treatment of systemic mycoses. Advances in medical technology, including organ and bone marrow transplantation, cytotoxic chemotherapy, widespread use of indwelling intravenous catheters, and the increased use of potent, broad-spectrum antimicrobial agents have all contributed to the dramatic increase in the incidence of fungal infections worldwide. Fungal infections have emerged as a major cause of death among cancer patients and transplant recipients.[1] In addition, patients with acquired immunodeficiency syndrome (AIDS) experience substantially more frequent and severe forms of cryptococcosis, histoplasmosis, coccidioidomycosis, and mucocutaneous (esophageal, oral, and vulvovaginal) candidiasis.[1–3]

Problems remain in the diagnosis, prevention, and treatment of fungal infections. Unlike the current availability of diagnostic techniques for most bacterial pathogens, there remain a host of unresolved issues regarding standardization of susceptibility testing methods, *in vitro* and *in vivo* models of infection, the utility of monitoring antifungal plasma concentrations, and the development and identification of resistant pathogens.[4–8] The emergence of new pathogens such as *Trichosporon beigelii, Alternaria* spp., and *Fusarium* spp., which were previously considered saprophytic organisms, is of concern. Current research focusing on newer diagnostic methods, combination therapy with antifungal agents, and the role of prophylactic and chronic suppressive therapy will help to clarify these concerns.[1–2]

The development of more potent, orally available antifungal agents has resulted in a wider selection of agents for the treatment of these infections. In addition, a number of promising new agents are currently under development. The results of controlled clinical trials evaluating the efficacy of these agents in comparison with older, established, but generally more toxic agents will help to establish the role of these newer compounds in the treatment of systemic fungal infections.

Current research in the diagnosis of mycoses includes the use of immunohistochemical and fluorescent antibodies and other techniques for the specific and rapid identification of fungi in tissues and body fluids. The use of exoantigen detection, detection of fungal antigen and fungal metabolites in patients with infection, and DNA/RNA gene probes and polymerase chain reactions offer promising new techniques for the diagnosis of infection.[1]

THE PATHOGEN

Fungi are eucaryotic organisms with a defined nucleus enclosed by a nuclear membrane, and a cytoplasmic membrane containing lipids, glycoproteins and sterols, mitochondria, Golgi apparatus, ribosomes bound to endoplasmic reticulum, and a cytoskeleton with microtubules, microfilaments, and intermediate filaments. Fungi have rigid cell walls composed of chitin, cellulose, or both, that stain with Gomori methenamine silver or periodic acid–Schiff reagent. Most fungi, except *Candida,* are too weakly gram positive to be seen well on Gram's stain. *Cryptococcus neoformans* has a polysaccharide capsule surrounding the cell wall.[9]

Morphologically, pathogenic fungi can be grouped as either filamentous *molds* or unicellular *yeasts.* Molds grow as multicellular branching, thread-like filaments (*hyphae*) that are either *septate* (divided by transverse walls) or *coenocytic* (multinucleate without cross walls) (Figure 113.1). On agar media, molds grow outward from the point of inoculation by extension of the tips of filaments, and then branch repeatedly, interweaving to form fuzzy, matted growths called *mycelium.* Yeasts are oval or spherically shaped unicellular forms that generally produce pasty or mucoid colonies on agar media, similar to those observed with bacterial cultures. Yeasts have rigid cell walls that reproduce by budding, a process in which daughter cells arise from pinching off a portion of the parent cell.

Fungi reproduce by forming spores asexually via mitosis to produce motile *sporangiospores* or nonmotile *conidia* (singular, *conidium*), or they reproduce sexually through meiosis to produce ascospores, basidiospores, oospores, or zygospores. Although terms such as *spore* and *conidia*

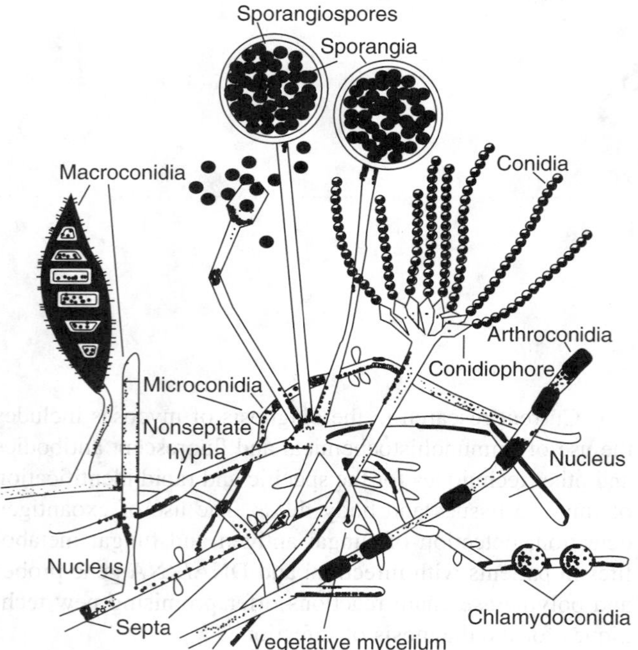

Figure 113.1. Forms of molds. The tubelike hyphae form their basic structure. Examples of spores and conidia and of the structures that bear them are shown. *(From Ryan KJ. Pathogenic fungi, in Sherris JC [ed]: Sherris Medical Microbiology, 3rd ed. Norwalk, CT, Appleton & Lange, 1994, p 574, with permission. Copyright 1994, Appleton & Lange.)*

should no longer be used interchangeably, some newer literature and much of the older medical literature continue to confuse these terms.

Most fungi produce both sexual *(teleomorph)* and asexual *(anamorph)* forms, although the pathogenic fungi classified as Deuteromycetes or *Fungi imperfecti* have no known sexual forms and produce only conidial spore formation. When no sexual stage is known, classification is based on the morphologic development of conidia, which may form on specialized *conidiophores,* on the sides or ends of nonspecialized hyphae, or from a hyphal cell. When more than one kind of conidium is produced within a given colony, the small, single-celled conidia are called *microconidia,* and the large, often multicellular conidia are called *macroconidia.* Three of the more common types of conidia include blastoconidia, aleurioconidia, and arthroconidia. *Blastoconidia* are simple structures that arise from budding, with subsequent separation of the bud from the parent cell (e.g., in *Candida* and *Cryptococcus*). *Aleurioconidia* (for example, *Blastomyces* and *Histoplasma*) describe conidia, with a broad base of attachment to a conidiogenous cell, that separate by lysis of the conidiogenous hyphal wall leaving a remnant attached to the conidium as an annular frill. *Arthroconidia* such as *Coccidioides immitis* result from hyphae fragmenting into individual cells.[9]

In the past, clinical identification and naming of fungi was based on observations of the fruiting structures (often the asexual form) associated with the development of conidia. In more recent years, complete life cycles of many clinically relevant fungi have been elucidated and additional names have been added to describe their sexual forms. However, many microbiology laboratories and clinicians continue to use the older names assigned to the asexual forms since most fungi isolated in the clinical laboratory are found in the asexual form, and the human diseases resulting from the pathogen are often based on this name. For example, *Blastomyces dermatitidis,* the etiologic agent of human blastomycosis, was named in 1898 based on its asexual (conidial) characteristics. In 1968, the life cycle of the fungus was found to include a meiotic stage that produces ascospores. A new name, *Ajellomyces dermatitidis,* was chosen to describe the sexual (ascomycetous) form. However, since the form isolated in clinical microbiology laboratories is *B. dermatitidis,* this name is retained for clinical use.

Many pathogenic fungi, termed *dimorphic fungi,* exist as either a yeast or a mold, depending on the pathogen, the site of growth (in the host or in the laboratory setting), and the temperature. Usually, yeasts are the parasitic form that invade human or animal host tissue while molds are the free-living form found in the environment. For example, *Histoplasma capsulatum* exists as a yeast in humans and as a mold in the laboratory.[9,10]

Currently, most laboratories do not routinely perform susceptibility tests on fungal isolates, and standardized methods for performing these tests are currently being developed. Similarly, the routine monitoring of plasma concentrations of antifungal agents to assess efficacy or toxicity of these agents is generally not available. Correlations between plasma concentrations of antifungal agents and therapeutic outcomes have been poorly studied. However, recent data demonstrating the emergence of azole-resistant *Candida albicans* in HIV-infected patients and the decreased bioavailability of ketoconazole and itraconazole in selected patient populations have prompted new studies addressing these issues.[7,11,12]

Risk of Acquiring a Fungal Infection

Systemic mycoses caused by primary or "pathogenic" fungi include histoplasmosis, coccidioidomycosis, cryptococcosis, blastomycosis, paracoccidioidomycosis, and sporotrichosis. Primary pathogens can cause disease in both healthy and immunocompromised individuals, although disease is generally more severe or disseminated in the immunocompromised host. In contrast, mycoses caused by opportunistic fungi such as *C. albicans, Aspergillus* species, *Trichosporon, Torulopsis (Candida) glabrata, Fusarium, Alternaria,* and *Mucor* are generally found only in the immunocompromised host.[9]

Most fungal infections are acquired as a result of accidental inhalation of airborne conidia. For example, *H. cap-*

sulatum is found in soil contaminated by bat, chicken, or starling excreta, and *C. neoformans* is associated with pigeon droppings. Although some fungi, including *C. albicans, C. neoformans,* and *Aspergillus* spp., are ubiquitous pathogens with worldwide distribution, other fungi have regional distributions associated with specific geographic environments.[9]

Systemic fungal infections are a major cause of morbidity and mortality in the immunocompromised patient.[9] Fungal infections account for 20–30% of fatal infections in patients with acute leukemia, 10–15% of fatal infections in patients with lymphoma, and 5% of fatal infections in patients with solid tumors. The frequency of fungal infections among transplant recipients ranges from 0–20% for kidney and bone marrow to 10–35% for heart and 30–40% for liver transplant recipients.

Approximately 2–4% of all hospitalized patients develop a nosocomial infection. Of these, bacteria comprise the most common etiologic agent.[9] However, fungi are becoming increasingly significant nosocomial pathogens. Although only limited data exist documenting the incidence and prevalence of nosocomial fungal infections, the Centers for Disease Control reported via its National Nosocomial Infections System (NNIS) that in 1990, fungi accounted for 9.9% of all bloodstream isolates. *Candida* spp. (primarily *C. albicans*) accounted for 78.3% of all nosocomial fungal infections.[10,13–15]

Nosocomially acquired fungal infections may arise from either exogenous or endogenous flora. Endogenous flora may include normal commensals of the skin, gastrointestinal, genitourinary or respiratory tract. *Candida albicans* is found as a normal commensal of the gastrointestinal tract in 20–30% of humans.[10,14]

A complex interplay of host and pathogen factors influences the acquisition and development of fungal infections. Intact skin or mucosal surfaces serve as primary barriers to infection. Desiccation, epithelial cell turnover, the fatty acid content, and the low pH of the skin are believed to be important factors in host resistance. Bacterial flora of the skin and mucous membranes compete with fungi for growth. Alterations in the balance of normal flora caused by the use of antibiotics or alterations in nutritional status can allow the proliferation of fungi such as *Candida,* increasing the likelihood of systemic invasion and infection.[9]

The growth of fungi within tissues is restrained by a number of mechanisms. For example, serum has fungistatic activity against *Candida* in part due to transferrins, the human iron-binding proteins, which deprive microbes of the iron needed for synthesis of respiratory enzymes. Serum also contains β globulins, which cause a nonimmunological clumping of *Candida,* facilitating their elimination by inflammatory cells.[9,10]

Tissue reaction in the presence of fungi varies with the fungal species, the site of proliferation, and the duration of infection. Phagocytosis by neutrophils and macrophages is the earliest mechanism that prevents the establishment of fungi. Consequently, patients with decreased neutrophil counts or decreased neutrophil function are at higher risk of infections, particularly those caused by *Candida* and *Aspergillus.* Some mycoses are characterized by a low-grade inflammatory response that does not eliminate the fungi. Fungal cells can sometimes persist within macrophages without being killed, perhaps due to resistance to the effects of lysosomal enzymes.[9]

Diagnosis of Invasive Fungal Infections

The diagnosis of invasive fungal infections is generally accomplished by careful evaluation of clinical symptoms, the results of serologic tests, and histopathologic examination and culture of clinical specimens. Skin tests are generally not useful diagnostically because they do not distinguish between active and past infection. They remain useful as screening tools and in epidemiologic studies to determine endemic areas. It is beyond the scope of this chapter to discuss the relative merits of each of the immunologic tests used in the diagnosis of invasive fungal infections. However, the interested reader is referred to several excellent reviews concerning this topic.[8,16,17]

Infections Caused by Pathogenic Fungi

Strategies for the prevention of invasive mycoses can be broadly classified as prophylaxis, early empirical therapy, empirical therapy, and secondary prophylaxis or suppression.[18] In patients undergoing cytotoxic chemotherapy, antifungal therapy is directed primarily at the prevention or treatment of infections caused by *Candida* and *Aspergillus. Prophylactic therapy* with topical, oral, or intravenous antifungal agents is administered prior to and throughout the period of granulocytopenia (absolute neutrophil count <1000/μL). The potential benefits of prophylactic therapy must be weighed against the potential risks inherent in each regimen. Perfect[19] has suggested that each clinician consider at least 6 criteria before justifying antifungal prophylaxis: (1) safety, (2) efficacy, (3) cost, (4) consequence, (5) prevalence, and (6) resistance. *Early empirical therapy* is the administration of systemic antifungal agents at the onset of fever and neutropenia. *Empirical therapy* with systemic antifungal agents is administered to granulocytopenic patients with persistent or recurrent fever despite the administration of appropriate antimicrobial therapy. *Secondary prophylaxis* (or *suppressive therapy*) refers to administration of systemic antifungal agents (generally prior to and throughout the period of granulocytopenia) to prevent relapse of a documented invasive fungal infection that was treated during a previous episode of granulocytopenia. Although these treatment classifications have also been applied to the treatment of fungal infections in AIDS, patients with AIDS rarely acquire systemic infections caused by *Candida* or *Aspergillus* spp. unless they become granulocytopenic due to disease or drugs. The use of antifungal prophylaxis is much less widely studied in this population, although recent studies have suggested that early antifungal prophylaxis may decrease the incidence of invasive cryptococcal disease.[20] Suppressive therapy is generally necessary following acute therapy for histoplasmosis, coccidioidomycosis, and cryptococcosis due to the high rates of relapse when antifungal therapy is discontinued.

HISTOPLASMOSIS

In humans, histoplasmosis is caused by inhalation of dust-borne microconidia of the dimorphic fungus *Histoplasma capsulatum.* Although there exist two dimorphic varieties of *H. capsulatum,* the small-celled (2- to 5-μm) form (variety *capsulatum*) occurs globally, while the large-celled (8- to 15-μm) form (variety *duboisii*) is confined to the African continent and Madagascar. *Histoplasma capsulatum* was originally named on the basis of intrahistiocytic plasmodia-like organisms recovered from tissues; however, the pseudo-encapsulated appearance proved to be an artifact caused by cytoplasmic shrinkage from the rigid cell wall during tissue fixation. In tissues stained by conventional techniques, *H. capsulatum* appears as an oval or round, narrow-pore budding, unencapsulated yeast.[3,21,22]

Although histoplasmosis is found worldwide, certain areas of North and Latin America are recognized as endemic areas; in the United States, most disease is localized along the Ohio and Mississippi river valleys. *Histoplasma capsulatum* is found in nitrogen-enriched soils, particularly those heavily contaminated by avian or bat guano, that accelerate sporulation. Blackbird or pigeon roosts, chicken coops, and sites frequented by bats, such as caves, attics, or old buildings, serve as "microfoci" of infections. Although birds are not infected because of their high body temperature, bats (mammals) may be infected and pass yeast forms in their feces, allowing the spread of *H. capsulatum* to new habitats.[3,22]

At ambient temperatures, *H. capsulatum* grows as a mold. The mycelial phase consists of septate branching hyphae with terminal micro- and macroconidia that range in size from 2–14 μm in diameter. When soil is disturbed, these conidia become aerosolized and reach the bronchioles or alveoli.[21,22]

Animal studies have demonstrated that within 2–3 days after reaching lung tissue, the conidia germinate, releasing yeast forms that begin multiplying by binary fission. During the next 9–15 days, organisms are ingested but not destroyed by large numbers of macrophages that are recruited to the infected site, resulting in small infiltrates. Infected macrophages migrate to the mediastinal lymph nodes and other sites within the mononuclear phagocyte system, particularly the spleen and liver. At this time, the onset of specific T-cell immunity in the nonimmune host activates the macrophages, rendering them capable of fungicidal activity. Tissue granulomas form, many of which develop central caseation and necrosis over the next 2–4 months. Over a period of several years, these foci become encapsulated and calcified, often with viable yeast trapped within the necrotic tissue.[21,22]

Cellular immunity, as measured by histoplasmin skin test reactivity, wanes in the absence of occasional reexposure. Although exposure to heavy inoculae may overcome these immune mechanisms, resulting in severe disease, reinfection occurs frequently in endemic areas. In the immune individual, the reactions of acquired immunity begin 24–48 hours after the appearance of yeast forms, resulting in milder forms of illness and little proliferation of organisms. Although viable organisms may be found within granulomas years after initial infection, the organisms appear to have little ability to proliferate within the fibrous capsules, except in immunocompromised patients.[21,22]

Clinical Presentation

The outcome of infection with *H. capsulatum* depends on a complex interplay of host, pathogen, and environmental factors. Host factors include the degree of immunosuppression, and the presence of immunity (from prior infection). Environmental factors include inoculum size, exposure within an enclosed area, and duration of exposure. In the vast majority of patients, low-inoculum exposure to *H. capsulatum* results in *asymptomatic infection* or an acute, self-limited illness with flu-like pulmonary symptoms, including fever, chills, headache, myalgia, and a nonproductive cough. A small percentage of patients will present with arthritis, erythema nodosum, pericarditis, or mediastinal granuloma, which may require the addition of anti-inflammatory agents to their therapy.[21,22]

Chronic pulmonary histoplasmosis generally presents as an opportunistic infection imposed on a preexisting structural abnormality such as lesions resulting from emphysema. Patients demonstrate chronic pulmonary symptoms and apical lung lesions that progress with inflammation, calcified granulomas, and fibrosis. Patients with early, noncavitary disease often recover without treatment. Progression of disease over a period of years, seen in 25–30% of patients, is associated with cavitation, bronchopleural fistulas, extension to the other lung, pulmonary insufficiency, and often death.[22]

In patients exposed to a large inoculum and in immunocompromised hosts, successful containment of the organism within macrophages may not occur, resulting in a progressive illness characterized by yeast-filled phagocytic cells and an inability to produce granulomas. This disease, termed *disseminated histoplasmosis,* is characterized by persistent parasitization of macrophages. The clinical severity of the four diverse forms of disseminated histoplasmosis (Table 113.1) generally parallels the degree of macrophage parasitization observed.[21]

Acute (infantile) disseminated histoplasmosis is characterized by massive involvement of the mononuclear phagocyte system by yeast-engorged macrophages. Classically, this severe type of infection is seen in infants and young children and (rarely) in adults with Hodgkin's disease or other lymphoproliferative disorders. In infants or children, acute disseminated histoplasmosis is characterized by unrelenting fever, anemia, leukopenia or thrombocytopenia, enlargement of the liver, spleen, and visceral lymph nodes, and gastrointestinal symptoms, particularly nausea, vomiting, and diarrhea. The chest roentgenogram often demonstrates remnants of the initiating acute pulmonary lesion. Untreated disease is uniformly fatal in 1–2 months. A less severe "subacute" form of the disease, which occurs in both infants and immunocompetent adults, is characterized by focal destructive lesions in various organs, weight loss, weakness, fever, and malaise. Untreated disease is generally fatal in approximately 10 months.[21]

Most adults with disseminated histoplasmosis demonstrate a mild, chronic form of the disease. Untreated patients are often ill for 10–20 years, demonstrating long asymptomatic periods interrupted by relapses of clinical illness, characterized primarily by weight loss, weakness, and fatigue. Although central nervous system (CNS) involvement occurs in 10–20% of patients with severe underlying immunosuppressive conditions, focal organ involvement is uncommon.[22]

TABLE 113.1. CLINICAL MANIFESTATIONS AND THERAPY OF HISTOPLASMOSIS

Type of Disease and Common Clinical Manifestations	Approximate Frequency (%)[a]	Therapy/Comments
Acute Pulmonary Histoplasmosis		
Asymptomatic histoplasmosis	50–99	Asymptomatic disease: No therapy generally required.
Self-limited disease	1–50	Self-limited disease: High-dose corticosteroids plus AmB[b] 0.3–0.5 mg/kg/d × 2–4 weeks or ketoconazole 400 mg orally daily × 3–6 months may be beneficial in patients with severe hypoxia following inhalation of large inoculae.
		Antifungal therapy generally not useful for arthritis, or pericarditis. NSAIDs[c] or corticosteroids may be useful in some cases.
		Mediastinal granulomas: Most lesions resolve spontaneously. Surgery or antifungal therapy with AmB 40–50 mg/d × 2–3 weeks or ketoconazole 400 mg/d orally × >30 months may be beneficial in some cases.
Inflammatory/fibrotic histoplasmosis	0.02	Fibrosing mediastinitis: Antifungal therapy generally not helpful; surgery may be of benefit if disease is detected early; late disease may not respond to therapy.
		Sarcoid-like: NSAIDs or corticosteroids may be of benefit for some patients.
Chronic Pulmonary Histoplasmosis	0.05	Chronic pulmonary histoplasmosis: Antifungal therapy generally recommended for immunosuppressed patients with either persistent cavitation, cavitary wall thickness >2 mm, or progressive symptoms (including weight loss, cough, sputum production, low-grade fever).
		Ketoconazole 400 mg/d orally for 1 year; increase to 600–800 mg/d if no favorable response or AmB >35 mg/kg over 10 weeks.
Disseminated Histoplasmosis	0.02–0.05	Disseminated histoplasmosis: Untreated mortality 83–93%; relapse 5–23% in non-AIDS patients.
Acute		Nonimmunosuppressed patients: Ketoconazole 400 mg/d orally × 6–12 months or AmB 35 mg/kg.
Subacute		Immunosuppressed patients (non-AIDS) or + endocarditis or CNS disease: AmB ≥35 mg/kg.
Chronic (adult-type)		
Progressive disease of AIDS	25–50[d]	AIDS patients: AmB 15–30 mg/kg (1–2 g over 4–10 weeks); followed by chronic itraconazole for initial therapy. Treat relapses with AmB.

[a]As a percentage of all patients presenting with histoplasmosis.
[b]AmB, amphotericin B.
[c]NSAIDs, nonsteroidal anti-inflammatory drugs.
[d]As a percentage of AIDS patients presenting with histoplasmosis as the initial manifestation of their disease. (Compiled from Refs. 9, 22, and 32.)

Adult patients with AIDS demonstrate an acute form of disseminated disease that resembles the syndrome seen in infants and children. *Progressive disseminated histoplasmosis* (PDH) can occur as the direct result of initial infection or due to the reactivation of dormant foci. In endemic areas, 50% of AIDS patients demonstrate PDH as the first manifestation of their disease. PDH is characterized by fever (75% of patients), weight loss, chills, night sweats, enlargement of the spleen, liver, or lymph nodes, and anemia. Pulmonary symptoms occur in only one-third of patients and do not always correlate with the presence of infiltrates on chest roentgenogram. A clinical syndrome resembling septicemia is seen in approximately 25–50% of patients.[21–25]

Diagnosis

Detection of single, yeast-like cells 2–5 μm in diameter with narrow-based budding in direct exam or histologic study of blood smears or tissues should raise strong suspicion of infection with *H. capsulatum.* Identification of mycelial isolates from clinical cultures can be made by conversion of the mycelium to the yeast form (requires 3–6 weeks), via commercially available exoantigen test kits, or by the more rapid (2 hours) and 100% sensitive DNA probe. In patients with suspected disseminated or chronic cavitary histoplasmosis, two to three blood, sputum, and bone marrow cultures and stains should be obtained utilizing the lysis centrifugation technique, and the cultures held for 14–21 days for optimal yield of *H. capsulatum.* In patients with acute self-limited histoplasmosis, extensive testing to verify the diagnosis may not be necessary.[16,21,22,24,25]

In most patients, serologic evidence remains the primary method in the diagnosis of histoplasmosis. Results obtained from commercially available complement fixation (CF), immunodiffusion (ID), and latex agglutination (LA) antibody tests are used alone or in combination. In general, the use of histoplasmin skin tests are of little value except in epidemiologic studies, since histoplasmin reactivity waxes in the absence of occasional reexposure. In addition, histoplasmin skin testing may result in a false increase in the CF titer for mycelial antigen (CF-M) to *H. capsulatum.* A fourfold rise in the CF titer is usually indicative of recent infection, although some patients with severe disease or profound immunosuppression may demonstrate a weaker antibody response. Since the immunodiffusion test is not as sensitive as CF, it should be used to assess the importance of weakly reactive results obtained by CF rather than as a screening procedure.[16,22] Radioimmunoassay (RIA), which measures IgM and IgG antibodies against a histoplasmin extract, is the most sensitive test, but may show a large number of false-positive reactions in patients living in an endemic area.[16,21,22]

In the AIDS patient with progressive disseminated histoplasmosis, the diagnosis is best established by bone marrow biopsy and culture, which yield positive cultures in >90% of patients, although blood cultures and histopathologic exam and culture of pulmonary tissue, sputum, skin, and lymph nodes may also be helpful. Detection of *H. capsulatum* polysaccharide antigen (HPA) in urine, blood, or cerebrospinal fluid (CSF) by enzyme-linked immunosorbent assay (ELISA) or a modified radioimmunoassay assay are promising new techniques for the rapid diagnosis of histoplasmosis. HPA (RIA) levels have also been used successfully to monitor the course of therapy and to detect relapses in patients with AIDS, and clearance of antigen from serum and urine correlates with clinical efficacy during maintenance therapy with itraconazole. Unfortunately, these tests are not yet available for clinical use.[16,22–26]

Treatment

Recommended therapy for the treatment of histoplasmosis is summarized in Table 113.1. In general, asymptomatic patients and patients with fibrosing mediastinitis or sarcoid-like disease do not benefit from antifungal therapy. Patients with mild, self-limited disease, chronic disseminated disease, or chronic pulmonary histoplasmosis who have no underlying immunosuppression can usually be treated with either oral ketoconazole or intravenous amphotericin B.

In AIDS patients, intensive primary (induction) antifungal therapy is followed by lifelong suppressive (maintenance) therapy. In patients with underlying immunosuppression, including AIDS patients with progressive disseminated histoplasmosis, amphotericin B remains the drug of choice for induction therapy, although The British Society for Antimicrobial Chemotherapy currently recommends oral itraconazole 400 mg daily for 6 weeks as an alternative to amphotericin B. Amphotericin B dosages of 50 mg/d (up to 1 mg/kg/d) should be administered to a cumulative dose of 15–35 mg/kg (1–2 grams) and until negative fungal cultures are achieved. Response to therapy should be measured by resolution of radiologic, serologic, and microbiologic parameters, and improvement in signs and symptoms of infection. Although investigators are limited by the lack of standardized criteria to quantify the extent of infection, degree of immunosuppression, or treatment response, response rates (based on resolution or improvement in presenting signs and symptoms) of >80% have been reported in case series in AIDS patients receiving varied dosages of amphotericin B. Rapid responses are reported, with resolution of symptoms in 25% and 75% of patients by day 3 and day 7 of therapy, respectively.

Limited data suggest that ketoconazole and fluconazole do not appear efficacious as primary therapy of disseminated histoplasmosis in AIDS, although inadequate dosages of fluconazole (<200 mg/d) were employed. Initial therapy with itraconazole 300 mg orally twice daily for 3 days followed by 200 mg twice daily for 12 weeks was successful in 51 of 61 AIDS patients. Fungemia was resolved in responders by week 8 of therapy. Microbiologic and/or clinical failures occurred in 6 patients. In another series, itraconazole 400 mg daily was successful (2 patients improved and 6 experienced remission) in 8 of 9 patients.[26]

Once the initial course of therapy for histoplasmosis is completed, lifelong suppressive therapy with oral azoles or amphotericin B (1–1.5 mg/kg weekly or biweekly) is recommended, because of the frequent recurrence of infection. Relapse rates in AIDS patients not receiving maintenance therapy range from 50–90%. Ketoconazole has been utilized with only limited success, with relapse rates of 50% following therapy. Limited data suggest that oral fluconazole 200–400 mg/d is successful in preventing relapse of disease. Itraconazole 200 mg orally twice daily for 3–12 weeks was successful in 39 of 42 (93%) AIDS patients, and only 1 patient was removed from the trial because of toxicity (hypokalemia). However, oral thrush was reported in 6 patients, 3 of whom had undetectable serum concentrations of itraconazole. Itraconazole may soon be recognized as the drug of choice for maintenance therapy because of the drug's ease of administration and favorable safety profile.[26] Patients failing suppressive therapy with itraconazole may benefit from plasma concentration monitoring of itraconazole.

BLASTOMYCOSIS

North American blastomycosis is a systemic fungal infection caused by *Blastomyces dermatitidis,* a dimorphic fungus that infects primarily the lung. However, patients may present with a variety of pulmonary and extrapulmonary clinical manifestations. Pulmonary disease may be acute or chronic and can mimic infection with tuberculosis, pyogenic bacteria, other fungi, or malignancy. Blastomycosis can disseminate to virtually every other body organ, and approximately 40% of patients with blastomycosis present with skin, bone and joint, or genitourinary tract involvement without any evidence of pulmonary disease.[27,28]

Blastomycosis was renamed "North American blastomycosis" in 1942 when Conant and Howell named a similar fungus endemic to South America *"Blastomyces braziliensis"* and the disease it caused "South American blastomycosis." The disease had previously been called paracoccidioidomycosis. Although the disease is now recognized to be endemic to the southeastern and south central states of the United States (especially those bordering on the Mississippi and Ohio river basins), and the midwestern states and Canadian provinces bordering on the Great Lakes, numerous cases of North American blastomycosis have been diagnosed in Africa, northern parts of South America, India, and Europe. Endemic areas have primarily been defined by analysis of sporadic cases and epidemics or clusters of disease, since the lack of a dependable skin or laboratory test makes wide-scale epidemiologic testing to determine the incidence of infection unfeasible at present.[27] Although initial review of sporadic cases suggested that males with outdoor occupations that exposed them to soil were at greatest risk for blastomycosis, more recent data suggest that there is no sex, age, or occupational predilection for blastomycosis.[27–29]

Although *B. dermatitidis* is generally considered to be a soil inhabitant, attempts to isolate the organism in nature have frequently been unsuccessful. *Blastomyces dermatitidis* has been isolated from soil containing decayed vegetation, decomposed wood, and pigeon manure, frequently in association with warm moist soil of wooded areas that is rich in organic debris.[27–29]

Pulmonary infection probably occurs by inhalation of conidia, which convert to the yeast form in the lung. A vigorous inflammatory response ensues, with neutrophilic recruitment to the lungs followed by the development of cell-mediated immunity and the formation of noncaseating granulomas.[13,27–29]

Clinical Presentation

Acute pulmonary blastomycosis is generally an asymptomatic or self-limited disease characterized by fever, shaking chills, and a productive cough in immunocompetent individuals that may be difficult to differentiate from other respiratory infections on the basis of clinical symptoms alone. Sporadic (nonepidemic) cases of pulmonary blastomycosis may present as a more chronic or subacute disease, with low-grade fever, night sweats, weight loss, and a productive cough that resembles tuberculosis rather than bacterial pneumonia.[27–29]

Chronic pulmonary blastomycosis is characterized by fever, malaise, weight loss, night sweats, and cough. Unlike patients with chronic pulmonary histoplasmosis, patients with chronic pulmonary blastomycosis often have evidence of disseminated disease that may appear 1–3 years after the primary pneumonia has resolved. Reactivation of disease may occur in the lungs or as the foci of new infection in other organs. However, in approximately 40% of patients dissemination is not accompanied by reactivation of pulmonary disease.[27–29] The most common sites for disseminated disease include the skin and bony skeleton, although less commonly the prostate, oropharyngeal mucosa, and abdominal viscera are involved. CNS disease, while exceedingly uncommon, is associated with the highest mortality rate.[29]

Diagnosis

The simplest and most successful method of diagnosing blastomycosis is by direct microscopic visualization of the large, multinucleated yeast with single, broad-based buds in sputum or other respiratory specimens, following digestion of cells and debris with 10% potassium hydroxide.[16,29] Histopathologic examination of tissue biopsies and culture of secretions should also be used to identify *B. dermatitidis,* although it may require up to 30 days to isolate and identify a small inoculum. Unfortunately, no reliable skin test exists to determine the incidence and prevalence of disease in endemic populations. Early and rapid definitive diagnosis of blastomycosis can be achieved by demonstration of *B. dermatitidis* in tissue or specimen culture or histopathology, or by a positive exoantigen or fluorescent antibody (FA) assay. Reliable serologic diagnosis of blastomycosis has long been hampered by lack of specific and standardized reagents. Some investigators recommend that a combination of ELISA and immunodiffusion tests be performed. An ELISA titer of 1:8 to 1:16 plus a positive immunodiffusion test or an ELISA of ≥32 plus a positive or negative immunodiffusion test is considered diagnostic for blastomycosis. Unfortunately, serologic response does not always correlate with clinical improvement, although some investigators have noted that a decline in the number of precipitins or in CF titers may offer evidence of a favorable prognosis in patients with established disease.[29,30]

Treatment

Acute pulmonary blastomycosis may not require therapy in patients with mild illness, but patients must be followed carefully for many years for evidence of reactivation or progressive disease.[29,31] Some authors recommend ketoconazole therapy for the treatment of self-limited pulmonary disease, with the hope of preventing late extrapulmonary disease; however, data supporting the efficacy of these regimens are lacking.[29] Ketoconazole appears to be as effective as amphotericin B for non–life-threatening, nonmeningeal, mild to moderate blastomycosis in immunocompetent hosts.[31,32] In a prospective, randomized, multicenter study conducted by the National Institute of Allergy and Infectious Diseases (NIAID) Mycoses Study Group,[32] high-dose (800 mg/d) oral therapy with ketoconazole was associated with a significantly higher cure rate than low-dose (400 mg/d) therapy (100% versus 79%, respectively) in 80 patients with blastomycosis. However, the increased frequency of adverse effects (primarily intolerable nausea and vomiting) associated with high-dose therapy prompted the NIAID's current recommendation of low-dose ketoconazole therapy for patients with nonmeningeal, non–life-threatening disease. The cure rate observed with low-dose therapy compares favorably with reported cure rates of 66–93% among patients treated with amphotericin B. The dosage of ketoconazole should be increased to 600–800 mg orally per day in the absence of a favorable clinical response.[31,32] Patients with CNS disease, progressive or life-threatening disease, or those experiencing toxicity while on ketoconazole should receive amphotericin B (40–50 mg/d) until clinical improvement is observed, followed by administration three times weekly until a total dose of 1.5–2 grams is achieved.[27]

All patients with chronic pulmonary blastomycosis and those with extrapulmonary disease require therapy. Ketoconazole 400 mg orally per day for 6 months cures more than 80% of patients with chronic pulmonary and nonmeningeal disseminated blastomycosis. Amphotericin B is more efficacious but more toxic, and therefore is reserved for severely ill patients, treatment failures, or noncompliant patients.[27–29] Patients with genitourinary tract disease should be treated initially with 600–800 mg/d of ketoconazole due to the low concentrations of drug achieved in the urine and prostate tissue. Patients should be monitored carefully for signs of clinical failure, and those who fail or are unable to tolerate ketoconazole therapy or develop CNS disease should be treated with amphotericin B for a total dose of 30–35 mg/kg.[29,31,32]

Itraconazole and fluconazole may offer equivalent or superior activity versus ketoconazole for the treatment of blastomycosis, but controlled clinical trials evaluating their use are not yet available.

For unclear reasons, blastomycosis is an uncommon opportunistic disease among immunocompromised individuals, including AIDS patients. However, blastomycosis may occur as a late (CD4+ lymphocytes <200/mm^3) and frequently fatal complication of HIV infection. In this population, overwhelming disseminated disease with frequent involvement of the CNS is common.[33] Following induction therapy with amphotericin B (total dose of 1 gram), HIV-infected patients should receive chronic suppressive therapy with an oral azole antifungal.[27,33]

COCCIDIOIDOMYCOSIS

Coccidioidomycosis is caused by infection with *Coccidioides immitis,* a dimorphic fungi found in the southwestern and western United States as well as parts of Mexico and South America. In North America, the endemic regions encompass the semi-arid regions of the southwestern United States from California to Texas known as the Lower Sonoran Zone, where there is scant annual rainfall, hot summers, and sandy, alkaline soil. *Coccidioides immitis* grows in the soil as a mold, and mycelia proliferate during the rainy season. During the dry season, resistant arthroconidia form and become airborne when the soil is disturbed. When individuals come in contact with contaminated soil during ranching, dust storms, or proximity to construction sites or archaeological excavations, arthroconidia are inhaled into the respiratory tree, where they transform into spherules, which reproduce by cleavage of the cytoplasm to produce endospores. The endospores are released when the spherules reach maturity. Similar to histoplasmosis, an acute inflammatory response in the tissue leads to infiltration of mononuclear cells, ultimately resulting in granuloma formation.[34–36]

Although generally considered to be a regional disease, coccidioidomycosis has increased in importance in recent years due to the increased tourism and population in endemic areas, the increased use of immunosuppressive therapy in transplantation and oncology, and the AIDS epidemic. Although there is no racial, hormonal, or immunologic predisposition for acquiring primary disease, these factors affect the risk of subsequent dissemination of disease.[34–36]

Clinical Presentation

Initial or primary infection with *C. immitis* almost always involves the lungs. Although approximately one-third of the population in endemic areas is infected, the average incidence of symptomatic disease is only approximately 0.43%.[35] Sixty percent of subjects are asymptomatic or have nonspecific symptoms that are often indistinguishable from ordinary upper respiratory infections, including fever, cough, headache, sore throat, myalgias, and fatigue. A fine diffuse rash may appear during the first few days of the illness. "Valley fever" is a syndrome characterized by erythema nodosum and erythema multiforme of the upper trunk and extremities in association with diffuse joint aches or fever. Valley fever occurs in approximately 25% of patients although, more commonly, a diffuse mild erythroderma or maculopapular rash is observed. Patients may have pleuritic chest pain and peripheral eosinophilia. Radiographic features tend to be quite variable; hilar adenopathy with alveolar infiltrates, tissue excavation of an infiltrate (resulting in a thin-walled cavity), or small pleural effusions are all commonly seen.[35] The development of erythema nodosum is thought to indicate the development of hypersensitivity to *C. immitis.*[34]

Some patients present with an acute pneumonia as the primary manifestation of disease. They have a productive cough that may be blood-streaked, and single or multiple soft or dense homogeneous hilar or basal infiltrates on chest roentgenogram. The disease usually lasts a few days to a few weeks and usually resolves spontaneously without therapy, although it can be fatal, particularly in patients who are immunocompromised.[34]

Although most primary pneumonias follow a benign course, pulmonary coccidioidomycosis can also develop into a chronic, persistent pneumonia complicated by hemoptysis, pulmonary scarring, and the formation of cavities or bronchopleural fistulas. Necrosis of pulmonary tissue with drainage and cavity formation occurs commonly in coccidioidal pneumonia. Most parenchymal cavities close spontaneously or form dense nodular scar tissue that may become superinfected with bacteria or spherules of *C. immitis*. These patients often have persistent cough, fevers, and weight loss.[34–36] Primary disease lasting more than 6 weeks is termed persistent pulmonary coccidioidomycosis. Rarely, chronic pulmonary (also known as "chronic progressive") pneumonia occurs, in which patients usually experience persistent cough, weight loss, chest pain, and intermittent fevers and hemoptysis. *Coccidioides immitis* can often be cultured from the sputum for a period of several years. Chest radiographs usually demonstrate apical fibronodular lesions or slowly progressive cavitation.[34,36]

Disseminated infection with *C. immitis* occurs in less than 1% of infected patients. The most common sites for dissemination are the skin, lymph nodes, bone, and meninges, although the spleen, liver, kidney, and adrenal gland may also be involved.[34] Occasionally, miliary coccidioidomycosis occurs, with rapid, widespread dissemination, often in concert with positive blood cultures for *C. immitis.* Patients with AIDS frequently present with miliary disease. Coccidioidomycosis in AIDS patients appears to be due to reactivation of disease in most patients.[34–37]

Risk factors for severe, disseminated infection include race (blacks, Hispanics, Native Americans, and Filipinos) and pregnancy, although these data have been disputed by several investigators. Older data suggest that race-related differences in the incidence of severe disease exist, while newer studies suggest that an exposure to dust containing high inocula of *C. immitis* played a more important role. Pregnancy may lead to a general depression in cell-mediated immunity (particularly during the third trimester) or to an increase in sex hormones that stimulate the growth of the fungus. Immunocompromised hosts, particularly patients with AIDS and those receiving corticosteroids or immunosuppressive agents, are also at an increased risk for disseminated disease.[37] For unclear reasons, males appear to be at higher risk than females for disseminated disease, as are neonates and patients with type B or AB blood type. Surprisingly, the risk of disseminated disease does not appear to increase with age or the presence of diabetes mellitus.[34,35]

CNS infection with *C. immitis* is a particularly devastating complication that develops in approximately 16% of patients with disseminated coccidioidomycosis.[38] Left untreated, coccidioidal meningitis is invariably fatal within 1–2 years. Early diagnosis is important, since early treatment appears to correlate with improved outcome. Patients may present with meningeal disease without previous symptoms of primary pulmonary infection, although disease usually occurs within 6 months after the primary infection. Signs of meningeal irritation common in bacterial meningitis are often absent. The signs and symptoms of coccidioidal meningitis are often subtle and nonspecific, including headache, weakness, changes in mental status (lethargy and confusion), neck stiffness, low-grade fever, weight loss, and occasionally hydrocephalus. Space occupying lesions are rare, and the main areas of involvement are the basilar meninges. CSF analysis generally reveals a lymphocytic pleocytosis with elevated protein, and a decreased glucose. Although serum is usually positive for coccidioidal CF antibodies, the coccidioidal skin test is often negative.[34,35]

Infection of the genitourinary system is an increasingly recognized site of disseminated disease. Although patients tend to have chronic disease at these sites, including endometritis, prostatitis, epididymitis, and coccidioidouria, these do not necessarily indicate disseminated disease or a poor prognostic sign. Therapy is generally not necessary, except in the AIDS population, in whom chronic suppressive therapy is usually required.[35,37]

Diagnosis

A number of tests have been developed to detect past or present infection with *C. immitis.* Most patients develop a positive skin test within 3 weeks of the onset of symptoms. Baseline evaluation of skin test reactivity and serology is essential in order to assess cell-mediated immunity. Patients who develop early positive skin test reactivity or whose coccidioidin skin test reactivity turns from negative to positive during therapy have an improved prognosis versus patients whose skin test reactivity develops later or does not change during therapy.[34,39] Patients with disseminated coccidioidomycosis whose skin tests are persistently negative are more likely to require prolonged therapy, and are more likely to relapse after completion of therapy.[39] The coccidioidal skin test also affects serologic tests for histoplasmosis but not those for coccidioidomycosis.[34]

Although cell-mediated immunity appears to be crucial in containing or resisting infection, the development of antibodies appears to have little effect on the course of disease. Patients with hypo- or agammaglobulinemia do not respond differently. However, antibody production can be used to follow the course of disease because most patients produce antibodies in response to infection with *C. immitis.* Early infection is characterized by the development of IgM antibody, which peaks within 2–3 weeks of infection then declines rapidly. IgM can be detected by either tube precipitin or immunodiffusion techniques.[34,36]

IgG antibody levels rise between 4 and 12 weeks after infection and decrease slowly over months to years. IgG can be detected in many body fluids, including serum, CSF, and pleural fluid by CF and immunodiffusion techniques. Quantitation of IgG is helpful in determining the prognosis of patients, except in patients with defective immunoglobulin synthesis, in whom complement fixation titers may be misleadingly low or negative. Although patients with mild primary disease may not develop a detectable antibody response by complement fixation assay, a positive response or a fourfold increase in titers can provide a valuable diagnostic tool. Higher titers (>1:16 or 1:32) occur more frequently with severe disease. Patients with disseminated coccidioidomycosis may have a negative skin test but a positive CF titer. Titers can be followed serially to evaluate the efficacy of antifungal therapy.[34,36]

The latex particle agglutination assay is a very sensitive test that detects the presence of both IgG and IgM. However, this test has a high rate of false positivity, and therefore a positive test should be confirmed with another methodology.[34,36]

Recovery of *C. immitis* from infected tissues or secretions for direct examination and culture provides an accurate and rapid method of diagnosis. Since the spherule–endospore phase of coccidioidomycosis found in tissue is not infective, transmission of coccidioidomycosis from person to person does not occur. However, the mycelial–arthroconidia phase of *C. immitis* is extremely infective, and laboratory-acquired disease due to inhalation of aerially transmitted infective arthroconidia has been documented in more than 200 cases. In the past, inoculation of laboratory animals to produce spherule-containing abscesses was utilized to definitively diagnose coccidioidomycosis. This has largely been replaced by detection of antigen from an extract of the mold phase.[34]

Direct microscopic examination and histopathologic studies of infected tissues will reveal the large, mature endosporulating spherules. However, young spherules without endospores may be confused with other fungi. Silver stains of body fluids or tissue biopsies are also helpful.[34,36]

Treatment

Therapy for coccidioidomycosis is difficult and the results unpredictable. The efficacy of antifungal therapy for coccidioidomycosis is often less certain than that for other fungal etiologies such as blastomycosis, histoplasmosis, or cryptococcus, even when *in vitro* susceptibilities and the sites of infections are similar. The refractoriness of coccidioidomycosis may relate to the ability of *C. immitis* spherules to release hundreds of endospores, maximally challenging host defenses.[39] Fortunately, only about 5% of infected patients require therapy. Candidates for therapy include those with severe primary pulmonary infection or increasing CF antibody titers (particularly ≥1:16 to 1:32), immunocompromised patients, and those with persistent (>6 weeks) fever, prostration, or worsening pulmonary disease. Any patient with evidence of disseminated disease should receive therapy.[35]

Although most patients with symptomatic primary pulmonary disease recover without therapy, severe infections should probably be treated, particularly in patients with high CF titers, in whom incipient or occult dissemination is likely.[36,39] Almost all patients with disease located outside the lungs should receive antifungal therapy.[36] Amphotericin B is usually administered intravenously in dosages of 1–1.5 mg/kg/d, tapering to 1–1.5 mg/kg three times a week to a total dose of 0.5–1.5 grams over 2–4 weeks, based on clinical response.[39,40] Some patients will require higher doses or more prolonged therapy; a minimum of 2–3 grams of amphotericin B is probably necessary for the treatment of persistent pulmonary infection or miliary coccidioidomycosis.[39] Approximately 50–75% of patients treated with amphotericin B for nonmeningeal disease achieve a sustained remission, and therapy is usually curative in patients with infections localized strictly to skin and soft tissues without extensive abscess formation or tissue damage.[39,40] The efficacy of local injection into joints or the peritoneum, as well as intra-articular or intradermal administration, remains poorly studied.[39] Amphotericin B appears to be most efficacious when cell-mediated immunity is intact (as evidenced by a positive coccidioidin or spherulin skin test or low CF antibody titer). However, controlled trials that document these clinical impressions are lacking.[36,39]

The introduction of the azole antifungal agents (miconazole, ketoconazole, fluconazole, and itraconazole) into practice has offered alternative therapy to amphotericin B. Miconazole was the first systemic azole to be utilized for the treatment of coccidioidomycosis. IV miconazole in a dosage of 0.6–1.2 grams three times daily was efficacious in a series of patients with skin and soft tissue or chronic pulmonary coccidioidomycosis who were unresponsive to amphotericin B. Although less toxic than amphotericin B, relapses following therapy are common. The role of miconazole in relation to other antifungal agents is unsettled and requires further comparative trials. The advent of orally available, less toxic alternatives such as ketoconazole, fluconazole, and itraconazole makes these studies unlikely to be performed.[36]

Ketoconazole, the first orally available azole, demonstrates variable absorption, particularly in patients with increased gastric pH due to H_2-receptor antagonists, antacids, or diseases (e.g., achlorhydria or AIDS).[41,42] Several noncomparative, open evaluations of ketoconazole for the treatment of progressive coccidioidomycosis have suggested that ketoconazole at a dosage of 400 mg orally per day is efficacious in patients with infiltrative pulmonary disease, soft tissue infection, or skeletal involvement.[31] However, the efficacy of ketoconazole in treatment of primary pulmonary coccidioidomycosis, vertebral osteomyelitis, and meningitis has not been established.[35] Dosages of 200–400 mg daily produce response rates in all forms of disease (with the exception of meningitis) comparable to those observed for amphotericin B or miconazole, even in patients unresponsive to other forms of therapy. Soft tissue infections improve more frequently following lower dosages of ketoconazole than do skeletal or pulmonary infections. However, relapse rates of ≥25% are disturbing. Dosages greater than 400 mg daily appear to be more toxic but no more efficacious than lower dosages.[43]

Limited data also suggest that fluconazole may prove beneficial in the treatment of coccidioidomycosis.[44–46] In open trials employing dosages of 50–100 mg/d for the treatment of persistent pulmonary or disseminated coccidioidomycosis, 12 of 14 patients responded to therapy, although 1 patient reactivated during therapy, and 6 patients experienced relapses after treatment was discontinued.[45] Galgiani and colleagues[44] administered 200 mg of fluconazole daily to 71 patients with chronic pulmonary, soft tissue, or skeletal lesions of *C. immitis*. Therapy was successful (any improvement within 4 months and ≥50% improvement by 8 months) in 61% of patients. Of 9 patients who failed therapy while receiving 200 mg daily, 4 responded when the dosage was increased to 400 mg daily. Toxicity with these dosages was negligible.

Initial studies suggest that itraconazole is effective in the treatment of nonmeningeal coccidioidomycosis.[40,47] In 49 patients with osteoarticular, chronic pulmonary, and soft tissue disease administered 100–400 mg of itraconazole orally per day, remission was achieved in 25 patients. Toxicity was minimal, even at the highest doses employed. However, therapy failed in 19 patients, and 4 of 25 achieving a remission experienced a relapse after discontinuation of therapy.[40]

Optimal therapy for the treatment of coccidioidal meningitis has not been established. The poor CSF penetration of amphotericin B has prompted investigators to initiate therapy with both intravenous and intrathecal amphotericin B for the treatment of meningitis. Intrathecal administration via the lumbar, cisternal, or ventricular routes has been utilized with varying rates of success and toxicity. Lumbar administration may not deliver drug to the basilar meninges, where maximal disease activity is found. Prolonged lumbar administration often results in lower extremity paresis, paresthesias, and other symptoms of arachnoiditis.[39] Addition of 10% glucose (hyperbaric therapy) and the use of a reverse Trendelenburg position to deliver drug to the base of the brain has resulted in acute toxic delirium and myelopathy due to local vascular damage to the spinal cord.[39] Administration of amphotericin B into the cisterna magna has the advantages of drug delivery to the site of maximal disease activity, and the presence of a larger pool of CSF in which to dilute drug, resulting in a decreased local inflammatory response. However, brainstem puncture and hemorrhage are potential risks of therapy that limit this route to those with training and experience in its use. Intraventricular administration of amphotericin B (usually via an Ommaya reservoir) is the most common route of administration of intrathecal amphotericin B despite the risk of complications due to the reservoir. Malplacement, obstruction, and secondary bacterial infections of the system can occur, as well as headache, nausea, vomiting, and fever.[39]

The optimal dose of intrathecal amphotericin B is unclear; therapy is generally initiated with very low dosages (0.025–1.5 mg) and increased cautiously to a maximum of 0.5–0.7 mg three to four times weekly. Although pharmacokinetic studies suggest that more frequent administration of amphotericin B is needed in order to maintain adequate concentrations of drug in the CSF, most patients experience headache and arachnoiditis with higher dosages.[39] Anecdotal reports suggest that administration of hydrocortisone or methylprednisolone with intrathecal amphotericin B may decrease inflammation. The addition of fentanyl to intracisternal amphotericin has also been reported to reduce post-treatment headache.[35] Therapy with systemic and intrathecal amphotericin B, which often must be continued for years, has decreased the mortality of this disease to approximately 30%.[38,39]

Ketoconazole cannot be routinely recommended for the treatment of coccidioidal meningitis due to its poor CNS penetration following oral administration. Chronic oral administration of 800–2000 mg of ketoconazole daily produced CSF concentrations of only 1.6–7.7% of concomitant serum concentrations.[43] Nevertheless, Craven et al.[48] reported control of infection with 800–1200 mg of ketoconazole daily in five patients unable to tolerate or receive intrathecal amphotericin B. Limited data suggest that combined therapy with intrathecal amphotericin B and ketoconazole has therapeutic benefit.[48,49]

Fluconazole also appears promising for the treatment of coccidioidal meningitis. Galgiani and colleagues[44] administered 400 mg of fluconazole daily to 38 patients with coccidioidal meningitis (19 as initial therapy; 10 patients with AIDS). Their initial results are promising; only 1 patient failed therapy, 4 patients died of unrelated causes, 1 patient was lost to follow-up, and the remaining patients were clinically stable on therapy. Tucker[50,51] administered 50–400 mg of fluconazole orally per day to 18 patients who had progression or relapse of their disease after previous therapy with amphotericin B. Ten (67%) of 15 assessable patients responded, 1 (7%) partially responded, and 4 (27%) did not respond to therapy. Five of 8 patients (63%) receiving fluconazole as sole therapy responded or partially responded to fluconazole therapy and three were unevaluable. Two patients experienced relapses once therapy was discontinued. Mean CSF to serum concentration ratios of 70.6, 83.8, and 82.6% were achieved following 50, 100, and 200 or 400 mg daily doses, respectively. Seven of the 15 patients received concomitant therapy with intrathecal amphotericin B or miconazole; these patients appeared to respond better than those not receiving concomitant intrathecal therapy, although the differences were not statistically significant. Toxicity was limited primarily to mild elevations of transaminases. Firm conclusions regarding the efficacy of fluconazole cannot be made at this time.

Itraconazole has been utilized in a prospective, nonrandomized open trial for the treatment of chronic coccidioidal meningitis. Tucker et al.[38] administered 300–400 mg of itraconazole daily for a median of 10 months to 10 patients with coccidioidal meningitis refractory to standard therapy. Of 8 assessable patients, 4 of 5 patients receiving itraconazole as sole therapy responded, and all 3 patients receiving concomitant intrathecal amphotericin B have discontinued intrathecal therapy with no evidence of active disease. Like amphotericin B, itraconazole appears efficacious in the treatment of some meningeal infections despite the poor penetration of drug into CSF. Itraconazole was not detectable in any of six CSF samples obtained more than 2 weeks into therapy.

CRYPTOCOCCOSIS

Cryptococcosis is a noncontagious, systemic mycotic infection caused by the ubiquitous encapsulated soil yeast *Cryptococcus neoformans,* which is found in soil, particularly in pigeon droppings, although disease occurs throughout the world, even in areas where pigeons are absent. Infection is acquired by inhalation of the organism. The incidence of cryptococcosis has risen dramatically in recent years, reflecting the increased numbers of immunocompromised patients, including those with malignancies, diabetes mellitus, chronic renal failure, and those receiving organ transplants or immunosuppressive agents. The AIDS epidemic has also contributed to the increased numbers of patients; cryptococcosis is the fourth most common infectious complication of AIDS and the second most common fungal pathogen.[52,53]

Although *C. neoformans* produces no toxins and evokes only a minimal inflammatory response in tissue, the polysaccharide capsule appears to allow the organism to resist phagocytosis by the host. The capsular polysaccharide of *C. neoformans* appears to comprise the major virulence factor for this pathogen. Four serotypes of *C. neoformans* (A through D) have been identified, that vary in their polysaccharide content, virulence, geographic foci, and response to antifungal therapy. Serotypes A and D are commonly associated with pigeon droppings and other environmental sites, and generally require shorter therapy than infections caused by serotypes B or C, which have been found only in infected humans and animals. Serotypes B and C appear more resistant to antifungal agents *in vitro.* AIDS patients are almost always infected with serotypes A and D, even in areas endemic for serotypes B and C.[53] There is no particular geographic area of endemic focus for *C. neoformans.*[52–55]

Cell-mediated immunity appears to play a major role in host defense against infection with *C. neoformans;* 29–55% of patients with cryptococcal meningitis have a predisposing condition. Many patients with disseminated cryptococcosis demonstrate defects in cell-mediated immunity. The predilection of *C. neoformans* for the CNS appears to be due to the lack of immunoglobulins and complement and excellent growth media afforded by CSF.[52–55]

Clinical Presentation

Primary cryptococcosis in humans almost always occurs in the lungs, although the pulmonary focus usually produces a subclinical infection. Symptomatic infections are usually manifested by cough, rales, and shortness of breath that generally resolve spontaneously. Disease may remain localized in the lungs or disseminate to other tissues, particularly the CNS, although the skin can also be affected.[53]

Hematogenous spread generally occurs in the immunocompromised host although it has also been seen in individuals with intact immune systems.[53] Cryptococcemia is the most common symptomatic extraneural infection associated with *C. neoformans.* Cryptococcemia can be documented in 5–22% of non-AIDS patients and CNS involvement of *C. neoformans* in 18–50% of AIDS patients.[54,55]

In the non-AIDS patient, the symptoms of cryptococcal meningitis are nonspecific. Headache, fever, nausea, vomiting, mental status changes, and neck stiffness are generally observed. Less common symptoms include visual disturbances (e.g., photophobia and blurred vision), papilledema, seizures, and aphasia. In AIDS patients, fever and headache are common, but meningismus and photophobia are much less common than in non-AIDS patients. Approximately 10–12% of AIDS patients have asymptomatic disease, similar to the rate observed in non-AIDS patients. Cryptococcal disease is present in 7.5–10% of AIDS patients. Therefore, patients with evidence of extraneural cryptococcosis should be evaluated for CNS disease.[54,55]

Once the CNS is involved, the usual course is weeks to months of progressive deterioration with 80% of untreated patients dying within the first year.[53] The prognosis of cryptococcal meningitis depends largely on the underlying predisposing factors of the host. Although cryptococcal antigen is positive in 90% of patients with cryptococcal meningitis, fewer than half of the patients with cryptococcal meningitis develop antibody to capsular polysaccharide. Those who produce antibody have a slightly improved prognosis.[53] In contrast, the presence of headache is a favorable symptom, presumably because it leads to an earlier diagnosis. A favorable outcome is also associated with a normal mental status upon diagnosis, and a CSF white blood cell (WBC) count of $>20/\text{mm}^3$. However, a poor outcome is predicted by the presence of one or more underlying diseases (including hematopoietic disorders and AIDS), corticosteroid or immunosuppressive therapy, pretreatment serum cryptococcal antigen titers of $\geq 1:32$, and post-therapy serum antigen titers of $\geq 1:8$. In non-AIDS patients, the cryptococcal antigen titer can be followed during therapy to assess response to antifungal therapy. In AIDS patients, decreasing titers are not necessarily predictive of success, and titers rarely become negative at the completion of therapy.

Diagnosis

Examination of CSF in patients with cryptococcal meningitis generally reveals an elevated opening pressure, CSF pleocytosis (usually lymphocytes), leukocytosis, a decreased CSF glucose, an elevated CSF protein, and a positive cryptococcal antigen.[53] Antigens to *C. neoformans* can be detected by latex agglutination. The test is rapid, specific, and extremely sensitive, but false-negatives can occur. False-positive tests can result from cross-reactivity with rheumatoid factor and *T. beigelii. Cryptococcus neoformans* can be detected in approximately 60% of patients by India ink smear of CSF, and cultured in more than 96% of patients. Occasionally, large volumes of CSF are required in order to confirm the diagnosis.[53] CSF parameters in patients with AIDS are similar to those seen in non-AIDS patients with the exception of a decreased inflammatory response to the pathogen, resulting in a strikingly low number of leukocytes in CSF and extraordinarily high cryptococcal antigen titers.[54,55]

Treatment

Prior to the introduction of amphotericin B, cryptococcal meningitis was an almost uniformly fatal disease; approximately 86% of patients died within 1 year. The use of large (1–1.5 mg/kg) daily doses of amphotericin B resulted in cure rates of approximately 64%.[52] When amphotericin B is combined with fluorocytosine, a smaller dose of amphotericin B can be employed due to the *in vitro* and *in vivo* synergy between the two antifungal agents. Resistance develops to fluorocytosine in up to 30% of patients treated with 5-fluorocytosine alone, limiting its usefulness as monotherapy.[52] In a randomized, comparative trial, amphotericin B in a dosage of 0.3 mg/kg/d plus oral fluorocytosine 150 mg/kg/d for 6 weeks was as effective as amphotericin B administered alone at a dosage of 0.4 mg/kg/d for 6 weeks, followed by 0.8 mg/kg every other day for 4 weeks. Combination therapy resulted in cure or improvement in 16 of 24 (67%) patients as compared to 11 of 27 (41%) patients treated with amphotericin B alone. In addition, the combination therapy resulted in less nephrotoxicity, fewer relapses, and more rapid sterilization of CSF cultures.[56] However, this study has been criticized for the low dosage of amphotericin B utilized in the amphotericin-B-alone arm of the study, which resulted in lower cure rates than those reported in earlier studies employing higher dosages. In addition, fluorocytosine toxicity (primarily bone marrow suppression) was observed in approximately one-third of patients.[56,57]

In a follow-up study,[58] a 4-week regimen of combination therapy was as effective as the 6-week regimen in patients with no underlying disease who were not receiving immunosuppressive therapy and had an uncomplicated course of disease. Unfortunately, these criteria exclude most patients with cryptococcal meningitis. This study also confirmed the relationship between peak serum concentrations of fluorocytosine and bone marrow suppression. The authors suggested that peak serum concentrations

>100 mg/L were associated with greater toxicity. In patients with impaired renal function, serum concentrations of fluorocytosine should be monitored and adjusted accordingly.[57,58]

Ketoconazole has been used successfully in the treatment of cutaneous cryptococcosis, but is not useful in the treatment of CNS disease, probably due to its poor penetration into the CNS. Despite low CSF concentrations of amphotericin B (2–3% of those observed in plasma), the use of intrathecal amphotericin B is not recommended for the treatment of cryptococcal meningitis except in patients who fail to respond to amphotericin B alone. Intraventricular therapy should be reserved for very ill patients or those with recurrent or progressive disease despite aggressive therapy with IV amphotericin B.[3,53,59] Preliminary evidence suggests that amphotericin B may interact with T lymphocytes to enhance the host's resistance. The dosage of amphotericin B employed is usually 0.5 mg administered via the lumbar, cisternal, or intraventricular (via an Ommaya reservoir) route two or three times weekly. Side effects of intrathecal amphotericin B include arachnoiditis and paresthesias. Intrathecal amphotericin B therapy should be administered in combination with intravenous amphotericin B.[3,53,59]

Treatment of cryptococcal meningitis in patients with AIDS has been discouraging. Although initial responses to therapy have been roughly equivalent for both combination (amphotericin B plus fluorocytosine) and single-drug (amphotericin B alone) therapies, it has become apparent that virtually all patients will suffer relapses if they are not administered chronic suppressive therapy. In the NIAID AIDS Clinical Trial Group (ACTG) Mycoses Study Group trial, IV amphotericin B 0.5 mg/kg daily was compared to oral fluconazole 200 mg daily. Of 99 evaluable patients, the proportion of responders was similar in each treatment group: 49% of patients receiving amphotericin B versus 53% of patients receiving fluconazole. The mortality of those patients surviving more than 2 weeks (23%) was the same in both groups. This study also defined those patients at risk for early deterioration and death. Patients with cryptococcal meningitis who have altered mental status, a CSF cryptococcal antigen titer >1:256, a CSF WBC count of <20/mm^3, or age <35 are "high-risk" patients. Serum cryptococcal antigen was a poor predictor of outcome.[60] At this time, amphotericin B with or without fluorocytosine remains the treatment of choice for acute therapy of cryptococcal meningitis in AIDS patients. Many clinicians will initiate therapy with amphotericin B 0.4–0.7 mg/kg/d IV (with or without oral fluorocytosine 75–100 mg/kg/d). After 1 week, therapy may be changed to oral fluconazole 400 mg daily for the remaining 9 weeks of therapy. Clinical trials evaluating the use of itraconazole as primary therapy of cryptococcal meningitis, higher dosages of fluconazole, and combination therapy with fluconazole plus fluorocytosine are presently under way; these studies may lead to less toxic and more convenient regimens for AIDS patients in the future.

Relapse of *C. neoformans* meningitis occurs in approximately 50% of AIDS patients after completion of primary therapy. Persistence of asymptomatic urinary *C. neoformans* has been documented in a high percentage of AIDS patients despite seemingly adequate courses of therapy for primary meningeal disease. The prostate appears to act as a sequestered reservoir of infection in these patients, resulting in systemic relapse. Fluconazole is currently recommended for chronic suppressive therapy of cryptococcal meningitis in AIDS patients. The recently completed ACTG 026 study demonstrated that oral fluconazole 200 mg daily was superior to IV administration of amphotericin B 1 mg/kg weekly in preventing relapse. In addition, the fluconazole-treated group showed a lower incidence of adverse drug reactions and bacterial infections.[20]

Infections Caused by Opportunistic Fungi

CANDIDA INFECTIONS

Candida species are yeasts that exist primarily as small (4- to 6-µm), unicellular, thin-walled, ovoid cells that reproduce by budding. On agar media, they form smooth, white, creamy colonies resembling staphylococci. Although there are more than 150 species of *Candida,* 8 species are regarded as clinically important pathogens in human disease, including *C. albicans, C. tropicalis, C. parapsilosis, C. krusei, C. stellatoidea, C. guilliermondi, C. lusitaniae,* and *C. rugosa.*[10,13,61] Yeast forms, hyphae, and pseudohyphae may be found in clinical specimens. A rapid presumptive identification of *C. albicans* can be made by incubation of the organism in serum; formation of a germ tube within 1–2 hours offers a positive identification of *C. albicans.* A negative germ tube test does not rule out the possibility of *C. albicans,* but further biochemical tests must be performed in order to differentiate between other non-*albicans* species.[10]

Candida albicans is a normal commensal of the skin, female genital tract, and the entire gastrointestinal tract of humans. Therefore, the mere presence of hyphae or pseudohyphae in a clinical specimen is not sufficient for the diagnosis of invasive disease. Thus, the majority of infections with *C. albicans* are acquired endogenously, although human-to-human transmission can also occur. Oral candidiasis in the newborn is probably acquired during passage through the birth canal, and balanitis in the uncircumcised male may be acquired through contact with a female with vaginal candidiasis.[10,61]

Although the term "fungemia" refers to the presence of fungi in the blood, the most commonly isolated organism is *C. albicans.* Candidiasis may cause mucocutaneous or systemic infection, including endocarditis, peritonitis, arthritis, and infection of the CNS. The role of an intact integument is crucial in the prevention of mucocutaneous or hematogenous candidiasis. Once *Candida* invades the dermis or enters the bloodstream, polymorphonuclear leukocytes (PMNs) play a major role in the defense of the patient, since PMNs are capable of damaging pseudohyphae and can phagocytize and kill blastoconidia.[10,61] In addition to neutrophils, lymphocytes, monocytes, macrophages, complement, and eosinophils play a role in the prevention of infection. The complex role of each of these components in the pathogenesis of infections with *Candida* has been reviewed by Odds.[61] Adherence of *C. albicans* is important in the pathogenesis of oral candidiasis and subsequent colonization of the gastrointestinal tract. Because evidence suggests that the GI tract is often the portal of entry for *Candida* in disseminated disease, factors that alter the adherence of *Candida* are crucial in the development of local and systemic infection. *Candida tropicalis* adheres to intravascular catheters at a higher rate than *C. albicans,* a factor that may help to account for the increased incidence of systemic infections caused by this pathogen.

Mucocutaneous Candidiasis

Mucocutaneous candidiasis can generally be divided into several categories: oropharyngeal candidiasis (thrush), esophageal candidiasis, gastrointestinal candidiasis, and vaginal candidiasis. Mucocutaneous candidiasis is generally caused by *C. albicans,* although other species of *Candida* (including *C. glabrata, C. tropicalis,* and *C. krusei*) are occasionally implicated. Oral candidiasis is often the first sign of infection in patients with AIDS; as many as 50% of AIDS patients with oral candidiasis who are not treated with antiretroviral therapy will develop an opportunistic infection within 3 months of the development of oral candidiasis.

Chronic Mucocutaneous Candidiasis

Chronic mucocutaneous candidiasis refers to a collection of syndromes characterized by chronic or recurrent infections of the skin, nails, and mucous membranes by *C. albicans.*[62] Most patients exhibit abnormalities in cell-mediated immunity. Although fungal infections in these patients generally respond to treatment with conventional antifungal agents, relapses are common after treatment is stopped.[62] Ketoconazole, itraconazole, and fluconazole have been used successfully as long-term therapy for this syndrome.[62]

Oral Candidiasis (Thrush)

A variety of local and systemic factors are generally necessary for the development of oral candidiasis. Precipitating factors include age, mucosal damage, the presence of host immune deficiencies (including malignancies, diabetes mellitus, and AIDS), nutritional deficiencies, radiation therapy, antineoplastic agents, and the use of local or systemic antibiotics or corticosteroids. Oral candidiasis occurs in as many as 5% of all newborn infants, >35% of patients with acute leukemia or those receiving chemotherapy for solid tumors, patients undergoing organ transplantation, and approximately 10% of all hospitalized, debilitated, elderly patients.[10,61]

Oral candidiasis is characterized by the presence of creamy, white plaques on the tongue and buccal mucosa that generally leave a painful, raw, ulcerated surface when scraped. The diagnosis of oral candidiasis is based on the clinical appearance of the lesions and by scraping of lesions, using either 10% potassium hydroxide digestion of this material to reveal the presence of pseudohyphae and yeast forms or the presence of gram-positive staining yeast forms.[10]

Although oral candidiasis is generally not life-threatening, it causes discomfort and in immunocompromised patients can spread to the esophagus, causing ulcerations and mucosal perforation. Colonization of the gastrointestinal tract with *C. albicans* increases the risk of invasive disease, particularly in patients with decreased numbers of neutrophils secondary to the administration of chemotherapy or immunosuppressive agents. When suspensions of *C. albicans* are administered into the gastrointestinal tract, they can migrate across intact endothelium by a process known as *persorption.*[63] Ulceration of the gastrointestinal tract secondary to chemotherapy may facilitate migration of *Candida* into the bloodstream. In addition a variety of factors including endotoxin, chemotherapy, and administration of adrenal corticosteroids can interfere with the elimination of *Candida* via the reticuloendothelial system. It is important to note that patients with defects in cell-mediated immunity (e.g., patients with chronic mucocutaneous candidiasis or AIDS) are generally predisposed to mucosal but *not* systemic infections with *Candida.*

Topical (local) therapy with a variety of antifungal agents, including nystatin suspension and clotrimazole troches are generally efficacious in the prophylaxis and therapy of oral candidiasis. The optimal dosage or agent has not been clearly defined. Nystatin has been utilized as a "swish and swallow" regimen in dosages ranging from 0.5 million units (MU) four times daily to 1.5 MU six times daily. However, some investigators have found nystatin therapy to be no more beneficial than placebo in the treatment of oral candidiasis or the prevention of systemic infection with *C. albicans.* The comparative efficacy of topical and systemic agents is also controversial. Although most agents have proven efficacious in controlled studies compared with a placebo, few comparative trials are available to assess the relative efficacy of these agents. In oncology patients, ketoconazole in dosages of 200–400 mg daily is as efficacious as nystatin in dosages of 0.5–3 MU four times daily for the treatment of oral candidiasis, but it is superior in the prevention of candidiasis at other mucocutaneous sites (e.g., *Candida* esophagitis and vaginal candidiasis) and in the prevention of systemic candidal infections.[64] Fluconazole 100 mg orally appears to be as efficacious as ketoconazole 400 mg daily, clotrimazole troches 10 mg five times daily, or amphotericin B 400 mg (as 200-mg tablets plus 200-mg suspension) administered four times daily in the prophylaxis or therapy of oropharyngeal candidiasis.[64–66]

In the AIDS patient, although few controlled trials have been performed, anecdotal data suggest that nystatin therapy is usually not well tolerated or efficacious for the prevention or treatment of oral candidiasis. The recurrent nature of oral candidiasis and the propensity for the development of esophageal candidiasis in the population suggests that topical agents such as clotrimazole may not be sufficient. Fluconazole in dosages of 50 mg daily is superior to ketoconazole 200 mg daily, and dosages of 100 mg daily are superior to clotrimazole 10 mg five times daily in the treatment of oral candidiasis in the AIDS patient.[67–69] Limited data suggest that single-dose regimens may provide safe, efficacious, and convenient regimens for the treatment and prophylaxis of oral candidiasis in AIDS patients. Initial studies suggest that a single, 150-mg oral dose of fluconazole provides a clinical and mycologic response equivalent to a 7-day course of therapy with 50 mg of fluconazole daily with equivalent relapse rates 2 weeks post-therapy.[70,71]

A number of studies have documented the emergence of resistant strains of *C. albicans* in HIV-infected patients treated with fluconazole for prolonged periods of time. Resistance to fluconazole generally confers resistance to ketoconazole and itraconazole. Some patients have responded to increased dosages of fluconazole or to an investigational formulation of itraconazole administered in cyclodextrin solution. Resistance to antifungal agents has been shown to occur by at least 3 separate mechanisms, including altered cell wall permeability, decreased affinity for fungal cytochrome P-450, and increased production of fungal cytochrome P-450.[11,72]

Esophageal Candidiasis

Candida esophagitis is most commonly associated with the treatment of malignancies and in AIDS patients, although it occasionally occurs in patients with no known underlying risk factors. Patients generally complain of pain and difficulty in swallowing, a feeling of obstruction, and occasionally substernal chest pain. Patients may occasionally have no symptoms until obstruction, bleeding, or perforation of the esophagus occurs.[10]

Although a definitive diagnosis is made by endoscopy with brush biopsy, a barium swallow can often reveal a characteristic "shaggy mucosa" appearance. Although the need for endoscopy is controversial, in patients with AIDS, a variety of bacterial, viral, and protozoal pathogens can also cause similar symptoms and may be present in association with *C. albicans*. Although the presence of oral thrush is often used as a "marker" for esophageal candidiasis, based on the theory that esophageal disease arises from "spread" of oral disease, as many as 20–50% of cancer patients with esophageal candidiasis have no associated oral candidiasis.[10]

The treatment of *Candida* esophagitis has not been well studied, particularly in patients with AIDS. Anecdotal evidence suggests that topical agents such as nystatin and clotrimazole are generally not efficacious due to a lack of contact time with the mucosa. Generally, systemic antifungal agents are required in this setting. Ketoconazole 200–400 mg daily has proven efficacious in small, noncomparative trials. A recent multicenter trial in predominantly AIDS patients demonstrated fluconazole 100–200 mg daily to be superior to ketoconazole 100–200 mg orally daily.[73] The decreased efficacy of ketoconazole in this population may be due to the hypochlorhydria observed in some AIDS patients, resulting in a decreased absorption of ketoconazole.[41] A lack of response to antifungal therapy can be due to altered absorption of drugs such as ketoconazole, or an inaccurate diagnosis. In patients who do not respond to oral therapy with ketoconazole or fluconazole, a low dose (10–15 mg) of IV amphotericin B is often successful.[74]

Vaginal Candidiasis

Vulvovaginal candidiasis is characterized by the presence of a thick, curdlike vaginal discharge, intense pruritus, and the presence of masses of epithelial cell, hyphae, and pseudohyphae on KOH smear of the vaginal discharge. Vulvovaginal candidiasis is a common infection in women; approximately one-fourth of women in their childbearing years develop an infection.[10] Factors thought to predispose toward the development of vulvovaginal candidiasis include the use of hormonal contraceptives, pregnancy, obesity, debilitation, diabetes, and drug therapy with systemic corticosteroids, antineoplastic agents, and systemic antibiotics.[10] Although treatment with 7-day topical regimens have been traditionally employed, recent studies have demonstrated success utilizing 1- and 3-day topical regimens. Several topical antifungal agents, including miconazole and clotrimazole, have recently become available as over-the-counter (OTC) preparations. A number of European studies have documented the efficacy of single oral doses (150 mg) of fluconazole.[75] Not surprisingly, most women prefer oral therapy with fluconazole or ketoconazole (200–400 mg daily) to topical therapy in the management of vaginal infections with *C. albicans*.

Women with AIDS appear to be very susceptible to the development of recurrent vaginal infections with *C. albicans*. These infections generally appear earlier in the course of disease than does oral candidiasis; infection may be seen before any significant decrease in CD4+ (T-helper) cells occurs.[76,77]

A variety of topical antifungal agents appear efficacious in the treatment of vaginal candidiasis. A review of currently available agents can be found in Ref. 78.

Hematogenous Candidiasis

The term *systemic candidiasis* has been used in the literature to describe any candidal infection that invades beyond the membranes of the skin or mucosa. This term does not differentiate hematogenously disseminated candidiasis (e.g., in a neutropenic transplant patient) from infections arising from the urinary tract. Accordingly, Edwards and Filler[79] have proposed that the term "systemic candidiasis" be eliminated, and the term "hematogenous candidiasis" be utilized to describe the clinical circumstances in which hematogenous seeding to deep organs such as the eye, brain, heart, and kidney occurs in a patient. Specific anatomic reference should be made to the site of the infection. For example, *Candida* infection of the peritoneum would be termed *Candida* peritonitis.

Hematogenous candidiasis is reported in significantly higher frequency due to the increased numbers of immunosuppressed patients, including those with lymphoreticular or hematologic malignancies, diabetes, immunodeficiency diseases, or those receiving immunosuppressive therapy with high-dose corticosteroids, immunosuppressants, antineoplastic agents, or broad-spectrum antimicrobial agents.[2,10,80] Patients who have undergone surgery (particularly surgery of the gastrointestinal tract) are increasingly susceptible to disseminated candidal infections.[81,82] Recent data from the Centers for Disease Control and Prevention's National Nosocomial Infection Survey implicated fungi as the cause of 7.9% of nosocomial pathogens implicated as a cause of infection. *Candida* species accounted for 79% of these nosocomial fungi.[79]

Candida is generally acquired via the gastrointestinal tract, although organisms may also enter the bloodstream via indwelling IV catheters. Risk factors for hematogenous disease include prior therapy with antibiotics, the presence of indwelling urinary or IV catheters, recent surgery, concomitant bacterial infections, extensive burns, and administration of total parenteral nutrition. In the postoperative group, patients with organ transplants, heart surgery, or GI tract surgery are at the greatest risk of infection.[10,14,82] A case-controlled study in patients with acute lymphocytic leukemia found previous bacteremia, prolonged neutropenia, prolonged fever, prolonged administration of antimicrobial agents, treatment with multiple antimicrobial agents, and a relatively high concentration of *Candida* in the stool to be significant risk factors for candidemia. In a logistic regression analysis, however, only administration of vancomycin and/or imipenem was identified as an independent risk factor for candidemia. Further analysis showed that administration of vancomycin promoted proliferation of *Candida* in the gastrointestinal tract and that this proliferation was associated with an increased risk of candidemia.[80]

Recognition of the role of the gastrointestinal tract in invasive *Candida* infections has led to efforts to decrease infections by prophylactic administration of topical or systemically absorbed antifungal agents in immunocompromised patients. This literature was recently reviewed by Reents et al.,[64] who concluded that the use of systemically absorbable agents such as azole antifungal agents appears to decrease the risk of invasive fungal infections. However, concerns have been raised by numerous investigators regarding the potential for selection of intrinsically resistant pathogens or the development of resistant strains with widespread use of these agents. For example, although administration of oral fluconazole appears to decrease the incidence of invasive *Candida* infections in patients undergoing bone marrow transplantation, some centers have reported an increase in the number of infections caused by *C. krusei,* a species of *Candida* that is intrinsically resistant to fluconazole.[64–66,83,84]

The diagnosis of hematogenous candidiasis remains a major stumbling block in the treatment of infectious diseases. Although a variety of serologic tests have been proposed for the detection of *Candida* protein antigens, serum antibodies to *Candida,* and antibodies to cell wall components such as mannan, no test has demonstrated reliable accuracy in the clinical setting for the diagnosis of disseminated infection with *Candida.*[8,10,85] The problem is often confounded by the absence of positive blood cultures; only 25–45% of neutropenic patients with disseminated candidiasis at autopsy have a positive blood culture with *C. albicans* prior to death. The interpretation of positive surveillance cultures of the skin, mouth, sputum, feces, or urine is hampered by their occurrence as commensal pathogens and in distinguishing colonization from invasive disease. Wingard et al.[86] performed surveillance cultures on patients with leukemia and bone marrow transplant recipients. *Candida albicans* was isolated from surveillance cultures in 67% of patients but disseminated infection occurred in only 5%. In contrast, *C. tropicalis* was cultured from only 28% of patients but disseminated disease was observed in 56% of positive patients. These results suggest that patients with positive blood cultures for *C. tropicalis* should receive serious consideration as candidates for systemic antifungal therapy.

Dissemination of *C. albicans* can result in infection in single or multiple organs, particularly the kidney, brain, myocardium, skin, eye, bone, and joints. Three distinct presentations of disseminated *C. albicans* have been recognized. In the first (and most common) type, patients present with the acute onset of fever, tachycardia, tachypnea, and occasionally chills or hypotension. The clinical presentation is generally indistinguishable from that seen with sepsis of bacterial origin. The second group of patients develops intermittent fevers, and are ill only when febrile. A third group of patients manifests progressive deterioration of their condition with or without fever.[13,61] In most patients, multiple, micro-, and macroabscesses are formed. Infection of the liver and spleen is becoming recognized as a particularly common and difficult to treat site of infection that characteristically occurs in patients undergoing chemotherapy for acute leukemia or lymphoma. Hepatosplenic candidiasis, which has been termed *chronic systemic candidiasis* by some investigators in order to distinguish this syndrome from acute, disseminated disease, is often manifested only as fever while the patient remains neutropenic (<1000 WBC/mm^3). As the WBC count increases to >1000 cells/mm^3, imaging studies can detect the presence of abscess or microabscesses in the liver and spleen, often found with acute suppurative and granulomatous reactions. Infection may persist for months and ultimately cause the patient's death despite aggressive systemic therapy with antifungal agents.[2]

The clinical management of suspected or documented candidemia also poses significant clinical dilemmas. Fraser and colleagues[81] documented the high rate of mortality in non-neutropenic patients with fungal blood cultures. Mortality was highest in those patients with sustained positive blood cultures, those who did not receive antifungal therapy, and in those infected with non-*albicans* strains of *Candida.* This study clearly documented the importance of early recognition and treatment of positive fungal blood cultures. Recent data suggest that administration of fluconazole 400 mg daily is as efficacious as intravenous amphotericin B 0.5 mg/kg/d in non-neutropenic patients with blood cultures with *C. albicans.*[81,87–90] No data are available for assessing the role of fluconazole as empiric therapy for fungemia. Since fluconazole has poor activity against *Aspergillus* spp. and some non-*albicans* strains of *Candida,* amphotericin B remains the therapy of choice in patients with suspected fungemia.

In some patients, particularly those patients with a relatively intact immune system and in whom candidemia is clearly associated with the presence of an indwelling venous catheter, removal of the catheter will result in spontaneous resolution. Edwards[13] has suggested that withholding treatment of catheter-associated candidemia may be considered in patients who meet the following criteria: (1) no unexplained fever, (2) improving clinical course, (3) no recurrence of candidemia following removal of the intravenous catheter, and (4) no clinical evidence consistent with disseminated candidiasis.

In immunocompromised patients, the presence of candidemia has been associated with evidence of disseminated disease in >70% of patients and a 70–80% fatality rate. Therapy should include removal of the catheter and administration of systemic antifungal therapy.[2] The optimal agent, dose, and duration of therapy is unclear, and patients must be carefully monitored with serial blood cultures and careful physical examinations, particularly of the retina. Currently, most clinicians recommend amphotericin B in total dosages of 0.5–1 gram administered over approximately 1–2 weeks in patients with *Candida* endophthalmitis and in all neutropenic patients with candidemia.[10,13,91] Longer courses of therapy may be needed in some patients.[13] The role of newer azole antifungals such as fluconazole and itraconazole is unclear at this time; clinical trials are currently under way to assess their efficacy. The decision to add fluorocytosine to therapy with amphotericin B remains controversial; although *in vitro* studies document synergy with these agents against *C. albicans,* the *in vivo* efficacy has not been well studied at this time. Similarly, the clinical utility of combinations of azole antifungal agents (ketoconazole, fluconazole, and itraconazole) with amphotericin B or fluorocytosine is also under investigation.

Many clinicians advocate early institution of empiric intravenous amphotericin B in patients with neutropenia and persistent (>5–7 days) fever.[91] Walsh et al.[92] recently reviewed the use of empiric therapy and pointed out that only two prospective randomized studies have examined the utility of this practice. Pizzo et al.[93] evaluated neutropenic patients with fever of unknown origin after receiving broad-spectrum antimicrobial therapy with cephalothin, carbenicillin plus gentamicin. After 1 week, patients were randomly assigned to discontinue antimicrobial therapy, continue antimicrobial therapy until resolution of fever and granulocytopenia, or continue antimicrobial therapy with the addition of amphotericin B (0.5 mg/kg daily). The results clearly favored administration of amphotericin B. The European Organization for Research on Treatment of Cancer (EORTC)[92] conducted a prospective, randomized trial to evaluate the efficacy of empiric amphotericin B 1.2 mg/kg every other day or 0.6 mg/kg daily in febrile neutropenic cancer patients. Patients who remained febrile after 4 days of antibacterial therapy were randomized to receive continued antibacterial therapy with or without the addition of IV amphotericin B 0.5 mg/kg daily. Although the response rates (69% versus 53%) for patients receiving amphotericin B versus no amphotericin B, respectively, were similar, fatality rates (16% versus 21%) were significantly lower, as were the frequencies of fungal infection at autopsy. The investigators concluded that empiric amphotericin B reduced the early mortality from fungal infection but appeared to have little effect on established infections, particularly in patients with progressive underlying diseases. Empiric therapy with amphotericin B was of particular benefit in patients who did not receive antifungal prophylaxis, those who were severely granulocytopenic, febrile patients with a clinically documented infection, and patients older than 15 years of age.

Although empiric amphotericin B is clearly indicated for some patients, the potential toxicities (particularly nephrotoxicity) of this agent preclude its routine use in all patients. Bodey[2] has suggested criteria for the empiric use of amphotericin B that include (1) fever of 5–7 days duration, unresponsive to antibacterial agents, (2) neutropenia of >7 days duration, (3) no other obvious cause for fever, (4) progressive debilitation, (5) chronic adrenal corticosteroid therapy, and (6) indwelling intravascular catheters.

Candiduria

Within the urinary tract, most common lesions are either *Candida* cystitis or hematogenously disseminated renal abscesses. *Candida* cystitis often follows catheterization or therapy with broad-spectrum antimicrobial therapy. The diagnosis of *Candida* cystitis may be problematic due to the frequent presence of *Candida* pseudohyphae and yeast cells in urine specimens secondary to urethral colonization. The usefulness of urine colony counts or antibody coating techniques is of questionable value. The recovery of ≥10,000 organisms or visualization of both yeast and pseudohyphae from fresh midstream urine or from bladder urine obtained by single catheterization (not indwelling) is suggestive of genitourinary candidiasis.[10] In most patients, the infection is asymptomatic and clears spontaneously without specific antifungal therapy.

Initial therapy of candidal cystitis should focus on removal of urinary catheters whenever possible. If this is not feasible, local irrigation may be used. Amphotericin B (50 mg in 500 mL of sterile water) can be instilled twice daily into the bladder via a three-way catheter. Minimal quantities (<3%) of amphotericin B are absorbed systemically from the bladder.[3] Alternatively, oral therapy with flucytosine or fluconazole can be considered for short courses of therapy; high urinary concentrations are achieved following oral administration. However, flucytosine may have serious hematopoietic side effects and resistance rapidly develops when the drug is used alone.[3] The role of ketoconazole and miconazole in urinary candidiasis remains unclear. Ketoconazole is excreted primarily by metabolic pathways and only 2–4% of the drug appears as active drug in the urine. However, Graybill and Galgiani[94] reported resolution of candiduria in 12 fungal urinary infections following therapy with ketoconazole 200 mg daily, despite urinary concentrations of <0.4 mg/L.

ASPERGILLUS

Aspergillus is an ubiquitous mold that grows well on a variety of substrates, including soil, water, decaying vegetation, moldy hay or straw, and organic debris. Although over 300 species of *Aspergillus* have been characterized, 3 species are most commonly pathogenic: *A. fumigatus, A. flavus,* and *A. niger.*[95] The varying degrees of pathogenicity of each species depend on their relative geographic prevalence, conidial size and shape, thermotolerance, and production of mycotoxins. For example, transport of *A. fumigatus* conidia into the lungs is facilitated by their smaller diameter in comparison to *A. flavus* and *A. niger.*[95,96]

The term "aspergillosis" may be broadly defined as a spectrum of diseases attributed to allergy, colonization, or tissue invasion caused by members of the fungal genus *Aspergillus.* A single satisfactory classification system for these disease entities is difficult because different populations of patients may develop the same type of infection. For example, osteomyelitis may result from local trauma or hematogenous dissemination in an immunocompromised host. Colonization in normal hosts can lead to allergic diseases ranging from asthma to allergic bronchopulmonary aspergillosis or, rarely, invasive disease.[95,97]

Aspergillosis is generally acquired by inhalation of airborne conidia that are small enough (2.5–3 µm) to reach alveoli or the paranasal sinuses.[95] Each conidiophore releases 10^4 conidia that remain suspended for long periods and are viable for months in dry locations. Although monitoring of hospital air for *Aspergillus* conidia has been advocated by some authors, guidelines for interpreting results do not exist. The use of high-efficiency particulate air (HEPA) filters in operating rooms and laminar flow rooms and removal of immunocompromised patients from hospital renovation sites may be helpful in preventing infection in this population.[95] Although the fate of *Aspergillus* conidia in the gastrointestinal tract has not been closely studied, limited evidence suggests that this route may provide an important portal of entry for disseminated infections in man.[98]

Superficial Infection

Superficial or locally invasive infections of the ear, skin, or appendages can often be managed with topical antifungal therapy. Skin infections in patients with burn wounds, while uncommon, may progress to deep tissue invasion despite the use of topical or parenteral antifungal agents. Risk factors for deep infection include extensive thermal injuries, malnutrition, cirrhosis, and previous infection with *Pseudomonas aeruginosa.*[95]

Allergic Bronchopulmonary Aspergillosis

Allergic manifestations of *Aspergillus* range in severity from mild asthma to allergic bronchopulmonary aspergillosis (BPA). BPA, which is almost always caused by *A. fumigatus,* is characterized by severe asthma with wheezing, fever, malaise, weight loss, chest pain, and a cough productive of blood-streaked sputum.[95] Following recurrent episodes of severe asthma, the disease usually progresses to fibrosis and bronchiectasis with granuloma formation. BPA develops when *Aspergillus* conidia become trapped in the viscous mucus of asthmatic patients. The fungus grows, releasing toxins and antigens. The resulting host sensitization results in a variety of immune reactions by the host. Early in the course of disease, an IgE-mediated (type I) immune reaction results in bronchospasm, eosinophilia, and immediate skin reactivity. The ensuing fibrosis and pulmonary infiltrates appear to be mediated by circulating or precipitating antibody complexes of IgG antibody, followed by granuloma formation and mononuclear infiltration due to a type IV delayed hypersensitivity reaction. Therapy is aimed at minimizing the quantity of antigenic material released in the tracheobronchial tree. Management of acute asthma attacks minimizes trapping of *Aspergillus* by bronchial secretions, and administration of parenteral corticosteroids clears lung infiltrates. Antifungal therapy is generally not indicated in the management of allergic manifestations of aspergillosis, although some patients have demonstrated a decrease in their corticosteroid dose following therapy with itraconazole.[95,99]

Aspergilloma

In the nonimmunocompromised host, *Aspergillus* infections of the sinuses most commonly occur as saprophytic colonization (aspergillomas or "fungus balls") of previously abnormal sinus tissue. Infection is usually localized in the maxillary sinus and is rarely associated with local invasion of adjacent bone or brain tissue. Treatment consists of removal of the aspergilloma. Sinus aspergillosis can also present as allergic sinusitis with nasal drainage of brownish mucus plugs. Therapy with corticosteroids and surgery is generally successful. In the immunocompromised host, subacute, chronic, or fulminant invasive disease can be seen, and a combination of antifungal and surgical therapy is generally required.[95]

Pulmonary aspergillomas are fungus balls arising in preexisting cavities due to tuberculosis, histoplasmosis, lung tumors, or radiation fibrosis, although occasionally no previous pulmonary disease is present.[95] Patients generally experience chest pain, dyspnea, and sputum production. Hemoptysis is observed in 50–80% of patients, probably due to ulceration of the epithelial lining of the cavity with formation of granulation tissue, and approximately 10% of patients have hemorrhage severe enough to cause death. Although *Aspergillus* can only be cultured in 50–60% of patients, precipitating antibodies are positive in virtually 100% of patients. Invasive disease rarely occurs, and therapy for this disease is controversial. Concern regarding the risk of severe hemorrhage has led some clinicians to utilize aggressive surgical excision of aspergillomas or pulmonary resection in patients with hemoptysis. However, complications including bronchopulmonary fistulas, hemorrhage, empyema, and persistent air space problems have led to the current recommendation that surgical intervention be reserved for patients with severe (>500 mL/24 hours) hemoptysis. Mild to moderate hemoptysis should be managed conservatively. Although intravenous amphotericin B is generally not useful in eradicating aspergillomas, intracavitary instillation of amphotericin B has been employed successfully in a limited number of patients. Hemoptysis generally ceases when the aspergilloma is eradicated.[95]

Invasive Aspergillosis

Although exposure to *Aspergillus* conidia is nearly universal, impaired host defenses are required for the development of invasive disease. Phagocytes (neutrophils, monocytes, and macrophages) rather than antibodies or lymphocytes constitute the primary host defense system against invasive disease with aspergillosis.[95,96] Macrophages prevent germination of conidia and also eradicate conidia, providing the first line of defense against invasive disease. Administration of corticosteroids appears to impair the killing of conidia by macrophages and impair mobilization of neutrophils. Neutrophils halt hyphal growth and dissemination and kill mycelia, constituting a second line of defense. Prolonged neutropenia appears to be the most important predisposing factor to the development of invasive aspergillosis, accounting for the high frequency of disease in patients with acute leukemia. Complement provides a source of chemotactic factor, and facilitates neutrophil damage to hyphae and monocyte killing of conidia. Complement is not necessary for the attachment or ingestion of conidia by human alveolar macrophages.[95,96]

Until recently, aspergillosis was an uncommon fungal infection in patients with AIDS. It has been suggested that AIDS patients are at less risk for aspergillosis than other fungal infections since the primary cellular defect in AIDS patients is in T lymphocytes, whereas neutrophils and macrophages constitute the primary lines of defense to infection with aspergillosis. Until recently, aspergillosis has been reported as a late complication of disease in AIDS patients with additional risk factors for aspergillosis, such as corticosteroid use, neutropenia, previous *Pneumocystis carinii* or cytomegalovirus pneumonia, marijuana smoking, or the use of broad-spectrum antibiotics. However, a recent study reported that approximately 50% of patients with aspergillosis had no classic risk factors. The majority of these patients had CD4+ counts <50/mm^3. Although some patients diagnosed early in their infection responded to treatment, most have not responded to therapy with amphotericin B 0.5 mg/kg daily or itraconazole 200 to 600 mg daily.[99–101]

Invasive disease with *Aspergillus* can arise *de novo* or from any of the allergic or colonizing forms of aspergillosis.[96] Predisposing factors to the development of invasive aspergillosis include glucocorticoid therapy, particularly following chronic administration or with higher dosages (30–200 mg of prednisone daily), cytotoxic agents, and recent or concurrent therapy with broad-spectrum antimicrobial agents. Patients with chronic hepatitis, alcoholism, diabetes mellitus, chronic granulomatous disease, leukopenia (<1000 cells/mm^3), leukemia (particularly acute lymphocytic or myelogenous leukemia), lymphoma, and acute rejection of an organ transplant are also at a higher risk of invasive disease. Although rare, invasive aspergillosis has been reported in apparently normal hosts.[95,96]

Clinical Presentation

Although the lung is the most common site of invasive disease, the liver, spleen, brain, heart, gastrointestinal tract, pericardium, and other body sites are involved in a substantial minority of cases. In neutropenic patients with *Aspergillus* pneumonia, hyphae invade the walls of bronchi and surrounding parenchyma, resulting in an acute necrotizing, pyogenic pneumonitis. As a result, patients often present with classic signs and symptoms of acute pulmonary embolus: pleuritic chest pain, fever, hemoptysis, a friction rub, and a wedge-shaped infiltrate on chest radiographs. Invasion of blood vessels causes thrombosis with resultant infarction, necrosis, and dissemination to other tissues and organs in the body. Survival beyond 2 or 3 weeks is uncommon. If bone marrow function returns, cavitation of the pulmonary lesion generally occurs and the spread of infection may be halted.[95,96]

Diagnosis

The diagnosis of *Aspergillus* is complicated by its presence as a normal commensal in the human gastrointestinal tract and respiratory secretions.[16,95] Though suggestive of infection, the presence of hyphae in a smear or biopsy specimen is not diagnostic. Demonstration of *Aspergillus* by repeated culture and microscopic examination of tissue provides the most firm diagnosis.[16,95,97] The appearance of *Aspergillus* in tissues varies with increasing host resistance, from the normal vegetative hyphae found with necrotic tissue and exudate in the alveoli of immunocompromised hosts to the compact tangled filaments ("granules") observed in fungal balls. Identification of *Aspergillus* is generally based on the appearance of 2- to 4-μm-wide septate hyphae that are dichotomously branched at 45-degree angles. *Aspergillus* hyphae are readily distinguished from *Candida* hyphae, which are generally smaller in diameter, and have yeast-like as well as filamentous forms, an absence of true branching, and constrictions at the septae. However, hyphae may appear indistinguishable in tissue from those of *Fusarium, Scopulariopsis, Pseudallescheria,* and *Penicillium,* which are increasingly common causes of infection in the immunocompromised host.[1,16] Sporulation is rarely observed in tissue.

In the immunocompromised host, aspergillosis is characterized by vascular invasion leading to thrombosis, infarction, and necrosis of tissue. Abundant hyphae in radially branching clusters can be observed in tissue. In contrast, vascular invasion is uncommon and there are sparse numbers of hyphae in patients with chronic granulomatous disease.[95,96] Although growth on Sabouraud dextrose or brain–heart infusion agar may be utilized for primary culture, bronchoscopy or bronchoalveolar lavage cultures are positive in only ~40% of histopathologically identified specimens.[96] Blood or bone marrow cultures are rarely positive for *Aspergillus.*

Many clinicians have treated positive respiratory cultures of *Aspergillus* as a common contaminant, and argued that a minimum of two to three positive cultures is necessary before antifungal therapy is indicated. However, recent studies suggest that any positive culture may be indicative of true infection in the immunocompromised host.[95,96] In a large series (98 patients) reported by the National Institutes for Health, 82% of patients had positive fungal cultures at some point during the course of their terminal illness. Despite these vigorous culturing methods, only 34% of patients had one antemortem culture positive for *Aspergillus* and only 9% had more than one positive culture.[97] Yu et al.[102] reported that isolation of *Aspergillus* from respiratory tract cultures correlated with proven aspergillosis in 100% of patients with acute leukemia, 94% of neutropenic patients, and 65% of patients receiving adrenal corticosteroids, but only 40% of patients receiving parenteral antibiotics. Similarly, Aisner et al.[103] correlated aspergillosis with isolation of *Aspergillus* from nasal cultures.

Serologic tests (immunoprecipitation, immunodiffusion, and counterimmunoelectrophoresis) to detect antibody production to *Aspergillus* are generally helpful only in the diagnosis of allergic BPA and aspergilloma. Unfortunately, their usefulness in invasive aspergillosis is limited due to the inability of these patients to elaborate antibodies.[8,95,96] Although serum precipitins are positive in 70–80% of patients with invasive pulmonary aspergillosis, the specificity and predictive value of single antibody titers is relatively low.[96] Serum antigen detection has shown promise in animal models of *Aspergillus* infection; however, results cannot be directly extrapolated to humans since these models employed IV injection of *Aspergillus* rather than acquisition via the respiratory tract, as occurs in human hosts.[8,95] Thus far, data from human studies suggest that serum antigen detection by radioimmunoassay may be valuable in the detection of pulmonary or disseminated infection, but less so in localized or sinus infections. However, these tests appear useful in determining the prognosis of disease and response to antifungal therapy.[8,95,96]

Treatment of Invasive Aspergillosis

Therapy for invasive aspergillosis is far from optimal at this time, in part due to the difficulties in establishing a diagnosis, and in part due to a lack of truly effective antifungal agents. Administration of amphotericin B appears to decrease mortality from >90% to approximately 45%. However, these data are difficult to interpret since many patients were diagnosed postmortem or amphotericin B therapy was not administered until the patient had very advanced disease. Mortality from pulmonary aspergillosis in bone marrow transplant recipients exceeds 94% regardless of therapy.[98] Although early diagnosis and administration of antifungal therapy may result in higher response rates, correction of underlying immune deficits (in particular, return of neutrophil counts) is of paramount importance in eradication of infection.[97,104]

Until the diagnosis of aspergillosis can be more rapidly and definitively determined, empiric therapy must be instituted when invasive disease is suspected. In patients at highest risk for invasive disease (acute leukemia and bone marrow transplant recipients), the most important predisposing factors include prolonged severe neutropenia (<100 cells/mm^3 for >1 week), graft rejection, chronic administration of corticosteroids, and tissue damage from preexisting infection. In these patients, antifungal therapy should be instituted in any of the following conditions: (1) persistent fever or progressive sinusitis unresponsive to antimicrobial therapy; (2) an eschar over the nose, sinuses, or palate; (3) the presence of characteristic radiographic findings, including wedge-shaped infarcts, nodular densities, new cavitary lesions; or (4) any clinical manifestation suggestive of orbital or cavernous sinus disease or an acute vascular event associated with fever. Isolation of *Aspergillus* spp. from nasal or respiratory tract secretions should be considered confirmatory evidence in any of the previously mentioned clinical settings.[95]

The optimal dosage or duration of amphotericin B therapy for the treatment of invasive aspergillosis has not been determined.[95,96,98] Since *Aspergillus* is only moderately susceptible to amphotericin B, full doses (1–1.5 mg/kg/d) are generally recommended, with response measured by defervescence and radiographic clearing.[95] The use of granulocyte transfusions or recombinant colony-stimulating factors to stimulate granulocyte production remains controversial, and controlled trials are lacking at this time. Although the addition of fluorocytosine and/or rifampin is advocated by some authors, controlled clinical studies verifying the efficacy of these combination therapies are lacking.[96,98] Amphotericin B (1 mg/kg daily) with fluorocytosine decreases mortality in neutropenic patients with pulmonary aspergillosis who did not receive a bone marrow transplant, but relapse is common. Response to therapy may be difficult to determine, since residual disease may remain for long periods of time and cavities may remain long after a patient becomes asymptomatic.[98] Although liposomal preparations of amphotericin B appear less toxic than standard preparations, only limited data regarding their relative efficacy are available at this time.[98]

Although earlier azole antifungal agents (miconazole and ketoconazole) possessed poor *in vitro* activity against *Aspergillus* species, newer triazoles have demonstrated improved activity both *in vitro* and in animal models of infection.[96,99] Itraconazole (100–500 mg daily for 11–192 days) has shown therapeutic benefit in patients with pulmonary, skeletal, and pericardial aspergillosis, particularly in those patients who are less immunocompromised.[98,99,105] The wide range of dosages, durations of therapy, and degree of immunosuppression in these trials makes selection of an appropriate regimen difficult. Jennings and Hardin[99] recently reviewed the role of itraconazole for aspergillosis and recommended that itraconazole be reserved as a second-line agent for patients intolerant or not responding to high-dose amphotericin B. If itraconazole is used, a loading dose of 200 mg three times daily with food for 2–3 days should be employed, followed by itraconazole 200 mg twice daily with food for a minimum of 6 months. Although early studies employing relatively low dosages (50–100 mg daily) of fluconazole demonstrated some activity against less invasive forms of aspergillosis, including chronic pulmonary disease and aspergillomas, data regarding the use of higher dosages (>100 mg daily) in patients with invasive disease are not available.

The use of prophylactic antifungal therapy to prevent primary infection or reactivation of aspergillosis during subsequent courses of chemotherapy is controversial.[99,104] Studies assessing the utility of intravenous administration of amphotericin B in low doses (0.1 mg/kg daily) as prophylactic therapy or with higher dosages of 0.5–0.6 mg/kg daily as empiric therapy for invasive fungal infections in patients with granulocytopenia have not included sufficient numbers of patients to enable detection of differences in the number of *Aspergillus* infections.[99] The prophylactic use of intranasal amphotericin B aerosol sprays (5 or 10 mg daily in three divided dosages) appeared beneficial in small studies in humans and in animal models. However, a larger randomized trial found that amphotericin B sprays reduced colonization of the nasal mucosa without any reduction in the frequency of invasive pulmonary infections with aspergillosis. Since failure of amphotericin B sprays may be due to the ability of small airborne conidia to access the alveolar spaces directly and establish infection, use of aerosolized forms of amphotericin B capable of reaching the alveolar spaces may be required.[99,106]

In granulocytopenic patients who recover from an episode of invasive aspergillosis, the risk of relapse of aspergillosis during subsequent courses of chemotherapy is >50%. Secondary prophylaxis of aspergillosis with empiric administration of high-dose amphotericin B decreases the risk of relapse. Amphotericin B 1 mg/kg daily is started 24–48 hours prior to the start of chemotherapy and continued throughout the period of granulocytopenia. Some investigators recommend the addition of fluorocytosine (dosed to achieve peak serum concentrations of 30–60 µg/mL) to the amphotericin B regimen.[18] Although the use of itraconazole (alone or in combination with amphotericin B or fluorocytosine) may be beneficial in this patient population, little is known regarding its efficacy in this setting. If itraconazole is administered, serum levels should be monitored to assess absorption, since poor absorption of drug has been documented in this patient population.[18,105]

SYSTEMIC ANTIFUNGAL THERAPY

AMPHOTERICIN B

Amphotericin B, introduced in 1957, acts by binding to ergosterol in the fungal cell membrane, disrupting the permeability and fluidity of the cell membrane. Despite its widespread and continued use as the "gold standard" agent for systemic antifungal therapy, a number of unanswered questions remain regarding its pharmacokinetics, efficacy, and toxicity. Amphotericin B remains the therapy of choice for many systemic fungal infections despite a lack of controlled clinical trials documenting the optimal dosage, duration of therapy, or relative efficacy of this agent in comparison to newer azole antifungal agents such as ketoconazole, itraconazole, or fluconazole.[3]

Recommendations for the administration of amphotericin B are largely empirical and in general, have not been tested in a controlled fashion. Most clinicians recommend administration of a 1-mg test dose of amphotericin B in 25–50 mL of 5% dextrose in water or as an aliquot of the initial daily dose infused over 1–2 hours, in order to detect the rare patient likely to experience an anaphylactic reaction to the drug. If tolerated, the remaining daily dose is prepared in a concentration of ≤0.1 mg/mL of 5% dextrose and infused over 2–4 hours. Amphotericin B is usually administered in gradually increasing dosages; most guidelines suggest daily increments of 5 mg or 0.1 mg/kg until the maximum daily dose of 0.5–0.75 mg/kg daily is achieved. However, many clinicians advocate the rapid escalation of doses in patients with documented infections or highly suspicious clinical symptoms; often therapy is instituted with 0.25 mg/kg on the first day of therapy, followed by full-dose therapy on subsequent days of treatment.[3]

Recent studies have suggested that infusion of amphotericin B over 2 hours is safe and may result in a lower incidence of fever and chills. The use of rapid infusions of amphotericin B should be avoided in patients with renal impairment, because they may be unable to tolerate the increased intracellular potassium released secondary to high serum concentrations of amphotericin B.[3]

Routine monitoring of serum concentrations of amphotericin B is not indicated. Most studies have been unable to document a correlation between serum concentrations of the drug and therapeutic efficacy.

The optimal total dosage or duration of amphotericin B therapy has not been determined for most fungal infections. For most deep-seated infections, therapy is often continued for 6–12 weeks. However, in severe infections, those caused by less susceptible pathogens (e.g., *Aspergillus* or *C. tropicalis*), infections in sites that are difficult to penetrate, or in immunocompromised hosts, the daily dosage of amphotericin B may range up to 1 mg/kg and total dosages of 2–4 g of amphotericin B may be administered over a period of months to years.

The side effects of amphotericin B are generally categorized as acute (infusion-related) or long-term side effects. Shaking chills, fever, myalgias, arthralgias, and headache are reported in >50% of patients receiving amphotericin B. A variety of premedications are routinely utilized in an effort to decrease the incidence and severity of these reactions; however, few have been studied in a controlled fashion. These medications include aspirin, acetaminophen, nonsteroidal anti-inflammatory agents, antihistamines, corticosteroids, pyridoxine, phenothiazines, and heparin. Evidence suggests that some of the infusion-related side effects may be due to induction of prostaglandins. Administration of oral ibuprofen (10 mg/kg) 30 minutes prior to administration of amphotericin B has been shown to reduce the incidence of chills from 87% to 49%. Meperidine has also been successful in terminating fever and chills in a randomized, double-blind trial. In another study, the administration of intravenous hydrocortisone (25 mg) at the beginning of amphotericin B infusions was significantly more effective than aspirin and diphenhydramine in reducing the incidence of fever, chills, and vomiting. Larger doses of hydrocortisone do not appear to offer any additional benefit.[3]

Thrombophlebitis is commonly reported in patients receiving amphotericin B therapy, probably as a result of the acidic pH of the reconstituted solution. Methods to reduce the problem include infusion into distal hand veins or in central venous lines in patients receiving long-term therapy, use of dilute solutions (<0.1 mg/mL), and the addition of 500–1000 units of heparin per liter of solution. The efficacy of heparin in reducing the incidence of phlebitis has not been studied in a controlled fashion.[3]

The relatively nonselective affinity of amphotericin B for ergosterol versus cholesterol is thought to provide the basis for many of the long-term side effects of amphotericin B. The most significant side effect of amphotericin B administration is renal toxicity. Although the exact mechanism of this adverse effect is unclear, amphotericin B appears to alter membrane permeability and to activate an intrarenal tubuloglomerular feedback mechanism that alters proximal and distal tubule delivery of ions, resulting in a decreased glomerular filtration and renal blood flow. Hypokalemia and hypomagnesemia may occur in association with decreased renal function, and the administration of supplemental potassium and magnesium may be required. Reversible impairment of renal function occurs within the first 2 weeks of amphotericin B therapy in up to 80% of patients. Irreversible renal dysfunction, while rare, occurs in some patients. It is unclear whether this effect is related to the total cumulative dosage of amphotericin B or to individual patient susceptibility. Amphotericin B can also produce a reversible renal tubular acidosis in patients receiving total dosages of 0.5–1 gram or more.[3] In an effort to decrease the incidence of nephrotoxicity, clinicians have tried several therapeutic modalities, including sodium loading, alternate-day therapy, and mannitol administration.

Amphotericin B can also produce a normochromic, normocytic anemia that is thought to result from a direct inhibition of erythrocyte or erythropoietin production. Hemoglobin concentrations generally return to normal within 2–3 months following discontinuation of amphotericin B. Thrombocytopenia has been rarely reported.

Combination therapy with amphotericin B and fluorocytosine may result in enhanced bone marrow suppression. The increased toxicity may result from enhanced cellular penetration of fluorocytosine or from accumulation of fluorocytosine resulting from amphotericin B-induced renal dysfunction. Serum concentrations of fluorocytosine should be monitored carefully to maintain peak concentrations (2 hours after oral administration) of <100 μg/mL.[57]

The association between increased pulmonary toxicity with the concomitant use of amphotericin B and granulocyte transfusions remains controversial. A tenfold increased risk of pulmonary toxicity, manifested as the development of worsening hypoxia, the appearance of new interstitial infiltrates, or acute dyspnea, has been reported in some studies when amphotericin B was administered in patients receiving granulocyte transfusions. This association has been disputed by other investigators on the basis of retrospective studies and prospective animal studies.[3] Nevertheless, slow administration of amphotericin B and avoidance of concomitant administration of amphotericin B and granulocytes is recommended in order to minimize the potential interaction.

LIPOSOMAL AMPHOTERICIN B

Recent interest has focused on the use of liposomally encapsulated preparations of amphotericin B. In these preparations, amphotericin B is incorporated into the phospholipid bilayer membrane, rather than in the enclosed aqueous phase. The preparation consists of both sheets and multilamellar spherical liposomes, ranging in size from ~0.5–6 μm. The sheets contain more amphotericin B than do the spheres. The optimal preparation and sterol composition of these compounds is still not known.[107–109] Amphotericin B has also been incorporated into lipid emulsions (such as Intralipid), cholesterol in dispersion or in lipoprotein, and detergents such as Triton X-100 and sucrose lauryl ester.[110–112]

The majority of liposomally encapsulated drug appears to be cleared by the reticuloendothelial system; amphotericin B is taken up by macrophages in the lung, liver, spleen, bone marrow, and circulating monocytes in plasma. In the lung, liposome-loaded monocytes migrate to alveoli to become alveolar macrophages. Although larger doses of these preparations are required to achieve similar pharmacologic effects as the desoxycholate form of amphotericin B, the toxicity appears to be much lower. More recent clinical studies have utilized 30 mol% of amphotericin B in the same phospholipid, which provides a formulation with only sheets and ribbons, rather than spherical particles.[107,108]

The use of liposomal preparations of amphotericin B has resulted in decreased toxicity in animal models of infection and in early human clinical trials. Although preliminary studies appear encouraging, controlled clinical trials evaluating the safety and efficacy of liposomal preparations of amphotericin B are incomplete.[109]

FLUOROCYTOSINE

Fluorocytosine (also known as 5-flucytosine or 5-FC) is a fluorinated pyrimidine analog that is highly water soluble. Fluorocytosine is transported into the cell and transformed into 5-fluorouracil (an antimetabolite) by cytosine deaminase, which then inhibits DNA synthesis by incorporation into RNA. Patients with creatinine clearances >40 mL/min should receive 100–150 mg/kg daily in four divided doses. The dosage should be reduced by 50% in patients with a creatinine clearance of 25–50 mL/min, and by 75% in patients with a clearance of 13–25 mL/min. Peak serum concentrations (2 hours after an oral dose) should be monitored in all patients (particularly those with a creatinine clearance of <10 mL/min) to maintain peak serum concentrations <100 mg/L.[6,113]

Fluorocytosine is generally associated with very few side effects in patients with normal renal, gastrointestinal, and hematologic function, although rash, gastrointestinal discomfort, diarrhea (5–10%), and reversible elevations in hepatic enzymes are occasionally observed. In patients with renal dysfunction or with concomitant amphotericin B therapy, leukopenia, thrombocytopenia, and (rarely) enterocolitis may occur. Although studies have suggested that little or no conversion of fluorocytosine to 5-fluorouracil occurs *in vitro,* serum concentrations of >1000 ng/mL (therapeutic for the treatment of malignancies) have been documented in some patients. Investigators have theorized that fluorocytosine may be secreted into the gastrointestinal tract, deaminated by intestinal bacteria, and reabsorbed as 5-fluorouracil.[113]

Fluorocytosine is used in the treatment of cryptococcosis, candidiasis, and chromomycosis. However, the rapid development of resistance to fluorocytosine precludes its use as single-agent therapy except perhaps in the treatment of chromomycosis. Mechanisms for drug resistance may include loss of deaminase and decreased permeability to the drug.[113]

SYSTEMIC AZOLE ANTIFUNGAL AGENTS

The introduction of the azole antifungal agents has rapidly expanded the armamentarium of agents useful in the treatment of systemic fungal infections. Clotrimazole, an early imidazole antifungal, proved inadequate for the treatment of systemic infections because it was found to rapidly induce its own metabolism after oral or intravenous administration. Its use is now largely confined to topical therapy, primarily for the treatment of vulvovaginal candidiasis and in the treatment and prophylaxis of mucocutaneous candidiasis. N-Substitution of imidazoles such as miconazole, clotrimazole, and ketoconazole has resulted in the triazole antifungal agents itraconazole and fluconazole. Although these agents have the same mechanism of action and spectrum of activity as imidazoles, they appear to interact much less with human cytochrome P-450. Consequently, they have less effect on human sterol metabolism.[105]

MICONAZOLE

Miconazole was the first systemically available imidazole antifungal agent. Miconazole is poorly soluble in aqueous solutions and is therefore administered in a polyethoxylated castor oil vehicle (Cremaphor EL) for intravenous administration. This vehicle appears to be responsible for many of the adverse effects associated with miconazole therapy, which include phlebitis and pruritis in more than 20% of patients; nausea, fever, and chills in 10–20%; and vomiting and anemia in >5%. With higher dosages of the drug, thrombocytosis, rouleaux formation of erythrocytes, and hyperlipidemia are reported. Rapid infusions of miconazole have resulted in cardiorespiratory arrest and anaphylactoid reactions, which are theorized to result from massive histamine release triggered by the solvent vehicle.

Although miconazole has been widely utilized for a variety of systemic fungal infections, including cryptococcosis, coccidioidomycosis, candidiasis, and paracoccidioidomycosis, its intravenous use has been largely supplanted by newer azoles. At this time, it remains the drug of choice for the treatment of infections caused by *Pseudallescheria boydii.* Miconazole is generally administered in dosages of 600–3600 mg daily in three or four doses as an intravenous infusion over 30–60 minutes. Miconazole is widely used in topical formulations for the treatment of vulvovaginal candidiasis and superficial skin infections.

Miconazole has been shown to prolong the prothrombin time in patients receiving warfarin therapy, presumably due to inhibition of the anticoagulant.

KETOCONAZOLE

Ketoconazole is a well-tolerated, orally available imidazole with a broad spectrum of activity against most fungal pathogens with the exception of *Aspergillus* spp.

Ketoconazole is poorly soluble in aqueous fluids; it is soluble only in acidic (pH <3) media. Consequently, the dissolution and absorption of ketoconazole is impaired in patients with elevated gastric pH. Patients with achlorhydria due to drugs (antacids or H_2-receptor antagonists) or disease (including AIDS patients) may not adequately absorb the drug.[41,42] In addition, sucralfate appears to interfere with the absorption of ketoconazole when they are administered simultaneously. This interaction can be avoided by separating the doses by 2 hours. For unclear reasons, some bone marrow transplant patients have also demonstrated a decreased absorption of ketoconazole. In achlorhydric patients, ketoconazole may be dissolved in 0.1 N HCl and the solution sipped through a straw (to avoid erosion of tooth enamel). Alternatively, administration of oral glutamic acid capsules (360–720 mg) may be employed to increase absorption.

Ketoconazole is extensively metabolized in the liver by oxidation, O-dealkylation, and aromatic hydroxylation and excreted primarily in the bile as inactive drug. Because less than 5% of an oral dosage is excreted as unchanged drug in the urine, dosage adjustments are not necessary in patients with renal dysfunction.

The most common adverse effect of ketoconazole is dose-related gastrointestinal discomfort. Nausea, vomiting, and anorexia have been reported in over 20% of patients receiving 200 mg daily; the incidence rises to >50% of patients when the dosage is increased to ≥400 mg daily.[32] Because most patients experience gastrointestinal discomfort with ketoconazole, administration with food is generally recommended. Asymptomatic, reversible elevations in hepatic transaminases are observed in 5–10% of patients, regardless of the dosage of ketoconazole administered. Hepatitis with hepatic necrosis is a rare, idiosyncratic reaction that occurs in <0.01% of patients.

Ketoconazole inhibits adrenal steroid synthesis by reversible, dose-dependent inhibition of the cytochrome P-450 dependent 11-β-hydroxylation of steroids. Although precipitation of adrenal crisis is rare, patients should be considered potentially unable to mount an adrenal stress response. Administration of ketoconazole as a single (rather than multiple) daily dose appears to minimize adrenal axis suppression. Gynecomastia, decreased libido, oligospermia, azospermia, and impotence secondary to decreased testosterone synthesis have been reported in males following high (>600 mg) daily dosages and during prolonged administration of lower dosages.[32]

ITRACONAZOLE

Itraconazole is an investigational triazole antifungal with a broad spectrum of antifungal activity. Despite its marked structural similarity to ketoconazole, itraconazole differs in several important respects. Itraconazole appears to have greater specificity against fungal versus mammalian cytochrome P-450, resulting in greater potency and a decrease in P-450 mediated side effects. In addition, itraconazole possesses excellent *in vitro* activity against *Aspergillus* and *Sporothrix* spp.

Like ketoconazole, itraconazole depends on the availability of low gastric pH for dissolution and absorption. Administration with food appears to enhance significantly the bioavailability of itraconazole. Since itraconazole exhibits pH-dependent dissolution and absorption, absorption is impaired in patients receiving antacids or H_2-receptor antagonists and in patients with achlorhydria. Plasma concentrations of itraconazole following a single oral dose in HIV-infected patients are approximately 50% lower than concentrations observed in healthy volunteers.[114]

The adverse effects of itraconazole appear to be similar to those observed with ketoconazole. Gastrointestinal disturbances (primarily nausea, vomiting, epigastric pain, and diarrhea) are the most common complaint, occurring in up to 20% of patients. Transient elevation of hepatic transaminases occurs in ~5% of patients, and reversible thrombocytopenia was reported in one patient. Sexual impotence despite normal testosterone levels has been reported in a small number of patients.[105]

FLUCONAZOLE

Fluconazole is a recently marketed triazole antifungal agent with markedly different pharmacologic features than previously marketed azole antifungals. The small molecular weight, low protein binding, and increased water solubility of fluconazole results in rapid, essentially complete absorption of drug following oral administration.

Fluconazole is excreted primarily (>80%) as unchanged drug in the urine, with the remainder of the dose excreted as glucuronide and N-oxide metabolites in the urine and as unchanged drug in the feces.

Side effects of fluconazole suggest that the drug is very well tolerated in most patients. Gastrointestinal side effects are the most frequently reported side effect (~7%), followed by CNS side effects (3%) and rash.

Relative to ketoconazole and itraconazole, fluconazole appears to be intermediate in its ability to inhibit human cytochrome P-450. Fluconazole appears to have minimal effects on steroid hormones. Clinically significant drug interactions have been documented with tolbutamide, warfarin, cyclosporine, phenytoin, cisapride, astemizole, terfenadine, and rifampin. Antacids and cimetidine do not affect the absorption or elimination of fluconazole.[105]

REFERENCES

1. Rinaldi MG. Problems in the diagnosis of invasive fungal diseases. Rev Infect Dis 1991;13:493–495.
2. Bodey GP. Fungal infections in cancer patients. Ann NY Acad Sci 1988;544:431–442.
3. Gallis HA, Drew RH, Pickard WW. Amphotericin B: 30 years of clinical experience. Rev Infect Dis 1990;12:308–329.
4. Powderly WG, Kobayashi GS, Herzig GP. Amphotericin B-resistant yeast infection in severely immunocompromised patients. Am J Med 1988;84:826–832.
5. Kobayashi GS, Spitzer ED. Testing of organisms for susceptibility to triazoles: Is it justified? Eur J Clin Microbiol Infect Dis 1989;8:387–389.
6. Galgiani JN. Susceptibility of *Candida albicans* and other yeasts to fluconazole: Relation between *in vitro* and *in vivo* studies. Rev Infect Dis 1990;12(suppl 3):S272–S275.
7. National Committee for Clinical Laboratory Standards. Reference method for broth dilution antifungal susceptibility testing of yeasts; proposed standard. Document M27-P. 1992;12:25.
8. de Repentigny L. Serodiagnosis of candidiasis, aspergillosis, and cryptococcosis. Clin Infect Dis 1992;14(suppl 1):S11–S22.
9. Bennett JE. Mycoses, in Mandell GL, Douglas RG, Bennett JE (eds): Principles and Practice of Infectious Diseases, 3rd ed. New York, Churchill Livingstone, 1990, p 1942.
10. Bennett JE. Pathogenic fungi, in Sherris JC (ed): Medical Microbiology, 2nd ed. New York, Elsevier, 1991, p 440.
11. Odds FC. Resistance of yeasts to azole-derivative antifungals. J Antimicrob Chemother 1993;31:463–471.
12. Pfaller MA, Rinaldi MG. Antifungal susceptibility testing. Current state of technology, limitations, and standardization. Infect Dis Clin North Am 1993;7:435–444.
13. Edwards JE. Candida species, in Mandell GL, Douglas RG, Bennett JE (eds): Principles and Practice of Infectious Diseases, 3rd ed. New York, Churchill Livingstone, 1990, p 1943.
14. Vazquez JA, Sanchez V, Dmuchowski C, et al. Nosocomial acquisition of *Candida albicans:* An epidemiologic study. J Infect Dis 1993;168:195–201.
15. Beck-Sague C, Jarvis WR. Secular trends in the epidemiology of nosocomial fungal infections in the United States, 1980–1990. National Nosocomial Infections Surveillance System. J Infect Dis 1993;167:1247–1251.
16. Kaufman L. Laboratory methods for the diagnosis and confirmation of systemic mycoses. Clin Infect Dis 1992;14(suppl 1):S23–S29.
17. Kappe R, Seeliger HP. Serodiagnosis of deep-seated fungal infections. Curr Top Med Mycol 1993;5:247–280.
18. Walsh TJ, Lee JW. Prevention of invasive fungal infections in patients with neoplastic diseases. Clin Infect Dis 1993;17(suppl 2):S468–S480.
19. Perfect JR. Antifungal prophylaxis: To prevent or not. Am J Med 1993;94:233–234.
20. Powderly WG, Saag MS, Cloud GA, et al. A controlled trial of fluconazole or amphotericin B to prevent relapse of cryptococcal meningitis in patients with the acquired immunodeficiency syndrome. N Engl J Med 1992;326:793–798.
21. Loyd JE, Des Prez RM, Goodwin RA. *Histoplasma capsulatum,* in Mandell GL, Douglas RG, Bennett JE (eds): Principles and Practice of Infectious Diseases, 3rd ed. New York, Churchill Livingstone, 1990, p 1989.
22. Wheat LJ. Diagnosis and management of histoplasmosis. Eur J Clin Microbiol Infect Dis 1989;8:480–490.

23. Wheat LJ, Connolly-Stringfield P, Kohler RB, et al. *Histoplasma capsulatum* polysaccharide antigen detection in diagnosis and management of disseminated histoplasmosis in patients with acquired immunodeficiency syndrome. Am J Med 1989;87:396–400.
24. Wheat LJ. Histoplasmosis in Indianapolis. Clin Infect Dis 1992;14(suppl 1):S91–S99.
25. Wheat LJ, Connolly-Stringfield PA, Baker RL, et al. Disseminated histoplasmosis in the acquired immune deficiency syndrome: Clinical findings, diagnosis and treatment, and review of the literature. Medicine 1990;69:361–374.
26. Drew RH. Pharmacotherapy of disseminated histoplasmosis in patients with AIDS. Ann Pharmacother 1993;27:1510–1518.
27. Chapman SW. Blastomyces dermatitidis, in Mandell GL, Douglas RG, Bennett JE (eds): Principles and Practice of Infectious Diseases, 3rd ed. New York, Churchill Livingstone, 1990, p 1999.
28. Bradsher RW. Blastomycosis. Clin Infect Dis 1992;14(suppl 1):S82–S90.
29. Davies SF, Sarosi GA. Blastomycosis. Eur J Clin Microbiol Infect Dis 1989;8:474–479.
30. Turner S, Kaufman L. Immunodiagnosis of blastomycosis. Semin Respir Infect 1986;1:22–28.
31. Bradsher RW, Rice DC, Abernathy RS. Ketoconazole therapy for endemic blastomycosis. Ann Intern Med 1985;103:872–879.
32. National Institute of Allergy and Infectious Diseases Mycoses Study Group. Treatment of blastomycosis and histoplasmosis with ketoconazole: Results of a prospective randomized clinical trial. Ann Intern Med 1985;103:861–872.
33. Pappas PG, Pottage JC, Powderly WG, et al. Blastomycosis in patients with the acquired immunodeficiency syndrome. Ann Intern Med 1992;116:847–853.
34. Bronnimann DA, Galgiani JN. Coccidioidomycosis: Clinical update. Eur J Clin Microbiol Infect Dis 1989;8:466–473.
35. Ampel NM, Wieden MA, Galgiani JN. Coccidioidomycosis. Rev Infect Dis 1989;6:897–910.
36. Stevens DA. *Coccidioides immitis*, in Mandell GL, Douglas RG, Bennett JE (eds): Principles and Practice of Infectious Diseases, 3rd ed. New York, Churchill Livingstone, 1990, p 2008.
37. Galgiani JN, Ampel NM. Coccidioidomycosis in human immunodeficiency virus-infected patients. J Infect Dis 1990;162:1165–1169.
38. Tucker RM, Denning DW, Dupont B, Stevens DA. Itraconazole therapy for chronic coccidioidal meningitis. Ann Intern Med 1990;112:108–112.
39. Drutz DJ. Amphotericin B in the treatment of coccidioidomycosis. Drugs 1983;26:337–346.
40. Graybill JR, Stevens DA, Galgiani JN, et al. Itraconazole treatment of coccidioidomycosis. Am J Med 1990;89:282–290.
41. Lake-Bakaar G, Tom W, Lake-Bakaar D, et al. Gastropathy and ketoconazole malabsorption in the acquired immunodeficiency syndrome (AIDS). Ann Intern Med 1988;109:471–473.
42. Lelawongs P, Barone JA, Colaizzi JL, et al. Effect of food and gastric acidity on absorption of orally administered ketoconazole. Clin Pharm 1988;7:228–235.
43. Sugar AM, Alsip SG, Galgiani JN, et al. Pharmacology and toxicity of high-dose ketoconazole. Antimicrob Agents Chemother 1987;31:1874–1878.
44. Galgiani JN, Catanzaro A, Cloud GA, et al. Fluconazole therapy for coccidioidal meningitis. Ann Intern Med 1993;119:28–35.
45. Catanzaro A, Fierer J, Friedman PJ. Fluconazole in the treatment of persistent coccidioidomycosis. Chest 1990;97:666–669.
46. Tucker RM, Denning DW, Dupont B, Stevens DA. Itraconazole therapy for chronic coccidioidal meningitis. Ann Intern Med 1990;112:108–112.
47. Tucker DW, Denning DW, Rinaldi MG, et al. Itraconazole (IZ) therapy (Rx) of progressive coccidioidomycosis (C) [Abstract 573]. 28th Interscience Conference for Antimicrobial Agents and Chemotherapy, 1988.
48. Craven PC, Graybill JR, Jorgensen JH, et al. High-dose ketoconazole for treatment of fungal infections of the central nervous system. Ann Intern Med 1983;98:160–167.
49. Graybill JR, Stevens DA, Galgiani JN, et al. Ketoconazole treatment of coccidioidal meningitis. Ann NY Acad Sci 1988;544:488–496.
50. Tucker RM, Williams PL, Arathoon EG, et al. Pharmacokinetics of fluconazole in cerebrospinal fluid and serum in human coccidioidal meningitis. Antimicrob Agents Chemother 1988;32:369–373.
51. Tucker RM, Galgiani JN, Denning DW, et al. Treatment of coccidioidal meningitis with fluconazole. Rev Infect Dis 1990;12(suppl 3):S380–S389.
52. Sugar AM, Stern JJ, Dupont B. Overview: Treatment of cryptococcal meningitis. Rev Infect Dis 1990;12(suppl 3):S338–S348.
53. Patterson TF, Andriole VT. Current concepts in cryptococcosis. Eur J Clin Microbiol Infect Dis 1989;8:457–465.
54. Chuck SL, Sande MA. Infections with *Cryptococcus neoformans* in the acquired immunodeficiency syndrome. New Engl J Med 1989;321:794–799.
55. Clark RA, Greer D, Atkinson W. Spectrum of *Cryptococcus neoformans* in 68 patients infected with human immunodeficiency virus. Rev Infect Dis 1990;12:768–777.
56. Bennett JE, Dismukes WE, Duma RJ, et al. A comparison of amphotericin B alone and combined with flucytosine in the treatment of cryptococcal meningitis. N Engl J Med 1979;301:126–131.
57. Stamm AM, Diasio RB, Dismukes WE, et al. Toxicity of amphotericin B plus flucytosine in 194 patients with cryptococcal meningitis. Am J Med 1987;83:236–242.
58. Dismukes WE, Cloud G, Gallis HA, et al. Treatment of cryptococcal meningitis with combination amphotericin B and flucytosine for four as compared with six weeks. N Engl J Med 1987;317:334–341.
59. Dismukes WE. Management of cryptococcosis. Clin Infect Dis 1993;17(suppl 2):S507–S512.
60. Saag MS, Powderly WG, Cloud GA, et al. Comparison of amphotericin B with fluconazole in the treatment of acute AIDS-associated cryptococcal meningitis. The NIAID Mycoses Study Group and the AIDS Clinical Trials Group. N Engl J Med 1992;326:83–89.
61. Odds FC. Pathogenesis of candidosis, in *Candida* and Candidosis. A Review and Bibliography, 2nd ed. London, Bailliere Tindall, 1988, p 236.

62. Kirkpatrick CH. Chronic mucocutaneous candidiasis. Eur J Clin Microbiol Infect Dis 1989;8:448–456.
63. Stone HH, Kolb LD, Currie CA, et al. *Candida* sepsis: Pathogenesis and principles of treatment. Ann Surg 1974;179:697–710.
64. Reents S, Goodwin SD, Singh V. Antifungal prophylaxis in immunocompromised hosts. Ann Pharmacother 1993;27:53–60.
65. Rozenberg-Arska M, Dekker AW, Branger J, Verhoef J. A randomized study to compare oral fluconazole to amphotericin B in the prevention of fungal infections in patients with acute leukaemia. J Antimicrob Chemother 1991;27:369–376.
66. Hathorn J, McCloskey R, Buell D. Fluconazole (FLU) vs Clotrimazole (CLO) in the treatment of oropharyngeal candidiasis in adults with malignancy [Abstract 267]. 30th Interscience Conference for Antimicrobial Agents and Chemotherapy, 1990.
67. Pons VG, Greenspan D, Koletar SL, et al. Fluconazole and clotrimazole troches for the treatment of oral thrush in AIDS [Abstract 1270]. 30th Interscience Conference for Antimicrobial Agents and Chemotherapy, 1990.
68. De Wit S, Weerts D, Goossens H, Clumeck N. Comparison of fluconazole and ketoconazole for oropharyngeal candidiasis in AIDS. Lancet 1989;1:746–747.
69. Koletar SL, Russell JA, Fass RJ, Plouffe JF. Comparison of oral fluconazole and clotrimazole troches as treatment for oral candidiasis in patients infected with human immunodeficiency virus. Antimicrob Agents Chemother 1990;34:2267–2268.
70. Chave JP, Cajot A, Bille J, Glauser MP. Single-dose therapy for oral candidiasis with fluconazole in HIV-infected adults: A pilot study. J Infect Dis 1989;159:806–807.
71. De Wit S, Fahir R, Weerts D, et al. Single dose versus 7 days fluconazole for treatment of oral candidiasis in HIV infected patients: A prospective randomized study [Abstract 1269]. 30th Interscience Conference for Antimicrobial Agents and Chemotherapy, 1990.
72. Sangeorzan JA, Bradley SF, He X, et al. Epidemiology of oral candidiasis in HIV-infected patients: Colonization, infection, treatment, and emergence of fluconazole resistance. Am J Med 1994;97:339–346.
73. Laine L, Dretler RH, Conteas CN, et al. Fluconazole compared with ketoconazole for the treatment of *Candida* esophagitis in AIDS. A randomized trial. Ann Intern Med 1992;117:655–660.
74. Deschamps MM, Pape JW, Verdier RI, et al. Treatment of candida esophagitis in AIDS patients. Am J Gastroenterol 1988;83:20–21.
75. Inman W, Pearce G, Wilton L. Safety of fluconazole in the treatment of vaginal candidiasis. A prescription-event monitoring study, with special reference to the outcome of pregnancy. Eur J Clin Pharmacol 1994;46:115–118.
76. Imam N, Carpenter CC, Mayer KH, et al. Hierarchical pattern of mucosal candida infections in HIV-seropositive women. Am J Med 1990;89:142–146.
77. Rhoads JL, Wright DC, Redfield RR, Burke DS. Chronic vaginal candidiasis in women with human immunodeficiency virus infection. JAMA 1987;257:3105–3107.
78. Doering PL, Santiago TM. Drugs for treatment of vulvovaginal candidiasis: Comparative efficacy of agents and regimens. Drug Intell Clin Pharm 1990;24:1078–1083.
79. Edwards JE Jr, Filler SG. Current strategies for treating invasive candidiasis: Emphasis on infections in nonneutropenic patients. Clin Infect Dis 1992;14(suppl 1):S106–S113.
80. Richet HM, Andremont A, Tancrede C, et al. Risk factors for candidemia in patients with acute lymphocytic leukemia. Rev Infect Dis 1991;13:211–215.
81. Fraser VJ, Jones M, Dunkel J, et al. Candidemia in a tertiary care hospital: Epidemiology, risk factors, and predictors of mortality. Clin Infect Dis 1992;15:414–421.
82. Wey SB, Mori M, Pfaller MA, et al. Risk factors for hospital-acquired candidemia. A matched case-control study. Arch Intern Med 1989;149:2349–2353.
83. Winston DJ, Chandrasekar PH, Lazarus HM, et al. Fluconazole prophylaxis of fungal infections in patients with acute leukemia. Results of a randomized placebo-controlled, double-blind, multicenter trial. Ann Intern Med 1993;118:495–503.
84. Goodman JL, Winston DJ, Greenfield RA, et al. A controlled trial of fluconazole to prevent fungal infections in patients undergoing bone marrow transplantation. N Engl J Med 1992;326:845–851.
85. Walsh TJ, Hathorn JW, Sobel JD, et al. Detection of circulating candida enolase by immunoassay in patients with cancer and invasive candidiasis. N Engl J Med 1991;324:1026–1031.
86. Wingard JR, Merz WG, Saral R. *Candida tropicalis:* A major pathogen in immunocompromised patients. Ann Intern Med 1979;91:539–543.
87. Rex JH, Bennett JE, Sugar AM, et al. A randomized trial comparing fluconazole with amphotericin B for the treatment of candidemia in patients without neutropenia. Candidemia Study Group and the National Institute. N Engl J Med 1994;331:1325–1330.
88. Anaissie EJ, Darwiche R, Mera J, et al. A prospective randomized multicenter comparing fluconazole to amphotericin B for nosocomial candidiasis [Abstract 808]. 33rd Interscience Conference on Antimicrobial Agents and Chemotherapy, 1993.
89. Edwards JE. Editorial response: Should all patients with candidemia be treated with antifungal agents? Clin Infect Dis 1992;15:422–423.
90. Wingard JR, Merz WG, Rinaldi MG, et al. Association of *Torulopsis glabrata* infections with fluconazole prophylaxis in neutropenic bone marrow transplant patients. Antimicrob Agents Chemother 1993;37:1847–1849.
91. Swerdloff JN, Filler SG, Edwards JE. Severe candidal infections in neutropenic patients. Clin Infect Dis 1993;17(suppl 2):S457–S467.
92. Walsh TJ, Lee J, Lecciones J, et al. Empiric therapy with amphotericin B in febrile granulocytopenic patients. Rev Infect Dis 1991;13:496–503.
93. Pizzo PA, Robichaud KJ, Gill FA, Witebsky FG. Empiric antibiotic and antifungal therapy for cancer patients with prolonged fever and granulocytopenia. Am J Med 1982;72:101–111.
94. Graybill JR, Galgiani JN. Ketoconazole therapy for fungal urinary tract infections. J Urol 1983;129:68–70.

95. Bodey GP, Vartivarian S. Aspergillosis. Eur J Clin Microbiol Infect Dis 1989;8:413–437.
96. Rinaldi MG. Invasive aspergillosis. Rev Infect Dis 1983;5:1061–1077.
97. Andriole VT. Infections with *Aspergillus* species. Clin Infect Dis 1993;17(suppl 2):S481–S486.
98. Denning DW, Stevens DA. Antifungal and surgical treatment of invasive aspergillosis: Review of 2,121 published cases. Rev Infect Dis 1990;12:1147–1181.
99. Jennings TS, Hardin TC. Treatment of aspergillosis with itraconazole. Ann Pharmacother 1993;27:1206–1211.
100. Lotholary O, Meyohas M, Dupont B, et al. Invasive aspergillosis in patients with acquired immunodeficiency syndrome: Report of 33 cases. Am J Med 1993;95:177–187.
101. Stansell JD. Pulmonary fungal infections in HIV-infected persons. Semin Respir Infect 1993;8(2):116–123.
102. Yu VL, Muder RR, Poorsattar A. Significance of isolation of *Aspergillus* from the respiratory tract in diagnosis of invasive pulmonary aspergillosis. Am J Med 1986;81:249–254.
103. Aisner J, Murillo J, Schimpff SC, Steere AC. Invasive aspergillosis in acute leukemia: Correlation with nose cultures and antibiotic use. Ann Intern Med 1979;90:4–9.
104. Perfect JR, Klotman ME, Gilbert CC, et al. Prophylactic intravenous amphotericin B in neutropenic autologous bone marrow transplant recipients. J Infect Dis 1992;165:891–897.
105. Como JA, Dismukes WE. Oral azole drugs as systemic antifungal therapy. N Engl J Med 1994;330:263–272.
106. Jeffery GM, Beard ME, Ikram RB, et al. Intranasal amphotericin B reduces the frequency of invasive aspergillosis in neutropenic patients. Am J Med 1991;90:685–691.
107. Lopez-Berestein G. Liposomes as carriers of antimicrobial agents. Antimicrob Agents Chemother 1987;31:675–678.
108. Mills W, Chopra R, Linch DC, et al. Liposomal amphotericin B in the treatment of fungal infections in neutropenic patients: a single-centre experience of 133 episodes in 116 patients. Br J Haematol 1994;86:754–760.
109. Berenguer J, Munoz P, Parras F, et al. Treatment of deep mycoses with liposomal amphotericin B. Eur J Clin Microbiol Infect Dis 1994;13:504–507.
110. de Marie S, Janknegt R, Bakker-Woudenberg IA. Clinical use of liposomal and lipid-complexed amphotericin B. J Antimicrob Chemother 1994;33:907–916.
111. Meunier F, Sculier JP, Coune A, et al. Amphotericin B encapsulated in liposomes administered to cancer patients. Ann NY Acad Sci 1988;544:598–610.
112. Moreau P, Milpied N, Fayette N, et al. Reduced renal toxicity and improved clinical tolerance of amphotericin B mixed with Intralipid compared with conventional amphotericin B in neutropenic patients. J Antimicrob Chemother 1992;30:535–541.
113. Francis P, Walsh TJ. Evolving role of flucytosine in immunocompromised patients: New insights into safety, pharmacokinetics, and antifungal therapy. Clin Infect Dis 1992;15:1003–1018.
114. Smith D, van de Velde V, Woestenborghs R, Gazzard BG. The pharmacokinetics of oral itraconazole in AIDS patients. J Pharm Pharmacol 1992;44:618–619.

Chapter 114

Infections in Immunocompromised Patients

S. Diane Goodwin, PharmD, and Douglas N. Fish, PharmD

An "immunocompromised host" is a patient with defects in host defenses that predispose to the development of infectious complications. Today, modern medical advances are creating larger numbers of immunocompromised hosts than ever before. Historically, many of these patients died from their underlying diseases. Improvements in survival resulting from current aggressive therapeutic management often render these patients profoundly immunosuppressed for extended periods, thus predisposing them to opportunistic infections. This chapter focuses on general risk factors for infection, common infecting organisms and infection sites, and prevention and management of suspected or documented infections in hematology–oncology patients (including bone marrow transplant patients), and solid organ transplant recipients. Infectious complications associated with human immunodeficiency virus (HIV) infection are discussed in Chapter 117.

Risk Factors for Infection

GRANULOCYTOPENIA

Granulocytopenia is an abnormal reduction in the number of granulocytes (primarily neutrophils) circulating in peripheral blood. The exact definition of granulocytopenia is controversial, but an absolute neutrophil count (ANC) of less than 1000/mm^3 indicates a reduction sufficient to predispose patients to infection.[1,2] The ANC is the sum of the absolute numbers of both mature neutrophils (polymorphonuclear cells, "PMNs," "polys," or "segs") and immature neutrophils (band forms or "bands"). The absolute number of polys and bands is determined by dividing the percentage of these cells (as obtained from the white blood cell [WBC] differential) by 100 and multiplying the quotient obtained by the total number of WBCs.

As early as 1966, it was reported that infection incidence and severity were inversely related to ANC.[1] Although patients at all levels of granulocytopenia may be at risk for infection, those patients with ANCs of less than 500/mm^3 are at highest risk. Incidence of bacteremia and death is greatest among patients with less than 100/mm^3 granulocytes.[1,3]

In addition to the degree of granulocytopenia, the rate of neutrophil decline and the duration of neutropenia are important risk factors for infection.[4] In patients with chemotherapy-induced neutropenia, the rapidity of ANC decline increases the patient's risk for infection. In fact, those patients whose neutrophil counts are falling rapidly and are expected to be below critical values within 24 hours are already considered to be neutropenic and treated accordingly. The longer the period of neutropenia, especially profound neutropenia (ANC less than 100/mm^3), the more likely the patient will become infected. Duration of chemotherapy-induced neutropenia varies considerably among subsets of cancer patients according to intensity of treatment, with the longest duration occurring in bone marrow transplant recipients who may have no detectable granulocytes on peripheral smear for up to 3–4 weeks.

Bacteria and fungi commonly cause infections in neutropenic patients. Gram-negative bacteria (*Escherichia coli, Klebsiella pneumoniae, Pseudomonas aeruginosa*) and gram-positive bacteria (*Staphylococcus aureus, S. epidermidis* and streptococci) are the most common causes of infection in this patient population. Patients who are neutropenic for extended periods of time and receive broad-spectrum antibiotics are at risk for fungal infection, usually due to *Candida* or *Aspergillus* species. Successful treatment of all infections in neutropenic patients is dependent on resolution of granulocytopenia.[5,6]

In immunocompromised patients, abnormalities may exist in granulocyte function as well as cell numbers. Defects in phagocyte function may be due to underlying disease or its treatment (e.g., corticosteroids, antineoplastic agents, or radiation).[7,8] Leukemic patients whose disease has relapsed are at increased risk of infection, even in the absence of neutropenia.[1]

IMMUNE SYSTEM DEFECTS

In addition to granulocytopenia, defects in T lymphocyte and macrophage function (cell-mediated immunity), B cell function (humoral immunity), or both predispose patients to infection. Cellular immune dysfunction is the result of underlying disease or immunosuppressive drug therapy. Defects in cell-mediated immunity result in a reduction in the ability of the host to defend against intracellular pathogens. Patients with Hodgkin's disease and transplant patients receiving immunosuppressive drugs such as cyclosporine, corticosteroids, antineoplastic agents, and azathioprine are at risk for bacterial, fungal, viral, and protozoal infections (Table 114.1). While some of these organisms are associated with asymptomatic or mild disease in normal hosts, they can cause disseminated, life-threatening infections in immunocompromised hosts.

Defects in humoral immune function are frequently due to underlying disease. Patients with multiple myeloma and chronic lymphocytic leukemia have progressive hypogammaglobulinemia.[10] Splenectomy performed as a part of the staging process for Hodgkin's disease places patients at risk for infectious complications. Disease states in which hypogammaglobulinemia, agammaglobulinemia, or splenic dysfunction occur predispose the patient to serious, life-threatening infection with encapsulated organisms such as *Streptococcus pneumoniae*, *Haemophilus influenzae*, and *Neisseria meningitidis*.

DESTRUCTION OF PROTECTIVE BARRIERS

Loss of protective barriers is a major factor predisposing immunocompromised patients to infection. Damage to the skin and mucous membranes via surgery, venipuncture,

TABLE 114.1. RISK FACTORS AND COMMON PATHOGENS IN IMMUNOCOMPROMISED PATIENTS

Risk Factor	Patient Conditions	Common Pathogens
Neutropenia	Acute leukemia Chemotherapy	Bacteria: *E. coli, K. pneumoniae, P. aeruginosa, S. aureus, S. epidermidis* Fungi: *Candida, Aspergillus, Zygomycetes* Viruses: Herpes simplex
Impaired cell-mediated immunity	Lymphoma Immunosuppressive therapy (steroids, cyclosporine, chemotherapy)	Bacteria: *Listeria, Nocardia, Legionella,* Mycobacteria Fungi: *Cryptococcus neoformans, Candida, Aspergillus, Histoplasma capsulatum* Viruses: Cytomegalovirus, Varicella-Zoster, Herpes simplex Protozoal: *Pneumocystis carinii*
Impaired humoral immunity	Multiple myeloma Chronic lymphocytic leukemia Splenectomy Immunosuppressive therapy (steroids, chemotherapy)	Bacteria: *S. pneumoniae, H. influenzae, N. meningitidis*
Loss of protective barriers		
Skin	Venipuncture, bone marrow aspiration, urinary catheterization, vascular access devices, radiation	Bacteria: *S. aureus, S. epidermidis, Bacillus* spp. Fungi: *Candida*
Mucous membranes	Respiratory support equipment, endoscopy, chemotherapy, radiation	Bacteria: *S. aureus, S. epidermidis,* Enterobacteriaceae, streptococci, *P. aeruginosa, Bacteroides* spp. Fungi: *Candida* Viruses: Herpes simplex
Surgery	Solid organ transplantation	Bacteria: *S. aureus, S. epidermidis,* Enterobacteriaceae, *P. aeruginosa, Bacteroides* spp. Fungi: *Candida* Viruses: Herpes simplex
Alteration of normal microbial flora	Antimicrobial therapy Chemotherapy Hospital environment	Bacteria: Enterobacteriaceae, *P. aeruginosa, Legionella, S. aureus, S. epidermidis* Fungi: *Candida, Aspergillus*
Blood products, donor organs	Bone marrow transplantation Solid organ transplantation	Fungi: *Candida* Viruses: Cytomegalovirus, Epstein–Barr virus, hepatitis B, hepatitis C Protozoal: *Toxoplasma gondii*

(Compiled from Refs. 4, 9, and 10.)

intravenous and urinary catheters, radiation, and chemotherapy disrupts the body's major host defense systems, leaving affected patients at high risk for infection. After chemotherapy with antimetabolites such as methotrexate, for example, mucous membranes of the oropharynx and gastrointestinal tract become eroded and establish a medium for subsequent infection by herpes simplex and *Candida.* Medical and surgical procedures such as transplant surgery, indwelling intravenous catheter placement, bone marrow aspiration, biopsies, and endoscopy further damage the integument and predispose patients to infection. Infections resulting from disruption of protective integumental barriers are usually a result of skin flora such as *S. aureus* or *S. epidermidis.*

ENVIRONMENTAL CONTAMINATION/ ALTERATION OF MICROBIAL FLORA

Infections in immunocompromised hospitalized patients are due to organisms colonizing the host or organisms acquired from the environment. Microorganisms may be transferred from patient to patient on the hands of hospital personnel unless strict infection control guidelines are followed. At one cancer center, 34% of hand cultures from hospital personnel revealed gram-negative rods or *S. aureus.*[11] Contaminated equipment such as nebulizers or ventilators and contaminated water supplies have been responsible for outbreaks of *P. aeruginosa* and *Legionella pneumophila* infections, respectively. Foods such as fruits and green leafy vegetables, often colonized with gram-negative bacteria and fungi, are also sources of microbial contamination and subsequent infection in immunocompromised hosts.[12]

Most infections in patients with cancer are due to organisms colonizing body sites such as the skin, oropharynx, and gastrointestinal tract.[11] Johanson et al.[13] reported shifts in oropharyngeal flora from normal flora to primarily gram-negative bacilli in hospitalized patients and correlated incidence and rapidity of gram-negative colonization with severity of underlying disease. Within 1 week after admission, 100% of seriously ill patients were colonized with gram-negative bacilli (as compared with 18% of moderately ill patients). Newman et al.[14] found that 33% of cancer patients were already colonized with gram-negative bacilli on admission, perhaps the result of frequent hospitalizations and clinic visits. However, about 50% of infections in hospitalized cancer patients are due to colonizing organisms acquired after admission.[11] Bacteria acquired in institutional settings are usually more resistant to antibiotic therapy and more difficult to eradicate than those acquired in the community.

Although hospital admission and severity of illness are risk factors for colonization by gram-negative bacilli, administration of broad-spectrum antimicrobial agents has the greatest impact on flora of immunocompromised hosts. Use of broad-spectrum antimicrobial agents for suspected or documented infection disrupts the delicate balance of gastrointestinal tract flora, thus predisposing the patient to infection with more virulent microbial pathogens. Dynamic interactions between microorganisms of the gastrointestinal tract determine risk of superinfection. If anaerobic flora are preserved, risk of infection and subsequent bacteremia from virulent gram-negative bacilli such as *P. aeruginosa* is decreased. Preservation of anaerobic flora is termed *colonization resistance.*[15] Attempts at maintaining colonization resistance are discussed in the section on antimicrobial prophylaxis. Administration of antineoplastic drugs such as cyclophosphamide, doxorubicin, fluorouracil, and methotrexate also may alter the gastrointestinal flora, leading to pseudomembranous colitis.[16] Alteration of gastrointestinal flora with H_2-receptor antagonists or antacids may also predispose patients to development of nosocomial pneumonias.[17]

Numerous factors such as underlying disease, immunosuppressive drug therapy, and antimicrobial administration determine the immunocompromised host's risk of developing infection. In many patients, several risk factors are present concomitantly (Table 114.1).

INFECTIONS IN NEUTROPENIC CANCER PATIENTS

Infection remains the leading cause of autopsy-determined death in neutropenic cancer patients (ANC less than 1000/mm^3).[4] In febrile neutropenic cancer patients, 6–30% of deaths are due to infection.[18,19] Patients with profound neutropenia are at greatest risk for systemic infection. Areas of impaired or damaged host defenses, such as the oropharynx, lungs, skin, sinuses, and gastrointestinal tract, are common sites of infection. While local infection in any site can progress to systemic infection and bacteremia, this is more likely with infections of the perirectal area, lung, and pharynx.[11] Febrile episodes in granulocytopenic cancer patients can be attributed to microbiologically or clinically documented infection in only about 30–40% of cases.[20] About 60% of bacteremic episodes in cancer patients are due to gram-positive organisms.[21] Gram-positive infections are becoming more prevalent due to increased use of vascular access devices for drug and blood product administration and blood withdrawal and increasing use of prophylaxis with drugs possessing relatively poor gram-positive coverage.[22,23]

ETIOLOGY

Table 114.1 lists organisms commonly infecting granulocytopenic cancer patients with various malignancies. Until the mid-1960s, the major causes of infectious complications in patients with acute leukemia were gram-positive bacteria, most often *S. aureus.* However, the incidence of fatal staphylococcal infections was dramatically reduced after the introduction of the antistaphylococcal penicillins in the mid- to late 1960s and the early 1970s.[10,19] The frequent use of indwelling intravenous catheters (e.g., Hickman, Broviac) and broad-spectrum antibiotics with relatively poor gram-positive coverage has led to the reemergence of staphylococci as important pathogens in cancer patients.[10,24,25] The incidence of pseudomonal infections has decreased during the past decade; however, morbidity and mortality associated with these infections remain very high.[19] Strains of bacteria such as group JK corynebacteria, *Clostridium* species, *Bacillus* species, *Enterobacter* species, *Serratia* species, alpha-hemolytic streptococci, and *Enterococcus fecaelis* are increasingly appearing as pathogens in immunocompromised patients.[4,9,20] Although the gastrointestinal tract is a common site of bacterial infection, septicemias due to anaerobic organisms are infrequent.[26] Polymicrobial infections accounted for only 10% of all septicemias over a 10-year period at M.D. Anderson Hospital and Tumor Institute, most often originating from gastrointestinal, soft tissue, or pulmonary sites.[27]

In addition to bacterial infections, neutropenic cancer patients are at risk for invasive fungal infections. Patients with extended periods of profound neutropenia who have been receiving broad-spectrum antibiotics are at highest risk for invasive fungal infection. Depending on the series, 8–69% of neutropenic cancer patients have histologic evidence of invasive fungal disease at autopsy.[28]

Candida albicans is the most common cause of fungal infections in neutropenic cancer patients. Up to 60% of immunocompromised cancer patients develop oral thrush, the most common clinical manifestation of fungal infection.[29] Candidal infections may be confined to the oropharynx or may disseminate to involve the esophagus, blood, and organs such as the liver. Mucous membranes damaged from cytotoxic chemotherapy and radiation serve as areas of candidal surface colonization and subsequent entry into the bloodstream, from which disease may disseminate throughout the body. Hepatosplenic candidiasis, commonly known as "chronic disseminated candidiasis," is an important infection in patients with hematologic malignancies at or after the time of bone marrow recovery.[30] Because candidal species are normal flora, alteration of body host defenses is an important risk factor for the development of these infections. *Candida* can be isolated from the blood in less than 25% of patients infected with these organisms; therefore, histopathologic identification from biopsy specimens is often required.[28]

Other species of *Candida* such as *Candida tropicalis, Candida parapsilosis,* and *Candida krusei* are being isolated with increasing frequency. An increase has also been noted in infections due to *Torulopsis glabrata, Trichosporon* species, *Fusarium* species, and *Curvularia.*[9,20]

Infections due to *Aspergillus* species are acquired via inhalation of airborne spores. After colonizing the lungs, *Aspergillus* invades the lung parenchyma and pulmonary vessels, resulting in hemorrhage, pulmonary infarcts, and a high mortality rate. *Aspergillus* species may also cause sinusitis in neutropenic patients. Prolonged granulocytopenia has been shown to be the primary risk factor for invasive pulmonary aspergillosis in neutropenic patients with acute leukemia.[31] Invasive *Aspergillus* should be suspected in those neutropenic cancer patients colonized with *Aspergillus* who remain persistently febrile despite a week or more of broad-spectrum antibiotic therapy.[32]

Chemotherapy-induced mucous membrane damage may predispose neutropenic cancer patients to the reactivation of herpes simplex virus (HSV), manifesting as gingivostomatitis or recurrent genital infections. Untreated, oropharyngeal HSV infections may spread to involve the esophagus, often coexisting with candidal infections. Clinical disease due to HSV occurs most often in patients with serologic evidence (e.g., serum antibodies to HSV) of prior infection. Both HSV-seropositive patients undergoing bone marrow transplantation and HSV-seropositive leukemics receiving intensive chemotherapy are at high risk for recurrent HSV disease during periods of immunosuppression.[33–35] In the past, *Pneumocystis carinii* pneumonia was a common pathogen in subsets of cancer patients, particularly those with acute lymphoblastic leukemia and lymphoma. However, routine use of trimethoprim–sulfamethoxazole (TMP–SMX) prophylaxis has substantially reduced the incidence of this infection.[36]

Because the majority of infecting organisms in cancer patients are from the host's own flora, some centers have employed routine surveillance cultures in an attempt to prospectively identify causes of fever and infection in patients with suspected infection. In a typical surveillance culture program, cultures of the nose, mouth, axillae, and perirectal area are performed twice weekly and culture results correlated with the clinical status of the patient. Risk of subsequent infection after colonization varies with virulence of the organism; approximately 50% of acute leukemics colonized with *P. aeruginosa* will develop bacteremias.[11] Presence of *Aspergillus flavus* from nasal cultures has been shown to correlate with risk of invasive aspergillosis.[32] Because surveillance cultures are costly and organisms other than those causing infection may be colonizing body sites, the utility of surveillance culture programs may be limited. However, surveillance cultures are useful as research tools and in certain clinical situations, such as in patients with prolonged profound neutropenia and in institutions with high rates of antimicrobial resistance or problems with virulent pathogens such as *P. aeruginosa* or *A. flavus.* Current opinion is that surveillance cultures are valuable in detecting colonization with methicillin-resistant *S. aureus* and *Aspergillus* species in the nasal area, *P. aeruginosa* in the rectal area, and the presence of antibiotic-resistant gram-negative rods and colonization with *Candida* or *Salmonella*.[2,12,14]

CLINICAL PRESENTATION

Because neutropenic cancer patients are at high risk for serious infections, frequent clinical assessments and physical examinations must be performed to search for possible signs of infection. The most important clinical finding in the neutropenic cancer patient is the presence of fever, defined as a single oral temperature of at least 38.3°C or multiple oral temperatures of at least 38.0°C persisting for over 1 hour in the absence of other causes.[2] Fever in the neutropenic cancer patient should be considered due to infection until proven otherwise. Infection can be documented clinically or microbiologically in only about 30–40% of febrile neutropenic cancer patients.[20] Other causes of fever unrelated to infection in this patient population include the administration of blood products, chemotherapeutic agents, and other drugs, including biologicals; cell lysis; and the underlying malignancy itself.

At the appearance of a febrile episode, the patient should be carefully evaluated for other signs and symptoms of infection. However, usual clinical signs and symptoms of infection may be absent or altered in neutropenic patients due to their relative reduction in leukocytes. For example, cough, sputum production and purulence, and dysuria, frequency, urgency, and pyuria were noted less commonly in granulocytopenic patients with pneumonia and urinary tract infections, respectively.[37] At the onset of fever, at least two sets of blood cultures should be obtained, including cultures both from peripheral veins and vascular access devices; other cultures (e.g., urine) should be obtained as clinically indicated.[2] Because the lungs are a common site of systemic infection in this patient population, a chest x-ray should be performed at the onset of a febrile episode.

MANAGEMENT OF FEBRILE EPISODES IN NEUTROPENIC CANCER PATIENTS

Management of febrile episodes in neutropenic cancer patients has remained an area of intense research and controversy for nearly 30 years. Much of the accumulated data in this area has been collected from patients with acute leukemia, because intensive chemotherapy usually renders these patients neutropenic for longer periods of time than patients being treated for other malignancies. While remission induction therapy for acute leukemia remains intense, therapy for other malignancies (e.g., solid tumors) has become increasingly aggressive, thus placing these cancer patients at high risk for infectious complications as well. Research conducted during the past 30 years has facilitated the development of guidelines for management of febrile episodes and documented infections in neutropenic cancer patients (Fig. 114.1).[2] A great deal of progress has been made in this area, as evidenced by the at least 50% reduction in infectious mortality rates during the past three decades.[19] However, many controversies remain regarding optimal management of these patients.

Because fever in the neutropenic cancer patient is considered a result of infection until proven otherwise, at the onset of fever or at the first signs/symptoms of infection, high-dose, parenteral, broad-spectrum, bactericidal, empiric antibiotic therapy should be initiated. The rationale for empiric antibiotic therapy in this clinical situation was established in the early 1970s when Schimpff and coworkers[38] demonstrated that withholding antibiotic therapy until isolation of an organism resulted in an unacceptably high mortality rate. The goal of empiric antibiotic therapy is to protect the neutropenic patient from death due to undiagnosed infection. In immunosuppressed patients, undiagnosed infection can rapidly disseminate from occult disease and result in fatal outcomes if left untreated or treated improperly. Failure to initiate appropriate antibiotic therapy for *P. aeruginosa* bacteremia at the onset of fever and collection of blood cultures in granulocytopenic cancer patients resulted in mortality rates of 15% and 70% within 12 and 48 hours, respectively.[39] Empiric antibiotic therapy has been able to reduce early morbidity and mortality.[19,38]

The optimal antibiotic regimen for empiric therapy in febrile neutropenic cancer patients remains controversial. However, the regimen should contain antimicrobial activity against the most likely pathogens. Although *P. aeruginosa* infections are decreasing in frequency, the significance of these infections demands that antipseudomonal antibiotic coverage still be included in empiric regimens. Because the first empiric regimens containing gentamicin plus carbenicillin provided poor activity against *S. aureus* and *K. pneumoniae*, three-drug antibiotic regimens were evaluated. To provide double antibiotic coverage for the most common organisms infecting cancer patients, three-drug regimens most often included gentamicin, cephalothin, and carbenicillin. Subsequent clinical trials, however, demonstrated that two-drug regimens were as effective, less toxic, and less costly than three-drug regimens.[40] In the past decade, researchers have shown that empiric monotherapy with antipseudomonal β-lactams (such as ceftazidime or imipenem) is as effective as combination antimicrobial therapy as long as the patient is carefully evaluated and therapy modified as needed.[41,42]

Basically, five different types of empiric antibiotic regimens are in use today: (1) aminoglycoside plus antipseudomonal penicillin (e.g., piperacillin, mezlocillin) or third-generation cephalosporin (ceftazidime); (2) monotherapy with an antipseudomonal β-lactam, aztreonam, or carbapenem (imipenem, meropenem); (3) addition of vancomycin to regimens (1) and (2); (4) double β-lactam therapy; and (5) fluoroquinolone (ciprofloxacin) in combi-

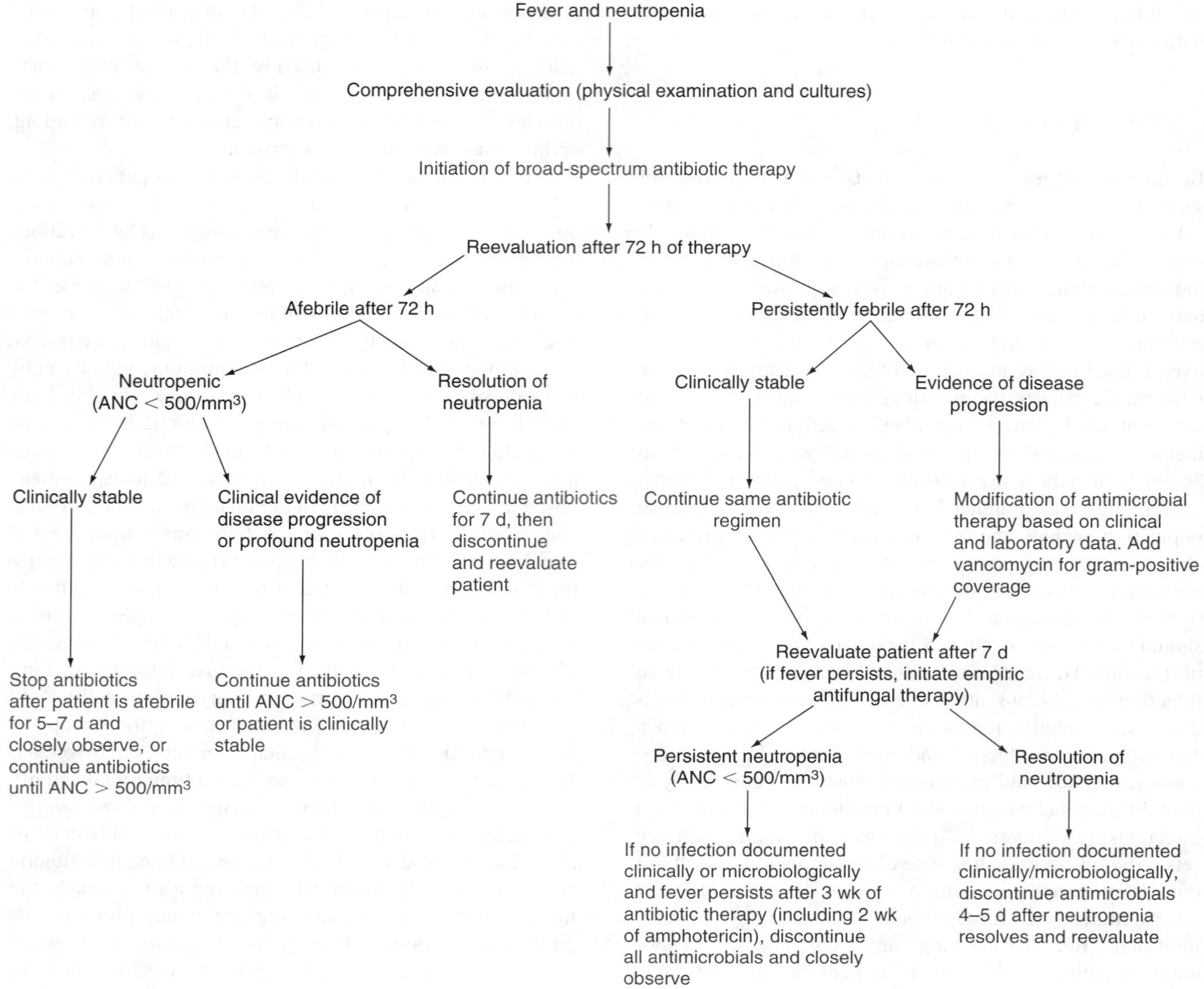

Figure 114.1. Management of febrile episodes in neutropenic cancer patients. *(Adapted from Hughes WT, Armstrong D, Bodey GP, et al. Guidelines for use of antimicrobial agents in neutropenic patients with unexplained fever. J Infect Dis 1990;161:381–396, with permission.)*

nation with β-lactam (ceftazidime), aminoglycoside, or vancomycin.[2,22,23] Each of these regimens is associated with both advantages and disadvantages, and there is no overwhelming evidence that any one of these regimens is superior to the others. The overall response to empiric antibiotic regimens in febrile neutropenic cancer patients is about 75–85%, regardless of whether or not a pathogen is isolated.[4] In a series of trials conducted by the European Organization for Research in the Treatment of Cancer (EORTC), response rate was primarily dependent on the activity of the β-lactam(s) against the infecting organism.[5,43] In designing optimal empiric antibiotic regimens for their cancer patient populations, clinicians must consider infection patterns and antimicrobial susceptibility trends in their respective institutions. Also, patient factors such as drug allergies and concomitant nephrotoxins should be considered.

Aminoglycoside Plus Antipseudomonal β-Lactam

Although regimens consisting of an aminoglycoside plus an antipseudomonal penicillin or third-generation cephalosporin may provide potential synergy against gram-negative bacteria, such regimens may have inadequate gram-positive activity. With the increasing incidence of gram-positive infections, including septicemias, this relative lack of activity remains a concern. However, the emergence of resistant gram-negative bacteria is lower in combination regimens of this type. Aminoglycoside toxicity may be a concern in patients receiving these regimens, because they may already be receiving other nephrotoxic drugs such as cisplatin and cyclosporine. Administration of aminoglycosides in large single daily doses may be as effective, while less costly and no more toxic than conventional dosing methods.[44] However, data on once-daily aminoglycoside therapy in neutropenic patients are lacking, so this practice cannot be recommended at this time. The choice of aminoglycoside and β-lactam for inclusion in empiric antibiotic regimens should be based on institutional epidemiology and antimicrobial susceptibility patterns. If *P. aeruginosa* is a common institutional pathogen, use of empiric tobramycin or amikacin should be considered since they are generally more active than gentamicin against this organism. Piperacillin or ceftazidime is frequently chosen as the β-lactam to be employed in this clinical situation.

Combinations of broad-spectrum β-lactams and aminoglycosides often provide synergistic activity against bacteria commonly infecting cancer patients. The role of synergy in outcome of febrile neutropenic patients treated with empiric antibiotic therapy remains controversial. Higher response rates have been reported in bacteremic granulocytopenic patients treated with synergistic antibiotic combinations.[45] However, in many studies demonstrating the value of synergistic antibiotic combinations, nonsynergistic antibiotic combinations often contained only a single agent to which an organism was sensitive, in many cases an aminoglycoside.[10] Because data from the EORTC demonstrate that response is related to the activity of β-lactam(s) in antibiotic treatment regimens, lack of this activity in the nonsynergistic combinations may help explain observed differences.[43] Synergistic combinations of antibiotics appear beneficial in patients with persistent profound neutropenia. In one series, 44% of patients receiving a synergistic combination responded to treatment, whereas no responses were noted in patients receiving nonsynergistic antibiotic combinations.[6]

β-Lactam Monotherapy

Several β-lactam antibiotics have been evaluated as monotherapy for management of febrile episodes in neutropenic cancer patients. These include third-generation cephalosporins (ceftazidime, cefoperazone), antipseudomonal penicillins (ticarcillin/clavulanic acid, piperacillin, mezlocillin), and imipenem/cilastatin.[2] Although the ureidopenicillins have excellent activity against *E. coli, K. pneumoniae,* and *P. aeruginosa,* response rates in febrile neutropenic cancer patients have been only about 50%, much lower than the 75% to 85% response rates usually noted.[19] However, responses with ceftazidime and imipenem/cilastatin have been much more promising.[41,42] In a large series of patients (550 episodes of fever and neutropenia) at the National Cancer Institute, Pizzo et al.[41] compared ceftazidime monotherapy with a three-drug combination (cephalothin, gentamicin, carbenicillin). These investigators found that monotherapy was as effective as combination therapy in initial empiric management (first 72 hours), but that additions or modifications were necessary in both groups in the case of documented infections. Overall, 78% of febrile patients with undocumented infections were managed successfully with one antibiotic, and no morbidity or mortality resulted from adding other antimicrobial agents only when clinically indicated. However, use of empiric monotherapy, as well as other empiric antibiotic regimens, requires a well-trained, attentive staff to evaluate the patient frequently and make additions and modifications to therapy as necessary. Although cost of monotherapy is lower and aminoglycoside toxicity is avoided, colonization and superinfection may occur more often with β-lactam monotherapy than when β-lactams are administered in combination with an aminoglycoside. Resistance due to β-lactamase induction and stable derepression may develop during β-lactam monotherapy for infections due to organisms such as *P. aeruginosa, Enterobacter* species, and *Serratia* species.[46,47] In addition, coverage for gram-positive organisms such as coagulase-negative staphylococci and methicillin-resistant *S. aureus* is poor with single β-lactams. Therefore, use of monotherapy may not be appropriate in institutions with high rates of gram-positive infections or infections due to gram-negative pathogens with resistance-conferring β-lactamases.

Empiric Regimens Containing Vancomycin

Concern over the lack of gram-positive coverage with empiric therapy with the first two regimens and increasing incidence of serious gram-positive infections has prompted a number of centers to include vancomycin in empiric antibiotic regimens. Basically, two general approaches are taken regarding empiric vancomycin therapy, each supported by the literature. The first approach is to include vancomycin in the initial empiric antibiotic regimen. In a randomized, double-blind, placebo-controlled study of acute leukemics, Karp et al.[48] noted no gram-positive infections in 33 patients who had vancomycin added to empiric regimens of gentamicin plus ticarcillin, whereas 16 of 22 (73%) patients randomized to placebo (plus gentamicin and ticarcillin) developed gram-positive infections. However, all patients randomized to the placebo group who developed gram-positive infections and subsequently required vancomycin treatment had prompt, successful responses to therapy. The second approach to the issue of empiric vancomycin therapy has been evaluated at the National Cancer Institute. Rubin et al.[49] found that the addition of vancomycin only when clinically indicated (and not as part of the initial empiric regimen) resulted in no mortality and no excessive morbidity. Only 20% of patients required the addition of vancomycin, thus resulting in tremendous cost savings. Moreover, the EORTC reported that febrile neutropenic patients not responding to empiric therapy can be successfully treated with vancomycin at the isolation of a gram-positive organism.[50] Whether vancomycin should be a part of the initial empiric antibiotic regimen in febrile, neutropenic cancer patients depends on gram-positive infection rates and antibiotic susceptibilities at each individual institution. At those centers with high rates of methicillin-resistant staphylococcal infections or infections due to clostridial species, addition of vancomycin to the initial regimen may be prudent. Empiric vancomycin use may also be warranted at institutions employing empiric antibiotic regimens without good activity against streptococci. The glycopeptide antibiotic teicoplanin may be a useful alternative to vancomycin in management of gram-positive infections in cancer patients.

Double β-Lactam Therapy

A still controversial regimen for empiric management of febrile episodes in neutropenic patients is double β-lactam therapy. Several combinations of β-lactams have been studied, including piperacillin in combination with cefoperazone, ceftazidime, or moxalactam; mezlocillin in combination with ceftazidime or cefoperazone; and carbenicillin plus cefamandole or ceftazidime.[2] Combinations of broad-spectrum β-lactams are as effective as aminoglycoside/β-lactam regimens.[2] Although double β-lactam combinations may be less toxic than aminoglycoside-containing regimens, double β-lactam regimens are expensive and have relatively poor activity against gram-positive organisms. In addition, theoretical concerns exist regarding possible antibiotic antagonism and the emergence of resistant organisms.[46,51] However, double β-lactam regimens yield response rates that are comparable to those obtained with an aminoglycoside plus an antipseudomonal β-lactam.[42]

Fluoroquinolone Plus Aminoglycoside, β-Lactam, or Vancomycin

Because the fluoroquinolone antibiotics have broad-spectrum activity (particularly versus gram-negative pathogens), rapid bactericidal activity, and favorable pharmacokinetic and toxicity profiles, these agents have been investigated as empiric therapy in febrile neutropenic cancer patients. Due to its good activity against *P. aeruginosa*, ciprofloxacin is the preferred quinolone for use in this clinical situation. Overall response rates of quinolone-containing regimens are comparable to those obtained with the other regimens previously described.[22,23] Due to the relatively poor activity of quinolones versus gram-positive pathogens, quinolone regimens yield lower response rates in patients with gram-positive infections. Due to the excellent pharmacokinetic profile of quinolones, conversion of intravenous therapy to oral therapy is possible and may allow for earlier patient discharges. Fluoroquinolones do not appear to retard bone marrow recovery after chemotherapy; however, at least seven cases of acute renal failure have been reported in cancer patients receiving ciprofloxacin.[52] Due to the limited data on the safety and efficacy of fluoroquinolones as empiric therapy, quinolone-containing regimens are not considered first-line therapy for cancer patients. Data on quinolone monotherapy regimens are insufficient to allow recommendation of these regimens at this time.

Of all the possible empiric regimens described previously, only those regimens containing antipseudomonal penicillins and imipenem/cilastatin have activity against gram-negative gut anaerobes such as *Bacteroides fragilis*. Therefore, use of regimens containing these agents may destroy the colonization resistance in the gut and predispose patients to infections with serious gram-negative pathogens.

MANAGEMENT OF ANTIMICROBIAL THERAPY AFTER INITIATION OF EMPIRIC THERAPY

After the administration of 72 hours of empiric antimicrobial therapy, the clinical status and culture results of febrile neutropenic cancer patients should be reevaluated to determine whether therapeutic modifications are necessary. Additions or modifications to the initial antimicrobial regimen will likely be required in patients with ANCs less than $500/mm^3$ for greater than a week. Modifications of antimicrobial therapy should be based on clinical and laboratory data; antibiotic therapy should be optimized based on culture results. However, during periods of neutropenia, patients should continue to receive broad-spectrum therapy due to the risk of secondary infections or breakthrough bacteremias when antimicrobial coverage is too narrow.[53]

Initiation of Antifungal Therapy

Neutropenic patients who remain febrile with undocumented infection after 4–7 days of broad-spectrum antibiotic therapy require the initiation of empiric antifungal therapy. A high percentage of febrile patients who die during prolonged neutropenia have evidence of invasive fungal infection on autopsy, even though many had no evidence of fungal disease before death.[28] Persistence of fever or development of a new fever during broad-spectrum antibiotic therapy may indicate the presence of fungal infection. Pizzo et al.[54] documented the value of empiric antifungal therapy in this clinical setting.

Because about one-third of febrile, neutropenic cancer patients not responding to 7 days of broad-spectrum antibiotic therapy are likely to have systemic fungal infections, empiric antifungal therapy should be initiated after 4–7 days of broad-spectrum antibiotic therapy to prevent fungal superinfection or treat undiagnosed fungal infection. The current lack of rapid, sensitive diagnostic tests for fungal organisms and the high morbidity and mortality associated with waiting for isolation of fungal organisms justify the empiric addition of antifungal therapy in this clinical setting. At present, the optimal empiric antifungal regimen is not known. However, amphotericin B or fluconazole are the antifungals most commonly used. Antifungal therapy should be continued for at least 2 weeks in the absence of signs and symptoms of active fungal disease; however, many clinicians will continue empiric antifungal therapy until resolution of granulocytopenia. In addition to fungal infections, other causes of persistent fever of unknown origin include resistant bacterial infection, tissue necrosis due to underlying tumor, nonbacterial and nonfungal infection (e.g., viral, mycobacterial, parasitic), and drug or blood product administration.

Cancer patients are at high risk for development of vascular access-related infections (incidence of 9–80%, depending on the series), most often due to *S. aureus* or coagulase-negative staphylococci.[55] The diagnosis of catheter-related bacteremia is made when blood cultures from both peripheral blood and the catheter itself are positive. Three types of catheter-related infections have been identified, including exit site infection, subcutaneous tunnel infection, and catheter-related bacteremia/fungemia.[54] Indwelling catheters are invaluable for providing continued vascular access for drug and blood product administration and blood withdrawal, so attempts at controlling catheter-related infections with antimicrobial therapy should be made in most cases prior to removing the vascular access device. Indications for catheter removal include subcutaneous tunnel infection, failure of bacteremia to clear within 72 hours after initiation of antibiotic therapy, persistence of fever, septic emboli, and bacteremia due to *Bacillus* species, group JK corynebacterium, and fungus (e.g., *Candida* species).[2,56] Removal of catheters in patients with fungemia may be adequate to achieve resolution of fungal infection, but 10–14 days of antifungal therapy with amphotericin B or fluconazole may avoid development of fungal abscesses or disseminated candidiasis. When multilumen catheters are involved, antimicrobial agent administration should be rotated among the ports to ensure eradication of the infecting organism from all catheter sites.

Duration of Therapy

The optimal duration of antimicrobial therapy in the neutropenic cancer patient remains controversial. Decisions regarding discontinuation of empiric antimicrobial therapy often are more difficult and complex than those regarding initiation of therapy. Pizzo et al.[57] randomized patients afebrile after 7 days (cephalothin, gentamicin, and carbenicillin [KGC]) to either continue or discontinue antibiotic therapy. Despite being afebrile when antibiotics were discontinued, 5 of 17 (41%) patients in this group developed infections, 2 of which were fatal. None of the patients who continued on the empiric KGC regimen developed infections. Therefore, these investigators recommended that patients with ANCs of less than 500/mm^3 be maintained on antimicrobial therapy until resolution of granulocytopenia, even if they became afebrile on antibiotic therapy.

Joshi et al.[58] discontinued antibiotic therapy after 5 days in 16 patients with persistent fever and neutropenia who were thought to have doubtful infections. Half of these patients required no further antibiotic therapy in the 2 weeks following antibiotic discontinuation. However, reinstitution of treatment was necessary (mean of 2.4 days) in the other 8 patients, 6 of whom had documented infections. Although 3 patients died, no deaths were attributed to infection. Based on these data, it appears that about 50% of persistently febrile neutropenic cancer patients with doubtful infections can be managed successfully by discontinuing empiric antibiotics after 1 week. However, because many patients will require the reinstitution of antibiotic therapy, these patients must be watched very closely for signs and symptoms of infection.

In patients with documented infections, antimicrobial therapy should be continued until the infecting organism is eradicated and signs and symptoms of infection have resolved (at least 10–14 days). If those neutropenic patients who become afebrile on empiric antibiotic therapy and have no signs and symptoms suggestive of infection can be closely watched, discontinuation of antibiotic therapy may be considered. However, many clinicians believe that all patients who remain febrile should be maintained on antimicrobial therapy until granulocytopenia resolves.

Preliminary data indicate that "low-risk" neutropenic patients (i.e., malignancy in remission, clinically stable with no evidence of serious infection, and evidence of marrow recovery) who become afebrile after 1–2 days of intravenous antibiotics could be successfully discharged without antibiotic therapy.[59] Some centers have opted to manage low-risk patients on oral antimicrobials administered on an outpatient basis. Advantages to both of these approaches include decreased exposure to nosocomial pathogens, increased quality of life, and decreased cost. In this era of health care reform, management of cancer patients on an outpatient basis will continue to be an area of intense research.

Resolution of granulocytopenia is the most important determinant of patient outcome from both febrile episodes and documented infections.[5,6] A number of investigations have evaluated the effect of myeloid growth factors (granulocyte-macrophage colony-stimulating factor, GM-CSF; granulocyte colony-stimulating factor, G-CSF; and macrophage colony-stimulating factor, M-CSF) on chemotherapy-induced neutropenia. In these studies, myeloid colony-stimulating factors were able to reduce the severity and duration of neutropenia and infectious complications associated with chemotherapy in a dose-related fashion, even in the setting of high-dose antineoplastic therapy with autologous bone marrow transplantation.[60] In addition to facilitating bone marrow recovery, colony-stimulating factors also enhance the function of neutrophils.[61] Although the effect of myeloid growth factors on overall survival remains to be determined, amelioration of neutropenia with subsequent administration of more optimal doses of chemotherapy is of great importance in this patient population. Therefore, colony-stimulating factors are important adjuncts to antimicrobial therapy in preventing and controlling infections in neutropenic cancer patients. Evaluation of colony-stimulating factors in the more challenging setting of allogeneic bone marrow transplantation is an area of intense research.

In the past, granulocyte infusions were used in patients not responding to antimicrobial therapy. With the continued expense and complications associated with these transfusions, the availability of more potent, broad-spectrum antibiotics, and increased use of colony stimulating factors, granulocyte infusions are rarely used in clinical practice.

PROPHYLAXIS OF INFECTIONS IN NEUTROPENIC CANCER PATIENTS

Because cancer patients are at risk for development of infections due to bacteria, fungi, and other pathogens during periods of neutropenia, efforts have been made to prevent these infectious complications with a number of environmental modifications and antimicrobial regimens.

Since Schimpff et al.[11] demonstrated that about 50% of pathogens infecting neutropenic cancer patients are acquired in the hospital, efforts at reducing acquisition of infectious organisms from the environment seem a logical place to begin in controlling nosocomial infection rates. Neutropenic patients should be placed on reverse isolation (isolation to protect patients from contracting infections from exposure to others), with strict adherence to infection control guidelines by hospital personnel. Because fresh fruits and vegetables are frequently colonized with bacteria and fungi, most centers exclude these foods from the diets of neutropenic cancer patients.

To reduce the risk of infection due to airborne pathogens such as *Aspergillus* species, laminar air flow rooms are in use at some cancer centers. Laminar air flow rooms work by directing filtered air away from the patient, thus minimizing risk of infection from airborne or environmental pathogens. When laminar air flow rooms are combined with dietary restrictions, infection control practices, and nonabsorbable antibiotics, incidence of infection in neutropenic cancer patients is reduced by at least 50%.[62] However, laminar air flow rooms are expensive, and use of these protective environments has not been shown to improve overall survival in bone marrow transplant recipients.[63]

Eighty-five percent of infections in neutropenic cancer patients are due to flora colonizing the patients themselves.[11] Early attempts at pharmacologic reduction of flora colonizing the gastrointestinal tract were made with combinations of nonabsorbable antibiotics, including gentamicin, nystatin, vancomycin, polymyxin B, and colistin. Combinations of nonabsorbable antibiotics are able to decontaminate the gut and destroy anaerobic flora as well as aerobic gram-negative rods. Therefore, colonization resistance is not preserved, and patients may be at risk for gram-negative infections. Animal studies by Deitch et al.[64] demonstrate that failure to preserve colonization resistance facilitates the translocation of virulent pathogens such as *P. aeruginosa* into the bloodstream.

Due to the unpalatable nature of nonabsorbable antibiotic combinations, patient acceptance and compliance with these regimens are poor. Poor compliance with nonabsorbable antibiotic regimens has been shown to result in suboptimal clinical results (e.g., failure to prevent infections) and rapid repopulation of the alimentary canal with gram-negative rods.[65] Furthermore, because aminoglycosides such as gentamicin are frequently employed to treat suspected or proven infections in cancer patients, use in prophylactic regimens may result in emergence of resistant strains of gram-negative bacilli and negate the value of aminoglycosides as treatment alternatives.[66] Because data regarding the efficacy of nonabsorbable antibiotic combinations outside the setting of protective environments are conflicting, routine use of these agents cannot be endorsed.[2]

Recognition of the value of preservation of colonization resistance has prompted numerous investigations of the absorbable antibiotic trimethoprim-sulfamethoxazole (TMP–SMX) for infection prevention in neutropenic cancer patients. With this drug combination, aerobic gram-negative bacilli and some gram-positive cocci are destroyed, while the anaerobic flora and colonization resistance are maintained. At doses commonly recommended (TMP–SMX 150 mg/750 mg per m^2/d in two divided doses, not to exceed 480 mg of TMP and 2400 mg of SMX per day), data from most placebo-controlled studies indicate that TMP–SMX is able to significantly reduce infection rates in cancer patients.[2] Although TMP–SMX is also effective as prophylaxis against *P. carinii,* its lack of activity against *P. aeruginosa* is worrisome, particularly in institutions where pseudomonal infections are a problem. Other concerns with the use of TMP–SMX prophylaxis include selection of resistant organisms, predisposition to development of fungal infections, and delay in bone marrow recovery.

Because of their oral administration and ability to preserve colonization resistance, the quinolone antibiotics have been evaluated for infection prophylaxis in immunocompromised hosts. Numerous studies have shown that the fluoroquinolones are more effective than placebo, nonabsorbable antibiotics, and TMP–SMX in preventing gram-negative infections in neutropenic cancer patients.[66] Although the quinolone antibiotics can reduce the risk of gram-negative bacteremia in neutropenic patients, use of these agents has led to the emergence of gram-positive organisms (viridans streptococci, *Streptococcus pneumoniae, Enterococcus fecaelis,* coagulase-negative *Staphylo-*

coccus), so combination prophylaxis with a macrolide may be required.[22] Since widespread quinolone prophylaxis may lead to the development of resistant gram-negative organisms and quinolones are quite useful for treatment of suspected or proven infections, the quinolones may need to be reserved for therapy of documented or suspected infections.

Although the use of antibacterial prophylaxis remains somewhat controversial due to poor patient tolerance, lack of consistent efficacy, development of resistant bacteria, high cost, and lack of impact on patient survival,[20,66] it is generally indicated for patients expected to remain profoundly neutropenic for greater than 1 week, such as bone marrow transplant patients. Granulocyte recovery will eliminate the need for continued prophylaxis, and recovery may be facilitated via use of colony-stimulating factors.[60]

Because most neutropenic cancer patients are at risk for mucocutaneous candidal infections that may disseminate and cause serious systemic illness, antifungal prophylaxis is administered during high-risk periods. Antifungal agents administered for both local effects (nystatin suspension, clotrimazole troches) and systemic activity (ketoconazole, fluconazole) have been employed to prevent fungal infections. Although the choice of antifungal prophylaxis agents remains controversial, azole compounds (clotrimazole, ketoconazole, fluconazole) appear to be more effective and better tolerated than nystatin suspension.[67] In a placebo-controlled trial in bone marrow transplant patients, fluconazole prophylaxis (400 mg/d orally) reduced the incidence of both superficial and systemic fungal infections and significantly decreased the mortality from fungal infections.[68] However, use of fluconazole prophylaxis has resulted in emergence of *Candida krusei* and *Torulopsis glabrata* infections.[68,69]

Strategies being investigated for *Aspergillus* prophylaxis in neutropenic patients include the oral azole itraconazole, reduced doses of amphotericin B, and intranasal/aerosol amphotericin B.[70] Currently, none of these interventions can be routinely recommended in clinical practice.

The use of TMP–SMX in cancer patients at risk for *P. carinii* pneumonia has substantially reduced the incidence of this infection.[36] Acyclovir prophylaxis is employed in most centers to reduce risk of HSV reactivation in patients with acute leukemia undergoing intensive chemotherapy.[33,71] Varicella vaccine provides good protection (90%) in leukemic children and may also be useful in seronegative adults, although the vaccine has been less well studied in this population.

Infections in Bone Marrow Transplant Patients

Along with graft-versus-host disease (GVHD), infection remains a major barrier to successful bone marrow transplantation. Bone marrow transplant recipients share risk factors discussed previously with other cancer patients. However, these patients are at enhanced risk of infection due to prolonged periods of granulocytopenia. In addition, patients receiving allogeneic transplants have added immune system insults imposed by immunosuppressive drug therapy for prevention and treatment of GVHD. Pretransplant conditioning regimens (high-dose cytotoxic chemotherapy and total body irradiation) as well as GVHD itself often disrupt protective barriers such as mucous membranes, skin, and gastrointestinal tract, placing patients at further risk of infection. Patients experiencing marrow graft failure have extended periods of profound neutropenia, often resulting in death due to infectious causes. GM-CSF is FDA-approved for bone marrow graft failure in both autologous and allogeneic transplants.

After the administration of intensive conditioning regimens to eliminate malignant cells and prevent rejection of donor marrow, patients remain profoundly neutropenic for 3–4 weeks. During this period, they are at risk for the same types of infectious complications noted in other granulocytopenic cancer patients (e.g., bacterial and fungal infections) and should be managed accordingly.

Due to the high incidence of gram-positive infections in patients undergoing bone marrow transplantation, some centers employ prophylactic parenteral vancomycin. At a dose of 15 mg/kg every 12 hours (given from 2 days prior to marrow infusion until neutropenia resolution or febrile episode), vancomycin was able to completely prevent the development of gram-positive infections in the treatment group, whereas 11/30 control patients (37%) developed gram-positive infections ($p < 0.002$).[72]

In addition to bacterial and fungal infections, bone marrow transplant recipients also are at risk for serious HSV infections during the first 6 weeks post-transplant. HSV infections, manifesting as severe gingivostomatitis, esophagitis, genital lesions, and, rarely, pneumonia are the most common viral infections in marrow recipients during the first month post-transplant. Clinical disease is more common in patients with serologic evidence (e.g., serum antibodies) of prior exposure and latent HSV infection pretransplant. Therefore, reactivation of latent disease during periods of immunosuppression is the most common etiology of HSV infection in these patients. Without prophylaxis, up to 80% of HSV-seropositive leukemics experience clinical mucocutaneous disease after receipt of intensive chemotherapy, compared to less than 25% of seronegative patients.[35,56,73] Oral and mucocutaneous HSV infections often coexist with candidal infection and mucositis secondary to chemotherapy or radiation. Painful swallowing associated with these infections makes it difficult for patients to take oral medications and maintain adequate nutritional intake. Due to the considerable morbidity associated with reactivation of HSV post-transplant, the serologic status (presence of serum antibodies to HSV) of patients should be determined prior to transplant.

A number of clinical studies employing a variety of dosage regimens have been performed to evaluate the benefit of acyclovir prophylaxis for HSV recurrence.[33–35] Depending on the series, 0–10% of HSV-seropositive patients receiving acyclovir experienced viral reactivation, whereas viral shedding and/or HSV-related clinical symptoms were noted in 60–80% of patients receiving placebo.[72] Acyclovir doses commonly used for prophylaxis are 250 mg/m^2 (5 mg/kg) intravenously every 8–12 hours or 200–400 mg orally four to five times daily.[33–35] Intravenous therapy will be necessary in most patients due to presence of severe mucositis from conditioning regimens. Although the duration of antiviral prophylaxis differs between centers, acyclovir is usually begun at the time of the conditioning regimen and continued for about 6 weeks or until resolution of neutropenia. In addition to preventing recurrence of HSV disease, acyclovir prophylaxis also may reduce the incidence of cytomegalovirus (CMV) reactivation.[74] High-dose oral acyclovir given for 6 months post-transplant significantly reduces reactivation of herpes zoster infections.[56]

After bone marrow engraftment has occurred, bone marrow transplant recipients remain at high risk for infection. Significant defects in neutrophil function and cell-mediated and humoral immunity, persisting for several months post-transplant, predispose patients to infectious complications. Acute and chronic GVHD result in prolonged periods of immunosuppression and increased infection rates. During the early postengraftment period, bone marrow transplant patients are at high risk for CMV infections, ranging in severity from asymptomatic viral shedding (urine, throat, lungs) to life-threatening disseminated disease and interstitial pneumonia.

As with HSV, patients seropositive for CMV pretransplant are at high risk for recurrent disease during periods of immunosuppression; about 70% of seropositive patients develop recurrent CMV disease after transplantation.[75] Other risk factors for CMV disease in bone marrow transplant patients include advanced age, HLA mismatch, total-body irradiation, multiagent conditioning regimens, and presence of GVHD.[56] Patients without serologic evidence of latent CMV infection (CMV-seronegative) pretransplant may develop primary CMV disease after receiving bone marrow and/or blood products from CMV-seropositive donors. Onset of both primary and recurrent CMV infection is 1–2 months post-transplant, and patients receiving allogeneic transplants are at highest risk for clinical infection. In an attempt to protect these patients from acquiring CMV infection, they should be given blood products and marrow from CMV-seronegative donors if possible.[76]

The most serious clinical manifestation of CMV disease and the leading cause of infectious death in bone marrow transplant recipients is interstitial pneumonia (IP), which is associated with an 85% mortality rate without treatment.[75,77] This severe clinical syndrome is characterized by fever, dyspnea, hypoxia, nonproductive cough, and diffuse pulmonary infiltrates. Overall, up to 40% of patients receiving allogeneic bone marrow transplants will develop IP, of which up to 40% of cases are due to CMV.[78] IP also may be due to other infectious (*P. carinii,* varicella-zoster virus) and noninfectious causes (pulmonary damage by radiation and chemotherapy).

Numerous single-agent treatments such as vidarabine, interferon, and ganciclovir have been employed unsuccessfully as treatment for CMV IP. However, the combination of high-dose intravenous immunoglobulin (IVIG) and the antiviral agent ganciclovir is able to decrease the mortality of this syndrome from 85% to only 30–50%, depending on the series.[79–81] The potential for ganciclovir-associated bone marrow suppression in patients just recovering from granulocytopenia remains a concern, especially in patients with unstable renal function.

Because the consequences of CMV disease, especially IP, are so severe in bone marrow transplant patients, prevention of CMV disease has been studied. If possible, CMV-seronegative patients should receive donor marrow and supportive blood products from seronegative donors only. Patients already CMV seropositive do not appear to be at additional risk by receiving blood or marrow from seropositive donors.

Pharmacologic prevention of CMV disease in both seronegative and seropositive patients has been attempted. A number of studies evaluating either IVIG or hyperimmune CMV-IVIG have been performed; however, results have been variable.[76,82,83] Reasons for lack of consistent findings include differences in doses and preparations of biologicals, differences in patient populations evaluated, and the number of blood transfusions received after transplantation. Because the benefit of immunoglobulins for CMV prophylaxis in bone marrow transplant patients is controversial and associated with considerable expense, no recommendations can be made at this time. However, this will continue to be an area of intense evaluation in the coming years.

Although acyclovir has relatively poor *in vitro* activity versus CMV, Meyers et al.[74] reported a decrease in CMV infection and clinical symptoms and an improvement in overall survival in HSV- and CMV-seropositive allogeneic bone marrow transplant recipients receiving intravenous acyclovir (500 mg/m^2 every 8 hours). In a randomized trial of allogeneic bone marrow transplant recipients with laboratory evidence of asymptomatic CMV pulmonary infection 35 days post-transplant, ganciclovir was more effective than placebo in preventing development of CMV IP in all patients able to tolerate full courses of therapy.[84] At first isolation of CMV from throat, urine, blood, or bronchoalveolar lavage fluid after successful marrow engraftment, Goodrich et al.[85] randomized allogeneic marrow transplant patients to treatment with ganciclovir (5 mg/kg twice daily for 7 days, then once daily) or placebo for the first 100 days post-transplant. These investigators found a 93% reduction in CMV disease and a significant reduction in mortality at both 100 and 180 days in patients on ganciclovir. Because CMV viremia was found to be highly predictive of subsequent CMV disease, early prophylactic ganciclovir therapy should be considered for these individuals. Ganciclovir-associated bone marrow suppression is a concern in allogeneic marrow transplant recipients. Colony-stimulating factors are beneficial in this setting, providing a benefit similar to that noted in neutropenic AIDS patients receiving ganciclovir therapy for CMV retinitis.

Another anti-viral agent, foscarnet, is effective in the treatment of sight-threatening CMV retinitis in AIDS patients and may be of benefit for treatment or prevention of CMV disease in bone marrow transplant patients. Foscarnet is also useful for the treatment of acyclovir-resistant herpes isolates. Foscarnet would be an attractive alternative to ganciclovir due to its relative lack of bone marrow toxicity. However, the nephrotoxicity associated with foscarnet may be problematic, especially in the period just after transplant when patients may be receiving numerous other nephrotoxic agents.

During the late transplant period (beginning about 4 months post-transplant) infections remain a major problem in those patients suffering from chronic GVHD. Additional immunosuppressive therapy for treatment of GVHD places these patients at risk for infection and infection-related deaths. Infections common during the late transplant period include those due to gram-positive cocci such as *S. aureus* and encapsulated organisms such as *S. pneumoniae* and *Haemophilus influenzae*.[56,86] Bone marrow transplant patients not suffering from chronic GVHD generally have few infections in the late post-transplant period.

Up to 50% of all patients surviving 6 months post-transplant develop clinical infections due to Varicella-Zoster virus (VZV).[87] Both primary (varicella) or recurrent disease (herpes zoster) usually present as skin lesions, most of which remain contained in the area of origin. However, 30–45% of these infections can spread to involve other cutaneous areas or body organs.[56,88] High-dose acyclovir (10 mg/kg IV every 8 hours) is effective and superior to vidarabine in the treatment of serious VZV infections in immunocompromised hosts.[89] Some centers use high-dose oral acyclovir prophylaxis for 6 months post-transplant to prevent reactivation of herpes zoster infections.

A variety of serious infections continues to plague patients undergoing bone marrow transplantation, particularly allogeneic transplantation. Discovery of methods to reduce GVHD without the use of immunosuppressive drug therapy will undoubtedly aid in the prevention and containment of infectious complications in this population. Biotechnologic research and evaluation of candidate antimicrobial agents for infection prevention and treatment should decrease mortality in all subsets of patients with neoplastic disease.

EVALUATION OF THERAPEUTIC OUTCOMES

The goals of antimicrobial drug use in cancer patients (including bone marrow transplant recipients) include (1) prevention of bacterial, fungal, viral, and protozoal infections during periods of neutropenia and postengraftment; (2) prevention of death from infectious causes in febrile neutropenic patients; and (3) effective treatment of established infections to reduce patient morbidity and mortality and allow for administration of optimal neoplastic therapy. All of these goals should be achieved at the lowest possible toxicity and cost. Close monitoring of febrile neutropenic cancer patients, including both clinical and laboratory data, is essential for early detection and treatment of infectious complications. The reader is referred to individual chapters within this textbook for more detailed discussions of monitoring parameters related to specific types of infections (e.g., pneumonia, urinary tract infections, etc).

INFECTIONS IN SOLID ORGAN TRANSPLANT RECIPIENTS

Since the introduction of cyclosporine in 1980, solid organ transplantation has become an established mode of treatment for end-stage diseases of the kidney, liver, heart, and lungs. Today, both patient and allograft survival rates greatly exceed those of the past. Reasons for improved survival include improvements in immunosuppressive drug therapy, candidate selection, transplant surgery techniques, as well as a growing experience in the management of complications (including infection) in these patients.[90] Major hindrances to successful transplantation and extended long-term survival include problems with allograft dysfunction and rejection and infectious complications. Despite advances in diagnostic techniques and antimicrobial therapy, infection remains an important cause of morbidity and mortality after solid organ transplantation.

RISK FACTORS

Many of the risk factors for infection discussed at the beginning of this chapter are present in solid organ transplant patients (Table 114.1). The most important risk factor for infection in this patient population is the immunosuppressive drug therapy that patients receive for prevention and treatment of allograft rejection. Risk of infection from immunosuppressive drug therapy is dependent on specific drug regimens, and dose and duration of immunosuppression. Most opportunistic infections in transplant patients occur during the time when the intensity and total cumulative doses of immunosuppressive therapy are very high (during the first 4 months post-transplant).[91,92] Drug regimens used for immunosuppression have evolved over the years. Combinations of corticosteroids and azathioprine ± antithymocyte globulins (ATG) were commonly used in the 1970s, and cyclosporine/corticosteroid regimens are commonly in use today. Tacrolimus (FK506) and mycophenolate, the most recently introduced immunosuppressive agents, provide additional alternatives for use in solid organ transplantation. A discussion of immunosuppressive drug regimens used in transplantation can be found in Chapter 9.

Since the introduction of cyclosporine-containing immunosuppressive regimens, the incidence, types, and severity of infectious complications associated with these regimens have been compared with those of past regimens.[93–96] In general, rates of infection and mortality from bacterial, viral, and fungal infectious complications are believed to be lower with cyclosporine/prednisone compared with azathioprine/prednisone.[93,94,96] This is probably due to the selective effect of cyclosporine on cell-mediated immunity. However, the risk of *P. carinii* pneumonia may be higher in renal transplant patients receiving cyclosporine regimens.[97,98] Early data from clinical trials suggest that tacrolimus may be associated with lower rates of serious bacterial and CMV infections than are currently seen with cyclosporine-based immunosuppressive regimens.[99,100] This has been attributed to a steroid-sparing effect of tacrolimus, which enables patients to be maintained on greatly reduced doses of corticosteroids; in many cases, steroids were completely discontinued.[99–101] It is currently too early to determine definitively comparative infection rates with new immunosuppressives such as tacrolimus. When evaluating published literature on infection patterns after solid organ transplantation, one must always consider the organ being transplanted and the nature of the immunosuppressive drug regimens in use at reporting centers.

In addition to prevention of allograft rejection, immunosuppressive drugs, often in escalated doses, are used to treat episodes of graft rejection. Drugs used to treat rejection include immunoglobulins directed against T cells (e.g., antithymocyte globulin [ATG]), murine monoclonal antibodies (OKT3), and high-dose intravenous or oral corticosteroids.[93,102,103] Rejection episodes generally occur during the post-transplant period when the overall cumulative dose or net state of immunosuppression is highest (2–4 months). Therefore, patients already at enhanced risk for infection become even more likely to become infected if additional immunosuppressive therapy is needed to treat one or more episodes of graft rejection. When infections occur, immunosuppressive drug therapy must be carefully evaluated because, in many cases, immunosuppression may have to be reduced in order for the patient to survive the infectious episode.

Risk of increased infectious complications from immunosuppressive therapy used to treat rejection episodes is determined, at least in part, by the type of immunosuppressive therapy employed. However, the wide array of drug combinations used to prevent and treat allograft rejection makes it difficult to determine the contribution of each immunosuppressant to the development of infectious complications. Use of ATG appears to be associated with significantly higher infection rates. In particular, an increased incidence of CMV infections has been reported in patients receiving ATG.[104,105] Mason et al.[102] reported a greater than 2.5-fold increase in infectious complications following administration of high-dose intravenous corticosteroids plus ATG for treatment of cardiac rejection (compared with oral prednisone therapy). Although the contribution of OKT3 to infection development is less well defined, patients receiving this agent may have increased rates of viral (HSV, CMV) and *P. carinii* infections.[103,106] However, because much of the data on the use of OKT3 for treatment of rejection is from patients failing standard antirejection therapy (i.e., steroids ± ATG), prior immunosuppression may have played a role in infection development.[107]

ETIOLOGY

As in cancer patients, microorganisms infecting organ transplant patients are present pretransplant or acquired from exogenous sources. All transplant recipients are at risk for mucocutaneous candidiasis from *Candida* species colonizing body sites. However, liver transplant patients are at greatest risk of developing serious invasive fungal disease.[108] Invasive fungal infection may occur in up to 40% of liver transplant recipients and carries a poor prognosis.[108] Abdominal surgery, especially the lengthy operations required for liver transplantation, has been shown to predispose patients to serious fungal disease, most likely as a consequence of entering an area highly colonized with *Candida* species.[106] Liver transplant recipients are also at risk for serious gram-negative bacterial infections originating in the abdomen.

Organisms present as latent tissue infections may reactivate and cause clinical disease post-transplant after the administration of immunosuppressive drug therapy for allograft survival. Clinical disease due to infection reactivation has been noted with viral (HSV I and II, CMV, VZV, Epstein–Barr virus), protozoal (*Toxoplasma gondii, P. carinii*), and mycobacterial (*Mycobacterium tuberculosis*) organisms. Serologic or immunologic tests are performed prior to transplantation to assess risk for infection due to reactivation and to identify other subclinical infections (e.g., hepatitis B, *Legionella*). Often, the only evidence of active infection from a latent tissue source is a rise in antibody titer from pretransplant baseline, a positive culture, or histologic evidence, because many patients with reactivated disease do not manifest clinical symptoms. However, reactivation of latent infection may occasionally result in severe, life-threatening disease.

Exogenous sources of infection in transplant patients include environmental contamination and transmission of microorganisms via transplanted organs and blood products. Environmental sources of infectious organisms are similar to those noted in other immunocompromised hosts such as cancer patients. Airborne pathogens, especially fungal organisms, such as *Aspergillus* and *Cryptococcus neoformans,* cause infections in transplant patients. Transplant patients are also at risk for common nosocomial infections and for infections occurring as hospital outbreaks, such as those due to *P. aeruginosa* and *Legionella.* Optimal prevention and management of nosocomial infections in transplant patients requires knowledge of current epidemiology of infections and susceptibility patterns in the institution.

Infections transmitted via donor organs or blood products are major causes of morbidity and mortality in transplant patients. Although a number of infections (including HSV, *T. gondii,* and hepatitis B) may be transmitted in this manner, the most important infections transmitted from the donor are CMV infections. In addition to causing serious syndromes themselves (pneumonia, hepatitis, fever, hematologic disorders, chorioretinitis), CMV infections also may predispose patients to other opportunistic infections and contribute to allograft dysfunction.[109] In contrast to reactivation disease, transplant patients contracting primary CMV disease are at increased risk for serious, life-threatening infections.[109,110] The most important source of primary CMV infection in transplant patients is the donor organ. Therefore, it is optimal to avoid transplanting organs from infected donors into CMV-seronegative patients. Evidence of latent infection in organ donors can be evaluated via serologic testing for such organisms as CMV, *T. gondii,* hepatitis B, HSV, and HIV. With the scarcity of suitable organs and the rapidity with which transplant decisions must often be made, it is not usually possible to "match" seronegative organ donors with seronegative organ recipients. However, efforts are made to avoid transplanting organs from CMV-seropositive donors into CMV-seronegative recipients due to the potentially severe consequences. The consequences of transplanting an organ from a CMV-seropositive donor into an already CMV-seropositive recipient are less clear. Evidence exists that CMV reinfection (as well as reactivation) syndromes may occur in these patients.[111] Organs from donors seropositive for *T. gondii* and HSV are generally not withheld from seronegative patients. However, organs from known HIV-seropositive donors are not used for transplantation. It has been recommended that asymptomatic HIV-seropositive individuals with a $CD4^+$ lymphocyte count greater than $400/mm^3$ may be considered for liver, heart, or lung transplantation without prohibitively high risk of acceleration of HIV disease.[112] Patients contracting primary Epstein–Barr virus (EBV) infections after transplant are more likely to have clinical symptoms and develop lymphoproliferative disease, including lymphoma, than are patients with reactivated disease.[113]

In addition to transmission from donor organs, primary CMV disease may also be transmitted from seropositive blood products, although this is a much less common mode of infection transmission. Risk of such transmission increases with administration of large numbers of blood products. If possible, CMV-seropositive blood products should not be used in CMV-seronegative liver, heart, and heart-lung transplant patients. Table 114.2 contains information on microbiology, clinical presentation, and treatment of infections in solid organ recipients. Although opportunistic viral, fungal, and protozoal infections may commonly occur, bacterial infections remain the most frequent infectious complications after transplantation in all allograft recipients.

TIMING OF INFECTIONS AFTER TRANSPLANTATION

Although risk of infection with particular pathogens varies with the type of transplant, the time course of infections is similar in all transplant recipients. Overall risk of infection is greatest during the first 3–4 months post-transplant. At this time, most risk factors (Table 114.1) for infection are present. Both daily doses and cumulative doses of immunosuppressive drug therapy are at high levels, and additional immunosuppression may be necessary for treatment of rejection episodes.

The time course of infections can be divided into three periods post-transplant. During the first month post-transplant, the patient is at risk for infections present and brought forward from the pretransplant period (e.g., hepatitis B), routine postoperative infections such as surgical wound and intravenous catheter infections, and reactivation of HSV.[92] Two to 4 months post-transplant, risk is highest for opportunistic infections, including primary and reactivated CMV disease.[110,114] After 4 months, the patient is at risk for persistent infections from earlier post-transplant periods, reactivation of VZV and *C. neoformans,* and routine infections affecting the general population.[90,92] Although Fig. 114.2 illustrates infection patterns after kidney transplantation, this infection time course can be applied to other types of solid organ transplants. However, the relative incidence and importance of a particular pathogen will vary according to the type of transplant.

TYPES OF INFECTIONS/ CLINICAL PRESENTATION

Transplant patients are at risk for infections occurring at a variety of sites, including skin, surgical wound, urinary tract, lungs, blood, abdomen, and central nervous system. However, most infections in the transplant patient occur at or near the site of the transplanted organ. For example, heart and heart–lung transplant recipients most often are afflicted with infections of the lungs or thoracic cavity. Uri-

TABLE 114.2. INFECTIOUS COMPLICATIONS AFTER SOLID ORGAN TRANSPLANTATION: SYNDROMES OF DISEASE AND TREATMENT GUIDELINES

Pathogen	Syndromes of Disease	Treatment
Bacterial		
Gram-negative aerobic rods (Enterobacteriaceae, *P. aeruginosa*, *H. influenzae*)	Blood, urinary tract, pulmonary, abdomen	According to culture and sensitivity results
Gram-positive cocci (*S. aureus*, *S. epidermidis*, *S. pneumoniae*, *Enterococcus fecaelis*)	Skin, blood, urinary tract, pulmonary, abdomen	According to culture and sensitivity results
Legionella spp.	Pulmonary	Erythromycin 0.5–1 g every 6 hours
Listeria monocytogenes	Central nervous system	Ampicillin 1–2 g every 4–6 hours/ gentamicin[a]; TMP–SMX 4 mg/kg every 12 hours[b]
Nocardia spp.	Skin, pulmonary, central nervous system	Sulfadiazine 1 g every 4–6 hours; TMP–SMX 4 mg/kg every 12 hours[b]
Fungal		
Candida spp.	Blood, urinary tract, mucous membranes, skin	Clotrimazole 10 mg five times daily; nystatin 100,000 units every 6 hours; ketoconazole 200 mg daily; fluconazole 100–200 mg daily; amphotericin B 0.5–0.7 mg/kg/d ± 5-flucytosine 100–150 mg/kg/d divided every 6 hours
Aspergillus spp.	Skin, pulmonary, central nervous system	Amphotericin B 1 mg/kg/d ± 5-flucytosine; itraconazole 200–400 mg daily
Cryptococcus neoformans	Skin, pulmonary, central nervous system	Amphotericin B 0.5 mg/kg/d ± 5-flucytosine; fluconazole 400 mg daily
Zygomycetes (Mucor)	Rhinocerebral disease	Amphotericin B 1 mg/kg/d

(continued)

nary tract infections remain an important cause of concern in the renal transplant patient, especially in the early post-transplant period. However, the practice of administering prophylactic antibiotics such as TMP–SMX to renal transplant patients has reduced the incidence and severity of bacterial urinary tract infections.[115] Serious, life-threatening bacterial and fungal infections originating from the abdomen and gastrointestinal tract are most common after liver transplantation and are related to such variables as length of surgery and surgical procedures performed.[106] Risk of bacteremia, usually originating from the gut, is highest in liver transplant patients. Data from the Pittsburgh Transplant Center indicate that renal transplant recipients are at lowest risk of infections and infectious deaths, while patients receiving heart–lung transplants are at highest risk of infections and death due to infections.[90,116]

Clinical presentation of infection in transplant patients is variable and depends on infecting organism, site of infection, present host immune status, time after transplantation, and dose and duration of immunosuppressive therapy.[109] History of prior exposure is important, because primary disease is usually more symptomatic and severe than disease due to reactivation. As in neutropenic cancer patients, fever is the single most important clinical sign indicating the presence of infection.[109,117,118] At the onset of fever, patients should be evaluated for other signs and symptoms of infection, especially at sites near the surgical incision and transplanted organ. Signs of allograft dysfunction may be related to infection, and distinguishing fever due to allograft rejection versus infection is often difficult and must be determined via allograft biopsy. Sources of fever in the transplant patient other than infection may include drug therapy (e.g., ATG) and medical/surgical problems such as embolic events and ischemic injury. Febrile responses to infection may be blunted by the administration of high-dose corticosteroids.

In contrast to febrile neutropenic cancer patients, the threshold for initiating empiric antimicrobial therapy is much higher in febrile transplant patients. As seen in Table 114.2, appropriate therapy for the large numbers of pathogens that may cause infections in transplant patients varies greatly from organism to organism. Therefore, careful attempts at definitive diagnosis of suspected infections should be made. If, after a comprehensive workup, no

TABLE 114.2. INFECTIOUS COMPLICATIONS AFTER SOLID ORGAN TRANSPLANTATION: SYNDROMES OF DISEASE AND TREATMENT GUIDELINES *(Continued)*

Pathogen	Syndromes of Disease	Treatment
Viral		
Herpes simplex virus	Skin, central nervous system, mucous membranes, pulmonary	Acyclovir 5–10 mg/kg every 8 hours; foscarnet 40 mg/kg every 8 hours
Cytomegalovirus	Pulmonary, blood, urinary tract, GI tract	Ganciclovir 5 mg/kg every 12 hours; foscarnet 60 mg/kg every 8 hours; hyperimmune globulins 100–500 mg/kg every 1–2 weeks
Varicella-zoster virus	Skin, disseminated disease	Acyclovir 10 mg every 8 hours, foscarnet 40 mg/kg every 8 hours
Epstein-Barr virus	Lymphoproliferative disease	No effective treatment
Papovaviruses (BK, JC)	Skin, central nervous system	No effective treatment
Protozoal/parasitic		
Pneumocystis carinii	Pulmonary	TMP–SMX 15–20 mg/kg/d divided every 6 hours[b]; atovaquone 750 mg every 12 hours; pentamidine 4 mg/kg daily; dapsone 100 mg daily + TMP 15–20 mg/kg/d divided every 6 hours; clindamycin 450–600 mg every 6 hours + primaquine 15 mg daily
Toxoplasma gondii	Central nervous system	Pyrimethamine 50–100 mg daily + sulfadiazine 1 g every 4–6 hours[c]; pyrimethamine 50–100 mg daily + clindamycin 450–600 mg every 6 hours[c]
Strongyloides stercoralis	Pulmonary, central nervous system	Thiabendazole 25 mg/kg every 12 hours (max 3.0 g/d)

[a]Gentamicin 2 mg/kg loading dose, then maintenance dose determined by serum concentrations.
[b]Based on the trimethoprim component of the combination.
[c]Folinic acid (5–10 mg/d) often recommended in conjunction with pyrimethamine-containing regimens for prevention of bone marrow toxicity.

source of infection is identified, careful observation of the febrile transplant patient (rather than empiric therapy) is common practice. Surveillance cultures may be useful during the first 3 months for detecting CMV and HSV infections.[91] Management and monitoring of documented infections such as urinary tract infections, pneumonias, and intra-abdominal infections is similar to that in other patient populations and is discussed in other chapters of this book.

PREVENTION OF INFECTION IN TRANSPLANT PATIENTS

Infection prevention in the transplant patient can be accomplished in a number of ways. First, risk of environmental contamination should be minimized. Immunocompromised transplant patients should be protected from institutional infectious outbreaks. Transplant patients should receive the pneumococcal vaccine once and the influenza vaccine yearly; however, their immunologic responses to these vaccines may be blunted by immunosuppressive therapy.[91,119]

Because the most important source of primary CMV disease is an infected donor organ, CMV-seronegative patients should not receive organs or blood products from seropositive donors if possible. A number of pharmacologic agents have been employed in an attempt to prevent CMV infection. Prophylactic ganciclovir (5 mg/kg every 12 hours) was demonstrated in a randomized, double-blind, placebo-controlled trial to reduce significantly the occurrence of CMV reactivation disease in a group of 112 patients undergoing heart transplantation.[120] In a group of 42 CMV-seropositive renal transplant recipients, Hirsch et al.[121] were able to reduce significantly the incidence of CMV reactivation with the use of a 14-week course of IFN-α. Balfour and coworkers,[122] in a randomized, placebo-controlled trial of oral high-dose acyclovir, were able to reduce the incidence of CMV infection and disease following renal transplantation. However, "preemptive" ganciclovir (initiated following isolation of virus from blood or urine) has been shown to be more effective than acyclovir in the prevention of both primary and reactivation CMV disease in liver transplant recipients. Although not initiated until the

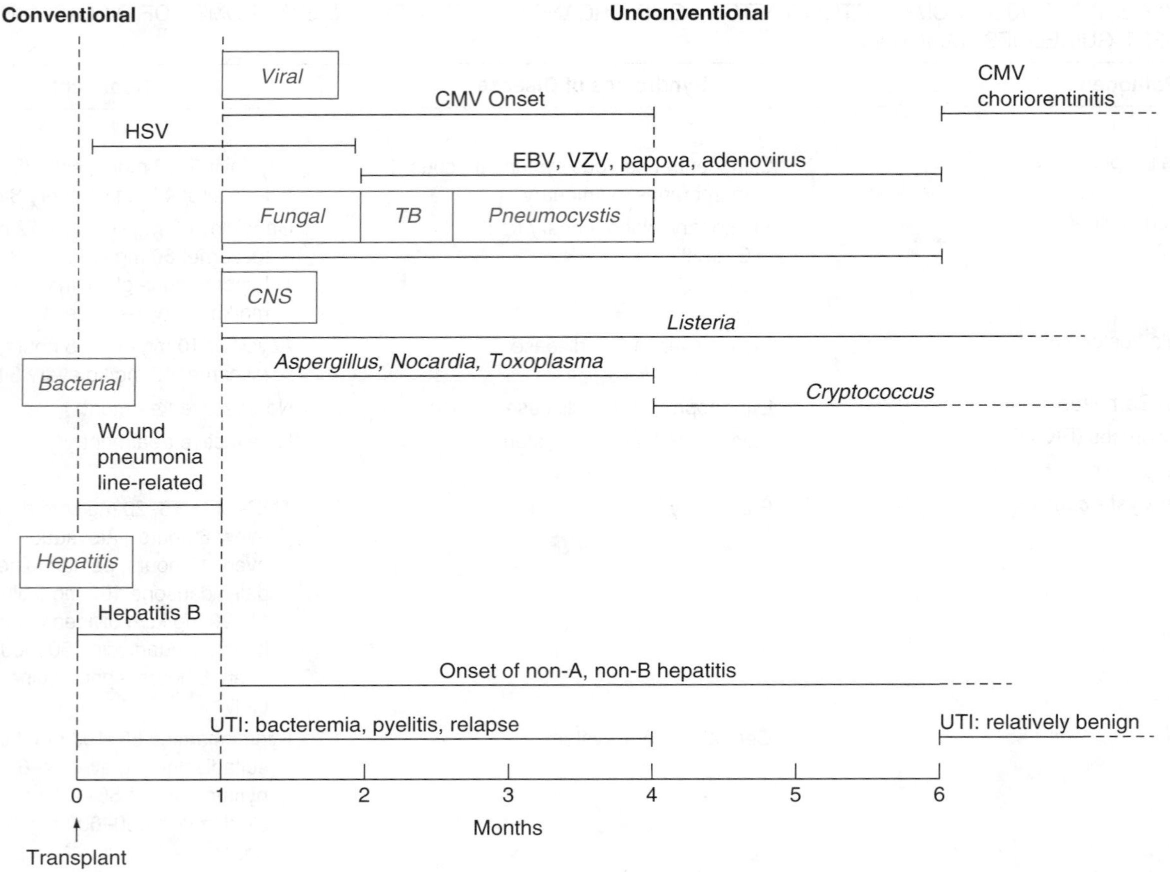

Figure 114.2. Timetable for the occurrence of infection in the renal transplant patient. CMV, cytomegalovirus; HSV, herpes simplex virus; EBV, Epstein–Barr virus; VZV, varicella-zoster virus; TB, tuberculosis; CNS, central nervous system; UTI, urinary tract infection. *(From Rubin RH, Wolfson JS, Cosimi AB, Tolkoff-Rubin NE. Infection in the renal transplant recipient. Am J Med 1981;70:405–411, with permission. Published by the University of Chicago Press.)*

first sign of viral shedding and continued for only 7 days, ganciclovir significantly reduced the occurrence of CMV disease compared to high-dose acyclovir begun shortly after surgery and administered continuously for 24 weeks.[123] Finally, with the prophylactic regimen of IVIG plus acyclovir, Stratta et al.[124] noted a reduction in the incidence of both primary and reactivated CMV disease.

A number of studies have demonstrated the value of CMV hyperimmune globulin (CMV-IVIG) in decreasing the incidence and severity of CMV disease following transplantation of kidneys,[125] hearts,[126] and livers.[127] Although prophylaxis with CMV-IVIG has been strongly recommended for CMV-seronegative renal and liver transplant recipients receiving organs from seropositive donors,[125] the benefits of CMV-IVIG in transplantation of other organs have not been well studied and no firm recommendations can be made.[128] Whether the combination of CMV-IVIG and ganciclovir offers substantial advantages over the use of either agent alone, either for primary prophylaxis or treatment of established CMV disease, is also unclear in solid organ transplantation.[128] Trials employing a combination of CMV hyperimmune globulin and ganciclovir are currently under way.

Although the use of prophylactic acyclovir in HSV-seropositive patients undergoing bone marrow transplantation is well accepted, prophylaxis in solid organ transplant recipients remains controversial. Acyclovir is currently being used at some centers due to the high incidence of clinical HSV infection, including pneumonias, occurring after transplantation.[129]

Prophylactic antibiotics and antifungal agents are of benefit to transplant patients in certain clinical situations. Use of perioperative antibiotic prophylaxis is controversial in renal transplant patients. However, prophylaxis with agents such as cefazolin, begun perioperatively and continued for less than 24 hours postoperatively, is considered by many to be effective in reducing wound infection rates.[128,130] In contrast to renal transplantation, surgical prophylaxis is considered mandatory in liver transplant patients who are at high risk of developing perioperative bacterial infections. In addition, post-transplant antibiotic prophylaxis has been shown to be effective in decreasing the number of bacterial infections in renal transplant patients. In a double-blind, placebo-controlled trial, Tolkoff-Rubin et al.[115] demonstrated the value of prophylactic TMP–SMX in reducing bacterial urinary tract infections in renal transplant patients. Other antibiotics such as the fluoroquinolones are also being evaluated for prevention of infection following renal transplant.[128] Prophylactic TMP–SMX also can reduce the incidence of *P. carinii* pneumonia in immunocompromised hosts.[36] Administration of oral low-dose TMP–SMX (one 160-mg TMP/800-mg SMX tablet daily) for 6–12 months for prevention of *P. carinii* infection following heart and lung transplantation is common, although the efficacy and optimal duration are still somewhat controversial.[131]

Preliminary data suggest that selective bowel decontamination consisting of nonabsorbable antibiotics in combination with a low bacterial diet (no fresh fruits and vegetables) is effective in reducing oropharyngeal and gastrointestinal colonization with gram-negative aerobes and *Candida* in liver transplant patients.[132] Because all immunosuppressed transplant recipients are at risk for mucocutaneous fungal infections, prophylactic oral or topical antifungal agents may be indicated in these patients.[68] Transplant patients, especially heart transplant recipients, without serologic evidence of prior exposure to *T. gondii* who receive organs from seropositive donors are at high risk for toxoplasmosis.[133] In a small series of patients, prophylactic pyrimethamine (25 mg orally daily for 6 weeks post-transplant) prevented clinical disease and seroconversion in seronegative patients receiving heart transplants from seropositive donors.[134] Although pyrimethamine prophylaxis is not routinely administered at all centers, this therapy may be justified in high-risk patients due to the delays in diagnosis and serious consequences associated with toxoplasmosis.[96]

The use of prophylactic isoniazid (INH) therapy for transplant patients with evidence of exposure to *M. tuberculosis* (e.g., those with a positive purified protein derivative skin test) remains controversial. Risk of reactivation and development of clinical tuberculosis is enhanced with post-transplant immunosuppression. However, some clinicians believe that the risk of INH-induced hepatotoxicity, especially in liver transplant recipients, outweighs the benefits of treatment.

EVALUATION OF THERAPEUTIC OUTCOMES

The goals of antimicrobial drug use in solid organ transplant recipients include (1) prevention of infectious complications in the immediate postoperative period; (2) prevention of late infectious complications associated with prolonged periods of immunosuppression; and (3) effective treatment of established infections in order to prevent graft rejection and decrease patient morbidity and mortality. All of these goals should be achieved at the lowest possible toxicity and cost. Close monitoring of transplant recipients, including both clinical and laboratory data, is essential for early detection and treatment of potentially severe opportunistic infections. The reader is referred to individual chapters within this textbook for more detailed discussions of monitoring parameters related to specific types of infections.

CONCLUSION

Despite advances in diagnosis and treatment, infectious complications continue to cause significant morbidity and mortality in immunocompromised hosts. Health care providers involved in the care of these patients must maintain vigilance for changes in the epidemiology of infections and susceptibility patterns of pathogens, both locally and on a global level. Research into new treatment modalities such as biotechnologic products and safer, more potent antimicrobial agents is ongoing. Until these new treatments are available, however, judicious selection of existing agents in combination with comprehensive patient monitoring for drug efficacy and safety will improve outcomes in immunocompromised hosts.

REFERENCES

1. Bodey GP, Buckley M, Sathe YS, Freireich EJ. Quantitative relationships between circulating leukocytes and infection in patients with acute leukemia. Ann Intern Med 1966;64:328–340.
2. Hughes WT, Armstrong D, Bodey GP, et al. Guidelines for use of antimicrobial agents in neutropenic patients with unexplained fever. J Infect Dis 1990;161:381–396.
3. The EORTC International Antimicrobial Therapy Research Project Group. Three antibiotic regimens in treatment of infection in febrile granulocytopenic patients with cancer. J Infect Dis 1978;137:14–29.
4. Brown AE. Neutropenia, fever, and infection. Am J Med 1984;76:421–428.
5. Klastersky J, Glauser MP, Schimpff SC, et al. Prospective randomized comparison of three antibiotic regimens for empirical therapy of suspected bacteremic infection in febrile granulocytopenic patients. Antimicrob Agents Chemother 1986;29:263–270.
6. DeJongh CA, Joshi JH, Newman KA, et al. Antibiotic synergism and response in gram-negative bacteremia in granulocytopenic cancer patients. Am J Med 1986;80(suppl C):96–100.
7. Tauber AI. Current views of neutrophil dysfunction. Am J Med 1981;70:1237–1246.
8. Mandell LA. Effects of antimicrobial and antineoplastic drugs on the phagocytic and microbicidal function of the polymorphonuclear leukocyte. Rev Infect Dis 1982;4:683–697.
9. Koll BS, Brown AE. Changing patterns of infections in the immunocompromised patient with cancer. Hematol Oncol Clin North Am 1993;7:753–769.
10. Bodey GP. Infections in cancer patients: A continuing association. Am J Med 1986;81(suppl 1A):11–26.

11. Schimpff SC, Young VM, Greene WH, et al. Origin of infection in acute nonlymphocytic leukemia. Ann Intern Med 1972;77:707–714.
12. Schimpff SC. Surveillance cultures. J Infect Dis 1981;144:81–84.
13. Johanson WG, Pierce AK, Sanford JP. Changing pharyngeal bacterial flora of hospitalized patients. N Engl J Med 1969;281:1137–1140.
14. Newman KA, Schimpff SC, Young VM, Wiernik PH. Lessons learned from surveillance cultures in patients with acute nonlymphocytic leukemia. Am J Med 1981;70:423–431.
15. Van der Waaij D, Berghuis JM, Lekkerkerk JEC. Colonization resistance of the digestive tract of mice during systemic antibiotic treatment. J Hyg 1972;70:605–610.
16. Gross MH. Management of antibiotic-associated pseudomembranous colitis. Clin Pharm 1985;4:304–310.
17. Prod'hom G, Leuenberger P, Koerfer J, et al. Nosocomial pneumonia in mechanically ventilated patients receiving antacid, ranitidine, or sucralfate as prophylaxis for stress ulcer. A randomized controlled trial. Ann Intern Med 1993;120:653–662.
18. Talcott JA, Finberg R, Mayer RJ, Goldman L. The medical course of cancer patients with fever and neutropenia. Arch Intern Med 1988;148:2561–2568.
19. Hathorn JW, Rubin M, Pizzo PA. Empirical antibiotic therapy in the febrile neutropenic cancer patient: Clinical efficacy and impact of monotherapy. Antimicrob Agents Chemother 1987;31:971–977.
20. Pizzo PA. Management of fever in patients with cancer and treatment-induced neutropenia. N Engl J Med 1993;328:1323–1332.
21. Awada A, Van der Auwera P, Meunier F, et al. Streptococcal and enterococcal bacteremia in patients with cancer. Clin Infect Dis 1992;15:33–48.
22. Maschmeyer G. Use of the quinolones for the prophylaxis and therapy of infections in immunocompromised hosts. Drugs 1993;45(suppl 3):73–80.
23. Van der Auwera P, Gerain J. Use of the quinolones in the prophylaxis and treatment of granulocytopenic immunocompromised cancer patients. Drugs 1993;45(suppl 3):81–90.
24. Press OW, Ramsey PG, Larson EB, et al. Hickman catheter infections in patients with malignancies. Medicine 1984;63:189–200.
25. Wade JC, Schimpff SC, Newman KA, Wiernik PH. *Staphylococcus epidermidis:* An increasing cause of infection in patients with granulocytopenia. Ann Intern Med 1982;97:503–508.
26. Brown EA, Talbot GH, Provencher M, Cassileth P. Anaerobic bacteremia in patients with acute leukemia. Infect Control Hosp Epidemiol 1989;10:65–69.
27. Elting LS, Bodey GP, Fainstein V. Polymicrobial septicemia in the cancer patient. Medicine 1986;65:218–225.
28. Commers JR, Pizzo PA. Empiric antifungal therapy in the management of the febrile-granulocytopenic cancer patients. Pediatr Infect Dis 1983;2:56–60.
29. Owens NJ, Nightingale CH, Schweizer RT, et al. Prophylaxis of oral candidiasis with clotrimazole troches. Arch Intern Med 1984;144:290–293.
30. Thaler M, Pastakia B, Shawker TH, et al. Hepatic candidiasis in cancer patients: The evolving picture of the syndrome. Ann Intern Med 1988;108:88–100.
31. Gerson SL, Talbot GH, Hurwitz S, et al. Prolonged granulocytopenia: The major risk factor for invasive pulmonary aspergillosis in patients with acute leukemia. Ann Intern Med 1984;100:345–351.
32. Aisner J, Murillo J, Schimpff SC, Steere AC. Invasive aspergillosis in acute leukemia: Correlation with nose cultures and antibiotic use. Ann Intern Med 1979;90:4–9.
33. Saral R, Ambinder RF, Burns WH, et al. Acyclovir prophylaxis against herpes simplex virus infection in patients with leukemia. Ann Intern Med 1983;99:773–776.
34. Wade JC, Newton B, Flournoy N, Meyers JD. Oral acyclovir for prevention of herpes simplex virus reactivation after marrow transplantation. Ann Intern Med 1984;100:823–828.
35. Saral R, Burns WH, Laskin OL, et al. Acyclovir prophylaxis of herpes-simplex-virus infections. N Engl J Med 1981;305:63–67.
36. Hughes WT, Rivera GK, Schell MJ, et al. Successful intermittent chemoprophylaxis for *Pneumocystis carinii* pneumonitis. N Engl J Med 1987;316:1627–1632.
37. Sickles EA, Greene WH, Wiernik PH. Clinical presentation of infection in granulocytopenic patients. Arch Intern Med 1975;135:715–719.
38. Schimpff S, Satterlee W, Young VM, Serpick A. Empiric therapy with carbenicillin and gentamicin for febrile patients with cancer and granulocytopenia. N Engl J Med 1971;284:1061–1065.
39. Bodey GP, Jadeja L, Elting L. *Pseudomonas* bacteremia: Retrospective analysis of 410 episodes. Arch Intern Med 1985;145:1621–1629.
40. International Antimicrobial Therapy Project Group of the EORTC. Combination of amikacin and carbenicillin with or without cefazolin as empirical treatment of febrile neutropenic patients. J Clin Oncol 1983;1:597–603.
41. Pizzo PA, Hathorn JW, Hiemenz J, et al. A randomized trial comparing ceftazidime alone with combination antibiotic therapy in cancer patients with fever and neutropenia. N Engl J Med 1986;315:552–558.
42. Winston DJ, Ho WG, Bruckner DA, Champlin RE. Beta-lactam antibiotic therapy in febrile, granulocytopenic patients. A randomized trial comparing cefoperazone plus piperacillin, ceftazidime plus piperacillin, and imipenem alone. Ann Intern Med 1991;115:849–859.
43. Klastersky J, Zinner SH, Calandra T, et al. Empiric antimicrobial therapy for febrile granulocytopenic cancer patients: Lessons from four EORTC trials. Eur J Cancer Clin Oncol 1988;24(suppl 1):S35–S45.
44. Gilbert DN. Once-daily aminoglycoside therapy. Antimicrob Agents Chemother 1991;35:399–405.
45. Klastersky J, Cappel R, Daneau D. Clinical significance of *in vitro* synergism between antibiotics in gram-negative infections. Antimicrob Agents Chemother 1972;2:470–475.
46. Livermore DM. Clinical significance of β-lactamase induction and stable derepression in gram-negative rods. Eur J Clin Microbiol 1987;6:439–445.

47. Chow JW, Fine MJ, Shlaes DM, et al. *Enterobacter* bacteremia: Clinical features and emergence of antibiotic resistance during therapy. Ann Intern Med 1991;115:585–590.
48. Karp JE, Dick JD, Angelopulos C, et al. Empiric use of vancomycin during prolonged treatment-induced granulocytopenia. Am J Med 1986;81:237–242.
49. Rubin M, Hathorn JW, Marshall D, et al. Gram-positive infections and the use of vancomycin in 550 episodes of fever and neutropenia. Ann Intern Med 1988;108:30–35.
50. EORTC International Antimicrobial Therapy Cooperative Group and the National Cancer Institute of Canada–Clinical Trials Group. Vancomycin added to empirical combination antibiotic therapy for fever in granulocytopenic cancer patients. J Infect Dis 1991;163:951–958.
51. Gutmann L, Williamson R, Kitzis M-D, Acar JF. Synergism and antagonism in double β-lactam antibiotic combinations. Am J Med 1986;80(suppl 5C):21–29.
52. Lo WK, Rolston KVI, Rubenstein ED, Bodey GP. Ciprofloxacin-induced nephrotoxicity in patient with cancer. Arch Intern Med 1993;153:1258–1262.
53. Pizzo PA, Ladisch S, Robichaud K. Treatment of gram-positive septicemia in cancer patients. Cancer 1980;45:206–207.
54. Pizzo PA, Robichaud KJ, Gill FA, Witebsky FG. Empiric antibiotic and antifungal therapy for cancer patients with prolonged fever and granulocytopenia. Am J Med 1982;72:101–111.
55. Hiemenz J, Skelton J, Pizzo PA. Perspective on the management of catheter-related infections in cancer patients. Pediatr Infect Dis 1986;5:6–11.
56. Sable CA, Donowitz GR. Infections in bone marrow transplant recipients. Clin Infect Dis 1994;18:273–284.
57. Pizzo PA, Robichaud KJ, Gill FA, et al. Duration of empiric antibiotic therapy in granulocytopenic patients with cancer. Am J Med 1979;67:194–200.
58. Joshi JH, Schimpff SC, Tenney JH, et al. Can antibacterial therapy be discontinued in persistently febrile granulocytopenic cancer patients? Am J Med 1984;76:450–457.
59. Mullen CA, Buchanan GR. Early hospital discharge of children with cancer treated for fever and neutropenia: Identification and management of the low-risk patient. J Clin Oncol 1990;8:1998–2004.
60. Lieschke GJ, Burgess AW. Granulocyte colony-stimulating factor and granulocyte-macrophage colony-stimulating factor. Part I. N Engl J Med 1992;327:28–35; Part II. N Engl J Med 1992;327:99–106.
61. Roilides E, Pizzo PA. Modulation of host defenses by cytokines: Evolving adjuncts in prevention and treatment of serious infections in immunocompromised hosts. Clin Infect Dis 1992;15:508–524.
62. Schimpff SC. Infection prevention during profound granulocytopenia. New approaches to alimentary canal microbial suppression. Ann Intern Med 1980;93:358–361.
63. Buckner CD, Clift RA, Sanders JE, et al. Protective environment for marrow transplant patients. Ann Intern Med 1978;89:893–901.
64. Deitch EA, Winterton J, Berg R. Effect of starvation, malnutrition, and trauma on the gastrointestinal tract flora and bacterial translocation. Arch Surg 1987;122:1019–1024.
65. Pizzo PA, Robichaud KJ, Edwards BK, et al. Oral antibiotic prophylaxis in patients with cancer: A double-blind randomized placebo-controlled trial. J Pediatr 1983;102:125–133.
66. Hathorn JW. Critical appraisal of antimicrobials for prevention of infections in immunocompromised hosts. Hematol Oncol Clin North Am 1993;7:1051–1099.
67. Reents S, Goodwin SD, Singh V. Antifungal prophylaxis in immunocompromised hosts. Ann Pharmacother 1993;27:53–60.
68. Goodman JL, Winston DJ, Greenfield RA, et al. A controlled trial of fluconazole to prevent fungal infections in patients undergoing bone marrow transplantation. N Engl J Med 1992;326:845–851.
69. Wingard JR, Merz WG, Rinaldi MG, et al. Increase in *Candida krusei* infection among patients with bone marrow transplantation and neutropenia treated prophylactically with fluconazole. N Engl J Med 1991;325:1274–1277.
70. Beyer J, Schwartz S, Heinemann V, Siegert W. Strategies in prevention of invasive pulmonary aspergillosis in immunocompromised or neutropenic patients. Antimicrob Agents Chemother 1994;38:911–917.
71. Gold D, Corey L. Acyclovir prophylaxis for herpes simplex virus infection. Antimicrob Agents Chemother 1987;31:361–367.
72. Attal M, Schlaifer D, Rubie H, et al. Prevention of gram-positive infections after bone marrow transplantation by systemic vancomycin: A prospective randomized trial. J Clin Oncol 1991;9:865–870.
73. Meyers JD, Flournoy N, Thomas ED. Infection with herpes simplex virus and cell-mediated immunity after marrow transplant. J Infect Dis 1980;142:338–346.
74. Meyers JD, Reed EC, Shepp DH, et al. Acyclovir for prevention of cytomegalovirus infection and disease after allogeneic marrow transplantation. N Engl J Med 1988;318:70–75.
75. Meyers JD, Flournoy N, Thomas ED. Risk factors for cytomegalovirus infection after human marrow transplantation. J Infect Dis 1986;153:478–488.
76. Bowden RA, Sayers M, Flournoy N, et al. Cytomegalovirus immune globulin and seronegative blood products to prevent primary cytomegalovirus infection after marrow transplantation. N Engl J Med 1986;314:1006–1010.
77. Meyers JD. Infection in bone marrow transplant recipients. Am J Med 1986;81(suppl 1A):27–38.
78. Meyers JD, Flournoy N, Thomas ED. Nonbacterial pneumonia after allogeneic marrow transplantation: A review of 10 years' experience. Rev Infect Dis 1982;4:1119–1132.
79. Schmidt GM, Kovacs A, Zaia JA, et al. Ganciclovir/immunoglobulin combination therapy for the treatment of human cytomegalovirus-associated interstitial pneumonia in bone marrow allograft recipients. Transplantation 1988;46:905–907.
80. Reed EC, Bowden RA, Dandliker PS, et al. Treatment of cytomegalovirus pneumonia with ganciclovir and intravenous cytomegalovirus immunoglobulin in patients with bone marrow transplants. Ann Intern Med 1988;109:783–788.
81. Emanuel D, Cunningham I, Jules-Elysee K, et al. Cytomegalovirus pneumonia after bone marrow transplan-

tation successfully treated with the combination of ganciclovir and high-dose intravenous immune globulin. Ann Intern Med 1988;109:777–782.
82. Winston DJ, Ho WG, Cheng-Hsien L, et al. Intravenous immune globulin for prevention of cytomegalovirus infection and interstitial pneumonia after bone marrow transplantation. Ann Intern Med 1987;106:12–18.
83. Sullivan KM, Kopecky KJ, Jocum J, et al. Immunomodulatory and antimicrobial efficacy of intravenous immunoglobulin in bone marrow transplantation. N Engl J Med 1990;323:705–712.
84. Schmidt GM, Horak DA, Niland JC, et al. A randomized, controlled trial of prophylactic ganciclovir for cytomegalovirus pulmonary infection in recipients of allogeneic bone marrow transplants. N Engl J Med 1991;324:1005–1011.
85. Goodrich JM, Mori M, Gleaves CA, et al. Early treatment with ganciclovir to prevent cytomegalovirus disease after allogeneic bone marrow transplantation. N Engl J Med 1991;325:1601–1607.
86. Atkinson K, Storb R, Prentice RL, et al. Analysis of late infections in 89 long-term survivors of bone marrow transplantation. Blood 1979; 53:720–731.
87. Atkinson K, Meyers JD, Storb R, et al. Varicella-zoster infection after marrow transplantation for aplastic anemia or leukemia. Transplantation 1980;29:47–50.
88. Locksley RM, Flournoy N, Sullivan KM, Meyers JD. Infection with varicella-zoster after marrow transplantation. J Infect Dis 1985;152:1172–1181.
89. Shepp DH, Dandliker PS, Meyers JD. Treatment of varicella-zoster infection in severely immunocompromised patients. N Engl J Med 1986;314:208–212.
90. Ho M, Dummer JS, Peterson PK, Simmons RL. Infections in solid organ transplant recipients, in Mandell GL, Douglas RG Jr, Bennett JE (eds): Principles and Practice of Infectious Diseases, 3rd ed. New York, Churchill Livingstone, 1990, pp 2294–2303.
91. Dummer JS. Infectious complications of transplantation. Cardiovascular Clinics 1988;20(2):163–178.
92. Rubin RH, Wolfson JS, Cosimi AB, Tolkoff-Rubin NE. Infection in the renal transplant patient. Am J Med 1981;70:405–411.
93. Najarian JS, Fryd DS, Strand M, et al. A single institution, randomized, prospective trial of cyclosporine versus azathioprine-antithymocyte globulin for immunosuppression in renal allograft recipients. Ann Surg 1985;201:142–157.
94. The Canadian Multicentre Transplant Study Group. A randomized clinical trial of cyclosporine in cadaveric renal transplantation. N Engl J Med 1983;309:809–815.
95. European Multicentre Trial. Cyclosporin A as sole immunosuppressive agent in recipients of kidney allografts from cadaver donors. Lancet 1982;2:57–60.
96. Hofflin JM, Potasman I, Baldwin JC, et al. Infectious complications in heart transplant patients receiving cyclosporine and corticosteroids. Ann Intern Med 1987;106:209–216.
97. Ho M, Wajszczuk CP, Hardy A, et al. Infections in kidney, heart, and liver transplant recipients on cyclosporine. Trans Proc 983;15:2768–2772.
98. Hardy AM, Wajszczuk CP, Suffredini AF, et al. *Pneumocystis carinii* pneumonia in renal-transplant recipients treated with cyclosporine and steroids. J Infect Dis 1984;149:143–147.
99. Hooks MA. Tacrolimus, a new immunosuppressant—a review of the literature. Ann Pharmacother 1994;28:501–511.
100. Uemoto S, Tanaka K, Honda K, et al. Experience with FK506 in living-related liver transplantation. Transplantation 1993;55:288–292.
101. Armitage JM, Kormos RL, Morita S, et al. Clinical trial of FK506 immunosuppression in adult cardiac transplantation. Ann Thorac Surg 1992;54:205–211.
102. Mason JW, Stinson EB, Hunt SA, Schroeder JS, Rider AK. Infections after cardiac transplantation: Relation to rejection therapy. Ann Intern Med 1976;85:69–72.
103. Singh N, Dummer JS, Kusne S, et al. Infections with cytomegalovirus and other herpesviruses in 121 liver transplant recipients: Transmission by donated organ and the effect of OKT3 antibodies. J Infect Dis 1988;158:124–131.
104. Bia MJ, Andiman W, Gaudio K, et al. Effect of treatment with cyclosporine versus azathioprine on incidence and severity of cytomegalovirus infection posttransplantation. Transplantation 1985;40:610–614.
105. Pass RF, Whitley RJ, Diethelm AG, et al. Cytomegalovirus infection in patients with renal transplants: Potentiation by antithymocyte globulin and an incompatible graft. J Infect Dis 1980;142:9–17.
106. Kusne S, Dummer JS, Singh N, et al. Infections after liver transplantation: An analysis of 101 consecutive cases. Medicine 1988;67:132–143.
107. Norman DJ, Barry JM, Bennett WM, et al. The use of OKT3 in cadaveric renal transplantation for rejection that is unresponsive to conventional anti-rejection therapy. Am J Kid Dis 1988;11:90–93.
108. Wajszczuk CP, Dummer JS, Ho M, et al. Fungal infections in liver transplant recipients. Transplantation 1985;40:347–353.
109. Ramsey PG, Rubin RH, Tolkoff-Rubin NE, et al. The renal transplant patient with fever and pulmonary infiltrates: Etiology, clinical manifestations, and management. Medicine 1980;59:206–222.
110. Dummer JS, White LT, Ho M, et al. Morbidity of cytomegalovirus infection in recipients of heart or heart-lung transplants who received cyclosporine. J Infect Dis 1985;152:1182–1191.
111. Chou S. Neutralizing antibody responses to reinfecting strains of cytomegalovirus in transplant recipients. J Infect Dis 1990;160:16–21.
112. Rubin RH, Tolkoff-Rubin NE. The impact of infection on the outcome of transplantation. Transplant Proc 1991;23:2068–2074.
113. Ho M, Miller G, Atchison RW, et al. Epstein–Barr virus infections and DNA hybridization studies in posttransplantation lymphoma and lymphoproliferative lesions: The role of primary infection. J Infect Dis 1985;152:876–886.
114. Peterson PK, Balfour Jr HH, Marker SC, et al. Cytomegalovirus disease in renal allograft recipients: A prospective study of the clinical features, risk factors, and impact on renal transplantation. Medicine 1980;59:283–300.

115. Tolkoff-Rubin NE, Cosimi AB, Russell PS, Rubin RH. A controlled study of trimethoprim–sulfamethoxazole prophylaxis of urinary tract infection in renal transplant recipients. Rev Infect Dis 1982;4:614–618.
116. Dummer JS, Montero CG, Griffith BP, et al. Infections in heart-lung transplant recipients. Transplantation 1986;41:725–729.
117. Hooper DC, Pruitt AA, Rubin RH. Central nervous system infection in the chronically immunosuppressed. Medicine 1982;61:166–188.
118. Peterson PK, Andersen RC. Infection in renal transplant recipients. Am J Med 1986;81(suppl 1A):2–10.
119. Huang K-L, Armstrong JA, Ho M. Antibody response after influenza immunization in renal transplant patients receiving cyclosporin A or azathioprine. Infect Immun 1983;40:421–424.
120. Merigan TC, Renlund DG, Keay S, et al. A controlled trial of ganciclovir to prevent cytomegalovirus disease after heart transplantation. N Engl J Med 1992;326:1182–1186.
121. Hirsch MS, Schooley RT, Cosimi AB, et al. Effects of interferon-α on cytomegalovirus reactivation syndromes in renal-transplant patients. N Engl J Med 1983;308:1489–1493.
122. Balfour Jr HH, Chace BA, Stapleton JT, et al. A randomized, placebo-controlled trial of oral acyclovir for the prevention of cytomegalovirus disease in recipients of renal allografts. N Engl J Med 1980;320:1381–1387.
123. Singh N, Yu VL, Mieles L, et al. High-dose acyclovir compared with short-course preemptive ganciclovir therapy to prevent cytomegalovirus disease in liver transplant recipients. Ann Intern Med 1994;120:375–381.
124. Stratta RJ, Shaefer MS, Cushing KA, et al. Successful prophylaxis of cytomegalovirus disease after primary CMV exposure in liver transplant recipients. Transplantation 1991;51:90–97.
125. Snydman DR, Werner BG, Tilney NL, et al. Final analysis of primary disease prevention in renal transplant recipients with a cytomegalovirus-immune globulin: Comparison of the randomized and open-label trials. Transplant Proc 1991;23:1357–1360.
126. Schaefers H-J, Milbradt H, Flik J, et al. Hyperimmunoglobulin for cytomegalovirus prophylaxis following heart transplantation. Clin Transplantation 1988;2:51–56.
127. Saliba F, Arulnaden JL, Gugenheim J, et al. CMV hyperimmune globulin prophylaxis after liver transplantation: A prospective randomized controlled study. Transplant Proc 1989;21:2260–2262.
128. Rubin RH, Tolkoff-Rubin NE. Antimicrobial strategies in the care of organ transplant recipients. Antimicrob Agents Chemother 1993;37:619–624.
129. Smyth RL, Higenbottam TW, Scott JP, et al. Herpes simplex virus infection in heart–lung transplant recipients. Transplantation 1990;49:735–739.
130. Tillegard A. Renal transplant wound infection: The value of prophylaxis antibiotic treatment. Scand J Urol Nephrol 1984;18:215–221.
131. Kramer MR, Stoehr C, Lewiston NJ, et al. Trimethoprim–sulfamethoxazole prophylaxis for *Pneumocystis carinii* infections following heart-lung and lung transplantation—how effective and for how long? Transplantation 1992;53:586–589.
132. Wiesner RH, Hermans PE, Rakela J, et al. Selective bowel decontamination to decrease gram-negative aerobic bacterial and *Candida* colonization and prevent infection after orthotopic liver transplantation. Transplantation 1988;45:570–574.
133. Luft BJ, Naot Y, Araujo FG, et al. Primary and reactivated toxoplasma infection in patients with cardiac transplants. Ann Intern Med 1983;99:27–31.
134. Wreghitt TG, Hakim M, Cory-Pearce R, et al. The impact of donor-transmitted CMV and *Toxoplasma gondii* disease in cardiac transplantation. Trans Proc 1986;18:1375–1376.

Chapter 115

Antimicrobial Prophylaxis in Surgery

Stephen W. Janning, PharmD, and Michael J. Rybak, PharmD, FCCP, BCPS

Approximately 23 million surgical procedures are performed annually in the United States. The reported postoperative infection rate is about 6%.[1] This number increases by 50% when data captured by postdischarge wound surveillance are included.[2] Surgical wound infections (SWIs) prolong hospital stays at an estimated direct cost of more than $1.5 billion per year and account for almost one-quarter of all nosocomial infections.[1] Prophylactic antibiotics have been shown to decrease the risk of infection for many different procedures and thus represent an important component of optimal management of the surgical patient.

By definition, *prophylactic* antibiotics are administered prior to contamination of previously sterile tissues or fluids. The goal is to *prevent* an infection from developing. Eradication of a preexisting distal infection lowers postoperative infection risk, but does not constitute a prophylactic regimen. In fact, surgical prophylaxis is often prescribed concurrently under these circumstances due to spectrum and timing issues (see section on Timing of Antibiotics). Similarly, the prevention and management of postoperative complications (non-SWI) such as catheter-related urinary tract infections and atelectasis are important and occasionally require antibiotics, but that is not the goal of surgical prophylaxis.

Antibiotics that are given when there is a strong possibility, but as yet unproven, of established infection are termed *presumptive.* Examples include acute cholecystitis and acute appendicitis of less than 24 hours' duration. If no signs of perforation or infection are found during surgery, then only perioperative antibiotics are indicated. Operative findings of a gangrenous gallbladder or a perforated appendix, for example, mean that an established infection is present and *therapeutic* antibiotics are required.[3]

SWIs are classified as either incisional or deep. Incisional SWI is diagnosed when purulent or culture positive drainage is isolated from any structure above the fascia in proximity to the initial wound. Deep SWIs are characterized by purulent drainage from subfascial drains, wound dehiscence, or abscess formation and involve adjacent sites manipulated during surgery. Both types by definition occur by postoperative day 30. This period extends to 1 year in case of deep infection associated with prosthesis implantation. While culture and sensitivity testing of drainage material can yield important information, a negative culture does not rule out SWI.[4]

Risk Factors for Surgical Wound Infection

The incidence of SWI depends on numerous factors specific to either the procedure itself or the individual patient. The traditional classification system developed by the National Research Council (NRC) stratifying surgical procedures by infection risk is reproduced in Table 115.1.[5] According to the NRC data, the risk of SWI depends on the microbiology of the surgical site, the presence of established infection, the risk of contaminating previously sterile tissue during surgery, and perioperative events.[5,6] In general, the procedure classification determines whether antibiotics are indicated. It should be emphasized that the NRC wound classification for a specific procedure is determined intraoperatively and is influenced by surgical findings (e.g., gangrenous gallbladder) and events (e.g., major technique breaks).[3]

INTRINSIC PATIENT RISK

While the NRC classification adequately categorizes the SWI risk for specific procedures, it does not account for underlying patient risk factors. Many underlying disease states and conditions are known to increase SWI risk. Several, such as diabetes mellitus, chronic immunosuppressed states, and extremes in age cannot be modified and will always influence SWI risk assessment. Others factors, such as recent corticosteroid use, prolonged hospitalization, and perhaps obesity can be minimized by simply delaying or

TABLE 115.1. NATIONAL RESEARCH COUNCIL WOUND CLASSIFICATION, RISK OF SURGICAL WOUND INFECTION, AND INDICATION FOR ANTIBIOTICS

Classification	SWI Rate (%)	Criteria	Antibiotics
Clean	<2	No acute inflammation or transection of gastrointestinal, oropharyngeal, genitourinary, biliary, or respiratory tracts. Elective case, no technique break	Not indicated unless high-risk procedure[a] (? high-risk patient)
Clean–contaminated	<10	Controlled opening of aforementioned tracts with minimal spillage/minor technique break. Clean procedures performed emergently or with major technique breaks	Prophylactic antibiotics indicated
Contaminated	20	Acute, nonpurulent inflammation present. Major spillage/technique break during clean–contaminated procedure	Prophylactic antibiotics indicated
Dirty	40	Obvious preexisting infection present (abscess, pus, or necrotic tissue present)	Therapeutic antibiotics required

[a]High-risk procedures include implantation of prosthetic materials and other procedures where surgical wound infection is associated with high morbidity (see text).

proper scheduling of elective procedures.[4] Preexisting distal infections increase SWI rates and should be resolved prior to surgery whenever possible. Underlying malnutrition is associated with an increased rate of postoperative complications, including SWI. Attempts to improve outcome in this population with perioperative total parenteral nutrition have not shown any benefit.[7]

INDIVIDUALIZING RISK FOR SURGICAL WOUND INFECTION

Two large epidemiologic studies have been published that objectively quantify SWI risk based on both patient and procedure specific factors. The Study on the Efficacy of Nosocomial Infection Control (SENIC) analyzed >100,000 surgery cases in order to identify and validate risk factors for SWI.[8] Abdominal operations, operations lasting >2 hours, contaminated or dirty procedures by NRC classification, and >3 underlying medical diagnoses were associated with increased incidence of SWI. When the NRC classification was stratified by the number of SENIC risk factors present, the infection rates varied by as much as a factor of 15 within the same operative category (Table 115.2).[2]

The National Nosocomial Infections Surveillance System (NNIS) published the results of a similar analysis of >84,000 cases that simplifies and refines the SENIC system.[9] Intrinsic patient risk was quantified using the American Society of Anesthesiologists (ASA) preoperative assessment score (Table 115.3).[10] An ASA score of ≥3 was associated with increased SWI risk. Other risk factors identified include operations classified as contaminated or dirty by NRC, and procedures longer than *T* hours, where *T* varies according to the specific procedure performed (for example, greater than 2 hours for a cholecystectomy). Again, the SWI rate was linked to the number of risk factors present and varied considerably within NRC class (Fig. 115.1).

Appropriate antimicrobial prophylaxis during surgery is best established by the results of randomized clinical trials. Studies currently available do not stratify according to overall SWI risk. Recognition of high-risk patients will help identify situations when antibiotic prophylaxis should be used for clean procedures. Future studies, particularly those involving clean procedures, should be stratified so high-risk patients who might benefit from prophylaxis can be identified.

REDUCING SURGICAL WOUND INFECTION RISK

Although appropriate antibiotics are crucial in lowering SWI risk for many surgical procedures, other effective measures can also be taken. Prolonged hospitalization is associated with colonization of (and, occasionally, infection with)

TABLE 115.2. SURGICAL WOUND INFECTION INCIDENCE (%) STRATIFIED BY NATIONAL RESEARCH COUNCIL WOUND CLASSIFICATION AND SENIC RISK FACTORS[a]

No. of SENIC Risk Factors	Clean	Clean–Contaminated	Contaminated	Dirty
0	1.1	0.6	N/A	N/A
1	3.9	2.8	4.5	6.7
2	8.4	8.4	8.3	10.9
3	15.8	17.7	11.0	18.8
4	N/A	N/A	23.9	27.4

[a]SENIC risk factors include abdominal operation, operations lasting >2 hours, contaminated or dirty procedures by NRC classification, and >3 underlying medical diagnoses.
(Adapted from Ref. 2.)

TABLE 115.3. AMERICAN SOCIETY OF ANESTHESIOLOGISTS PHYSICAL STATUS CLASSIFICATION

Class	Description
1	Normal healthy patient
2	Mild systemic disease
3	Severe systemic disease that is not incapacitating
4	Incapacitating systemic disease that is a constant threat to life
5	Not expected to survive 24 hours with or without operation

(From Ref. 10, with permission.)

nosocomial bacteria, which increases the incidence of SWI. For this reason, elective surgery is often postponed if the patient is hospitalized for an unrelated medical problem. Shaving the incision site with a razor the day before surgery is associated with higher infection rates. Clipping the operative site just prior to the procedure is preferred. Preoperative showering with an antiseptic soap may also lower infection rates.[4]

Recognizing the importance of maintaining sterile technique was a major advance in the evolution of surgery.

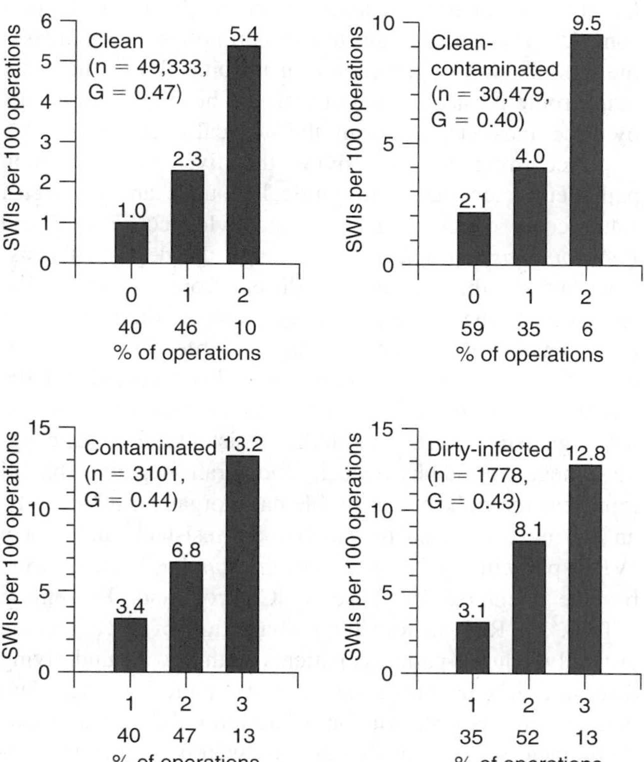

Figure 115.1. SWI rates, by traditional wound classification and risk index. G, Goodman–Kruskal correlation coefficient. *(From Culver DH, Horan TC, Gaynes RP, et al. Surgical wound infection rates by wound class, operative procedure, and patient risk index. Am J Med 1991;91(suppl 3B):155S. Reprinted with permission from American Journal of Medicine Supplement.)*

Enhancing the sterility of the operating room by using ultraviolet light or a laminar air flow system has been attempted but does not consistently reduce infection risk. Unnecessary prolongation of the surgical procedure results in a higher incidence of SWI, possibly due to subtherapeutic antibiotic concentrations.[11] Placement of open (Penrose) drains instead of closed suction drains (Jackson–Pratt) increases SWI rates.

Microbiology

Since the premise for surgical prophylaxis is protection from infection, the type of antibiotic prophylaxis required depends on the most likely anticipated pathogens. Organisms involved in SWI are either acquired from the patient's normal flora (endogenous) or from contamination during the surgical procedure (exogenous). Based on the type of procedure, NRC classification (Table 115.1), and body location, resident flora can be anticipated (Fig. 115.2) and appropriate antibiotic choices can be made.

The ability of an organism to cause SWI depends on a variety of factors that include the virulence of the organism, the number of organisms involved, and the general condition of the host immune system. The majority of organisms that make up the commensal flora are generally not pathogenic and in fact serve the host as a form of protection against more invasive organisms that would otherwise colonize the tissue site. These opportunistic organisms, although more problematic to the host in large numbers, are kept in check by the normal flora. Therefore, loss of these protective flora via antibiotics can upset the balance and allow pathogenic bacteria to proliferate and increase infectious risk. Normal flora can become pathogenic when translocated to a normally sterile tissue site or fluid during surgical procedures. Examples of this phenomenon would be the translocation of *Staphylococcus aureus* or *S. epidermidis* from the surface of the skin to deeper tissues and *Escherichia coli* from the colon to the peritoneal cavity, bloodstream, or urinary tract. Studies in animals and healthy volunteers have shown that the number of organisms acquired during bacterial contamination of the surgical wound is important in determining the incidence of secondary infection.[12–14] In the past, animal models of infection have demonstrated that more than 1,000,000 *S. aureus* per square centimeter or gram of tissue are required to produce infection in a small clean wound site. However, less than 100,000 of *Streptococcus pyogenes* per square centimeter or gram are required to produce infection because of its more virulent nature.[13,14]

Compromises in host defenses reduce the number of bacteria required to establish infection. Obviously, any alteration of normal host defenses through surgical intervention (i.e., breach of skin or mucous membrane barriers, prosthetic devices) may potentiate the ability of organisms

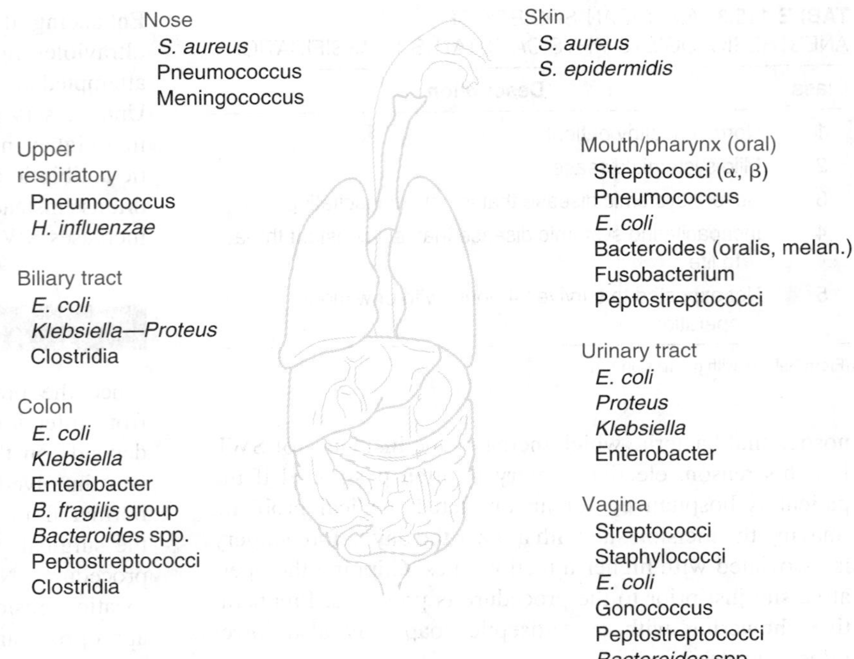

Figure 115.2. Pathogens regularly found at various body sites. *(From Condon RW, Wittman DH. The use of antibiotics in general surgery. Curr Probl Surg 1991;28:802–907, with permission.)*

to cause infection. Loss of specific immune factors such as complement activation, tissue-derived inhibitors, cell-mediated response (T cell, etc.) and granulocytic or phagocytic function (neutrophils, macrophages) can greatly increase the risk of SWI.[15,16] In addition, vascular occlusive states from the surgical procedure or those occurring from hypovolemic shock and/or the use of vasopressors can greatly affect the blood flow to the surgical site, diminishing much of the host's ability to defend against microbial invasion.[17] The presence of traumatized tissue, hematomas, and foreign material also enhances the potential infection.[17,18] When a foreign body is introduced during a surgical procedure, fewer than 100 bacterial colony-forming units (CFUs) are required to cause a wound infection.[18] Recent experiments with polytetrafluoroethylene tissue cages and vascular grafts have demonstrated the ability of *S. aureus* to produce wound infections when given a suitable niche sequestered from normal host defenses.[14,18,19] Studies carried out with *S. aureus* contaminated sutures in the skin of healthy volunteers demonstrated a 10,000-fold reduction in the amount of organism required to establish a wound infection compared to wound induced without sutures.[12]

Resistant Microorganisms

All organisms have the potential to become antibiotic resistant. Resistant organisms causing surgical infections can be acquired from the hospital setting prior to the surgical intervention through recolonization of the host with antibiotic resistant hospital flora. Epidemiologic studies have indicated that nosocomial acquired multiresistant organisms are largely transmitted to patients via the hands of hospital personnel.[20] The concomitant use of antibiotics also increases the colonization of patients with hospital flora. The other major route for acquisition of resistant hospital flora occurs by direct introduction during the surgical intervention.

According to the NNIS, the five most common pathogens encountered in surgical wounds are *S. aureus,* Enterococci, coagulase-negative staphylococci, *E. coli,* and *Pseudomonas aeruginosa.*[21] Although the degree of resistance among these pathogens differs from one institution to another, the increased frequency of these resistant pathogens being implicated in surgical infections is of concern. Since the cephalosporins have been considered the workhorse for prophylactic antibiotics, cephalosporin-resistant organisms such as methicillin-resistant *S. aureus,* coagulase-negative staphylococci, and gram-negative bacilli represent the bulk of the problematic organisms. Recently, an alarming increase in vancomycin-resistant enterococci (VRE) particularly *Enterococcus faecium* has been reported by the Centers for Disease Control and Prevention (CDC).[21,22] Risk factors for colonization of VRE include critically injured patients, patients with severe underlying diseases, immunosuppression, ICU patients, transplant patients, and patients who have had intra-abdominal or cardiothoracic surgical procedures, indwelling catheters, central venous lines, and prolonged courses of antimicrobials including vancomycin.[22,23] The CDC has published recommendations to control the spread of VRE including the restriction of routine prophylaxis with vancomycin.[22] Vancomycin may be substituted for cefazolin in institutions where methicillin-resistant *S. aureus* are prevalent.[24] Caution must be observed with the routine use of vancomycin as a prophylactic agent, however, since there are a number of drawbacks associated with this antibiotic, including the lack of broad-spectrum coverage, potential for resistance development, and the increased prevalence of adverse reactions including infusion-related problems.[24]

In cases involving methicillin-sensitive *S. aureus,* cefazolin failure has been reported in patients undergoing cardiac surgery. In a comparison trial with cefamandole and cefuroxime, significantly more failures were attributed to cefazolin even though the primary pathogen was methicillin-sensitive *S. aureus.* It has been proposed that the β-lactamase expressed by these organisms hydrolyzes cefazolin more readily than cefuroxime or cefamandole. Although this information is disturbing, the overall incidence of cefazolin failure is low. Cefazolin remains a mainstay in cardiovascular surgical procedures.[25,26] Lastly, an increased frequency of fungal infections in surgical patients has drawn increasing concern. The increased incidence of fungal infections in surgical patients is likely due to overzealous use of broad-spectrum antibiotics. There are no current recommendations for the use of prophylactic antifungal agents at this time.[27,28]

Timing of Antibiotics

The basic principles for the use of antimicrobial surgical prophylaxis include (1) antimicrobials should be delivered to the targeted tissue site prior to the initial incision, (2) bactericidal antibiotic tissue concentrations should be maintained throughout the length of the surgical procedure, and (3) distal infections should be eradicated prior to the procedure. Animal and human models have demonstrated the efficacy of a single dose of an antibiotic when administered just prior to bacterial contamination.[29,31] However, considerable debate exists over the importance of administering subsequent postoperative doses.[30,31] It is difficult to predict the exact moment of bacterial contamination during a procedure, however, the greatest risk probably occurs during the closing of the wound. Studies in patients undergoing

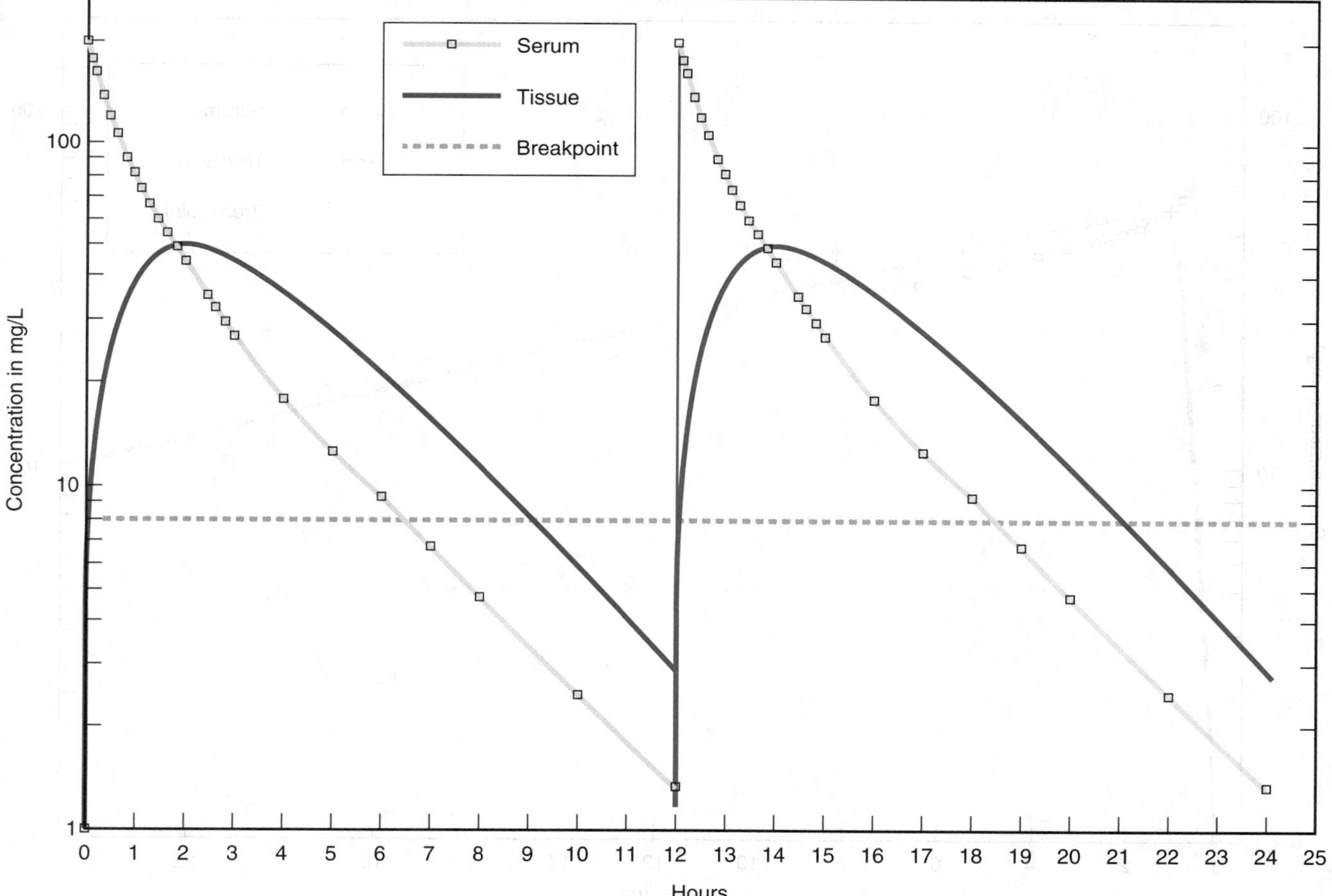

Figure 115.3. Serum and tissue fluid concentrations of cefazolin following short IV infusions of 2 grams every 12 hours. *(From Condon RW, Wittman DH. The use of antibiotics in general surgery. Curr Probl Surg 1991;28:802–907, with permission.)*

cardiac surgery have demonstrated a higher infection rate among patients with undetectable antibiotic serum concentrations at the close of surgery.[32]

The question of whether a single or multiple preoperative doses are required to ensure adequate protection depends on a number of factors. The ideal prophylactic antibiotic would rapidly achieve tissue concentrations well above the minimum inhibitory concentration (MIC) of the potential contaminating pathogens and maintain therapeutic concentrations throughout the procedure after a single preoperative dose. Therefore, theoretically, antimicrobials with long half-lives would be preferable to ensure sustained tissue concentrations. Antimicrobials with short serum half-lives may require multiple dosing at frequent dosing intervals, especially if the surgery is prolonged or in instances of massive blood loss. Studies examining serum concentrations secondary to intravenous administration of antibiotics with different pharmacokinetic profiles have demonstrated variability in achieved and sustained antimicrobial concentrations.[11]

Figures 115.3 and 115.4 illustrate typical serum and tissue concentrations after cefazolin and vancomycin IV administration to a patient with normal renal function. MIC breakpoints of 8 μg/mL for cefazolin and 5 μg/mL for vancomycin were chosen to represent a reasonable target tissue concentration that would provide protection against most common pathogens. Under ideal conditions, the antibiotic chosen for surgical prophylaxis would achieve its highest tissue concentrations at the time of initial skin incision during surgery. Antibiotics administered too early or after skin incision would likely achieve subtherapeutic concentrations putting the patient at high risk of infection.[11,30] In a recent study examining the timing of antibiotics in 2847 patients receiving prophylaxis, Classen et al.[30] evaluated patients who received prophylaxis early (2–24 hours), preoperative (0–2 hours) prior to surgery, perioperative (up to 3 hours after incision), and postoperatively (>3 hours after incision). The risk of infection was lowest (0.6%) for those patients who received preoperative prophylaxis, moderate (1.4%) for those who received perioperative antibiotics, and greatest for those who received postoperative antibiotics (3.3%) or too early preoperatively (3.8%). The results indicated that the risk of infection increased dramatically with each hour postsurgical incision until antibiotics are admin-

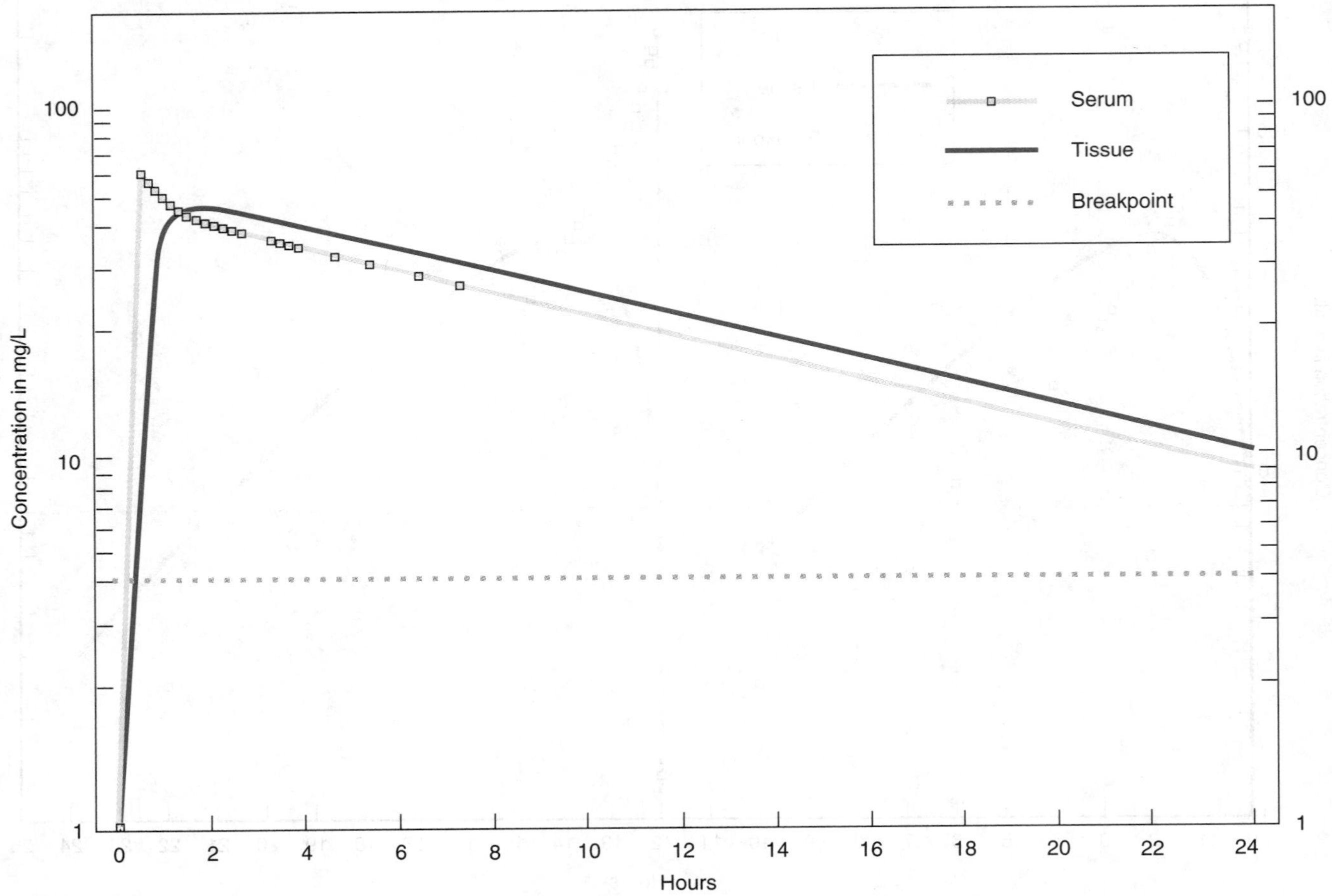

Figure 115.4. Serum and tissue fluid concentrations following a short IV infusion of 1 gram of vancomycin. *(From Condon RW, Wittman DH. The use of antibiotics in general surgery. Curr Probl Surg 1991;28:802–907, with permission.)*

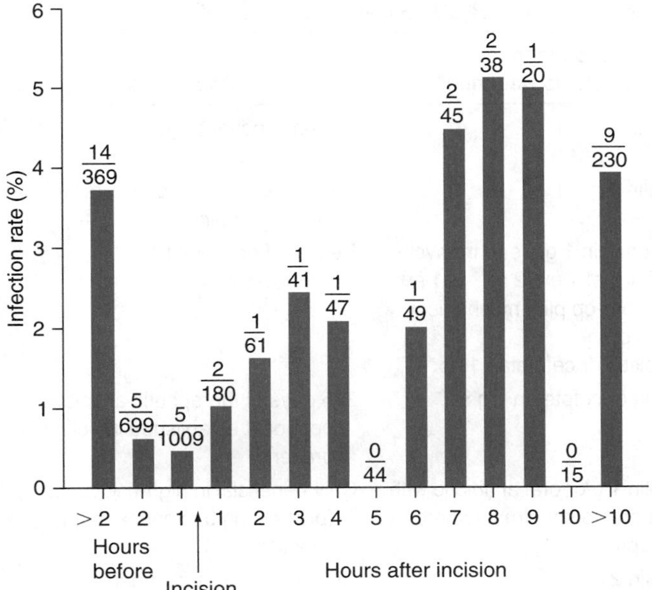

Figure 115.5. Rates of SWI corresponding to the temporal relation between antibiotic administration and the start of surgery. The number of infections and the number of patients for each hourly interval appear as the numerator and denominator, respectively, of the fraction for that interval. The trend toward higher rates of infection for each hour that antibiotic administration was delayed after the surgical incision was significant (z score = 2.00; $P < 0.05$ by the Wilcoxon test). *(From Classen DC, Evans RS, Pestotnik SL, et al. The timing of prophylactic administration of antibiotics and the risk of surgical wound infection. N Engl J Med 1992;326:281–286. Reprinted by permission of* The New England Journal of Medicine. *Copyright 1992, Massachusetts Medical Society.)*

istered (Fig. 115.5).[30] Additional considerations in the selection and timing of antibiotic administration should include the underlying disease states of the patient with regards to circulation, metabolism, and elimination of antibiotics. Patients with thermal burn and spinal cord injuries have been shown to eliminate certain classes of antibiotics, primarily the aminoglycosides and β-lactams, at unusually high rates compared to controls.[33–35] Individuals undergoing cardiac bypass may have altered antibiotic disposition and may require special consideration.[36–38]

Antimicrobial Selection

The choice of the prophylactic antimicrobial depends on a multitude of factors, including the type of surgical procedure, most likely pathogenic organisms, the safety and efficacy of the antimicrobial, the track record for success based on published literature, and costs. Although most surgical infections involve the patient's own flora, the selection of the antimicrobial must also take into account the susceptibility patterns of nosocomial-derived pathogens associated with the specific institution. Typically gram-positive coverage is included in the choice of surgical prophylaxis since organisms such as *S. aureus* and *S. epidermidis* are commonly encountered as skin flora. The decision to broaden coverage to gram-negatives and anaerobic organisms is site specific (e.g., upper respiratory tract, gastrointestinal tract, genitourinary tract etc., Table 115.4) and depends on whether the operation will transect a hollow viscous or mucous membrane containing resident flora.[39]

Although a variety of antimicrobial prophylactic administration routes (oral, topical, intramuscular, etc.) are advocated, intravenous is favored because of its reliability in achieving suitable tissue concentrations.[11] As previously mentioned, the cephalosporin class of compounds is by far the most often prescribed class of agents for surgical prophylaxis. This is justified by the antimicrobial spectrum, the favorable pharmacokinetic profile, the low incidence of unwanted side effects, and the pharmacoeconomic advantages. It is commonly accepted that first-generation cephalosporins are the preferred choice (as good as second- or third-generation cephalosporins) for surgical prophylaxis. Cefazolin continues to dominate as the drug of choice for most clean surgical procedures.[26] Although there are some reports of failure with cefazolin in cardiac procedures associated with methicillin-sensitive *S. aureus,* the majority of concern is due to the increasing incidence of methicillin-resistant *S. aureus* (MRSA) infections.[26,40,41] Vancomycin would seem to be a logical alternative to cefazolin in institutions with a high incidence of MRSA. However, its narrow spectrum of coverage, increased potential for toxicities, resistance development, and cost should limit its use to those procedures at highest risk or for patients with β-lactam allergy. In cases where broader gram-negative and anaerobic coverage is desired, the antianaerobic cephalosporins such as cefoxitin, cefotetan, and cefmetazole are appropriate. Although third-generation cephalosporins (e.g., ceftriaxone) have been advocated for prophylaxis because of the increased gram-negative coverage and prolonged half-lives, inferior gram-positive, anaerobic coverage, and high cost discourage widespread utilization of these agents for prophylaxis.[26,39,41] As previously mentioned, the side effects of cephalosporins are relatively minor in comparison to the overall benefit from their routine use. Side effects encountered include allergic reactions ranging from minor skin manifestations at the site of infusion, rash, and pruritus to anaphylaxis. Cross-reactivity from penicillins to cephalosporins is approximately 5%. Therefore, caution should be used when administering cephalosporin agents to individuals with history of a penicillin anaphylactic reaction.

The overall incidence of pseudomembranous colitis secondary to cephalosporins is infrequent and generally manageable with a short course of metronidazole or vancomycin. Although the incidence is relatively low, bleeding abnormalities secondary to cephalosporin use has been reported.[42] The primary hematologic effect appears to be an inhibition of normal platelet function and the coagulation cascade. These effects are reflected by changes in bleeding times and increases in prothrombin time and activated par-

TABLE 115.4. MOST LIKELY PATHOGENS AND SPECIFIC RECOMMENDATIONS FOR SURGICAL PROPHYLAXIS

Type of Operation	Likely Pathogens	Recommended Prophylaxis Regimen[a]	Comments
Gastroduodenal	Enteric gram-negative bacilli, gram-positive cocci, oral anaerobes	Cefazolin 1 g × 1	High-risk patients only
Biliary tract	Enteric gram-negative bacilli, enterococci, clostridia	Cefazolin 1 g × 1	Bactobilia does not correlate well with pathogens
Colorectal	Enteric gram-negative bacilli, anaerobes	PO: neomycin 1 g + erythromycin base 1 g at 1 PM, 2 PM, + 11 PM 1 day pre-op plus mechanical bowel prep IV: cefoxitin or cefotetan 1 g × 1	Benefit of oral plus IV is controversial
Appendectomy	Enteric gram-negative bacilli, anaerobes	Cefoxitin or cefotetan 1 g × 1	3–5 days of therapeutic antibiotics post-op if established infection present
Urologic	*E. coli*	Cefazolin 1 g or oral antibiotic with comparable spectrum (where appropriate) × 1	Only beneficial in high-risk cases (preexisting bacteriuria, high infection rate)
Cesarean section	Enteric gram-negative bacilli, anaerobes, group B streptococci, enterococci	Cefazolin 2 g × 1	Give after cord is clamped
Hysterectomy	Same as Cesarean section	Vaginal: cefazolin 1 g × 1, may repeat q8h × 2 doses Abdominal: cefazolin 1 g × 1	Beneficial in abdominal hysterectomy regardless of risk
Head and neck	*S. aureus,* streptococci, oral anaerobes	Cefazolin 2 g or clindamycin 600 mg at induction and q8h × 2 more doses	Addition of gentamicin to clindamycin is controversial
Cardiac	*S. aureus, S. epidermidis,* corynebacterium, enteric gram-negative bacilli	Cefazolin 1 g q8h × 48 hours beginning at induction	Second-generation cephalosporins have been advocated; controversial
Vascular	*S. aureus, S. epidermidis,* enteric gram-negative bacilli	Cefazolin 1 g at induction and q8h × 2 more doses	Abdominal and lower extremity procedures have highest infection rate
Orthopedic	*S. aureus, S. epidermidis*	Joint replacement: cefazolin 1 g × 1 pre-op, then q8h × 2 more doses Hip fracture repair: same except continue for 48 hours total	Open fractures assumed contaminated with gram-negative bacilli; aminoglycosides often used—see text
Neurosurgery	*S. aureus, S. epidermidis*	Cefazolin 1 g × 1	Use in CSF shunting procedures is controversial

[a]One-time doses are optimally infused at induction of anesthesia except as noted. Repeat doses may be required for long procedures. See text for references.

tial thromboplastin time. The mechanism is thought to be related to α-carboxyl substitution on the β-lactam molecule or the methylthiotetrazole (NMTT) side chain of some agents, particularly cefamandole and cefotetan. Most data indicate that patients at greatest risk have received multiple doses of these agents and have underlying risk factors such as vitamin K-deficient hypoprothrombinemia.[43] Infusion-related side effects such as thrombophlebitis and hypotension, particularly with vancomycin, can usually be controlled by adequate dilution and slower administration rates.[44–46] Since prophylactic antibiotic use represents a major potential for antibiotic resistance development and usually accounts for most of the antibiotic budget, curtailing inappropriate prophylactic use has become a focus point for most institutions. Inappropriate antibiotic prophylaxis includes the use of broader spectrum antimicrobials when a specific targeted spectrum is preferred, continuing prophylaxis beyond the standard recommendations of one to three doses of antibiotic coverage, and the use of more costly antibiotics when equivalent, less expensive agents are available. The most effective tools for control of prophylactic antibiotics are knowledge of the institution's post-surgical infection rate for each type of procedure, bacterial epidemiology studies, protocols which focus on control of problem pathogens, and institution-based antibiotic susceptibility data broken down for each surgical area within the hospital. With this information in hand, formulary selection, criteria for use, and policies governing surgical prophylaxis can be drafted with surgical attending staff involvement.

Recommendations for Specific Types of Surgery

Traditionally, recommendations for surgical prophylaxis have been grouped according to which tissues will be manipulated during surgery. This is a logical approach because, although many different surgical procedures can be performed at a given location, features such as endogenous flora and the pharmacokinetics, pharmacodynamics, and spectrum of selected antimicrobials are constant (see section on Antimicrobial Selection). The reader is reminded that prophylactic regimens are best evaluated through the results of properly conducted clinical trials. In the absence of data specific to the procedure in question, regimens appropriate for the anatomic site involved should suffice. Subsequent modifications are based on intraoperative findings or events.

A comprehensive review of the surgical prophylaxis literature is beyond the scope of this chapter. What follows is a brief discussion of the issues pertinent to the types of surgical procedures most frequently encountered. Specific recommendations are summarized in Table 115.4. The reader is also referred to the reviews published by the Surgical Infection Society[3] and the American Society of Hospital Pharmacists Commission on Therapeutics.[41] The latter document includes a comprehensive bibliography with primary references.

GASTRODUODENAL SURGERY

Due to their relative acidity, the stomach and the duodenum normally contain insignificant numbers of bacteria. Therefore, the rate of SWI is generally low ("clean" procedure). The risk rises with concurrent conditions associated with abnormally alkaline pH and subsequent bacterial overgrowth such as obstruction, hemorrhage, malignancy, or acid suppression therapy ("clean–contaminated").[47] Antimicrobial prophylaxis has been shown to be beneficial. A single dose of intravenous cefazolin will provide adequate prophylaxis for most cases.[48,49] Postoperative antibiotics may be indicated if perforation is detected during surgery, depending on whether an established infection is present.

BILIARY TRACT SURGERY

Antibiotic prophylaxis has been proven beneficial for surgery involving the biliary tract. The bile is normally sterile and in the absence of any other underlying risk factors, the SWI rate is low. However, bile contamination (bactobilia) occurs with many concurrent conditions such as acute cholecystitis, biliary obstruction, and advanced age. Bactobilia is associated with a higher frequency of SWI.[50] Most frequently encountered organisms include *E. coli, Klebsiella,* and *enterococci. Pseudomonas* is an uncommon finding in the absence of cholangitis. The correlation between bactobilia in surgical specimens and subsequent pathogens implicated in SWI is poor and may explain the lack of a detectable difference in comparative studies involving antibiotics with different spectrums.[51] Single-dose prophylaxis with cefazolin is currently recommended.

Some surgeons use *presumptive* antibiotics for cases of acute cholecystitis or cholangitis and defer surgery until the patient is afebrile in an attempt to decrease infection rates further, but this practice is controversial. Detection of an active infection during surgery (gangrenous gallbladder, suppurative cholangitis) is an indication for *therapeutic* postoperative antibiotics. In either case, antibiotics with additional antianaerobic activity (e.g., cefoxitin or cefotetan) are indicated.[52]

COLORECTAL SURGERY

Bacterial counts in fecal material present in the colon frequently exceed 10^9 per gram. Anaerobes and gram-negative aerobes predominate, although gram-positive aerobes are also important (Table 115.4). Therefore, the risk of SWI in the absence of an adequate prophylactic regimen is substantial. Reducing this bacteria load with a thorough bowel preparation regimen (4 liters of polyethylene glycol solution administered orally the day before surgery) is the single most important method to prevent SWI.

Effective antibiotic prophylaxis reduces SWI risk even further. Specific recommendations are listed in Table 115.4. Several oral regimens designed to reduce bacterial counts in the colon have been studied. The combination of 1 gram of neomycin plus 1 gram of erythromycin base given orally 19, 18, and 9 hours preoperatively is the most commonly used regimen in the United States. Neomycin is poorly absorbed and provides high intralumen concentrations effective against most gram-negative aerobes. Oral erythromycin is partially absorbed, but still produces concentrations in the colon sufficient to suppress the involved anaerobes. If surgery is postponed, the antibiotics must be redosed to maintain efficacy. It is worth noting that elective colorectal surgery is the only procedure where oral antibiotics have consistently been shown to provide effective prophylaxis.[53] Patients who cannot take oral medications should receive parenteral antibiotics (Table 115.4). Whether perioperative parenteral antibiotics, in addition to the standard preoperative oral antibiotic regimen, will lower SWI rates further still is controversial.[54,55] Postoperative antibiotics are unnecessary in the absence of any untoward events or findings during surgery.

APPENDECTOMY

Appendectomy is one of the most frequently performed abdominal procedures. A multitude of different antibiotic regimens with activity against gram-positive and gram-negative aerobes plus anaerobes have been studied and found to be effective in reducing the incidence of SWI. A cephalosporin with antianaerobic activity such as cefoxitin or cefotetan is currently recommended as first-line therapy.[56] Selection of an antibiotic with an unnecessarily broad spectrum (i.e., *Pseudomonas*) does not further reduce SWI risk,[57] but may increase cost of therapy and promote resistance. Single-dose therapy is adequate as long as the appendix is not found to be gangrenous or perforated during surgery.[56] Established intra-abdominal infections require appropriate *therapeutic* postoperative antibiotics.

UROLOGIC PROCEDURES

The most important risk factor for development of a SWI after urologic surgery is the presence of preoperative bacteriuria. It is therefore imperative to test for bacteriuria prior to the procedure and to administer *therapeutic* antibiotics as necessary. As long as the urine is sterile preoperatively, the risk of SWI after urologic procedures is very low and the benefit of *prophylactic* antibiotics in this setting is controversial.[58] This is further obscured by the frequent presence of urinary catheters in the postoperative period and the subsequent risk of bacteriuria independent of any risk accrued from the surgery itself. Specific recommendations are listed in Table 115.4. *Escherichia coli* is the most frequently encountered organism. Routinely expanding the spectrum by using a third-generation cephalosporin or a fluoroquinolone does not lower SWI rates any further and is not recommended. Single-dose therapy is adequate: Regimens as long as 3 weeks have been reported, but this is probably unnecessary. Urologic procedures requiring an abdominal approach such as a nephrectomy or cystectomy require prophylaxis appropriate for a clean–contaminated abdominal procedure.[3]

CESAREAN SECTION

Cesarean section is the most frequently performed surgical procedure in the United States. Previously, antibiotics were felt to be beneficial only in patients considered at "high risk," such as in emergency cases, premature rupture of membranes, or those who did not receive prenatal care. However, several large trials and a recent meta-analysis have documented the efficacy of antibiotics for all women undergoing cesarean section regardless of underlying risk factors. Prophylactic antibiotics are given to avoid SWI and prevent endometritis. Several types of bacteria have been implicated (Table 115.4). Despite this, cefazolin remains the drug of choice. Providing a broader spectrum by using cefoxitin against anaerobes or piperacillin for better coverage against *Pseudomonas* or *enterococci,* for example, does not lower postoperative infection rates any further in comparative studies.

Unlike most surgical procedures, a single 2-gram dose of cefazolin has been found to be superior to a 1-gram dose and is thus recommended.[59] Another distinctive feature is that unlike most operations (see section on Timing), antibiotics are given *after* the incision is made. Administering the antibiotic just after the umbilical cord is clamped avoids exposing the infant to the drug and may actually lower rates of neonatal sepsis. Longer durations of therapy do not result in lower infection rates.

HYSTERECTOMY

The incidence of SWI after hysterectomy depends on the type of procedure performed. Due to the polymicrobial flora normally present at the operative site (Table 115.4), vaginal hysterectomies are associated with a high rate of postoperative infection when performed without the benefit of prophylactic antibiotics. As with cesarean sections, cefazolin is the drug of choice in spite of the involved microbiology.[60] Single-dose therapy should be adequate, but most reports used a 24-hour regimen.

Abdominal hysterectomy is not associated with bacterial contamination from the vaginal flora, and SWI rates are correspondingly lower. However, prophylactic antibiotics are still recommended regardless of underlying risk factors. Both cefazolin and antianaerobic cephalosporins (e.g., cefoxitin, cefotetan) have been studied extensively.[61,62] It is unclear which is superior, but in either case a course not exceeding 24 hours' duration is sufficient and, in fact, single-dose therapy has been effective.[62] As with other procedures, perioperative events and findings may require the use of *therapeutic* antibiotics after surgery.

HEAD AND NECK SURGERY

The use of prophylactic antibiotics during head and neck surgery depends on the type of procedure performed. Many, such as parotidectomy or a simple tooth extraction, are clean procedures by NRC definition and are associated with very low rates of SWI. As expected, surgical prophylaxis has not been proven to be beneficial in these circumstances.[63] However, head and neck procedures involving an incision through a mucosal layer (and therefore breaching primary immune system barriers) carry a high risk of SWI. The normal mouth flora is polymicrobic (see Table 115.4) as are SWIs after head and neck surgery. Anaerobes and gram-positive aerobes predominate. Specific recommendations for prophylaxis are listed in Table 115.4. While typical doses of cefazolin are ineffective for anaerobic infections, the 2-gram dose recommended produces concentrations high enough to be inhibitory to these organisms. A combination of clindamycin plus gentamicin has also been described.[64] It is unclear whether the addition of an aminoglycoside further reduces SWI risk since clindamycin alone has been shown to be effective.[65] A 24-hour duration has been used in most studies, but single-dose therapy may also be effective. There is no additional benefit in extending therapy beyond 24 hours.[64]

CARDIAC SURGERY

Although most cardiac surgeries are technically "clean" procedures, prophylactic antibiotics have been shown to lower rates of SWI. The substantial morbidity associated with SWI after cardiac surgery and the use of prosthetic implants further justify routine prophylaxis. The usual pathogens are skin flora (see Table 115.4) and, rarely, gram-negative enteric organisms. Cefazolin has been extensively studied and is currently considered the drug of choice.[66] Several studies and a recent meta-analysis have been published that advocate preferential use of a second-generation cephalosporin (cefuroxime, cefamandole) instead of cefazolin.[67] However, the significance of these findings is controversial due to numerous problems with study design, and cefazolin remains the standard of care (see section on Resistant Microorganisms). The accepted duration of prophylactic antibiotics after cardiac surgery is currently 48 hours. There is some evidence that 24 hours is sufficient. Extending therapy for 3–5 days does not lower SWI rates further.[66]

It may be necessary to use vancomycin in hospitals with a high incidence of SWI with MRSA. The need for vancomycin should be evaluated carefully as previously discussed.

NONCARDIAC VASCULAR SURGERY

As with cardiac surgery, most vascular surgery is considered "clean" by NRC criteria. Similarly, SWI in this setting results in extensive morbidity and mortality, especially when a prosthetic graft is involved. Prophylactic antibiotics are beneficial, especially in procedures involving the abdominal aorta and the lower extremities.[68,69] Again, *Staphylococci* and gram-negative enterics are the most likely pathogens. Twenty-four hours of prophylaxis with IV cefazolin is adequate. Topical therapy has also been proven to be effective, but is not currently considered first-line therapy.[68]

ORTHOPEDIC SURGERY

Although most orthopedic surgery is "clean" by definition, prophylactic antibiotics have been shown to be beneficial in cases involving implantation of prosthetic material (pins, plates, artificial joints).[70,71] Late-occurring infectious complications in particular result in substantial morbidity (and often require prosthesis removal for definitive management), further justifying prophylaxis. The most likely pathogens mirror those of other clean procedures and include *Staphylococci* and, infrequently, gram-negative aerobes. Again, cefazolin is the best studied antibiotic and is thus the drug of choice. Rates of SWI after total joint replacement are reduced with 24 hours of prophylactic antibiotics. They are also indicated for hip fracture surgery, but the current accepted duration is 48 hours. Patients suffering open (compound) fractures are especially susceptible to infection since contamination is almost always present. The use of antibiotics is *presumptive* under these circumstances. Cefazolin is often combined with an aminoglycoside in this setting, but controlled trials are lacking.[72] The duration of therapy is highly variable and depends on surgical findings during debridement and results of intraoperative cultures.[73] Established joint infections or osteomyelitis requires an extended course of *therapeutic* antibiotics.

NEUROSURGERY

The use of prophylactic antibiotics in neurosurgery is controversial. The rates of SWI after these clean operations are very low, but are associated with significant morbidity and mortality. Consequently, in contrast to the other clean procedures discussed previously, data demonstrating the benefit of prophylactic antibiotics in this setting are equivocal. A recent review and meta-analysis concluded that single doses of cefazolin or, where required, vancomycin (see section on Antimicrobial Selection) appear to lower SWI risk after craniotomy.[74,75] Conversely, studies performed on shunting procedures do not consistently show lower infection rates with antibiotic prophylaxis, although a recent meta-analysis suggests efficacy.[76]

CONCLUSION

Antimicrobial prophylaxis remains an important component of optimal surgical care. When prescribed properly, the incidence of SWIs can be substantially reduced. The following points need to be considered when designing appropriate regimens for surgical prophylaxis:

1. Intrinsic patient risk and type of surgical procedure performed determine the indication for prophylaxis. Further modifications may be necessary due to intraoperative events.
2. Proper timing of prophylactic antibiotics is crucial for efficacy.
3. Prolonged regimens increase cost and adverse effects without lowering SWI rates further.

4. First-generation cephalosporins remain the mainstay for antimicrobial prophylaxis for the vast majority of procedures (with the exception of abdominal surgery). Single-dose prophylaxis appears to be effective for many types of surgery.

REFERENCES

1. Wenzel RP. Preoperative antibiotic prophylaxis. N Engl J Med 1992;326:337–339.
2. Weigelt JA, Dryer D, Haley RW. The necessity and efficiency of wound surveillance after discharge. Arch Surg 1992;127:77–82.
3. Page CP, Bohnen JMA, Fletcher JR, et al. Antimicrobial prophylaxis for surgical wounds. Guidelines for clinical care. Arch Surg 1993;128:79–88.
4. Nichols RL. Surgical wound infection. Am J Med 1991;91(suppl 3B):54S–64S.
5. National Academy of Sciences—National Research Council. Postoperative wound infections: The influence of ultraviolet irradiation of the operating room and of various other factors. Ann Surg 1964;160:32–135.
6. Cruse PJE, Foord R. A five-year prospective study of 23,649 surgical wounds. Arch Surg 1973;107:206–210.
7. The Veterans Affairs Total Parenteral Nutrition Cooperative Study Group. Perioperative total parenteral nutrition in surgical patients. N Engl J Med 1991;325:525–532.
8. Haley RW, Culver DH, Morgan WM, et al. Identifying patients at high risk of surgical wound infection. A simple multivariate index of patient susceptibility and wound contamination. Am J Epidemiol 1985;121:206–215.
9. Culver DH, Horan TC, Gaynes RP, et al. Surgical wound infection rates by wound class, operative procedure, and patient risk index. Am J Med 1991;91(suppl 3B):152S–157S.
10. Owens WD, Felts JA, Spitznagel EL. ASA physical status classifications: A study of consistency of ratings. Anesthesiology 1978;49:239–243.
11. Condon RW, Wittman DH. The use of antibiotics in general surgery. Curr Probl Surg 1991;28:802–907.
12. Elek SD, Conen PE. The virulence of *Staphylococcus pyogenes* for man. A study of the problems of wound infection. Br J Exp Pathol 1958;38:573–586.
13. Burke JF. Identification of the sources of staphylococci contaminating the surgical wound during operation. Ann Surg 1963;158:898–904.
14. Kaiser AB, Kernodle DS, Parker RA. Low-inoculum model of surgical wound infection. J Infect Dis 1992;166:393–399.
15. Meakins JL, Pietsch JB, Bubenick O, et al. Delayed hypersensitivity: Indicator of acquired failure of host defenses in sepsis and trauma. Ann Surg 1977;186:241–250.
16. Christou NV, McLean APH, Meakins JL. Host defense in blunt trauma: Interrelationships of kinetics of anergy and depressed neutrophil function, nutritional status and sepsis. J Trauma 1980;20:833–841.
17. Richet HM, Chidiac C, Prat A, et al. Analysis of risk factors for surgical wound infections following vascular surgery. Am J Med 1991;91:(suppl 3b):170S–172S.
18. Zimmerli W, Waldvogel FA, Vaudaux P, et al. Pathogenesis of foreign body infection: Description and characteristics of an animal model. J Infect Dis 1987;146:487–497.
19. Arbeit RD, Dunn RM. Expression of capsular polysaccharide during experimental focal infection with *Staphylococcus aureus*. J Infect Dis 1987;156:947–952.
20. Schaberg D. Major trends in the microbial etiology of nosocomial infection. Am J Med 1991;91(suppl 3B):72S–75S.
21. Jarvis WR, Martone WJ. Predominant pathogens in hospital infections. J Antimicrob Chemother 1992;29(suppl A):19–24.
22. Centers for Disease Control and Prevention. Recommendations for preventing the spread of vancomycin resistance: Hospital Infection Control Practice Advisory Committee. Infect Control Hosp Epidemiol 1995;16:105–113.
23. Handwerger S, Raucher B, Altarac D, et al. Nosocomial outbreak due to *Enterococcus faecium* highly resistant to vancomycin, penicillin, and gentamicin. Clin Infect Dis 1993;16:750–755.
24. Ena J, Dick RW, Jones RN, et al. The epidemiology of intravenous vancomycin usage in a university hospital: A 10 year study. JAMA 1993;269:598–602.
25. Kaiser AB, Petracek MR, Lea JW IV, et al. Efficacy of cefazolin, cefamandole, and gentamicin as prophylactic agents in cardiac surgery. Ann Surg 1987;206:791–797.
26. Abramowicz M (ed). Antimicrobial prophylaxis in surgery. Med Lett 1993;35:91–94.
27. Fraser VJ, Jones M, Dunkel J, et al. Candidemia in a tertiary care hospital: Epidemiology, risk factors and predictors of mortality. Clin Infect Dis 1992;15:414–421.
28. Pittet D, Monod M, Suter PM, et al. Candida colonization and subsequent infections in critically ill surgical patients. Ann Surg 1994;220:751–758.
29. Burke JF. The effective period of preventive antibiotic action in experimental incisions and dermal lesions. Surgery 1961;50:161–168.
30. Classen DC, Evans RS, Pestotnik SL, et al. The timing of prophylactic administration of antibiotics and the risk of surgical wound infection. N Engl J Med 1992;326:281–286.
31. DiPiro JT, Cheung RPF, Bowden TA, Mansberger JA. Single dose systemic antibiotic prophylaxis of surgical wound infections. Am J Surg 1986;152:552–559.
32. Goldman DA, Hopkins CC, Karchmer AW. Cephalothin prophylaxis in cardiac valve surgery. A prospective, double-blind comparison of two-day and six-day regimen. J Thorac Cardiovasc Surg 1977;73:470–479.
33. Sawchuk RJ. Drug absorption and disposition in burn patients, in Benet LZ, Massoud N, Gambertoglio JG (eds): Pharmacokinetic Basis for Drug Treatment. New York, Raven Press, 1984, pp 333–348.
34. Rybak MJ, Albrecht LM, Berman J, et al. Vancomycin pharmacokinetics in burn patients and intravenous drug abusers. Antimicrob Agents Chemother 1990;34:792–795.
35. Segal JL, Gray DR, Gordon SK, et al. Gentamicin disposition in humans with spinal cord injury. Paraplegia 1985;23:47–55.
36. Miller KW, McCoy HG, Chan KHK, et al. Effect of cardiopulmonary bypass on cefazolin disposition. Clin Pharmacol Ther 1980;27:550–556.
37. Klamerus KJ, Rodvold KA, Silverman NA, Levitsky S. Effect of cardiopulmonary bypass on vancomycin and netilmicin disposition. Antimicrob Agents Chemother 1988;32:631–635.

38. Jungbluth GL, Pasko MT, Beam TR, Jusko WJ. Ceftriaxone disposition in open-heart surgery patients. Antimicrob Agents Chemother 1989;33:850–856.
39. Alexander JW, Dellinger PE. Surgical infections and choice of antibiotics. In Sabiston (ed). Textbook of Surgery, 14th ed. 1990, W. B. Saunders, Philadelphia, Chap 13, pp 221–236.
40. Kernodole DS, Classen DC, Burke JP, et al. Failure of cephalosporins to prevent *Staphylococcus aureus* surgical wound infections. JAMA 1990;263:961–966.
41. ASHP Commission on Therapeutics. ASHP therapeutic guidelines on antimicrobial prophylaxis in surgery. Clin Pharm 1992;11:483–513.
42. Sattler FR, Weitekamp MR, Ballard JO. Potential for bleeding with the new beta lactam antibiotics. Ann Intern Med 1986;105:924–931.
43. Babiak LM, Rybak MJ. Hematological effects associated with beta-lactam use. Drug Intell Clin Pharm 1986;20:833–836.
44. Romanelli VA, Howie MB, Myerowitz PD, et al. Intraoperative and postoperative effects of vancomycin administration in cardiac surgery patients: A prospective, double-blind, randomized trial. Crit Care Med 1993;21:1124–1131.
45. Polk RE. Anaphylactoid reactions to glycopeptide antibiotics. J Antimicrob Chemother 1991;27(suppl B):17–29.
46. O'Sullivan TL, Ruffing MJ, Lamp KC, et al. Prospective evaluation of Red Man syndrome in patients receiving vancomycin. J Infect Dis 1993;168:773–776.
47. LoCicero J, Nichols RL. Sepsis after gastroduodenal operations: Relationship to gastric acid, motility, and endogenous microflora. South Med J 1980;73:878–880.
48. Pories WJ, vanRij AM, Burlingham BT, et al. Prophylactic cefazolin in gastric bypass surgery. Surgery 1981;90:426–432.
49. Lewis RT, Goodall RG, Marien B, et al. Efficacy and distribution of single-dose preoperative antibiotic prophylaxis in high-risk gastroduodenal surgery. Can J Surg 1991;34:117–122.
50. Meijer WS, Schmitz PIM, Jeekel J. Meta-analysis of randomized controlled clinical trials of antibiotic prophylaxis in biliary tract surgery. Br J Surg 1990;77:283–290.
51. Garibaldi RA, Skolnick D, Maglio S, et al. Postcholecystectomy wound infection: The impact of prophylactic antibiotics on the epidemiology of infections. Ann Surg 1986;204:650–654.
52. Lee WJ, Chang KJ, Lee CS, Chen M. Surgery in cholangitis: Bacteriology and choice of antibiotic. Hepatogastroenterology 1992;39:347–349.
53. Bartlett JG, Condon RE, Gorbach SL, et al. Veterans administration cooperative study on bowel preparation for elective colorectal operations: Impact of oral antibiotic regimen on colonic flora, wound irrigation cultures and bacteriology of septic complications. Ann Surg 1978;188:249–254.
54. Condon RE, Bartlett JG, Greenlee H, et al. Efficacy of oral and systemic antibiotic prophylaxis in colorectal operations. Arch Surg 1983;118:496–502.
55. Stellato TA, Gordon NH, Danziger LH. Addition of parenteral cefoxitin to regimen of oral antibiotics for elective colorectal operations [letter]. Ann Surg 1991;213:375–376.
56. Bauer T, Vennits B, Holm B, et al. Antibiotic prophylaxis in acute nonperforated appendicitis. Ann Surg 1989;209:307–311.
57. Lau WY, Fan ST, Chu KW, et al. Randomized, prospective, and double-blind trial of new β-lactams in the treatment of appendicitis. Antimicrob Agents Chemother 1985;28:639–642.
58. Childs SJ, Wells WG, Mirelman S. Antibiotic prophylaxis for genitourinary surgery in community hospitals. J Urol 1983;130:305–308.
59. Faro S, Martens MG, Hammill HA, et al. Antibiotic prophylaxis: Is there a difference? Am J Obstet Gynecol 1990;162:900–909.
60. Hemsell DL, Bawdon RE, Hemsell PG, et al. Single-dose cephalosporin for prevention of major pelvic infection after vaginal hysterectomy: Cefazolin versus cefoxitin versus cefotaxime. Am J Obstet Gynecol 1987;156:1201–1205.
61. Hemsell DL, Hemsell PG, Heard ML, Nobels BJ. Preoperative cefoxitin prophylaxis for elective abdominal hysterectomy. Am J Obstet Gynecol 1985;153:225–226.
62. Hemsell DL, Johnson ER, Bawdon RE, et al. Ceftriaxone and cefazolin prophylaxis for hysterectomy. Surg Gynecol Obstet 1985;161:197–203.
63. Tabet JC, Johnson JT. Wound infection in head and neck surgery: Prophylaxis, etiology, and management. J Otolaryngol 1990;19:197–200.
64. Johnson JT, Wagner RL. Infection following uncontaminated head and neck surgery. Arch Otolaryngol Head Neck Surg 1987;113:368–369.
65. Johnson JT, Myers EN, Wagner RL. An assessment of the need for Gram-negative coverage in antibiotic prophylaxis for oncological head and neck surgery. J Infect Dis 1987;155:331–333.
66. Ariano RE, Zhanel GG. Antimicrobial prophylaxis in coronary bypass surgery: A critical appraisal. DICP Ann Pharmacother 1991;25:478–484.
67. Kreter B, Woods M. Antibiotic prophylaxis for cardiothoracic operations. A metaanalysis of thirty years of clinical trials. J Thorac Cardiovasc Surg 1992;104:590–599.
68. Pitt HA, Postier RG, MacGowan WAL, et al. Prophylactic antibiotics in vascular surgery—topical, systemic, or both? Ann Surg 1980;192:356–364.
69. Hasselgren PO, Ivarsson L, Risberg B, Seeman T. Effects of prophylactic antibiotics in vascular surgery; a prospective, randomized double-blind study. Ann Surg 1984;200:86–92.
70. Pollard JP, Hughes SPF, Scott JE, et al. Antibiotic prophylaxis in total hip replacement. B Med J 1979;1:707–709.
71. Hill C, Mazas F, Flamant R, Evrard J. Prophylactic cefazolin versus placebo in total hip replacement. Lancet 1981;1:795–797.
72. Patzakis MJ, Wilkins J, Wiss DA. Infection following intramedullary nailing of long bones. Clin Orthop 1986;212:182–191.
73. Dellinger EP, Caplan ES, Weaver LD, et al. Duration of preventive antibiotic administration for open extremity fractures. Arch Surg 1988;123:333–339.
74. Haines SJ. Efficacy of antibiotic prophylaxis in clean neurosurgical operations. Neurosurgery 1989;24:401–405.
75. Barker FG. Efficacy of prophylactic antibiotics for craniotomy: A meta-analysis. Neurosurgery 1994;35:484–492.
76. Haines SJ, Walters BC. Antibiotic prophylaxis for cerebrospinal fluid shunts: A metaanalysis. Neurosurgery 1994;34:87–93.

Chapter 116

Vaccines, Toxoids, and Other Immunobiologics

Joseph S. Bertino, Jr, PharmD, FCCP, and Daniel T. Casto, PharmD, FCCP

The discovery and introduction of vaccines, toxoids, and immunoglobulins has resulted in a significant decline in worldwide morbidity and mortality. In addition, they have been shown to be generally safe and cost effective.[1,2] This chapter is aimed at introducing the reader to three groups of agents: vaccines, toxoids, and immune sera (together known as immunobiologics). These groups will be defined and related agents will be dealt with concurrently in an attempt to illustrate total immunotherapy. Obscure agents and agents used only by the military have been eliminated from this discussion in the interest of brevity.

Principles of Immunization

THE IMMUNE RESPONSE TO IMMUNIZATION

Immunization can be explained on a molecular level much more specifically than ever before. T lymphocytes play a central role in the immune response. With vaccines, T lymphocytes help B lymphocytes make antibodies. T-cell receptors recognize antigens as a complex of a short peptide bound to a major histocompatibility complex (MHC) molecule on the surface of an antigen presenting cell (Lanzavecchia). MHC molecules are polymorphic with a distinct ability to bind peptides. Vaccines are designed to elicit a protective response to the organism being vaccinated against. The choice of antigen to be used for vaccination relates to the varability of the host and the pathogen. Although the ability of the host to respond to the antigen being used can be influenced by the general health of the host, immune response is primarily determined by genetic MHC polymorphism.[3] Different individuals will recognize different epitopes in a complex protein antigen. Thus, a vaccine must contain enough epitopes that can be recognized by at least one allele in every individual in order to be effective in the majority of people.

Vaccines that contain epitopes that can be processed and bind to alleles (alternative forms of the same gene) commonly found in the majority of the population are very effective in inducing protective response in most individuals. Some epitopes can bind to several alleles thus eliciting an immune response in the majority of individuals. However, when vaccines contain epitopes that bind to few alleles, they may fail to elicit an immunologic response in the majority of individuals or they may allow mutations of the antigen to escape and cause disease. This is the case for human immunodeficiency virus (HIV) and hepatitis C virus.

Immunizing agents elicit their response through antibody production and/or the T-cell system. Parenterally administered agents may elicit a rise in immunoglobulin M (IgM) titers, which fall over a few weeks as IgG rises. This bimodal immunoglobulin response requires the cooperation of both B and T cells. Certain agents (i.e., pneumococcal type III polysaccharide) cause pure B–cell-mediated antibody production. Other agents stimulate effector T cells, resulting in cell-mediated immunity (i.e., BCG vaccine). Revaccination (use of a second dose) results in heightened immune response as a result of invoking immunologic memory. Other agents may not invoke immune memory.

Orally and intranasally administered agents generally cause production of IgA antibodies resulting in high local concentrations of antibodies.

The process of inducing or providing immunity artificially by administering an immunobiologic agent is known as immunization. The term *immunization* is considered more specific than the term *vaccination.*

PRODUCTS TO PRODUCE IMMUNIZATION

Vaccines and toxoids are separate and distinct products. Both types of products, however, act to induce active immunity; that is, immunity generated by a natural immunologic response to an antigen. Vaccines are derived from the infecting organism itself. Viral vaccines can be either live attenuated or killed. Killed viral vaccines may consist of whole or split viral particles or specific viral fragments (subunits) as in the case of hepatitis B vaccine. Bacterial vaccines are generally killed whole bacteria or specific bacterial wall antigens. Live attenuated vaccines induce an immunologic response more consistent with that occurring with natural infection. Because the organisms in live attenuated vaccines multiply in the body after injection, they may confer lifelong immunity with one dose (as does a primary natural infection). However, this is not an absolute (as evidenced by the need for an additional dose of measles vaccine at some time after the initial dose in infancy). Killed vaccines, on the other hand, do not induce permanent immunity and require additional doses at varying time intervals (booster doses).

Toxoids are inactivated bacterial toxins that are generally combined with aluminum salts (i.e., alum) to enhance their antigenicity by prolonging antigen absorption. These adjuvants also increase local tissue irritation when injected. Toxoids retain the ability to stimulate the formation of antitoxin.

Immune sera are sterile solutions containing antibody derived from human (immune globulin) or equine (horse) [antitoxin] sources. Immune globulins are derived from donor pools of blood plasma and are processed using cold ethanol fractionation in order to inactivate any potentially infecting agent. Antitoxins are made by immunizing animals with an antigen and then harvesting the antibodies (antitoxins) made against the antigens. These sera are indicated for induction of passive immunity (temporary immunity to infection as a result of the administration of antibodies not produced by the host). Human immune sera is preferred due to its lower incidence of serum sickness and other allergic reactions as compared to equine-derived sera (see section on Other Immunobiologics).

In addition to the active component in an immunobiologic, other active and inert ingredients are often present in an immunobiologic. Suspending agents such as water, saline, or complex fluids containing proteins or antigens are used as the vehicle for the immunobiologic agent. Preservatives, stabilizers, and antibiotics are often added to help maintain sterility. Finally, adjuvants to enhance immunologic response are used (aluminum salts). Keep in mind that patients may respond with allergic reactions, not to the immunobiologic agent itself, but to the other components of the pharmaceutical preparation. Different manufacturers of the same immunobiologic may have different active and inert ingredients in their product.[4]

Certain vaccines manufactured by various companies are considered interchangeable. Hepatitis B vaccine produced by two different companies (Merck & Co. Inc. and SmithKline Beecham) are considered interchangeable.[4] Both human diploid cell vaccine and rabies vaccine adsorbed are fully interchangeable with intramuscular use only. DPT, oral polio, and inactivated polio vaccines are interchangeable between manufacturers. Finally, all licensed *Haemophilus influenzae* type b conjugate vaccines are considered interchangeable, with the primary series being three doses of vaccine.

In general, vaccines and toxoids must be kept refrigerated, because breaking the "cold chain" may result in loss of potency. Certain vaccines such as measles–mumps–rubella (MMR) may also be frozen. Immune sera generally should be kept refrigerated and not frozen except for lyophilized intravenous human immune globulin, which can be stored at room temperature. Certain vaccines such as yellow fever and oral polio vaccine (OPV) are very sensitive to increased temperature. While some vaccines may be stored below 0°C, toxoids in general tend to aggregate upon freezing, leading to increased adverse local effects. On the other hand, some vaccines when stored under incorrect conditions may not be easily distinguished from potent vaccine.

FACTORS AFFECTING RESPONSE TO IMMUNIZATION

Various factors are known to affect response to vaccines and toxoids. Viability of the antigen is an important factor (i.e., live attenuated versus killed) as previously discussed. Total dose is also important, because a threshold dose seems to exist above which no further increase in antibody titer is seen.[5] However, the use of split doses or multiple reduced doses of a vaccine (such as those used in patients with allergies to some immunobiologic component as both a desensitization and immunization program) may result in inadequate protection. In such instances, serologic testing should be performed to ascertain whether protection to the antigen had been attained. The interval between immunization doses and/or the number of doses given may change immune response to an agent. For hepatitis B vaccine, giving the third dose (in a three-dose series) at 12 months (after the first dose) has been shown to result in increased antibody titers compared to giving the third dose at 6 months.[6] Alternatively, additional doses of influenza vaccine have been shown to be minimally effective in immunocompetent, non–HIV-infected patients, HIV-infected patients, and in patients with acquired immunodeficiency syndrome (AIDS)-related complex (ARC).[7] Generally, intervals longer than those recommended between vaccine doses do not reduce immune response.[8]

The route and site of administration of the immunobiologic is also important. This is best illustrated by the hepatitis B vaccine, which elicits a satisfactory antibody response when given into the deltoid muscle but not consistently when administered in the gluteal area.9 Injections should be administered in a site where there is little likehood of site damage. Immunobiologics containing adjuvants should be given into muscle mass because they can cause irritation when given subcutaneously or intradermally. Subcutaneous injections should be administered into the thigh of infants and in the deltoid area of older children and adults. At ⅝- to ¾-inch, 23- to 25-gauge needle should be used, being careful not to administer the dose intradermally or intramuscularly. For intramuscular injection, the anterolateral aspect of the upper thigh (infants and toddlers) or the deltoid muscle of the upper arm (children and adults) should be used. The buttock should not be used because of the potential for inadequate immunologic response and because of the potential risk of injury to the sciatic nerve. When the buttock must be used (as for large doses of immune globulin), only the upper, outer quadrant should be used with the needle being inserted anteriorly. Intradermal injections should be administered on the volar surface of the forearm except for human cell rabies vaccine (HDCV), which should be given into the deltoid area to reduce reactions. A ⅜- to ¾-inch, 25- or 27-gauge needle should be used with care being taken not to inject the immunobiologic into the subcutaneous tissue.

Jet injectors are considered safe and effective for multiple person immunization despite the fact that the nozzle tip is used over and over again. No reports exist in the United States of transmission of blood-borne pathogens (i.e., HIV or hepatitis B or C) with the use of jet injectors.[4] Generally, it is suggested that if a jet injector is used and contamination of the nozzle is noted, the device should be cleaned or the tip changed. In addition, the swabbing of the nozzle with alcohol or acetone between patients is routinely suggested.

For orally administered vaccines (i.e., typhoid or oral polio), the general recommendation is to readminister the vaccine at the same visit if the vaccine is regurgitated within 5–10 minutes of administration. If the second dose is not retained, neither dose should be counted and the vaccine should be readministered at the next visit.

Questions often arise concerning the simultaneous administration of vaccines. In general, inactivated vaccines can be simultaneously administered at separate sites. If single-site administration must be done, the thigh muscle is the preferred site of injection. If two or more killed antigens cannot be administered simultaneously, they may be administered with no regard to spacing between doses. Killed and live antigens may be administered simultaneously or, if they cannot be administered simultaneously, at any interval between doses with the exception of cholera (killed) and yellow fever (live) vaccine, which should be given at least 3 weeks apart. Simultaneous administration of live attenuated vaccines should be avoided if possible unless specified (i.e., measles, mumps, rubella). Theoretically, live vaccines should be given at least 1 month apart; however, oral polio vaccine may be given at the same time as measles, mumps, and rubella vaccine. The data on simultaneous administration of live attenuated viral vaccines should be prefaced with the knowledge that simultaneous administration of these vaccines has been performed with no resultant decrease in immunity to any of the agents used, when compared to single vaccine administration alone. Oral polio vaccine and oral typhoid vaccine (both live vaccines) may be administered simultaneously. Live viral vaccines may interfere with the purified protein derivative (PPD) response and thus tubercular testing should be postponed 4–6 weeks after live virus vaccine administration.

The simultaneous administration of immune globulin (general or disease specific) and live attenuated vaccines (but not inactivated vaccines) may inhibit host antibody response due to impairment of viral replication. Guidelines state that there is a dose relationship between administration of immune globulin and inhibition of immune response to a vaccine (Table 116.1). Whole blood and other blood products containing antibodies may interfere with the response to MMR vaccine. For women who have experienced a birth and have received a blood product in the last trimester or anti Rh_o(D) IG at the time of delivery, vaccination with MMR should be done immediately with antibody testing at least 3 months later to determine response. In any patient, if vaccination with MMR and immune globulin administration must be done, separate injection sites are recommended with seroconversion to the viral antigens confirmed at 3 months with reimmunization if necessary. Immune globulin does not interfere with the response to oral vaccines or to yellow fever vaccine.

For killed vaccines, administration of these along with immune globulins simultaneously is not contraindicated. Different sites are recommended, however, for killed vaccine and immune globulin administration. It is not recommended to increase the dose or number of vaccines used in this circumstance.

IMMUNIZATION OF SPECIAL POPULATIONS

NEONATES, INFANTS, AND PREGNANT WOMEN

The age of the recipient is another important determining factor in vaccine/toxoid response. In the first few months of life, passive immunity (temporary immunity to infection as a result of the acquisition of antibodies via maternal–fetal passage) both protects an infant and prevents adequate vaccine/toxoid response to certain agents.

Premature infants should be vaccinated at the same chronological age using the same schedule and precautions as full-term infants. Full recommended doses of vaccines should be used regardless of age or birthweight. Hepatitis B vaccine should be administered if the infant weighs 2000 grams or be held until the infant is 2 months of age. Breastfed infants should be vaccinated according to standard pediatric schedules.

TABLE 116.1. SUGGESTED INTERVALS BETWEEN ADMINISTRATION OF IMMUNE GLOBULIN PREPARATIONS FOR VARIOUS INDICATIONS AND VACCINES CONTAINING LIVE MEASLES VIRUS[a]

Indication	Dose (including mg IgG/kg)	Suggested Interval Before Measles Vaccination (months)
Tetanus (TIG)	250 units (10 mg IgG/kg) IM	3
Hepatitis A (IG)		
Contact prophylaxis	0.02 mL/kg (3.3 mg IgG/kg) IM	3
International travel	0.06 mL/kg (10 mg IgG/kg) IM	3
Hepatitis B prophylaxis (HBIG)	0.06 mL/kg (10 mg IgG/kg) IM	3
Rabies prophylaxis (HRIG)	20 IU/kg (22 mg IgG/kg) IM	4
Varicella prophylaxis (VZIG)	125 units/10 kg (20–40 mg IgG/kg) IM (maximum 625 units)	5
Measles prophylaxis (IG)		
Normal contact	0.25 mL/kg (40 mg IgG/kg) IM	5
Immunocompromised contact	0.50 mL/kg (80 mg IgG/kg) IM	6
Blood transfusion		
Red blood cells (RBCs), washed	10 mL/kg (negligible IgG/kg) IV	0
RBCs, adenine-saline added	10 mL/kg (10 mg IgG/kg) IV	3
Packed RBCs (Hct 65%)[b]	10 mL/kg (60 mg IgG/kg) IV	6
Whole blood (Hct 35–50%)[b]	10 mL/kg (80–100 mg IgG/kg) IV	6
Plasma/platelet products	10 mL/kg (160 mg IgG/kg) IV	7
Replacement of humoral immune deficiencies	300–400 mg/kg IV[c] (as IGIV)	8
Treatment of:		
ITP[d]	400 mg/kg IV (as IGIV)	8
ITP[d]	1000 mg/kg IV (as IGIV)	10
Kawasaki disease	2 grams/kg IV (as IGIV)	11

[a]This table is not intended for determining the correct indications and dosage for the use of immune globulin preparations. Unvaccinated persons may not be fully protected against measles during the entire suggested interval and additional doses of immune globulin and/or measles vaccine may be indicated following measles exposure. The concentration of measles antibody in a particular immune globulin preparation can vary by lot. The rate of antibody clearance following receipt of an immune globulin preparation can also vary. The recommended intervals are extrapolated from an estimated half-life of 30 days for passively acquired antibody and an observed interference with the immune response to measles vaccine for 5 months following a dose of 80 mg IgG/kg.
[b]Assumes a serum IgG concentration of 16 mg/mL.
[c]Measles vaccination is recommended for children with HIV infection but is contraindicated in patients with congenital disorders of the immune system.
[d]ITP, Immune (formally, idiopathic) thrombocytopenic purpura. (From Centers for Disease Control and Prevention. General recommendations on immunization: Recommendations of the Advisory Committee on Immunization Practices (ACIP). MMWR 1994;43 (RR-1):1–38.)

Pregnant women present a particularly difficult problem in deciding on vaccination. In general, administration of live attenuated vaccines should not be done during pregnancy, and inactivated vaccines should not be given until the second trimester; however, inactivated vaccines have not been shown to be teratogenic during the first trimester.[10,11] Administration of rubella vaccine during pregnancy is not a reason to routinely interrupt pregnancy.[11] Diphtheria and tetanus vaccination should be carried out with the use of a booster dose or a complete series of vaccines in unimmunized women. Hepatitis B, oral polio, influenza, and pneumococcal vaccine are all recommended in pregnant women if indicated.

IMMUNOCOMPROMISED HOSTS

Vaccination in compromised hosts (i.e., those with chronic disease such as diabetes, connective tissue disease, alcoholicism, or those with cancer or HIV disease) must be individualized based on the disease state and its treatment. The Centers for Disease Control and Prevention (CDC) has classified persons with immunocompromising conditions into three groups[12]:

1. Persons with conditions that cause limited immune deficiency (i.e., renal disease, diabetes, liver disease, asplenia).
2. Individuals who are severely immunocompromised not as a result of HIV infection (i.e., congenital immunodeficiency, drug- or radiation-induced disease, hematologic or solid tumor).
3. Persons with HIV infection.

Patients with chronic pulmonary, renal, hepatic, or metabolic disease who are not receiving immunosuppressants may receive both live attenuated and killed vaccines and toxoids to induce active immunity. These patients may often need higher doses of vaccines or more frequent dosing to induce immunity. Generally, immunization should be considered early in the course of the disease in an attempt to induce immunity at a point when the disease is less severe.

Those patients with active malignant disease may receive killed vaccines or toxoids but should not be given live vaccines. In addition, OPV should not be administered to household contacts of these patients. MMR is not contraindicated for close contacts however. Live virus vaccines may be administered to persons with leukemia who have not received chemotherapy for at least 3 months. Vaccines should be given at times to avoid coinciding with the start of chemotherapy or radiation therapy (i.e., at least 2 weeks in advance of the start of these therapies). If vaccines cannot be given before at least 2 weeks or more before the start of these therapies, immunization should be postponed until 3 months after the therapy has been completed. Passive immunization with immune globulin may be used in place of active immunization, regardless of the history of immunization.

The role of glucocorticoids in causing immunosupression is an interesting one. It is generally believed that when therapy duration is ≤2 weeks (low to moderate dose, that is <20 mg or 2 mg/kg/d, whichever is less), no contraindication to immunization exists.[12] In addition, long-term alternate-day steroid therapy with short-acting agents, maintenance physiologic doses, topical, aerosol, intra-articular, bursal, or tendon injections are not considered contraindications to immunization. If patients have been receiving high-dose corticosteroids, or have had a course lasting ≥2 weeks, then a 3-month period of time should pass before immunization with live virus vaccines.

The patient with HIV infection requires special consideration. Responses to live and killed antigens is generally suboptimal and decreases as the disease progresses. HIV produces defects in cell-mediated immunity and in humoral immunity. This results in increased morbidity for measles infection. Consequently, measles vaccine (given as MMR) is recommended in all children and adult patients regardless of HIV status using standard schedules. There is no suggestion that serious adverse events are seen more frequently in these individuals. Enhanced inactivated polio vaccine (eIPV) should be used as an alternative to OPV in these patients; however, full response may not be assured. If OPV is inadvertently administered to a household contact, close contact between the individual immunized and the patient should be avoided for 30 days. Pneumococcal vaccine is recommended for HIV-infected persons ≥2 years of age. Children <2 years of age should receive *H. influenzae* vaccine according to the recommended schedule for nonimmunocompromised children. Diphtheria–tetanus–pertussis (DTP) vaccination is also recommended. There is no suggestion that larger doses or more frequent dosing of vaccine is of benefit.

Other killed vaccines may be used without concern for increased risk. Live typhoid vaccine should be avoided. Yellow fever vaccine may be used if absolutely necessary, but may pose a theoretical risk of encephalitis.

MISCONCEPTIONS ON THE USE OF IMMUNIZATION

There are very few contraindications to the use of vaccines except as outlined previously. These contraindications include a history of anaphylactic reactions to the vaccine or a component of the vaccine, immunosupression (as specified for each group above), pregnancy (for MMR), and administration of immunoglobulin or blood products. For agents such as DTP, history of encephalopathy or hypotonic–hyporesponsive episode with a previous dose and fever of ≥40.5°C within 48 hours of a previous dose are contraindications. Generally, history of mild to moderate local reactions, mild acute illnesses, concurrent antibiotic use, prematurity, family history of adverse events, diarrhea, and breast feeding are not contraindications to immunization.

IMMUNIZATION HISTORY

The history of immunization should be obtained from each patient, preferably by review of the written record. If this is not available, patient characteristics (i.e., military service, travel history, occupation) may provide clues as to the immunization history. Serology testing for immunity against certain diseases can provide specific information. In the event a written record does not exist, one should be generated at the time of initiation of immunization. For persons who have no record, these persons should be considered susceptible and an immunization program started and completed unless a serious adverse reaction occurs (more commonly to DPT or diphtheria–tetanus [Td]).

VACCINE DELIVERY

None of the currently used vaccines is perfect with regard to efficacy and safety. However, all of them have had tremendous impact on reducing the number of cases of serious communicable diseases. Even more lives could be saved, however, if the available vaccines were administered to more patients for whom they are indicated.[13–15]

Shortfalls in vaccine coverage exist in both the adult and pediatric populations.[16,17] Among children, those of preschool age are often the most neglected. Because entry into public school is contingent on having completed immunizations, vaccine coverage rates are above 97% in children 6 years and older. However, the lack of an enforcement mechanism in younger patients has contributed to immunization rates below 50%, particularly in children less than 2 years of age. In many instances, unvaccinated individuals have been seen by health care providers, but have not been administered indicated vaccines either due to oversight, because of inappropriate "contraindications" to vaccination, or because of reluctance to administer multiple vaccines at the same visit. These "missed opportunities" to immunize patients have been shown to occur in patients of all ages and in a variety of practice settings.[16,18–21]

According to the CDC, every health care visit, regardless of its purpose, should be viewed as an opportunity to review a patient's immunization status and administer needed vaccines. Immunization is perhaps the most cost-effective medical practice available.[22] Pharmaceutical care should encompass assessment of individuals' vaccine needs, administration of indicated agents, and documentation of immunization histories. The outcome measure of what percentage of patients in a particular practice site is completely immunized may be one of the most important ones that can be identified. The benefits of optimal vaccine use extend beyond the individual patient to the public as a whole.

The National Vaccine Injury Compensation Act

In 1986, the National Vaccine Injury Act (NVIA) was passed by the U.S. Congress and signed into law by President Reagan.[23] Four parts compose the act. Part A (effective October 1, 1988) outlines compensation for vaccine-related injuries per a Vaccine Injury Table. Awards are limited to $250,000 for pain and suffering, and the same amount for a death benefit, along with attorney's fees. Part B is the "no-fault" provision, which frees the manufacturer from liability for damage if adequate warnings for vaccine use are provided. Part C provides that adverse reactions to vaccines must be reported to the Food and Drug Administration (FDA) by health care providers and vaccine manufacturers within 7 days of any adverse reaction. Part D gives legal recourse against the Secretary of the Department of Health and Human Services for not performing duties as outlined by the act.[23] The bill also instituted mandatory record keeping by health care providers in the permanent medical record. Specifically, the manufacturer and lot number of the vaccine, the date of administration, and the name, address, and title of the person giving the vaccine must be recorded. In addition, the act mandates that health care providers report to their local health department or the FDA any occurrence of the adverse events listed in Table 116.2. This table is subject to periodic review and modification. To facilitate reporting of any adverse events suspected of being vaccine related, the Vaccine Adverse Event Reporting System (VAERS) was established.[24] The toll-free telephone number for information and ordering report forms is 1-800-822-7967.

Use of Vaccines and Toxoids

The recommended schedules for routine immunization of children and adults are shown in Appendixes 116.1 and 116.2, respectively. Appendix 116.3 lists the minimum age for initial vaccination and minimum interval between vaccine doses. Children should be fully immunized before 6 years of age. This is a legal requirement in many states. Adults should be fully immunized against diphtheria, tetanus, measles, mumps, and rubella. If this is not the case, a complete series of immunizations should be given. Certain high-risk individuals should be vaccinated against other agents as outlined in Appendix 116.2.

Toxoids and Their Immunobiologics

DIPHTHERIA TOXOID ADSORBED AND DIPHTHERIA ANTITOXIN

Diphtheria toxoid adsorbed (DTA) is a sterile suspension of toxoids of *Corynebacterium diphtheriae,* which induce immunity against the exotoxin of *C. diphtheriae*. The use of DTA has essentially eliminated diphtheria from the United States.

Primary immunization with DTA is indicated for children older than 6 weeks of age.[25] The usual dose is 0.5 mL intramuscularly at rotating sites. Generally, DTA is given along with pertussis and tetanus vaccine at ages 2, 4, and 6–12 months of age. Additional doses of DTA are given at 18 months and 4–6 years of age. Three doses of DTA induce immunity in 90% of persons for at least 10 years. Booster doses of DTA should be given every 10 years. Recent data from Great Britain indicate that DPT may be given in a 2-, 3-, and 4-month immunization schedule and induce immunity in an equal number of children which lasts until the preschool booster dose.[26] This schedule is not approved for use in the United States. Immunization prior to 6 weeks of age should not be given due to the possible inhibiting effect of maternal antibodies.

If primary immunization is given to an immunosuppressed patient, an additional dose of DTA should be administered 1 month following the return to normal immune status. DTA may be administered to persons with mild febrile illnesses and with other live or killed vaccines.[27]

For nonimmunized adults, a complete three-dose series of diphtheria toxoid should be administered with the first two doses given at least 4 weeks apart and the third dose given 6–12 months after the second. The combined preparation, Td, is recommended in adults since it contains less diphtheria toxoid than DPT with fewer reactions seen to the diphtheria preparation. Booster doses are given every 10 years.

TABLE 116.2. REPORTABLE EVENTS FOLLOWING IMMUNIZATION

Vaccine/Toxoid	Event[a]	Interval from Immunization
DTP, P, DTP/poliovirus combined	A. Anaphylaxis or anaphylactic shock	24 hours
	B. Encephalopathy (or encephalitis)[b]	7 days
	C. Shock-collapse or hypotonic-hyporesponsive collapse[b]	7 days
	D. Residual seizure disorder[b]	[b]
	E. Any acute complication or sequela (including death) of above events	No limit
	F. (See package insert)[c]	(See package insert)
Measles, mumps, and rubella; DT, Td, T toxoid	A. Anaphylaxis or anaphylactic shock	24 hours
	B. Encephalopathy (or encephalitis)[b]	15 days for measles, mumps, and rubella vaccines; 7 days for DT, Td, and T toxoids
	C. Residual seizure disorder[b]	[b]
	D. Any acute complication or sequela (including death) of above events	No limit
	E. (See package insert)[c]	(See package insert)
Oral poliovirus vaccine	A. Paralytic poliomyelitis	
	—in a nonimmunodeficient recipient	30 days
	—in an immunodeficient recipient	6 months
	—in a vaccine-associated community case	No limit
	B. Any acute complication or sequela (including death) of above events	No limit
	C. (See package insert)[c]	(See package insert)
Inactivated poliovirus vaccine	A. Anaphylaxis or anaphylactic shock	24 hours
	B. Any acute complication or sequela (including death) of above event	No limit
	C. (See package insert)[c]	(See package insert)

[a]Events listed are required by law to be reported to the U.S. Department of Health and Human Services; however, VAERS will accept *all* reports of suspected adverse events after the administration of *any* vaccine.

[b]Aids to Interpretation:

- Shock-collapse or hypotonic-hyporesponsive collapse may be evidenced by signs or symptoms such as decrease in or loss of muscle tone, paralysis (partial or complete), hemiplegia, hemiparesis, loss of color or change of color to pale white or blue, unresponsiveness to environmental stimuli, depression of or loss of consciousness, prolonged sleeping with difficulty arousing, or cardiovascular or respiratory arrest.
- Residual seizure disorder may be considered to have occurred if no other seizure or convulsion unaccompanied by fever or accompanied by a fever of <102°F occurred before the first seizure or convulsion after the administration of the vaccine involved,
  AND, if in the case of measles-, mumps-, or rubella-containing vaccines, the first seizure or convulsion occurred within 15 days after vaccination OR in the case of any other vaccine, the first seizure or convulsion occurred within 3 days after vaccination,
  AND, if two or more seizures or convulsions unaccompanied by fever or accompanied by a fever of <102°F occurred within 1 year after vaccination.
- The terms seizure and convulsion include grand mal, petit mal, absence, myoclonic, tonic-clonic, and focal motor seizures and signs.
- Encephalopathy means any substantial acquired abnormality of, injury to, or impairment of brain function. Among the frequent manifestations of encephalopathy are focal and diffuse neurologic signs, increased intracranial pressure, or changes lasting ≥6 hours in level of consciousness, with or without convulsions. The neurologic signs and symptoms of encephalopathy may be temporary with complete recovery, or they may result in various degrees of permanent impairment. Signs and symptoms such as high-pitched and unusual screaming, persistent unconsolable crying, and bulging fontanel are compatible with an encephalopathy, but in and of themselves are not conclusive evidence of encephalopathy. Encephalopathy usually can be documented by slow wave activity on an electroencephalogram.

[c]Refer to the Contraindication section of the manufacturer's package insert for each vaccine. (From Centers for Disease Control. VAERS program. MMWR 1990;39:730–731.)

Adverse effects of DTA include mild to moderate tenderness, erythema, and induration at the injection site. Rarely do systemic reactions occur.[28]

Diphtheria antitoxin (DA) is a sterile antitoxin derived from hyperimmunized horses and is indicated for immediate use in patients with diphtheria. It should be stored at 2–8°C but may be frozen without affecting potency. DA is rarely indicated for diphtheria prophylaxis. DA is given intramuscularly or intravenously in a dosage related to the site and size of the diphtheric membrane, degree of toxicity, and duration of illness. Sensitivity testing by performing an intradermal or scratch test and a conjunctival test should be performed before administration. The intradermal test entails injecting 0.1 mL of a 1:100 dilution of DA in 0.9% sodium chloride. The test is read after 20 minutes. A positive test is the formation of a wheal and flare with or without pseudopods. The test can be done as a scratch skin test. The conjunctival test is performed by placing 1 drop of a

1:10 dilution of DA into the lower conjunctival sac of one eye. A positive test mimicks an allergic reaction with redness, burning, itching, and lacrimation. These tests do not rule out systemic allergic reactions in 100% of the cases.

The usual dose of DA is 20,000–40,000 U for pharyngeal disease, 40,000–60,000 U for nasopharyngeal lesions, and 80,000–120,000 U for extensive disease of 3 or more days. When given intravenously, the dose should be diluted 1:20 in 0.9% saline or dextrose 5% in water and infused at 1 mL/min after being warmed to 32–34°C.

Adverse reactions to DA include anaphylactic reactions in 7% of patients and/or serum sickness occurring 12 days postadministration. Serum sickness may be accelerated (7–12 days) in persons previously sensitized. Fortunately, the widespread use of DTA vaccine has greatly reduced the incidence of the disease and thus the use of DA.

TETANUS TOXOID, TETANUS TOXOID ADSORBED, AND TETANUS IMMUNE GLOBULIN

Tetanus toxoid (TT) and tetanus toxoid adsorbed (TTA) (adsorbed onto aluminum hydroxide, phosphate, or potassium sulfate to increase antigenicity) are sterile suspensions of the toxoid from *Clostridium tetani.*

Both toxoids are used to promote immunization against tetanus; however, TTA is the preferred agent. While single doses in a nonimmunized individual do not produce sufficient antibody response, three 0.5-mL doses of TTA or four doses of TT produce protection in 90% of vaccinees older than 6 weeks of age. Primary vaccination provides protection for at least 10 years. Additional doses of TTA are recommended as part of traumatic wound management if a patient has not received a dose of TTA or TT over the preceding 5 years. For minor or clean wounds, no dose is given. These recommendations are summarized in Table 116.3. In certain situations tetanus immune globulin should also be given. TIG should be used with TTA using separate syringes and separate sites.

In children, primary immunization against tetanus is usually done in conjunction with diphtheria and pertussis vaccination. The trivalent vaccine, DPT, containing TTA is given intramuscularly at a dose of 0.5 mL at 2, 4, 6, and 18 months of age.[27,29] In adults or children where primary immunization against tetanus alone is needed, a series of three 0.5-mL doses of TTA is administered intramuscularly initially, followed by repeat doses at 4–8 weeks and 6–12 months. Boosters are recommended every 10 years. TT and TTA may be given to immunosuppressed patients if needed. TT or TTA may be simultaneously given with other killed and live vaccines.

Adverse reactions to TT and TTA include mild to moderate local reactions at the injection site such as warmth, erythema, and induration. Rarely, fever, malaise, aches and pains, or neurologic disorders have been reported. In general, major local reactions occur within 2–8 hours after administration to patients with high serum tetanus antitoxin levels. This type of reaction suggests a high level of protection. Local reactions do not limit the use of the toxoid for further dosing. While safe use during pregnancy has not been definitely established, TT and TTA have been administered to pregnant women for the prevention of neonatal tetanus. Generally, waiting until the second trimester is suggested.

TABLE 116.3. SUMMARY GUIDE TO TETANUS PROPHYLAXIS IN ROUTINE WOUND MANAGEMENT[a]

	Clean, Minor Wounds		All Other Wounds[b]	
	Td[c]	TIG[d]	Td[c]	TIG[d]
Uncertain or <3	Yes	No	Yes	Yes
>3[e]	No[f]	No	No[g]	No

[a]Refer also to text on specific vaccines or toxoids for contraindications, precautions, dosages, side effects, adverse reactions, and special considerations. Important details are in the text and in the ACIP recommendations on diphtheria, tetanus, and pertussis (DTP) (MMWR 1991: 40 [RR-10]).
[b]Such as, but not limited to, wounds contaminated with dirt, feces, and saliva; puncture wounds; avulsions; and wounds resulting from missiles, crushing, burns, and frostbite.
[c]Td, tetanus and diphtheria toxoids, adsorbed (for adult use). For children <7 years old, DTP (DT, if pertussis vaccine is contraindicated) is preferred to tetanus toxoid alone. For persons ≥7 years old, Td is preferred to tetanus toxoid alone.
[d]TIG, tetanus immune globulin.
[e]If only three doses of fluid toxoid have been received, a fourth dose of toxoid, preferably an adsorbed toxoid, should be given.
[f]Yes, >10 years since last dose.
[g]Yes, >5 years since last dose. (More frequent boosters are not needed and can accentuate side effects.) (From Centers for Disease Control. Update on adult immunization: Recommendations of the Advisory Committee on Immunization Practices (ACIP). MMWR 1991;40 (RR-12):1–95.)

Tetanus immune globulin (TIG) is a sterile, concentrated, nonpyrogenic solution of immunoglobulins prepared from hyperimmunized humans. TIG is used to provide passive tetanus immunization following the occurrence of traumatic wounds in nonimmunized or suboptimally immunized persons (see Table 116.3). A dose of 250–500 U should be administered intramuscularly. When administered with TTA, separate sites for administration should be used. TIG is also used for the treatment of tetanus. In this setting a single dose of 3000–6000 U is administered intramuscularly.

Adverse effects of TIG include pain, tenderness, erythema, and muscle stiffness at the injection site, which may persist for several hours. Rarely do systemic reactions occur. Intravenous administration has been associated with severe adverse reactions and is not recommended.

VACCINES AND THEIR IMMUNOBIOLOGICS

BACILLUS CALMETTE–GUÉRIN VACCINE (BCG)

BCG vaccine is derived from a live attenuated strain of *Mycobacterium bovis,* and is used for vaccination against tuberculosis. While the use of the vaccine has been shown to result in a positive tuberculin skin test in the majority of recipients, field trials in India have led to doubts concerning its efficacy.[10,30] A recent meta-analysis suggests that the use of BCG gives an overall protection rate of 50% with a protective effect in pulmonary TB of 78%, TB meningitis of 64%, and death reduction of 71%.[31] The vaccine is considered to be approximately 50–77% effective over a 10- to 20-year period in some populations.[32,33] No data are available as to the total duration of protection, however. Generally, tuberculin tests stay positive for 7–10 years following BCG administration.

Because the incidence of tuberculosis in the United States is low, the indications for this vaccine are few. The vaccine is recommended for (1) health care workers with an annual attack rate of greater than 1% in the face of other tuberculosis control measures, (2) groups with an excessive new infection rate in whom surveillance and treatment cannot be accomplished or have failed, and (3) individuals in close contact with infected patients who have been ineffectively treated.

Within 6 weeks of vaccine administration (either before or after vaccination), a negative Mantoux skin test should be assured. It is difficult to distinguish active disease from vaccine effect in patients with positive skin tests who have received BCG and, thus, any patient with a positive purified protein derivative (PPD) should be considered to have active infection unless known to be previously negative.

The vaccine is administered in a dose of 0.2–0.3 mL for patients over 1 month of age, and 0.1 mL for infants less than 1 month of age. The vaccine is administered percutaneously using a bifurcated needle. When percutaneous administration is performed, 0.2–0.3 mL of the vaccine is placed on the skin and then at least 20 punctures are made to administer the agent. In neonates (less than 1 month of age), if the 0.1-mL dose does not produce a positive PPD and if still indicated, an additional 0.2–0.3 mL dose should be administered after 1 year of age. Repeat vaccination is not recommended and does not seem to be guided by the use of skin tests.

Following correct percutaneous vaccination, a small red papule should appear within 7–10 days. This lesion may reach 8 mm in size within 5 weeks. Within the next 6 months, the lesion should ulcerate and scar.

The agent is contraindicated in immunosuppressed individuals regardless of the cause because it is a live vaccine. The vaccine should not be given to burn patients, patients who have recently received smallpox vaccines, or patients on isoniazid, due to inhibition of bacterial replication. The use of the vaccine in pregnant women is discouraged unless there is an excessive risk of exposure. Even then, the vaccine should not be used in the first trimester.

Adverse effects of BCG vaccine have been noted with varying frequencies. Excessive skin ulceration, disseminated *M. bovis* infection, and generalized adenitis have been reported, but for the most part are unusual. Disseminated infection occurs in 1–10 per million doses. Localized or limited adenitis and ulceration may occur in 1–10% of patients receiving the vaccine. These effects probably occur in patients who have previously received the vaccine and are transient. Late-onset adverse reactions are usually in the form of granulomas, which may occur 4–6 weeks following injection. These granulomas may persist for months and often go on to form keloid scars.

While the major use of BCG vaccine has been as immunoprophylaxis of tuberculosis, other uses of the agent in neoplastic disease have been studied. In these circumstances, the agent has been used in various dosages and routes of administration. Specific protocols are generally followed. This form of immunotherapy in neoplastic disease has been met with limited success.

HAEMOPHILUS INFLUENZAE TYPE B VACCINES

Haemophilus influenzae type b (Hib) is a gram-negative bacillus capable of causing life-threatening illness, primarily in children less than 5 years of age. Until recently this organism was the leading cause of bacterial meningitis in infants and children in the United States, causing approximately 10,000 cases annually. Hib meningitis has a 5–10% mortality rate, and up to 40% of survivors are left with neurologic deficits. Annually Hib was also responsible for thousands of cases of other serious illnesses (e.g., epiglottitis, pneumonia, sepsis, septic arthritis). The incidence of Hib disease has declined significantly, however, since the introduction of vaccines based on the organism's capsular substance, polyribosylribitol phosphate (PRP).

The first Hib vaccines introduced consisted of purified PRP; however, they lacked immunogenicity in the highest risk patients, those under the age of 18 months. Hib vaccines currently in use are conjugate products, consisting of either a polysaccharide or oligosaccharide of PRP covalently linked to a protein carrier (Table 116.4). The protein carrier is important because it provides for T-lymphocyte-dependent immunologic response, whereas earlier Hib vaccines that consisted of only unconjugated PRP elicited a response that was T-cell independent. T-cell involvement in the response provides for (1) a greater antibody response, regardless of the age of the patient receiving the vaccine, (2) immunologic response at an earlier age (including infants), and (3) a booster effect on subsequent exposure to the Hib capsule, whether through revaccination or natural exposure.

Hib conjugate vaccines are stable at 2–8°C and should not be frozen. They are indicated for routine use in all infants and children less than 5 years of age. All of the conjugate products are more immunogenic than the earlier nonconjugated vaccines, but only three of the four commer-

TABLE 116.4. ***HAEMOPHILUS INFLUENZAE*** **VACCINES CURRENTLY AVAILABLE IN THE UNITED STATES**

Manufacturer	Abbreviated Name	Trade Name	Protein Carrier
Connaught Labs	PRP-D	ProHIBit	Diphtheria toxoid
Lederle-Praxis	HbOC[a]	HIBTITER	CRM_{197} (diphtheria toxin)
Merck	PRP-OMP	PedvaxHIB	OMP (from *N. meningitidis*)
Pasteur Merieux	PRP-T	ActHIB/OmniHIB	Tetanus toxoid

Note: PRP-D is recommended by the American Academy of Pediatrics for infants age ≥12 months only. HbOC, PRP-OMP, and PRP-T are recommended for infants age ≥2 months.
[a]Available as Tetramune, a combination vaccine with DPT. (Abstracted from Pediatrics 1993;92:480–488.)

cially available products are suitable for use in infants. Additionally, the three products indicated for use in children less than 1 year of age differ in their immunogenicity and schedule of administration. The primary series of Hib vaccination consists of a 0.5–mL IM dose at ages 2, 4, and 6 months, if HbOC (HibTITER) or PRP-T (OmniHIB) is used. If PRP-OMP is being used, the primary series consists of doses given at 2 and 4 months of age. It is likely that use of more than one product for the primary series will provide adequate protection, but until more data are available, it is recommended that the same product be used for the entire primary series. A booster dose is recommended at age 12 months. Any of the four Hib conjugate products, including PRP-D (Pro HIBit), is suitable for the booster dose, regardless of which conjugate was used for the primary series of doses.[34,35] DTP and Hib vaccines may be given simultaneously at different sites.

For infants 7–11 months who have not been vaccinated, three doses of HbOC, PRP-OMP, and PRP-T should be given: two doses, spaced 8 weeks apart, and then a booster dose at age 12–18 months (but at least 8 weeks since dose 2). For unvaccinated children ages 12–14 months, two doses should be given, with an interval of 2 months between them. In a child older than 15 months, a single dose of any of the four conjugate vaccines is indicated.[34,35]

The vaccine should only be used in patients greater than 5 years of age if they have underlying conditions (HIV infection, IgG_2 subclass deficiency, sickle cell disease, splenectomy, bone marrow transplants, and those receiving chemotherapy for malignancies) that place them at higher than normal risk for Hib infection. Antibody response is less in individuals with these conditions and, based on limited data, two doses of Hib vaccine are recommended.

Adverse reactions to Hib vaccine are uncommon. Erythema and induration at the injection site occur in approximately 10–12% of children and resolve within 24 hours. Fever, diarrhea, and vomiting are occasionally reported. Fever of greater than 38°C is reported in 2.4% of children.

HEPATITIS A VACCINE

Hepatitis A (HAV) is a small RNA virus classified in the picronavirus group. HAV is spread through the fecal–oral route. It has been suggested that the annual cost of cases in the United States is $200 million.[36]

Late in 1993, the Biologic Advisory of the FDA suggested approval of a hepatitis A vaccine (SmithKline Beecham). One other manufacturer (Merck & Co., Inc.) was also investigating a hepatitis A vaccine at the time of this writing.

Hepatitis A vaccine is a formalin inactivated whole virus product adsorbed to alum. The vaccine has been investigated in one-, two-, and three-dose regimens.[36] The two-dose regimen has been given at 0 and 6 months, and the three-dose regimen at 0, 1, and 6 months. The single-dose regimen has been shown in children to induce levels of antibodies exceeding that seen with the use of immune globulin at 3 months.[36] The vaccine also has been shown to have an estimated protection rate of 100% of vaccine recipients.[36] When administered with immune globulin, antibody response is blunted but mimics levels seen without immune globulin use when booster doses are given.[37]

The suggested dose of HAV vaccine is 1440 units (HAVRIX) IM given 24 weeks apart. Adverse effects include pain at the injection site and fever. No cases of HAV disease have been noted.

HEPATITIS B VACCINE

Hepatitis B continues to be a major pathogen worldwide. In the United States, approximately 300,000 hepatitis B infections occur each year, leading to 10,000 hospitalizations, 250 acute deaths, and 4000 cirrhosis-related deaths. It is estimated that there are 800 cases of liver cancer associated with hepatitis B each year in the United States.[38,39] In 1981, a safe, immunogenic vaccine for the prevention of hepatitis B was licensed. The first commercially available hepatitis B vaccine (Heptavax) was derived from plasma of carefully screened and monitored human, high-titer hepatitis B carrier/donors. In 1986, a recombinantly produced hepatitis B vaccine (RecombivaxHB) was introduced in the United States followed by an additional recombinant vaccine introduced in 1989 (Engerix-B). These recombinant vaccines have been shown to be as effective (albeit produce lower geometric mean titers) as human-derived vaccine. The plasma-derived vaccine is now only indicated with persons who have a known allergy to yeast and for hemodialysis and immunocompromised patients.

The vaccine consists of hepatitis B surface antigen (HBsAg) subunit particles and does not include the preS1 or preS2 particles. The vaccine induces only anti-hepatitis B surface antibody (anti-HBs) in recipients.[40]

Clinical trials in healthy individuals have demonstrated antibody conversion rates of approximately 90% after completion of the three-dose series[41] and a protective effect in vaccinees subsequently exposed to hepatitis B virus (HBV).[40] The 10% of subjects who are considered unprotected fall into the categories of nonresponders (anti-HBs <2.1 mIU/mL) and hyporesponders (anti-HBs >2.1 and <10 mIU/mL). It is not clear what percentage of patients are nonresponders, and what percentage are hyporesponders. Lack of development of a protective response is seen in older individuals, with nonresponse rates increasing with increasing age.[42] Other factors that have been identified as leading to poor vaccine response include increased body mass index, being a smoker, and male gender.[41,43,44] When protective antibody concentrations are seen, this protective response lasts 6–10 years in 40–75% of patients.[44] While the two currently available vaccines are considered equivalent in inducing protection to hepatitis B, some data suggest that Recombivax-HB may lead to a higher failure rate than Engerix-B.[42,43,45] The true significance of this is still unclear. A normal immune response has also been seen in patients with Down's syndrome.[40] Response rates in hemodialysis and immunocompromised patients have been lower, requiring higher vaccine dosages to achieve protective levels. The vaccine protects against all hepatitis B serotypes (including delta viroid) but does not cross-react with other hepatitis viruses (i.e., hepatitis A, C, E).

In the preexposure setting, the vaccine has been recommended for persons with occupational risk (health care workers, public safety workers), persons in training for health care fields, clients and staff of institutions for the developmentally disabled, hemodialysis patients, recipients of clotting factor concentrate, household contacts and sex partners of hepatitis B carriers, adoptees from countries where hepatitis B is endemic, international travelers (those spending more than 6 months in areas with high rates of hepatitis B infection or high-risk, short-term travelers), injecting drug users, sexually active homosexual/bisexual men, sexually active heterosexual men and women, and inmates of long-term correctional facilities.[38,40] In addition, the American Academy of Pediatrics recommends universal immunization of all newborns.[39]

Hepatitis B vaccine is also used with hepatitis B immune globulin (HBIG) in the postexposure setting. Persons for whom this regimen is recommended include susceptible individuals having percutaneous or permucosal exposure to blood containing HBsAg, sexual contacts of HBsAg carriers who will continue to be exposed, and infants born of mothers who are HBsAg carriers.[40,46–48] HBIG does not interfere with induction of neutralizing antibody and the combination has been shown to be more protective than when two doses of HBIG alone have been given (85–90% efficacy versus 70–75%).

For neonates born to mothers who are not positive for HBsAg, the primary vaccination series is 2.5 μg of RecombivaxHB or 10 μg of Engerix-B. The first dose should be given at 0–2 days of age, the second dose at 1–2 months of age, and the third dose at 6–18 months of age. An alternative schedule of the three doses administered at 2, 4, and 6–18 months of age may be used. In addition, the appropriate pediatric dose of either brand of hepatitis B vaccine may be used at 2, 4, and 6 months of age for primary immunization.[49] This schedule corresponds more closely with the immunization schedule for other vaccines in infancy. In infants born to HBsAg-positive mothers, immunization should proceed on a different dosing regimen. In addition to administration of HBIG, vaccination with 5 μg of RecombivaxHB or 10 μg of Engerix-B should be given at 12 hours after birth (but no more than 7 days after birth), 1 month, and 6 months of age. These infants should be tested for anti-HBs at 9 months of age or later. A fourth dose of vaccine should be administered to infants who are anti-HB nonresponders or hyporesponders and are HBsAg negative. These children should be tested 1 month after the fourth dose for anti-HBs. If titers of >10 mIU/mL are still not achieved, two additional doses, 1 month apart, may be given with testing for anti-HBs 1 month after the last dose.

For children <11 years old who are not born of mothers who are HBsAG positive, 2.5 μg of RecombivaxHB or 10 μg of Engerix-B should be administered at 0, 1, and 6 months. Children and adolescents ages 11–19 should receive 5 μg of RecombivaxHB or 20 μg of Engerix-B at 0, 1, and 6 months. An alternate four-dose schedule (0, 1, 2, and 12 months) may be used for Engerix-B.

Adults ≥20 years of age should receive 10 μg of RecombivaxHB or 20 μg of Engerix-B at 0, 1, and 6 months. An alternative schedule of 20 μg at 0, 1, 2, and 12 months may be used for Engerix-B only.

Hemodialysis patients are considered poor responders to hepatitis B vaccine; thus, the dose of vaccine is escalated in this population. These patients should receive either 40 μg of RecombivaxHB or 40 μg of Engerix-B in a 0-, 1-, and 6-month schedule. Anti-HBs should be determined and if the value is <10 mIU/mL, one to three booster doses should be administered. In addition, these persons should be tested yearly and boosted with a single dose of 40 μg if anti-HBs <10 mIU/mL.[38,48]

The preferred site of administration is the deltoid muscle in adults (immunogenicity is significantly lower in adults who receive injection in the buttock)[9] and the anterolateral thigh in infants.

Patients who should receive postvaccination serologic testing include immunocompromised patients (due to any cause), persons at occupational risk of exposure, and infants born of HBsAG-positive mothers.

The question arises as to the approach to normal hyporesponders and nonresponders. Approximately 5–15% of normals will not mount a sufficient antibody titer. In some instances, this may be due to measuring the anti-HBs level too long after the last vaccination in the primary series. Generally, while measurement of anti-HBs is suggested 1–6 months after the last dose of vaccine, in reality, measurement of anti-HBs 1–3 months after the last dose is probably wiser.[44] Some data in gay men suggest that 15–25% respond (with development of protective anti-HBs levels) to a single additional dose of vaccine with 30–50% responding to three additional doses.[50] However, these data were generated for the plasma-derived vaccine. Our own data suggest that three doses of 40-μg RecombivaxHB results in development of protective antibody response in 100% of normal hypo- and nonresponders.[51] Non- and hyporesponse may be determined genetically (on the HLA locus); however, the data to assure this are limited.

The need for booster doses of vaccine has not been established.[52] Of persons who develop protective antibody (≥10 or more sample ratio units by radioimmunoassay or positive antibody by enzyme immunoassay), 10–15% will have lost detectable antibody within 4 years with 40–75% of patients having protective antibody level after 6–10 years. Protection against serious infection and liver inflammation appears to persist.[50,53–55] Controversy continues, however, for individuals with normal immune function. Some authors recommend checking antibody status 3–5 years after initial vaccination and administering a single booster dose if antibody concentration is less than 10 mIU/mL.[56] Other authors note that data suggest that protection is in force for at least 7–9 years and, thus, they do not recommend repeat doses before then.[38,57] Further studies are needed to elucidate this.

The same dosage schedule used for primary immunization is used in the postexposure setting. The hepatitis B vaccine series should be initiated as soon as possible after HBIG administration. Table 116.5 illustrates the specifics of vaccine use.

Side effects following vaccine administration have been minimal, with soreness at the injection site being the primary complaint in approximately 25% of vaccinees. Arthralgias and neurologic side effects are exceedingly rare.[3] The incidence of Guillain–Barré syndrome temporally related to administration of the vaccine does not appear to be above the expected case rate in adults and no etiologic association with the vaccine has been made. The vaccine does not adversely or therapeutically affect hepatitis B carriers or persons who are already antibody positive.[58]

HEPATITIS B IMMUNE GLOBULIN

HBIG is used for postexposure, and rarely preexposure, prophylaxis for hepatitis B infection. The product is prepared from pooled plasma obtained from a small group of healthy donors who have high titers of hepatitis B surface antibody (anti-HBs) as a result of hyperimmunization with hepatitis B vaccine.

Indications for the use of HBIG include passive immunization following exposure to hepatitis B virus via percu-

TABLE 116.5. RECOMMENDATIONS FOR HEPATITIS B PROPHYLAXIS FOLLOWING PERCUTANEOUS EXPOSURE

	Treatment When Source Is Found to Be		
Exposed Person	**HBsAg Positive**	**HBsAg Negative**	**Unknown or Not Tested**
Unvaccinated	Administer HBIG × 1[a] and initiate hepatitis B vaccine	Initiate hepatitis B vaccine	Initiate hepatitis B vaccine
Previously Vaccinated			
Known responder	Test exposed person for anti-HBs 1. If adequate, no treatment 2. If inadequate, hepatitis B vaccine booster dose	No treatment	No treatment
Known nonresponder	HBIG × 2 or HBIG × 1, plus 1 dose of hepatitis B vaccine	No treatment	If known high-risk source, may treat as if source were HBsAg positive
Response unknown	Test exposed person for anti-HB[b] 1. If inadequate HBIG × 1, plus hepatitis B vaccine booster dose 2. If adequate, no treatment	No treatment	Test exposed person for anti-HBs[b] 1. If inadequate hepatitis B vaccine booster dose 2. If adequate, no treatment

[a]Hepatitis B immune globulin (HBIG) dose 0.06 mL/kg intramuscularly.
[b]Adequate anti-HBs is ≥10 mIU. (From Centers for Disease Control. Hepatitis B virus: A comprehensive strategy for eliminating transmission in the United States through universal childhood vaccination: Recommendations of the Immunization Practices Advisory Committee (ACIP). MMWR 1991:40(RR-13):1–25.)

taneous, permucosal, or oral ingestion routes (e.g., needlesticks, accidental splash, sexual contact, mouth pipetting) and for infants born to mothers who are hepatitis B carriers. HBIG has also been used for preexposure prophylaxis in the dialysis setting. However, with the advent of hepatitis B vaccine and the use of erythropoietin, a decline in the incidence of hepatitis B in dialysis units has been noted and, thus, HBIG is not generally recommended.

Reports on the use of HBIG have confirmed a significant protective effect of this product (70–75% efficacy) and, in general, superior efficacy when compared to standard immune globulin.[40,59–62] However, there is evidence that HBIG may prolong the incubation period in situations where protective efficacy is not achieved.[63]

The timing of HBIG prophylaxis regarding both frequency of dosing and proximity to the time of exposure has not been completely defined. It is currently recommended by the CDC that HBIG be given as soon as possible after acute exposures (percutaneous, permucosal, oral ingestion), preferably within 24 hours. It is not recommended that HBIG be given beyond 14 days after acute exposure. Variations in the recommendations reflect the relative risk associated with the type of exposure that exists.[64] Generally, the use of HBIG (single dose) with initiation of the hepatitis B vaccine series is thought to be 70–95% effective in preventing infection with hepatitis B.[65]

INFLUENZA VIRUS VACCINE

Influenza virus vaccine (IVV) was first introduced in 1945. Currently, IVV is an inactivated (killed), trivalent whole or split virus vaccine. The virus is grown in antibiotic-free chick embryos and is formaldehyde inactivated for use. Currently available preparations generally contain 45 μg of antigen, in 15-μg trivalent units per 0.5 mL.

Influenza is classified as type A or B, with influenza A further subtyped based on hemaglutinin (H) and neuraminidase (N) surface antigens. Influenza A causes significant disease in humans and the virus is subject to mutation by a phenomenon known as antigenic drift and shift, resulting in the development of different influenza strains. Influenza B, also a significant cause of human disease, is less likely to mutate. The antigenic composition of IVV from year to year is determined by the predominant circulating strains worldwide and may change on a yearly basis.

Issues pertaining to dose, composition, number of doses, route of administration, reactogenicity (adverse effects), antibody response, and efficacy have been debated. IVV efficacy and reactogenicity may be related to the dose of the antigen and the immune status of the individual.[66] Split virus vaccine is felt to be less reactogenic than whole virus vaccine, particularly in children.[67] Antigenic superiority of whole versus split virus vaccine is controversial. In patients who are immunologically "unprimed" (previously unexposed to the antigen), whole and split virus vaccines are likely to induce equal rises in antibody titer.[68,69] However, in "primed" individuals, split virus vaccine may be more effective than whole.[70]

Response to IVV is generally measured in terms of antibody response and, more importantly, efficacy. Generally, an antibody titer of greater than or equal to 1:40 is considered protective.[68–70] Efficacy in a high-risk nursing home population has been proven; vaccinated individuals are significantly less likely to develop influenza, be hospitalized, develop radiologically proven pneumonia, or die.[71] Noted, however, that while IVV has been shown to be cost effective,[72] not all individuals respond with a significant antibody titer rise and thus acquired protection. Generally, sufficient titer rises (greater than fourfold) are determined by the age of the patients and whether or not they have been previously exposed to the antigen.[69] Younger individuals (ages 16–25 years) generally have a lower response to a single dose than those 26 years or older.[67] These differences have led to vaccine dose standardization to facilitate response in the majority of subjects. Antibody titers that generally decline at least twofold by 6 months postvaccination are not changed significantly by the use of booster doses.[73] HIV-positive patients may have an inadequate response to a one- or two-dose IVV regimen (less than 50%).[7] Individuals with HIV should be vaccinated however.

Indications for current split and whole virus influenza vaccines are as follows: (1) adults with chronic cardiovascular or pulmonary diseases, (2) residents of nursing home facilities, (3) health care personnel dealing with high-risk patients, (4) healthy adults older than age 65, (5) adults with chronic metabolic disease, and (6) children with chronic metabolic or cardiopulmonary diseases. In addition, groups that can transmit influenza to high-risk people should be vaccinated. These groups include health care personnel, employees of nursing homes or chronic care facilities who have patient contact, providers of home care to high-risk patients, and household members (including children) of persons in high-risk groups.[74] Individuals who should not be vaccinated are those with anaphylactic hypersensitivity to eggs or other components of the vaccine or adults with febrile illness (until the fever abates).

IVV (split or whole virus) is given as a single 0.5-mL IM injection to persons >12 years of age. Because the availability of split virus vaccine is greater, it is the more commonly used vaccine. In persons 3–12 years of age, one or two 0.5-mL doses of split virus vaccine given 1 month apart are recommended. For ages 6–35 months, 0.25 mL of the split virus vaccine is administered.[75] Two doses are given to children less than 9 years of age who are receiving influenza vaccine for the first time. Influenza vaccine may be administered simultaneously with most other vaccines, especially childhood vaccines.

Adverse reactions to the vaccine include local tenderness or low-grade fever in 3–5% beginning 6–12 hours post-immunization and lasting 1–2 days. Treatment with salicylates or acetaminophen is recommended. Immediate allergic reactions are rare but may occur in patients with hypersensitivity to eggs. Guillain–Barré syndrome was associated only with the 1976 swine influenza vaccine and has not been associated with subsequent vaccines.

Cold-adapted, live attenuated influenza vaccines are under development, and may offer an alternative to the currently used inactivated vaccine. To date, these live vaccines appear to be safe and effective, particularly in young children.[76] Whether the live attenuated vaccine will have great enough safety or efficacy advantages to warrant its use over the inactivated vaccine remains to be determined.

LYME DISEASE VACCINE

Lyme disease is a spirochetal-induced disease, transmitted by a tick vector, *Ixodes dammini.* The causative agent is *Borrelia burgdorferi.* This disease has received much publicity in the lay press with a large amount of anecodotal information and hysteria accompanying it. In mid-1994, the first published trial of a vaccine for Lyme disease appeared.[77] This pilot study of a recombinant outer surface lipoprotein Lyme vaccine in healthy adults showed the vaccine to be immunogenic with relatively mild adverse effects (i.e., local pain and tenderness, mild joint pain). Further trials are ongoing to determine the optimal dose and dosing interval and to ascertain efficacy of this vaccine.

MEASLES VACCINE

Measles vaccine is a live attenuated virus vaccine that produces a subclinical, noncommunicable infection. Approximately 95% of vaccine recipients seroconvert after a single dose, and most are protected for life.[78] However, some data suggest that 9–15% of children may experience primary or secondary vaccine failure, with failure determined by homogenosity in the HLA locus. The vaccine is available as a lyophilized powder derived from a virus grown in chick embryo cell cultures.

Measles vaccine is administered in the arm (or in the thigh if the patient is less than 15 months of age), via subcutaneous injection only, as a 0.5-mL dose. The vaccine is administered for primary immunization to persons 15 months of age or older, usually as MMR (measles–mumps–rubella). A second dose is recommended prior to entry into elementary school or junior high school.[4,79] The second dose of vaccine results in seroconversion in 95% of individuals who were first dose nonresponders, and also boosts immunity in those who had a measurable immunologic response to the first dose.[80]

The vaccine should not be given to immunosuppressed patients (except those infected with HIV), pregnant women, or to patients with a history of egg allergy. In addition, the vaccine should not be given within 6 weeks (preferably 3 months) of IM immune globulin administration, or within 8 months of IGIV given as replacement therapy for humoral immune deficiencies.[79] It is recommended that the vaccine not be given within 1 month of any other live vaccine except mumps, rubella, and oral polio. In allergic patients with a history of anaphylaxis to eggs, skin testing and desensitization is recommended. Allergy to chickens or feathers is not a contraindication to use. In addition, these patients are not at increased risk for anaphylaxis. Known neomycin sensitivity is a contraindication to use, because each 0.5-mL dose contains 25 μg of neomycin. Finally, mild febrile illness is not a contraindication to vaccination. Although seroconversion rates following a single dose of measles vaccine may be lower in patients who have a concurrent upper respiratory tract infection, mild illness is not a reason to postpone vaccination.[81] "Missed opportunities" to administer vaccine to children at an appropriate age contributed greatly to the nationwide measles epidemic of 1989–1991.

Measles vaccine is indicated in all persons born after 1956 or in those who lack documentation of wild virus infection either by history or antibody titers. Persons who received killed measles vaccine alone, were given live vaccine within 3 months of receiving killed vaccine, or who have received a vaccine of unknown type between 1963 and 1967 should be revaccinated. Revaccination should be considered for students entering college and health care workers. If two doses are needed, they should be given at least 1 month apart.[10] Following vaccination, antibodies may be detected within 2–3 weeks in patients 12 months of age or older.

For postexposure prophylaxis, the vaccine is effective if given within 72 hours of exposure. In addition, immune globulin may be administered intramuscularly at a dose of 0.25 mg/kg (maximum dose, 15 mL), if given within 6 days of exposure. In children under 1 year of age, postexposure vaccination may be given as early as 6 months of age, but should be repeated at 12–15 months of age.[78,82,83]

Adverse effects to measles vaccine are limited. Febrile reactions (rarely above 39.4°C) may occur in the month following immunization. Transient rash (generalized) may also occur. These reactions generally appear 5–12 days postvaccination and last 2–5 days. Febrile seizures rarely occur. Other adverse effects such as headache, cough, sore throat, eye pain, malaise, and transient thrombocytopenia may occur. Local reactions at the injection site, while rare, may occur in subjects who have previously been vaccinated with killed vaccine. The vaccine may suppress a positive tuberculin skin test for up to 6 weeks postadministration.

MENINGOCOCCAL POLYSACCHARIDE VACCINE

Meningococcal polysaccharide vaccine (MPV) containing purified capsular polysaccharide antigen from *Neisseria meningitidis* is licensed for use in the United States. Serotypes currently available include groups A, C, Y, and W-135. MPV is available for use as a bivalent (50 μg each, serotypes A and C) or quadrivalent preparation.

MPV is indicated in high-risk populations such as those exposed to the disease, those in the midst of uncontrolled outbreaks, or travelers to an area with epidemic or hyperendemic meningococcal disease. In the United States, serotype B, a strain not contained in the current vaccine, causes the majority of disease, thus routine vaccination is not recommended. The vaccine should not be given to pregnant women unless there is a substantial risk of infection.

MPV (bivalent or quadrivalent) is administered subcutaneously as a single 0.5-mL dose. Subjects should be over 2 years of age[84,85]; however, younger children can produce sufficient antibody levels if given two doses 3 months apart.[84] Antibody levels are attained within 10–14 days.[86] Revaccination may be reconsidered in 2–3 years in children who on initial vaccination are less than 4 years old.[85,87] Antibody decline is more rapid in infants and children.[85] The vaccine shows documented effectiveness in preventing meningococcal disease in 85% to 95% of recipients for serotypes A and C.[86,87] Efficacy of the vaccine for serotypes Y and W-135 is presumed but not documented.

Adverse effects of MPV include fever and erythema at the injection site lasting 1–2 days. Occasionally, headache occurs.

MUMPS VACCINE

The current mumps vaccine is a lyophilized live attenuated vaccine prepared from chick embryo cultures. Each 0.5-mL dose of the vaccine also contains 25 μg of neomycin. The vaccine is available alone or in combination with measles and rubella.

Mumps vaccine is used to produce active immunity while producing a subclinical, noncommunicable infection. A single dose induces antibody formation in 97% of children older than 12 months of age and in 93% of adults. Clinical efficacy approaches 75–90%.[88] Although protection may last a lifetime,[89] outbreaks have been reported in previously vaccinated young adults, suggesting the possibility of waning immunity.[90]

The vaccine (usually given in conjunction with measles and rubella) is given as a 0.5-mL subcutaneous injection in the upper arm. Dosing recommendations coincide with those for measles vaccine, with the first dose being administered at age 12–15 months, and the second one prior to entry into elementary school (or alternatively, prior to entry into junior high school).[91] If the vaccine is given before 12 months of age, revaccination is necessary and should be given after reaching 1 year of age.[89] The vaccine is also indicated in previously unvaccinated adults and in those in whom a poor history of wild virus infection or previous administration of killed mumps exists. Postexposure vaccination is of no benefit.

Mumps vaccine should not be given to pregnant women or immunosuppressed patients. Additionally, conception should be avoided for 3 months following vaccination. In patients with a history of anaphylaxis to eggs, the same schema as in the case of measles should be used. The vaccine should not be given within 6 weeks (preferably 3 months) of administration of immune globulin. Finally, the vaccine should not be given to neomycin-sensitive individuals.

Serious adverse reactions to the vaccine are rarely reported. Parotitis, rash, pruritus, and purpura rarely occur. Local reactions including soreness, burning, and stinging may occur at the injection site.

PERTUSSIS VACCINE

Vaccines for the prevention of pertussis (whooping cough) have been available since 1948. Whole-cell pertussis vaccine is a suspension of killed, whole *Bordetella pertussis* organisms. It is usually administered in combination with diphtheria and tetanus toxoids (as DTP). The primary immunization series for pertussis vaccine consists of four 0.5-mL intramuscular doses given at ages 2, 4, 6, and 15–18 months. A booster dose is recommended at age 4–6 years. The efficacy of pertussis vaccine is approximately 80%. Because disease-related risks decline and vaccine-related side effects increase after age 7, whole-cell pertussis vaccine is not recommended for use beyond this age.

Significant controversy has surrounded pertussis vaccine use in recent years because adverse effects are greater with this vaccine than with other vaccines. Local reactions (pain, redness, and swelling at the site of injection) and febrile reactions occur after approximately 50% of doses. More worrisome events reportedly having a temporal relationship to pertussis vaccine administration include prolonged crying (3%), unusual high-pitched cry (0.1%), convulsions (0.06%), and acute neurologic illness (0.00005%).[92] Other authors have reported mortality in 0.05–0.1% and permanent brain damage of 0.005% of vaccine recipients.[93,94] Recent data on the vaccine currently licensed in the United States indicate that the vaccine carries with it no increased risk of afebrile seizures, encephalopathy, or acute symptomatic seizures.[95,96] A large population-based case control study designed to overcome some of the methodologic flaws of earlier studies failed to find an increased risk of serious acute neurologic illness within 7 days of DTP administration.[97]

Advocates of pertussis vaccine cite the increased incidence of pertussis in Great Britain following decreased use of vaccine after 1975. Vaccination levels decreased from 70–90% in 1975 to 30% by 1978,[98–100] while pertussis disease reached epidemic proportions in 1977–1979 and 1982–1983.[98–100] These advocates also stress the decline in mortality due to pertussis in the United States and England prior to and following vaccine institution. Between 1926 and 1930, there were 36,013 whooping cough deaths in the United States. Between 1979 and 1981, however, only seven deaths were reported in the United States.[101] Finally, 1984 data suggest a significant decrease in pertussis among household contacts ages 6 months to 9 years vaccinated with three or more doses of the vaccine versus nonvaccinated individuals.[101]

The American Academy of Pediatrics and the Immunization Practices Advisory Committee continue to recommend routine pertussis vaccine. There are only two absolute contraindications to pertussis administration: an immediate anaphylactic reaction to a previous dose, or encephalopathy within 7 days of a previous dose, with no evidence of other cause. A convulsion within 3 days of DTP, persistent inconsolable screaming for 3 or more hours within 2 days of DTP, hypotonic–hyporesponsive episode within 48 hours, and a temperature of 40.5°C or greater, unexplained by another cause, within 48 hours once were considered contraindications, but are now identified as precautions. None of these events has been proven to cause permanent sequelae. The decision of whether to administer additional doses of pertussis vaccine to patients who have experienced one of these events should be based on the possible risks of the disease (i.e., during a pertussis outbreak).

Whether patients with a seizure disorder should receive pertussis vaccine has been a matter of debate; but a history of a seizure disorder is not itself a contraindication. In patients with a recent onset of seizures, vaccine should be withheld until it is determined whether a neurologic disorder is evolving and, if not, pertussis vaccine may be continued.[102]

Recently, the FDA approved the use of diphtheria and tetanus toxoids and acellular pertussis (aP) vaccine (DTaP) for the fourth (ages 15–18 months) and fifth dose (age 4–6 years).[103] These acellular vaccines contain only components of the *B. pertussis* organism, rather than the intact, killed microbe. Two acellular products are licensed, one containing equal amounts of pertussis toxin (PT) and filamentous hemagglutinin (FHA), the other one containing a predominance of FHA and small amounts of PT, pertactin (a 69-kD outer membrane protein), and agglutinins. Although it is unknown which components are essential to inducing a protective immunologic response, antibody development to the components of aP is at least equivalent to that of pertussis vaccine, when used as the fourth and fifth doses of the DTP series. They also appear to be immunogenic in infants, but FDA approval for DTaP use in the first three doses of the series has not been granted.

Based on experience with aP in other countries, it appears that aP and P are of equal efficacy. The acellular products are safer, though, in that they cause fewer local reactions and febrile responses. The same contraindications and precautions apply to both the whole-cell and acellular pertussis vaccines.[104,105]

PNEUMOCOCCAL VACCINE

Pneumococcal vaccine is a mixture of highly purified capsular polysaccharides from 23 of the 83 most prevalent or invasive types of *Streptococcus pneumoniae* seen in the United States. These 23 types represent 90% of all blood isolates and 85% of pneumococcal isolates from other generally sterile sites seen in the United States. Each 0.5-mL dose of vaccine contains 25 μg of each polysaccharide type dissolved in isotonic saline solution, for a total of 575 μg of polysaccharide, and contains 0.25% phenol as preservative. Significant cross-reactivity with other pneumococcal capsular antigens not represented in the vaccine does not occur.

Following vaccination of healthy adults, antibody levels to these strains remain elevated for at least 5 years. In certain individuals, these levels decline within 10 years. Children may be protected only 3–5 years.[106] Patients with AIDS may respond poorly to the vaccine; however, asymptomatic HIV-infected patients respond sufficiently.

The pneumococcal vaccine is recommended for persons at high risk of acquiring the disease. Data have demonstrated an increased incidence of serious pneumococcal infection in patients who are immunosuppressed (e.g., Hodgkin's disease and other lymphoproliferative disorders, multiple myeloma, renal failure) and those with splenic dysfunction or anatomic asplenia. Patients with chronic illnesses of the cardiovascular and pulmonary systems, alcoholism, and the elderly, particularly those who are institutionalized, are also felt to be at increased risk. Previous hospitalization can help define high-risk individuals, because two-thirds of patients with serious disease have been hospitalized within the previous 5 years, generally with an underlying condition that would predispose to pneumococcal disease.[107] Recommendations for pneumococcal vaccine include adults and children over the age of 2 who are at high risk for pneumococcal disease, and otherwise healthy adults over the age of 65.[10,11,25,108,109] An antibody rise of 1.4- to 2-fold or 200–300 ng of antibody nitrogen per milliliter is often used to define an adequate immune response to this vaccine.[110–112] Most immunocompetent groups of patients have demonstrated at least a twofold rise in antibody within 2–3 weeks after immunization. Children over the age of 2 and young adults with sickle cell anemia and splenectomy have also had adequate responses. However, certain groups have not demonstrated an adequate response, including children less than 2 years of age, asplenic Hodgkin's disease patients on chemotherapy, and persons with impaired immunoglobulin synthesis and multiple myeloma.[112,113]

Studies demonstrating decreases in the incidence of pneumococcal disease are more difficult to carry out due to low and variable attack rates and the need for large study populations. In controlled studies of African goldminers, immunization resulted in a 76–78.5% reduction in pneumonia and an 82.3–92% reduction in bacteremia.[110] In patients with sickle cell disease and patients with splenectomy, a protective effect against vaccine-specific organisms has been suggested.[114,115] An octavalent vaccine was demonstrated to reduce the incidence of otitis media in immunized black children aged 6–11 months, but had no effect on a similar white population.[116] Efficacy studies in both noninstitutionalized and institutionalized elderly patients and those in a psychiatric facility were inconclusive.[117,118] Conflicting opinions also exist with regard to the use of the vaccines in patients with chronic lung disease. It is not clear if this group is at significant risk of pneumococcal disease, or if preexisting high antibody levels in these patients affect vaccine response.[119] As a result, considerable controversy exists over widespread use of the vaccine, particularly in healthy elderly populations. Recent data suggest that efficacy of the vaccine varies in different patient groups. Overall efficacy is approximately 60%, and in immunocompetent persons older than 65 years of age it is around 75%.[120]

Pneumococcal vaccine is recommended for routine use in immunocompetent adults and immunocompromised adults at increased risk of pneumococcal disease (including HIV infection).[106] Children 2 years and older with chronic disease (including HIV infection) that places them at increased risk for pneumococcal disease should be vaccinated.[104] This does not include children with recurrent otitis media, sinusitis, or upper respiratory infection. When possible the vaccine should be administered at least 2 weeks before the administration of immunosuppressive therapy or splenectomy.

In adults who have had a documented or suspected pneumococcal infection, some authorities recommend an interval of 2–3 months between the episode before immunization. However, this suggestion is not supported by literature data, and thus each case should be individually assessed as to whether the patient will return for immunization.

Revaccination has been a controversial issue. The duration of clinical protection afforded by a single injection is not known; however, it is known that type-specific antibodies decline with time, at different rates. Additionally, early studies indicated that local adverse effects occurred more commonly and were more severe than after the first dose, if there was too short an interval between the two doses. Currently recommendations suggest limiting revaccination to the following individuals: (1) persons who received the 14-valent vaccine and who are at highest risk of fatal infection (e.g., asplenic patients); (2) adults at high risk who received the 23-valent vaccine 6 years or more previously and who may have significant declines in antibody levels; and (3) children at high risk who would be 10 years or younger at revaccination (3–5 years after initial vaccination).[106,121]

Pneumococcal vaccine safety is well documented. Local reactions occur frequently and are generally mild. Local erythema and induration (30%), local discomfort (40%), and local swelling (3%) are the side effects most commonly observed. Rarely, severe systemic reactions can occur and they consist of weakness, myalgia, headache, photophobia, chills, and fever.

POLIOVIRUS VACCINES

Two types of trivalent poliovirus vaccines are currently licensed for distribution in the United States.[122,123] An inactivated vaccine (IPV), developed by Salk was licensed for use in 1955. In 1987, an enhanced-potency inactivated vaccine was introduced (eIPV), and this has replaced the original IPV. Since 1962, a live attenuated, oral vaccine (OPV), developed by Sabin, has been available and is currently the primary immunizing agent for poliovirus infection. Both vaccines are produced from three approved, attenuated, seed strains of poliovirus: type I Mahoney, type II MEF-1, and type III Saukett.

OPV is administered in a series of three oral 0.5-mL doses with a second dose given 6–8 weeks after the first and the third dose 6 to 8 weeks after the second. In children, OPV immunization generally begins at 6–12 weeks of age, commonly with the first DTP immunization.

OPV closely parallels natural infection, stimulating humoral antibody and secretory IgA in lymphatic tissues surrounding the intestinal tract within 7–10 days of ingestion. Virus replicates within the gastrointestinal tract and can be found in pharyngeal secretions and stool for several weeks. This shedding of virus can result in immunization of some contacts of vaccinees, as well as risk of infection in contacts with compromised immune status. Immunity is achieved in 95% of vaccine recipients.

There are no immediate side effects of OPV. Rarely, vaccine-associated poliomyelitis will develop in vaccinees (1 out of 9 million doses) or contacts (1 out of 7 million doses).[11] Individuals with primary immune deficiency are at increased risk for this adverse reaction and for this reason OPV is not recommended for persons who are immunodeficient or for normal individuals who reside in a household where another person is immunodeficient. It is recommended that HIV-infected patients receive eIPV in place of the live vaccine; however, in other countries of the world the live product has been used. OPV should not be given during pregnancy because of the small but theoretical risk to the fetus.

Primary immunization with eIPV consists of a series of three 1-mL subcutaneous injections given 4–8 weeks apart with a similar booster dose 6–12 months after the third injection. If interruption of the series occurs, a sufficient immune response can be obtained by administration of only those doses which had been omitted. Following immunization, humoral antibodies are induced in 95% of recipients. The duration of protection following immunization has not been definitively determined.

There are no serious side effects or contraindications to IPV except pregnancy, where IPV should be given only if clearly needed (e.g., women who will be traveling or living in an area with endemic or epidemic poliovirus).

Primary poliomyelitis immunization is recommended for all children and young adults up to age 18. OPV is the vaccine of choice in this age group unless an immunodeficiency exists in the patient or a household contact, in which case eIPV is recommended. Primary immunization of adults over the age of 18 is not routinely recommended because a high level of immunity already exists in this age group and the risk of exposure in developed countries is small. However, unimmunized adults who are at increased risk for exposure because of travel, residence, or occupation should receive primary immunization with eIPV, because there is a small but increased risk of vaccine-induced paralysis following OPV administration in adults. HIV-positive patients should receive eIPV.

Incompletely immunized adults or children should complete the series of eIPV or OPV regardless of the interval since initiation of primary immunization. Booster doses of OPV or eIPV are recommended for children before entering school. In adults, booster doses are not routinely recommended unless an increased risk of exposure (e.g., travel) exists, in which case a single dose of OPV or eIPV should be given.

It appears that poliomyelitis has been eradicated in the United States. There have been no cases due to wild-type poliovirus since 1982. Each year approximately 10 cases of paralytic disease are reported to the CDC, but these are due to vaccine strains of the virus. Because of the low risk of natural polio in the United States, and the risk of vaccine-associated disease, some people feel that eIPV should become the routine product. Others feel that use of eIPV for the first two doses (when risk of vaccine-associated polio is greatest), followed by booster doses of OPV would be preferable, since this regimen provides the greatest systemic immunity.[124] It is unlikely that eIPV use in the United States will become routine, however, until a vaccine containing it in combination with DTP is commercially available, due to concern over the large number of injections required to immunize infants and children.

RABIES VACCINE

Human diploid cell vaccine (HDCV) and rabies vaccine adsorbed (RVA) are killed vaccines used for preexposure and postexposure rabies virus prophylaxis. These agents are successors to previous vaccines, including duck embryo vaccine, and are more immunogenic with fewer side effects than their predecessors.

Transmission of rabies can occur via percutaneous, permucosal, or airborne exposure to the rabies virus. Circumstances favoring such transmission include animal bites or attacks, and contamination of scratches, cuts, abrasions, or mucous membranes with saliva or other infectious material (e.g., brain tissue). Airborne acquisition in laboratories and in bat-infested caves has been reported. Unprovoked attacks and daytime attacks by nocturnal animals are considered highly suspect. Common wild animal transmitters include skunks, foxes, and raccoons. Rabies in domestic animals in the United States varies among regions. Dog rabies is very common in certain foreign countries (e.g., India, African nations). Rabies kills more than 25,000 people each year in India.[125] Rodents, rabbits, and hares are rarely infected. There have been four reports of person-to-person transmission via corneal transplant.[126] Reports of rabid animals has increased over the past decade in the United States.

Preexposure indications for using HDCV or RVA include persons whose vocation or avocation place them at high risk for rabies exposure, for example, veterinarians, animal handlers, laboratory workers in rabies research labs, and field personnel (trappers, hunters, cave explorers). Travelers who will be in a country or area of a country where there is a constant threat of rabies, whose stay is likely to extend beyond 1 month, and who may not have readily available medical services (e.g., Peace Corps workers, missionaries) should also be considered for preexposure prophylaxis. The population at large need not be vaccinated.[127]

Postexposure prophylaxis should be given after percutaneous or permucosal exposure to saliva or other infectious material from a high-risk source. Each case needs to be considered individually. Consideration needs to be given to the geographic area, species of animal, circumstances of the incident, and type of exposure. Local or state health departments may be able to provide guidelines.

HDCV for preexposure prophylaxis is administered in three doses of 1.0 mL intramuscularly or 0.1 mL intradermally on days 0 and 7 and between days 21 and 28.[128,129] HDCV for intradermal prophylaxis must be given using the specific intradermal dosage form and syringe. Although literature suggests that intradermal vaccine gives protective titers in equal number of patients compared to intramuscular dosing,[130–132] recent field reports suggest that intradermal HDCV may give a nonprotection rate of 7.5%.[133] This observation has led the New York State Department of Health to recommend the routine use of intramuscular HDCV. If intradermal injection is used, it is suggested that rabies antibody titers be checked 30 days after the last dose of vaccine (NYS Memo). RVA may be used intramuscularly but not intradermally for preexposure prophylaxis. Pregnancy is not a contraindication if the risk of rabies is great. The vaccine is not recommended for persons who are immunocompromised. An intramuscular booster dose every second year is recommended for persons who will have continued exposure. Some authors recommend testing rabies antibody with booster doses deferred if the rapid fluorescent focus inhibition test (RFFIT) is >1:5. Intradermal boosters doses, while recommended by some groups,[127] are not recommended by the New York State Department of Health.[134] Suboptimal responses have been documented in persons receiving chloroquine chemoprophylaxis for malaria,[135] and thus vaccine should be administered 1 month prior to the institution of chloroquine therapy. If this is not possible, intramuscular HDCV or RVA should be used. For individuals who have received the duck embryo vaccines in the past, a single intramuscular booster dose of HDCV or RVA may be used.

Preexposure prophylaxis does not eliminate the need for postexposure prophylaxis. The regimen for postexposure prophylaxis is determined by whether or not a person has previously received HDCV or RVA. Persons previously immunized with HDCV or RVA or those who have received postexposure prophylaxis previously should receive two 1.0-mL intramuscular doses of HDCV or RVA on postexposure days 0 and 3. Rabies immune globulin should not be given to this group. Individuals who have not been previously immunized should receive the recommended regimen of rabies immune globulin (see later section) and five doses of HDCV or RVA, 1.0-mL intramuscularly on days 0, 3, 7, 14, and 28 after exposure.[10,11,127] The intradermal route should not be used for postexposure prophylaxis.

Adverse reactions to HDCV and RVA are not uncommon. Approximately 20% will experience pain, erythema, swelling, and itching at the injection site. Another 20% may have headache, nausea, abdominal pain, muscle aches, and/or dizziness.[10,131] Systemic allergic reactions ranging from hives to anaphylaxis occur in an estimated 11 out of 10,000 vaccinees.[136] It is recommended that persons exposed to rabies who do have adverse reactions continue the vaccine series in a setting with medical support services. In persons receiving booster doses of HDCV or RVA, an immune complex-like disease has been seen in up to 7% of vaccinees.[136]

Antibody conversion occurs in virtually 100% of HDCV of RVA recipients. The CDC considers titers of 1:5 by RFFIT testing as being protective. The World Health Organization uses a value of 0.5 IU/mL as evidence of protective antibody. Persons who are receiving corticosteroids or other immunosuppressant agents and who receive postexposure prophylaxis should have their antibody status determined.

RABIES IMMUNE GLOBULIN

Human rabies immune globulin is an immunoglobulin used in conjunction with rabies vaccine as part of postexposure rabies management for previously unvaccinated individuals. The product is derived from plasma obtained from donors who have been hyperimmunized with rabies vaccine and have high titers of circulating antibody.

In persons who have not been previously immunized against rabies, rabies immune globulin is given simultaneously with rabies HDCV to provide optimal coverage in the interval before immune response to the vaccine occurs. The efficacy of this regimen has been clearly demonstrated. In situations where vaccine has been used alone, mortality rates of 50–60% have been observed. Mortality after the combination vaccine/rabies immune globulin regimens is an exceedingly rare event.[10,137,138]

Rabies immune globulin does not interfere with vaccine-induced antibody formation. However, its use is not recommended beyond 8 days after initiation of the vaccine series nor in persons previously immunized to rabies.

Human rabies immune globulin is administered in a dose of 20 IU/kg (0.133 mL/kg), half to be given intramuscularly and the other half infiltrated around the wound site. This product should never be administered by the intravenous route. Because other antibodies in the rabies immune globulin may interfere with the response to live virus vaccines (e.g., MMR), it is recommended that these immunizations be delayed for 3 months.

Side effects are rare, but may include local soreness at the wound or intramuscular injection site and mild temperature elevations. Caution is advised when administering this product to persons with known systemic allergies to immune globulin or thimerosal. Pregnancy is not a contraindication for its use.

RUBELLA VACCINE

Rubella vaccine contains lyophilized live attenuated rubella (German measles) virus grown in human diploid cell culture. The vaccine is available alone or in combination with measles and/or mumps vaccine. Each 0.5-mL dose also contains 25 μg of neomycin.

Rubella vaccine induces antibodies to the virus that are thought to be protective against wild virus infection.[139] Following a single 0.5-mL subcutaneous dose, 95% of children 1 year of age become rubella antibody positive within 2–6 weeks.[140,141] The duration of immunity has not been established and booster doses are not recommended. However, a second dose is recommended at the same time measles vaccine is administered (i.e., as a second dose of MMR). The vaccine is indicated for children greater than 1 year of age, persons 12 years or older without evidence of wild virus infection, women of childbearing potential for whom serologic testing is unavailable, and to persons at a substantial risk for exposure.[142,143] The vaccine should not be given to immunosuppressed individuals nor used within 6 weeks (preferably 3 months) of immune globulin administration. Additional immune globulin should not be given within 14 days of vaccine. The vaccine should not be given to neomycin-sensitive patients.

Adverse effects of rubella virus vaccine tend to increase with the age of the recipient. Symptoms are similar to wild virus infection and include lymphadenopathy, rash, urticaria, fever, malaise, sore throat, headache, myalgias, and paresthesias of the extremities. These occur 11–20 days after vaccination and last 1–5 days. Joint symptoms occur at 1–10 weeks in 20–40% of adult women and their incidence is greater in adolescent women than in children.[143] Overt arthritis occurs in less than 1% of recipients. Symptoms last 1–3 days and rarely recur. The vaccine may cause suppression of tuberculin skin tests for up to 6 weeks postvaccination. While the vaccine virus may be excreted in nose and throat secretions, it is not contagious.

While the vaccine has been shown to be safe to the fetus, its use in pregnancy is discouraged.[143] Women should be counseled not to become pregnant for 3 weeks following vaccination. Termination of pregnancy is not indicated in women who are accidentally given the vaccine.[10]

VARICELLA VACCINE

Live attenuated varicella vaccine has been under development for about two decades. It is licensed in Japan and several European countries, and the United States experience with this vaccine has led to anticipation of its licensure sometime in 1994. Takahashi, in 1974, developed a vaccine using an OKA strain of varicella-zoster (VZ) virus. Most subsequent vaccines have also used the OKA strain but a KMcC strain has also been studied. It is only recently that the existence of multiple VZ strains has been recognized and no comparison of the strains has been made. However, there is evidence that the OKA strain may not be cross-protective against some other wild virus strains.

Studies to date indicate that OKA VZ vaccine is safe and immunogenic in healthy adults and children, as well as severely immunocompromised patients.[144–146] A single dose will result in seroconversion in greater than 94% of healthy children, and over 90% have persisting antibodies 1 year later. Studies in normal, healthy adults have shown inconsistent results, with seroconversion rates of as low as 80% following a single dose. Use of a two-dose regimen, with a 3-month interval between doses, results in antibody response in approximately 95% of recipients. Similar results have been observed in immunocompromised children: 88% response rate with one dose, >95% seroconversion after two doses.[147]

Although VZ vaccine has been approximately 80% effective in preventing chickenpox in leukemic children, the target group for varicella vaccine is expected to be VZ-susceptible normal healthy children, and normal healthy adults, in whom the vaccine's efficacy is about 90%. It is desirable to protect immunocompromised children in whom VZ infection may be a life-threatening event (e.g., those with leukemia), but use of VZ vaccine in these individuals likely will be restricted to compassionate protocol, under the guidance of specialists.[148]

The duration of immunity induced by VZ vaccine is unknown, but is of concern since chickenpox in adults is typically more severe than it is in children. Although antibody titers may decline with time, VZ vaccine stimulates both humoral and cell-mediated immune response.[149] Humoral and cell-mediated immunity persist for a minimum of 6 years in vaccinated children, suggesting that protection is long lasting.[150] Additionally, children who are immunized against varicella and then develop asymptomatic reinfection from wild virus experience an immunologic boost.[151] Thus, protection may persist following immunization as a result of asymptomatic reinfection. The necessity of routine administration of booster doses will be the subject of study for a number of years.

Individuals who develop chickenpox despite having been vaccinated typically experience milder disease, with a lower incidence of fever and fewer skin lesions, many of which do not vesiculate.[152] Similarly, the secondary spread of virus following vaccination occurs at a low rate and results in mild disease, confirming attenuation of the virus.[2]

Because VZ vaccine is a live virus vaccine, there has been concern regarding the occurrence of zoster in vaccinees, as a result of latent VZ infection with the vaccine virus. Although this risk is present, zoster appears to develop no more frequently following vaccination than it does as a sequela to natural VZ infection. In fact, among patients with leukemia, zoster occurs less frequently in vaccinated individuals.[153] VZ-specific immunologic response can be boosted in the elderly, yet the vaccine has not been shown to reduce clinical zoster infection.[147]

No severe side effects to the vaccine have been reported. Mild to moderate delayed-onset rashes have occurred in approximately 4% of normal healthy vaccine recipients and in up to 50% of vaccinees with leukemia. Pain, local swelling, and erythema at the injection site are reported in up to 25% of patients, fever in 4–10%, and mild upper respiratory symptoms in a smaller number.

Whether VZ vaccine becomes a routinely recommended vaccine for healthy children remains to be seen. Recent cost-effectiveness analysis suggested that routine vaccination of healthy children would be cost effective from a societal perspective, which includes work loss costs as well as medical costs. However, from a health payer's perspective (medical costs only) the same degree of cost effectiveness would not be realized.[154] The economic benefit of vaccinating pediatric patients prior to solid organ transplantation, however, has been estimated to be much greater.[155] In 1995, the American Academy of Pediatrics recommended routine immunization with varicella vaccine for all children.

VARICELLA-ZOSTER IMMUNE GLOBULIN

Varicella-zoster immune globulin (VZIG) is used for passive immunization of susceptible immunodeficient patients exposed to VZ infection. It is prepared by Cohn cold ethanol fractionation from plasma found in routine screening of normal volunteer blood donors to contain high titers of VZ antibody.[156,157] On the average, VZIG has been found to contain 10–20 times more VZ antibody than immune globulin.[158]

Use of VZIG should be considered in exposed children and certain adults who are immunocompromised and susceptible to VZ. Criteria for its use in children are listed in Table 116.6 and take into consideration underlying disease, type of exposure, prior varicella history, age, and interval since exposure. Criteria for its use in immunocompromised adults are less clear because of difficulties in determining susceptibility status. A positive history of varicella infection eliminates the need for VZIG. However, a negative infection history is not a valid indicator because 85–95% of persons with negative or unknown varicella infection histories are serologically positive for VZ antibodies. Individuals with a previous household exposure (siblings or children) and those who have attended an urban school or have had previous occupational exposure (e.g., nursery school, kindergarten) are likely to be immune.[158] Positive serologic tests on immunocompromised patients can be misleading because VZ antibody may be transiently acquired from blood products. In such cases it is best to consult with the regional Red Cross Blood Distribution Center regarding the appropriate course of action.

Varicella can cause congenital malformation early and, rarely, late in pregnancy. While VZIG may attenuate maternal infection, its efficacy in preventing intrauterine infection has not been demonstrated. There is an increased risk of serious infection and an associated 30% mortality in infants whose mothers develop varicella 4 days prior to or 2 days after delivery or whose onset of infection is between 5 and 10 days of age. Normal, full-term infants exposed postnatally are not at increased risk for complications. Use of VZIG perinatally is therefore aimed at the critical period for complications (see Table 116.6).[157]

TABLE 116.6. INDICATIONS FOR VARICELLA-ZOSTER IMMUNE GLOBULIN[a]

1. Susceptible to VZ infection
2. Significant exposure within 96 hours
   a. Household contact
   b. Playmate contact (more than 1 hour of play indoors)
   c. Hospital contact (in adjacent beds or same two- to four-bed room)
   d. School contact (adjacent desks in same classroom or same carpool)
   e. Transplacental contact (newborn born to mother who developed varicella less than 5 days prior to or 48 hours after delivery)
3. Age <15, with administration to immunocompromised adolescents, adults, and other older patients on an individual basis
4. One of the following underlying illnesses or conditions:
   a. Leukemia or lymphoma
   b. Congenital or acquired immunodeficiency
   c. Immunosuppressive treatment
   d. Newborn of mother with varicella (2e above)
   e. Premature infant (≥28 week gestation) whose mother lacks a prior history of chicken pox
   f. Premature infants (<28 weeks gestation or ≤1000 grams) regardless of maternal history

[a]Patients should meet all four criteria. (Compiled from Ref. 8.)

The efficacy of VZIG has been measured by three parameters: clinical attack rates, severity of illness, and incidence of subclinical disease. Clinical attack rates after VZIG have varied from 20–65% compared to normal attack rates of 80–90% after household exposures without prophylaxis. However, the severity of illness has been significantly affected with VZIG, and the majority of cases have been mild with complications occurring in only 7%. Subclinical infections commonly occur after VZIG. In one study, 33% of leukemic patients had evidence of subclinical infection after VZIG compared to a 5% incidence after natural infections.[159–161]

For maximum effectiveness, VZIG must be given within 48 hours and not more than 96 hours following exposure. Because this agent may only attenuate infection, patients who receive VZIG may still have a period of communicability. VZIG may prolong the incubation period to 28 days.

VZIG is distributed by the American Red Cross Services. Contact with the distribution centers must be made within 72 hours of exposure and specific criteria met in order for the product to be released.

Administration of VZIG is by the intramuscular route (never intravenously) at doses of 125 U per 10 kg of body weight up to 625 U (5 vials) for patients more than 40 kg. The dose for newborn infants is 125 U. Side effects include local soreness at the site of injection. VZIG should be avoided in persons with bleeding diathesis. There are no other contraindications for the use of this product. Duration of antibody protection is not known, but is felt to be at least one half-life of the immune globulin, approximately 3 weeks.

OTHER IMMUNOBIOLOGICS

CYTOMEGALOVIRUS IMMUNE GLOBULIN

Cytomegalovirus immune globulin intravenous (CMV-IGIV) contains IgG antibodies obtained from healthy persons with high titers of antibodies to cytomegalovirus (CMV).[162] The agent is currently available commercially.

CMV-IGIV is only indicated at present for attenuation of primary CMV disease associated with kidney transplantation in seronegative recipients of seropositive kidneys.[163] CMV-IVIG is dosed using a tapering schedule. Dosage is 150 mg/kg preoperatively or within 72 hours postoperatively; 100 mg/kg at 2, 4, 6, and 8 weeks; and 50 mg/kg at weeks 12 and 16. These doses are for all ages. The use of

CMV-IVIG has resulted in a 50% reduction of CMV-related syndromes.[162] CMV-IVIG has been investigated for use with gancyclovir in treating CMV infection in liver and bone marrow transplant patients. Data in this area are preliminary and its routine use is not recommended.

Adverse effects of CMV-IGIV are seen in less than 5% of recipients and include flushing, chills, muscle cramps, back pain, chest tightness, fever, nausea, vomiting, hypotension, and tachycardia. Anaphylaxis rarely occurs.

Since CMV-IVIG contains other antibodies, it has been suggested that vaccination with live viral vaccines be withheld until 3 months after CMV-IVIG administration.

IMMUNE GLOBULIN

Immune globulin (IG) is available as both intramuscular (IGIM) and intravenous preparations (IGIV). IGIM, or the Cohn fraction II, is prepared from pooled plasma of several thousand donors by cold ethanol fractionation.[164] IGIM typically contains greater than 95% IgG and trace amounts of IgM, IgA, and other plasma proteins. Because IG is harvested from a large donor pool, it contains a wide spectrum of IgG antibodies to the pathogens prevalent in the area from which the donors were obtained. In the fractionation process, high molecular weight IgG aggregates are formed, which can activate complement in the absence of antigen and precipitate anaphylactoid reactions. For this reason, intramuscular IG is unsuitable for intravenous administration. Intramuscular IG typically contains 15–18% protein and not less than 90% IgG.

A number of intravenous preparations of IG are commercially available in the United States.[165] Generally, these preparations contain greater than 90% IgG monomers and trace to small amounts of IgA.[166] These agents are rendered suitable for intravenous use because their anticomplement activity is removed either by selective reduction and alkylation of interchain disulfide bonds, or by treatment at low pH in the presence of small amounts of pepsin which removes the IgG aggregates and/or IgA. These products are available as lypholized powders or solutions.

When administered either intravenously or intramuscularly, IG distributes in approximately 5% of the body weight of the recipient.[165] The plasma half-life of IG averages 18–32 days. This range of half-life is probably attributable to the variation in the half-life of IgG subclasses. Peak serum concentrations occur relatively immediately with intravenous IG whereas intramuscular IG produces peak concentrations within 2 days. After the initial period of equilibration, circulating IgG levels are superimposable between intravenous and intramuscular equivalent dosages. No dosage adjustment is necessary in patients with renal and/or hepatic insufficiency, in dialysis patients, or in geriatric patients. Serum IgG levels increase approximately 250 mg% for each 100 mg/kg of intravenous IG infused.[167,168]

IG is indicated in a wide variety of circumstances to provide passive immunity to individuals.[165] The indications for IGIM differ from those of IGIV.

IGIM is indicated for providing passive immunity in hepatitis A infections, as an alternative to HBIG in hepatitis B exposures (however, HBIG is significantly more effective), hepatitis C (but not hepatitis E), measles, varicella zoster, and primary immunodeficiency diseases. IGIM is not indicated for prevention of rubella, mumps, or poliomyelitis. Table 116.7 lists the suggested dosages for IGIM in various disease states.

IGIV has been studied in many disease states. Currently there are many approved indications and other non-approved disease states for which IGIV is used. Dosages vary based on the preparation used.[166,169]

In primary immunodeficiency states, monthly doses of between 100–800 mg/kg are administered, with the average dose being 200 mg/kg. These immunodeficiency states include both antibody deficiencies and combined deficiencies. HIV disease is not in this class.

For the treatment of idiopathic thrombocytopenia purpura (ITP), doses of 400 mg/kg daily for 2–5 days are indicated. Some manufacturers recommend 1 g/kg for 1–2 days. Others recommend 2 g/kg/d for 2–7 days. IGIV is acceptable for treatment of both chronic and acute ITP. IGIV has been used in ITP associated with pregnancy with-

TABLE 116.7. INDICATIONS AND DOSAGE OF INTRAMUSCULAR IMMUNE GLOBULIN IN INFECTIOUS DISEASES

Primary immunodeficiency states	1.2 mL/kg IM then 0.6 mL/kg IM every 2–4 weeks
Hepatitis A exposure	0.02 mL/kg IM within 2 weeks
Hepatitis A prophylaxis	0.0 2 mL/kg IM if exposure <3 months 0.06 mL/kg if exposure >3 months, every 4–6 months
Hepatitis B	0.06 mL/kg IM (HBIG is preferred in known exposures) as soon as possible
Non-A/non-B hepatitis	0.06 mL/kg IM as soon as possible (questionable effectiveness)
Measles	0.25 mL/kg IM within 6 days (maximum dose = 15 mL)
Rubella	0.55 mL/kg, single dose
Primary immunodeficiency states	1.2 mL/kg IM then 0.6 mL/kg IM every 2–4 weeks

out adverse effects on the fetus.[166] It should be noted that corticosteroids are the drugs of choice for adult ITP.

Chronic lymphocytic leukemia (CLL) is a disease state for which IGIV has been used. IGIV is used in CLL patients who have had a serious bacterial infection. Doses of 400 mg/kg every 3–4 weeks are used.

A number of other proposed uses of IGIV can be identified. It is important to note that generally these are not approved indications and are not generally accepted in the medical community for routine treatment. These uses include the following:

- *Kawasaki disease (mucocutaneous lymph node syndrome):* This disease, which generally occurs in children, carries the hallmark of development of coronary artery abnormalities. Generally, it is recommended by the American Academy of Pediatrics that if the strict criteria for Kawasaki disease are met, an IGIV dose of 400 mg/kg/d for 4 consecutive days be used. The dose should be administered within 10 days of disease onset. Other dosage levels are currently under investigation including doses as high as 2 g/kg/d. Aspirin should also be administered.[166]
- *Neonatal sepsis:* Neonatal sepsis can cause significant morbidity within 24 hours of birth. While Group B streptococcus and *Escherichia coli* remain the primary infecting organisms, other bacteria and fungi may be associated with sepsis. IGIV appears to be effective in neonates <34 weeks gestational age or <1500 g. Doses of 500–900 mg/kg have been used.[166,169]
- *Autoimmune diseases:* IGIV may be effective in self-limited immunoregulatory diseases but less effective in chronic diseases such as systemic lupus erythematosus. Definite conclusions about the use of IGIV cannot be made in this category.
- *Cystic fibrosis:* Only one study exists that has examined the use of IGIV in this disease. At this time, no firm recommendations can be made on its use.[68]
- *Intractable epilepsy:* In patients who have confirmed IgG_2 deficiency, IGIV may be useful. Otherwise, it is not indicated.[68]
- *Thermal injury:* Not indicated.
- *Cytomegalovirus infection:* The use of CMV-IVIG is recommended versus the use of IGIV.
- *HIV infection:* The FDA recently approved the use of IGIV for reducing the incidence of infections in children with HIV.[170] Dosages of 400 mg/kg each month are recommended.
- *Bone marrow transplant:* In 1994 the FDA approved the use of IGIV for reducing graft-versus-host disease and infections in patients over the age of 20. Patients received 500 mg/kg each week from 7 days before transplantation to 3 months after. At 100 days post-transplant, patients received a monthly dose of IGIV for 1 year. Infection decreased from 51% to 34%.[170]

Other diseases in an uncontrolled setting for which IGIV has been used include Guillain–Barré syndrome, myasthenia gravis, epilepsy, amyotrophic lateral sclerosis, rheumatoid arthritis, and factor VIII inhibition due to autoantibody. In addition, recent data suggest the efficacy of IGIV in severe IgA nephropathy and Henoch–Schonlein purpura.[171]

Adverse effects of IG vary with the route of administration. Following IGIM, pain, tenderness, and muscle stiffness persisting for hours or days are seen. Repeat courses may cause sensitization with resultant allergic reactions. With IGIV, adverse effects are seen in less than 1% of immunocompetent patients and in less than 10% of others. Most adverse effects are related to the rate of the infusion. Infusion should be given at a rate of 0.01–0.02 mL/kg/min for 30 minutes and then, if no reactions occur, increased to 0.02–0.04 mL/kg/min. While infusion rate recommendations vary slightly depending on the preparation, the guidelines presented can be followed for the various intravenous preparations.

ANTILYMPHOCYTE IMMUNE GLOBULINS

Antilymphocyte immune globulins are either equine or murine derived IgG directed against human thymocytes. One polyclonal (Atgam, lymphocyte immune globulin [LIG]) and one monoclonal preparation (Orthoclone-OKT3, murononab-CD3) are currently available. These preparations are used to either reduce the number of circulating thymus-dependent lymphocytes (LIG) or alter cell function (OKT3). These pharmacologic actions result in immunosuppression. All antilymphocyte immune globulins, whether from an equine, caprine, or murine source cause the development of human neutralizing antibodies with continued use.

LYMPHOCYTE IMMUNE GLOBULIN

This preparation is a polyclonal IgG derived from an equine source. Antibody contamination of LIG occurs and may result in leukopenia, thrombocytopenia, or red blood cell hemolysis. Additionally, LIG may act to alter the myelosupressive activity of supressor T cells in patients with aplastic anemia, allowing marrow recovery. The preparation is given intravenously over a 4- to 6-hour period, diluted in 0.9% saline.

The main indications for LIG are limited to the prevention and treatment of renal transplant rejection,[172,173] along with treatment of moderate to severe aplastic anemia. As a preventive agent, LIG when combined with standard immunosuppressive therapy results in significantly fewer rejection episodes.[173] In acute renal transplant rejection, LIG is also effective when used along with conventional therapy.[174] LIG is also used in reversing acute and resistant rejection in heart, bone marrow, liver, pancreatic, and other solid organ transplantation. Additionally, LIG has been used successfully in the treatment of myasthenia gravis[175] and multiple sclerosis.[176]

LIG is available as a 50 mg/mL solution. The normal adult dose is 10–30 mg/kg/d infused over a minimum of 4 hours. The usual pediatric dose is 5–25 mg/kg/d. For rejection prophylaxis, 15–30 mg/kg/d for 14 days has been used or 15 mg/kg/d for 14 days followed by 15 mg/kg every other day for seven doses. Therapy should be instituted within 24 hours of transplant. In acute transplant rejection, 10–15 mg/kg/d (adults and children) for 14 days is recommended. This may be followed by 10–15 mg/kg/d every other day for seven doses. In aplastic anemia, 10–20 mg/kg/d for 8–14 days, followed by the same dosage every other day for seven doses is recommended (adults and children).

Additional uses include skin allotransplantation; 10 mg/kg is administered 24 hours prior to allograft, followed by 5–40 mg/kg/d. The dose is adjusted to help rosette forming at all levels at 10% of pretreatment level.

A 0.1-mL intradermal test dose of a 1:1000 dilution (5 grams equine LIG) is recommended prior to the first infusion of LIG along with a saline control. If systemic reactions occur, no LIG should be administered. If a wheal or erythema greater than 10 mm occurs, LIG may be given with caution.

Adverse effects of LIG are numerous. These include fever (33%), leukopenia (14%), chills (14%), rash (12.5%), thrombocytopenia (11%), pain in the chest or back (1–5%), hypotension (1–5%), and others. The concurrent use of steroids may reduce allergic reactions.

MUROMONAB-CD3

This preparation is a monoclonal IgG_{2a} antibody derived from a murine source. The antibody acts by binding to a glycoprotein on the surface of CD3 T lymphocytes, blocking their role in acute rejection. The preparation is available as 1 mg/mL, 5-mL ampules. This agent is given as an intravenous bolus over a period of less than 1 minute.

OKT3 is indicated for prevention or treatment of renal transplant rejection. It has also been studied in preventing rejection in liver and heart transplants, but is not currently indicated for this.[177]

Dosage of OKT3 for treatment of acute renal transplant rejection is 5 mg/d for 10–14 days. Methylprednisolone, 1 mg/kg IV, should be given prior to OKT3 administration with hydrocortisone sodium succinate, 100 mg, given 30 minutes after injection to reduce the incidence of adverse effects (first dose only).

Adverse reactions to OKT3 include fever, chills, headache, dyspnea, chest pain, neck stiffness, vomiting, wheezing, nausea, diarrhea, tremor, and photophobia. Severe pulmonary edema has been reported in fluid-overloaded patients, and this has been fatal.

Rh_o(D) IMMUNE GLOBULIN

Rh_o(D) immune globulin (RDIG) is a sterile solution of immunoglobulins prepared from human sera with high titers of Rh_o(D) antibody. Plasma or serum used to prepare RDIG is negative for hepatitis B surface antigen.

RDIG suppresses the antibody response and formation of anti-Rh_o(D) in Rh_o(D)-negative, D^u-negative women exposed to Rh_o(D)-positive blood. Administration of RDIG prevents the future chance of erythroblastosis fetalis in subsequent pregnancies with a Rh_o(D)-positive fetus. RDIG, when administered within 72 hours of delivery of a full-term infant, reduces active antibody formation from 12% to 1–2%. Reduced antibody formation is less when it is given 72 hours postpartum. Additionally, smaller doses of RDIG are used after abortion, miscarriage, amniocentesis, or abdominal trauma. In addition, RDIG is also used in the case of a premenopausal woman who is Rh_o(D)-negative or D^u-negative and has inadvertently received Rh_o(D)-positive or D^u-positive blood or blood products.

The dosage of RDIG varies with the indication. A standard dose of 300 μg is given within 72 hours of a term delivery. Occasionally, where the fetus is known to be Rh_o(D)-positive, a 300-μg dose is given at 28 weeks gestation and within 72 hours after delivery. For postpregnancy termination occurring up to 13 weeks gestation, one microdose (50-μg) vial is given within 72 hours. For pregnancy termination after 13 weeks, one standard dose (300 μg) is given within 72 hours. In other circumstances such as in abdominal trauma, amniocentesis, or transfusion accidents, the dosage (number of standard dose vials) is based on the estimated packed red blood cell volume of the fetal/maternal hemorrhage divided by 15. RDIG is administered intramuscularly only.

When considering RDIG for use, one must be certain of the mother's Rh_o(D) and D^u antigen status. RDIG should not be given to individuals positive for either of these antigens or to those with anti-Rh_o(D) antibodies. Occasionally, a large fetal bleed of Rh_o(D)- or D^u-positive blood may make cross-matching of the mother difficult. In those cases, RDIG should only be given if previous tests have shown the mother to be $Rh_o(D)$-negative and D^u-negative with no anti-$Rh_o(D)$ antibody.

Adverse reactions to RDIG include injection site tenderness and fever.

Vaccines for Travel

Persons who are planning travel to underdeveloped parts of the world where unsanitary conditions or unusual disease exposures exist need to be evaluated for additional vaccines or immunobiologics. The yearly publication *Health Information for International Travel,*[178] published by the CDC, provides country-specific information on required and recommended immunization for travel. The following sections review three vaccines commonly used for foreign travel to prevent cholera, typhoid, and yellow fever. Based on the nature of the travel, other vaccines previously discussed may need to be considered. These include polio, tetanus, rabies, hepatitis B, measles, and meningococcal vaccines. Also, immune globulin is frequently administered for hepatitis A prophylaxis.

CHOLERA VACCINE

The currently available vaccine for cholera consists of a suspension of killed whole cell *Vibrio cholerae* bacteria from two bacterial strains: Ogawa and Inaba.

Cholera vaccine is approximately 25–50% effective in reducing the incidence of disease but does not prevent transmission of infection. The vaccine provides greater efficacy in persons who have previously had the disease. The duration of antibody following vaccination is 3–6 months compared to 3 years following natural infection. Frequent booster doses (every 6 months) are therefore needed to sustain protection. The vaccine may be used in immunocompromised individuals.

The primary use of cholera vaccine is in travelers who will be visiting countries that require health department validation of cholera vaccination. Some clinicians also administer it to persons who will be traveling in endemic areas. However, the risk of cholera to tourists is exceedingly low and therefore does not warrant routine vaccination.

The primary immunization series in adults consists of two 0.5-mL intramuscular or subcutaneous doses or two 0.2-mL intradermal doses administered 1 week to 1 month apart. Intramuscular doses in children under 10 years are modified accordingly: 0.2 mL ages 6 months to 4 years; 0.3 mL ages 5–10 years. Similar booster doses are recommended every 6 months.

Side effects are common and consist of local reactions (pain, erythema, induration, tenderness), fever, malaise, and headache. The systemic reactions such as fever, malaise, and headache occur in <1% of individuals and may last 1–2 days. Serious reactions including neurologic complications are rare. No data are available on its use in pregnancy but it is not believed to be contraindicated. The only contraindication is a history of previous severe systemic reaction to the vaccine. A 3-week interval between administrations of cholera and yellow fever vaccine is recommended because of reported decreased antibody response with their simultaneous administration. However, there is no evidence that protection is affected by simultaneous administration and when necessary it may be done.[10]

JAPANESE ENCEPHALITIS VIRUS VACCINE

Japanese encephalitis (JE) is an arboviral infection spread by mosquitoes. JE affects 50,000 people annually in Asia and Oceania and causes viral encephalitis. Transmission is seasonal with the highest times of transmission occuring in the summer and early fall. While the risk for the most travelers is quite low, the risk for individuals depends on the season, location, and duration of travel. It is estimated that the risk of acquiring JE is <1 person per million travelers, however, this may be a low estimate.[179]

Monovalent inactivated JE virus vaccine has been commercially available in the United States since 1992. Three doses are needed to provide protective levels of neutralizing antibodies. The vaccine is more immunogenic when administered in a 0-, 7-, 30-day schedule rather than in a 0-, 7-, 14-day regimen (GMTs higher at 6 months for the 30-day schedule). Duration of antibody protection is unknown. Protective titers have been reported for up to 3 years after primary immunization. Additionally, single booster doses given 1 year after primary immunization have resulted in substantial rises in antibody titers.

Adverse reactions include pain and tenderness at the injection site (20%), and systemic side effects such as fever, headache, malaise, rash, chills, dizziness, myalgia, nausea, vomiting, and abdominal pain in 10%.[179] In addition, there are sporadic reports of hypersensitivity reactions to the vaccine. The manifestations of this type of reaction includes urticaria, angioedema, and respiratory distress. These reactions generally have occurred after a medicam of 12 hours after the first dose of vaccine with 88% of reactions within 3 days. After a second dose, these hypersensitivity reactions may occur 3–14 days after injection.

JE virus vaccine is recommended for U.S. expatriates residing in areas where JE is endemic or epidemic. The vaccine is not routinely recommended for travelers to Asia.

JE vaccine is administered to individuals >3 years of age as 1-mL doses given subcutaneously on days, 0, 7, and 30. The 0-, 7-, and 14-day schedule can be used if time is a constraint. In addition, a 0-, 7-day schedule can be used if absolutely necessary and provide protection for 80% of persons. The last dose should be administered at least 10 days before traveling to watch for adverse reactions. For children ages 1–3, 0.5 mL of vaccine are administered subcutaneously using the above schedules. No data are available for children <1 year of age. Pregnant women who travel to an epidemic or endemic area should be vaccinated. No data are available for immunocompromised patients. JE vaccine can be administered simultaneously with DPT vaccine. No data are available for concurrent administration with other vaccines or antimalarial agents.

TYPHOID VACCINE

Typhoid vaccine consists of a saline suspension of killed *Salmonella typhi* bacteria. It is recommended for travelers to underdeveloped areas where there is poor sanitation and where typhoid is often endemic. It is also recommended for use in household contacts of *S. typhi* carriers. The vaccine is 50–90% effective, depending in part on levels of existing natural immunity and size of inocula exposures.[10,180] Hence, careful selection of food and water is still a very important part of disease prevention.

The recommended primary immunization schedule for adults is two 0.5-mL subcutaneous doses of heat- or phenol-inactivated typhoid vaccine given 4 or more weeks apart or, where time does not permit, three 0.5-mL doses given weekly. A single booster dose (0.5 mL subcutaneously or 0.1 mL intradermally) is recommended every 3 years for persons traveling to or remaining in endemic areas. If a period longer than 3 years has passed since immunization, a single booster dose is still recommended. For children less than 10 years of age, 0.25 mL given subcutaneously in the same schedule as for adults is recommended. Booster doses in children are 0.25 mL subcutaneously or 0.1 mL intradermally. The intradermal dose is not recommended for primary immunization nor is it recommended if an acetone or dried vaccine is used (as occurs in the military population).[11] Vi capsular polysaccharide typhoid vaccine is given as a single 0.5 mL (25 μg) IM injection in children 2 years of age and younger. Booster doses are indicated every 2 years.

Side effects are common and include local reactions (pain, induration, and erythema at the injection site), malaise, headache, and fever starting within 24 hours of receiving the vaccine and lasting 1–2 days, usually responsive to mild analgesia. No studies have been done during pregnancy but the vaccine, being composed of killed bacteria, is not felt to pose any fetal risk. The vaccine should not be given during acute viral respiratory infections nor to persons who have a known hypersensitivity to the vaccine.

Oral typhoid vaccine (Ty-21a) has been shown to be as effective as the parenteral vaccine.[181] This vaccine became available in the United States in 1990. Although field trials used a three-dose oral regimen,[182] a four-dose regimen is approved for use in the United States. The oral vaccine may be used in persons as young as 6 years of age.[183] The recommended dose is one enteric-coated capsule on days 1, 3, 5, and 7. Booster doses consist of a repeat course of primary immunization given every 5 years. The vaccine is without significant adverse reactions.[182] Oral typhoid vaccine should not be used in immunocompromised individuals. Parenteral typhoid vaccine may be used in the immunocompromised person since it is an inactivated agent.

YELLOW FEVER VACCINE

Live, attenuated, yellow fever virus vaccine is recommended for persons who will be traveling or living in areas where yellow fever infection occurs—currently parts of Africa and South America—and is required for entry into certain countries.[10] Vaccination should also be considered for laboratory workers who may be exposed to the virus. The reconstituted vaccine is thermolabile and unused portions must be discarded 1 hour after reconstitution.

The recommended dose is 0.5 mL subcutaneously given once with similar booster doses recommended every 10 years. However, the vaccine has been shown to be highly immunogenic with antibodies persisting for at least 40 years and perhaps for life. Mild side effects consisting of headache, myalgias, and low-grade fever 1–2 weeks after vaccination occur in less than 10% of vaccinees; treatment should be symptomatic. Immediate hypersensitivity reactions are rare (1 per million doses) and occur primarily in persons who have anaphylactic reactions to eggs. Neurologic accidents are rare (20 cases to date) and have occurred primarily in infants less than 6 months of age, in whom the vaccine is not recommended. The French neurotropic vaccine (Dakar strain) was associated with meningoencephalitis in children and is no longer manufactured. This has not occurred with the 17D strain.

On theoretical grounds, the vaccine should be avoided during pregnancy unless travel to a high-risk area is imperative. It is also not recommended for persons who are immunocompromised or immunosuppressed. In addition, it should not be given to infants less than 4 months of age and, in general, should be used only if a child is 9 months of age or older. Children 4–9 months must be considered on an individual basis. It is contraindicated in persons with a history of an anaphylactic reaction to eggs. Where the history is in question, intradermal testing consisting of 0.02-mL doses of vaccine and normal saline control applied to the volar surface of the forearm should be done. The demonstration of an erythematous, urticarial wheal and negative control constitutes a positive response and contraindicates vaccination. This intradermal testing may be sufficient to produce antibodies; however, serologic testing should be done to confirm this.

Yellow fever vaccine may be simultaneously administered with all other vaccines except cholera, with which a 3-week interval between vaccines is recommended. Simultaneous administration of immune globulin does not interfere with the immune response to this agent.

Future Vaccine Research

To date, vaccines have been used for prevention of disease. Research in this area continues, with potential research in the areas of respiratory syncytial virus, parainfluenza and adenoviruses, Epstein–Barr virus, hepatitis C virus, cytomegalovirus, malaria, HIV, herpes simplex type 2, chlamydia, *Helicobacter pylori,* and parasites such as schistosomiasis, to name a few.[184] However, exciting data are being uncovered concerning the use of vaccines in patients already having the diseases that the vaccine should prevent. Straus et al.[185] showed, in a population with genital herpes, that a recombinant glycoprotein D of herpes simplex virus type 2 reduced the number of recurrences of genital herpes within the first 4 months of vaccination. In addition, the HSV-2 neutralizing antibody titers and the gD2 titers rose fourfold and sevenfold, respectively, with the vaccine. This was the first investigation to show that a vaccine can modify the course of a viral infection.

Finally, the search for a vaccine against HIV continues. Two uses of the vaccine are proposed, prevention of disease and treatment of already established disease. The types of vaccines under investigation fall into various categories: recombinant proteins, synthetic peptides, different viral vectors, whole killed inactivated virus, and psuedovirons.[186] In addition, microencapsulated antigens, designed to stimulate mucosal immunity, are being investigated. New adjuvants such as saponin and monophosphoryl-lipid A are also under investigation to increase immune response to HIV vaccines.

It is clear that, with our increased knowledge of molecular biology, more understanding about the immune response is known. Genetic factors appear to play an important role in vaccine response, along with immunizing agent factors. The next decade may bring major advances in the use of vaccines for disease prevention and treatment.

References

1. Willems JS, Sanders CR. Cost-effectiveness and cost–benefits analysis of vaccines. J Infect Dis 1981;144:486–493.
2. Koplan JP, Axnick MW. Benefits, risks and costs of viral vaccines. Prog Med Virol 1982;28:180–191.
3. Lanzavecchia A. Identifying strategies for immune intervention. Science 1993;260:937–944.
4. Advisory Committee on Immunization Practices. General recommendations on immunization. MMWR 1994;43(RR-1):1–38.
5. Edsall G. Immunoprophylaxis of bacterial diseases, in Gell PGH, Coombs RRA, Lachmann PJ (eds): Clinical Aspects of Immunology. Oxford, Blackwell Scientific, 1975, p 1601.
6. Jilg W, Schmidt M, Deinhardt F. Prolonged immunity after late booster doses of hepatitis B vaccine. J Infect Dis 1988;157:1267–1269.
7. Miotti P, Nelson KE, Dallabetta GA, et al. The influence of HIV infection on antibody response to a two-dose regimen of influenza vaccine. JAMA 1989;262:779–783.
8. Immunization Practices Advisory Committee. General recommendations on immunization. MMWR 1989;38:205–228.
9. Centers for Disease Control. Suboptimal response to hepatitis B vaccine given by injection into the buttock. MMWR 1985;34:105–113.
10. Guide for Adult Immunization 1990, 2nd ed. Philadelphia, American College of Physicians, 1990, pp 19–35.
11. Centers for Disease Control. Adult Immunization. Recommendations of the Immunization Practices Advisory Committee. MMWR 1991;40:1–94.
12. Advisory Committee on Immunization Practices. Use of vaccines and immune globulins in persons with altered immunocompetence. MMWR 1993;42(RR-4):1–19.
13. Milgrom F, Abeyounis CJ, Kano K. Principles of Immunological Diagnosis in Medicine. Philadelphia, Lea and Febiger, 1981.
14. Beal AJ. Immunoprophylaxis of viral disease, in Gell PGH, Coombs RRA, Lachmann PJ (eds): Clinical Aspects of Immunology. Oxford, Blackwell Scientific, 1975, p 1631.
15. Gardner P, Schaffner W. Immunization of adults. N Engl J Med 1993;328:1252–1258.
16. Williams WW, Hickson MA, Kane MA, et al. Immunization policies and vaccine coverage among adults. The risk for missed opportunities. Ann Intern Med 1988;108:616–625.
17. Centers for Disease Control. Retrospective assessment of vaccination coverage among school-aged children—selected U.S. cities, 1991. MMWR 1992;41:103–107.
18. Farizo KM, Stehr-Green PA, Markowitz LE, Patriarca PA. Vaccination levels and missed opportunities for measles vaccination: A record audit in a public pediatric clinic. Pediatrics 1992;89:589–592.
19. Szilagyi PG, Rodewald LE, Humiston SG, et al. Missed opportunities for childhood vaccinations in office practices and the effect on vaccination status. Pediatrics 1993;91:1–7.
20. Centers for Disease Control. Early childhood vaccination in two rural counties—Nebraska, 1991–1992. MMWR 1992;41:688–691.
21. Centers for Disease Control. Standards for pediatric immunization practices. Recomended by the National Vaccine Advisory Committee. Approved by the U.S. Public Health Service. MMWR 1993;42(RR-5):1–13.
22. Peter G. Childhood immunizations. N Engl J Med 1992;327:1794–1800.
23. Bartell LH, Charney SA. National Vaccine Injury Compensation Act: A viable alternative to litigation? J Pharm Pract 1989;2:36–44.
24. Centers for Disease Control. Vaccine Adverse Event Reporting System—United States. MMWR 1990;39:730–733.
25. Committee on Infectious Diseases, 21st ed. Elk Grove Village, IL, American Academy of Pediatrics, 1988, pp 15–16.
26. Ramsay MEB, Rao M, Begg NT, et al. Antibody response to accelerated immunization with diphtheria, tetanus, pertussis vaccine. Lancet 1993;342:203–205.

27. Centers for Disease Control. Recommendation of the Immunization Practices Advisory Committee: Diphtheria, tetanus and pertussis. Guidelines for vaccine prophylaxis and other preventive measures. MMWR 1981;30:392–396, 401–407.
28. Middaugh JP. Side effects of diphtheria-tetanus toxoid in adults. Am J Public Health 1979;69:246–249.
29. Eckmann L. Active and passive tetanus immunization. N Engl J Med 1964;271:1087–1090.
30. Clemens JD, Chuong JJH, Feinstein AR. The BCG controversy: A methodological and statistical reappraisal. JAMA 1983;249:2362–2369.
31. Colditz GA, Brewer TF, Berkey CS, et al. Efficacy of BCG vaccine in the prevention of tuberculosis. JAMA 1994;271:698–702.
32. Hart PDA, Sutherland I. BCG and the role of bacillus vaccines in the prevention of tuberculosis in adolescence and early adult life. Br Med J 1977;2:293–295.
33. US Department of Health, Education, and Welfare. Status of immunization in tuberculosis in 1971: Report of a conference on progress to date, future trends and research needs. DHEW publication (NIH) 72–68, 1971.
34. American Academy of Pediatrics Committee on Infectious Diseases. Haemophilus influenzae type b conjugate vaccines: Recommendations for immunization with recently and previously licensed vaccines. Pediatrics 1993;92:480–482.
35. Centers for Disease Control. General recommendations on immunization. Recommendations of the Advisory Committee on Immunization Practices (ACIP). MMWR 1994;43(RR-1):1–38.
36. Werzberger A, Mensch B, Kuter B, et al. A controlled trial of a formalin-inactivated hepatitis A vaccine in healthy children. N Engl J Med 1992;327:453–457.
37. Green MS, Cohen DM, Lerman Y, et al. Depression of the immune response to an inactivated hepatitis A vaccine administered concomitantly with immune globulin. J Infect Dis 1993;168:740–743.
38. Advisory Committee on Immunization Practices. Hepatitis B virus: A comprehensive strategy for eliminating transmission in the United States through universal childhood vaccination. MMWR 1991;40(RR-13):1–25.
39. Committee on Infectious Diseases. Universal hepatitis B immunization. Pediatrics 1992;89:795–800.
40. Centers for Disease Control. Recommendations for protection against viral hepatitis. MMWR 1985;34:313.
41. Roome AJ, Walsh SJ, Cartter ML, Hadler JL. Hepatitis B vaccine responsiveness in Connecticut public safety personnel. JAMA 1993;270:2931–2934.
42. West D. Personal communication, Merck & Co, April 6, 1994.
43. Wood RC, MacDonald KL, White KE, et al. Risk factors for lack of detectable antibody following hepatitis B vaccination of Minnesota health care workers. JAMA 1993;270:2935–2939.
44. Margolis, HS, Presson, AC. Host factors related to poor immunogenicity of hepatitis B vaccine in adults. JAMA 1993;270:2971–2972.
45. Treadwell TL, Keeffe EB, Lake J, et al. Immunogenicity of two recombinant hepatitis B vaccines in older individuals. Am J Med 1993;95:584–588.
46. Seef L, Koff. Passive and active immunoprophylaxis of hepatitis B. Gastroenterology 1984;86:958–981.
47. Tada H, Mosohiko Y, Mishira J, et al. Combined passive and active immunization for preventing perinatal transmission of hepatitis B virus carrier state. Pediatrics 1982;70:613–619.
48. Beasley R, Hwang L, Lee G, et al. Prevention of perinatally transmitted hepatitis B virus infections with hepatitis B immune globulin and hepatitis B vaccine. Lancet 1983;2:1099–1102.
49. Smithkline Beecham's Engerix-B new dosing schedule gets go-ahead from FDA committee: AAP/ACIP flexible dose recommendations okayed for all HBV vaccines. Pink Sheet 1994;56:(5)12.
50. Hadler SC, Francis DP, Maynard JE, et al. Long-term immunogenicity and efficacy of hepatitis B vaccine in homosexual men. N Engl J Med 1986;315:209–214.
51. Bertino JS Jr, Tirrell P, Greenberg R, et al. Preliminary results of a comparative trial of standard 10 μg or high dose recombinant hepatitis B vaccine versus 10 μg mixed particle vaccine to induce protective anti-HBs in normal nonresponders. Clin Pharm Ther 1994;55:191.
52. Recommendations of the Immunization Practices Advisory Committee. Hepatitis B virus: A comprehensive strategy for eliminating transmission in the United States through universal childhood vaccination. MMWR 1992;40:1–25.
53. Troisi C, Heiberg D, Hollinger F. Normal immune response to hepatitis B vaccine in patients with Down's syndrome: A basis for immunization guidelines. JAMA 1985;254:3196–3199.
54. Wainwright RB, McMahon BJ, Bulkow LR, et al. Duration of immunogenicity and efficacy of hepatitis B vaccine in a Yupik Eskimo population. JAMA 1989;261:2362–2366.
55. Lo KJ, Lee SD, Tsai YT, et al. Long-term immunogenicity and efficacy of hepatitis B vaccine in infants born to HBeAG-positive HBsAG-carrier mothers. Hepatology 1988;8:1647–1650.
56. Anonymous. New recombinant hepatitis B vaccine offers safe and effective immunoprophylaxis. Hosp Formul 1990(suppl C);25:2–7.
57. Lanphear BP. Hepatitis B immunoprophylaxis: Developing a cost-effective program in the hospital setting. Infect Control Hosp Epidemiol 1990;11:47–50.
58. Dienstag JL, Stevens CO, Bhan AK, et al. Hepatitis B vaccine administered to chronic carrier of hepatitis B surface antigen. Ann Intern Med 1982;96:575–579.
59. Prince AM, et al. Hepatitis B immune globulin: Final report of a controlled multicenter trial of efficacy in prevention of dialysis-associated hepatitis. J Infect Dis 1978;137:131–144.
60. Seef LB et al. Type B hepatitis after needle-stick exposure: Prevention with hepatitis B immune globulin. Ann Intern Med 1978;88:285–293.
61. Frosner G, Frosner H, Dienhardt F, et al. Failure of hyperimmune serum globulin, given several days after exposure, to protect against hepatitis B. Lancet 1977;2:1023.
62. Masuko K, Mitsui T, Iwano K, et al. Factors influencing postexposure immunoprophylaxis of hepatitis B virus infection with hepatitis B immune globulin. Gastroenterology 1985;88:151–155.

63. Grady GF, Lee VA. Hepatitis B immune globulin—prevention of hepatitis from accidental exposure among medical personnel. N Engl J Med 1975;293:1067–1070.
64. Perillo R, Campbell C, Strang S, et al. Immune globulin and hepatitis B immune globulin: Prophylactic measures for intimate contacts exposed to acute type B hepatitis. Arch Intern Med 1984;144:81–85.
65. Centers for Disease Control. Update on hepatitis B prophylaxis. MMWR 1987;36:353–360.
66. LaMontagne JR, Noble GR, Quinnan GV, et al. Summary of clinical trials of inactivated influenza vaccine—1978. Rev Infect Dis 1983;5:723–736.
67. Gross RA, Ennis FA. Influenza vaccine: Split product versus whole virus types—How do they differ? N Engl J Med 1977;296:567–568.
68. Waldman RH, Mann JJ, Small PA Jr. Immunization against influenza. Prevention of illness in man by aerosolized inactivated vaccine. JAMA 1969;207:520–524.
69. Hobson D, Curry RL, Beare AS. Hemoglutinin-inhibiting antibody titers as a measure of protection against influenza in man, in Perkins FT, Regamey RH (eds): Symposia Series in Immunological Standardization, No. 20. Basel, S Karger AG, 1973, pp 164–168.
70. Quinnan GV, Schooley R, Dolin R, et al. Serologic responses and systemic reactions in adults after vaccination with monovalent A/USSR/77 and trivalent A/USSR/77, A/Texas/77, B/Hong Kong/72 influenza vaccines. Rev Infect Dis 1983;5:748–757.
71. Feery BJ, Evered MG, Morrison EI. Different protection rates in various groups of volunteers given subunit influenza virus vaccine in 1976. J Infect Dis 1979;139:237–241.
72. Riddiough MA, Sisk JE, Bell JC. Influenza vaccination cost-effectiveness and public policy. JAMA 1983;249:3189–3195.
73. Cate TR, Caulh RB, Parker D, et al. Reactogenicity, immunogenicity, and antibody persistence in adults given inactivated influenza virus vaccines—1978. J Infect Dis 1983;5:737–747.
74. Advisory Committee on Immunization Practices. Prevention and control of influenza: Part I, vaccines. MMWR 1994;43:1–21.
75. Advisory Committee on Immunization Practices. Influenza prevention. MMWR 1990;39:1–15.
76. Couch RB. Advances in influenza virus vaccine research. Ann NY Acad Sci 1993;685:803–812.
77. Keller D, Koster FT, Marks DH, et al. Safety and immunogenicity of a recombinant outer surface protein A Lyme vaccine. JAMA 1994;271:1764–1768.
78. American Academy of Pediatrics. Measles, in Peter G (ed): 1994 Red Book: Report of the Committee on Infectious Diseases, 23rd ed. Elk Grove Village, IL, American Academy of Pediatrics, 1994, pp 308–323, 355–367.
79. Centers for Disease Control. General recommendations on immunization. Recommendations of the Advisory Committee on Immunization Practices (ACIP). MMWR 1994;43(RR-1):1–38.
80. Cote TR, Sivertson D, Horan JM, et al. Evaluation of a two-dose measles, mumps, and rubella vaccination schedule in a cohort of college athletes. Public Health Rep 1993;108:431–435.
81. Krober MS, Stracener CE, Bass JW. Decreased measles antibody response after measles–mumps–rubella vaccine in infants with colds. JAMA 1991;265:2095–2096.
82. Linnemann CC, Dine MS, Roselle GH, et al. Measles immunity after revaccination: Results in children vaccinated before 10 months of age. Pediatrics 1982;69:332–335.
83. Centers for Disease Control. Measles prevention: Recommendations of the Immunization Practices Advisory Committee (ACIP). MMWR 1989;38(S-9):1–18.
84. Gold R, Lepow ML, Goldschneider I, et al. Kinetics of antibody production to group A and group C meningococcal polysaccharide vaccines administered during first 6 years of life: Prospects for routine immunization of infants and children. J Infect Dis 1979;140:690–697.
85. ACIP. Meningococcal vaccines. MMWR 1985;34:255.
86. Binkin N, Bond J. Epidemic of meningococcal meningitis in Banako, Mali: Epidemiological features and analysis of vaccines efficacy. Lancet 1982;2:315–318.
87. Reingold A, Broome CV, Hightower AW, et al. Age-specific differences in duration of clinical protection after vaccination with meningococcal polysaccharide a vaccine. Lancet 1985;2:114–118.
88. Centers for Disease Control. Mumps prevention. MMWR 1989;38:388–400.
89. Advisory Committee on Immunization Practices. Mumps vaccine: Recommendation of the Immunization Practices Advisory Committee. MMWR 1982;31:617–620, 625.
90. Briss PA, Fehrs LJ, Parker RA. Sustained transmission of mumps in a highly vaccinated population: Assessment of primary vaccine failure and waning vaccine-induced immunity. J Infect Dis 1994;169:77–82.
91. Centers for Disease Control. Diphtheria, tetanus, and pertussis: Recommendations for vaccine use and other preventive measures. recommendations of the Immunization Practices Advisory Committee (ACIP). MMWR 1991;40(RR-10):1–28.
92. Miller DL, Ross EM, Alderslade R, et al. Pertussis immunization and serious acute neurological illness in children. Br Med J 1981;282:1595.
93. Cherry JD. The epidemiology of pertussis and pertussis immunization in the United Kingdom and the U.S.: A comparative study. Curr Probl Pediatr 1984;14:7–77.
94. Leung A. Pertussis vaccine production [letter]. Am J Dis Child 1985;139:9.
95. Griffin MR, Ray WA, Mortimer EA, et al. Risk of seizures and encephalopathy after immunization with the diphtheria–tetanus–pertussis vaccine. JAMA 1990;263:1641–1645.
96. Cherry JD. Pertussis vaccine encephalopathy: Is it time to recognize it as the myth that it is? JAMA 1990;263:1679–1680.
97. Gale JL, Thapa PB, Wassilak SGF, et al. Risk of serious acute neurological illness after immunization with diphtheria–tetanus–pertussis vaccine. A population-based case-control study. JAMA 1994;271:37–41.
98. Johnstone T. Whooping cough in the United States and Britain [letter]. N Engl J Med 1983;309:108–109.
99. Fulginitti VA. Pertussis vaccine [letter]. Am J Dis Child 1984;183:890–891.
100. CDC. Pertussis surveillance, 1979–1981. MMWR 1982;31:333–335.

101. CDC. Pertussis—United States, 1982–1983. MMWR 1984;33:573–575.
102. CDC. Supplementary statement of contraindications to receipt of pertussis vaccine. MMWR 1984;33:169–171.
103. Advisory Committee on Immunization Practices. Food and Drug Administration approval of use of diphtheria and tetanus toxoids and acellular pertussis vaccine. MMWR 1991;40:881–882.
104. American Academy of Pediatrics. Pertussis, in Peter G (ed): 1994 Red Book: Report of the Committee on Infectious Diseases, 23rd ed. Elk Grove Village, IL, American Academy of Pediatrics, 1994, pp 355–367.
105. Centers for Disease Control. Pertussis vaccination: Acellular pertussis vaccine for reinforcing and booster use—supplementary ACIP statement. Recommendations of the Immunization Practices Advisory Committee (ACIP). MMWR 1992;41(RR-1):1–10.
106. Advisory Committee on Immunization Practices. Pneumococcal polysaccharide vaccine. MMWR 1989;38:64–76.
107. Fedson D, Chiarello L. Previous hospital care and pneumococcal bacteremia: Importance for pneumococcal immunization. Arch Intern Med 1983;143:885–889.
108. Hirschman J, Lipsky B. Pneumococcal vaccine in the United States. JAMA 1981;246:1428–1431.
109. American Academy of Pediatrics. Pneumococcal infections, in Peter G (ed): 1994 Red Book: Report of the Committee on Infectious Diseases, 23rd ed. Elk Grove Village, IL, American Academy of Pediatrics, 1994, pp 371–375.
110. Smit P, Oberholzer D, Hayden-Smith S, et al. Protective efficacy of pneumococcal polysaccharide vaccines. JAMA 1977;238:2613–2626.
111. Hilleman M, Carlson A, McLean A, et al. *Streptococcus pneumoniae* polysaccharide vaccine: Age and dose responses, safety, persistence of antibody, revaccination, and simultaneous administration of pneumococcal and influenza vaccines. Rev Infect Dis 1981;3:S31–S42.
112. Schwartz S. Pneumococcal vaccine: Clinical efficacy and effectiveness. Ann Intern Med 1982;96:208–220.
113. Broome C. Efficacy of pneumococcal polysaccharide vaccines. Rev Infect Dis 1981;3(suppl):S82–S96.
114. Bolan G, Broome C, Facklam R, et al. Pneumococcal vaccine efficacy in selected populations in the United States. Ann Intern Med 1986;104:1–6.
115. Ammann A, Addiego J, Wara D, et al. Polyvalent pneumococcal-polysaccharide immunization of patients with sickle cell anemia and patients with splenectomy. N Engl J Med 1977;297:897–900.
116. Howie V, Ploussard J, Sloyer J, et al. Use of pneumococcal polysaccharide vaccine in preventing otitis media in infants: Different results between racial groups. Pediatrics 1984;73:79–81.
117. Bentley D, Ha K, Mamot K, et al. Pneumococcal vaccine in the institutionalized elderly: Design of a nonrandomized trial and preliminary results. Rev Infect Dis 1981;3(suppl):S71–S81.
118. Bentley D. Pneumococcal vaccine in the institutionalized elderly: Review of past and recent studies. Rev Infect Dis 1981;3:S61–S70.
119. Williams J, Moser K. Pneumococcal vaccine and patients with chronic lung disease. Ann Intern Med 1986;104:106–109.
120. Butler JC, Breiman RF, Campbell JF, et al. Pneumococcccal polysaccharide vaccine efficacy. An evaluation of current recommendations. JAMA 1993;270:1826–1831.
121. Giebink GS, Le CT, Schiffman G. Decline of serum antibody in splenectomized children after vaccination with pneumococcal capsular polysaccharides. J Pediatr 1984;105:576–584.
122. Poliovirus vaccine live oral, in McEvoy GK (ed): AHFS Drug Information 1994. Bethesda, MD, American Society of Hospital Pharmacists, 1994, pp 2223–2226.
123. Centers for Disease Control. Poliomyelitis prevention: Enhanced potency inactivated poliomyelitis vaccine—supplementary statement. MMWR 1987;36:795–798.
124. Faden H, Duffy L, Sun M, Shuff C. Long-term immunity to poliovirus in children immunized with live attenuated and enhanced-potency inactivated trivalent poliovirus vaccines. J Infect Dis 1993;168:452–454.
125. Dutta JK, Dutta TK. Rabies in endemic countries. Br Med J 1994;1:488–489.
126. Advisory Committee on Immunization Practices. Rabies prevention—United States, 1984. MMWR 1984;33:393–402, 407–408.
127. Advisory Committee on Immunization Practices. Rabies prevention. MMWR 1991;40(RR-3):1–19.
128. Ajjan M, Soulebat JP, Triau R, et al. Intradermal immunization with rabies vaccine: Inactivated Wistar strain cultivated in human diploid cells. JAMA 1980;244:2528–2531.
129. Bernhard KW, Roberts MA, Samner J, et al. Human diploid cell rabies vaccine: Effectiveness of immunization with small intradermal or subcutaneous doses. JAMA 1982;247:1138–1142.
130. Bernard KW, Roberts MA, Sumner J, et al. Human diploid cell rabies vaccine. Effectiveness of immunization with small intradermal or subcutaneous doses. JAMA 1982;247:1138–1142.
131. Bernard KW, Mallonnee J, Wright JC, et al. Preexposure immunization with intraderal human diploid cell rabies vaccine. JAMA 1987;257:1059–1063.
132. Fishbein DB, Pacer RE, Holmes DF, et al. Rabies preexposure prophylaxis with human diploid cell rabies vaccine: A dose-response study. J Infect Dis 1987;156:50–55.
133. Trimarchi CV, Safford M Jr. Poor response to rabies vaccination by the intradermal route. JAMA 1992;268:874.
134. State of New York, Department of Health Memorandum, Public Health Series H-28, PH-11, Series 92-93. Rabies control update. November 25, 1992.
135. Pappaioanou M, Fishbein D, Dressen D, et al. Antibody response to pre-exposure human diploid cell rabies vaccine given concurrently with chloroquine. N Engl J Med 1986;314:280–284.
136. Centers for Disease Control. Systemic allergic reactions following immunization with human diploid cell rabies vaccine. MMWR 1984;33:185.
137. Nicholson KG, Turner GS, Aoki EY. Immunization with a human diploid cell strain of rabies virus vaccine: Two-year results. J Infect Dis 1978;137:783–788.
138. Bahmanyar M, Fayaz A, Nour-Salehi S, et al. Successful protection of humans exposed to rabies infection: Postexposure treatment with the new human diploid cell rabies vaccine and antirabies serum. JAMA 1976;236:2751–2754.

139. Greaves WI, Orenstein WA, Hinman AZ, et al. Clinical efficacy of rubella vaccine. Pediatr Infect Dis 1983;2:284–286.
140. Advisory Committee on Immunization Practices. Rubella prevention. MMWR 1984;33:301–310.
141. Centers for Disease Control. Rubella vaccine. Recommendations of the Immunizations Practice Advisory Committee (ACIP). MMWR 1990;39(RR-15):1–18.
142. Advisory Committee on Immunization Practices. Rubella prevention. MMWR 1984;33:315–318.
143. CDC. Rubella vaccination during pregnancy—United States, 1971–1982. MMWR 1983;32:429–432.
144. Gershon A. Immunoprophylaxis of varicella zoster infections. Am J Med 1984;76:672–677.
145. Gershon A, Steinberg S, Geld L, et al. Live attenuated varicella vaccine: Efficacy for children with leukemia in remission. JAMA 1984;252:355–362.
146. Weibel R, Neff B, Kuter B, et al. Live attenuated varicella vaccine: Efficacy trial in healthy children. N Engl J Med 1984;310:1409–1415.
147. Gershon AA, LaRussa P, Steinberg SP. Live attenuated varicella vaccine: Current status and future uses. Semin Pediatr Infect Dis 1991;2:171–177.
148. Centers for Disease Control. Change in source of information: Availability of varicella vaccine for children with acute lymphocytic leukemia. MMWR 1993;42:499.
149. Starr SE. Status of varicella vaccine for children. Pediatrics 1989;84:1097–1098.
150. Watson B, Gupta R, Randall T, Starr S. Persistence of cell-mediated and humoral immune responses in healthy children immunized with live attenuated varicella vaccine. J Infect Dis 1994;169:197–199.
151. Johnson C, Rome LP, Stancin T, et al. Humoral immunity and clinical reinfections following varicella vaccine in healthy children. Pediatrics 1989;84:418–421.
152. Watson BM, Piercy SA, Plotkin SA, Starr SE. Modified chickenpox in children immunized with the Oka/Merck varicella vaccine. Pediatrics 1993;91:17–22.
153. Gershon AA, LaRussa P, Hardy I, et al. Varicella vaccine: The American experience. J Infect Dis 1992;166(suppl 1):S63–68.
154. Lieu TA, Cochi SL, Black SB, et al. Cost-effectiveness of a routine varicella vaccination program for US children. JAMA 1994;271:375–381.
155. Kitai IC, King S, Gafni A. An economic evaluation of varicella vaccine for pediatric liver and kidney transplant recipients. Clin Infect Dis 1993;17:441–447.
156. Berger R, Leuscher D, Just M. Enhancement of varicella-zoster-specific immune responses in the elderly by boosting with varicella vaccine. J Infect Dis 1984;149:647.
157. Advisory Committee on Immunization Practices. Varicella-zoster immune globulin for the prevention of chicken pox. MMWR 1984;33:84.
158. Committee on Infectious Diseases. Expanded guidelines for use of varicella-zoster immune globulin. Pediatrics 1983;72:886–889.
159. Zaia JA, Levin NJ, Preblud SR, et al. Evaluation of varicella-zoster immune globulin: Protection of immunosuppressed children after household exposure to varicella. J Infect Dis 1983;147:737–743.
160. Gershon AA. Immunoprophylaxis of varicella-zoster infection. Am J Med 1984;76:672–677.
161. Orenstein WA, et al. Prophylaxis of varicella in high-risk children: Dose-response effect of zoster immune globulin. J Pediatr 1981;98:368–373.
162. Snydman DR, et al. Use of cytomegalovirus immune globulin to prevent cytomegalovirus disease in renal transplant recipients. N Engl J Med 1987;312:1049–1054.
163. Young FE, Nightingale SL. FDA's newly designated treatment INDs. JAMA 1988;260:224–225.
164. Cohn E, Strong L, Hues W. Preparation and properties of serum plasma proteins. IV: A system for the separation into fractions of the protein and lipoprotein components of biological tissues and fluids. J Am Chem Soc 1946;68:459–675.
165. Berkman SA, Lee ML, Gale RP. Clinical uses of intravenous immunoglobulins. Ann Intern Med 1990;112:278–292.
166. ASHP Commission on Therapeutics. ASHP therapeutic guidelines for intravenous immune globulin. Clin Pharm 1992;11:117–136.
167. Morell A, Schurch B, Ryser D, et al. *In vivo* behaviour of γ-globulin preparations. Vox Sang 1980;38:272–283.
168. Ochs HD, Fischer SH, Wedgwood RJ, et al. Comparison of high-dose and low-dose intravenous immunoglobulin therapy in patients with primary immunodeficiency diseases. Am J Med 1984;76:78–82.
169. Siber, GR, Snydman, DR. Use of immune globulins in the prevention and treatment of infections. Curr Clin Topics Infect Dis 1992;12:1–40.
170. Miles' gamimmune N IVIG gains BMT and pediatric HIV infection indication. Pink Sheet 1994;56(No. 1):6.
171. Rostoker G, Desvaux-Belghiti D, Pilatte Y, et al. High-dose immunoglobulin therapy for severe IgA nephropathy and henoch-schonlein purpura. Ann Intern Med 1994;120:476–484.
172. Cosimi AB. The clinical value of antilymphocyte antibodies. Transplant Proc 1981;13:462–468.
173. Butt KMH, Zielinksi CM, Parsa I, et al. Trends in immunosuppression for kidney transplantation. Kidney Int 1978;13(suppl 8):595–598.
174. Hardy MD, Nowygrod R, Elberg A, et al. Use of ATG in treatment of steroid-resistant rejection. Transplantation 1980;29:162–164.
175. Pirofsky B, et al. Myasthenia gravis treated with purified antithymocyte antiserum. Neurology 1979;29:112–116.
176. Martin J et al. Double-blinded controlled trial of immunosuppression in treatment of multiple sclerosis. Lancet 1980;2:949–951.
177. Grabenstein JD. Isoantibodies: II. Comparison of antilymphocyte antibodies. Hosp Pharm 1993;28:42–49.
178. Centers for Disease Control. Health Information for International Travel, 1990.
179. Advisory Committee on Immunization Practices. Inactivated Japanese encephalitis virus vaccine. MMWR 1993;42(RR-1):1–15.
180. Hook E. *Salmonella* species (including typhoid fever), in Mandell G, Douglas RG, Bennett J (eds): Principles and Practice of Infectious Diseases, 3rd ed. New York, John Wiley and Sons, 1990, pp 1700–1715.
181. Levene MM, Ferreccio C, Black RE, et al. Progress in vaccines against typhoid fever. Rev Infect Dis 1989(suppl 3);11:S552–S567.

182. Anonymous. Advice for travelers. Med Lett 1990;32:33–36.
183. Levine MM, Ferreccio C, Black RE, et al. Large-scale field trial of TY21A live oral typhoid vaccine in enteric coated capsule formulation. Lancet 1987;1:1049–1052.
184. Plotkin SA. Vaccination in the 21st century. Journ Infect Dis 1993;168:29–37.
185. Straus SE, Corey L, Burke RL, et al. Placebo-controlled trial of vaccination with recombinant glycoprotein D of herpes simplex virus type 2 for immunotherapy of genital herpes. Lancet 1994;343:1460–1463.
186. Chang NT. The search for an AIDS vaccine. AIDS Reader, March/April 1994, pp 45–49.

Appendix 116.1

Immunization Schedules in Children

Vaccine	At Birth (Before Hospital Discharge)	1–2 Months	2 Months[a]	4 Months	6 Months	6–18 Months	12–15 Months	15 Months	4–6 Years (Before School Entry)
Diphtheria-tetanus-pertussis[b]			DTP	DTP	DTP			DTaP/DTP[c]	DTaP/DTP
Polio, live oral			OPV	OPV	OPV[d]				OPV
Measles-mumps-rubella							MMR		MMR[e]
Haemophilus influenzae type b conjugate									
HbOC/PRP-T[b,f]			Hib	Hib	Hib		Hib[g]		
PRP-OMP[f]			Hib	Hib			Hib[g]		
Hepatitis B[h]									
Option 1	HepB	HepB[i]				HepB[i]			
Option 2		HepB[i]		HepB[i]		HepB[i]			

[a]Can be administered as early as 6 weeks of age.

[b]Two DTP and Hib combination vaccines are available (DTP/HbOC [TETRAMUNE]; and PRP-T [ActHIB, OmniHIB] which can be reconstituted with DTP vaccine produced by Connaught).

[c]This dose of DTP can be administered as early as 12 months of age provided that the interval since the previous dose of DTP is at least 6 months. *Diphtheria and tetanus toxoids and acellular pertussis vaccine (DTaP) is currently recommended only for use as the fourth and/or fifth doses of the DTP series among children aged 15 months through 6 years (before the seventh birthday).* Some experts prefer to administer these vaccines at 18 months of age.

[d]The American Academy of Pediatrics (AAP) recommends this dose of vaccine at 6–18 months of age.

[e]The AAP recommends that two doses of MMR should be administered by 12 years of age with the second dose being administered preferentially at entry to middle school or junior high school.

[f]HbOC: [HibTITER] (Lederle Praxis). PRP-T: [ActHIB, OmniHIB] (Pasteur Merieux). PRP-OMP: [PedvaxHIB] (Merck, Sharp, and Dohme). A DTP/Hib combination vaccine can be used in place of HbOC/PRP-T.

[g]After the primary infant Hib conjugate vaccine series is completed, any of the licensed Hib conjugate vaccines may be used as a booster dose at age 12–15 months.

[h]For use among infants born to HBsAg-negative mothers. The first dose should be administered during the newborn period, preferably before hospital discharge, but no later than age 2 months. Premature infants of HBsAg-negative mothers should receive the first dose of the hepatitis B vaccine series at the time of hospital discharge or when the other routine childhood vaccines are initiated. (All infants born to HBsAg-positive mothers should receive immunoprophylaxis for hepatitis B as soon as possible after birth.)

[i]Hepatitis B vaccine can be administered simultaneously at the same visit with DTP (or DTaP), OPV, Hib, and/or MMR. (From Centers for Disease Control and Prevention. General recommendations on immunization: Recommendations of the Advisory Committee on Immunization Practices (ACIP). MMWR 1994;43 (RR-1):1–38.)

Appendix 116.2

Immunization Schedules in Adults

Age Group (years)	Vaccine/Toxoid[a]					
	Td[b]	Measles	Mumps	Rubella	Influenza	Pneumococcal Polysaccharide
18–24	X	X	X	X		
25–64	X	X[c]	X[c]	X		
≥65	X				X	X

[a]Refer also to sections in text on specific vaccines or toxoids for indications, contraindications, precautions, dosages, side effects, adverse reactions, and special considerations.

[b]Td = Tetanus and diphtheria toxoids, adsorbed (for adult use), which is a combined preparation containing <2 flocculation units of diphtheria toxoid.

[c]Indicated for persons born after 1956. (From Centers for Disease Control. Update on adult immunization: Recommendations of the Advisory Committee on Immunization Practices (ACIP). MMWR 1991;40(RR-12):1–95.)

Minimum Age for Pediatric Vaccination

Vaccine	Minimum Age for First Dose[a]	Minimum Interval from Dose 1 to 2[a]	Minimum Interval from Dose 2 to 3[a]	Minimum Interval from Dose 3 to 4[a]
DTP (DT)[b]	6 weeks[c]	4 weeks	4 weeks	6 months
Combined DTP-Hib	6 weeks	1 month	1 month	6 months
DTaP[b]	15 months			6 months
Hib (primary series)				
HbOC	6 weeks	1 month	1 month	[d]
PRP-T	6 weeks	1 month	1 month	[d]
PRP-OMP	6 weeks	1 month	[d]	
OPV	6 weeks[c]	6 weeks	6 weeks[f]	
IPV[e]	6 weeks	4 weeks	6 months[f]	
MMR	12 months[g]	1 month		
Hepatitis B	Birth	1 month	2 months[h]	

DTP Diphtheria–tetanus–pertussis
DTaP Diphtheria–tetanus–acellular pertussis
Hib *Haemophilus influenzae* type b conjugate
IPV Inactivated poliovirus vaccine
MMR Measels–mumps–rubella
OPV Live oral polio vaccine

[a]These minimum acceptable ages and intervals may not correspond with the optimal recommended ages and intervals for vaccination.

[b]DTaP can be used in place of the fourth (and fifth) dose of DTP for children who are at least 15 months of age. Children who have received all four primary vaccination doses before their fourth birthday should receive a fifth dose of DTP (DT) or DTaP at 4–6 years of age before entering kindergarten or elementary school and at least 6 months after the fourth dose. The total number of doses of diphtheria and tetanus toxoids should not exceed six each before the seventh birthday.

[c]The American Academy of Pediatrics permits DTP and OPV to be administered as early as 4 weeks of age in areas with high endemicity and during outbreaks.

[d]The booster dose of Hib vaccine which is recommended following the primary vaccination series should be administered no earlier than 12 months of age and at least 2 months after the previous dose of Hib vaccine.

[e]See text to differentiate conventional inactivated poliovirus vaccine from enhanced-potency IPV.

[f]For unvaccinated adults at increased risk of exposure to poliovirus with <3 months but >2 months available before protection is needed, three doses of IPV should be administered at least 1 month apart.

[g]Although the age for measles vaccination may be as young as 6 months in outbreak areas where cases are occurring in children <1 year of age, children initially vaccinated before the first birthday should be revaccinated at 12–15 months of age, and an additional dose of vaccine should be administered at the time of school entry or according to local policy. Doses of MMR or other measles-containing vaccines should be separated by at least 1 month.

[h]This final dose is recommended no earlier than 4 months of age. *(From Centers for Disease Control and Prevention. General recommendations on immunization: Recommendations of the Advisory Committee on Immunization Practices (ACIP). MMWR 1994;43(RR-1):1–38.)*

Chapter 117

Principles and Management of Human Immunodeficiency Virus Infection

Courtney V. Fletcher, PharmD, and Ann C. Collier, MD

The acquired immunodeficiency syndrome (AIDS) was first recognized by the medical community as a distinct clinical entity in 1981. This syndrome was initially described in healthy young homosexual men and was characterized by profound immunologic deficits, multiple opportunistic infections, and malignant neoplasms.[1–4] By 1991, more than 200,000 persons in the United States had been diagnosed with AIDS.[5] A retrovirus, human immunodeficiency virus type one (HIV-1) [formerly called lymphadenopathy-associated virus (LAV) or human T lymphotropic virus type III (HTLV-III)] is the major cause of AIDS.[6–8] A second retrovirus, HIV-2, has been recognized to cause AIDS although it is far less common than HIV-1. HIV-1 and HIV-2 may have some differences in clinical manifestations, antiretroviral susceptibilities, and necessitate development of different vaccines.[9]

Evidence has shown that these retroviruses are transmitted by sexual contact and by contact with contaminated blood or blood products. Several risk behaviors for acquisition of HIV infection have been identified, most notably the practice of anorectal intercourse (by homosexual men and heterosexuals) and the sharing of blood-contaminated needles by injection drug users. Transmission of HIV between heterosexuals and from childbearing women to their offspring is an increasing problem.[10] The development of serologic tests to detect the presence of antibodies to HIV-1 in the blood was a major advancement and prerequisite for both prevention and treatment strategies. Statistics on the prevalence and incidence of this disease remain grim, and all treatments to date have been unsuccessful in eradicating HIV from infected persons. However, several therapies have been able to suppress HIV replication *in vitro* and *in vivo,* and one treatment, zidovudine, an inhibitor of viral reverse transcriptase, has been shown to prolong survival in patients with AIDS and advanced HIV infection. This chapter provides a discussion of the epidemiology and manifestations of HIV infection, therapeutic strategies directed at inhibition of the virus, and management of HIV-associated opportunistic infections.

EPIDEMIOLOGY

The total number of reported cases of AIDS in the United States [meeting the surveillance definition of the Centers for Disease Control and Prevention (CDC)] at the beginning of 1995 was more than 400,000: More than half of these individuals have died. The CDC estimates that 800,000 to 1.2 million people in the United States are currently infected with HIV and that 40,000 new HIV infections occur annually among adults and adolescents.[11] In addition, an estimated 1500–2000 newborns are infected by HIV perinatally each year.[12] HIV infection, however, is a worldwide epidemic. In early 1993, the World Health Organization (WHO) estimated that of the approximately 2.5 million cases of AIDS in the world, 80% occurred in the developing world. By the year 2000, WHO has estimated that 30–40 million persons worldwide will be infected with HIV.

AIDS cases reported to the CDC meet the surveillance case definition and are reported by a health care provider to a public health department. A case definition of AIDS was first established in 1981 and underwent modifications in 1985, 1987, and 1992. The current case definition became effective January 1, 1993. This latest version expands the definition of AIDS to include not only persons with serious symptomatic disease, but also all HIV-infected people who have <200 CD4 lymphocytes/μL, or a CD4 T-lymphocyte percentage of total lymphocytes <14. The 1993 definition retained the 23 clinical conditions (e.g., *Pneumocystis carinii* pneumonia, cytomegalovirus retinitis) that had been part of previous definitions and added three additional: pulmonary tuberculosis, recurrent pneumonia, and invasive cervical cancer. Table 117.1 is a listing of the clinical conditions included in the 1993 defi-

TABLE 117.1. CONDITIONS INCLUDED IN THE CENTERS FOR DISEASE CONTROL AND PREVENTION 1993 AIDS SURVEILLANCE CASE DEFINITION

Candidiasis of bronchi, trachea, or lungs	Lymphoma, Burkitt's
Candidiasis, esophageal	Lymphoma, immunoblastic
Cervical cancer, invasive[a]	Lymphoma, primary, of brain
Coccidioidomycosis, disseminated or extrapulmonary	*Mycobacterium avium* complex or *M. kansasii,* disseminated or extrapulmonary
Cryptococcosis, extrapulmonary	*Mycobacterium tuberculosis,* any site (pulmonary or extrapulmonary)
Cryptosporidiosis, chronic intestinal (>1 month duration)	*Mycobacterium,* other species or unidentified species, disseminated or extrapulmonary
Cytomegalovirus disease (other than liver, spleen, or nodes)	*Pneumocystis carinii* pneumonia
Cytomegalovirus retinitis (with loss of vision)	Pneumonia, recurrent[a]
Encephalopathy, HIV-related	Progressive multifocal leukoencephalopathy
Herpes simplex: chronic ulcer(s) (>1 month duration); or bronchitis, pneumonitis, or esophagitis	*Salmonella* septicemia, recurrent
Histoplasmosis, disseminated or extrapulmonary	Toxoplasmosis of brain
Isosporiasis, chronic intestinal (>1 month duration)	Wasting syndrome due to HIV
Kaposi's sarcoma	

[a]Added in the 1993 expansion of the AIDS surveillance case definition.

nition, and Table 117.2 presents the 1993 classification system for HIV infection.[13]

There are three major modes for the transmission of HIV: sexual, parenteral (injection drug use, receipt of infected blood, blood products, or organs), and perinatal transmission from an HIV-infected mother. Of these, sexual contact is the most common route of HIV transmission and is estimated to account for almost 90% of the cases of HIV worldwide. No sexual act between two persons can be considered absolutely safe. Sexual practices well established as modes of HIV transmission include receptive anal intercourse and receptive vaginal intercourse. The risk of receptive oral intercourse is less well established. Data suggest that male-to-female sexual transmission is more efficient that female-to-male sexual transmission.[14] The probability of HIV transmission from heterosexual or homosexual intercourse has been estimated at 0.1–0.2 per sexual contact.[15] A number of factors may be associated with increased risk of HIV sexual transmission, including the presence of other sexually transmitted diseases (e.g., syphilis, herpes simplex virus, chancroid, gonorrhea) and possibly circumcision.[16] In the United States, heterosexually acquired HIV represents the exposure category with the largest proportionate increase in new AIDS cases. Whereas heterosexual transmission represented 1.9% of total AIDS cases in 1985, 9% in 1993 were linked to this mode of transmission.[17] Persons at highest risk for heterosexual transmission include sexual partners of injection drug users, individuals with multiple sex partners, and persons with ulcerative sexually transmitted diseases. HIV has been transmitted through artificial insemination.[18] Casual contact with AIDS patients or persons with HIV (e.g., as occurs with household contacts) does not appear to be a significant risk factor for HIV transmission. A large number of studies have shown no household transmission of HIV infection among adults, children, and friends with nonsexual contact with AIDS or AIDS-related complex patients although a few isolated cases have been reported.[19]

HIV can be transmitted through parenteral exposure, including contaminated blood or blood products, donated organs or tissues, and through the sharing of contaminated needles or other drug-related paraphernalia. In the United

TABLE 117.2 CENTERS FOR DISEASE CONTROL AND PREVENTION 1993 REVISED CLASSIFICATION SYSTEM FOR HIV INFECTION IN ADULTS

	Clinical Categories		
CD4+ T-cell Categories (absolute number and percentage)	**(A) Asymptomatic, Acute (Primary) HIV or PGL[a]**	**(B) Symptomatic, Not (A) or (C) Conditions**	**(C) AIDS-Indicator Conditions**
1. ≥500/μL or ≥29%	A1	B1	C1
2. 200–499/μL or 14–28%	A2	B2	C2
3. <200/μL or <14% (AIDS-indicator T-cell count)	A3	B3	C3

[a]PGL, persistent generalized lymphadenopathy.

States and other developed countries, blood donor screening and viral inactivation procedures for many clotting factor products have dramatically reduced transfusion-acquisition of HIV. There is a small but definite occupational risk of parenteral HIV transmission among health care workers through accidental injury. Most cases of occupationally acquired HIV in health care workers have been a result of percutaneous injury. Studies indicate that the risk of HIV infection following percutaneous exposure is approximately 0.4%.[20] Guidelines to be followed by health care workers, referred to as "universal blood and body substance isolation techniques," to minimize the potential for acquisition of HIV have been published by the CDC and other organizations and have been widely adopted.[21] However, compliance with these precautions is less than ideal.[22]

As the number of women that are HIV infected has increased, so has the number of children who have acquired HIV infection from their mother. The exact timing of perinatal transmission and the factors that determine the transmission are not completely understood. HIV appears to be transmitted during pregnancy, during delivery, and postpartum by breast-feeding; most perinatal transmission occurs close to delivery. The risk of mother-to-child HIV transmission has been reported to range from 14 to 40%.[23] Mothers who have AIDS or low CD4 cell counts appear to be at an increased risk of transmitting HIV to their infants. In countries where safe and available alternatives to breast-feeding exist, HIV-infected mothers are strongly recommended not to breast-feed.

Origin and Detection of HIV

The origin of HIV is not firmly elucidated. The virus is a member of the lentivirus subfamily of human retroviruses. Nucleotide sequencing has demonstrated that there are two types of HIV, HIV-1 and HIV-2, and that they are related but distinct (a possible third type, currently called "O", for others, has recently been suggested).[24] Both HIV types are associated with AIDS. In addition, each person infected with HIV harbors multiple strains that can be identified through molecular cloning. It appears that a primate retrovirus in sub–Saharan Africa was transmitted to the human population and was the source for HIV-1 and HIV-2 infection. The earliest identified infection with HIV occurred in central Africa in 1959.[25]

Once the viral etiology of AIDS was established in 1984, the availability of screening tests to detect antibodies directed against HIV became of critical importance. The current commercial enzyme-linked immunosorbent assays (ELISAs) are excellent for detecting HIV-1 antibodies, although there are occasional false-negative and false-positive results.[26] Currently licensed ELISA tests have sensitivities for detection of antibodies to HIV-1 of 93–99%, and have above 99% specificity.[26] Use of a confirmatory test, such as the Western blot or radioimmunoprecipitation assay (RIP), is important since the ELISA was developed as a screening test. The positive predictive value of any test, even a highly sensitive and specific test, is related to the disease prevalence for which it is being tested. Because of the widely variable prevalence of HIV-1 in different populations some have suggested that different criteria for negative and positive results of the ELISA be used in populations with different disease prevalence, although logistically this may be problematic. However, based on the low prevalence of HIV-2 in the United States today, and the failure to detect HIV-2 infections in surveys of large blood donor populations, the Food and Drug Administration (FDA) has determined that routine HIV-2 screening of blood is not necessary.[27] Polymerase chain reaction (PCR) testing is a relatively new technique that amplifies, via *in vitro* enzymatic methods, selected fragments of a genome, and can detect very low amounts of viral RNA.[28] Although this test is not yet widely available for clinical use, PCR may be useful when licensed tests are discordant or to quantitate the effects of antiretroviral therapy.

Natural History of HIV Disease

HIV is an infection that attacks cells of the immune system, and a wide number of immunologic abnormalities (both immune activation and immunosuppression) have been described in persons with HIV.[29] The progressive loss of immune system function leads to the opportunistic infections and malignancies associated with AIDS. Although the course of HIV infection varies among individuals, a general pattern has emerged (Fig. 117.1).[30] Primary infection is associated with a high viral burden and development of an immune response that for a period of time suppresses, but may not eliminate, viral replication. During the primary infection period, HIV becomes widely disseminated. This period is followed by a prolonged phase of clinical latency. The median time from initial infection with HIV to the development of an opportunistic infection and AIDS is 10 years. The phase between primary infection and symptomatic disease is referred to as clinical latency. The clinically latent period, however, is not virologically latent because viral replication and gradual immune system deterioration are ongoing. A persistent decrease in CD4 lymphocytes is the most obvious and measurable aspect of this immune system destruction. Recently, it has been shown that during this clinically latent period, HIV accumulates and actively replicates in lymphoid tissues despite a low viral burden in peripheral blood mononuclear cells.[31,32]

A brief review of T lymphocyte differentiation and function and a discussion of the immunologic abnormalities associated with HIV infection may be useful. In the initial developmental stages of T lymphocytes, both CD4 and CD8 antigens are expressed simultaneously on the same cell. Later in development, T cells usually express either the CD4 or the CD8 antigen; occasionally, neither or both are

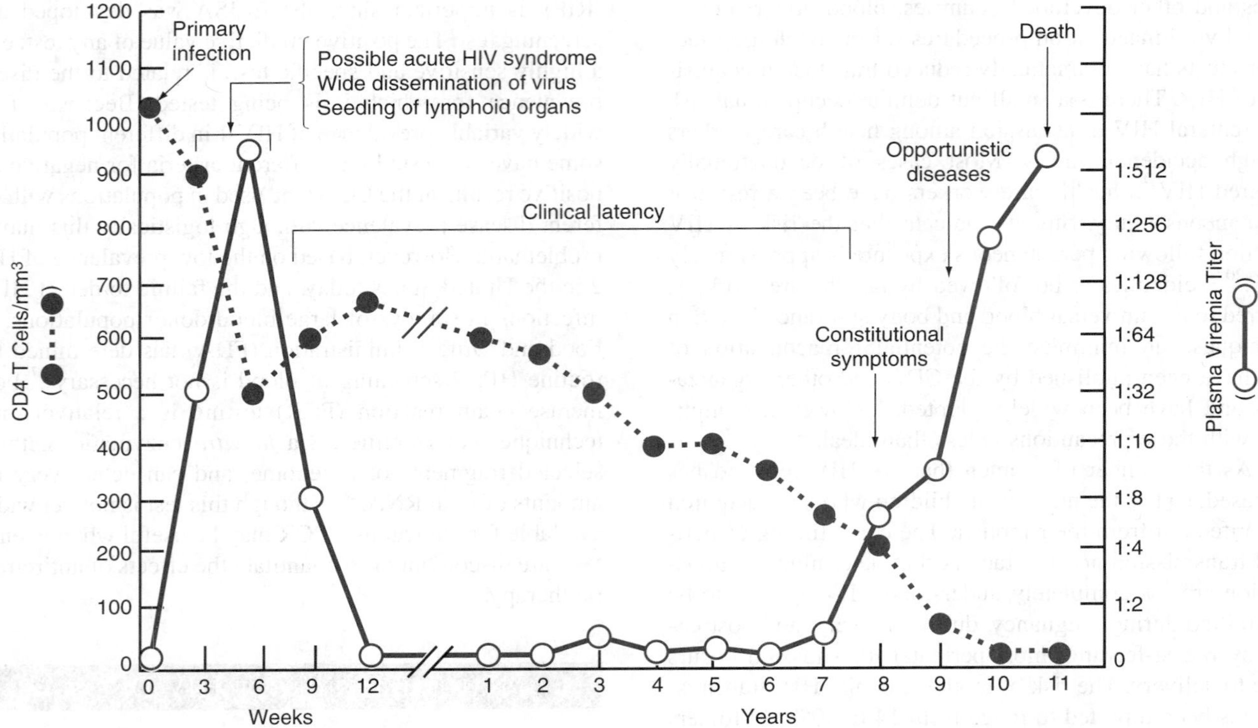

Figure 117.1. Typical course of HIV infection. *(From Pantaleo G, Graziosi C, Fauci AS. The immunopathogenesis of human immunodeficiency virus infection. N Engl J Med 1993;328:329. Reprinted by permission of* The New England Journal of Medicine. *Copyright 1993, Massachusetts Medical Society.)*

expressed. Functionally speaking, CD4 lymphocytes have been commonly called "helper" cells because of their role in assisting in antibody production by B lymphocytes, whereas CD8 lymphocytes are associated with suppressor cytotoxic activity. However, more correctly, it must be recognized that CD4 lymphocytes are heterogeneous and may be occasionally cytotoxic cells as well as suppressor, inducer, and effector cells. Accordingly, CD8 lymphocytes also occasionally "help" or amplify the interaction of CD4 lymphocytes with B cells. Patients with HIV infection show decreased numbers and percentages of CD4 cells, often increased CD8 cells, and decreased CD4 : CD8 ratios. The absolute number of CD4 cells is a more variable number than percent CD4 cells since the number is derived using the WBC differential. The absolute number of CD4 cells is widely used clinically. The normal number of CD4 cells is approximately 800, the percent of CD4 lymphocytes is 31–61% and 18–39% for CD8 lymphocytes. HIV may reduce the number of detectable CD4 cells by a variety of mechanisms including direct lysis or by blocking the CD4 receptor (on the T cell) such that the cell becomes unrecognizable as a CD4 cell.[29]

Functional abnormalities of T lymphocytes in HIV-infected patients with AIDS are numerous and are discussed in detail elsewhere.[29,30] B-cell lymphocytes also do not appear to have normal function in patients with advanced HIV infection. There is often a depressed response to pure B-cell mitogens, as well as an inability to mount a response to new antigens.[33] There is spontaneous secretion of immunoglobulin, increased spontaneous lymphocyte proliferation, elevated circulatory immune complexes, and numerous autoimmune phenomena. Finally, monocyte and macrophage function (e.g., chemotaxis) also may be abnormal in advanced HIV infection.[34]

Most patients with advanced HIV infection are anergic. Regardless of the mechanism, patients with AIDS have inadequate immune responsiveness to specific antigens and eventually lose the ability to respond to nonspecific mitogens.[29] Characteristically, they also have a moderate anemia (hemoglobin of 7–12 g/dL), moderate leukopenia (1000–3000/mm^3), and moderate thrombocytopenia. Antiplatelet antibodies are sometimes detectable. Lymphocyte counts are frequently less than 1500/µL with a disproportionate decrease in T lymphocytes compared with B lymphocytes. The abnormalities discussed appear more pronounced in patients who have had opportunistic infections than in persons who present only with Kaposi's sarcoma.[29] Of most direct clinical relevance is the association of low CD4 counts with the development of symptomatic or clinical disease.[35] Other immunologic markers (i.e., β_2-microglobulin, neopterin interleukin-2 [IL-2] receptors) are useful as prognostic markers for progression of HIV especially when combined with CD4, and in determining the time for therapeutic intervention. Several approaches are currently under investigation to restore the immune system in persons with advanced HIV including adoptive cellular immunotherapy, passive antibody administration, active vaccination with envelope vaccines, and cytokine therapy. Except for a brief discussion of vaccine development, immunologic treatments are not addressed further in this chapter.

The clinical manifestations of infection with HIV are an inevitable consequence of an ongoing immune dysfunction measured by destruction of CD4 lymphocytes. A broad spectrum of conditions, including severe persistent constitutional signs and symptoms, opportunistic infections, or neoplasms, characterize the late symptomatic phase of HIV disease. The earliest manifestation of HIV infection is the acute retroviral syndrome. Several classification schemes have been proposed to describe HIV disease. The CDC's 1993 classification scheme divides HIV infection into a matrix of nine categories based on CD4 cell count and clinical condition. The three categories based on CD4 T lymphocyte count are >500, 200–500, and <200 cells/μL (Table 117.2).[13] Clinical conditions in this classification system are also divided into three categories. Category A consists of asymptomatic infection, persistent generalized lymphadenopathy, and the acute retroviral syndrome. Category B consists of mild to moderate symptomatic conditions that are not included among the AIDS-defining conditions: bacillary angiomatosis, oropharyngeal candidiasis, vulvovaginal candidiasis that is persistent, frequent, or poorly responsive to therapy, cervical dysplasia, unexplained constitutional symptoms (fever >38.5°C, diarrhea lasting >1 month), oral hairy leukoplakia, recurrent or multidermatomal varicella-zoster, idiopathic thrombocytopenia purpura, Listeriosis, pelvic inflammatory disease, and peripheral neuropathy. This category includes the entity referred to as AIDS-related complex (ARC). Category C includes the clinical conditions in the AIDS surveillance case definition (Table 117.1), which are generally severe, life-threatening opportunistic diseases.

The signs and symptoms in patients infected with HIV may be due to infectious or neoplastic complications, in addition to HIV itself. Clinical presentation of HIV infection varies. Following initial infection with HIV (1–12 weeks postinfection), the patient may be asymptomatic or may experience a mononucleosis-like syndrome with fever, malaise, lymphadenopathy, rash, headache, arthralgias/myalgias, or may have, less commonly, aseptic meningitis. The patient who appears clinically asymptomatic may demonstrate lymphopenia, a depressed CD4 lymphocyte count and CD4 : CD8 cell ratio, cutaneous anergy, and/or reduced *in vitro* immunologic responses to various antigens. The previously asymptomatic patient may present *de novo* with opportunistic infections or malignancies, such as respiratory failure from *P. carinii* infection or disseminated Kaposi's sarcoma. The incidence of Kaposi's sarcoma in AIDS patients has decreased from the early to late 1980s for unexplained reasons.[36] Other patients complain of ill-defined persistent constitutional symptoms or a variety of symptoms involving the gastrointestinal or central nervous systems. Some individuals develop persistent generalized lymphadenopathy (usually anterior or posterior cervical, and axillary) with or without constitutional symptoms (lymph node biopsy reveals reactive hyperplasia). Another presentation may be that of a single mucocutaneous lesion of Kaposi's sarcoma in the absence of any systemic symptoms. A small number of studies have been performed that define manifestations of HIV that may be unique to women. Several have suggested that esophageal candidiasis may be more frequent. There is an increased incidence of cervical dysplasia, a precursor lesion for cervical cancer in HIV-infected women.[37] Invasive cervical cancer is considered an AIDS-defining disease. Persistent or recurrent vaginal candidiasis and severe pelvic inflammatory disease may also occur in HIV-infected women.

HIV IN CHILDREN

HIV infection has been recognized in children since before the 1980s. The major route of virus transmission to children is perinatal. More than 5000 children with AIDS have been reported in the United States; from 1992–1993 there was a 24% increase in children (<13 years) reported with AIDS.[38] The pediatric AIDS case definition includes children from birth through 12 years and has similarities to the adult surveillance definition, yet also includes clinical conditions unique to children. Table 117.3 outlines the CDC classification of HIV infection in children under 13 years of age.

HIV-related illnesses in children often present with unexplained physical signs such as hepatomegaly, failure to thrive and weight loss, unexplained fever, splenomegaly,

TABLE 117.3. CENTERS FOR DISEASE CONTROL AND PREVENTION 1994 REVISED CLASSIFICATION SYSTEM FOR HIV INFECTION IN CHILDREN LESS THAN 13 YEARS OF AGE

Immunologic Categories	N: No Signs/ Symptoms	A: Mild Signs/ Symptoms	B: Moderate Signs/Symptoms	C: Severe Signs/Symptoms
1. No evidence of suppression	N1	A1	B1	C1
2. Evidence of moderate suppression	N2	A2	B2	C2
3. Severe suppression	N3	A3	B3	C3

unexplained lymphadenopathy, low birth weight (in prenatally exposed infants), eczema, and parotitis.[39] Laboratory findings include anemia, hypergammaglobulinemia, altered mononuclear cell function, and altered T-cell subset ratios. Of note, the normal range for CD4 cell counts in young children is much different than adults. The following age-adjusted absolute CD4+ counts are also indicative of immunosuppression: children 1–11 months, <1500 cells/μL; children 1–5 years, <1000/μL; and children 6–12 years, <500/μL. Bacterial infections, including *Streptococcus pneumonia, Salmonella* species, and *Mycobacterium tuberculosis* may be more prevalent in children with AIDS than in adults with the disease. Kaposi's sarcoma is rare in children. Children with HIV infection may develop lymphocytic interstitial pneumonitis without evidence of *P. carinii* or other pathogens on lung biopsy.[39] Some children present with progressive, unexplained, neurologic deterioration, including late-onset seizures, loss of developmental milestones, cessation of brain growth, and diffuse, unexplained encephalopathy.[39] A history of recurrent or persistent bacterial, viral, or fungal infections, which may be chronic, and initially subclinical, or slowly progressive, has been observed. Included in this group are children with recurrent bacterial sepsis, meningitis, and chronic otitis media, and children with chronic oral candidiasis and presumed disseminated histoplasmosis.[39] The CDC's current pediatric AIDS surveillance definition excludes children with congenital or perinatally acquired cytomegalovirus or other identified causes of congenital immunodeficiency. Other children present with unexplained immune thrombocytopenia and neutropenia.[40] In part, because of reporting bias, the majority of children reported with HIV infection have had opportunistic infections with the organisms seen most often in adults, especially *P. carinii* and *Mycobacterium avium* complex.[39] Medical management of the HIV-infected child involves principles similar to those for adults: antiretroviral therapy, treatment and prophylaxis of opportunistic infections, and supportive care.[41]

The Life-Cycle of HIV and Strategies to Inhibit Replication

Since the discovery of HIV as the causative agent of AIDS, numerous advancements have been made with respect to understanding the complex life cycle of this retrovirus and the potential therapies directed toward its suppression. Deciphering the HIV life cycle and its genomic organization has revealed unique points of attack by which replication can be selectively inhibited. There are several potential targets where replication may be interrupted. These sites can be divided into four major categories: binding and entry, reverse transcriptase, transcription and translation, and viral maturation and budding. As of the date this was written, only the inhibition of reverse transcriptase by compounds such as zidovudine, didanosine, and zalcitabine has proven clinically beneficial.

Rational development and application of antiretroviral compounds requires knowledge of the life cycle of the virus (Fig. 117.2). The first step in the process of replication is virion access to the host through exposure to HIV-infected blood or body fluid. The virion envelope glycoprotein (gp120) selectively binds to specific cell-surface proteins located on a subpopulation of T-helper lymphocytes, called the CD4 receptor.[42] HIV has also been shown to infect monocytes and macrophages, and targets other than the CD4 receptor may be involved.[43] Enormous effort is directed toward the development of a vaccine that will elicit an immune response to protect against infection with HIV. The gp120 envelope glycoprotein of HIV is the primary target of virus-neutralizing antibodies. Unfortunately, there is sequence variation of gp120 not only between individuals, but even within an individual. The consequence of this variation is that antibodies induced by one immunogen may lack the ability to neutralize other HIV isolates. The likelihood that a preventive vaccine using a single antigen will have 100% efficacy is small. However, numerous strategies are being used in the development of vaccines. Types of vaccines against HIV under investigation include a live-attenuated vaccine, inactivated vaccine, individual and multivalent HIV protein subunit vaccines, and subunit immunogens in live vectors.[44] The traditional approaches to vaccine development, inactivated whole virus or live attenuated virus vaccines, both have potential drawbacks because of safety concerns. The most extensively studied vaccines have been subunits of HIV envelope proteins such as gp120 or gp160. Preliminary clinical trials have been conducted or are ongoing for several vaccines to establish safety and immunogenicity. For example, Dolin and coworkers[45] evaluated a recombinant envelope glycoprotein (rgp160) vaccine in 72 HIV-1-seronegative individuals. Following four doses of rgp160, neutralizing activity and complement-mediated antibody-dependent enhancement was observed in five (21%) and six (25%) participants, respectively. In all patients, rgp160 was well tolerated and safe at the doses tested. Other candidate vaccines have also been only marginally successful at producing a durable antibody response. Recent reports of the inability of vaccine-induced neutralizing antibodies to neutralize clinical HIV isolates have been discouraging.[46] The potential of using vaccines as a therapeutic intervention for HIV infection is also under consideration. Several studies have demonstrated the feasibility of modulating the immune response to HIV in HIV-infected persons with relatively preserved CD4 cells. Currently, there are several phase I/II trials of subunit and inactivated vaccines under way evaluating this approach. A 1-year, double-blind trial in 103 HIV-infected persons has been completed using a gp120-depleted, inactivated HIV-1 preparation in incomplete Freund's adjuvant.[47] Preliminary data from this study suggest that vaccine immunotherapy may alter the rate of increase of

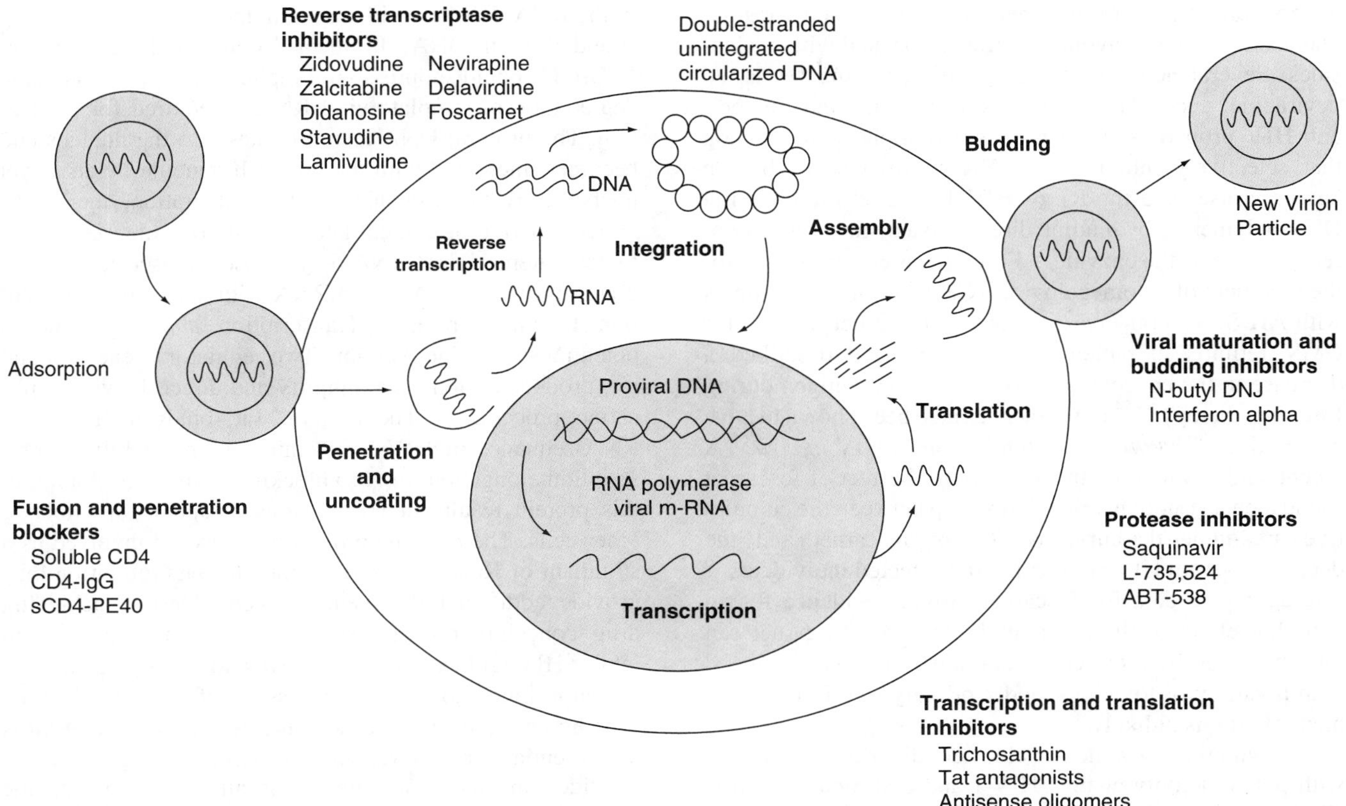

Figure 117.2. Life cycle of HIV with potential targets where replication may be interrupted and known or putative antiretroviral agents. *(Reprinted with permission, © Courtney V. Fletcher, 1995.)*

HIV in peripheral blood mononuclear cells and decrease the rate of decline in CD4 lymphocytes. Vaccine development for both prevention and treatment of HIV is a national priority and, historically, vaccines have been our most potent weapon against viral pathogens.

Binding of the virion to the host-cell surface and subsequent fusion into the target cell represent potential areas of therapeutic intervention. Compounds such as low molecular weight sulfated polysaccharides, antibodies to HIV or host-cell receptors, soluble CD4, and CD4 conjugated exotoxins are examples of agents that have been targeted at impeding the viral entry process. Recombinant soluble CD4 (rCD4) has been shown to inhibit HIV-1 binding and replication *in vitro* by attaching to gp120 on the viral capsid.[48] Two published studies of rCD4 found the compound well tolerated, but the evidence for antiretroviral properties was equivocal.[49,50] A more recent explorative study of very high-dose rCD4 suggested a possible antiviral effect.[51] Additionally, recombinant soluble CD4 at best provides only passive defense against HIV-1. It may block transmission from infected to uninfected cells but it does not facilitate destruction of the virus. In an attempt to overcome this limitation, conjugates of CD4 have been created. These immunoadhesions are rCD4 molecules linked either to an antibody (IgG, IgM) or a toxin (*Pseudomonas* exotoxin). The theoretical advantage of these immunoadhesions is a prolonged circulating half-life and an ability to kill HIV-infected cells. Trials of CD4-IgG suggested the compound was well tolerated, but no efficacy was demonstrated. Trials of sCD4-PE40 (CD4 linked to *Pseudomonas* exotoxin A) are ongoing. The theoretical strategy represented by rCD4 remains quite attractive, however the clinical usefulness of rCD4 at this time has not been demonstrated.

After binding and fusion of the virion into the host cell, it is uncoated within the cytoplasm yielding viral genomic RNA. Reverse transcriptase (RT), located in the core of the virus and released upon entry, uses the viral RNA as a template to form single-stranded DNA. RT is a unique enzyme in that it catalyzes the synthesis of DNA from RNA, contrary to the more typical genetic transferring process of DNA to RNA. RT, for practical purposes, is unique to the family of retroviruses and thus is a pivotal target for antiretroviral agents. Nucleoside agents such as zidovudine, didanosine, zalcitabine, and stavudine exert their antiretroviral effect through the inhibition of RT. A discussion of the clinical use of these agents follows. Nucleoside compounds may affect human DNA polymerases by competing with naturally occurring nucleotides; this likely explains certain of their adverse effects. There has been an active search for non-nucleoside agents to avoid toxicities associated with nucleosides. Several non-nucleoside agents, including foscarnet, nevirapine, and delavirdine, have been evaluated for their anti-HIV properties. Foscarnet is a pyrophosphate analog that selectively inhibits the DNA polymerase of human herpes viruses and the RT of HIV. Foscarnet inhibits viral DNA polymerase by binding directly to a distinct but similar receptor site on the enzyme.[52] Foscarnet is currently used for the treatment of cytomegalovirus (CMV) retinitis in patients with AIDS. Several investigations of foscarnet therapy for CMV retinitis in patients with AIDS have described a decrease in the concentration of serum HIV antigen during foscarnet therapy.[53,54] Foscarnet has also been shown to have an additive effect with zidovudine against HIV *in vivo.*[55] A recent study evaluating the antiretroviral effect of foscarnet found a pharmacodynamic relationship between the cumulative area-under-the-curve (AUC) of foscarnet and the decline in serum HIV antigen in HIV-infected individuals.[56] The aggregate data for foscarnet provide evidence for an anti-HIV effect of the compound. However, foscarnet can only be given by intravenous administration, is associated with a variety of toxicities, and a primary role in the treatment of HIV is unlikely.

Nevirapine is a non-nucleoside dipyridodiazepinone with potent activity against HIV-1 and oral bioavailability. Clinical trials of nevirapine alone and in combination with zidovudine have been undertaken. Nevirapine has a plasma half-life of at least 20 hours, which may allow once-daily dosing, and has no pharmacokinetic interactions with zidovudine.[57] Alone or in combination with zidovudine, nevirapine administration in doses of 12.5–400 mg has been associated with reductions in HIV antigen levels in HIV-infected individuals.[58] However, the rapid emergence of nevirapine-resistant isolates of HIV resulted in the HIV antigen suppression rarely persisting beyond 6 weeks.[59] Additional investigation of nevirapine in combination with nucleoside analogs is under way.

Delavirdine is a bisheteroaryl piperadine (BHAP) non-nucleoside RT inhibitor shown to inhibit HIV-1 replication *in vitro.* The drug has a wide therapeutic index *in vitro* with 50% inhibitory concentration (IC_{50}) values against HIV-1 of 2.6 μM and values of >440 μM for DNA polymerases alpha and gamma.[60] Clinical evaluations of delavirdine, in combination with one or two nucleoside agents, are currently under way. The rapid emergence of HIV-1 resistance to non-nucleoside RT inhibitors such as nevirapine seems to preclude a role for these agents alone in the treatment of HIV infection. Whether they have a role as part of combination regimens remains to be established through carefully controlled clinical investigations.

Single-stranded DNA is duplicated with the aid of RT to form unintegrated, circularized double-stranded DNA (proviral DNA). The conversion to proviral DNA is accomplished through the activity of ribonuclease H (RNase H). This enzyme is responsible for degrading the RNA template of the RNA–DNA hybrid, allowing the synthesis of double-stranded viral DNA. In theory, compounds that inhibit RNase H should suppress viral replication, since systematic degradation of template viral RNA is required for replication. The proviral DNA then migrates into the nucleus and becomes integrated with the host-cell genome by an as-yet uncharacterized mechanism. After integration, there is a variable period of clinical latency, but no evidence of virological latency. Host RNA polymerases transcribe the integrated proviral DNA into mRNA with subsequent translation to viral proteins. Transcription also represents a potential site for intervention. Two regulatory genes, *tat* and *rev,* produce proteins that amplify and direct the viral replication process.[61,62] The protein, Tat, binds to a specific RNA sequence of HIV-1 that initiates and stabilizes transcription elongation. *In vitro* blocking of the presentation of this protein results in HIV virions incapable of infecting other cells. The *tat* gene protein may also be involved as a stimulant of Kaposi's sarcoma, therefore its inhibition may provide additional therapeutic benefit. Despite achieving drug concentrations in excess of those hypothesized to inhibit HIV replication, one *in vivo* study of a putative TAT inhibitor failed to show suppression of viral replication. This finding may support the contention of some that *tat* is not essential for HIV replication. Synthetic oligodeoxynucleotides are antisense compounds aimed at blocking the expression of these specific retroviral genes.[63] If gene expression could be selectively manipulated, it would be possible to turn off viral replication by preventing the production of critical proteins necessary for the construction of new viruses. Human trials of one antisense compound directed at inhibition of the HIV *gag* gene are under way.

Following translation, further modification of precursor polyproteins is required to produce functional peptides. HIV-1 protease is a virus-specific enzyme responsible for cleavage of the p55 Gag protein precursor into structural core proteins and for cleavage of the gp160 Gag-Pol precursor into at least four additional proteins, including RT and the HIV-1 protease itself.[64] Protease inhibitors are an encouraging approach to anti-HIV therapy due to the virus-specific nature of the enzyme and the integral role it plays in the production of infectious virions. Several peptide-based protease inhibitors have now been developed.[65,66] Peptidomimetic compounds, however, may exhibit low biologic activity due to factors such as poor oral absorption and decreased stability. Compounds have been designed that exhibit fewer peptide-like characteristics and appear more stable to degradation, but in preclinical studies oral absorption was still inadequate for certain compounds.[67,68] Phosphate prodrugs of peptide HIV protease inhibitors and nonpeptidyl inhibitors have been developed. Three protease inhibitors (L-735,524, saquinavir, and ABT-538) are currently in or about to enter phase III clinical trials; mutations conferring resistance to protease inhibitors have already been described.[69–71]

In addition to the viral protease, post-translational modification of viral proteins is also accomplished by cellular enzymes through glycosylation and myristoylation processes. Glycosidases are enzymes involved with the normal processing of oligosaccharides on the envelope glycoprotein gp120. Castanospermine and *N*-butyldeoxynojirimycin (*N*-butyl DNJ) are prototype examples of trimming glycosidase inhibitors. The safety and efficacy of *N*-butyl DNJ (SC-48334) has been evaluated in combination with zidovudine in 60 patients with 200–500 CD4 cells.[72] The combination of *N*-butyl DNJ (1000 mg q 8 h) and zidovudine (100 mg q 8 h) was not superior to therapy with zidovudine alone. The mean increase in CD4 cells was 74 and 52 cells at week 4, respectively, for combination and zidovudine only groups. Diarrhea, flatulence, abdominal pain, and weight loss were more common in the combination therapy group. Pharmacokinetic data indicate that trough concentrations of *N*-butyl DNJ were below the *in vitro* inhibitory concentration for HIV. This trial does provide a rationale for further study of *N*-butyl DNJ because of the evidence for an anti-HIV effect. A prodrug of *N*-butyl DNJ has been developed with the goal of minimizing the gastrointestinal toxicity observed with the parent compound. Clinical studies with this prodrug (SC-49483) are now under way. Myristoylation inhibitors prevent viral particle assembly by halting the addition of myristic acid to the gag proteins. Myristic acid analogs have been developed and examined *in vitro*.[73] After assembly of the viral proteins in the cytoplasm, the virus buds from the cell surface and proceeds to infect other cells. Interferon-α has been shown to inhibit the late stage of HIV-1 replication and is under study for its potential utility in HIV infection.[74]

Antiretroviral Agents

ZIDOVUDINE (ZDV, AZIDOTHYMIDINE)

Since 1985, numerous studies have demonstrated the virologic, immunologic, and clinical improvements observed with zidovudine therapy in patients with AIDS and ARC and in HIV-infected asymptomatic persons. The active form of zidovudine, zidovudine triphosphate, is formed intracellularly by the enzymes thymidine kinase, thymidylate kinase, and nucleoside diphosphate kinase. Zidovudine is a competitive inhibitor of RT and causes chain termination when incorporated into a growing viral strand. In addition, zidovudine monophosphate may contribute to HIV inhibition as a result of its ability to suppress RNase H activity.[75] Zidovudine is well absorbed orally but is subject to first-pass hepatic glucuronidation. Zidovudine and its inactive glucuronide metabolite are renally eliminated with approximately 20% of the parent drug excreted unchanged in the urine. Zidovudine significantly penetrates the cerebrospinal fluid (CSF) with an average CSF:plasma ratio of 0.6 although this ratio can be quite variable (9–120%) and is correlated with time since last dose.[76,77] The plasma elimination half-life is 1.1 hours but the intracellular half-life of the active triphosphate form is 3 hours.[78] Table 117.4 presents select pharmacologic parameters for zidovudine and other known or putative antiretroviral compounds.[79]

Placebo-controlled trials have demonstrated that zidovudine prolongs survival in patients with AIDS and advanced ARC. Fischl et al.[80] and Volberding et al.[81] have demonstrated that zidovudine therapy transiently delays the onset of AIDS-defining events in symptomatic and asymptomatic HIV-infected individuals, respectively. The latter trial (ACTG 019) randomized individuals to receive placebo, 500 mg/d or 1500 mg/d of zidovudine and stratified participants according to CD4 cell count (<200 or 200–500 cells/μL). Disease progression, defined as the development of AIDS or advanced ARC, was the primary endpoint. Individuals receiving 500 mg/d of zidovudine had significantly lower rates of disease progression compared to placebo after a mean follow-up of 55 weeks ($p = 0.01$).

A European–Australian Collaborative Group has also examined the effects of zidovudine in asymptomatic persons with HIV infection who had >400 CD4 cells/μL.[82] Zidovudine therapy (1000 mg/d) was again shown to delay

TABLE 117.4. PHARMACOLOGIC PARAMETERS OF ANTIRETROVIRAL COMPOUNDS

Drug	*In Vitro* Susceptibility (Range, μM)	*F* (%)	V_d (L/kg)	$T_{1/2}$ (h)	CL (mL/min)	Adult Dose	Approximate Plasma C_{max}/ C_{min} (μM)
Zidovudine	0.05–1.0	63	1.40	1.1	1200	100 mg 5 times per day	2/0.2
Didanosine	1.0–10.0	40	1.00	1.4	800	200 mg twice daily	4/0.02
Zalcitabine	0.01–0.05	85	0.60	1.2	200	0.75 mg three times daily	0.05/0.001
Stavudine	2.0	82	0.53	1.2	500	40 mg twice daily	4/0.004
Lamivudine	0.0025–0.09	82	1.3	2.5	400	150 mg twice daily	7.5/0.22
Nevirapine[a,b]	0.04	50	1.40	40	35	200 mg once daily	5.5/3.0
Delavirdine[a]	0.0001–0.69	NA	1.0	4.7	70+	400 mg three times daily	35/14

Key: *F*, bioavailability; V_d, distribution volume; $T_{1/2}$, elimination half-life; CL, total body clearance; C_{max}, maximum plasma concentration; C_{min}, minimum plasma concentration; NA, not available.

[a]Investigational agent.

[b]After oral administration.

overall disease progression ($p = 0.001$) as defined by the study protocol after a period of approximately 2 years. Hamilton and colleagues demonstrated that earlier treatment with zidovudine delayed progression to AIDS, but found no effect of earlier therapy on patient survival.[83]

The French–English Concorde trial evaluated the survival and/or progression of disease benefits of immediate zidovudine use compared to deferred therapy in asymptomatic individuals.[84] The mean follow-up period was 3 years and data from 1749 patients were analyzed: The 3-year survival rates were 92% (90–94%) in the immediate treatment group and 93% (92–95%) in the deferred treatment group ($p = 0.15$). This study did observe a delay in the clinical progression to AIDS or severe ARC at short-term follow-up periods. However, the results indicate no delay in disease progression after a longer period of time (3 years). The duration of the benefits of zidovudine therapy has been evaluated in a long-term follow-up of ACTG 019. During follow-up of up to 4.5 years, zidovudine use in this population remained associated with a significant decrease in the risk of progression to AIDS or death.[85] This prolonged follow-up, however, clearly demonstrated that the effect of zidovudine was not permanent because benefit decreased with increased duration of use. Additionally, no significant differences in survival were found between those randomized to receive zidovudine or placebo. Last, the recently released results from the third arm of ACTG 019, which evaluated zidovudine therapy in persons with >500 CD4 cells, found similar efficacy results to those in persons with CD4 cells <500 (Executive Summary, August 9, 1994). Thus no basis presently exists to initiate zidovudine therapy while CD4 cells remain above 500/μL.

A recent placebo-controlled trial of zidovudine (ACTG 076) evaluated the risk of HIV transmission in 477 HIV-infected pregnant women (14–34 weeks gestation) to their babies. The zidovudine regimen consisted of antepartum zidovudine (100 mg five times daily) plus continuous infusion zidovudine during labor (2 mg/kg IV load followed by 1 mg/kg/h), and zidovudine for the newborn (2 mg/kg orally every 6 hours for 6 weeks). This study found that the HIV transmission rate was 7.9% when the mothers and their babies received zidovudine, but was 27.7% among those that received placebo.[86] This difference corresponds to a two-thirds reduction in the risk of maternal-to-infant HIV transmission. Adverse reactions associated with zidovudine therapy in the study were minimal: Hemoglobin concentrations were significantly lower in infants at birth whose mothers received zidovudine but this difference disappeared by 12 weeks of age; there was no difference in minor or major structural abnormalities in the two groups. All HIV-infected pregnant women should receive counseling informing them of the potential risks and benefits of zidovudine therapy.

The major toxicities associated with zidovudine are anemia and neutropenia[87] while less significant, but potentially drug or dose limiting, adverse effects include headache, insomnia, and nausea. Earlier studies that used higher doses of zidovudine (up to 1500 mg/d) and enrolled patients in later stages of disease, found a greater incidence of hematologic toxicities than studies utilizing lower doses and commencing earlier in the disease course.[87,88] Fischl et al. reported a 34% overall incidence of anemia and a 44% incidence of neutropenia in patients with AIDS who received 1500 or 600 mg/d.[80] Significantly less anemia (29% versus 39%) and neutropenia (37% versus 51%) was observed in patients receiving 600 mg/d and this regimen was at least as effective as 1500 mg/d in the treatment of patients with advanced HIV disease. Similarly, Volberding et al.[85] conducted a study in patients with asymptomatic HIV infection using zidovudine doses of 500 or 1500 mg/d. The patients in the low-dose group had a lower incidence of anemia (1.1%) and neutropenia (1.8%) than those in the high-dose regimen (6.3% for both); both regimens were equally effective. Preliminary data regarding zidovudine doses of 300 mg/d suggest clinical and virologic effects similar to standard therapy, although further assessment is necessary.[89] We would not recommend zidovudine doses less than 300 mg/d for adults. Virologic results of a 150 mg/d regimen, which was included in a study of zidovudine and zalcitabine, suggested this dose was suboptimal.[90]

The widespread chronic use of antiretroviral agents for HIV disease raises concern about the potential for development of resistance of HIV to zidovudine and other agents. The IC_{50} of HIV-1 to zidovudine has been examined in isolates from both zidovudine naive individuals and persons who had been treated with zidovudine for 6 months.[91] The IC_{50} was between 0.01 and 0.05 μM for those who never received zidovudine, but many-fold higher, 2 to 5.6 μM, for those receiving treatment. Isolates with an IC_{50} of less than 0.05 μM were considered to be sensitive to zidovudine and those greater than 1 μM resistant. HIV resistance also develops to other 2′,3′-dideoxynucleosides, such as didanosine and zalcitabine. Several mutations of the HIV-1 RT have been shown to be responsible for HIV resistance to these 2′,3′-dideoxynucleosides.[92] The cumulative development of mutations from prolonged treatment is associated with a highly resistant virus. The clinical importance of resistance is becoming more clear with some studies, suggesting a relationship between zidovudine-resistant viruses and disease progression. A study in 19 children receiving zidovudine monotherapy found a significant association between zidovudine resistance and poor clinical outcome.[93] In this trial, those children who remained stable had a median IC_{50} of 0.57 μM while those who deteriorated or died had a median IC_{50} of 3.5 μM. Several factors may contribute to the development of resistant isolates of HIV-1. These include increased viral burden during advanced disease, length of therapy, low CD4+ lymphocyte counts, and increased virulence as a result of RT mutations.[94] One additional mode of acquiring resistant isolates that has recently been reported is via direct transmission of zidovudine-resistant HIV-1 strains.[95] Strategies to prevent or delay emergence of HIV resistance are not clear.

DIDANOSINE (ddI)

Didanosine was the second nucleoside RT inhibitor to be approved by the FDA for the treatment of HIV infection. Didanosine is rapidly metabolized intracellularly to its active form, dideoxyadenosine (ddA) triphosphate, and shares a similar mechanism of action with other nucleoside analogs. Select pharmacologic characteristics of didanosine are presented in Table 117.4.[96,97] The bioavailability of didanosine varies considerably among patients as a result of its susceptibility to stomach acid, the dosage form administered, and the presence of food in the gastrointestinal tract. An additional factor may be the influence of disease conditions, such as HIV enteropathy, which are known to affect gastrointestinal motility and absorption. The bioavailability may reach 40% by fasting-state administration and the addition of a buffer or concomitant use of antacids.[96] Oral bioavailability in children is lower (19%) and more variable (range, 2–89%) than in adult patients.[98] The tablet form of didanosine is approximately 25% more bioavailable than the powder form (sachet), hence the dose of the powder for oral solution is proportionately increased. While the plasma half-life of didanosine averages 1.43 hours, the intracellular half-life of the active drug is 12 hours or more, forming the basis for less frequent dosing compared to zidovudine and zalcitabine.[99,100] Data are limited about the CSF/plasma ratio of didanosine; this value has been estimated to be 0.21, which is less than zidovudine and similar to zalcitabine. Approximately 50% of an intravenous didanosine dose is excreted unchanged in the urine and an unknown amount is either eliminated in the bile or is hepatically metabolized via as-yet uncharacterized mechanisms.

The initial approval of didanosine was based on small uncontrolled phase I trials and an expanded access program, which provided information about didanosine toxicity. In the phase I trials of didanosine, approximately 170 patients were evaluated for antiviral effects utilizing changes in CD4 lymphocyte counts as endpoints. At 4 weeks, the CD4 count had increased by 29% from baseline, and there was still a 14% increase after 12 weeks of therapy. These data were compared to historical controls who had progressive declines in CD4 lymphocyte counts throughout the 12-week period.[91] Forty-three children received didanosine orally in doses ranging from 60–540 mg/m^2 divided three times daily for 24 weeks.[92] The median CD4 lymphocyte count increased from 218 cells/μL at baseline to 327 cells/μL after 20–24 weeks ($p = 0.001$). In addition, the median p24 antigen concentration in 27 children with detectable levels at entry decreased from 272 to 77 pg/mL at 20–24 weeks ($p = 0.005$). Furthermore, a concentration–effect relationship was observed; children who had a p24 antigen response had a significantly higher AUC than the nonresponders (1.93 versus 0.79 μM • h, $p = 0.002$). A significant pharmacodynamic response was also noted with respect to didanosine AUC and change in IQ score ($p = 0.05$, $r = 0.39$). The safety and efficacy of didanosine has also been evaluated in 913 patients with advanced HIV disease who had received at least 16 weeks of previous zidovudine therapy.[101] Patients were randomized to either continue zidovudine therapy at 600 mg/d or change therapy to 500 or 750 mg/d of didanosine. The average length of follow-up from randomization was 55 weeks; the median duration of prior zidovudine therapy was 13.9 months. Those that received 500 mg/d of didanosine had significantly fewer new or recurrent AIDS events or deaths ($p = 0.02$), and the time to development of a new AIDS event was also significantly prolonged ($p = 0.015$) compared to the zidovudine arm. The progression rates for these same endpoints in the 750-mg didanosine group showed a similar trend but did not differ significantly from the zidovudine group. There was no significant difference in survival between the three groups. This study led to the indication of didanosine for persons who have received prior zidovudine therapy.

The major adverse reactions associated with didanosine therapy include painful peripheral neuropathy and pancreatitis. Peripheral neuropathy appears to be more common at higher daily doses (>12 mg/kg/d) and with prolonged exposure. The true incidence of didanosine-associated peripheral neuropathy is difficult to assess due to the nature of HIV-related complications, which can include peripheral neuropathy, and concomitant drug therapy. More than 20,000 patients have received didanosine in expanded access protocols and the manufacturer states that up to 16% of the patients who received doses similar to what is currently recommended experienced peripheral neuropathy.[96] In a blinded study, Kahn et al. found no significant difference in the rate of peripheral neuropathy between the two doses of didanosine (14% at 750 mg/d and 13% at 500 mg/d) and zidovudine (14% at 600 mg/d).[101] The incidence of pancreatitis, however, was significantly higher in persons receiving 750 mg/d (13%) versus those on 500 mg/d (7%) and also higher than the rate in persons taking zidovudine (3%).[101] According to analyses of patients in the didanosine expanded access program, the incidence of pancreatitis ranged from 5–13.8%, with fatal pancreatitis developing in 0.35% of patients without a prior history of pancreatitis.[96] Risk factors for didanosine-associated pancreatitis include a history of pancreatitis and advanced HIV. HIV-infected patients are at higher risk for developing pancreatitis as a result of concurrent drug therapy (i.e., trimethoprim–sulfamethoxazole [TMP–SMX] and pentamidine) and opportunistic infections involving the pancreas, such as CMV and Kaposi's sarcoma.[102] Other less severe but commonly observed adverse reactions include diarrhea (due to the antacid in the buffered powder for oral solution), bloating, rash, and nausea and vomiting.

ZALCITABINE (ddC)

Zalcitabine is a synthetic analog of the naturally occurring nucleoside 2′-deoxycytidine in which the 3′-hydroxyl group has been replaced by hydrogen. Zalcitabine is sequentially converted intracellularly to its active form, ddC triphosphate, by cellular kinases and becomes a natural substrate for DNA polymerase. Once it is incorporated into the growing end of DNA, chain elongation is terminated as a result of the absent 3′-hydroxyl group. Zalcitabine also competitively inhibits RT (viral DNA polymerase) by serving as an analog of the natural substrate required for viral DNA synthesis. Table 117.4 gives select pharmacologic data for zalcitabine. *In vitro,* zalcitabine is one of the most potent dideoxynucleosides tested against HIV. Zalcitabine is well absorbed orally, is primarily excreted unchanged in the urine, and has a CSF : plasma ratio of 0.14, which is considerably less than that of zidovudine.[103]

Zalcitabine monotherapy has been evaluated against zidovudine monotherapy in a randomized, double-blind study.[104] Adults with AIDS or ARC who had received ≤3 months of previous zidovudine therapy received either zalcitabine 0.75 mg every 8 hours or zidovudine 200 mg every 4 hours for a median duration of 44 weeks. The study was terminated early based on 1-year survival results, which showed a significant difference favoring the zidovudine group. Of the 635 patients enrolled, there were 59 deaths in the zalcitabine group versus 33 deaths in the zidovudine group ($p = 0.007$). In addition, 41% of the patients in the zalcitabine group had progressed to death or a new opportunistic infection at the 1-year interim analysis, compared to 30% of the zidovudine recipients. Toxicities that required drug discontinuation were primarily peripheral neuropathy (10%) in the zalcitabine group and hematologic toxicity (7%) in the zidovudine group. CPCRA 002 was a randomized, open-label study that examined zalcitabine versus didanosine in HIV-infected patients intolerant of or failing zidovudine therapy.[105] A total of 467 patients were randomized to receive didanosine or zalcitabine. The median baseline CD4 lymphocyte count on entry was ≤40 cells/μL for both groups. After a mean follow-up period of 16 months, 157 patients taking didanosine demonstrated disease progression or death compared to 152 patients receiving zalcitabine ($p = 0.56$). There was a survival advantage for patients receiving zalcitabine after adjustments between groups were made for minor differences in baseline Karnofsky scores, CD4 cell counts, and previous AIDS-defining conditions. By 12 months after randomization, 62% of those receiving didanosine and 52% of those randomized to zalcitabine had permanently discontinued taking their assigned drug. The results of this study indicate that zalcitabine and didanosine are equally effective in slowing disease progression in this population of patients with very advanced AIDS.

Two strategies conceived to extract the antiretroviral benefits but minimize toxicities were alternating and combination therapy. One hundred thirty-one patients were enrolled in a phase II trial of zalcitabine alternating with zidovudine and randomized to one of seven different treatment arms: weekly or monthly alternating zalcitabine (0.01 or 0.03 mg/kg every 4 hours) and zidovudine (200 mg every 4 hours); weekly intermittent zidovudine, 200 mg every 4 hours, or zalcitabine, 0.03 mg/kg every 4 hours; and continuous zidovudine.[106] The median follow-up period was 40 weeks. The regimens that produced acceptable toxicity while maintaining a sustained antiretroviral effect were the weekly alternating regimen of zidovudine and 0.01 mg/kg zalcitabine, and the monthly alternating regimen of zidovudine and 0.03 mg/kg zalcitabine. Hematologic toxicity was significantly less in the weekly or monthly alternating zidovudine groups compared to the continuous zidovudine arm ($p = 0.02$), and peripheral neuropathy occurred in 10–21% of the patients receiving weekly or monthly alternating zalcitabine at both doses. These data indicate that the alternating approach allowed use of a zidovudine dose twice as high as usual, and a zalcitabine dose of two to six times usual with acceptable rates of toxicity. The clinical utility of alternating therapy is unknown and, in fact, a small study of simultaneous or alternating zidovudine and didanosine found the simultaneous regimen produced more sustained elevations in CD4 count over 1 year.[107] The role of zalcitabine in combination with zidovudine is included in the combination therapy section of this chapter.

Toxicities associated with zalcitabine include a painful, dose-dependent peripheral neuropathy, fever, rash, and oral and esophageal aphthous ulcers. The latter reactions often subside with continued therapy. In addition, rare cases of pancreatitis have been associated with the use of zalcitabine and reports of possible esophageal ulceration and cardiomyopathy have been described.[104]

STAVUDINE (D4T, 2′,3′-DIDEOXY-2′,3′-DIDEHYDROTHYMIDINE)

Stavudine is a newer nucleoside that is less potent *in vitro* than zidovudine and appears to cause less myelosuppression. This decreased toxicity relative to zidovudine may be the result of their different mechanisms of activation. Stavudine has a much lower affinity for thymidine kinase, the enzyme that transfers phosphate groups to purine or pyrimidine bases and produces the mono-, di-, and triphosphorylated nucleotides. As a result, the monophosphate intermediate of stavudine does not accumulate and no significant inhibition of pyrimidine synthesis occurs.[108] Zidovudine, however, has a high affinity for thymidine kinase, which leads to excessive accumulation of its monophosphate form. This results in thymidine kinase enzyme saturation and reduced production of deoxythymidine triphosphate, the natural and essential DNA component. Depletion of the cellular stores of deoxythymidine triphosphate via thymidine kinase saturation is thought to be one mechanism by which zidovudine induces bone marrow suppression. The pharmacokinetics of stavudine were evaluated in a dose-ranging study of 22 patients with AIDS or AIDS-related complex.[109] Oral absorption of stavudine was rapid with peak concentrations generally occurring within 1 hour and the bioavailability was 82% in six of the patients who received both oral and intravenous drug. The plasma elimination half-life ranged from 1.0–1.6 hours and 34–43% of an oral dose was excreted unchanged in the urine. Stavudine was detected in the cerebrospinal fluid of two patients.

Phase I/II dose-ranging trials (0.1–12 mg/kg/d) of stavudine have been completed. The primary findings were an increased CD4 lymphocyte count, weight gain, and decreased HIV antigen load.[110] Dose modification was required in 29% of the patients and 16% discontinued therapy within 6 months. Adverse effects associated with stavudine were peripheral neuropathy and increased hepatic transaminases. A double-blind comparison of stavudine (40 mg twice daily) versus zidovudine (200 mg three times daily) in 822 HIV-infected individuals with CD4 counts of 50–500 and less than 6 months of prior zidovudine therapy is under way. Preliminary results indicate that stavudine produced consistent and sustained improvements in surrogate markers (CD4 cells, HIV antigen, body weight). Stavudine has not been shown to be superior to zidovudine in terms of delay in progression of HIV disease.[111]

The safety, virologic, and immunologic efficacy of stavudine have been evaluated in 18 HIV-infected children (7 months to 12.3 years) in a phase I, open-label dose-ranging study.[112] The doses ranged from 0.125 to 2.0 mg/kg/d divided twice daily. The drug was well tolerated and no adverse events occurred at the 36-week median follow-up point. No child required a dose reduction or drug discontinuation and the mean CD4 lymphocyte count increased from 18.8% to 19.7% at 12 weeks at doses of at least 0.5 mg/kg/d. No subject with a negative HIV p24 antigen test upon entry became positive, and among the 7 children with positive HIV p24 antigen tests at entry, the median levels decreased from 59 to 35 pg/mL at 12 weeks. Dose escalation is expected to increase to 4 and 8 mg/kg/d for newly enrolled children.

Stavudine is currently approved for treatment of adults with advanced HIV infection who are no longer responsive to, or intolerant of, other antiretroviral drugs. Adverse reactions associated with stavudine therapy were peripheral neuropathy and elevation of liver function tests.

COMBINATION ANTIRETROVIRAL THERAPY

The complex life cycle of HIV provides many potential targets for antiretroviral therapy. Reasons for combination therapy are to use agents that exploit the various targets of HIV replication, to minimize toxicities associated with these compounds, and to decrease the emergence of antiretroviral resistance. Several different approaches to combination therapy have been and are continuing to be evaluated. These include use of a nucleoside RT inhibitor with an immunomodulator, such as interferon-α; a nucleoside RT inhibitor with another antiretroviral agent that has a different mechanism of action such as a protease inhibitor; a nucleoside RT inhibitor with a non-nucleoside RT inhibitor; two nucleoside RT inhibitors; and a nucleoside RT inhibitor with a colony-stimulating growth factor. There are no published data at this time to indicate that combination therapy is superior to monotherapy with zidovudine.

Zidovudine and Interferon-α

Interferon-α (IFN-α) is a protein produced by peripheral blood mononuclear cells, which has at least 15 different subtypes. It has been known for some time that IFN-α exerts an antiretroviral effect, in addition to an immunomodulatory effect, as a result of studies that examined its use as treatment for Kaposi's sarcoma.[113] Toxicities associated with IFN-α, however, have generally precluded its use as a single agent for the treatment of HIV infection. Zidovudine and IFN-α are promising candidates for combination therapy because both have anti-HIV activity, they share two different mechanisms of action, and IFN-α is effective against Kaposi's sarcoma. The drugs also have some differences in toxicity profiles. Zidovudine causes bone marrow suppression and, although IFN-α may contribute to myelosuppression, its major toxicities are flu-like symptoms. As a result, lower doses of each agent may be successful at reducing adverse events and increasing response. Several studies have been completed that examined the effects of this combination. Initial trials using zidovudine and IFN-α for the treatment of AIDS-related Kaposi's sarcoma suggest that this strategy can be safely employed in doses that elicit antitumor and antiretroviral responses.[114,115] More recent data suggest that low-dose IFN-α (3×10^6 units three times weekly) with zidovudine (500 mg/d) may help sustain T-lymphocyte counts longer than zidovudine alone in symptomatic HIV-infected individuals.[116] This combination versus each agent alone has also been evaluated in asymptomatic HIV infection, but definitive conclusions about efficacy cannot be made at this time.[117]

Zidovudine and Zalcitabine

The regimen of zidovudine and zalcitabine has been the most extensively investigated combination therapy for HIV infection to date. A phase I/II study (ACTG 106) evaluated zidovudine plus zalcitabine in 56 patients with advanced HIV disease who had never received previous antiretroviral therapy.[90] Patients were randomized to one of six treatment arms: zidovudine 50 mg and zalcitabine 0.005 mg/kg every 8 hours; zidovudine 100 or 200 mg every 8 hours paired with zalcitabine 0.005 or 0.01 mg/kg every 8 hours; or zidovudine 50 mg every 8 hours as monotherapy. Forty-eight patients completed at least 10 weeks of treatment with a median follow-up period of 43.1 weeks. Results indicated that combination therapy at the doses tested did not result in unexpected toxicities and was well tolerated by patients. Also, the higher dose zidovudine regimens (300 or 600 mg/d) along with zalcitabine (0.01 or 0.005 mg/kg orally every 8 hours) produced greater and more persistent effects in patients with advanced HIV infection when compared to other protocol regimens and to the results of previous zidovudine monotherapy trials. The rates of toxicity were not significantly different among the six treatment arms ($p = 0.15$) and the regimen that produced the best overall response was zidovudine 200 mg every 8 hours plus zalcitabine 0.01 mg/kg every 8 hours. This combination regimen was selected for further evaluation in a trial of 991 patients with advanced HIV disease who had received ≥24 weeks of prior zidovudine therapy (ACTG 155).[118] Participants were randomized to receive continued zidovudine therapy, zalcitabine monotherapy, or a combination of both agents. Neither the combination of 2.25 mg/d (~0.03 mg/kg/d) zalcitabine with 600 mg/d zidovudine, nor the switch to zalcitabine monotherapy was superior to continued zidovudine monotherapy in terms of delay in disease progression or survival. A preplanned subgroup analysis, however, suggested that the combination regimen appeared to be more effective in patients with CD4 lymphocyte counts between 150 and 300 cells/μL, leading to a 50% reduction in the risk of disease progression or death compared with continued zidovudine. Similarly, a trend analysis found that as the CD4 count increased, combination therapy produced a significantly lower rate of disease progression compared to monotherapy. Participants who had CD4 lymphocyte counts of <150 cells/μL did not demonstrate significant differences in study endpoints. Toxicity associated with the combination was considerably higher than that of the monotherapy regimens, especially in patients with lower CD4 counts, because interruption of study medications was twice as likely in the former group.

Zidovudine and Didanosine

The safety, pharmacokinetics, and virologic activity of five different zidovudine and didanosine combination regimens has been evaluated in an open-label, dose-ranging study.[119] Sixty nine HIV-infected individuals with CD4 counts less than 400 cells/μL and fewer than 121 days of previous zidovudine therapy received either one of five different combination regimens or zidovudine alone. Fifty-five patients received combination therapy and 14 received zidovudine alone (600 mg/d). The combination regimens included 150 and 90 mg/d, 300 and 334 mg/d, 600 and 334 mg/d, 300 and 500 mg/d, and 600 and 500 mg/d of zidovudine and didanosine, respectively. Primary outcome measures included CD4 cell counts, HIV-1 RNA plasma titers, and toxicity. The combination regimens produced a higher and more sustained increase in CD4 cell counts compared to zidovudine alone ($p < 0.001$); there was no significant difference between the five combination regimens. The median CD4 cell increase was 166 cells/μL with combination therapy and 77 cells/μL in the zidovudine only group ($p = 0.001$) after 24 weeks of treatment. Eighty-three percent of patients receiving combination therapy demonstrated decreases in HIV-1 RNA titers compared to 29% in the zidovudine-alone group ($p = 0.017$). No additive toxic effects of the combinations were observed and neither agent affected the other's plasma pharmacokinetic profile. This trial was not designed to detect differences in rates of disease progression or survival, but it does provide the impetus to evaluate further this combination regimen.

Other Combinations

Several combination regimens of antiretroviral agents are under study including immunologically based therapies such as interleukin-2 (IL-2), monoclonal antibodies and cytotoxic T lymphocyte infusions, and inhibitors of cytokine-mediated virus activation. A cogent rationale, that being the *in vitro* additive/synergistic anti-HIV effect of double and triple combination regimens, forms the basis for large-scale ongoing clinical trials sponsored by the AIDS Clinical Trials Group such as ACTG 175, 193, and 241. The therapeutic regimens in ACTG 175 are zidovudine alone, didanosine alone, zidovudine plus didanosine, and zidovudine plus zalcitabine. Participants have between 200–500 CD4 cells/μL.

ACTG 193A is a randomized, double-blind four-arm study comparing zidovudine plus didanosine or zalcitabine, monthly alternating zidovudine with didanosine, and zidovudine plus didanosine and nevirapine. ACTG 241 is a randomized, double-blind trial comparing zidovudine and didanosine versus zidovudine, didanosine, and nevirapine in HIV-infected persons with CD4 cell counts <350/μL. A three-drug combination was reported to inhibit HIV-1 replication *in vitro* by forcing mutations on the reverse transcriptase enzyme that render the virus inviable.[120] The combinations examined were zidovudine, didanosine, and non-nucleoside RT inhibitors including pyridinone, nevirapine, and foscarnet. Unfortunately, it was later discovered upon further DNA sequencing that an unintentional mutation had been introduced into the reverse transcriptase clones in addition to the intended mutations. This unintended mutation was adequate to describe why viruses derived from these clones were not viable.

MANAGEMENT OF HIV INFECTION

Current guidelines suggest the initiation of antiretroviral therapy in HIV-infected asymptomatic adults with a CD4 cell count between 200–500 cells/μL (Fig. 117.3). Clinical observation and monitoring without therapy is also an acceptable strategy in the asymptomatic group because the best time to initiate therapy with currently available agents is unknown. Persons with HIV-related symptoms, regard-

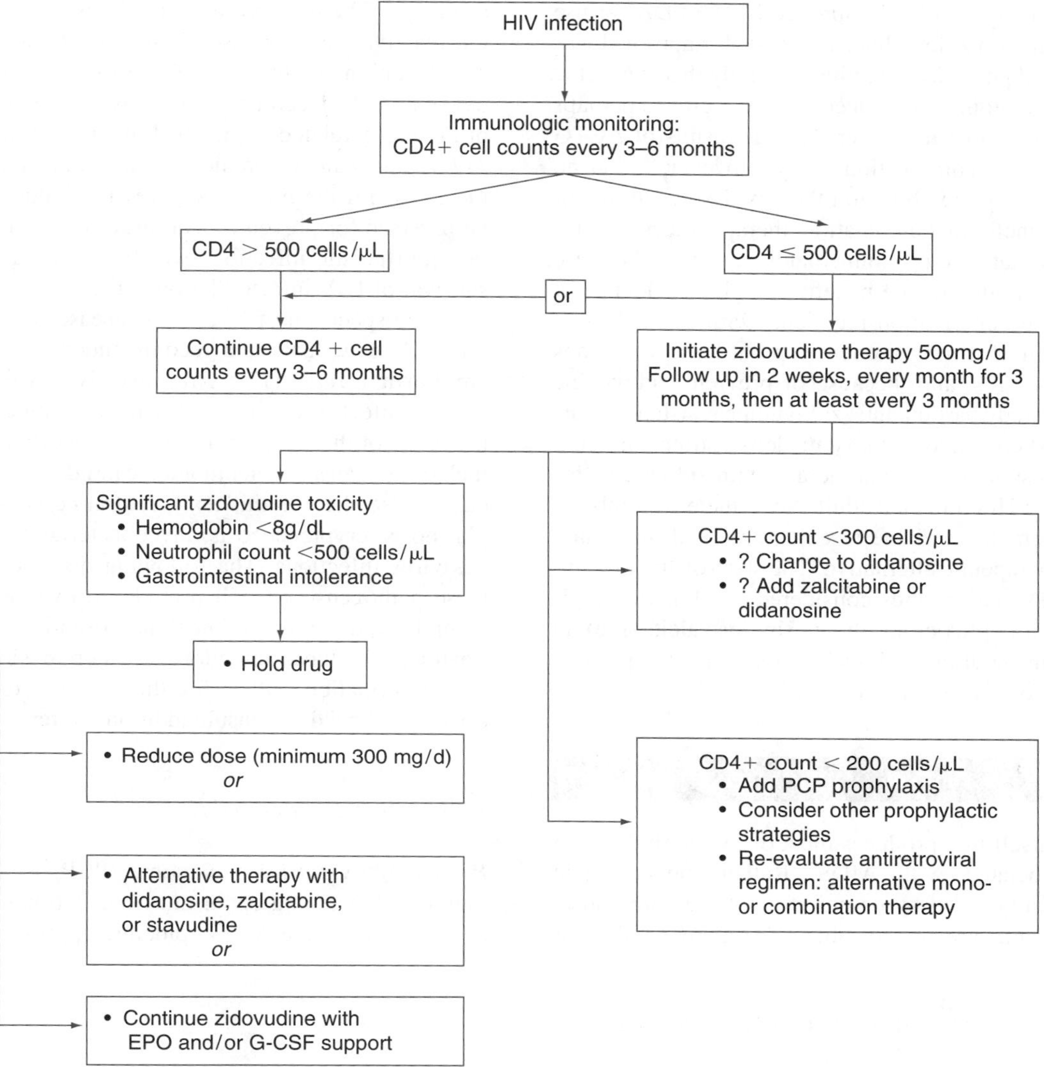

Figure 117.3. Management of HIV infection. *(Reprinted with permission, © Courtney V. Fletcher, 1995.)*

less of their CD4 cell count, and all HIV-infected individuals with a CD4 count below 200 cells/μL should receive antiretroviral therapy. At this time, persons with a CD4 cell count >500 should continue to receive clinical and immunologic monitoring; there are no recommendations for antiretroviral therapy in this population. Zidovudine has been available for use since 1987 and is the drug with which we have the greatest experience. Two controlled trials of zidovudine versus didanosine and zidovudine versus zalcitabine provide support for zidovudine as the initial drug of choice for asymptomatic or symptomatic HIV-infected adults who have not received previous antiretroviral therapy. The recommended dose for zidovudine is 500–600 mg/d.[121] Following initiation of zidovudine, several clinical scenarios warrant the reevaluation of this therapy: drug intolerance, usually anemia, neutropenia, or gastrointestinal upset, prolonged use without toxicity, therapeutic failure, and disease progression.

Didanosine is currently considered a second-line agent, indicated for the treatment of HIV infection in patients who have experienced disease progression while receiving zidovudine therapy, who are unable to tolerate zidovudine because of adverse effects, or who have simply received at least 4 months but in practice usually at least 1 year of zidovudine therapy. The recommended dose of didanosine is 200 mg of the tablet formation twice daily. Based on the results of CPCRA 002, zalcitabine monotherapy appears as effective as didanosine monotherapy in patients (with CD4 cells <50/μL) intolerant or failing zidovudine and can appropriately be considered as an alternative. Zalcitabine is also indicated for combination therapy with zidovudine in adult patients with advanced HIV infection (CD4 count ≤300 cells/μL) who have demonstrated significant clinical or immunologic deterioration on zidovudine alone. The recommended adult dose of zalcitabine is 0.75 mg orally every 8 hours.

Zalcitabine was initially approved by the FDA for use in combination with zidovudine. The basis for approval was largely the small phase I/II combination study that suggested the combination regimen produced anti-HIV effects perhaps superior to zidovudine monotherapy. The results of ACTG 155, the first large combination study, however, found no overall advantage to combination therapy. Explanations for the lack of benefit to combination therapy despite compelling *in vitro* data are not immediately apparent. Possible explanations include no true benefit, a higher incidence of toxicities in the combination recipients with clinical management actually favoring monotherapy at least in persons with <50 CD4 cells, and, because of previous zidovudine therapy in the study participants, zidovudine resistance. Currently, we must conclude that no data demonstrate combination therapy is superior to monotherapy with zidovudine for treatment of the HIV-infected adult. Nevertheless, combination therapy remains a viable research area and, in certain situations, a therapeutic alternative. The state-of-the-art conference on HIV therapeutics considered combination regimens (zidovudine plus either didanosine or zalcitabine) an option for consideration as initial therapy and for persons showing signs of disease progression.

Infectious Complications

It is not HIV itself that produces most of the morbidity and mortality associated with AIDS. Rather, opportunistic infections, many caused by organisms that are common in the environment, are responsible for almost 90% of deaths.[122] These opportunistic diseases usually represent the reactivation of quiescent infections and thus are overt manifestations of the loss of cell-mediated immunity. The development of certain opportunistic infections is directly or indirectly related to the level of CD4+ lymphocytes (Fig. 117.4) and can be predicted with some degree of accuracy.[123] Until the immunosuppression induced by HIV can be reversed, or prevented, the prevention and management of opportunistic infections will be essential for improving survival of HIV-infected individuals.

The spectrum of infectious diseases observed in HIV-infected individuals and recommended first-line therapies are shown in Table 117.5. An exhaustive review of all opportunistic infections associated with HIV infection is beyond the scope of this chapter. The major opportunistic infections include *P. carinii* pneumonia, candidal esophagitis (discussed elsewhere in this text), central nervous system toxoplasmosis, cryptococcosis, mycobacterial disease, and herpes virus infections. The following discussion emphasizes these pathogens and will provide an overview of the epidemiology, diagnosis, clinical manifestations, and results of treatment for these infections. Readers desiring more specific information, either for the diseases or agents mentioned, will need to consult additional references.

PNEUMOCYSTIS CARINII

Pneumocystis carinii pneumonia (PCP) is the most common life-threatening opportunistic infection in patients with AIDS. Early in the AIDS epidemic approximately 60% of

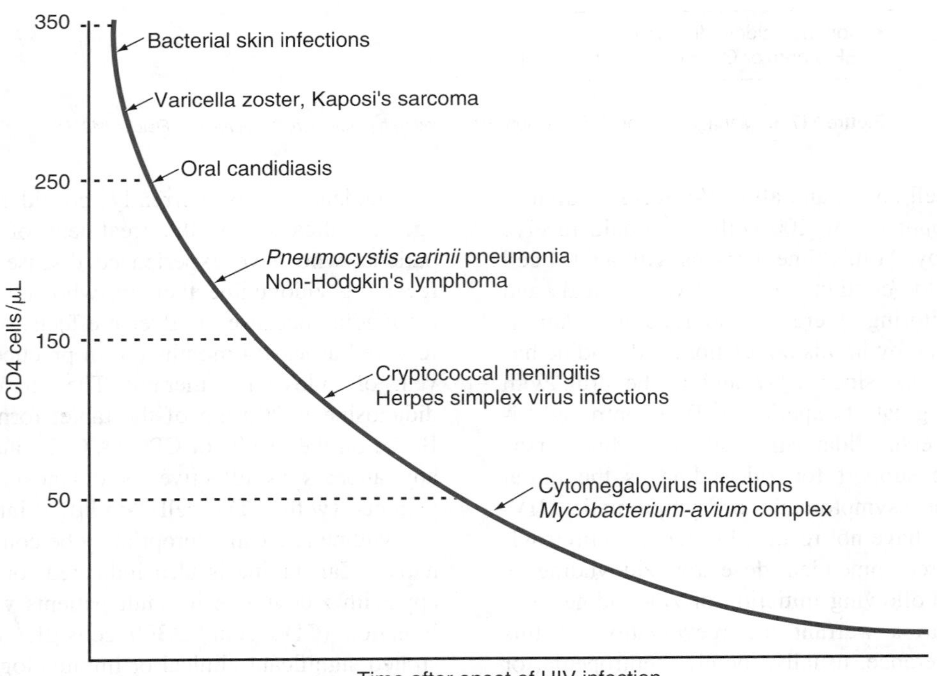

Figure 117.4. Natural history of opportunistic infections associated with HIV infection. *(Reprinted with permission, © Courtney V. Fletcher, 1995.)*

patients with AIDS had PCP as their AIDS-defining event and 80% experienced PCP at some point during their lifetime.[124] The advent of effective prophylaxis for PCP has decreased the relative incidence of PCP. Prophylaxis has not eliminated the disease because of persons unaware of their HIV infection, breakthrough PCP in those receiving prophylaxis, and variable compliance with prophylaxis. The taxonomy of the organism is unclear, having been classified as both protozoan and fungal. Recent evidence based on genomic sequences suggests that *P. carinii,* however, is a fungus.[125] Exposure to *P. carinii* is widespread with most children developing antibody by the age of 4 years. The organism appears to reside without consequence in the human unless the host becomes immunologically compromised; immunosuppression allows the organism to multiply, giving rise to clinical disease. A report of a cluster of PCP in the elderly without a specific underlying immunosuppressive illness suggests a potential for other patients being at risk for this disease.[126]

PCP in patients with AIDS differs in clinical presentation from patients with other immunosuppressive conditions, such as malignant neoplasms. In AIDS patients, the presentation is often more subacute. Characteristic symptoms include fever and dyspnea; clinical signs are tachypnea with or without rales or rhonchi, and a nonproductive or mildly productive cough. Chest radiographs may show florid or subtle infiltrates or occasionally be normal, although, infiltrates are usually interstitial and bilateral. Arterial blood gases may show minimal hypoxia (Pa_{O_2} 80–95 mm Hg), but in more advanced disease may be markedly abnormal. The onset of PCP is often insidious, occurring over a period of weeks, although more fulminant presentations can occur. The diagnosis of PCP is usually made by identification of the organism in induced sputum or in specimens obtained from bronchoalveolar lavage. Less commonly, transbronchial biopsy is used for diagnosis.

Untreated PCP has a mortality of nearly 100%. Treatment with agents such as TMP–SMX or parenteral pentamidine is associated with a 60–100% response rate. Controversy exists as to which is the preferred first-line agent. Historically, pentamidine was the drug of choice for PCP until the 1970s when Hughes compared the efficacy and tolerance of TMP–SMX and pentamidine in children with PCP.[127] Both agents were found to be equally efficacious, however, TMP–SMX was less toxic. TMP–SMX became the regimen of choice for treatment and subsequently prophylaxis of non–HIV-associated PCP. TMP–SMX is currently considered to be the therapy of choice for HIV-associated PCP as well.[128]

TMP–SMX, when used for the treatment of PCP, is usually given in doses of 15–20 mg/kg/d (based on the TMP component) as three to four divided doses. Doses of 12–15 mg/kg/d may be as effective and perhaps reduce the incidence of toxicity. TMP–SMX is usually initiated by the intravenous route, although oral therapy (as oral absorption is high) may suffice in mildly ill and reliable patients, or to complete a course of therapy after a response has been achieved with intravenous administration. If oral therapy is utilized, it would be prudent to document absorption with serum concentrations of TMP or SMX because gastrointestinal disturbances or a malabsorption syndrome are known to alter drug absorption in patients with AIDS. Target concentrations for TMP are between 5–8 μg/mL.

For treatment of HIV-associated PCP, pentamidine isethionate is administered intravenously usually in doses of 4 mg/kg/d, although a pilot study has reported successful treatment with 3 mg/kg/d.[129,130] The elimination half-life is 6–10 hours and renal elimination accounts for the majority of drug clearance.[131] Aerosolized pentamidine has also been utilized for the treatment of PCP. Comparative studies with intravenous pentamidine indicate that aerosolized pentamidine treatment is associated with a slower clinical response, higher rates of therapeutic failure, and PCP relapse.[131,132]

The efficacy of TMP–SMX or pentamidine for treatment of an initial episode of PCP in HIV-infected individuals is similar, with published response rates between 60–80%. While comparative studies between the two regimens are few, one prospective, randomized trial found that oxygenation improved more quickly and survival was better in those that received TMP–SMX.[133] The optimum length of therapy for treatment of PCP with either agent is not known, but 21 days is commonly recommended. Clinical improvement in patients with AIDS is often slower than in non-AIDS patients. One study demonstrated improvement in chest radiograph or gallium scan in only two-thirds of patients at the end of treatment.[134] Thus, the lack of prompt clinical improvement is not necessarily an indication of no response. In fact, patients frequently may worsen before they improve. However, continued worsening after 4 days or lack of improvement after 7–10 days is an indication for a change in therapy, regardless of which agent was started initially. There are no data regarding the utility of concurrent therapy with both TMP–SMX and pentamidine, and this approach is not recommended.

Adverse reactions to both TMP–SMX and pentamidine are common and range between 20–85% in this setting. The more common adverse reactions seen with TMP–SMX are rash, fever, leukopenia, elevated transaminases, and thrombocytopenia. Mild rashes should be watched closely for progression to more severe reactions, but are not an absolute contraindication to continuing therapy. The incidence of these adverse reactions is higher in HIV-infected individuals than in those not infected with HIV.[135] For pentamidine, side effects include hypotension, tachycardia, nausea, vomiting, severe hypoglycemia or hyperglycemia, pancreatitis, irreversible diabetes mellitus, elevated transaminases, nephrotoxicity, leukopenia, and cardiac arrhythmias. Some of these reactions appear to be infusion-rate related (hypotension, tachycardia) and can be minimized by infusion durations of 1 hour. The overall incidence of adverse reactions to pentamidine appears similar

TABLE 117.5. THERAPIES FOR COMMON OPPORTUNISTIC PATHOGENS IN HIV-INFECTED INDIVIDUALS

Clinical Disease	Selected Therapies for Acute Infection in Adults	Common Drug or Dose Limiting Adverse Reactions
Fungi		
Candidiasis, oral	Nystatin 500,000 units PO swish 4–6 times daily for 7–10 days	Taste, patient acceptance
	or	
	Clotrimazole 10 mg (1 troche) PO 5 times daily for 7–10 days	
Candidiasis, esophageal	Ketoconazole 400 mg/d PO for 10–14 days	Elevated liver function tests, hepatotoxicity, nausea and vomiting
	or	
	Fluconazole 200 mg PO or IV on the first day then 100 mg/d for 10–14 days	Elevated liver function tests,hepatotoxicity, rash, nausea and vomiting
Pneumocystis carinii pneumonia	Trimethoprim–sulfamethoxazole IV or PO 12–20 mg/kg/d as TMP component in 3–4 divided doses for 21 days[a]	Skin rash, fever, leukopenia, thrombocytopenia
	or	
	Pentamidine IV 3–4 mg/kg/d for 21 days[a]	Azotemia, hypoglycemia, hyperglycemia
	Mild episodes: Atovaquone 750 mg PO thrice daily for 21 days[a]	Rash, elevated liver enzymes, diarrhea
Cryptococcal meningitis	Amphotericin B IV 0.5–0.7 mg/kg/d for minimum of 2 weeks *with or without*	Nephrotoxicity, hypokalemia, anemia, fever, chills
	Flucytosine 100–150 mg/kg/d PO in 4 divided doses	Bone marrow suppression, elevated liver enzymes
	followed by	
	Fluconazole 100–200 mg/d, PO[a]	Same as above
Histoplasmosis	Amphotericin B 0.5–1 mg/kg/d IV for 6–8 weeks[a]	Same as above
	or	
	Itraconazole 200–400 mg/d for 3 months[a]	Elevated liver function tests, hepatotoxicity, nausea and vomiting, hypertension
Coccidiodomycosis	Amphotericin B 0.5–1 mg/kg/d IV for 6–8 weeks[a]	Same as above
Protozoa		
Toxoplasmic encephalitis	Pyrimethamine 200 mg PO once then 50–100 mg/d	Bone marrow suppression
	plus	
	Sulfadiazine 1–1.5 g PO four times daily	Allergy, rash, drug fever
	and	
	Folinic acid 10–20 mg PO daily for a minimum of 28 days[a]	
Isosporiasis	Trimethoprim and sulfamethoxazole: 640 mg TMP and 3200 mg SMX per day PO in 2–4 divided doses per day for 2–4 weeks	Same as above

(continued)

between individuals infected with HIV and those not infected. Dosage modification or pharmacokinetic monitoring can reduce somewhat the toxicity of both pentamidine and TMP–SMX.[134] Dose reductions of pentamidine from 4 to 3 mg/kg/d appears successful in minimizing further rises in serum creatinine. Maintenance of serum TMP concentrations between 5 and 8 μg/mL may help prevent severe myelosuppression.

The early addition of adjunctive corticosteroid therapy to anti-PCP regimens has been shown to decrease the risk of respiratory failure and improve survival in patients with AIDS and moderate to severe PCP ($Pao_2 \leq 75$ mm Hg or A-a gradient ≥ 35 mm Hg).[136,137] The adverse effects associated with corticosteroid therapy in these patients were minimal, primarily an increased incidence of herpetic lesions, although some concerns exist about the potential for reactivation of tuberculosis. The optimal dose and duration of corticosteroid therapy have not been identified. The regimen currently recommended is 40 mg of prednisone orally twice daily during days 1–5; 40 mg once daily on days 6–10; and 20 mg once daily on days 11–21, or for the duration of therapy.[138] In general, adjunctive corticosteroid therapy should be initiated when antipneumocystis therapy is started, because the data supporting the use of corticosteroids are based on initiation within the first 24–72 hours of the start of antipneumocystis therapy.

Dapsone and dapsone plus trimethoprim have been studied as alternatives for the treatment of PCP. Dapsone in

TABLE 117.5. THERAPIES FOR COMMON OPPORTUNISTIC PATHOGENS IN HIV-INFECTED INDIVIDUALS *(Continued)*

Clinical Disease	Selected Therapies for Acute Infection in Adults	Common Drug or Dose Limiting Adverse Reactions
Bacteria		
Organisms associated with T-cell defects		
Mycobacterium avium complex	Clarithromycin 0.5–1 g PO twice daily	Gastrointestinal intolerance
	plus	
	Ethambutol 15 mg/kg/d PO to a maximum of 1000 mg/d	Optic neuritis, peripheral neuritis
	may also add	
	Rifampin 10 mg/kg/d PO to a maximum of 600 mg/d for 12 weeks	Hepatitis, discoloration of secretions
	or	
	Clofazimine 100–200 mg PO daily	Discoloration of skin and eyes, gastrointestinal intolerance
	or	
	Ciprofloxacin 500–750 mg PO twice daily	Gastrointestinal intolerance
Salmonella enterocolitis or bacteremia	Ciprofloxacin 500–750 mg PO twice daily for 14 days	Same as above
	or	
	Trimethoprim (320 mg)–sulfamethoxazole (1600 mg) PO in 2 divided doses/d for 14 days	Same as on previous page
Organisms associated with B-cell defects		
Campylobacter enterocolitis	Ciprofloxacin 500 mg PO twice daily for 7 days	Same as above
	or	
	Erythromycin 250–500 mg PO four times daily for 7 days	Gastrointestinal intolerance, colitis, ototoxicity
Shigella enterocolitis	Ciprofloxacin 500 mg PO twice daily for 5 days	Same as above
Viruses		
Mucocutaneous herpes simplex	Acyclovir 1–2 g/d PO in 3–5 divided doses, for 7–10 days	Gastrointestinal intolerance
Varicella-zoster	Acyclovir 30 mg/kg/d IV in 3 divided doses or 4 g/d PO for 7–10 days	Obstructive nephropathy, CNS symptomatology
Cytomegalovirus	Ganciclovir 7.5–10 mg/kg/d in 2–3 divided doses for 14 days[a]	Neutropenia, thrombocytopenia
	or	
	Foscarnet 180 mg/kg/d in 2–3 divided doses for 14 days[a]	Nephrotoxicity, hypo–hypercalcemia, hypo–hyperphosphatemia, anemia

[a]Maintenance therapy is recommended.

doses of 100 mg/d orally for 21 days when compared to historical controls was less effective than standard therapy and should not be used alone for the treatment of PCP.[139] The combination of dapsone plus trimethoprim compared to TMP–SMX was found to have similar efficacy in a small controlled trial of patients with AIDS and first episode PCP.[140] Treatment failures were 7% and 10%, respectively, for the dapsone–trimethoprim group versus the TMP–SMX group. However, major adverse reactions (neutropenia and elevation of liver function tests) were significantly more common in the TMP–SMX group and necessitated a change to alternate therapy more frequently. The group that received dapsone–trimethoprim had a higher incidence of methemoglobinemia, a known complication of dapsone. The existence of a drug interaction between dapsone and trimethoprim resulting in increased concentrations of each in the presence of the other may have contributed to the incidence of methemoglobinemia.[141] Oral administration of dapsone–trimethoprim does appear to represent a satisfactory alternative for mild to moderately ill patients with PCP. Candidates for this regimen should be screened for glucose-6-phosphate dehydrogenase deficiency before therapy is initiated; individuals deficient in this enzyme should not receive dapsone. Malaise, fatigue, cyanosis, and decreased hemoglobin are suggestive of methemoglobinemia and methemoglobin concentrations should be obtained.

Other alternative therapies for PCP are available. Regimens include the combination of clindamycin and primaquine, and the hydroxynaphthoquinone compound atovaquone.[142] Atovaquone was found to be less effective than TMP–SMX in a study of 322 patients with AIDS and mild or moderately severe PCP; however, treatment-limiting adverse reactions were less in the atovaquone recipients.[143] Trimetrexate also is useful for "salvage" therapy in patients who do not respond or cannot tolerate standard PCP therapies. The use of trimetrexate is complicated by myelosuppression, and simultaneous leucovorin must be administered during treatment and for 48–72 hours after trimetrexate is administered. In an open trial of trimetrexate–leucovorin, the survival rate appeared equivalent to that of TMP–SMX and pentamidine.[144]

HIV-infected individuals who have had PCP are at high risk for recurrent PCP if no prophylactic measures are taken. Even though the treatment of PCP is becoming increasingly successful, the mortality rate from first episode PCP is still between 5–20%, and therapy is often complicated by adverse reactions. Prevention of PCP is clearly a preferable strategy to treatment. A retrospective study of 100 HIV-infected individuals found the circulating CD4+ lymphocyte counts were less than 200 cells/μL within 60 days before 46 of 49 episodes of PCP.[145] The relative risk of PCP in 1665 HIV-infected participants who did not have AIDS was 4.9 in those with CD4+ lymphocyte counts <200/μL.[146] These data indicate that HIV-infected adults with a CD4+ count <200 cells/μL, or whose CD4+ cells are <20% of total lymphocytes, are at high risk to develop PCP and are especially likely to benefit from prophylactic therapy. Prophylactic therapy for PCP is necessary despite treatment with antiretroviral agents, such as zidovudine. Currently, in the United States, PCP prophylaxis is recommended for all HIV-infected individuals who have already had previous PCP and for any HIV-infected person who has a CD4+ lymphocyte count <200 cells/μL or if their CD4+ cells are <20% of total lymphocytes.[147]

TMP–SMX and aerosolized pentamidine are both effective for primary and secondary prophylaxis of PCP. However, TMP–SMX has been found to be more effective than aerosolized pentamidine as secondary prophylaxis, is less expensive, and is considered the therapy of choice for PCP prophylaxis. The earliest controlled study of TMP–SMX for PCP prophylaxis in patients with AIDS used a regimen of 160 mg TMP and 800 mg SMX orally, given twice daily with 5 mg of leucovorin given once daily.[148] No patient (0 of 30) developed PCP while taking TMP–SMX. In addition, the use of TMP–SMX was associated with an increase in the mean survival time compared with those patients who received no prophylaxis. The addition of leucovorin to the TMP–SMX regimen was an attempt to reduce the incidence of adverse reactions (primarily neutropenia and rash). The effectiveness of leucovorin for this use is unknown, however, because no group received TMP–SMX without leucovorin, and 50% of patients who received the TMP–SMX plus leucovorin combination still experienced some type of adverse reaction. This study established that PCP prophylaxis in patients with AIDS could have a high degree of efficacy.

Subsequently, a study of TMP–SMX versus aerosolized pentamidine in 310 adults with AIDS recently recovered from an episode of PCP found the 1-year estimated recurrence rate was 3.5% for TMP–SMX but was 18.5% for aerosolized pentamidine.[149] Results of an evaluation comparing TMP–SMX, dapsone, and aerosolized pentamidine for primary PCP prophylaxis in 843 patients with HIV infection and <200 CD4 cells indicate that all three treatment strategies have similar efficacy.[150] However, the lowest rates of PCP breakthrough among all subgroups were in those individuals currently taking TMP–SMX. TMP–SMX and dapsone were more effective than aerosolized pentamidine in patients with fewer than 100 CD4 cells. These data provide additional support for the selection of TMP–SMX as the first-line agent for PCP prophylaxis. The recommended dose in adults and adolescents is one double-strength tablet daily, although other regimens, such as one double-strength tablet thrice weekly, have been used in an attempt to reduce the incidence of adverse reactions.[151]

TMP–SMX is also the recommended therapy of choice for PCP prophylaxis in children.[152] As previously described, the normal range for CD4+ lymphocytes is very different for children than for adults. Both the absolute CD4+ count and CD4+ cells as a percentage of the total should be determined. A CD4+ percentage <25% is an indication of immunosuppression. The utility of TMP–SMX for prophylaxis is well established for children not HIV-infected receiving myelosuppressive therapy.[153] The TMP–SMX regimen recommended (although other acceptable alternatives exist) is 150 mg/m^2/d of TMP and 750 mg/m^2/d of SMX given in divided doses twice daily, three times weekly on consecutive days (e.g., Monday–Tuesday–Wednesday).[153] The total daily dose of TMP–SMX in children should not exceed 320 mg of TMP with 1600 mg of SMX. PCP prophylaxis in HIV-exposed/infected children is recommended for (1) all HIV-exposed infants between 4 weeks and 12 months of age if infection status is unknown, (2) all HIV-infected infants 4 weeks to 12 months of age, and (3) all HIV-infected children greater than 1 year with severe immunosuppression (Guidelines for Preventing Opportunistic Infections, U.S. Public Health Service, Infectious Disease Society of America, in press).

Aerosolized pentamidine has efficacy in the prevention of PCP. A three-arm study of HIV-infected persons found that recipients of 300 mg of pentamidine via a Respirgard II nebulizer every 4 weeks had fewer confirmed episodes of PCP compared to those that received 30 mg every 2 weeks or 150 mg every 2 weeks.[154] A placebo-controlled study demonstrated that aerosolized pentamidine (300 mg every 28 d) was 60–70% effective in preventing first episode PCP.[155]

The most frequent adverse event related to aerosolized pentamidine use is cough. Pretreatment with a bronchodilator is widely used and may help alleviate this problem. Additional issues to be considered with the use of aerosolized pentamidine include potential for upper lobe pneumonia, presumably secondary to decreased drug deposition in these areas; late breakthrough disseminated disease (extrapulmonary pneumocystosis)[156]; and cost, because aerosolized pentamidine is considerably more expensive than TMP–SMX. Other agents, which could be considered for prophylaxis of PCP when neither TMP–SMX, dapsone, or aerosolized pentamidine can be administered, include pyrimethamine–sulfadoxine, pyrimethamine–clindamycin, clindamycin–primaquine, and atovaquone. Their actual role in the prophylaxis of PCP awaits completion of rigorous clinical trials.

TOXOPLASMA GONDII

Toxoplasma gondii is a protozoan that seroepidemiologic studies indicate infects up to one-third of the general population in the United States; infection rates are much higher in some European countries. The parasite is passed to humans from raw or undercooked meat, and contact with feces from infected cats. *Toxoplasma gondii* can infect any organ of the body and cause an acute infection; it has a predilection for the brain and the eye. Once infected, the organism can replicate forming tissue cysts that persist for the life of the host. Many individuals will not have symptoms of disease. Immunosuppression, however, allows the release of tachyzoites from tissue cysts that produce a necrotic foci of infection, most often the brain. In the patient with AIDS, *T. gondii* is an important opportunistic pathogen, responsible for most focal intracerebral lesions.[157]

The seroprevalence of *T. gondii* in HIV-infected individuals from major urban areas of the United States varies from 10–45%, but is considerably higher in countries such as France. A retrospective study suggested that 30% of AIDS patients seropositive for *T. gondii* will ultimately develop toxoplasmic encephalitis.[158] The clinical signs and symptoms of toxoplasmosis are most frequently associated with involvement of the central nervous system (CNS), and less commonly the lungs and eyes although any organ can be affected. Clinical presentation often includes fever, headache, seizures (in approximately 10–25% of patients), focal neurologic abnormalities (in approximately 60–90%), and mental status changes. Brain biopsy is required to make a definitive diagnosis of toxoplasmic encephalitis although presumptive diagnosis is commonly made in *T. gondii* seropositive patients with typical CNS lesions. Radiographic abnormalities found by computer tomography (CT) or magnetic resonance imaging (MRI) have also been valuable in the diagnosis of CNS toxoplasmosis.

The initial treatment of CNS toxoplasmosis is often empiric. Brain biopsy in the patient with AIDS may be complicated by potential morbidity, location of lesion(s), or thrombocytopenia. Anti-*Toxoplasma* therapy is usually initiated in patients with AIDS who are seropositive for *Toxoplasma,* have clinical symptoms suspicious for toxoplasmosis, and have characteristic findings on neuroradiographic studies (multiple ring-enhancing lesions). In this setting, brain biopsy is usually not undertaken unless the patient fails to respond clinically or radiologically to 10–14 days of therapy, or clinically deteriorates. Brain biopsy is an initial consideration in the *T. gondii* seronegative patient or in patients with atypical lesions.

The combination of pyrimethamine and sulfadiazine is considered the most effective regimen for acute therapy of AIDS-related CNS toxoplasmosis.[159,160] This regimen works synergistically by sequentially inhibiting two steps in folic acid synthesis of the proliferative form of *T. gondii.* No widespread agreement exists regarding the optimal doses of pyrimethamine and sulfadiazine. Pyrimethamine loading doses of 75 mg orally on the first day, followed by 25 mg/d thereafter, have been commonly used. The erratic concentrations of pyrimethamine found in patients with AIDS and toxoplasmic encephalitis at lower doses (25 mg/d) have prompted some investigators to use larger doses.[161] Loading doses of 100–200 mg followed by daily oral doses of 1–1.5 mg/kg/d (50–100 mg/d) have been recommended.[162] The usual dose of sulfadiazine is 1–1.5 grams every 6 hours (4–8 g/d). Folinic acid, in doses of 5–10 mg/d (although doses as high as 50 mg/d have been used), is usually added to the combination to reduce the pyrimethamine-induced bone marrow toxicity. Acute therapy with this combination should be continued for at least 3 weeks, but 6 weeks of treatment is recommended for more severely ill patients. Response rates (combined partial and complete) of approximately 85% have been observed following a minimum of 4 weeks of therapy. Adverse reactions, primarily bone marrow suppression associated with pyrimethamine, and sulfadiazine hypersensitivity reactions, may limit therapy in as many as 40% of AIDS patients.[161] A regimen of pyrimethamine plus clindamycin (300–1200 mg PO or IV every 6 hours) appears approximately equivalent to the combination of pyrimethamine and sulfadiazine and may be regarded as an acceptable alternative in patients unable to tolerate sulfadiazine.[163] Unfortunately, the combination of pyrimethamine plus clindamycin is no less toxic than that of pyrimethamine plus sulfadiazine. Other investigational alternative regimens include TMP–SMX, and pyrimethamine and leucovorin plus either clarithromycin, azithromycin, atovaquone, or dapsone.

The discontinuation of pyrimethamine–sulfadiazine after successful initial therapy is associated with a relapse rate that may approach 100%.[164] Thus, lifelong maintenance therapy/secondary prophylaxis is recommended for AIDS patients to prevent recrudescence of the disease.

Again, there is no general agreement on the doses of pyrimethamine and sulfadiazine to be used but it is likely that lower doses may be satisfactory if patients have had a favorable outcome from primary therapy. A regimen of pyrimethamine (25–50 mg/d with folinic acid) plus 2 g/d (1 gram every 12 hours) of sulfadiazine has been recommended.[163] Pyrimethamine plus clindamycin can also be considered for maintenance therapy but this regimen may be associated with a higher relapse rate. A further advantage to the combination of pyrimethamine plus sulfadiazine is that an additional agent for prophylaxis for PCP is unnecessary, which is not the case with the pyrimethamine plus clindamycin combination.[165]

Only limited information about primary prophylaxis of *T. gondii* in the HIV-infected person is available from carefully controlled prospective studies. However, data from several sources do suggest that it may be possible to prevent reactivation of latent toxoplasmosis. Regimens that have been found to have some efficacy in the primary prophylaxis of toxoplasmosis include TMP–SMX, pyrimethamine plus dapsone, and pyrimethamine plus sulfadoxine (Fansidar). A double-blind placebo-controlled comparison of clindamycin and pyrimethamine was halted prematurely because adverse reactions (primarily diarrhea and rash) were significantly higher in the clindamycin group.[166] Concern regarding pyrimethamine for primary prophylaxis has been raised because of a study that found patients receiving 25 mg three times weekly had a higher death rate than placebo recipients. At this time, the most appropriate population to receive prophylaxis and which regimen to use are not clear.

CRYPTOCOCCUS NEOFORMANS

Infection with *Cryptococcus neoformans* occurs in up to 7% of individuals with AIDS in the United States.[167] Infections are probably originally contracted through inhalation, and the respiratory tract is believed to be the first infected site. Cryptococcal infection is the fourth most common infection in patients with AIDS and is the most common life-threatening fungal infection. The usual clinical presentation of cryptococcal infection is meningitis, although recognition of pneumonia and disseminated disease may be increasing. The clinical features of cryptococcal meningitis may be subtle, nonspecific, and not localized to the CNS.[167] Fever, headache, and malaise are the most frequent symptoms. Meningeal features, mental status changes, and other focal neurologic signs only occur in a minority of patients. The diagnosis of cryptococcal meningitis should always be considered when HIV-infected individuals with advanced disease or low CD4+ lymphocyte count present with nonspecific symptoms, pulmonary, or CNS findings.

Methods for diagnosis of cryptococcal infection include serum and CSF fungal cultures and testing for cryptococcal antigen. Detection of cryptococcal antigen in serum and CSF is the most sensitive and specific test; an antigen titer greater than 1:8 should be regarded as evidence for infection. Identification of *C. neoformans* on India ink examination of the CSF or from culture may also be used to confirm the diagnosis when antigen is unavailable. Factors suggestive of a poor prognosis in patients with cryptococcal meningitis include alteration in mental status, CSF antigen >1:1024, a low CSF leukocyte count, and age <35 years.

The goals of therapy for cryptococcal meningitis in patients with AIDS are to induce a remission and maintain a high quality of life. The standard therapeutic approach has been amphotericin B for both acute and maintenance therapy, although the introduction of azole compounds is changing the therapeutic approach for clinically stable patients. One retrospective evaluation supports the effectiveness of amphotericin B for the treatment of cryptococcal meningitis in patients with AIDS and the value of long-term suppressive therapy.[167] The addition of flucytosine to the amphotericin B regimen was not found to enhance survival in this retrospective evaluation of patients with AIDS, which is in marked contrast to data on this combination in non-AIDS patients with cryptococcal meningitis.[168] Early uncontrolled evaluations of the triazole compound, fluconazole, suggested efficacy of this drug for cryptococcal infections in AIDS patients.[169] The combination of amphotericin B and flucytosine, however, was found to be superior to fluconazole in one small randomized trial in patients with AIDS and cryptococcal meningitis.[170]

The largest controlled clinical trial of amphotericin B (mean daily dose ≈ 0.4 mg/kg) plus flucytosine at physician discretion versus fluconazole for cryptococcal meningitis in 194 patients with AIDS found treatment was successful in 40% of the amphotericin recipients and in 34% of fluconazole.[171] The death rate in the first 2 weeks of treatment was 18% in the fluconazole arm, and 14% in the amphotericin arm. The death rate after 2 weeks was 4% and 6%, respectively in the fluconazole and amphotericin groups. The median time to sterilization of CSF cultures was 42 days in amphotericin B recipients but was 64 days in those that received fluconazole. These data suggest that while fluconazole is effective for treatment of cryptococcal meningitis, amphotericin B is moderately superior because of its lower rates of early death and disease progression. Most patients with cryptococcal meningitis should probably receive amphotericin B in an intravenous dose of at least 0.5 mg/kg/d for a minimum of 2 weeks as acute therapy. Flucytosine in doses of 100–150 mg/kg/d can be considered for combination with amphotericin B; serum concentrations should be monitored and peak levels kept below 100 μg/mL to minimize hematologic adverse reactions.

Once the acute treatment of cryptococcal meningitis is completed, maintenance therapy is necessary to prevent relapse. A retrospective review found that long-term suppressive therapy with either ketoconazole or amphotericin

B was associated with improved survival in patients with AIDS.[167] Placebo-controlled trials of 100–200 mg/d of fluconazole, as well as controlled trials versus 1 mg/kg/week of amphotericin B have been undertaken to prevent recurrence of cryptococcal disease in patients who completed acute therapy.[172,173] Compared to patients receiving amphotericin B maintenance therapy, the probability of remaining relapse free at 1 year was higher for fluconazole recipients (97% versus 78%) and the rate of serious drug toxicity was lower (7% versus 31%). These data indicate that fluconazole is superior to either placebo or amphotericin for maintenance therapy and can be considered the drug of choice to prevent relapse of cryptococcal meningitis. It is not known whether there is any advantage to combined fluconazole and amphotericin B therapy, but there are theoretical reasons to avoid this combination.

Other triazole compounds, like itraconazole, are undergoing evaluation for treatment of cryptococcal disease. In addition to treatment strategies, investigations are under way to determine whether fungal infections can be prevented. Results of a controlled trial of fluconazole (200 mg/d) versus clotrimazole troches (10 mg five times daily) suggest that fluconazole recipients after a median follow-up of 35 months had a significant benefit in terms of reduced rate of invasive fungal infection (primarily cryptococcosis) and esophageal candidiasis.[174] For example, of 32 total invasive fungal infections, 17 were cryptococcosis. Two cases occurred in fluconazole recipients while 15 developed in clotrimazole recipients. The benefit of fluconazole therapy was greater for patients with <50 CD4 cells. The 2-year cumulative risk of cryptococcosis was 1.6% in the fluconazole group and 9.9% in the clotrimazole group, in contrast to risks of 0.8% and 4.3%, respectively in patients with higher CD4 counts. There was, however, no survival difference between the two groups. Despite fluconazole therapy, 10.6% of recipients developed proved or presumed candidiasis raising the possibility of emergence of resistance to fluconazole. Drug-resistant candidiasis caused by *Candida albicans* and *C. krusei* has been observed in patients infected with HIV who are receiving fluconazole. The central question of whether the benefit of fluconazole and other agents for prophylaxis of fungal infections outweighs the risks, including resistance, remains to be clearly delineated.

MYCOBACTERIUM INFECTIONS

Mycobacterium tuberculosis infection is a well-recognized and treatable complication of HIV infection and AIDS. A discussion of the clinical presentation and treatment is found elsewhere in this book.

Infections with nontuberculous mycobacterial organisms especially *Mycobacterium avium* complex (MAC) were recognized early in the AIDS epidemic. Disseminated MAC infections are among the most common systemic bacterial infections, occurring in up to 43% of patients with AIDS.[175,176] MAC is the index diagnosis of AIDS in approximately 3–4% of HIV-infected individuals. The major risk factor for MAC is advanced immunosuppression; the mean CD4+ lymphocyte count in patients with disseminated MAC is usually less than 50 cells/μL, and infection is rare in individuals with >100 cells/μL. The organism is a common water and soil saprophyte; the routes of acquisition in patients with AIDS are thought to be gastrointestinal and/or respiratory. In patients with advanced HIV disease, MAC causes a widely disseminated infection. Local colonization can also occur and precede disseminated disease, although cultures of sputum or gastrointestinal tract have a poor predictive value for subsequent disseminated MAC. The clinical syndrome associated with MAC includes high spiking fevers, diarrhea, night sweats, malaise, weight loss, anemia, and neutropenia. Persistent diarrhea and abdominal pain, a malabsorption syndrome, and extrahepatic biliary obstruction are manifestations associated with MAC gastrointestinal infection. Diagnosis of MAC infection is usually based on culture of the organisms from the blood, although biopsies of the liver, bone marrow, and lymph nodes are also highly sensitive and specific. Diagnosis of disseminated MAC in advanced HIV disease suggests a poor long-term prognosis without therapy.

Unfortunately, MAC is resistant to the standard drugs used for tuberculosis like isoniazid and pyrazinamide. Multiple agents such as rifampin, rifabutin (ansamycin), clofazimine, imipenem, amikacin, ethambutol, ciprofloxacin, clarithromycin, and azithromycin have varying degrees of *in vitro* anti-MAC activity.[176] Controversy formerly existed as to whether treatment for MAC is beneficial, but recent data have been supportive that an aggressive therapeutic approach decreases symptoms and prolongs survival.[175,176] For example, 15 of 17 patients treated with amikacin, ciprofloxacin, ethambutol, and rifampin had a marked reduction in their blood mycobacterial counts, and an associated reduction in clinical manifestations such as fever and night sweats after 4 weeks of therapy.[177] These microbiologic and clinical results were maintained in 8 of 10 patients who received oral therapy with ciprofloxacin, ethambutol, and rifampin for at least 12 weeks. Drug-limiting adverse reactions in this regimen included gastrointestinal intolerance and hepatotoxicity. Forty-one HIV-infected persons with two consecutive blood cultures positive for MAC were enrolled in a trial of four drugs: rifampin (600 mg/d), ethambutol (15 mg/kg/d), clofazimine (100 mg qd), and ciprofloxacin (750 mg twice daily) administered orally for 12 weeks.[178] Amikacin, 7.5 mg/kg daily for 4 weeks, was allowed at physician discretion after the first 4 weeks of oral therapy had been completed. Among the 31 evaluable patients, 13 (42%) became culture negative, and 19 patients (61%) completed 12 weeks of therapy. The mean MAC colony count decreased significantly after 2 weeks of therapy in evaluable patients and temperature fell from 38.9

to 38°C ($p < 0.01$) after 1 week of therapy. These data suggested that the regimen had an anti-MAC effect and reduced systemic symptoms, although an effect on survival is uncertain.

A clearer indication of the benefit of antimycobacterial therapy for MAC comes from a prospective evaluation of the treatment of MAC bacteremia in 367 patients with AIDS and CD4+ cells ≤50/μL.[179] In this study, treatment was initiated within 60 days of positive mycobacterial culture; the treatment regimen was left to the discretion of the physician. MAC bacteremia was found to be associated with an increased risk of death and those patients who were treated had a longer median survival (263 versus 139 days) than those who were not. A role for clarithromycin in the treatment of MAC is derived from a randomized, double-blind dose ranging study in 154 patients with HIV infection, positive blood cultures for MAC, and symptomatic MAC disease.[180] After 6 weeks of clarithromycin therapy, mycobacterial quantitative blood cultures were significantly decreased; there was no difference in the reduction between the three regimens (500, 1000, and 2000 mg twice daily). Patients receiving 500 mg twice daily had a longer survival (median 249 days) and a lower death rate in the first 12 weeks.

There are several important issues regarding therapy of MAC, most notably who to treat, which drugs to use and for how long, and how to assess response to therapy. A U.S. Public Health Service Task Force has constructed a series of recommendations to address these issues.[181] First, treatment regimens should contain at least two antimycobacterial agents. Second, every regimen should contain either clarithromycin or azithromycin. Of these agents, and of this writing, clarithromycin is the preferred agent based on greater clinical experience. It is the only one of the two agents FDA-approved for this indication. For the second agent numerous choices are available, although ethambutol is preferred by many experts. Many clinicians would add a third and some a fourth drug to this regimen. Clinical responses usually occur within 2–8 weeks of the start of therapy. If a clinical and microbiologic response is observed, therapy would then continue for the duration of the patient's life.

Disseminated MAC infection contributes significantly to morbidity and mortality in the HIV-infected person, therapy is not uniformly successful, and a high-risk population can be identified. Therefore, a basis for prophylaxis of MAC exists. Two trials of rifabutin for prophylaxis have been conducted in patients with AIDS and CD4 cell counts ≤200/μL.[182] In both, rifabutin significantly reduced the incidence of MAC bacteremia, 17% for placebo versus 8% for rifabutin in the first, and 18% for placebo versus 9% for rifabutin in the second. These data indicate that rifabutin can decrease by about 50% the incidence of MAC bacteremia. Guidelines for use of rifabutin from the task force described above suggest that persons considered for prophylaxis should have a CD4+ cell count less than 100/μL and should be assessed to be sure they do not have active disease due to MAC or *M. tuberculosis*. The recommended dose of rifabutin is 300 mg PO qd, and therapy should continue for the patient's lifetime unless disseminated MAC develops. Clarithromycin has also been reported to reduce the risk of disseminated MAC.[183] In a double-blind placebo-controlled study, 684 persons with AIDS and CD4 lymphocyte counts <100 were randomized to receive clarithromycin, 500 mg twice daily, or placebo. MAC bacteremia developed nearly three times as often in placebo as in clarithromycin recipients: There were 15 (4.5%) breakthrough MAC infections in the clarithromycin group versus 42 (12.5%) in the placebo arm. Clarithromycin-resistant strains of MAC were detected in some patients. There were 74 deaths in those that received clarithromycin compared to 97 deaths in the placebo group.

HERPESVIRUS INFECTIONS

Cytomegalovirus

CMV is the most common life-threatening viral infection in patients with AIDS. Like other herpes group viruses, infection with CMV is ubiquitous; seropositivity among homosexual men with AIDS approaches 100%.[184] There are numerous manifestations of CMV infection including retinitis, esophagitis, hepatitis, gastrointestinal involvement, and less commonly radiculopathy, encephalitis, and pneumonitis. CMV may occur in up to 30–40% of patients with advanced HIV infection. Significant CMV disease is rarely seen in patients with CD4+ cells >50/μL.

CMV retinitis, the most commonly recognized CMV disease associated with AIDS, occurs in approximately 20–25% (range 6–38%) of patients with AIDS.[185,186] CMV retinitis is usually associated with a painless progressive loss of vision. Patients may initially complain of blurry vision, loss of visual acuity, or "floaters." CMV retinitis usually begins unilaterally, but bilateral involvement may occur. Untreated, CMV retinitis invariably leads to blindness. The diagnosis of CMV retinitis is made by funduscopic examination and identification of characteristic findings. Lesions characteristic of CMV retinitis include a fluffy white perivascular exudate frequently associated with hemorrhage. Early diagnosis and treatment is crucial to prevent further visual deterioration.

CMV infection of the gastrointestinal tract can involve sites ranging from the esophagus and stomach to the colon and rectum. In one series of AIDS patients with gastrointestinal tract infection, the colon was the most common site of infection followed by the stomach or esophagus.[187] CMV colitis may be characterized by abdominal pain, fever, weight loss, and diarrhea—symptoms quite common among patients with HIV disease even in the absence of CMV infection. Characteristic symptoms of CMV esophagitis are dysphagia and substernal chest pain. Barium contrast studies may demonstrate abnormalities, but will not distinguish between other etiologic agents such as *Candida* or HSV, both of which are more common. The definitive diagnosis of CMV gastrointestinal infection requires endoscopy and biopsy with histologic identification of CMV inclusions or *in situ* antigen detection.

The first approved agent of treatment for CMV diseases was ganciclovir. Structurally ganciclovir differs from acyclovir only by a single hydroxyl side chain, but it is 30–50 times more active *in vitro* against CMV. The use of ganciclovir therapy has traditionally been divided into two phases, induction and maintenance, because high relapse rates are found after discontinuation of the drug following successful completion of a 2- to 3-week course of initial therapy. Induction regimens are typically 7.5–10 mg/kg/d intravenously in two or three equally divided doses for 14 days or longer if there is a slow clinical response. Maintenance therapy is usually 5–6 mg/kg once daily, 5–7 days/week for an indefinite period of time. Initial response rates for retinal CMV disease range from 60–90%.[188,189] Unfortunately, even with intravenous maintenance therapy, relapse of CMV retinitis is common and occurs at a median of approximately 55–80 days.

Despite the poor oral bioavailability of ganciclovir, oral regimens are being evaluated as a possible alternative to long-term intravenous maintenance administration. Indeed, oral ganciclovir is now available for maintenance therapy of CMV retinitis. Three randomized trials have evaluated intravenous or oral ganciclovir as maintenance therapy for CMV retinitis. In all three studies, the time to progression of CMV retinitis was longer in those that received intravenous administration of ganciclovir than in those that received oral drug.[190] The differences in mean time to progression ranged from 5–12 days and indicate that oral ganciclovir maintenance therapy is associated with a more rapid rate of disease progression. The convenience of oral administration, however, may favor use of oral drug in certain individuals. The recommended dose of oral ganciclovir for maintenance therapy of CMV retinitis is 1000 mg three times daily taken with food. CMV isolates resistant to ganciclovir have been recovered from immunocompromised patients; the incidence and prevalence remains to be determined.[191]

The therapy of CMV gastrointestinal disease has been more controversial. The only placebo-controlled study of ganciclovir for CMV colitis in persons with AIDS found no significant differences between evaluable patients in the severity of diarrhea, changes in body weight, or colonoscopy scores.[192] Ganciclovir treatment did significantly decrease viral excretion in this study. Other uncontrolled trials of ganciclovir for CMV gastrointestinal disease have found a favorable response to ganciclovir therapy.[189] Symptomatic CMV gastrointestinal disease warrants therapy, although the role of maintenance is less clear.

Neutropenia and thrombocytopenia are the most common drug- or dose-limiting adverse reactions associated with use of ganciclovir. Up to 50% of patients with AIDS receiving ganciclovir (alone) may need a dose reduction or interruption of therapy as a result of hematologic toxicity. The combination of zidovudine and ganciclovir is poorly tolerated by HIV-infected individuals due to additive hematologic toxicity.[193] Little data are available on the combination of ganciclovir with other antiretroviral agents. Erythropoietin and GM–CSF offer some potential amelioration of the adverse hematologic effects of ganciclovir. Intravitreal administration of ganciclovir has also been used as salvage therapy in an attempt to circumvent these adverse reactions.[194] Sustained-release intraocular ganciclovir implants represent another strategy developed not only to overcome systemic toxicity but to reduce the frequency with which intravitreal injections would need to be given.[195] Twenty-six patients (30 eyes) were enrolled in an evaluation of immediate therapy with a ganciclovir intraocular implant intended to release drug over an 8-month period, or deferred treatment until progression of retinitis. The median time to progression of retinitis was 15 days in the deferred group but was 226 days in the immediate implant recipients. This small study presents compelling evidence that the ganciclovir implant has efficacy for the treatment of CMV retinitis. However, an assessment of morbidity and mortality relative to systemic therapy is necessary to clearly delineate the role of intraocular implants for treatment of CMV retinitis.

Foscarnet is a pyrophosphate analog with both anti-HIV and anti-CMV activity; it has been under evaluation for herpes virus infections in Europe for several years. Uncontrolled data indicate the initial response rate to foscarnet, at least for CMV retinitis, appears to be similar to that associated with ganciclovir.[196] Controlled trials to evaluate immediate versus delayed foscarnet therapy of CMV retinitis in HIV-infected individuals found immediate foscarnet therapy more effective than delayed in preventing progression of CMV disease.[197] Furthermore, prolonged survival and an anti-HIV effect (as assessed by a decline in HIV or p24 antigen) was observed.[198] An unblinded randomized trial comparing ganciclovir with foscarnet therapy of CMV retinitis was conducted in 234 patients with AIDS.[199] Both drugs were administered in standard 14-day induction regimens followed by maintenance therapy. Ganciclovir and foscarnet were equally effective in delaying the progression of CMV disease. The median time to progression of retinitis was 56 days in the ganciclovir groups and 59 days in the foscarnet group. There was a difference, however, in survival between these two groups. Median survival was 8.5 months for ganciclovir recipients, whereas it was 12.6 months for those that received foscarnet. The explanation for this survival difference is unknown. It is conceivable that the difference in mortality was due to the anti-HIV effect of foscarnet. Adverse reactions that necessitated a switch in therapy were more common among the foscarnet recipients. Currently, the choice of whether to use ganciclovir or foscarnet for initial therapy of CMV retinitis is largely dictated by the adverse reaction profiles of the two agents, concomitant medications being taken by the patient, and underlying disease states.

While foscarnet appears less likely to cause neutropenia than ganciclovir, it has a variety of potential adverse effects. The most common side effects are renal insufficiency, and metabolic disturbances (both increases and decreases) in calcium and phosphorus. Other adverse reactions include anemia, thrombocytopenia, infusion site reactions, nausea and vomiting, penile ulcerations, and seizures. Hydration has been demonstrated to reduce the incidence of serum creatinine elevations from 66% in a nonhydrated control group to 13% in hydrated individuals.[200] Foscarnet, like ganciclovir, is currently administered in two phases, induction and maintenance. Induction doses are 180 mg/kg/d intravenously in two or three divided doses for 14 days, followed by maintenance therapy in doses of 90–120 mg/kg intravenously once daily; foscarnet doses must be adjusted in individuals with renal insufficiency.

Various strategies are under evaluation to determine whether CMV disease in HIV-infected individuals can be prevented. High-dose oral acyclovir has been shown effective in reducing the incidence of CMV infection and disease in bone marrow and renal transplant recipients.[201,202] Uncontrolled observations in patients with AIDS have suggested similar benefits, and a controlled trial in HIV-infected patients is under way to assess whether CMV disease can be suppressed. A randomized, double-blind, placebo-controlled study of oral ganciclovir (1000 mg every 8 hours) in CMV seropositive patients with AIDS found that oral ganciclovir significantly reduced the incidence of CMV disease.[203] CMV disease occurred in 30% of placebo recipients versus 16% of ganciclovir recipients. However, there was no difference in survival between the two groups: Death occurred in 29% of placebo versus 22% of ganciclovir recipients.

Herpes Simplex Virus

Herpes simplex viruses (HSV) types 1 and 2 cause significant morbidity in patients with AIDS. Seropositivity for HSV is widespread among adults with AIDS, and clinical disease is usually the result of reactivation of latent virus. The manifestations of HSV disease observed in persons with AIDS include orolabial, genital, anorectal mucocutaneous disease, esophagitis, and, less commonly, encephalitis. Ulcerative HSV lesions present for longer than 1 month in an individual with laboratory evidence for HIV infection, or no other apparent cause for immunodeficiency, are considered an AIDS-defining condition.

Anorectal lesions are the most common clinically evident HSV disease causing morbidity in homosexual men with AIDS, and likely reflect the common risk factors for acquisition (sexual contact) of both HSV and HIV. Chronic perianal HSV lesions were among the first opportunistic infections associated with AIDS.[204] Symptoms include pain, itching, and painful defecation. The clinical presentation of anal, orolabial, and genital herpes in the patient with AIDS are similar to that in other immunosuppressed individuals. The severity of the episode can range from mild to severely destructive. The severity of mucocutaneous HSV disease increases with progressive immunosuppression. Other HSV manifestations such as encephalitis are rare in the patient with AIDS, but are life threatening. Differentiation from other CNS infections such as those caused by *C. neoformans* or *T. gondii* is important, and prompt treatment is essential.

Acyclovir is the initial drug of choice for treatment of HSV disease. For mild to moderate mucocutaneous disease oral acyclovir in doses of 200 mg five times daily or 400 mg three times daily are used, although regimens of 400 mg 5 times daily have occasionally been described as clinically necessary. Intravenous acyclovir (15 mg/kg/d) should be used in those settings where absorption of oral drug is questionable, or oral tolerance is unlikely (HSV esophagitis) or perhaps when severe mucocutaneous disease is present. Treatment of mucocutaneous disease should be continued until all lesions have crusted. Intravenous acyclovir (30 mg/kg/d) should also be used for viscerally disseminated disease, and for HSV encephalitis.

Recurrent HSV disease is common in many patients with AIDS following discontinuation of therapy. These individuals can often be managed with low-dose suppressive oral acyclovir therapy, as have other immunosuppressed patients at risk for frequently recurring HSV diseases.[205] Regimens commonly used include 200 mg four times daily and 400 mg twice daily. Daily doses of 400 mg four times daily, however, have been necessary to control recurrences in some individuals.

Acyclovir-resistant HSV has been isolated from patients with AIDS.[206] The primary mechanism of resistance appears to be a deficiency in viral thymidine kinase. Strategies that have been employed for management of severe, acyclovir-resistant HSV infections include increasing the dose of acyclovir, discontinuation of acyclovir, and use of an alternative antiviral agent. Vidarabine and foscarnet, because they do not require phosphorylation by thymidine kinase, are examples of potential alternative agents.[207,208] A randomized comparison of foscarnet and vidarabine indicates that foscarnet is more effective and associated with fewer adverse reactions than vidarabine.[209]

Varicella-Zoster Virus

Most adults with AIDS have been previously infected with varicella-zoster virus (VZV) and thus are not susceptible to primary infection (chickenpox) but may develop recurrent infection (zoster). The prevalence of zoster in HIV-infected individuals appears higher than in other age-matched immunocompetent persons, and seems to reliably herald the loss of cell-mediated immunity and progression to AIDS.[210,211]

Zoster usually begins as radicular pain followed by localized erythematous rash and characteristic vesicles. Zoster will usually remain confined to a limited number of dermatomes, but complications such as widespread cutaneous involvement and disseminated visceral zoster may occur. Like the treatment of HSV infections, acyclovir is the drug of choice for VZV infections. While an oral acyclovir regimen of 4 g/d has been shown effective for the treatment of zoster in immunocompetent adults, the drug has not been fully evaluated in immunocompromised patients such as those with AIDS.[212] For practical reasons, oral acyclovir is often used for localized zoster. However, careful monitoring for signs of progression of zoster is essential. AIDS patients with disseminated cutaneous or visceral zoster should receive treatment with intravenous acyclovir in doses of 30 mg/kg/d for at least 7 days or until all lesions are crusted. Acyclovir-resistant VZV infections have been reported in patients with AIDS.[213]

Conclusion

Irrefutable progress has been made in the management of HIV. Four antiretroviral agents are now available for clinical use and additional compounds are likely to follow. However, therapy is still suboptimal and only moderately effective. There are significant deficits in our understanding of the virologic and immunologic processes associated with HIV infection and the clinical pharmacology of anti-HIV compounds. Critical issues include the emergence of drug-resistant viral isolates and the inexorably progressive nature of HIV infection despite antiretroviral therapy. There is a clear need for more selective and potent inhibitors of HIV.

The medical management of opportunistic infections associated with HIV disease has changed dramatically since the recognition of AIDS early in the 1980s, and has improved survival. The approach to PCP is most illustrative. The transition from an era marked by only treatment of established disease to one where primary and secondary prophylaxis based on CD4 lymphocyte count are standards of care reflects both progress in understanding the risk factors for opportunistic infections and in pharmacologic therapy. These lessons have been learned from the management of PCP: prospective immunologic monitoring and early recognition; concurrent use of antiretroviral agents; and primary and secondary prophylaxis are relevant to other opportunistic infections. Emphasis on these principles coupled with carefully controlled investigations of novel agents and therapeutic strategies will offer definite benefit and improve the quality of life for HIV-infected individuals, and yield an advantage over this pernicious virus that causes AIDS.

ACKNOWLEDGMENTS

We thank Teresa A. Tartaglione for her invaluable contributions to this chapter in the first and second editions of this textbook. Grant support came from RO1 AI 33835, UO1 AI 27551, and UO1 AI 27661 from the National Institute of Allergy and Infectious Disease.

References

1. Gottlieb MS, Schroff R, Schauber HM, et al. *Pneumocystis carinii* pneumonia and mucosal candidiasis in previously healthy homosexual men. N Engl J Med 1981;305:1425–1431.
2. Masur H, Michelis MA, Greene JB, et al. An outbreak of community acquired *Pneumocystis carinii* pneumonia—initial manifestation of cellular immune dysfunction. N Engl J Med 1981;305:1431–1438.
3. Siegal FP, Lopez C, Hammer GS, et al. Severe acquired immunodeficiency in male homosexuals manifested by chronic perianal ulcerative herpes simplex lesions. N Engl J Med 1981;305:1439–1444.
4. Friedman-Kien AE, Laubenstein LJ, Rubinstein P, et al. Disseminated Kaposi's sarcoma in homosexual men. Ann Intern Med 1982;96:693–700.
5. Centers for Disease Control. The second 100,000 cases of acquired immunodeficiency syndrome—United States, June 1981–December 1991. MMWR 1992;41:28–29.
6. Gallo RC, Salahuddin SZ, Popovic M, et al. Frequent detection and isolation of cytopathic retroviruses (HTLV-III) from patients with AIDS and at risk for AIDS. Science 1984;224:500–503.
7. Barre-Sinoussi F, Chermann JC, Rey F, et al. Isolation of a T-lymphotropic retrovirus from a patient at risk for acquired immunodeficiency syndrome (AIDS). Science 1983;220:868–871.
8. Levy JA, Hoffman AD, Kramer SM, et al. Isolation of lymphocytopathic retroviruses from San Francisco patients with AIDS. Science 1984;225:840–842.
9. Centers for Disease Control. AIDS due to HIV-2 infection—New Jersey. MMWR 1988;37:33–35.
10. Centers for Disease Control. Update: Heterosexual transmission of AIDS and HIV infection—United States. MMWR 1989;38:423–434.
11. Steele FR. A moving target: CDC still trying to estimate HIV-1 prevalence. J NIH Res 1994;6:25–26.
12. Centers for Disease Control. HIV prevalence estimate and AIDS projections for the United States: Report based upon a workshop. MMWR 1990;39:1–31.
13. Centers for Disease Control. 1993 revised classification system for HIV infection and expanded surveillance case definition for AIDS among adolescents and adults. MMWR 1992;41(RR-17):1–19.

14. Haverkos HW, Battjes RJ. Female-to-male transmission of HIV. JAMA 1992;268:1855.
15. Anderson RM, May RM. Epidemiological parameters of HIV transmission. Nature (London) 1988;333:514–519.
16. Piot P, Laga M. Genital ulcers, other sexually transmitted diseases, and the sexual transmission of HIV. Br Med J 1989;298:623–634.
17. Centers for Disease Control. Heterosexually acquired AIDS—United States, 1993. MMWR 1994;43:155–160.
18. Wofsy CB, Cohen JB, Hauer LB, et al. Isolation of AIDS-associated retrovirus from genital secretion of women with antibodies to the virus. Lancet 1986;1:527–529.
19. Friedland GH, Saltzman BR, Rogers MF, et al. Lack of transmission of HTLV-III/LAV infection to household contacts of patients with AIDS or AIDS-related complex with oral candidiasis. N Engl J Med 1986;314:344–349.
20. Centers for Disease Control. Public Health Service statement on management of occupational exposure to human immunodeficiency virus, including considerations regarding zidovudine postexposure use. MMWR 1990;39(RR-1):1–14.
21. Centers for Disease Control. Guidelines for prevention of transmission of human immunodeficiency virus and hepatitis B virus to health care and public safety workers. MMWR 1989;38(S6):1–37.
22. Hammond JS, Eckes J, Gomez GA, et al. HIV, trauma, and infection control: Universal precautions are universally ignored. J Trauma 1990;30:555–561.
23. Anonymous. Maternal factors involved in mother-to-child transmission of HIV-1. Report of a consensus workshop. J Acq Immune Def Syn 1992;5:1019–1029.
24. World Health Organization. Recommendations for the interpretation of HIV-2 Western blot results. Wkly Epidemiol Rec 1990;65:69–76.
25. Nahamias AJ, Weiss J, Yao X, et al. Evidence for human infection with an HTLV-III LAV-like virus in Central Africa, 1959. Lancet 1986;1:1279–1280.
26. Petricciani JC. Licensed tests for antibody to human T-lymphotropic virus type III: Sensitivity and specificity. Ann Intern Med 1985;103:726–729.
27. Centers for Disease Control. Surveillance for HIV-2 infection in blood donors—United States, 1987–1989. MMWR 1990;39:829–831.
28. Kwok S, Mack DH, Mullis KB, et al. Identification of human immunodeficiency virus sequences by using *in vitro* enzymatic amplification and oligomer cleavage detection. J Virol 1987;61:1690–1694.
29. Edelman AS, Zolla-Pazner S. AIDS: A syndrome of immune dysregulation, dysfunction, and deficiency. FASEB J 1989;3:22–30.
30. Pantaleo G, Graziosi C, Fauci AS. The immunopathogenesis of human immunodeficiency virus infection. N Engl J Med 1993;328:327–335.
31. Embretson J, Zupancic M, Ribas JL, et al. Massive covert infection of helper T lymphocytes and macrophages by HIV during the incubation period of AIDS. Nature 1993;362:359–362.
32. Pantaleo G, Graziosi C, Demarest JF, et al. HIV infection is active and progressive in lymphoid tissue during the clinically latent stage of disease. Nature 1993;362:355–358.
33. Lane HC, Masur H, Edgar LC, et al. Abnormalities of B-cell activation and immunoregulation in patients with the acquired immunodeficiency syndrome. N Engl J Med 1983;309:453–458.
34. Smith P, Ohura K, Masur H, et al. Monocyte function in the acquired immunodeficiency syndrome: Defective chemotaxis. J Clin Invest 1984;74:2121–2128.
35. Munoz A, Carey V, Saah A, et al. Predictors in the decline in CD4 lymphocytes in a cohort of homosexual partners infected with the human immunodeficiency virus. J Acq Immune Def Syn 1988;1:396–404.
36. Rutherford GW, Schwarcz SK, Lemp GF, et al. The epidemiology of AIDS-related Kaposi's sarcoma in San Francisco. J Infect Dis 1989;159:569–571.
37. Schafer A, Friedmann W, Mielke M, et al. The increased frequency of cervical dysplasia–neoplasia in women infected with the human immunodeficiency virus is related to the degree of immunosuppression. Am J Obstet Gynecol 1991;164:593–599.
38. Centers for Disease Control. Update: Impact of the expanded AIDS surveillance case definition for adolescents and adults on case reporting—United States, 1993. MMWR 1994;43:160–170.
39. Pahwa S. Human immunodeficiency virus infection in children: Nature of immunodeficiency, clinical spectrum, and management. Pediatr Infect Dis J 1988;7:S61–S71.
40. Wykoff RF, Pearl ER, Saulsbury FT. Immunologic dysfunction in infants infected through transfusions with HTLV-III. N Engl J Med 1985;312:294–296.
41. Working Group on Antiretroviral Therapy: National Pediatric HIV Resource Center. Antiretroviral therapy and medical management of the human immunodeficiency virus-infected child. Pediatr Infect Dis J 1993;12:513–522.
42. Dalgeish AG, Beverly PCL, Clapham PR, et al. The CD4 (T4) antigen is an essential component of the receptor for the AIDS retrovirus. Nature 1984;312:763–767.
43. Tateno M, Gonzalez-Scarano F, Levy JA. Human immunodeficiency virus can infect CD4-negative human fibroblastoid cells. Proc Natl Acad Sci USA 1989;86:4287–4290.
44. Haynes BF. Scientific and social issues of human immunodeficiency virus vaccine development. Science 1993;260:1279–1286.
45. Dolin R, Graham BS, Greenberg SB, et al. The safety and immunogenicity of a human immunodeficiency virus type 1 (HIV-1) recombinant gp160 candidate vaccine in humans. Ann Intern Med 1991;114:119–127.
46. Cohen J. Jitters jeopardize AIDS vaccine trials. Science 1993;262:980–981.
47. Trauger RJ, Ferre F, Daigle AE, et al. Effect of immunization with inactivated gp120-depleted human immunodeficiency virus type 1 (HIV-1) immunogen on HIV-1 immunity, viral DNA, and percentage of CD4 cells. J Infect Dis 1994;169:1256–1264.
48. Smith DH, Byrn RA, Masters SA, et al. Blocking of HIV-1 infectivity by a soluble, secreted form of the CD4 antigen. Science 1987;238:1704–1706.
49. Schooley RT, Merigan TC, Gault P, et al. Recombinant soluble CD4 therapy in patients with the acquired immunodeficiency syndrome (AIDS) and AIDS-related complex. Ann Intern Med 1990;112:247–253.

50. Kahn JO, Allan JD, Hodges TL, et al. The safety and pharmacokinetics of recombinant soluble CD4 (rCD4) in subjects with the acquired immunodeficiency syndrome (AIDS) and AIDS-related complex. Ann Intern Med 1990;112:254–261.
51. Schaker T, Coombs RW, Collier AC, et al. The effects of high-dose recombinant soluble CD4 on human immunodeficiency virus type 1 viremia. J Infect Dis 1994;169:37–40.
52. Derse D, Bastow KF, Cheng Y-C. Characterization of the DNA polymerases induced by a group of herpes simplex virus type I variants selected for growth in the presence of phosphonoformic acid. J Biol Chem 1982;257:10251–10260.
53. Jacobson MA, Crowe S, Levy J, et al. Effect of foscarnet therapy on infection with human immunodeficiency virus in patients with AIDS. J Infect Dis 1988;158:862–865.
54. Palestine AG, Polis MA, de Smet MD, et al. A randomized controlled trial of foscarnet in the treatment of cytomegalovirus retinitis in patients with AIDS. Ann Intern Med 1991;115:665–673.
55. Jacobson MA, van der Horst C, Causey DM, et al. In vivo additive antiretroviral effect of combined zidovudine and foscarnet therapy for human immunodeficiency virus infection (ACTG protocol 053). J Infect Dis 1991;163:1219–1222.
56. Fletcher CV, Collier AC, Rhame FS, et al. Foscarnet for suppression of HIV replication. Antimicrob Agents Chemother 1994;38:604–607.
57. Cheeseman SH, Hattox SE, McLaughlin MM, et al. Pharmacokinetics of nevirapine: Initial single-rising-dose study in humans. Antimicrob Agents Chemother 1993;37:178–182.
58. Cheesman SH. Nevirapine (NVP) alone and in combination with zidovudine (ZDV): safety and activity [abstract], in Proceedings of the Eighth International Conference on AIDS. July 20, 1992. Amsterdam, The Netherlands.
59. Richman DD. Loss of nevirapine activity associated with the emergence of resistance in clinical trials [abstract], in Proceedings of the Eighth International Conference on AIDS. July 20, 1992. Amsterdam, The Netherlands.
60. Dueweke TJ, Poppe SM, Romero DL, et al. U-90152, a potent inhibitor of human immunodeficiency virus type 1 replication. Antimicrob Agents Chemother 1993;37:1127–1131.
61. Goh WC, Rosen C, Sodroski J, et al. Identification of a protein encoded by the *trans* activator gene *tat* III of human T-cell lymphotrophic retrovirus type III. J Virol 1986;59:181–184.
62. Feinberg MB, Jarrett RF, Aldovini A, et al. HTLV-III expression and production involve complex regulation at the levels of splicing and translation of viral RNA. Cell 1986;46:807–817.
63. Zamecnik PC, Stephenson ML. Inhibition of rous sarcoma virus replication and cell transformation by a specific oligodeoxynucleotide. Proc Natl Acad Sci USA 1978;75:280–284.
64. Jacks T, Power MD, Masiarz FR, et al. Characterization of ribosomal frameshifting in HIV-1 gag-pol expression. Nature 1988;331:280–283.
65. McQuade TJ, Tomasselli AG, Liu L, et al. A synthetic HIV-1 protease inhibitor with antiviral activity arrests HIV-like particle maturation. Science 1990;247:454–456.
66. Roberts NA, Martin JA, Kinchington D, et al. Rational design of peptide-based HIV proteinase inhibitors. Science 1990;248:358–361.
67. Erickson J, Neidhart DJ, VanDrie J, et al. Design, activity, and Å crystal structure of a C2 symmetric inhibitor complexed to HIV-1 protease. Science 1990; 249:527–533.
68. Kempf D, Marsh K, Paul DA, et al. Antiviral and pharmacokinetic properties of C2 symmetric inhibitors of the human immunodeficiency virus type 1 protease. Antimicrob Agents Chemother 1991;35:2209–2214.
69. Mellors J, Steigbiegel R, Gulick R, et al. A randomized, double-blind study of the oral HIV protease inhibitor, L-735,524 vs zidovudine in p24 antigenemic HIV-1 infected patients with <500 CD4 cells/mm^3 [abstract], in 2nd National Conference on Human Retroviruses and Related Infections. The American Society for Microbiology. January 29, 1995. Washington, DC.
70. Markowitz M, Jalil L, Hurley A, et al. Evaluation of the antiviral activity of orally administered ABT-538, an inhibitor of HIV-1 protease [abstract], in 2nd National Conference on Human Retroviruses and Related Infections. The American Society for Microbiology. January 29, 1995. Washington, DC.
71. Condra JH, Schleif WA, Blahy OM, et al. Mutations in HIV protease conferring resistance to inhibitor L-735,524 [abstract], in 2nd National Conference on Human Retroviruses and Related Infections. The American Society for Microbiology. January 29, 1995. Washington, DC.
72. Fischl MA, Resnick L, Coombs R, et al. The safety and efficacy of combination *N* butyl deoxynojirimycin (SC-48334) and zidovudine in patients with HIV-1 infection and 200–500 CD4 cells/mm^3. J Acq Immune Def Syn 1994;7:139–147.
73. Bryant ML, Ratner L, Duronio RJ, et al. Incorporation of 12-methoxydecanoate into the human immunodeficiency virus 1 gag polyprotein precursor inhibits its proteolytic processing and virus production in a chronically infected human lymphoid cell line. Proc Natl Acad Sci USA 1991;88:2055–2059.
74. Smith MS, Thresher RJ, Pagano JS. Inhibition of human immunodeficiency virus type 1 morphogenesis in T cells by alpha interferon. Antimicrob Agents Chemother 1991;35:62–67.
75. Tan CK, Cival R, Mian AM, et al. Inhibition of RNase activity of HIV reverse transcriptase by azidothymidylate. Biochemistry 1991;30:4831–4835.
76. Yarchoan R, Mitsuya H, Myers CE, et al. Clinical pharmacology of 3′-azido-2′,3′-dideoxythymidine (zidovudine) and related dideoxynucleosides. N Engl J Med 1989;321:726–738.
77. Tartaglione TA, Collier AC, Coombs RW, et al. Acquired immunodeficiency syndrome cerebrospinal fluid findings in patients before and during long-term oral zidovudine therapy. Arch Neurol 1991;48:695–699.
78. Furman PA, Fyfe JA, St Clair MH, et al. Phosphorylation of 3′-azido-3′-deoxythymidine and selective interaction of the 5′-triphosphate with human immunodeficiency virus reverse transcriptase. Proc Natl Acad Sci USA 1986;83:8333–8337.

79. Klecker RW, Collins JM, Yarchoan R, et al. Plasma and cerebrospinal fluid concentrations of 3′-azido-3′-deoxythymidine: A novel pyrimidine analog with potential application for the treatment of patients with AIDS and related diseases. Clin Pharmacol Ther 1987;41:407–412.
80. Fischl MA, Richman DD, Hansen N, et al. The safety and efficacy of zidovudine (AZT) in the treatment of mildly symptomatic human immunodeficiency virus type I (HIV) infection: A double-blind, placebo-controlled trial. Ann Intern Med 1990;112:727–737.
81. Volberding PA, Lagakos SW, Koch MA, et al. Zidovudine in asymptomatic human immunodeficiency virus infection: A controlled trial in persons with fewer than 500 CD4-positive cells per cubic millimeter. N Engl J Med 1990;322:941–949.
82. Cooper DA, Gatell JM, Kroon S, et al. Zidovudine in persons with asymptomatic HIV infection and CD4 cell counts greater than 400 per cubic millimeter. N Engl J Med 1993;329:297–303.
83. Hamilton JD, Hartigan PM, Simberkoff MS, et al. A controlled trial of early versus late treatment with zidovudine in symptomatic human immunodeficiency virus infection. N Engl J Med 1992;326:437–443.
84. Concorde Coordinating Committee. MRC/ANRS randomized double-blind controlled trial of immediate and deferred zidovudine in symptom-free HIV infection. Lancet 1994;343:871–881.
85. Volberding PA, Lagakos SW, Grimes JM, et al. The duration of zidovudine benefit in persons with asymptomatic HIV infection. JAMA 1994;272:437–442.
86. CDC. Zidovudine for the prevention of HIV transmission from mother to infant. MMWR 1994;43:285–287.
87. Richman DD, Fischl MA, Grieco MH, et al. The toxicity of azidothymidine (AZT) in the treatment of patients with AIDS and AIDS-related complex. A double-blind, placebo controlled trial. N Engl J Med 1987;317:192–197.
88. Fischl MA, Parker CB, Pettinelli C, et al. A randomized controlled trial of a reduced daily dose of zidovudine in patients with the acquired immunodeficiency syndrome. N Engl J Med 1990;323:1009–1014.
89. Collier AC, Bozzette S, Coombs RW, et al. A pilot study of low-dose zidovudine in human immunodeficiency virus infection. N Engl J Med 1990;323:1015–1021.
90. Meng TC, Fischl MA, Boota AH, et al. Combination therapy with zidovudine and dideoxycytidine in patients with advanced human immunodeficiency virus infection: A phase I/II study. Ann Intern Med 1992;116:13–20.
91. Larder BA, Darby G, Richman DD. HIV-1 with reduced sensitivity to zidovudine (AZT) isolate during prolonged therapy. Science 1989;243:1731–1734.
92. De Clercq E. HIV resistance to reverse transcriptase inhibitors. Biochemical Pharmacol 1994;47:155–169.
93. Tudor-Williams G, St. Clair MH, McKinney RE, et al. HIV-1 sensitivity to zidovudine and clinical outcome in children. Lancet 1992;339:15–19.
94. Richman DD, Grimes JM, Lagakos SW. Effect of stage of disease and drug dose on zidovudine susceptibilities of isolates of human immunodeficiency virus. J Acq Immun Def Syn 1990;3:473–476.
95. Erice A, Mayers DL, Strike DG, et al. Primary infection with zidovudine-resistant human immunodeficiency virus type 1. N Engl J Med 1993;328:1163–1165.
96. Videx (didanosine) package insert. New York, Bristol-Myers Squibb, October 1991.
97. Hartman NR, Yarchoan R, Pluda JM, et al. Pharmacokinetics of 2′,3′-dideoxyadenosine and 2′,3′-dideoxyinosine in patients with severe human immunodeficiency virus infection. Clin Pharmacol Ther 1990;47:647–654.
98. Butler KM, Husson RN, Balis FM, et al. Dideoxyinosine in children with symptomatic human immunodeficiency virus infection. N Engl J Med 1991;324:137–144.
99. Knupp CA, Shyu WC, Dolin R, et al. Pharmacokinetics of didanosine in patients with acquired immunodeficiency syndrome or acquired immunodeficiency syndrome-related complex. Clin Pharmacol Ther 1991;49:523–535.
100. Ahluwahlia G, Jonson MA, Fridland A, et al. Cellular pharmacology of the anti-HIV agent 2′,3′-dideoxyadenosine [abstract]. Proc Am Acad Cancer Res 1988;29:349.
101. Kahn JO, Lagakos SW, Richman DD, et al. A controlled trial comparing continued zidovudine with didanosine in human immunodeficiency virus infection. N Engl J Med 1992;327:581–587.
102. Schwartz MS, Brandt LJ. The spectrum of pancreatic disorders in patients with the acquired immunodeficiency syndrome. Am J Gastroenterol 1989;84:459–462.
103. Klecker RW, Collins JM, Yarchoan RC, et al. Pharmacokinetics of 2′,3′-dideoxycytidine in patients with AIDS and related disorders. J Clin Pharmacol 1988;28:837–842.
104. HIVID (Zalcitabine) package insert. Nutley, NJ, Roche Laboratories, June 1992.
105. Abrams DI, Goldman AI, Launer C, et al. A comparative trial of didanosine or zalcitabine after treatment with zidovudine in patients with human immunodeficiency virus infection. N Engl J Med 1994;330:657–662.
106. Skowron G, Bozzette SA, Lim L, et al. Alternating and intermittent regimens of zidovudine and dideoxycytidine in patients with AIDS or AIDS-related complex. Ann Intern Med 1993;118:321–330.
107. Yarchoan R, Lietzau JA, Nguyen BY, et al. A randomized pilot study of alternating or simultaneous zidovudine and didanosine therapy in patients with symptomatic human immunodeficiency virus infection. J Infect Dis 1994;169:9–17.
108. Ho HT, Hitchcock MJM. Cellular pharmacology of 2′,3′-dideoxy-2′,3′-didehydrothymidine: A nucleoside analogue active against human immunodeficiency virus. Antimicrob Agents Chemother 1989;33:844–849.
109. Dudley MN, Graham KK, Kaul S, et al. Pharmacokinetics of stavudine in patients with AIDS or AIDS-related complex. J Infect Dis 1992;166:480–485.
110. Dunkle L, Anderson R, McLaren C, et al. Stavudine (d4t) a promising antiretroviral agent [abstract], in Proceedings of the Eighth International Conference on AIDS. July 20, 1992. Amsterdam, The Netherlands.
111. Dunkle LM, Pavia A, Messina M, Cross A, BMS-019 Study Group. Stavudine (d4T) vs. zidovudine for the treatment of HIV-infected patients with CD4 counts of 50–500 cells/mm^3 following at least 6 months of zidovudine [abstract], in 34th Interscience Conference on Antimicrobial Agents and Chemotherapy. October 4, 1994. Orlando, FL.

112. Kline MW, Dunkle LM, Federici ME, et al. Safety and preliminary virologic and immunologic efficacy of stavudine (d4T) in children with HIV infection [abstract], in 33rd Interscience Conference on Antimicrobial Agents and Chemotherapy. October 17, 1993. New Orleans, LA.
113. Lane HC, Kovacs JA, Feinberg J, et al. Anti-retroviral effects of interferon alfa in AIDS-associated Kaposi's sarcoma. Lancet 1988;2:1218–1222.
114. Krown SE, Gold JWM, Niedzwiecki D, et al. Interferon alpha with zidovudine: safety, tolerance, and clinical and virological effects in patients with Kaposi sarcoma associated with the acquired immunodeficiency syndrome (AIDS). Ann Intern Med 1990;112:812–821.
115. Kovacs JA, Deyton L, Davey R, et al. Combined zidovudine and interferon alpha therapy in patients with Kaposi sarcoma and the acquired immunodeficiency syndrome (AIDS). Ann Intern Med 1989;111:280–287.
116. Frissen PH Jos, Weverling GJ. Zidovudine and interferon-alpha versus zidovudine in symptomatic HIV-1 infection [abstract], in Proceedings of the Eighth International Conference on AIDS. July 20, 1992. Amsterdam, The Netherlands.
117. Lane HC, Herpin B, Banks S, et al. Zidovudine vs alpha interferon vs the combination in patients with early HIV infection [abstract], in Proceedings of the Eighth International Conference on AIDS. July 20, 1992. Amsterdam, The Netherlands.
118. Fischl MA, Stanley K, Collier AC, et al. Combination and monotherapy with zidovudine and zalcitabine in patients with advanced HIV disease. Ann Intern Med 1995;122:24–32.
119. Collier AC, Coombs RW, Fischl MA et al. Combination therapy with zidovudine and didanosine compared to zidovudine alone in HIV-1 infection. Ann Intern Med 1993;119:786–793.
120. Chow Y-K, Hirsch MS, Merril DP, et al. Use of evolutionary limitations of HIV-1 multidrug resistance to optimize therapy. Nature 1993;361:650–654.
121. Sande MA, Carpenter CCJ, Cobbs CG, et al. Antiretroviral therapy for adult HIV-infected individuals. JAMA 1993;270:2583–2589.
122. Masur H. Problems in the management of opportunistic infections in patients infected with human immunodeficiency virus. J Infect Dis 1990;161:858–864.
123. Centers for Disease Control. Public Health Service Task Force on antipneumocystis prophylaxis in human immunodeficiency virus-infected individuals. MMWR 1989;38:1–9.
124. Centers for Disease Control. AIDS Weekly Surveillance Report. January 30, 1989.
125. Davey RT, Masur H. Recent advances in the diagnosis, treatment, and prevention of Pneumocystis carinii pneumonia. Antimicrob Agents Chemother 1990;34:499–504.
126. Jacobs JL, Libby DM, Winters RA, et al. A cluster of *Pneumocystis carinii* pneumonia in adults without predisposing illness. N Engl J Med 1991;324:246–250.
127. Hughes WT, Feldman S, Chaudary S, et al. Comparison of pentamidine isethionate and trimethoprim-sulfamethoxazole in the treatment of Pneumocystis carinii pneumonia. J Pediatr 1978;92:285–291.
128. Masur H. Prevention and treatment of Pneumocystis pneumonia. N Engl J Med 1992;327:1853–1860.
129. Conte JE Jr, Hollander H, Golden JA. Inhaled pentamidine or reduced dose intravenous pentamidine for *Pneumocystis carinii* pneumonia: A pilot study. Ann Intern Med 1987;107:495.
130. Conte JE, Chernoff D, Feigal DW, et al. Intravenous or inhaled pentamidine for treating Pneumocystis carinii pneumonia in AIDS. Ann Intern Med 1990;113:203–209.
131. Conte JE, Upton RA, Phelps RT, et al. Use of a specific and sensitive assay to determine pentamidine pharmacokinetics in patients with AIDS. J Infect Dis 1987;156:923–929.
132. Hoo GWS, Mohsenifar Z, Meyer R. Inhaled or intravenous pentamidine therapy for Pneumocystis carinii pneumonia. Ann Intern Med 1990;113:195–202.
133. Sattler FR, Cowan R, Nielsen DM, Ruskin J. Trimethoprim–sulfamethoxazole compared with pentamidine for treatment of *Pneumocystis carinii* pneumonia in the acquired immunodeficiency syndrome. Ann Intern Med 1988;109:280–287.
134. Wharton JM, Coleman DL, Wofsy CB, et al. Trimethoprim–sulfamethoxazole or pentamidine for *Pneumocystis carinii* pneumonia in the acquired immunodeficiency syndrome. Ann Intern Med 1986;105:37–44.
135. Wofsy CB. Use of trimethoprim–sulfamethoxazole in the treatment of *Pneumocystis carinii* pneumonia in patients with acquired immunodeficiency syndrome. Rev Infect Dis 1987;9(suppl 2):S184–S194.
136. Gagnon S, Boota AM, Fischl MA, et al. Corticosteroids as adjunctive therapy for severe Pneumocystis carinii pneumonia in the acquired immunodeficiency syndrome. N Engl J Med 1990;323:1444–1450.
137. Bozzette SA, Sattler FR, Chiu J, et al. A controlled trial of early adjunctive treatment with corticosteroids for *Pneumocystis carinii* pneumonia in the acquired immunodeficiency syndrome. N Engl J Med 1990;323:1451–1457.
138. The National Institutes of Health–University of California Expert Panel for Corticosteroids as Adjunctive Therapy for *Pneumocystis Carinii* Pneumonia. Consensus statement on the use of corticosteroids as adjunctive therapy for Pneumocystis pneumonia in the acquired immunodeficiency syndrome. N Engl J Med 1990;323:1500–1504.
139. Mills J, Leoung G, Medina I, et al. Dapsone treatment of *Pneumocystis carinii* pneumonia in the acquired immunodeficiency syndrome. Antimicrob Agents Chemother 1988;32:1057–1060.
140. Medina I, Mills J, Leoung G, et al. Oral therapy for *Pneumocystis carinii* pneumonia in the acquired immunodeficiency syndrome: A controlled trial of trimethoprim–sulfamethoxazole versus trimethoprim–dapsone. N Engl J Med 1990;323:776–782.
141. Lee BL, Medina I, Benowitz N, et al. Dapsone, trimethoprim, and sulfamethoxazole plasma levels during treatment of pneumocystis pneumonia in patients with the acquired immunodeficiency syndrome. Ann Intern Med 1989;110:606–611.
142. Toma E, Poisson M, Phaneuf D, et al. Clindamycin with primaquine for pneumocystis carinii pneumonia. Lancet 1989;1046–1048.

143. Hughes W, Leoung G, Kramer F, et al. Comparison of atovaquone (566C80) with trimethoprim–sulfamethoxazole to treat *Pneumocystis carinii* pneumonia in patients with AIDS. N Engl J Med 1993;328:1521–1527.
144. Allegra CJ, Chabner BA, Tuazon CU, et al. Trimetrexate for the treatment of Pneumocystis carinii pneumonia in patients with the acquired immunodeficiency syndrome. N Engl J Med 1987;317:978–985.
145. Masur H, Ognibene FP, Yarchoan R, et al. CD4 counts as predictors of opportunistic pneumonias in human immunodeficiency virus (HIV) infection. Ann Intern Med 1989;111:223–231.
146. Phair J, Munoz A, Detels R, et al. The risk of *Pneumocystis carinii* pneumonia among men infected with human immunodeficiency virus type 1. N Engl J Med 1990;322:161–165.
147. Centers for Disease Control. Recommendation for prophylaxis against *Pneumocystis carinii* pneumonia for adults and adolescents infected with human immunodeficiency virus. MMWR 1992;41(RR-4):1–11.
148. Fischl MA, Dickinson GM, La Voie L. Safety and efficacy of sulfamethoxazole and trimethoprim chemoprophylaxis for *Pneumocystis carinii* pneumonia in AIDS. JAMA 1988;259:1185–1189.
149. Hardy WD, Feinberg J, Finkelstein DM, et al. A controlled trial of trimethoprim–sulfamethoxazole or aerosolized pentamidine for secondary prophylaxis of *Pneumocystis carinii* pneumonia in patients with the acquired immunodeficiency syndrome. N Engl J Med 1992;327:1842–1848.
150. Bozzette SA, Finkelstein DM, Spector SA, et al. A randomized trial of three antipneumocystis agents in patients with advanced human immunodeficiency virus infection. N Engl J Med 1995;332:693–699.
151. Stein DS, Weems JJ, Williams CL. Use of low dose trimethoprim–sulfamethoxazole thrice weekly for primary and secondary prophylaxis of *Pneumocystis carinii* pneumonia in patients with AIDS. Antimicrob Agents Chemother 1991;35:1705–1709.
152. Centers for Disease Control. Guidelines for prophylaxis against *Pneumocystis carinii* pneumonia for children infected with human immunodeficiency virus. JAMA 1991;265:1637–1644.
153. Hughes WT, Kuhn S, Chaudhary S, et al. Successful chemoprophylaxis for *Pneumocystis carinii* pneumonitis. N Engl J Med 1977;297:1419–1426.
154. Leoung GS, Feigal DW, Montgomery BA, et al. Aerosolized pentamidine for prophylaxis against *Pneumocystis carinii* pneumonia. N Engl J Med 1990;323:7690–7775.
155. Hirschel B, Lazzarin A, Chopard P, et al. A controlled study of inhaled pentamidine for primary prevention of Pneumocystis carinii pneumonia. N Engl J Med 1991;324:1079–1083.
156. Northfelt DW, Clement MJ, Safrin S. Extrapulmonary pneumocystosis: Clinical features in human immunodeficiency virus infection. Medicine 1990;69:392–398.
157. Tuazon CU. Toxoplasmosis in AIDS patients. J Antimicrob Chemother 1989;23(suppl A):77–82.
158. Grant IH, Gold JWM, Rosenblum M, et al. Toxoplasma gondii serology in HIV-infected patients: The development of central nervous system toxoplasmosis. AIDS 1990;4:519–521.
159. Luft BJ, Brooks RG, Conley FK, et al. Toxoplasmic encephalitis in patients with acquired immunodeficiency syndrome. JAMA 1984;252:913–917.
160. Leport C, Raffi F, Matheron S, et al. Treatment of central nervous system toxoplasmosis with pyrimethamine/sulfadiazine combination in 35 patients with the acquired immunodeficiency syndrome: Efficacy of long-term continuous therapy. Am J Med 1988;84:94–100.
161. Weiss LM, Harris C, Berger M, et al. Pyrimethamine concentrations in serum and cerebrospinal fluid during treatment of acute *Toxoplasma* encephalitis in patients with AIDS. J Infect Dis 1988;157:580–583.
162. Wong SY, Remington JS. Toxoplasmosis in the setting of AIDS, in Broder S, Merigan TC Jr, Bolognesi D (eds): Textbook of AIDS Medicine. Baltimore, Williams and Wilkins, 1994.
163. Dannemann B, McCutchan A, Israelski D, et al. Treatment of toxoplasmic encephalitis in patients with AIDS, a randomized trial comparing pyrimethamine plus clindamycin to pyrimethamine plus sulfadiazine. Ann Intern Med 1992;116:33–43.
164. Luft BJ, Remington JS. Toxoplasmic encephalitis. J Infect Dis 1988;157:1–6.
165. Herald A, Flepp M, Chave J-P, et al. Treatment for cerebral toxoplasmosis protects against *Pneumocystis carinii* pneumonia in patients with AIDS. Ann Intern Med 1991;115:760–763.
166. Jacobson MA, Besch CL, Child C, et al. Toxicity of clindamycin as prophylaxis for AIDS-associated toxoplasmic encephalitis. Lancet 1992;339:333–334.
167. Chuck SL, Sande MA. Infections with *Cryptococcus neoformans* in the acquired immunodeficiency syndrome. N Engl J Med 1989;321:794–799.
168. Bennett JE, Dismukes WE, Duma RJ, et al. A comparison of amphotericin B alone and combined with flucytosine in the treatment of cryptococcal meningitis. N Engl J Med 1979;301:126–131.
169. Robinson PA, Knirsch AK, Joseph JA. Fluconazole for life-threatening fungal infections in patients who cannot be treated with conventional antifungal agents. Rev Infect Dis 1990;12(suppl 3):S349–S363.
170. Larsen RA, Leal MAE, Chan LS. Fluconazole compared with amphotericin B plus flucytosine for cryptococcal meningitis in AIDS. Ann Intern Med 1990;113:183–187.
171. Saag MS, Powderly WG, Cloud GA, et al. Comparison of amphotericin B with fluconazole in the treatment of acute AIDS-associated cryptococcal meningitis. N Engl J Med 1992;326:83–89.
172. Bozzette SA, Larsen RA, Chiu J, et al. A placebo-controlled trial of maintenance therapy with fluconazole after treatment of cryptococcal meningitis in the acquired immunodeficiency syndrome. N Engl J Med 1991;324:580–584.
173. Powderly WG, Saag MS, Cloud GA, et al. A controlled trial of fluconazole or amphotericin B to prevent relapse of cryptococcal meningitis in patients with the acquired immunodeficiency syndrome. N Engl J Med 1992;326:793–798.

174. Powderly WG, Finkelstein DM, Feinberg J, et al. A randomized trial comparing fluconazole with clotrimazole troches for the prevention of fungal infections in patients with advanced human immunodeficiency virus infection. N Engl J Med 1995;332:700–705.
175. Horsburgh CR, Jr. Mycobacterium avium complex infection in the acquired immunodeficiency symdrome. N Engl J Med 1991;324:1332–1338.
176. Benson CA, Ellner JJ. Mycobacterium avium complex infection and AIDS: Advances in theory and practice. Clin Infect Dis 1993;17:7–20.
177. Chiu J, Nussbaum J, Bozzette S, et al. Treatment of disseminated *Mycobacterium avium* complex infection in AIDS with amikacin, ethambutol, rifampin, and ciprofloxacin. Ann Intern Med 1990;113:358–361.
178. Kemper CA, Meng TC, Nussbaum J, et al. Treatment of *Mycobacterium-avium* complex bacteremia in AIDS with a four drug oral regimen. Ann Intern Med 1992;116:466–472.
179. Chin DP, Reingold AL, Stone EN, et al. The impact of *Mycobacterium avium* complex bacteremia and its treatment on survival in AIDS patients—a prospective study. J Infect Dis 1994;170:578–584.
180. Chaisson RE, Benson CA, Dube MP, et al. Clarithromycin therapy for bacteremic *Mycobacterium avium* complex disease. Ann Intern Med 1994;121:905–911.
181. Masur H. Recommendations on prophylaxis and therapy for disseminated *Mycobacterium-avium* complex disease in patients infected with the human immunodeficiency virus. N Engl J Med 1993;329:898–904.
182. Nightengale SD, Cameron DW, Gordin FM, et al. Two controlled trials of rifabutin prophylaxis against *Mycobacterium avium* complex infection in AIDS. N Engl J Med 1993;329:828–833.
183. Pierce M, Lamarca A, Jablonowski H, et al. A placebo-controlled trial of clarithromycin prophylaxis against MAC infection in AIDS patients, in Program and Abstracts, 34th Interscience Conference on Antimicrobial Agents and Chemotherapy. October 4, 1994, Orlando, FL.
184. Quinnan GV, Masur H, Rook AH, et al. Herpes virus infections in the acquired immunodeficiency syndrome. JAMA 1984;252:72–77.
185. Jabs DA, Enger C, Bartlett JG. Cytomegalovirus retinitis and acquired immunodeficiency syndrome. Arch Ophthalmol 1989;107:75–80.
186. Jacobson MA, Mills J. Serious cytomegalovirus disease in the acquired immunodeficiency syndrome. Ann Intern Med 1988;108:585–594.
187. Dietrich DT, Chachoua A, LaFleur F, et al. Ganciclovir treatment of gastrointestinal infections caused by cytomegalovirus in patients with AIDS. Rev Infect Dis 1988;10(suppl 3):S532–S537.
188. Fletcher CV, Balfour HH Jr. Evaluation of ganciclovir for cytomegalovirus disease. DICP Ann Pharmacother 1989;23:5–12.
189. Buhles WC, Mastre BJ, Tinker AJ, et al. Ganciclovir treatment of life- or sight-threatening cytomegalovirus infection: Experience in 314 immunocompromised patients. Rev Infect Dis 1988;10(suppl 3):S495–S504.
190. Cytovene (ganciclovir) package insert. Nutley, NJ, Roche Laboratories, 1994.
191. Erice A, Chou S, Biron KK, et al. Progressive disease due to ganciclovir-resistant cytomegalovirus in immunocompromised patients. N Engl J Med 1989;320:289–293.
192. Dietrich D, Kotler D, Busch D, et al. Randomized, placebo-controlled study of ganciclovir treatment of cytomegalovirus colitis in AIDS patients [abstract], in 6th International Conference on AIDS. June 23, 1990, San Francisco, CA.
193. Hochster H, Dieterich D, Bozzette S, et al. Toxicity of combined ganciclovir and zidovudine for cytomegalovirus disease associated with AIDS. Ann Intern Med 1990;113:111–117.
194. Cantrill HL, Henry K, Melroe NH, et al. Treatment of cytomegalovirus retinitis with intravitreal ganciclovir: Long-term results. Ophthalmology 1989;96:367–374.
195. Martin DF, Parks DJ, Mellow SD, et al. Treatment of cytomegalovirus retinitis with an intraocular sustained-release ganciclovir implant. Arch Ophthalmol 1994;112:1531–1539.
196. Jacobson MA, O'Donnell JJ, Mills J. Foscarnet treatment of cytomegalovirus retinitis in patients with the acquired immunodeficiency syndrome. Antimicrob Agents Chemother 1989;33:736–741.
197. Palestine AG, Polis MA, DeSmet MD, et al. A randomized controlled trial of foscarnet in the treatment of cytomegalovirus retinitis. Ann Intern Med 1991;115:665–673.
198. Polis MA, DeSmet MD, Bard BF, et al. Increased survival of a cohort of patients with acquired immunodeficiency syndrome and cytomegalovirus retinitis who received sodium phosphonoformate (foscarnet). Am J Med 1993;94:175–180.
199. Studies of the Ocular Complications of AIDS Research Group. Mortality in patients with the acquired immunodeficiency syndrome treated with either foscarnet or ganciclovir for cytomegalovirus retinitis. N Engl J Med 1992;326:213–220.
200. Deray G, Katlama C, Dohin E. Prevention of foscarnet nephrotoxicity. Correspondence. Ann Intern Med 1990;113:332.
201. Meyers JD, Reed EC, Shepp DH, et al. Acyclovir for prevention of cytomegalovirus infection and disease after allogeneic marrow transplantation. N Engl J Med 1988;318:70–75.
202. Fletcher CV, Englund JA, Edelman CK, et al. Pharmacologic basis for high-dose oral acyclovir prophylaxis of cytomegalovirus disease in renal allograft recipients. Antimicrob Agents Chemother 1991;35:938–943.
203. Spector SA, McKinley G, Drew L, Stempien MJ. A randomized, double-blind study of the efficacy and safety of oral ganciclovir for the prevention of cytomegalovirus disease in HIV-infected persons, in Abstracts of the 2nd National Conference on Human Retroviruses. American Society for Microbiology. January 29, 1995, Washington, DC.
204. Siegel FP, Lopez C, Hammer BS, et al. Severe acquired immunodeficiency in male homosexuals, manifested by chronic perianal ulcerative herpes simplex lesions. N Engl J Med 1981;305:1439–1444.

205. Wade JC, Newton B, Flournoy N, et al. Oral acyclovir for prevention of herpes simplex virus reactivation after marrow transplantation. Ann Intern Med 1984;100:823–828.
206. Erlich KS, Mills J, Chatis P, et al. Acyclovir-resistant herpes simplex virus infections in patients with the acquired immunodeficiency syndrome. N Engl J Med 1989;320:293–296.
207. Fletcher CV, Englund JA, Bean B, et al. Continuous infusion high-dose acyclovir for serious herpes virus infections. Antimicrob Agents Chemother 1989;33:1375–1378.
208. Erlich KS, Jacobson MA, Koehler JE, et al. Foscarnet therapy for severe acyclovir-resistant herpes simplex virus type-2 infections in patients with the acquired immunodeficiency syndrome. Ann Intern Med 1989;110:710–713.
209. Safrin S, Crumpacker C, Chatis P, et al. A controlled trial comparing foscarnet with vidarabine for acyclovir-resistant mucocutaneous herpes simplex virus in the acquired immunodeficiency syndrome. N Engl J Med 1991;325:551–555.
210. Rogers MF, Morens DM, Stewart JA, et al. National case control study of Kaposi's sarcoma and *Pneumocystis carinii* pneumonia in homosexual men: Part 2, laboratory results. Ann Intern Med 1983;99:151–158.
211. Melbye M, Grossman RJ, Goedert JJ, et al. Risk of AIDS after herpes zoster. Lancet 1987;1:728–731.
212. Huff JC, Bean B, Balfour HH Jr, et al. Therapy of herpes zoster with oral acyclovir. Am J Med 1988;85(suppl 2A):84–89.
213. Jacobson MA, Berger TG, Fikrig S, et al. Acyclovir-resistant varicella-zoster virus infection after chronic oral acyclovir therapy in patients with the acquired immunodeficiency syndrome. Ann Intern Med 1990;112:187–191.

Chapter 118

Nosocomial and Device-Related Infections

Robert P. Rapp, PharmD, Sean P. Gorman, PhD, and Colin G. Adair, PhD

Infections that occur in an institutional setting are known as nosocomial infections. Institutional refers to any health care facility where patients are housed for a period of time such as hospitals, nursing homes, or convalescent care centers. Most epidemiologic studies exclude infections that occur in the first 48–72 hours after admission to the institution, because such infections were most likely acquired before admission. Infections that become apparent months after discharge are considered "nosocomial" and will be missed unless there is sufficient follow-up after discharge.

Historic Overview

Before the days of Joseph Lister and Louis Pasteur, the rate of infection in both traumatic and surgical wounds was virtually 100%. Because of high mortality rates, modern medicine and surgery gained slow acceptance during the first half of the nineteenth century. During his tenure at the Royal Infirmary in Glasgow from 1861 to 1869, Joseph Lister developed the principles and practice of antisepsis. Using "carbolic acid," Lister sprayed operating room suites, instruments, and wounds and noted a significant reduction in postoperative infection rates. Unfortunately, instruments dropped on floors, hands wiped on dirty aprons, and other less-than-acceptable practices continued to lead to an unacceptably high rate of fatal infections in patients.

Lister, during the latter part of his work on antiseptic surgery, gave full credit to the work of Louis Pasteur, a French scientist who worked out the germ theory of disease. Using the groundwork laid by both Lister and Pasteur in the 1880s, German physicians and scientists developed the ritual of aseptic surgery. Surgical gowns and instruments were sterilized prior to use. Wound infections, urinary tract infections, and septicemia continued to occur, however, and as surgeons operated on older patients or more debilitated patients and entered areas of the body containing natural endogenous flora, postoperative and post-traumatic infections remained a problem between 1900 and the 1930s.

Prior to the antibiotic era (1940) the cause of most nosocomial infections remained relatively constant, with gram-positive aerobic cocci constituting the majority of infections. Commonly encountered organisms included coagulase-positive staphylococci, β-hemolytic nongroup D streptococci, and *Streptococcus pneumoniae.* Prior to the late 1950s the only important gram-negative aerobic bacilli were *Escherichia coli* and a few infections caused by *Salmonella.*[1] The scarcity of nosocomial infections caused by fungal species, other Enterobacteriaceae (*Klebsiella, Enterobacter, Serratia* species), enterococcus species, and coagulase-negative staphylococci should be noted and duly appreciated by every student and practitioner with an interest in infectious disease.

The antibiotic era ushered in major changes in the species of bacteria causing nosocomial infections. Other major factors in the changing etiology of hospital-acquired infections were the development of intensive care units (ICUs), specialized critical care units, life support systems with respirators, arterial catheters, access to the central veins, immunosuppressive therapy, and organ transplant surgery as well as the aging of the U.S. population. Many organisms including bacteria, fungus, and viral species play an important role in modern hospitalization. Some of these organisms are either not treatable or treatable only with difficulty or with toxic chemotherapeutic agents. For a complete review of the changing face of infectious disease the reader is referred to reviews of this area and to studies of the incidence and etiology of nosocomial bacteremia and fungemia in hospital populations over extended periods of time.[2–5]

The Antibiotic Era

Coagulase-positive staphylococci (*Staphylococcus aureus*) were the most important pathogens encountered in U.S. hospitals in the 1940s and became epidemic in the 1950s and early 1960s. Introduction of the penicillinase-resistant penicillins (methicillin) and the first-generation cephalosporins were responsible for the decreasing importance of this bacteria in the 1970s. *Staphylococcus aureus* continues to be the great "true pathogen" and is still responsible for some 10–20% of nosocomial infections. The isolation of methicillin-resistant *S. aureus* (MRSA), which is not susceptible to other β-lactam antibiotics, represents one of the major events in infectious disease practice and research in the twentieth century.[6,7] Instead of producing an enzyme that destroys the antibiotic, MRSA is generally not inhibited by virtue of alterations in its penicillin-binding protein characteristics. This feature also has been found in penicillin-resistant *S. pneumoniae* in the past 10 years.

One of the most interesting developments of the past several years has been the emergence of coagulase-negative staphylococci as a significant pathogen. This is covered later in this chapter in the section on Device-Related Infections. During the 1980s, the Centers for Disease Control and Prevention (CDC) in Atlanta reported a 133% increase in nosocomial bacteremias.[8] Regardless of hospital type or size this trend held true. The major pathogens implicated in all nosocomial infections and those responsible for primary bloodstream infections are listed in Table 118.1 (National Nosocomial Infections Surveillance data [NNIS], 1990–1992).[9] Coagulase-negative staphylococci were responsible for virtually all of the observed increases in primary bacteremias. The CDC has stated "clearly, coagulase-negative staphylococci is emerging as the most important contributor to primary nosocomial infection rates." This 133% increase in nosocomial bacteremias in real numbers increased from 1.8 in 1980 to 4.2 infections per 1000 patient discharges in 1989.[10] This trend has continued in the 1990–1992 data. Coagulase-negative staphylococci are also important pathogens for renal and bone marrow transplant services, and in the 1980s infectious disease specialists frequently include vancomycin in their presumptive regimen in the febrile neutropenic patient as the only effective therapy against coagulase-negative staphylococci. At the University Hospital, University of Kentucky Medical Center, in 1993 only 11% of isolates of *S. aureus* were methicillin/oxacillin resistant, whereas 69% of coagulase-negative staphylococci were methicillin/oxacillin resistant.

TABLE 118.1. PATHOGENS CAUSING NOSOCOMIAL ENDEMIC INFECTIONS

Pathogen	% of Isolates
Escherichia coli	12
Staphyloccocus aureus	12
Coagulase-negative staphylococci	11
Enterococci	10
Pseudomonas aeruginosa	9
Candida species	7
Klebsiella species	6
Enterobacter species	6
Proteus mirabilis	3
All others	24

(Data from Ref. 9.)

A new threat in nosocomial infections has emerged in the 1990s. From 1989–1993 the percentage of nosocomial enterococcal infections reported to the CDC NNIS system that were resistant to vancomycin increased from 0.3% to 7.9%. Although a trend in this increasing resistance was seen in non-ICU patients, a majority of the increase came from patients in ICU areas. This alarming increase in enterococcal vancomycin resistance comes at the same time as an increasing incidence of high-level penicillin and aminoglycoside resistance. Obviously, the treatment op-tions in patients with bacteremia or endocarditis from these highly resistant enterococci are very limited and include totally experimental combinations of various antibiotics.[11–13] Further, in the laboratory, the *vanA* gene in the *Enterococcus* can be plasmid mediated and has been transferred *in vitro* to *S. aureus.* Although vancomycin resistance has not yet been reported in either *S. aureus* or *S. epidermidis,* vancomycin resistant *S. haemolyticus* has been reported. The CDC Subcommittee on the Prevention and Control of Antimicrobial Resistance Microorganisms in Hospitals has recently suggested that stringent measures are necessary to control the use of vancomycin in the hospital setting.[14]

With the exception of *Escherichia coli,* few gram-negative organisms appeared in nosocomial infection surveys prior to the mid-1950s. With the introduction of the penicillins and the first-generation cephalosporins, gram-negative organisms became important pathogens. Common isolates included species of *Klebsiella, Enterobacter, Serratia,* and indole-positive *Proteus, Pseudomonas aeruginosa,* and nonfermenting bacteria such as *Citrobacter* and *Acinetobacter.* During the 1970s anaerobic culture techniques were further developed and refined, leading to the recognition that specific anaerobes were an important component of polymicrobial pelvic and abdominal infections. The *Bacteroides fragilis* group of organisms and *Clostridium* species were the most prominent anaerobic pathogens recognized. In the late 1970s, pseudomembranous colitis was recognized after therapy with many antibiotics. This disease was subsequently found to result from overgrowth of the anaerobic bacteria *Clostridium difficile* in the lumen of the large intestine.[15] Prior to the antibiotic era fungi caused few infections in hospitalized patients and virtually no cases of fungemia are found in bacteremia/fungemia surveys prior to 1953. Today, as a result of broad-spectrum antibiotic therapy and suppression of anaerobic gut flora, fungi (primarily *Candida albicans*) are responsible for 7–8% of cases of septicemia with positive blood cultures.[16] Nosocomial fungal infection rates showed dramatic increases in the 1980s. A comparison of the types of fungal infections seen in the 1980s is shown in Table 118.2.[17]

TABLE 118.2. TYPES OF NOSOCOMIAL FUNGAL INFECTIONS SEEN IN THE 1980s

Fungal Species	% of Isolates
Candida species	79
C. albicans (76%)	
C. tropicalis (7%)	
C. parapsilosis (2.5%)	
Torulopsis species	8
Aspergillus species	1.3
Others	11.7

(Data from Ref. 16.)

COMMON NOSOCOMIAL INFECTIONS

Approximately 3.35% (33.5 per 1000 hospital discharges) of all general medical and surgical patients admitted to U.S. hospitals suffer a nosocomial infection (over 1 million patients per year). Further, some 18% of patients with nosocomial infections have more than one infection.[17]

The most common site of nosocomial infection is the urinary tract, which accounts for 33.1% of reported infections (Table 118.3); 15.5% are lower respiratory infections, 14.9% surgical wound infections, and 13.1% bacteremias.[9] For differences in nosocomial infections between surgical and medical patients see Table 118.4. Although surgical patients constitute only about 42% of hospital admissions they have 71% of all nosocomial infections. Nosocomial infections generally increase with increasing age at all sites of infection; patients older than 84 years have two to five times the risk of infection of 18- to 24-year-old patients. Sexual differences are also noted, with women being more susceptible to surgical wound infections, pneumonia, and bacteremia. Surgical specialty has a predictable effect on the site of nosocomial infections; neurosurgical and urology patients have high rates of urinary tract infection (indwelling Foley catheters); surgical wound infection rates are highest for general surgery and obstetrics; and bacteremias are highest for cardiothoracic surgery patients. Many other factors have major effects on the occurrence of nosocomial infections. Factors known to increase the risk include immunosuppressive therapy, longer hospital stay, previous infections, longer duration of surgery, and mechanical ventilatory support.

TABLE 118.3. NOSOCOMIAL INFECTIONS BY SITE: ALL PATIENTS

Site	%
Urinary tract	33.1
Pneumonia	15.5
Surgical wound	14.9
Bacteremia	13.1
Other	23.4

(Data from Ref. 9.)

TABLE 118.4. NOSOCOMIAL INFECTIONS BY SITE: MEDICAL VERSUS SURGICAL PROCEDURES

Site	Medical (%)	Surgical (%)
Urinary tract	42.1	30.2
Surgical wound	2.3	24.5
Pneumonia	17.0	16.4
Bacteremia	14.8	9.5
Other sites	23.8	19.4

(Data from Ref. 9.)

Nosocomial infections are caused by a wide variety of microorganisms but about one-half dozen are most prevalent (Table 118.1). *Escherichia coli* and *S. aureus* are the most common pathogens in most hospitals, each causing 12% of all nosocomial infections. Other pathogens falling into the top 10 category of causative microorganisms include coagulase-negative staphlococci, *Enterococcus* species, *P. aeruginosa, Enterobacter* species, *Candida* species, *Klebsiella pneumoniae,* and *Proteus mirabilis.* These "endemic" hospital infections are quite different from epidemic infections that occur in clusters from a definable reservoir. Reports of epidemic infections show that *S. aureus* is the most common organism (19%), followed by *Salmonella* (13%), tribe Klebsielleae (12%), and hepatitis B (8%). Infectious disease practitioners should note and have a great deal of respect for the ability of these nosocomial pathogens to survive and persist within the hospital environment. This will continue to be a major challenge in the decade of the 1990s.

NEW NOSOCOMIAL ORGANISMS

VIRAL INFECTIONS

The transmission and identification of the virus causing the acquired immunodeficiency syndrome (AIDS) is one of the most significant occurrences in the history of infectious disease (human immunodeficiency virus [HIV]). Concern over the transmission of this virus has led to the introduction of "universal precautions" at all U.S. hospitals to protect both patients and employees. Recent evidence that health care workers with AIDS can transmit the virus to their patients has created another ethical and moral dilemma relative to required HIV testing and disclosure of such test results to patients.[18] Accidental needle sticks from discarded needles occurring in hospital employees represent another major ethical and legal dilemma for hospitals. Studies that demonstrate the effectiveness of taking prophylactic antiviral drugs such as zidovudine (AZT) following accidental needle sticks are badly needed.[19] However, given the fatal outcome of HIV infection, such studies may be difficult even in the face of significant drug toxicity that occurs from drugs such as AZT.

Other nosocomial viral infections also are recognized as an increasing and significant problem in hospitals. Viruses are particularly important relative to transplant services where treatment includes immunosuppressive therapy. Cytomegalovirus, varicella, herpes zoster, rotavirus, herpes simplex, and hepatitis virus are seen with increasing frequency.[20–23] In immunocompromised patients cytomegalovirus acquired either exogenously (from a transplanted organ, granulocyte transfusions, etc.) or by activation of endogenous latent viruses can involve the liver and lungs and be rapidly associated with a fatal outcome. Better diagnostic methods and viral chemotherapeutic agents will play important roles in transplant centers in the future.

METHICILLIN-RESISTANT *STAPHYLOCOCCUS AUREUS*

MRSA has been a clinical problem since the early 1960s and has reached epidemic proportions in some large U.S. hospitals since 1980.[24] Recent work, primarily by Hartman and Tomasz,[25] has attributed the resistance to alteration of the penicillin-binding proteins, which have a low affinity for methicillin and other β-lactam antibiotics. MRSA has significant clinical and financial implications for the hospital pharmacy. Even though standard sensitivity tests might indicate that MRSA is sensitive to cephalosporin antibiotics, therapeutic failures are common.[26] The drug of choice for MRSA is vancomycin.[27] It is abundantly clear that MRSA are virulent nosocomial pathogens that can be transmitted to patients from the hands of health care workers. The reservoir for MRSA includes patients who are both colonized and infected with the major sites of concern being wounds and secretions of intubated and mechanically ventilated patients.[28] Most infectious disease practitioners believe that rigid hand-washing procedures and the isolation of patients with MRSA are effective ways to control the spread of the organism.[29,30] MRSA also can cause bacteremia, pneumonia, endocarditis, and wound infections.

CEPHALOSPORIN-TOLERANT STAPHYLOCOCCI

An emerging controversy in infectious disease concerns the use of specific cephalosporins for surgical prophylaxis. Cefazolin, an extended half-life first-generation cephalosporin, has become the preferred agent for surgical prophylaxis in many hospitals. The knowledge that *S. aureus* and coagulase-negative staphylococci are the most important pathogens in postoperative prosthetic valve endocarditis, cause over one-half of all vascular graft infections, and are the most frequently isolated pathogens in infected orthopedic implants, combined with the safety and favorable pharmacokinetics of cefazolin, appeared to make this drug an excellent choice.[31] Several recent studies, however, have called into question the choice of cefazolin as the preferred antibiotic for such surgical procedures.[32–34] These trials compared second-generation cephalosporins (cefamandole and cefuroxime) to cefazolin and results seemed to indicate the second-generation agents were more effective prophylactic agents. Patients receiving cefazolin continued to have postoperative infectious morbidity from *S. aureus* and coagulase-negative staphylococcus. Although the reasons for such prophylactic failures with cefazolin have not been clearly documented, there is laboratory evidence and animal data suggesting that cefazolin, in comparison with other first-generation cephalosporins and the second-generation drugs cefamandole and cefuroxime, might be more susceptible to inactivation by some β-lactamase-producing strains of staphylococci.[35] Strains of staphylococci isolated from patients receiving cefazolin prophylaxis seem to document this "more rapid hydrolysis" theory. Also very interesting is the fact that the older and somewhat forgotten first-generation cephalosporin, cephalothin, is overall still the most resistant cephalosporin to staphylococcal β-lactamase hydrolysis and this probably warrants a reexamination of this agent for surgical prophylaxis. Unfortunately, the short biologic half-life of cephalothin would make more frequent dosing a necessity. This controversy will continue to grow in importance and the effect will more than likely spill over into other areas where cefazolin is still used for surgical prophylaxis.

INCREASING ROLE OF THE ENTEROCOCCI AND EMERGING RESISTANCE

Enterococci (formerly group D streptococci) are commensal organisms well suited to survival in the intestinal and vaginal tract and in the oral cavity. Enterococci also possess virulence factors that can allow the bacteria to become pathogenic. Frequent sites of isolation include the urinary tract, abdominal and pelvic surgical wounds, and the bloodstream. When isolated from the blood, infective endocarditis must be suspected.[36] Surveys of causative organisms in endocarditis show that the enterococcus is responsible for 15% of such cases. Even excluding endocarditis, enterococcus bacteremia is associated with high mortality.[37] The usual source of most enterococcal bacteremia is the genitourinary area. *Enterococcus faecalis* is the most common enterococcus isolated from clinical specimens. *Enterococcus faecium* is less frequently isolated.

All cephalosporin antibiotics exhibit either total resistance or poor activity against enterococcus; thus, when these agents are used prophylactically or therapeutically the enterococcus frequently colonizes and sometimes infects the patient. In a study in which either a second- or third-generation cephalosporin was used in either a one- or three-dose regimen as prophylaxis in vaginal hysterectomy, *Enterococcus* colonized the vaginal cuff in over 60% of patients.[38] This selection process may explain why the rate of superinfection has increased since cephalosporins were introduced in the 1960s. When serious infections, especially bacteremia, occur with enterococcus, treatment is difficult; combinations of penicillins or vancomycin with an aminoglycoside are used to achieve a synergistic killing effect. For urinary tract infections (uncomplicated) the use of ampicillin alone may be effective in eradicating the organism.

The use of single agents to treat serious enterococci infections has resulted in a high failure rate. Therefore, combination therapy primarily with an aminoglycoside and penicillin has been the standard therapeutic regimen. For patients with penicillin allergy, vancomycin served as the replacement agent, and demonstrated synergy with aminoglycosides in a similar fashion to penicillins. Unfortunately, recent evidence has accumulated that "high-level" resistance to aminoglycosides, increasing tolerance to penicillins, and, in the 1990s, vancomycin resistance are major clinical problems. Such resistance may require the use of special clinical microbiology laboratory procedures to document that antibiotic combinations will remain effective in serious enterococcal infections.[39] Further, in isolates of enterococci resistant to all three primary agents, there may not be effective therapy for serious infections.[40,41]

CONTINUING ROLE OF ENTEROBACTERIACEAE

Escherichia coli has always been an important nosocomial pathogen but it was not until the late 1960s and early 1970s that other members of this group of organisms were recognized as prominent pathogens. In many hospitals, *K. pneumoniae,*[42] *Enterobacter* species,[43] and *Serratia marcescens*[44] are now among the most frequent causes of gram-negative sepsis. Fever, hypotension, complement activation, and disseminated intravascular coagulation (activation of factor XII) are seen when these organisms invade the bloodstream.

Antibiotic resistance of hospital-associated Enterobacteriaceae is an ever-increasing problem. In major teaching hospitals resistance to aminoglycosides and first-, second-, and even third-generation cephalosporins is common. Methods of resistance include both plasmid and chromosomally mediated β-lactamases, cell wall permeability barriers, and the production of aminoglycoside-altering enzymes.[44] Recent reviews indicate that Enterobacteriaceae cause greater than 40% of all nosocomial infections in the United States. See Table 118.5 for a classification of the Enterobacteriaceae. Beginning in 1983 in Europe, a new plasmid-mediated β-lactamase capable of hydrolyzing even the newer cephalosporins such as ceftazidime and cefotaxime and even carbapenams such as imipenam were reported.[45] The major bacteria implicated in the production of the extended spectrum β-lactamases has been *K. pneumoniae.* By 1994 these enzymes have been reported from around the world and over 20 varieties have been identified.[46,47] It is clear that these enzymes result from antibiotic selection pressure and they can emerge wherever antibiotic use favors their selection.

TABLE 118.5. CLASSIFICATION OF THE ENTEROBACTERIACEAE

Tribe Klebsielleae	Tribe Proteae
Klebsiella pneumoniae	*Proteus mirabilis* (indole-negative)
Klebsiella oxytoca	*Proteus vulgaris*
Enterobacter aerogenes	*Proteus morganii*
Enterobacter cloacae	*Providencia rettgeri*
Enterobacter agglomerans	*Providencia stuartii*
Serratia marcescens	
Serratia liquefaciens	Tribe Salmonelleae
Tribe Escherichieae	*Citrobacter freundii*
Escherichia coli	*Citrobacter diversus*
Shigella dysenteriae	*Salmonella typhi*
	Salmonella paratyphi
	Salmonella arizona

Pseudomonas aeruginosa is a major nosocomial pathogen in trauma, immunocompromised, and cystic fibrosis patients. As with the enterococcus, the differentiation between colonization and infection with *P. aeruginosa* is sometimes difficult. Many ventilator-dependent patients who are receiving antibiotics colonize their bronchial–tracheal secretions with *P. aeruginosa.* When actual pneumonia does occur, usually with lower lobe infiltrates, the organisms must be treated with vigorous antibiotic therapy (usually aminoglycoside/antipseudomonal penicillin combinations). In patients with pneumonia who develop bacteremia the prognosis is grave, with some reports of mortality approaching 100%.[48] One of the pathologic features of *P. aeruginosa* infections is the ability to invade the walls of blood vessels, leading to ecthyma gangrenosum, a grave clinical sign with massive tissue infection. A notorious antibiotic-resistant organism, *P. aeruginosa* produces both chromosomally and plasmid-mediated β-lactamases.[49] Present in the environment of many hospitals are *P. aeruginosa* that are resistant to the aminoglycosides, antipseudomonal penicillins, third-generation cephalosporins, and even the newer monobactams, carbapenams, and fluoroquinolone antibiotics. Aminoglycoside resistance can result from enzymatic alteration or from an inability of the antibiotic to penetrate the cell wall. Resistance to β-lactams can result from hyperproduction of β-lactamases or decreases

TABLE 118.6. *PSEUDOMONAS AERUGINOSA*—SELECTED ANTIBIOTIC SENSITIVITIES

Antibiotic	Number of Isolates	% Sensitive
Amikacin	461	78
Ceftazidime	461	77
Aztreonam	461	58
Ciprofloxacin	461	79
Gentamicin	461	42
Imipenem	461	83
Mezlocillin	461	66
Piperacillin	461	85
Tobramycin	461	75

(Data from *Clinical Microbiology,* University Hospital, University of Kentucky, September–December 1993.)

in cell wall drug permeability in the case of imipenem.[50] See Table 118.6 for antibiotic sensitivities against *P. aeruginosa.*

Aminoglycoside antibiotics continue to be required in a majority of life-threatening *P. aeruginosa* infections. Because resistance to the newer cephalosporins such as ceftazidime and the carbapenems such as imipenem is already a problem, single agents are not totally reliable, and monotherapy continues to be a subject of great debate among infectious disease physicians. An unusual feature of *P. aeruginosa* is its ability to flourish in a variety of environments and supposedly bactericidal solutions. Hospital soap dispensers, benzalkonium chloride, and povidone–iodine solutions have been found to be contaminated with this organism.

STENOTROPHOMONAS (XANTHOMONAS) MALTOPHILIA AND BURKHOLDERIA (PSEUDOMONAS) CEPACIA

These two gram-negative bacteria are now frequently encountered as nosocomial pathogens. They present with a different clinical picture, have differing metabolic requirements and a different antibiotic sensitivity pattern than that of *P. aeruginosa.* They have been reported in association with contaminated hospital products such as disinfectants,[51] lymphokine activated killer (LAK) cells used in cancer chemotherapy,[52] ventilator temperature probes,[53] blood components, and arterial pressure transducers. Both organisms are resistant to many currently available antibiotics. *Xanthomonas maltophilia* is usually resistant to all aminoglycosides and even has been found to be resistant to newer agents such as imipenem.[54] An even rarer clinical pathogen, *Pseudomonas pickettii,* was recently associated with bacteremia traced to a narcotic tampering episode by health care personnel.[55]

COAGULASE-NEGATIVE STAPHYLOCOCCI

Coagulas-negative staphylococci (CNS) are frequent contaminants in positive blood cultures obtained in adults. Unfortunately, methods for distinguishing between contaminants and pathogens remain poorly defined and disappointing. However, CNS recovered from the bloodstream should not be ignored and clinical judgment must be used in determining the significance of positive CNS blood cultures.[56]

As a cause of invasive disease, CNS infections usually occur in clinical situations where patients are granulocytopenic,[57] and in patients with prosthetic heart valves, intravenous or intra-arterial catheters, ventriculoperitoneal shunts, or other implantable devices.[58] Persistent recovery of *S. epidermidis* from multiple blood cultures must lead the clinician to suspect infection and not contamination. Methicillin-resistant CNS constitutes 25–50% of all isolates of this organism in larger hospitals. Further, 70–85% of *S. epidermidis* organisms causing prosthetic valve endocarditis are methicillin resistant. Like MRSA the drug of choice for this organism is vancomycin because of the high rate of methicillin resistance.[59] Coagulase-negative staphylococcus bacteremia has been associated with the use of intravenous lipid emulsions in the neonatal ICU.[60,61]

LEGIONELLA PNEUMOPHILA

Legionnaire's disease is now considered in cases of unresponsive nosocomial pneumonia. The prevalence of this organism depends on its presence in the hospital's water supply.[62] The organism can grow and proliferate in standing water such as cooling or holding tanks. *Legionella* spreads through aerosolization of the contaminated water supply and its subsequent inhalation by patients. Parenteral erythromycin is presently the suggested drug for Legionnaire's disease although some of the newer fluoroquinolone antibiotics may be effective. In addition to causing pneumonia, *Legionella* has recently been implicated in other types of nosocomial infections including sternal wounds and prosthetic valve endocarditis coming from contaminated tap water used for bathing of patients in the hospital.[63]

ATYPICAL MYCOBACTERIUM

Prior to 1970 *Mycobacterium fortuitum* and *M. chelonei* caused only an occasional nosocomial infection. Since 1970 there has been an increase in infections caused by these organisms. Wound infections are reported in increasing frequency after cardiac surgery, vascular surgery, and breast implants.[64,65] Severe disseminated infection is seen most frequently in the immunocompromised host. Unfortunately, the antimicrobial drugs presently available are for the most part ineffective against the atypical Mycobacterium, and a satisfactory response requires a combination of drugs. Imipenem and some of the newer fluoroquinolones and macrolides may prove useful against these two organisms in the future.

INCREASING ROLE OF FUNGI

Hospital-acquired nosocomial fungal infections increased dramatically in the decade of the 1980s and now comprise some 7.9% of all isolates.[10] In addition, candida bloodstream infections have increased 300% during the 1980s. Patients at risk include those who receive parenteral nutrition, have indwelling urinary catheters or intravascular catheters, or are dialysis patients, particularly when broad-spectrum antibiotics are prescribed as a part of their hospital care. Such therapy leads to a marked increase in *Candida albicans* in the stool flora.[66] This phenomenon is particularly seen for drugs with a high degree of biliary elimination such as cefoperazone and ceftriaxone where *C. albicans* becomes the predominant aerobic flora. It is reasonable to expect that as more broad-spectrum drugs are used, fungi will play an increasing role, with *C. albicans* being the most frequently encountered pathogen.[67]

Transplantation procedures, intensive cancer chemotherapy, and AIDS, all of which severely depress the cellular immune system, can lead to fungal infections not only with *Candida* species but with a wide variety of opportunistic and dermatophyte fungi that were rarely or never known to cause infections in patients prior to 1975, including aspergillus, cryptococcus, trichophyton, pseudallescheria, and Mucoraceae.[68] Transmission of some of these fungi can be quite dramatic and include environmental sources. For example, pigeon feces on the window ledge adjacent to room air-intake ducts has been known to lead to aspergillus infections. Hospital construction and renovation that cause soil dust to contaminate air conditioning and venting systems have caused clusters of aspergillus in transplant and neonatal patients. A number of excellent reviews on nosocomial fungal infections have been published.[69]

Treatment of serious systemic fungal infections has generally required the use of intravenous amphoterocin B with resultant systemic and renal toxicities. The recent introduction of the new "triazole" antifungal drugs such as fluconazole and itraconazole may make the treatment of such infections more effective without the toxicity seen with amphotericin B. Several comparative studies in patients with documented candidiasis have demonstrated equal outcome.[70] See Table 118.2 for a list of nosocomial fungal pathogens.

INFUSION-RELATED NOSOCOMIAL BACTEREMIAS AND HOSPITAL PHARMACY PREPARED, CONTAMINATED PRODUCTS

Between 1970 and 1971, hospitals using a certain company's intravenous fluids experienced a significant occurrence of primary bacteremia caused by *Enterobacter* species.[71] Subsequent studies indicated that members of the tribe Klebsielleae have been responsible for over 90% of infusion-related bacteremias. *Klebsiella pneumoniae, E. cloacae, E. agglomerans,* and *S. marcescens* are uniquely capable of growing in crystalloid intravenous fluids containing dextrose.[72] These organisms do well because they can (1) fix atmospheric nitrogen for use as a protein source; (2) grow at room temperature; and (3) survive the low acidity of dextrose-containing intravenous fluids. Interestingly, even though these organisms can survive in intravenous fluids they reach a concentration of only 10^5–10^6 organisms per 1 mL of fluid, which is below the concentration necessary to cause turbidity; thus, heavily contaminated solutions are usually crystal clear by visual inspection. A review of the world literature between 1965 and 1978 shows 97 epidemics of hospital-acquired bacteremia; one-third of these resulted from some aspect of infusion therapy.[73] *Burkholderia capacia* has also been implicated in infusion-related bacteremia in recent years (Table 118.7).

When total parenteral nutrition (TPN) solutions were manufactured using protein hydrolysates as the nitrogen source, the incidence of primary bacteremia/fungemia from use of these TPN solutions increased.[74] Most bacteria and fungi could grow to turbidity in these solutions in 48–72 hours with inocula greater than 10^7 colony-forming units per milliliter of fluid.[75] In the late 1970s and early 1980s, TPN fluids contained, as the nitrogen source, mainly synthetic amino acids that were solubilized as the acetate salts. The high concentration of acetate ion in the final solution acts as a "bacteriostatic" agent in synthetic amino acid/dextrose TPN fluids, because most bacteria and fungal organisms do not grow well or at all in these fluids. The failure of these fluids to support microbiologic growth has resulted in a significant decrease in primary infusate-related sepsis in patients receiving TPN.

Pharmacy-run intravenous admixture programs have been responsible for a number of infusion-related infections.[76] All instances of contamination resulted from poor or nonexistent quality control procedures in the pharmacy department.[77] Errors included (1) failure to include a

TABLE 118.7. MICROORGANISMS ASSOCIATED WITH INFUSION-RELATED INFECTIONS

Contaminated intravenous fluids	*Klebsiella* species *Enterobacter* species *Serratia* species *Citrobacter* species *Pseudomonas cepacia*
Parenteral nutrition (synthetic amino acids as protein source)	*Candida albicans* (most septicemia related to catheter sepsis: solutions with synthetic amino acids are a poor growth medium)

preservative in a multiple-dose vial stored at room temperature, leading to fungal infection; (2) failure to clean the vacuum system used in preparing TPN solutions, leading to contaminated solutions; and (3) failure to follow aseptic practice in preparing large-volume potassium chloride admixtures, leading to septicemia.[78] The issue of contaminated products coming from hospital pharmacy controlled intravenous admixture and manufacturing facilities is certainly a major issue of the 1990s and the subject of recent concerns in the hospital pharmacy literature.[79] A Food and Drug Administration alert letter was sent to hospital pharmacists on November 29, 1990, citing the use of incorrect methods in the batch production of drug products as the cause of contamination and subsequent nosocomial infections. Certainly advanced training and knowledge in infectious disease and related topics is one step toward avoiding such catastrophes.

Control of Nosocomial Infections in the Hospital

The Joint Commission on Accreditation of Health Care Organizations states, as a principle, "There shall be an effective hospitalwide program for the surveillance, prevention, and control of infection."[80] The program includes the following basic elements directed toward the control of nosocomial infections:

1. There are written policies and procedures that describe the types of surveillance carried out to monitor the rates of nosocomial infections, the systems used to collect and analyze data, and the activities to prevent and control infections.
2. There is ongoing review and analysis of nosocomial infection data, risk factors, and, as needed, special studies that relate to infection prevention and control.
3. A multidisciplinary committee oversees the program for surveillance, prevention, and control of infection.
4. Committee membership includes representatives from at least the medical staff, nursing staff, administration, and the person(s) directly responsible for management of the infection surveillance, prevention, and control program.
5. Representation from housekeeping, central services, laundry, the dietetic department, the engineering and maintenance department, pharmacy, and the operating suite is available on at least a consultative basis.
6. There are written policies and procedures for infection surveillance, prevention, and control for all patient care departments.
7. The annual report of the committee includes studies of organisms of epidemiologic significance (for example, trends in antibiotic resistance patterns).

The pharmacist is a key individual in aiding the Hospital Infection Committee to implement many of the preceding elements. A member of the pharmacy clinical staff who is familiar with the practice of infectious disease should represent the pharmacy department on the committee. In addition, the pharmacy department must have written policies and procedures relating to infection control for all areas where aseptic technique, sterilization, or manufacture of parenteral solutions occurs. Pharmacists serving on Infection Control Committees also should review all infection control procedures from other hospital departments where sterile drug products are used or admixed. Examples include the operating room, the emergency room, radiology, and anesthesiology holding areas.

Antibiotic Use and Nosocomial Infections

Hospitalized patients become colonized with a variety of bacteria during any admission period. Surveillance studies indicate that inpatients acquire new organisms at the rate of 0.5 organisms per patient per week. Most of these organisms are gram-negative bacilli of the type most likely to cause nosocomial infections. Colonizing bacteria or fungi in patients receiving antibiotics are frequently resistant to the drug or drugs the patient is receiving. Examples are easy to identify. *Candida albicans* colonizes the vaginal tract, urinary tract, and bronchial tree of patients receiving broad-spectrum antibiotics, and becomes more prominent in the colonic flora. Enterococci frequently colonize the vaginal cuff in patients receiving cephalosporin antibiotics as prophylaxis for vaginal hysterectomy. *Pseudomonas aeruginosa* colonizes bronchial secretions in patients receiving cephalosporins not effective against this organism. Third-generation cephalosporins are capable of inducing β-lactamase production in members of the Enterobacteriaceae.[81] These enzymes accumulate in the periplasmic space of the organism and can cause slow hydrolysis of even the most β-lactamase-stable cephalosporins.[82] The use of antibiotics can of course save a patient's life; by the same token, the misuse of antibiotics can have a devastating effect on both the patient and the hospital environment. It is mandatory that antimicrobial drugs be prescribed with both knowledge and restraint if therapy is to be maximized and adverse effects are to be minimized.

Device-Related Infection

The availability of medical devices for temporary or permanent implantation constitutes a major advance in modern medicine. It is estimated that several millions of various kinds of medical devices are implanted annually into patients in the United States. With the continuing rapid development of biocompatible synthetic materials or biomaterials, the prediction that "ultimately, almost every human in technologically advanced societies will host a biomaterial" appears to be pertinent. Unfortunately, as the use of such devices becomes increasingly common, so does the incidence of complications associated with their use—infection being the most common. Table 118.8 gives examples of implanted devices and associated infection rates.

The body is protected from invasion of pathogenic bacteria by the formation of boundaries of bacterial colonization such as the laryngopharynx, the lower third of the urethra, and the cervical canal.[83] Devices that bypass these boundaries allow migration of bacteria to normally uncolonized areas. Infection may arise at the time of device placement because it is already colonized with potential pathogens, or after implantation as a result of microbial migration from an outside source. Epidemiological studies have revealed that skin flora such as *S. epidermidis* (CNS) are commonly found to be associated with device-related infections. These CNS adhere readily to devices inserted through the skin or implanted beneath it. In contrast, infections caused by gram-negative bacilli (GNB) such as *P. aeruginosa* are often found to be associated with prostheses that are partially or fully exposed to the environment.

TABLE 118.8. INCIDENCE OF INFECTION AND PATHOGENS ASSOCIATED WITH IMPLANTED MEDICAL DEVICES

Medical Device	Incidence of Infection (%)	Commonly Associated Pathogens
CAPD catheters	100[a]	CNS
Central lines	10	*S. epidermidis*
CSF shunts	1.5–6	*S. epidermidis* *S. aureus*
Endotracheal tubes	9–70	*Pseudomonas aeruginosa* *Proteus* species *S. aureus*
Prosthetic heart valves	0.4–2	*S. epidermidis* *S. aureus* *Enterococcus* species
Orthopedic	1–2	CNS, *S. aureus*
Urinary catheters	20[b]	*Escherichia coli* *Klebsiella* species *Proteus* species
Vascular grafts	1.5–6	*S. aureus* Gram-negative species

[a]Long-term catheters also used at home.
[b]Incidence varies according to type of patient.

TABLE 118.9. FACTORS INFLUENCING MICROBIAL COLONIZATION OF MEDICAL DEVICES

Patient	Skin preparation Catheter site and position Diameter of vessels vs. catheter Type of insertion, e.g., tunneled
Medical personnel	Hand washing Insertion technique, site care Therapy via catheter
Medical device	Design and biomaterial Protein deposition on biomaterial, e.g., fibrinogen Surface roughness Surface hydrophobicity and charge Leachable substances
Microorganism	Surface hydrophobicity and charge Absence/presence of bacterial slime Proximity of microorganism to biomaterial

MICROBIAL ADHERENCE AND BIOFILM FORMATION

The initial important step in the infection process is for the infecting microorganism to adhere to the biomaterial. (A list of factors influencing microbial colonization is given in Table 118.9.) Once adhered, the bacteria may exude extracellular polysaccharides so that their progeny can attach firmly to the surface and be enveloped by this adhesive glycocalyx (sometimes referred to as slime) to form a biofilm. Bacteria encased in this matrix are relatively resistant to the action of antimicrobial agents and host defenses. Three reasons have been proposed to explain this resistance:

1. The glycocalyx is presented as a physical barrier to antibiotics, preventing their access to microorganisms within the biofilm. However, the glycocalyx does not appear to impede antibiotic penetration significantly, although some antibiotics are more affected than others.[84,85] It is, however, known that the extracellular polysaccharide matrix is essentially negatively charged and can bind with positively charged agents such as those of the aminoglycoside group.[86] However, this mechanism does not explain the resistance to neutral and negatively charged agents.
2. Biofilm has also been presented as an enzymatic barrier where degradative enzymes within the biofilm, such as β-lactamases, can inactivate antibiotics along the diffusion pathways, thereby reducing the concentrations of antibiotics reaching the inner cells.[86,87] It has been demonstrated that *P. aeruginosa* adherent to catheter material within a biofilm

can produce 32 times more β-lactamase than the same cells when in suspension[88] and therefore has a greater potential to inactivate antibiotic than the suspended microorganisms.

3. The microenvironment set up within the biofilm has high concentrations of enzymes, but limited oxygen and nutrient supply, resulting in a slow rate of microbial growth. Bacteria growing in such nutrient-depleted conditions can undergo physiologic changes that alter their susceptibility to antibiotics.[89] Therefore, the successful eradication of biofilm may require antibiotics that have sufficient effect on slow growing microorganisms.

A distinction must be made between "colonization" and "infection" of medical devices because this may determine the course of action needed. For example, almost all urethral catheters in long-term catheterized patients are expected to become colonized, although not all of these patients will develop clinical infection. Therefore treatment should be reserved for those with symptomatic urinary tract infection. This may be in tandem with catheter removal or replacement.

TREATMENT OF DEVICE-ASSOCIATED INFECTION

As medical devices have evolved, so also has the treatment of device-associated infection. The emphasis of treatment still errs on the side of device removal but increasing success has been achieved with antibiotic combinations. Device removal in the case of urinary catheters or endotracheal tubes is relatively uncomplicated, however, removal of other implanted devices may present dangers. Cerebrospinal fluid shunt removal, for example, will induce hydrocephalus as pressure is no longer released and hemorrhage may occur.

The major risk of device retention is that a nidus of continuing infection remains with the potential for bacteremia and abscess formation.[90] Whereas common sense tells us that early action is appropriate to counter colonization of devices placed in normally sterile sites, immediate action is not always required. For instance, if gram-negative enterobacterial colonization of endotracheal tubes occurs in intensive care patients the situation is usually observed closely for several days. If there is no evidence of pneumonia or bacteremia, no further action is normally necessary.

The most important factors in the prevention of intravascular catheter sepsis are careful aseptic technique and subsequent care of the catheter. This advice should apply to all medical devices. Prosthetic heart valves, for example, become infected from direct contamination of the site at the time of surgery or as a result of subsequent contamination. The bacteria infecting during the first 2 months following surgery closely resemble the skin flora with CNS representing approximately 30% of infections. In contrast, with delayed infection, the types of infecting organisms are quite different and include viridans streptococci and enterococci. Similar patterns have been observed in medical devices where manipulations subsequent to insertion or implantation are necessary in their use.

Antibiotics have been used successfully to eliminate free-floating bacteria, but they frequently fail to completely eradicate adherent bacteria within glycocalyx-protected biofilms. An important study by Anwar et al.[91] showed that young biofilm cells, 2 days old, of *P. aeruginosa* were still susceptible to tobramycin, suggesting that young biofilms may be treatable. In contrast, 7-day-old cells of the bacterium were highly resistant to the antibiotic. Similarly, young (4 days) biofilm cells of *S. aureus* were sensitive to a combination of 100 μg of cephalexin and 5 μg of tobramycin while aging (13 days) biofilms were resistant to these antibiotics. It is important to recognize that minimum inhibitory concentrations of antibiotics should be determined with biofilm populations of bacteria. The best strategy, therefore, for controlling biofilm-associated infections is to initiate the antibiotic therapy as early as possible.

The best antibiotics for treatment of CNS infections associated with intravascular catheters are those of the glycopeptide group—vancomycin and teicoplanin.[92] Response rates of 80% and 69% were observed with vancomycin and teicoplanin, respectively, in the treatment of infections associated with Hickman catheters without device removal.[93] The virulence of the infecting microorganism is, obviously, a major determinant in deciding treatment. Therefore, where *S. aureus* infection of a centrally sited intravascular catheter arises, device removal is advisable and at least 2 weeks of treatment with an antistaphylococcal penicillin such as flucloxacillin or oxacillin, preferably by the intravenous route. Device removal is required if there is candidal vascular catheter infection, and systemic antifungal therapy is advised because of the high mortality associated with candidemia. Similar action should be followed if gram-negative bacterial infection is present, particularly if this is by *P. aeruginosa.*

The major cause of technique failure and morbidity in patients on CAPD treatment is peritonitis. Peritonitis due to touch contamination during bag exchanges has been reduced greatly by the development of improved connecting sets, although peritonitis due to catheter site-related infections is still of considerable concern.[94] The catheter exit site frequently becomes colonized by skin bacteria such as *S. aureus* and *S. epidermidis.* Recurrent peritonitis from catheter-related infection is resistant to common antibiotics and frequently requires removal of the catheter. Catheter removal is still recommended where *S. aureus* or

P. aeruginosa infection of the catheter tunnel occurs. We have reported viable microbial biofilm on 87% of CAPD catheters retrieved from renal transplant patients and on 100% of CAPD catheters removed due to recurrent peritonitis.[95] Biofilm encased bacterial microcolonies remain protected from host defense antibodies, cytokines, and phagocytes. However, when host defenses are poor, biofilm bacteria can disseminate into the peritoneal cavity and produce clinical peritonitis.

The failure of joint prostheses is a major concern in orthopedic surgery and the problem of loosening of the device with subsequent mechanical failure is associated with low-grade infection. Antibiotic therapy with retention of the device is successful in about 20% of cases, therefore device removal is recommended. Flucloxacillin plus fusidic acid has shown some success against the common staphylococcal infections of this area but less effect has been observed with ciprofloxacin and rifampicin. This is somewhat surprising because this combination displays good pharmacokinetic properties; however, CNS rapidly develop resistance to fluoroquinolones.

A WORD OF CAUTION

One of the difficulties in eradicating microorganisms associated with device-related infection is that susceptibility testing of these pathogens is usually performed when they are in suspension. *In vivo,* however, the microorganism may exist within a biofilm. Therefore, while microorganisms in suspension are susceptible to a range of antimicrobials, those within biofilm may effectively be resistant to antibiotic action. It is important to appreciate that susceptibility can vary and that failure to eradicate the infecting microorganism may lead to treatment failure or relapsing infection.

REFERENCES

1. McGowan JE. Changing etiology of nosocomial bacteremia and fungemia and other hospital-acquired infections. Rev Infect Dis 1985;7(suppl 3):5357–5379.
2. Eickhoff TC. Nosocomial infections—a 1980 view: Progress, priorities and prognosis, in Dixon RE (ed): Nosocomial Infections. New York, Yorke Medical Books, 1981, pp 1–9.
3. Finegold SM, Kirby WM. Changing pattern of hospital infections: Implications for therapy. Am J Med 1984;77:1–2.
4. Neu HC. Changing mechanisms of bacterial resistance. Am J Med 1984;77:11–23.
5. Decker MD. Changing trends in infection control and hospital epidemiology. Infect Dis Clin North Am 1989;3(4):671–682.
6. Dunkle LM, Naqvi SH, Callum R, et al. Eradication of epidemic methicillin-gentamicin-resistant *Staphylococcus aureus* in an intensive care nursery. Am J Med 1981;70:455–458.
7. Boyce JM, White RL, Spruell EY. Impact of methicillin-resistant *Staphylococcus aureus* on the incidence of nosocomial staphylococcal infections. J Infect Dis 1983;148:763.
8. Maki DG. Nosocomial bloodstream infections [abstract]. 3rd International Conference on Nosocomial Infections, Centers for Disease Control, Atlanta, July 31–August 3, 1990.
9. Emori TG, Gaynes RP. An overview of nosocomial infections, including the role of the microbiology laboratory. Clin Microb Rev 1993;6:428–442.
10. Banerjee S, Emori TG, Culver DH, et al. Secular trends in nosocomial primary bloodstream infections in the United States, 1980–1989. Am J Med 1991;91(suppl 3B):86S–94S.
11. Bradley DJ, Huycke MM, Gilmore MS. Virulence of enterococci. Clin Microb Rev 1994;7:462–478.
12. Eliopoulos GM. The 10 most common questions about resistant enterococcal infections. Infect Dis Clin Prac 1994;3:125–129.
13. Johnson AP. The pathogenicity of enterococci. J Antimicrob Chemother 1994;33:1083–1089.
14. Anonymous. Preventing the spread of vancomycin resistance—report from the hospital control practices advisory committee. Fed Reg 1994;59(May 17):25758–25763.
15. Riley TV, Bowman RA, Carroll SM. Diarrhea associated with *Clostridium difficile* in a hospital population. Med J Aust 1983;19:166–169.
16. Jarvis WR. Nosocomial fungal infections in the United States [abstract]. 3rd International Conference on Nosocomial Infections, Centers for Disease Control, Atlanta, July 31–August 3, 1990.
17. Horan TC. Nosocomial infection surveillance, 1984. MMWR 1986;35:17ss–29ss.
18. Anonymous. Update: Transmission of HIV infection during an invasive dental procedure—Florida. MMWR 1991;40:21–27.
19. Lange JMA, et al. Failure of zidovudine prophylaxis after accidental exposure to HIV. N Engl J Med 1990;322:1375–1377.
20. Dworsky ME, Welch K, Cassady G, et al. Occupational risk for primary cytomegalovirus infection among pediatric health care workers. N Engl J Med 1983;309:950–953.
21. Hammerberg O, Watts J, Chernesky M, et al. An outbreak of herpes simplex virus type I in an intensive care nursery. Pediatr Infect Dis 1983;2:290–294.
22. Hall CB. The nosocomial spread of respiratory syncytial viral infection. Ann Rev Med 1983;34:311–319.
23. Graman PS, Hall CB. Epidemiology and control of nosocomial viral infections. Infect Dis Clin North Am 1990;3(4):815–841.
24. Haley RW, Hightower AW, Khobbaz RF, et al. The emergence of methicillin-resistant *Staphylococcus aureus* infections in the United States hospitals. Ann Intern Med 1982;97:297–308.
25. Hartman B, Tomasz A. Altered penicillin binding protein in methicillin-resistant strains of *Staphylococcus aureus.* Antimicrob Agents Chemother 1981;19:726–735.
26. Sabath LD, Wallace SJ. Factors influencing methicillin resistance in staphylococci. Ann NY Acad Sci 1971;182:258–266.
27. Sorrell TC, Packman DR, Shanker S, et al. Vancomycin therapy for methicillin-resistant *Staphylococcus aureus.* Ann Intern Med 1983;97:344–350.

28. Boyce JM. Methicillin-resistant *Staphylococcus aureus* detection, epidemiology, and control measures. Infect Dis Clin North Am 1990;3(4):901–913.
29. Cohen SH, Morita MM, Bradford M. Control of MRSA: A 7-year experience [abstract]. 3rd International Conference on Nosocomial Infections, Atlanta, July 31–August 3, 1990.
30. Faoagali JL, Thong ML, Grant D. Ten years' experience with methicillin-resistant *Staphylococcus aureus* (MRSA) [abstract]. 3rd International Conference on Nosocomial Infections, Atlanta, July 31–August 3, 1990.
31. Anonymous. Choice of cephalosporins. Med Lett 1990;32(832):107–110.
32. Kaiser AB, Petracek JW, Lea IV DS, et al. Efficacy of cefazolin, cefamandole, and gentamicin as prophylactic agents in cardiac surgery: Results of a prospective, randomized, double-blind trial in 1030 patients. Ann Surg 1987;206:791–797.
33. Meszaros RM, Windisch C, Koltai C, et al. Comparative study of cefamandole versus cephalothin as antibiotic prophylaxis for open heart surgery. Cor Vasa 1986;29:61–66.
34. Slama TG, Slkar SJ, Misinski J, et al. Randomized comparison of cefamandole, cefazolin, and cefuroxime prophylaxis in open-heart surgery. Antimicrob Agents Chemother 1986;29:744–747.
35. Sabath LD. Reappraisal of the antistaphylococcal activities of first-generation (narrow-spectrum) and second-generation (expanded-spectrum) cephalosporins. Antimicrob Agents Chemother 1989;33:407–411.
36. Mandell GL, Kaye D, Levison ME, et al. Enterococcal endocarditis: An analysis of 38 patients. Arch Intern Med 1970;125:258–264.
37. Wells V, Wong ES, Coudron P, et al. Outbreak of nosocomial infections due to β-lactamase producing, gentam icin-resistant *Enterococcus faecalis:* A case control study. 3rd International Conference on Nosocomial Infections, Atlanta, July 31–August 3, 1990.
38. Rapp RP, Connors JE, Hager WD, et al. Comparison of single-dose moxalactam and a three-dose regimen of cefoxitin for prophylaxis in vaginal hysterectomy. Clin Pharm 1986;5:988–993.
39. Herman DJ, Gerding DN. Antimicrobial resistance among enterococci. Antimicrob Agents Chemother 1991;35:1–4.
40. Hayden MK, Koenig GI, Trenholme GM. Bactericidal activities of antibiotics against vancomycin-resistant *Enterococcus faecium* blood isolates and synergistic activities of combinations. Antimicrob Agents Chemother 1994;38:1225–1229.
41. Feldman RJ, Paul S, Cody R, et al. Analysis of treatment for patients with vancomycin-resistant enterococcal bacteremia [abstract]. ICAAC 34th Meeting, Orlando, Florida, October, 1994.
42. Meyer KS, Urben C, Eagan JA, et al. Nosocomial outbreak of *Klebsiella* infection resistant to late-generation cephalosporins. Ann Intern Med 1993;119:353–358.
43. Nordmann P, Mariotte S, Naas T, et al. Biochemical properties of a carbapenam-hydrolyzing beta-lactamase from *Enterobacter cloacae* and cloning of the gene into *Escherichia coli.* 1993;37:939–946.
44. Naas T, Vandel L, Sougakoff W, et al. Cloning and sequence analysis of the gene for a carbapenem-hydrolyzing class A beta-lactamase, Sme-1, from *Serratia marcesens* S6. Antimicrob Agents Chemother 1994;38:1262–1270.
45. Jacoby GA, Archer GL. New mechanisms of bacterial resistance to antimicrobial agents. N Engl J Med 1991;324:601–611.
46. Chanal C, Sirot D, Malaure H, et al. Sequences of CAZ-3 and CTX-2 extended spectrum beta-lactamase genes. Antimicrob Agents Chemother 1994;38:2452–2453.
47. Urban C, Meyer KS, Mariano N, et al. Identification of TEM-26 beta-lactamase responsible for a major outbreak of ceftazidime-resistant *Klebsiella pneumoniae.* Antimicrob Agents Chemother 1994;38:392–395.
48. Neu HC. Current mechanisms of resistance to antimicrobial agents in microorganisms causing infection in the patient at risk for infection. Am J Med 1984;76(5A):11–27.
49. Lodge JM, Piddock JV. The control of class I beta-lactamase expression in Enterobacteriaceae and *Pseudomonas aeruginosa.* J Antimicrob Chemother 1991;28:167–172.
50. Neu HC. The crisis in antibiotic resistance. Science 1992;257:1064–1073.
51. Newman KA, Tenney JH, Oken HA, et al. Persistent isolation of an unusual *Pseudomonas* species from a phenolic disinfectant system. Infect Control 1984;5:219–222.
52. Stolz S, Alvarado C, Maki DG. Pseudomonas bacteremia from contaminated LAK cells used in cancer chemotherapy: A new nosocomial problem [poster]. 3rd International Conference on Nosocomial Infections, Atlanta, July 31–August 3, 1990.
53. Cole CB, Weems JJ. Nosocomial *Pseudomonas cepacia* outbreak in intensive care due to contaminated ventilator temperature probes [poster]. 3rd International Conference on Nosocomial Infections, Atlanta, July 31–August 3, 1991.
54. Krapp H, Gerchens L, Sundelof JG, et al. Antibacterial activity of imipenem: The first thienamycin antibiotic. Rev Infect Dis 1985;7(suppl 3):S389–S410.
55. Maki DG, Klein BS, McCormick RD, et al. Nosocomial *Pseudomonas pickettii* bacteremias traced to narcotic tampering. JAMA 1991;265:981–986.
56. Rupp ME, Archer GL. Coagulase-negative staphylococci: Pathogens associated with medical progress. Clin Infect Dis 1994;19:231–245.
57. Wade JC, Schempff SC, Newman KA, et al. *Staphylococcus epidermidis:* An increasing cause of infection in patients with granulocytopenia. Ann Intern Med 1982;97:503–508.
58. Karchmer AW, Archer GL, Dismukes WE. *Staphylococcus epidermidis* causing prosthetic valve endocarditis: Microbiologic and clinical observations as guides to therapy. Ann Intern Med 1983;98:447–455.
59. Lowy FD, Chang D, Lash P. Synergy studies using combinations of vancomycin, gentamicin, or rifampin against methicillin-resistant coagulase-negative staphylococci. Antimicrob Agents Chemother 1983;23:932–934.
60. Freeman J, Goldman DA, Smith NE, et al. Association of intravenous lipid emulsion and coagulase-negative staphylococcal bacteremia in neonatal intensive care units. N Engl J Med 1990;323:301–308.
61. Klein JO. From harmless commensal to invasive pathogen—coagulase-negative staphylococci. N Engl J Med 1990;323:339–340.
62. Meyer RD. Legionnaires' disease: Aspects of nosocomial infection. Am J Med 1984;76:657–663.

63. Lowry PW, Blankenship R, Gridley W, et al. Transmission of *Legionella* extrapulmonary infections by bathing with contaminated tap water [abstract]. 3rd International Conference on Nosocomial Infections, Atlanta, July 31–August 3, 1990.
64. Hand WL, Sanford JP. *Mycobacterium fortuitum*—a human pathogen. Ann Intern Med 1970;73:971–977.
65. Levy C, Curtin JA, Watkins A, et al. *Mycobacterium chelanei* infection of porcine heart valves. N Engl J Med 1977;197:667–668.
66. Guggenbichler JP, Kofler J, Allerberger F. The influence of third-generation cephalosporins on the aerobic intestinal flora. Infections 1985;13(suppl):S137–S139.
67. Mulligan ME, Citron DM, McNamara BT, et al. Impact of cefoperazone therapy on fecal flora. Antimicrob Agents Chemother 1982;22:222–230.
68. Anaissie E, Bodey GP. Nosocomial fungal infections: Old problems and new challenges. Infect Dis Clin North Am 1990;3(4):867–882.
69. Walsh TJ, Pizzo PA. Nosocomial fungal infections: A classification for hospital-acquired fungal infections and mycoses arising from endogenous flora or reactivation. Ann Rev Microbiol 1988;42:517–545.
70. Rex JH, Benett JE, Sugar AM, et al. A randomized trial comparing fluconazole with amphotericin B for the treatment of candidemia in patients without neutropenia. N Engl J Med 1994;331:1325–1330.
71. Maki DG, Rhames FS, Mackel DC, et al. Nationwide epidemic of septicemia caused by contaminated intravenous products. I. Epidemiologic and clinical features. Am J Med 1976;60:471–485.
72. Goldman DA, Fuederson CC, Dixon RE, et al. Nationwide epidemic of septicemia caused by contaminated intravenous products. II. Assessment of the problem by a national nosocomial infection surveillance system. Am J Epidemiol 1978;108:207–213.
73. Maki DG. Nosocomial bacteremia, an epidemiologic overview, in Dixon RE (ed): Nosocomial Infection. New York, Yorke Medical Books, 1981, pp 183–196.
74. Ashcroft KW, Leape LL. Candida sepsis complicating parenteral feeding. JAMA 1970;212:454–456.
75. Goldman DA, Martin WT, Worthington JW. Growth of bacteria and fungi in total parenteral nutrition solutions. Am J Surg 1973;126:314–318.
76. Plouffe JF, Brown DG, Silva J, et al. Nosocomial outbreak of *Candida parapsilosis* fungemia related to intravenous infusion. Arch Intern Med 1977;137:1686–1689.
77. Zellmer W. Quality control in admixture services. Am J Hosp Pharm 1978;35:527.
78. Anonymous. ASHP gears up multistep action plan regarding sterile drug products. Am J Hosp Pharm 1991;48:386–388.
79. Anonymous. Draft technical assistance bulletin on quality assurance for pharmacy-prepared sterile products. Amer J Hosp Pharm 1993;50:1440–1461.
80. Anonymous. Accreditation Manual for Hospitals. Chicago, Joint Commission on Accreditation of Health Care Organizations, 1994, Volume II, Scoring Guidelines, Section 4, Infection Control, pp 1–21.
81. Sanders CC. Novel resistance selected by the new expanded spectrum cephalosporins: A concern. J Infect Dis 1983;147:585–589.
82. Livermore DM. Do β-lactamases "trap" cephalosporins? J Antimicrob Chemother 1985;14:511–521.
83. Costerton JW, Cheng K-J, Ladd TI, et al. Bacterial biofilms in nature and disease. Ann Rev Microbiol 1987;41:435–464.
84. Nichols WW. Biofilms, antibiotics and penetration. Rev Med Microbiol 1991;2:177–181.
85. Brown MRW, Gilbert P. Sensitivity of biofilms to antimicrobial agents. J Appl Bacterial Symp Suppl 1993;74:87S–97S.
86. Nichols WW, Dorrington SM, Slack MPE, Walmsley HL. Inhibition of tobramycin diffusion by binding to alginate. Antimicrob Agents Chemother 1988;32:518–523.
87. LeChevalier MW, Cawthon CD, Lee RG. Inactivation of biofilm bacteria. Appl Envir Bacteriol 1988;54:2492–2499.
88. Giwercman B, Jensen ET, Pedersen SS, Holby N. Induction of β-lactamase production in *Pseudomonas aeruginosa* biofilm. Antimicrob Agents Chemother 1990;35:1008–1010.
89. Costerton JW, Cheng KJ, Geesey KG, et al. Bacterial biofilms in nature and disease. Ann Rev Microbiol 1987;41:435–464.
90. Gorman SP, Adair CG, O'Neill F, et al. Influence of selective decontamination of the digestive tract on microbial biofilm on endotracheal tubes from artificially ventilated patients. Eur J Clin Microbiol Infect Dis 1993;12:9–17.
91. Anwar H, Dasgupta M, Lam K, Costerton JW. Tobramycin resistance of mucoid *Pseudomonas aeruginosa* biofilm grown under iron limitation. J Antimicrob Chemother 1988;24:647–655.
92. Elliott TSJ, Faroqui MH. Infections and intravascular devices Br J Hosp Med 1992;4:496–503.
93. Smith SR, Cheesbrough J, Spearing R, Davies JM. Randomized prospective study comparing vancomycin and teicoplanin in the treatment of infections associated with Hickman catheters. Antimicrob Agents Chemother 1989;33:1193–1197.
94. Mawhinney WM, Adair CG, Gorman SP. Development and treatment of peritonitis in continuous peritoneal dialysis. Int J Pharm Pract 1991;1:10–18.
95. Gorman SP, Adair CG, Mawhinney WM. Incidence and nature of peritoneal catheter biofilm determined by electron and confocal scanning laser microscopy. Epidemiol Infect 1994;112:551–559.

PART FOUR

Oncologic Disorders

Chapter 119

Basic Principles of Cancer Treatment and Cancer Chemotherapy

Carol Balmer, PharmD, and Amy Wells Valley, PharmD

Cancer is a group of more than 100 different diseases, characterized by uncontrolled cellular growth, local tissue invasion, and distant metastases.[1,2] It is second only to cardiovascular disease in causes of mortality in Americans. More than 1.2 million cases of cancer are diagnosed annually, and cancer claims more than 500,000 lives in the United States each year.[3] The estimated incidence of common cancers and cancer-related deaths is illustrated in Figs. 119.1 and 119.2. In 1995, the three most common cancers in men were prostate, lung, and colorectal cancer. In women, breast, lung, and colorectal cancers were most common. The most common cause of cancer-related deaths in both men and women in the United States is lung cancer, which claims more than 153,000 lives each year. These cancers are discussed in further detail in the chapters that follow.

The role of the pharmacist in the management of the cancer patient can be very diverse. Thorough knowledge of antineoplastic drug pharmacology and pharmacokinetics is essential in order to prevent and manage many drug-induced toxicities. Supportive care issues such as nutritional support, pain management, infection, and nausea and vomiting require application of both clinical and pharmacologic principles. Investigational drugs are employed at many institutions to further the search for effective treatment options. The pharmacist is often involved in the procurement, maintenance, and dispensing of these new agents. Provision of drug information is another critical role for the oncology pharmacist. This service is provided to other health professionals and to patients and their families. Experienced pharmacists are well equipped to fulfill these roles and make valuable contributions to patient care in the oncology setting.

This chapter (1) introduces the basic concepts of carcinogenesis, tumor growth, and cancer treatment; (2) provides general information on the pharmacology and clinical use of the antineoplastic agents; and (3) presents an overview of supportive care issues in the oncology patient.

Etiology of Cancer

CARCINOGENESIS

The mechanism by which cancers occur is not completely understood. A cancer, or neoplasm, is thought to develop from a cell in which the normal mechanisms for control of growth and proliferation are altered. Current evidence supports the concept of carcinogenesis as a multistage process that is genetically regulated (Fig. 119.3).[2,4,5] The first step in this process is *initiation,* which requires exposure of normal cells to carcinogenic substances. These carcinogens produce genetic damage that, if not repaired, results in irreversible cellular mutations. This mutated cell has an altered response to its environment and a selective growth advantage, giving it the potential to develop into a clonal population of neoplastic cells. During the second phase, known as *promotion,* carcinogens or other factors alter the environment to favor growth of the mutated cell over normal cells. The primary difference between initiation and promotion is that promotion is a reversible process. In fact, because it is reversible, the promotion phase may be the target of future chemoprevention strategies, including changes in lifestyle and diet. At some point, however, the mutated cell becomes cancerous (conversion). Depending on the type of cancer, months to years may elapse between the two carcinogenic phases and the development of a clinically detectable cancer. The final stage of neoplastic growth, called *progression,* involves further genetic changes leading to increased cell proliferation. The critical elements of this phase include tumor invasion into local tissues and the development of metastases.

Substances that may act as carcinogens or initiators include chemical, physical, and biologic agents. Exposure to chemicals may occur by virtue of occupational and environmental means, as well as lifestyle habits. The association of aniline dye exposure and the subsequent develop-

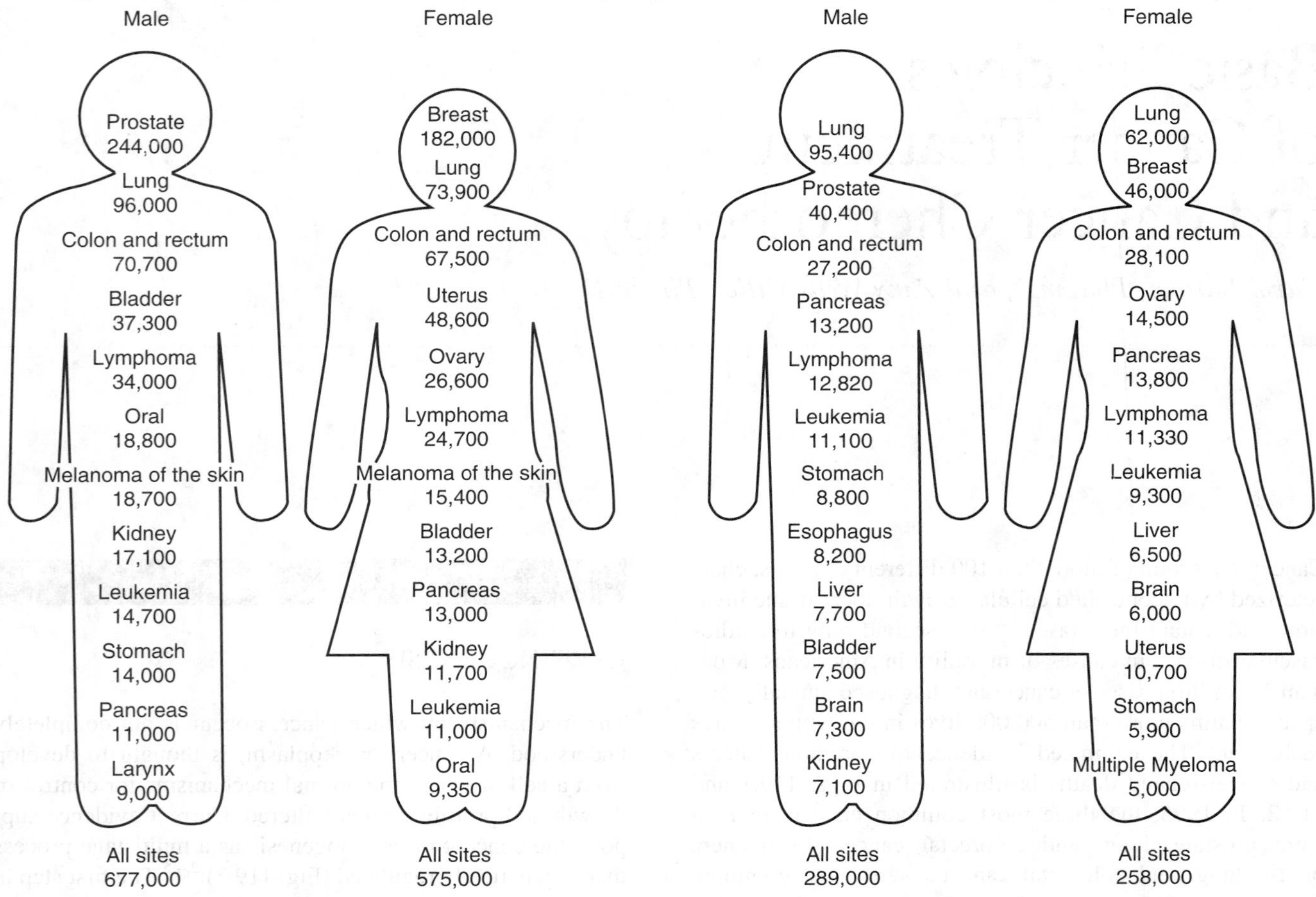

Figure 119.1. Cancer incidence by site and sex. *(From Cancer Facts and Figures—1995. American Cancer Society, Atlanta, 1995, with permission.)*

Figure 119.2. Cancer deaths by site and sex. *(From Cancer Facts and Figures—1995. American Cancer Society, Atlanta, 1995, with permission.)*

ment of bladder cancer is one such example. Sufficient data exist to support the role of benzene in the development of some leukemias.[6] Some drugs and hormones may also be classified as carcinogenic chemicals (Table 119.1).[4,6–8] Physical agents that may act as carcinogens include ionizing radiation and ultraviolet light. These types of radiation induce mutations by forming free radicals that damage DNA and other cellular components. Viruses are considered biologic agents and have also been associated with certain cancers.[8] The Epstein–Barr virus is believed to be an important factor in the initiation of African Burkitt's lymphoma. Likewise, infection with hepatitis B virus is known to be a major cause of hepatocellular cancer. All the aforementioned carcinogens, as well as age, sex, diet, growth factors, and chronic irritation, are among the factors considered to be promoters of carcinogenesis.[4,5,8]

ONCOGENES

Recent explorations into the etiology of cancer have centered on the role of oncogenes, or genes that cause cancer.[2,9–14] There are two major classes of genes involved in carcinogenesis, oncogenes and tumor suppressor genes, which are compared in Table 119.2. Oncogenes develop from normal genes, termed proto-oncogenes, and may have important roles in all of the four phases of carcinogenesis (i.e., initiation, promotion, conversion and progression) previously outlined.[2,9] Proto-oncogenes are present in all cells and are essential regulators of normal cellular functions, including the cell cycle. Genetic alteration of the proto-oncogene through point mutations, insertions, deletions, or chromosomal translocations may activate the oncogene. These genetic alterations may be caused by carcinogenic agents such as radiation, chemicals, or viruses (Fig. 119.3). Once activated, the oncogene may produce excessive amounts of the normal gene product, or an aberrant gene product. The result is dysregulation of normal cell growth and proliferation, which imparts a distinct growth advantage to the cell and increases the probability of neoplastic transformation. An example is the *myc* family of oncogenes. The normal gene product of *myc* acts as a signal for cellular proliferation. As an oncogene, the gene product is overexpressed or amplified, resulting in excessive cellular

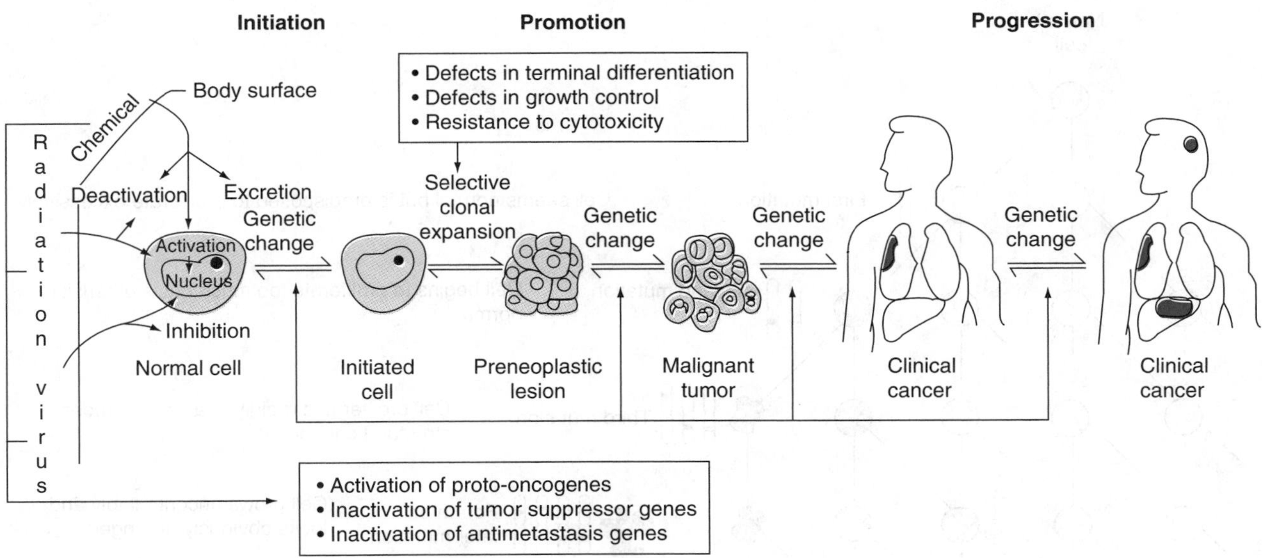

Figure 119.3. Multistage model of carcinogenesis. *(Adapted from Shields PG, Harris CC. Principles of carcinogenesis: chemical, in DeVita VT, Jr, Hellman S, Rosenberg SA, [eds]: Cancer: Principles and Practice of Oncology, 4th ed. Philadelphia, JB Lippincott, 1993, p 201.)*

proliferation. Expression of *myc* has been noted in Burkitt's lymphoma, and carcinomas of the breast, lung, and cervix.

Another type of oncogene has recently been identified. These oncogenes interfere with the normal mechanisms involved in programmed cell death, also known as apoptosis.[13,15] Apoptosis (pronounced "ay-puh-TOE-sis") is a normal mechanism of cell death required for tissue homeostasis and is distinct from cell necrosis. This process is regulated by oncogenes and tumor suppressor genes and is also a mechanism of cellular death after exposure to cytotoxic agents. Overexpression of oncogenes responsible for apoptosis may produce an "immortal" cell, which has increased potential for malignancy. The *bcl-2* oncogene is an example. The most common chromosomal abnormality found in lymphoid malignancies is the t(14;18) translocation. The *bcl-2* proto-oncogene is normally located on chromosome 18. Translocation of this proto-oncogene to chromosome 14 in proximity to the immune globulin heavy gene leads to overexpression of *bcl-2,* which decreases apoptosis and confers a survival advantage to the cell.

TABLE 119.1. SELECTED DRUGS AND HORMONES THAT ARE KNOWN OR POTENTIAL CARCINOGENS

Chemical or Drug	Associated Malignancy
Alkylating agents (cyclophosphamide, melphalan, chlorambucil, carmustine, thiotepa)	Leukemia, bladder
Coal tars	Skin
Diethylstilbestrol	Vagina (clear cell carcinoma), cervix
Epipodophyllotoxins (etoposide, teniposide)	Leukemia
Estrogen	Liver (premenopausal) Endometrium (postmenopausal)
Immunosuppressive drugs (cyclosporine, azathioprine)	Lymphoma, skin
Procarbazine	Skin
Tamoxifen	Endometrium

(Adapted from Refs. 4 and 6.)

TABLE 119.2. CHARACTERISTICS OF ONCOGENES AND TUMOR SUPPRESSOR GENES

Characteristic	Proto-Oncogenes	Tumor Suppressor Genes
Normal function	Transcription factors or signal transduction	Inhibit growth and proliferation, negative regulation of cell cycle
Gene expression	Dominant	Recessive
Number of mutations for carcinogenesis	One	Two
Function of mutated allele	Gain of function	Loss of function
Tissue specificity	Some, but may be present in many tissues	Extensive tissue specificity
Germline inheritance	Rarely involved in carcinogenesis	Frequently involved in carcinogenesis
Examples	Myc, Ras, Abl	Rb (retinoblastoma gene), p53

(Adapted from Refs. 6, 12, and 13.)

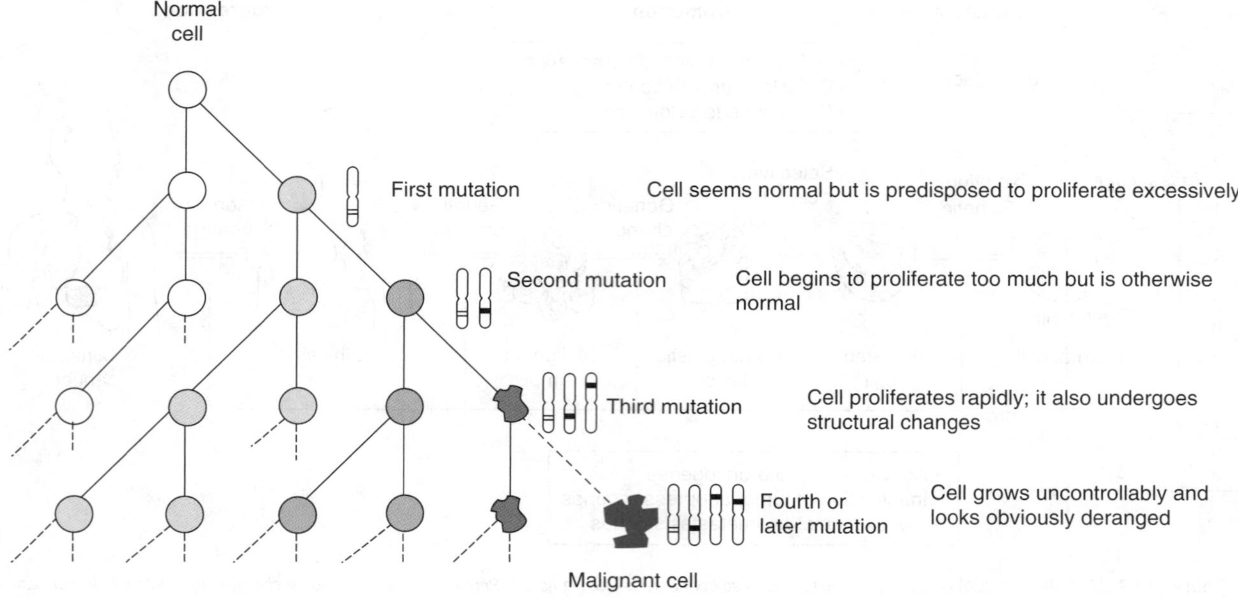

Figure 119.4. Emergence of a cancer cell from a normal cell is thought to occur through a process known as clonal evolution. First, one daughter cell inherits or acquires a cancer-promoting mutation and passes the defect to its progeny and all future generations. At some point, one of the descendants acquires a second mutation, and a later descendant acquires a third and so on. Eventually, some cell accumulates enough mutations to cross the threshold to cancer. *(From Cavenee WK, White RL. The genetic basis of cancer. Scientific American, March 1995, pp 72–79, with permission.)*

Tumor suppressor genes are another category of genes involved in carcinogenesis.[10–12,14] The normal function of these genes is to regulate and inhibit inappropriate cellular growth and proliferation. Gene loss or mutation can result in loss of control over normal cell growth. Two common examples of tumor suppressor genes are the retinoblastoma *(Rb)* and *p53* genes. Mutation of *p53* is one of the most common genetic changes associated with cancer. The normal gene product of *p53* is responsible for negative regulation of the cell cycle, allowing the cell cycle to halt for repairs, corrections, and responses to other external signals. Inactivation of *p53* by various mechanisms removes this checkpoint, allowing mutations to occur. Studies have also shown that *p53* may be a regulator of apoptosis. Loss of *p53* disrupts normal apoptotic pathways, imparting a survival advantage to the cell. Another important function of *p53* may be in modulation of cytotoxic drug effects. Loss of *p53* has been associated with antineoplastic drug resistance. Mutation of *p53* has been linked to a variety of malignancies, including brain tumors (astrocytoma); carcinomas of the breast, colon, and lung; and osteosarcoma. Antimetastasis genes have also recently been detected. Loss of these genes results in increased potential for metastasis. An example of this type of gene is the *nm23* gene.

As information regarding the role of oncogenes and tumor suppressor genes accumulated, it became evident that a single mutation was probably not sufficient to initiate cancer. Scientists postulated that combinations of mutations were required for carcinogenesis and that each mutation was inherited by the next generation of cells (Figs. 119.3 and 119.4). Thus, in an established tumor there may be several detectable genetic mutations. Early mutations are found in both premalignant lesions and established tumors, while later mutations are found only in the established tumor. This theory of sequential genetic mutations resulting in cancer has been best demonstrated in colon cancer and in brain tumors.[14] In colon cancer, the initial genetic mutation is believed to be loss of the *APC* (adenomatous polyposis coli) gene, which results in formation of a small benign polyp. Oncogenic mutation of the *ras* gene is often the next step, leading to enlargement of the polyp. Loss of the *p53* gene and another gene, believed to be the *DCC* (deleted in colorectal cancer) gene, complete the transformation into a malignant lesion.

Identification of genes involved in carcinogenesis has several important clinical implications. In the future, they may be used in cancer screening to identify individuals at increased risk for cancer and in cancer treatment to design new anticancer agents and gene therapies. If the presence of these genes is found to predict reliably the clinical course or response to certain cancer therapies, then genetic analysis may become an important prognostic and treatment decision tool.

Principles of Tumor Growth

TUMOR GROWTH

The study of tumor growth forms the foundation for many of the basic principles of modern cancer chemotherapy. The growth of most tumors is characterized by the Gompertzian tumor growth curve (Fig. 119.5).[16–18] Gompertz was a German insurance actuary who described the relationship between age and expected death. This mathematical model also approximates tumor cell proliferation. In the early stages, tumor growth is exponential, which means that the tumor takes a constant amount of time to double its size. During this early phase, a large portion of the tumor cells is actively dividing. This population of cells is called the growth fraction. The doubling time, or time required for the tumor to double in size, is very short. Because most anticancer drugs have a greater activity on rapidly dividing cells, tumors are most sensitive to the effects of chemotherapy when the tumor is small, and the growth fraction is high.[17] However, as the tumor grows, the doubling time is slowed.[18] The growth fraction is decreased, probably due to the tumor outgrowing its blood and nutrient supply, or the inability of blood and nutrients to diffuse throughout the tumor mass. Wide variability exists in measured doubling times for different cancers. The doubling time of most solid tumors is approximately 2–3 months. However, Burkitt's lymphoma, a very aggressive tumor, has a doubling time of only 1 day.[19,20]

TUMOR BURDEN

The impact of tumor burden is also illustrated by Fig. 119.5. It takes 10^9 cancer cells (1 gram mass, 1 cm in diameter) in order for the tumor to be clinically detectable by palpation or radiography. Such a tumor has undergone approximately 30 doublings in cell number. It only takes 10 additional doublings for this 1 gram mass to reach 1 kg in size. A tumor possessing 10^{12} cancer cells (1 kg mass) is considered lethal. Thus, a tumor is clinically undetectable for most of its life span. As the tumor grows beyond 10^9 cells, doubling time declines. Tumor burden also relates to response to chemotherapy. The cell kill hypothesis states that a certain *percentage* of cancer cells (not a certain *number* of cells) will be killed with each course of chemotherapy. For example, if a tumor consists of 1000 cancer cells and the chemotherapy regimen kills 90% of the cells, then 10% or 100 cancer cells would remain. The second chemotherapy course kills another 90% of cells, and again only 10% or 10 cells remain. According to this hypothesis, the tumor burden will never reach absolute zero. Tumors consisting of less than 10^4 cells are believed to be small enough for elimination by host factors, including immunologic mechanisms, and these factors must be in place for a cure to be possible. The limitations of this theory are that it assumes all cancers are equally responsive, and that drug resistance and metastases do not occur.[18,20]

Metastasis is the spread of neoplastic cells from the primary tumor site to distant sites. Despite advances in diagnostic techniques and screening for cancer, an average of 30% of patients will have detectable metastatic disease at diagnosis. Once clinically evident distant metastases are present, cancers are seldom curable. Another 30% of newly diagnosed cancer patients have microscopic cancer metastases.[21,22] Although undetectable, these small clusters of disease must be present, as many patients subsequently relapse at distant sites despite removal of the primary tumor. Some patients with micrometastatic disease may be cured with systemic chemotherapy. All totaled, at least 60%

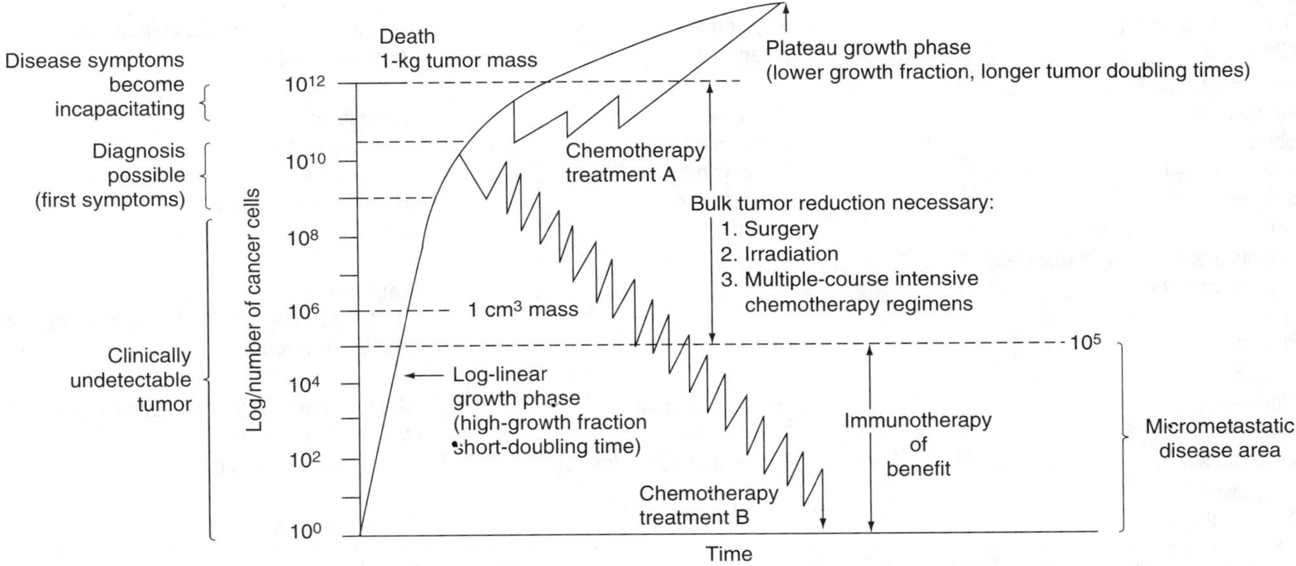

Figure 119.5. Gompertzian kinetics tumor growth curve. Relationship to symptoms, diagnosis, and various treatment regimens. *(From Buick RN. Cellular basis of chemotherapy, in Dorr RT, Von Hoff DD [eds]: Cancer Chemotherapy Handbook, 2nd ed. New York, Elsevier, 1994, p 8, with permission.)*

of cancer patients will have some form of metastatic disease at diagnosis.

The two primary pathways of metastasis are hematogenous and lymphatic. Tumors are constantly shedding neoplastic cells into the systemic circulation or surrounding lymphatics. This process may begin early in the life of the tumor and often increases with time. The time course for metastasis depends largely on the biology of the tumor. Breast cancer, for example, tends to metastasize very early. Not all of the shed cancer cells, or "seeds," result in a metastatic lesion. The "seed" must first find the appropriate "soil," or an environment suitable for growth. This process is illustrated in the diverse patterns of metastasis that are characteristic of individual types of cancer. An example is prostate cancer, which commonly metastasizes to bone, but rarely to the brain. To form a successful metastasis, the disseminated cell must first attach to the vascular endothelium and invade the basement membrane. This new colony of cancer also will stimulate the formation of new blood vessels to provide oxygen and nutrients, a process known as angiogenesis. Because angiogenesis has been recognized as a critical element in tumor growth as well as metastasis, it has become a target for development of new anticancer agents. At every step of the way, the potential metastatic cell must fight the host immune system. Other less common modes of disease spread include dissemination via cerebrospinal fluid, and transabdominal spread within the peritoneal cavity.

Pathology of Cancer

TUMOR CHARACTERISTICS

Tumors may be either benign or malignant. Benign tumors are noncancerous growths that are often encapsulated, localized, and indolent. Cells of benign tumors resemble the cells from which they developed. These masses seldom metastasize and, once removed, they rarely recur. In contrast, malignant tumors invade and destroy the surrounding tissue. In fact, the name "cancer" arose from the first descriptions of malignancies in which claw-like projections were noted to be extending from the central tumor. These claws resembled those of a crab, or cancer. The cells of malignant tumors are genetically unstable and loss of normal cell architecture results in cells that are atypical of their tissue or cell of origin. These cells lose the ability to perform their usual functions. This loss of structure and function is defined as anaplasia. Malignant tumors tend to metastasize and, consequently, recurrences are common after removal or destruction of the primary tumor.

TUMOR ORIGIN

Tumors may arise from any of four basic tissue types: epithelial tissue, connective tissue (i.e., blood, bone, and cartilage), muscle tissue, and nerve tissue. Although some

TABLE 119.3. TUMOR CLASSIFICATION BY TISSUE TYPE

Tissue of Origin	Benign	Malignant
Epithelial		
Surface epithelium	Papilloma	Carcinoma (squamous, epidermoid)
Glandular	Adenoma	Adenocarcinoma
Connective tissue		
Fibrous tissue	Fibroma	Fibrosarcoma
Bone	Osteoma	Osteosarcoma
Smooth muscle	Leiomyoma	Leiomyosarcoma
Striated muscle	Rhabdomyoma	Rhabdomyosarcoma
Fat	Lipoma	Liposarcoma
Lymphoid tissue and hematopoietic cells		
Bone marrow elements		Leukemias
Lymphoid tissue		Hodgkin's disease, non-Hodgkin's lymphoma
Plasma cell		Multiple myeloma
Neural tissue		
Glial tissue	"Benign" gliomas	Glioblastoma multiforme, astrocytoma
Nerve sheath	Neurofibroma	Neurofibrosarcoma
Melanocytes	Pigmented nevus (mole)	Malignant melanoma
Mixed tumors		
Gonadal tissue	Teratoma	Teratocarcinoma

(From Robbins SL, Cotran RS, Kumar V. Pathologic Basis of Disease, 3rd ed. Philadelphia, WB Saunders, 1984, with permission.)

malignant cells are atypical of their cells of origin, the involved cells usually retain enough of their parent's traits to identify their origin. Benign tumors are named by adding the suffix *-oma* to the name of the cell type. Hence, adenomas are benign growths of glandular origin, or growths that exhibit a glandular pattern. A list of common tumor nomenclature by tissue type is presented in Table 119.3.[23]

Some cancers are preceded by cellular changes that are abnormal, but not yet malignant. Detection of these early changes could potentially prevent the occurrence of a cancer. Precancerous lesions may be described as consisting of either hyperplastic or dysplastic cells. Hyperplasia is an increase in the number of cells in a particular tissue or organ, which results in an increased size of the organ. It should not be confused with hypertrophy, which is an increase in the size of the individual cells. Hyperplasia occurs in response to a stimulus and reverses when the stimulus is removed. Dysplasia is defined as an abnormal change in the size, shape, or organization of cells or tissues. Hyperplasia and dysplasia may precede the appearance of a cancer by several months or years.

Malignant cells are divided into those of epithelial origin or the other tissue types. Carcinomas are malignant growths arising from epithelial cells. Malignant growths of muscle or connective tissue are called sarcomas. Therefore, an adenocarcinoma is a malignant tumor arising from glandular origin. Another term used frequently in the description of malignancy is the term carcinoma *in situ.* In this instance, the cancer is limited to the epithelial cells of origin; it has not yet invaded the basement membrane. Carcinoma *in situ* is a preinvasive stage of malignancy, and most tumors have progressed well beyond this stage at diagnosis. Like all classification systems, there are exceptions to these rules. Malignancies of hematologic origin are separately classified. Leukemias and lymphomas are discussed in later chapters.

Diagnosis and Staging

SCREENING

Because cancers are most curable with surgery or radiation before they have metastasized, early detection and treatment have obvious benefit. In addition, small tumors are more responsive to chemotherapy, as discussed previously. Early diagnosis is difficult for many cancers because they do not produce clinical signs or symptoms until they have become large or have metastasized. Lack of effective screening methods for some cancers and inaccessibility of some anatomic sites further complicate the process. Education of the public on the early warning signs of common cancers is extremely important in order to facilitate early detection. For some cancers, effective screening procedures do exist. The Pap smear test, for example, has been proven to be an effective tool to detect cervical cancer in its early stages. Self-examination of the breasts in women and of the testicles in men may lead to early diagnosis of cancers in these organs. The American Cancer Society has published guidelines for routine screening examinations. These recommendations are listed in Table 119.4.[24]

DIAGNOSIS

The presenting signs and symptoms of cancer vary widely and depend on the type of cancer. The presentation in adults may include one of cancer's seven warning signs, as well as pain and loss of appetite (Table 119.5).[25] The warning signs of cancer in children are different, and reflect the types of tumors more common in this patient population (Table 119.6).[26] Even with increased public awareness, the fear of a cancer diagnosis can deter patients from seeking medical attention. The definitive diagnosis of cancer relies on the procurement of a sample of the tissue or cells suspected of malignancy and pathologic assessment of this sample. This sample can be obtained by biopsy, exfoliative cytology, or fine needle aspiration. A tissue diagnosis is essential, since many benign conditions can masquerade as cancer. Definitive treatment should not begin without a pathologic diagnosis.

STAGING

In addition to tissue diagnosis, all tumors should be staged to determine the extent of disease before any definitive treatment is initiated.[27] The process is dictated by knowledge of the biology of the tumor and patient signs and symptoms elicited in the history and physical examination. Staging provides information on prognosis and dictates treatment selection. Once treatment is begun, the initial staging workup may be repeated in order to evaluate the effectiveness of the treatment. Uniform staging criteria are imperative in clinical research aimed at developing and evaluating cancer treatment regimens. Staging has been valuable in learning more about the biology of various tumor types. A staging workup may involve x-rays, computed tomography (CT) scans, magnetic resonance imaging (MRI), ultrasounds, bone marrow biopsies, bone scans, lumbar puncture (LP), and a variety of laboratory tests, including appropriate tumor markers. Some cancers produce antigens, or other substances, which are characteristic of that particular cancer. These so-called tumor markers are often nonspecific and may be elevated in patients with more than one type of cancer, or in nonmalignant diseases. As a result, tumor markers are generally more useful for monitoring response and detecting recurrence than as diagnostic

TABLE 119.4. RECOMMENDATIONS FOR EARLY DETECTION OF CANCER IN AN ASYMPTOMATIC PERSON

Test or Procedure	Sex	Age (yr)	Frequency
Sigmoidoscopy	M and F	Over 50	Every 3–5 years
Stool guaiac test	M and F	Over 50	Every year
Digital rectal exam	M and F	Over 40	Every year
Prostate-specific antigen (PSA)	M	Over 50 Under 50 if high risk[a]	Every year
Pap test and pelvic exam	F	18–65 Under 18 if sexually active	Every year[b]
Endometrial biopsy	F	At menopause or at high risk[c]	At menopause
Breast self-examination	F	Over 20	Monthly
Breast physical examination	F	20–40 Over 40	Every 3 years Every year
Mammography	F	By age 40 40–49 Over 50	Baseline Every 1–2 years Every year
Chest x-ray			Not recommended
Sputum cytology			Not recommended
Health counseling and cancer checkup[d]	M and F	20–40 Over 40	Every 3 years Every year

[a]High risk includes African-Americans and men with strong familial predisposition.
[b]After three negative annual examinations, the Pap test may be done at less frequent intervals, as determined by the physician.
[c]High risk includes patients with history of infertility, obesity, failure to ovulate, abnormal uterine bleeding, or estrogen or tamoxifen therapy.
[d]To include examination for cancers of the mouth, thyroid, testicles, skin, lymph nodes, prostate, and ovaries. (From The American Cancer Society Recommendation for the Early Detection of Cancer in Asymptomatic People, No. 3251, Revised 11/92, with permission.)

tools. Examples are the measure of human chorionic gonadotropin (HCG) and alpha-fetoprotein (AFP) in patients with testicular cancer, or prostate-specific antigen (PSA) in prostate cancer.

The most commonly applied staging system for solid tumors is the TNM classification, where T = tumor, N = node, and M = metastases. A numerical value is assigned to each letter to indicate the size or extent of disease. The designated rating for tumor describes the size of the primary mass and ranges from T_1 to T_4. Carcinoma *in situ* is designated T_{is}. Nodes are described in terms of the extent and quality of nodal involvement (N_0 to N_3). Metastases are scored depending on their presence or absence (M_0 or M_1). Using this system, any tumor could have possibly 24 TNM categories (e.g., $T_1N_1M_0$, $T_2N_1M_0$, $T_3N_1M_0$, etc.). To simplify the staging process, most cancers are classified according to extent of disease by a numerical system involving stages I through IV. In this system, stage I is localized tumor, stages II/III represent local and regional extension of disease, and stage IV denotes the presence of distant metastases. The criteria for classifying disease extent are quite specific for each different type of cancer. The assigned TNM rating translates into a particular stage classification. For example, in general, a $T_3N_1M_0$ tumor is a moderate to large sized primary mass, with regional lymph node involvement, and no distant metastases, and for most cancers is stage III. An example of the staging system for colon cancer is outlined in Table 119.7.[27]

TABLE 119.5. CANCER'S SEVEN WARNING SIGNS

Change in bowel or bladder habits
A sore that does not heal
Unusual bleeding or discharge
Thickening or lump in breast or elsewhere
Indigestion or difficulty in swallowing
Obvious change in wart or mole
Nagging cough or hoarseness

If YOU have a warning signal, see your doctor!

TABLE 119.6. CANCER'S WARNING SIGNS IN CHILDREN

Unexplained or persistent **lump**
Unexplained or persistent **limp**
Unexplained normocytic **anemia**
Unexplained thrombocytopenic **bruising**
Unexplained **weight loss**
Abdominal **mass**
Unexplained persistent **headache** and/or **vomiting** on awakening

(Adapted from Ref. 26.)

TABLE 119.7. TNM STAGING CLASSIFICATION SYSTEM FOR COLORECTAL CANCER

Primary Tumor (T)

T_x Primary tumor cannot be assessed
T_0 No evidence of primary tumor
T_{is} Carcinoma in situ
T_1 Tumor invades submucosa
T_2 Tumor invades muscularis propria
T_3 Tumor invades through the muscularis propria into the subserosa, or into nonperitonealized pericolic or perirectal tissues
T_4 Tumor perforates the visceral peritoneum, or directly invades other organs or structures

Regional Lymph Nodes (N)

N_x Regional lymph nodes cannot be assessed
N_0 No regional lymph node metastasis
N_1 Metastasis in one to three pericolic or perirectal lymph nodes
N_2 Metastasis in four or more pericolic or perirectal lymph nodes
N_3 Metastasis in any lymph node along the course of a named vascular trunk

Distant Metastasis (M)

M_x Presence of distant metastasis cannot be assessed
M_0 No distant metastasis
M_1 Distant metastasis

Stage Grouping				**Dukes**
Stage 0	T_{is}	N_0	M_0	
Stage I	T_1	N_0	M_0	A
	T_2	N_0	M_0	
Stage II	T_3	N_0	M_0	B
	T_4	N_0	M_0	
Stage III	Any T	N_1	M_0	C
	Any T	N_2,N_3	M_0	
Stage IV	Any T	Any N	M_1	

(From the American Joint Committee on Cancer. Manual of Staging of Cancer, 3rd ed. Philadelphia, JB Lippincott, 1988, with permission.)

Modalities of Cancer Treatment

Four primary modalities are employed in the approach to cancer treatment: surgery, radiation, chemotherapy, and immunotherapy. The oldest of these is surgery, which plays a major role in the diagnosis and treatment of cancer. Surgery remains the treatment of choice for many solid tumors diagnosed in the early stages.[28] Radiation therapy was first used for cancer treatment in the late 1800s, and remains a mainstay in the management of cancer. More than one-half of patients with cancer will receive radiation therapy at some point in their illness.[29] Although very effective for treating many types of cancer, surgery and radiation are local treatments. These modalities are likely to produce a cure in patients with truly localized disease. However, since the majority of patients with cancer have metastatic disease at diagnosis, localized therapies often fail to completely eliminate the cancer. In addition, systemic diseases such as leukemia cannot be treated with a localized modality. Chemotherapy and hormonal therapy access the systemic circulation and can theoretically treat the primary tumor, as well as any metastatic disease. The 1990s have seen rapid advances in biotechnology and the application of immunologic principles to cancer treatment. Immunotherapy provides another means to deliver systemic anticancer therapy. This modality usually involves stimulating the host's immune system to fight against the cancer. Most of the agents in this category are naturally occurring cytokines, which have been produced using recombinant DNA technology. Agents used in immunotherapy include BCG vaccine, levamisole, interferons, and interleukins. These drugs are discussed in detail elsewhere in this chapter.

Many cancers may be apparently eliminated by surgery or radiation. However, the high incidence of later recurrence implies that the primary tumor begins to metastasize before it is removed. These early metastases are too small to detect with currently available diagnostic tests and are known as micrometastases. Adjuvant chemotherapy is defined as chemotherapy that is given to eradicate micrometastatic disease, following localized modalities such as surgery or radiation, or both. The hope is that chemotherapy given in this setting will reduce subsequent recurrence rates and prolong long-term survival. Thus, adjuvant chemotherapy is given to patients with potentially curable malignancies, who have no clinically detectable disease after surgery or radiation. Because adjuvant therapy is given at a time that the cancer is undetectable, its effectiveness cannot be measured by response rates. Instead, it is evaluated by recurrence rates and survival. Adjuvant chemotherapy has been most extensively studied in the management of breast cancer. Chemotherapy may also be given in the neoadjuvant preoperative setting. The goal in this instance is to make other treatment modalities more effective by reducing tissue damage or by decreasing tumor burden, as well as destroying micrometastases. In head and neck cancer, neoadjuvant chemotherapy is employed in an attempt to shrink large tumors and make them more amenable to later surgical resection.

The management of most types of cancer involves the use of combined modalities. Breast cancer is a good example of the use of a combined modality approach. The primary tumor is removed surgically, and radiation therapy is delivered to the remaining breast (after lumpectomy) or to the axilla (if there is marked lymph node involvement). Adjuvant chemotherapy with or without hormonal therapy is then administered to eradicate any micrometastatic disease. Figure 119.6 illustrates the principles of combined modality therapy and rationale for adjuvant and neoadjuvant chemotherapy.[30]

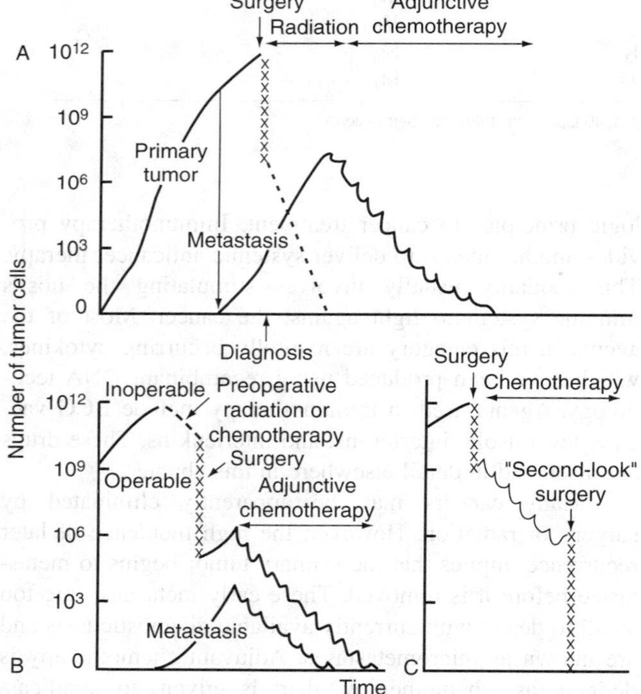

Figure 119.6. Rationale for combined modality approach. (A) Effect of combination surgery, radiation, and adjuvant chemotherapy. Example: breast cancer. (B) Effect of neoadjuvant chemotherapy in an inoperable tumor, followed by surgery and adjuvant chemotherapy. Example: head and neck cancer. (C) Effect of second look surgery following surgery and chemotherapy. Example: ovarian cancer. *(From Bleyer WA. Antineoplastic drugs, in Yaffe SJ [ed]: Pediatric Pharmacology: Therapeutic Principles in Practice. New York, Grune and Stratton, 1980, pp 349–378, with permission.)*

PRINCIPLES OF CHEMOTHERAPY

PURPOSES OF CHEMOTHERAPY

The era of modern cancer chemotherapy was born in 1941, when Goodman and Gilman first administered nitrogen mustard to patients with lymphoma.[31] Since that time, numerous antineoplastic agents have been developed, and a variety of chemotherapy regimens have been investigated in every type of cancer. The responsiveness of common tumors to chemotherapy is summarized in Table 119.8.[32] Cancer chemotherapy may be indicated as a primary, palliative, adjuvant, or neoadjuvant treatment modality. Treatment with cytotoxic drugs is the primary curative modality for a few diseases, including leukemias, choriocarcinomas, and testicular cancer. Most solid tumors are not curable with chemotherapy alone, either because of the biology of the tumor or because of advanced disease. Chemotherapy in this setting is often initiated for palliative purposes. It is often possible to decrease tumor size or retard growth enough to reduce untoward symptoms caused by the tumor. Adjuvant and neoadjuvant chemotherapy are defined in the previous section.

RESPONSE CRITERIA

The response to chemotherapy and other treatment modalities may be described as a *cure, complete response, partial response, stable disease,* or *progression.*[33] These terms are used routinely in oncology to define the response to chemotherapy and other treatment modalities. A cure implies that the patient is entirely free of disease and has the same life expectancy as a cancer-free individual. Although there is no way to be absolutely certain that an individual patient is cured, a stable plateau in the survival curve after cancer treatment is taken as evidence of cure. For most cancers, the survival curves have plateaued by approximately 5 years. Thus, 5 years of survival without disease recurrence is equated with a cure. However, there are some malignancies, such as breast cancer and melanoma, for example, in which patients are still at significant risk for relapse after 5 years.

Complete response (CR) means complete disappearance of all cancer and no evidence of new disease for at least 1 month after treatment. The terms "cure" and "CR" are not synonymous. Although an individual must have a CR in order to be cured, many individuals who achieve a CR will eventually relapse from growth of clinically undetectable disease. A partial response (PR) is defined as a 50% or greater decrease in the tumor size or other objective disease markers, and no evidence of any new disease for at least 1 month. Overall objective response rates for a given

TABLE 119.8. RESPONSIVENESS OF SPECIFIC TUMORS TO CHEMOTHERAPY

Tumors Curable in Advanced Stages by Chemotherapy	
Choriocarcinoma	Wilm's tumor
Acute lymphocytic leukemia (in children and adults)	Burkitt's lymphoma
Hodgkin's disease	Embryonal rhabdomyosarcoma
Intermediate grade lymphomas	Ewing's sarcoma
Lymphoblastic lymphoma (in children and adults)	Neuroblastoma
Acute myelogenous leukemia	Testicular cancer
Tumors Curable in the Adjuvant Setting by Chemotherapy	
Breast cancer	Soft tissue sarcoma
Osteogenic sarcoma	Colorectal cancer
Tumors Responsive in Advanced Stages But Not Yet Curable	
Bladder cancer	Endometrial cancer
Chronic myelogenous leukemia	Adrenocortical cancer
Chronic lymphocytic leukemia	Prostate cancer
Hairy cell leukemia	Breast cancer
Multiple myeloma	Carcinoid tumors
Low-grade lymphomas	Glioblastoma multiforme
Gastric carcinoma	Head and neck cancer
Cervical carcinoma	Soft tissue sarcoma
Small cell lung cancer	
Tumors Poorly Responsive in Advanced Stages to Chemotherapy	
Osteogenic sarcoma	Colorectal cancer
Pancreatic cancer	Non–small cell lung cancer
Renal cancer	Metastatic melanoma
Thyroid cancer	Hepatocellular carcinoma
Carcinoma of the vulva or penis	

(Adapted from Devita VT, Jr. Principles of chemotherapy, in DeVita VT Jr, Hellman S, Rosenberg SA (eds): Cancer: Principles and Practice of Oncology, 3rd ed. Philadelphia, JB Lippincott 1989, pp 276–300, with permission.)

treatment are determined by adding the CR and PR rates. A patient whose tumor size neither grows nor shrinks significantly has stable disease. Despite the small changes in tumor size, some patients may experience subjective improvement in the symptoms caused by their cancer. While clinically important, this does not indicate a true response. Progression of disease is defined as a 25% increase in the tumor size or the development of any new lesions while receiving treatment. These definitions are applicable for solid tumors, but diseases such as the leukemias and multiple myeloma are not characterized by discrete, measurable masses. Responses in these diseases are measured by elimination of abnormal cells (e.g., return to normal hematology parameters and normal bone marrow in leukemia), return of tumor markers to normal levels (e.g., normal serum protein electrophoresis in multiple myeloma), disappearance of pleural or peritoneal effusions, or improved function of affected organs (e.g., improved renal function after obstructive uropathy).

FACTORS AFFECTING RESPONSE TO CHEMOTHERAPY

These include tumor burden, tumor cell heterogeneity, drug resistance, dose intensity, and patient-specific factors. The significance of tumor burden has been discussed earlier. Tumors consist of a heterogenous population of cell types. Because of the genetic instability of cancer cells compared to normal cells, mutations commonly occur during cell division. Large tumors have undergone multiple cell divisions and, hence, multiple cell mutations resulting in genetically varied cell populations.[34] In 1979, Goldie and Coldman[35] proposed that these cytogenetic changes were not completely random and were highly associated with the development of the ability to resist drug action. The probability of developing resistant cell populations increases as tumor size increases. It is believed that a small percentage of resistant cancer cells may exist in a tumor and survive initial chemotherapy. This resistant population later proliferates and eventually may become the dominant cell type. This explains the relative frequency of an initial response to chemotherapy, followed by progressive tumor regrowth despite continuing the same treatment regimen.

Drug resistance may be either an acquired or inherited property of a neoplastic cell. Mechanisms of drug resistance include decreased activation of prodrugs, decreased uptake of drugs secondary to alterations in drug transport systems, change in the target enzymes, alterations in the cell's ability to repair drug-induced damage, and increased drug inactivation.[36] Research in the area of drug resistance currently focuses on pleiotropic drug resistance, or multidrug resistance (MDR).[36,37] When some cancer cells are exposed to increasing concentrations of an antineoplastic agent *in vitro,* they become resistant to this agent. Surprisingly, these same cells also become resistant to other structurally unrelated antineoplastic agents. Cytotoxic agents derived from natural products, such as the anthracyclines, actinomycin D, mitomycin C, the vinca alkaloids, the epipodophyllotoxins, and the taxanes, have been shown to produce MDR. The resistant cancer cells have been shown to possess a membrane associated protein known as P170 or P-glycoprotein, which appears to enhance the export of toxins, such as chemotherapy agents, out of the cell (Fig. 119.7). The gene that encodes for P-glycoprotein is known as the *MDR1* gene. Expression of this gene is amplified in cells that are resistant to the natural products listed previously. P-glycoprotein is also found in high concentrations in tumors that are traditionally resistant to chemotherapy (e.g., renal cell and lung cancers), and thus may also be an important mechanism of intrinsic or inherited drug resistance. Several drugs are being investigated as possible inhibitors of this efflux pump, such as the calcium channel blockers, quinidine, cyclosporine, and the phenothiazines. Another efflux pump, known as the multidrug resistance-

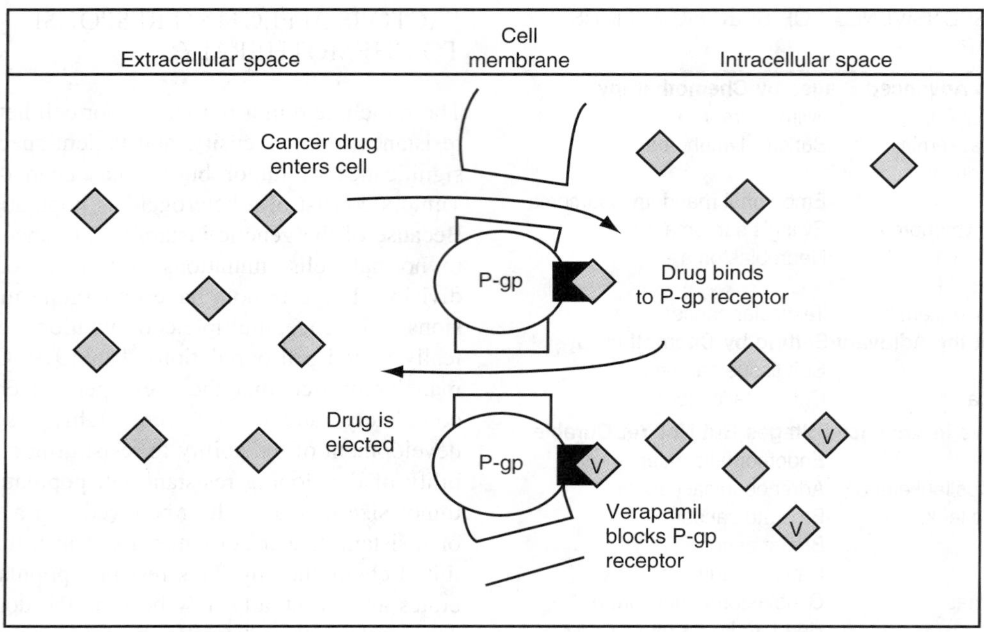

Figure 119.7. P-glycoprotein (P-gp) is a membrane associated protein which acts as a drug efflux pump. Anticancer agents enter the cell, bind to the P-gp receptor and are ejected. Some agents which modify multidrug resistance, like verapamil, block the P-gp receptor, allowing the anticancer agent to remain in the cell. *(Adapted from Refs. 36 and 37.)*

associated protein (MRP) has also recently been identified. Other potential mechanisms of drug resistance include inactivation of chemotherapy agents by glutathione metabolism and decreased apoptosis after exposure to chemotherapy. The latter mechanism is mediated by *bcl-2* oncogene overexpression or loss of the *p53* gene, as discussed in the oncogene section.

The relationship between dose and response has been extensively explored in the arena of cancer chemotherapy. Dose is believed to be a critical factor in determining response for many types of cancers.[38] The concept of dose intensity is defined as the dose delivered to the patient over a specified period of time.[39,40] The delivery of optimal dose intensity is compromised by the toxicities of the oncologic drugs. Treatment cycles are commonly delayed due to inadequate recovery from drug toxicity, especially myelosuppression. Subsequent doses of chemotherapy are often reduced to prevent or reduce the severity of these toxicities. The impact of this issue on patient outcome has been proven in studies showing reduced rates of response and survival in individuals receiving less than optimal chemotherapy doses.[41,42] The development of drug- and toxicity-specific chemoprotective agents may aid in the application of the dose intensity principles.[43] The colony-stimulating factors avert myelosuppression and permit delivery of dose-intensive regimens that are usually compromised by this toxicity. Monitoring of antineoplastic drug concentrations may also improve the therapeutic index. Pharmacokinetic and pharmacodynamic modeling has been associated with improved responses and decreased toxicity in children with acute leukemia.[44] The issue of dose intensity is brought into a new light in the era of high-dose chemotherapy with autologous bone marrow support. Although lethal myelosuppression is avoided by administration of bone marrow, other severe end-organ toxicities emerge as the antineoplastic doses are increased.

Patient-specific factors create unpredictable variables in predicting response to chemotherapy. The biology of cancer is strongly affected by host characteristics and genetics. Interindividual variations in drug absorption or metabolism, for example, may lead to sub- or supertherapeutic levels of antineoplastic agents and their metabolites.[45] As a result, both drug efficacy and drug toxicity can be affected. Underlying nononcologic disease states may also affect response to treatment by limiting treatment options. The overall functional status of a patient may be assessed using performance status scales, such as the Karnofsky and ECOG scales (Table 119.9).[46,47] These scales can be used to predict patient tolerance of chemotherapy, as well as to assess the effects of chemotherapy on the patient's level of activity and quality of life. In many cancers, performance status is the most important prognostic indicator.

COMBINATION CHEMOTHERAPY

Although single-agent therapy is sometimes employed, more commonly the approach to chemotherapy involves

TABLE 119.9. PERFORMANCE STATUS SCALES

Description: Karnofsky Scale	Karnofsky Scale %	Zubrod Scale (ECOG)[a]	Description: ECOG Scale
No complaints; no evidence of disease	100	0	Fully active, able to carry on all predisease activity
Able to carry on normal activity; minor signs or symptoms of disease	90		
Normal activity with effort, some signs or symptoms of disease	80	1	Restricted in strenuous activity, but ambulatory and able to carry out work of a light or sedentary nature
Cares for self; unable to carry on normal activity or to do active work	70		
Requires occasional assistance but is able to care for most personal needs	60	2	Out of bed more than 50% of time; ambulatory and capable of self-care, but unable to carry out any work activities
Requires considerable assistance and frequent medical care	50		
Disabled; requires special care and assistance	40	3	In bed more than 50% of time; capable of only limited self-care
Severely disabled; hospitalization indicated, although death not imminent	30		
Very sick; hospitalization necessary; requires active supportive treatment	20	4	Bedridden; cannot carry out any self-care, completely disabled
Moribund; fatal processes progressing rapidly	10		
Dead	0		

[a]ECOG, Eastern Cooperative Oncology Group. (Adapted from Refs. 46 and 47.)

administration of multiple agents.[48] This approach is based on the Goldie–Coldman hypothesis, which addresses the issue of tumor cell heterogeneity and the inevitable development of drug resistance. Combination chemotherapy is employed to target as many types of cells in the tumor as possible. Selection of agents for combination chemotherapy regimens involves consideration of drug-specific factors such as mechanism of action, antitumor activity, and toxicity profile. Drugs that possess minimally overlapping mechanisms of action and toxicities are combined, when possible. Myelosuppressive combinations are sometimes alternated with nonmyelosuppressive combinations to allow bone marrow recovery, but still gain additive antitumor effects. The selected agents should each have significant activity against the tumor that is to be treated. If a synergistic reaction is known to exist for two agents, they may be combined in various treatment regimens.

CLINICAL PHARMACOLOGY OF CANCER CHEMOTHERAPY AGENTS

CELL CYCLE

Both cancer cells and normal cells reproduce themselves in a series of steps known as the cell cycle.[19,49] Figure 119.8 depicts the cell cycle and the phases of activity for commonly used antineoplastic agents. The first phase is mitosis (M). Mitosis lasts for approximately 30–60 minutes and during this phase, cell division occurs. After mitosis, the cell may enter a dormant phase (G_0), or proceed to the first gap phase (G_1). G_0 is the largest variable in the cell cycle, and during this resting phase, the cell is not actively committed to cell division. Some stimulus results in the cell entering the first gap phase (G_1). During G_1, the cell prepares for DNA synthesis by manufacturing necessary enzymes. DNA synthesis (S) occurs next, and this phase lasts 10–20 hours. The percentage of cells in the S phase can be measured by flow cytometry and is an indicator of the rate of tumor cell proliferation. Tumors with a high percentage of S-phase cells are aggressively growing. The synthesis phase is followed by a second gap or premitotic phase (G_2), lasting 2–10 hours. During this second gap, the cell prepares for mitosis by producing RNA and specialized proteins, as well as the mitotic spindle apparatus. The cycle then begins again with the M phase. Most normal human cells exist in the G_0 phase, and most cancer cells are not sensitive to the effects of chemotherapy when in this stage. The cell cycle is regulated by external mitogens, including lymphokines, hormones, and growth factors. As mentioned earlier, some of the genes that regulate the cell cycle are known to be proto-oncogenes and tumor suppressor genes.

All cancer cells do not proliferate faster than normal cells; some cancer cells reproduce more rapidly, and others are more indolent. Many anticancer drugs target rapidly proliferating cells (both normal and cancerous cells) and these agents may act at selective or multiple sites of the cell cycle. Agents with major activity in a particular phase of the cell cycle are known as cell cycle

1. Vinca alkaloids
   Vincristine, vinblastine, vinorelbine
2. Taxanes
   Paclitaxel, docetaxel

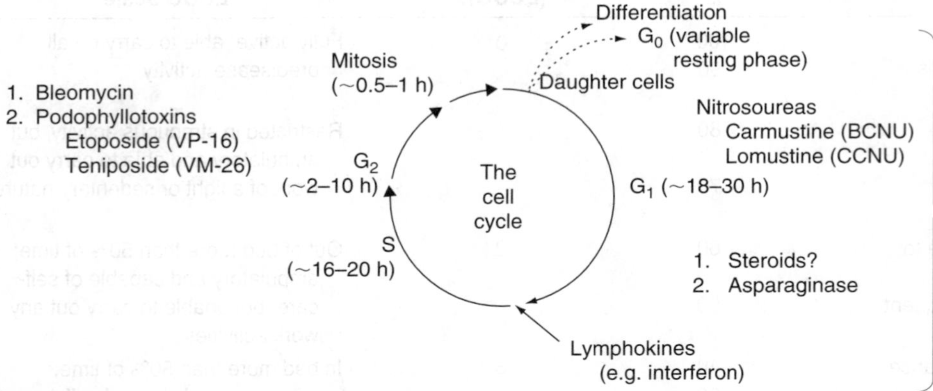

Cell cycle (phase) nonspecific agents
1. Classic alkylating agents (mechlorethamine, melphalan, busulfan, chlorambucil cyclophosphamide, ifosfamide)
2. Anthracycline antibiotics (doxorubicin, daunorubicin, idarubicin)
3. Miscellaneous (dacarbazine, cisplatin)
4. Nitrosoureas (also G0)
5. Mitomycin C
6. Dactinomycin

Antimetabolites
1. Antifolates (methotrexate)
2. Antipyrimidines (cytarabine, fluorouracil)
3. Antipurines (mercaptopurine, thioguanine, fludarabine, chlorodeoxyadenosine)
4. Miscellaneous (hydroxyurea, procarbazine)
5. Steroids? (also G1)

Figure 119.8. Cell cycle activity for anticancer drugs. Cell cycle (phase)-specific agents appear to be most active during a particular phase, but may also be active in another phase. Cell cycle (phase)-nonspecific agents may have greater activity in one phase than another, but not to the degree of cell cycle (phase)-specific agents. In many cases, it is likely that drug cytotoxicity involves multiple intracellular sites of action, and may not be linked to specific cell cycle events.

phase-specific agents. The antimetabolites exert their major effect during the S phase. Cell cycle phase-specific agents may also be active to a lesser extent in other phases of the cycle. Cell cycle phase-nonspecific agents are those with significant activity in multiple phases. The alkylating agents, such as nitrogen mustard, are examples. In many cases, the cytotoxic effect of a drug may be due to interactions with other intracellular activities and is not related to specific cell cycle events. Hormonal agents are an example of this type of drug.

Knowledge of cell cycle specificity has been applied to the scheduling of chemotherapy administration. By definition, phase-specific agents exert their major activity when cells are in a particular phase of the cell cycle. At any given time, the heterogenous cell populations within a tumor are at various stages in the cell cycle. By giving phase-specific agents as a continuous infusion or in multiple repeated fractions, it is theoretically possible to target more cells by allowing them to progress to the drug-sensitive phase. Thus, phase-specific agents are also termed schedule dependent. In contrast, cell cycle phase-nonspecific drugs are active at any stage and, consequently, are not schedule dependent. The activity of this group of drugs is dependent on the magnitude of the dose, and these drugs are termed dose dependent.[17]

MOLECULAR BIOLOGY

Because many antineoplastic agents interfere with the cellular synthesis of DNA, RNA, and proteins, it is important to review the basic principles of molecular biology.[50,51] Each normal human cell contains 46 chromosomes, which are composed of DNA (deoxyribonucleic acid). Hereditary information is carried by DNA in units called genes. A single chromosome can contain 20,000 genes. Genes code for specific proteins that regulate cellular activity and inherited traits. The genetic information is encoded in DNA by precise sequencing of subunits known as nucleotides. Each nucleotide consists of a sugar (deoxyribose), phosphoric acid, and a base. Four bases exist in DNA: adenine, thymine, guanine, and cytosine. Adenine and guanine are purine type bases; thymine and cytosine are pyrimidine type bases (Fig. 119.9). These nucleotides are connected linearly to form a chain. Each DNA molecule is made up of two chains of nucleotides, which wind around each other to form a double helix (Fig. 119.10). The two strands are held together by chemical bonding between the bases. The bonding process is very specific; adenine binds only with thymine, and guanine binds only with cytosine. This is known as complementary base-pairing. RNA (ribonucleic acid) is important in the DNA-directed synthesis of proteins

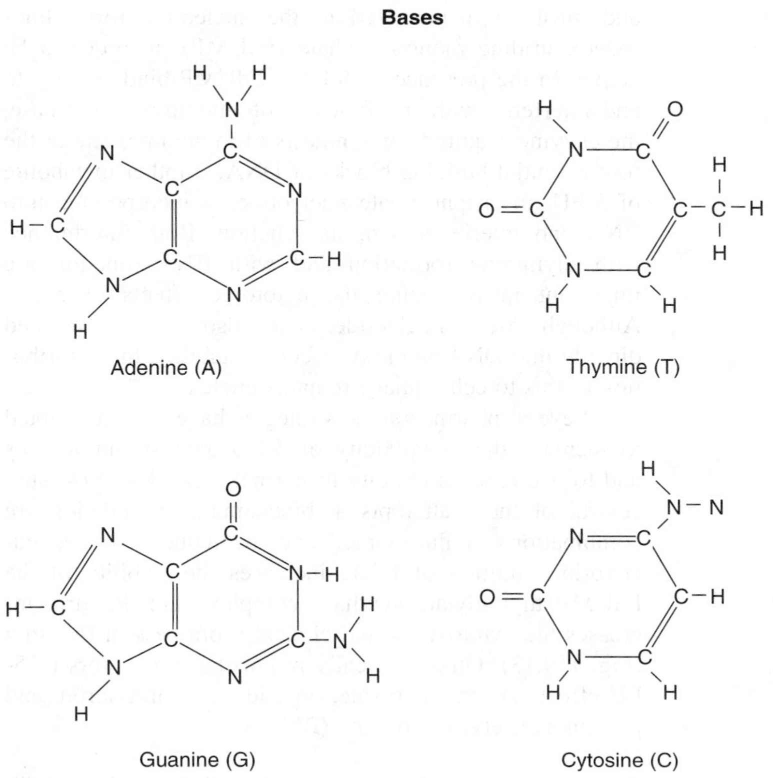

Bases

Adenine (A) Thymine (T)

Guanine (G) Cytosine (C)

Figure 119.9. Structures of DNA constituents.

or enzymes. RNA differs from DNA in that it is composed of a single strand of nucleotides; the sugar is ribose, and the base uracil is substituted for thymine. There are three known types of RNA, messenger RNA (mRNA), transfer RNA (tRNA), and ribosomal RNA (rRNA).

DNA SYNTHESIS

During the DNA synthesis phase, which takes place in the cell nucleus, the DNA unwinds and exposes its nucleotides. When DNA unwinds for replication or protein synthesis, only the portion of the molecule containing the needed nucleotides needs to be exposed. Rather than unwinding the entire strand, topoisomerase I and II enzymes cleave the DNA strands to facilitate unwinding of the section in demand. The enzyme DNA polymerase matches free complementary nucleotides from the environment to the exposed nucleotides of the DNA (Fig. 119.9). The newly created strands rewind, resulting in two complete double helices. The topoisomerase enzymes are responsible for resealing the cleaved DNA strands.

PROTEIN SYNTHESIS

Proteins consist of chains of amino acids in a very specific sequence. The synthesis of proteins is a more complex process. As in DNA synthesis, the double helix must unwind. However, in protein synthesis, only the portion of the DNA molecule that codes for the desired protein is exposed. The enzyme RNA polymerase matches free complementary RNA nucleotides to the exposed DNA nucleotides, and the resultant chain of nucleotides is called mRNA. This process is called *transcription.* The mRNA travels to ribosomes in the cytoplasm, where protein synthesis occurs. Each three nucleotides of the mRNA chain compose a codon, whose sequence is specific for a particular amino acid. The codon is recognized by tRNA, which then carries the amino acid to the ribosome where it is added to the growing peptide chain. This process is known as *translation.* The completed protein is then ready for its intended use as an enzyme or as a structural component.

CATEGORIES OF ANTICANCER AGENTS

Agents used in cancer chemotherapy are commonly categorized by their mechanism of action or by their origin. The alkylating agents exert their effects on DNA and protein synthesis by binding to DNA and preventing the unwinding of the DNA molecule. The antimetabolites resemble naturally occurring metabolites, such as the nucleotide bases, or inhibit enzymes involved in the synthesis of DNA and proteins. Antitumor antibiotics gain their name from their

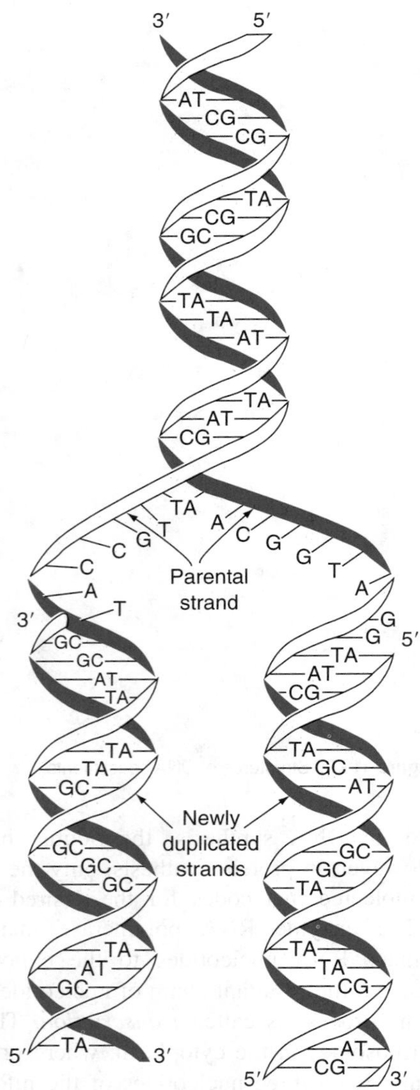

Figure 119.10. Structure of DNA. *(Adapted from Ref. 51.)*

source of derivation; they are fermentation products of *Streptomyces* species. Figure 119.11 depicts the sites of activity of common categories of antineoplastic agents.[31] The following section discusses these classes of agents and the most commonly used cytotoxic agents in the treatment of cancer.

ANTIMETABOLITES

Fluorinated Pyrimidines

Fluorouracil

Fluorouracil (5-FU) is a fluorinated analogue of the naturally occurring pyrimidine, uracil, and was originally synthesized in the late 1950s (Fig. 119.12).[52] It is a prodrug and must be metabolized to the nucleotide form, fluorodeoxyuridine monophosphate (FdUMP), in order to be active. In the presence of folates, FdUMP binds tightly to and interferes with the function of thymidylate synthase, the enzyme required for synthesis of thymidine, one of the four essential building blocks of DNA. Another metabolite of 5-FU, the triphosphate nucleotide, is incorporated into RNA and interferes with its function. Both interference with thymidine formation and with RNA function are important in producing the cytotoxic effects of 5-FU. Although 5-FU nucleotides can also be incorporated directly into DNA and may affect its stability, the contribution of this to cell damage remains unclear.[52–54]

Several pharmacologic strategies have been attempted to increase the cytotoxicity of 5-FU against tumor cells and to decrease its toxicity to normal cells. The most successful of these attempts at biochemical modulation are combinations of fluorouracil and the reduced folate, leucovorin. Addition of folate increases the stability of the FdUMP–thymidylate synthase complex, and, in turn, increases the cytotoxicity and clinical usefulness of the drug (Fig. 119.13). Other clinically promising modulators of 5-FU effects are methotrexate, dipyridamole, interferon, and phosphonoacetyl-L-aspartate (PALA).[54,55]

Pharmacokinetics. Fluorouracil is distributed rapidly throughout the body and also is cleared rapidly from the plasma. Ninety percent of its elimination is accounted for by metabolism. It is catabolized by the enzyme dihydropyrimidine dehydrogenase. Deficiency of this enzyme has recently been associated with increased toxicity (and potentially efficacy) of 5-FU.[56] Catabolism takes place primarily in the liver and in the kidneys, although lung tissue is also an important site of 5-FU metabolism. Because some of the clearance of 5-FU is extrahepatic and only small amounts of drug are excreted unchanged in the urine, dose adjustment is not known to be necessary in hepatic or renal dysfunction. The kinetics of fluorouracil are nonlinear, and clearance is more rapid in women than in men. With such potential variability in kinetic behavior of 5-FU, adaptive control of drug exposure using therapeutic drug monitoring techniques is proving to be increasingly useful in targeting 5-FU doses, especially during continuous infusions.[53,54,57]

Clinical Uses. Fluorouracil is useful systemically in the treatment of several solid tumors, especially breast cancer, colorectal carcinomas, and other gastrointestinal tumors, and squamous cell cancers of the head and neck. Regional delivery of 5-FU via the hepatic artery can produce sustained responses in patients with colorectal cancer metastasized to the liver. 5-FU is also administered topically for treatment of actinic keratoses and noninvasive skin cancers.[54,58]

Toxicity and Management. Clinical toxicity of 5-FU is a function of the schedule, dose, and route of administration. It

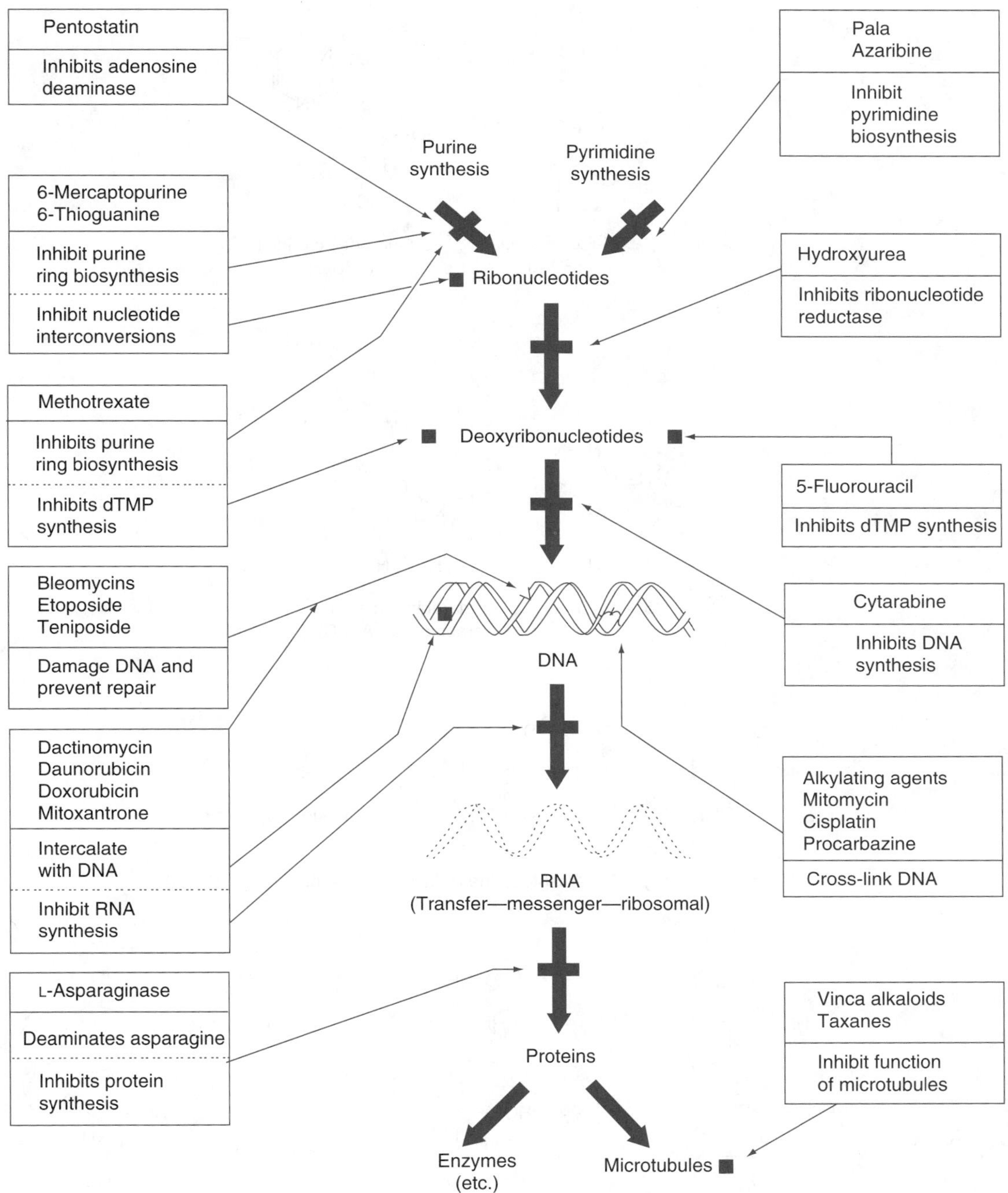

Figure 119.11. Summary of the mechanism and sites of action of selected chemotherapeutic agents useful in neoplastic disease. *(From Calabresi P, Chabner BA. Chemotherapy of neoplastic diseases, in Gilman AG, Rall TW, Nies AS, et al [eds]: Goodman & Gillman's The Pharmacologic Basis of Therapeutics, 8th ed. New York, Pergamon Press, 1990, p 1208, with permission.)*

is most typically administered either as an intravenous bolus or as continuous intravenous infusion. Higher total doses are tolerated by continuous infusion compared with bolus regimens. The toxicity pattern differs by the schedule of administration. The dose-limiting toxicity after bolus administration is myelosuppression, which especially affects white blood cells and platelets. In continuous infusion regimens, and in combination regimens with leucovorin, mucosal damage is dose limiting, and myelosuppression is less prominent. Diarrhea and stomatitis secondary to mucosal damage can be life threatening, with elderly women at greatest risk.[59] Severe diarrhea necessitates dose reduction, but octreotide may be useful in symptomatic treatment of 5-FU–induced diarrhea.[60] Dermatologic toxicities, including hyperpigmen-

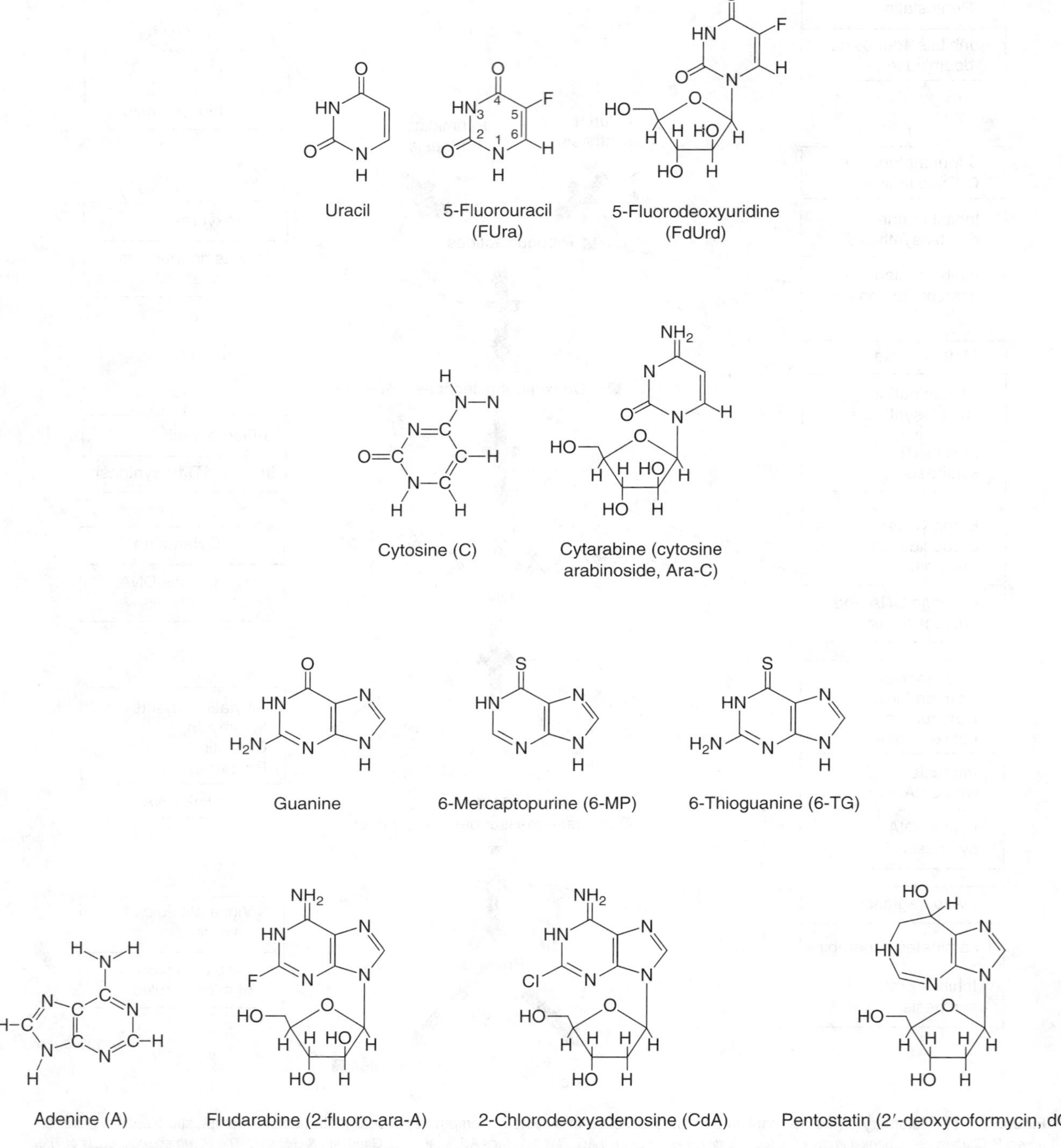

Figure 119.12. Structures of natural purines and pyrimidines, and their structural analogues. *(Adapted from Pratt WB, Ruddon RW, Ensminger WD, Maybaum J, eds. The Anticancer Drugs, 2nd ed. New York, Oxford University Press, 1994, pp 82, 87, 92, 93, 96, with permission.)*

tation, alopecia, photosensitivity, and nail banding, can also occur. Ocular toxicity manifests as excessive tearing, itching, and burning, all of which are well-recognized effects. Application of ocular ice packs before and during the 5-FU bolus administration may decrease the severity of this toxicity.[61] Nausea and vomiting are generally mild and easily controlled with antiemetics. Major organ toxicity has been increasingly recognized with 5-FU administration. Cardiac toxicity, most commonly manifest as myocardial ischemia, occurs in about 2% of patients receiving 5-FU and may exceed 5% in patients receiving high-dose continuous infusions.[62,63] Recently, mild and reversible hepatic toxicity has been noted in nearly 40% of patients receiving 5-FU and levamisole as adjuvant therapy for colorectal cancer. Asymp-

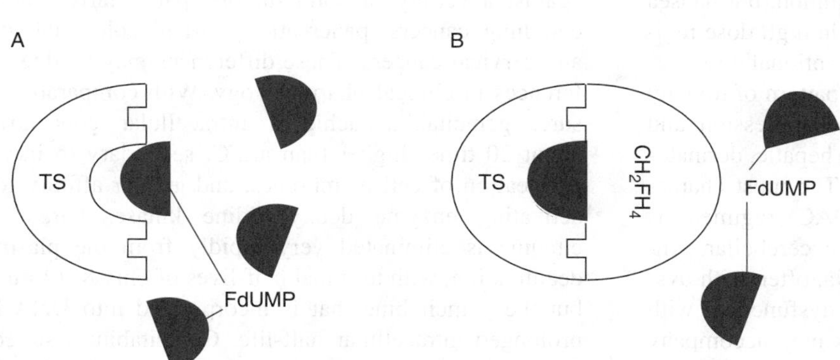

Figure 119.13. Interaction of leucovorin and 5-fluorouracil. (A) Binding of FdUMP to thymidylate synthase (TS) in the absence of folate cofactor. In the absence of the folate cofactor, which is supplied by leucovorin, FdUMP binds poorly to the enzyme TS. Therefore, DNA synthesis is not adequately inhibited, resulting in poor cytocidal outcome. (B) Binding of FdUMP to TS in presence of folate cofactor. In the presence of the folate cofactor, a very stable ternary complex is formed, made up of FdUMP, TS, and the folate cofactor methylenetetrahydrofolate (CH_2-FH_4 folate.) By binding available TS and making it unavailable for DNA synthesis, the cytocidal outcome is significantly enhanced. *(From Bertino JR, Knobf T, Remington JS. Leucovorin: Interaction of leucovorin with 5-fluorouracil. Burroughs Wellcome, 1985, monograph WE-49, pp 1–6, with permission.)*

tomatic elevations of alkaline phosphatase are the most common abnormalities.[64]

Floxuridine

Floxuridine (FUDR) is the deoxyribonucleoside derivative of fluorouracil, and is converted to 5-FU in the body. Its mechanisms are believed to be identical to those of 5-FU, although it is a more potent inhibitor of thymidylate synthase activity. Its toxicities, especially mucosal damage, are also similar.

Clinical use of FUDR was limited for many years to regional administration, particularly intra-arterial infusions into the liver, where dosing is limited by biliary toxicity.[52–54,65] Now systemic administration is more widely used, particularly in treatment of renal cell cancer. Mucosal toxicity of FUDR infusion can be decreased by administration of time-modified rate-adjusted infusions, according to circadian patterns of drug metabolism.[66]

Cytidine Analogues

Cytarabine

Cytarabine (arabinosyl cytosine, cytosine arabinoside, ara-C) is an arabinose analogue of cytosine, one of the four key nucleoside bases that make up DNA. Arabinose nucleosides differ from the normal human nucleosides only by the orientation of one hydroxyl group in the sugar portion of the nucleoside (Fig. 119.12). Cytarabine was originally isolated from sponges, but is now produced synthetically.

Ara-C has many effects on DNA synthesis. It penetrates cells by a carrier-mediated process and is phosphorylated to its active triphosphate form (ara-CTP) within tumor cells by a series of enzymatic steps. Once within the cell, ara-CTP inhibits the enzyme DNA polymerase, responsible for strand elongation. It is also incorporated directly into DNA, where it inhibits the replication of DNA and acts as a chain terminator to prevent DNA elongation. The extent of formation of ara-CTP and/or the ability of leukemic cells to retain ara-CTP may correlate with response rates and duration in patients with acute nonlymphocytic leukemias. Activation of ara-C is opposed by deaminase enzymes, particularly cytidine deaminase, which degrades ara-C to an inactive form, ara-U.[52,54,67]

Pharmacokinetics. Ara-C is water soluble and distributes rapidly into total body water after administration. It enters the central nervous system (CNS) readily and achieves concentrations equal to 20–40% of simultaneous plasma levels. Cytidine deaminase, which degrades ara-C, is present in only very low levels in the brain and cerebral spinal fluid, resulting in a prolonged half-life of ara-C elimination of 2–3 hours in the CNS after intrathecal administration. Cytidine deaminase is widely present in the liver, plasma, white blood cells, and the gastrointestinal tract, however, and disappears rapidly from plasma after intravenous administration, with a half-life of only a few minutes. Its metabolite, ara-U, has a longer elimination half-life of 3–6 hours. Increased concentrations of deaminase enzymes present in tumor cells may account for the resistance of some cancers to the antitumor effects of ara-C. Cytarabine is well absorbed after subcutaneous injection, but has very low oral bioavailability, because it is rapidly destroyed by enzymes in the gastrointestinal tract.[57,68]

Clinical Uses. Cytarabine is an antitumor agent of narrow specificity. It is most useful clinically in the treatment of acute leukemias, especially acute nonlymphocytic leukemia (ANLL), in combination with anthracene derivatives. The standard doses for ANLL induction therapy are 100–200 mg/m^2 for 5–7 days, administered by continuous infusion to provide sustained levels. A dose-response effect is evident in management of ANL, and high-dose regimens—2–3 g/m^2 as a short (1–3 hour) infusion twice daily for 3–6 days—may be effective in patients who are refractory or resistant to standard dose regimens, and as intensive postremission therapy.[69] Cytarabine is also valuable in management of lymphomas, and intraperitoneally for ovarian cancers, but does not have significant activity against most solid tumors. Direct CNS administration is valuable for treatment of meningeal involvement with leukemias and lymphomas.[67,68]

Toxicity. The dose-limiting toxicity of cytarabine in conventional schedules is myelosuppression, which particularly affects granulocytes. Alopecia is common, but nausea is dose related, and becomes severe only in high-dose regimens. Major organ damage is rare in conventional dose regimens, but at high doses, a very different pattern of toxicity emerges. In addition to profound myelosuppression and severe nausea, characteristic CNS, ocular, hepatic, dermatologic, and pulmonary toxicities emerge. The most characteristic toxicity of high-dose ara-C (HDAC) regimens is CNS damage, typically manifesting as a cerebellar syndrome of dysarthria, nystagmus, and ataxia, often with dysdiadochokinesia and dysmetria. Cerebral dysfunction, with generalized encephalopathy, and seizures may accompany the cerebellar syndrome or occur independently. CNS toxicity has been documented in up to 40% of patients receiving HDAC, although severe toxicity is estimated to occur in 10–14%. Cerebellar toxicity is usually reversible, resolving over several days after cytarabine discontinuation, but may be permanent, and is occasionally fatal. Risk of CNS toxicity is most convincingly correlated with advanced age. Hepatic dysfunction, high cumulative doses, and renal insufficiency may also increase the risks of neurotoxicity.[68,70–72] It is possible that renal insufficiency permits accumulation of high levels of ara-CTP, which is believed to be neurotoxic. Dose reductions are advised in patients with renal insufficiency, but optimal dosing in these patients has not been determined.[73,74] Intrathecal administration of cytarabine can also produce CNS dysfunction, particularly when administered in conjunction with high systemic ara-C doses or cranial radiation.

Other toxicities characteristic of HDAC are chemical conjunctivitis, which can be prevented or managed by application of steroid eye drops or saline eye washes, intrahepatic cholestasis, and dermatologic toxicity consisting most characteristically of plantar-palmar or acral erythema.[70] Pulmonary toxicity may be related to a capillary leak syndrome. Respiratory distress and noncardiogenic pulmonary edema typically present suddenly, a few days to a month after treatment with HDAC. It may be particularly common in pediatric patients, and more frequently fatal.[75,76]

Gemcitabine

Gemcitabine (difluorodeoxycytidine, LY-188011) is a fluorine-substituted deoxycytidine analogue closely related structurally to cytarabine. Its activation and mechanism of action are similar to cytarabine, with phosphorylation to the active diphosphate and triphosphate forms necessary for antitumor effect. Gemcitabine is incorporated into DNA, where it causes inhibition of DNA polymerase activity. It also inhibits ribonucleotide reductase, blocking conversion of ribonucleotides to their deoxy forms, and inhibiting *de novo* nucleotide production. Gemcitabine demonstrates important differences from ara-C in schedule dependency and activity. Intermittent dosing is more effective than continuous dosing schedules, and gemcitabine has efficacy against a variety of solid tumors, particularly non–small cell lung cancers, pancreatic, ovarian, colorectal, breast, and cervical cancers. These differences may be due to differences in clinical pharmacology. With comparable exposure, gemcitabine achieves intracellular concentrations about 20 times higher than ara-C, secondary to increased permeation of cell membranes, and greater affinity for the activating enzyme deoxycytidine kinase. Parent gemcitabine is eliminated very rapidly from the plasma by deamination, with terminal half-lives of only 8–14 minutes, but the gemcitabine that is incorporated into DNA has a prolonged intracellular half-life. Gemcitabine's stereoconfiguration causes another normal base pair to be added subsequent to the fraudulent gemcitabine base pair in the DNA strand. This "masked chain termination" protects the gemcitabine from excision. The gemcitabine deamination product, difluorodeoxyuridine (dFdU) demonstrates a long terminal phase of 14–24 hours, and is eliminated primarily by the kidneys. Women clear gemcitabine more slowly than males.[77–80]

Toxicity. Gemcitabine is usually administered on a weekly schedule for 3 weeks, followed by a week of rest. Given this way, it is very well tolerated. It is myelosuppressive, but neutropenia is usually mild to moderate. Thrombocytopenia or thrombocythemia may occur. Elevations in liver transaminases are common. Although these abnormalities rarely necessitate stopping treatment, gemcitabine should be used with caution in patients with impaired liver function. Mild proteinuria and hematuria are reported in about half of patients, but are rarely clinically significant. However, caution is recommended in patients with impaired renal function, since a few cases of renal failure of uncertain etiology have been reported in patients receiving gemcitabine. Generalized rashes occur in about 25% of patients. The rashes are typically erythematous, pruritic, and maculopapular, and develop 2–3 days after drug administration. These are reversible and respond to local therapy, and only rarely require discontinuation of drug. Fevers and flu-like symptoms, which usually occur within 6–12 hours of drug administration, are also common, especially following administration of the first dose. Nausea and vomiting are mild, but peripheral edema may be clinically important. In contrast to cytarabine, gemcitabine is not known to be neurotoxic.[77–79]

Purines and Purine Antimetabolites

6-Mercaptopurine and 6-Thioguanine

Some of the oldest and newest anticancer agents are synthetic analogues of the naturally occurring purines, guanine and adenine (Fig. 119.12). 6-Mercaptopurine (6-MP) was the first purine analogue to be used in cancer chemotherapy since its introduction for treatment of acute lymphocytic leukemia (ALL) about 40 years ago. Its major clinical application today is in combination with methotrexate for remission maintenance of ALL. Recently, high-dose continuous infusions have shown promise in relapsed or unresponsive ANLL, when given in combination regimens with cytarabine or methotrexate. Thioguanine (6-TG) is the 2-amino analogue of 6-mercaptopurine. Its clinical utility is limited to remission consolidation or maintenance therapy in patients with acute ANLL.[81–83] These two purine analogues are believed to act similarly, although the true mechanism of their cytotoxicity is still unclear. Neither agent is active in its administered form but both are rapidly converted to ribonucleotides, which inhibit purine biosynthesis, and also various purine interconversion reactions which are needed to supply purine precursors for synthesis of nucleic acids. Although both compounds may be incorporated into DNA as "false" purines, this is only believed to be a major mechanism of action for 6-thioguanine. Clinical cross-resistance is generally observed between these two agents and probably results from decreased activation to active forms within resistant cells.[52,81]

Pharmacokinetics. The pharmacokinetics of the two drugs are similar as well. Both compounds are rapidly activated and distributed into most peripheral compartments, although neither enters the CNS in therapeutically useful concentrations following conventional doses. 6-MP demonstrates rapid clearance after oral administration, secondary to extensive first-pass metabolism. Oral bioavailability of both drugs is variable and incomplete, and is reduced by food intake.[54,57,81] Variability in absorption can result in significant differences in systemic exposure to a given dose of 6-MP and has been suggested as a prognostic consideration affecting the risk of relapse in children with ALL.[84] Despite this unreliable oral absorption, 6-MP and 6-TG are currently only available commercially for oral use. Parenteral 6-MP remains investigational, but permits greater systemic exposure, which is associated with longer remissions in ALL, and which may produce therapeutic effects against CNS disease.[83]

After conventional doses both 6-MP and 6-TG are eliminated primarily by metabolism in the liver and other tissues, although renal excretion of intact drug may become significant when high doses of 6-MP are administered. Metabolites are eliminated renally, and consideration should be given to decreasing doses in patients with hepatic or renal disease, although criteria for dose adjustment have not been defined.[57,83]

An important difference between these agents is the pathway of metabolic inactivation. 6-MP depends on the enzyme xanthine oxidase for an initial oxidation step. Because of this dependence, metabolism is markedly decreased by concomitant administration of the xanthine oxidase inhibitor, allopurinol, and serious toxicity may result. This drug interaction is of major clinical significance, and oral 6-MP doses must be reduced by at least 50% when allopurinol is administered together with 6-MP. Because xanthine oxidase is *not* involved in the elimination of 6-TG, no interaction with allopurinol occurs, and no dose reduction is necessary.[52,57,85]

Toxicity. Both 6-MP and 6-TG are relatively well tolerated. Gastrointestinal toxicity occurs more commonly with 6-MP than 6-TG, but even with 6-MP, it occurs in less than one-third of patients. Bone marrow suppression is mild with typical oral doses of 6-MP, but is dose limiting for 6-TG, and for high-dose infusional 6-MP. Chronically administered mercaptopurine produces hepatic injury in 6–40% of patients, which most typically manifests as jaundice after 1–2 months of treatment. Hepatic injury is dose related and is more common in adults than children. 6-TG has also caused hepatocellular damage, as well as rare hepatic veno-occlusive disease.[81,83,86]

Fludarabine Monophosphate

Fludarabine monophosphate (FAMP) is an analog of the purine adenine that incorporates two structural changes from the parent molecule (Fig. 119.12). The arabinose analog of adenine (ara-A or vidarabine) was first developed in an attempt to design new antineoplastics using the structural alterations of the effective anticancer drug, cytarabine. Ara-A demonstrated some antineoplastic activity, as well as antiviral activity, but was rapidly inactivated by deaminase enzymes. It is marketed as an antiviral drug. The fluorinated analog, fludarabine or F-ara-A, proved to be both resistant to deamination and to have significant antitumor activity.[87,88]

Pharmacology and Pharmacokinetics. Fludarabine monophosphate is rapidly dephosphorylated in plasma to F-ara-A by first-pass metabolism, then enters cells, where it is rephosphorylated to its pharmacologically active triphosphate form (F-ara-ATP) by the enzyme deoxycytidine kinase. The intracellular accumulation of F-ara-ATP results in inhibition of DNA synthesis. Like cytarabine, fludarabine interferes with DNA polymerase, causing chain termination. Unlike ara-C, fludarabine is incorporated into RNA, resulting in inhibited transcription. It is inactivated by deaminase enzymes. The dephosphorylated form is eliminated with a terminal half-life of about 10 hours. Renal excretion accounts for the major clearance of metabolites, and renal failure predisposes patients to increased toxicity. Guidelines for dose modification (Table 119.10) are not yet available.[52,88]

Clinical Uses and Toxicity. Fludarabine has proven to be a very active agent in management of hematologic malignancies, especially chronic lymphocytic leukemia (CLL), low-grade non-Hodgkin's lymphomas, and mycosis fungoides. It is not effective in solid tumors. Although high doses of

TABLE 119.10. EMPIRIC DOSE MODIFICATIONS IN PATIENTS WITH RENAL AND HEPATIC DISEASE[a]

Agent	Organ Dysfunction	Suggested Dose Modification
Methotrexate	Renal impairment	In proportion to lowered creatinine clearance (normal 60 mL/min/m^2)
Cisplatin	Renal impairment	In proportion to creatinine clearance
Carboplatin	Renal impairment	See Table 119.13 for dosing guideline
Cyclophosphamide	Renal failure (creatinine clearance < 25 mL/min)	50% decrease
Bleomycin	Renal failure (creatinine clearance < 25 mL/min)	50–75% decrease
Fludarabine	Renal impairment	In proportion to creatinine clearance
Pentostatin	Renal impairment	In proportion to creatinine clearance
Hydroxyurea	Renal impairment	In proportion to creatinine clearance
Streptozotocin	Renal failure (creatinine clearance < 25mL/min)	50–75% decrease
Doxorubicin Daunorubicin Vincristine Vinblastine	Hepatic dysfunction	1. Only approximate guidelines can be offered. 2. For bilirubin > 1.5 mg/100 mL, reduce initial dose by 50%. 3. For bilirubin > 3.0 mg/100 mL, reduce initial dose by 75%.
Idarubicin Mitoxantrone	Hepatic dysfunction	Consider dose reductions
Taxol	Hepatic dysfunction	Dose reductions required; see text

[a]Only approximate guidelines can be given. See text for explanations and limitations. (Adapted from Chabner BA. Clinical strategies for cancer treatment: The role of drugs, in Chabner BA, Collins JM (eds): Cancer Chemotherapy: Principles and Practice. Philadelphia, JB Lippincott, 1990, pp 1–15.)

fludarabine were extremely effective in inducing remissions in patients with ANLL during phase I trials, its use was limited by a syndrome of delayed CNS toxicity, characterized by blindness, paralysis, and coma. Fortunately, fludarabine is effective at doses in CLL (25 mg/m^2/d × 5 days) at which serious CNS toxicity is rare. About 15% of patients treated with this dose of fludarabine experience some degree of neurotoxicity, most commonly somnolence, mild peripheral neuropathy, paresthesias, and mild visual disturbances.[89] The usual dose-limiting toxicity at these lower doses is myelosuppression, with associated opportunistic infections. Pulmonary toxicity consistent with interstitial pneumonitis has been documented, with a usual onset after several courses of therapy, and is slowly reversible. Tumor lysis syndrome may occur secondary to effective cell kill. Prophylactic use of allopurinol, hydration, and alkalinization of urine are recommended in patients with large tumor burdens during initiation of fludarabine therapy. Nausea and vomiting are mild and easily controlled.[75,87,88]

Cladribine

Cladribine (2-chlorodeoxyadenosine, 2-CDA) is another recently developed purine nucleoside analog. Cladribine is resistant to inactivation by adenosine deaminase. Like fludarabine, the drug is sequentially phosphorylated intracellularly by deoxycytidine kinase. The triphosphate form of this agent is incorporated into DNA, resulting in inhibition of DNA synthesis and early chain termination. Cladribine's antitumor activity is unusual in that it affects both actively dividing and resting cancer cells. This drug also appears to be involved in induction of apoptosis.[90,91]

Pharmacokinetics. In contrast to the other purine nucleoside analogs, cladribine is well absorbed following oral administration, with a bioavailability of approximately 50%, although it is not currently available in an oral preparation. After subcutaneous dosing, the drug is 100% bioavailable. The terminal elimination half-life approaches 7 hours. The metabolic fate of cladribine is unknown, although approximately 20% of the drug is eliminated unchanged in the urine.[90,91]

Clinical Uses. Cladribine is approved for the treatment of hairy cell leukemia. In this type of leukemia, a single course of cladribine at a dose of 0.1 mg/kg/d by continuous intravenous infusion for 7 days is sufficient to induce a durable complete remission in most patients. The drug also has significant activity in several other lymphoid malignancies, including low-grade non-Hodgkin's lymphomas, chronic lymphocytic leukemia, and cutaneous T-cell lymphoma.[90–92]

Toxicity. The dose-limiting toxicity of cladribine is myelosuppression. Like fludarabine, cladribine possesses immunosuppressive effects that place patients at risk for serious opportunistic infections. The most common toxicity noted in clinical trials was culture-negative fever, usually beginning on the fifth to seventh day of therapy.[90,91]

Pentostatin

Pentostatin, or deoxycoformycin, is an unrelated purine analogue that is also useful in management of hairy cell leukemia, chronic lymphocytic leukemia, and other lymphoproliferative disorders. It is a potent inhibitor of adenosine deaminase, the enzyme responsible for breakdown of adenosine and deoxyadenosine. Triphosphate forms of the nucleosides accumulate intracellularly, inhibiting ribonucleotide reductase, and ultimately causing a relative deficiency of other deoxyribonucleotides that are needed for normal DNA and RNA synthesis. Other mechanisms may also be involved in pentostatin's cytotoxicity. Pentostatin has a large volume of distribution following intravenous administration. It crosses the blood–brain barrier, reaching concentrations within the cerebrospinal fluid (CSF) that are about 10% of serum concentrations, and is cleared from the CSF slowly compared with systemic clearance. Pentostatin is eliminated largely unchanged in the urine and may require dose adjustment in patients with impaired renal function (Table 119.10).[93]

Toxicity. In the doses currently recommended (4 mg/m^2 every 2 weeks), the most common toxicities of pentostatin are nausea and vomiting, which are delayed in onset. Symptoms usually begin 12–24 hours after drug administration and may persist for 2–3 days, making several days of antiemetic therapy advisable. Reversible elevation of liver transaminases is very common, with rare incidence of severe hepatotoxicity. Nephrotoxicity was common in earlier higher dose studies, but is rare at approved doses. Similarly, severe neurotoxicity is uncommon with standard-dose therapy. Mild to moderate paresthesias, lethargy, and transient confusion are the most common neurologic effects. They occur in about 15% of patients and are usually transient and reversible.[89,93,94]

Folate Antagonists

The folate vitamins are essential cofactors in many reactions important for the synthesis of DNA. They carry one-carbon groups in transfer reactions that are required for purine and thymidylic acid synthesis and, in turn, for formation of DNA and for cell division. Structurally, the folates consist of a multiring pteridine group, attached to *para*-aminobenzoic acid, with one or more glutamic acid groups attached. Natural folates circulating in the blood have a single glutamic acid group, but within cells they are converted to polyglutamates, which are more efficient cofactors and which are preferentially retained inside the cells.[95–97]

Dietary folates must be chemically reduced to their tetrahydro forms, with four hydrogens on the pteridine ring, in order to be active. The enzyme responsible for this reduction is dihydrofolate reductase, and it is this enzyme whose actions methotrexate and other antifolates inhibit. The result of this inhibition is depletion of intracellular pools of reduced folate (tetrahydrofolates) essential for thymidylate and purine synthesis. Lack of either thymidylate or purines prevents synthesis of DNA. The effects of antifolate drugs on normal and probably cancerous cells may be counteracted by supplying reduced folates exogenously. The reduced folate used clinically for "rescue" is leucovorin (folinic acid). Leucovorin bypasses the metabolic block induced by antifolate drugs (Fig. 119.14).[95–97]

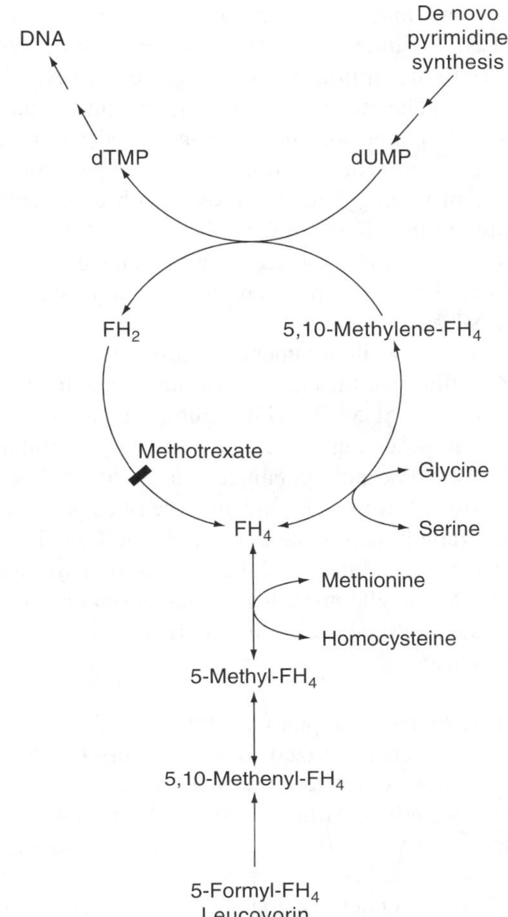

Figure 119.14. The folate cycle, the site of action of methotrexate, and the activation and entry "bypass" site of leucovorin. *(From Bleyer WA. Clinical pharmacology and therapeutic drug monitoring. Am Assoc Clin Ther Drug Monit-Toxicology 1985;6[11]:1–14, with permission.)*

Methotrexate

The folic acid analogue methotrexate (MTX) is the most widely used and best understood of all drugs in the broad category of "antimetabolites." It has activity in many different cancer types, and also has several nononcology applications. MTX has been in clinical use for more than 40 years, since its original success for remission induction in childhood acute leukemias in the 1950s. It differs from folic acid by substitution of an amino group for a hydroxyl group on the pteridine ring, and in an additional methyl group.[98]

Clinical Pharmacology. Like physiologic folates, methotrexate is transported intracellularly by an active transport system. In high doses, passive diffusion becomes important in transport, and may therefore overcome tumor cell resistance based on limited or saturated active transport systems. Resistance to the antifolates can also occur by several other mechanisms. The most clinically significant of these, in addition to impaired transport, are increased production of the target enzyme dihydrofolate reductase, or inherently slow rates of thymidylate synthesis, which make cells less susceptible to the effects of antifolate drugs. Like impaired transport mechanisms, increased production of dihydrofolate reductase may also be overcome by administering high doses of MTX.

Other, less well-documented causes of resistance are decreased affinity of the enzyme for methotrexate or lack of polyglutamation of MTX within tumor cells.[96,97,99] MTX, like naturally occurring folates, is normally polyglutamated within cells. These polyglutamated forms of MTX are not readily extruded from cells, and are at least as potent as and likely less rapidly reversible than MTX itself as dihydrofolate reductase inhibitors. Malignant cells may achieve greater MTX polyglutamate levels than normal cells, which may provide relative protection of normal cells from MTX-induced damage.[97]

Pharmacokinetics. The pharmacokinetics of methotrexate have been well characterized. Bioavailability of oral doses is variable and incomplete. Low doses (up to 30 mg/m^2) are completely absorbed. At higher doses, absorption is significantly less, and varies from 12–77%. MTX is rapidly distributed into total body water and is 40–50% bound to plasma proteins. Other organic acids such as sulfonamides can displace MTX from binding sites, although the clinical significance of this interaction is not proven. Distribution of MTX into abnormal fluid accumulations, such as ascites or pleural effusions, can have important clinical effects. These "third-space" fluids act as depots from which MTX is slowly released. This may result in prolonged exposure to concentrations above those required to cause both tumor cell effects and toxicity to normal cells. Careful monitoring of serum MTX levels and prolonged duration of leucovorin rescue may be required in these patients. In conventional oral or parenteral doses, levels of MTX achieved in the CNS are low, and direct instillation into the CNS is necessary for therapeutic effects. High-dose MTX regimens (greater than 1 g/m^2) may produce therapeutic levels and avoid the need for intrathecal or intraventricular administration.[57,97,100]

Methotrexate is metabolized to 7-hydroxy-methotrexate (7-OH-MTX) by the liver, to diamino-methylpteroic acid (DAMPA) by intestinal bacteria during enterohepatic cycling, and to methotrexate polyglutamates. DAMPA usually accounts for less than 5% of an administered dose. Both MTX and its metabolites are eliminated renally, by glomerular filtration and tubular secretion. At high doses, concentrations in the renal tubules may exceed MTX solubility and result in renal damage from crystallization. The distribution half-life is 0.45–2 hours, and the $t_{1/2}$ β ranges from 3–5 hours in patients with normal renal function. A terminal phase half-life of 8–26 hours represents redistribution from deep tissue sites. Elimination may be greatly prolonged in patients with renal insufficiency, mandating dose reduction and careful therapeutic drug monitoring (Table 119.10).[2] Presence of third-space fluids (as described above), or gastrointestinal obstruction, which can increase enterohepatic cycling, can also delay elimination.[57,97,100]

Both DAMPA and 7-OH-MTX have only very modest cytotoxic potential, and do not contribute significantly to MTX's antineoplastic effects. However, 7-OH-MTX concentrations may exceed those of the parent drug and may alter MTX's therapeutic and toxic effects. 7-OH-MTX may decrease elimination of MTX by competing for tubular secretion. It is less soluble in the urine than is MTX and may contribute to crystallization damage in high-dose regimens. 7-OH-MTX may also compete with MTX for polyglutamation within cells.[100]

Accurate and readily available assays for MTX levels in the serum have made therapeutic drug monitoring of MTX a practical and useful tool. The threshold for cytotoxic effects of MTX is approximately 5×10^{-8} *M*. Toxicity and, it appears, efficacy are related not only to achievement of therapeutic drug concentrations but, more importantly, to duration of time that concentrations are above this threshold level. With MTX doses requiring leucovorin rescue (generally greater than 100 mg/m^2), leucovorin must be administered until levels fall below this cytotoxic threshold (Fig. 119.15). Several excellent reviews are available which

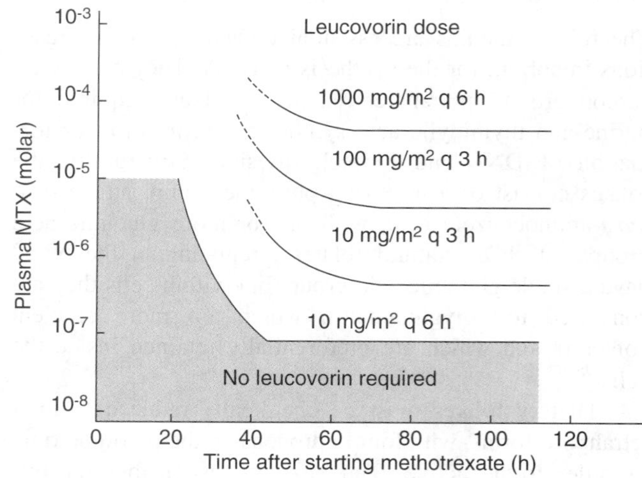

Figure 119.15. Leucovorin dosing based on monitored serum methotrexate (MTX) levels. Note that the level for discontinuation of leucovorin in this nomogram is 1.0×10^{-7} *M*. The actual value recommended may be lower, depending on the MTX assay used, patient age, prior or concurrent therapy, whether or not the patient has had a bone marrow transplant, and other factors. *(From Bleyer WA. New vistas for leucovorin in cancer chemotherapy. Cancer 1989;63:995–1007, with permission.)*

detail the appropriate therapeutic monitoring of MTX and determination of leucovorin rescue regimens.[57,100,101] Therapeutic drug monitoring is useful not only for prevention and management of potential toxicity, but has also been established as an effective means of increasing the likelihood of therapeutic success, by individualizing doses based on target parameters. This has been best applied in the treatment of children with ALL.[102]

Clinical Uses. Methotrexate is broadly useful in the management of both hematologic and solid malignancies. It is very effective in ALL, meningeal involvement from a wide range of tumors, non–Hodgkin's lymphomas, choriocarcinoma, breast and bladder cancers, osteosarcoma in high-dose regimens, and, occasionally, for lung and head and neck cancers. Nononcology applications include management of ectopic pregnancy and rheumatic disorders, especially rheumatoid arthritis, prevention of graft-versus-host disease secondary to allogeneic bone marrow transplantation, management of psoriasis, and steroid-dependent asthma. Many of these nononcology applications take advantage of MTX's established immunosuppressive effects.[97,103–106]

Toxicity. The normal cells most sensitive to MTX damage are the rapidly growing cells of the bone marrow and the gastrointestinal mucosa, making myelosuppression and mucositis the most common dose-limiting toxicities. Toxicity is dose and schedule dependent (Table 119.11).[95] Mucositis usually precedes myelosuppression, and occurs 3–7 days after drug administration. Stomatitis is the most common manifestation of mucosal damage, but diarrhea may also occur. Mucosal ulceration can be life threatening and requires dose interruption. Granulocytes and platelets are the most sensitive blood cells to MTX's effects. Myelosuppression and mucositis can both be prevented with leucovorin rescue, but cannot be reversed with leucovorin after they have occurred.[95,97,100]

Major organ toxicity from MTX includes hepatic, renal, neurologic, and pulmonary damage. Hepatic toxicity, which manifests as portal fibrosis and occasionally cirrhosis, is common in patients treated with chronic low-dose oral daily regimens, such as those used for psoriasis. "Pulse" dosing decreases the risk of severe toxicity. Hepatic damage is uncommon with intermittent intravenous dosing, even with high-dose regimens. Nephrotoxicity, as discussed above, is a result of exceeding drug solubility in the renal tubules during high-dose MTX infusions. It can be prevented by alkaline hydration with bicarbonate solutions to maintain the urine pH above 7 for 1–2 days after drug administration to increase the solubility of methotrexate in urine. Vigorous hydration can also alter the disposition of MTX and reduce the frequency of high MTX concentrations and toxicity in high-dose MTX regimens. Pulmonary toxicity, which can be fatal, generally presents as fever, dry cough, dyspnea, and chest pain. It is not clearly dose related and is variably responsive to corticosteroids.[75,97,107]

CNS toxicity may occur either secondary to direct instillation of MTX into the CNS, or from concentrations achieved by diffusion into the CNS during high-dose infusions. Neurotoxicity secondary to intrathecal administration includes three distinct syndromes. Chemical arachnoiditis, which presents with headache, nuchal rigidity, vomiting, and fever is both most acute in onset and most common. A subacute syndrome of motor paralysis, cranial nerve palsy,

TABLE 119.11. METHOTREXATE TOXICITIES

	Myelotoxicity	Nephrotoxicity	Hepatotoxicity	Mucositis	Pulmonary Toxicity	Neurotoxicity
Intermediate IV (50–100 mg/m^2)	+++	+	+ (transaminasemia)	++	±	–
High-dose IV with leucovorin (100–12,000 mg/m^2)	+	+++ (requires urinary alkalinization and hydration)	++ (transaminasemia)	++	±	++ (acute and chronic)
Low-dose PO daily dose (5–25 mg/m^2)	–	–	+++ (up to 25% cirrhosis)	–	±	–
Low-dose PO pulse therapy (5–25 mg/m^2)	–	–	++ (rarely cirrhosis)	–	+	–
Intrathecal	–	–	–	–	–	++ (acute, subacute, and chronic)

Key: +, low risk; ++, moderate risk; +++, high risk; ±, inconclusive association. (From Allegra CJ. Antifolates, in Chabner BA, Collins JM (eds): Cancer Chemotherapy: Principles and Practice. Philadelphia, JB Lippincott, 1990, p 137, with permission.)

seizures, or coma may occur during the second or third week of treatment, most typically in adult patients with active meningeal leukemia. In patients receiving higher than currently recommended doses (12–15 mg), incidence is approximately 10%. The last syndrome is a chronic demyelinating encephalopathy with associated dementia, spasticity, and sometimes coma, which is usually seen months or years after MTX treatment, and which is not reversible. Most patients who develop encephalopathic symptoms have also received cranial irradiation. Encephalopathy also occurs subacutely after high-dose MTX regimens, and generally presents 2 or 3 months after treatment. High-dose regimens may also cause an acute, readily reversible syndrome of paralysis, aphasia, behavior abnormalities, or seizures. This occurs a few days after MTX administration, reverses in 2–3 days, and rarely occurs on rechallenge. The etiology of CNS toxicity from MTX is not known, but it is not preventable with leucovorin.[72,95,97]

Other toxicities from MTX include mild nausea and vomiting, photosensitivity, eye discomfort, and hypersensitivity reactions which can include anaphylaxis. It is highly teratogenic, especially when administered during the first trimester of pregnancy.[97,108]

Drug Interactions. Several pharmacokinetic and pharmacodynamic drug interactions with MTX are of clinical importance. The most clinically important interactions are those with cisplatin, probenecid, and nonsteroidal anti-inflammatory drugs (NSAIDs). Cisplatin is an established nephrotoxin which may decrease the elimination of methotrexate, even when patients fail to show laboratory evidence of renal insufficiency. Probenecid also delays methotrexate elimination by inhibiting renal tubular transport. Therapeutic as well as toxic effects of methotrexate may be increased. Aspirin and other NSAIDs may decrease elimination by effects on renal function.[85,100,109]

Other Folate Analogues

Several folate analogues have been developed which are lipid soluble and therefore do not depend on active transport mechanisms for entry into cells. These include piritrexim, trimetrexate, and 10-ethyl-10-deazoaminopterin (10-EDAM, or edatrexate). All have shown some activity against solid tumors. Edatrexate is a promising agent in management of non–small cell lung cancer.[77,97]

Plant Alkaloids

Vincristine and Vinblastine

Vincristine and vinblastine are natural alkaloids derived from the periwinkle (vinca) plant. They act as mitotic inhibitors, or "spindle poisons." Although the two alkaloids are very similar structurally (Fig. 119.16), they have different activities and patterns of toxicity.

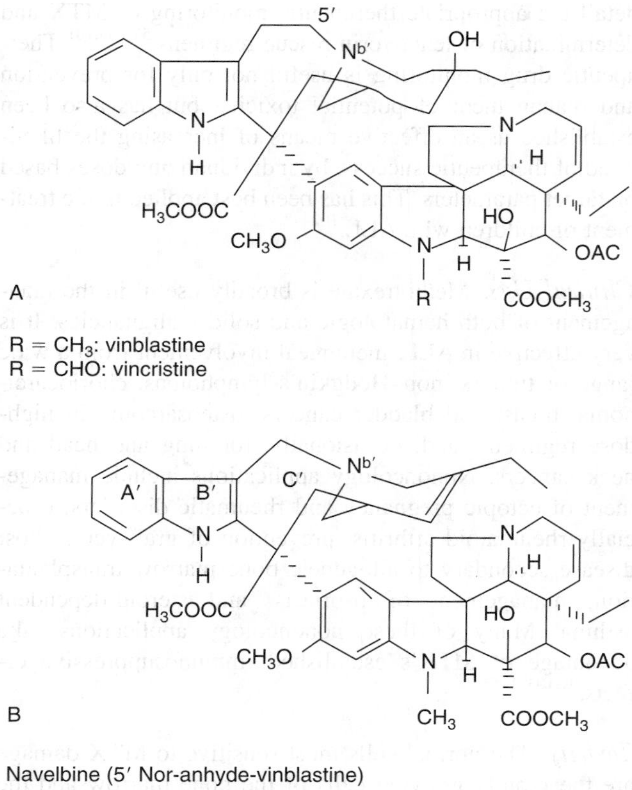

A

R = CH_3: vinblastine
R = CHO: vincristine

B

Navelbine (5′ Nor-anhyde-vinblastine)

Figure 119.16. Structures of vinca alkaloids. *(From Jones AL, Smith IE. Navelbine and the anthrapyrazoles. Hematol Oncol Clin North Am 1994;8:141–152.)*

Mechanism and Clinical Pharmacology. Both vincristine and vinblastine are believed to function as antineoplastic agents by binding to tubulin, the structural protein that polymerizes to form microtubules. These are the hollow tubes that make up the mitotic spindle and that are also important in nerve conduction and neurotransmission. Vincas disrupt the normal balance between polymerization and depolymerization of microtubules. The result is inhibition of *assembly* of the microtubules (Fig. 119.17). This interferes with formation of the mitotic spindle and causes cells to accumulate in the mitosis phase of the cell cycle. Resistance to the vinca alkaloids develops from pP-glycoprotein mediated MDR, or secondary to alterations in tubulin, which lead to decreased drug binding.[110–112]

Pharmacokinetics. Oral absorption of these alkaloids is unpredictable, and they are administered intravenously. They bind tightly to blood elements, especially platelets, and do not enter the CNS in significant amounts. Vincristine and vinblastine are both metabolized, although vinblastine is metabolized to a greater extent than is vincristine. Both are eliminated primarily by biliary excretion and may require dose modification in patients with biliary obstruction (Table 119.10). Their elimination is triexponential. Vincristine is eliminated much more slowly than vinblastine, with a terminal half-life of approximately 85

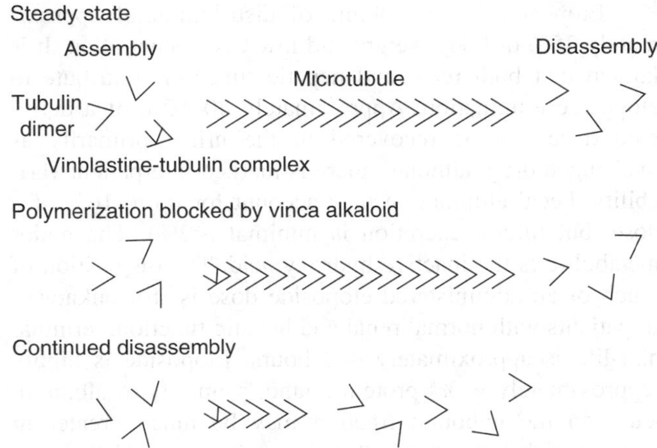

Figure 119.17. Mechanism of action of vinca alkaloids. *(From Pratt WB, Ruddon RW. The Anticancer Drugs. New York, Oxford University Press, 1979, p 225, with permission.)*

hours, compared with 24 hours for vinblastine. The long half-life of vincristine may partially explain why its maximum tolerated dose is lower than other vincas.[110,111,113] There is evidence that clearance of vincristine may be significantly decreased in patients receiving H_2 antagonists.[114]

Clinical Uses and Dosing. Vincristine is an agent with broad clinical activity against hematologic neoplasms, but limited activity against solid tumors. Its primary uses are treatment of acute lymphocytic leukemias and lymphomas (both Hodgkins and non-Hodgkins types), multiple myeloma, and a few solid tumors such as small cell lung and breast cancers and Kaposi's sarcoma. It is usually administered by intravenous bolus in doses of 1–2 mg/m^2. Although doses are traditionally capped at 2 mg to decrease the risk of neurotoxicity, the justification for this is controversial.[115] Nononcology use of vincristine is limited to management of platelet disorders, such as idiopathic thrombocytopenic purpura (ITP). Vinblastine is also active against lymphomas, most particularly as a component of the Hodgkin's disease regimen "ABVD" (Adriamycin, bleomycin, vinblastine, and dacarbazine). It is a first-line agent for treatment of bladder and testicular cancers and Kaposi's sarcoma, where it is sometimes used in dilute concentrations for direct injection into oral lesions. Vinblastine is also useful in management of breast and non–small cell lung cancers.[111,112,116]

Toxicity. The dose-limiting toxicity of vincristine is neurotoxicity. This is probably an extension of its therapeutic effects, because microtubules are involved in nerve conduction as well as formation of the mitotic spindle. The neuropathy is usually distal and symmetrical, and affects both sensation and motor function. Depressed deep tendon reflexes are the earliest objective signs of neurotoxicity, and paresthesias of the fingers and toes are the most common clinical manifestations. These changes are generally reversible and are not reasons to discontinue therapy unless they are disabling. Cranial nerves may also be affected and their damage may present as hoarseness, facial palsies, or jaw pain. Autonomic neuropathy also occurs, usually manifesting as constipation or colicky abdominal pain, but occasionally as orthostatic hypotension. Vincristine generally is not myelosuppressive, and is therefore frequently used in combination regimens with myelosuppressive drugs. It may produce inappropriate antidiuretic hormone secretion (SIADH). Vinblastine dosing, in contrast, is limited by myelosuppression. Neurotoxicity is not common from vinblastine, but when it occurs, it most commonly manifests as muscle aching.[72] Both agents are vesicants and may cause tissue damage if extravasated. No antidote has been demonstrated to be effective in humans, but hyaluronidase use is supported by animal data.[117]

Vinorelbine

Vinorelbine (Navelbine) is a semisynthetic vinca alkaloid analog that differs from vinblastine by modification of the catharanthine ring and broader antitumor activity (Fig. 119.16). The mechanism of action is identical to that of vincristine and vinblastine. The drug is also eliminated via hepatic metabolism and biliary excretion, and is extensively bound to plasma proteins. Unlike the other vincas, vinorelbine exhibits 40% bioavailability and an oral formulation is under investigation. In non–small cell lung cancer (NSCLC), vinorelbine has shown response rates comparable to those seen with single-agent cisplatin, and FDA approval for this indication was granted early in 1995. Other responsive malignancies include breast and ovarian carcinomas and Hodgkin's disease.[118,119]

Toxicity. The dose-limiting toxicity for both the oral and intravenous routes is myelosuppression, especially neutropenia. Thrombocytopenia is rarely seen. Neurotoxicity, including constipation, is not as common with vinorelbine as with other vincas, possibly due to differences in tubulin binding between mitotic microtubules and other types of microtubules, such as axonal nerve microtubules. Paresthesias occur in only 2–7% of vinorelbine recipients, as compared to 50% of patients receiving vincristine. The incidence of nausea and vomiting, alopecia, and extravasation reactions is similar to that seen with naturally occurring vincas.[118,119]

Etoposide and Teniposide

Etoposide (VP-16) and teniposide (VM-26) are semisynthetic podophyllotoxin derivatives. Podophyllin is extracted from the mayapple or mandrake plant and, like the vincas, binds to tubulin and interferes with microtubule formation. Unlike the parent compound, however, the cell damage produced by etoposide and teniposide is caused by strand breakage, which they produce by inhibiting the enzyme

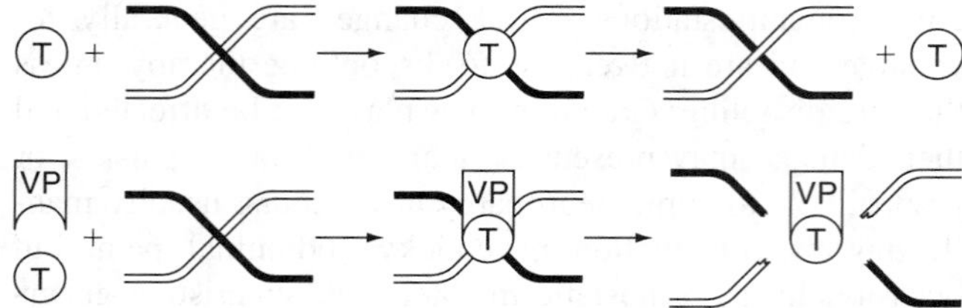

Figure 119.18. Topoisomerase II (T) interaction with DNA and etoposide (VP). T normally interacts with DNA to produce breakage–cleavage reactions required for normal cellular function *(upper panel).* The epipodophyllotoxins seem to cause DNA strand breakage by forming a complex with DNA and T *(lower panel). (From Bender RA, Hamel E, Hande KR. Plant alkaloids, in Chabner BA, Collins JM [eds]: Cancer Chemotherapy: Principles and Practice. Philadelphia, JB Lippincott, 1990, pp 253–275, with permission.)*

topoisomerase II. This is the "unwinding" enzyme responsible for creation and repair of strand breaks essential for DNA replication processes. As shown in Fig. 119.18, DNA topoisomerases cleave DNA strands and form intermediates with the strands, which makes a gap for passage of DNA strands, then reseals the breaks. Etoposide and teniposide both form complexes with the topoisomerase II and DNA, which inhibit strand rejoining after breakage. Teniposide differs from etoposide by the addition of a sulfur-containing group in place of a methyl group on its sugar ring. It is several times more potent than etoposide in stimulating DNA cleavage. Resistance to either etoposide or teniposide drugs may be caused by cellular differences in topoisomerase II levels, by increased cell ability to repair strand breaks, or by increased levels of P-glycoproteins. They are usually clinically cross-resistant. Etoposide and teniposide are cell cycle phase specific, and arrest cells in the S or early G_2 phase.[110,112,120]

Pharmacokinetics. Etoposide and teniposide are not soluble in water. Etoposide is formulated in a polyethylene glycol solution for parenteral administration, and teniposide is solubilized for parenteral use in a formulation containing polyoxyethylated castor oil (Cremophor® EL). These formulations result in concentration-dependent stability, and contribute to hypotension with rapid infusions and to hypersensitivity reactions. Etoposide phosphate is a water-soluble derivative which is rapidly converted to etoposide. This formulation permits bolus dosing and treatment at high drug concentrations. It is pharmacokinetically and biologically equivalent to etoposide.[121] Etoposide is available for oral use in liquid-filled gelatin capsules. Oral bioavailability is dose dependent. Mean bioavailabilities of 76–86% have been reported after administration of a 100-mg oral dose, compared with 45–48% following a 400-mg dose. At both dose levels, interpatient variability is marked, producing a range of bioavailability that can have serious clinical consequences if either significantly more or less drug is absorbed than predicted.[122,123]

Etoposide has a volume of distribution of approximately 25% of body weight and low CNS penetration. It is known that both renal and hepatic function contribute to etoposide elimination. Approximately 40–60% of a delivered dose can be recovered in the urine, primarily as unchanged drug, although there is marked interpatient variability. Fecal elimination may account for up to 16% of a dose, but biliary excretion is minimal (<2%). The major metabolite is the inactive hydroxy acid. The disposition of much of an administered etoposide dose is still unknown. In patients with normal renal and hepatic function, terminal half-life is approximately 4–8 hours. Etoposide is highly (approximately 95%) protein bound, primarily to albumin, although the unbound fraction may be much greater in patients with low serum albumin, as is commonly seen in cancer patients. Binding may also be altered in patients with elevated serum bilirubin levels.[112,124–126]

The pharmacologic effects resulting from a particular dose depend on a complex interplay of protein binding, renal, and hepatic function. All these are important in dosing considerations in cancer patients.[127] Unfortunately, no validated guidelines for dose changes in patients with abnormal renal or hepatic function or hypoalbuminemia currently exist. Dose reductions are recommended in patients with impaired renal function. One guideline of a 30% dose reduction in patients with serum creatinine levels above 1.5 mg/dL has been recommended, but has not been prospectively validated.[125] Pharmacologic effects may or may not be increased in patients with impaired hepatic function, depending on the binding status, so no dosing guidelines can be given.[127] Etoposide is not significantly removed by dialysis.

Teniposide is even more highly protein bound than is etoposide (>97%). Teniposide has a lower systemic clearance, a longer elimination half-life of about 9 hours, and less urine elimination of parent drug than etoposide. Renal elimination accounts for only about 10% of teniposide clearance; therefore, renal insufficiency is unlikely to be important in dose considerations. Hepatic metabolism is the predominant route of teniposide elimination, but dose modification guidelines are not yet available for patients with impaired hepatic function. As with etoposide, serum albumin and factors that affect protein binding must also be taken into consideration in dosing decisions.[112,124,128]

Drug interactions with drugs that affect hepatic function and protein binding may be clinically significant in patients receiving etoposide or teniposide. This has been best described with anticonvulsants.[124,129]

Clinical Uses. Etoposide is a broad-spectrum antineoplastic, with activity in a wide variety of hematologic malignancies as well as solid tumors. It is particularly valuable in the treatment of testicular carcinomas, lung cancers, non-Hodgkin's lymphomas, acute leukemias, and Kaposi's sarcoma, and has value in high doses as a preparative regimen before bone marrow transplantation.[112,120] It demonstrates synergistic cytotoxicity with cisplatin, both *in vitro* and clinically, and is most frequently administered with platinum derivatives in combination regimens.[120,130] Activity is dramatically greater in divided doses over several days than in large single doses, probably because of the cycle specificity of this agent.[124] Chronic daily administration of oral etoposide and prolonged low-dose infusional schedules are being studied to take advantage of this schedule dependency.[123,131] Clinical use of teniposide is limited to treatment of patients with ALL.[112]

Toxicity. Both etoposide and teniposide are well-tolerated drugs. Their dose-limiting toxicity is myelosuppression. Nausea and vomiting are usually mild, although more likely after oral administration of etoposide than parenteral. Alopecia is common, and mucositis may be limiting at high doses. Orthostatic hypotension occurs with either drug, but is generally preventable by a slow infusion time over 30 minutes to 1 hour. Etoposide phosphate may be administered as a rapid bolus without producing cardiovascular effects. Hypersensitivity reactions have occasionally been reported, although the mechanism of these reactions is not established.[108,112] Major organ toxicity is rare, although etoposide has occasionally been implicated as a cause of hepatotoxicity.[132]

Secondary leukemias associated with etoposide and teniposide use have recently been recognized.[133] Most of the secondary leukemias have been acute nonlymphocytic leukemias identified in children receiving these agents for treatment of acute lymphocytic leukemia. Most patients demonstrate characteristic chromosomal translocations involving the long arm of chromosome 11 and the short arm of chromosome 9, and have leukemias of the myelomonocytic or monocytic subtypes. These iatrogenic leukemias typically occur after a short latency period between drug administration and diagnosis of the leukemia (<5 years) and do not demonstrate a preleukemic or myelodysplastic phase, in contrast to leukemias induced by alkylating agents. Like those leukemias, however, the leukemias secondary to etoposide and teniposide are characterized by low response rates to treatment and short remission durations. Dose and schedule response relationships with these agents are being evaluated.[134–136]

Paclitaxel and Docetaxel

Paclitaxel and docetaxel are novel taxoid plant alkaloids with antimitotic activity (Fig. 119.19). Paclitaxel (Taxol) was isolated from the bark of the Pacific yew tree, *Taxus brevifolia,* in 1971. Development of the drug was hindered by inadequate drug supplies. The yew is a slow-growing plant, and once the bark is harvested, the tree dies. It is estimated that the bark from more than 2000 trees is currently required to produce 1 kilogram of Taxol. The complex taxane ring structure proved difficult to synthesize, and efforts

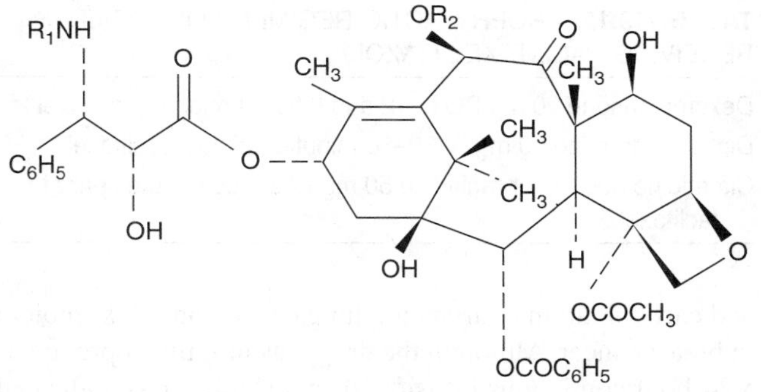

Paclitaxel $R_1 = COC_6H_5$, $R_2 = CH_3CO$
Docetaxel $R_1 = COOC(CH_3)_3$, $R_2 = H$

Figure 119.19. The chemical structures of paclitaxel and docetaxel. *(From Pazdur R, Kudelka AP, Kavanagh JJ, et al. The taxoids: Paclitaxel (Taxol) and Docetaxel (Taxotere). Cancer Treat Rev 1993;19:351–386.)*

turned to more readily available and renewable resources than yew tree bark. The search led to the discovery of docetaxel (Taxotere) from the needles of the European yew, *Taxus baccata.* Docetaxel is a semisynthetic taxoid extracted from 10-deacetyl baccatin III, a noncytotoxic precursor.[137–140]

Clinical Pharmacology. Paclitaxel and docetaxel both act by binding to tubulin, but unlike the vincas, do not interfere with tubulin assembly. Instead, the taxoids promote microtubule assembly and interfere with microtubule disassembly. This is accomplished by induction of tubulin polymerization, resulting in formation of stable, but nonfunctional, microtubules. Preliminary studies indicate that docetaxel is twice as potent as paclitaxel in binding to tubulin.[138,140]

Pharmacokinetics. The taxoids are widely distributed after administration, and bind extensively to plasma and tissue proteins. As expected, this results in large volumes of distribution for both agents and plasma protein binding that exceeds 90%. Elimination half-lives range from 1.3–8.6 hours for paclitaxel and 11.4–18.5 hours for docetaxel and are not dose dependent.[137–140] Elimination is primarily through hepatic metabolism and biliary excretion; less than 10% of parent drug is found unchanged in the urine. The optimal dose for patients with hepatic impairment has not been established, but dose reduction is necessary in patients with moderate or severely elevated bilirubin or serum aminotransferase concentrations.[140,141]

Clinical Uses. Both agents have shown extensive activity in clinical trials, especially against ovarian cancers refractory to cisplatin-based regimens, breast cancer, and non–small cell lung cancers. Paclitaxel has also shown activity against melanoma. Currently, only paclitaxel is commercially available. Ongoing trials are evaluating the activity of paclitaxel in combination with other antineoplastic agents like cisplatin

TABLE 119.12. PROPHYLACTIC REGIMEN FOR PATIENTS RECEIVING PACLITAXEL (TAXOL)

Dexamethasone 20 mg PO at 12 and 6 hours prior to paclitaxel
Diphenhydramine 50 mg IV 30–60 minutes prior to paclitaxel
Cimetidine 300 mg or ranitidine 50 mg IV 30–60 minutes prior to paclitaxel

and carboplatin in ovarian and lung cancer, and doxorubicin in breast cancer. Although the drug was initially approved as a 24-hour continuous infusion, recent studies have indicated that a 3-hour infusion is also safe and is associated with a lower incidence of neutropenia.[137–140]

Toxicity. The dose-limiting side effect of the taxoids is myelosuppression, particularly neutropenia. Anemia and thrombocytopenia are uncommon. For paclitaxel, the incidence of neutropenia may be related to the duration of infusion, with longer durations producing more profound neutropenia. For docetaxel, neutropenia is not schedule dependent. Other common shared toxicities include mucositis, total alopecia, none to mild nausea and vomiting, cumulative neurotoxicity (predominantly peripheral neuropathy), and hypersensitivity reactions. The hypersensitivity reactions were noted early in the development of paclitaxel, occurring in 30–60% of patients. The duration of infusion was prolonged to 24 hours and a prophylactic regimen of corticosteroids, and H_1- and H_2-receptor antagonists was adopted (Table 119.12). Subsequently, the incidence of serious reactions was reduced to 2–4%. The hypersensitivity reactions may be due, in part, to the Cremophor EL (castor oil and absolute ethanol) vehicle used in its formulation. Docetaxel is much more water soluble than paclitaxel, and is formulated in a polysorbate 80 vehicle. However, docetaxel is also associated with hypersensitivity reactions in 18% of patients (4% serious reactions), suggesting that the taxane ring structure, rather than the vehicle, may be the cause of hypersensitivity.[108,137–140]

Docetaxel, but not paclitaxel, is known to cause cumulative fluid retention, which may result in edema, weight gain, and pleural effusions. A corticosteroid premedication regimen is often used with docetaxel to prevent fluid retention and hypersensitivity reactions. Docetaxel also commonly causes dermatologic reactions, which usually consist of a maculopapular rash affecting the hands and feet, with occasional desquamation.[138,139] Toxicities unique to paclitaxel include myalgias and cardiac toxicity. Cardiac rhythm disturbances were noted in early clinical trials of the drug, and routine telemetry monitoring was initiated. Asymptomatic bradycardia is the most common adverse cardiac effect, although heart block and ventricular dysrhythmias can also occur. However, serious cardiac effects are uncommon, and routine cardiac monitoring is no longer recommended. Cardiotoxicity may be more likely to occur in individuals with a prior history of cardiac disease.[137,140]

Drug Interactions. Studies of paclitaxel in combination with cisplatin indicate that administration of paclitaxel after cisplatin results in a 25% reduction in paclitaxel clearance and more severe neutropenia than when paclitaxel precedes cisplatin. Since taxoid metabolism may be mediated by hepatic P-450 enzymes, agents which interact with these enzymes could theoretically alter taxoid pharmacokinetics and clinical effects.

Irinotecan and Topotecan

Camptothecin is a plant alkaloid derived from *Camptotheca acuminata,* and is a potent inhibitor of DNA topoisomerase I. Although camptothecin showed significant activity in preclinical testing, clinical trials failed to show activity, and the drug produced severe unpredictable toxicity. As a result, the camptothecin analogs irinotecan (CPT-11) and topotecan were synthesized in an attempt to reduce toxicity and improve therapeutic effects.

Clinical Pharmacology. Topoisomerases are essential enzymes involved in maintaining DNA topologic structure during replication and transcription. The enzymes relieve torsional strain during DNA unwinding by producing strand breaks, thus permitting one or more strands to pass through the gap. The enzymes then reseal or religate the strand breaks. Topoisomerase I produces single strand breaks (Fig. 119.20), while topoisomerase II produces double strand breaks. Topoisomerase I inhibitors act by stabilizing the single strand breaks, and inhibiting religation.[142,143]

Pharmacokinetics. Irinotecan is rapidly converted by carboxylesterases to an active metabolite known as SN-38, which has 250- to 1000-fold greater antitumor activity than irinotecan. Irinotecan, SN-38, and topotecan undergo pH-dependent hydrolysis of the E-ring lactone to an open-ringed hydroxy acid (Fig. 119.21). Only the closed lactone form, which is favored in an acidic environment, exerts antitumor effects. The preferred diluent for these agents is 5% dextrose, which has a more acidic pH than saline, and slows hydrolysis of the lactone ring. However, once administered systemically, hydrolysis occurs rapidly; at equilibrium approximately 50% of drug exists in the closed lactone form. The major route of elimination of irinotecan and SN-38 is biliary excretion. Topotecan undergoes renal excretion, with 45% of the drug eliminated in the urine in the first 24 hours. Dosing guidelines in patients with impaired organ function have not been established.[142,143]

Clinical Uses. Irinotecan has significant activity in advanced colorectal cancer, possibly due to the presence of 14- to 16-fold higher concentrations of topoisomerase I, as compared to normal mucosa. Additional activity has been noted in several tumors, including lung, gastric, cervical, and ovarian cancers. Topotecan also exhibits broad antitu-

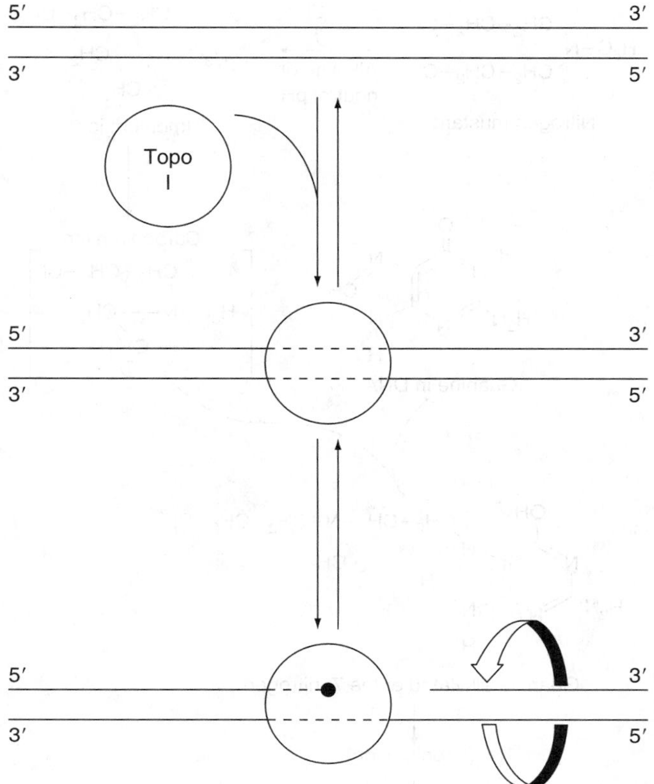

Figure 119.20. Topoisomerase I becomes covalently bound to DNA, creating a DNA protein cross-link and a nick in the phosphodiester backbone. DNA relaxation results from swiveling at this nick. *(From Creemers GJ, Lund B, Verweij J. Topoisomerase I inhibitors: Topotecan and irinotecan. Cancer Treat Rev 1994;20:73–96.)*

mor effects, including lung cancer, ovarian cancer, and myelogenous leukemias.[142,143]

Toxicity. The dose-limiting toxicity of both agents is myelosuppression. Neutrophils are most profoundly affected, and neutropenia is often accompanied by mild to moderate thrombocytopenia. For irinotecan, diarrhea also proved a severe toxicity, occurring in 20% of patients. The diarrhea may have two different presentations—either an acute onset occurring during or immediately after irinotecan administration, or a delayed onset occurring several days later. The acute form is often accompanied by facial flushing and abdominal cramping and responds to scopolamine or atropine. Premedication with serotonin-receptor antagonists and antihistamines largely prevents this complication. The chronic form is a secretory diarrhea, which may result in life-threatening dehydration. Prompt initiation of loperamide (given every 2 hours) at the first sign of diarrhea has minimized the consequences of this toxicity and permitted dosage escalation. Mild diarrhea is sometimes observed with topotecan. Pneumonitis has been associated following irinotecan administration. Other side effects common to both agents include alopecia, mild to moderate nausea and vomiting, rash, low-grade fevers, malaise, mucositis, and mild elevations in liver function tests.[142,143]

ALKYLATING AGENTS

The alkylating agents are among the oldest and most useful of antineoplastic drugs. Their clinical use evolved from observed shrinkage of lymph nodes in victims of sulfur mustard gas warfare during World War I. On the possibility that similar agents might be useful in overgrowths of lymphoid tissues such as lymphomas, less reactive derivatives

	R_1	R_2	R_3
CPT	H	H	H
TPT	OH	$(CH_3)_2NHCH_2$	H
CPT-11	(piperidinopiperidine carbonyloxy)	H	C_2H_5
SN-38	OH	H	C_2H_5

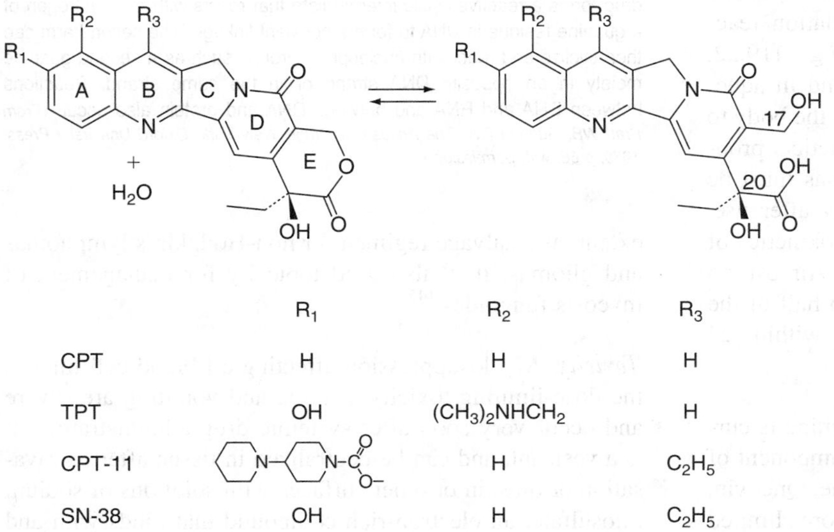

Figure 119.21. Structure of camptothecin (CPT), topotecan (TPT), irinotecan (CPT-11), and SN-38 lactone and the hydroxy acid form. *(Adapted from Creemers GJ, Lund B, Verweij J. Topoisomerase I inhibitors: Topotecan and irinotecan. Cancer Treat Rev 1994;20:73–96.)*

were synthesized. Their effectiveness as anticancer agents was confirmed by clinical trials in the middle 1940s.[144]

All of the alkylating agents are highly reactive compounds which work through the covalent bonding of alkyl groups or substituted alkyl groups with nucleophilic groups of cell components. Some of these nucleophilic groups are phosphates, or amino, carboxyl, sulfhydryl, or imidazole groups of proteins and nucleic acids. The most common site of binding for alkylating agents is the 7-nitrogen group of guanine. These covalent reactions can result in cross-linking between two DNA strands, or between bases in the same strand of DNA. Reactions between DNA and RNA, and between drug and proteins may also occur, but the main insult that results in cell death is inhibition of DNA replication. Because the alkylating agents can damage DNA during any phase of the cell cycle, they are considered cell cycle nonphase specific. However, their greatest effect is seen in rapidly dividing cells.[144,145] The several chemical classes of alkylators (e.g., nitrogen mustard derivatives, nitrosoureas, aziridines, sulfonic acid esters) differ in their spectrum of activity, pharmacologic characteristics, and toxicity patterns, but all of the alkylators are cytotoxic, mutagenic, teratogenic, carcinogenic, and myelosuppressive. Resistance to these agents can occur from increased DNA repair capabilities, or from decreased entry into cells. Various degrees of clinical cross-resistance among the alkylators exist.[144,145]

Nitrogen Mustard Derivatives

The best understood and most commonly used alkylating agents are the nitrogen mustard derivatives: mechlorethamine, chlorambucil, melphalan, cyclophosphamide, and ifosfamide.

Mechlorethamine

Mechlorethamine (also referred to as "nitrogen mustard" or HN_2) was the first mustard derivative to be used extensively. It is a bifunctional alkylating agent, that is, it has two reactive groups. A schematic of the alkylation reaction of mechlorethamine is illustrated in Fig. 119.22. Mechlorethamine is a highly unstable compound in aqueous solutions, and is degraded within minutes in the body to its alkylating intermediate. This also creates practical problems in patient care, because parenteral solutions must be freshly prepared and administered immediately after use. Because of this rapid degradation, the pharmacokinetics of mechlorethamine are not well characterized. Almost no intact drug is detectable in urine, but more than half of the inactive metabolites are excreted in urine within 24 hours.[145,146]

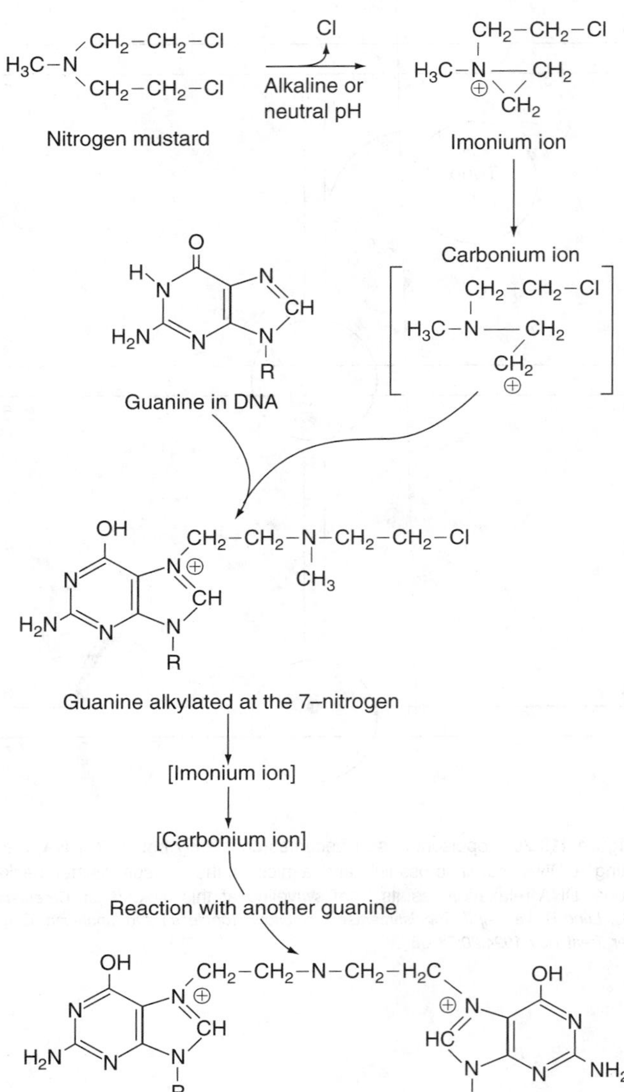

Figure 119.22. Alkylation reaction of nitrogen mustard. In solution, the drug forms a reactive cyclic intermediate that reacts with the 7-nitrogen of a guanine residue in DNA to form a covalent linkage. The second arm can then cyclize and react with nucleophilic groups such as a second guanine moiety in an opposite DNA strand or in the same strand. Reactions between DNA and RNA and between DNA and protein also occur. *(From Pratt WB, Ruddon RW. The Anticancer Drugs. New York, Oxford University Press, 1979, p 66, with permission.)*

Clinical Uses. The clinical use of mechlorethamine is currently limited to Hodgkin's lymphomas, as a component of the first-line "MOPP" regimen (mechlorethamine, Oncovin, procarbazine, and prednisone), and to a more limited extent, as a salvage regimen for non-Hodgkin's lymphomas and gliomas. It is also used topically for management of mycosis fungoides.[145]

Toxicity. Myelosuppression affecting all blood cell lines is the dose-limiting toxicity. Nausea and vomiting are severe and occur very soon after systemic drug administration. It is a vesicant, and can be neutralized in tissue after extravasation or on skin or other surfaces with solutions of sodium thiosulfate, an electron-rich compound that binds with and inactivates the reactive groups of nitrogen mustard. The most serious long-term consequences of this agent are development of second cancers, especially when it is used in combination with radiation therapy, and sterility.[117,144]

Melphalan

Melphalan, or phenylalanine mustard (L-PAM), was developed in an attempt to create an alkylating agent that would preferentially accumulate in melanoma tumor cells, since phenylalanine is a precursor of melanin. The compound did not prove to have the desired selectivity for melanocytes, but is useful in several tumors, especially multiple myeloma, breast and ovarian cancers, and in high doses with bone marrow support or stem-cell rescue for treatment of various solid tumors. Parenteral melphalan is also administered for treatment of limb lesions in malignant melanoma by isolated regional limb perfusion techniques.[144,147]

Pharmacokinetics. Melphalan is less reactive than the parent compound, mechlorethamine, and can be given orally, or by infusion of the parenteral form. Bioavailability after oral administration is quite variable, but approximates 70%. It is decreased by food. Following intravenous administration, melphalan is distributed into total body water, and eliminated with a half-life of 1–2 hours. The disposition half-life is affected by hydration status of the patient. Spontaneous degradation is believed to be the main route of elimination. Although only about 15% of an administered intravenous dose is detectable in urine within 24 hours, toxicity of intravenous melphalan may be increased in patients with renal dysfunction, and may require dose reduction. Dose considerations are affected by variations in the percentage of unbound drug in plasma.[144,146,148]

Toxicity. Dose-limiting toxicity of melphalan is myelosuppression, which is characterized by damage to marrow stem cells, resulting in slow recovery of blood counts, and sometimes cumulative marrow damage. It does not usually cause nausea, vomiting, or alopecia in conventional low daily doses. Hypersensitivity reactions have been documented in fewer than 5% of patients receiving intravenous melphalan, but have not been reported with oral use. In high doses administered as part of marrow transplant regimens, gastrointestinal toxicity with mucositis, nausea, vomiting, and diarrhea become dose limiting, and alopecia is also reported.[144,145,148]

Chlorambucil

Chlorambucil is a nitrogen mustard derivative with selective cytotoxicity for lymphocyte cell lines. As such, its major application is for treatment of chronic lymphocytic leukemia, although it has some application in lymphomas, breast cancers, and ovarian cancer. It is available only for oral use and is more rapidly and completely absorbed than melphalan, although its absorption is also decreased by food. Elimination is mainly by metabolic degradation, and the half-life is about 1.5 hours. An active metabolite, phenylacetic acid mustard, may contribute to both therapeutic and toxic effects. Chloramubucil is well tolerated, with dose-limiting myelosuppression and little nausea. Chronic therapy has been associated with a high incidence of secondary acute leukemias.[144,146]

Cyclophosphamide and Ifosfamide

Cyclophosphamide is the most widely used of the nitrogen mustard derivatives and of all the alkylating agents. Ifosfamide is closely related in structure, clinical use, and toxicity. Neither agent is active in its parent form and must be activated by mixed hepatic oxidase enzymes to the alkylating moieties. The active metabolite of cyclophosphamide is probably phosphoramide mustard. Another metabolite, 4-hydroxycyclophosphamide, is cytotoxic, but is not an alkylating agent, and probably acts as a transport form to deliver phosphoramide mustard into cells. Another metabolite of both drugs, acrolein, does not have antitumor activity, but may be responsible for some of the toxicity seen with these drugs. Ifosfamide undergoes hepatic activation to its active alkylating metabolite, ifosfamide mustard, and to acrolein, but this activation process occurs more slowly than with cyclophosphamide.[144,145,149]

Pharmacokinetics. Characterization of the pharmacokinetic behavior of these compounds is complicated by the existence of multiple active and inactive metabolites. Cyclophosphamide is well absorbed orally, with a systemic availability approaching 100%, although it is variable among patients. The terminal phase half-life is about 7 hours, and the major metabolic site is the liver. About 15% of unchanged drug and most of the metabolites are eliminated in the urine. Empiric dose reductions have been recommended in patients with creatinine clearance below 30 mL/min. Although cyclophosphamide is largely metabolized, there has been no consistent pattern of altered metabolism in patients with hepatic dysfunction, and dose reductions are not known to be necessary. Significant amounts of an administered cyclophosphamide dose can be cleared by dialysis. It does not enter the CNS in significant concentrations.[144,146]

Pharmacokinetics of ifosfamide are similar. Because of the slower rate of activation, ifosfamide must be used in greater doses (approximately three to four times) than the cyclophosphamide dose required to achieve similar alkylating activity. More unchanged drug is excreted in the urine (20–50%) than is true for cyclophosphamide. The half-life is schedule dependent, and is about 6 hours if divided daily doses are administered, but increases to 16 hours with single large doses. Unchanged drug is detectable in the CNS in significant quantities, but only very small amounts of the active metabolites are detectable. It is unlikely that ifosfamide will therefore be active in CNS tumors, but this limited penetration may account for its CNS toxicity.[146,149]

Clinical Uses. Cyclophosphamide is a broad-spectrum antineoplastic agent, with activity against acute leukemias, lymphomas, and a variety of solid tumors, especially breast cancer, sarcomas, ovarian and endometrial cancers, small cell lung cancer, and multiple myeloma. It is widely used as part of preparative regimens for both autologous and allogeneic bone marrow transplantation. Cyclophosphamide is also a potent immunosuppressive agent, and has several nononcology applications, including management of rheumatic disorders and autoimmune-mediated nephritis. Ifosfamide is primarily used for testicular cancers refractory to first-line treatment, soft tissue sarcomas, non-Hodgkin's lymphomas, and small cell lung cancers.[144,149]

Toxicity. Myelosuppression occurs with both agents and is dose limiting for cyclophosphamide. White blood cells are particularly sensitive to these drugs, but platelets are uncommonly reduced to hazardous levels, making these drugs relatively platelet sparing. Recovery from leukopenia is rapid, indicating little stem-cell damage. Myelosuppression from ifosfamide is much less severe from divided daily doses than from a single large dose. Both agents are potent emetogens. The nausea and vomiting from cyclophosphamide, but not ifosfamide, is characterized by a delay in onset of up to 8 hours. Alopecia is dose related.[144,149]

The classic toxicity of these drugs, and the dose-limiting toxicity for ifosfamide, is hemorrhagic cystitis. This is a syndrome of blood loss from the bladder accompanied by symptoms of frequency and irritation, which can cause sclerosis of the bladder, massive hemorrhage, and occasionally bladder carcinoma. The toxic metabolite common to both cyclophosphamide and ifosfamide, acrolein, is believed to be responsible for this cystitis, by binding to critical thiols in the bladder wall. Damage is proportional to dose and to duration of exposure, and may be minimized by hydration with frequent voiding to decrease acrolein contact with the bladder mucosa. Patients receiving conventional doses of cyclophosphamide should be counseled to drink 3 L of fluids on the day of cyclophosphamide administration, and for 2 days after dosing. In most cases, this will successfully prevent mucosal damage. However, in high-dose cyclophosphamide regimens, such as those used in bone marrow transplant programs, or for conventional ifosfamide dosing, hydration is typically inadequate prevention. Either high-volume bladder irrigations, or systemic administration of sulfhydryl compounds is recommended in addition to hydration. The approved sulfhydryl compound is "mesna" (mercapto ethane sulfonate sodium). The sulfhydryl groups of mesna bind preferentially with acrolein, forming a nontoxic complex which can be voided from the bladder, preventing mucosal acrolein attachment and damage. Mesna does not interfere with the cytotoxic activity of cyclophosphamide or ifosfamide. When ifosfamide is administered in fractionated daily doses, mesna is given before and at 4 and 8 hours after the ifosfamide dose, in doses equal to 20% of the ifosfamide dosage.[145,149,150] Prostaglandins have been used anecdotally in the management of cyclophosphamide-induced cystitis.[151]

Although bladder toxicity is most characteristic of these compounds, damage to the renal tubules may also occur. Nephrotoxicity has been best documented in children receiving ifosfamide and in high-dose regimens. Damage may involve any part of the nephron and may result in clinically relevant glomerular and/or renal tubular impairment, such as Fanconi's syndrome. The risk of nephrotoxicity is increased by nephrectomy and by concomitant cisplatin. Toxicity may be mediated by a similar mechanism to bladder toxicity, or through the effects of the ifosfamide metabolite, chloroacetaldehyde. Although mesna may be able to detoxify the toxic metabolites, it may not reach the renal tubules in a high enough concentration to provide adequate protection.[152–155]

One toxicity that is common from ifosfamide but does not occur with cyclophosphamide is CNS toxicity, which typically presents as decreased level of arousal, with occasional progression to somnolence, coma, and death. Confusion, hallucinations, and seizures may also occur. Assessment of CNS status is complicated by the effects of antiemetic therapy which is required in conjunction with ifosfamide. CNS toxicity is less severe with fractionated doses of ifosfamide than with single large doses. Rare toxicities from cyclophosphamide include pulmonary fibrosis and cardiac toxicity, especially in bone marrow transplant doses. Inappropriate antidiuretic hormone release may also occur from cyclophosphamide therapy.[144,149,155]

Nitrosoureas

The nitrosoureas are alkylating agents characterized by lipophilicity and ability to cross the blood–brain barrier. Carmustine or bischloroethylnitrosourea (BCNU), lomustine (CCNU), and a closely related methylnitrosourea, streptozotocin, are commercially available. Methyl CCNU (semustine) remains an investigational agent. The nitrosoureas decompose to reactive alkylating metabolites as well as to isocyanate compounds which have several effects on reproducing cells and which may be involved in the toxicity of these drugs.[144,145]

Pharmacokinetics. The nitrosoureas are extensively and rapidly biotransformed after administration, and the degradation products demonstrate a prolonged elimination, perhaps from binding to cellular components. Metabolites and a small percentage of intact drug are excreted in urine. Because of the lipophilic nature of these compounds, they enter the CNS readily, and achieve concentrations of about 30% of simultaneous plasma levels. Lomustine and methyl–CCNU are administered orally and are well absorbed. Some enterohepatic circulation may occur. Streptozotocin disposition is similar to that of the other nitrosoureas.[144–146]

Clinical Uses. Because of their excellent CNS penetration, the nitrosoureas have been studied in the treatment of primary brain tumors. Carmustine and lomustine are indicated for the palliative treatment of this disease. They also have activity in multiple myeloma, refractory Hodgkin's disease, and melanoma. Lomustine and methyl–CCNU have some activity in gastrointestinal tract tumors. Methyl–CCNU has been most extensively studied in the adjuvant treatment of rectal cancers, where it demonstrates some modest benefit. Clinical use of streptozotocin is limited to pancreatic tumors, especially of islet cell origin, and carcinoid tumors.[144]

Toxicity. Myelosuppression is the dose-limiting toxicity of the nitrosoureas in conventional doses. The myelosuppression is unusually delayed and prolonged, and complete recovery typically takes 6–8 weeks. Thrombocytopenia occurs earlier and is generally more pronounced than leukopenia. Streptozotocin, however, is not myelosuppressive. All these compounds, particularly streptozotocin, cause severe nausea and vomiting. They are also renal toxins, and produce dose-related damage, which consists of glomerulosclerosis, severe tubular loss, and interstitial fibrosis. Renal toxicity correlates with cumulative doses. Carmustine commonly causes facial flushing and pain along the vein during infusion, which may be related to the alcohol vehicle.[144,145]

In long-term treatment or in the high doses used with bone marrow transplantation, pulmonary toxicity of carmustine can be dose limiting. Incidence may be as high as 30% in patients with brain tumors treated with carmustine as a single agent. Patients typically present with shortness of breath, tachypnea, and nonproductive cough, and may improve clinically with administration of corticosteroids. Histologic damage is usually characterized as interstitial pneumonitis and fibrosis. Lomustine has also occasionally produced pulmonary damage.[75,144]

Other Alkylating Agents

Thiotepa

Thiotepa is the only member of the aziridine group of alkylating agents currently in clinical use. The aziridines are analogues of the closed-ring intermediates of the nitrogen mustards, and are believed to alkylate through opening of the aziridine ring. Thiotepa, or triethylenethiophosphoramide, is poorly absorbed from the gastrointestinal tract, is lipid soluble, achieves therapeutic levels in the CNS, and is primarily excreted unchanged in the urine. It is administered intravesically, intravenously, or, occasionally, intrathecally. Thiotepa is active locally for superficial bladder cancers, and is a second- or third-line agent for treatment of breast cancer as a component of the "VATH" regimen (vinblastine, Adriamycin, thiotepa, Halotestin) and for ovarian cancer. Recently, it has received increased interest as a component of regimens for autologous bone marrow transplantation, because its main toxicity is hematopoietic. Bone marrow depression may occur even after bladder instillation. Paresthesias can occur when thiotepa is administered intrathecally in hypertonic solutions, so sterile water rather than saline is the recommended diluent for CNS administration. However, because of the ready entry of thiotepa and its active metabolite into the CNS after systemic administration, there is no pharmacokinetic advantage to intrathecal injection.[144,146]

Busulfan

The last of the classic alkylating agents to be discussed is busulfan, an alkyl alkane sulfonate. Busulfan, like other alkylators, is toxic to the bone marrow, but, unlike the other agents, produces greater myelosuppressive damage to myeloid than lymphoid cells. This relative specificity has made it a useful agent for treatment of chronic myelogenous leukemia. It is not active against solid tumors in conventional doses, but has activity in high-dose alkylating regimens with bone marrow transplant rescue. Busulfan is well absorbed orally in low doses, and the intact drug disappears very rapidly from the plasma. Metabolites are excreted in the urine. Pharmacokinetics of high-dose busulfan are age dependent, with lower systemic exposure in children than adults. In contrast to most cytotoxic drugs, busulfan enters the CSF readily after systemic administration, achieving concentrations at least equal to those in plasma, and persisting in the CSF for several hours.[146,156]

Toxicity. The most common toxicity of busulfan is an extension of its therapeutic effects—bone marrow suppression. It appears to damage bone marrow stem cells and can produce prolonged myelosuppression. Busulfan also causes skin hyperpigmentation, especially at skin creases, and occasionally, Addisonian symptoms. Nausea and vomiting are uncommon at standard doses, but may occur in high-dose regimens. Neurotoxicity characterized by generalized tonic–clonic seizures is associated with high-dose regimens administered as preparation for bone marrow transplantation, but can be prevented by prophylactic anticonvulsant administration. High doses of busulfan are also believed to contribute to the occurrence of hepatic veno-occlusive disease (VOD) in bone marrow transplant patients, although the cause of VOD is multifactorial.[156] The most classic toxicity of busulfan is pulmonary fibrosis, or "busulfan lung." Clinical incidence is estimated at 4% of patients overall, although the incidence of subclinical damage is probably much higher. The mechanism of pulmonary damage is unknown, but increased epithelial sensitivity to the drug may be a factor. The best established risk factor is duration of busulfan treatment, with an average time to onset of more than 3 years. Radiation exposure also increases risk. Onset of symptoms is insidious and characteristically includes development of nonproductive cough, shortness of breath, weight loss, and sometimes fevers. Chest x-ray usually shows a reticular pattern in the lung bases, and histologically, interstitial pulmonary fibrosis is prominent. No treatment has been proven effective by controlled trials, but anecdotally, corticosteroids may be helpful. The mean survival after diagnosis, however, is only 5 months.[75,156]

Nonclassic Alkylating Agents

Several other cytotoxic agents appear to act as alkylators, although their structures do not include the classic alkylation chloroethyl group. They are capable of binding covalently to cellular components, and include procarbazine, dacarbazine, and hexamethylmelamine. In addition, some antitumor antibiotics have been proposed to function as alkylators.[157]

Procarbazine

Procarbazine was originally synthesized as a monoamine oxidase (MAO) inhibitor, but was shown in routine screening to have antitumor activity. It is a prodrug, and must be converted to cytotoxic intermediates, probably by liver cytochrome P-450. These intermediates are believed to have alkylating activity, although several other cellular damaging effects have been detected. Ultimately, procarbazine inhibits DNA, RNA, and protein synthesis.[145,157]

Pharmacokinetics. Pharmacokinetic information for procarbazine is incomplete despite its many years of use. Procarbazine is administered orally, and is rapidly and completely absorbed. A "first-pass" effect is likely. It is rapidly metabolized, with metabolites eliminated primarily in the urine. Procarbazine enters the CNS very readily and achieves concentrations comparable to those in plasma.[146,157]

Clinical Uses. Procarbazine's clinical use is limited primarily to treatment of Hodgkin's disease as a component of the "MOPP" regimen, although it has some activity in non-Hodgkin's lymphomas, and in brain tumors because of its ready entry into the CNS.[157]

Toxicity. The most common toxicities of procarbazine administration are protracted myelosuppression and gastrointestinal symptoms of anorexia, nausea, and vomiting. Tolerance often occurs to these gastrointestinal symptoms with continued use. Occasional neurotoxic and hypersensitivity reactions also occur. Procarbazine is highly toxic to reproductive organs and commonly produces sterility, particularly in males. It is highly mutagenic and carcinogenic, and is associated, with mechlorethamine, in the increased risk of secondary malignancies after MOPP therapy.[157,158] There are also several drug–drug and drug–food interactions of potential consequence. Because procarbazine is a MAO inhibitor, therapy with tricyclic antidepressants, sympathomimetic drugs, and foods containing high levels of tyramine, such as red wines, aged cheeses, yogurt, and bananas, can precipitate acute hypertensive reactions. A disulfiram-like reaction can occur with alcohol, and the effects of other CNS depressants may be potentiated.[157]

Dacarbazine

Dacarbazine, or dimethyl triazeno imidazole carboxamide (DTIC) is a nonclassic alkylating agent with activity in malignant melanoma, Hodgkin's disease, and soft tissue sarcomas. It was synthesized in an attempt to make purine antimetabolites, as an analogue of the carboxamide intermediate in purine synthesis, but it does not interfere with purine synthesis. Its exact mechanism of action is unknown, but the parent molecule does undergo demethylation to active intermediates which can alkylate nucleic acids *in vitro*. In cell culture, dacarbazine also inhibits DNA, RNA, and protein synthesis. It appears to be active in all phases of the cell cycle and may cause delays in the G_2 phase.[145,157]

Pharmacokinetics. Dacarbazine is not well absorbed orally and is administered by intravenous infusion. It disappears from the plasma biphasically with an alpha phase half-life of about 19 minutes and a beta phase half-life of 5 hours. About half of an administered dose is recoverable in urine as parent drug; tubular secretion is believed to be involved. Hepatobiliary excretion may also occur, but effects of renal and hepatic dysfunction on drug elimination are not defined. Dacarbazine penetrates poorly into the CNS, but does have modest activity against brain tumors. It decomposes in the presence of light, but this is not clinically relevant in usual administration schedules.[146,157]

Toxicity. Toxicity to dacarbazine is characterized by severe nausea and vomiting, which tends to decrease with successive doses on multiple-day schedules, and mild to moderate myelosuppression. It also produces a flu-like syndrome, which occurs near the end of dacarbazine treatment and persists for several days, burning pain along the injection site, and photosensitivity. Hepatic toxicity has been reported, with rare instances of VOD.[157]

Hexamethylmelamine

Hexamethylmelamine (altretamine, HMM) was synthesized in the 1950s and began clinical trials in the 1960s, but has only very recently been approved for clinical use. Its mechanism of action is unknown. It is structurally similar to the alkylating agent triethylenemelamine, but it is not currently recognized as an alkylator. It is believed that methyl groups and metabolic activation are essential for cytotoxic activity. There is also some evidence that HMM inhibits RNA and DNA synthesis. Little is known about resistance to HMM, except that clinical cross-resistance with other alkylators is inconsistent.[157,159,160]

Pharmacokinetics. Clinical tests of HMM have used an oral capsule, because the compound has poor water solubility, but oral bioavailability is extremely variable. Peak plasma levels, which may vary 100-fold among patients, are achieved at an average 1–3 hours after oral administration. Plasma disappearance is also variable, with a half-life of 3–13 hours. It is metabolized in liver microsomes and metabolites are excreted in urine. CSF penetration of HMM is low, but metabolites may enter the CNS as well.[159,160]

Clinical Uses. The main clinical utility and only approved use of HMM is in treatment of ovarian cancer, particularly cancers resistant to first-line therapy. In that situation, HMM as a single agent has an objective response rate of about 20%, with occasional complete responses. It also has activity in lung cancers and endometrial carcinoma. The recommended dose as a single agent is 260 mg/m^2 daily for 14 days each month.[157,159,160]

Toxicity. At conventional 2-week doses, the main toxicity of HMM is gastrointestinal, with symptoms of nausea, vomiting, anorexia, and diarrhea. Peripheral neuropathy also occurs. Longer dose schedules are associated with an increased incidence of neurotoxicity, which typically presents as paresthesias, hyporeflexia, motor weakness, and decreased sensation. Myelosuppression occurs with prolonged administration, but is rarely dose limiting.[159,160]

ANTHRACENE DERIVATIVES

The anthracene derivatives are very useful anticancer drugs with a broad spectrum of anticancer activity among the group members. The most widely used and best understood of the group is doxorubicin, also commonly known by its earliest trade name, Adriamycin or "adria," although it is now available from several manufacturers. Other members of the anthracene group include daunorubicin (daunomycin), idarubicin, the investigational agent epirubicin, and mitoxantrone. Most members of the group share a common, four-membered anthracene ring complex. The ring complex is a chromophore and accounts for the intense colors of these compounds. Most also have an attached aglycone or sugar portion. Doxorubicin differs from the parent compound daunorubicin by the addition of a hydroxyl group on the attached sugar, and it is sometimes consequently referred to as hydroxydaunorubicin. A hydroxyl group on epirubicin is in the *epi* conformation compared with doxorubicin (epidoxorubicin); and idarubicin is demethoxydaunorubicin. Mitoxantrone is an anthracenedione rather than an anthracycline, and has no sugar group attached to the three-membered anthracene ring complex.[161,162]

Doxorubicin, Daunorubicin, and Idarubicin

The mechanism of action of the anthracyclines is not yet completely defined. It is known that they bind tightly to double-stranded DNA, and that binding is essential for their cytotoxic action. Traditionally they have been considered as intercalating agents, that is, compounds that insert between base pairs of DNA, causing deformation and local uncoiling of the DNA. Although it is well established that the planar groups of the anthracene ring complex do intercalate with DNA, this is not believed to be the direct mechanism of cytotoxicity. The anthracycline intercalators cause protein-associated breaks, from interference with the actions of topoisomerase II, the enzyme that regulates the three-dimensional structure of DNA as the strands open and close. The anthracyclines bind to the DNA–topoisomerase II complex, making a "dead-end" ternary complex that prevents the broken DNA from resealing.[161–163]

Another consideration in the mechanism of anthracycline-induced cytotoxicity is that of free radical formation. The anthracyclines can undergo electron reductions to reactive compounds that can damage DNA and cell membranes. Free radicals formed from reduction of the anthracyclines donate electrons to oxygen to make superoxide, which can react with itself to make hydrogen peroxide. Cleavage of this produces the highly reactive and destructive hydroxyl radical. This last step is believed to require iron, and the anthracyclines bind iron very powerfully. Iron–anthracycline complexes can bind to DNA, and react rapidly with hydrogen peroxide to produce the hydroxyl radicals that actually cleave DNA. Human cells have natural defenses against oxygen radical damage, specifically enzymes that can convert the radicals to less reactive compounds, or which can repair DNA damage. Differences in distribution of these defensive enzymes may account for characteristic sites of toxicities of the anthracyclines. For example, heart muscle has low levels of defensive enzymes, and high levels of enzymes which activate anthracyclines (see Toxicity discussion). Oxygen radical formation is firmly established as a cause of toxicity such as cardiac damage and extravasation injury, but is less likely as a cause of tumor cell kill.[161–163] Other potential mechanisms of cytotoxicity include interactions with helicases, enzymes that separate double-stranded DNA, and interactions with the cell membranes.[163]

Resistance to the anthracyclines is usually secondary to P-glycoprotein-dependent multidrug resistance, which causes active pumping of drug from the cells. Verapamil, cyclosporin, tamoxifen, and other agents may be used clinically to reverse the resistance. Encapsulation of anthracyclines in liposomes and treatment with targeted antibodies are other strategies that are being evaluated. Altered topoisomerase II activity or altered free radical chemistry may also be clinically important mechanisms of resistance to the anthracyclines.[161–163]

Pharmacokinetics. The most important factor in the pharmacokinetic behavior of doxorubicin is its extensive tissue binding. Doxorubicin distributes rapidly to all body tissues except those of the CNS and binds primarily to DNA, accounting for its very large volume of distribution of about 1000 L/m^2. It is only slowly released from tissues, with a half-life of 30 hours. Doxorubicin has been detected in tissue even months after administration. It is metabolized by cytoplasmic aldoketoreductases to doxorubicinol, an active metabolite, and 50% is excreted in bile. Less than 10% is eliminated in the urine, although this is enough to discolor the urine a characteristic orange-red color, and much of the elimination remains unaccounted for. Ability of the liver to metabolize the drug is much greater than the rate of release of drug from tissues, and brings into question the validity of empiric guidelines for dose modification based on elevated liver function tests (Table 119.10). Elevated bilirubin levels in association with primary liver cancer have recently been confirmed to alter doxorubicin pharmacokinetics and pharmacodynamics. The presence of large or diffuse liver metastases may alter anthracycline pharmacokinetics, even in the absence of bilirubin elevations. There is some evidence that aspartate aminotransferase levels may be more useful than bilirubin in adjustment of anthracycline doses. Until dosing guidelines can be validated, dose modification in patients with elevated bilirubins remains the accepted, but cautious, recommendation.[115,162–164]

Daunorubicin's pharmacokinetics are similar to those of doxorubicin. It is rapidly and extensively metabolized to daunorubicinol. The elimination is believed to be biphasic, with terminal half-lives of 15–20 hours for daunorubicin and about 30 hours for daunorubicinol. As with doxorubicin, tissue binding is extensive, but similar empiric dose modifications should be considered in patients with hepatic dysfunction (Table 119.10).[162,164]

Idarubicin is more lipophilic than the other anthracyclines and is taken up into cells more rapidly. Its primary metabolite, idarubicinol, is as active as the parent drug. The concentration of idarubicinol in plasma is typically more than double that of the parent compound. Elimination is poorly defined. Renal excretion is greater than for doxorubicin, but accounts for <5% of idarubicin elimination and about 10% of idarubicinol. The role of hepatic elimination also has been questioned, and much of the elimination is uncertain. The half-life of idarubicin is 15–20 hours, but that of idarubicinol is 40–60 hours. An oral formulation is under investigation.[165,166]

Clinical Uses. Doxorubicin is a very broad-spectrum and useful anticancer agent. It is one of the most active single drugs available against breast cancer, and is also useful in treatment of sarcomas, gastrointestinal tumors, bladder cancer, gynecologic malignancies, multiple myeloma, and lung cancer, as well as Hodgkin's and non-Hodgkin's lymphomas and acute leukemias. Its efficacy is not schedule dependent, but seems to correlate with total exposure expressed as area under the curve (AUC). Clinical use of daunorubicin and idarubicin is limited to induction and consolidation therapy in patients with ANLL. Idarubicin achieves slightly higher response rates and longer median survival than daunorubicin regimens in ANLL.[162,163,166]

Toxicity. Although the anthracyclines are very active drugs, they are also very toxic. The most common dose-limiting toxicity in the short term is myelosuppression. They also cause moderate to severe dose-related nausea and vomiting, alopecia, and mucositis. Mucositis may be dose limiting in doxorubicin infusion protocols.[162,163] Recently, secondary acute myeloid leukemia with chromosome translocations similar to epipodophyllotoxin-associated leukemia has been recognized in patients receiving anthracyclines in combination with alkylating agents.[167] However, the anthracyclines are most famous for their cardiac toxicity and for extravasation injuries.

There are two main components of anthracycline-induced cardiac damage: acute and chronic. Acute toxicity consists primarily of rhythm disturbances, especially nonspecific ST/T-wave changes, sinus tachycardia, and increased frequency of ventricular premature beats. Typically, these occur within the first 24 hours after drug administration. They are usually self-limited and do not appear to increase the risks of future cardiac events. However, a pericarditis–myocarditis syndrome of fever, pericarditis, and congestive heart failure can also occur at low cumulative doses and may be fatal.[163,168]

More serious than the acute cardiac changes is the risk of congestive cardiomyopathy, which effectively limits the cumulative dose of anthracycline that can be administered. Cardiomyopathy is believed to be secondary to free radical formation within the heart muscle, which results in damage to the sarcoplasmic reticulum and gradual loss of myofibrils from the cells. Damage to the sarcoplasmic membrane results in loss of its ability to bind calcium, and disrupts the link between electrical excitation and muscle contraction. Clinical evidence of cardiac damage is clearly dose related and depends on the extent of myofibril loss. Although there is a real but very low incidence in patients with cumulative doxorubicin dose less than 550 mg/m^2, the incidence approaches 50% in doses that are double that, in bolus dosing (Fig. 119.23). Risk is greater and deterioration occurs at lower cumulative doses in patients with previous cardiac irradiation. The elderly, the very young, females, and those with preexisting hypertension or cardiac disease are also at increased risk.[163,168–170]

Incidence is also closely associated with dose schedule, and schedule changes are currently the most effective

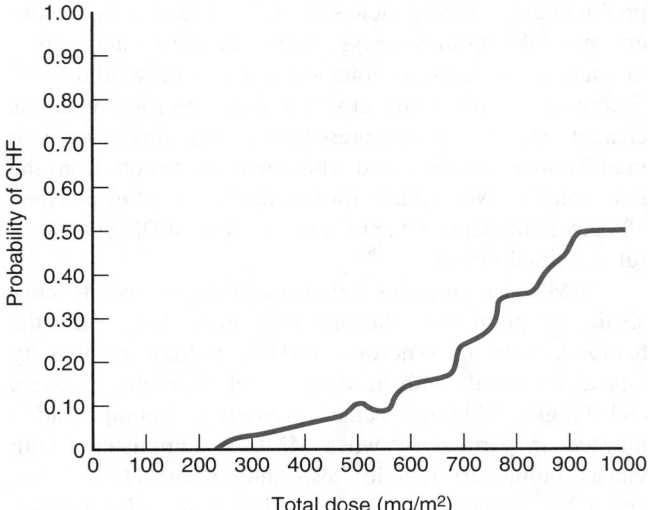

Figure 119.23. Risk of cardiac toxicity with cumulative doxorubicin dose. CHF, congestive heart failure. *(From Von Hoff DD, Layard MW, Basa P, et al. Risk factors for doxorubicin-induced congestive heart failure. Ann Intern Med 1979;91:710–717, with permission.)*

interventions readily available to decrease risk of cardiac toxicity. The risk estimates outlined above and in Fig. 119.23 refer to traditional doxorubicin dosing, that is, 60 mg/m^2 by intravenous bolus every 3–4 weeks. It has been established that cardiac damage correlates with *peaks* of drug concentration achieved, rather than with total exposure to the drug (AUC). Administering the same total dose in small weekly doses[171] or by continuous infusion over 2–4 days[172] markedly improves the cardiology risk-to-benefit ratio of doxorubicin administration, but continuous infusion leads to more severe stomatitis. Serial endomyocardial biopsies or evaluations of left ventricular ejection fraction such as multigaited acquisition ("MUGA") scans may be useful in assessing extent of cardiac muscle injury and the individualized risk of continuing anthracycline therapy in patients who are responding to treatment but approaching the recommended dose, or in those with coexisting risk factors. Unfortunately, the appearance of cardiac toxicity may be delayed until many months or years after completion of therapy, which may decrease the utility of prospective monitoring.[163,168,170]

Although many different pharmacologic interventions to prevent cardiac damage have been attempted, the only FDA-approved agent is dexrazoxane (ICRF-187). The carboxylamine metabolite of dexrazoxane is a potent chelator of divalent ions, including iron in its ferric state. Anthracycline complexation with iron is known to be essential for the free radical formation which initiates cardiac damage. Dexrazoxane's ability to disrupt the iron–anthracycline complex and prevent reactive radical formation may be responsible for its cardioprotective effects. It is indicated for reducing the incidence and severity of doxorubicin-induced cardiomyopathy. FDA approval for its use is currently limited to women with breast cancer who have received a cumulative dose of 300 mg/m^2 of doxorubicin who are expected to benefit from continued doxorubicin therapy. Formulation of anthracyclines in liposomal delivery systems may also decrease cardiotoxicity of these compounds, since liposomes are not taken up as readily by cardiac tissue as free drug.[170,173]

Daunorubicin and doxorubicin have similar potential for cardiac toxicity, but, because of the limited use of daunorubicin and the rarity of high cumulative doses in the leukemic population, clinically important cardiomyopathy is uncommonly seen. Doses of 900–1000 mg/m^2 are approximately equivalent in risk to doxorubicin doses of 550 mg/m^2. Idarubicin may be less cardiotoxic than doxorubicin or daunorubicin in equivalent doses.[166,168]

The other classic toxicity of the anthracycline drugs is tissue damage on extravasation. Deep ulceration with tissue necrosis may occur and progress over many weeks. Ulcers typically have raised red edges and necrotic centers, and heal very slowly if at all. Drug may be detected in the ulcer tissue for months after extravasation. At present, no remedy of well-documented efficacy exists to prevent or reverse tissue damage, although application of ice to the extravasation site is the current standard of care. Topical application of dimethylsulfoxide (DMSO) to the extravasation site is inconsistently useful in some animal models and anecdotally useful in humans, but DMSO has not been studied systematically and is not considered standard treatment for anthracycline extravasation.[117] Doxorubicin may also cause a "flare" reaction that presents during or immediately after injection, with redness and urticaria extending up the vein. It is self-limiting and usually subsides within 30 minutes. Doxorubicin may also reactivate skin damage in sites of previous radiation therapy, the so-called "radiation recall" reaction.

Mitoxantrone

Mitoxantrone is an anthracendione, a compound that shares a similar ring structure with the anthracyclines, but does not possess the attached sugars. It was synthesized in attempts to develop compounds with comparable antitumor activity to doxorubin but with a better safety profile. Mitoxantrone is a reasonably broad-spectrum antitumor agent, with good activity against breast cancer, lymphomas, acute leukemias, and ovarian cancer. It is less active as a single agent against breast cancer than is doxorubicin. In ANLL, its overall activity as an induction agent is comparable to that of daunorubicin, but a higher percentage of patients will achieve complete remission with one cycle of induction therapy than with a single daunorubicin cycle. ANLL induction, in combination with cytarabine, is the only approved indication for mitoxantrone.[162,174]

The mechanisms of action of mitoxantrone are similar to the anthracyclines and include intercalation with production of single- and double-strand DNA breaks, but its potential for free radical formation is much less than that of the anthracycline drugs. Pharmacokinetics are characterized by extensive tissue binding and slow elimination, with metabolism and biliary excretion accounting for most of the known elimination. Perhaps because of the decreased tendency for free radical formation, the nonmarrow toxicity of mitoxantrone is markedly less than the traditional anthracyclines. Nausea and vomiting, mucositis, and alopecia are substantially less common and severe than with doxorubicin, and the risks of cardiac toxicity and ulceration after extravasation, although still present, are markedly reduced. Mitoxantrone's intense blue color produces a blue-green discoloration of urine, and may give a blue tint to sclera and skin. In high doses, hyperbilirubinemia may be dose limiting.[162,174–176]

ANTITUMOR ANTIBIOTICS

Mitomycin C

Mitomycin C (MMC) is an antitumor antibiotic first produced as a fermentation product from *Streptomyces caespitosus* in the late 1950s. It has been commercially available for about 25 years. It is believed to function as an alkylating agent. MMC itself is a prodrug, and must be activated by reduction reactions to the alkylating species. Ultimately, strand breakage and inhibition of DNA synthesis occur. MMC activation may also result in the production of superoxide free radicals, which can contribute to the cytotoxic effects by causing lipid peroxidation or nucleic acid damage.[177,178]

Pharmacokinetics. Plasma concentrations of MMC decline in a biexponential manner, with a distribution half-life of less than 10 minutes, and a terminal half-life of 0.5–1.5 hours. Only 1–20% of drug is recoverable from urine, and the liver is believed to be the main site of biotransformation. Hepatic dysfunction, however, does not alter MMC pharmacokinetics, and it is possible that MMC is cleared from the plasma by a biodegradation process.[177,179] Very little MMC is absorbed into the systemic circulation after intravesical administration.

Clinical Uses. MMC is primarily used in treatment of solid tumors, especially as salvage therapy for breast cancers in combination with vinblastine, for non–small cell lung cancers, gastrointestinal tumors, and intravesically for treatment of superficial transitional cell carcinomas of the bladder. It may also be useful in squamous cell cancers, especially cancers of the uterine cervix. It is increasingly used as a chemoembolization agent for tumors localized to the liver.[177,180]

Toxicity. The dose-limiting toxicity of MMC is myelosuppression, which is characteristically delayed in onset, prolonged in duration, dose related, cumulative, and which preferentially affects platelets and white blood cells. Recovery may take up to 8 weeks. Anorexia, nausea and vomiting, and alopecia are uncommon and generally mild.[177,178] Extravasation may result in severe tissue necrosis, which is characterized by delayed presentation, sometimes weeks or months after injection, and which may be remote from the injection site. No antidote for this damage is of established efficacy in humans, but application of topical DMSO is useful in animal models.[117,181]

MMC also produces serious major organ toxicity, consisting of pulmonary damage and, more frequently, the hemolytic–uremia syndrome (HUS). Pulmonary toxicity typically presents with insidious onset of dyspnea, cough, and fatigue, although acute respiratory decompensation may occur, particularly when MMC is administered with vincas. Pulmonary function tests show a restrictive defect, and CXR commonly shows a diffuse reticular pattern. Known risk factors are previous or concurrent thoracic radiation, and exposure to high oxygen concentrations, but it is not known to be dose related. Mortality of MMC-induced pulmonary damage is high, although corticosteroids may produce dramatic responses, and anecdotally may decrease the risk of pulmonary toxicity when administered concurrently with MMC therapy.[75,182]

Cancer-associated HUS (C-HUS) consists of microangiopathic hemolytic anemia, renal dysfunction, and thrombocytopenia. It occurs in patients with adenocarcinoma who have received MMC and who most commonly are in remission from their disease at the time of presentation, or have stable disease. Pulmonary edema in the setting of blood transfusions is also characteristic. C-HUS usually develops within 4 months after the last MMC dose in patients who have received at least 60 mg of drug, and is fatal in over half of cases, usually because of renal failure. The most successful treatment strategy is early diagnosis through careful monitoring of renal function and hematologic parameters, avoidance of transfusions and immunopheresis over staphylococcal protein A columns. Immunoperfusion is believed to alter or deplete circulating immune complexes which may be involved in development of the syndrome.[154,177,183]

Actinomycin D

Actinomycin D (Act-D, DACT, or Dactinomycin) is an antitumor antibiotic isolated from *Streptomyces* species whose clinical utility is limited almost exclusively to pediatric tumors, gestational trophoblastic disease, and salvage therapy for testicular cancers. The pediatric tumors responsive to actinomycin D include Wilms' tumor, neuroblastoma, Ewing's sarcoma, and rhabdomyosarcoma.[162,177]

Pharmacology and Pharmacokinetics. Actinomycin D contains a chromophore ring and, like the anthracene derivatives, inserts itself either between bases of a single DNA strand (intercalation) or between bases in nonpaired strands (pseudointercalation). Binding to DNA inhibits RNA and protein synthesis. Act-D accumulates in tissues by passive diffusion and is susceptible to P-170 glycoprotein-mediated resistance. Plasma elimination is slow, with a half-life of 36 hours, likely secondary to extensive tissue binding. Only about 35% of drug is accounted for by urinary and fecal excretion.[161,177]

Toxicity. Myelosuppression is common and is usually the dose-limiting toxicity, although severe nausea and vomiting may be acutely dose limiting. Diarrhea, mucositis, and alopecia are also common. Actinomycin D is a severe vesicant if extravasated. No antidote to extravasation damage from this drug is known. It may also cause inflammatory radiation recall reactions in previously irradiated sites.[117,161,177]

Bleomycin

Bleomycin or "bleo" is one of the most widely used of the antitumor antibiotics. It has significant activity against Hodgkin's and non-Hodgkin's lymphomas, testicular cancer, head and neck cancers, Kaposi's sarcoma, and squamous cell cancers of the cervix, and is widely used by intracavitary injection for management of malignant effusions. Nononcology use is limited to management of plantar warts.[161,184]

Bleomycin is a mixture of peptides from fungal *Streptomyces* species, and as such, its strength is expressed in units of drug activity. One unit is roughly equal to one milligram of polypeptide protein.[185] The predominant peptide is bleomycin A_2, which makes up approximately 70% of the commercial product. Bleomycin's cytotoxicity is secondary to DNA strand breakage, or scission, which it produces via free radical formation. Cytotoxicity depends on binding of an iron–bleomycin complex to DNA. There is some evidence that intercalation between opposing DNA strands might occur. The bleomycin–iron complex then reduces molecular oxygen to free oxygen radicals, which primarily cause single-strand breaks in the DNA. Bleomycin has greatest effect on cells in the G_2 phase of the cell cycle and in mitosis.[161,185,186]

Pharmacokinetics. Bleomycin is taken up slowly by cells and is inactivated within cells by the enzyme aminohydrolase. This enzyme is widely distributed, but is present in only low concentrations in the skin and the lungs, which may account for the predominant toxicities of bleomycin in those sites. The presence of hydrolase enzymes in the cytosol is probably the primary mechanism of resistance to bleomycin as well. Cells can also become resistant by repairing the DNA breaks produced by bleomycin, and resistance has been correlated with increased repair capacity. Bleomycin is eliminated renally; 45–70% of the dose is excreted in the urine within 24 hours. Half-life of elimination is 2–4 hours in patients with normal renal function, and may increase to more than 20 hours in the presence of renal failure. Clearance may also be decreased in patients receiving concurrent cisplatin. Increased toxicity, especially pulmonary toxicity, has been associated with renal impairment. Dose reduction proportional to the degree of impairment is recommended in patients with severely compromised renal function (i.e., creatinine clearance less than 25–35 mL/min), although no validated guidelines exist (Table 119.10).[161,185,186] Following intracavitary administration, cavitary levels are about 10–20 times higher than corresponding plasma levels, although nearly half of an intracavitary dose eventually reaches the systemic circulation.[187]

Toxicity. Unlike most antineoplastic agents, bleomycin is not myelosuppressive and, consequently, is frequently given in combination with agents that are toxic to bone marrow. Nausea and vomiting are also mild. Bleomycin does produce fevers within hours to 2 days of administration in one-fourth to one-half of patients, which may be prevented or managed with antipyretics. Rarely, high fevers occur which can produce tachypnea, hypotension, delirium, and even death. Although these reactions have sometimes been characterized as anaphylactic reactions, they probably are not true hypersensitivity reactions. They are believed to be caused by the direct release of pyrogens in unusually sensitive patients. Patients with lymphoma who have preexisting disease-related fevers are most susceptible to these hyperpyrexial episodes. Administering a test dose (1 U) of bleomycin before the first dose has only limited utility in predicting which patients are at risk for this reaction.[108,186]

The most important toxicities of bleomycin are to the lungs and the skin. Characteristic pulmonary toxicity is interstitial pneumonitis, which can progress to fibrosis and cause death from hypoxia. It is related both to high single doses (greater than 30 U) and to cumulative dose, with an incidence of about 3% up to a total dose of 450 U, and 10% in patients receiving higher doses. Advanced age, preexisting pulmonary disease, previous chest irradiation, exposure to high oxygen concentrations, and renal impairment also increase risk. The clinical features are usually dyspnea with pulmonary infiltrates. Deterioration may be sudden and severe, and may occur months after completing therapy. Chest radiograph findings are nonspecific, and lung biopsy is required for definitive diagnosis. Measurement of carbon monoxide diffusing capacity has been recommended as a means of monitoring toxicity and predicting risk, although the utility of this is controversial. Treatment of pulmonary damage is drug discontinuation, but pulmonary symptoms may continue to progress after discontinuation. The value of corticosteroids has not been proven, except in patients with pulmonary reactions secondary to hypersensitivity. In patients who survive bleomycin pneumonitis, the pulmonary symptoms may reverse with long-term follow-up.[75,161,186,188,189]

Mucocutaneous toxicity is less serious than pulmonary damage, but more common. It includes mild stomatitis, hyperpigmentation over the elbows, knees, and small joints of the hands, thickening of the nail beds, alopecia, and a syndrome of skin erythema and edema.[161,186]

Heavy Metal Compounds

Cisplatin

Cisplatin is a platinum complex with a broad spectrum of antitumor activity and remarkable usefulness in cancer treatment. Recognition of its cytotoxic activity was the result of a serendipitous observation that bacterial growth in culture was altered when current was delivered to the media through platinum electrodes. The growth change was noted to be similar to that produced by alkylating agents and radiation, and it was found that a platinum chloride complex, now known as cisplatin, generated by the current was responsible for the changes. In clinical trials, cisplatin was found to have desirable efficacy but unacceptable serious toxicity, especially gastrointestinal and renal toxicities. Later, successful attempts were made to improve the therapeutic index by hydration and vigorous antiemetic therapy, which led to cisplatin's approval for commercial use in the late 1970s.[189,190]

Mechanism of Action. The main cytotoxic target of cisplatin is believed to be DNA, although the type of DNA lesion produced by platinum compounds is not conclusively established. Cytotoxicity in culture and probably *in vivo* depends on platinum binding to DNA and the formation of intrastrand cross-links between neighboring guanines. These intrastrand links cause a major bending of the DNA, and may cause cellular damage by distorting the normal DNA conformation and preventing bases which are normally paired from lining up with each other. Interstrand cross-links also occur, although with much lower frequency than intrastrand links. It is known that *cis* forms of platinum compounds are much more cytotoxic than those in a *trans* configuration. Although the reasons for this are not clearly established, it may be related to the ability to form strand linkages.[145,189]

The cytotoxic form of cisplatin is the aquated species, that is, that in which the two chloride groups have been replaced by hydroxyl groups of or water molecules (Fig. 119.24). This reaction occurs readily in low concentrations of chloride, such as the concentrations present within cells, and produces a positively charged compound which can react with DNA. The aquated species is responsible for both the efficacy and toxicity of cisplatin. Resistance to the therapeutic effects of cisplatin may occur through several mechanisms. Transmembrane transport of drug may be altered, the ability to repair DNA damage increased, or cisplatin may be neutralized by intracellular glutathione or sulfhydryl-containing proteins.[145,189–191]

Pharmacokinetics. Assessment of cisplatin pharmacokinetics following intravenous infusion is complicated by the existence of three major compartments, which include free or unbound drug, protein-bound drug, and drug bound to erythrocytes. It is characterized by a triphasic removal pattern. The first two phases represent removal of free drug, with elimination half-lives of 20–30 minutes, and of about 1 hour. This elimination is primarily renal and represents a combination of glomerular filtration and tubular secretion. Protein-bound drug is removed much more slowly, with a terminal half-life of 1–3 days. Although renal excretion is important in elimination of protein-bound drug, protein catabolism and biliary excretion also contribute. In addition to depending on renal function for its elimination, cisplatin is also nephrotoxic; thus dose reduction is recommended in patients with preexisting or therapy-induced renal dysfunction (Table 119.10). Clearance has been demonstrated to decrease and exposure to drug (AUC) to increase with successive cisplatin courses, even in the absence of significant changes in creatinine clearance. These changes correlate with increased drug toxicity and make guidelines for dose changes based on serum creatinine or creatine clearance undependable. More accurate dosing systems based on individual kinetic behavior are not widely available at present.[145,189,191–193]

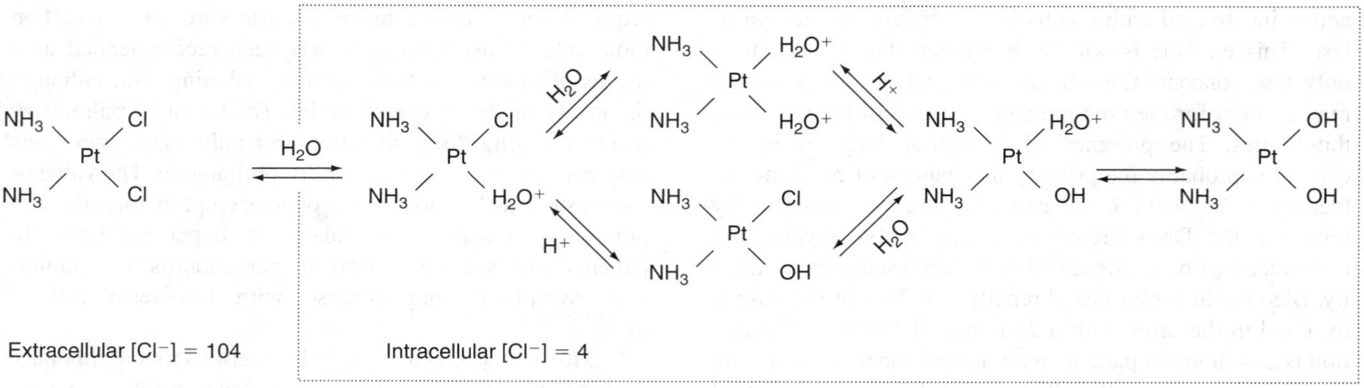

Extracellular $[Cl^-] = 104$

Intracellular $[Cl^-] = 4$

Figure 119.24. The aquation reaction of cisplatin. *(From Loehrer PJ, Einhorn LH. Cisplatin. Ann Intern Med 1984;100:705, with permission.)*

Cisplatin is also administered regionally, especially in the peritoneal cavity. Peak peritoneal cavity concentrations of free drug exceed plasma levels by at least 20-fold. This regional pharmacokinetic advantage may be increased by simultaneous intravenous infusion of the sulfhydryl compound sodium thiosulfate, which neutralizes the cytotoxic activity of cisplatin and reduces systemic exposure.[192,194,195]

Clinical Uses. Cisplatin is a versatile drug with efficacy against a wide range of solid tumors as well as lymphomas. It is a first-line agent for management of testicular cancer, ovarian cancer, metastatic bladder carcinoma, small cell and non–small cell lung cancers, head and neck cancers, and cervical cancer. It also has activity in non-Hodgkin's lymphomas, sarcomas, melanoma, brain tumors, esophageal cancers, and breast cancer. Because of its broad activity, cisplatin is a key agent in regimens designed for cancers of unknown primary.[189,190]

Toxicity. Cisplatin is a highly toxic antineoplastic agent, with potential for serious nephrotoxicity, ototoxicity, peripheral neuropathy, emesis, and anemia. The significant efficacy of cisplatin against many tumor types makes it a valuable agent despite these toxicities, many of which can be prevented or managed with aggressive supportive care measures.

Nephrotoxicity and emesis were previously the most common dose-limiting toxicities of cisplatin administration, but these have been problems most amenable to preventive measures. The proximal tubules are most sensitive to cisplatin-induced damage, but distal tubular function is also affected. Nephrotoxicity is characterized clinically by reduced glomerular filtration rates, electrolyte losses, especially potassium and magnesium, or renal failure, which may occur acutely even in the first day after drug administration. Hypomagnesemia and reduced filtration rate are most characteristic of the acute phase of toxicity. Stable reduced creatinine clearance, which may not produce elevated serum creatinine, occurs chronically. Renal damage from cisplatin is often slowly reversible, although hypomagnesemia and reduced creatine clearance may persist in one third or more of patients for many years. Risk of nephrotoxicity correlates with high single doses, cumulative doses, dehydration, preexisting renal impairment, and administration of other renal toxins. Advanced age and presence of only one functioning kidney are not known to increase the risk of nephrotoxicity.[154,196–198]

The incidence of nephrotoxicity can be decreased by careful diuresis and by aggressive hydration with chloride-containing solutions, which help to keep the cisplatin in the renal tubules in the nonaquated and therefore nontoxic form. Drug administration in hypertonic saline solutions may also be helpful, but is not clearly established as superior to providing large amounts of chloride via hydration fluids, and is probably not necessary at conventional cisplatin doses. Diuretics, especially mannitol and furosemide, have been used to increase urine flow and reduce contact time of the cisplatin with the renal tubule. It is possible that mannitol may protect the kidney by delaying cisplatin binding onto renal tubular proteins. Furosemide has not been convincingly shown to decrease nephrotoxicity, but diuretics are useful in patients with cardiovascular compromise.[196,197,199] Sodium thiosulfate has also been used to decrease nephrotoxicity in combination with both intraperitoneal and systemic administration of cisplatin. Sodium thiosulfate accumulates in the renal tubules in high concentrations where it rapidly neutralizes the cytotoxic activity of cisplatin. In the concentrations achieved in plasma, the half-life of the neutralization reaction is much slower; therefore thiosulfate does not interfere with the therapeutic effect of the drug. It is not effective in ameliorating any toxicity except nephrotoxicity.[195–197] A variety of other chemoprotective agents have been studied in attempts to decrease the nephrotoxic potential of cisplatin. Amifostine (WR-2721) is a thiol ester which can protect normal tissues against radiotherapy and alkylating agent-induced damage. It is moderately effective against cisplatin nephrotoxicity.[196,197,200] Diethyldithiocarbamate (DDTC), a chelating agent, has the potential of removing platinum from binding sites, but has been disappointing in controlled studies.[201] Some of the other antidotes under evaluation are selenium compounds, glutathione, probenecid, bismuth, and corticosteroids.[196,197]

Cisplatin is one of the most severe emetogens known among marketed antineoplastic agents. Acute nausea and vomiting are nearly universal without prophylactic interventions, but can be prevented or limited with aggressive antiemetic therapy. Regimens containing corticosteroids and either seretonin antagonists, such as ondansetron or granisetron, or dopamine antagonists such as metoclopramide, droperidol, or high-dose chlorpromazine have been very successful in controlling acute cisplatin-induced emesis. About 60% of patients receiving cisplatin will also experience delayed nausea and vomiting, 2–4 days after drug administration, which is less easily prevented by conventional antiemetic therapy, and which can have a serious impact on fluid and nutritional status.[202]

Neuropathy, which includes ototoxicity, peripheral neuropathy, and, rarely, ocular toxicity, has emerged as a dose-limiting toxicity of cisplatin with current effective management of renal damage and emesis. Ototoxicity most commonly affects the high-frequency hearing ranges and may be associated with loss of outer hair cells from the cochlea. Hearing loss is usually permanent, but associated vestibular toxicity generally reverses over time. Concurrent ifosfamide administration may exacerbate cisplatin-induced hearing loss. Effective means of preventing these toxicities are not known.[203,204]

Peripheral neuropathy is characteristically distal and sensory, in a "stocking-and-glove" distribution, and may begin and progress after cisplatin is discontinued. The dorsal root ganglia is the neural structure most sensitive to cisplatin damage. Peripheral neuropathy is associated with cumulative dose and is usually reversible, although complete resolution may take more than a year.[72,189,205] Chemoprotectors such as amifostine may limit neural damage[200] and some information suggests that an adrenocorticotropic-hormone analogue (Org 2766) might prevent or delay cisplatin neuropathy.[206]

Although significant granulocytopenia or thrombocytopenia are unusual from cisplatin administration, normocytic, normochronic anemia is common. This anemia can be corrected with erythropoietin treatment. Hemolytic anemia also occurs.[207] Other toxicities of cisplatin include disturbances in color perception, hypersensitivity reactions, Raynaud's phenomenon, hypercholesterolemia, and rare hepatic toxicity.[108,189,208,209]

Carboplatin

Carboplatin is a structural analogue of cisplatin in which the chloride groups of the parent compound are replaced by a carboxycyclobutane moiety. It shares the same mechanism of action as cisplatin, although it generates an aquated reactive form much more slowly than cisplatin. The spectrum of activity is similar, although carboplatin only has FDA approval for treatment of ovarian cancer. Cross-resistance between the two agents is common. Carboplatin differs markedly from cisplatin, however, in its pharmacokinetics and toxicity.[145]

Pharmacokinetics. Many pharmacokinetic differences between carboplatin and cisplatin may be accounted for by differences in plasma protein binding. Carboplatin binds to plasma protein more slowly and less extensively than does cisplatin, which results in a much longer plasma half-life of unbound carboplatin platinum in comparison with cisplatin. Carboplatin's pharmacokinetics are linear, with a steady-state volume of distribution approximately equal to total body water, and clearance of ultrafilterable carboplatin platinum is more than double that of creatinine clearance. The reduced protein binding also results in a much larger percentage of carboplatin than cisplatin being excreted in urine (60–80%).[192,210,211] In patients with compromised renal function, doses of carboplatin must be reduced to limit myelosuppressive toxicity. Several guidelines for dose modification in patients with impaired renal function have been developed,[212] but the most clinically useful dosage schema uses a target AUC and renal function parameters to estimate the carboplatin dose. This schema was developed by Calvert and colleagues, and is referred to as the "Calvert formula" (Table 119.13). Estimated or measured creatinine clearance is typically used to represent glomerular filtration rate (GFR) in this formula, but may underpredict the GFR.[213] Similar dose guidelines have been developed for children.[214]

Toxicity. Unlike cisplatin, whose dose-limiting toxicities include nephrotoxicity and neurotoxicity, carboplatin administration is limited by hematologic toxicity. It causes suppression of white blood cells, but more particularly, platelets, with characteristic delayed recovery that can prevent retreatment more often than every 4–5 weeks. In contrast, however, its potential to cause renal damage, peripheral neuropathy, and ototoxicity is much less than that of comparative cisplatin doses, and it has proven to be a very useful alternative to cisplatin therapy in patients with preexisting compromise to these organs or at high risk of damage. The emetogenic potential of carboplatin is also substantially less than that of cisplatin, although it is still a moderate to severe emetogen.[210,211] Hypersensitivity reactions are rare, but may be more common in children.[215,216]

MISCELLANEOUS AGENTS

Hydroxyurea

Hydroxyurea is a drug that falls broadly into the category of antimetabolites, but which is not a nucleoside analogue. It inhibits ribonucleotide reductase, the enzyme required to convert ribonucleotides into the deoxyribonucleotide forms which are required for both DNA synthesis and repair. Consequently, hydroxyurea stops DNA synthesis without interfering with formation of RNA or protein. Cells accumulate in the S phase because DNA synthesis is inhibited, and only abnormally short DNA strands are produced.[52,217]

Pharmacokinetics. Hydroxyurea is well absorbed orally and is administered by that route, with peak concentrations achieved in 1–2 hours. The main route of elimination is renal excretion, although the percent detected in urine varies markedly from patient to patient. Guidelines for dose reduction in patients with impaired renal function are not available, but hydroxyurea should be used cautiously in these patients. It distributes rapidly to tissues and enters both the CNS and "third-space" fluids readily.[217]

TABLE 119.13. CARBOPLATIN DOSE MODIFICATIONS IN PATIENTS WITH IMPAIRED RENAL FUNCTION

Dose = AUC × (GFR + 25)

where

Dose =	**Total** dose in milligrams
AUC =	Desired area under the curve in mg/mL × min: Target AUC is 5–7 for single-agent carboplatin. Target AUC is 4–5 for carboplatin in combination with other myelosuppressive drugs.
GFR =	Glomerular filtration rate (not normalized for surface area). Estimated or measured creatinine clearance is usually substituted for true GFR, but may underestimate carboplatin dose.
25 =	Average nonrenal clearance for adults.

(From Ref. 213.)

Clinical Use and Toxicity. Clinical oncologic use of hydroxyurea is limited to the myeloproliferative diseases, especially chronic myelogenous leukemia. It is also used to rapidly reduce elevated blood cell counts in myelogenous leukemias, polycythemia vera, and thrombocytosis, and may have some utility in high doses in malignant lymphomas.[217,218] Hydroxyurea is useful in sickle cell anemia, in decreasing the frequency of sickle cell crises by elevating the concentration of fetal hemoglobin.[219] Toxicity is primarily marrow suppression of rapid onset, which is sometimes a desired therapeutic effect of the drug. It produces significant nausea, vomiting, anorexia, and mucositis, particularly in high-dose regimens. Chronic therapy produces skin hyperpigmentation, erythema especially of the face and hands, and rashes. Radiation recall reactions may occur.[217–219]

L-Asparaginase

L-Asparaginase is unique among antineoplastics in its unusual mechanism of action, pattern of toxicity, and source. It is an enzyme produced by bacteria. It is commercially available in two forms, both of *Escherichia coli* origin. The first is an unconjugated form of the enzyme, available under the trade name Elspar which is sometimes called native protein. L-Asparaginase has also recently been marketed as pegaspargase (Oncospar), in which polyethylene glycol (PEG) has been covalently conjugated to L-asparaginase. L-Asparaginase has very limited clinical application, and is used almost exclusively for treatment of acute lymphocytic leukemia.[220,221]

Mechanism of Action. L-Asparagine is a nonessential amino acid which can be synthesized by most mammalian cells, except for those of certain human malignancies, which lack or have very low levels of the synthetase enzyme required for L-asparagine formation. L-Asparagine is degraded by the enzyme L-asparaginase, which depletes existing supplies and inhibits protein synthesis, with secondary block of nucleic acid synthesis. Malignant cells of lymphocyte origin are most likely to lack the capacity to synthesize new supplies of asparagine, and are therefore most affected by L-asparagine depletion. Increased L-asparagine synthetase activity within tumor cells causes resistance to L-asparaginase treatment.[220,221]

Pharmacokinetics. The metabolic fate and elimination of L-asparaginase are not known, but are believed to be mediated, at least in some patients, by antibody reactions with the L-asparaginase protein. The half-life of elimination of the native protein form of L-asparaginase is slightly longer than 1 day. Conjugation with PEG reduces uptake by the reticuloendothelial system and antibody formation in response to the protein, resulting in significant prolongation of the half-life to about 6 days. PEG protection of L-asparaginase permits both lower doses and less frequent drug administration. Clearance of either preparation is markedly accelerated in patients who develop hypersensitivity to the drug. Peak levels after intramuscular administration of native asparaginase are approximately half of levels after equal doses given intravenously. Asparaginase distributes within the intravascular space and achieves low but useful levels within the CNS. No L-asparaginase activity is detectable in urine.[220–222]

Toxicity. Toxicity of L-asparaginase consists primarily of hypersensitivity reactions to the antigenic protein, and reactions which are effects of its therapeutic inhibition of protein synthesis. Hypersensitivity reactions occur in about 25% of patients receiving unconjugated L-asparaginase, and are most common in those receiving intravenous doses, single-agent therapy, or repeated courses of treatment. True anaphylaxis occurs in 5–9% of patients, is fatal in about 1%, and requires allergic precautions during administration. Skin testing may be helpful in selecting patients at high risk for reactions, but is not uniformly predictive of allergic reactions, which occasionally occur even on first drug administration. PEG-asparaginase is less immunogenic than the native form, and is indicated in patients who have experienced hypersensitivity reactions to conventional L-asparaginase. Hypersensitivity reactions are still common in patients receiving the PEG conjugated form of L-asparaginase, but are rarely severe.[108,223]

Inhibition of protein synthesis results in several toxicities, particularly hemorrhage or thrombosis from impaired synthesis of clotting factors and/or naturally occurring anticoagulants, particularly protein C and antithrombin III. Hyperglycemia secondary to decreased insulin synthesis is also common, and can be abrupt in onset. Pancreatic toxicity may manifest as acute pancreatitis and occasionally progresses to hemorrhagic pancreatitis. Liver toxicity is common, with increases in transaminases, bilirubin, alkaline phosphatase, and hypoalbuminemia, and is sometimes dose limiting. Cerebral dysfunction, which most typically manifests as somnolence or confusion, but which may progress to coma, occurs in about 25% of patients. This may be secondary to low amino acid levels within the CNS. Nausea occurs in more than half of patients. L-Asparaginase, however, does not produce myelosuppression, mucositis, or alopecia. The incidence of nonhypersensitivity-related adverse reactions is not affected by conjugation of L-asparaginase with PEG.[221,223]

One drug interaction with L-asparaginase is of established clinical significance. L-Asparaginase administered after methotrexate can stop both methotrexate's therapeutic and toxic actions—perhaps by interfering with protein synthesis and the entry of cells into the S phase—which are important for methotrexate's cytotoxic effects. This effect has been used to advantage in some combination regimens.[220,221]

All *Trans*-Retinoic Acid

All *trans*-retinoic acid (ATRA, tretinoin) is a naturally occurring derivative of vitamin A (retinol). Vitamin A and its metabolites, collectively referred to as the retinoids, are known to play important roles in numerous biologic processes, including cellular differentiation. The promotion of normal differentiation of squamous cells prompted extensive investigation of the retinoids as chemoprevention agents in several malignancies, including head and neck cancer and lung cancer. The retinoids also stimulate differentiation of erythroid and myeloid progenitor cells. Since leukemias are often defined as a failure of normal hematopoietic differentiation, the retinoids have also been studied as potential antileukemic agents.[224] This section focuses on that application.

Clinical Pharmacology. ATRA has recently been reported to produce high complete remission rates in patients with acute promyelocytic leukemia (APL). APL accounts for approximately 10% of cases of acute nonlymphocytic leukemia. It is often characterized by the presence of a severe, and sometimes fatal, hemorrhagic coagulopathy. In the past few years, researchers have discovered that the genetic defect characteristic of APL seems to be a 15;17 chromosomal translocation. The gene for nuclear retinoic acid receptor alpha (RAR-α) is located on chromosome 17, and the translocation is associated with production of an abnormal RAR-α fusion protein. Administration of ATRA reverses the effects of abnormal RAR-α, and promotes terminal myeloid differentiation. Complete response rates in APL range from 69–84%. Unlike standard chemotherapeutic agents, which produce rapid antileukemic effects, the complete responses to ATRA are delayed, usually occurring at 1–2 months. Duration of response has been variable, and averages 4 months. Interestingly, ATRA therapy is also associated with resolution of APL-related coagulopathies. The most commonly used dose is 45 mg/m^2/d, administered in two equally divided doses.[225,226]

Pharmacokinetics. Following oral administration, peak plasma concentrations occur at 1–2 hours, but vary significantly among patients. This retinoid is heavily protein bound to albumin. Unlike its stereoisomer *cis*-retinoic acid, ATRA is rapidly cleared from the systemic circulation, with a half-life of approximately 1 hour. ATRA undergoes hydroxylation by P-450 enzymes. Its metabolites are conjugated and secreted via the biliary system into the gastrointestinal tract, where they may undergo enterohepatic recycling. Over time, plasma concentrations of ATRA markedly diminish, and this effect may be associated with loss of clinical response in APL.[224–226]

Toxicity. The most commonly reported adverse effect is headache, which usually responds to mild analgesics. However, intracranial hypertension (pseudotumor cerebri) has also been reported. These patients present with severe headache, nausea, and papilledema, and may require serial lumbar punctures, high-dose corticosteroids, and narcotic analgesics. Other toxicities are common to vitamin A derivatives in general, and affect the skin and mucous membranes (i.e., xerostomia, cheilitis, skin desquamation), the eyes (i.e., dryness, blepharoconjunctivitis, corneal erosion), musculoskeletal system (i.e., myalgias, arthralgias, bone pain), and hypertriglyceridemia. Dry skin and mucous membranes respond well to topical emollients. Tolerance usually develops to headache and musculoskeletal symptoms with continued dosing. ATRA does not accumulate in the liver as does vitamin A, and chronic liver damage has not been reported. However, reversible elevations in serum transaminases and bilirubin may occur. ATRA also shares the teratogenic properties of theretinoids, and all patients should be counseled to avoid pregnancy.[224–226]

Hyperleukocytosis (white blood count > 20,000/mm^3) may occur in up to 50% of APL patients who receive ATRA. This requires no specific intervention if unaccompanied by other symptoms, and may indicate a positive response to ATRA therapy. However, hyperleukocytosis may also be an early indicator of the "retinoic acid syndrome," a syndrome that occurs in up to 25% of patients and is characterized by fever and respiratory distress in addition to hyperleukocytosis. Patients may develop pulmonary infiltrates, pleural or pericardial effusions, weight gain, edema, and hypotension. The clinical scenario is comparable to the capillary leak syndrome seen with administration of some cytokines such as interleukin-2. This syndrome usually occurs during the first 2–3 weeks of ATRA administration, but has occurred as early as the second day of therapy. Progressive respiratory deterioration may require mechanical ventilation. Multiorgan failure and death have occurred in up to a third of affected patients. The most effective known treatment is early institution of high-dose corticosteroids (dexamethasone 10 mg every 12 hours for three days).[225,226]

Endocrine Therapies

Endocrine manipulation is an option for management of cancers from tissues whose growth is under gonadal hormonal control, especially breast, prostate, and endometrial cancers. These cancers may regress if the "feeding" hormone is eliminated or antagonized. Major organ system toxicity is uncommon from hormonal treatment, making it the least toxic of systemic anticancer therapies. The clinical applications and toxicity of individual agents are detailed in the breast and prostate cancer chapters.[227,228] Tamoxifen, long known as an effective antiestrogen for the treatment of breast cancer, is finding increasing use in the treatment of other solid tumors, especially malignant melanoma. Although its activity as a single agent in this disease is minimal, response rates are markedly improved when tamoxifen is added to chemotherapy regimens. This anticancer action may be independent of tamoxifen's antiestrogen effects.[229]

Corticosteroids are also useful anticancer agents because of their lymphocytotoxic effects. Their primary use is

TABLE 119.14. APPLICATION OF CORTICOSTEROIDS IN SUPPORTIVE CARE OF CANCER PATIENTS

Nausea and vomiting
Cerebral edema secondary to brain metastases or cranial irradiation
Spinal cord compression
Hypercalcemia
Transfusion reactions
Appetite stimulation
Radiation or drug-induced pneumonitis
Anaphylactic reactions
Graft-versus-host disease after bone marrow transplantation
Pain secondary to nerve compression or edema

in management of hematologic malignancies, especially lymphomas, lymphocytic leukemias, and the plasma cell cancer, multiple myeloma. In addition to their cytotoxic effects, corticosteroids have many other applications in supportive care of cancer patients as outlined in Table 119.14. The corticosteroids have diverse toxicities in chronic or high-dose use, but are generally well tolerated in short-term therapy.[230]

All steroid hormones share the same four-ring cyclopentane–perhydrophenanthrene structural nucleus, and all are derived from cholesterol. Despite their greatly diverse actions, all steroid hormones are believed to act by a similar mechanism (Fig. 119.25). Hormones diffuse passively across cell membranes and are trapped by protein receptors in the cytoplasm. The hormone/receptor complex is then "activated," and transferred into the nucleus, where it binds to DNA and ultimately alters gene expression. These gene alterations in turn change protein synthesis, and through this, change cell function and produce the hormone's biologic effects. The secretion of steroid hormones is under hypothalamic and pituitary control.[227,228]

BIOLOGIC RESPONSE MODIFIERS

Interferons

The interferons (IFN) are a family of proteins produced by nucleated cells, and now also by means of recombinant DNA technology, which have antiviral, antiproliferative, and immunoregulatory activities. They are classified as alpha, beta, or gamma interferons based on antigenic, biologic, and pharmacologic properties. Many subtypes of IFN-α are known, and three IFN-α preparations are commercially available in the United States. IFN-α-2a and α-2b are each single species recombinant products, and are very similar both structurally and biologically. These are the only interferons approved for anticancer indications. Alpha-n3 interferon is a purified mixture of IFN-α species produced in leukocytes. IFN-α, also known as immune IFN, is known to be a potent macrophage-activating factor, and is approved for the treatment of chronic granulomatous disease. Recombinant IFN-β was recently approved by the FDA for the treatment of multiple sclerosis.[231]

The mechanism of IFN-α's antitumor action remains speculative. Although IFN administration increases the activity of various cytotoxic cells within the immune system, direct antiproliferative effects certainly play a role as

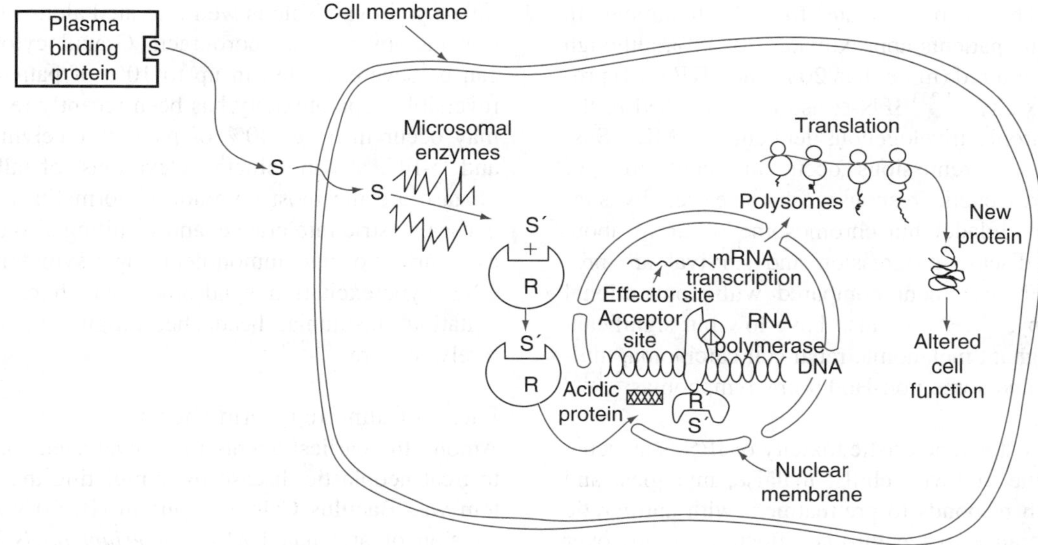

Figure 119.25. Schematic representation of the mechanism of steroid hormone action. Hormones diffuse into cells (S), bind to receptors (R), and are translocated to the nucleus, where they bind to DNA and alter expression of specific genes and, in turn, change protein production and alter cell function. *(From Lipman ME, Eil C. Steroid therapy of cancer, in Chabner BA [ed]: Pharmacologic Principles of Cancer Treatment. Philadelphia, WB Saunders, 1982, pp 132–182, with permission.)*

well. These actions may be an extension of IFN's antiviral actions, in which a protein kinase is activated, which in turn alters the activity of other factors needed for protein synthesis. IFN-α also inhibits ornithine decarboxylase production, which may result in overall cell cycle slowing. Interferons can inhibit new blood vessel formation in tumors, and can increase the expression of antigens on tumor cell surfaces, making them more easily recognized by the cells of the immune system, and can inhibit or block certain oncogenes.[232,233]

Pharmacokinetics. The interferons are not absorbed orally, because they are proteins destroyed by digestive enzymes. The bioavailability of IFN-α after intramuscular or subcutaneous administration is nearly complete, however. Total body clearance is nearly double normal creatinine clearance, suggesting that renal secretion and catabolism or extrarenal elimination occurs. Little or no IFN is excreted into the urine, and hepatic metabolism of IFN-α is minor. Animal data indicate that proteolytic degradation in renal tubules may be the major method of elimination. The half-life of plasma elimination is 4–5 hours, but biologic effects may persist for several days, permitting convenient three-times-weekly dosing schedules.[233]

Clinical Uses. Labeled indications for IFN-α in cancer treatment include hairy cell leukemia, acquired immunodeficiency disease (AIDS)-associated Kaposi's sarcoma, and malignant melanoma. Low-dose IFN therapy produces clinical response in approximately 70% of patients with hairy cell leukemia, and symptomatic improvement in about 90%. Most patients relapse following discontinuation of interferon therapy but may respond to retreatment.[92,231,233] The response rate to IFN treatment in Kaposi's sarcoma patients approximates 30–40%, although the high doses required (more than 20 million IU/m^2/d) produce serious toxicity.[231,233] IFN-α use is established in the treatment of chronic myelogenous leukemia (CML). Sustained hematologic remissions occur in about 70% of patients and cytogenetic responses characterized by suppression of the Philadelphia chromosome occur in about 30%. Time to disease progression and survival are prolonged with IFN treatment compared with conventional cytotoxic therapy.[234] IFN-α's also have low but significant activity in malignant melanoma, renal cell carcinoma, multiple myeloma, and some non-Hodgkin's lymphomas.[231,233]

Toxicity. The most characteristic toxicity of IFN is an acute flu-like syndrome of fever, chills, malaise, myalgias, and headache, which responds to pretreatment with antipyretic analgesics. Tolerance to the flu-like effects develops over several days to weeks, but does not develop to fatigue, which is dose related and is the most common dose-limiting toxicity of IFN-α. Gastrointestinal toxicities, myelosuppression, increased liver function tests, and neurologic toxicities (e.g., vertigo, decreased mental status, confusion, depression, paresthesias) are rarely troublesome at low doses, but increase in incidence and severity as doses increase. Permanent major organ toxicity is rare.[231,233,234] Drug interactions with IFN use may be clinically important, and may be due to inhibition of cytochrome P-450 enzymes.[233]

Levamisole

Levamisole is an antihelminthic agent which has been used for more than 25 years for treatment of human and veterinary parasitic worm infections. In the 1970s it was also discovered to have immunologic activity, which is best described as immunorestorative in nature. Levamisole has multiple and diverse effects on the immune system which may be responsible for its antitumor activity. Levamisole is for the adjuvant treatment of colorectal cancer, in combination with 5-fluorouracil. Its clinical use for colorectal cancer is detailed in Chapter 122.[235–237]

Pharmacokinetics. Levamisole is rapidly and well absorbed, with peak levels achieved in 1–3 hours, although the absolute bioavailability has not yet been determined. It is extensively metabolized by the liver, primarily by hydroxylation and subsequent glucuronidation, and demonstrates a terminal half-life of about 4 hours. Renal elimination within 24 hours accounts for less than 15% of an administered dose. Pharmacokinetic behavior in patients with impaired renal or hepatic function have not been studied, but the relatively low renal clearance suggests that dose adjustment in patients with impaired renal function is unnecessary.[235]

Toxicity. Levamisole is well tolerated alone or in combination therapy with 5-fluorouracil. Granulocytopenia, which can be severe, occurs in up to 10% of patients. Mild and reversible hepatotoxicity has been recently recognized, and may occur in up to 40% of patients receiving levamisole and 5-FU. Asymptomatic elevations of alkaline phosphatase are the most common abnormalities. Skin rashes, nausea, gastric intolerance, and vomiting also occur, as well as a variety of uncommon neurologic symptoms, including CNS hyperexcitation syndromes, which can manifest as agitation, insomnia, headache, fatigue, nightmares, and, rarely, seizures.[64,235,237]

Bacillus Calmette Guérin Vaccine

Among the earliest agents to be evaluated for its potential to treat neoplastic disease by stimulating the immune system was Bacillus Calmette Guérin (BCG) vaccine, a suspension of attenuated *Mycobacterium bovis* long used to promote active immunity against tuberculosis infection. BCG vaccine administration is known to stimulate cell-mediated immunity and is considered to be a nonspecific immune stimulant. It was extensively studied during the

1970s and early 1980s in a variety of tumors, for both systemic and local effects, alone and in combination with conventional antineoplastics, and as adjuvant therapy as well as treatment of metastatic disease. BCG vaccine's efficacy as a systemic anticancer agent in these trials was uniformly modest, but its effectiveness in local administration has justified its approval for management of superficial bladder cancers. Approximately 80% of patients with carcinoma *in situ* of the bladder will respond to repeated intravesical administration of BCG vaccine. It is also effective in treatment of superficial transitional cell bladder tumors. The mechanism of action of BCG vaccine is not known. It is postulated that localized inflammatory reactions or nonspecific immune stimulation are responsible for its antitumor effects.[238,239]

Toxicity. The toxicity of intravesical BCG vaccine administration is usually limited to irritative bladder effects such as hematuria, dysuria, and frequency, which occur in more than half of patients. Symptoms usually begin within a few hours of administration and persist for 1–3 days. However, systemic reactions also occur. Malaise, fever, and chills are most common, but rare cases of fatal disseminated tuberculosis infection have occurred following bladder administration of BCG vaccine.[240,241] Because of this risk, severely immunocompromised patients should not be given BCG vaccine, and precautions to avoid inadvertent exposure should be exercised during preparation and administration.[242]

Interleukin-2 (Aldesleukin)

Interleukin-2 (IL-2, aldesleukin), formerly known as T-cell growth factor, is a lymphokine which is now produced recombinantly and has diverse immunologic effects. IL-2 promotes B- and T-cell proliferation and differentiation and initiates a cytokine cascade with multiple interacting immunologic effects. The IL-2 receptor is expressed in increased amounts on activated T cells, and mediates most of IL-2 effects. Antitumor effects depend on proliferation of a variety of cytotoxic cells which have the ability to recognize and destroy tumor cells without damaging normal cells. Some of these cytotoxic cells are natural killer (NK) cells, lymphokine activated killer (LAK) cells, and tumor-infiltrating lymphocytes (TIL). The growth of these cells may be stimulated *in vivo* or harvested from patients, grown in culture with IL-2, and reinfused into the patient as a form of adoptive immunotherapy.[243–245]

Pharmacokinetics. Like the interferons, IL-2 preparations are proteins which are not absorbed after oral administration. Bioavailability after intramuscular injection is approximately 35%. Serum concentrations following intravenous administration are proportional to dose and decline biexponentially, with a terminal half-life of 30–120 minutes. Elimination is longer after subcutaneous administration, but peak concentrations achieved are 10–100 times lower than those immediately after intravenous bolus. Clearance is estimated at 120 mL/min, suggesting that renal tubular filtration is the major means of elimination.[243,246]

Clinical Uses. IL-2 has demonstrated clinical activity both alone and in combination with transferred cytotoxic cells. Most of the clinical trials with IL-2 have been in patients with metastatic renal cell cancer, malignant melanoma, and colorectal cancers, which are relatively resistant to treatment with conventional antineoplastic drugs. In renal cell cancer patients, IL-2 produces objective responses in about 20% of patients, some of which may persist for several years without further IL-2 therapy. Patients with prior nephrectomy and low tumor burden are most likely to respond to IL-2 treatment. The objective response rate in malignant melanoma is about 15% as a single agent, although IL-2 may produce higher response rates in combination with conventional antineoplastics known to have activity in this disease. The objective response rate in colorectal cancer is 10%, but responses are typically brief.[243–245] IL-2 is under evaluation in acute leukemia patients to control minimal residual disease.[247] Low-dose regimens of IL-2 alone, or in combination with IFN or cytotoxic agents are currently under investigation.[243,244]

Toxicity. The toxicity of IL-2 is related to dose, route, and duration of therapy, but, in general, IL-2 is toxic therapy which requires vigorous supportive care in conventional dose regimens. Low doses may be well tolerated, even in outpatient administration.

The most common dose-limiting toxicities are hypotension, fluid retention, and renal dysfunction. IL-2 decreases peripheral vascular resistance with peripheral vasodilation and tachycardia, which produce hypotension. A characteristic vascular or capillary leak syndrome results in fluid retention often greater than 10% of body weight, which in turn can cause respiratory compromise. These toxicities require administration of vasopressors, judicious use of fluid support and diuretics, and supplemental oxygen in most patients. Patients with underlying cardiovascular or renal abnormalities are more susceptible to these adverse effects.[243–245,248,249]

In addition to the hemodynamic and renal effects, most patients treated with IL-2 in full doses experience thrombocytopenia, anemia, eosinophilia, reversible cholestasis, and skin erythema with burning and pruritus. Neuropsychiatric changes, hypothyroidism, and bacterial infections, particularly staphylococcal infections, are also common.[243,244,250] In general, the toxicities from IL-2 therapy are reversible, and can be managed or prevented by careful prospective monitoring and pharmacologic supportive care. Although many of the IL-2 adverse effects can be ameliorated by corticosteroid administration,[229,251] it is possible that steroids may decrease the antitumor effects of

IL-2. A variety of dose regimens and schedules have been evaluated to decrease the toxicity associated with IL-2 administration. Prolonged low-dose regimens and continuous infusion regimens may be effective, with less toxicity than high-dose bolus injection.[243,244]

General Supportive Care Issues

The treatment of cancer with antineoplastic drugs is complicated by the incidence of multiple serious toxicities, many of which are life threatening. Drug-specific toxicities, such as doxorubicin-induced cardiotoxicity and bleomycin-related pulmonary toxicity, have been discussed in the previous sections. Several adverse effects are common among the antineoplastic agents. These include nausea and vomiting, myelosuppression, mucositis, alopecia, infertility, and carcinogenesis. Nutritional support and pain management are also important supportive care issues, although they are not specifically the result of drug-induced toxicity. The management of chemotherapy-induced nausea and vomiting and the basic principles of nutritional support and pain management are discussed in detail in other sections of this text.

Cancer cells do not necessarily proliferate faster than normal cells. Since many antineoplastic drugs affect DNA synthesis, any cell with a high turnover rate will be more sensitive to the toxic effects of chemotherapy. Normal tissues which consist of rapidly proliferating cells are targets for the toxicities of many anticancer drugs.[252] The bone marrow, intestinal mucosa, and hair follicles are such tissue sites where drug effects are manifested. Although not seen with all antineoplastic agents, myelosuppression is the most common dose-limiting side effect of cytotoxic agents.

MYELOSUPPRESSION

Bone marrow suppression does not usually occur immediately after chemotherapy administration. Blood components that have already been produced must be consumed before the effect is evident. White blood cells (WBCs), especially granulocyte precursors, are most significantly affected because of their rapid proliferation and short life span (6–12 hours). Platelets (5- to 10-day life span) are also affected, but to a lesser degree than granulocytes. Erythrocytes have a 120-day life span and are affected the least. Usual nadirs, or lowest blood cell counts, occur at 10–14 days following chemotherapy administration, with recovery by 3–4 weeks. There are some exceptions to this general rule. The nitrosoureas and mitomycin C exhibit a delayed pattern of nadir (4–6 weeks) and recovery (6–8 weeks). Planned courses of chemotherapy may be delayed while waiting for the granulocyte count to return to normal. In order for a patient to safely receive another cycle of chemotherapy, a WBC $\geq 3000/\text{mm}^3$ or absolute neutrophil or granulocyte count (ANC, AGC) of $\geq 1500/\text{mm}^3$, and a platelet count of $\geq 100{,}000/\text{mm}^3$ is usually required.

Myelotoxicity is an expected phenomenon in leukemia patients during induction chemotherapy. However, myelosuppression is an undesirable side effect during chemotherapy for other malignancies. If undesirable myelosuppression has occurred with prior courses of chemotherapy, the doses of the offending agent(s) in subsequent courses may be reduced. However, dosage reduction may also compromise antitumor response. The magnitude of dose reduction is dictated by the degree of myelosuppression incurred and the incidence and severity of infection or bleeding. Empiric dosage reductions may be made for the first chemotherapy treatment if the patient has a low baseline WBC or platelet count, has a diminished bone marrow reserve, has impaired drug elimination capabilities, or is to receive a combination of several drugs which cause myelosuppression. Patients who have received multiple prior courses of other myelotoxic chemotherapy regimens or extensive radiation therapy may have a decreased bone marrow reserve. They are more sensitive to the myelosuppressive effects of chemotherapy, and normal doses may produce profound marrow toxicity. The pharmacokinetic profile of a myelosuppressive agent is also important in determining the appropriate dose. For example, the anthracyclines exhibit bone marrow suppression as an acute dose-limiting toxicity, and these agents depend on biliary excretion as their primary route of elimination. A patient with biliary obstruction may have compromised elimination of anthracyclines and is at increased risk for severe bone marrow suppression.

NEUTROPENIA

When the ANC falls below 500, infection risk increases.[253,254] The ANC may be calculated by multiplying the percentage of granulocytes (segmented plus banded neutrophils) by the total WBC count. The duration of neutropenia is also directly proportional to the risk for infection. Other risk factors for infection include alteration in the integrity of physical defense barriers, and the functional integrity of WBCs. The patient's underlying cancer, as well as treatment with cytotoxic drugs and radiation, can affect neutrophil function. The diagnosis of infection in the neutropenic patient is complicated by the lack of WBCs. Usual signs and symptoms of infection, such as pus, abscesses, and infiltrates on chest x-ray depend on the presence of WBCs. The only reliable indication of infection in these patients is fever. Definitive culture results may take days, and a septic neutropenic cancer patient can die within hours if not treated. Therefore, the basic approach to the management of the febrile neutropenic cancer patient is prompt initiation of empiric antibiotics. The antibiotics are chosen based on reliable coverage of the most likely organisms, antibiotic sensitivities at the institution, the patient's signs

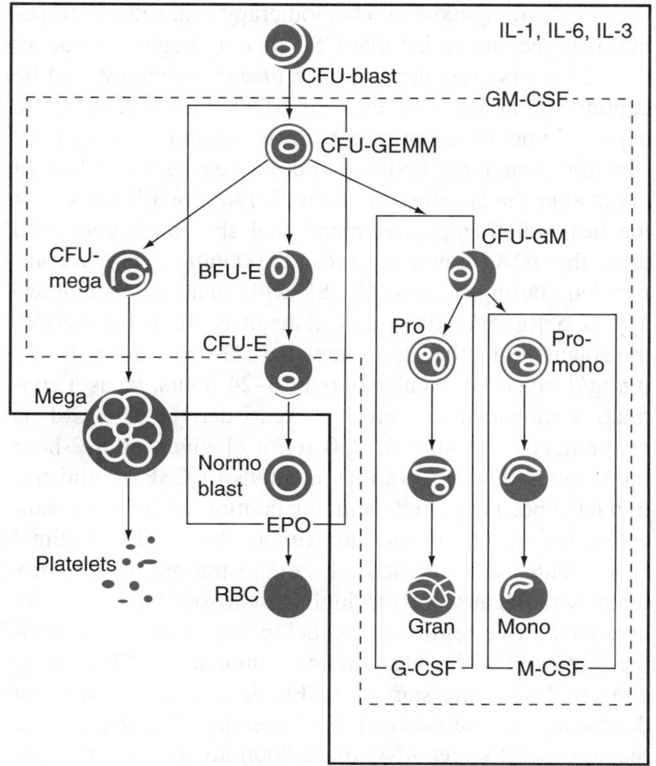

Figure 119.26. Regulation of hematopoietic cell development. IL, interleukin; CSF, colony-stimulating factor; CFU, colony-forming unit; CFU-GEMM, CFU-granulocyte erythroid macrophage-megakaryocyte; Mega, megakaryocyte; CFU-GM, CFU-granulocyte macrophage; BFU-E, burst-forming unit-erythroid; CFU-E, CFU-erythroid; EPO, erythropoietin; blast, immature cell; Pro, promyelocyte; Mono, monocyte; Gran, granulocyte. *(From Gabrilove JL. Introduction and overview of hematopoietic growth factors. Semin Hematol 1989;26(suppl 2):104, with permission.)*

and symptoms (if present), side-effect profiles, and cost.[255] The most common source of infection in these patients is self-infection with body flora, which includes both gram-positive and gram-negative bacteria. Although most early infections are due to bacteria, fungi become important pathogens as the course of neutropenia is prolonged. Traditionally, all febrile neutropenic cancer patients have received intravenous antibiotics in the hospital setting until full recovery of neutrophils. However, it is possible to identify patients at low risk for infection who may be candidates for alternative treatment strategies, including early discharge from the hospital and outpatient oral or intravenous antibiotics.[256]

Numerous methods have been explored to prevent infections in cancer patients.[257] Colony-stimulating factors (CSFs) are commonly employed for this reason.[258–260] These hormones are naturally occurring proteins which are essential for the normal growth and maturation of blood cell components (Fig. 119.26).[261] The CSFs have the ability to enhance the production and also the function of their target cells. Two agents, G-CSF (granulocyte colony-stimulating factor) and GM-CSF (granulocyte-macrophage colony-stimulating factor) are commercially available.[262–264] Several interleukins (e.g., IL-1, IL-6, IL-11, and IL-3 [also known as multi-CSF]) and other growth factors (e.g., macrophage CSF [M-CSF], stem-cell factor [S-CSF], and pixy321 [GM-CSF/IL-3 fusion protein]) are currently being investigated in clinical trials.[265] G-CSF (filgrastim, Neupogen) specifically stimulates the production of neutrophilic granulocytes. GM-CSF (sargramostim, Leukine) promotes the proliferation of granulocytes (neutrophils and eosinophils), as well as monocytes/macrophages. Although GM-CSF has been shown to stimulate megakaryocytes *in vitro,* no consistent effect on platelet production has been defined in clinical trials. Both agents initially enhance demargination and mobilization of mature cells from the marrow, then provide constant stimulation on stem-cell progenitors. The two CSFs have contrasting effects on neutrophil migration: G-CSF enhances this process, while GM-CSF inhibits it. The clinical implications of this difference are unknown. Another effect unique to GM-CSF is an increase in neutrophil adhesion to capillary endothelial cells. This process may account for some of the side effects seen more commonly with GM-CSF. Several host sources have been employed in the recombinant DNA technology used to produce CSFs, including bacteria (*E. coli*), yeast, and mammalian cells (Chinese hamster ovary or CHO cells) (Table 119.15). Products derived from yeast or mammalian sources are glycosylated to varying degrees, as are naturally occurring CSFs, while those derived from *E. coli*

TABLE 119.15. G-CSF AND GM-CSF PRODUCTS AND SOURCES

CSF	Generic Name	Brand Name	Manufacturer	r-DNA Source
G-CSF	Filgrastim	Neupogen	Amgen	*E. coli*
	Lenograstim	Neutrogin[a] (Investigational)	Chugai-Rhone Poulenc	CHO[b] cells
GM-CSF	Sargramostim	Leukine	Immunex	*Saccharomyces cetevisiae*
Yeast	Molgramostim	Leucomax[a] (Investigational)	Schering-Plough/Sandoz	*E. coli*

[a]Available outside the United States.
[b]CHO, Chinese hamster ovary.

are nonglycosylated. It is unclear if this difference results in any clinically significant effects.

The CSFs have been shown to reduce the incidence, magnitude, and duration of neutropenia following a variety of standard chemotherapy regimens.[258–263] These effects have been accompanied by a decrease in febrile days, fewer infections, and fewer days on antibiotics. An unexpected benefit in some G-CSF studies has been a decrease in the incidence of mucositis. Growth factors have also permitted the administration of subsequent chemotherapy courses on schedule, resulting in enhanced dose intensity. Whether the increased dose intensity provided by the CSFs will translate into improved tumor response remains to be demonstrated. Although there is experience with both G-CSF and GM-CSF in prevention of febrile neutropenia after administration of standard doses of chemotherapy, at this time only G-CSF is FDA-approved for this indication.

Only a few studies have addressed the role of CSFs in the treatment of established neutropenia.[264] These initial studies suggest no or only minimal clinical benefit from use of CSFs. Future studies will determine the true cost effectiveness of this strategy. Both CSFs have also proven effective in acceleration of hematopoietic engraftment and in treatment of graft failure following bone marrow transplantation.[266] Other uses for the CSFs include peripheral blood stem-cell mobilization, neutropenia in AIDS patients, myelodysplastic syndromes, congenital neutropenia, and aplastic anemia.

At currently recommended doses, the CSFs are well tolerated. Side effects are more commonly seen with GM-CSF, and may be related to the drug's ability to enhance binding of neutrophils to endothelial cells. Another theory points to the GM-CSF's activation of monocytes/macrophages, which may stimulate the release of cytokines, such as IL-1 and TNF.[261] The most common toxicity of the CSFs is bone pain (20–25% of patients), which can be treated with acetaminophen or NSAIDs. Bone pain was the most significant toxicity seen in clinical trials with G-CSF. Other side effects of G-CSF include an increase in lactate dehydrogenase, alkaline phosphatase, and uric acid levels. Additional toxicities of GM-CSF include constitutional symptoms, such as fever, myalgias, arthralgias, lethargy, and mild headache. GM-CSF may also produce an elevation in liver transaminase enzymes. At higher doses of GM-CSF, pleural and pericardial effusions, capillary leak syndrome, and thrombus formation may occur. A first-dose reaction has been described after GM-CSF administration, and has been reported more commonly with the *E. coli*-derived product (molgramostim), which is investigational. This reaction is more common after intravenous infusion, and consists of dyspnea, facial flushing, hypotension, hypoxia, and tachycardia. Both G-CSF and GM-CSF may produce mild erythema at subcutaneous injection sites, as well as a generalized maculopapular rash with either subcutaneous or intravenous administration.

For prophylaxis of chemotherapy-induced neutropenia, it is recommended that CSF therapy begin not sooner than 24 hours after the last dose of chemotherapy, and be continued until the ANC exceeds 10,000/mm^3 following the expected chemotherapy nadir. In the setting of bone marrow transplantation, CSFs should not begin sooner than 24 hours after the last dose of chemotherapy (or 12 hours after the last radiotherapy treatment) and should be continued until the ANC count exceeds 20,000/mm^3. The recommended starting dose of G-CSF with standard chemotherapy is 5 μg/kg/d given subcutaneously. In bone marrow transplantation, the recommended G-CSF dose is 10 μg/kg/d given intravenously over 4–24 hours, or as a continuous subcutaneous infusion. Yeast-derived GM-CSF is recommended to start at 250 μg/m^2/d given as a 2-hour intravenous infusion. Various methods of CSF administration have been explored including continuous infusion, subcutaneous injection, and intravenous bolus. The optimal dose, route, and method of administration is currently unknown. Because of the high cost associated with CSF use, alternative regimens are being explored. These regimens attempt to decrease the total amount of CSF used by either delaying the start of CSFs, decreasing the dose or decreasing the duration of CSF therapy. Specifically, the recommended target ANC of 10,000/mm^3 is often reduced to an ANC of greater than 5000/mm^3 in clinical practice.

ANEMIA AND THROMBOCYTOPENIA

Chemotherapy-induced thrombocytopenia puts the patient at risk for significant bleeding. To date, platelet transfusions remain the mainstay of management. Other CSFs, such as interleukins-3, -6, and -11 and pixy-321, may be able to stimulate platelet production, but these agents are still under development.[267] Pixy-321 is a fusion protein which combines GM-CSF and IL-3 in a single molecule. The recent discovery of thrombopoietin (megakaryocyte growth and development factor) may represent the most significant factor in the future of thrombocytopenia treatment.[268]

Anemia is a common finding in cancer patients, and may have multiple contributing factors, including anemia of chronic disease, chronic gastrointestinal blood loss, chemotherapy and radiation therapy, and bone marrow invasion by the tumor. Chemotherapy-induced anemias may be due to a direct effect on the bone marrow, but some anticancer drugs have the potential to cause other types of anemia. Cisplatin-induced anemia is a common finding, and may be due to stem-cell damage, but hemolysis has also been documented.[190] Until recently, the only option for the treatment of chemotherapy-related anemia was red blood cell transfusions. This intervention is still the mainstay of management, but the availability of human recombinant erythropoietin has provided another option. Recent studies have documented the efficacy of erythropoietin in the anemia of malignancy[269] and in treating chemotherapy-induced anemias.[270] Recombinant human erythropoietin was the first CSF to be approved for clinical use. Erythropoietin in doses of 100–150 U/kg given subcutaneously three times per week results in increases in hematocrit, decreases in transfusion requirements, and improved quality of life. Further studies will attempt to identify those patients most likely to benefit from this agent.

MUCOSITIS

The gastrointestinal (GI) mucosa is composed of epithelial cells with a high mitotic index and rapid turnover rate, making it a common site of chemotherapy-induced toxicity.[271–273] The subsequent inflammation, or mucositis, can lead to painful ulcerations, local infection, and inability to eat, drink, and swallow. The disruption of the GI mucosal barrier may also provide an avenue for systemic microbial invasion. The time course for development and resolution of mucositis often parallels that seen with neutropenia. Agents most commonly associated with mucositis include 5-fluorouracil (5-FU) and methotrexate. The most effective means of preventing mucositis is through good oral hygiene. Patients at high risk for this toxicity should be evaluated by a dentist prior to chemotherapy and should be instructed to rinse their mouths frequently with baking soda and salt water, or chlorhexidine (Peridex) rinses following chemotherapy.[272] For patients receiving 5-FU treatment, the use of ice (oral cryotherapy) may decrease the risk for mucositis by decreasing drug delivery to the oral mucosa.[273] Once mucositis has developed, treatment is mainly supportive, including use of topical or systemic analgesics, and oral hygiene (including the rinses described above). Viscous lidocaine, diphenhydramine liquid, and dyclonine are topical anesthetics commonly employed. Severe cases may lead to dehydration and require intravenous hydration. Local infections due to *Candida* species and herpes simplex viruses are common in these patients. Suspicious lesions should be cultured, and appropriate antifungal and/or antiviral treatment should then be instituted. Antifungal therapy may be delivered topically for mild infections (thrush), using clotrimazole (Mycelex) troches or nystatin (Nilstat, others) oral suspension. For more severe oral or esophageal fungal infections, systemic treatment with oral ketoconazole (Nizoral), fluconazole (Diflucan), or intravenous amphotericin B is indicated.[274]

Mucosal damage can occur at any point along the entire length of the GI tract. In the lower portion of the GI tract, this damage can be manifested as diarrhea (mild to life threatening in nature) and abdominal pain. Support with intravenous fluids and electrolyte supplementation should be initiated promptly in severe cases. Once infectious causes have been ruled out, diarrhea can safely be treated with antispasmodics, like Lomotil or loperamide (Imodium). Recently, the somatostatin-analog octreotide has been used successfully to treat severe cases of 5-FU-induced diarrhea.[60]

ALOPECIA

Although not a life-threatening side effect of chemotherapy, the toxicity that patients often find most distressing is alopecia. Alopecia from chemotherapy is usually temporary, and the degree of hair loss varies widely.[275] The loss of hair is not limited to the scalp; any area of the body may be affected. Hair loss usually beings 1–2 weeks after chemotherapy, and regrowth may begin before the chemotherapy courses are completed. Cryotherapy (local application of ice) and scalp tourniquets have both been investigated as methods of preventing alopecia. Both techniques produce vasoconstriction, resulting in decreased exposure of hair follicles to the chemotherapy agents. These techniques have not been found to be uniformly effective, and are contraindicated in patients with cancers that may metastasize to the scalp, such as leukemia and lymphoma.

EXTRAVASATION

Certain antineoplastic agents have the ability to cause severe tissue damage if they escape from the vasculature, and are called vesicants.[117,276] These agents include the anthracyclines, actinomycin D, the vinca alkaloids, mitomycin C, and nitrogen mustard. The anthracyclines are the most notorious agents, and most extensively investigated. The tissue damage may result in prolonged pain, tissue sloughing, infection, and loss of mobility. Prompt initiation of the appropriate interventions is important to minimize morbidity. Unfortunately, most information on extravasation management is anecdotal; few controlled clinical studies have been conducted to determine optimal intervention strategies. Therefore, prevention has become the focus of extravasation management. The most important method of prevention is good administration technique,[276] but even then, extravasations may occur. The vein selected for administration should be on the distal portion of the arm. The large veins of the forearm are desirable because if a drug does extravasate, there is maximum soft-tissue coverage to protect crucial structures like nerves and tendons. The vesicants should be administered slowly via intravenous injection (IV push) through the side-arm of a running IV. Vesicants should not be administered by intravenous infusion unless the patient has a central venous catheter. The person administering the vesicant should verify needle stability and adequate blood return after each 1–2 mL of drug is injected. For extravasation of vesicants, one of the most important interventions is the application of ice packs to the affected area. One exception to this rule is the vinca alkaloids, which are better managed with application of heat. Only a few antidotes to vesicant agents are employed clinically. Sodium thiosulfate is used to neutralize nitrogen mustard extravasations, and hyaluronidase has been shown to improve the outcome after vinca alkaloid extravasation. Topical application of dimethyl sulfoxide (DMSO) may be an effective method for managing anthracycline and mitomycin C extravasations.[117]

INFERTILITY

Advances in the treatment of some cancers, such as Hodgkin's disease and testicular cancer, have produced long-term survivors and the opportunity to examine the late consequences of chemotherapy administration. Infertility and secondary cancers have emerged as important late effects. The gonadal toxicities of chemotherapy have not received much attention in the past because they are not life threatening. High rates of fertility deficits and sexual dysfunction have been noted for both men and women.[277] In men, the antitumor drugs have been shown to produce severe oligospermia or azoospermia, and infertility. Serum testosterone levels are only rarely altered. The recovery of spermatogenesis after completion of chemotherapy is unpredictable. Men receiving combination chemotherapy appear to have more long-lasting adverse effects on fertility than men receiving single-agent therapy. Age, total dose, duration of therapy, and type of drug are other important variables. In women, toxic effects on the ovaries result clinically in amenorrhea, vaginal epithelial atrophy, and menopausal symptoms. These effects are related to dose and age. Younger patients appear to be more resistant to the effects on the ovaries. As with men, the recovery of fertility is unpredictable, but women younger then 25 years of age appear to have the best outcomes. The effects of the alkylating agents on fertility have been extensively studied. This group of drugs exerts profound and consistently detrimental effects on reproductive function. Less is known about commonly used agents such as doxorubicin, methotrexate, and bleomycin. Patients with potentially curable tumors, who desire to have children in the future, should be informed about the risk for infertility and sperm or oocyte banking options.

SECONDARY MALIGNANCIES

Secondary cancers induced by chemotherapy and radiation pose a serious long-term complication.[278] Although many types of solid tumors have been reported as chemotherapy-induced malignancies, ANLL accounts for more than 50% of secondary cancers. ANLL has been reported following successful treatment of Hodgkin's disease, acute leukemias, non-Hodgkin's lymphomas, multiple myeloma, breast cancer, and advanced ovarian cancer. For curable cancers, the relatively small risk for occurrence of secondary malignancies is far outweighed by the benefits of survival in large numbers of patients. However, for cancers such as ovarian cancer, the risk of leukemia is not offset by improved survival in chemotherapy recipients. The issue of secondary malignancies is of particular concern in patients receiving adjuvant chemotherapy. As with the late complication of infertility, the group of antineoplastic agents primarily associated with secondary cancers is the alkylating agents. Etoposide has also recently been linked to secondary leukemias.

SAFETY AND HANDLING ISSUES

As discussed previously, the cytotoxic drugs used to treat cancer are carcinogenic, mutagenic, and teratogenic. Consequently, these drugs should be handled with care to avoid inadvertent exposure of health care professionals.[279] All pharmacies should have written standard procedures for handling these drugs, and all personnel should be oriented to these procedures. The most common avenue of exposure is via inhalation of aerosolized drug. Individuals preparing chemotherapy should work in a Class II biologic safety cabinet and wear gowns and powder-free disposable latex gloves. The gowns should be made of lint-free, low-permeability fabric with a solid front, long sleeves, and tight-fitting elastic cuffs. Negative pressure techniques should be employed in drug preparation to minimize aerosolization. Health care workers administering these agents should take similar precautions to avoid exposure. Kits for cleaning up chemotherapy spills should be located in all areas of the institution in which chemotherapy is handled. Cytotoxic waste should be disposed of properly, and patients should be informed of proper methods of disposing of potentially contaminated body excreta and cytotoxic waste.

CANCER PREVENTION

DIET

The relationship between diet and cancer is the subject of intense investigation. Although controversy exists over the true role of dietary factors in carcinogenesis, some general recommendations have been developed by the National Cancer Institute (Table 119.16).[280] Consumption of a high-fat diet appears to increase the risk for breast, colorectal, and prostate cancers. The average American consumes 36–38% of daily calories as fat. A decrease in fat intake to less than 30% of daily calories may decrease the risk for developing cancer, as well as heart disease. Obese individ-

TABLE 119.16. AMERICAN CANCER SOCIETY DIETARY RECOMMENDATIONS

1. Maintain a desirable body weight. Avoid obesity.
2. Eat a varied diet, in moderation.
3. Include a variety of both vegetables and fruits each day.
4. Eat more high fiber foods, such as whole grain cereals, legumes, vegetables, and fruits.
5. Reduce total fat intake.
6. Limit consumption of alcoholic beverages, if you drink at all.
7. Limit consumption of salt-cured, smoked, and nitrite-preserved foods.

Weinhouse S, Bal DG, Adamson R, The Work Study Group on Diet, Nutrition, and Cancer. (From American Cancer Society guidelines on diet, nutrition, and cancer. CA 1991;41:334–338.)

uals have been shown to have an increased risk of several cancers, including colorectal, breast, biliary, and uterine cancers. The inverse relationship between dietary fiber and colon cancer has received much attention.[281] The American diet is typically low in fiber (11 grams per day). High fiber intake (20–30 grams per day) may decrease the risk of colon cancer. A high alcohol intake has been shown to increase the risk for many upper aerodigestive tract malignancies, especially in smokers.

CHEMOPREVENTION

This is defined as the systemic use of natural or synthetic products to reverse, suppress, or prevent carcinogenesis. Several agents have been studied in chemoprevention. Beta-carotene, vitamin A and related retinoids, and vitamins C and E may prevent, halt, or reverse the carcinogenic process. These vitamins are present in fresh fruits and vegetables. The known effects of these agents on the cancer process have resulted in several trials to determine their effectiveness as chemoprotective agents.[282] To date, the most encouraging results have been in the area of oral leukoplakia and squamous cell head and neck cancer. Oral leukoplakia is a white, patchy, premalignant lesion of the oral mucosa associated with tobacco use, and is also related to carcinogenesis at other sites within the aerodigestive tract. Patients with smoking-related malignancy have acquired a so-called field cancerization defect, meaning that any part of the aerodigestive tract exposed to the tobacco carcinogens is at risk for development of cancer. For example, patients cured of head and neck cancer commonly present several years later with a second primary cancer of the upper aerodigestive tract. Clinical trials of vitamin A and the retinoids have shown significant activity against oral leukoplakia and the development of second primary tumors in patients with head and neck cancer. In addition to smoking cessation, patients cured of their head and neck malignancy should be considered candidates for chemoprevention.

Hormonal therapy may represent another effective mechanism of chemoprevention. It is known that certain hormones play a role in the initiation, promotion, and progression of malignancy. For example, estrogen is known to stimulate breast cancer cell growth and testosterone stimulates prostate cancer growth. The antiestrogen tamoxifen effectively blocks this stimulatory effect in breast cancer. A large clinical trial sponsored by the National Surgical Adjuvant Bowel and Breast Project (NSABP) is currently under way to assess tamoxifen's efficacy in breast cancer prevention in high-risk individuals. The Prostate Cancer Prevention Trial will assess the efficacy of the 5-alpha-reductase inhibitor finasteride, which inhibits the conversion of testosterone to its active form, dihydrotestosterone. The results of these trials will not be available for many years, but will provide valuable information on the utility of hormonal manipulation on cancer prevention.

TOBACCO

In 1990, almost 413,000 deaths (20% of all deaths) in the United States were due to smoking-related illnesses.[283] Cigarette smoking remains the most preventable cause of premature death in the United States. For many types of cancer, the underlying etiology is unknown. One notable exception is lung cancer; cigarette smoking is the major cause of this disease.[284] More than 90% of all cases of lung cancer are diagnosed in smokers. Tobacco smoking also increases the relative risk for development of many other types of cancer, including cancers of the mouth, pharynx, larynx, esophagus, and bladder. Passive inhalation of exhaled tobacco by-products and cigarette smoke represents a significant risk factor for lung cancer in the nonsmoking population. Smokeless tobacco has been connected to the development of oral cancers. Abstinence from chewing and smoking tobacco is believed to be a major factor in the prevention of these malignancies.

SUN EXPOSURE

The association between sun exposure and skin neoplasms is also well established. The incidence of both nonmelanomatous skin cancer and melanoma has steadily increased in past decades, paralleling the increase in recreational sun exposure.[285] During this same time period, protection from the ultraviolet light exposure normally provided by the ozone layer has been compromised. Fair-skinned individuals who sunburn easily are particularly at high risk. Melanoma and skin cancers can be largely prevented by minimizing exposure to the sun, and by applying strong sunscreens and sunblocks to sun-exposed areas (SPF $\geq$ 15).

REFERENCES

1. Chabner BA. Clinical strategies for cancer treatment: The role of drugs, in Chabner BA, Collins JM (eds): Cancer Chemotherapy: Principles and Practice. Philadelphia, JB Lippincott, 1990, pp 1–15.
2. Perkins AS, VandeWoude GF. Principles of molecular cell biology of cancer: Oncogenes, in DeVita VT Jr, Hellman S, Rosenberg SA (eds): Cancer: Principles and Practice of Oncology, 4th ed. Philadelphia, JB Lippincott, 1993, pp 35–59.
3. Cancer facts and figures—1995. American Cancer Society, Atlanta, 1995.
4. Shields PG, Harris CC. Principles of carcinogenesis: Chemical, in DeVita VT Jr, Hellman S, Rosenberg SA (eds): Cancer: Principles and Practice of Oncology, 4th ed. Philadelphia, JB Lippincott, 1993, pp 200–212.
5. Pitot HC. The molecular biology of carcinogenesis. Cancer 1993;72:962–970.
6. Schilsky RL, Erlichman C. Infertility and carcinogenesis: Late complication of chemotherapy, in Chabner BA, Collins JM (eds): Cancer Chemotherapy: Principles and Practice. Philadelphia, JB Lippincott, 1990, pp 32–58.
7. Rieche K. Carcinogenicity of antineoplastic agents in man. Cancer Treat Rev 1984;11:39–67.
8. Howley PM. Principles of carcinogenesis: Viral, in Devita VT Jr, Hellman S, Rosenberg SA (eds): Cancer: Principles and Practice of Oncology, 4th ed. Philadelphia, JB Lippincott, 1993, pp 182–199.
9. Smith MR, Matthews NT, Jones KA, Fung HF. Biologic actions of oncogenes. Pharmacol Ther 1993;58:211–236.
10. Friend SH, Dryja TP, Weinberg RA. Oncogenes and tumor-suppressing genes. N Engl J Med 1988;318:618–622.
11. Yamamoto T. Molecular basis of cancer: Oncogenes and tumor suppressor genes. Microbiol Immunol 1993;37: 11–22.
12. Levine AJ. The tumor suppressor genes. Ann Rev Biochem 1993;62:623–651.
13. Korsmeyer SJ. Bcl-2 initiates a new category of oncogenes: Regulators of cell death. Blood 1992;80:879–886.
14. Cavanee WK, White RL. The genetic basis of cancer. Sci Am 1995;72–79.
15. Stewart BW. Mechanisms of apoptosis: Integration of genetic, biochemical, and cellular indicators. J Natl Cancer Inst 1994;86:1286–1296.
16. Schabel FM. The use of tumor growth kinetics in planning "curative" chemotherapy of advanced solid tumors. Cancer Res 1969;29:2384.
17. Dorr RT, Von Hoff DD, eds. Cancer Chemotherapy Handbook, 2nd ed. New York, Elsevier, 1994.
18. Norton L, Simon R. The Norton–Simon hypothesis revisited. Cancer Treat Rep 1986;70:163–169.
19. Baserga R. Principles of molecular cell biology of cancer: The cell cycle, in DeVita VT Jr, Hellman S, Rosenberg SA (eds): Cancer: Principles and Practice of Oncology, 4th ed. Philadelphia, JB Lippincott, 1993, pp 60–66.
20. Skipper HE. The effects of chemotherapy on the kinetics of leukemic cell behavior. Cancer Res 1965;25:1544.
21. Liotta LA, Stetler-Stevenson WG. Principles of molecular cell biology of cancer: Cancer metastasis, in Devita VT Jr, Hellman S, Rosenberg SA (eds): Cancer: Principles and Practice of Oncology, 4th ed. Philadelphia, JB Lippincott, 1993, pp 134–149.
22. Schirrmacher V. Cancer metastasis: Experimental approaches, theoretical concepts, and impacts for treatment strategies. Adv Cancer Res 1985;43:1.
23. Robbins SL, Cotran RS, Kumar V. Pathologic Basis of Disease, 3rd ed. Philadelphia, WB Saunders, 1984.
24. Recommendations for the early detection of cancer in asymptomatic people. American Cancer Society No. 3251, Atlanta, Georgia, Revised 1992.
25. Seven warning signs of cancer. American Cancer Society, Atlanta, Georgia.
26. Fernbach DJ, Vietti TJ, eds. Clinical Pediatric Oncology, 4th ed. St. Louis, Mosby-Year Book, 1991, pp 1–10.
27. American Joint Committee on Cancer. Manual for Staging of Cancer, 3rd ed. Philadelphia, JB Lippincott, 1988.
28. Rosenberg SA. Principles of surgical oncology, in Devita VT Jr, Hellman S, Rosenberg SA, (eds): Cancer: Principles and Practice of Oncology, 4th ed. Philadelphia, JB Lippincott, 1993, pp 238–247.
29. Coia LR, Moylan DJ, eds. Therapeutic Radiology for the House Officer. Baltimore, MD, Williams & Wilkins, 1984.
30. Bleyer WA. Antineoplastic drugs, in Yaffe SJ (ed): Pediatric Pharmacology: Therapeutic Principles in Practice. New York, Grune and Stratton, 1980, pp 349–378.
31. Calabresi P, Chabner BA. Chemotherapy of neoplastic diseases, in Gilman AG, Rall TW, Nies AS, Taylor P (eds): Goodman & Gilman's the Pharmacologic Basis of Therapeutics, 8th ed. New York, Pergamon Press, 1990, pp 1202–1263.
32. DeVita VT Jr. Principles of chemotherapy, in Devita VT Jr, Hellman S, Rosenberg SA, (eds): Cancer: Principles and Practice of Oncology, 3rd ed. Philadelphia, JB Lippincott, 1989, pp 276–300.
33. Haskell CM. Principles of Cancer Chemotherapy, in Haskell CM (ed): Cancer Treatment, 2nd ed. Philadelphia, WB Saunders, 1985, p 37.
34. Skipper HE, Simpson-Herren L. Relationship between tumor stem cell heterogeneity and responsiveness to chemotherapy. In Devita VT Jr, Hellman S, Rosenberg SA (eds): Important Advances in Oncology 1985. Philadelphia, JB Lippincott, 1985, pp 63–77.
35. Goldie JH, Coldman AJ. A mathematical model for relating drug sensitivity of tumors to spontaneous mutation rate. Cancer Treat Rep 1979;63:1727–1733.
36. Leighton JC, Goldstein LJ. P-glycoprotein in adult solid tumors: Expression and prognostic significance. Hematol/Oncol Clin North Am 1995;9:251–273.
37. Fisher GA, Sikic BI. Clinical studies with modulators of multidrug resistance. Hematol/Oncol Clin North Am 1995; 9:363–382.
38. Frei E III, Canellos GP. Dose: A critical factor in cancer chemotherapy. Am J Med 1980;69:585–594.
39. Hryniuk W, Bush H. The importance of dose intensity in chemotherapy of metastatic breast cancer. J Clin Oncol; 1984;2:1281–1287.

40. Stewart CF. Pharmacodynamics and cancer: Practical aspects of dose intensity for pharmacists. J Pharm Practice 1991;4:11–19.
41. Hryniuk WM, Figuerdo A, Goodyear M. Applications of dose-intensity to problems in chemotherapy of breast and colorectal cancer. Sem Oncol 1987;14(suppl 4):3–11.
42. Hryniuk WM, Levine MN. Analysis of dose intensity for adjuvant chemotherapy trials. J Clin Oncol 1986;4:1162–1170.
43. Dorr RT. Chemoprotectants for cancer chemotherapy. Sem Oncol 1991;18(suppl 2):48–58.
44. Rodman JH, Relling MV, Stewart CF, et al. Clinical pharmacokinetics and pharmacodynamics of anticancer drugs in children. Sem Oncol 1993;20:18–29.
45. Collins JM. Pharmacokinetics and clinical monitoring, in Chabner BA, Collins JM (eds): Cancer Chemotherapy: Principles and Practice. Philadelphia, JB Lippincott, 1990, pp 16–31.
46. Casciato DA, Lowitz BB, eds. Manual of Clinical Oncology, 2nd ed. Boston, Little, Brown, 1988, p 584.
47. Skeel RT. Systemic assessment of the patient with cancer, in Skeel RT (ed): Handbook of Cancer Chemotherapy. Boston, Little, Brown, 1991, pp 55–70.
48. Capizzi RL, Keiser LW, Sartorelli AC. Combination chemotherapy: Theory and practice. Semin Oncol 1977;4:277–253.
49. Tannock I. Cell kinetics and chemotherapy: A critical review. Cancer Treat Rep 1978;62:1117.
50. Rosenthal N. DNA and the genetic code. N Engl J Med 1994;331:39–41.
51. Vande Woude S, Vande Woude GF. Principles of molecular cell biology of cancer: Introduction to methods in molecular biology, in Devita VT Jr, Hellman S, Rosenberg SA (eds): Cancer: Principles and Practice of Oncology, 4th ed. Philadelphia, JB Lippincott, 1993, pp 3–22.
52. Pratt WB, Ruddon RW, Ensminger WD, Maybaum J. The Anticancer Drugs, 2nd ed. New York, Oxford University Press, 1994, pp 69–107.
53. Grem JL. Fluorinated pyrimidines, in Chabner BA, Collins JM (eds): Cancer Chemotherapy: Principles and Practice. Philadelphia, JB Lippincott, 1990, pp 180–224.
54. Handschumacher RE, Cheng YC. Purine and pyrimidine antimetabolites, in Holland JF, Frei E III, Bast RC, et al (eds): Cancer Medicine, 3rd ed. Philadelphia, Lea & Febiger, 1993, pp 712–754.
55. Advanced colorectal cancer meta-analysis project. Meta-analysis of randomized trials testing the biochemical modulation of fluorouracil by methotrexate in metastatic colorectal cancer. J Clin Oncol 1994;12:960–969.
56. Diasio, RB, Lu Z. Dihydropyrimidine dehydrogenase activity and fluorouracil chemotherapy. J Clin Oncol 1994;12: 2239–2242.
57. Peters GJ, Schornagel JH, Milano GA. Clinical pharmacokinetics of antimetabolites. Cancer Survey 1993;17:123–156.
58. deTakats PG, Kerr DJ, Poole CJ, et al. Hepatic artery chemotherapy for metastatic colorectal cancer. Br J Cancer 1994;69:372–378.
59. Stein BN, Petrelli NJ, Douglass HO, et al. Age and sex are independent predictors of 5-fluorouracil toxicity. Cancer 1995;75:11–17.
60. Cascinu S, Fedeli A, Fedeli SL, Catalano G. Octreotide versus loperamide in the treatment of fluorouracil-induced diarrhea: A randomized trial. J Clin Oncol 1993;11:148–151.
61. Loprinzi CL, Wender DB, Veeder MH, et al. Inhibition of 5-fluorouracil-induced ocular irritation by ocular ice packs. Cancer 1994;74:945–948.
62. deForni M, Malet-Martino MC, Jaillais P, et al. Cardiotoxicity of high-dose continuous infusion fluorouracil: A prospective clinical study. J Clin Oncol 1992;10:1795–1801.
63. Anand AJ. Fluorouracil cardiotoxicity. Ann Pharmacotherapy 1994;28:374–378.
64. Moertel CG, Fleming TR, Macdonald JS, et al. Hepatic toxicity associated with fluorouracil plus levamisole adjuvant therapy. J Clin Oncol 1993;11:2386–2390.
65. Stagg RJ, Venook AP, Chase JL, et al. Alternating hepatic intra-arterial floxuridine and fluorouracil: A less toxic regimen for treatment of liver metastases from colorectal cancer. J Natl Cancer Inst 1991;83:423–428.
66. Von Reomeling R, Hrushesky WJM. Determination of the therapeutic index of floxuridine by its circadian infusion pattern. J Natl Cancer Inst 1990;82:386–393.
67. Chabner BA. Cytidine analogues, in Chabner BA, Collins JM (eds): Cancer Chemotherapy: Principles and Practice. Philadelphia, JB Lippincott, 1990, pp 154–179.
68. Balis FM, Poplack DG. Central nervous system pharmacology of antileukemic drugs. Am J Pediatr Hematol Oncol 1989;11:74–86.
69. Mayer RJ, Davis RB, Schiffer CA, et al. Intensive post-remission chemotherapy in adults with acute myeloid leukemia. N Engl J Med 1994;331:896–903.
70. Graves T, Hooks M. Drug-induced toxicities associated with high-dose cytosine arabinoside infusions. Pharmacotherapy 1989;9:23–28.
71. Baker WJ, Royer GL Jr, Weiss RB. Cytarabine and neurologic toxicity. J Clin Oncol 1991;9:679–693.
72. Tuxen MK, Hansen SW. Neurotoxicity secondary to antineoplastic drugs. Cancer Treat Rev 1994;20:191–214.
73. Damon LE, Mass R, Linker CA. The association between high-dose cytarabine neurotoxicity and renal insufficiency. J Clin Oncol 1989;7:1563–1568.
74. Jolson HM, Bosco L, Bufton MG, et al. Clustering of adverse drug events: Analysis of risk factors for cerebellar toxicity with high dose cytarabine. J Natl Cancer Inst 1992;84:500–505.
75. Kreisman H, Wolkove N. Pulmonary toxicity of antineoplastic therapy. Semin Oncol 1992;19:508–520.
76. Shearer P, Katz J, Bozeman P, et al. Pulmonary insufficiency complicating therapy with high dose cytosine arabinoside in five pediatric patients with relapsed acute myelogenous leukemia. Cancer 1994;74:1953–1958.
77. Lilenbaum RC, Green MR. Novel chemotherapeutic agents in the treatment of non–small-cell lung cancer. J Clin Oncol 1993;11:1391–1402.
78. Kaye SB. Gemcitabine: Current status of phase I and II trials [editorial]. J Clin Oncol 1994;12:1527–1531.

79. Protocol B9E-MC-JHEW(c). Treatment IND of Gemzar® (gemcitabine) for patients with pancreatic cancer. Lilly Research Laboratories, Indianapolis, Indiana, December 1994.
80. Grunewald R, Kantarjian H, Du M, et al. Gemcitabine in leukemia: A phase I clinical, plasma, and cellular pharmacology study. J Clin Oncol 1992;10:406–413.
81. McCormack JJ, Johns DG. Purine and purine nucleoside antimetabolites, in Chabner BA, Collins JM (eds): Cancer Chemotherapy: Principles and Practice. Philadelphia, JB Lippincott, 1990, pp 234–252.
82. Lockhart S, Plunkett W, Jeha S, et al. High-dose mercaptopurine followed by intermediate-dose cytarabine in relapsed acute leukemia. J Clin Oncol 1994;12:587–595.
83. Pinkel D. Intravenous mercaptopurine: Life beings at 40. J Clin Oncol 1993;11:1826–1831.
84. Koren G, Ferrazini G, Sulh H, et al. Systemic exposure to mercaptopurine as a prognostic factor in acute lymphocytic leukemia in children. N Engl J Med 1990;323:17–21.
85. Balis FM. Pharmacokinetic drug interactions of commonly used anticancer drugs. Clin Pharmacokinet 1986;11:223–235.
86. Perry MC. Chemotherapeutic agents and hepatotoxicity. Semin Oncol 1992;19:551–565.
87. Hood MA, Finley RS. Fludarabine: A review. DICP, Ann Pharmacother 1991;25:518–524.
88. Chun HG, Leyland-Jones B, Cheson BD. Fludarabine phosphate: A synthetic purine antimetabolite with significant activity against lymphoid malignancies. J Clin Oncol 1991;9:175–188.
89. Cheson BD, Vena DA, Foss FM, Sorensen JM. Neurotoxicity of purine analogs: A review. J Clin Oncol 1994;12:2216–2228.
90. Bryson HM, Sorkin EM. Cladribine: A review of its pharmacodynamic and pharmacokinetic properties and therapeutic potential in haematological malignancies. Drugs 1993;46:872–894.
91. Saven A, Piro LD. 2-chlorodeoxyadenosine: A newer purine analog active in the treatment of indolent lymphoid malignancies. Ann Intern Med 1994;120:784–791.
92. Piro LD, Carrera CJ, Carson DA, et al. Lasting remissions in hairy-cell leukemia induced by a single infusion of 2-chlorodeoxyadenosine. N Engl J Med 1990;322: 1117–1121.
93. Kane BJ, Kuhn JG, Roush MK. Pentostatin: An adenosine deaminase inhibitor for the treatment of hairy cell leukemia. Ann Pharmacotherapy 1992;26:939–946.
94. Grever M, Kopecky K, Foucar MK, et al. Randomized comparison of pentostatin versus interferon alfa-2a in previously untreated patients with hairy cell leukemia: An intergroup study. J Clin Oncol 1995;13:974–982.
95. Allegra CJ. Antifolates, in Chabner BA, Collins JM (eds): Cancer Chemotherapy: Principles and Practice. Philadelphia, JB Lippincott, 1990, pp 110–153.
96. Jolivet J, Cowan KH, Curt GA, et al. The pharmacology and clinical use of methotrexate. N Engl J Med 1983;309: 1094–1104.
97. Bertino JR, Romanini A. Folate antagonists, in Holland JF, Frei E III, Bast RC Jr, et al. (eds): Cancer Medicine, 3rd ed. Philadelphia, Lea and Febiger, 1993, pp 698–711.
98. Bertino JR. Ode to methotrexate. J Clin Oncol 1993;11:5–14.
99. Ackland SP, Schilsky RL. High-dose methotrexate: A critical reappraisal. J Clin Oncol 1987;5:2017–2031.
100. Madden T, Eaton VE. Methotrexate, in Schumacher GE (ed): Therapeutic Drug Monitoring. Norwalk, CT, Appleton and Lange, 1995, pp 527–552.
101. Bleyer WA. New vistas for leucovorin in cancer chemotherapy. Cancer 1989;63:995–1007.
102. Evans WE, Crom WR, Abramowitch M, et al. Clinical pharmacodynamics of high-dose methotrexate in acute lymphocytic leukemia: Identification of a relation between concentration and effect. N Engl J Med 1986;314:471–477.
103. Floridon C, Thomsen SG. Methotrexate treatment of ectopic pregnancy. Acta Obstet Gynecol Scand 1994;73:746–752.
104. Reid DJ, Segars LW. Methotrexate for the treatment of chronic corticosteroid-dependent asthma. Clin Pharm 1993;12:762–767.
105. Schwinghammer TL, Bloom EJ. Pharmacologic prophylaxis of acute GVHD after allogeneic marrow transplantation. Clin Pharm 1993;12:736–761.
106. Salach RH, Cash JM. Methotrexate: The emerging drug of choice for serious rheumatoid arthritis. Clin Ther 1994;16:912–922.
107. Relling MV, Fairclough D, Ayers D, et al. Patient characteristics associated with high-risk methotrexate concentrations and toxicity. J Clin Oncol 1994;12:1667–1672.
108. Weiss R. Hypersensitivity reactions. Semin Oncol 1992;19:458–477.
109. Tracy TS, Jones DR, Hall SD. The effect of NSAIDs on methotrexate disposition in patients with rheumatoid arthritis [abstract]. Clin Pharmacol Ther 1990;47:138.
110. Pratt WB, Ruddon RW, Ensminger WD, Maybaum J. The Anticancer Drugs, 2nd ed. New York, Oxford University Press, 1994, pp 183–198.
111. Beck WT, Cass CE, Houghton PJ. Anticancer drugs from plants: Vinca alkaloids and taxol, in Holland JF, Frei E III, Bast RC Jr, et al (eds): Cancer Medicine, 3rd ed. Philadelphia, Lea and Febiger, 1993, 782–795.
112. Bender RA, Hamel E, Hande KR. Plant alkaloids, in Chabner BA, Collins JM (eds): Cancer Chemotherapy: Principles and Practice. Philadelphia, JB Lippincott, 1990, pp 253–275.
113. Rahmani R, Zhou XJ. Pharmacokinetics and metabolism of vinca alkaloids. Cancer Survey 1993;17:269–281.
114. Crom WR, deGraaf SSN, Synold T, et al. Pharmacokinetics of vincristine in children and adolescents with acute lymphocytic leukemia. J Pediatr 1994;125:642–649.
115. Sulkes A, Collins JM. Reappraisal of some dosage adjustment guidelines. Cancer Treat Rep 1987;71:229–233.
116. Epstein JB. Treatment of oral Kaposi's sarcoma with intralesional vinblastine. Cancer 1993;71:1722–1725.
117. Dorr RT. Antidotes to vesicant chemotherapy administration. Blood Rev 1990;4:41–60.
118. Jones AL, Smith IE. Navelbine and the anthrapyrazoles. Hematol/Oncol Clin North Am 1994;8:141–152.
119. Toso C, Lindley C. Vinorelbine: A novel vinca alkaloid. Am J Health-Syst Pharm 1995;52:1287–1304.

120. Fleming RA, Miller AA, Stewart CF. Etoposide: An update. Clin Pharm 1989;8:274–293.
121. Schacter LP, Igwemezie LN, Seyedsadr M, et al. Cancer Chemotherapy and Pharmacology 1994;34(suppl):S58–S63.
122. Hande KR, Krozely MG, Greco FA, et al. Bioavailability of low-dose oral etoposide. J Clin Oncol 1993;11:374–377.
123. Greco FA. Chronic etoposide administration: Overview of clinical experience. Cancer Treat Rev 1993;19(suppl C):35–45.
124. McLeod HL, Evans WE. Clinical pharmacokinetics and pharmacodynamics of epipodophyllotoxins. Cancer Surveys 1993;17:253–268.
125. Joel SP, Shah R, Slevin ML. Etoposide dosage and pharmacodynamics. Cancer Chemotherapy Pharmacol 1994;34(suppl):S69–S75.
126. Stewart CF, Arbuck SG, Fleming RA, et al. Changes in the clearance of total and unbound etoposide in patients with liver dysfunction. J Clin Oncol 1990;8:1874–1879.
127. Stewart CF. Use of etoposide in patients with organ dysfunction: Pharmacokinetic and pharmacodynamic considerations. Cancer Chemotherapy Pharmacol 1994;34(suppl):S76–S83.
128. Rodman JH, Furman WL, Sunderland M, et al. Escalating teniposide systemic exposure to increase dose intensity for pediatric patients. J Clin Oncol 1993;11:287–293.
129. Rodman JH, Murry DJ, Madden T, Santana VM. Altered etoposide pharmacokinetics and time to engraftment in pediatric patients undergoing autologous bone marrow transplantation. J Clin Oncol 1994;12:2390–2397.
130. Durand RE, Goldie JH. Interaction of etoposide and cisplatin in an *in vitro* tumor model. Cancer Treat Rep 1987;71:673–679.
131. Thompson DS, Hainsworth JD, Hande KR, et al. Prolonged administration of low-dose, infusional etoposide in patients with etoposide-sensitive neoplasms: A phase I/II study. J Clin Oncol 1993;11:1322–1328.
132. Tran A, Housset C, Boboc B, et al. Etoposide (VP-16-213) induced hepatitis. Report of three cases following standard-dose treatments. J Hepatology 1991;12:36–39.
133. Pui CH, Ribeiro RC, Hancock ML, et al. Acute myeloid leukemia in children treated with epipodophyllotoxins for acute lymphoblastic leukemia. N Engl J Med 1991;325:1682–1687.
134. Kobayashi K, Ratain MJ. Pharmacodynamics and long-term toxicity of etoposide. Cancer Chemotherapy Pharmacol 1994;34(suppl):S64–S68.
135. Winick NJ, McKenna RW, Shuster JJ, et al. Secondary acute myeloid leukemia in children with acute lymphoblastic leukemia treated with etoposide. J Clin Oncol 1993;11:209–217.
136. Smith MA, Rubinstein L, Cazenave L, et al. Report of the cancer therapy evaluation program monitoring plan for secondary acute myeloid leukemia following treatment with epipodophyllotoxins. J Natl Cancer Inst 1993;85:554–558.
137. Kohler DR, Goldspiel BR. Paclitaxel (Taxol). Pharmacother 1994;14:3–34.
138. Pazdur R, Kudelka AP, Kavanagh JJ, et al. The taxoids: Paclitaxel (Taxol) and docetaxel (Taxotere). Cancer Treat Rev 1993;19:351–386.
139. Bissett D, Kaye SB. Taxol and taxotere—current status and future prospects. Eur J Cancer 1993;29A:1228–1231.
140. Rowinsky EK, Donehower RC. Paclitaxel (Taxol). N Engl J Med 1995;332:1004–1014.
141. Venook AP, Egorin M, Brown TD, et al. Paclitaxel (Taxol) in patients with liver dysfunction (CALGB 9264) [abstract]. Proc Am Soc Clin Oncol 1994;13:139.
142. Creemers GJ, Lund B, Verweij J. Topoisomerase I inhibitors: Topotecan and irenotecan. Cancer Treat Rev 1994;20:73–96.
143. Burris HA III, Fields SM. Topoisomerase I inhibitors: An overview of the camptothecin analogs. Hematol/Oncol Clin North Am 1994;8:333–355.
144. Colvin M, Chabner BA. Alkylating agents, in Chabner BA, Collins JM (eds): Cancer Chemotherapy: Principles and Practice. Philadelphia, JB Lippincott, 1990, pp 276–313.
145. Pratt WB, Ruddon RW, Ensminger WD, Maybaum J. The Anticancer Drugs, 2nd ed. New York, Oxford University Press, 1994, pp 108–154.
146. Lind MJ, Ardiet C. Pharmacokinetics of alkylating agents. Cancer Surveys 1993;17:157–188.
147. Lejeune FJ, Lienard D, Leyvraz S, Mirimanoff RO. Regional therapy of melanoma. Eur J Cancer 1993;29A:606–612.
148. Sarosy G, Leyland-Jones B, Soochan P, et al. The systemic administration of intravenous melphalan. J Clin Oncol 1988;6:1768–1782.
149. Schoenike SE, Dana WJ. Ifosfamide and mesna. Clin Pharm 1990;9:179–191.
150. Stillwell TJ, Benson RC. Cyclophosphamide-induced hemorrhagic cystitis: A review of 100 patients. Cancer 1988;61: 451–457.
151. Miller LJ, Chandler SW, Ippoliti CM. Treatment of cyclophosphamide-induced hemorrhagic cystitis with prostaglandins. Ann Pharmacotherapy 1994;28:590–594.
152. Skinner R, Sharkey IM, Pearson ADJ, Craft AW. Ifosfamide, mesna, and nephrotoxicity in children. J Clin Oncol 1993;11:173–190.
153. Rossi R, Godde A, Kleinbrand A, et al. Unilateral nephrectomy and cisplatin as risk factors of ifosfamide-induced nephrotoxicity: Analysis of 120 patients. J Clin Oncol 1994;12:159–165.
154. Patterson WP, Reams GP. Renal toxicities of chemotherapy. Semin Oncol 1992;19:521–528.
155. Fields KK, Elfenbein GJ, Lazarus HM, et al. Maximum-tolerated doses of ifosfamide, carboplatin, and etoposide given over 6 days followed by autologous stem-cell rescue: Toxicity profile. J Clin Oncol 1995;13:323–332.
156. Buggia I, Locatelli F, Regazzi MB, Zecca M. Busulfan. Ann Pharmacotherapy 1994;28:1055–1062.
157. Averbuch SD. Dacarbazine, procarbazine, hexamethylmelamine, in Holland JF, Frei E III, Bast RC Jr, et al (eds): Cancer Medicine, 3rd ed. Philadelphia, Lea and Febiger, 1993, pp 755–764.
158. Tucker MA, Coleman CN, Cox RS, et al. Risk of second cancers after treatment for Hodgkin's disease. N Engl J Med 1988;318:76–81.
159. Foster BJ, Harding BJ, Leyland-Jones B, et al. Hexamethylmelamine: A critical review of an active drug. Cancer Treat Rev 1986;13:197–217.

160. Hansen LA, Hughes TE. Altretamine. DICP, Ann Pharmacother 1991;25:146–152.
161. Pratt WB, Ruddon RW, Ensminger WD, Maybaum J. The Anticancer Drugs, 2nd ed. New York, Oxford University Press, 1994, pp 155–182.
162. Myers C. Anthracyclines and DNA intercalators, in Holland JF, Frei E III, Bast RC Jr, et al (eds): Cancer Medicine, 3rd ed. Philadelphia, Lea and Febiger, 1993, pp 764–773.
163. Booser DJ, Hortobagyi GN. Anthracycline antibiotics in cancer therapy: Focus on drug resistance. Drugs 1994;47:223–258.
164. Robert J, Gianni L. Pharmacokinetics and metabolism of anthracyclines. Cancer Surveys 1993;17:219–252.
165. Robert J. Clinical pharmacokinetics of idarubicin. Clin Pharmacokinetics 1993;24:275–288.
166. Cersosimo RJ. Idarubicin: An anthracycline antineoplastic agent. Clin Pharm 1992;11:152–167.
167. Sandoval C, Pui CH, Bowman LC, et al. Secondary acute myeloid leukemia in children previously treated with alkylating agents, intercalating topoisomerase II inhibitors, and irradiation. J Clin Oncol 1993;11:1039–1045.
168. Hale JP, Lewis IJ. Anthracyclines: Cardiotoxicity and its prevention. Arch Dis Children 1994;71: 457–462.
169. Von Hoff DD, Layard MW, Basa P, et al. Risk factors for doxorubicin-induced congestive heart failure. Ann Intern Med 1979;91:710–717.
170. Basser RL, Green MD. Strategies for prevention of anthracycline cardiotoxicity. Cancer Treat Rev 1993;19:57–77.
171. Torti FM, Bristown MR, Howes AE. Reduced cardiotoxicity of doxorubicin delivered on a weekly schedule. Ann Intern Med 1983;99:745–749.
172. Legha SS, Benjamin RS, Mackay B. Reduction of doxorubicin cardiotoxicity by prolonged continuous intravenous infusion. Ann Intern Med 1982;96:133–139.
173. Seifert CF, Nesser ME, Thompson DF. Dexrazoxane in the prevention of doxorubicin-induced cariotoxicity. Ann Pharmacotherapy 1994;28:1063–1072.
174. Koeller J, Eble M. Mitoxantrone: A novel anthracycline derivative. Clin Pharm 1988;7:574–581.
175. Estorch M, Carrio I, Martinez-Duncker D, et al. Myocyte cell damage after administration of doxorubicin or mitoxantrone in breast cancer patients assessed by indium 111 antimyosin monoclonal antibody studies. J Clin Oncol 1993;11:1264–1268.
176. Feldman EJ, Alberts DS, Arlin Z, et al. Phase I clinical and pharmacokinetic evaluation of high-dose mitoxantrone in combination with cytarabine in patients with acute leukemia. J Clin Oncol 1993;11:2002–2009.
177. Verweij J, den Hartigh J, Pinedo HM. Antitumor antibiotics, in Chabner BA, Collins JM (eds): Cancer Chemotherapy: Principles and Practice. Philadelphia, JB Lippincott, 1990, pp 382–396.
178. Doll DC, Weiss RB, Issell BF. Mitomycin: Ten years after approval for marketing. J Clin Oncol 1985;3:276–286.
179. Dorr RT. New findings in the pharmacokinetics, metabolic, and drug-resistance aspects of mitomycin c. Semin Oncol 1988;15(suppl 4):32–41.
180. Farmer DG, Rosove MH, Shaked A, Busuttil RW. Current treatment modalities for hepatocellular carcinoma. Ann Surg 1994;219:236–247.
181. Dorr RT. Pharmacologic management of vesicant chemotherapy extravasations, in Dorr RT, Von Hoff DD. Cancer Chemotherapy Handbook, 2nd ed. Norwalk, CT: Appleton and Lange, 1994, pp 109–118.
182. Yuang-Chi A, Kuebler JP, Pandya KJ, et al. Pulmonary toxicity induced by mitomycin c is highly responsive to glucocorticoids. Cancer 1986;57:2285–2290.
183. Lesesne JB, Rothschild N, Erickson B, et al. Cancer-associated hemolytic-uremic syndrome: Analysis of 85 cases from a national registry. J Clin Oncol 1989;7:781–789.
184. Andrews CO, Gora ML. Pleural effusions: Pathophysiology and management. Ann Pharmacotherapy 1994;28:894–902.
185. Dorr RT. Bleomycin pharmacology: Mechanism of action and resistance, and clinical pharmacokinetics. Semin Oncol 1992;19(2, suppl 5):3–8.
186. Chabner BA. Bleomycin, in Chabner BA, Collins JM (eds): Cancer Chemotherapy: Principles and Practice. Philadelphia, JB Lippincott, 1990, pp 341–355.
187. Ostrowski MJ. Intracavitary therapy with bleomycin for the treatment of malignant pleural effusions. J Surg Oncol Suppl 1989;1:7–13.
188. Van Barneveld PWC, Sleijer D TH, Van Der Mark THW, et al. Natural course of bleomycin-induced pneumonitis: A follow-up study. Am Rev Respir Dis 1987;135:48–51.
189. Reed E, Kohn KW. Platinum analogues, in Chabner BA, Collins JM (eds): Cancer Chemotherapy: Principles and Practice. Philadelphia, JB Lippincott, 1990, pp 465–490.
190. Loehrer PJ, Einhorn LH. Cisplatin. Ann Intern Med 1984;100:704–713.
191. Colvin M. Alkylating agents and platinum antitumor compounds, in Holland JF, Frei E III, Bast RC Jr, et al (eds): Cancer Medicine, 3rd ed. Philadelphia, Lea and Febiger, 1993, pp 733–754.
192. Calvert H, Judson I, Van Der Vijgh WJF. Platinum complexes in cancer medicine: Pharmacokinetics and pharmacodynamics in relation to toxicity and therapeutic activity. Cancer Surveys 1993;17:189–218.
193. Desoize B, Dumont P, Manot L, et al. Comparison of two dose prediction models for cisplatin. Anticancer Res 1994;14:2285–2290.
194. Howell SB, Pfeifle CL, Wung WE, et al. Intraperitoneal cisplatin with systemic thiosulfate protection. Ann Intern Med 1982;97:845–851.
195. Goel R, Cleary SM, Horton C, et al. Effect of sodium thiosulfate on the pharmacokinetics and toxicity of cisplatin. J Natl Cancer Inst 1989;81:1552–1560.
196. Pinzani V, Bressolle F, Haug IJ, et al. Cisplatin-induced renal toxicity and toxicity-modulating strategies: A review. Cancer Chemother Pharmacol 1994;35:1–9.
197. Anand AJ, Bashey B. Newer insights into cisplatin nephrotoxicity. Ann Pharmacotherapy 1993;27:1519–1525.
198. Thyss A, Saudes L, Otto J, et al. Renal tolerance of cisplatin in patients more than 80 years old. J Clin Oncol 1994;12:2121–2125.
199. Ozols RF, Corden BJ, Jacob J, et al. High-dose cisplatin in hypertonic saline. Ann Intern Med 1984;100:19–24.
200. Capizzi RL. Protection of normal tissues from the cytotoxic effects of chemotherapy by amifostine (ethyol): Clinical experience. Semin Oncol 1994;21(suppl 11):8–15.

201. Gandara DR, Nahhas WA, Adelson MD, et al. Randomized placebo-controlled multicenter evaluation of diethyldithiocarbamate for chemoprotection against cisplatin-induced toxicities. J Clin Oncol 1995;13:490–496.
202. Grunberg SM, Hesketh PJ. Control of chemotherapy-induced emesis. N Engl J Med 1993;329:1790–1796.
203. Kobayashi H, Ohashi N, Watanabe Y, et al. Clinical features of cisplatin vestibulotoxicity and hearing loss. Otolaryngology 1987;49:67–72.
204. Meyer WH, Ayers D, HcHaney VA, Roberson P, Pratt CB. Ifosfamide and exacerbation of cisplatin-induced hearing loss [letter]. Lancet 1993;341:754–755.
205. Gregg RW, Molepo JM, Monpetit VJA, et al. Cisplatin neurotoxicity: The relationship between dosage, time, and platinum concentration in neurologic tissues, and morphologic evidence of toxicity. J Clin Oncol 1992;10:795–803.
206. Gerritsen van der Hoop R, Vecht CJ, van der Burg MEL, et al. Prevention of cisplatin neurotoxicity with and ACTH (4-9) analogue in patients with ovarian cancer. N Engl J Med 1990;322:89–94.
207. Gietema JA, Sleijfer DT, Willemse PHB, et al. Long-term follow-up of cardiovascular risk factors in patients given chemotherapy for disseminated nonseminomatous testicular cancer. Ann Intern Med 1992;116:709–715.
208. Cascinu S, Fedeli A, DelFerro E, et al. Recombinant human erythropoietin treatment in cisplatin-associated anemia: a randomized, double-blind trial with placebo. J Clin Oncol 1994;12:1058–1062.
209. Cersosimo RJ. Hepatotoxicity associated with cisplatin chemotherapy. Ann Pharmacotherapy 1993;27:438–441.
210. Woloschuk DMM, Pruemer JM, Cluxton RJ Jr. Carboplatin: A new cisplatin analog. DICP, Ann Pharmacother 1988;22:843–849.
211. Van Echo DA, Egorin MJ, Aisner J. The pharmacology of carboplatin. Semin Oncol 1989;16(suppl 5):1–6.
212. Egorin MJ, Van Echo DA, Olman EA, et al. Prospective validation of a pharmacologically based dosing schema for *cis*-diamminedichlorplatinum (II) analogue diamminecyclobutanedicarboxylato-platinum. Cancer Res 1985;45:6502–6506.
213. Calvert AH. Dose optimisation of carboplatin in adults. Anticancer Res 1994;14:2273–2278.
214. Newell DR, Pearson ADJ, Balmanno K, et al. Carboplatin pharmacokinetics in children: The development of a pediatric dosing formula. J Clin Oncol 1993;11:2314–2323.
215. Weidmann B, Mulleneisen N, Bojko P, Niederle N. Hypersensitivity reactions to carboplatin. Cancer 1994;73:2218–2222.
216. Chang SM, Fryberger S, Crouse V, et al. Carboplatin hypersensitivity in children. Cancer 1995;75:1171–1175.
217. Donehower RC. Hydroxyurea, in Chabner BA, Collins JM (eds): Cancer Chemotherapy: Principles and Practice. Philadelphia, JB Lippincott, 1990, pp 225–233.
218. Vaughan WP, Kris E, Vose J, et al. Phase I/II study incorporating intravenous hydroxyurea into high-dose chemotherapy for patients with primary refractory or relapsed and refractory intermediate-grade and high-grade malignant lymphoma. J Clin Oncol 1995;13:1089–1095.
219. Charache S, Terrin ML, Moore RD, et al. Effect of hydroxyurea on the frequency of painful crises in sickle cell anemia. N Engl J Med 1995;332:1317–1322.
220. Chabner BA. Enzyme therapy: L-asparaginase, in Chabner BA, Collins JM (eds): Cancer Chemotherapy: Principles and Practice. Philadelphia, JB Lippincott, 1990, pp 397–407.
221. Capizzi RL, Holcenberg JS. Asparaginase, in Holland JF, Frei E III, Bast RC Jr, et al (eds): Cancer Medicine, 3rd ed. Philadelphia, Lea and Febiger, 1993, pp 796–805.
222. Asselin BL, Whitin JC, Coppola DJ, et al. Comparative pharmacokinetic studies of three asparaginase preparations. J Clin Oncol 1993;11:1780–1786.
223. Ettinger LJ, Kurtzberg J, Woute PA, et al. An open-label, multicenter study of polyethylene glycol-L-asparaginase for the treatment of acute lymphoblastic leukemia. Cancer 1995;75:1176–1181.
224. Smith MA, Parkinson DR, Cheson BD, Friedman MA. Retinoids in cancer therapy. J Clin Oncol 1992;10:839–864.
225. Warrell RP Jr, de The H, Wang AY, Degos L. Acute promyelocytic leukemia. N Engl J Med 1993;329:177–189.
226. Frankel SR, Eardley A, Heller G, et al. All-trans retinoic acid for acute promyelocytic leukemia. Ann Intern Med 1994;120:278–286.
227. Pratt WB, Ruddon RW, Ensminger WD, Maybaum J. The Anticancer Drugs, 2nd ed. New York, Oxford University Press, 1994, pp 199–231.
228. Swain SM, Lippman ME. Endocrine therapies of cancer, in Chabner BA, Collins JM (eds): Cancer Chemotherapy: Principles and Practice. Philadelphia, JB Lippincott, 1990, pp 59–109.
229. McClay EF, McClay MET. Tamoxifen: Is it useful in the treatment of patients with metastatic melanoma? J Clin Oncol 1994;12:617–626.
230. Cidlowski JA, Schwartzman RA. Corticosteroids, in Holland JF, Frei E III, Bast RC Jr, et al (eds): Cancer Medicine, 3rd ed. Philadelphia, Lea and Febiger, 1993, pp 845–857.
231. Balmer CM. Clinical use of biologic response modifiers in cancer treatment: An overview. Part I: The interferons. DICP, Ann Pharmacotherapy 1990;24:761–767.
232. Pratt WB, Ruddon RW, Ensminger WD, Maybaum J. The Anticancer Drugs, 2nd ed. New York, Oxford University Press, 1994, pp 285–305.
233. Dorr RT. Interferon-alpha in malignant and viral diseases: A review. Drugs 1993;45:177–211.
234. The Italian Cooperative Study Group on Chronic Myeloid Leukemia. Interferon alfa-2a as compared with conventional chemotherapy for the treatment of chronic myeloid leukemia. N Engl J Med 1994;330:820–825.
235. Mutch RS, Hutson PR. Levamisole in the adjuvant treatment of colon cancer. Clin Pharm 1991;10:95–109.
236. Janik J, Kopp WC, Smith JW II, et al. Dose-related immunologic effects of levamisole in patients with cancer. J Clin Oncol 1993;11:125–135.
237. Moertel CG, Fleming TR, Macdonald JS, et al. Fluorouracil plus levamisole as effective adjuvant therapy after resection of stage III colon carcinoma: A final report. Ann Intern Med 1995;122:321–326.
238. Herr HW, Schwalb DM, Zhang Z-F, et al. Intravesical Bacillus Calmette-Guérin therapy prevents tumor progression and death from superficial bladder cancer: Ten-year follow-up of a prospective randomized trial. J Clin Oncol 1995;13:1404–1408.

239. Sarosdy MF. Principles of intravesical chemotherapy and immunotherapy. Urol Clin North Amer 1992;19:509–519.
240. Lamm DL, Stogdill VD, Stogdill BJ, et al. Complications of bacillus Calmette-Guérin immunotherapy in 1278 patients with bladder cancer. J Urol 1986;135:272–274.
241. Rawls WH, Lamm DL, Lowe BA, et al. Fatal sepsis following intravesical bacillus Calmette-Guérin administration for bladder cancer. J Urol 1990;144:1328–1330.
242. Brosman SA, Lamm DL. The preparation, handling, and use of intravesical bacillus Calmette-Guérin for the management of stage T_a, T_1, carcinoma *in situ* and transitional cell cancer. J Urol 1990;144:313–315.
243. Bruton JK, Koeller JM. Recombinant interleukin-2. Pharmacotherapy 1994;14:635–656.
244. Whittington R, Faulds D. Interleukin-2: A review of its pharmacological properties and therapeutic use in patients with cancer. Drugs 1993;46:446–514.
245. Rosenberg SA, Lotze MT, Muul LM, et al. Observations on the systemic administration of autologous lymphokine-activated killer cells and recombinant interleukin-2 to patients with metastatic cancer. N Engl J Med 1985;313:1485–1492.
246. Konrad MW, Hemstreet G, Hersh EM. Pharmacokinetics of recombinant IL-2 in humans. Cancer Res 1990;50:2009–2017.
247. Foa R. Does interleukin-2 have a role in the management of acute leukemia? J Clin Oncol 1993;11:1817–1825.
248. Lee RE, Lotze MT, Skibber JM, et al. Cardiorespiratory effects of immunotherapy with interleukin-2. J Clin Oncol 1989;7:7–20.
249. Guleria AS, Yang JC, Topalian SL, et al. Renal dysfunction associated with the administration of high-dose interleukin-2 in 199 consecutive patients with metastatic melanoma or renal carcinoma. J Clin Oncol 1994;12:2714–2722.
250. Pockaj BA, Topalian SL, Steinbeg SM, et al. Infectious complications associated with interleukin-2 administration: A retrospective review of 935 treatment courses. J Clin Oncol 1993;11:136–147.
251. Vetto JT, Papa MZ, Lotze MT, et al. Reduction of toxicity of interleukin-2 and lymphokine-activated killer cells in humans by the administration of corticosteroids. J Clin Oncol 1987;5:496–503.
252. Chabner BA. Anticancer drugs, in Devita VT Jr, Hellman S, Rosenberg SA (eds): Cancer: Principles and Practice of Oncology, 4th ed. Philadelphia, JB Lippincott, 1993, pp 325–417.
253. Lee JW, Pizzo PA. Management of the cancer patient with fever and prolonged neutropenia. Hematol/Oncol Clin North Am 1993;7:937–960.
254. Rubin M, Hathorn JW, Pizzo PA. Controversies in the management of febrile neutropenic cancer patients. Cancer Investigations. 1988;6:167–184.
255. Hughes WT, Armstrong D, Bodey GP, et al. Guidelines for the use of antimicrobial agents in neutropenic patients with unexplained fever. J Infect Dis 1990;161:381–396.
256. Buchanan GR. Approach to the treatment of the febrile cancer patient with low-risk neutropenia. Hematol/Oncol Clin North Am 1993;7:919–936
257. Pizzo PA. Considerations for the prevention of infectious complications in patients with cancer. Rev Infect Dis 1989;11(suppl 7):S1551–S1563.
258. Wallerstein R, Jr, Deisseroth A. Hematopoietic growth factors in cancer treatment. Principles Practice Oncol Updates 1990;9:1–16.
259. Demetri GD. Hematopoietic growth factors: Current knowledge, future prospects. Curr Prob Cancer 1992;16:179–259.
260. Groopman JE, Molina JM, Scadden DT: Hematopoietic growth factors: Biology and clinical applications. N Engl J Med 1989;321:1449–1459.
261. Gabrilove JL. Introduction and overview of hematopoietic growth factors. Sem Hematol 1989;26(suppl 2):1–4.
262. Lieschke GJ, Burgess AW. Granulocyte colony-stimulating factor and granulocyte-macrophage colony-stimulating factor. N Engl J Med 1992;327:28–35, 99–106.
263. Harmenberg J, Hoglund M, Hellstrom-Lindberg E. G- and GM-CSF in oncology and oncological haematology. Eur J Haematol 1994;52:1–28.
264. ASCO Ad Hoc Colony-Stimulating Factor Guideline Expert Panel. American Society of Clinical Oncology recommendations for the use of hematopoietic colony-stimulating factors: Evidence-based, clinical practice guidelines. J Clin Oncol 1994;12:2471–2508.
265. Vose JM, Armitage JO. Clinical applications of hematopoietic growth factors. J Clin Oncol 1995;13:1023–1035.
266. Aurer I, Ribas A, Gale RP. What is the role of recombinant colony stimulating factors in bone marrow transplantation? Bone Marrow Transplantation 1990;6:79–87.
267. Gordon MS, Hoffman R. Growth factors affecting human thrombopoiesis: Potential agents for the treatment of thrombocytopenia. Blood 1992;80:302–307.
268. Metcalf D. TPO: At last. Nature 1994;369:519–520.
269. Oster W, Herrmann F, Gamm H, et al. Erythropoeitin for the treatment of anemia of malignancy associated with neoplastic bone marrow infiltration. J Clin Oncol 1990;8:956–962.
270. Henry DH, Abels RI. Recombinant human erythropoietin in the treatment of cancer and chemotherapy-induced anemia: Results of double-blind and open label follow-up studies. Sem Oncol 1994;21:21–28.
271. Stonis ST. Oral complications of cancer therapy, in Devita VT Jr, Hellman S, Rosenberg SA (eds): Cancer: Principles and Practice of Oncology, 4th ed. Philadelphia, JB Lippincott, 1993, pp 2385–2394.
272. National Institutes of Health Consensus Development Conference Statement. Oral complications of cancer therapies: Diagnosis, prevention, and treatment. US Department of Health and Human Services, April 17–19, 1989.
273. Mahood DJ, Dose AM, Loprinzi CL, et al. Inhibition of fluorouracil-induced stomatitis by oral cryotherapy. J Clin Oncol 1991;9:449–452.
274. Sonis S, Clark J. Prevention and management of oral mucositis induced by antineoplastic therapy. Oncology 1991;5:11–18.
275. Seipp CA. Hair loss, in Devita VT Jr, Hellman S, Rosenberg SA (eds): Cancer: Principles and Practice of Oncology, 4th ed. Philadelphia, JB Lippincott, 1993, pp 2394–2395.
276. Cancer chemotherapy guidelines: Recommendations for the management of vesicant extravasation, hypersensitivity, and anaphylaxis. Oncology Nursing Society 1992.
277. Myers SE, Schilsky RL. Prospects for fertility after cancer chemotherapy. Sem Oncol 1992;19:597–604.

278. Tucker MA. Secondary cancers, in Devita VT Jr, Hellman S, Rosenberg SA (eds): Cancer: Principles and Practice of Oncology, 4th ed. Philadelphia, JB Lippincott, 1993, pp 2407–2416.
279. ASHP technical assistance bulletin on handling cytotoxic and hazardous drugs. Am J Hosp Pharm 1990;47:1033–1049.
280. Weinhouse S, Bal DG, Adamson R, The Work Study Group on Diet, Nutrition, and Cancer. American Cancer Society guidelines on diet, nutrition, and cancer. American Cancer Society 1991;41:334–338.
281. Greenwald P, Lanza E, Eddy GA. Dietary fiber in the reduction of colon cancer risk. J Am Dietetic Assoc 1987;87(9):1178–1188.
282. Lippman SM, Benner SE, Hong WK, et al. Cancer chemoprevention. J Clin Oncol 1994;12:851–873.
283. Boring CC, Squires TS, Tong T, et al. Mortality trends for detected smoking-related cancers and breast cancer—United States, 1950–1990. MMWR 1993;42:857–866.
284. Blum A. Curtailing the tobacco pandemic, in Devita VT Jr, Hellman S, Rosenberg SA (eds): Cancer: Principles and Practice of Oncology, 4th ed. Philadelphia, JB Lippincott, 1993, pp 480–491.
285. Balch CM, Houghton A, Peters LJ. Cutaneous melanoma, in Devita VT Jr, Hellman S, Rosenberg SA (eds): Cancer: Principles and Practice of Oncology, 4th ed. Philadelphia, JB Lippincott, 1993, pp 1612–1661.

Chapter 120

Breast Cancer

Celeste Lindley, PharmD, MS, FCCP, FASHP

Incidence and Mortality Trends

Breast cancer is the most common cancer site and second only to lung cancer as a cause of cancer death in women. Estimates were that 182,000 new cases of breast cancer would be diagnosed and that 46,000 women would die of breast cancer in 1994. These projections are based on the Surveillance, Epidemiology, and End Results (SEER) program of the National Cancer Institute. Since 1973, the SEER program has collected cancer incidence, mortality, and survival data each year for residents in nine metropolitan areas (or entire states), comprising about 10% of all the cancers diagnosed in the United States.[1]

A great deal of public and health professional concern currently surrounds the increasing incidence of breast cancer. The Connecticut Tumor Registry demonstrated a 1% per year increase in breast cancer incidence between 1940 and 1980. SEER program estimates also show an increase of about 1% per year from 1973 to 1980. In 1980, the breast cancer incidence rate started to rise more sharply. Between 1980 and 1987, cancer incidence rate grew from 84.4 per 100,000 to 112.4 per 100,000. This represents an increase of 32.5% according to SEER data or more than 4% per year. After reaching a peak in 1987, breast cancer incidence rates in the subsequent 3 years leveled off (Fig. 120.1).[2]

The increase in breast cancer incidence in the 1980s is characterized by an increase in the detection of small sized lesions, and carcinoma *in situ.*[3] As shown in Fig. 120.2, the incidence rate for invasive cancers smaller than 1 centimeter grew from 9 per 100,000 in 1982 to 36 per 100,000 in 1988, and to 35 per 100,000 in 1989. The number of cancers 1–1.9 centimeters detected increased from 40 per 100,000 in 1982 to 84 per 100,000 in 1988, and then dropped to 80 in 1989. On the other hand, the rate of detection for tumors 2–2.9 centimeters remained about the same from 1982–1989, while the number of large cancers found at diagnosis (i.e., those of 3 centimeters) decreased. Although not reflected in the SEER data, the rate of detection of carcinoma *in situ* increased greatly from 4 per 100,000 in 1973 to a high of 15 per 100,000 in 1987.

Increased public awareness and increased use of screening mammography are largely responsible for increased detection of breast cancers in the small or localized stage. The cause of the increased incidence of breast cancer observed during the 1980s is subject to continued debate. The increase in breast cancer incidence coincides with an increased use of mammography in asymptomatic women in the 1980s. As the increase in mammography usage levels off in the late 1980s and early 1990s, indications are that the incidence rate also may fall to about the levels seen in the early 1980s. However, the long-term trend prior to the 1980s was for a 1% annual increase in breast cancer. It is possible that changes in risk factors may be at least partially responsible for the increased incidence seen not only during the 1980s, but during the past four decades.

It is well recognized that breast cancer in the early stages is potentially curable in the majority of patients and that metastatic breast cancer is usually incurable. Thus, increased detection of localized and small breast cancer seen in the 1980s should have an impact on mortality rate from breast cancer. The number of cases of breast cancer and deaths from breast cancer have both risen sharply in the decades from 1970–1990. Cases have increased by 117%, whereas deaths have increased by nearly 50%. These increases are due partly to a change in the demographics of the population of American women that include an increase in the number of women alive, an increase in the average length of life, and an increase in the absolute number of older women. Age adjustment (to the base year 1970) is designed to remove the effects of a shift in the age distribution of the population and allows one to focus on changes other than those due solely to changing demographics. With age adjustment, the incidence of breast cancer has increased by 21%, whereas the mortality rate has been essentially flat, increasing only 3%. Of note, mortality, since 1973, has declined by 11% for women younger than 50, and increased by 6% for women ages 50 and over for the overall yield of a 3% increase in mortality. The decline in mortality for women less than 50 years of age has been attributed to the use of adjuvant systemic therapy following primary local-regional therapy.

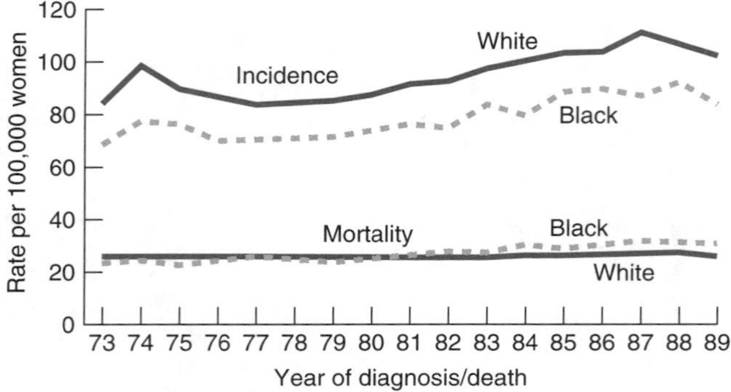

Figure 120.1. Breast cancer incidence and mortality rates by race, SEER, 1973–1989.

The numbers presented thus far have shown the risk of breast cancer for all races combined. There are differences in incidence and mortality breast cancer among ethnic groups in the United States. Young women, less than 50 years of age, have approximately the same incidence rates regardless of race, but black women in this same age group have much higher mortality rates. White women, older than 50 years have a considerably increased risk of developing cancer (approximately 20%), whereas mortality rates for white and black women are nearly equal.[4] These figures are consistent with earlier detection in whites leading to higher survival and a corresponding lower mortality.

Epidemiology and Etiology

The two variables most strongly associated with the occurrence of breast cancer are gender and age. Although one commonly thinks of breast cancer as a disease confined to women, approximately 1000 cases of male breast cancer were projected to be diagnosed in the United States in 1994. Although male gender had been considered a poor prognostic factor in some investigations, it is now believed that higher mortality rates in men are attributable to more advanced disease at the time of diagnosis. When stage and other known prognostic factors are controlled for, men do not fare differently from their female counterparts. Similarly, treatment of male breast cancer is not different from treatment of breast cancer in females.

The incidence of breast cancer increases with advancing age. Perhaps the most frequently quoted breast cancer statistic is that 1 in 8 women will develop breast cancer during their lifetime. If risk of developing breast cancer is truncated at age 85, the risk is 1 in 9. It should be emphasized that this is a cumulative lifetime risk of developing the disease. The risk of developing cancer from birth based on SEER data from 1987 and 1988 is shown in Table 120.1.[5] It is apparent from this table that although the cumulative probability of developing breast cancer increases with increasing age, the greatest probability of developing the disease occurs in women 50–60 years of age.

Aside from female gender and age, a number of additional risk factors have been identified. Complex experimental and epidemiologic evidence points to an association between breast cancer and endocrine factors, environment, and genetics. Although the exact nature of the association is unclear, the majority of factors recognized as increasing a woman's risk above the average are related to one or more of these influences. The strength of the association between a given risk factor and the development of breast cancer is indicated by a "relative risk ratio" or "odds ratio." These are derived from epidemiological studies, which can be described as case control or cohort studies where the incidence of disease among persons possessing a characteristic in question is divided by the incidence of disease among otherwise similar persons without the characteristic. Computation of "relative risk ratios" through epidemiological research is complex and inexact. This area of research is hindered by many fundamental methodologic problems such as selection bias, recall bias, incomplete data, and, most impor-

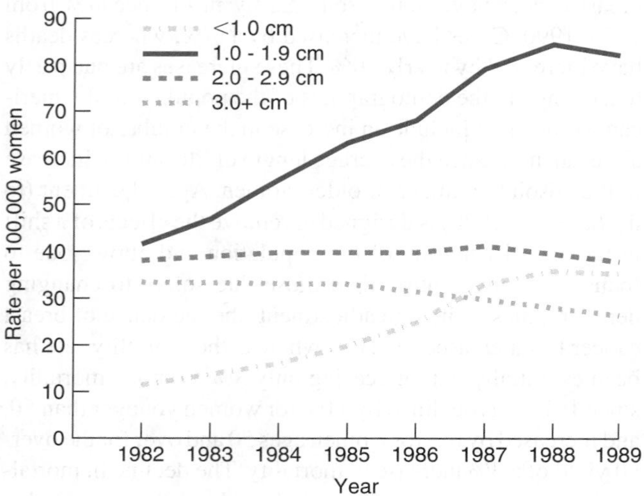

Figure 120.2. Breast cancer incidence rates by size at diagnosis, SEER, 1982–1989.

TABLE 120.1. RISK OF DEVELOPING BREAST CANCER IN SEER AREAS, WOMEN, ALL RACES 1987–1988

Age Interval	Probability (%) of Developing Invasive Breast Cancer During the Interval		
Before 40	0.46	or	1 in 217
40–50	1.58	or	1 in 63
50–60	2.41	or	1 in 41
60–70	3.59	or	1 in 28
70–80	4.13	or	1 in 24
70–death	7.08	or	1 in 14
From birth–death	12.57	or	1 in 8

(Data from Fuer EJ, Wun LM, Boring CC, Flanders WD, Timmel MJ, Tong T. The lifetime risk of developing breast cancer. J Natl Cancer Inst 1993;85:892–897.)

tant, the presence of confounding factors. A large number of case control and cohort studies that examine the relationship between certain factors and risk of developing breast cancer have been conducted and often have yielded conflicting results. However, it is important to review established and probable risk factors for cancer and to continue to conduct research in this area. Through these efforts, the etiology of breast cancer can be further elucidated, women who would benefit from intensified surveillance or prophylactic treatment may be identified, and recommendations for modifiable risk factors that will ultimately reduce the incidence of breast cancer can be established.

An understanding of the relationship between age and the incidence of breast cancer is particularly relevant when one discusses "risk factors" or factors other than age that increase a woman's probability of developing breast cancer. The "relative risk" of developing breast cancer for an individual woman in a defined risk group is usually multiplied by the probability of any woman developing breast cancer during a lifetime, and this figure is taken as the cumulative lifetime risk of that individual developing breast cancer. However, the risk of developing breast cancer is age dependent.[6] Thus, a more meaningful way to counsel patients regarding their risk of developing breast cancer based on the presence of a known risk factor incorporates an age-specific incidence rate, not cumulative lifetime risk. For example, if a 40-year-old woman with a strong family history of breast cancer is thought to have a "relative risk ratio" of 2.0, her risk of developing breast cancer by the age of 50 is only 3.17% (2 × 1.58) not 25.14% (2 × 12.57). It is also important to note that recognized risk factors are not "additive" in a simple mathematical sense and that the observed cumulative lifetime risk has rarely exceeded 30% (1 in 3) in any study regardless of the number and significance of individual risk factors.[6]

ENDOCRINE FACTORS

A number of endocrine factors have been linked to the incidence of breast cancer.[6,7] Many of these relate to the total duration of menstrual life. Early menarche, generally defined as menstruation beginning before age 12, has been shown by a number of investigators to increase the cumulative lifetime risk of breast cancer development compared to menarche at age 16 or greater. Conversely, early age of natural menarche has been shown to result in a reduction of risk. Similarly, investigators have reported that bilateral oophorectomy prior to age 35 reduces the relative risk of developing breast cancer.

Nulliparity and a late age at first birth (greater or equal to 30 years) have been reported to increase the lifetime risk of developing breast cancer twofold. Women who have their first child after the age of 35 have a slightly higher risk than a nulliparous woman. It has been suggested that the period between the onset of menses and the age of first pregnancy provides a "window of initiation" for the development of breast cancer. This is a time when an unbalanced hormonal environment reacts with the abundant and highly responsive breast tissue. Investigators have postulated that international differences in age of menarche, age at menopause, and childbearing may account for a substantial part of the international differences in the incidence of breast cancer. In underdeveloped countries where the incidence of breast cancer is low compared to the United States, a late onset of menarche is the rule and frequently there is a decreased interval between puberty and first pregnancy followed by several pregnancies and early menopause.

A large number of investigators have evaluated the relationship between exogenous hormones and development of breast cancer. Postmenopausal estrogen replacement therapy has been the subject of several recent meta-analyses. A report from investigators from the Harvard School of Public Health concluded that women who have used estrogens in the past are not at an increased risk of breast cancer, but that current use may be associated with a 40% increased risk (i.e., RR = 1.4). This meta-analysis also suggested that long-term use might lead to a slight increase in risk.[8] Another meta-analysis has suggested that the combined results from multiple studies provide evidence that menopausal therapy (consisting of 0.625 mg or less of conjugated estrogen per day) does not increase breast cancer risk.[9] A report from the Centers for Disease Control and Prevention evaluating that proportional increase in risk of breast cancer for each year of estrogen use reported that the risk did not appear to increase until after at least 5 years of estrogen use.[10] These data are encouraging and suggest that a large effect of hormone therapy on breast cancer risk may be excluded and that the use of low doses of estrogen for short periods as replacement therapy in postmenopausal women is relatively safe. The National Institutes of Health recently began a prospective randomized trial of estrogen replacement therapy to more definitively address this important question.

The use of postmenopausal estrogen replacement therapy in women with a history of breast cancer is generally considered contraindicated. Because of the association of estrogen and risk of breast cancer, many physicians believe that patients with a strong family history of breast cancer should not receive postmenopausal estrogen replacement therapy. This dogma has recently been challenged in the medical literature.[11] Proponents of estrogen replacement therapy in patients with successfully treated operable breast cancer often state that the benefits of replacement therapy in terms of cardiovascular health and reduction of morbidity and mortality from osteoporosis and subsequent fractures outweigh an unknown but potential increased risk of breast cancer development. At the current time, there is not enough information to state confidently that estrogen replacement therapy has any significant impact, positive or negative, on prognosis in women with a personal or family history of breast cancer.

There are more than 20 epidemiologic studies of the potential carcinogenic effect of oral contraceptives and most of these studies have shown no relationship between birth control pills and breast cancer incidence. However, results are conflicting and assessment of the studies necessitates consideration of the particular oral contraceptive products involved, daily and cumulative doses of the hormones administered, and the latency for development of breast cancer. A review and meta-analyses suggest that, overall, there has been no increase in the risk of breast cancer for women who had ever received oral contraceptive drugs; however, women who had used these agents for a prolonged period of time or prior to a first pregnancy were at a higher risk of developing breast cancer.[12] It should be pointed out that early use of oral contraceptives may be associated with early menarche and result in late age of first birth, both of which are recognized risk factors for breast cancer. However, other investigators have also suggested that use of oral contraceptives in young women is associated with an increased risk of developing breast cancer. Although it is not entirely possible to rule out a promotional effect of oral contraceptives in young patients, most experts believe that the safety and benefits of low-dose oral contraceptives currently outweigh the potential risks and that changes in the prescribing practice for the use of oral contraceptives are not warranted.

GENETICS

Both personal and family history influence a woman's risk of developing breast cancer. A past medical history for breast cancer is associated with the relative risk of 5.0 for the development of a contralateral breast cancer. Cancer of the uterus and ovary have also been associated with an increased risk of the development of breast cancer. Breast cancer is observed as part of cancer family syndromes in association with other tumors. Only 5% of breast cancer patients are thought to have a pedigree consistent with hereditary breast cancer.

A topic that bears some discussion due to its prevalence in the general population is the relationship of fibrocystic breast disease to the development of invasive breast cancer. As many as 85% of American women have "lumpy breasts" and may bear a clinical diagnosis of fibrocystic breast disease or benign breast disease. The risk of breast cancer in patients with a history of fibrocystic breast disease has ranged from 1.5 to 2.0 in reported studies. However, fibrocystic disease involves a heterogeneous group of pathologic changes associated with various degrees of breast cancer risk. Thus, a clinical diagnosis of fibrocystic or benign breast disease has little practical significance for counseling patients regarding individual risk of breast cancer. A useful system for classifying benign breast disease was recently adapted by the American College of Pathologists.[13] Benign breast conditions are classified as nonproliferative or proliferative and on the basis of review of more than 10,000 breast biopsies, relative risks of breast cancer were determined. Women with proliferative disease were found to have a relative risk of 1.9 and the subcategory of women with atypical hyperplasia was found to have a relative risk of 4.4. Nonproliferative breast disease was associated with no excess risk of breast cancer. Approximately 78% of the reviewed biopsies were found to have nonproliferative breast disease, and of those demonstrating proliferation, only 3.6% were "atypical." This suggests that benign breast disease or fibrocystic disease is most often not associated with proliferation and that the majority of women with this condition are not at increased risk for developing breast cancer. However, it must be noted that "lumpy breasts" may lead to a delay in diagnosis of breast cancer due to the inability of the patient or physician to detect a true malignant lesion.[13]

It has been recognized for some time that a family history of breast cancer is associated rather strongly with the woman's own risk for developing the disease. Empirical estimates of the risks associated with particular patterns of family history of breast cancer indicate the following[14]:

1. Having any first-degree relative with breast cancer increases a woman's risk of breast cancer 1.5- to 3-fold, depending on age.
2. The higher relative risk is associated with breast cancer with onset younger than age 45 in one or more first-degree relatives.
3. Having multiple first-degree relatives affected has been inconsistently associated with elevated risks.
4. Having a second-degree relative affected increases a woman's risk of developing breast cancer by approximately 50% (relative risk 1.5).
5. Affected family members on the maternal side and the paternal side contribute similarly to the risk.

The relative risk ratios given in Table 120.2 indicate that although certain patterns of family history are associated with substantial elevations in the risk of breast cancer, these high-risk patterns occur only infrequently in the general population. The percentage of all breast cancers in the population that can be attributed to family history range between 6% and 12%. Thus, it appears that for a sizable minority of the breast cancer that occurs in the population, some sort of genetically transmitted susceptibility contributes to their etiology.

Pedigree analysis of population-based data on familial patterns provides evidence for a rare autosomal dominant

TABLE 120.2. ESTABLISHED AND PROBABLE RISK FACTORS FOR BREAST CANCER

Risk Factor	Comparison Category	Risk Category	Typical Relative Risk
Family history of breast cancer	No first-degree relatives affected	Mother affected before the age of 60	2.0
		Mother affected after the age of 60	1.4
		Two first-degree relatives affected	4–6
		Breast cancer in one or more second-degree relatives	1.36
		Breast cancer in two or more second-degree relatives	1.49
		Ovarian cancer in one or more first-degree relatives	1.59
Age at menarche	16 year	11 yr	1.3
Age at birth of first child	Before 20 yr	20–24 yr	1.3
		25–29 yr	1.6
		≥30 yr	1.9
Age at menopause	45–54 yr	After 55 yr	1.5
		Before 45 yr	0.7
		Oophrectomy before 35 yr	0.4
Benign breast disease	No biopsy or aspiration	Any benign disease	1.5
		Proliferation only	2.0
		Atypical hyperplasia	4.0
		Lobular carcinoma *in situ*	7.2
Obesity	10th percentile	90th percentile;	
		Age, 30–49 yr	0.8
		Age, ≥50 yr	1.2
Oral contraceptive use	Never used	Ever use	1.0
		≥4 yr before first pregnancy	1.7
Postmenopausal estrogen replacement	Never used	Current use all ages	1.4
		15+ years	1.3
		Past use	1.0
Alcohol use	Nondrinker	1 drink/day	1.10
		2 drinks/day	1.25
		3 drinks/day	1.50

(Adapted from Harris JR, Lippman ME, Veronesi U, Willett W. Breast cancer. Part 1. N Engl J Med 327(5):319–328, with permission.)

allele that increases a carrier's susceptibility to breast cancer. Carriers of this breast cancer susceptibility gene develop breast cancer at an early age. Ovarian cancer has been shown to be associated with breast cancer in families, and genetic linkage has provided strong evidence for a breast–ovarian cancer gene located on chromosome 17q 12-21 (BRCA1). Isolation of the BRCA1 gene was initially reported in 1994. BRCA2, the second susceptibility gene for breast cancer, has recently been localized to a portion of chromosome 13 but it remains to be isolated. Recent data support the hypothesis that BRCA1 is a tumor suppressor gene that may be important in the development of not only inherited but also sporadic breast and ovarian cancers. Although breast cancer that can be attributed to a BRCA1 and BRCA2 germline mutation probably accounts for a small percent of all breast cancers, identification of these breast cancer susceptibility genes likely will have far-reaching consequences. For example, loss of BRCA1 region may occur in up to 30–60% of sporadic breast cancers (i.e., breast cancers arising in women without a significant family history). Thus, the specific abnormality is likely to be an uncommon inherited trait, but may be an acquired defect in the majority of sporadic cases. Now that at least one of the responsible genes has been identified, screening of high-risk patients for its presence will be possible within the next 3 years. If the gene is found to be present, the risk of developing breast cancer is approximately 85%, and breast cancer will develop in more than half of these women before the age of 50 years. Prophylactic bilateral mastectomy in early adulthood of carriers of the BRCA1 gene would circumvent future development of disease and possibly death. Most importantly, isolation and cloning of BRCA1 and BRCA2 will ultimately lead to a greater understanding of the biology of malignant transformation of mammary epithelium, and to major advances in diagnostic and therapeutics benefiting all breast cancer patients. It is hoped that an improved basic understanding of the molecular mechanisms involved in breast cancer development and the discovery of novel approaches to reverse or prevent these processes will lead ultimately to the ability to cure this extremely common and often fatal disease.[15]

ENVIRONMENTAL AND LIFESTYLE FACTORS

The observation of large differences in breast cancer rates between countries has led to the observation that environmental factors may play an important role in the etiology of breast cancer. Perhaps the most compelling evidence that environment plays a role in breast cancer incidence was derived from studies of Japanese women who migrated from Japan to the San Francisco Bay area. The incidence of breast cancer in Japanese women who live in Japan is quite low, however, the incidence of breast cancer in Japanese women who were first-generation U.S. born, or who migrated from Japan to the United States, was found to be nearly equal to that of the white population in the same area.

Diet is an obvious environmental factor and possible relations between fat or cholesterol intake and steroid hormone metabolism have led to an emphasis on dietary fat as a possible etiologic agent. International studies relating age-adjusted cancer mortality rate and national per capita fat intake demonstrate a positive correlation.[16] The correlation is stronger in postmenopausal than in premenopausal women. Studies in laboratory animals provide further evidence of a relationship between dietary fat intake and breast cancer.[17] Despite these compelling indirect data, case control and perspective studies performed in the United States have generally failed to show an association between dietary fat and breast cancer risk. In the largest epidemiologic survey, 89,538 nurses between the ages of 34 and 59 were studied. There was no relation between the relative risk of breast cancer and calorie-adjusted total fat, saturated fat, linoleic acid, or cholesterol intake. In fact, the relative risk of developing breast cancer among the women with the highest quintile of total fat intake was 0.85 compared with women in the lowest quintile. However, the difference in fat intake among women in these two extremes was only 25%.[18] Practically, this suggests that women who reduce fat intake in the context of the usual American diet are not likely to reduce their breast cancer risk. The possible benefits of lowering fat intake to levels substantially below 30% of caloric intake will need to be tested in randomized trials.

Dietary factors in addition to fat content that have been investigated include micronutrients and food-derived heterocyclic amines. Many of the studies which have examined the relative risk for breast cancer for high fat intake have also examined the association between breast cancer and intake of fiber beta-carotene and vitamins C, E, and A. The relationship between vitamin A and breast cancer risk is varied. In contrast, most studies support some benefit from beta-carotene, vitamin C, and/or dietary fiber.[16] It should be cautioned that these studies are limited by very small numbers of breast cancer cases, as well as the many difficulties in inherent cohort and case control studies.[16] Experimental and epidemiological evidence suggests an association between breast cancer and the Western diet, which typically includes a high amount of cooked meats and fat, as well as a high caloric intake. One group of compounds that may play a role in human breast cancer is heterocyclic amines found in commonly cooked beef, fish, and chicken. At least 19 heterocyclic amines with mutagenic activity have been identified in grilled, broiled, and fried meat and fish. Among these, 10 have been examined for long-term carcinogenicity and all were proven to be positive.[19] Experimental studies examining the interaction between heterocyclic amines and other dietary factors with respect to mammary carcinogenesis are warranted.

Both body weight and height are associated with breast cancer. Indices of obesity are related to breast cancer risks in a complex way that differs by age and menopausal status. Most studies on the premenopausal period show either no relationship with body weight or slightly declining breast cancer risks with increasing body weight. No plausible biological mechanisms have been proposed to explain this phenomenon. Most studies in postmenopausal women, however, show increasing breast cancer risks with increasing body weight. Not only obesity but the distribution of body fat also may play an independent role in breast cancer. Upper body (central or abdominal) adiposity increases the risk of breast cancer independent of overall obesity. This association has been proposed to be caused by the excess levels of free-circulating estrogen resulting from the conversion of androstenedione to estradiol in peripheral adipose tissue in conjunction with suppressed levels of circulating sex hormone binding globulin in women with central adiposity.[20] Studies that have examined breast cancer mortality tend to show stronger relationships with body weight in postmenopausal age groups than do studies of breast cancer incidence, suggesting that body weight exerts an influence on tumor behavior rather than on cancer etiology.[16]

Reports of more than 50 epidemiologic investigations of the relationship between alcohol and breast cancer have appeared in the literature. A recent meta-analysis[21] of these studies indicates both a modest positive association between alcohol and breast cancer (an approximately 25% increase in risk with daily intake of the equivalent of two drinks) and a dose–response relation. Data suggest that risk increases with consumption of alcohol in general, regardless of the beverage type. Several factors, including age, weight, and estrogen usage, have been shown to modify this relation in some studies. The mechanism of the alcohol breast cancer hypothesis may include increased levels of estradiol or other reproductive steroid hormones; altered hepatic mechanism of carcinogens; production of cytotoxic protein products; diminished immunological surveillance; impaired DNA repair; or possibly an influencing effect of alcohol on cell membrane integrity and/or metabolism of conjugers.[21,22] A series of methodological issues in the study of alcohol and breast cancer are apparent from the meta-analysis and these include inherent errors in alcohol assessment, the relatively small relative risk demonstrated, the presence of confounding variables in women who drink alcohol, and the lack of consistency of positive findings for the relationship between alcohol and the development of breast cancer. In addition, animal studies, which have been a relatively recent development in this area, have yielded mixed results regarding the influence of alcohol on the incidence of breast cancer. Although a causal relationship between alcohol consumption and breast cancer has not been proven, the weight of the epidemiologic and other types of evidence suggest that the relationship, direct or indirect, may exist.

Radiation is associated with an increased risk of breast cancer in survivors of the atomic bomb, in patients given radiation for postpartum mastitis, in women receiving multiple fluoroscopes during therapy for tuberculosis, and in animal models. Interestingly, this risk appears to be confined to exposure to radiation prior to the age of 40, which again suggests that a "window of initiation" for breast cancer occurs at a relatively early age. Exposure to diagnostic x-rays including annual screening mammography does not impart a sufficient dose of radiation for clinical concern.[6]

Cigarette smoking does not appear to increase the risk of breast cancer. Augmentation mammoplasty does not increase the risk of breast cancer. Blood pressure medications, reserpine, and other drugs that increase prolactin levels have not been shown to increase the risk of breast cancer. Caffeine also has no predisposing effect on breast cancer, but may play a role in exacerbation of benign breast disease. The role of environmental carcinogens has not been systematically evaluated.[6]

CLINICAL PRESENTATION

The initial sign in more than 90% of women with breast cancer is a painless lump. The typical malignant mass is solitary, unilateral, solid, hard, irregular, and nonmobile. In approximately 10% of cases, stabbing or aching pain is the first symptom. Less commonly, nipple discharge, retraction, or dimpling may herald the onset of the disease. In more advanced cases, prominent skin edema, redness, warmth, and induration of the underlying tissue may be observed.

It should be emphasized that the breast is a complex organ composed of skin, subcutaneous tissue, fatty tissue, and branching ductal and glandular structures. Various diseases that affect these structures can produce a palpable mass. In addition, the physiologic changes associated with the menstrual cycle can cause abnormalities of the breast that produce a three-dimensional mass. The foremost common causes of breast masses in young women are fibroadenoma, fibrocystic disease, carcinoma, and fat necrosis.

Approximately 90% of women first detect some breast abnormalities themselves, underscoring the importance of breast self-examination. In the United States, it is increasingly common for breast cancer to be detected during routine screening mammography in asymptomatic women. It is widely accepted that the smaller the mass, the higher the likelihood of cure, and the more conservative the treatment options offered to the patient. Thus, as the number of breast cancer cases found by screening mammography increases, overall survival of breast cancer patients is expected to improve significantly.

Breast cancer that is confined to a localized breast lesion is often referred to as *early, primary, localized,* or *curable.* Unfortunately, as is discussed shortly, breast cancer cells often spread by contiguity, lymph channels, and through the blood to distant sites. As discussed in subsequent sections, this often occurs early in the breast cancer growth, and deposits of tumor cells in distant sites (micrometastases) cannot be detected with current diagnostic methods and equipment. When breast cancer cells can be detected in sites distant from the breast, the disease is referred to as *advanced* or *metastatic* breast cancer. Tissues most commonly involved with metastases are lymph nodes, skin, bone, liver, lungs, and brain. Symptoms of bone pain, difficulty breathing, abdominal enlargement, jaundice, and mental status changes may herald the clinical presentation of metastatic breast cancer. Approximately 10% of women have signs and symptoms of distant metastases when they first seek treatment. In virtually all of them, a breast mass has been present for a relatively long period of time. In addition, approximately one-half of all patients who initially are treated for localized disease develop signs and symptoms of metastatic breast cancer; most commonly 3–5 years following local potentially curative therapy with surgery, radiation, and systemic adjuvant therapy.

Diagnosis

Initial work-up for a woman presenting with a localized lesion or other symptoms suggestive of breast cancer should include a careful history and physical examination of the breast and three-dimensional mammography, and also may include other breast imaging techniques such as ultrasound. Most (80–85%) breast cancers can be visualized on a mammogram as a mass, a cluster of calcifications, or a combination of both. The detection of a mass smaller than 2 millimeters is the ideal, but realistically, it is difficult to detect most tumors smaller than 5 millimeters. Large, noncalcified masses may be difficult to detect in the dense glandular breast, which is common in women of childbearing age. The threshold for the detection of a cancer is variable and depends on the radiographic abnormality, the fat to glandular tissue ratio of the breast, the technical quality of the examination, and the diligence and expertise of the radiologist.

Interpretations of mammography obtained either for screening or to evaluate a new breast mass generally fall into one of three categories: (1) the radiologist notes nothing suspicious for malignancy; (2) something of concern is seen and follow-up or further testing is advised; and (3) something clearly suspicious is present and a biopsy is indicated. A detailed discussion of abnormal mammogram radiographic findings and their significance is beyond the scope of this chapter, however, excellent references are available.[23,24] However, it should be noted that well-circumscribed x-ray masses are benign in 98% of cases; such lesions may not require a biopsy, but may be followed radiographically at 6-month intervals. Masses that are interpreted as "suspicious and a biopsy should be performed" have a 20–30% probability of malignancy. Masses that are interpreted as "highly suspicious radiographically" are malignant in 75–90% of cases. The overall probability of malignancy when a biopsy is performed on a nonpalpable mammographic abnormality ranges from 20–35%.

Breast biopsy is indicated for a mammographic abnormality that suggests malignancy or for a mass that is palpable on physical examination. The type of biopsy used depends on the mass size and characteristics. Excisional biopsy is the standard biopsy technique for clinically benign lesions or for malignant lesions less than 2 centimeters in diameter. This term indicates the complete removal of the abnormal tissue. Excisional biopsy may be performed either under a local or general anesthesia. It is usually done as an outpatient procedure.

Mammographically guided needle biopsy is a promising technique for the diagnosis of breast lesions. This procedure is associated with minimal discomfort and anxiety, few complications, no disfigurement, and could represent significant cost-savings when compared to conventional surgical excisional biopsy. Needle biopsies have included both core biopsy and fine-needle aspiration. These procedures require experienced mammographers and cytopathologists. Numerous studies have shown that the accuracy of core breast biopsy is at least equal to that of traditional localization and open-surgical breast biopsy. The accuracy of fine-needle aspiration is quite good in experienced hands. Results of a fine-needle aspiration can be used as the basis for mastectomy when the physical examination and mammographic abnormality coincide with the cytological diagnosis. However, many of the large series have reported at least one case of false-negative cancer diagnosis. For this reasons, many surgeons will not depend on fine-needle aspiration as the only biopsy prior to mastectomy. Other limitations of fine-needle aspiration include false-negatives (range 1–10%) and specimens with material insufficient for diagnosis (1–10% of aspirates). It should be pointed out that needle localization biopsy, with fine needle or core, is used only to establish the diagnosis. Following confirmation of malignancy, subsequent surgical procedures are performed to assure complete removal of the abnormal tissue.

Staging and Prognosis

Few malignant diseases illustrate the importance of stage (anatomic extent of disease) at the time of diagnosis and overall survival more clearly than breast cancer. Stage is defined on the basis of the size of the primary tumor (T1–4), presence and extent of lymph node involvement (N1–3), and presence, or absence of distant metastases (M) (Fig 120.3 and Table 120.3). Although many possible combinations of T and N are possible within a given stage, simplistically, stage 0 represents carcinoma *in situ* or disease that has not invaded the basement membrane. Stage I represents small primary tumor without lymph node involvement, and the majority of stage II disease involves regional lymph nodes. Stages 0, I, and II are often referred to as *early breast cancer.* It is in these early stages that the disease is curable. Stage III, also referred to as *locally advanced disease,* usually represents a large tumor with extensive nodal involvement in which either node or tumor is fixed to the chest wall. Stage IV disease is characterized by the presence of metastases to organs distant from the primary tumor. Stages III and IV are often referred to as *advanced disease.* Although a small number of patients with stage III disease may be cured, locally advanced breast cancers, as well as all metastatic breast

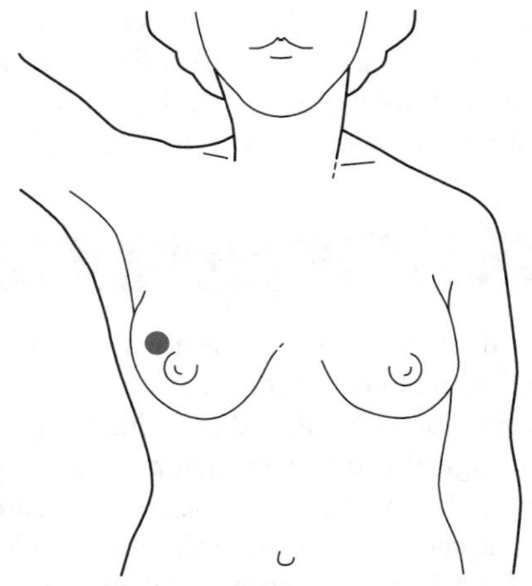

Tumor (T)

T_0 No evidence of tumor

T_{is} Carcinoma in situ or Paget's disease of nipple with no tumor

T_1 ≤ 2 cm

- T_{1a} ≤0.5 cm
- T_{1b} >0.5 cm–1 cm
- T_{1c} >1 cm–2 cm

T_2 >2 cm–5 cm

T_3 >5 cm

T_4 Any size; direct extension to chest wall (excluding pectoral muscle); skin infiltration; *peau d'orange;* satellite nodules

- T_{4a} Extension to chest wall
- T_{4b} Edema or ulceration of skin or presence of satellite nodules
- T_{4c} Both T_{4a} and T_{4b}
- T_{4d} Inflammatory carcinoma

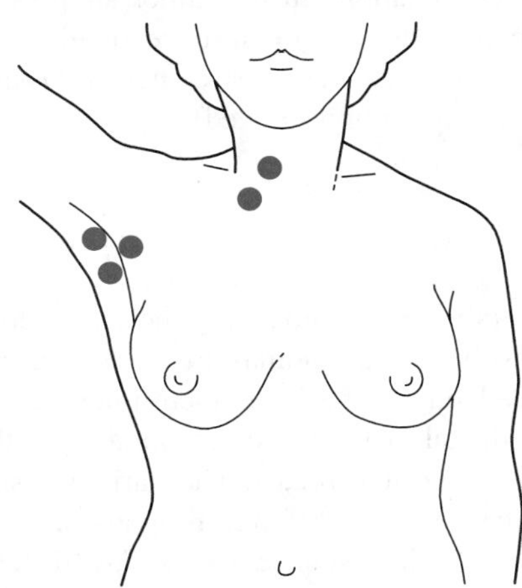

Nodes (N)

N_0 No regional lymph node metastasis

N_1 Metastasis to movable ipsilateral axillary lymph node or nodes

N_2 Metastasis to ipsilateral axillary node or nodes fixed to one another or other structures

N_3 Metastasis to ipsilateral internal mammary node or nodes

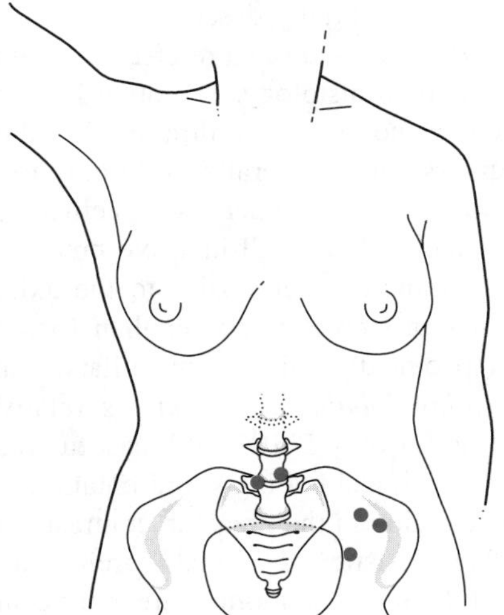

Metastasis (M)

M_0 No distant metastases

M_1 Distant metastasis, including metastasis to ipsilateral supraclavicular lymph node or nodes

Figure 120.3. TNM four-stage system. (See Table 120.3.) *(Adapted with permission from Stockdale FE. Breast cancer, in Rubenstein E, Federman DD (eds): Scientific American Medicine. New York, Scientific American, 1991, pp. 1–17.)*

TABLE 120.3. STAGES OF PRIMARY BREAST CANCER[a]

	T	N	M
Stage 0	T_{is}	N_0	M_0
Stage I	T_1	N_0	M_0
Stage IIA	T_0	N_1	M_0
	T_1	N_1	
	T_2	N_0	
Stage IIB	T_2	N_1	M_0
	T_3	N_0	
Stage IIIA	T_0	N_2	M_0
	T_1	N_2	
	T_2	N_2	
	T_3	N_1, N_2	
Stage IIIB	T_4	Any N	M_0
	Any T	N_3	
Stage IV	Any T	Any N	M_1

[a]See Fig. 120.3. (Adapted from Stockdale FE. Breast cancer, in Rubenstein E, Federman DD (eds): Scientific American Medicine. New York, Scientific American, 1991, pp 1–17, with permission.)

cancers, are usually incurable with standard treatment approaches.

The approximate percent of patients presenting with each stage of breast cancer and an estimate of their 5-year disease-free survival (DFS) is shown in Table 120.4. Five-year DFS is not synonymous with cure; however, 10-year DFS rates are on average 10% lower for each stage. It is important to recognize that many subsets exist within each stage and that both presentation and treatment of breast cancer is evolving at a rapid rate and therefore these estimates may vary among reference sources. Current estimates suggest that the majority of women present with early breast cancer and that a significant number of these women are cured with today's treatment approaches. As is discussed in subsequent sections, adjuvant systemic therapy has improved absolute survival rates by up to 10% in selected populations of patients with early breast cancer (stages I and II). Combined modality approaches utilizing neoadjuvant chemotherapy, surgery and/or radiation, followed by adjuvant chemotherapy has resulted in benefits of a similar magnitude in patients with locally advanced breast cancer (stage III). Unfortunately, a still significant percentage of women in both of these categories do experience recurrence, usually manifested in lungs, bone, liver, skin, or brain following treatment of the primary disease.

TABLE 120.4. ESTIMATED STAGE AT PRESENTATION AND 5-YEAR DISEASE-FREE SURVIVAL: BREAST CANCER 1994

	Percent of Total Cases	5-Year DFS[a] (%)
Stage I	40	70–90
Stage II	40	50–70
Stage III	15	20–30
Stage IV	5	0–10[b]

[a]With current conventional local and systemic therapy.
[b]Patients in stage IV are rarely free of disease, however, 10–20% of these patients may survive with minimal disease for 5–10 years.

PATHOLOGY

The pathological evaluation of breast lesions serves to establish the histological diagnosis and to confirm the presence or absence of other factors believed to influence prognosis. These nonhistological prognostic factors include the presence of necrosis, lymphatic or vascular invasion, nuclear grade, hormone receptor status, proliferative index, amount of aneuploidy, presence or absence of oncogenes, presence or absence of mutations in the tumor suppressor *p53* gene, and, perhaps, presence or absence of elevated growth factor levels, as well as enzymes (cathepsin D) and proteins (stress-related haptoglobin-related).

INVASIVE CARCINOMA

Invasive breast cancers are a histologically, heterogeneous group of lesions. Most breast carcinomas are adenocarcinomas and are classified on the basis of their microscopic appearance as either ductal or lobular corresponding to the ducts and lobules of the normal breast. The various histologic types of breast cancer have different prognoses, but it is not known whether their response to therapy differs, since patients in therapeutic trials are not typically stratified according to histological type. The five most common types of invasive breast cancer are briefly described.

Infiltrating ductal carcinoma (also referred to as intraductal) is the most common histology. The other histological patterns can occur alone or with infiltrating ductal carcinoma. These tumors are generally referred to as infiltrating ductal carcinoma "not otherwise specified" and account for approximately 75% of all invasive breast cancers. These tumors commonly metastasize to the axillary lymph nodes and their prognosis is poorer than for other histological types (specifically tubular, medullary, mucinous/colloid). *Infiltrating lobular carcinoma* is relatively uncommon, accounting for only 5–10% of breast tumors in most series. The typical clinical finding at presentation is an area of ill-defined thickening in the breast in contrast to the prominent lump characteristic of ductal carcinoma. A greater proportion of lobular carcinomas are multicentric tumors, either in the same or opposite breast, as compared with infiltrating ductal carcinoma. Overall, infiltrating lobular carcinoma and infiltrating ductal carcinoma have similar likelihoods of axillary node involvement and similar prognosis. However, the sites of metastases of these two types tend to differ. Ductal carcinoma is more frequently metastasized to the bone or to the liver, lung or brain, whereas lobular carcinoma is more metastasized to meningeal and serosal surfaces, and other unusual sites.

The three most common special types of invasive cancer are *tubular, medullary,* and *mucinous. Medullary carcinoma* is a well-defined lesion with characteristic microscopic appearance that includes a well-circumscribed border, intense infiltration with small lymphocytes, and other factors. It accounts for 5–7% of all breast carcinomas and is believed to have a better prognosis than infiltrating ductal carcinoma. *Mucinous* (or *colloid*) *carcinoma* constitutes about 3% of all mammary carcinomas and is characterized by the abundant accumulation of extracellular mucin around clusters of tumor cells. It is slow growing and can be bulky. When the tumor is predominantly mucinous, the prognosis tends to be more favorable. *Tubular carcinoma* is a type of carcinoma in which tubule formation is conspicuous. Tubular carcinoma constitutes about 2% of all breast cancers. Axillary metastases are uncommon and the prognosis is considerably better than for infiltrating ductal carcinomas. Histologies rarely reported include adenocystic carcinoma, carcinosarcomas, and papillary. In some pathology reports, infiltrating ductal carcinoma may include small areas containing these special tumor types.

Special situations seen clinically and histologically include Paget's disease of the breast and inflammatory breast cancer. Paget's disease of the breast occurs in 1–4% of all patients with breast cancer. Clinically, the patient presents with a relatively long history of eczematous changes in the nipple with itching, burning, oozing, bleeding, or some combination of these. The nipple changes are associated with an underlying carcinoma in the breast that is usually palpable. The histology of the tumor type is either ductal carcinoma *in situ* or invasive ductal carcinoma. Prognosis is related to the histological type of the associated tumor.

Inflammatory breast cancer is characterized clinically by prominent skin, edema, redness and warmth, visible erysipeloid margin, and induration of the underlying tissue. Biopsies of the involved skin reveal cancer cells in the dermal lymphatics. Prognosis of patients with inflammatory breast cancer is poor, even if the disease is apparently localized.

NONINVASIVE BREAST CARCINOMA

As with invasive carcinoma, the noninvasive lesions may be divided broadly into ductal and lobular categories. *In situ* carcinoma (ductal and lobular) has also been referred to as intraductal carcinoma. These lesions histologically appear as their invasive counterparts, however invasion through the basement membrane by light microscopy is absent.

The widespread use of routine screening mammography and the increased recognition of noninvasive breast carcinoma by pathologists has increased the diagnosis of *in situ* breast cancer significantly during the past decade. There has been a fivefold increase in the incidence of *in situ* breast cancer between 1973 and 1987 in the United States.[25] Ductal carcinoma *in situ* is seen more frequently than lobular carcinoma *in situ* at a rate of about 6:1. Most cases of ductal carcinoma *in situ* are now small, nonpalpable lesions unlike its presentation in prior years as a palpable mass in more than 50% of cases. Recent studies of nonpalpable breast lesions discovered by mammography document that ductal carcinomas *in situ* currently comprise about 7% of all breast biopsies and 30% of all breast malignancies.[26] Autopsy studies show that up to 16% of asymptomatic women have ductal carcinoma *in situ.*[27] This lesion now imparts a significant impact on society, emphasizing the importance of understanding its biology and ascertaining its appropriate management. Although a detailed discussion of the biology and appropriate management of noninvasive breast cancer is beyond the scope of this review, some of the more salient characteristics of ductal carcinoma *in situ* and lobular carcinoma *in situ* are described below and the reader is referred to a number of excellent reviews for a more comprehensive discussion.[28–30]

As previously eluded to, our knowledge of the natural history and incidence of ductal carcinoma *in situ* (DCIS) is evolving. Today, most cases of DCIS are found on biopsy performed for clustered calcifications seen on screening mammographies. The high rate of characteristic microcalcifications renders DCIS more amenable to detection by screening mammography compared to lobular carcinoma *in situ* (LCIS). DCIS has the same age distribution as invasive carcinoma. There are four distinct histological patterns of DCIS, which probably represent successive steps in its evolution toward invasive carcinoma. The biological characteristics are consistent with the direct precursor to invasive carcinoma, which develops in the majority of cases if left untreated generally within 10 years of diagnosis. Axillary lymph node dissection generally is not considered necessary in the treatment of DCIS in view of its low yield (1–2% of positive results). Mastectomy has been the standard treatment of DCIS for several decades due in part to extensive multicentricity and to the known danger of DCIS evolving into an invasive carcinoma. The combined data from 1061 women who underwent mastectomy for DCIS reported in 14 published studies with the follow-up ranging from 2 to more than 15 year shows an overall local recurrence rate of only 0.75% and an overall cancer mortality rate of only 1.7%.[26–28] Breast conservation, i.e., wide local excision followed by irradiation of breast tissue, may be an effective alternative to mastectomy although the safety and efficacy of breast conservation is not quite as certain in DCIS as in invasive carcinoma. There is currently no proven benefit for the use of cytotoxic chemotherapy or hormonal manipulation in this disease, although clinical trials are currently under way to test these regimens. Follow-up of women who have been treated with DCIS should be as comprehensive as that of women with invasive breast carcinoma to facilitate early detection of any subsequent malignancy.

LCIS, like DCIS, is frequently nonpalpable. It is virtually impossible to make the diagnosis of LCIS by clinical examination. Unlike DCIS, LCIS does not produce calcifications on mammography and, thus, conventional mammography is likewise not usually helpful. LCIS is most frequently diagnosed in biopsy specimens that were obtained due to symptoms caused by benign lesions such as fibrocystic breast disease. Multicentricity is common (greater than 30%) with LCIS and the opposite breast is affected in up to 50% of patients. It is unclear whether or not LCIS proceeds to invasive carcinoma or serves as a marker for a higher chance of invasive carcinoma elsewhere in the breast. Thus, the management of LCIS is controversial. Some authorities favor a program of breast self-examination, periodic physician examination, and mammography as management of LCIS. In selected patients who are particularly anxious about the development of cancer, bilateral total mastectomies and prompt reconstruction are a reasonable approach. Radiation therapy, systemic chemotherapy, or hormonal therapy currently have no role in the management of LCIS.

PATHOLOGICAL PROGNOSTIC FACTORS

Tumor size and the presence and number of involved axillary lymph nodes are established primary factors in assessing the risk for breast cancer recurrence and subsequent metastatic disease. Table 120.5 shows the 5-year relapse rate according to size of primary tumor and axillary node involvement with results of three investigations.[31–33] It should be clear from the data presented that the major factor that influences the likelihood of recurrence is the presence of positive axillary nodes. However, in both axillary node negative and axillary node positive groups, the size of the primary tumor remains an independent prognostic factor for disease recurrence. In axillary node negative patients, a tumor size of less than 2 centimeters is associated with a very favorable prognosis. However, there does not appear to be a large difference between prognosis in patients with large (greater than 5-centimeter) tumors and negative nodes compared to patients with 2- to 5-centimeter tumors and negative nodes. Thus, the size of the primary tumor in patients with negative axillary lymph nodes may not provide as much information regarding prognosis as in node positive patients. The number of affected nodes is directly related to disease recurrence. Estimates are that 35% of patients with one to three positive nodes will relapse within 5 years compared to 75% of patients with greater than or equal to four positive nodes.[34,35]

TABLE 120.5. FIVE-YEAR RELAPSE RATE (%) BASED ON SIZE OF PRIMARY TUMOR AND AXILLARY NODAL STATUS

	Size of Primary (cm)		
Axillary Status	<2	2–5	>5
Axillary Nodes Negative			
Fisher et al.[31]	12	24	27
Nemoto et al.[32]	13	19	25
Valagussa et al.[33]	8	24	19
Axillary Nodes Positive			
Fisher et al.[31]	50	60	79
Nemoto et al.[32]	39	50	65
Valagussa et al.[33]	37	64	74

The natural history of breast cancer varies greatly between patients. Some patients have extremely aggressive disease that progresses rapidly, while others are diagnosed with a disease that follows a more indolent course. The ability to predict which patients have a better disease prognosis is extremely important in designing treatment recommendations to maximize quantity and quality of life. A number of potential pathologic prognostic factors have been identified and intense research in this area is ongoing.

Aside from axillary lymph node involvement and tumor size, the presence or absence of hormone receptors has received the most attention in the characterization of primary breast cancer. Hormone receptors are used clinically as indicators of prognosis and to predict response to hormone therapy. Hormone receptors are cytoplasmic proteins that transmit signals to the nucleus of the cell for growth and proliferation. The hormone receptors clinically useful in discussions of breast cancer include the estrogen receptor (ER) and the progesterone receptor (PR). The presence of these proteins in the primary tumor (or less often metastases) is routinely measured by enzyme-linked immunochemical assays and radioassays. Concentrations of hormone receptors less than 3 fentamoles per milligram of cytosol protein are considered negative, 3–10 fentamoles per milligram of cytosol protein are "intermediate," and concentrations of hormone receptors greater than 10 fentamoles per milligram of cytosol protein are positive. It appears that the level (i.e., quantitative) of hormone receptor and the methodology used to assess hormone receptors are important for predictive ability. Although the estrogen receptor has received the most attention to date, more recent data suggest that the presence of the progesterone receptor protein is required for the functional effects of the estrogen receptor protein to occur. This is evidenced by a large number of studies that have found that response to hormonal manipulation and prognosis are highly correlated with the presence of both positive estrogen receptor protein and positive progesterone receptor protein. Hormone receptors are most valuable in predicting response to hormone therapy. Approximately 70–80% of patients who are ER positive and PR positive will respond to hormonal manipulation. PR negative patients rarely respond to hormonal manipulation. Patients that are ER negative and PR positive lie somewhere in between.

Approximately 50–70% of patients with primary or metastatic breast cancer have hormone positive tumors. The median level and frequency of hormone receptor positive tumors are higher in postmenopausal patients compared with premenopausal patients. This difference is likely responsible for the variance in recommendations for adjuvant and metastatic treatment of breast cancer between premenopausal and postmenopausal patients discussed in later sections of this chapter. A number of prominent authorities in the area of breast cancer research have suggested that breast cancer which occurs in postmenopausal women is substantively different than that occurring in premenopausal women. Breast cancer is predominantly a disease of the elderly. When it occurs in younger patients, the course of the disease is more aggressive. This is observed with many of the other common tumor types. Hormone receptor positivity, more common in postmenopausal women, is associated with not only and most importantly a superior response to hormone therapy, but also with a longer disease-free interval between primary and subsequent metastatic disease, and overall a more favorable prognosis. The presence of hormone receptors in tumors has been associated with a favorable disease-free interval and perhaps an overall survival difference of 5–10% (compared to hormone receptor negative patients). The value of hormone receptors as a prognostic factor is being eroded by increasing new knowledge of newer prognostic factors such as epidermal growth factor receptor, proliferative capacity, nuclear grade, and expression of the HER-2/*neu* oncogene.[36]

The rate of tumor cell proliferation also has prognostic significance in breast cancer recurrence. Rate of cell proliferation can be determined using either the tritiated-thymidine labeling index (TLI) or DNA flow cytometry, which determines the percentage of tumor cells actively dividing (S-phase fraction). Both techniques have shown that patients with rapidly proliferating tumors have a decreased DFS compared with patients with slowly proliferating tumors.[37–39] A number of investigators have demonstrated that patients with rapidly proliferating tumors are those that benefit most from administration of adjuvant chemotherapy.[40–42] In addition to growth fraction of tumor cell population, flow cytometry can also detect abnormal DNA content, or aneuploidy, in breast cancer cells. Although there are conflicting reports regarding the clinical significance of ploidy status, a number of studies report that patients with aneuploid tumors have significantly shorter relapse-free survival times than do patients with diploid tumors.

Nuclear grade and tumor (histologic) differentiation are known, independent prognostic indicators. Several histological grading systems have been developed and shown to have prognostic value in the evaluation of breast cancer. Fisher et al.[43] have shown a 5-year survival of 93% for patients with good nuclear grade compared with 79% for patients with poor nuclear grade. LeDoussal et al.[44] demonstrated a recurrence rate ranging from 0–19% among the five nuclear grades based on the modified Scarff–Bloom–Richardson system. However, interobserver lack of concordance has thwarted the use of this prognostic indicator in clinical trials.

A number of additional potential prognostic factors have been identified in the past 5 years. These include overexpression of the HER-2/*neu* oncogene and the c-ERB-B2 protein, the epidermal growth factor receptor (EGFR), cathepsin-D, angiogenic growth factors, mutations in the tumor suppresser *p53* gene, and others. Research in this area is proceeding at a rapid rate and the reader is referred to several excellent reviews for more detailed information.[36,45,46] A number of the new potential prognostic factors have been shown to be strongly correlated with established risk factors. For example, ER positive tumors are commonly EGFR and cathepsin-D negative as well, thus making it difficult to discern from clinical trials the relative importance of potential prognostic factors. Thus, it is unclear at the present time which of these serve as independent prognostic factors. Identification of these numerous factors and the presence of correlations between these and known prognostic factors that affect clinical outcome is of interest because each correlation allows basic mechanistic insights into disease processes. Practically, they allow prediction of probable clinical outcomes that can guide therapeutic decision making.

Although there is a growing understanding of the prognostic significance of individual factors, the topic of how practically to use multiple prognostic factors in concert is largely unexplored. The development of decision-making systems for clinical applications will require improvements in the areas of (1) standardization of methodologies and interlaboratory quality control for prognostic factor determinations, (2) definition of a limited set of prognostic markers that are independently predictive, and (3) staging systems or pools that integrate this information.

Treatment of Early Breast Cancer

LOCAL-REGIONAL THERAPY

The majority of patients presenting with breast cancer today, as previously discussed, have either an *in situ* tumor, a small tumor with negative lymph nodes, or a small stage II cancer. Surgery alone can cure most, if not all, patients with *in situ* cancers, and approximately half of all patients with stage II cancers. The choice of surgical procedures has changed drastically over the past 5 decades. This is in part due to our changing understanding of the biology of breast cancer, and in part due to a series of elegant and well-conducted trials that were performed during this time period.

The Halstedian theory and concept of tumor growth, formulated at the end of the nineteenth century, held that breast cancer was a local regional disease that spread to involve larger contiguous areas of the breast, chest wall, and adjacent lymph nodes. This hypothesis gave rise to emphasis throughout most of the twentieth century on the Halsted radical mastectomy, the hallmark of an approach holding that cure of early diseases could best be achieved with expansive, meticulously performed surgical procedures. The *radical mastectomy* involves removal of the breast and both major and minor pectoralis muscles. The axillary nodes on the same side (ipsilateral) as the breast lesion are also removed. Substantial morbidity is associated with this procedure. Muscle resection decreases strength and range of motion, and removal of axillary lymph nodes can produce edema of the arm and resected breast area. This procedure was often followed by external beam radiation therapy to the involved area.

During the 1960s, it was recognized that breast cancer is usually disseminated microscopically at the time of initial diagnosis. The evolutionary concept that breast cancer is not only a local, but also a systemic disease has resulted in major changes in the local treatment, as well as systemic therapy of this illness. In 1980, the Commission on Cancer of the American College of Surgeons reported on its breast cancer survey, which began in 1978.[47] This report recognized that there had been an apparent gradual shift of operation from a radical mastectomy to modified radical mastectomy since December of 1972. The modified radical mastectomy, also termed *total mastectomy with axillary lymph node dissection,* is not as precisely defined or standardized as the radical mastectomy. The pectoralis minor muscle may be excised or divided or left intact, and more importantly there may be variation in the extent of axillary lymph node dissection ranging from sampling to full dissection. It was recognized during this time period that a major factor in prognosis was involvement of axillary lymph nodes rather than the type of initial surgical procedure performed.

Results of a large trial conducted in the United States by the National Surgical Adjuvant Breast and Bowel Project (NSABP) repudiated the Halsted theory and principle theory and supported the alternative systemic hypothesis. NSABP B-04 published in 1977 randomized almost 2000 women among three treatment regimens: radical mastectomy, simple mastectomy with local-regional irradiation, and simple mastectomy and removal of nodes if they later became clinically positive.[48] Forty percent of patients who underwent the radical mastectomy had pathologically positive lymph nodes, thus, it can be assumed that 40% of patients in the groups treated with simple mastectomy alone or with local-regional irradiation had positive axillary nodes that were not removed. Despite the disparity in local-regional treatment, no significant difference in treatment failure, distant metastases, or overall survival were observed through more than 14 years of follow-up.

With negation of the primacy radical mastectomy, the NSABP instituted a second trial (B-06) the results of which were published in 1985.[49] In this landmark paper, patients with stage I or II breast cancer, in which the tumor size was 4 centimeters or less, were treated with either total mastectomy or lumpectomy with or without radiation therapy. In this study, lumpectomy followed by radiation resulted in a 5-year survival of 85% compared to 76% for total mastectomy. A subsequent study reported on the 8-year results of the study. Their observation at 8 years was consistent with the previous findings at 5 years, which continue to support the use of lumpectomy in patients with stage I or II breast cancer. This study also found that radiation therapy reduced the probability of local recurrence of tumor in patients treated with lumpectomy. In this study, breast irradiation after lumpectomy decreased the likelihood of tumor recurrence in the involved breast by approximately 30%. The local failure rate of total mastectomy was 8.1% compared to 7.2% for lumpectomy alone and 1.1% for lumpectomy and radiation therapy. The 8-year data confirmed the previous observation that lumpectomy followed by breast irradiation in all patients and adjuvant systemic therapy in patients with positive nodes was appropriate treatment for stages I and II breast cancer. Neither the rate or development of distant metastases or contralateral breast cancer were different in the treatment groups.

The National Institutes of Health (NIH) Consensus Conference on the Treatment of Early Stage Breast Cancer addressed the roles of modified radical mastectomy versus breast conservation and concluded that primary therapy for breast cancer stages I and II should be *breast conservation.*[50] Breast conservation consists of lumpectomy, also referred to as segmental mastectomy or partial mastectomy, and is defined as excision of the primary tumor and adjacent breast tissue followed by radiation therapy to reduce the risk of local recurrence. Sampling of axillary lymph nodes is recommended for completeness of staging and prognostic information. The reason given for favoring breast conservation therapy is that it achieved similar results to more extensive surgical procedures with cosmetically superior results.

The majority of patients with breast cancer can be treated by partial mastectomy and radiation therapy. Several factors should be considered in selecting patients for breast conservation therapy. Multiple sites of cancer within the breast and the inability to attain negative pathological margins on the excised breast specimen are predictive for an increased risk of recurrence with breast conserving therapy and indications for mastectomy. Preexisting collagen vascular disease is a contraindication for the use of breast-conserving radiation and surgery. Although local recurrence following breast conservation therapy is not associated with increased mortality, it is disturbing to the patient and requires surgical removal of the breast. In addition, reconstructive therapy is often not feasible in a breast that has previously received irradiation. Another major consideration in selecting patients for breast conserving therapy is the expected cosmetic result. Although the size of the tumor is not an important consideration for breast cancer recurrence, the relationship of the size of the tumor to the total breast volume is an important cosmetic consideration. If the volume of the tissue removed is large in a woman with small breasts, better results can often be obtained with mastectomy and reconstruction. Despite the desire of the patient and the willingness of the surgeon to avoid mastectomy, in some circumstances, a lumpectomy will approximate so closely a mastectomy that both the patient and the physician will agree that preservation of a very limited amount of breast tissue would not justify the inconvenience of radiation therapy. Aside from the probability of local recurrence and the ability to achieve a satisfactory cosmetic result, consideration must be given to the availability of an external beam radiation facility and the patient's willingness to comply with the prescribed course of radiotherapy. In most instances, external beam radiation therapy used in conjunction with breast conserving procedures involves 4–6 weeks of radiation therapy directed to the breast tissue (total of 5000 cGy administered as 200-cGy doses daily to eradicate residual disease). Complications associated with radiation therapy to the breast are minor and include reddening and erythema of the breast tissue, and subsequent shrinkage of total breast mass beyond that predicted on the basis of breast tissue removal.

Simple or *total mastectomy* involves removal of the entire breast without resection of the underlying muscle or axillary nodes. The major disadvantage of this procedure is that axillary nodal status is not determined and, thus, important prognostic information may be lost. This procedure is used in patients with carcinoma *in situ* where there is a 1% incidence of axillary node involvement, or in cases of local recurrence following breast conservation therapy. However, the importance of determining axillary lymph node involvement is being challenged by the identification of new prognostic pathological factors which bear concordance with axillary nodal status and with the new and evolving recommendations for systemic adjuvant therapy for all patients regardless of nodal status. Thus, simple mastectomy may be a reasonable alternative for women who wish to avoid the inconvenience of radiation therapy and preserve their option for breast reconstruction in the future.

The NSABP B-04 and B-06 trials are most commonly credited with the finding that breast conservation is an appropriate primary therapy for the majority of women with stages I and II disease, and preferable in that it provides survival rates equivalent to that of modified radical mastectomy. However, these trials were no less important for the valuable information they provide regarding the natural history of the disease and the identification of pathological prognostic factors associated with early cancer spread. The preponderance of information available regarding predicting women most likely to benefit from systemic adjuvant therapy was derived from pathological evaluation of the archives of these trials.

SYSTEMIC ADJUVANT THERAPY

Systemic adjuvant therapy is defined as the administration of systemic therapy following definitive therapy (surgery, radiation, or a combination of these) when there is no evidence of metastatic disease, but a high likelihood of disease recurrence. The concept of breast cancer being a systemic disease and the rationale of adjuvant chemotherapy was based on a series of laboratory and clinical investigations conducted during the 1960s and 1970s and directed primarily toward achieving a better understanding of tumor metastases. The laboratory findings, clinical abnormalities, and biologic hypothesis that lead to recognition of breast cancer as a systemic disease and documented the value of adjuvant chemotherapy are illustrated in Table 120.6. The very earliest adjuvant trials in breast cancer consisted of perioperative administration of alkylating agents with the intent of eradicating micrometastases that were disseminated at the time of surgical excision of the tumor. Large numbers of collaborative research groups, both in the United States and abroad, have conducted step-

TABLE 120.6. LABORATORY FINDINGS, CLINICAL OBSERVATIONS, AND BIOLOGIC HYPOTHESIS OF BREAST CANCER AS A SYSTEMIC DISEASE AND THE VALUE OF ADJUVANT CHEMOTHERAPY

- By the time cancer becomes clinically detectable, it is advanced (about 30 doublings) and has had ample opportunity to establish distant micrometastases.
- There is no orderly pattern of tumor cell dissemination, and the bloodstream is of considerable importance in tumor spread.
- Operable breast cancer is often a systemic disease and variations in local-regional therapy have not substantially affected survival. Only by control of distant disease can there be an improvement in the outcome of breast cancer patients.
- Likelihood of disease recurrence is related to size of tumor mass and axillary node involvement at diagnosis.
- Recurrence of breast cancer following local-regional therapy is most commonly at sites distant from the breast.
- Tumor growth fraction is inversely related to tumor population site. Therefore, optimal kinetic conditions to achieve cure with chemotherapy exist in the setting of micrometastatic disease.
- Efficacy of chemotherapy is dose dependent and optimal doses of combination chemotherapy can be more safely and effectively administered in the adjuvant setting as opposed to the setting of advanced diseases.

wise series of studies designed to identify appropriate candidates for systemic adjuvant therapy, as well as optimal regimens and duration of systemic adjuvant therapy. Several hundred randomized clinical trials evaluating various systemic adjuvant modalities have been reported. Most published results confirmed that chemotherapy, hormonal therapy, or a combination of the two result in advantages in DFS or overall survival for all treated patients, or more commonly for patients in specific prognostic subgroups (i.e., nodal involvement, menopausal status, hormonal receptor status, growth fraction, nuclear grade, etc.). The huge amount of data generated by these trials has resulted in a great deal of controversy with different conclusions being reached by different experts.

A number of factors make interpretation of results of systemic adjuvant therapy trials difficult. These include differences in the patient populations studied, the variation in natural history of breast cancer, the absence of information regarding pathological prognostic factors in many studies, differences in treatment approach, and methods of analysis. It is important to remember that the goal of systemic adjuvant therapy is cure. Therefore, patients in these studies must be followed for long periods of time before results can be determined. In addition, since the majority of patients with early breast cancer (50–90%) in the various trials are cured with local-regional therapy alone, large numbers of patients are required to show a statistically significant difference that can be attributed to systemic adjuvant therapy. For these reasons, combined analysis, or meta-analysis, of all breast cancer trials has been conducted and is the most frequently referred to information regarding systemic adjuvant therapy. This effort, organized by the Early Breast Cancer Trialists Collaborative Group, is based on a worldwide collaboration involving 133 randomized trials conducted between 1957 and 1985 with 31,000 recurrences of disease, and 24,000 deaths among 75,000 women. The most recent publication of this overview was in 1992.[51] The majority of women in these trials were node positive (70%). Data on hormone receptor status and many of the newer pathological prognostic factors were not available in many of the trials.

The 10-year results of the overview are described in Table 120.7. As can be seen in this table, in women less than 50 years of age, adjuvant chemotherapy alone reduces the annual odds of recurrence by 37%, and the annual odds of death by 27%. This is in contrast to tamoxifen alone, which reduced the annual odds of recurrence by 27% and the annual odds of death by 17%.

When one compares the results of trials that compared tamoxifen plus chemotherapy versus chemotherapy alone, or chemotherapy and tamoxifen versus tamoxifen alone, it is apparent that the combination offered very little benefit in women less than or equal to 50 years of age. An interesting theory with some laboratory and clinical support holds that tamoxifen antagonizes the beneficial effects of chemotherapy in women less than or equal to 50 years of age. Chemotherapy acts by inhibiting DNA synthesis and thereby causing death of tumor cells, whereas tamoxifen is believed to have a static effect on tumor cell growth. The growth inhibitory effect of tamoxifen may thereby diminish the

TABLE 120.7. TEN-YEAR RESULTS OF THE OVERVIEW ANALYSIS

		Reduction in Annual Odds of (% + Standard Deviation)	
	No. Patients	**Recurrence**	**Death**
Women ≤50 Years			
Tamoxifen	8578	12 ± 4	6 ± 5
Tam alone vs. no treatment	2216	27 ± 7	17 ± 10
Tam + chemo vs. chemo	6362	7 ± 4	3 ± 5
Chemotherapy	3362	36 ± 5	25 ± 5
Chemo alone vs. no treatment	2976	37 ± 5	27 ± 6
Chemo + tam vs. tam	386	32 ± 16	6 ± 23
Ovarian ablation	1817	26 ± 6	25 ± 7
Ablation alone vs. no treatment	878	30 ± 9	28 ± 9
Ablation + chemo vs. chemo	939	21 ± 9	19 ± 11
Women >50 Years			
Tamoxifen	21,262	29 ± 2	20 ± 2
Tam alone vs. no treatment	13,114	30 ± 2	19 ± 3
Tam + chemo vs. chemo	8148	28 ± 3	20 ± 4
Chemotherapy	7677	23 ± 3	12 ± 4
Chemo alone vs. no treatment	3745	22 ± 4	14 ± 5
Chemo + tam vs. tam	3932	26 ± 5	10 ± 7

(Adapted from Gelber RD, Goldhirsch A, Coates AS: Adjuvant therapy for breast cancer: Understanding the overview. J Clin Oncol 1993;11:580–585, with permission.)

cytotoxic effect of chemotherapy, resulting in subsequent recurrence of disease in women that received the two agents together. This has led to controversy regarding the optimal way to administer chemo–endocrine therapy in the adjuvant setting with some experts favoring sequential use (chemotherapy followed by tamoxifen) while others continue to use concurrent (chemotherapy plus tamoxifen) therapy.

Interestingly, results of the meta-analysis suggest that ovarian ablation has approximately the same magnitude of effects in women less than or equal to 50 years of age as chemotherapy. These findings have renewed interest in adjuvant ovarian ablation in women less than or equal to 50 years of age. It is incorrect to infer from the overview that chemotherapy and ovarian ablation are equivalent. These are "indirect comparisons" between the results of the chemotherapy trials and ovarian ablation trials. Patient selection factors and other aspects of the early ablation trials may have differed from those in the more recent chemotherapy trials, so these trials are not comparable. The relative value of chemotherapy and ovarian ablation must be evaluated in direct comparison using randomized trials.

Of note, premenopausal women treated with adjuvant chemotherapy often develop amenorrhea. The potential therapeutic importance of chemotherapy-induced amenorrhea has been recognized for many years, leading some to speculate that the effects of adjuvant chemotherapy are mediated by the endocrine effects of ovarian ablation. Supporting this view is the observation that chemotherapy-induced amenorrhea is associated with superior DFS in some adjuvant trials, although not in others. An alternative hypothesis is that amenorrhea is merely a marker that identifies patients for whom the chemotherapy is more effective. Although this debate is difficult to resolve precisely, it seems likely that patients with hormonally responsive cancers will benefit from both the cytotoxic effects of chemotherapy and the estrogen deprivation of ovarian ablation.

In women 50 years of age or older, adjuvant tamoxifen reduces the annual odds of recurrence by 30% and the annual odds of death by 19%. Chemotherapy offers smaller benefits in this group reducing the annual odds of recurrence and death by 22% and 14%, respectively. In the tamoxifen in combination with chemotherapy trials, the avoidance of recurrence is chiefly during the first 5 years, but the avoidance of mortality is highly significant during both the first and second 5 years; therefore, the cumulative differences in survival are large, both at 5 and then at 10 years.[52] Between the ages of 50 and 69, direct comparisons show that chemotherapy plus tamoxifen is superior to chemotherapy alone for both recurrence and mortality and better than tamoxifen alone for recurrence.

The overview also demonstrated that the proportional benefits of chemotherapy in node negative and node positive patients are comparable, combination chemotherapy is superior to single agents, and adjuvant treatment duration of 12–24 months is no more effective than 6 months of treatment. Indirect comparisons showed that long-term tamoxifen (2–5 years) is significantly more effective than tamoxifen treatment programs of shorter duration and that tamoxifen doses greater than 20 mg are not associated with better responses than 20-mg daily doses.

Proportional reductions in the annual odds of recurrence or death describe the treatment benefit only in those who might have had recurrences or those who died during the observation period. It is important to consider that the underlying risk of death or recurrence varies in breast cancer patients and, hence, the absolute benefits of adjuvant therapy will also vary accordingly. For example, in a group of untreated axillary node positive patients, perhaps 50% or more would be expected to die within 10 years. A 25% reduction in the annual odds of death amounts to about 10 fewer deaths per 100 treated patients at the end of 10 years or an absolute increase in the 10-year survival from 50 to 60%. However, the absolute benefits of treatment are much smaller in node negative patients with a favorable prognosis. For example, if 25% of a group of node negative patients were expected to die within 10 years, a 25% reduction in the annual odds of death amounts to about 5 fewer deaths per 100 treated patients at the end of 10 years or an absolute increase in the 10-year survival from 75 to 80%. Hence, the benefit of adjuvant therapy expressed as a reduction in the annual odds of recurrence or death must be put into perspective with the likelihood of death without treatment.

Despite the very large number of clinical trials conducted in women with early stage breast cancer, optimal therapy has not been defined. To assist in identifying optimal treatment guidelines, all women with early stage breast cancer are encouraged to participate in randomized cooperative group clinical trials. Current estimates are that less than 5% of women in the United States and Europe with early breast cancer are currently enrolled in cooperative group research studies. This is unfortunate because optimal treatment cannot be defined in the absence of data derived from well-designed, well-conducted clinical investigations. From a practical standpoint, it is also unfortunate that this leaves the medical oncologist, as well as the patient, with a dilemma in selecting treatment outside of the context of clinical trials. To assist in these situations, the NIH conducted consensus conferences in 1985 and 1990 on the treatment of early stage breast cancer. In 1992, an international group of researchers met at St. Gallen and also developed treatment recommendations for treatment of women with early stage breast cancer outside of the context of clinical trials.[52] A comparison of the 1990 NIH Consensus Conference and the St. Gallen recommendations is found in Table 120.8. The timing of the 1992 St. Gallen conference was fortunate in that the 10-year data from the overview had recently been published. In addition, the role of currently accepted and new prognostic factors was a subject of intense debate at the St. Gallen conference. Thus, the treat-

TABLE 120.8. COMPARISON OF THE TREATMENT GUIDELINES FOR PREMENOPAUSAL AND POSTMENOPAUSAL WOMEN

Node Status	1990 NIH	1992 St. Gallen
Premenopausal Women		
Node negative		
Low/minimal[a]	No treatment	No treatment or tamoxifen
Good risk[b]	No treatment	Tamoxifen
High risk[c]		
ER+	CT or tamoxifen	CT ± Tamoxifen
ER–	CT or tamoxifen	CT
Node positive		
ER+	CT	CT ± Tamoxifen
ER–	CT	CT
Postmenopausal Women		
Node negative		
Low/minimal risk[a]	No treatment	No treatment or tamoxifen
Good risk[b]	No treatment	Tamoxifen
High risk[c]		
ER+	CT or tamoxifen	Tamoxifen ± CT
ER–	CT or tamoxifen	CT ± Tamoxifen
Node positive		
ER+	Tamoxifen or CT	Tamoxifen ± CT
ER–	Tamoxifen or CT	CT ± Tamoxifen

Key: CT, chemotherapy.
[a]Small (≤1 cm) invasive carcinoma, *in situ*, or good histopathology (colloid, tubular, papillary).
[b]ER+, low nuclear grade, or tumor size 1–2 cm.
[c]ER–, cancers of ≥1 cm; ER+, cancers ≥ 2 cm, and all cancers with nuclear grade III.
(Adapted from Clin Oncol Alert 1993;2:15, with permission.)

ment recommendations put forward at St. Gallen differ from the NIH conference in that they attempt to define low-risk, good-risk, and high-risk groups of women with node negative disease, and they are also more aggressive in use of combined chemohormonal therapy in hormone receptor negative patients, as well as in postmenopausal patients in general.

The absolute benefits of adjuvant therapy are primarily related to the patient's risk of metastases and ultimately cancer death. The risks are of a sufficient magnitude to justify the use of adjuvant chemotherapy for all node positive, premenopausal women, and adjuvant tamoxifen for all node positive, ER positive, postmenopausal women. The options are less certain for node positive, ER negative, postmenopausal women. Chemotherapy is strongly favored by the St. Gallen recommendations. Tamoxifen may also represent a possible treatment because the benefits of treatment of the postmenopausal patients with estrogen receptor values of less than 10 fmol/mg may be of similar magnitude to those from chemotherapy. Since the risk of metastases and death is lower in node negative patients, there is more uncertainty regarding the benefits of adjuvant therapy in this group. Node negative patients with primary breast tumors of less than 1 centimeter have an excellent prognosis and there is general agreement that the absolute benefits of adjuvant therapy may be too small to justify its use outside the clinical trial. Intensive research efforts are directed toward identifying those characteristics of the primary tumor (pathological prognostic factors) that may predict for a higher or lower likelihood of metastases and death in node negative patients. Although a multitude of prognostic factors are being investigated, no single factor or combinations of factors sufficiently identifies those at risk of metastases or is sufficiently standardized to be reproducibly applicable to all patients. Furthermore, it cannot be assumed that patients with a poor prognosis have the same or greater likelihood of benefiting from adjuvant therapy. In some cases, the "poor prognostic factor" will be associated with resistance to adjuvant therapy. Certainly decisions regarding adjuvant therapy in node-negative patients should be individualized based on the estimated risk of relapse and death, the expected benefits of treatment, the toxicity of treatment, and the impact of therapy on quality of life. There is an increasing trend in clinical decision making to take hormone receptor status, nuclear grade, and tumor size into consideration in recommending adjuvant therapy. For a more in-depth discussion of the issues and controversies regarding adjuvant therapy of breast cancer, the reader is referred to several excellent references.[53–55] Adjuvant therapy of breast cancer is an emerging treatment; therefore, the most up-to-date information will be found only in the primary literature.

Adjuvant Chemotherapy

Cytotoxic drugs that have been used alone and in combination as adjuvant therapy in breast cancer include doxorubicin, cyclophosphamide, methotrexate, fluorouracil, melphalan, prednisone, and vincristine. The most common combination chemotherapy regimens employed in the adjuvant setting are listed in Table 120.9.

Combination chemotherapy regimens used in the adjuvant setting are essentially the same as regimens used for metastatic breast cancer. The basic principle of adjuvant therapy for any cancer type is that the regimen with the highest response rate in advanced disease is the optimal regimen for use in the adjuvant setting. Early administration of effective combination chemotherapy at a time when the tumor burden is low should increase the likelihood of cure and minimize the emergence of drug-resistant tumor cell clones. Doxorubicin is often referred to as the most active single agent in the treatment of metastatic breast cancer. This has led to the assumption that doxorubicin-containing regimens are associated with a higher cure rate than non–adriamycin-containing regimens when used in the adjuvant setting. In an indirect comparison of the effects of adjuvant chemotherapy in trials that used doxorubicin-containing regimens with results of trials in which CMF-type regimens were used failed to show any significant advantage for the doxorubicin

TABLE 120.9. COMBINATION CHEMOTHERAPY OF BREAST CANCER

Abbreviation	Regimen
FAC	5-Fluorouracil, 400–500 mg/m^2 IV, days 1 and 8 Adriamycin, 40–50 mg/m^2 IV, day 1 Cyclophosphamide, 400–500 mg/m^2 IV, day 1 Repeat every 28 days as tolerated
CMFVP (Cooper)	Cyclophosphamide, 80–100 mg PO per day Methotrexate, 20–25 mg IV per week 5-Fluorouracil, 500 mg IV per week Vincristine, 1.0 mg IV per week Prednisone, 45 mg PO per day × 14 days, then 30 mg PO per day × 14 days, then 15 mg PO per day
CAF	Cyclophosphamide, 500 mg/m^2 IV, day 1 Adriamycin, 50 mg/m^2 IV, day 1 5-Fluorouracil, 500 mg/m^2 IV, day 1 Repeat every 21 days as tolerated
CMF (original)	Cyclophosphamide, 100 mg/m^2 PO, per day × 14 days Methotrexate, 40 mg/m^2 IV days 1 and 8 5-Fluorouracil, 600 mg/m^2 IV days 1 and 8 Repeat every 28 days as tolerated
CMF (revised)	Cyclophosphamide, 600 mg/m^2 IV, day 1 Methotrexate, 40 mg/m^2 IV, day 1 5-Fluorouracil, 600 mg/m^2 IV, day 1 Repeat every 21 days as tolerated
AC	Adriamycin, 30–40 mg/m^2 IV, day 1 Cyclophosphamide, 150–200 mg/m^2 PO, days 3–6 Repeat every 21 days as tolerated

Note: Doses are modified for leukopenia, thrombocytopenia, impaired renal and liver function, etc. Maximum tolerated doses should be used.

regimens.[53] The results from at least 12 trials that enrolled almost 9000 patients to receive either a doxorubicin- or non-doxorubicin-containing regimen have been published. Significant survival advantage for patients randomized to the doxorubicin arm were seen in only one of these studies.[56] One important trial clearly demonstrated the value of adding doxorubicin in patients with four or more positive lymph nodes.[57] Several of these trials have demonstrated a disease-free survival benefit although it appears at the current time that doxorubicin-containing regimens may not be clearly superior to non-doxorubicin-containing regimens in the adjuvant setting. Additional follow-up of these trials is required for definitive analysis.

Although the optimal duration of adjuvant chemotherapy administration is unknown, it appears to be on the order of 4–6 months. Chemotherapy should be initiated within 3 weeks of surgical removal of the primary. "Dose response" and "dose intensity" appear to be critical factors in achieving optimal outcomes. *Dose response* refers to a direct relationship between the amount of chemotherapy administered and observed antitumor effect. *Dose intensity* is defined as the amount of drug administered per unit of time, typically reported in mg/m^2/week. Retrospective analysis and prospective randomized trials suggest the importance of dose response and dose intensity in the treatment of breast cancer. The relative importance of dose response versus dose intensity is unclear at the present time. It is similarly unclear what subset of patients benefit from administration of high-dose or dose-intense regimens.

A major focus in clinical investigation is the use of more high-dose chemotherapy regimens as adjuvant therapy. Since bone marrow suppression is the dose-limiting toxicity for most chemotherapeutic agents, high-dose chemotherapy regimens followed by colony-stimulating factors (CSFs) or transplantation of autologous bone marrow and/or peripheral blood progenitor cells have recently been developed. Trials to define the specific usefulness of high-dose regimens, as well as autologous bone marrow transplantation in conjunction with dose-intense regimens, appear justified given the positive response rates seen in the metastatic breast cancer setting and the very poor prognosis associated with stage II disease with 10 or more positive axillary lymph nodes and/or other negative pathological prognostic factors. Four prospective randomized trials currently under way in North America are testing the concept of high-dose chemotherapy following a period of standard dose chemotherapy. Two are targeted to patients with 10 or more positive lymph nodes in the adjuvant setting and two are examining patients with poor prognosis stage IV disease.[58]

The short-term toxic effects of chemotherapy used in the adjuvant setting are generally well tolerated. Although a number of investigators have demonstrated a reduction in quality of life, most patients are able to maintain a reasonable level of function and emotional and social well-being during treatment.[59] In general, supportive therapy of the patient receiving systemic adjuvant chemotherapy has improved in the past decade. Increased attention to the impact of symptoms on quality of life may account for some of this improvement. In addition, serotonin-antagonist antiemetics have become available to assist in managing chemotherapy-induced nausea and vomiting, and CSFs are often helpful in preventing febrile neutropenia, particularly in elderly patients or patients receiving high-dose and dose-intense chemotherapy regimens. However, a number of side effects are common with the regimens employed and patients should be appropriately counseled regarding the likelihood of alopecia, weight gain, and fatigue. Patients who are menstruating will experience a cessation of menses that may or may not return. Along with cessation of menses are accompanying signs and symptoms of menopause. Deep vein thrombosis has been reported in women receiving combination chemotherapy regimens.[60] A recent study estimated that about 1–10 of 10,000 patients treated for 6 months with cyclophosphamide-based regimens might be expected to have leukemia within 10 years of diagnosis of breast cancer.[61]

Cardiomyopathy induced by doxorubicin occurs less than 1% of the time in women whose total dose is less than 320 mg/m^2 of body surface area.[62] Toxicities associated with the chemotherapy regimens employed in the experimental autologous bone marrow transplant and/or peripheral blood progenitor cell transplant programs are likely to be greater than those incurred with the standard adjuvant chemotherapy regimens described.

Adjuvant Hormonal Therapy

Hormonal therapies that have been studied in the treatment of primary or early breast cancer include oophorectomy, ovarian irradiation, tamoxifen, and luteinizing hormone-releasing hormone (LHRH) agonists.

Tamoxifen is currently the adjuvant hormonal therapy of choice. Tamoxifen has been used in the adjuvant setting for three decades. Tamoxifen is antiestrogenic in breast cancer cells, however, it appears to have estrogenic properties in other tissues and organs.[63,64] Although its major mechanism of action has been attributed to its ability to block hormone receptors, studies have shown that the drug is capable of stimulating the production of transforming growth factor beta, an inhibitory growth factor that could in fact inhibit not only estrogen receptor positive cancer cells, but also estrogen receptor negative cancer cells.[65,66] In the laboratory, tamoxifen has also been shown to reduce angiogenesis.[66] It does this presumably by decreasing local stimulatory growth factors, thus creating a hostile environment for tumor cells. Women receiving adjuvant tamoxifen therapy have a reduced incidence of development of contralateral breast cancer compared to women not receiving adjuvant tamoxifen therapy.[51] This, coupled with evidence of tamoxifen's beneficial estrogenic effects on the cardiovascular system and bone density, has led to tamoxifen being the hormonal agent of choice, not only in the adjuvant setting but in the treatment of metastatic disease as well.

The optimal dose of tamoxifen appears to be 20 mg/d. Due to the long biological half-life of tamoxifen, this can be administered as a single daily dose. Adjuvant tamoxifen therapy is generally initiated shortly after surgery or as soon as pathology results are known and the decision to administer tamoxifen as adjuvant therapy is made. An exception to this may be in women who receive combined chemo–endocrine therapy where, for the reasons described earlier, tamoxifen therapy is postponed until chemotherapy is completed. The optimal duration of tamoxifen therapy in the adjuvant setting has not been defined. Although most current recommendations suggest 2–5 years of tamoxifen therapy, there is a growing trend in practice toward continuing tamoxifen for more than 5 years. Data do not exist to support the use of prolonged courses of tamoxifen in the adjuvant setting. However, as discussed in a subsequent section, tamoxifen is currently being studied for its value as a chemopreventive agent in women at high risk for developing breast cancer (see section on Prevention and Early Detection). Women with a personal history of breast cancer are clearly at high risk for the development of a subsequent breast cancer. If the results of the chemoprevention trials under way are positive, it may become standard to continue the administration of adjuvant tamoxifen therapy for life.

Tamoxifen is usually well tolerated. Symptoms of estrogen withdrawal (hot flashes and vaginal bleeding) are the most troublesome but will decrease in frequency and intensity over time. When used in the metastatic setting, a flare of bone pain and hypercalcemia occasionally occur, particularly in patients with bone metastases. This does not occur in the adjuvant setting. Of particular importance are concerns about carcinoma of the liver and uterus in women receiving tamoxifen.[65,66] Proliferation of the endometrium, an estrogenic effect of tamoxifen, appears to be dose dependent and related to the duration of therapy. The incidence of endometrial cancer has been highest in patients receiving doses of 40 mg/d for at least 2 years. However, the results of six trials using tamoxifen doses of 20 mg/d, continuously for 5 years, found a twofold increase in endometrial cancer in women receiving tamoxifen compared to women receiving placebo.[66] This twofold increase in risk of endometrial cancer is similar in magnitude to that associated with postmenopausal estrogen replacement therapy. Arguments have been made that this was acceptable because the endometrial cancer induced by tamoxifen is low stage and low grade, is easily treated with surgery or other means, and does not pose a life-threatening risk to women. There have been no reports of liver cancer in patients receiving 20 mg/d dose and only two in patients receiving 40 mg/d. The carcinogenic potential of tamoxifen is of some concern in the adjuvant and chemoprevention settings. These would not be concerns in the metastatic breast cancer setting due to the length of survival associated with metastatic breast cancer.

Treatment of Locally Advanced Breast Cancer (Stage III)

"Locally advanced cancer of the breast" refers to breast carcinomas with significant primary tumor and nodal disease but where distant metastases cannot be documented. This stage of breast cancer has been shown to be poorly controlled by radical surgery alone and also to have a poor prognosis. Patients may present with a wide spectrum of disease, ranging from large tumors to skin or chest wall involvement, sometimes associated with advanced regional lymph node tumor involvement. Many patients with stage III breast cancer have disease that is technically unresectable at diagnosis. Inflammatory breast cancer with pathological evidence of dermal lymphatic tumor permeation with clinical findings of diffuse erythema in duration and edema of at least 30% of the breast usually without a palpable mass is a special type of locally advanced breast cancer.

Local regional therapy of locally advanced breast cancer consists of surgery, radiation, or a combination of the two. With mastectomy alone, the reported local recurrence rate ranges from 6–40%, and with radiation alone 25–50%. Survival with either modality is about 40–50% at 5 years and 30% at 10 years.[67,68] Radiation therapy can be effective in controlling these locally advanced cancers, however, doses greater than that used to treat early stage tumors are required. Whereas 5000 cGy is effective in irradicating microscopic amounts of tumor in breast conservation techniques, doses in excess of 6000 cGy are required for gross tumor. These higher doses of radiation therapy are associated with moderate to severe arm edema, brachial plexopathy, and adverse cosmetic effects such as breast retraction and telangiectasia. The results from a number of nonrandomized and randomized trials suggest that there is no advantage for mastectomy over primary radiation therapy in patients with stage III disease. The benefit of combining mastectomy and postoperative radiation for patients with locally advanced breast cancer is controversial. Retrospective studies of patients treated with a combination of mastectomy and radiation have shown excellent local tumor control (local-regional recurrence 10–20%) in 5 years compared with mastectomy or radiation alone (15–40%), but demonstration of a definitive impact on survival is lacking. Addition of radiation to mastectomy to improve local tumor control must be balanced against the possible increase and likelihood of complications. Unfortunately, similar to early breast cancer, distant metastases are the ultimate cause of death.

In the early 1980s, reports began to appear in the literature describing improvement in local-regional tumor control, DFS, and, in some instances, overall survival with combinations of multiagent chemotherapy, surgery, and radiation.[69–71] The natural history of locally advanced breast cancer suggested that even when local-regional control was accomplished, systemic relapse and death from breast cancer were eventually observed in the majority of patients. This led to interest in the use of "neoadjuvant" or "primary" chemotherapy in locally advanced breast cancer. Neoadjuvant or primary chemotherapy is the administration of systemic chemotherapy prior to a definitive local-regional procedure. Early aggressive systemic therapy has been used to control micrometastases, reduce tumor bulk, and allow for more limited procedures for local control. Primary or neoadjuvant chemotherapy followed by surgery with radiation therapy or both, and adjuvant systemic therapy has become the treatment choice for locally advanced breast cancer, including inflammatory breast cancer. Most tumors respond with more than a 50% decrease in tumor size, approximately 70% of patients experience downstaging through neoadjuvant chemotherapy. Breast conservation is possible for many patients with locally advanced breast cancer, and almost all patients initially are rendered disease free.

Although it is clear that neoadjuvant chemotherapy should be the initial choice of treatment for patients with locally advanced breast cancer, it is unclear what the optimal sequence of subsequent therapies should be, whether one or two local treatment modalities are necessary, and whether the addition of hormonal therapy to chemotherapy has significant benefit. The use of neoadjuvant treatment strategies for early breast cancer is currently under evaluation. One of the research directions to improve the survival of patients with locally advanced breast cancer is dose intensification of neoadjuvant or postoperative (adjuvant) chemotherapy. Several reports of open phase II trials have suggested an early benefit in DFS. No definite survival benefits have been reported; however, comparative trials are necessary to assess the relative value of dose intensification in this group of patients.

Treatment of Metastatic Breast Cancer (Stage IV)

The goal of therapy with early breast cancer, as well as locally advanced breast cancer, is to cure the disease. However, once breast cancer has advanced beyond a local-regional disease, it is currently incurable. Treatment of metastatic breast cancer with either cytotoxic or endocrine therapy often results in regression of disease and improvements in quality of life. In patients who respond to therapy with either endocrine or cytotoxic therapy, duration of survival is also increased. The goal of treatment of metastatic breast cancer is to improve symptoms and quality of life. Thus, it is important to choose therapy with good activity while minimizing toxicities. The choice of therapy for metastatic disease is based on the site of disease involvement and presence or absence of certain characteristics. For example, patients who experience a long DFS following local-regional therapy, or have disease that is primarily located in the bone or soft tissue, or are late premenopausal or postmenopausal will likely respond to endocrine therapy. The most important factor predicting response to endocrine therapy, however, is the presence of estrogen and progesterone receptors in the primary tumor tissue. Fifty to 60% of ER positive patients and 75–80% of ER and PR positive patients will respond to hormonal therapy, while those with ER and PR negative tumors have a less than 10% response rate. Thus, the largest factor determining choice of endocrine versus cytotoxic chemotherapy is the presence of hormone receptors in the primary breast tumor. Site of disease is also important in that numerous studies have shown that endocrine therapy is more likely to be effective in patients with bone and soft tissue metastases. Visceral involvement (i.e., liver) and central nervous system involvement are generally nonresponsive to hormonal therapy and seldom respond to chemotherapy. Endocrine therapy is the treatment of choice for patients who are hormone receptor positive and exhibit the first sign of metastatic disease in soft tissue, bone, or pleura due to the equal probability of response to hormonal compared chemotherapy and the lower toxicity profile of endocrine therapy.

Patients who respond to initial endocrine therapy often respond to a second hormonal manipulation. Response rate is lower and duration of response is shorter with secondary hormonal manipulations. Patients are sequentially treated with endocrine therapy until they have progressive symptoms resulting from rapidly growing metastatic disease, at which time cytotoxic chemotherapy can be given. Women with hormone receptor negative tumors, with rapidly progressive lung, liver, or bone marrow involvement, or those having failed initial endocrine therapy, are not likely to benefit from endocrine therapy and are usually treated initially with cytotoxic chemotherapy.

ENDOCRINE THERAPY

In general, there is little evidence that the response or survival benefit from one endocrine therapy is superior to that achieved with other therapies. Tamoxifen, progestins, aminoglutethimide, estrogens, and androgens, as well as surgical procedures including oophorectomy, adrenalectomy, and hypophysectomy, have been shown to be equivalent in many randomized trials. Because most endocrine therapies are equally effective, the choice of a particular one is based primarily on toxicity (Table 120.10). In women who received tamoxifen as adjuvant therapy, tamoxifen is still usually the preferred initial agent in the metastatic setting. An exception to this occurs when the patient is currently receiving adjuvant tamoxifen at the time of diagnosis of metastatic disease. In these cases, either a progestin or chemotherapy is generally employed.

Tamoxifen is generally considered to be the agent of choice in both premenopausal and postmenopausal women with metastatic breast cancer who are also hormone receptor positive. Tamoxifen is usually administered in doses of 10 mg twice daily or 20 mg once daily. There is no advantage for higher doses of tamoxifen. Moreover, long-term administration of very high doses of tamoxifen (e.g., 12 months of 60–100 mg/m^2 twice daily) have been associated with decreased visual acuity and retinopathy.

With a dose schedule of 20 mg/d, serum tamoxifen levels gradually rise to reach a steady state at about week 16. The half-life of a single dose of tamoxifen is 9–12 hours, but the half-life after chronic dosing is 7 days. Serum tamoxifen levels can be detected 6 weeks after discontinuation of therapy. Thus, the maximum beneficial effects of tamoxifen are not observed for at least 2 months following initiation of therapy and it is unlikely that symptoms of metastatic disease will return if patients miss several doses. The toxicities of tamoxifen are described in the adjuvant endocrine therapy section of this chapter. The only additional toxicity that one might expect to find in the setting of metastatic breast cancer is a tumor flare or hypercalcemia, which occurs in approximately 5% of patients following the initiation of endocrine therapy. Tumor flare or hypercalcemia is not an indication to discontinue tamoxifen therapy. This phenomenon has also been associated with other endocrine therapies. It is generally accepted that this is a positive indication that the patient will respond to endocrine therapy.

The effectiveness of tamoxifen in premenopausal women has been compared with oophorectomy in two randomized trials. In general, there was no difference in the overall response rate. However, the secondary response rate to oophorectomy after tamoxifen treatment was somewhat higher than to tamoxifen after primary oophorectomy (33% versus 11%).[72] This has been interpreted by some experts as suggesting that tamoxifen does not completely antagonize estrogen production, particularly in premenopausal women.

TABLE 120.10. ENDOCRINE THERAPIES USED FOR METASTATIC BREAST CANCER

Class	Drug	Dose	Side Effects
Antiestrogen	Tamoxifen	10–20 mg PO bid	Disease flare, hot flashes, nausea, vomiting, edema
LHRH analogs	Leuprolide	7.5 mg sq q28d	Amenorrhea, hot flashes, occasional nausea
	Goserelin	3.6 mg sq q28d	
Progestins	Medroxyprogesterone acetate	400–1000 mg IM qwk	Weight gain, hot flashes, vaginal bleeding
	Megestrol acetate	40 mg PO qid	
Aromatase inhibitors	Aminoglutethimide	250 mg PO bid × 2 weeks then qid with hydrocortisone 40 mg/d	Lethargy, rash, postural dizziness, ataxia, nystagmus
Estrogens	Diethylstilbestrol	5 mg PO tid	Nausea/vomiting, fluid retention, hot flashes, anorexia, thromboembolism, hepatic dysfunction
	Ethinylestradiol	1 mg PO tid	
	Conjugated estrogens	2.5 mg PO tid	
Androgens	Fluoxymesterone	10 mg PO bid	Deepening voice, alopecia, hirsutism, facial/truncal acne, fluid retention, menstrual irregularities, cholestatic jaundice

Ovarian ablation is still commonly used in some parts of the United States and is considered by many specialists to be the endocrine therapy of choice in premenopausal women. The mortality rate with surgical oophorectomy is low, usually less than 2–3% in appropriately selected patients. The response rate in postmenopausal patients was less than 6%, thus, oophorectomy should never be employed in this group.[6]

Medical castration with LHRH analogues has been used in premenopausal metastatic breast cancer patients and found to induce remissions in about one-third of unselected cases. The mechanism of action of LHRH analogues in breast cancer is thought to result from down-regulation of LHRH receptors in the pituitary. Decreased levels of luteinizing-hormone subsequently led to a decrease in estrogen to castrate levels. Thus, the effect of LHRH analogs on circulating estrogen levels in premenopausal breast cancer simulates oophorectomy. The two agents that are available in the United States include leuprolide and goserelin. Both of these agents are administered as a subcutaneous injection every 4 weeks and are associated with minimal side effects including amenorrhea, hot flashes, and occasional nausea. Studies using oophorectomy, tamoxifen, or LHRH analogues as first-line therapy in premenopausal patients with metastatic breast cancer are necessary to determine the definitive choice for initial therapy. Combination endocrine therapy with tamoxifen plus an LHRH analog is also under investigation. The rationale behind this combination is that tamoxifen interferes with peripheral estradiol production and the LHRH analogue interferes with ovarian estradiol production.

Progestins such as megesterol acetate (Megace) and medroxyprogesterone acetate (Provera) have been compared with tamoxifen in randomized trials and have been found to yield equal or equivalent response rates. Although there were no direct comparisons of these two forms of progestational therapy, they appear to be equally effective. Medroxyprogesterone acetate is more frequently used in Europe and megesterol acetate in the United States. A number of recent trials have suggested progestins may be an alternative to first-line therapy with tamoxifen. The side-effect profile of progestins is generally very good. The most common dose used for Megace is 160 mg/d, but doses as high as 1600 mg/d have been used. Currently, several randomized trials are being conducted with high-dose megesterol therapy in an attempt to increase response rates. The higher dose regimens may be associated with both better response rates and better quality of life although this is yet to be widely accepted in the scientific community. Side effects are more frequent with high-dose regimens. The most common side effects include weight gain, which may occur in 20–50% of patients. Patients experiencing weight gain may have fluid retention, but fluid retention is not responsible for total weight gain. In cachectic cancer patients, the weight gain may be desirable, however, this is not uniformly true of all patients with metastatic breast cancer. Additional side effects associated with progestins include vaginal bleeding in 5–10% of patients either while patients are taking the progestational agent or when it is discontinued, and somewhat less than a 10% incidence of hot flashes.[6]

Aminoglutethimide given with corticosteroids is among the more effective and less toxic forms of endocrine therapy. Aminoglutethimide decreases peripheral estrogen concentrations by inhibiting cytochrome P-450-dependent conversion of androstenedione to estrone in target tissues. At higher doses, it also inhibits the adrenal conversion of cholesterol to pregnenolone, resulting in a decrease in androstenedione. The standard dose of aminoglutethimide is 250 mg orally four times per day. Hydrocortisone 40 mg/d divided into three doses is usually administered with aminoglutethimide. Hydrocortisone is generally administered at the dose of 10 mg at 3:00 PM and 10 mg at 6:00 PM and 20 mg at 10:00 PM. The rationale behind this dosage administration of hydrocortisone is that it mimics the natural cortisol production, and thereby prevents suppression of the hypothalamic pituitary axis. This should, in theory, prevent the development of Addisonian crises. More recently, aminoglutethimide doses as low as 250 mg twice daily have been reported to be effective in postmenopausal metastatic breast cancer. Low doses of aminoglutethimide may selectively inhibit peripheral conversion of androstenedione to estrone without significantly inhibiting any adrenal function. Consequently, it might not be necessary to add hydrocortisone in order to avoid adrenal insufficiency. However, death secondary to Addisonian crises after a low-dose aminoglutethimide without hydrocortisone has been reported. Neither dose has been specifically approved by the Food and Drug Administration for use in the treatment of breast cancer in the United States.

Aminoglutethimide has been compared to tamoxifen in adrenalectomy and hypophysectomy in randomized trials. In general, response rates are equivalent, but in several trials, aminoglutethimide plus hydrocortisone appeared to be more effective than tamoxifen.[73,74] Aminoglutethimide is somewhat more toxic than tamoxifen oophorectomy or progestins, although most of the toxicities disappear within 6 weeks after initiation of therapy. Aminoglutethimide is chemically related to the sedative glutethimide (Doriden). Therefore, it is not surprising that approximately one-third of patients experience lethargy. Approximately 20% of patients will develop a rash during the first weeks of aminoglutethimide therapy. This is not an indication for discontinuation of aminoglutethimide and it can be alleviated by a transient doubling of the steroid dose. Additional side effects include nystagmus, ataxia, lethargy, dizziness, and nausea. Aminoglutethimide and hydrocortisone are generally considered third-line hormonal therapy in the treatment of metastatic breast cancer.[6]

Estrogens and androgens are used rarely today because these agents are more toxic than the other drugs discussed thus far. The estrogens used most frequently are diethylstilbestrol (DES) 5 mg three times a day, ethinyl estradiol 1 mg three times a day, or Premarin 2.5 mg three times a day. Approximately one-third of patients placed on estrogens will discontinue them because of toxic side effects, the most important of which are vomiting and fluid retention. Less common side effects include areolar hyperpigmentation, breast tenderness and engorgement, vaginal discharge, incontinence, hot flashes, and phlebitis. It is appropriate to use half doses of estrogen during the first month of therapy with a gradual increase in dose as the patient experiences fewer side effects. Although there is speculation, there is little evidence that estrogens stimulate tumor growth in premenopausal patients with breast cancer. However, it is generally accepted that estrogens are not effective in premenopausal patients. About one-third of patients who respond to estrogens will have a withdrawal response if estrogens are discontinued at the first evidence of tumor regrowth. Estrogens are not infrequently associated with a disease flare. This may manifest as the appearance of flu symptoms or an exacerbation of disease symptoms beginning several days after initiating therapy and subsiding spontaneously within a month. Most commonly, these symptoms consist of a diffuse achiness or increase in pain at sites of metastases. Hypercalcemia is the most serious side effect associated with the tumor flare and is seen most commonly in women with metastatic bone disease.

Androgens have been shown in randomized trials to be less effective than estrogens.[75] All the effective androgens have masculinizing effects including hirsutism and acne in more than 50% of patients. Androgens are the endocrine therapy most associated with the "flare" and androgen therapy is occasionally useful in older women with congestive heart failure because androgen use is not accompanied by fluid retention whereas both progestins and estrogens can exacerbate congestive heart failure.

CYTOTOXIC THERAPY

Cytotoxic chemotherapy will eventually be required in most patients with metastatic breast cancer. Patients with hormone receptor negative tumors usually require chemotherapy at the first sign of symptomatic metastases. As previously stated, even patients who initially respond to hormone manipulations will eventually cease to respond and go on to require and benefit from chemotherapy. Combination chemotherapy will result in an objective response in approximately two-thirds of patients previously unexposed to chemotherapy. The majority of patients have partial responses and complete disappearance of disease occurs in less than 20% of patients treated. The median duration of response is 5–12 months, however, some patients will have an excellent response to an initial course of chemotherapy and may live 5 to more than 10 years without evidence of disease. In general, survival of patients after treatment with commonly used drug combinations for metastatic breast cancer is a median of 14–33 months. The median time to response has ranged from 2–3 months in most studies, but this period is dependent in large part on the site of measurable disease. The median time to appearance of response is between 3–6 weeks in patients whose disease is primarily in the skin and lymph nodes, 6–9 weeks for patients with metastatic lung involvement, 15 weeks with hepatic involvement, and nearly 18 weeks in patients with bone involvement. Thus, it is oftentimes the case that an immediate response to therapy is not apparent and, in general, once a chemotherapy regimen has been initiated, it is continued until there is unequivocal evidence of progressive disease.

There are no well-defined clinical characteristics or established tests to identify patients likely to benefit from chemotherapy. Factors associated with an increased probability of response which have been identified include a good performance status, a limited number (one to two) of disease sites, and patients who respond to chemotherapy or hormonal therapy with a long disease-free interval. Patients whose disease progresses during chemotherapy have a lower probability of response to a different type of chemotherapy. However, this is not necessarily true for patients who are given chemotherapy after some interval during which they have received no chemotherapy. Patients who do not respond to endocrine therapy are as likely to respond to chemotherapy as patients who are treated with chemotherapy as their initial treatment modality. Age, menopausal status, site of disease, and receptor status have not been associated with favorable or unfavorable response to chemotherapy.

A number of chemotherapeutic agents have demonstrated activity in the treatment of breast cancer, including doxorubicin, cyclophosphamide, fluorouracil, methotrexate, mitozantrone, vinblastine, mitomycin-C, thiotepa, and melphalan. The objective response rates reported with these drugs as single-agent therapy range from 20–40%. The drug discovery program of the National Cancer Institute and the pharmaceutical industry have recently provided oncologists with a wide array of new chemotherapeutic agents that have considerable potential for breast cancer treatment.[76] Foremost among these new agents are paclitaxel and vinorelbine, which have been associated with impressive response rates of up to 50% in patients with metastatic breast disease. In spring 1994, paclitaxel (Taxol) was approved by the FDA for single-agent treatment of metastatic breast cancer for patients who had relapsed following therapy with a doxorubicin-containing regimen. The recommended dose of paclitaxel is 175 mg/m^2 every 21 days, which is considerably higher than the dose used for treatment of ovarian cancer, the other disease for which paclitaxel has obtained FDA approval for use. Efforts are now being directed toward optimizing dose and schedule of paclitaxel in the metastatic setting and its integration into combination regimens. Vinorelbine (Navelbine), a microtubule interactive agent, has also shown impressive response rates in metastatic breast cancer. Navelbine was approved by the FDA in December 1994, for the treatment of non–small cell lung cancer. It is not yet approved for breast cancer; however, response rates in patients with advanced breast cancer to weekly IV doses of 30 mg/m^2 of vinorelbine range from 30–50% with an overall 5% complete response rate in the phase I/II studies reported. As has been observed with paclitaxel, patients with less prior treatment fare better than those who are more heavily pretreated. Importantly, both paclitaxel and vinorelbine display evidence of not being cross-resistant with anthracyclines, which are currently considered the most active agents in metastatic breast cancer.

Other agents that have undergone phase II testing in breast cancer include edatrexate, losoxantrone, docetaxol, as well as several others. It remains to be determined, however, whether these drugs possess substantial advantages over other members of their class.

Combination chemotherapy regimens have been associated with higher response rates than single-agent therapy in the treatment of metastatic breast cancer. The chemotherapy regimens which are frequently used first line in the metastatic setting are similar, if not identical, to the ones previously described for the adjuvant setting. If doxorubicin was included in the first-line regimen, second-line combinations in common use include mitomycin-C (10 mg/m^2) on day 1 and vinblastine (5 mg/m^2) on days 1 and 15 repeated every 4 weeks; VATH (vinblastine 4.5 mg/m^2 IV D1, doxorubicin 45 mg/m^2 IV D1, thiotepa 12 mg/m^2 IV D1, fluoxymesterone [Halotestin] 10 mg PO TID); or single-agent treatment with paclitaxel, vinorelbine, nitrosurea derivatives, platinum derivatives, or mitoxantrone. Recent investigation has focused on designing combination regimens which include vinorelbine or paclitaxel.

The probability of a response to chemotherapy among patients whose disease worsens while they are receiving a first combination regimen is, in general, between 20–40%. Patients who have been treated with chemotherapy whose disease progresses after an interval during which chemotherapy was not given (6 months or more) have a much higher probability of a secondary response including a secondary response to the regimen to which they previously responded. In the past, the benchmark for gauging response to secondary chemotherapy was whether they had previously been exposed to doxorubicin. For example, patients who had not been previously exposed to doxorubicin were said to have a higher probability of responding to doxorubicin-containing regimens compared to patients who had been previously exposed to doxorubicin. However, the availability of the newer antineoplastic agents, paclitaxel and vinorelbine, may make these comparisons less pivotal in the future. Other issues that remain to be determined in the management of metastatic breast cancer with systemic chemotherapy include optimal duration of treatment and the combination chemotherapy regimen of first, second, and third choice. Use of combination chemotherapy in conjunction with hormonal therapies is also being investigated for the treatment of metastatic disease.

Research innovations designed to improve the efficacy of combination chemotherapy have included the use of high doses of drugs. There is an undeniable dose response effect for most of the drugs used to treat breast cancer. Very high doses of single agents or combinations have been used with autologous bone marrow transplant to circumvent dose-limiting myelosuppression. Autologous bone marrow transplantation has developed during the past decade as a treatment for solid tumors responsive to, but not currently cured by, chemotherapy. Metastatic breast cancer has been the model for solid tumors in a number of large autologous bone marrow transplant research programs. A recent review of the results of these programs suggest that patients with refractory metastatic disease have a high response rate, but the duration of response is brief.[77,78] However, patients with metastatic breast cancer who obtain a complete response or a near complete response to conventional combination chemotherapy regimens may derive a far greater benefit from participation in high-dose chemotherapy with autologous bone marrow transplantation programs. From the limited data available, it would appear that approximately 10–20% of patients who receive high-dose chemotherapy with autologous bone marrow transplant following, obtaining a complete or near complete response to conventional chemotherapy, may in fact be cured of their disease or at least derive the benefit of a prolonged disease-free interval.

RADIATION THERAPY

Radiation is an important modality in the treatment of symptomatic metastatic disease. The most common indication for the treatment with radiation therapy is painful bone metastases or other localized sites of disease refractory to systemic therapy. Approximately 90% of patients treated for painful bone metastases will obtain significant pain relief. Radiation is also an important modality in the palliative treatment of metastatic brain lesions and spinal cord lesions which respond poorly to systemic therapy, as well as eye or orbit lesions and other sites where significant accumulation of tumor cells occurs.

PREVENTION AND EARLY DETECTION OF BREAST CANCER

Current efforts at breast cancer prevention are directed toward the identification and removal of risk factors. Unfortunately, a number of risk factors associated with development of breast cancer do not lend themselves to modification. For example, family history of breast cancer or personal history of breast or other gynecological malignancies cannot be modified. Women with a very high risk of breast cancer based on family history or personal history may sometimes be considered for a prophylactic bilateral mastectomy. Isolation and cloning of breast cancer susceptibility genes will allow screening of women with histories suggestive of "breast cancer families" in the near future and identification of appropriate candidates for prophylactic bilateral mastectomy. There are currently no absolute indications for prophylactic bilateral mastectomy. This surgery is considered for women at very high risk for the development of breast cancer, particularly if the women's breast are difficult to evaluate by both physical examination and mammography, and she has persistent disabling fears that she will have the disease.

In the past 5 years, there has been increasing interest in "chemoprevention" of breast cancer. These include interventions directed at inhibiting neoplastic development through pharmacological measures. Two important agents being studied in research on breast cancer chemoprevention are retinoids and tamoxifen. Retinoids (all vitamin A [Retinol] and its isomers derivatives and synthetic analogs) are biological regulators of orderly epithelial cell development and are therefore potentially ideal agents for controlling abnormal epithelial proliferation which occurs in carcinogenesis. The agent that is currently receiving the most attention as a chemoprevention agent is tamoxifen. Although we traditionally think of tamoxifen as an antiestrogen, it appears that it has estrogenic activity in other areas of the body and systems other than the breast. For example, early results of several trials suggest that tamoxifen can prevent or retard loss of bone density which occurs in osteoporosis thereby mimicking the effect of postmenopausal estrogen replacement.[63,64] In addition, it appears that tamoxifen, like estrogens, has a favorable effect on lipoproteins.[79] As previously described, tamoxifen is useful as an adjunct after treatment of primary breast cancer, especially in postmenopausal women. In randomized trials of tamoxifen as an adjuvant treatment for breast cancer, women who received tamoxifen were also found to have a reduced incidence of contralateral primary breast carcinomas.[51] This coupled with laboratory evidence that tamoxifen can inhibit carcinogen-induced mammary tumors and spontaneously occurring mammary carcinomas in laboratory animals has been the basis for the development and implementation of randomized trials to evaluate the benefits of tamoxifen as a chemoprevention agent in this country as well as in several European countries.

The NSABP is currently conducting a trial in the United States that compares 5 years of tamoxifen therapy to placebo in 16,000 women aged 35 and older who are at increased risk for breast cancer (The Breast Cancer Prevention Trial [BCPT]). This trial is the first large chemoprevention trial conducted in the United States and has generated a great deal of controversy. Controversy largely surrounds the unknown benefit of tamoxifen therapy as a chemoprevention agent, and the potential for risk associated with its administration. Tamoxifen has been repeatedly shown to be a relatively safe drug with an acceptable toxicity profile when used to treat patients with breast cancer. Tamoxifen therapy is associated with several manageable toxicities such as hot flashes, menstrual irregularities, and vaginal discharge, as well as with more serious side effects such as thromboembolic events and endometrial tumors. The ultimate benefit and costs associated with use of tamoxifen as a chemoprevention agent in breast cancer awaits the results of the NSABP trial as well as trials that are ongoing in several European countries. Unfortunately, even if the design of these trials proves to be sufficient to answer the research question, the results will still not be available until the late 1990s or early 2000s.

The association of early childbirth and menopause with decreased breast cancer risk and the finding that the use of oral contraceptives for 5 years reduces the incidence of endometrial and ovarian cancer suggest that pharmacological hormone interventions during the reproductive years may have a beneficial impact on reducing breast cancer risks as well as the risk of other gynecological malignancies.[80] Reversible elimination of ovarian function via the use of LHRH analogs has been suggested as a way of reducing breast cancer risks. Another theoretical approach would be to use an oral contraceptive during the teenage years that would simulate pregnancy. Although such approaches may seem radical, it is important to point out that most young women employ some form of oral contraceptive during the childbearing years, and that epidemiological and animal evidence suggests that these types of hormonal manipulations could potentially reduce the incidence of breast cancer.

The rationale for early detection of breast cancer is based on the clear relationship between stage of breast cancer at diagnosis and the probability for cure. Thus, if all breast cancer could be detected at a very early stage of the disease (i.e., small primary tumor and negative lymph nodes), then more patients with the disease could be cured. Screening guidelines for early detection of breast cancer have been put forward by the American Cancer Society, the U.S. Preventive Task Force, and the National Cancer Institute (Table 120.11). Currently, the American Cancer Society recommends that all women over the age of 20 perform monthly breast self-examinations. There is evidence to support this recommendation and at least one investigator has demonstrated that women who perform breast self-examinations were generally diagnosed with an earlier stage of the disease and had a higher 5-year survival rate when compared to women who did not perform self-examinations.[81] Numerous brochures are available which outline the

TABLE 120.11. GUIDELINES FOR EARLY DETECTION OF BREAST CANCER

	U.S. Preventive Task Force	American Cancer Society	National Cancer Institute
Breast self-exam (BSE)	NR	Monthly (20+)	NR
Clinical breast exam (CBE)	Every year (40+)[a]	3 years (20–40) Annual (40+)	3 years (20–40) Annual (40+)
Mammogram	NR (40–49) 1–2 years (50+)	1–2 years (40–49) Annual (50+)	NR (40–49) Annual (50+)

Key: NR, no recommendation.
[a]For high-risk women, start CBE at age 35.

current methodology for performing breast examinations. It is generally agreed that for this to be an effective screening tool, the examination should be thorough and conducted at approximately the same time in a woman's monthly cycle. Recommendations for breast examination by a physician (clinical breast exam) vary among the three groups. A large majority of breast cancers are discovered by patients during regular self-examinations. Therefore, the value of the clinical breast exam recommendation for women who perform regular self-examinations is questionable. However, since many women fail to perform monthly self-examinations, an annual physician examination may be of value to them.

Clearly, the largest area of controversy in screening recommendations for breast cancer surrounds annual mammography. Most, if not all, guidelines recommend annual mammography for women 50 years old and older. Nearly 75% of all breast cancer occurs in women 50 years of age or greater and it has been conclusively demonstrated by a large number of independent studies that regular use of screening mammography can reduce mortality from breast cancer from 20–40% in this age group. Controversy regarding the use of screening mammography is largely confined to women less than 50 years of age. The American Cancer Society recommends that a baseline mammography be performed between 35 and 40 years of age, and that screening mammography occur every 1–2 years in the 40- to 50-year age group. However, in December 1993, the National Cancer Institute withdrew its support of the use of screening mammography in women less than 50 years of age. This was based on a report of the National Cancer Institute's, International Workshop on Screening for Breast Cancer, held in February 1993.[82] Data from eight major randomized control trials of breast cancer screening performed over the last 30 years were reviewed and it was concluded that no benefit from screening women between the ages of 40 and 49 years was apparent 5–7 years after enrollment into any of these studies. Possible reasons for these findings include the much lower incidence of breast cancer in women 40–49 years of age, as well as the increased density of breast tissue found in menstruating women, which renders detection of lesions by mammography more difficult.

Opponents of screening women less than 50 years of age suggest that multiple studies have failed to prove a benefit among women 40–49 years of age. However, proponents for screening women 40–49 years of age claim that the studies were not designed to detect a difference of 25–30% decrease in mortality for women 40–49 years. A recent review of these trials concluded that none of the trials included in the analysis conducted by the National Cancer Institute had the statistical power to be able to provide clear proof of benefit for screening women ages 40–49 years because none of the trials involved sufficient numbers of women in these age groups.[83] These authors suggest that the conclusion from these trials is a benefit from screening was demonstrated that lacked statistical significance. Five of the eight trials with all their performance and design flaws (insufficient numbers of women ages 40–49 years, poor quality mammography, single-view mammography, 2-year screening interval, high contamination rate, and high intervention threshold) are showing a benefit, which indicates the benefit would be significant if the number of women in these trials had been sufficiently large to permit statistical significance. The debate regarding the value of screening mammography in women less than 50 years of age continues among various health care providers and is the source of great confusion for the health care consumer.[84,85]

Significant advances in the safety and efficacy of screening mammography have occurred during the past two decades. This has allowed superior visualization of breast and breast tissue with a concurrent reduction in the dose of radiation that is delivered. Approximately 10% of all palpable masses are not detected by mammography. This is most commonly observed in premenopausal women and is felt to be directly related to the increased density of breast tissue in this estrogen-rich environment. Current estimates are that for women ages 40–50 years, the effect of 10 mammographies would cause 60 mammography-related breast cancers in 1 million women.[86] As women age, incidence for developing mammography-related breast cancer is lower because of the lower carcinogenic effects of radiation in older women. Although the safety and efficacy of screening mammography in terms of image quality and dosimetry are very acceptable, the American College of Radiology (ACR) has recognized for some years the need for greater quality control in mammography. A voluntary accreditation program developed by this organization and adopted by various state and federal agencies has greatly improved the overall quality of mammography in the majority of facilities in this country.[87] Many of the details of the accreditation process have recently been adopted for use by governmental agencies culminating in the Mammography Quality Standards at QS of 1992. This act, which essentially codifies the ACR program, assures that all mammographic facilities will now be required to achieve a common high standard of quality assurance. Responsibility for operation of the act has been given to the FDA. As of October 1, 1994, all facilities that offer mammography must be FDA-certified to remain open. Passage of this landmark legislation, as well as provision of appropriate levels of funding to conduct this program, represents an important contribution to the health of women.

Evaluation of Therapeutic Outcomes

The desired therapeutic outcome of adjuvant therapy of breast cancer differs significantly from that of metastatic disease. Adjuvant therapy—chemotherapy, hormonal therapy, or both—is administered with curative intent. The rational behind adjuvant therapy in breast cancer is that breast cancer, even when diagnosed in early stages where clinical evidence of distant spread is not apparent, is a systemic disease that spreads early to distant sites. Adjuvant therapy is intended to eradicate these micrometastases and thus cure the patient of breast cancer. Therefore, the overall goal of adjuvant therapy is to cure the disease, which is something that cannot be fully evaluated for years following initial diagnosis and treatment. In addition, since there is no clinical evidence of disease at the time adjuvant therapy is administered, assessment of disease response is not possible. Instead, a predetermined number of cycles of adjuvant therapy and/or years of hormonal therapy is administered. Oftentimes, adjuvant chemotherapy is associated with significant toxicity. Maintaining dose intensity has been demonstrated to be important in cure of disease and, therefore, optimizing supportive care measures such as antiemetics and growth factors is highly recommended.

Palliation is the therapeutic outcome in treatment of metastatic breast cancer. In general, the least toxic therapies are used initially with increasingly aggressive therapies applied in a sequential fashion and in a manner that doesn't significantly compromise the quality of the patient's life. Tumor response to a particular treatment regimen may be measured by clinical chemistry such as liver enzyme elevation in a patient with hepatic metastases, or imaging techniques such as bone scans or chest x-rays. However, assessment of the patient's clinical status and symptom control is often adequate to evaluate response to the therapy administered. In the patient with metastatic breast cancer, it is common to initiate hormonal therapy or chemotherapy and continue administration until signs and symptoms of disease progress or new signs and symptoms present. Optimizing quality of life is the therapeutic endpoint in the treatment of patients with metastatic breast cancer. A number of valid and reliable tools are available for objective assessment of quality of life in patients with breast cancer.

Conclusion

Breast cancer is the most commonly occurring cancer in women in the United States and is second only to lung cancer as the most common cancer cause of death. The incidence of breast cancer has been increasing during the past 50 years and has increased rapidly since the early 1980s. It is unclear whether the recent increase in the incidence of breast cancer reflects a true increase in the new cases of this disease or, instead, increased detection of the disease by screening mammography. The etiology of breast cancer is unknown; however, a number of factors have been identified that increase a woman's chances of developing the disease. These risk factors, as well as information regarding the biology of the disease, suggest that a complex interplay between hormones, genetic factors, and environmental and lifestyle influences all contribute to the etiology of this disease. The recent identification of the BRCA1 gene, a tumor suppresser gene important in the development of inherited and perhaps sporadic breast and ovarian cancer, holds promise in identifying patients at high risk, as well as improving our basic understanding of the causes of breast and ovarian cancer.

The majority of breast cancers are diagnosed in early stages before the disease has disseminated to sites distant from the breast. Treatment consists of local management, as well as systemic adjuvant therapy with either chemotherapy, hormonal therapy, or a combination of these. Breast conservation therapy, which consists of complete removal of the tumor (lumpectomy), combined with breast irradiation and axillary lymph node sampling, is currently the preferred method of treatment for most patients with localized breast cancer. Patients who are not candidates for breast conservation or who do not choose this local therapy will generally receive the modified radical mastectomy.

It is apparent from clinical and laboratory experiments and observation that the spread of breast cancer via the bloodstream occurs early in the course of the disease. This results in patients relapsing with systemic metastatic disease following local curative therapy. The likelihood of later development of metastatic disease is related to the size of the primary tumor, presence or absence of lymph node involvement, and a number of additional pathological prognostic factors, which include proliferative capacity, nuclear grade, hormone receptor status, and presence or absence of oncogenes and other protein products. Systemic adjuvant therapy is commonly administered to patients with localized breast cancer following surgical procedures to diminish the risk or delay disease recurrence. Specific recommendations for adjuvant therapy are determined by stage of the disease, age of the patient, presence of hormone receptors in the primary tumor, as well as other pathological prognostic factors. Adjuvant therapy treatment recommendations have been developed by an NIH consensus conference, as well as an international consensus group and these treatment recommendations continue to evolve as new data become available.

Advanced breast cancer includes locally advanced breast cancer (stage III) and metastatic breast cancer (stage IV). Treatment of stage III breast cancer generally consists of a combination of surgery, radiation, and chemotherapy administered in an aggressive approach. Although response rates and survival have improved, there is still much progress to be made in stage III breast cancer. Metastatic breast cancer is, in the majority of cases, incurable. The only exception to this is that some promising long-term response rates have been observed in a subset of patients with metastatic disease who have a complete response to conventional chemotherapy and then receive autologous bone marrow transplant with high-dose chemotherapy. Unfortunately, this represents a small number of the total population of patients with metastatic breast cancer. Metastatic breast cancer is treated with endocrine therapy or combination chemotherapy. Patients who are hormonal receptor positive will generally receive initial endocrine therapy followed by combination chemotherapy when endocrine therapy fails. Patients who are hormone receptor negative or have disease involving the liver or central nervous system will generally receive combination chemotherapy as first-line therapy of metastatic disease. Combination chemotherapy will result in an objective response in approximately 70% of patients previously unexposed to chemotherapy. The majority of patients have partial response and complete disappearance of disease occurs in less than 20% of patients treated. Median duration of response is 5–12 months, however, some patients will have an excellent response to an initial course of chemotherapy and may live 5–10 years without evidence of disease. In general, survival of patients after treatment with commonly used drug combinations for metastatic breast cancer is a median of 14–33 months. Response to second- and third-line combination chemotherapy has been on the order of 20–40%. This is in large part dependent on previous chemotherapy regimens the patient has received. The availability of paclitaxel and vinorelbine offers the promise of more successful second- and third-line treatment of metastatic breast cancer in the future.

Current efforts at breast cancer prevention are directed toward the identification and removal of risk factors. In addition, two agents, the retinoids and tamoxifen, are being evaluated for their ability to prevent breast cancer. Any statement regarding the value of these modalities awaits the results of ongoing clinical trials. Early detection of breast cancer remains an important modality for decreasing breast cancer mortality. The rationale for early detection of breast cancer is based on the clear relationship between stage of breast cancer at diagnosis and the probability of a cure. Screening guidelines for early detection of breast cancer have been developed by the American Cancer Society, the U.S. Preventive Task Force, and the National Cancer Institute. Although all these agencies agree that annual clinical breast exam and screening mammographies should be performed in women older than 50, controversy exists regarding the value of screening women in the 40–50 age group. This controversy has, unfortunately, created a great deal of confusion in the general public.

Intensive research efforts are ongoing in all aspects of breast cancer etiology, detection, prevention, and treatment. Efforts in the past have resulted in substantial reduction in mortality in selected patient subsets. Hopefully, the information obtained in the next decade will result in the knowledge required to significantly reduce mortality from breast cancer for all women.

References

1. Boring CC, Squires TS, Tong T, Montgomerie S. Cancer statistics 1994. CA Cancer J Clin 1994;44:7–26.
2. Miller BA, Ries LAG, Hankey BF, et al (eds). Cancer Statistics Review: 1973–1990. Bethesda, MD, National Cancer Institute, Report NIH 93-2789, 1993.
3. Miller BA, Feuer EJ, Hankey BF. Recent incidence trends for breast cancer in women and the relevance of early detection: An update. CA Cancer J Clin 1993;43:27–41.
4. Sondik EJ. Breast cancer trends: Incidence mortality and survival. Cancer 1994;74:995–999.
5. Feuer EJ, Wun LM, Boring CC, et al. The lifetime risk of developing breast cancer. J Natl Cancer Inst 1993;85:892–897.
6. Henderson IC, Harris JR, Kinne DW, Hellman S. Cancer of the breast, in DeVita VT Jr, Hellman S, Rosenberg SA (eds): Cancer Principles and Practice of Oncology, 3rd ed. Philadelphia, JB Lippincott, 1989, pp 1197–1034.
7. Harris JR, Lippman ME, Veronesi U, Willett W. Breast Cancer. Part 1. N Engl J Med 327(5):319–328.
8. Colditz GA, Stampfer MJ, Willett WC. Prospective study of estrogen replacement therapy and risk of breast cancer in postmenopausal women. JAMA 1990;264:2648–2653.
9. Dupont WD, Page DL. Menopausal estrogen replacement therapy and breast cancer. Arch Intern Med 1991;151:67–72.
10. Steinberg KK, Thacker SB, Smith SJ, et al. A meta-analysis of the effect of estrogen replacement therapy on the risk of breast cancer. JAMA 1991;265:1985–1990.
11. DiSaia PJ. Hormone-replacement therapy in patients with breast cancer. Cancer 1993;71(4):1490s–1500s.
12. Romieu I, Berlin JA, Colditz G. Oral contraceptives and breast cancer: Review and meta-analysis. Cancer 1990;66:2253–2263.

13. Harris JR, Morrow M, Bonadonna G. Cancer of the breast, in DeVita VT Jr., Hellman S, Rosenberg SA (eds): Cancer: Principles of Oncology, 4th ed. Philadelphia, JB Lippincott, 1993, pp 1264–1324.
14. Thompson WD. Genetic epidemiology of breast cancer. Cancer 1994;74(1):279–287.
15. Weber BL, Abel JK, Brody LC, et al. Familial breast cancer. Cancer 1994;74(3):1013–1020.
16. Byers T. Nutritional risk factors for breast cancer. Cancer 1994;74(1):288–295.
17. Howe GR. Dietary fat and breast cancer risks. Cancer 1994;74(3):1078–1084.
18. Howe GR, Friedenreich CM, Jain M, Miller AB. A cohort study of fat intake and risk of breast cancer. J Natl Cancer Inst 1991;83:336–340.
19. Nagao M, Ushijima T, Wakabayashi K, et al. Dietary carcinogens and mammary carcinogenesis. Cancer 1994;74(3):1063–1069.
20. Schapira DV, Kumar NB, Lyman GH. Obesity, body fat distribution and sex hormones in breast cancer patients. Cancer 1991;67:2215–2218.
21. Longnecker MP. Alcohol consumption in relation to risk of breast cancer. Cancer Causes Control 1994;5(1):73–82.
22. Schatzkin A, Longnecker MP. Alcohol and breast cancer. Cancer 1994;74:1101–1110.
23. McKenna RJ. The abnormal mammogram radiographic findings, diagnostic optional, pathology, and stage of cancer diagnosis. Cancer 1994;79(1):244–255.
24. Kopans DB. The Breast Imaging Report. Philadelphia, JB Lippincott, 1989, pp 351–353.
25. Frykberg ER, Bland KI. Overview of the biology and management of ductal carcinoma in situ of the breast. Cancer 1994;74(1):350–361.
26. Frykberg ER, Bland KI. *In situ* breast carcinoma. Adv Surg 1993;26:29–72.
27. Neilsen M, Jensen J, Andersen JA. Precancerous and cancerous breast lesions during lifetime and at autopsy: A study of 83 women. Cancer 1984;54:612–615.
28. Frykberg ER, Ames FC, Bland KI. Current concepts for management of early (in situ and occult invasive) breast carcinoma, in Bland KI, Copeland EM (eds): The Breast: Comprehensive Management of Benign and Malignant Diseases. Philadelphia, WB Saunders, 1991, pp 731–751.
29. Hutchins L, Broadwater R Jr, Lang N, et al. Breast cancer. DM 1990;35:63–125.
30. Harris JR, Lippman ME, Veronesi U, Willett W. Breast cancer. N Engl J Med 1992;327(6):390–398.
31. Fisher B, Slack NH, Bross IDJ. Cancer of the breast: Size of neoplasm and prognosis. Cancer 1969;24:1071–1080.
32. Nemoto T, Vana T, Bedwani RN, et al. Management and survival of female breast cancer. Cancer 1980;45:2917–2924.
33. Valagussa P, Bonadonna G, Veronesi U. Patterns of relapse and survival in operable breast carcinoma with positive and negative axillary nodes. Tumori 1978;64:241–258.
34. McGuire WL, Clark GM. Prognosis in breast cancer. Recent Results Cancer Res 1989;115:170–174.
35. Osborne CK. Prognostic factors in breast cancer. Princ Pract Oncol Updates 1990;4:1–11.
36. Mansour EG, Ravdin PM, Dressler L. Prognostic factors in early breast cancer. Cancer 1994;74(1):381–400.
37. Dressler LG, Bartow SA. DNA flow cytometry in solid tumors: Practical aspects and clinical applications. Semin Diagn Pathol 1989;6:55–82.
38. Hedley DW, Clark GM, Cornelisse CJ, et al. Consensus review of the clinical utility of DNA cytometry in carcinoma of the breast. Cytometry 1993;14:482–485.
39. Hedley DW, Rugg CA, Gelber RD. Association of DNA index and S-phase fraction with prognosis of nodes positive early breast cancer. Cancer Res 1987;47:4729–4735.
40. Brifford M, Spyratos F, Tubiana-Hulin M, et al. Sequential cytopunctures during pre-operative chemotherapy for breast cancer: Cytomorphologic changes, initial tumor ploidy and tumor regression. Cancer 1989;63:631–637.
41. Spyrotas F, Brifford M, Tubiana-Hulin M, et al. Sequential cytopunctures during pre-operative chemotherapy for primary breast carcinoma: II. DNA flow cytometry changes during chemotherapy, tumor regression and short-term follow-up. Cancer 1992;69:470–475.
42. Remvikos Y, Beuzobon P, Zadjela A, et al. Correlation of pre-treatment proliferative activity with response to cytotoxic chemotherapy. J Natl Cancer Inst 1989;81:1383–1387.
43. Fisher B, Redmond C, Fisher E, et al. Relative worth of estrogen or progesterone receptor and pathologic characteristics of differentiation as indicators of prognosis in node-negative breast and Bowel Project Protocol B-06. J Clin Oncol 1988;6:1076–1087.
44. LeDoussal V, Tubiana-Hulin M, Hacene K, et al. Nuclear characteristics as indicators of prognosis in node-negative breast cancer patients. Breast Cancer Res 1989;14:207–216.
45. Gasparini G, Pozza F, Harris AL. Evaluating the potential usefulness of new prognostic and predictive indicators in node-negative breast cancer patients. J Natl Canc Inst 1993;85(15):1206–1219.
46. Oza AM, Tannock IF. Clinical relevance of breast cancer biology. Hem/Onc Clin North Am 1994;8(1):1–11.
47. Nemoto T, Vana J, Bedwani RN, et al. Management and survival of female breast cancer: Results of a national survey by the American College of Surgeons. Cancer 1980;45:2917–2924.
48. Fisher B, Redmond C, Fisher ER, et al. Ten-year results of a randomized clinical trial comparing radical mastectomy and total mastectomy with or without radiation. N Engl J Med 1985;312:674–681.
49. Fisher B, Redmond C, Poisson R, et al. Eight-year results of a randomized clinical trial comparing total mastectomy and lumpectomy with or without irradiation in the treatment of breast cancer. N Engl J Med 1989;320:822–828.
50. NIH Consensus Conference. Treatment of early-stage breast cancer. JAMA 1991;265:391–395.
51. Early Breast Cancer Trialists' Collaborative Group T. Systemic treatment of early breast cancer by hormonal, cytotoxic, or immune therapy: 133 randomized trials involving 31,000 recurrences and 24,000 deaths among 75,000 women. Lancet 1992;339:1–15, 1–85.
52. Adjuvant Therapy of Primary Breast Cancer: The Saint Gallen conference. Recent Results Cancer Res 1993;127:1–300.
53. Henderson JC. Adjuvant systemic therapy for early breast cancer. Cancer 1994;74(1):401–409.

54. Shapiro CL, Henderson IC. Adjuvant therapy of breast cancer. Hem/Onc Clin North Am 1994;8(1):213–231.
55. Ravdin PM. A practical view of prognostic factors for staging, adjuvant treatment planning, and as baseline studies for possible future therapy. Hem/Onc Clin North Am 1994;8(1):197–211.
56. Misset JL, Gil-Delgado M, Fomoleau P, et al. Ten-year results of the French Adjuvant Trial for node positive breast cancer comparing CMF to a combination of Adriamycin, vincristine, cyclophosphamide, and 5-fluorouracil, in Salmon SE (ed): Adjuvant Therapy of Cancer VII. Philadelphia, JB Lippincott, 1993, pp 75–80.
57. Buzzoni R, Bonadonna G, Valagussa P, Zambetti M. Adjuvant chemotherapy with doxorubicin plus cyclophosphamide, methotrexate, and fluorouracil in the treatment of resectable breast cancer with more than three positive axillary nodes. J Clin Oncol 1991;9:2134–2140.
58. Livingston RB. Dose intensity and high dose therapy. Two different concepts. Cancer 1994;74:1177–1183.
59. Winer EP. Quality-of-life research in patients with breast cancer. Cancer 1994;74:410–415.
60. Levine MN, Gent M, Hirsh J, et al. The thrombogenic effect of anticancer drug therapy in women with stage II breast cancer. N Engl J Med 1988;318:404–407.
61. Curtis RE, Boice JD Jr, Stovall M, et al. Risk of leukemia after chemotherapy and radiation treatment for breast cancer. N Engl J Med 1992;326:1745–1751.
62. Henderson IC, Sloss JL, Jaffe N, et al. Serial studies of cardiac function in patients receiving adriamycin. Cancer Treat Rep 1978;62:923–929.
63. Love RR, Mazess RB, Barden HS, et al. Effects of tamoxifen on bone mineral density in postmenopausal women with breast cancer. N Engl J Med 1992;326:852–856.
64. Love RR, Wiebe DA, Newcomb PA, et al. Effects of tamoxifen on cardiovascular risk factors in postmenopausal women. Ann Intern Med 1992;115:860–864.
65. Catherino WH, Jordan VC. A risk-benefit assessment of tamoxifen therapy. Drug Safety 1993;8(5):381–397.
66. Nayfield SG, Karp JE, Ford LG, et al. Potential role of tamoxifen in prevention of breast cancer. J Natl Cancer Inst 1991;83:1450–1459.
67. Fowble B, Goodman RL, Glock JH, Rosato EF, editors. Breast Cancer Treatment: A Comprehensive Guide to Management. St. Louis, Mosby Year Book, 1991.
68. Monyak D, Levitt SH. Breast: Locally advanced (T3 and T4) and recurrent tumors, in Perez CA, Brady LW (eds): Principles and Practice of Radiation Oncology, 2nd ed. Philadelphia, JB Lippincott, 1992, pp 948–969.
69. De Lena M, Varini M, Zucali R, et al. Multimodal treatment for locally advanced breast cancer: Results of chemotherapy-radiotherapy versus chemotherapy-surgery. Cancer Clin Trials 1981;4:229–236.
70. Perez CA, Graham ML, Taylor ME, et al. Management of locally advanced carcinoma of the breast. Cancer 1994;74(1):453–465.
71. Hortobagyi GN. Multidisciplinary management of advanced primary and metastatic breast cancer. Cancer 1994;74:416–423.
72. Ingle JN, Krook JE, Green SJ, et al. Randomized trial of bilateral oophrectomy versus tamoxifen in premenopausal women with metastatic breast cancer. J Clin Oncol 1986;4:178–185.
73. Abrams JS, Moore TD, Friedman M. New chemotherapeutic agents for breast cancer. Cancer 1994;74:1164–1176.
74. Lipton A, Harvey HA, Santen RJ, et al. Randomized trial of aminoglutethimide versus tamoxifen in metastatic breast cancer. Cancer Res 1982;42:3434s–3435s.
75. Smith JE, Harris AL, Morgan M, et al. Tamoxifen versus aminoglutethimide versus combined tamoxifen and aminoglutethimide in the treatment of advanced breast carcinoma. Cancer Res 1982;42:3430s–3433s.
76. Henderson IC. Endocrine therapy of metastatic breast cancer, in Harris JR, Hellman S, Henderson IC, Kinne DW (eds): Breast Diseases. Philadelphia, JB Lippincott, 1987, pp 398–428.
77. Ayash LJ. High dose chemotherapy with autologous stem cell support for the treatment of metastatic breast cancer. Cancer 1994;74(1):532–535.
78. Gilbert C. The role of autologous bone marrow transplantation in breast cancer. Highlights on antineoplastic drugs. 1991;9(3):48–52.
79. Rössner S, Wallgren A. Serum lipoproteins and proteins after breast cancer surgery and effects of tamoxifen. Atherosclerosis 1984;52:339–346.
80. Bernstein L, Ross RK, Henderson BE. Prospects for the primary prevention of breast cancer. Am J Epidemiol 1992;135:142–152.
81. Huguley CM, Brown RL, Greenberg RS, Clark WS. Breast self-examination and survival from breast cancer. Cancer 1988;62:1389–1396.
82. Fletcher SW, Black W, Harris R, et al. Report of the international workshop on screening for breast cancer. J Natl Cancer Inst 1993;85:1644–1656.
83. Kopans DB, Halpern E, Hulka CA. Statistical power in breast cancer screening trials and mortality reduction among women 40–49 years of age with particular emphasis on the National Breast Screening Study of Canada. Cancer 1994;74(4):1196–1203.
84. Dupont WD. Evidence of efficacy of mammographic screening for women in their forties. Cancer 1994;74(4):1204–1206.
85. Kopans DB, Halpern E, Hulka CA. Mammography screening for breast cancer. Cancer 1994;74(4):1212–1216.
86. Rosato FE, Rosenberg AL. Examination techniques: Role of the physician and patient in evaluating breast disease, in Bland KI, Copeland EM (eds): The Breast. Philadelphia, WB Saunders, 1991, pp 409–418.
87. Osuch JR, Camburn JF, Sienko DG, Potchen EJ. The history and the effect of the mammography quality assurance legislation in Michigan. Cancer 1994;74(1):270–263.

Chapter 121

Lung Cancer

Rebecca S. Finley, PharmD, MS

Lung cancer is a major cause of morbidity and mortality that has reached epidemic proportions in many industrialized countries. The American Cancer Society estimated that 169,000 new cases of lung cancer were diagnosed in the United States during 1995 and that 157,000 deaths were attributed to this disease during the same year.[1] Despite major advances in the understanding and management of the disease, the overall 5-year survival rate for all types of lung cancer remains 13%.[1]

Lung cancer accounts for 14% of all cancer in men and 13% of all cancer in women.[1] It is the leading cause of cancer death in men ages 35 years and older (accounting for 32% of all cancer deaths in men) and the leading cause of cancer death in women (24% of all cancer deaths).[1] In 1987, for the first time, lung cancer surpassed breast cancer as the primary cause of cancer death among American women.[1] The incidence of lung cancer increases with age; the peak age of diagnosis is between 55 and 65 years. Among patients 40 years of age and older, the likelihood that a solitary pulmonary nodule seen on chest x-ray is a carcinoma is high, and this probability increases proportionally with age.[2]

ETIOLOGY

Lung carcinomas arise from pluripotent epithelial cells, which are capable of expressing a variety of phenotypes.[3] The natural history of lung cancer begins with exposure of these cells to carcinogens, which causes chronic inflammation and eventually leads to genetic and cytologic changes that progress to carcinoma.[4] Hereditary phenotypes that influence activation or detoxification of carcinogens may influence the risk of lung cancer.[4] Activation of protooncogenes and uncontrolled secretion of growth factors also contribute to cellular proliferation and this malignant transformation.[5,6] Numerous studies have established the relationship between tobacco exposure and lung cancer. The American Cancer Society estimates that cigarette smoking is responsible for about 83% of all lung cancer cases and studies have established a dose–response relationship between the number of cigarettes smoked, the duration of smoking, tar and nicotine content of cigarettes, and the development of lung cancer.[4,7] Mattson et al.[8] estimated that a 35-year-old man who smokes 25 cigarettes per day or more has a 13% risk of dying of lung cancer before age 75. The increased rate of lung cancer deaths among women has also been attributed to increased smoking.[1] Cessation of smoking is associated with a gradual decrease in the risk, but a long period of time (more than 6 years) is necessary before an appreciable diminution of the risk occurs.[9,10] Passive exposure to cigarette smoke is believed to contribute to the increased risk of lung cancer in nonsmokers living with smokers.[11–13]

Other carcinogens also increase the risk of lung cancer and may act synergistically with cigarette smoking.[4] Occupational or environmental exposure to asbestos, chloromethyl ethers, various heavy metals, polycyclic aromatic hydrocarbons, and radon has also been associated with the development of lung cancer.[4] In addition, the incidence of lung cancer is higher in urban than in rural areas and air pollution has been implicated as a possible causative agent.[14] Observational epidemiologic data have suggested that intake of β-carotene and carotene (vitamin A) are inversely associated with lung cancer risk.[15,16] The first prospective randomized chemoprevention trial using antioxidants in a large, well-nourished population was reported in 1994.[17] This trial randomized more than 29,000 middle-age male smokers to receive dietary supplementation with β-carotene, alpha-tocopherol, or both for 6 years. Interestingly, the trial failed to detect any significant protective effect of either vitamin and, in fact, there were significantly more new cases of lung cancer in the group treated with β-carotene.

HISTOLOGIC CLASSIFICATION

The World Health Organization lung cancer classification is accepted worldwide (Table 121.1).[18] Four major cell types of carcinomas (i.e., squamous cell carcinoma, adenocarcinoma, and large cell and small cell carcinomas) account for more than 90% of all lung tumors.[19] Histologic confirmation of cell type is usually made by light microscopy and is essential in treatment planning because of differences in the

TABLE 121.1. WORLD HEALTH ORGANIZATION CLASSIFICATION OF LUNG CANCER

I. Benign
II. Dysplasia and carcinoma *in situ*
III. Malignant
  A. Squamous cell carcinoma (epidermoid)
  B. Small cell carcinoma
    1. Oat cell
    2. Intermediate cell
    3. Combined oat cell
  C. Adenocarcinoma
    1. Acinar
    2. Papillary
    3. Bronchoalveolar
    4. Mucus secreting
  D. Large cell carcinoma

(From Ref. 4.)

natural histories, clinical features, and response to therapy of the various types. Several additional biologic and cytogenetic characteristics (e.g., secretion of peptide hormones, autocrine growth factor receptors, specific mutations, or chromosomal deletions of lung tumors) are currently being evaluated for their prognostic significance. In terms of management strategy and overall prognosis, adenocarcinoma and squamous cell, and large cell carcinomas are frequently grouped together and referred to as non–small cell lung cancers (NSCLCs).

Although once the most common type of NSCLC, squamous cell (or epidermoid) carcinoma now accounts for less than 30% of all lung cancers and is distinguished histologically by evidence of squamous differentiation.[4,17] This tumor tends to be central in origin, arising from metaplastic bronchial epithelium, and frequently extends into the bronchial lumen resulting in obstruction. Squamous cell carcinomas (along with small cell lung cancers) have a much higher incidence among smokers and among males.[4] Although they can grow rapidly, most squamous cell carcinomas tend to be slow growing and confined to the lungs (especially early in the disease course). Such tumors may eventually metastasize to the hilar and mediastinal lymph nodes, liver, adrenal glands, kidneys, bone, and gastrointestinal tract.[19]

Adenocarcinoma is now the most common type of lung cancer in North America, accounting for about 40%. This is partly due to the increased incidence of lung cancer in women who tend to have more adenocarcinomas than epidermoid cancers. These tumors are usually located in the peripheral sections of the lung and are distinguished pathologically by a glandular or papillary pattern and mucin production.[4] Adenocarcinomas may present as a single nodule, multifocal nodules, or rapidly progressing, bilateral, diffuse processes. However, they are likely to metastasize at an early stage (often before the diagnosis of the primary tumor) and spread widely to distant sites including the contralateral lung, liver, bone, adrenal glands, kidneys, and central nervous system.[19]

Large cell carcinomas are anaplastic tumors that show no evidence of differentiation.[19] These tumors account for only about 15% of all lung cancers.[4] The large cell carcinomas tend to be large and bulky tumors arising in the periphery of the lung and tend to have a propensity to metastasize in a pattern quite similar to that of adenocarcinomas.[19]

Small cell carcinomas (sometimes called oat cell carcinoma) account for about 25% of all lung tumors[19] and epidemiologic evidence suggests that it is the most rapidly increasing type of lung cancer, especially in women.[20] They are distinguished by a proliferation of neoplastic cells with round to oval nuclei.[19] These tumors tend to arise in the central portion of the lung but may also be found in the lung periphery. Small cell lung carcinoma (SCLC) is a very aggressive and rapidly growing tumor with about 60–70% of patients initially presenting with disseminated disease outside of the hemithorax.[4] SCLC secretes gastrin-releasing peptide that acts as an autocrine growth factor.[21] Secretion of other peptide hormones, cytogenetic abnormalities, and amplification and increased expression of oncogenes are also common. This disease has a propensity to metastasize to the lymph nodes, opposite lung, liver, adrenal glands and other endocrine organs, bone, bone marrow, and central nervous system.[19]

Lung tumors frequently exhibit more than one histology. Occasionally patients also have multiple lung nodules arising in different lobes or the contralateral lung. This is referred to as *synchronous tumors* and the nodules may be of similar or different cell types.[22] This usually worsens the patient's overall prognosis.

CLINICAL PRESENTATION

Location and extent of the tumor will determine the presenting signs and symptoms. If the lesion is in the central portion of the bronchial tree, it is likely to cause symptoms at an earlier stage than a lesion in the periphery of the lung, which may remain asymptomatic until the lesion is quite large or has spread to other areas. The most common initial signs and symptoms include cough, dyspnea, chest pain, sputum production, and hemoptysis. Unfortunately, many patients with lung cancer also have chronic pulmonary and/or cardiovascular diseases (usually related to smoking), and such symptoms may go unnoticed or be attributed to the concomitant disease. Many patients also exhibit systemic symptoms such as anorexia, weight loss, and fatigue that are suggestive of a malignancy.[4,23] Other signs and symptoms that may be associated with the primary tumor or its spread within the thorax are listed in Table 121.2. Such symptomatology may occur at the tumor's initial presentation or at any point during its recurrence or progression.

Disseminated disease also may be responsible for extrapulmonary signs and symptoms such as neurologic deficits resulting from central nervous system (CNS) metastases, bone pain or pathologic fractures secondary to bone metastases, or liver dysfunction resulting from tumor involvement in the liver.

Paraneoplastic syndromes are signs and symptoms which occur at sites away from the primary tumor or its metastases and are not associated with "direct" tumor involvement. They may be due to the production of biologically active substances (e.g., peptide hormones) or antibodies, or other undefined mechanisms. Paraneoplastic syndromes occur more frequently with lung cancer than any other tumor. These syndromes may be the first signs of a tumor and may prompt the search for an underlying malignancy. Paraneoplastic syndromes that commonly occur in association with lung cancers include cachexia, hypercalcemia, syndrome of inappropriate hormone secretion, and Cushing's syndrome.[4,23]

TABLE 121.2. COMMON SIGNS AND SYMPTOMS OF LUNG CANCER

- Local signs and symptoms associated with primary tumor or regional spread within the thorax
  - Cough
  - Hemoptysis
  - Dyspnea
  - Rust-streaked or purulent sputum
  - Chest, shoulder, or arm pain
  - Wheeze and stridor
  - Superior vena caval obstruction
  - Pleural effusion or pneumonitis
  - Dysphagia (secondary to esophageal compression)
  - Hoarseness (secondary to laryngeal nerve paralysis)
  - Horner's syndrome
  - Phrenic nerve paralysis
  - Pericardial effusion/tamponade
  - Tracheal obstruction
- Extrapulmonary signs and symptoms associated with metastatic involvement
  - Bone pain and/or pathologic fractures
  - Liver dysfunction
  - Neurologic deficits
  - Spinal cord compression
- Paraneoplastic syndromes
  - Weight loss
  - Cushing's syndrome
  - Hypercalcemia
  - Syndrome of inappropriate antidiuretic hormone (SIADH)
  - Pulmonary hypertrophic osteoarthropathy
  - Clubbing
  - Anemia
  - Eaton–Lambert myasthenic syndrome

SCREENING

At the time of initial diagnosis, many patients with lung cancer have advanced disease and unfortunately the prognosis is poor. In an attempt to detect lung tumors earlier and improve the cure rate, screening studies have been conducted in high-risk populations (e.g., men over age 40 who smoke).[24–26] Chest x-rays and sputum cytology have been the most commonly used screening techniques in these studies. Although several of these studies have demonstrated that lung cancers may be detected at an earlier stage, actual mortality rates are not affected.[25,26] Furthermore, chest x-rays and sputum cytology are associated with false-positive results in approximately 5% and 0.5% of these high-risk individuals, respectively, leading to needless and costly workups and anxiety.[27] Currently, no biochemical markers (tumor markers) have been identified with sufficient sensitivity and specificity to reliably screen for early lung cancer.

DIAGNOSIS

Once signs and symptoms of lung cancer have been recognized, chest x-rays and computed tomography (CT) scans are the most valuable diagnostic tests. Chest x-ray is the primary method of lung cancer detection and may also be useful in measuring tumor size, establishing gross lymph node enlargement, and aiding in detection of other tumor-related findings such as pleural effusion, lobar collapse, and metastatic bone involvement of ribs, spine, and shoulders. CT is helpful in all of the above as well as in evaluation of parenchymal lung abnormalities, detection of masses only suspected on the chest x-ray, and assessment of mediastinal and hilar lymph nodes.

Clinical characteristics of a lung nodule may also help to differentiate benign from malignant nodules[28] and thus determine when invasive diagnostic tests are warranted. For example, benign lesions usually have sharp borders, whereas malignant lesions usually have irregular or radiating borders.

When there is clinical and radiologic evidence of a tumor, pathologic confirmation must be established. This may be accomplished by examination of sputum cytology and/or tumor biopsy by fiber optic bronchoscopy, percutaneous needle biopsy, or open-lung biopsy. All patients must also have a thorough history and physical examination with emphasis on detecting signs and symptoms of the primary tumor, regional spread of the tumor, distant metastases, and paraneoplastic syndromes. The physical examination also aids in determining whether or not a patient may be able to withstand aggressive surgery or chemotherapy.

Unfortunately, by the time the tumor is diagnosed, dissemination has already occurred in many patients. Determination of the extent (or stage) of the tumor involvement is important because it will aid in the selection of treatment, and estimation of the probability of cure and survival, as well as facilitating comparison of the individual patient to large-scale clinical trials.

STAGING

NON-SMALL CELL LUNG CANCER

The American Joint Committee[29] has established a TNM staging classification for lung cancer based on the primary tumor size and extent (T), regional lymph node involvement (N), and the presence or absence of distant metastases (M). Table 121.3 outlines this staging system. For comparison of various therapeutic modalities, a more simple stage grouping system is also used in which stage I refers to tumors confined to the lung without lymphatic spread, stage II refers to large tumors with ipsilateral peribronchial or hilar lymph node involvement, stage III includes other lymph node and regional involvement, and stage IV includes any tumor with distant metastases.[29]

The primary tumor is assessed using chest x-rays and fiber optic bronchoscopy while lymphatic spread is usually assessed by mediastinoscopy, gallium-67 citrate scanning, or CT.[4] If the history and physical examination or other routine clinical studies (e.g., CBC, liver functions tests) suggest the possibility of metastatic disease, then special scans (e.g., bone, brain, or liver) or biopsies (e.g., bone marrow or liver) may be necessary for staging.[4]

SMALL CELL LUNG CANCER

A two-stage classification established by the Veterans Administration Lung Cancer Study Group is widely used in the United States to stage SCLS.[23] Limited disease is classified as disease confined to one hemithorax and to the regional lymph nodes. All other disease is classified as extensive. Approximately 70% of patients initially present with extensive disease. Because of this high frequency of disseminated disease at diagnosis (bone 38%, liver 22–28%, bone marrow 17–23%, CNS 8–14%), radionuclide scans of the bone and liver, CT scans of the brain, and bone marrow biopsies are generally recommended prior to initiation of therapy.[23,30] In addition, any suspicious signs or symptoms detected during the physical examination should be carefully investigated.

TABLE 121.3. TUMOR (T), NODE (N), AND METASTASIS (M) STAGING FOR LUNG CANCER

T_X	Positive malignant cell; no lesion seen
T_1	≤3 cm surrounded by lung or visceral pleura
T_2	>3 cm or involvement of main bronchus 2 cm or more distal to the carina, or invasion of visceral pleura, or associated atelectasis or obstructive pneumonitis extending to hilar region
T_3	Direct invasion of chest wall, diaphragm, mediastinal pleura, or parietal pericardium; or tumor in main bronchus less than 2 cm distal to the carina; or associated atelectasis or obstructive pneumonitis of the entire lung
T_4	Invasion of mediastinum, heart, great vessel, trachea, esophagus, vertebral body, carina; or tumor with a malignant pleural effusion
N_0	No regional lymph node involvement
N_1	Metastasis in ipsilateral peribronchial and/or ipsilateral hilar lymph nodes, including direct extension
N_2	Metastasis in ipsilateral mediastinal and/or subcarinal lymph node(s)
N_3	Metastasis in contralateral mediastinal, contralateral hilar, ipsilateral or contralateral scalene, or supraclavicular lymph node(s)
M_0	No distant metastases
M_1	Distant metastases

Stage Groupings

Stage I	T_1	N_0	M_0
	T_2	N_0	M_0
Stage II	T_1	N_1	M_0
	T_2	N_1	M_0
Stage III_A	T_1	N_2	M_0
	T_2	N_2	M_0
	T_3	N_0,N_1,N_2	M_0
Stage III_B	Any T	N_3	M_0
	T_4	Any N	M_0
Stage IV	Any T	Any N	M_1

(From Ref. 29.)

MANAGEMENT

NON-SMALL CELL LUNG CANCER

Currently only surgery and to a lesser extent, radiation therapy offers an opportunity for long-term survival in a significant percentage of patients; however, only about 30% of unselected patients have localized disease (stage I or II) that is amenable to local therapy.[4] Curative therapy in this disease is determined by the anatomic stage of the disease (it must be localized with no evidence of distant metastases) and the ability of the patient to withstand the therapy. If untreated, most patients die within 1 year of diagnosis.[2]

Surgery

Surgical resection is the treatment of choice for patients with clinical stage I and II disease (disease that by all evidence is stage I or II before surgical dissection of mediastinal lymph nodes).[2] Overall, more than 50% of patients with stage I and 35% of patients with stage II disease who undergo surgical resection survive 5 years without disease recurrence.[4] The single most important prognostic factor in patients undergoing curative resection is the presence or absence of lymph node involvement. In one series of 216 patients that had clinical stage I disease before surgery only 125 patients were found to have stage I disease after surgery and lymph node dissection.[31] Therefore, it is apparent that mediastinal lymph node dissection at the time of surgery is of great importance. Klingman and DeMeester[32] reported that only 25% of patients with T_1N_0 or T_2N_0 disease that underwent lobectomy had recurrences. Other series have reported 5-year survival rates of 73–90% for patients with stage I disease.[33,34] Stage II disease (N_1) has a poorer prognosis. In one series, patients with stage II disease had only a 34% 2-year survival versus 62–72% for patients with stage I disease.[35] Pneumonectomy (versus lobectomy) is indicated in patients found to have lymph node involvement at the time of surgery and such patients may benefit from postoperative radiation therapy or radiation plus chemotherapy.[2,36] Even if no residual disease is evident at surgery, 50% of patients die within 2 years as a result of recurrent disease.[4]

The size of the tumor in stage I and II disease also has prognostic importance. In patients with stage I disease (old staging system), Martini and Beattie[31] reported a 5-year survival rate of 80% when the primary tumor was 3 cm or less but only 50% when the tumor was larger than 3 cm. It has been suggested that pneumonectomy, rather than lobectomy, also may reduce the rate of local recurrences in patients with larger stage I tumors.[32]

Stage III_A tumors also are considered surgically resectable with 5-year survival rates ranging from 20–50% depending on tumor size and lymph node involvement.[37–40]

Radiation

Radiation therapy is considered an alternative modality in patients with stage I or II disease who decline surgery or are considered high surgical risks because of concomitant illness or restrictive pulmonary reserve.[4] In addition, radiation therapy may also be utilized when the tumor is not resectable because of fixation to a major blood vessel, the trachea, or esophagus. The 2- and 5-year survival rates appear to be highest for patients whose tumors would otherwise be considered resectable.[41] Local control of tumor growth may be achieved in up to 60% of patients with stage III disease; however, the overall 5-year survival is only about 6%.[4] When radiation therapy is given after surgery it may reduce the incidence of local recurrences; however, it does not appear to improve survival because distant metastases still occur.[4]

In situations when radiation is used with curative intent, relatively higher doses and large treatment volumes are required and there are significant risks to the normal tissue surrounding the tumor (see section on Complications and Supportive Care).

Chemotherapy

Because many patients with NSCLC are inoperable at diagnosis (e.g., locally advanced stage III_B or metastatic disease stage IV), and because systemic dissemination occurs in the majority of patients who are initially surgically resected or radiated for potential cure, there is clearly a definite need for effective systemic therapy (i.e., chemotherapy) in this disease.

Metastatic or Recurrent Disease

Unfortunately, the response rates for chemotherapy in NSCLC have been disappointingly low and overall survival benefits have not been clearly demonstrated; thus there is no standard chemotherapy regimen for NSCLC. However, it does appear that patients who respond to chemotherapy are likely to have a survival benefit over nonresponders.[42] It is unclear if this survival advantage is related to the chemotherapy or some biologic characteristic of the disease that would permit prolonged survival independent of any treatments.[4] Several factors have been suggested as having prognostic importance in terms of response and survival in patients receiving chemotherapy. These factors include the patient's initial performance status, weight loss, and extent of disease.[43,44] Among these factors, an initial favorable performance status of the patient appears to be the most consistent factor predicting a better response and improved survival.[43,44] There is no evidence of the usefulness of chemotherapy in persons with a Karnofsky performance status of less than 50%.[4]

Direct comparison of response rates between clinical trials is difficult and interpretation of the results requires careful analysis of the methodology. Two factors that must be considered are the method of patient selection and the criteria for response that were used. As previously mentioned, several factors are believed to have prognostic significance and it is necessary to know the status of such factors (i.e., performance status, extent of disease prior to therapy) in the study population when comparing clinical trials. Likewise, it is important to know if patients with an unfavorable prognosis were intentionally excluded from the trial. In addition, to compare results of clinical trials, it is imperative that both trials utilize the same response criteria. In most series a complete response is defined as the complete disappearance of all evidence of the tumor while a partial response is defined as a reduction in measurable tumor mass of greater than 50% lasting longer than 1 month. Because many lung tumors do not have definite margins to measure, the term *objective response* is used to describe disease where there has been a definite decrease in the size of the lesion without appearance of any new lesions.[4]

Single-agent chemotherapy has generally demonstrated objective response rates of 5–15% with no significant effect on overall survival. When responses do occur after single-agent chemotherapy the duration of the response is usually quite brief (2–4 months) and complete responses are rare.[4] Among the most active single agents in NSCLC are cisplatin, carboplatin, vinblastine, vinorelbine, ifosfamide, etoposide, mitomycin, and paclitaxel and the investigational drugs vindesine, gemcitabine, docetaxel, irinotecan, topotecan, edetrexate, and epirubicin.

Combination chemotherapy has been utilized in the management of NSCLC since the late 1960s and, although response rates for combination therapy generally have been better than those for single-agent therapy, consistent improvement in overall survival rates has been more difficult to demonstrate. Therefore, the use of combination chemotherapy in advanced NSCLC remains controversial.

The introduction of cisplatin hailed the most significant development in combination therapy in NSCLC. Today it is included in the most widely studied and recommended regimens. Table 121.4 describes some of the cisplatin-containing regimens studied in NSCLC. The most widely studied of these combinations are the "CAP" regimens, cyclophosphamide (C), doxorubicin (A), and cisplatin (P) and the various cisplatin-etoposide regimens. In general, response rates have been in the range of 20–40% with responders surviving longer than nonresponders and complete responses occurring only rarely.

Preclinical studies demonstrated that cisplatin and etoposide were synergistic against some experimental leukemia cell lines and subsequent highly successful results of this combination in testicular cancer led to its evaluation in lung cancer and other tumors. Two randomized studies comparing single-agent cisplatin to the cisplatin and etoposide regimen reported higher response rates for the combination; however, no overall survival benefits were realized.[57,66]

Active regimens that have commonly reported response rates exceeding 30% have used various combinations of cisplatin, ifosfamide, mitomycin, and vinblastine, vinorelbine, or vindesine. Table 121.4 describes some of these combinations; however, at the present time no single regimen is considered standard therapy for NSCLC. Evidence suggests that the dose of cisplatin may have an impact on response. Single-agent cisplatin trials in NSCLC demonstrated higher response rates for increasing doses and a meta-analysis of 100 chemotherapy regimens showed that cisplatin 100 mg/m^2 (in combination with other agents) had higher response rates than trials using 70 mg/m^2.[4] Despite modest improvements in response rates in many trials, most responses continue to be only partial and brief in duration. Furthermore, response rates and survival durations have varied widely between clinical trials using the same regimen, suggesting wide variations in the patient populations and supportive care. In general, patients with stage III disease are more likely to respond than those with stage IV. Because of the questionable benefits of chemotherapy in terms of overall survival advantage in NSCLC and the toxic effects associated with its use, it is common practice to reserve chemotherapy for patients with a good performance status and otherwise favorable prognosis. Several randomized trials have demonstrated that survival is modestly improved in such patients that received chemotherapy when compared to patients receiving only supportive care.[67–70] Interestingly, a companion study to one of these trials[67] demonstrated that chemotherapy was associated with cost savings over best supportive care alone. This was largely because patients receiving only supportive care spent more time in the hospital.[71] Patients with an unfavorable prognosis (weight loss, poor performance status) and/or significant concomitant diseases should be given supportive care and palliative radiation when necessary.

In patients receiving chemotherapy, a minimum of two courses of therapy is usually given before evaluating the patient for response. If no objective response is seen, the regimen should be discontinued. Patients responding to chemotherapy should continue therapy until disease progression has been documented.

Locally Advanced Disease

Because of the poor long-term survival rates following surgery alone or surgery followed by radiation therapy in locally advanced disease (stage III) and because recurrence at distant sites is a major problem,[72] chemotherapy has also been investigated in such patients. When administered prior to surgery (neoadjuvant), the goals of chemotherapy are to (1) deliver chemotherapy to the tumor site prior to destruction of the local vasculature by surgery and/or radiation, (2) reduce the size of the tumor to increase the likelihood of successful local therapy (e.g., complete surgical resection), and (3) eradicate undetectable micrometastases. In addition, neoadjuvant chemotherapy may allow for less extensive resections and therefore conservation of normal lung tissue.[4] Conversely, potential disadvantages of neoadjuvant chemotherapy include (1) a risk that toxicities due to the chemotherapy may decrease the patient's ability to tolerate subsequent surgery and/or radiation, (2) a risk that if the tumor does not respond to the chemotherapy that it will continue to grow and become unresectable, and (3) a significant prolongation of the duration of treatment.

The preceding rationale coupled with the identification of newer chemotherapy regimens with apparent increased activity in NSCLC stimulated several pilot studies of neoadjuvant chemotherapy in patients with locally advanced disease.[73] The highest response rates have been observed with regimens that include cisplatin 100 mg/m^2 Results of these studies indicated that most patients with stage III disease were able to tolerate two or three courses of aggressive chemotherapy followed by definitive surgery and/or radiation. Although several of these studies reported encouraging response rates (>50%), survival advantages could not be appropriately addressed in these nonrandomized trials. The Cancer and Leukemia Group B randomized

TABLE 121.4. COMBINATION CHEMOTHERAPY IN NON–SMALL CELL LUNG CANCER

Combination	Dosages	Schedule	Overall Response Rate (%)	Ref.
CAP				
CTX	400 mg/m^2 IV day 1			
ADR	40 mg/m^2 IV day 1	Repeat course every 4 weeks	6–39	45–52
DDP	40 mg/m^2 IV day 1			
CE				
DDP	60–100 mg/m^2 IV day 1			
ETOP	80–120 mg/m^2 IV × 3 days	Repeat course every 3–4 weeks	19–41	53–59
CAVP (or PACE)				
CTX	400 mg/m^2 IV day 3			
ADR	40 mg/m^2 IV day 2			
ETOP	50 mg/m^2 IV days 1–3	Repeat course every 4 weeks	46	60
DDP	20 mg/m^2 IV days 1–3			
or				
CTX	800 mg/m^2 IV day 1	Repeat course every 3 weeks	28	61
ADR	45 mg/m^2 IV day 1			
ETOP	100 mg/m^2 IV days 1, 3, and 5			
DDP	40 mg/m^2 IV day 1			
PEV				
DDP	60 mg/m^2 IV day 1	Repeat course every 3 weeks	40	62
ETOP	120 mg/m^2 IV days 3, 5, and 7			
VCR	1.5 mg/m^2 IV days 1 and 7			
DDP/VIN				
DDP	120 mg/m^2 IV days 1 and 29	Then repeat every 6 weeks	40	63
VIN	3 mg/m^2 IV Q week × 6	Then repeat course every 2 weeks		
or				
DDP	60 mg/m^2 IV days 1 and 29	Then repeat every 6 weeks		
VIN	3 mg/m^2 IV Q week × 6	Then repeat every 2 weeks	46	63
or				
DDP	100 mg/m^2 IV day 1	Repeat course every 4 weeks	33	64
VIN	3 mg/m^2 IV days 1, 8, and 15			
MV				
MIT	15–20 mg/m^2 IV day 1	Repeat dose every 6 weeks		
VIN	3 mg/m^2 IV Q week × 6	Repeat dose every 2 weeks	36	65
MVP				
MIT	8 mg/m^2 IV days 1 and 29			
VIN	3 mg/m^2 IV days 1, 8, 29, and 36		43	64
DDP	80 mg/m^2 IV days 1 and 29, then Q every weeks			

Key: CTX, cyclophosphamide; ADR, doxorubicin or Adriamycin; MTX, methotrexate; PRO, procarbazine; BLE, bleomycin; CCNU, lomustine; VCR or ONC, vincristine or Oncovin; HN_2, mechlorethamine; DDP, cisplatin; ETOP, etoposide; VIN, vindesine; MIT, mitomycin.

155 evaluable patients with unresectable NSCLC to receive either radiation alone or two courses of cisplatin and vinblastine followed by radiation. Forty-three percent of patients receiving radiation alone responded versus 56% of patients receiving the combined modality. At a median follow-up of 19 months, the median survival for combined modality therapy was 16.5 months versus 8.5 months for radiation alone, thus demonstrating a survival advantage for the combination.[74] Follow-up at 5 years continued to show this survival advantage.[75] It is important to note that this study and a similar trial reported by Sause et al.[76] included only fully ambulatory patients with less than 5% weight loss and no malignant pleural effusions prior to treatment. Therefore, these results may not be applicable for patients with poor prognostic disease characteristics. A meta-analysis of 11 trials including 1780 patients receiving chest radiation with or without cisplatin-based chemotherapy also indicated that mortality was reduced by 13% in patients randomized to receive chemotherapy.[77]

Other investigators have evaluated the use of concurrent radiation and chemotherapy in patients with locally advanced unresectable NSCLC. This strategy allows for micrometastases to be treated at the earliest possible time and maximizes the additive effects of radiation and chemotherapy. Although encouraging response rates have been reported (51–74%), most initial trials have reported median survival durations in the range expected for radiation alone (10–16 months).[78–81]

SMALL CELL LUNG CANCER

Chemotherapy

In contrast to NSCLC, the use of aggressive combination chemotherapy regimens in SCLC has demonstrated a four- to fivefold increase in median survival.[82] Without treatment, survival is generally less than 12 weeks. Because SCLC has the propensity to disseminate early in the disease, surgery is almost never indicated, except possibly in the rare patient who presents with a small, isolated lesion.

A number of factors have been identified that appear to have prognostic importance in SCLC.[83] Patients who initially present with limited disease and are treated with aggressive chemotherapy regimens demonstrate a significantly longer median survival than patients presenting with extensive disease treated with the same regimens.[30,82,84–86] Patients presenting with a better (i.e., ambulatory) performance status[30,82,84,86,87] and no weight loss[82] also appear to have an improved prognosis. Females appear to have a better prognosis than males as do patients younger than age 60.[82,85,87] Patients with normal pretreatment serum lactate dehydrogenase are also more likely to have limited disease, higher complete response rates, and longer median survivals.[87,88]

A number of cytotoxic agents have demonstrated significant single-agent activity in SCLC. Among the active agents are cyclophosphamide, doxorubicin, etoposide, carboplatin, vincristine, lomustine, cisplatin, ifosfamide, procarbazine, methotrexate, altretamine, and teniposide with response rates from 15–45%.[89] Investigational drugs with single-agent activity in SCLC include vindesine and epirubicin. Combination chemotherapy is clearly superior to single-agent therapy and the best results are generally observed when three or more active agents are combined. In recent years it has been observed that aggressive chemotherapy regimens appear to produce higher response rates, longer median survivals, and a higher percentage of long-term survivals.[4] Some of the more frequently used regimens are (1) CAV—cyclophosphamide (C) + doxorubicin (A) + vincristine (V); (2) CAE—C-A-etoposide (E); and (4) CE—cisplatin + E. These regimens are described in Table 121.5. Overall response rates and survival durations are generally superior in patients with limited disease versus those with extensive disease (Table 121.6); however, there are very few long-term survivors in either group (about 8–10% of patients survive longer than 3 years). Unfortunately, when the disease recurs, it is usually less sensitive to chemotherapy. Restaging to determine the effects of chemotherapy is usually done after three courses of treatment. At this point therapy is continued in patients responding to therapy and discontinued or changed in patients demonstrating evidence of disease progression. In patients achieving a complete response the optimal duration to continue therapy remains unknown with recommendations ranging from 6–24 months.

Several new strategies have been also investigated to try to improve long-term survival rates.

Dose Intensity

Experimental animal and human tumor data have suggested that the amount of drug administered over a unit of time may be critical to the degree of tumor cell kill.[97] This influence of dose intensity has been evaluated in many types of human cancer, particularly those like SCLC that are initially responsive to chemotherapy, but not usually curable with conventional therapies. Randomized trials using increased dosages of the CAV or CE regimens failed to improve overall survival.[98–100] A meta-analysis of 60 reported clinical trials failed to establish consistent dose-intensity-outcome correlations for most SCLC chemotherapy regimens.[101] For example, increasing the dose intensity of the CAE or CAVE regimen in patients with extensive disease was associated with a longer median survival; however, no effects could be identified for the CE regimen.

Alternating Non–Cross-Resistant Regimens

Because the duration of response is usually brief (less than 1 year) in patients achieving a complete response, it appears that drug-resistant cells continue to grow during treatment and eventually constitute a major portion of the tumor. The Goldie–Coldman theory[102] predicts that the cycling of two separate active chemotherapeutic regimens may overcome this problem. Although theoretically it would seem ideal to administer all the drugs simultaneously, the treatment-related toxic effects would be prohibitive. A number of trials have used alternating, non–cross-resistant regimens in the management of SCLC and most have failed to demonstrate substantial benefits.[103,104] Examples of such regimens include cyclophosphamide, methotrexate, and lomustine alternating with vincristine, doxorubicin, and procarbazine; vincristine, doxorubicin, and cyclophosphamide alternating with etoposide; and cyclophosphamide, doxorubicin, and etoposide alternating with vincristine, methotrexate, lomustine, and procarbazine. Note, however, that in many of these trials the second regimen was not cross-resistant and subtherapeutic doses were administered.[105] In at least one large trial the National Cancer Institute of Canada demonstrated a higher overall response rate (80% versus 63%, $p < 0.002$) and longer progression-free survivals and overall survivals for patients randomized to receive CAV alternating with CE versus CAV only.[106]

TABLE 121.5. COMBINATION CHEMOTHERAPY IN SMALL CELL LUNG CANCER

Combination	Dosages	Schedule	Overall Response Rate (%)	Ref.
CAV				
CTX	750–1500 mg/m^2 IV day 1			
ADR	45–50 mg/m^2 IV day 1	Repeat course every 3 weeks	63–100	90
VCR	2 mg IV day 1			
CAE				
CTX	1000 mg/m^2 IV day 1			
ADR	45 mg/m^2 IV day 1	Repeat course every 3 weeks	63–100	65,83,85,89–93
ETOP	50 mg/m^2 IV days 1–5 *or* 80 mg/m^2 IV days 103			
CEV				
CTX	1000 mg/m^2 IV day 1			
ETOP	50 mg/m^2 IV day 1, then 100 mg/m^2 PO days 2–5	Repeat course every 3 weeks	80	94
VCR	1.4 mg/m^2 IV day 1			
CE				
DDP	80 mg/m^2 IV day 1	Repeat course every 3 weeks	65	95
ETOP	150 mg/m^2 IV days 3–5			
CBDCA/ETOP				
CBDCA	100 mg/m^2 IV days 1–3	Repeat course every 4 weeks	77	96
ETOP	120 mg/m^2 IV days 1–3			

Key: CTX, cyclophosphamide; ADR, doxorubicin or Adriamycin; VCR, vincristine; ETOP, etoposide; CBDCA, carboplatin.

Combination Chemotherapy Plus Colony-Stimulating Factor

Most of the chemotherapy regimens are associated with a significant degree of toxicity, especially granulocytopenia, which increases the risk of serious infections; therefore, aggressive SCLC regimens have been combined with a colony-stimulating factor (CSF) such as filgrastim to reduce the incidence and severity of infectious complications. When patients receiving CAE therapy were randomized to receive either filgrastim or placebo, those receiving the CSF experienced shorter durations of severe neutropenia (5.2 versus 1.8 days), fewer febrile neutropenic episodes, and required fewer days of antibiotics or hospitalization.[107]

TABLE 121.6. RESPONSES TO OPTIMAL CHEMOTHERAPY REGIMENS BASED ON STAGE OF DISEASE

	Limited Disease	Extensive Disease
Overall response (CR + PR)	85–95%	75–85%
CR	50–60%	15–30%
Median survival (months)	12–16	7–11
Two-year disease-free survival	15–20%	Rare

(Adapted from Ref. 23.)

Other modalities also under investigation include total-body irradiation[108] or high-dose chemotherapy followed by autologous bone marrow transplantation. Because there exists a small, but definite, cure rate in SCLC, extensive research efforts such as these are warranted in the hope that this rate will improve.

Radiotherapy

SCLC is a very radiosensitive tumor and radiotherapy has been used in combination with chemotherapy to treat tumors limited to the thoracic cavity. The rationale for combined-modality therapy is that radiotherapy and chemotherapy together will fight bulk disease in the chest primary site and that chemotherapy will fight systemic metastases.[23] This combined-modality therapy may decrease the incidence and delay the onset of local tumor recurrences.[109] In most randomized trials, combined modality therapy has only modestly improved the overall duration of survival (e.g., 1–4 months) over that achieved with chemotherapy alone. A meta-analysis of 13 randomized studies including more than 2100 patients with limited stage SCLC reported that chemotherapy plus radiation significantly reduced the death rate by 14% and improved the 3-year survival by 5.4%.[110] The optimal dose and scheduling of radiation therapy in combination with chemotherapy is not yet defined. However, it appears that radiation therapy given concurrently or alternating with chemotherapy is more likely to produce favorable responses versus administration of radiation after completion of chemotherapy. Unfortunately, these studies of combined-modality therapy also have been associated with increased morbidity when compared to chemotherapy alone or radiation after chemotherapy. When radiation therapy is combined with radiosensitizing drugs like doxorubicin the incidence of radiation esophagitis and pneumonitis may increase.[111] Clinical trials currently under way are evaluating various dosages and schedules of radiation therapy in combination with a variety of chemotherapeutic agents in an attempt to maximize tumor control with an acceptable degree of toxicity.

CNS metastases are present in about 10% of patients initially and occur at some point in the disease process in 20–30% of patients.[23] For this reason, prophylactic cranial irradiation has been commonly recommended in all patients achieving a complete response to chemotherapy.[84] In a review of randomized trials evaluating prophylactic whole-brain irradiation, Bleehan et al.[112] reported that the incidence of brain metastases was 20% in patients not receiving prophylactic whole-brain irradiation compared with 6% in patients who did receive it. Neurologic and cognitive impairment and abnormalities on brain CT scans have been reported in long-term survivors following prophylactic cranial irradiation (PCI).[23,113–116] This has led to increased controversy regarding whether patients achieving a complete response should receive PCI. Some experts now recommend that cranial radiation be withheld until brain metastases manifest, while others recommend PCI, but only in lower dose fractions (200–300 cGy versus 400 cGy) after chemotherapy has been completed.[23] In patients with persistent disease, despite chemotherapy, the tumor may continue to seed the CNS, therefore negating any effects of prophylactic irradiation.[117] In patients with intracranial metastases, therapeutic cranial irradiation usually controls the CNS disease and patients generally die from progressive systemic disease.[118] Adrenocorticosteroids (to decrease intracranial pressure) and anticonvulsants (to prevent seizures) are routinely administered to patients with CNS metastases.

COMPLICATIONS AND SUPPORTIVE CARE

Patients with lung cancer frequently have many medical problems. Such problems may be related to the primary tumor and its metastases (see section on Clinical Presentation), the antitumor therapy, or concomitant diseases.

Many of the chemotherapy regimens used in the management of lung cancer are very intense (Tables 121.4 and 121.5) and are associated with a wide variety of toxic effects. Nausea and vomiting may be severe (especially in the cisplatin-containing regimens) and require aggressive antiemetic regimens. Patients experiencing protracted nausea and vomiting may require intravenous hydration and nutritional support. Myelosuppression is often the dose-limiting toxic effect associated with these combinations and granulocytopenia following many of the more aggressive regimens places patients at high risk of serious infections. Other toxic effects associated with these regimens include mucositis, peripheral neuropathies, nephrotoxicity, and ototoxicity.

Likewise, patients receiving radiation therapy may experience complications including fatigue, esophagitis, radiation pneumonitis, and cardiac toxicity.[41] When combined with chemotherapy these toxicities are often enhanced.[119]

As previously mentioned, patients with lung cancer frequently suffer from concomitant medical problems including chronic obstructive pulmonary diseases and cardiovascular disorders (probably related to smoking), which require pharmacologic interventions.

It is apparent that many patients with lung cancer often receive complex pharmacologic regimens that may include chemotherapeutic agents, antiemetics, antibiotics, analgesics, bronchodilators, corticosteroids, anticonvulsants, and cardiovascular agents. Such regimens necessitate intensive therapeutic monitoring in order to avoid drug-related toxic effects and to optimize patient management.

CONCLUSION

Lung cancer is currently the leading cause of cancer death in the United States although the American Cancer Society has estimated that up to 83% of all cases could be prevented if cigarette smoking were eliminated. Unfortunately, even with application of the current best diagnostic and therapeutic strategies the overall cure rate is only about 10%.

Surgery, and radiation therapy to a lesser extent, offers the only chance of cure in patients with NSCLC; however, the majority of patients are inoperable at diagnosis. Unfortunately, the response rates to combination chemotherapy in this disease are disappointingly low and it is controversial whether such therapy offers significant benefit to the patient in terms of quality of life or survival. Research endeavors continue to look for new effective agents and regimens in NSCLC in the hope of improving response rates and survival.

In contrast, combination chemotherapy has demonstrated dramatic response rates and clearly improved survival in patients with SCLC; however, the percentage of long-term survivors remains low. Research endeavors in SCLC continue to look for new agents, improved combinations, and new modalities that will enhance the cure rate.

Despite progress during the last decade in the management of advanced lung cancer the only clear-cut hope for control of this devastating disease lies in the elimination of cigarette smoking.

References

1. 1995 Cancer facts and figures. Atlanta, GA, American Cancer Society, 1995.
2. Martini N. Preoperative staging and surgery for non-small cell lung cancer, in Aisner JA (ed): Lung Cancer. New York, Churchill Livingstone, 1985, pp 101–130.
3. Linnoila I. Pathology of non-small cell lung cancer. Hematol Oncol Clin North Am 1990;4:1027–1051.
4. Ginsberg RJ, Kris MG, Armstrong JG. Non-small cell lung cancer, in DeVita VT, Hellman S, Rosenberg SA (eds): Cancer. Principles and Practice of Oncology. Philadelphia, JB Lippincott, 1993, pp 673–723.
5. Minna J, Battey J, Birrer M, et al. Genetic changes involved in the pathogenesis of human lung cancer including oncogene activation, chromosomal deletions, and autocrine growth factor production, in Fortner JG, Rhoads JE (eds): Accomplishments in Cancer Research 1987. Philadelphia, JB Lippincott, 1988, pp 155–182.
6. Aaronson SA. Growth factors and cancer. Science 1991;254:1146–1153.
7. Stanley KE. Lung cancer and tobacco: A global problem. Cancer Detect Prevent 1986;9:83–89.
8. Mattson ME, Pollack ES, Cullen JW. What are the odds that smoking will kill you? Am J Pub Health 1987;77:525–531.
9. Wynder EL. Etiology of lung cancer: Reflections on 2 decades of research. Cancer 1972;30:1332–1339.
10. Damber LA, Larson LG. Smoking and lung cancer with special regard to type of cancer: A case-control study in north Sweden. Br J Cancer 1986;53:673–681.
11. Janerich DT, Thompson WD, Varela LR, et al. Lung cancer and exposure to tobacco smoke in the household. NEJM 1990;323:632–636.
12. Garfinkel L, Auerbach O, Joubert L. Involuntary smoking and lung cancer. A case-control study. JNCI 1985;75:4463–4469.
13. Pershagen G, Hrubec Z, Svensson C. Passive smoking and lung cancer in Swedish women. Am J Epidemiol 1987;125:17–24.
14. Menck HR, Casagrande JT, Henderson BE. Industrial air pollution. Possible effect on lung cancer. Science 1974;183:210–212.
15. Menkes MS, Comstock GW, Vulleumier JP, et al. Serum beta-carotene, vitamin A and E, selenium and the risk of lung cancer. N Engl J Med 1986;315:1250–1254.
16. Ziegler RG, Mason TJ, Stemhagen A, et al. Carotenoid intake, vegetables, and the risk of lung cancer among white men in New Jersey. Am J Epidemiol 1986;123:1080–1093.
17. The Alpha-Tocopherol, Beta Carotene Cancer Prevention Study Group. The effect of vitamin E and beta carotene on the incidence of lung cancer and other cancers in male smokers. N Engl J Med 1994;330:1029–1035.
18. Sobin LH. The World Health Organizations Histological Classification of Lung Tumors: A comparison of the first and second editions. Cancer Detect Prevent 1982;5:391–406.
19. Aisner SC, Matthews MJ. The pathology of lung cancer, in Aisner JA (ed): Lung Cancer. New York, Churchill Livingstone, 1985, pp 1–23.
20. El-Torky M, El-Zeky F, Hall JC. Significant changes in the distribution of histologic types of lung cancer. Cancer 1990;65:2361–2367.
21. Cuttitta F, Carney DN, Mulshine J, et al. Bombensin-like peptides can function as autocrine growth factors in human small-cell lung cancer. Nature 1985;316:823–826.
22. Ferguson MK, DeMeester TR, Deslauries J, et al. Diagnosis and management of synchronous lung cancer. J Thorac Cardiovasc Surg 1985;89:378–383.
23. Ihde DG, Pass HI, Glatstein EJ. Small cell lung cancer, in DeVita VT, Hellman S, Rosenberg SA (eds): Cancer. Principles and Practice of Oncology. Philadelphia, JB Lippincott, 1993, pp 723–758.
24. Fontana RS, Sanderson DR, Woolner LB, et al. Lung cancer screening: The Mayo program. J Occup Med 1986;28:746–750.
25. Melamed MR, Flehinger BJ, Zaman MB, et al. Screening for early lung cancer. Results of the Memorial Sloan–Kettering study in New York. Chest 1984;86:44–53.
26. Tockman MS. Survival and mortality from lung cancer in a screened population. The Johns Hopkins Study. Chest 1986;89(suppl):324S–325S.
27. Eddy DM. Screening for lung cancer. Ann Intern Med 1989;111:232–237.
28. Theros EG. Varying manifestations of peripheral pulmonary neoplasm: A radiologic–pathological correlative study. Am J Roentgenol 1977;128:893–
29. Mountain CF. A new international staging system for lung cancer. Chest 1986(suppl):225S–233S.
30. Ihde DC, Makuch RW, Carney DN, et al. Prognostic implication of sites of metastases in patients with small cell carcinoma of the lung given intensive combination chemotherapy. Am Rev Respir Dis Chest 1981;123:500–507.
31. Martini R, Beattie EJ. Results of surgical treatment in stage I lung cancer. J Thorac Cardiovasc Surg 1977;74:499–506.
32. Klingman RR, DeMeester TR. Surgical approach to non-small cell lung cancer. Stage I and II. Hematol Oncol Clin North Am 1990;4:1079–1091.
33. Gail MH, Eagan RT, Feld R, et al. Prognostic factors in patients with resected stage I non–small cell lung cancer. Cancer 1984;54:1802–1813.
34. Martini N, Flehinger BJ, Nagasaki F, et al. Prognostic significance of N_1 disease in carcinoma of the lung. J Thorac Cardiovasc Surg 1983;86:646–653.
35. Kayser K, Bulzerbruch H, Probst G, et al. Retrospective and prospective tumor staging evaluating prognostic factors in operated bronchus carcinoma patients. Cancer 1987;59:355–361.
36. Ferguson MK, Little AG, Golomb HM, et al. The role of adjuvant therapy after resection of $T_1N_1M_0$ and $T_2N_1M_0$ non–small cell lung cancer. J Thorac Cardiovasc Surg 1986;91:344–349.

37. McCaughan BC, Martini N, Bains MS, McCormack P. Chest wall invasion of carcinoma of the lung: Therapeutic and prognostic implication. J Thorac Cardiovasc Surg 1985;89:836–841.
38. Martini N, Ginsberg RJ. Surgical approach to non–small cell lung cancer stage III_A. Hematol Oncol Clin North Am 1987;67:1121–1131.
39. Martini N, Flehinger BJ. The role of surgery in N_2 lung cancer. Surg Clin North Am 1987;67:1037–1049.
40. Mountain CF. The biological operability of Stage II non–small cell lung cancer. Ann Thorac Surg 1985;40:60–64.
41. Seagren SL. Radical radiation therapy for lung cancer. Hematol Oncol Clin North Am 1990;4:1093–1109.
42. Aisner J, Hansen HH. Commentary: Current status of chemotherapy for non–small cell lung cancer. Cancer Treat Rep 1981;65:979–986.
43. Stanley KE. Prognostic factors for survival in patients with inoperable lung cancer. J Natl Cancer Inst 1980;65:25–32.
44. O'Connell JP, Kris MG, Gralla RJ, et al. Frequency and prognostic importance of pretreatment clinical characteristics in patients with advanced non–small cell lung cancer treated with combination chemotherapy. J Clin Oncol 1986;4:1604–1614.
45. Eagan RT, Ingle JN, Frytak S, et al. Platinum-based polychemotherapy versus dianhydrogalactitol in advanced non–small cell lung cancer. Cancer Treat Rep 1977;61:1339–1345.
46. Ruckdeschel JC, Mason B, Ettinger D, et al. Chemotherapy of metastatic non–oat cell bronchogenic carcinoma: The Eastern Cooperative Group experience, in The III World Conference on Lung Cancer, 1978, pp 1207–1210.
47. Krook JE, Fleming TR, Eagen RT, et al. Comparison of combination chemotherapy programs in advanced adenocarcinoma-large cell carcinoma of the lung: A North Central Cancer Treatment Group study. Cancer Treat Rep 1984;68:493–498.
48. Knost JA, Greco FA, Hande KR, et al. Cyclophosphamide, doxorubicin and cisplatin in the treatment of advanced non–small cell lung cancer. Cancer Treat Rep 1981;65:941–945.
49. Britell JC, Eagan RT, Ingle JN, et al. Cis-dichlorodiammineplatinum (11) alone followed by adriamycin plus cyclophosphamide at progression versus cis-dichlorodiammineplatinum (11), adriamycin, and cyclophosphamide in combination for adenocarcinoma of the lung. Cancer Treat Rep 1978;62:1207–1210.
50. Evans WK, Feld R, DeBoer G, et al. Cyclophosphamide, doxorubicin and cisplatin in the treatment of non–small bronchogenic carcinoma. Cancer Treat Rep 1981;65:947–954.
51. Gralla RJ, Cvitkovic E, Goldberg RB, et al. Cis-dichlorodiammineplatinum (II) in non–small cell carcinoma of the lung. Cancer Treat Rep 1979;63:1585–1588.
52. Davis S, Rambotti P, Park YK. Combination cyclophosphamide, doxorubicin and cisplatin (CAP) chemotherapy for extensive non–small cell carcinomas of the lung. Cancer Treat Rep 1981;65:955–958.
53. Longeval E, Klastersky J. Combination chemotherapy with cisplatin and etoposide in bronchogenic squamous cell carcinoma and adenocarcinoma: A study by the EORTC Lung Cancer Working Party. Cancer 1982;50:2751–2756.
54. Dhingra HM, Valdivieso M, Booser DJ, et al. Chemotherapy for advanced adenocarcinoma and squamous cell carcinoma of the lung with etoposide and cisplatin. Cancer Treat Rep 1984;671–673.
55. Dhingra HM, Valdivieso M, Carr DT, et al. Randomized trial of three combinations of cisplatin with vindesine or VP-16-12 in the treatment of advanced non–small-cell lung cancer. J Clin Oncol 1985;3:176–183.
56. Cavalli F, Goldhirsch A, Joss R. Cis-dichlorodiammineplatinum (11) and VP-16-213 combination chemotherapy for non–small cell lung cancer. Chemotherapia 1982;1:164–167.
57. Crino L, Tonato M, Darwish S, et al. A randomized trial of three cisplatin (CDDP)-containing chemotherapy regimens in advanced non–small cell lung cancer (NSCLC): A study of the Umbrian Lung Cancer Group [abstract]. Proc Am Soc Clin Oncol 1987;6:716.
58. Klastersky J, Sculier JP, Ravez P, et al. A randomized study comparing a high and a standard dose cisplatin in combination with etoposide in the treatment of advanced non–small cell lung carcinoma. J Clin Oncol 1986;4:1780–1786.
59. Klastersky J, Longeval E, Nicaise C, Weerts D. Etoposide and cis-platinum in non–small-cell bronchogenic carcinoma. Cancer Treat Rev 1982;9(suppl A):133–138.
60. Eagan RT, Frytak S, Nichols WC, et al. Evaluation of VP-16-213, cyclophosphamide, doxorubicin and cisplatin (V-CAP) in advanced large cell lung cancer. Cancer Treat Rep 1981;65:715–717.
61. Fuks JZ, Aisner JA, VanEcho DA, et al. Randomized study of cyclophosphamide, doxorubicin and etoposide (VP-16-213) with or without cisplatinum in non–small cell lung cancer. J Clin Oncol 1983;1:295–301.
62. Klastersky J, Sculier JP, Nicaise C, et al. Combination chemotherapy with cisplatin, etoposide, and vindesine in non–small cell lung carcinoma: A clinical trial of the EORTC Lung Cancer Working Party. Cancer Treat Rep 1983;67:727–730.
63. Gralla RJ, Casper ES, Kelsen DP, et al. Cisplatin and vindesine combination chemotherapy for advanced carcinoma of the lung: A randomized trial investigating two dosage schedules. Ann Intern Med 1981;95:414–420.
64. Fukouka M, Masuda N, Furuse K, et al. A randomized trial in inoperable non–small cell lung cancer: Vindesine and cisplatin versus mitomycin, vindesine, and cisplatin versus etoposide and cisplatin alternating with vindesine and mitomycin. J Clin Oncol 1991;9:606–613.
65. Luedke D, Luedke S, Martello O, et al. Response of non–small cell lung cancer to vindesine and mitomycin: A Southeastern Cancer Study Group Pil Study [abstract]. Proc Am Soc Clin Oncol 1983;2:190.
66. Rosso R, Salvati F, Ardizzoni A, et al. Etoposide (E) vs E plus cisplatin (P) in the treatment of advanced non–small cell lung cancer (NSCLC). A FONICAP randomized trial [abstract]. Proc Am Soc Clin Oncol 1987;6:186.
67. Rapp E, Pater J, Willan A, et al. Chemotherapy can prolong survival in patients with advanced non–small cell lung cancer. Report of a Canadian multicenter randomized trial. J Clin Oncol 1988;6:633–641.

68. Woods R, Williams C, Levi J, et al. A randomized trial of cisplatin and vindesine versus supportive care only in advanced non–small cell lung cancer. Br J Cancer 1990;61:608–611.
69. Cormier Y, Bergeron D, La Forge J, et al. Benefits of polychemotherapy in advanced non–small cell bronchogenic carcinoma. Cancer 1982;50:845–849.
70. Cellerino R, Tummarello D, Guidi F, et al. A randomized trial of alternating chemotherapy versus best supportive care in advanced non–small cell lung cancer. J Clin Oncol 1991;9:1453–1461.
71. Jaakimainen L, Goodwin J, Pater J, et al. Counting the costs of chemotherapy in National Cancer Institute of Canada randomized trial in non–small lung cancer. J Clin Oncol 1990;8:1301–1309.
72. Stanley KE, Cox JD, Petrovich Z, et al. Patterns of failure with inoperable carcinoma of the lung. Cancer 1981;47:2725–2729.
73. Vokes EE. Sequential combined modality therapy for stage III non–small cell lung cancer. Hematol Oncol Clin North Am 1990;4:1133–1142.
74. Dillman RO et al. A randomized trial of induction chemotherapy plus high-dose radiation versus radiation alone in stage III non–small-cell lung cancer. N Engl J Med 1990;323:940–945.
75. Dillman RO et al. Randomized trial of induction chemotherapy plus radiation therapy vs RT alone in stage III non–small cell lung cancer (NSCLC): Five-year follow-up of CALGB 84-33. Proc Am Soc Clin Oncol 1993;12:329.
76. Sause W et al. Preliminary analysis of phase III trial in regionally advanced unresectable non–small cell lung cancer [abstract]. Proc Am Soc Clin Oncol 1994;13:325.
77. Stewart LA et al. A meta-analysis using individual patient data from randomised clinical trials of chemotherapy in non–small cell lung cancer: (3) Survival in the locally advanced setting [abstract]. Proc Am Soc Clin Oncol 1994;13:334.
78. Eagan RT, Ruud C, Lee RE, et al. Pilot study of induction therapy with cyclophosphamide, doxorubicin and cisplatin (5-CAP) and chest irradiation prior to thoracotomy in initially inoperable stage III M_0 non–small cell lung cancer. Cancer Treat Rep 1987;71:895–900.
79. Rowland K, Bonomi P, Taylor SG, et al. Phase II trial of etoposide, cisplatin, 5-FU and concurrent split course radiation in stage III_A, and III_B non–small cell lung cancer [abstract]. Proc Am Soc Clin Oncol 1988;7:203.
80. Strauss G, Sherman L, Matthiesen O, et al. Concurrent chemotherapy and radiotherapy followed by surgery in marginally resectable stage III_A non–small cell lung cancer: A Cancer and Leukemia Group B study [abstract]. Proc Am Soc Clin Oncol 1988;7:203.
81. Weiden P, Pinatodosi S. Preoperative chemoradiotherapy in stage III non–small cell lung cancer: A phase II study of the lung cancer study group (LCSG) [abstract]. Proc Am Soc Clin Oncol 1988;7:197.
82. Hansen HH, Rorth M, Aisner JA. Management of small-cell carcinoma of the lung, in Aisner JA (ed): Lung Cancer. New York, Churchill Livingstone, 1985, pp 269–285.
83. Armstrong JG. Long-term outcome of small cell lung cancer. Cancer Treat Rev 1990;17:1–13.
84. Bunn PA, Cohen MH, Ihde DC, et al. Advances in small cell bronchogenic carcinoma. Cancer Treat Rep 1977;61:333–342.
85. Spiegelman D, Maurer L, Ware J, et al. Prognostic factors in small-cell carcinoma of the lung: An analysis of 1251 patients. J Clin Oncol 1989;7:334–354.
86. Cerny T, Blair V, Anderson H, et al. Pretreatment prognostic factors and scoring system in 497 small-cell lung cancer patients. Int J Cancer 1987;39:146–149.
87. Albain K, Crowley JJ, LeBlanc M, Livingston RB. Determinants of improved outcome in small-cell lung cancer: An analysis of the 2,580-patient Southwest Oncology Group Database. J Clin Oncol 1990;8:1563–1574.
88. Sagman U, Feld R, Evans WK, et al. The prognostic significance of pretreatment serum lactate dehydrogenase in patients with small-cell lung cancer. J Clin Oncol 1991;9:954–961.
89. Aisner J, Alberto P, Comis R, et al. Role of chemotherapy in small cell lung cancer. A consensus report of the IASLC Workshop. Cancer Treat Rep 1983;67:37–43.
90. Aisner J, Wiernik PH. Chemotherapy versus chemoimmunotherapy for small-cell undifferentiated carcinoma of the lung. Cancer 1980;46:2543–2549.
91. Broder LE, Cohen MH, Selawry OS. Treatment of bronchogenic carcinoma II small cell. Cancer Treat Rev 1977;4:219–260.
92. Greco FA, Richardson RL, Snell JD, et al. Small cell lung cancer: Complete remission and improved survival. Am J Med 1979;66:625–630.
93. Hansen HH, Dombernowsky P, Hansen M. Chemotherapy of advanced small-cell anaplastic carcinoma: Superiority of a four-drug combination to a three-drug combination. Ann Intern Med 1978;89:177–181.
94. Issell B, Rudolph A, Lawson R, et al. The substitution of etoposide for doxorubicin in small cell lung cancer combination chemotherapy, in Proc 13th Int Congress of Chemother, 1983.
95. Wolf M, Havemann K, Holle R, et al. Cisplatin/etoposide versus isosfamide/etoposide combination chemotherapy in small cell lung cancer; a multicenter German randomized trial. J Clin Oncol 1987;5:1880–1889.
96. Bishop JF, Raghavan D, Stuart-Harris R, et al. Carboplatin (CBDCA, JM-8) and VP-16-213 in previously untreated patients with small cell lung cancer. J Clin Oncol 1987;5:1574–1578.
97. Schabel FM, Griswold DP, Corbett TH, et al. Increasing the therapeutic response rates to anticancer drugs by applying the basic principles of pharmacology. Cancer 1984;54:1160–1167.
98. Johnson DH, Einhorn LH, Birch R, et al. A randomized comparison of high-dose versus conventional-dose cyclophosphamide, doxorubicin, and vincristine for extensive stage small cell lung cancer. J Clin Oncol 1987;5:1731–1738.
99. Figuerdo AT, Hryniuk WM, Straufmanis I, et al. Co-trimoxazole prophylaxis during high-dose chemotherapy of small cell lung cancer. J Clin Oncol 1985;2:54–64.
100. Ihde DC, Johnson BE, Mulshine JL, et al. Randomized trial of high dose versus standard dose etoposide and cisplatin in

extensive stage small cell lung cancer. Proc Am Soc Clin Oncol 1987;6:181.

101. Klasa RJ, Murray N, Coldman AJ. Dose-intensity meta-analysis of chemotherapy regimens in small-cell carcinoma of the lung. J Clin Oncol 1991;9:499–508.
102. Goldie JH, Coldman AJ, Gudauskas GA. Rationale for the use of alternating non-cross resistant chemotherapy. Cancer Treat Rep 1982;66:439–449.
103. Goodman GE, Crowley JJ, Blasko JC, et al. Treatment of limited small-cell lung cancer with etoposide and cisplatin alternating with vincristine, doxorubicin, and cyclophosphamide versus concurrent etoposide, vincristine, doxorubicin, and cyclophosphamide and chest radiotherapy: A Southwest Oncology Group study. J Clin Oncol 1990;8:39–47.
104. Wolf M, Pritsch M, Drings P, et al. Cyclic-alternating versus response-oriented chemotherapy in small-cell lung cancer: A German multicenter randomized trial of 321 patients. J Clin Oncol 1991;9:614–624.
105. Greco FA, Johnson DH, Hainsworth JD, Wolff SN. Chemotherapy of small-cell lung cancer. Sem Oncol 1985;4(suppl 6):31–37.
106. Evans WK, Feld R, Murray N, et al. Superiority of alternating non-cross-resistant chemotherapy in extensive small cell lung cancer. Ann Intern Med 1987;107:451–458.
107. Crawford J, Ozer H, Johnson D, et al. Granulocyte colony stimulating factor: Prevention of chemotherapy induced febrile neutropenia (FN) in patients with small cell lung cancer (SCLC) [abstract]. Proc Am Soc Clin Oncol 1990;9:229.
108. Spitzer G, Dicke KA, Litam J, et al. High-dose combination chemotherapy with autologous bone marrow transplantation in adult solid tumors. Cancer 1980;45:3075–3085.
109. Wilson HE, Stanley K, Vincent RG, et al. Comparison of chemotherapy alone versus chemotherapy and radiation therapy of extensive small cell carcinoma of the lung. J Surg Oncol 1983;23:181–184.
110. Johnson DH, Arriagada R, Ihde DC, et al. Meta-analysis of randomized trials evaluating the role of thoracic radiotherapy in limited-stage small cell lung cancer. Proc Am Soc Clin Oncol [abstract]. 1992;11:288.
111. Phillips TL. Acute and late effects of multi therapy on normal tissues. Cancer 1977;40:489–494.
112. Bleehen NM, Bunn PA, Cox JD, et al. Role of radiation therapy in small anaplastic carcinoma of the lung. Cancer Treat Rep 1983;67:11–19.
113. Fleck JF, Einhorn LH, Lauer RC, et al. Is prophylactic cranial irradiation indicated in small-cell lung cancer? J Clin Oncol 1990;8:209–214.
114. Johnson BE, Becker B, Goff WB, et al. Neurologic, neuropsychologic, and cranial computed tomography scan abnormalities in 2–10 year survivors of small cell lung cancer. J Clin Oncol 1985;3:1659–1667.
115. Laukkanen E, Klonoff J, Allan B, et al. The role of prophylactic brain irradiation in limited stage small cell lung cancer: Clinical, neuropsychologic, and CT sequelae. Int J Rad Oncol Biol Phys 1988;14:1109–1114.
116. Lee JS, Umsawasdi T, Lee Y, et al. Neurotoxicity in long-term survivors of small cell lung cancer. Int J Rad Oncol Biol Phys 1986;12:313–321.
117. Qasim MM. Combined total body irradiation and local radiation therapy in oat cell carcinoma of the bronchus. Clin Radiol 1979;30:161–163.
118. Bunn PA, Rosen ST. Central nervous system manifestations of small cell lung cancer, in Aisner JA (ed): Lung Cancer. New York, Churchill Livingstone, 1985, pp 287–305.
119. Payne DG, Feld R. Concurrent radiotherapy and chemotherapy in lung cancer at the Princess Margaret Hospital. Antibiot Chemother 1988;41:96–101.

Chapter 122

Colorectal Cancer

Lisa E. Davis, PharmD, and Motria M. Krawczeniuk, PharmD

Colorectal cancer involves the colon, rectum, and the anal canal. It is one of the three most common cancers occurring in adult men and women in the United States and accounts for about one out of eight cancer diagnoses. In 1996, an estimated 133,500 new cases will be diagnosed of which 94,500 will involve the colon and 39,000 the rectum.[1]

For both adult men and women, colorectal cancer is the third leading cause of cancer-related deaths in the United States. An estimated 55,300 deaths occurred during 1995. Mortality associated with colorectal cancer has decreased during the past 30 years; the rate of decline is greatest for females.

Mortality rates associated with colorectal cancer in the United States are comparable to those of other industrialized areas such as North America, certain areas of Northern and Western Europe, Australia, and New Zealand. Deaths attributed to cancer of the colon or rectum in less developed areas such as South America and rural Africa are less frequent than in the United States.

Multiple factors are associated with the development of these malignancies, including acquired and inherited genetic susceptibility, environmental elements, and lifestyle. Overall, approximately 37% of affected individuals undergo a surgical procedure alone intended for cure. An additional 35% can potentially be cured by undergoing surgery followed by radiation therapy, chemotherapy, or both. Curability is influenced primarily by extent of tumor invasion into adjacent tissues or organs and presence of metastatic disease. Five-year survival rates are close to 93% and 87% for persons with early stages of colon and rectal cancer, respectively. Once tumor has spread regionally to adjacent organs or lymph nodes, survival rates drop to 63% for colon cancer and 53% for cancer of the rectum. Five-year survival for individuals with metastatic disease is less than 7%.

Treatment modalities include surgery, radiation therapy, chemotherapy, and immunotherapy. Surgery is the most important and definitive procedure associated with cure; radiation therapy can be used to improve curability following surgical resection and to reduce symptoms and complications associated with advanced disease. Chemotherapy and immunotherapy (levamisole) are used in adjuvant treatment regimens. Chemotherapy—either a single agent, a combination of agents, or a combination of chemotherapy and immunotherapy—can be used for advanced stages of disease. Although the efficacy of a standard postoperative monitoring program for patients with resected colorectal cancer has not been established, elements of such a program may include physical examination, colonoscopy, chest and abdominal imaging studies, serum carcinoembryonic (CEA) measurements, liver function tests, and fecal occult blood testing.

Epidemiology

Worldwide, the highest incidence rates occur in highly industrialized areas such as North America, certain areas of Northern and Western Europe, Australia, and New Zealand. Less developed areas such as South America and rural Africa report the lowest incidence rates of colorectal cancer. Rates have increased substantially, however, in previously lower risk countries such as Japan and China, as well as among persons migrating from low-risk areas to the United States.

The incidence of colon cancer is greatest among males, who have an age-adjusted incidence rate of 40.7 per 100,000 as compared to females in which the rate is 29.9 per 100,000.[2] Cancer of the rectum occurs less frequently. Although the total number of new cases continues to rise due to population growth, the overall incidence of colon and rectal cancers in the United States has declined since 1985. This decline is greater in the female population than for males. Incidence and mortality rates and recent trends among white males and females in the United States can be compared in Table 122.1. These rates are somewhat higher for black males and females.

The median age at diagnosis is about 69 years.[4] Fewer than 3% of affected persons are under the age of 40. An individual's risk, however, increases with increasing age. Sixty-two percent of cases develop in adults greater than 60 years of age. Hispanics and African Americans have a younger mean age at diagnosis and tend to present with later stage disease at diagnosis than do non-Hispanic whites.

Approximately 1 of every 10 cancer deaths is due to cancer of the colon or rectum. Roughly 55,300 deaths were

TABLE 122.1. INCIDENCE AND MORTALITY TRENDS FOR COLORECTAL CANCER AMONG WHITE MALES AND FEMALES, 1975–1979 TO 1987–1991

	Incidence Rate[a] (%) 1987–1991	Incidence Rate Change (%) Since 1975–1979	Mortality Rate[a] (%) 1987–1991	Mortality Rate Change (%) Since 1975–1979
White males				
Colon	40.4	5	20.0	–2.9
Rectum	18.3	–5.7	3.4	–34.6
White females				
Colon	29.5	–6.6	13.7	15.4
Rectum	10.4	–12.6	1.9	–36.7

[a]Rates are per 100,000 person-years and are age-adjusted to the 1970 U.S. standard population. (From Ref. 3.)

estimated in 1995, despite a decline in overall combined mortality for both colon and rectal cancer observed during the last 30 years by almost 30% for women and 7% for men. Differences exist, however, among specific racial and gender populations. The greatest decline has been experienced within white females, whereas mortality rates among black males continue to rise. These trends in mortality are similar to those of other countries such as Spain, Italy, Portugal, and Greece between 1975–1988.[5] Factors contributing to the overall decline in mortality are unclear but may reflect the impact of decreasing incidence rates, better treatment, a decrease in treatment-related complications, changes in dietary habits, screening programs, and, possibly, other contributing factors such as nonsteroidal anti-inflammatory drug (NSAID) use.

PATHOGENESIS

ANATOMY AND BOWEL FUNCTION

The large intestine consists of the cecum, ascending, transverse, descending, and sigmoid colon, and the rectum (Fig. 122.1). In adults it extends approximately 1.5 m and has a diameter ranging from 8 cm in the cecum to 2 cm in the sigmoid colon. The function of the large intestine is to receive 500 to 2000 mL of ileal contents per day. Absorption of fluid and solutes occurs in the right colon or the segments proximal to the middle of the transverse colon with movement and storage of fecal material in the left colon and distal segments of the colon. Mucus secretion from goblet cells into the intestinal lumen lubricates the mucosal surface and facilitates movement of the dehydrated feces. It also serves to protect the luminal wall from bacteria and colonic irritants such as bile acids.

Four major tissue layers, from the lumen outward, form the large intestine: the mucosa, submucosa, muscularis externa, and serosa (Fig. 122.2). Embedded in the submucosa and muscularis externa is a rich lymphatic capillary system. Lymphatic channels do not extend into the mucosa. The muscularis externa consists of circular smooth muscle and three outer longitudinal smooth muscle bands. Contraction of these muscle groups moves colonic material toward the anal canal. The outermost layer of the colon, the serosa, secretes a fluid which allows the colon to slide easily over nearby structures within the peritoneum. The serosa covers only the anterior and lateral aspects of the upper third of the rectum. The lower third lies completely extraperitoneal and is surrounded by fibrofatty tissue as well as adjacent organs and structures.

The surface epithelium of the colonic mucosa undergoes continual renewal, and complete replacement of epithelial cells occurs every 4–8 days. Cell replication normally takes place within the lower third of crypts, the tubular glands located within the intestinal mucosa. The cells then mature and differentiate to either goblet or absorptive cells as they migrate toward the bowel lumen. The total number of epithelial cells remains relatively constant as the number of cells migrating from the crypts is balanced by the rate of exfoliation of cells from the mucosal surface. This two-phase process is critical to the malignant transformation of the epithelial cells.

ETIOLOGIC FACTORS

Numerous studies suggest that the development of colorectal cancer can be caused or promoted by dietary or environmental factors that affect the bowel.[6–10] An understanding of these processes has formed the basis for several interventional and preventive trials, which are discussed later in this chapter. Key areas of study include dietary fat, fiber, and micronutrient intake.[11]

Epidemiologic studies of worldwide incidence of colorectal cancer suggest that economic development and dietary habits strongly influence its development. Inhabitants of affluent societies are more likely to have more fat and less fiber in their diets. In western countries, fat consumption typically accounts for approximately 40% of total caloric intake.[12] Although prospective studies thus far have failed to support a direct causal relationship between

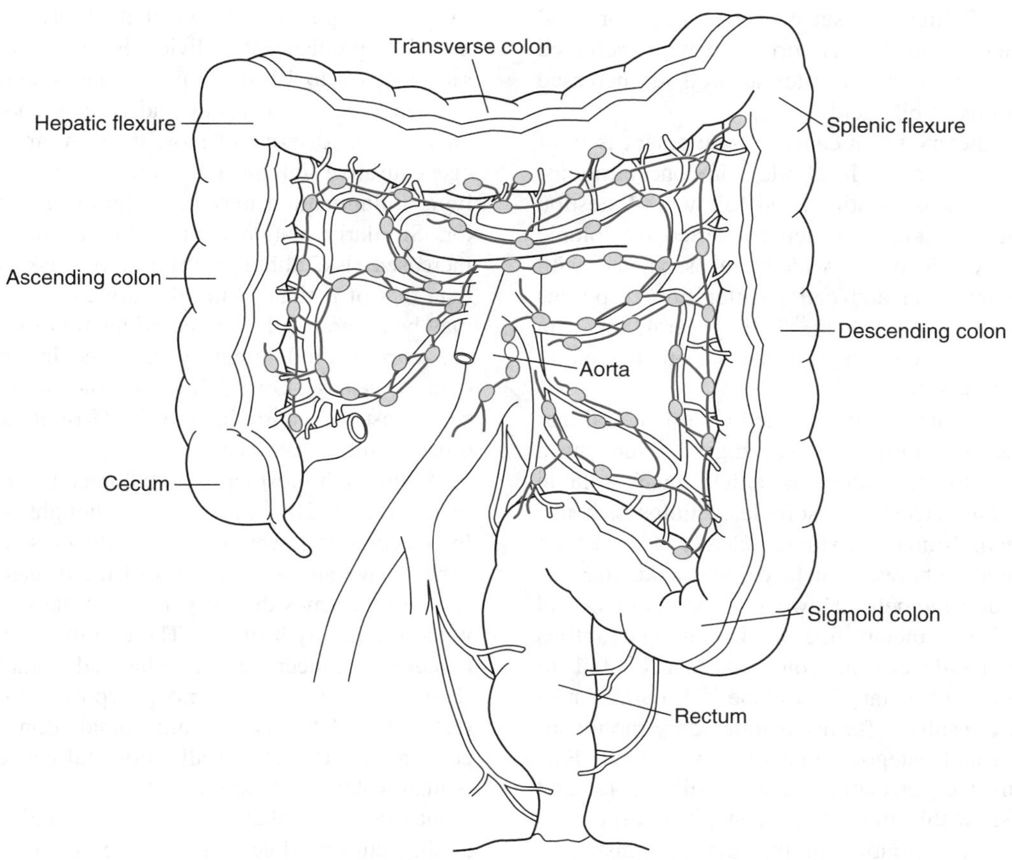

Figure 122.1. Colon and rectum anatomy. *(Modified from Miller TA. Colonic anatomy and physiology, in Greenfield LJ, Mulholland MW, Oldham KT, Zelenock GB [eds]: Surgery: Scientific Principles and Practice. Philadelphia, JB Lippincott, 1993, p 981, with permission.)*

dietary fat consumption and cancer, numerous studies suggest that a relationship exists between dietary fat intake and colorectal cancer risk. Whether the source of the fat is important is unclear since most of the fat in many of these studies was derived from ingested animal meat. Results from case-control studies are somewhat inconsistent but also provide evidence supporting a relationship between dietary fat intake and colorectal cancer. In addition, animal studies demonstrate an influence of type, timing, and amount of dietary fat consumed on carcinogenesis.[12]

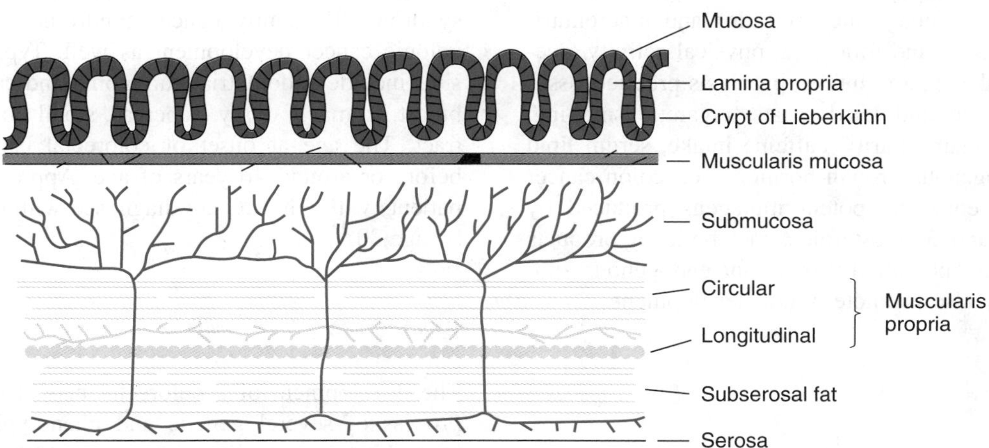

Figure 122.2. Cross section of bowel wall. *(Modified from Cole PP. The intramural spread of rectal carcinoma. BMJ 1993;432, with permission.)*

Administration of high-fat substances (e.g., corn oil boluses) to human volunteers is correlated with increased colonic crypt cell proliferation rates as well as increased fecal concentrations of bile acids.

The role of dietary fat in cancer development is most likely due to its influence on fecal bile acid concentrations. The release of bile acids is stimulated following ingestion of dietary fat. These acids are then converted by colonic flora to secondary bile acids, which are associated with bowel mucosal irritation and cell proliferation responses and may promote tumor growth.[9,10] In general, the data suggest that dietary fat consumption plays a greater role in tumor promotion than in initiation.

Dietary fiber is the part of ingested plant material that is not processed by normal human digestive enzymes. Fibers are frequently classified as either water soluble (pectins, gums, mucilages) or insoluble (celluloses, hemicellulose, lignins). Numerous studies clearly demonstrate an inverse association between dietary fiber intake and colorectal cancer development. However, comparative and case-control studies of dietary fiber intake among countries with dissimilar incidences of colorectal cancer fail to demonstrate the role of dietary fiber alone.[12] Accurate interpretation of these results is further hampered by the inconsistent definition and categorization of dietary fiber. Furthermore, an inverse correlation between dietary fat and fiber intake exists within most diets. Thus, it is difficult to ascertain the true contribution of this dietary constituent alone toward cancer development. Postulated protective effects of dietary fiber include dilution of carcinogens in the bowel, reduction of fecal pH, and enhanced bowel transit time. These effects may also reflect an associated concomitant reduction in dietary fat intake. Fiber from fruit and vegetable sources may be more desirable than cereal fiber.[13]

More recently, postmenopausal hormone replacement therapy has been shown to significantly decrease colon cancer risk.[14] The risk is reduced in postmenopausal women receiving both estrogen only and combined estrogen and progestin therapy. Less well recognized are the effects of various dietary micronutrients and macronutrients such as calcium and folic acid, physical activity, obesity, alcohol intake, energy intake, pyrolysis products associated with broiled and fried meats, cigarette smoking, occupational exposure, parity, caffeine intake, serum lipid levels, and endogenous growth hormones on colon cancer risk.[9,15–18] Fecapentaenes, potent mutagens produced by gut microflora, and 3-ketosteroids, metabolic by-products of cholesterol, are potentially important endogenous substances that may also promote tumor development.

CLINICAL RISK FACTORS

Several clinical conditions and genetic disorders increase one's risk of developing colorectal cancer. Chronic ulcerative colitis, particularly when it involves the entire large intestine, predisposes individuals to colorectal cancer at a rate that is 4 to 10 times higher than average.[19,20] The risk is even greater for young individuals and for those who have had the disease for more than 8 years. Although a precise causative link has not been established, chronic underlying inflammation may be a significant predisposing factor. Similarly, patients with Crohn's disease are also at increased risk, although the relative risk is slightly lower than that of patients with ulcerative colitis. This difference may be related to the decreased length of bowel affected by the chronic inflammatory process in individuals with Crohn's disease. Overall, persons diagnosed with either disease constitute approximately 1–2% of all new cases of colorectal cancer each year.

Although most cases of colorectal cancer are sporadic in nature, 10–20% of cases are thought to be hereditary. First-degree relatives of patients diagnosed with colorectal cancer have an increased risk of the disease that is at least two to four times that of persons in the general population without a family history.[21] The two most common forms of hereditary cancer are familial adenomatosis polyposis (FAP) and hereditary nonpolyposis colorectal cancer (HNPCC). FAP is an autosomal dominant trait that accounts for 0.5–1% of all colorectal cancers. The disease is manifested by hundreds to thousands of tiny sessile adenomatous polyps that carpet the colon and rectum, typically arising during adolescence.[22] The risk of developing colorectal cancer for individuals with untreated FAP is virtually 100%; most will develop colorectal cancer by their fourth decade of life.[23]

HNPCC, also referred to as Lynch syndromes I or II, is an autosomal dominantly inherited syndrome that probably accounts for at least 10% of colon cancer cases. In contrast to FAP, adenomatous polyps generally number only up to 100 and tend to be located primarily in the proximal (cecum, ascending, transverse) colon. Type I or Lynch syndrome I is characterized by the aggregation of colorectal cancer within a particular family, whereas type II (Lynch syndrome II, family cancer syndrome) represents extracolonic cancer development as well. Typical extracolonic sites include endometrial carcinoma and carcinomas of the breast, stomach, ovary, pancreas, small bowel, and urinary tract. The age at onset of colorectal cancer is typically before or around 40 years of age. Approximately 50% of patients with HNPCC are diagnosed with colorectal cancer by age 80.[24]

PATHOLOGY

The development of a colorectal neoplasm is a multistep process of several genetic and phenotypic alterations of normal bowel epithelium structure and function.[25] Since the majority of colorectal cancers develop sporadically, efforts have been directed toward identifying these alterations, determining if they develop in any type of sequential order, and learning whether discovery of the presence of such changes may lead to improved cancer detection and/or treatment outcomes.

A genetic model has been proposed for colorectal tumorigenesis that describes a process of transformation from adenoma to carcinoma.[26,27] An overview of the model is depicted in Fig. 122.3. The adenoma–carcinoma sequence of tumor development reflects a sequential series of mutations within colonic epithelium, each of which results in cellular replication or enhanced invasiveness. Key elements of this process include hyperproliferation of epithelial cells to form a small benign neoplasm or adenoma in conjunction with cellular gene mutations. These mutations occur early and frequently in sporadic cases of both adenomas and colorectal cancer.[23,28] Genetic changes include mutational activation of oncogenes as well as inactivation of tumor suppressor genes. Both types of genetic alterations are required to produce the malignant tumor.

Oncogenes are mutated forms of normal cellular genes, or protooncogenes, that induce many of the aberrant features of malignant cells. Activating mutations of *ras* protooncogenes, primarily involving the K-*ras* and N-*ras* genes, occur frequently in colorectal cancer.[27] The *ras* family of genes is responsible for encoding proteins involved in signal transduction. Although the effects of these mutated genes are not completely understood, their activation is believed to be important in tumor progression.

Tumor suppressor genes are normal cellular genes that are capable of transforming normal cells to cancerous cells through their deletion or inactivation. One of the earliest genetic changes in colorectal tumorigenesis involves the mutation or loss of the adenomatous polyposis coli (*APC*) gene, a tumor suppressor gene, localized on the long arm of chromosome 5q21. The *APC* gene encodes for a protein that is believed to be involved in regulation of cell shape and cell-to-cell communication. This alteration leads to abnormal epithelial proliferation and differentiation of cells. Inactivation of the *APC* gene is the single gene defect responsible for FAP.

Mutational inactivations of two additional important tumor suppressor genes, *p53*, located on chromosome 17p, and the *DCC* (deleted in colorectal carcinoma) gene, located on chromosome 18q, occur later during the adenoma–carcinoma sequence. Normal *p53* gene expression is responsible for apoptosis, an irreversible cell process resulting in cell death. Loss of *p53* activity through mutation is the most common genetic abnormality associated with human tumors and may contribute toward their growth advantage.[29] The protein encoded by the normal *DCC* gene is believed to share similar structural features to certain types of cell-adhesion molecules and, as such, may interact with various proteins. Loss of specific cell-adhesive properties could contribute toward tumor invasion and metastasis.

A distinct group of genetic traits has also been identified for individuals with HNPCC. "Replication errors" occur frequently and represent widespread alterations in the length of a series of repeated nucleotides within tumor DNA.[30] Mutations of genes that appear to recognize and regulate DNA replication errors, *hMSH2, hMLH1, hPMS1,* and *hPMS2*, may contribute to colorectal tumorigenesis.[31] Tumor progression may then be facilitated through a link between DNA repair defects and a loss of inhibitory growth control. Inactivation of a receptor for type II transforming growth factor-β (TGF-β), a protein that inhibits epithelial cell growth, has been demonstrated in cells with replication errors.[32]

Adenocarcinomas account for greater than 90% of tumors of the large intestine.[8] Other histologic types such as mucinous adenocarcinoma, signet ring adenocarcinoma, carcinoid simplex, and carcinoid tumors occur less frequently. Adenocarcinomas are assigned one of three tumor grade designations based on the degree of cellular differentiation, the degree to which the tumor resembles the structure, and function of its cell of origin. The most differentiated adenocarcinomas, or grade I tumors, generally resemble adenomas, whereas grade III tumors are considered "high grade," the most undifferentiated, and have frequently lost the characteristics of mature normal cells. Features of well-differentiated tumors include relatively normal tubule and glandular formation and low numbers of mitoses. Poorly differentiated or high-grade tumors contain

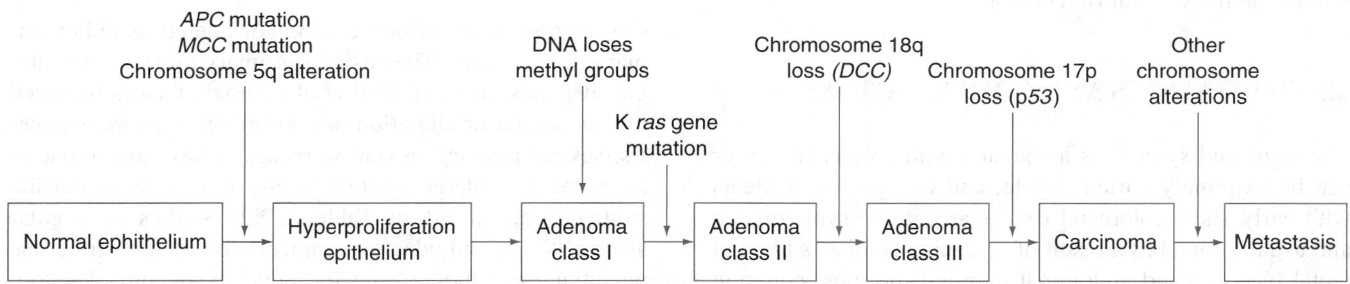

Figure 122.3. Adenoma–carcinoma sequence. *(Modified from Fearon ER, Vogelstein B. A genetic model for colorectal tumorigenesis. Cell 1990; 61:756–767, with permission.)*

few or no glandular structures and have an increased nuclear to cytoplasmic ratio, large nuclei, and dark staining due to increased DNA content. Poorly differentiated tumors are associated with a worse prognosis than those that are better differentiated.[33,34]

Mucinous adenocarcinomas possess the same basic structure as adenocarcinomas but differ in that they secrete an abundant quantity of extracellular mucus. They account for only about 10% of colorectal carcinomas but tend to be most frequent in patients with HNPCC and patients with coexisting ulcerative colitis.[35] Signet-ring adenocarcinomas have a characteristic appearance due to the displacement of the nucleus to one side by large vacuoles of intracellular mucin. Patients tend to present with a more advanced stage of disease and have a highly invasive tumor. Both mucinous and signet-ring adenocarcinoma histologies confer a poor prognosis.

DNA content of the tumor is also related to overall prognosis.[36,37] This is easily and reliably measured using flow cytometry. Tumors with DNA content equal to normal are referred to as *diploid;* tumors with abnormal DNA content are referred to as *aneuploid.* Aneuploid tumors are more likely to recur following primary resection and patients with aneuploid tumors have decreased survival compared to patients with diploid tumors.

The frequencies at which cancer occurs in the various areas of the colon vary. The proportion of tumors occurring in the right (cecum, ascending, and transverse colon) side of the colon has increased during the past 30 years with fewer occurring in the rectum and left (descending and sigmoid colon) side. For example, the percentage of colon cancer cases detected in the ascending colon/cecum in 1990 increased to 36.3 from 28.6 in 1971.[4] About 33.7% of tumors arise in the sigmoid colon area. Seventeen percent are detected in the area of the transverse colon and splenic flexure and 7.7% develop in the descending colon. In addition, the tendency for tumors to shift to the proximal (right) side increases with increasing patient age.[38] Whether this is due to more frequent and better access to the proximal area of the bowel or rather a shift in the biology of the disease is unknown. The implications of this phenomenon suggest that fewer lesions are accessible to sigmoidoscopy, a standard screening program procedure that only allows evaluation of the more distal (left) colon.

MANIFESTATIONS AND COMPLICATIONS

The signs and symptoms associated with colorectal cancer can be extremely varied, subtle, and nonspecific. Patients with early stage colorectal cancer are often asymptomatic and usually found as a result of screening studies. Although rectal bleeding and abdominal pain are the most common signs, any change in bowel habits (e.g., constipation, diarrhea, alteration in size or shape of stool), vague abdominal discomfort, or distention may all be warning signs of a malignant process.

Colorectal lesions tend to involve the bowel in a circular rather than longitudinal fashion, thereby narrowing and compressing the lumen. The presence or absence of symptoms is therefore often related to the location and size of the primary tumor and extent of disease involvement.[39] Tumors of the cecum and ascending colon are usually not associated with significant changes in bowel habits; however, watery diarrhea sometimes develops. In contrast, obstructive symptoms and changes in bowel habits frequently develop with tumors located in the transverse and descending colon. This is where the stool is the driest.

Nausea, vomiting, and abdominal discomfort are often secondary signs of a larger underlying problem such as obstruction, perforation, and/or bleeding. Bleeding may be acute or chronic and most commonly appears as bright, red blood mixed with stool. Iron deficiency anemia, presenting as weakness and occasionally high-output congestive heart failure, frequently develops as a result of chronic occult blood loss.

Approximately 20–25% of patients with colorectal cancer present with metastatic disease.[2,4] Metastatic spread occurs as a result of direct tumor invasion of adjacent tissues or by lymphatic or hematogenous spread. The venous drainage of the colon and rectum influence the pattern of metastases most commonly seen. The most common site of metastasis is the liver, often the only site of metastatic disease in 40% of patients, followed by the lungs and then bones, specifically the sacrum, coccyx, pelvis, and lumbar vertebrae. Hepatomegaly, obstruction, weight loss, and jaundice are indicative of liver metastases which are present in 5–10% of patients at presentation. Other evidence of widespread disease may include leg edema due to lymph node involvement, thrombophlebitis, fistula formation, jaundice, weight loss, or pain, especially in the lower back or radiating down the legs.[39] Pain associated with hepatic metastases is sometimes localized in the right upper quadrant of the abdomen, right posterior chest or right shoulder, and characterized as a continuous ache.

PREVENTION AND SCREENING

Cancer prevention efforts can be considered as either primary or secondary. The basis for primary prevention strategies depends on identification of etiologic factors followed by eradication or alteration of their effects on carcinogenesis. Several primary preventive measures have undergone or are currently undergoing study; some of the most promising strategies are listed in Table 122.2. Studies of regular aspirin[43,44] or sulindac[45] administration demonstrate the potential use of these agents for reducing adenoma development, inducing adenoma regression, and determining colorectal cancer risk. Clinical application of much of these

TABLE 122.2. PRIMARY PREVENTION STRATEGIES FOR COLORECTAL CANCER

Intervention	Proposed Beneficial Effects
Dietary Supplementation[7,17]	
Fiber	Decreases fecal bile acid concentrations; increases bowel transit time
Calcium	Reduces the cellular proliferative response to fatty acids and bile acids; dietary supplementation decreases epithelial cell proliferation in high-risk individuals
Vitamin A, beta-carotene	Antioxidative activities; ? direct suppression of tumor growth
Chemoprevention	
α-difluoromethylornithine (DFMO)[42]	Inhibition of ornithine decarboxylase reduces polyamine synthesis, thereby suppressing carcinogenesis
Aspirin, NSAIDs[43]	Interference with prostaglandin synthesis which may be essential for tumor development; ? immune enhancement, inhibit metabolism of substances that activate carcinogens; reduce ornithine decarboxylase activity

data is hampered by the lack of definitive associations between intermediate biomarkers commonly employed in chemoprevention trials (tritiated thymidine incorporation for colonic epithelial proliferation; abnormal crypts, microadenomas, protein kinase C) and frank cancer development.[20]

Secondary prevention includes procedures that range from colonoscopic removal of precancerous polyps (colonoscopic polypectomy) to total colectomy for individuals with FAP or in other high-risk settings.[23,46]

Based on the recognized incidence of colorectal cancer, identification of high-risk individuals, and the high rate of curability associated with localized lesions, cancer screening recommendations have been established. The current American Cancer Society guidelines for average-risk individuals are outlined in Table 122.3. More rigorous screening recommendations have been established for high-risk individuals.[48,49]

The digital rectal examination has been a traditional part of the annual physical examination in patients older than 40 years of age and accounts for the detection of approximately 10% of all cancers that are within reach of

TABLE 122.3. AMERICAN CANCER SOCIETY SCREENING RECOMMENDATIONS FOR COLORECTAL CANCER

Annual digital rectal examination starting at age 40 years
Annual occult fecal blood testing starting at age 50 years
Sigmoidoscopic examination starting at age 50 years and repeated at one year; if each of the two examinations is negative, then repeat every 3–5 years

(From Ref. 47.)

7–10 cm of the anus.[49] The use of fecal occult blood tests results further in an increased number of asymptomatic individuals with early stages of disease discovered.[35] Three major methods are available to detect occult blood in the feces: guaiac dye or derivative, heme-porphyrin, and immunochemical. Guaiac-based tests utilize paper impregnated with a guaiac resin which contains α-guaiaconic acid, a phenolic compound that responds to peroxidases in the blood. When a solution containing hydrogen peroxide is poured over paper which has previously been exposed to absorbed peroxidases from blood in the stool, the phenolic compound is oxidized and a blue colorization develops.

The sensitivity of the test, a positive result in the setting in which blood is present, can be influenced by several factors. Since hemoglobin is degraded by bacteria in the stool, test sensitivity is diminished when samples are stored or when the lesion is located in the proximal area of the bowel. Although the sensitivity can be improved by rehydrating the stool sample, the specificity of the test is reduced. Ascorbic acid ingestion in excess of 250 mg/d, failure to ingest a high-residue diet for several days prior to testing, and assays of dry stools may also yield false-negative results.[50] Conversely, foods containing pseudoperoxidase or peroxidase activity can cause a false-positive reaction: rare red meat and uncooked fruits and vegetables such as broccoli, turnips, cauliflower, cantaloupe, and radishes. These foods should be avoided for 3 days prior to and during testing. Other sources of potential false-positive results include the use of iron supplements, rectal medications, or any medications that may potentially alter the integrity of the gastrointestinal lining. Anti-inflammatory agents should be avoided for 7 days prior to and during testing. Approximately 2 mL of blood must be present in the stool to produce a positive test result.[35] Since tumors bleed intermittently, multiple stool specimens should be sampled to minimize false-negative results.

Heme-porphyrin and immunochemical assays were developed to reduce the rate of false-positive results associated with fecal guaiac blood tests. The heme-porphyrin assay quantifies the conversion of heme to fluorescent porphyrins. Since it also measures fecal heme that has been degraded by bacteria, test sensitivity is not altered significantly by the site of bleeding or fecal storage. Immunochemical tests react with the globin moiety of hemoglobin and are therefore affected less by dietary influences. However, test sensitivity is influenced by bleeding site and stool storage. Both of these assays are more complex and labor intensive to perform. Several comparative trials of fecal occult blood tests have been performed.[35,46,50,51] Both HemeSelect and Hemoccult SENSA appear to provide the best combination of sensitivity and specificity compared to HemoQuant.

The limitations associated with fecal occult blood screening remain an issue of active concern. Many early stage tumors do not bleed and therefore the false-negative rates are approximately 70% for cancer and 90% for polyps. The overall detection rate for asymptomatic colorectal cancer using fecal occult blood testing is only about 33%.[50] Even though false-positive rates are only between 2–10%, a false-positive result can prove to be very expensive and inconvenient for a patient due to the follow-up tests required for a positive result.[48,50] Nevertheless, two studies evaluating the effects of fecal occult blood screening tests have established that their use is associated with a reduction in mortality due to colorectal cancer by approximately one-third.[31]

Sigmoidoscopy is useful for examining the lower 35–60% of the bowel, depending on the instrument, and thus increases the detection rate by approximately two- to threefold. A 60-cm flexible sigmoidoscope can be used to reach the splenic flexure in order to detect 50–60% of cancers but it requires more operator training, is associated with increased risk, and patient tolerance is less than with the 35-cm instrument.[49] Studies suggest that screening sigmoidoscopy, according to currently recommended guidelines, could effectively reduce mortality from colorectal cancer by about 60%.[51,52] These data, however, have yet to be validated through randomized, prospective trials.

A colonoscope facilitates examination of the bowel to the cecum in the majority of patients. However, its use is not routinely recommended for current screening practices for average risk individuals. An air-contrast barium enema is less sensitive than colonoscopy in the area of the distal rectum and is therefore not routinely included in screening programs of asymptomatic patients. It may be useful, however, for certain high-risk individuals due to its ability to identify small abnormalities of the mucosa.[31] In the future, analysis of stool samples for the presence of specific chromosomal point mutations, such as K-*ras,* may offer an effective screening alternative.[53]

Workup and Diagnosis

When a patient is suspected of having colorectal carcinoma, a careful history and physical examination should be performed. The patient history should include a past medical history and family history, especially noting the presence of colorectal cancer, polyps, and cancers of the breast, ovary, and endometrium. A complete physical examination includes careful abdominal examination for the presence of masses or ascites, a rectal examination, and an assessment for possible hepatomegaly and lymphadenopathy. In all women, a breast and pelvic examination is recommended, especially in women with a history of breast, ovarian, or endometrial cancer.

An unexplained anemia in an older patient requires surveillance of the entire large bowel, especially the right colon. Red blood cell indices (e.g., hemoglobin, hematocrit, mean corpuscular volume, reticulocyte count) and a workup of iron status (e.g., serum ferritin, serum iron, and TIBC) may be useful to confirm acute or chronic blood loss and/or iron-deficiency anemia. An evaluation of the entire large bowel is undertaken with either colonoscopy or sigmoidoscopy and an air-contrast barium enema. A barium enema may be preferred in situations in which a partially obstructing lesion prohibits passage of the endoscope; however, it should be avoided if complete obstruction or perforation of the bowel is suspected. A characteristic finding indicative of colon cancer seen on barium enema is an apple core-shaped lesion with tumor involving the circumference of the bowel. When possible, the endoscope is used to collect tissue for a histologic evaluation and provide a preliminary diagnosis following the procedure.

Baseline laboratory tests should be obtained and include a complete blood cell count, platelet count, prothrombin time (PT), activated partial thromboplastin time (aPTT), liver function tests, and serum CEA. Abnormal liver function tests may suggest liver involvement with tumor. However, patients with metastatic disease to the liver may have normal liver function tests and abnormal liver function tests are not always indicative of metastatic disease.

CEA belongs to a group of cell-surface glycoproteins, termed "oncofetal proteins," which are expressed during embryonic development and reexpressed on the cell surfaces of many carcinomas, particularly those of the gastrointestinal tract. While the function of CEA is not well understood, it is proposed to be a cellular adhesion molecule and possibly contribute toward tumor invasion and metastasis. The concentration of CEA can be measured in the blood and can therefore potentially serve as a "marker" for colorectal cancer. Approximately 28% of patients with stage A and 45% of patients with B colorectal cancer will have an elevated serum CEA level at time of diagnosis.[54] Elevated concentrations are even more frequent in patients with metastatic disease. It is important to recognize, however, several concomitant disease states that can artificially elevate CEA: alcoholic and chronic hepatitis, diverticulitis, renal failure, cholelithiasis, fibrocystic breast disease, and smoking.[55] Although CEA measurement is too insensitive and nonspecific to be used as a screening test for early-stage colorectal cancer, it may be useful for monitoring colorectal cancer response to treatment, particularly if the pretreatment concentration is elevated.[56,57] The CEA test also has preoperative prognostic implications because it has been shown to correlate with the size and degree of differentiation of the carcinoma.[55] Elevated preoperative CEA levels correlate with a poor survival, regardless of tumor stage upon diagnosis. After a potentially curative resection, CEA levels should return to normal within 1 month. Persistently elevated CEA levels may indicate residual disease.

Radiographic imaging studies help evaluate the extent of disease involvement. A chest x-ray should be performed to rule out the presence of metastatic spread to the lungs. A bone scan can also be helpful in evaluating the extent of disease involvement in a symptomatic patient. A computed tomography (CT) scan or ultrasound of the abdomen is often performed to evaluate hepatic and retroperitoneal involvement, occult abdominal and pelvic disease, and to determine the depth of tumor penetration into the bowel wall and/or invasion to adjacent organs. Detection of lymph node involvement with either study is limited by the difficulty distinguishing inflammatory or reactive lymph nodes from those infiltrated with tumor. Since peritoneal seeding, small distant lymph node metastasis, or liver metastasis in colon cancer may not be adequately detected by CT scan, an occasional patient may need to undergo a laparotomy in order to confirm metastatic disease. This is infrequent, however, since most patients eventually undergo surgical resection for colorectal cancer unless the procedure is contraindicated.

Intrarectal or transrectal ultrasonography is a technique that is becoming more widely available for the evaluation of patients with rectal cancer. It is excellent for detecting the depth of tumor penetration and, like pelvic CT scans, is fair to good in determining lymph node involvement.[58] Cystoscopy or intravenous pyelography studies are rarely indicated except for very large rectal tumors found on examination, if the patient exhibits symptoms, or if a CT scan suggests bladder involvement. Intraluminal and hepatic magnetic resonance imaging (MRI) studies may also provide useful information.

Immunodetection of tumors using tumor-directed antibodies is receiving greater recognition as an imaging technique for the early detection and imaging of colorectal cancers. Several tumor-associated proteins have been identified within or on the surface membrane of colorectal malignant cells to which monoclonal antibodies have been targeted.[59] Of these, CEA and TAG-72 antigen have undergone the greatest amount of study. Radiolabeled monoclonal antibodies directed against these antigens have been used in clinical studies for both external immunoscintography as well as intraoperative localization of tumor. OncoScint CR/OV, an indium-111-labeled monoclonal antibody targeted to the TAG-72 antigen, is an FDA-approved diagnostic imaging agent available for determining the location and extent of extrahepatic disease in patients with colorectal cancer. The use of OncoScint CR/OV is generally reserved for those patients who have completed standard diagnostic imaging tests but may still require additional information regarding the extent of disease. While these approaches are helpful for addressing some of the limitations of current radiographic techniques, they are limited somewhat by the heterogeneity associated with antigen expression at different sites of tumor within individual patients.[59] More recently, clinical trials have focused on the therapeutic use of immunoconjugates against tumors with linkage of monoclonal antibodies to radioactive isotopes, toxins, and chemotherapeutic agents.[60]

STAGING

The purpose of the staging examinations is to describe precisely the malignancy at a point in its natural history that is germane to patient treatment options and overall prognosis. Traditionally, the Dukes' classification, originally published in 1932, has been used in the staging of colorectal cancers.[61] Since then, it has undergone several modifications; a modified Astler–Coller version is used more extensively.[62] Prognosis and survival data associated with each stage of disease in this classification system have been collected extensively. However, since multiple staging systems exist and have been used for various clinical trials, the literature is often difficult to evaluate. Therefore, in an effort to standardize the staging system for colorectal cancer, the American Joint Committee on Cancer (AJCC) and the International Union Against Cancer (IUAC) jointly agreed to utilize and recommend the TNM classification system. This classification takes three aspects of cancer growth—T = *t*umor size, N = lymph *n*ode involvement, and M = presence or absence of *m*etastases—into account for determining the disease stage. The TNM classification allows for various subdivisions within each of the three categories.[63] A schematic representing the relationship between both staging systems can be found in Fig. 122.4.

The stage of colorectal cancer upon diagnosis, identified primarily by depth of tumor invasion of the bowel wall and presence or absence of involved lymph nodes, is the most important independent prognostic factor for survival and disease recurrence. A comparison of the stage of disease upon presentation and relative survival rates for individuals with colon and rectum cancer is provided in Table 122.4. The stage of disease also provides the basis for determining the most appropriate initial treatment. However, additional clinical and pathologic variables may affect the prognosis of patients with colorectal cancer. Consideration of these factors plays an important role in determining optimal strategies for treatment as well as appropriate follow-up. The patient's overall health status will also influence treatment tolerability and therapeutic options. Clinical factors present at time of diagnosis that are associated with

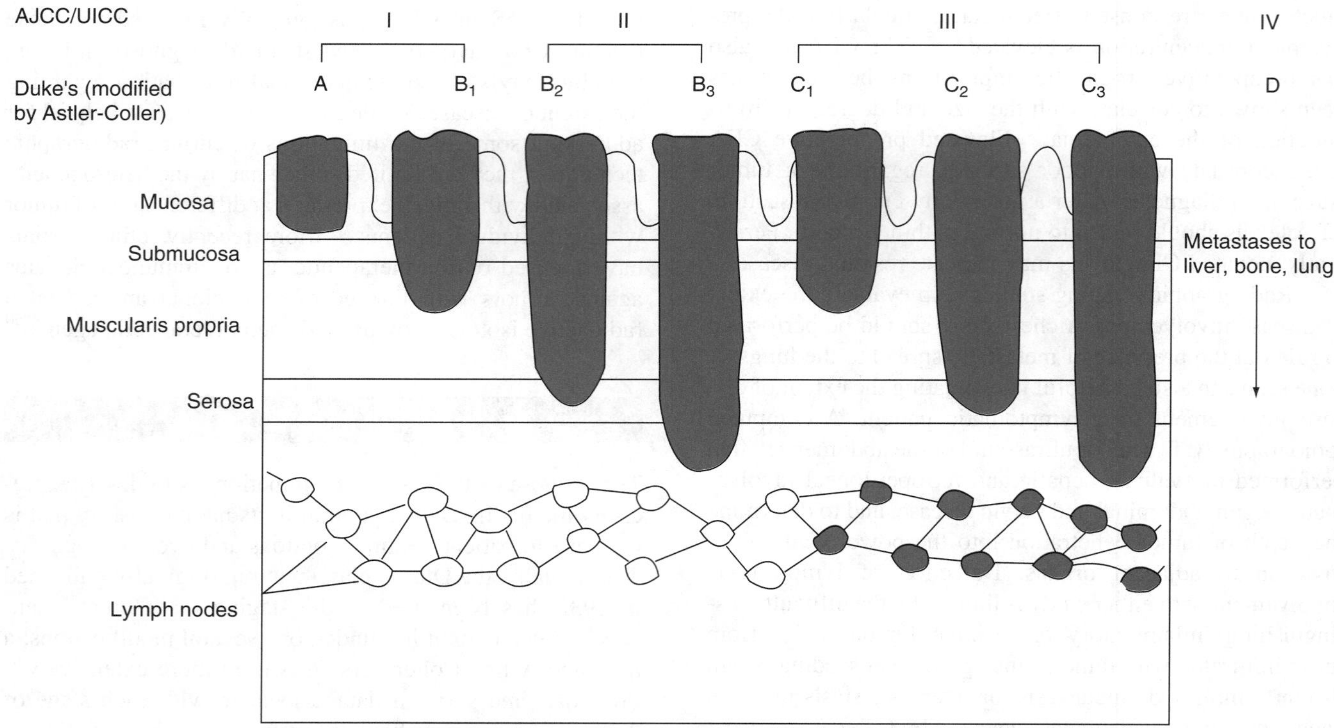

Figure 122.4. Staging system for colorectal cancer.

a poor prognosis and decreased survival include bowel obstruction or perforation, high preoperative CEA level, distant metastases, and location of the primary tumor in the rectum or rectosigmoid area.[8,35] Pathologic variables associated with a negative influence on prognosis include depth of muscular invasion, venous, lymphatic, or perineural invasion, number of involved lymph nodes, high proliferation indices, increased aneuploidy, mucinous or signet-ring histology, and poor tumor differentiation. Data from recent and ongoing studies demonstrate that *p53* overexpression and genetic alterations on certain oncogenes and tumor suppressor genes further influence prognosis.[65] Allelic loss of chromosome 18q, which is located on the *DCC* gene, is predictive of mortality, independent of tumor differentiation, vascular invasion, and TNM stage. Five-year survival rates of approximately 93% are associated with stage II colorectal cancer; survival rates for patients with stage II disease and allelic loss of chromosome 18q drop to approximately 54%, similar to that of patients with stage III disease and intact chromosome 18q.[66] These factors may provide important clues as to which patients with intermediate-stage disease should require additional therapy after surgical resection.

TABLE 122.4. COLON AND RECTUM CANCER DISEASE STAGE AND SURVIVAL RATES

AJCC Stage at Diagnosis	% Patients Presenting		% 5-Year Relative Survival	
	Colon	Rectum	Colon	Rectum
0	7.6	8.4	90+	90+
I	22.4	29.8	70–95	70–93
II	29.6	23.4	63–80	55–71
III	23.5	23.9	25–60	28–41
IV	16.9	14.5	12	9

(From Refs. 4, 8, and 64.)

TREATMENT MODALITIES

SURGERY

Surgical removal of the primary tumor is the treatment of choice for most patients with colorectal cancer. The surgical approach for colon cancer generally involves a complete resection of the tumor with an appropriate margin of tumor-free bowel and a regional lymphadenectomy. In the elective setting, a temporary colostomy is rarely required.[67] A total colectomy may, however, be indicated for selected patients with FAP or chronic ulcerative colitis. Surgery for rectal cancer depends on the region of tumor involvement.[35,67] Patients with lesions in the lower portion of the rectum may require an abdominoperineal resection if either the amount of unaffected bowel is insufficient for a resection far enough away from the tumor or too close to areas that cannot permit an anastomosis. Newer surgical techniques have been developed in an attempt to retain function of the rectal sphincter and still achieve complete tumor resection. Individuals who are not candidates for sphincter-sparing resections or have extensive local spread of tumor will require an abdominoperineal resection. This involves removal of the distal sigmoid, rectosigmoid, rectum, and anus with the establishment of a permanent sigmoid colostomy. Only about 1 in 7 patients will require a permanent colostomy for rectal cancer.[67] The American Cancer Society, United Ostomy Association, and the International Association of Enterostomal Therapy offer ostomy rehabilitation services. Other complications associated with colorectal surgery can include infection, adhesion formation, and malabsorption syndromes.

RADIATION THERAPY

Radiation therapy (XRT) can be administered in conjunction with curative surgical resection and in the setting of advanced or metastatic disease. In patients undergoing surgery, XRT is used to reduce local tumor recurrence. Symptom reduction is the primary goal of XRT for patients with advanced or metastatic disease. XRT is given prior to or following surgery and can be delivered using a variety of dosing regimens, administration schedules, and techniques that expose different amounts of body surface area.[68]

Retrospective data suggest that preoperative XRT may be used to reduce the initial size of the tumor to such an extent that the tumor could be reclassified to a lower stage, or "downstaged," and therefore rendered more resectable. This might then lead to improved patient survival or require that a less extensive surgical procedure be performed. Preoperative XRT is also administered to reduce the amount of tumor seeding that can occur during surgery; however, this approach is more likely to affect a greater area than is necessary.[64] Postoperative administration of XRT may more adequately treat a defined area, but is associated with more toxicity due to a greater amount of bowel being present in the treatment field.

Adverse effects associated with XRT can be acute or chronic. Acute effects primarily include hematologic depression, dysuria, diarrhea, abdominal cramping, and proctitis. Chronic symptoms that sometimes persist for months following discontinuation of XRT may involve persistent diarrhea, proctitis, or enteritis, small bowel obstruction, perineal tenderness, and impaired wound healing.

CHEMOTHERAPY

Since the mid-1950s, 5-FU has been the most active and widely used chemotherapeutic agent for colorectal cancer. Biochemical modulation is an alternative approach to single-agent 5-FU therapy that involves the addition of another agent in an attempt to modify or change its activity in order to improve response rates and, ultimately, patient survival. Examples of biochemical modulating agents used for colorectal cancer include leucovorin, interferon, methotrexate, hydroxyurea, PALA, dipyridamole, and thymidine. Proposed mechanisms for their influence on 5-FU effects are described in Table 122.5. The pharmacology of the key agents used for colorectal cancer is discussed in the following sections.

TABLE 122.5. DRUGS AND MECHANISMS OF BIOCHEMICAL MODULATION OF 5-FLUOROURACIL

Agent	Proposed Mechanism of Modulation
Leucovorin	Increased intracellular levels of reduced folates enhance FdUMP-mediated inhibition of thymidylate synthase.
Methotrexate	Blocks purine nucleotide synthesis, resulting in increased levels of intracellular phosphoribosylpyrophosphate (PRPP), a substrate that promotes the synthesis of FdUMP and 5-FUTP.
Interferon-α	Decreases 5-FU clearance, decreases thymidine kinase activity, inhibits thymidine incorporation into DNA, decreases rate of thymidine phosphorylation, increases FdUMP formation, and may inhibit thymidylate synthase.
(*N*-phosphonacetyl)-L-aspartic acid (PALA)	Inhibits pyrimidine synthesis by blocking aspartate carbamyl transferase, an enzyme that competes with and depletes uridine and cytidine nucleotide stores. As a result, the ratio of FUTP to uridine triphosphate (UTP) is increased, thereby increasing the incorporation of FUTP into RNA.
Hydroxyurea	Inhibits ribonucleotide reductase, which then lowers levels of a substance that competes with FdUMP for thymidylate synthase, deoxyuridine monophosphate (dUMP).
Dipyridamole	Inhibits efflux of FdUDR, leading to increased retention of intracellular FdUMP.
Thymidine	Lowers 5-FU plasma clearance and enhances incorporation of FUTP into RNA.

(From Refs. 69–71.)

5-Fluorouracil (5-FU) and 5-Fluoro-2′-Deoxyuridine (FUDR; Floxuridine)

5-FU, the most common fluorinated pyrimidine used clinically, is a member of the only group of cytotoxics whose development is based on rational predicted biochemical action. FUDR produces the same cytotoxic effect as 5-FU through its conversion in a single-step reaction by deoxyuridine kinase to an active metabolite, FdUMP.

As a prodrug, 5-FU undergoes anabolism to two primary products, 5-fluorouridine-5′-triphosphate (FUTP) and 5-fluorodeoxyuridine-5′-monophosphate (FdUMP), to exert its antitumor effects[72] (Fig. 122.5). FUTP is incorporated into RNA, thereby impairing protein synthesis. FdUMP forms a tight but reversible covalent bond with thymidylate synthase (TS) in the presence of methylenetetrahydrofolate (CH_2-THF), one of the intracellular metabolites of folinic acid. TS is the key enzyme necessary for *de novo* synthesis of thymidylate through conversion of deoxyuridine monophosphate (dUMP) to 2′-deoxythymidine-5′-monophosphate (dTMP). The lack of available TS therefore reduces the rate of DNA synthesis, replication, and repair. When combined with folinic acid, the antitumor effects of 5-FU are enhanced through stabilization of the ternary complex of TS, FdUMP, and CH_2-THF. A recent study has suggested that determination of TS activity and duration of TS inhibition may be predictive for response to 5-FU therapy.[70] These findings may help identify which patients will benefit from 5-FU therapy for colorectal cancer.

Used alone and in combination, 5-FU forms the basis for many chemotherapy regimens used in the adjuvant setting and metastatic treatment of colorectal cancer. 5-FU is typically administered as an intravenous (IV) bolus injection, generally once weekly or daily for 5 days each month, or via a continuous IV infusion. Although the duration of continuous IV infusions is usually 5 days, it can extend for several weeks. FUDR can be administered intravenously but intrahepatic use is more common. It is preferable to 5-FU for intrahepatic administration because a much greater percentage of FUDR is removed from the systemic circulation with one pass through the liver.

Clinical studies comparing efficacy of bolus and continuous infusion schedules consistently appear to favor continuous infusion of 5-FU. This is consistent with evidence that suggests that the duration of infusion may be an important determinant of the biologic activity of 5-FU.[73] The primary cytotoxic effect associated with bolus 5-FU is on RNA synthesis, whereas interference with DNA is the predominant effect of continuous 5-FU infusion.

Toxicity patterns also differ based on the dose, route, and schedule of 5-FU administration. Leukopenia is the primary dose-limiting toxicity of IV bolus 5-FU, although diarrhea, stomatitis, and nausea and vomiting can also occur.[74] The incidence and severity of stomatitis can be significantly reduced with the use of oral cryotherapy.[75] In this approach, the patient is required to chew and hold ice chips in the mouth during the period between 5 minutes prior to and 30 minutes following the bolus injection of 5-FU. The basis for the protective effects of this procedure is based on the premise that local vasoconstriction caused by the ice chips temporarily reduces blood flow to the oral mucosa, thereby reducing drug exposure to the oral mucosa.

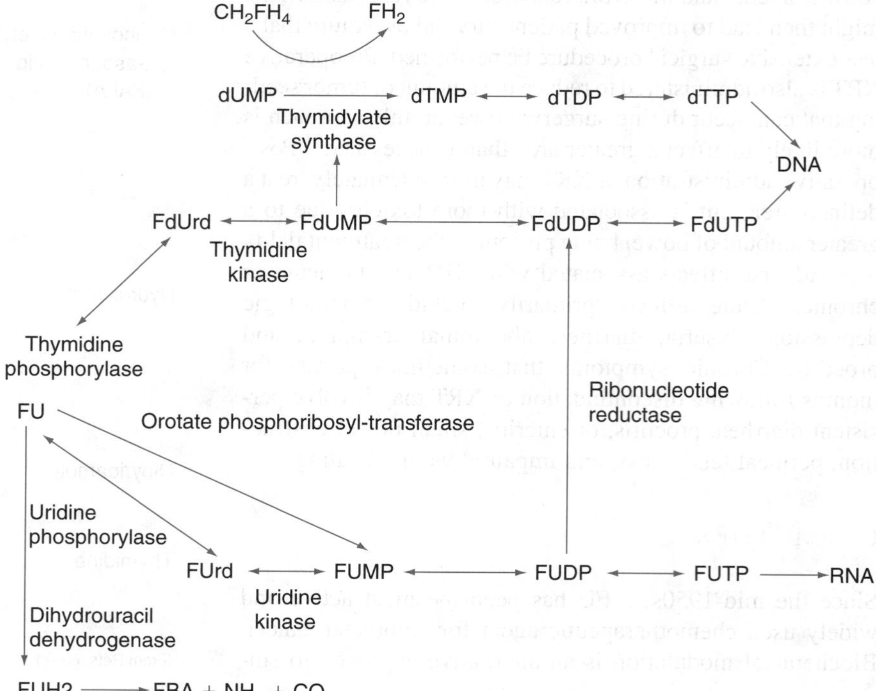

Figure 122.5. Metabolic pathways and sites of 5-FU. *(Reprinted from Zhang AG, Harstrick A, Rustum YM. Mechanisms of resistance to fluoropyrimidines. Semin Oncol 1992;19:5, with permission.)*

Although continuous IV infusion 5-FU is generally well tolerated, dose-limiting toxicities can be substantial. A distinct toxicity, palmar-plantar erythrodysesthesia ("hand–foot syndrome") and stomatitis occur most frequently with this route of administration.[71,74,76] Hand–foot syndrome occurs in 24–40% of patients receiving extended continuous IV infusions and is characterized by painful swelling and erythroderma of the soles of the feet, palms of the hands, and distal fingers. This type of skin toxicity is fully reversible upon interruption of therapy or dose reduction, and is not life threatening; however, it can be acutely disabling. The incidence of stomatitis, diarrhea, and hematologic toxicity is not substantial at standard doses but increases with increasing doses of 5-FU.

Levamisole (Ergamisol)

Levamisole is a synthetic, oral anthelmintic drug with immunomodulatory properties. Some of its stimulatory effects on the immune system include T-cell activation, augmentation of macrophage activity, and enhancement of the chemotactic response of polymorphonuclear cells and monocytes. Despite its synergy with 5-FU *in vitro,* levamisole alone does not produce direct cytotoxicity at levels achieved clinically. Although the mechanism of its synergistic effect with 5-FU is unknown, various proposed mechanisms have recently been summarized.[77] Effects of levamisole or its metabolites may be related to its immune effects, biochemical modulation independent of immunomodulatory activity, or possibly inhibition of cellular phosphatases, such as tyrosine phosphatase.[78]

Toxicities due to levamisole are generally mild, infrequent, and clinically tolerable. Levamisole is associated with taste abnormalities (described as metallic and occasionally associated with an altered sense of smell), arthralgias, and myalgias.[79] Central nervous system (CNS) toxicities expressed as anxiety, irritability, somnolence, depression, insomnia, agitation, confusion, or cerebellar ataxia occur in fewer than 5% of patients and resolve upon discontinuation of therapy.[79] Significant hematologic depression develops in less than 1% of patients receiving levamisole alone; however, agranulocytosis has been reported which, in a few cases, has been fatal. Up to 40% of patients treated with levamisole plus 5-FU show laboratory abnormalities consistent with hepatic toxicity: elevations in alkaline phosphatase, transaminases, or serum bilirubin.[80] These laboratory changes are mild, rarely symptomatic, and reversible on discontinuation of therapy.

Leucovorin Calcium (Folinic Acid, Citrovorum Factor)

The administration of leucovorin increases intracellular concentrations of reduced folate, which stabilizes the ternary complex between FdUMP and TS. As a result, there is a reduction in the availability of free TS, which catalyzes the conversion of dUMP to dTMP, a rate-limiting step in DNA synthesis. As a result, inhibition of TS activity is more complete and prolonged, thereby enhancing 5-FU cytotoxicity.

Leucovorin is generally nontoxic in therapeutic doses, although hypersensitivity reactions, such as anaphylaxis and urticaria, have been reported. The combination of 5-FU with either low- or high-dose leucovorin, however, produces greater toxicity to the gastrointestinal epithelium, the primary dose-limiting toxicity. An increase in the incidence and severity of stomatitis (25–30%) and diarrhea is most commonly observed.[81,82] Serious toxic effects develop in 3–6% of patients.[83,84]

Severe diarrhea develops in 25% of patients more often receiving high-dose leucovorin regimens, and has resulted in a 5% mortality rate due to diarrhea-related events or cardiovascular collapse.[81] Early treatment of diarrhea-related dehydration with bowel rest, IV fluids, and discontinuation of chemotherapy until resolution of all symptoms is recommended. Loperamide and diphenoxylate can also be used for symptomatic treatment. For those patients who do not respond to these treatment measures, the use of octreotide acetate should be considered. Several studies have demonstrated the safety and efficacy of octreotide acetate, administered subcutaneously at a dosage of 100 μg two or three times daily or 50–150 μg/h via continuous IV infusion, for controlling refractory, 5-FU-induced diarrhea.[85,86]

Occasionally, stomatitis and conjunctivitis develop. Significant hematologic toxicity is uncommon, although severe leukopenia (white blood cells [WBCs] < 2000/mm^3) has been noted in approximately 20% of patients treated with 5-FU/leucovorin combination therapy.[82] Seizures have infrequently developed in association with both low- and high-dose leucovorin administration regimens.[87] The mechanism may be similar to that between anticonvulsants and folic acid. The dose-limiting toxicity for low-dose leucovorin is usually stomatitis as compared to diarrhea with high-dose regimens.[88]

Interferon

In vitro studies combining interferon (IFN) with 5-FU have shown that IFN-α, -β, and -γ enhance the cytotoxic activity of 5-FU in cell culture lines, including colon cancer.[89] This is accomplished by augmenting the binding of the active 5-FU metabolite to the target site in the tumor cell. Several potential mechanisms by which IFN modulates 5-FU activity and metabolism have been identified.[89] *In vivo* data have demonstrated that the administration of IFN-α alters the pharmacokinetics of 5-FU, causing a dose-dependent decrease in 5-FU clearance, an increased 5-FU half-life, and a 30% increase in 5-FU area under the concentration-versus-time curve. This may be due to an inhibition of dihydropyrimidine dehydrogenase, the key enzyme responsible for regulating 5-FU degradation.[90] IFN-α has also been shown to increase FdUMP formation, thereby elevating intracellular levels of FdUMP and enhancing TS inhibition.

The toxicities related to IFN-α and 5-FU include flu-like symptoms that resolve either spontaneously or upon dose reduction or discontinuation of the IFN. Lethargy has also been problematic for some individuals. Stomatitis and leukopenia can develop and may require a reduction in the dose of 5-FU.

Primary Treatment of Colorectal Cancer

Adjuvant therapy in colorectal cancer is administered after complete tumor resection in an attempt to eliminate residual local or metastatic microscopic disease, thereby decreasing tumor relapse and improving patient survival. Adjuvant radiation therapy plus chemotherapy is considered standard treatment for patients with stage II/III rectal cancer and adjuvant chemotherapy is standard therapy for patients with stage III colon cancer.[91] The approach to adjuvant therapy requires different treatment strategies for colon and rectal cancer because the natural history and patterns of recurrence following resection are uniquely different. Since tumors arising in the rectum are technically more difficult to resect with wide circumferential margins, local recurrences occur more frequently than with colon cancers. Therefore, radiation therapy is an important aspect of adjuvant therapy to reduce risk of local tumor recurrence.

The stage of disease is the most important prognostic factor for risk of relapse and survival and is therefore the primary determinant for the selection of patients into adjuvant treatment trials. Because approximately 80–95% of patients with stage I colorectal cancer are cured by surgical resection alone, adjuvant therapy is not indicated.[92] Also, by definition, adjuvant therapy is not given to patients with metastatic disease. The administration of agents with proven activity at maximally tolerated doses is most effective when the tumor burden is minimal and tumor growth kinetics is optimal. An additional factor, the risk-to-benefit ratio for therapy, must be favorable for individuals who remain asymptomatic for their natural life expectancy after tumor resection.

Although numerous trials have been conducted to improve the results of curative surgery, this chapter focuses on prospective randomized controlled trials with adequate long term follow-up. In order for adjuvant therapy to be beneficial for a specific malignancy, clinical trials need to demonstrate a significant improvement in the rates of local recurrence, survival, or quality of life. Once a benefit of adjuvant therapy has been established, additional trials need to evaluate the optimal duration of treatment.

ADJUVANT THERAPY FOR COLON CANCER

The presence of lymph node involvement with tumor places patients with stage III colon cancer at highest risk for relapse. The value of adjuvant therapy is less clear for patients with stage II colon cancer. Although there is no lymph node involvement, these tumors can penetrate through the muscle wall, into surrounding structures, or through the visceral peritoneum. Even though the relative 5-year survival rates are more favorable than for stage III disease, an intermediate risk of relapse still exists due to the invasive nature of stage II disease. Thus far, analyses of clinical trial results have been unable to identify patients with stage II colon cancer who may benefit from adjuvant therapy. However, the status of chromosome 18q may provide important prognostic information for patients with stage II disease and possibly identify a subset of patients for whom adjuvant therapy should be administered.[66]

Radiation Therapy

There is currently no definitive role for adjuvant XRT in extrapelvic colon cancer. Although tumors above the peritoneal reflection have a higher incidence of failure within the abdominal cavity, effective doses of whole abdominal XRT are limited by considerable toxicity. Although postoperative local XRT reduces risk of local recurrence, it does not improve 5-year survival.[8]

Single-Agent Chemotherapy

Alkylating agents such as nitrogen mustard and thiotepa were the first chemotherapeutic drugs used in the adjuvant setting in the late 1950s.[92] Their use, however, failed to improve results associated with surgery alone. During the 1970s, interest centered around the use of single-agent 5-FU and FUDR based on their activity against metastatic colorectal cancer. Although not statistically significant, four large randomized trials demonstrated a small improvement in disease-free survival with a 5–10% increase in overall survival rates for patients receiving single-agent adjuvant 5-FU or FUDR.[93]

Combination Chemotherapy

5-FU and Levamisole

In 1990, the NIH Consensus Development Conference recommended that the use of 5-FU and levamisole be considered standard therapy for patients with surgically treated stage III colon cancer. In a study sponsored by the Mayo Clinic and the North Central Cancer Group, surgery alone was compared with postoperative levamisole and postoperative levamisole plus 5-FU in patients with surgically treated stage II and stage III colorectal cancer.[94] 5-FU, 450 $mg/m^2/d$, was administered by IV bolus injection for 5 consecutive days, starting within 21–35 days following surgery. Starting 1 month later, patients received 5-FU, 450 mg/m^2, as a single IV bolus injection each week for 48 weeks. Levamisole was administered 50 mg orally every 8 hours each day for 3 consecutive days. Each 3-day cycle was repeated every 2 weeks and continued for 1 year. Although the combination of levamisole and 5-FU significantly reduced recurrence rates, it did not confer a statistically significant survival advantage. A potential survival benefit for patients with stage III disease was, however, identified through subset analysis of the data. Results of a larger trial first published in 1990 and later updated in 1995 demonstrated that the combination of 5-FU plus levamisole following surgical resection for stage III colon cancer reduced the recurrence rate by 40% and the death rate by 33%.[79] Levamisole alone provided no significant reduction in either recurrence or deaths. Toxicities from postoperative levamisole or levamisole plus 5-FU were clinically tolerable.

5-FU and Leucovorin

Based on the observation that 5-FU plus leucovorin substantially improves response rates associated with 5-FU alone for metastatic disease, this combination has undergone study in the adjuvant setting. Several randomized trials have evaluated the efficacy of 5-FU plus leucovorin as adjuvant therapy for patients with stage II or III colon cancer and are summarized in Table 122.6. In each of the studies, rates of recurrence and survival improved substantially for patients receiving 5-FU plus either high-dose or low-dose leucovorin. The optimal doses, administration schedule, and duration of therapy have yet to be determined. Although the efficacy and toxicity associated with each of the regimens are relatively similar, the costs of leucovorin doses ranging from 20–500 mg/m^2 are significantly different.[96] Based on the results of longer patient follow-up, overall cost of regimens may ultimately play a role in influencing therapeutic decisions.

TABLE 122.6. ADJUVANT CHEMOTHERAPY REGIMENS FOR STAGES II AND III COLON CANCER

Standard Regimen for Stage III[96]:
5-FU + levamisole (begin simultaneously 3–5 weeks after surgery)
  5-FU 450 mg/m^2 rapid IV injection (IVP) for 5 days, then weekly starting at day 28 for 1 year
Levamisole 50 mg orally (PO) three times daily for 3 days, repeated every 2 weeks for 1 year
Regimens with Potential Value[83,84,95]:
Intensive course of 5-FU + low-dose leucovorin
  5-FU 425 mg/m^2 IVP + leucovorin 20 mg/m^2 IVP on days 1–5, repeated every 4–5 weeks for 6 months
Intensive course of 5-FU + high-dose leucovorin
  5-FU 370–400 mg/m^2 IVP + leucovorin 200 mg/m^2 IVP on days 1–5, repeated every 5 weeks for 6 months
Weekly 5-FU + high-dose leucovorin (begin within 6 weeks after surgery)
  5-FU 500 mg/m^2 IVP + leucovorin 500 mg/m^2 IVP weekly during 6 of every 8 weeks for 1 year

Perioperative Portal Vein Chemotherapy

Because the liver is the site of recurrence in approximately 40% of patients, infusion of chemotherapy via the portal vein provides an additional adjuvant treatment approach. The rationale for this is based on a belief that intraoperative manipulation of the tumor provides emboli of tumor that travel directly into the portal vein circulation, ultimately developing into hepatic micrometastasis.[92] Historically, 5-FU has been the most common agent used for hepatic portal vein infusion. Because greater than 80% of a dose of 5-FU administered systemically is metabolized by the liver, direct hepatic infusion of 5-FU provides high local concentrations of the drug at the most common site of recurrence and minimizes systemic toxicity. Perioperative portal vein chemotherapy administration might then destroy cells before they can establish tumor growth.

An early trial evaluated the effect of a postoperative infusion of 1 gram of 5-FU infused via the portal vein daily for 7 days as compared to no further therapy following surgical resection to patients with stage I, II, or II colorectal cancer. Heparin was also infused to reduce thrombosis.[97] Those patients who received 5-FU and heparin experienced a significant benefit in the reduction of hepatic metastasis and a dramatic improvement in survival. Results from a larger trial of patients with stage I, II or III colon cancer who were randomized to receive either a continuous infusion of 5-FU 600 mg/m^2/d for 7 days with heparin via the portal vein or no therapy following surgical resection were recently updated.[98] Although there was no significant difference in hepatic metastases between the two groups, a modest but statistically significant improvement in disease-free survival and overall survival was observed in the chemotherapy group. Complications are generally mild and include nausea, vomiting, hematologic depression, hepatotoxicity, and infection. Several additional trials conducted thus far have failed to demonstrate a significant effect of hepatic portal vein infusion on disease recurrence or survival.[99] At this time, therefore, the value of portal vein infusion of 5-FU for colon cancer remains unproven and controversial.

Immunotherapy

A variety of agents with immunomodulating effects have undergone or are currently under study in adjuvant treatment regimens, including bacillus Calmette Guérin (BCG), autologous tumor cell vaccines, IFN-α, and monoclonal antibodies.[93,100] Early results from some studies of autologous tumor cell vaccines and monoclonal antibodies suggest that they may help reduce the rates of tumor recurrence and, perhaps, influence survival.[8,101] A recent study evaluated the effect of a murine IgG2a antibody directed against 17-1A antigen on disease recurrence and patient survival following curative surgery for stage III colorectal cancer.[101] Patients were randomized to receive five monthly intravenous infusions of 17-1A antibody or postoperative observation alone. After a median follow-up of 5 years, a reduction in the recurrence rate by 27% and the overall death rate by 30% was observed in the antibody-treated group. Patients in whom distant metastases developed as the first site of relapse appeared to benefit most. Although the most common toxicities were gastrointestinal and general flu-like symptoms, they were infrequent. Anaphylactic reactions were rare and could be managed with intravenous steroids. Based on these results, the use of monoclonal antibodies in adjuvant treatment regimens appears promising and may provide an alternative to the use of chemotherapeutic agents.

Adjuvant Treatment Options For Rectal Cancer

Rectal cancer is very distinct from colon cancer in that it has a propensity for both local and distant recurrence. The higher incidence of local failure and poorer overall prognosis associated with rectal cancer is due to anatomic limitations in excising adequate radial margins around the rectal tumor. The local recurrence rate following surgery alone is approximately 25% for patients with stage II and 50% for patients with stage III disease. Since treatment with surgery, radiation therapy, or systemic chemotherapy at the time of the recurrence is often suboptimal, adjuvant therapy after tumor resection is an important aspect of treatment of the primary tumor.

RADIATION THERAPY

The goal of adjuvant radiation therapy for rectal cancer is to decrease local tumor recurrence after surgery as opposed to improving survival. In general, pre- or postoperative XRT administered in conventional doses effectively decreases local recurrence rates for rectal cancer by up to 50% compared to rates with surgery alone.[68] Prospective data for postoperative XRT are limited but suggest that this approach decreases local failure. Preoperative XRT may be more likely to improve survival; however, data regarding this approach are mostly retrospective. There are no prospective randomized trials comparing preoperative and postoperative XRT. Currently, postoperative delivery of XRT is the standard approach in the United States for rectal tumors.

XRT PLUS CHEMOTHERAPY

Combination regimens of XRT and systemic chemotherapy have been developed to improve the results of adjuvant therapy for rectal cancer. Similar to adjuvant therapy for colon cancer, 5-FU provides the basis for chemotherapy regimens for rectal cancer. In addition, 5-FU may also sensitize rectal tumor cells to the cytotoxic effects of XRT.[96] Although postoperative systemic chemotherapy alone can reduce disease recurrence in distant sites and increase survival, local recurrence rates are not improved. Systemic chemotherapy in combination with XRT, however, reduces local tumor recurrence and improves patient survival in high-risk patients.[102–107] The details of some of these regimens are provided in Table 122.7. Results from the Gastrointestinal Tumor Study Group (GITSG) and the North Central Cancer Treatment Group (NCCTG) studies form the basis for the current recommendations that all patients receive combined modality adjuvant therapy for stage II or III rectal cancer.[91,103,104,106–108]

The GITSG evaluated patients with stage II or III rectal cancer who were randomized into one of four groups: (1) observation only (control), (2) postoperative XRT alone, (3) postoperative chemotherapy consisting of 5-FU and semustine (methyl-CCNU) for 18 months, or (4) postoperative combination of XRT and chemotherapy.[103] The XRT was administered over 4–5.5 weeks. Despite a substantial number of protocol violations and a median follow-up of only 80 months, the study finished earlier than anticipated due to the statistically significant results favoring the combined modality treatment. The patients receiving the combination therapy had a reduced rate of both local (6.5 versus 21%) and distant (22 versus 31%) recurrence rates as compared to the control group. Local recurrence rates for patients receiving chemotherapy or XRT were similar (19 versus 18%) whereas distant recurrence was more frequent in the XRT group (28 versus 19%). Although overall survival did not differ significantly among the four treatment groups at the time of initial data analysis, a subsequent reestimate of survival probabilities at a median follow-up of 94 months demonstrated that the combination treatment was associated with a 24% survival advantage over the control group.[107] As expected, combined modality therapy resulted in severe hematologic toxicity, enteritis, and diarrhea as compared to either chemotherapy or XRT alone.

The NCCTG trial evaluated postoperative XRT with or without combination chemotherapy of 5-FU and semustine in a similar population of 204 patients with rectal cancer.[106] The decision to consider XRT therapy as the control

TABLE 122.7. ADJUVANT CHEMOTHERAPY REGIMEN FOR STAGES II AND III RECTAL CANCER

5-FU 500 mg/m^2 IVP for 5 days, starting on days 1 and 28, begin 22–70 days after surgery
XRT 5040 cGy in 180-cGy fractions for 5 days each week for 6 weeks, begin on day 56 after initiation of therapy
5-FU 500 mg/m^2 IVP for 3 days, begin simultaneously with XRT and repeated on the first 3 days of the last week of XRT
5-FU 400 mg/m^2 IVP for 5 days, beginning 1 month after XRT and followed in 4 weeks by 5-FU 500 mg/m^2 IVP for 5 days

(From Refs. 96 and 106.)

group was based on the acknowledgment that, in many centers, XRT alone was considered standard therapy. In addition, the failure of the GITSG trial to demonstrate a significant advantage for combination therapy over XRT alone might be attributed to the relatively low XRT doses employed and the high deviation rate (39%) from the XRT treatment protocol.

The postoperative treatment, XRT or XRT plus 5-FU, was both preceded and followed by one cycle of 5-FU plus semustine. This was the first randomized trial in which one cycle of combination chemotherapy was given before and after XRT in addition to the administration of 5-FU during XRT. This is sometimes referred to as a "sandwich" treatment regimen. The use of combined chemotherapy and XRT significantly affected local recurrence, relapse-free survival, and overall survival as compared to XRT alone. Patients receiving combined therapy experienced a 42% recurrence rate at 5 years compared to a 63% recurrence rate in the XRT only group for an overall relative reduction of 34%. Similarly, local recurrence was decreased by 46% in the combined group compared to XRT alone (14 versus 25%) and distant recurrence was reduced by 37% (29 versus 46%). Both disease-free (59 versus 37%) and overall survival (58 versus 48%) at 5 years were significantly improved for the combined group.

Acute complications such as severe hematologic toxicity (leukopenia and thrombocytopenia), enteritis, and diarrhea were commonly observed in the combined group. Hematologic toxicity was more noticeable during postradiation chemotherapy, despite reduced doses. Although small bowel complications were uncommon, four deaths were reported as a result of complications due to small bowel obstruction, fistulas, septicemia resulting from perforation, and hemorrhage. There was a 6% incidence of primary cancers, equally divided between the XRT and combined groups. Due to the leukemogenic potential associated with semustine and results from prospective comparative trials that demonstrate that it does not contribute to overall treatment efficacy, semustine is not included in current standard adjuvant treatment regimens outside of clinical trial.[96] This regimen without semustine represents the current standard adjuvant regimen for rectal cancer.

Based on preclinical studies that suggest continuous infusions of 5-FU provide more effective radiosensitization than intravenous bolus injections, a third trial was undertaken to compare protracted intravenous 5-FU infusion to intermittent bolus injections.[108] Six hundred and sixty patients with stage II or III rectal cancer received either administration regimen during postoperative pelvic XRT with either 5-FU plus semustine or 5-FU alone both before and after XRT. With a median follow-up of 46 months, both disease-free and overall survival were significantly improved among the patients receiving protracted 5-FU infusion. The incidence of leukopenia (WBC $< 2000/mm^3$) was greater in the 5-FU bolus group whereas diarrhea was more frequent in the protracted infusion group. Longer follow-up of these results is needed to determine whether this regimen will replace the current standard adjuvant therapy for rectal cancer.

Further work is needed to establish the best combination of surgery, XRT, and chemotherapy since neither modality alone provides satisfactory efficacy for both disease recurrence and survival from rectal cancer. Interest in preoperative adjuvant therapy has resurfaced based on advances in both imaging techniques (transrectal ultrasound and MRI) and more accurate preoperative staging of rectal tumors. Studies evaluating the contribution of levamisole and leucovorin to the efficacy of adjuvant therapy for rectal cancer are also under way.

Treatment Options for Metastatic Disease

Significant improvements have been made in developing efficacious treatment options for metastatic colorectal cancer. Whereas surgery and radiation therapy are most often used to manage isolated sites of tumor, chemotherapy is most useful for patients with disseminated disease and is the primary treatment modality for unresectable metastatic colorectal cancer. The site(s) of tumor involvement and presence of symptoms help to define an appropriate initial management strategy. A general management scheme is described in Fig. 122.6. In general, treatment options are similar for metastatic cancer of the colon and rectum.

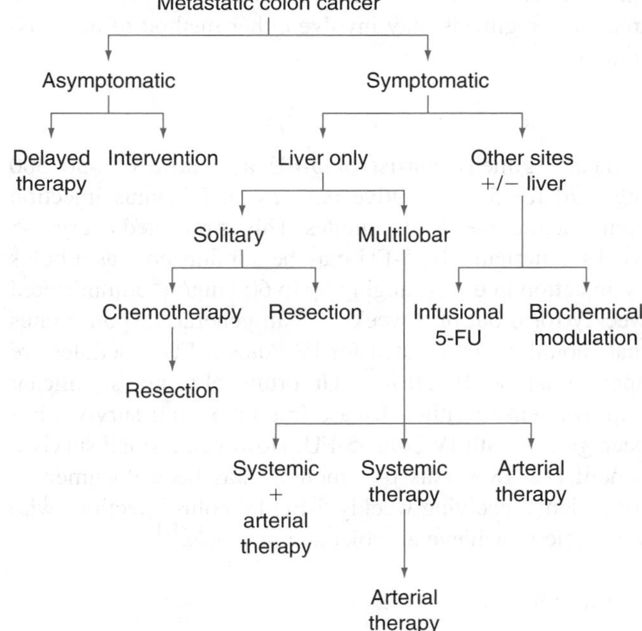

Figure 122.6. Algorithm for the methodic approach to the patient with metastatic colorectal cancer. *(Reprinted from Kemeny N, Lokich JJ, Anderson N, et al. Recent advances in the treatment of advanced colorectal cancer. Cancer 1993;71:16, with permission.)*

SURGERY

Several studies have shown that surgical resection of isolated hepatic and pulmonary metastases can be accomplished and may offer selected patients an opportunity to experience extended disease-free survival.[25] Retrospective and prospective investigations have confirmed that curative resection of isolated hepatic metastases improves median survival.[109] Patients with no significant general medical risk factors, fewer than four hepatic lesions, CEA levels less than 200 ng/mL, small tumor size, lack of extrahepatic tumor, and adequate surgical margins have the best opportunity for an improved long-term outcome. For these patients, 5-year survival rates may approach 36%. Since modalities other than surgical resection have not consistently improved survival in patients with isolated hepatic metastases and operative morbidity and mortality risks are acceptable, this approach should be considered for patients with potentially resectable disease. Although resection of pulmonary metastases has been studied to a lesser extent, patients with three or fewer metastases confined to the lungs are most likely to benefit from pulmonary metastectomy; overall 5-year survival rates are about 43%.[110]

CHEMOTHERAPY

5-FU is the most active single chemotherapeutic agent against metastatic colorectal cancer. Despite the evidence that suggests that continuous IV infusion schedules are more effective than IV bolus injections of 5-FU, effective treatment regimens may involve either method of administration.

Intravenous (IV) 5-FU Bolus Injection

Typical regimens consist of 5-FU at a dose of 450–500 mg/m^2/d for 5 consecutive days as an IV bolus injection administered over 5–10 minutes. This is repeated every 4–5 weeks. Alternatively, 5-FU may be administered as a bolus IV injection in doses ranging up to 600 mg/m^2 administered weekly for 6 out of 8 weeks.[74,76] In general, response rates that should be anticipated for IV bolus 5-FU schedules are approximately 10–20%.[71] Unfortunately, no significant improvement in either disease-free or overall survival has been gained with IV bolus 5-FU. However, a small survival benefit (12–18 versus 6–8 months) has been documented for patients receiving weekly 5-FU IV bolus injections who were able to achieve an objective response.[111]

Continuous Intravenous (IV) 5-FU Infusion

The relatively low response rates achieved with bolus 5-FU administration can perhaps be explained based on our understanding of tumor cell and drug kinetics.[112] Slow-growing colorectal cancer cells are found primarily in the resting or G_0 phase of the cell cycle. Since 5-FU primarily kills actively dividing tumor cells and has a short plasma half-life, many susceptible tumor cells may not be exposed to 5-FU for an adequate period of time. A variety of continuous IV infusion regimens have therefore been developed to increase the duration of drug exposure and hopefully improve efficacy. Some of these schedules include 8- to 24-hour, 4- to 5-day, and most recently very high 24-hour infusions (1000 mg/m^2/d for 4 days repeated every 28 days).[74] Protracted continuous infusions have utilized 5-FU at doses of 250–300 mg/m^2 IV over 24 hours each day for up to 10 weeks without a substantial amount of toxicity.[76,112] Currently, 300 mg/m^2/d is the maximally tolerated dose for long-term continuous infusion 5-FU. Several phase II trials of patients receiving continuous infusions of 5-FU for up to 12 weeks have reported improved response rates of up to 31–53%.[76,112] Although only a small number of patients were studied, comparative investigations have shown statistically greater overall response rates associated with continuous infusion versus IV bolus 5-FU (30–44 versus 7–22%).[69,76,112] Dose intensification may account for some differences seen in efficacy. As yet, however, these increased response rates have not translated into significant survival advantages.

Continuous infusion of 5-FU is one of the most efficacious methods of dose intensification, based on the assumption that a dose–response relationship exists for colorectal cancer. The maximum cumulative 5-FU dose that can be administered via continuous IV infusion in a 28-day period is approximately 4000–7400 mg/m^2 as compared to 2400–2500 mg/m^2 with IV bolus 5-FU.[74] Technologic advancement in venous access devices and portable infusion pumps has made continuous IV infusion of 5-FU both possible and practical. For now, however, the current trend favors IV bolus schedules because of inexpensive cost, ease of administration, and documented efficacy.

5-FU Plus Leucovorin (High Versus Low Dose)

Numerous studies have evaluated various doses of leucovorin in an attempt to improve the response rates and survival of single-agent 5-FU given via IV bolus or continuous IV infusion. Response rates of 10–60% have been noted with a variety of doses of 5-FU with leucovorin doses between 20–500 mg/m^2.[113] Leucovorin can be given by IV bolus, prolonged infusion, and orally. A schedule for administering leucovorin prior to 5-FU is the most effective approach to enable the level of intracellular reduced folates to accumulate prior to 5-FU administration. However, the maximum tolerated dose of 5-FU when given in combination with leucovorin is lower than that when given alone. In addition, a qualitative alteration of the toxicity pattern has been noted.

In a phase III trial conducted by the GITSG, a 5-day course of IV bolus 5-FU (500 mg/m^2) repeated every 4 weeks was compared to a combination of 5-FU (600 mg/m^2) and low-dose (25 mg/m^2) or high-dose (500 mg/m^2) leucovorin, administered for 6 out of 8 weeks.[81] The 5-FU and low-dose leucovorin regimen was no more effective than 5-FU alone (19 versus 12% response rate) whereas a 30% response rate was observed in patients who received weekly 5-FU and high-dose leucovorin. Conflicting results have been published by the Mayo Clinic NCCTG which found 5-FU (425 mg/m^2/d by IV bolus injection for 5 days, repeated every 4–5 weeks) and low-dose leucovorin (20 mg/m^2) to be more effective than either 5-FU alone or 5-FU (370 mg/m^2/d for 5 days) with high-dose leucovorin (200 mg/m^2/d) (43, 10, and 26% response rate, respectively).[82] These results were recently confirmed.[113] Although the low-dose leucovorin regimen was more effective than the high-dose regimen, the difference in response could be attributed to the higher doses of 5-FU that were administered in combination with low-dose leucovorin.

A recent meta-analysis of nine randomized clinical studies comparing weekly and monthly 5-FU plus leucovorin confirmed that the addition of leucovorin to 5-FU provided a treatment benefit in terms of objective tumor response only.[114] Despite the improvement in response rates, only two trials thus far have demonstrated an improvement in survival. In a study of patients with nonmeasurable metastatic disease, the addition of either low- or high-dose leucovorin increased survival from 7.7 to 12.0 and 12.2 months, respectively.[82] Other studies, however, have noted a trend toward survival benefit with high-dose leucovorin only.[81] A direct comparison of the GITSG and NCCTG trials was unable to identify a significant difference in tumor response rates (28 versus 33%) or median survival (10 months for each group) for patients receiving high-dose versus low-dose leucovorin.[88]

Phase III trials evaluating 5-FU and leucovorin for metastatic colorectal cancer have been criticized because doses of 5-FU used in control groups have been below the maximum-tolerated dose.[81] As a result, the addition of leucovorin may appear to produce a greater antitumor effect when in fact it is being compared to a suboptimal control group. Thus, the dose of 5-FU must also be evaluated.

5-FU plus low-dose leucovorin is currently recommended as standard systemic treatment for metastatic colorectal cancer based on response rates, toxicity, lower estimated drug costs, and quality of life indices such as performance status, weight gain, and symptoms.[82,96,113] The most common dosing regimens for 5-FU and leucovorin are described in Table 122.8.

TABLE 122.8. 5-FU/LEUCOVORIN THERAPY FOR METASTATIC COLORECTAL CANCER

Standard Regimen[82,88,113]:

5-FU + low-dose leucovorin

5-FU 425 mg/m^2 IVP + leucovorin 20 mg/m^2 IVP on days 1–5, repeated at 4 and 8 weeks and every 5 weeks thereafter.

Other Regimens:

5-FU + high-dose leucovorin[81,88]

5-FU 500 mg/m^2 IVP + leucovorin 500 mg/m^2 IV weekly for 6 weeks, followed by a 2-week rest period prior to repeating the cycle

5-FU + high-dose leucovorin[82,113]

5-FU 370 mg/m^2 IVP + leucovorin 200 mg/m^2 IVP on days 1–5, repeated at 4 and 8 weeks, and every 5 weeks thereafter

5-FU and IFN-α ± Leucovorin

Most published studies in metastatic colorectal cancer have employed a variety of intermediate doses of IFN-α, such as 5–10 × 10^6 units administered subcutaneously (SQ) three times weekly to 5 × 10^6 units/m^2/d administered SQ for 1–7 days or 18 × 10^6 units administered SQ on days numbered 1 through 3.[71] The routes of 5-FU administration have also varied. One of the most common 5-FU dosing regimens involves 5-FU 750 mg/m^2/d via continuous IV infusion for 5 days, followed by a weekly IV bolus at the same dose. An overall response rate of 26–63% using IFN-α and 5-FU in previously untreated patients with metastatic colorectal cancer has been reported. Complete responses to IFN-α in patients previously treated for advanced disease have not been reported. Larger studies comparing 5-FU plus IFN-α to 5-FU alone have only been published in abstract form but suggest that response rates (31 versus 19–21%) are not significantly different.

Promising activity has been reported in a phase II study evaluating 5-FU, leucovorin, and IFN-α in previously untreated patients with good performance status and measurable metastatic disease.[115] IFN-α (5 × 10^6 units/m^2 via SQ injection) was administered on days 1–7 and on days 2–6, 5-FU (370 mg/m^2/d IV bolus injection) was infused 1 hour after a 30-minute IV infusion of leucovorin (500 mg/m^2/d). IFN-α was administered immediately prior to leucovorin on concomitant days of therapy and cycles were repeated at 3-week intervals. An overall response rate of 54% was noted and included some complete responses. After a median follow-up of 19 months, disease-free recurrence and overall survival was 8 and 16 months, respectively. Although 5-FU doses were escalated to 425 mg/m^2/d, only 40% of patients could tolerate the higher doses. Dose-limiting toxicity occurred in 61% of patients and 26% of patients required a significant IFN-α dose reduction because of flu-like symptoms.

PALA (*N*-(Phosphonacetyl)-L-Aspartate)

As a single agent, PALA is inactive against human malignancies; however, the combination of 5-FU and PALA has undergone extensive clinical testing. Controlled studies have failed to show any significant advantage of the combination of PALA with 5-FU compared to 5-FU alone, although complete and partial responses have been reported in previously untreated patients with advanced disease.[116] The role of PALA in the management of colorectal cancer remains under investigation.

COMBINATION CHEMOTHERAPY

Attempts to improve response rates to chemotherapy by combining 5-FU with either cisplatin or methotrexate have been generally disappointing, although both cisplatin and methotrexate have some activity against colorectal cancer. Response rates are higher when cisplatin is administered with continuous IV infusion 5-FU as compared to bolus IV 5-FU, but they are not significantly better than those of 5-FU alone.[71,112] Furthermore, myelosuppression, primarily of the granulocytic cell line, also appears to be enhanced by the combination of cisplatin and IV bolus 5-FU. The timing between sequential administration of methotrexate and 5-FU appears to be an important determinant of efficacy. Intervals of as much as 24 hours between methotrexate and 5-FU administration, as well as duration of 5-FU infusions, have been studied. It is unclear, however, whether this combination provides any particular advantage to the combination of 5-FU and leucovorin.

Salvage Chemotherapy Regimens

Options for patients who no longer respond to standard treatments for metastatic colorectal cancer are limited. Response rates of approximately 10% can be expected with nitrosoureas. Mitomycin-C in combination with 5-FU has been used to induce response rates in patients with metastatic disease, primarily rectal cancer. A recent study of patients with progressive disease following 5-FU/leucovorin reported a partial response rate of 17% with a median duration of response of 9.5 months.[117] The regimen consisted of 5-FU, leucovorin, and a bolus injection of mitomycin-C, 10 mg/m^2. Although a small number of patients participated, this may represent a viable option for refractory disease.

REGIONAL THERAPEUTIC APPROACHES

Hepatic Artery Infusion

The rationale for hepatic artery infusion (HAI) is based on the principle that normal liver hepatocytes and early micrometastases obtain their primary blood supply from the portal vein. In contrast, tumors in the liver are thought to receive most of their blood supply via the hepatic artery.[118] FUDR and 5-FU have undergone the most study for infusion via the hepatic artery either via continuous infusion or IV bolus injection. The majority of hepatic arterial infusions have been directed at patients with unresectable liver metastases.[119]

The pharmacokinetic properties of FUDR in particular provide for rapid systemic clearance and high liver drug extraction. Delivery of FUDR via the hepatic artery therefore results in increased local drug concentrations at the tumor site that may translate into improved response rates. 5-FU is used less frequently because of a much lower hepatic extraction rate. Also, since approximately 80% of the administered FUDR dose is metabolized by the liver, systemic toxicity due to exposure of normal extrahepatic tissues is minimized.[71]

Early trials of HAI revealed objective response rates of 50% or higher, many of which were observed in previously treated patients.[76] The greatest problems encountered were related to complications of external catheters such as arterial thrombosis, catheter dislodgement, bleeding, bulky pump equipment limiting patient mobility, and hospitalization. The availability of implantable, portable infusion devices has significantly decreased complications and renewed interest in hepatic arterial infusional chemotherapy.[120] As a result, randomized trials comparing HAI with systemic therapy in patients with liver metastases were initiated in the 1980s. Their results have been summarized in several general review articles.[71,76,96]

FUDR via HAI has been compared to IV infusion of 5-FU and FUDR. The dose is typically 0.3 mg/kg/d administered as a continuous 24-hour infusion for a total of 14 days. This is in contrast to a comparable IV dose equal to 0.125 mg/kg/d. Heparin, in doses ranging from 10,000–17,500 units/50 mL of solution, is often added to the HAI mixture in an attempt to decrease the incidence of arterial thromboses. Prospective randomized studies have consistently demonstrated significantly higher response rates of 50–60% with HAI as compared to 20% response rates observed with IV therapy.[71,76,96] Median survival rates also are slightly higher for patients receiving HAI as compared to systemic therapy (17–20 versus 11–12 months). In addition, a general trend toward a superior 2-year survival rate appears to exist for patients who receive HAI, whether is it administered initially or following failure with systemic therapy. Patients with minimal liver involvement and lack of extrahepatic disease are most likely to benefit from therapy. Studies evaluating HAI therapy must be interpreted with caution, however, because complicating features such as crossover treatment design and presence of extrahepatic disease may account for differences in response rates and survival.[71]

The primary limitations of HAI include development and/or progression of extrahepatic disease and treatment toxicities. Common toxicities include gastric ulceration and hepatobiliary toxicity. The degree of hepatobiliary toxicity ranges from an elevation in hepatic enzymes resulting in a chemical hepatitis to sclerosing cholangitis (bile duct strictures). Elevation of liver function enzymes occurs in

35–70% of patients and is manifested by an elevation of transaminase enzymes or increased serum bilirubin levels, noted in 25% of patients. Bile duct toxicity resulting in biliary sclerosis (8–25%) is most often seen with higher doses (≥0.3 mg/kg/d) and prolonged infusions (≥2 weeks) and should be suspected when alkaline phosphatase and bilirubin levels are elevated. Hepatobiliary toxicity often resolves on discontinuation of therapy, although permanent damage to the biliary tree has been reported.[71] Various approaches have been suggested in an attempt to limit hepatobiliary toxicity and include regimens alternating FUDR with 5-FU, decreasing the FUDR dose, or by combining FUDR with dexamethasone.[120] Gastritis and gastrointestinal ulceration have been reported in 25–40% of patients and are reversible upon discontinuation of therapy. They are believed to occur because of perfusion of chemotherapy into the stomach and duodenum via small vessels branching from the hepatic artery.[71] This toxicity may be ameliorated by surgical ligation of the blood vessels supplying the stomach and duodenum or H_2-antagonist therapy. Because of toxicities associated with HAI, most patients require some transient interruption of therapy, a decrease in dosage, or discontinuation of therapy. Rest periods between therapy have also been recommended in an attempt to prevent or minimize toxicity. Although increased response rates and a trend toward improved survival have been reported, the costs and toxicities with this approach are significant. Until more data become available, HAI should be reserved for palliative treatment of isolated liver metastases and in patients who have failed systemic therapy.

Hepatic Arterial Chemoembolization

The largest experience with hepatic arterial chemoembolization has been seen in patients with metastatic carcinoid tumors or primary hepatocellular carcinomas. Most recently, small trials have been expanded to include hepatic metastases caused by colorectal cancer.[118] Hepatic arterial chemoembolization delivers high concentrations of cytotoxic agents directly to the tumor and results in the embolization or devascularization of the liver, which blocks perfusion of the tumor and eliminates its blood supply. This procedure involves the instillation of a mixture that incorporates chemotherapeutic agents, radioactive contrast dye, and/or an embolic agent directly into the hepatic artery. Agents and doses most commonly studied have included doxorubicin (40–60 mg), mitomycin (10–20 mg), and cisplatin (100–150 mg), which are usually dissolved in approximately 10–15 mL of a radiographic contrast dye. Addition of an embolic agent to the mixture, such as a gelatin sponge (Gelfoam), polyvinyl alcohol particles, bovine collagen, or iodized poppyseed oil (Lipiodol, Ethiodol), results in either a temporary or permanent occlusion of the hepatic artery. Although approximately 80% of patients in one trial experienced a response, the number of patients with colorectal cancer that have undergone this procedure thus far is relatively low. A detailed review describing the procedure, complications, and patient selection criteria has recently been published.[118] Other novel organ-targeted approaches for colorectal cancer that are under current investigation include HAI of leucovorin with IFN-α or FUDR, direct intralesional chemotherapy using ethanol or cisplatin, and cryosurgery via ultrasound-guided cryoprobe placement.

Investigational Agents

Investigational treatments include administration of monoclonal antibodies directed against tumor associated antigens, such as TAG-72 or murine MoAb B72.3 conjugated to ^{90}Y; biologic modifier therapy; and gene therapy techniques. Newer chemotherapeutic agents such as CPT-11, a topoisomerase I inhibitor, and Tomudex, a thymidylate synthase inhibitor, have demonstrated encouraging activity in both previously treated and untreated patients with metastatic colorectal cancer.[121–124]

CPT-11 (irinotecan) is a water-soluble camptothecin derivative that inhibits topoisomerase I, an enzyme necessary for DNA replication. The majority of the phase II studies have been conducted in patients with advanced colon and lung cancer. Preliminary results indicate that single-agent CPT-11 appears to be an effective salvage therapy for patients with 5-FU refractory colorectal cancer.[122] Various dosing schedules are currently being evaluated ranging from 100–150 mg/m^2 weekly, 150 mg/m^2 biweekly, 125 mg/m^2 weekly × 4 every 6 weeks to 350 mg/m^2 every 3 weeks.[124] Response rates have ranged from 14–33%, with median response rates of 25% for both untreated and previously treated patients with metastatic colorectal cancer. Diarrhea is the most common dose-limiting toxicity and may necessitate aggressive use of antidiarrheal agents or early withdrawal of therapy. Leukopenia is less common, but can also be dose-limiting.

Tomudex (ZD1694) is a folate analogue that acts as a potent and selective inhibitor of TS. In a phase II trial of previously untreated patients receiving Tomudex, 3 mg/m^2 IV every 3 weeks for metastatic colorectal cancer, a 26% objective response rate was observed.[123] The most common toxicities included neutropenia, nausea, vomiting and diarrhea, fatigue, and a reversible elevation of serum transaminases. Studies comparing Tomudex with combination 5-FU and leucovorin therapy for metastatic colorectal cancer are currently ongoing.

MONITORING THERAPEUTIC OUTCOMES

The goal of monitoring is to evaluate whether the patient is receiving any benefit from the management of their disease or to detect recurrence. Similarly, follow-up examinations help to determine whether preventive interventions or screening studies effectively reduce an individual's risk for developing colorectal cancer or presenting with an advanced stage of disease.

Symptoms of recurrence such as pain syndromes, changes in bowel habits, rectal or vaginal bleeding, pelvic masses, anorexia, and weight loss develop in less than 50% of patients.[125] A greater percentage of recurrences are detected in asymptomatic patients due to increased serum CEA levels that lead to further examination. However, the value of CEA monitoring for asymptomatic disease recurrence is questionable due to the related expense and emotional stress associated with false-positive elevations.[56] Patients who undergo curative surgical resection, with or without adjuvant therapy, require close follow-up based on the premise that early detection and treatment of recurrence could still render them cured. In addition, early treatment for asymptomatic metastatic colorectal cancer may be superior to observation only in improving median survival and prolonging the asymptomatic interval.[126] Although specific tests and the time intervals at which they should be performed are somewhat controversial, general guidelines have been reported (Table 122.9).

Recommendations for the management of colorectal cancer are reviewed in Table 122.10. The goals of adjuvant therapy for both stage II colon cancer and stages II and III rectal cancer are to reduce local and distant recurrence and improve patient survival. These endpoints represent the key therapeutic outcomes for which treatments should be evaluated. Although some regimens may not provide a substantial improvement in overall patient survival, an improvement in disease-free survival may still be a viable therapeutic outcome. Similarly, treatment approaches for metastatic colorectal cancer are assessed by their ability to produce a partial tumor response (generally considered as at least a 50% reduction in the tumor mass) or a complete response (total absence of any remaining measurable tumor). Some measurable tumor response is usually necessary for any treatment to improve disease-free or overall patient survival. In the absence of the ability of a specific treatment to improve survival, important outcome measures should include the effects of the treatment on patient symptoms, daily activities and performance status, and other quality of life indicators. Since metastatic colorectal cancer is incurable, a specific decision regarding an individual patient's care will ultimately be required; this should be based on a careful assessment of the balance between risks associated with treatment (or lack thereof) and benefits of treatment. Effort should also be made to ensure that the costs of screening, diagnostic tests, treatments, and follow-up procedures for colorectal cancer are consistent with their value in improving patient outcomes.

TABLE 122.9. GENERAL GUIDELINES FOR FOLLOW-UP AFTER CURATIVE RESECTION

Procedure or Test	Frequency
History and physical exam Fecal occult blood testing CEA Sigmoidoscopy	Every 3–4 months for 3 years, then every 6 months for 2 years, then annually
Colonoscopy or sigmoidoscopy + barium enema	Annually for several years, then every 2–3 years
Chest x-ray	Annually
Liver function tests Chest, abdominal, or pelvic CT scan Liver ultrasound Liver–spleen scan Bone scan Laparotomy	As indicated by above findings

(Modified from Ref. 8, with permission.)

TABLE 122.10. CURRENT RECOMMENDATIONS FOR TREATMENT OF CANCER OF THE COLON AND RECTUM

Stage I (Dukes' A)	Surgical resection of primary tumor and regional mesenteric lymph nodes
Stage II (Dukes' B)	
Colon	Surgery as above
Rectum	Surgery + postoperative radiation therapy + chemotherapy radiosensitization (5-FU)
Stage III (Dukes' C)	
Colon	Surgery + adjuvant chemotherapy (5-FU + levamisole)
Rectum	Surgery + postoperative radiation therapy + chemotherapy radiosensitization (5-FU)
Stage IV (Dukes' D)	Radiation therapy, systemic chemotherapy, hepatic chemotherapy, surgical resection of isolated pulmonary or hepatic metastases, symptom management

(From Ref. 91.)

References

1. Parker SL, Tong T, Bolden S, Wingo PA. Cancer statistics, 1996. CA Cancer J Clin 1996;65:5–27.
2. Ries LAG, Miller BA, Hankey BF, et al (eds). SEER cancer statistics review: 1973–1991: Tables and graphs, National Cancer Institute. NIH Publication 94-2789, Bethesda, MD, 1994.
3. Devesa SS, Blot WJ, Stone BJ, et al. Recent cancer trends in the United States. J Natl Cancer Inst 1995;87:175–182.
4. Steele GD. The national cancer data base report on colorectal cancer. Cancer 1994;74:1979–1989.

5. Coleman MP, Esteve J, Damiecki P, et al. Trends in cancer incidence and mortality. IARC Sci Publ 1993;121:1–806.
6. Burkitt DP. Epidemiology of cancer of the colon and rectum. Cancer 1971;28:3–13.
7. Milsom JW. Pathogenesis of colorectal cancer. Surg Clin North Am 1993;73:1–11.
8. Cohen AM, Minsky BD, Schilsky RL. Colon cancer, in DeVita VT, Hellman S, Rosenberg SA (eds): Cancer: Principles and Practice of Oncology, 4th ed. Philadelphia, JB Lippincott, 1993, pp 939–945.
9. Peipins LA, Sandler RS. Epidemiology of colorectal adenomas. Epidemiol Rev 1994;16:273–297.
10. Hill MJ. Metabolic epidemiology of dietary factors in large bowel cancer. Cancer Res 1975;35:3398–3402.
11. Bruce WR. Recent hypotheses for the origin of colon cancer. Cancer Res 1987;47:4237–4242.
12. Burnstein MJ. Dietary factors related to colorectal neoplasms. Surg Clin North Am 1993;73:13–29.
13. Trock B, Lanza E, Greenwald P. Dietary fiber, vegetables, and colon cancer: Critical review and meta-analyses of the epidemiologic evidence. J Natl Cancer Inst 1990;82:650–661.
14. Newcomb PA, Storer BE. Postmenopausal hormone use and risk of large-bowel cancer. J Natl Cancer Inst 1995;87:1067–1071.
15. Levin B. Nutrition and colorectal cancer. Cancer 1992;70:1723–1726.
16. Wynder EL, Reddy BS, Weisburger JH. Environmental dietary factors in colorectal cancer: Some unresolved issues. Cancer 1992;70:1222–1228.
17. Giovannucci E, Ascherio A, Rimm EB, et al. Physical activity, obesity, and risk for colon cancer and adenoma in men. Ann Intern Med 1995;122:327–334.
18. Potter JD, Slattery ML, Bostick RM, Gapstur SM. Colon cancer: A review of the epidemiology. Epidemiol Rev 1993;15:499–545.
19. Eckbom A, Helmick C, Zack M, Adami HO. Ulcerative colitis and colorectal cancer: A population-based study. N Engl J Med 1990;323:1228–1233.
20. Levin B. Inflammatory bowel disease and colon cancer. Cancer 1992;70:1313–1316.
21. Fuchs CS, Giovannucci EL, Colditzs GA, et al. A prospective study of family history and the risk of colorectal cancer. N Engl J Med 1994;331:1669–1674.
22. Lynch HT, Watson P, Smyrk T, et al. Colon cancer genetics. Cancer 1992;70:1300–1312.
23. Rustgi AK. Hereditary gastrointestinal polyposis and nonpolyposis syndromes. N Engl J Med 1994;331:1694–1702.
24. Lynch HT, Smyrk TC, Watson P, et al. Genetics, natural history, tumor spectrum, and pathology of hereditary nonpolyposis colorectal cancer: An updated review. Gastroenterol 1993;104:1535–1549.
25. Steele G. Accomplishment and promise in the understanding and treatment of colorectal cancer. Lancet 1993;342:1092–1096.
26. Vogelstein B, Fearon ER, Hamilton SR, et al. Genetic alterations during colorectal-tumor development. N Engl J Med 1988;319:525–532.
27. Fearon ER, Vogelstein B. A genetic model for colorectal tumorigenesis. Cell 1990;61:759–767.
28. Hamilton SR. Molecular genetics of colorectal carcinoma. Cancer 1992;70:1216–1221.
29. Cho KR, Vogelstein B. Genetic alterations in the adenoma–carcinoma sequence. Cancer 1992;70:1727–1731.
30. Aaltonen LA, Peltomäki P, Leach FS, et al. Clues to the pathogenesis of familial colorectal cancer. Science 1993;260:812–816.
31. Toribara NW, Sleisenger MH. Screening for colorectal cancer. N Engl J Med 1995;332:861–867.
32. Markowitz S, Wang J, Myeroff L, et al. Inactivation of the type II TGF-β receptor in colon cancer cells with microsatellite instability. Science 1995;268:1336–1338.
33. Dukes CE. The classification of cancer of the rectum. J Pathol 1932;35:323–332.
34. Spratt JS, Spuitt HJ. Prevalence and prognosis of individual clinical and pathological variables associated with colorectal carcinoma. Cancer 1967;20:1976–1985.
35. Bresalier RS, Kim YS. Malignant neoplasms of the large intestine, in Sleisenger MH, Fordtran (eds), Scharschmidt BE, Feldman (assoc eds): Gastrointestinal Disease: Pathophysiology, Diagnosis, Management, 5th ed. Philadelphia, WB Saunders, 1993, p 1449.
36. Armitage NC, Robins RA, Evans DF, et al. The influence of tumor cell DNA abnormalities on survival in colorectal cancer. Br J Surg 1985;72L:828–830.
37. Kokal W, Sheibani K, Terz J, Harada JR. Tumor DNA content in the prognosis of colorectal carcinoma. JAMA 1986;255:3123–3127.
38. Cooper GS, Yuan Z, Landefeld CS, et al. A national population-based study of incidence of colorectal cancer and age. Cancer 1995;75:775–781.
39. Silverman AL, Desai TK, Dhar R, et al. Clinical features, evaluation and detection of colorectal cancer. Gastroenterol Clin North Am 1988;17:713–725.
40. Greenberg ER, Baron JA, Tosteson TD, et al. A clinical trial of antioxidant vitamins to prevent colorectal adenoma. N Engl J Med 1994;331:141–147.
41. Vargas PA, Alberts DS. Primary prevention of colorectal cancer through dietary modification. Cancer 1992;70:1229–1235.
42. Meyskens FL, Emerson SS, Pelot D, et al. Dose de-escalation chemoprevention trial of α-difluoromethylornithine in patients with colon polyps. J Natl Cancer Inst 1994;86:1122–1130.
43. Thun MJ, Namboodiri MM, Heath CW. Aspirin use and reduced risk of fatal colon cancer. N Engl J Med 1991;325:1593–1596.
44. Giovannucci E, Rimm EB, Stampfer MJ, et al. Aspirin use and the risk for colorectal cancer and adenoma in male health professionals. Ann Intern Med 1994;121:241–246.
45. Giardiello FM, Hamilton SR, Krush AJ, et al. Treatment of colonic and rectal adenomas with sulindac in familial adenomatous polyposis. N Engl J Med 1993;328:1313–1316.
46. Winawer SJ, Zauber AG, Ho MN, et al. Prevention of colorectal cancer by colonoscopic polypectomy. N Engl J Med 1993;329:1977–1981.
47. Cancer facts and figures—1995. Atlanta, GA, American Cancer Society, 1995.
48. Lynch PM, Skibber JM. Screening guidelines for colorectal cancer. Cancer Bull 1994;46:359–364.

49. Winawer SJ, Schottenfeld D, Flehinger BJ. Colorectal cancer screening. J Natl Cancer Inst 1991;83:243–253.
50. Ahlquist DA. Occult blood screening: Obstacles to effectiveness. Cancer 1992;70(suppl 5):1259–1265.
51. Selby JV, Friedman GD, Quesenberry CP, Weiss NS. A case-control study of screening sigmoidoscopy and mortality from colorectal cancer. N Engl J Med 1992;326:653–657.
52. Ransohoff DF, Lang CA. Sigmoidoscopic screening in the 1990s. JAMA 1993;269:1278–1281.
53. Sidransky D, Tokino T, Hamilton SR, et al. Identification of *ras* oncogene mutations in the stool of patients with curable colorectal tumors. Science 1992;256:102–105.
54. Bates SE. Clinical applications of serum tumor markers. Ann Intern Med 1991;115:623–638.
55. Vignati PV, Roberts PL. Preoperative evaluation and postoperative surveillance for patients with colorectal carcinoma. Surg Clin North Am 1993;73:67–84.
56. Moertel CG, Fleming TR, Macdonald JS, et al. An evaluation of the carcinoembryonic (CEA) test for monitoring patients with resected colon cancer. JAMA 1993;270:943–947.
57. McCall JL, Black RB, Rich CA, et al. The value of serum carcinoembryonic antigen in predicting recurrent disease following curative resection of colorectal cancer. Dis Colon Rectum 1994;37:857–881.
58. Cohen A. Preoperative evaluation of patients with primary colorectal cancer. Cancer 1992;70:1328–1332.
59. Kuhn JA, Thomas G. Monoclonal antibodies and colorectal carcinoma: A clinical review of diagnostic applications. Cancer Invest 1994;12:314–323.
60. Mellstedt, Frödin JE, Masucci G, et al. The therapeutic use of monoclonal antibodies in colorectal carcinoma. Semin Oncol 1991;18:462–477.
61. Dukes CE. The classification of cancer of the rectum. J Pathol 1932;35:2310–2314.
62. Thompson WM, Trenkner SW. Staging colorectal carcinoma. Radiol Clin North Am 1994;32:25–37.
63. American Joint Committee on Cancer. In Behars OH, Henson D, Hutter RVP, et al (eds): Manual for Staging of Cancer, 3rd ed. Philadelphia, JB Lippincott, 1987.
64. Cohen AM, Minsky BD, Friedman MA. Rectal cancer, in DeVita VT, Hellman S, Rosenberg SA (eds): Cancer: Principles and Practice of Oncology, 4th ed. Philadelphia, JB Lippincott, 1993, p 978.
65. Skibber JM, Curley SA, Lotan R. Colon tumor markers for prognosis and therapy. Cancer Bull 1994;46:331–335.
66. Jen J, Kim H, Plantadosi S, et al. Allelic loss of chromosome 18q and prognosis in colorectal cancer. N Engl J Med 1994;331:213–221.
67. DeCosse JJ, Cennerazzo W. Treatment options for the patient with colorectal cancer. Cancer 1992;70:1342–1345.
68. Cummings BJ. Radiation therapy for colorectal cancer. Surg Clin North Am 1993;1:167–181.
69. Lokich JJ, Ahlgren JD, Gullo JJ, et al. A prospective randomized comparison of continuous infusion fluorouracil with a conventional bolus schedule in metastatic colorectal carcinoma: A Mid-Atlantic Oncology program study. J Clin Oncol 1989;7:425–432.
70. Peters GJ, van der Wilt CL, van Groeningen CJ, et al. Thymidylate synthase inhibition after administration of fluorouracil with or without leucovorin in colon cancer patients: Implications for treatment with fluorouracil. J Clin Oncol 1994;12:2035–2042.
71. Vaughn DJ, Haller DG. Nonsurgical management of recurrent colorectal cancer. Cancer 1993;71:4278–4292.
72. Schalhorn A, Kühl M. Clinical pharmacokinetics of fluorouracil and folinic acid. Semin Oncol 1992;19(suppl 3):82–92.
73. Kemeny N, Conti JA, Niedzwiecki D, et al. Biochemical modulation of bolus fluorouracil by PALA in patients with advanced colorectal cancer. J Clin Oncol 1992;10:747–752.
74. Leichman CG. Prolonged infusion of fluorinated pyrimidines in gastrointestinal malignancies: A review of recent clinical trials. Cancer Invest 1994;12:166–175.
75. Mahood DJ, Dose AM, Loprinzi CL, et al. Inhibition of fluorouracil-induced stomatitis by oral cryotherapy. J Clin Oncol 1991;9:449–452.
76. Kemeny N. Current approaches to metastatic colorectal cancer. Semin Oncol 1994;21(4 suppl 7):67–75.
77. Takimoto CH. Enigma of fluorouracil and levamisole. J Natl Cancer Inst 1995;87:471–472.
78. Kovach JS, Svingen PA, Schaid DJ. Levamisole potentiation of fluorouracil antiproliferative activity mimicked by orthovanadate, an inhibitor of tyrosine phosphatase. J Natl Cancer Inst 1992;84:515–519.
79. Moertel CG, Fleming TR, Macdonald JS, et al. Fluorouracil plus levamisole as effective adjuvant therapy after resection of stage III colon carcinoma: A final report. Ann Intern Med 1995;122:321–326.
80. Moertel CG, Fleming TR, Macdonald JS, et al. Hepatic toxicity associated with fluorouracil plus levamisole adjuvant therapy. J Clin Oncol 1993;11:2386–2390.
81. Petrelli N, Douglass HO, Herrera L, et al. The modulation of fluorouracil with leucovorin in metastatic colorectal carcinoma: A prospective randomized phase III trial. J Clin Oncol 1989;7:1419–1426.
82. Poon MA, O'Connell MJ, Moertel CG, et al. Biochemical modulation of fluorouracil: Evidence of significant improvement of survival and quality of life in patients with advanced colorectal carcinoma. J Clin Oncol 1989;7:1407–1418.
83. Wolmark N, Rockette H, Fisher B, et al. The benefit of leucovorin-modulated fluorouracil as postoperative adjuvant therapy for primary colon cancer: Results from National Surgical Adjuvant Breast and Bowel Project Protocol C-03. J Clin Oncol 1993;11:1879–1887.
84. International Multicentre Pooled Analysis of Colon Cancer Trials (IMPACT) Investigators. Efficacy of adjuvant fluorouracil and folinic acid in colon cancer. Lancet 1995;345:939–944.
85. Wadler S, Haynes H, Wiernik PH. Phase I trial of somatostatin analog octreotide acetate in the treatment of fluoropyrimidine-induced diarrhea. J Clin Oncol 1995;13:222–226.
86. Petrelli NJ, Rodrigues-Bigas M, Rustum Y, et al. Bowel rest, intravenous hydration, and continuous high-dose infusion of octreotide acetate for the treatment of chemotherapy-induced diarrhea in patients with colorectal carcinoma. Cancer 1993;72:1543–1546.
87. Meropol NJ, Creaven PJ, Petrelli NJ, et al. Seizures associated with leucovorin administration in cancer patients. J Natl Cancer Inst 1995;87:56–58.

88. Gerstner J, O'Connell MJ, Wieand HS, et al. A prospectively randomized clinical trial comparing 5-FU combined with either high or low dose leucovorin for the treatment of advanced colorectal cancer. Proc Am Soc Clin Oncol 1991;10:134.
89. Wadler S, Schwartz EL. Biologic agents as biochemical modulators: Pharmacologic basis for the interaction of cytotoxic chemotherapeutic drugs and interferon. Cancer Chemother Pharmacol 1994;35:21–30.
90. Milano G, Fischel JL, Etienne MC, et al. Inhibition of dihydropyrimidine dehydrogenase by α-interferon: Experimental data on human tumor cell lines. Cancer Chemother Pharmacol 1994;34:147–152.
91. National Institutes of Health Consensus Development Conference. Adjuvant therapy for patients with colon and rectal cancer. JAMA 1990;84:515–519.
92. Kane MJ. Adjuvant systemic treatment for carcinoma of the colon and rectum. Semin Oncol 1991;18(5):421–442.
93. Sinicrope FA, Sugarman SM. Adjuvant therapy for colon carcinoma: Current status and future directions. Cancer Bull 1994;46:344–351.
94. Laurie JA, Moertel CG, Fleming TR, et al. Surgical adjuvant therapy of large bowel carcinoma: An evaluation of levamisole and combination of levamisole and 5-fluorouracil. J Clin Oncol 1989;7:1447–1456.
95. O'Connell MJ, Mailliard J, Macdonald J, et al. An intergroup trial of intensive course 5FU and low dose leucovorin as surgical adjuvant therapy for high risk colon cancer. Proc Am Soc Clin Oncol 1993;12:190.
96. Moertel CG. Chemotherapy for colorectal cancer. N Engl J Med 1994;330:1136–1142.
97. Taylor I, Machin D, Mullee M, et al. A randomized controlled trial of adjuvant portal vein cytotoxic perfusion in colorectal cancer. Br J Surg 1985;72:359–363.
98. Wolmark N, Rockette H, Petrelli N, et al. Long-term results of the efficacy of perioperative portal vein infusion of 5-FU for treatment of colon cancer: NSABP C-02. Proc Am Soc Clin Oncol 1994;13:194.
99. O'Connell MJ. Is portal-vein fluorouracil hepatic infusion effective colon cancer surgical adjuvant therapy? J Clin Oncol 1990;1454–1456.
100. Beatty JD. Immunotherapy of colorectal cancer. Cancer 1992;70:1425–1433.
101. Riethmüller G, Schneider-Gädicke E, Schlimok G, et al. Randomised trial of monoclonal antibody for adjuvant therapy of resected Dukes' C colorectal carcinoma. Lancet 1994;343:1177–1183.
102. Schnall SF, Macdonald JS. Adjuvant therapy in colorectal carcinoma. Semin Oncol 1991;18:560–570.
103. Gastrointestinal Tumor Study Group. Prolongation of the disease-free interval in surgically treated rectal carcinoma. N Engl J Med 1985;312:1465–1472.
104. Schneebaum S, Arnold MW, Martin EW. Adjuvant treatment for rectal cancer: Current status. Oncology 1993;7:84–98.
105. Moertel CG. Accomplishments in surgical adjuvant therapy for large bowel cancer. Cancer 1992;70:1364–1371.
106. Krook JE, Moertel CG, Gunderson LL, et al. Effective surgical adjuvant therapy for high-risk rectal carcinoma. N Engl J Med 1991;324:709–715.
107. Douglass HO, Moertel CG, Mayer RJ, et al. Survival after postoperative combination treatment of rectal cancer. N Engl J Med 1986;315:1294–1295.
108. O'Connell MJ, Martenson JA, Wieand HS, et al. Improving adjuvant therapy for rectal cancer by combining protracted infusion fluorouracil with radiation therapy after curative surgery. N Engl J Med 1994;331:502–507.
109. Ballantyle GH, Quin J. Surgical treatment of liver metastases in patients with colorectal cancer. Cancer 1993;71:4252–4266.
110. van Halteren HK, van Geel AN, Hart AAM, Zoetmulder FAN. Pulmonary resection for metastasis of colorectal origin. Chest 1995;107:1526–1531.
111. Ansfield F, Klotz J, Nealon T, et al. A phase III study comparing the clinical utility of four regimens of 5-fluorouracil. A preliminary report. Cancer 1977;39:34–40.
112. Köhne-Wompner CH, Schmoll HJ, Harstrick A, Rustum YM. Chemotherapeutic strategies in metastatic colorectal cancer: An overview of current clinical trials. Semin Oncol 1992;19(2 suppl 3):105–125.
113. Poon MA, O'Connell MJ, Wieand HS, et al. Biochemical modulation of fluorouracil with leucovorin: Confirmatory evidence of improved therapeutic efficacy in advanced colorectal cancer. J Clin Oncol 1991;9:1967–1972.
114. The Advanced Colorectal Cancer Meta-Analysis Project. Modulation of fluorouracil by leucovorin in patients with advanced colorectal cancer: Evidence in terms of response rate. J Clin Oncol 1992;10:896–903.
115. Grem JL, Robson ME, Binder RA, et al. Phase II study of fluorouracil, leucovorin, and interferon alfa-2a in metastatic colorectal carcinoma. J Clin Oncol 1993;11:1737–1745.
116. Kemeny N, Conti JA, Seiter K, et al. Biochemical modulation of bolus fluorouracil by PALA in patients with advanced colorectal cancer. J Clin Oncol 1992;10:747–752.
117. Conti JA, Kemeny NE, Saltz LB, et al. Continuous infusion fluorouracil/leucovorin and bolus mitomycin-C as a salvage regimen for patients with advanced colorectal cancer. Cancer 1995;75:769–774.
118. Soulen MC. Chemoembolization of hepatic malignancies. Oncology 1994;8:77–84.
119. Patt YZ, Mavligit GM. Arterial chemotherapy in the management of colorectal cancer: An overview. Semin Oncol 1991;18:478–490.
120. Patt, YZ. Regional hepatic arterial chemotherapy for colorectal cancer metastatic to the liver: The controversy continues. J Clin Oncol 1993;11(5):815–819.
121. Conti JA, Kemeny NE, Saltz LB, et al. Irinotrecan is an active agent in untreated patients with metastatic colorectal cancer. J Clin Oncol 1996;14:709–715.
122. Shimada Y, Yoshino M, Wakui A, et al. Phase II study of CPT-11, a new camptothecin derivative in metastatic colorectal cancer. J Clin Oncol 1993;11:909–913.
123. Zaleberg JR, Cunningham D, Van Cutsem E, et al. ZD1694: A novel thymidylate synthase inhibitor with substantial activity in the treatment of patients with advanced colorectal cancer. J Clin Oncol 1996;14:716–721.
124. Slichenmeyer WJ, Rowinsky EK, Donehower RC, et al.

The current status of camptothecin analogues as antitumor agents. J Natl Cancer Inst 1993; 85:271–291.
125. Steele G. Standard postoperative monitoring of patients after primary resection of colon and rectum cancer. Cancer 1993;71:4225–4235.
126. The Nordic Gastrointestinal Tumor Adjuvant Therapy Group. Expectancy or primary chemotherapy in patients with advanced asymptomatic colorectal cancer: A randomized trial. J Clin Oncol 1992;10:904–911.

Chapter 123

Prostate Cancer

Barry R. Goldspiel, PharmD, Jill M. Kolesar, PharmD, and John G. Kuhn, PharmD, FCCP

Prostate cancer is the most frequent cancer among American men and represents the second leading cause of cancer-related deaths in all males.[1] In the United States alone, it was estimated that 244,000 new cases of prostatic carcinoma would be diagnosed and more than 40,400 men would die from this disease in 1995.[1] The rise in incidence over the past decade may be attributable to an aging population or better detection methods. The endocrine dependence of this tumor is well documented and hormonal manipulation to decrease circulating androgens remains the basis for the treatment of advanced disease.

Epidemiology/Etiology

Table 123.1 summarizes the possible risk factors associated with prostate cancer.[2–5] The only widely accepted risk factors are age, race-ethnicity, and family history of prostate cancer.[2,3,6] The disease is rare under the age of 40, but the incidence sharply increases with each subsequent decade.[2,3] The incidence of clinical prostate cancer varies across geographic regions. Scandinavian countries and the United States report the highest incidence of prostate cancer, while in Japan and other Eastern countries the disease is relatively rare.[2,3,6] African American men have the highest rate of prostate cancer in the world and in the United States; overall 5-year survival is approximately 15% less for African Americans compared to Caucasians.[1] Both hormonal and genetic differences may contribute to the altered susceptibility to prostate cancer in these populations.[6] Testosterone, commonly implicated in the pathogenesis of prostate cancer, is 15% higher in African-American men when compared to Caucasian males. 5-α-Reductase activity, the enzyme that converts testosterone to its more active form, dihydrotestosterone, in the prostate, is decreased in Japanese men compared to African Americans and Caucasians. In addition to hormonal differences, genetic variations in the androgen receptor exist. The androgen receptor gene contains a variable trinucleotide repeat (CAG) sequence and there is evidence to suggest that an increased number of trinucleotide repeats results in decreased androgen receptor activity. There is a significant difference in androgen receptor trinucleotide repeats between African-American, Caucasian, and Asian-American populations in the United States. African Americans have the least number of trinucleotide repeats while Asian Americans have the most androgen receptor trinucleotide repeats.[2]

Hereditary prostate cancer is estimated to account for 9% of all prostate cancer and 45% of disease reported in men under the age of 55.[6] Carter and colleagues[4] have demonstrated that familial clustering of prostate cancer can be explained by Mendelian inheritance of a rare autosomal dominant allele. Efforts are under way to identify the gene in the candidate regions of BRCA1, 8p22, and 16q22.

Other factors thought to be associated with prostate cancer include occupational exposure, diet, benign prostatic hyperplasia, and vasectomy.[3,6–8] Workers exposed to alkaline batteries come into contact with cadmium, a trace mineral that may be antagonistic to zinc. Zinc is found in very high levels in the prostate and is required in several enzymes involved in the repair and synthesis of DNA and RNA. Farm workers and workers in the rubber industry may also be at increased risk for prostate cancer. High-fat, low-fiber diets seem to be associated with an increase in prostate cancer, although the mechanism remains unclear. Because fat intake is a modifiable risk factor, dietary intervention may be promising in the prevention of prostate cancer. Increased theobromine intake has been associated with a higher prostate cancer incidence.[9] The precise relationship between benign prostatic hyperplasia and prostate carcinoma is unclear, although some evidence suggests a relative risk of 5.1–13.5.[3] Vasectomy has emerged as a possible risk factor for prostate cancer. A number of case-control studies have shown an increased incidence of prostate cancer in men who have had vasectomies, although similarly designed studies have also shown no association.[8] A prospective cohort study of U.S. health professionals reported an age-adjusted relative risk of 1.56 in men with vasectomies and a relative risk of 1.85 in men who had vasectomies more than 20 years ago.[8]

Smoking has not been associated with an increased risk of prostate cancer.[9] The relationships between prostate

TABLE 123.1. ETIOLOGIC FACTORS ASSOCIATED WITH PROSTATE CANCER

Factor	Possible Relationship
Environmental	Clinical carcinoma incidence varies worldwide Latent carcinoma similar between regions Nationalized males adopt intermediate incidence rates between that of the United States and their native country
Occupational	Increased risk associated with cadmium exposure
Genetic	Familial prostate cancer inherited in an autosomal dominant manner Mutations in *p53, Rb,* E-cahedrin, α-catenin, androgen receptor, *KAI1,* microsatellite instability, loss of heterozygocity at 10q, 16q, 8p, 17p
Diet	Increased risk associated with high-meat and high-fat diets
Vasectomy	Relative risk: 1.56–1.85
Hormonal	Does not occur in eunuchs Low incidence in cirrhotic patients Up to 80% are hormonally dependent African-Americans have 15% increased testosterone Japanese have decreased 5-α-reductase activities Polymorphic expression of the androgen receptor

(From Refs. 3, 5, 6–8, and 11–15.)

cancer and sexually transmitted diseases and sexual activity remains unclear.[3]

MOLECULAR GENETICS

Malignancy is generally accepted to be a multistep process involving a number of molecular events that can lead to the development of prostate cancer (Fig. 123.1).[10] The initial step in cancer progression involves early mutations in stability genes. Hypermethylation, associated with gene inactivation, has been reported frequently in prostate cancer.[5] *p53* is thought to function by halting cell cycle progression in cells with DNA damage, resulting in cell death via apoptotic pathways. The loss of functional *p53* may result in replication of damaged DNA and subsequently unregulated cell growth. Point mutations in *p53* thought to be caused by environmental toxins have been identified in 42% of prostate carcinomas. Mutations were present in stages B to D, although not in latent prostate carcinomas studied.[11] *Rb* mutations, also thought to be important in cell cycle regulation, have been identified in patients with prostate cancer.[5] Microsatellite instability, a marker for genetic instability and the inability to repair damaged DNA, has also been reported in prostate cancer.[12] Loss of the ability to repair damaged DNA predisposes the cell to an increased frequency of mutation.

The metastasic potential of the cell is likely to involve the E-cahedrin gene, which is located on chromosome 16.22.1 and is mutated in 36% of prostate carcinomas. Aberrant E-cahedrin immunohistochemical staining is associated with high-grade prostate tumors and poor outcome in terms of disease progression and overall survival in patients with prostate cancer.[5] In addition, E-cahedrin interacts with α-catenin to link with the microfilament cytoskeleton. This interaction is required for cell–cell adhesion. α-Catenin is located at 5q22 and approximately 25% of prostate cancers are mutated at this location.[5] *KAI1,* or Kang ai, which is Chinese for anticancer, is a recently isolated antimetastatic gene. The gene codes for a protein belonging to a family of leukocyte surface glycoproteins that function in cell–cell interactions and cell–extracellular matrix interactions.[13] Mutations in the androgen receptor gene, altering the hormone binding activity, have been reported in metastatic androgen-independent prostate cancer.[14]

Despite the great variance in the clinical incidence of prostate cancer, the incidence of latent or histological low-grade prostate cancer is similar in Japan and the United States. Interestingly, androgen receptor mutations may contribute to this difference. A significant number of latent prostatic carcinomas in Japanese men contain an inactivating mutation in the androgen receptor while no such mutations were found in latent carcinomas of American men.[15] It appears that the stage in which an androgen receptor mutation occurs (latent versus metastatic) as well as the functional significance of the mutation, can alter the clinical course of prostate cancer. Additional genetic analysis has identified mutations in *Ha-ras* in less than 4% of American prostate carcinomas and up to 25% of Japanese carcinomas. Mutations in late stage clinical carcinoma were identified in *Ha-ras;* however latent prostate carcinoma had mutations in *Ka-ras,* possibly indicating a protective mutation.[5]

Although the molecular characterization of prostate carcinoma is just evolving, this area of study represents a major advance in our understanding of disease pathology and may represent future avenues for diagnosis, staging, and treatment of prostate cancer.

PATHOPHYSIOLOGY

The prostate gland is a solid, rounded, heart-shaped organ positioned between the neck of the bladder and the urogenital diaphragm (Fig. 123.2). The organ consists of single anterior, posterior, and median lobes with two lateral lobes. The posterior lobe is palpable by anterior rectal examination at 2–5 cm from the anal verge. Within the four morphologically defined areas of the prostate gland, 95% of the carcinomas arise from the glandular epithelium of the peripheral zone.[16] In contrast, benign prostatic hyperplasia

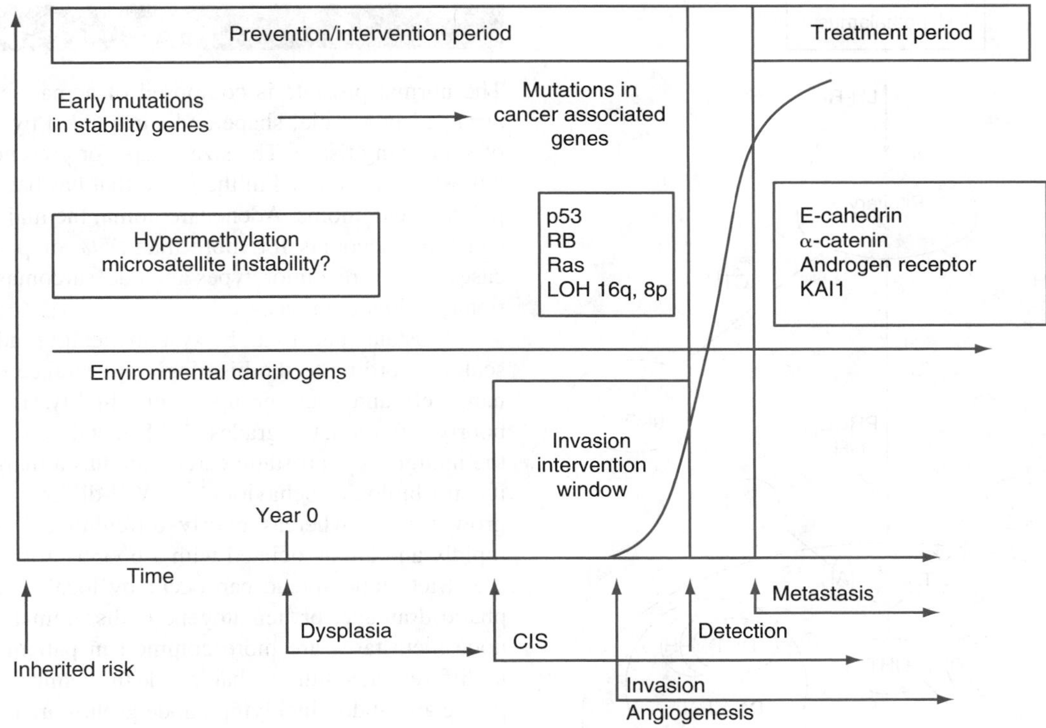

Figure 123.1. Molecular events in prostate cancer. *(From Isaacs WB, Bova SG, Morton RA, et al. Molecular genetics and chromosomal alterations in prostate cancer. Cancer 1995;75:2004–2012 and Kohn EC, Liotta LA. Molecular insights into cancer invasion: Strategies for prevention and intervention. Cancer Res 1995;55:1856–1862.)*

arises from the central or periurethral regions of the prostate gland.

Normal growth and differentiation of the prostate depends on the presence of androgens, specifically dihydrotestosterone (DHT).[17,18] The testes and the adrenal glands are the major sources of circulating androgens. Hormonal regulation of androgen synthesis is mediated through a series of biochemical interactions between the hypothalamus, pituitary, adrenal glands, and the testes (Fig. 123.3). Luteinizing hormone-releasing hormone (LHRH) released from the hypothalamus stimulates the release of luteinizing hormone (LH) and follicle-stimulating hormone (FSH) from the anterior pituitary gland. Luteinizing hormone complexes with receptors on the Leydig cell testicular membrane and stimulates the production of testosterone and small amounts of estrogen. FSH acts on the Sertoli cells within the testes to promote the maturation of LH receptors and to produce an androgen-binding protein. Circulating testosterone and estradiol influence the synthesis of LHRH, LH, and FSH by a negative feedback loop operating at the hypothalamic and pituitary level.[6,17–19] Prolactin, growth hormone, and estradiol appear to be important accessory regulators for prostatic tissue permeability, receptor binding, and testosterone synthesis. However, a precise relationship between these hormones and prostate growth has not been defined.[6,17–19]

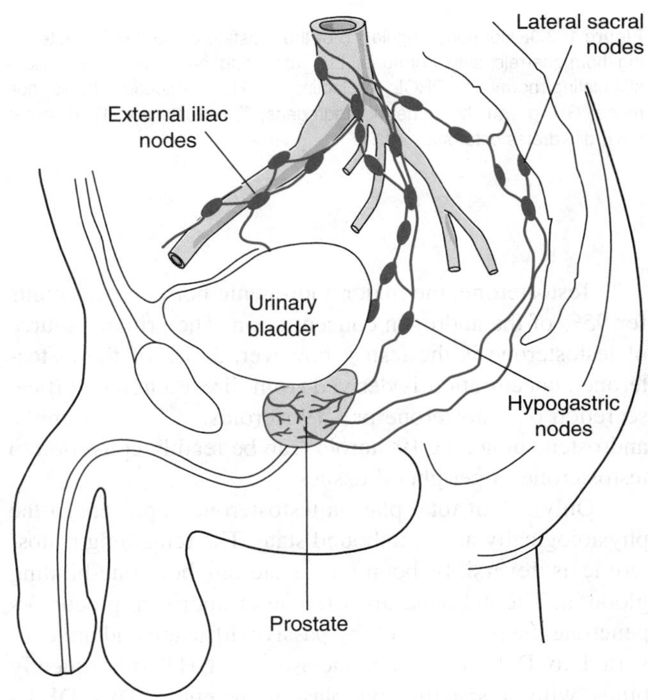

Figure 123.2. The prostate gland. *(From Spirnak JP, Kesnick MI. Clinical staging of prostatic cancer: New Modalities. Urol Clin North Am 1984;11:224, with permission.)*

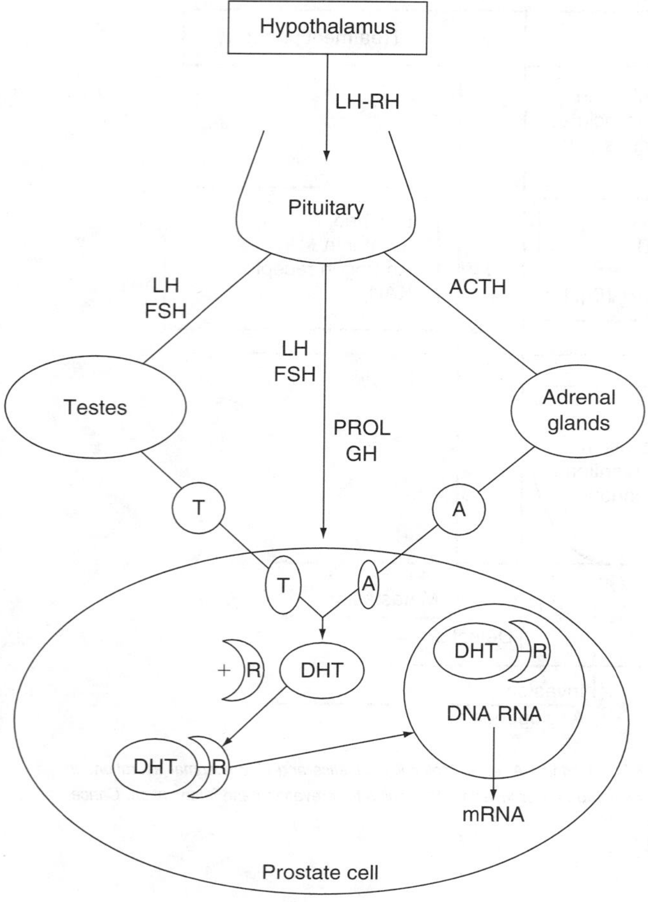

Figure 123.3. Hormonal regulation of the prostate gland. LH-RH, luteinizing hormone-releasing hormone; LH, luteinizing hormone; FSH, follicle-stimulating hormone; PROL, prolactin; ACTH, adrenocorticotropic hormone; GH, growth hormone; A, androgens; T, testosterone; R, receptor; DHT, dihydrotestosterone.

Testosterone, the major androgenic hormone, accounts for 95% of the androgen concentration. The primary source of testosterone is the testes; however, 3–5% of the testosterone concentration is derived from direct adrenal cortical secretion of testosterone or C19 steroids.[17,20] For example, androstenedione, a C19 steroid, can be readily converted to testosterone in peripheral tissues.

Only 2% of total plasma testosterone is present in the physiologically active unbound state. The remaining testosterone is reversibly bound to a steroid hormone-binding globulin. The unbound testosterone or androgen precursors penetrate the prostatic cell by passive diffusion and are converted to DHT by 5-α-reductase.[20,21] DHT subsequently binds with a specific cytoplasmic receptor. This DHT–receptor complex is then transported to the nucleus of the cell where transcription and ultimately translation of stored genetic material occurs.[17,18]

Pathology

The normal prostate is composed of acinar secretory cells arranged in a radial shape and surrounded by a foundation of supporting tissue. The size, shape, or presence of acini is almost always altered in the gland that has been invaded by prostatic carcinoma. Adenocarcinoma, the major pathologic cell type, accounts for more than 95% of prostate cancer cases.[22,23] Rare tumor types include sarcomas and transitional cell carcinomas.

Prostate cancer can be systematically graded (Gleason scale) according to the histologic appearance of the malignant cell and then grouped into highly, moderately, or poorly differentiated grades.[24,25] Depending on the grade of the malignancy, prostatic carcinoma has a marked variability in biologic behavior.[24,25] Well-differentiated tumors grow slowly, whereas poorly differentiated tumors grow rapidly and are associated with a poorer prognosis.

Metastatic spread can occur by local extension, lymphatic drainage, or hematogenous dissemination.[23] Lymph node metastases are more common in patients with large, undifferentiated tumors that invade the seminal vesicles. The pelvic and abdominal lymph node groups are the most common sites of lymph node involvement (Fig. 123.2). Skeletal metastases from hematogenous spread are the most common sites of distant spread. Typically, the bone lesions are osteoblastic or a combination of osteoblastic and osteolytic. The most common site of bone involvement is the lumbar spine. Other sites of bone involvement include the proximal femurs, pelvis, thoracic spine, ribs, sternum, skull, and humerus. The lung, liver, brain, and adrenal glands are the most common sites of visceral involvement; however, these organs are not usually involved initially. Twenty-five percent to 35% of patients will have evidence of lymphangitic or nodular pulmonary infiltrates at autopsy. The prostate is a rare site for metastatic involvement from other solid tumors.

Clinical Presentation

While prostatic carcinoma may be asymptomatic in patients with localized disease, most patients with signs and symptoms have advanced disease at presentation. In patients with locally invasive disease, the most common complaints arise from ureteral dysfunction or impingement. Patients complain of alterations in micturation manifested by urinary frequency, hesitancy, and dribbling.[22,26] New onset impotence or less firm penile erections in an elderly male may indicate prostate cancer. Most commonly, patients with advanced disease present with back pain and stiffness due to osseous metastases. Eventually, spinal cord lesions may lead to cord compression if not properly treated. Rarely, pathologic fractures can occur. Lower extremity edema can occur as a result of lymphatic obstruction. Anemia and weight loss are nonspecific signs of advanced disease.

Screening/Diagnosis/Staging

Digital rectal exam (DRE) is a commonly employed method for the detection of prostate cancer with a sensitivity of 55–69%, specificity of 89–97%, positive predicative value of 11–26%, and a negative predictive value of 85–96%.[27] Estimated sensitivity, specificity, and positive predictive values for prostate-specific antigen (PSA) as a single screening test are 67, 97, and 43%, respectively.[27] Since PSA screening is able to identify nonpalpable cancers, it increases the detection rate of prostate cancer in asymptomatic men older than 50 by 50% compared to DRE alone. Most of the detected tumors are organ confined and greater than 0.5 mL in volume, representing clinically significant, yet curable disease. Unfortunately, only 38–48% of men with clinically significant prostate cancer have a serum PSA outside the reference range.[28] Neither DRE or PSA is sensitive or specific enough to be used alone as a screening test. While the relative predictability of DRE and PSA is similar, the tumors identified by each method are different. Catalona and associates[29] confirmed that the combination of a rectal examination plus a PSA with ultrasonography performed on patients with abnormal findings is a better method of detecting prostate cancer than rectal examination alone. The PLCO (prostate, lung, colorectal, and ovarian) Cancer Screening Trial of the National Cancer Institute is currently under way with the primary objective of determining whether screening 60- to 74-year-old men with DRE and serum PSA decreases mortality.[27]

Although discovered more than 20 years ago, PSA is the most sensitive biochemical marker available for the diagnosis, staging, and monitoring of prostate cancer. In addition to its value as a tumor marker, PSA may be involved in cancer growth. PSA is a prostate-specific glycoprotein produced only in the cytoplasm of benign and malignant prostate cells.[28] PSA functions as a serine protease, which liquefies seminal fluid after ejaculation. In addition to its biological activity, PSA may also enhance cellular growth by its ability to cleave insulin-like growth factor binding proteins (IGFBPs). Cleavage activates insulin-like growth factor (IGF), which can then bind to IGF receptors and stimulate growth in the prostate.[30]

The major form of measurable PSA in the serum is as a complex of PSA and α_1-anti-chymotrypsin or α_2-macroglobulin. PSA may also complex with a variety of other acute phase proteins or it may exist in an uncomplexed form that is enzymatically inactive. Patients with prostate cancer have higher levels of PSA complexes, which may be diagnostically useful.[31]

New ultrasensitive immunoassays for PSA allow detectability as low as 0.1 ng/mL, although they are not yet in routine use. Currently, the Tandem-R by Hybritech and the IM_x assay by Abbott Laboratories are two FDA-approved PSA immunoassays available in the United States. The IM_x assay was designed using the same calibration standard as the Tandem-R assay and PSA results are considered interchangeable. There are a number of assays both within and outside the United States that are not currently FDA approved and PSA levels obtained with these assays are not interchangeable.[31]

Unlike acid phosphatase, PSA levels are not influenced by ambient conditions nor subject to diurnal variation but are influenced by sedentary conditions. Therefore, it is recommended that all PSA measurements be made on sera collected from ambulatory patients.[32] PSA levels not only rise with prostatic manipulation such as transrectal ultrasound and/or biopsy but remain above normal for several weeks thereafter. The reported serum half-life of PSA is 2–3 days.[33] Although PSA is prostate specific, it is not cancer specific. Benign conditions, including acute urinary retention, acute prostatitis, prostatic ischemia, or infarction and benign prostatic hypertrophy (BPH), will cause an elevation of PSA.[28]

Despite the ability of serum PSA levels to predict early prostate cancer, an elevated PSA does not always indicate prostate cancer. Efforts to increase specificity include the use of age-specific PSA levels, PSA density, and PSA velocity.

An increase in serum PSA with increasing age in the absence of clinically detectable prostate cancer has been documented by a number of investigators in studies including more than 6000 healthy males.[34] The age-specific PSA reference ranges (upper limit defined by the 95th percentile) is reported to be 0–2.5 ng/mL for men aged 40–49, 0–3.5 ng/mL for those 50–59, 0–4.5 ng/mL for those 60–69, and 0–6.5 ng/mL for men 70–79 (Table 123.2).[28] Prostate volume is the most significant factor responsible for increases in PSA with advancing age. Some investigators recommend determining the prostate volume by transurethral ultrasonography (TRUS). PSA density (PSAD) is calculated by dividing the serum PSA level by the prostatic gland volume ($l \times w \times h \times 0.52$), as measured by TRUS. The overall agreement between prostate volume and age-specific reference ranges of serum PSA concentration is 96%. This suggests that the determination of prostate volume by TRUS for early detection of prostate cancer probably does not provide any greater information than PSA alone.[28] PSA velocity (PSAV), which evaluates the rate of change of PSA over time, is another method that may improve accuracy of PSA screening for prostate cancer. Increases of PSAV of 0.75 ng/mL/y or more using at least three PSA levels may indicate the presence of prostate cancer and a workup should be initiated even if serum PSA remains in the normal range.

The American Cancer Society currently recommends that all men older than 50 years of age should have an annual PSA and DRE.[35] If both tests are normal, no further diagnostic action is required; however, if either is abnormal, further workup by TRUS is indicated (Table 123.2).[28,34,35]

TABLE 123.2. DIAGNOSTIC ALGORITHM FOR PROSTATE CANCER

PSA[a]	DRE[b]	Diagnostic Action
≤Age-specific range[c]	Neg	Annual PSA and DRE
>Age-specific range[c]	Neg	TRUS: Biopsy visible lesions. Sextant biopsy of remaining prostate, with 2 cores containing transition zone tissue
Any value	Pos	TRUS: Biopsy palpable and visible lesions; sextant biopsy of remaining prostate

[a]Tandem-R or IM_x PSA.
[b]Digital rectal exam.
[c]40–49: 0–2.5 ng/mL
50–59: 0–3.5 ng/mL
60–69: 0–4.5 ng/mL
70–79: 0–6.5 ng/mL (From Oesterling JE, Cooner WH, Jacobsen SJ, et al. Influence of patient age on the serum PSA concentration. An important clinical observation. Urol Clin North Am 1993;20:671–680.)

African-American men, or younger men who are at higher risk due to a significant family history of prostate cancer, should have both these tests performed earlier.

Prostatic carcinoma produces a specific hypoechogenic pattern by ultrasound imaging.[36] Sagittal and axial imaging by transrectal ultrasound enables the identification of the prostatic capsule, seminal vesicles, and intraprostatic extent of the disease. Ultrasound-guided transrectal biopsies can be used to obtain histologic specimens and accurately define the extraprostatic extension of the tumor. This provides both a method for determining the precise local extent of disease and a parameter to follow for treatment.[36] Transrectal ultrasonography appears to have little utility in the early diagnosis of prostate cancer if both the rectal examination and the PSA are normal.

Although the rectal examination combined with PSA constitutes the best method for detecting prostate cancer, the actual diagnosis and histologic grading can only be established by biopsy. The transperianal or transrectal routes are the most common approaches for needle biopsy. Patients with abnormalities by TRUS should undergo biopsies of hypoechoic areas as well as systemic biopsies. Those with PSA >10 ng/mL but normal TRUS should undergo random, systematic biopsies of the prostate.

Table 123.3 summarizes the diagnostic staging workup, which should include a thorough history and physical examination. Physical examination should include careful digital inspection of the rectum and palpation of regional lymph nodes, abdomen, and spine. The posterior lobe of the prostate is palpated for size, configuration, and consistency. Classically, prostatic carcinoma is characterized by a rock-hard nodule or mass in the gland, whereas in BPH, the gland is smooth and rubbery. The lower extremities should

TABLE 123.3. DIAGNOSTIC AND STAGING WORKUP FOR PROSTATE CANCER

Routine tests
Physical examination with digital rectal palpation
Prostate-specific antigen
Transrectal ultrasonography
Excretory urogram
Chest x-ray
Serum phosphatases (acid/alkaline)
Liver function tests
Bone scan
Additional tests for staging
Skeletal films
Lymph node evaluation
Bipedal lymphangiogram
Pelvic CT scan
Pelvic lymphadenectomy
Transrectal MRI

be tested for strength and reflex symmetry. Initial laboratory tests should include a complete blood chemistry, liver function tests, serum creatinine, serum acid phosphatase, serum alkaline phosphatase, and a urinalysis.

Alkaline phosphatase is frequently increased in prostate cancer due to the metabolic activity of the bone surrounding the bone metastases.[22,23] The source of an elevated alkaline phosphatase can be determined by the reaction of the sample to heat. Alkaline phosphatase derived from bone is heat labile, whereas the fraction derived from the liver is heat stable.

The bone scan is more sensitive than a skeletal survey in detecting early metastatic disease.[22,23] Thirty percent to 50% of bone must be replaced by tumor before it can be detected by routine radiologic procedures. Up to 50% of patients with a positive bone scan can have a normal skeletal radiograph.[22,23,26] The bone scan is highly sensitive, but also detects other bone abnormalities. Due to the low specificity, the bone scan should be reviewed along with skeletal films or tomograms directed at the radioisotopic-positive areas.[22,26] PSA levels are the best overall predictor of bone scan findings, and may make a staging radionucleotide bone scan unnecessary for patients with (1) newly diagnosed, previously untreated prostate cancer, (2) serum PSA 10 ng/mL or less, or (3) no skeletal symptoms.[28,34]

Several techniques are used to evaluate lymph node involvement.[22,23,26] Bipedal lymphangiography determines the extent of periaortic and pelvic node involvement. This technique is associated with a false-negative rate of 40–50% because all places of metastatic involvement are not opacified by the contrast media. Pelvic computerized tomography scanning is useful in determining the local extension of the tumor and the appearance of the seminal vesicles.[26,37] This scan fails to discriminate lesions within

TABLE 123.4. STAGING AND CLASSIFICATION SYSTEMS FOR PROSTATE CANCER

AUS[a] Stage (A–D)	AJC–UICC[b] Classification (TNM)
A (occult, nonpalpable)	$T_xN_xM_x$ (cannot be assessed)
	$T_0N_0M_0$ (nonpalpable)
A_1: Focal	T_0: Focal or diffuse
A_2: Diffuse	
B (confined to prostate)	$T_1N_0M_0$, $T_2N_0M_0$
B_1: single nodule in 1 lobe, <1.5 cm	T_1 (Clinically inapparent tumor not palpable or visible by imaging)
	T1a: Tumor incidental histologic finding in 5% or less of tissue resected
	T1b: Tumor incidental histologic finding in 5% or more of tissue resected
	T1c: Tumor identified by needle biopsy (e.g., because of elevated PSA)
B_2: Diffuse involvement of whole gland, >1.5 cm	T_2: (Tumor confined within the prostate[c])
	T2a: Tumor involves half of a lobe or less
	T2b: Tumor involves more than half a lobe, but not both lobes
	T2c: Tumor involves both lobes
C (localized to periprostatic area)	$T_3N_0M_0$, $T_4N_0M_0$
C_1: No seminal vesicle involvement, <70 grams	T_3: (Tumor extends through the prostatic capsule[d])
	T3a: Unilateral extracapsular extension
	T3b: Bilateral extracapsular extension
	T3c: Tumor invades the seminal vesicle(s)
C_2: Seminal vesicle involvement, >70 grams	T_4: (Tumor is fixed or invades adjacent structures other than the seminal vesicles)
	T4a: Tumor invades any of bladder neck, external sphincter, or rectum
	T4b: Tumor invades levator muscles and/or is fixed to the pelvic wall
D (metastatic disease)	Any T,N_{1-4}, M_0, or N_{0-4}, M_1
D_1: Pelvic lymph nodes or ureteral obstruction	N_1: Metastasis in a single lymph node, 2 cm or less in greatest dimension
D_2: Bone, distant lymph node, organ, or soft tissue metastases	N_2: Metastasis in single lymph node more than 2 cm but not more than 5 cm in greatest dimension; or multiple lymph node metastases, none more than 5 cm in greatest dimension
	N_3: Metastasis in lymph node more than 5 cm in greatest dimension
	M_{1a}: Nonregional lymph node(s)
	M_{1b}: Bone(s)
	M_{1c}: Other site(s)

[a]American Urologic System or Whitmore classification.
[b]American Joint Committee–International Union Against Cancer.
[c]Tumor found in one or both lobes by needle biopsy, but not palpable or visible by imaging, is classified as T_{1c}.
[d]Invasion into the prostatic apex or into (but not beyond) the prostatic capsule is not classified as T_3 but as T_2. (From Beahrs OH, D.E. H, Hutter RVP, et al. Manual for Staging Cancer, 4th ed. Philadelphia, JB Lippincott, 1992, with permission.)

the lymph nodes unless the lymph nodes are greater than 2 cm in diameter.

Pelvic lymph node dissection is used in conjunction with definitive radiation therapy or as a staging procedure prior to radical prostatectomy. Pelvic lymph node dissection is associated with a high morbidity and this procedure is reserved for patients in whom the information obtained will directly affect treatment decisions.[22,26]

Serum PSA level appears to be the best predictor of pelvic lymph node metastasis. Patients with low grade, low stage, and a serum PSA concentration less than 16 ng/mL will have less than a 10% likelihood of pelvic disease. In combination with the primary and clinical grade, PSA may eliminate the need for pelvic lymph node dissection in 61% of men with stage T_{1a}-T_{2b} and 30% of those with stage T_{1a}-T_{2c}.[28]

Although further study is required, PSA monitoring appears to have utility in the screening, detection, staging, and monitoring of prostate cancer. The use of a simple and noninvasive laboratory value may decrease the need for invasive procedures and contribute to the earlier detection of prostate cancer.

The information obtained from the diagnostic tests is used to stage the patient. There are two commonly recognized staging classification systems (Table 123.4). The formal international classification system (TNM) adopted by the International Union Against Cancer (UICC) in 1974 was updated in 1992 in an effort to provide congruence with the classical Whitmore staging system for prostate cancer.[38] The Whitmore classification is the most commonly used staging system in the United States (Table 123.4). Patients are assigned to stages A through D based on size of the tumor, local or regional extension, presence of involved lymph node groups, and presence of metastases.[38] An additional subclassification system has been proposed that further divides each of the major stages into subcategories.[38] Some studies classify patients that have progressed after hormonal therapy as stage D_3.[26,38] Stage A_1, A_2 to B_2, and C patients comprise 10, 30, and 10% of cases, respectively.[39] Stage D accounts for the majority of patients with prostate cancer, representing 50% of newly diagnosed prostatic carcinoma cases.[39]

Prognosis

The prognosis for patients with prostate cancer depends on the histologic grade, the tumor size, and local extent of the primary tumor.[24,25] The most important prognostic criterion appears to be the histologic grade because the degree of differentiation ultimately determines the stage of disease. Poorly differentiated tumors are highly associated with both regional lymph node involvement and distant metastases.[23–25,40] For stages B and C, poorly differentiated tumors are associated with a 5-year survival of approximately 40% and highly differentiated tumors with an 80% 5-year survival rate.[41] Other prognostic factors that are being explored include DNA content, cell proliferative activity, epidermal growth factor (EGF), transforming growth factor-α, EGF receptor, *ERBB2* oncogene, *ras* oncogene, *RB1* tumor suppressor gene, and *p53* tumor suppresor gene.[42]

With treatment, the 5-year survival rates for patients with stages A, B, C, and D are 77, 65, 48, and 21%, respectively.[22,26] In another study, 10-year cancer-specific survival estimates were 95% for stage A_1, 80% for stages A_2 to B_2, 60% for stage C, and 40% for stage D_1 and 10% for stage D_2.[39] It is estimated that more than 85% of patients with stage A_1 can be cured, whereas less than 1% of patients with stage D_2 will be cured.

Treatment

The treatment for prostate cancer depends on the stage of the disease (Table 123.5). Patients with incidental carcinoma found at the time of a transurethral resection for BPH (stage A_1) require only careful observation due to slow progression of the disease to more advanced stages.[26,43] Approximately 2% of patients progress within 7 years; however, up to 25% may progress by 10 years.[22,26,43] Still, the 10-year mortality rate for these patients is less than 1%. Surgery may be considered in the young patient with stage A_1 disease.

For select patients with either stage A_2 or B disease, radical prostatectomy with staging pelvic lymphadenectomy or interstitial irradiation therapy may be used.[22,26,43]

TABLE 123.5. TREATMENT OF PROSTATE CANCER BY STAGE OF DISEASE

Stage	Treatment
A_1	Transurethral resection followed by close observation
A_2	Radical prostatectomy or radiation therapy
B	Radical prostatectomy Radiation therapy
C	Radiation therapy Hormonal manipulation[a]
D_0	Treat local symptoms if necessary If urinary obstruction present Transurethral prostatectomy or radiation therapy
D_1	Systemic treatment[a] Close observation alone or early endocrine therapy Radical prostatectomy, lymph node dissection, and orchiectomy
D_2	Pharmacotherapy Hormonal manipulation Combination hormonal therapy Cytotoxic chemotherapy Combination hormonal/chemotherapy Palliative radiation therapy for symptomatic areas

[a]Under investigation. (From Garnick, M. Urologic cancer. In Rubenstein E, Federman DD, eds. Scientific American Medicine, Sec. 12, Vol. IX. New York: Scientific American, 1993.)

Complications from radical prostatectomy include blood loss, stricture formation, incontinence, lymphocele, fistula formation, anesthetic risk, and impotence.[26,43] However, recent identification of important nerve bundles responsible for erection and better surgical techniques have led to newer potency-sparing procedures and less blood loss during surgery. Using these new techniques, potency may be regained in 50–80% of patients within the first year, and only two units of autologous blood may be needed for the entire procedure.[44,45] Younger patients with limited disease have the best sexual recovery. PSA falls rapidly after successful surgical removal of prostate cancer. Historically, both iodine-125 or gold-198 have been used for interstitial radiotherapy. The radioactive implants may be placed percutaneously via the transperianal route under ultrasound guidance to avoid the need for an extensive surgical procedure. Interstitial radiotherapy is used less frequently than external beam techniques.

For stage A_2 or B patients who are not surgical candidates, external beam irradiation is the more common treatment.[46] Acute complications from radiation therapy include cystitis, proctitis, hematuria, urinary retention, penoscrotal edema, and impotence.[26,43] Chronic complications include proctitis, diarrhea, cystitis, enteritis, impotence, urethral stricture, and incontinence.[26,43] In contrast to surgery, radiation therapy causes impotence in 30% of patients treated for locally advanced prostate cancer. There is a slower decline in PSA values after successful radiation therapy, but

PSA still remains a useful marker to follow patients. Rising PSA values can indicate either a failure of local therapy or development of new metastatic disease.

Ongoing studies are attempting to define the best treatment for patients with stage C disease.[26,43] The failure rate for stage C patients is much higher than for either stage A or B, and better diagnostic techniques have demonstrated that some stage C patients have occult disease dissemination at presentation. While external beam radiotherapy has been the primary treatment option, some investigators feel there is also a role for androgen deprivation.[26,43]

The treatment of patients with localized prostate cancer (stages A_2, B, or C) remains controversial because many of the studies used inadequate methods to properly define the patient populations treated.[26,47] Treatment complications can easily be compared; however, relative outcomes of watchful waiting, radiation therapy, or radical prostatectomy are difficult to assess.[26,47] Results from a pooled analysis from nonrandomized studies suggest that initial conservative management followed by delayed hormone therapy is an effective strategy for patients with grade 1 or 2 localized prostate cancer especially in those with a life expectancy of less than 10 years.[48]

There is controversy about the best approach to treating patients with stage D prostate cancer because the majority of therapy is palliative and cure is not possible. Patients with stage D_0 prostate cancer may be carefully watched and appropriate local therapy (surgery or radiation) may be instituted when symptoms appear. The majority of these patients will develop metastatic disease and will then require systemic therapy.[26,43] Stage D_1 patients may be treated in a similar fashion; however, some clinicians feel that early hormonal intervention in these cases is warranted based on the observations that stage D_2 patients with minimal disease have better overall survival with hormonal therapy compared to those patients with a large tumor burden.[43,49]

The major treatment modality for advanced prostate cancer (stage D_2) is pharmacotherapy in the form of hormonal manipulation or cytotoxic chemotherapy.[26,43,50–52] Local radiation therapy also is commonly used to palliate painful skeletal metastases in patients who have relapsed following endocrine therapy.

PHARMACOTHERAPY OF ADVANCED PROSTATE CANCER

Hormonal Manipulation

The observation by Huggins and Hodges[53] that both normal and malignant prostatic tissues contain a high level of acid phosphatase suggests that prostatic malignancy represents an overgrowth of prostate tissue. Both Huggins and Hodges[53] and Nesbit and Baum[54] demonstrated that a decrease in serum acid phosphatase along with symptomatic relief occurred in patients with metastatic prostate cancer treated with either estrogens or orchiectomy, therapies known to reduce circulating androgens. Hormonal manipulation is used in the treatment and palliation of advanced prostate cancer because prostatic epithelium undergoes atrophy when the normal physiologic effect of androgens is reduced.[17,18]

Hormonal manipulations to ablate or reduce circulating androgens can occur through several mechanisms (Table 123.6). The organs responsible for androgen production can be surgically removed. Hormonal pathways that modulate prostatic growth can be interrupted at several steps (Fig. 123.3). Interference with LHRH or LH can reduce testosterone secretion by the testes. Androgen synthesis can be inhibited in the testes or in the adrenal gland. Direct interference at the target tissue level by antiandrogens offers yet another treatment alternative. Finally, the conversion of testosterone to DHT may be inhibited by 5-α-reductase inhibitors.

Androgen Source Ablation

Bilateral orchiectomy, adrenalectomy, and hypophysectomy can reduce circulating androgens, although orchiectomy is still the preferred surgical procedure.[43,55] Unfortunately, many patients are not surgical candidates due to their advanced age and other patients find this procedure psychologically unacceptable.[26,43] Subcapsular orchiectomy promptly produces castration levels of testosterone (<50 ng/dL), yet it preserves the outer integrity of the testicles.

TABLE 123.6. HORMONAL MANIPULATIONS IN ADVANCED PROSTATE CANCER

Androgen source ablation
Orchiectomy
Adrenalectomy
Hypophysectomy
LHRH or LH inhibition
Estrogens
LHRH agonists
Progestogens[a]
Cyproterone acetate[b]
Androgen synthesis inhibition
Aminoglutethimide
Ketoconazole
Progestogens[a]
Antiandrogens
Flutamide
Biclutamide
Dilutamide[b]
Cyproterone acetate[b]
Progestogens
5-α-Reductase inhibition
Finasteride[b]

[a]Minor mechanisms of action.
[b]Investigational compounds or use.

Orchiectomy is the preferred initial treatment in patients with impending spinal cord compression or ureteral obstruction. While adrenalectomy and hypophysectomy can remove the extratesticular sources of androgens, these procedures are not commonly performed due to the high mortality and availability of medical alternatives.

LHRH or LH Inhibition

Several pharmacologic agents suppress the release of LH from the pituitary gland resulting in reduced testosterone production.[19,56,57] These agents include estrogens, LHRH agonists, progestogens, and cyproterone acetate.

Estrogen administration reduces androgens by directly inhibiting LH release, interfering with hormone synthesis, or by acting directly on the prostate cell. Further information suggests that estrogens increase the steroid-binding globulin level thereby reducing the amount of free circulating androgens.[23,55] The onset of response is usually 1–2 weeks after initiation of therapy. Several Veterans Administration Cooperative Urological Research Group (VACURG) trials have assessed the role of estrogen therapy in the treatment of advanced prostate cancer.[58,59] In one trial, patients were randomized to receive diethylstilbestrol (DES) 5 mg/d, orchiectomy, both treatments simultaneously, or placebo.[58] Fewer deaths from cancer were observed in patients treated with estrogens, but there was an increased incidence of death due to cardiovascular complications. The excess mortality from cardiovascular-related deaths offset any therapeutic advantage of estrogen administration. The cardiovascular deaths were more common in patients over 75 years of age and in those with a prior history of cardiovascular disease.

In a second VACURG trial,[59] DES doses of 5, 1, and 0.2 mg/d were compared with placebo. Compared with the 0.2-mg dose or placebo, both the 1- and 5-mg doses reduced cancer-related deaths. The 5-mg dose was superior to the 1-mg dose in suppressing acid phosphatase and testosterone levels. Nevertheless, the clinical responses observed with either of these doses were similar, suggesting that the lower estrogen dose (1 mg) maintains antitumor activity. Again, cardiovascular-related deaths occurred more frequently in patients treated with DES 5 mg/d. The incidence of cardiovascular-related deaths in the DES 1-mg group was not different from placebo. Other complications from DES therapy include fluid retention, nausea, vomiting, impotence, and painful gynecomastia. Gynecomastia can be attenuated with bilateral breast irradiation if instituted prior to estrogen therapy.

The results of the VACURG trials demonstrated that estrogen therapy should be withheld from a patient with advanced prostate cancer until he becomes symptomatic. Several investigators argue that treatment should be initiated early in the course of the disease when the suspected tumor burden is low.[51,55] Reanalysis of the data from the VACURG studies has suggested that the young, good performance-status patient subpopulation may benefit from early hormonal intervention.[60] Estrogen therapy provides symptomatic relief in 60–80% of previously untreated patients.[50,61] The response is manifested by decreased bone pain and relief of urinary symptoms. The usual duration of response is 1–2 years and almost all patients progress and present with bone pain due to metastatic disease.[50,56,61] There is no benefit to using orchiectomy and estrogens simultaneously.

Investigators do not agree on the proper initial DES dose. Some investigators use DES 3 mg/d in three divided doses to uniformly suppress testosterone production. The relative incidence of cardiovascular complications for DES 3 mg compared with 1 or 5 mg has not been assessed in direct comparative clinical trials, although it is suspected that there is a dose–response relationship reflecting higher cardiovascular risk from higher estrogen doses. Other clinicians may institute therapy with DES 1 mg/d recognizing that incomplete testosterone suppression may occur in up to 70% of patients. Testosterone concentrations and PSA should be carefully monitored in patients treated with DES 1 mg/d.

Ethinyl estradiol, conjugated estrogens, chlorotrianisene, and polyestradiol phosphate have been used as alternatives to DES.[56,57] In general, no therapeutic advantage over DES can be expected with any of the alternate estrogen products, and all of these products are considerably more expensive than DES. These estrogenic substances can be used, however, if patients cannot tolerate DES administration.

The isolation of the naturally occurring hypothalamic decapeptide hormone, gonadotropin hormone-releasing hormone, or LHRH, has provided a new class of effective agents for the treatment of advanced prostate cancer.[19,62–64] The physiologic response to LHRH depends on both the dose and the mode of administration. Intermittent pulsed LHRH administration, which mimics the endogenous release pattern, causes sustained release of both LH and FSH.[62,63] However, high-dose or continuous intravenous administration of LHRH inhibits gonadotropin release due to a decrease both in number and sensitivity of pituitary receptors, a physiologic process termed *down-regulation.*[19,62,65] Structural modification of the naturally occurring LHRH at the sixth and tenth positions has produced a series of LHRH agonists that possess supraphysiologic potency and longer plasma half-lives.[19,62,63] The longer duration of action provided by these agonists causes a similar down-regulation of pituitary receptors and a decrease in testosterone production.

In the first multicenter leuprolide trial, 94 evaluable patients with stage D_2 prostate cancer received a daily subcutaneous injection of either 1 or 10 mg of leuprolide.[66] The clinical response rate reported for previously untreated patients was 76% and for patients who had prior endocrine therapy, 23%. These values are similar to those seen with estrogen administration.[50,61] During the first week of treatment, 10% of patients reported a "flare-up" in their disease manifested by increased bone pain. This drug-induced disease flare corresponds to the initial increase in both LH and FSH and resolves by the second week of continued therapy. Other adverse effects noted in this trial included hot flashes, sexual dysfunction manifested by erectile impotence and decreased libido, and minor irritation at the injection site.

In a multicenter randomized trial of untreated patients with stage D_2 prostate cancer, leuprolide 1 mg subcutaneously daily was compared with DES 3 mg daily.[67] Responses, as evaluated by the National Prostatic Cancer Project (NPCP) criteria, were similar for both groups. Of 92 evaluable patients in the leuprolide group, the total response rate was 86%, and of 94 evaluable patients in the DES-treated group, the total response rate was 85%. Neither the median time to disease progression nor the median survival time was significantly different between the two groups.

Substantial differences in drug-related toxicity were demonstrated in this trial. Patients assigned to the leuprolide group had a significantly higher incidence of hot flashes, and 7% experienced a transient exacerbation of their disease during the first week of therapy. Patients in the DES group had a higher incidence of gynecomastia and breast tenderness despite pretreatment breast irradiation in 50% of patients. Cardiovascular complications, which included peripheral edema, thrombosis, phlebitis, and pulmonary embolus, were more common in estrogen-treated patients.

These studies demonstrated that the LHRH agonist leuprolide is a suitable alternative to estrogen administration and is not associated with cardiovascular toxicity. Further development of several other LHRH agonists was initiated to provide a drug delivery system that allowed an extended duration of action.[19,62,63]

Two additional LHRH agonists, leuprolide depot and goserelin acetate implant, are available and allow the LHRH agonist to be given on a once-monthly schedule.[68–71] The leuprolide depot formulation contains leuprolide acetate in coated pellets. The dose is administered intramuscularly and the coating dissolves at different rates to allow sustained levels of leuprolide and testosterone suppression throughout the dosing interval. Goserelin acetate implant contains goserelin acetate dispersed in a matrix of D,L-lactic and glycolic acids copolymer and is administered subcutaneously. Hydrolysis of the copolymer material provides continuous release of goserelin over a 28-day period.

Clinical studies with both leuprolide depot and goserelin acetate implant have demonstrated similar efficacy and toxicity to that of the regular leuprolide acetate formulation.[67,71] The extended duration of action is a distinct advantage for these LHRH agonists and they are the preferred LHRH therapy. However, because there are no direct comparative trials between leuprolide depot and goserelin acetate implant, and they appear to be therapeutically equivalent, the choice between the two is usually made by cost, and patient and physician preference. The disease flare with both products also manifests within the first week of therapy similar to the regular leuprolide formulation.

If LHRH agonists are used as initial therapy, similar response rates to orchiectomy and estrogen administration can be expected. There is a lower incidence of cardiovascular-related adverse effects associated with LHRH therapy than with estrogen administration. Patients should be counseled to expect worsening symptoms during the first week of therapy and caution should be exercised when initiating LHRH agonist therapy in patients with widely metastatic disease involving the spinal cord or having the potential for ureteral obstruction. Irreversible complications may occur.

Both megestrol acetate, a progestational agent, and cyproterone acetate, a progestogenic antiandrogen, inhibit the release of LH from the pituitary in addition to their antiandrogen action at the target tissue level.[20,40]

Androgen Synthesis Inhibition

Several compounds interfere with the synthesis of androgens by the testes or adrenal gland. These agents include aminoglutethimide, ketoconazole, and the progestational agents.

As the majority of patients with advanced prostate cancer progress after initial hormonal therapy, surgical adrenalectomy has been used to reduce extratesticular sources of androgens. Response rates observed with surgical adrenalectomy are from 20–40%.[55,56] However, the operative morbidity and mortality with this procedure is high. Medical adrenalectomy using aminoglutethimide is now the preferred alternative to surgery.

Aminoglutethimide inhibits the desmolase enzyme complex in the adrenal gland, thereby preventing the conversion of cholesterol to pregnenolone. Pregnenolone is the precursor substrate for all adrenal-derived steroids including androgens, glucocorticoids, and mineralocorticoids.[56,57] Concurrent glucocorticoid administration is necessary to prevent negative feedback increases in ACTH production, which could competitively overcome the adrenal blockade. Mineralocorticoid replacement may be necessary in select patients.

In clinical trials, aminoglutethimide can delay disease progression and produce symptomatic relief for a short time in up to 50% of patients with progressive disease despite previous estrogen administration or orchiectomy.[72,73] If the patient is currently taking an estrogen, it is continued to suppress the testicular source of androgen production. Due to central nervous system-related adverse effects, therapy is usually initiated with aminoglutethimide 250 mg orally twice daily and increased gradually to 250 mg orally three or four times daily depending on patient tolerance. Supplementation with physiologic doses of hydrocortisone or cortisone acetate is begun concomitantly. Dexamethasone should be avoided because of the variability in dexamethasone metabolism induced by aminoglutethimide.[74] Care should be taken in patients already on oral anticoagulants, because aminoglutethimide increases the rate of warfarin clearance. The duration of therapy should be at least 4–6 weeks to properly assess the efficacy of aminoglutethimide.

Adverse effects during aminoglutethimide therapy occur in approximately 50% of patients.[72–74] Central nervous system effects that include lethargy, ataxia, and dizziness are the major adverse reactions. A generalized morbilliform pruritic rash has been reported in up to 30% of patients treated. The rash is usually self-limiting and resolves within 5–8 days with continued therapy.

Ketoconazole, an imidazole antifungal agent, has been used in the treatment of advanced prostate cancer based on the observation that it produces gynecomastia in select individuals. Subsequent investigations have determined that ketoconazole administration results in a dose-related, reversible reduction in serum cortisol and testosterone concentration by inhibiting both adrenal and testicular steroidogenesis.[75,76]

In several uncontrolled nonrandomized trials, ketoconazole 400 mg given orally every 8 hours relieved symptoms in previously untreated patients with stage D prostate cancer.[76,77] Responses were manifested by a rapid diminution of pain and discontinuation of narcotic analgesics, decrease in prostatic acid phosphatase, and decrease in prostate size. The rapidity of response appears to be the major therapeutic advantage and is similar to that seen after orchiectomy. Adverse effects included gastrointestinal intolerance, transient rises in liver and renal function tests, and hypoadrenalism.

As a secondary mechanism to its antiandrogen action, megestrol acetate inhibits the synthesis of androgens. This inhibition appears to occur at the adrenal level, but circulating levels of testosterone also are reduced, suggesting that inhibition at the testicular level also may occur.[20,40]

Antiandrogens

Antiandrogens inhibit the formation of the DHT–receptor complex and thereby interfere with androgen-mediated action at the cellular level.[78] Flutamide and biclutamide are currently available. Megestrol acetate, a progestational agent, also is available and has antiandrogen actions. Cyproterone acetate and nilutamide are antiandrogens under clinical investigation.

In a study of 72 previously untreated patients with advanced prostate cancer, flutamide 250 mg orally three times a day produced a favorable response in 88% of patients.[79] Response was manifested by improvement in bone pain, decrease in prostate size, or improvement in performance status. Adverse effects were minimal. Gynecomastia was the major adverse reaction that occurred in 72% of patients. Of 37 patients who claimed sexual potency prior to study entry, 32 patients (86%) were able to maintain potency during treatment. Other studies have demonstrated similar results with flutamide monotherapy; however, the approved use for flutamide is in combination with an LHRH agonist.[80] Liver function test abnormalities and the possible development of methemoglobinemia are also possible adverse effects.[80]

Megestrol acetate, a progestational antiandrogen, blocks both androgen production and androgen action at doses of 120–160 mg orally per day.[20,81] The possible mechanisms of action for megestrol include weak competition with DHT, inhibition of nuclear and cytosol androgen receptor formation, and moderate inhibition of 5-α-reductase.[20] With doses of 80 mg/d, megestrol can maintain castration levels of testosterone for up to 5 months.[20,81]

5-α-Reductase Inhibition

Testosterone is reduced to DHT by 5-α-reductase. DHT has a greater receptor binding affinity than testosterone in androgen-dependent cells. Theoretically, compounds that inhibit 5-α-reductase action can block the formation of DHT–receptor complex and prevent receptor activation. Finasteride, a 4-aza-steroid, has demonstrated 5-α-reductase blocking activity resulting in inhibition of DHT–receptor complex formation, but not testosterone–receptor complex formation.[82] Testosterone functions, such as muscle mass, libido, and sperm production, continue while DHT functions, such as prostatic growth, are inhibited. Clinical studies with finasteride in patients with BPH have demonstrated efficacy and reduction in prostate volume. Clinical trials in patients with advanced prostate cancer are ongoing.[82,83] 5-α-Reductase inhibitors may prove useful in combination with other agents such as flutamide[84] or as part of a chemoprevention program.[85]

Combined Hormonal Blockade

Although up to 80% of patients with advanced prostate cancer will respond to initial hormonal manipulation, almost all patients will relapse within 2 years after initiating therapy. Two mechanisms have been proposed to explain this tumor resistance.[20,50,51] The tumor could be heterogeneously composed of cells that are hormone dependent and hormone independent, or the tumor could be stimulated by extratesticular androgens that are converted intracellularly to DHT. The rationale for combination hormonal therapy is to interfere with multiple hormonal pathways to completely eliminate androgen action. In clinical trials, combination hormonal therapy, sometimes also referred to as “maximal androgen deprivation” or “total androgen blockade,” has included an agent or therapy that suppresses testosterone synthesis and an agent that either interferes with androgen synthesis or blocks androgen action. The combination of an LHRH agonist with flutamide or of low-dose estrogen with megestrol are examples of this approach.

Labrie et al.[86] provided information for the initial reports combining an LHRH agonist with flutamide and has subsequently provided follow-up for 363 patients. Response rates, the main endpoint of these studies, have been greater than 90% in previously untreated patients.[86]

However, response rates of less than 35% have been observed with this combination in patients previously treated with initial hormonal manipulation.

These studies, although quite encouraging, have been criticized for lack of a concurrent control arm and for using response rather than survival as the final endpoint. For these reasons, the National Cancer Institute sponsored a randomized, placebo-controlled, double-blind, multicenter trial comparing leuprolide with leuprolide plus flutamide 250 mg orally three times a day in newly diagnosed patients with stage D prostate cancer.[49,86] This well-designed study used median progression-free survival and overall median survival as the main endpoints, although best response as judged by NPCP criteria was also reported.

Both median progression-free survival (16.5 versus 13.9 months; $p = 0.039$) and overall median survival (35.6 versus 28.3 months; $p = 0.035$) were significantly longer in the 303 evaluable patients treated with leuprolide plus flutamide than in the 300 evaluable patients treated with leuprolide alone. The best response to combination therapy was observed in patients with minimal disease (no disease in ribs, long bones, or soft tissue other than lymph nodes) and a good performance status. An update of this trial has demonstrated that median survival was 61 months in the combination arm and 41 months in the leuprolide alone arm in patients with minimal disease.[87] The addition of flutamide to leuprolide reduced the symptoms from the flare phenomenon associated with LHRH agonist therapy. Patients in both groups experienced common adverse effects associated with LHRH agonist treatment. Diarrhea was the only additional adverse effect attributable to flutamide administration. The results of this study provided the data necessary to approve flutamide for use in combination with an LHRH agonist for the treatment of advanced prostate cancer. No survival benefit was demonstrated when flutamide was added at the time of progression in those patients that received only leuprolide initially.[88]

Several other studies comparing combined androgen blockade to conventional medical or surgical castration have been performed (Table 123.7).[89–92] In one of the few studies comparing two different antiandrogens combined with a LHRH agonist, Schellhammer et al.[93] reported that the time to treatment failure was significantly better for biclutamide plus goserelin compared to flutamide plus goserelin ($p = 0.05$). Results for the secondary endpoints, survival, quality of life, and subjective response were similar between the two groups. Diarrhea occurred more frequently in patients treated with flutamide.

A meta-analysis of 22 randomized trials in 5710 patients comparing maximal androgen blockade to conventional medical or surgical castration failed to show any additional survival benefit for maximal androgen blockade.[94]

While some investigators now consider combined androgen ablation to be the initial therapy of choice for newly diagnosed patients, the clinician is left to weigh the costs of combined therapy against potential benefits in light of conflicting results in the randomized trials.[26,43,95,96] Thus far, studies have demonstrated a major benefit in patients with minimal disease[87,97] and this may be the ideal population for combined androgen ablation. Further carefully designed studies, which use survival as the main endpoint, and response, time to progression, quality of life, and patient preference as secondary endpoints, should be conducted.

Hormone Withdrawal Syndromes

Objective and subjective responses have been noted following the discontinuation of flutamide[98] or biclutamide[99] in patients receiving these agents as part of combined androgen ablation with an LHRH agonist. Responses in these patients were manifested as PSA declines of approximately 50% for an average of 6 months postdiscontinuation and improved clinical symptoms. Mutations in the androgen receptor have been described where antagonist compounds,

TABLE 123.7. SUMMARY OF RANDOMIZED COMBINED ANDROGEN BLOCKADE TRIALS

Ref.	Treatment	N	Disease-Free Survival (months)		Overall Median Survival (months)	
49	Leuprolide 1 mg SQ qd	300	13.9		28.3	
	Leuprolide + flutamide	303	16.5	$p = 0.039$	35.6	$p = 0.035$
89	Orchiectomy	208	14.7		29.8	
	Orchiectomy + nilutamide	202	20.8	$p = 0.0041$	37.1	$p = 0.0041$
90	Goserelin	282			26.9	
	Goserelin + flutamide	287			29	NS
91	Orchiectomy	133	16.8		27.6	
	Goserelin + flutamide	129	16.5	NS	22.7	NS
92	Orchiectomy	148			27.1	
	Goserelin + flutamide	149			34.4	$p = 0.02$

such as flutamide or biclutamide, or their metabolites become agonists.[100–104] This may partially explain the reason for clinical progression in patients receiving hormonal therapy who are labeled as "hormone refractory" whereby a portion of the prostate cancer cells have become refractory to the antiandrogen. Clinically, antiandrogen withdrawal might be useful in a patient progressing on combined androgen blockade and is usually required before a patient is enrolled on a clinical trial.

Chemotherapy

Extensive testing of both single agents and combination chemotherapy regimens for advanced prostate cancer has demonstrated that no currently approved antineoplastic agents or combinations prolong survival in patients with advanced prostate cancer. Most of these trials have evaluated the use of chemotherapeutic agents in patients with progressive disease after hormonal therapy—a situation in which the expected response based on cell kinetic principles and resistance mechanisms should be low. Although no clear benefit has been established, androgen ablation is usually continued when chemotherapy is initiated.[43,105]

Single Agents

Agents that have demonstrated modest activity in prostate cancer include cyclophosphamide, estramustine, 5-fluorouracil, methotrexate, DTIC, doxorubicin, and cisplatin.[106–109] Cyclophosphamide is used as the standard agent for comparison in NPCP trials. The reported response range is 26–41% if stable disease is included as a favorable response.

Combinations

Several trials have evaluated the use of combination therapy containing the single agents that demonstrate activity.[106–108,110,111] The combination of two tubulin-active agents, estramustine and vinblastine, has been reported to produce an overall 31% objective response rate, a 50% or more decline in PSA in 80% of patients, and pain relief in 43% of patients.[110,111] In NPCP-sponsored trials, however, randomized comparison of single agents versus combination therapy failed to demonstrate a marked difference in response rates, although the intensity of combination treatment as measured by nadir leukocyte count was questioned.[108]

Studies using currently available cytotoxic chemotherapy agents for advanced prostate cancer have produced marginal clinical benefits and no survival advantage. This indicates a need to further investigate new compounds in this disease. Of all investigational compounds, suramin, a growth factor antagonist, has proceeded furthest in clinical trials.[112,113] In 38 patients, the initial trial reported a median survival of 42 weeks.[112] Of 21 patients with bone only disease, PSA declined by more than 75% with five patients returning to a normal PSA value.[112] In the initial trials, suramin was dosed according to a Bayesian pharmacokinetic adoptive control model.[114] To simplify the dosing schedule, several investigators have developed dosing schemes that do not require intensive pharmacokinetic monitoring.[115,116]

Cytotoxic chemotherapy should be used in the investigational setting and it is justified to use either second-line hormonal therapy or supportive therapy as the control arm. Future developments will focus on therapies and/or agents with nontraditional mechanisms of action, such as growth factor inhibition oncogene regulation, biologic response modification, or gene therapy.[107,117–119]

Combination Cytotoxic Chemotherapy/Hormonal Therapy

Because prostate cancer is a heterogeneous disease based on response, it is likely that the tumor is composed of cells sensitive to hormonal therapy, chemotherapy, both therapies, or neither therapy. It would then seem rational to combine endocrine therapy and chemotherapy to produce an additive effect.

In an NPCP-sponsored prospective randomized trial, standard therapy (DES or orchiectomy) and DES plus cyclophosphamide were compared in newly diagnosed patients with stage D prostate cancer.[120] The response rate, median survival, and time to progressive disease were similar between the two treatment groups. In another trial, initial hormonal therapy plus chemotherapy was compared with hormone therapy followed at progression by chemotherapy.[121] Although the response rate was greater for patients treated initially with the combination, overall median survival was similar.

Because androgenic hormones cause growth of prostate malignancies, it is possible that stimulation of the tumor prior to administering chemotherapy would produce better results. This relies on the hypothesis that chemotherapeutic agents have greater cytotoxicity in the more rapidly growing cells. In several studies, androgen priming with fluoxymesterone before chemotherapy has produced variable results. While objective and subjective response has been reported in a small number of patients, fatal tumor stimulation resulting in spinal cord compression has occurred. The preliminary results suggest that the risks of androgen priming outweigh the benefits.[121]

APPROACH TO THE PATIENT WITH ADVANCED PROSTATE CANCER

The initial recommendation that the patient with stage D prostate cancer be offered hormonal manipulation when symptoms appear was based on the VACURG trials demonstrating no survival advantage for early hormonal intervention. As the more recent analysis suggests, some subpopulations may benefit from hormonal therapy initiated before symptoms appear.[60] Also, the major contributing factor to the equivalent survival rates was the excess cardiovascular toxicity associated with estrogens. Now that suitable estrogen alternatives are available that are not associated with cardiovascular toxicity (LHRH agonists and flutamide), the issue of when best to start hormonal therapy is unclear and the subject of several clinical trials.[96,122]

The initial hormonal manipulation should be based on physician assessment, patient preference, cost, and adverse effects. Orchiectomy is the preferred initial manipulation, especially in the patient with cardiovascular disease or in the emergent setting of impending spinal cord compression or ureteral obstruction. Orchiectomy is a one-time procedure associated with relatively low morbidity and mortality. The addition of flutamide to orchiectomy has become common practice by many clinicians, although there are still ongoing studies assessing the possible benefits of this combination.

If the patient refuses orchiectomy or is not a surgical candidate, other forms of androgen ablation may be tried. They vary considerably in cost (Table 123.8).[123] Some clinicians prefer DES 1 mg three times per day as initial therapy due to its low cost. DES 1 mg/d can be used if serum testosterone levels and PSA are monitored to ensure that castration levels are achieved. LHRH agonists, due to the low cardiovascular toxicity, are suitable alternatives to DES although they are considerably more expensive. However, they should not be used as initial therapy in patients with impending urinary obstruction or spinal cord compression. The sustained-action formulations have almost completely replaced those that must be given daily.

Adding an antiandrogen (flutamide or biclutamide) to LHRH agonist therapy is considered by some clinicians to be the "gold standard" hormonal therapy for patients with stage D prostate cancer.[95,124] However, not all clinical trials have demonstrated a clear survival advantage for combination therapy and the use of this combined androgen blockade approach is quite costly. The maximal benefit appears to be in patients with minimal disease and good performance status. In several trials, antiandrogens have been shown to lessen the symptoms associated with the flare reaction seen during the first week of LHRH agonist therapy.

When disease progression from hormonal manipulation occurs, compliance with the initial therapy should be assessed and a testosterone level should be checked to ensure that castrate levels have been achieved. If the patient has progressed despite adequate testosterone suppression, a second hormonal manipulation can be attempted; however, if the patient is currently receiving an antiandrogen, the antiandrogen should first be discontinued and PSA monitored. Chemotherapy can be instituted at this point and, if possible, should be performed as part of a research protocol. Also, earlier institution of chemotherapy or the use of combined chemotherapy plus hormonal therapy should be

TABLE 123.8. COMPARATIVE COSTS OF HORMONAL THERAPY FOR ADVANCED PROSTATE CANCER

Drug	Dose	Average Wholesale Price per Month of Therapy ($)
Diethylstilbestrol	3 mg/d	8.22
Leuprolide	1 mg/d	535.00
Leuprolide depot	7.5 mg/mo	472.50
Goserelin implant	3.6 mg every 28 days	358.55
Flutamide	750 mg/d	268.64
Biclutamide	50 mg/d	307.50

(From Drug Topics: Annual Pharmacists' Reference (Redbook). Oradell, NJ, Medical Economics, 1995, with permission.)

performed as part of a clinical trial. Adjunctive therapy for bone pain palliation often becomes the major therapeutic goal and includes reassessment of current therapy, radiation therapy, and analgesics.

Chemoprevention Efforts

Prostate cancer is a significant health concern with few modifiable risk factors. Because androgens are involved in prostate cancer development, it would seem that prolonged administration of drugs that block androgens may prevent subclinical disease from becoming clinically apparent.[85,125] As part of an NCI chemoprevention effort, a large double-blind, randomized trial comparing finasteride 5 mg/d to placebo has been initiated.[125] This trial will accrue 18,000 participants 55 years or older with a normal PSA and digital rectal examination. Drug administration will be for 7 years. Enrollees will be followed with an annual DRE and PSA determination. Sextant biopsies will be performed in patients if the PSA rises above 4 ng/mL or the DRE becomes abnormal. In addition to determining whether this intervention will reduce the prostate cancer incidence, it will also provide information about the epidemiology, risk factors, natural history, screening, and diagnosis of prostate cancer and will collect important quality of life data.

Evaluation of Therapeutic Outcomes

Localized prostate cancer is curable and treatment modalities (surgery and radiation) should be performed with an effort to reduce any postprocedure complications (impotence, stricture, and incontinence).[26,43] Advanced prostate cancer (stage D) is not currently curable and treatment should focus on providing symptom relief and maintaining quality of life.[126]

Clinical trials in prostate cancer should include homogenous populations[127] and adequate staging criteria. Age-adjusted overall survival and disease-free survival should be the ultimate outcome measures; however, subjective and objective responses, standardized according to NPCP guidelines, should also be included.[128] The objective parameters include assessment of the primary tumor size, evaluation of involved lymph nodes, and the response of tumor markers to treatment. Subjective parameters include a scale for activity grading, an assessment of weight change, alterations in analgesic requirement, and general patient symptoms. After each of these criteria is evaluated, the response is judged to be a complete objective response, partial objective response, stable disease, objective progression, or subjective response. Including stable disease as a favorable response is controversial. PSA reductions greater than 50%[129] to 75%[112] have been associated with improved survival and thus PSA has become a surrogate marker to evaluate new agents in clinical trials. Quality of life evaluations are essential to include in clinical trials.

Conclusion

Prostate cancer occurs in older males and is curable when local disease is present. Efforts are under way to better define screening and early detection approaches and how best to use PSA as a screening, diagnostic, and therapeutic monitoring test. Proper staging at initial patient presentation is essential because the therapy intensity will depend on the disease stage. For patients with advanced disease, there are many treatment options. Hormonal manipulations to decrease circulating androgen concentrations are very effective for symptom palliation. These therapies include orchiectomy, DES, LHRH agonists, and/or antiandrogens. Combined androgen blockade with either orchiectomy or an LHRH agonist and an antiandrogen is routinely used despite equivocal studies and cost. Studies are still ongoing to define the best initial therapy, and research efforts are focusing on identifying which patient subpopulation might benefit best from a given treatment modality.

The role of cytotoxic chemotherapy is undefined. Single-agent therapy is as effective as combination therapy and neither produces many complete objective responses or prolongs survival. Research efforts are concentrating on developing new agents, many with novel mechanisms of action.

Several areas still require further investigation including the appropriate time to institute both hormonal therapy and chemotherapy. Further insight into the molecular basis for prostate cancer development may lead to some new therapeutic approaches.

References

1. Wingo PA, Tong T, Bolden S. Cancer Statistics—1995. CA Cancer J Clin 1995;45:8–30.
2. Ross R, Coetzee GA, Reichardt J, et al. Does the racial-ethnic variation in prostate cancer have a hormonal basis? Cancer 1995;75:1778–1882.
3. Pienta KJ, Esper PS. Risk factors for prostate cancer. Ann Int Med 1993;118:793–803
4. Carter BS, Beaty TH, Steinberg GD, et al. Mendelian inheritance of familial prostate cancer. Proc Natl Acad Sci USA 1992;89:3367–3372.
5. Isaacs WB, Bova SG, Morton RA, et al. Molecular genetics and chromosomal alterations in prostate cancer. Cancer 1995;75:2004–2012.
6. Newling DWW. The molecular basis for prostatic cancer: How it may influence treatment choice. Eur J Surg Oncol 1995;21:310–315.
7. Bostwick DG, Cooner WH, Denis L, et al. The association of benign prostatic hyperplasia and cancer of the prostate. Cancer 1992;70:291–301.
8. Giovannucci E, Ascherio A, Rimm EB, et al. A prospective cohort study of vasectomy and prostate cancer in US men. JAMA 1993;269:873–877.
9. Slattery ML, West DW. Smoking, alcohol, coffee, tea, caffeine, and theobromine: Risk of prostate cancer in Utah (United States). Cancer Causes Cont 1993;4:559–563.
10. Kohn EC, Liotta LA. Molecular insights into cancer invasion: Strategies for prevention and intervention. Cancer Res 1995;55:1856–1862.
11. Chi SG, deVere RW, White FJ. *p53* in prostate cancer: Frequent expressed transition mutations. JNCI 1994;86:926–933.
12. Uchida T, Wada C, Wang C, et al. Microsatellite instability in prostate cancer. Oncogene 1995;10:1019–1022.
13. Dong JT, Lamb PW, Rinker-Schaeffer CW, et al. *KAI1,* a metastasis suppressor gene for prostate cancer on human chromosome 11p11.2. Science 1995;268.
14. Taplin ME, Bubley GJ, Shuster TD, et al. Mutation of the androgen receptor gene in metastatic androgen independent prostate cancer. N Engl J Med 1995;332:1393–1398.
15. Takahashi H, Furusato M, Allsbrook WC, et al. Prevalence of androgen receptor gene mutations in latent prostatic carcinomas from Japanese men. Cancer Res 1995;55:1621–1624.
16. McNeal JE. The prostate gland. Monogr Urol 1983;4:3–33.
17. McConnell JD. Physiologic basis of endocrine therapy for prostatic cancer. Urol Clin North Am 1991;18:1–3.
18. Sanberg AA. Endocrine control and physiology of the prostate. Prostate 1980;1:169–184.
19. Eisenberger MA, O'Dwyer PJ, Friedman MA. Gonadotropin hormone-releasing hormone analogues: A new therapeutic approach for prostatic carcinoma. J Clin Oncol 1986;4:414–424.
20. Geller J. Rationale for blockade of adrenal as well as testicular androgens in the treatment of advanced prostate cancer. Semin Oncol 1985;12(suppl 1):28–35.
21. Aumuller G. Morphologic and endocrine aspects of prostatic function. Prostate 1983;4:195–214.
22. Gittes RF. Carcinoma of the prostate. N Engl J Med 1991;324:236–245.
23. Slack NH, Lane WW, Priore RL, et al. Prostate cancer. Urology 1986;27:205–213.
24. Bostwick DG. Grading prostate cancer. Am J Clin Pathol 1994;102(suppl 1):S38–S56.
25. Gleason DF. Histologic grade, clinical stage, and patient age in prostate cancer. NCI Monogr 1988;7:15–18.
26. Garnick MB. Prostate cancer: Screening, diagnosis, and management. Ann Intern Med 1993;118:804–818.
27. Gohagan JK, Prorok PC, Kramer BS, et al. The Prostate, Lung, Colorectal, and Ovarian Cancer Screening Trial of

the National Cancer Institute. Cancer 1995;75(suppl):1869–1873.
28. Oesterling JE, Cooner WH, Jacobsen SJ, et al. Influence of patient age on the serum PSA concentration. An important clinical observation. Urol Clin North Am 1993;20:671–680.
29. Catalona WJ, Smith DS, Ratliff TL, et al. Measurement of prostate-specific antigen in serum as a screening test for prostate cancer. N Engl J Med 1991;324:1156–1161.
30. Peehl DM. Prostate specific antigen role and function. Cancer 1995;75(suppl):2021–2026.
31. Vessella RL, Lange PH. Issues in the assessment of PSA immunoassays. Urol Clin North Am 1993;20:607–620.
32. Brauer MK. Laboratory studies for the detection of carcinoma of the prostate. Urol Clin North Am 1990;77:759–768.
33. Oesterling JE. Prostate-specific antigen: A valuable clinical tool. Oncology 1991;5:107–122.
34. Oesterling JE. Prostate specific antigen: Its role in diagnostics and staging of prostate cancer. Cancer 1995;75(suppl):1795–1804.
35. Mettlin C, Jones G, Averette H, et al. Defining and updating the ACS guidelines for the cancer-related checkup: Prostate and endometrial cancer. CA Cancer J Clin 1993;43:42–46.
36. Lee F, Gray JM, McLeary RD, et al. Transrectal ultrasound in the diagnosis of prostate cancer: Location, echogenicity, histopathology, and staging. Prostate 1985;7:117–129.
37. Anonymous. Advances in urologic ultrasound. Urol Clin North Am 1989;16:617–762.
38. Beahrs OH, D.E. H, Hutter RVP, et al. Manual for Staging Cancer, 4th ed. Philadelphia, JB Lippincott, 1992.
39. Scardino PT, Weaver R, Hudson MA. Early detection of prostate cancer. Hum Pathol 1992;23:211–222.
40. Jones GW. Diagnosis and management of prostate cancer. Cancer 1983;51:2456–2459.
41. Perez CA, Hanks GE, Leibel SA, et al. Localized carcinoma of the prostate (stages T_{1B}, T_{1C}, T_2, and T_3). Review of management with external beam radiation therapy. Cancer 1993;72:3156–3173.
42. Visakorpi T, Kallioniemi OP, Kaivula T, et al. New prognostic factors in prostatic carcinoma. Eur Urol 1993;24:438–449.
43. Catalona WJ. Management of cancer of the prostate. N Engl J Med 1994;331:996–1003.
44. Walsh PC, Partin AW. Treatment of early stage prostate cancer: Radical prostatectomy. In DeVita VT, Hellman S, Rosenberg SA, eds. Important Advances in Oncology—1994. JB Lippincott: Philadelphia. 1994:211–223.
45. Walsh PC, Partin AW, Epstein JI. Cancer control and quality of life following anatomical radical retropubic prostatectomy: Results at 10 years [see comments]. J Urol 1994;152:1831–1836.
46. Perez CA, Hanks GE, Leibel SA, et al. Localized carcinoma of the prostate (stages T_{1B}, T_{1C}, T_2, and T_3). Review of management with external beam radiation therapy. Cancer 1993;72:3156–3173.
47. Wasson JH, Cushman CC, Bruskewitz RC, et al. A structured literature review of treatment for localized prostate cancer. Prostate Disease Patient Outcome Research Team [published erratum appears in Arch Fam Med 1993 Oct;2(10):1030]. Arch Fam Med 1993;2:487–493.
48. Chodak GW, Thisted RA, Gerber GS, et al. Results of conservative management of clinically localized prostate cancer [see comments]. N Engl J Med 1994;330:242–248.
49. Crawford ED, Eisenberger MA, McLeod DG, et al. A controlled trial of leuprolide with and without flutamide in prostatic carcinoma. N Engl J Med 1989;321:419–424.
50. Crawford ED, Nabors W. Hormone therapy of advanced prostate cancer: Where we stand today. Oncology 1991;5:21–30.
51. Labrie F. Medical treatment of prostate cancer. Drug Ther 1989;11:22–37.
52. Labrie F, Dupont A, Simard J, et al. Intracrinology: The basis for the rational design of endocrine therapy at all stages of prostate cancer. Eur Urol 1993;2:94–105.
53. Huggins C, Hodges CV. Studies on prostatic cancer. 1. The effect of castration, of estrogen, and of androgen injection on serum phosphatases in metastatic carcinoma of the prostate. Cancer Res 1941;1:293–297.
54. Nesbit RM, Baum WC. Endocrine control of prostatic carcinoma: Clinical and statistical survey of 1818 cases. JAMA 1950;143:1317–1320.
55. Waxman J. Hormonal aspects of prostatic cancer: A review. J R Soc Med 1985;78:129–135.
56. Creaven PJ, Madajewicz S, Mittelman A. New potential treatment modalities for disseminated prostatic cancer. Urol Clin North Am 1984;11:343–356.
57. Soloway MS. Newer methods of hormonal therapy for prostate cancer. Urology 1984;24:30–39.
58. The Veterans Administration Cooperative Urological Research Group. Carcinoma of the prostate: Treatment comparisons. J Urol 1967;98:516–522.
59. Blackard CE. The Veterans' Administration Cooperative Urological Research Group. Studies of carcinoma of the prostate: A review. Cancer Chemother Rep 1975;59:225–227.
60. Byar DP, Corle DK. Hormone therapy for prostate cancer: Results of the Veterans Administration Cooperative Urologic Research Group studies. NCI Monogr 1988;7:165–170.
61. Scott WW, Menon M, Walsh PC. Hormonal therapy of prostatic cancer. Cancer 1980;45:1929–1936.
62. Conn PM, Crowley WF. Gonadotropin-releasing hormone and its analogues. N Engl J Med 1991;324:93–103.
63. Santen RJ, Bourguignon JP. Gonadotropin-releasing hormone: Physiologic and therapeutic aspects, agonists, and antagonists. Hormone Res 1987;28:88–103.
64. Waxman J. Gonadotropin-releasing hormone analogues for prostatic cancer: An overview. Semin Oncol 1988;15:366–370.
65. Santen RJ, Warner B. Evaluation of synthetic agonist analogue of gonadotropin-releasing hormone (leuprolide) on testicular androgen production in patients with carcinoma of the prostate. Urology 1985;25:53–59.
66. Smith JA, Glode LM, Max DT, et al. Clinical effects of gonadotropin-releasing hormone analogue in metastatic carcinoma of the prostate. Urology 1985;25:112–114.
67. Garnick MR, Glode LM. Leuprolide versus diethylstilbestrol for metastatic prostate cancer. N Engl J Med 1984;311:1281–1286.

68. O'Brien A, Hibbard M. Clinical efficacy and safety of a new leuprorelin acetate depot formulation in patients with advanced prostatic cancer. J Int Med Res 1990;18(suppl 1):57–68.
69. Sharifi R, Soloway M, and the Leuprolide Study Group. Clinical study of leuprolide depot formulation in the treatment of advanced prostate cancer. J Urol 1990;143:68–71.
70. Chrisp P, Goa K. Goserelin: A review of its pharmacodynamic and pharmacokinetic properties, and clinical use in sex hormone-related conditions. Drugs 1991;41:254–288.
71. Peeling WB. Phase III studies to compare goserelin (Zoloadex) with orchiectomy and with diethylstilbesterol in treatment of prostatic cancer. Urology 1989;33(suppl 5):45–52.
72. Drago JR, Santen RJ, Lipton A, et al. Clinical effect of aminoglutethimide, medical adrenalectomy, in treatment of 43 patients with advanced prostatic carcinoma. Cancer 1984;53:1447–1450.
73. Crawford ED, Ahmann FR, Davis MA, et al. Aminoglutethimide in metastatic adenocarcinoma of the prostate. Prog Clin Biol Res 1987;243A:283–288.
74. Sanford EJ, Drago JR, Rohner TJ, et al. Aminoglutethimide medical adrenalectomy for advanced prostatic carcinoma. J Urol 1976;115:170–172.
75. Trachtenberg J, Halpern N, Pont A. Ketoconazole: A novel and rapid treatment for advanced prostatic cancer. J Urol 1983;130:152–153.
76. Trump DL, Havlin KH, Messing EM, et al. High-dose ketoconazole in advanced hormone-refractory prostate cancer: Endocrinologic and clinical effects. J Clin Oncol 1989;7:1093–1098.
77. Jubelirer SJ, Hogan T. High-dose ketoconazole for the treatment of hormone refractory metastatic prostate cancer: 16 cases and review of the literature. J Urol 1984;132:61–63.
78. McLeod DG. Antiandrogenic drugs. Cancer 1993;71(suppl):1046–1049.
79. Sogani PC, Vagaiwala MR, Whitmore WF. Experience with flutamide in patients with advanced prostatic cancer without prior endocrine therapy. Cancer 1984; 54:744–750.
80. Brogden RN, Chrisp P. Flutamide: A review of its pharmacodynamic and pharmacokinetic properties, and therapeutic use in advanced prostate cancer. Drugs Aging 1991;1:104–115.
81. Bonomi P, Pessis D, Bunting N, et al. Megestrol acetate used as primary hormonal therapy in stage D prostate cancer. Semin Oncol 1985;12(suppl 1):36–39.
82. Rittmaster RS. Finasteride. N Engl J Med 1994;330:120–125.
83. Gormley GJ. Role of 5-α-reductase inhibitors in the treatment of advanced prostatic carcinoma. Urol Clin North Am 1991;18:93–98.
84. Fleshner NE, Trachtenberg J. Treatment of advanced prostate cancer with the combination of finasteride plus flutamide: Early results. Eur Urol 1993;2:106–112.
85. Brawley OW, Thompson IM. Chemoprevention of prostate cancer. Urology 1994;43:594–599.
86. Labrie F, Dupont A, Cusan L, et al. Combination therapy with flutamide and medical (LH-RH agonist) or surgical castration in advanced prostate cancer: 7-year clinical experience. J Steroid Biochem Molec Biol 1990;37:943–950.
87. Eisenberger M, Crawford ED, Blumenstein B, et al. National Cancer Institute Intergroup Study 0036. Prognostic factors in stage D_2 prostate cancer; important implications for future trials: Results of a cooperative intergroup study (int 0036). Semin Oncol 1994;21:613–619.
88. McLeod DG, Benson R Jr., Eisenberger MA, et al. The use of flutamide in hormone-refractory metastatic prostate cancer. Cancer 1993;72:3870–3873.
89. Janknegt RA. Total androgen blockade with the use of orchiectomy and nilutamide (Anandron) or placebo as treatment of metastatic prostate cancer. Anandron International Study Group. Cancer 1993;72:3874–3877.
90. Tyrrell CJ, Altwein JE, Klippel F, et al. Multicenter randomized trial comparing Zoladex with Zoladex plus flutamide in the treatment of advanced prostate cancer. Survival update. International Prostate Cancer Study Group. Cancer 1993;72:3878–3879.
91. Iversen P, Rasmussen F, Klarskov P, et al. Long-term results of Danish Prostatic Cancer Group trial 86. Goserelin acetate plus flutamide versus orchiectomy in advanced prostate cancer. Cancer 1993;72:3851–3854.
92. Denis LJ, Carnelro de Moura JL, Bono A, et al. Goserelin acetate and flutamide versus bilateral orchiectomy: A phase III EORTC trial (30853). EORTC GU Group and EORTC Data Center. Urology 1993;42:119–129.
93. Schellhammer P, Sharifi R, Block N, et al. A controlled trial of bicalutamide versus flutamide, each in combination with luteinizing hormone-releasing hormone analogue therapy, in patients with advanced prostate cancer. Casodex Combination Study Group. Urology 1995;45:745–752.
94. Maximum androgen blockade in advanced prostate cancer: An overview of 22 randomised trials with 3283 deaths in 5710 patients. Prostate Cancer Trialists' Collaborative Group. Lancet 1995;346:265–269.
95. Labrie F. Endocrine therapy of prostate cancer: Optimal form and timing. J Clin Endocrinol Metab 1995;80:1066–1071.
96. Crawford ED, DeAntonio EP, Labrie F, et al. Endocrine therapy of prostate cancer: Optimal form and appropriate timing. J Clin Endocrinol Metab 1995;80:1062–1066.
97. Denis L, Murphy GP. Overview of phase III trials on combined androgen treatment in patients with metastatic prostate cancer. Cancer 1993;72:3888–3895.
98. Scher HI, Kelly WK. Flutamide withdrawal syndrome: Its impact on clinical trials in hormone refractory prostate cancer. J Clin Oncol 1993;11:1566–1572.
99. Nieh PT. Withdrawal phenomenon with the antiandrogen casodex. J Urol 1995;153:1070–1072.
100. Veldscholte J, Berrevoets CA, Ris-Stalpers C, et al. The androgen receptor in LNCaP cells contains a mutation in the ligand binding domain which affects steroid binding characteristics and response to antiandrogens. J Steroid Biochem Mol Biol 1992;41:665–669.
101. Klocker H, Culig Z, Hobisch A, et al. Androgen receptor alterations in prostatic carcinoma. Prostate 1994;25:266–273.
102. Newmark JR, Hardy DO, Tonb DC, et al. Androgen receptor gene mutations in human prostate cancer. Proc Natl Acad Sci USA 1992;89:6319–6323.

103. Culig Z, Hobisch A, Cronauer MV, et al. Mutant androgen receptor detected in an advanced-stage prostatic carcinoma is activated by adrenal androgens and progesterone. Mol Endocrinol 1993;7:1541–1550.
104. Gaddipati JP, McLeod DG, Heidenberg HB, et al. Frequent detection of codon 877 mutation in the androgen receptor gene in advanced prostate cancers. Cancer Res 1994;54:2861–2864.
105. Hussain M, Wolf M, Marshall E, et al. Effects of continued androgen-deprivation therapy and other prognostic factors on response and survival in phase II chemotherapy trials for hormone-refractory prostate cancer: A Southwest Oncology Group report. J Clin Oncol 1994; 12:1868–1875.
106. Eisenberger MA. Chemotherapy for prostate cancer. NCI Monogr 1988;7:151–163.
107. Kreis W. Current chemotherapy and future directions in research for the treatment of advanced hormone-refractory prostate cancer. Cancer Invest 1995;13:296–312.
108. Tannock IF. Is there evidence that chemotherapy is of benefit to patients with carcinoma of the prostate? J Clin Oncol 1985;3:1013–1021.
109. Walzer Y, Oswalt J, Soloway MS. Estramustine phosphate-hormone, chemotherapeutic agent, or both? Urol 1984;24:53–58.
110. Seidman AD, Scher HI, Petrylak D, et al. Estramustine and vinblastine: Use of prostate specific antigen as a clinical trial end point for hormone refractory prostatic cancer. J Urol 1992;147:931–934.
111. Hudes GR, Greenberg R, Krigel RL, et al. Phase II study of estramustine and vinblastine, two microtubule inhibitors, in hormone-refractory prostate cancer. J Clin Oncol 1992;10:1754–1761.
112. Myers C, Cooper M, Stein C, et al. Suramin: A novel growth factor antagonist with activity in hormone-refractory metastatic prostate cancer [see comments]. J Clin Oncol 1992;10:881–889.
113. Eisenberger MA, Sinibaldi V, Reyno L. Suramin. Cancer Pract 1995;3:187–189.
114. Cooper MR, Lieberman R, LaRocca RV, et al. Adoptive control with feedback strategies for suramin dosing. Clin Pharmacol Ther 1992;52:11–23.
115. Reyno LM, Egorin MJ, Eisenberger MA, et al. Development and validation of pharmokinetically based fixed dosing scheme for suramin. J Clin Oncol 1995; 13:2187–2195.
116. Kobayashi K, Vokes EE, Vogelzang NJ, et al. Phase I study of suramin given by intermittent infusion without adaptive control in patients with advanced cancer. J Clin Oncol 1995;13:2196–2207.
117. Warner JA, Heston WDW. Future developments of nonhormonal systemic therapy for prostatic carcinoma. Urol Clin North Am 1991;18:25–33.
118. Sanda MG, Simons JW. Gene therapy for urologic cancer. Urology 1994;44:617–624.
119. Sanda MG, Ayyagari SR, Jaffee EM, et al. Demonstration of a rational strategy for human prostate cancer gene therapy. J Urol 1994;151:622–628.
120. Murphy GP, Beckley S, Brady MF, et al. Treatment of newly diagnosed metastatic prostate cancer patients with chemotherapy agents in combination with hormones versus hormones alone. Cancer 1983;51:1264–1272.
121. Osborne CK, Blumenstein B, Crawford ED, et al. Combined versus sequential chemo-endocrine therapy in advanced prostate cancer: Final results of a randomized southwest oncology group study. J Clin Oncol 1990;8:1675–1682.
122. Cookson MS, Sarosdy MF. Hormonal therapy for metastatic prostate cancer: Issues of timing and total androgen ablation. South Med J 1994;87:1–6.
123. Drug Topics: Annual Pharmacists' Reference. Oradell, NJ, Medical Economics, 1995.
124. Labrie F, Belanger A, Simard J, et al. Combination therapy for prostate cancer: Endrocrine and biologic basis of its choice as new standard first-line therapy. Cancer 1993;71:1059–1067.
125. Ford LG, Brawley OW, Perlman JA, et al. The potential for hormonal prevention trials. Cancer 1994; 74 (suppl 9):2726–2733.
126. Fossa SD, Opjordsmoen S. Assessment of quality of life in patients with prostate cancer. Semin Oncol 1994;21:657–661.
127. Scher HI, Steineck G, Kelly WK. Hormone-refractory (D3) prostate cancer: Refining the concept. Urology 1995;46:142–148.
128. Slack NH, Murphy GP, et al. Criteria for evaluating patient responses to treatment modalities for prostatic cancer. Urol Clin North Am 1984;11:337–342.
129. Kelly WK, Scher HI, Mazumdar M, et al. Prostate-specific antigen as a measure of disease outcome in metastatic hormone-refractory prostate cancer [see comments]. J Clin Oncol 1993;11:607–615.

Chapter 124

Malignant Lymphomas

Jim Koeller, MS, and Val Adams, PharmD

HODGKIN'S DISEASE

Thomas Hodgkin first described the mysterious disease of the lymph system that bears his name more than 150 years ago. Hodgkin's disease is a form of lymphoma, the cause of which is still unknown, and is invariably fatal if left untreated. Studies have demonstrated the orderly spread of this disease. Hodgkin's disease is classified into four histologic subtypes that differ somewhat in their natural history and treatment. The stage of Hodgkin's disease influences prognosis as well as therapy. The pathologic stage represents the best approximation of extent of disease and is based on histopathologic examination of the specimen obtained from biopsy of appropriate tissue during staging laparotomy. Dramatic advances have been made in the understanding and treatment of Hodgkin's disease during the past three decades. Today, many of the newly diagnosed patients with Hodgkin's disease will be cured. This extraordinary success has not been without cost. The programs are intense and technically demanding and are associated with significant acute toxicity and long-term complications. The long-term effects of standard chemotherapy regimens have been more fully documented in recent years and could shape therapy for the future.

INCIDENCE/EPIDEMIOLOGY/ETIOLOGY

It was estimated that there would be nearly 7800 new cases of Hodgkin's disease diagnosed in the United States in 1995, which represents just more than 1% of all known cancers.[1] This disease occurs slightly more frequently in males than in females (56 versus 44%). Once thought to be only a disease of the young, it is now recognized that Hodgkin's disease exhibits a bimodal distribution in industrialized countries.[2,3] The first peak occurs between the ages of 15 and 34 and again in those older than 55.[4] In recent years, there has been an increased incidence seen in the younger age bracket and a declining incidence in those older than 40.[5] The 10-year survival rates for Hodgkin's disease for the different stages are given in Table 124.1.

The etiology of Hodgkin's disease has not been fully elucidated. Infection has long been considered a potential cause ever since the disease was first described. Initially, organisms such as *Mycobacterium tuberculosis* were suspect due to the high incidence of tuberculosis seen in Hodgkin's patients. However, these have not withstood careful scrutiny over the years. Instead, viruses have emerged as the leading candidates for an infectious etiology. Studies have suggested an increased risk of Hodgkin's disease in patients who have had mononucleosis caused by the Epstein–Barr virus (EBV).[6,7] Reed–Sternberg cells (which are associated with Hodgkin's disease) have, in fact, been found in mononucleosis patients.[7] Both serologic and molecular methods have now linked the EBV to Hodgkin's disease.[8,9]

BIOLOGY/HISTOPATHOLOGY/ CLASSIFICATION

Lymphocytes, the principal cellular component of lymphoid tissue, are widely distributed throughout the body and in aggregated centers. The bone marrow and thymus are the primary organs of lymphopoiesis, with secondary sites being the lymph nodes, spleen, lamina propria of the gastrointestinal tract, and Waldeyer's ring.

Hodgkin's disease is unique among the lymphomas because only a very small percent of cells from the involved tissue actually contains malignant cells; the vast majority are normal reactive hematopoietic cells. The exact cellular origin of the malignant cell has yet to be determined. Many believe that it is derived from either a B lymphocyte or a macrophage/reticulum cell lineage. More recent availability of monoclonal antibodies and molecular genetic analysis have greatly improved our understanding of the immunohistology and histopathology of Hodgkin's disease. Although the *BCL2* oncogene had been identified in Hodgkin's tissue samples (which would suggest a B-cell origin), more recent work has associated the t(14;18) chromosomal translocation to a bystander normal lymphocyte and not the Reed–Sternberg cell.[10] Another study found the expression of the *p53* suppressor oncogene in all types of Hodgkin's disease, except lymphocyte-predominant disease.[11] An explanation

TABLE 124.1. 10-YEAR HODGKIN'S DISEASE SURVIVAL

Stage	Survival (%)[a]
I	84
II	78
III	62
IV	42

[a]Based on deaths due only to the Hodgkin's disease. Overall survival = 65%.
(Compiled from Kennedy BJ, Loeb V, Peterson VM, et al. National survey of pattern of care for Hodgkin's disease. Cancer 1985;56:2547–2556.)

for the apparent multilineage origin of the Reed–Sternberg cell is that the malignant cell represents an *in vivo* clonal population that occurs in response to viral stimuli (EBV) that promotes fusion of the interdigitating reticular cell, B cells, T cells, or both lymphocytes.[12]

Lukes, Hicks, and Butler introduced a histopathologic classification of Hodgkin's disease (known as the Lukes–Butler classification) that was modified at the Rye conference in 1965 and is today called the Rye classification.[13,14] This classification is still widely accepted by both pathologists and clinicians. The Rye classification divides Hodgkin's disease into four subtypes: lymphocyte-predominant, nodular sclerosis, mixed cellularity, and lymphocyte-depleted (Table 124.2). The subtypes in this classification are based on characteristics of the Reed–Sternberg cell and the surrounding cells and connective tissue. They differ somewhat in natural history and response to treatment. With the introduction of extensive staging, sophisticated megavolt radiotherapy, and effective combination chemotherapy, the true prognostic value of these subtypes is much less clear.

Lymphocyte-Predominant

Lymphocyte-predominant Hodgkin's disease (LPHD) has characteristic benign-appearing lymphocytes that have a more diffuse growth pattern. LPHD is generally associated with localized, indolent disease. The lymph nodes are usually partially to completely destroyed. Reed–Sternberg cells are uncommon, while the predominant cell appears to be a B lymphocyte (expressed by the L and H variant) that lacks expression of the characteristic R3 marker, Leu-M1. Fibrosis is also uncommon. This subtype can account for 6% of all Hodgkin's disease, is slightly more common in males than females, and represents a more favorable prognosis.

TABLE 124.2. THE RYE (LUKES–BUTLER) CLASSIFICATION

Histologic Subtype	Incidence (%)
Lymphocyte-predominant	46
Nodular sclerosis	60
Mixed cellularity	24
Lymphocyte-depleted	4
Unclassified	6

(Compiled from Glaser SL, Swartz WG. Time trends in Hodgkin's disease incidence. Cancer 1990;66:2196–2204.)

Nodular Sclerosis

Nodular sclerosis Hodgkin's disease has two features that distinguish it from all other forms: the presence of the lacunar cell, which is a variant of the Reed–Sternberg cell, and the presence of a capsule that divides the lymphoid tissue into distinct nodules. Actually, Reed–Sternberg cells are rare. This subtype can represent up to 60% of all Hodgkin's disease, is usually more localized, is equally divided between females and males, and again is associated with a more favorable prognosis.

Mixed Cellularity

Mixed cellularity Hodgkin's disease occupies a position between the lymphocyte-predominant and lymphocyte-depleted subtypes with regard to the number of neoplastic cells present. It can be mistaken for high-grade non-Hodgkin's lymphoma. Reed–Sternberg cells are more common in this subtype. Diffuse fibrosis is uncommon. This subtype can account for 24% of all Hodgkin's disease, is slightly more common in males than females, and is associated with an intermediate prognosis.

Lymphocyte-Depleted

Lymphocyte-depleted Hodgkin's disease (LDHD) is associated with an abundance of Reed–Sternberg cells and their variants. It also can be easily mistaken for high-grade non-Hodgkin's lymphoma. Diffuse fibrosis and necrosis are commonly seen. This subtype accounts for 4% of all Hodgkin's disease, is more common in males than females, is often widespread at the time of diagnosis, and may be associated with a less favorable prognosis. This category is also most commonly associated with the acquired immunodeficiency syndrome for which prognosis is very poor.

Unclassified

Up to 6% of Hodgkin's cases are difficult to subclassify.

CLINICAL PRESENTATION

Most patients with lymphomas present with some form of adenopathy. The clinical presentations of Hodgkin's disease and the non-Hodgkin's lymphomas have some striking differences (Table 124.3). It is generally not possible to differentiate the various lymphomas by the physical characteristics of the lymph node itself, but the distribution can offer useful information.

Patients with Hodgkin's disease may have adenopathy that waxes and wanes for an average of 5 months before diagnosis. This adenopathy is usually localized to the cervical region and is painless and rubbery. Adenopathies of the inguinal and axillary regions may be present at diagnosis but are less common, whereas involvement of Waldeyer's ring and the epitrochlear nodes occurs in roughly 1% of patients

TABLE 124.3. CLINICAL FEATURES OF THE LYMPHOMAS

	Hodgkin's Disease	Non-Hodgkin's Lymphoma
Lymph node disease	Centripetal	Centrifugal
Contiguous spread	Common	Uncommon
Mediastinal disease	50%	20%[a]
Abdominal disease	Uncommon	Common
Bone marrow involvement	Uncommon	Common
Liver involvement	Uncommon (if present, spleen usually involved)	Common in follicular, uncommon in diffuse
Extranodal disease	Uncommon	Gastrointestinal tract, Waldeyer's ring, testes, epitrochlear nodes, brain
Systemic "B" symptoms	40%	20%

[a]With the exception of T-cell lymphobastic lymphoma.

(Fig. 124.1).[15] Other common sites of nodal involvement include the mediastinal, hilar, and retroperitoneal regions. Up to 40% of patients with Hodgkin's disease may also present with constitutional symptoms including fever, night sweats, weight loss, and pruritis.[15] Hodgkin's disease, similar to other lymphomas, can also present as superior vena cava syndrome, acute spinal cord compression, a solitary thyroid nodule, a tumor nodule of the skin, or an unexplained anemia.

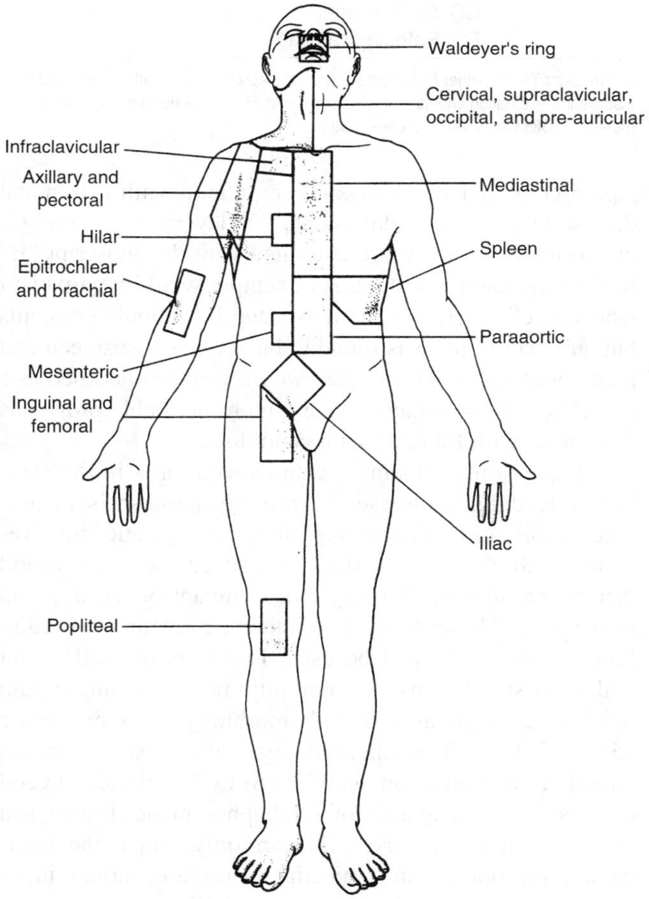

Figure 124.1. Schematic representation of the anatomic regions used in the staging of Hodgkin's disease. *(From Rosenberg SA. The staging of Hodgkin's disease. [Letter to the Editor] Radiology 1966; 87:145, with permission.)*

DIAGNOSIS/STAGING

The diagnosis and pathological classification of Hodgkin's disease can only be made by biopsy of the enlarged node and histopathologic examination under a microscope. Occasionally, additional biopsies may be needed for proper diagnosis. There are four major reasons why a full evaluation for extent of disease is necessary with Hodgkin's disease. First, the information is necessary for making an accurate diagnosis. Because of the toxic effects associated with the treatment (chemotherapy and radiotherapy), it is important to avoid unnecessary treatment if possible. Second, it is still believed by many that certain patterns of organ involvement have prognostic implications. Third, staging is based on the diagnostic evaluation. Fourth, specific knowledge of the involved sites can be used to determine response. As mentioned earlier, certain features may imply a poor prognosis for a given patient. These specific features are listed in Table 124.4.

The Ann Arbor staging classification, which was developed at the 1970 Ann Arbor conference, has proven to be a good workable scheme.[16] The Ann Arbor version modified the Rye staging classification of 1965. In 1989 a modified Ann Arbor classification was proposed. It was called the Cotswald system and was developed as a result of the increased use of new diagnostic techniques (e.g., computed tomography [CT] scanning and magnetic resonance imaging [MRI]). The Cotswald classification is outlined in Table 124.5. After careful staging, roughly half the patients have localized disease (stages I, II, and IIE) and the remainder have advanced disease, of which 10–15% are stage IV. One of the most important factors to remember is that Hodgkin's disease appears to follow a predictable pattern of nodal spread that is not seen with the non-Hodgkin's lymphomas.

TABLE 124.4. FEATURES THAT IMPLY A POOR PROGNOSIS

Hodgkin's disease
- Advanced age
- Male sex
- Presence of "B" symptoms
- Lymphocyte-depleted histology
- Large mediastinal or abdominal involvement
- Three to five involved sites
- Extranodal extension
- Subdiaphragmatic, lower abdominal, mensenteric, or pelvic lymph node involvement

Non-Hodgkin's lymphoma
- Advanced age
- Elevated LDH
- Large tumor burden
- Stage II disease or greater
- Lymphoblastic or Burkitt's lymphoma
- Presence of "B" symptoms
- Bone marrow and gastrointestinal involvement
- Richter's syndrome (conversion of low-grade to high-grade lymphoma)

The appropriate diagnostic and staging procedures are shown in Table 124.6. These are based on recommendations made at the Ann Arbor conference and new scientific advances. Clinical staging begins with a thorough history to evaluate possible symptoms including fever, night sweats, and weight loss; greater than 10% weight loss has been associated with a poor prognosis. A complete physical exam is done to determine nodal and extranodal involvement. Laboratory tests assess bone marrow, renal, and hepatic function. As stated previously, a true diagnosis can be made only with an adequate surgical biopsy, not aspiration. A chest roentgenogram and thoracic CT are necessary to evaluate mediastinal involvement. Abdominal involvement is evaluated using the lower extremity lymphogram and abdominal CT. With the advent of the abdominal CT, some experts now question the usefulness of the lymphogram. Skeletal films are used to evaluate the thoracic and lumbar vertebrae, pelvis, and proximal extremities. A bone marrow biopsy (not aspiration) is especially helpful in patients that are symptomatic or have an elevated alkaline phosphatase, hypercalcemia, or unexplained anemia.

Other diagnostic procedures including intravenous pyelogram, whole-lung tomography, pelvic CT, gallium scanning, isotope scanning, and MRI are now reserved for special situations or until a true definitive use can be determined.

Staging can be based on clinical or pathologic findings. Clinical staging is based on the history, physical exam, initial diagnostic biopsy, laboratory tests, and radiologic findings. Pathologic staging is based on the biopsy findings of strategic sites (e.g., muscle, bone, skin, spleen, abdominal nodes) using an invasive procedure such as a

TABLE 124.5. ANN ARBOR STAGING CLASSIFICATION FOR HODGKIN'S DISEASE

Stage I	Involvement of single lymph node region or structure (e.g., spleen, thymus).
Stage II	Involvement of two or more lymph node regions on the same side of the diaphragm (i.e., the mediastinum is a single site, hilar nodes are laterized). The number of anatomic sites should be indicated by a subscript (e.g., II_2).
Stage III	Involvement of lymph node regions on both sides of the diaphragm: III_1: with or without splenic hilar, celiac, or portal nodes III_2: with paraortic, iliac, or mesenteric nodes.
Stage IV	Involvement of one or more extranodal site(s) beyond that designated E: A: No symptoms B: Fever (greater than 38°C for 3 consecutive days), sweats, weight loss (greater than 10%) X: Bulky disease >⅓ the width of the mediastinum >10 cm maximal dimension of nodal mass E: Involvement of a single extranodal site, contiguous or proximal to a known nodal site CS: Clinical stage PS: Pathological stage.

(From Lister TA, Crowther D, Sutcliffe SB, et al. Report of a committee convened to discuss the evaluation and staging of patients with Hodgkin's disease: Cotswald meeting. J Clin Oncol 1989;7:1630–1636.)

laparoscopy or laparotomy. Those patients with extranodal disease (e.g., muscle, skin, bone, Waldeyer's ring) contiguous to involved nodes are classified with the subscript "E" in the Rye staging system. An example would be a patient who was clinically classified as stage II without symptoms but, at laparotomy, was found to have a positive spleen and para-aortic nodes. This patient would then be classified as a PS $IIIA_{SE}$. These patients have a more favorable prognosis than those with frank disseminated disease.

Laparotomy remains a controversial area in the staging of Hodgkin's disease. Its primary purpose is to provide information concerning subdiaphragmatic involvement, such that if the stage is altered, so then would therapy be altered. The major determinant of the decision to perform a laparotomy is whether treatment with radiation therapy alone will be used. Laporatomy itself is not without risk; the overall mortality rate can range from 0.5% to as high as 6% with morbidity rates exceeding 25%.[17,18] The CT scan, MRI and gallium single-photon emission computed tomography (SPECT) provide several options for the diagnosis of subdiaphragmatic disease and should decrease the use of laparotomy. Thus, the treatment philosophies of a specific institution should influence the decision for laparotomy. Differences over the use of laparotomy will continue until a clear survival advantage can be demonstrated.

TABLE 124.6. DIAGNOSIS AND STAGING PROCEDURES

Required
- Thorough history
- Complete physical examination
- Laboratory studies
  - Complete blood count
  - Serum chemistries
- Renal and liver function
- Adequate surgical biopsy
- Radiologic studies
  - Chest roentgenogram (posterior–anterior and lateral)
  - Chest and abdominal computed tomography scan
  - Bilateral lower extremity lymphangiogram
  - Skeletal survey
- Bone marrow biopsy (needle or open)

May Be Required in Specific Circumstances
- Intravenous pyelogram
- Whole-lung tomography
- Pelvic computed tomography
- Gallium scan
- Isotope scanning
- Magnetic resonance imaging

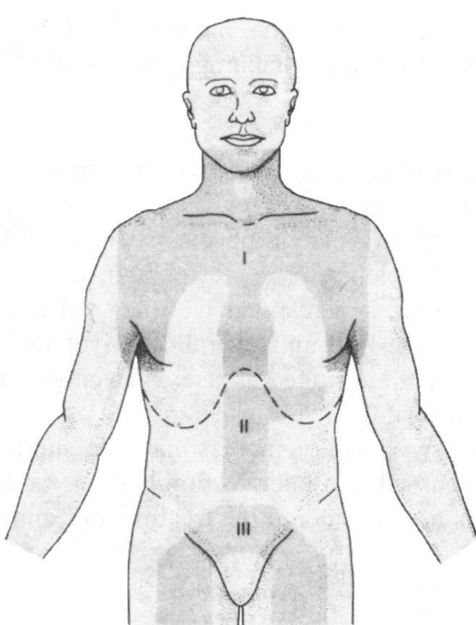

Figure 124.2. Radiation fields (shaded) commonly employed in Hodgkin's disease. I = mantle, II = para-aortic–splenic pedicle, III = pelvic, I + II = subtotal nodal irradiation (STNI), I + III = total nodal irradiation (TNI). *(From Rubin P [ed]. Clinical Oncology, 6th ed. Washington, DC, American Society, 1983, p 352, with permission.)*

TREATMENT

The current goal in the treatment of Hodgkin's disease is to maximize curability while minimizing short- and long-term treatment-related complications. The development of effective therapies for all stages of Hodgkin's disease remains one of the most remarkable achievements and success stories in modern cancer care. This has been brought about by the introduction of modern linear accelerators providing radiation beams in the range of <10 MeV, effective combination chemotherapy regimens, and new methods of combining these two modalities.

Radiation Therapy Alone

Radiation therapy alone is still the cornerstone of treatment for a majority of patients with localized Hodgkin's disease (stages IA and IIA). The types of fields used are shown in Fig. 124.2. Therapeutic doses of radiation to involved sites range from 40–44 Gy, which are fractionated with daily treatments of 1.5–2.0 Gy (depending on field size and patient tolerance).[15] Just as important for curative radiotherapy can be the treatment of adjacent uninvolved areas, which typically require a minimum of 30–35 Gy.

Stage IA and IIA (Supradiaphragmatic)

Patients with stage I–IIA supradiaphragmatic (above the diaphragm) disease can be successfully treated with radiation therapy. Mantle irradiation utilizing doses ranging from 40–44 Gy is employed. This may be followed with treatment of the para-aortic splenic pedicle field alone, or including the area below the bifurcation of the aorta including the iliac nodes (which is called the spade field), with radiation doses ranging from 30–40 Gy. Treating uninvolved areas such as these is called *extended-field radiotherapy*. Extended-field radiotherapy (also called subtotal nodal irradiation) is still considered by many to be the treatment of choice for stage I–IIA disease. This treatment produces disease-free survival rates ranging from 65–85% and overall survival rates ranging from 75–93%,[19–22] although some data indicate that there is no difference in both disease-free survival and overall survival when involved-field (mantle) radiation is given versus extended-field radiation.[15,23] These studies also revealed pelvic relapse rates of less than 5%, indicating that total nodal irradiation may not be necessary.

Stage IB and IIB

Roughly, 15–20% of patients with stage I or II disease will present with B symptoms. Data from Stanford University and the Joint Center for Radiation Therapy indicate that subtotal nodal irradiation is as effective as combined modality (radiation + chemotherapy).[24] Pelvic irradiation or chemotherapy added no benefit in terms of disease-free survival or overall survival. At 20 years following the use of irradiation alone, disease-free survival is 67% and the overall survival is 79%.

Stage IA and IIA (Subdiaphragmatic)

Nodal involvement below the diaphragm is seen in only 10% of stages I and II patients. Patients who do not have splenic involvement (60% of patients) can receive extended-field or total nodal irradiation (see Fig. 124.2).

With these approaches, the outcome will be similar to patients treated for supradiaphragmatic disease.[25]

Stage IIIA

Only a subset of patients with IIIA disease should be considered for radiation therapy alone. Thirty percent of patients belong to a subgroup classified as $IIIA_1$ (limited spleen, celiac, splenic, or portal nodes), have a favorable disease outcome, and respond well to total nodal irradiation. The disease-free and overall survival rates compare favorably to earlier stage disease.[26] Twenty-year disease-free survival is 65%.

Patients with bulky mediastinal and stage $IIIA_2$ disease are discussed in a later section because radiation therapy alone is not considered the treatment of choice.

Chemotherapy

In 1963, the first pilot study using four drugs in combination (mechlorethamine, vincristine, methotrexate, prednisone) was carried out in patients with Hodgkin's disease.[27] In 1964, by substituting procarbazine for methotrexate, the four-drug combination of MOPP was formed. MOPP chemotherapy has been the mainstay of treatment for patients with stage IIIB and IV advanced Hodgkin's disease. The MOPP regimen is shown in Table 124.7. MOPP has produced complete remissions (disappearance of all measurable disease) in 80% of patients and has a 10-year cure rate of 54%.[28] This is in contrast to single-agent therapy, where remissions occur less rapidly and are not as durable. Several other trials reviewed by Coltman have reported similar results, with complete response rates ranging from 40–80% and survival rates ranging from 54–80%.[29] A 20-year follow-up of the National Cancer Institute's (NCI's) durable remissions shows that 54% of patients remained disease free and that 48% of the original 198 patients are still alive.[30] These studies indicate that patients should receive two cycles of therapy beyond that required to produce a complete response; a minimum of six cycles should be administered. Maintenance therapy has not been shown to increase survival and may contribute to the long-term complications seen with therapy. Delivering full or nearly full doses of chemotherapy is extremely important. This is now referred to as dose intensity. Dose reduction within the various studies is probably the single most important factor, explaining the differences in response rates between institutions administering seemingly similar regimens. Dosage reductions based on toxicity can be made, but significant reductions can alter response and survival.[31]

TABLE 124.7. MOPP REGIMEN[a]

Drug	Full Dose (mg/m^2)	Route	Days
Mechlorethamine (nitrogen mustard)	6	IV	1, 8
Vincristine (Oncovin)	1.4	IV	1, 8
Procarbazine	100	PO	1–14
Prednisone	40	PO	1–14

[a]One cycle is 28 days. Prednisone is given in cycle 1 and every subsequent third cycle.

MOPP Variations and Other Alternative Regimens

In the 25 years since MOPP therapy was created and the efficacy confirmed, researchers have been modifying the regimen in an attempt to improve efficacy and possibly decrease toxicity. Some MOPP variations and their outcomes are shown in Table 124.8.[32–39] MVPP, CVPP, BVCPP and ChlVPP are attractive alternatives to MOPP because they offer equal efficacy and differing or less severe toxicities. ChlVPP is especially attractive due to its equal activity and because it causes less nausea, vomiting, and neurotoxicity. The various combination chemotherapy regimens appear to produce initial complete response rates in over 80% of the patients treated and result in roughly a 55–65% cure rate for advanced Hodgkin's disease.

One of the first alternative regimens was ABVD (doxorubicin, bleomycin, vinblastine, dacarbazine) developed by Bonadonna. In one of the first comparisons of ABVD to MOPP in advanced disease, 72 and 63% response rates were reported, respectively. No major differences in disease-free or overall survival were noted, although ABVD was shown to be effective in MOPP failures.[40]

Alternating and Hybrid Regimens

The Goldie–Coldman hypothesis concerning spontaneous mutation rates and the development of resistant clones can explain many clinical findings related to cancer chemotherapy, including chemotherapy failure.[41] Their findings have led to the investigation of alternating non-cross-resistant drug combinations.[42] One of the key requirements in such a concept is that each alternating regimen possess equal activity. Another reason for using alternating or hybrid regimens is to decrease cumulative toxicities. In alternating and hybrid regimens including MOPP and ABVD, the sterilizing and leukemogenic doses of procarbazine and nitrogen mustard are cut in half and the cardiotoxic dose of doxorubicin is cut by one-half in the alternating and one-third in the hybrid regimen. In addition, the potential for pulmonary toxicity from bleomycin will also be reduced.

The Milan Cancer Institute was one of the first groups to apply the Goldie–Coldman hypothesis to the treatment of Hodgkin's disease. They began a prospective randomized trial of MOPP versus MOPP/ABVD (doxorubicin, bleomycin, vinblastine, dacarbazine).[37] The 8-year follow-up on that trial revealed a disease-free survival of 36% for MOPP and 65% for the MOPP/ABVD alternating regimen.[43] The overall survival rates of 62 versus 76%, respectively, were not significantly different. This is one of the

TABLE 124.8. RESULTS OF TREATMENT WITH MOPP VARIATIONS AND OTHER REGIMENS

Regimen	N	Prior Therapy	Complete Response (%)	Disease-Free Survival (%/yr)	Overall Survival (%/yr)	Author
MVPP	133	PR	82	60/5	76/5	Sutcliffe et al.[32]
MVPP	114	None	74	86/5	70/5	Wagstaff et al.[33]
BVCPP	188	RT	68	55/4	—	Gams et al.[34]
ChlVPP	59	None	73	63/5	66/5	Dady et al.[35]
ChlVPP	44	None/RT	76	97/3	—	Vose et al.[36]
ABVD	35	RT	72	80/5	73/5	Bonadonna[37]
MOPP-ABV	76	None	97	91/4	94/4	Klimo et al.[38,39]

Key: MVPP, mechlorethamine, vinblastine, procarbazine, prednisone; BVCPP, BCNU, vinblastine, cyclophosphamide, procarbazine, prednisone; ChlVPP, chlorambucil, vinblastine, procarbazine, prednisone; ABVD, doxorubicin, bleomycin, vinblastine, dacarbazine; MOPP-ABV, mechlorethamine, vincristine, procarbazine, prednisone, doxorubicin, bleomycin, vinblastine; RT, radiation therapy.

few randomized trials that has actually shown a true advantage for the alternating regimen. However, only 7% of MOPP refused to complete treatments versus 22% for the alternating regimen; many have argued that the single-regimen MOPP doses were markedly reduced in this study and thus tainted the positive result.

Based on these data, other groups initiated alternating regimen trials. Table 124.9 lists some of the regimens considered non-cross-resistant with MOPP. The NCI randomized 79 patients to a trial comparing MOPP with alternating cycles of MOPP/CABS (CCNU, doxorubicin, bleomycin, streptozotocin). With initial complete response rates being 92 and 87%, respectively, the 6-year follow-up demonstrated a disease-free survival of 73 versus 80%, respectively, and the overall survival for both arms was 76%.[44] Although the outcomes of the two arms were equivalent, the alternating arm did have more toxicity. The Cancer and Leukemia Group B (CALGB) has reported on a randomized, prospective trial of MOPP versus ABVD versus MOPP/ABVD.[45] In this study, once again, dose modifications to the MOPP-alone arm were significant (capping the vincristine dose and allowing for 50% reductions in the doxorubicin and procarbazine doses by course 3). The complete response rates were 69, 81, and 82%, respectively, whereas disease-free survival was 48, 64, and 64%, respectively, at 3 years. These data contend that the four-drug

TABLE 124.9. NON–CROSS-RESISTANT ALTERNATIVES TO MOPP

ABVD	Doxorubicin, bleomycin, vinblastine, dacarbazine
B-CAVe	Bleomycin, CCNU, doxorubicin, vinblastine
EVAP	Etoposide, vinblastine, cytarabine, cisplatin
CABS	CCNU, doxorubicin, bleomycin, streptozotocin
MOP-BAP	Mechlorethamine, vincristine, bleomycin, doxorubicin, prednisone
VABCD	Vinblastine, doxorubicin, bleomycin, CCNU, dararbazine
BVDS	Bleomycin, vinblastine, doxorubicin, prednisone
CEP	CCNU, etoposide, prednimustine

regimen of ABVD is equivalent to the alternating regimen and superior to attenuated doses of MOPP. The Eastern Cooperative Oncology Group (ECOG) has compared MOPP/ABVD to their BVCPP regimen alone and with low-dose radiation. In an analysis of 294 patients, complete response rates were 68 versus 75% for the BVCPP-alone arm and there was no difference in projected 3-year disease-free survival for the complete responders (66%). Finally, the Italians have initiated a study comparing MOPP/ABVD to a regimen called MA/MA in which the drugs of MOPP and ABVD are consolidated into one monthly cycle (this results in patients being exposed to their ABVD drugs 2 weeks sooner). The complete response rate was 91 and 90%, respectively, and at 30 months, 76 and 79%, respectively, remained relapse free.[46]

In the MOPP-ABV hybrid regimen of Klimo and Connors, MOPP and ABVD (omitting the dacarbazine and increasing doxorubicin from 25 to 35 mg/m^2) are given in a single monthly cycle.[38,39] Their 97% complete response rate with less than 10% recurrence at 4 years is remarkable. The relapse-free survival at more than 5 years is 90%. It must be realized that 13% of their patients did receive localized radiation. The Canadians have reported equivalency between MOPP/ABVD and the hybrid MOPP/ABV, although the hybrid is less difficult to give.

None of the alternating regimen trials have clearly demonstrated an advantage over a fully dosed four-drug (e.g., ABVD) program. In addition, the alternating regimens have been given more than 12 months versus 6–8 months for the other regimens. The problem may also be that many of the alternating regimens used are not truly non–cross-resistant with MOPP. Few data are available that truly establish a non–cross-resistant antitumor effect for any regimen. Until further data are available, alternating regimens will probably not replace well-established single regimens.

Combined Modality Treatment

Controversy remains as to the true role radiotherapy plays when added to chemotherapy for the treatment of Hodgkin's disease. In settings where radiation therapy alone demonstrated poor results (disease with large mediastinal involvement, bulky disease, stage $IIIA_2$ disease, stage IV disease), chemotherapy alone or a combination of chemotherapy and radiation therapy remains the only other option. Some groups have routinely added radiation, either prior to or after chemotherapy, to sites of known disease. One group, in a nonrandomized fashion, studied 50 advanced-stage patients in whom MOPP was alternated with CAVmP (cyclophosphamide, doxorubicin, VM-26, prednisone) for six cycles followed by radiotherapy to involved sites.[47] Following chemotherapy, 68% of patients achieved a complete response. This was increased to 87% following radiation. Three-year follow-up showed a disease-free survival of 73%. No direct comparison to chemotherapy alone was made. Prosnitz and colleagues provided 15-year follow-up data on a trial involving 102 previously untreated advanced-stage patients and 82 who had recurrence following radiotherapy alone.[48] Initially, MVVPP (mechlorethamine, vincristine, vinblastine, pro-carbazine, prednisone) was administered for three courses and then followed by radiation to involved sites. The chemotherapy regimen was later changed to alternating MOPP-ABVD and, ultimately, randomized between MOPP and MVVPP. The 15-year overall survival rate is 54%. Overall survival is 71% if one considers only Hodgkin's disease as the cause of death. Twelve of the 17 non-Hodgkin's-related deaths were due to secondary malignancies. The three different drug programs proved to be clinically equivalent. The authors stated that this combined treatment regimen offered a 20% improvement in survival when compared to the NCI's MOPP-alone data. In a follow-up to some earlier data, the Memorial group has reported no difference in outcome for patients treated with MOPP/ABVD or CAD (CCNU, phenylalanine mustard, vindesine) alternated with MOPP/ABVD combined with low-dose radiation to involved sites.[49] The disease-free and overall survival data were no different than those reported for MOPP alone.

Combined modality therapy has also been used in early-stage Hodgkin's disease, especially stage IIIA. Dutcher and coworkers[50] have reported 14-year results of their trial in patients with IA or B, IIA or B or IIIA Hodgkin's disease randomized to receive extended-field radiation alone, or involved-field radiotherapy followed by 6 courses of MOPP. Significant improvement in disease-free survival and overall survival were only seen in patients with large mediastinal masses and stage $IIIA_2$ disease.

Discord over the appropriate treatment of stage IIIA patients continues. Most would agree that radiation therapy alone is not effective for stage IIIA disease, except possibly for disease restricted to the upper abdomen (stage $IIIA_1$). Either chemotherapy alone or, in some specific cases, combination therapy should be used for most stage IIIA disease. The NCI has reported a 96%, 15-year survival for patients with IIIA or IVA disease.[51] Crowther and coworkers[52] randomized patients to receive MVPP alone or followed by radiation to involved sites. No significant difference in outcome was demonstrated. The Southwest Oncology Group (SWOG) also reported a study comparing MOPP–bleomycin to MOPP–bleomycin plus radiation for stage IIIA or B disease.[53] The chemotherapy-alone regimen proved just as effective as the combination treatment. One other group has recently tried using only two cycles of MOPP with radiotherapy for stage $IIIA_2$ or B disease.[54] The 10-year disease-free and overall survival rates were 86 and 84%, respectively. The authors concluded that this regimen was as effective as intensive chemotherapy, preserves some gonadal function, and has a 1% incidence of acute leukemia at 15 years.

The only patients that may benefit from combined modality therapy are those patients with early stage disease and massive mediastinal involvement (mediastinal masses larger than one-third the greatest chest diameter on x-ray). Normally, up to 75% of these patients can expect to relapse if treated with radiation alone. The rationale for combined modality therapy in this setting is clear. Neither radiation therapy nor chemotherapy alone is particularly successful. One group randomized 94 patients with massive mediastinal involvement to receive CVPP alone or in combination with mantle irradiation.[55] At 7 years in the chemotherapy-alone arm, there was only a 34% disease-free survival rate compared to 75% for the combination arm. In addition, the NCI has reported recent data on patients with large mediastinal involvement being treated with MOPP/ABVD plus mantle radiation.[56] They report only a 13% relapse rate at 3 years.

Combination chemotherapy appears the optimal therapy for most stage IIIA disease. Only in specific settings, such as large mediastinal involvement does combined modality therapy show benefit in early stage disease.

Salvage Chemotherapy

MOPP or one of its variants can cure roughly 50–60% of patients treated for advanced Hodgkin's disease. The other 40–50% of patients will either not respond initially or will relapse after achieving a complete response.[31] For patients who relapse after an initial complete response to MOPP, reinduction is possible. The NCI has reported on their long-term follow-up of MOPP-retreated patients.[47] Patients with long initial remissions had a 45% relapse-free sur-vival rate at 10 years. However, it is doubtful if a regimen that was unable to cure when used as first-line therapy should be used for salvage when other effective regimens with less chance of cross-resistance are available. The choice of salvage treatment, then, should be guided by the estimation of the patient's tolerance for a particular set of agents. Examples of salvage regimens and their response data can be found in Table 124.10.[57–62] Although roughly 40% of patients will achieve a complete response, only 10–15% of those treated will, in fact, be cured by their salvage regimen.

Patients who relapse following salvage chemotherapy are candidates for bone marrow transplantation. Bone marrow transplantation in Hodgkin's disease is fully reviewed in Chapter 129.

TABLE 124.10. SALVAGE THERAPY FOR MOPP FAILURES

Regimen	*N*	Complete Response (%)	Median Duration (mo)	Ref.
ABVD	54	59	17	57
ABDIC	34	35	47	58
B-CAVe	48	44	24	59
CEP	58	40	15	60
CABS	17	35	>8	61
VABCD	18	44	>30	62

Key: ABVD, doxorubicin, bleomycin, vinblastine, dacarbazine; ABDIC, doxorubicin, bleomycin, dacarbazine, CCNU, prednisone; B-CAVe, bleomycin, CCNU, doxorubicin, vinblastine; CEP, CCNU, etoposide, prednimustine; CABS, CCNU, doxorubicin, bleomycin, streptozotocin; VABCD, vinblastine, doxorubicin, bleomycin, CCNU, dacarbazine.

Complications

A variety of side effects can occur during radiation therapy for Hodgkin's disease. Most are transient and seldom produce significant morbidity. Anorexia, xerostomia, odynophagia, skin burns, and changes in taste perception are quite common. Myelosuppression can also be seen.

More serious toxic effects involving the mantle and the heart can occur during radiation therapy for Hodgkin's disease. Paramediastinal pulmonary densities, radiation pneumonitis and fibrosis, pericardial complications, and abnormal ventricular function have been reported.

The most common neurologic complication seen as a result of radiation therapy for Hodgkin's disease is Lhermitte's syndrome, which occurs in up to 15% of patients. This syndrome consists of numbness and tingling caused by head flexion. Spinal cord transections have been reported with overlap of mantle and para-aortic fields. As the techniques for radiation therapy improve, the significant complications associated with its use will continue to be reduced.

Side effects of chemotherapy can be acute or long term. Acute toxic effects seen with the treatment of Hodgkin's disease are similar to those seen with most combination regimens. Myelosuppression is the major dose-limiting toxic effect of most of these regimens. With the advent of the colony-stimulating factors (e.g., G-CSF, GM-CSF), myelosuppression can be lessened, and dose-intensification may be possible. It is anticipated that many of the leading regimens (e.g., MOPP, ABVD, ChlVPP, MOPP-ABV) will all be restudied with the addition of hematopoietic growth factors.

Nausea and vomiting are frequently seen with the use of dacarbazine, doxorubicin, and mechlorethamine, although with the availability of the new $5HT_3$ antagonists, this may become much less of a factor. A significant number of patients experience neurotoxicity secondary to the vincristine used in MOPP therapy. Other acute toxic effects include alopecia, dermatitis, mucositis, phlebitis, malaise and fatigue, pulmonary reactions, cardiomyopathy, and renal dysfunction.

The achievement of cures in Hodgkin's disease with radiation therapy, chemotherapy, or combined modality programs has provided the unique opportunity to observe long-term complications of cancer treatment in patients. The mutagenic, carcinogenic, and teratogenic potential of chemotherapy has long been recognized.

Gonadal dysfunction and secondary malignancies have become important considerations in the treatment of Hodgkin's disease. It is now recognized that these are major long-term complications. Almost all men and up to 50% of premenopausal women treated with six full cycles of regimens containing alkylating agents (e.g., MOPP, BVCPP, ChlVPP) will become sterile.[63,64] This does appear to be a dose-related phenomenon. Some males who received only two to three cycles of MOPP regain their gonadal function.[65] In addition, more than 40% of MOPP/ABVD-treated men recover spermatogenesis 2 years following treatment.[66] For men, there does not appear to be a safe nonsterilizing dose of nitrogen mustard or chlorambucil, so if fertility is a major concern, ABVD may be the best alternative. For patients who have received full-dose radiation to their mediastinum, ABVD can be started, but the patient must be informed that there is an increased risk of bleomycin pulmonary toxicity, although groups at Nebraska and the Royal Marsden Hospital report minimal secondary leukemia effects with ChlVPP use.[67,68]

Now that 10- and 15-year survival data are available, evaluation of secondary malignancy can be made. Secondary malignancies fit two general categories: (1) solid tumors and (2) leukemias. Looking at numbers only, solid tumors are the most common. Radiation therapy is most often implicated as the causative agent.[69] If chemotherapy was also used, solid tumor incidence did not seem to increase significantly. This may imply that secondary solid tumors could be reduced if radiation was only used for those patients with large mediastinal masses and not as part of routine treatment.

The overall risk of developing acute leukemia (most commonly acute nonlymphocytic leukemia) ranges from 3–6%, but in certain subsets of patients may be as high as 20%.[70–72] More recent data confirm these rates with overall leukemia rates ranging from 3.5–4.1%.[73–76] Rates were low for patients treated with radiation therapy or chemotherapy alone, but when radiation therapy and chemotherapy were combined, that secondary leukemia rate ranged from 3.5–12.5%. In radiation therapy patients treated with MOPP as salvage therapy, the rate was 15.5%.[74] These studies also demonstrated that the cumulative amount of chemotherapy (the alkylating agents mechlorethamine, procarbazine, and BCNU) was also important. Patients receiving six cycles or more of these agents had the highest risk.

An international collaborative group of cancer registries and hospitals recently reported on 163 cases of leukemia in 29,552 patients with Hodgkin's disease.[77] This is the largest report of its kind. They presented their results in terms of relative risk instead of percent chance. Chemotherapy alone produced a relative risk of leukemia of 9 when compared to radiation therapy alone. For patients treated with greater than six cycles of combinations containing mechlorethamine or procarbazine, the risk of leukemia was 14 times higher than for radiation alone. For patients treated with both chemotherapy and radiation, the relative risk was 7.7, or roughly equal to that of chemotherapy alone. The incidence of leukemia peaked at 5 years following chemotherapy, with development lasting for at least 8 years after finishing treatment.

Besides these known long-term effects, radiation therapy plus ABVD is associated with an increased risk of cardiac and pulmonary complications. Future trials must try to maintain the high cure rates while lowering the long-term complications.

Current Recommendations

With radiation therapy, chemotherapy, and salvage bone marrow transplantation, more than 75% of patients with advanced Hodgkin's disease can now be cured. Although specific treatment recommendations are influenced by the special circumstances of the patient, available resources, technologies, and the skill of the practitioners, the following general recommendations can be made.

For patients with laparotomy-staged, supradiaphragmatic stage IA or IIA disease, mantle radiation with paraaortic fields should be used. If exploratory laparotomy or radiation is not desirable, combination chemotherapy can be recommended. The routine use of radiation therapy following combination chemotherapy cannot be recommended with currently available data. Only in the instance of large bulky mediastinal disease can combined modality therapy be recommended (combination chemotherapy followed by radiation to the mediastinum). Patients who have laparotomy-stage IIB disease may be treated with subtotal nodal radiation therapy. Again, if a laparotomy has not been performed, stage IIB disease may be best treated with combination chemotherapy. Radiation therapy alone may not be appropriate for stage IIIA disease, except in the instance of $IIIA_1$ disease with a few splenic nodes. For all other patients, combination chemotherapy is the choice. The treatment of choice for stage IV patients is also combination chemotherapy. The choice should be based on expected toxicity and physician treatment habits. Toxicities of MOPP and ABVD are roughly equivalent, but different. Fears of nausea and vomiting and neurotoxicity generally lead to larger dose reductions of MOPP than with ABVD. Based on the recent CALGB data (discussed earlier) and issues related to sterility, ABVD may be a reasonable initial regimen (although the cardiopulmonary toxicities of doxorubicin and bleomycin cannot be taken lightly). If fertility is not an issue, the MOPP alternative, ChlVPP, may be the best choice. It is very well tolerated and does not generally cause alopecia or neuropathy. Its leukemogenic effects are likely less than those seen with MOPP, but higher than ABVD. Of the alternating programs, the MOPP/ABV hybrid is less emetogenic, leukemogenic, and given over 8 months versus MOPP/ABVD alternating regimens given over 12 months.

In advanced-stage disease for patients who fail or have relapsed from combination chemotherapy, salvage therapy may be tried or patients may be treated with conventional-dosed salvage chemotherapy prior to high-dose therapy with bone marrow support (see Chapter 129).

Non-Hodgkin's Lymphoma

The non-Hodgkin's lymphomas are a heterogeneous group of lymphoproliferative disorders involving the lymphatic and immune systems that affect people from early childhood to late adulthood. Advances in molecular biology techniques and our understanding of the human immune system have led to major progress in understanding the pathogenesis of the lymphomas. An increased incidence of lymphomas has been seen over the past years. This is partially due to the acquired immunodeficiency syndrome (AIDS) epidemic, in which lymphoma has become one of the many manifestations. A better understanding of human immunodeficiency virus (HIV) infections may add further insight into the development of malignant lymphomas. Non-Hodgkin's lymphoma can be classified into three broad prognostic groups that differ in morphologic appearance, natural history, clinical presentation, and approach and response to treatment. Significant advances have been made in the treatment of non-Hodgkin's lymphoma. The use of extensive combination chemotherapeutic regimens has shown dramatic improvement in survival, and actual cure in patients with a disease that once was considered incurable. The 5-year survival rate for patients with non-Hodgkin's lymphomas has increased from 31% to 52% during the past 30 years.[1] Further improvement in survival is anticipated with the continued expansion of our therapeutic armamentarium, including bone marrow transplantation and biologic therapy.

INCIDENCE/EPIDEMIOLOGY/ETIOLOGY

Non-Hodgkin's lymphoma is the seventh most common cause of newly diagnosed cancer in the United States and accounts for approximately 3% of all cancers. An estimated 50,900 new cases were diagnosed in 1995 (56% male and 44% female), and it is estimated that 22,700 people died from non-Hodgkin's lymphomas during this same period.[1] The median age of patients at the time of diagnosis is about 55 years. However, non-Hodgkin's lymphoma can occur at any age, from childhood (especially lymphoblastic and Burkitt's lymphoma) through age 80. The incidence of lymphoma has increased by greater than 65% since the early 1970s. The reason for this is unclear, although the increasing number of patients with AIDS, and its association with the development of lymphoma, is one contributing factor. However, increased incidence rates have also been seen in non–HIV-positive groups.[1]

The etiology of non-Hodgkin's lymphoma is still unknown. A relationship between certain viral infections and the development of lymphoma has been seen. There is a strong association between infections with the EBV and the development of Burkitt's lymphoma in Africa. However, this association with EBV and the diagnosis of Burkitt's lymphomas in the United States does not appear to be as strong.[78] Further evidence for a viral etiology appears to be as strong. Further evidence for a viral etiology comes from the isolation of human T-cell leukemia/lymphoma virus (HTLV-1), a type C-RNA retrovirus from the cells of certain patients with an aggressive form of T-cell lymphoma, also known as adult T-cell leukemia/lymphoma (ATL).[79,80] HTLV-1 is endemic in southwestern Japan, the Caribbean, and the southeastern United States.

An increased incidence of lymphoma is seen in many congenital and acquired immunodeficiency states, supporting the role of immune dysregulation in the etiology of lymphoma.[81] Patients with congenital immunodeficiency disorders (Wiskott–Aldrich syndrome, ataxia telangiectasia), acquired immunodeficiency disorders (AIDS, acquired hypogammaglobulinemia, graft-versus-host disease), autoimmune diseases (Sjögren's syndrome, systemic lupus erythematosus, rheumatoid arthritis), and chronic pharmacologic immunosuppression (organ transplantation, especially renal) are predisposed to the development of lymphoma, namely, diffuse aggressive lymphomas with central nervous system involvement. Chronic antigen stimulation may play a role in the development of lymphoma in these situations. An association with EBV also has been proposed in these immunodeficient patients (T-lymphocyte deficiency may allow autonomous proliferation of EBV-infected B cells).[82] Other diseases that predispose a patient to the development of lymphoma include Klinefelter's syndrome and Chediak Higashi syndrome. A hereditary influence also has been suggested as a possible cause of lymphoma, because patients with inherited immunodeficiency diseases and families of patients with immunologic disorders show an increased incidence of non-Hodgkin's lymphoma.[81]

Recently, cytogenetic analyses have shown that chromosomal rearrangements may play a role in the malignant transformation of cells in lymphoma.[81] Small noncleaved cell lymphomas (Burkitt's and non-Burkitt's types) are associated with cytogenetic translocations involving the immunoglobulin gene loci located on chromosomes 2, 14, and 22, and chromosome 8 near the site of the cellular oncogene *c-myc*. The t(8;14) translocations are most common. Approximately 85% of follicular lymphomas and 20% of diffuse lymphomas contain a translocation involving chromosome 14 and chromosome 18, where the oncogene *bcl2* is located.[81] These translocations appear to lead to a disruption in the expression of the *c-myc* or *bcl2* oncogenes, possibly resulting in neoplastic transformation and subsequent uncontrolled proliferation of the lymphoma cells. The translocation involving *bcl2* leads to the expression of a *bcl2*-IGH, mRNA which codes for a protein that appears to inhibit programmed cell death. *bcl2* positivity is likely part of the pathogenesis of certain lymphomas and may also provide a way to detect residual disease. Patients who are *bcl2* positive at diagnosis and become *bcl2* negative after treatment are more likely to remain disease free than those who do not become *bcl2* negative.[83] Research is being done to determine if patients that have achieved a complete remission, but remain *bcl2* positive through treatment, would benefit from more treatment.[84] Continued research of these and other chromosomal abnormalities will contribute to our understanding of the development, treatment, and prevention of lymphoma. Other possible etiologic factors in the development of non-Hodgkin's lymphoma include exposure to ionizing radiation and environmental factors, such as pesticide or herbicide exposure.[81]

HISTOPATHOLOGY/CLASSIFICATION

The non-Hodgkin's lymphomas are neoplasms derived from the monoclonal proliferation of B or T lymphocytes and their precursors. Lymphomas of B-cell origin are more common than T-cell lymphomas. The proliferation of the malignant cells results in the replacement of the normal cells and architecture of lymph nodes or bone marrow with a relatively uniform population of lymphoid cells. In 1956, Rappaport and coworkers[85] proposed a classification scheme based on the architecture of the lymph node and cytologic differentiation of the predominant cell. The Rappaport classification characterizes lymphomas as being either nodular or diffuse, depending on the presence or absence of clusters of malignant cells, and either lymphocytic (small cells) or histiocytic (large cells).

Nodular (also called follicular) lymphomas are neoplasms of the proliferative regions of the B-lymphocyte system, the lymphoid follicle (Fig. 124.3). These neoplasms form circumscribed aggregates that may involve only a portion of the nodal architecture. In contrast, the diffuse non-Hodgkin's lymphomas develop from the medullary cord region of the lymph node, which relates to the secretory compartment of the B-lymphocyte system.

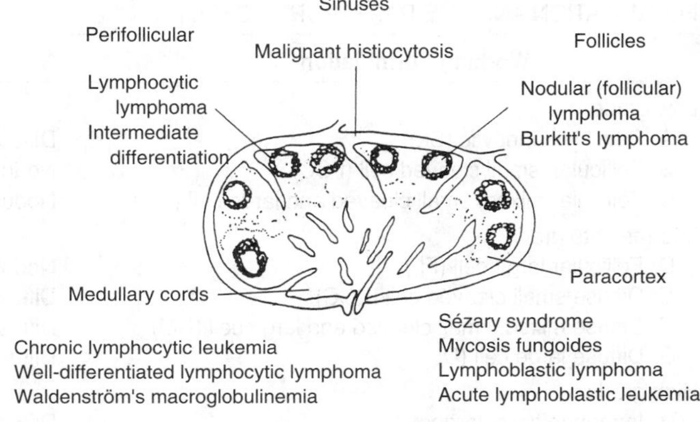

Figure 124.3. Classification of non-Hodgkin's lymphoma according to functional anatomy. *(From Mann RB, Jaffe ES, Berard CW. Am J Pathol 1979;94:103–192, with permission.)*

Lymphoid neoplasms derived from T lymphocytes are much less common. Malignant transformation of T lymphocytes, found predominantly in the paracortical region of the lymph node, gives rise to mycosis fungoides/Sezary syndrome and to approximately one-quarter of the diffuse aggressive non-Hodgkin's lymphomas.

The classification by Rappaport has been the most widely used and valuable scheme for clinicopathologic studies. However, this system is limited because it includes some imprecise terms ("histiocytic" for a tumor derived from transformed lymphoid cells) and, with the recent advancement in the understanding of the immune system, lacks immunologic classification. New classifications were proposed that attempted to classify the lymphomas more precisely, and included both the immunologic and morphologic characteristics of the malignant cells. There are currently at least six different pathologic classification systems (modified Rappaport, Dorfman, Lukes and Collins, Bennet, Kiel, and WHO) for non-Hodgkin's lymphomas used worldwide, posing much controversy and confusion in the comparison of clinical trials. An international study to compare the six classification systems was undertaken and new terminology for defining the lymphomas was proposed.[86] The Working Formulation for clinical usage was developed to serve as a common language and aid in the translation between the different classification systems. Many pathologists and investigators in clinical trials now utilize the Working Formulation as their primary classification system. Recent long-term follow-up of the original patients in the international study has verified the utility of the Working Formulation nomenclature.[87] A comparison of the Working Formulation and the Rappaport classification is found in Table 124.11. The Working Formulation divides non-Hodgkin's lymphomas into three major groups: low, intermediate, and high grade. This grading system is based not only on morphologic features of the malignant cells, but also on the aggressiveness of the tumor and survival characteristics.

Low-Grade Lymphomas

Malignant lymphoma, small lymphocytic (previously termed diffuse well-differentiated lymphocytic), is the solid tumor counterpart of chronic lymphocytic leukemia (CLL). It is the only low-grade lymphoma with a diffuse pattern. This lymphoma appears if an arrest in the process of lymphocyte transformation has occurred at the level of site a, as shown in Fig. 124.4.[14] The malignant cells are monoclonal B lymphocytes, which is the case for the majority of low-grade lymphomas. At presentation, bone marrow, liver, and other visceral organ involvement, along with generalized asymptomatic lymphadenopathy, are seen. With time, a progression to CLL is usually seen with this disease. A small number of patients show an emergence and proliferation to larger lymphoid cells, indicating a progression to a diffuse large cell lymphoma. This transformation is known as Richter's syndrome.[81]

Malignant lymphoma, follicular, predominantly small cleaved cell (previously termed nodular poorly differentiated lymphocytic), is one of the most common non-Hodgkin's lymphomas and accounts for approximately 60% of the cases of follicular lymphoma.[81] An accumulation of these small cleaved cells occurs when lymphocyte transformation is arrested at site b (Fig. 124.4). The monoclonal lymphocytes present in the involved lymph nodes also are found in the peripheral blood of many patients and could account for the widespread involvement of extranodal organs, including the bone marrow, liver, and spleen, commonly seen at diagnosis. Of interest, spontaneous regression of this lymphoma has been reported in a small number of cases.[88]

Malignant lymphoma, follicular mixed, small cleaved, and large cell (previously termed nodular mixed lymphocytic-histiocytic), is an infiltration of both small and large cells, with no clear preponderance of either cell type. Diffuse areas of cellular proliferation may be present in addition to the follicular pattern found in the lymph node. The prognosis of patients whose lymphoma shows a mixed fol-

TABLE 124.11. COMPARISON OF SYSTEMS OF CLASIFICATION OF NON-HODGKIN'S LYMPHOMAS: THE WORKING FORMULATION AND THE RAPPAPORT SCHEME

Working Formulation	Rappaport Classification	Incidence (%)
Low grade		
A. Small lymphocytic (SL)	Diffuse well-differentiated lymphocytic (DWDL)	5
B. Follicular, small cleaved cell (FSC)	Nodular poorly differentiated lymphocytic (NPDL)	25
C. Follicular mixed, small cleaved and large cell (FM)	Nodular mixed, lymphocytic–histiocytic (NM)	10
Intermediate grade		
D. Follicular large cell (FL)	Nodular histicytic (NH)	4
E. Diffuse small cleaved cell (DSC)	Diffuse poorly differentiated lymphocytic (DPDL)	8
F. Diffuse mixed, small cleaved and large cell (DM)	Diffuse mixed lymphocytic–histiocytic (DM)	8
G. Diffuse large cell (DL)	Diffuse histiocytic (DH)	20
High grade		
H. Immunoblastic, large cell	Diffuse histiocytic (DH)	10
I. Lymphoblastic	Diffuse lymphoblastic (DL)	5
J. Small noncleaved cell (SNC)	Diffuse undifferentiated (DU) (Burkitt's and non-Burkitt's)	5

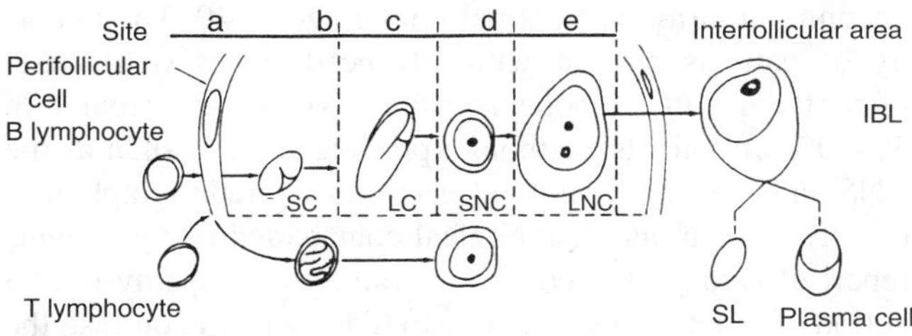

Figure 124.4. Process of lymphocyte transformation and theoretical sites for development of non-Hodgkin's lymphoma. SNC, small noncleaved cell; LNC, large noncleaved cell; SC, small cleaved cell: LC, large cleaved cell; IBL, immunoblast; SL, small lymphocyte—often with plasmacytoid features. *(Modified from Lukes RJ. Am J Clin Pathol 1979;72:657, with permission.)*

licular and diffuse pattern appears to be worse than for patients who have a purely follicular lymphoma, especially if the diffuse component exceeds 50% of the affected node.[89] Disseminated disease is usually present in patients at diagnosis. Interestingly, the disseminated sites of disease, such as the bone marrow and liver, frequently contain only the small cleaved cells.[81]

Intermediate-Grade Lymphomas

Malignant lymphoma, follicular, predominantly large cell (previously termed nodular histiocytic), is the least common type of follicular lymphoma. An arrest at site c (Fig. 124.4) would result in accumulation of these large cleaved cells, although noncleaved cells also may be found. Like the follicular lymphomas, it is usually a B-cell lymphoma, but it tends to have a more diffuse pattern within the node compared with the other follicular lymphomas. Prognosis for this lymphoma is worse than for other follicular lymphomas and actually is similar to that of the diffuse lymphomas if even a focal diffuse component is present.[81] Because its natural history tends to be more aggressive than the low-grade lymphomas, follicular large cell lymphoma is classified as an intermediate-grade lymphoma.

Malignant lymphoma, diffuse small cleaved cell (previously termed diffuse poorly differentiated lymphocytic) is a B-cell lymphoma and, histologically, is the diffuse counterpart of follicular small cleaved cell lymphoma. This diffuse lymphoma may arise *de novo* or, less commonly, as a consequence of progression of the follicular lymphoma. There has been some question raised as to whether diffuse small cleaved cell lymphoma is actually a distinct clinicopathologic category, or if it would more appropriately be classified as lymphocytic lymphoma of intermediate differentiation/mantle zone lymphoma.[90] This disease occurs more often in males than females (2:1), and involvement of extranodal sites such as the skin, gastrointestinal tract, and Waldeyer's ring is frequently seen. The clinical behavior of this lymphoma appears to be heterogeneous, with some patients having an indolent course of disease while others may manifest as more aggressive lymphoma. Despite the aggressive nature, sustained complete remissions are infrequently seen.

Malignant lymphoma, diffuse mixed, small and large cell (previously termed diffuse mixed lymphocytic-histiocytic), includes the diffuse counterpart of follicular mixed lymphoma (likely secondary to progression of the follicular lymphoma, and usually of B-cell origin), as well as diffuse, mixed lymphomas that originate from T cells, such as Lennert's lymphoma (epitheloid cell).[90] Atypical large and small lymphoid cells are usually present, and a misdiagnosis of Hodgkin's disease is possible if the binucleated large lymphocytes are mistaken for Reed–Sternberg cells.

Malignant lymphoma, diffuse large cell (previously termed diffuse histiocytic), results from a block in lymphocyte transformation at site e (Fig. 124.4). The neoplastic cells usually originate from B lymphocytes and may be either large cleaved or large noncleaved cells; the clinical significance of this morphologic difference is uncertain. In the Rappaport classification, both diffuse large cell and immunoblastic large cell lymphoma would be categorized as "diffuse histiocytic" lymphoma. In the Working Formulation study, large cell lymphomas originating from follicular center cells (diffuse large cell) were noted to have a significant survival advantage compared with those of nonfollicular center cell origin (immunoblastic). For this reason, the Working Formulation divides the diffuse large cell lymphomas into intermediate-grade (diffuse large cell lymphoma) and high-grade (immunoblastic large cell lymphoma) categories. Of note, significant differences in survival could no longer be detected between patients with diffuse large cell and immunoblastic lymphomas in a recent long-term follow-up analysis of the original patients in the Working Formulation study.[87]

High-Grade Lymphomas

Malignant lymphoma, large cell, immunoblastic (previously termed diffuse histiocytic), occurs with an apparent arrest at the level of the immunoblast (Fig. 124.4). Several subtypes are recognized, including plasmacytoid, clear cell, polymorphous, and epithelioid cell. Lymphomas with plasmacytoid features are usually of B-cell origin. A wide variety of T-cell lymphomas, such as the Japanese T-cell lymphoma, HTLV-1 associated adult T-cell lymphoma, and T-cell immunoblastic sarcoma, are included in the polymorphous category; the clear cell and epithelioid subtypes are usually associated with lymphomas originating from T cells as well. The immunoblastic lymphomas tend to be very aggressive, especially the Japanese and HTLV-1 associated T-cell lymphoma. Generalized lymphadenopathy and widespread organ involvement, including the liver, spleen, gastrointestinal tract, and central nervous system (CNS), are frequently seen. Invasion of the lymphoid sinuses by a variant of immunoblastic lymphoma also has been reported.[81]

Malignant lymphoma, lymphoblastic (previously termed diffuse lymphoblastic), is usually a T-cell lymphoma and commonly presents in adolescent males. The malignant cells resemble acute lymphoblastic leukemia (ALL) cells, and are usually positive for the enzyme terminal deoxynucleotidyl transferase (TdT).[81] A progression to ALL frequently occurs. Approximately 75% of patients with lymphoblastic lymphoma present with a large mediastinal mass, an uncommon feature among the other types of non-Hodgkin's lymphoma. Patients also commonly present with bone marrow and cerebrospinal fluid (CSF) involvement. Neoplastic cells in the CSF place these patients at high risk for meningeal infiltration. Approximately 10–20% of cases of lymphoblastic lymphoma originate from precursor B lymphocytes and have a phenotype closely related to that of common ALL or pre-B-cell ALL.[91] Unlike the T-cell lymphoblastic lymphomas, these patients usually do not present with mediastinal masses, and in some cases lytic bone lesions have been observed.

Malignant lymphoma, small noncleaved cell (previously termed diffuse undifferentiated), is a B-cell lymphoma that occurs secondary to an arrest in lymphocyte transformation at site d (Fig. 124.4). This aggressive lymphoma includes both Burkitt's and non-Burkitt's subtypes. Burkitt's cells are moderately sized with round nuclei, several prominent nucleoli, a distinct cytoplasmic rim, and numerous mitoses with a characteristic "starry sky" pattern.[81] Non-Burkitt's cells are more variable in size and shape. Burkitt's lymphoma usually presents in children. Bulky disease in extranodal sites such as the face and jaw bones (endemic cases in Africa) or the abdomen (nonendemic cases in the United States and other areas) are frequently seen. Lymph node involvement at presentation is rare. Non-Burkitt's lymphomas usually present in adults (median age 34 years) and commonly in nodal regions. Small noncleaved cell lymphoma also is one of the most common forms of lymphoma associated with HIV infections.

CLINICAL PRESENTATION

Patients with non-Hodgkin's lymphoma present with a wide variety of symptoms, which depend on the site of involvement and whether tumor involvement is nodal or extranodal. Sites of involvement and dissemination of the malignant cell can, in some cases, be predicted based on the lymphoma's cell of origin and the fact that the tumor frequently disseminates to areas where the normal counterparts of the lymphoma cells are located. For example, lymphomas of B-cell origin involve areas of the lymphoid system normally populated by B lymphocytes, such as lymph nodes, spleen, and bone marrow. T-cell lymphomas commonly disseminate to various extranodal sites, such as the skin and lungs. In contrast to Hodgkin's disease, the bone marrow is commonly involved in non-Hodgkin's lymphoma.

Clinical presentation also is dependent on the type of non-Hodgkin's lymphoma and the stage of disease at presentation. Low-grade lymphomas usually arise in middle-aged or older individuals (median age, 55 years), and are uncommon in individuals before the age of 40. The majority of patients present with advanced stages of disease, often the result of bone marrow involvement (found in 30–70% of patients), although privileged sites, such as the CNS and testes, are rarely affected. Low-grade lymphomas usually have an indolent clinical course, and many patients report a history of waxing and waning adenopathy over a period of months to years prior to diagnosis. In contrast, the intermediate- and high-grade lymphomas occur over a broader age range and are more aggressive in their clinical behavior. Patients present at various stages of disease. Although bone marrow involvement is not as common, occurring in only 10–30% of patients (except lymphoblastic lymphoma, in which bone marrow is affected in 50% of patients), the lymphoma tends to disseminate rapidly and often involves extranodal and privileged sites.

In general, patients may have either localized or generalized adenopathy, with the involved nodes being painless, rubbery, and discrete, and usually located in the cervical and supraclavicular regions as in Hodgkin's disease. The liver or spleen may be enlarged in patients with generalized adenopathy. Patients with mesenteric or gastrointestinal involvement may present with signs and symptoms of nausea, vomiting, obstruction, abdominal pain, a palpable abdominal mass, or gastrointestinal bleeding. Patients with bone marrow involvement may have symptoms related to anemia (fatigue, pallor, tachycardia, dyspnea on exertion), neutropenia (recurrent infections), or thrombocytopenia (easy bruising, epistaxis, petechiae). Non-Hodgkin's lymphoma has a greater tendency to involve the testes, epitrochlear nodes, and Waldeyer's ring than Hodgkin's disease. The incidence of solitary brain lymphoma is increasing, especially in patients with AIDS. Infrequently, patients with non-Hodgkin's lymphoma may present with acute renal failure from retroperitoneal adenopathy causing ureteral obstruction or from metabolic abnormalities such as hyperuricemia with uric acid nephropathy.

In contrast to Hodgkin's disease, only 20% of patients with non-Hodgkin's lymphoma have the constitutional symptoms of fevers, night sweats, and weight loss of greater than 10%. The clinical features of Hodgkin's lymphomas are compared in Table 124.3.

DIAGNOSIS/STAGING

As with Hodgkin's disease, the diagnosis of non-Hodgkin's lymphoma must be established by an appropriate biopsy to provide tissue for pathologic review. An entire involved lymph node should be removed carefully for evaluation to preserve its architecture and prevent distortional artifact of the architecture, which could lead to an inaccurate diagnosis. Likewise, needle biopsy of the node prevents architecture evaluation and is not adequate in the diagnosis of non-Hodgkin's lymphoma. When adenopathy is not present, diagnosis may be established by biopsy of cutaneous lesions, bone marrow biopsy, and aspiration in patients with unexplained myelosuppression, liver biopsy in patients with hepatomegaly or elevated liver function transaminases, or biopsy of involved extranodal organs, such as bone, Waldeyer's ring, lung, and testis.

Further diagnostic procedures and staging are not indicated in patients whose age or underlying medical problems limit treatment to palliative therapy. Otherwise, the extent of the investigative workup required prior to therapy is determined by the histopathology and available treatment for the subtype of non-Hodgkin's lymphoma. Table 124.6 outlines evaluation and staging procedures for non-Hodgkin's lymphoma.

Clinical staging always begins with a thorough history and physical examination. Patients should be questioned about the presence or absence and extent of fever, night sweats, and weight loss. A detailed history of lymphadenopathy also should be obtained, including when and where the lymph nodes were first noted, and their rate of growth. A complete physical examination is performed to assess the extent of disease involvement with special attention given to all nodal areas. All patients should have a complete blood count, serum chemistries including liver and renal profiles, a chest x-ray, and bone marrow aspiration and biopsy. Bone marrow biopsy from each posterior iliac crest should be performed early in evaluation of all patients because a positive result, given further confirmation of the diagnosis, establishes stage IV disease and eliminates the need for more extensive and invasive tests.

Lumbar puncture to evaluate the CSF is recommended as part of the initial staging in patients who are at risk for CNS involvement, including patients with lymphoblastic lymphoma and small noncleaved cell lymphomas (Burkitt's and non-Burkitt's). Although bone marrow involvement is not as common in diffuse large cell lymphomas (including diffuse mixed and immunoblastic types), its presence is associated with the development of CNS lymphoma. Up to 25% of patients with diffuse large cell lymphoma and a positive bone marrow biopsy may develop CNS disease.[81] Patients with lymphoma involving the testes or epidural space also are at high risk for CNS involvement. Evaluation of the CSF is therefore recommended in patients with diffuse large cell lymphomas with bone marrow, epidural, or testicular involvement.

Various radiologic studies are utilized in the staging of non-Hodgkin's lymphoma, but recommendations for their use are sometimes controversial. Abdominal CT is very useful in the evaluation of the upper abdominal lymph nodes, including mesenteric, splenic, and hepatic nodes, and always is recommended. The use of chest CT is not as well established, and is usually unnecessary if chest x-rays are normal. Exceptions to this are in the unusual cases where chest radiotherapy is to be given alone or to rule out mediastinal disease in patients with stage I disease.[81] Lymphangiography is the most sensitive test for evaluating the para-aortic, iliac, and retroperitoneal nodes, and allows easy follow-up of abnormal nodes. However, an advance in stage with a positive lymphangiogram is infrequent because most patients already have palpable adenopathy at the time. The use of lymphangiography varies among institutions, and may not be necessary unless less invasive studies, such as the abdominal CT, are negative. MRI has not been shown superior to CT, and its use is not routinely recommended.[92] Other tests, such as liver–spleen scan, bone scan, upper gastrointestinal series, and intravenous pyelogram are useful in patients with organ symptomology or serum chemistry abnormalities.

Staging laparotomy is of limited use in non-Hodgkin's lymphoma as the treatment of stages II, III, and IV disease of a specific subtype of lymphoma is essentially the same (i.e., chemotherapy alone) and the majority of patients will have documented advanced disease by less invasive studies. Staging laparotomy is reserved for patients with clinical stage I disease, where the discovery of intra-abdominal disease would mandate a change in therapy from localized radiation therapy to combination chemotherapy.

The Ann Arbor staging classification developed for the clinical staging of Hodgkin's disease also is useful in staging and defining patient composition in non-Hodgkin's lymphoma (Table 124.5). After staging, the majority of patients have advanced disease (stages III and IV). In fact, truly localized disease usually is seen in only three histologic subtypes (diffuse mixed, diffuse large cell, and immunoblastic lymphoma), in which approximately 50% of patients will present with stage I or II disease.[87] Stage is more important prognostically in Hodgkin's disease than in non-Hodgkin's lymphoma. As an example, the distinction between stage III and IV non-Hodgkin's lymphoma is of little importance in the determination of treatment, because stage III non-Hodgkin's lymphoma is not commonly treatable with total nodal irradiation as it can be in some stage III patients with Hodgkin's disease. The prognosis of non-Hodgkin's lymphoma is more dependent on the histologic subtype and the presence of a variety of clinical factors found to affect prognosis. These are outlined in Table 124.4.

TREATMENT

The primary goals in the treatment of non-Hodgkin's lymphoma are to relieve symptoms and cure the patient of disease whenever possible, and to do this with acceptable toxicity. The treatment strategy depends on many factors including patient's age, concomitant disease, histologic subtype, and stage of disease. With the introduction and improvement of megavoltage radiotherapy, combination chemotherapy regimens and, most recently, bone marrow transplantation, complete remission and cure can be achieved in a number of patients, namely, those with intermediate and high-grade aggressive lymphomas.

Traditionally, non-Hodgkin's lymphoma has been classified by the clinical behavior and degree of aggressiveness it exhibits. The terms *good risk, favorable,* and *indolent* have been applied to low-grade lymphomas by virtue of their relatively indolent behavior. Patients with low-grade lymphoma usually have a relatively long disease-free survival (measured in years), with or without aggressive chemotherapy. Although these lymphomas are responsive to a wide range of therapeutic approaches, response is often transient, relapse is common, and patients are rarely cured of their disease.

In contrast, the intermediate and high-grade lymphomas have been termed unfavorable due to their aggressive behavior and short survival (measured in months), if appropriate therapy is not initiated. Two of the high-grade lymphomas, lymphoblastic and small noncleaved cell, are considered highly aggressive lymphomas, with survival measured in weeks if left untreated. Because of their high growth fractions and rapid tumor doubling times, these aggressive lymphomas can be cured with intensive combination chemotherapy. Thus, the terminology for the non-Hodgkin's lymphomas represents a paradox, where "good" is bad and "bad" is good. In other words, the favorable (good) lymphomas are relatively indolent tumors that respond to chemotherapy but cannot be cured. On the other hand, the unfavorable (bad) lymphomas generally are more aggressive but in certain instances can be cured.

Different lymphoma histologies can be seen within an individual lymph node or at a separate anatomic site. For example, a follicular pattern may be observed in one area while a diffuse pattern is seen in another. Low-grade lymphomas also have the ability to progress over time to a higher grade lymphoma. In these situations, treatment should be based on the more aggressive subtype.

The therapeutic approach to non-Hodgkin's lymphoma involves radiation therapy and chemotherapy, as well as the use of biologic agents. The role of radiation therapy in the treatment of non-Hodgkin's lymphoma differs from the role already discussed for the treatment of Hodgkin's disease. Although the disease is responsive to radiation therapy, only a small percentage of patients with non-Hodgkin's lymphoma are amenable to remission induction and cure with local and/or regional irradiation. This is because truly localized disease at diagnosis is rare. Radiation therapy is used more commonly in advanced disease, but mainly as a palliative measure to control local bulky disease.

Effective chemotherapy for non-Hodgkin's lymphoma ranges from single-agent therapy in the low-grade lymphomas to aggressive, complex combination chemotherapy regimens in the intermediate and high-grade lymphomas. The most active agents used in the treatment of non-Hodgkin's lymphoma include the alkylating agents (e.g., cyclophosphamide, chlorambucil), bleomycin, doxorubicin, etoposide, methotrexate, vincristine, and corticosteroids (e.g., prednisone, dexamethasone). The rationale for intensive combination chemotherapy regimens is based, in part on the somatic mutation theory of Goldie and Coldman[41] discussed previously.

Appropriate therapy for non-Hodgkin's lymphoma is dependent on the tumor histology and the stage of disease. In general, the therapeutic approach can be divided into limited disease and advanced disease. Limited disease includes those patients with localized disease (Ann Arbor stages I and II). Advanced disease is defined as all Ann Arbor stage III or IV patients, and also frequently includes Ann Arbor stage II patients with one or more of the poor prognostic features listed in Table 124.5. For the purpose of treatment, immunoblastic lymphoma will be grouped with the intermediate-grade lymphomas because the treatment of these lymphomas is essentially the same.

Limited Disease (Stages I and II)

Low-Grade Lymphoma

As stated earlier, localized disease is uncommon and accounts for only 10–20% of patients with low-grade lymphoma. Most patients have painless lymph node enlargement, often waxing and waning in size, and tolerate the disease despite its usual widespread dissemination. Although only a small percentage of patients have early-stage disease, it is important to identify these patients due to the potential for cure with therapy.

Radiation therapy is the standard treatment for early-stage low-grade lymphoma. Involved-field, extended-field, and total nodal irradiation have been used. Carefully staged patients with either stage I or contiguous stage II disease treated with radiation therapy can achieve up to an 85% disease-free survival rate at 10 years. In a retrospective study from Stanford University, 54% of patients with stage I or II follicular lymphoma treated with radiation therapy were disease free after 10 years of follow-up.[81,93] A significant improvement in freedom from relapse was seen in patients who received total nodal irradiation compared with those who received involved-field radiation. However, overall survival was similar regardless of the extent of radiation fields. To further evaluate the extent of radiation therapy required for the treatment of low-grade follicular lymphoma, the Stanford group conducted a small prospective randomized trial comparing involved-field with total nodal irradiation. No significant difference in either disease-free survival (more than 80% at 5 years) or overall survival (more than 75% at 5 years) was seen between the two groups. Both involved-field and total nodal irradiation appear potentially curative, although some still feel an increased risk of relapse remains with the use of limited-field radiation, and suggest that total nodal irradiation is the treatment of choice in patients with stage I or II low-grade lymphoma (especially the follicular lymphomas).[81] Unlike treatment for Hodgkin's disease, there are no data to support the use of extended-field irradiation to clinically uninvolved contiguous lymph node chains. This is due to the fact that in non-Hodgkin's lymphoma, the spread of disease is frequently noncontiguous and less certain than the usual contiguous spread seen in Hodgkin's disease.

The role of adjuvant chemotherapy in the management of localized stage I or II disease is unclear. The use of combination chemotherapy (namely CVP, or cyclophosphamide, vincristine, and prednisone) plus radiation has not been shown superior to radiation alone in several small randomized trials.[81] A significant improvement in relapse-free survival was found when CHOP (cyclophosphamide, doxorubicin, vincristine, prednisone) rather than CVP was combined with radiation therapy compared with radiation alone.[94] The CHOP regimen is shown in Table 124.12. Currently, the role of combined chemotherapy and radiation therapy remains unresolved.

Intermediate-Grade Lymphoma

Although relatively uncommon for intermediate-grade lymphomas, up to 40% of patients with diffuse mixed, diffuse large cell, and immunoblastic lymphoma will have localized disease. Intermediate-grade lymphomas are more aggressive and usually have slightly worse 5-year survival rates compared with low-grade lymphomas.

Radiation therapy was the first therapeutic approach used to produce long-term survival in patients with localized aggressive lymphoma. The efficacy of radiation therapy in these patients is dependent on the extent of disease and the aggressiveness of the staging procedures (e.g., laparotomy). Patients with unfavorable prognostic factors, such as B symptoms, three or more sites of involvement, or bulky disease have higher relapse rates (up to 90%) compared with those without these features (25%).[95] When staging includes laparotomy, greater than 90% of patients with stage I disease may have long-term survival.[96] In contrast, patients who undergo less intensive staging without laparotomy (clinical staging) have decreased 5-year survival rates of 65 and 25% for stage I and II patients, respectively.[97] Therefore, radiation therapy alone appears most effective in patients with less bulky disease and who have undergone a laparotomy as part of their staging workup.

Staging laparotomy has been associated with various surgical complications and may lead to delays in therapy, which is an important point considering that these tumors are aggressive and have the potential for rapid growth and dissemination. For this reason, investigators began to evaluate the role of combination chemotherapy in addition to radiation therapy in patients with localized aggressive lymphoma not undergoing laparotomy. Several randomized trials have confirmed a significant improvement in treatment outcome with the use of combined modality therapy compared with radiation therapy alone.[81,98] Overall, the 5-year disease-free survival with combined modality therapy is 80–90% in stage I patients and 70–75% in stage II patients. Chemotherapy regimens that contain doxorubicin, such as CHOP or BACOP (CHOP plus bleomycin), appear superior to non doxorubicin-containing regimens.[99] In the Milan study, the use of BACOP resulted in significantly higher 5-year survival rates (approximately 80% in both stages I and II disease) compared with the CVP regi-men (69% in stage I and 49% in stage II).[81] In most series, six cycles of chemotherapy are combined with radiation therapy, although shorter courses of chemotherapy (three cycles) have achieved similar results.[100] Excellent results also have been obtained with a modified ProMACE- MOPP regimen (prednisone, methotrexate, doxorubicin, cyclophosphamide, etoposide, MOPP), in which 75% of the normal doses of myelosuppressive drugs and four treatment cycles, rather than six, are used.[101] The question has been raised as to whether combined modality therapy is really necessary or if the use of chemotherapy alone may be just as effective. Cabanillas[102] has demonstrated a 91 and 70% 5-year relapse-free survival rate in stage I and II disease, respectively, with the use of chemotherapy (mainly CHOP) alone. Randomized trials suggest that chemotherapy alone is as effective as combined modality treatment, with less toxicity.[99,103]

It is currently recommended that patients with early-stage aggressive lymphoma without poor prognostic features not undergo exploratory laparotomy, but rather receive four to six cycles of combination chemotherapy followed by involved-field radiation therapy. In the presence of poor prognostic features, patients should be treated in the same manner as patients with advanced disease. The role of chemotherapy alone in the treatment of localized aggressive lymphoma requires further evaluation.

TABLE 124.12. CHOP REGIMEN[a]

Drug	Dose (mg/m^2)	Route	Treatment Days
Cyclophosphamide	750	IV	1
Doxorubicin	50	IV	1
Vincristine	1.4	IV	1
Prednisone	100	PO	1–5

[a]One cycle is 21 days.

High-Grade Lymphoma

Lymphoblastic lymphoma and small noncleaved cell lymphoma (Burkitt's and non-Burkitt's diseases) are much more common in children and young adults. These lymphomas are extremely aggressive due to their rapid tumor doubling times, and prompt initiation of appropriate therapy is required. Acute leukemia-like protocols are used in the treatment of both lymphoblastic lymphoma and small noncleaved cell lymphoma, and include high-dose induction, consolidation, and maintenance regimens, along with CNS prophylaxis. Treatment of limited and advanced disease is essentially the same.

Advanced Disease (Stages III and IV)

Low-Grade Lymphoma

The management of stage III and IV low-grade lymphoma remains controversial because standard therapeutic approaches have not been shown curative despite the high complete remission rates. Therapeutic options for these patients are diverse, ranging from no therapy to combination chemotherapy with radiation. Total lymphoid irradiation using 35 Gy has been used as the sole modality for stage III low-grade lymphoma, with 40% relapse-free survival at 10 years.[104] Most patients had their relapses in nonirradiated sites, suggesting that extended treatment fields might have produced increased disease-free survival. Total-body irradiation therefore has been investigated, but results have not been found superior to those for total lymphoid irradiation or chemotherapy alone.[81,93] In addition, a 12% incidence of secondary acute nonlymphocytic leukemia was noted in the irradiated group. Several randomized trials have shown equivalent efficacy of single alkylating agents (chlorambucil or cyclophosphamide) versus CVP,[105] and CVP versus CVP plus total lymphoid irradiation.[106] Regardless of the treatment modality, a majority of patients respond but relapse at a rate of 10–15% per year. Use of more intensive regimens, such as BACOP, COPP (cyclophosphamide, vincristine, procarbazine, prednisone), or M-BACOD (methotrexate, bleomycin, doxorubicin, cyclophosphamide, vincristine, dexamethasone) again show high response rates but no significant survival advantage.[93] Overall, complete response can be achieved in 60–80% of patients with single-agent, combination chemotherapy, or combined modality therapy. Median remission durations range from 12–26 months. Five-year survival rates exceed 80%, but fall to 30–50% by 10 years.

Because various treatment regimens have not produced convincing data supporting improved survival, it has been suggested that initial therapy be withheld from patients who are asymptomatic. This "watchful waiting" strategy was first proposed by Horning and Rosenberg.[107] Selected patients were followed without initial therapy until they became symptomatic. The median time until therapy was required was 3 years. The 10-year survival was 73%, which does not differ significantly from patients who receive therapy at the time of diagnosis. Of interest, disease progression was significantly more rapid for patients with follicular mixed lymphoma (16.5 months) compared with the other low-grade lymphomas (48–72 months). In addition, complete remissions following chemotherapy appear to be more durable in follicular mixed lymphoma (approximately 7 years) than in follicular small cleaved cell lymphoma (4.5 years). Therefore, watchful waiting may not be appropriate for patients with follicular mixed histologies.

Advantages of treatment deferral include prevention of exposure to agents that may induce drug resistance, prevention of drug-induced toxicity, possible spontaneous regression, administration of appropriate palliative therapy when the disease progresses, and potential evolution to a potentially curable lymphoma. Potential disadvantages of withholding treatment include disease progression in threatening sites, which may compromise palliative therapy, and evolution of the disease to a lymphoma that is more aggressive and more resistant to therapy.

The NCI is currently conducting a randomized prospective trial comparing no initial treatment with intensive combination chemotherapy (MACE-MOPP) plus low-dose total nodal irradiation given at diagnosis.[108] Palliative radiation therapy is used for the control of local adenopathy. If systemic symptoms arise, patients are crossed over to the treatment group. At 6 years, only 44% of the patients in the observation group have required systemic therapy. Median time to initiation of combined modality therapy was 34 months. Fifty percent of these patients achieved a complete remission with therapy and 71% of these continue to be disease free at 4 years. This is compared with a 78% complete remission rate in patients initially treated at diagnosis, and 86% of these are free of disease at 4 years of follow-up. Continued follow-up will be required to answer the question of whether or not it is necessary to treat asymptomatic patients at diagnosis. Heinz and colleagues[109] report their institution's experience involving 1520 non-Hodgkin's lymphoma patients. They found no improvement in prognosis with early aggressive chemotherapy, and support a "watch and wait" approach.

An important feature of low-grade lymphoma is its propensity to evolve to a more aggressive intermediate- or high-grade lymphoma. The actuarial risk of histologic transformation appears to increase over time, with a 10% risk reported at 5 years and increasing up to 40% at 10 years, occurring with equal frequency in both treated and untreated patients.[107] Rapid disease progression and short median survival (less than 1 year) are common following transformation. The use of combination chemotherapy may eradicate the aggressive clone, although these patients remain at risk for relapse with either a low-grade or more aggressive lymphoma.

Intermediate-Grade Lymphoma

Among the heterogeneous group of non-Hodgkin's lymphomas, the most important therapeutic advances have been made with intensive chemotherapy regimens for the intermediate- and high-grade lymphomas. There are several important points to consider in the treatment of these lymphomas. First, the intermediate- and high-grade non-Hodgkin's lymphomas are potentially curable diseases, even when they are widely metastatic. Therefore, unlike the patient with low-grade non-Hodgkin's lymphoma, "no treatment" is not an option. These tumors, when left untreated, are almost universally fatal within 2 years. Second, because it is uncommon to achieve a complete remission with single-agent therapy and long-term survival is not possible without induction of a complete remission, intensive combination chemotherapy should be used. In other words, the treatment regimen with the highest likelihood of cure should be administered first, because durable responses with salvage therapy (other than bone marrow transplantation) are less likely. Third, dosage and administration schedules for these intensive regimens, which are often accompanied by severe toxic effects, must be rigidly adhered to. Dose reduction or prolongation of the interval between cycles can be associated with rapid regrowth of the tumor and the inability to produce cure. Patients receiving greater than 70% of planned dose intensity (measured in mg/m^2/week) have a better prognosis than those receiving less than 70% of the planned dose intensity.[110] Last, the use of long-term maintenance therapy following a complete response has not been shown to improve survival (excluding lymphoblastic and small noncleaved cell lymphomas). Two cycles of chemotherapy following attainment of a complete response are usually recommended, with the majority of current regimens lasting 6–9 months. There are exceptions, however, such as MACOP-B, which requires only 12 weeks of therapy.

Diffuse large cell lymphoma is the most common subtype of intermediate-grade lymphomas and therefore is the most widely studied (along with immunoblastic large cell lymphoma). Patients with follicular large cell, diffuse small cleaved cell, or diffuse mixed cell lymphomas appear to have a poorer response to chemotherapy compared with patients with large cell lymphoma. Although complete response rates of 60–75% have been reported, relapse is common and overall long-term disease-free survival drops to approximately 40%.[81,111]

Advanced-stage large cell lymphoma was considered an incurable disease 25 years ago. Initial combination regimens using CVP produced a plateau on the survival curve of just 10%, with a median survival of less than 1 year. During this same period, DeVita and colleagues demonstrated improved response, survival, and cure rates in the treatment of patients with Hodgkin's disease with MOPP. As an outgrowth of this trial, DeVita et al.[112] developed the C-MOPP (cyclophosphamide, vincristine, procarbazine, prednisone) regimen and demonstrated a complete remission rate of approximately 40% in large cell lymphoma. Based on the activity of single-agent doxorubicin, McKelvey and associates[113] developed the CHOP regimen, which gained widespread popularity because it had the highest complete remission rate (67%) of any regimen reported at that time. Relapses within the first 2 years were common, and durability of the complete responses was questioned. A review of the SWOG's 12-year experience with CHOP-based regimens in more than 400 patients reported a complete remission rate of 53%, with an overall survival of 30%.[114] The use of additional agents, such as bleomycin (CHOP-Bleo, BACOP) or methotrexate (COMLA), did not significantly affect treatment outcome.[81,115] Results from trials with these first-generation regimens are listed in Table 124.13. Overall, these regimens produce complete remissions in 40–60% of patients and about one-third of all patients appear to be cured with their use.

Various approaches taken by different investigators led to the development of the second-generation chemotherapy regimens in the late 1970s. These regimens are characterized by the use of six or more antineoplastic agents, with the myelosuppressive agents being cycled more frequently, generally every 3 weeks, and the nonmyelosuppressive agents administered during weeks of cytopenias. These additional chemotherapy agents are frequently cell-cycle active and/or marrow-sparring, are generally non–crossresistant to the myelosuppressive agent, and provide continuous tumor suppression even during periods of cytopenia. COP-BLAM I, M-BACOD (high-dose methotrexate = 3 g/m^2), m-BACOD (moderate-dose methotrexate = 200 mg/m^2), and ProMACE-MOPP are examples of second-generation regimens (Table 124.14).[115–118] The ProMACE-MOPP flexitherapy combination is based in part on the Norton–Simon hypothesis on the development of drug resistance.[119] The Norton–Simon hypothesis incorporates Gompertzian kinetics (as the tumor size increases, the fraction of cells contributing to the growth of the tumor decreases) and proposes that as the tumor burden is reduced the number of chemotherapy-sensitive cells also is reduced (increased fraction of drug-resistant tumor cells). To achieve the maximal probability of cure, therapy should be initiated to decrease the tumor burden and the rate of tumor response monitored. As the tumor cells become resistant to the chemotherapeutic agents, the response rate slows. At this point, therapy should be switched to a combination regimen to which the tumor has not been exposed. With the ProMACE-MOPP flexitherapy, ProMACE is administered for a flexible number of cycles until the rate of tumor response appears to slow, and then therapy is switched

TABLE 124.13. FIRST-GENERATION CHEMOTHERAPY TREATMENT REGIMENS FOR ADVANCED INTERMEDIATE- AND HIGH-GRADE LYMPHOMAS

Regimen[a]	Author	*N*	Complete Reponse (%)	Long-Term Survival (B)[b]
C-MOPP	DeVita (1973)	27	41	37
CHOP	McKelvey (1976)	115	67	50% (22 mo)
	Coltman (1986)	418	53	30
CHOP-Bleo	Rodriguez (1977)	26	69	—
	Lee (1986)	28	75	53
BACOP	Schein (1976)	32	48	37
COMLA	Sweet (1980)	42	55	—
	Gaynor (1985)	72	40	30

[a]C-MOPP = cyclophosphamide, vincristine, procarbazine, prednisone; CHOP = cyclophasphamide, doxorubicin, vincristine, prednisone; CHOP-Bleo = cyclophosphamide, doxorubicin, vincristine, prednisone, bleomycin; BACOP = bleomycin, doxorubicin, cyclophosphamide, vincristine, prednisone; COMLA = cyclophosphamide, vincristine, methotrexate, leucovorin, cytarabine.
[b]Greater than 3 years. Data from Refs. 81, 114, 115, and 118.

TABLE 124.14. SECOND-GENERATION CHEMOTHERAPEUTIC INTERMEDIATE- AND HIGH-GRADE LYMPHOMAS

Regimen	*N*	Complete Response (%)	Long-Term Survival (%)[a]	Author
COP-BLAM-I	33	73	55	Laurence
M-BACOD	81	72	63	Skarin
m-BACOD	134	61	63	Shipp
m-BACOD	78	65	61	Dana
ProMACE-MOPP	99	74	53	Fisher
CHOP/HOAP-Bleo/IMVP-16	56	82	—	Cabanillas

Key: COP-BLAM I, cyclophosphamide, vincristine, prednisone, bleomycin, doxorubicin, procarbazine; M/m-BACOD, methotrexate, bleomycin, doxorubicin, cyclophosphamide, vincristine, dexamethasone; ProMACE-MOPP, prednisone, methotrexate, doxorubicin, cyclophosphamide, etoposide, MOPP; CHOP/HOAP-Bleo/IMVP-16, CHOP, doxorubicin, vincristine, cytarabine, bleomycin, ifosfamide, methotrexate, etoposide.
[a]2–3 years. (Data from Refs. 115–118.)

TABLE 124.15. RANDOMIZED TRIALS COMPARING CHOP TO OTHER REGIMENS

Regimen	*N*	Complete Response (%)	Long-Term Survival (%)[b]	Author
CHOP	33	61	52	Mathews[124]
MATCOP[a]	47	66	45	
CHOP	225	44	54	Fisher[123] (SWOG)
m-BACOD	223	48	52	
ProMACE-CytaBOM	233	56	50	
MACOP-B	218	51	50	
CHOP	174	51	48	Gordon[120] (ECOG)[c]
m-BACOD	151	56	49	
CHOP	125	59	51	Cooper[125]
MACOP-B	111	51	56	

[a]MATCOP, methotrexate, doxorubicin, teniposide, cyclophosphamide, vincristine, prednisone.
[b]Greater than or equal to 3 years.
[c]Australian and New Zealand Lymphoma Group. (Data from Refs. 120, 123–125.)

to MOPP. After the rate of response to MOPP slows, or a complete response is achieved, patients are switched back to ProMACE for consolidation. This approach resulted in a complete response rate of 74%, and after more than 9 years of follow-up, approximately half of the patients appeared to be cured.[115]

Overall, second-generation regimens have produced complete remission rates of 75% and long-term survival in approximately 50% of patients. These regimens appear to be superior to the first-generation regimens. However, a randomized comparative trial that controls for length of follow-up and differences in patient populations is the appropriate method of comparing regimens. A randomized prospective trial comparing a first-generation (CHOP) to a second-generation (m-BACOD) regimen has been conducted.[120] Results show no difference in the complete response rates and the impact of these regimens on survival (Table 124.15).

The Goldie–Coldman hypothesis[41] and the Hryniuk and Bush dose-intensity hypothesis[121] have aided in the design of the third-generation treatment regimens. These chemotherapy regimens focus on alterations in schedules (the use of more drugs and early exposure to non–cross-resistant agents) and doses (increasing relative dose intensity) rather than the addition of new drugs. Hryniuk and Bush[121] observed that the treatment outcome of patients with metastatic breast cancer was related to the dose intensity (amount of drug delivered per unit time) of the treatment regimens. In short, the best chance for cure can be achieved by using more drugs at higher doses as frequently as possible. The importance of dose-intensity in the treatment outcome of patients with non-Hodgkin's lymphoma has recently been reviewed.[122]

The third-generation treatment regimens—MACOP-B, ProMACE-CytaBOM, COP-BLAM III, and F-MACHOP—have produced complete remissions in 70–80% of patients and cures in 55–65% of patients (Table 124.16).[115,118] These regimens use higher doses of more drugs early in intensive short-course treatment. For example, the MACOP-B regimen emphasizes dose intensity, and treatment lasts for only 12 weeks, during which combinations of myelosuppressive agents and nonmyelosuppressive agents are alternated and administered weekly. The COP-BLAM III regimen differs from the other regimens in that it uses infusional vincristine and bleomycin (prolonged exposure to cell cycle-specific agents) and dose escalation of doxorubicin and cyclophosphamide, allowing maximum dose intensity.

TABLE 124.16. THIRD-GENERATION CHEMOTHERAPY REGIMENS FOR ADVANCED INTERMEDIATE- AND HIGH-GRADE LYMPHOMAS

Regimen	*N*	Complete Response (%)	Long-Term Survival (%)[a]	Author
MACOP-B	126	84	69	Klimo
MACOP-B	109	50	51	Levy and Miller
ProMACE-CytaBOM	94	86	n/a	Longo
ProMACE-CytaBOM	78	65	57	Gilewski and Richards
COP-BLAM III	43	86	70	Boyd
F-MACHOP	s56	77	60	Guglielmi

Key: MACOP-B, methotrexate, doxorubicin, cyclophosphamide, vincristine, prednisone, bleomycin; ProMACE-CytaBOM, ProMACE, cytarabine, bleomycin, vincristine; COP-BLAM III, cyclophosphamide, vincristine, prednisone, bleomycin, doxorubicin, procarbazine; F-MACHOP, fluorouracil, methotrexate, cytarabine, cyclophosphamide, doxorubicin, vincristine, prednisone.
[a]2–3 years minimum. (Data from Refs. 115 and 118.)

The third-generation regimens appear to be superior to the first- and second-generation regimens. However these observations are from separate studies and not randomized comparative trials that take into account the length of follow-up and differences in patient populations. Recently, SWOG reported a prospective trial in which 899 patients were randomized to treatment with either CHOP, m-BACOD, ProMACE-CytaBOM, or MACOP-B.[123] Complete response and survival rates were not significantly different between these regimens (Table 124.15).[120,123–125] Fatal toxicity, however, occurred in 1% of the CHOP group, 3% of the ProMACE-CyaBOM group, 5% of the m-BACOD group, and 6% of the MACOP-B group. The CHOP and ProMACE-CytaBOM groups had significantly fewer life-threatening and fatal reactions compared to m-BACOD and MACOP-B groups. This large, randomized, controlled trial concludes that CHOP is the therapy of choice based on response and survival rates, toxicity and cost.

Some observations can be made concerning the treatment of advanced intermediate-grade lymphomas: (1) The incidence of complete remission and of long-term survival has been improved greatly with the use of combination chemotherapy regimens; (2) a rapid response to chemotherapy (i.e., a complete response achieved in the first three treatment cycles) is associated with a more durable remission compared with patients requiring longer treatment; (3) relapse usually occurs within the first 2 years of induction of a complete remission (although relapses up to 7 years are reported), such that the vast majority of 2- to 3-year disease-free survivors are probably cured; and (4) while no regimen has improved response rates compared to CHOP, treatment with full doses of effective cytotoxic agents (CHOP) on schedule provides the best responses. With the use of the colony-stimulating factors (e.g., G-CSF, GM-CSF), this goal may be more easily achieved and allow for the safer use of even further dose-intensified regimens, which may result in a new superior regimen.

High-Grade Lymphoma

As mentioned previously, the treatment of limited and advanced-stage lymphoblastic and small noncleaved cell lymphoma is essentially the same.

Salvage Chemotherapy

While long-term remissions for non-Hodgkin's lymphoma are possible with intensive treatment regimens, 20–30% of patients do not enter a complete remission with initial therapy. Of those patients achieving a complete response, 20–40% subsequently relapse and die within a few months. Patients who relapse following a complete response to chemotherapy are more likely to respond to salvage therapy than patients with resistant or partially responding disease. Unfortunately, second-line salvage therapies are not capable of consistently inducing remission in relapsed or refractory non-Hodgkin's lymphoma, in contrast to effective salvage regimens available for Hodgkin's disease. A possible reason for the failure of salvage regimens might be the use of nearly all effective agents in the primary treatment regimens in the hope of improving the chance for cure. Several clinical trials are now evaluating the utility of newer investigational agents, alone and in combination, or the use of commercially available agents in high doses, with or without bone marrow rescue.

A wide variety of salvage chemotherapy regimens have been used in patients with relapsed or refractory non-Hodgkin's lymphoma, including single-agent therapy (e.g., mitoxantrone, high-dose cytarabine) and combination chemotherapy (e.g., MINE, mitoguazone, ifosfamide, methotrexate, etoposide; DHAP, cisplatin, high-dose cytarabine, dexamethasone). Results of several trials are listed in Table 124.17.[118,126–128] At best, complete responses are obtained in approximately 30% of patients, the median remission duration is 1–2 years, and only 5–10% of the patients will have long-term disease-free survival.[118]

To improve this situation, investigators began to evaluate the role of high-dose chemotherapy and/or radiation with bone marrow transplantation (BMT). Initial studies reported an improvement in the outlook for patients failing primary treatment. In the late 1970s, Appelbaum and colleagues[129] were the first to report high response rates and long-term survival in a small proportion of patients with Burkitt's lymphoma following high-dose chemotherapy and autologous BMT. Since that time, various studies have been published utilizing different high-dose regimens followed by autologous (most common), allogeneic, or syngeneic BMT. Survival rates are similar regardless of the source of

TABLE 124.17. SALVAGE CHEMOTHERAPY IN NON-HODGKIN'S LYMPHOMA

Regimen	N	Complete Response (%)	Median Duration of CR (mo)	Author
MINE	123	32	15	Cabanillas
DHAP	74	32	24	Velazquez
IMVP-16	38	37	12	Cabanilas
CAMP	30	27	~35	Ruit
NOAC	66	26	7	Ho
EPOCH	70	27	6.8	Jaffe
IMEVC Ara C	30	53	15	Buzzoni
DICEP	23	52	7.7	Neidhart

Key: MINE, mitoguazone, ifosfamide, methotrexate, etoposide; DHAP, cisplatin, high-dose cytarabine, dexamethasone; IMVP-16, ifosfamide, methotrexate, etoposide; CAMP, lomustine, cytarabine, mitoxantrone, prednisone; NOAC, mitoxantrone, high-dose cytarabine; EPOCH, etoposide, vincristine, doxorubicin, cyclophosphamide, prednisone; IMEVC Ara C, ifosfamide, mitoxantrone, etoposide, vindesine, cisplatin, cytarabine; DICEP, cyclophosphamide, etoposide, cisplatin. (Data from Refs. 118, 126–128.)

hematopoietic stem cells. BMT has been used at various stages of disease in patients with non-Hodgkin's lymphoma (e.g., initial, consolidation, or salvage therapy). Results in over 500 autologous BMT patients have documented long-term survival rates of 20–70%. Non-Hodgkin's lymphoma, namely, diffuse large cell lymphoma, has become one of the most common diseases to be treated with autologous BMT. A thorough review of BMT can be found in Chapter 129.

Biologic Response Modifiers

Conventional therapy of non-Hodgkin's lymphoma has consisted primarily of radiation and chemotherapy agents. However, biologic response modifiers are emerging as important agents in the investigational treatment of non-Hodgkin's lymphoma. Interferons (INFs), interleukin-2 (IL-2) with or without lymphokine activated killer (LAK) cells, and monoclonal antibodies all have been evaluated individually or in combination with each other or with chemotherapy.[81,93,130] The most promising results of these agents have been seen in the low-grade lymphomas, namely, the follicular lymphomas (Table 124.18).[93,130] Interferon has been the most extensively studied biologic agent. As a single agent, recombinant INF-α yields objective response rates of approximately 40% in low-grade lymphoma and 10–15% in intermediate- and high-grade lymphoma.[93,130] The majority of responses are partial, with median durations of 6–12 months. Responses are similar in previously treated and untreated patients. The most effective dose and schedule have not been determined, although lower doses appear to achieve similar results compared with higher doses. The role of continued maintenance therapy has not been fully evaluated.

Interferon and chemotherapy have been combined to evaluate the potential additive or synergistic effect between these two treatments. Interferon has been used with both single-agent therapy (usually chlorambucil) and combination chemotherapy (e.g., COPA, ProMACE-CytaBOM).[130] Preliminary results do not suggest dramatic improvements with this combined therapy, but most of the studies have included small numbers of patients. Myelosuppression appears to be the dose-limiting toxicity. Several large prospective trials are currently under way to further evaluate the use of interferon with chemotherapy, including one study in which interferon is administered to complete responders in an attempt to prolong their remission duration.

Few reports of IL-2 therapy of non-Hodgkin's lymphoma exist and it is not clear what role IL-2 will play in the treatment of lymphoma. High-dose IL-2 and LAK cells result in a low response rate of short duration in patients with intermediate- to high-grade non-Hodgkin's lymphoma and is not considered effective treatment.[131] In contrast, high-dose IL-2 and LAK cells can be effective treatment for patients with relapsed low-grade lymphoma.[132] Further studies are evaluating IL-2 alone versus IL-2/LAK to determine if any benefit is derived from the LAK cells.

Unlike the nonspecific biologic agents already discussed, monoclonal antibodies are a form of specific immunotherapy. Monoclonal antibodies directed against a specific immunoglobulin molecule on the surface of B-cell lymphomas are known as anti-idiotype antibodies.[133] Because the particular immunoglobulin molecule is unique to the B-cell tumor, anti-idiotype antibodies are able to distinguish between the tumor and normal B cells. The normal function of the surface immunoglobulin molecule is to serve as a receptor for antigens that trigger cell growth, so antibodies against that molecule may be able to dampen cellular proliferation. The majority of clinical trials with anti-idiotype monoclonal antibodies have included patients with follicular low-grade lymphoma. Responses to therapy are usually partial, but complete responses have been reported, with remission durations of 2 to more than 32 months (longest duration to date is 6 years).[133] Toxicity of this therapy is usually mild, the most frequent side effects including fever and chills. Other potential problems include the development of a human anti-mouse antibody (HAMA) response, the binding of the anti-idiotype antibody to circulating immunoglobulin that has been shed from the B-cell tumor, thereby impairing the ability of the antibody to reach the tumor cells, and the development of somatic variants no longer expressing the original surface immunoglobulin (idiotype-negative cells). Other therapeutic approaches now under study include conjugating monoclonal antibodies to

TABLE 124.18. BIOLOGIC RESPONSE MODIFIERS IN LOW-GRADE LYMPHOMAS

Therapy[a]	Dose[b]	*N*	Response[c]	Duration (mo)	Author
IFN alfa-2a	50 MU/m^2 TIW	24	4 CR, 9 PR	8	Foon
IFN alfa-2a	12 MU/m^2 TIW	16	1 CR, 6 PR	2–20+	O'Connell
IFN alfa-2b	10 MU/m^2 TIW	16	3 CR, 7 PR	1–24	Leavitt
IFN alfa-2b	2 MU/m^2 TIW	34	2 CR, 15 PR	11	Wagstaff
IL-2 + LAK cells	100,000 U/kg q 8 h	7	1 CR, 3 PR	—	Rosenberg
IL-2	3–6 MU/m^2	7	0 CR, 3 PR	—	Allison
anti-I MoAb	—	11	1 CR, 4PR	36+	Meeker
anti-I MoAb + IFN alfa	—	12	2 CR, 7 PR	1–32+	Brown

[a]IFN, interferon; IL-2, interleukin-2; anti-I MoAb, anti-idiotypic monoclonal antibody.
[b]MU, Million units; TIW, three times per week.
[c]CR, complete response; PR, partial reponse. Data from Refs. 93 and 130.

radioisotopes, toxins, and chemotherapy agents.[134–136] Further clinical trials are needed to define ultimately the role of biologic response modifiers and infusion toxins in the treatment of non-Hodgkin's lymphoma.

AIDS-Associated Non-Hodgkin's Lymphoma

The association between congenital and acquired states of immunodeficiency and the development of B-cell non-Hodgkin's lymphoma is well established. An increased incidence of non-Hodgkin's was seen early in the acquired immunodeficiency syndrome (AIDS) epidemic. In 1985, the Centers for Disease Control included the appearance of B-cell non-Hodgkin's lymphoma in the diagnostic criteria for AIDS.[137] Approximately 5–10% of patients infected with HIV will develop non-Hodgkin's lymphoma. Lymphomas occurring in immunodeficiency states are predominantly of B-cell origin and nearly 75% are classified as high grade, either immunoblastic or small noncleaved cell subtypes. The majority of patients present with Ann Arbor stage III or IV disease. Involvement of extranodal sites of disease, especially the bone marrow, CNS, gastrointestinal tract, and liver, is seen in 75–95% of patients. Primary CNS lymphoma has been reported in up to 25% of patients with AIDS-associated lymphomas. Survival is generally poor (2–5 months) in AIDS patients with CNS lymphoma. The total number of CD4-positive lymphocytes also may be an important predictor of survival, with a median survival of 24 months being reported in patients with a CD4 count greater than 100 cells/mm^3, in contrast to a median survival of 4 months in those with CD4 counts of less than 100 cells/mm^3.[138]

The treatment of patients with AIDS-associated lymphoma presents quite a therapeutic challenge. Because myelosuppression is the most common adverse effect of chemotherapy and these patients are usually immunocompromised at the time of diagnosis, the risks of both morbidity and mortality following therapy are high, primary due to the occurrence of opportunistic infections. For a patient with good immune function and without a history of an opportunistic infection, standard-dose chemotherapy may be appropriate. A lower dose chemotherapy regimen, or even a decision to withhold therapy, may be more appropriate for severely immunocompromised patients. The results of treatment with standard chemotherapy regimens, including CHOP, BACOP, m-BACOD, and MACOP-B, have been disappointing. Complete response rates range from 30–50%, relapse frequently occurs, and the median duration of survival ranges from only 4 to 7 months.[137] The most common causes of death are uncontrolled lymphoma and opportunistic infection. The use of intensive leukemia-like regimens normally employed in the treatment of small noncleaved cell lymphoma results in particularly high mortality rates. The current approach to therapy is the use of reduced doses of standard chemotherapy regimens or standard-dose combination chemotherapy with concurrent administration of a colony-stimulating factor. CNS prophylaxis and *Pneumocystis carinii* prophylaxis should be incorporated into either approach. A randomized multicenter trial is currently in progress to evaluate the efficacy of reduced-dose m-BACOD compared with standard-dose m-BACOD plus GM-CSF.

The treatment of primary CNS lymphoma usually consists of whole-brain radiation.[137] Despite complete response rates up to 70%, survival duration remains short (2–5 months). Opportunistic infection is the most common cause of death in AIDS patients with lymphoma, especially patients who are severely immunocompromised at the time of diagnosis.

Due to advances in antiretroviral therapy and treatment or prophylaxis against opportunistic infection, the average life span of patients with AIDS has continued to increase since the beginning of the epidemic. Although survival may be prolonged with these interventions, they are not able to improve the poor immune function of the AIDS patient. As patients live longer without an increase of CD4 cells, an increase in the incidence of non-Hodgkin's lymphoma is likely to result. Continued research into the optimal therapeutic management of these patients is necessary.

Evaluation of Therapeutic Outcomes

Establishing the correct diagnosis and stage for lymphomas is critical if an appropriate pharmaceutical care plan is to be created. Pathologic evaluation of tissue, presenting symptoms evaluated through a thorough physical examination, and corresponding laboratory work and additional procedures are all necessary to select appropriate treatment and establish a prognosis.

For Hodgkin's disease, all medical decisions revolve around the stage of the disease. Treatment decisions and prognosis hinge heavily on stage. Early-stage disease can be managed with radiation therapy alone, while more advanced disease requires chemotherapy or a combination of chemotherapy and radiotherapy. Keep in mind that with appropriate treatment over half the patients treated for Hodgkin's disease can be cured.

Chemotherapy remains the mainstay of treatment for all but early-stage Hodgkin's patients. Data support thinking that it is not so much *what* regimen the patient receives but *how* the patient receives that regimen. The single most important predictor of a positive outcome for the treatment of Hodgkin's disease is the dose intensity of chemotherapy received. Patients who receive full doses of chemotherapy on time do significantly better than those who do not. However, it must be understood that MOPP therapy (considered the standard for Hodgkin's disease) is not benign treatment. It is rigorous, toxic, and demands full cooperation of patient and treatment team. ABVD is a major alternative to MOPP therapy and, although the toxicities are different, they are nonetheless just as taxing to the patient.

To optimize chemotherapy administration, toxicity management is key. From a pharmaceutical care standpoint, the pharmacist must identify, monitor, treat, and proactively prevent or minimize treatment-related toxicity. A thorough understanding of the patient's medical history and a review of systems (from a physical examination standpoint) is essential. Pertinent laboratory data and a review of other procedures will help establish a baseline to use for monitoring purposes. Major organ and system toxicities that need to be followed include hematologic (blood work), neurologic, skin, pulmonary, gastrointestinal, renal, and cardiac. Long-term toxicities and complications including gonadal function (if reproduction is an issue) and secondary malignancies must also be addressed when treatment decisions are made.

Myelosuppression is a constant concern with aggressive chemotherapy treatment of Hodgkin's disease. The risk of neutropenic fever with infection is a real threat and appropriate patient education and monitoring are critical. Treatment-related anemia must also be monitored.

Nutritional assessment should also be undertaken. Patients may require enteral and/or parenteral nutritional supplementation during their treatment to maintain their physical state and keep up their performance status.

The primary patient outcome to be identified is tumor response. Physical examination and other diagnostic procedures will be necessary to determine response. Complete response is the desired outcome. For only with a complete response will the patient have a chance for cure. Patients typically receive two cycles of chemotherapy beyond achieving a complete response, with a minimum of six cycles of treatment.

Patients are generally monitored at 3- to 6-month intervals for the first year or two following treatment, with longer intervals instituted when appropriate.

SUMMARY

Approximately 25 years ago, non-Hodgkin's lymphoma was considered a fatal disease. Today, at least half of all patients with certain types of lymphoma are cured. Although all malignant lymphomas may be responsive to chemotherapy and/or radiation, only the aggressive intermediate- or high-grade lymphomas are curable at this time. Our current capacity to cure these patients is the result of many factors, including development of an accurate and reproducible classification system, a more uniform approach to staging of lymphoma, and advances in the treatment strategies. The goal for the future is to develop treatment modalities to achieve cure in a larger number of patients, including those with low-grade lymphomas, while at the same time avoiding excessive treatment-related morbidity and mortality. The use of bone marrow transplantation already supports the administration of more dose-intensified chemotherapy regimens, and the colony-stimulating factors may represent the next phase of treatment development. A better understanding of the pathogenesis of non-Hodgkin's lymphoma through continued research in molecular biology and immunology will allow further exploration of other treatment modalities, including immune modulation with biologic response modifiers and monoclonal antibodies.

REFERENCES

1. Cancer facts and figures—1995. Atlanta, GA, American Cancer Society, 1995.
2. MacMahon B. Epidemiological evidence of the nature of Hodgkin's disease. Cancer 1957;10:1045–1054.
3. Gutensohn NM. Social class and age at diagnosis of Hodgkin's disease: New epidemiologic evidence for the "two-disease hypothesis." Cancer Treat Rep 1982;66:689–695.
4. Glaser SL, Swartz WG. Time trends in Hodgkin's disease incidence. Cancer 1990;66:2196–2204.
5. Rosdahl N, Larsen SO, Clemmensen J. Hodgkin's disease in patients with previous mononucleosis, 30 years experience. Br Med J 1974;2:253–256.
6. Munoz N, Davidson RJ, Witthoff B, et al. Infectious mononucleosis and Hodgkin's disease. Int J Cancer 1978;22:10–13.
7. Lukes RJ, Tindle BH, Parket JW. Reed–Sternberg-like cells in infectious mononucleosis. Lancet 1969;2:1000–1004.
8. Kadin ME. Hodgkin's disease: Immunobiology and pathogenesis, in Knowles DM (ed): Neoplastic Hematopathology. Baltimore, MD, Williams and Wilkins, 1992, pp 535–554.
9. Gaffey MJ, Weiss LM. Association of Epstein–Barr virus with human neoplasia. Pathol Ann 1992;27:55–74.
10. Poppema S, Kaleta J, Hepperle B. Chromosomal abnormalities in patients with Hodgkin's disease. JNCI 1992;84:1789–1993.
11. Doglioni C, Pelosio P, Mombella A, et al. Immunohistochemical evidence of abnormal expression of the antioncogene-encoded *p53* phosphoprotein in Hodgkin's disease and CD30+ anaplastic lymphoma. Hematol Pathol 1991;5:67–73.
12. Sinkovics JG. Hodgkin's disease revisited: Reed–Sternberg cells as natural hybridomas. Crit Rev Immunol 1991;11:33–63.
13. Lukes RF, Butler JJ, Hicks ED. Natural history of Hodgkin's disease as related to its pathological picture. Cancer 1966;19:319.
14. Lukes RJ, Craver LF, Hall TC, et al. Report of the nomenclature committee. Cancer Res 1966;26:1311.
15. Kaplan HS. Hodgkin's Disease, 2nd ed. Cambridge, MA, Harvard University Press, 1980.
16. Carbone PP, Kaplan HS, Musshoff K, et al. Report of the committee on Hodgkin's disease staging classification. Cancer Res 1970;31:1860–1861.
17. Dresser RL, Ultmann JE. Risk of severe infection in patients with Hodgkin's disease or lymphoma after diagnostic laparotomy and splenectomy. Ann Intern Med 1972;77:143–147.
18. Meeker WR, Richardson JD, West W, et al. Critical evaluation of laparotomy and splenectomy in Hodgkin's disease. Arch Surg 1972;105:222.

19. Mauch P, Tarbell N, Weinstein, et al. Stage IA and IIA supradiaphragmatic Hodgkin's disease: Prognostic factors in surgically staged patients treated with mantle and paraaortic irradiation. J Clin Oncol 1988;6:1576–1583.
20. Hoppe RT, Coleman CN, Cox RS, et al. The management of stage I–II Hodgkin's disease with irradiation alone or in combined modality therapy: The Stanford experience. Blood 1982;59:455–465.
21. Hellman S, Mauch P. Role of radiation therapy in the treatment of Hodgkin's disease. Cancer Treat Rep 1982;66:915–923.
22. Zagars G, Rubin P. Hodgkin's disease stage IA and IIA: A long-term follow-up study on the gains achieved by modern therapy. Cancer 1985;56:1905–1912.
23. Collaborative study. Survival and complications of radiotherapy following involved and extended field therapy of Hodgkin's disease: Stage I–IIA collaborative study. Cancer 1976;38:288–305.
24. Crnkovich MJ, Leopold K, Hoppe RT, et al. Stage I to VIB Hodgkin's disease: The combined experience at Stanford University and the Joint Center for Radiation Therapy. J Clin Oncol 1987;5:1041–1049.
25. Krikorian JG, Portlock SC, Mauch PM. Hodgkin's disease presenting below the diaphragm: A review. J Clin Oncol 1986;4:1551–1562.
26. Hoppe RT, Cos RS, Rosenberg SA, et al. Prognostic factors in pathologic stage III Hodgkin's disease. Cancer Treat Rep 1982;66:743–749.
27. DeVita, Moxley JH, Brance K, et al. Intensive combination chemotherapy and x-irradiation in the treatment of Hodgkin's disease. Proc Am Assoc Cancer Res 1965;6:15.
28. DeVita, Simon RM, Hubbard SM, et al. Curability of advanced Hodgkin's disease with chemotherapy: Long-term follow-up of MOPP-treated patients at the National Cancer Institute. Ann Intern Med 1980;92:587–595.
29. Coltman CA. Chemotherapy of advanced Hodgkin's disease. Semin Oncol 1980;7:155–173.
30. Longo DL, Young RC, Wesley M, et al. Twenty years of MOPP chemotherapy for Hodgkin's disease. J Clin Oncol 1986;4:1295–1306.
31. Carde P, MacKintosh FR, Rosenburg SA. A dose and time response analysis of the treatment of Hodgkin's disease with MOPP chemotherapy. J Clin Oncol 1983;1:146–153.
32. Sutcliffe SB, Wrigley PM, Pet J, et al. MVPP chemotherapy regimen for advanced Hodgkin's disease. Br Med J 1978;1:679–683.
33. Wagstaff J, Steward W, Jones M, et al. Factors affecting remission and survival in patients with advanced Hodgkin's disease treated with MVPP. Hematol Oncol 1986;4:135–147.
34. Gams RA, Durant JR, Bartolucci AA. Chemotherapy for advanced Hodgkin's disease: Conclusions from the Southeastern Cancer Study Group. Cancer Treat Rep 1982;66:899–905.
35. Dady PJ, McElwain TJ, Auston DE, et al. Five year experience with ChlVPP effective low-toxicity combination chemotherapy for Hodgkin's disease. Br J Cancer 1982;45:851–859.
36. Vose J, Armitage J, Weisenburger D, et al. ChlVPP: An effective and well tolerated alternative to MOPP therapy for Hodgkin's disease. Am J Clin Oncol 1988;11:423–426.
37. Bonadonna G. Chemotherapy strategies to improve the control of Hodgkin's disease. Cancer Res 1982;42:4309–4320.
38. Klimo P, Connors JM. An update on the Vancouver experience in the management of advanced Hodgkin's disease treated with MOPP-ABV hybrid program. Sem Hematol 1988;25(suppl 2):34–40.
39. O'Reilly SE, Hoskins P, Klimo P, et al. MACOP-B and VACOP-B in diffuse large cell lymphomas and MOPP/ABV in Hodgkin's disease. Ann Oncol 1991;2(suppl 1):17–23.
40. Santoro A, Bonfante V, Bonadonna G. Salvage chemotherapy with ABVD in MOPP-resident Hodgkin's disease. Ann Intern Med 1982;96:139–143.
41. Goldie JH, Coldman AJ. The genetic origin of drug resistance in neoplasms, implications for systemic therapy. Cancer Res 1984;44:3643–3653.
42. Goldie JH, Coldman AJ, Gudauskas GA. Rationale for the use of alternating non-cross-resistant chemotherapy. Cancer Treat Rep 1982;66:439–450.
43. Bonadonna G, Valagussa P, Santoro A. Alternating non-cross-resistant combination chemotherapy with ABVD or MOPP in stage IV Hodgkin's disease: A report of eight year results. Ann Intern Med 1986;104:739–746.
44. Longo D. The use of chemotherapy in the treatment of Hodgkin's disease. Semin Oncol 1990;17:716–735.
45. Canellos GP, Anderson JR, Propert K, et al. Chemotherapy of advanced Hodgkin's disease with MOPP, ABVD, or MOPP alternating with ABVD. N Engl J Med 1992;327:1478–1484.
46. Bonadonna G, Valagussa P, Santoro A, et al. The Milan cancer institute experience with MOPP and ABVD. Rec Results Cancer Res 1989;117:168–174.
47. Longo DL, Duffey PL, Young RC, et al. Conventional-dose salvage combination chemotherapy in patients relapsing with Hodgkin's disease after combination chemotherapy: The low probability of cure. J Clin Oncol 1992;10:210–218.
48. Prosnitz LR, Farber LR, Kapp DS, et al. Combined modality therapy for advanced Hodgkin's disease: 15-year follow-up data. J Clin Oncol 1988;6:603–612.
49. Straus DJ, Myers J, Gaynor J, et al. Long-term results of treatment of advanced Hodgkin's disease with potentially non-cross-resistant drug combinations and moderate-dose radiation therapy. Proc Am Soc Clin Oncol 1987;6:202.
50. Dutcher JP, Wiernik PH. Combined modality treatment of Hodgkin's disease confined to lymph nodes: Results 14 years later, in Cavalli F, Bonadonna G, Rozeneweig M (eds): Malignant Lymphomas and Hodgkin's Disease: Experimental and Therapeutic Advances. Boston, Martinus Nijhoff, 1985, pp 317–328.
51. Long DL, Young RC, Wesley M, et al. Twenty years of MOPP therapy for Hodgkin's disease. J Clin Oncol 1986;4:1295–1306.
52. Crowther D, Wagstaff J, Deakin D, et al. A randomized study comparing chemotherapy alone with chemotherapy followed by radiotherapy in patients with pathologically staged IIIA Hodgkin's disease. J Clin Oncol 1984;2:892–897.

53. Grozea PN, DePersio EJ, Coltman CA, et al. A Southwest Oncology Group study: Chemotherapy versus chemotherapy plus radiotherapy in the treatment of stage III Hodgkin's disease. Rec Results Cancer Res 1982;80:83–91.
54. Henkleman GC, Hagemeister FB, Fuller LM. Two cycles of MOPP and radiation for stage III_1A and III_1B Hodgkin's disease. J Clin Oncol 1988;6:1293–1302.
55. Pavlovsky S, Maschio M, Santarelli MT, et al. Randomized trial of chemotherapy versus chemotherapy plus radiotherapy for stage I-II Hodgkin's disease. J Natl Cancer Inst 1988;80:1466–1473.
56. Longo D, Glatstein E, Young R, et al. Combined modality therapy for stage II, III or IV massive mediastinal Hodgkin's disease: The NCI experience. Proc Am Soc Clin Oncol 1988;7:226.
57. Santoro A, Bonfante V, Bonadonna G. Salvage chemotherapy with ABVD in MOPP-resistant Hodgkin's disease. Ann Intern Med 1982;96:139–143.
58. Tannir N, Hagemeister F, Velasquez W, et al. Long-term follow-up with ABDIC salvage chemotherapy of MOPP-resistant Hodgkin's disease. J Clin Oncol 1983;1:432–439.
59. Harker GW, Kushlan P, Rosenberg SA. Combination chemotherapy for advanced Hodgkin's disease after failure of MOPP: ABVD and B-CAVe. Ann Intern Med 1984;10:440–446.
60. Santoro A, Viviani SS, Valagussa P, et al. CCNU, etoposide and prednimustine (CEP) in refractory Hodgkin's disease. Semin Oncol 1986;13:23–26.
61. Levi JA, Wiernik PH, Diggs CH. Combination chemotherapy of advanced previously treated Hodgkin's disease with streptozotocin, CCNU, adriamycin, and bleomycin. Med Pediatr Oncol 1977;3:33–40.
62. Einhorn LH, Williams SD, Stevens EE, et al. Treatment of MOPP-refractory Hodgkin's disease with vinblastine, doxorubicin, bleomycin, CCNU, and dacarbazine. Cancer 1983;51:1348–1352.
63. DeVita VT. The consequences of the chemotherapy of Hodgkin's disease. The 10th David A. Karnofsky memorial lecture. Cancer 1981;47:1–13.
64. Whitehead E, Shalit SM, Blackledge G, et al. The effect of combination chemotherapy on ovarian function in women treated for Hodgkin's disease. Cancer 1983;52:988–993.
65. DaCunha MF, Meistrich ML, Fuller ML, et al. Recovery of spermatogenesis after treatment of Hodgkin's disease: Limiting the dose of MOPP chemotherapy. J Clin Oncol 1984;2:571–577.
66. Viviani S, Santoro A, Ragni G, et al. Pre- and post-treatment testicular dysfunction in Hodgkin's disease. Proc Am Soc Clin Oncol 1988;7:227.
67. Vose JM, Bierman PJ, Anderson JR, et al. ChlVPP chemotherapy with involved-field irradiation for Hodgkin's disease: Favorable results with acceptable toxicity. J Clin Oncol 1991;9:1421–1425.
68. Selby P, Patel P, Milan S, et al. ChlVPP combination chemotherapy for Hodgkin's disease: Long-term results. Br J Cancer 1990;62:279–285.
69. Tucker MA, Coleman CN, Cox RS, et al. Risk of second cancers after treatment of Hodgkin's disease. N Engl J Med 1988;318:76–81.
70. Pedersen-Bjergaard J, Larsen SO. Evidence of acute nonlymphocytic leukemia, preleukemia, and acute myeloproliferative syndromes up to 10 years after treatment of Hodgkin's disease. N Engl J Med 1982;307:965–971.
71. Coltman CA, Dixon DO. Second malignancies complicating Hodgkin's disease: A Southwest Oncology Group 10-year follow-up. Cancer Treat Rep 1982;66:1023–1034.
72. Aisenberg AC. Acute nonlymphocytic leukemia after treatment of Hodgkin's disease. Am J Med 1983;75:449–454.
73. Valagussa P, Sontoro A, Fossati-Bellani F, et al. Second acute leukemia and other malignancies following treatment for Hodgkin's disease. J Clin Oncol 1986;4:830–837.
74. Henry-Amar M, Pellae-Cosset B, Bayle-Weisgerber C, et al. Risk of secondary acute leukemia and preleukemia after Hodgkin's disease: The Institute Gustave-Roussy experience. Rec Results Cancer Res 1989;117:270–283.
75. Andrieu JM, Ifrah N, Payen C, et al. Increased risk of secondary acute nonlymphocytic leukemia after extended-field radiation therapy combined with MOPP chemotherapy for Hodgkin's disease. J Clin Oncol 1990;8:1148–1154.
76. VanderVelden JW, VanPatten WLJ, Guinee VF, et al. Subsequent development of acute nonlymphocytic leukemia in patients treated for Hodgkin's disease. Int J Cancer 1988;42:252–255.
77. Kaldor JM, Day NE, Clarke A, et al. Leukemia following Hodgkin's disease. N Engl J Med 1990;233:7–13.
78. Lindahl T, Klein G, Reedman BM, et al. Relationship between Epstein–Barr virus (EBV) DNA and the EBV-determined nuclear antigen (EBNA) in Burkitt lymphoma biopsies and other lymphoproliferative malignancies. Int J Cancer 1974;13:764–772.
79. Poiesz BJ, Ruscetti FW, Gazdar AF, et al. Detection and isolation of type C retrovirus particles from fresh and cultured lymphocytes of a patient with cutaneous T cell lymphomas. Proc Natl Acad Sci USA 1980;77:7415–7419.
80. Broder S, Bunn PA, Jaffe ES, et al. T cell lymphoproliferative syndrome associated with human T cell leukemia/lymphoma virus. Ann Intern Med 1984;100:543–557.
81. Longo DL, DeVita VT, Jaffe ES, et al. Lymphocytic lymphomas, in DeVita VT, Hellman S, Rosenberg SA (eds): Cancer: Principles and Practice of Oncology, 4th ed. Philadelphia, JB Lippincott, 1993, pp 1859–1927.
82. List AF, Greco FA, Vogler LB. Lymphoproliferative diseases in immunocompromised hosts: The role of Epstein–Barr virus. J Clin Oncol 1987;5:1673–1689.
83. Gribben GJ, Neuberg D, Freedman AS, et al. Detection by polymerase chain reaction of residual cells with the *bcl-2* translocation is associated with increased risk of relapse after autologous bone marrow transplantation for B-cell lymphoma. Blood 1993;81:3449–3457.
84. Hardingham JE, Kotasek D, Sage RE, et al. Molecular detection of residual lymphoma cells in peripheral blood stem cell harvests and following autologous transplantation. Bone Marrow Transplantation 1993;11:15–20.
85. Rappaport H, Winter WJ, Hicks EB. Follicular lymphoma: A reevaluation of its position in the scheme of malignant lymphoma based on a survey of 253 cases. Cancer 1956;9:792–821.

86. The Non-Hodgkin's Lymphoma Pathologic Classification Project: National Cancer Institute-sponsored study of classifications of non-Hodgkin's lymphomas: Summary and description of a working formulation for clinical usage. Cancer 1982;49:2112–2135.
87. Simon R, Durrleman S, Hoppe RT, et al. The non-Hodgkin lymphoma pathologic classification project: Long-term follow-up of 1153 patients with non-Hodgkin lymphomas. Ann Intern Med 1988;109:939–945.
88. Krikorian JG, Portlock CS, Cooney DP, et al. Spontaneous regression of non-Hodgkin's lymphomas. A report of nine cases. Cancer Res 1980;46:2093–2099.
89. Ezdinli EZ, Costello WG, Kucuk O, et al. Effect of the degree of nodularity on the survival of patients with nodular lymphomas. J Clin Oncol 1987;5:413–418.
90. Burke JS. The histopathologic classification of non-Hodgkin's lymphomas: Ambiguities in the working formulation and two newly reported categories. Semin Oncol 1990;17:3–10.
91. Cossman J, Chused T, Fisher R, et al. Diversity of immunologic phenotypes of lymphoblastic lymphoma. Cancer Res 1983;43:4486–4490.
92. Skillings JR, Bramwell V, Nicholson R, et al. A prospective study of magnetic resonance imaging in lymphoma staging. Cancer 1991;67:1838–1843.
93. Portlock CS. Management of the low-grade non-Hodgkin's lymphomas. Semin Oncol 1990;17:51–59.
94. McLaughlin P, Fuller LM, Velasquez WS, et al. Stage I–II follicular lymphoma: Treatment results for 76 patients. Cancer 1986;58:1596–1602.
95. Sutcliffe SB, Gospodarowicz MK, Bush RS, et al. Role of radiation therapy in localized non-Hodgkin's lymphoma. Radiother Oncol 1985;4:211–223.
96. Vokes EE, Ultmann JE, Golomb HM, et al. Long-term survival of patients with localized diffuse histiocytic lymphoma. J Clin Oncol 1985;3:1309–1317.
97. Jones SE, Fuks Z, Kaplan HS, et al. Non-Hodgkin's lymphoma versus results of radiotherapy. Cancer 1973;32:682–691.
98. Mauch P, Leonard R, Skarin A, et al. Improved survival following combined radiation therapy and chemotherapy for unfavorable prognosis stage I–II non-Hodgkin's lymphomas. J Clin Oncol 1985;3:1301–1308.
99. Jones SE, Miller TP, Connors JM. Long-term follow-up and analysis for prognostic factors for patients with limited stage diffuse large-cell lymphoma treated with initial chemotherapy with or without adjuvant radiotherapy. J Clin Oncol 1989;7:1186–1191.
100. Connors JM, Klimo P, Fairey RN, et al. Brief chemotherapy and involved field radiation for limited-stage, histologically aggressive lymphoma. Ann Intern Med 1987;107:25–30.
101. Longo DL, Glatstein E, Duffey PL, et al. Treatment of localized aggressive lymphomas with combination chemotherapy followed by involved-field radiation therapy. J Clin Oncol 1989;7:1295–1302.
102. Cabanillas F. Chemotherapy as definitive treatment of stage I–II large cell and diffuse mixed lymphomas. Hematol Oncol 1985;3:25–31.
103. Link MP, Donaldson SS, Benard CW, et al. Results of treatment of childhood localized non-Hodgkin's lymphoma with combination chemotherapy with or without radiotherapy. N Engl J Med 1990;322:1169–1174.
104. Paryani SB, Hoppe RT, Cox RS, et al. The role of radiation therapy in the management of stage II follicular lymphomas. J Clin Oncol 1984;2:841–848.
105. Lister TA, Cullen MH, Beard MEJ, et al. Comparison of combined and single-agent chemotherapy in non-Hodgkin's lymphoma of favorable histologic type. Br Med J 1978;1:533–537.
106. Portlock CS, Rosenberg SA, Glatstein E, et al. Treatment of advanced non-Hodgkin's lymphomas with favorable histologies: Preliminary results of a prospective trial. Blood 1976;47:474–476.
107. Horning SJ, Rosenberg SA. The natural history of initially untreated low-grade non-Hodgkin's lymphoma. N Engl J Med 1984;311:1471–1475.
108. Young RC, Longo DL, Glatstein E, et al. The treatment of indolent lymphomas: Watchful waiting versus aggressive combined modality treatment. Semin Hematol 1988;25(suppl 2):11–16.
109. Heinz R, Fortelny A, Schneider B, et al. Long-term follow-up of 1520 NHL patients classified according to the kiel classification—Experiences of a single institution. Fourth International Conference on Malignant Lymphoma. June 6–9, 1990, Lugano, Switzerland, p 79.
110. Lepage E, Gisselbrecht C, Haioun C, et al. Prognostic significance of received relative dose intensity in non-Hodgkin's lymphoma patients: Application to LNH-87 protocol. The GELA (Groupe d'Etude des Lymphomes de l'Adulte). Annals Oncol 1993;4:651–656.
111. Al-Katib A, Koziner B, Kurland E, et al. Treatment of diffuse poorly differentiated lymphocytic lymphoma. Cancer 1984;53:2404–2412.
112. DeVita VT, Cannelos GP, Chabner BA, et al. Advanced diffuse histiocytic lymphoma, a potentially curable disease. Lancet 1975;1:248–250.
113. McKelvey EM, Gottleib JA, Wilson HE, et al. Hydroxyldaunomycin (Adriamycin) combination chemotherapy in malignant lymphoma. Cancer 1976;38:1484–1493.
114. Coltman CA, Dahlberg S, Jones SE, et al. CHOP is curative in 30% of patients with large cell lymphomas: A 12-year Southwest Oncology Group follow-up, in Skarin AT et al (eds): Advanced in Cancer Chemotherapy: Update on Treatment for Diffuse Large-Cell Lymphoma. New York, Park Row, 1986, pp 71–78.
115. Urba WJ, Duffey PL, Longo DL. Treatment of patients with aggressive lymphomas: An overview. J Natl Cancer Inst Monogr 1990;10:29–37.
116. Yi PI, Coleman M, Saltz L, et al. Chemotherapy for large cell lymphoma: A status update. Semin Oncol 1990;17:60–73.
117. Shipp MA, Yeap BY, Harrington DP, et al. The m-BACOD combination chemotherapy regimen in large-cell lymphoma: Analysis of the completed trial and comparison with the M-BACOD regimen. J Clin Oncol 1990;8:84–93.

118. Salles G, Shipp MA, Coiffier B. Chemotherapy of non-Hodgkin's aggressive lymphomas. Semin Oncol 1994;31:46–69.
119. Norton L, Simon R. Tumor size, sensitivity to therapy and design of treatment schedules. Cancer Treat Rep 1977;61:1307–1317.
120. Gordon LI, Harrington D, Andersen J, et al. Comparison of a second-generation combination chemotherapeutic regimen (m-BACOD) with a standard regimen (CHOP) for advanced diffuse non-Hodgkin's lymphoma. N Engl J Med 1992;327:1342–1349.
121. Hryniuk W, Bush H. The importance of dose intensity in chemotherapy of metastatic breast cancer. J Clin Oncol 1984;2:1281–1288.
122. Meyer RM, Hryniuk WM, Goodyear MDE. The role of dose intensity in determining outcome in intermediate-grade non-Hodgkin's lymphoma. J Clin Oncol 1991;9:339–347.
123. Fisher RI, Gaynor ER, Dahlberg S, et al. Comparison of a standard regimen (CHOP) with three intensive chemotherapy regimens for advanced non-Hodgkin's lymphoma. N Engl J Med 1993;328:1002–1006.
124. Mathews JRD, Mathews JP, Cooper IA, ChongDing J. Failure of intensive chemotherapy in poor prognosis non-Hodgkin's lymphoma. Aust NZ J Med 1992;22:123–128.
125. Cooper IA, Wolf MM, Robertson TI, et al. Randomized comparison of MACOP-B with CHOP in patients with intermediate-grade non-Hodgkin's lymphoma. The Australian and New Zealand Lymphoma Group. J Clin Oncol 1994;12:769–778.
126. Wilson WH, Bryant G, Bates S, et al. EPOCH chemotherapy: Toxicity and efficacy in relapsed and refractory non-Hodgkin's lymphoma. J Clin Oncol 1993;11:1573–1582.
127. Buzzoni R, Colleoni M, Bajetta E, et al. Effective salvage chemotherapy in relapsed or refractory non-Hodgkin's lymphoma. Ann Oncol 1993;4:251–253.
128. Neidhart JA, Kubica R, Stidley C, et al. Multiple cycles of dose-intensive cyclophosphamide, etoposide, and cisplatinum (DICEP) produce durable responses in refractory non-Hodgkin's lymphoma. Cancer Invest 1994;12:1–11.
129. Appelbaum FR, Diesseroth AB, Graw RG, et al. Prolonged complete remission following high-dose chemotherapy of Burkitt's lymphoma in relapse. Cancer 1978;41:1059–1063.
130. Gilewski TA, Richards JM. Biologic response modifiers in non-Hodgkin's lymphomas. Semin Oncol 1990;17:74–87.
131. Margolin KA, Aronson FR, Sznol M, et al. Phase II trial of high-dose interleukin-2 and lymphokine-activated killer cells in Hodgkin's disease and non-Hodgkin's lymphoma. J Immunother 1991;10:214–220.
132. Weber J, Yang JC, Topalian SL, et al. Interleukin-2 and LAK for the treatment of patients with non-Hodgkin's lymphoma. Proc Ann Meet Am Soc Clin Oncol 1992;11:A844.
133. Levy R, Miller RA. Therapy of lymphoma directed at idiotypes. J Natl Cancer Inst Monogr 1990;10:61–68.
134. Czuczman MS, Straus DJ, Divgi CR, et al. Phase I dose-escalation trial of iodine 131-labeled monoclonal antibody OKB7 in patients with non-Hodgkin's lymphoma. J Clin Oncol 1993;11:2021–2029.
135. Hesketh P, Caguioa P, Koh H, et al. Clinical utility of a cytotoxic fusion protein (DAB486IL-2) in the treatment of cutaneous non-Hodgkin's lymphoma. Proc Ann Meet Am Soc Clin Oncol 1992;11:A1076.
136. LeMaistre CF, Craig FE, Meneghetti C, et al. Phase I trial of a 90-minute infusion of the fusion toxin DAB486IL-2 in hematological cancers. Cancer Res 1993;53:3930–3934.
137. Freter CE. Acquired immunodeficiency syndrome-associated lymphoma. J Natl Cancer Inst Monogr 1990;10:45–54.
138. Kaplan LD, Abrams DI, Feigal L, et al. AIDS-associated non-Hodgkin's lymphoma in San Francisco. JAMA 1989;261:719–724.

Chapter 125

Ovarian Cancer

William C. Zamboni, PharmD, and Barry R. Goldspiel, PharmD

Ovarian cancer is the fourth most common noncutaneous malignancy diagnosed in women.[1] Overall, it is the fourth leading cause of cancer-related death and most common death from gynecologic malignancy in this group. In the United States alone, it was estimated that 26,600 new cases of ovarian cancer would be diagnosed and more than 14,500 females would die from this disease in 1995.[1] A woman has a 1 in 70 lifetime chance of developing ovarian cancer. Based on SEER data collected from 1983 to 1987, overall 5-year survival approximates 42%; however, survival dramatically increases to 90% in patients with localized disease.[1] Unfortunately, the majority of patients have disseminated disease at diagnosis because symptoms usually do not appear until late in the disease course.

Epidemiology/Risk Factors

Ovarian cancer usually occurs in postmenopausal Caucasian women during the sixth decade.[2–4] The most important risk factor appears to be genetics. The risk for developing ovarian cancer markedly increases in women with a family history involving two or more first-degree relatives.[4–7] The risk for ovarian cancer is decreased in women who have had several pregnancies, especially in women who first became pregnant before age 25, and is increased in nulliparous women or women who first became pregnant after age 35, suggesting that uninterrupted ovulation may be a contributing factor.[3,4,8] Women of North American or North European descent are at a higher risk for ovarian cancer development compared to other nationalities. Prolonged oral contraceptive use or breast-feeding lowers the risk for developing ovarian cancer.[3,9,10] A higher risk has been associated with environmental exposure to asbestos or talc.[3,11]

Several hereditary ovarian cancer syndromes have been described which include the development of breast and ovarian cancers or ovarian, endometrial, and nonpolyposis colon cancers.[2,7,12] These syndromes tend to occur at an earlier age than the usual development for each of the individual malignancies and account for about 5% of the total ovarian cancer incidence.[4,12]

A number of genetic abnormalities have been detected in patients with ovarian cancer.[13] These include *p21* expression, amplification, and mutation; *c-myc* overexpression; epithelial growth factor receptor expression; *HER-2/neu* overexpression and amplification; *p53* overexpression and amplification; *Rb* loss of heterozygosity; and chromosome 6, 11, and 17 loss of heterozygosity. Although it is still too early for this information to be clinically useful, understanding the molecular basis for ovarian cancer development might help to discover methods for early detection and chemoprevention.

Pathology

Most ovarian tumors (85–90%) are derived from the epithelial surface of the ovary.[2,3] The histologic types (percent incidence) of epithelial ovarian cancer are serous cystadenocarcinoma (≈40%), endometrioid (≈15%), mucinous cystadenocarcinoma (≈12%), clear cell (≈6%), and undifferentiated carcinoma (≈17%).[3,14] Epithelial ovarian cancers can be classified as benign, malignant, or borderline (low malignant potential). The remaining ovarian tumors are derived from germ, sex chord, and stromal cell origin.[15]

Clinical Presentation

The majority of women with ovarian cancer have no symptoms until the malignancy has spread outside the pelvis.[3,14] Patients with early ovarian cancer can present with nonspecific, vague abdominal symptoms such as nausea, discomfort, dyspepsia, flatulence, bloating, fullness, early satiety, and digestive disturbances.[3,14] These symptoms can easily be confused with symptoms that happen normally throughout the menstrual cycle. Late symptoms can include pain, abdominal distention, ascites, and abdominal or pelvic masses.[3,14,16] A palpable ovary in a postmenopausal woman should be promptly evaluated as functional cysts do not usually occur in this age group.[14]

Diagnosis

The diagnostic workup for suspected ovarian cancer includes a careful physical examination including a thorough breast examination, a PAP smear, and a rectovaginal examination.[11,14,17] A careful family history should be taken especially noting the rate and pattern of relatives with malignancies.

A complete blood count, chemistry profile including liver and renal function tests, and a CA-125 assay should be performed.[3,11] CA-125 is an antigen common to most nonmucinous epithelial ovarian cancers and is detected in the laboratory by using OC-125, a monoclonal antibody directed at this antigen.[18–20] CA-125 is a useful tumor marker in that it is found in more than 80% of ovarian tumors and rising (or falling) titers correlate with disease extent.[18–22] Normal CA-125 values are less than 35 U/mL.[18,19,21]

Refractory disease is often associated with a CA-125 level that does not return to normal[19,21] or that remains elevated after completion of chemotherapy.[18–20] A new elevation in the CA-125 level may be the first sign of relapse.[19,23]

Other diagnostic tests should include a chest x-ray, an intravenous pyelogram, cystoscopy, proctoscopy, and a barium enema. Depending on clinical evaluation, computed tomography (CT), magnetic resonance imaging (MRI), or ultrasound may be indicated. An upper GI series is indicated in patients with gastrointestinal symptoms or in those with bowel obstruction.

The approach to diagnosing an adnexal mass discovered on pelvic examination depends on several factors including the patient's reproductive age, adnexal mass size, menopausal status, and symptoms.[15] Exploratory laparotomy is indicated in premenarchal women, women with masses greater than 8 cm or those that increase or persist through several menstrual cycles or those that are fixed to peritoneal surfaces, women with bilateral masses, or in women with intra-abdominal pain or ascites.[15]

Screening

Ovarian cancer would be an ideal malignancy for early screening efforts because greater than 65% of cases are currently diagnosed with advanced disease.[24–26] However, in order for screening efforts to be successful, suitable sensitive, specific, cost-effective screening tests with an adequate positive predictive value must be available. Also, there must be a detectable preclinical phase, and the disease must be amenable to therapy.[24–26] Three screening tests have been used to detect ovarian cancer: bimanual rectovaginal pelvic examination; CA-125 determination; and transvaginal ultrasonography (TVS).[11,25,26] Bimanual rectovaginal pelvic examination is inadequate for screening purposes because it lacks useful sensitivity and specificity.[24–26] CA-125 is only elevated in 50% of stage I cases and a significant number of women with benign ovarian disease have abnormal CA-125 values.[24–26] TVS is not specific enough to use as the sole screening modality.

At a recent National Institutes of Health (NIH) consensus conference,[26,27] the following guidelines for screening were developed:

- All women should have a comprehensive family history taken focusing on all the known ovarian cancer risk factors. Rectovaginal pelvic exam should be performed as part of ordinary medical care.
- For women without a family history of ovarian cancer or with a family history of ovarian cancer in one relative, routine screening with ultrasound or CA-125 is not recommended because current evidence does not support any benefit. Participation in ovarian cancer screening trials would be appropriate.
- In women with a family history of ovarian cancer in two or more relatives, the risk for developing ovarian cancer is 7%. No conclusive data support the thinking that screening in these patients will produce additional benefit. However, since this situation carries a 3% risk of having a hereditary ovarian cancer syndrome, these women should be counseled by a gynecologic oncologist or other qualified specialist regarding their individual risk.
- Women from families with hereditary ovarian cancer syndromes have a 40% lifetime risk of developing ovarian cancer. While no data indicate that screening will reduce mortality, annual rectovaginal pelvic examination, CA-125 determinations, and TVS are recommended in these women until age 35 or when childbearing is complete. Prophylactic bilateral oophorectomy should then be considered to reduce the overall risk.

Staging

The stage of ovarian cancer depends on the extent of disease found at surgical exploration (Table 125.1). Epithelial ovarian cancer spreads by peritoneal surface shedding and lymphatic dissemination (Fig. 125.1).[11,28] At diagnosis, 23% of ovarian cancers are localized, 26% present with regional metastases, and 46% present with distant metastases.[1] A careful and accurate surgical staging laparotomy is necessary to properly stage the patient; it is therefore recommended that a gynecologic–oncologic surgeon[29] do this procedure to prevent understaging (Table 125.2).[15] Total abdominal hysterectomy, bilateral salpingo-oophorectomy, and partial omentectomy are performed.[11,14,17] A careful

TABLE 125.1. FIGO[a] STAGING FOR EPITHELIAL OVARIAN CANCER

I Confined to the ovaries
IA: One ovary, no ascites, intact capsule
IB: Both ovaries, no ascites, intact capsule
IC: Ruptured capsule, capsular involvement, positive peritoneal washings, or malignant ascites
II Ovarian tumor with pelvic extension
IIA: Extension to uterus or tubes
IIB: Extension to other pelvic organs (bladder, rectum, or vagina)
IIC: Pelvic extension, plus findings for IC
III Tumor outside the pelvis or with positive nodes
IIIA: Microscopic seeding outside true pelvis
IIIB: Gross deposits ≤2 cm
IIIC: Gross deposits >2 cm or positive nodes
IV Distant organ involvement, including liver parenchyma or pleural space

[a]International Federation of Gynecologic Oncologists.

examination of all serosal surfaces is done and biopsies of any grossly involved areas are taken. Ovarian capsule rupture, if present, is noted. Ascites is collected and peritoneal washings are done. Integral to the initial surgical staging procedure, the surgeon attempts to debulk as much gross tumor as possible because the amount of residual disease in patients with stage III ovarian cancer correlates with survival.[11,30]

Prognosis

The prognosis for patients with epithelial ovarian cancer is related to disease stage, pathologic grade, and cell histology. Patients with well-differentiated stage IA or IB tumors have a 5-year survival of greater than 90% with no additional benefit derived from adjuvant therapy.[3,11,15,17,27] With adjuvant therapy, patients with any poorly differentiated stage I, stage IC, or stage II disease have an 80% 5-year survival rate.[3,11,17,31] Survival in patients with stage III disease is poorer than in earlier stages and is directly related to the size of residual tumors present after debulking surgery. Patients with implants under 0.5 cm have a median survival of 40 months, those with implants 0.5–2 cm have a median survival of 18 months, and those with residual tumor greater than 2 cm have a median survival of 6–12 months.[3,30,32,33] The 5-year survival rate for stage IV patients is only 5–10%.[3] Patients with borderline ovarian cancer have an excellent prognosis with a 5-year survival rate of 93% and a 10-year survival rate of 91%.[3]

Treatment

Ovarian cancer management depends primarily on the disease stage at initial presentation, the histological type, and pathologic grade (Table 125.3). In general, the treatment of patients with ovarian cancer initially involves surgical debulking at the time of staging laparotomy and adjunctive or consolidation chemotherapy therapy. However, the effect of debulking on outcome in stage IV patients is questionable.[34] If residual disease is found after consolidative chemotherapy, then second-line therapy is recommended. Many clinical trials are ongoing to determine the optimum therapeutic modalities for each disease stage; entering patients with any disease stage onto clinical trials is appropriate.

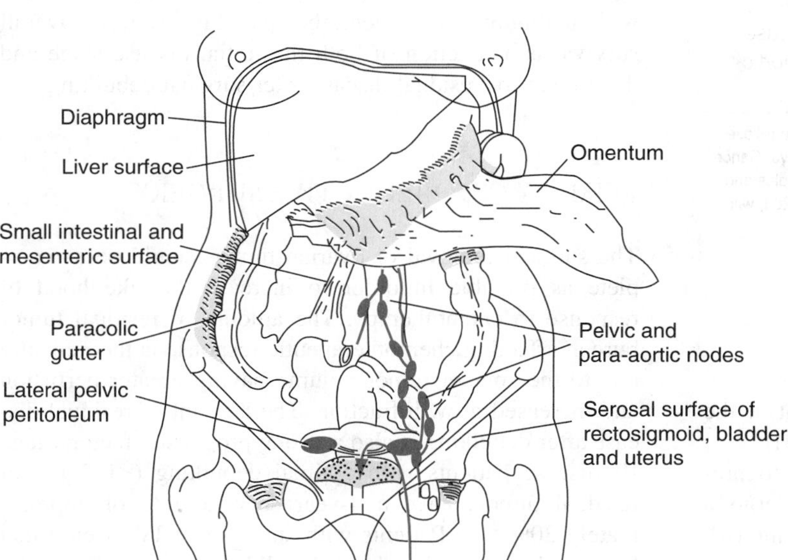

Figure 125.1. Staging laparotomy for ovarian cancer. *(From Young RC, Perez CA, Hoskins WJ. Cancer of the ovary, in Devita VT, Hellman S, Rosenberg SA (eds): Cancer—Principles and Practice of Oncology, 4th ed. Philadelphia, JB Lippincott, 1993, pp 1226–1263, with permission.)*

TABLE 125.2. SURGICAL STAGING FOR OVARIAN CANCER

Step 1.	If ascites is present, remove as much as possible for cytology. If no ascites is present, obtain cell washings from the pelvis, both abdominal gutters, and both subdiaphragmatic areas.
Step 2.	Determine whether the mass is malignant; if malignant, perform appropriate pelvic procedure (total abdominal hysterectomy and bilateral salpingo-oophorectomy unless patient desires additional childbearing, and there is no evidence of spread beyond the ovary).
Step 3.	Carefully examine pelvic peritoneum; if lesions are present, remove as much as possible and biopsy any lesion that cannot be removed. If no lesions are seen, sample at a minimum the peritoneum of the lateral pelvic sidewalls, the bladder, the rectosigmoid, and the cul-de-sac.
Step 4.	Examine the paracolic gutters, and remove any lesions seen. If no lesions are seen, obtain a 1- × 3-cm strip of peritoneum on either side.
Step 5.	Examine the omentum, and remove any that contains visible tumor (including the supracolic omentum if involved by tumor). If no lesions are seen, remove the infracolic omentum.
Step 6.	Examine and palpate both diaphragms and the surface of the spleen and liver. If lesions are present, remove as much as possible; biopsy if they cannot be removed. If no lesions are seen, a strip of peritoneum 1 × 2 cm should be carefully excised from the right hemidiaphragm. (*Note:* only peritoneum is needed, and care should be taken not to create a pneumothorax.)
Step 7.	Beginning at either the rectum or cecum, carefully inspect the entire large colon and remove and/or biopsy any suspicious lesion of the intestine or mesentery.[a]
Step 8.	Beginning at either the ileocecal valve or ligament of Treitz, carefully inspect the entire small bowel and mesentery, removing and/or biopsing any lesions.[a]
Step 9.	If, after all of the above procedures, no gross disease larger than 1 or 2 cm is left, the pelvic and para-aortic lymph nodes should be sampled.

[a]If resection of intestine is necessary to cytoreduce the tumor optimally or to relieve obstruction, it should be performed. (From Young RC, Perez CA, Hoskins WJ. Cancer of the ovary, in Devita VT, Hellman S, Rosenberg SA (eds): Cancer—Principles and Practice of Oncology, 4th ed. Philadelphia, JB Lippincott, 1993, pp 1226–1263, with permission.)

TREATMENT BY STAGE

Local/Limited Disease (Stages I and II)

About one-third of ovarian cancer patients present at the initial diagnosis with localized disease (stage I or II).[1,11,27] Women with stage IA ovarian tumors who wish to preserve ovarian and reproduction function can undergo a unilateral salpingo-oophorectomy without significant risk of decreased survival.[11,35] The beneficial effects of adjuvant chemotherapy in localized disease depend on the stage and subtype of the disease. Postoperative adjuvant chemotherapy is not required in stage IA grade 1 ovarian cancer, whereas patients with stage I grade 3 and stage IC ovarian cancer do require adjuvant chemotherapy.[15,27] It is currently unclear whether other types of stage I disease will benefit from adjuvant chemotherapy.[11,27] Patients with stage II disease should receive adjuvant treatment.[15,27]

TABLE 125.3. MANAGEMENT OF EPITHELIAL OVARIAN CANCER

Stage	Therapy
IA, IB (low grade)	TAH, BSO, omen
IA, IB (high grade)	TAH, BSO, omen + (chemotherapy or IP ^{32}P or total abdomino-pelvic radiation)
II (minimal disease <2 cm)	TAH, BSO, tumor debulking + (chemotherapy or total abdomino-pelvic radiation or IP ^{32}P)
II (macroscopic disease >2 cm)	TAH, BSO, tumor debulking + chemotherapy
III	TAH, BSO, omen, tumor debulking + chemotherapy
IV	TAH, BSO, tumor debulking[a] + platinum-based chemotherapy

Key: TAH, total abdominal hysterectomy; BSO, bilateral salpingo-oophorectomy; omen, omentectomy.
[a]Controversial, although commonly done.

Advanced Disease (Stages III and IV)

The majority of women with ovarian cancer present with stage III or IV disease.[3,11] The approach to advanced ovarian cancer is initial surgical debulking and then treatment with platinum-based chemotherapy (Fig. 125.2). Overall survival is a function of both the initial disease stage and the amount of residual disease after surgical debulking.

PRIMARY CYTOREDUCTIVE SURGERY

The surgical removal of ovarian tumor should be as complete as possible in order to increase the likelihood of response to chemotherapy. The amount of residual tumor burden affecting chemotherapeutic response is theoretically due to the smaller tumor volume having greater perfusion and increased growth fraction. The amount of residual disease after debulking is also a strong prognostic factor. Stage III disease patients with optimal debulking (<1–2 cm of residual tumor) have a 4-year survival rate of approximately 30%.[2,3,11] Patients with stage III or IV disease that have undergone suboptimal debulking (>2 cm of residual tumor) have less than a 10% chance of long-term survival.[11,30,33]

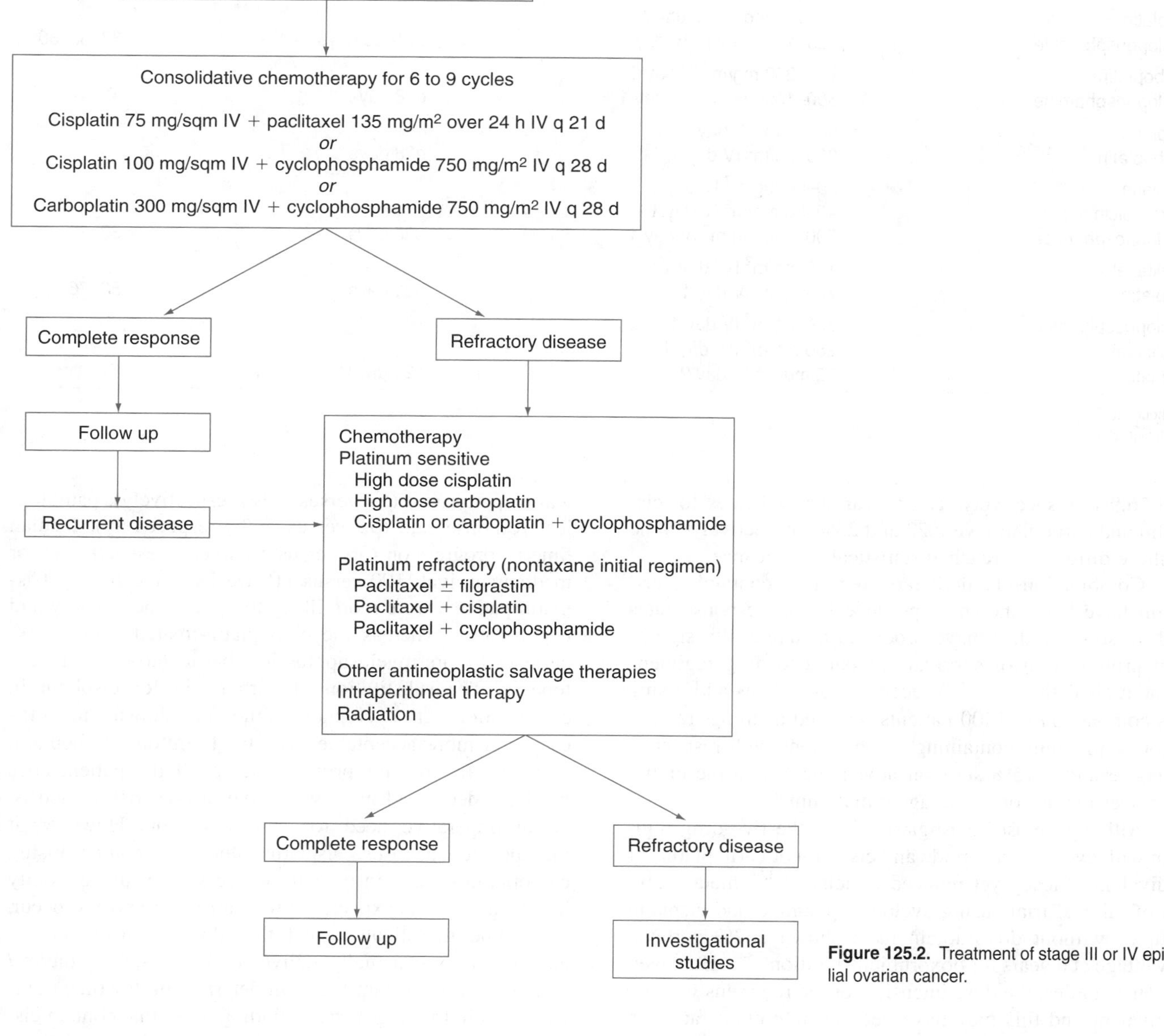

Figure 125.2. Treatment of stage III or IV epithelial ovarian cancer.

SYSTEMIC CHEMOTHERAPY CONSOLIDATION

Systemic chemotherapy following optimal surgical debulking is a cornerstone of first-line treatment of advanced epithelial ovarian cancer. A summary of chemotherapeutic regimens used as the initial treatment of newly diagnosed ovarian cancer can be found in Table 125.4. For many years, the "standard" chemotherapy for newly diagnosed patients was a regimen containing a platinum analog (cisplatin or carboplatin) plus a DNA alkylating agent (cyclophosphamide).[33,36] However, new first-line regimens are being developed that include paclitaxel (Taxol, Bristol-Myers, Squibb, Princeton, New Jersey).

Cisplatin and carboplatin have been used as single-agent therapy in previously untreated stage III and IV ovarian cancer.[37] Cisplatin 100 mg/m^2 was administered for courses 1 through 5 and 30 mg/m^2 for courses 6 through 10 scheduled every 4 weeks. Carboplatin was administered every 4 weeks at 400 mg/m^2 for the entire 10 courses. The complete remissions for cisplatin and carboplatin were 30.8

TABLE 125.4. INITIAL CHEMOTHERAPEUTIC REGIMENS FOR EPITHELIAL OVARIAN CANCER

Drugs	Dose(s)	Cycle Frequency	Ref.
Cisplatin	100 mg/m^2 IV day 1	q28 days	42
Carboplatin	400–600 mg/m^2 IV day 1	q28–35 days	37
Cisplatin Cyclophosphamide	50–100 mg/m^2 IV day 1 500–1000 mg/m^2 IV day 1	q21–28 days	32, 33, 36
Carboplatin Cyclophosphamide	200–300 mg/m^2 IV day 1 500–1000 mg/m^2 IV day 1	q28 days	41, 42
Cisplatin Carboplatin	50 mg/m^2 IV day 1 300 mg/m^2 IV day 1	q28 days	46
Cisplatin Doxorubicin Cyclophosphamide	50–60 mg/m^2 IV day 1 40–50 mg/m^2 IV day 1 500–750 mg/m^2 IV day 1	q28 days	33, 36
Paclitaxel Cisplatin	135 mg/m^2 IV[a] day 1 75 mg/m^2 IV day 1	q21 days	52, 76
Cyclophosphamide Paclitaxel Cisplatin	750 mg/m^2 IV day 1 250 mg/m^2 IV[a] day 1 75 mg/m^2 IV day 2	q21 days[b]	57

[a]24-hour infusion.
[b]With filgrastim.

and 26.9%, respectively. The 5-year survival rates for cisplatin and carboplatin were 22 and 25%, respectively. None of these differences reached statistical significance.

Combination chemotherapy regimens containing cisplatin have been shown to produce higher response rates and, in some studies, have produced a statistically significant prolongation of survival compared to drug regimens without cisplatin.[3,11,17,38] A recent meta-analysis addressing this comparison in 1400 patients revealed a strong trend in favor of platinum-containing combinations with respect to response and a 15% survival advantage out to the eighth year over the use of single-agent platinum.[38]

Although most investigators favor the two-drug regimen with cyclophosphamide and cisplatin or carboplatin for equivalent efficacy yet reduced toxicity,[32,33,36] meta-analyses of clinical trials using cyclophosphamide and cisplatin with or without doxorubicin have shown a 7% survival advantage at 6 years for doxorubicin addition.[38–40] However, in some studies, the dose intensity for the regimens was not equivalent and this may have been an important factor in determining the overall response and survival rate.[39]

The toxic effects of cisplatin, such as renal insufficiency, peripheral neuropathy, ototoxicity, and nausea, have stimulated the study of less toxic platinum analogs such as carboplatin. In trials comparing cyclophosphamide in combination with cisplatin or carboplatin for the initial treatment of advanced ovarian cancer, the carboplatin regimen caused less nausea, less renal toxicity, and less neurotoxicity.[38,41,42] Swenerton et al.[42] randomized patients with newly diagnosed stage III or IV ovarian cancer to either cisplatin or carboplatin in combination with cyclophosphamide. There were no significant differences in clinical response rate (57 versus 59%, respectively), pathological response rate (52 versus 54%, respectively), median time to progression (56 versus 58 weeks, respectively), or median survival (100 versus 110 weeks, respectively). Cisplatin patients were more likely to develop neuropathy and nephropathy, whereas the carboplatin-treated patients experienced more myelosuppression, particularly thrombocytopenia. The substitution of carboplatin for cisplatin in combination with cyclophosphamide has shown equal efficacy and more acceptable toxicity. Therefore, carboplatin might be favored for primary therapy if the patient does not have decreased marrow reserve, a high risk of sepsis, or an imperative need for anticoagulation. However, it may be prudent to use cisplatin rather than compromising carboplatin dosage in patients where severe myelotoxicity has occurred or is expected (low marrow reserve) to occur.

Some investigators feel that dose intensity, or the amount of drug actually delivered (expressed as mg/m^2/week), is an important factor in determining treatment outcomes with drug regimens, including those that contain cisplatin, in patients with ovarian cancer.[43] Most of these analyses were performed retrospectively and the patient populations varied considerably. A retrospective review of 45 randomized trials found no correlation between cisplatin dose and treatment outcome.[38]

To answer this question properly, McGuire et al.[44] performed a prospective randomized trial in patients with suboptimally debulked stage III (>1-cm residual masses) and any stage IV disease. Four hundred fifty-eight patients were randomized to receive cyclophosphamide 500 mg/m^2 IV plus either cisplatin 50 mg/m^2 (n = 235) or 100 mg/m^2 IV (n = 223) every three weeks. Patients in the cisplatin 50 mg/m^2 group received eight cycles and patients in the cisplatin 100 mg/m^2 group received four cycles. Clinical and pathologic response rates, response duration, and survival were similar in both groups. Hematologic, gastrointestinal, febrile events, septic events, and renal toxicities were significantly more common and severe in the patients receiving the higher cisplatin dose. This observation is consistent with other investigators' views that dose intensity may not be as important as cumulative dose received.[45]

Cisplatin has also been studied in combination with carboplatin. In a phase II study, patients with advanced ovarian cancer received low doses (50 mg/m^2) of cisplatin plus moderate doses (300 mg/m^2) of carboplatin.[46] The overall response rate was 71 with 57% achieving a complete response. The primary toxicities encountered were nausea, vomiting, and myelosuppression. In addition, there was no significant renal toxicity, neurotoxicity, or ototoxicity observed. This platinum analogue combination may be a practical alternative to high-dose cisplatin in the initial treatment of advanced ovarian cancer.

Paclitaxel is a relatively new chemotherapeutic agent found to have significant activity in ovarian cancer.[47–51] McGuire et. al.[52] reported that the combination of paclitaxel (135 mg/m^2 over 24 hours) and cisplatin (75 mg/m^2) achieved better response rates and survival outcomes compared to cyclophosphamide (750 mg/m^2) and cisplatin (75 mg/m^2) in patients with newly diagnosed suboptimally debulked stages III and IV ovarian cancer. The objective response in the paclitaxel–cisplatin group was 73%, with 51% complete responses; in the cyclophosphamide–cisplatin group, the objective response was 60%, with 31% complete responses ($p = 0.01$). The median progression-free survival was 18 months and 13 months, and the median survival was 38 months and 24 months for the paclitaxel–cisplatin and cyclophosphamide–cisplatin treated groups, respectively ($p < 0.001$ for both comparisons). Cisplatin dose-intensity was similar for both treatment groups. Neutropenia, alopecia, and peripheral neuropathy were more severe in the paclitaxel–cisplatin group. These results provide strong evidence that paclitaxel–cisplatin is more effective than cyclophosphamide–cisplatin as initial therapy in patients with newly diagnosed advanced ovarian cancer.

Other paclitaxel-containing combination regimens are being developed.[53–55] Ozols[53] have completed a phase I study of paclitaxel administered as a 3-hour infusion and carboplatin pharmacokinetically dosed by the Calvert formula[56] to various systemic exposures (area under the concentration–time curve, AUC). These investigators recommend the combination of paclitaxel 175 mg/m^2 over 3 hours plus carboplatin dosed to an AUC of 7.5 for further evaluation. Preliminary results with a cyclophosphamide, paclitaxel, cisplatin combination regimen are encouraging.[55,57]

Myleosuppression is the dose-limiting toxicity (DLT) associated with paclitaxel when given at doses of 135–175 mg/m^2 over 3 or 24 hours every 21 days.[49,50,58] The duration of administration of paclitaxel dramatically affects the incidence of grade 4 neutropenia and febrile neutropenia, with a substantially greater incidence occurring with 24-hour infusion compared to 3-hour infusion.[58] The use of granulocyte colony-stimulating factors (filgrastim) has allowed paclitaxel dose intensification.[59–62] At doses of 200–250 mg/m^2 given over 24 hours every 21 days the DLT becomes neuromuscular and neurotoxicity.[49,59] Neurotoxicity appears to be related to cumulative dose, and symptoms may persist for an extended period of time after paclitaxel is discontinued.

Cardiotoxicity and hypersensitivity reactions are two acutely occurring adverse reactions associated with paclitaxel.[63–65] Cardiac toxicity has been described as a transient sinus bradycardia, in addition to more severe conduction abnormalities.[63,64] It is currently unknown whether the cardiac toxicity associated with paclitaxel is due to the drug itself, or its Cremophor-based solvent. It is also unknown whether certain drug combinations or patient risk factors predispose patients to the cardiotoxicity. The hypersensitivity reactions occur at a high frequency when paclitaxel is administered by short infusion over 1–3 hours without premedication, and some reactions may be due to the Cremophor-based solvent used in the paclitaxel formulation.[49,50,65] To decrease the frequency of the hypersensitivity reactions with paclitaxel infusions of 24 hours duration or less, it is recommended that premedications such as steroids, H_1 and H_2 histamine antagonists be used.[47,49,50,65,66] At almost every infusion duration, paclitaxel alone rarely causes nausea or emesis.[49,50]

The duration of consolidative chemotherapy for advanced ovarian cancer has been evaluated in several studies. In a study by Hainsworth et al.,[33] the administration of a cisplatin-containing regimen repeated at 4-week intervals for 6 months produced results comparable to prolonged treatment. In advanced ovarian cancer, the administration of 5 cycles of cyclophosphamide, cisplatin, and doxorubicin was equally effective and less toxic compared to 10 cycles of chemotherapy.[67] Six to 9 cycles of chemotherapy have become the standard approach and result in clinical response rates of approximately 60–70% and 5-year survivals of 10–20%. Since approximately 50% of patients with a confirmed pathologic response will ultimately relapse,[2,3,14] some clinicians continue chemotherapy for 2 to 3 cycles beyond best response.[11,24]

Many questions still need to be answered about initial therapy for stages of ovarian cancer. Ongoing clinical trials are addressing whether some of the paclitaxel-containing regimens are better than current regimens for early-stage disease. There are also several comparative trials for advanced-stage ovarian cancer. These studies include determining the optimal paclitaxel dose, schedule, and treatment duration; comparing paclitaxel plus cisplatin to paclitaxel plus carboplatin in optimally debulked stage III patients; comparing these same combinations in suboptimally debulked stage III or IV patients; and determining whether dose intensification aided by growth factor support will produce higher response rates and improve survival.

SECONDARY CYTOREDUCTIVE SURGERY

The role of secondary cytoreduction (or interval debulking) after consolidative chemotherapy is currently unclear. A Gynecologic Oncology Group symposium debated the role of secondary cytoreduction.[68] Several conflicting studies exist with regard to the survival advantages of secondary cytoreduction. The overall effect of this treatment is probably significantly influenced by several factors including initial response to chemotherapy, the amount of residual disease before and after second-look surgery, and the presence of microscopic residual disease. The role of secondary cytoreductive surgery should optimally be determined by a randomized trial.

RECURRENT/REFRACTORY DISEASE

Approximately 20–50% of patients without evidence of residual disease on second-look laparotomy will relapse.[2,3,11] Patients with recurrent or refractory disease after initial chemotherapy historically have had a poor short-term and overall prognosis. Improved outcomes have been achieved in recurrent and refractory ovarian cancer with the use of high-dose chemotherapeutic agents such as cisplatin, carboplatin, paclitaxel, and the use of combination regimens containing these agents. A summary of chemotherapeutic regimens used in the treatment of recurrent or refractory ovarian cancer can be found in Table 125.5.

The choice of chemotherapy depends on the time frame in which the disease recurs.[3,11] Patients with disease that is refractory to the initial platinum-containing chemotherapy or that which recurs within 6 months after treatment (often termed "platinum-refractory") are unlikely to benefit from additional standard-dose platinum, whereas patients in which the disease recurs more than 6 months after the initial treatment (termed "platinum-sensitive") have a response rate of 27–59% with a second-line platinum regimen.[69]

In addition, cisplatin has shown a steep dose–response curve in ovarian carcinoma.[43,70] The major cisplatin toxicities when it is administered at doses of 50–100 mg/m^2 per cycle are nausea, vomiting, electrolyte disturbances including prolonged magnesium wasting, and nephrotoxicity. The development of improved antiemetic agents and aggressive hydration has allowed for the cisplatin dose escalation. Increasing the dose of cisplatin to 200 mg/m^2 per cycle results in myelosuppression and significant, long-lasting neurotoxicity.[71]

Paclitaxel has shown significant activity in platinum resistant-refractory ovarian cancer.[49,58,62,66,72,73] In a study by Trimble et al.,[72] platinum-resistant, heavily pretreated ovarian cancer patients were administered paclitaxel 135 mg/m^2 as a 24-hour continuous infusion every 21 days. The therapy achieved complete and partial response rates of 4 and 18%, respectively. The median survival duration and time to progression were 8.8 and 7.1 months, respectively. Thigpen et al.[73] treated patients with persistent or progressive ovarian carcinoma following cisplatin-based chemotherapy with paclitaxel 170 mg/m^2 as a 24-hour continuous infusion every 21 days. Among those accessible for response, the complete and partial responses were each 18%. The median survival and progression-free interval were 16 and 4.2 months, respectively. The primary toxicity associated with paclitaxel at these doses was frequent and severe, but manageable, myelosuppression.

The use of granulocyte colony-stimulating factors (filgrastim) to offset the DLT of myelosuppression has allowed for the dose escalation of paclitaxel in platinum-resistant ovarian cancer.[60,61] In a phase II trial, 44 patients received paclitaxel 250 mg/m^2 over 24 hours every 21 days and filgrastim 10 mcg/kg/d given subcutaneously.[62]

TABLE 125.5. CHEMOTHERAPEUTIC REGIMENS FOR RELAPSED OR REFRACTORY EPITHELIAL OVARIAN CANCER

Drugs	Dose(s)	Cycle Frequency	Ref.
Altretamine	260 mg/m^2 PO (divided in four daily doses) × 14–21 days	q28 days	83, 84
Cisplatin	100–150 mg/m^2 IV (total course dose usually given over 1–5 days)	q21 days	43, 70, 71
Paclitaxel	135–250^a mg/m^2 IV^b day 1	q21 days	59, 61, 62, 66, 72
Carboplatin	400–600 mg/m^2 IV day 1	q28–35 days	37
Paclitaxel Cisplatin	135 mg/m^2 IV^a day 1 75 mg/m^2 IV day 1	q21 days	52, 76
Paclitaxel Cyclophosphamide	250^a mg/m^2 IV^c day 1 1000 mg/m^2 IV day 2	q21 days	75

^{a}Filgrastim used with 250 mg/m^2 dose.
^{b}3- or 24-hour infusion.
^{c}24-hour infusion.

The clinical response, defined as greater than 50% reduction in the measurable tumor mass, was 48%. This is higher than the 24% response seen when paclitaxel is administered at 117–135 mg/m^2.[2,48,66,73] Sensory peripheral neuropathy emerged as the new DLT when paclitaxel was administered at 250 mg/m^2 over 24 hours.[62] The results of dose-intensive paclitaxel have been duplicated by the ovarian cancer group at MD Anderson[74] and are currently being evaluated in a Gynecological Oncology Group randomized trial. Therapy with dose-intensive paclitaxel and filgrastim should be considered for patients with advanced platinum-refractory ovarian cancer.

Several studies have evaluated two- and three-drug combinations of cisplatin, cyclophosphamide and paclitaxel.[75,76] Theoretically, the increased cytotoxic activity of these chemotherapeutic combinations lies in the understanding of their mechanisms of action and the process of DNA repair. Platinum analogues inhibit DNA synthesis through the formation of platinum–DNA cross-links or adducts. In mammalian cells, platinum–DNA adduct repairs are made via the nucleotide-excision-repair pathway. Paclitaxel has been shown to inhibit the repair of platinum–DNA adducts by up to 90%, and is associated with enhanced cell kill.[51,77,78] The synergistic effects of paclitaxel and cisplatin have been shown to be specific to the sequence of drug administration.[55,79] The combination was highly effective when paclitaxel was administered prior to cisplatin. The interaction was antagonistic when cisplatin was administered prior to paclitaxel and when the combination was infused concurrently. It is also hypothesized that the enhanced effect of paclitaxel with cyclophosphamide is related to inhibition of alkylator–DNA repair, similar to that demonstrated for cisplatin. The ability of paclitaxel to inhibit both DNA-repair pathways supports the hypothesis that a combination of paclitaxel, cisplatin, and cyclophosphamide should result in enhanced clinical efficacy.

Since many patients will receive paclitaxel or another taxane-derivative as initial therapy or salvage therapy and many of these will unfortunately relapse, it is important to know which agents or regimens can then be used to provide some benefit in these patients. Kavanagh et al.[80] treated 33 platinum-refractory ovarian cancer patients who also had progressed after taxane salvage therapy with carboplatin 300 mg/m^2 every 28 days. These investigators noted a 21% partial response rate with a median response duration greater than 7 months. However, all responding patients had a platinum-free interval of at least 12 months. "Cessation of progression" was noted in 39% of patients.

Other agents that have shown an overall 15–25% response rate include etoposide, ifosfamide, 5-fluorouracil, and altretamine.[11,81] Altretamine (hexamethylmelamine) is a chemotherapeutic agent that undergoes metabolic activation to form alkylating intermediates.[82] Altretamine has shown activity in resistant-refractory advanced ovarian cancer.[83,84] In this setting, altretamine has achieved objective response rates of up to 33% and disease stabilization in 8–78% of patients. Altretamine is approved as single-agent therapy, at a total daily dose of 260 mg/m^2/d administered in four divided doses for 14–21 days given every 28 days. When administered in combination with other bone marrow suppressive agents, the dose is reduced to 150 mg/m^2/d for 14 days given every 28 days. Tamoxifen has also been used in the salvage setting and usually produces responses in patients with positive estrogen receptors.[85]

BORDERLINE OVARIAN CANCER

Borderline (low malignant potential) ovarian cancers account for approximately 15% of all epithelial ovarian cancers; the majority (75%) are stage I at the time of diagnosis.[13,86] These tumors must be recognized, since their prognosis and treatment is clearly different from malignant invasive carcinomas. Kurman and Trimble reviewed 953 patients with a mean follow-up of 7 years and found a survival rate of 92% for advanced-stage tumors with the usual cause of death being benign disease complications (e.g., small bowel obstruction) and therapy-related complications. Malignant transformation was rarely the cause of death. In one series, the 5-, 10-, 15-, and 20-year survival rates of patients with all stages of low malignant potential tumors were 97, 95, 92, and 89%, respectively.[87]

In patients with stage I or II disease, no additional chemotherapy or radiation treatment is indicated for a completely resected tumor of low malignant potential.[86,88] In the presence of bilateral ovarian cystic neoplasms or a single ovary involvement, partial oophorectomy or a unilateral salpingo-oophorectomy can be performed if childbearing potential is to be maintained. When childbearing is not a consideration, a total abdominal hysterectomy and bilateral salpingo-oophorectomy are appropriate therapy as most clinicians favor removing the remaining ovarian tissue, which is at risk for recurrence of a borderline tumor or rarely developing invasive carcinoma.

Patients with advanced borderline ovarian cancer should undergo a total hysterectomy, bilateral salpingo-oophorectomy, omentectomy, node sampling, and aggressive cytoreductive surgery; however, there is little evidence that adjuvant chemotherapy or radiotherapy alters disease course.[86,88] There have been no controlled studies comparing postoperative treatment with no treatment.

INTRAPERITONEAL CHEMOTHERAPY

Significant advances have occurred in the understanding, advantages, limitations, and administration methods of intraperitoneal (IP) chemotherapy for ovarian cancer treatment.[89–92] The theoretical advantages of IP administration are increasing the intensity and duration of tumor exposure, while decreasing the systemic exposure and possible toxicity.[90–92] Studies have shown potential value in IP administration for initial, consolidation, and salvage therapy. It appears that patients with small volume tumors (i.e., minimal disease <2 cm) are optimally suited for IP drug administration because these patients have had the best outcomes for both initial therapy or relapsed-disease treatment.[91,93,94] Drugs that have been given IP include cisplatin, carboplatin, cytarabine, etoposide, doxorubicin, mitoxantrone, paclitaxel, 5-fluorouracil, melphalan, and methotrexate.[90,91] A summary of IP chemotherapeutic regimens can be found in Table 125.6.

Alberts et al.[95] randomized patients with optimally debulked (<2-cm residual masses) stage III ovarian cancer to six courses of either cisplatin 100 mg/m^2 IP plus cyclophosphamide 600 mg/m^2 IV (IP/IV) or cisplatin 100 mg/m^2 IV plus cyclophosphamide 600 mg/m^2 IV (IV/IV) given at 3-week intervals. Complete response as determined by second-look laparotomy was 40% in the IP/IV group and 31% in the IV/IV group ($p = 0.1$). However, estimated median survival in the IP/IV cohort (49 months) was significantly better than in the IV/IV group (41 months; $p = 0.03$). Clinical hearing loss and neutropenia were more common and more severe with IV/IV administration.

To determine if the pharmacologic advantage of IP chemotherapy as the initial treatment of advanced ovarian cancer could be translated into greater response and survival rate, a phase III study compared IP cisplatin (200 mg/m^2) plus IP etoposide (350 mg/m^2) with intravenous (IV) sodium thiosulfate protection administered every 4 weeks versus IV cisplatin (100 mg/m^2) plus IV cyclophosphamide (600 mg/m^2) administered every 3 weeks in patients with stage III or IV ovarian cancer.[96] Patients were entered regardless of their postsurgical disease status. The complete response rate in evaluable patients was 48% in the IP group and 52% in the IV group. There was no difference in response rates between the groups as a function of size of residual disease (i.e., <1 or >1 cm). There was also no difference between IP and IV therapy with regards to time to reoccurrence in those who relapsed (i.e., 12 and 14 months, respectively) or survival (i.e., 44 and 50%, respectively) at a median follow-up of 46 months. Both regimens were well tolerated with similar hematologic and nonhematologic toxicities.

Intraperitoneal cisplatin and carboplatin have achieved documented complete responses in relapsed patients initially treated with systemic platinum-containing regimens.[93,97] In a prospective study, patients with stage III or IV recurrent or persistent ovarian cancer after first-line cisplatin-based chemotherapy were treated with an IP chemotherapy regimen consisting of cisplatin 200 mg/m^2, cytarabine 1.2 g/m^2, and bleomycin 2 U/m^2 plus systemic protection with IV sodium thiosulfate repeated every 28 days for six cycles. Twenty-four percent of patients had a surgically documented complete response. The median survival from the time of initial diagnosis was 42.7 months, the 2-year survival was 76%, and the 5-year survival was 27%.

Studies have tried to determine which group of patients may have the best response to IP therapy. A retrospective study evaluated the results of IP cisplatin with etoposide or cytarabine as salvage therapy.[93] Forty-one percent of patients with microscopic disease at the time of IP therapy achieved a surgically defined complete response, whereas only 29% of patients with macroscopic disease (i.e., largest residual tumor mass less than 0.5 cm in diameter) had a surgically definable complete response. Patients whose largest residual tumor mass was greater than 1 cm only achieved a 5% complete response rate. This is similar to data showing a 1- to 2-cm depth of penetration of IP cisplatin into tumor or normal tissue.[98] An objective response rate of less than 10% is anticipated for IP cisplatin in patients who have failed to demonstrate at least a partial response to initial systemic cisplatin.[94] Thus, IP cisplatin should not be used in patients who are initially cisplatin

TABLE 125.6. INTRAPERITONEAL CHEMOTHERAPEUTIC REGIMENS FOR OVARIAN CANCER

Drugs	Dose(s)	Cycle Frequency	Ref.
Cisplatin	50–100 mg/m^2 IP day 1	q21–28 days	91, 93, 95
Cisplatin Cyclophosphamide	100 mg/m^2 IP day 1 600 mg/m^2 IV day 1	q21 days	95
Etoposide Cisplatin Sodium Thiosulfate	200–350 mg/m^2 IP[a] day 1 100–200 mg/m^2 IP day 1 12–16 g/m^2 IV day 1	q28 days	93, 96
Cisplatin Cytarabine	100–150 mg/m^2 IP day 1 600–1200 mg/m^2 IP day 1	q28 days	97
Paclitaxel	125 mg/m^2 IP day 1	q28 days	90, 100
Mitoxantrone	20–30 mg/m^2 IP day 1	q28 days	99

[a]IP, intraperitoneally.

refractory. The primary toxicity associated with IP cisplatin was bone marrow suppression.

Mitoxantrone IP achieved surgically definable results and limited systemic toxicity, but had a high incidence of severe abdominal pain, and several patients developed abdominal adhesions and bowel obstructions that required surgical treatment.[99] The administration of mitoxantrone with large volumes of 0.9% sodium chloride reduced the severity and frequency of the local adverse effects.[99]

Intraperitoneal paclitaxel has also been studied.[100,101] A phase I trial of IP paclitaxel resulted in a DLT of abdominal pain at doses greater than 125 mg/m^2.[100] The exposure of the peritoneal cavity after IP paclitaxel was approximately 30 times higher than plasma exposure.[100,101] Further study is needed to determine the role of IP paclitaxel in the management of ovarian cancer.

Complications from IP therapy may be related to catheter function, infection, or bowel problems.[90,91] Mechanical obstruction to fluid inflow has been reported in approximately 5% of patients.[90,91] Most commonly this results from fibrin sheath formation around the catheter tip.[89] In some cases, peritoneal adhesions obstruct fluid entry into the abdominal cavity causing uneven distribution of the chemotherapeutic agent. Infections are the most prevalent IP-related complication and are reported in approximately 10% of patients.[89–91,101] Infections range from superficial cellulitis around the catheter entry site to deep tissue infections to peritonitis. In most cases, catheter removal is required to eradicate the infection.[89] Bowel-related complications (approximate 3% incidence) include obstruction, ileus, and perforation.[89,91] IP administration may also result in a false CA-125 elevation.[91]

The results thus far of IP chemotherapy for ovarian cancer treatment have been very encouraging, but additional well-designed comparative trials are needed to define the role of IP versus systemic chemotherapy ovarian cancer management.

SALVAGE THERAPIES

Radiation Therapy

The use of radiation therapy in the treatment of ovarian cancer is controversial. The two forms of radiation therapy used in ovarian cancer are external beam whole abdominal irradiation and intraperitoneal isotopes (^{32}P). The two therapeutic uses of radiation therapy have been as adjuvant therapy in patients with no residual disease and as consolidation therapy in patients with minimal residual disease.

Abdominal irradiation[102,103] and intraperitoneal isotopes[104,105] have not shown improvements in response and have been associated with greater toxicity. In one study, ovarian cancer patients treated with abdomino-pelvic radiation were analyzed for post-treatment complications.[103] The incidence of acute complications associated with treatment were vomiting (61%) and diarrhea (68%). Serious late complications presented as bowel obstruction in 4.2% of patients; 64% required surgical intervention. The incidence of bowel obstruction was significantly higher in the intraperitoneal ^{32}P versus the cisplatin-treated groups (11 and 2% respectively, $p = 0.004$).[105] There is currently no study reporting the use of radiation therapy to be superior to chemotherapy in any treatment setting.

Autologous Bone Marrow Transplant (ABMT)

The use of high-dose myeloablative chemotherapy followed by bone marrow rescue has been used as salvage therapy in hematologic and solid tumor malignancies. The most common ablative regimens used in ovarian cancer contain platinum analogs (i.e., cisplatin or carboplatin), alkylating agents (i.e., melphalan, thiotepa, or cyclophosphamide), and/or etoposide.[106–110] These agents are used because of proven activity in ovarian cancer and bone marrow suppression as the DLT.

Shpall et al.[106] evaluated the use of IP cisplatin and high-dose systemic cyclophosphamide and thiotepa followed by autologous bone marrow support in advanced ovarian cancer. Seventy-five percent of patients evaluated had pathologically documented partial response (i.e., >75% reduction in tumor mass). Mulder et al.[109] reports two long-term survivors (i.e., 43 and 75 months) after treatment with high-dose cyclophosphamide and etoposide followed by ABMT. Based on the minimal and short-duration of response in patients that have been extensively treated without considerable response and the severe chemotherapy-related toxicity, ABMT should probably only be used in patients with persistent nonbulky disease that have had a significant response to initial platinum-based chemotherapy. The role of bone marrow transplantation in the treatment of advanced refractory ovarian cancer is unclear due to the small number of patients treated.

TREATMENT OF NONEPITHELIAL OVARIAN CANCER

Ovarian Stromal Tumors

Ovarian stromal tumors normally have an indolent natural history and rarely occur bilaterally. They are managed by unilateral salpingo-oophorectomy and usually do not require additional treatment.[2,11,14] Stage II stromal tumors require more extensive surgery due to the lack of effective adjuvant therapy. Due to the low overall number of granulosa-theca cell tumor patients treated, the role of chemotherapy is unclear.

Ovarian Germ Cell Tumors

Germ cell tumors are rare and may have a mixed histology. Thus, treatment should be directed toward the most malignant component of the tumor. Surgery alone has not been very effective, producing 2-year survival rates of 13–16%.[111] Combination chemotherapy has produced high cure rates and improved prognosis in patients with germ cell tumors.[111]

Endodermal sinus and dysgerminoma are two subtypes of germ cell tumors. Endodermal sinus tumors are aggressive tumors and usually occur unilaterally. Without chemotherapy, almost all patients die from their disease; thus patients with all stages of disease should receive combination chemotherapy. The most common combination chemotherapeutic regimens used are vincristine, dactinomycin, and cyclophosphamide; and cisplatin and bleomycin in combination with vincristine or etoposide.[111] Dysgerminoma tumors have a high cure rate and are highly sensitive to radiation therapy; however, the sterility associated with abdominal irradiation has resulted in systemic chemotherapy becoming first-line therapy. The treatment of choice for newly diagnosed disease is a platinum-containing regimen.[111–113] A report of 35 cases of germ cell tumors, half of which were advanced-stage or recurrent or progressive disease, demonstrated a 97% sustained remission at 10–54 months after the start of bleomycin/etoposide/cisplatin (BEP) chemotherapy.[114] Also, two Gynecologic Oncology Group trials demonstrated that 89 of 93 patients with stages I, II, and III disease with completely resected tumors were disease free after three BEP cycles.[112–114] Patients with recurrent or refractory disease after cisplatin-based chemotherapy can be treated with radiation therapy.[111]

Evaluation of Patient Outcomes

Localized ovarian cancer is highly curable by surgery and chemotherapy where appropriate. The goals of therapy should be to maintain the patient's quality of life and, if possible and desired, preserve reproductive capabilities.

Newly diagnosed advanced ovarian cancer is highly responsive to surgical debulking and subsequent consolidative chemotherapy; however, cure rates are much lower than with localized disease. The goals of therapy in advanced ovarian carcinoma are to cure the disease, to extend disease-free survival, and to prolong overall survival. Patients with recurrent or refractory disease are generally not curable and have a poor long-term prognosis. Thus, the primary direction of therapy may be symptom management, quality of life maintenance, and treatment-related toxicity minimization.

When applied mainly to clinical trials, complete response is defined as complete resolution (CR) of all disease and can be further categorized either as a pathologic or clinical complete response.[3,11,14] A pathologic complete response is defined as no detectable disease on second-look laparotomy. A clinical complete response is defined as no detectable disease by radiologic imaging techniques. The recent NIH consensus conference on ovarian cancer concluded that second-look laparotomy should only be performed in clinical trials.[11,27] Partial response (PR) is defined as a greater than 50% decrease in all measurable disease. Stable disease is defined as disease maintenance progression. In addition, general definitions for response duration and survival apply to ovarian cancer. Disease-free survival is defined from the point of achieving a complete response to the time of disease recurrence. Overall survival is defined from the point of diagnosis to time of death. Since a proportion of patients with newly diagnosed or recurrent disease do not achieve complete responses, the goal of therapy is usually palliation. Thus, maintaining quality of life by relieving symptoms such as abdominal pain, bloating, and constipation is the desired outcome.

Conclusion

Although the number of women in the United States dying from ovarian cancer continues to increase, substantial treatment progress has been made. There are still several therapeutic questions that need to be asked and problems that need to be solved. Further investigation is needed to determine if the combination of platinum and paclitaxel is the treatment of choice in newly diagnosed advanced stage ovarian cancer. New approaches to the treatment of advanced primary as well as recurrent and refractory ovarian cancer, such as agents to overcome resistance, should be studied. The optimum adjuvant and consolidation treatment modalities should be determined. The role of IP chemotherapy in all stages of disease is unclear as is the most appropriate salvage therapy. Answering these therapeutic questions and solving these therapeutic problems may increase the complete response rate and prolong the long-term survival.

References

1. Wingo PA, Tong T, Bolden S. Cancer Statistics—1995. CA Cancer J Clin 1995;45:8–30.
2. Makar APH, Trope CG. Endometrial and ovarian malignancies: Epidemiology, etiology, and prognostic factors. Acta Obstet Gynecol Scand 1992;71:331–336.
3. Leung Y, DePetrillo AD. Etiology, epidemiology, risk and prognostic factors, screening, and imaging of gynecologic cancers. Curr Opin Oncol 1993;5:869–876.
4. Daly MB. The epidemiology of ovarian cancer. Hematol Oncol Clin North Am 1992;6:729–738.
5. Schildkraut JM, Thompson WD. Familial ovarian carcinoma: A population-based case-control study. Am J Epidemiol 1989;13:1071–1073.
6. Koch M, Gaedke H, Jenkins H. Family history of ovarian cancer patients: A case control study. Int J Epidemiol 1989;18:782–.
7. Daly MB, Lerman C. Ovarian cancer risk counseling: A guide for the practitioner. Oncology 1993;7:27–34.
8. Green MH, Clark JW, Blayney DW. The epidemiology of ovarian cancer. Oncology 1984;11:209–226.

9. Cramer DW, Hutchinson GE, Welch WR, et al. Factors affecting the association of oral contraceptives and ovarian cancer. N Engl J Med 1982;307:1047–1051.
10. Woutersz TB. Benefits of oral contraception: Thirty years' experience. Int J Fertil 1991;3:26–31.
11. Cannistra SA. Cancer of the ovary [published erratum appears in N Engl J Med 1994 Feb 10;330(6):448]. N Engl J Med 1993;329:1550–1559.
12. Lynch HT, Watson P, Lynch JF, et al. Hereditary ovarian cancer: Heterogeneity in age at onset. Cancer 1993;71(suppl 2):573–581.
13. Taylor RR, Tenerillo MG, Nash JD, et al. The molecular genetics of gyn malignancies. Oncology 1994;8:63–70.
14. Young RC, Perez CA, Hoskins WJ. Cancer of the ovary, in Devita VT, Hellman S, Rosenberg SA (eds): Cancer—Principles and Practice of Oncology, 4th ed. Philadelphia, JB Lippincott, 1993, pp 1226–1263.
15. Young RC, Walton LA, Ellenberg SS, et al. Adjuvant therapy in stage I and stage II epithelial ovarian cancer: Results of two prospective randomized trials. N Engl J Med 1990;322:1021–1027.
16. Kent SN, McKay DG. Primary cancer of the ovary. Am J Obstet Gynecol 1960;80:430–438.
17. Hand R, Fremgen A, Chmiel JS, et al. Staging procedures, clinical management, and survival outcome for ovarian carcinoma. JAMA 1993;269:1119–1122.
18. Kenemans P, Yedema CA, Bon GG, von Mensdorff-Pouilly S. CA 125 in gynecologic oncology—a review. Eur J Obstet Gynecol Repro Biol 1993;49:115–124.
19. Hempling RE. Tumor markers in epithelial ovarian cancer. Obstet Gynecol Clin North Am 1994;21:41–61.
20. Niloff JM. The role of the CA 125 assay in the management of ovarian cancer [see comments]. Oncology 1988;2:67–76.
21. Lavin PT, Knapp RC, Malkasian G, et al. CA 125 for the monitoring of ovarian carcinoma during primary therapy. Obstet Gynecol 1987;69:223–227.
22. Willemse PH, Aalders JG, de Bruyn HW, et al. CA-125 in ovarian cancer: Relation between half-life, doubling time and survival. Eur J Cancer 1991;27:993–995.
23. Niloff JM, Bast Jr RC, Schaetzl EM, Knapp RC. Predictive value of CA-125 antigen levels in second-look procedures for ovarian cancer. Am J Obstet Gynecol 1985;151:981–986.
24. Mackey SE, Creasman WT. Ovarian cancer screening. J Clin Oncol 1995;13:783–793.
25. van Nagell JR, DePriest PD, Gallion HH, Pavlik EJ. Ovarian cancer screening. Cancer 1993;71:1523–1528.
26. Carlson KJ, Skates S, Singer DE. Screening for ovarian cancer. Ann Intern Med 1994;121:124–132.
27. Ovarian Cancer Screening, Treatment and Followup. NIH Consensus Statement 1994;12:1–30.
28. Fuks Z. Patterns of spread of ovarian carcinoma: Relation to therapeutic strategies. Adv Biosci 1980;26:39–51.
29. Nguyen HN, Averette HE, Hoskins W, et al. National survey of ovarian carcinoma. Part V. The impact of physician's specialty on patients' survival. Cancer 1993;72:3663–3670.
30. Louie KG, Ozols RF, Myers CE, et al. Long-term results of a cisplatin-containing combination chemotherapy regimen for the treatment of advanced ovarian carcinoma. J Clin Oncol 1986;4:1579–1585.
31. Kawai M, Kikkawa F, Hattori S, et al. Long-term follow-up of patients with epithelial carcinoma of the ovary. Int J Gynaecol Obstet 1994;44:259–266.
32. Omura GA, Brady MF, Homesley HD, et al. Long-term follow-up and prognostic factor analysis in advanced ovarian carcinoma: The Gynecologic Oncology Group experience. J Clin Oncol 1991;9:1138–1150.
33. Hainsworth JD, Grosh WW, Burnett LS, et al. Advanced ovarian cancer: Long-term results of treatment with intensive cisplatin-based chemotherapy of brief duration. Ann Intern Med 1988;108:165–170.
34. Goodman HM, Harlow BL, Sheets EE, et al. The role of cytoreductive surgery in the management of stage IV epithelial ovarian carcinoma. Gynecol Oncol 1992;46:367–371.
35. Miyazaki T, Tomoda Y, Ohta M, et al. Preservation of ovarian function and reproductive ability in patients with malignant ovarian tumors. Gynecol Oncol 1988;30:329–341.
36. Neijt JP, ten Bokkel Huinink WW, van der Burg ME, et al. Randomized trial comparing two combination chemotherapy regimens (CHAP-5 v CP) in advanced ovarian carcinoma. J Clin Oncol 1987;5:1157–1168.
37. Taylor AE, Wiltshaw E, Gore ME, et al. Long-term follow-up of the first randomized study of cisplatin versus carboplatin for advanced epithelial ovarian cancer. J Clin Oncol 1994;12:2066–2070.
38. Advanced Ovarian Cancer Trials Group. Chemotherapy in advanced ovarian cancer: An overview of randomized clinical trials. BMJ 1991;303:884–893.
39. Cyclophosphamide plus cisplatin versus cyclophosphamide, doxorubicin, and cisplatin chemotherapy of ovarian carcinoma: A meta-analysis. The Ovarian Cancer Meta-Analysis Project. J Clin Oncol 1991;9:1668–1674.
40. A'Hern RP, Gore ME. Impact of doxorubicin on survival in advanced ovarian cancer. J Clin Oncol 1995;13:726–732.
41. Alberts DS, Green S, Hannigan EV, et al. Improved therapeutic index of carboplatin plus cyclophosphamide versus cisplatin plus cyclophosphamide: Final report by the Southwest Oncology Group of a phase III randomized trial in stages III and IV ovarian cancer [published erratum appears in J Clin Oncol 1992 Sep;10(9):1505] [see comments]. J Clin Oncol 1992;10:706–717.
42. Swenerton K, Jeffrey J, Stuart G, et al. Cisplatin–cyclophosphamide versus carboplatin–cyclophosphamide in advanced ovarian cancer: A randomized phase III study of the National Cancer Institute of Canada Clinical Trials Group [see comments]. J Clin Oncol 1992;10:718–726.
43. Levin L, Hryniuk WM. Dose intensity analysis of chemotherapy regimens in ovarian carcinoma. J Clin Oncol 1987;5:756–767.
44. McGuire WP, Hoskins WJ, Brady MF, et al. Assessment of dose-intensive therapy in suboptimally debulked ovarian cancer: A Gynecologic Oncology Group study. J Clin Oncol 1995;13:1589–1599.
45. Alberts DS, Garcia DJ. Total platinum dose versus platinum dose intensification in ovarian cancer treatment. Semin Oncol 1994;21:11–15.
46. Segelov E, Stuart-Harris R, Bell D, et al. A phase II study of carboplatin and cisplatin in advanced ovarian cancer. Eur J Gynaecol Oncol 1994;15:277–282.

47. McGuire WP. Taxol: A new drug with significant activity as a salvage therapy in advanced epithelial ovarian carcinoma. Gynecol Oncol 1993;51:78–85.
48. McGuire WP, Rowinsky EK, Rosenshein NB, et al. Taxol: A unique antineoplastic agent with significant activity in advanced ovarian epithelial neoplasms. Ann Intern Med 1989;111:273–279.
49. Rowinsky EK, Donehower RC. Paclitaxel (Taxol) [published erratum appears in N Engl J Med 1995 Jul 6;333(1):75]. N Engl J Med 1995;332:1004–1014.
50. Kohler DR, Goldspiel BR. Paclitaxel (Taxol). Pharmacotherapy 1994;14:3–34.
51. Horwitz SB. Taxol (paclitaxel): Mechanisms of action. Ann Oncol 1994;5:S3–S6.
52. McGuire WP, Hoskins WJ, Brady MF, et al. Cyclophosphamine and cisplatin compared with paclitaxel and cisplatin in patients with stage III and stage IV ovarian cancer. N Engl J Med 1996;334:1–6.
53. Ozols RF. Carboplatin and paclitaxel in ovarian cancer. Semin Oncol 1995;22:78–83.
54. ten Bokkel Huinink W, Veenhof C, Helmerhorst T, et al. Paclitaxel plus carboplatin in the treatment of ovarian cancer. Semin Oncol 1995;22:97–100.
55. Reed E, Kohn EC, Sarosy G, et al. Paclitaxel, cisplatin, and cyclophosphamide in human ovarian cancer: Molecular rationale and early clinical results. Semin Oncol 1995;22:90–96.
56. Calvert AH, Newell DR, Gumbrell LA, et al. Carboplatin dosage: Prospective evaluation of a simple formula based on renal function. J Clin Oncol 1989;7:1748–1756.
57. Kohn E, Reed E, Link C, et al. A pilot study of Taxol, cisplatin, cyclophosphamide and GCSF in newly diagnosed stage III/IV ovarian cancer patients [abstract]. Proc Am Soc Clin Oncol 1993;12:257.
58. Eisenhauer EA, ten Bokkel Huinink WW, Swenerton KD, et al. European–Canadian randomized trial of paclitaxel in relapsed ovarian cancer: High-dose versus low-dose and long versus short infusion. J Clin Oncol 1994;12:2654–2666.
59. Sarosy G, Kohn E, Stone DA, et al. Phase I study of Taxol and granulocyte colony-stimulating factor in patients with refractory ovarian cancer. J Clin Oncol 1992;10:1165–1170.
60. Sarosy G, Reed E. Taxol dose intensification and its clinical implications. J Natl Med Assoc 1993;85:427–431.
61. Seewaldt VL, Greer BE, Cain JM, et al. Paclitaxel (Taxol) treatment for refractory ovarian cancer: Phase II clinical trial. Am J Obstet Gynecol 1994;170:1666–1670.
62. Kohn EC, Sarosy G, Bicher A, et al. Dose-intense Taxol: High response rate in patients with platinum-resistant recurrent ovarian cancer. J Natl Cancer Inst 1994;86:18–24.
63. Arbuck SG, Strauss H, Rowinsky E, et al. A reassessment of cardiac toxicity associated with Taxol. Monogr Natl Cancer Inst 1993;15:117–130.
64. Rowinsky EK, McGuire WP, Guarnieri T, et al. Cardiac disturbances during the administration of Taxol. J Clin Oncol 1991;9:1704–1712.
65. Weiss RB, Donehower RC, Wiernik PH, et al. Hypersensitivity reactions from Taxol. J Clin Oncol 1990;8:1263–1268.
66. Einzig AI. Review of phase II trials of Taxol (paclitaxel) in patients with advanced ovarian cancer. Ann Oncol 1994;5:S29–S32.
67. Hakes TB, Chalas E, Hoskins WJ, et al. Randomized prospective trial of 5 versus 10 cycles of cyclophosphamide, doxorubicin, and cisplatin in advanced ovarian carcinoma. Gynecol Oncol 1992;45:284–289.
68. Potter ME. Secondary cytoreduction in ovarian cancer: Pro or con? Gynecol Oncol 1993;51:131–135.
69. Markman M, Rothman R, Hakes T, et al. Second-line platinum therapy in patients with ovarian cancer previously treated with cisplatin. J Clin Oncol 1991;9:389–393.
70. Kaye SB, Lewis CR, Paul J, et al. Randomised study of two doses of cisplatin with cyclophosphamide in epithelial ovarian cancer [see comments]. Lancet 1992;340:329–333.
71. Rothenberg ML, Ozols RF, Glatstein E, et al. Dose-intensive induction therapy with cyclophosphamide, cisplatin, and consolidative abdominal radiation in advanced-stage epithelial ovarian cancer [see comments]. J Clin Oncol 1992;10:727–734.
72. Trimble EL, Adams JD, Vena D, et al. Paclitaxel for platinum-refractory ovarian cancer: Results from the first 1,000 patients registered to National Cancer Institute Treatment Referral Center 9103. J Clin Oncol 1993;11:2405–2410.
73. Thigpen JT, Blessing JA, Ball H, et al. Phase II trial of paclitaxel in patients with progressive ovarian carcinoma after platinum-based chemotherapy: A Gynecologic Oncology Group study. J Clin Oncol 1994;12:1748–1753.
74. Kavanaugh JJ, Kudelka AT, Edwards RS, et al. A randomized crossover trial of parenteral hydroxyurea v. high dose taxol in cisplatin/carboplatin resistant epithelial ovarian cancer [abstract]. Proc Am Soc Clin Oncol 1993;12:259.
75. Reed E, Sarosy G, Kohn E, et al. Phase I study of paclitaxel and cyclophosphamide in reccurrence adenocarcinoma of the ovary [abstract]. Proc Am Assoc Cancer Res 1994;34:234.
76. McGuire WP, Hoskins WJ, Brady MF, et al. A phase III trial comparing cisplatin/taxol (PT) in advanced ovarian cancer (AOC) [abstract]. Proc Am Soc Clin Oncol 1993;12:254.
77. Schiff PB. Taxol assembles tubulin in the absence of exogenous guanosine 5′-triphosphate of microtubule-associated protein. Biochem 1981;20:3247–3252.
78. Parker RJ, Dabholkar MD, Lee KB, et al. Taxol effects on cisplatin sensitivity and cis cellular accumulation in human ovarian cancer cells. Monogr Natl Cancer Inst 1993;15:83–88.
79. Jekunen AP, Christen RD, Shalinsky DR, Howell SB. Synergistic interaction between cisplatin and taxol in human ovarian carcinoma cells *in vitro.* Br J Cancer 1994;69:299–306.
80. Kavanagh J, Tresukosol D, Edwards C, et al. Carboplatin reinduction after taxane in patients with platinum-refractory epithelial ovarian cancer. J Clin Oncol 1995;13:1584–1588.
81. McGuire WP. Primary treatment of epithelial ovarian malignancies. Cancer 1993;71:1541–1550.
82. Lee CR, Faulds D. Altretamine. A review of its pharmacodynamic and pharmacokinetic properties, and therapeutic potential in cancer chemotherapy. Drugs 1995;49:932–953.
83. Manetta A, MacNeill C, Lyter JA, et al. Hexamethylmelamine as a single second-line agent in ovarian cancer. Gynecol Oncol 1990;36:93–96.
84. Rosen GF, Lurain JR, Newton M. Hexamethylmelamine in ovarian cancer after failure of cisplatin-based multiple-agent chemotherapy. Gynecol Oncol 1987;27:173–179.

85. Hatch KD, Beecham JB, Blessing JA, Creasman WT. Responsiveness of patients with advanced ovarian carcinoma to tamoxifen. A Gynecologic Oncology Group study of second-line therapy in 105 patients. Cancer 1991;68:269–271.
86. Trimble CL, Trimble EL. Management of epithelial ovarian tumors of low malignant potential. Gynecol Oncol 1994;55:S52–S61.
87. Leake JF. Tumors of low malignant potential. Curr Opin Obstet Gynecol 1992;4:81–85.
88. Trope C, Kaern J, Vergote IB, et al. Are borderline tumors of the ovary overtreated both surgically and systemically? A review of four prospective randomized trials including 253 patients with borderline tumors. Gynecol Oncol 1993;51:236–243.
89. Brandner P, Neis KJ. Use of an implantable catheter system for intraperitoneal chemotherapy in ovarian cancer. Artif Organs 1994;18:328–330.
90. Markman M. Intraperitoneal therapy for treatment of malignant disease principally confined to the peritoneal cavity. Crit Rev Oncol Hematol 1993;14:15–28.
91. Schneider JG. Intraperitoneal chemotherapy. Obstet Gynecol Clin North Am 1994;21:195–212.
92. Myers CE, Collins JM. Pharmacology of intraperitoneal chemotherapy. Cancer Invest 1983;1:395–407.
93. Markman M, Reichman B, Hakes T, et al. Responses to second-line cisplatin-based intraperitoneal therapy in ovarian cancer: Influence of a prior response to intravenous cisplatin. J Clin Oncol 1991;9:1801–1805.
94. Markman M, Berek JS, Blessing JA, et al. Characteristics of patients with small-volume residual ovarian cancer unresponsive to cisplatin-based ip chemotherapy: Lessons learned from a Gynecologic Oncology Group phase II trial of IP cisplatin and recombinant alpha-interferon [see comments]. Gynecol Oncol 1992;45:3–8.
95. Alberts DS, Liu PY, Hannigan EV, et al. Phase III study of intraperitoneal (IP) cisplatin (CDDP)/intravenous (IV) cyclophosphamide (CPA) vs IV CDDP/IV CPA in patients (PT) with optimal disease stage III ovarian cancer: A SWOG–GOG–ECOG Intergroup study (INT 0051) [abstract]. Proc Am Soc Clin Oncol 1995;14:273.
96. Kirmani S, Braly PS, McClay EF, et al. A comparison of intravenous versus intraperitoneal chemotherapy for the initial treatment of ovarian cancer. Gynecol Oncol 1994;54:338–344.
97. Piver MS, Recio FO, Baker TR, Driscoll D. Evaluation of survival after second-line intraperitoneal cisplatin-based chemotherapy for advanced ovarian cancer. Cancer 1994;73:1693–1698.
98. Los G, Mutsaers PH, Vijgh WJ, et al. Direct diffusion of cis-diamminedichloroplatinum(II) in intraperitoneal rat tumors after intraperitoneal chemotherapy: A comparison with systemic chemotherapy. Cancer Res 1989;49:3380–3384.
99. Markman M, Hakes T, Reichman B, et al. Phase II trial of weekly or biweekly intraperitoneal mitoxantrone in epithelial ovarian cancer. J Clin Oncol 1991;9:978–982.
100. Markman M, Francis P, Rowinsky E, et al. Intraperitoneal Taxol (paclitaxel) in the management of ovarian cancer. Ann Oncol 1994;5:S55–S58.
101. Markman M, Francis P, Rowinsky E, Hoskins W. Intraperitoneal paclitaxel: A possible role in the management of ovarian cancer? Semin Oncol 1995;22:84–87.
102. Chiara S, Conte P, Franzone P, et al. High-risk early-stage ovarian cancer. Randomized clinical trial comparing cisplatin plus cyclophosphamide versus whole abdominal radiotherapy. Am J Clin Oncol 1994;17:72–76.
103. Fyles AW, Dembo AJ, Bush RS, et al. Analysis of complications in patients treated with abdomino-pelvic radiation therapy for ovarian carcinoma. Int J Radiat Oncol Biol Phys 1992;22:847–851.
104. Soper JT, Berchuck A, Dodge R, Clarke-Pearson DL. Adjuvant therapy with intraperitoneal chromic phosphate (^{32}P) in women with early ovarian carcinoma after comprehensive surgical staging. Obstet Gynecol 1992;79:993–997.
105. Vergote IB, Vergote-De Vos LN, Abeler VM, et al. Randomized trial comparing cisplatin with radioactive phosphorus or whole-abdomen irradiation as adjuvant treatment of ovarian cancer. Cancer 1992;69:741–749.
106. Shpall EJ, Clarke-Pearson D, Soper JT, et al. High-dose alkylating agent chemotherapy with autologous bone marrow support in patients with stage III/IV epithelial ovarian cancer. Gynecol Oncol 1990;38:386–391.
107. Shea TC, Flaherty M, Elias A, et al. A phase I clinical and pharmacokinetic study of carboplatin and autologous bone marrow support. J Clin Oncol 1989;7:651–661.
108. Shpall EJ, Jones RB, Bearman S. High-dose therapy with autologous bone marrow transplantation for the treatment of solid tumors. Curr Opin Oncol 1994;6:135–138.
109. Mulder PO, Willemse PH, Aalders JG, et al. High-dose chemotherapy with autologous bone marrow transplantation in patients with refractory ovarian cancer. Eur J Cancer Clin Oncol 1989;25:645–649.
110. Dauplat J, Legros M, Condat P, et al. High-dose melphalan and autologous bone marrow support for treatment of ovarian carcinoma with positive second-look operation. Gynecol Oncol 1989;34:294–298.
111. Williams SD. Chemotherapy of ovarian germ cell tumors. Hematol Oncol Clin North Am 1991;5:1261–1269.
112. Segelov E, Campbell J, Ng M, et al. Cisplatin-based chemotherapy for ovarian germ cell malignancies: the Australian experience [see comments]. J Clin Oncol 1994;12:378–384.
113. Williams S, Blessing JA, Liao SY, et al. Adjuvant therapy of ovarian germ cell tumors with cisplatin, etoposide, and bleomycin: A trial of the Gynecologic Oncology Group. J Clin Oncol 1994;12:701–706.
114. Gershenson DM. Update on malignant ovarian germ cell tumors. Cancer 1993;71:1581–1590.

Chapter 126

Acute Leukemias

Steven P. Smith, PharmD, BCPS, and Mary E. Teresi, PharmD

The leukemias are heterogenous hematologic malignancies characterized by unregulated proliferation of the blood-forming cells of the bone marrow. These immature proliferating leukemia cells (blasts) physically "crowd out" or inhibit normal cellular maturation in bone marrow, resulting in anemia, granulocytopenia, and thrombocytopenia. Leukemic blasts may also leave the bone marrow and infiltrate a variety of tissues such as lymph nodes, skin, liver, spleen, kidney, and the central nervous system (CNS).

The term *leukemia* was coined by Virchow to describe the "white blood" of some patients that he saw under the microscope in 1847.[1] Ehrlich later developed cellular staining techniques that led to Naegeli's classification of the disease into lymphocytic and myelocytic types in 1900.[1] Historically, leukemia has also been classified as acute or chronic based on differences in cell of origin and cell line maturation, patient life expectancy, clinical presentation, rapidity of progression of the untreated disease, and response to therapy. Using these categories, four major leukemias are recognized: acute lymphocytic leukemia (ALL), acute nonlymphocytic leukemia (ANLL), chronic lymphocytic leukemia (CLL), and chronic myeloid leukemia (CML). Acute leukemias are characterized by undifferentiated, immature cells that autonomously proliferate. Chronic leukemias also autonomously proliferate but the cells are more differentiated and mature.[2,3] Untreated, the acute leukemias are rapidly progressive, resulting in death in 2–3 months.

Approximately 25,700 new cases of acute and chronic leukemias are diagnosed per year in the United States, accounting for 2% of the total cancer incidence. The incidence has been relatively stable for 30 years. An estimated 20,400 deaths per year and 3.7% of all cancer deaths are due to leukemias. It is the seventh most common cause of cancer-related death in women and sixth in men. In adults, acute and chronic leukemias occur at equal rates. There are approximately 5 cases of acute leukemia per 100,000 individuals. More than 90% of these cases occur in adults. Each year, the total number of cases diagnosed in adults exceeds 10,400 of ANLL and 2600 of ALL. Most adult ALL appears between 20 and 40 years of age while ANLL appears between ages 35 and 65.[2,4] The incidence of ANLL rises with age from 1 in 100,000 individuals under 30 to 14 per 100,000 older than age 75.[3] Acute leukemia is slightly more common in males than in females. In the United States, acute leukemia is slightly more common among whites than blacks.[2,4–6]

Despite the low overall leukemia incidence rate, in children less than 15 years old, the acute leukemias are the most common malignancy, and rank second only to accidents in mortality.[7] Of the 2600 new cases each year, 2000 of them are ALL, 500 are ANLL, and 100 are chronic leukemias.[7] The annual incidence of the childhood acute leukemias is 40 and 24 per 1,000,000 in white and black children under 15 years of age, respectively. Unlike adult leukemia, ALL accounts for about 75% of the pediatric leukemias. Childhood ALL has a slight male dominance (1.4:1) and peaks at age 4 years.[9] ANLL has not displayed any gender or racial preference and occurs throughout childhood without any peak age periods. Acute leukemia during the first 4 weeks of life is usually ANLL.[10]

Chemotherapy has dramatically improved the outlook of patients with acute leukemia. More than 80% of children and young adults with acute leukemia achieve an initial complete remission from their disease. Overall, only 65% of adults achieve an initial complete remission.[4,9] Long-term survival in children ranges from 30–90% depending on the type of leukemia and patient risk factors. The prognosis of adult acute leukemia is generally worse than that of childhood leukemia, with only 20–40% of patients becoming long-term survivors.[4,9]

ETIOLOGY

The exact cause of the acute leukemias is not known. A multifactorial process is likely, involving genetics, environmental factors, toxins, immunologic status, and viral exposures. Table 126.1 summarizes the major factors that have been linked to acute leukemias.[1,3–5,10–13] In pediatric ALL, a number of factors have been investigated as possible causes: the electromagnetic fields of high-voltage power lines; maternal use of alcohol; parental exposure to drugs or chemicals; or chemical contamination of groundwater.[9] In

TABLE 126.1. CONDITIONS ASSOCIATED WITH AN INCREASED FREQUENCY OF ACUTE LEUKEMIA

Drugs	**Chemicals**
Alkylating agents	Benzene
Epipodophyllotoxins	**Radiation**
Chloramphenicol	Electromagnetic radiation
Phenylbutazone	**Viruses**
Genetic Conditions	HTLV-1
Down syndrome	**Smoking**
Bloom's syndrome	Cigarette
Fanconi's anemia	Maternal marijuana use
Kleinfelter's syndrome	
Ataxia telangiectasia	
Wiskott–Aldrich syndrome	
Turner's syndrome	
Severe combined immunodeficiency	
Kostman's syndrome	
Neurofibromatosis	

most patients who develop leukemia, a causative agent cannot be identified.

PATHOGENESIS

A basic understanding of normal hematopoiesis is needed before one can understand the pathogenesis of leukemia. Normal hematopoiesis consists of multiple, well-orchestrated steps of cellular development. A pool of pluripotent stem cells undergoes differentiation, maturation, and proliferation to form the mature blood cells seen in the peripheral circulation. These pluripotent stem cells initially differentiate to form two distinct stem-cell pools. The myeloid stem cell gives rise to six types of blood cells (erythrocytes, platelets, monocytes, basophils, neutrophils, and eosinophils), whereas the lymphoid stem cell differentiates to form circulating B and T lymphocytes. Leukemia may develop at any stage and within any cell line. As an example, Fig. 126.1 illustrates sites along the development of the myeloid cell at which myeloid leukemias could arise.

Two features are common to both ANLL and ALL. Both arise from a single leukemic cell that proliferates (monoclonality). Secondly, there is a failure to maintain a relative balance between proliferation and differentiation, so that the cells do not differentiate past a particular stage of hematopoiesis but then proliferate uncontrollably. Proliferation and differentiation are under genetic control and when the balance between the two is altered in favor of proliferation, leukemia occurs. New antileukemia drug therapies are being developed that are specifically targeted at restoring differentiation.[1]

ANLL affects the hematopoietic cell population and probably arises from a defect in the pluripotent stem cell or a more committed myeloid precursor resulting in partial

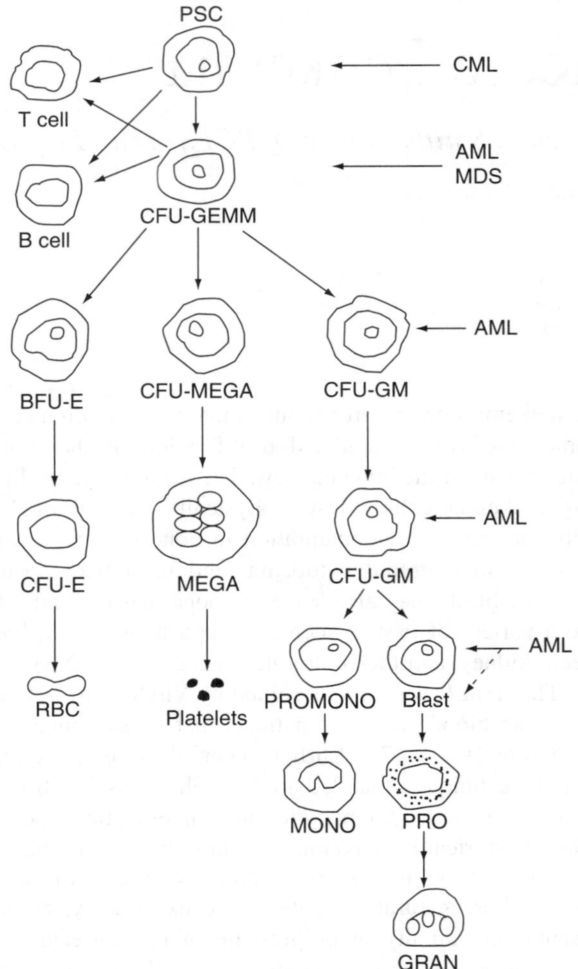

Figure 126.1. Cells of origin for ANLL. Acute nonlymphocytic leukemia may develop at different levels of differentiation and maturation of the myeloid cell line. ALL is synonymous with ANLL in this figure. The sites of development of chronic myelogenous leukemia (CML) and myelodysplastic syndrome (MDS) are also indicated. *(Adapted from Griffin JD, Lowenberg B. Clonogenic cells in acute myeloblastic leukemia. Blood 1986:68:1189.)*

differentiation and proliferation of immature precursors of the myeloid blood-forming cells.[4] One cell type usually dominates and results in the different morphologic and histochemical classifications of ANLL. The French–American–British (FAB) classification system outlined in Table 126.2 identifies eight different morphologic subtypes of ANLL. As an example, in acute promyelocytic leukemia, the leukemia cells mature and differentiate up to the stage of the promyelocyte, but no further. They then proliferate as promyelocytes without differentiation or maturation into mature neutrophils.[16,17]

ALL is a disease characterized by proliferation of immature lymphoblasts. In this type of acute leukemia, the defect is probably at the level of the lymphopoietic stem cell or a very early lymphoid precursor.[4,9] Markers on the cell surface or membrane of the lymphoblast can be used to

TABLE 126.2. MORPHOLOGIC (FAB) CLASSIFICATION OF ACUTE NONLYMPHOCYTIC LEUKEMIA

Subtype	Morphologic Features
M_1 Acute myeloblastic leukemia with minimal differentiation	Myeloblasts with scant granules
M_2 Acute myeloblastic leukemia with maturation	Myeloblasts with granules, promyelocytes, few myelocytes
M_3 Acute promyelocytic leukemia	Promyelocytes with prominent granules
M_4 Acute myelomonocytic leukemia	Myeloblasts, promyelocytes, monoblasts, promonoblasts
M_{5a} Acute monoblastic leukemia without differentiation	Large monoblasts with lacy nuclear chromatin and abundant cytoplasm
M_{5b} Acute monoblastic leukemia with differentiation	Monoblasts, promonocytes, monocytes, blood monocytosis
M_6 Acute erythroleukemia	Megaloblastic erythroid precursors, myeloblasts
M_7 Megakaryocytic leukemia	Megakaryocytes, lymphoid morphology, cytoplasmic budding

(Adapted from Lukens JN. Classification and differentiation of the acute leukemias, in Lee GR, Bithell TC, Foerster J, et al (eds): Wintrobe's Clinical Hematology, 9th ed. Philadelphia, Lea and Febiger, 1993, pp 1873–1891.)

classify ALL (Table 126.3). Advances in the use of monoclonal antibodies for surface markers led to the recognition of subclasses of B- and T-cell lineages. ALL may also be described by cytogenetic abnormalities. Chromosomes may be too many (hyperploidy) or too few (hypoploidy) or exhibit specific translocations.[8]

Leukemic cells have a growth advantage over normal cells, leading to a "crowding out" phenomenon in the bone marrow. This growth advantage is not due to more rapid proliferation as compared with normal cells,[18] but is probably due to a factor produced by leukemic cells that inhibits normal cellular proliferation and differentiation or to a lower rate of leukemic cell loss compared with normal blood cells.[19]

The exact genetic alterations that lead to leukemia have only recently become evident. The defect may be activation of a normally suppressed gene to create an oncogene that signals unregulated proliferation, differentiation, or survival. All normal cells are programmed to die at some time, but in cancer cells, the appropriate programmed signal is interrupted, leading to continued survival and replication. There are four types of genetic defects that lead to inappropriate proliferation and differentiation. The leukemia genes may send either (1) a growth stimulation signal from the cell membrane to the nucleus, (2) a signal to enhance transcription of DNA to RNA, (3) a signal for differentiation, or (4) a signal to prevent programmed death. A second genetic cause of leukemia is the loss or disturbance of genes that suppress cancer's development.[20] These genes are referred to as tumor suppressor genes. The tumor suppressor gene *p53* is found in some hematologic malignancies. Alterations in *p53* are found in 15% of ANLL patients and 3% of common ALL patients.[21] Some forms of ALL have a *p53* frequency of 50%.[21] Normal *p53* allows cells to stop in the G_1 phase of the cell cycle. Mutant *p53* does not stop the cells in G_1, but allows cells to proliferate unregulated, a characteristic of leukemia. The net effect of these genetic changes is to give either the leukemia cell a proliferative advantage over normal hematopoietic cells or to prevent normal differentiation and cell death of the leukemia cell.[20] Certain antileukemia drugs such as doxorubicin can actually induce normal *p53* production.[22]

TABLE 126.3. MORPHOLOGIC (FAB) CLASSIFICATION OF ACUTE LYMPHOCYTIC LEUKEMIA

Subtype	Cells of Origin	Morphologic Features
L_1	Early pre-B cell Pre-B cell B cell T cell	Small cell with indistinct nucleoli, scant cytoplasm, regular nucleus shape
L_2	Early pre-B cell Pre-B cell B cell T cell	Large cell with prominent nucleoli, abundant cytoplasm, irregular nucleus shape
L_3	B cell	Large cell with prominent nucleoli, abundant cytoplasm, regular nucleus shape

(Adapted from Lukens JN. Classification and differentiation of the acute leukemias, in Lee GR, Bithell TC, Foerster J, et al (eds): Wintrobe's Clinical Hematology, 9th ed. Philadelphia, Lea and Febiger, 1993, pp 1873–1891.)

Another example of a genetic defect leading to acute leukemia is the *ras* gene. This gene is involved in cell signal pathways for proliferation and differentiation. Point mutations in the *ras* gene lead to unregulated proliferation and differentiation. Thirty percent of ANLL patients demonstrate a defect in the *ras* gene. It is less common in ALL.[20]

Last, in one form of ANLL, acute promyelocytic leukemia (APL), there is a specific chromosomal aberration that leads directly to the cessation of cell differentiation.[16] In APL, there is a reciprocal translocation between chromosomes 15 and 17. The rearrangement leads to formation of an oncogenic retinoic acid receptor gene. Normally the retinoic acid receptor gene codes for a protein that serves as a receptor for retinoids—vitamin A analogues—that promote differentiation of the promyelocyte to its mature myeloid form. The oncogenic retinoic acid receptor gene codes instead for a protein that impairs differentiation of the promyelocyte and impairs programmed cell death.[16]

Clinical Presentation

SIGNS AND SYMPTOMS

The signs and symptoms of acute leukemia are nonspecific and can be attributed to replacement of normal functional blood cells with immature dysfunctional leukemic cells and to leukemic infiltration of a specific organ or site.[4] Anemia often manifests as lassitude, malaise, and pallor. Fatigue is the most common symptom, and is usually worse than expected for the degree of anemia. Less commonly, palpitations or dyspnea on exertion may be noted. Granulocytopenia may present as fever with or without frank infection. Thrombocytopenia may manifest as simple petechiae or frank bleeding or bruising, often involving the gums, skin, or gastrointestinal tract. Menorrhagia may be seen in premenopausal women. Because leukemic infiltrates may involve any organ, unusual presenting symptoms such as seizures, gum hypertrophy, loss of vision, the presence of an abnormal mass, or bone pain may also be observed. Leukemic meningitis occurs at presentation in fewer than 5% of patients. Headache, diplopia, nausea, or vomiting may be reported or the patient with meningeal involvement may be asymptomatic. As is frequently seen with many types of cancer, mild weight loss may be present. Patients with acute leukemia in 10% of cases can be diagnosed by routine blood analysis without any significant history of physical findings.[5,9,17]

PHYSICAL AND LABORATORY FINDINGS

Physical findings are compatible with anemia (pallor, tachycardia, cardiac murmurs), granulocytopenia (infection, fever), thrombocytopenia (bruising, frank bleeding, petechiae, ecchymoses, purpura, menorrhagia), and leukemic infiltration (lymphadenopathy, splenomegaly, hepatomegaly, sternal tenderness). Petechiae and ecchymoses are more common in ANLL. Bone pain, hepatomegaly, and splenomegaly are more common in ALL. Lymphadenopathy is rare in ANLL but is common in ALL. Other physical findings related to leukemia cell infiltration include cervical lymphadenopathy, gingival hypertrophy, cranial palsies, and skin infiltration. Skin or soft tissue infiltration by myeloid leukemia creates a chloroma, so named because intracellular enzymes create a greenish discoloration, similar to chlorophyll.[4,5]

Anemia and decreased reticulocytes are nearly always present because of decreased red blood cell production. The anemia is usually normocytic and normochromic. The hemoglobin is usually reduced to about 8 gm/dL.[4] The platelet count is reduced in nearly all patients; the median being 40,000–50,000/μL. The white blood cell (WBC) count is normal or elevated in about 85% of patients with ALL; in some patients, the white blood cell count is greatly elevated (>50,000/μL).[4,9,17] Hyperleukocytosis can be life threatening, especially in ANLL, because blasts can occlude small vessels in the brain, heart, lungs, or elsewhere.[4] A high WBC count is often associated with T-cell ALL.[2] In adults with ANLL, the WBC count at the time of diagnosis will be elevated in one-third, normal in one-third, and low in one-third. The peripheral blood smear usually demonstrates a decrease in normal granulocytes, with an increase in blasts.[4,17]

Serum uric acid is mildly elevated in about one-half of patients with adult leukemia. Occasionally, patients may present with renal failure secondary to uric acid nephropathy. Serum calcium imbalances may be noted. In patients with mild renal failure, hypocalcemia may be seen and is usually accompanied by hyperphosphatemia. Hypercalcemia is often due to ectopic parathyroid hormone production by leukemic cells, or rapid destruction of large numbers of leukemic cells. Hyperkalemia may also occur secondary to rapid cell kill. Hypoalbuminemia occurs in up to 40% of acute leukemia patients. Hypogammaglobulinemia is also present in some patients.[5,9]

APL or M_3 ANLL is characterized by many of the same signs and symptoms as other types of ANLL. One important difference is the propensity of APL to cause disseminated intravascular coagulation. This syndrome is characterized by thrombocytopenia, hypofibrinoginemia, depletion of clotting factors, and a bleeding diathesis. The unusual laboratory values are helpful to identify this subtype of ANLL so that therapy specific for it may be instituted (see section on Acute Promyelocytic Leukemia).[23]

Marrow biopsy and aspirate are necessary to establish a diagnosis and follow disease progression and response to therapy. At diagnosis, the marrow is usually hypercellular with a predominance of blasts. Leukemia is diagnosed if more than 30% of the marrow cells are blasts. If the percentage is less than 5%, then the marrow is considered normal. If the marrow has 5–30% leukemic blasts, the term "myelodysplasia" is used and the latter condition is considered a preleukemic state that will eventually evolve into frank ANLL.[5]

Risk Factors

Many clinical and laboratory features at diagnosis have been associated with response to treatment. Identification of these risk factors may allow the oncologist to better understand the disease and to tailor treatment according to the predicted response. They aid to identify patients most likely to attain a complete remission, maintain that remission, and experience long-term survival. For example, if a patient has many clinical and laboratory features that are associated with a good response to chemotherapy ("good risk"), then the oncologist may choose to give less intensive therapy to

TABLE 126.4. PROGNOSTIC FACTORS IN ACUTE LYMPHOCYTIC LEUKEMIA RISK FOR LEUKEMIC RELAPSE

Factor	Low	High
Morphology[a]	L_1	L_2, L_3
Immunologic phenotype	Early pre-B cell	Null cell, T cell, pre-B cell, B cell
Philadelphia chromosome	Absent	Present
Cytogenetics	Normal karyotype	Abnormal karyotype
Myeloid markers	Absent	Present
WBC count at diagnosis[a]	$<10,000/mm^3$	$>50,000/mm^3$
Hemoglobin	<7 gm/dL	>10 gm/dL
Platelets[a]	$>100,000/mm^3$	$<30,000/mm^3$
Patient age[a]	3–7 yr	<1 yr or >10 yr
Patient gender[a]	Female	Male
Race	White	Black
CNS leukemia	Absent	Present
Node/liver[a]/spleen enlargement	Absent	Massive
Mediastinal mass[a]	Absent	Present
Time to remission[a]	<14 days	>14 days

[a]Factors with greatest relative importance. (Adapted from Lukens JN. Acute lymphocytic leukemia, in Lee GR, Bithell TC, Foerster J, et al (eds): Wintrobe's Clinical Hematology, 9th ed. Philadelphia, PA, Lea and Febiger, 1993, 1892–1919, and Poplack DG. Acute lymphoblastic leukemia, in Pizzo PA, Poplack DG (eds): Principles and Practice of Pediatric Oncology, 2nd ed. Philadelphia, JB Lippincott, 1993, pp 431–481.)

reduce the risk of long-term toxic effects. Conversely, if a patient is not likely to respond well to therapy ("high or poor risk"), then the oncologist may choose to give more intensive chemotherapy.

In adults with ALL, recent studies have identified several risk factors that correlate with prognosis (Table 126.4). Because most patients with ALL achieve a complete clinical remission, these factors refer to the risk of leukemic relapse rather than the risk of not achieving a complete remission. Adult patients generally have a poorer prognosis than children. Several characteristics of the disease, drug activity, and patient tolerance of treatment make for a poorer outcome in adult ALL (Table 126.5).

In childhood ALL, similar prognostic factors apply (Table 126.4). Analysis of these factors in a large series of children revealed that the most important factors were the WBC, gender, presence of a mediastinal mass, no evidence of disease in day 14 bone marrow, age, platelet count, liver size, and morphologic type. Several chromosomal translocations and abnormalities have been recognized as specifically denoting good or poor risk. The number of chromosomes is also important, with hyperploidy (more than 50 per cell) being a good risk factor and hypoploidy (less than 45 per cell) being a poor risk factor.[8] Prognostic factors are routinely used to categorize pediatric patients according to their likelihood of cure from chemotherapy.[9]

Prognostic factors in adult ANLL have not been as well defined as in adult ALL, but several patient- and disease-related factors have been reported to influence prognosis. The most important patient factor is age, with younger patients more likely to achieve a complete remission than older patients (older than age 60).[11] The lower complete remission rate in older patients appears to result from increased frequency of fatal infectious and bleeding complications as well as chemotherapy resistance.[4] The duration of remission is also shorter in older patients compared to younger ones. Other patient-specific prognostic factors include overall performance status and any major organ impairment.[5] FAB morphologic subtype may be a factor, with types M_6 and M_7 having the worst outcome.[11] Patients with extramedullary disease, CNS involvement, or underlying myelodysplastic syndrome have a worse prognosis.[11] Certain cytogenetic abnormali-

TABLE 126.5. FEATURES OF ADULT ALL THAT CONTRIBUTE TO POORER PROGNOSIS COMPARED WITH CHILDHOOD ALL

Disease Biology

1. Increased frequency of cytogenetic abnormalities
2. Increased incidence of expression of myeloid antigens
3. Less frequent early pre-B immunophenotype
4. Decreased formation of methotrexate polyglutamates
5. Increased incidence of specific resistance mechanisms (e.g., P-glycoprotein)
6. Increased incidence of high WBC at presentation
7. Slower response to therapy
8. Increased frequency of mediastinal masses

Treatment Tolerance

1. Poorer tolerance by the bone marrow to treatment
2. Increased extramedullary intolerance (e.g., heart, liver)
3. Poorer tolerance to specific drugs (e.g., asparaginase)
4. Poorer compliance with intensive protocols

(Adapted from Copelan EA, McGuire EA. The biology and treatment of acute lymphoblastic leukemia in adults. Blood 1995;85:1151–1168.)

ties are also known to worsen the response rate and survival of patients with ANLL.[11] In addition, patients who develop a "secondary" leukemia after treatment of another malignancy usually have a very poor response to antileukemic chemotherapy, depending on the cytogenetic abnormality that develops.[5,17]

In pediatric ANLL, some prognostic factors have been identified but not consistently from study to study.[10] Factors that reduce the chances of a complete remission include an initial WBC greater than 100,000/mm^3, FAB classification M_1 without Auer rods present, having underlying myelodysplasia and having ANLL secondary to prior chemotherapy or radiation therapy. Remission duration is affected by the same factors as well as age under 2 years, a high fraction of cells in S phase at any time, requiring two or more courses of chemotherapy to achieve a complete remission, and, finally, having the M_5 subtype.[10] Some genetic abnormalities have been recognized for prognostic significance such as translocation of chromosomes 9 and 11 (good prognosis) and monosomy 7 (poor prognosis). Unlike pediatric ALL in which several prognostic factors clearly can be used to assess risk of relapse, the prognostic factors associated with pediatric ANLL lack the strong relationship to predict outcome from therapy.

TREATMENT

The short-term goal of treatment for acute leukemia is to rapidly achieve a complete clinical and hematologic remission. In the absence of a complete remission, a rapid and fatal outcome is inevitable. Complete remission is defined as the disappearance of all clinical and bone marrow evidence (normal cellularity with <5% blasts) of leukemia, with restoration of normal hematopoiesis. Partial remission is a significant response to treatment, although evidence of residual disease (5–25% blasts) in the bone marrow remains.

After a complete remission is achieved, the goal is to maintain the patient in continuous complete remission. As discussed later, the occurrence of leukemic relapse in the bone marrow usually removes any hope of cure of the disease. Of those patients who will die from acute leukemia, most die within the first 5 years and survival beyond the fifth year after therapy does not continue to decline as rapidly.

ACUTE LYMPHOCYTIC LEUKEMIA

Treatment of adult ALL has been modeled after treatment of childhood ALL. Although treatment results with adult ALL are worse than those with childhood ALL, recent use of aggressive therapy in adult ALL has increased the complete remission rate to 65–85% and the proportion of 5-year disease-free survivors to 20–30%.[4] In adults, the median remission duration is 19–27 months and the median survival time is approximately 2 years.[5] Therapy for adult ALL has been designed after treatment for childhood ALL and was historically divided into four phases: (1) remission induction, (2) CNS prophylaxis, (3) consolidation therapy, and (4) maintenance therapy (Fig. 126.2). Recently more complex regimens have been explored and the lines between phases of therapy are less clear. All adult patients still receive some form of initial induction therapy but it may require 2 months to administer two separate phases of induction. Some form of postremission therapy is needed to treat microscopic disease and may include some intensive inpatient therapy (consolidation or intensification therapy) followed by less aggressive outpatient therapy (maintenance). CNS prophylaxis is needed at some time during therapy in all adult ALL patients to prevent leukemic

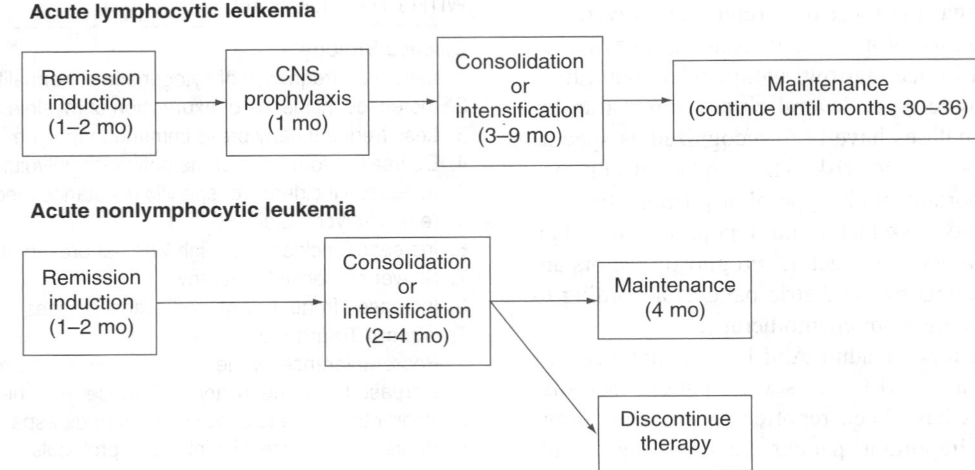

Figure 126.2. Therapy for acute lymphocytic and nonlymphocytic leukemias.

meningitis. Table 126.6 shows several representative treatment regimens for adult ALL.

Remission Induction Therapy

The goal of remission induction is to rapidly induce a complete clinical and hematologic remission. The combination of vincristine and prednisone forms the foundation for induction therapy. Together these two drugs induce complete remission in about 50% of adults with ALL. The addition of an anthracycline (daunorubicin or doxorubicin) to vincristine and prednisone increases the complete remission rate to 83% and carries a treatment-related mortality rate of only 3–17%.[29,30] Substituting asparaginase for an anthracycline may yield a similar complete remission rate and disease-free survival rate but substitutes coagulopathies for congestive heart failure.[31] The addition of a fourth agent to the combination of vincristine, prednisone, and an anthracycline does not dramatically improve the response rate.[32] As seen in Table 126.6, prednisone, vincristine, daunorubicin, and asparaginase are a common combination for remission induction therapy. Asparaginase is often included although few data exist that it significantly improves response in adult ALL patients above that of the other three drugs together. The dosing of prednisone and vincristine is fairly similar from regimen to regimen, but the doses of daunorubicin or asparaginase are diverse. Other agents that are sometimes included in remission induction regimens are cyclophosphamide, cytarabine (high dose or standard dose), mercaptopurine, methotrexate (standard dose or high dose), and mitoxantrone, although it appears that they do not contribute significantly to the efficacy of the remission induction regimen.[33]

Few prospective studies have compared remission induction regimens. The value of adding more drugs to the basic three- or four-drug regimen is unclear. Equally unclear is the value of higher doses of the standard combination of drugs for remission induction. Some data suggest that high-dose methotrexate with cyclophosphamide and cytarabine may improve response and survival in patients with B-cell ALL and that higher doses of cytarabine or cyclophosphamide may be indicated for patients with T-cell ALL.[25,32–34]

In pediatric ALL, therapy is based on the relative risk of relapse. Lower risk patients commonly receive only a glucocorticoid, vincristine, and asparaginase for remission induction. The complete remission rate is near 99%.[8] The induction remission rate for high-risk patients is less than that for low-risk patients (approximately 84% in one study), however, with intensified chemotherapy for induction and postremission therapy, the long-term survival of even the high-risk patients can equal that of lower risk patients.[8,35] In high-risk patients, the induction regimen may include the same three drugs plus two or three others. One approach adds daunorubicin and cyclophosphamide to the combination of a steroid, vincristine, and asparaginase.[35] A second approach uses etoposide, cytarabine, and high-dose methotrexate with the basic three drugs.[36] The important aspect of induction therapy in pediatric ALL is that therapy must be tailored to the relative risk and that a glucocorticoid, vincristine, and asparaginase must be included in the induction regimen.

Central Nervous System Prophylaxis

After patients achieve complete remission, they usually receive CNS prophylaxis. This phase may overlap with or be incorporated into induction or consolidation. The rationale for CNS prophylaxis is based on two observations. First, many chemotherapeutic agents do not readily cross the blood–brain barrier. Second, many patients with ALL with no evidence of CNS involvement at diagnosis experience a relapse of their leukemia in the CNS. The CNS relapse rate without prophylaxis in adult ALL patients is approximately 21–50% and in children it exceeds 50%.[10,33] Current treatment approaches have reduced the incidence to 10–15%.[33,37] These observations indicate that the CNS is a potential sanctuary for leukemic cells and that undetectable leukemic cells are present in the CNS in many patients. CNS involvement is more common in ALL than ANLL. CNS involvement at the time of diagnosis is relatively uncommon (5–10%) in ALL.[5] Factors that have been associated with an increased risk of CNS involvement at diagnosis include a high initial WBC count, rapid leukemic cell proliferation rate (high S fraction), high plasma lactic dehydrogenase, T-cell phenotype, and B-cell phenotype.[33]

The goal of CNS prophylaxis is to eradicate residual but undetectable leukemic cells present in the CNS after remission induction. Leukemic meningitis is more easily prevented than treated. Once CNS relapse has occurred, patients are at increased risk of bone marrow relapse and death from refractory leukemia. It is important to note that the benefit of CNS prophylaxis is not apparent until after 2 years of continuous complete remission. Although CNS prophylaxis has been shown to significantly decrease the risk of CNS relapse in adults, survival in the CNS prophylaxis group was not significantly longer compared with patients not given CNS prophylaxis.[38,39]

Although CNS prophylaxis has not been shown to improve survival in adults with ALL, some form of CNS prophylaxis is usually included in ALL treatment protocols. CNS prophylaxis usually includes cranial irradiation and intrathecal methotrexate to eradicate undetectable leukemia in the cranial region and spinal column, respectively. Cranial irradiation is typically given in 2-Gy fractions to a total dose of 18–24 Gy. Methotrexate 10–15 mg is given intrathecally once or twice weekly for four to six doses. In some protocols, intrathecal cytosine arabinoside (20–100 mg), hydrocortisone (10–35 mg) and methotrexate (12–15 mg) are given together for CNS prophylaxis.[33]

TABLE 126.6. REPRESENTATIVE CHEMOTHERAPY REGIMENS FOR ADULT ACUTE LYMPHOCYTIC LEUKEMIA

Remission Induction		CNS Prophylaxis		Consolidation		Maintenance (Drug, Dose, & Schedule)
(Drug & Dose)	(Days)	(Drug & Dose)	(Days)	(Drug & Dose)	(Days)	
German Regimen[26]						
PRED (PO) 60 mg/m^2	1–28	Cranial irradiation &		DEX (PO) 10 mg/m^2	1–28	MP (PO) 60 mg/m^2 QD
VCR (IV) 1.5 mg/m^2[a]	1,8,15,22	MTX (IT) 10 mg/m^2[b]	31,38,45,52	VCR (IV) 1.5 mg/m^2[a]	1,8,15,22	and
DNR (IV) 25 mg/m^2	1,8,15,22			DOX (IV) 25 mg/m^2	1,8,15,22	MTX (PO/IV) 20 mg/m^2
ASP (IV) 5000 U/m^2	1–14			CTX (IV) 650 mg/m^2[c]		weekly
CTX (IV) 650 mg/m^2[c]	29,43,57				29	Weeks 10–18 and 29–130
ARA-C (IV) 75 mg/m^2	31–34,38–41,			ARA-C (IV) 75 mg/m^2	31–34,38–41	
	45–48,52–55			TG (PO) 60 mg/m^2	29–42	
MP (PO) 60 mg/m^2	29–57					
University of California–San Francisco, Stanford University, and City of Hope Medical Center[27]						
DNR (IV) 50 mg/m^2	1–3	Cranial irradiation &		*Cycles 1,3,5,7*		MTX (PO) 20 mg/m^2
VCR (IV) 2 mg	1,8,15,22	MTX (IT) 12 mg	Weekly × 6			weekly
				DNR (IV) 50 mg/m^2	1,2	MP (PO) 75 mg/m^2 daily
PRED (PO) 60 mg/m^2	1–28			VCR (IV) 2 mg	1,8	until 30 months in
ASP (IM) 6000 U/m^2	17–28			PRED (PO) 60 mg/m^2	1–14	continuous complete
				ASP (IM) 12,000 U/m^2	2,4,7,9,11,14	remission
If day 14 bone marrow has leukemia						
DNR (IV) 50 mg/m^2	15			*Cycles 2,4,6,8*		
				TEN (IV) 165 mg/m^2	1,4,8,11	
If day 28 bone marrow has leukemia				ARA-C (IV) 300 mg/m^2	1,4,8,11	
DNR (IV) 50 mg/m^2	29,30					
VCR (IV) 2 mg	29,36			*Cycle 9*		
PRED (PO) 60 mg/m^2	29–42			MTX (IV) 690 mg/m^2 over 42 h		
ASP (IM) 6000 U/m^2	29–35			LEUC (IV) 15 mg/m^2 Q6h × 12 doses, beginning at 42 h		

CALGB 8811[28]

Course I

CTX (IV) 1200 mg/m^2	1
DNR (IV) 45 mg/m^2	1,2,3
VCR (IV) 2 mg	1,8,15,22
PRED (PO) 60 mg/m^2	1–21
ASP (SC) 6000 U/m^2	5,8,11,15,18,22

For patients ≥ 60 yr old, use:

CTX 800 mg/m^2	day 1
DNR 30 mg/m^2	days 1,2,3
PRED 60 mg/m^2	days 1–7

Course II: Early Intensification

MTX (IT) 15 mg	1
CTX (IV) 1000 mg/m^2	1
MP (PO) 60 mg/m^2	1–14
ARA-C (SC) 75 mg/m^2	1–4,8–11
VCR (IV) 2 mg	15,22
ASP (SC) 6000 U/m^2	15,18,22,25

Course III

Cranial irradiation	
MTX (IT) 15 mg	1,8,15,22,29
MP (PO) 60 mg/m^2	1–70
MTX (PO) 20 mg/m^2	36,43,50,57,64

Course IV: Late Intensification

DOX (IV) 30 mg/m^2	1,8,15
VCR (IV) 2 mg	1,8,15
DEX (PO) 10 mg/m^2	1–14
CTX (IV) 1000 mg/m^2	29
TG (PO) 60 mg/m^2	29–42
ARA-C (SC) 75 mg/m^2	29–32,36–39

Course V

VCR (IV) 2 mg day 1 monthly

PRED (PO) 60 mg/m^2 days 1–5 monthly

MTX (PO) 20 mg/m^2 days 1,8,15,22 monthly

MP (PO) 60 mg/m^2 days 1–28 monthly

Key: ARA-C, cytarabine; ASP, asparaginase; CTX, cyclophosphamide; DEX, dexamethasone; DNR, daunorubicin; DOX, doxorubicin; MP, mercaptopurine; MTX, methotrexate; PRED, prednisone; TEN, teniposide; TG, thioguanine; VCR, vincristine.

[a]Maximum single dose, 2 mg.

[b]Maximum single dose, 15 mg.

[c]Maximum single dose, 1000 mg.

In children, initial trials employed cranial irradiation and intrathecal methotrexate. Subsequent efforts have examined the need for radiation because of long-term effects on cognitive function. Low-risk ALL patients can probably be treated with a combination of cytarabine, methotrexate, and hydrocortisone. High-risk patients require chemotherapy and radiation.[40] The doses of chemotherapeutic agents used in pediatric ALL patients must be individualized by age due to differences in the volume of cerebrospinal fluid between ages 1 and 3 (Table 126.7).

Cranial irradiation and/or chemotherapy has been associated with significant acute and chronic neurotoxic effects in children but in adults the effects are less common and less serious. In children, cranial irradiation has been recognized to cause neuropsychological deficits, growth impairment, and endocrine changes.[9,41] Adults typically experience somnolence, headache, meningismus, transient paraplegia, arachnoiditis, or injection site infections.[17,33] Cranial irradiation can also compromise the dose of total body irradiation used to prepare patients for allogeneic bone marrow transplant as well as limit the amount of subsequent systemic chemotherapy that can be given because of an increased incidence of adverse effects.[28] This latter problem presumably occurs because cranial irradiation increases permeability of the blood–brain barrier to toxic chemotherapeutic agents.[42] In an effort to reduce the neurotoxicity of CNS prophylaxis, several trials have examined the use of systemic chemotherapy or intrathecal methotrexate alone without cranial irradiation as CNS prophylaxis.[43,44] Intrathecal methotrexate alone yielded a CNS relapse rate of 3% in one trial.[44] Patients who receive high-dose methotrexate (100–300 mg/kg/d monthly for 12 months) may have a CNS relapse rate as low as 8.3%, and with high-dose cytarabine (2 g/m^2 every 12 hours for 12 doses) with systemic methotrexate (200–800 mg/m^2), the rate is 11%.[43,45] Recent prospective studies have demonstrated that intravenous high-dose methotrexate alone or intermediate-dose methotrexate with intrathecal triple chemotherapy can offer equal protection against CNS relapse as standard cranial irradiation and intrathecal methotrexate.[9]

TABLE 126.7. INTRATHECAL THERAPY IN PEDIATRIC ALL[a]

Age (yr)	Cytarabine (mg)	Methotrexate (mg)	Hydrocortisone (mg)
0–1	20	6	10
1–2	30	8	15
2–3	50	10	25
>3	70	12	35

[a]If all three drugs are to be administered concurrently, a 3 to 1 to 2 ratio of cytarabine, methotrexate, and hydrocortisone could be used to simplify preparation.

The selection of a CNS prophylactic regimen must consider efficacy, toxicity, and risk of CNS disease. Patients with low risk of ALL relapse may be adequately treated with only intrathecal therapy. Those with high-risk ALL may need a combination of intrathecal and systemic chemotherapy. Because few randomized studies have compared different CNS regimens in ALL, it is not possible to recommend any one regimen over another. Based on the experience with childhood ALL, CNS prophylaxis should be included in treatment protocols for both childhood and adult ALL and should include intrathecal methotrexate either alone or combined with cranial irradiation, or intravenous infusions of intermediate-dose methotrexate with intrathecal triple chemotherapy, or intravenous high-dose methotrexate or high-dose cytarabine alone.

Consolidation Therapy

Consolidation therapy in adult ALL is started after a complete remission has been achieved and refers to continued intensive chemotherapy in an attempt to eradicate clinically undetectable disease. Many regimens usually incorporate either non-cross-resistant drugs different from the induction regimen or else high-dose chemotherapy.[32] The specific benefit of any one consolidation therapy is difficult to demonstrate because of the overall complexity of therapy in ALL. Randomized trials have been equivocal in demonstrating a survival benefit.[33] The three regimens listed in Table 126.6 offer three different approaches to consolidation with similar results. The German regimen mostly imitates the induction regimen, but substitutes dexamethasone for prednisone (better CNS penetration to prevent leukemic meningitis), doxorubicin for daunorubicin, and thioguanine for mercaptopurine.[26] The study from California employs teniposide, cytarabine, and intermediate-dose methotrexate with drugs also used in induction.[27] Finally, the CALGB (Cancer and Leukemia Group B) trial uses a consolidation regimen far more complicated than the induction regimen. The latter includes different drugs and higher doses, at least with the cyclophosphamide dose.[28] The outcomes from these distinctly different trials are similar. The German investigators found a median survival of 27.5 months and the estimated 5-year survival to be 39%.[26] The California group reported, after a median follow-up of 77 months, that 35% of patients could expect long-term disease-free survival.[27] The CALGB study reported a short follow-up time (median 43 months) so that only 3-year estimates were available; however, the results included a median survival of 36 months and an overall survival of 39% for those 30–59 years old.[28] A consolidation phase in adult ALL therapy appears necessary, although specific questions remain about drug selection, duration of therapy, dosing, and timing of administration.

A phase of dose-intensified chemotherapy usually follows induction in pediatric ALL therapy, especially in patients with recognized poor risk factors. The drugs chosen are similar to those used in adults and no specific combination can be considered standard care. Clinical trials incorporating consolidation in the treatment of high-risk ALL have reported long-term survival for 65–70% of patients.[9]

Maintenance Therapy

Many patients relapse shortly after completion of remission induction and consolidation therapy, presumably because of residual disease. The goal of maintenance therapy is, therefore, to further eradicate residual leukemic cells and prolong remission duration. While maintenance therapy is clearly beneficial in childhood ALL, the possible benefit in adults has only recently been suggested. In some adult ALL trials that included induction and consolidation, but omitted maintenance, the disease-free survival at 2 years was only 18–35% compared to a survival rate of almost 40% in trials that included maintenance.[46,47]

As with childhood ALL, maintenance therapy usually consists of mercaptopurine and methotrexate, at doses that produce minimal myelosuppression, with or without intermittent "pulses" of vincristine and prednisone.[4] The typical doses for these agents in this phase are listed in Table 126.6. Some of the best results have been reported with a complicated treatment program that includes intensive consolidation and maintenance phases[44]; however, similar results were reported with two other treatment protocols that included standard mercaptopurine and low-dose methotrexate as maintenance therapy.[26,27] As discussed previously, both of those treatment programs included an intensive consolidation phase, suggesting that standard low-dose maintenance therapy may be adequate when an intensive consolidation phase is included.

The optimal duration of maintenance therapy in adults and children is unknown, but most treatment programs continue maintenance therapy for at least 30 months. Most recently, clinicians have begun to make decisions about maintenance therapy based on what subtype of ALL is found. Common pre-B-cell ALL does benefit from conventional maintenance therapy with methotrexate and mercaptopurine. Patients with B-cell ALL or Philadelphia chromosome positive ALL probably gain greater benefit from intensive induction and consolidation and little from maintenance.[33]

One final issue in maintenance therapy of pediatric ALL has been the recognition that interpatient variability in the pharmacokinetics of oral methotrexate and mercaptopurine can affect outcome. Slow absorbers of either drug have higher relapse rates. Similarly, rapid eliminators are at risk of treatment failure because of decreased exposure to methotrexate or mercaptopurine.[48–50] To account for the interpatient variability, some clinicians titrate the dose of either agent to maintain a WBC of 1500–4000/mm^3. The importance of pharmacokinetics in adults is less well defined.

ALL in the Elderly

ALL occurs rarely in patients older than age 60 and no specific treatment recommendations can be made. Recent trials including patients older than age 60 demonstrated that the 3-year survival rate could be up to 20%.[34] In CALGB 8811 (Table 126.6), 9% of the patients were over age 60. The complete remission rate was approximately 65%, but the 3-year survival was only 17%.[28] In general, older patients have a lower complete remission rate and, when achieved, the duration of remission is shorter than that of younger patients.

ACUTE NONLYMPHOCYTIC LEUKEMIA

ANLL accounts for the majority of acute leukemia in adults and occurs with increasing frequency in elderly patients. It accounts for only 20% of the acute leukemias in children. With recent advances in chemotherapy and supportive care, 60–80% of all patients achieve complete remission and 15–30% become long-term survivors.[6,51] Overall, the median duration of remission is 1–2 years.[51] In patients older than age 60, the median duration of remission is shorter than 1 year. In contrast to ALL, all of the active drugs in ANLL are marrow suppressive, with the exception of *trans*-retinoic acid. As a result, patients with ANLL, particularly elderly patients (older than age 60), are at greater risk for treatment-related fatal infectious and bleeding complications.

Treatment of ANLL, unlike that of ALL, usually consists only of induction and intensive postremission therapy. Occasionally a maintenance phase is administered, although this phase is less commonly used today (Fig. 126.2). CNS prophylaxis is not routinely given for ANLL because the risk of CNS relapse is lower than in patients with ALL. Several representative chemotherapeutic regimens for treatment of ANLL are presented in Table 126.8.

Remission Induction Therapy

As with ALL, the goal of remission induction for ANLL is to rapidly induce a complete remission. Compared with ALL, fewer patients with ANLL achieve complete remission. The lower complete remission rate in ANLL is related in part to differences in the toxicity of the drugs in remission induction regimens. In ALL, several active agents are relatively nonmyelosuppressive (prednisone, vincristine, L-asparaginase), whereas in ANLL, every active agent (except *trans*-retinoic acid) is myelosuppressive. As a result, patients with ALL may achieve complete remission without severe and prolonged marrow hypoplasia. In contrast, since the complete remission rate in ANLL is related

TABLE 126.8. REPRESENTATIVE CHEMOTHERAPY REGIMENS FOR ADULT ACUTE NONLYMPHOCYTIC LEUKEMIA

Remission Induction	Intensive Postremission Therapy	Maintenance Therapy
Southeastern Cancer Study Group[52]		
Cytarabine 100 mg/m^2/d continuous infusion days 1–7 Idarubicin 12 mg/m^2/d days 1–3	Cytarabine 100 mg/m^2 every 12 h × 10 doses Thioguanine 100 mg/m^2 PO every 12 h for 10 doses Idarubicin 15 mg/m^2/d on day 1 (3 courses)	None
CALGB[53]		
Cytarabine 200 mg/m^2/d continuous infusion days 1–7 Daunorubicin 45 mg/m^2/d days 1–3	Cytarabine 3 g/m^2 every 12 h days 1,3,5 (4 courses) every 12 h days 1–5	Cytarabine 100 mg/m^2 SC Daunorubicin 45 mg/m^2 day 1 (4 courses)
Boston Group[54]		
Daunorubicin 45 mg/m^{2}d days 1–3 Cytarabine 100 mg/m^2/d continuous infusion days 1–7 Cytarabine 2 g/m^2 every 12 h days 8–10	*Cycle 1,3* Daunorubicin 60 mg/m^2/d days 1–2 Cytarabine 200 mg/m^2/d continuous infusion days 1–5 *Cycle 2* Cytarabine 2 g/m^2 every 12 h days 1–3 Etoposide 100 mg/m^2/d days 4–5	

to the intensity of the remission induction regimen, the drugs used in ANLL are given at doses that uniformly cause severe marrow hypoplasia. One reason for the lower complete remission rate in ANLL compared with ALL is the inability to give optimal doses of chemotherapy because of marrow toxicity. With continued improvement of supportive care for patients undergoing chemotherapy, more intensive treatment regimens are being given in an effort to reduce the high rate of leukemic relapse and increase the proportion of long-term survivors.

The most active single agents in ANLL are the anthracycline antibiotics (daunorubicin, doxorubicin, and idarubicin) and the antimetabolite cytarabine (ara-C). The complete remission rate with a combination of cytarabine and an anthracycline is 60–80%.[51–53] The remission rate is lower (approximately 50%) in patients older than age 60.[53] Because daunorubicin has similar antileukemic activity but causes less gastrointestinal toxicity (necrotizing colitis) than doxorubicin, daunorubicin has historically been the preferred anthracycline for remission induction regimens.[55] The optimal dosage schedules for daunorubicin and ara-C are not known, but one randomized study showed that patients who received 7 days of ara-C by continuous intravenous infusion and 3 days of daunorubicin (7 + 3) had a significantly higher complete remission rate than patients who received 5 days of ara-C and 2 days of daunorubicin (5 + 2).[56] This study also showed that patients who received ara-C by continuous intravenous infusion had a higher response rate than those who received ara-C by intravenous bolus. Another study compared the 7 + 3 regimen to a 10 + 3 design with 10 days of cytarabine or to a 7 + 3 regimen with 7 days of 6-thioguanine concurrent with the 7 days of cytarabine.[57] No statistical difference was found between the three induction regimens.

The use of idarubicin has been the most significant advance in adult ANLL induction therapy in recent years. Some studies have shown a significant improvement in complete remission rate over daunorubicin. In the Southeastern Cancer Study Group trial comparing these two drugs, complete remission was achieved in 69% of patients receiving idarubicin/cytarabine compared to 55% of patients receiving conventional daunorubicin/cytarabine. Median survival in this study was not significantly improved (297 days versus 277 days for idarubicin and daunorubicin, respectively).[52] In a similar study with similar complete remission rates, the median time of survival in this study was significantly longer with patients reaching 328–508 days with idarubicin/cytarabine versus 277–435 days for daunorubicin/cytarabine.[58] Idarubicin has replaced daunorubicin as the anthracycline of choice for remission induction in adult ANLL in many protocols. Idarubicin has not been as well tested in pediatric ANLL patients; therefore, daunorubicin or doxorubicin and cytarabine are still commonly used.[8]

The third regimen in Table 126.8 illustrates another maneuver to improve the complete remission rate in adults. Mitus et al.[54] added high-dose cytarabine to conventional 7 & 3. The remission rate after induction therapy in this trial was 89%, which is higher than that achieved in the Southeastern Cancer Study group or the CALGB trial reported in Table 126.8. The validity of this result and the possible impact of substituting idarubicin for daunorubicin in the therapy reported by Mitus et al. remain to be confirmed by other trials.

Most patients achieve a complete remission after one or two courses of chemotherapy. Patients who require additional chemotherapy to achieve a complete remission have been reported to have a poor prognosis, even if remission is ultimately achieved.

Intensive Postremission Therapy

Although most adults with ANLL achieve a complete remission, the duration of remission is short (4–8 months) if no further treatment is given. Relapse is presumably due to the presence of residual but clinically undetectable leukemic cells after remission induction therapy. The goal of intensive postremission therapy (IPRT) is to eradicate these residual leukemic cells and to prevent the emergence of drug-resistant disease. The need for IPRT is based on postmortem analysis and cell kinetic data suggesting that nearly 10^8–10^9 residual leukemic cells remain after effective remission induction therapy.[59]

In the treatment of ANLL, IPRT is often referred to as consolidation or intensification. Consolidation is instituted after a complete remission is achieved but involves the administration of drugs that the patient has not previously received. Intensification therapy is defined as the administration of one or two courses of high doses of the same drugs used for remission induction, immediately after a complete remission is achieved. Intensification may be started early (within a few months of achievement of remission) or late (complete remission longer than 6–12 months). Because consolidation and intensification are sometimes defined differently by different investigators, both phrases are referred to as IPRT throughout this section. IPRT may be defined as the administration of high-dose combination chemotherapy to a patient in complete remission in an attempt to eradicate clinically undetectable disease.

Most centers incorporate some form of IPRT into ANLL therapy. No consensus exists regarding the best drugs, doses, or duration of treatment. The three regimens in Table 126.8 offer three distinctly different approaches to postremission therapy. The Southeastern Group used a consolidation regimen similar to the induction regimen, in terms of dose intensity and drug selection.[52] The median duration of remission in the idarubicin patients was 433 days. CALGB compared three doses of cytarabine: 100 mg/m^2, 400 mg/m^2, and 3 g/m^2.[53] At 4 years, the disease-free survival for all patients was 21, 25, and 39% for the three doses, respectively. Disease-free survival was statistically superior for the 3 g/m^2 dose compared to the other two doses for all patients combined and for patients under age 60. For patients over age 60, disease-free survival at 4 years was not different between the three consolidative regimens. Finally, in the study from Boston, IPRT included a combination of standard-dose cytarabine and daunorubicin for two cycles with a combination of intensified cytarabine with etoposide given in between.[54] Many of the patients later underwent bone marrow transplant. The overall survival at 5 years was 55%.

IPRT using high-dose cytarabine alone or in combination appears promising and is commonly a part of leukemia therapy. High-dose cytarabine refers to doses of 1–3 g/m^2 given by short infusion every 12 hours for 8–12 doses. The toxicity of high-dose cytarabine is discussed in Chapter 119. The emphasis on consolidation evolved from evidence that repeating the induction regimen with the same drugs would only lengthen remission duration from 4–8 months to 10–15 months.[60] The UCLA group compared patients receiving high-dose cytarabine and daunorubicin to an historical control group receiving azacytidine and doxorubicin for IPRT. The control group had a median remission duration of 9 months and a 5-year survival of 24%. Using high-dose cytarabine with daunorubicin, the UCLA group observed a median remission duration of 23 months, with 32% of the patients alive after 5 years.[61]

It is not clear whether the same agents (cytarabine and an anthracycline) given for remission induction should be used for IPRT in higher doses or whether different agents altogether should be given. If leukemic relapse is caused by a resistant cell line, then the use of agents different from and non–cross-resistant with drugs used in induction would appear to be beneficial. The Seattle group used high-dose cytarabine with L-asparaginase, amsacrine, and etoposide in six cycles, but could only achieve a 3-year survival of 34%.[62] The survival rate was similar to the UCLA study.

High-dose cytarabine appears to be a key part of IPRT today. How many grams per square meter of cytarabine to give, how many doses per cycle, or how many cycles of cytarabine to give remain unanswered questions. The only generally accepted practice is that induction alone is insufficient and that some form of IPRT prolongs survival.

Maintenance Therapy

After induction followed by IPRT, most patients receive no further treatment. Selected patients may go on to bone marrow transplantation (see as follows). Occasionally, a maintenance phase is included and usually employs low-dose subcutaneous cytarabine as illustrated in the CALGB trial in Table 126.8.[53] Other trials have concluded that the maintenance phase is of no benefit over placebo.[63]

ANLL in the Elderly

Many older patients tolerate ANLL induction and consolidation as well as younger patients, but often therapy fails because of fatal infections and bleeding. Patients older than age 60 tend to have more cytogenetic abnormalities, underlying myelodysplasia, and a poorer performance status, all of which compromise the long-term success of therapy.[64] The complete remission rate varies from as low as 31% to as high as 65%.[65,66] Concern exists about the value of chemotherapy and decreased quality of life when treating older patients. Three approaches have been examined: (1) no therapy, (2) standard anthracycline/cytarabine induction, and (3) low-dose cytarabine. Löwenberg et al.[67] prospectively randomized patients to either a conventional chemotherapy arm or an observation arm on which patients could receive modest doses of chemotherapy for symptom palliation. The chemotherapy group survived a median of 21 weeks versus 11 weeks for the observation group. The quality of life of each group was similar, each spending approximately 50% of the study time in the hospital.

Chemotherapy may prolong survival without significantly decreasing the quality of life for elderly patients.

Standard anthracycline/cytarabine therapy has been tried in older patients with less positive results than in younger patients.[64–66] The complete response rate may be only near 33% compared to twice that for younger patients. The mortality rate during induction, usually due to infections, is approximately 9% higher. For the patients that achieve a remission, the median disease-free survival is less than 1 year. The studies performed in elderly ANLL patients demonstrate less frequent complete remissions and less durable remissions compared to younger patients.

A third approach uses low-dose cytarabine 10 mg/m^2 subcutaneously for up to 6 weeks. Low-dose cytarabine is believed to work as a differentiating agent that promotes the normal development of a leukemic blast to a normal myeloid cell. Although the experience with low-dose cytarabine is limited, the complete remission rate, the duration of remission, and survival may be comparable to that achieved by conventional chemotherapy in this age group. In one trial, patients were randomized between low-dose cytarabine and conventional chemotherapy and no difference was found in survival or remission duration. Patients receiving chemotherapy had more infections and required more blood product transfusions.[68] In contrast, in a case series using only low-dose subcutaneous cytarabine, the complete response rate was 23% compared to perhaps 65% with conventional chemotherapy in younger patients.[68] This low-dose regimen yielded a median duration of remission of 9.9 months, but even those who maintained remission had a median survival of only 19.5 months.[69] Compared to younger patients with ANLL, in this study, the remissions in elderly ANLL patients were less frequent and durable.

No specific recommendations can be made to treat ANLL in the elderly. Some patients will tolerate conventional chemotherapy, but identifying such patients is difficult. Low-dose cytarabine appears to be an option. It can induce a remission in some cases, can be given at home, and is less toxic, but probably does not lead to long-term survival.

ACUTE PROMYELOCYTIC LEUKEMIA

APL is one subclass of ANLL and makes up 10% of all cases. It has historically been diagnosed by the distinctive cytoplasmic granules seen on light microscopy and treatment has been the same as other subclasses of ANLL. Most recently, the genetic abnormality and pathophysiology of the disease have become better understood. Concurrently, a new treatment modality has been developed, that of differentiation therapy with all-*trans*-retinoic acid (TRA), which allows induction of remission without life-threatening pancytopenia.[23] The pharmacology, pharmacokinetics, and toxicity of TRA are reviewed in Chapter 119.

In APL, differentiation and maturation are arrested at the level of the promyelocyte. Examination of the chromosomes reveals a translocation between numbers 15 and 17. Chromosome 15 carries the gene for the retinoic acid receptor. Normal binding of retinoids to this receptor leads to cell proliferation and differentiation, among other functions. The retinoic acid receptor gene clusters on chromosome 17 near a second gene named *PML*. The fusion of the these two genes leads to production of a protein that presumably impairs differentiation. The discovery of the t(15,17) translocation now provides a cytogenetic marker of the disease. It is a prognostic marker in favor of response to TRA.[23]

TRA was first reported in 1987 to induce remission in patients with APL.[70] Subsequently more than 1500 patients worldwide have been treated with this new therapy.[23] TRA is usually given orally in a dose of 45 mg/m^2 as a single dose or divided into two doses, given after a meal. The complete remission rate can be as high as 95% in patients with the t(15,17) translocation. The time to achieve remission may be 1–3 months. TRA does not cross the blood–brain barrier; therefore, leukemic meningitis should be treated with conventional intrathecal chemotherapy. TRA is usually only given for initial induction because continuous use leads to autoinduction of cytochrome P-450 enzymes, enhanced metabolism, and declining blood concentrations. An alternative explanation is that leukemic cells overexpress cellular retinoic acid binding proteins that bind and trap TRA in the cell, thus lowering plasma concentrations necessary to promote differentiation. The median duration of remission when TRA is given alone is only 3.5 months.[23] As a result, TRA induction is followed now with conventional chemotherapy consolidation.

Several clinical trials have now reported positive results with TRA. Fenaux et al.[71] randomized 101 patients with newly diagnosed APL to either induction and consolidation with conventional chemotherapy or to induction with TRA and consolidation with conventional chemotherapy. The major endpoint was event-free survival defined as time without disease or death. The complete response rate was 91% on TRA and was not statistically different from the chemotherapy arm. The mortality rate was also similar, 5 with TRA and 4 with chemotherapy induction. The major difference between the two arms was the much higher relapse rate after only 22 months, resulting in early discontinuation of this trial. The event-free survival at 12 months was 79% for TRA and 50% for chemotherapy. Kanamaru et al.[72] also reported on newly diagnosed patients and found that 89% of 109 patients achieved a complete remission. At 23 months, the disease-free survival for those achieving a complete remission was 81%, which was better than an historical control group given chemotherapy and obtaining a survival rate of 65%. Both studies demonstrate that TRA can induce durable remissions in newly diagnosed patients without any frequent and serious adverse events. The studies by Fenaux and Kanamuru only examined newly diagnosed APL patients. Frankel et al.[73] studied TRA in 56 patients with either new or relapsed APL and achieved a complete remission rate of 86%. The median survival was more than 31 months. Frankel's case series demonstrated that TRA was also highly effective to induce remission even in patients who present in relapse. All three trials demonstrate the benefits of TRA: complete remission rate equal to or better than that achieved with conventional chemotherapy, disease-free survival longer than that of chemotherapy, and less life-threatening toxicity than conventional chemotherapy. The major adverse reactions to TRA included headache, skin and mucuous membrane reactions, bone pain, and nausea.

TRA induces remission in most patients, with newly diagnosed or relapsed APL. It is safer than conventional induction chemotherapy, except for the retinoic acid syndrome explained in Chapter 119. TRA is currently an investigational agent in the United States, but has been recommended for approval by the Food and Drug Administration Advisory Committee. The rapid evolution in understanding APL and the role of TRA should enable more patients to achieve a rapid remission without the complications of conventional chemotherapy.

Relapse

Most adult patients with acute leukemia who achieve complete remission eventually experience a leukemic relapse. In children, the relapse rate in ANLL is approximately the same as adults, but less frequent in pediatric ALL. Relapse usually occurs in the bone marrow, but may also occur in the CNS or other extramedullary sites. Treatment and outcome depend primarily on whether relapse occurred during or after completion of treatment. Duration of the initial remission is probably the most important factor associated with the ability to achieve a second remission.[74] After the first relapse the median survival is 6–8 months with only 7% of patients alive at 3 years.[75]

About one-half of patients with ALL or ANLL who experience a leukemic relapse while receiving chemotherapy achieve a second complete remission with chemotherapy, but remission duration usually lasts only several months and long-term survivors are uncommon. Some patients with ALL who relapse after chemotherapy is discontinued, however, can experience prolonged survival with chemotherapy. There is no consensus regarding appropriate drugs for reinduction or consolidation after relapse has occurred. Bone marrow transplantation may be undertaken if the patient is a suitable candidate (see Chapter 129).

Salvage therapy for ALL has involved similar drugs used during initial induction administered on different schedules. The VAD regimen reported by the M. D. Anderson group used a 4-day continuous infusion of vincristine and doxorubicin with intensive dexamethasone therapy. IPRT followed for 24–30 months. Overall, 39% of patients achieved a remission and 20% were disease free at 2 years.[76] Another reported regimen uses prednisone, intermediate-dose cytarabine, mitoxantrone, and etoposide in relapsed or refractory ALL. Seventy percent achieved remission with a median survival of 7 months.[77] Combinations with high-dose cytarabine or methotrexate are also commonly employed.

Several agents, including high-dose cytarabine, etoposide, intermediate- or high-dose methotrexate, L-asparaginase, carboplatin, mitoxantrone, and idarubicin have been useful in the treatment of relapsed or resistant ANLL. If the relapse occurs 6 months or more beyond the initial remission, then induction with the original chemotherapy may be successful. Single-agent therapy with high-dose cytarabine can yield a complete response rate of 12–70%. High-dose cytarabine with etoposide can produce a response rate of 70%.[75] Most recently, the combination of mitoxantrone, etoposide, and cytarabine has yielded a complete remission rate of 60%.[78] Some patients went on to bone marrow transplantation as postremission therapy. The patients who received conventional chemotherapy as consolidation had a median survival of only 7 months.

Of recent interest is our understanding of leukemic cell resistance. One mechanism identified has been the P-glycoprotein, a membrane protein capable of removing certain antineoplastics from the intracellular space into the extracellular space. Antileukemic drugs affected by this resistance mechanism include vincristine, doxorubicin, daunorubicin, etoposide, and teniposide. This protein is encoded by the *MDR* gene (multidrug resistance gene). Certain substances have been recognized as antagonists of the P-glycoprotein, among them cyclosporine and its analogs. Considerable research is now under way to develop compounds that, when administered with conventional drugs such as daunorubicin or etoposide, would overcome resistance to these agents.[79]

Bone Marrow Transplantation

For both ALL and ANLL, bone marrow transplantation (BMT) is yet another viable treatment option once remission is induced. The specific role of either allogeneic or autologous BMT in the treatment of acute leukemia is still being developed; however, its acceptance for high-risk patients and patients in relapse is fairly high. The reader is referred to Chapter 129 for specific details regarding BMT techniques, toxicities, and supportive care.

A number of confounding variables make comparison of chemotherapy and BMT in acute leukemia difficult. For example, the remission induction regimen used is usually different between studies or even within a single study.

Conventional consolidation may or may not be given after induction and before BMT. The BMT preparative regimen used can vary from study to study. The source of stem cells, the application of purging techniques to the marrow, the use of colony-stimulating factors, and advances in supportive care all influence the comparison of chemotherapy and BMT. Not all patients are equally eligible for allogeneic BMT since only 30% of the patients will have an HLA-matched sibling donor. Eligibility for bone marrow transplant is frequently limited by age (e.g., under age 50) while the median age for ANLL patients is 62–64 years old. Last, the timing of transplantation can vary from study to study. In some studies, patients are transplanted immediately after initial remission and, in other studies, transplanted at the point of early relapse. The difficulties in comparing chemotherapy alone to BMT arise from a lack of consensus on what constitutes the best chemotherapy and best BMT care.

ANLL

In the treatment of ANLL, allogeneic BMT has been compared to chemotherapy and, in general, disease-free survival is longer. At 4 to 5 years beyond transplantation, 45–50% of BMT patients are alive compared to 19–30% of patients receiving conventional chemotherapy.[80,81] Chemotherapy has never been shown superior to BMT but, in some studies, BMT has been statistically better than chemotherapy.[82] Leukemic relapse is less with BMT. In BMT patients, the risk is 13–34% compared with 60–88% of patients receiving chemotherapy and this difference has been statistically significant in some studies.[80,81]

When given as IPRT, allogeneic BMT for ANLL has been shown to improve disease-free survival over chemotherapy alone. Overall survival may also have been improved. Patients who relapse after an initial remission should be offered allogeneic BMT if a donor is available. The benefit of allogeneic BMT over chemotherapy or autologous BMT after first remission is currently being studied.

Autologous BMT is available to a larger number of patients because the patient serves as the donor and because patients up to age 60 can undergo such a transplant, unlike allogeneic transplants. Most clinicians agree that autologous marrow should be harvested early in remission, when any possible leukemic burden will be low. Results indicate that long-term survival is similar with autologous BMT compared with allogeneic BMT. Whether to purge the autologous marrow of leukemic cells remains an unresolved issue. For patients in second or third remission receiving unpurged marrow, the survival rate is 27–52%, and with purged marrow, it is 30–53%.[82] When used in first remission the survival with unpurged marrow is 23–58% and with purged marrow, 40–76%.[82] Purged marrow has not been shown clinically superior to unpurged marrow, but many patients still receive purged marrow. The general consensus at this time is that ANLL patients in second or later remission who do not qualify for an allogeneic BMT should be offered autologous BMT as soon as possible after achieving remission.[82–84]

ALL

Allogeneic BMT has also been attempted in the treatment of ALL. As a general approach, allogeneic BMT is equivalent to IPRT for patients in first remission and superior to chemotherapy once a relapse has occurred. Horowitz et al.[85] conducted a retrospective review of 484 patients in first remission who received conventional IPRT and 250 patients in first remission who received an allogeneic BMT. The 5-year probability of leukemia-free survival was 38% for patients receiving chemotherapy and 44% for patients undergoing BMT. This difference was not statistically significant. The probability of relapse was higher for the chemotherapy group (59%) than the BMT group (26%). BMT patients died more often from transplant-related complications such as graft-versus-host disease, interstitial pneumonitis, or infection. Because the initial remission is usually easily achieved in ALL and no benefit to BMT has been demonstrated in immediate postremission BMT, allogeneic BMT is not recommended in first remission for most patients.

Once a relapse has occurred, an allogeneic BMT should be performed if a donor is available. According to data from the International Bone Marrow Transplant Registry, the 5-year disease-free survival for patients undergoing allogeneic BMT in second or later remission is 30% and the probability of relapse is 50%, based on a population of more than 750 reported patients.[80] A study specifically done in children demonstrated that in second remission ALL, an allogeneic BMT could reduce the risk of relapse at 5 years from 80 to 45% regardless of prognostic risk factors.[86] The risk of leukemic relapse after BMT increases if BMT is delayed to later remissions.

A number of risk factors have been identified that may determine who with ALL should be transplanted while in first remission. Transplantation during first remission should be considered for patients with an L_3 marrow, Philadelphia chromosome positive cytogenetics and certain other cytogenetic findings, a WBC of more than 30,000, age older than 35, an initial marrow recovery greater than 4 weeks, relapse which occurs during chemotherapy, and having T-cell ALL.[80,87]

Autologous BMT has not been applied as often in ALL but is currently receiving more attention. As with ANLL, various purging techniques have been tried and the value of purging remains debatable. When used in first remission, autologous BMT yields an overall survival of 20–65%. In second or later remission the survival is

18–38%.[82] Compared to conventional postremission chemotherapy, autologous BMT offers no survival advantage after an initial remission is achieved. After a relapse occurs, autologous BMT does lead to longer disease-free survival than could be gained from conventional chemotherapy. Compared to allogeneic BMT for patients in second remission or later, overall survival is similar, but the relapse rate is greater with autologous BMT (79 versus 56%).[82] Autologous BMT remains an option for patients after relapse when a suitable donor is not available.

USE OF HEMATOPOIETIC GROWTH FACTORS IN ACUTE LEUKEMIA

Neutropenia with risk of serious infection is one of the most critical complications of acute leukemia therapy. In patients with solid tumors receiving myelosuppressive chemotherapy, the hematopoietic growth factors (HGF) have reduced infectious morbidity. In the acute leukemia patients, the utilization of these drugs has only recently become acceptable. Specific discussion of these drugs can be found in Chapter 119.

The original package inserts listed myeloid malignancies as contraindications to the use of G-CSF or GM-CSF. Myeloid blast cells carry receptors for G-CSF or GM-CSF, and the fear initially existed that using these factors would stimulate regrowth of the myeloid leukemia. Subsequent studies have shown this not to be true. When using the HGF with ANLL therapy, refractory or relapse leukemia has not been more frequent than in historical or concurrent control groups. Several studies now show that the duration of neutropenia can be reduced by up to 7 days after using a HGF. This reduction in the period of neutropenia has not, however, consistently reduced infectious morbidity. Mortality has also not been reduced in the studies reported, except one.[88]

The use of HGF in elderly ANLL patients has received particular attention but the results to date are not conclusive that this subset of patients will benefit. A recent randomized, blinded, placebo-controlled trial used yeast-derived GM-CSF with induction and consolidation chemotherapy in ANLL patients older than 55 years of age. There was a statistically significant improvement in overall survival with GM-CSF but the difference was only marginal and the survival rate in the placebo arm was unusually low. The incidence and mortality from infections as well as duration of neutropenia were also reduced with GM-CSF. An economic analysis has yet to be published that might demonstrate that these benefits exceed the cost of GM-CSF therapy.[89]

A number of unanswered questions remain. Which HGF should be used, at what dose, starting on what day after chemotherapy, and continuing for how long? The economic benefit of these factors in the ANLL patient also is unknown. Recently, GM-CSF was recommended for approval by the Food and Drug Administration for use in ANLL.

The role of CSF in care of the ALL patient is also being defined. Chemotherapy given to this population is often given frequently with little time in between courses. CSF might need to be given with chemotherapy to support the neutrophil count. CSFs are not typically given with chemotherapy, but in this population, it is difficult not to administer CSF without overlapping with chemotherapy. Large studies in ALL patients have not been performed but preliminary results indicate that G-CSF given during ALL therapy can reduce the depth and duration of neutropenia, but not the incidence of febrile neutropenia. Perhaps most important, the CSF may allow chemotherapy in ALL to be given on time.[90,91] Given during induction or consolidation chemotherapy, G-CSF does not worsen the marrow suppression. An improvement in survival or a reduction in infectious morbidity and mortality have not been demonstrated when CSFs are used with ALL chemotherapy.[91]

SUPPORTIVE CARE

The most common and significant toxic effect of antileukemic agents is marrow suppression. With the exception of prednisone, L-asparaginase, and vincristine, antineoplastic agents used to treat acute leukemias cause a rapid fall in peripheral platelet and WBC counts. During ANLL remission induction therapy, daily monitoring of the complete blood count and the absolute neutrophil count is necessary to determine when red cell and platelet transfusions are needed and when neutropenia is achieved. Less frequent monitoring than daily may be sufficient during ALL induction. Marrow hypoplasia usually reaches its lowest point (nadir) after 1–2 weeks of beginning therapy and lasts for another 1–2 weeks. During this period of hypoplasia, infectious and bleeding complications are major causes of death in leukemic patients. As typical signs and symptoms of infection may be absent in the neutropenic host, frequent monitoring of vital signs and daily physical examination are important. Infection control strategies include routine hand washing; dietary restrictions; reverse isolation and laminar airflow rooms; routine surveillance cultures; fungal, pneumocystis, and bacterial prophylaxis; and the empiric use of broad-spectrum antibiotics (see Chapter 114). Patients are often seen by a dentist prior to induction therapy to identify and treat potential infectious sources in the mouth. Chlorhexidine mouthwash may be used to maintain good oral hygiene.

Acute leukemia patients, particularly those with an initial elevated WBC count, should receive allopurinol prior to and during chemotherapy to prevent the development of urate nephropathy from rapid destruction of white cells. In adults, 300 mg of allopurinol once daily, started 1–2 days prior to chemotherapy, is usually adequate. Once marrow hypoplasia ensues, allopurinol may be discontinued. Tumor lysis syndrome may lead not only to hyperuricemia, but also hyperkalemia, hyperphosphatemia, and hypocalcemia. Hypercalcemia has been observed in some patients secondary to ectopic parathyroid production by leukemia cells.

Hematologic support consists primarily of platelet and packed red cell transfusion. Platelet transfusions are often given for peripheral counts less than 5000/μL or clinical signs of bleeding. Transfusions of packed red cells for a hematocrit less than 20%, profound fatigue, or for chest pain, may also be indicated. Promyelocytic leukemia can release procoagulants, which can cause disseminated intravascular coagulation, necessitating heparin therapy. Because of the gastrointestinal toxic effects of chemotherapy, parenteral nutrition should be used liberally. Patients are frequently receiving infusions of antibiotics, fluids, hyperalimentation, and blood products simultaneously. To provide the total support needed for these patients, a triple lumen central venous access device such as a Hickman catheter is placed at the start of therapy.

The reader is referred to other chapters for discussions of the individual antineoplastic agents, care of the febrile neutropenic patient, and bone marrow transplantation.

Evaluation of Therapeutic Outcomes

Appropriate development of a pharmaceutical care plan for the acute leukemia patient begins with establishing the diagnosis and prognosis for the patient. Examination of the bone marrow will identify the diagnosis and genetic abnormalities. Initial information from the physical examination and laboratory reports will provide other information to allow the pharmacist to determine the patient's prognosis.

The diagnosis and prognosis determine which chemotherapeutic agents are selected and for how long. High-risk patients will be directed toward bone marrow transplantation for postremission therapy. Patients without high-risk factors will receive conventional therapy.

During induction and postremission therapy, monitoring focuses on reducing infectious and hemorrhagic complications. Intense monitoring of hematologic and chemistry laboratory values, microbiology reports, and the patient's physical condition are necessary to identify infections early. Frequent culturing and early institution of antibiotics will prevent infectious deaths. Close monitoring of the patient's condition and laboratory values also allows appropriate blood product support as well as nutritional support.

During therapy, the pharmacist can be an important agent in patient education. Patients should receive information regarding acute and chronic toxicities of the chemotherapy being administered as well as possible treatments for those toxicities. The pharmacist can be an important resource for information regarding antibiotics, antiemetics, nutritional support, and other supportive care issues.

The chief outcome to be identified initially is the establishment of remission. The return of hematologic values to normal and a repeat bone marrow biopsy that demonstrates no evidence of disease serve as documentation that remission has been achieved. Monitoring guidelines for induction or consolidation are similar. After the appropriate postremission therapy has been completed, the patient may return on a regular basis to check hematologic values. If no evidence of disease exists after 5 years from the diagnosis and the patient has been in continuous complete remission, the patient is considered cured.

Several late sequelae from leukemia therapy have been recognized. CNS irradiation may lead to several different neurologic problems but the most common is cortical atrophy. Intellectual function and perceptual motor function can be disturbed. Growth hormone production from the pituitary in children may reduce the rate of growth. Secondary gliomas after cranial radiation have been reported. Long-term cardiomyopathy with symptomatic congestive heart failure has been observed months or years later in some patients receiving anthracyclines during acute leukemia therapy. Most recently has been the observation that secondary ANLL can occur in pediatric ALL patients after receiving etoposide or teniposide.[10,11] Pharmacists caring for leukemia patients after acute therapy is completed should monitor for these effects and initiate any supportive care. The long-term consequences of bone marrow transplantation are discussed in Chapter 129.

References

1. Sullivan AK. Classification, pathogenesis, and etiology of neoplastic diseases of the hematopoietic system, in Lee GR, Bithell TC, Foerster J, et al (eds): Wintrobe's Clinical Hematology, 9th ed. Philadelphia, Lea and Febiger, 1993, pp 1725–1791.
2. Lukens JN. Classification and differentiation of the acute leukemias, in Lee GR, Bithell TC, Foerster J, et al (eds): Wintrobe's Clinical Hematology, 9th ed. Philadelphia, Lea and Febiger, 1993, pp 1873–1891.
3. Mitus AJ, Rosenthal DS. Adult leukemias, in Holleb AI, Fink DJ, Murphy GP (eds): American Cancer Society Textbook of Clinical Oncology, 2nd ed. Atlanta, GA, American Cancer Society, 1991, p 411.
4. Schiffer CA. Acute myeloid leukemia in adults, in Holland JF, Frei E, Bast RC, et al (eds): Cancer Medicine, 3rd ed. Philadelphia, Lea and Febiger, 1993, pp 1907–1933.
5. Cancer facts and figures—1995. Atlanta, GA, American Cancer Society, 1995.
6. Keating MJ, Estey E, Kantarjian H. Acute leukemia, in Devita VT, Hellman S, Rosenberg SA (eds): Cancer—Principles and Practice of Oncology, 4th ed. Philadelphia, JB Lippincott, 1993, pp 1938–1964.

7. Wingo PA, Tong T, Bolden S. Cancer Statistics—1995. CA Cancer J Clin 1995;45:8–30.
8. Pui CH. Childhood leukemias. N Engl J Med 1995;332:1618–1630.
9. Poplack DG. Acute lymphoblastic leukemia, in Pizzo PA, Poplack DG (eds): Principles and Practice of Pediatric Oncology, 2nd ed. Philadelphia, JB Lippincott, 1993, pp 431–481.
10. Grier HE, Weinstein HJ. Acute myleogenous leukemia, in Pizzo PA, Poplack DG (eds): Principles and Practice of Pediatric Oncology, 2nd ed. Philadelphia, JB Lippincott, 1993, pp 483–500.
11. Greer JP, Kinney MC. Acute nonlymphocytic leukemia, in Lee GR, Bithell TC, Foerster J, et al (eds): Wintrobe's Clinical Hematology, 9th ed. Philadelphia, Lea and Febiger, 1993, pp 1920–1945.
12. Cohen T, Creger WP. Acute myeloid leukemia following seven years of aplastic anemia induced by chloramphenicol. Am J Med 1967;43:762–770.
13. Jensen MK, Roll K. Phenylbutazone and leukemia. Acta Med Scand 1965;178:505–513.
14. Smith SP, Yee GC. Hematopoiesis. Pharmacotherapy 1992;12(2 part 2):11s–19s.
15. Griffin JD, Lowenberg B. Clonogenic cells in acute myeloblastic leukemia. Blood 1986;68:1185.
16. Grignani F, Fagioli M, Alcalay M, et al. Acute promyelocytic leukemia: From genetics to treatment. Blood 1994;83:10–25.
17. McCauley DL. Treatment of adult acute leukemias. Clin Pharm 1992;11:767–796.
18. Kantarijian HM, Barlogie B, Keating MJ, et al. Pretreatment cytokinetics in acute myelogenous leukemia. Age-related prognostic implications. J Clin Invest 1985;76:319–324.
19. Broxmeyer HE, Grossbard E, Jacobsen N, et al. Persistence of inhibitory activity against normal bone marrow cells during remission of acute leukemia. N Engl J Med 1979;30:346–351.
20. Cline MJ. The molecular basis of leukemia. N Engl J Med 1994;330:328–336.
21. Inamura J, Miyoshi I, Koeffler HP. *p53* in hematologic malignancies. Blood 1994;84:2412–2421.
22. Prokocimer M, Rotter V. Structure and function of *p53* in normal cells and their aberrations in cancer cells: Projection on the hematologic cell lineages. Blood 1994;84:2391–2411.
23. Warrell RP, de Thé H, Wang Z, Degos L. Acute promyelocytic leukemia. N Engl J Med 1993;329:177–189.
24. Lukens JN. Acute lymphocytic leukemia, in Lee GR, Bithell TC, Foerster J, et al (eds): Wintrobe's Clinical Hematology, 9th ed. Philadelphia, Lea and Febiger, 1993, pp 1892–1919.
25. Copelan EA, McGuire EA. The biology and treatment of acute lymphoblastic leukemia in adults. Blood 1995;85:1151–1168.
26. Hoelzer D, Thiel E, Löffler H, et al. Prognostic factors in a multicenter study for treatment of acute lymphoblastic leukemia in adults. Blood 1988;71:123–131.
27. Linker CA, Levitt LJ, O'Donnell M, et al. Treatment of adult acute lymphoblastic leukemia with intensive cyclical chemotherapy: A follow-up report. Blood 1991;78:2814–2822.
28. Larson RA, Dodge RK, Burns CP, et al. A five-drug remission induction regimen with intensive consolidation for adults with acute lymphoblastic leukemia: Cancer and Leukemia Group B Study 8811. Blood 1995;85:2025–2037.
29. Gottleib AJ, Weinberg V, Ellison RR, et al. Efficacy of daunorubicin in the therapy of adult acute lymphocytic leukemia: A prospective randomized trial by Cancer and Leukemia Group B. Blood 1984;64:267–274.
30. Kantarjian HM. Adult acute lymphocytic leukemia: Critical review of current knowledge. Am J Med 1994;97:176–184.
31. Wiernik PH, Dutcher JP, Gucalp R, et al. MOAD therapy for adult acute lymphocytic leukemia. Proc Am Soc Clin Oncol 1990;9:205.
32. Preti A, Kantarjian HM. Management of adult acute lymphocytic leukemia: Present issues and key challenges. J Clin Oncol 1994;12:1312–1322.
33. Hoelzer D. Treatment of acute lymphoblastic leukemia. Semin Hematol 1994;31:1–15.
34. Ong ST, Larson RA. Current management of acute lymphoblastic leukemia in adults. Oncology 1995;9:433–441.
35. Gaynon PS, Steinherz PG, Bleyer WA, et al. Intensive therapy for children with acute lymphoblastic leukemia and unfavorable presenting features. Early conclusions of study CCG106 by the Children's Cancer Study Group. Lancet 1988;2:921–924.
36. Rivera GK, Raimondi SC, Hancock ML, et al. Improved outcome in childhood acute lymphoblastic leukemia with reinforced early treatment and rotational combination chemotherapy. Lancet 1991;337:61–66.
37. Pocheldly C. Prevention of meningeal leukemia. Review of 20 years of research and current recommendations. Hematol Oncol Clin North Am 1990;4:951–969.
38. Omura GA, Moffitt S, Vogler WR, et al. Combination chemotherapy of adult acute lymphoblastic leukemia with randomized central nervous prophlaxis. Blood 1987;55:199–204.
39. Omura GA, Raney M. Long-term survival in adult acute lyphoblastic leukemia: Follow-up of a Southeastern Cancer Study Group Trial. J Clin Oncol 1985;3:1053–1058.
40. Miller DR, Coccia PF, Bleyer WA, et al. Early response to induction therapy as a predictor of disease-free survival and late recurrence of childhood acute lymphoblastic leukemia: A report from the Children's Cancer Study Group. J Clin Oncol 1989;7:1807–1815.
41. Byrd R. Late effects of treatment of cancer in children. Pediatr Clin North Am 1985;32:835–857.
42. Storm AJ, Van Der Kogel AJ, Nooter K. Effect of x-irradiation on the pharmacokinetics of methotrexate in rats: Alteration of the blood–brain barrier. Eur J Cancer Clin Oncol 1985;21:759–764.
43. Esterhay RJ, Wiernik PH, Grove WR, et al. Moderate dose methotrexate, vincristine, asparaginase, and dexamethasone for treatment of adult acute lymphocytic leukemia. Blood 1982;59:334–345.
44. Schauer P, Arlin ZA, Mertelsmann R, et al. Improved results of treatment of adult acute lymphoblastic leukemia. Blood 1987;69:1242–1248.
45. Kantarjian HM, Walters RS, Keating MJ, et al. Results of the vincristine, doxorubicin, and dexamethasone regimen in adults with standard- and high-risk acute lymphocytic leukemia. J Clin Oncol 1990;8:994–1004.
46. Cuttner J, Mick R, Budman DR, et al. Phase III trial of brief intensive treatment of adult acute lymphoblastic leukemia

comparing daunorubicin and mitoxantrone-A CALGB study. Leukemia 1991;5:425–431.

47. Cassileth PA, Anderson JW, Bennett JM, et al. Adult acute lymphocytic leukemia: The Eastern Cooperative Oncology Group experience. Leukemia 1992;6(suppl 2):178–181.
48. Borsi JD, Moe PJ. Systemic clearance of methotrexate in prognosis of acute lymphoblastic leukemia in children. Cancer 1987;60:3020–3024.
49. Koren G, Ferrazini G, Sulhlt D, et al. Systemic exposure to mercaptopurine as a prognostic factor in acute lymphoblastic leukemia in children. N Engl J Med 1990;323:17–21.
50. Bostrom B, Erdmann G. Cellular pharmacology of 6-mercaptopurine in acute lymphoblastic leukemia. Am J Pediatr Hematol Oncol 1993;15:80–86.
51. Mastrianni DM, Tung NM, Tenen DG. Acute myelogenous leukemia: Current treatment and future directions. Am J Med 1992;92:286–295.
52. Vogler WR, Velez-Garcia E, Weiner RS, et al. A phase III trial comparing idarubicin and daunorubicin in combination with cytarabine in acute myelogenous leukemia: A Southeastern Cancer Study Group study. J Clin Oncol 1992;10:1103–1111.
53. Mayer RJ, Davis RB, Schiffer CA, et al. Intensive postremission chemotherapy in adults with acute myeloid leukemia. N Engl J Med 1994;331:896–903.
54. Mitus AJ, Miller KB, Schenkein DP, et al. Improved survival for patients with acute myelogenous leukemia. J Clin Oncol 1995;13:560–569.
55. Yates J, Glidewell O, Wiernik P, et al. Cytosine arabinoside with daunorubicin or adriamycin for therapy for acute myelocytic leukemia: A CALGB study. Blood 1982;60:454–462.
56. Rai KR, Holland JF, Glidewell OJ, et al. Treatment of acute myelocytic leukemia: A study by Cancer and Leukemia Group B. Blood 1981;58:1203–1211.
57. Priesler H, Davis RB, Kirshner J, et al. Comparison of three remission induction regimens and two postinduction strategies for the treatment of acute nonlymphocytic leukemia: A Cancer and Leukemia Group B study. Blood 1987;69:1441–1449.
58. Berman E, Heller G, Santorsa J, et al. Results of a randomized trial comparing idarubicin and cytosine arabinoside with daunorubicin and cytosine arabinoside in adult patients with newly diagnosed acute myelogenous leukemia. Blood 1991;77:1666–1674.
59. Mayer RJ, Weinstein HJ, Coral FS, et al. The role of intensive postinduction chemotherapy in the management of patients with acute myelogenous leukemia. Cancer Treat Rep 1982;66:1455–1462.
60. Mayer RJ. Current chemotherapeutic treatment approaches to the management of previously untreated adults with *de novo* acute myelogenous leukemia. Semin Oncol 1987;14:384–396.
61. Champlin R, Gajewski J, Nimer S, et al. Postremission chemotherapy for adults with acute myelogenous leukemia: Improved survival with high-dose cytarabine and daunorubicin consolidation treatment. J Clin Oncol 1991;8:1199–1206.
62. Tallman MS, Appelbaum FR, Amos DA, et al. Evaluation of intensive postremission chemotherapy for adults with acute nonlymphocytic leukemia using high-dose cytosine arabinoside with L-asparaginase and amsacrine with etoposide. J Clin Oncol 1987;5:918–926.
63. Toronto Leukemia Study Group. Survival in acute myeloblastic leukemia is not prolonged by remission maintenance or early reinduction chemotherapy. Leuk Res 1988; 12:195–200.
64. Baudard M, Marie JP, Cadiou M, Zittoun R. Acute myelogenous leukaemia in the elderly: Retrospective study of 235 consecutive patients. Brit J Haematol 1994;86:82–91.
65. Ryan DH, Kopecky KJ, Head D, et al. Analysis of treatment failure in acute nonlymphocytic leukemia patients over fifty years of age. Am J Clin Oncol 1992;15:69–75.
66. Heyll A, Aul C, Gogolin F, et al. Results of conventional-dose cytosine arabinoside and idarubicin in elderly patients with acute myeloid leukemia. Ann Hematol 1994;68:279–283.
67. Löwenberg B, Zittoun R, Kerkhofs H, et al. On the value of intensive remission-induction chemotherapy in elderly patients of 65+ years with acute myeloid leukemia: A randomized phase III study of the European Organization for Research and Treatment of Cancer Leukemia Group. J Clin Oncol 1989;7:1268–1274.
68. Tilly H, Castaigne S, Bordessoule D, et al. Low-dose cytarabine versus intensive chemotherapy in the treatment of acute nonlymphocytic leukemia in the elderly. J Clin Oncol 1990;8:272–279.
69. Powell BL, Capizzi RL, Muss HB, et al. Low-dose Ara-C therapy for acute myelogenous leukemia in elderly patients. Leukemia 1989;3:23–28.
70. Menger H, Yu-chun Y, Shu-rong C, et al. All-trans retinoic acid with or without low dose cytosine arabinoside in acute promyelocytic leukemia. Chin Med J 1987;100:949–953.
71. Fenaux P, Le Deley MC, Castaigne S, et al. Effect of all transretinoic acid in newly diagnosed acute promyelocytic leukemia. Results of a multicenter randomized trial. Blood 1993;82:3241–3249.
72. Kanamaru A, Takemoto Y, Tanimoto M, et al. All-trans retinoic acid for the treatment of newly diagnosed acute promyelocytic leukemia. Blood 1995;85:1202–1206.
73. Frankel SR, Eardley A, Heller G, et al. All-trans retinoic acid for acute promyelocytic leukemia. Ann Intern Med 1994;120:278–286.
74. Keating MJ, Kantarjian H, Smith TL, et al. Response to salvage therapy and survival after relapse in acute myelogenous leukemia. J Clin Oncol 1989;7:1071–1080.
75. Hiddemann W, Büchner T. Treatment strategies in acute myeloid leukemia (AML). Blut 1990;60:163–171.
76. Kantarjian HM, Walters RS, Keating MJ, et al. Experience with vincristine, doxorubicin, and dexamethasone (VAD) chemotherapy in adults with refractory acute lymphocytic leukemia. Cancer 1989;64:16–22.
77. Milpied N, Gisselbrecht C, Harousseau J, et al. Successful treatment of adult acute lymphoblastic leukemia after relapse with prednisone, intermediate-dose cytarabine, mitoxantrone, and etoposide (PAME) chemotherapy. Cancer 1990;66:627–631.
78. Archimbaud E, Thomas X, Leblond V, et al. Timed sequential chemotherapy for previously treated patients with acute myeloid leukemia: Long-term follow-up of the etoposide, mitoxantrone, and cytarabine-86 trial. J Clin Oncol 1995;13:11–18.

79. Arceci RJ. Clinical significance of P-glycoprotein in multidrug resistance malignancies. Blood 1993;81:2215–2222.
80. Christiansen NP. Allogeneic bone marrow transplantation for the treatment of adult acute leukemias. Hematol Oncol Clin North Am 1993;7:177–200.
81. Long GD, Blume KG. Allogeneic bone marrow transplantation for acute myeloid leukemia, in Forman SJ, Blume KG, Thomas ED (eds): Bone Marrow Transplantation. Boston, Blackwell Scientific Publications, 1994, pp 607–617.
82. Ball ED, Rybka WB. Autologous bone marrow transplantation for adult acute leukemia. Hematol Oncol Clin North Am 1993;7:201–231.
83. Yeager AM. Autologous bone marrow transplantation for acute myeloid leukemia, in Forman SJ, Blume KG, Thomas ED (eds): Bone Marrow Transplantation. Boston, Blackwell Scientific Publications, 1994, pp 709–730.
84. Stuart RK. Autologous bone marrow transplantation for leukemia. Semin Oncol 1993;20(suppl 6):40–54.
85. Horowitz MM, Messerer D, Hoelzer D, et al. Chemotherapy compared with bone marrow transplantation for adults with acute lymphoblastic leukemia in first remission. Ann Int Med 1991;115:13–18.
86. Barrett AJ, Horowitz MH, Pollock BH, et al. Bone marrow transplants from HLA-identical siblings as compared with chemotherapy for children with acute lymphoblastic leukemia in a second remission. N Engl J Med 1994;331:1253–1258.
87. Storb R, Buckner CD. Human marrow transplantation. Eur J Clin Invest 1990;20:119–132.
88. Estey EH. Use of colony-stimulating factors in the treatment of acute myeloid leukemia. Blood 1994;83:2015–2019.
89. Rowe JM, Anderson JW, Mazza JJ, et al. A randomized placebo-controlled phase III study of granulocyte-macrophage colony-stimulating factor in adult patients (>55 to 70 years of age) with acute myelogenous leukemia: A study of the Eastern Cooperative Oncology Group (E1490). Blood 1995;86:457–462.
90. Scherrer R, Geissler K, Kyrle PA, et al. Granulocyte colony-stimulating factor (G-CSF) as an adjunct to induction chemotherapy of adult acute lymphoblastic leukemia (ALL). Ann Hematol 1993;66:283–289.
91. Ottman OG, Hoelzer D, Gracien E, et al. Concomitant granulocyte colony-stimulating factor and induction chemoradiotherapy in adult lymphoblastic leukemia: A randomized phase III trial. Blood 1995;86:444–450.

Chapter 127

Chronic Leukemias

Timothy R. McGuire, PharmD, and Peter W. Kazakoff, PharmD

Chronic leukemia includes at least four recognized disease entities: chronic myelogenous leukemia (CML), chronic lymphocytic leukemia (CLL), prolymphocytic leukemia, and hairy cell leukemia. Because CML and CLL occur far more frequently, this chapter deals with these two cancers, which represent about half of all new cases of leukemias occurring in the United States during 1994.[1]

Chronic Myelogenous Leukemia

CML, also known as chronic granulocytic leukemia, is one of a group of hematologic cancers known as myeloproliferative disorders and is one of the most carefully researched and well understood of the human malignancies. CML results from the malignant transformation of a pluripotent stem cell leading to the clonal proliferation and accumulation of both progenitor and mature myeloid and lymphoid cells.[2] CML is characterized by hematologic and cytogenetic abnormalities involving the myeloid and B-lymphoid elements of bone marrow.[3] The clinical course of CML has multiple phases beginning as an indolent chronic phase in which signs and symptoms can be controlled with conventional chemotherapy, followed by an acute phase known as blast crisis, which, similar to acute leukemia, leads to rapid degeneration and death of the patient. An accelerated phase can usually be identified in the interval between the chronic phase and blastic phase, and although the definition of the accelerated phase is vague, it is generally recognized as the stage where CML becomes more resistant to maintenance chemotherapy.[3,4]

CML was first described in 1845, but the extensive research into the genetic and molecular aspects of the disease began with the discovery of the Philadelphia chromosome (Ph[1]) in 1960 by Nowell and Hungerford.[5] Research in the 1980s identified the molecular changes that occur as a result of the Ph[1] and an oncogenic protein product resulting from the Ph[1] was identified and implicated in the pathophysiology of CML.[5,6]

INCIDENCE AND ETIOLOGY

It is estimated that about 5000 new cases of CML occurred in the United States in 1994, representing about 15–20% of all leukemias.[1,7] CML is predominantly a neoplasm of middle-aged adults, with the median age at diagnosis in the fifth decade of life. A "juvenile" variant of CML that occurs in young children is rare and is not discussed in this chapter.[8]

Although ionizing radiation and heavy occupational exposure to benzene are known to be exogenous causes, the etiology of CML is largely unknown.[3,4] Only rarely does a newly diagnosed patient have an identifiable risk factor for the development of CML. There was a 20- to 25-fold increase in the incidence of all leukemias in atomic bomb survivors. The incidence of leukemia was highest in those who were youngest at the time of exposure, with more CML cases than acute lymphocytic leukemia cases.[9] There are only case reports of CML after radiotherapy for malignancies or ankylosing spondylitis.[3,4] There are no known oncogenic viruses associated with CML.

PATHOPHYSIOLOGY

Molecular Biology

Ph[1] was the first karyotypic abnormality specifically implicated in the pathogenesis of cancer, and has resulted in extensive research into the molecular biology of CML.[4,5] This chromosomal abnormality is characteristic of CML and is present in 90–95% of patients with a presumptive diagnosis of the disease. It can also occur in up to 20% of adults and 5% of children with acute lymphocytic leukemia, and 5% of adults and children with acute myelogenous leukemia.[10]

Ph[1] is identified as a shortened long arm of chromosome 22, and is found in granulocyte and erythrocyte progenitors, macrophages, megakaryocytes, and some lymphocytes.[11] This anomaly is the consequence of breaks in chromosomes 9 and 22, resulting in a transposition that relocates the 3′ end of the c-*abl* protooncogene from its normal site on chromosome 9 at band 34 to the 5′ end of the breakpoint cluster region *(bcr)* on chromosome 22 at band 11.[12,13] This reciprocal translocation is usually symbolized as t(9;22)(q34;q11), and results in the formation of the hybrid *bcr-abl* fusion gene (Fig. 127.1). Through this chromosomal translocation, the c-*abl* protooncogene is able to escape the normal genetic controls on its expression and is activated into a functional oncogene, directing the transcription of an 8.5-kilobase mRNA molecule that is translated into a 210-kDa protein.[14] This protein, known as $p210^{BCR\text{-}ABL}$, is unique to Ph^1-positive leukemia, and although its precise role in CML is not clear, there is mounting evidence for its importance in CML pathogenesis. The $p210^{BCR\text{-}ABL}$ protein has a higher tyrosine phosphokinase activity than the 145-kDa protein translated by the mRNA of the normal c-*abl* gene.[14,15] The higher kinase activity of $p210^{BCR\text{-}ABL}$ may be essential in the development of CML since the phosphorylation of tyrosine residues on growth factor receptors is believed to be a critical intracellular signal in cell proliferation.[16] The $p210^{BCR\text{-}ABL}$ protein has also been shown to transform hematopoietic cells *in vitro* and to induce a CML-like myeloproliferative disorder in mice after infection of their bone marrow with a retrovirus that encodes the $p210^{BCR\text{-}ABL}$ protein.[13,17]

Natural History of CML

Advances in understanding the cellular events associated with CML have led to the development of a multistep model of disease pathogenesis, beginning with a period of monoclonal hematopoiesis, followed by the chronic phase and ending with the blastic phase.

It is generally accepted that carcinogenesis begins with the transformation of a single cell. In CML, this alteration gives the transformed progenitor cell an inheritable selective growth advantage, leading to the proliferation of a neoplastic, monoclonal population of pluripotent stem cells.[18] These cells initially lack the Ph^1 but soon the disease evolves into a Ph^1-positive chronic phase. The Ph^1 can be found in both myeloid and lymphoid cells suggesting that the transformed cell of CML is a totipotent stem cell.[2,19]

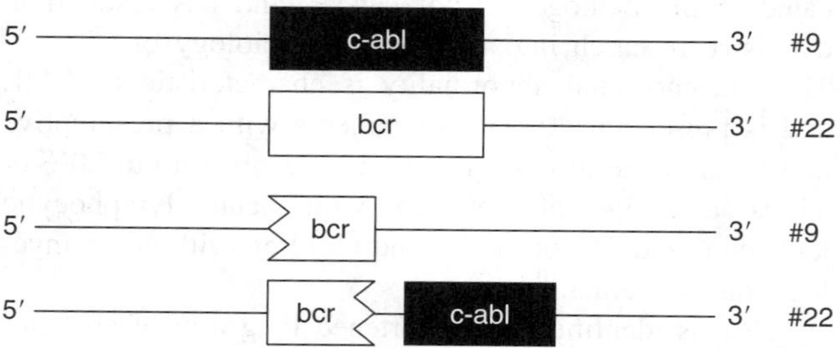

Figure 127.1. Diagram of the chromosomal translocation that results in the Philadelphia chromosome. This abnormality is encountered in 90–95% of patients who have chronic myelogenous leukemia. *(Reproduced from Fishleder AJ. Oncogenes and cancer: Clinical applications. Cleve Clin J Med 1990;57:723, with permission.)*

Granulocytosis is usually present in CML and results from the increased growth rate of the transformed clone and disruption of normal hematopoietic cell maturation. Disrupted maturation leads to additional divisions by CML progenitor cells before reaching a nonproliferative stage; the resulting number of circulating granulocytes may be many times higher than normal.[20,21] Immature CML progenitors are also less responsive to cellular and molecular controls that inhibit growth and proliferation in normal hematopoietic cells, such as the induction of programmed cell death, or apoptosis.[20,21] Later in the clinical course of CML, cytopenias may occur corresponding to fibrotic changes in the bone marrow.[2,4]

The silent monoclonal growth phase of CML evolves into the clinically recognized chronic phase when the malignant cells acquire Ph^1. The chronic phase is not simply a period of increasing granulocytosis; it is common for the white blood cell (WBC) count to oscillate, and the immature myeloid cells begin to lose the ability to differentiate into mature functioning cells.[18] At this stage therapeutic intervention can effectively control the expansion of these clonal cells and normalize the WBC count.[18,22] As CML progresses, the genetic instability of the malignant clone increases, and chromosomal abnormalities other than Ph^1 begin to occur.[19,23] Clinical evidence of the accelerated phase of CML begins to emerge as the patient's WBC count becomes increasingly difficult to manage. The rate of progression of CML is subject to wide variability; in some instances blastic phase can erupt without any apparent accelerated phase. The relative mass of the chronic phase cell populations, genetic predetermination, and differences in either genetic stability or proliferative state of the leukemic cells are possible explanations for this variability.[2,24]

The final stage of CML, known as the acute phase or blastic phase, is marked by the presence of rapidly proliferating blast cells that have lost the ability to differentiate into nonproliferating cells.[4,24] The proliferative advantage of blast cells over normal hematopoietic cells is even greater than chronic phase leukemic cells. CML in blastic phase is resistant to treatment. This poor response to chemotherapy is not exclusively due to drug resistance; it also results from the high proliferative rate of blastic phase CML and the replacement of malignant cells eliminated by chemotherapy.[25] The increased proliferative rate of blastic phase CML is the consequence of a number of factors, one of which may be the high levels of cytokines produced by CML cells. For example, interleukin-1 (IL-1) beta is produced in large quantities by CML cells in culture and IL-1 beta antibody is able to inhibit the clonal expansion of blastic phase CML cells *in vitro*. IL-1 beta may also indirectly stimulate blastic phase CML cells by inducing endothelial cells and fibroblasts to secrete hematopoietic growth factors.[26]

Philadelphia Chromosome-Negative CML

In about 5–10% of patients diagnosed with CML, the Ph^1 cannot be identified. These patients can be divided into two populations; the first group (Ph^1–,*bcr*+) where the *bcr-abl* fusion gene and $p210^{BCR\text{-}ABL}$ can be demonstrated using molecular techniques, and the second group of patients where there is no evidence of karyotype or fusion gene product (Ph^1–,*bcr*–). Ph^1–,*bcr*+ CML is indistinguishable from Ph^1-positive CML in its clinical course. These similarities have led investigators to consider Ph^1–,*bcr*+ CML and its Ph^1-positive counterpart to be the same disease entity and subject to the same therapeutic strategies.[11] Patients in the other group (Ph^1–,*bcr*–) have no evidence of either the karyotype or fusion gene but early in the disease display many of the same clinical signs and symptoms of classical CML. This variant has a somewhat different clinical course than Ph^1+,*bcr*+ and Ph^1–,*bcr*+ CML in that the blastic phase is usually absent. Rather than having the large number of circulating immature cells, the late terminal stage of this variant manifests with leukocytosis, organomegaly, blast counts of less than 20%, and bone marrow failure with resulting anemia and thrombocytopenia. An alternative view of *bcr*– CML is that it is not a true disease entity but is a result of laboratory misdiagnosis. Because of the very small number of CML patients who are *bcr*– this is difficult to assess.[11,27]

CLINICAL PRESENTATION AND PROGNOSIS

The diagnosis of CML is usually made during the chronic phase following an abnormal peripheral blood smear. Occasionally the blood sample is obtained during a routine physical examination or more commonly after the patient presents with symptoms such as weight loss, fatigue, malaise, night sweats, and fever. Splenomegaly and hepatomegaly are found in 30–40% of patients. Typical laboratory findings of the peripheral blood during the chronic phase include leukocytosis, thrombocytosis, basophilia, and abnormal leukocyte alkaline phosphatase levels. In one series of newly diagnosed CML, the most common feature of the peripheral blood was a highly elevated WBC count (>100,000/μL) occurring in about 70% of patients.[3,28]

Before the advent of modern therapeutic strategies, CML patients had a median survival after diagnosis of about 3 years with only about 20% of patients alive at 5 years. With the use of current therapies including single-agent and combination chemotherapy, interferon, and bone marrow transplantation (BMT) the 5-year survival ranges between 40–70%.[29] To date, only allogeneic BMT has been able to cure patients by permanently eliminating the Ph^1-positive clone.

Due to the wide variability in survival among CML patients, there has been disagreement in the use of prognostic systems. Two commonly used systems are those by Sokal et al.[30] and the newer synthesis staging system proposed by Kantarjian et al.[28] The synthesis system identifies poor prognostic characteristics from both chronic phase and accelerated phase CML. A summary of the synthesis system is given in Table 127.1.

The accelerated phase of CML is clinically the least distinct of the three phases of CML and may be difficult to recognize in some patients. Hematologic signs and symptoms reflect a progression in myeloproliferative acceleration and the approach of fatal blast crisis. Physical symptoms of acceleration include a resurgence of splenic enlargement, unexplained fever, and persistent bone pain. WBC counts and other signs and symptoms begin to be increasingly difficult to control with conventional oral chemotherapeutic agents. Accelerated phase usually lasts from 3–6 months, and it is in this phase that BMT is the only method of achieving long-term disease-free survival.

The prognosis for patients not eligible for BMT is extremely poor.[3,8] The clinical course of CML terminates in blastic phase in which patients have peripheral blood and bone marrow findings very similar to acute leukemia. The one laboratory parameter that is used by most investigators to confirm this phase is the presence of greater than 20% blasts in the bone marrow or peripheral blood.[3,4] A proposal by Arlin et al.[31] uses 30% myeloid blasts plus promyelocytes or 20% lymphoblasts in the bone marrow as diagnostic criteria for blastic phase. The median survival for patients in the blastic phase is 4–6 months, with most treatment options providing no survival advantage.

TABLE 127.1. SYNTHESIS PROGNOSTIC SYSTEM FOR CML

		Estimated % Survival		
Stage	**Definition**	**1 year**	**2 year**	**4 year**
I	0 or 1 element from List A	94	87	62
II	2 elements from List A	94	78	46
III	≥3 elements from List A	91	68	25
IV	≥1 element from List B	71	57	25

List A	List B
Age ≥ 60 years	Cytogenetics: clonal evolution
Spleen ≥ 10 cm below costal margin	Blasts in blood ≥ 15%
Blasts ≥ 3% in blood or 5% in marrow	Blasts + promyelocytes ≥ 30% in blood
Basophils ≥ 7% blood or ≥ 3% marrow	Basophils ≥ 20% in blood
Platelets ≥ 700 × 10^3/μL	Platelets < 100 × 10^3/μL

(Adapted from Ref. 28.)

TREATMENT

Cure of CML can only be achieved by eradication of the Ph[1]-positive cells. Conventional cytotoxic chemotherapy can be used in chronic phase CML to attain hematologic remission, which is defined as normalization of WBC count. Use of conventional chemotherapy in chronic phase has no significant cytogenetic effects and has only marginally improved median survival in CML. Interferon can produce hematologic and cytogenetic responses which lead to longer median survivals but it has been unable to eliminate the malignant clone as evidenced by recurrence of the Ph[1] clone after stopping interferon therapy.[32] Cytogenetic remission has been defined as the elimination of Ph[1] from bone marrow, while major cytogenetic response is defined as less than 35% Ph[1]-positive cells in the bone marrow. To date, only through allogeneic BMT has the Ph[1]-positive malignant clone been permanently eliminated. Table 127.2 illustrates the effect of various treatment modalities on median survival in CML.[29]

Conventional Chemotherapy

Although there have been many chemotherapeutic agents used to treat chronic phase CML, two have been employed most frequently, busulfan (Myleran) and hydroxyurea (Hydrea). These agents can be taken orally, are inexpensive, have a reasonable side-effect profile, and are able to rapidly normalize elevated WBC counts in chronic phase CML. Although both agents produce predictable declines in WBC count and hematologic remissions in 70–80% of chronic phase CML patients, busulfan and hydroxyurea have very little effect on Ph[1]-positive cells in bone marrow.[32] Despite the fact that busulfan has historically been considered the drug of choice, recent results from a randomized study of nearly 500 CML patients by the German CML Study Group showed that hydroxyurea treatment provided a significant survival advantage of more than 1 year over busulfan therapy.[33] Combination cytotoxic chemotherapy has not been shown to provide any improvement in survival over single-agent therapy (see Table 127.2).

TABLE 127.2. EFFECT OF VARIOUS TREATMENT MODALITIES ON SURVIVAL IN CML

Therapy	Median Survival (months)
No treatment	37 (mean)
Splenic irradiation	42 (mean), 28 (median)
Busulfan	35–47
Hydroxyurea	48–69
Combination chemotherapy	45–55
Bone marrow transplantation	40–70% alive at 5 years[a]
IFN-α	50–60% alive at 5 years

[a]Only therapy to eliminate Ph[1] clone. (Adapted from Ref. 29.)

Hydroxyurea inhibits the enzyme ribonucleotide reductase, leading to suppression of DNA synthesis and in cell culture the elimination of cells in the S phase of the cell cycle and the synchronization in the G_1 or pre-DNA synthesis phase.[34] Hydroxyurea is administered either daily or intermittently. In the daily schedule, hydroxyurea is initiated at 50 mg/kg/d in divided doses until the WBC count falls below 10,000/μL. At this point, the dose can be decreased to a maintenance level of 20 mg/kg/d, or temporarily discontinued and reinitiated at the daily maintenance dose when the WBC count begins to climb. With hydroxyurea therapy, the WBC count rarely continues to fall if the drug is discontinued. Because prolonged daily administration of hydroxyurea has been associated with adverse dermatologic effects, an intermittent maintenance dose of 20 mg/kg twice daily (40 mg/kg/d) 2 days each week has been proven effective in controlling the WBC count while minimizing cutaneous toxicity.[34] Occasional dose adjustments may be required in both maintenance dose schedules.

Because of its toxicity, busulfan may not be the preferred drug for the initial treatment of CML. Initial doses of busulfan are 4–8 mg/d; this regimen is continued until the WBC count approaches 20,000/μL, then discontinued. The WBC count will continue to fall after the drug is discontinued and appropriate WBC counts can be maintained for several weeks without continuous drug therapy. Toxicities include prolonged myelosuppression, pulmonary fibrosis, and skin hyperpigmentation. Patients who have received busulfan therapy followed later with allogeneic BMT appear to have a greater incidence of complications.[35] For this reason, and because of the possibility of inducing drug resistance in the malignant clone, busulfan is not considered first-line therapy in patients who are candidates for BMT. A comparison of hydroxyurea and busulfan can be seen in Table 127.3.

Interferons

The interferons are a family of glycoproteins involved in many of the functional aspects of the hematopoietic system. Recombinant DNA technology has provided new methods by which sufficient quantities of these cytokines can be produced for therapeutic use. Alpha interferon (IFN-α) and beta interferon (IFN-β) bind to the same cell-surface receptor on target cells, while gamma interferon (IFN-γ) binds to a separate receptor. Although all have been studied in the treatment of chronic phase CML, IFN-α has been most intensely investigated in the management of CML.[36] IFN-α was first isolated from leukocytes after viral exposure; two recombinant forms are presently marketed: IFN-α-2a (Roferon) and IFN-α-2b (Intron A). Fibroblasts are the primary source of IFN-β; and although this form has potent inhibitory activity on CML cells *in vitro,* no effect has been shown in normalizing blood counts and differentials *in*

TABLE 127.3. COMPARISON OF HYDROXYUREA AND BUSULFAN IN CHRONIC PHASE CML

Effect of Therapy	Hydroxyurea	Busulfan
Rate of WBC decline	Rapid	Slower
Myelosuppression	Uncommon at usual dose	Common
Side-effect profile	Mild—skin	Severe—lung
Effect on platelet count	No effect	Decreased
Effect on splenomegaly	Significant reversal	Significant reversal
Effect on Ph^1-positive marrow	None	After prolonged myelosuppression
BMT eligible patients	Recommended	Not recommended

vivo.[37] IFN-γ, originally found in T-lymphocytes, has been used in combination therapy with IFN-α in the treatment of chronic phase CML with disappointing results.[38]

The exact mechanism of IFN-α activity in CML is not known. The numerous and complex activities of IFN-α include antiproliferative, immunoregulatory, antiviral, and differentiation-inducing effects. One proposed mechanism for IFN-α in the treatment of CML is the binding of IFN-α to its receptor, initiating a cascade of biochemical processes that can result in direct cytotoxicity to leukemic cells. For example, synthesis of the enzyme 2′-5′-oligoadenylate-synthetase is enhanced by IFN-α receptor binding and results in the activation of RNAse, which may lead to the degradation of CML growth factor and oncogene transcripts.[39] Leukemic cells have a reduced expression of cell-surface molecules such as histocompatibility antigens that allow them to escape surveillance by the immune system. It has been suggested that IFN-α binding corrects this abnormality by increasing histocompatibility antigen expression, resulting in the recognition of CML cells as "foreign" and leading to the removal of the malignant clone by immune mechanisms.[39] Perhaps the most important site of action of IFN-α occurs in the bone marrow microenvironment. A reduced expression of cell-adhesion molecules on CML progenitor cells may be responsible for their propensity to enter the circulation rather than adhering to the bone marrow stroma as do normal cells. This decreased adhesion could also be a mechanism by which the leukemic cells escape normal hematopoietic regulation. In co-culture experiments performed using bone marrow-derived stromal cells and CML cells, it was found that cell adhesion was increased sixfold in the presence of IFN-α over control.[40] Finally, there is evidence from patient data and *in vitro* experiments that IFN-α suppresses the production of interleukins 1 and 8 (both are elevated in the serum of CML patients) and increases the production of tumor necrosis factor-alpha. These effects can result in inhibition of leukemic cell proliferation.[41]

The enthusiasm regarding the use of human IFN-α in the treatment of chronic phase CML is based on the observation that some patients achieve cytogenetic response (a decrease or loss of Ph^1-positive cells) along with hematologic remissions.[42] Studies performed with the two forms of recombinant IFN-α (IFN-α-2a and IFN-α-2b) have demonstrated similar results. Long-term follow-up results from M. D. Anderson Cancer Center in early chronic phase CML patients (<12 months from diagnosis to treatment) with partially pure human IFN-α, recombinant IFN-α-2a, and IFN-α-2b showed complete hematologic remissions (normalization of blood count) in 70–80% of patients. Major cytogenetic response (suppression of Ph^1-positive metaphases to <35% of total) occurred in 20–40%, and a major durable cytogenetic response in 10–25% of patients. Median survival was 65 months, with 60% of patients alive at 5 years.[43] Separate studies done in Italy and Spain resulted in hematologic remission rates of about 50–70% with about 30–50% of patients obtaining some form of cytogenetic response.[44,45] The doses used in all studies ranged from 2×10^6 to 5×10^6 U/m^2 administered daily either subcutaneously or intramuscularly.[42–45]

It is difficult to compare IFN-α studies because of variations in the type of pretreatment, variation in IFN-α dosing, and disease status at the time of treatment. Patients who achieve any cytogenetic response exhibit a distinct survival advantage over those with no decrease in the percentage of Ph^1-positive cells. Patients who have undergone pretreatment with other agents or are in accelerated phase CML appear to respond poorly to IFN-α therapy. The optimal dose schedule appears to be 5×10^6 U/m^2/d with doses above 5×10^6 U/m^2/d being unlikely to improve response rates while increasing the incidence of toxicities.[4,42–45]

The importance of achieving a 5×10^6 U/m^2/d dose may be illustrated by a randomized study of IFN-α versus hydroxyurea in which the average dose was lower than other studies. Hehlmann et al.[46] reported equivalent survival rates between patients receiving IFN-α versus those receiving hydroxyurea. In addition, they reported major hematologic and cytogenetic responses that were lower than those reported by several other groups.[42–44,47] Other explanations for response differences between the various IFN-α studies other than dose include differences in baseline prognostic factors, differences in adjunctive therapies, and frequency of determining cytogenetic responses.

Adverse effects of IFN-α therapy consist of short-term constitutional effects and potentially dose-limiting long-term effects. The most predictable early toxicity is a flu-like syndrome involving fever, chills, myalgias, headache, and anorexia. These dose-dependent effects are a result of IFN-α-induced leukocytosis and release of cytokines. This acute flu-like syndrome can be ameliorated by starting IFN-α dosing at 50% of the final dose during the first week, by giving the drug at bedtime, and by coadministering acetaminophen or indomethacin. Reduction of initial WBC counts to around 10,000/μL with hydroxyurea may also reduce these symptoms.[3,4] Despite these methods of ameliorating toxicity, the flu-like syndrome is an important source of morbidity occasionally requiring termination of therapy. Cardiovascular toxicities (tachycardia, hypotension) are seen in about 15% of patients in the first 1–2 weeks. Long-term adverse effects include weight loss, alopecia, neurologic effects (paresthesias, cognitive impairment, depression), and immune-mediated complications (hemolysis, thrombocytopenia, nephrotic syndrome, systemic lupus erythematosus, hypothyroidism), which can be dose limiting in 10–25% of patients.[3,4] Recently, Beelen et al.[48] reported that using IFN-α prior to allogeneic BMT is deleterious to outcomes. There was a higher graft failure rate and slower engraftment time in patients receiving IFN-α therapy leading to reduced 5-year survival rates.

To date, enough clinical data are not available on combination therapy of IFN-α with cytotoxic chemotherapy to draw any important conclusions. In several small studies, IFN-α has been used in combination with busulfan, intensive chemotherapy regimens, hydroxyurea, and cytosine arabinoside (ara-C). Results from IFN-α/busulfan studies reported cytogenetic responses at least as frequently as with IFN-α alone, but at the price of myelosuppression as a dose-limiting toxicity.[49] Three cycles of intensive chemotherapy consisting of daunorubicin, ara-C, vincristine, and prednisone followed by daily maintenance IFN-α resulted in significant cytogenetic responses. These responses proved to be transient in most patients and survival rates were equivalent to patients treated with IFN-α alone.[43]

The combination of hydroxyurea and IFN-α has some promise in treating CML. Hydroxyurea was started first at a dose of 50 mg/kg/d and titrated to keep WBC counts at a normal level; IFN-α was then initiated at a dose of 5×10^6 $U/m^2/d$. The incidence of cytogenetic response was not significantly different from IFN-α therapy alone. In this small study the investigators reported an 82% complete hematologic remission rate and a 62% cytogenetic response compared to 58% complete hematologic remission rate and 48% cytogenetic response in an IFN-α alone group.[45] The advantage of this combination is the rapid normalization of blood counts and differentials, lower incidence of IFN-α-induced symptoms associated with leukocytosis, and higher complete hematologic remission rates.[43]

Favorable outcomes have resulted from a combination of low-dose ara-C and IFN-α. This combination has been studied in early chronic phase CML by Guilhot,[50] and in late chronic phase and accelerated phase CML by the M. D. Anderson follow-up study group.[43] In all the following studies, the dose of IFN-α was 5×10^6 U/m^2 daily. Patients with early chronic phase CML were given ara-C at 10 mg/m^2 subcutaneously for 10 days of each month or at 15 mg/m^2 subcutaneously daily in divided doses for 2 weeks during the first cycle then for 7 days of each month thereafter. These regimens were compared with IFN-α therapy alone. This group found no difference in complete hematologic remission rates, which approached 80%, between the IFN-α/low-dose ara-C and IFN-α alone groups. Major cytogenetic responses occurred in 33% of IFN-α-treated patients and in 45% of combination therapy patients; complete cytogenetic response was 14 versus 23%. In late chronic phase, complete hematologic remission rates were 28% for IFN-α-treated patients and 55% in combination therapy patients; cytogenetic response was 5 versus 15%. Accelerated phase patients had similar response rates, although this study had a smaller number of patients.[43]

Nonpharmacologic Therapy

Nondrug therapy for CML includes leukopheresis and splenectomy. Leukopheresis can be used to maintain safe WBC counts when pregnancy prevents the use of potentially teratogenic chemotherapy. Leukopheresis may be used when WBC counts become high enough (>100,000/μL) to cause symptoms of hyperleukocytosis and rapid reduction of WBC count is required. Leukopheresis is accompanied by allopurinol (300 $mg/m^2/d$) and, where possible, hydroxyurea (1000 mg/m^2 every 8 hours).[3,4]

Because splenomegaly is often a painful consequence of the disease, splenectomy has occasionally been a useful therapeutic intervention in CML. However, controlled studies have shown that splenectomy does not delay the appearance of blastic phase, does not provide any augmentation of chemotherapy, and does not improve survival.[51] If performed before allogeneic BMT, splenectomy may speed hematopoietic recovery, but may also increase the incidence of graft-versus-host disease.[52] The role of splenectomy is limited and should be used for symptomatic relief in patients unresponsive to other treatments (chemotherapy, radiation).[3,4]

Treatment in Blastic Phase

The terminal phase of CML known as the blastic phase presents as one of two different forms. In about two-thirds of cases the blast cells are of myeloid origin; the remaining instances are of a lymphoid phenotype, nearly always represented as a B-lymphocyte form.[53] Different acute leukemia induction protocols are used in each form of the blastic phase.

The more common myeloid form has been most responsive to high-dose ara-C. The usual protocol for this treatment is ara-C 3000 mg/m^2 every 12 hours for up to 12 doses. This regimen has resulted in complete responses of 25–40%.[3,4]

Bauder et al.[54] investigated the addition of amsacrine to ara-C. The dose of ara-C was reduced to 500–1000 mg/m^2 every 12 hours as a 2-hour infusion on days 1–6, with amsacrine given at 120 mg/m^2 once daily (also as a 2-hour infusion) on days 5–7. Complete response rates were in the range of 40%, with a median survival of 37 weeks compared to 7 weeks for partial responders and resistant disease patients. Prolonged bone marrow aplasia occurred in all patients leading to nearly a 20% mortality from infection.

The most effective treatment of the lymphoid form of blastic phase is a combination vincristine–prednisone regimen; the dose of vincristine is usually 2 mg intravenously each week and prednisone 60 mg/m^2/d. The addition of doxorubicin to this protocol may enhance complete response to around 50%. As with the myeloid form, complete responders survive longer than resistant patients, although this period is still typically less than 1 year.[3,4]

Bone Marrow Transplantation

After reviewing all of the treatment modalities used for CML, the practitioner is left with the fact that with conventional chemotherapy CML is invariably fatal. The only therapeutic option that can result in cure, achieved only through eradication of the Ph^1-positive clone, is allogeneic BMT. BMT is discussed in detail in Chapter 129. We cover only special aspects of BMT that relate to the treatment of CML.

Approximately 60% of CML patients in chronic phase undergoing BMT from an (HLA)-identical sibling donor can be cured of their disease. Results with this type of transplant can be optimized by transplanting patients within the first year of diagnosis with 5-year survival rates approaching 80%.[55] For patients with an HLA-matched sibling donor, BMT must be considered the treatment of choice and should be performed shortly after diagnosis.[56] Unfortunately, less than 30% of patients diagnosed with CML will have this ideal donor and alternative forms of transplantation must be considered. Studies have demonstrated that related one-antigen-mismatch transplants have survival rates which approach HLA-matched transplants. The mortality associated with the higher incidence of severe acute graft-versus-host disease (GVHD) and graft rejection is offset by a reduction in relapse rates as a result of graft-versus-leukemia effect. However, the use of one-antigen-mismatched related donors only increases the donor pool by 5–10%. Attempts to use related donors with two to three antigen mismatches has led to high mortality from graft rejection and acute GVHD. Another potential donor is an unrelated individual who is HLA matched. The results from the National Marrow Donor Program are promising with about 40% of patients alive and in remission at 2 years.[57] The use of matched unrelated BMT to treat CML has the potential to offer this curative therapy to all patients able to tolerate the procedure.[54]

One method of reducing the morbidity and mortality associated with acute GVHD in patients undergoing allogeneic BMT is by T-cell depletion of the donor marrow. Unfortunately, this increases the relapse rates in CML patients due to the loss of a graft-versus-leukemia effect. Soiffer et al.[58] used low-dose IL-2 ($2–6 \times 10^5$ U/m^2/d) starting a median of 60 days after transplant in a group of patients without acute GVHD. IL-2 effectively stimulated immune-related tumor surveillance, leading to significantly lower rates of disease relapse without high rates of severe acute GVHD.[58] Immunostimulants like IL-2 hold promise in reducing relapses in patients with minimal residual disease.

The importance of detecting the *bcr-abl* fusion gene product after BMT has been controversial. A recent study has clarified this issue in patients undergoing allogeneic BMT for CML. Radich et al.[59] studied 346 patients and collected 634 blood samples for polymerase chain reaction (PCR) analysis of *bcr-abl.* This group found that a positive PCR 3 or 36 months after transplant did not predict for relapse of their CML but a positive PCR at 6 or 12 months was highly predictive. With this tool it may be possible to identify patients who are at high risk for relapse after transplant and place them on interferon or IL-2 in an attempt to suppress or irradicate residual disease.[59]

The use of autologous BMT has recently received attention as a result of the observation that there is a reduction in the Ph^1 clone in marrow harvested in chronic phase and stored prior to transplantation.[60] Autologous transplantation of bone marrow or peripheral blood stem cells has resulted in transient loss of the Ph^1 positive clone for several years in a few patients.[61] Relapse rates remain very high and methods for successfully purging CML marrow have been elusive because of the similarity between CML cells and normal stem cells. It is likely that purging CML cells would also eliminate normal marrow stem cells required for bone marrow engraftment. New molecular methods of purging such as the *in vitro* use of antisense oligonucleotide directed against *bcr-abl* mRNA may be more successful. Antisense oligonucleotides with sequences which are "antisense" and complimentary to mRNA for the p210$^{BCR\text{-}ABL}$ have been shown to suppress leukemic cell growth by 95% with no effect on the growth of normal and immature bone marrow cells.[62]

In a recent study using unpurged autologous marrow in patients with chronic phase CML, there was a 58% survival after 7 years of follow-up. The plateau in the survival curve would suggest that autologous BMT is disease modifying. To determine whether patients free of disease several years after autologous BMT are cured, longer follow-up is required.[63]

Chronic Lymphocytic Leukemia

CLL is a lymphoproliferative disorder resulting in a progressive accumulation of functionally incompetent lymphocytes.[64] CLL is an indolent disorder which usually results from malignant transformation of a B lymphocyte with subsequent clonal proliferation. CLL is the most common leukemia in the United States but is rare in Japan and China. Occasional family clusters have been recognized and first-degree relatives of patients with CLL are at three times the risk compared to the general population of developing a lymphoid malignancy. CLL is a disease of the elderly with a median age of onset in the sixth decade of life, although about 10% of CLL occurs in patients less than 50 years of age. There is a male predominance of approximately 2:1. Etiologic factors have not been identified in CLL and there are no data supporting either radiation or viral oncogenesis.[64–66]

CLINICAL PRESENTATION AND STAGING

The diagnosis of CLL is often made after the patient complains of various constitutional symptoms (e.g., fatigue, fever, etc.). These symptoms result from reduction in normal hematopoiesis and the production of dysfunctional lymphocytes.[4,67] Often an abnormal CBC is characterized by high numbers of mature-looking small lymphocytes. A lymphocytosis is nearly always present and a bone marrow aspirate usually shows infiltration with mature-appearing lymphocytes making up 30% of nucleated cells. Diagnosis can be confirmed by analyzing phenotypic characteristics of the peripheral blood lymphocytes. The presence of a monoclonal B lymphocytosis is often sufficient to confirm the diagnosis.[67,68] Rarely, it becomes difficult to differentiate between CLL and a leukemic phase of indolent non-Hodgkins lymphoma, which explains the occasional misdiagnosis of these disease entities.[69] In about 60% of patients, there is lymphadenopathy usually in the cervical, axillary, or inguinal areas. Intra-abdominal nodes may also be palpable and about 50% of patients have spleen and liver enlargement. In addition to these relatively common presentations lymphoid infiltrates can uncommonly be detected at other anatomic sites including, skin, lung, gastrointestinal tract, and central nervous system.[67–69]

A number of laboratory abnormalities can be identified at the time of diagnosis. As stated earlier, lymphocytosis in the peripheral blood and lymphocytic infiltration of the bone marrow are usually seen at diagnosis. Frequently, anemia, thrombocytopenia, and neutropenia are evident either at the time of diagnosis or sometime during the course of the disease. The underlying reason for these cytopenias is not clear but most likely results from infiltration of the bone marrow by malignant lymphocytes. Other potential causes of cytopenias include autoimmune consumption of red blood cells and platelets and excessive T-suppressor cell or diminished T-helper cell function.[69,70] Hypogammaglobulinemia is often present at diagnosis and develops in nearly all patients as the disease progresses. Unlike the Ph^1 in CML, there are no cytogenetic markers for CLL. While no single chromosomal rearrangement identifies CLL, more than 50% of patients with CLL have abnormal karyotypes.[71] A number of the chromosomal rearrangements have predictive value in determining prognosis for a given patient.

There is a wide variability in survival times with some patients dying within 1 year of diagnosis with others living two decades with CLL. The Rai staging system has helped to design appropriate management strategies for CLL.[72] Table 127.4 gives the staging system and median survival time for each stage. The staging system attempts to measure tumor burden. For example, the difference between stage I CLL and stage II CLL is the involvement of abdominal organs rather than more superficial lymph nodes. Prognosis is poorer with increasing stage and it can be concluded that duration of survival is directly related to tumor burden at diagnosis. There remains variability in disease course within each stage so that one patient may have an indolent course with long survival time while another patient may have more aggressive disease and have relatively short survival times.[72,73]

The Rai staging system has been combined into a risk classification with low-risk consisting of stage 0; intermediate risk, stages I and II; and high risk, stages III and IV.[74]

TABLE 127.4. RAI STAGING SYSTEM AND 10-YEAR SURVIVAL

	Lymph[a]	Lymphadenopathy	Organomegaly[b]	Hgb[c]	Platelets[d]
Low Risk (Median Survival, 7–10 Years)					
Stage 0	+	–	–	–	–
Intermediate Risk (Median Survival, 5–6 Years)					
Stage I	+	+	–	–	–
Stage II	+	+/–	+	–	–
High Risk (Median Survival, 2–3 Years)					
Stage III	+	+/–	+/–	+	–
Stage IV	+	+/–	+/–	+/–	+

[a] $>15 \times 10^9$/L blood lymphocytes.
[b] Enlarged liver and spleen.
[c] Hemoglobin < 11 g/dL.
[d] Platelets $< 100{,}000 \times 10^9$/L.

TREATMENT

There are no curative treatments for CLL and therapy is designed to improve quality of life.[75] Without a method to cure this disease, it is not surprising that management of CLL patients is highly variable and somewhat physician specific. Some clinicians delay drug therapy after diagnosis to obtain several weeks of baseline information on signs and symptoms of the disease.[71,76] The decision on whether drug therapy should be initiated after this baseline period is based on several parameters. If there are signs and symptoms of progressive disease, worsening of blood dyscrasias, autoimmune complications, symptomatic splenomegaly, bulky lymph nodes, severe lymphocytosis (greater than 100–200,000/μL), and increased infectious complications, treatment is instituted.

Most stage 0 patients do not require treatment and are usually managed with close observation. In patients with stage I or II disease, management is controversial since studies performed in this group of patients have not found a consistent survival benefit from drug therapy.[77] The use of cytotoxic chemotherapy in early-stage CLL may be reserved for patients who have disease characteristics consistent with more aggressive disease such as short lymphocyte doubling times and diffuse lymphocytic infiltrates in the bone marrow biopsy. In stage III and IV disease, treatment is required with the intention of achieving a partial or complete remission. Median survival times for patients who achieve some form of remission exceed 4 years, while those who do not achieve remission have a median survival of less than 2 years.[77,78] Usually drug therapy is begun with chlorambucil and corticosteroids; chlorambucil can be replaced with cyclophosphamide without compromising response rates. Splenic radiation or splenectomy is often recommended in patients with stage III and IV disease to reduce symptoms and to improve autoimmune blood dyscrasia.[77]

Corticosteroid Therapy

Prednisone has been studied alone and combined with chlorambucil. Response rates are low when prednisone is used alone, rarely resulting in complete remission.[79] When combined with chlorambucil, response rates can approach 70% with about 40% complete responses.[80] Prednisone is particularly helpful when treating patients with autoimmune thrombocytopenia and anemia, both relatively frequent complications of CLL. Splenomegaly, anemia, and thrombocytopenia often improve under corticosteroid therapy.[79,80]

Cytotoxic Chemotherapy

Chlorambucil and prednisone continue to be the standard for treatment of CLL. The use of this combination is based on a small study which showed that prednisone added to chlorambucil was better than chlorambucil alone.[81] However, subsequent experience suggests that the addition of prednisone does not significantly increase response rates but is important in decreasing the morbidity associated with autoimmune blood dyscrasias.[79,80] Chlorambucil is dosed either on a daily basis or intermittently every 2–4 weeks. One study showed that chlorambucil given intermittently reduced marrow toxicity without compromising response rates.[82]

Cyclophosphamide gives a similar response to chlorambucil and can be used in patients who have difficulty tolerating chlorambucil or where response is not optimal. Some patients refractory to chlorambucil will respond to cyclophosphamide. Cyclophosphamide is less commonly used because of its risk of hemorrhagic cystitis with prolonged treatment.[79,80]

Inadequate initial response to chemotherapy or the development of refractory disease after chronic treatment results in subsequent response rates which are half those seen with chlorambucil and prednisone in newly diagnosed patients. In these patients, more intensive combination chemotherapy resulted in response rates that range between 30 and 40% with median durations of response of less than 1 year.[83] The new purine nucleoside analogues, fludarabine, 2-chlorodeoxyadenosine (2-Cda) and 2-deoxycoformycin (pentostatin) may have an important role in the management of patients who have become resistant to chlorambucil plus prednisone.

Fludarabine has been used in patients refractory to standard chlorambucil and prednisone. Keating et al.[84] describe the outcome of 369 patients with previously treated CLL; treatment with fludarabine produced about a 30% complete remission rate and a 15% partial remission rate for an overall response rate of 45%. In general, responses of significant duration occurred in patients with lower stage disease.[84,85] Patients receiving prior alkylating therapy who do not respond to the purine nucleosides have a poor survival. With the superior response rates in patients with refractory disease, fludarabine was investigated in chemotherapy naive patients resulting in response rates of about 80%.[86] While it is difficult to compare these results with alkylating therapy because of different definitions of response, results with fludarabine appear to be similar to chlorambucil.

2-Cda and pentostatin inhibit adenosine deaminase, leading to lethal accumulation of deoxyadenosine in lymphocytes. Pentostatin has only moderate activity in CLL with under 30% of patients achieving a response. It is unlikely that pentostatin alone will have a significant role in the treatment of CLL.[87] 2-Cda does have good activity in CLL with overall response rates in the range of 45% in previously treated patients.[88] Despite equivalent overall response to fludarabine, complete remission with 2-Cda was only 4%, much lower than that reported with fludarabine therapy.[84] Larger studies are required to investigate

2-Cda in previously treated CLL to determine if complete remission rates are comparable to fludarabine.

Juliusson et al.[89] have reported on four patients who responded to 2-Cda after failing fludarabine therapy, suggesting non-cross resistance between these two agents.[89] This observation led to a study in 28 fludarabine-resistant CLL patients. Only 2 patients had a partial remission with 2-Cda without normalization of anemia or thrombocytopenia. It is unlikely that patients who fail fludarabine therapy will benefit from 2-Cda.[90]

Allogeneic Bone Marrow Transplantation

BMT is an important curative therapy for several hematologic malignancies including CML and acute leukemias. In general, BMT is most effective in malignant diseases where there is a relationship between dose of chemotherapy and disease response. While the dose–response relationship with CLL has not been extensively evaluated, there is evidence that it may exist. A regimen of high-dose chlorambucil resulted in a higher number of complete remissions of longer duration compared to standard chemotherapy.[4] In addition, the European Bone Marrow Transplant Group has reported a promising 53% 2-year survival for patients receiving BMT for refractory CLL.[91]

Experience regarding BMT in CLL is limited. Review of the literature and the International Bone Marrow Registry show that a total of 26 patients have been treated with BMT for refractory CLL (24 allogeneic, 2 syngeneic). Median age of the patients was 38 years. The conditioning regimens used contained cyclophosphamide and total body irradiation. Of the 22 patients that could be evaluated for disease status, 19 achieved complete remission. Despite this high complete remission rate, only two patients were free from disease after transplant as measured by molecular studies.[91]

Clearly, dose intensification of CLL therapy is an area of growing interest. While this modality of treatment holds some promise, difficulties will arise given the advanced age of most CLL patients. The median age of onset of 60 years of age eliminates allogeneic transplant as an acceptable option for most CLL patients. The role of dose intensification of conventional chemotherapy has yet to be determined in CLL but is likely to be of moderate application given the morbidity and mortality associated with aggressive chemotherapy in an elderly population.

Biologic Response Modifiers

The mechanism by which IFN-α has its beneficial effects on B-cell malignancies (hairy cell leukemia, CLL, and B-cell lymphomas) is not well understood. It may involve the disruption of tumor necrosis factor-alpha (TNF-α) stimulation of the B-lymphocyte clone. This is supported by the preliminary observation that TNF-α antibodies can produce effects similar to IFN-α in patients with CLL.[92]

The current role of IFN-α is limited. Unlike low-grade non-Hodgkins lymphoma or hairy cell leukemia where IFN-α responses range from 50–90%, the response in advanced CLL is well under 20%.[93] In one study, there was a 50% response with low-dose IFN-α (2×10^6 U/m^2 three times per week) in patients with untreated low-risk CLL.[3,4] The relevance of this finding is unclear given the good quality of life and long-term survival of these patients. It is estimated that it would take 10–15 years to determine if IFN-α offered a survival benefit in patients with newly diagnosed CLL.

A potentially useful application of low-dose IFN-α is following cytotoxic chemotherapy to increase the duration of response. Ferrara et al.[94] demonstrated a significant reduction in relapse in patients given IFN-α after cytotoxic chemotherapy. In addition, two patients who received a partial remission with chemotherapy subsequently had a complete remission with IFN-α therapy. This experience is consistent with observations that IFN-α works best in patients with low tumor burden.

Intravenous Immunoglobulin

Infection as a result of hypogammaglobulinemia is a major cause of morbidity and mortality in patients with CLL.[4] Low IgG levels have been reported in up to 70% of unselected patients with CLL. The decline in IgG concentrations correlates with the stage and duration of disease, patients with advanced disease or disease of long duration having the lowest IgG levels. The efficacy of administering intravenous IgG preparations to CLL patients with hypogammaglobulinemia was well illustrated in a randomized, placebo-controlled, double-blind clinical trial of intravenous IgG dosed at 400 mg/kg every 3 weeks for 1 year.[95] There was a significant reduction in bacterial infections with the intravenous IgG group having 14 bacterial infections versus 36 infections in the placebo arm. However, a cost-effectiveness analysis based on this study demonstrated that its routine use is difficult to justify on a quality of life or economic basis.[96]

Infections cause morbidity and mortality in about 50% of CLL patients. Severe and persistent autoimmune-related decline in red blood cells and platelets is a significant source of morbidity and mortality in about 20–30% of CLL patients.[4] While corticosteroids are considered the therapy of choice for autoimmune blood disorders associated with CLL, intravenous IgG may be helpful in patients who are not receiving benefit from prednisone or are unable to receive prednisone.[3,4]

Intravenous IgG has demonstrated the ability to improve disease parameters in CLL, leading to a reduction in lymphocyte numbers and lymphadenopathy and organomegaly. These are preliminary observations and require further study to determine any definite role of intravenous IgG in the treatment of this malignancy.[97]

Evaluation of Therapeutic Outcomes

For the last 15 years allogeneic BMT has been the only curative therapy for CML. Recently, cytogenetic responses have been obtained with IFN-α leading to an improved duration of survival. However, there is no indication that IFN-α can permanently eliminate the malignant clone. Chemotherapy in chronic phase CML is used to maintain a normal WBC count and consists of oral doses of hydroxyurea or busulfan with patients who are candidates for BMT receiving hydroxyurea. While chemotherapy can produce hematologic remissions, it is unable to produce permanent cytogenetic responses. It is likely that improved cure rates in CML will come by increasing the number of patients who can receive BMT by using matched unrelated donors and by improving supportive care post-transplant so BMT can be offered to the older patient. Since CLL is often an indolent disease that occurs in older patients, an important goal should be to optimize quality of life rather than using aggressive relatively toxic therapy. Chemotherapy which initially involves the administration of chlorambucil and prednisone combinations is used to reduce tumor bulk and relieve symptoms. Later, as the tumor becomes less responsive to initial chemotherapy, fludarabine is able to achieve a second response. In younger patients with more aggressive CLL, dose intensification including BMT may offer long-term disease-free survival.

References

1. Cancer facts and figures—1994. Atlanta, GA, American Cancer Society, 1994.
2. Gale RP. Chronic myelogenous leukemia: Molecule to man. Henry Ford Hosp Med J 1991;39:108–111.
3. Goldman JM. Chronic myelogenous leukemias, in Moossa AR, Schimpff SC, Robson MC, et al. (eds): Comprehensive Textbook of Oncology, 2nd ed., Baltimore, Williams and Wilkins, 1991.
4. Deisseroth AB, Andreeff M, Champlin R, et al. Chronic leukemias, in Devita VT, Hellman S, Rosenberg SA (eds): Cancer: Principles and Practice of Oncology. Philadelphia, JB Lippincott, 1993, pp 1965–1980.
5. Rowley JD. Molecular cytogenetics: Rosetta stone for understanding cancer—twenty-ninth G.H.A. Clowes Memorial Award Lecture. Cancer Res 1990;50:3816–3825.
6. Goldman JM. Chronic myeloid leukemia. Leuk Lymphoma 1993;11:7–9.
7. Boring C, Squires T, Tong T. Cancer statistics—1994. CA Cancer J Clin 1994;41:19–36.
8. Busque L, Gilliland G, Prchal J, et al. Clonality in juvenile CML. Blood 1995;85:21–30.
9. Butturini A, Gale RP. Age of onset and type of leukemia. Lancet 1989;2:789–791.
10. Carabasi MH. Chronic myelogenous leukemia. Cancer Invest 1993;11:408–419.
11. Kurzrock R, Moshe Talpaz. The molecular pathology of chronic myelogenous leukemia. Br J Hemaetol 1991;79:34–37.
12. Westbrook CA. The role of molecular techniques in the clinical management of leukemia. Cancer 1992;70:1695–1700.
13. Leibowitz D, Young KS. The molecular biology of CML: A review. Cancer Invest 1989;7:195–203.
14. Fishleder AJ. Oncogenes and cancer: Clinical applications. Cleveland Clin J Med 1990;57:721–726.
15. Epner DE, Koeffler HP. Molecular genetic advances in chronic myelogenous leukemia. Ann Intern Med 1990;113:3–6.
16. Nowell PC. Chromosomal and molecular clues to tumor progression. Semin Oncol 1989;16:116–127.
17. Daley GQ, Van Etten RA, Baltimore D. Induction of chronic myelogenous leukemia in mice by the *p210 bcr-abl* gene of the Philadelphia chromosome. Science 1990;247:824–830.
18. Preisler H, Raza A. An overview of some studies of chronic myelogenous leukemia: Biological–clinical observations and viewing the disease as a chaotic system. Leuk Lymphoma 1993;11:145–150.
19. Mitelman F. The cytogenetic scenario of chronic myeloid leukemia. Leuk Lymphoma 1993;11:11–15.
20. Eaves AC, Eaves CJ. Growth control in leukemia, in Effects of Therapy on Biology and Kinetics of Residual Tumor, Part A: Pre-Clinical Aspects, 1990, pp 223–236.
21. Clarkson B, Strife A. Cytokinetic considerations relevant to development of a successful therapeutic strategy in chronic myelogenous leukemia. Leuk Lymphoma 1993;11:101–107.
22. Feldman EJ, Arlin ZA. Modern management of chronic myelogenous leukemia. Cancer Invest 1988;6:737–742.
23. Feinstein E, Cimino G, Gale RP, et al. Initiation and progression of chronic myelogenous leukemia. Leukemia 1992;6:37–43.
24. Canellos GP. Clinical characteristics of the blast phase of chronic granulocytic leukemia. Hematol Oncol Clin North Am 1990;4:359–367.
25. Preisler HD, Raza A, Baccarani M. Proliferative advantage rather than classical drug resistance as the cause of treatment failure in chronic myelogenous leukemia. Leukemia Lymphoma 1993;11:303–306.
26. Estrov Z, Kurzrock R, Talpaz M. Role of interleukin-1 inhibitory molecules in therapy of acute and chronic myelogenous leukemia. Leukemia Lymphoma 1993;10:407–411.
27. Kantarijian HM, Deisseroth A, Kurzrock R, et al. Chronic myelogenous leukemia: A concise update. Blood 1993;82:691–703.
28. Kantarjian HM, Keating MJ, Smith TL, et al. Proposal for a simple synthesis prognostic staging system in chronic myelogenous leukemia. Am J Med 1990;88:1–8.
29. Hehlmann R, Ansari H, Hasford J, et al. Chronic myelogenous leukemia: Progress in chemotherapy and evaluation of prognostic score. Semin Hematol 1993;30:44–48.
30. Sokal JE, Baccarani M, Russo D, et al. Staging and prognosis in chronic myelogenous leukemia. Semin Hematol 1988;25:49–61.
31. Arlin ZA, Silver RT, Bennett JM. Blastic phase or chronic myeloid leukemia: A proposal for standardization of diagnostic and response criteria. Leukemia 1990;4:755–757.

32. Rogers S. Current trends in the management of chronic myeloid leukemia. Br J Hosp Med 1992;47:817–823.
33. Hehlmann R, Heimpel H, Kolb HJ, et al. The German CML study, comparison of busulfan versus hydroxyurea versus interferon-alpha and establishment of prognostic score 1. Leuk Lymphoma 1993;11:159–168.
34. Kennedy BJ. The evolution of hydroxyurea therapy in chronic myelogenous leukemia. Semin Oncol 1992;19:21–26.
35. Clift RA, Appelbaum FR, Thomas ED. Treatment of chronic myeloid leukemia by marrow transplantation. Blood 1993;82:1954–1956.
36. Griesshammer M, Hehlmann R, Hochhaus A, et al. Interferon in chronic myeloid leukemia. Ann Hematol 1993;67:101–106.
37. Aulitzky WE, Despres D, Rudolf G, et al. Recombinant interferon beta in chronic myelogenous leukemia. Semin Hematol 1993;30:14–16.
38. Kloke O, Wandl U, Opalka B, et al. A prospective randomized comparison of single-agent interferon-alpha with the combination of interferon-alpha and low-dose interferon-gamma in CML. Eur J Hematol 1992;48:93–98.
39. Freund M, Huber C. Interferon alpha has become a standard in the treatment of chronic myelogenous leukemia. Semin Hematol 1993;30:1–5.
40. Dowding C, Gordon M, Guo A, et al. Potential mechanisms of action of interferon-alpha in CML. Leuk Lymphoma 1993;11:185–191.
41. Peschel C, Aman MJ, Rudolf G, et al. Regulation of the cytokine network by interferon: A potential mechanism of interferon in chronic myelogenous leukemia. Semin Hematol 1993;30:28–31.
42. Kantarjian HM, Smith TL, O'Brien S, et al. Prolonged survival in CML after cytogenetic response to interferon-alpha therapy. Ann Intern Med 1995;122:254–261.
43. Kantarhian HM, Talpaz M. Long-term follow-up results of alpha interferon therapy in chronic myelogenous leukemia at M.D. Anderson Cancer Center. Leuk Lymphoma 1993;11:169–174.
44. Fernandez-Ranada JM, Lavilla E, Odriozola J, et al. Interferon alpha 2A in the treatment of chronic myelogenous leukemia in chronic phase. Results of the Spanish group. Leuk Lymphoma 1993;11:175–179.
45. Morra E, Alimena G, Lazzarino M, et al. Evolving approaches with interferon alpha in chronic myelogenous leukemia. Semin Hematol 1993;30:26–27.
46. Hehlmann R, Heimpel H, Hasford J, et al. Randomized comparison of interferon-alpha with busulfan and hydroxyurea in CML. Blood 1994;84:4064–4077.
47. The Italian Cooperative Study Group on Chronic Myeloid Leukemia: Interferon-alpha-2a as compared with conventional chemotherapy for the treatment of CML. N Engl J Med 1994;330:820–825.
48. Beelen DW, Graeven U, Elmaagacli, et al. Prolonged administration of interferon-alpha in patients with chronic phase philadelphia chromosome positive CML before allogeneic bone marrow transplantation may adversely affect transplant outcome. Blood 1995;85:2981–2990.
49. Freund M, Hild F, Grote-Metke A, et al. Combination of chemotherapy and interferon alpha-2b in the treatment of chronic myelogenous leukemia. Semin Hematol 1993; 30:11–13.
50. Guilhot F. Interferon alpha and low-dose cytosine arabinoside for the treatment of patients with chronic myelogenous leukemia in chronic phase. Semin Hematol 1993;30:24–25.
51. The Italian Cooperative Study Group on Chronic Myeloid Leukemia. Results of a prospective randomized trial of early splenectomy in chronic myeloid leukemia. Cancer 1984;54:333–338.
52. Gratwohl A, Goldman J, Gluckman E, et al. Effect of splenectomy before bone marrow transplantation on survival in chronic granulocytic leukemia. Lancet 1985;2:1290–1291.
53. Advani SH, Malhotra H, Kadam PR, et al. T-lymphoid blast crisis in chronic myeloid leukemia. Am J Hematol 1991;36:86–92.
54. Bauder F, Delmer A, Blanc MC, et al. Treatment of chronic myelogenous leukemia in blast crisis and in accelerated phase with high or intermediate dose cytosine arabinoside and amsacrine. Leukemia and Lymphoma 1993;10:195–200.
55. Goldman JM, Szydlo R, Horowitz MM, et al. Choice of pretransplant treatment and timing of transplants for chronic myelogenous leukemia in chronic phase. Blood 1993;82:2235.
56. Thomas ED, Clift RA, Fefer A, et al. Marrow transplantation for the treatment of chronic myelogenous leukemia. Ann Intern Med 1986;104:155–163.
57. McGlave P, Bartsch G, Anasetti A, et al. Unrelated donor marrow transplantation therapy for chronic myelogenous leukemia: Initial experience of the National Marrow Donor Program. Blood 1993;81:543.
58. Soiffer R, Murray C, Fairclough D, et al. Low-dose IL-2 following T-cell depleted allogeneic bone marrow transplantation for chronic myelogenous leukemia. Blood 1994;84:213a.
59. Radich JP, Gehly G, Gooley T, et al. Polymerase chain reaction detection of the *BCR-ABL* fusion transcript after allogeneic bone marrow transplantation for chronic myelogenous leukemia: Results and implications in 346 patients. Blood 1995;85:2632–2638.
60. Coulombel L, Kalousek D, Eaves CJ, et al. Long-term marrow culture reveals chromosomally normal hematopoietic progenitor cells in patients with Philadelphia chromosome positive chronic myelogenous leukemia. N Engl J Med 1983;308:1493–1498.
61. Daley DQ, Goldman JM. Autologous transplant for CML revisited. Exper Hematol 1993;21:734–737.
62. DeFabritiis P, Amadori S, Calabretta B, Mandelli F. Elimination of clonogenic Philadelphia-positive cells using *BCR-ABL* antisense oligodeoxynucleotides. Bone Marrow Trans 1993;12:261–265.
63. McGlave PB, DeFabritiis P, Deisseroth A, et al. Autologous transplants for CML: Results from eight transplant groups. Lancet 1994;343:1486–1488.
64. Foon KA, Rai KR, Gale RP. Chronic lymphocytic leukemia: New insights into biology and therapy. Ann Intern Med 1990;113:525–539.
65. Dighiero G, Travade P, Chevret S, et al. B-cell chronic lymphocytic leukemia: Present status and future directions. Blood 1991;78:1901–1914.
66. Mulligan SP, Catovsky. The chronic B-cell leukemias. Aust NZ J Med 1993;23:42–50.
67. Karmiris TD, Lister A, Rohatiner ZS. Chronic lymphocytic leukemia. Br J Hosp Med 1991;46:379–385.

68. Tefferi A, Phyliky RL. Clinical update on chronic lymphocytic leukemia. Mayo Clin Proc 1992;67:349–353.
69. Pangalis GA, Boussiotis VA, Kittas C. Malignant disorders of small lymphocytes. Hematopathology 1993; 99:402–408.
70. Juttner CA. Changing concepts in the management of leukemia. Med J Aus 1989;151:43–51.
71. O'Brien S, Giglio AD, Keating M. Advances in the biology and treatment of B-cell CLL. Blood 1995;85:307–318.
72. Geisler C, Hansen MM. B cell chronic lymphocytic leukemia: Recent concepts in classification and treatment. Eur J Hematol 1989;42:31–37.
73. Rai KR, Han T. Prognostic factors and clinical staging in chronic lymphocytic leukemia. Hematol Oncol Clin North Am 1990;4:447–457.
74. Geisler CH. Chronic lymphocytic leukemia newer prognostic approaches in relation to clinical stage. Danish Med J 1993;40:190–207.
75. Mughal T, Goldman JM. Chronic leukemias: Can they be cured? BCJP 1989;43:353–356.
76. Cheson BD. Current approaches to the chemotherapy of B-cell chronic lymphocytic leukemia: A review. Am J Hematol 1989;32:72–77.
77. Rozman C, Montserrat E. Chronic lymphocytic leukemia: When and how to treat. Blut 1989;59:467–474.
78. Schrek R. Chronic lymphocytic leukemic patients, resistant to chemotherapy. Medical Hypothesis 1988;26:227–228.
79. Han T, Rai KR. Management of chronic lymphocytic leukemia. Hematol Oncol Clin North Am 1990;4:431–445.
80. Robertson LE, Keating MJ. Therapeutic approaches to chronic lymphocytic leukemia. Texas Med 1991;87:68–74.
81. Han T, Ezdinli EZ, Shimaoka K, Desai DV. Chlorambucil versus combined chlorambucil–corticosteroid therapy in chronic lymphocytic leukemia. Cancer 1973;31:502.
82. Sawitsky A, Rai KR, Glidewell O, et al. Comparison of daily versus intermittent chlorambucil and prednisone therapy in the treatment of patients with chronic lymphocytic leukemia. Blood 1977;50:1049.
83. Tefferi A, Phyliky RL. Clinical update on chronic lymphocytic leukemia. Mayo Clin Proc 1992;67:457–461.
84. Keating MJ, O'Brien S, Kantarjian H, et al. Nucleoside analogs in treatment of chronic lymphocytic leukemia. Leuk Lymphoma 1993;10:139–145.
85. Feldman EJ, Keating MJ. Fludarabine in the treatment of lymphoproliferative malignancies. Cancer Invest 1993;11:314–318.
86. Keating MJ. Fludarabine phosphate in the treatment of chronic lymphocytic leukemia. Semin Oncol 1990;17:49–62.
87. Gribbon TE. New purine analogues for the treatment of chronic B-cell malignancies. Henry Ford Hosp Med J 1991;39:98–102.
88. Saven A, Carrera CJ, Carson DA, et al. 2-chlorodeoxyadenosine treatment of refractory chronic lymphocytic leukemia. Leuk Lymphoma 1991;5:133–138.
89. Juliusson G, Elmhorn-Rosenborg A, Liliemark J. Response to 2-chlorodeoxyadenosine in patients with B-cell chronic lymphocytic leukemia resistant to fludarabine. N Engl J Med 1992;327:1056–1061.
90. O'Brien S, Kantarjian H, Estey E, et al. Lack of effect of 2-chlorodeoxyadenosine therapy in patients with chronic lymphocytic leukemia refractory to fludarabine therapy. N Engl J Med 1994;330:319–322.
91. Bandini G, Michallet M, Rosti G, Tura S. Bone marrow transplantation for chronic lymphocytic leukemia. Bone Marrow Trans 1991;7:251–253.
92. Heslop HE, Brenner MK, Ganeshagaru K, et al. Possible mechanism of action of interferon-alpha in chronic B-cell malignancies. Br J Hemaetol 1991;79:14–19.
93. Montserrat E, Villamor N, Urbano-Ispizua A, et al. Alpha interferon in chronic lymphocytic leukemia. Eur J Cancer 1991;27:S74–S77.
94. Ferrara F, Rametta V, Mele G, et al. Recombinant interferon-α2A as maintenance treatment for patients with advanced stage chronic lymphocytic leukemia responding to chemotherapy. Am J Hematol 1992;41:45–49.
95. Cooperative Group for the Study of Immunoglobulin in Chronic Lymphocytic Leukemia. Intravenous immunoglobulin for the prevention of infection in chronic lymphocytic leukemia. A randomized, controlled clinical trial. N Engl J Med 1988;319:902–907.
96. Weeks JC, Tierney MR, Weinstein MC. Cost effectiveness of prophylactic intravenous immune globulin in chronic lymphocytic leukemia. N Engl J Med 1991;325:81–86.
97. Besa EC. Recent advances in the treatment of chronic lymphocytic leukemia: Defining the role of intravenous immunoglobulin. Semin Hematol 1992;29:14–23.

Chapter 128

Melanoma

Rowena N. Schwartz, PharmD

Cutaneous melanoma is increasingly becoming a more common disease. It is one of the few cancers in which both the incidence and mortality is increasing every year. In the late 1970s, the incidence of cutaneous melanoma in the United States took a dramatic leap, and the current lifetime risk of melanoma in the United States is approximately 1 in 100. Considering the rapid increase in incidence it is projected that 1 in 90 Americans will develop melanoma by the year 2000.[1] The incidence of melanoma has increased by greater than 80% between 1973 and 1987, and the mortality has increased by almost 30%.[2] The incidence of melanoma has increased during the past decade at a rate faster than that of any other malignancies except lung cancer in women.

Worldwide the incidence of cancer varies. The incidence is approximately 1 per 100,000 per year in the non-Caucasian population, but is as high as 30 per 100,000 per year for fair-skinned people living in the Queensland Province of Australia. The increase in incidence has most affected industrialized countries.

ETIOLOGY

The precise cause of melanoma is not fully understood. A number of host factors and environmental factors have been identified and are likely to combine effect to increase the occurrence of cutaneous melanomas. These factors are listed in Table 128.1.

Genetic factors have been strongly linked to the development of melanoma, but accounts for a small percentage of the overall incidence. Familial atypical multiple mole syndrome (FAMMM) or hereditary dysplastic nevus syndrome (HDNS) is a hereditary disease transmitted by an autosomal dominant gene, and is characterized by a predisposition to develop dysplastic nevi and cutaneous melanoma. In individuals with dysplastic nevus and a family history of cutaneous melanoma, the cumulative lifetime incidence approaches 100%.[4] Approximately 10% of cases of melanoma are associated with family history or HDNS. Dysplastic nevi are thought to be precursors of 20–40% of sporadic melanoma precursors.

Sunlight is one of the most important environmental factors in the pathogenesis of melanoma, and radiation in the ultraviolet B range (280–320 nm) is proposed to be a critical factor. Whites with a tendency to burn who rarely tan with exposure to sunlight are especially at risk. Non-melanoma skin cancers, such as squamous cell and basal cell cancer, have long been shown to be directly related to total sun exposure, and it was thought that melanoma was similarly related to lifetime exposure to the sun. Epidemiologic research has not been able to demonstrate such a relationship between cumulative exposure to sunlight and the occurrence of cutaneous melanoma. Studies have demonstrated a lower risk for the development of melanoma in outdoor workers when compared to indoor workers.[5] These findings suggest that the relationship of the sun to cutaneous melanoma is more complex than that of total exposure. Intermittent overexposure to sunlight, blistering sunburns, and the time of life exposure to sun are now believed to be the more critical factors for development of cutaneous melanoma.[3] Individuals that have a history of severe sunburns appear to have a higher risk of the development of melanoma than those individuals that have had chronic sun exposure without a history of burning. The risk with sunlight and ultraviolet radiation seems to be most active during childhood and adolescence. Intensive exposure to sunlight during infancy and early adolescence is more hazardous than exposure during adult life.

Patients who are immunocompromised are at increased risk for the development of cutaneous melanoma. Immunodeficiency includes those individuals with ataxia telangiectasia, chronic lymphocytic leukemia, Hodgkin's disease, and immunosuppression following organ transplant. Acquired immunodeficiency syndrome also has been shown to increase the risk of developing cutaneous melanoma.

PATHOGENESIS

The pathogenesis of melanoma has not been fully elucidated. Melanocytes are dendritic pigmented cells that arise from the neural-crest tissue during early fetal development and then migrate by 4–6 weeks to a variety of sites within the

TABLE 128.1. RISK FACTORS FOR MELANOMA

Host Risk Factors
Adulthood (>15 years)
History of cutaneous melanoma
Dysplastic nevi
Cutaneous melanomas in first-degree relative
Immunodeficiency/immunosuppression
High density of nevi
High degree of freckling
Sunburn easily/tan rarely
Blond or red hair
Blue or green or gray eyes
Socioeconomic status (higher > lower)
White (versus black) race
External Risk Factors
Intense intermittent sun exposures
History of sunburn
>4 Painful sunburns before the age of 15
Outdoor leisure

(From Refs. 1 and 3.)

body. Melanocytes migrate to the skin, uveal tract, meninges, and ectodermal mucosa. In the adult the majority of melanocytes are located at the epidermal–dermal junction of the skin and the choroid of the eye. Melanocytes are found in a variety of other tissues, such as the meninges and the alimentary and respiratory tract. Primary melanoma can, therefore, arise in any area of the body with melanocytes. The skin is the most frequent site of melanoma; cutaneous melanoma constitutes 90% of all melanoma. Primary melanoma can also arise in the eye, and less frequently in the meninges, respiratory tract, and gallbladder.

Melanocytes synthesize melanin to protect various tissues, such as the skin, from ultraviolet radiation-induced damage. Tyrosinase is the enzyme that is used in the melanosomes to synthesize melanin. Melanoma results from the malignant transformation of skin melanocytes or from the transformation of preexisting nevocellular nevus. Melanoma is a disorder of cell differentiation and proliferation.

Normal melanocytes arise from melanoblasts and undergo a series of differentiation events before reaching a final end-cell differentiation state. Normal melanocytes can be arrested in their differentiation process at any give state of maturation without loss of their proliferation capacity. The pathologic components of the progression in human melanoma appear to involve a series of morphologic stages: (1) an acquired or congenital melanocytic nevus, (2) melanocytic nevus with architectural atypia, (3) histologically dysplastic nevus with cytologic atypia and architectural atypia, (4) primary melanoma in radial growth phase, (5) primary melanoma in vertical growth phase with or without transit metastases, (6) regional lymph node metastatic melanoma (lymphatic), and (7) distant metastatic melanoma (hematogenous).[6] Primary melanoma is characterized by radial growth and limited vertical thickness (<0.75 mm). Primary melanoma demonstrate little tendency to metastasize. Melanoma has a potential for metastasis formation with the onset of a vertical growth phase. Metastatic melanoma is seen with an increase in vertical thickness. Therefore the thickness of a primary melanoma is an important prognostic indicator and is used in the staging classification of cutaneous melanoma.

Normal melanocytes require growth factors for proliferation, but melanoma cells are able to proliferate in the absence of growth factor supplementation. Melanoma cells secrete a variety of growth autocrine and paracrine factors that facilitate proliferation. The types of products that have been isolated from melanoma include various growth factors, proteases, protease inhibitors, cell adhesion proteins, and host response modifiers.[7] The identification of these biologically active substances has led to potential targets for cytotoxic and immunotherapy of melanoma.

Immune factors appear to be involved in the progression of melanoma more than in most other solid tumors. Spontaneous cancer regressions are rare, but are a well-documented phenomenon seen in melanoma.[1] Focal regression in primary melanoma has also been reported. The regression of tumor appears to be associated with host immunity.

A number of different tumor antigens have been identified on melanoma cells by the use of monoclonal antibodies in both human and murine models. Melanoma-associated antigens (MAAs) have been identified in the cellular membrane and cytoplasm of melanoma cells. Ganglioside antigens have been of particular interest in the development of immunotherapy for melanoma. A large number of murine monoclonal antibodies have been developed to MAA and are currently being used in clinical trials for the diagnosis and therapy of melanoma.

The humoral and the cellular responses of individuals with MAA have been described and offer insight into the potential of immunotherapy in the management of metastatic melanoma. Melanoma-directed antibodies have been isolated in the sera of patients with melanoma. The presence of antimelanoma antibodies in the sera of patients correlates with the clinical status of the patients, and the antibodies disappear from the serum as the disease progresses. This phenomenon may be explained by the possible formation of anti-idiotype antibody directed against the anti-melanoma antibody, increase in the circulation of soluble tumor antigens that saturate all the antibody combining sites, increased levels of immunosuppression, or absorption of the antibodies on the tumor mass.

In recent years interest has focused on the role of cell-mediated immune response in melanoma. Specific cell-mediated responses may play a role in tumor regression, but the role of specific cells such as cytotoxic T lymphocytes (CTL) are not fully understood. Tumor-infiltrating lymphocytes (TILs) have been shown *in vivo* and *in vitro* to possess antitumor reactivity. TILs contain a high frequency of mature tumor-specific lymphocytes and have been a target for manipulation in immunotherapeutic approaches for melanoma.

Specific genetic alterations have been demonstrated in the pathogenesis of melanoma. At least four genes have been identified on chromosomes 1, 6, 7, and 9. Alterations in other genes located on other chromosomes may also contribute to the progression of melanoma. Alterations of chromosome 1 are seen in many forms of human cancer. The region of chromosome 1 that is involved in melanoma involves tumor suppressor gene. The alterations seen in chromosome 6 potentially link melanoma and the major histocompatibility complex (MHC). A number of oncogenes have also been found to be activated in melanoma. The genetic influence to melanoma progression appears to involve a series of complex interactions. As these interactions are understood, the potential for gene therapy in melanoma expands.

HISTOLOGIC SUBTYPES OF MELANOMA

Cutaneous melanoma are categorized by growth patterns. The four histologic subtypes of cutaneous melanoma are distinctive in developmental phases and clinical features. The four major subtypes of cutaneous melanoma are superficial spreading melanoma, nodular melanoma, lentigo maligna melanoma, and acral lentiginous melanoma.[8] The is no difference in the clinical outcome of the four subtypes, if the comparison is controlled for depth of penetration.

Superficial spreading melanoma is the most common morphologic type of cutaneous melanoma and accounts for about 70% of all melanoma. The lesions usually arise from a preexisting nevus, and evolve slowly over 1–5 years. At some point superficial spreading melanoma may progress to a more rapid growth phase. Early in the lesion development the superficial spreading melanoma is flat, but as the lesion develops the surface becomes irregular and asymmetrical. As the lesion develops a vertical growth phase, it enlarges and the edges appear notched. This subtype of melanoma is more common in women. Superficial spreading melanoma usually occur after puberty.

Nodular melanoma is the second most common growth pattern of melanoma and occurs in 15–30% of patients. Nodular melanoma is a "pure" vertical growth phase disease. In nodular melanoma a small expansile nodule in the papillary dermis invades the reticular dermis and subcutis. Radial growth phase is absent at all times. Nodular melanomas are more aggressive, and they develop more rapidly than superficial spreading melanoma. Nodular melanoma are dark blue-black and often uniform in color, although a small percentage of nodular melanomas are amelanotic and have a fleshy appearance. Nodular melanoma are raised and are often symmetrical. They occur at any age, and are most common on the trunk or head and the neck. Nodular melanoma are more common in men.

Lentigo maligna melanoma represent a small percentage of melanomas and are unique from other histologic subtypes because lentigo maligna melanomas do not have the same propensity to metastasize. Lentigo maligna melanoma are generally large (>3 cm), flat, tan-colored lesions with shades of brown and black. This subtype of melanoma occurs in an older age group, and they are typically located on the face of elderly Caucasians. Lentigo maligna melanoma are uncommon before the age of 50 and may have been present for more than 5 years.

Acral lentiginous melanoma are characteristically seen on the palms of the hands, soles of the feet, and beneath the nailbeds. Most acral lentiginous melanoma are located on the sole of the foot and look like a large (>3 cm) tan or brown stain. The lesions often have irregular, convoluted borders. Acral lentiginous melanoma include subungual melanoma, and may present as a brown or black line in the great toe or the thumb nail. The acral lentiginous melanoma occur in less than 10% of Caucasians with melanoma, but is the most common type of melanoma reported in blacks, Asians, and Hispanics.

CLINICAL PRESENTATION

The initial clinical presentation of melanoma is often a melanoma lesion. The lesion can be located anywhere on the body, but is most common on the lower extremities in women, and the back and trunk of men. The clinical features used to describe or evaluate a questionable lesion are called the ABCDs of melanoma. Unlike benign pigmented lesions the shape of a melanoma lesion is often (A) asymmetric. Benign lesions tend to have regular margins, whereas melanoma lesions often have irregular (B) borders. The (C) color of melanoma lesions are often variegated, ranging in colors from tan to blue-black, and at times the lesion is intermingled with colors of red, purple, and white. The size or (D) diameter of a melanoma lesion is frequently 6 mm or greater when identified, whereas benign lesions are usually smaller. Early melanoma lesions may be diagnosed at a smaller size. Another warning sign of a potential melanoma is a change in a preexisting nevi. Changes such as the sudden or continuous enlargement of a lesion, an elevation of a lesion, or any changes in the skin surrounding a nevi including redness or swelling are important clinical signs. Uncommonly the sensation of the lesion may become itchy, or tender and painful. Friability of the lesion resulting in bleeding or oozing is also a danger sign.[9] Perhaps the most important warning sign of danger is the evolution in any characteristic of a lesion.

The clinical appearance of a melanoma depends on the histogenesis and the stage of development of the lesion. It is usually possible to distinguish three variants of cutaneous melanoma including flat melanoma, nodular melanoma, and a flat melanoma with a nodular area. Flat melanoma usually corresponds to the histologic classification of superficial spreading melanoma.

The diagnosis of melanoma is complicated by a number of pigmented moles (melanocytic nevi) and nonmelanocytic lesions that resemble melanoma. Ordinary nevi, found on the skin of white adults, average between 10 and 40 lesions. These lesions are usually absent at birth and increase in number through adult life, then gradually decline in number. They appear as tiny pinpoint macules and are usually uniform in color, but increase in size to a maximum of 4–6 mm. Nonmelanocytic pigmented lesions such as seborrheic keratoses, pigmented basal cell carcinoma, and vascular lesions can also appear similar to a melanoma lesion.

SCREENING

The evidence of improved survival rates for melanoma has been the result of the treatment of the lesion at an earlier stage in the development. Efforts to improve survival rates are concentrated on the diagnosis and treatment of the primary lesion. The cost effectiveness of massive screening for all adults by physicians has never been demonstrated. A number of agencies, such as the American Academy of Dermatology and the American Cancer Society, have sponsored free annual screenings. Routine examination of the skin by physicians is recommended for individuals at high risk. The entire cutaneous surface should be examined including the scalp.

Self-examination of the skin places the responsibilities of identification on the individual. Identification of the early melanoma allows the opportunity to treat the lesions when they are thin and curable. Educational pamphlets describing the method of self-examination for the public are available through the American Cancer Society, the American Academy of Dermatology, and the Skin Cancer Foundation. If a newly discovered pigmented lesion is identified or if a preexisting pigmented lesion changes, the patient should see a physician immediately.

DIAGNOSIS

A biopsy is critical in establishing the diagnosis of melanoma. The subsequent histologic interpretation of the biopsy will determine the therapy and prognosis. An excisional biopsy with a margin of normal-appearing skin is recommended for suspicious lesion, and should include a portion of underlying subcutaneous fat for microstaging.[10] Although a biopsy is recommended for large lesions where an excisional biopsy is impractical, an incisional biopsy can be performed but should include a core of full thickness of skin and subcutaneous tissue.

Evaluation of any individual with a suspected melanoma includes a complete history and total body skin examination. The focus of the evaluation is to identify potential risk factors and must include a complete family history. Additionally, any signs or symptoms suggestive of metastatic disease should be completely evaluated.

STAGING

There is a definite association between the size of a primary melanoma lesion and the likelihood of metastases. The prognostic factor originally used to determine survival was based on the cross-sectional profile of the primary tumor, which could be evaluated if the deepest invasive tumor cells lay above or below the sweat glands.[11] This assessment was further clarified by Clark[12] who described the relationship of depth of invasion of the cancer cells to the standard anatomic landmarks of the skin (Table 128.2). Clark's classification is a practical approach for patients with more superficial tumors, because tumors classified as Clark's level I through III seldom metastasize. Criticism of the Clark classification system is related to problems associated with practical measurements. Melanoma lesions that occur in the presence of lymphoid infiltration, fibrosis, or even the cells of preexisting nevus are difficult to assess with classical reference landmarks.

Breslow[13] replaced Clark's classification of reference landmarks with the use of thickness of the primary melanoma lesion. Tumor thickness is quantified to the nearest tenth of a millimeter with an ocular micrometer, measuring from the top of the granular layer of the overlying epidermis to the deepest contiguous invasive melanoma cell. The correlation between tumor thickness and probability of tumor metastases is strong, but does not include aspects such as tumor satellites and vascular invasion.

The American Joint Committee on Cancer (AJCC) has developed a staging system[14] for melanoma that divides patients with localized melanoma into groups according to the microstaging criteria of Breslow and Clark. Table 128.3 compares these three systems. In addition to the considera-

TABLE 128.2. CLARK LEVEL

Clark Level	Anatomic Landmark
N	Epidermis
I	Dermoepidermal junction
II	Papillary dermis
III	Interface between papillary dermis and reticular dermis
IV	Reticular dermis and the subcutaneous fat

(From Ref. 12.)

TABLE 128.3. STAGING OF CUTANEOUS MELANOMA

Stage	Description	TNM	Breslow (mm)	Clark
IA	Localized	$T_1N_0M_0$	≤0.75	II
IB	Localized	$T_2N_0M_0$	0.76–1.5	III
IIA	Localized	$T_3N_0M_0$	1.51–4.0	IV
IIB	Localized	T_4	>4.1 mm	V
III	Limited nodal or <5 in-transit metastases but without nodal involvement	Any TN_1M_0		
IV	Advanced regional or distance metastases	Any TN_2M_0 or any M		

Primary Tumor (T)

T_1: Tumor <0.75 mm thick, invading papillary dermis
T_2: Tumor 0.76–1.5 mm thick, invading papillary reticular dermal interface
T_3: Tumor 1.51–4.00 mm thick, invading reticular dermis
T_4: Tumor >4.00 mm thick, invading subcutaneous tissue, or satellites within 2 cm of primary tumor

Regional Lymph Nodes (N)

N_0: No regional lymph node metastasis
N_1: Metastasis ≤3 cm in greatest dimension in any regional lymph node
N_2: Metastasis >3 cm in greatest dimension in any regional lymph node, or in-transit metastasis

Metastasis (M)

M_0: No distant metastasis
M_1: Distant metastasis

Note: When the thickness and level of invasion criteria do not coincide within a T classification, thickness should take precedence.

tion of primary lesion, the AJCC staging system includes aspects of the tumor satellites, lymph node involvement, and distant metastases.

TREATMENT

The treatment and management of a patient with cutaneous melanoma is decided according to stage of the disease. Local disease is managed and cured with surgical ablation. Regional disease involves the surgical management of the lesion and, with results of recent trials, may incorporate adjuvant immunotherapy. Treatment for disseminated melanoma remains a challenge. Although the literature provides details on numerous clinical trials with single-agent and combination chemotherapy, endocrine manipulations, and immunotherapy, no standard treatment regimen exists for metastatic melanoma.

SURGERY

Melanoma that is determined to be localized can be cured, in most cases, with surgical excision. The extent of margin to excise is important in the prevention of local recurrence and ultimate survival. Primary tumors ≥1 mm require a 1-cm margin.[15] This recommendation is a significant reduction from the 5-cm margin recommended in the past. Large primary tumors between 1 and 4 mm thick can also be surgically excised, but appear to require a more extensive margin up to 2 cm.[16]

When isolated regional lymph nodes are detected via physical exam, therapeutic lymphadenectomy is recommended. The question of lymphadenectomy is not as clear in situations in which the regional lymph nodes do not appear to be involved by clinical examination. A subgroup of patients with clinically staged stage I melanoma will have microscopic metastatic disease in nonpalpable lymph nodes.[17] Clinical evaluation of a lymph node is certainly not a foolproof method to determine if a primary cutaneous melanoma has spread beyond the initial lesion. While prophylactic regional lymph node dissection has not been shown to affect the rate of relapse or survival, its role is still being evaluated. At the present time routine lymphadenectomy is not recommended for all patients with a melanoma lesion. It will be important to determine which patients are at an increased risk for micrometastases and further define the role of lymph node evaluation.

One of the most important aspects of the surgical management of cutaneous melanoma is the role of patient follow-up. Postsurgical follow-up for patients that have had a melanoma excised is essential. Even after excision there remains a risk of undetected metastatic disease and the risk of the development of an additional primary cutaneous melanoma. Scheduled screening in addition to routine surgical follow-up is required for any patient that has had a melanoma.

The role of surgery as curative is limited to that of early-stage disease in cutaneous melanoma. The role of surgery beyond that of cure is less defined, because surgery may offer a mechanism of palliation of isolated metastases. Resection of isolated lesions in the brain[18] and the lungs[19] may be appropriate in certain cases, and should be evaluated based on individual patient criteria. Surgery can be an option in situations when the lesion is accessible, and when the resection may cause problems if not removed. Melanoma in the gastrointestinal tract can lead to obstruction, and appropriate resection may allow the patient significant relief of symptoms. Despite the lack of controlled clinical trials the impact on palliative surgery should be viewed in the context of a patient's comfort and quality of life. Surgery may be considered if the outcome is to provide patient comfort. However, surgery may constitute a significant physical challenge or financial burden to a patient with a limited life expectancy. The clinical scenarios involving surgical resection should be fully evaluated in terms of overall quality of life.

CHEMOTHERAPY

A number of cytotoxic drugs have been found to be effective against melanoma in a small percentage of cases. Although, rarely, chemotherapy has cured a patient, in clinical practice the aim of chemotherapy is to palliate. The results of clinical trials are generally expressed in the term of response rates. The response rate often signifies the fraction of patients that experience a partial response plus those who experience a complete response. Partial response criteria vary, but may require a 50% reduction of the tumor for a minimum of 1 month. A complete response would require a total regression of all metastases for at least 1 month. It is essential to realize these response rates do not reflect survival, and do not evaluate benefit to the patient. Response rates do not incorporate the toxicities and the complications of therapy.

Dacarbazine (DTIC), a cytotoxic drug thought to exert its antitumor effect through alkylation, as a single agent is currently the most effective agent for the treatment of melanoma. In prospective controlled clinical trials response rates of 20–25% have been seen.[20] Early clinical trials demonstrate that patients with skin, subcutaneous tissue, and lymph node involvement respond most frequently, whereas metastatic disease to the liver, bone, and central nervous system (CNS) is often unresponsive.[8] Complete responses are uncommon, with a dismal 2% of patients treated with single-agent dacarbazine sustaining long-term complete responses.[21] Common side effects of dacarbazine therapy include moderate myelosuppression, severe nausea and vomiting, and a flu-like syndrome after large doses. The nausea and vomiting can be prevented and managed with available antiemetics and is not a major complication at this time.

Temozolomide is one of a series of imidazoletetrazine derivatives that was developed as a potential alternative to dacarbazine. Temozolomide is a prodrug of the active metabolite of dacarbazine. At physiologic pH, temozolomide chemically degrades to the cytotoxic triazene monomethyl5-triazenoimidazolecarboxamide (MTIC). Temozolomide is administered orally and appears to be less emetogenic than dacarbazine. Initial phase II trials in chemotherapy-naive metastatic melanoma suggest response rates similar to those seen with dacarbazine.[22]

The *nitrosoureas* have also been shown to be active against melanoma. Again, response rates for this group of alkylating agents tend to fall between 10–20%. Sites of response are similar to those seen with dacarbazine.[23] It was initially thought that there may be an added benefit to the use of the lyophilic nitrosoureas in a malignancy that can metastasize to the brain. Unfortunately, despite the ability of these agents to cross the blood–brain barrier the commercially available nitrosoureas have not been shown to produce an increased response in melanoma in the CNS. Fotemustine, an investigational nitrosourea, has shown preliminary responses in a limited number of patients with cerebral metastases.[24] The most common toxicity of the nitrosoureas is myelosuppression that can be delayed in occurrence and recovery. Leukopenia and thrombocytopenia may be seen as long as 3–5 weeks postdrug administration.

Cisplatin[25] and related compounds[26,27] have also been evaluated in the management of metastatic melanoma. The effectiveness of platinum compounds as single agents is limited, with response rates reported to be less than 10%.[28] The toxicities of cisplatin can be problematic and include acute and delayed nausea and vomiting, renal toxicity, and neurotoxicity.

COMBINATION CHEMOTHERAPY

In an attempt to extend the efficacy of dacarbazine, DTIC has been combined with other chemotherapeutic agents and, most recently, immunotherapy. The combination of dacarbazine with other chemotherapy, most commonly cisplatin, has been able to increase response rates, but the survival benefit has been minimal.[28–30] Again, responses were often limited to metastases in soft tissue, lymph nodes, and the lung—the sites most likely to respond to single-agent dacarbazine. The concern with combination chemotherapy is the cost of therapy in terms of toxicity. Cisplatin and dacarbazine combinations have been extremely toxic. At this time, the risks of combination chemotherapy do not justify the modest response benefit over dacarbazine alone.

ENDOCRINE THERAPY

In an attempt to improve the response rate with dacarbazine, alone or in combination with other chemotherapy, the antiestrogen tamoxifen has been combined with preliminarily positive results. *Tamoxifen* was shown to be beneficial in one randomized trial[31] in terms of response and survival when combined with dacarbazine in 117 patients with metastatic melanoma. The benefit seen with the dacarbazine and tamoxifen combination was most pronounced in women.

The mechanism of action of tamoxifen in melanoma is not understood. Estrogen receptors have been reported in melanoma, but the concentration is usually low. It has been suggested that estrogens may modulate the biology of some tumors, such as melanoma.[32] In addition, the immunologic mechanism that appears to be important in melanoma can be influenced by estrogens. T-lymphocyte activity is suppressed, and the activities of B lymphocytes, macrophages, and natural killer cells can be suppressed or stimulated with estrogens.[33]

Megestrol acetate, a synthetic progestin, has also been combined with chemotherapy in an attempt to influence patient responses and survival. In a small study of 19 patients with melanoma, the addition of megestrol 160 mg/d to dacarbazine, cisplatin, and carmustine suggests a response benefit.[34] Unfortunately, the trial was small and further investigation is warranted.

IMMUNOTHERAPY

Melanoma appears to interact and to respond to the immune system of the host in which it arises. The immune system can influence the pathogenesis of melanoma. In addition, because melanoma is one of the tumors most resistant to standard modalities of radiation and chemotherapy, immunotherapy may offer an avenue of treatment if surgery fails or is not an option. The development of recombinant DNA technology combined with a growing understanding of the molecular basis of the immunologic defenses of melanoma give rise to new opportunities for the development of immune-based treatment for melanoma. Melanoma was an early target for immunotherapeutic trials, and has been a target for a variety of therapeutic approaches to the management of melanoma. Biologic response modifiers have been evaluated for treatment of metastatic disease, and more recently for the postoperative adjuvant treatment for high-risk melanoma patients.

The *interferons* (IFNs) consist of a group of antigenically and genetically distinct species and subspecies; the interferon have differing immunomodulations and are directly cytostatic and cytotoxic. A number of studies have looked at various doses and schedules of recombinant interferon for the treatment of metastatic melanoma as indicated in Table 128.4. Response rates range from 10–30%, but overall response rates are approximately 15% for IFN-α and IFN-β. Unfortunately, the optimal dose, treatment schedule, and treatment combination have not been established for the management of metastatic melanoma.

Initial clinical trials with interferon in metastatic cutaneous melanoma demonstrate the response rates are best in those patients with minimal disease. In addition, responses are most frequent in subcutaneous and lymph node metastases and in pulmonary lesions but have been seen in all sites of disease. These facts initiated the study of IFN-α in the adjuvant treatment of patients after surgical resection.

Interferon is currently being evaluated in the management of patients with high-risk melanoma following the surgical resection. It is clear that the survival rates of patients is dependent on the stage and extent of the primary lesion. In has also been demonstrated in the clinical studies of interferon that there is a negative correlation between the tumor mass and the likelihood of response to interferon therapy. A number of cooperative groups are conducting large multicenter trials to determine the role of interferon in the management of micrometastatic disease.

Toxicities seen with interferon consist of flu-like syndrome including fevers, chills, headache, malaise, myalgias,

TABLE 128.4. IFN-α THERAPY OF MELANOMA

IFN	Dose (mU/m^2)	Route	Weekly Schedule	Response Rates (%)	Ref.
α-2a	12	IM	3 × week	20	35
α-2a	50	IM	3 × week	23	36
α-2a	20	IV	Daily × 5	0	37
α-2a	50	IM	3 × week	11	38
α-2a	3–36	IM	Daily × 7	10	39
α-2a	18	IM	—	14	40
α-2a	18	IM	Daily × 7	8	41
α-2b	10–100	IM/IV	Daily × 7	22	42
α-2b	10	SC	3 × week	27	43
α-2b	30	SC/IV	3 × week	25	44
α-2b	10	IM	3 × week	14	45

and arthralgias. Other toxicities that may be exacerbated by concomitant chemotherapy include renal insufficiency and neurologic toxicities. Hematologic toxicity is generally not dose limiting and it correlates with dosage, schedule, and route of administration. In an attempt to limit systemic toxicity and to optimize local benefit the regional administration of interferon has been evaluated in a variety of settings. Intralesional and perilesional application of interferon have been shown to have some efficacy and appear to be well tolerated.[46]

Interleukin-2 (IL-2), a glycoprotein that is produced by activated lymphocytes, has been extensively studied in the management of metastatic melanoma. IL-2 stimulates the production and release of many secondary cytokines including IL-1, IL-2, tumor necrosis factor (TNF), and interferons. In addition IL-2 appears to stimulate the cytotoxic activities of NK cells, monocytes, and cytotoxic T cells. As is seen with the interferons, IL-2 monotherapy has not been well characterized for the management of melanoma.

Initial studies with IL-2 used relatively high doses of the drug.[47] The response rates were about 20%, but did not provide significant survival benefit. In addition, the toxicities associated with high doses of IL-2 are significant and limit the practicality of therapy. At high doses, capillary leak syndrome is seen, and may be accompanied by hypotension, visceral edema, dyspnea, tachycardia, and arrhythmias. In an attempt to provide the benefit of IL-2 therapy without the limiting side effect, a number of studies have evaluated lower dose IL-2 alone[48] or with chemotherapy[49] and with interferon therapy.[50–52] Response rates have been promising, but survival rates have not been significantly affected.

Active immunization has been a strategy for immunomodulation for melanoma. Vaccines from viable autologous or allogeneic tumor cells or tumor-derived products can be used to elicit a response targeted for the melanoma. A variety of different vaccine preparations have been tested,[53] but survival benefit has not been demonstrated in a controlled clinical trial.

Monoclonal antibodies have been used for the diagnosis and the treatment of melanoma. Two strategies have been pursued: treatment with a monoclonal antibody to activate the host immune system[54,55] and treatment with a conjugated monoclonal antibody. Monoclonal antibodies have been conjugated to cytotoxic agents, radioisotopes, and toxins such as ricin A. Trials of monoclonal antibodies where initially limited secondary to the production of the monoclonal antibody. A problem that is seen in current studies is the induction of neutralizing antibodies to the murine monoclonal antibodies. Humanized murine or pure human monoclonal antibodies against melanoma-associated

TABLE 128.5. CHEMOIMMUNOTHERAPY IN MELANOMA

Ref.	Regimen	Pt (N)	Objective Response (%)
49	DTIC 1000 mg/m^2 CI day 1 IL-2 12–30 mIU IV days 15–19 + 22–26 Q4 weeks	32	22
59	CDDP 40 mg/m^2 IV days 1 + 8 IFN-α 3 mU/m^2 SQ days 1–5 + 8–12 Q3–4 weeks	42	24
60	DTIC 200 mg/m^2 IV days 1–5 VCR 1 mg/m^2 IV days 1 + 4 Bleo 15 mg IV days 2 + 5 CCNU 80 mg PO day 1 IFN-α 3 × 10^6 IU/day SQ × 6 weeks, then 6 × 10^6 IU 3 × week	45	62
63	CDDP 135–150 mg/m^2 IV days 32 + 53 (+ WR 2721) *or* CDDP 50 mg/m^2 IV days 32–35 + 53–55 IL-2 6 × 10^5 IU/kg IV Q 8 h days 1–5 + 15–19 Q 10 weeks	27	37
67	CDDP 100 mg/m^2 IV day 1 IL-2 18 × 10^6 IU/m^2/d CI days 3–6 + 17–21 IFN-α 9 × 10^6 IU SQ 3 × week Q28 days	39	53.8
68	DTIC 800 mg/m^2 IV day 1 Q3 weeks IFN-α 9 mIU days 1–6 × 10 weeks, then 9 mIU 3 × week	75	25
69	DTIC 200 mg/m^2 IV days 22–26 Q4 weeks IFN-α 15 mIU days 1–5 × 3 weeks, then 10 mIU 3 × week	30	53
70	VDS 3 mg/m^2 IV Q3 weeks IFN-α 3–9 mIU SQ daily	19	26

antigens could potentially avoid the problem with the human antimouse antibody (HAMA).

Gene therapy of human melanoma is still in its infancy but suggests several exciting approaches to the management of metastatic melanoma. Several strategies for gene therapy are currently under investigation for the treatment of melanoma.[56] One approach to gene therapy for melanoma is the modification of melanoma cells with the insertion of one or more cytokine genes, and then administering these altered allogeneic or autologous cells as a vaccine. Cytokine gene transduction has been accomplished with a number of cytokines including IL-2, TNF, IL-4, and IFN. The insertion of cytokine genes into melanoma cells is hoped to significantly increase the cells' immunogenicity.

Genes can also be transferred *in vitro* into tumor infiltrating lymphocytes (TILs) associated with melanoma in an attempt to potentiate the cytotoxicity of these cells. Rosenberg and colleagues[57,58] were the first to attempt to transduce the gene coding for resistance to neomycin into human TILs. This approach has since been used to transfer the TNF gene into TILs.

COMBINATION IMMUNOTHERAPY AND CHEMOTHERAPY

The use of chemotherapy and immunotherapy alone have been limited by low overall response rates and toxicity. A new generation of multidrug combinations includes IFN-α and/or IL-2 with chemotherapy and they have provided higher response rates. The initial phase I and II trials of chemoimmunotherapy approaches include combinations of interferon and chemotherapy,[59,60] IL-2 and chemotherapy,[61–65] or the combination of IL-2, chemotherapy, and interferon[66,67] (Table 128.5). The problem with most of the published trials is the lack of comparison of drug regimens to a standard or control. Results, to date, suggest response rates greater than those seen with dacarbazine alone, but the regimens have not yet been evaluated against single-agent dacarbazine. Toxicities can be severe and are consistent with the individual agents in the regimen.

LIMB PERFUSION

For recurrent melanoma of the limbs, one approach to therapy is regional isolated perfusion with cytostatic drugs.[71–73] After regional perfusion, objective response rates have been reported to be as high as 80%. The role of hyperthermia (39–40°C) with regional isolated perfusion is not clearly defined. Although most clinical trials have used melphalan[72–74] it is not known whether a combination of melphalan with other agents may improve results. Recent work with the biological response modifiers such as TNF has been encouraging.[75]

CONCLUSION

Cutaneous melanoma is becoming a common cancer, but it is a cancer that can be prevented and cured if detected early. Early stage melanoma has excellent complete response rates with surgical resection. It is the dilemma with metastatic disease that remains a clinical challenge. At this time there is no standard therapy choice. The results of chemoimmunotherapy look promising, but the definitive drug combination and schedule is not defined; this is the challenge of future comparative clinical trials. The role of IFN in an adjuvant setting is promising. Results from cooperative studies suggest a definitive role will soon be available.[76]

The results of early treatment emphasize the role for early detection and prevention.[77,78] Education and re-education about the importance of sunscreens and sun protection has the potential to help decrease the rising incidence of this disease.

REFERENCES

1. Koh HK. Cutaneous melanoma. N Engl J Med 1991;325:171–182.
2. Rigel DS, Kopf AW, Friedman RJ. The rate of malignant melanoma in the United States: Are we making an impact? J Am Acad Dermatol 1987;17:1050–1053.
3. Autier P. Epidemiology of melanoma, in Lejeune FJ, Chaudhuri PK, Das Gupta TK (eds): Malignant Melanoma: Medical and Surgical Management. New York, McGraw-Hill, 1994, pp 1–7.
4. Greene MH, Clark WH, Tucker M, et al. Acquired precursors of cutaneous malignant melanoma. N Engl J Med 1985;312:91–94.
5. Gallagher RP, Elwood JM, Yang P. Is chronic sunlight exposure important in accounting for increases in melanoma incidence? Int J Cancer 1989;44:813–815.
6. Kirkwood JM, Lotze MT. Melanoma, in Kirkwood JM, Lotze MT, Yasko JM (eds): Current Cancer Therapeutics. Philadelphia, Current Medicine, 1994, p 131.
7. Dore JF, Carrel S. Biology of melanoma differentiation and progression, in Lejeune FJ, Chaudhuri PK, Das Gupta K (eds): Malignant Melanoma: Medical and Surgical Management. New York, McGraw-Hill, 1994, pp 9–26.
8. Balch CM, Houghton AN, Peters LJ. Cutaneous melanoma, in DeVita, Hellman S, Rosenberg SA (eds): Cancer: Principles and Practice of Oncology, 4th ed. Philadelphia, JB Lippincott, 1993, pp 1613–1614.
9. Friedman RJ, Rigel DS, Silverman MK, et al. Malignant melanoma in the 1990's: The continued importance of early detection and the role of physician examination and self-examination of the skin. CA Cancer J Clin 1991;41:201–227.
10. NIH Consensus Development Panel on Early Melanoma. Diagnosis and treatment of early melanoma. NIH Consensus Conference. J Am Med Assoc 1992;268:1314–1319.

11. Cochran AJ. Histology and prognosis in malignant melanoma. J Pathol 1969;97:459–468.
12. Clark WH, Jr. A classification of malignant melanoma in man correlated with histogenesis and biologic behavior, in Montagna W, Hu F (eds): Advances in Biology of the Skin. The Pigmentary System. London, Pergamon Press, 1967, pp 621–645.
13. Breslow A. Thickness, cross-sectional areas and depth of invasion in the prognosis of cutaneous melanoma. Ann Surg 1970;1902–1908.
14. Melanoma of the skin (excluding eyelid), in Beahrs OH, Henson DE, Hutter RVP, Myers MH (eds): Manual for Staging Cancer, 3rd ed. Philadelphia, JB Lippincott, 1988, pp 139–144.
15. Veronesi U, Cascineli N. Narrow excision (1-cm margin). Arch Surg 1991;126:438–441.
16. Balch CM, Urist MM, Karakousis CP, et al. Efficiency of 2-cm surgical margins for intermediate-thickness melanomas (1-4 mm): Results of a multi-institutional randomized surgical trial. Ann Surg 1993;218:262–269.
17. Cay CL, Sober AJ, Lew RA, et al. Malignant melanoma patients with positive nodes and relatively good prognosis: Microstaging retains prognostic significance in clinical stage I melanoma patients with metastases to regional nodes. Cancer 1981;47:955–962.
18. Somoza S, Kondziolka D, Lansford D, et al. Stereostatic radiosurgery for cerebral metastatic melanoma. J Neurosurg 1993;79:661–666.
19. Harpole DH, Johnson CM, Wolfe, et al. Analysis of 945 cases of pulmonary metastatic melanoma. J Thorac Cardiovasc Surg 1992;103:743–750.
20. Comis RL. DTIC in malignant melanoma. A perspective. Cancer Treat Rep 1976;64:1123.
21. Hill GJ, Krementz ET, Hill HZ. Dimethyl traiazenoimidazole carboxamide and combination therapy for melanoma. IV. Late results after complete responses to chemotherapy. Cancer 1984;53:1299–1305.
22. Bleehen NM, Newlands ES, Lee SM, et al. Cancer research campaign phase II trial of temozolomide in metastatic melanoma. J Clin Oncol 1995;13:910–913.
23. Ahmann DL. Nitrosoureas in the management of disseminated malignant melanoma. Cancer Treat Rep 1976;60:747.
24. Jacquillat C, Khayat D, Banzet P, et al. Final report of the French multicenter phase II study of the nitrosourea fotemustine in 153 evaluable patients with disseminated malignant melanoma including patients with cerebral metastases. Cancer 1990;66:1873–1878.
25. Mechl Z, Kreja P. *Cis*-diamminedichloroplatinum in the treatment of disseminated malignant melanoma. Neoplasia 1983;30:371–377.
26. Olver I, Green M, Peters W, et al. A phase II trial of zeniplatin in metastatic melanoma. Am J Clin Oncol 1995;18:56–58.
27. Evans L, Casper ES, Rosenbluth R. Phase II trial of carboplatin in advanced melanoma. Cancer Treat Rep 1987;71:171.
28. Steffens TA, Bajorin D, Chapman PB, et al. A phase II trial of high-dose cisplatin and dacarbazine: Lack of efficacy of high-dose, cisplatin-based therapy for metastatic melanoma. Cancer 1991;68:1230–1237.
29. Luger SM, Kirkwood JM, Ernstoff MS, Vlock DR. High-dose cisplatin and dacarbazine in the treatment of metastatic melanoma. J Natl Cancer Inst 1990;82:1934–1937.
30. Murren JR, DeRosa W, Durivage HJ, et al. High-dose cisplatin plus DTIC in the treatment of metastatic melanoma. Cancer 1991;67:1514–1517.
31. Cocconi G, Bella M, Calabresi F, et al. Treatment of metastatic malignant melanoma with dacarbazine plus tamoxifen. N Engl J Med 1992;327:516–523.
32. Adami HO, Bergstrom R, Holmberg L, et al. The effect of female sex hormones on cancer survival. J Am Med Assoc 1990;263:2189–2193.
33. Paavonen T, Andersson LC, Adlercreutz H. Sex hormone regulation of *in vitro* immune response: Estradiol enhances human B cell maturation via inhibition of suppressor T cells in pokeweed mitogen-stimulated cultures. Exp Med 1981;154:1935–1945.
34. Nathanson L, Meelu MA, Losada R. Chemohormone therapy of metastatic melanoma with megestrol acetate plus dacarbazine, carmustine, and cisplatin. Cancer 1994;73:98–102.
35. Creagan ET, Ahmann DL, Green SJ, et al. Phase II study of low dose recombinant leukocyte A interferon in disseminated malignant melanoma. J Clin Oncol 1984;2:1002–1005.
36. Creagan ET, Ahmann DL, Green SJ, et al. Phase II study of recombinant leukocyte A interferon (rIFN-alpha A) in disseminated malignant melanoma. Cancer 1984;54:2844–2849.
37. Coates A, Rallingsm, Hersey P, Swanson C. Phase II study of recombinant alpha 2-interferon in advanced malignant melanoma. J Interferon Res 1986;6:1–4.
38. Hersey P, Hasic E, MacDonald M, et al. Effects of recombinant leukocytes interferon (rIFN-alpha a) on tumor growth and immune responses in patient with metastatic melanoma. Br J Cancer 1985;51:815–826.
39. Legha SS, Papadopoulos NE, Plager C, et al. Clinical evaluation of recombinant interferon alfa-2a (Roferon-a) in metastatic melanoma using two different schedules. J Clin Oncol 1987;5:1240–1246.
40. Elsasser-Beile U, Drews H. Interferon in the treatment of malignant melanoma. Results of clinical studies. Fortschr Med 1987;105:401.
41. Steiner A, Wolf C, Pehamberger H. Comparison of the effects of three different treatment regimens of recombinant interferons (r-IFN alpha, r-IFN gamma, and r-IFN-alpha + cimetidine) in disseminated malignant melanoma. J Cancer Res Clin Oncol 1987;113:459–465.
42. Kirkwood JM, Ernstoff MS, Davis CA, et al. Comparison of intramuscular and intravenous recombinant alpha-2 interferon in melanoma and other cancers. Ann Intern Med 1985;103:32–36.
43. Dorval T, Palangie T, Jouve M, et al. Clinical phase II trial of recombinant DNA interferon (interferon alfa 2b) in patients with metastatic malignant melanoma. Cancer 1986;58:215–218.
44. Robinson WA, Mughal TI, Thomas MR, et al. Treatment of metastatic malignant melanoma with recombinant interferon alpha-2. Immunobiol 1986;172:275–282.
45. Sertoli MR, Bernengo MG, Ardizzoni A, et al. Phase II trial of recombinant alfa-2b interferon in the treatment of metastatic skin melanoma. Oncology 1989;46:96–98.

46. von Wussow P, Bock B, Hartmann F, Deicher H. Intralesional interferon-alpha therapy in advanced malignant melanoma. Cancer 1988;61:1071–1074.
47. Parkinson DR, Abrams JS, Wiernik PH, et al. Interleukin-2 therapy in patients with metastatic malignant melanoma: A phase II study. J Clin Oncol 1990;8:1650–1656.
48. Whitehead RP, Kopecky KJ, Samson MK, et al. Phase II study of intravenous bolus recombinant interleukin-2 in advanced malignant melanoma: Southwest Oncology Group study. J Nat Cancer Inst 1991;83:1250–1252.
49. Flaherty LE, Redman BG, Chabot G, et al. A phase I–II study of dacarbazine in combination with outpatient interleukin-2 in metastatic malignant melanoma. Cancer 1990;65:2471–2477.
50. Richards JM, et al. Sequential chemotherapy in the treatment of metastatic melanoma. J Clin Oncol 1992;1338–1343.
51. Keilholz U, Scheibenbogen, Tilgen W, et al. Interferon-alpha and interleukin-2 in the treatment of metastatic melanoma. Cancer 1993;72:607–614.
52. Atzpodien J, Korfer A, Fanks CR, et al. Home therapy with recombinant interleukin-2 and interferon-alpha 2b in advanced human malignancies. Lancet 1990;335:1509–1512.
53. Morton DL, Foshag LJ, Dave SB, et al. Prolongation of survival in metastatic melanoma after active specific immunotherapy with a new polyvalent melanoma vaccine. Ann Surg 1992;216:463–482.
54. Carrasquillo JA, Abrams PG, Schroff RW, et al. Effect of antibody dose on the imaging and biodistribution of indium-111 9.2.27 anti-melanoma monoclonal antibody. J Nucl Med 1988;29:39–47.
55. Murray JL, Rosenblum MG, Lamki L, et al. Clinical parameters related to optimal tumor localization of indium-111-labeled mouse antimelanoma monoclonal antibody ZME-018. J Nucl Med 1987;28:25–33.
56. Parmiani G, Colombo MP. Somatic gene therapy of human melanoma: Preclinical studies and early clinical trials. Melan Res 1995;5:295–301.
57. Rosenberg ST, Aebersold P, Cornetta K. Gene transfer into humans—immunotherapy of patients with advanced melanoma, using tumor-infiltrating lymphocytes modified by retroviral gene transduction. N Engl J Med 1990;323:570–578.
58. Rosenberg AS, Anderson F, Blaese, Hwu P. The development of gene therapy for the treatment of cancer. 1993;218:455–464.
59. Margolin KA, Doroshow JH, Akman ST. Phase II trial of cisplatin and alpha-interferon in advanced malignant melanoma. J Clin Oncol 1992;10:1574–1578.
60. Pyrhonen S, Hahka-Kemppinen M, Muhonen T. A promising interferon plus four-drug chemotherapy regimen for metastatic melanoma. J Clin Oncol 1992;10:1919–1926.
61. Mitchell MS, Kempf RA, Harel W, et al. Effectiveness and tolerability of low-dose cyclophosphamide and low-dose intravenous interleukin-2 disseminated melanoma. J Clin Oncol 1988;6:409–424.
62. Shiloni E, Pouillart P, Janssens J, et al. Sequential dacarbazine chemotherapy followed by recombinant interleukin-2 in metastatic melanoma. A pilot multicenter phase I–II study. Eur J Cancer Clin Oncol 1989;25(suppl 3):S45–S49.
63. Demchak PA, Mier JW, Robert NJ, et al. Interleukin-2 and high-dose cisplatin in patients with metastatic melanoma: A pilot study. J Clin Oncol 1991;9:1821–1830.
64. Stoter G, Aamdal S, Rodenhuis S, et al. Sequential administration of recombinant human interleukin-2 and dacarbazine in metastatic melanoma: A multicenter phase II study. J Clin Oncol 1991;9:1687–1691.
65. Flaherty LE, Robinson W, Redman BG, et al. A phase II study of dacarbazine and cisplatin in combination with outpatient administered interleukin-2 in metastatic malignant melanoma. Cancer 1993;71:3520–3525.
66. Richards JM, Mehta N, Ramming K, Skosey P. Sequential chemoimmunotherapy in the treatment of metastatic melanoma. J Clin Oncol 1992;10:1338–1343.
67. Khayat D, Tourani JM, Benhammouda A, et al. Sequential chemoimmunotherapy with cisplatin, interleukin-2, and interferon alfa-2a for metastatic melanoma. J Clin Oncol 1993;11:2173–2180.
68. Bajetta E, Negretti E, Giannotti B, et al. Phase II study of interferon-2a and dacarbazine in advanced melanoma. Am J Clin Onc 1990;13:405–409.
69. Falkson CI, Falkson G, Falkson HC. Improved results with the addition of recumbent interferon alpha-2b to dacarbazine in treatment with patients with metastatic malignant melanoma. J Clin Oncol 1991;9:1403–1408.
70. Smith KA, Green JA, Eccles JM. Interferon alpha-2a and vindesine in the treatment of advanced malignant melanoma. Eur J Cancer 1992;28:438–441.
71. Kroon BBR. Regional isolation perfusion in melanoma of the limbs; accomplishments, unsolved problems, future. Eur J Surg Oncol 1998;14:101–110.
72. Klaase JM, Kroon BBR, van Geel AN, et al. Prognostic factors for tumor response and limb recurrence-free interval in patients with advanced melanoma of the limbs treated with regional isolated perfusion with melphalan. Surgery 1994;115:39–45.
73. Klaase JM, Kroon BBR, van Geel AN, et al. A retrospective comparative study evaluating the results of a single perfusion versus double-perfusion schedule with melphalan in patients with recurrent melanoma of the lower limb. Cancer 1993;71:2990–2994.
74. Edwards MJ, Soong SJ, Boddie AW, et al. Isolated limb perfusion for localized melanoma of the extremity. Arch Surg 1990;125:317–321.
75. Lejeuene FJ, Lienard D. Isolation perfusion of the limbs for in transit melanoma metastased with cytokines and chemotherapy, in Lejeune FJ, Chaudhuri PK, Das Gupta TK (eds): Malignant Melanoma: Medical and Surgical Management. New York, McGraw-Hill, 1994, pp 233–240.
76. Kleeberg UR. Adjuvant treatment of melanoma, in Lejeune FJ, Chaudhuri PK, Das Gupta TK (eds): Malignant Melanoma: Medical and Surgical Management. New York, McGraw-Hill, 1994, pp 271–286.
77. Lober CW. Dysplastic (atypical) nevi: Significance and management. S Med J 1992;85:870–877.
78. Koh HK, Geller AC, Miller DR, Lew RA. Screening for melanoma and skin cancer in the United States, in Miller AB, Chamberlain J, Day NE, et al (eds): Cancer Screening. New York, Cambridge University Press, 1990.

Chapter 129

Bone Marrow Transplantation

Gary C. Yee, PharmD, FCCP

Bone marrow transplantation (BMT) is a process that involves intravenous infusion of hematopoietic stem cells from a compatible donor into a recipient with a life-threatening disease. Because of the widespread acceptance of peripheral blood rather than bone marrow as a source of hematopoietic stem cells for autologous transplants, BMT is sometimes referred to as hematopoietic stem-cell transplantation (HSCT) and autologous BMT is sometimes referred to as autologous blood or marrow transplantation (ABMT) or blood cell transplantation (BCT). The rationale for BMT in the treatment of malignant disease is based on studies that show that most anticancer drugs have a steep dose–response relationship and that bone marrow suppression limits the chemotherapy dosage that can be safely administered. Although standard-dose chemotherapy can prolong survival in many cancer patients, most patients are not cured of their disease (Fig. 129.1). The infusion of hematopoietic stem cells allows oncologists to administer very high chemotherapy doses (as much as tenfold higher). Tumor cell kill will therefore be greatly increased, and the likelihood of cure higher, if we assume that most tumor cells that are resistant to standard doses would be sensitive to higher doses. Chemotherapy dose cannot be escalated indefinitely, however, because of the risk of death due to nonhematopoietic toxicity.

BMT has become an important treatment modality for a variety of malignant and nonmalignant diseases. There are more than 100 active BMT programs in the United States. It was estimated that 20,000 patients would be transplanted in 1995 worldwide (12,000 autologous, 8000 allogeneic), and the number is expected to increase 15–20% each year. Historically the most common type of donor was a genetically nonidentical individual (referred to as allogeneic BMT) such as a histocompatible sibling. But the number of autologous transplants—in which the patient serves as his or her own donor—has increased dramatically, and the number of autologous transplants performed each year currently exceeds the number of allogeneic transplants. The rapid growth in the number of autologous transplants is related to the observation that this treatment modality results in long-term survival and probably cure in many patients with lymphoma and breast cancer. Although the use of high-dose chemotherapy with autologous rescue in women with breast cancer remains controversial, this issue has greatly increased the awareness of the lay public and health care professionals to BMT as a treatment modality. Insurance coverage for BMT in women with breast cancer is now required in some states, and other states are considering similar mandates. Although this chapter focuses on the application of BMT in the treatment of malignant disease, it is important to note that many nonmalignant diseases—including aplastic anemia, thalassemia, sickle cell anemia, immunodeficiency disorders, and other genetic disorders—are potentially curable with allogeneic BMT.

This chapter summarizes the current use of BMT in the treatment of acute and chronic leukemia, lymphoma, multiple myeloma, breast cancer, and other solid tumors. More detailed information on BMT can be found in recently published reviews and books.[1–7]

Selection of Donors

Three types of donors are used in BMT. In autologous BMT, patients receive their own hematopoietic stem cells, which were collected and stored before intensive cytotoxic therapy. In syngeneic BMT, an identical twin serves as the donor. In allogeneic BMT, the donor is genetically not identical to the recipient but shares some common tissue antigens. Immunologic compatibility is evaluated with studies of cell surface antigens encoded by genes of the major histocompatibility complex (MHC), which in humans is located on the sixth chromosome and is referred to as the HLA (human leukocyte antigen) complex.[8,9] The genes of the HLA system are clustered in three distinct regions designated class I, class II, and class III. Class I and class II antigens function as major transplantation antigens while products of class III genes play important roles in the immune system. The major class I loci in humans are referred to as HLA-A, HLA-B, and HLA-C. There is one major class II locus (HLA-D); this region is comprised of three sets of genes encoding HLA-DR, HLA-DQ, and HLA-DP molecules. HLA-D antigens are primarily DR specific, and the two are strongly correlated. Class I and class

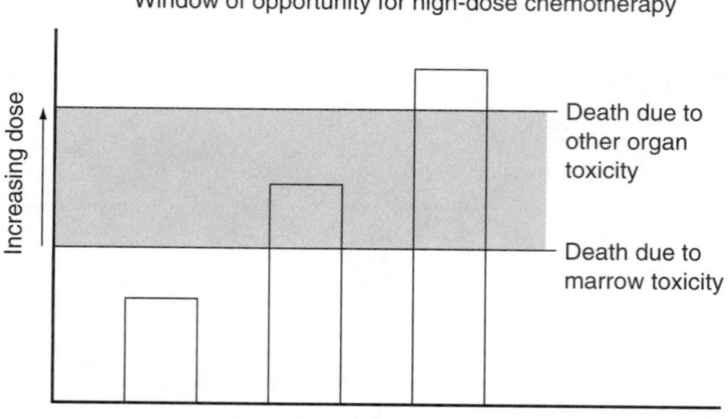

Figure 129.1. Patients represented by the middle column are the best candidates for bone marrow transplantation because this technique allows administration of chemotherapy or radiation in doses that would otherwise be intolerable due to severe myelosuppression. *(From Bierman PJ, Armitage JO. Autologous bone marrow transplantation for non-Hodgkin's lymphoma, in Forman SJ, Blume KG, Thomas ED (eds): Bone Marrow Transplantation. Boston, Blackwell, 1994, p 687. Reprinted by permission of Blackwell Science, Inc.)*

II antigens differ in their tissue distribution, structure, and function. Class I antigens are expressed on virtually all nucleated cells and serve as the primary targets for cytotoxic T lymphocytes. In contrast, class II antigens are expressed only on macrophages, B lymphocytes, and activated T lymphocytes, and serve as the primary targets for helper T lymphocytes. The relative importance of class I versus class II antigens as determinants of risk of acute graft-versus-host disease (GVHD) or graft failure is not clear.

The most important HLA loci in BMT appear to be HLA-A, HLA-B, and HLA-D or HLA-DR. Typing for HLA-A, HLA-B, and HLA-DR is usually performed by serologic typing with standard microcytotoxicity assays. HLA types determined by this method are reported as the loci (A, B, or DR), followed by a number. A lowercase "w" is sometimes added before the number to indicate "workshop" or tentative designation based on American or international histocompatibility workshops. Typing for the HLA-D region also can be performed with cellular typing methods, such as the mixed lymphocyte reaction (MLR) or mixed lymphocyte culture (MLC). A "positive" MLR or MLC indicates incompatibility somewhere in the HLA-D region. Individuals who have a small degree of reactivity in the MLR or MLC (expressed as a low percent relative response) and who meet other selection criteria could serve as marrow donors. However, recent studies indicate that MLR or MLC reactivity does not correlate significantly with the risk of acute GVHD and some BMT centers no longer use this method to determine HLA compatibility.[10,11] In addition to serologic typing, some BMT centers use DNA-based techniques (e.g., polymerase chain reaction [PCR]) for HLA-DR typing because of the extensive polymorphism in the HLA-DR subregion and the high error rate in serologic HLA-DR typing.[9] For example, although there are more than 100 DRB1 alleles, serologic reagents can distinguish no more than 15 different DR serotypes. Preliminary results indicate that the use of these DNA-based techniques to select unrelated donors may reduce the risk of severe acute GVHD in that setting.[12]

Historically, the most common donor for allogeneic BMT was an HLA-identical sibling. However, only about 30% of Americans have an HLA-identical sibling. In an effort to offer allogeneic BMT to patients who lack an HLA-identical sibling donor, there is increasing interest in the use of alternative donors: a related donor who is partially HLA matched or a fully or closely HLA-matched unrelated donor.[11] Rarely, a parent can be HLA identical with his or her child. It is estimated, however, that only an additional 10% of patients will have a closely HLA-matched, related donor. A relative who serves as a marrow donor can be a zero- (rare), one-, two-, or three-loci mismatch (assuming testing for HLA-A, -B, and -DR antigens).

The most common type of alternative donor is an individual who is fully or closely HLA matched. To facilitate identification of these donors, the National Marrow Donor Program (based in Minneapolis) was started in 1986 with initial funding from a U.S. Navy contract.[13,14] Similar programs outside of the United States also have been started. By the end of 1994, the number of potential donors in the National Marrow Donor Program had increased to more than 1.5 million. If we assume that testing is performed at three HLA loci (A, B, and DR) and that each patient has two phenotypes for each locus (one from each parent), matching is required for a total of six antigens. Therefore, a "completely" matched (i.e., 6/6 antigen match) unrelated donor is matched for HLA-A, -B, and -DR and is also MLC nonreactive. A "closely" matched unrelated donor is usually incompatible at one or two HLA antigens or is MLC reactive. The likelihood of any one unrelated individual being a match ranges from 1 in 100 to 1 in 1,000,000, depending on the prevalence of the patient's HLA type and their ethnic background. With the current number of potential donors, the overall likelihood of finding an HLA-A, -B, and -DR identical donor is about 50%. This figure is lower than that predicted, probably because there appear to be more HLA types than previously recognized. Because most minorities are poorly represented in the program, the likelihood of finding a donor for patients from certain ethnic groups is lower. Another limitation is the long time (i.e., several months) needed to search for a potential donor. Many patients with advanced leukemia will therefore relapse while waiting for completion of the search. To date, more than 3000 allogeneic transplants from matched unrelated donors have been performed with assistance from this program. The most common diagnoses for matched unrelated BMT are chronic myelogenous leukemia (34%), acute lymphocytic leukemia (20%), and acute nonlymphocytic leukemia (18%). Early results of matched unrelated transplants indicate that some patients can be cured of their disease.[15]

With the increasing availability of donors other than HLA-identical siblings, patients with some types of leukemia who do not have an HLA-identical sibling donor often must choose between allogeneic or autologous BMT. Each approach has advantages and disadvantages. Patients treated with allogeneic BMT have a lower risk of leukemic relapse because of the graft-versus-leukemia effect but they are at higher risk for GVHD and its associated complications. Patients treated with autologous BMT have a lower risk of transplant-related complications but may have a higher risk of leukemic relapse because of the lack of graft-versus-leukemia and the use of marrow that is potentially contaminated with residual leukemic cells.

Collection of Hematopoietic Stem Cells

The most important transplanted cells in BMT are hematopoietic stem cells, which serve as "mother" cells for all blood cells including erythrocytes, leukocytes, and platelets (see Chapter 92, Hematopoiesis).[16] Stem cells have varying degrees of "stemness"; true totipotent stem cells are capable of replicating indefinitely and can differentiate into any of the different blood cells. Because of their capacity for self-renewal, these stem cells are capable of repopulating the marrow of the recipient. There is intense interest in stem cells because a single totipotent stem cell should be capable of permanently reconstituting the entire blood-producing and immune systems. Hematopoietic stem cells are also attractive targets for gene therapy of inherited hematologic diseases, because genes introduced into stem cells would persist for long periods, possibly as long as the patient's lifetime. Totipotent stem cells are rare cells, comprising less than 0.01% of all bone marrow cells. It has been extremely difficult to isolate stem cells because of their rarity, their similarity in appearance to other cells, and the lack of a rapid and direct method to quantitate the number of stem cells.

Figures 129.2 and 129.3 show the schemes for autologous and allogeneic BMT, respectively. Bone marrow from the donor is obtained by more than 100 separate aspirations from the anterior and posterior iliac crests.[17] The procedure takes about a hour and yields 200–1500 mL depending on the size of the donor. The marrow is transferred into tissue culture medium containing preservative-free heparin. The pooled marrow is then passed through a series of stainless steel screens to break up aggregated particles, resulting essentially in a single-cell suspension. In allogeneic BMT, the marrow stem cells are given to the recipient within 12–24 hours after harvest. In autologous BMT, the marrow is frozen and stored until needed. After intravenous infusion over several hours, the marrow stem cells enter the systemic circulation and find their way to the bone marrow cavity, where they reseed and grow in the bone marrow microenvironment. Although the donor experiences local soreness for a few days, the procedure is usually well tolerated, with no delayed complications resulting from the marrow aspiration. The major risk of serving as a marrow donor is that of undergoing general anesthesia.

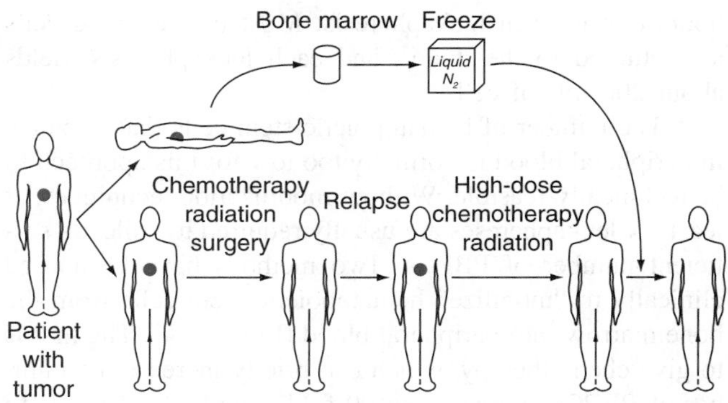

Figure 129.2. Scheme for autologous bone marrow transplantation. The patient with cancer typically undergoes marrow collection and cryopreservation early in the course of the disease. At a time when the disease is resistant to conventional treatment, intensive combined modality therapy is administered followed by reinfusion of the stored autologous bone marrow cells. *(From Champlin RE, Gale RP. Role of bone marrow transplantation in the treatment of hematologic malignancies and solid tumors: Critical review of syngeneic, autologous, and allogeneic transplants. Cancer Treat Rep 1984;68:146.)*

Because hematopoietic stem cells can also circulate in peripheral blood, there has been recent interest in the use of peripheral blood progenitor cells (PBPCs) (also referred to as peripheral blood stem cells [PBSCs]) for autologous transplantation.[18–20] PBPCs are found in the mononuclear (lymphocytes and monocytes) fraction of white blood cells (WBCs) and are collected by a procedure called *leukapheresis.* In this outpatient procedure, about 9–14 liters of blood are processed over several

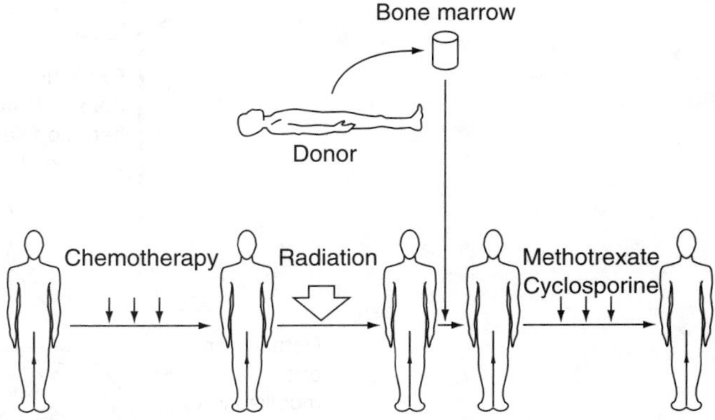

Figure 129.3. Scheme for allogeneic bone marrow transplantation in the treatment of cancer. The patient typically receives marrow ablative chemotherapy and/or total body irradiation to eradicate the malignancy and as immunosuppression to prevent transplant rejection. The bone marrow is administered as an intravenous infusion followed by post-transplant immunosuppression to prevent GVHD. *(From Champlin RE, Gale RP. Role of bone marrow transplantation in the treatment of hematologic malignancies and solid tumors: Critical review of syngeneic, autologous, and allogeneic transplants. Cancer Treat Rep 1984;68:146.)*

hours during each leukapheresis. Most of the blood cells are returned to the donor, and each leukapheresis yields about 200 mL of cells.

The number of hematopoietic stem cells that circulate in peripheral blood is normally too low for this approach to be technically feasible. Without mobilization techniques, at least six leukaphereses are usually required to collect a sufficient number of PBPCs. Two methods have been used clinically to "mobilize" hematopoietic stem cells from the bone marrow into peripheral blood (Fig. 129.4). The first is to give chemotherapy, which can briefly increase the number of PBPCs as much as 100-fold. Another method is to give a recombinant hematopoietic growth factor such as G-CSF or GM-CSF. The combination of chemotherapy followed by administration of a recombinant growth factor appears to increase the number of PBPCs to a greater extent than either method alone. With these mobilization techniques, the number of leukaphereses is reduced, and many centers collect sufficient PBPCs with three or fewer leukaphereses. Figure 129.5 shows a representative protocol for mobilization and collection of PBPCs.

PBPCs can be given either as an alternative or in addition to bone marrow stem cells for autologous rescue. The use of peripheral blood instead of bone marrow as a source of hematopoietic stem cells for high-dose chemotherapy with autologous rescue offers several advantages.[18–20] The most clinically important advantage is that patients who receive mobilized PBPCs experience more rapid hematopoietic engraftment. Although engraftment of all lineages is more rapid when PBPCs are used, the most significant effect is observed with platelet recovery. Patients who receive mobilized PBPCs experience platelet recovery as much as 2–3 weeks earlier than those who receive BMT. Another advantage is that the donor does not experience the discomfort associated with marrow aspirations and is not exposed to the risk associated with undergoing general anesthesia. For those patients who cannot donate marrow stem cells because of bone marrow abnormalities such as marrow metastases or fibrosis, collection of PBPCs allows these patients to potentially benefit from high-dose chemotherapy with autologous rescue. Another theoretical advantage is that PBPCs may be less likely to be contaminated with malignant cells compared with marrow stem cells. Finally, since PBPCs are collected from the mononuclear cell fraction, a fraction that also contains immunocompetent cells, some investigators believe that infusion of PBPCs may represent a form of "adoptive immunotherapy." In this model, lymphocytes targeted against tumor cells would help to kill residual tumor cells.

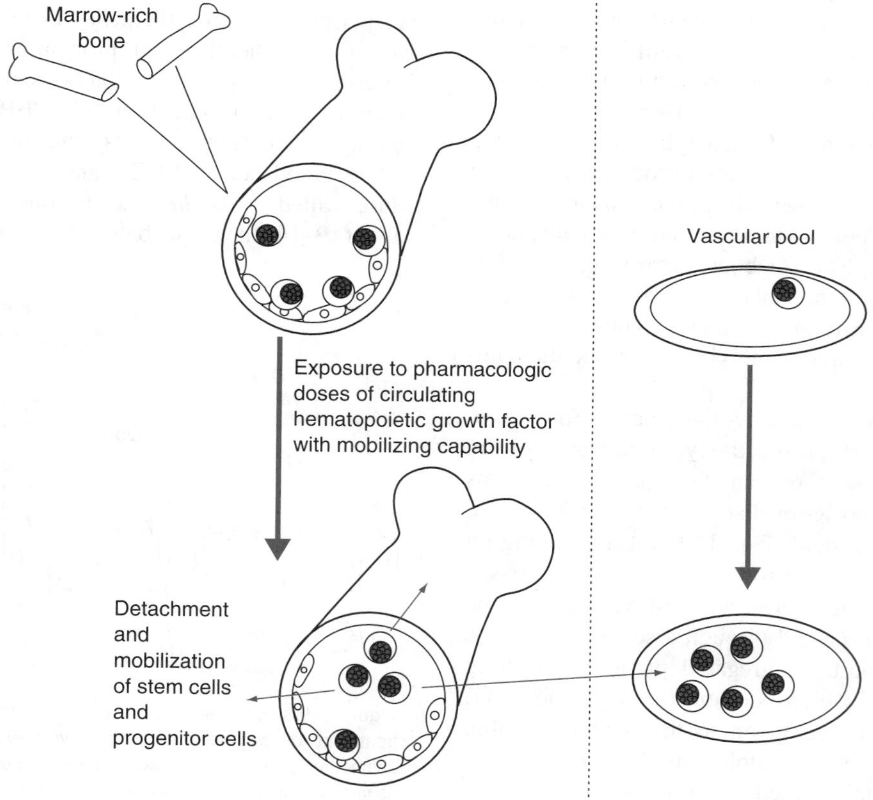

Figure 129.4. Hematopoietic growth factor-mediated mobilization of hematopoietic progenitor cells into the circulation. Many hematopoietic growth factors (G-CSF, GM-CSF, IL-1, IL-3, SCF, and likely others) have the ability to redistribute hematopoietic progenitor cells (and presumably true stem cells) from the bone marrow into the peripheral blood. *(Reprinted with permission from Demetri GD. Hematopoietic growth factors. Curr Probl Cancer 1992;16:238.)*

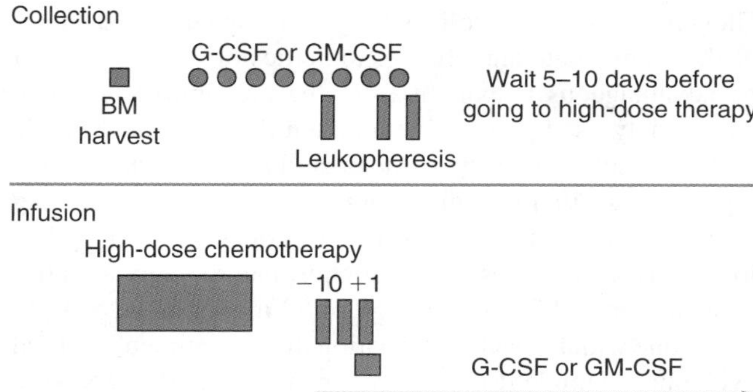

Figure 129.5. Schema for collection of PBPCs after full hematopoietic recovery from a previous course of chemotherapy. BM, bone marrow.

Most studies have not reported a difference in disease-free survival between patients who receive PBPCs and those who receive BMT. One study, however, found that patients with good-risk non-Hodgkin's lymphoma who received high-dose chemotherapy with PBPCs had significantly better disease-free survival at three years (70 versus 32%) than those who received high-dose chemotherapy with autologous BMT.[21] The use of PBPCs and growth factors is associated with other benefits. As a result of more rapid neutrophil and platelet recovery, patients who receive PBPCs and a recombinant growth factor are usually discharged earlier from the hospital. Many patients are discharged as early as 10–14 days post-transplant and some BMT centers with intensive clinic support discharge patients as early as 2 days post-transplant.[22] The overall cost of high-dose chemotherapy with autologous rescue has been dramatically reduced with the use of PBPCs. With PBPCs and recombinant growth factors, the overall cost of HSCT at some centers has decreased from about $90,000–$125,000 to about $50,000–$75,000.[22]

Although peripheral blood is rapidly replacing bone marrow as a source of hematopoietic stem cells for autologous rescue, bone marrow remains the major source of hematopoietic stem cells for allogeneic BMT, primarily because the large number of T lymphocytes present in peripheral blood makes the risk of GVHD unacceptably high. Since there is no rapid and direct method to quantitate the number of stem cells, another concern is that PBPCs do not contain sufficient numbers of "totipotent" hematopoietic stem cells, which are needed for permanent, multilineage engraftment. A higher risk of late graft failure has not been observed in patients receiving PBPCs alone, but longer follow-up is needed to determine if the infusion of PBPCs alone results in permanent, multilineage engraftment.

Another source of hematopoietic stem cells is umbilical cord blood.[16,23] Umbilical cord blood is an attractive source for several reasons. Since the stem cells are collected from placental blood, there is no risk to the mother or the baby. There is also very low risk of transmissible infectious diseases, such as cytomegalovirus and Epstein–Barr virus. Although the stem cells collected from umbilical cord blood could theoretically be used for either autologous or allogeneic transplants, they have been used primarily for allogeneic transplants. Most of the transplants have used HLA-identical sibling donors, although programs have been established to bank umbilical cord blood for possible use in unrelated transplants. As of late 1994, more than 3500 umbilical cord blood grafts had been collected, HLA typed, tested for transmissible infectious diseases, and cryopreserved at the New York Blood Center. Preliminary results have been encouraging. In the first 44 recipients of umbilical cord blood transplantation reported to the International Cord Blood Transplant Registry, more than 80% of patients engrafted and only 3% developed grades II–IV acute GVHD.[23] The apparently lower risk of acute GVHD with umbilical cord blood suggests that cells from umbilical cord blood are less likely to mediate GVHD and that greater HLA disparities between donor and recipient may be tolerated. All of the recipients of umbilical cord blood transplants to date have been children, with the largest successful recipient weighing about 35 kg. It is not clear whether the numbers of stem and progenitor cells in umbilical cord blood are sufficient for engraftment of larger recipients.

APPROACHES TO ERADICATE MALIGNANT CELLS

PRETRANSPLANT CHEMOTHERAPY

Nearly all patients undergoing BMT must be prepared (or "conditioned") before infusion of hematopoietic stem cells.[24] In patients with malignant disease, the goal of the preparative regimen is to kill as many malignant cells as possible. Preparative regimens usually include commonly used anticancer drugs given at very high doses—doses that would be associated with severe and life-threatening bone marrow suppression if hematopoietic stem cells were not infused. In patients undergoing allogeneic BMT, another purpose of the preparative regimen is to suppress the immune system of the recipient so that the graft is not rejected.

In some preparative regimens, the only drug given is cyclophosphamide, a drug with both immunosuppressive and cytotoxic effects. Because of the inadequate antitumor activity of cyclophosphamide in some types of cancers, other drugs are often added to the basic cyclophosphamide regimen. Examples of drugs that often are included in preparative regimens are cytarabine (ara-C), busulfan, thiotepa, etoposide (VP-16), carboplatin, cisplatin, and carmustine (BCNU).[25–28] Specific drug regimens are discussed in detail below.

Many BMT patients also receive total body irradiation (TBI). In patients with malignant disease, the rationale is to eradicate malignant cells located in areas inaccessible to the systemic circulation. TBI also has significant immunosuppressive activity. Historically, the standard total body irradiation regimen involves the administration of a midline tissue dose of about 1000 cGy (1 cGy = 1 rad), which is more than twice the lethal dose of radiation for a normal person. Many centers currently give fractionated rather than single-dose TBI to patients with malignant disease. The rationale for this approach is an improved therapeutic ratio—to destroy more leukemic cells and marrow stem cells while sparing other normal tissues.[29] One randomized trial has demonstrated improved antileukemic activity with fractionated-dose TBI compared with single-dose TBI.[30] The nonmarrow acute toxicities of total body irradiation are generally mild, consisting of low-grade fever, nausea, vomiting, diarrhea, and tender swelling of the parotid gland.[31]

The administration of high-dose chemotherapy, either alone or combined with TBI, is associated with serious and sometimes life-threatening toxicities to organs other than the bone marrow (see discussion on regimen-related toxicities).

Leukemia

In patients with leukemia undergoing allogeneic BMT, the standard regimen is cyclophosphamide and TBI. Cyclophosphamide is usually given first, as two 60 mg/kg doses, followed by TBI. TBI can be given as a single dose or fractionated over several days. Fractionated TBI appears to increase the therapeutic index compared with single-dose TBI.[29,30] The maximally tolerated dose of fractionated TBI is 1200 cGy, given as 200-cGy fractions daily for 6 days. Although higher TBI doses provide additional antileukemic activity, one randomized trial showed that survival is not improved because of increased mortality from causes other than relapse.[32] The cyclophosphamide–TBI regimen provides adequate antileukemic activity in patients with acute nonlymphocytic leukemia (ANLL) in first remission or chronic myelogenous leukemia (CML) in chronic phase, but it is associated with an unacceptably high relapse rate in patients with acute lymphocytic leukemia (ALL) or those with more advanced disease.

One variation of that regimen is to give hyperfractionated TBI first, followed by cyclophosphamide.[33] In that regimen, 11 TBI doses of 120 cGy are given; doses are given three times a day on days –7 to –5 (*note:* day 0 is designated as the day of transplant), and twice a day on the last day (day –4). After TBI, two doses of cyclophosphamide are given intravenously once a day at a dosage of 60 mg/kg on days –3 and –2. As described below, this regimen appears to be more effective than the standard cyclophosphamide and TBI regimen in patients with ALL. It is not clear whether the increased effectiveness is related to the hyperfractionated TBI or the change in the sequence of TBI and cyclophosphamide administration.

Because many anticancer drugs do not have adequate immunosuppressive activity, most preparative regimens in allogeneic BMT include TBI or cyclophosphamide. Because of the many acute and chronic toxicities of TBI,[31] it would be advantageous to omit it from the preparative regimen. One widely used preparative regimen that does not include TBI is busulfan and cyclophosphamide.[27] In that original regimen, busulfan was given orally at a dosage of 1 mg/kg every 6 hours (4 mg/kg/d) for 16 doses on days –9 to –6, followed by four doses of cyclophosphamide, given intravenously once daily at a dosage of 50 mg/kg on days –5 to –2. In one widely used modification of that regimen, the total cyclophosphamide dosage is reduced from 200 (50 × 4) to 120 (60 × 2) mg/kg.

Several prospective randomized studies have compared cyclophosphamide (120 mg/kg) and either TBI or busulfan (16 mg/kg) in patients with leukemia. In patients with CML in first chronic phase, the busulfan–cyclophosphamide regimen had similar or greater antileukemic activity and was better tolerated than cyclophosphamide and TBI.[34,35] But in patients with ANLL in first remission or advanced leukemia (e.g., patients beyond first remission or first chronic phase), the cyclophosphamide–TBI regimen was associated with significantly better disease-free survival than busulfan and cyclophosphamide.[36,37] In contrast to the results of the study conducted by the Seattle BMT team,[34] one of those studies also reported that busulfan and cyclophosphamide was associated with more regimen-related toxicity than cyclophosphamide and TBI.[36]

Other allogeneic BMT groups have given other drugs in addition to or instead of cyclophosphamide in the preparative regimen, particularly in patients with ALL. Examples of other drugs that have been included in combination with TBI are cytarabine[38,39] or etoposide.[26,40] There are no convincing data to indicate that any of these regimens are superior to the standard regimen of cyclophosphamide combined with either TBI or busulfan. The same preparative regimens are usually given in patients undergoing autologous BMT.[41]

Lymphoma

Based on experience in patients with leukemia, the initial regimen used in many patients with lymphoma was cyclophosphamide and TBI, particularly in allogeneic BMT. Most preparative regimens used in autologous BMT for lymphoma include cyclophosphamide and at least one other drug.[42,43] TBI is usually not included in the conditioning regimen. One widely used regimen in autologous BMT is the CBV regimen, which consists of cyclophosphamide, carmustine (BCNU), and etoposide (VP-16). In that original regimen, cyclophosphamide was given at a dosage of 1.5 g/m^2 on days –6 to –3, carmustine was given at a dosage of 300 mg/m^2 on day –6, and etoposide was given at a dosage of 100 mg/m^2 every 12 hours for six doses on days –6 to –4.[44] Various BMT groups have modified the original CBV regimen by changing the dosage of some of the drugs. Other BMT groups have added or substituted other drugs to the CBV regimen, including cytosine arabinoside, etoposide, melphalan, lomustine, and thioguanine.[42,43] Other widely used regimens are BEAC (BCNU, etoposide, ara-C, and cyclophosphamide) and BEAM (BCNU, etoposide, ara-C, and melphalan). No one preparative regimen has been shown to be clearly superior to other regimens in the treatment of lymphoma.

Although TBI is usually not included in the conditioning regimen, some form of radiation therapy is often given, depending on the type of disease and the location and extent of disease. Instead of TBI, some patients receive localized radiation in high doses to areas of residual or bulky disease. Because many patients with Hodgkin's disease have received thoracic radiation as primary therapy for their disease, TBI is usually avoided in patients with Hodgkin's disease. Conversely, most patients with indolent non-Hodgkin's lymphoma receive TBI as part of their preparative regimen because of the known sensitivity of these tumors to low doses of radiation.

One novel approach is to substitute targeted radiotherapy for TBI. The goal of this approach is to deliver higher doses of radiotherapy to tumor sites, while exposing normal tissues to lower doses of irradiation. Monoclonal antibodies to antigens expressed on the malignant cells are used to deliver the irradiation (i.e., radioimmunotherapy). In studies conducted by the Seattle BMT team, ^{131}I-labeled anti-CD20 (B1) antibody was used to deliver maximally tolerated doses of radiotherapy (without chemotherapy) followed by autologous stem-cell rescue.[45,46] Results of phase I and II studies have been encouraging.

Solid Tumors

Initially, the conditioning regimens used in patients with solid tumors were similar to those used in patients with leukemia. Many patients with refractory disease also participated in phase I–II trials of single agents, in an attempt to determine the maximally tolerated dosage in the setting of BMT and the dose–response relationship in a selected solid tumor.[47–49]

Breast cancer has served as a model for the development of intensive conditioning regimens in autologous BMT. Based on preclinical and clinical models, Frei et al.[49] have listed seven strategies for the development of an optimal conditioning regimen: (1) Three or more agents should be used, (2) agents should be individually effective in the treatment of metastatic disease, (3) agents should have a steep dose–response curve, (4) agents should be minimally or non–cross-resistant, (5) agents should ideally exhibit synergism in preclinical or clinical models, (6) agents should have a tolerated dosage in the autologous BMT setting that is at least fivefold higher than the standard maximally tolerated dosage, and (7) agents should have sufficiently different nonhematologic dose-limiting toxicities to allow their use in combination in the autologous BMT setting without significant compromise in dose of individual agents. Several agents were identified that satisfied their criteria, including cyclophosphamide, thiotepa, carmustine, melphalan, and carboplatin. Other anticancer drugs that modulated the activity of alkylating agents, such as etoposide, were also attractive drugs to include in high-dose preparative regimens. Most conditioning regimens in autologous BMT include at least one alkylating agent, because of their steep dose–response curve and other favorable characteristics. Many BMT groups include more than one alkylating agent, based on preclinical studies that show that resistance to a specific alkylating agent does not impart cross-resistance to other alkylating agents.

Table 129.1 shows the evolution of conditioning regimens at the Dana–Farber Cancer Institute.[28] STAMP I (Solid Tumor Autologous Marrow Program) combined three alkylating agents at nearly full BMT dosages. Although that regimen continues to be used in some autologous BMT centers, the low activity of carmustine in breast cancer and its variable pharmacokinetics led investigators at the Dana-Farber Cancer Institute to develop a new conditioning regimen. Based on preclinical studies, STAMP III was developed, which combined cyclophosphamide, thiotepa, and melphalan. Because of severe mucositis, the dosage of melphalan could not be significantly escalated. This led to the development of STAMP V, where carboplatin is substituted for melphalan. In an effort to increase efficacy, decrease toxicity, and facilitate pharmacokinetic studies, these drugs are given as a continuous intravenous infusion. Based on phase I studies, the maximally tolerated dosages of these drugs in the autologous BMT setting are 6 g/m^2 of cyclophosphamide, 500 mg/m^2 of thiotepa, and 800 mg/m^2 of carboplatin. Clinical results in breast cancer are discussed below.

MARROW PURGING

One disadvantage of the use of the patient as the marrow donor (autologous BMT) is that the marrow may be contaminated with residual malignant cells. Marrow harvest is usually performed when the patient has no evidence of tumor cells in the bone marrow by standard diagnostic techniques. However, because of our inability to detect small numbers of malignant cells, residual malignant cells are probably present in most patients who serve as marrow donors. Several BMT teams are developing newer, more sensitive methods to detect "minimal residual disease."[50,51] Some of these methods can detect as few as one in a million cells.

Infusion of these malignant cells may theoretically result in tumor relapse. Many approaches are used by BMT teams to eliminate ("purge") the marrow of these tumor cells. The most common approach is to add substances, such as chemicals or monoclonal antibodies, to the marrow

TABLE 129.1. SCHEMATA FOR STAMP[a] I, III, AND V

	Day from Marrow Reinfusion								
Bone Marrow Reinfusion	**−8**	**−7**	**−6**	**−5**	**−4**	**−3**	**−2**	**−1**	**0**
STAMP I									
Cyclophosphamide		↑	↑	↑	↑				
Cisplatin	-------	-------	-------	-------	-------				
BCNU					↑[b]				
Melphalan[c]				↑					
STAMP III									
Cyclophosphamide	-------	-------	-------	-------	-------				
Thiotepa	-------	-------	-------	-------	-------				
Melphalan		↑	↑	↑	↑				
STAMP V									
Cyclophosphamide	-------	-------	-------	-------	-------				
Thiotepa	-------	-------	-------	-------	-------				
Carboplatin	-------	-------	-------	-------	-------				

[a]STAMP, Solid Tumor Autologous Marrow Program.
[b]The last 12 patients were given same total dose, divided over 4 days (administered twice a day).
[c]Dose levels 5–6 only. (Reproduced from Ahtman K, Eder JP, Elias A, et al. High-dose thiopeta alone and in combination regimens with bone marrow support. Semin Oncol 1990;17(suppl 3):35, with permission.)

while it is outside of the body (*ex vivo*) (Fig. 129.6). Because the substances are removed before marrow infusion, the advantage of this approach is that nonhematopoietic tissues are not exposed to the substances and therefore are not damaged. However, these substances can remove or damage pluripotent hematopoietic stem cells, which are essential for complete and rapid engraftment. *Ex vivo* marrow purging also is performed in allogeneic BMT in an attempt to eliminate T cells believed to be responsible for acute GVHD (Fig. 129.6). Results with this approach are discussed in the Graft-Versus-Host Disease section.

One approach is to add one or more monoclonal antibodies directed against specific antigens present on the tumor cells but absent on nearly all other cells.[52,53] Killing of tumor cells is usually achieved with the addition of complement. One novel approach is to add a monoclonal antibody against the cell surface product of the multidrug resistant (MDR) gene, in an attempt to purge multidrug-resistant tumor cells.[54] Another method to kill tumor cells is to use immunotoxins (monoclonal antibodies linked to a toxin). Although these approaches are theoretically attractive, they are limited by the observation that not all cells from

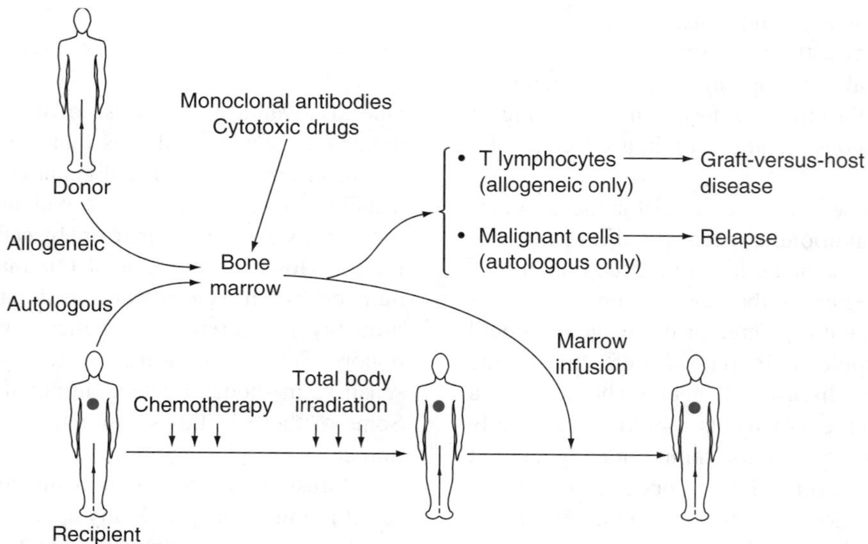

Figure 129.6. The use of *ex vivo* marrow purging to remove or destroy T lymphocytes (allogeneic only) or residual malignant cells (autologous only).

patients with the same type of cancer will express a specific antigen. Furthermore, for some types of cancers, it has been difficult to identify antigens distinct from those present on normal hematopoietic progenitor cells. To date, this approach has been used most commonly in patients with lymphoid malignancies, either ALL or non-Hodgkin's lymphoma. Results are discussed in the Clinical Results section.

Another approach is to add chemicals or drugs to kill the tumor cells.[55] The advantage of this approach is that it can be used for a broader range of tumor types. However, this approach is not completely selective for tumor cells, and it is therefore important to add the precise amount of chemical or drug that kills sufficient numbers of tumor cells while sparing the largest number of hematopoietic stem cells. The chemical that is most commonly used for marrow purging is 4-hydroperoxycyclophosphamide (4-HC), a congener of cyclophosphamide. 4-HC is a stable compound that enters cells and is rapidly reduced to 4-hydroxycyclophosphamide, which serves as the precursor to the reactive phosphoramide mustard. The level of aldehyde dehydrogenase, the enzyme that inactivates 4-hydroxycyclophosphamide, appears to be highest in early hematopoietic progenitors and decreases as these cells differentiate. This observation may explain why 4-HC appears to have an acceptable therapeutic index. Other analogues of cyclophosphamide and drugs such as etoposide also are being investigated as chemical purging agents.

A novel method to purge malignant cells is to identify, select, and concentrate hematopoietic stem cells, a process known as positive selection. Several different techniques are being commercially developed, but all technologies use anti-CD34 monoclonal antibodies.[56] In this process, cells collected from marrow or peripheral blood are treated *ex vivo* with monoclonal antibodies against CD34, an antigen expressed on hematopoietic stem cells and early progenitor cells. CD34 positive cells are therefore separated from those that are CD34 negative, including most malignant cells. The final volume of enriched cells that is infused back into the patient is remarkably small—only about 5 mL. Preliminary results with one of these techniques show that a one- to four-log depletion of tumor cells can be achieved without any evidence of delayed hematopoietic recovery.[57]

POST-TRANSPLANT IMMUNOTHERAPY

The rationale for post-transplant immunotherapy is based on observations that recovery of immune function can be impaired for months to years post-transplant and that the T lymphocytes that mediate GVHD can be directed toward leukemic cells.[58–60] This effect is referred to as the "graft-versus-leukemia" effect. Evidence for a graft-versus-leukemia effect is based on retrospective studies that show that patients who developed acute or chronic GVHD had a lower risk of leukemic relapse than those who did not develop GVHD. However, because of the direct and indirect effects of GVHD, GVHD is usually associated with increased nonrelapse mortality during the early post-transplant period.

Based on these retrospective studies, the Seattle BMT team initiated a prospective, randomized study to determine if a reduction in the intensity of acute GVHD prophylaxis or infusion of donor leukocytes (e.g., T lymphocytes) would reduce the risk of leukemic relapse in patients with advanced hematologic malignancies treated with allogeneic BMT.[61] Although the risk of acute GVHD was increased in patients randomized to receive short methotrexate or long methotrexate plus donor buffy coat cells, the risk of relapse was not decreased and survival was not improved. The incidence of chronic GVHD was similar in each of the three treatment groups. Donor leukocyte infusions, either alone or in combination with interferon (IFN)-α, have also been given in an attempt to induce a graft-versus-leukemia reaction in patients who have relapsed after allogeneic BMT.[62,63] Complete remissions have been reinduced with this approach, although about 20% of patients die of treatment-related complications including GVHD and graft failure.

Recently, based on reports that GVHD developed after cyclosporine was withdrawn in rats after syngeneic or autologous BMT, some BMT groups have induced autologous GVHD in an attempt to induce a graft-versus-leukemia effect.[64,65] The mechanism by which cyclosporine causes autologous GVHD is unknown, but the effector cells appear to be cytotoxic T cells aimed against MHC class II antigens. More recent studies show that the antitumor effect can be enhanced with IFN-γ administration. In human studies, autologous GVHD is induced with administration of low doses of cyclosporine (1 mg/kg, given intravenously) for 28 days, beginning on the day of marrow infusion. With this regimen, about two-thirds of patients develop autologous GVHD of the skin while receiving the drug. Although generalized GVHD is observed in animals, autologous GVHD in humans does not appear to develop in extracutaneous organs. The skin rash either resolved spontaneously or with systemic corticosteroids. Preliminary results with this approach have been encouraging.[66,67]

Another approach is to administer a cytokine with immunomodulatory activity, such as interleukin (IL)-2 or interferons.[60,68,69] Early clinical experience indicates that IL-2 can be safely administered post-transplant and results in significant activation of immune effector cells and may reduce the risk of leukemic relapse.

Post-transplant immunotherapy would be particularly useful in patients undergoing autologous blood or marrow transplantation because these patients would not benefit from graft-versus-tumor reactions. Cytokines that directly or indirectly stimulate lymphocytes should be used cautiously in recipients of allogeneic BMT because they may exacerbate GVHD.

Clinical Results

Because of the high cost and the morbidity and mortality associated with the procedure, high-dose chemotherapy with BMT should only be performed in cancer patients who have little chance of long-term survival with standard-dose chemotherapy. Table 129.2 lists the most common types of cancer treated with BMT. Many potential indications for BMT are controversial, and coverage for BMT is often denied if the payer believes that the likelihood for long-term survival and cure is low. High-dose chemotherapy with BMT can be used at different times in the disease course (Table 129.3). Although high-dose chemotherapy with autologous or allogeneic BMT can cure a few patients with refractory disease, it is most effective when the tumor burden is low (i.e., when the patient is in remission). BMT is currently most often used as intensive consolidation therapy in patients who have responded to standard-dose chemotherapy but who have a low likelihood of long-term survival or cure. One example of this strategy is patients with ANLL who undergo BMT during their first remission. BMT is also commonly used in patients who experience relapse or recurrence of their cancer and respond to salvage chemotherapy (i.e., sensitive relapse). These patients undergo high-dose chemotherapy with BMT during their remission. Examples of this strategy include patients with acute lymphocytic leukemia or lymphoma who undergo BMT during their second remission or patients with metastatic breast cancer who undergo BMT after responding to standard-dose chemotherapy. Finally, high-dose chemotherapy with BMT is sometimes used as part of intensive adjuvant chemotherapy in high-risk patients, such as women with breast cancer with ≥10 positive lymph nodes.

TABLE 129.3. POSSIBILITIES FOR TIMING OF BONE MARROW TRANSPLANTATION IN THE TREATMENT OF CANCER

- Primary treatment
- Partial responders or slow responders (before progression)
- Initial complete remission (i.e., consolidation)
- Nonresponders (primary treatment failure)
- Relapse
  - Untested (i.e., no other salvage therapy)
  - Tested (i.e., after other salvage therapy)
    - Sensitive relapse (i.e., complete or partial remission)
    - Resistant relapse (i.e., no response or progression)
- End-stage patients

(Modified from Armitage JO. Bone marrow transplantation in the treatment of patients with lymphoma. Blood 1989;73:1750, with permission.)

ACUTE NONLYMPHOCYTIC LEUKEMIA

In ANLL, high-dose chemotherapy with autologous or allogeneic BMT is the only curative option for patients who fail initial induction therapy or those who have experienced leukemic relapse. The proportion of long-term survivors after allogeneic BMT when patients are transplanted while in untreated first relapse or in second remission is about 20–35% (Table 129.4).[70–72] The proportion of long-term survivors decreases to about 20% when patients are transplanted while in chemotherapy-resistant first relapse or to

TABLE 129.2. THE USE OF BONE MARROW TRANSPLANTATION IN SELECTED MALIGNANT DISEASES

	Bone Marrow Transplantation		
Disease	**Preferred Type**	**Potentially Curative in Advanced Disease**	**Standard Therapy**[a]
Acute leukemia	Allogeneic in most cases	Yes	Yes
Chronic myelogenous leukemia	Allogeneic	Yes	Yes
Chronic lymphocytic leukemia	Allogeneic in most cases	Uncertain	No
Multiple myeloma	Controversial	Uncertain	No
Non-Hodgkin's lymphoma			
Histologically aggressive	Autologous in most cases	Yes	Yes
Histologically indolent	Autologous in most cases	Uncertain	Yes
Hodgkin's disease	Autologous in most cases	Yes	Yes
Breast cancer	Autologous	Uncertain	No
Testicular cancer	Autologous	Yes	Yes
Neuroblastoma	Uncertain	Probably	Yes

[a]Standard therapy is defined as treatment that is widely accepted by physicians and routinely reimbursed by most third-party payers at some point in the course of the disease. As noted in the text, the designation of bone marrow transplantation as standard therapy is controversial. For example, although transplantation in patients with breast cancer is not routinely reimbursed by most third-party payers, the rate of reimbursement is approximately 75% at Duke University Hospital and 50% at the University of Nebraska Medical Center. (From Armitage JO. Bone marrow transplantation. N Engl J Med 1994;330:832. Reprinted by permission of The New England Journal of Medicine. Copyright 1994, Massachusetts Medical Society.)

TABLE 129.4. LONG-TERM RESULTS OF HIGH-DOSE CHEMOTHERAPY WITH ALLOGENEIC BONE MARROW TRANSPLANTATION (BMT) VERSUS INTENSIVE CHEMOTHERAPY IN THE TREATMENT OF LEUKEMIAS

		Long-Term Survival (%)	
Disease[a]	**Status**	**BMT**	**Chemotherapy**
ANLL	1st remission	40–60	20–30
	2nd remission	20–30	0
	Multiple relapses	10–15	0
ALL	1st remission (high risk)	30–50	30–50
	2nd remission	25–40	<10
	Multiple relapses	10–15	0
CML	Chronic phase	50–60	0
	Accelerated/blast phase	15–30	0

[a]ANLL, acute nonlymphocytic leukemia; ALL, acute lymphoblastic leukemia; CML, chronic myelogenous leukemia.

10–15% when allogeneic BMT is performed after patients have had multiple relapses. In patients who achieve a complete remission with standard remission-induction therapy, however, the role of BMT is not clear. Response rates and median survival have steadily improved in patients with ANLL treated with intensive chemotherapy. About 20–40% of patients with ANLL survive for more than 5 years and are probably cured of their disease (see Chapter 126). In contrast, long-term survival is observed in 40–60% of patients with ANLL treated with allogeneic BMT from an HLA-identical sibling while in first remission (Table 129.4).[70,72] This difference in disease-free survival between patients treated with intensive chemotherapy versus allogeneic BMT has been confirmed in several prospective studies, but the difference is not statistically significant in all studies. In the largest series of more than 600 patients with ANLL, patients in the allogeneic BMT group had significantly better disease-free survival at 4 years than those in the intensive chemotherapy group (55 versus 30%).[73] Overall survival, however, was not significantly different between the two groups. Some investigators argue that the better results reported with BMT are related to patient selection. For example, patients undergoing allogeneic BMT are usually less than 50 years of age. Survival for patients treated with either intensive chemotherapy or allogeneic BMT is related to age, with better survival in younger patients.

Since patients treated with high-dose chemotherapy with BMT as intensive postremission therapy have a longer disease-free survival than those treated with standard intensive chemotherapy, some investigators argue that all eligible patients should be offered high-dose chemotherapy with allogeneic BMT during first remission (Fig. 129.7). Other investigators argue that BMT should be delayed until the patient experiences a leukemic relapse. This approach also would spare patients cured with standard chemotherapy from the risks of BMT. Because 20–35% of patients transplanted while in first relapse or second remission can be cured with high-dose chemotherapy and BMT, the overall proportion of patients cured of their ANLL is similar regardless of whether BMT is offered to all patients as intensive postremission therapy or only after they have experienced leukemic relapse.[73]

The leukemic relapse rate with either cyclophosphamide and TBI or busulfan and cyclophosphamide is about 20% in patients with ANLL who undergo allogeneic BMT while in first remission. Patients with more advanced disease have higher relapse rates. Variations of that regimen or the addition of other drugs do not appear to provide superior antileukemic activity.[25]

Results with high-dose chemotherapy with autologous BMT appear to be similar to those with allogeneic BMT.[71,72] Preparative regimens used in autologous BMT are similar to those used in allogeneic BMT. Marrow is sometimes "purged" in an effort to remove residual leukemic cells before infusion. One common approach is to add a chemical

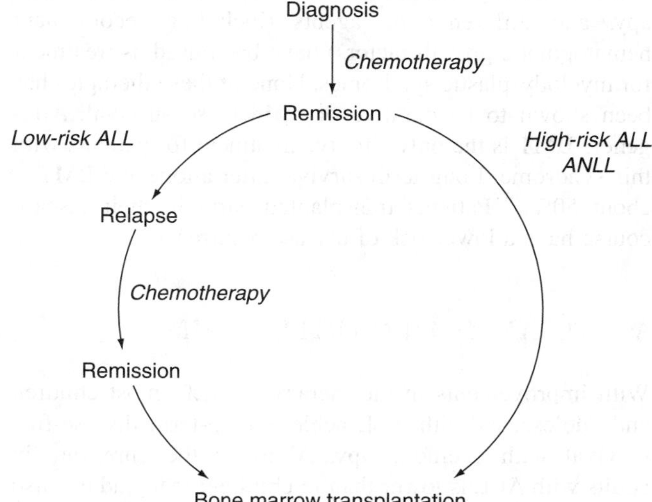

Figure 129.7. Current application of allogeneic bone marrow transplantation in the treatment of ANLL and ALL. *(Modified from Yee GC, McGuire TR. Allogeneic bone marrow transplantation in the treatment of hematologic diseases. Clin Pharm 1985;4:152. © 1985 American Society of Health-System Pharmacists, Inc. All rights reserved. Reprinted with permission.)*

such as 4-HC.[55] Although the value of marrow purging with 4-HC has not been proven in a controlled study, some investigators believe that this approach reduces the risk of leukemic relapse. This is supported by the observation that patients with adequate marrow purging, as measured by the number of hematopoietic progenitor cells, had significantly longer disease-free survival than those with inadequate marrow purging.[74]

Another controversy in the use of BMT as treatment for ANLL is whether patients should undergo allogeneic or autologous BMT. As discussed earlier in the chapter, each approach has advantages and disadvantages. In one prospective study of more than 600 patients with ANLL transplanted while in first remission, disease-free survival at 4 years was similar in patients assigned to either autologous or allogeneic BMT.[73] The causes of death, however, differed depending on the type of transplant. The risk of leukemic relapse was higher in the autologous BMT group while the risk of nonrelapse mortality—primarily related to GVHD—was higher in the allogeneic BMT group. Most of the patients in the autologous BMT group did not receive purged marrow. Ongoing trials for patients with ANLL compare allogeneic BMT from an HLA-identical sibling donor with autologous BMT with 4-HC purged marrow.

Allogeneic BMT with closely or fully HLA-matched unrelated donors has been used to treat ANLL.[11,12,15] The major difficulty with this approach is that many patients will relapse during the time needed to find a donor.

MYELODYSPLASTIC SYNDROME

Myelodysplastic syndromes are a heterogeneous group of disorders associated with an increased risk of transformation to acute myeloid leukemia.[75,76] Hormones, chemotherapy, and differentiating agents (including recombinant hematopoietic growth factors) have been used as treatment for myelodysplastic syndromes. None of these therapies has been shown to be curative or to increase survival. Allogeneic BMT is the only curative treatment for patients with this syndrome. Long-term survival after allogeneic BMT is about 50%.[76] Patients transplanted early in their disease course have a lower risk of disease recurrence.

ACUTE LYMPHOBLASTIC LEUKEMIA

With improvements in the therapy of ALL, most children and adolescents with ALL achieve long-term disease-free survival with chemotherapy. Although the cure rate in adults with ALL is lower than in children, many adults also can be cured of their disease with conventional chemotherapy (see Chapter 126). Therefore, BMT is usually reserved for patients with ALL who have experienced leukemic relapse, particularly if the duration of the first remission is short (less than 18 months) (Fig. 129.7).[77,78] Although many studies show that chemotherapy can often induce a second or subsequent remission, the duration of remission is usually short and long-term survival is uncommon. In comparison, about 25–40% of patients with ALL transplanted while in second remission become long-term survivors (Table 129.4). In a large matched-pair analysis of children with ALL in second remission, children who received allogeneic BMT had significantly better disease-free survival at 5 years than those who received continued chemotherapy (40 versus 17%).[79] The difference in survival was related to a marked difference in the risk of relapse. Long-term survival after allogeneic BMT decreases to about 10–15% in patients who have had multiple relapses.

The application of allogeneic BMT as intensive consolidation during first remission in patients with ALL who are at high risk for leukemic relapse is controversial. Examples of patients in this high-risk group are most adults and some children with high-risk features, such as those with high WBC counts or certain immunophenotypes or cytogenetic abnormalities, or those who require repeated courses to induce a complete remission. Long-term, disease-free survival is about 60% in children and 40% in adults transplanted while in first remission (Table 129.4).[77] Most of these patients were prepared with cyclophosphamide and TBI. In a prospective comparison of chemotherapy versus allogeneic BMT for adults with ALL in first remission, disease-free survival was higher in the BMT group (45 versus 31%), although the difference was of borderline statistical significance ($p = 0.1$).[80] In that study, significantly better survival was observed in those patients with high-risk ALL (39 versus 14%), which suggests that allogeneic BMT may be preferred over chemotherapy in certain patient groups. There is limited experience with closely or fully matched unrelated BMT in the treatment of ALL.[14] One of the difficulties with this approach in ALL is that many patients will relapse during the time needed to find a donor.

Most patients transplanted in these early studies were prepared with high-dose cyclophosphamide, followed by TBI. Because of the unacceptably high relapse rate with this regimen, some BMT groups are investigating new preparative regimens. As described earlier, preliminary results with the use of hyperfractionated TBI before cyclophosphamide in allogeneic BMT are encouraging.[33] With this regimen, estimated disease-free survival at 5 years is about 60% and 40% in children and adolescents with ALL transplanted while in second and third remission, respectively. Other BMT groups have reported promising results with preparative regimens that include high-dose cytarabine or etoposide, usually combined with TBI.[38–40]

Although there is less experience with autologous BMT, studies suggest that long-term survival with autologous BMT is slightly lower compared with allogeneic BMT.[78,81] Because of the widespread availability of monoclonal antibodies against antigens expressed on malignant lymphocytes, many patients have their marrow purged with monoclonal antibodies. Some also received 4-HC-purged marrow. Long-term survival is about 20–30% in children and adults with ALL treated with autologous BMT while in remission (primarily second or subsequent remission). High-dose chemotherapy with autologous BMT has also been used as intensive postremission therapy in adults with ALL. Preliminary results of one study did not show a survival benefit of autologous BMT over maintenance chemotherapy.[82]

As with ANLL, there is controversy whether eligible patients with high-risk ALL should be treated with high-dose chemotherapy with BMT as soon as possible after complete remission is achieved, or to delay BMT until leukemic relapse occurs. Because of the effectiveness of current chemotherapy protocols, many investigators recommend delaying BMT until leukemic relapse occurs.

CHRONIC MYELOGENOUS LEUKEMIA

With the possible exception of IFN-α, no currently available therapy is capable of eradicating the malignant clone, measured clinically by the presence of cytogenetic markers (see Chapter 127). In contrast, many studies indicate that high-dose chemotherapy with allogeneic BMT from HLA-identical sibling donors can cure 60–70% of patients with chronic-phase CML (Table 129.4).[83] As a result, CML is currently the most common indication for allogeneic BMT in many BMT centers. In some series, the best results are achieved when BMT is performed early after diagnosis and in younger patients. For example, long-term survival in patients transplanted within 1 year of diagnosis is about 80%, compared with 40–50% when BMT is performed 1–3 years from diagnosis.[84] Because busulfan may increase the risk of post-transplant interstitial pneumonitis and hepatic veno-occlusive disease, it has been recommended that pretransplant busulfan be avoided if patients are eligible for and considering BMT. Prolonged administration of IFN-α before BMT may adversely affect transplant outcome.[85] When allogeneic BMT is delayed until the patient is in accelerated or blast phase, survival is worse, but 15–30% of patients still can be cured (Table 129.4).[83]

The leukemic relapse rate is 10–30% in patients prepared with either cyclophosphamide and TBI or busulfan and cyclophosphamide and who are transplanted while in chronic phase.[83] Randomized studies show that busulfan and cyclophosphamide has similar or better antileukemic activity than cyclophosphamide and TBI.[34,35] When BMT is delayed until accelerated or blast phase, the relapse rate exceeds 50% in patients prepared with standard preparative regimens.[83]

Because of the relatively long duration of the chronic phase, there is usually adequate time to perform a search for a fully or closely matched unrelated donor for those patients with CML who lack an HLA-identical sibling donor. Therefore, CML has become the most common indication for allogeneic BMT from unrelated donors.[11,12,15] In a study of 102 patients with CML treated with allogeneic BMT from matched unrelated donors, survival at 2.5 years was about 30%.[86] Survival in patients who had an HLA-matched donor was slightly better than in those who had a closely HLA-matched donor (39 versus 27%), although longer follow-up will be needed to compare long-term survival in subgroups of patients.

Experience with autologous BMT is limited but it appears that autologous BMT is less effective in eradication of the malignant clone than allogeneic BMT.[87] Because the major cause of treatment failure is leukemic relapse, many BMT centers are investigating new preparative regimens and pharmacologic or immunologic approaches to purge marrow of malignant cells.

LYMPHOMA

Although most patients with Hodgkin's disease and some with aggressive NHL are cured with combination chemotherapy, the prognosis for those who relapse is poor. Similarly, most patients with indolent NHL are not cured of their disease with chemotherapy. In the United States alone, it is estimated that more than 10,000 patients with lymphoma are not cured with standard chemotherapy and are less than 60 years old. Although lymphoma is currently the second most common indication for autologous rescue, it is estimated that only a small proportion of the eligible patients are currently treated with this procedure.

Based on the success of allogeneic BMT in leukemia, allogeneic or syngeneic BMT was used initially as salvage therapy in patients with relapsed or refractory Hodgkin's disease or aggressive NHL. Long-term results of these early studies show that some of these patients can be cured with high-dose chemotherapy and BMT.[42,43] Although a graft-versus-lymphoma effect has been reported, there is no convincing evidence that survival is higher with allogeneic BMT compared with autologous BMT. Moreover, allogeneic BMT is not feasible in most patients and is associated with a higher risk of transplant-related complications due to GVHD. As a result, most eligible patients with lymphoma currently are treated with high-dose chemotherapy and autologous rescue, usually with PBPCs.

High-dose chemotherapy with autologous rescue can be used at different times in the disease course (Table 129.3). It is most commonly used as initial salvage therapy in patients with Hodgkin's disease or aggressive NHL who experience their first relapse or as intensive consolidation therapy in relapsed patients who demonstrate a response to conventional-dose salvage chemotherapy. In that setting, high-dose chemotherapy with autologous rescue produces a complete remission rate of 25–80%, with many patients in unmaintained, continuous complete remission for more than 5 years.[42,43] The best results have been observed in patients who had responded to conventional-dose salvage therapy and who received autologous rescue as intensive consolidation therapy. Results indicate that more than one-half of patients transplanted at a time when minimal disease was present are alive; many of these patients are likely to be cured of their disease. Although high-dose chemotherapy with autologous rescue has a high complete remission rate in newly diagnosed patients who never attained a complete remission or in those who had experienced multiple relapses, long-term survival in patients with refractory disease is poor. Results from uncontrolled trials with the use of high-dose chemotherapy and autologous rescue as intensive consolidation therapy (i.e., during first complete remission) in high-risk patients are encouraging.[42,43] However, in a large prospective randomized trial of patients with aggressive non-Hodgkin's lymphoma in first complete remission, disease-free survival and overall survival at 3 years were not significantly improved in patients who received high-dose chemotherapy compared with those treated with standard-dose consolidation therapy.[88] Fewer patients with indolent NHL have been treated with autologous BMT. Early results are encouraging, and most patients have achieved a complete remission.[89] Because of the indolent nature of the disease, longer follow-up is required before high-dose chemotherapy with autologous rescue can be recommended for this group of patients.

One of the major problems in this group of patients is disease relapse. A variety of conditioning regimens have been used in these studies, and no one conditioning regimen has been shown to be clearly superior to other regimens.[41,42] One novel approach is targeted radiotherapy with a radiolabeled monoclonal antibody (i.e., radioimmunotherapy) in an attempt to deliver higher doses of irradiation to tumor sites.[45,46] Results of a phase II study in 25 patients given myeloablative doses of ^{131}I-labeled anti-CD20 (B1) antibody (without chemotherapy) show that targeted radiotherapy can produce complete responses of long duration in most patients with relapsed B-cell lymphomas.[46] Disease-free survival was significantly higher in patients who received more than 2000 cGy to the dose-limiting normal organ (with higher doses to tumor sites). Another approach is to eliminate residual malignant cells. Many patients treated with high-dose chemotherapy and autologous BMT had their marrow purged with monoclonal antibodies, sometimes combined with 4-HC. The role of marrow purging is controversial. One retrospective study reported that *ex vivo* purging had no significant effect on disease-free survival.[90] Another study, however, recently reported that patients who had no detectable residual lymphoma cells after immunologic marrow-purging had increased disease-free survival compared with those who had residual lymphoma in their marrow.[91] In that study, a sensitive PCR method was used to detect the presence of residual lymphoma cells in the marrow.

BREAST CANCER

Breast cancer has served as the model for the study of high-dose chemotherapy with autologous BMT in the treatment of chemotherapy-responsive solid tumors.[49,92] That tumor was selected because of its high incidence and studies that demonstrated a correlation between dose intensity and objective response rate or median survival. Breast cancer is currently the most common indication for high-dose chemotherapy with autologous rescue.

Table 129.3 shows the possibilities for timing of high-dose chemotherapy with autologous rescue. Initially, high-dose chemotherapy with autologous BMT was used in patients with metastatic disease who had failed prior chemotherapy. In that setting, the overall response rate was about 60%, which was about twofold higher than that achieved with conventional-dose salvage chemotherapy.[92] When high-dose chemotherapy with autologous BMT was used as initial treatment for metastatic disease, the objective response rate was about 80%, of which 40–50% were complete responses. Some of the complete responders have remained in unmaintained remission for several years.

Based on the experience in leukemia and lymphoma, it was likely that high-dose chemotherapy with autologous BMT would be most effective when used in patients with early or minimal disease (i.e., as consolidation therapy). This approach has been used in patients with metastatic disease or high-risk primary disease. In patients with metastatic disease, high-dose chemotherapy with autologous BMT is given after the patient has received induction with standard-dose chemotherapy. In that setting, the objective response rate is about 90% and the complete response rate is about 60%.[92] About one-half of the complete responders remain alive in unmaintained, continuous, complete remission with several years of follow-up. High-dose chemotherapy with autologous BMT is also used in patients with high-risk primary disease. Women in these studies usually have stage II or III disease involving 10 or more axillary lymph nodes. Historical data indicate that 55–87% of these patients will relapse within 5 years, despite standard-dose adjuvant chemotherapy.[92] Patients usually receive several courses of standard-dose adjuvant chemotherapy, followed by high-dose chemotherapy with autologous rescue as intensive consolidation. Uncontrolled studies conducted at Duke University show that about 70% of women with high-risk primary disease treated with this approach are alive at 3 years.[93] Based on these encouraging results, the role of high-dose chemotherapy with autologous BMT as intensive consolidation in women with high-risk primary disease is currently being evaluated by several cooperative oncology groups.[92]

Because of the large number of women with breast cancer, the use of high-dose chemotherapy with autologous rescue has greatly increased the awareness of the lay public and health care professionals to BMT as a treatment modality. Although early results are encouraging, its use is controversial and there is variability in insurance coverage for the treatment.[94,95]

MULTIPLE MYELOMA

Multiple myeloma is a relatively rare hematologic malignancy characterized by uncontrolled proliferation of plasma cells derived from a single malignant clone. Although combination chemotherapy induces a response in most patients, complete responses are uncommon and the disease is not curable with standard-dose chemotherapy. High-dose chemotherapy with autologous rescue induces a complete or partial response in 70–80% of newly diagnosed patients with multiple myeloma, and some of these patients may be cured of their disease.[96–98] Several factors were predictive of response to high-dose chemotherapy with autologous rescue: response to standard therapy, age ≤ 50 years old, β^2 microglobulin levels ≤ 2.5 mg/L, and time from diagnosis (≤12 months). The most commonly used preparative regimen is high-dose melphalan, given either alone or combined with TBI. Some aggressive protocols include two transplants.

OTHER SOLID TUMORS

High-dose chemotherapy with autologous rescue has been used as salvage therapy for many adults with solid tumors, particularly chemotherapy-responsive tumors such as germ cell tumors and small cell lung cancer.[47,48] Some patients with solid tumors not usually responsive to chemotherapy, such as colorectal cancer and malignant melanoma, also have been treated. Many children with neuroblastoma, Ewing's sarcoma, rhabdomyosarcoma, and brain tumors also have been treated, with varying success.[48,99]

COMPLICATIONS OF BONE MARROW TRANSPLANTATION

Although many patients with cancer treated with high-dose chemotherapy and autologous or allogeneic BMT experience long-term survival and cure of their disease, this modality is associated with many serious and potentially life-threatening complications. In the early 1970s, early post-transplant mortality was extremely high, and most BMT patients did not survive beyond 100 days. During those early years of allogeneic BMT, death was usually related to infection, GVHD, interstitial pneumonia, and leukemic relapse. The therapeutic armamentarium available at that time was limited. Today, largely because of the availability of new and potent drugs such as broad-spectrum antibiotics, immunosuppressive drugs, antiviral drugs, and hematopoietic growth factors and other biotechnology drugs, transplant-related mortality has been greatly reduced. For example, about 90% of patients with CML who undergo allogeneic BMT from an HLA-identical sibling donor during their chronic phase are alive at 1 year.[33] Until recently, allogeneic BMT was usually restricted to patients less than 50 years old with an HLA-identical sibling donor. With advances in the prevention and treatment of transplant-related complications, allogeneic BMT is now being offered to more high-risk patients such as those who lack an HLA-identical sibling donor and those older than 50 years of age. Patients treated with high-dose chemotherapy with autologous rescue have a very low risk for immune-mediated complications. The risk of transplant-related mortality after high-dose chemotherapy with autologous rescue for lymphoma or breast cancer is less than 10% at most centers and less than 5% at some centers.

Unfortunately, similar progress has not been made in the eradication of malignant cells and tumor relapse remains the major cause of death post-transplant. The use of more sensitive methods to detect tumor cells, novel purging techniques, more effective conditioning regimens, and adoptive immunotherapy may lead to more effective tumor control.

REGIMEN-RELATED TOXICITY

Because myelosuppression is not a concern, dosages of anticancer drugs can be increased many times above those used in conventional chemotherapy. As a result, most patients undergoing BMT experience regimen-related toxicity in nonhematopoietic tissues and some patients experience early death as a result of these toxicities. In the BMT setting, these nonhematologic toxicities are dose limiting. Because of the severity of these regimen-related toxicities, toxicity grading scales used in cooperative oncology group trials are not appropriate. A toxicity grading system has recently been developed by the Seattle BMT team.[24] In that grading system, toxicities in eight different organs are graded on a scale of 0 (none) to 4 (fatal). If a toxicity is related to another cause other than the preparative regimen, it is not considered regimen-related toxicity. After toxicity to individual organs is graded, the patient is assigned an overall grade of toxicity equivalent to the highest grade achieved in any organ.

In patients with leukemia, regimen-related toxicity is usually more severe in allogeneic BMT recipients compared with autologous BMT recipients, which suggests that GVHD or post-transplant immunosuppression contributes to regimen-related toxicity. Severe regimen-related toxicities are also more common in patients with advanced disease at the time of BMT. In the setting of autologous BMT, where graft rejection and GVHD do not occur, the mortality associated with severe regimen-related toxicity is about

10–20%. The dose-limiting nonhematologic toxicity varies according to the drugs included in the conditioning regimen. Table 129.5 lists the dose-limiting nonhematologic toxicity for several drugs commonly included in conditioning regimens. These toxicities may be uncommon or rare with the administration of conventional doses of a specific drug. Several unusual and severe manifestations of regimen-related toxicities are discussed in detail below.

The management of specific toxicities is supportive. The mechanism of toxicity probably varies according to the conditioning regimen and the organ involved. The clinical expression of regimen-related toxicity may be related to the release of tumor necrosis factor (TNF)-α and other inflammatory cytokines. Drugs that inhibit the release of inflammatory cytokines are being investigated to reduce regimen-related toxicity after BMT. Results of randomized controlled trials with pentoxifylline, an inhibitor of TNF-α production, have been disappointing.[100,101]

Hepatic Veno-Occlusive Disease

Hepatic veno-occlusive disease (VOD), defined as an obliteration of the small intrahepatic central venules, is one of the most severe regimen-related toxicities.[102,103] Clinical signs of hepatic VOD include sudden weight gain, ascites, hepatomegaly, and increased serum bilirubin concentrations occurring within the first 3 weeks after transplant. The incidence of hepatic VOD ranges from 5–20% in most series. Factors reported to increase the risk of hepatic VOD include the use of TBI-containing conditioning regimens and the presence of elevated liver function tests or metastatic liver disease pretransplant. The use of some drugs, such as busulfan or carmustine, also may increase the risk of hepatic VOD. In one study, busulfan concentrations correlated with the risk of hepatic VOD.[104] Patients with a high area-under-the-curve (AUC) for busulfan concentration had a greater risk of hepatic VOD than those with a low AUC. Based on these studies, some BMT centers adjust busulfan doses based on plasma concentrations. Hepatic VOD is frequently progressive, leading to death in 50–75% of patients. At many BMT centers, hepatic VOD is one of the leading causes of transplant-related mortality after high-dose chemotherapy with autologous rescue. Treatment is supportive. Some studies suggest that prostaglandin E_1, heparin, or ursodiol may be partially effective in the prevention of hepatic VOD.[102,103]

Pulmonary Complications

Idiopathic interstitial pneumonitis also is a severe form of regimen-related toxicity.[105,106] Patients with idiopathic interstitial pneumonitis are clinically indistinguishable from those with interstitial pneumonitis related to infection. The risk is similar in recipients of autologous or allogeneic marrow, but appears higher in patients who are conditioned with a TBI-containing regimen. Mortality is as high as 50% in some studies. Diffuse alveolar hemorrhage has been described recently after autologous BMT.[107] It is diagnosed by examination of bronchoalveolar lavage fluid. Mortality also is high. Prompt treatment with high doses of corticosteroids has been reported to be beneficial.[108]

GRAFT FAILURE

Initial engraftment usually occurs in the first 2–4 weeks post-transplant and is evidenced by rising peripheral blood counts and the presence of hematopoietic precursor cells in the marrow. In allogeneic BMT, the presence of donor cells is confirmed with cytogenetic markers. In most patients, engraftment is sustained with complete recovery of hematopoiesis.

Graft failure can occur after autologous, syngeneic, and allogeneic BMT. Two syndromes have been observed.[109,110]

TABLE 129.5. DOSE-LIMITING NONHEMATOLOGIC TOXICITIES FOR SELECTED CHEMOTHERAPEUTIC AGENTS INCLUDED IN CONDITIONING REGIMENS IN AUTOLOGOUS BONE MARROW TRANSPLANTATION

Drug	Conventional Dose[a] (mg/m²)	ABMT[b] Dose (mg/m²)	Dose-Limiting Toxicity
Busulfan	2	450	Hepatic
Carboplatin	400	2000	Hepatic, renal
Carmustine	200	1200	Pulmonary, hepatic
Cisplatin	100	200	Renal, peripheral neuropathy
Cyclophosphamide	1000	7500	Cardiomyopathy
Etoposide	300–600	2400	Mucositis
Ifosfamide	5000	18000	Renal
Melphalan	40	225	Mucositis
Thiotepa	20–50	1125	Mucositis, CNS

[a]Doses are approximate and are for drugs as single agents. When combinations are used, doses may need to be decreased.
[b]ABMT, autologous bone marrow transplantation. (Modified from Eder JP, Elias A, Shea TC, et al. A phase I–II study of cyclophosphamide, thiotepa, and carboplatin with autologous bone marrow transplantation in solid tumor patients. J Clin Oncol 1990;8:1242, with permission.)

Early graft failure is diagnosed clinically when the rate of neutrophil recovery is delayed (also referred to as primary graft failure or delayed engraftment), whereas late graft failure is characterized by a decline in the neutrophil count after temporary engraftment (also referred to as secondary graft failure). When graft failure occurs after allogeneic BMT and is characterized by the regrowth of immunocompetent host cells and a simultaneous loss of donor cells, it is referred to as graft rejection. Graft rejection occurs rarely in recipients of unmodified marrow from HLA-identical sibling donors who are conditioned with cyclophosphamide and TBI.[111] An increased risk of graft rejection has been observed in several groups of patients undergoing allogeneic BMT: recipients of marrow from partially HLA-mismatched donors, recipients of T-cell–depleted marrow (HLA-identical sibling donors), recipients of marrow from matched unrelated donors, and patients with severe aplastic anemia. With widespread use of PBPCs and post-transplant growth factors, graft failure is rare after autologous transplantation.

Graft failure not immunologically mediated also can occur in allogeneic BMT. It is usually difficult to determine the precise cause, although potential causes include infusion of low numbers of hematopoietic stem cells, viral infection (i.e., cytomegalovirus), or drug toxicity. Drug-induced graft failure can be caused not only by drugs that are known to be myelosuppressive (e.g., methotrexate, ganciclovir), but also by drugs that are not usually associated with neutropenia (e.g., ranitidine).[112] The use of chemicals or drugs, such as 4-HC, in *ex vivo* marrow purging in autologous BMT may damage hematopoietic stem cells and also increase the risk of graft failure.[55]

Regardless of the cause, the long-term prognosis in patients with graft failure is poor.[113] Despite supportive care, death usually occurs from infection or bleeding. In some patients with an HLA-identical sibling donor, a second marrow transplant can be beneficial. The most effective therapy for graft failure is recombinant growth factors, such as G-CSF or GM-CSF. In one uncontrolled study, more than one-half of patients with marrow graft failure responded within 2 weeks to recombinant GM-CSF.[113] In many cases, responses were sustained without maintenance GM-CSF therapy. GM-CSF-treated patients had a better survival than historic controls.

The use of recombinant G-CSF or GM-CSF post-transplant dramatically reduces the incidence of early graft failure after autologous BMT.[114,115] Before the availability of recombinant growth factors, most patients required 3–4 weeks to engraft after autologous BMT. Recombinant G-CSF or GM-CSF given during the early post-transplant period significantly accelerates the rate of myeloid recovery in patients undergoing autologous BMT, defined as the number of days needed to reach a neutrophil count of 500 or $1000/mm^3$.[116,117] The usual dosage of recombinant GM-CSF is 250 mg/m^2/d. Higher dosages (e.g., 10 μg/kg/d) of recombinant G-CSF can be given because of its more favorable adverse effect profile compared with recombinant GM-CSF. Neither recombinant G-CSF or GM-CSF, however, has a significant effect on platelet recovery. Although recombinant growth factors were initially not given to patients undergoing allogeneic BMT because of concern that they may exacerbate GVHD, recent studies suggest that they may accelerate the rate of hematopoietic recovery.[118,119]

Although recombinant G-CSF or GM-CSF clearly accelerates myeloid recovery after autologous BMT, its role is less clear in patients who receive mobilized PBPCs instead of bone marrow as a source of hematopoietic stem cells. Some investigators believe that PBPCs are primarily responsible for the rapid neutrophil and platelet recovery observed after high-dose chemotherapy and that post-transplant administration of recombinant G-CSF or GM-CSF is less important and may not be necessary. However, in a prospective randomized trial, patients who received mobilized PBPCs and post-transplant recombinant G-CSF had significantly more rapid neutrophil recovery than those who received mobilized PBPCs alone.[120]

GRAFT-VERSUS-HOST DISEASE

GVHD is caused by immunocompetent donor T lymphocytes reacting against antigens on host tissues.[109,121–123] In that setting, donor T lymphocytes recognize histocompatibility antigens of the host as genetically foreign, become activated, proliferate, and attack recipient tissue, thereby producing the clinical syndrome of GVHD. Excessive or dysfunctional production of inflammatory cytokines such as IL-1 and TNF-α is probably responsible at least in part for the clinical syndrome of GVHD.[65,124] This hypothesis is supported by the observation that some patients with refractory acute GVHD respond to treatment with inhibitors of these cytokines (discussed below). Graft rejection can be viewed as a host-versus-graft reaction, an immune-mediated reaction in the opposite direction as GVHD. Two different clinical syndromes have been recognized, depending on the onset of GVHD. Acute GVHD occurs early while chronic GVHD occurs late in the post-transplant course.

Acute Graft-Versus-Host Disease

Acute GVHD usually becomes clinically evident during the first 60 days post-transplant and is characterized by selective epithelial damage of target organs. The principal target organs for acute GVHD are the skin, liver, and gastrointestinal tract. Acute GVHD is classified into four grades, depending on the number of organs involved and the degree of involvement of each organ (Fig. 129.8).[121–123] Grade I disease involves only the skin while grades II through IV involve the skin and either the liver or gastrointestinal tract, or both. The initial sign of acute GVHD is usually a gener-

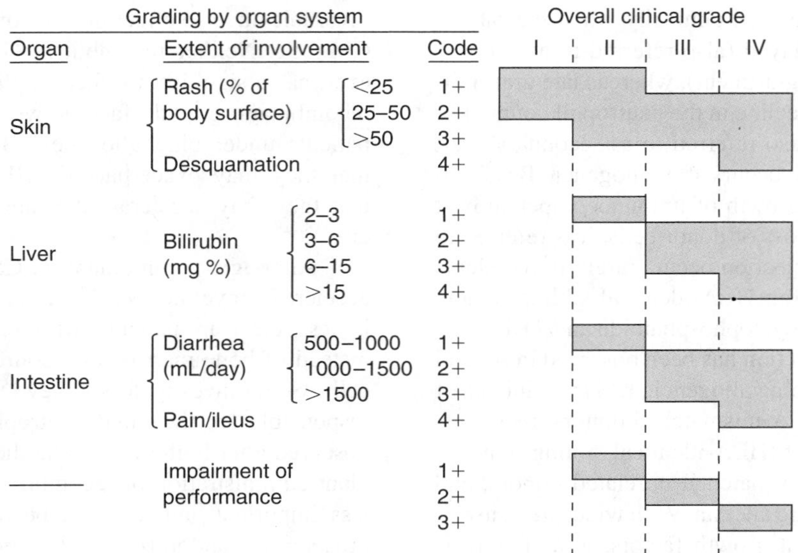

Figure 129.8. Clinical grading of acute GVHD. The left panel of the figure summarizes the grading by organ system; the right panel shows the overall clinical grade. With grade I, only the skin can be involved. With more extensive involvement of the skin or involvement of liver and intestinal tract and impairment of the clinical performance status, either alone or in any combination, the severity grade advances from II to IV. *(Reproduced, with permission, from the* Annual Review of Medicine, *Volume 35, © 1984, by Annual Reviews Inc.)*

alized maculopapular rash. Acute GVHD usually progresses, involving the liver, gastrointestinal tract, or both. Intestinal GVHD is manifested as diarrhea but may progress to abdominal pain and ileus. Hepatic GVHD is usually asymptomatic, consisting of hyperbilirubinemia and increases in serum aminotransferase and alkaline phosphatase levels.

The overall incidence of moderate to severe (grades II–IV) GVHD ranges from 10% to more than 80% after allogeneic BMT, depending on the degree of histocompatibility, number of T lymphocytes in the graft, patient age, and prophylactic regimen.[121,122] Other factors associated with an increased risk for acute GVHD in some studies are donor:recipient sex mismatch and the parity of female donors; the highest risk was observed in male recipients who received marrow from a previously pregnant female donor.[125] This observation suggests that alloimmunization against minor histocompatibility antigens may be important in the pathogenesis of acute GVHD. The reasons for the increased risk in older patients are not known, although many investigators believe that it is related to the gradual reduction in thymic function with increasing age. The most severe acute GVHD is observed in allogeneic BMT with non-HLA-identical related or HLA-identical unrelated donors. In that setting, the incidence of grades II–IV acute GVHD exceeds 50%, despite aggressive prophylactic immunosuppression with two or more drugs, sometimes combined with immunologic purging of T cells from donor marrow.[11,14]

Multiorgan acute GVHD and the drugs given to prevent or treat it are associated with delayed immunologic recovery and increased susceptibility to infections, particularly cytomegaloviral infection. Because treatment of established acute GVHD is unsatisfactory, aggressive preventive treatment is usually given. The most common strategy used to prevent acute GVHD is to block the activation of T lymphocytes by administration of immunosuppressive agents.[121–123] Several immunosuppressive agents have been used, including cyclophosphamide, methotrexate, cyclosporine, antithymocyte globulin, corticosteroids, and most recently tacrolimus or monoclonal antibodies directed at T lymphocytes. Most GVHD prophylaxis regimens combine two or more immunosuppressive agents that affect different stages of T-cell activation. Another strategy is to remove or deplete most T lymphocytes from donor bone marrow by physical separation (i.e., lectin agglutination) or by treatment with monoclonal antibodies directed at T cells (Fig. 129.6).[126]

In allogeneic BMT with HLA-identical sibling donors, the combination of cyclosporine and either methotrexate or corticosteroids reduces the incidence of grades II–IV acute GVHD to 25–40%.[125,127–129] Intravenous cyclosporine is usually started around day 0 at an initial dosage of 3–5 mg/kg/d, given in two divided doses. Dosages are adjusted based on trough cyclosporine concentrations. Patients are converted to oral cyclosporine when they can tolerate oral medications. Cyclosporine is given at full doses until about day 50, gradually tapered thereafter, and discontinued by day 180. "Short" methotrexate is given intravenously on days 1, 3, 6, and 11 post-transplant.[127] The methotrexate dosage is 10 mg/m^2, except for the first dose given on day 1 (15 mg/m^2). Some protocols omit the day 11 dose because of adverse effects. When cyclosporine is given in combination with corticosteroids, methylprednisolone is usually started during the first 2 weeks post-transplant, given at full dosages for several weeks, and gradually tapered. Although the efficacy of cyclosporine–methotrexate and cyclosporine–corticosteroids appears to be similar, the use of methotrexate may increase the risk of early graft failure.[118] It is not clear whether three-drug regimens are more effective than two-drug regimens. In one prospective randomized study conducted by the Seattle BMT team, the addition of methylprednisolone did not further increase the efficacy of the cyclosporine and methotrexate regimen.[130] Unexpectedly, patients who received cyclosporine, methotrexate, and methylprednisolone had a higher incidence of acute and chronic GVHD than those given cyclosporine and methotrexate. Subsequent analysis of that trial showed that patients who received three drugs as GVHD prophylaxis also had a significantly higher risk of infection early post-transplant compared with those who received cyclosporine and methotrexate.[131] But in another prospective randomized study, the three-drug combination of cyclosporine, methotrexate, and corticosteroids further reduced the incidence of grades II–IV acute GVHD to about 10%, compared with a 20% incidence in those randomized to receive cyclosporine and glucocorticoids.[132] It is not clear why the two trials reached different conclusions. In the trial conducted by the Seattle BMT team, methylprednisolone was given from days 0–35 post-transplant. In contrast, methylprednisolone was not started in the other trial until day 7 post-transplant. Some investigators speculate that early administration of methylprednisolone may have interfered with the antiproliferative effects of methotrexate on T lymphocytes.[130]

Newer approaches may increase the efficacy of GVHD prophylaxis after allogeneic BMT. Tacrolimus, given either alone or combined with methotrexate or methylprednisolone, is also being studied as GVHD prophylaxis after BMT from HLA-identical siblings.[133] Systemic monoclonal antibodies are also being studied in some clinical trials. Although uncontrolled trials suggest possible benefit, results of a controlled trial showed that addition of a monoclonal antibody directed against the IL-2 receptor to standard GVHD prophylaxis was associated with significantly lower disease-free survival, primarily because of an increased risk of late relapses.[134] Another interesting observation is that high doses of commercially available intravenous immunoglobulin appear to reduce the risk of acute GVHD in certain subsets of allogeneic BMT recipients.[135]

The role of T-cell depletion from donor bone marrow is controversial (Fig. 129.6). Although the use of T-cell-depleted marrow can reduce the incidence and severity of acute GVHD, it is associated with an increased risk of graft failure and leukemic relapse.[109,123,126] As a result, survival in recipients of HLA-identical sibling donor marrow is not improved with this approach. However, because of the higher risk of GVHD in allogeneic BMT with HLA-mismatched or matched unrelated donors, T-cell depletion is often included as part of the GVHD prophylaxis regimen in that setting (see below).

With allogeneic BMT with HLA-mismatched or HLA-identical unrelated donors, the risk of moderate to severe (grades II–IV) acute GVHD is 50% or higher with conventional prophylaxis with two immunosuppressive agents.[11,12,15] The combination of cyclosporine and corticosteroids is preferred by some investigators because of the bone marrow toxicity of methotrexate.[14] Several approaches are generally used to reduce the risk of acute GVHD in this high-risk group of patients: three-drug GVHD prophylaxis (cyclosporine, methotrexate, and corticosteroids), T-cell depletion of donor bone marrow (Fig. 129.6), or the addition of an intravenously administered monoclonal antibody directed at T cells to standard GVHD prophylaxis. In recipients of matched unrelated transplants, T-cell depletion has been associated with a significantly lower incidence of early graft failure and acute GVHD, with apparent preservation of the graft-versus-leukemia effect.[15,136]

Initial treatment of established acute GVHD usually consists of high-dose corticosteroids, given as intravenously administered methylprednisolone. The usual dosage is 2.0 mg/kg/d, given in two divided doses. The initial dosage is as high as 10 mg/kg/d in some protocols, although there is no convincing evidence that higher dosages are more effective. Results of one study suggest that a cumulative dose of 2000 mg/m^2 (about 50 mg/kg) of prednisone (or methylprednisolone) is needed for complete resolution of acute GVHD in most patients.[137] Antithymocyte globulin appears to be as effective as methylprednisolone, but difficulties in supply and toxicities have limited its usefulness. Overall complete or partial responses are observed in about 40% of patients.[123,138,139] Nonrelapse mortality is strongly correlated to response to initial treatment; mortality ranged from about 25% in patients who had a complete response to about 80% in those who had no response or progressive disease. Octreotide has been reported effective in some patients with severe diarrhea related to intestinal GVHD.[140] In patients who fail initial treatment with corticosteroids, antithymocyte globulin or monoclonal antibodies directed at T lymphocytes can be given with some success.[141] In patients who experience a flare in their GVHD during the taper phase of corticosteroid therapy, therapy consists of increasing the steroid dose. A variety of biotechnology drugs have been shown to be effective in the treatment of refractory acute GVHD. Encouraging results have been reported with an immunotoxin targeted against an antigen found on mature T lymphocytes (CD5),[142] a humanized monoclonal antibody that binds to the IL-2 receptor,[143] a monoclonal anti–TNF-α antibody,[144] and recombinant IL-1 receptor antagonist.[145]

Chronic Graft-Versus-Host Disease

Chronic GVHD usually occurs after day 100 and is the major determinant of late transplant-related morbidity and mortality.[122,146] Chronic GVHD is classified as limited or extensive, depending on pathologic findings and the extent of systemic involvement. Limited chronic GVHD indicates either localized skin involvement, mild hepatic dysfunction, or both. Most patients have extensive disease, with involvement of the skin, liver, eyes, mouth, esophagus, or other organs. The clinicopathologic findings of chronic GVHD are similar to those observed in various autoimmune diseases. Screening studies such as skin and lip biopsies and Schirmer's testing for lacrimal function done on day 100 have been shown to predict for the subsequent development of chronic GVHD.

The incidence of chronic GVHD in patients who survive more than 150 days ranges from 15–65%.[122,146] The risk of chronic GVHD increases with increasing patient age, and is higher in recipients of marrow from HLA-nonidentical related or unrelated donors, and in patients who had prior acute GVHD. In patients with aplastic anemia, the administration of donor buffy-coat transfusions also is associated with an increased risk of chronic GVHD. Most patients who develop chronic GVHD have a previous history of acute GVHD, although 20–30% develop the disease *de novo*.

If no functional impairment is present, patients with limited disease are not treated. Many patients with extensive chronic GVHD, if left untreated, will die of infections or become disabled. Long-term survival is worse in certain subgroups of patients, such as patients with thrombocytopenia or progressive onset of chronic GVHD, and those who fail to respond to immunosuppressive therapy.[147] Chronic GVHD is treated with immunosuppressive agents such as corticosteroids, cyclosporine, cyclophosphamide, or azathioprine. In patients without thrombocytopenia, treatment with prednisone alone (initial dosage: 1.0 mg/kg/d) is superior to prednisone and azathioprine.[147] Although control of chronic GVHD was similar between the two groups, patients treated with prednisone and azathioprine had more frequent bacterial and viral infections, which resulted in higher nonrelapse mortality (40 versus 21%). In patients with thrombocytopenia, an alternating-day cyclosporine and prednisone regimen appears superior to prednisone alone in the treatment of chronic GVHD.[148] In patients who fail initial treatment, azathioprine or alternating cyclosporine and prednisone have been used with some success. Thalidomide appears effective in some patients who fail initial treatment and is being investigated as primary treatment for high-risk chronic GVHD.[149] Oral trimethoprim–sulfamethoxazole is usually given as infection prophylaxis in all patients receiving treatment for chronic GVHD.

Treatment is continued until signs and symptoms of the disease have resolved, usually over a period of several months. As chronic GVHD improves, the immunosuppressive drug is discontinued, followed by gradual tapering of corticosteroid therapy. Because patients are usually leading fairly normal lives at this stage, it is important to minimize any unnecessary side effects of therapy.

INFECTION

Patients undergoing autologous or allogeneic BMT are severely immunocompromised and therefore at high risk for bacterial, fungal, and viral infection. Management of these infections is discussed in detail in Chapter [114].

LATE COMPLICATIONS

With the success of BMT, the number of long-term survivors has grown. Many survivors experience delayed complications of BMT. Major late complications include restrictive and obstructive pulmonary disease; cataract formation; endocrine dysfunction, including sterility; impaired growth; infections; and secondary malignancies.[146,150]

REFERENCES

1. Champlin R (ed). Bone Marrow Transplantation. Boston, Kluwer Academic Publishers, 1990.
2. Forman SJ (ed). Bone marrow transplantation. Hematol/Oncol Clin North Am 1990;4:507–714.
3. Williams SF (ed). Autologous bone marrow transplantation. Hematol/Oncol Clin North Am 1993;7:501–752.
4. Gulati S, Yahalow J, Portlock C. Autologous bone marrow transplantation. Curr Prob Cancer 1991;15:1–57.
5. Armitage JO. Bone marrow transplantation. N Engl J Med 1994;330:827–838.
6. Forman SJ, Blume KG, Thomas ED (eds). Bone Marrow Transplantation. Boston, Blackwell, 1994.
7. Atkinson K (ed). Clinical Bone Marrow Transplantation. Cambridge, Cambridge University Press, 1994.
8. Dupont B, Yang SY. Histocompatibility, in Forman SJ, Blume KG, Thomas ED (eds): Bone Marrow Transplantation. Boston, Blackwell, 1994, pp 22–40.
9. Begovich AB, Erlich HA. HLA typing for bone marrow transplantation. J Am Med Assoc 1995;273:586–591.
10. Mickelson EM, Bartsch GE, Hansen JA, Dupont B. The MLC assay as a test for HLA-D region compatibility between patients and unrelated donors: Results of a national marrow donor program involving multiple centers. Tissue Antigens 1993;42:465–472.
11. Anasetti C, Hansen J. Bone marrow transplantation from HLA-partially matched related donors and unrelated volunteer donors, in Forman SJ, Blume KG, Thomas ED (eds): Bone Marrow Transplantation. Boston, Blackwell, 1994, pp 665–679.
12. Petersdorf EW, Longton GM, Anasetti C, et al. The significance of HLA-DRB1 matching on clinical outcome after HLA-A, B, DR identical unrelated donor marrow transplantation. Blood 1995;86:1606–1613.

13. McCullough J, Hansen JA, Perkins H, et al. Establishment of the National Bone Marrow Donor Registry, in Gale RP, Champlin R (eds): Bone Marrow Transplantation: Current Controversies. New York, Alan R. Liss, 1989, pp 641–658.
14. Stroncek D, Bartsch G, Perkins HA, et al. The National Marrow Donor Program. Transfusion 1993;33:567–577.
15. Kernan NA, Bartsch G, Ash RC, et al. Analysis of 462 transplantations from unrelated donors facilitated by the National Marrow Donor Program. N Engl J Med 1993;328:593–602.
16. Golde DW. The stem cell. Sci Am 1991;Dec:86–93.
17. Thomas ED, Storb R. Technique for human marrow grafting. Blood 1970;36:507–515.
18. Lowry PA, Tabbara IA. Peripheral hematopoietic stem cell transplantation: Current concepts. Exper Hematol 1992;20:937–942.
19. Kessinger A. Utilization of peripheral blood stem cells in auto-transplantation. Hematol/Oncol Clin North Am 1993;7:535–545.
20. Lasky LC. Hematopoietic reconstitution using progenitors recovered from blood. Transfusion 1989;29:552–557.
21. Vose JM, Anderson JR, Kessinger A, et al. High-dose chemotherapy and autologous hematopoietic stem-cell transplantation for aggressive non-Hodgkin's lymphoma. J Clin Oncol 1993;11:1846–1851.
22. Peters WP, Ross M, Vredenburgh JJ, et al. The use of intensive clinic support to permit outpatient autologous bone marrow transplantation for breast cancer. Semin Oncol 1994;21(suppl 7):25–31.
23. Wagner JE, Kernan NA, Steinbuch M, et al. Allogeneic sibling umbilical-cord blood transplantation in children with malignant and non-malignant disease. Lancet 1995;346:214–219.
24. Petersen FB, Bearman SI. Preparative regimens and their toxicity, in Forman SJ, Blume KG, Thomas ED (eds): Bone Marrow Transplantation. Boston, Blackwell, 1994, pp 79–95.
25. Aurer I, Gale RP. Are new conditioning regimens for transplants in acute myelogenous leukemia better? Bone Marrow Transplant 1991;7:255–261.
26. Blume KG, Forman SJ. High-dose etoposide (VP-16)-containing preparatory regimens in allogeneic and autologous bone marrow transplantation for hematologic malignancies. Semin Oncol 1992;19(suppl 13):63–66.
27. Santos GW. The development of busulfan/cyclophosphamide preparative regimens. Semin Oncol 1993;20(suppl 4):12–16.
28. Antmann K, Eder JP, Elias A, et al. High-dose thiotepa alone and in combination regimens with bone marrow support. Semin Oncol 1990;17(suppl 3):33–38.
29. Peters LJ, Withers HR, Cundiff JH, et al. Radiobiological considerations in the use of total body irradiation for bone-marrow transplantation. Radiology 1979;131:243–247.
30. Thomas ED, Clift RA, Hersman J, et al. Marrow transplantation for acute nonlymphoblastic leukemia in first remission using fractionated or single-dose irradiation. Int J Radiat Oncol Biol Phys 1982;8:817–821.
31. Deeg HJ. Acute and delayed toxicities of total body irradiation. Int Radiat Oncol Biol Phys 1983;9:133–139.
32. Clift RA, Buckner CD, Appelbaum FR, et al. Allogeneic marrow transplantation in patients with chronic myelogenous leukemia in the chronic phase: A randomized trial of two irradiation regimens. Blood 1991;77:1660–1665.
33. Brochstein JA, Kernan NA, Groshen S, et al. Allogeneic bone marrow transplantation after hyperfractionated total-body irradiation and cyclophosphamide in children with acute leukemia. N Engl J Med 1987;317:1618–1624.
34. Clift RA, Buckner CD, Thomas ED, et al. Marrow transplantation for chronic myeloid leukemia: A randomized study comparing cyclophosphamide and total body irradiation with busulfan and cyclophosphamide. Blood 1994;84:2036–2043.
35. Devergie A, Blaise D, Attal M, et al. Allogeneic bone marrow transplantation for chronic myeloid leukemia in first chronic phase: A randomized trial of busulfan–cytoxan versus cytoxan–total body irradiation as preparative regimen: A report from the French Society of Bone Marrow Graft. Blood 1995;85:2263–2268.
36. Ringden O, Ruutu T, Remberger M, et al. A randomized trial comparing busulfan with total body irradiation as conditioning in allogeneic marrow transplant recipients with leukemia: A report from the Nordic Bone Marrow Transplantation Group. Blood 1994;83:2723–2730.
37. Blaise D, Maraninchi D, Archimbaud E, et al. Allogeneic bone marrow transplantation for acute myeloid leukemia in first remission: A randomized trial of a busulfan–cytoxan versus cytoxan–total body irradiation as preparative regimen: A report from the group d'Etudes de la Greffe de Moelle Osseuse. Blood 1992;79:2578–2582.
38. Woods WG, Ramsay NKC, Weisdorf DJ, et al. Bone marrow transplantation for acute lymphocytic leukemia utilizing total body irradiation followed by high doses of cytosine arabinoside: Lack of superiority over cyclophosphamide-containing conditioning regimens. Bone Marrow Transplant 1990;6:9–16.
39. Coccia PF, Strandjord SE, Warkentin PI, et al. High-dose cytosine arabinoside and fractionated total-body irradiation: An improved preparative regimen for bone marrow transplantation of children with acute lymphoblastic leukemia in remission. Blood 1988;71:888–893.
40. Snyder DS, Chao NJ, Amylon MD, et al. Fractionated total body irradiation and high-dose etoposide as a preparatory regimen for bone marrow transplantation in 99 patients with acute leukemia in first complete remission. Blood 1993;82:2920–2928.
41. Champlin R. Preparative regimens for autologous bone marrow transplantation. Blood 1993;81:277–280.
42. Bierman PJ, Armitage JO. Autologous bone marrow transplantation for non-Hodgkin's lymphoma, in Forman SJ, Blume KG, Thomas ED (eds): Bone Marrow Transplantation. Boston, Blackwell, 1994, pp 683–695.
43. Philips GL. Transplantation for Hodgkin's disease, in Forman SJ, Blume KG, Thomas ED (eds): Bone Marrow Transplantation. Boston, Blackwell, 1994, pp 696–708.
44. Jagannath S, Dicke K, Armitage JO, et al. High-dose cyclophosphamide, carmustine, and etoposide and autologous bone marrow transplantation for relapsed Hodgkin's disease. Ann Intern Med 1986;104:163–168.

45. Press OW, Eary JF, Appelbaum FR, et al. Radiolabelled-antibody therapy of B-cell lymphoma with autologous bone marrow support. N Engl J Med 1993;329:1219–1224.
46. Press OW, Eary JF, Appelbaum FR, et al. Phase II trial of ^{131}I-B1 (anti-CD20) antibody therapy with autologous stem cell transplantation for relapsed B cell lymphomas. Lancet 1995;346:336–340.
47. Ayash LJ, Antman K, Cheson BD. A perspective on dose-intensive therapy with autologous bone marrow transplantation for solid tumors. Oncology 1991;5:25–33.
48. Antman K, Elias A, Fine HA. Dose-intensive therapy with autologous bone marrow transplantation in solid tumors, in Forman SJ, Blume KG, Thomas ED (eds): Bone Marrow Transplantation. Boston, Blackwell, 1994, pp 767–788.
49. Frei E, Antman K, Teicher B, et al. Bone marrow autotransplantation for solid tumors—prospects. J Clin Oncol 1989;7:515–526.
50. Gribben JG, Nadler LM. Monitoring minimal residual disease. Semin Oncol 1993;20:143–155.
51. Negrin RS, Cleary ML. Laboratory evaluation of minimal residual disease, in Forman SJ, Blume KG, Thomas ED (eds): Bone Marrow Transplantation. Boston, Blackwell, 1994, pp 179–188.
52. Gribben JG, Nadler LM. Antibody-mediated purging, in Forman SJ, Blume KG, Thomas ED (eds): Bone Marrow Transplantation. Boston, Blackwell, 1994, pp 149–163.
53. Anderson KC, Nadler LM, Takvorian T, et al. Monoclonal antibodies: Their use in bone marrow transplantation. Prog Hematol 1987;15:137–181.
54. Aihara M, Aihara Y, Schmidt-Wolf G, et al. A combined approach for purging multidrug-resistant leukemic cell lines in bone marrow using a monoclonal antibody and chemotherapy. Blood 1991;77:2079–2084.
55. Rowley SD. Pharmacological purging of malignant cells, in Forman SJ, Blume KG, Thomas ED (eds): Bone Marrow Transplantation. Boston, Blackwell, 1994, pp 164–178.
56. Edgington SM. New horizons for stem-cell bioreactors. Biotechnology 1992;10:1099–1106.
57. Shpall EJ, Jones RB, Bearman SI, et al. Transplantation of enriched CD34-positive autologous marrow into breast cancer patients following high-dose chemotherapy: Influence of CD34-positive peripheral-blood progenitors and growth factors on engraftment. J Clin Oncol 1994;12:28–36.
58. Sullivan KM, Weiden PL, Storb R, et al. Influence of acute and chronic graft-versus-host disease on relapse and survival after bone marrow transplantation from HLA-identical siblings as treatment of acute and chronic leukemia. Blood 1989;73:1720–1728.
59. Horowitz MM, Gale RP, Sondel PM, et al. Graft-versus-leukemia reactions after bone marrow transplantation. Blood 1990;75:555–562.
60. Fefer A. Graft-versus-tumor responses: Adoptive cellular therapy in bone marrow transplantation, in Forman SJ, Blume KG, Thomas ED (eds): Bone Marrow Transplantation. Boston, Blackwell, 1994, pp 231–241.
61. Sullivan KM, Storb R, Buckner CD, et al. Graft-versus-host disease as adoptive immunotherapy in patients with advanced hematologic malignancies. N Engl J Med 1989;320:828–834.
62. Giralt SA, Champlin RE. Leukemia relapse after allogeneic bone marrow transplantation: A review. Blood 1994;84:3603–3612.
63. Porter DL, Roth MS, McGarigle C, et al. Induction of graft-versus-host disease as immunotherapy for relapsed chronic myeloid leukemia. N Engl J Med 1994;330:100–106.
64. Hess AD, Jones RJ, Morris LE, et al. Autologous graft-versus-host disease: A novel approach for antitumor immunotherapy. Hum Immunol 1992;34:219–224.
65. Vogelsang GB, Hess AD. Graft-versus-host disease: New directions for a persistent problem. Blood 1994;84:2061–2067.
66. Yeager AM, Vogelsang GB, Beveridge RA, et al. Induction of cutaneous graft-versus-host disease by administration of cyclosporine to patients undergoing autologous bone marrow transplantation for acute myeloid leukemia. Blood 1992;79:3031–3035.
67. Kennedy MJ, Vogelsang GB, Beveridge RA, et al. Phase I trial of cyclosporine to induce graft-versus-host disease in women undergoing autologous bone marrow transplantation for breast cancer. J Clin Oncol 1993;11:478–484.
68. Fefer A, Benyunes MC, Massumoto C, et al. Interleukin-2 therapy after autologous bone marrow transplantation for hematologic malignancies. Semin Oncol 1993;20(suppl 9):41–45.
69. Bilgrami S, Silva M, Cardoso A, et al. Immunotherapy with autologous bone-marrow transplantation: Rationale and results. Exper Hematol 1994;22:1039–1050.
70. Long GD, Blume KG. Allogeneic bone marrow transplantation for acute myeloid leukemia, in Forman SJ, Blume KG, Thomas ED (eds): Bone Marrow Transplantation. Boston, Blackwell, 1994, pp 607–617.
71. Yeager AM. Autologous bone marrow transplantation for acute myeloid leukemia, in Forman SJ, Blume KG, Thomas ED (eds): Bone Marrow Transplantation. Boston, Blackwell, 1994, pp 709–730.
72. Geller RB. Post-remission therapy of acute myelocytic leukemia in adults: Curability breeds controversy. Leukemia 1992;6:915–925.
73. Zittoun RA, Mandelli F, Willemze R, et al. Autologous or allogeneic bone marrow transplantation compared with intensive chemotherapy in acute myelogenous leukemia. N Engl J Med 1995;332:217–223.
74. Rowley SD, Jones RJ, Piantadosi S, et al. Efficacy of *ex vivo* purging for autologous bone marrow transplantation in the treatment of acute nonlymphoblastic leukemia. Blood 1989;74:501–506
75. Cheson BD. The myelodysplastic syndromes: Current approaches to therapy. Ann Intern Med 1990;112:932–941.
76. Appelbaum FR. Allogeneic bone marrow transplantation for myelodysplastic and myeloproliferative disorders, in Forman SJ, Blume KG, Thomas ED (eds): Bone Marrow Transplantation. Boston, Blackwell, 1994, pp 629–639.
77. Chao NJ, Forman SJ. Allogeneic bone marrow transplantation for acute lymphoblastic leukemia, in Forman SJ, Blume KG, Thomas ED (eds): Bone Marrow Transplantation. Boston, Blackwell, 1994, pp 618–628.
78. Ritz J, Ramsay NK, Kersey JH. Autologous bone marrow transplantation for acute lymphoblastic leukemia, in

Forman SJ, Blume KG, Thomas ED (eds): Bone Marrow Transplantation. Boston, Blackwell, 1994, pp 731–742.

79. Barrett AJ, Horowitz MM, Pollock BH, et al. Bone marrow transplants from HLA-identical siblings as compared with chemotherapy for children with acute lymphoblastic leukemia in a second remission. N Engl J Med 1994;331:1253–1258.
80. Sebban C, Lepage E, Vernant J-P, et al. Allogeneic bone marrow transplantation in adult acute lymphoblastic leukemia in first complete remission: A comparative study. J Clin Oncol 1994;12:2580–2587.
81. Kersey JH, Weisdorf D, Nesbit ME, et al. Comparison of autologous and allogeneic bone marrow transplantation for treatment of high-risk refractory acute lymphoblastic leukemia. N Engl J Med 1987;317:461–467.
82. Fiere D, Lepage E, Sebban C, et al. Adult acute lymphoblastic leukemia: A multicentric randomized trial testing bone marrow transplantation as postremission therapy. J Clin Oncol 1993;11:1990–2001.
83. Champlin R, McGlave P. Allogeneic bone marrow transplantation for chronic myeloid leukemia, in Forman SJ, Blume KG, Thomas ED (eds): Bone Marrow Transplantation. Boston, Blackwell, 1994, pp 595–606.
84. Thomas ED, Clift RA, Fefer A, et al. Marrow transplantation for the treatment of chronic myelogenous leukemia. Ann Intern Med 1986;104:155–163.
85. Beelen DW, Graeven U, Elmaagacli AH, et al. Prolonged administration of interferon-α in patients with chronic-phase Philadelphia chromosome-positive chronic myelogenous leukemia before allogeneic bone marrow transplantation may adversely affect transplant outcome. Blood 1994;85:2981–2990.
86. McGlave PB, Beatty P, Ash R, et al. Therapy for chronic myelogenous leukemia with unrelated donor bone marrow transplantation: Results in 102 cases. Blood 1990;75:1728–1732.
87. Butturini A, Keating A, Goldman J, et al. Autotransplants in chronic myelogenous leukaemia: Strategies and results. Lancet 1990;335:1255–1258.
88. Haioun C, Lepage E, Gisselbrecht C, et al. Comparison of autologous bone marrow transplantation with sequential chemotherapy for intermediate-grade and high-grade non-Hodgkin's lymphoma in first complete remission: A study of 464 patients. J Clin Oncol 1994;12:2543–2551.
89. Armitage JO. Bone marrow transplantation for indolent lymphomas. Semin Oncol 1993;20(suppl 5):136–142.
90. Weisdorf DJ, Haake R, Miller WJ, et al. Autologous bone marrow transplantation for progressive non-Hodgkin's lymphoma: Clinical impact of immunophenotype and in vitro purging. Bone Marrow Transplant 1991;8:135–142.
91. Gribben JG, Freedman AS, Neuberg D, et al. Immunologic purging of marrow assessed by PCR before autologous bone marrow transplantation for B cell lymphoma. N Engl J Med 1991;325:1525–1531.
92. Peters WP. Autologous bone marrow transplantation for breast cancer, in Forman SJ, Blume KG, Thomas ED (eds): Bone Marrow Transplantation. Boston, Blackwell, 1994, pp 789–801.
93. Peters WP, Ross M, Vredenburgh JJ, et al. High-dose chemotherapy and autologous bone marrow support as consolidation after standard-dose adjuvant therapy for high-risk primary breast cancer. J Clin Oncol 1993;11:1132–1143.
94. Peters WP, Rogers MC. Variation in approval by insurance companies of coverage for autologous bone marrow transplantation for breast cancer. N Engl J Med 1994;330:473–477.
95. Hillner BE, Smith TJ, Desch CE. Efficacy and cost-effectiveness of autologous bone marrow transplantation in metastatic breast cancer. J Am Med Assoc 1992;267:2055–2061.
96. Barlogie B, Jagannath S. Autologous bone marrow transplantation for multiple myeloma, in Forman SJ, Blume KG, Thomas ED (eds): Bone Marrow Transplantation. Boston, Blackwell, 1994, pp 754–766.
97. Barlogie B, Jagannath S, Vesole D, Tricot G. Autologous and allogeneic transplants for multiple myeloma. Semin Hematol 1995;32:31–44.
98. Anderson KC. Who benefits from high-dose therapy for multiple myeloma? J Clin Oncol 1995;13:1291–1296.
99. Seeger RC, Reynolds CP. Treatment of high-risk solid tumors of childhood with intensive therapy and autologous bone marrow transplantation. Ped Clin North Am 1991;38:393–424.
100. Clift RA, Bianco JA, Appelbaum FR, et al. A randomized controlled trial of pentoxifylline for the prevention of regimen-related toxicities in patients undergoing allogeneic bone marrow transplantation. Blood 1993;82:2025–2030.
101. Attal M, Huguet F, Rubie H, et al. Prevention of regimen-related toxicities after bone marrow transplantation by pentoxifylline: A prospective, randomized trial. Blood 1993;82:732–736.
102. Shulman HM, Hinterberger W. Hepatic veno-occlusive disease—liver toxicity syndrome after bone marrow transplantation. Bone Marrow Transplant 1992;10:197–214.
103. Bearman SI. The syndrome of hepatic veno-occlusive disease after marrow transplantation. Blood 1995;85:3005–3020.
104. Grochow LB. Busulfan disposition: The role of therapeutic drug monitoring in bone marrow transplantation induction regimens. Semin Oncol 1993;20(suppl 4):18–25.
105. Krowka MJ, Rosenow EC, Hoagland HC. Pulmonary complications of bone marrow transplantation. Chest 1985;87:237–246.
106. Ettinger NA, Trulock EP. Pulmonary considerations of organ transplantation—part 2. Am Rev Resp Dis 1991;144:213–223.
107. Robbins RA, Linder J, Stahl MG, et al. Diffuse alveolar hemorrhage in autologous bone marrow transplant recipients. Am J Med 1989;87:511–518.
108. Chao NJ, Duncan SR, Long GD, et al. Corticosteroid therapy for diffuse alveolar hemorrhage in autologous bone marrow transplant recipients. Ann Intern Med 1991;114:145–146.
109. Martin PJ, Hansen JA, Storb R, et al. Human marrow transplantation: An immunological perspective. Adv Immunol 1987;40:379–438.
110. Quinones RR. Hematopoietic engraftment and graft failure after bone marrow transplantation. Am J Ped Hematol/Oncol 1993;15:3–17.

111. Anasetti C, Amos D, Beatty PG, et al. Effect of HLA compatibility on engraftment of bone marrow transplants in patients with leukemia or lymphoma. N Engl J Med 1989;320:197–204.
112. Agura ED, Vila E, Petersen FB, et al. The use of ranitidine in bone marrow transplantation. Transplantation 1988;46:53–56.
113. Nemunaitis J, Singer JW, Buckner CD, et al. Use of recombinant human granulocyte-macrophage colony-stimulating factor in graft failure after bone marrow transplantation. Blood 1990;76:245–253.
114. Aurer I, Ribas A, Gale RP. What is the role of recombinant colony-stimulating factors in bone marrow transplantation? Bone Marrow Transplant 1990;6:79–87.
115. Mertelsmann R, Herrmann F, Hecht T, et al. Hematopoietic growth factors in bone marrow transplantation. Bone Marrow Transplant 1990;6:73–77.
116. Sheridan WP, Morstyn G, Wolf M, et al. Granulocyte colony-stimulating factor and neutrophil recovery after high-dose chemotherapy and autologous bone marrow transplantation. Lancet 1989;2:891–895.
117. Nemunaitis J, Rabinowe SN, Singer JW, et al. Recombinant granulocyte-macrophage colony-stimulating factor after autologous bone marrow transplantation for lymphoid cancer. N Engl J Med 1991;324:1773–1778.
118. Nemunaitis J, Buckner CD, Appelbaum FR, et al. Phase I/II trial of recombinant human granulocyte-macrophage colony-stimulating factor following allogeneic bone marrow transplantation. Blood 1991;77:2065–2071.
119. Schriber JR, Chao NJ, Long GD, et al. Granulocyte colony-stimulating factor after allogeneic bone marrow transplantation. Blood 1994;84:1680–1684.
120. Klumpp TR, Mangan KF, Goldberg SL, et al. Granulocyte colony-stimulating factor accelerates neutrophil engraftment following peripheral-blood stem-cell transplantation: A prospective, randomized trial. J Clin Oncol 1995;13:1323–1327.
121. Ferrara JLM, Deeg HJ. Graft-versus-host disease. N Engl J Med 1991;324:667–674.
122. Sullivan KM. Graft-versus-host disease, in Forman SJ, Blume KG, Thomas ED (eds): Bone Marrow Transplantation. Boston, Blackwell, 1994, pp 339–362.
123. Pietryga D. Prevention and treatment of acute graft-versus-host disease. Am J Ped Hematol/Oncol 1993;15:28–48.
124. Antin JH, Ferrara JLM. Cytokine dysregulation and acute graft-versus-host disease. Blood 1992;80:2964–2968.
125. Nash RA, Pepe MS, Storb R, et al. Acute graft-versus-host disease: Analysis of risk factors after allogeneic marrow transplantation and prophylaxis with cyclosporine and methotrexate. Blood 1992;80:1838–1845.
126. Kernan NA. T-cell depletion for prevention of graft-versus-host disease, in Forman SJ, Blume KG, Thomas ED (eds): Bone Marrow Transplantation. Boston, Blackwell, 1994, pp 124–135.
127. Storb R, Deeg HJ, Whitehead J, et al. Methotrexate and cyclosporine compared with cyclosporine alone for prophylaxis of acute graft-versus-host disease after marrow transplantation for leukemia. N Engl J Med 1986;314:729–735.
128. Santos GW, Tutschka PJ, Brookmeyer R, et al. Cyclosporine plus methylprednisolone versus cyclophosphamide plus methylprednisolone as prophylaxis for graft-versus-host disease: A randomized double-blind study in patients undergoing allogeneic marrow transplantation. Clin Transplant 1987;1:21–28.
129. Forman SJ, Blume KG, Krance RA, et al. A prospective randomized study of acute graft-versus-host disease in 107 patients with leukemia: Methotrexate/prednisone versus cyclosporine A/prednisone. Transplant Proc 1987;19:2605.
130. Storb R, Pepe M, Anasetti C, et al. What role for prednisone in prevention of acute graft-versus-host disease in patients undergoing marrow transplants? Blood 1990;76:1037–1345.
131. Sayer HG, Longton G, Bowden R, et al. Increased risk of infection in marrow transplant patients receiving methylprednisolone for graft-versus-host disease prevention. Blood 1994;84:1328–1332.
132. Chao NJ, Schmidt GM, Niland JC, et al. Cyclosporine, methotrexate, and prednisone compared with cyclosporine and prednisone alone for prophylaxis of acute graft-versus-host disease. N Engl J Med 1993;329:1225–1230.
133. Nash RA, Etzioni R, Storb R, et al. Tacrolimus (FK506) alone or in combination with methotrexate or methylprednisolone for the prevention of acute graft-versus-host disease after marrow transplantation from HLA-matched siblings: A single-center study. Blood 1995;85:3746–3753.
134. Blaise D, Olive D, Michallet M, et al. Impairment of leukaemia-free survival by addition of interleukin-2 antibody to standard graft-versus-host prophylaxis. Lancet 1995;345:1144–1146.
135. Sullivan KM, Kopecky KJ, Jocom J, et al. Immunomodulatory and antimicrobial efficacy of intravenous immunoglobulin in bone marrow transplantation. N Engl J Med 1990;323:705–712.
136. Drobyski WR, Ash RC, Casper JT, et al. Effect of T-cell depletion as graft-versus-host disease prophylaxis on engraftment, relapse, and disease-free survival in unrelated marrow transplantation for chronic myelogenous leukemia. Blood 1994;83:1980–1987.
137. Hings IM, Filipovich AH, Miller WJ, et al. Prednisone therapy for acute graft-versus-host disease: Short- versus long-term treatment. Transplantation 1993;56:577–580.
138. Martin PJ, Schoch G, Fisher L, et al. A retrospective analysis of therapy for acute graft-versus-host disease: Initial treatment. Blood 1990;76:1464–1472.
139. Weisdorf D, Haake R, Blazar B, et al. Treatment of moderate/severe acute graft-versus-host disease after allogeneic bone marrow transplantation: An analysis of clinical risk features and outcome. Blood 1990;75:1024–1030.
140. Bianco JA, Higano C, Singer J, et al. The somatostatin analog octreotide in the management of the secretory diarrhea of the acute intestinal graft-versus-host disease in a patient after bone marrow transplantation. Transplantation 1990;49:1194–1195.
141. Martin PJ, Schoch G, Fisher L, et al. A retrospective analysis of therapy for acute graft-versus-host disease: Secondary treatment. Blood 1991;77:1821–1828.
142. Byers VS, Henslee PJ, Kernan NA, et al. Use of an anti-pan T lymphocyte ricin A chain immunotoxin in steroid-resistant acute graft-versus-host disease. Blood 1990;75:14256.

143. Anasetti C, Hansen JA, Waldmann TA, et al. Treatment of acute graft-versus-host disease with humanized anti-Tac: An antibody that binds to the interleukin-2 receptor. Blood 1994;84:1320–1327.
144. Herve P, Flesch M, Tiberghien P, et al. Phase I–II trial of a monoclonal anti-tumor necrosis factor α antibody for the treatment of refractory severe acute graft-versus-host disease. Blood 1992;79:3362–3368.
145. Antin JH, Weinstein HJ, Guinan EC, et al. Recombinant human interleukin-1 receptor antagonist in the treatment of steroid-resistant graft-versus-host disease. Blood 1994;84:1342–1348.
146. Sullivan KM, Agura E, Anasetti C, et al. Chronic graft-versus-host disease and other late complications of bone marrow transplantation. Semin Hematol 1991;28:250–259.
147. Sullivan KM, Witherspoon RP, Storb R, et al. Prednisone and azathioprine compared with prednisone and placebo for treatment of chronic graft-versus-host disease: Prognostic influence of prolonged thrombocytopenia after allogeneic marrow transplantation. Blood 1988;72:546–554.
148. Sullivan KM, Witherspoon RP, Storb R, et al. Alternating-day cyclosporine and prednisone for treatment of high-risk chronic graft-versus-host disease. Blood 1988;72:555–561.
149. Vogelsang GB, Farmer ER, Hess AD, et al. Thalidomide for the treatment of chronic graft-versus-host disease. N Engl J Med 1992;326:1055–1058.
150. Deeg HJ. Delayed complications and long-term effects after bone marrow transplantation, in Forman SJ, Blume KG, Thomas ED (eds): Bone Marrow Transplantation. Boston, Blackwell, 1994, pp 538–544.

PART FIVE

Nutrition and Nutritional Disorders

Chapter 130

Assessment of Nutrition Status and Nutrition Requirements

Kathleen M. Teasley-Strausburg, MS, RPh, BCNSP, and Jan D. Anderson, PharmD, BCNSP

The assessment of a patient's nutrition status initially involves the identification of the presence of risk factors for malnutrition. If the patient is at risk for malnutrition, a more comprehensive nutrition assessment is performed to identify the type and extent of malnutrition. This comprehensive evaluation includes a medical and dietary history, physical examination, anthropometric measurements, and laboratory data,[1] and provides a basis for determining the patient's nutrition requirements, the optimal type of nutrition intervention, and when nutrition therapy should be initiated. Nutrition requirements will be dependent on the need for chronic maintenance versus acute repletion of nutrition status as well as the effect of organ function (e.g., renal function) on nutrient utilization. Nutrition assessment requires clinical skills, knowledge of objective measurements that reflect nutrition status, and the ability to apply general guidelines for nutrition requirements with a consideration for patient-specific factors.

This chapter is a critical review of the current markers used for nutrition screening and assessment. It is also provides guidelines for developing a scheme for accurate, relevant, and cost-effective nutrition assessment including the determination of patient-specific nutritional requirements.

Classification of Nutrition Diseases

Malnutrition, or more specifically undernutrition, is usually the result of starvation (inadequate nutrition intake) or altered metabolism (inappropriate utilization of ingested nutrients). In starvation states the problem is one of not getting adequate amounts of appropriate nutrients to the cells for tissue repair or new tissue synthesis. An alteration in metabolism exists when the cell has altered substrate demands or utilization characteristics. A clinically useful definition of malnutrition, therefore, is a state induced by alterations in dietary intake or nutrient utilization resulting in changes in subcellular, cellular, and/or organ function that expose the individual to increased risks of morbidity and mortality and that can be reversed by appropriate nutrition support.[2] In general, deficiency states can be categorized as those involving protein and calories [protein-calorie malnutrition (PCM)] or those resulting from single nutrients such as individual vitamins or trace minerals. The three types of PCM are marasmus, kwashiorkor, and mixed marasmus–kwashiorkor (Table 130.1)[3,4]:

1. *Marasmus* is a chronic condition resulting from a deficiency in total energy intake. Consequently, the individual's reserves of protein and energy are depleted. There is wasting of both somatic protein (skeletal muscle) and adipose stores, but visceral protein production (e.g., serum albumin and transferrin concentration) is preserved. When severe, cell-mediated immunity (measured by delayed cutaneous hypersensitivity) and muscle function are impaired. Patients with wasting diseases such as cancer commonly have marasmus and a starved, cachectic appearance. The relative weight loss threshold for marasmus is 85% of ideal body weight.
2. *Kwashiorkor* is common in patients who have adequate calorie intake but a relative protein deficiency. These patients are often catabolic, usually secondary to trauma, infection, or burns. There is depletion of visceral (and to some degree somatic) protein pools with relative preservation of adipose tissue. Kwashiorkor is classically characterized by hypoalbuminemia and edema. This condition may develop rapidly in response to protein deprivation in the setting of metabolic stress and may be accompanied by impaired immune function.

TABLE 130.1. INDICATORS OF PROTEIN AND ENERGY MALNUTRITION (PEM)

Condition	Primary Deficit	Indicators				
		Body Weight	Body Fat	Somatic Protein	Visceral Protein	Immune Function
Marasmus	Energy	↓	↓	↓	slightly ↓ or WNL	↓
Kwashiorkor	Protein	↓	WNL	WNL	↓	↓
Mixed marasmus–kwashiorkor	Protein and energy	↓	↓	↓	↓	↓

Key: ↓, decreased; WNL, within normal limits. (Reprinted with the permission of Simon & Schuster, Inc., from the Macmillan College text CLINICAL NUTRITION AND DIETETICS 2/E by Frances J. Zeman. Copyright © 1991 by Macmillan College Publishing Company, Inc.)

3. *Mixed marasmus–kwashiorkor* is a form of severe PCM in chronically ill, starved patients who are undergoing hypermetabolic stress. It manifests as reduced visceral protein synthesis superimposed on wasting of somatic protein and energy (adipose tissue) stores. Immunocompetence is lowered, the incidence of infection is increased, and there is poor wound healing.

Single-nutrient deficiencies can and often do occur in combination with any of the preceding diagnoses. Depletion of individual nutrients leads to symptoms related to that nutrient's function. Therefore, all potential nutritional deficiency states should be evaluated before an acute or chronic repletion plan is developed.

Nutrition Screening

Nutrition screening provides a systematic way of identifying an individual at risk for PCM. Risk factors for malnutrition include any disease state, complicating condition, treatment and socioeconomic condition that result in a decreased nutrient intake, altered metabolism, and/or malabsorption.[5,6] Nutrition screening can be done in the home by home health care professionals, in long-term care facilities, or in the hospital. Various rating and classification systems have been proposed to assess nutritional risk and guide subsequent interventions.[5–7] Checklists are often utilized to characterize a person's food and alcohol consumption habits, physical capability of buying and preparing food, and weight history. Depending on the specific criteria evaluated, three to four risk factors may put a person at risk for malnutrition.[8]

Nutrition screening in the hospital utilizes clinical and laboratory parameters obtained from the patient's medical record.[7,8] Diagnosis and treatment plans can also be factored in to categorize and determine nutrition risk. Even in stable patients in the hospital setting, nutrition status should be reevaluated every 7–14 days to avoid deterioration secondary to changes in food intake during their hospitalization. By identifying individuals at risk for malnutrition, nutrition screening can be a cost-effective way to help decrease complications and length of hospital stay.[9]

Nutrition Assessment

Nutrition assessment is "a comprehensive evaluation to define nutrition status, including medical history, dietary history, physical examination, anthropometric measurements and laboratory data."[1]

CLINICAL EVALUATION

Clinical evaluation with a medical and dietary history and a physical examination remains the oldest, simplest, and probably most widely used method of evaluating nutrition status. Clinical evaluation of nutrition status has been well correlated with objective evaluations (e.g., laboratory parameters, anthropometric measurements).[10] When clinical evaluation is used as the sole method for identifying nutrition-related disease it is referred to as subjective global assessment (SGA).[10] Laboratory parameters, however, provide additional objective data to confirm the diagnosis, quantify the degree of malnutrition, and identify the end-organ changes that occur with malnutrition. These objective parameters also provide a baseline from which to evaluate the response to nutrition therapy.

The medical and dietary history components of the clinical evaluation provide information about factors that predispose the patient to developing malnutrition (e.g., chronic diseases, gastrointestinal malfunction, alcohol abuse). The clinician should focus the evaluation to elicit any history of weight loss, anorexia, vomiting, diarrhea, and decreased or unusual food intake (Table 130.2). The physical examination focuses on an assessment of lean body mass and the physical findings of vitamin, trace mineral, and essential fatty acid deficiency. The assessment should characterize the presence and degree of muscle wasting, edema, loss of subcutaneous fat, dermatitis, glossitis, cheilosis, and/or jaundice (Table 130.3).

ANTHROPOMETRIC MEASUREMENTS

Anthropometric measurements are gross measurements of body cell mass. The most common measurements are

TABLE 130.2. PERTINENT DATA FROM MEDICAL AND DIETARY HISTORY FOR NUTRITION ASSESSMENT

Nutrition Intake and Dietary Habits
- Anorexia; changes in taste
- Actual intake; special diets
- Supplemental vitamin or mineral intake
- Food allergies or intolerance

Underlying Pathology with Nutritional Effects
- Chronic infections or inflammatory states
- Neoplastic diseases
- Endocrine disorders
- Chronic illnesses including pulmonary disease, cirrhosis, renal failure
- Hypermetabolic states: trauma, burns, sepsis
- Digestive or absorptive diseases
- Hyperlipidemia

End-Organ Effects
- Weight changes
- Skin or hair changes
- Exercise tolerance, fatigue
- Obesity
- Gastrointestinal tract symptoms: diarrhea, vomiting, constipation

Miscellaneous
- Catabolic medications or therapies: steroids, immunosuppressive agents, radiation, or chemotherapy
- Other medications: diuretics, laxatives
- Genetic background: body habitus of parents, siblings, and family
- Alcohol or drug abuse

TABLE 130.3. PHYSICAL FINDINGS SUGGESTIVE OF MALNUTRITION

General Appearance
- Edema
- Cachexia or obesity
- Ascites
- Signs and symptoms of dehydration: skin turgor, sunken eyes, orthostasis, dry mucous membranes

Skin and Mucous Membranes
- Thin, shiny, or scaling skin
- Decubitus ulcers
- Ecchymoses, perifollicular petechiae
- Poorly healing surgical or traumatic wounds
- Pallor or redness of gums, fissures at mouth edge
- Glossitis; stomatitis; cheilosis

Musculoskeletal
- Retarded growth
- Bone pain or tenderness, epiphyseal swelling
- Muscle mass less than expected for habitus, genetic history, and level of exercise

Neurologic
- Ataxia, positive Romberg test, decreased vibratory or position sense
- Nystagmus
- Convulsions, paralysis
- Encephalopathy

Hepatic
- Jaundice
- Hepatomegaly

height, weight, and measurements of limb size, such as midarm muscle circumference, skinfold thickness, and wrist circumference. These parameters are used in two ways—to compare an individual with a population and as repeated measurements in an individual to indicate the response to changes in their nutritional environment. Nutrition-related changes in anthropometric measurements occur slowly; several weeks are often required before detectable changes are noted. Acute changes in anthropometric measurements, specifically weight and skinfold thickness, usually reflect changes in fluid status, and fluid must be considered in the interpretation of these parameters.

Body weight is a nonspecific measure of body cell mass, representing skeletal mass, body fat, and the energy-utilizing component referred to as "lean body mass."[11] Changes in weight over time, particularly in the absence of edema, ascites, and voluntary losses, are an important indicator of altered lean body mass. Interpretation of any actual body weight (ABW) measurement should take into consideration ideal weight for height, usual body weight, fluid status, and age.

The ideal body weight for height (IBW) provides a population reference standard against which the ABW can be compared. The ideal weight for a given height is that weight correlating with maximum longevity. Numerous reference tables have been generated based on various population statistics.[12–14] The most commonly accepted table of ideal weight for height was derived from Metropolitan Life Insurance data.[15,16] Desirable weight tables were published in 1959 and revised in 1983. The revised table reflects an increase in the average weight associated with the lowest mortality rate (Table 130.4).[16]

The degree of change in weight over time can be calculated as the percentage of IBW or usual body weight (UBW) where % change = (ABW/IBW) × 100 or (ABW/UBW) × 100. Use of the patient's UBW as a reference point provides a more accurate reflection of clinically and nutritionally significant change in weight. Determining a patient's UBW, however, depends on patient recall, which may be inaccurate.[17] The use of UBW avoids the problems of normative tables, and it documents comparative changes in body weight. The degree of change in weight must be interpreted relative to time (Table 130.5). An absolute unintentional weight loss of more than 10 pounds in less than 6 months has been correlated with an increased incidence of mortality in adult surgical patients.[18]

Body Mass Index

Body mass index (BMI), defined as body weight in kilograms/height in meters squared, is another way to compare weight to height. BMI has been used to categorize obesity

TABLE 130.4. IDEAL WEIGHT FOR HEIGHT

Female		Male	
Height (cm)	**Weight (kg)**	**Height (cm)**	**Weight (kg)**
147.3	55.0	157.5	64.1
149.9	55.9	160.0	65.0
152.4	57.3	162.6	65.9
154.9	58.6	165.1	67.3
157.5	60.0	167.6	68.6
160.0	61.4	170.2	70.0
162.6	62.7	172.7	71.4
165.1	64.1	175.3	72.7
167.6	65.5	177.8	74.1
170.2	66.8	180.3	75.4
172.7	68.2	182.9	77.3
175.3	69.5	185.4	79.1
177.8	70.9	188.0	80.9
180.3	72.3	190.5	82.7
182.9	73.6	193.0	85.0

Note: This table represents Metropolitan Life Insurance's 1983 data for medium frame; men wearing clothing weighing 2.3 kg, shoes with 2.54-cm heels; women wearing clothing weighing 1.4 kg, shoes with 2.54-cm heels. (From Metropolitan Life Insurance Company. Statistical Bulletin, New Weights and Standards for Men and Women. Chicago, Metropolitan Life, 1983, vol 64, pp 2–9, with permission.)

and malnutrition. BMI values within a range of 18.5–25 have been associated with the least risk of early death, whereas values greater than 25 are associated with obesity and values less than 18.5 are indicative of malnutrition.[19] It has been observed that BMI increases with age and that the ideal BMI for a 65 year old is approximately 27.[20] This index is not a reflection of body composition, as demonstrated in the situation of a very muscular person who has a high BMI but a low percentage of total body fat. In this setting, the person may be falsely categorized as obese based solely on BMI.

Interpretation of a body weight measurement also is dependent on knowledge of the patient's hydrational status. Dehydration from nausea, vomiting, or other fluid losses results in a decreased body weight but not a loss in body cell mass. The presence of edema or ascites indicates excess total body water, which will increase body weight. More subtle changes in fluid status may be detected by monitoring the patient's daily fluid intake and output and should be evaluated coincident with weight changes.

TABLE 130.5. WEIGHT CHANGES REFLECTING SIGNIFICANT LOSS OF BODY MASS

Time	Significant Weight Loss (%)	Severe Weight Loss (%)
1 wk	1–2	>2
1 mo	5	>5
3 mo	7.5	>7.5
6 mo	10	>10

(From Blackburn GL, Bistrian BR, Maini BS, et al. Nutritional and metabolic assessment of the hospitalized patient. J Parenter Enter Nutr 1977;1:17, with permission.)

Skinfold thickness measurement provides an estimate of subcutaneous fat. More than half of the total body fat is subcutaneous, and changes in subcutaneous fat have been assumed to reflect changes in body fat.[21] The measurement of skinfold thickness is relatively insensitive to short-term changes in tissue composition, but serial measurements in a given patient performed by the same trained observer on the same body side are reproducible.[22] Triceps skinfold thickness (TSF) is the most common site of measurement, although reference standards also exist for subscapular and iliac sites. Careful technique and the use of pressure-regulated calipers (Lange, Halipern) are essential for reproducibility and reliability in measuring TSF.[23] The value measured is compared with population standards.[14] Values between the 35th and 40th percentiles indicate mild depletion, between the 25th and 35th percentiles, moderate depletion, and below the 25th percentile, severe depletion.[24] Interpretation of results must include consideration of differences in body build, particularly extremes such as obesity or muscle hypertrophy associated with weight training. Body fat measurements do not necessarily correlate with muscle mass and body protein status.

Midarm-Muscle Circumference

Midarm-muscle circumference (MAMC) is a noninvasive, easy, inexpensive method of assessing skeletal muscle mass. MAMC is calculated as follows, where MAC is midarm circumference.[25]

$$\text{MAMC (cm)} = \text{MAC (cm)} - \pi\text{TSF (mm)}/10$$

This calculation assumes the muscle compartment is round, that TSF is accurate and consistent about the circumference, and that the bone is of constant cross-sectional area. The calculated value for MAMC is compared with population standards.[14] A decrease from the expected value at the 20th percentile suggests a significant reduction in somatic protein mass.[24]

Anthropometric measurements are safe, simple, and easy tests for both population analysis and individual long-term monitoring. However, the results of individual anthropometric measurements should be cautiously interpreted because (1) standards do not account for individual variations in bone size, hydrational status, or skin compressibility; (2) reference standards do not account for obesity, ethnicity, and increased age; (3) technique is critical and interobserver error may be as high as 30%; and (4) these parameters are slow to change, often requiring weeks before significant alterations from baseline can be observed.

BIOCHEMICAL PARAMETERS OF LEAN BODY MASS

Lean body mass is representative of both structural proteins (skeletal muscle, somatic protein compartment) and functional proteins (circulating proteins, visceral protein compartment). It can be assessed by creatinine-height index and serum visceral protein concentrations in addition to body weight and MAMC measurements.

Creatinine-Height Index

Creatinine-height index (CHI) is based on creatinine, which is the metabolic end product of creatine, a complex molecule synthesized in the liver and concentrated mainly in body muscle. Creatinine is excreted unchanged in the urine; therefore, collection of a timed urine with measurement of total creatinine excreted indirectly reflects the total muscle mass.[26] For clinical assessment, the creatinine production of an individual patient (obtained by the measurement of creatinine in 24-hour urine collection) is compared with the expected excretion by a healthy individual of similar height and ideal weight. Expected creatinine excretion is derived from the product of the mean creatinine excretion in healthy young men (23 mg/kg/d) and women (18 mg/kg/d), and the ideal weight for height (Table 130.6).[27] The CHI is the percentage the actual 24-hour creatinine represents of the expected value:

$$\text{CHI} = \frac{\text{Actual 24-hour creatinine excretion}}{\text{Ideal 24-hour creatinine excretion}} \times 100\%$$

A CHI of 80% or greater indicates no or mild somatic muscle depletion, a CHI of 60–80% indicates moderate depletion, and a CHI of less than 60% represents severe depletion.[28] The CHI does not accurately reflect muscle mass in patients with impaired renal function or dehydration, and may be affected by a high dietary protein intake, steroids, age, or stress. It also is dependent on the accuracy of the 24-hour urine collection and the appropriateness of the ideal weight for height standards.

The visceral protein compartment is assessed by measuring the concentration of serum transport proteins synthesized in the liver. It is assumed that a low serum protein concentration in states of malnutrition reflects the hepatic protein synthetic mass[29] and, therefore, indirectly the functional protein mass of other organs such as heart, lung, kidney, and intestines. The visceral proteins currently thought to be of greatest relevance for nutritional assessment are serum albumin, transferrin, retinol-binding protein, and thyroxine-binding prealbumin (transthyretin).[30–33] Many factors besides nutrition affect the serum concentration of these proteins, such as abnormal losses via the kidney (e.g., nephrotic syndrome) or gastrointestinal (GI) tract (e.g., protein-losing enteropathy), hydration status (e.g., dehydration may result in hemoconcentration, overhydration in hemodilution), and renal and hepatic function and metabolic stress (e.g., sepsis, trauma, surgery, and/or infection). Therefore, visceral protein data must be interpreted relative to the clinical status of the individual (Table 130.7).[34–36]

TABLE 130.6. IDEAL 24-HOUR URINARY CREATININE EXCRETION BY ADULTS OF VARIOUS HEIGHTS (FOR USE IN CALCULATION OF THE CREATININE-HEIGHT INDEX)

Height		Ideal Creatinine Excretion (mg)	
(in.)	(cm)	Adult Women[a]	Adult Men[b]
58	147.3	830	—
59	149.9	851	—
60	152.4	875	—
61	154.9	900	—
62	157.5	925	1288
63	160	949	1325
64	162.6	977	1359
65	165.1	1006	1386
66	167.6	1044	1426
67	170.2	1076	1467
68	172.7	1109	1513
69	175.3	1141	1555
70	177.8	1174	1596
71	180.3	1206	1642
72	182.9	1240	1691
73	185.4	—	1739
74	188	—	1785
75	190.5	—	1831
76	193	—	1891

[a]Creatinine coefficient (women) = 18 mg/kg of ideal body weight.
[b]Creatinine coefficient (men) = 23 mg/kg of ideal body weight. (From Blackburn GL, Bistrian RB, Maini BS, et al. Nutritional and metabolic assessment of the hospitalized patient. J Parenter Enter Nutr 1977;1:15, with permission.)

Albumin

Albumin was one of the first biochemical markers of malnutrition and has long been used in population studies. Because of a large body pool size (4–5 g/kg body weight), a high extravascular distribution (60%), and a long biologic half-life (18–20 days), albumin is a relatively insensitive index of early protein malnutrition. However, chronic protein deficiency in the setting of adequate nonprotein caloric intake leads to marked hypoalbuminemia because of a net loss of albumin from the intravascular and extravascular pools (kwashiorkor malnutrition). Serum albumin concentrations also are affected by zinc deficiency, caloric deficiency, hepatic disease, renal disease, and infection. Although interpretation of serum albumin concentrations is difficult, data consistently indicate a positive correlation between depressed albumin levels and poor clinical outcome.[37–41]

TABLE 130.7. SUMMARY OF VISCERAL PROTEINS USED FOR ASSESSMENT OF LEAN BODY MASS

Serum Protein	Biosynthetic Site	Normal Value (range)[a]	Half-life (days)	Function	Factors Resulting in Increased Values[b]	Factors Resulting in Decreased Values[b]
Albumin	Hepatocyte	3.5–5.0 g/dL	18–20	Maintain plasma oncotic pressure; carrier for small molecules	Dehydration, anabolic steroids, insulin, infection	Overhydration, edema, renal insufficiency, nephrotic syndrome, poor intake, impaired digestion, burns, congestive heart failure, cirrhosis, thyroid/adrenal/pituitary hormones, trauma, sepsis
Fibronectin	Hepatocyte, fibroblasts, endothelial cells	210–300 μg/mL	0.5–1.0	A glycoprotein which in blood has opsonic activity; may exert chemotactic activity and facilitate wound healing	None currently described	Trauma, shock, burns, sepsis, disseminated intravascular coagulation; inappropriate specimen handling
Prealbumin (Transthyretin)	Hepatocyte	10–40 mg/dL	1–2	Binds T_3 and to a lesser extent T_4; carrier for RBP	Renal dysfunction	Cirrhosis, hepatitis, stress, inflammation, surgery, hyperthyroidism, cystic fibrosis, renal dysfunction
Retinol-binding protein (RBP)	Hepatocyte	2.0–6.0 mg/dL	0.5	Transports vitamin A in plasma; binds noncovalently to prealbumin	Renal dysfunction, vitamin A supplementation	Same as prealbumin; also vitamin A deficiency
Somatomedin C (IGF-1)	Hepatocyte	0.4–2.0 IU/mL	0.1–0.3	An insulin-like peptide that has anabolic actions on fat, muscle, cartilage and cultured cells	None currently described	Growth hormone deficiency; psychosocial growth failure; hypothyroidism; renal failure; cirrhosis; drugs (estrogens, prednisolone)
Transferrin	Hepatocyte	200–400 mg/dL	8	Binds Fe in plasma and transports to bone	Iron deficiency, pregnancy, hypoxia, chronic blood loss, estrogens	Chronic infection, cirrhosis, enteropathies, nephrotic syndrome, burns, cortisone, testosterone

[a]Normal values represent pooled subjects; ranges vary between centers; check local values.
[b]All of the listed proteins are influenced by hydration and the presence of hepatocellular dysfunction. (From Refs. 24, 33–35.)

Transferrin

Transferrin is the glycoprotein that binds and transports ferric iron. It is more likely to respond to protein depletion before alterations in albumin are manifest because of its shorter biologic half-life (8 days) and smaller body pool (less than 100 mg/kg body weight).[42] Transferrin concentrations may be determined by direct measurement or can be estimated indirectly from measurement of total iron-binding capacity (TIBC). Several formulas for the estimation of transferrin from TIBC have been proposed. For example,[28]

$$\text{Serum transferrin} = (0.8 \times \text{TIBC}) - 43$$

It is recommended, whenever possible, that each laboratory establish a formula relating the measurement of TIBC to the results of immunodiffusion radioassay for transferrin.[28,43] The serum transferrin concentration is affected by the same factors affecting serum albumin and by iron stores. In iron deficiency, transferrin concentrations are elevated.[44]

Thyroxine-Binding Prealbumin

Thyroxine-binding prealbumin (TBPA) is also referred to as prealbumin or transthyretin. It is the transport protein for thyroxine and a carrier protein for retinol-binding protein. It has a short biologic half-life (1–2 days) and a small body pool size (10 mg/kg body weight). TBPA may be reduced in as few as 3 days after calorie and protein intake is decreased.[42,45,46] Because of its short half-life, it is useful in monitoring the short-term effects of nutrition support.[47] However, TBPA concentrations also rapidly decline in acute stress, such as trauma or sepsis, in which there is increased protein catabolism. As with albumin and transferrin, TBPA concentrations are depressed with liver disease because of decreased hepatic synthesis. Increased TBPA concentrations have been noted in patients with renal disease and are thought to result from impaired degradation of TBPA by the kidney.[48]

Retinol-Binding Protein

Retinol-binding protein (RBP) is a specific protein for vitamin A alcohol (retinol) transport. It is filtered by the glomeruli and is metabolized by the kidney. RBP has a very short biologic half-life (12 hours) and a small body pool size (2 mg/kg body weight). As a nutrition assessment parameter it has the same limitations as TBPA, i.e., its levels are dependent on the degree of stress, hepatic, and renal function. Vitamin A deficiency results in depressed RBP concentrations, whereas vitamin A supplementation may result in elevated amounts in the serum.[49]

These four serum proteins (albumin, transferrin, TBPA, and RBP) are of greatest value in assessing uncomplicated semistarvation and recovery. In the setting of acute stress (e.g., trauma, burn injury, sepsis), these proteins become poor markers of nutrition status. Their synthesis is down-regulated as the liver reprioritizes hepatic protein synthesis in response to systemic injury. In this setting, the liver produces acute phase reactants (APR), which are proteins such as C-reactive protein, α_1-acid glycoprotein, and α_1-antitrypsin.[50,51] Other serum proteins, such as fibronectin (an opsonic protein)[36,52] and somatomedin-C (insulin-like growth factor-1, IGF-1),[36,53,54] have been suggested as indicators of nutritional status. However, the clinical availability of tests that measure these proteins is limited, and their relevance to nutrition status and the outcome of hospitalization has not been determined.

Plasma amino acid concentrations also have been used to assess lean body mass. Altered amino acid patterns have been identified in the setting of PCM and are characterized by a slight decrease in essential amino acid concentrations and an increase or no change in the nonessential amino acid concentrations.[12,55–57] Consequently, the ratio of essential to nonessential amino acid concentrations decreases and has been used to characterize PCM. However, unless the nutritional depletion is severe, plasma amino acid concentrations are maintained fairly constant by the body's homeostatic mechanisms. The depletion state is clinically apparent before changes in amino acid concentrations become significant. Furthermore, plasma amino acid concentrations are altered in various disease states such as hepatic failure, renal failure, and sepsis. In addition to the lack of sensitivity and specificity, the measurement of plasma amino acid concentrations is not widely available and is expensive. Therefore, plasma amino acid concentrations are of limited usefulness in the assessment of lean body mass.

INDICES OF IMMUNE FUNCTION

The frequency with which immunocompetence is impaired and the high incidence of infection in malnutrition led to the suggestion that tests of immune function be used as markers of nutrition status[58,59] and as predictors of outcome.[60] The manner in which nutrition factors interact with immune status may be either direct, affecting primarily the lymphoid system; or indirect, affecting cellular metabolism or another organ system that is in turn involved with the regulation of immunocompetence.

The tests of immune function most frequently used in nutrition assessment are total lymphocyte count (TLC) and delayed cutaneous hypersensitivity (DCH) reactions. Both are simple, readily available, and inexpensive tests. TLC reflects the number of circulating lymphocytes, most of which are T cells. Tissues generating T cells are very sensitive to malnutrition and undergo involution with a decrease in the production of T cells.[61] This eventually leads to lymphopenia. The circulating lymphocyte count can be calculated from the peripheral white blood cell (WBC) count and differential:

$$\text{Total lymphocyte count (cells/mm}^3) = \text{WBC (cells/mm}^3) \times \frac{\%\text{lymphocyte}}{100}$$

A TLC of 1200–2000/mm³ correlates with mild malnutrition, 800–1200/mm³ with moderate malnutrition, and <800/mm³ with severe malnutrition.[24]

DCH reactions represent an *in vivo* test of cell-mediated immunity. DCH may be assessed as a primary response to a mitogen such as phytohemagglutinin (PHA) or a chemical irritant such as dinitrochlorobenzene (DCNB). However, DCNB is no longer recommended because it leaves a scar in those with normal immunity. DCH is more commonly assessed as a secondary response using antigens to which the patient has been previously sensitized. The recall antigens used in nutrition assessment are mumps, *Candida albicans,* streptokinase–streptodornase (SKSD), *Trichophyton,* coccidioidin, and purified protein derivative (PPD). Usually a battery of three to five antigens is applied. The inflammatory reaction, marked by dermal erythema and induration, is evaluated at 24 and 48 hours. A positive response is defined as induration at the site of antigen injection of at least 5 mm at 24–48 hours.[24] Interpretation of the degree of anergy or failure of DCH response varies somewhat with different investigators.[62,63] If three of five tests are nonresponsive, the individual is generally considered anergic. Numerous studies have correlated anergy with malnutrition in hospitalized patients,[64–66] and with aggressive nutrition support a positive DCH response has been restored.[65,67]

TABLE 130.8. NON-NUTRITIONAL FACTORS AFFECTING TESTS OF IMMUNE FUNCTION

Category	Specific Factor
Patient factors	Age, race, geographic location, circadian rhythm, psychological state
Immune system diseases	Congenital (DiGeorge's syndrome, thymic aplasia); acquired (systemic lupus erythematosus, rheumatoid arthritis)
Other nonmalignant diseases	Infectious (viral [HIV], bacterial, fungal); metabolic (renal failure, liver failure); inflammatory (Crohn's disease, ulcerative colitis)
Malignancies	Most solid tumors (especially advanced stages), lymphomas, leukemias
Iatrogenic and other causes	Radiation, general anesthesia, surgery; trauma, burns, hemorrhage; medications (e.g., corticosteroids, many chemotherapeutic agents)

Both TLC and DCH may be affected by non-nutrition factors and, therefore, at best are nonspecific indicators of malnutrition (Table 130.8). Non-nutrition factors that affect TLC include infection, immunosuppressant drugs, steroids, and the presence of neoplasia. Factors that affect DCH include fever, critical illness, drugs (e.g., immunosuppressive agents such as corticosteroids, cyclosporine), and surgery. While this lack of specificity currently limits the usefulness of these and other tests of immune function as markers of nutrition status and predictors of outcome, there may be a future role for these tests when a nutrition regimen includes nutritional immunotherapy.[68] Nutrients such as arginine, omega-3 fatty acids, and nucleic acids given in pharmacologic doses have been shown to improve immune function in a variety of settings.[69–73] Monitoring the efficacy of nutrition regimens that include these immunomodulating nutrients may need to include tests of immune function.

SPECIFIC NUTRIENT DEFICIENCIES

The assessment of nutrition status should include an evaluation of possible trace mineral, vitamin, and essential fatty acid deficiencies. Because of their key role in metabolic processes (e.g., as coenzymes and cofactors), the deficiency of any single nutrient may result in altered metabolism and cell dysfunction and may interfere with processes necessary for repletion of PCM. The assessment of single-nutrient-deficiency states includes an accurate history to evaluate symptoms and the existence of factors predisposing the patient to developing a deficiency state, a physical examination for signs of deficiencies, and biochemical assessment to confirm the diagnosis. Ideally, biochemical assessment should be based on the function of the nutrient, e.g., metalloenzyme activity, rather than simply measuring the concentration present in the assay sample. Unfortunately, few practical methods to assess micronutrient function are currently available, and most assays measure tissue or fluid concentration of a nutrient.

TRACE MINERALS

The trace minerals identified as essential to humans and for which deficiency states have been described are zinc, copper, manganese, selenium, chromium, iodine, molybdenum, and iron. Each of these minerals participates in a variety of biologic functions and is necessary for normal metabolism (see Chapter 132). The absorption, distribution, and excretion characteristics of these trace minerals are summarized in Table 130.9.[74] Other trace minerals essential to humans but for which deficiency states have not been recognized include nickel, vanadium, cobalt, and silicon.

TABLE 130.9. TRACE MINERAL ABSORPTION, DISTRIBUTION, AND EXCRETION CHARACTERISTICS

Trace Mineral	Absorption[a] (%)	Distribution[b]	Excretion
Chromium	0.5–2	Transferrin	0.2–0.6 μg/L urine
Copper	30–60	Ceruloplasmin; transcuprein, albumin; amino acids	Bile (80%); intestinal wall (16%); urine (4%)
Iodine	>50–100 from gut; also absorbed from skin	Mainly T_3 and T_4	Urine; 2/3 of iodine is excreted within 2–3 days
Molybdenum	40–100 in duodenum	Protein bound	Principally urine but also feces
Manganese	3–4; inhibited by iron, cobalt	Transferrin, transmanganin, β_1-globulin	Bile (>99%); excretion rather than absorption regulates homeostasis
Selenium	35–85 in duodenum	Protein bound	Principally urine but also feces
Zinc	10–40; absorbed in duodenum and proximal jejunum; excess copper intake will suppress zinc absorption	Albumin, transferrin, ceruloplasmin, gammaglobulin	Biliary and pancreatic losses may account for up to 25% of daily losses; GI tract; sweat

[a]Percent of orally ingested amount.
[b]Substance to which trace mineral is bound. (Adapted from Baumgartner TG (ed). Clinical Guide to Parenteral Micronutrition. Deerfield, IL, Fujisawa, 1991, pp 219–220, 239–240, 257–258, 270–271, 292–295, 314–315, 327–328, with permission.)

Zinc deficiency is clinically characterized by the development of a moist eczematous dermatitis most apparent in the nasolabial folds and around orifices.[75] Other presenting signs and symptoms may include hypogeusia (blunted sense of taste), alopecia, diarrhea, rash (which may vary from papular, scaly lesions to weeping, open erosions), apathy, and depression. Clinical zinc deficiency occurs most frequently in the setting of abnormal losses, such as in Crohn's disease, malabsorption states, and fistula losses, or from prolonged inadequate intake, such as with zinc-free parenteral nutrition. Zinc deficiency can be documented by the presence of low serum zinc concentrations (Table 130.10).[35,72,74] However, since zinc is a normal contaminant of most blood collection tubes, special zinc-free collection tubes (e.g., Bio/Rad polypropylene micro test tube) must be used for serum assays. Zinc status also can be assessed by red cell zinc content, urinary zinc concentration, or zinc content in hair, but these assays are not widely available.

Copper deficiency may present as hematologic changes (anemia, leukopenia, and neutropenia) and skeletal demineralization. In severe cases, such as in Menkes' syndrome, copper deficiency is further manifested as hypothermia, depigmentation of hair and skin, progressive mental deterioration, and growth retardation. Factors predisposing to copper deficiency include malabsorption states, protein-losing enteropathy, nephrotic syndrome, copper-free parenteral nutrition, and copper-deficient enteral nutrition.[76,77] Laboratory diagnosis of copper deficiency is made most frequently on the basis of serum concentrations, although urinary concentrations also may be assessed. As with zinc, serum copper concentrations may be altered by a variety of conditions and, therefore, may not accurately reflect copper nutrition (Table 130.10). Copper function may be assessed by measuring activity of cuproenzymes (e.g., erythrocyte superoxide dismutase or cytochrome c oxidase in platelets or leukocytes). Enzyme activity is significantly decreased in copper deficiency. However, measurements of the activity of these enzymes are method and technique sensitive and not readily available.[78]

Chromium deficiency is characterized by glucose intolerance but also may include neuropathy, increased free fatty acid concentrations, and a low respiratory quotient (Table 130.10). Chromium deficiency has been identified in the setting of long-term, chromium-free parenteral nutrition.[79] Serum chromium concentrations do not reflect chromium nutrition, presumably because the biologically active form of chromium is an organic chromium-containing substance known as *glucose tolerance factor*. Furthermore, laboratory tests measuring chromium content of tissue and fluids have not been established due to the difficulty of accurately determining very low concentrations.[80]

Manganese deficiency has been reported only in association with chemically defined manganese-deficient oral diets.[80] The symptoms include nausea, vomiting, dermatitis, color changes in hair, hypocholesterolemia, and growth retardation (Table 130.10). As with chromium, laboratory tests to measure tissue and fluid concentrations of manganese have not been established. The effect of clinical conditions or specific diseases on manganese nutriture is unknown.

Selenium deficiency has been described in patients receiving long-term selenium-free total parenteral nutrition.[81–83] Myopathy and abnormal glutathione peroxidase concentrations are most frequently observed (Table 130.10). In one case a fatal cardiomyopathy was seen.[82] Selenium status may be assessed by plasma or serum concentrations. Reduced concentrations may indicate selenium deficiency, but reductions have also been observed in patients with malignancies, liver failure, and pregnancy.

TABLE 130.10. ASSESSMENT OF TRACE MINERAL STATUS

Trace Mineral	Signs of Deficiency	Normal Serum Concentration[a]	Factors Resulting in Altered Plasma Concentrations
Chromium	Glucose intolerance, peripheral neuropathy, increased free fatty acid levels, low respiratory quotient	0.12–2.1 μg/L	Not known
Copper	Neutropenia, hypochromic anemia, osteoporosis, decreased hair and skin pigmentation; dermatitis, anorexia, diarrhea	80–155 μg/L (female) 70–140 μg/L (male)	Decreased: serum ceruloplasmin concentrations, corticosteroid therapy, Wilson's disease Increased: infection, rheumatoid arthritis, pregnancy, birth control pills
Iodine	Hypothyroid goiter, hypothyroidism	(Assessed by T_4, TSH and free T_4 index)[b]	Assays are specific to hypo- and hyperthyroid states
Manganese	Nausea, vomiting, dermatitis, color changes in hair, hypocholesterolemia, growth retardation	0.6–2.0 ng/mL (plasma)	Not known
Molybdenum	Tachycardia, tachypnea, altered mental status, visual changes, headache, nausea, vomiting	0.1–3.0 μg/L	Varies with assay method used
Selenium	Muscle weakness and pain, cardiomyopathy	46–143 μg/dL	Decreased: malignancy, liver failure, pregnancy Increased: reticuloendothelial neoplasia
Zinc	Dermatitis, hypogeusia, alopecia, diarrhea, apathy, depression	70–150 μg/dL	Decreased: infection, hypoalbuminemia, corticosteroid therapy, stress, inflammation, pregnancy Increased: tissue injury, hemolysis, contaminated collection tubes

[a]Normal values may vary between laboratories and will also depend on assay procedure.
[b]See Chapter 73, Thyroid Disorders. (From Refs. 35 and 74.)

Measurement of the activity of the selenium-containing enzyme glutathione peroxidase in platelets is a more sensitive measurement of selenium status, although not widely available.

Molybdenum deficiency in humans has rarely been observed.[84] The presenting symptoms included tachycardia, tachypnea, headache, night blindness, nausea, vomiting, central scotomas, lethargy, disorientation, and ultimately coma (Table 130.10). Biochemical assessment has revealed amino acid intolerance, particularly of methionine, and low serum uric acid concentrations. Serum molybdenum concentrations were not assessed. Predisposing factors to molybdenum deficiency appear to be excessive loss via the gastrointestinal tract, as with short-bowel syndrome, and long-term inadequate intake, as with molybdenum-free parenteral nutrition. Assays of molybdenum concentration in tissues or fluids are not readily available.

Iodine deficiency may result in goiter formation (see Chapter 73, Thyroid Disorders). However, not everyone will experience goiter formation with an iodine-deficient diet. Iodine is needed for synthesis of the thyroid hormones thyroxine (T_4) and triodothyronine (T_3). Laboratory assessment of thyroid function is used to assess iodine status (Table 130.10). During parenteral nutrition iodine needs are generally adequately met by cutaneous absorption of iodine from germicides (e.g., povidone iodine) used in catheter care.[85,86] Therefore, intravenous supplements of iodine are not usually given during short-term courses of parenteral nutrition.

Patients with iron deficiency anemia present with fatigue, weakness, and pallor, and possibly also with glossitis, headache, dysphagia, fingernail changes, gastric atrophy, and paresthesias. Inadequate intake of iron, malabsorption, and blood loss from any origin are the principal causes of iron deficiency anemia. Iron deficiency is confirmed on the basis of an assessment of body iron stores as reflected indirectly by measurement of hemoglobin, serum iron, iron-binding capacity, and serum ferritin, or directly by marrow staining and liver biopsy. The direct methods are the most accurate but are invasive. Therefore, the indirect measurements are more commonly used (see Chapter 93, Anemias). Each indirect parameter may be altered by chronic illness independent of iron stores; thus, concomitant illness must be considered in their interpretation (Table 130.11).[35]

VITAMINS

A carefully performed history and physical examination may be the most valuable means of screening patients for

TABLE 130.11. INDIRECT ASSESSMENT OF BODY IRON STORES

Parameter	Normal Values (Adult)[a] Women	Men	Value in Iron Deficiency	Value in Specific Medical States
Hemoglobin (mg/dL)	11.7–15.5	13.2–17.3	Decreased	Decreased value in chronic illness
Serum iron (μg/dL)	50–170	65–170	Decreased	Decreased value in infection, nephrosis Increased value in hemolytic disorders, hemochromatosis, oral contraceptive use, acute liver disease
Total iron-binding capacity (μg/dL)	150–450	250–400	Increased	Decreased value in chronic disease, protein deficiency, liver disease Increased value in pregnancy
Serum ferritin (ng/mL)	10–120	20–250	<15	Decreased value in reticuloendothelium cell damage Increased value in inflammation

[a]Normal values may vary between laboratories. (From Ref. 35.)

risk factors as well as identifying symptoms that suggest physical findings of vitamin deficiency (Table 130.12).[35,87] Laboratory assessment is useful in confirming clinical suspicions. Laboratory assessment also identifies subclinical vitamin deficiencies; the first indication of a deficiency is usually a fall in circulating amounts of the vitamin or its coenzyme. Subsequently, there is a decrease in urinary excretion of the vitamin, which in turn is followed by diminished concentrations of the vitamin in tissue.

The most common measurements of vitamin status are assays of circulating amounts in plasma or serum. Assays also may be performed to determine biochemical or metabolic function of the vitamin and are more likely to reflect body stores than are serum assays. Most of these functional assays use extracts of erythrocytes or leukocytes to determine activity of an apoenzyme, which is dependent on the vitamin coenzyme. Vitamin assays are summarized in Table 130.12.

ESSENTIAL FATTY ACIDS

In general, essential fatty acid (EFA) deficiency, or more specifically linoleic acid deficiency, is rare but can occur during prolonged use of continuously infused parenteral nutrition that does not include long-chain fatty acids. It also may occur with severe PCM. Symptoms of EFA deficiency include dermatitis (e.g., dry, cracked, scaly skin), alopecia, and impaired wound healing. In severe cases neurologic deficits, abnormal liver function, respiratory insufficiency, cardiac arrhythmias, and hemolysis may occur. A deficiency may appear as early as within 1 week of fat-free parenteral nutrition.

Laboratory assessment of EFA deficiency is expensive and not readily available. Fatty acid composition of plasma may be measured: 5,8,11-eicosatrienoic acid and arachidonic acid are the primary fatty acids of interest. Eicosatrienoic acid is not normally present. With a deficiency of linoleic acid and, hence, decreased synthesis of arachidonic acid from linoleic acid, oleic acid metabolism to 5,8,11-eicosatrienoic acid becomes the primary metabolic pathway. The ratio of 5,8,11-eicosatrienoic (triene) acid to arachidonic acid (tetraene) reflects this derangement in metabolism. Normally, this ratio of triene to tetraene is less than 0.4. Values of 0.5 or greater define a deficiency state.

CARNITINE

Carnitine is a substance with vitamin-like properties, however, in states of normal nutriture there is no specific dietary requirement. Carnitine plays a role in lipid oxidation as the transport substance for the intramitochondrial transfer of long-chain fatty acids. Carnitine is available from dietary sources and can be endogenously synthesized from lysine and methionine. A deficiency of carnitine has been described in the setting of severe protein malnutrition, inborn errors of metabolism, and in newborn infants with insufficient dietary carnitine intake.[88–91] Other predisposing factors to carnitine deficiency include kidney disease, liver disease, and vitamin C deficiency.[91,92] The clinical presentation of carnitine deficiency includes generalized skeletal muscle weakness, fatty liver, and reactive hypoglycemia.[93] Carnitine status may be assessed by measuring plasma, urine, or red blood cell concentrations using a radioisotope assay method.[92]

OTHER METHODS OF NUTRITION ASSESSMENT

Bioelectric impedance analysis (BIA) is one of the newer and perhaps more promising methods of body composition

TABLE 130.12. ASSESSMENT OF VITAMIN STATUS

Vitamin	Signs of Deficiency	Laboratory Assay	Normal Values	Comments
Niacin (B_5)	Pellagra: dermatitis, dementia, glossitis, diarrhea, loss of memory, and headaches	Urinary niacin metabolites	2.4–6.4 mg/d	Varies with age, sex, pregnancy; blood levels not done
Folate (B_9)	Megaloblastic anemia, diarrhea, and glossitis	Serum folate	3–16 ng/mL	Levels may be decreased in cases of increased cellular or tissue turnover (pregnancy, malignancy, hemolytic anemia)
Cyanocobalamin (B_{12})	Pernicious anemia, glossitis, spinal cord degeneration, and peripheral neuropathy	Serum B_{12}	100–700 pg/mL	
Thiamine (B_1)	Paresthesias, nystagmus, impaired memory, congestive heart failure, lactic acidosis, Wernicke–Korsakoff syndrome	Red blood cell transketolase activity	850–1000 μg/mL/h	
Riboflavin (B_2)	Mucositis, dermatitis, cheilosis; vascularization of cornea, photophobia, lacrimation, and decreased vision, impaired wound healing, normocytic anemia	Urinary riboflavin	80–120 μg/g creatinine	Varies with age, pregnancy, exercise, nitrogen balance
Pyridoxine (B_6)	Dermatitis, neuritis, and convulsions, microcytic anemia	Plasma B_6	5–30 ng/mL	Varies with age, sex
Pantothenic acid (B_3)	Fatigue, malaise, headache, insomnia, vomiting, and abdominal cramps	Serum pantothenic acid	1.03–1.83 μg/mL	
Biotin	Dermatitis, depression, alopecia, lassitude, somnolence	Urinary biotin	6–50 μg/d	
Ascorbic acid (C)	Enlargement and keratosis of hair follicles; impaired wound healing; anemia, lethargy, depression, bleeding, ecchymosis	Plasma ascorbic acid	0.5–1.5 mg/dL	
A	Dermatitis, night blindness, keratomalacia, xerophthalmia	Serum vitamin A	30–80 μg/dL	
D	Rickets and osteomalacia, muscle weakness	Plasma 25-hydroxy-vitamin D	13–50 ng/mL	Decreased in uremia, in cirrhosis, in individuals greater than 60 years old; may be decreased in winter
E	Hemolysis	Serum vitamin E	5.0–13 μg/mL	Decreased with low blood lipoprotein concentrations
K	Bleeding	Serum phylloquinone	0.13–1.19 ng/mL	Decreased with hepatic disease, anticoagulants

(From Refs. 35 and 87.)

and fluid assessment.[94,95] It is a simple, noninvasive technique used to measure lean body mass. By placing electrodes on the wrist and ankle and applying an electrical current, impedance (resistance) to flow is measured. Lean tissue has a higher electrical conductivity (less resistance) because of its greater fluid and electrolyte content, while fat is a poor conductor of current. Assessment of body water and its distribution can also be determined with BIA.[96–99] Decreased impedance is seen with increased total body water. Therefore, it is important to evaluate fluid status along with BIA data. The potential limitations of the use of BIA include variability with electrolyte imbalance, interference by large fat masses, and the need for standards that reflect variations in individual body sizes.

Hand grip strength, or forearm muscle dynamometry, and stimulation of the ulnar nerve have been measured as indicators of muscle function and correlated with patient outcome.[100,101] Forearm muscle dynamometry is a relatively simple, noninvasive, and inexpensive procedure. Ulnar nerve stimulation causes measurable muscle contraction. In the setting of malnutrition, increased fatigability and a slowed muscle relaxation rate have been noted, with these indices returning to normal after refeeding.[102] Both of these parameters have the advantage of being an indicator of tissue function rather than composition. Their utility in clinical practice is currently hampered by a lack of appropriate reference standards and limited data confirming their sensitivity and specificity as nutrition assessment tools.

Various methods to determine body composition have been utilized in the clinical research setting. These methods are generally complex, require expensive technology, and at present are limited mainly to experimental studies. Ultrasound and infrared interactance can be applied to measure subcutaneous fat. The latter utilizes an inexpensive and portable device, but the results of measurements have not been used extensively for nutritional assessment.[102] Dual photon and dual energy radiography, magnetic resonance imaging (MRI), and computed tomography (CT) can measure subcutaneous, intra-abdominal and regional fat distribution.[103] Neutron activation is a means of measuring body nitrogen, calcium, sodium, chloride, and phosphorus. These measurements can then be used to calculate total body fat, bone, and protein.[96] Isotope dilutional methods determine total body water and underwater weighing determines density. In addition, these methods can be used to estimate lean body mass and body fat. Furthermore, lean body mass can also be estimated via total body conductivity (TOBEC) and by measuring the naturally occurring isotope ^{40}K.[103]

Assessment of Nutrient Requirements

Nutrient requirements vary with age, sex, size, disease state, clinical condition, nutrition status, and level of physical activity. An assessment of nutrient requirements must, therefore, be made using guidelines interpreted in the context of these patient-specific factors. As a general reference point the U.S. recommended dietary allowances (RDAs) should be considered.[104] However, the RDAs are intended to represent the nutritional needs of healthy individuals.

ENERGY

There are numerous methods for determining an individual's energy, or calorie (kcal), requirement.[105] The most commonly used methods are to determine energy requirements on the basis of calories per body weight (i.e., kcal/kg), to calculate the Harris–Benedict equation or to use indirect calorimetry.

The simplest method is to determine energy requirements on the basis of calories per body weight. This method requires that assumptions be made about the energy requirements associated with various disease states or clinical conditions as well as the additional requirements for repletion of a malnourished individual. It does not take into consideration age- or sex-related differences in energy metabolism in adults. In general, adult requirements determined by this method, using lean body weight, are as follows:

Healthy, normal nutrition status	~25 kcal/kg
Malnourished or mildly metabolically stressed	~30 kcal/kg
Critically ill, hypermetabolic	30–35 kcal/kg
Major burn injury	40+ kcal/kg

Clinical judgment as well as close monitoring is essential to ensure that the desired nutrition outcomes are attained.

The Harris–Benedict equation (HBE) has become a popular method to assess calories during the last two decades. It has the advantage of taking into consideration the age, height, weight, sex, and clinical condition of the patient. The HBE was derived from oxygen consumption measurements made on normally nourished individuals who were in a fasting, resting state.[106] The HBE calculates basal energy expenditure (BEE), which is the amount of energy expended to perform only basal functions such as breathing, pumping blood, and fasting metabolic processes. The HBE is:

$$\text{BEE (females)} = 655 + 9.6\,(\text{wt}) + 1.8\,(\text{ht}) - 4.7\,(\text{age})$$

$$\text{BEE (males)} = 66 + 13.7\,(\text{wt}) + 5\,(\text{ht}) - 6.8\,(\text{age})$$

where BEE is kcal/d, wt is weight in kilograms, ht is height in centimeters, and age is in years. Since this equation merely represents energy requirements to perform basal functions, it must be further modified by a "stress factor" and an "activity factor" to estimate actual energy requirements. Clinical judgment is required to evaluate the clinical condition of the patient so that the appropriate factors can be chosen (Table 130.13).[105]

TABLE 130.13. FACTORS BY WHICH TO MODIFY BASAL ENERGY EXPENDITURE (BEE) TO DETERMINE ADULT ENERGY REQUIREMENTS

Condition	Increase Above BEE (%)
Activity	
Confined to bed	20
Out of bed	30
Minor surgery	30
Fracture	30
Peritonitis	40
Trauma	40–50
Sepsis	40–75
Severe burn injury	80–130

The most accurate clinical tool for estimating energy requirements is indirect calorimetry.[107] Indirect calorimetry is based on the measurement of the oxygen and carbon dioxide content in expired air. In a noninvasive procedure, oxygen consumption (Vo_2, mL/min) and carbon dioxide production (Vco_2, mL/min) are determined. Using the abbreviated Weir equation, resting energy expenditure (REE, kcal/d) can be calculated:

$$REE = [3.9(Vo_2) + 1.1\,(Vco_2)] \times 1.44$$

This measured energy expenditure represents the actual energy expended by the patient for the point in time that the measurement was taken. It is extrapolated to a 24-hour period to represent approximate daily energy requirements. This measurement will reflect any alterations in energy requirements due to disease or clinical condition but does not include a requirement for repletion of nutrition status in a malnourished individual. Increasing energy intake by 20–25% may accommodate the need for additional calories for repletion.

The data obtained from indirect calorimetry can also be used to determine a respiratory quotient (RQ). The RQ reflects substrate oxidation and is calculated as follows:

$$RQ = Vco_2/Vo_2$$

Each type of substrate produces a different RQ value. The following RQ values reflect the net substrate oxidation: fat, 0.7; carbohydrate, 1.0; mixed substrate (fat, carbohydrate, and protein), 0.85; and protein, 0.80. An RQ value of greater than 1.0 represents either lipogenesis or patient hyperventilation; an RQ value of less than 0.7 may indicate a ketogenic diet, fat gluconeogenesis, or ethanol oxidation. Values that fall outside of the 0.67–1.3 range would raise serious doubts as to the validity of the test. Clinically, the RQ is used to determine if a patient is being overfed, which is indicated by an RQ value greater than 1.0.

PROTEIN

Adult protein requirements are based on nutrition status, disease state, and clinical condition (Table 130.14).[105] Protein metabolism is dependent on both kidney and liver function. Therefore, protein requirements will be altered with decreased kidney or liver function. Critical illness (e.g., sepsis, burns, trauma) will result in a hypermetabolic state in which there is increased protein synthesis and degradation. Consequently, protein requirements will be increased. The application of these guidelines requires both clinical judgment and frequent monitoring of renal and liver function, clinical condition, and nutrition outcomes.

An alternative method for determining protein requirements is to measure urinary nitrogen excretion. This measurement indirectly reflects an individual's protein utilization or protein catabolic rate (PCR). An increase in PCR is one of the characteristics of hypermetabolism.[108] As the stress level increases, the concomitant increase in protein catabolism results in an increase in urinary nitrogen.[109] Usually in clinical practice the amount of urea nitrogen is measured in a 24-hour urine collection (UUN). The quantity of UUN accounts for 60–90% of the total urinary nitrogen (TUN) excreted.[33,110] Therefore, total nitrogen output is approximated by:

$$\text{Nitrogen output (g/d)} = (UUN \times 1.20) + 1$$

where 1 represents the estimated nitrogen losses from skin, fecal, and respiratory sources.[111] Alternatively, if it is available, TUN can be measured and may be more accurate.[112] In the setting of renal failure where measured urinary nitrogen does not represent nitrogen generation, protein turnover can be approximated by using equations based on the kinetics of urea to estimate the rate at which urea is being produced.[113–115]

TABLE 130.14. APPROXIMATE PROTEIN REQUIREMENTS IN ADULTS

Clinical Condition	Daily Protein Intake, g/kg (range)
Recommended daily allowance	0.8–1.0
Low stress	
Maintenance	1.0–1.2
Anabolic	1.3–1.7
Hypermetabolic stress	1.5–2.5
Renal failure	
No dialysis	0.6–1.0
With dialysis[a]	1.2–2.7
Severe hepatic failure	0.5–1.5

[a] Varies with type of dialysis; patients undergoing peritoneal dialysis generally require a higher protein intake than patients undergoing hemodialysis (Adapted from Mandt JM, Teasley-Strausburg KM, Shronts EP. Nutritional requirements, in Teasley-Strausburg KM (ed): Nutrition Support Handbook: A Compendium of Products with Guidelines for Usage. Cincinnati, OH, Harvey Whitney Books Company, 1992, p 30, with permission.)

FLUID

Daily adult fluid requirements are dependent on many factors but in general can be estimated as approximately 30 mL/kg or can be based on energy requirements and calculated as 1 mL/kcal. Increased fluid requirements are observed in individuals with increased insensible losses [e.g., fever, excessive sweating, increased metabolism (e.g., hyperthyroidism)] or with increased gastrointestinal losses (e.g., vomiting, diarrhea, high-output fistula). Decreased fluid requirements have been observed in patients with renal failure or with an expanded extracellular fluid volume (e.g., congestive heart failure) and in hypoproteinemia with starvation. When estimating fluid intake via a nutrition regimen, all non-nutrition sources of fluid intake must be taken into consideration (e.g., the fluid vehicle for intravenous medications) (see Chapter 51).

MICRONUTRIENTS

Requirements for the micronutrients (i.e., electrolytes, trace minerals and vitamins) vary with the route by which the nutrient is ingested (Table 130.15).[116] The variability is dependent on the extent to which the nutrient is absorbed via the GI tract versus intravenously. Nutrients which are administered intravenously bypass absorption, and their absorption is equivalent to 100%. Those micronutrients that are poorly absorbed via the GI tract usually will be required in greater doses enterally than parenterally. However, many water-soluble micronutrients are more rapidly excreted via the kidneys when administered IV versus being ingested enterally. In these situations the IV nutrient dose will be greater than the enteral dose. Other factors that affect micronutrient requirements include GI losses via diarrhea, vomiting, high-output fistula, and hypermetabolism. The electrolytes sodium, potassium, magnesium, and phosphorus are particularly dependent on renal function, and in the setting of renal failure intake may need to be restricted. Patients who are severely malnourished will have increased electrolyte requirements during early refeeding due to preexisting deficiencies and/or rapid intracellular uptake with anabolism.[117] Failure to provide adequate electrolytes during refeeding has resulted in death.[118]

TABLE 130.15. RECOMMENDED ADULT DAILY MAINTENANCE DOSES FOR ELECTROLYTES, TRACE MINERALS, AND VITAMINS

Nutrient	Enteral	Parenteral
Electrolytes		
Calcium	800–1200 mg	10–15 mEq
Chloride	1700–5100 mg	—
Fluoride	1.5–4.0 mg	—
Magnesium	280–350 mg	10–20 mEq
Phosphorus	800–1200 mg	20–45 mmol
Potassium	1875–5625 mg	60–100 mEq
Sodium	1100–3300 mg	60–100 mEq
Trace Minerals		
Chromium	50–200 μg	10–15 μg[a]
Copper	1.5–3 mg	0.5–1.5 mg
Iodine	150 μg	70–140 μg
Iron	10–15 mg	0.5 mg
Manganese	2–5 mg	0.15–0.8 mg
Molybdenum	75–250 μg	100–200 μg
Selenium	55–70 μg	40–80 μg
Zinc	12–15 mg	2.5–4.0 mg[b]
Vitamins		
Biotin	30–100 μg	60 μg
Cyanocobalamin (B_{12})	2.0 μg	5.0 μg
Folic acid	200 μg	400 μg
Niacin	13–19 mg NE	40 mg NE
Pantothenic acid (B_3)	4.7 mg	15 mg
Pyridoxine (B_6)	1.6–2.0 mg	4 mg
Riboflavin (B_2)	1.2–1.7 mg	3.6 mg
Thiamin (B_1)	1.0–1.5 mg	3 mg
Vitamin A	800–100 μg RE	600 μg RE (3300 IU)
Vitamin C	60 mg	100 mg
Vitamin D	5–10 μg	5 μg (200 IU)
Vitamin E	8–10 mg TE	10 mg TE (10 IU)
Vitamin K	60–80 μg	0.7–2.5 mg

Key: NE, niacin equivalents; RE, retinol equivalents; TE, tocopherol equivalent.
[a]An additional 20 μg chromium/d is recommended in patients with intestinal losses.
[b]An additional 12.2 mg zinc/L of small-bowel fluid lost and 17.1 mg zinc/kg of stool or ileostomy output is recommended; an additional 2.0 mg zinc/d for acute catabolic stress. (Adapted from Shronts EP, Lacey JA. Metabolic support, in Gottschlich MM, Matarese LE, Shronts EP (eds): Nutrition Support Dietetics—Core Curriculum, 2nd ed. Silver Spring, MD, ASPEN, 1993, p 358, with permission.)

PRACTICAL GUIDELINES FOR NUTRITION ASSESSMENT

The value of any given marker or group of markers used for nutrition assessment is only as great as its ability to accurately identify the patient with malnutrition and to correlate with malnutrition-associated complications. Most of the currently available markers of nutrition status were first used in epidemiologic studies to define large populations suffering from malnutrition caused by famine. The response of the various markers of nutrition status to nutrition therapy and the correlation between improvement in these markers and decreased morbidity and mortality further support their validity. However, when applied to an individual, most of these markers lack specificity and sensitivity, which makes the development of a clinically useful, cost-effective approach to individual patient nutrition assessment challenging.

The importance of the history and physical examination in both nutrition screening and nutrition assessment cannot be overemphasized. The least amount of objective data that can further substantiate the clinical impression and provide a baseline for subsequent monitoring are those markers that show the best correlation with outcome: *weight* and *serum albumin concentration.* The cost effectiveness of the addition of further biochemical parameters is yet to be determined. The assessment of other anthropometric measures is probably most useful in the setting of anticipated long-term nutrition support in which these measurements will serve as a longitudinal marker of the individual response to therapy.

The assessment of nutrition requirements is best achieved with ongoing reassessment of nutrition goals and nutrition status. Initially, nutrition requirements are determined on the basis of assumptions made about clinical condition and the nutrition needs associated with repletion. Once nutrition intervention has been initiated, a periodic reassessment of nutrition status will determine the accuracy of the initial estimate of nutrition requirements. Also, nutrition requirements may be dynamic in the setting of acute or critical illness—as the patient's clinical status changes so may protein and energy requirements. This further emphasizes the need for periodic reassessment.

Better markers of nutrition status and methods for determining patient-specific nutrition requirements are definitely needed. Functional tests and simple, noninvasive tests for body composition analysis hold promise for the future. However, until better methods of assessment become clinically available and are demonstrated to be cost effective, the currently available battery of tests will continue to be the mainstay of nutrition assessment.

References

1. ASPEN Board of Directors. Revised definition of terms used in ASPEN guidelines and standards. Nutr Clin Prac 1995;10:1–3.
2. Grant JP. Nutritional assessment in clinical practice. Nutr Clin Prac 1986;1:3–11.
3. Teasley-Strausburg KM. Nutritional/metabolic assessment, in Teasley-Strausburg KM (ed): Nutrition Support Handbook: A Compendium of Products with Guidelines for Usage. Cincinnati, OH, Harvey Whitney Books Company, 1992, pp 1–18.
4. Hopkins B. Assessment of nutritional status, in Gottschlich MM, Matarese LE, Shronts EP (eds): Nutrition Support Dietetics—Core Curriculum, 2nd ed. Silver Spring, MD, ASPEN, 1993, pp 15–70.
5. White JV, Ham RJ, Lipschitz DA. Report of nutrition screening: Toward a common view. Washington, DC, The Nutrition Screening Initiatve, 1991.
6. Council on Practice Quality Management Committee. Identifying patients at risk: ADA's definitions for nutrition screening and nutrition assessment. J Am Diet Assoc 1994;94(8):838–839.
7. Nagel MR. Nutrition screening: Identifying patients at risk for malnutrition. Nutr Clin Prac 1993;8:171–175.
8. Ford DA, Fairchild MM. Managing inpatient clinical nutrition services: A comprehensive program assures accountability and success. J Am Diet Assoc 1990;90(5):695–704.
9. Reilly JJ, Hull SF, Albert N, et al: Economic impact of malnutrition: A model system for hospitalized patients. J Parenter Enter Nutr 1988;12(4):371–376.
10. Baker JP, Detsky AS, Wesson DE, et al. Nutritional assessment: A comparison of clinical judgment and objective measurement. N Engl J Med 1982;306:969–972.
11. Goode AW. The scientific basis of nutritional assessment. Br J Anaesth 1981;53:161–167.
12. Jeliffe DB. The Assessment of Nutritional Status of the Community. World Health Organization Monograph No. 53. Geneva, World Health Organization, 1966.
13. Weight by Height and Age of Adults 18–74 Years: United States, 1971–74. Atlanta, GA, National Center for Health Statistics, 1979, series 11, no 9.
14. Bishop CW, Bowen PE, Ritchey SJ. Norms for nutritional assessment of American adults by upper arm anthropometry. Am J Clin Nutr 1981;31:2530–2539.
15. Metropolitan Life Insurance Company. Statistical Bulletin, New Weights and Standards for Men and Women. Chicago, Metropolitan Life, 1959, vol 40, 1–4.
16. Metropolitan Life Insurance Company. Statistical Bulletin, New Weights and Standards for Men and Women. Chicago, Metropolitan Life, 1983, vol 64, 2–9.
17. Morgan DB, Hill GL, Burkinshaw L. The assessment of weight loss from a single measurement of body weight: The problems and limitations. Am J Clin Nutr 1980;33:2101–2105.
18. Seltzer MH, Slocum BA, Cataldi-Betcher EL, et al. Instant nutritional assessment; absolute weight loss and surgical morbidity. J Parenter Enter Nutr 1982;6:218–221.
19. Heymsfield SB, Tighe A, Wang Z. Nutritional assessment by anthropometric and biochemical methods, in Shils ME, Olson JA, Shike M (eds): Modern Nutrition in Health and Disease, 8th ed. Philadelphia, Lea & Febiger, 1994, pp 827–828.
20. Mason JB, Russell RM. Parenteral nutrition in the elderly, in Rombeau JL, Caldwell MD (eds): Clinical Nutrition: Parenteral Nutrition, 2nd ed. Philadelphia, WB Saunders, 1993, pp 738–739.
21. Bastow MD. Anthropometrics revisited. Proc Nutr Soc 1982;41:381–388.
22. Edwards DAW, Hammond WH, Healey MJR, et al. Design and accuracy of calipers for measuring subcutaneous tissue thickness. Br J Nutr 1955;9:133–143.
23. Jensen TG, Dudrick SJ, Johnston DA. A comparison of triceps skinfold and upper arm circumference measurements taken in standard and supine positions. J Parenter Enter Nutr 1981;5:519–521.
24. Grant JP, Custer PB, Thurlow J. Current techniques of nutritional assessment. Surg Clin North Am 1981;61:437–463.
25. Buzby GP, Mullen JL. Nutritional assessment, in Rombeau J, Caldwell MD (eds): Clinical Nutrition, Philadelphia, WB Saunders, 1984, vol 1, pp 127–128.
26. Forbes GB, Bruining GJ. Urinary creatinine excretion and lean body mass. Am J Clin Nutr 1976;29:1359–1366.
27. Bistrian RB, Blackburn GL, Sherman M, et al. Therapeutic index of nutritional depletion in hospital patients. Surg Gynecol Obstet 1975;141:512–516.
28. Blackburn GL, Bistrian RB, Maini BS, et al. Nutritional and metabolic assessment of the hospitalized patient. J Parenter Enter Nutr 1977;1:11–22.
29. Travill AS. The synthesis and degradation of liver-produced proteins. Gut 1972;13:225–241.
30. Benjamin DR. Laboratory tests and nutritional assessment. Ped Clin North Am 1989;36:139–161.
31. Boosalis MG, Ott L, Levine AS, et al. Relationship of visceral proteins to nutritional status in chronic and acute illness. Crit Care Med 1989;17:741–747.
32. Church JM, Hill GL. Assessing the efficacy of intravenous nutrition in general surgical patients: Dynamic nutritional assessment with plasma proteins. JPEN 1987;11:135–139.
33. Konstantinides FN, Kaproth PL, Cerra FB. Other aspects of metabolic monitoring in critically ill patients. Clin Chem 1990;36:1596–1603.

34. Veldee MS. Nutrition, in Burtis CA, Ashwood ER (eds): Tietz Textbook of Clinical Chemistry, 2nd ed. Philadelphia, WB Saunders, 1994, pp 1236–1274.
35. Painter PC, Cope JY, Smith JL. Appendix: Table 41–20. Clinical chemistry and toxicology, in Burtis CA, Ashwood ER (eds): Tietz Textbook of Clinical Chemistry, 2nd ed. Philadelphia, WB Saunders, 1994, pp 2176–2211.
36. Mattox TW, Brown RO, Boucher BA, et al. Use of fibronectin and somatomedin-C as markers of enteral nutrition support in traumatized patients using a modified amino acid formula. J Parenter Enter Nutr 1988;12:592–596.
37. Mullen JL, Germer MH, Buzby GP, et al. Implications of malnutrition in the surgical patient. Arch Surg 1979;114:121–125.
38. Bienia R, Ratcliff S, Barbour GL, et al. Malnutrition and hospital prognosis in the alcoholic patient. J Parenter Enter Nutr 1982;6:301–303.
39. Anderson CF, Wochos DN. The utility of serum albumin values in nutritional assessment of hospitalized patients. Mayo Clin Proc 1982;57:181–184.
40. Rudman D, Feller AB, Nagraj HS, et al. Relation of serum albumin concentration to death rate in nursing home men. JPEN 1987;11:360–363.
41. Bernstein LH, Leukhardt-Fairfield CJ, Pleban W, et al. Usefulness of data on albumin and prealbumin concentrations in determining effectiveness of nutritional support. Clin Chem 1989;35:271–274.
42. Spiekerman AM: Proteins used in nutritional assessment. Clin Lab Med 1993;13(2):353–369.
43. Weisberg HF. Evaluation of nutritional status. Ann Clin Lab Sci 1983;13:95–106.
44. Fairbanks VF. Iron in medicine and nutrition, in Shils ME, Olson JA, Shike M (eds): Modern Nutrition in Health and Disease, 8th ed. Philadelphia, Lea & Febiger, 1994, pp 190–191.
45. Ingenbleek Y, Van Den Schriek HC, DeNayer P, et al. The role of retinal-binding protein in protein calorie malnutrition. Metabolism 1975;24:633–641.
46. Winkler MF, Gerrior SA, Pomp A, et al. Use of retinol-binding protein and prealbumin as indicators of the response to nutrition therapy. J Am Diet Assoc 1989;89:684–687.
47. Erstad BL, Campbell DJ, Rollins CJ, Rappaport WD. Albumin and prealbumin concentrations in patients receiving postoperative parenteral nutrition. Pharmacotherapy 1994;14(4):458–462.
48. Smith FR, Goodman DS, Zaklama MS, et al. Serum vitamin A, retinol-binding protein, and prealbumin concentrations in protein calorie malnutrition. 1. A functional defect in hepatic retinol release. Am J Clin Nutr 1973;26:973–981.
49. Large S, Neal G, Glover J, et al. The early changes in retinol-binding protein and prealbumin concentrations in plasma of protein energy malnourished children after treatment with retinol and an improved diet. Br J Nutr 1980;43:393–402.
50. Sganga G, Siegel JH, Brown G, et al. Reprioritization of hepatic plasma protein release in trauma and sepsis. Arch Surg 1985;120:187–199.
51. Peterson VM, Moore EE, Jones TN, et al. Total enteral nutrition versus total parenteral nutrition after major torso injury: Attenuation of hepatic protein reprioritization. Surgery 1988;104:199–207.
52. Sandstedt S, Dederblad G, Larsson J, et al. Influence of total parenteral nutrition on fibronectin in malnourished subjects with or without inflammatory response. J Parenter Enter Nutr 1984;8:493–496.
53. Clemmons DR, Underwood LE, Dickerson RN, et al. Use of plasma somatomedin-C/insulin-like growth factor 1 measurements to monitor the response to nutritional repletion in malnourished patients. Am J Clin Nutr 1985;41:191–198.
54. Donahue ST, Phillips LS. Response of IGF-1 to nutritional support in malnourished hospital patients: A possible indicator of short-term changes in nutritional status. Am J Clin Nutr 1989;50:962–969.
55. Arroyave G, Wilson D, de Funes C, et al. The free amino acids in blood plasma of children with kwashiorkor and marasmus. Am J Clin Nutr 1962;11:517–524.
56. Edozien JC, Phillips EJ, Collis WRF. The free amino acids of plasma and urine in kwashiorkor. Lancet 1960;1:615–618.
57. Holt LE, Snyderman SE, Norton PM, et al. The plasma aminogram in kwashiorkor. Lancet 1963;2:1343–1348.
58. Chandra RK. Immunocompetence as a functional index of nutritional status. Br Med Bull 1981;89–94.
59. Dominioni L, Dionigi R. Immunologic function and nutritional assessment. J Parenter Enter Nutr 1987;11:705–725.
60. Peck MD, Alexander JW. The use of immunologic tests to predict outcome in surgical patients. Nutrition 1990;6:16–19.
61. Smythe PM, Schonland M, Brereton-Stiles GC, et al. Thymolytic deficiency and depression of cell-mediated immunity in protein-calorie malnutrition. Lancet 1971;2:939–943.
62. Twomey R, Ziegler D, Rombeau J. Utility of skin testing in nutritional assessment: A critical review. J Parenter Enter Nutr 1982;6:50–58.
63. Miller CL. Immunologic assays as measurements of nutritional status: A review. J Parenter Enter Nutr 1978;2:554–566.
64. Bistrian BR, Blackburn GL, Scrimshaw NS, Flatt J. Cellular immunity in semi-starved states in hospitalized patients. Am J Clin Nutr 1975;28:1148–1155.
65. Law DK, Dudrick SJ, Abdou NI. Immunocompetence of patients with protein-calorie malnutrition. The effects of nutritional repletion. Ann Intern Med 1973;79:545–550.
66. Jensen TG, Englert DM, Dudrick SJ, et al. Delayed hypersensitivity skin testing: Response rates in a surgical population. J Am Diet Assoc 1983;82:17–23.
67. Nuwer N, Cerra FB, Shronts EP, et al. Does modified amino acid total parenteral nutrition alter immune response in high level surgical stress? J Parenter Enter Nutr 1983;7:521–524.
68. Alexander JW, Peck MD. Future prospects for adjunctive therapy: Pharmacologic and nutritional approaches to immune system modulation. Crit Care Med 1990;18:S159–S164.
69. Moore FA, Moore EE, Kudsk KA et al. Clinical benefits of an immune-enhancing diet for early postinjury enteral feeding. J Trauma 1994;37:607–615.
70. Daly JM, Reynolds J, Thom A, et al. Immune and metabolic effects of arginine in the surgical patient. Ann Surg 1988;208:512–522.

71. Barbul A, Lazarou SA, Efron DT, et al. Arginine enhances wound healing and lymphocyte immune responses in humans. Surgery 1990;108:331–337.
72. Gottschlich MM. Selection of optimal lipid sources in enteral and parenteral nutrition. Nutr Clin Prac 1992;7:152–165.
73. Rudolph FB, Kulkarni AD, Fanslow WC, et al. Role of RNA as a dietary source of pyrimidines and purines in immune function. Nutrition 1990;6(suppl):45–52.
74. Baumgartner TG. Trace elements in clinical nutrition. Nutr Clin Prac 1993;8:251–263.
75. Fawaz F. Zinc deficiency in surgical patients: A clinical study. J Parenter Enter Nutr 1985;9:364–369.
76. Tamura H, Hirose S, Watanabe O, et al. Anemia and neutropenia due to copper deficiency in enteral nutrition. J Parenter Enter Nutr 1994;18:185–189.
77. Wasa M, Satani M, Tanano H, et al. Copper deficiency with pancytopenia during parenteral nutrition. J Parenter Enter Nutr 1994;18:190–192.
78. Milne DB. Trace elements, in Burtis CA, Ashwood ER (eds): Tietz Textbook of Clinical Chemistry, 2nd ed. Philadelphia, WB Saunders, 1994, pp 1317–1353.
79. Jeejeebuoy KW, Chu RC, Marliss EB. Chromium deficiency, glucose intolerance, and neuropathy reversed by chromium supplementation in a patient receiving long-term total parenteral nutrition. Am J Clin Nutr 1977;30:531–538.
80. Jacob RA, Milne DB. Biochemical assessment of vitamins and minerals. Clin Lab Med 1993;18:371–386.
81. King WW. Reversal of selenium deficiency with oral selenium. N Engl J Med 1981;304:1304–1305.
82. Fleming CR. Selenium deficiency and fatal cardiomyopathy in a patient on home parenteral nutrition. Gastroenterology 1982;83:689–693.
83. Abrams CK, Siram SM, Galsim C, et al. Selenium deficiency in long-term total parenteral nutrition. Nutr Clin Prac 1992;7:175–178.
84. Abumrad NN, Schneider AJ, Steel D, Rogers LS. Amino acid intolerance during prolonged parenteral nutrition reversed by molybdate therapy. Am J Clin Nutr 1981;34:2551–2559.
85. Clugston GA, Hetzel. Iodine, in Shils ME, Olson JA, Shike M (eds): Modern Nutrition in Health and Disease, 8th ed. Philadelphia, Lea & Febiger, 1994, pp 252–263.
86. Nichoalds GE. Iodine, in Baumgartner TG (ed): Clinical Guide to Parenteral Micronutrition, 2nd ed. Deerfield IL, Lyphomed, Division of Fujisawa, 1991, pp 289–309.
87. McCormick DB, Greene HL. Vitamins, in Burtis CA, Ashwood ER (eds): Tietz Textbook of Clinical Chemistry, 2nd ed. Philadelphia, WB Saunders, 1994, pp 1275–1316.
88. Borum PR. Clinical Aspects of Human Carnitine Deficiency. New York, Pergamon Press, 1986.
89. Slonim AE, Borum PR, Tanaka K, et al. Dietary dependent carnitine deficiency as a cause of nonketotic hypoglycemia in an infant. J Pediatr 1981;99:551–556.
90. Tao RC, Yoshimura NN. Carnitine metabolism and its application in parenteral nutrition. J Parenter Enter Nutr 1980;4:469–486.
91. Broquist HP. Carnitine, in Shils ME, Olson JA, Shike M (eds): Modern Nutrition in Health and Disease, 8th ed. Philadelphia, Lea & Febiger, 1994, pp 459–465.
92. Borum PR. Carnitine, in Baumgartner TG (ed): Clinical Guide to Parenteral Micronutrition, 2nd ed. Deerfield IL, Lyphomed Division of Fujisawa, Inc, 1991, pp 591–604.
93. Worthley LIG, Fishlock RC, Snoswell AM. Carnitine deficiency with hyperbilirubinemia, generalized skeletal muscle weakness and reactive hypoglycemia in a patient on long-term total parenteral nutrition: Treatment with intravenous L-carnitine. J Parenter Enter Nutr 1983;7:176–180.
94. Schroeder D, Christie PM, Hill GL. Bioelectrical impedance analysis for body composition: Clinical evaluation in general surgical patients. J Parenter Enter Nutr 1990;14:129–133.
95. Lukaski HC, Johnson PE, Bolonchuk WW, Lykken GL. Assessment of free mass using bioelectrical impedance measurements of the human body. Am J Clin Nutr 1985;41:810–814.
96. Jacobs DO, Scheltinga MRM. Metabolic assessment, in Rombeau JL, Caldwell MD (eds): Clinical Nutrition: Parenteral Nutrition, 2nd ed. Philadelphia, WB Saunders, 1993, pp 253–259.
97. Scheltinga MR, Jacob DO, Kimbrough TD. Alterations in body fluid content can be detected by bioelectrical impedance analysis. J Surg Res 1991;50:461–468.
98. Robert S, Zarowitz BJ, Hyzy R, et al. Bioelectrical impedance assessment of nutritional status in critically ill patients. Am J Clin Nutr 1993;57:840–844.
99. Zarowithz BJ, Pilla AM. Bioelectrical impedance in clinical practice. Drug Intell Clin Pharm 1989;23:548–555.
100. Kalfarentzos F, Spiliotis J, Velimezis G, et al. Comparison of forearm muscle dynamometry with nutritional prognostic index, as a preoperative indicator in cancer patients. J Parenter Enter Nutr 1989;13:34–36.
101. Shizgal HM, Vasileusky CA, Gardiner PF. Nutritional assessment and skeletal muscle function. Am J Clin Nutr 1986;44:761–771.
102. Lipkin EW, Bell S. Assessment of nutritional status. Clin Lab Med 1993;13(2):329–351.
103. Forbes GB. Body composition: Influence of nutrition, disease, growth and aging, in Shils ME, Olson JA, Shike M (eds): Modern Nutrition in Health and Disease, 8th ed. Philadelphia, Lea & Febiger, 1994, pp 781–801.
104. Food and Nutrition Board, National Research Council. Recommended Dietary Allowances, 10th ed. Washington, DC, National Academy of Sciences, 1989.
105. Mandt JM, Teasley-Strausburg KM, Shronts EP. Nutritional requirements, in Teasley-Strausburg KM (ed): Nutrition Support Handbook: A Compendium of Products with Guidelines for Usage. Cincinnati, OH, Harvey Whitney Books Company, 1992, pp 19–36.
106. Harris JA, Benedict FG. A Biometric Study of Basal Metabolism in Man, publication 279. Washington, DC, Carnegie Institute, 1919.
107. McClave SA, Snider HL. Use of indirect calorimetry in clinical nutrition. Nutr Clin Prac 1992;7:207–221.
108. Long CL, Lowry SR. Hormonal regulation of protein metabolism. J Parenter Enter Nutr 1990;14:555–562.
109. Barton RG. Nutrition support in critical illness. Nutr Clin Prac 1994;9:127–139.

110. Loder PB, Kee AJ, Horsburgh R, et al. Validity of urinary urea nitrogen as a measure of total urinary nitrogen in adult patients requiring parenteral nutrition. Crit Care Med 1989;17:309–312.
111. Valesco N, Long CL, Otto DA, et al. Comparison of three methods for the estimation of total nitrogen losses in hospitalized patients. J Parenter Enter Nutr 1990;14:517–522.
112. Konstantinides FN, Konstantinides NN, Li JC, et al. Urinary urea nitrogen: Too insensitive for calculating nitrogen balance studies in surgical clinical nutrition. J Parent Enter Nutr 1991;15:189–193.
113. Sargent JA. Urea mass balance: Nutrition and treatment of the acutely ill. Nutr Supp Serv 1982;2:38–39.
114. Kosanovich JM, Dumler F, Horst M, et al. Use of urea kinetics in the nutritional care of the acutely ill patient. J Parenter Enter Nutr 1985;9:165–169.
115. Shronts EP, Teasley KM. Clinical utility of urea kinetics for calculating nitrogen balance in acutely ill patients. Nutr Supp Serv 1988;8:12–15.
116. Shronts EP, Lacey JA. Metabolic support, in Gottschlich MM, Matarese LE, Shronts EP (eds): Nutrition Support Dietetics—Core Curriculum, 2nd ed. Silver Spring, MD, ASPEN, 1993, p 358.
117. Solomon SM, Kirby DF. The refeeding syndrome: A review. J Parent Enter Nutr 1990;14:90–97.
118. Weinsier R, Krumdieck C. Death resulting from overzealous total parenteral nutrition: The refeeding syndrome revisited. Am J Clin Nutr 1981;34:393–399.

Chapter 131

Prevalence and Significance of Malnutrition

Kathleen M. Teasley-Strausburg, MS, RPh, BCNSP

Malnutrition is recognized as a contributing factor in the poor outcome of many disease states. In this chapter the *prevalence* of malnutrition as defined by a variety of nutrition assessment parameters is documented, and the *significance* of observed abnormalities in these nutrition assessment parameters is evaluated in selected disease states relative to morbidity and mortality. Strategies for the management of malnutrition and the economic consequences of malnutrition are also presented.

Effect of Malnutrition on Organ and Cellular Function

The outcome of malnutrition is an inappropriate reduction in lean body mass resulting in loss of structure and/or function (Table 131.1). Essentially every organ system is affected by malnutrition. The clinical significance of the effect will depend on the specific anatomic structure or system and on the degree of malnutrition. For example, with mild malnutrition, loss of skeletal muscle mass may be apparent as weakness or a decreased level of physical activity. However, alterations in cardiac function usually are not apparent until severe malnutrition is present.

Alterations in the immune system (Table 131.2) represent an end-organ or functional response to malnutrition and may reflect a decline in lean body mass as well as a deficiency in specific nutrients such as zinc.[1,2] Clinically, this is manifested as an increased incidence of infection.

Malnutrition also has an adverse effect on wound healing. Although wounds have biologic priority and, thus, wound healing will occur at the expense of other tissues in the setting of protein-energy malnutrition (PEM), the rate at which the wound heals and the tensile strength of the wound are decreased.[3] Wound healing is further disrupted in the setting of malnutrition due to the increased incidence of wound infection from altered immunity. Deficiency of an individual nutrient may also affect wound healing. Those nutrients that are most critical to wound healing include arginine, copper, vitamin C, vitamin A, and zinc (Table 131.3). When given in pharmacologic doses, vitamin A and arginine have been shown to promote earlier wound healing.[3,4] Other nutrients, when ingested in excessive amounts, may impair wound healing. For example, excess vitamin E antagonizes the promotion of wound healing by vitamin A, and excess zinc will displace copper and interfere with lysyl oxidase (the enzyme necessary for collagen cross-link formation).[3]

Prevalence of Malnutrition

The recognition of malnutrition in the hospital setting resulted from astute clinical observation of the association of complications with clinically debilitated patients. The systematic application of nutrition assessment techniques to populations of hospitalized individuals has only come about in recent years. In the mid-1970s to mid-1980s, surveys of patients from varying socioeconomic backgrounds hospitalized in a variety of institutions on numerous specialty services detected a high prevalence (25–50%) of previously unrecognized malnutrition.[5–14] Several of these surveys also found an association between malnutrition and length of stay.[7,15–17] Recently, similar surveys have reported a 29–38% prevalence of malnutrition on admission to the hospital.[15,18] Although these data indicate minimal or no improvement in the nutrition status of patients on admission, Coats et al.[15] found that patients were less likely to develop malnutrition during hospitalization in 1993 when compared to their survey results reported in 1979. These authors conclude that the heightened awareness of nutritional disease has resulted in better in-hospital nutrition management and, hence, the lower prevalence of hospital-acquired malnutrition.

TABLE 131.1. END-ORGAN RESPONSES IN MALNUTRITION

Organ	Anatomic Responses	Physiologic Response
Heart	Four-chamber dilation; atrophic degeneration with necrosis and fibrosis; myofibrillar disruption	QT prolongation, low voltage, bradycardia; decreased cardiac output, stroke volume, and contractility; preload intolerance; diminished responsiveness to drugs
Lung	Emphysematous changes; pulmonary infarcts; reduced bacterial clearance; muscle atrophy	Pneumonia; decreases in functional residual capacity, vital capacity, and maximum breathing capacity; depressed hypoxic/hypercarbic drives
Hematologic system	Failure of stem-cell production; depressed erythropoietin synthesis; decreased PMN chemotaxis; decreased lymphocyte count with reduced helper T and increased suppressor T and killer cells; decreased blastogenesis to phytohemagglutinin	Anemia; anergy; decreased granuloma formation; impaired response to chemotherapy; increased infection rate
Renal system	Epithelial swelling; atrophy; mild cortical calcification	Reduced glomerular filtration rate and inability to handle sodium loads; polyuria; metabolic acidosis
Gastrointestinal tract	Disproportionate mass loss; hypoplastic and atrophic changes; decrease in total mucosal height	Depressed enzymatic activity; shortened transit time; impaired motility; propensity for bacterial overgrowth; maldigestion and malabsorption
Liver	Mass loss; periportal fat accumulation	Decreased visceral protein synthesis; depressed microsomal activity; eventual hepatic insufficiency

(From Cerra FB (ed.). Manual of Surgical Nutrition. St Louis, MO, CV Mosby, 1984, p 6, with permission.)

Disease-Specific Consequences of Malnutrition

Malnutrition seldom exists as an isolated disease state but rather is usually found in patients with other preexisting illnesses. Often the primary disease or complications of the disease predispose an individual to the development of malnutrition. The primary factors that contribute to the likelihood of developing malnutrition include decreased dietary intake (e.g., due to nausea, vomiting, anorexia), malabsorption (e.g., due to short bowel syndrome, severe diarrhea, high-output fistula), and altered metabolism (e.g., hypermetabolic and catabolic states due to sepsis, trauma, cancer, AIDS). Those disease states or clinical conditions which are most likely to have associated malnutrition are discussed below. Malnutrition is also associated with major

TABLE 131.2. IMMUNE RESPONSE MECHANISMS IN MALNUTRITION

Parameter	Observation in Malnutrition
Cell-Mediated Immune Response	
Delayed cutaneous hypersensitivity	Decreased
Lymphocyte transformation	Decreased
Polymorphonuclear leukocyte response	
Phagocytosis	Normal or decreased
Metabolism	Decreased
Bactericidal capacity	Decreased
Chemotaxis	Decreased
Total lymphocyte count	Decreased
T cells	
CD4+	Decreased
CD8+	Decreased
Helper: suppressor	Decreased
Humoral Response	
Complement activity (CH50)	Decreased
Secretory IgA	Decreased
Serum complement	Decreased or normal
Serum immunoglobulins	Normal
Serum opsonization	Normal

TABLE 131.3. NUTRITIONAL DISORDERS AND WOUND HEALING

Nutritional Disorder	Effect on Wound Healing
Arginine deficiency	Altered collagen formation
Copper deficiency	Impaired lysyl oxidase activity
Protein-energy malnutrition	Decreased wound strength via decreased hydroxyproline content of wound; decreased rate of wound healing; increased incidence of wound infection
Vitamin C deficiency	Decreased fibroblast maturation with failure of collagen synthesis; decreased angiogenesis
Vitamin A deficiency	Decreased collagen accumulation; formation of abnormal collagen
Zinc deficiency	Impaired DNA and protein synthesis; impaired mitosis and cell proliferation

organ failure, e.g., renal, hepatic, cardiac, and pulmonary failure and multisystem organ failure (see Chapter 136).

CANCER

Patients with cancer have many factors that contribute to the likelihood of developing malnutrition (Table 131.4). Malnutrition associated with cancer occurs with varying frequency depending on the type of cancer.[19] Data describing the frequency of weight loss in different types of cancer illustrate this variability (Table 131.5). A relationship between weight loss and survival has also been demonstrated (Table 131.6).[19] Theoretically, early recognition and management of malnutrition in cancer patients may minimize the nutritional consequences, improve tumor response to therapy, reduce side effects of therapy, and improve survival. Cancer patients treated with bone marrow transplantation have shown improved tumor response and clinical outcome with parenteral nutrition (PN) compared to control groups not receiving PN.[20] Malnutrition due to simple starvation, characterized by normal metabolism but inadequate nutrient intake or malabsorption, appears to be responsive to nutrition intervention.[21] However, malnutrition due to cancer cachexia, characterized by altered nutrient utilization in spite of adequate supply, does not.[22,23] Treatment of malnutrition due to cancer cachexia is controversial, especially in the absence of data showing an improved quality of life with nutrition therapy.

TABLE 131.4. RISK FACTORS FOR MALNUTRITION IN CANCER PATIENTS

Risk Factor	Nutritional Consequence
Primary Disease	
Tumor type	Weight loss, anorexia, altered taste, altered metabolism
Complicating Conditions	
Malabsorption	Impaired absorption of all or selected nutrients, diarrhea
Bowel obstruction	Nausea and vomiting, inability to ingest nutrients orally or by enteral nutrition
Infection	Increased energy expenditure and protein requirements, altered metabolism, anorexia, malabsorption
Psychological response	Anorexia, food aversion
Treatments	
Chemotherapy	Taste and appetite alterations, nausea and vomiting, mucositis, esophagitis, diarrhea, constipation
Surgery	
Radical resection of oropharyngeal region	Problems with chewing and swallowing
Esophageal reconstruction	Gastric stasis and hypochlorhydria secondary to vagotomy; diarrhea and steatorrhea
Gastrectomy	Dumping syndrome, malabsorption, lack of intrinsic factor, hypoglycemia
Intestinal resection	Malabsorption, renal oxilate stones, metabolic acidosis, diarrhea
Pancreatectomy	Malabsorption, diabetes mellitus
Radiation	
Head and neck	Stomatitis, dysgeusia, xerostomia
Abdomen and pelvis	Bowel obstruction, fistulae, radiation enteritis (diarrhea, protein-losing enteropathy, malabsorption)

TABLE 131.5. FREQUENCY OF WEIGHT LOSS IN CANCER PATIENTS

Tumor Type	Frequency of Weight Loss (% of patients with weight loss during the 6 months prior to diagnosis)
Measurable gastric	87
Nonmeasurable gastric	83
Pancreas	83
Lung, non–small cell	61
Lung, small cell	57
Prostate	56
Colon	54
Unfavorable non-Hodgkin's lymphoma	52
Sarcoma	40
Acute nonlymphocytic leukemia	39
Breast	36
Favorable non-Hodgkin's lymphoma	31

(Data adapted from Dewys WD, Begg C, Lavin PT, et al. Prognostic effect of weight loss prior to chemotherapy in cancer patients. Am J Med 1980;69:493, with permission.)

AIDS

One of the well-known characteristics of AIDS is the wasting and malnutrition that occur with the disease.[24] In many cases weight loss and wasting are the earliest symptoms along with opportunistic infection. The malnutrition is often progressive and may lead to death in some patients.[25,26] Poor nutrition status as indicated by weight loss and decreased serum albumin concentrations has been shown to be a predictor of survival in AIDS patients.[26–28] Many risk factors contribute to the seemingly inevitable malnutrition

TABLE 131.6. EFFECT OF WEIGHT LOSS ON SURVIVAL IN CANCER PATIENTS

	Median Survival (weeks)	
Tumor Type	No Weight Loss	Weight Loss
Measurable gastric	18	16
Nonmeasurable gastric	41	27[a]
Pancreas	14	12
Lung, non–small cell	20	14[a]
Lung, small cell	34	27[a]
Prostate	46	24[a]
Colon	43	21[a]
Unfavorable non-Hodgkin's lymphoma	107	55[a]
Sarcoma	46	25[a]
Acute nonlymphocytic leukemia	8	4
Breast	70	45[a]
Favorable non-Hodgkin's lymphoma	[b]	138

[a]A statistically significant difference in survival exists between patients without weight loss and patients with weight loss.
[b]At the time of publication, data were not available. (Data adapted from Dewys WD, Begg C, Lavin PT, et al. Prognostic effect of weight loss prior to chemotherapy in cancer patients. Am J Med 1980;69:493, with permission.)

in AIDS (Fig. 131.1), and the response to nutrition intervention has been variable. Kotler and associates[29] evaluated the effect of prolonged parenteral nutrition on body composition in 12 patients with AIDS. Body composition was determined by measuring total body potassium. All patients gained body weight and increased body fat content. However, body cell mass improved only in the 5 patients with altered intake or absorption. The 7 patients with systemic disease, e.g., systemic infection, did not have an improvement in body cell mass. Kottler and associates[30] have also demonstrated body-cell-mass repletion with enteral nutrition in AIDS patients with weight loss and inadequate food intake. In a retrospective review of home parenteral nutrition in 22 AIDS patients with weight loss greater than 10% of usual body weight, 15 patients gained weight, 6 stabilized, and 2 continued to lose weight.[31]

CRITICAL ILLNESS/TRAUMA/BURN INJURY

One of the characteristics of critical illness is hypermetabolism. Trauma, burn injury, and sepsis are all catalysts for the release of mediators that initiate and regulate the hypermetabolic response. The metabolic consequences of this mediator response include altered carbohydrate metabolism, increased protein synthesis and degradation, and increased lipid oxidation.[32] The result of hypermetabolism and altered substrate utilization is a loss of protein and lean body mass. In a previously well-nourished individual, critical illness can result in the rapid onset of kwashiorkor-like malnutrition within 3–5 days. In a previously malnourished individual, critical illness can precipitate severe mixed marasmus–kwashiorkor. The goal of nutrition support in this setting is to prevent the development or worsening of malnutrition. Studies indicate that enteral nutrition initiated within 24–48 hours of injury may attenuate the hypermetabolic response.[33,34] Enteral nutrition has also been shown to result in fewer septic complications when compared to parenteral nutrition.[35–38]

INFLAMMATORY BOWEL DISEASE

Inflammatory bowel disease (IBD) includes Crohn's disease and ulcerative colitis. Crohn's disease typically affects the terminal ileum but may occur anywhere in the gastrointestinal tract. Two-thirds to three-fourths of patients hospitalized with Crohn's disease are malnourished and exhibit weight loss, hypoalbuminemia, and vitamin deficiencies (Table 131.7).[39] Growth failure occurs in 15–40% of prepubertal patients and is characterized by retarded skeletal maturation (which may be irreversible) and delayed development of secondary sex characteristics.[40] The nutritional consequences of ulcerative colitis tend to be less severe than Crohn's disease. Approximately 25–50% of patients with ulcerative colitis are hypoalbuminemic and 2–20% experience growth failure. The specific factors contributing to the risk of malnutrition in IBD are numerous (Table 131.8).[39] Nutrition management of IBD may include enteral and/or parenteral nutrition.[41] Enteral is the preferred route except in patients with a high-output fistula or obstruction or if it exacerbates pain. Enteral or parenteral nutrition is likely to facilitate remission in 60–80% of patients with acute Crohn's disease. However, the course of ulcerative colitis is not influenced by the use of nutrition support, although nutrition status may be maintained in an acute exacerbation.

CHRONIC INTESTINAL PSEUDO-OBSTRUCTION

Pseudo-obstruction refers to a disorder of the gastrointestinal tract that presents with the symptoms of bowel obstruction but no mechanical obstruction exists. The cause is thought to be due to a neuromuscular disorder of the smooth muscle and/or its innervation, which leads to hypomotility or dysmotility. Prolonged dysmotility can result in malnutrition and also in growth failure in children.[42] The primary factors contributing to a risk of malnutrition are anorexia, nausea, vomiting, and obstruction which may recur over years. Approximately 15–30% of patients with pseudo-obstruction require nutrition support with either parenteral or enteral nutrition.[42]

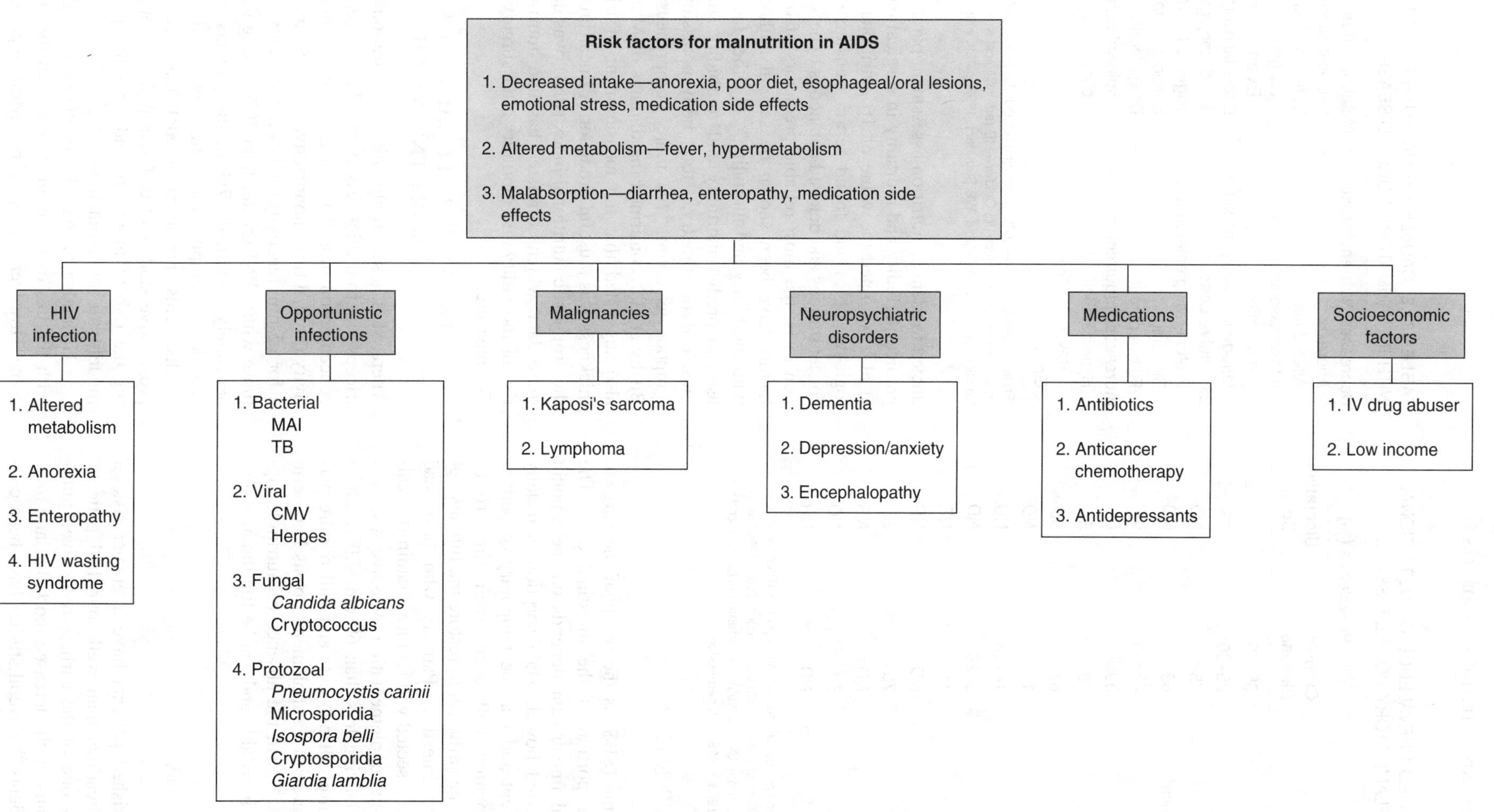

Figure 131.1. Risk factors for malnutrition in AIDS.

TABLE 131.7. REPORTED PREVALENCE OF NUTRITIONAL DEFICIENCIES IN INFLAMMATORY BOWEL DISEASE

	Prevalence (%)	
Deficiency	**Crohn's Disease**	**Ulcerative Colitis**
Weight loss	65–75	18–62
Hypoalbuminemia	25–80	25–50
Intestinal protein loss	75	ND
Negative nitrogen balance	69	ND
Anemia	25–85	66
Iron deficiency	39	81
Vitamin B_{12} deficiency	48	5
Folic acid deficiency	67	30–40
Calcium deficiency	13	ND
Magnesium deficiency	14–33	ND
Potassium deficiency	5–20	ND
Vitamin A deficiency	11	NR
Vitamin C deficiency	ND	NR
Vitamin D deficiency	75	35
Vitamin K deficiency	ND	NR
Zinc deficiency	50	ND
Copper deficiency	ND	NR

Key: ND, reported but incidence not described; NR, not reported. (From Afonso JJ, Rombeau JL. Parenteral nutrition for patients with inflammatory bowel disease, in Rombeau JL and Caldwell MD (eds): Clinical Nutrition: Parenteral Nutrition, 2nd ed. Philadelphia, WB Saunders, 1993, p 428, with permission.)

SHORT BOWEL SYNDROME

Short bowel syndrome (SBS) is the result of the surgical resection of a large portion of the intestinal tract. The degree of nutritional impairment depends on the amount and location of excised bowel. Malabsorption is usually present to some extent and may be temporary or permanent.[43] Bowel adaptation will occur over time (6–12 months) but may not be sufficient to restore the full absorptive capacity of the intestine. Patients who have had 100–200 cm of ileum resected will require vitamin B_{12}, calcium, and magnesium supplementation. Massive resection of the small bowel leaving less than 60 cm will result in severe malabsorption of all nutrients and will require parenteral nutrition on at least a supplemental basis long term or even permanently.[44,45] In the absence of nutrition support, malnutrition is inevitable and can be life threatening.

SURGICAL PATIENTS

In general, malnourished patients have a greater risk of postoperative complications than well-nourished patients. Loss of weight was one of the earliest recognized nutritional factors associated with increased morbidity and mortality in surgical patients.[46] Several studies have been conducted to identify nutrition assessment parameters that may predict morbidity and mortality in surgical patients. Mullen et al.[5] examined the value of 16 nutritional and immunologic variables and found serum transferrin and albumin concentrations and delayed cutaneous hypersensitivity reaction to be the most reliable predictors of outcome. These factors have been shown by several authors to correlate with morbidity and mortality.[47–50] Other factors have been used to predict mortality and morbidity such as forearm muscle dynamometry,[51] total body potassium,[52] and total lymphocyte count.[53] A more comprehensive study by Buzby et al.[52] confirmed the findings of Mullen et al.[5] and also suggested that the measurement of triceps skinfold thickness was a useful predictor. A linear predictive model, the prognostic nutritional index (PNI), was developed from these data, which correlated baseline nutrition status with risk of morbidity and mortality after surgery as a quantitative measure:

$$\text{PNI}\ (\%) = 158 - 1.66\ (\text{ALB}) - 0.78\ (\text{TSF}) - 0.02\ (\text{TFN}) - 5.8\ (\text{DH})$$

where ALB is serum albumin concentration (g/dL), TSF is triceps skinfold thickness (mm), TFN is serum transferrin concentration (mg/dL), and DH is maximal skin test reactivity (graded 0 for nonreactive, 1 for 5-mm reactivity, and 2 for >5-mm reactivity). High-risk patients were defined as those with a PNI greater than 50%. Using this model, they accurately identified 87% of the patients who developed significant complications and 96% of the postoperative deaths. This predictive model has been validated in prospective studies of different patient groups by comparing the risk of morbidity and mortality predicted by the model with actual outcome.[54–56]

No studies have evaluated the effect of altering the PNI with the use of nutrition support and the subsequent outcome. However, the use of preoperative parenteral nutrition

TABLE 131.8. CAUSES OF MALNUTRITION IN PATIENTS WITH INFLAMMATORY BOWEL DISEASE

Decreased Nutrient Intake	Malabsorption
Anorexia	Mucosal abnormalities
Altered taste	Diminished absorptive surface
Intake-associated pain or discomfort	Surgery
Iatrogenic dietary restrictions	Extensive disease
Excessive Losses	Bacterial overgrowth and bile
Protein-losing enteropathy	Salt deconjugation
Bleeding	**Iatrogenic Factors**
Fistula output	Surgical complications
Increased Requirements	Drugs (corticosteroids, sulfasalazine, cholestyramine)
Hypercatabolic states (fever, sepsis)	
Growth	

(From Afonso JJ, Rombeau JL. Parenteral nutrition for patients with inflammatory bowel disease, in Rombeau JL, Caldwell MD (eds): Clinical Nutrition: Parenteral Nutrition, 2nd ed. Philadelphia, WB Saunders, 1993, p 429, with permission.)

in patients with malnutrition, particularly when associated with a low albumin concentration, has been demonstrated to reduce the incidence of major postoperative complications in several patient populations.[49,57–60] Furthermore, early postoperative parenteral nutrition has been shown to improve convalescence coincident with improvement in nutritional status after esophagogastrectomy[61] and radical bladder cystectomy.[62] Conflicting data were found in the multi-institutional VA Cooperative Study.[63] This prospective, randomized clinical trial in 395 malnourished patients evaluated perioperative parenteral nutrition versus no perioperative parenteral nutrition. Nutrition status was defined by the nutrition risk index (NRI), which was based on serum albumin concentration and current weight relative to ideal body weight. A NRI of >97.5 was defined as borderline malnutrition, 83.5–97.5 as mild malnutrition, and <83.5 as severe malnutrition. Overall, the rates of postoperative complications at 30 and 90 days were similar in the parenteral nutrition and no parenteral nutrition groups. However, the types of complications in the two groups were different. The parenteral nutrition group had a higher incidence of infectious complications, and the no parenteral nutrition group had a higher incidence of noninfectious complications. Complications after stratification according to baseline nutrition status indicated that the incidence of noninfectious complications increased with increasing severity of malnutrition. In the parenteral nutrition group, the highest incidence of infectious complications was in the borderline or mildly malnourished patients. Differences in mortality at 30 and 90 days were not statistically significant. The overall conclusions from the study were that preoperative parenteral nutrition did not result in an improved postoperative course except in patients who were severely malnourished preoperatively. In patients who were mild to moderately malnourished, the incidence of infectious complications associated with the use of parenteral nutrition outweighed the benefits.

PEDIATRIC DISEASES

Regardless of the disease process, pediatric patients in general are at greater risk for nutritional disorders and the more severe consequences associated with malnutrition. Not only does the nutritional deficiency affect existing organs and cells, but it also impacts development and may result in permanent, irreversible damage.

Necrotizing enterocolitis (NEC) is a disease characterized by intestinal mucosal injury secondary to decreased mesenteric blood flow. NEC typically occurs in premature infants (<38 weeks gestational age), low birth weight infants (weighing <2500 grams) and in the first 1–10 days of life. The severe inflammation of the intestinal tract caused by the mucosal injury results in malabsorption of nutrients. Total bowel rest is the treatment of choice; hence, in order to prevent malnutrition, parenteral nutrition is indicated.[64] If NEC results in bowel performation or necrosis of the bowel, surgery is required to resect the injured portion of the bowel. SBS may be a consequence if a large portion of bowel is resected, and long-term home parenteral nutrition will be required.[64]

The predominant clinical findings of cystic fibrosis (CF) are related to altered pulmonary function and altered pancreatic exocrine function. Growth retardation and failure to thrive are classic features of CF. The factors that contribute to the nutritional disorders associated with CF include an increased energy expenditure, malabsorption, anorexia, and treatments with medications and pulmonary toilet.[65] Increased energy requirements in CF patients are the result of the increased amount of work required to breath. In addition to this factor, the CF patient may have frequent respiratory infections, which further exacerbate the work of breathing and may create a hypermetabolic response. It is also theorized that the genetic defect that causes CF affects metabolism, causing an increase in energy requirements. The altered pancreatic function of CF manifested as pancreatic insufficiency occurs in about 85% of patients with CF. There is an insufficiency of the enzymes normally secreted by the pancreas into the intestines which are necessary for digestion. This primarily affects the absorption of fat and fat-soluble vitamins. The treatment of CF patients includes "pulmonary toilet." This treatment is the physical pounding on the back of the patient while in a partially inverted position in an attempt to loosen the thickened bronchial secretions which impair breathing. It may be performed numerous times throughout the day and may result in an increase in energy expenditure. It also interferes with the feeding schedule, which needs to be designed to ensure that the stomach is empty or nearly empty before the pulmonary toilet begins in order to prevent pulmonary aspiration of stomach contents. Finally, the disease itself contributes to the development of anorexia in patients with CF. Nutritional management typically focuses on the use of oral pancreatic enzymes (e.g., Viokase, Pancrease), supplemental fat-soluble vitamins, and a high-protein, high-calorie diet.[65] If nutrition status cannot be maintained with these measures, supplemental enteral or parenteral nutrition may be indicated.

Chronic protracted diarrhea of infancy is a major cause of fluid and electrolyte imbalance as well as malnutrition in infants younger than 3 months of age. Chronic protracted diarrhea of infancy is defined as persistent diarrhea for more than 2 weeks with stool cultures negative for enteropathogens. The primary factor contributing to the risk of malnutrition is malabsorption.[66] The extent of malabsorption will depend on the severity of the diarrhea and the underlying cause. The child may also develop anorexia due to the relationship between eating and the onset of the diarrhea. Nutrition support, enterally or parenterally as tolerated, is indicted to prevent malnutrition and consequent growth failure.[66]

Management of Malnutrition

The increased awareness of the prevalence and significance of untreated protein-calorie malnutrition has provided a strong clinical incentive for a more rigorous approach to identifying abnormalities of nutrition status and for the nutrition support of malnourished patients. A stepwise approach to nutrition management is recommended (Fig. 131.2).[67] In general, if nutrition assessment (see Chapter 130) reveals no malnutrition, then the patient should merely be counseled on appropriate maintenance goals for nutritional intake. If mild to moderate malnutrition is present, an anabolic feeding regimen should be initiated using oral supplements. If anorexia is a major contributing factor, enteral

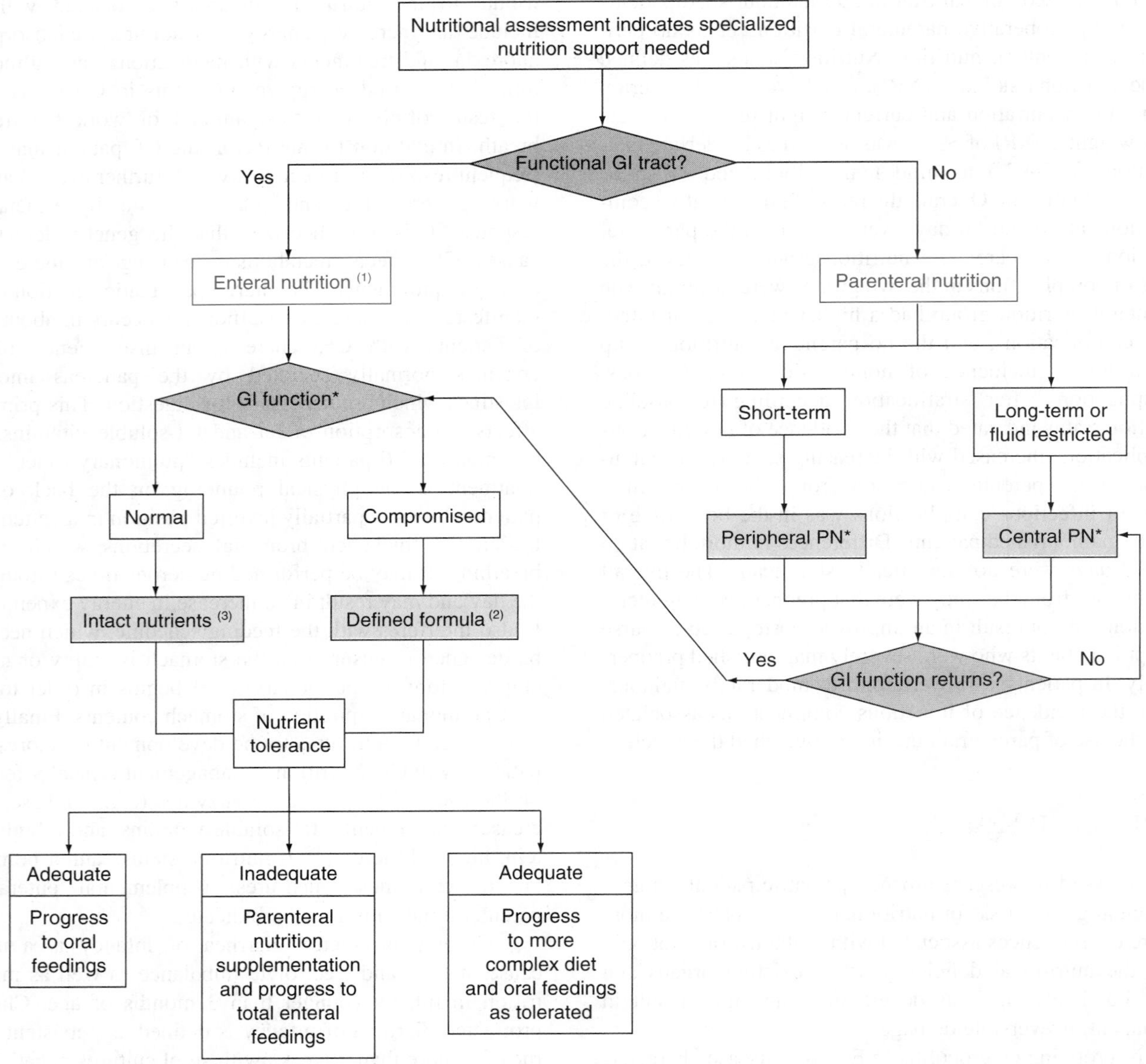

Figure 131.2. Clinical decision algorithm: route of nutrition support. *(From ASPEN Board of Directors. Section III: Routes to deliver nutrition support in adults. J Parenter Enter Nutr 1993;17(suppl):7SA, with permission.)*

tube feeding may be indicated. If malabsorption is a major contributing factor, tube feeding using a disease-specific formula or, alternatively, supplemental or total parenteral nutrition may be indicated. In the presence of severe malnutrition an anabolic feeding regimen should be initiated either enterally or parenterally depending on intestinal function and malabsorption. Routine reevaluation of the response to nutrition therapy and attainment of nutrition goals should be incorporated into the overall patient care plan.

Economic Consequences of Malnutrition

Malnourished patients have increased complications during their hospital course, an increased length of stay (LOS), and increased health care costs.[15–17] They are among the 10% of patients who disproportionately consume health care resources.[68] Robinson and associates[16] conducted a prospective study of 100 general medical patients with similar "diagnosis severity" based on diagnosis-related groups (DRGs) to determine the relationship between nutrition status on admission to the hospital and length of stay and hospital costs. Nutrition status was defined using dietary history, history of weight loss, anthropometrics, visceral protein measurements, and delayed cutaneous hypersensitivity. Forty of the 100 patients were identified as malnourished, 44 were well-nourished, and 16 were borderline. The diagnoses of malnutrition included kwashiorkor (12 patients), marasmus (1 patient), and mixed kwashiorkor–marasmus (27 patients). Malnourished patients had a significantly prolonged LOS compared to normal or borderline patients (Table 131.9). Hospital charges were also significantly greater in the malnourished patients than the normal patients (Table 131.9).

In a retrospective study, Reilly and associates[17] evaluated the effect of the likelihood of malnutrition (LOM) at admission on hospital length of stay, costs, and charges in medical and surgical patients. LOM was determined using dietary history of inadequate intake, physical examination, height for weight measurement <80% of ideal body weight, serum albumin concentration ≤3.5 g/dL, and total lymphocyte count <1500 mm^3. The presence of any one of the objective, subjective, or historical criteria was cause for LOM. LOM was present in 59% of the medical patients and 48% of the surgical patients on admission. Across all major medical and surgical DRGs, patients with a LOM had a greater LOS than patients with no LOM. Consequently, hospital charges which were also converted to direct variable costs were greater for patients with LOM than with no LOM.

While the evidence is strong that malnutrition is associated with increased health care costs, little data exist to define the cost–benefit or cost savings of nutrition intervention. Based on assumptions derived from the literature, Twomey and Patching[69] concluded that preoperative parenteral nutrition could be cost saving in patients undergoing surgery for gastrointestinal cancer. A similar conclusion applied to a broader patient population is supported by a model that examines the financial implications of malnutrition and nutrition therapy.[68] This model takes into consideration the increased costs associated with an increased LOS, morbidity and mortality due to malnutrition as well as the costs of identifying patients at risk for malnutrition, providing nutrition support, and managing the complications associated with the nutrition support.

Patient Outcomes

While the cost–benefit debate goes unresolved, the issue which seems clear is that malnutrition is associated with a significant morbidity and mortality in numerous disease states and clinical settings. Furthermore, it is likely that improved patient outcomes can be achieved by a systematic approach to the early recognition of risk factors for malnutrition, the diagnosis of malnutrition and its nutritional management.[70] The pharmacist's responsibilities in the management of nutrition disease include the following:

1. Assist in identifying patients at risk for malnutrition and/or candidates for nutrition intervention.

TABLE 131.9. IMPACT OF NUTRITION STATUS ON LENGTH OF STAY (LOS) AND HOSPITAL CHARGES

	Malnourished	Normal	Borderline
Actual LOS (days) mean ± SEM	15.6 ± 2.2[a]	8.2 ± 0.7	10.2 ± 1.7
Allowed LOS (days) mean ± SEM	10.7 ± 0.6	10.0 ± 0.6	10.3 ± 1.0
Hospital charges mean ± SEM	$16,691 ± 4389[a]	$7692 ± 687	$14,118 ± 4962[a]
DRG allowance mean ± SEM	$4631 ± 238	$4352 ± 222	$5124 ± 852

[a]$p < 0.01$ by analysis of variance. (Adapted from Robinson G, Goldstein M, Levine GM. Impact of nutritional status on DRG length of stay. J Parenter Enter Nutr 1987;11:49–51, with permission.)

2. Assist in the design of patient-specific nutrition support regimens.
3. Evaluate and manage all drug–nutrient interactions.
4. Evaluate laboratory data, especially parameters used to determine safety and efficacy of nutrition support.

REFERENCES

1. Chandra RK. Nutrition and immunity: Lessons from the past and new insights into the future. Am J Clin Nutr 1991;53:1087–1101.
2. Bower RH. Nutrition and immune function. Nutr Clin Prac 1990;5:189–195.
3. Albina JE. Nutrition and wound healing. J Parenter Enter Nutr 1994;18:367–376.
4. Orgill D, Demling RH. Current concepts and approaches to wound healing. Crit Care Med 1988;16:8899–8908.
5. Mullen JL, Gertner MH, Buzby GP, et al. Implications of malnutrition in the surgical patient. Arch Surg 1979;114:121–125.
6. Bistrian BR, Blackburn GL, Hallowell E, Heddle R. Protein status of general surgical patients. JAMA 1974;230:858–860.
7. Weinsier RL, Hunker EM, Krumdieck CL, Butterworth CE. Hospital malnutrition: A prospective evaluation of general medical patients during the course of hospitalization. Am J Clin Nutr 1979;32:418–426.
8. Bistrian BR, Blackburn GL, Vitale J, et al. Prevalence of malnutrition in general medical patients. JAMA 1976;235:1567–1570.
9. O'Leary JP, Dunn GD, Basil S, et al. Incidence of malnutrition among patients admitted to a VA hospital. South Med J 1982;75:1095–1098.
10. Willard MD, Gilsdorf RB, Price RA. Protein-calorie malnutrition in a community hospital. JAMA 1980;243:1720–1722.
11. Merritt RJ, Suskind RM. Nutritional survey of hospitalized pediatric patients. Am J Clin Nutr 1979;32:1320–1325.
12. Guarnieri G. Nutritional assessment in hospital malnutrition. J Parenter Enter Nutr 1987;11:34S–35S.
13. Kamath SK, Lawler M, Smith AE, Olson R. Hospital malnutrition: A 33-hospital screening study. JADA 1986;86:203–206.
14. Reinhardt GR, Mayscofski JW, Wilkens BD, et al. Incidence and mortality of hypoalbuminemic patients in hospitalized veterans. J Parenter Enter Nutr 1980;4:357–359.
15. Coats KG, Morgan SL, Bartolucci AA, Weinsier RL. Hospital-associated malnutrition: A re-evaluation 12 years later. JADA 1993;93:27–33.
16. Robinson G, Goldstein M, Levine GM. Impact of nutritional status on DRG length of stay. J Parenter Enter Nutr 1987;11:49–51.
17. Reilly JJ, Hull SF, Albert N, et al. Economic impact of malnutrition: A model system for hospitalized patients. J Parenter Enter Nutr 1988;12:371–376.
18. Sayarath VG. Nutrition screening for malnutrition: Potential economic impact at a community hospital. JADA 1993;93:1440–1442.
19. Dewys WD, Begg C, Lavin PT, et al. Prognostic effect of weight loss prior to chemotherapy in cancer patients. Am J Med 1980;69:491–497.
20. Weisdorf SA, Lysne J, Wind D, et al. Positive effect of prophylactic total parenteral nutrition on long-term outcome of bone marrow transplantation. Transplantation 1987;43:833–838.
21. Klein S, Simes J, Blackburn G. TPN and cancer clinical trials. Cancer 1986;58:1378–1386.
22. Brennan MF. Uncomplicated starvation versus cancer cachexia. Cancer Res 1977;37:2359–2364.
23. Kern KA, Norton JA. Cancer cachexia. J Parent Enter Nutr 1988;12:286–298.
24. Raiten DJ. Nutrition and HIV. Nutr Clin Pract 1991;6(suppl):16S–52S.
25. ASPEN Board of Directors. Acquired immune deficiency syndrome. J Parenter Enter Nutr 1993;17(suppl):13SA–14SA.
26. Kotler D, Tierney A, Wang J, et al. Magnitude of body-cell-mass depletion and the timing of death from wasting in AIDS. Am J Clin Nutr 1989;50:444–447.
27. Chlebowski RT, Grosvenor MB, Bernhard NH, et al. Nutritional status, gastrointestinal dysfunction, and survival in patients with AIDS. Am J Gastroent 1989;84:1288–1292.
28. Trujillo EB, Borlase BC, Bell SJ, et al. Assessment of nutritional status, nutrient intake, and nutrition support in AIDS patients. JADA 1992;92:477–478.
29. Kotler DP, Tierney AR, Culpepper-Morgan JA, et al. Effect of home total parenteral nutrition on body composition in patients with acquired immuno-deficiency syndrome. J Parenter Enter Nutr 1990;14:454–458.
30. Kotler DP, Tierney AR, Ferraro R, et al. Enteral alimentation and repletion of body cell mass in malnourished patients with acquired immunodeficiency syndrome. Am J Clin Nutr 1991;53:149–154.
31. Singer P, Rothkopf MM, Kvetan V, et al. Risks and benefits of home parenteral nutrition in the acquired immunodeficiency syndrome. J Parenter Enter Nutr 1991;15:75–79.
32. Barton RG. Nutrition support in critical illness. Nutr Clin Prac 1994;9:127–139.
33. Peterson VM, Moore EE, Jones TN, et al. Total enteral nutrition versus total parenteral nutrition after major torso injury: Attenuation of hepatic protein reprioritization. Surgery 1988;104:199–207.
34. Chiarelli A, Enzi G, Casadei A, et al. Very early nutrition supplementation in burned patients. Am J Clin Nutr 1990;51:1035–1039.
35. Moore EE, Jones TN. Benefits of immediate jejunostomy feeding after major abdominal trauma—a prospective, randomized study. J Trauma 1986;26:874–881.
36. Moore FA, Moore EE, Jones TN, et al. TEN versus TPN following major abdominal trauma—reduced septic morbidity. J Trauma 1989;29:916–923.
37. Moore FA, Feliciano DV, Andrassy RJ, et al. Early enteral feeding, compared with parenteral, reduces postoperative septic complications. The results of a meta-analysis. Ann Surg 1992;216:172–183.
38. Kudsk KA, Croce MA, Fabian TC, et al. Enteral versus parenteral feeding. Effects on septic morbidity after blunt and penetrating abdominal trauma. Ann Surg 1992;215:503–513.

39. Afonso JJ, Rombeau JL. Parenteral nutrition for patients with inflammatory bowel disease, in Rombeau JL, Caldwell MD (eds): Clinical Nutrition: Parenteral Nutrition, 2nd ed. Philadelphia, WB Saunders, 1993, pp 427–441.
40. Seidman EG, LeLeiko N, Ament M, et al. Nutritional issues in pediatric inflammatory bowel disease. Symposium report. J Pediatr Gastroenterol Nutr 1991;12:424–438.
41. ASPEN Board of Directors. Inflammatory bowel disease. J Parenter Enter Nutr 1993;17(suppl):18SA–20SA, 45SA.
42. Vargas JH, Sachs P, Ament ME. Chronic intestinal pseudo-obstruction syndrome in pediatrics. Results of a national survey by members of the North American Society for Pediatric Gastroenterology and Nutrition. J Pediatr Gastroenterol Nutr 1988;7:323–332.
43. Allard JP, Jeejeebuoy KN. Nutritional support and therapy in the short bowel syndrome. Gastroenterol Clin North Am 1989;18:5899–5901.
44. Bernard DKH, Shaw MJ. Principles of nutrition therapy for short-bowel syndrome. Nutr Clin Prac 1993;8:153–162.
45. ASPEN Board of Directors. Short bowel syndrome. J Parent Enter Nutr 1993;17(suppl):19SA–20SA.
46. Studley HO. Percentage of weight loss: A basic indicator of surgical risk in patients with chronic septic ulcer. JAMA 1936;106:458–460.
47. Rudman D, Feller AB, Nagraj HS, et al. Relation of serum albumin concentration to death rate in nursing home men. J Parenter Enter Nutr 1987;11:360–363.
48. Meakins JL, Pietsch JB, Bubenick O, et al. Delayed hypersensitivity: An indicator of acquired failure of host defenses in sepsis and trauma. Ann Surg 1977;186:241–250.
49. Harvey KB, Ruggiero JA, Regan CS, et al. Hospital morbidity–mortality risk factors using nutritional assessment. J Clin Nutr 1978;26:251–257.
50. Kaminsky MV, Fitzgerald MJ, Murphy RJ, et al. Correlation of mortality with serum transferrin and anergy. J Parenter Enter Nutr 1977;1(4):27A.
51. Kalfarentzos F, Spiliotis J, Velimezis G, et al. Comparison of forearm muscle dynamometry with nutritional prognostic index, as a preoperative indicator in cancer patients. J Parenter Enter Nutr 1989;13:34–46.
52. Buzby GP, Mullen JL, Mathews DC, et al. Prognostic nutritional index in gastrointestinal surgery. Am J Surg 1980;139:160–166.
53. Halliday AW, Benjamin IS, Blumgart LH. Nutritional risk factors in major hepatobiliary surgery. J Parenter Enter Nutr 1988;12:43–48.
54. Yamanaka H, Nishi M, Kanemaki T, et al. Preoperative nutritional assessment to predict postoperative complication in gastric cancer patients. J Parenter Enter Nutr 1989;13:286–291.
55. Smale BF, Mullen JL, Buzby GP, Rosato EF. The efficacy of nutritional assessment and support in cancer surgery. Cancer 1981;47:2375–2381.
56. Dempsey DT, Buzby GP, Mullen JL. Nutritional assessment in the seriously ill patient. J Am Coll Nutr 1983;2:15–23.
57. Holler AR, Fischer JE. The effects of perioperative hyperalimentation on complications in patients with carcinoma and weight loss. J Surg Res 1977;23:31–34.
58. Mullen JL, Buzby GP, Mathews DC, et al. Reduction of operative morbidity and mortality by combined preoperative and postoperative nutritional support. Ann Surg 1981;192:604–613.
59. Muller JM, Brenner U, Dienst C, et al. Preoperative parenteral feeding in patients with gastrointestinal carcinoma. Lancet 1982;1:68–71.
60. Starker PM, Lasala PA, Askanazi J, et al. The response to TPN—a form of nutritional assessment. Ann Surg 1983;198:720–724.
61. Moghissi K, Hornshaw J, Teasdale PR, Dawes EA. Parenteral nutrition in carcinoma of the oesophagus treated by surgery: Nitrogen balance and clinical studies. Br J Surg 1977;64:125–128.
62. Askanazi J, Starker PM, Olsson C, et al. Effect of immediate postoperative nutritional support on length of hospitalization. Ann Surg 1986;203:236–239.
63. The Veterans Affairs Total Parenteral Nutrition Cooperative Study Group. Perioperative total parenteral nutrition. N Engl J Med 1991;325:525–532.
64. ASPEN Board of Directors. Necrotizing enterocolitis. J Parent Enter Nutr 1993;17(suppl):SA37.
65. Ramsay BW, Farrell PM, Penchartz P, et al. Consensus report: Nutritional assessment and management of cystic fibrosis. Am J Clin Nutr 1992;55:108–116.
66. Kleinman RE, Galeano NF, Ghishan F, et al. Nutritional management of chronic diarrhea and/or malabsorption. J Pediatr Gastroenterol Nutr 1989;9:407–415.
67. ASPEN Board of Directors. Routes to deliver nutrition support in adults. J Parenter Enter Nutr 1993;17(suppl):7SA–11SA.
68. Bernstein LH, Shaw-Stiffel TA, Schorow M, Brouillette R. Financial implications of malnutrition. Clin Lab Med 1993;13:491–507.
69. Twomey PL, Patching SC. Cost-effectiveness of nutritional support. J Parenter Enter Nutr 1985;9:3–10.
70. ASPEN Board of Directors. Rationale for adult nutrition support guidelines. J Parenter Enter Nutr 1993;17(suppl):5SA–6SA.

Chapter 132

Nutrient Metabolism and Regulation

Jay M. Mirtallo, MS, RPh, FASHP, BCNSP

Nutrition is defined as a function of living plants and animals, consisting of the taking in and assimilation of material through chemical changes (metabolism) whereby tissue is built up and energy liberated. Its successive stages, that is, metabolism, are known as digestion, absorption, assimilation, and excretion. In humans, digestion is preceded by mastication and deglutition. Excretion is effected by expiration, perspiration, urination, and defecation.[1] Not all of the materials involved with human metabolism can be synthesized by the body. Therefore, these essential materials—nutrients—must be provided by the diet.

Malnutrition is either primary (lack of food) or conditioned (potentially adequate diet but inefficient nutrient utilization related to chronic or acute disease and its treatment).[2] As a result of the multiplicity of variables causing conditioned malnutrition, this form is more complicated to manage successfully but, unfortunately, is the most common type of malnutrition encountered in clinical practice. Nutritional therapeutics is defined as management of the nutritional state of the patient. The purpose of nutritional therapeutics is the prevention, recognition, and management of malnutrition during the course of medical and pharmacologic management of disease.

The information required to practice nutritional therapeutics is not easily retained by most, even by those specializing in this area of professional practice. This chapter summarizes those principles of nutrient metabolism most frequently encountered by the clinical pharmacist and is intended to be comprehensive but not totally inclusive. As such, this chapter provides a scientific and biochemical basis for the clinically oriented chapters in this section. It is organized as energy metabolism, normal metabolism, and malnutrition including starvation, stress, and altered metabolism of nutrients in specific diseases.

Energy Metabolism

The body needs a constant source of fuel (energy) for growth and maintenance. The major function of metabolic pathways is to process this fuel into energy that can be used for synthetic reactions, for locomotion, for pumping ions or molecules against concentration gradients, and for other cell processes.[3] Energy is most commonly stored and provided by the high energy phosphate bond, that is, adenosine triphosphate (ATP, Fig. 132.1). Energy is stored in the two terminal high-energy phosphate bonds and is released or transferred to support reactions requiring energy. Most of the high-energy phosphate available to the cells is produced in the mitochondria[3] via the citric acid cycle, also known as the trichloroacetic acid (TCA) or Krebs cycle. The production of ATP requires adequate amounts of oxygen, acetyl coenzyme A (Fig. 132.2), and the presence of adenosine diphosphate (ADP). Thus, the presence of ADP in the mitochondria increases oxygen consumption, with the production of 3 ATP molecules per molecule of oxygen consumed. This is accomplished via the citric acid cycle as illustrated in Fig. 132.3. During the complete oxidation of the acetyl group of acetyl coenzyme A, the high-energy yield is 12 molecules of ATP. The source of the ATP is the conversion of acetyl coenzyme A to oxaloacetate (1 ATP), three NADH via oxidative phosphorylation (9 ATP), and oxidative phosphorylation of ubiquinone (2 ATP).[4] Note that one NADH yields 3 molecules of ATP during oxidative phosphorylation. This occurs when there is a perfect coupling of oxidation and phosphorylation, and consumes 4 molecules of oxygen.[4] "Uncoupled" oxidative phosphorylation occurs when the electron transfers in the mitochondria are dissociated from phosphorylation, thereby impairing the supply of ATP. This causes an increased oxygen consumption without a further increase in ATP production or utilization.[3]

High-energy bonds are only generated from the citric acid cycle within the cell. The conversion of glucose to pyruvate during oxidation reactions is a source of cellular ATP, as are anaerobic sources via the Cori cycle[3] as discussed later. Nutrient sources of fuel for energy metabolism (production of ATP) are fat, carbohydrate, and protein. The biochemical processes by which these fuel sources are used by the body to produce ATP are discussed in the next sections.

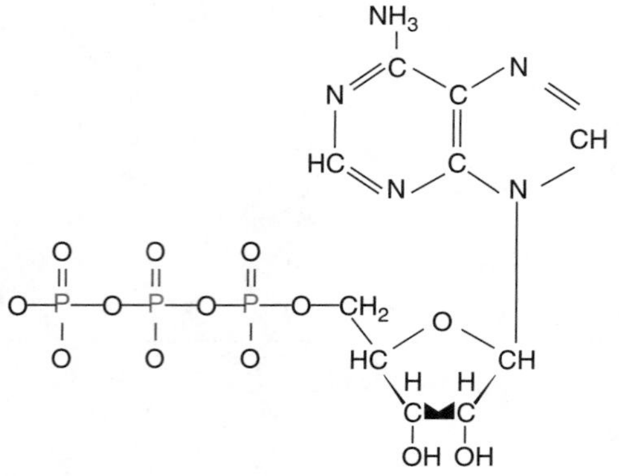

Figure 132.1. Structure of adenosine triphosphate (ATP).

FAT METABOLISM

The major storage form of energy in the body is in adipose (fat) tissue.[5] This endogenous source of energy is of significance during periods of starvation and stress, when it is used as a major fuel for the preservation of life.

Fat oxidation occurs when free fatty acids (FFAs) are present within the cell. Rapid uptake of FFAs by various cells occurs by diffusion across cell membranes. Another source of intracellular FFAs is the hydrolysis of triglycerides (Fig. 132.4). Once within the cell cytosol, FFAs are converted to long-chain acyl coenzyme A and transported into the mitochondria along with carnitine.[6] Acyl coenzyme A (Fig. 132.5) differs from acetyl coenzyme A in that an acyl (derived from the fatty acid) group, rather than an acetyl group, is attached to the coenzyme A molecule. Once formed within the cell, acyl coenzyme A requires transport into the mitochondria for beta-oxidation and ultimately ATP production. As the mitochondrial membrane is nearly impermeable to coenzyme A (CoA) and its derivatives, carnitine is required to facilitate transport of acyl CoA into the mitochondrial matrix in the following manner (Fig. 132.6). Carnitine at the inner surface of the mitochondrial membrane picks up the acyl groups of acyl CoA and transports these to the mitochondrial matrix, where acyl carnitine equilibrates with CoA to form acyl CoA within the mitochondria. The transfer of acyl groups is governed by carnitine palmitoyl transferase and is facilitated by a carnitine-O-acylcarnitine antiport carrier.[6] An antiport car-

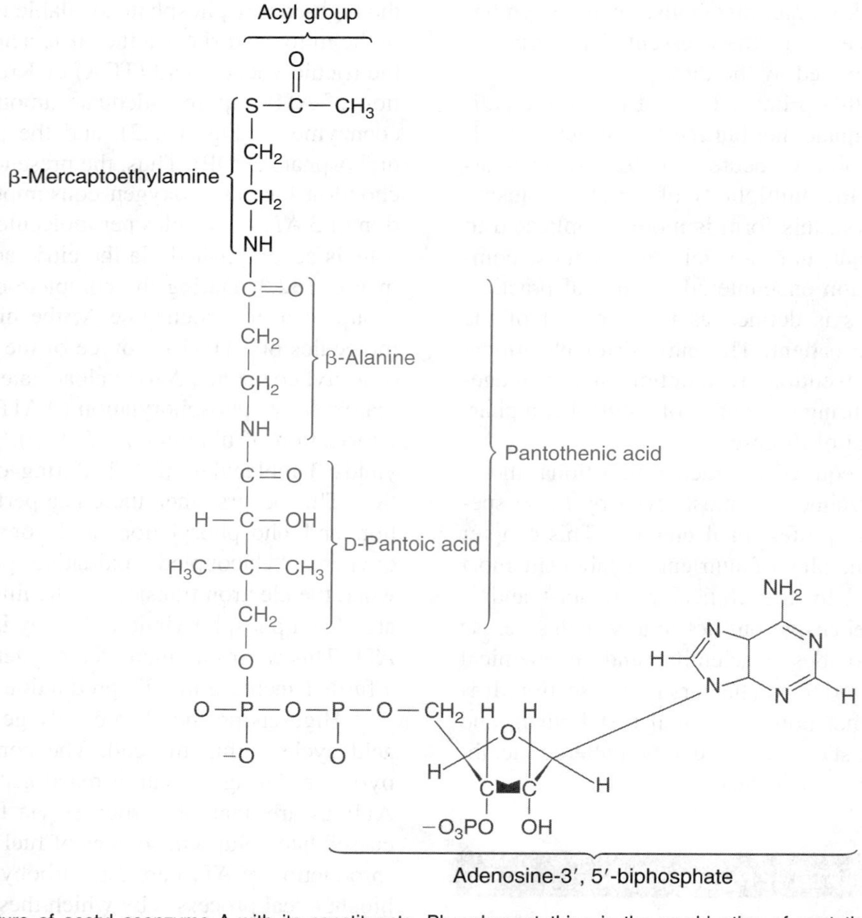

Figure 132.2. Structure of acetyl coenzyme A with its constituents. Phosphopantethine is the combination of pantothenic acid and beta-mercaptoethylamine.[4] *(From McGilvey, RW [ed]. Biochemistry, A Functional Approach, 3rd ed. Philadelphia, WB Saunders, 1983, p. 423, with permission.)*

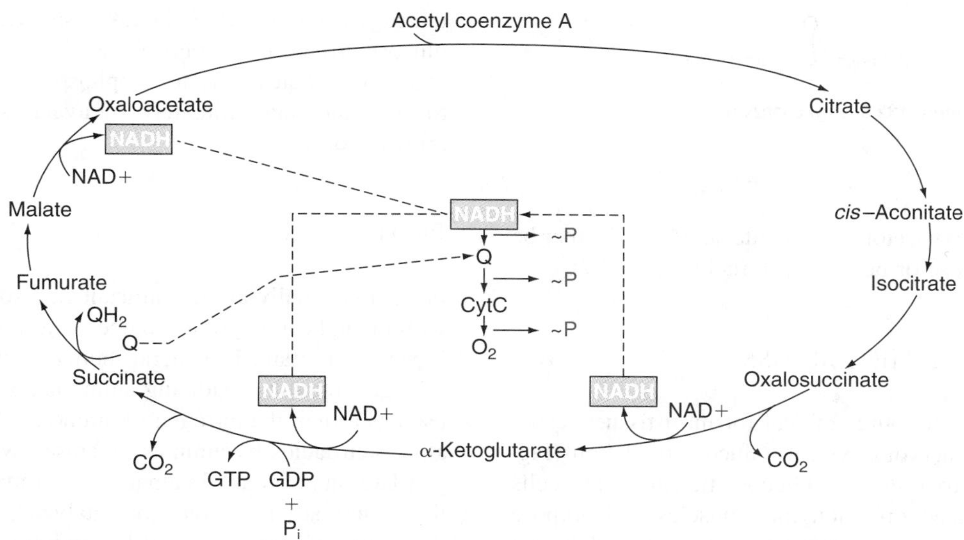

Figure 132.3. The citric acid cycle. The enzymes required for the citric acid cycle are present in the aqueous phase of the mitochondria and are responsible for the transfer of the energy of the carbon–hydrogen bonds from acetyl coenzyme A to specific carriers; NADH enters the solid phase of the mitochondria where the energy is converted into high-energy phosphate through the process of oxidative phosphorylation. In the oxidation of succinate to fumurate, flavin adenine dinucleotide is a coenzyme that transfers electrons directly to ubiquinone (Q) thereby bypassing the first phosphorylation site of oxidative phosphorylation.[3,4]

rier facilitates the movement of two compounds, each in opposite direction to the other (see Fig. 132.6). This carnitine-dependent transport is required only for long-chain fatty acids, because shorter chain (4–12 carbons) fatty acids are sufficiently water soluble to pass freely across membranes.[5] The short-chain fatty acids are then acted on by butyl CoA synthetase for further oxidation within the mitochondria.

Once inside the mitochondrial matrix, beta-oxidation—the process by which acyl CoA is reduced by two carbons to form acetyl CoA—occurs. Each acetyl CoA molecule may then enter the citric acid cycle. For palmitate, the most abundantly used fatty acid for oxidation, a total of five high-energy phosphate bonds are generated per molecule of acetyl CoA cleaved through beta-oxidation of the fatty acid (acyl) CoA and its residual parts. This occurs before energy (ATP) production by the acetyl CoA via the citric acid cycle.[5] Oxidation of fatty acids differs in the following ways:

1. *Saturated fatty acids:* Carbons are cleaved two at a time until the entire fatty acid is used to produce acetyl CoA.
2. *Odd-numbered fatty acids:* Oxidation results in a three-carbon fragment (proprionyl CoA), which does not yield substantial energy when metabolized.
3. *Unsaturated fatty acids:* Oxidation follows the general route of saturated fatty acids, with the addition of two more reactions: the isomerization of the double bond and racematization of a D-isomer product of unsaturated fatty acid oxidation to its metabolically active L-isomer.

The short-chain fatty acids (SCFAs)—acetate, propionate, and butyrate—are produced during metabolism of pyruvate (generated during glucose oxidation via the Embden–Meyerhof pathway, Fig. 132.7). A major source of glucose in the colon is the bacterial fermentation of carbohydrate. Carbohydrates reach the colon in three forms: (1) nonstarch polysaccharides such as dietary fiber, including that found in some enteral nutrition products; (2) starch polysaccharides; and (3) simple carbohydrates that avoided absorption in the small bowel. The quantity of SCFAs produced in the colon is dependent on anaerobic bacterial activity and the amount and type of dietary fiber ingested. Once produced, SCFAs are metabolized by cecal and colonic mucosal epithelial cells and may contribute from 5–30% of the daily energy requirements.[7]

Glycerol, which is released by the hydrolysis of fats, is another source of energy derived from fat. It may be taken up by the liver and converted to glycerol 3-phosphate by a reaction catalyzed by a glycerokinase. This glycerol 3-phosphate may then be used to form new triglycerides or

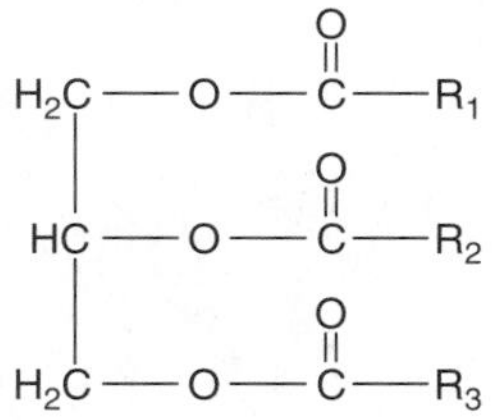

$H_2C—O—C(=O)—R_1$
$HC—O—C(=O)—R_2$
$H_2C—O—C(=O)—R_3$

Figure 132.4. Chemical structure of triglycerides. R_1, R_2, and R_3 are fatty acids. Mono- and diglycerides contain one or two fatty acids, respectively.

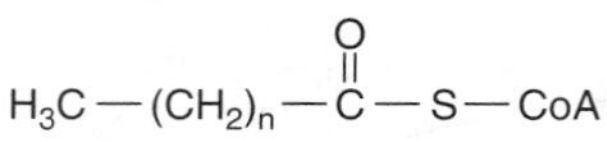

$$H_3C-(CH_2)_n-\overset{\overset{\displaystyle O}{\|}}{C}-S-CoA$$

Figure 132.5. Acyl coenzyme A.

add to the dihydroxyacetone phosphate supply and either be converted to glucose or be used as a fuel (Fig. 132.7).[6]

CARBOHYDRATE METABOLISM

Glucose is the major source of fuel for most tissues; especially the central nervous system. Glucose oxidation (Fig. 132.7) occurs in four steps.[8,9] Glucose transport into cells occurs by facilitated diffusion into muscles and adipose tissue in a reaction that is governed by insulin. Glucose phosphorylation, a process that uses 1 mole of ATP, is regulated by the enzyme, hexokinase. The phosphorylated glucose, fructose 1,6-phosphate, then splits to yield two triose phosphates. The triose phosphate is then converted to pyruvate and ultimately pyruvate is oxidized in the mitochondria.

PROTEIN AS A FUEL

Protein is usually an insignificant fuel source as compared with fat and carbohydrate sources, but in some conditions it is very important. In general, humans obtain only 10% of ATP generated by oxidizing amino acids (protein).[10] When used as a fuel, the nitrogen of amino acids is transferred to alpha-keto acids by aminotransferases. Much of this nitrogen later appears as glutamate, which may undergo oxidative deamination, in a reaction catalyzed by glutamate dihydrogenase. Carbon atoms of the amino acids are processed to make other constituents and appear as either carbon

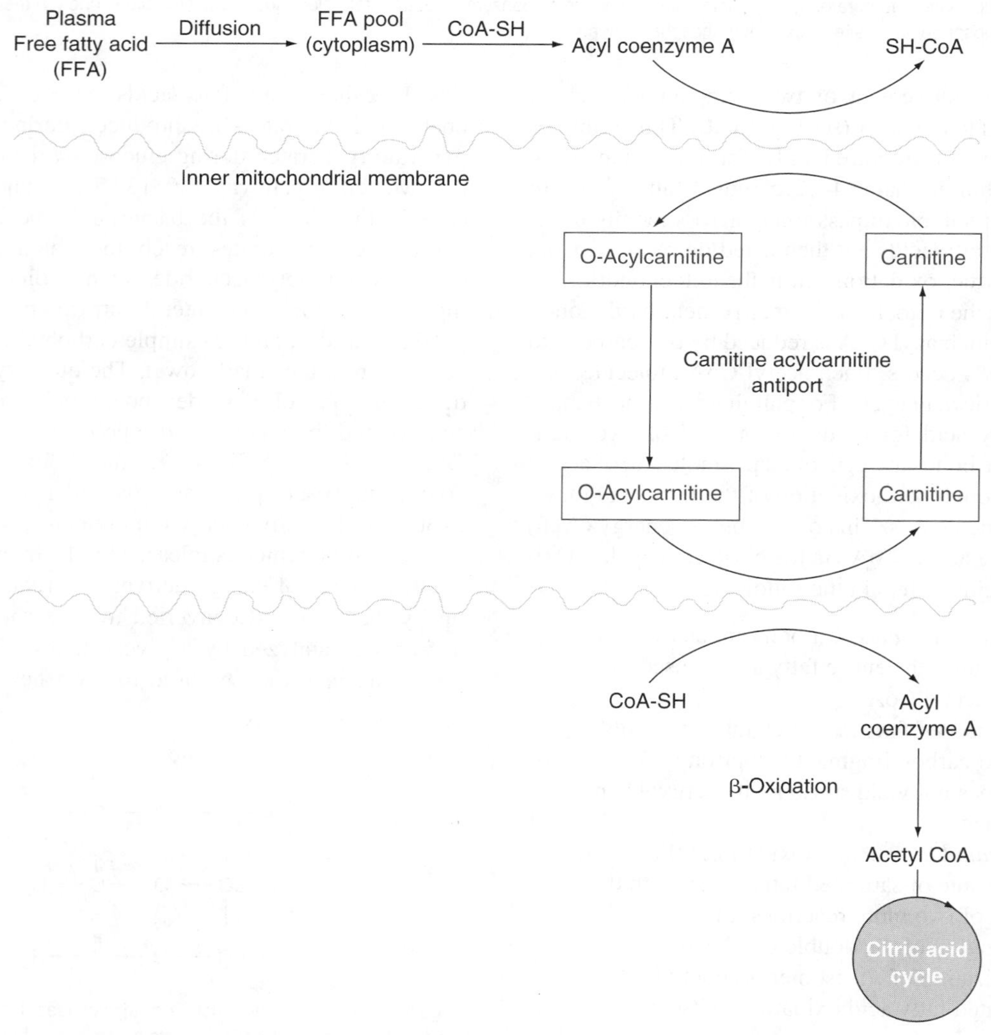

Figure 132.6. Schematic representation of fatty acid oxidation.

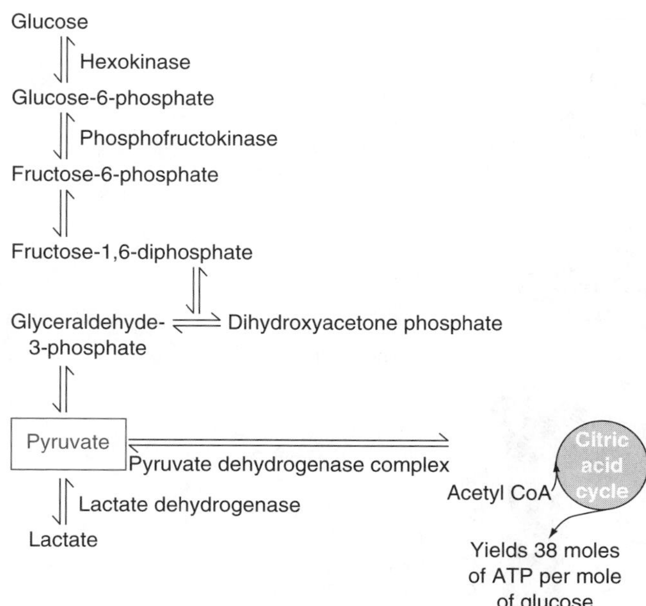

Figure 132.7. Glucose oxidation via glycolysis with the production of pyruvate (Embden–Meyerhof pathway) for entry into the citric acid cycle or as a precursor to lactate under anaerobic conditions. Glycerol oxidation also depicted is a reaction that occurs only within the liver.

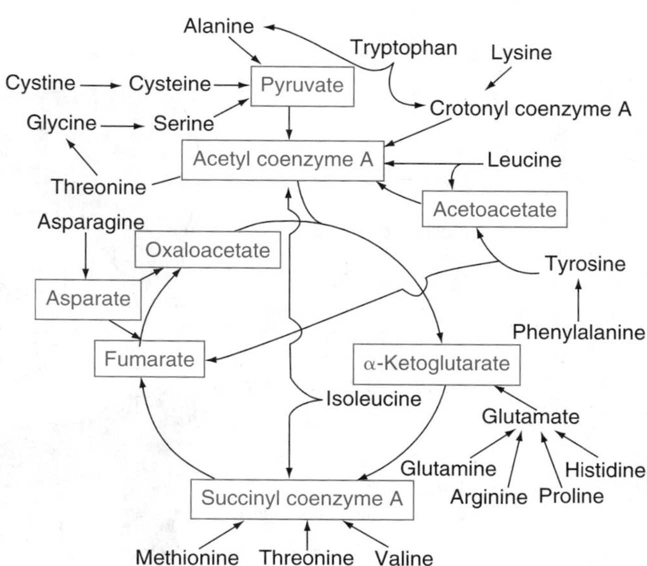

Figure 132.8. Outline of the fate of the carbon skeletons of the amino acids when used as fuels with possible conversions to any of eight intermediates of fuel metabolism.

dioxide or as eight familiar intermediates of fuel metabolism (Fig. 132.8).[11]

Normal Metabolism

In fed humans, the availability of substrate (nutrients) for cellular reactions is accomplished by the enteral or parenteral intake of nutrients. The metabolic fate of these nutrients depends on the nutrient needs of individual cells or tissues; the body's recognition and normal reaction to these needs; nervous system and hormonal regulatory mechanisms; substrate (nutrient) availability; and the appropriate ratio of nutrients in the diet.[12] The net result of these factors could be that the nutrient becomes a component of cellular material, influences synthetic reactions, is used as energy, is stored for use as a fuel or substrate during periods of excess need or nutrient deprivation (starvation), or is metabolized and subsequently disposed of by the body. The following discussion of normal metabolism focuses on the source and assimilation of carbohydrates, fats, proteins, trace elements, and vitamins by the body.

NUTRIENT ABSORPTION

For an oral diet, foodstuffs are presented to the alimentary tract where they are processed for absorption. Through chewing, enzymes and neurochemical control of organ function and enzyme secretion, foodstuffs are broken down to substrates that can be absorbed via either active or passive processes in the small intestine. Subsequently, these water-soluble substrates pass into the circulation via the portal vein. Fat-soluble molecules are taken up by the lymphatics and made available to the circulation where the lymph channels join the blood vessels in the thoracic duct.[13] Protein is absorbed in the jejunum, the rate of which is more limited by gastric emptying than the rate of hydrolysis. Hydrolysis of protein yields di- and tripeptides as well as free amino acids with the peptides being more efficiently absorbed.[14] This may have important clinical implications when selecting an enteral tube feeding formula for patients with compromised gastrointestinal absorption. The major sites of nutrient absorption are depicted in Fig. 132.9.[15]

Normally, the absorptive and digestive surface area of the small intestine exceeds that required to maintain adequate nutrition. Major surgical resection and other gastrointestinal disorders, however, may significantly alter the absorptive capacity of the intestinal tract, leading to single and/or multiple nutrient deficiencies.[16] Resection of the ileum has a more profound effect than gastric, jejunal, duodenal, or colonic resection on one's ability to maintain adequate gastrointestinal absorptive capacity. Resection of 50% or more of the ileum results in a significant decrease in absorptive capacity and a shorter small intestinal transit time. This disrupts bile salt recirculation, increasing the delivery of bile salts to the colon where they are deconjugated and cause a watery cholerrheic diarrhea. If extensive ileal resection occurs, the bile salt pool is diminished and this may result in fat malabsorption. This increased delivery

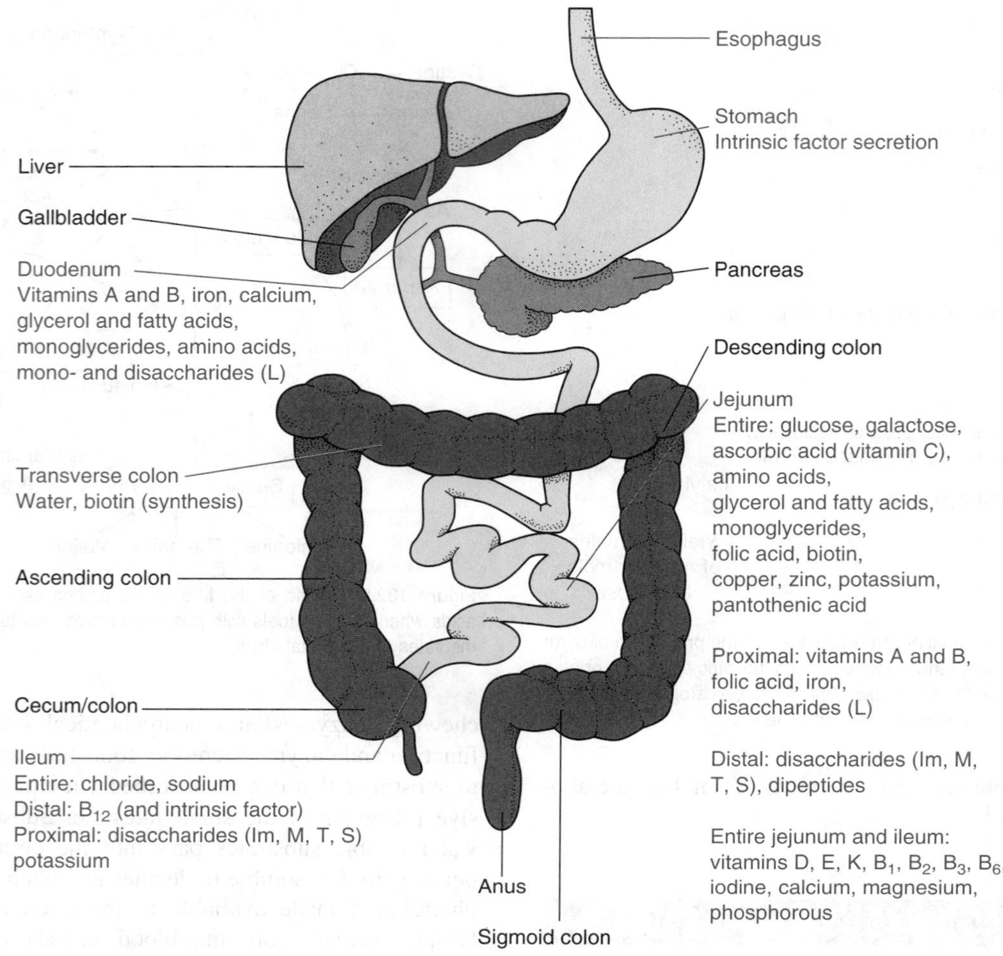

Figure 132.9. The sites of absorption of nutrients are shown. The exact sites for absorption of manganese, cobalt, selenium, chromium, molybdenum, and cadmium are unknown. L, lactose; Im, isomaltase; M, maltase; T, trehalose; S, sucrose.

of fatty acids to the colon causes steatorrhea.[16] Gastrointestinal fistulas, by bypassing significant areas of small intestine, or inflammatory processes created by intra-abdominal infections limit the absorptive capacity of the gastrointestinal tract. Inflammatory bowel disease (IBD) also decreases mucosal absorptive surface area due to inflammation and surgical resection(s). Small intestinal bacterial overgrowth, fistulas, partial obstruction, and the presence of deconjugated bile salts also indirectly alter the normal absorptive capacity of IBD patients.[17] Finally, the presence of one or more enteric pathogens is a major cause of malabsorption and diarrhea in the patient with acquired immunodeficiency syndrome.

CARBOHYDRATE METABOLISM

Starch is the principal source of carbohydrate from the diet. It is digested to monosaccharides such as dextrose and fructose and oligosaccharides such as sucrose, maltose, dextrin, and lactose.[13] Clinical nutrition is concerned primarily with glucose or dextrose metabolism. Glucose is absorbed either by diffusion or by active processes. Oral rehydration solutions prescribed for the treatment of acute diarrhea or improved electrolyte balance in patients with short-bowel syndrome relies on active absorption of glucose.[18] In these cases, active uptake of glucose creates a solvent drag that facilitates fluid and electrolyte absorption in the small bowel proximal to the diseased area.

The use of glucose as a fuel has been discussed previously. The major storage form of glucose is glycogen. Normally, glycogen stores in the liver are 65 grams (or 400 moles) per kilogram of tissue, whereas skeletal muscle contains 14 grams (or 85 moles) per kilogram of tissue.[19] Glycogen synthesis is dependent on the balance of the levels of insulin and glucagon in various tissues. In the liver, insulin produces glycogenesis and glucagon causes glycogenolysis. In the muscle, receptors for glucagon are absent,[19] and the hormone therefore exerts no regulatory effect in this tissue. Glycogen synthesis in the muscle is favored when insulin and also glucose are available. In this setting, glycogen synthase and pyruvate dehydrogenase activity is increased and phosphorylation of glycogen is suppressed. This results in net glycogen synthesis and increased conversion of pyruvate to acetyl CoA. In contrast, phosphorylation of glycogen and subsequent glycogenolysis are facilitated by catecholamines that activate "phosphorylase a" via the second messenger cyclic AMP.[19] Elevated levels of ionized calcium in the skeletal muscle cell may also activate "phosphorylase a."[19]

Since the storage of glucose as glycogen in the body is limited, any excess glucose not oxidized or stored as glycogen is converted to and stored as fat. In this process, glucose is converted to acetyl CoA, which may then be processed into fatty acids (described in next section). Also, if glucose intake exceeds the body's ability to transport it intracellularly, increased extracellular levels in excess of the renal threshold for glucose reabsorption will result in glucosuria and, if left unrecognized, could lead to excessive free water losses and hyperosmolar coma.[20]

Gluconeogenesis

Endogenous sources of glucose via gluconeogenesis (Fig. 132.10) consist of lactate, protein, and sorbitol. The Cori cycle provides a cyclical turnover of glucose[21] whereby 6.5 moles of ATP is consumed for each mole of glucose produced from 2 moles of lactate. Lactate is the end product of glycolysis during anaerobic conditions; it is released from the muscle and carried by the bloodstream to the liver where it is available for conversion to glucose.

In general, amino acids are gluconeogenic during periods of starvation[11] (Fig. 132.8), but one of the most important protein sources of glucose is the glucose–alanine cycle (Fig. 132.11).[22] Alanine and glutamine serve as nitrogen carriers in the body. Uptake of glutamine occurs in the small bowel, where it is metabolized. It then appears in the liver as either ammonium ions, alanine, and citrulline. Further, glutamine may be preferentially oxidized by the gastrointestinal tract in place of glucose during catabolic states.[23] In contrast, alanine produced in the muscle from the nitrogen of branched-chain amino acids (leucine, isoleucine, valine) and pyruvate is taken up by the liver. The nitrogen of alanine is transferred to glutamate, in a reaction catalyzed by alanine aminotransferase to yield glutamine plus pyruvate. Pyruvate may then be converted to glucose. The glutamine, in the presence of aspartate aminotransferase, is converted to aspartate, which may enter either the urea cycle or the citric acid cycle as either oxaloacetate or fumurate (Fig. 132.3).

The oxidation of sorbitol produces glucose in a process that allows fructose to become a glucose source as well.[24] However, enzymes in the body do not favor this metabolic process. Side effects of this process include increased production of lactate and uric acid in addition to loss of body water and electrolytes. These effects have limited the usefulness of sorbitol as an energy source in clinical practice.

FAT METABOLISM

Lipids are responsible for many metabolic and structural functions. They are the major source of stored energy and are precursors to the eicosanoids, prostaglandins, and leukotrienes. Structurally, lipids are components of cell membranes, pad vital organs, and insulate against physical injury and heat loss. Dietary lipids, as the major source of fat to the body, are ingested as long-chain triglycerides,

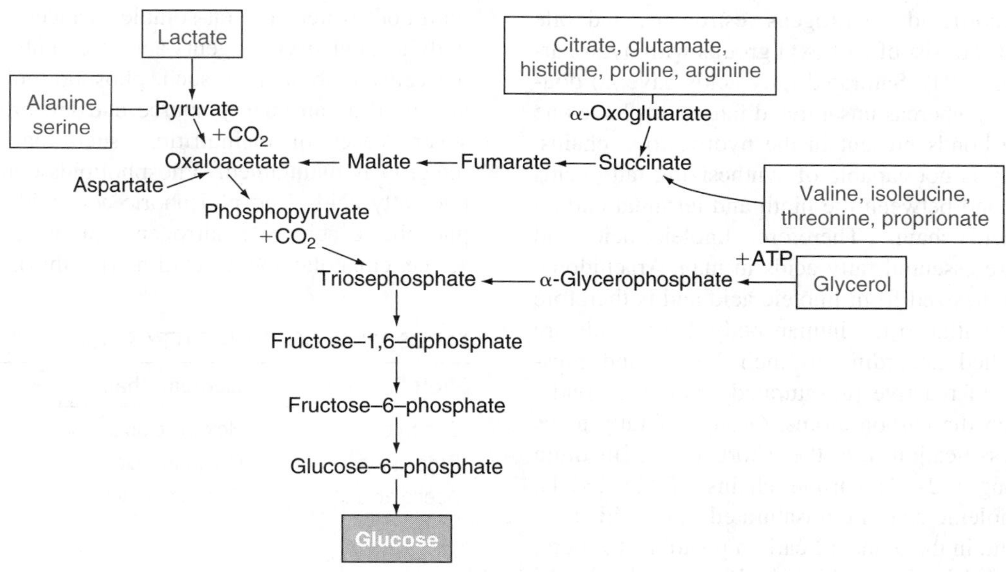

Figure 132.10. Pathways of gluconeogenesis from various precursors.

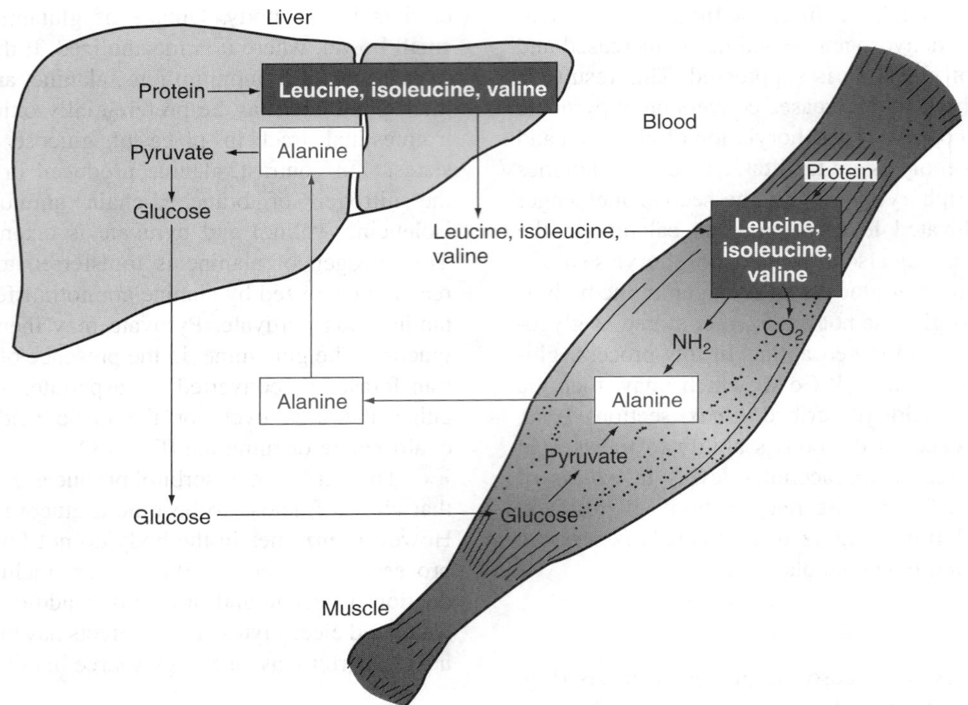

Figure 132.11. The glucose–alanine cycle. A major gluconeogenic pathway from protein.

phospholipids (lecithin predominantly), and cholesterol.[5] Long-chain triglycerides are fatty acid esters of glycerol, the hydroxyl groups of which are esterified with either one, two, or three fatty acids to form monoglycerides, diglycerides, or triglycerides, respectively. Triglycerides are the predominant dietary, storage, and transport form of lipids.

The fatty acids of the triglyceride molecule are a source of acetyl CoA, which is the precursor to cholesterol and therefore to prostaglandins, leukotrienes, glucocorticoids, mineralocorticoids, androgens, estrogens, and bile acids. Fatty acids consist of carboxyl groups with hydrocarbon chains (R–COOH). Saturated fatty acids have no double bonds present, whereas unsaturated fatty acids have one or more double bonds present in the hydrocarbon chains. The human body is not capable of synthesizing fatty acids with a double bond between the ninth and terminal carbon of the fatty acid chain.[5] Therefore, linoleic acid and linolenic acid are essential fatty acids in man. Arachidonic acid may be synthesized from linoleic acid and is therefore conditionally essential to the human body. Fatty acids are generally classified according to their length and presence/or absence of reactive (unsaturated or double bonds) linkages between the carbon atoms. Groups of fatty acids within this classification are the short (1–6), medium (6–10), and long (12–24) carbon chains (Table 132.1). Linoleic and linolenic acid are unsaturated fatty acids having a double bond in the 9 and 12 carbon positions for both, with linolenic acid having a third double bond in the 15 position. Therefore, linolenic acid is classified as an omega 3 while linoleic acid is an omega 6 fatty acid. This is important since intravenous fat emulsions are predominantly omega 6 fatty acids (50–66% of fat content), which increase the production of endogenous prostaglandins.[5] An imbalance in eicosanoid production and resultant effects on inflammatory and immune responses may thus be dependent on the type and quantity of fatty acid ingested.[25]

Phospholipids have both hydrophobic (fatty acids) and hydrophilic (phosphoryl) ends, which allow for interaction with both water- and fat-soluble surfaces.[5] These serve the body as emulsifying agents and as essential components of the cell membrane. As such, phospholipids are not generally used as an energy source and are preserved, even in severe cases of malnutrition, such that cell membrane integrity is maintained.[5] Phospholipids consist of glycerol, two fatty acids, and phosphoric acid with esterification of phosphoric acid to a nitrogen-containing moiety such as serine, ethanolamine, or choline (lecithin).

TABLE 132.1. COMMON FATTY ACIDS

Short Chain	Medium Chain	Long Chain
Butyrate	Hexanoic acid	Palmitic acid
Propionate	Octanoic acid	Stearic acid
Acetic acid	Decanoate acid	Oleic acid
		Linoleic acid
		Linolenic acid
		Arachidonic acid

Oral lipids are acted on by gastric lipase, pancreatic enzymes, biliary lecithin, and bile salts. This results in the hydrolysis and emulsification of the lipids for absorption.[13] Hydrolysis by gastrointestinal lipase yields medium-chain fatty acids that are available for absorption via passive diffusion across the gastrointestinal mucosa in the jejunum (Fig. 132.9). Long-chain triglycerides require hydrolysis and emulsification with lecithin and bile salts for gastrointestinal mucosal uptake. Once within the mucosal cell, long-chain fatty acids are recombined with glycerol to form triglycerides, which are then packaged in a chylomicron consisting of triglyceride (80%), cholesterol (9%), phospholipid (7%), and coated with lipoprotein (4%).[5] Lipoproteins serve as solubilizing agents for lipid transport through an aqueous medium and consist of a triglyceride and cholesterol ester core surrounded by a surface coat of apoproteins, phospholipids, and free cholesterol.[5] Lipoproteins are classified as chylomicrons, very low density lipoproteins (VLDLs), low-density lipoproteins (LDLs), and high-density lipoproteins (HDLs) with each having specific proteins or apoproteins that direct the lipoprotein's metabolism via interaction with key enzymes and receptors.[26] In the final process of lipid absorption, chylomicrons are secreted into the lymph and transported into the blood via the thoracic duct.

Fatty acids are made available to the liver via the enterohepatic circulation for medium-chain triglycerides or the systemic circulation for long-chain fatty acids and remnants of chylomicrons. Once in the liver, the triglyceride may enter the hepatocyte and be available for hydrolysis to its glycerol and fatty acid components.[5] Glycerol is either oxidized as a carbohydrate or is synthesized into a new triglyceride molecule, whereas the fatty acid may become a triglyceride or phospholipid or undergo beta-oxidation. Excess fatty acids have various metabolic fates including synthesis of phospholipids, resynthesis of triglycerides, complete degradation with the production of energy, or ketogenesis (the production of ketones for use as energy substrate in the muscle).

Cellular deposition of fat occurs from chylomicrons made available from the small intestine or from VLDLs released by the liver.[5] Fatty acids are removed from chylomicrons and VLDLs circulating in the bloodstream by lipoprotein lipase, which is present in muscle and adipose tissue. The fatty acids released by lipoprotein lipase move freely into the cell, where they are converted to triglycerides in preparation for storage as fat. This process occurs in situations of excess for the muscle and normally in adipose tissue. Lipoprotein lipase is activated by contact with specific proteins present in the chylomicron or VLDLs and is also activated by heparin and insulin. The metabolism of parenteral fat emulsions resembles that of the endogenous chylomicron. There are, however, differences in the composition of the lipid emulsion and chylomicrons that influence the manner in which the lipid emulsion is metabolized by the body (Table 132.2).[5] Lipid emulsions have a greater quantity of triglyceride and phospholipid. They are very low in cholesterol and have no cholesterol esters or protein. As a result, lipid emulsion triglycerides must acquire apoproteins in order to activate lipoprotein lipase and be hydrolyzed.[5] Also, the high phospholipid content creates two distinctly different particle populations in the lipid emulsion: triglyceride-rich particles resembling chylomicrons and phospholipid-rich particles resembling liposomal phospholipid bilayers. The phospholipid-rich particles are probably responsible for the increase in free cholesterol levels observed during lipid infusions.[5] Since lipid emulsions have no cholesterol, this must originate from endogenous sources interacting with phospholipid-rich particles to create cholesterol–phospholipid complexes. These complexes may also acquire apoproteins and interfere with triglyceride hydrolysis and LDL metabolism. Lipid emulsions having a high phospholipid: triglyceride ratio (the 10% emulsion has a fourfold greater quantity of phospholipid than the 20% emulsion) induce a high level of phospholipids, free cholesterol, and plasma triglycerides.[5] Also, the free fatty acid composition of lipid emulsions influences the rate of hydrolysis. Medium-chain triglycerides are metabolized faster than long-chain triglycerides due to their high degree of water solubility. Thus, medium-chain triglycerides (MCTs) are a readily available energy source, but metabolism may be too rapid and lead to ketosis. The reaction to hydrolyze MCTs is slowed in the presence of long-chain triglycerides (LCTs) thereby improving the safety of MCT administration. Currently, 50/50 mixtures of LCT/MCT emulsions are under clinical investigation. These may provide more appropriate fats for energy (MCT), structure (LCT), and function (reduced LCT and omega 6 fatty acid administration).

TABLE 132.2. COMPOSITION (WEIGHT %) OF PARENTERAL LIPID EMULSIONS COMPARED WITH THE ENDOGENOUS CHYLOMICRON

		Parenteral Lipid Emulsion	
	Chylomicron	**10%**	**20%**
Triglyceride	68.8	89.0	94.2
Phospholipids	4.5	10.7	6.7
Free cholesterol	2.0	0.3	0.1
Cholesterol ester	3.0	0	0
Protein	1.7	0	0

Fat is mobilized and released (lipolysis) from adipose tissue by a hormone-sensitive lipase that hydrolyzes any and all bonds in the triglyceride molecule. The fatty acids are then bound to albumin for transport and the glycerol is transported to the liver for processing. Lipolysis is regulated by insulin and catecholamine levels. Insulin favors fat storage, blocks fat release, favors fat synthesis from glucose in the liver, and permits the use of glucose as a fuel in skeletal muscle rather than fat. Simply, insulin promotes fat

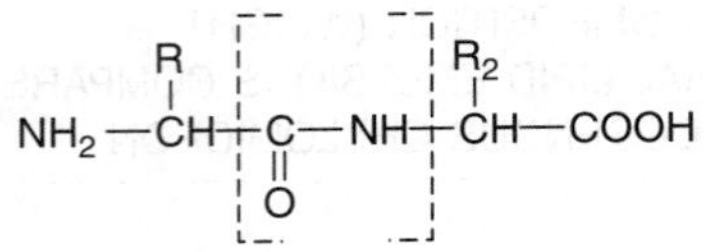

$$NH_2-\underset{}{\overset{R}{\overset{|}{CH}}}-\underset{\underset{O}{\|}}{C}-NH-\overset{R_2}{\overset{|}{CH}}-COOH$$

Figure 132.12. Peptide linkage of two amino acids.

storage and use of glucose as the principal fuel. In contrast, catecholamines mediate the release of fatty acids from the adipocyte. Subsequently, increased levels of fatty acids in the blood will increase their utilization by muscle tissue as an energy source. In addition, hepatic uptake of fatty acids is increased. The diet is the major source of fatty acids, but fatty acids may be made available and synthesized from endogenous (glucose and amino acids) sources.[5]

PROTEIN METABOLISM

Proteins are complex polymers of alpha-amino acids joined by a peptide linkage (Fig. 132.12) from the amino group of one amino acid to a carboxyl group of another. Proteins consist elementally of carbon, hydrogen, oxygen, nitrogen, and sometimes sulfur.[27] Proteins function as structural components and in regulatory, movement, immunologic, transport, and repair processes. Proteins are an essential component of the nucleus, cytoplasm, and membrane of the cell[28] and are the "machinery" of the body and as such are vital to life-sustaining processes.[29] Alterations in protein metabolism are common and may be partially responsible for death in some common diseases.[27]

Dietary protein is hydrolyzed to amino acids, dipeptides, and tripeptides before absorption into the portal system. No intact protein enters the human body; therefore, all body protein is synthesized *de novo*.[27] Most amino acids entering the liver from the portal vein are extracted by this organ except the branched-chain amino acids, which become available to the systemic circulation. The metabolic fate of amino acids is determined by the nutritional state and clinical condition of the patient. Metabolic processes are present for protein catabolism in which the carbon skeleton (ketoacid) of the amino acid is removed and used for energy. The ammonia component of the amino acid may be either transaminated to a new ketoacid, producing another amino acid, or discarded as urea. Protein synthetic processes are also available to utilize the amino acids in the production of structural, enzymatic, and transport proteins.

Amino acids released into the circulation from the liver or from "endogenous" sources (protein breakdown) are rapidly taken up by metabolically active tissues (kidney, pancreas, and intestinal mucosa). Uptake by the skeletal muscle is slow but the large mass of this tissue makes it the largest reservoir or pool of "labile" amino acids.[27] This "labile" or "free" amino acid pool represents only about 1% of total body amino acids, but provides for movement of amino acids between various organs, and supports the dynamic state of protein metabolism. The dynamic state of protein metabolism is referred to as "protein flux,"[29] meaning that the quantities of amino acids entering the pool (from either exogenous or endogenous sources) or leaving the pool (via synthesis or catabolism and excretion of protein) are in equilibrium. Thus, protein flux refers to the turnover of protein such that a bal-

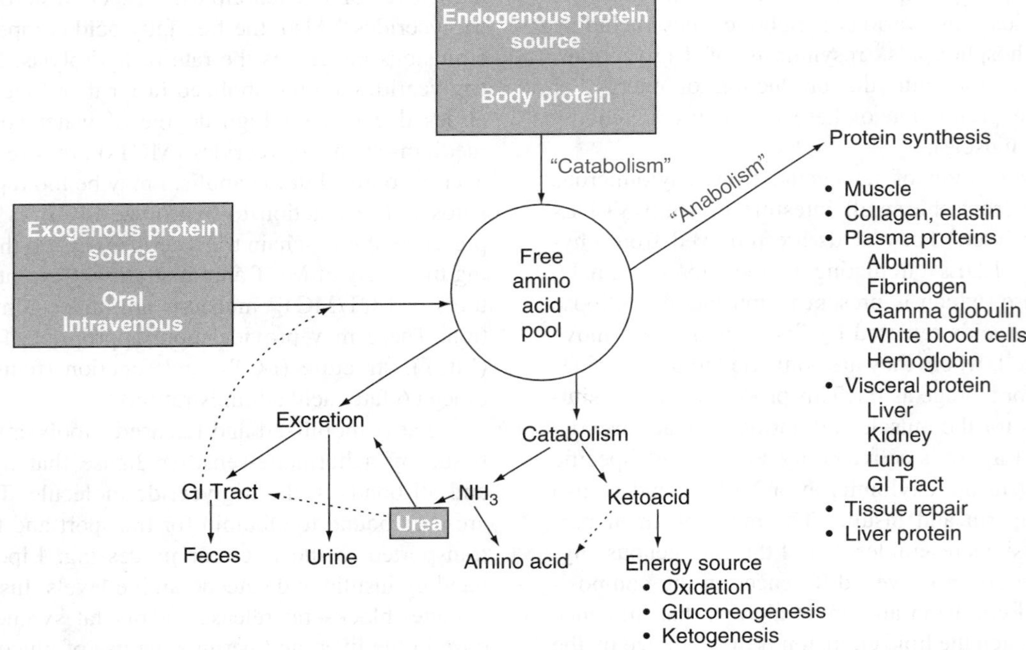

Figure 132.13. Body protein dynamics. Under normal homeostatic conditions, anabolic and catabolic protein processes are in equilibrium ("protein flux"), leaving the size of the free amino acid pool constant.

ance exists between synthetic and catabolic processes (Fig. 132.13). The state of this dynamic equilibrium determines the state of the overall protein balance of the body.

Whether an amino acid is incorporated into new protein or is catabolized is determined by a number of factors. These factors include the amino acid supply, hormonal milieu present in the body, and the state of protein deprivation. Essential amino acids (EAAs) are those that the body is incapable of producing in sufficient quantities to prevent deficiency symptoms in healthy individuals when exogenous sources of the amino acid are absent. The essential amino acids in man are isoleucine (Iso), leucine (Leu), lysine (Lys), methionine (Meth), phenylalanine (Phe), threonine (Thr), tryptophan (Trp), and valine (Val) (Table 132.3). Histidine (Hist) and arginine (Arg) are "semiessential" or conditionally essential in some clinical states such as renal or hepatic insufficiency.[30]

A classification scheme for amino acids is provided in Table 132.3[31] and the chemical structures of selected amino acids important to nutritional therapeutics are depicted in Fig. 132.14. Branched-chain amino acids (BCAAs) are used by muscle for energy and are the only amino acids that are not metabolized by the liver. The ammonia from BCAAs may become a precursor along with pyruvate for alanine and also glutamine, both of which are nitrogen carriers in the body and gluconeogenic precursors. The aromatic amino acids (AAAs), metabolized by the liver, may accumulate in patients with liver disease and contribute to encephalopathic symptoms. The disulfide bridges of the sulfur-containing amino acids, cysteine (Cys) and methionine (Meth), provide the configuration and structure of protein.

Glutamine is the most abundant amino acid in the body and constitutes more than 60% of the free amino acid pool.[32] Nearly all tissues are capable of synthesizing glutamine, explaining its classification as a nonessential amino acid. Several organs, including the kidney and gastrointestinal tract, have a large capacity to extract glutamine from the circulation where it serves as a principal fuel for replicating cells such as endothelial cells, lymphocytes, renal tubular cells, fibroblasts, and small intestinal mucosa. Glutamine's functions[32] support its importance to the maintenance of body physiology and metabolism despite being considered nonessential as an amino acid.

The semiessential amino acid arginine (Arg) is an essential component of the urea cycle and thus nitrogen disposal by the body. It is also a potent stimulator of pituitary growth hormone and insulin release. The trophic and stimulatory effects of arginine on the immune system may be beneficial during injury or critical illness. Arginine has been shown to enhance immunity in the laboratory by preserving thymic mass, increasing thymic lymphocyte content following injury, and improving lymphocyte blastogenesis in

TABLE 132.3. CLASSIFICATIONS OF AMINO ACIDS

Amino Acid	Essential	Gluconeogenic	Ketogenic	Cationic	Anionic
Iso	o	o	o		
Leu	o		o		
Lys	o	o	o	o	
Meth	o	o			
Phe	o	o	o		
Thr	o				
Trp	o	o	o		
Val	o	o			
His				o	
Arg		o		o	
Cys		o			
Pro		o			
Glu				o	
Ala		o			
Asp		o			o
Asparagine					o
Gly		o			
Glutamate					o
Hydroxypro		o			
Ser		o			
Tyr		o	o		
Citr				o	
Orn				o	

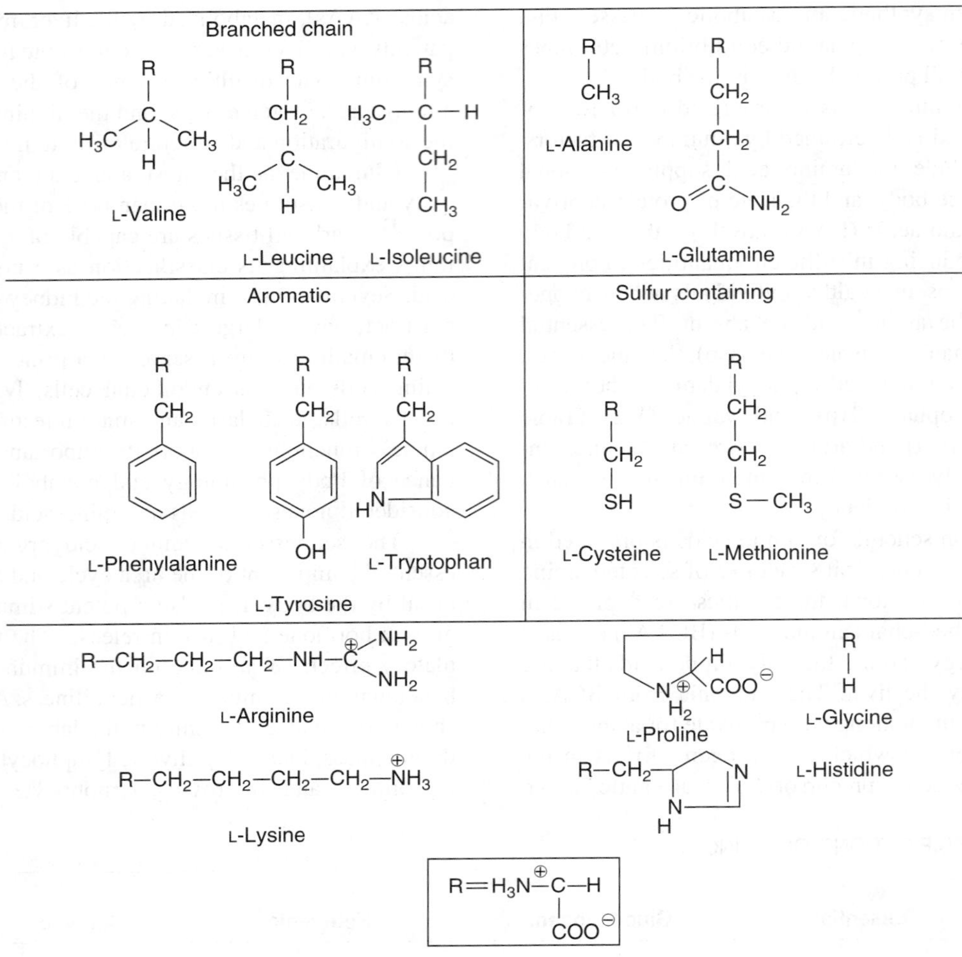

Figure 132.14. Chemical structures of selected amino acids important to nutritional therapeutics.

response to mitogens.[33] Of note is the fact that the guanidine component of arginine may be oxidized under certain cellular conditions to the highly reactive molecule, nitrous oxide. This may produce both harmful and beneficial effects; it inhibits tumor and bacterial growth but has negative effects on vascular tone.[34] Proline provides a source of hydroxyproline and is a major component of collagen along with glycine. Glutamic acid and lysine are also important to collagen synthesis.[34] In the classification of amino acids, gluconeogenic refers to glucose precursors, whereas ketogenic compounds are the precursors to fatty acids and ketones.

In anabolic pathways, amino acids are linked by peptide bonds in a predetermined sequence involving a complex interaction with nucleic acids in the ribosome, and result in the synthesis of a specific protein.[27] The detailed steps in protein synthesis have been outlined elsewhere.[35] Protein metabolism occurs by removal of amino groups, decarboxylation, or transmethylation.[36] The primary site of amino group removal is in the liver, although other tissues may participate. One type of amino group removal is transamination; a process that transfers an amino group to another alpha-ketoacid, forming a new amino acid plus the ketoacid residue of the original amino acid. This reaction requires a transaminase enzyme, which exerts its activity only in the presence of pyridoxal phosphate and a metal ion.[36] The most active exchange of transamination occurs between glutamate and aspartate. More than one-half of total nitrogen in amino acids passes through glutamate, which undergoes transamination to aspartate or oxidative deamination to ammonia that goes into either the production of urea, pyrimidines, or glutamine. Most ketoacids of amino acids are available in the body for transamination except for lysine and methionine.[37] Oxidative deamination has been previously described; oxidases required for this reaction are available in the liver and kidney and catalyze the oxidation of all amino acids except serine, threonine, and di- and tricarboxylic acids. Amino groups may also be removed from amino acids by pyridoxal-dependent dehydrases and desulfurases that are responsible for the deamination of threonine, serine, and cysteine.

Protein metabolism via decarboxylation involves the conversion of amino acids to a corresponding amine such as histamine from histidine, tyramine from tyrosine, and norepinephrine and epinephrine from phenylalanine. This reaction requires pyridoxal phosphate as a coenzyme and a specific decarboxylase for each amino acid.[36]

TABLE 132.4. TRACE ELEMENTS WITH ASSOCIATED COENZYME

Trace Element	Metalloenzymes
Zinc	Carbonic anhydrase, alcohol dehydrogenase, alkaline phosphatase, lactic dehydrogenase
Copper	Cytochrome C oxidase, tyrosinase, monoamine oxidase, ascorbic acid oxidase
Chromium	Glucose tolerance factor
Manganese	Pyruvate carboxylase, activates—alkaline phosphatase, arginase, carboxylase, and cholinesterase
Selenium	Glutathione peroxidase
Molybdenum	Aldehyde oxidase, sulfite oxidase, xanthine oxidase

Finally, certain methyl donors such as methionine and choline have a "labile" methyl group attached to the sulfur or nitrogen group that allows for transmethylation as a means of protein metabolism. The primary methyl donor is S-adenosyl methionine, the transfer of which is regulated by the enzyme methyl transferase. The methyl transfers of importance include the formation of phosphatidylcholine, a component of the cell membrane, and the synthesis of creatine, used for energy transfer in the muscle.[36]

TRACE ELEMENTS AND VITAMINS

The discussion of nutrient metabolism thus far has been restricted to the macronutrients, but micronutrients such as trace elements and vitamins serve several important functions in the homeostatic regulatory mechanisms of the body. The metabolism of trace elements and vitamins is an extensive topic covered in many texts. The purpose of this section is to provide an overview of the essential functions of trace elements and vitamins and, specifically, the enzymatic processes in which these elements are involved. Trace elements are substances present in human tissue in minute amounts and constitute microgram or even picogram amounts of wet tissue weight.[38] Trace elements function as nonprotein cofactors in metalloenzymes required for proper catalytic activity, cofactors in protein and nucleic acid synthesis, and structural stabilizers of some proteins. Essential trace elements are chromium, manganese, selenium, molybdenum, vanadium, nickel, tin, silicon, fluorine, and arsenic. Four trace elements with functional roles in metabolism include cobalt, iodine, zinc, and copper. The trace elements and their associated metalloenzymes of importance to nutritional therapeutics are provided in Table 132.4.[38]

Vitamins are organic compounds that are neither carbohydrate, protein, nor fat that are necessary in minute quantities for the maintenance of normal biological activity. Vitamins function primarily as coenzymes in the metabolism of energy-yielding nutrients. In this manner, they coordinate growth and maintenance and assist in storage and utilization of energy. Vitamins cannot be synthesized by the body, making dietary supplementation necessary. The 13 vitamins may be classified as either fat or water soluble and serve many coenzyme functions (Table 132.5).[39]

TABLE 132.5. COENZYME FUNCTIONS OF VITAMINS

Vitamin	Coenzyme Function
Fat Soluble	
A, retinol	Rhodopsin, visual cycle, night vision
K, menadiol	Blood clotting factors II, VII, IX, X
D, calciferal	Calcium and phosphorous homeostasis
E, tocopherol	Antioxidant, glutathione oxidase
Water Soluble	
C, ascorbate	Antioxidant, regulation of intracellular oxidation–reduction potentials, certain hydroxylation reactions that require copper or iron, i.e., hydroxylation of proline in collagen synthesis
B_1, thiamin	Oxidative decarboxylation of amino acids, transketolase
B_2, riboflavin	Flavin mononucleotide and flavin adenine dinucleotide, essential for oxidative systems and oxygen transport
B_3, pantothenic	As coenzyme A precursor, necessary for acid acyl transfers
B_5, niacin	Endogenous source from tryptophan. Component of nicotinamide adenine dinucleotide (NAD) and its phosphorylate (NADP); assists in hydrogen transfer of glycolysis, fatty acid synthesis and tissue respiration
B_6, pyridoxine	Nitrogen metabolism: transamination, racemization, decarboxylation, cleavage, synthesis, dehydration and desulfhydration
B_{12}, cyanocobalamin	Methylation of homocysteine to methionine, conversion of methyl malonyl–coenzyme A to succinyl–coenzyme A
Biotin	Cofactor for some carboxylases: acetyl COA carboxylase, pyruvate carboxylase, B-methylcrotonyl carboxylase and methylmalonyle carboxylase
Folic acid	Transport of single carbon fragments, especially nucleic acid synthesis and metabolism of some amino acids

MALNUTRITION

Malnutrition is the impaired nutrient utilization that results from malassimilation, poor diet, overeating, or altered metabolism by disease. Types of malnutrition discussed in this section are starvation, stress metabolism, and obesity. Included in the section on stress metabolism is the presentation of altered metabolism caused by some common diseases (i.e., sepsis and cancer).

STARVATION

Humans have the ability to go without food for sustained periods with minimal impairment of mobility and thus survival. The change in the availability of substrate elicits a metabolic response involving changes in hormonal concentrations in an attempt to maintain glucose homeostasis during acute stages of starvation and a gradual adaptation to fat as the primary fuel for the purposes of preserving body protein mass during prolonged periods of a fast.[40] The stages of starvation are summarized as brief, uncomplicated starvation; prolonged starvation; and stressed starvation. During starvation, the body calls on its body stores of energy and protein (Table 132.6).[28,40] for the maintenance of vital body functions. Significant adaptations occur during a fast to minimize losses of vital body elements, a process regulated by the balance of hormones in the plasma of starved patients. This hormonal milieu alters the metabolism of protein, glucose, and fat.

Protein Metabolism

The initial response to a fast is a decrease in protein synthetic rate with either no change or a slight increase in protein catabolism. The increase in protein catabolism is accomplished via oxidative deamination and gluconeogenesis to preserve glucose levels in the circulation via the alanine cycle. With prolonged starvation, an adaptation to fat as an energy source occurs and the need for glucose and therefore gluconeogenesis from protein is reduced. Protein catabolism then decreases accordingly (Table 132.6). The clinical observation of this process is the decrease in appearance of urea nitrogen in the urine of fasting subjects from 12 g/d in the first 3–5 days of starvation to a minimal level of 3–4 g/d in 1–2 weeks.[40] This energy adaptation to fat as a fuel is depicted by the use of 2 grams of fat per gram of protein catabolyzed early in starvation to a level of 7.5 grams of fat per gram of protein in late stages of starvation.[41]

Glucose Metabolism

During a fast, insulin concentrations are depressed favoring glycogenolysis, and glycogen stores are rapidly depleted.[42] Key organs that usually use glucose as a primary energy source are the brain, central nervous system, red blood cells, white blood cells, active fibroblasts, and certain phagocytes.[43] This need for glucose is met by gluconeogenesis from protein after glycogen stores are depleted. The sources of glucose include alanine from muscle (only 8% of muscle protein is alanine) or pyruvate (muscle glycogen), incomplete oxidation of blood glucose, and other amino acids, especially the BCAAs. Under the hormonal influence of decreased insulin and increased glucagon concentrations in the circulation, glycogenolysis, hepatic glucose release, gluconeogenesis from amino acids, breakdown of ketogenic amino acids with an increase in peripheral FFAs, enhanced fatty acid oxidation, and ketone body production occur.

TABLE 132.6. ENERGY STORES (kcal), EXPENDITURE AND PROTEIN METABOLISM DURING PERIODS OF STARVATION

	Overnight		8 Days		40 Days	
	Stores	Daily Loss	Stores	Daily Loss	Stores	Daily Loss
Total	125,000	1700	111,380	1600	60,380	1425
Fat	100,000	1200	88,000	1400	42,000	1350
CHO	680	300	380	0	300	0
Protein	25,000	200	23,000	200	18,500	75
Energy Expenditure (kcal/h)						
Total	70		65		60	
Fat	50		58		56	
Glucose[a]	20		7		4	
Protein Metabolism (g/kg/d)						
Synthesis	300		150		150	
Catabolism	300		170		150	

[a]Includes glycogen and gluconeogenic sources of glucose.

Fat Metabolism

FFAs are released from triglycerides in the presence of low insulin concentrations and transported to the remainder of the body to be consumed as a fuel. Fat provides the greater proportion of calories for the human body during starvation (Table 132.6). The oxidation of fatty acids in the liver leads to ketone body production and release into the circulation. This is important, because fatty acids are not available to the central nervous system as an energy source, whereas ketone bodies are capable of passage across the blood-brain barrier and are available as a source of fuel for the brain.

In summary, the metabolic adaptation to acute starvation is (1) conservation of protein mass by decreasing proteolysis, increasing the availability and use of ketone bodies as an energy source, with subsequent decreased levels of amino acids in the plasma, a decline in amino acid efflux in the muscle, and a decreased splanchnic uptake of amino acids; and (2) a gradual decrease in energy expenditure (Table 132.6). With prolonged starvation, there is an enhanced oxidation of fat, and the use of ketones as primary fuels by the brain with a decreased need for and production of glucose by the body. The kidney increases its production of glucose to equal that synthesized by the liver. The gluconeogenic source as protein decreases but remains the same for lactate and glycerol. Hopefully, the loss of nitrogen is minimized for preservation of life-sustaining processes, but if more than 30–50% of body nitrogen stores (Table 132.6) are lost, death will ensue.[44]

An important consideration in early starvation is that the liver is geared for fatty acid oxidation and gluconeogenesis, because the enzymes required for these processes are preserved at this time. Concurrently, urea cycle enzymes are decreased. Therefore, the ammonia generated from the alanine–glucose cycle does not necessarily appear in urea and may need to be eliminated by the kidney. The other major source of ammonia in the kidney is from glutamine, which facilitates acid elimination by the kidney by producing ammonia under the regulation of the enzyme glutaminase. The ammonia thus produced may accept a hydrogen molecule, thereby neutralizing the acidic products of metabolism. This is important in starvation because ketones produced by the body at this time in excess of body need will be eliminated in the kidney and will need to be neutralized by the ammonia of glutamine. At this time, urine urea nitrogen excretion may decrease to 1–2 g/d while ammonia nitrogen excretion increases from 0.5 to 2.5 g/d.[44] Therefore, the conservation of protein is compromised to the extent that body protein (via proteolysis of muscle) is made available to provide for sufficient synthesis of glutamine in the kidney, which will be used for renal ammoniagenesis.

STRESS METABOLISM

Injury or stress generates a vigorous metabolic response designed to establish the metabolic priorities required for the repair of injured tissues.[45] The hormones secreted in response to stress elicit various metabolic effects (Table 132.7). Cuthbertson[45] has described two metabolic periods during acute stress: the "ebb" phase almost immediately after the injury, which is a period of diminished vitality or shock; and the "flow" phase, the subsequent period of increased metabolism or traumatic inflammation that facilitates the healing process. Both anabolic and catabolic processes increase during injury. Catabolism occurs predominantly in the carcass (as opposed to vital organ muscle such as liver, kidney, heart, lungs, etc.) with skeletal muscle being the major source of extra nitrogen excreted in the urine after injury. Anabolism occurs predominantly in the liver at this time.[45] With this elevated turnover and disposal of nitrogen, only 12–22% of total body energy expenditure is from protein while 80–90% is from fat oxidation.[46]

The overall effects of stress metabolism are the appearance of hyperglycemia with insulin resistance, increased protein synthesis, breakdown and catabolism, mobilization, and utilization of FFAs for energy; increased energy expenditure; and urinary nitrogen losses as urea that are quantitatively proportional to the extent of injury.[45] Gluconeogenesis occurs via the glucose–alanine cycle and contributes to lactate production due to the anaerobic conditions in hypoxic tissues. Hypoxia may further contribute to increases in beta-hydroxybutyrate levels, ketone bodies, and the lactate:pyruvate ratio. Energy expenditure (as nitrogen losses[47]) is increased in proportion to the severity of illness (Fig. 132.15).[48] The nitrogen loss during stress is increased not

TABLE 132.7. METABOLIC EFFECTS OF HORMONES SECRETED IN RESPONSE TO STRESS

Hormone	Metabolic Effect
Catecholamines	Increased glycogenolysis, inhibited pancreatic release of insulin, increased fatty acid oxidation
Corticosteroids	Increased gluconeogenesis, inhibition of insulin activity, increased muscle catabolism, inhibition of protein synthesis, mobilization of fatty acids, increased protein turnover in the liver and kidney, increased amino acid release from muscle
Growth hormone	Increased gluconeogenesis, inhibition of insulin activity, mobilization of fatty acids
Glucagon	Increased glycogenolysis, inhibition of insulin activity, increased muscle protein catabolism (proteolysis), inhibition of protein synthesis, mobilization of fatty acids, increased hepatic fatty acid oxidation

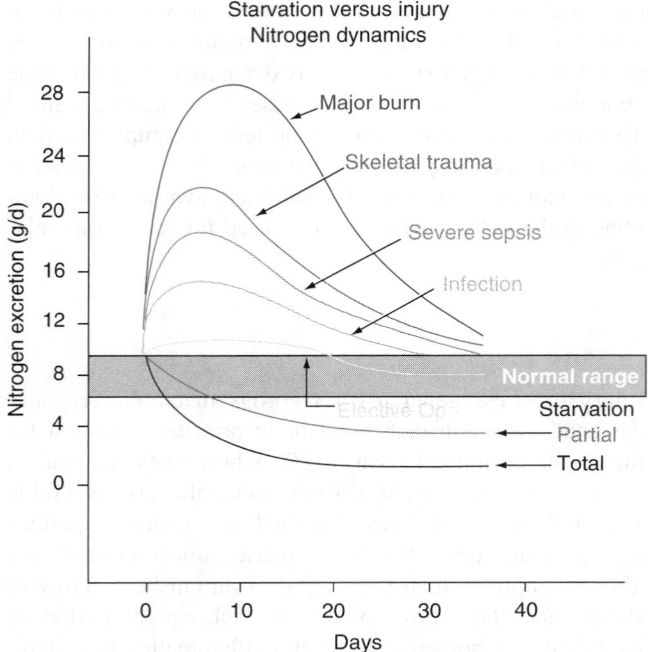

Figure 132.15. Increase in urinary nitrogen losses in the six patient groups with time.

just from disposal of injured or infected tissue but is derived from skeletal muscle (proteolysis) as well.[49]

Sepsis

Sepsis is a severe metabolic derangement culminating in multiorgan failure and death, apparently as a result of the inhibition of ATP production.[50] The metabolic response is mediated by a leukocyte endogenous mediator, resulting in a fuel deficit appearing as resistance to insulin, carnitine deficiency, and possibly intracellular metabolic blocks that lead to decreased substrate utilization and low oxygen consumption.[51] On muscle biopsy, decreased ATP and increased ADP concentrations have been reported, suggesting an inhibition of substrate entry into the citric acid cycle in muscle during sepsis.[52] This decreased oxygen consumption results in physiologic and hemodynamic abnormalities characteristic of sepsis. The cause of these metabolic blocks may be an alteration in the redox potential and alteration of processes that require oxidized NAD at the mitochondrial level.[51] In comparison to other forms of stress, sepsis is intermediate to traumatic injuries, such as multiple fractures and severe burns.[53]

Starvation During Stress

Injury blocks the normal adaptation to starvation and its protein conservation effect. Therefore, the protein catabolism of stress is unaltered,[54] hastening protein losses of the body and substantially decreasing the lethal starvation period. In stress, injured tissue, the brain, and kidneys use glucose as a fuel, while the skeletal muscle uses fatty acids for energy. In the injured tissue or wound, glucose undergoes anaerobic metabolism resulting in lactate production. The lactate then becomes a gluconeogenic precursor via the Cori cycle in the liver. The source of the nitrogen loss in injury is the result of an imbalance of protein catabolism and anabolism. Some evidence exists that during stress there may be a decrease in protein synthesis with no change in catabolic rates,[55,56] while others have found an increase in both synthetic and catabolic protein processes.[57,58] These processes are mediated by increased circulating concentrations of catecholamines, glucocorticoids, and glucagon and an inappropriately low insulin concentration in relation to serum glucose concentration.[59] With sepsis as the source of injury, the response is mediated by the release of endogenous pyrogens. Leukocyte endogenous mediator has a direct action on organ metabolism and an indirect effect on central nervous system and neuroendocrine responses. In contrast to starvation, gluconeogenesis is not turned off by the exogenous administration of glucose in infection and sepsis.[53]

HORMONAL REGULATION

Periods of starvation and stress are hormonally mediated. The specific effects of hormones such as catecholamines, glucagon, glucocorticoids, growth hormone, and insulin have been tabulated (Table 132.7). Catecholamines increase hepatic gluconeogenesis, stimulate glycogenolysis, and stimulate the conversion of three carbon precursors such as lactate and pyruvate to glucose. In skeletal muscle, the mobilization of glycogen stores with subsequent lactate production is stimulated, while in adipose tissue, FFAs are mobilized. Meanwhile, glucagon release is stimulated and insulin secretion by the pancreas is suppressed. The release of glucagon accentuates glycogenolysis, gluconeogenesis, and ureagenesis in the liver and has little effect on skeletal muscle. Glucocorticoids and growth hormone enhance the hormonal effects observed during the injury response. Glucocorticoids potentiate hepatic and skeletal muscle effects of catecholamines by stimulating intracellular enzymes, while growth hormone increases FFA release from adipose tissue and increases peripheral insulin resistance.[34] Insulin concentrations in the circulation are elevated in stress, as the major storage hormone of the body facilitates glycogenesis, lipogenesis, and protein synthesis; however, the differential resistance of adipose and muscle tissue to elevated insulin concentration results in inadequate insulin activity to reverse the muscle breakdown and might possibly inhibit lipolysis while allowing the release of amino acids into the bloodstream.

Cytokines, principally elaborated by inflammatory cells, are a diverse group of endogenous mediators of the stress and septic response. They are biologically active in very small concentrations and regulate metabolism via several mechanisms. Some are primarily immune modulating and others have effects on cellular proliferation, growth, and differentiation. The effects of cytokines may be classified according to the manner by which they elicit a metabolic response.[60] Although cytokines elicit many responses to injury, the effect on nutrient metabolism is difficult to determine since it is likely that they do not act alone but rather with multiple mediators. Two of the better known cytokines are tumor necrosis factor (TNF) and interleukin-1 (IL-1). TNF is produced by the stimulated macrophage and elicits various effects on protein, carbohydrate, and fat metabolism. It accelerates skeletal muscle breakdown, redistributing this amino acid supply to the liver for hepatic production of acute-phase proteins.[61] In the liver, it acts synergistically with glucagon to increase uptake of amino acids. TNF influences glucose metabolism by increasing transport of glucose in muscle cells where it also depletes glycogen stores and increases the efflux of lactate. Although not confirmed as yet, it is suspected that TNF influences lipid metabolism by inhibiting the activity of lipoprotein lipase. Also, TNF increases the release of IL-1, which acts synergistically with TNF. IL-1 release from the activated macrophage is augmented by increased plasma levels of corticosteroids, catecholamines, and glucagon.[60] IL-1 stimulates glucocorticoid release by affecting the pituitary–adrenal axis.[61] Finally, the hepatic synthesis of albumin is inhibited while the production of fibrinogen, haptoglobin, c-reactive protein, serum amyloid A, and ceruloplasmin is stimulated by IL-1.[60] With the identification of these substances that mediate the inflammatory response, it is apparent that the mechanisms of this response are very complex, probably involving multiple mediators, some of which affect inflammatory and immune events while others act primarily on metabolic processes. In any case, the response and utilization of exogenously administered nutrients during this injury response are profoundly influenced by these inflammatory response mediators.

The combined effects of starvation and clinical disease create a complex clinical situation in which the response and tolerance to infused nutrients are altered. In this situation, the metabolic fate of infused glucose and fat may not be reliably predicted. Stress metabolism expands the available glucose pool by stimulating endogenous glucose production (gluconeogenesis) and decreasing glucose utilization as a result of impaired insulin secretion and activity.[62] Infused glucose contributes to this "glucose pool," the quantity of which may easily exceed the body's ability to oxidize it appropriately as a fuel source. In fact, at an infusion rate of 4 mg/kg/min, less than 50% of the administered glucose is directly oxidized.[9] The amount of glucose that is directly oxidized does not increase at higher glucose infusion rates, leaving proportionally greater amounts of glucose to be disposed of by the body. The hyperglycemia that ensues may respond to exogenous insulin administration but this increased delivery of glucose within the cell has little effect on glucose oxidation. Therefore, there is a lack of correlation between glucose clearance and oxidation when the maximal rate of glucose oxidation (~4 mg/kg/min) is exceeded. When this occurs, detrimental effects may be observed (Table 132.8).[9]

TABLE 132.8. PHYSIOLOGIC EFFECTS OF EXCESS GLUCOSE ADMINISTRATION

- Triglyceride synthesis and deposition in the liver, leading to fatty infiltration and cholestasis
- Increased metabolic rate due to increased energy required for triglyceride synthesis
- CO_2 production increased in excess of elevated oxygen consumption, resulting in an increased respiratory quotient
- Increased water production during conversion of glucose to fat

During stress, the mobilization of FFAs from adipose tissue leads to an increased hepatic uptake of FFAs with subsequent increased production and release of triglycerides. The triglycerides released by the liver are a source for extrahepatic tissue oxidative metabolism. However, these triglycerides require enzymatic hydrolysis by lipoprotein lipase (LPL) to release FFAs, thereby making them available to the cell. LPL is located in the luminal surface of capillary endothelial cells in various tissues. The metabolic fate of the FFAs released by LPL is dependent on the tissue where the LPL resides.[63] LPL activity may be suppressed during sepsis, limiting the capacity of extrahepatic tissues to clear triglycerides.[61] The significance of this to clinical nutrition and to the use of fat as a calorie source during sepsis has not been determined.

In summary, the hormonal profile of injury produces a rapid breakdown of body protein and a rapid increase in the rate of fat oxidation. The body favors endogenous stores of fuel while the "biologic importance of the wound," prevails whereby net negative nitrogen balance occurs for the body *in toto* and positive nitrogen balance exists in the injured tissue.[34] This adaptation of body protein turnover is well tolerated for short periods (Table 132.9) but with extension of this period along with starvation, significant decreases in body cell mass (BCM) could occur (Table 132.9).

TABLE 132.9. PERCENT LOSS OF MUSCLE MASS[a] DURING STARVATION AND TRAUMA

Condition	Duration (days)	% Muscle Lost
Starvation	1	0.6
Starvation	5	3.1
Mild trauma	5	4.1
Severe trauma	10	12.4
Severe trauma	30	36.8

[a]Assumes all nitrogen loss is from muscle mass as explained in text.

BIOLOGICAL IMPORTANCE OF THE WOUND

The composite process of wound healing is made up of various components including epithelialization, contraction, establishment of full thickness continuity, and restoration of tensile strength through collagen synthesis.[34] The biochemical events of collagen synthesis are sensitive to certain nutritional deficiencies.[64,65] Protein deficiency causes a decrease in proteoglycan and collagen synthesis. Methionine is essential for the reversal of the negative influence of protein deficiency on collagen production. Its conversion to cysteine allows for appropriate cofactor activity in the presence of a cation or provides a disulfide bond essential for alignment and triple helix formation of tropocollagen. Vitamins have various effects on collagen synthesis. Ascorbic acid is required for hydroxylation of proline and lysine, whereas vitamin A is reported to counteract the inhibitory action of corticosteroids on collagen synthesis and may be a cofactor for collagen synthesis and cross-linkage. Vitamin E interferes with collagen synthesis and cross-linkage. Vitamin E interferes with collagen synthesis and wound repair; the vitamins pyridoxine, riboflavin, and thiamine may act as cofactors in collagen cross-linking reactions.

The major components of collagen are glycine, proline, alanine, and hydroxyproline. Hydroxyproline and hydroxylysine are not found in significant quantities in any other protein than collagen. Approximately every third amino acid in collagen is glycine and 25% of collagen is hydroxyproline. Collagen is low in content of tyrosine and tryptophan (aromatic amino acids). The amino acid sequence of collagen is highly repetitive with alternating polar (glutamic acid, lysine) and nonpolar compounds. The fibroblast is the active cell of collagen formation.[34]

CANCER

There are many nutrient metabolic abnormalities in cancer patients. Anorexia related to an altered taste and smell sensation is common.[66] Metabolic abnormalities may also be created by the stress of cancer treatment, be it surgery, chemotherapy, radiation therapy, or their combined complications. Altered metabolism includes increased energy metabolism, glucose intolerance, change in fatty acid metabolism with increased oxidation and lipolysis, and increased protein breakdown and gluconeogenesis from protein as well as lactate.[67] The cancer cell creates a demand for glucose as a fuel at a high rate of anaerobic metabolism. This elevated gluconeogenic activity drains the body's ATP; as 6 moles of ATP is required per mole of synthesized glucose, as the body loses 8 moles of ATP per mole of glucose recycled. In contrast, the complete oxidation of glucose via the citric acid cycle forms 30 moles of ATP.

The cancer cell depends on glucose as a fuel, even though fatty acids are available from lipolysis created by a deranged insulin-to-glucagon ratio. (Lipolysis will, however, make fat available as an energy source for normal tissues.[68]) Protein turnover and synthesis increase, with an increase in hepatic synthesis, but skeletal muscle synthesis declines.[69] Also, cancer tissue may act as a "nitrogen trap," because protein taken up by the cancer cell may not be influenced by hormonal and neuroendocrine protein control and therefore not be available to support the dynamic protein state that normally exists.

Alterations in cytokine production in response to tumor have been proposed to explain the anorexia and metabolic derangements found in cancer.[68] If the proposed immunologic defense to rapidly growing tumors is ineffective, secretion of cytokines will continue. In addition to influencing nutrient metabolism, these substances may also be responsible for the anorexia commonly observed in cancer. While cytokine effects are of profound clinical significance in the acutely injured patient, the persistent response found in cancer patients results in severe depletion of the host body cell mass, i.e., cancer cachexia.

OBESITY

Obesity, a common condition, is the excessive accumulation of fat in the storage areas of the body. Adipose cell enlargement, hyperplasia of the cell, or both may lead to fat accumulation. Obese individuals have a higher likelihood of mortality than individuals of "ideal" body weight.

Obesity is difficult to define, and is usually based on weight, percentage over normal or as weight relates to Metropolitan Life Table definitions of ideal weight. An accepted definition is a body mass index greater than 25 kg/m^2. Gross obesity is a body mass greater than 40 kg/m^2.[70]

Metabolic abnormalities during obesity relate to insulin homeostasis.[70] Insulin secretion is increased while growth hormone is decreased. Also, cortisol secretion and turnover are increased, which, combined with the insulin status, lead to increased lipogenesis and decreased lipolysis. The pathogenesis of this abnormality may be related to beta cell hypersensitivity to carbohydrate loading to a postprandial hyperinsulinism, hypoglycemia, and hypercorticism. Tissue resistance to insulin along with the resultant hyperglycemia will then cause beta cell hyperplasia. This energy imbalance, along with an excessive energy intake, results in an intensive lipogenesis caused by the hyperinsulin state.[70]

Excess caloric intake also can result in fat accumulation in the liver (fatty infiltration). This fatty liver is the result of increased fatty acid synthesis, accumulation of acetyl CoA from glucose metabolism, and fat storage. This rate of fat synthesis may exceed the liver's normal capacity to mobilize newly synthesized fat, leading to hepatic steatosis.[71] Also, excess energy intake and the resultant lipogenesis may exceed the pulmonary capacity to expire the carbon dioxide that is produced during lipogenesis, a situation significant in patients with underlying lung disease.

PHARMACOTHERAPEUTIC CONSIDERATIONS

The pharmacologic management of disease leads to various abnormalities in nutrient metabolism. Drugs may induce specific nutrient deficiencies, suppress one's appetite, alter taste perception, or impair nutrient absorption, metabolism, and excretion. Nutritional deficiencies induced by medications may develop slowly without clinically apparent symptoms and may require sophisticated laboratory analysis or radiologic examination to diagnose and therefore are oftentimes not identified.[72]

Drug effects on appetite and taste and smell sensations impair nutrient intake.[73] Phenothiazines and antidiabetic agents are the most common drugs that increase appetite. Other examples of drugs that increase the desire for food are chlorpromazine, insulin, lithium carbonate, thioridazine, cyproheptadine, prednisone, and other corticosteroids. These effects may be beneficial in dementia patients who are at risk of protein-energy malnutrition but may lead to obesity in older adults or poor glycemic control in the diabetic.[74] Selected medications may result in decreased nutrient intake because of side effects such as taste dysfunction or dry mouth.[75] Digoxin imposes the risk of severe anorexia leading to weight loss and contributing to cardiac cachexia.[74] Dry mouth occurs frequently in patients receiving drugs having anticholinergic properties. Other effects such as gastric irritation (indomethacin and dipyridamole), appetite suppression (anticonvulsants, lithium, and procainamide) and altered sense of smell may decrease the acceptability and intake of food.[75] Nutrient absorption can also be modified if antacids, laxatives, or cathartics are taken. Other drugs such as mineral oil, cholestyramine, and clofibrate may cause fat malabsorption. Loss of efficacy and toxicity of specific drugs is frequently related to timing of drug administration in conjunction with meals or snacks.[74] The rate and efficiency of absorption of theophylline, phenytoin, nifedipine, and cyclosporine are highly influenced by the presence of food or liquid enteral formulas.[74] Phenytoin absorption has been shown to be diminished by concomitant administration of enteral tube feedings. Absorption was improved when continuous feedings were stopped 2 hours before and 2 hours after drug administration.[75]

Maintaining patency of the feeding tube is important in sustaining this route of nutrient administration. Incompatibilities of drugs with enteral tube feeding products is a common cause of clogged enteral feeding tubes.[75] Most commonly, drugs that are incompatible with enteral feedings are those that are oleaginous, have a low pH, or are syrups. One should avoid administering incompatible drugs with tube feedings and if drugs are to be administered via the feeding tube, appropriate procedures should be followed in order to maintain patency of the tube.[75]

Gastrointestinal disturbances caused by appropriate or toxic doses of drugs may interfere with nutrient intake or gastrointestinal absorption (Table 132.10). Drugs with a low therapeutic index whose side effects or toxicities influence nutritional health are lithium, digoxin, theophylline, and phenytoin. For metabolic disorders such as diabetes, uncontrolled or noncompliance with diet may lead to frequent adjustments of drug dosages or large fluctuations in blood sugar that could lead to potentially dangerous clinical conditions such as hyperosmolar coma and diabetic ketoacidosis. Hyperosmolar liquid drug preparations may exceed the body's osmolality by as much as 10-fold and induce gastrointestinal cramping, pain, nausea, vomiting, and diarrhea. Dilution of these preparations is sometimes required prior to administration in order to avoid symptoms.[76]

DRUG–NUTRIENT INTERACTIONS

Drug–nutrient interactions are defined as interactions of drugs and nutrients or non-nutrient components of food that alter drug or nutrient disposition, action, or toxicity.[77] A drug–nutrient interaction occurs when the drug interferes with nutrient metabolism. In particular, protein stores may become depleted due to the use of glucocorticoids (enhances gluconeogenesis) or antibiotics and antineoplastics that may inhibit protein synthesis. Hyper- or hypoglycemia may be induced by anabolic steroids, monoamine oxidase inhibitors, propranolol, salicylates, furosemide, and others (Table 132.11). Electrolyte imbalances can result from altered renal or gastrointestinal excretion induced by drugs.[78] Cancer chemotherapeutic agents have many effects on nutrient metabolism which may affect nutrient intake, absorption, assimilation, and excretion.

Review of the patient's medication profile may identify drug–nutrient and drug–drug interactions that may impede their nutritional status. These activities are based on the premise that medication use may do the following:

- Alter an individual's nutrient needs.
- Alter the body's response to nutrients.
- Impair an individual's ability to perform certain nutrition-related functions as a result of drug reactions or improper use of medications.
- Potentiate drug-related problems influencing the nutritional condition of the elderly caused by age, multiple drug use, and the presence of one or more chronic, debilitating diseases.

The medication profile review should include the assessment of information related to drug and food allergies and sensitivities; current weight; special diets or dietary restrictions prescribed for control of disease, i.e., low-

TABLE 132.10. SOME EFFECTS OF DRUGS IN RELATION TO VITAMINS

Drug	Possible Vitamin Effect
Antacids	Thiamine deficiency
Antibiotics	Vitamin K deficiency
Antineoplastics	Folic acid antagonism and malabsorption
Cathartics	Increased requirements for vitamin D, C, and pyridoxine
Anticonvulsants	Vitamin D and folic acid impaired absorption
Isoniazid	Pyridoxine deficiency

sodium, low-fat, low-sugar, or postgastrectomy diets; an assessment of weight changes over time; and patient loss of appetite, taste, smell, or interest in eating. Drug-related symptoms that limit mobility place the patient at risk due to the inability to prepare nutritionally adequate meals.[74] Common health problems that frequently limit an individual's ability to obtain food and prepare meals may be an indication that drugs being administered are not controlling the disease symptomatology.[74] These symptoms are manifested as susceptibility to falls, fatigue, chest pain, breathlessness on exertion, back and joint pain, incontinence, impaired visual acuity, and confusion.[76] These symptoms may be due to drug misuse or ineffectiveness of drug action when drugs are taken inappropriately in relation to meals. Also, multiple drug use has the potential to lead to adverse drug reactions or drug–drug interactions that limit food shopping ability.

Drug–nutrient interactions may result in both beneficial and undesired outcomes. Most frequently, the effects of food on drug absorption need to be considered. Food influences drug absorption by any or all of the following mechanisms: changing gastric and intestinal transit time, changing gastric pH, binding drugs to food, becoming a physical barrier to drug contact with the intestinal mucosa, and changing splanchnic blood flow.[79] Food decreases gastric emptying, which may cause excess degradation of acid-labile drugs such as penicillins when retained for prolonged periods of time in the stomach. However, retention of drug in the stomach may also increase the amount of drug dissolved when it reaches the small intestine, thereby increasing its absorption. Impaired drug absorption may also result from chelation with heavy metals (tetracycline) or by complexing with protein present in food. In general, solutions and suspensions of drugs are less susceptible to interactions with food than other drug formulations.[79] Enteric-coated preparations, however, are more susceptible to food interactions since retention in the stomach will delay drug release from the dosage form.[79] Drugs whose absorption is enhanced in the presence of food are nitrofurantoin, metoprolol, propranolol, and diazepam.[80] Food impairs the absorption of ampicillin, tetracycline, penicillin, captopril, and hydrochlorthiazide. These are only a few examples of alterations that food causes in drug absorption. It is important to note that drug absorption is commonly affected by the presence of food, the result of which is dependent on many variables. The drug, its dosage form, chemical nature (acidic or basic), the type and amount of food ingested, and the volume of fluid taken with the meal affect the extent, if any, of the drug–nutrient absorption interaction to occur. Beneficial effects of drug–nutrient interactions occur when nitrofurantoin absorption is enhanced by food, or when vitamin K antagonists (warfarin) are used to prevent thrombosis, or when the antifolic drug, methotrexate, is used as a cancer chemotherapy agent.[73] Undesired outcomes of drug–nutrient interactions appear as loss of efficacy, nutritional deficiencies (fat-soluble vitamins with mineral oil and cholestyramine use), and acute or toxic reactions that may be life threatening. Other iatrogenic disorders induced by drug–nutrient interactions are hyperglycemia (thiazide diuretics, corticosteroids) and hyperlipidemia (thiazides, adrenergic blocking agents, cyclosporine, and corticosteroids).

TABLE 132.11. DRUGS THAT ALTER GLUCOSE METABOLISM

Hyperglycemia	Hypoglycemia
Chlorpramazine	Anabolic steroids
Corticosteroids	Disopyramide
Dopamine	Clofibrate
Furosemide	Haloperidol
Phenytoin	Insulin
Theophylline	Oral hypoglycemics
Somatostatin	Propranolol
	Somatostatin

MALNUTRITION AND DRUG DISPOSITION

Protein-energy malnutrition results in derangements in gastrointestinal, cardiovascular, renal, hepatic, endocrine, and immunologic functions (Table 132.12). The individual and combined effects of these diminished body system functions may affect all aspects of drug disposition. Although massive resection of the gastrointestinal tract has no effect on oral digoxin absorption,[81] the dose of coumadin may require particularly careful monitoring in short bowel syndrome.[82] The distribution of drugs may be affected as a result of an increase in plasma volume with an associated decrease in hematocrit.[83] This results in varied effects on free drug levels.[84] Patients at high risk of malnutrition are reported to have a significantly elevated gentamicin volume of distribution (0.443 ± 0.18 L/kg) than those not at risk (0.286 ± 0.102 L/kg).[85]

Altered pharmacokinetics of drugs have been reported in patients with kwashiorkor.[83] For drugs relying on renal

TABLE 132.12. EFFECTS OF PROTEIN-ENERGY MALNUTRITION ON BODY FUNCTIONS

Edema	
Gastrointestinal	Atrophy of bowel, especially the jejunal mucosa
Cardiovascular	Diminished cardiac output, prolonged circulation time
Renal	Diminished glomerular filtration rate and renal blood flow
Total body water	Increased in proportion to the degree of malnutrition
Extracellular fluid	Proportional increase with total body water
Potassium	Depressed serum and total body stores
Liver	Fatty infiltration with abnormal liver function tests and sodium sulfobromophthalein retention, decreased urea cycle enzymes
Endocrine	Normal or elevated growth hormone, elevated thyroid stimulating hormone, atrophic adrenal glands, abnormal insulin secretion
Immunity	Depressed, increased incidence of pulmonary, renal, gastrointestinal, and bloodstream infections

excretion, methods used to estimate creatinine clearance from serum creatinine levels may be reliable but have large individual variations in malnourished patients, thereby limiting their utility.[86] In obesity, the apparent volume of distribution is greatly increased for some drugs (benzodiazepines, thiopentone, phenytoin, verapamil, and lidocaine), modestly increased for others (methylxanthines, aminoglycosides, vancomycin, ibuprofen, prednisolone, and heparin), while others are not affected (digoxin, cimetidine, procainamide).[87] Protein binding and oxidative drug metabolism do not appear to be influenced by obesity.[87] Drug disposition appears to be altered in patients with protein-energy malnutrition. The clinical significance of these effects, however, remains to be proven. At present, it is important to recognize that the effectiveness or toxicity of a medication may be influenced by the nutritional state of the patient.

CONCLUSION

Nutrition affects every metabolic and organ process in the body. As such, the provision of nutrients by either the oral or parenteral route makes available essential nutrients for metabolic purposes; however, it is the capability of the organ, tissue, or cell and the influences of the regulatory systems present at the time of nutrient availability that dictate the metabolic fate of that nutrient. This discussion presents the various possible metabolic fates that a nutrient may undergo following ingestion during both health and disease. Normal metabolism and, therefore, the treatment of malnutrition during disease processes are impaired. As a result, rehabilitation of the malnourished patient requires the stabilization of disease as well. Simply, the provision of nutrients to the body does not necessarily effect a cure for malnutrition unless a favorable metabolic status exists for efficient nutrient utilization.

REFERENCES

1. Stedman's Medical Dictionary, 22nd ed. Baltimore, Williams and Wilkins, 1972, p 865.
2. Van Itallie TB. Malnutrition: Concepts of pathogenesis and treatment, in Thorn WG, Adams RO, Braunwald E, et al (eds): Harrison's Principles of Internal Medicine, 8th ed. New York, McGraw-Hill, 1977, pp 442–445.
3. Cahill GF. Intermediary metabolism of protein, fat, and carbohydrate, in Thorn GW, Adams RO, Braunwald E. et al (eds): Harrison's Principles of Internal Medicine, 8th ed. New York, McGraw-Hill, 1977, pp 352–363.
4. The citric acid cycle, in McGilvery RW (ed): Biochemistry, A Functional Approach, 3rd ed. Philadelphia, WB Saunders, 1983, pp 421–439.
5. Wolfe BM, Ney DM. Lipid metabolism in parenteral nutrition, in Rombeau JL, Caldwell MD (eds): Clinical Nutrition, vol 2, Parenteral Nutrition. Philadelphia, WB Saunders, 1986, pp 72–99.
6. The oxidation of fatty acids, in McGilvery RW (ed): Biochemistry, A Functional Approach, 3rd ed, Philadelphia, WB Saunders, 1983, pp 440–458.
7. Rombeau JL, Kripke SA. Metabolic and intestinal effects of short-chain fatty acids. J Parent Enter Nutr 1990; 14(suppl):181S–185S.
8. The oxidation of glucose, in McGilvery RW (ed): Biochemistry, A Functional Approach, 3rd ed, Philadelphia, WB Saunders, 1983, pp 459–483.
9. Wolfe RR. Carbohydrate metabolism and requirements, in Rombeau JL, Caldwell MD (eds): Clinical Nutrition, vol 2, Parenteral Nutrition. Philadelphia, WB Saunders, 1986, pp 53–71.
10. Amino acids: Disposal of nitrogen, in McGilvery RW (ed): Biochemistry, A Functional Approach, 3rd ed. Philadelphia, WB Saunders, 1983, pp 572–592.
11. Amino acids: Disposal of the carbon skeletons, in McGilvery RW (ed): Biochemistry, A Functional Approach, 3rd ed. Philadelphia, WB Saunders, 1983, pp 593–617.
12. Rudman D, Mikkikan WJ, Richardson TJ, et al. Elemental balances during intravenous hyperalimentation of underweight adult subjects. J Clin Invest 1975;55:99–104.
13. Digestion, absorption and metabolism of food, in Hui YH (ed): Human Nutrition and Diet Therapy. Monterey, CA, Wadsworth Health Sciences, 1983, pp 193–226.
14. Howard L, Michalek AV, Alger SA. Enteral nutrition and gastrointestinal, pancreatic, and liver disease, in Rombeau JL, Caldwell MD (eds): Clinical Nutrition, vol 2, Parenteral Nutrition. Philadelphia, WB Saunders, 1993, pp 416–449.
15. Caldwell MD, Kennedy-Caldwell C. Normal nutritional requirements. Surg Clin North Am 1981;61:489–508.

16. Hiyama DT, Rolandelli RH. Short bowel syndrome, in Rombeau JL, Caldwell MD (eds): Clinical Nutrition, vol 2, Parenteral Nutrition. Philadelphia, WB Saunders, 1993, pp 498–511.
17. Afonso JJ, Rombeau JL. Parenteral nutrition for patients with inflammatory bowel disease, in Rombeau JL, Caldwell MD (eds): Clinical Nutrition, vol 2, Parenteral Nutrition, Philadelphia, WB Saunders, 1993, pp 427–441.
18. MacMahon RA. The use of the World Health Organization's oral rehydration solution in patients on home parenteral nutrition. J Parenter Enter Nutr 1984;8:720–721.
19. Storage of glucose as glycogen, in McGilvery RW (ed): Biochemistry, A Functional Approach, 3rd ed. Philadelphia, WB Saunders, 1983, pp 500–526.
20. Bivins BA, Hyde BL, Sachatello CR, et al. Physiopathology and management of hyperosmolar hyperglycemic nonketotic dehydration. Surg Gynecol Obstet 1982;154:434–440.
21. Glycolysis and gluconeogenesis, in McGilvery RW (ed): Biochemistry, A Functional Approach, 3rd ed. Philadelphia, WB Saunders, 1983, pp 484–499.
22. Felig P. The glucose-alanine cycle. Metabolism 1973;22:179.
23. Souba WW, Smith RJ, Wilmore DW. Glutamine metabolism by the intestinal tract. J Parenter Enter Nutr 1985;9:608–617.
24. Zollner N. Evaluation of non-glucose carbohydrates in parenteral nutrition, in Johnston ID (ed): Advances in Parenteral Nutrition. Lancaster, England, MTP Press Limited, 1978, p 64.
25. Wan JM-F, Teo TC, Babayan VK, Blackburn GL. Invited comment: Lipids and the development of immune dysfunction and infection. J Parenter Enter Nutr 1988; 12(suppl):43S–52S.
26. Mahley RW. Atherogenic hyperlipoproteinemia—the cellular and molecular biology of plasma lipoproteins altered by dietary fat and cholesterol. Med Clin North Am 1982; 66:375–403.
27. Stein TP, Buzby GP. Protein metabolism in surgical patients. Surg Clin North Am 1981;61:519–528.
28. Stein TP. Protein metabolism and parenteral nutrition, in Rombeau JL, Caldwell MD (eds): Clinical Nutrition, vol 2, Parenteral Nutrition. Philadelphia, WB Saunders, 1986, pp 100–134.
29. Blackburn GL, Bistrian BR, Hemsy FN. Protein metabolism in the surgical patient, in Kirkpatrick JR (ed): Nutrition and Metabolism in the Surgical Patient. Mount Kisco, NY, Futura Publishing, 1983, pp 59–88.
30. Wolfe BM, Ruderman RL, Pollard A. Basic principles of surgical nutrition: Metabolic response to starvation, trauma, and sepsis, in Dietel M (ed): Nutrition in Clinical Surgery, 2nd ed. Baltimore, Williams and Wilkins, 1985, pp 14–23.
31. Amino acids and peptides, in McGilvery RW (ed): Biochemistry, A Functional Approach, 3rd ed. Philadelphia, WB Saunders, 1983, pp 3–23.
32. Souba WW, Herskowitz K, Austgen TR, et al. Glutamine nutrition: Theoretical considerations and therapeutic impact. J Parenter Enter Nutr 1990;14(suppl):237S–243S.
33. Barbul A. Arginine biochemistry, physiology, and therapeutic implications. J Parenter Enter Nutr 1986;10:227–238.
34. Moore FD, Brennan MF. Surgical injury: Body composition, protein metabolism and neuroendocrinology, in Ballinger WF, Collins JA, Saucker WR, et al (eds): Manual of Surgical Nutrition, Philadelphia, WB Saunders, 1975, pp 169–222.
35. Ribonucleic acids and formation and function, in McGilvery RW (ed): Biochemistry, A Functional Approach, 3rd ed. Philadelphia, WB Saunders, 1983, pp 60–99.
36. Coon WW, Kowalczyk RS. Protein metabolism, in Ballinger WF, Collins JA, Drucker WR, et al (eds): Manual of Surgical Nutrition. Philadelphia, WB Saunders, 1975, pp 50–72.
37. Jackson AA. Aminoacids: Essential and non-essential? Lancet 1983;1:1034–1037.
38. Minerals, in Alpers DA, Clouse RE, Starson WF (eds): Manual of Nutritional Therapeutics. Boston, Little, Brown, 1983, pp 53–110.
39. Gann DS, Robinson HB. Salt, water and vitamins, in Ballinger WF, Collins JA, Drucker WR, et al (eds): Manual of Surgical Nutrition. Philadelphia, WB Saunders, 1975, pp 73–92.
40. Mequid MM, Collin MP, Howard LJ. Uncomplicated and stressed starvation. Surg Clin North Am 1981;61:529–544.
41. Aoki TT, Finley RJ. The metabolic response to fasting, in Rombeau JL, Caldwell MD (eds): Clinical Nutrition, vol 2, Parenteral Nutrition. Philadelphia, WB Saunders, 1986, pp 9–28.
42. Cahill GF. Starvation in man. N Engl J Med 1978; 282:668–675.
43. Levenson SM, Crowley LV, Seifter E. Starvation, in Ballinger WF, Collins JA, Drucker WR, et al (eds): Manual of Surgical Nutrition. Philadelphia, WB Saunders, 1975, pp 236–266.
44. Felig P, Owen OE, Wahren J, et al. Amino acid metabolism during prolonged starvation. J Clin Invest 1969;48:584–594.
45. Cuthbertson DP. Alterations in metabolism following injury: Part 1. Injury 1979;11:175–189.
46. Duke JG, Jorgenson SB, Broell JR, et al. The contribution of protein to caloric expenditure following injury. Surgery 1970;68:168.
47. Long CL, Kinney JM, Broell JR, et al. Contribution of protein to caloric expenditure. Surgery 1970;68:168–174.
48. Long CL, Schaffel N, Geiger JW, et al. Metabolic response to injury and illness: Estimation of energy and protein needs from indirect calorimetry and nitrogen balance. J Parenter Enter Nutr 1979;3:452–456.
49. Airlick LH, Wilmore DW. Increased peripheral amino acid release following burn injury. Surgery 1979;85:560–565.
50. Freund HR. Parenteral nutrition in the septic patient, in Rombeau JL, Caldwell MD (eds): Clinical Nutrition, vol 2, Parenteral Nutrition. Philadelphia, WB Saunders, 1986, pp 533–554.
51. Cerra FB, Caprioli J, Siegel JH, et al. Proline metabolism in sepsis, cirrhosis and general surgery. Ann Surg 1979;190:577–581.
52. Bergstrom J, Bostrous H, Furst R, et al. Pulmonary studies of energy rich phosphorous in critically ill patients. Crit Care Med 1976;4:197–204.
53. Long CL. Energy balance and carbohydrate metabolism in infection and sepsis. Am J Clin Nutr 1977;30:1301–1310.
54. Kinney JM. Clinical biochemistry: Implications for nutritional support. J Parenter Enter Nutr 1990;14:148S–156S.
55. O'Keefe SJD, Sculler PM, James WPT. "Catabolic" loss of body nitrogen in response to surgery. Lancet 1974; 2:1035–1037.

56. Crane CW, Pilou D, Smith R, et al. Protein turnover in patients before and after elective orthopedic operations. Br J Surg 1977;64:129–133.
57. Kien CL, Young VR, Rohrbaugh DK, et al. Increased rates of whole body protein synthesis and breakdown in children recovering from burns. Ann Surg 1978;187:383–391.
58. Wolfe RR, Goodenough RD, Burke JF, et al. Response of protein and urea kinetics in burn patients to different levels of protein intake. Ann Surg 1983;197:163–171.
59. Kudsk KA, Mirtallo JM. Nutritional support of the critically ill patient. Drug Intell Clin Pharm 1983;17:501–506.
60. Bessey PQ. Parenteral nutrition and trauma, in Rombeau JL, Caldwell MD (eds): Clinical Nutrition, vol 2, Parenteral Nutrition. Philadelphia, WB Saunders, 1993, pp 538–565.
61. Frankel WL, Evans NJ, Rombeau JL. Scientific rationale and clinical application of parenteral nutrition in critically ill patients, in Rombeau JL, Caldwell MD (eds): Clinical Nutrition, vol 2, Parenteral Nutrition. Philadelphia, WB Saunders, 1993, pp 597–616.
62. Knapke CM, Owens JP, Mirtallo JM. Management of glucose abnormalities in patients receiving parenteral nutrition. Clin Pharm 1989;8:136–144.
63. Eckel RH. Lipoprotein lipase. A multifunctional enzyme relevant to common metabolic disease. N Engl J Med 1989; 320:1060–1068.
64. Ruberg RL. Role of nutrition in wound healing. Surg Clin North Am 1984;64:705–714.
65. Kanke Y, Bashey RI, Mori Y. Biochemistry of collagen. NY State Med J 1981;81:1045–1052.
66. Brennan MF. Total parenteral nutrition in the cancer patient. N Engl J Med 1981;305:375–382.
67. Wesdorp RIC, Krause R, Von Meyenfeldt MF. Cancer cachexia and its nutritional implications. Br J Surg 1983; 70:352–355.
68. Kern KA, Norton JA. Cancer cachexia. J Parenter Enter Nutr 1988;12:286–298.
69. Lowry SF, Brennan MF. Intravenous feeding of the cancer patient, in Rombeau JL, Caldwell MD (eds): Clinical Nutrition, vol 2, Parenteral Nutrition. Philadelphia, WB Saunders, 1986, pp 445–470.
70. Mazansky H. A review of obesity and its management in 203 cases. S Afr Med J 1975;49:1955–1962.
71. Wolfe BM, Chock E. Energy sources, stores and hormonal controls. Surg Clin North Am 1981;61:509–518.
72. Niemiec PW, Vanderveen TW: Pharmacotherapeutic considerations during nutrition support, in Brown TR, Smith ML (eds): Handbook of Institutional Pharmacy Practice. Baltimore, Williams and Wilkins, 1986, pp 288–311.
73. Schiffman SS. Taste and smell in desease: Part 1. N Engl J Med 1983;308:1275–1279.
74. Nutrition Interventions Manual for Professionals Caring for Older Americans. Nutrition Screening Initiative, Washington, DC, 1992, pp 71–84.
75. Gora ML, Tschampel MM, Visconti JA. Considerations of drug therapy in patients receiving enteral nutrition. Nutr Clin Pract 1989;4:105–110.
76. Dickerson RN, Melnick G. Osmolality of oral drug solutions and suspensions. Am J Hosp Pharm 1988;45:832–834.
77. Roe DA. Drug effects on nutrient absorption, transport and metabolism. Drug–Nutrient Interact 1985a;4:117–135.
78. Nanji AA. Drug-induced electrolyte disorders. Drug Intell Clin Pharm 1983;17:175–185.
79. Welling PG. Interactions affecting drug absorption. Clin Pharmacokin 1984;9:404–434.
80. Skaar DJ. Drug–nutrient interactions: Implications for pharmaceutical care. Partners Pharmaceut Care 1991; (Oct):11–20.
81. Krausz MM, Berry E, Freund U, Levy M. Absorption of orally administered digoxin after massive resection of the small bowel. Am J Gastroenterol 1979;71:220–223.
82. Owens JP, Mirtallo JM, Murphy CC. Oral anticoagulation in patients with short-bowel syndrome. DICP Ann Pharmacother 1990;24:585–589.
83. Buchanan N. Drug kinetics in protein energy malnutrition. S Afr Med J 1978;53:327–330.
84. Buchanan N. Drug-protein binding and protein energy malnutrition. S Afr Med J 1977;52:733–737.
85. Zarowitz BJ, Pilla AM, Popovich J. Expanded gentamicin volume of distribution in patients with indicators of malnutrition. Clin Pharm 1990;9:40–44.
86. Boyce EG, Dickerson RN, Cooney GF, et al. Creatinine clearance estimation in protein-malnourished patients. Clin Pharm 1989;8:721–726.
87. Abernethy DR, Greenblatt DJ. Drug disposition in obese humans. An update. Clin Pharmacokin 1986;11:199–213.

Chapter 133

Parenteral Nutrition

Todd W. Mattox, PharmD, BCNSP

Maintenance of a sound nutrition status during illness has long been recognized as an integral part of the medical treatment plan for patients who are unable to utilize normal physiologic means of nourishment.[1,2] Successful techniques for providing intravenous nutrition support were introduced for clinical use in humans during the early 1960s.[3] Dilute nutrient solutions containing glucose with or without hydrolyzed protein were infused peripherally along with intravenous fat emulsion to provide adequate calories. However, fat emulsions were withdrawn from commercial availability in the United States in 1965 following several reports of serious adverse effects associated with infusions of the cottonseed oil products. Without lipid emulsions, larger volumes of nutrient solutions were required to provide the patient's energy requirements. Patients receiving intravenous nutrition solution volumes of up to 5 L/d were often given concomitant diuretic therapy to manage fluid status.[3] Metabolic complications associated with fluid overload and electrolyte imbalances stimulated the investigation of central venous access. These larger vessels permitted infusion of more concentrated formulas which decreased the fluid volume required and avoided the phlebitis that commonly occurred when hypertonic infusions were given peripherally.

By the late 1960s, Rhoads and Dudrick[3] had documented continued growth and improvement in nutritional markers in humans with the use of central intravenous nutrition. As the use of intravenous nutrition became more widespread, reports of complications increased. During the subsequent 15–20 years, clinical experience and research resulted in the development of standard protocols which promoted better patient care and a decline in complications associated with parenteral nutrition (PN) therapy.[4,5] The scope of practice for nutrition support clinicians has broadened as a result of increasing knowledge about the metabolic consequences associated with acute injury or chronic disease states and the subsequent increase in the number of products, techniques, and equipment designed for use in providing nutritional care. Nutrition support clinicians who practice specialized nutrition support may utilize specially formulated parenteral or enteral nutrients to maintain or restore optimal nutrition status depending on the level of nutritional intervention required based on a patient's nutrition assessment.[6] The pharmacist's role in providing nutrition support has been recently defined (Table 133.1).[118] A clear understanding of the principles of patient selection, initial therapy design, and outcome monitoring is essential to provide safe and effective care to those who require nutrition support.[119] This chapter addresses indications for PN, components of PN formulations, routes of intravenous administration, practical aspects of regimen design, solution admixture considerations, outcome monitoring, and management of complications.

Goals of Nutrition Support

The overall objective of nutrition support therapy is to promote positive clinical outcomes of an illness or improve a patient's quality of life. Four fundamental steps are key to providing optimal care for patients who require nutrition support. They are definition of nutrition goals, determination of nutrient requirements for achievement of the nutrition goals, delivery of the required nutrients, and subsequent assessment of the nutrition regimen.[8] Definition of a patient's nutrition goals can be established after a thorough nutritional assessment (see Chapter 130). Nutrient requirements and an appropriate route for delivery of the required nutrients can then be determined. Goals of nutrition support include correction of caloric and nitrogen imbalances, fluid or electrolyte abnormalities, and any known vitamin or trace element abnormalities without causing or worsening other metabolic complications. Specific caloric goals include energy equilibrium and preservation of fat calorie stores in well-nourished individuals and positive energy balance in malnourished patients with depleted endogenous fat stores. Obese patients with excess endogenous fat stores (>120% ideal body weight) likely require less caloric support than nonobese patients within a range of negative energy balance to energy equilibrium depending on the clinical condition of the patient.[9–11] Specific nitrogen goals are positive nitrogen balance or nitrogen equilibrium and improvement in the serum concentration of a short half-life visceral protein marker such as transferrin or prealbumin.

TABLE 133.1. SCOPE OF PRACTICE FOR NUTRITION SUPPORT PHARMACISTS

Activities	Description
Assessment of the patient's nutrition care needs	• Determine nutrient requirements based on patient's data. • Prevent and/or identify nutrient–nutrient, drug–nutrient, drug–drug, and drug–disease/condition interactions. • Assess suitability for specialized nutrition support.
Development of a nutrition care plan	• Define goals and objectives of specialized nutrition support therapy. • Select the preferred route for administration of nutrition support therapy. • Design patient-specific feeding formulations.
Implementation of the nutrition care plan	• Obtain or write prescriptions for feeding formulations. • Be proficient with techniques of compounding feeding formulations. • Perform or supervise the compounding and dispensing of parenteral feeding formulations.
Monitoring the patient's response to the nutrition therapy	• Evaluate laboratory data to determine the patient's clinical, nutritional, and metabolic responses to specialized nutrition support. • Prevent and or identify nutrient–nutrient, drug–nutrient, drug–drug, and drug–disease/condition interactions. • Evaluate continued need for specialized nutrition support.
Administrative management	• Participate in development of policy and procedures for patient care and operational aspects of specialized nutrition support.
Quality of care	• Develop and implement quality improvement activities directed at the process of nutritional and metabolic care.
Advancement of nutrition support pharmacy practice	• Contribute to the professional development of pharmacists and other health care professionals and to the education of patients through presentations, publications, and research.

(Adapted from Ref. 118.)

The clinical decision algorithm (see Chapter 131, Fig. 131.2) outlines the process for choosing the route of nutrition support for adult patients.[12] The gastrointestinal (GI) tract is the optimal route for providing nutrients unless obstruction, pancreatitis, or other GI complications are present. Other considerations that may impact determination of an appropriate route for nutrition support include expected duration of nutrition therapy and risk of aspiration. Patients who have a nonfunctional GI tract or are otherwise not a candidate for enteral nutrition (EN) may benefit from PN. Use of the intravenous route for nutrition support is also commonly referred to as total parenteral nutrition (TPN) or hyperalimentation. Routine monitoring is necessary to ensure the nutrition regimen is suitable for a given patient as his or her clinical condition changes and to minimize or treat complications early.

Indications for Parenteral Nutrition

Although improvement in nutrition status as defined by various clinical nutrition markers has been reported in patients who received PN, the impact on clinical outcome has been difficult to demonstrate. Several investigations have reported a positive effect of PN on complications and mortality while others have failed to demonstrate any difference.[13] Early studies have been criticized for defects in study design such as small sample sizes, inappropriate randomization, and inconsistent nutrition status among the study group, which hindered demonstration of the effectiveness of PN therapy. However, the association between malnutrition and development of complications and mortality has been well documented.[14] These conflicting data have complicated identification of the patient who is most likely to benefit from PN. Reports from a variety of health professional groups are evidence for the controversy concerning the appropriate role of PN in clinical care.[15–18] One of the earliest statements regarding indications for PN was the initial American Society for Parenteral and Enteral Nutrition (ASPEN) guidelines for use of TPN in hospitalized patients.[15] However, because of the generalized nature of these guidelines, they were not a useful tool for identification of the ideal candidate for PN therapy. More recent guidelines are based on expanded clinical experience and investigations of PN in specific patient populations where PN therapy is often prone to misuse, such as presurgical patients or patients receiving chemotherapy.[19–21] These investigations have demonstrated that some patients who previously may have been considered candidates for PN may not necessarily benefit from the intervention.

TABLE 133.2. INDICATIONS FOR TPN

1. Inability to absorb nutrients via the gastrointestinal tract because of one or more of the following:
   a. Massive small bowel resection.
   b. Intractable vomiting when adequate enteral intake is not expected for 5–7 days.
   c. Severe diarrhea not expected to resolve in 5–7 days.
   d. Inflammatory bowel disease (Crohn's disease, ulcerative colitis)
      PN may benefit patients with acute exacerbations of ulcerative colitis when surgery is being considered and when preservation of lean body mass and functional capacity with enteral nutrition is impossible.
   e. Bowel obstruction
2. Cancer—antineoplastic therapy, radiation therapy, bone marrow transplantation
   Enteral tube feeding and parenteral nutrition support may benefit some severely malnourished cancer patients or those in whom gastrointestinal or other toxicities are anticipated to preclude adequate oral nutritional intake for more than 1 week. Patients who are candidates for nutrition intervention under these circumstances should receive nutrition support, if possible, in conjunction with the initiation of oncologic therapy.
   Specialized nutrition support is not routinely indicated for well-nourished or mildly malnourished patients undergoing surgery, chemotherapy, or radiation treatment and in whom adequate oral intake is anticipated.
   PN is unlikely to benefit patients with advanced cancer whose malignancy is documented as unresponsive to chemotherapy or radiation therapy.
3. Moderate to severe pancreatitis when adequate enteral intake is not expected for 5–7 days.
   PN should be used when enteral feeding exacerbates abdominal pain, ascites, or fistula output in patients with pancreatitis and limited oral intake.
4. Severe malnutrition[a] with a temporary (5–7 days) nonfunctional gastrointestinal tract.
5. Critical care
   Moderate to severe catabolism with or without malnutrition when the gastrointestinal tract is nonfunctional for 5–7 days (e.g., major surgery, trauma, sepsis).
6. Organ failures—liver, renal, respiratory
   Moderate to severe catabolism with or without malnutrition when enteral feeding is contraindicated.
7. Preoperative malnutrition[a] when the gastrointestinal tract is not functional and surgery is not expected for at least 7 days.
8. Hyperemesis gravidarum
9. Eating disorders
   PN should be considered for patients with anorexia nervosa who require nonvolitional feeding but who cannot tolerate enteral support for physical or emotional reasons.

[a]Malnutrition (upon initial assessment):
Ref. 21:
- 0–5% weight loss over past 6 months and serum albumin <3.0 g/%.
- 10–15% weight loss over past 6 months and serum albumin <3.5 g/%.

Ref. 18:
- Loss of ≥10% pre-illness weight, decreased serum albumin concentration.

A recent report from the Technology Assessment and Practice Guidelines Forum was a major step toward development of more comprehensive guidelines for identifying patients who may benefit from PN therapy.[17] The forum panel that produced these guidelines consisted of health care practitioners from a variety of backgrounds including surgery, pediatrics, internal medicine, nursing, nutrition, statistics, research methodology, and policy analysis. The most current statement regarding indications for PN is the revised guidelines published by the ASPEN Board of Directors.[18] This statement includes detailed background information concerning the development of the practice guidelines and specific patient criteria characteristics or clinical situations when PN is indicated (Table 133.2). Although many of the consensus reports from various health professional groups do not fully agree and lack specificity in describing appropriate candidates for PN, the ASPEN guidelines provide a degree of specificity, which should facilitate institutional development of appropriate, specific PN usage guidelines.

Parenteral Nutrition Components

Parenteral nutrition solutions should provide the optimal combination of macronutrients and micronutrients to meet the specific nutritional requirements of the patient. Macronutrients include water, protein, dextrose, and intravenous lipid emulsion. Micronutrients include vitamins, trace elements, and electrolytes. Both macronutrients and micronutrients are necessary for maintenance of normal metabolism. In general, macronutrients are utilized for energy (dextrose, fat) and as structural substrates (protein, fats). Micronutrients are usually required in smaller amounts to support a variety of metabolic activities necessary for cellular homeostasis such as enzymatic reactions, fluid balance, and regulation of electrophysiologic processes. These components usually require individualized adjustments as the patient's clinical condition dictates changes in metabolic stress, organ function, fluid and electrolyte balance, and acid–base status.

AMINO ACIDS

Protein in PN solutions is provided in the form of crystalline amino acids (CAAs). This nutritional substrate is utilized primarily for protein synthesis (see Chapter 132). The caloric contribution from protein is usually not considered in calculating total calories provided by the PN regimen. Sufficient energy substrate should be provided to allow utilization of amino acids for protein synthesis rather than an energy source. However, oxidation of amino acids for energy has been demonstrated in critically ill patients and is thought to occur because of metabolic derangements seen during severe metabolic stress.[22] Hence, some institutions may include the caloric contribution from amino acids when determining the total daily calories provided by a PN regimen. When oxidized for energy, 1 gram of protein yields 4 kilocalories (kcal).

Commercially available CAA solutions may be categorized as standard amino acid solutions or modified amino acid solutions. Standard amino acid solutions are designed for use in patients with "normal" organ function and nutritional requirements (Table 133.3). These solutions contain a balanced profile of essential, semiessential, and nonessential L-amino acids. Although the optimal proportion of different amino acids in CAA solutions has not been clearly defined, use of currently available standard CAA products has resulted in similar effects on markers of protein utilization.[23,24] These products also differ in total nitrogen content, electrolyte content, and commercially available concentrations. Differences in nitrogen content per gram weight of amino acids among CAA products may affect

TABLE 133.3. MACRONUTRIENT COMPONENTS OF PARENTERAL NUTRITION SOLUTIONS

Nutritional Substrate	Intravenous Source	Commercial Product (Manufacturer)		Concentrations Available (%)
Fluid	Sterile water for injection USP	Various manufacturers		
Nitrogen	Crystalline amino acids	Aminosyn	(Abbott)	3.5, 5, 7, 8.5, 10
		Aminosyn II	(Abbott)	3.5, 5, 7, 8.5, 10, 15
		FreAmine III	(McGaw)	3, 8.5, 10
		Travasol	(Travenol)	5.5, 8.5, 10
		Novamine	(KabiVitrum)	15
	Intravenous dipeptides	Investigational		
	L-alanyl-L-glutamine			
	Glycyl-L-tyrosine			
	L-alanyl-L-tyrosine			
	N-acetyl-L-tyrosine	Used in Trophamine	(McGaw)	
Energy				
Carbohydrate	Dextrose	Various manufacturers		5, 10, 20, 25, 30, 50, 60, 70
	Glycerol	Used in Procalamine	(McGaw)	3% amino acids/3% glycerol
	Xylitol	Investigational		
Fat	Intravenous fat emulsion			
	LCT emulsions {oil source}	Intralipid {soybean}	(Clintec)	10, 20, 30[a]
		Liposyn II {soybean/safflower}	(Abbott)	10, 20
		Liposyn III {soybean}	(Abbott)	10, 20
		Neutrilipid {soybean}	(McGaw)	10, 20
		Soyacal {soybean}	(Alpha Therapeutic)	10, 20
	LCT/MCT combination	Investigational		
	Short-chain fatty acids	Investigational		
	Omega 3 fatty acids	Investigational		

Key: LCT, long-chain triglycerides; MCT, medium-chain triglycerides; { }, source of triglycerides.
[a]Approved only for use in the preparation of total nutrient admixtures and is not intended for direct administration.

$$\text{Nitrogen balance} = \text{nitrogen}_{in} - \text{nitrogen}_{out}$$

$$\text{Nitrogen}_{in}\ (g/d) = \text{protein}_{in}\ (g/d) \div 6.25\ \text{g protein/g nitrogen}$$

$$\text{Nitrogen}_{out}\ (g/day) = \text{urinary nitrogen} + (\text{nonurea nitrogen} + \text{insensible losses} + \text{integumentary losses})^*$$

*Clinically, these measurements are usually estimated to be 2–7 g/d depending on the clinical condition of the patient (see chapter 130).

Figure 133.1. Calculation of nitrogen balance.

calculation of nitrogen amounts infused when determining nitrogen balance (Fig. 133.1).[25] Because dietary protein consists of approximately 16% by weight nitrogen, 6.25 is commonly accepted as the conversion figure for calculating the amount of nitrogen provided by CAA protein. However, the nitrogen content of commercially available CAA solutions varies from approximately 11–17% per gram weight of amino acid.[25] The clinical significance of the difference in calculations is not known. Use of 6.25 g protein/g nitrogen is commonly recommended for routine clinical calculation of nitrogen balance.[25–27]

Electrolyte composition of standard CAA solutions varies from small, obligatory amounts to the provision of maintenance requirement of most electrolytes for an adult. The contribution of electrolytes from CAA solutions must be considered when determining a patient's individual requirements. CAA solutions are available in several concentrations, which facilitates compounding of patient-specific PN regimens. The higher concentrated solutions, the 10 and 15% products, are attractive for use in critically ill patients who typically require fluid restriction but have large protein needs.[28] Modified amino acid solutions are designed for use in patients who have altered protein requirements such as those with hepatic encephalopathy, renal failure, metabolic stress/trauma, and neonates and pediatric patients (Table 133.4). These solutions tend to be more expensive than standard CAA solutions. In addition, the rationale for and clinical role of modified amino acids in disease-specific PN regimens is controversial (see Chapter 136). Commercially available CAA solutions have been altered by some to provide conditionally essential amino acids (CEAAs) in PN solutions.[29] CEAAs are considered nonessential because they are produced from other amino acids during health. However, under certain physiologic conditions such as the perinatal period, or pathophysiologic conditions such as sepsis, these amino acids cannot be synthesized in sufficient quantities.[24] Some alterations of the composition of CAA solutions may not be clinically feasible, since some amino acids are relatively unstable or poorly soluble. To overcome these limitations, dipeptide amino acids have been investigated as a potential parenteral source for CEAAs. Dipeptides are synthesized by combin-

TABLE 133.4. MODIFIED CRYSTALLINE AMINO ACID SOLUTIONS

Clinical Condition	Amino Acid Solution (Manufacturer)	Characteristics
Hepatic encephalopathy	Hepatamine 8% (McGaw)	Amino acid profile includes higher concentrations of BCAA and lower concentrations of AAA and methionine.
Renal failure	Aminosyn RF 5.2% (Abbott) NephrAmine 5.4% (McGaw) RenAmine 6.5% (Clintec) Aminess 5.2% (Clintec)	Amino acid profile includes higher concentrations of EAA and histidine.
Metabolic stress/trauma	Aminosyn HBC 7% (Abbott) FreAmine 6.9% HBC (McGaw) BranchAmin 4%[a] (Clintec)	Amino acid profile includes standard essential, semiessential, and nonessential amino acids with higher concentrations of BCAA.
Pediatrics	Aminosyn PF 7%, 10% Trophamine 6%, 10%	Amino acid profile includes standard essential, semiessential, and nonessential amino acids with lower concentrations of methionine, phenylalanine, and glycine. These solutions also contain taurine, glutamate and aspartate.

Key: BCAA, branched-chain amino acids (leucine, isoleucine, valine); AAA, aromatic amino acids (includes phenylalanine and tyrosine); EAA, essential amino acids (leucine, isoleucine, valine, phenylalanine, tryptophan, methionine, threonine, and lysine).

[a]Used as a supplement to a standard amino acid solution to increase BCAA content.

ing two amino acids with a peptide bond. The resulting protein is more soluble and stable than the individual amino acids alone.[30] Examples of those amino acid combinations currently under investigation in humans or present in current CAA products are listed in Table 133.3. Intravenous dipeptide formulations would be clinically advantageous since they incorporate higher concentrations of some specific amino acids, as well as some low solubility, low stability amino acids that are omitted or present in small quantities in current CAA solutions. In addition, use of dipeptides would allow formulation of CAA solutions with a higher nitrogen content. Further studies are needed to assess long-term safety and optimal combinations of amino acids in different disease states.[31]

DEXTROSE

The primary energy source in PN solutions is carbohydrate, usually in the form of dextrose monohydrate. This nutritional substrate is available in a variety of concentrations ranging from 5–70%, which allows compounding of patient-specific PN regimens. When oxidized, each gram of hydrated dextrose provides 3.4 kcal. Dextrose is oxidized at a maximum rate of 4–7 mg/kg/min in humans receiving TPN.[32] Dextrose infused in amounts beyond this rate are used by the liver for repletion of glycogen stores and lipid synthesis. Higher infusion rates may also contribute to development of metabolic complications such as hyperglycemia, excess carbon dioxide production, lipogenesis, and increased liver function tests secondary to fatty liver.[33] Recommended doses for routine clinical care rarely exceed 5 mg/kg/min.[34,35] Dextrose requires insulin for transport into many cells such as skeletal muscle for oxidation. Because critically ill patients tend to develop stress-related hyperglycemia, which may complicate providing PN, other non-insulin-dependent sources of carbohydrate have been investigated.[36] Those that have received the most attention are xylitol, sorbitol, fructose, and glycerol. Of these nutrients only glycerol is approved for clinical use in humans. Glycerol is a sugar alcohol that provides 4.3 kcal/g and is commercially available as a 3% solution in combination with 3% amino acids and supplemental electrolytes (Procalamine, McGaw). This product is nearly isotonic so it may be infused peripherally. A major disadvantage with the use of this formula is the dilute concentrations of amino acids and carbohydrate. Most patients may require up to 3–4 L/d of Procalamine solution together with lipid emulsion as a caloric source to provide minimum energy requirements.[37]

LIPID EMULSION

Intravenous lipid emulsion (IVLE) may also be used as a concentrated source of calories in a PN regimen as well as a source of essential fatty acids. When oxidized, 1 gram of fat yields 9 kcal. Current IVLE products differ in source of triglycerides, fatty acid content, and commercially available concentrations. IVLEs are derived from soybean oil or a combination of soybean oil and safflower oil. The source of triglycerides is emulsified with egg phospholipids and glycerol is added to make the emulsion isotonic. Finally water is added to make final concentrations of either 10, 20, or 30% emulsion (Table 133.3). Because of the caloric contribution from the egg phospholipid and glycerol, the caloric content of IVLE is 1.1 kcal/mL for 10% emulsion, 2 kcal/mL for 20% emulsion, and 3 kcal/mL for 30% emulsion.[38,39] The sources of triglyceride in IVLE differ in fatty acid composition. Soybean oil emulsions contain approximately 50–60% linoleic acid and 4–11% linolenic acid, while IVLEs that contain safflower oil are made of approximately 66% linoleic acid and 4% linolenic acid.[39,40] Linolenic is an omega 3 fatty acid and linoleic acid is an omega 6 fatty acid. They are both polyunsaturated long-chain triglycerides (LCTs). Both types of emulsions are effective in the treatment or prevention of essential fatty acid deficiency (EFAD). EFAD is the result of a biochemical deficiency of linoleic acid and arachidonic acid, which are considered essential in humans. Linolenic acid may be essential although the data are not conclusive. However, all commercially available IVLEs contain soybean oil as a predominant source of linolenic acid. These fatty acids are important for a variety of functions such as cellular integrity, platelet function, and wound healing.[41] Normally, linoleic acid is converted to the tetraene arachidonic acid. EFAD occurs when linoleic acid is not present in sufficient amounts to drive the preferred reaction to arachidonic acid. Instead, oleic acid is converted to the triene 5,8,11-eicosatrienoic acid, a fatty acid of lesser physiologic integrity. EFAD may be prevented by providing 2–5% of total calories as linoleic acid. This may be achieved in most patients by giving 500 mL of 10% fat emulsion two to three times weekly. Patients with clinical manifestations of EFAD usually respond after a 2-week course of lipid emulsion given in amounts to provide 25% of the total daily caloric requirements.[38,41]

As a caloric source, lipid emulsion is probably most useful in metabolic stress, pancreatitis or diabetes, and carbon dioxide-retaining ventilator dependency. The use of lipid emulsion may facilitate provision of adequate calories and minimize complications of nutrition therapy such as hyperglycemia, hepatotoxicity, or increased production of carbon dioxide (see Chapter 136). In the past, general recommendations for use of IVLEs as part of a PN regimen have been 25–50% of total nonprotein calories, not to exceed 60% of the total caloric intake. Thus, the daily dosage should not exceed 2.5 g/kg/d in adults and 4 g/kg/d in infants.[38,41] Lipid emulsion may be infused over 4–6 hours. However, recent data in animals and humans suggest that rapid infusion of the current long-chain fatty acid formulations may negatively impact immunocompetence by saturating the reticuloendothelial system.[42,43] Provision of approximately 1–1.5 g/kg/d not to exceed 30–40% of total calories infused over 24 hours appears to be a reasonable compromise in view of the lack of clear data concerning effects on morbidity and mortality in humans and the clinical utility of lipid emulsion as a noncarbohydrate source.[34,35,38,44]

The manufacturer's guidelines suggest initiating lipid emulsion infusions with a test dose. However, in most patients, this is probably not necessary because of the relatively low incidence and benign nature of acute adverse reactions. In addition, infusions over 24 hours eliminate the need for a test dose because the infusion rate is less than the test dose rate recommended by the manufacturer. Commercially available 10 and 20% IVLE products may be administered either by central or peripheral vein. They may be added directly to the parenteral nutrition solution as a total nutrient admixture (TNA) or 3-in-1 system (lipids, protein, glucose, and additives) or they may be piggybacked with the CAA/dextrose solution.[38] The more concentrated 30% IVLE is approved only for use in the preparation of TNA and is not intended for direct intravenous administration.[39] In general, the use of IVLE is contraindicated in patients with an impaired ability to clear lipid emulsion.[38,41]

A history of egg allergy is a relative contraindication to the use of IVLE. However, patients with a reported egg allergy should be carefully evaluated for the nature and severity of the reaction before deciding to initiate a lipid-based PN regimen. Most of the more toxic reactions such as impaired liver function, thrombocytopenia, prolonged clotting time, and spontaneous bleeding were reported in the early 1960s with the intravenous use of Lipomul, a cottonseed oil emulsion that was subsequently withdrawn from the market.[45] Although the frequency of immediate or early adverse effects has been reported to be less than 1% with current formulations, patients receiving their first dose of lipid emulsion should be monitored for acute adverse reactions such as dyspnea, tightness of chest, palpitations, and chills. Headache, nausea, and fever have also been reported and may be associated with a rapid infusion rate. Hepatic abnormalities such as elevated transaminases, hepatomegaly, and intrahepatic cholestasis have been reported with multiple infusions although these alterations are transient and are usually associated with excessive doses.[38,41]

The negative effects of LCT on immune function have stimulated a search for new sources of lipids.[42,43] Medium-chain triglycerides (MCTs) have been investigated in humans and may offer several advantages especially for critically ill patients. MCTs are more rapidly hydrolyzed and cleared than LCTs and they do not accumulate in the liver. In addition, MCTs do not require carnitine for entrance into mitochondria for oxidation. However, MCTs are not a source of essential fatty acids. Furthermore, in early studies of pure MCTs in animals and humans, central nervous toxicities and other significant adverse effects such as dyspnea and vomiting that appeared to be dose related were reported.[42,46] Subsequent studies of intravenous MCT/LCT mixtures in a variety of patients have demonstrated safety and efficacy comparable to standard LCT emulsions.[42,43,46] Several MCT/LCT products are available in Europe although no intravenous MCT formulations are currently commercially available in the United States. Other intravenous lipid formulations currently being investigated contain omega 3 polyunsaturated fatty acids (PUFAs).[47,48] Current IVLE contains omega 6 PUFAs as linoleic acid and omega 3 PUFAs as linolenic acid. Omega 3 PUFAs are metabolized to cytokine mediators, which may be less inflammatory and immunosuppressive than those derived from omega 6 PUFAs.[49] Use of enteral solutions with a higher concentration of omega 3 PUFAs has been associated with decreased infections and improvement in *in vitro* immunological indices in critically ill patients.[42,50] However, the optimal balance of omega 3 and omega 6 PUFAs required to achieve the greatest desired change in metabolism for different disease states is not known.[42,51]

VITAMINS

Vitamins are important components of a PN regimen since they are necessary for the maintenance of normal metabolism and cellular function. Fat soluble vitamins are extensively stored in the body's fat tissue, while water-soluble vitamins are stored in limited amounts by the body. Maintenance guidelines for daily parenteral vitamin supplements have been established by the Nutrition Advisory Group of the American Medical Association (NAG–AMA) for adults, children, and infants.[52] These guidelines are based on the recommended daily allowances (RDAs), which are designed to meet requirements of healthy people. Vitamin requirements during metabolic stress or specific organ failures have not been fully agreed upon.[53–55] The most current NAG–AMA recommendations for parenteral vitamin requirements in infants and children reflect data reported in pediatric patients who received currently available formulations.[56] In general, the revised recommendations focused on changes for preterm infants requiring PN.

Several commercially available adult and pediatric multiple vitamin products have been formulated to comply specifically with the NAG–AMA guidelines (Table 133.5). Parenteral multiple vitamin products for adults do not contain vitamin K in order to avoid a drug–nutrient interaction in patients receiving anticoagulants, which antagonize vitamin K. The NAG–AMA recommendation for vitamin K in adults is 2–4 mg weekly. However, others have recommended larger doses of 5–10 mg weekly.[55] Vitamin K may be given intramuscularly or subcutaneously or added to the PN solution.[57] Vitamin requirements may be altered in malnutrition and other specific disease states or with certain drug therapies. Individual and combination products are

TABLE 133.5. MICRONUTRIENT COMPONENTS OF PARENTERAL NUTRITION SOLUTIONS: VITAMINS[a]

Intravenous Source	Commercial Product (Manufacturer)	How Supplied
Fat soluble	Adult	Multiple vitamin products are available as complete solutions or as individual nutrient solutions. Those listed to the left are multiple vitamin solutions for adults and pediatric patients. Vitamin K is not included in commercially prepared adult intravenous multiple vitamin products but is included in pediatric solutions. Refer to manufacturers' product information for specific vitamin composition.
A, D, E, K	MVI-12 (Astra)	
Water soluble	MVC 9 + 3 (Lyphomed)	
Thiamine (B_1)	Pediatric	
Riboflavin (B_2)	MVI-Pediatric (Astra)	
Pyridoxine (B_6)		
Cyanacobalamin (B_{12})		
Vitamin C (ascorbic acid)		
Folic acid		
Nicotinic acid (niacin, B_3)		
Pantothenic acid		
Biotin		

[a]This is not a complete listing of all commercially available formulations of intravenous multiple vitamin solutions at the time of publication.

available to provide additional or tailored supplementation, which may be necessary to prevent development of vitamin toxicities or deficiencies caused by altered metabolism or drug therapy.

TRACE ELEMENTS

Trace elements are minerals that are required in very small amounts for a variety of biochemical and physiologic functions. Many trace elements are an important part of metalloenzymes and also function as cofactors in a variety of regulatory metabolic pathways.[58,59] Although 17 trace elements have demonstrated biologic importance, clear deficiency syndromes in humans have been described only for iron, iodine, cobalt (as vitamin B_{12}), zinc, and copper.[58–61] The NAG–AMA recognized zinc, copper, and chromium as being essential for intravenous supplementation in patients receiving PN.[62] While a clear deficiency syndrome for manganese has not been reported in humans, the NAG–AMA considered manganese essential based on data from case reports of patients receiving PN with metabolic complications that corrected after manganese supplementation.[59,60,62] More recent reports of deficiency syndromes associated with selenium and molybdenum deficiency suggest they may also be essential. However, recommendations for supplemental dosing of the two do not agree.[58,60,63] Recommendations for trace elements in pediatric patients receiving PN have been revised as well.[56]

Commercially prepared intravenous trace elements are available as single mineral, multiple mineral, and multiple mineral with electrolytes solutions for adult and pediatric patients (Table 133.6). These products are designed to provide approximate daily requirements for zinc, copper, chromium, and manganese according to the NAG–AMA recommendations. Other products contain iodide, molybdenum, or selenium in addition to the NAG–AMA essential trace elements. Routine use of these trace elements during short-term PN is controversial. Currently little evidence exists to support routine supplementation of the other trace elements in patients receiving PN. Requirements for trace elements are age specific and may change depending on the clinical condition of the patient. For example, higher doses of supplemental zinc are likely necessary in patients with high-output ostomies or diarrhea because the normal route of excretion for zinc is predominantly via the GI tract. Manganese and copper are excreted through the biliary tract, whereas chromium, molybdenum, and selenium are excreted renally. Hence, these trace elements should be restricted or withheld from PN solutions in patients with cholestatic liver disease and renal failure, respectively. Because requirements of these trace elements during organ failure are not clearly defined, a clinically practical method of empirically reducing trace element doses when using a multiple trace element solution is to give the recommended daily dose two to three times weekly instead of daily.[64]

ELECTROLYTES

Electrolytes such as sodium, potassium, calcium, magnesium, phosphorus, chloride, and acetate are necessary components of PN for the maintenance of numerous cellular functions including acid–base balance and cellular growth. Electrolytes may be given to maintain normal serum concentrations or to correct deficits. Patients who have "normal" organ function and relatively normal serum concentrations of any electrolyte should receive normal maintenance doses of electrolytes on initiation of PN and daily thereafter. Requirements for specific electrolytes will vary according to the patient's disease state, organ function (see Chapter 136), previous and current drug therapy, nutrition status, and extrarenal losses such as nasogastric suction, vomiting, diarrhea, or fistulas (see Table 133.11 in a

TABLE 133.6. MICRONUTRIENT COMPONENTS OF PARENTERAL NUTRITION SOLUTIONS: TRACE ELEMENTS[a]

Intravenous Source	Commercial Product (Manufacturer)	How Supplied
Trace elements associated with a defined clinical deficiency Zinc Copper Chromium Manganese Iodine Selenium Molybdenum Iodine Iron[b]	Adults Multiple Trace Element Multiple Trace Element with Selenium (American Regent) MulTE-PAK-4 MulTE-PAK-5 ConTE-PAK-4 (Smith and Nephew SoloPak) MTE-4 MTE-5 MTE-6 MTE-7 Tracelyte Tracelyte with Double Electrolytes Tracelyte II Tracelyte II with Double Electrolytes (Lyphomed) Pediatrics Multiple Trace Element Neonatal Multiple Trace Element Pediatric (American Regent) PedTE-Pak-4 (Smith and Nephew SoloPak) Neotrace-4 Pedtrace-4 PTE-4 PTE-5 (Lyphomed)	Trace element products are available as complete solutions or as individual nutrient solutions. Some trace element products include limited supplemental electrolytes. Those listed to the left are multiple trace element solutions for adults and pediatric patients. Refer to manufacturers' product information for specific trace element composition.
Ultra trace elements Vanadium Nickel Silicon Tin Lithium Boron	Not commercially available in single or multiple trace element solutions	Daily requirements are not well defined. Routine supplementation is not recommended at this time.

[a]This is not a complete listing of all commercially available formulations of intravenous trace mineral solutions at the time of publication.
[b]Iron is not included in commercially prepared multiple trace element solutions.

later section). Electrolytes are commercially available as single nutrient and multiple nutrient solutions (Table 133.7). Multiple electrolyte solutions are useful in stable patients with normal organ function who are receiving PN. Concentrated multiple electrolyte solutions designed for addition to PN solutions generally contain only sodium, potassium, calcium, and magnesium. Phosphorus must be added as a separate additive. Detailed information regarding metabolism and requirements of vitamins, trace elements, and electrolytes is given elsewhere.[65]

DESIGNING A PN REGIMEN

Designing a PN regimen requires several considerations including available venous access, fluid status of the patient, and amounts of macronutrients and micronutrients required by the patient as determined by a nutrition assessment. A patient's venous access will determine how concentrated the PN solution may be compounded. The fluid status of the patient will also determine how concentrated the PN solution may be and, hence, will impact the amount of nutrient that may be provided.

ROUTES OF PARENTERAL NUTRITION ADMINISTRATION

Parenteral nutrition solutions may be administered by central or peripheral venous access. The clinical condition of the patient will determine which route is most appropriate.

Peripheral Route

Peripheral PN (PPN) is infused through a peripheral vein, usually a large vein in the forearm area. Because of physical limitations of peripheral veins, PPN regimens are usu-

TABLE 133.7. MICRONUTRIENT COMPONENTS OF PARENTERAL NUTRITION SOLUTIONS: ELECTROLYTES[a]

Intravenous Source	Commercial Product (Manufacturer)	How Supplied (Concentration per mL)
Sodium salts	Various manufacturers	
Na chloride		2 mEq Na; 2 mEq chloride 4 mEq Na; 4 mEq chloride
Na acetate		2 mEq Na; 2 mEq acetate 4 mEq Na; 4 mEq acetate
Na phosphate[b]		4 mEq Na; 3 mmol phosphate
Potassium salts	Various manufacturers	
K chloride		2 mEq K; 2 mEq chloride
K acetate		2 mEq K; 2 mEq acetate 4 mEq K; 4 mEq acetate
K phosphate[b]		4.4 mEq K; 3 mmol phosphate
Calcium salts	Various manufacturers	
Calcium gluconate (10% solution)		0.465 mEq Ca
Calcium chloride (10% solution)		1.36 mEq Ca
Calcium gluceptate	Abbott	0.9 mEq Ca
Magnesium salts	Various manufacturers	
Magnesium sulfate (10% solution)		0.8 mEq Mg
Magnesium sulfate (12.5% solution)		1 mEq Mg
Magnesium sulfate (50% solution)		4 mEq Mg
Magnesium chloride (20% solution)		1.97 mEq Mg
Multiple electrolyte solutions		Multiple electrolyte products are concentrated solutions designed to provide standard daily amounts of selected electrolytes when diluted in an appropriate volume of diluent. Refer to manufacturers' product information for electrolyte composition.
Hyperlyte Concentrate	McGaw	
Hyperlyte CR Concentrate	McGaw	
Hyperlyte R Concentrate	McGaw	
Nutrilyte concentrate	American Regent	
Nutrilyte II Concentrate	American Regent	
TPN Electrolytes	Abbott	
TPN II Electrolytes	Abbott	
TPN III Electrolytes	Abbott	

[a]This is not a complete listing of all commercially available formulations of intravenous electrolyte solutions at the time of publication.
[b]Phosphorous should always be dosed in terms of millimoles. The milliequivalent dose of sodium or potassium being administered as a part of a phosphate dose may be calculated by multiplying the millimolar amount of sodium phosphate by 1.3 and potassium phosphate by 1.5.

ally dilute solutions of amino acids, dextrose, and other micronutrients. Early PPN studies supported the use of amino acids alone as "protein-sparing" therapy. The rationale for protein-sparing PPN was based on the theory that the provision of dextrose in the setting of altered metabolism or stress would promote further increases in serum insulin concentrations, and thereby hinder the utilization of endogenous fat stores and promote nitrogen catabolism.[66,67] Subsequent investigations have challenged this theory.[66–68] Thus, protein-sparing PPN is now used for patients with marginal nutrition status and inadequate oral intake who are not candidates for central catheter placement and when PN is anticipated only for a brief period of approximately 1 week. However, two recent investigations of patients receiving postoperative PN suggest that some patients who meet criteria for protein-sparing PPN may not benefit from PN support.[19,21]

The addition of IVLE to PPN is referred to as the lipid system. The lipid system is designed for use in mild to moderately stressed patients where central access is unavailable or undesirable and enteral feeding is expected to return within 5–7 days. The addition of IVLE increases caloric support to levels more consistent with PN regimens administered centrally. Advantages of using PPN are primarily associated with avoiding the risk of infectious, metabolic, and technical complications that may occur with central vein catheterization. However, several other factors may complicate use of PPN in many patient populations. Patients who have received multiple courses of chemotherapy, malnourished patients, elderly patients, and others with an illness of long duration who have already been subjected to multiple venous accesses for administration of fluids and medications are likely to have limited peripheral venous access. Use of PPN is also limited by relatively poor tolerance of peripheral veins to hypertonic solutions. Thrombophlebitis is a commonly reported complication in patients receiving PPN. Although the risk of developing phlebitis is greater with solution osmolarities greater than 600–900 mOsm/L,[66,67] peripherally administered total nutrient admixtures with much higher osmolarities have been associated with low infusion site complications in some centers.[69] Efforts to minimize development of phlebitis in patients receiving PPN include addition of IVLE to the regimen as a possible venous lumen protectant, subtherapeutic doses of heparin (1000 U/L) to prevent formation of a thrombus, and/or small doses of hydrocortisone (5 mg/L) to minimize inflammation of the access site.[67] The osmolarity of a PN solution may be estimated by using the guidelines for osmolarities of selected PN components in Table 133.8. Because lower osmolarity solutions are relatively dilute, much larger volumes of solution are generally required to meet estimated nutritional requirements. Finally, patients with large nutrition requirements who receive PPN will likely require the use of IVLE as a caloric source so these patients should also be evaluated for lipid tolerance.

In summary, PPN is a relatively safe and simple method of nutritional support when patients are appropriately selected. Candidates for PPN include patients who do not have large nutritional requirements, are not fluid restricted, and are expected to begin enteral intake within 7–10 days.[68]

Central Route

Central PN (CPN) solutions are highly concentrated, hypertonic solutions. They are administered through a large central vein. Unlike peripheral veins, central veins have a much more rapid rate of blood flow, which quickly dilutes the hypertonic PN solutions. Central venous catheters are most commonly inserted percutaneously into the subclavian vein and advanced so that the tip is at the superior vena cava. If this approach is not possible, the internal jugular vein may be used. Radiographic verification of correct placement is necessary prior to infusion of the CPN solution. Catheterization may be performed either in the operating suite or in the patient's hospital room. Strict adherence to established protocols and catheter placement by an experienced clinician lessens the risk of complications (Table 133.9).[70]

Central venous catheters vary in composition, lumen size, number of injection ports, and other special features that affect ease or convenience of care and maintenance.

TABLE 133.8. OSMOLARITIES OF SELECTED PARENTERAL NUTRIENTS

Nutrient	Osmolarity
Amino acid	100 mOsm/%
Dextrose	50 mOsm/%
Lipid emulsion	1.7 mOsm/%
Sodium (acetate, chloride, phosphate)	2 mOsm/mEq
Potassium (acetate, chloride, phosphate)	2 mOsm/mEq
Magnesium sulfate	1 mOsm/mEq
Calcium gluconate	1.4 mOsm/mEq

TABLE 133.9. COMPLICATIONS OF CENTRAL VENOUS CATHETERS

Complication	Description
Arterial injury	Puncture of subclavian or carotid artery during catheter insertion.
Pneumothorax	Perforation of the pleura or lung during insertion, which results in air collection in the pleural space.
Air embolism	Introduction of air into the catheter, which subsequently enters the venous circulation.
Catheter embolism	A portion of the catheter fragments and enters the venous circulation.
Venous thrombosis	Formation of thrombosis inside the lumen of the catheter and/or inside the vessel around the catheter, which may result in catheter or vessel occlusion.
Chylothorax	Injury to the thoracic duct during catheter insertion.
Brachial plexus injury	Injury to the nerve during catheter insertion, or injury secondary to catheter malposition or extravasation of a hypertonic solution.

(Adapted from Ref. 70.)

Central venous catheters may be placed for short-term access or long-term access. Catheters are usually inserted by percutaneous venipuncture when therapy is expected to last less than 4 weeks. When therapy is expected to last longer than 4 weeks in either the hospital or at home, the catheter is usually tunneled subcutaneously before entering the central vessel, secured initially with retaining sutures,[71] and anchored in place with a felt cuff that promotes the growth of subcutaneous fibrotic tissue around the catheter. The injection port may remain external or be entirely concealed beneath the skin. Implanted central venous catheters have a larger port or reservoir which is surgically placed beneath the skin surface and anchored in the muscle of the chest wall.

Central PN is useful in patients who may require PN for periods of greater than 7–10 days during hospitalization or indefinitely at home. Central PN is also useful in patients with large nutrient requirements and in those where fluid volume is of concern. CPN is most useful for patients with major organ failure and metabolically stressed patients such as those with extensive surgery, trauma, sepsis, or malignancy. Central venous administration is also necessary for patients who receive home PN. Disadvantages of CPN include risks of catheter insertion, routine use of the catheter, and care of the access site. Relative to peripheral venous access, central venous catheter access is associated with a greater potential for infection. In addition, the risk of more serious catheter-induced trauma and related sequelae and other serious technical or mechanical problems is greater than with peripheral access.

Once the route of delivery has been chosen, components of the PN regimen are decided based on the patient's nutritional assessment. The patient's clinical condition and the compounding practices of an institution will impact decisions concerning PN infusion rates. For example, some institutions prepare PN solutions using a "standard formula" format. This approach offers a variety of base formulas (CAA/dextrose combination) with a fixed nonprotein calorie-to-nitrogen ratio (NPC:N). The standard formula format usually includes different formulas designed for mild to moderately stressed patients, renal failure patients, fluid-restricted patients, and liver failure patients. Because the NPC:N is fixed, the amount of nutrient delivered depends solely on the infusion rate. Other institutions may compound "individualized" formulas. This approach permits compounding of patient-specific solutions. Compounding of the PN solution is limited only by the concentrations of stock solutions and stability concerns. The amount of nutrient delivered is dependent on daily volume of the PN solution infused and the nutrient concentrations in the PN solution. The total daily amount of PN solution may be prepared in multiple, 1-liter bags or more cost effectively in a single container.[72,73]

CALCULATING THE PN REGIMEN

Although computer software for calculating volumes of base solutions for PN regimens is now widely available, the steps for manual calculations are briefly reviewed. There are several guidelines or clinical "rules of thumb" that may help the pharmacist calculate a PN regimen after a patient's nutritional requirements have been decided. For example, patients receiving only PN therapy will likely need larger volumes of fluid to provide maintenance requirements and replace extrarenal losses. However, patients requiring other intravenous drug therapy will likely receive adequate fluids through the use of a standard intravenous maintenance solution such as 0.45% NaCl in 5% dextrose and piggybacked medications. Depending on individual institutional practices, maximally concentrating the PN solution and utilizing an inexpensive maintenance fluid to manage hydration may provide a cost-effective regimen that requires fewer adjustments. Another guideline that may be helpful in designing a PN regimen where the CAA/dextrose base is infused separately from the IVLE is to allow a volume of approximately 50–100 mL/L of base solution for electrolytes and other additives. Given this guideline, two clinically useful and highly concentrated base solutions are (final concentration) 7% CAA/15% dextrose, which can be prepared from 10% CAA and 70% dextrose stock solutions, or (final concentrations) 8% CAA/25% dextrose, compounded from 15% CAA and 70% dextrose stock solutions. Parenteral nutrition regimens for patients who require very small amounts of additives such as those with renal failure, may be further concentrated. The example in Fig. 133.2 illustrates how volumes of solutions for a PN regimen can be calculated.

ORDERING THE PN REGIMEN

Ordering PN solutions may be accomplished by several methods that are generally institution specific. Some institutions may require the entire formula to be written in individual components and additives. More commonly, institutions have simplified the ordering process by implementing order forms designed specifically for parenteral nutrition. These standardized order forms promote education of practitioners by providing brief guidelines for initiating PN and foster cost-efficient nutrition support by minimizing errors in ordering, compounding, and administration.[74,75] Standardized order forms may also include options for ordering certain related procedures, laboratory tests, protocols for patient management or consultations with other medical services related to the patient's nutrition support (Fig. 133.3). Standardized forms and protocols should be reviewed and updated periodically to reflect changes in the practices and patient population of an institution and also advances in technology that may affect provision of nutrition support.

COMPOUNDING, STORAGE AND INFECTION CONTROL

Several considerations are necessary when preparing and storing PN solutions. In general, the type of solution being prepared will dictate methods of compounding, storage, and infusion. Currently, the two major types of PN solutions most commonly used are the traditional CAA/dextrose combination with or without IVLE piggybacked into the PN line, and TNAs. Use of TNA solutions offers several potential advantages including reduced inventory (infusion pumps, tubing, and other related supplies), decreased time for compounding and administration, potential decrease in manipulations of the infusion line, which should correspond with a decreased risk of catheter contamination, and ease of delivery and storage for patients receiving home PN.[76] Potential disadvantages are associated with infectious, stability, and compatibility concerns. For example, stability of TNA solutions may be less predictable compared to CAA/dextrose solutions. In addition, the opaque solution that results after the addition of IVLE makes detection of particulate matter difficult, and TNA solutions cannot be filtered with a bacterial retentive 0.22-μm filter.[76–78] Methods for compounding PN solutions vary based on an

The total daily volume of a PN solution may be determined based upon a patient's maintenance fluid requirements or an approximation of the minimum volume may be determined by calculating the volumes of stock solutions required to provide the daily nutrients desired as illustrated below.

> Pt. Case: A patient's estimated nutritional requirements have been assessed at approximately 95–105 grams protein/day and 1800–2100 nonprotein kcal/day. The patient has no history of hyperlipidemia or allergy to eggs and is not fluid restricted. The PN solution will be compounded as an individualized regimen utilizing a single bag, 24-hour infusion of a crystalline amino acid (CAA)/dextrose combination with intravenous lipid emulsion (IVLE) piggy-backed into the PN infusion line. The stock solutions used to compound this regimen are 10% CAA and 70% Dextrose.

- Step 1: Determine the volume of IVLE required

$$2000 \text{ kcal/day} \times 30\text{–}40\% \text{ of total as fat} = 600\text{–}800 \text{ kcal*}$$

The most clinically reasonable choice of IVLE product for this regimen is IVLE 20% 250 mLs/day or IVLE 10% 500 mLs/day.

IVLE 20% 250 mLs/day × 2 kcal/mL= 500 kcal/day; IVLE 10% 500 mLs/day × 1.1 kcal/mL = 550 kcal/day

2000 kcal/day	Estimated daily nonprotein calorie requirements
−500 kcal/day	IVLE calories
1500	kcal needed from dextrose

- Step 2: Calculate the volume of 10% CAA stock solution required to provide 100 g protein

$$\frac{100 \text{ g protein}}{\mathbf{X} \text{ mLs}} = \frac{10 \text{ g protein}}{100 \text{ mLs}} \qquad \mathbf{X} = 1000 \text{ mLs } 10\% \text{ CAA}$$

- Step 3: Calculate the volume of 70% dextrose required to provide 1500 calories

$$1500 \text{ kcal/day} \div 3.4 \text{ kcal/g dextrose} = 441 \text{ g dextrose}$$

$$\frac{441 \text{ g dextrose}}{\mathbf{X} \text{ mLs}} = \frac{70 \text{ g dextrose}}{100 \text{ mLs}} \qquad \mathbf{X} = 630 \text{ mLs } 70\% \text{ dextrose}$$

- Step 4: Determine the infusion rate

Total base volume:	1000 mLs 10% CAA
	+ 630 mLs 70% dextrose
	1630 mLs base solution
	+ 50–100 mLs/L for additives
Total PN volume =	1700–1800 mLs/day or 70–75 mLs/hr

- Step 5: Calculate the PN order

Choose 75 mL/hr or 1800 mLs/day for PN volume

$$\frac{100 \text{ g Protein}}{1800 \text{ mLs}} = \frac{\mathbf{X} \text{ g protein}}{100 \text{ mLs}} \qquad \mathbf{X} = 5.6\% \text{ CAA (round down to 5.5\%)}$$

$$\frac{441 \text{ g Dextrose}}{1800 \text{ mLs}} = \frac{\mathbf{X} \text{ g Dextrose}}{100 \text{ mLs}} \qquad \mathbf{X} = 24.5\% \text{ (round up to 25\%)}$$

Final PN order (base solution): 5.5% CAA/25% dextrose at 75 mLs/hr + IVLE 20% 250 mLs/day

This regimen provides approximately 99 g protein/day and 2030 nonprotein calories/day

* See text for IVLE dosing guidelines.

Figure 133.2. Calculations for compounding a parenteral nutrition regimen.

ROUTE OF ADMINISTRATION ☐ Central ☐ Peripheral

RATE:
(check one)
☐ Continuous Infusion ______ ml/hour
☐ Cyclic Infusion ______ ml/hour X ____ hrs Start Time: ______

BASE FORMULA

Final Concentrations

Amino Acids:
(check one)
☐ Amino Acids (Standard Base) 10% ______ %
* ☐ Amino Acids (Vol. Restricted Base) 15% ______ %
* ☐ Hepatamine ______ %

Dextrose: ______ %

* Use of these solutions requires consultation from the Nutrition Support Team

ELECTROLYTES

(check one) **Per Liter Concentrations**

☐ Standard

Na Cl	50 mEq/L
K Ace	40 mEq/L
Ca Gluc	4.7 mEq/L
Mg SO_4	8 mEq/L
Na Phos	15 mMol/L

☐ Individualized
Na Cl ______ mEq/L Mg SO_4 ______ mEq/L
Na Ace ______ mEq/L Ca Gluc ______ mEq/L
Na Phos ______ mMol/L
(1 mMol Na Phos = 1.3 mEq Na)
K Cl ______ mEq/L
K Ace ______ mEq/L
K Phos ______ mMol/L
(1 mMol K Phos = 1.5 mEq K)

MICRONUTRIENTS / OTHER ADDITIVES

☐ MVI-12 (Vitamins) 10 ml/day
☐ MTE-6 (Trace Elements) 1 ml/day
☐ Aquamephyton (Vitamin K) ______ mg/day
☐ Ranitidine ______ mg/day
☐ Additional Zinc ______ mg/day
☐ Insulin ______ units/L

Other Additions
______
______
______
______

LIPID EMULSION:

(check one) ☐ 10% ☐ 20%
(check one) ☐ 250 mls ☐ 500 mls
RATE: ______ ml/hour over ______ hours

ORDERING GUIDELINES

- **TPN ORDERS MUST BE WRITTEN DAILY AND RECEIVED IN THE PHARMACY BY 12:00 NOON.**
- Routine "Parenteral Nutrition Clinical Orders" should be ordered upon initiation of TPN

BASE FORMULA GUIDELINES

PROTEIN:	1-2	g/kg/day
CARBOHYDRATE:	2-5	g/kg/day
FAT:	0.5-1	g/kg/day

- An appropriate solution to initiate Central TPN would be AMINO ACIDS 5% and Dextrose 15% (Final Concentrations).
- Maximum substrate concentrations for Peripheral TPN are Amino Acids 5% and Dextrose 5%.

ELECTROLYTE GUIDELINES

- USUAL ADULT REQUIREMENTS/24 HOURS

Na	60-100	mEq
K	60-100	mEq
Mg	10-20	mEq
Ca	10-15	mEq
Phos	20-45	mMol
Cl	As needed to maintain	
Ace	acid/base balance	

- Max. K concentration in Peripheral TPN is 40 mEq/L
- Max. Phos/Ca concentrations: no more than 45 mMol/L Phos in combination with no more than 10 meq/L Ca

MICRONUTRIENT GUIDELINES

- Usual Adult Vitamin Requirements /24 hrs - provided in 10 mls/d MVI-12
- Usual Adult trace element Requirements /24 hrs - provided in 1 ml/d MTE-6
- Usual Adult Vitamin K requirements - 10-25 mg/week

LIPID INFUSION GUIDELINES

- Lipid emulsion should be infused over 12-24 hours; 24-hour continuous infusion is recommended in critically ill patients

DATE/TIME ______ PHYSICIAN'S SIGNATURE ______ MD

Patient Addressograph

H. LEE MOFFITT CANCER CENTER & RESEARCH INSTITUTE
At the University of South Florida

PARENTERAL NUTRITION ORDERS (PN)

699-4-002 (5/95) WHITE - CHART; YELLOW - PHARMACY

Figure 133.3. Adult parenteral nutrition order form.

institution's size, patient population, and medical practices. Some institutions prepare PN base solutions by transferring CAA stock solutions to partially filled bags of concentrated dextrose stock solutions. Other institutions may use commercially prepared CAA/dextrose products that are separated in a single bag and then mixed prior to use. Recent advances in compounding technology have facilitated use of automated compounders in the hospital setting. Automated compounders are computer-based systems that perform the calculations necessary to determine volumes of nutrient stock solutions for preparation of PN solutions. In addition, most automated compounder systems include software that directly communicates the determined calculations to a transfer pump device. The pump delivers appropriate volumes of stock solutions to an empty intravenous bag by converting volume to weight based on the specific gravity of the stock solution. Advantages associated with automated compounders include reduction in personnel time and compounding materials and improved accuracy of compounding.[79] Disadvantages include the potential for equipment failure and power outages.

Assurance of solution sterility during compounding, storage, and administration is very important in reducing the risk of infection and related complications in patients receiving PN.[80] Several studies of microbial growth in CAA/dextrose PN solutions have demonstrated that these solutions are poor media for bacterial growth.[78] The acidic pH and hypertonicity of CAA/dextrose solutions hinder bacterial growth. However, fungi such as *Candida albicans* may continue to proliferate in CAA/dextrose solutions for 7–10 days. Refrigeration at 4°C suppresses growth of both bacteria and *C. albicans* and should be the routine storage temperature.[78] The National Coordinating Committee on Large Volume Parenterals (NCCLVP) recommends immediate refrigeration of admixed solutions that are not administered within 1 hour after admixing. If refrigerated, admixed solutions should be used within 24 hours of compounding.[81] The addition of albumin to PN solutions also increases the potential for fungal and bacterial growth.[82] Intravenous lipid emulsions support growth of gram-positive and gram-negative bacteria as well as fungi. Visual changes may or may not occur even with high concentrations of microbial contamination.[78,83] Currently the Centers for Disease Control and Prevention recommends a maximum hang time of 12 hours for IVLE except when used within a TNA system based on reports of substantial microbial growth in contaminated IVLE after 12 hours.[84] However, in a recent investigation of IVLE solutions infused for up to 24 hours in patients receiving PN, no correlation was observed between risk of infection and length of hang time.[85] In view of these findings, many institutions now allow expiration times up to 24 hours for IVLE infusions. Results from investigations of microbial growth in TNA solutions do not agree.[77,78] In general, TNA solutions appear to support growth of bacteria less than IVLE but more than CAA/dextrose solutions. However, investigations of TNA used in a clinical setting have demonstrated safe administration over 24 hours without greater risk of contamination than is reported with CAA/dextrose solutions.[76,77]

Use of aseptic technique during compounding and administration is prerequisite for assuring that the patient receives an uncontaminated PN solution. Solutions should be prepared in the aseptic environment provided by a properly maintained laminar flow hood. The hood should be situated such that the contaminant potential of normal work traffic and air currents is minimized. Personnel must be adequately trained and must practice strict aseptic technique. Supervision by a pharmacist experienced in compounding intravenous solutions and knowledgeable about stability, compatibility, and storage of PN solutions is also necessary. Quality assurance procedures should be developed to maintain safe and accurate admixture preparation. The potential risk of sepsis associated with PN solution contamination can be greatly decreased when pharmacy-based admixture programs follow specific guidelines developed to ensure proper compounding of PN solutions.[80,86]

Stability and Compatibility

Because of their complex compositions, PN solutions are prone to problems with stability and compatibility. Comprehensive sources of current information about compatibilities and stability of PN solutions are *Trissel's Handbook on Injectable Drugs,* which is published every 2 years with supplements during alternating years, and the *Guide to Parenteral Admixtures,* which is updated quarterly.[87,88] In many cases, the exact answer to a compatibility question may not be readily available and a review of the primary literature may be necessary. When information is not available, clinical judgment and experience must be used carefully to resolve the situation.

CAA/dextrose solutions are generally stable for 1–2 months if refrigerated at 4°C and protected from light.[89] Many studies have investigated stability of solutions containing various amounts of CAA, dextrose, and IVLE.[78] Several factors affect stability of TNA solutions including pH, electrolyte charges, temperature, and time after compounding. Because of differences in pH among various CAA products and differences in phospholipid content among IVLE products, specific manufacturers should be consulted for compatibility and stability information prior to routine mixing of components. In general, electrolytes (except phosphorus) and trace elements should be added to the dextrose solution, phosphate should be added to the CAA solution, and, finally, the amino acid solution should be added to the IVLE prior to or simultaneously with the dextrose solution. While TNA solutions should be infused within 24–48 hours after compounding, investigations of certain TNA solutions have reported acceptable stability for 10–28 days when refrigerated at 4–5°C.[78]

The precipitation of calcium and phosphorus is a common interaction that is potentially life threatening.[90] Factors that enhance the risk of precipitate formation include high concentrations of calcium and phosphorus salts, use of the chloride salt of calcium, decreased amino acid concentrations, increased solution temperature, increased solution pH, use of an improper sequence when mixing calcium and phosphorus salts, and the presence of other additives including IVLE.[87] Specific guidelines for avoiding a calcium–phosphorus interaction have been published elsewhere.[78,87] Electrolyte stability in TNA solutions is of greater concern because of poor visualization of a precipitate should one occur. Alternative methods of delivering electrolytes or other medications should be pursued in clinical situations where compatibility information involving a TNA solution is lacking. Although some published compatibility data suggest otherwise, the addition of sodium bicarbonate to PN solutions is not recommended.[87,91] Addition of bicarbonate to acidic PN solutions may result in the formation of carbon dioxide gas and insoluble calcium and magnesium carbonates. Use of a bicarbonate precursor salt such as acetate is usually preferred.

Vitamins may be adversely affected by changes in solution pH, presence of other additives, storage time, solution temperature, and exposure to light.[65] Variable but significant losses of vitamin A have been reported secondary to adsorption to intravenous administration tubing and polyvinyl chloride intravenous bags.[78] Thiamine may be subject to degradation in solutions containing bisulfite. Because of variable stabilities of individual vitamins, intravenous vitamin solutions should be added to the PN solution as near to the time of administration as is clinically feasible and should not be in the PN solution longer than 24 hours.

Many patients receiving PN at home or in a hospital also receive other intravenous medications. The compatibility of PN and other intravenous solutions is an important concern in delivering safe and effective drug and nutritional therapy. Intravenous medications are most often infused as a separate admixture piggybacked in the PN line. However, some medications may be added directly to the PN solution and administered at the same rate as the PN infusion. Because of the potential for ineffective drug therapy or other complications associated with physiochemical incompatibility and stability of the PN solution, specific criteria should be considered before one adds a medication directly to the PN solution.[92] The dosage regimen should be stable for each 24-hour period and should have pharmacokinetic properties appropriate for continuous infusion. There should be documented chemical and physical compatibility of the medication with PN mixture components and other medications that may be concomitantly piggybacked into the PN line. Finally, the PN regimen should be infused continuously over 24 hours. Advantages of using PN admixtures as drug vehicles include consolidation of dosage units, improved pharmacotherapy for certain drugs, conservation of fluid in volume-restricted patients, fewer venous catheter violations and decreased compounding and administration time.[92] However, a major disadvantage to use of PN solutions as drug delivery vehicles is the lack of compatibility and stability data in the PN solutions, which are commonly used in clinical practice. Original research reports should be carefully reviewed for experimental conditions and assay determination methods before extrapolating data into institution-specific guidelines.[78] Medications frequently added to PN solutions include albumin, aminophylline, hydrochloric acid, regular insulin, and histamine-2 antagonists such as cimetidine, ranitidine, and famotidine.[87,88,92]

ADMINISTRATION

The PN solution is infused through special tubing for intravenous administration that connects the PN bag or bottle with the intravenous catheter. PN solutions should be administered with an infusion pump to ensure consistent and controlled delivery of the solution. The intravenous administration line may include an in-line filter at a point prior to connection to the catheter. A 0.22 μm filter is recommended for use with CAA/dextrose solutions to remove particulate matter, air, and any microorganism that may be present in the solution from prior manipulations of the admixture or the administration line. Because the average size of IVLE particles is approximately 0.5 μm, IVLE administered separately from the CAA/dextrose solution must be piggybacked into the PN line at a site beyond the in-line filter.[93] Routine use of in-line filters (>0.22 μm) with TNA solutions is controversial.[94] However, the Food and Drug Administration recommends use of a 1.2-μm filter, which may be effective in preventing catheter occlusion due to precipitates or lipid aggregates.[90] This filter size is also reported to remove *C. albicans.*[95] Others support use of a 5-μm filter to minimize occlusion alarms from infusion pumps while maintaining filtration of particles capable of obstructing pulmonary capillaries.[96]

CONTINUOUS VERSUS INTERMITTENT INFUSIONS

Parenteral nutrition solutions may be infused continuously or intermittently. The concentration of dextrose in the formula and the patient's history of glucose tolerance will dictate the infusion rate at which the PN solution should be initiated. Protocols for initiating PN differ widely among institutions. Many institutions begin infusions slowly and gradually increase the rate over 24–48 hours to the desired rate. The rate is also lowered in a stepwise fashion when PN therapy ends. This protocol is used to prevent development of hyperglycemia and rebound hypoglycemia, respectively. However, Krzyda et al.[97] investigated 18 patients who were initiated on PN solutions at the desired rate and discontinued without a taper schedule. Patients were monitored for clinical evidence of hyperglycemia or hypoglycemia at the initiation and discontinuation of a lipid-based PN regimen given over 24 hours continuous infusion. The severity of illness of the patients ranged from stable condition postoperatively to multiple-system organ failure. Six patients had diabetes mellitus. None of the patients demonstrated clinical signs of hyperglycemia or hypoglycemia during the study period. The blood glucose concentrations of patients who received insulin from the PN infusion were less predictable when the PN infusion was stopped compared to those from patients who did not require insulin. While these investigators observed no adverse effects from abruptly initiating and discontinuing PN infusions, tapered scheduling has been recommended for patients receiving intermittent subcutaneous regular insulin, patients with severe renal or hepatic disease, patients with other disease states that may increase risk for development of hypoglycemia such as severe diabetes or pancreatic malignancy, and patients who are receiving concurrent drug therapy that may predispose development of hypoglycemia (oral hypoglycemics) or mask the cardiovascular symptoms of hypoglycemia (beta blockers).[98]

Cyclic PN is the infusion of PN over a period of time less than 24 hours, usually for 12- to 18-hours each day.[99] Cyclic PN is useful in hospitalized patients with limited venous access where administration of multiple other medications requires interruption of the PN infusion. Cyclic PN may also prevent or treat hepatotoxicities associated with continuous PN therapy. In addition, cyclic PN allows patients receiving PN at home the ability to resume a relatively normal lifestyle.[99] Recommendations for administration of cyclic PN are similar to those for continuous PN. Various protocols have been reported that suggest incremental increases to the maximum infusion rate for a desired period of time followed by a gradual taper to discontinue the solution. However, metabolically stable patients receiving lipid-based PN regimens are likely candidates for abrupt initiation and discontinuation of the cyclic PN regimen.[97,98] Cyclic PN may not be well tolerated by patients with severe glucose intolerance or diabetes, or by those patients with unstable fluid balance.

Assessment of Outcomes

Thorough and consistent monitoring of patients receiving PN is necessary to ensure that the desired nutritional outcomes are achieved and to prevent the occurrence of adverse effects or complications associated with PN therapy. Routine evaluation should include the assessment of the patient's clinical condition with a focus on nutritional and metabolic effects of the PN regimen. Serial documentation of a patient's response to a particular regimen is a helpful guide for determining appropriate adjustments in fluid, electrolyte, and nutrient therapies.

A variety of biochemical and clinical measurements are necessary for effective monitoring of patients receiving PN. Important clinical laboratory measurements include serum concentrations of electrolytes, hematologic indices, and biochemical markers for renal function, liver function, and nutrition status. Other important clinical measurements include vital signs, weight, total fluid intake and losses, and nutritional intakes. The frequency of clinical laboratory measurements is usually dependent on the stability of a patient's clinical condition. Monitoring parameters considered important for patients receiving PN and the suggested frequency of measurement for each are outlined in Table 133.10.

TABLE 133.10. ROUTINE MONITORING DATA FOR PARENTERAL NUTRITION

Every Day	2–3 Times/Wk	Every Week
Weight	Complete blood count	Nitrogen balance
Vital signs (temperature, pulse, respirations)	Clotting studies (PT/PTT, platelets)	Total protein
Fluid	Creatinine	Albumin
Nutritional intake	Calcium	Transferrin or prealbumin
kcal, protein, fat	Phosphorus	Liver biochemical tests
Electrolytes, vitamins	Magnesium	Alkaline phosphatase
Trace elements		AST
Serum electrolytes		ALT
Sodium		LDH
Potassium		Bilirubin
Chloride		Other tests as warranted
Bicarbonate		
Glucose		
BUN		
Urine glucose, acetone (every 6 h)		
Output		
Urine		
Gastrointestinal		
Other losses		

Key: PT, prothrombin time; PTT, partial thromboplastin time; AST, aspartate aminotransferase (SGOT); ALT, alanine aminotransferase (SGPT); LDH, lactate dehydrogenase; BUN, blood urea nitrogen.

Appropriate assessment and evaluation of patient data can identify impending complications that may be avoided or treated early. Monitoring protocols should be developed and tailored for a specific institution's patient population, medical practices, and resources.

COMPLICATIONS OF PARENTERAL NUTRITION

Parenteral nutrition can be a safe and effective therapy when appropriate patients have been selected and the course of therapy is correctly monitored and adjusted as a patient's metabolic condition dictates. However, PN support is a complex therapy that is associated with numerous complications. These complications may be divided into four categories: mechanical or technical, infectious, metabolic, and nutritional.[80]

MECHANICAL/TECHNICAL

Mechanical or technical complications include malfunctions in the system used for intravenous delivery of the solution. Examples of such malfunctions include infusion pump failure, problems with administration sets or tubing, and problems with the catheter. Catheter-related complications are often of concern because they are potentially life-threatening (Table 133.9). Pneumothorax, catheter misdirection into the wrong vein or ill-positioned within the cardiac chambers, arterial puncture, bleeding, and hematoma formation may occur during surgical placement of the catheter. Many of these complications in addition to venous thrombosis and air embolism may occur after insertion as well. Catheters occasionally occlude or break during use. If these problems cannot be easily rectified, the catheter may need to be surgically replaced.[70,100]

INFECTIONS

Infectious complications can be a major hazard in patients receiving central PN. Often these patients are predisposed to infection as a result of compromised immunity and/or concomitant infection already present in the urinary tract, wounds, or lungs. Frequent use of broad-spectrum antibiotic therapy and malnutrition are also predisposing factors for development of infection. Bacterial translocation across the wall of the GI tract has also been implicated as a source of sepsis in patients receiving PN for prolonged periods without enteral feeding.[101] Infection may develop secondary to solution contamination. However, strict adherence to specific protocols for preparation of PN solutions has minimized this occurrence.[80] A more common source of infection is catheter-related infections. Catheter-related sepsis is defined as the presence of bacterial or fungal growth from the catheter tip and peripheral blood cultures. Catheter infection is defined as microbial growth from the catheter tip or from a blood culture drawn from the catheter with no growth of the same organism in the peripheral blood culture.[102] Patients with catheter-related infections may exhibit signs of sepsis syndrome such as fever, chills, mental status changes, hypotension, or glucose intolerance. These infections occur when the catheter becomes colonized by direct microbial invasion of the skin at the insertion site or at the infusion site of the catheter. For example, colonization may occur after multiple manipulations of the line used for PN administration, which can occur when the PN line is used to administer other medications. Other examples include failure of in-line bacterial filters, poor technique used in placement of the catheter, and poor care of the insertion site.[100]

When no other source of infection is apparent in symptomatic patients, the catheter should be evaluated as the potential source. Blood cultures are drawn from a peripheral site and from the central catheter. In many institutions the suspected catheter is removed, the tip is quantitatively cultured, and a new central catheter is inserted. If bacterial or fungal growth of the same organism occurs from the catheter tip and the peripheral blood culture, the exchanged catheter is removed and another is placed in a different anatomic site. If bacterial or fungal growth occurs from the catheter tip or from a blood culture drawn from the catheter with no growth of the same organism in the peripheral culture, the catheter may be removed and replaced with another in the same anatomic location.[102] However, because the clinical value of frequent central catheter replacement in patients with sepsis secondary to catheter-related infection is controversial, other treatment protocols have been suggested.[103]

METABOLIC/NUTRITIONAL

Metabolic complications associated with PN therapy are numerous and, if left untreated, may be potentially fatal. Common metabolic abnormalities related to substrate intolerance and fluid, electrolyte, and acid–base disorders are presented in Tables 133.11 and 133.12. Predisposing factors and general strategies for intervention are also included.[104] The etiology, mechanisms, and implications of individual metabolic abnormalities are multifactorial and have been summarized.[103–106]

Hepatic dysfunction, as evidenced by elevations in serum liver function measurements such as total bilirubin, AST, ALT, and alkaline phosphatase, is well documented in the literature. The most commonly reported abnormalities are fatty liver, cholelithiasis, and cholestasis.[107,108] In most patients, these complications are reversible by manipulations of substrate intake. Progressive liver injury in patients who have received long-term PN has been reported in a small number of patients.[108] However, the relationship

TABLE 133.11. SUBSTRATE INTOLERANCE IN PARENTERAL NUTRITION

Complication	Possible Causes	Intervention
Hyperglycemia	Stress, infection, corticosteroids, pancreatitis, diabetes mellitus, peritoneal dialysis, excessive dextrose administration	Decrease dextrose load by decreasing infusion rate or dextrose concentration (may substitute fat calories); administer insulin
Hypoglycemia (rare)	Abrupt withdrawal of dextrose, insulin overdose	Increase dextrose intake; decrease exogenous insulin
Excess of carbon dioxide production	Excess dextrose intake	Decrease dextrose intake; balance calories from fat and dextrose
Hyperlipidemia (elevated cholesterol and triglyceride)	Stress, familial hyperlipidemia, pancreatitis	Decrease intake of fat or discontinue if indicated
Serum amino acid imbalance	Stress, hepatic failure	Modify amino acid intake if possible or decrease intake of amino acids
Abnormal liver function tests (elevated AST, alkaline phosphatase, and bilirubin)	Stress, infection, cancer, excess carbohydrate intake, excess caloric intake, essential fatty acid deficiency	Decrease dextrose load (substitute fat); decrease total calories; provide essential fatty acids

Key: AST, aspartate aminotransferase (SGOT). (Adapted from Teasley-Strausburg KM, Shronts EP. Metabolic and gastrointestinal complications, in Teasley-Strausburg KM (ed): Nutrition Support Handbook: A Compendium of Products with Guidelines for Usage. Cincinnati, OH, Harvey Whitney Books Company, 1992, pp 298–299, with permission.)

between long-term PN and development of chronic liver disease is not clear.

Nutritional complications of parenteral nutrition therapy generally develop over a prolonged course of therapy (weeks to months) as a result of inappropriate intake of a particular nutrient. Certain conditions, such as metabolic stress in a previously malnourished patient, may elicit symptoms of deficiency much earlier if a nutrient is not appropriately provided. For this reason, at least maintenance doses of vitamins, trace elements, and essential fatty acids should be provided to all patients receiving PN.

Clinical symptoms of trace element deficiencies, although rare, have been reported in patients receiving PN. More commonly, decreased serum trace element concentrations have been reported in a variety of patient populations. However, the clinical significance of decreased concentrations of many trace elements is not known because serum concentrations often do not correlate with total body

TABLE 133.12. FLUID, ELECTROLYTE, AND ACID–BASE ABNORMALITIES

Problem	Possible Causes	Intervention
Hypovolemia	Gastrointestinal fluid losses, osmotic diuresis	Increase fluid intake
Hypervolemia	Renal failure, excess fluid intake	Decrease fluid intake and diuretics
Hyponatremia	Gastrointestinal losses, fluid overload, diuretics	Varies with cause
Hypernatremia	Dehydration	Increase fluid intake
Hypokalemia	Gastrointestinal losses, diuretics, anabolism	Increase potassium intake
Hyperkalemia	Renal failure	Decrease potassium intake
Hypophosphatemia	Phosphate-binding antacids, anabolism, phosphate-free dialysate	Discontinue phosphate binders; increase phosphorus intake
Hyperphosphatemia	Renal failure	Decrease phosphorus intake
Hypomagnesemia	Diarrhea, malabsorption, anabolism	Increase magnesium intake
Hypermagnesemia	Renal failure	Decrease magnesium intake
Hypocalcemia	Hypoalbuminemia, chronic renal failure	Increase calcium intake (with chronic renal failure only)
Hypercalcemia	Rare	Decrease calcium intake
Metabolic acidosis	Diarrhea, high-output fistulae, renal failure, excess amino acid intake	Treat underlying causes; increase acetate and decrease Cl in TPN solution; decrease amino acid intake
Metabolic alkalosis	Gastric losses	Treat underlying cause; increase Cl and decrease acetate in TPN solution

(Adapted from Teasley-Strausburg KM, Shronts EP. Metabolic and gastrointestinal complications, in Teasley-Strausburg KM (ed):. Nutrition Support Handbook: A Compendium of Products with Guidelines for Usage. Cincinnati, OH, Harvey Whitney Books Company, 1992, pp 298–299, with permission.)

stores.[58,60] Zinc deficiency has been observed in both children and adults who have received shorter courses of PN and long-term PN.[58] Patients with large ostomy losses or severe chronic diarrhea are at highest risk for development of zinc deficiency. Clinical signs of zinc deficiency include hair loss, periorbital seborrheic dermatitis, dysgeusia, and sometimes ileus.[58,60,109] Chromium deficiency presents as a diabetes-like syndrome, while copper deficiency may appear as a hypochromic, normocytic anemia with neutropenia. Selenium deficiency may develop during the course of PN therapy as cardiomyopathy and muscle pain.[58,60,63]

Patients receiving PN regimens without IVLE for extended periods of weeks to months are at risk for development of EFAD. Clinical signs of EFAD include hair loss, desquamative dermatitis, thrombocytopenia, and malabsorption and diarrhea resulting from changes in intestinal mucosa.[41,42] These manifestations may occur 1–3 weeks after initiation of fat-free TPN.[41] Biochemical evidence of EFAD as demonstrated by a triene:tetraene ratio ≥ 0.4 may occur as early as 1 week after PN initiation in metabolically stressed patients.[41]

Occasionally patients may develop nutrient-induced toxicities, most commonly as a result of the accumulation of fat-soluble vitamins or trace elements. Toxic accumulation may be caused by either excessive intake or decreased excretion. Certain disease states (for example, renal failure) may necessitate reduction in vitamin and trace element intake.[110] Patients receiving PN should be monitored closely by clinical observation and laboratory measurements, if indicated, to detect signs and symptoms of nutrient deficiency or excess. In either case, the PN regimen should be appropriately adjusted.

Home Parenteral Nutrition

Advances in technology for the delivery of intravenous solutions have allowed patients who require extended PN therapy to be maintained indefinitely on intravenous nutrition. Usually these patients are medically stable and continued hospitalization is not needed. An increasing concern for cost containment of health care services has fostered utilization of sophisticated infusion devices to provide PN at home. Numerous programs are now available to support patients with various long-term or permanent medical conditions outside the traditional health care setting. Standards have been developed to promote safe and effective care.[111,112] Home PN services may be coordinated and administered through a hospital, by a commercially operated corporation, or through a joint venture between the two.[113]

Many factors are considered in selecting candidates for home PN therapy. Significant benefit must be expected from placing a patient into the program. Additionally, the patient and his or her caregiver must be willing to successfully complete training and assume numerous other responsibilities that are important for managing a new daily routine in the home. Other logistics such as funding, procurement of solutions and supplies, and clinical management and follow-up must be evaluated, resolved, and implemented for each patient in order to achieve the desired outcomes.[112,114]

Patients with Crohn's disease, ischemic bowel disease, severe GI motility disorders, extensive intestinal obstruction, radiation enteritis, and congenital bowel function have been successfully maintained with home PN.[115] Although patients with active cancer are the largest group of patients on home PN, the number of patients with AIDS on home PN is increasing rapidly.[115,116] Home PN is administered through a central catheter placed specifically for long-term use. In the past, patients or their caregiver may have been trained to mix PN solutions in the home. Today patients commonly receive premixed PN solutions from the hospital or a commercial vendor. Intravenous vitamins or other additives may be added daily by the patient or caregiver depending on the arrangement with the PN provider. The solution is generally administered through the night by infusion pump over 10–18 hours. A cycled regimen allows the patient time away from the pump during daylight hours and provides many patients with the freedom to have a reasonably normal daily routine. Clinical management and follow-up are performed periodically according to the needs of the patient and the protocol of the care provider. A coordinated effort among several health care professionals including physicians, pharmacists, nurses, social workers, and the patient and his or her caregiver, as well as the suppliers is paramount to providing safe and effective management. Home PN affords some patients the potential for an ambulatory lifestyle while maintaining an intravenous feeding regimen previously only available in the hospital setting. For others, home PN may contribute to a better quality of life in the comfort of their home. As growth of home health care programs continues, further study will be needed to better define those patients who benefit from extended home PN therapy, especially within the groups of patients with cancer and AIDS.[115]

Conclusion

Parenteral nutrition is not a benign therapy. Appropriate patient selection, assessment, and monitoring are key to successful nutritional therapy and prevention of unnecessary complications or harm to the patient. Standardized order forms and monitoring protocols are useful tools to ensure appropriate administration and monitoring of PN therapy. Pharmacists have been involved in the provision of PN at many levels including direct patient care, education, and research. The field of pharmacy nutrition support has grown into a well-defined area of pharmacy practice with formally defined standards of practice.[7] These standards, while broad in scope, were considered to be focused and the demand for the services sufficient that specialty recognition by the Board of Pharmaceutical Specialties is now available for pharmacists.[117] The use of PN therapy and the role of the nutrition support pharmacist will be affected primarily by new insights from clinical research and economic challenges in the health care environment.

REFERENCES

1. Meguid MM, Campos AC, Hammond WG. Nutritional support in surgical practice: Part I. Am J Surg 1990;159:358.
2. Meguid MM, Campos AC, Hammond WG. Nutritional support in surgical practice: Part II. Am J Surg 1990;159: 427–443.
3. Rhoads JE, Dudrick SJ. History of intravenous nutrition, in Rombeau JL, Caldwell MD (eds): Clinical Nutrition: Parenteral Nutrition, 2nd ed. Philadelphia, WB Saunders, 1993, pp 1–10.
4. Mirtallo JM, Powell CR, Campbell SM, et al. Cost-effective nutrition support. Nutr Clin Prac 1987;2:142–151.
5. Dalton MJ, Schepers G, Gee JP, et al. Consultative total parenteral nutrition teams: The effect on the incidence of total parenteral nutrition-related complications. J Parenter Enter Nutr 1984;8:146–152.
6. ASPEN Board of Directors. Definitions of terms used in ASPEN guidelines and standards. J Parenter Nutr 1995;19:1–2.
7. American Society for Parenteral and Enteral Nutrition. Standards for nutrition support pharmacists. Nutr Clin Pract 1993;8:124–127.
8. Foster GD, Knox LS, Dempsey DT, Mullen JL. Caloric requirements in total parenteral nutrition. J Am Coll Nutr 1987;6:231–253.
9. Burge JC, Goon A, Choban PS, Flancbaum L. Efficacy of hypocaloric total parenteral nutrition in hospitalized obese patients: A prospective double-blind randomized trial. J Parenter Enter Nutr 1994;18:203–207.
10. Dickerson RN, Rosate EF, Mullen JL. Net protein anabolism with hypocaloric parenteral nutrition in obese stressed patients. Am J Clin Nutr 1986;44:747–755.
11. Ireton-Jones CS, Turner WW. Actual or ideal body weight: Which should be used to predict energy expenditure? J Am Diet Assoc 1991;91:193–195.
12. ASPEN Board of Directors. Routes to deliver nutrition support in adults. J Parenter Enter Nutr 1993; 17:7SA–8SA.
13. Buzby GP, Williford WO, Peterson OL, et al. A randomized clinical trial of total parenteral nutrition in malnourished surgical patients: The rationale and impact of previous clinical trials and pilot study on protocol design. Am J Clin Nutr 1988;47:357–365.
14. Dempsey DT, Mullen JL, Buzby GP. The link between nutritional status and clinical outcome: Can nutritional intervention modify it? Am J Clin Nutr 1988;47:352–356.
15. ASPEN Board of Directors. Guidelines for the use of total parenteral nutrition in the hospitalized adult patient. J Parenter Enter Nutr 1986;10:441–445.
16. Sitzmann JV, Pitt HA, The Patient Care Committee of the American Gastroenterological Association. Statement on the guidelines for total parenteral nutrition. Dig Dis Sci 1989;34:489–496.
17. Technology Assessment and Practice Guidelines Forum Panel. Evaluating total parenteral nutrition: Core statement of the technology assessment and practice guidelines forum. Nutrition 1990;6:475–489.
18. ASPEN Board of Directors. Guidelines for the use of parenteral and enteral nutrition in adults and pediatric patients. J Parenter Enter Nutr 1993;17:12SA–49SA.
19. Detsky AS, Baker JP, O'Rourke K, Goel V. Perioperative parenteral nutrition: A meta-analysis. Ann Int Med 1987; 107:195–203.
20. American College of Physicians. Position paper: Parenteral nutrition in patients receiving cancer chemotherapy. Ann Int Med 1989;110:734–736.
21. Veterans Affairs Total Parenteral Nutrition Cooperative Study Group. Perioperative total parenteral nutrition in surgical patients. N Engl J Med 1991;6:336–337.
22. Douglas RG, Shaw JHF. Metabolic response to sepsis and trauma. Br J Surg 1989;76:115–122.
23. Mirtallo JM, Schneider PJ, Mavco K, Ruberg RL. Clinical comparison of two 8.5% amino acid injection products. Am J Hosp Pharm 1981;38:83–89.
24. Furst P, Stehle P. Are intravenous amino acid solutions unbalanced? New Horizons 1994;2:215–223.
25. Miller SJ. The nitrogen balance revisited. Hosp Pharm 1990;25:61–65, 70.
26. Grant JP. Administration of parenteral nutrition solutions, in Handbook of Total Parenteral Nutrition, 2nd ed. Philadelphia, WB Saunders, 1992, pp 171–202.
27. Teasley-Strausburg KM. Nutritional/metabolic assessment, in Teasley-Strausburg KM (ed): Nutrition Support Handbook: A Compendium of Products with Guidelines for Usage. Cincinnati, OH, Harvey Whitney Books Company, 1992, pp 1–18.
28. Broyles JE, Brown RO, Vehe KL, et al. Pharmacist interventions improve fluid balance in fluid restricted patients requiring parenteral nutrition. DICP Ann Pharmacotherapy 1991;25:119–122.
29. Ziegler TR, Young LS, Benfell K, et al. Clinical and metabolic efficacy of glutamine-supplemented parenteral nutrition after bone marrow transplantation. Ann Int Med 1992;116:821–828.
30. Vasquez JA, Daniel H, Adibi SA. Dipeptides in parenteral nutrition: From basic science to clinical applications. Nutr Clin Prac 1993;8:95–105.
31. Furst P, Stehle P. The potential use of parenteral dipeptides in clinical nutrition. Nutr Clin Prac 1993;8:106–114.
32. Wolfe RR. Carbohydrate metabolism and requirements, in Rombeau JL, Caldwell MD (eds): Clinical Nutrition: Parenteral Nutrition, 2nd ed. Philadelphia, WB Saunders, 1993, pp 113–131.
33. Freund HR. Abnormalities of liver function and hepatic damage associated with total parenteral nutrition. Nutrition 1991;7:1–5.

34. Goins WA, Wiles CE III, Cerra FB. Pharmacology, monitoring and nutritional support. Crit Care Clin 1993; 9:689–713.
35. Cerra FB, Holman RT, Bankey PE, Mazuski JE. Nutritional pharmacology: Its role in the hypermetabolism-organ failure syndrome. Crit Care Med 1990;18:S154–S158.
36. Dudrick PS, Souba WW. Special fuels in parenteral nutrition, in Rombeau JL, Caldwell MD (eds): Clinical Nutrition: Parenteral Nutrition, 2nd ed. Philadelphia, WB Saunders, 1993, pp 209–222.
37. Waxman K, Day AT, Stellin GP, et al. Safety and efficacy of glycerol and amino acids in combination with lipid emulsion for peripheral parenteral nutrition support. J Parenter Enter Nutr 1993;16:374–378.
38. Dickerson RN. Clinical utility of intravenous lipid emulsion. Hosp Pharm 1986;21:564–566, 568–569.
39. Intralipid 30% package insert. Deerfield, IL, Clintec Nutrition Company, January 1994.
40. Fat emulsions, in McEvoy GK (ed): AHFS Drug Information 95. Bethesda, MD, American Society of Hospital Pharmacists, 1995, pp 1774–1775.
41. Pelham LD. Rational use of intravenous fat emulsion. Am J Hosp Pharm 1981;38:198–208.
42. Gottschlich MM. Selection of optimal lipid sources in enteral and parenteral nutrition. Nutr Clin Pract 1992; 7:152–165.
43. Jensen GL, Mascioli EA, Seidner DL, et al. Parenteral infusion of long- and medium-chain triglycerides and reticuloendothelial system function in man. J Parenter Enter Nutr 1990;14:467–471.
44. Ota DM, Jessup JM, Babcock GF, et al. Immune function during intravenous administration of a soybean oil emulsion. J Parenter Enter Nutr 1985;9:23–27.
45. Wretlind A. Development of fat emulsions. J Parenter Enter Nutr 1981;5:230–235.
46. Ball MJ. Hematological and biochemical effects of parenteral nutrition with medium-chain triglycerides: Comparison with long-chain triglycerides. Am J Clin Nutr 1991;53:916–922.
47. Manner T, Katz DP, Askanazi J, et al. Parenteral fish-oil administration in patients with cystic fibrosis. J Parenter Enter Nutr 1993;17:24S.
48. Mashima Y, Tashiro T, Yamamori Y, et al. Effect of intravenous fish-soybean oil emulsion in serum fatty acid composition in total parenteral nutrition. J Parenter Enter Nutr 1992;16:28S.
49. Kinsella JE, Lokesh B. Dietary lipids, eicosanoids and the immune system. Crit Care Med 1990;18:S94–S113.
50. Bower RH, Cerra FB, Bershadsky B, et al. Early enteral administration of a formula (Impact) supplemented with arginine, nucleotides, and fish oil in intensive care unit patients: Results of a multicenter, prospective, randomized, clinical trial. Crit Care Med 1995;23:436–449.
51. Sanders TAB. Marine oils: Metabolic effects and role in human nutrition. Proc Nutr Soc 1993;52:457–472.
52. American Medical Association Department of Foods and Nutrition. Multivitamin preparations for parenteral use. A statement by the nutritional advisory group. J Parenter Enter Nutr 1979;3:258–262.
53. Boosalis MG, Edlund D, Moudry B, et al. Circulating blood and twenty-four hour urinary levels of water-soluble vitamins: Are current intravenous multivitamin preparations adequate? Nutrition 1988;4:431–438.
54. Dempsy DT, Mullen JL, Rombeau JL, et al. Treatment effects of parenteral vitamins in total parenteral nutrition patients. J Parenter Enter Nutr 1987;11:229–237.
55. Demetriou AA, Keck-Jones L. Vitamins, in Rombeau JL, Caldwell MD (eds): Clinical Nutrition: Parenteral Nutrition, 2nd ed. Philadelphia, WB Saunders, 1993, pp 184–202.
56. Green HL, Hambidge KM, Schanler R, Tsang RC. Guidelines for the use of vitamins, trace elements, calcium, magnesium, and phosphorus in infants and children receiving total parenteral nutrition: Report of the subcommittee on pediatric parenteral nutrient requirements from the committee on clinical practice issues of the American Society for Clinical Nutrition. Am J Clin Nutr 1988;48:1324–1342.
57. Schepers GP, Dimitry AR, Eckhauser FE, et al. Efficacy and safety of low-dose intravenous versus intramuscular vitamin K in parenteral nutrition patients. J Parenter Enter Nutr 1988;12:174–177.
58. Solomons NW. Trace elements, in Rombeau JL, Caldwell MD (eds): Clinical Nutrition: Parenteral Nutrition, 2nd ed. Philadelphia, WB Saunders, 1993, pp 150–183.
59. Leichtmann GA, Sitrin MD. Update on trace elements. Comp Ther 1991;17:42–48.
60. Fleming CR. Trace element metabolism in adult patients requiring total parenteral nutrition. Am J Clin Nutr 1989; 49:573–579.
61. Mertz W. The essential trace elements. Science 1981; 213:1332–1338.
62. American Medical Association. Guidelines for essential trace element preparations for parenteral use. A statement by the Nutrition Advisory Group. J Parenter Enter Nutr 1979;3:263–267.
63. Levander OA, Burk RF. Report on the 1986 ASPEN Research Workshop on Selenium in Clinical Nutrition. J Parenter Enter Nutr 1986;10:545–549.
64. Cerra FB. Parenteral nutrition, in Pocket Manual of Surgical Nutrition. St Louis, MO, CV Mosby, 1984, pp 120–142.
65. Baumgartner TG (ed). Clinical Guide to Parenteral Micronutrition, 2nd ed. Deerfield, IL, Fujasawa USA, 1991.
66. Miller SJ. Peripheral parenteral nutrition: Theory and practice. Hosp Pharm 1991;26:796–801.
67. Payne-James JJ, Khawaja HT. First choice for total parenteral nutrition: The peripheral route. J Parenter Enter Nutr 1993;17:468–478.
68. Daly JM, Long JM III. Intravenous hyperalimentation: Technique and potential complications. Surg Clin North Am 1981;61:583–604.
69. Hoffman E. A randomized study of central versus peripheral intravenous nutrition in the perioperative period. Clin Nutr 1989;8:179–180.
70. Grant JP. Vascular access for total parenteral nutrition: Techniques and complications, in Handbook of Total Parenteral Nutrition, 2nd ed. Philadelphia, WB Saunders, 1992, pp 107–138.
71. Lehmann S. Parenteral and enteral access devices, in Teasley-Strausburg KM (ed): Nutrition Support Handbook: A Compendium of Products with Guidelines for Usage.

Cincinnati, OH, Harvey Whitney Books Company, 1992, pp 205–259.
72. Mirtallo JM, Jozefczyk KG, Hale KM, et al. Providing 24-hour nutrient infusions to critically ill patients. Am J Hosp Pharm 1986;43:2205–2208.
73. Raebel MA, McDonald JB. Twenty-four-hour single-container system for parenteral nutrient admixture. Am J Hosp Pharm 1985;42:1355–1358.
74. Krenek G, Maxwell K, Foulks C. A quality assurance recommended TPN order form design results in a decrease in overfeeding and enhances compliance with nutrition support service (NSS) recommendations. J Parenter Enter Nutr 1994;18:32S.
75. Miller SJ, North GLT, Anderson WD. Parenteral nutrition order form to improve dextrose and lipid use. Am J Hosp Pharm 1990;47:2515–2518.
76. Campos ACL, Paluzzi M, Meguid MM. Clinical use of total nutritional admixtures. Nutrition 1990;6:347–356.
77. Warshawsky KY. Intravenous fat in clinical practice. Nutr Clin Prac 1992;7:187–196.
78. Dickerson RN, Brown RO, White KG. Parenteral nutrition solutions, in Rombeau JL, Caldwell MD (eds): Clinical Nutrition: Parenteral Nutrition, 2nd ed. Philadelphia, WB Saunders, 1993, pp 310–333.
79. Dickson LB, Somani SM, Hermann G, Abramowitz PW. Automated compounder for adding ingredients to parenteral nutrient base solutions. Am J Hosp Pharm 1993; 50:678–682.
80. Williams WW. Infection control during parenteral nutrition therapy. J Parenter Enter Nutr 1985;9:735–746.
81. National Coordinating Committee on Large Volume Parenterals. Recommendations to pharmacists for solving problems with large-volume parenterals. Am J Hosp Pharm 1976;33:231–236.
82. Mirtallo JM, Caryer K, Schneifer PJ, et al. Growth of bacteria and fungi in parenteral nutrition solutions containing albumin. Am J Hosp Pharm 1981;38:1907–1910.
83. Keammerer D, Mayhall CG, Hall GO, et al. Microbial growth patterns in intravenous fat emulsions. Am J Hosp Pharm 1983;40:1650–1653.
84. Brown DH, Simkover RA. Maximum hang times for i.v. fat emulsions. Am J Hosp Pharm 1987;44:282, 284.
85. Ebbert ML, Farraj M, Hwang LT. The incidence and clinical significance of intravenous fat emulsion contamination during infusion. J Parenter Enter Nutr 1987;11:42–45.
86. National Coordinating Committee on Large Volume Parenterals. Recommended guidelines for quality assurance in hospital centralized intravenous admixture services. Am J Hosp Pharm 1980;37:645–655, 660–667.
87. Trissel LA. Handbook on Injectable Drugs, 8th ed. Bethesda, MD, American Society for Hospital Pharmacists, 1994.
88. King JC. Guide to Parenteral Admixtures. St. Louis, MO, Pace Marq, 1994.
89. Parr MD, Bertch KE, Rapp RP. Amino acid stability and microbial growth in total parenteral nutrient solutions. Am J Hosp Pharm 1985;42:2688–2691.
90. Lumpkin MM, Burlington DB. FDA safety alert: Hazards of precipitation associated with parenteral nutrition. April 18, 1994.
91. Henann NE, Jacks TT. Compatibility and availability of sodium bicarbonate in total parenteral nutrient solutions. Am J Hosp Pharm 1985;42:2718–2720.
92. Driscoll DF, Baptista RJ, Mitrano FP, et al. Parenteral nutrient admixtures as drug vehicles: Theory and practice in the critical care setting. DICP Ann Pharmacother 1991; 25:276–283.
93. Driscoll DF. Clinical issues regarding the use of total nutrient admixtures. DICP Ann Pharmacotherapy 1990; 24:296–303.
94. Mirtallo JM. The complexity of mixing calcium and phosphate. Am J Hosp Pharm 1994;51:1535–1536.
95. Mershon J, Nogami W, Williams JM, et al. Bacterial/fungal growth in a combined parenteral nutrition solution. J Parenter Enter Nutr 1986;10:498–502.
96. Driscoll DF, Bacon M, Provost PS, Bristrian BR. Automated compounders for parenteral nutrition admixtures. J Parenter Enter Nutr 1994;18:385–386.
97. Krzyda EA, Andris DA, Whipple JK, et al. Glucose response to abrupt initiation and discontinuation of total parenteral nutrition. J Parenter Enter Nutr 1993;17:64–67.
98. Dickerson RN. Question: How fast can I taper TPN in a hospitalized patient? Hosp Pharm 1985;20:620–621.
99. Bennett KM, Rosen GH. Cyclic total parenteral nutrition. Nutr Clin Prac 1990;5:163–165.
100. Evans NJ, Bamba M, Rombeau JL. Care of central venous catheters, in Rombeau JL, Caldwell MD (eds): Clinical Nutrition: Parenteral Nutrition, 2nd ed. Philadelphia, WB Saunders, 1993, pp 353–366.
101. Alexander JW. Nutrition and translocation. J Parenter Enter Nutr 1990;14:170S–174S.
102. Cahill SL, Benotti PN. Catheter infection control in parenteral nutrition. Nutr Clin Prac 1991;6:65–76.
103. Grant JP. Septic and metabolic complications: Recognition and management, in Handbook of Total Parenteral Nutrition, 2nd ed. Philadelphia, WB Saunders, 1992, pp 239–274.
104. Teasley-Strausburg KM, Shronts EP. Metabolic and gastrointestinal complications, in Teasley-Strausburg KM (ed): Nutrition Support Handbook: A Compendium of Products with Guidelines for Usage. Cincinnati, OH, Harvey Whitney Books Company, 1992, pp 295–303.
105. Apovian CM, McMahon MM, Bistrian BR. Guidelines for refeeding the marasmic patient. Crit Care Med 1990; 18:1030–1033.
106. Knapke CM, Owens JP, Mirtallo JM. Management of glucose abnormalities in patients receiving total parenteral nutrition. Clin Pharm 1989;8:136–144.
107. Freund HR. Abnormalities of liver function and hepatic damage associated with total parenteral nutrition. Nutrition 1991;7:1–5.
108. Fischer RL. Hepatobiliary abnormalities associated with total parenteral nutrition. Gastroent Clin North Am 1898; 18:645–666.
109. Wolman SL, Anderson H, Marliss EB, Jeejeebhoy KN. Zinc in total parenteral nutrition: Requirements and metabolic effects. Gastroenterology 1979;76:458–467.
110. Shuler CL, Wolfson M. Nutrition in acute renal failure, in Rombeau JL, Caldwell MD (eds): Clinical Nutrition: Parenteral Nutrition, 2nd ed. Philadelphia, WB Saunders, 1993, pp 667–675.

111. American Society for Parenteral and Enteral Nutrition. Standards for home nutrition support. Nutr Clin Prac 1992;7:65–69.
112. Joint Commission on Accreditation of Healthcare Organizations. 1995 Accreditation Manual for Home Care. Oakbrook Terrace, IL, Joint Commission on Accreditation of Healthcare Organizations, 1994.
113. Crocker KS. Current status of home infusion therapy. Nutr Clin Prac 1992;7:256–263.
114. Evans MA, Liffrig TK, Nelson JK, Compher C. Home nutrition support patient education materials. Nutr Clin Prac 1993;8:43–47.
115. Howard L, Heaphey L, Fleming CR, et al. Four years of North American registry home parenteral nutrition outcome data and their implications for patient management. J Parenter Enter Nutr 1991;15:384–393.
116. Howard L, Blackburn G, Broviac J, et al. National trends in the use of home parenteral and enteral nutrition (HPEN) therapy [abstract]. J Parenter Enter Nutr 1994;18:22S.
117. Task Force on Specialty Recognition and Certification of Nutritional Support Pharmacists. Executive summary of petition requesting recognition of nutritional support pharmacy as a specialty. Am J Hosp Pharm 1988;45:162–170.
118. Holcombe BJ, Thorne DB, Strausburg KM, et al. Pharmacy practice insights. Analysis of the practice of nutrition support pharmacy specialists. Pharmacotherapy 1995;15:806–813.
119. American Society for Parenteral and Enteral Nutrition. Standards for nutrition support: Hospitalized patients. Nutr Clin Pract 1995;10:208–218.

Chapter 134

Enteral Nutrition

Douglas D. Janson, PharmD

Oral ingestion of food or the delivery of liquid formulas by a tube placed beyond the oral cavity are forms of enteral nutrition. Enteral nutrition and tube feeding are often used interchangeably to describe an artificial feeding method that includes the use of specialized feeding formulas, tubes, and pumps. Patients who are unable to eat or swallow because of a GI obstruction, advanced neurologic or psychiatric diseases, or prolonged unconsciousness associated with critical illness benefit from nutrient delivery to the gut by tube feedings.

In this chapter the principles and practices related to the successful use of enteral nutrition support are described. Included herein is a review of digestive and absorptive physiology, the rationale for the use of the enteral feeding route whenever possible, indications for enteral nutrition, and a description of various enteral access and administration methods. Characteristics of commercially available formulas are presented, as well as initiation and monitoring guidelines to prevent complications. In addition, issues of drug compatibility, drug–nutrient interaction, and drug administration during enteral nutrition are discussed. Lastly, the effectiveness of enteral nutrition to enhance nutrition and disease outcome goals is reviewed.

Gastrointestinal Tract Physiology

Digestion and absorption are important and inseparably associated gastrointestinal (GI) processes which generate the usable fuels for the body. Digestion consists of the stepwise conversion of a complex chemical and physical nutrient form into a molecular form acceptable to the intestinal mucosa. Absorption from the GI tract (GIT) consists of transfer of a nutrient across an intestinal cell membrane. The nutrient ultimately reaches the systemic circulation through the portal venous or splanchnic lymphatic systems provided that it is not excreted by the GI or biliary tract. Since the molecular forms of ingested nutrients are primarily large polymers which cannot be absorbed by the mucosal membrane unless they are broken down or transformed into an absorbable molecular form, digestion and absorption are inseparable. In addition, a coordinated interplay of gastrointestinal motility and neurohormonal secretion is required to facilitate adequate digestion and absorption.[1,2]

Nutrient digestion involves the complex coordination of multiple mechanical, enzymatic, and physicochemical processes. Mechanical dissolution of food occurs by chewing, mixing, and grinding of the stomach contents. Food stimulates the secretion of numerous neurohormones and enzymes from the salivary glands, stomach, liver and biliary system, pancreas, and intestines (Table 134.1). As food passes along the gut lumen, these neurohormones control GI motility and secretion among the organs of the digestive system. Nutrient digestion occurs within the gut lumen and also on the intestinal mucosa membrane. Absorption is a specific function of the intestinal mucosal membrane. The basic absorptive unit is a finger-like projection called the villus, which is made up of epithelial cells called enterocytes. The enterocyte surface contains special luminal projections called microvilli, which provide an increased surface area that is referred to as the brush border membrane.[1,2]

Digestible carbohydrates are presented to the small intestine as polysaccharides (starches) and oligosaccharides (sucrose and lactose). Enzymatic digestion within the gut lumen and at the surface of the brush border membrane produce simple sugars which are translocated across the membrane via active and passive transport mechanisms and are eventually released into the portal vein as shown in Fig. 134.1. Undigestible polysaccharides such as cellulose complexes and other fiber components are digested within the colon by bacterial hydrolases, disaccharidases, and enzymes to short-chain fatty acids (SCFAs). Subsequent to their rapid colonic absorption, SCFAs stimulate sodium and water reabsorption, serve as an energy source, and are trophic or nourishing to the cells of the intestinal mucosa.[3] Fat is primarily presented to the gut as long-chain triglycerides (LCTs) containing 14–24 carbons. LCT digestion includes lypolysis and the formation of mixed bile salt micelles to facilitate solubility and absorption across the mucosal membrane. Within the enterocyte cytosol, triglycerides are re-esterified and packaged into chylomicrons for release into the lymphatic system as shown in Fig. 134.1. Chylomicrons eventually reach the

TABLE 134.1. GASTROINTESTINAL ENZYMES AND HORMONES

Enzyme/Hormone	Site of Secretion	Main Actions
Amylase	Salivary glands	Converts carbohydrates, starch, and glycogen to simple disaccharides
Cholecystokinin (CCK)	Duodenum, jejunum	Stimulates pancreatic enzyme secretion and gallbladder contraction
Chymotrypsinogen	Pancreas	Breaks down proteins into proteases and peptides
Enteroglucagon	Duodenum, small intestine	Inhibits pancreatic enzyme secretion and bowel motility
Gastric inhibitory peptide (GIP)	Small intestine	Decreases gastric motility and stimulates insulin secretion
Gastrin	Stomach, duodenum	Stimulates gastric acid secretion and mucosal growth
Glucagon	Pancreas	Stimulates hepatic glycogenolysis and inhibits motility
Lipase	Pancreas	Hydrolyzes short-chain and medium-chain triglycerides, involved in fat absorption
Pancreatic polypeptide	Pancreas	Inhibits gallbladder contraction and pancreatic and biliary secretion
Pepsinogen	Stomach	Converts large proteins into polypeptides
Secretin	Small intestine	Stimulates hepatic and pancreatic water and bicarbonate
Trypsinogen	Pancreas	Breaks down proteins into proteases and peptides
Vasoactive inhibitory peptide (VIP)	Small intestine, pancreas	Vasodilator; stimulates water and bicarbonate secretion, release of insulin and glucagon, and production of small intestinal juice

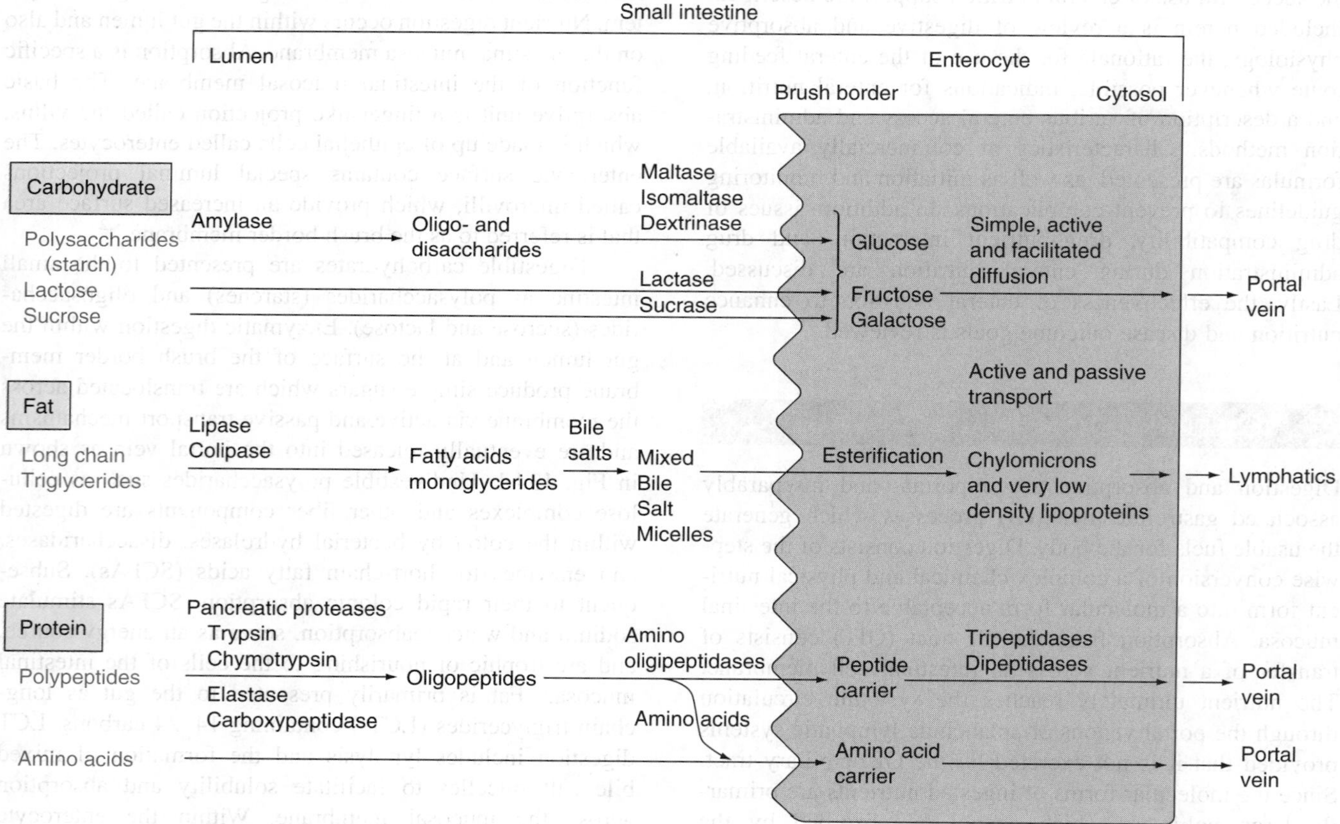

Figure 134.1. Schematic representation of carbohydrate, fat, and protein digestion and absorption within the small intestine. Subsequent to mechanical and enzymatic digestion of these substrates within the lumen and/or brush border of the enterocyte, smaller molecular forms are absorbed into the cytosol by numerous transport mechanisms. Then, nutrients are released from the enterocyte into the systemic circulation.

venous system after transport through the thoracic duct. Medium-chain triglycerides (MCTs) containing 8–12 carbons do not require luminal lipolysis and can be absorbed intact by the mucosal membrane. Within the enterocyte, MCTs are acted on by intracellular lipase and the resultant free fatty acids pass directly into the portal vein.[4]

Protein is primarily presented to the gut as large polypeptides and to a small extent as amino acids due to the denaturation of protein within the stomach. Subsequent to the luminal digestion of polypeptides to oligopeptides of two to eight amino acids, brush border membrane amino-oligopeptidases generate dipeptides and tripeptides. Membrane translocation of the resultant peptides occurs via a peptide-transport system and free amino acids are carried via specific amino acid transport systems. Amino acids and dipeptides are then passed into the portal vein as shown in Fig. 134.1. The digestive and absorptive physiology of these and other nutrients such as water, electrolytes, vitamins, and trace elements are discussed in detail in Chapter 132 on Nutrient Metabolism and Regulation. Under normal circumstances, almost 100% of carbohydrates and more than 80% of amino acids are absorbed within the proximal jejunum. The majority of fat absorption occurs within the jejunum and is completed in the ileum. The absorptive location of these and other nutrients within the GI tract is depicted in Fig. 132.9 of the Nutrient Metabolism and Regulation chapter.

Understanding the mechanisms of digestive and absorptive physiology can greatly enhance the rational use of enteral nutrition support during conditions of normal or altered GI function. Several circumstances may alter the efficacy of nutrient digestion and absorption (Table 134.2). These factors, as they relate to successful enteral nutrition practice, are discussed in greater detail throughout this chapter.

GUT HOST DEFENSE MECHANISMS

Besides digesting and absorbing nutrients to maintain nutritional health, the GI tract is actively involved in defending the host from toxins and antigens by means of nonimmunologic and immunologic mechanisms (Table 134.3). These gut host defense mechanisms are also collectively referred to as the "gut barrier function."[5,6] The gut barrier acts to prevent the spread of intraluminal bacteria and endotoxin to systemic organs and tissues. Hydrochloric acid secreted by the stomach kills the majority of the bacteria ingested with food. Under normal circumstances a mucus gel layer coats the intestinal epithelium and thereby alters the adherence of bacteria to the cells of the GI tract, and provides a favorable environment for anaerobic bacteria. Anaerobic bacteria, which normally colonize the mucus layer, aid in preventing tissue colonization by potential pathogens. Small bowel peristalsis further prevents bacterial stasis and overgrowth. The gut barrier function is also maintained by the intestinal immune system, known as the gut-associated lymphoid tissue (GALT). GALT regulates the local immune response to antigens within the GI tract. Specific immunoglobulins are secreted to kill remaining organisms and neutralize any toxins they produce. Lastly, the hepatic Kupffer's cells help to maintain gut barrier function by clearing the portal blood of gut-derived bacteria and endotoxin. The integrity of gut barrier function may be affected by numerous pathogenic insults such as physiologic stress, ischemia, and a variety of drugs including chemotherapeutic agents. The nutritional aspects that influence the maintenance of the gut barrier are discussed in the next section.

TABLE 134.2. FACTORS AFFECTING INTESTINAL NUTRIENT ABSORPTION

Method of ingestion
Digestibility
Gastric emptying
Intraluminal digestive capacity of the pancreas and the bile
Transit time
Contact surface
Length
Surface of villi
Brush border enzyme content
Carrier function
Diffusion barrier thickness (unstirred layer)

TABLE 134.3. GUT HOST DEFENSE MECHANISMS

Nonimmunologic	Immunologic
Mechanical	Gut-associated lymphoid tissue (GALT)
Epithelial cell	
Epithelial mucus gel layer	Secretory immunoglobulin A
Peristalsis	Hepatic Kupffer's cells
Gastric acid	
Bile salts	
Salivary secretions	
Indigenous microflora	
Limits microbial proliferation	
Microbial antagonism	

RATIONALE FOR ENTERAL NUTRITION

Enteral nutrition is the preferred route of nourishment if the GI tract is functioning and accessible. A considerable body of laboratory and clinical evidence supports the importance and potential advantages of using enteral over parenteral nutrition. Advantages of enteral nutrition include maintaining the structure and function of the GI tract, fewer metabolic and infectious complications, and lower costs.

Experimental data derived predominantly from animal studies suggest that the maintenance of GI tract structure and function is dependent on the presence and composition of luminal nutrients as well as the presence of trophic hormones. A frequently cited benefit of enteral nutrition is that it preserves the process of intestinal crypt cell renewal necessary for the support of normal villi structure and associated enzymatic functions which are required for normal digestion and absorption. Rats who underwent an experimental small bowel bypass from the nutrient stream demonstrated a decrease in mucosal weight, protein, RNA, and enzyme activity.[7] Rats fed parenteral nutrition without enteral feeding for 7 or 12 days were also found to have a significant reduction in small bowel mucosal weight, height, protein, DNA content, and disaccharidase activity.[8,9] Mucosal atrophy and deficient disaccharidase and trypsin activities have also been documented in small bowel biopsies obtained from 16 malnourished infants with protracted diarrhea and malnutrition.[10] The data from these studies suggest that the absence of luminal nutrients induces "gut atrophy" or mucosal hypoplasia and decreased enzymatic activity. Clinically, the gut atrophy that occurs during a prolonged absence of enteral feeding may be responsible for the development of symptoms such as cramping and diarrhea when enteral nutrition is reintroduced.

The nutrient complexity of the enteral diet also appears to have an effect on the maintenance of intestinal mucosa mass. The small intestinal mucosa segment weights, DNA, and protein content of rats were best maintained when rats were fed a complex intact diet instead of an isocaloric hydrolyzed (partially digested) diet.[11,12] Furthermore, the colonic mucosal mass in rats fed a complex diet was better maintained than those who received a hydrolyzed diet; this suggests that there may be some contribution of the fiber contained in the rat chow.[11] Young and coworkers also noted that the maintenance of intestinal mucosa was dependent on whether the animals were fed by the oral, gastric, or jejunal route.[12] The presence of luminal nutrients in animals also has been shown to stimulate the production of enteric hormones such as gastrin and enteroglucagon, which are trophic to the gut mucosa.[13–15] These hormones are found in humans, but have not been studied as intensively in humans as they have in animal models.

The intestine is an organ of protein synthesis as well as one of digestion and absorption. It therefore utilizes nutritional substrates directly. Glucose, glutamine, and L-leucine are examples of fuels used more efficiently when given via the enteral route as opposed to parenterally.[16,17] L-Leucine yields greater protein synthesis when given orally and is incorporated into the intestinal structure differently depending on the route of ingestion. Serum glutamine levels fall during stress, while intestinal uptake rises.[18] Glutamine and ketones are absent from parenteral solutions and may account for some of the intestinal structural deterioration seen during the administration of parenteral nutrition. The results from the aforementioned studies and others have stimulated several investigations into the effects of specific types of enteral diets, specific nutrients such as glutamine and fiber, and the interaction of trophic hormones on their ability to maintain the GI mucosa.

Maintenance of the functional integrity of the GI tract is intimately linked to proper gut barrier function. The immunologic and barrier functions listed in Table 134.3 prevent antigenic invasion of the gut mucosa, induction of local inflammation, and translocation of gut bacteria to the portal or lymphatic circulation. It has been suggested that bacterial translocation, the appearance of enteric organisms in the mesenteric lymph nodes, spleen, and liver, is promoted by parenteral nutrition and bowel rest. Since enteral nutrition better maintains the functional integrity of the gut, it may also prevent gut bacterial translocation. Animal studies comparing parenteral and enteral nutrient delivery supporting the theory of gut bacterial translocation include the following: enteral nutrition resulted in higher secretary IgA and biliary tract secretions,[19] less bacterial leak through intestinal mucosa,[20] greater maintenance of mucosal weight and thickness with lower secretion of catabolic hormones following a burn injury,[21] and reduced mortality following septic[22] or hypotensive insult.[23] The results of one human study among healthy volunteers also suggest the potential role of enteral nutrition in maintaining the gut mucosal barrier and preventing bacterial translocation. Subjects receiving total parenteral nutrition (TPN) and complete bowel rest for 7 days, compared to subjects receiving enteral feedings, had significantly higher levels of arterial epinephrine, glucagon, and hepatic venous tumor necrosis factor when given an equivalent dose of enteral endotoxin. Additionally, the parenterally fed subjects also had enhancement of acute-phase protein response, increased peripheral amino acid mobilization, and increased peripheral lactate production, a metabolic response expected to occur with systemic endotoxin effect.[24] The 1990 summary guidelines for the scientific review of enteral food products by the Life Sciences Research Office, Federation of American Societies for Experimental Biology, concluded that although available human data are insufficient to establish whether the atrophic changes in the gut that are associated with a lack of enteral nutrition lead to clinically significant translocation of gut bacteria, endotoxins, and antigenic macromolecules, these considerations seem to justify the use of at least partial enteral nutrition as one means of maintaining the gut mucosa or reducing such complications.[25] Prospective, randomized clinical trials among critically ill patients comparing enteral and parenteral delivery are unable to substantiate a direct cause and effect between the parenteral route and gut bacterial translocation. However, a recent critical review of several studies suggests that enteral nutrition may have a favorable impact on GI immunologic function and infectious morbidity.[26]

A metabolic advantage of enteral feeding compared to the parenteral route is improved glucose tolerance and markedly less hyperinsulinemia.[27,28] It has been proposed that better control of peripheral blood glucose levels occurs during enteral administration because the insulin released is absorbed with the glucose via the portal vein and is handled by the liver. The enteral feeding route is also as effective as the parenteral route in maintaining or promoting repletion of nutritional indices among several patient populations.[28–31] An additional physiologic benefit of enteral feeding is that it stimulates bile flow through the biliary tract and, hence, reduces the development of gallbladder sludge and stone formation, which has been associated with long-term parenteral nutrition and bowel rest.[32] Finally, enteral nutrition removes the potential infectious or technical complications associated with the placement and use of a central venous access device required for parenteral nutrition. In addition to the reduced complications of enteral over parenteral nutrition, the reported cost of tube feeding is 36–44% that of TPN.[29,30]

INDICATIONS FOR ENTERAL NUTRITION

Subsequent to assessing the nutritional state of a patient and the need for initiating specialized nutrition support, the clinician must assess the functional status of the GI tract and the optimal access site for tube placement as shown in Fig. 133.1 of the Parenteral Nutrition chapter. Although enteral nutrition is indicated for many conditions or disease states (Table 134.4), its use is contraindicated for patients with a mechanical obstruction of the GI tract, diffuse peritonitis, severe diarrhea that makes metabolic management difficult, severe GI hemorrhage, intractable vomiting, chronic intestinal pseudo-obstruction, or severe malabsorption.

TABLE 134.4. POTENTIAL INDICATIONS FOR ENTERAL NUTRITION

Neoplastic Disease	**Gastrointestinal Disease**
Chemotherapy	Inflammatory bowel disease
Radiotherapy	Short bowel syndrome
Upper gastrointestinal tumors	Esophageal motility disorder
Cancer cachexia	Pancreatitis
	Fistulas
Organ Failure	**Neurologic Impairment**
Hepatic	Comatose state
Renal	Cerebrovascular accident
Cardiac cachexia	Demyelinating disease
Pulmonary	Severe depression
Multiple organ system failure	Failure to thrive
Hypermetabolic States	**Other Indications**
Closed head injury	Acquired immune deficiency syndrome
Burns	Anorexia nervosa
Trauma	Complications during pregnancy
Postoperative major surgery	Geriatric patients with multiple chronic disease
Sepsis	Organ transplantation

FUNCTIONAL STATUS OF THE GI TRACT

An assessment of the length, anatomy, and motility of the GI tract is required prior to the initiation of enteral therapy (Table 134.2). The minimum length of functional small bowel required for nutrient absorption is approximately 100–150 cm of jejunum and/or ileum.[33] Enteral nutrient delivery may be effective with less than 100 cm of small bowel especially if the ileocecal valve and the colon are present and intact. Increased small bowel motility, also referred to as an increase in transit time, occurs when the ileum and/or ileocecal valve are removed. The ileocecal valve acts as a brake and reduces the transit of the GI contents through the small bowel and into the colon. The presence of the colon maintains fluid and electrolyte balance in an enterally fed patient.

Hospitalized patients may have reduced gastric motility and emptying due to sepsis, postoperative anesthetic agents, opioid analgesics, and underlying pathology such as diabetic gastroparesis. Reduced gastric emptying can place a gastrically fed patient at risk for nausea, vomiting, and subsequent pulmonary aspiration of gastric contents. Rather than resorting to parenteral nutrition, successful enteral nutrition can be initiated by placing the tip of the feeding tube beyond the pylorus into the duodenum or, preferably, more distal into the jejunum. Although there is some evidence that continuous feeding into the stomach or the duodenum increases the small bowel transit time, intestinal nutrient absorption is complete for either route.[34] Early enteral feedings started within 12–24 hours for the postoperative patient via the small bowel are frequently given, even in the absence of bowel sounds. However, during states of shock, borderline tissue oxygenation, and unstable cardiopulmonary hemodynamics, initiation of early GI feedings should be withheld since nutrient delivery and its associated oxygen requirement can further compromise oxygen tissue perfusion. Anecdotal reports and animal studies suggest that early enteral nutrition can be provided to the GI tract of a patient who has recently undergone a GI anastomosis without compromising the integrity of the anastomosis.[35]

Guidelines for the use of enteral nutrition have been established and published by the American Society of Parenteral and Enteral Nutrition.[36] Patients with neurologic impairment or psychological diseases who will not or cannot eat, but have functioning GI tracts, are candidates for enteral nutrition. Patients with organ failure, GI diseases, and patients in hypermetabolic states such as burns or trauma are frequently candidates for enteral nutrition. Enteral feeding is indicated during some clinical situations of GI fistulous disease such as colocutaneous or low-output ileal fistulas. Enteral nutrition is also favored for patients with an esophageal, gastric, duodenal, and proximal jejunal fistula when distal GI tract tube feeding access is possible. The use of enteral nutrition during severe pancreatitis or associated complications has increased over recent years. Human studies have confirmed the results of animal studies that continuous jejunal feeding does not significantly increase exocrine pancreatic secretion. Therefore, clinicians have utilized the placement of a feeding tube into the jejunum for administering specialized enteral formulas to those patients with severe and complicated pancreatitis. Of the published data, no aggravation of disease has been reported when utilizing this route of enteral nutrition in pancreatitis.[37] Unfortunately, there is a lack of objective and prospective studies in this area that make clear and concise recommendations for the use of enteral nutrition during pancreatitis. It has been recommended that TPN should be used when enteral feeding exacerbates abdominal pain, ascites, or fistulous output in patients with pancreatitis and limited oral intake.[36] Several clinical trials have shown that enteral nutrition is effective in supporting Crohn's patients with exacerbations of their disease. However, enteral nutrition is contraindicated in Crohn's disease with concomitant high-output fistula or high-grade obstruction, or when enteral feeding fails to normalize the nutritional status or results in unacceptable GI symptoms.[36] In patients with acquired immune deficiency syndrome (AIDS), enteral nutrition should be utilized unless situations of severe malabsorption develop because of GI infections such as cryptosporidium or cytomegalovirus or during complications of lymphoma involving the small bowel.[38]

Enteral Access

Enteral nutrition support is distinguished in part from normal eating by the routes of nutrient intake and the equipment needed to administer it. Because the conditions necessitating specialized nutrition support are varied, multiple options are available to provide the therapy. All routes involve placement of a tube through which a liquid formula is infused. As the site of nutrient delivery moves further away from the mouth, the tube insertion becomes more difficult and invasive but, at the same time, more permanent. The technique and selection of enteral routes and access devices have recently been extensively reviewed in the literature.[39–41] The indications, placement options, advantages, and disadvantages associated with the different tube feeding routes are summarized in Table 134.5.

The most frequently used short-term enteral feeding routes are those accessed by inserting a tube through the nose and threading it into the stomach or upper small bowel (Fig. 134.2). The names of these routes are nasogastric (NG), nasoduodenal (ND), and nasojejunal (NJ), indicating both the tube insertion point and the termination point. The oral gastric (OG) route is reserved for patients in whom the nasopharyngeal area is unaccessible or in infants unable to take food by mouth. These routes do not require surgical intervention and, therefore, are the least invasive. They are also temporary, because the tubes are frequently held in place by a piece of tape on the nose. One disadvantage is that they can easily be pulled out during routine patient care. Undesired tube removal has been reported to occur in up to 60% of patients receiving enteral nutrition via the nasoenteric route.[40]

Dobbie and Hoffmeister[42] were the first to describe feeding through a flexible, weighted tube. Prior to their report, all enteral feedings were infused through heavy, large-bore, rigid rubber tubes. The use of the rigid tube was associated with loss of lower esophageal sphincter tone, otitis media, esophagitis, esophageal perforations, and mucosal injury.[43] Modern tubes patterned after Dr. Dobbie's prototype generally consist of small-bore pliable silicone rubber or polyurethane, which makes them lightweight and comfortable for the patient. The tube tip is either unweighted or weighted, frequently with inert tungsten. The weighted end is intended to help facilitate successful tube passage via peristalsis through the pylorus and into the small intestine after entering the stomach. Modern feeding tubes are available in varying lengths of 16–60 inches and small-bore sizes of 6–12 French, allowing for numerous options among pediatric and adult populations. A disadvantage of the small-bore tube is that it may become clogged, due to improper medication administration or tube flushing techniques.

In general, the stomach is the least expensive and the least labor-intensive access site to use for enteral feeding; however, it is not necessarily the best. Patients who have delayed gastric emptying from complications of diabetes or gastric atony during the postoperative period are at a higher risk for aspiration of gastric contents into the pulmonary system. Therefore, postpyloric tube placement may be required to enable successful enteral feeding. Studies have yet to prove definitively whether postpyloric tube feedings actually do decrease the risk of aspiration and pneumonia.[39] The NG, OG, ND, and NJ tubes can all be placed manually at the patient's bedside. Greater skill is required to place the feeding tube beyond the pylorus at the bedside. Several techniques have been described in the literature to help facilitate manual placement at the bedside. These include the use of styletted tubes, that is, a wire in the tube to help guide its placement, weighted tubes, patient placement onto their right side, and/or use of metoclopramide. Even though success rates of 80–90% have been quoted in the literature using such techniques for postpyloric tube placement, this degree of success is not experienced by all clinicians.[39] Alternatively, it may be necessary to move the tube physically through the pylorus by utilizing fluoroscopy or endoscopy, which also increases the cost of enteral therapy. X-ray veri-

TABLE 134.5. OPTIONS AND CONSIDERATIONS IN THE SELECTION OF TUBE FEEDING ACCESS

Access	Indications	Tube Placement Options	Advantages	Disadvantages
Nasogastric or orogastric	Short-term Intact gag reflex Normal gastric emptying	Manually at bedside	Ease of placement Allows for intermittent bolus or continuous feeding Inexpensive Multiple commercially available tubes and sizes	Potential tube displacement Increased aspiration risk Cosmetically unappealing Small bore tube
Nasoduodenal or nasojejunal	Short-term Delayed gastric emptying (early postoperative period or diabetic neuropathy) High risk gastroesophageal reflux or aspiration	Manually at bedside Fluoroscopic Endoscopic	Reduced aspiration risk Allows for early postoperative feeding Multiple commercially available tubes and sizes	Manual transpyloric passage requires greater skill Potential tube displacement Continuous (and cyclic) feeding only Cosmetically unappealing Attendant risks of complication for endoscopic placement Small bore tube
Esophagostomy or pharyngostomy	Long-term Nasopharyngeal access contraindicated Tumors or trauma of head or neck region	Bedside with local anesthesia or during surgery	Large bore tube Easy tube replacement	Dressing changes by patient more difficult due to location Cosmetically unappealing Requires stoma site care
Gastrostomy	Long-term Normal gastric emptying Swallowing dysfunction due to neuromuscular disease or central nervous system disorders Esophageal stricture or neoplasm	Surgically Endoscopically (percutaneous endoscopic gastrostomy [PEG]) Laparoscopically Fluoroscopically	Allows for intermittent, bolus, or continuous feeding Large bore tube Multiple commercially available tubes and sizes Low-profile buttons available	Cosmetically appealing Attendant risks for complication for each method of placement Higher cost, particularly with surgical placement Aspiration risk potential Requires stoma site care
Jejunostomy	Long-term Impaired gastric emptying (diabetic neuropathy) Facilitate postoperative enteral feeding in trauma, malnourished or upper GIT surgery Inability to access upper GIT	Surgically Endoscopically (accessing jejunum via PEG) Laparoscopically Fluoroscopically	Allows for early postoperative feeding Reduced aspiration risk Multiple commercially available tubes and sizes	Cosmetically appealing Attendant risks for complication for each method of placement Continuous (and cyclic) feeding only Requires stoma site care

fication of nasogastric or nasoenteric feeding tubes placed by manual techniques must be obtained routinely on all patients with altered consciousness, altered cough or gag reflex, or those who are mechanically ventilated.[40]

More invasive, yet more permanent enteral feeding access includes esophagostomy or pharyngostomy, gastrostomy, and jejunostomy placement (Fig. 134.2). Pharyngostomies and esophagostomies are indicated in patients with head and neck malignancies or maxillofacial anomalies that contraindicate nasopharyngeal access. Cervical pharyngostomy and esophagostomy are invasive as the tube is located in the neck and passes through the skin into the esophagus or the pharynx. Therefore, they are generally considered long-term enteral access devices. These routes use large-bore tubes and tube replacement can be accomplished quite easily. As with any ostomy, site care is required. Dressing changes may be more difficult to perform by the patient due to the location. Complications of these routes, though infrequent, include recurrent laryngeal nerve damage, aspiration, and infection.[40,41]

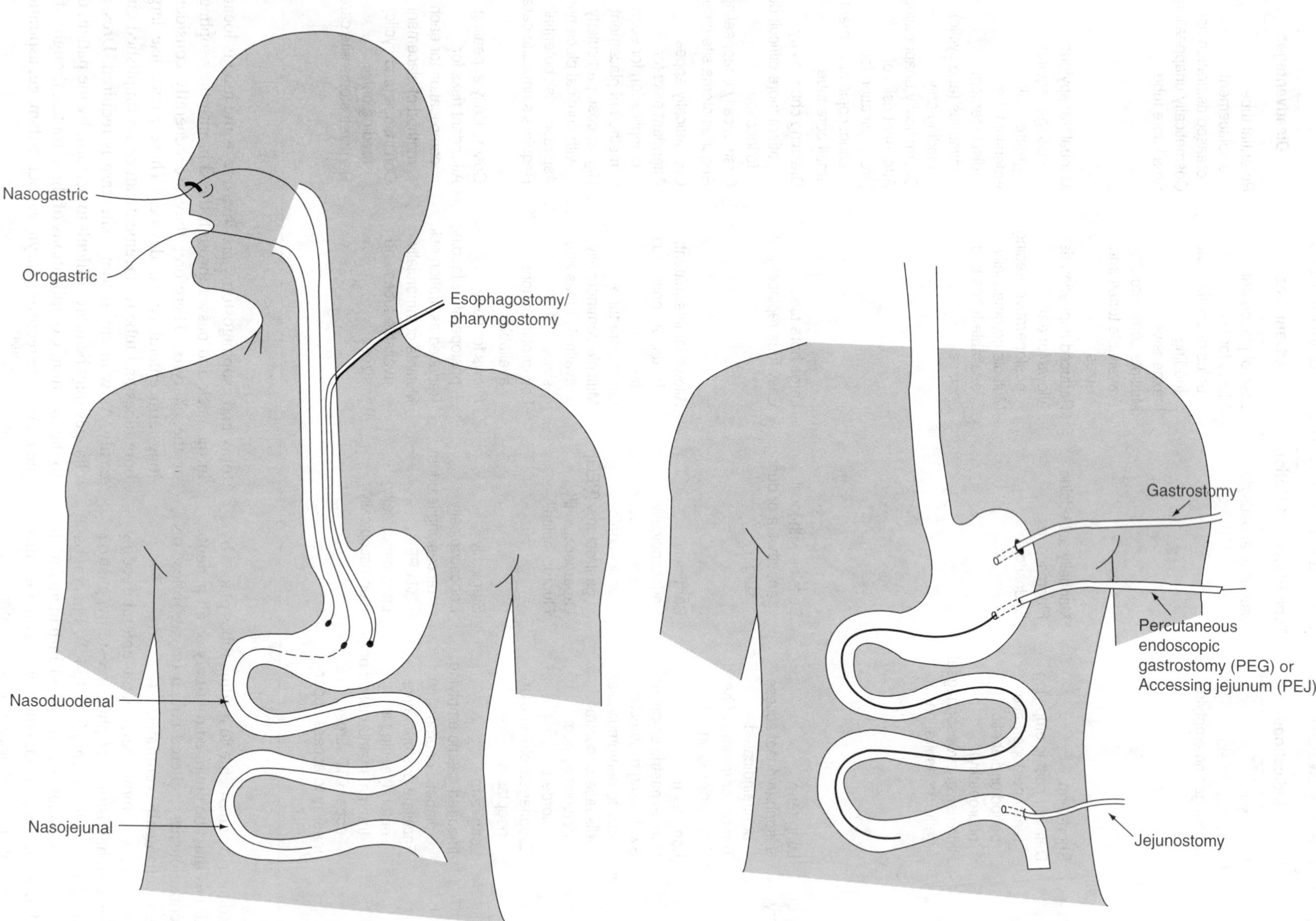

Figure 134.2. Access sites for tube feeding. Nasogastric, orogastric, nasoduodenal, and nasojejunal are generally short-term (less than 6 weeks) enteral feeding routes. Esophagostomy/pharyngostomy, gastrostomy, PEG, percutaneous endoscopic jejunostomy (PEJ), and jejunostomy are longer term (months to years) enteral feeding routes.

A feeding gastrostomy is another long-term enteral access device indicated for a patient with esophageal obstruction or impaired swallowing; however, the patient must have adequate gastric emptying. A gastrostomy can be placed surgically, under general anesthesia. The attendant risks of general anesthesia are hypotension and aspiration. However, if the patient requires surgery for another reason, a gastrostomy tube can also be placed at the time of surgery. The complication rates of surgical gastrostomy placement average less than 2% for such complications as wound infection or dehiscence, tube site problems including infection, continuous drainage or fistula formation, tube dislodgement or subsequent peritoneal contamination, and GI bleeding.[39] The percutaneous endoscopic gastrostomy (PEG) is a popular nonoperative procedure that can be performed safely and cost effectively using local anesthesia. PEGs are generally placed in an endoscopy suite, eliminating costly operating room time. The results of a prospective randomized comparison between PEG and operative gastrostomy demonstrated similar complication rates, but the PEG had greater cost–benefit. More recently, two other techniques for gastrostomy placement have been described in the literature. They are laparoscopically and fluoroscopically placed gastrostomy tubes. Further investigation will be required to define the role of these two techniques. Gastrostomies utilize large-bore tubes, are associated with less tube clogging, and allow for all methods of tube feeding administration. Subsequent to the maturity of the surgical tract where the gastrostomy tube lies, a low-profile skin-level gastrostomy button may be placed for patient convenience and comfort. Gastrostomy sites require general stoma site care to prevent inflammation and infection.

Lastly, jejunostomies are long-term enteral access devices indicated during stomach or duodenal obstruction, impaired gastric emptying from diabetic neuropathy, or for the same situations as a gastrostomy tube. Frequently, jejunostomies are placed during a surgical procedure when the small bowel is readily accessible. This may allow for early postoperative enteral feeding since the small bowel is least affected by surgical manipulation, whereas gastric atony and colonic ileus may persist for a long time postoperatively. Delayed gastric emptying has been observed in 50% of patients undergoing pylorus-preserving pancreaticoduodenectomies.[44] Successful early enteral feeding of these patients requires gastric decompression while feeding into the small bowel through a jejunostomy tube. A jejunostomy tube may be placed surgically and has a complication rate of less than 1% with intraperitoneal leakage of infusion as the major complication. Further, a jejunostomy tube may be created by conversion of a PEG to a jejunostomy (PEJ) by passing a feeding tube through the lumen of the PEG and then beyond the pylorus and into the jejunum.[40] In addition, laparoscopically and fluoroscopically placed jejunostomies are also described in the literature.[39] Administration of enteral feeding into the jejunum should only be done by a continuous or a continuous-cyclic method of tube feeding. This is done to reduce the potential incidence of GI bloating, cramping, and diarrhea from tube feeding formula administered into the small capacity of the intestinal lumen.

ADMINISTRATION METHODS

The administration methods for tube feeding are continuous, continuous-cyclic, intermittent, and intermittent-bolus (Table 134.6). The choice of administration method is dependent on the anatomic location of the feeding tube, the clinical condition of the patient, the environment in which the patient resides, the intestinal function, and the patient's tolerance to the tube feeding.

CONTINUOUS

Continuous tube feeding is characterized by the administration of enteral nutrition formula via a delivery system over 16–24 h/d. The delivery system includes a feeding reservoir or bag attached to an extension set that is connected to a pump. The delivery system is then attached to the patient's enteral access tube. Even though continuous infusion may increase nursing time to routinely check the enteral infusion, it does provide maximal tolerance by minimizing the side effects of abdominal distention or diarrhea. Infusion rates usually range from 50–125 mL/h, although rates of 150 mL/h have been reported without complications. Continuous delivery of nutrients is mandatory when the tube is placed in the duodenum or the jejunum. Continuous enteral feeding is widely practiced among critically ill patients.[44] A survey of nutritional support services compared the different techniques of administration of enteral feedings. The results indicated that 83% of enteral nutrition is given continuously while 17% is delivered by intermittent or bolus methods.[45] Continuous feeding is also beneficial for patients who have limited absorption capacity because of a rapid GI transit time or severely impaired digestion. Slow continuous administration in such patients allows greater time for digestion and absorption of nutrients as they pass through the intestine.

CONTINUOUS CYCLIC

Continuous-cyclic tube feeding utilizes the same delivery system as continuous feeding but the formula is administered over 10–14 h/d at the desired rate as specified by the tolerance of the patient and his or her nutrient requirements. Continuous-cyclic therapy is generally recommended for the noncritically ill patient, home tube feeding patient, or patients who are in rehabilitation settings. Cyclic enteral feedings allow a patient a physical and psychological break

TABLE 134.6. ADMINISTRATION METHODS FOR TUBE FEEDING

Method	Equipment	Indication	Infusion Example
Continuous	Infusion pump generally recommended Enteral formula container Administration set	Gastric tube feeding Postpyloric tube feeding Critically ill patient Limited absorption capacity Limited feeding tolerance via intermittent and bolus methods	Full strength isotonic formula infused at 20 cc/h, advanced by 20 cc/h increments every 8 hours to desired goal rate as tolerated
Continuous-cyclic	Infusion pump generally recommended Enteral formula container Administration set	Gastric or postpyloric tube feeding Home tube feeding Rehabilitation patient Nocturnal tube feeding Potential transition to oral intake during daytime Limited feeding tolerance via bolus or intermittent method	Formula infused over 10–14 h daily at desired goal rate to achieve nutrient requirements
Intermittent	Infusion pump or gravity flow Enteral formula container Administration set	Gastric tube feeding Home tube feeding Rehabilitation patient Patient unlikely to transition to oral intake Limited feeding tolerance via bolus method	240–480 cc formula infused over 20–40 min 4–6 times daily
Intermittent-bolus	Large syringe (60 cc)	Gastric tube feeding Home tube feeding Rehabilitation patient Patient unlikely to transition to oral intake	240–280 cc formula infused over <10 min 4–6 times daily

from being connected to the enteral infusion system and allow for greater rehabilitation and return to the activities of daily living. Frequently, continuous-cyclic enteral feeds are administered nocturnally, which may allow for transitioning a patient's diet to more oral intake during the day time. Continuous-cyclic tube feedings may be administered into the stomach or small bowel. Cyclic feedings may require formulas of higher nutrient densities or higher infusion rates to compensate for the periods when the tube feedings are discontinued.[44] Therefore monitoring for GI tolerance is particularly important when patients are being initiated on a continuous-cyclic enteral feeding protocol.

INTERMITTENT

Intermittent feeding consists of the administration of 240–480 cc of formula infused over 20–40 min four to six times daily. This method of delivery should only be administered to patients with feeding tube tips that lie within the stomach, because the stomach is capable of handling large and more rapid volumes of feeding formula. Since the stomach is the natural nutrient reservoir that controls the volume and osmolality reaching the small intestine, this prevents the dumping syndrome. The dumping syndrome occurs when a large quantity of a hyperosmolar solution is introduced too rapidly into the small bowel. Clinically this syndrome manifests as nausea, cramping, lightheadedness, and diarrhea. Intermittent enteral feeds may be administered by an infusion pump or via gravity flow with a roller clamp. Many authors advocate pump-assisted rate control, because roller clamps used to adjust the rate manually are known to be inaccurate and some patients may be acutely sensitive to even small variances.[46] However, gastric installation generally does not require such meticulous titration as long as gastric motility and the pyloric sphincter are intact. Intermittent enteral feeding is indicated for home tube feeding patients or patients in rehabilitation-type settings. Intermittent feeding is frequently selected for patients who are not able to eat normally on their own such as patients who have altered mental or cognitive function. Therefore, the tube feeding is given intermittently and is more physiologically consistent with normal eating patterns. Patients who receive intermittent feeding may be at higher risk for complications such as nausea, vomiting, and aspiration.

BOLUS

Bolus feeding consists of the administration of 240–480 cc of formula infused over less than 10 min four to six times daily. It is used primarily for esophagostomy, pharyngostomy, or gastrostomy patients who have intact stomachs.

The stomach then regulates the flow of formula into the intestine. Bolus feedings have the advantage of requiring little administration time and minimal equipment. Many times, only a large 60-cc syringe or bulb is needed to instill the feeding into the appropriate tube. Alternatively, they can be infused via a complete infusion system consisting of an infusion reservoir, tubing, and possibly a feeding pump. Unfortunately, bolus feedings may not be well tolerated and can result in cramping, nausea, vomiting, aspiration, and diarrhea.

Feeding Equipment

Feeding containers, administration tubing, and pumps should all be evaluated prior to their use. Feeding containers should be leakproof, unbreakable, and easy to clean. They should be equipped with a reliable closure and have easy-to-read volume markings. The adaptability of the container to multiple infusion sets, volume capacity, and distinguishability from an intravenous container should also be examined.[47]

Administration sets consist of tubing that connects the feeding container to the feeding tube. These sets should be distinctly different from intravenous sets and adaptable to many feeding containers and feeding tubes. In addition, they should be long enough to connect the feeding container and patient easily. Lastly, the administration set should be equipped with an infusion control regulator that allows a reasonably accurate flow rate to within 20% of the expected rate.

Pharmacists are sometimes asked to assist in evaluating enteral feeding pumps because of their familiarity with intravenous infusion pumps. Many considerations are the same for both types of pumps. They should be lightweight, easy to operate, have reasonably long battery life, and require little maintenance. The pump should have a useful alarm system that indicates low battery power, an empty container or that the pressure in the set is rising. Rising pressure indicates set occlusion. Lastly, the pump should be easy to operate by hospital or nursing home personnel and patients alike. Although delineation of the specific features of several manufacturers' enteral infusion pumps is beyond the scope of this chapter, they have been recently reviewed.[48]

Characteristics of Enteral Formulas

Since the introduction of enteral formulas in the 1940s, the composition and nutrient profile of enteral formulas have become highly sophisticated. Initially, enteral formulas were created to provide essential nutrients, then formula enhancements were made such as including fiber, or modifying the specific amino acids to optimize the biological value and utilization. Recently, enteral formulas have been modified in nutrient composition by changing the content of the amino acids, such as glutamine and arginine, changing the omega 3 polyunsaturated fatty acid content and adding ribonucleic acid, to promote a favorable physiologic effect that improves the disease outcome. Modifying the enteral formula's nutrient content to improve the disease outcome for a patient has been coined "nutritional pharmacology."[49] Currently, the U.S. Food and Drug Administration (FDA) describes enteral formulas as medical foods. The use of a medical food product is based on a need to provide energy and/or specific nutrients because of an underlying medical condition.[50] A lack of consensus exists as to whether medical foods should be components of supportive care and/or whether they ought to be categorized as pharmacologic treatment.[51] The Life Sciences Research Office has suggested that medical foods should "have documented evidence supporting claims of maintenance or improvement of nutritional status of patients . . . and or improvement of one or more specific nutrient-related disease manifestations significantly more than that observed from use of commercially available nutritionally complete formulas."[25] Currently the FDA has not developed any specific regulations for enteral formulas as to current food labeling requirements or to rules governing their health claims other than the regulatory statutes which are designed to ensure good manufacturing practices for all processed foods.

The macronutrient content of enteral formulas (namely, protein, carbohydrate, and fat) varies in nutrient complexity (Table 134.7). Nutrient complexity refers to the amount of hydrolysis and digestion a substrate source requires prior to intestinal absorption. Polymeric or intact substrates are of similar molecular form as the food we eat. Those enteral formulas, which contain partially hydrolyzed or elemental substrates, are characterized as defined formula diets. The caloric contribution of each of the macronutrients is as follows: carbohydrates, 4 kcal/g; protein, 4 kcal/g; and fat, 9 kcal/g. The micronutrients, including electrolytes, vitamins, trace elements, and water, do not contribute to caloric content.

PROTEIN COMPOSITION

Important factors concerning the protein within enteral formulas are the quantity, quality, and the molecular form of protein. The essential amino acid content of the protein source determines the quality of the protein. The protein quality is frequently expressed in two standard ways, the biological value and chemical score. It is desirable to have a protein source which is of high biological value and chemical score because then less protein will be required to meet the patient's nitrogen requirements. Most of the readily available formulas contain proteins of high quality.[52] The molecular form of the protein source in enteral formulas will determine the amount of digestion that is required

TABLE 134.7. ENTERAL FORMULA NUTRIENT COMPLEXITY

Nutrient	Polymeriic or Intact	Partially Hydrolyzed	Elemental
Carbohydrate	Starches Fruit, vegetable, cereal solids Glucose polymers Corn syrup solids Polysaccharides	Oligosaccharides Maltodextrins Dissacharides Maltose, sucrose, lactose	Monosaccharides Glucose Galactose
Fat	Long-chain triglycerides Polyunsaturated fatty acids Corn oil Safflower oil Soybean oil Butter fat Menhaden Fish oils	Medium-chain triglycerides Coconut oil Palm kernel Free fatty acids Linoleic	
Protein	Whole Egg, milk, meat, whey Isolates Caseinate salts Lactalbumin	Oligopeptides Dipeptides Tripeptides	L-Amino acids

for adequate absorption within the small bowel. Polymeric or intact protein sources require complete digestion to smaller peptides and free amino acids before they are absorbed from the GI tract. Therefore, enteral formula protein sources such as meat, milk, eggs, and caseinates require complete digestion by hydrochloric acid, specific protein enzymes, and pancreatic enzymes. Subsequent to these digestive processes, amino acids, oligopeptides, dipeptides, and tripeptides are presented to the enterocytes of the small bowel (Fig. 134.1). The protein sources within enteral solutions have also been formulated with partially hydrolyzed proteins as peptides or elemental protein as L-amino acids (Table 134.7). The carriers for the peptides have proven to be very efficient in that they do not depend on sodium to function properly. Free amino acids, on the other hand, are absorbed via sodium-dependent mechanisms that appear to be slower and less efficient than peptide ones. Therefore, partially digested protein entities are the most readily absorbable form of nitrogen substrate.[2,34] As the molecular form of protein is reduced in size, the osmotic load within the enteral formula is increased. Also, as simplicity of the protein molecule increases, so does the prevalance of amino acids containing free sulfur; this in turn imparts a bitter flavor and foul odor to feeding solutions, making them less desirable for oral consumption.[53] Many commercially available enteral solutions contain combinations of intact and partially hydrolyzed protein sources.

Conditionally Essential Amino Acids

Recently, glutamine and arginine have been added to some enteral formulas. These amino acids are normally nonessential amino acids. However, during disease states of high physiologic stress, glutamine and arginine may become deficient and, therefore, have been characterized as conditionally essential. Glutamine is synthesized mostly in muscle and is used as the primary fuel for the enterocytes.[3] Therefore, during glutamine-deficient states, the utilization of glutamine increases beyond the synthesis or release of glutamine from the muscle tissue. Since glutamine is the primary fuel for the enterocyte, it has undergone investigation to determine its role in maintaining the integrity of the gut mucosa. Furthermore it has been postulated that glutamine may play a role in preventing bacterial translocation. Free glutamine is not normally contained in TPN solutions. Two prospective, randomized clinical investigations of 0.57 g/kg of intravenous glutamine supplemented in TPN among bone marrow transplant patients have demonstrated conflicting results relative to the nutritional response and infectious complications. However, both demonstrated reduced length of hospital stay.[54,55] Glutamine-supplemented TPN in animals has been shown to increase the gut mass based on duodenal biopsies and reduced bowel permeability. Also in animal studies, glutamine-supplemented enteral amino acid diets have shown improved gut mass and function, while other investigators have found little benefit in supplementing glutamine to enteral diets.[3,56] The glutamine content of selected enteral formulas varies in the range of 1.8–14.2 g/L of formula. Enteral formulas containing glutamic acid also serve as an immediate precursor and eventually result in an increased production of glutamine. It has been questioned whether free glutamine is required to have a beneficial effect on the gut.[57] Some investigators have raised the concern whether glutamine may actually enhance some tumors in that it may act as a tumor stimulator. Obviously further research and investigation are required as to the potential benefits and harm associated with glutamine-enriched specialized nutrient formulas.[58]

Arginine is also a conditionally essential amino acid, in that it may not be synthesized in sufficient quantity during states of trauma or stress.[59] Data from animal investigations have demonstrated that arginine may have an antitumor effect, and among healthy subjects it has been shown to stimulate T-cell blastogenesis. In addition, supplemental arginine has been shown to decrease protein catabolism, enhance nitrogen retention following injury, and also accelerate wound healing. Arginine has been supplemented in selected enteral formulas in the range of 4.5–14 g/L of enteral formula. Diets enhanced with arginine have been studied in burn, cancer, and septic patients.

CARBOHYDRATE COMPOSITION

The carbohydrate content of enteral formulas is the major source of nonprotein calories. Polymeric or intact enteral formulas contain starches and numerous types of glucose polymers, which require complete digestion to the monosaccharide moieties prior to intestinal absorption (Fig. 134.1). As the hydrolysis of carbohydrate increases within an enteral formula, the osmolality of the formula is also further increased. Elemental carbohydrates such as glucose and galactose contribute significantly to the osmolality of enteral formulas, which is directly correlated to enteral feeding intolerance. Therefore, partially digested entities, rather than elemental sugars, are the choice for inclusion in enteral formulas. Glucose polymers provide an especially useful carbohydrate source that is tolerated by most individuals (Table 134.7). The polymers are large chains that provide a minimal osmotic load, yet are easily absorbed in the intestine. The one shortcoming of glucose polymers and oligosaccharides is that they are not as sweet as simple glucose and thus may decrease the palatability of orally consumed products. Finally, most commercially available enteral formulas are lactose free because some ethnic populations are lactose deficient and disaccharidase production within the gut lumen is reduced during illness or bowel rest.

FAT COMPOSITION

Fat is an important constituent in the diet because it provides a concentrated calorie source and serves as a carrier for fat-soluble vitamins. Sufficient linoleic acid is required to prevent essential fatty acid deficiency (EFAD), and should approximate 1–3% of total daily calories.[60] The most frequent sources of polymeric intact fat are vegetable oils (soy or corn) rich in polyunsaturated fatty acids. The digestion and absorption of LCTs are more complicated than those of either protein or carbohydrates. Fat digestion requires pancreatic enzyme release and formation of mixed bile salt micelles, which then facilitate absorption across the intestinal enterocyte as depicted in Fig. 134.1. The concentration of fat in enteral feeding formulas varies from less than 2–45% of total calories. The LCT fat sources have carbon chain lengths of 12 carbons. An alternative source of fat within enteral formulas is the MCTs, derived from palm kernel or coconut oils. MCTs are of 6–12 carbon lengths and have a caloric density between 8.2–8.4 kcal/g. MCTs do not contain the essential fats or linoleic acid. Therefore, most formulas contain some LCTs to provide essential fatty acids. Potential advantages of MCTs over LCTs are that they are more water soluble, they undergo rapid hydrolysis, and they require little to no pancreatic lipase or bile salt for absorption. They also do not require chylomicron formation for small bowel enterocyte absorption.

Recently, some manufacturers have changed the source of long-chain fat (from omega 6 to 3 fatty acids) within enteral formulas to reduce the amount of the resultant physiologic products (i.e., prostaglandins, thromboxanes, and leukotrienes).[57,59] The omega 6 fatty acids are high in linoleic acid and are derived from vegetable oil, whereas the omega 3 fatty acids, derived from coldwater fish oils, are high in linolenic acid. The eicosanoid products of the omega 6 fatty acids have been shown to be potent inflammatory mediators and also decrease cell-mediated immunity. Therefore, if the fat content delivered from omega 3 is increased, the patient should experience less inflammation and immunosuppression.

NUTRITIONALLY COMPLETE FORMULAS

Most commercially prepared formulas contain micronutrients, including electrolytes, vitamins, trace elements, and water, to make them nutritionally complete. Nutritionally complete commercial formulas provide the recommended daily allowances (RDAs) of micronutrients for a patient receiving a sufficient volume of formula to meet their daily energy and macronutrient needs. Such a predetermined nutrient complement, however, may not fit an individual's need because electrolyte, vitamin, and trace element requirements vary with disease state and organ function. One fairly common electrolyte abnormality occurring with enteral nutrition is hyponatremia.[61] Most formulas are made to mimic a low-salt diet, so hyponatremia could arise due to the limited sodium concentration. A low salt intake appears reasonable, because many patients who receive enteral nutrition are elderly and may have compromised cardiac function. However, patients who do not receive a sufficient volume of enteral formula to meet their RDA for micronutrients due to complications of fluid restriction or volume intolerance may require supplemental minerals and vitamins. Based on the adequate or high levels of vitamins in the blood of patients who have received long-term enteral therapy, the stability and absorption of vitamins which are contained in complete enteral formulas are felt to be adequate.[62] Patients who are fed enterally and have significant fat malabsorption may, over a long-term period, develop deficiencies of fat-soluble vitamins and therefore may need further supplementation of these vitamins. Most enteral feeding formulas contain the RDA of trace elements including iron, zinc, copper, and iodine, again based on receiving a sufficient volume of formula to meet the macronutrient needs of the patient. Selected enteral formulas also contain the RDA of selenium, molybdenum, and chromium. During deficiency states such as when diarrhea persists, supplementation of trace elements, namely, zinc, may be warranted.

FIBER CONTENT

Fiber, in the form of soy polysaccharide fiber, has been added to several enteral formulas in doses of 10–24 g of dietary fiber/L. Subsequent to bacterial degradation of fiber within the colon the end products of fiber ingestion are SCFAs. Potential benefits of fiber are the trophic effects on the large bowel mucosa as well as promotion of sodium and water absorption within the colon, as well as an energy source from the resultant SCFAs. Fiber also has the ability to regulate bowel function by moderating intestinal transit time in individuals with altered motility conditions. The experimental evidence and clinical implications of fiber-enhanced enteral nutrition among healthy volunteers and several patient populations has been recently reviewed.[63] These authors concluded that even though there is good experimental evidence that fiber may play an integral role in normal human nutrition, the results of clinical studies have been disappointing. Fiber supplementation may be beneficial in long-term tube feeding of constipated patients. In intensive care units, however, drugs and stress seem to be more powerful determinates of bowel function than the addition of fiber to formulas.

OSMOLALITY AND RENAL SOLUTE LOAD

In addition to the macro- and micronutrient content within enteral formulas, the physical characteristics of formulas are important to the successful use of enteral nutrition in a patient. Patient tolerance and response to enteral formulas can be affected by the osmolality and the renal solute load. The osmolality of a given enteral formula is a function of the size and quantity of ionic and molecular particles primarily related to the protein, carbohydrate, electrolyte, and mineral content within a given volume of formula. The unit of measure of osmolality is milliosmoles/kg (mOsm/kg). Enteral formulas with greater amounts of partially hydrolyzed or elemental substrates have a higher osmolality than formulas containing only polymeric or intact substrate forms. Therefore, formulas that contain sucrose or glucose, dipeptides and tripeptides, and amino acids are hyperosmolar. In general, enteral formulas range in osmolality from 300–900 mOsm/kg. Increased caloric density increases the hyperosmolar profile of an enteral formula. Symptoms of gastric retention, diarrhea, abdominal distention, nausea, and vomiting have been ascribed to the relative osmolality of the enteral feeding product. The results of clinical investigation to assess the relationship between osmolality and the incidence of GI side effects are conflicting.[64–66] Hospitalized patients administered hypotonic, isotonic, or hypertonic enteral formulas at a constant infusion rate demonstrated no significant differences in GI tolerance.[64] Other factors such as concurrent antibiotic therapy, which may alter the intestinal microflora; the method of delivery such as continuous versus bolus; and the appropriate selection of an enteral feeding formula for its composition play as much a role in the associated tolerance to the formula as the osmolality of the formula alone.[67]

The renal solute load is collectively made up of the protein, sodium, potassium, and chloride content of the enteral formula. Formulas that contain a greater solute load increase the obligatory water loss via the kidney. It is estimated that 40–60 mL of water is the minimal amount necessary to excrete 1 gram of nitrogen.[52] Those receiving high nitrogen enteral formulas, such as a geriatric patient or a patient with altered mental status unable to ingest more water, may be at risk for significant dehydration. Dehydration may be clinically detected as thirst, dry mucous membranes, depressed skin tugor, or an increased serum blood urea nitrogen or sodium level.

The rapid administration of hyperosmolar formulas reduces the gastric emptying rate.[52] Continuous administration into the stomach allows the pylorus to regulate the delivery of nutrient content into the duodenum and, hence, reduce gastric retention and associated symptoms of nausea and vomiting. When administering enteral formulas into the small bowel, products that are iso-osmolar can be initially administered at slow rates and advanced incrementally based on tolerance. Hyperosmolar formulas may require slower advancement to prevent the development of the dumping syndrome. As the lumen of the small bowel receives hypertonic enteral feedings, the small bowel secretes water to effectively dilute the formula and make it iso-osmotic, hence, contributing to the diarrhea and further fluid and electrolyte depletion.

SELECTING AN ENTERAL FORMULA

The selection of an appropriate enteral feeding formula requires knowledge of several patient characteristics. First, the patient's medical history should be obtained. The length of small bowel, nutrient digestibility, and functional capacity help determine the appropriate formula complexity (Table 134.7). In addition, the patient's underlying diseases, nutritional status, and fluid tolerance are required in order to determine nutritional goals. Knowledge of the feeding site will allow the selection of the appropriate delivery method of enteral feeding and reduce potential complications of therapy.

CHARACTERISTICS OF ENTERAL NUTRITION FORMULAS

The proliferation of new enteral nutrition products continues and it is easy to become overwhelmed with the variety of formulations available. Development of an enteral nutrition product formulary has been shown to be cost effective and to minimize confusion by identifying the rational use of prototype products.[68] Different criteria have been proposed to evaluate and categorize enteral nutrition products based on their unique characteristics.[25,57,58] The enteral formulas listed in Table 134.8 are categorized on the basis of the composition of the enteral formula with an emphasis on the general indication for product prototypes.

Polymeric Formulas

Polymeric solutions contain macronutrients in the form of intact protein, triglycerides, and carbohydrate polymers. They can be used orally or through a tube and provide complete nutrition.[58] An enteral formula is described as a "complete" product when it contains all of the micro- and macronutrients necessary to meet the RDAs for a patient. The majority of enteral products commercially available are lactose free, although there are enteral formulas available as oral supplements that do contain lactose. Frequently, the polymeric lactose-free tube feeding products are referred to as complete, "standard" enteral products. Describing enteral products as "standard" infers that these products require normal GI digestive and absorptive function for maintaining the nutritional status of a patient. Polymeric enteral feeding products are used in numerous settings including the critically ill, the noncritically ill, rehabilitation patients, and home enteral nutrition support patients. These polymeric enteral formulas or standard formulas are manufactured with variable caloric and protein densities ranging from 1–2 kcal/cc and 35–60 g/L protein, and have osmolalities ranging from 300–900 mOsm/kg. Products that are calorically concentrated generally have higher osmolalities. Fiber has also been supplemented in some of the standard formulas. The commercially available blenderized diets are made from natural whole foods. They are complete products with variable amounts of fiber and lactase. These products, due to the nature of their composition, may have a higher viscosity and generally require an infusion pump and access through a large-bore feeding tube for successful administration.

Monomeric Formulas

Monomeric enteral formulas have partially hydrolyzed and/or elemental components of protein, carbohydrate, and fat and, therefore, require less digestive and absorptive capacity. The major difference between polymeric and monomeric formulas is that monomeric formulas contain protein in small molecular forms. The chemically defined enteral formulas are those in which the protein is in the form of oligopeptides, dipeptides, and tripeptides. The elemental products are those that can generally contain L-amino acids as the protein source (Table 134.8). Carbohydrates are frequently in the form of oligosaccharides, sucrose, and glucose while fat sources are usually in the form of MCTs with small amounts of LCTs to provide essential fatty acid requirements. In general, the osmolality of monomeric products is higher, ranging from 500–700 mOsm/kg. The caloric density of monomeric formulas is generally 1.0 kcal/cc and they contain approximately 40–50 g protein/L. The intact protein of polymeric products must be digested to lower molecular weight peptides and/or free amino acids prior to absorption, whereas the monomeric enteral products, which already contain dipeptides and tripeptides, are more readily absorbed by the enterocyte.

The physiologic basis and clinical relevance for the use of monomeric enteral formulas in the clinical setting have been extensively reviewed.[34,58] The results from human and animal intestinal perfusion studies indicate that the partially hydrolyzed sources of protein have an absorptive advantage over those formulas that contain free amino acid. However, there are few controlled data on the nutritional efficacy of the protein hydrolysates or free amino acid formulations in humans. Even among pancreatectomized patients or those with severe short bowel, only slight differences in improved absorption have been shown to occur with the use of peptide-based diets. It has been hypothesized that the great reserve and adaptive capacity of the absorptive mucosa of the small bowel will still promote an adequate amount of nutrient absorption irrespective of the form of protein substrate delivered. Therefore, the relative indication for these products is currently controversial. Monomeric diets cannot be recommended for routine use in patients with normal GI function, those requiring early postoperative enteral feeding, or those with only mildly impaired pancreatic exocrine function, partial gastrectomy, and minor small intestinal resections. However, in pancreatectomized patients or those with markedly reduced GI surface area, the potential clinical benefit for the use of monomeric products warrants a therapeutic trial.[34,58] Monomeric prod-

TABLE 134.8. ENTERAL FORMULA CLASSIFICATION SYSTEM

Category	Subcategories	Indication	Features	Product Examples
Polymeric (normal GIT digestive and absorptive capacity required)	Lactose-free	Standard oral supplement Complete tube feeding	Iso-osmolar, high nitrogen, fiber enhanced, and highly concentrated formulas available	Osmolite Resource IsoSource VHN Ultracal Deliver 2.0
	Lactose-containing	Oral supplement Lactose tolerant	Palatable; hyperosmolar	Sustogen Meritene
	Blenderized	Complete tube feeding	May contain lactose, high viscosity and may require infusion pump	Complete modified
Monomeric (less digestion and absorption required)	Chemically defined	Complete tube feeding and some use as oral supplements Disease states that alter digestive or absorptive surface capacity	Nutrients hydrolyzed to varying degrees Osmolarity varies	Peptamen Reabilan HN
	Elemental	Complete tube feeding, rarely as an oral supplement Disease states that alter digestive or absorptive surface capacity Fat malabsorption	Free amino acids, >80% of kcal as oligosaccharides, <15% fat content as long-chain fat	Vivonex Plus Tolerex
Specialized (monomeric or polymeric)	Organ failure	Complete (±[a]) tube feeding, rarely as an oral supplement Specific products for pulmonary, renal, hepatic, and endocrine failure	Composition varies; nutrient requirements modified to a specific disorder	Pulmocare Travasorb Renal Nutrihep DiabetiSource
	Metabolic disorders	Complete (±) tube or oral feeding Management of inherited metabolic disorders such as tyrosinemia, phenylketonuria		Lofenalac Maxamaid XP
	Immune support	Complete tube feeding, rarely as an oral supplement Enhance immune competency during critical illness or sepsis	Specific nutrients modified for immunopharmacologic function	Immun-Aid Impact
Modular (majority are polymeric)	Protein Carbohydrate Fat	Generally feeding tube, can be used to compound complete (±) formulas or to supplement enteral or oral feeding	May be labor intensive Micronutrients available to make complete formulas	ProMod Polycose MCT oil
Hydration	Glucose Electrolytes	Feeding tube or oral Dehydration, severe or chronic diarrhea		Equalyte

[a]±: May or may not be complete nutrient composition.

ucts that have higher percentages of MCTs and small amounts of LCTs are generally recommended for patients with severe pancreatic insufficiency such as chronic pancreatitis and cystic fibrosis or severe abnormalities of the intestinal mucosa such as untreated celiac disease or extensive small bowel resection.[34]

Disease State-Specific Formulas

A third descriptive category of enteral feeding formulas is the specialized formulas based on specific metabolic needs such as organ failure, inborn errors of metabolism, and immune dysfunction. These specialized enteral formulas vary in their nutrient complexity composition (Table 134.8). Specific nutrient concerns during organ failure are discussed in Chapter 136, Nutritional Considerations in Major Organ Failure. The specialized enteral formulas that have been formulated to enhance immune competency during critical illness or sepsis provide substrates in pharmacologic doses which have experimentally been shown to enhance immune function.[59,69] These products contain more arginine and ribonucleic acids and an increased proportion of omega 3 polyunsaturated fatty acids. Glutamine has also been supplemented in some of these formulas to promote intestinal mucosal integrity and reduce infectious complications. A recent prospective, randomized, double-blind multicenter clinical trial compared an immune enhanced enteral product to a polymeric enteral product among patients in intensive care units after an event such as trauma, surgery, or sepsis.[70] Extensive statistical analysis of the aggregate data revealed that within a highly stratified subgroup of 37 septic patients, the intervention group had a decreased median length of hospital stay by 10 days (28 versus 18 days) and fewer infectious complications. Immune enhanced products have also been studied among 85 patients who had major operations for cancer.[71] The length of hospital stay for the specialty formula group was reduced (15.8 ± 5.1 versus 20.2 ± 9.4 days), and favorable results from the *in vitro* tests of immune function were demonstrated. The nitrogen intake between the experimental and control populations in both of these studies was not controlled, and it is possible that the endpoints may have been affected by the nitrogen disparity between the groups. These study results also do not address which nutrient(s) may have contributed to the improvement in clinical outcome.

Modular Formulas

A fourth category of enteral products is the modular nutrient components. Occasionally it is desirable or necessary to achieve a nutrient mix not supplied by a single commercially available product. Therefore, a single nutrient component such as carbohydrate, protein, and fat can be added to readily available solutions to enhance the specific substrate content. Protein modules may be singularly added to ready-made formulas when a higher nitrogen content is desired. These modules are marketed in powder form and may contain free amino acids, caseinates, or whole protein such as egg whites, solids, or whey. The module's nutrient complexity added to a commercial formula should be based on a patient's digestive capacity. Caloric enhancement of ready-made formulas may also be done by adding carbohydrate modules. Carbohydrate products such as glucose polymers are available in either solid or liquid forms and their caloric content varies.

Hydration Formulas

The last descriptive category of enteral products is hydration formulas. Oral rehydration formulas may be used in dehydrated patients to reduce diarrheal sequelae or replenish ostomy drainage fluid and electrolyte losses. Such formulas do not require intravenous access, are economical, and can be either purchased commercially or extemporaneously compounded. These formulas have been successfully used to manage mild to moderate dehydration in both children and adults. The oral rehydration solution is successful because of its glucose content. Glucose stimulates active transport systems, which in turn stimulate passive sodium and water uptake simultaneously with the glucose. Therefore, oral administration of several liters may actually decrease fecal water loss and generate a positive electrolyte balance.

FORMULARY AND DELIVERY SYSTEM CONSIDERATIONS

A practical issue that affects the enteral product selected for use in a patient is the product formulary of an institution. Obviously the selection of product should be based on the patient characteristics and the product features as previously discussed. However, such administrative concerns as cost, shelf life, ordering policies, product form, administration systems, and contract opportunities are frequently taken into account when an institution develops an enteral formulary. The majority of enteral products are available as ready-to-use, prepackaged liquids, whereas others are in a dehydrated, powdered state and require reconstitution prior to use. Advantages of ready-to-use liquid formulas are convenience and low susceptibility to microbiologic contamination. One of the disadvantages is that more storage space is required. The ease or convenience of packaging is especially important for patients involved in self-care, the disabled, and those who have difficulty receiving or following printed instructions.

Another practical issue that affects an institution's choice of an enteral delivery system is the potential complication of bacterial contamination. Both animal and human studies have demonstrated that contaminated enteral feeding formulas have been directly associated with infectious complications.[72–74] The GI tract may serve as a port of entry for bacteria into the systemic circulation, especially in patients who are receiving multiple antibiotics or who have undergone a surgical procedure. The contamination of enteral feeding formulas has been associated with the lack of attention to proper handling techniques, inability to disinfect preparation equipment, and nonsterile or contaminating tube feeding additives. Controversy exists as to how stringent handling procedures must be in order to ensure that the enteral feeding is safe for administration.[75] Nonetheless, controlling bacterial populations found in enteral feedings is warranted. Sterile enteral diets have been available in the form of the closed-administration systems, which are prefilled containers in volumes of 1–1.5 liters of ready-to-feed enteral formula. This is in contrast to the more conventional open systems, which require cans or mixed powders to be decanted into larger volume delivery bags by institution personnel. The closed-administration system offers the advantage of requiring no mixing of formula and therefore lowers the risk of contamination and reduces time and labor required in preparing the formula.[76] Numerous types of enteral formulas are now available in the closed-administration system. The closed-administration system also offers the advantage of allowing hang times beyond 24–36 hours, whereas the conventional delivery system had hang times of generally 6–12 hours. A disadvantage of the closed-administration system is the inability to add minerals or color additives without breaking the closed system.[57]

Initiating an Enteral Nutrition Regimen

Subsequent to selecting the appropriate enteral access and feeding formula, the rate and strength of formula advancement must be determined. Schedules for progression of tube feeding delivery from initial to target rates are important and influence the maximum rate the patient can tolerate.[44] Frequently in the institutional setting, feeding into either the stomach or small bowel is begun with an infusion pump for slow continuous feeding. Although the advancement of enteral feeding should be individualized to specific patient issues, one may start half-strength dilution of the formula and administer it at a rate of 25–50 cc/h, regardless of the actual formula employed. This practice is used to prevent GI complications of enteral feeding such as diarrhea, abdominal cramping, bloating, and nausea. The rate is increased in 25 cc/h increments every 6–8 hours to a maximal rate with subsequent increase of the formula strength in the next day(s).[44] Such a progression should take no more than 3 days before the patient is at target feeding goals. However, many patients will tolerate more rapid advancement of a full-strength feeding formula from a rate of 20–25 cc/h with increments of 20–25 cc/h every 6–8 hours until the desired goal is achieved.

Drug Compatibility with Enteral Formulas

Mixing of commercially available liquid medications with selected enteral nutrition products has been associated with several types of physical incompatibilities: granulation, gel formation, separation, and precipitation.[77,78] Not only can these physical incompatibilities inhibit the drug absorption within the small bowel of a patient, gel formation may potentially clog small-bore enteral feeding tubes. Physical incompatibility with medications is more common in formulas that contain intact protein than those with hydrolyzed protein. Also medication and enteral formula incompatibilities are more common with the use of acidic pharmaceutical syrups. Liquid medications have osmolalities that range from 500–5000 mOsm/kg.[79] Subsequent admixture of liquid medications into enteral formulas can thus greatly enhance the final osmolality and result in the development of diarrhea. The most prudent recommendation for the mixing of commercial liquid medications and enteral nutrition formulas is to avoid the routine admixture whenever possible, especially the nonaqueous preparations and syrups. In the clinical setting, exceptions do exist, such as adding electrolyte injections of potassium or sodium to enteral formulas to assist in maintaining or repleting the electrolyte requirements for a patient.

Complications of Concomitant Drug Administration

Enteral feeding tubes are frequently used as a route for the delivery of medications. However, the pharmacologic agent and its mode of delivery are modified when a feeding tube is placed. Concomitant administration of medications with enteral feedings delivered directly into the stomach through nasogastric or gastrostomy tubes allows the stomach to function in its normal capacity for drug dissolution. However, placement of enteral tubes beyond the pylorus, such as with nasoduodenal, nasojejunal, and jejunostomy, alters drug dissolution because the stomach is bypassed. Therefore one must consider the anatomic location of the feeding tube tip when administering medications such as antacids or sucralfate, because their therapeutic effect is designed to occur within the stomach. Because many drugs are best absorbed in the fasted state, medications should be administered on an empty stomach as much as possible. Patients receiving bolus intragastric feedings may receive medications appropriately spaced between the feedings.[80,81] For those patients receiving continuous enteral feeding, the feedings may require interruption for drug administration, followed by prudent flushing of the tube with water. Pharmacists need to be aware of potential problems which may arise when medications are administered through enteral feeding tubes such as the degradation and/or inactivation of nutrient components or altered bioavailability of a drug that may compromise therapeutic efficacy[82–84] (Table 134.9).

Selecting the proper medication dosage form for administration by enteral feeding tubes is crucial to avoid drug inactivation and altered bioavailability (Table 134.10). Medications in sublingual form, sustained-released capsules or tablets, and enteric-coated tablets are designed not to be crushed and therefore should not be administered via enteral feeding tubes. An extensive list of oral dosage forms that should not be crushed is available in the literature.[85] For the most part, liquid drug preparations are the preferred dosage form when administering medications via enteral feeding tubes. In situations where a liquid medication is unavailable, compressed tablets or the contents of hard or soft gelatin capsules can be admixed with water and admin-

TABLE 134.9. GENERAL CONSIDERATIONS FOR MEDICATION ADMINISTRATION BY ENTERAL FEEDING TUBES

1. Administer medications by mouth when feasible; consider enteral feeding tube as an alternative route.
2. Determine location of the feeding tube tip, because pre- or postpyloric drug instillation can alter effectiveness.
3. Liquid dosage forms should be used if available. Dosage and frequency adjustment are required if changing from a sustained-release drug to administer a non-sustained-release liquid form.
4. Hyperosmolar medications require dilution.
5. The contents of hard or soft gelatin capsules reconstituted with 10–15 mL of water and crushed compressed tablets reconstituted with 15–30 mL of water can be administered when a liquid form is unavailable.
6. Do not crush and administer sustained-release or enteric-coated medications.
7. Flush the feeding tube with water prior to administering a medication. Do not mix medications. Administer each medication separately, flushing with water between medications. Flush with water after medication administration completed.
8. In general, do not add medications to the enteral formula. Exceptions exist for the adding of hypertonic electrolyte injection to enteral formulas. Be aware of specific drug–enteral product incompatibilities.

istered down enteral feeding tubes. Adherence to proper technique for administering the contents of tablets or capsules down feeding tubes such as flushing of the tube with water prior to and following the administration of medication is important to prevent clogging of the feeding tube.

DRUG–NUTRIENT INTERACTIONS

The most significant drug and nutrient interactions that can occur during continuous enteral nutrition are those in which the bioavailability of the drug is reduced and the desired pharmacologic effect is not achieved. Unfortunately, limited clinical studies are available to document the extent of this problem with enteral feeding. Most of the observations are anecdotal case reports among few patients. A reduction in bioavailability of phenytoin has been demonstrated during continuous tube feeding, with subsequent subtherapeutic drug levels.[86] The exact cause for reduced phenytoin bioavailability during continuous enteral feeding is unclear; however, the results of *in vitro* studies suggest that protein and calcium chloride may bind the drug. A variety of methods to minimize this interaction for patients receiving continuous tube feedings have been suggested (Table 134.11). Little consensus exists as to the best method to prevent or reduce the impact of this interaction. Pharmacists must be aware that patients may require higher than normal doses of phenytoin while on enteral nutrition. The patient's clinical response and serum phenytoin levels should be closely monitored during continuous enteral feeding and after the discontinuation of enteral feeds.

Clinical studies documenting altered bioavailability with antibiotics during continuous enteral feeding are lacking. However, based on case reports and theoretical concerns, holding the tube feeding for 30 minutes before and 30 minutes after a selected antibiotic is administered is recommended (Table 134.11). Warfarin resistance has also been documented during enteral feeding due to the vitamin

TABLE 134.10. GUIDELINES FOR MEDICATION ADMINISTRATION BY ENTERAL FEEDING TUBES

Dosage Form	Administered by Enteral Feeding Tube	Comment
Sublingual or buccal tablets	No	Low dosage of drug not designed for gastric or intestinal administration Altered drug bioavailability and potency due to first-pass effect
Sustained-release capsules or tablets	Not preferred Do not crush	Crushing a sustained release dosage from destroys its time-release effect Altered therapeutic drug response and gastrointestinal irritation can occur
Enteric-coated tablets	Not preferred Do not crush	Crushing can result in gastrointestinal irritation and drug inactivation
Compressed tablets (sugar or film coated)	Yes	May be crushed and administered without altering therapeutic drug response May clog small-bore feeding tubes
Hard or soft gelatin capsules	Yes	Powders from hard capsules and oils from soft capsules may be administered without altering therapeutic drug response
Liquid preparations Solutions Suspensions Elixirs Emulsions	Yes Preferred	Frequently recommended, however, drug form can be hyperosmolar requiring dilution Strong acid syrups may interact with enteral formulas and clog tubes

TABLE 134.11. MEDICATIONS WITH SPECIAL CONSIDERATIONS FOR ENTERAL FEEDING TUBE ADMINISTRATION

Drug	Interaction	Comments
Phenytoin	Reduced bioavailability demonstrated when administered during continuous tube feeding. Results of *in vitro* studies suggest that protein (caseinate salts) and calcium chloride may reduce phenytoin bioavailability.[87]	Limited data from clinical studies and case reports provide basis for suggestions to overcome incompatibility. Suggestions include holding tube feeding 2 h before and after phenytoin[86]; administering phenytoin capsules rather than the suspension during continuous feeding[88]; and using a meat-based enteral formula rather than a protein hydrolysate containing formula.[89] Monitor patient's clinical response and serum drug level closely.
Antibiotics (selected)	Reduce bioavailability demonstrated between food and penicillin, tetracycline, isoniazid, rifampin, enoxacin, norfloxacin, and ofloxacin.[90] Interaction also theoretically applied to continuous tube feeding.	Existence of clinical studies documenting enteral formula interaction with selected antibiotics is lacking. Holding tube feeding administration for specified time periods before and after drug administration has been recommended.[91] Monitor patients clinical response closely.
Warfarin	Pharmacologic interaction demonstrated between warfarin and the vitamin K contained in enteral feeding formulas, resulting in reduced anticoagulation effect.	Vitamin K is contained in most enteral products in doses less than 200 μg per 1000 kcal. Adjust warfarin dose based on monitoring the INR and observing the vitamin K content of the enteral formula.
Antacids	Altered pharmacologic effect of antacid if administered into the small bowel. A physical incompatibility has been reported with aluminum-containing antacids causing an esophageal plug formation.	Administer antacids only into feeding tubes with the tip placed in the stomach. Administering aluminum-containing antacids after holding the tube feeding formula may prevent physical incompatibility formation.[92]

K content contained within the enteral feeding products. Prior to 1980, it was thought that the content of vitamin K in dosages of up to 1330 μg/1000 kcal of enteral feeding formula was contributing to the pharmacologic interaction with warfarin. Subsequently, the vitamin K content within formulas has been reformulated to less than 200 μg/1000 kcal. However, warfarin resistance has continued to be reported. Pharmacists should be observant of the vitamin K content within enteral formulas and adjust the warfarin dose based on the monitoring of the patient's coagulation parameters.

Complications and Monitoring of Enteral Nutrition

A major advantage of enteral nutrition over that of parenteral nutrition is a reduced complication rate.[67] Major complications and potential causes for metabolic, GI, technical, and infectious complications associated with enteral tube feeding are listed in Table 134.12. Several of the factors responsible for the metabolic complications seen among enteral nutrition patients are similar to those seen during parenteral nutrition. However, the GI, technical, and infectious complications seen during enteral nutrition are unique to this route of therapy.

METABOLIC COMPLICATIONS

The metabolic complications related to hydration and electrolyte and glucose control are more frequently observed in patients with underlying illnesses that cause organ dysfunction. The micronutrient and water content within enteral feeding formulas are in fixed amounts (RDAs) intended for the average patient. Therefore, the frequency of clinical and laboratory assessment to adequately monitor hydration, electrolyte, organ function, and glucose control for a patient who is critically ill is greater than for a stable patient residing in a rehabilitation unit or at home (Table 134.13). It is important to evaluate the actual content of water and micronutrients provided by the enteral formula for a patient at high risk for metabolic complications such as the critically ill. Additional hydration and electrolytes may need to be provided for patients being inadequately supported with an enteral formula. Conversely, for patients who have excessive fluid retention or increased serum electrolytes, the enteral formula may need to be changed to one that is more concentrated or provide less of a particular nutrient(s).

TABLE 134.12. COMPLICATIONS OF TUBE FEEDING

Complications	Causes
Metabolic	
Dehydration	Insufficient fluid intake
	Excessive fluid losses
	Overusage of diuretics
Hyperglycemia	Underlying disease response
	Diabetes mellitus
	Infection
	Metabolic stress
	Drug induced (corticosteroids)
	Overfeeding
Increased serum electrolytes	Organ dysfunction
	Hepatic
	Renal
	Cardiac
	Dehydration
	Excess intake (antacids)
Decreased serum electrolytes	Fluid overload due to excessive intake or organ dysfunction (hepatic, renal, cardiac)
	Drug induced (cisplatin, amphotericin B, diuretics)
	Extraordinary fluid losses (diarrheal, nasogastric)
	Refeeding syndrome
Decreased trace elements	Extraordinary fluid losses (diarrheal)
	Drug induced (diuretics)
Gastrointestinal	
Diarrhea	Drug related
	Antibiotic-induced bacterial overgrowth
	Hyperosmolar medications administered via feeding tubes
	Antacids containing magnesium
	Malabsorption
	Hypoalbuminemia/gut mucosal atrophy
	Pancreatic insufficiency
	Inadequate GIT surface area
	Rapid GIT transit
	Radiation enteritis
	Tube feeding related
	Rapid formula administration
	Formula hyperosmolality
	Low-residue (fiber) content
	Lactose intolerance
	Bacterial contamination
Nausea and vomiting	Gastric dysmotility (surgery, anticholinergic drugs, diabetic gastroparesis)
	Rapid infusion of hyperosmolar formula
Constipation	Dehydration
	Drug induced (anticholinergics)
	Inactivity
	Low residue (fiber) content
	Obstruction/fecal impaction
Abdominal distention/cramping	Too rapid formula administration
Technical	
Occluded feeding tube lumen	Insoluble complexation of enteral formula and medication(s)
	Inadequate flushing of feeding tube
	Undissolved feeding formula
Tube displacement	Self extubation
	Vomiting or coughing
	Inadequate fixation (jejunostomy)
Nasolabial, nasopharyngeal, or esophageal irritation	Prolonged local pressure of large-bore polyvinylchloride tube
Aspiration	Improper patient position
	Gastroparesis/atony causing regurgitation
	Feeding tube malpositioned
	Compromised lower esophageal sphincter
	Diminished gag reflex
Peristomal excoriation	Improper skin and tube care
	GIT secretions leaking peristomally
Infectious	
Aspiration pneumonia	Same as technical-aspiration comments
Acute otitis media or sinusitis	Prolonged use of large-bore polyvinylchloride tube
Microbial contamination of enteral formula and delivery system	Improper preparation, storage, or administration

TABLE 134.13. SUGGESTED MONITORING OF ENTERAL NUTRITION (EN) TO PREVENT COMPLICATIONS

Parameter	During Initiation of EN or for a Critically Ill Patient	During Stable EN Therapy or for a Rehabilitating Patient	During Long-Term Home EN Therapy
Vital signs Temperature respirations, pulse, blood pressure	Every 4–6 h	Every 12–24 h	Tailored to patient's clinical state, routinely done once or twice weekly
Physical exam[a] Abdomen, lung fields, extremities, mucous membranes, skin turgor	Every 4–6 h	Every 12–24 h	Tailored to patient's clinical state, routinely done once or twice weekly
Clinical assessment Weight Total intake/output Urine, gastrointestinal and extraordinary fluid losses Stool frequency/consistency/volume Nausea or vomiting	Daily	Daily	Tailored to patient's clinical state, routinely done once or twice weekly
Concurrent medications and administration route	Daily	Daily	Tailored to patient's clinical state, routinely done once or twice weekly
Verification of nasal or oral tube placement with x-ray	Done prior to initiating EN	N/A[b]	N/A
Ongoing assessment by tube placement	Every 6 h	Every 12 h	Tailored to patient's clinical state, routinely done once or twice weekly
Gastric residual checks	Every 8–12 h	Every 8–12 h	Daily by patient and/or caregiver
Enterostomy tube site assessment for leakage and/or skin irritation/redness	Daily	Daily	Daily by patient and/or caregiver
Patient compliance with feeding procedures and feeding tube/ostomy care	N/A	Daily	Tailored to patient's clinical state, routinely done once or twice weekly
Serum electrolytes, BUN/Cr, serum glucose[c]	Daily	2–3 times/wk	Tailored to patient's clinical state, routinely done weekly
Serum calcium, magnesium, and phosphorus	4–5 times/wk	2–3 times/wk	Tailored to patient's clinical state, routinely done weekly
Liver function tests	Weekly	Monthly	Tailored to patient's clinical state, routinely done monthly
Urine glucose/acetone[c]	Every 6 h	Daily	Tailored to patient's clinical state, routinely done 2–3 times/wk
Trace elements, vitamins	Frequency tailored to patient-specific situations	Frequency tailored to patient-specific situations	Frequency tailored to patient-specific situations

[a]Includes eyes, ear, nose, and throat exam for patients with nasoenteric feeding tubes.
[b]Not applicable.
[c]Frequency of glucose assessment for the nondiabetic patient.

GI COMPLICATIONS

The GI complications associated with tube feeding include diarrhea, nausea and vomiting, constipation, abdominal distention, and cramping. In general, these GI side effects can be attributed to either drug-related, patient-related, or tube feeding-related factors. Diarrhea has been reported to occur in 2.3–30.6% of enterally fed patients.[67] It is speculated that the wide variability in incidence is due, in part, to the multiplicity of clinical definitions for diarrhea. Monitoring of the patient for diarrhea includes evaluating stool frequency, consistency, and volume (Table 134.13) and taking into consideration the patient's previous bowel habits and underlying disease state.[93] Drug-related causes of diarrhea include the administration of hyperosmolar medications or elixirs which contain high concentrations of sorbitol. Infectious causes, such as antibiotic-induced bacterial overgrowth by *Clostridium difficile* need to be considered when diarrhea develops. Diarrhea may also occur as a result of malabsorption, due to such circumstances as severe malnutrition and related gut mucosal atrophy, exocrine failure such as chronic pancreatitis or cystic fibrosis, inadequate surface area or too rapid transit through the small bowel due to radiation enteritis, short bowel syndrome, or celiac disease. During such clinical circumstances, a continuous infusion of chemically defined feeding formula may help improve the symptoms of malabsorption. Of the tube feeding-related factors which may contribute to diarrhea (Table 134.12), the rate of infusion is a primary factor. Even hyperosmolar solutions can be infused without diarrhea or abdominal distention if the feeding is infused at a constant rate and incrementally titrated according to the tolerance of the patient.[67,93]

Occasionally pharmacologic intervention is indicated to control severe diarrhea. The primary agents employed are opiates, diphenoxylate, and loperamide.[94] Diphenoxylate acts by the same mechanism as the opioids, by decreasing GI motility and secretions. These actions decrease the amount of fluid to be reabsorbed in the small intestine and colon and increase the transit time to allow more absorption of exogenous fluids. Loperamide decreases GI motility and decreases small bowel output via the ileum. It is two to three times as potent as diphenoxylate and thus may be administered less frequently. Use of these agents should be limited, because overuse may produce constipation and paralytic ileus.

Nausea and vomiting in a patient receiving nasogastric tube feeding may be due to gastric atony subsequent to recent surgery, anticholinergic side effect of drugs, and/or an underlying disease such as diabetic gastroparesis. Advancement of the feeding tube beyond the pylorus may reduce the associated symptoms of nausea and vomiting and enable successful enteral feeding. Constipation may also occur with tube feeding, particularly in the elderly and the long-term enteral nutrition patient. Multiple causes may contribute to the constipation (Table 134.12). Using enteral formulas with enhanced fiber may improve the symptoms of constipation; however, the exact amount as well as the optional source of fiber is yet to be established.[63,95]

TECHNICAL COMPLICATIONS

The technical complications of enteral nutrition are frequently associated with the feeding tube. Occluded feeding tubes have been reported to occur in 10% of patients.[67] It is a common cause for feeding tube replacement and increases the cost of enteral feeding. Different techniques for clearing obstructed tubes have included instillation of water, meat tenderizer, pancreatic enzymes,[44] and passing of an endoscopic cytology brush.[67] Adherence to appropriate flushing protocols of the feeding tube during continuous tube feeding and medication administration is an extremely important variable in prevention of occluded feeding tubes (Table 134.9). Inadvertent tube displacement has been reported to occur in >50% of patients receiving enteral tube feeding.[67] Securing the tube and ongoing assessment of its appropriate placement may prevent tube displacement.

ASPIRATION OF GASTRIC CONTENTS

Bronchopulmonary aspiration of gastric contents is a potentially fatal complication of tube feeding. Patients who are mechanically ventilated or those with swallowing disorders are at higher risk for this complication. The incidence has been reported to be as high as 46%.[67] The use of small-bore feeding tubes preserves the lower esophogeal sphincter and, hence, patients are less prone to develop reflux in the esophagus with potential for aspiration. Aspiration can be further minimized by not allowing a large volume to accumulate in the stomach. The amount of liquid residing in the stomach is called the gastric residual. After holding the tube feeding for at least 30 minutes, gastric residuals can be checked by attaching a syringe to the open end of the tube and filling it with the liquid. In adults, the residuals should be less than 200 mL.[96] Small tubes often collapse easily when back pressure is applied, making it difficult to measure residuals. Additionally, the risk of aspiration can be reduced by keeping the patient's head of the bed at 30–45° during feeding and for 30–60 minutes after intermittent infusion. This makes it more difficult for fluid to migrate up the esophagus against gravity. Lastly, the aspiration risk may be decreased by infusing the feedings into the small intestine instead of the stomach. The passage of a small-bore feeding tube into the tracheobronchial passage with subsequent infusion of an enteral diet can also be fatal. Obviously patients with a diminished gag reflex are at risk for this complication. The small-bore tubes may not trigger the gag reflex, which indicates proper placement, therefore the tube position should always be verified with an x-ray to reduce the chance of infusion into the lung. Alleviation or prevention of bronchopulmonary aspiration involves meticulous tube insertion and tube maintenance. Other infectious complications besides bronchopulmonary aspiration, however less frequent, are acute otitis media or sinusitis. This complication has been associated with long-term use of polyvinylchloride tubes.[43]

THERAPEUTIC NUTRITION AND DISEASE OUTCOMES

Nutrition outcome goals of enteral tube feeding are to reverse protein calorie malnutrition, promote growth and development of infants and children, or maintain an adequate nutritional state. Assessing the outcome of enteral nutrition includes monitoring objective measures of body composition, protein and energy balance as well as subjective outcome for physiologic muscle function and wound

TABLE 134.14. SUGGESTED MONITORING OF ENTERAL NUTRITION (EN) TO PROMOTE NUTRITIONAL EFFICACY

Parameter	During Initiation of EN or for a Critically Ill Patient	During Stable EN Therapy or for a Rehabilitating Patient	During Long-Term Home EN Therapy
Anthropometrics			
Weight	Daily	Weekly	Weekly
Triceps skinfold	N/A[a]	N/A	Every 1–2 months
Midarm muscle circumference	N/A	N/A	Every 1–2 months
Muscle function			
Level of physical endurance	N/A	Weekly	Weekly to monthly, then frequency tailored to the patient situation
Metabolic			
Albumin	Monthly	Monthly	Monthly, then frequency tailored to the patient response
Transferrin	Weekly	Weekly	Once to twice monthly, then frequency tailored to the patient response
24-h urine urea nitrogen	Weekly	Once or twice monthly	Frequency tailored to patient-specific situations
Indirect calorimetry	Frequency tailored to patient-specific situations	Frequency tailored to patient-specific situations	Frequency tailored to patient-specific situations
Nutritional intake			
Calories	Daily	2–3 times weekly	Weekly, then frequency tailored to the patient situation
Protein, fluid, electrolytes, trace elements, vitamins	Daily	2–3 times weekly	Weekly, then frequency tailored to the patient situation
Skin integrity	Daily	Daily	Weekly
Wound healing			
Pressure sore(s)			

[a]Not applicable.

healing (Table 134.14). These nutritional outcome indices have improved with enteral feedings among critically ill,[31] rehabilitation,[97] and long-term home enteral patients.[98] Besides an improvement in nutrition outcome, another goal of enteral nutrition is to reduce disease-related morbidity and mortality (Fig. 134.3).[51] Measures of disease-related morbidity include the length of hospital stay, infectious complications, and the patient's sense of well-being. Such clinical outcome goals are extremely difficult to document with the use of enteral nutrition, in part, because other factors such as age, underlying comorbidities, extent of injury, immunocompetence, and end-organ complications affect disease outcome.

Only a few prospective randomized controlled trials have demonstrated a change in disease outcome with the use of enteral nutrition. However, the results of clinical investigations of enteral nutrition in specific diseases such as Crohn's and acute alcoholic liver disease suggest an improvement in some indices of clinical outcome. Historically, TPN and bowel rest were prescribed for patients with an active flare of their Crohn's disease. However, clinical investigation has established that for most patients with disease flare, bowel rest is not necessary to induce a clinical remission.[99] Short courses of nutrition support in hospitalized patients often demonstrate remission rates of 60% and 80% with either TPN or defined enteral diets. Polymeric and partially hydrolyzed formulas appear to be equivalent to the elemental formulas in clinical efficacy.[36,100] The results of a randomized controlled clinical trial involving the effectiveness of tube feeding supplementation during acute alcoholic liver disease demonstrated an improvement

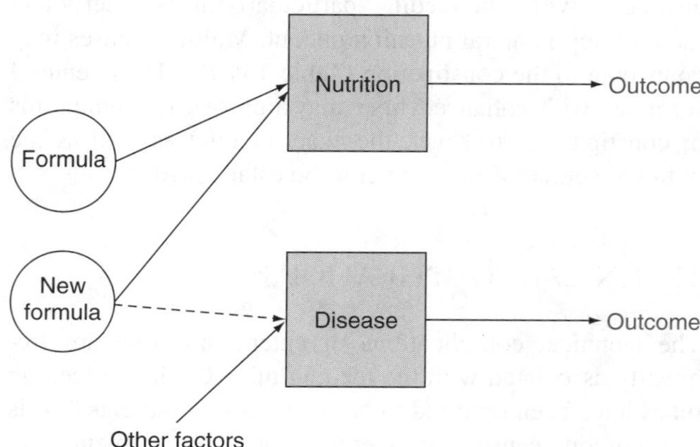

Figure 134.3. Goals of enteral nutrition support are to effect favorable nutritional and disease-related outcomes. Specialized (new) formulas with nutrient enhancements purported to have direct effects on disease outcomes are under investigation. The independent effects of new formulations on disease outcome may be diminished because of other factors, thus the complexity and cost of quality study designs will be increased. *(Reprinted from Heymsfield SB. Enteral solutions: Is there a solution? NCP 1995; 10(1):4–7, with permission.)*

in nutritional parameters as well as significantly faster improvement in encephalopathy, serum bilirubin levels, and antipyrine clearance.[101]

The use of enteral nutrition over that of TPN has been evaluated for its effectiveness in reducing morbidity and mortality in critically ill patients. Heyland and colleagues[26] evaluated the role of enteral nutrition, particularly early enteral nutrition, on morbidity and mortality in critically ill patients. Of the eight randomized nonblinded clinical trials, three studies used objective criteria to define infectious outcomes. Although no differences were seen in the incidence of multiple organ failure syndrome or mortality in the enteral versus the parenteral group,[102] patients who received enteral nutrition had a 17% sepsis rate, which included a 3% rate of major septic complications, compared to the parenteral group, which had a septic complication rate of 37% and a 20% rate of major septic complications.[31] In the third study, the septic complication rate was 15.7% in the enteral nutrition group compared to 40% in the parenteral group.[103] The enteral and parenteral study groups were comparable with respect to age, injury type, and their severity of illness scores.[31,103] Based on the results of the aforementioned studies and others reviewed, Heyland and colleagues conclude that sufficient data exist to suggest that critically ill patients benefit from early enteral nutrition and that enteral nutrition should be commenced as early as possible in the course of a patient's illness. Even if enteral nutrition may not meet all of the nutrient goals immediately, the role of tube feeding should be as a stimulant to the patient's GI immunologic function and mucosal integrity. Enteral nutrition may thus result in reduction of infectious complications in the critically ill patient. No prospective randomized controlled studies evaluating enteral nutrition in the critically ill have resulted in reduced mortality. Further clinical investigations are needed to establish the effect of specific nutrients on length of hospital stay and infectious complications. New enteral formulas with altered nutrient composition which include different enhancements of hydrolyzed protein sources (dipeptides, tripeptides), ribonucleic acid, increased omega 3 fatty acids, arginine and glutamine may improve disease-related morbidity. Further prospective randomized clinical trials are warranted to assess the benefits and safety of these costly specialized formulas, in order to determine what components are most beneficial in reducing morbidity within specific disease states.

REFERENCES

1. Cashman MD. Principles of digestive physiology for clinical nutrition. Nutr Clin Prac 1986;1(5):241–249.
2. Caspary WF. Physiology and pathophysiology of intestinal absorption. Am J Clin Nutr 1992;55:299S–308S.
3. O'Dwyer ST, Smith RJ, Kripke SA, et al. New fuels for the gut, in Rombeau JL, Caldwell MD (eds): Clinical Nutrition: Enteral and Tube Feeding, 2nd ed. Philadelphia, WB Saunders, 1990, p 548.
4. Record KE, Kolpek JH, Rapp RP. Long chain versus medium chain length triglycerides, a review of metabolism and clinical use. Nutr Clin Prac 1986;1:279–287.
5. Mainous MR, Block EFJ, Dietch EA. Nutritional support of the gut: How and why. New Horizons 1994;2:193–201.
6. Langkamp-Henken B, Glezer JA, Kudsk KA. Immunologic structure and function of the gastrointestinal tract. Nutr Clin Prac 1992;7:100–114.
7. Gleeson MH, Dowling RH, Peters TJ. Biochemical changes in intestinal mucosa after experimental small bowel by-pass in the rat. Clin Sci 1972;43:743–757.
8. Levine GM, Deren JJ, Steiger E, et al. Role of oral intake in maintenance of gut mass and disaccharide activity. Gastroenterology 1974;67:975–982.
9. Thompson JS, Vaughan WP, Forst CF, et al. The effect of route on nutrient delivery on gut structure and diamine oxidase levels. J Parenter Enter Nutr 1987;11:28–32.
10. Greene HL, McCabe DR, Merenstein GB. Protracted diarrhea and malnutrition in infancy: Changes in intestinal morphology and disaccharidase activities during treatment with total intravenous nutrition or oral elemental diets. J Pediatr 1975;87:695–704.
11. Morin CL, Ling V, Bourassa D. Small intestine and colonic changes induced by a chemically defined diet. Dig Dis Sci 1980;25:123–128.
12. Young EA, Cioletti LA, Winborn WB, et al. Comparative study of nutritional adaptation to defined formula diets in rats. Am J Clin Nutr 1980;33:2106–2118.
13. Johnson LR, Copeland EM, Dudrick SJ, et al. Structural and hormonal alterations in the gastrointestinal tract of parenterally fed rats. Gastroenterology 1975;68:1177–1183.
14. Sagor GR, Ghatei MA, Al-Mukhtar MYT, et al. Evidence for a humoral mechanism after small intestinal resection. Gastroenterology 1983;84:902–906.
15. Lickley HLA, Track NS, Vranic M, Bury KD. Metabolic responses to enteral and parenteral nutrition. Am J Surgery 1978;135:172–176.
16. Adibi SA. Leucine absorption rate and net movements of sodium and water in human jejunum. J Appl Phys 1970; 28:753–757.
17. Souba WW, Scott TE, Wilmore DW. Intestinal consumption of intravenously administered fuels. J Parenter Enter Nutr 1985;9:18–22.
18. Souba WW, Wilmore DW. Postoperative alteration of arteriovenous exchange of amino acids across the gastrointestinal tract. Surgery 1983;94:342–350.
19. Alverdy J, Chi HS, Sheldon G. The effect of parenteral nutrition on gastrointestinal immunity: The importance of enteral immunity. Ann Surg 1985;202:681–684.
20. Alverdy JC, Aoys E, Moss GS. TPN promotes bacterial translocation from the gut. Surgery 1988;104:185–190.
21. Saito H, Trocki O, Alexander JW, et al. Effect of route of administration on the nutritional state, catabolic hormone secretion and gut mucosal integrity after burn injury. J Parenter Enter Nutr 1987;11:1–7.
22. Kudsk KA, Stone JM, Carpenter G, Sheldon GF. Enteral and parenteral feeding influences mortality after hemoglobin. *E. coli* peritonitis in normal rats. J Trauma 1983;23:605–609.
23. Zaloga GP, Knowles R, Black KW, Prielipp R. Total parenteral nutrition increases mortality after hemorrhage. Crit Care Med 1990;19:54–59.

24. Fong Y, Marano MA, Barber A, et al. Total parenteral nutrition and bowel rest modify the metabolic response to endotoxin in humans. Ann Surg 1989;210:449–457.
25. Talbot JM. Guidelines for the scientific review of enteral food products for special medical purposes. J Parenter Enter Nutr 1991;15(suppl):99S–173S.
26. Heyland DK, Cook DJ, Guyatt GH. Enteral nutrition in the critically ill patient: A critical review of the evidence. Inten Care Med 1993;19:435–442.
27. Vernet O, Christin L, Schultz Y, et al. Enteral versus parenteral nutrition: Comparison of energy metabolism in healthy subjects. Am J Physiol 1986;250:E47–E54.
28. McArdle AH, Palmason C, Morency I, Brown RA. A rationale for enteral feeding as the preferable route for hyperalimentation. Surgery 1981;100:616–621.
29. Hamaoui E, Lefkowitz R, Olender L, et al. Enteral nutrition in the early postoperative period: A new semi-elemental formula versus total parenteral nutrition. J Parenter Enter Nutr 1990;14:501–507.
30. Bower RH, Talamini MA, Sax HC, et al. Postoperative enteral vs parenteral nutrition. Arch Surg 1986; 121:1040–1045.
31. Kudsk KA, Groce MA, Fabian TC, et al. Enteral versus parenteral feeding—effects on septic morbidity after blunt and penetrating abdominal trauma. Ann Surgery 1992; 215:503–513.
32. Messing B, Bories C, Kunstlinger F, Bernier JJ. Does total parenteral nutrition induce gall bladder sludge formation and lithiasis? Gastroenterology 1983;84:1012–1019.
33. Freeman HJ, Kim YS, Sleisinger MH. Protein digestion and absorption in man: Normal mechanisms and protein-energy malnutrition. Am J Med 1979;67:1030–1036.
34. Silk DBA, Grimble GK. Relevance of physiology of nutrient absorption to formulation of enteral diets. Nutrition 1992;8(1):1–12.
35. McClave SA, Lowen CC, Snider HL. Immunonutrition and enteral hyperalimentation of critically ill patients. Dig Dis Sci 1992;37:1153–1161.
36. American Society of Parenteral and Enteral Nutrition Board of Directors. Guidelines for the use of parenteral and enteral nutrition in adult and pediatric patients. J Parenter Enter Nutr 1993;17(suppl):1SA–52SA.
37. Marulendra S, Kirby DF. Nutrition support in pancreatitis. Nutr Clin Prac 1995;10:45–53.
38. Bell SJ, Mascioli EA, Forse RA, Bistrian BR. Nutrition support and the human immunodeficiency virus (HIV). Parasitology 1993;107(suppl):63S–67S.
39. Minard G. Enteral access. Nutr Clin Prac 1994;9:172–182.
40. Payne-James J. Enteral nutrition: Accessing patients. Nutrition 1992;8(4):223–231.
41. Lehman S. Parenteral and enteral access devices, in Teasley-Strausburg KM (ed): Nutrition Support Handbook: A Compendium of Products with Guidelines for Usage. Cincinnati, OH, Harvey Whitney Books Company, 1992, pp 205–257.
42. Dobbie RP, Hoffmeister JA. Continuous pump-tube enteric hyperalimentation. Surg Gynecol Obstet 1976;143:273–276.
43. Torosian MH, Rombeau JL. Feeding by tube enterostomy. Surg Gynecol Obstet 1980;150:918–927.
44. Clevenger FW, Rodriguez DJ. Decision-making for enteral feeding administration: The why behind where and how. Nutr Clin Prac 1995;10:104–113.
45. Martin D, Jastram CW. Enteral nutrition. Part II. Nutr Supp Serv 1987;7:8–10.
46. Leider Z, Sullivan L, Mullen MA, et al. Intermittent tube feedings: Pros and cons. Nutr Supp Serv 1984;4(3):59–62.
47. Orvieto A, Kirsch J, Goldberger J. Evaluation of enteral delivery systems. Nutr Supp Serv 1983;3(4):44–48.
48. Lehman S. Nutrient infusion devices, in Teasley-Strausberg KM (ed): Nutrition Support Handbook: A Compendium of Products with Guidelines for Usage. Cincinnati, OH, Harvey Whitney Books Company, 1992, pp 259–282.
49. Cerra FB, Holman RT, Bankey PE, et al. Omega-3 polyunsaturated fatty acids as modulators of cellular function in the critically ill. Pharmacotherapy 1991;11:71–76.
50. Mueller C, Nestle M. Regulation of medical foods: Toward a rational policy. Nutr Clin Prac 1995;10:8–15.
51. Heymsfield SB. Enteral solutions: Is there a solution? Nutr Clin Prac 1995;10:4–7.
52. MacBurney MM, Russell C, Young LS. Formulas, in Rombeau JL, Caldwell MD (eds): Clinical Nutrition: Enteral and Tube Feeding, 2nd ed. Philadelphia, WB Saunders, 1990, pp 149–173.
53. Smith JL, Heymsfield SB. Enteral nutrition support: Formula preparation from modular ingredients. J Parenter Enter Nutr 1983;7:280–288.
54. Schloerb PR, Almar M. Total parenteral nutrition with glutamine in bone marrow transplantation and other clinical applications (a randomized, double-blind study). J Parenter Enter Nutr 1993;17:407–413.
55. Ziegler TR, Young LS, Benfell K, et al. Clinical and metabolic efficacy of glutamine-supplemented parenteral nutrition after bone marrow transplantation (a randomized, double-blind, controlled study). Ann Intern Med 1992; 116:821–828.
56. Zaloga GP, MacGregor DA. What to consider when choosing enteral or parenteral nutrition. J Crit Illness 1990; 5:1180–1200.
57. Shronts EP, Havala T. Formulas, in Teasley-Strausberg KM (ed): Nutrition Support Handbook: A Compendium of Products with Guidelines for Usage. Cincinnati, OH, Harvey Whitney Books Company, 1992, pp 147–186.
58. Shike M. Enteral feeding, in Shils ME, Olson JA, Shike M (eds): Modern Nutrition in Health and Disease, 8th ed. Philadelphia, Lea and Febiger, 1994, pp 1417–1429.
59. Kudsk KA. Clinical applications of enteral nutrition. Nutr Clin Prac 1994;9:165–171.
60. Mead J. Nutrients with special functions: Essential fatty acids, in Alfin-Slater R, Kritchervsky D (eds): Human Nutrition. New York, Plenum, 1980, vol 3A, pp 213–238.
61. Vanlandingham S, Simpson S, Daniel P, et al. Metabolic abnormalities in patients supported with enteral tube feeding. J Parenter Enter Nutr 1981;5:322–324.
62. Berner YN, Morse R, Frank D, et al. Vitamin plasma levels in long-term enteral feeding patients. J Parenter Enter Nutr 1989;13:525–528.
63. Scheppach WM, Bartram HP. Experimental evidence for and clinical implications of fiber and artificial enteral nutrition. Nutrition 1993;9(5):399–405.
64. Keohane PP, Attrill H, Love M, et al. Relation between osmolality of diet and gastrointestinal side effects in enteral nutrition. Br Med J 1984;288:678–681.
65. Zimmaro DM, Rolandelli RH, Koruda MJ, et al. Isotonic tube feeding formula induces liquid stool in normal sub-

jects: Reversed by pectin. J Parenter Enter Nutr 1989; 13:117–123.
66. Jones TN, Moore FA, Moore EE, McCroskey BL. Gastrointestinal symptoms attributed to jejunostomy feeding after major abdominal trauma—a critical analysis. Crit Care Med 1989;17:1146–1150.
67. Cabre E, Gassull MA. Complications of enteral feeding. Nutrition 1993;8(6):1–9.
68. Durfee DD, Skinner-Domet VM. Cost effectiveness of an enteral product's formulary. Am J Hosp Pharm 1984; 41:2352–2354.
69. Gottschlick MM, Jenkins M, Warden GD, et al. Differential effects of three enteral dietary regimens on selected outcome variables in burn patients. J Parenter Enter Nutr 1990;14:225–235.
70. Bower RH, Cerra FB, Bershadsky B, et al. Early enteral administration of a formula (Impact) supplemented with arginine, nucleotides, and fish oil in intensive care unit patients: Results of a multicenter, prospective, randomized, clinical trial. Crit Care Med 1995;23:436–449.
71. Daly JM, Lieberman MD, Goldfine J, et al. Enteral nutrition with supplemental argenine, RNA, and omega-3 fatty acids in patients after operation: Immunologic metabolic, and clinical outcome. Surgery 1992;112:56–67.
72. Levy J, Laethen T, Verhaegen G, et al. Contaminated enteral nutrition solutions as a cause of nosocomial bloodstream infection: A study using plasmid fingerprinting. J Parenter Enter Nutr 1989;13:228–234.
73. Thurn J, Crossley K, Gerdts A, et al. Enteral hyperalimentation as a source of nosocomial infectin. J Hosp Infect 1990;15:203–217.
74. VanEnk R, Furtado D. Bacterial contamination of enteral nutrient solutions: Intestinal colonization and sepsis in mice after infection. J Parenter Enter Nutr 1986; 10:503–507.
75. Havala T, Shronts EP. Formula compounding, in Teasley-Strausberg KM (ed): Nutrition Support Handbook: A Compendium of Products with Guidelines for Usage. Cincinnati, OH, Harvey Whitney Books Company, 1992, pp 187–204.
76. Wagner DR, Emore MF, Knoll DM. Evaluation of "closed" vs "open" systems for the delivery of peptide-based enteral diets. J Parenter Enter Nutr 1994;18:453–457.
77. Cutie AJ, Altman E, Lenkel L. Compatability of enteral products with commonly employed drug additives. J Parenter Enter Nutr 1983;7:186–191.
78. Hardin TC, Reed M (eds). Nutrition and Drug Therapy: Clinical Pharmacology Drug Compatability and Stability—An Annotated Bibliography. Silver Spring, MD, ASPEN, 1992.
79. Dickerson RN, Melnik G. Osmolality of oral drug solutions and suspensions. Am J Hosp Pharm 1988;45:832–834.
80. Kumpf VJ, Barber JR. Enteral nutrition. US Pharm 1987; (June):H–1, 2, 5, 8–10, 15.
81. Bradley J. Principles of enteral nutrition. Hosp Pharm 1994;23:197–204.
82. Strom JG, Miller SW. Stability of drugs with enteral nutrient formulas. Drug Intell Clin Pharm 1990;24:130–134.
83. Gora ML, Tschampel MM, Visconti JA. Considerations of drug therapy in patients receiving enteral nutrition. Nutr Clin Prac 1989;4:105–110.
84. Thompson CT, Rollins C. Enteral feeding and medication incompatibilities. Support Line-Dietitians Nutr Support 1991;13(3):9–12.
85. Mitchell JF, Pavlicki KS. Oral dosage forms that should not be crushed: 1990 revision. Hosp Pharm 1990;25:329–335.
86. Bauer LA. Interference of oral phenytoin absorption by continuous nasogastric feedings. Neurology 1982;32:570–572.
87. Melnick G. Pharmacologic aspects of enteral nutrition, in Rombeau JL, Caldwell MD (eds): Clinical Nutrition: Enteral and Tube Feeding, 2nd ed. Philadelphia, WB Saunders, 1990, pp 472–509.
88. Nishimura LY, Armstrong RP, Plezia PM, Iacono RP. Influence of enteral feedings on phenytoin sodium absorption from capsules. Drug Intell Clin Pharm 1988;22:130–133.
89. Guidry JR, Eastwood TF, Curry SC. Phenytoin absorption in volunteers receiving selected enteral feeds. West J Med 1989;150(6):659–661.
90. Drug Facts and Comparisons. St. Louis, MO, Wolters Kluwer Company, 1995.
91. Gora ML, Tschampel MM, Visconti JA. Considerations of drug therapy in patients receiving enteral nutrition. Nutr Clin Prac 1989;4:105–110.
92. Valli C, Schulthess HK, Asper R, et al. Interaction of nutrients with antacids: A complication during enteral tube feeding. Lancet 1986;8483:747–748.
93. Eisenberg PG. Causes of diarrhea in tube-fed patients: A comprehensive approach to diagnosis and management. Nutr Clin Prac 1993;8:119–123.
94. Mirtallo JM, Fabri PJ. Concurrent therapy for complications of enteral nutrition support. Hosp Form 1982; 17(July):945–953.
95. Shankardass K, Chuchmach S, Chelswick K, et al. Bowel function of long-term tube-fed patients consuming formulae with and without dietary fiber. J Parenter Enter Nutr 1990; 14:508–512.
96. McClave SA, Snider HL, Lowen CC, et al. Use of residual volume as a marker for enteral feeding intolerance: Prospective blinded comparison with physical examination and radiographic findings. J Parenter Enter Nutr 1992; 16:99–105.
97. Hebuterne X, Broussard JF, Rampal P. Acute renutrition by cyclic enteral nutrition in elderly and younger patients. J Am Med Assoc 1995;273:638–643.
98. Newmark SR, Simpson MS, Beskitt MP, et al. Home tube feeding for long-term nutritional support. J Parenter Enter Nutr 1981;5:76–79.
99. Greenberg GR, Fleming CR, Jeejeebhoy KN, et al. Controlled trial of bowel rest and nutritional support in the management of Crohn's disease. Gut 1988;29:1309–1315.
100. Fleming CR. Nutrition in patients with Crohn's disease: Another piece of the puzzle. J Parenter Enter Nutr 1995; 19:93–94.
101. Kearns PJ, Young H, Garcia G, et al. Accelerated improvement of alcoholic liver disease with enteral nutrition. Gastroenterology 1992;102:200–205.
102. Cerra FB, McPherson JP, Konstantinides FN, et al. Enteral nutrition does not prevent multiple organ failure syndrome (MOFS) after sepsis. Surgery 1988;104:727–733.
103. Moore FA, Moore EE, Jones TN, et al. TEN versus TPN following major abdominal trauma-reduced septic morbidity. J Trauma 1989;29:916–923.

Chapter 135

Pediatric and Geriatric Nutrition Support

Katherine Hammond Chessman, PharmD, BCNSP, BCPS, and Jan Dalke Anderson, PharmD, BCNSP

Pediatric Nutrition

Children have unique physiologic needs that make provision of nutritional support to them distinctly different than adults. The high incidence of protein-calorie malnutrition reported in hospitalized children[1,2] necessitates that all pediatric health care providers be familiar with pediatric nutrition support. With insufficient oral intake, normally nourished children should, in general, be given appropriate specialized nutrition support after 5–7 days of suboptimal intake, term infants after 3–5 days, and preterm infants within 1–3 days.[3] Children with preexisting malnutrition may warrant earlier intervention.

PHYSIOLOGY

Body composition varies with age. A young child's body contains a higher percentage of water and lower calorie and protein reserves than an adult's. The percentage of body weight that is protein is approximately the same as an adult; however, only about 50% of the protein is deposited in skeletal muscle compared to 90% in adults.

Caloric requirements per kilogram are higher because a child's basal metabolic rate (BMR) is higher since the major metabolic organs, especially the brain, constitute a larger portion of the body. BMR is approximately 50–55 kcal/kg/d in infancy and declines to about 20–25 kcal/kg/d during adolescence. Equations used to estimate BMR in children are shown in Table 135.1.[4–6] For children less than age 3, a modification of the Harris–Benedict equation has been developed (Table 135.1).[7] When compared to measured resting energy expenditure (mREE) determined by indirect calorimetry in normal children, all these equations predicted BMR within 10%. The BMR calculated using the Schofield and FAO/WHO/UNU equations was not statistically significantly different from mREE in any group. Using the Harris–Benedict equations, calculated BMR was statistically different from mREE in males only.[8] Extrapolation of these values to sick children may not be appropriate. Chwals et al.[9] found that measured energy expenditure was only 52.6% of predicted energy requirements in 20 critically ill infants and children.

In children, normal growth and development is critical and depends on adequate nutrition, making growth a primary screening and monitoring tool for nutrition adequacy. Two critical growth periods necessitate increased caloric intake: the first 3 years of life and the adolescent growth spurt. In healthy infants, 35–40% of energy is used for growth but by 2 years of age, only 2–5% is used for this purpose. Severe stress may impair growth even if adequate calories and protein are provided due to increased production of catecholamines and "counterregulatory hormones," which oppose insulin's anabolic effects, resulting in decreased endogenous tissue stores of protein, fat, and carbohydrate.[9,10]

Due to immature renal, hepatic, and gastrointestinal tract function, nutrients may be digested, absorbed, or metabolized differently, especially during the neonatal period. Neonates, especially premature ones, are more prone to hyperglycemia due to reduced insulin secretion, failure of glucose to suppress hepatic glucose output, and peripheral insulin resistance. Preterm infants also have a low renal threshold for glucose excretion; therefore, glycosuria may occur even at "normal" serum glucose concentrations.[11] Certain amino acids including cysteine, taurine, and tyrosine are considered essential in newborns due to their immature enzyme systems. These same enzyme systems allow for accumulation of potentially toxic amino acids such as methionine and phenylalanine if given in large concentrations. Plasma amino acid concentrations 2 hours postprandial in normally growing, 30-day-old breast-fed infants have been characterized and used for evaluating nutritional products.[12] Gastrointestinal tract immaturity may lead to decreased absorption of nutrients including lactose, protein, and fat.

TABLE 135.1. EQUATIONS TO ESTIMATE BASAL ENERGY EXPENDITURE IN CHILDREN

Harris–Benedict[4] (kcal/d):

Males: BEE = 66 + (13.7*W*) + [5*H*(cm)] − (6.8*A*)

Females: BEE = 655 + (9.6*W*) + [1.8*H*(cm)] − (4.7*A*)

Caldwell–Kennedy (kcal/d)[7]:

Infants: BEE = 22 + (31*W*) + [1.2*H*(cm)]

Schofield[6] (MJ/d) (to convert to kcal/d multiply by 239.2):

3–10 years of age

Males: BMR = (0.08*W*) + [0.55*H*(m)] + 1.74

Females: BMR = (0.07*W*) + [0.68*H*(m)] + 1.55

10–18 years of age

Males: BMR = (0.07*W*) + [0.57*H*(m)] + 2.16

Females: BMR = (0.04*W*) + [1.95*H*(m)] + 0.84

FAO/WHO/UNU[5] (kcal/d)

3–10 years of age

Males: BMR = 22.7*W* + 495

Females: BMR = 22.5*W* + 499

10–18 years of age

Males: BMR = 17.5*W* + 651

Females: BMR = 12.2*W* + 746

Key: *W*, weight in kilograms; *H*, height in centimeters (cm) or meters (m), as indicated; *A*, age in years; BEE, basal energy expenditure; BMR, basal metabolic rate; FAO/WHO/UNU, Food and Agriculture Organization/World Health Organization/United Nations University.

NUTRITION ASSESSMENT

Nutrition assessment is a crucial aspect of pediatric patient care. The goals of assessment are to screen for existing malnutrition, identify children at risk for developing malnutrition and its complications, and monitor the outcome of nutritional support regimens. Appropriate assessment includes a complete physical examination, medical and dietary history, anthropometric measurements, and appropriate laboratory studies. None of these tools is sensitive or specific enough for use alone. More sophisticated techniques, such as measuring body composition and energy expenditure, are used in some settings but are not available to most practitioners.

Growth is evaluated by comparison of recumbent length (children less than 2 years of age), height (children older than 2 years of age), weight, head circumference (children less than 3 years of age), and growth rate to age- and gender-related standards as well as to previous measurements. Accurate measurement is important. Weight and height are evaluated by percentile according to age, by the weight-for-height percentile, and by growth velocity. These data are obtained by plotting measurements on an appropriate National Center for Health Statistics (NCHS) growth curve developed from data obtained from 1962–1974 in a large population of normal children.[13] Special curves are available for assessment of short-term[14] and long-term growth[15] of premature infants and children with Down syndrome.[16] For premature infants with corrected age of 40 weeks or more, the NCHS growth charts can be used; however, weight-for-age and height-for-age should be plotted according to corrected age until 2 years of age and 3.5 years of age, respectively.[17] Appropriate time intervals between measurements necessary for meaningful evaluation of growth are as follows: weight, 7 days; length, 4 weeks; height, 8 weeks; and head circumference, 7 days in infants and 4 weeks in children up to 3 years of age.[18] Adequate weight gain is 10–12 g/kg/d in a term newborn and two to three times that rate in a premature infant. Weight gain per kilogram declines considerably after 2–3 months of age.

Growth failure or "failure to thrive" is defined as weight-for-age or weight-for-height at less than 5th percentile or a "fall-off" of two or more major percentiles (major percentiles are defined as 95th, 90th, 75th, 50th, 25th, 10th, and 5th). Weight-for-height evaluation is age independent and helps differentiate the stunted child (chronic malnutrition) from the wasted child (acute malnutrition). Short stature, which is associated with many chronic diseases, is a manifestation of chronic undernutrition. Common classifications of undernutrition are shown in Table 135.2.[19] Use of these methods to categorize nutrition status gives varying results. They are best used to define risk of possible adverse effects of undernutrition rather than to label a child as "malnourished."[20] Catch-up growth can be initiated within 2 days to 2 weeks with appropriate refeeding.[21,22] Height usually lags behind weight but will recover if dietary treatment is not stopped prematurely because of an unwarranted fear of obesity.

A medical and dietary history may identify variations from normal intake such as vegetarian diets, meal-skipping, sports "fad" diets, anorexia/bulimia, and medications. In children, primary malnutrition or inadequate intake may be due to an altered maternal–child relationship, lack of parental education, poverty, restricted allergy diets, and food fads. Secondary malnutrition is often due to congenital malformation, infectious disease, trauma, malignancy, and chronic disease. The most accurate approach to a diet history is a 3- to 5-day diet diary. Parental 24-hour recall without warning has been called "no more than a test of memory."[23]

Laboratory studies used for nutrition assessment of children are similar to those used for adults; however, normal values may vary with age. Nitrogen balance studies are less reliable in infants and young children. It is often difficult to get a complete 24-hour urine collection that is not

TABLE 135.2. COMMON CLASSIFICATIONS OF UNDERNUTRITION

		Degree of Malnutrition		
	Normal	**Mild**	**Moderate**	**Severe**
Weight-for-height	>90	80–90	70–80	<70
Weight-for-age	>90	75–90	61–75	<60
Weight-for-height	110–90	85–90	75–85	<75

contaminated with stool, unless the child has a urinary catheter. Shorter collection times have been found to correlate well with 24-hour collections.[24] Additionally, in infants, urine urea nitrogen represents an extremely variable proportion of total urine nitrogen.

NUTRIENT REQUIREMENTS

Although recommended dietary allowances (RDAs) for various nutrients have been established for normal healthy children,[25] these may be altered by disease or injury. Furthermore, premature infants were not included in the RDAs because desired intakes are less well defined for this population. Children should be encouraged to eat a variety of foods to ensure provision of RDAs and other nutrients for which no RDA has been established.

Fluid Intake

Fluid requirements per kilogram are higher in newborns due to the higher percentage of body water and higher BMR (Table 135.3).[26] Premature neonates have increased fluid requirements due to greater insensible losses and the kidney's inefficiency in concentrating urine. The Holliday–Segar method[27] is a commonly employed, quick, and simple method for estimating the minimum daily fluid needs of infants and children. Using this method, 100 mL/kg/d is given for the first 1–10 kg body weight plus an additional 50 mL/kg/d for each kilogram between 11 and 20 kg plus an additional 20 mL/kg/d for each kilogram above 20 kg. For example, maintenance fluid needs for a child weighing 17 kg would be 1350 mL/d. Alternatively, maintenance fluids may be estimated as 1500 mL/m^2/24 h in children weighing more than 10 kg. Factors that alter fluid needs are shown in Table 135.4.

Fluid status can be assessed by monitoring urine output and specific gravity, serum electrolytes, and weight changes. A urine output of 1.0–2.0 mL/kg/h or more is considered adequate. Urine output should be higher if large fluid volumes or high renal solute loads are being administered. Urine specific gravity depends on the kidney's concentrating and diluting capabilities. The neonatal kidney has limited ability to concentrate urine. A urine specific gravity of greater than 1.020 (1.015 in neonates) may indicate a need for more fluid while a urine specific gravity of 1.008 or less suggests fluid overload. Diuretic therapy limits the usefulness of urine specific gravity due to increased solute excretion.

TABLE 135.3. RECOMMENDED FLUID INTAKES FOR NEWBORNS (mL/kg/d)

Birth Weight (g)	Days 1–2	Day 3	Days 15–20
751–1000	105	140	150
1001–1250	100	130	140
1251–1500	90	120	130
1501–1750	80	110	130
1751–2000	80	110	130
Term infant	70	80	90–100

(Adapted from Ref. 26, p. 255, with permission.)

TABLE 135.4. FACTORS THAT ALTER FLUID REQUIREMENTS IN CHILDREN

Increased Requirements	Decreased Requirements
Fever	Fluid overload
Radiant warmers	Cardiac failure
Diuretics	Decreased urinary output
Vomiting	Heat shields
Nasogastric suction	Relatively high humidity
Ostomy/fistula drainage	Humidified air via endotracheal tube
Diarrhea	
Glycosuria	
Phototherapy	
Increased ambient temperatures	
Hyperventilation	

Caloric Intake

Suggested caloric intakes for maintenance and normal growth of children are shown in Table 135.5. Maintenance energy requirements are approximately 150% of BMR. An alternative method to estimate maintenance caloric need is to use the value calculated with the Holliday–Segar method since it was derived using BMR. To maintain positive nitrogen balance, premature infants should receive at least 60 nonprotein kcal/kg/d with at least 2.5 g protein/kg/d; term infants at least 80 nonprotein kcal/kg/d with at least 2.5 g protein/kg/d. To attain postnatal growth rates approximately equal to *in utero* growth of 10–15 g/kg/d, premature infants must receive 120–150 kcal/kg/d.[28]

Caloric requirements increase with fever, severe stress, sepsis, major surgery, trauma, burns, long-term growth failure, and in the presence of chronic conditions such as bron-

TABLE 135.5. SUGGESTED DAILY CALORIC INTAKE FOR MAINTENANCE OF BODY MASS AND NORMAL GROWTH OF CHILDREN

Age	kcal/kg/d
Premature	120–150
0–1 years	100
1–7 years	75–90
7–12 years	60–75
12–18 years	30–60

chopulmonary dysplasia (BPD) and congenital heart disease. Caloric needs may decrease with obesity and neurologic disability (e.g., cerebral palsy). The response to stress in children is similar to that seen in critically ill adults[29] and stress factors have been suggested for various conditions in children (Table 135.6).[30] Although several formulas are available for determining caloric requirements in burned children, the Hildreth–Carvajal formula[31] (i.e., kcal/d = 1800 kcal/m^2 BSA + 2200 kcal/m^2 × % BSA burned) appears to correlate most closely with measured energy expenditure. Of note is that with the use of these stress factors, with the exception of severe burns and severe sepsis, energy needs during stress (stress factor times BMR) may be slightly less than maintenance energy needs of 150% of BMR. Acute stress is a catabolic state. Counterregulatory hormones present may diminish and even stop growth, which would decrease energy expenditure.[9] Pharmacologic paralysis and sedation also decrease energy expenditure by decreasing activity. Premature infants with BPD require a minimum of 120–150 kcal/kg/d. Energy needs may increase with concomitant disease and decline as pulmonary function improves. Children with BPD often have limited physical activity, and caloric needs after 6 months corrected age may be as low as 70–80 kcal/kg/d.[17] Guidelines for energy needs in children with developmental disabilities are shown in Table 135.7.[32]

Overfeeding may increase the risk of obesity, diabetes, cardiovascular disease, and carbon dioxide production. A more accurate characterization of the stress response in children is needed. Measuring energy expenditure via indirect calorimetry is preferred but not widely available due to technical problems encountered with measurements in small children. No studies to date, however, show an improved patient outcome with the use of indirect calorimetry compared to traditional methods of estimating caloric need.

To achieve "catch-up" growth after long-term growth failure, a child must receive nutrients in excess of normal requirements. Caloric needs for catch-up growth may be estimated using Eq. (1)[33] or Eq. (2).[34] In general, children will require 1.5–2 times their age-appropriate intake to achieve optimal "catch-up" growth.[34]

TABLE 135.6. STRESS FACTORS[a] FOR USE IN CHILDREN

Condition	Stress Factor
Simple starvation	1.0
Postoperative recovery, uncomplicated surgery	1.0
Sepsis (moderate)	1.3
Sepsis (severe)	1.6
Trauma, mild (e.g., long bone fracture)	1.2
Trauma, central nervous system (sedated)	1.3
Trauma, moderate to severe	1.5
Burns (proportionate to burned area)	Up to 2.0

[a]Multiply BMR by stress factor for approximate energy requirements. (Reprinted from Ref. 30, p. 214, with permission.)

TABLE 135.7. ESTIMATED CALORIC NEEDS IN CHILDREN WITH DEVELOPMENTAL DISABILITIES

Condition	Caloric Recommendations
Ambulatory, ages 5–12 yr	13.9 kcal/cm height
Nonambulatory, ages 5–12 yr	11.1 kcal/cm height
Cerebral palsy with severely restricted activity	10 kcal/cm height[a]
Cerebral palsy with mild to moderate activity	15 kcal/cm height
Athetoid cerebral palsy, adolescence	Up to 6000 kcal/d
Down syndrome, boys, ages 1–14 yr	16.1 kcal/cm height
Down syndrome, girls, ages 1–14 yr	14.3 kcal/cm height
Myelomeningocele	Approximately 50% of RDA for age after infancy. May need as little as 7 kcal/cm height to maintain normal weight.

[a]May need to decrease to 7 kcal/cm height once growth stops. (Adapted from Ref. 32, p. 457, with permission.)

$$\text{kcal/kg/d} = \frac{\text{kcal/kg for wt age} \times \text{ideal wt (kg) for age}}{\text{actual wt (kg)}} \quad (1)$$

$$\text{kcal/kg/d} = \frac{120\ \text{kcal/kg} \times \text{ideal wt for actual ht}}{\text{actual wt (kg)}} \quad (2)$$

where "wt age" is the age at which present weight is 50th percentile; "ideal wt for age" is the 50th percentile weight for current age; and "ideal wt for actual ht" is 50th percentile weight for actual height.

Energy must be provided as both glucose and fat. Glucose requirements per kilogram are higher in children due to the increased percentage of metabolic activity contributed by the brain per kilogram. Dietary guidelines limiting fat intake should not be imposed on children until after 2 years of age to avoid compromising central nervous system development. After that, fat should not exceed 30% of the total calories.[35] As in adults, children require approximately 1–2% of calories as linoleic acid to prevent essential fatty acid deficiency (EFAD).[36] Arachidonic and linoleic acid requirements, however, are not well established. Newborns and small infants have limited fat stores; therefore, EFAD may develop more rapidly than in adults. Biochemical EFAD, evidenced by a rise in the triene:tetraene ratio, has been demonstrated within 72 hours after birth in preterm infants receiving fat-free intravenous solutions.[37]

Protein Intake

Daily protein needs are based on age and factors such as injury, hypermetabolism, and malnutrition (Table 135.8).[38]

TABLE 135.8. PROTEIN REQUIREMENTS IN INFANTS, CHILDREN, AND ADOLESCENTS

	Daily Protein Intake (g/kg body wt)		
Clinical Condition	**Infants (0–1 yr)**	**Children (1–10 yr)**	**Children (≥ 10 yr)**
RDA	1.6–2.2	1.0–1.2	0.8–1.0
Low stress			
Maintenance	2.0–2.5	2.0–2.5	1.0–1.2
Anabolism	2.5–3.0	2.5–3.0	1.3–1.7
Hypermetabolism	2.5–3.5	2.5–3.5	1.5–2.5
Severe burn injury	2.5–3.5	2.5–3.5	2.0–3.0
Renal failure			
No dialysis	1.6–2.0	1.0–1.8	0.6–1.0
Dialysis[a]	3.0–4.0	1.5–3.6	1.2–2.7
Severe hepatic failure	—	2.0–3.0	0.5–1.5

[a]Varies with type of dialysis; peritoneal dialysis usually necessitates a higher protein intake than hemodialysis. (From Ref. 38, p. 30, with permission.)

Protein must be increased in similar proportions to energy during catch-up growth. Protein intake for catch-up growth can be calculated using Eq. (3)[33]:

$$\text{Protein g/kg/d} = \frac{\text{g/kg for wt age} \times \text{ideal wt (kg) for age}}{\text{actual wt (kg)}} \quad (3)$$

In health, RDAs for most vitamins and trace elements are met with a well-balanced diet so that supplementation is not needed.[39] Therapeutic supplementation may be needed in certain disease states and conditions including pregnancy, cystic fibrosis,[40] hepatic disease,[41] prematurity,[42] and malabsorption syndromes.

ENTERAL NUTRITION

Most children have a sufficiently intact gastrointestinal tract to enable them to be fed enterally, and, whenever possible, oral intake is preferred. If oral intake is not possible or insufficient to meet nutrient needs then placement of a feeding tube is the next logical step. Gastric tubes (e.g., nasogastric, gastrostomy) are preferred if no contraindication exists to gastric feedings. Alternatively, transpyloric feeding tubes may be used. Table 135.9 lists common indications for tube feedings in children. Contraindications to enteral feedings include severe acute pancreatitis, bowel obstruction, and intestinal atresia. A number of formulas are available to supply enteral nutrition (EN) to children. Formulas are classified according to the age group for which they are indicated: premature infants, term infants to 1 year of age, children 1–10 years of age, and children older than 10 years of age. Formula selection also depends on gastrointestinal tract function, metabolic needs, fluid requirements, viscosity, and diagnosis.

Formulas for Infants

Human breast milk is the food of choice for newborns. Human milk contains unique biochemical, immunologic, and cellular components. Contraindications to breast-feeding include galactosemia, phenylketonuria, urea cycle defects, and a few other rare inborn errors of metabolism. Maternal diseases, including tuberculosis, hepatitis, and AIDS, may also preclude breast-feeding. Furthermore, some drug therapies may prevent a mother from nursing.

TABLE 135.9. COMMON INDICATIONS FOR TUBE FEEDINGS IN CHILDREN

Oral Intake Contraindicated	Inadequate Oral Intake	Malabsorption/Altered Metabolism
Prematurity (<34 weeks)	Anorexia nervosa	Intractable vomiting
Cerebral palsy	Cancer	Short bowel syndrome
Head injury	Cystic fibrosis	Chronic diarrhea
Coma	Chronic renal/hepatic disease	Pancreatitis
Facial trauma	Inflammatory bowel disease	Inflammatory bowel disease
Esophageal injury	Congenital heart disease	Inborn errors of metabolism
	Bronchopulmonary dysplasia	Gastroesophageal reflux
	Burns	Pseudo-obstruction
	Trauma	
	Sepsis	

Briggs et al.[43] have published an excellent reference guide for the use of drugs in pregnancy and lactation.

The first modified cow's milk-based formula was developed in 1915 and marketed in 1919 as SMA® (synthetic milk adapted). Today, many formulas are available in powder, concentrate, or ready-to-feed form to provide an alternative to human breast milk when mothers do not or cannot breast feed (Table 135.10). These formulas are all very similar and provide approximately 67 kcal/dL with 1.5 g/dL protein as either whey or casein, 3.5 g/dL fat (45% of total calories) as a mixture of vegetable oils, and carbohydrate as lactose. Added vitamins and minerals provide RDAs.

Protein intake provided by human milk is lower than formula. Human milk contains a high percentage (70%) of whey protein, a more easily digestible protein than casein, which is the primary (80%) cow's milk protein. Whey protein also includes carriers for immunoglobulins, albumin, lysozyme, enzymes such as amylase, transaminases, proteases, lipases, vitamins, and minerals.

Iron absorption from human milk (20–50%) is significantly higher than from formula (4–7%) probably due to iron-binding proteins in human milk, lower protein and phosphorus content, or its lactose and ascorbate content. Historically, low iron formulas were recommended until approximately 4–6 months of age due to concerns that iron-fortified formulas contributed to colic, constipation, diarrhea, and regurgitation. Scientific investigations do not support these concerns.[44,45] The American Academy of Pediatrics (AAP) now recommends iron-fortified formulas starting from birth in all non-breast-fed infants including preterm infants.[46] Whole cow's milk should not be introduced until 1 year of age to avoid milk protein sensitization, gastrointestinal blood loss, iron deficiency, dehydration due to high renal solute load, and nutrient deficiencies.[47]

Special Needs Formula

A number of formulas are available for infants with special needs (Table 135.10). Soy-based formulas are lactose free and indicated for the treatment of uncomplicated primary lactase deficiency, secondary lactose intolerance after gastroenteritis, protein-calorie malnutrition or other causes of mucosal injury, galactosemia, and cow's milk protein allergy[48] except in cases where soy protein allergy coexists. Soy formulas are nutritionally equivalent to cow's milk-based formulas.

Hydrolyzed formulas or semielemental formulas (Table 135.11) are indicated for infants or children with altered digestion, absorption, or metabolism. Common indications include cow's milk and soy protein allergy, generalized malabsorption (e.g., short bowel syndrome), pancreatic insufficiency (e.g., cystic fibrosis), chylothorax, biliary atresia, chronic diarrhea, and AIDS. Hydrolysate formulas cost two to three times or more the cost of standard cow's milk- or soy-based formulas.

Neither human milk nor cow's milk-based formulas are adequate to supply the premature infant's needs. Human milk fortifiers (Table 135.12) are available to add additional nutrients to human milk. Formulas designed for premature infants (Table 135.11) are modified to compensate for alterations in digestion and absorption. In these formulas, carbohydrate is provided as both lactose and glucose polymers, protein in higher quantities and a higher whey-

TABLE 135.10. INFANT FORMULAS

Formula Type	Products (Mfr[a])	Indications
Cow's milk-based	Enfamil (MJ) 20, 24 kcal/oz; Similac (R) 20, 24, 27 kcal/oz; Gerber Baby Formula (G); Carnation Good Start (C)	Normal, healthy infants
Soy-based	Isomil, Isomil DF,[b] Isomil SF[c] (MJ); Prosobee (R); Gerber Soy Formula (G); Soyalac, I-Soyalac (LL)	Lactase deficiency; lactose intolerance; galactosemia; cow's milk allergy
Premature	Similac Special Care (R) 20, 24 kcal/oz; Enfamil Premature (MJ) 20, 24 kcal/oz	Preterm infant less than 2–3 kg
Transition	Advance (R); Carnation Follow-Up (C)	Transition from formula to cow's milk
Special diets	MSUD Diet Powder (MJ)	Maple syrup urine disease or branched-chain amino acid disorders
	Phenyl-Free (MJ)	Phenylketonuria
	Similac PM 60/40 (R)	Renal, cardiac, or endocrine disorders
	Protein Free Diet Powder (MJ) (Product 80056)	Altered amino acid metabolism
	Ross Carbohydrate-free (RCF) (R)	Intractable diarrhea; carbohydrate intolerance
	Product 3232-A (MJ)	Intractable diarrhea; carbohydrate intolerance

[a]Manufacturers: R, Ross Laboratories; MJ, Mead Johnson Nutritionals; C, Carnation Nutritional Products; G, Gerber; LL, Loma Linda.
[b]Diarrhea formula—contains g/100 mL fiber.
[c]Sucrose free.

TABLE 135.11. SEMI-ELEMENTAL INFANT FORMULAS

Product (Mfr[a])	Carbohydrate	Fat	Protein
Nutramigen (MJ)	Sucrose, modified tapioca starch	Corn oil	Hydrolyzed casein
Pregestimil (MJ)	Corn syrup solids, modified tapioca starch	MCT 60%, sunflower oil	Hydrolyzed casein
Alimentum (R)	Sucrose, modified tapioca starch	MCT 50%; coconut, safflower and soy oil	Hydrolyzed casein; free amino acids
Portagen (MJ)	Sucrose, corn syrup solids	MCT 86%; corn oil	Sodium caseinate
Vivonex Pediatric (S)	Maltodextrin, modified starch	MCT; soybean oil	Free amino acids
Peptamen Junior (C)	Maltodextrin, corn starch	MCT; soybean oil; canola oil	Hydrolyzed whey

[a]Manufacturers: MJ, Mead Johnson Nutritionals; R, Ross Laboratories; S, Sandoz; C, Clintec.

to-casein ratio (60:40), and fat partially as medium-chain triglycerides (MCTs). Calcium, phosphorus, sodium, and vitamin content is also higher. These formulas are safe and produce improved growth rates, bone mineralization, and nitrogen retention compared to standard infant formulas.[28,49] Healthy preterm infants may be weaned from premature formulas at approximately 2 kg. With fluid restriction, increased energy needs, and diuretic therapy, preterm infants with BPD may benefit from preterm formulas until their weight reaches 3 kg.[17]

Formulas for Older Children

Several products are available specifically to meet the mineral, vitamin, trace element, and protein needs of children 1–10 years of age: Pediasure and Pediasure with Fiber (Ross Laboratories), Nutren Junior and Nutren Junior with Fiber (Clintec), Kindercal (Mead Johnson Nutritionals), Vivonex Pediatric (Sandoz), and Peptamen Junior (Clintec). Standard products are essentially lactose and gluten free but are not predigested and, therefore, not suitable for children with malabsorption. They are also contraindicated in children with galactosemia. Both Vivonex Pediatric and Peptamen Junior are semielemental formulas, which may be useful in children with malabsorption or intolerance to standard formulas.

TABLE 135.12. MODULAR ENTERAL PRODUCTS

Primary Nutrient Supplied	Example Products (Mfr[a])
Carbohydrate	LC (C), PC (C), Moducal (MJ), Polycose (R), Sumacal (SM)
Protein	ProMod (R), Propac (SM), ProMix RDP (C), Casec (MJ), Gevral Protein (L), ProViMin (R)
Fat	High MCT Supplement (C), MCT Oil (MJ), Lipomul (RO), Microlipid (SM)
Human milk fortifier	Enfamil Human Milk Fortifier (MJ), Similac Natural Care (R)
Pectin/carbohydrate/potassium	Banana Flakes (K)

[a]Manufacturers: R, Ross Laboratories; MJ, Mead Johnson Nutritionals; SM, Sherwood Medical; L, Lederle; RO, Roberts Pharmaceutical Corporation; C, Corpak; K, Kanana.

Formulas intended for adults (see Chapter 134, Enteral Nutrition) have also been used for children older than 6–10 years of age or in children older than 1 year of age with nutrition needs not met by age-specific formulas. Use of the newer pediatric-specific products will decrease the need to use adult products in children.

Occasionally, commercial formulas fail to meet nutrient needs. Adding less water or a modular product (Table 135.12) is an option for increasing nutrient delivery to children who have increased caloric or protein needs, who cannot tolerate the volume necessary to receive sufficient calories with standard products, or who have malabsorption of one or more nutrients. Generally, infant formulas are first concentrated to 24 kcal/oz by adding less water or, if available, using the ready-to-use 24 or 27 kcal/oz product, and then one or more modular components is added to further increase the desired nutrient. Adding modules to 20 kcal/oz formula is usually avoided due to dilution of other nutrients to suboptimal levels. Mixing powdered or concentrated formulas with less water increases delivered quantities of all nutrients and may increase the renal solute load predisposing to dehydration since insufficient water may be provided. Modules may also be added to any of the pediatric or adult enteral formulas.

Enteral Feeding Regimens

A number of approaches to initiating and advancing feedings are practiced, most of which are based on strong feelings and experience rather than controlled trials. In a stable, closely monitored child, it is reasonable to select an appropriate formula and to administer 100% of the therapeutic goal either by continuous or bolus feedings immediately.[50] This approach may be well tolerated and preferable to approaches that taper either concentration or volume since it is the fastest way to initiate feedings and may shorten hospital stay. Many, however, prefer a more gradual advancement usually by advancing volume over hours to days depending on the child's condition. When feeding intolerance is documented or when intolerance is expected (e.g., short bowel syndrome), gradual tapering with a combination of parenteral and enteral nutrition is preferred. In premature infants, slow advancement of dilute enteral feedings has been suggested as a means of decreasing the incidence of necrotizing enterocolitis; however, this has not been proven scientifically.

Intermittent bolus feedings are preferred because they simulate normal feeding, are less expensive, and allow greater flexibility and mobility. However, children with severe intestinal disease usually tolerate continuous infusion better than bolus.[51]

Tolerance is monitored by assessing the development of vomiting, abdominal distention, or diarrhea. Checking residuals, that is, the volume remaining in the stomach immediately prior to the next feeding, is not routinely recommended except in children at risk for aspiration.[52] When aspiration is a concern, residuals should be checked every 2–4 hours initially, then less often as tolerance is documented. Acceptable residual volume is variable. One rule of thumb often employed is that the residual volume should be less than one-half of the previously administered volume. A single high residual should not result in feeding discontinuation. Holding a feeding or decreasing the rate for several hours may be adequate. Stool character is highly variable even in normal children and is often related to formula type. Stool volume less than 15–20 mL/kg/d and absence of fecal reducing substances (i.e., unabsorbed sugars) or fat are indications of tolerance despite frequency, consistency, or color of stool.

Complications of Enteral Nutrition

Complications of EN in children are similar to those seen in adults (see Chapter 134). Diarrhea is frequently associated with concomitant medications, carbohydrate malabsorption, or viral illness. Addition of glucose in large amounts may result in loose stools. Large quantities of added fat, especially MCTs, may result in diarrhea or delayed gastric emptying and gastroesophageal reflux. Constipation is frequently associated with long-term use of liquid formulas and may develop due to lack of sufficient fluid or bulk in the diet, medications, decreased muscle tone, or inactivity. Increased fluid intake, avoidance of constipating medications, and use of fiber-containing formulas or fiber supplements may be helpful if constipation develops.

Children fed exclusively via tube for extended periods, especially during the first year of life, may develop oral hypersensitivity, poor oral-motor skills, and food aversions. Transitioning from tube to oral nutrition often requires the involvement of an occupational therapist, behavioral psychologist, or other trained individual. Avoidance of a strict nothing by mouth (NPO) status, if possible, is recommended.

PARENTERAL NUTRITION

Early parenteral nutrition (PN) techniques could not provide sufficient calories to support normal development due to the inability of peripheral veins to tolerate highly osmolar solutions or for the patients to tolerate large fluid volumes. In 1963, Wilmore and Dudrick[53] reported the first successful use of central venous PN in a child. Central venous PN has since provided a means to support normal growth and has resulted in decreased mortality for a number of patient populations, particularly those infants with surgical or other catastrophic gastrointestinal defects or diseases.[54] PN is indicated only when a trial of EN has failed or when severely diminished intestinal function is anticipated due to underlying disease or treatment.[55] Common diagnoses necessitating the use of PN in children are similar to those of adults with the exception of extreme prematurity.

Central versus Peripheral Administration

Route selection, peripheral versus central, depends on expected length of therapy, caloric stores and needs, peripheral vein access, and inpatient or outpatient status. Peripheral administration is limited by the solution osmolality. The AAP recommends that peripherally administered solutions not exceed 900 mOsm/L.[56] Central administration is limited primarily by catheter complications including infection and thrombosis.

Caloric Needs

Carbohydrate is generally administered as dextrose and, due to osmolality limitations, the maximum dextrose concentration recommended for peripheral PN is 10%. Phlebitis and other catheter complications are increased with higher concentrations. Dextrose is usually advanced over several days to provide 40–60% of nonprotein calories. In neonates, dextrose is initiated at 5–6 mg/kg/min and advanced by 1–2 mg/kg/min daily to approximately 10–14 mg/kg/min. Older children less than 16 years of age usually tolerate larger daily increases in dextrose. Increases of 2–4 mg/kg/min up to 6–9 mg/kg/min are generally well tolerated. Children older than 16 years of age should receive dextrose at 2–5 mg/kg/min as recommended in adults.[57] Dextrose tolerance can be monitored by checking serum and urine glucose every 8–24 hours initially and less frequently once tolerance is documented.

Insulin must be used with caution since children, especially neonates, may have variable reactions to insulin administration that can result in hypoglycemia.[57,58] If persistent hyperglycemia is present, it is prudent to administer insulin as a separate continuous infusion, 0.05–0.1 unit/kg/h initially, or as a sliding scale, which will allow more careful titration of glucose concentrations until daily needs are established. Addition to PN solutions is usually reserved until a chronic daily need has been established.

Protein Sources

Amino acid solutions used in children are the same as those used in adults (see Chapter 133, Parenteral Nutrition) with the exception of two products marketed specifically for neonates and infants: Aminosyn-PF (Abbott Laboratories) and TrophAmine (McGaw Laboratories). Studies comparing outcomes with the use of these products versus standard amino acid solutions demonstrate improved weight gain and nitrogen balance and "normal" amino acid patterns in neonates who receive them.[59,60] Experience with the use of other specialty amino acids such as HepatAmine (McGaw Laboratories) and FreAmine HBC (McGaw Laboratories) is limited in children.

The optimal initiation and advancement protocol for intravenous protein remains controversial. Starting at 0.25–1.0 g/kg/d and advancing by an equal amount daily has been recommended by some, but others initiate amino acid intake at full protein requirements. There is little evidence that tapering is necessary; however, tapering may be appropriate for very low birth weight neonates and in children with renal or severe hepatic dysfunction.

Carnitine, an amino acid required for transport of free fatty acids into the mitochondria for β-oxidation and energy production, can be synthesized from lysine and methionine. Synthesis is decreased in premature infants, and low plasma carnitine concentrations and/or overt carnitine deficiency have been documented in premature or surgical infants receiving PN or other carnitine-free diets.[61–63] Additionally, the carnitine content of protein hydrolysate formulas may not be adequate. Routine carnitine supplementation is not yet recommended but doses of 8–16 mg/kg/d intravenously have been shown to improve utilization of intravenous fat emulsions in premature infants.[64] Higher doses may be needed for documented carnitine deficiency; oral doses of 50–100 mg/kg/d have been recommended for correction of carnitine deficiency.

Fat Formulations

Intravenous fat emulsions provide both essential fatty acids and a concentrated iso-osmolar calorie source and have been shown to prolong viability of peripheral intravenous lines when co-infused with dextrose and amino acid solutions.[65] Neonates, with the possible exception of low and very low birth weight infants, are able to use fat as an energy source on the first day of life.[66] Fat emulsions are usually started at 0.25–0.5 g/kg/d in neonates and 0.5–1 g/kg/d in older children and increased daily by an equal amount to a maximum of 3–4 g/kg/d[67] as long as triglycerides are not elevated above 150–200 mg/dL. Tapering may increase tolerance by allowing time for increased lipoprotein lipase production although many children will tolerate higher initial lipid doses. A test dose of 1 mL/kg given over 1 hour for children less than 5 kg and 0.1 mL/min for 10–15 minutes for children greater than 5 kg have been recommended due to the potential for an immediate hypersensitivity reaction. Many institutions omit the test dose but monitor the patient's vital signs carefully during the first hour of the initial lipid infusion. Fat emulsions generally supply 30–50% of calories but should not exceed 60% to prevent ketosis.

Adverse effects of intravenous fat emulsions are similar to those seen in adults. Hyperlipemia is uncommon and is minimized by infusion rates that do not exceed 0.25 g/kg/h.[28,67] Brans et al.[68] demonstrated no adverse effects on pulmonary function when lipids were infused at 4 g/kg/d over 24 hours. There is a potential risk of kernicterus with the use of fat emulsions in neonates with hyperbilirubinemia since fat emulsions are hydrolyzed to triglycerides which are converted to free fatty acids (FFAs). These FFAs compete with bilirubin for albumin binding sites. Displacement depends on the relative concentrations of albumin, bilirubin, and unesterified fatty acids.[69] Gutcher et al.[70] found that infants approximately 24 hours of age receiving 1 g/kg/d of intravenous lipid experienced a significant rise in free bilirubin concentration associated with increased FFAs. The measured FFA-to-albumin ratio, however, never exceeded six, the level at which significant displacement is expected.[71] Caution is warranted in infants whose bilirubin concentration exceeds 12 mg/dL. In these newborns, fat infusions should be limited to 0.5–1.0 g/kg/d, doses sufficient to prevent EFAD, and increased once the bilirubin is consistently less than 12 mg/dL.[72]

Electrolyte and Vitamin Requirements

Parenteral electrolyte requirements are shown in Table 135.13. Requirements may be altered with pathologic states such as necrotizing enterocolitis, peritonitis, prematurity, renal and hepatic dysfunction, and drug therapy such as diuretics, amphotericin B, and corticosteroids. Of particular interest in pediatrics is the conditional solubility in solution of calcium and phosphorus. Factors determining solubility include pH, time, temperature, order of mixing, and concentration of the two minerals. Pediatric-specific amino acid solutions have a lower pH and are useful in neonates since they allow for improved delivery of calcium and phosphorus.

Current recommendations for intravenous vitamin intake in children are based on revisions[73] of the American Medical Association Nutritional Advisory Group's 1979 guidelines.[74] The appropriateness of these guidelines has been questioned. MVI-Pediatric (Lyphomed) is the only product marketed specifically to meet these needs. For children greater than 3 kg to 11 years of age, the recommended daily dose is 5 mL/d. Preterm infants should receive

TABLE 135.13. INTRAVENOUS ELECTROLYTE REQUIREMENTS FOR NEONATES, INFANTS, AND CHILDREN

Recommended Intake	Preterm Neonates	Full-Term and Infants	Children
Sodium (mEq/kg/d)	3–6[a]	2–5	2–5
Potassium (mEq/kg/d)	2–3[a]	2–5	2–5
Chloride (mEq/kg/d)	3–6[a]	2–5	2–5
Phosphorus (mmol/kg/d)	1.5–2	1–2	1–1.5
Magnesium (mEq/kg/d)	0.5–1	0.5–1	0.25–0.5
Calcium (mEq/kg/d)	2–4	1–2	0.5–1
Acetate	b	b	b

[a]Higher requirements may be needed for newborns and low birth weight or very low birth weight infants or with concomitant disease (e.g., necrotizing enterocolitis).
[b]As needed to maintain acid–base balance.

2 mL/kg (i.e., 40% of the 5-mL vial/kg) up to 5 mL/d.[73] Children older than 11 years of age may receive an adult vitamin preparation.

Recommended parenteral intakes of essential trace elements are shown in Table 135.14.[73,75] Combination products are available specifically for children which provide manganese, copper, chromium, zinc, and selenium. Usual recommended intake is 0.3 mL/kg for children weighing less than 3 kg and 0.2 mL/kg for children weighing more than 3 kg with a maximum recommended intake of 5 mL/d.[75] Children weighing more than 25 kg may receive the recommended adult dose and product. Due to decreased elimination, trace element intake may need to be decreased in renal disease (zinc, selenium, chromium) and cholestatic liver disease (copper, manganese). Children with high ostomy or stool output and burns will need extra zinc.

Prematurity, acute illness, chronic gastrointestinal losses, and long-term, selenium-free total PN are associated with low selenium levels and decreased glutathione peroxidase activity.[76] The clinical significance of reduced selenium levels is unclear. Selenium supplementation is recommended for preterm and term infants after 2 weeks of PN[77] and for older children after 4 weeks[73] (see Table 135.14).

TABLE 135.14. RECOMMENDED DAILY INTAKE OF PARENTERAL TRACE ELEMENTS

Trace Element	Preterm Neonate	Term	Children
	mcg/kg/d (maximum daily dose μg/d)		
Zinc	300–400	250 (<3 months) 100 (>3 months)	50 (5000)
Copper	20	20	20 (300)
Chromium	0.14–0.2	0.14–0.2	0.14–0.2 (5)
Manganese	1	1	1 (50)
Selenium	1.5–2	2–3	2–3 (30)
Molybdenum[a]	0.25	0.25	0.25 (5)
Iodide[a]	1	1	1

[a]Long-term PN only.

Iodine is not routinely added to PN solutions, but children have been maintained on iodine-free total PN without developing evidence of hypothyroidism. Iodine absorption from topical povidone iodine used during catheter dressing changes and the iodide contaminant in PN solutions is apparently adequate.[78–80] Periodic assessment for signs of hypothyroidism is suggested but routine monitoring of thyroid hormone levels is not recommended.

Oral iron supplementation is preferred to the use of parenteral iron since iron absorption from the proximal small intestine may occur even with bowel impairment. When oral therapy is not possible, intravenous or intramuscular iron may be given. Local muscular reactions, pain, and skin staining with intramuscular injection make the intravenous route preferred. Iron has been administered daily in PN solutions but monthly administration with the total monthly requirement given over several days is effective, less time consuming, and less expensive.[81] Iron doses required for iron-deficiency anemia can be calculated using Eq. (4), where hemoglobin (g/dL) desired (Hgb_d) is 12 if < 15 kg or 14.8 if > 15 kg and Hgb_a is measured hemoglobin (g/dL).

$$\text{Dose (mg Fe)} = \text{wt (kg)} \times 4.5 \times (Hgb_d - Hgb_a) \quad (4)$$

The maximum recommended daily dose of iron dextran is 25 mg for children weighing less than 5 kg, 50 mg for children weighing 5–10 kg, and 100 mg for children weighing more than 10 kg infused no faster than 50 mg/min. Anaphylaxis is uncommon but may occur with iron dextran. A test dose of 0.5 mL (0.25 mL for infants) given over 1 hour has been recommended. When iron dextran is added to PN solutions, many practitioners institute anaphylactic precautions for 1 hour after the infusion is started in lieu of a test dose.

Metabolic and electrolyte abnormalities experienced in children receiving PN are similar to those in adults. Two complications with unique presentations in children are metabolic bone disease and cholestatic jaundice. The etiology of PN-associated cholestatic jaundice remains unclear. Toxic effects of amino acids and lipids have been proposed but not substantiated. Excess energy intake probably contributes to cholestasis. Nutrient deficiencies (e.g., taurine, carnitine) have also been linked to the development of cholestatic jaundice. Liver toxicity is apparent generally only after several weeks or more on total PN. In the early stages, liver dysfunction is reversible but may be progressive, leading to fulminant hepatic failure. Premature infants, especially those experiencing necrotizing enterocolitis or sepsis, appear to develop liver dysfunction more commonly than others receiving long-term PN. Preventive strategies include early provision of enteral nutrients, cycling of PN solutions, and avoidance of overfeeding.

Due to the relative insolubility of calcium phosphate in PN solutions, the amount of calcium provided to premature infants may not be adequate for normal bone mineralization. However, serum calcium concentrations will remain normal despite inadequate intake due to calcium release from bone. Osteopenia, rickets, and collapsed vertebrae have been reported in both low birth weight and term infants requiring prolonged PN. Alkaline phosphatase activity is a good marker for metabolic bone disease.

Cyclic PN is used commonly in children especially in the home, although there is little published information on the practice. Collier et al.[82] reported the use of cyclic PN in 10 infants less than 6 months of age (range 37–124 days). Cycling is usually begun with 1–2 hours "off" each day in infants and 2–4 hours "off" for older children. The time "off" is advanced to 4–6 hours for infants and 12–14 hours for older children as tolerated. Tapering on and off in three steps by beginning at one-third to one-fourth the final rate for 30 minutes, increasing to two-thirds to one-half the final rate for 30 minutes, and then increasing to the final rate is well tolerated. Serum glucose should be evaluated 30–60 minutes after discontinuation or advancement to full rate. Hyperglycemia is uncommon; hypoglycemia, if it occurs, is usually transient and asymptomatic.

Besides the increased mobility offered by cycling, a decreased incidence of cholestatic jaundice may be associated with its use. Collier et al.[82] reported a decrease in total bilirubin concentration after 2 weeks of cycling although this difference was not statistically significant. Others have noted improved hepatic function with cycling. If PN is expected to be used for more than 1 month, early cycling may delay or decrease liver disease.

PHARMACIST'S CONTRIBUTION TO PATIENT OUTCOMES

The pharmacist involved with the care of children must be aware of the importance of adequate nutrition to normal growth and development. Pharmacists practicing in any setting should be comfortable with nutrition assessment techniques which allow for identification of over- and undernutrition as well as those at risk for malnutrition. Drug therapies with potential negative effects on nutrition must be identified and appropriate steps taken to prevent or correct the effects. Once a child has been found to be either malnourished or at risk, the pharmacist, along with other members of an interdisciplinary patient care team, can participate in the development and monitoring of an appropriate nutrition support plan individualized for the patient to ensure that the desired outcomes are met. Desired outcomes will vary from patient to patient. In children, the pharmacist can monitor adequacy of calorie, protein, and other nutrient intake by monitoring growth and development as well as appropriate laboratory tests. The pharmacist, both inpatient and outpatient, can be a vital resource to patients, families, and other health care professionals.

GERIATRIC NUTRITION

The elderly population in the United States is the fastest growing segment of our population. It is estimated that by the year 2000, 13% of the population will be older than 65 years old, with those older than 85 being in the highest proportion.[83,84] The elderly are the most heterogeneous group in our society encompassing all levels in terms of socioeconomic status, health status, marital status, and educational background. It is estimated that 85% of all older Americans are at risk of malnutrition[84] and its associated adverse effects such as increased rate of infection, poor wound healing, and increased morbidity and mortality (see Chapter 131, Prevalence and Significance of Malnutrition). Although an increasing number of elderly are leading vigorous lifestyles, those that are at risk of poor health will have a greater likelihood of dependence, which is estimated to have an enormous impact on our health care systems.[83]

PHYSIOLOGIC CHANGES

The human aging process is a continuum of biological alterations. Changes in organ function, body composition, and physical performance are all part of this process and occur at varying rates in each individual. Factors that influence these changes include disease pathology, genetics, socioeconomic status, diet, and the environment. Nutrition plays a key role in maintaining biologic processes, preventing diseases, and aiding in the recovery from acute illness.

Body composition changes are the most obvious of the aging process. They include decreases in lean body mass, total body water, and bone density and an increase in total body fat. Unequivocally, the decrease in lean body mass (LBM) or muscle tissue, which includes both skeletal muscle (somatic tissue) and smooth muscle (visceral/organ tissue), is the most outstanding. There is a progressive decline in LBM through the years. From the ages of 25–70 years, males will lose 16–19% of their LBM while females will lose 12%.[85] This decrease in muscle mass is secondary to decreases in protein synthesis and physical activity. Exercise can help minimize the amount of muscle lost as well as aid in rebuilding muscle mass in the elderly.

Corresponding with the decrease in LBM is an increase in adipose (fat) tissue. This occurs slowly from the ages of 25–70 years. During this time, body fat will increase by 18% in males and 12% in females.[85] Along with the increase in fat proportion there is also an alteration in fat distribution. As people age, fat tends to be located on the trunk of the body with internal fat deposited around the vital organs. This type of fat distribution has been associated with increased risk for cardiovascular disease, stroke, and cancer.[86]

Total body water (TBW) decreases 10–20% by age 70–80 years.[85] Seventy-two percent of TBW is found in LBM as the intracellular compartment, hence, with a decrease in LBM there is a subsequent decrease in TBW. Decreases in TBW contribute to an increased likelihood of rapid dehydration under conditions of inadequate fluid intake.

Bone mass peaks at age 35 years and is determined by genetics, age, gender, exercise, and calcium intake. Bone loss occurs gradually over time, commencing between the ages of 40–50 years, with the degree of loss varying according to gender and anatomic site.[87]

Organ function declines with age. Changes in cardiovascular, pulmonary, hepatic, renal, and gastrointestinal function ultimately affect nutrient and substrate requirements, tolerance, and utilization. Of these, gastrointestinal changes may be the most obvious to have an impact on nutrition status. A reduced rate of gastric emptying, with accompanying reductions in gastric acid, intrinsic factor, and pepsin secretion, all have a potential impact on nutrient utilization. Small intestinal changes include a diminished production of enzymes and a decline in absorptive capacity. In addition, large intestine motility is frequently slowed with constipation being a chief complaint of the elderly. This constipative state is enhanced by a low-fiber diet, lack of exercise, and insufficient fluid intake. Finally, other age-related transformations of importance to nutrition include insulin resistance, depressed response to thirst, a decreased ability to sense odor, and an altered taste sensitivity.[88]

NUTRITION ASSESSMENT

Nutrition status plays an important role in the function of all muscle groups and organ systems and can be a factor in the length of hospital stay, wound healing, immune function, and mental status. However, accurately assessing the nutrition status of the elderly presents many challenges. Several factors, including those related to age, need to be evaluated and considered during the assessment process. Older adults tend to have chronic disease states, multiple drug regimens, and physiologic changes which have the potential to alter nutrition status. Body composition changes and lack of established anthropometric measurement standards all influence nutrition assessment parameters and their interpretation.

An accurate assessment combines data gathered from dietary, medical, drug and social histories, physical exam, and appropriate anthropometric and laboratory measurements. During the process of evaluating nutrition status, risk factors associated with malnutrition can also be identified. Risk factors include inappropriate food intake, poverty, social isolation, dependency/disability, acute/chronic diseases or conditions, chronic medication use, and advanced age.[89,90] Furthermore, a nutrition assessment has a predictive or prognostic value in certain settings. Elderly people with a subjective clinical diagnosis of malnutrition along with below-normal values in anthropometric measurements, visceral proteins (albumin, prealbumin, and transferrin), and vitamin A and C concentrations were shown to have increased mortality.[91] Nutrition assessments and screenings are of particular importance in the elderly because once malnutrition or the risk factors of malnutrition are identified, early intervention may preclude a poor response to injury or disease.

The National Health and Nutrition Examination Surveys (NHANES) are conducted by the National Center for Health Statistics of the Centers for Disease Control and Prevention. NHANES I (1971–1975) and NHANES II (1976–1980) gathered data from people aged 1–74 years and 0.5–74 years of age, respectively. These surveys included interviews, physical examinations, and biochemical assessments of more than 20,000 people. From these data, reference materials such as growth and weight/height charts are produced. Unfortunately, no data were collected for the over-75-year-old age group, a group which is at risk for malnutrition. However, NHANES III (1988–1994) set no upper age limit on the participants and planned an oversampling of older people.[92] The oversampling process is to ensure that enough people are surveyed to allow for nonresponders. Furthermore, the National Institute on Aging funded the NHANES III Supplemental Nutrition Survey of Older Americans. This includes gathering 24-hour diet recall information via telephone interviews on people older than 50 years of age who completed parts of the NHANES III survey. Our knowledge of the nutrition status and dietary habits of the elderly should be greatly enhanced once this information is published.[93]

Anthropometric Measurements

Anthropometric measurements are used to estimate body fat and LBM. Typically they include weight, height, limb circumference, and various skinfold thickness measurements. These parameters are used to compare an individual with a population standard, and repeated measurements in the same person can indicate response of an individual to changes in nutrition. Limitations of their utility in the heterogeneous elderly population include lack of age-appropriate norms and standards to interpret the data and reliability in the measurement process.[86,94,95] There are standards, based on frame size, for skinfold thickness (triceps and subscapular) and bone-free upper arm muscle area for people ages 55–74 years.[96] However, the current national standards for those older than 74 years of age are extrapolations of data from younger populations. With no national standards, researchers have focused on defining anthropometric values and reference ranges in the elderly population. One group studied elderly males and females, ages 65–90 years, and published limited reference data for recumbent measurements of subscapular and triceps skinfold thickness and calf and midarm circumference.[97]

The reliability of triceps skinfold thickness measurements in the elderly is compromised. They may be difficult to obtain since skin becomes less resilient and muscle becomes softer with advancing age, making it difficult to differentiate from the fat fold. Furthermore, triceps fat folds tend to decline in elderly women due to redistribution of adipose tissue with less redistribution in men.

Midarm muscle circumference is reflective of somatic protein stores. However, neuropathology and unilateral wasting secondary to stroke may present problems with this measurement.

Weight history should include weight changes over time and as a percentage of ideal body weight. Ideal body weight is generally based on height, which may be difficult to determine in the elderly. Accurate measurement of height depends on the person's ability to stand erect, and older people may be bedridden or have spinal curvature, which prevents this upright posture. In these situations, estimating height, or stature, is based on the measurement of long bones. Measuring from the knee to the heel, with the knee flexed at a 90° angle, the measurement begins 2 inches proximal to the patella. Stature can then be determined by Eq. (5) and Eq. (6).[98]

$$\text{Stature for men (cm)} = [2.02 \times \text{knee ht (cm)}] - [(0.04 \times \text{age (yr)}] + 64.19 \quad (5)$$

$$\text{Stature for women (cm)} = [1.83 \times \text{knee ht (cm)}] - [(0.24 \times \text{age (yr)}] + 84.88 \quad (6)$$

Clinical Assessment

Physical exam and medical history should focus on the identification of major and minor indicators of poor nutritional status (Tables 135.15 and 135.16, respectively). These indicators were developed to allow for prioritization and categorization of observations, and are not absolute indicators of malnutrition.[89] The physical exam should focus on assessing muscle wasting, edema, loss of subcutaneous fat, and physical findings of vitamin, trace element, and essential fatty acid deficiencies (see Chapter 130). Examining the mouth is a crucial part of the physical exam.[88] Poor dentition, mouth lesions, or infections have an impact on the type and quantity of food selected and consumed.

TABLE 135.15. MAJOR INDICATORS OF POOR NUTRITIONAL STATUS IN OLDER AMERICANS

Weight loss over time	5.0% in 1 month 7.5% in 3 months 10% or 10 pounds in 6 months
Low or high weight for height	20% below or above desired body weight
Reduced serum albumin	Serum albumin concentration <3.5 g/L
Change in functional status	Change to "dependent" in 2 of the ADLs or 1 of the nutrition-related IADLs
Inappropriate food intake	Failure to eat minimum U.S. dietary guidelines from more than one basic food group Failure to observe moderation in salt and sugar intake Failure to observe saturated fat limitation Alcohol consumption above 1 oz/d (women) or 2 oz/d (men)
Reduction in midarm circumference	<10th percentile of NHANES standard
Increase or decrease in skinfold	<10th percentile >95th percentile
Obesity	>120% of desirable weight
Nutrition-related disorders	Osteoporosis Osteomalacia Folate deficiency Vitamin B_{12} deficiency

(Reprinted with permission by the Nutrition Screening Initiative, a project of the American Academy of Family Physicians, the American Dietetic Association, and the National Council on the Aging, Inc., and funded in part by a grant from Ross Products Division, Abbott Laboratories.)

A complete medication history to include nonprescription medications (e.g., vitamin/mineral supplements and laxatives) and prescription drugs must be taken. Drug–nutrient interactions are a serious problem in this population since the use of multiple drugs increases the potential for such interactions. Drugs that are of importance include those agents that induce gastrointestinal changes (e.g., narcotics) and/or that alter electrolyte concentrations (e.g., diuretics) and nutrient absorption (e.g., cholestyramine, antacids).[99]

Activities of daily living (ADLs) and instrumental activities of daily living (IADLs) are a general means of assessing functional status. ADLs include bathing, dressing, toileting, and feeding. IADLs are the skills needed to buy and prepare food. A change from independent to dependent in these activities is a potential indicator of poor nutrition status.[89] Chronic disease states such as arthritis and Parkinson's and Alzheimer's diseases have detrimental effects on functional status as well.

TABLE 135.16. MINOR INDICATORS OF POOR NUTRITIONAL STATUS IN OLDER AMERICANS

Concurrent syndrome	Alcoholism Cognitive impairment Chronic renal insufficiency Multiple concurrent medications Malabsorption syndromes
Symptoms	Anorexia Nausea Early satiety Dysphagia Change in bowel habits Fatigue, apathy, memory loss, and new onset falling
Physical signs	Cheilosis, angular stomatitis Glossitis Dehydration Poor dental status Poor wound healing, skin ulcerations Loss of subcutaneous fat Loss of muscular mass Fluid retention
Laboratory deficiencies and decreases	Serum albumin, transferrin or prealbumin Folate Iron Ascorbic acid Zinc

(Reprinted with permission by the Nutrition Screening Initiative, a project of the American Academy of Family Physicians, the American Dietetic Association, and the National Council on the Aging, Inc., and funded in part by a grant from Ross Products Division, Abbott Laboratories.)

Biochemical Parameters

Visceral protein status indicators are albumin, transferrin, prealbumin (transthyretin), and retinol-binding protein. As with the anthropometric standards, normal values for those older than 74 years of age are unknown with the exception of serum albumin, which decreases slightly with increasing age.[100] Hepatic function, stress metabolism, trauma, and hydration status need to be considered when interpreting serum albumin concentrations. Albumin concentrations appear to be a strong prognostic indicator in the elderly and increased mortality has been associated with decreased albumin concentrations.[101,102] However, values appear to be maintained in the elderly who are well and are responsive to nutritional repletion over time. Transferrin values are not reliable nutrition markers in the elderly. They tend to have increased iron stores and therefore less circulating transferrin.[88] Prealbumin and retinol-binding protein concentrations are maintained in the elderly, with prealbumin being the more discriminant biochemical marker of nutrition status.[103]

Other Markers of Protein Status

Creatinine height index is a measure of somatic muscle mass. It is dependent on a 24-hour urine collection, which may be problematic in the elderly without catheterization of the bladder. It is not an accurate reflection of muscle mass in cachectic individuals, those with impaired renal function, or in states of dehydration. It is also important to consider that creatinine excretion declines as age increases and LBM decreases, both of which occur in the elderly.

Nitrogen balance studies rely on a 24-hour urine collection to determine urine urea nitrogen and total urinary nitrogen excretion. Inactivity (immobility, bedridden) leads to an increase in nitrogen excretion secondary to muscle breakdown. Providing increased protein may not reverse this process, thus a negative nitrogen balance results. To preserve muscle mass, or at least decrease the loss, exercise and adequate protein intake are required.

Hematologic Indicators

Nutrition-related anemias secondary to deficiencies in iron, folate, and vitamin B_{12} are more prevalent in the elderly and appear to be related to dietary intake, pathology, and malabsorption. Chronic iron deficiency is often caused by gastrointestinal blood loss as the result of peptic ulcer disease or carcinoma of the colon or stomach. Medications such as aspirin, nonsteroidal anti-inflammatory drugs, or anticoagulants also increase the risk of bleeding and thus iron loss. Folic acid deficiency is caused by low dietary intake, malabsorption, or altered folate metabolism as seen with alcoholism.[104] Common causes of vitamin B_{12} deficiency in the elderly are decreased absorption secondary to atrophic gastritis or ileal resection. Megaloblastic anemia is characteristic of vitamin B_{12} deficiency.[105]

Immunologic Markers

Immune status indicators are affected similarly by age and malnutrition. It is thus difficult to separate the effects of nutrition on the immune system from the normal effects of aging. Quantitative assessments of cell-mediated immunity include skin testing or delayed cutaneous hypersensitivity (see Chapter 130). The incidence of anergy does increase with age, but anergy due to malnutrition can be reversed in the elderly with nutritional repletion over time. These markers are generally not used in routine monitoring but serve as additional indicators of nutrition status.

NUTRIENT REQUIREMENTS

Age, gender, stature, physical activity, health status, and environment all influence individual nutrient and energy (kcal) requirements. There is a decrease in basal metabolic rate with a decline in LBM and less physical activity.

Therefore, total caloric requirements may be reduced in the elderly. Basal energy expenditure (BEE) can be estimated from the Harris–Benedict equations which utilize weight, height, and age in gender-specific equations. These equations were developed over 75 years ago and their application in clinical settings has been questioned.[106,107] Therefore, other equations have been developed for individuals over age 60:

$$\text{Men: BEE (kcal/d)} = 8.8W + 1128H - 1071 \quad (7)$$

$$\text{Women: BEE (kcal/d)} = 9.2W + 637H - 302 \quad (8)$$

where W is actual weight in kilograms and H is the height in meters.[107] Increases in energy requirements above the BEE are estimated to be 1.2–1.5 times the calculated BEE in active healthy elderly.[106,108]

The utility of the RDAs in accurately reflecting the requirements of the elderly is controversial.[109,110] The controversy arises because the RDAs are stated as categories based on age and gender. The uppermost age category is "51 years and older" thus, there is no differentiation between a 51-year-old and a 90-year-old. The RDAs state that both males and females ages 51 years and older require 30 kcal per kg body weight.[25] The RDAs should be viewed as a guideline with modifications employed based on disease state and activity level of the individual.[25]

Unlike energy requirements, protein requirements do not decrease with age. The RDA for protein for ages 15–51 years and older is 0.8 g/kg/d.[25] However, there is some controversy as to whether this is an adequate estimation in the setting of normal renal function. Therefore, protein intake may need to be greater than the RDA to help decrease the loss of LBM. It appears that 1 g protein/kg/d is appropriate in the elderly increasing up to 1.5–2.0 g/kg/d in states of metabolic stress such as infection, trauma, and surgery.[111] In general, protein intake should be 12–14% of total calories in the diet.

Carbohydrate is the major component of the American diet and should be 50–60% of total calories. Glucose tolerance decreases with age and simple sugars are not well tolerated, hence, complex carbohydrates (e.g., starch) should be utilized whenever possible. Fiber is a form of carbohydrate which adds bulk, not calories, to the diet. With fluids and exercise, fiber aids in the normalization of bowel function. As with the younger population, dietary fat requirements should be 30% of total calories to provide energy, essential fatty acids, and fat-soluble vitamins. Limiting the saturated fat to less than 10%, monounsaturated to 10–15%, and polyunsaturated fatty acids to 10% appears to be a prudent recommendation.[112]

Dehydration is likely to occur with increased fluid loss secondary to a compromised urine concentrating ability, an increased insensible fluid loss via fragile skin, and a decreased thirst response. Hence, water is of importance in the elderly. Fluid requirements are estimated to be 30 mL/kg body weight/d or 1.5 to 2.0 L/d.[111]

Vitamin and mineral requirements change slightly with increasing age. Decreases in thiamine, riboflavin, and niacin needs in healthy adults correspond with the decrease in total kilocalories for both males and females 51 years and older.[25] Iron requirements for postmenopausal women also decrease. Vitamin A requirements may need to be decreased to avoid toxicities in the setting of decreased renal and hepatic function, but specific doses have not been determined. Vitamin A toxicity may present as dry skin, bone pain, cracking at the corners of the mouth, and anorexia. Vitamin D requirements increase if exposure to sunlight is decreased since a large part of vitamin D is synthesized by the skin upon exposure to sunlight. Vitamin B_6 deficiency has been noted in several elderly populations, hence requirements may need to be higher than what is stated in the RDAs.[113] Finally, vitamin B_{12} requirements may need to be increased as absorption is decreased in the elderly who have atrophic gastritis, which leads to the inability to digest protein substances which contain vitamin B_{12}.[113]

PHARMACIST'S CONTRIBUTIONS TO PATIENT OUTCOMES

The pharmacist will have several opportunities to assess, establish, and monitor nutrition care. The exact role of the pharmacist will depend on the practice site. Hospitals may employ pharmacists as nutrition support team members to consult on critically ill and/or ambulatory patients. Home care companies may rely on the pharmacist to provide expertise in home parenteral nutrition management. Nursing home consultant pharmacists may find themselves monitoring enteral therapy. In any setting, the pharmacist needs to be cognizant of the indicators of poor nutrition and of the treatment options available for malnutrition in the elderly.

Before nutrition therapy is initiated, the goals of such support need to be identified. The decision to initiate nutrition for the elderly person should be the same as for a younger individual in similar circumstances. Nutrition support in the setting of terminal disease states may require ethical decisions on whether to institute or withdraw nutrition care. In this situation, living wills and advance directives are of value in knowing the patient's attitude toward such endeavors. Once nutrition support is indicated, the route of administration needs to be decided (see Chapters 133 and 134, respectively). To ensure optimal patient outcomes, the pharmacist needs to ensure that adequate calories and protein are provided and harm is not caused by underfeeding or overfeeding of the patient. The elderly require close attention to fluid status and drug–nutrient interactions; therefore, good clinical skills in assessing and monitoring tolerance to therapy are required.

References

1. Merritt RJ, Suskind RM. Nutritional survey of hospitalized pediatric patients. Am J Clin Nutr 1979;32:1320–1325.
2. Pollack MM, Wiley JS, Holbrook PR. Early nutritional depletion in critically ill children. Crit Care Med 1981; 9:580–583.
3. American Society for Parenteral and Enteral Nutrition. Standards for nutrition support: Hospitalized pediatric patients. Nutr Clin Prac 1989;4:33–37.
4. Harris J, Benedict F. A biometric study of basal metabolism in man. Washington, DC, Carnegie Institute of Washington, publication no 279, 1919.
5. World Health Organization. Energy and protein requirements: Report of a joint FAO/WHO/UNU expert consultation. Geneva, World Health Organization, WHO technical report series, no 724, 1985.
6. Schofield C. Predicting basal metabolic rate, new standards and review of previous work. Hum Nutr Clin Nutr 1985;39c(suppl 1):5–42.
7. Caldwell MO, Kennedy CC. Normal nutritional requirements. Surg Clin North Am 1981;61:491–498.
8. Firouzbakhsh S, Mathis RK, Dorchester WL, et al. Measured resting energy expenditure in children. J Pediatr Gastroenterol Nutr 1993;16:136–142.
9. Chwals WJ, Lally KP, Woolley MM, Mahour GH. Measured energy expenditure in critically ill infants and young children. J Surg Res 1988;44:467–472.
10. Marks KH, Maisels MJ, Moore E, et al. Head growth in sick premature infants—a longitudinal study. J Pediatr 1979;94:282–285.
11. Kien CL. Carbohydrates, in Tsang RC, Lucas A, Uauy R, Zlotkin S (eds): Nutritional Needs of the Preterm Infant: Scientific Basis and Practical Guidelines. Baltimore, Williams and Wilkins, 1993, pp 47–64.
12. Wu PYK, Edwards NB, Storm MC. The plasma amino acid pattern of normal term breast-fed infants. J Pediatr 1986;109:347–349.
13. Hamil PVV, Drizd TA, Johnson CL, et al. Physical growth: National Center for Health Statistics percentages. Am J Clin Nutr 1979;32:607–629.
14. Shaffer SG, Quimoro CL, Anderson JV, Hall RT. Postnatal weight changes in low birth weight infants. Pediatrics 1987;79:702–705.
15. Babson SG. Growth of low birthweight infants. J Pediatr 1970;77:11–18.
16. Cronk C, Crocker AC, Pueschel SM, et al. Growth charts for children with Down syndrome: 1 month to 18 years of age. Pediatrics 1988;81:102–110.
17. Reimers KJ, Carlson SJ, Lombard KA. Nutritional management of infants with bronchopulmonary dysplasia. Nutr Clin Prac 1992;7:127–132.
18. Klish WJ. Nutritional assessment, in Wyllie R, Hyams JS (eds): Pediatric Gastrointestinal Disease: Pathophysiology, Diagnosis, Management. Philadelphia, WB Saunders, 1993, pp 1090–1109.
19. Hendricks K. Nutritional assessment, in Baker SB, Baker RD, Davis A (eds): Pediatric Enteral Nutrition. New York, Chapman & Hall, 1994, pp 105–118.
20. Wright JA, Ashenburg CA, Whitaker RC. Comparison of methods to categorize undernutrition in children. J Pediatr 1994;124:944–946.
21. Casey PH, Arnold WC. Compensatory growth in infants with severe failure to thrive. South Med J 1985;78:1057–1060.
22. Ellerstein NS, Ostrov BE. Growth patterns in children hospitalized because of caloric-deprivation failure to thrive. Am J Dis Child 1985;139:164–166.
23. Figueroa-Colon R. Clinical and laboratory assessment of the malnourished child, in Suskind RM, Lewinter-Suskind L (eds): Textbook of Pediatric Nutrition, 2nd ed. New York, Raven Press, 1993, pp 191–205.
24. Lopez AM, Wolfsdorf J, Raszynski A, Contijoch-Serrano V. Estimation of nitrogen balance based on a six-hour urine collection in infants. JPEN 1986;10:517–518.
25. Food and Nutrition Board. Recommended Dietary Allowances, 10th ed. Washington, DC, National Academy Press, 1989.
26. Nash MA. The management of fluid and electrolyte disorders in the neonate. Clin Perinatol 1981;8(2):251–262.
27. Holliday MA, Segar WE. The maintenance need for water in parenteral fluid therapy. Pediatrics 1957;19:823–832.
28. Committee on Nutrition, American Academy of Pediatrics. Nutritional needs of low-birth-weight infants. Pediatrics 1985;75:976–986.
29. Weise K, Zaritsky A. Endocrine manifestations of critical illness in the child. Pediatr Clin North Am 1987;34:119–130.
30. Pollack MM. Nutritional support of children in the intensive care unit, in Suskind RM, Lewinter-Suskind L (eds): Textbook of Pediatric Nutrition, 2nd ed. New York, Raven Press, 1993, pp 207–216.
31. Hildreth M, Carvajal HF. Caloric requirements in burned children. A simple formula to estimate daily caloric requirements. J Burn Care Rehabil 1980;3:78–80.
32. Other nutritional considerations, in Nelson JK, Moxness KE, Jensen MD, Gastineau CF (eds): Mayo Clinic Diet Manual. A Handbook of Nutrition Practices, 7th ed. St. Louis, CV Mosby, 1994, p 457.
33. Udall JN. Malnutrition and re-feeding, in Baker SB, Baker RD, Davis A (eds): Pediatric Enteral Nutrition. New York, Chapman & Hall, 1994, pp 205–216.
34. MacLean WC, de Romana GL, Masse E, Graham GG. Nutritional management of chronic diarrhea and malnutrition: Primary reliance on oral feeding. J Pediatr 1980;97:316–323.
35. American Academy of Pediatrics, Committee on Nutrition. Statement on cholesterol. Pediatrics 1992;90:469–473.
36. Paulsrud JR, Pensler L, Whitten CF, et al. Essential fatty acid deficiency in infants induced by fat-free intravenous feeding. Am J Clin Nutr 1972;25:897–904.
37. Foote KD, MacKinnon MJ, Innis SM. Effect of early introduction of formula versus fat free parenteral nutrition on essential fatty acid status of preterm infants. Am J Clin Nutr 1991;54:93–97.
38. Mandt JM, Teasley-Strausburg KM, Shronts EP. II. Nutritional requirements, in Teasley-Strausburg KM (ed): Nutrition Support Handbook: A Compendium of Products with Guidelines for Usage. Cincinnati, OH, Harvey Whitney Books Company, 1992, pp 19–36.

39. American Academy of Pediatrics, Committee on Nutrition. Vitamin and mineral supplement needs in normal children in the United States. Pediatrics 1980;66:1015–1021.
40. Cystic Fibrosis Foundation (CCF). Consensus conference report: Nutritional assessment and management in cystic fibrosis. vol 1, section V, April 1990. Available upon request from the CCF, 6931 Arlington Road, Bethesda, MD 20814.
41. Kaufman SS, Murray ND, Wood RP, et al. Nutritional support for the infant with extrahepatic biliary atresia. J Pediatr 1987;110:679–686.
42. Orzalesi M, Colarizi P. Critical vitamins for low birthweight infants. Acta Paediatr Scand 1982;(suppl 296):104–109.
43. Briggs GG, Freeman RK, Yaffe SJ. A Reference Guide to Fetal and Neonatal Risk: Drugs in Pregnancy and Lactation, 4th ed. Baltimore, Williams and Wilkins, 1994.
44. Oski FA. Iron-fortified formulas and gastrointestinal symptoms in infants: A controlled study. Pediatrics 1980;66:168–170.
45. Nelson SE, Ziegler EE, Copeland AM, et al. Lack of adverse reactions to iron-fortified formula. Pediatrics 1988;81:360–364.
46. American Academy of Pediatrics, Committee on Nutrition. Iron-fortified infants formulas. Pediatrics 1989;84:1114–1115.
47. American Academy of Pediatrics, Committee on Nutrition. The use of whole cow's milk in infancy. Pediatrics 1992;89:1105–1109.
48. American Academy of Pediatrics, Committee on Nutrition. Soy-protein formulas: Recommendations for use in infant feeding. Pediatrics 1983;72:359.
49. Brady MS, Rickard KA, Ernst JA, et al. Formulas and human milk for preterm infants: A review and update. J Am Diet Assoc 1982;81:547–552.
50. Fuchs GJ, III. Enteral support of the hospitalized child, in Suskind RM, Lewinter-Suskind L (eds): Textbook of Pediatric Nutrition, 2nd ed. New York, Raven Press, 1993, pp 239–246.
51. Thureen PJ, Hay WW, Jr. Conditions requiring special nutritional management, in Tsang RC, Lucas A, Uauy R, Zlotkin S (eds): Nutritional Needs of the Preterm Infant: Scientific Basis and Practical Guidelines. Baltimore, Williams and Wilkins, 1993, pp 243–265.
52. Davis A. Indications and techniques for enteral feeds, in Baker SB, Baker RD, Davis A (eds): Pediatric Enteral Nutrition. New York, Chapman & Hall, 1994, pp 67–94.
53. Wilmore DW, Dudrick SV. Growth and development of an infant receiving all nutrients exclusively by vein. JAMA 1963;203:140–144.
54. Heird WC, Kashyap S, Gomez MR. Parenteral alimentation of the neonate. Semin Perinatol 1991;15:493–502.
55. American Society for Parenteral and Enteral Nutrition. Guidelines for the use of parenteral and enteral nutrition in adult and pediatric patients. J Parenter Enter Nutr 1993; 17(suppl):1SA–52SA.
56. American Academy of Pediatrics, Committee on Nutrition. Commentary on parenteral nutrition. Pediatrics 1983;71:547–552.
57. Teasley-Strausburg KM. Parenteral nutrition. II. Carbohydrate solutions, in Teasley-Strausburg KM (ed): Nutrition Support Handbook: A Compendium of Products with Guidelines for Usage. Cincinnati, OH, Harvey Whitney Books Company, 1992, pp 73–79.
58. American Academy of Pediatrics, Committee on Nutrition. Nutritional needs of preterm infants, in Barness LA (ed): Pediatric Nutrition Handbook, 3rd ed. Elk Grove Village, IL, American Academy of Pediatrics, 1993.
59. Heird WC, Dell RB, Helms RA, et al. Amino acid mixture designed to maintain normal plasma amino acid patterns in infants and children requiring parenteral nutrition. Pediatrics 1987;80:401–408.
60. Helms RA, Christensen ML, Mauer EC, Storm MC. Comparison of a pediatric versus standard amino acid formulation in preterm neonates requiring parenteral nutrition. J Pediatr 1987;110:466–470.
61. Schmidt-Sommerfeld E, Penn D, Wolf H. Carnitine deficiency in premature infants receiving total parenteral nutrition: Effect of L-carnitine supplementation. J Pediatr 1983;102:931–935.
62. Smith RB, Sachan DS, Plattsmier J, et al. Plasma carnitine alterations in premature infants receiving various nutritional regimens. J Parenter Enter Nutr 1988;12:37–42.
63. Tibboel D, Delemarre FMC, Przyrembel H, et al. Carnitine deficiency in surgical neonates receiving total parenteral nutrition. J Pediatr Surg 1990;25:418–421.
64. Helms RA, Mauer EC, Hay WW. Effect of intravenous L-carnitine on growth parameters and fat metabolism during parenteral nutrition in neonates. J Parenter Enter Nutr 1990;14:448–453.
65. Phelps SJ, Cochran EB. Effect of the continuous administration of fat emulsion on the infiltration of intravenous lines in infants receiving peripheral parenteral nutrition solutions. J Parenter Enter Nutr 1989;13:628–632.
66. Andrew F, Chan G, Schiff D. Lipid metabolism in the neonate. J Pediatr 1976;88:273–278.
67. Committee on Nutrition, American Academy of Pediatrics. Use of intravenous fat emulsions in pediatric patients. Pediatrics 1981;68:738–743.
68. Brans YW, Dutton EB, Andrew DS, et al. Fat emulsion tolerance in very low birth weight neonates: Effect on diffusion of oxygen in the lungs and on blood pH. Pediatrics 1986;78:79–84.
69. Starinsky R, Shafrir E. Displacement of albumin-bound bilirubin by free fatty acids. Implications for neonatal hyperbilirubinemia. Clin Chim Acta 1970;29:311–318.
70. Gutcher GR, Farrell PM. Intravenous infusion of lipid for the prevention of essential fatty acid deficiency in premature infants. Am J Clin Nutr 1991;54:1024–1028.
71. Andrew G, Chan G, Schiff D. Lipid metabolism in the neonate. II. The effect of intralipid on bilirubin binding *in vitro* and *in vivo*. J Pediatr 1976;88:279–284.
72. Innis SM. Fat, in Tsang RC, Lucas A, Uauy R, Zlotkin S (eds): Nutritional Needs of the Preterm Infant: Scientific Basis and Practical Guidelines. Baltimore, Williams and Wilkins, 1993, pp 65–86.
73. Greene HL, Hambridge KM, Schanler R, et al. Guidelines for the use of vitamins, trace elements, calcium, magnesium, and phosphorus in infants and children receiving total parenteral nutrition: Report of the subcommittee on Pediatric Parenteral Nutrient Requirements from the Committee

on Clinical Practice Issues of the American Society for Clinical Nutrition. Am J Clin Nutr 1988;48:1324–1342.

74. American Medical Association, Department of Foods and Nutrition, 1975. Multivitamin preparations for parenteral use: A statement by the Nutrition Advisory Group. J Parenter Enter Nutr 1979;3:258–262.
75. American Medical Association. Guidelines for essential trace element preparations for parenteral use: A statement by the Nutrition Advisory Group. J Parenter Enter Nutr 1979;3:263–267.
76. Lockitch G, Jacobson B, Quigley G, et al. Selenium deficiency in low birth weight neonates: An unrecognized problem. J Pediatr 1989;114:865–870.
77. Heird WC, Gomez MR. Parenteral nutrition, in Tsang RC, Lucas A, Uauy R, Zlotkin S (eds): Nutritional Needs of the Preterm Infant: Scientific Basis and Practical Guidelines. Baltimore, Williams and Wilkins, 1993, pp 225–242.
78. Pyati SP, Ramamurthy RS, Krauss MT, Pildes RS. Absorption of iodine in the neonate following topical use of povidone iodine. J Pediatr 1977;91:825–828.
79. Gough DSC, Laing I, Astley P. Thyroid function on short term total parenteral nutrition without iodine supplements. J Parenter Enter Nutr 1982;6:439–440.
80. Moukarzel AA, Buchman AL, Salas JS, et al. Iodine supplementation in children receiving long-term parenteral nutrition. J Pediatr 1992;121:252–254.
81. Cochran EB, Phelps SJ, Helms RA. Parenteral nutrition in pediatric patients. Clin Pharm 1988;7:351–366.
82. Collier S, Crouch J, Hendricks K, Caballero B. Use of cyclic parenteral nutrition in infants less than 6 months of age. Nutr Clin Prac 1994;9:65–68.
83. Randall T. Demographers ponder the aging of the aged and await unprecedented looming elder boom. JAMA 1993;269:2331–2332.
84. Dwyer JT. Screening older Americans' nutritional health: Current practices and future possibilities. Washington, DC, Nutrition Screening Initiative, 1991.
85. Kuczmarski RJ. Need for body composition information in elderly subjects. Am J Clin Nutr 1989;50:1150–1157.
86. Forbes GB. Body composition: Influence of nutrition, disease, growth and aging, in Shils ME, Olson JA, Shike M (eds): Modern Nutrition in Health and Disease, 8th ed. Philadelphia, Lea & Febiger, 1994, pp 781–801.
87. Johnston CC, Slemenda CW. Changes in skeletal tissue during the aging process. Nutr Rev 1992;50:385–387.
88. Chernoff R. Physiologic aging and nutritional status. Nutr Clin Prac 1990;5:8–13.
89. White JV, Ham RJ, Lipschitz DA. Report of nutrition screening: Toward a common view. Washington, DC, Nutrition Screening Initiative, 1991.
90. Posner BM, Jette AM, Smith KW, Miller DR. Nutrition and health risks in the elderly: The Nutrition Screening Initiative. Am J Pub Health 1993;83:972–978.
91. Volkert D, Kruse W, Oster P, Schlierf G. Malnutrition in geriatric patients: diagnostic and prognostic significance of nutritional parameters. Ann Nutr Metab 1992; 36:97–112.
92. Harris T, Woteki C, Briefel RR, Kleinman JC. NHANES III for older persons: Nutrition content and methodological considerations. Am J Clin Nutr 1989;50:1145–1149.
93. McDowell MA. The NHANES III supplemental nutrition survey of older Americans. Am J Clin Nutr 1994;59(suppl):224S–226S.
94. Sullivan DH, Patch GA, Baden AL, Lipschitz DA. An approach to assessing the reliability of anthropometrics in elderly patients. J Am Geri Soc 1989;37:607–613.
95. Chumlea WC, Baumgartner RN. Status of anthropometry and body composition data in elderly subjects. Am J Clin Nutr 1989;50:1158–1166.
96. Frisancho AR. New standards of weight and body composition by frame size and height for assessment of nutritional status of adults and the elderly. Am J Clin Nutr 1984;40:808–819.
97. Chumlea WC, Steinbaugh ML, Roche AF, et al. Nutritional anthropometric assessment in elderly persons 65 to 90 years of age. J Nutr Elderly 1985;4:39–51.
98. Chumlea WC, Roche AF, Mukherjee D. Nutritional assessment of the elderly through anthropometry. Columbus, OH, Ross Laboratories, 1987.
99. Roe DA. Drugs and nutrition in the elderly, in Roe DA (ed): Geriatric Nutrition, 3rd ed. Englewood Cliffs, NJ, Prentice-Hall, 1992, pp 182–207.
100. Morrow FD. Assessment of nutritional status in the elderly: Application and interpretation of nutritional biochemistries. Clin Nutr 1986;5:112–120.
101. Rudman D, Feller AG, Nagari HS, et al. Relation of serum albumin concentrations to death rate in nursing home men. J Parenter Enter Nutr 1987;11:360–336.
102. Corti MC, Guralnik JM, Salive ME, Sorkin JD. Serum albumin level and physical disability as predictors of mortality in older persons. JAMA 1994;272:1036–1042.
103. Kergoat MJ, Leclerc BS, PetitClerc C, Imbach A. Discriminant biochemical markers for evaluating the nutritional status of elderly patients in long-term care. Am J Clin Nutr 1987;46:849–861.
104. Lipschitz DA. Impact of nutrition on the age-related declines in hematopoiesis, in Chernoff R (ed): Geriatric Nutrition. Gaithersburg, MD, Aspen Publishers, 1991, pp 271–287.
105. Klein S, Rogers R. Nutritional requirements in the elderly. Gastroenter Clin North Am 1990;19:473–491.
106. Mason JB, Russell RM. Parenteral nutrition in the elderly, in Rombeau JL, Caldwell MD (eds): Clinical nutrition: Parenteral nutrition, 2nd ed. Philadelphia, WB Saunders, 1993, p 741.
107. Makk LJK, McClave SA, Creech PW, et al. Clinical application of the metabolic cart to the delivery of total parenteral nutrition. Crit Care Med 1990;18:1320–1327.
108. Young VR. Macronutrient needs in the elderly. Nutr Rev 1992;50:454–462.
109. Hegsted DM. Recommended dietary intakes of elderly subjects. Am J Clin Nutr 1989;50:1190–1194.
110. Blumberg JB. Changing nutrient requirements in older adults. Nutrition Today 1992;(Sept/Oct):15–20.
111. Carter WJ. Macronutrient requirements for elderly persons, in Chernoff R (ed): Geriatric Nutrition. Gaithersburg, MD, Aspen Publishers, 1991, pp 11–24.
112. Ausman LM, Russell RM. Nutrition in the elderly, in Shils ME, Olson JA, Shike M (eds): Modern Nutrition in Health and Disease, 8th ed. Philadelphia, Lea & Febiger, 1994, pp 770–780.
113. Russell RM. Micronutrient requirements of the elderly. Nutr Rev 1992;50:463–464.

Chapter 136

Nutritional Considerations in Major Organ Failure

Rex O. Brown, PharmD, and Gordon S. Sacks, PharmD

Organ failure may alter the absorption, utilization, and excretion of essential nutrients. Therefore, administration of "standard" macronutrients and micronutrients to patients with significant organ dysfunction may be inappropriate or harmful. Preparation of a rational nutrition support formula for these patients often requires a carefully planned, disease-specific approach. The monitoring of these patients often requires different markers and laboratory tests, or more frequent use of traditional markers to ensure that the nutrients are being administered in utilizable forms. Also, meticulous assessment of the patient with organ dysfunction is needed to ensure that the nutrition formula is not causing harm. Monitoring the efficacy of nutrition support in patients with organ failure also may be very difficult. For example, it would be impossible to collect a 24-hour urine specimen for urea nitrogen measurement to calculate nitrogen balance in an anuric patient. An alternative method of calculating urea nitrogen appearance or protein catabolic rate is required in this situation.

Alterations in the metabolism or excretion of macronutrients can have a major impact on the preparation of an appropriate nutrition formula, whereas altered homeostasis of a micronutrient may require little adjustment in the nutrition support formula. In this chapter, specific nutritional alterations in patients with hepatic, renal, pulmonary, cardiac, and gastrointestinal failure are presented. Recommendations for nutrition support in patients with multiple organ dysfunction syndrome are also addressed. Approaches to ensure delivery of safe and efficacious macronutrients and micronutrients to patients with these disorders are discussed.

Most patients with acute organ dysfunction or failure will be hospitalized, with a majority of them receiving treatment in an intensive care unit. There is substantial documentation that pharmacists can provide an important service through metabolic monitoring of these types of patients.[1–3] To be effective in providing appropriate nutrition support to these patients, the pharmacist should have a thorough understanding of the pathophysiology of organ failure, fluid and electrolyte balance, acid–base status, hemodynamic monitoring, types of dialysis, and critical care pharmacotherapy. This knowledge coupled with basic pharmacy skills such as compatibility and drug delivery issues can result in the pharmacist being a very effective practitioner for these patients.

Hepatic Failure

The liver is the primary organ involved in the digestion, metabolism, and storage of nutrients. It contains many enzymes and receives, processes, and prepares nutrients for the periphery. Therefore, when functional capacity is depressed, profound macronutrient and micronutrient intolerance may result. Other sequelae that may accompany the failing liver are fluid and electrolyte imbalances, vitamin deficiencies, and undernutrition. The challenge of providing nutrition support in utilizable forms during severe liver failure is thus formidable. Patients whose liver disease has progressed to cirrhosis or hepatic fibrosis will be considered to have hepatic failure. A comprehensive review of this subject contains additional information.[4]

MACRONUTRIENT CONSIDERATIONS

Energy

The increased availability of mobile metabolic carts has allowed researchers to study the energy needs (resting energy expenditure) of specific patient populations. These are instruments that measure oxygen consumption (V_{O_2}) and carbon dioxide production (V_{CO_2}) by indirect calorimetry. These data are particularly valuable in patients who have disease states associated with a poor nutritional status (e.g., hepatic failure). It appears that patients with alcoholic hepatitis or cirrhosis are hypermetabolic (up to 50% greater than expected) when their resting energy expenditure is normalized for lean body mass and compared with normal controls.[5–8]

Carbohydrate

The liver is of critical importance in carbohydrate homeostasis because of its ability to remove and release glucose into the intravascular compartment. In healthy adults, approximately 60% of absorbed glucose is taken up by the liver and utilized for glycogen synthesis, triglyceride synthesis, and glycolysis. In general, glycogen synthesis and glycolysis are enhanced by insulin, while gluconeogenesis and glycogen breakdown are controlled by glucagon.

Hyperglycemia is quite common in patients with cirrhosis, most likely as a result of peripheral insulin resistance.[9] It has been suggested that this disorder is mediated by a decreased binding to insulin receptors and defective postreceptor signal handling in peripheral tissues.[9] Plasma concentrations of insulin are usually elevated with or without a glucose stimulus. This may make administration of large doses of glucose questionable, because administration of insulin to control hyperglycemia may not improve utilization substantially.

Patients with fulminant hepatitis are prone to hypoglycemia. There is depressed hepatic glucose production secondary to decreased glycogen stores and diminished gluconeogenesis. Also, impaired degradation of insulin by the damaged liver may contribute to this disorder. A continuous intravenous infusion of glucose usually prevents hypoglycemia in acute hepatitis, but concentrations greater than 10% glucose in water may be needed in the more severe forms of this disease.

Fat

The liver is responsible for synthesis of cholesterol, high-density lipoproteins, and very low density lipoproteins. The enzymes lipoprotein lipase and lecithin–cholesterol acyltransferase also are synthesized in this organ. Increased serum triglyceride and free fatty acid (FFA) concentrations often are encountered in patients with hepatic dysfunction or failure. Alcohol ingestion has been shown to increase circulating triglycerides, and chronic intake has caused fatty infiltration of the liver. The patient with liver failure may not tolerate standard doses of intravenous fat secondary to elevations in serum triglyceride concentrations during or after fat infusion. Monitoring serum triglyceride concentration and FFA oxidation (using carbon-labeled fat emulsion experimentally) to ensure that intravenously administered lipid is both cleared from the bloodstream and oxidized appropriately has been suggested. Most institutions are not able to measure FFA oxidation, leaving serum triglyceride concentrations as the only available marker. Although not an indicator of utilization, this can help prevent marked hypertriglyceridemia and associated disorders (e.g., pancreatitis) if followed closely. Intravenous fat should be used in patients with liver failure only to prevent essential fatty acid deficiency when serum triglyceride concentrations exceed 300 mg/dL. If serum triglyceride concentrations are low or normal, intravenous fat also may be used as a calorie source. A preliminary report suggests that high-fat parenteral nutrition may improve hepatic encephalopathy when compared with parenteral nutrition, with glucose providing the entire dose of nonprotein calories.[10] Objective tests assessing mental status were better in the group receiving the high-fat parenteral nutrition; however, encephalopathy grade was not improved and mortality was high in all patients. Further research will be required to ascertain if high-fat parenteral nutrition provides any beneficial effect.

Steatorrhea is very common in patients with hepatic cholestasis because inadequate bile acids and pancreatic enzymes are secreted into the gastrointestinal tract lumen. Micelle formation is impeded and thus the long-chain fatty acids pass through the colon, resulting in a foul-smelling, soapy diarrhea. Therefore, assessment of the gastrointestinal tract is necessary before large amounts of lipid are administered by the oral route. Oral medium-chain triglycerides (MCTs) have been used occasionally with success because they do not require pancreatic enzymes or micelle formation before absorption.[11] These products do not, however, provide essential fatty acids.

Protein

Nitrogen requirements for the patient with liver failure are not unlike those of normal subjects, but intolerance to protein is well described in patients with cirrhosis, and protein restriction has been used rather successfully as part of the therapy. A dilemma arises when the diet becomes so restrictive that undernutrition inevitably results and the patient becomes susceptible to infection and other complications. Overzealous use of protein to correct nutritional deficits invariably results in hepatic encephalopathy. Therefore, careful monitoring and recognition that a therapeutic window for protein intake exists (40–80 g/d) are essential.

Because the liver metabolizes the aromatic amino acids (phenylalanine, tyrosine, tryptophan), methionine, and glutamine, the plasma concentrations of these amino acids often are elevated in cirrhotic patients. Plasma concentrations of the branched-chain amino acids (valine, leucine, isoleucine) often are depressed because these amino acids are metabolized by the skeletal muscle. This altered plasma aminogram is thought to be involved in the etiology of hepatic encephalopathy. In health the ratio of branched-chain amino acids to aromatic amino acids is 3–3.5:1, while ratios of 1:1 have been associated with hepatic encephalopathy in patients with cirrhosis.[4]

Therapy directed at the normalization of this altered plasma aminogram has prompted the clinical testing and marketing of both parenteral and enteral nutrition products with modified amino acid profiles.[12] Modified amino acid products may also suppress protein breakdown, stimulate protein synthesis, and serve as a preferential calorie source. While altered plasma amino acid concentrations have been normalized with these products, improvement in encephalopathy or outcome has not been universal. These conflicting results may be explained in part by the complexity of the disease process, the sample size studied, and the length of the evaluation period. Other etiologies of hepatic encephalopathy include excessive ammonia production from conversion of protein in the gastrointestinal tract and increased concentrations of glutamine, free tryptophan, or γ-aminobutyric acid in the central nervous system. Most likely, hepatic encephalopathy is a multifactorial disorder that includes several of these etiologies.

In most cases, parenteral nutritional support in the patient with liver failure can be accomplished via the administration of standard mixed amino acids (Fig. 136.1). If the gastrointestinal tract is functioning, the enteral route should be used. In those patients with grade III or IV encephalopathy (see Alcoholic Liver Disease, Chapter 37) who have decompensated or have not attained nitrogen equilibrium while receiving moderate doses of standard amino acids, use of a modified amino acid should be considered. This provides amino acid nitrogen in high concentrations of branched-chain amino acids and low concentrations of aromatic amino acids and methionine. Because this modified amino acid product costs considerably more than standard amino acids, the strict criteria described before should be used to prevent inappropriate use leading to unnecessary expense.

Fluid and Electrolytes

Patients with severe cirrhosis often have ascites and peripheral edema. This represents excess total body sodium with an even greater excess in total body water. Hyponatremia invariably results from this disorder. Increased sympathetic activity has been shown to correlate well with the impaired sodium and water excretion in cirrhotic patients. Stimulation of arginine vasopressin secretion secondary to a decrease in effective blood volume also has been demonstrated. Generally, salt and fluid restriction is required so as not to exacerbate this overhydrated state. It is not uncommon for patients who require parenteral nutrition to have sodium eliminated from the formulation. Severe sodium and fluid restriction during intravascular depletion may cause or exacerbate hepatic encephalopathy. Therefore, during fluid and salt restriction, patients should be observed closely for symptoms of volume depletion (e.g., pulse rate, blood pressure, dry mucous membranes). Severe hypernatremia and volume depletion have been reported in association with lactulose therapy in patients with portal-systemic encephalopathy.[13]

Hypokalemia is very common in the patient with liver failure who has normal renal function. Poor intake and frequent vomiting may cause this disorder. If vomiting is severe enough, contraction alkalosis may occur, which results in increased renal excretion of potassium. Secondary hyperaldosteronism, which is frequently seen in the liver failure patient with intravascular depletion, also increases renal excretion of potassium. Loop-diuretic therapy can increase renal excretion of potassium, while diarrhea secondary to lactulose or antacid therapy may increase fecal excretion of this essential ion. All these conditions can lead to profound hypokalemia. Therefore, potassium requirements in the liver failure patient receiving specialized nutrition support are often increased twofold over standard amounts.

Treating patients with upper gastrointestinal hemorrhages with vigorous antacid therapy can lead to hypophos-

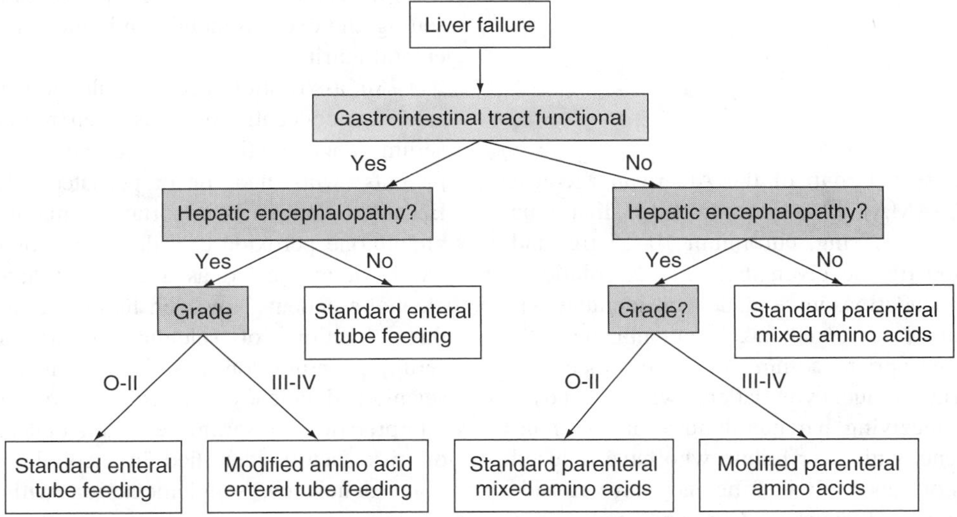

Figure 136.1. Nutrition support approach for the patient with liver failure (selection of amino acid).

phatemia and, potentially, phosphate depletion. Patients with liver failure are very susceptible to upper gastrointestinal hemorrhage and frequently are treated with these drugs. During nutrition support, requirements for intracellular ions such as phosphorus may be supranormal as synthesis of lean body mass occurs (refeeding). Therefore, this patient population is at particular risk of developing hypophosphatemia from concomitant antacid administration and refeeding.

Poor intake and increased excretion of magnesium secondary to diuretic therapy or alcohol ingestion contribute to depletion of magnesium and hypomagnesemia in the liver failure patient.[14] Magnesium repletion is usually part of standard care of the alcoholic patient with liver failure early in the hospital course; however, needs may become supranormal during aggressive nutrition support. The dose of magnesium should be individualized to maintain serum concentrations in the normal range during nutrition support. This often results in magnesium concentrations as high as 24 mEq/L in parenteral nutrition (PN), which results in doses of two to three times standard amounts.

Acid–Base Disorders

Liver failure patients who have excessive diarrhea will lose considerable quantities of bicarbonate in the stool, leading to metabolic acidosis. Replacement therapy with bicarbonate may be required. Acetate or citrate will be ineffective because the diseased liver often cannot convert these ions to bicarbonate. Excessive losses of gastrointestinal fluid secondary to vomiting or nasogastric suction can result in considerable loss of acid, and lead to metabolic alkalosis. Replacement therapy in these patients should include volume, potassium, and chloride. It would be common in these types of patients to require from 80–100 mEq of KCl/L in PN until the potassium deficit is corrected.

MICRONUTRIENT CONSIDERATIONS

Trace Elements

The Nutrition Advisory Group of the American Medical Association (NAG-AMA)[15] has recommended that zinc 2.5–4 mg, copper 0.5–1.5 mg, chromium 10–15 μg, and manganese 150–800 μg, be given daily in PN solutions. Since these recommendations were made, considerable evidence that selenium is essential has been published.[16,17] Data addressing appropriate administration of trace elements and monitoring frequency in patients with organ dysfunction who are receiving parenteral nutrition are relatively scarce. Patients with liver failure who have reduced bile acid synthesis or pancreatic insufficiency have considerable malabsorption and diarrhea. Chronic diarrhea has been shown to cause zinc deficiency because stool contains substantial quantities of zinc.[18] Other potential mechanisms associated with hypozincemia in liver disease include altered zinc metabolism, increased urinary losses, and decreased absorption secondary to elevated cytokine concentrations. Cytokines such as tumor necrosis factor (TNF)-α, interleukin (IL)-1, and IL-6 may stimulate metallothionein, an intestinal zinc-binding protein, thereby inhibiting zinc absorption.[19] Considering the importance of zinc in metalloenzyme reactions, wound healing, immunocompetence, and the senses of taste and smell, patients with chronic diarrhea or large ostomy losses should be suspected of having zinc deficiency if replacement therapy has not been administered. This may be very difficult in a patient receiving a protein-restricted diet because substantial amounts of zinc are found in red meat. Oral supplementation of zinc as zinc sulfate capsules or intravenous zinc as zinc chloride can be used to prevent deficiency or correct deficits. Oral supplementation with zinc acetate in a small group of cirrhotic patients has been reported to improve hepatic encephalopathy.[20] The authors suggested that correction of an underlying zinc deficiency allowed appropriate conversion of ammonia to urea nitrogen in these patients. Further work in this area is required.

Because copper and manganese are excreted in the bile, it has been recommended that these two trace elements not be administered or be administered in reduced doses to patients with serous cholestasis.[15] Although manganese toxicity is rare, copper overload or toxicity causes symptoms such as severe nausea and vomiting. Administration of copper should, therefore, be addressed in the parenteral nutrition patient with cholestasis. It is prudent to withhold copper from the PN solution until a copper serum concentration in the normal range is documented or the cholestasis resolves (e.g., sepsis). Patients who have chronic cholestasis may require copper in reduced doses (e.g., 0.6 mg/d); however, they should have serum copper concentrations checked regularly (once per month in the acute care setting and every 6 months in home patients receiving parenteral nutrition).

An association between alcoholism and low serum selenium concentrations has been reported.[21] The lowest serum concentrations of selenium were reported in patients who had decompensated alcoholic cirrhosis. Because selenium is important in maintaining the enzyme glutathione peroxidase, a deficiency of this trace element has been implicated as a cause of hepatic injury in the alcoholic patient. However, human serum contains at least three fractions of selenium, complicating the use of serum selenium concentrations as an accurate marker for selenium deficiency. Therefore, care must be used in the interpretation of serum selenium concentrations.[19] Based on risk factors identified in alcoholic patients for selenium deficiency, supplementation with selenium should be considered during parenteral nutrition in this patient population.

Vitamins

Deficiencies of vitamins are common in patients with chronic liver disease. Poor intake and malabsorption are the principal causes of these nutrient disorders. Depletion of hepatic stores of vitamin A, pyridoxine, folic acid, riboflavin, pantothenic acid, vitamin B_{12}, and thiamine have been reported in patients with hepatic failure. Folic acid deficiency, the most common vitamin deficiency, may lead to megaloblastic anemia, while thiamine deficiency may result in Wernicke's encephalopathy after rehydration with intravenous glucose. When dextrose-based parenteral nutrition is started in these patients, additional thiamine may be needed to prevent Wernicke's encephalopathy, especially if thiamine was not replaced after admission to the hospital.[4]

Hepatic stores of vitamin A have been reported to be depleted in the patient with alcoholic liver injury.[22] Because vitamin D is metabolized to one of the active forms, 25-hydroxyvitamin D, in the liver, low concentrations of this vitamin are seen in patients with biliary cirrhosis. Impaired absorption of dietary vitamin D also may contribute to these low serum concentrations. It is unclear whether vigorous supplementation of these fat-soluble vitamins should be given to these patients during nutrition support, but therapeutic doses are indicated when a deficiency has been documented.

ADMINISTRATION ROUTES AND PRODUCTS

Parenteral Therapy

Generally, the indications for parenteral nutrition in the patient with liver failure would be similar to those for general hospitalized patients. Patients with liver failure may have periods of acute malabsorption and maldigestion requiring parenteral nutrition or specialized enteral nutrition support. Concomitant sepsis, which may cause a prolonged ileus, also would require the parenteral route for nutrient administration. If the gastrointestinal tract is functional and accessible, enteral nutrition support should be attempted. A recent prospective study demonstrated a more rapid improvement in median encephalopathy scores and serum bilirubin concentrations in alcoholic liver disease patients receiving a regular diet supplemented with specialized enteral nutrition support.[23]

The major controversy in nutrition support of the patient with liver failure has centered around the use of protein products. The package insert of intravenous standard amino acids lists hepatic coma as a contraindication, but these products have been cautiously administered for years. A modified amino acid solution for parenteral nutrition (Hepatamine, McGaw Laboratories) is now marketed for patients with liver failure and hepatic encephalopathy. It is enriched with branched-chain amino acids (BCAAs) and has reduced amounts of aromatic amino acids (AAAs) and methionine. The product was formulated on the basis of the false neurotransmitter hypothesis where AAAs become elevated in the serum and pass into the central nervous system (CNS) resulting in hepatic encephalopathy.

Administration of Hepatamine during parenteral nutrition has normalized plasma profiles of amino acids, which correlated with improved encephalopathy in some studies.[24] One prospective, randomized clinical trial involved comparison of neomycin/glucose with modified amino acids/ glucose and found decreased encephalopathy scores and mortality in the amino acid group.[24] Currently, this is the best controlled study available evaluating amino acids in liver failure; however, it is not clear whether the benefit in the treatment group was derived from the modified amino acid formula or simply the administration of amino acid nitrogen. Interestingly, a study from France failed to show improvement in hepatic encephalopathy when modified amino acids were compared with standard amino acids during parenteral nutrition in cirrhotic patients.[25] Likewise, a study from Japan demonstrated no difference in prevalence of hepatic encephalopathy between standard and modified amino acids in postoperative cirrhotics.[26] The patients in the latter study did not have hepatic encephalopathy before surgery and the prevalence of it was very low in both groups after surgery. Therefore, this may not have been an appropriate group of patients to study with this specialized formulation. A meta-analysis of the benefits of parenteral modified amino acids suggests a significant benefit in mental recovery from high-grade encephalopathy.[27]

Other studies with modified amino acids in liver failure have shown efficacy comparable with that of lactulose,[28] improvement in plasma aminograms without improvement in encephalopathy,[29] and very low tyrosine and cystine concentrations without improvement in encephalopathy.[30] These studies either had few subjects, used an intravenous formula with only BCAAs (i.e., not a complete nutritional formula), or attempted comparison of this nutritional product with standard pharmacologic therapy. Table 136.1 gives an example of a central PN formula for a patient in liver failure. These patients need a very individualized approach based on fluid and electrolyte balance, acid–base status, grade of encephalopathy, and concurrent pharmacotherapy.

Enteral Therapy

Currently, two products are being marketed as food supplements for patients with hepatic encephalopathy (Hepatic-Aid II, McGaw Laboratories; NutriHep, Clintec Nutrition Company). Both supplements have increased amounts of BCAAs and reduced amounts of AAAs and methionine, but differ with regards to micronutrient composition. Hepatic-Aid II is virtually electrolyte and vitamin free, necessitating supplementation in appropriate amounts if tube feeding is

TABLE 136.1. EXAMPLES OF PN FORMULAS FOR PATIENTS WITH ORGAN FAILURE

	Hepatic Failure	Hepatic Transplantation	Acute Renal Failure	Chronic Renal Failure	Respiratory Failure	Cardiac Failure	Short Bowel Syndrome
Dextrose, %[a]	25	20	40	30	15	30	25
CAAs, %	5[b]	5	3	4	5	6[c]	5
Lipid, %	2	2	1	2	4	2	1.5
0.45% sodium chloride injection, mL	—	—	—	—	—	—	500
Na Chloride-, mEq/L	0	0	0	0	0	0	80[d]
Na acetate, mEq/L	0	0	0	30	0	0	0
Na phosphate, mM/L	15	15	0	7.5	30	15	15
K acetate, mEq/L	50	40	0	0	50	40	60
Acetate, mEq/L	0	0	0	10	0	0	0
Magnesium sulfate, mEq/L	16	20	0	6	12	12	20
Calcium gluconate, mEq/L	5	10	0	5	5	5	10
Multivitamins, mL/d	10	10	10	10	10	10	10
Zinc, mg/d	3	8	3	3	3	3	10
Copper, mg/d	1.2	1.2	1.2	1.2	1.2	1.2	12
Manganese, µg/d	300	300	300	300	300	300	300
Chromium, µg/d	12	12	12	12	12	12	20
Selenium, µg/d	40	40	—	40	40	40	60

[a]Final concentrations after admixture.
[b]Hepatamine 4% when criteria for use are met.
[c]Amino acid 15% product would be needed to make this formulation.
[d]Does not include 0.45% sodium chloride injection or lipid.

used as the sole source of nutrient intake. NutriHep meets the U.S. RDA vitamin and mineral requirements, contains a high percentage of MCTs and is supplemented with carnitine. The clinical trials using these products have been inconsistent.[31] Comparative studies (dietary protein versus dietary protein/BCAA supplement) have demonstrated benefit by improving nitrogen balance, encephalopathy grade, and mortality.[32–34] A cooperative study demonstrated improved nutritional status in patients with alcoholic hepatitis who were given BCAA supplementation with their normal hospital diet.[35] It appears that the chronic use of these enteral diets is beneficial in cirrhotic patients, especially those who become encephalopathic with normal doses of dietary protein. Restriction of these modified amino acid supplements is suggested as outlined in Fig. 136.1.

Recently, there has been considerable interest in the use of vegetable-protein diets in the chronic management of patients with cirrhosis and hepatic encephalopathy. Enthusiasm for this therapy is based on the reduced amounts of phenylalanine, tyrosine, methionine, and tryptophan in vegetable protein. Some authors propose that the beneficial effects of vegetable protein may also result from decreased nitrogen absorption in response to increased gastrointestinal transit or an increased fecal nitrogen excretion by colonic bacterial flora.[36] Dried beans are an example of a vegetable high in protein. Although these diets are somewhat more difficult to adhere to, preliminary results justify further study of this concept.[36]

FUTURE DIRECTIONS

Some work has been completed in patients with hepatic encephalopathy who received ketoanalogues of essential or branched-chain amino acids.[37,38] Benefit from this therapy has been marginal at best and interest in this theory may be waning. Certainly, more studies demonstrating which patients with liver failure need modified amino acids for optimal therapy are required.

HEPATIC TRANSPLANTATION

Orthotopic liver transplantation has become an important intervention for the patient with end-stage liver disease.[39] Many patients receive PN support following this operation because of their poor preoperative nutritional status and the postoperative stress. Although hypermetabolism [36–38% above the basal energy expenditure (BEE)] in the early postoperative period has been previously reported,[40] a recent study demonstrated that a caloric intake 1.2 times BEE would achieve caloric requirements immediately post-transplantation and up to 28 days after transplantation. Increased protein catabolism and urinary 3-methylhistidine have also been noted in response to the stress of liver transplantation and the administration of large doses of corticosteroids following surgical intervention.[41]

MACRONUTRIENT CONSIDERATIONS

Carbohydrate

Postoperative hyperglycemia is very common during the first 24 hours after orthotopic hepatic transplantation. Therefore, it is recommended to wait 24 hours before starting parenteral nutrition or begin very slowly with a relatively low concentration of dextrose (e.g., $D_{15}W$). Cyclosporine, which is routinely given to these patients to prevent organ rejection, has been reported to suppress insulin synthesis and secretion as well as increase insulin clearance.[42] Administration of this drug may thus contribute to the hyperglycemia observed during the postoperative period.

Protein

Most patients will tolerate standard amino acids following orthotopic hepatic transplantation because the new liver is functioning properly and hepatic encephalopathy will not be a problem. The excessive nitrogen losses associated with this procedure warrant that the provision of protein exceed at least 1.2 g/kg/d.[41] Modified amino acids should be reserved for those patients with marginal hepatic function associated with rejection or hepatic encephalopathy.

Fluid/Electrolytes/Acid–Base Disorders/ Trace Elements

Patients undergoing orthotopic liver transplantation receive a substantial amount of crystalloid and blood products during the operative procedure. This often results in an edematous state in the postoperative period, especially in patients who had ascites in the preoperative period. Sodium rarely needs to be added to the PN solution in patients with this condition. The large citrate load from administered blood products has been implicated in causing hypocalcemia (citrate binding of ionized calcium) and metabolic alkalosis (conversion of citrate to bicarbonate) in the postoperative period. This would require supplemental doses of calcium and the addition of anions as the chloride salt in the PN formulation. Low serum concentrations of zinc and magnesium are very common in the postoperative period. Restricted diets before surgery, hyperzincuria secondary to liver disease, and postoperative stress all can contribute to hypozincemia in this patient population. Supplementation of zinc above standard amounts should be considered in the PN formula. Reduced intake from restricted diets and increased urinary excretion secondary to cyclosporine therapy contribute to hypomagnesemia. These patients often require magnesium in amounts that exceed standard doses during postoperative nutrition support. Patients who have severe cholestasis before and after orthotopic hepatic transplantation should have copper and manganese restricted as they are excreted in the bile and serum concentrations may thus be elevated. An example of a PN formula for the patient who has received an orthotopic liver transplant appears in Table 136.1.

RENAL FAILURE

The kidney is responsible primarily for excretion of water, nonmetabolized solute from the diet, and the end products of nitrogen metabolism. Impairment of these processes results in overhydration, urea nitrogen accumulation, and impaired protein synthesis. Patients who have chronic renal failure (CRF) and receive dialysis therapy have impaired host-defense mechanisms and increased risk of infection.[43] Undernourished patients with CRF have decreased skeletal muscle function.[44] However, many patients compliant with diet and drug therapy during maintenance dialysis demonstrated no substantial loss of nutritional status during a 24-month study period.[45] The adequacy of dialysis and the serum albumin concentration are strong predictors of mortality.[46] This relationship appears to be valid for patients receiving peritoneal dialysis too.[47] There is also some evidence that serum insulin-like growth factor 1 (IGF-1) is a good indicator of early undernutrition in dialysis patients.[48] Also, energy expenditure in these patients appears to be similar to normal subjects and nondialyzed patients with chronic renal failure.[49,50] Renal failure may be acute or chronic and oliguric or nonoliguric, making provision of appropriate nutrition support very challenging. As in hepatic failure, nutrition support in renal failure requires provision of substrate in utilizable forms in an appropriate volume while limiting accumulation of nitrogen waste. Major differences in the nutrition management of acute renal failure (ARF) and CRF exist and are therefore discussed separately. Excellent reviews are available which discuss in greater depth than space will allow the nutritional management of ARF and CRF.[51,52]

MACRONUTRIENT CONSIDERATIONS IN ACUTE RENAL FAILURE

Carbohydrate

Hyperglycemia and peripheral insulin resistance are common in the patient with ARF. These patients usually have a superimposed illness (sepsis or major injury), which may cause glucose intolerance. The etiology of glucose intolerance in renal failure is thought to be an interaction between glucagon, growth hormone, and the catecholamines, all known antagonists of insulin. Other proposed mechanisms include an elevated glucagon-to-insulin ratio secondary to impaired degradation of these hormones and elevated secretion of inflammatory cytokines.

Occasionally, patients with ARF are treated with intermittent peritoneal dialysis (IPD), which may exacerbate glucose intolerance already present from the stress of illness secondary to peritoneal absorption of glucose. Excessive absorption of dextrose (more than 1700 kcal per 24-hour period) during IPD with 4.25% dextrose has been reported.[53] Based on 12 exchanges per 24 hours, this means that approximately 45% of the dextrose was absorbed. The patients in this study demonstrated increased carbon dioxide production presumedly from excessive glucose intake. Addition of regular insulin to the dialysate has been advocated during IPD to prevent or minimize hyperglycemia. This may be particularly beneficial in the diabetic nephropathy patient, because it may prevent frequent intravenous or subcutaneous dosing of insulin during dialysis therapy. During hemodialysis there may be some carbohydrate loss but it is not clinically important. Net uptake of infused glucose (up to 300 g/d) has been reported with the use of continuous arteriovenous hemofiltration (CAVH) in patients with acute oliguric renal failure.[54]

Fat

Intolerance to intravenous fat emulsions is very common in patients with ARF. Elevated serum concentrations of triglycerides are thought to be caused by decreased catabolism of triglycerides and possibly increased synthesis from FFAs.[55] Current practice dictates measurement of a triglyceride concentration before administration of intravenous fat emulsions to patients with this disease state. FFA concentrations have been reported to be elevated in ARF. This aberration, however, could not be appreciated by measurement of the triglyceride concentration. Therefore, low doses of intravenous fat (3–7 kcal/kg/d infused over 24 h) should be used to prevent essential fatty acid deficiency and to provide lipid calories when the serum triglyceride concentration is less than 300 mg/dL. Intravenous fat emulsions containing a combination of MCTs and long-chain triglycerides (LCTs) are available in Europe and most likely will be available in this country in the future. MCTs are readily used for energy, not stored, and are carnitine independent, all features that make them an attractive fuel substrate. The elimination of MCTs in patients with ARF appears to be impaired like LCTs are.[56] Therefore, they will undoubtedly need to be used with caution in patients with ARF when they become available.

Protein

Urea, the end product of nitrogen metabolism, accumulates rapidly in patients with ARF. As discussed earlier, most patients with ARF have an underlying illness that causes significant stress resulting in ureagenesis. The composition and dose of protein during nutrition support in ARF have been the subject of considerable investigation and controversy. The appropriate nitrogen intake is determined by the interventions being used. Even the type of dialysis has an influence on the appropriate amount of nitrogen.[57,58] For example, a patient with ARF could be receiving no dialysis, hemodialysis, peritoneal dialysis, CAVH, or continuous arterial venous or veno-venous hemodialysis (CAVHD or VVHD) (see Chapter 43, Acute Renal Failure). Clark et al.[59] have demonstrated superior control of azotemia over intermittent hemodialysis with continuous venovenous hemofiltration in patients with ARF. Druml et al.[60] have reported on the alterations of the plasma aminogram and clearance of amino acids in ARF and CRF. In general, the clearances of histidine and tryptophan were enhanced while the clearances of phenylalanine and valine were reduced in these patient groups when compared to controls.[60]

In early acute renal failure, the nutrition support formula needs to be protein restricted (20–30 g/d) while the patient is being evaluated for etiologic factors and dialysis need. A low protein intake during ARF minimizes urea nitrogen accumulation from exogenous protein. Urea nitrogen appearance also is determined by endogenous breakdown of protein, which is very important in a stressed patient with sepsis or major trauma. Therefore, in this type of patient, endogenous catabolism certainly contributes more to nitrogen accumulation when a restricted dose of exogenous protein is given. If dialysis is instituted, the protein intake can be liberalized somewhat. Generally, the patient receiving hemodialysis can tolerate 1–1.2 g of protein/kg/d. If IPD is used, the protein intake may be liberalized to 1.2–1.5 g/kg/d. CAVH removes large quantities of extracellular fluid by extracorporeal ultrafiltration. This procedure may allow infusion of the required nutritional substrates in a reasonable volume and avoid the hypotensive effects of hemodialysis.[61] CAVHD, which combines the advantages of both CAVH and hemodialysis, has been referred to as nutritional dialysis.[54] Adequate nutrition support usually can be infused without volume restriction while the clearance of urea is markedly increased over CAVH alone. Frequency and effectiveness of dialytic therapy are the final determinants of the protein-infusion ranges.

Some investigations have suggested that dialysis therapy be instituted early in ARF so that aggressive nutrition support can be started. In patients with severe injury or sepsis plus ARF, attainment of protein requirements (1.5–2.5 g/kg/d) may not be possible, even with early institution of dialysis. Four commercially available intravenous preparations of primarily essential amino acids are marketed for nutrition support of ARF and are discussed later in this chapter.

Fluid and Electrolytes

The patient with oliguric ARF will have impaired excretion of sodium and water. In these situations, the nutrition support formula should be concentrated in as small a volume as possible and contain little or no sodium. In the patient with nonoliguric ARF, considerable quantities of sodium may be lost in the urine, necessitating replacement to maintain sodium balance. This also may apply to the patient who is losing considerable quantities of gastric fluid from suction. Patients receiving CAVH or CAVHD will be given sodium via intravenous fluid and losing it from the hemofiltration or dialysis. Therefore, standard amounts of sodium can be given and fluid restriction is unnecessary.

Hyperkalemia is frequently observed in patients with ARF secondary to protein catabolism and intracellular potassium release. Hyperkalemia also results from the impaired secretion and excretion of potassium by the kidney, and the endogenous release from tissue breakdown. If this disorder is severe enough, emergency dialysis may be required. PN formulas in patients with ARF and hyperkalemia should not contain potassium salts. After several days of feeding, the serum potassium concentration decreases, often necessitating cautious addition of this electrolyte to the PN formula. If the enteral route can be used for nutritional support, formulas void or reduced in potassium may be required initially.

Because phosphorus is excreted renally, hyperphosphatemia is very common in patients with ARF. Like potassium, large amounts of phosphorus may be released into the circulation secondary to tissue breakdown during ARF, compounding the problem. Control of hyperphosphatemia is extremely important during ARF because when the product of serum phosphorus (in mg/dL) and serum calcium (in mg/dL) exceeds 70, metastatic calcification of the renal tubules can occur. Therefore, for patients with ARF, phosphorus should be omitted from the nutrition formula until serum concentrations have normalized. This may take anywhere from a few days to 2 weeks. Phosphorus should be added to the PN solution cautiously in small doses when the serum concentration is less than 4.0 mg/dL. Failure to add phosphorus at this time can eventually lead to severe hypophosphatemia, even with continued renal failure.

Hypermagnesemia is very common in patients with ARF secondary to impaired renal excretion and endogenous release from tissue breakdown. Serum magnesium concentrations do not decrease as quickly as potassium and phosphorus do during electrolyte-free parenteral nutrition. As renal function returns and/or serum concentrations decrease to the low–normal range, magnesium should be added cautiously to the parenteral nutrition solution in less-than-standard doses (e.g., 4–6 mEq/L). Overzealous use of magnesium resulting in hypermagnesemia may require emergent dialysis.

Acid–Base Disorders

Patients with ARF usually have metabolic acidosis because of impaired excretion of waste products and organic acids. If potassium and sodium additions are needed in the PN formula for patients with ARF, they should be added as acetate salts. This may help treat or at least not worsen the acid–base disorder. The metabolic acidosis usually improves during dialytic intervention.

MICRONUTRIENT CONSIDERATIONS IN ACUTE RENAL FAILURE

Trace Elements

The requirements for trace elements during nutrition support of ARF are not well established. Zinc and chromium are excreted mainly by the kidney in the absence of ostomy output or diarrhea. Indeed, some investigators have advocated elimination of trace elements from the PN formula of patients with ARF. Because manganese and copper are excreted in the bile and zinc may be lost in the dialysis bath, patients with ARF receiving parenteral nutrition should be treated according to NAG-AMA guidelines for trace elements.[15]

Vitamins

Very few data are available concerning vitamin requirements in patients with ARF receiving parenteral nutrition. Currently, it seems prudent to administer vitamins as recommended by the NAG-AMA. If the enteral route can be used for nutritional support during ARF, vitamin administration to meet the RDAs is reasonable.

ADMINISTRATION ROUTES AND PRODUCTS IN ACUTE RENAL FAILURE

Parenteral Therapy

Most patients with ARF have a superimposed illness (septic shock or trauma with hypotension and ileus) that requires nutrition support by the parenteral route. An early study by Abel et al.[62] showed both improved survival rate and return of renal function when essential amino acids (EAAs) plus glucose were compared with glucose alone in patients with ARF. Consequently, intravenous amino acids containing only or predominantly EAAs (Nephramine, McGaw Laboratories; RenAmin, Clintec Nutrition Co., Aminosyn-RF, Abbott Laboratories; Aminess, Clintec Nutrition Co.) were marketed. These products are usually mixed with dextrose 70% resulting in a final concentration of 30–45% dextrose. These products were formulated on the hypothesis that substantial nitrogen reutilization occurs during ARF (i.e., circulating urea can be used to synthesize nonessential amino acids). This reutilization of nitrogen does not occur in patients with uremia. Thereafter, investigators began to question whether EAAs were any more effective than general mixed amino acids (MAAs). This led to several controlled and uncontrolled studies comparing different amino acid products in patients with ARF.[62–66] A summary of these studies appears in Table 136.2.

TABLE 136.2. STUDIES COMPARING EAAs AND MAAs IN NUTRITIONAL SUPPORT FOR ACUTE RENAL FAILURE PATIENTS

Authors	Study Design	Patients	Nutritional Regimen	Results
Blackburn et al.[63]	Prospective	19 (11 unstressed) (8 stressed)	EAAs + 73% glucose MAAs + 37% glucose MAAs + 52% glucose	No significant difference in decreased BUN in the unstressed patients; 5 of 8 died in the stressed group
Freund et al.[64]	Retrospective	50	EAAs + 46% glucose MAAs + 46% glucose	91% mortality in the group receiving MAAs versus 25% in the group receiving EAAs
Feinstein et al.[65]	Prospective Double-blind	30	46% glucose[a] EAAs + 46% glucose MAAs + 46% glucose	No significant difference in mortality and return of renal function
Mirtallo et al.[66]	Prospective Double-blind Randomized	45	EAAs + 46% glucose[b] MAAs + 46% glucose[b]	No significant difference in mortality, urea nitrogen appearance, and nitrogen balance

Key: EEA, essential amino acid; MAA, mixed amino acid; BUN, blood urea nitrogen.
[a]70% glucose and 20% glucose were used to deliver 2050 or 2800 kcal/d.
[b]70% glucose was used to administer 1.75 × basal energy expenditures.

The studies by Feinstein et al.[65] and Mirtallo et al.[66] were prospective and well controlled. Freund et al.[64] studied a group of very ill patients with ARF who received parenteral nutrition and MAAs. These patients were then compared with a group of retrospective controls who had ARF and received parenteral nutrition with EAAs.[62] The patients in the Freund et al.[64] study had concomitant trauma, burns, or cardiac disease, which were exclusions in the control group. The poor study design makes any conclusions from these data very questionable. The type of intravenous protein for parenteral nutrition in ARF remains somewhat controversial, but the well-controlled studies do not indicate clinically significant advantages when EAAs are used. See Table 131.2 for an example of a parenteral nutrition solution in ARF. Note that dextrose 70% is the energy substrate of choice when fluid restriction is required.

There is evidence that arginine is a conditionally essential amino acid in ARF because there is a report of hyperammonemia associated with the infusion of a formula containing only EAAs.[67] It is known that arginine is needed to convert ammonia to urea. Based on the available data, it appears prudent to use MAAs in patients who require PN and have ARF (Fig. 136.2).

Enteral Therapy

Continuous-pump tube feeding should be considered when patients with ARF have functioning gastrointestinal tracts and will not or cannot ingest sufficient nutrients. The products used most frequently during enteral nutrition (EN) support of ARF are the electrolyte-free or electrolyte-reduced formulas that appear in Table 136.3. The formulas are most useful in patients with hyperkalemia, hyperphosphatemia, or hypermagnesemia. Unfortunately, most patients with ARF are critically ill and have an ileus making enteral nutrition support impossible (Fig. 136.2).

MACRONUTRIENT CONSIDERATIONS IN CHRONIC RENAL FAILURE

Carbohydrate

In general, CRF patients are not as stressed as patients with ARF; however, more than one-half of patients with CRF have insulin resistance and hyperglycemia. This can be attributed in part to the increased glucagon-to-insulin ratio, resulting in protein breakdown and gluconeogenesis. Patients with CRF who require parenteral nutrition and receive continuous ambulatory peritoneal dialysis (CAPD) absorb a substantial amount of glucose. This can worsen existing hyperglycemia and contribute significantly to the patient's energy intake. One study found that more than 180 grams of glucose (approximately 600 kcal) were absorbed per day during CAPD.[68] This provided 12–34% of these patients' energy intake. It is, therefore, not uncommon for these patients to have kwashiorkor-type malnutrition. Insulin can be added to CAPD bags to control hyperglycemia[69]; however, glucose control usually is not a major problem in CRF unless the patient is diabetic, infected, or subjected to operative stress. Insulin is adsorbed to plastic CAPD bags; thus, not all drug added to the bag is delivered to the patient.

Fat

Type IV hypertriglyceridemia is present in more than one-half of all CRF patients. This is thought to be caused mainly by decreased catabolism of triglycerides secondary to decreased hepatic lipoprotein lipase activity.[55] For this reason, currently marketed fat emulsions must be administered cautiously in CRF patients. Most patients receiving hemodialysis would receive heparin, which should activate lipoprotein lipase and convert triglycerides to FFAs and glycerol. If FFAs are not utilized by the body properly (e.g., as in carnitine deficiency), serum triglyceride mea-

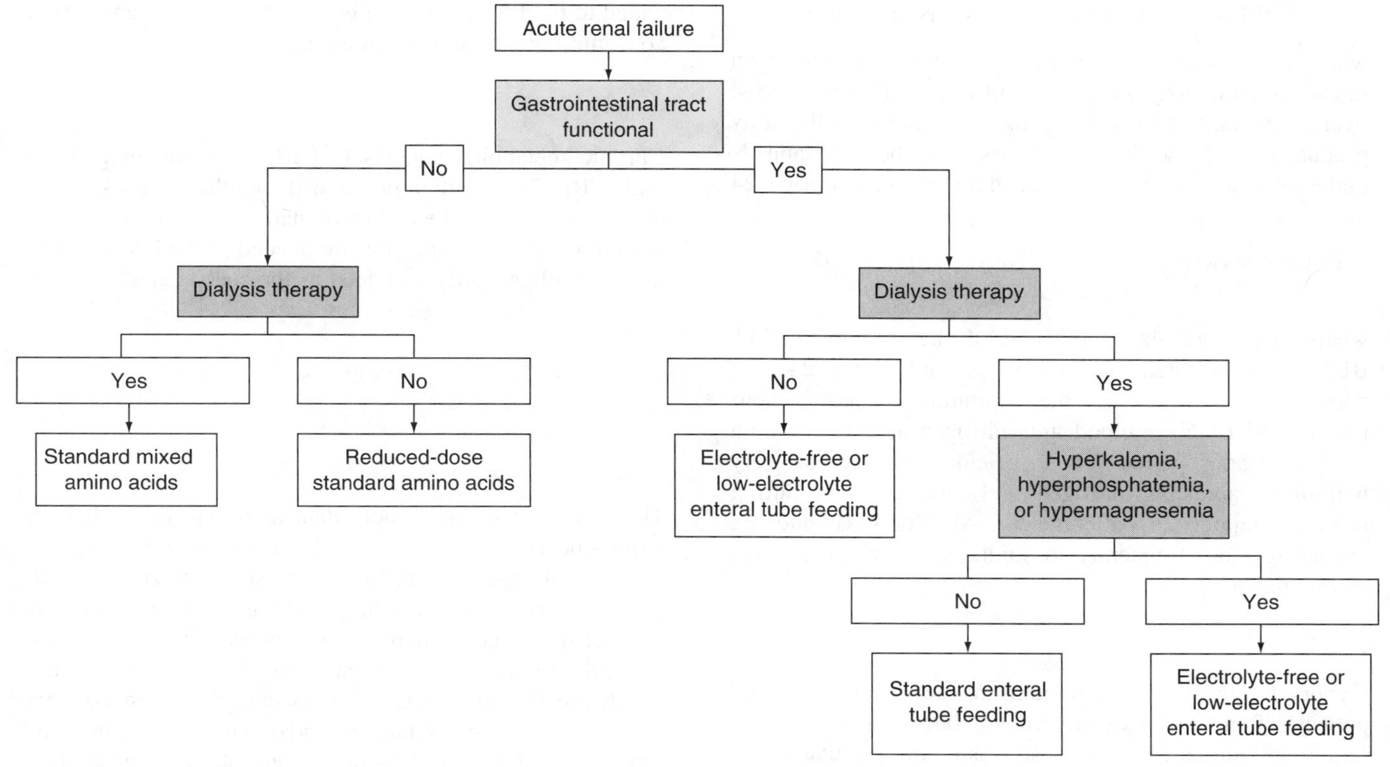

Figure 136.2. Nutrition support approach for the patient with acute renal failure (selection of amino acid).

surements will not identify this defect. Also, patients receiving long-term dialysis treatment have been shown to accumulate remnants of triglyceride-rich lipoproteins. This lipoprotein abnormality can result in type III hyperlipidemia with increased intermediate density lipoprotein.

Protein

With respect to nitrogen requirements in CRF, patients should be divided into two groups: those receiving and those not receiving dialysis. Protein intake can be liberalized to approximately 1 g/kg/d for CAPD patients.[70] When nutritional status is adequate, 1 g/kg/d usually maintains nitrogen equilibrium with either hemodialysis or CAPD. The original studies on protein losses during CAPD were conducted during the day's first exchange. Because protein losses during this exchange are higher than subsequent exchanges, total daily losses were somewhat overestimated and protein doses may have been too liberal.

Preliminary data suggested that protein restriction in patients with chronic renal dysfunction would delay the institution of dialysis.[71–73] More recently, data from large controlled trials have not supported this dietary intervention.[74,75] Hence patients with chronic renal insufficiency can be given a diet with normal amounts of protein (e.g., 1 g/kg/d) based on available information.

Because urine collections for assessing nitrogen balance often are impossible in patients with renal failure, a method for determination of nitrogen balance that estimates urea nitrogen appearance has been developed. This method estimates protein catabolism by measuring losses in the urine and/or the dialysate fluid and the urea nitrogen that remains in the body. When nitrogen intake is known, an estimated nitrogen balance can be calculated:

TABLE 136.3. ENTERAL NUTRITION PRODUCTS USED IN RENAL FAILURE

Product	AminAid (McGaw)	Travasorb Renal (Clintec Nutrition Company)	Suplena (Ross)	Nepro (Ross)	Isocal-HCN (Bristol-Myers)	TwoCal (Ross)	Magnacal (Sherwood Medical)
Caloric density (kcal/mL)	2.0	1.2	2.0	2.0	2.0	2.0	2.0
Electrolytes	None	None	Low	Low	Low	Normal	Low
Vitamins	None	Water soluble	Yes	Yes	Yes	Yes	Yes
Osmolality (mOsm/kg H_2O)	700	590	615	635	690	690	590

$$ENB = Ni - (UUN + 4 + UNA + N\ dialysate)$$

where ENB = estimated nitrogen balance, Ni = nitrogen intake for 24 hours, UUN = urea nitrogen collected in urine over 24 hours, UNA = urea nitrogen remaining in the body produced over the last 24 hours (see below), and N dialysate = urea nitrogen lost in dialysate fluid during 24 hours.[76]

$$UNA = [wt_2\ (kg) \times 0.6 \times BUN_2\ (g/L)] - [wt_1\ (kg) \times 0.6 \times BUN_1\ (g/L)]$$

where wt_2 = weight at the end of the 24-hour period, BUN_2 = blood urea nitrogen at the end of the 24-hour period, wt_1 = weight at the beginning of the 24-hour period, and BUN_1 = blood urea nitrogen at the beginning of the 24-hour period. These calculations may be very helpful in adjusting nitrogen and caloric doses during nutrition support in patients with ARF or CRF and are appearing more frequently in studies of nutrition support of this patient population.

Fluid and Electrolytes

Hyponatremia is very common in the chronic dialysis patient, often due to overhydration, but usually does not require additional administration of sodium. Regular dialysis is the principal means for control of body water and serum sodium concentration. Generally, sodium should be administered to CRF patients during nutrition support only to replace losses.

Patients with CRF who develop hyperkalemia have usually ingested potassium in excess of what the kidneys or dialysis can handle. The undernourished CRF patient receiving parenteral nutrition may require considerable potassium as new lean body tissue is synthesized. When inappropriately low amounts of potassium are given during refeeding, hypokalemia may develop. Once anabolism is attained in CRF patients, potassium requirements may be as high as 40–80 mEq/d. This dose would need to be given carefully and requires frequent serum potassium concentration monitoring.

Patients with CRF are often treated for hyperphosphatemia chronically with aluminum- or calcium-containing antacids or phosphorus-restricted diets (see Chapter 44 on chronic renal failure). When these patients receive aggressive nutrition support, the combination of refeeding (cellular uptake of phosphorus for synthesis of lean body mass) and vigorous antacid therapy can result in moderate to severe hypophosphatemia fairly quickly. Therefore, conservative amounts of phosphorus usually need to be administered during parenteral nutrition. If the CRF patient is being dialyzed regularly and has a functioning gastrointestinal tract, enteral nutrition should be used (Table 136.3).

Hypermagnesemia is less common in patients with CRF when compared with those with ARF. It is usually added to the PN solution daily in reduced doses, and serum concentrations need to be monitored frequently.

Acid–Base Disorders

Chronic metabolic acidosis is fairly common in patients with CRF. This will improve with regular dialysis, especially when an acetate or bicarbonate dialysis bath is used. If sodium or potassium salts are needed in the PN solution, they should generally be added as the acetate salt.

MICRONUTRIENT CONSIDERATIONS IN CHRONIC RENAL FAILURE

Trace Elements

There are considerably more data involving trace element requirements in patients with CRF than those with ARF.[77] It has been reported that total body stores of zinc in CRF were increased, but skeletal muscle and serum concentrations of this trace element were decreased. This suggests a redistribution of zinc or increased need to maintain normal enzymatic function in CRF. It appears that most patients with CRF being hemodialyzed have depressed serum concentrations of zinc and elevated concentrations of copper. The clinical relevance of these disorders is difficult to interpret; however, universal zinc supplementation of CRF patients cannot be recommended at this time. Interestingly, zinc absorption has been reported to be impaired in patients with uremia, especially in those receiving hemodialysis.[78]

The most severe trace element disorder in patients with CRF is aluminum toxicity. This has been caused by aluminum in the dialysate or excessive use of aluminum-containing antacids. Consequently, significant quantities of aluminum have been removed from currently available dialysis solutions and calcium antacids have replaced aluminum as phosphate binders.[79] The older protein solutions for PN (protein hydrolysates) contained considerable aluminum, but the change to crystalline amino acid products has eliminated that problem.

Vitamins

Patients with CRF are very prone to develop water-soluble vitamin deficiencies because many foods that contain these vitamins are restricted because of their potassium content. Specifically, CRF patients should receive ascorbic acid 70–100 mg/d, pyridoxine 5–10 mg/d, and folic acid 1 mg/d in addition to the other essential vitamins. During short-term parenteral nutrition in patients with CRF, elimination or reduction of the dose of vitamin A has been recommended. Vitamin A concentrations are often elevated in CRF patients and exogenous administration is unwarranted in the short term.

ADMINISTRATION ROUTES AND PRODUCTS IN CHRONIC RENAL FAILURE

Parenteral Therapy

Patients with CRF who require nutrition support rarely need parenteral nutrition because their gastrointestinal tract is functional. If there is superimposed illness that prevents enteral administration of nutrients, parenteral nutrition is indicated. Because many of these patients are already receiving hemodialysis or peritoneal dialysis, MAAs can be used as the protein component of parenteral nutrition.

Enteral Therapy

As mentioned earlier, most patients with CRF have accessible and functioning gastrointestinal tracts so enteral therapy should always be considered first in this patient population. The calorically dense low-electrolyte formulas listed in Table 136.3 are particularly useful in these patients. Even though these patients receive regular dialysis, most of them are anuric so excess fluid intake is always a potential problem. Nepro (Ross Laboratories) is marketed specifically for the patient with CRF who receives regular dialysis. Suplena (Ross Laboratories), which is lower in protein and some electrolytes than Nepro, can be used in patients with renal insufficiency without dialysis or occasionally in patients with ARF who can tolerate enteral nutrition.

FUTURE DIRECTIONS

The association between poor nutritional status and increased morbidity and mortality in patients with CRF is quite compelling.[47,80,81] Some data exist that support infusion of glucose/amino acid/lipid admixtures to patients receiving dialysis.[82–85] This is referred to as intradialytic parenteral nutrition (IDPN). This method is particularly attractive because these patients have intravenous access for the infusion of concentrated PN admixtures. Also, many patients come to a dialysis unit on a regular schedule, such as three times per week, allowing short time intervals for the infusion of PN. Capelli et al.[84] have reported reduced mortality in undernourished hemodialysis patients who received IDPN. This study, however, was retrospective and nonrandomized. Also, control patients had their enteral supplements discontinued after 3 months while the treated group continued to receive IDPN throughout the 2-year study. Other problems with IDPN include expense and the provision of relatively low intakes of calories and protein because of the limited time for PN infusion. Because of these low nutrient intakes, a substantial period of time would be needed to demonstrate meaningful, positive outcomes in this patient population receiving IDPN. Until these data are available, IDPN should be reserved for severely undernourished patients who clearly have failed a trial of oral supplements or enteral tube feeding. Patients with CRF who have severe gastrointestinal compromise requiring PN generally will need it on a daily basis and not just during dialysis.

There has also been some use of amino acids as a peritoneal dialysis solution.[86] One method in a descriptive study was to use a 1% amino acid solution in place of two of the dextrose exchanges. This 8-week trial resulted in an improved plasma aminogram, however, no real clinical benefit was obvious.[86] Ketoanalogues of EAAs have been given with a phosphorus-restricted diet (20–30 g protein/d) to patients with chronic renal dysfunction and either slowed or halted the progression of renal insufficiency.[87] Products such as epoeitin alfa and human growth hormone are being used in patients with CRF. The effects these drugs have on nutritional status are currently being studied.[88]

Bioelectrical impedance (BIA) is starting to be used in patients with ARF and CRF. This a noninvasive measurement of total body water and body cell mass. Because body water fluctuates in these patients, BIA needs to be validated in this patient population. It could potentially be very useful in documenting the adequacy of dialysis and changes in nutritional status.

PULMONARY FAILURE

The lung is responsible primarily for gas exchange. Oxygen is inhaled through the lung and absorbed into the circulatory system while carbon dioxide is exhaled. Substantial information exists that emphasizes the interaction between nutrition and respiratory function.[89–91] For example, decreased pulmonary function and survival were associated with decreased body weight in the National Institutes of Health Intermittent Positive-Pressure Breathing Trial.[90] Impaired gas exchange has been associated with depressed visceral protein markers of nutritional status (e.g., albumin, prealbumin).[89] Also, undernourished patients with chronic tracheostomy have demonstrated increased bacterial binding in the lower respiratory tract with enteric gram-negative bacilli.[91]

The deleterious effects of overfeeding the patient with pulmonary compromise have received a great amount of attention, and this has led to newer methods to determine resting energy expenditure (REE). Mobile metabolic carts using the technique of indirect calorimetry are more prevalent. Recent investigations using indirect calorimetry have demonstrated a state of hypermetabolism (increased REE) in stable, undernourished patients with chronic obstructive pulmonary disease or emphysema.[92–94] This state of hypermetabolism appears to exist without accompanying hypercatabolism. In most other disease states, undernutrition and weight loss results in hypometabolism. This may account in part for the nearly universal weight loss seen in patients with these pulmonary disease states, even when nutritional intake appears adequate. Patients with emphysema had a markedly increased rate of carbohydrate oxidation compared with undernourished controls.[94] Nonsurgical patients who have acute respiratory failure requiring mechanical ventilation and sepsis have demonstrated a 20% increase in REE over that predicted by the Harris–Benedict equations.[95] Other patients in this report who required mechanical ventilation and were not septic did not demonstrate hypermetabolism.[95]

Although patients with pulmonary failure do not have the severe metabolic alterations observed in patients with renal or hepatic failure, there is substantial information to aid the practitioner in providing safe and efficacious nutrition support. The reader also is referred to in-depth reviews of nutrition support in patients with respiratory disease.[96,97]

MACRONUTRIENT CONSIDERATIONS

Carbohydrate

Semistarvation in normal subjects (500 kcal of carbohydrate per day) has been shown to blunt the normal response to hypoxia, and refeeding restored this response to normal.[98] Depression of the hypoxic ventilatory response correlated well with decreases in all of the following: body weight, oxygen consumption (Vo_2), carbon dioxide production (Vco_2), resting minute ventilation, and heart rate. These data suggest that early feeding of the mechanically ventilated patient may improve the hypoxic response.

Oxidation of the major nutritional substrates can be represented by a respiratory quotient (RQ) determined by dividing Vco_2 by Vo_2. Carbohydrate oxidation, protein oxidation, and fat oxidation have RQs of 1.0, 0.8, and 0.7, respectively. The RQ for fat synthesis from carbohydrate is 8.0. Oxidation of carbohydrate generates 1 mole of carbon dioxide for every mole of oxygen consumed. When a subject is overfed with glucose (net fat synthesis), the Vco_2 markedly exceeds the Vo_2. When this occurs, the RQ for that period of time will exceed 1.0.

Much interest has been generated from reports of the inability to wean mechanically ventilated patients because of overfeeding with glucose-based parenteral nutrition.[99] It is presumed that excessive infused carbohydrate is used for fat synthesis, resulting in substantial liberation of carbon dioxide. This would make weaning impossible secondary to respiratory acidosis. Despite this potential problem, the percentage of patients with spontaneous ventilation does increase as calories are increased in mechanically ventilated patients.[100] One group has reported significant increases in Vco_2 and RQ when glucose-based parenteral nutrition was administered to both depleted and severely stressed patients at approximately 50% above measured REE.[101] From these data, glucose-based parenteral nutrition should be administered in moderate doses (25–30 kcal/kg/d) to patients with respiratory disease or mechanical ventilation.

Fat

Because fat is oxidized at a lower RQ than glucose, intravenous fat emulsion at 30–50% of the nonprotein calories has been suggested in patients with respiratory failure who require parenteral nutrition.[102] As discussed before, patients who are overfed with glucose synthesize fat, which increases carbon dioxide production. Decreases of 18% and 24% in Vco_2 were recorded when ventilated patients were switched from glucose-based parenteral nutrition to a formulation containing 33% and 50% intravenous fat emulsion, respectively.[102] These data are supported by other investigations.[103] There has been some concern with the reduction in pulmonary membrane diffusion capacity, increased pulmonary artery pressure, and increased venous admixture during intravenous fat emulsion administration.[104] Most of these potential problems have occurred with rather large doses of intravenous fat during short periods of infusion (e.g., 500 mL 10% intravenous lipid over 4 hours). Rapid infusion of lipid emulsion is associated with synthesis of prostaglandin $F_2\alpha$, a known pulmonary vasoconstrictor, while slow-continuous infusion results in synthesis of prostaglandin E_2 and prostaglandin I_2, known pulmonary vasodilators. The infusion rate and dose of intravenous fat emulsion may explain some of the ventilation/perfusion inequalities observed in patients during lipid administration. It is unclear what the clinical significance of these aberrations will be as more institutions convert to total nutrient admixtures where the lipid dose is infused over a 24-hour period. Many institutions infuse the lipid dose over a 24-hour period, even when it is not admixed with the PN solution. The clearance of triglycerides from intravenous fat emulsions is actually increased in critically ill patients when compared with normal subjects.[105] One report suggested that patients who have adult respiratory distress syndrome (ARDS) with a disrupted alveolar capillary membrane are more prone to develop ventilation/perfusion inequalities during intravenous fat emulsion.[106] Further studies of intravenous fat emulsion administration have been conducted in septic patients with ARDS.[107] After administration of 500 mL of 20% intravenous fat emulsion given over 8 hours, significant decreases in po_2/Fio_2 (an index of oxygenation), and significant increases in mean pulmonary arterial pressure and pulmonary vasculature resistance were reported in the septic patients. Patients with sepsis and ARDS should be monitored closely during intravenous lipid administration. Moderate doses of lipid (e.g., 1 g/kg/d) should preferably be infused over a 24-hour period each day in these type of patients. The reader is referred to an excellent review on the use of intravenous fat emulsion and its effect on lung function.[108]

Protein

Undernourished patients have demonstrated a blunted response to hypercapnia that improves after 1 week of adequate nutrition support. This response is thought to result from protein administration as evidenced by decreased P_{CO_2}, increased minute ventilation, and improved breathing patterns after the start of parenteral nutrition. One group reported a significant increase in neuromuscular ventilatory drive following protein administration preceded by 7 days of semistarvation.[109] It appears that increasing protein intake beyond standard doses significantly improves this response.[110] Even though increased neuromuscular drive from protein administration can be beneficial, it also can be detrimental in patients who are unable to increase their minute ventilation. In other words, excessive protein intake might increase pulmonary workload, resulting in muscle fatigue and respiratory failure. Therefore, only moderate doses of protein (1.0–1.5 g/kg/d) can be recommended for the patient with stable chronic obstructive pulmonary disease (COPD). Patients who are mechanically ventilated with superimposed illness (e.g., sepsis) may require higher doses of protein (1.5–2.5 g/kg/d). A preliminary report suggested an improved response to hypercapnia following administration of mainly BCAAs compared with a standard amino acid in normal volunteers.[111] It is unclear what the clinical significance of this effect would be in patients with respiratory failure.

Fluid and Electrolytes

Ill patients with COPD or patients with pneumonia receiving mechanical ventilation should have intake and output recorded daily. In most cases, it is desirable to keep these patients slightly "dry." Mortality has been reported to be significantly lower in patients who have ARDS and demonstrate a negative fluid balance when compared with those ARDS patients who retained fluid.[112] Similar results have been reported in patients with pulmonary edema.[113] Therefore, excessive infusions of salt and water should be avoided because they may exacerbate already compromised pulmonary function, and parenteral and enteral formulas should be relatively low in sodium. Losses of sodium from nasogastric suction or abdominal drains should, of course, be replaced.

The incidence of hypophosphatemia is higher in patients with pulmonary disease than in the general hospitalized population.[114] This is particularly true in patients with pneumonia. Fiaccadori et al.[115] reported phosphorus depletion in external intercostal and quadricep femoris muscles in patients with COPD. It is well known that phosphorus is essential for adenosine triphosphate (ATP) and 2,3-diphosphoglycerate (2,3-DPG). Hypophosphatemia can cause reduced erythrocyte concentrations of these two compounds. Hemoglobin does not release oxygen during hypoxia appropriately without adequate 2,3-DPG and respiratory muscles may be weakened without adequate stores of ATP. It has been shown that hypophosphatemia impairs diaphragmatic contractility in patients with acute respiratory failure. Correction of this disorder with intravenous potassium phosphate improved diaphragmatic contractility significantly.[116] These data, combined with the problems of hypophosphatemia from refeeding, emphasize the importance of phosphorus homeostasis in this patient population during nutrition support.

Acid–Base Disorders

Ventilator-dependent patients and those with stable COPD often have respiratory acidosis. As mentioned earlier, excessive administration of carbohydrate results in net fat synthesis and liberalization of large quantities of carbon dioxide. This can make weaning from the ventilator extremely difficult and even induce respiratory failure in a stable COPD patient. The acid–base status of the patient with pulmonary compromise receiving nutrition support should be monitored very closely.

MICRONUTRIENT CONSIDERATIONS

There are no known significant alterations in trace element and vitamin metabolism in patients with pulmonary disease. Patients receiving parenteral nutrition should receive vitamins and trace elements as recommended by the NAG-AMA. Patients receiving enteral nutrition should receive the RDAs for vitamins, zinc, and selenium, and the recommended amounts for the other trace elements.

ADMINISTRATION ROUTES AND PRODUCTS

Parenteral Therapy

Patients with pulmonary failure should receive nutrition support by the enteral route unless the gastrointestinal tract is not functional or accessible. Patients with pulmonary failure from severe pneumonia or septicemia may have a prolonged ileus, necessitating PN support. Because there are no major substrate alterations in pulmonary failure, moderate doses of intravenous carbohydrate, fat, and protein are appropriate in most clinical conditions. A review of nutrition support of ventilator-dependent patients suggests that nonprotein calories be administered as glucose and fat in a range from 55–80% carbohydrate and 20–45% lipid.[96] The protein dose recommended was 1.5 g/kg/d. As emphasized earlier, excessive carbohydrate administration increases carbon dioxide production, which may impair weaning of patients from the ventilator. As a result of this well-published concept, many investigators are advocating the use of lipid as a daily caloric source in PN regimens. The availability of total nutrient admixtures has made it very convenient to administer intravenous lipid to patients on a daily basis. Overfeeding with total calories is probably as important to avoid as overfeeding with carbohydrate. Talpers et al.[117] demonstrated a significant rise in V_{CO_2} in mechanically ventilated patients as total calories were increased from 1.0 to 1.5 and 2.0 times the BEE. When total calories were fixed at 1.3 times BEE, caloric composition (40–70% carbohydrate, 5–40% fat) had little effect on V_{CO_2}. Table 136.1 gives an example of a PN formula using lipid as a caloric source. While intravenous fat emulsions are certainly not reserved for only the patient with pulmonary failure, their use as a daily caloric source is being advocated. In patients where fluid restriction is essential (e.g., severe ARDS) and parenteral nutrition is required, the use of the more expensive concentrated amino acids may be indicated. The use of dextrose 70%, Aminosyn-II 15% (Abbott Laboratories), or Novamine 15% (Clintec Nutrition Co.), and lipid 20 or 30% can deliver substantial calories in 1.5 L/d.

Enteral Therapy

Most general tube feeding products contain a balance of nonprotein energy between carbohydrate and fat. Elemental or chemically defined products are the exception as they are intended as high-carbohydrate, low-fat formulas. Comparison of high-carbohydrate with high-fat enteral tube feeding in undernourished patients revealed a significant increase in minute ventilation, heat production, and carbon dioxide production when the high-carbohydrate formula was administered.[118] Also, outpatients with COPD and hypercapnia demonstrated a significant decrease in V_{CO_2}, RQ, and p_{CO_2} when changed from a high-carbohydrate, low-fat to a low-carbohydrate, high-fat liquid diet.[119] It appears the principles of energy expenditure calculated from V_{CO_2} and V_{O_2} also apply during EN support. Because most general formulas contain balanced nonprotein calories, moderate doses of these products are appropriate in most patients with pulmonary disease.

Investigators have begun to measure changes in pulmonary function and respiratory muscle strength in patients with lung diseases receiving nutrition support.[120,121] Undernourished patients with COPD who received supplemental tube feeding (1000 kcal/d) for a mean of 16 days demonstrated significant weight gain, increases in maximal expiratory pressure, and increases in mean sustained inspiratory pressure.[120] This short-term study showed overall improvement in respiratory muscle function with refeeding. Contrary to the previous study, undernourished patients with emphysema who were given a 400-kcal supplement daily for 13 weeks demonstrated weight gain but no improvement in pulmonary function or immunologic status compared with controls.[121] While the study period seemed adequate, the supplemental dose of nutrients may have been too small in the latter study.

Because most patients with acute respiratory failure would be hospitalized in an intensive care unit, the risk of developing stress ulceration exists. An initial report suggested that concurrent enteral feeding during mechanical ventilation afforded adequate stress ulcer prophylaxis.[122] Subsequent reports have not confirmed these initial observations,[123] so these patients should still receive pharmacologic therapy, even when being fed enterally.

Several enteral products (Pulmocare, Ross Laboratories; Nutrivent, Clintec Nutrition Company; Respilor, Bristol-Myers) are marketed for the patient with pulmonary failure. These products contain a substantial amount of fat and a lower amount of carbohydrate than standard enteral products. Further studies with enteral nutrition in pulmonary failure patients are needed before high-fat formulas can be recommended universally. Concentrated enteral formulas (e.g., 2 kcal/mL) would be helpful in feeding patients with severe ARDS, pulmonary edema, and others who may require fluid restriction.

FUTURE DIRECTIONS

Sophisticated methods for assessing energy expenditure of hospitalized patients now commercially available include indirect calorimetry with metabolic carts. Indirect calorimetry employs the collection of expired air from the patient by placing a canopy over the patient's head or by collecting expired air from the mechanically ventilated patient. The measured V_{CO_2} and V_{O_2} can then be used to calculate resting energy expenditure (REE, kcal/d):

$$\text{REE} = [(V_{O_2} \times 3.9) + (V_{CO_2} \times 1.1)](1.44)$$

These instruments are very expensive, precluding most hospitals from purchasing them for use in nutrition support, but their use in research protocols is becoming essential.

Growth hormone plus nutrition support has been used in two pilot studies of undernourished patients with COPD.[124,125] Improved nitrogen retention, weight gain, and increased concentrations of insulin-like growth factor-1 have been reported in some of the patients receiving growth hormone. Studies focusing on improved clinical outcome will need to be conducted before expensive biotechnology products can be used as adjunctive therapy to nutrition support in undernourished patients with respiratory disease.

CARDIAC FAILURE

A significant relationship exists between cardiac function and protein-calorie deprivation.[126] In starvation, cardiac muscle is not spared and the loss roughly parallels loss of lean body mass. Cardiac output and stroke volume are reduced in undernutrition, resulting in hypotension and bradycardia. This allows the heart to function at a reduced V_{O_2}.

Refeeding the starved patient disrupts the cardiovascular dynamics of starvation.[127] There is usually a marked increase in metabolic rate and only gradual restoration of myocardial contractile proteins with refeeding. Consequently, excessive administration of nutrients or fluid volume could overwhelm the heart, resulting in failure. The goal of nutrition support in the patient with cardiac disease should be to improve gradually or maintain nutrition status. Also, improvement in serum albumin concentrations should decrease edema in this patient population.

MACRONUTRIENT CONSIDERATIONS

Carbohydrate/Fat/Protein

Patients with cardiac failure should be able to handle the major nutrition substrates without problems. However, because it is usually beneficial to restrict fluid intake in these patients, the most concentrated substrates are the optimal means of providing nutrition support. Administration of concentrated intravenous fat emulsion (20%) has been reported to have a myocardial depressant effect when infused rapidly (120 mL/h) into patients following coronary bypass surgery.[128] This adverse effect was not observed when the concentrated lipid was infused at a slower rate (60 mL/h).[128] It is therefore reasonable to infuse the intravenous lipid component of parenteral nutrition cautiously (preferably over a 24-h period) to cardiac patients.

Fluid and Electrolytes

Generally, the patient with cardiac disease is at risk of developing congestive heart failure (CHF). Salt and water restriction continues to be an important part of the management of these patients and the nutrition formula should reflect these restrictions. Overzealous addition of sodium to the PN formula can exacerbate CHF and worsen edema. Hyponatremia in this patient population usually signifies fluid and sodium overload and should be treated with fluid restriction. Loop-diuretic therapy is frequently used to increase excretion of salt and water.

It is well known that loop-diuretic therapy increases the urinary excretion of potassium, often resulting in hypokalemia. This can be particularly significant in the undernourished patient receiving nutrition support because potassium requirements increase as lean body mass is synthesized. Patients receiving concomitant digoxin therapy need to have serum potassium concentrations maintained in the normal range to prevent ventricular arrhythmias. Patients receiving angiotensin-converting enzyme inhibitors for CHF are prone to develop mild hyperkalemia and may not require a standard dose of potassium during concomitant nutrition support.

Hypophosphatemia and cardiopulmonary decompensation have been associated with refeeding the undernourished patient.[127] Phosphorus shifts from the serum to the intracellular space as new lean body mass is synthesized. Energy is shifted from fat metabolism (which does not require phosphate-containing intermediates) to glucose (which does). There also is an association between profound hypophosphatemia and severe congestive cardiomyopathy. It would seem prudent to treat the severely undernourished patient conservatively by increasing the nutrient infusion slowly, administering a portion of the energy as fat, checking heart rate regularly, and assessing the patient for edema or rales.

Homeostasis of magnesium may be affected by aggressive loop-diuretic therapy in that renal excretion of this cation is markedly enhanced. Poor magnesium intake secondary to anorexia of CHF coupled with increased excretion from diuretic therapy may compound existing hypomagnesemia. Magnesium depletion has been associated with the development of atherosclerotic disease, coronary artery spasms, and myocardial irritability.[129] Low serum and intracellular magnesium concentrations have also been reported in patients suffering acute myocardial infarction.[130] Serum concentrations need to be checked two to three times weekly during nutrition support of these patients.

MICRONUTRIENT CONSIDERATIONS

Patients with cardiac failure receiving PN should receive the vitamins and trace elements as recommended by the NAG-AMA. Those receiving EN support should receive the RDAs for vitamins, zinc, and selenium. Theoretically, urinary excretion of zinc may be increased by vigorous loop-diuretic therapy, but routine supplementation above suggested intake is not recommended unless a deficiency is documented.

Selenium deficiency has been shown to cause Keshan's disease, a dilated congestive cardiomyopathy, in geographic areas where the selenium content of the soil is extremely low (e.g., China). Selenium deficiency has been reported in patients on long-term parenteral nutrition without selenium supplementation.[131] Some of these case studies reported deaths from cardiomyopathy, presumed to be secondary to selenium deficiency. Because this cardiomyopathy has been reported to be irreversible, selenium supplementation of 40–80 μg/d should be considered in long-term parenteral nutrition patients. Patients receiving long-term parenteral nutrition have demonstrated improvement in serum concentrations of selenium after supplementation but not in functional activity, as measured by erythrocyte glutathione peroxidase.[132]

ADMINISTRATION ROUTES

Parenteral Therapy

Patients with cardiac disease need parenteral nutrition only when a superimposed illness prevents use of the gastrointestinal tract. Currently, there are no disease-specific products marketed for this patient population; however, a 15% amino acid and 30% intravenous fat emulsion are available for patients who require severe fluid restriction. A sodium-free parenteral nutrition solution would be appropriate in many clinical conditions. An example of a parenteral nutrition solution for this patient type is given in Table 136.1.

Enteral Therapy

Most patients with cardiac failure have functioning gastrointestinal tracts so that EN support can be used. Both poor palatability of a salt-restricted diet and anorexia secondary to CHF may impede adequate ingestion of nutrients. If dietary intervention with oral liquid supplements is unsuccessful and the patient is either undernourished or at risk of becoming so, enteral tube feeding should be strongly considered. Because fluid restriction is often desirable in cardiac failure, enteral products delivering 1.5–2.0 kcal/mL may be indicated. Also, most commercially available enteral formulas are relatively low in sodium (20–50 mEq/L). Undernourished patients with CHF have been managed with concentrated EN formulas given via nasoenteric infusion, and demonstrated loss of weight as extracellular fluid and gain of lean body mass without exacerbating cardiac function.[133]

SHORT-BOWEL SYNDROME

Because the gastrointestinal tract is essential for absorption and digestion of nutrients, dysfunction or malabsorption can have a significant impact on nutritional status. Gastrointestinal failure secondary to the short bowel syndrome (SBS) is a disease state in which morbidity and mortality have been significantly improved by parenteral nutrition.[110] Parenteral nutrition also has had a major impact on the treatment of patients with severe inflammatory bowel disease, enterocutaneous fistulas, and radiation enteritis. The goal of nutrition support in patients with SBS should be to maintain nutritional status or correct nutritional deficiencies by the appropriate route. Both parenteral and enteral nutrition support are used extensively in patients with gastrointestinal failure.[134]

MACRONUTRIENT CONSIDERATIONS

Carbohydrate/Fat/Protein

Once absorbed, the macronutrients should be processed normally in patients with gastrointestinal failure. If enteral nutrients cannot be absorbed appropriately, parenteral nutrition will be required temporarily or, in patients with extreme SBS, indefinitely. Enteral nutrition can often be used for provision of part of the required nutrients, with parenteral nutrition supplying the balance.

Fat malabsorption has received the most attention in SBS because this process is very complex. It involves both pancreatic secretion of lipase, and micelle formation with bile acids. Some patients with fat malabsorption have been treated with medium-chain triglycerides that do not require pancreatic enzymes or bile acids for absorption. This product, however, does not provide essential fatty acids, and thus patients may develop essential fatty acid deficiency. Long-chain fatty acids would need to be given orally or parenterally to prevent this disorder. More recently, the malabsorption of carbohydrate in SBS has been shown to be a major cause of the watery diarrhea universally seen in this disease state.[135]

Traditionally, enteral nitrogen in its simplest form (free amino acids) has been recommended in patients with moderate to severe SBS because it was assumed that this absorptive pathway was most efficient. Enteral formulas containing partially hydrolyzed protein as small peptides are absorbed better than formulas containing nitrogen only as free amino acids.[136] It appears that the absorption of free amino acids by the enteral route is a saturable process, whereas the absorption of small peptides is not. This suggests theoretically that the products with small peptides would be absorbed better in SBS; however, further clinical research is needed in this area. Studies will need to be designed so that the contribution of each macronutrient can be assessed individually.

Fluid and Electrolytes

Fluid and sodium balance are extremely important in patients with gastrointestinal failure because of the large amounts of extrarenal losses. Often, the appropriate parenteral or enteral nutrition regimen includes extra fluid to replace losses and maintain urine output. Substantial losses of any body fluids (e.g., from jejunostomy or colostomy) need to be considered when preparing the nutritional formula. Diarrhea is a hallmark disorder of SBS and losses may be difficult to measure. Stool frequency and consistency may aid in the calculation of the amount of replacement needed. Serum sodium concentration may not reflect sodium status, especially in the dehydrated state in which hypernatremia can result.

Losses of potassium from an ostomy in SBS can be as high as 200 mEq/d. If these losses are stable, they can be replaced by adding supplemental potassium into the PN formula. Metabolic alkalosis, which occurs when a patient becomes dehydrated, can accelerate the renal excretion of potassium, because all hydrogen ions will be conserved in an attempt to correct the acid–base disorder. As bicarbonate ions are excreted renally, potassium is taken with them to maintain osmotic balance. Diarrheal fluid also is concentrated in potassium and requires fluid and potassium replacement if it cannot be controlled.

Patients with severe SBS invariably have some fat malabsorption. Complexation of both dietary and secreted calcium in the remaining bowel by unabsorbed FFAs renders the ion unabsorbable, leading to negative calcium balance. Patients on long-term parenteral nutrition will need calcium added to their nutrition formula to maintain calcium balance. Also, long-term parenteral nutrition has been associated with metabolic bone disease resulting in osteomalacia and osteoporosis. Excessive aluminum loading from protein hydrolysates (no longer used), parenteral vitamin D, and excessive infusion of protein all have been shown to cause hypercalciuria, a potential etiology of this disorder. It therefore appears reasonable to measure a 24-hour urine collection for calcium before a patient is sent home with parenteral nutrition. This will help identify patients who may have trouble maintaining calcium balance. For patients with SBS who are able to maintain nutrition status on oral nutrition, calcium supplementation (1–4 g/d) as the gluconate or carbonate salt often is required.

Considerable losses of magnesium occur with diarrhea and ostomy losses. Like the other electrolytes, magnesium is usually replaced in the PN formula in patients with severe SBS. Oral replacement of magnesium with gluconate or oxide salts may be used in less severe cases of SBS, but excessive use of oral magnesium results in diarrhea, which may exacerbate a magnesium deficit.

Acid–Base Disorders

Patients with severe SBS are at great risk of developing dehydration and metabolic alkalosis. They can lose substantial amounts of chloride (60–140 mEq/L) and sodium (80–160 mEq/L) from ostomies, and daily losses of fluid may vary from 0.5–10 L/d. Dehydration occurs when there are stable losses from an ostomy that are not replaced or when the patient is noncompliant with a restricted diet resulting in loss of more fluid than is taken in. Patients who have SBS complicated by a pancreatic fistula lose considerable bicarbonate and may develop metabolic acidosis. Quantifying fluid losses with particular attention to the sources of loss will aid in the acid–base management of these complex patients.

MICRONUTRIENT CONSIDERATIONS

Trace Elements

Much of the information that has been gained about trace element balance during specialized nutrition support has come from patients on long-term parenteral nutrition. This can, in part, be explained by the length of time required for a deficiency in trace elements to develop or be recognized (months to years). Also, signs or symptoms of deficiency may be underappreciated, and biochemical analysis is not available in all hospitals.

Zinc is the trace element that has been studied most often during parenteral nutrition. Twenty-four patients with gastrointestinal disease who were receiving parenteral nutrition had zinc metabolism studied.[18] These patients were given three separate doses of parenteral zinc during three 1-week periods while zinc balance was done. It was shown that small bowel fluid, colostomy fluid, and diarrheal fluid contained considerable quantities of zinc. An equation to estimate zinc requirements was developed:

$$\text{Zn replacement (mg/d)} = 2.0 + 17.1\text{SIO} + 12.2\text{SBF}$$

where SIO = kilograms of stool or ileostomy output and SBF = liters of small bowel fluid lost. Therefore, patients who have SBS and require parenteral nutrition should have zinc added to their formula. Doses above the NAG-AMA recommendations should be given when excessive losses of gastrointestinal fluids occur.[15]

Because copper is excreted primarily in the bile, excessive losses of gastrointestinal fluid can have a substantial impact on copper balance. Copper balance during parenteral nutrition also has been studied in a group of patients with gastrointestinal disease.[137] Although requirements for patients with excessive gastrointestinal losses were higher (0.4–0.5 mg/d) than those for patients with normal gastrointestinal losses (0.3 mg/d), recommendations by the NAG-AMA exceed both of these doses. It is clear, however, that administration of parenteral nutrition without copper will result in depressed serum copper concentrations and eventually copper deficiency, which can lead to anemia.

Two of the three patients reported in the literature who have developed chromium deficiency during long-term parenteral nutrition had excessive gastrointestinal fluid losses after enterectomy.[138,139] It was suggested that these losses contributed to the chromium deficiency and glucose intolerance experienced by these patients. These data, although scant, suggest that patients with excessive gastrointestinal fluid losses need a supplemental dose of chromium (20 μg/d).[138]

Selenium should be administered to all patients receiving chronic PN since an RDA has been established and there are several cases of cardiomyopathy reported in association with documented or presumed deficiency of this trace element. Decreased absorption of oral selenium has been reported in patients with SBS.[140]

Vitamins

Most water-soluble vitamins (except vitamin B_{12}) are absorbed in the jejunum, so unless the patient has severe SBS, these usually can be maintained with an oral diet. Because patients with resection of the distal ileum cannot absorb vitamin B_{12}, the parenteral form of this vitamin needs to be administered. Patients with SBS who have fat malabsorption are prone to malabsorb the fat-soluble vitamins (A, D, E, and K). These vitamins often can be supplemented orally if there is sufficient gastrointestinal tract left. The patients with severe SBS who will be receiving PN should receive intravenous vitamins in virtually all cases.

ADMINISTRATION ROUTES AND PRODUCTS

Parenteral Therapy

Patients who have had a major resection of the gastrointestinal tract usually require a period of central PN to maintain nutritional status while the remaining small bowel is undergoing hypertrophy. There are usually no substrate alterations in these patients, so standard crystalline amino acids, glucose, and intravenous lipids may be used in conventional doses either to maintain nutrition status or to correct nutritional deficits in these patients. An example of a parenteral nutrition formula for the patient with SBS is given in Table 136.1. If the patient has had major enterectomy, home parenteral nutrition may be needed for the rest of the patient's life. Gouttebel et al.[141] reported a significant negative correlation between the length of bowel remaining and the duration of parenteral nutrition following the surgery. Specifically, patients who had less than 150 cm but more than 80 cm of small bowel required 1–6 months of parenteral nutrition; patients with 50–70 cm of small bowel also required 1–6 months of parenteral nutrition if they had an intact colon and rectum; patients with 40–70 cm of small bowel with a hemicolectomy required 6–12 months of parenteral nutrition; and patients with less than 60 cm of small bowel without a colon or patients with less than 30 cm of small bowel with a colon needed parenteral nutrition indefinitely.[141]

Enteral Therapy

After major gastrointestinal resection, enteral therapy should be introduced soon, because food is the stimulus for secretion of pancreatic enzymes and other trophic hormones thought essential for small bowel hyperplasia. Elemental diets or chemically defined formulas have been used initially during enteral therapy in selected patients because the substrates are in the simplest or an easily digestible form. One group reported that most patients with severe SBS can be converted to enteral nutrition therapy.[142] If other studies verify these data, the need for long-term home parenteral nutrition would be reduced considerably. Another report suggests using energy malabsorption as a measure of gastrointestinal failure in patients with SBS and a guide for appropriate long-term therapy.[143] For instance, a patient with SBS could have sequential measurements of total energy, carbohydrate, fat, and protein absorption to determine the dose of parenteral nutrition to meet nutritional needs. As small bowel adaption occurs, some patients could be weaned from parenteral nutrition appropriately (i.e., maintaining nutritional status). Weaning of chronic PN is best accomplished by gradually decreasing the volume of PN and IV solutions over several days to weeks. Once the patient has been weaned to 1 liter, the frequency of administration can be decreased (e.g., every other day) until the patient can support him- or herself entirely by the oral route.[134]

Traditionally, patients with SBS who can maintain nutritional status by the oral route have been prescribed low-fat diets because fat malabsorption is a common disorder in these patients. More recent studies have challenged this traditional approach and the patients were given regular diets.[144,145] Five end jejunostomy patients who were studied on three diets with different percentages of fat demonstrated no significant increases in loss of ostomy volume or monovalent cations with the high-fat diet.[144] In this study, only divalent cations (copper, zinc, calcium, magnesium) were lost in significantly greater quantities when the high-fat diet was used. Likewise, other investigators found that stable patients with SBS for at least 1 year were able to be switched to a high-fat diet without affecting absorption of major substrates and most divalent cations.[145]

FUTURE DIRECTIONS

The identification of other essential trace elements needed by these patients who are receiving long-term parenteral nutrition remains to be determined. Specific fuels for the gastrointestinal tract such as glutamine and short-chain fatty acids are the subject of intense investigation and may provide a therapy to preserve the gut mass or induce gastrointestinal hypertrophy following major enterectomy. Currently, small bowel transplantation in humans is in its infancy and many patients with SBS will become potential candidates for this operative procedure as more experience is gained.[146]

Several major problems exist during transplantation of the small bowel. First, the gastrointestinal graft is very sensitive to ischemia, with the villi becoming denuded of epithelial cells only a couple of hours after harvest. Hypothermic storage and flushing with crystalloid solutions improves the viability of the graft. Because the gastrointestinal tract is very immunocompetent, graft-versus-host disease is very common. Immunosuppressive agents like cyclosporine and tacrolimus have been successful in a few series of patients receiving transplanted small bowel. Also, combining this procedure with a liver transplant appears to have a protective effect on the graft that is currently not understood. Some centers have patients who have had gastrointestinal grafts in place for over 2 years.

As more patients with SBS survive with the administration of specialized nutrition support or are treated with small bowel transplantation, the management of these patients' pharmacotherapy will need to be addressed and studied. There will undoubtedly be a period immediately postoperative in which the patient will require parenteral nutrition. As oral nutrients are introduced and the gastrointestinal graft becomes "functional," medications will invariably be changed to oral dosage forms. Currently, the amount of information addressing pharmacotherapy in patients with SBS is limited.[147]

MULTIPLE ORGAN DYSFUNCTION SYNDROME

Several critically ill patients develop the multiple organ dysfunction syndrome (MODS), which has been defined at a critical care consensus conference as the "presence of altered organ function in an acutely ill patient, such that homeostasis cannot be maintained without intervention."[148] MODS can result in impairment of the pulmonary, renal, hepatic, CNS, and gastrointestinal systems.[149] Primary MODS results from a well-defined insult (e.g., trauma) in which organ dysfunction occurs early in the patient's course. Secondary MODS develops as a result of a host response, usually the systemic inflammatory response syndrome (SIRS).[148]

The mortality rate is quite high in MODS and it increases proportionally to the number of involved organs and the length of time of organ failure.[150] Originally it was believed that infection was the cause of MODS in all patients, however, many of these patients have SIRS and MODS with no evidence of an infection. Involvement of cytokines, including IL-1, IL-6, TNF, and IL-8, has been implicated as a mediator in the development of sepsis, organ dysfunction, and immune suppression.[151] One popular hypothesis for the development of MODS in a critically ill patient is the gastrointestinal tract's involvement with this disorder. It is thought that a systemic insult upsets the balance of indigenous bacteria of the gastrointestinal tract, resulting in an overgrowth of gram-negative organisms and fungi.[152] The host becomes immunologically suppressed and the gastrointestinal barrier becomes compromised through loss of physical or functional mass. Nutritional management of these patients is extremely complex because of multiple organs requiring supportive interventions.

MACRONUTRIENT CONSIDERATIONS IN MODS

Carbohydrate/Fat/Protein

Virtually all critically ill patients are hypermetabolic and hypercatabolic, making them suitable candidates for specialized nutrition support.[153,154] Patients with MODS would have at least the same obligate requirements for glucose that all humans have. Burke et al.[155] demonstrated that maximum glucose oxidation rates in convalescing thermally injured patients were achieved at a dose of 25 kcal/kg/d (5 mg/kg/min). To date there is no evidence that this dose of glucose should be exceeded in any patient with MODS.

Generally, intravenous fat should provide between 20–30% of calories in the critically ill patient receiving PN or EN. This provides both essential fatty acids and an energy source that is readily utilized. Some patients with MODS have extremely elevated serum concentrations of triglycerides without infusion of exogenous lipids. Most practitioners hold intravenous fat until triglyceride serum concentrations are <300 mg/dL. The primary fear of elevated triglycerides in this patient population is the development of acute pancreatitis. Furthermore, since immune dysfunction caused by long-chain triglycerides has been reported, many practitioners limit intravenous lipid dosages to 1 g/kg/d.[154] Serum triglycerides should therefore be monitored at least once per week in a patient with MODS who is receiving intravenous fat.

Patients with MODS are hypercatabolic and usually require between 1.5–2.5 g protein/kg/d. The major problem with administering this dose is the residual function of the affected organs. For instance, a patient with ARF and dialysis is usually limited in the protein that can be infused to 1.2–1.5 g/kg/d. Severe hepatic failure may also be a factor that would lead one to administer less protein than is actually needed. Nitrogen balance would be very helpful in these patients and should be possible because urine can be collected accurately in an intensive care setting. Therefore, renal and hepatic function, frequency and type of dialysis, and nitrogen balance results all need to be considered when suggesting a protein dose for patients with MODS.

Fluid and Electrolytes

Patients who have oliguric ARF or ARDS as part of their MODS complex will need to have nutrient formulas concentrated. This can be done with either PN or EN. These patients are often edematous and would not require sodium. Like all critically ill patients, acute fluctuations in potassium, calcium, phosphorus, and magnesium can occur. Frequent monitoring of these with judicious replacement is prudent. Patients with MODS and ARF undoubtedly would need these electrolytes restricted initially during the administration of PN or EN.

Acid–Base/Vitamins/Trace Elements

Metabolic and/or respiratory acidosis is quite common in patients with MODS. Acetate ions should be used in PN for patients with metabolic acidosis. A mixture of chloride and acetate ions in PN is usually appropriate with respiratory acidosis because excessive chloride ions can worsen the acidosis, and excessive acetate ions could lead to increased carbon dioxide retention. Standard vitamins and trace elements are usually given to patients with MODS. If ARF or hepatic cholestatsis is present, the guidelines provided earlier in this chapter should be used.

ADMINISTRATION ROUTES AND PRODUCTS

Parenteral/Enteral Therapy

Patients who have developed MODS often have an ileus and gastrointestinal failure. Even though there is an emphasis on using the gastrointestinal tract in the critically ill, PN is often the only effective way to deliver nutrients to patients who have already developed MODS. Dextrose, intravenous lipids, and standard amino acids are appropriate for these patients. The volume of the PN is extremely important especially in patients who are overhydrated or edematous. Frequently 70% dextrose, 15% amino acids, and 30% intravenous fat emulsion are used for PN admixtures in these patients. Currently, this concentrated fat emulsion is only approved for total nutrient admixtures in the United States, not for direct intravenous infusion into patients.

It is extremely difficult to successfully administer EN to patients who have MODS since ileus, poor gastric emptying, and gut ischemia frequently occur. Clearly, if critically ill patients can be fed enterally early in their hospital course, it should be done.[156] Infectious complications have been reduced in critically ill trauma patients fed with EN via jejunostomy when compared to those given PN. The effect of this intervention on the development of MODS has not been studied in a sufficient number of patients to see if it is decreased.

FUTURE DIRECTIONS

Several nutrients known to stimulate immune function or prevent bacterial translocation have been studied in critically ill patients who are prone to develop sepsis and MODS.[157,158] Some of these include glutamine, arginine, omega 3 fatty acids, and soluble fiber. PN and EN formulas enhanced with these nutrients may stimulate immune function, preserve gastrointestinal mass, decrease infection, and actually prevent MODS. A preliminary clinical study using a formula with some of these nutrients in critically ill trauma patients demonstrated a small but significant decrease in the development of MODS when compared to a similar group of patients receiving standard EN.[159]

REFERENCES

1. Matsunaga S, Wolk R. Role of clinical pharmacy specialist in metabolically managing nutrition patients. Nutrition 1992;8:149–154.
2. Gales BJ, Riley DG. Improved total parenteral nutrition therapy management by a nutritional support team. Hosp Pharm 1994;29:469–470, 473–475.
3. Dickerson RN. Clinical pharmacy specialist in nutritional support. Nutrition 1994;10:351–352.
4. Marsano L, McClain CJ. Nutrition and alcoholic liver disease. J Parenter Enter Nutr 1991;15:337–344.
5. Shanbhogue RL, Bistrian BR, Jenkins RL, et al. Resting energy expenditure in patients with end-stage liver disease and in normal population. J Parenter Enter Nutr 1987; 11:305–308.
6. John WJ, Phillips R, Ott L, et al. Resting energy expenditure in patients with alcoholic hepatitis. J Parenter Enter Nutr 1989;13:124–127.
7. Muller MJ, Loyal S, Schwarze M, et al. Resting energy expenditure and nutritional state in patients with liver cirrhosis before and after liver transplant. Clin Nutr 1994;13:145–152.
8. Muller MJ, Boker KH, Selberg O. Are patients with liver cirrhosis hypermetabolic? Clin Nutr 1994;13:131–144.
9. Petrides AS, DeFrenzo RA. Glucose and insulin metabolism in cirrhosis. J Hepatol 1989;8:107–114.
10. Glynn MJ, Powell-Tuck J, Reaveley DA, Murray-Lyon IM. High lipid parenteral nutrition improves portasystemic encephalopathy. J Parenter Enter Nutr 1988;12:457–461.
11. Record KE, Kolpek JH, Rapp RP. Long chain versus medium chain length triglycerides. Nutr Clin Prac 1986; 1:129–136.
12. Mizock BA. Branched-chain amino acids in sepsis and hepatic failure. Arch Intern Med 1985;145:1284–1288.
13. Nelson DC, McGrew WR, Hoyumpa AM. Hypernatremia and lactulose therapy. JAMA 1983;249:1295–1298.
14. Salem M, Muhoz R, Chernow B. Hypomagnesemia in critical illness: A common and clinically important problem. Crit Care Clin 1991;7:225–252.
15. Anonymous. Guidelines for essential trace element preparations for parenteral use. JAMA 1979;241:2051–2054.
16. Dworkin B, Rosenthal WS, Jankowski RH, et al. Low blood selenium levels in alcoholics with and without advanced liver disease. Dig Dis Sci 1985;30:838–844.
17. Lane HW, Lotspeich CA, Moore CE, et al. The effect of selenium supplementation on selenium status of patients receiving chronic total parenteral nutrition. J Parenter Enter Nutr 1987;11:177–182.
18. Wolman SL, Anderson H, Marliss EB, Jeejeebhoy KN. Zinc in total parenteral nutrition: Requirements and metabolic effects. Gastroenterology 1979;76:458–467.
19. McClain CJ, Marsano L, Burk RF, Bacon B. Trace metals in liver disease. Sem Liv Dis 1991;11:321–339.
20. Reding P, Duchateau J, Bataille C. Oral zinc supplementation improves hepatic encephalopathy. Lancet 1984; 1:493–495.
21. Korpela H, Kumpulainen J, Luoma PV, et al. Decreased serum selenium in alcoholics as related to liver structure and function. Am J Clin Nutr 1985;42:147–151.
22. Leo MA, Lieber CS. Hepatic vitamin A depletion in alcoholic liver injury. N Engl J Med 1982;307:597–601.
23. Kearns PJ, Young H, Carcia G, et al. Accelerated improvement of alcoholic liver disease with enteral nutrition. Gastroenterology 1992;102:200–205.

24. Cerra FB, Cheung NK, Fischer JE, et al. Disease-specific amino acid infusion (F080) in hepatic encephalopathy: A prospective, randomized, double-blind, controlled trial. J Parenter Enter Nutr 1985;9:288–295.
25. Michel H, Bories P, Aubin JP, et al. Treatment of acute hepatic encephalopathy in cirrhotics with a branched-chain amino acids enriched versus a conventional amino acids mixture. Liver 1985;5:282–289.
26. Kanematsu T, Koyanagi N, Matsumata T, et al. Lack of preventive effect of branched-chain amino acid solution on postoperative hepatic encephalopathy in patients with cirrhosis: A randomized, prospective trial. Surgery 1988; 104:482–488.
27. Naylor CD, O'Rourke K, Detsky AS, Baker JP. Parenteral nutrition with branched-chain amino acids in hepatic encephalopathy. Gastroenterology 1989;97:1033–1042.
28. Rossi-Fanelli F, Riggio O, Cangiano C, et al. Branched-chain amino acids versus lactulose in the treatment of hepatic coma. Dig Dis Sci 1982;27:929–935.
29. Wahren J, Denis J, Desurmont P. Is intravenous administration of branched-chain amino acids effective in the treatment of hepatic encephalopathy? A multicenter study. Hepatology 1983;3:475–480.
30. Rudman D, Kutner M, Ansley J, et al. Hypotyrosinemia, hypocystinemia, and failure to retain nitrogen during total parenteral nutrition of cirrhotic patients. Gastroenterology 1981;81:1025–1035.
31. Mattox TW, Brown RO. Use of modified amino acid formulas in the enteral nutritional support of patients with portosystemic encephalopathy: A review. Nutrition 1988; 4:7–12.
32. Egberts EH, Schomerus H, Hamster W, Jurgens P. Branched-chain amino acids in the treatment of latent portosystemic encephalopathy. Gastroenterology 1985;88:887–895.
33. Cabre E, Gonzalez-Hiux F, Abad-Lacruz A, et al. Effect of total enteral nutrition on the short-term outcome of severely malnourished cirrhotics. Gastroenterology 1990;98:715–720.
34. Marchesini G, Dioguardi FS, Bianchi GP, et al. Long-term oral branched-chain amino acid treatment in chronic hepatic encephalopathy. J Hepatol 1990;11:92–101.
35. Medenhall C, Bongiovanni G, Goldberg S, et al. VA cooperative study on alcoholic hepatitis. III: Changes in protein-calorie malnutrition associated with 30 days of hospitalization with and without enteral nutritional therapy. J Parenteral Enter Nutr 1985;9:590–596.
36. Bianchi GP, Marchesini G, Fabbri A, et al. Vegetable versus animal protein diet in cirrhotic patients with chronic encephalopathy: A randomized cross-over comparison. J Intern Med 1993;233:385–392.
37. Herlong HF, Maddrey WC, Walser M. The use of ornithine salts of branched-chain ketoacids in portal-systemic encephalopathy. Ann Intern Med 1980;93:545–550.
38. Maddrey WE, Weber FL, Coulter AW, et al. Effects of keto analogues of essential amino acids in portal-systemic encephalopathy. Gastroenterol 1976;71:190–195.
39. Wood RP, Ozaki CF, Katz SM, et al. Liver transplantation: The last ten years. Surg Clin North Am 1994; 74:1133–1154.
40. Delafosse B, Faure JL, Bouffard Y, et al. Liver transplantation—energy expenditure, nitrogen loss, and substrate oxidation rate in the first 2 postoperative days. Trans Proceed 1989;21:2453–2454.
41. Plevak DJ, DiCecco Sr, Wiesner RH, et al. Nutritional support for liver transplantation: Identifying caloric and protein requirements. Mayo Clin Proc 1994;69:225–230.
42. Dresner LS, Andersen DK, Kahng KU, et al. Effects of cyclosporine on glucose metabolism. Surgery 1989; 106:163–170.
43. Mattern WD, Hak LJ, Lamanna RW, et al. Malnutrition altered immune function, and the risk of infection in maintenance hemodialysis patients. Am J Kid Dis 1982; 1:206–218.
44. Berkelhammer CH, Leiter LA, Jeejeebhoy KN, et al. Skeletal muscle function in chronic renal failure: An index of nutritional status. Am J Clin Nutr 1985;42:845–854.
45. Carvounis CP, Carvounis G, Hung M. Nutritional status of maintenance hemodialysis patients. Am J Clin Nutr 1986;43:946–954.
46. Owen WF, Lew NL, Liu Y, et al. The urea reduction ratio and serum albumin concentration as predictors of mortality in patients undergoing hemodialysis. N Engl J Med 1993; 329:1001–1006.
47. Spiegel DM, Breyer JA. Serum albumin: A predictor of long-term outcome in periotoneal dialysis patients. Am J Kid Dis 1994;23:283–285.
48. Sanaka T, Shinobe M, Ando M, et al. IGF-1 as an early indicator of malnutrition in patients with end-stage renal disease. Nephron 1994;67:73–81.
49. Monteon FJ, Laidlaw SA, Shaib JK, Kopple JD. Energy expenditure in patients with chronic renal failure. Kidney Int 1986;30:741–747.
50. Schneeweiss B, Graninger W, Stockenhuber F, et al. Energy metabolism in acute and chronic renal failure. Am J Clin Nutr 1990;52:596–601.
51. Druml W. Nutritional support in acute renal failure. Clin Nutr 1993;12:196–207.
52. Walser M. Nutritional management of chronic renal failure. Am J Kidney Dis 1982;1:261–275.
53. Manji N, Shikora S, McMahon M, et al. Peritoneal dialysis for acute renal failure: Overfeeding resulting from dextrose absorbed during dialysis. Crit Care Med 1990;18:29–31.
54. Monaghan R, Walters JM, Clancey SM, et al. Uptake of glucose during continuous arteriovenous hemofiltration. Crit Care Med 1993;21:1159–1163.
55. Keane WF. Lipids and the kidney. Kidney Int 1994; 46:910–920.
56. Druml W, Fischer M, Sertl S, et al. Fat elimination in acute renal failure: Long chain versus medium chain triglycerides. Am J Clin Nutr 1992;55:468–472.
57. Seidner DL, Matarese LE, Steiger E. Nutritional care of the critically ill patient with renal failure. Sem Nephrol 1994;14:53–63.
58. Hynote ED, McCamish MA, Depner TA, Davis PA. Amino acid losses during hemodialysis: Effects of high-solute flux and parenteral nutrition in acute renal failure. J Parenter Enter Nutr 1995;19:15–21.
59. Clark WR, Mueller BA, Alka KJ, Macias WL. A comparison of metabolic control by continuous and intermittent

therapies in acute renal failure. J Am Soc Nephrol 1994; 4:1413–1420.
60. Druml W, Fischer M, Liebisch B, et al. Elimination of amino acids in renal failure. Am J Clin Nutr 1994; 60:418–423.
61. Goldstein DJ. Nutrition for acute renal failure patients on continuous hemofiltration. Nutr Clin Prac 1988;3:238–241.
62. Abel RM, Beck CH, Abbott WM, et al. Improved survival from acute renal failure after treatment with intravenous essential L-amino acids and glucose. N Engl J Med 1973; 288:695–699.
63. Blackburn GL, Etter G, Mackenzie T. Criteria for choosing amino acid therapy in acute renal failure. Am J Clin Nutr 1978;31:1841–1853.
64. Freund H, Atamian S, Fischer JE. Comparative study of parenteral nutrition in renal failure using essential and non-essential amino acid containing solutions. Surg Gynecol Obstet 1980;151:652–656.
65. Feinstein EI, Blumenkrantz MJ, Healy M, et al. Clinical and metabolic responses to parenteral nutrition in acute renal failure. Medicine 1981; 60:124–137.
66. Mirtallo JM, Schneider PJ, Mavko K, et al. A comparison of essential and general amino acid infusions in the nutritional support of patients with compromised renal function. J Parenter Enter Nutr 1982;6:109–113.
67. Rapp RP, Bivins BA, McRoberts JW. Hyperammonia encephalopathy in a patient receiving essential amino acid/dextrose parenteral nutrition. Clin Pharm 1982; 1:276–280.
68. Grodstein GP, Blumenkrantz MJ, Kopple JD, et al. Glucose absorption during continuous ambulatory peritoneal dialysis. Kidney Int 1981;19:564–567.
69. Chan E, Montgomery PA. Administration of insulin by continuous ambulatory peritoneal dialysis. Pharmacother 1993;13:455–460.
70. Blumenkrantz MJ, Kopple JD, Moran JK, Coburn JW. Metabolic balance studies and dietary protein requirements in patients undergoing continuous ambulatory peritoneal dialysis. Kidney Int 1982;21:849–861.
71. Giovannetti S. Dietary treatment of chronic renal failure: Why is it not used more frequently. Nephron 1985; 40:1–12.
72. Ihle BU, Becker GJ, Whitworth JA, et al. The effect of protein restriction on the progression of renal insufficiency. N Engl J Med 1989;321:1773–1777.
73. Maschio G, Oldrizzi L, Tessitore N. Effects of dietary protein and phosphorus restriction on the progression of early renal failure. Kidney Int 1982;22:371–376.
74. Klahr S, Levey AS, Beck GJ, et al. The effects of dietary protein restriction and blood pressure control on the progression of chronic renal disease. N Engl J Med 1994; 330:877–884.
75. Locatelli F, Buccianti G, Alberti D, et al. Prospective randomized multicenter trial of effect of protein restriction on progression of chronic renal insufficiency. Lancet 1991; 337:1299–1304.
76. Mitrallo JM, Schneider PJ, Ruberg RL, Fabri PJ. Monitoring protein requirements of the patient receiving hemodialysis and total parenteral nutrition. Am J Hosp Pharm 1981; 38:1483–1486.
77. Wolk R. Micronutrition in dialysis. Nutr Clin Prac 1993; 8:267–276.
78. Grekas D, Nicolaides P, Tsakalos N, Tourkantonis A. Pharmacokinetics of zinc in chronic renal failure patients. Trace Elements Med 1985;4:139–142.
79. Slatopolsky E, Weerts C, Lopez-Hilker S, et al. Calcium carbonate as a phosphate binder in patients with chronic renal failure undergoing dialysis. N Engl J Med 1986; 315:157–161.
80. Lindsay RM, Heidenheim P, Sapnner E, et al. Adequacy of hemodialysis and nutrition—important determinants of morbidity and mortality. Kidney Int 1994;45(suppl):S85–S90.
81. Iseki K, Kawazoe N, Fukiyama K. Serum albumin is a strong predictor of death in chronic dialysis patients. Kidney Int 1993;44:115–119.
82. Wolfson M, Jones MR, Kopple JD. Amino acid losses during hemodialysis with infusion of amino acids and glucose. Kidney Int 1982;21:500–506.
83. Cano N, Labastie-Coeyrehourq J, Lacombe P, et al. Perdialytic parenteral nutrition with lipids and amino acids in malnourished hemodialysis patients. Am J Clin Nutr 1990; 52:726–730.
84. Capelli JP, Kushner H, Camiscioli TC, et al. Effect of intradialytic parenteral nutrition on mortality rates in end-stage renal disease care. Am J Kid Dis 1994;23:808–816.
85. Chertow GM, Ling J, Lew NL, et al. The association of intradialytic parenteral nutrition administration with survival in hemodialysis patients. Am J Kid Dis 1994; 24:912–920.
86. Arfeen S, Goodship TH, Kirkwood A, Ward MK. The nutrition/metabolic and hormonal effects of 8 weeks of continuous ambulatory periotoneal dialysis with a 1% amino acid solution. Clin Nephrol 1990;33:192–199.
87. Mitch WE, Walser M, Steinman IT, et al. The effect of a keto acid-amino acid supplement to a restricted diet on the progression of chronic renal failure. N Engl J Med 1984; 311:623–629.
88. Hakim RM, Levin N. Malnutrition in hemodialysis patients. Am J Kid Dis 1993;21:125–137.
89. Schols A, Mostert R, Soeters P, et al. Inventory of nutritional status in patients with COPD. Chest 1989; 96:247–249.
90. Wilson DO, Rogers RM, Wright EC, Anthonisen NR. Body weight in chronic obstructive pulmonary disease. Am Rev Resp Dis 1989;139:1435–1438.
91. Niederman MS, Merrill WW, Ferranti RD, et al. Nutritional status and bacterial binding in the lower respiratory tract in patients with chronic tracheostomy. Ann Intern Med 1984; 100:795–800.
92. Wilson DO, Donahue M, Rogers RM, Pennock BE. Metabolic rate and weight loss in chronic obstructive lung disease. J Parenter Enter Nutr 1990;14:7–11.
93. Schols AM, Soeters PB, Mostert R, et al. Energy balance in chronic obstructive pulmonary disease. Am Rev Resp Dis 1991;413:1246–1252.
94. Goldstein SA, Thomashow BM, Kvetan V, et al. Nitrogen and energy relationships in malnourished patients with emphysema. Am Rev Resp Dis 1988;138:636–644.
95. Liggett SB, Renfro AD. Energy expenditure of mechanically ventilated nonsurgical patients. Chest 1990;98:682–686.

96. Mowatt-Larssen CA, Brown RO. Specialized nutrition support in respiratory disease. Clin Pharm 1993;12:276–292.
97. Pingleton SK, Harmon GS. Nutritional management in acute respiratory failure. JAMA 1987;257:3094–3099.
98. Doekel RC, Zwillich CW, Scoggin CH, et al. Clinical semistarvation. Depression of hypoxic ventilatory response. N Engl J Med 1976;295:358–361.
99. Dark DS, Pingleton SK, Kerby GR. Hypercapnia during weaning. A complication of nutritional support. Chest 1985;88:141–153.
100. Laaban JP, Lemaire F, Baron JF, et al. Influence of caloric intake on the respiratory mode during mandatory minute volume ventilation. Chest 1985;87:67–72.
101. Askanazi J, Rosenbaum SH, Hyman AI, et al. Respiratory changes induced by the large glucose loads of total parenteral nutrition. JAMA 1980;243:1444–1447.
102. Askanazi J, Nordenstrom J, Rosenbaum SH, et al. Nutrition for the patient with respiratory failure: Glucose versus fat. Anesthesiology 1981;54:373–377.
103. Herve P, Simonneau G, Girard P, et al. Hypercapnic acidosis induced by nutrition in mechanically ventilated patients: Glucose versus fat. Crit Care Med 1985;13:537–540.
104. Venus B, Prager R, Chandrakant BP, et al. Cardiopulmonary effects of intralipid infusion in critically ill patients. Crit Care Med 1988;16:587–590.
105. Jarnberg PO, Lindholm M, Eklund J. Lipid infusion in critically ill patients. Crit Care Med 1981;9:27–31.
106. Hwang TL, Huang SL, Chen MF. Effects of intravenous fat emulsion on respiratory failure. Chest 1990;97:934–938.
107. Venus B, Smith RA, Patel C, Sandoval E. Hemodynamic and gas exchange alterations during intralipid infusion in patients with adult respiratory distress syndrome. Chest 1989;95:1278–1281.
108. Skeie B, Askanazi J, Rothkopf MM, et al. Intravenous fat emulsion and lung function: A review. Crit Care Med 1988;16:183–194.
109. Weissman C, Askanazi J, Rosenbaum S, et al. Amino acids and respiration. Ann Intern Med 1983;98:41–44.
110. Askanazi J, Weissman C, LaSala PA, et al. Effect of protein intake on ventilatory drive. Anesthesiology 1984; 60:106–110.
111. Takala J, Askanazi J, Weissman C, et al. Changes in respiratory control induced by amino acid infusions. Crit Care Med 1988;16:465–469.
112. Simmons RS, Berdine GG, Seidenfeld JJ, et al. Fluid balance and the adult respiratory distress syndrome. Am Rev Resp Dis 1987;135:924–929.
113. Schuller D, Mitchell JP, Calandrino FS, Schuster DP. Fluid balance during pulmonary edema. Is fluid gain a marker or a cause of poor outcome? Chest 1991; 100:1068–1075.
114. Fisher J, Magid N, Kallman C, et al. Respiratory illness and hypophosphatemia. Chest 1983;83:504–508.
115. Fiaccadori E, Coffrini E, Fracchia C, et al. Hypophosphatemia and phosphorus depletion in respiratory and peripheral muscles of patients with respiratory failure due to COPD. Chest 1994;105:1392–1398.
116. Aubier M, Murciano D, Lecocguic Y, et al. Effect of hypophosphatemia on diaphragmatic contractility in patients with acute respiratory failure. N Engl J Med 1985; 313:420–424.
117. Talpers SS, Romberger DJ, Bunce SB, Pingleton SK. Nutritionally associated increased carbon dioxide production. Excess total calories vs. high proportion of carbohydrate calories. Chest 1992;102:551–555.
118. Heymsfield SB, Head A, McManus CB, et al. Respiratory, cardiovascular, and metabolic effects of enteral hyperalimentation: Influence of formula dose and composition. Am J Clin Nutr 1984;40:116–130.
119. Angelillo VA, Sukhdarshan B, Durfee D, et al. Effects of low and high carbohydrate feedings in ambulatory patients with chronic obstructive pulmonary disease and chronic hypercapnia. Ann Intern Med 1985;103:883–885.
120. Whittaker JS, Ryan CF, Buckley PA, Road JD. The effects of refeeding on peripheral and respiratory muscle function in malnourished chronic obstructive pulmonary disease patients. Am Rev Resp Dis 1990;142:283–288.
121. Otte KE, Ahlburg P, D'Amore F, Stellfeld M. Nutritional repletion in malnourished patients with emphysema. J Parenter Enter Nutr 1989;13:152–156.
122. Pingleton SK, Hadzima SK. Enteral alimentation and gastrointestinal bleeding in mechanically ventilated patients. Crit Care Med 1983;11:13–16.
123. Rigaud D, Chastre J, Accary JP, et al. Intragastric pH profile during acute respiratory failure in patients with chronic obstructive pulmonary disease. Chest 1986;90:58–63.
124. Suchner U, Rothkopf MM, Stanislaus G, et al. Growth hormone and pulmonary disease: Metabolic effects in patients receiving parenteral nutrition. Arch Intern Med 1990;150:1225–1230.
125. Pape GS, Friedman M, Underwood LE, Clemmons DR. The effect of growth hormone on weight gain and pulmonary function in patients with chronic obstructive lung disease. Chest 1991;99:1495–1500.
126. Heymsfield SB, Smith J, Redd S, Whitworth HB. Nutritional support in cardiac failure. Surg Clin North Am 1981;61:635–652.
127. Solomon SM, Kirby DF. The refeeding syndrome: A review. J Parenter Enter Nutr 1990;14:90–97.
128. Abel RM, Fisch D, Grossman ML. Hemodynamic effects of intravenous 20% soy oil emulsion following coronary bypass surgery. J Parenter Enter Nutr 1983;7:534–540.
129. Iseri LT. Magnesium in coronary artery disease. Drugs 1984;18(suppl 1):151–160.
130. Tsutsui M, Shimokawa H, Yoshihara S, et al. Intracellular magnesium deficiency in acute myocardial infarction. Jpn Heart J 1993;34:391–401.
131. Lane HW, Barroso AO, Englert D, et al. Selenium status of seven chronic intravenous hyperalimentation patients. J Parenter Enter Nutr 1982;6:426–431.
132. Baptista RJ, Bistrian BR, Blackburn GL, et al. Utilizing selenious acid to reverse selenium deficiency in total parenteral nutrition patients. Am J Clin Nutr 1984;39:816–820.
133. Heymsfield SB, Casper K. Congestive heart failure: Clinical management by use of continuous nasoenteric feeding. Am J Clin Nutr 1989;50:539–544.
134. Purdam PP, Kirby DF. Short-bowel syndrome: A review of the role of nutrition support. J Parenter Enter Nutr 1991;15:93–101.

135. Ameen VZ, Powell GK, Jones LA. Quantitation of fecal carbohydrate excretion in patients with short bowel syndrome. Gastroenterology 1989;92:493–500.
136. Smith JL, Arteaga C, Heymsfield SB. Increased ureagenesis and impaired nitrogen use during infusion of a synthetic amino acid formula. N Engl J Med 1982;306:1013–1018.
137. Shike M, Roulet M, Kurian R, et al. Copper metabolism and requirements in total parenteral nutrition. Gastroenterology 1981;81:290–297.
138. Jeejeebhoy KN, Chu RC, Marliss EB, et al. Chromium deficiency, glucose intolerance, and neuropathy revised by chromium supplementation, in a patient receiving long-term total parenteral nutrition. Am J Clin Nutr 1977;30:531–538.
139. Brown RO, Forloines-Lynn S, Cross RE, Heizer WD. Chromium deficiency after long-term total parenteral nutrition. Dig Dis Sci 1986;31:661–664.
140. Sandstrom B, Davidsson L, Bosaeus I, et al. Selenium status and absorption of zinc (^{65}Zn), selenium (^{75}Se), and manganese (^{54}Mn) in patients with short bowel syndrome. Eur J Clin Nutr 1990;44:697–703.
141. Gouttebel MC, Saint-Aubert B, Astre C, Joyeux H. Total parenteral nutrition needs in different types of short bowel syndrome. Dig Dis Sci 1986;31:718–723.
142. Cosnes J, Gendre JP, Evard D, Quintrec YL. Compensatory enteral hyperalimentation for management of patients with severe short bowel syndrome. Am J Clin Nutr 1985; 41:1002–1009.
143. Rodrigues CA, Lennard-Jones JE, Thompson DG, Farthing MJ. Energy malabsorption as a measure of intestinal failure in the short bowel syndrome. Gut 1989;30:176–183.
144. Ovesen L, Shu R, Howard L. The influence of dietary fat on jejunostomy output in patients with severe short bowel syndrome. Am J Clin Nutr 1983;38:270–277.
145. Woolf GM, Miller C, Kurian R, Jeejeebhoy KN. Nutritional absorption in short bowel syndrome. Dig Dis Sci 1987; 32:8–15.
146. Hiyama DT. The current role of small-bowel transplantation in intestinal failure. Nutr Clin Prac 1993;8:5–11.
147. McFadden MA, DeLegge MH, Kirby DF. Medication delivery in the short-bowel syndrome. J Parenter Enter Nutr 1993;17:180–186.
148. Bone RC, Balk RA, Cerra FB, et al. Definitions for sepsis and organ failure and guidelines for the use of innovative therapies in sepsis. Chest 1992;101:644–655.
149. Deitch EA. Multiple organ failure: Pathophysiology and potential future therapy. Ann Surg 1992;216:117–134.
150. Knaus WA, Draper EA, Wagner DP, Zimmerman JE. Prognosis in acute organ-system failure. Ann Surg 1985; 202:685–693.
151. Molloy RG, Mannick JA, Rodrick ML. Cytokines, sepsis, and immunomodulation. Br J Surg 1993;80:289–297.
152. Marshall JC, Christou NV, Meakins JL. The gastrointestinal tract: The undrained abscess of multiple organ failure. Ann Surg 1994;218:111–119.
153. McMahon MM, Farnell MB, Murray MJ. Nutritional support of critically ill patients. Mayo Clin Proc 1993; 68:911–920.
154. Baron RG. Nutrition support in critical illness. Nutr Clin Prac 1994;9:127–139.
155. Burke JF, Wolfe RR, Mullany CJ, et al. Glucose requirements following burn injury. Ann Surg 1979; 190:274–283.
156. Lowry SF. The route of feeding influences injury responses. J Trauma 1990;30(suppl):S10–S15.
157. Ahrendt GM, Barbul A. Nutrition and multiple organ dysfunction syndrome. Curr Opin Gastroenterol 1994; 10:203–209.
158. Deitch EA. Bacterial translocation: The influence of dietary variables. Gut 1994;1(suppl):S23–S27.
159. Moore FA, Moore EE, Kudsk KA, et al. Clinical benefits of an immune enhancing diet for early postinjury enteral feeding. J Trauma 1994;37:607–615.

Index

Note: Page numbers followed by *f* refer to illustrations; page numbers followed by *t* refer to tables.

C

D

G

H

J

K

L

M

O

Q

R

S

T

AVERAGE PHARMACOKINETIC PARAMETERS FOR SELECTED DRUGS IN ADULTS WITH NORMAL RENAL AND HEPATIC FUNCTION

Drug	Oral Availability (F) (%)	Urinary Excretion (%)	Bound in Plasma (%)	Clearance (L/h/70 kg)	Volume of Distribution (L/70 kg)	Half-life (h)	Effective Concentrations	Toxic Concentrations
Acetaminophen	88	3	0	21	67	2	10–20 mg/L	>300mg/L
Acyclovir	23	75	15	19.8	42	2.4	…	…
Amikacin	…	98	4	5.5	19	2.3	15–30 mg/L peak	>8 mg/L trough
Amoxicillin	93	86	18	10.8	15	1.7	…	…
Amphotericin	…	4	90	1.9	53	18	…	…
Ampicillin	62	82	18	16.2	20	1.3	…	…
Amrinone	93	25	45	157[a]/70.6[b]	91	2.0[a]/4.4[b]	3.7 mg/L	…
Aspirin	68	1	49	39	11	0.25	200–300 mg/L analgesia	>500 mg/L
Atropine	50	57	18	24.6	120	4.3	…	…
Azathioprine	60	<2	…	239.4	57.4	0.16	…	…
Azlocillin	…	65	28	Conc-dependent	15.2	1.4	…	…
Bumetanide	81	62	99	10.9	9.1	0.8	…	…
Caffeine	100	<2	36	5.9	43	4.9	…	…
Captopril	65	38	30	50.4	57	2.2	50 ng/mL	…
Carbamazepine	>70	<1	74	5.3	98	15	4–10 mg/L	>10 mg/L
Cefazolin	…	80	89	4.0	8.4	1.8	…	…
Cefoperazone	…	29	89–93	5.0	6.3	2.1	…	…
Cefoxitin	…	78	73	103.0	21.7	0.65	…	…
Ceftazidime	…	84	21	34.0	16.1	1.6	…	…
Ceftriaxone	…	46	Conc-dependent	1.0	11.2	7.3	…	…
Cephalexin	90	91	14	18	18	0.9	…	…
Chloramphenicol	80	25	53	10.2	66	3–4	10–25 mg/L	>25 mg/L
Chlordiazepoxide	100	<1	97	2.3	21	10	>0.7 mg/L	…
Chloroquine	89	61	61	7.6	8050	738	15–30 ng/mL	250 ng/mL
Chlorpropamide	90	20	96	0.13	6.8	33	…	…
Cimetidine	84	62	19	32.4	70	2.0	0.5–0.9 mg/L	…
Ciprofloxacin	60	65	40	25.2	130	4.1	…	…
Clonazepam	98	<1	86	6.5	224	23	5–70 μg/L	…
Codeine	50	Negligible	7	46.2	182	2.9	65 μg/L	…
Cyclosporine	23	<1	93	24.6	85	5.6	Assay specific	Assay specific
Diazepam	100	<1	99	1.6	77	43	300–400 ng/mL	…
Diclofenac	54	<1	>99.5	17.6	11.9	1.1	…	…
Digitoxin	90	32	97	0.23	38	161	>10 ng/mL	>35 ng/mL
Digoxin	70	60	25	7.8	440	39	>0.8 ng/mL	>2 ng/mL
Diltiazem	44	<4	78	50.4	220	3.7	…	…
Disopyramide	83	55	Conc-dependent	5.0	41	6	3 mg/L	>8 mg/L
Doxorubicin	5	<15	79–85	71.4	425	30	…	…
Enalapril	41	90	55	9	40	11	5–20 μg/L	…
Erythromycin	35	12	84	38.2	55	1.6	…	…
Ethambutol	77	79	<5	36	110	3.1	…	>10 mg/L
Ethosuximide	…	25	0	0.80	50	45	40–100 mg/L	…
Flucytosine	84	99	4	7.2	48	4.2	35–70 mg/L	>100 mg/L
Fluoxetine	>60	<2.5	94	40.3	2450	53	<500 ng/mL	…
Foscarnet	17	82	15	140	30.1	3.3	100–500 μmol/L	…
Gentamicin	…	90	10	5.4	21	2.5	4–10 mg/L peak	>2 mg/L trough
Heparin	…	Negligible	Extensive	Conc-dependent	4.0	Conc-dependent	…	…
Imipramine	40	2	90	63	1260	12–16	100–300 ng/mL	>1 mg/L
Indomethacin	98	15	90	8.4	18	2.4	0.3–3 mg/L	>5 mg/L

(continued)